MOSBY'S
Medical, Nursing, and Allied Health
DICTIONARY

MOSBY'S
Medical, Nursing, and Allied Health
DICTIONARY

FOURTH EDITION

Illustrated in full color throughout

Revision Editor

Kenneth N. Anderson

Consulting Editor and Writer

Lois E. Anderson

Consulting and Pronunciation Editor

Walter D. Glanze

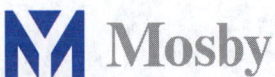 Mosby

St. Louis Baltimore Boston Chicago London Madrid Philadelphia Sydney Toronto

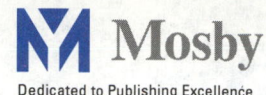
Mosby
Dedicated to Publishing Excellence

Senior Vice President and Publisher: Alison Miller
Executive Editor: N. Darlene Como
Senior Developmental Editor: Laurie Sparks
Developmental Editors: Rebecca Sweeney, Lin Dempsey,
Terry Eynon, Diane Lofshult
Illustration Researchers: Rebecca Sweeney, Elaine Steinborn,
Terry Eynon, Tracy Diamond, Rina Steinhauer
Project Managers: Peg Fagen, Kathleen L. Teal
Production Editor: Kathleen L. Teal
Production Editing Assistant: Theresa Silvey
Designer: Betty Schulz
Manufacturing Supervisor: Theresa Fuchs

Cover illustrations:
Retina from *Selected Topics in Ophthalmology,* Medcom Clinical
Lecture Guides, Garden Grove, California, 1973, Medcom, Inc.
Blood cells from Hayhoe FGJ and Flemans RJ *Color Atlas of
Hematological Cytology,* ed. 3. London, 1992, Wolfe Publishing,
Ltd.
Chest tube drainage system and **triceps skinfold calipers** from
Potter PA and Perry AG, *Fundamentals of Nursing: Concepts,
Process, and Practice,* ed. 3. St. Louis, 1993, Mosby–Year Book,
Inc.
Positron emission tomography from Perkin GD, Rose FC,
Blackwood W, and Shawdon HH. *Atlas of Clinical Neurology.*
London, 1986, Gower Medical Publishing.

FOURTH EDITION
Copyright © 1994 by Mosby–Year Book, Inc.

Previous editions copyrighted 1982, 1986, 1990

Printed in the United States of America
Composition by The Clarinda Company
Printing/binding by Rand McNally

Mosby–Year Book, Inc.
11830 Westline Industrial Drive
St. Louis, Missouri 63146

Library of Congress Cataloging in Publication Data
Mosby's medical, nursing, and allied health dictionary / revision editor, Kenneth N.
  Anderson; consulting editor and writer, Lois E. Anderson; consulting and pronunciation
  editor, Walter D. Glanze.—4th ed.
     p.   cm.
   Includes bibliographical references.
   ISBN 0-8016-7225-2 (Professional).—ISBN 0-8151-6113-1.—ISBN 0-8151-6111-5
(Trade)
    1. Medicine—Dictionaries. 2. Nursing—Dictionaries.
I. Anderson, Kenneth, 1921–   . II. Anderson, Lois E. III. Glanze, Walter D.
IV. Title: Medical, nursing, and allied health dictionary.
  [DNLM: 1. Nursing—dictionaries.   W 13 M8941 1993]
R121.M89 1993
610′.3—dc20
DNLM/DLC
for Library of Congress   93-39959
                                            CIP

93 94 95 96 97 / 9 8 7 6 5 4 3 2 1

STAFF

Revision Editor:
Kenneth N. Anderson

Consulting Editor and Writer:
Lois E. Anderson

Consulting and Pronunciation Editor:
Walter D. Glanze

Programing and Composition by:
The Clarinda Company

Artists and Photographers:
Molly Babich, Ernest W. Beck, Joan Beck, Scott Bodell,
G. David Brown, Lisa Chuck, Barbara Cousings, John Daugherty,
Marsha J. Dohrmann, Ronald J. Ervin, Jody L. Fulks, Kathy Mitchell Gray,
Andrew Grivas, John V. Hagen, Marcia Hartsock, R.T. Hutchings,
Christy Krames, David J. Mascaro, Rebecca S. Montgomery,
William Ober, Donald O'Connor, Christine Oleksyk,
David M. Phillips, Jeanne Robertson, Michael Schenk, Elizabeth D. Sims,
Nadine Sokol, Kevin Somerville, George J. Wassilchenko,
Patrick Watson, Marcia Williams

CONTENTS

PUBLISHER'S FOREWORD

Medical and biological science and technology are advancing at a staggering rate. The language of health care and biology evolves to keep pace with these changes. To master the body of knowledge essential to their professional practice and to communicate effectively with their colleagues in various disciplines, health professionals must have access to the language of this vast and vital field.

Mosby's Medical, Nursing, and Allied Health Dictionary was developed to provide a single source of authoritative, up-to-date information concerning health and health care terminology. Now in its fourth edition, *Mosby's Dictionary* has been praised by educators, students, and practitioners for its clarity, comprehensiveness, reliability, and currency. The hallmarks of our dictionary include the use of a large, easy-to-read typeface, encyclopedic definitions for many key terms, comprehensive entries for numerous drugs, the detailed Color Atlas of Human Anatomy, and a wealth of useful reference information provided in the appendixes.

To reflect new developments in many different facets of health care, approximately 6,000 entirely new entries have been added to the fourth edition. Further, all new and former entries were thoroughly reviewed by experts and revised, as needed, to reflect current knowledge and practice. To accomplish this ambitious goal, we expanded our consultant board to over 150 individuals, representing not only diverse specialties and disciplines, but Canadian and international interests as well. We are indebted to our consultants for their invaluable advice and assistance.

Many refinements have been made in developing the fourth edition. However, the most noticeable change is the addition of nearly 2,000 high-quality illustrations, most in full color, throughout the dictionary to enhance and clarify definitions. Now, for the first time in a medical, nursing, or allied health dictionary in the English language, disorders, anatomical features, and essential equipment are shown in full color to assist in understanding and using terminology. Readers of the fourth edition will have a new appreciation of the adage "a picture is worth a thousand words." A list of illustrations appears on p. xv to assist in locating these valuable resources. In addition, the 43-page Color Atlas of Human Anatomy is presented once again in full color and is placed in the front of the dictionary for easy access.

Over 60 new and updated tables appear throughout the dictionary to provide key reference information to supplement the definitions. A list of tables is included on p. xxvii to facilitate quick reference.

The appendixes offer an extensive compendium of additional useful reference information, including normal laboratory values for adults and children, units of measurement, complete anatomy tables, common drug interactions and trade and generic equivalents, nutrition guidelines, directories of key health organizations, Spanish translations for commonly used vocabulary, immunizations, contagious and sexually transmitted diseases, diagnosis-related groups, and the latest NANDA-approved nursing diagnoses. All appendixes have been updated to include the latest available information.

In addition, new appendixes have been added to provide essential information on advance directives, OSHA guidelines for bloodborne pathogens (in addition to universal precautions guidelines), clinical calculations, French equivalents of common medical terms and phrases, assessment guides, guidelines for relating to patients from different cultures, and an extensive listing of nursing diagnoses related to numerous diseases, disorders, and procedures. The appendixes alone make our dictionary an indispensable resource for students and professionals in the health sciences.

All the virtues of the first three editions have been retained. Word roots and pronunciations are provided for principal entries to assist in learning and using vocabulary. Among the entries on diseases, drugs, and procedures, at least 1,000 include practical information presented under separate headings such as "methods," "adverse effects," "nursing considerations," and "outcome criteria." The rationale for all procedures is given due attention. The inclusion of numerous prefixes and suffixes gives the reader additional access not only to the meanings of defined terms but also to terms that are not included in this dictionary and that, to a large extent, are not found in other reference works. The myriad cross references from definition to definition are well chosen and contribute to the dictionary's encyclopedic dimensions. As with the prior editions, *Mosby's Dictionary* continues to serve nursing and allied health students and professionals as the most comprehensive, authoritative, and up-to-date dictionary available.

It is impossible to acknowledge specifically the many individuals who have contributed to the fourth edition of *Mosby's Dictionary*. However, we would particularly like to thank Ken and Lois Anderson for their dedication, patience, professionalism, and flexibility in writing and rewriting new and existing entries and Walter D. Glanze for his insight, attention to detail, and commitment to quality in reviewing all proofs and for writing pronunciations. Our board of consultants graciously gave of their time and expertise to help ensure that the new edition of our dictionary would be a comprehensive, reliable, up-to-date resource for students and professionals in the health sciences. We appreciate their important contribution. We are especially grateful to the many Mosby, Wolfe, and Gower authors and artists whose photographs and line drawings appear in this new edition of our dictionary. We thank our team of illustration researchers who tirelessly pursued the daunting challenge of selecting nearly 2,000 high-quality, relevant illustrations to enhance and clarify definitions. Fiona Foley, Elizabeth Horne, Jane Hunter, and Pauline Manton of Mosby's London and New York offices were of invaluable assistance in contacting authors and obtaining approval for the use of these illustrations. These people and many others played important roles in the development and publication of our new edition. We appreciate their contributions and trust that they will be proud to be associated with the landmark fourth edition of *Mosby's Medical, Nursing, and Allied Health Dictionary*.

Mosby

CONSULTANTS

Betty J. Ackley, MSN, EdS, RN
Professor of Nursing
Jackson Community College
Jackson, Michigan

Beth Arnold
Department of Nursing
Vernon Regional Junior College
Vernon, Texas

Emilie J. Aubert, MA, PT
Assistant Professor of Physical
Therapy
Marquette University
Milwaukee, Wisconsin

Addison Ault, PhD
Department of Chemistry
Cornell College
Mount Vernon, Iowa

Miriam G. Austrin, RN, BA
Consultant
Austrin Associates
St. Louis, Missouri

Deborah Bartnick
Department of LPN
Ivy Tech College
Lafayette, Indiana

Edward S. Bennett, OD, MS, MEd
Associate Professor of Optometry
School of Optometry
University of Missouri, St. Louis
St. Louis, Missouri

Diane M. Billings, EdD, RN, FAAN
Professor of Nursing & Assistant
Dean of Learning Resources
Indiana University School of Nursing
Indianapolis, Indiana

Jackie Birmingham, RN, BSN, MS
Director
Discharge Planning
Hartford Hospital
Hartford, Connecticut

Joseph Bittengle, MEd, RT(R) (ARRT)
Assistant Professor/Chairman
Department of Radiologic
Technology
University of Arkansas for Medical
Sciences
Little Rock, Arkansas

Christine Bolwell, RN, MSN
Consultant
Diskovery: Computer-Assisted
Healthcare Education
Saratoga, California

Edward T. Bope, MD
Riverside Methodist Hospital
Columbus, Ohio

Violet Breckbill, PhD, RN
Nursing Consultant, Biological
Sciences
Vero Beach, Florida

Frances R. Brown, RN, PhD
Assistant Professor
Decker School of Nursing
State University of New York at
Binghamton
Binghamton, New York

Lynda Burroughs, BSN, MAN
Associate Professor of Nursing
Broward Community College
Broward, Florida

Katharine G. Butler, PhD
Research Professor
Communication Sciences and
Disorders
Syracuse University
Syracuse, New York

Mary Butts, RN, CSN, MEd
School of Practical Nursing
Franklin County Area Vocational-
Technical School
Chambersburg, Pennsylvania

Deborah Cameron, RN, BAAN, MEd
(pending)
Nursing Professor
School of Health Sciences
Centennial College of Applied Arts
and Technology
Scarborough, Ontario, Canada

Gayle Kathleen Campbell, RN, BSN,
BHSA
Programme Co-ordinator
School of Applied Arts and Health
Sciences
Georgian College of Applied Arts and
Technology
Orillia, Ontario, Canada

Toni Cascio, RN, MN, CCRN
Clinical Educator - Adult Critical Care
Department of Nursing Education and
Research
Ochsner Foundation Hospital
New Orleans, Louisiana

Carol J. Chancey, RN, MS
Nursing Faculty
St. Petersburg Junior College
St. Petersburg, Florida

Jane C. Clark, MN, RN, OCN
Clinical Nurse Specialist, Oncology
Emory University Hospital
Atlanta, Georgia

Jacqueline J. Clibourn, RN, HP
(ASCP)
Manager, Clinical Research Programs
Haemonetics Corporation
Braintree, Massachusetts

Charlene D. Coco, RN, MN
Louisiana State University Medical
Center
School of Nursing
Associate Degree Program
New Orleans, Louisiana

Jeffrey A. Cokely, PhD
Assistant Professor of Audiology
Department of Communication
Disorders
Baylor University
Waco, Texas

Bruce Colbert, MS, RRT
Respiratory Care Program
University of Pittsburgh at
Johnstown
Johnstown, Pennsylvania

Mary Boudreau Conover, RN, BS
Director of Education
Critical Care Conferences
Santa Cruz, California

Patricia Dardis, MS, RNC, CNS, FNP
Assistant Professor of Nursing
University of North Dakota
Statewide Psychiatric Nursing
Education Program
Jamestown, North Dakota

Mardell Davis, RN, MSN, CETN
University of Alabama School of
Nursing
University of Alabama at Birmingham
Birmingham, Alabama

Hetty L. DeVroom, RN, BSN, CNRN
Clinical Research Nurse
Surgical Neurology Branch
NINDS, National Institutes of Health
Bethesda, Maryland

Clarice L. Dietrich, RDH, MA
Associate Professor
Program Coordinator, Dental Hygiene
Onondaga Community College
Syracuse, New York

Marcelline Eachus, RN, BSN
Department of Health Occupation
Gloucester County Vocational-
   Technical School
Sewell, New Jersey

Jody A. Eckler, RN BSN
Huron County Health Department
School Nurse & Maternal-Child
   Health Division
Director, Phoenix Health & Education
   Services
Castalia, Ohio

Janet E. Edens, MSN, RN
Department of Nursing
Eastern Kentucky University
Richmond, Kentucky

Irene Eskildsen, RN, BSN
School of Nursing
Royal Alexandra Hospital
Edmonton, Alberta, Canada

Ann Fagerness, RN, BSN, CNRN,
   CCRN, RNC
Health Education Network
Seattle, Washington

Neil B. Ford, PhD
Professor
Department of Biology
University of Texas at Tyler
Tyler, Texas

Stephanie Fox-Young
Head of Programme Nursing
Division of Nursing and Health
   Sciences
Gold Coast University College of
   Griffith University
Southport, Queensland, Australia

Kerry E. George
School of Respiratory Therapy
Des Moines Area Community College
Ankeny, Iowa

M.A. Gray, MEd, BA, DipNEd
Associate Professor
Faculty of Nursing
University of Technology
Sydney, New South Wales, Australia

Patty Hale, RN, MSN
Assistant Professor
University of Virginia
Health Sciences Center
School of Nursing
Charlottesville, Virginia

Mark Hamelink, CRNA, MSN
Lakeshore Anesthesia, P.C.
South Haven, Michigan

Wendy B. Hamilton, RN, BA, MEd
Professor
School of Nursing
Ryerson Polytechnical University
Toronto, Ontario, Canada

Mildred L. Hamner, RNC, EdD
Professor of Nursing
University of Alabama School of
   Nursing
University of Alabama at Birmingham
Birmingham, Alabama

Mary Barb Haq, PhD, RN, CS
Assistant Professor
Seton Hall University
College of Nursing
South Orange, New Jersey

Janice Hausauer, RN, MS, CCRN
College of Nursing
Montana State University
Bozeman, Montana

E. Charles Healey, PhD
Associate Professor of
   Speech-Language Pathology
Department of Special Education and
   Communication Disorders
University of Nebraska-Lincoln
Lincoln, Nebraska

Susan R. Herman, MSN, RN
Associate Professor, Nursing
Chaffey College
Rancho Cucamonga, California

Marcia J. Hill, RN, MSN
Manager, Dermatologic Therapeutics
The Methodist Hospital
Clinical Assistant Professor
Baylor College of Medicine
Houston, Texas

Shirley P. Hoeman, PhD, RN
Health Systems Consultations
Long Valley, New Jersey

Michael S. Hudecki, PhD, DSc
Research Associate Professor
Department of Biological Science
State University of New York at
   Buffalo
Buffalo, New York

Terry Karapas, RN, MS
Neuroscience Clinical Nurse Specialist
University of Chicago Hospitals
Chicago, Illinois

Larita Norris Kaspar, MSN, RN
Assistant Professor
Division of Allied Health & Nursing
Lorain County Community College
Elyria, Ohio

Jerry H. Kennedy, MN, RNCS
Instructor
Associate Degree Nursing
Midlands Technical College
Columbia, South Carolina

Patricia T. Ketcham, MSN, RN
Assistant Professor
Undergraduate Program Director
Oakland University School of Nursing
Rochester, Michigan

Marjorie Knox, MPA, MA, RN
Professor of Nursing
Community College of Rhode Island
Nursing Program
Warwick, Rhode Island

Kathy Kozak, RN, BA, BScN
Nursing Instructor
Kelsey Diploma Nursing Program
Saskatchewan Institute of Applied
   Science and Technology
Saskatoon, Saskatchewan, Canada

Thomas Kraker, MEd, RT(R)
Chairman/Associate Professor
Boise State University
Department of Radiologic Sciences
Boise, Idaho

Joan M. Kulpa, EdD, MSN, RN
Associate Professor
Department of Nursing
Bradley University
Peoria, Illinois

Mavis Kyle, RN, BScN, MHSA
College of Nursing
University of Saskatchewan
Saskatoon, Saskatchewan, Canada

Gail B. Ladwig, MSN, RN
Professor of Nursing
Jackson Community College
Jackson, Michigan

Diane Langevin, CDA, RDH, MA
Dental Technologies Department
  Manager
York Technical College
Rock Hill, South Carolina

Linda Armstrong Lazure, RN, MSN
School of Nursing
Creighton University
Omaha, Nebraska

Elaine Lee
Department of Nursing
Australian Catholic University
North Sydney, New South Wales,
  Australia

Donna M. Lewis-Stevens, RN, CMNP
Washington University School of
  Medicine
Department of Rheumatology
St. Louis, Missouri

Maxine E. Loomis, RNCS, PhD, FAAN
College of Nursing
University of South Carolina
Columbia, South Carolina

Carolyn Loop, BSRT, RT
Radiology School Coordinator
School of Radiologic Sciences
St. Francis Regional Medical Center
Wichita, Kansas

Brad Lopez, BA, MS
Instructor Health Sciences
Respiratory Therapy Program
Fresno City College
Fresno, California

Ruth Ludwick, RNC, PhD
Assistant Professor
Kent State University
School of Nursing
Kent, Ohio

Lois Irby Mack, MS, RN, CMAC
Assistant Professor MA/MLT
Cuyahoga Community College
Cleveland, Ohio

Jannetta MacPhail, PhD, MSN, FAAN, LLD(Hon)
Professor Emeritus and Retired Dean
Faculty of Nursing
University of Alberta
Edmonton, Alberta, Canada

Ann Marriner-Tomey, RN, BS, MS, PhD, FAAN
Dean and Professor
School of Nursing
Indiana State University
Terre Haute, Indiana

Lori Martell, BS, PhD
Section of Neurosurgery
The University of Michigan Medical
  Center
Ann Arbor, Michigan

Sheryl A. Martz, RN, MSN
Associate Professor
Brookdale Community College
Lincroft, New Jersey

Edwina A. McConnell, RN, PhD
Independent Nurse Consultant
Madison, Wisconsin

Linda McLeod, RegN, BSN, MContEd
Nursing Instructor
Kelsey Diploma Nursing Program
Sasketchewan Institute of Applied
  Science and Technology
Saskatoon, Saskatchewan, Canada

Bozena B. Michniak, BSc, PhD, MRPharmSoc
College of Pharmacy
University of South Carolina
Columbia, South Carolina

Christina M. Mumma, CRRN, PhD
University of Alaska, Anchorage
School of Nursing and Health
  Sciences
Anchorage, Alaska

Helen K. Mussallem, CC, BN, MA, EdD, LLD, DSc, DStJ, FRCN, MRSH
Special Adviser to National and
  International Health Organizations
Ottawa, Ontario, Canada

Dennis R. Myers, BA, RT(R)
Academic Director
St. Francis Regional Medical Center
School of Radiologic Sciences
Wichita, Kansas

Kim A. Neudorf, RN, BSN
Instructor
Kelsey Diploma Nursing Program
Saskatchewan Institute of Applied
  Science and Technology
Saskatoon, Saskatchewan, Canada

Susan Jenkinson Neuman, RN, AS, BA
Nursing Practice Adviser
College of Nurses of Ontario
Toronto, Ontario, Canada

Donna Ortega, RN, MSN
School of Nursing
Community College of Denver
Denver, Colorado

Martin Owen
Faculty of Nursing
Deakin University
Geelong, Victoria, Australia

Kathleen Deska Pagana, PhD, RN
Associate Professor of Nursing
Lycoming College
Williamsport, Pennsylvania

Michael A. Pagliarulo, EdD, PT
Physical Therapy Program
Ithaca College
Ithaca, New York

Glenda Paisley, BA, RN, BSCN
School of Nursing
Royal Alexandra Hospital
Edmonton, Alberta, Canada

Emma Ree Pelham, RN
Coordinator, Nursing Skills Lab
Fresno City College
Fresno, California

Cindy A. Peternelj-Taylor, RN, BScN, MSc
Assistant Professor
College of Nursing
University of Saskatchewan
Saskatoon, Saskatchewan, Canada

Olga Carol Petrozella, RN, BSN, MSEd, MSN
Associate Professor, Senior
Miami Dade Community College
Nursing Education, Medical Center
  Campus
Miami, Florida

Timothy Philipp, RN, PhD
Chicago, Illinois

Victoria Poole, RN, DSN
Assistant Professor
University of Alabama School of
  Nursing
University of Alabama at Birmingham
Birmingham, Alabama

Joyce Powers, RN, MSN, CS
Veterans Administration Medical
Center
Albuquerque, New Mexico

Joanne Profetto-McGrath, RN,
BAPsych, BScN, MEd
Facilitator-Curriculum
Royal Alexandra Hospital
School of Nursing
Edmonton, Alberta, Canada

Dale Rajacich, MSCN, RN
Assistant Professor
University of Windsor
Windsor, Ontario, Canada

William G. Rector Jr, MD
Associate Clinical Professor of
Medicine
University of Colorado School of
Medicine
Denver, Colorado

Diana Reding, RN, BS, MS
Dallas County Community College
El Centro College/ADN
Dallas, Texas

Kathlyn L. Reed, PhD, OTR, MLIS
Information Services/Education
Librarian
Houston Academy of Sciences
Texas Medical Center Library
Houston, Texas

Malvin E. Ring, DDS, MLS, FACD
Clinical Associate Professor (Ret)
School of Dental Medicine
State University of New York at
Buffalo
Buffalo, New York

Janet T. Robuck, MS, RD
Associate Professor of Nutrition
University of Alabama School of
Nursing
University of Alabama at Birmingham
Birmingham, Alabama

Elizabeth A. Schenk, MSN, CRRN,
RNCS
Vice President of Nursing
Heather Hill, Inc.
Chardon, Ohio

Sister Mary Arthur Schramm,
CRNA, PhD
Director/Professor
Mount Mary College
Graduate Program in Nurse
Anesthesiology
Yankton, South Dakota

Charlotte Searle, RN, RM, BA, MA,
LLD, DCur, DLitt et Phil
Professor Extraordinarius
University of Namibia
Windhoek, Republic of Namibia

Kay See-Lasley, MS, RPh
Medical Writer/Editor
Kay See-Lasley Associates
Even Better Publishing
Tulsa, Oklahoma

Brenda K. Shelton, MS, RN, CCRN,
OCN
The Johns Hopkins Oncology Center
Baltimore, Maryland

Kim Sherer, RN, MN
Department of Nursing
Northern Oklahoma College
Tonkawa, Oklahoma

Dan Shock, MA, RT(T)
West Virginia University Hospitals
Morgantown, West Virginia

Sandra L. Siehl, RN, BA, BSN, MSN
Barnes Hospital
St. Louis, Missouri

Nancy Simmons, RN, MS, CNA
School of Nursing
St. Xavier College
Chicago, Illinois

Kathleen Simpson, RNC, MSN
Perinatal Clinical Nurse Specialist
St. John's Mercy Medical Center
Lecturer
University of Missouri–St. Louis
School of Nursing
St. Louis, Missouri

Candace Skrapek, RegN, BN
Kelsey Diploma Nursing Program
Saskatchewan Institute of Applied
Science and Technology
Saskatoon, Saskatchewan, Canada

Ida L. Slusher, MSN
Assistant Professor
Department of Nursing
Eastern Kentucky University
Richmond, Kentucky

Donna Phillips Smith, MS, RN
Genetic Counselor
Chapman Institute of Medical
Genetics
Children's Medical Center
Tulsa, Oklahoma

Robert R. Smith, BS, MS, PhD
Professor
Science Department
Forest Park Community College
St. Louis, Missouri

Joanne Spaide, PhD, RD, LD
University of Northern Iowa
Associate Professor and Director
Didactic Program in Dietetics
Cedar Falls, Iowa

Sandra Mason Spengler, RN, MSN
George C. Wallace Community
College
Dothan, Alabama

Annette Smith Stacy, MSN, RN, CS,
OCN
Assistant Professor of Nursing
College of Nursing and Health
Professions
Arkansas State University
Jonesboro, Arkansas

Kaye L. Stanek, PhD, RD, CN
University of Nebraska
Department of Nutritional Science and
Dietetics
Lincoln, Nebraska

Ruth Anderson Stephens, RN, PhD
Professor of Nursing
Florida Community College at
Jacksonville
Department of Associate Degree
Nursing
Jacksonville, Florida

Bernice D. Stiansen, RN, BScN
Instructor
Grant MacEwan Community College
Edmonton, Alberta
Canada

Stephen P. Storfer, MD
Chief, Infectious Diseases
Incarnate Word Hospital
St. Louis, Missouri

Michael Strysick
Consultant and R&D Research
Sheboygan, Wisconsin

Patricia Greb Sullivan, RN, MS
Instructor
Associate Degree Nursing
Midland College
Midland, Texas

Dorothy Thomas, RN, MSN
Associate Professor of Nursing
St. Louis Community College at
  Florissant Valley
St. Louis, Missouri

June D. Thompson, RN, MS
Prairie View A & M University
  (formerly)
Prairie View, Texas

Catherine A. Trombly, ScD OTR/L,
  FAOTA
Professor
Department of Occupational Therapy
Sargent College of Allied Health
  Professions
Boston University
Boston, Massachusetts

Mary L. Turgeon, EdD
Associate Director of Medical
  Education
Guthrie HealthCare System
Sayre, Pennsylvania

Jean Urick, RN, MN
Southeastern Louisiana University
School of Nursing
Hammond, Louisiana

Margaret Uyeda
Department of Nursing
Charles Stuart University
North Wagga Wagga, North South
  Wales, Australia

Louis Verardo, MD
Associate Director of Family Practice
  Residency Program
Director CME
North Shore University Hospital at
  Glen Cove
Glen Cove, New York
Clinical Assistant Professor of Family
  Medicine
State University of New York at
  Stony Brook
Stony Brook, New York

Carole J. Petrosky Vozel, RN, C,
  PhD
The Western Pennsylvania Hospital
  School of Nursing
Pittsburgh, Pennsylvania

Pamela Becker Weilitz, MSN(R), RN
Barnes Hospital at Washington
  University Medical Center
St. Louis, Missouri

Patricia Wells, AB
Program Director
School of Nuclear Med Technology
Overlook Hospital
Summit, New Jersey

O.T. Wendel, PhD
Assistant Dean of Medical Education
College of Osteopathic Medicine of
  the Pacific
Pomona, California

John R. White Jr, PharmD
Assistant Professor
Washington State University
College of Pharmacy
Spokane, Washington

Jo Wiggens, RN, BSN, CEN
University of Kentucky Hospital
Clinical Nurse III
Emergency Deparment
Lexington, Kentucky

P. Sharon Wilson, RN, MEd, MN
Professor, School of Nursing
Ryerson Polytechnical Institute
Toronto, Ontario, Canada

William Wojciechowski, MS, RRT
Chairman & Associate Professor
Department of Respiratory Care and
  Cardiopulmonary Sciences
University of South Alabama
Mobile, Alabama

Gale Woolley, EdD, ARNP
Professor
Miami-Dade Community College
Medical Center Campus
Miami, Florida

Caroline M. Wright, RN, CM,
  DipTeach(Nurs), MA(Hon), PhD
Senior Lecturer
Faculty of Nursing and Community
  Studies
University of Western Sydney,
  Hawkesbury
Richmond, New South Wales,
  Australia

Bonnie Young, RN, BSN
Sharon Regional Health System
School of Nursing
Sharon, Pennsylvania

Katherine E. Yutzy, RN, MSN
Associate Professor
Department of Nursing
Goshen College
Goshen, Indiana

Hana Zemplenyi, MSc
Los Angeles County School of
  Nursing
Los Angeles, California

LIST OF ILLUSTRATIONS

LIST OF TABLES

GUIDE TO THE DICTIONARY

A. ALPHABETIC ORDER

The entries are alphabetized in dictionary style, that is, letter by letter, disregarding spaces or hyphens between words:

analgesic   artificial lung
anal membrane   artificially acquired immunity
analog   artificial pacemaker

(Alphabetized in telephone-book style, that is, word by word, the order would be different: **anal membrane / analgesic / analog; artificial lung / artificial pacemaker / artificially acquired immunity.**)

The alphabetization is alphanumeric; that is, words and numbers form a single list, numbers being positioned as though they were spelled-out numerals: **Nilstat/90-90 traction/ninth nerve.** (An example of the few exceptions to this rule is the sequence **17-hydroxycorticosteroid / 11-hydroxyetiocholanolone / 5-hydroxyindoleacetic acid,** which can be found between the entries **hydroxochloroquine sulfate** and **hydroxyl,** not, as may be expected, **17-** . . . in letter "S," **11-.** . . in letter "E," and **5-.** . . in letter "F.").

Small subscript and superscript numbers are disregarded in alphabetizing: **No / N₂O / nobelium**

For the alphabetization of prefixes and suffixes, see F below.

B. COMPOUND HEADWORDS

Compound headwords are given in their natural word order: **abdominal surgery,** not **surgery, abdominal; achondroplastic dwarf,** not **dwarf, achondroplastic.**

When appropriate, a reference is made elsewhere to the nonalphabetized element; the entry **dwarf,** for example, shows this indirect cross-reference: ". . . Kinds of dwarfs include **achondroplastic dwarf,** . . ." (followed by additional terms ending in "dwarf").

There are few exceptions to this natural word order; nearly all of these concern formal classifications, for example: "**comfort, alteration in: pain,** a nursing diagnosis accepted by the Fourth National Conference on the Classification of Nursing Diagnoses . . ."

(NOTE: In this guide, the term "headword" is used to refer to any alphabetized and nonindented definiendum, be it a single-word term or a compound term.)

C. MULTIPLE DEFINITIONS

If a headword has more than one meaning, the meanings are numbered and are often accompanied by an indication of the field in which a sense applies: "**fractionation, 1.** (in neurology) . . . **2.** (in chemistry) . . . **3.** (in bacteriology) . . . **4.** (in histology) . . . **5.** (in radiology) . . ."

Smaller differences in meaning are occasionally separated by semicolons: "**enervation, 1.** the reduction or lack of nervous energy; weakness; lassitude, languor. **2.** removal of a complete nerve or of a section of nerve."

Words that are spelled alike but have entirely different meanings and origins are usually given as separate entries, with superscript numbers: "**aural**[1], of or pertaining to the ear or hearing . . ." followed by "**aural**[2], of or pertaining to an aura."

For reference entries that appear in the form of numbered senses, see the example of **hyperalimentation** at E below.

D. THE BOLDFACE ELEMENTS OF AN ENTRY

After the entry headword, which has large boldface type, the following elements may occur in boldface, in this order.

In boldface:

■ HEADWORD ABBREVIATIONS: **central nervous system (CNS)**
A corresponding abbreviation entry is listed: "**CNS,** abbreviation for **central nervous sytem.**" (For abbreviation entries, see F below.)

Occasionally the order is reversed: "**DDT (dichlordiphenyltrichloroethane),**" with a corresponding reference entry: "**dichlordiphenyltrichloroethane.** See **DDT.**" (For reference entries, see E below.)

■ PLURAL OR SINGULAR FORMS that are not obvious. The first form shown is the more common except when plurals are of more or less equal frequency: "**carcinoma,** *pl.* **carcinomas, carcinomata**"; **cortex,** *pl.* **cortices**"; "**data,** *sing.* **datum**"

A reference entry is listed only when the terms are alphabetically separated; for example, there are several entries between **data** and "**datum.** See **data.**"

■ HIDDEN ENTRIES, that is, terms that can best be defined in the context of a more general entry. For example, the definition of the entry **equine encephalitis** continues as follows: ". . . **Eastern equine encephalitis (EEE)** is a severe form of the infection . . . **western equine encephalitis (WEE),** which occurs . . . **Venezuelan equine encephalitis (VEE),** which is common in . . ."

The corresponding reference entries are **"eastern equine encephalitis. See equine encephalitis."; "western equine encephalitis. See equine . . .";** and so forth. For further reference, from the abbreviations **EEE, WEE,** and **VEE,** see F below.

■ INDIRECT CROSS-REFERENCES to other defined entries, shown as part of the definition and usually introduced by "Kinds of": **"dwarf, . . .** Kinds of dwarfs include **achondroplastic dwarf, asexual dwarf, . . . ,** and **thanatophoric dwarf."**

The entry referred to may or may not show a reciprocal reference, depending on the information value.

■ SYNONYMOUS TERMS, preceded by "Also called," "Also spelled," or, for verbs and adjectives, "Also": **"abducens nerve, . . .** Also called **sixth nerve."**

A corresponding reference entry is usually given: **"sixth nerve. See abducens nerve."**

Occasionally the synonymous term is accompanied by a usage label: **"abdomen, . . .** Also called *(informal)* **belly."**

If a synonymous term applies to only one numbered sense, it precedes rather than follows the definition, to avoid ambiguity: **"algology, 1.** the branch of medicine that is concerned with the study of pain. **2.** also called **phycology.** the branch of science that is concerned with algae." (Whenever a synonymous term *follows* the last numbered sense, it applies to all senses of the entry.)

■ (DIRECT) CROSS-REFERENCES, preceded by "See also" or "Compare," referring to another defined entry for additional information: **"abdominal aorta, . . .** See also **descending aorta."**

The cross-reference may or may not be reciprocal.

Cross-references are also made to illustrations, to tables, to the color atlas, and to the appendixes.

For cross-references from an abbreviation entry (with "See"), see F below.

■ PARTS OF SPEECH related to the entry headword, shown as run-on entries that do not require a separate definition: **"abalienation, . . . —abalienate,** *v.,* **abalienated,** *adj.*"

E. REFERENCE ENTRIES

Reference entries are undefined entries referring to a defined entry. There, they usually correspond to the boldface terms for which reference entries are mentioned at D above.

However, many of the less frequently used synonymous terms are listed as a reference only; at the entry referred to, the reader's attention is not drawn to them with "Also called."

A reference entry may also refer to a defined entry for other reasons: A particular lightface term in the definition is occasionally referred to: **"motion sickness, . . .** air sickness . . ."—with the reference entry **"air sickness: See motion sickness."** Or a reference is made to give additional

access to a definition or to part of a definition: **"congenital condition. See congenital anomaly."**—although the latter entry does not literally mention "congenital condition," and is not a synonymous term.

Some reference entries appear in the form of a numbered sense of a defined entry: **"hyperalimentation, 1.** overfeeding or the . . . in excess of the demands of the appetite. **2.** See **total parenteral nutrition."** The latter entry says "Also called **hyperalimentation."**

If two or more alphabetically adjacent terms refer to the same entry or entries, they are styled as one reference entry: **"coxa adducta, coxa flexa. See coxa vara."**

A reference entry that would be derived from a boldface term in an immediately adjacent entry is not listed again as a headword; it becomes a "hidden reference entry": **"acardius amorphus, . . .** Also called **acardius anceps."** But **acardius anceps** is not listed again as a reference entry because it would immediately *follow* the entry, the next entry being **acariasis.** Likewise: **"acoustic neuroma, . . .** Also called **acoustic neurilemmoma, acoustic neurinoma, acoustic neurofibroma."** But the three synonymous terms are not listed again as reference entries because they would immediately *precede* the entry, the entry ahead being **acoustic nerve.** Therefore:

> **If a term is not listed at the expected place, the reader might find it among the boldface terms of the immediately preceding or the immediately following entry.**

F. OTHER KINDS OF ENTRIES

■ ABBREVIATION ENTRIES: Most abbreviation entries, including symbol entries, show the full form of the term in boldface: **"ABC,** abbreviation for **aspiration biopsy cytology." "H,** a symbol for **hydrogen."** Implied reference is made to the entries **aspiration biopsy cytology** and **hydrogen** respectively.

Abbreviation entries for which there is no corresponding entry show the full form in italics: **"CBF,** abbreviation for *cerebral blood flow."* **"f,** symbol for *respiratory frequency."*

A combination of abbreviation entry and reference entry occurs when the abbreviation is that of a boldface or lightface term appearing under another headword. For example, the hidden entries at D above (in addition to the reference entries shown there) are also referred to in the following manner: **"EEE,** abbreviation for **eastern equine encephalitis. See equine encephalitis."** An example with a lightface term: **"HLA-A,** abbreviation for *human leukocyte anti-*

gen A. See **human leukocyte antigen.**" The latter entry says ". . . They are HLA-A, HLA-B, HLA-C . . ."

■ PREFIXES AND SUFFIXES: The large amount and the nature of prefix and suffix entries are an important feature of this dictionary. Through these entries the reader has additional access to the meanings of headwords and the words used in defining them. But such entries also give access to thousands of terms that are not included in this dictionary (and, to a large extent, are not found in any other reference work). For example, the entries **xylo-** and **-phage** (plus **-phagia, phago-,** and **-phagy**) may lead to the meaning of "xylophagous," namely, "wood-eating."

Prefix and suffix headwords consisting of variants are alphabetized by the first variant only. For example, **"epi-, ep-,** a prefix meaning 'on, upon' . . ." is followed by **epiblast** (notwithstanding **"ep-"**). The other variant or variants are listed in their own alphabetical place as reference entries referring to the first variant: **"ep-.** See **epi-."**

■ ENTRIES WITH SPECIAL PARAGRAPHS: Among the entries on diseases, drugs, and procedures, at least 1000 feature special paragraphs, with headings such as:

observations, intervention, and *nursing considerations.* (for disease entries),

indications, contraindications, and *"adverse effects."* (for drug entries),

"method," "nursing interventions," and *"outcome criteria."* (for procedure entries).

G. FURTHER COMMENTS

■ EPONYMOUS TERMS THAT END IN "SYNDROME" OR "DISEASE" are given with an apostrophe (and "s" where appropriate) if they are based on the name of one person: **Adie's syndrome; Symmers' disease; Treacher Collins' syndrome** (the ophthalmologist Edward Treacher Collins). If they are based on the names of several people, they are without apostrophe: **Bernard-Soulier syndrome; Brill-Symmers disease.**

■ ABBREVIATIONS AND LABELS IN ITALIC TYPE: The abbreviations are *pl.* (plural), *npl.* (noun plural), *sing.* (singular); *n.* (noun), *adj.* (adjective), *v.* (verb). The recurring labels are *slang, informal, nontechnical, obsolete, archaic; chiefly British, Canada, U.S.*

■ DICTIONARY OF FIRST REFERENCE for general spelling preferences is *Webster's New Collegiate Dictionary;* thereafter: *Webster's Third New International Dictionary.*

H. PRONUNCIATION

■ SYSTEM: See the Pronunciation Key on p. xxxiii. The pronunciation system of this dictionary is basically a system that most readers know from their use of popular English dictionaries, especially the major college or desk dictionaries. All

symbols for English sounds are ordinary letters of the alphabet with few adaptations, and with the exception of the schwa, /ə/ (the neutral vowel).

■ ACCENTS: Pronunciation, given between slants, is shown with primary and secondary accents, and a raised dot shows that two vowels or, occasionally, two consonants, between the slants are pronounced separately:

anoopsia /an′ō·op′sē·ə/
cecoileostomy /sē′kō·il′ē·os′təmē/
methemoglobin /met′hēməglō′bin, met·hē′məglōbin/

Without the raised dot, the second /th/ in the last example would be pronounced as in "thin." (The pronunciation key lists the following paired consonant symbols as representing a single sound: /ch/, /ng/, /sh/, /th/, *th/*, /zh/, and the foreign sounds /kh/ and *kh*/—if no raised dot intervenes.)

■ TRUNCATION: Pronunciation may be given in truncated form, especially for alternative or derived words:

defibrillate /difī′brilāt, difib′-/
bacteriophage /baktir′ē·əfāj′, . . .—**bacteriophagy** /-of′əjē/, *n.*

In the last example, the reader is asked to make the commonsense assumption that the primary accent of the headword becomes a secondary accent in the run-on term: /baktir′ē·of′əjē/.

■ LOCATION: Pronunciation may be given for any boldface term and may occur anywhere in an entry:

aura /ôr′ə/, **1.** *pl.* **aurae** /ôr′ē/, a sensation . . . **2.** *pl.* **auras,** an emanation of light . . .
micrometer, 1. /mīkrom′ətər/, an instrument used for . . . **2.** /mī′krōmē′tər/, a unit of measurement . . .

Occasionally it is given for a lightface term:

b.i.d., (in presecriptions) abbreviation for *bis in die* /dē′ā/, a Latin phrase meaning . . .
boutonneuse fever. . ., an infectious disease . . . a tache noire /täshnô·är′/ or black spot . . .

■ LETTERWORD VERSUS ACRONYM: Letterwords are abbreviations that are pronounced by sounding the names of each letter, whereas acronyms are pronounced as words. If the pronunciation of an abbreviation is not given, the abbreviation is usually a letterword:

ABO blood groups [read /ā′bē′ō′/, not /ā′bō/]

If the pronunciation is an acronym, this is indicated by pronunciation:

AWOL /ā′wôl/

Some abbreviations are used as both:

JAMA /jä′mä, jam′ə, jā′ā′em′ā′/

■ FOREIGN SOUNDS: Non-English sounds do not occur often in this dictionary. They are represented by the following symbols:

/œ/   as in (French) **feu** /fœ/, **Europe** /œrôp'/; (German) **schön** /shœn/, **Goethe** /gœ'tə/

/Y/   as in (French) **tu** /tY/, **déjà vu** /dāzhävY'/; (German) **grün** /grYn/, **Walküre** /vulkY'rə/

/kh/   as in (Scottish) **loch** /lokh/; (German) **Rorschach** /rôr'shokh/, **Bach** /bokh, bäkh/

/kh/   as in (German) **ich** /ikh/, **Reich** /rīkh/ (or, approximated, as in English **fish:** /ish/, rīsh/)

/N/   This symbol does not represent a sound but indicates that the preceding vowel is a nasal, as in French **bon** /bôN/, **en face** /äNfäs'/, or **international** /aNternäsyōnäl'/.

/nyə/ Occurring at the end of French words, this symbol is not truly a separate syllable but an /n/ with a slight /y/ (similar to the sound in "onion") plus a near-silent /ə/, as in **Bois de Boulogne** /boolō'nyə/, **Malgaigne** /mälgā'nyə/.

Because this work is a subject dictionary rather than a language dictionary, certain foreign words and proper names are rendered by English approximations. Examples are **Müller** /mil'ər/ (which is closer to German than /mY'lər/), **Niemann** /nē'mon/ (which is closer than /nē'män/), **Friedreich** /frēd'rīsh/ (which is close enough for anyone not used to pronouncing /kh/), or **jamais vu,** for which three acceptable pronunciations are given: /zhämävY'/ (near-French) and the approximations /zhämävē'/ and /zhämävoo'/ (/-vē'/ being much closer to French than /-voo'/). Depending on usage, a foreign word or name may be given with near-native pronunciation, with entirely assimilated English pronunciation (as in **de Quervain's fracture** /də kərvänz'/), or with both (as **Dupuytren's contracture** /dYpY·itraNs', dēpē·itranz'/ or **Klippel-Feil syndrome** /klipel'fel', klip'əlfīl'/).

At any rate, the English speaker should not hesitate to follow whatever is usage in his or her working or social environment.

Many of the numerous *Latin* terms in this dictionary are not given with pronunciation, mainly because there are different ways (all of them understood) in which Latin is pronounced by the English speaker and may be pronounced by speakers elsewhere. However, guidance is given in many cases, often to reflect common usage.

■ LATIN AND GREEK PLURALS: The spelling of Latin and Greek plurals is shown in most instances. However, when the plural formation is regular according to Latin and Greek rules, the pronunciation is usually not included. Therefore, the following list shows the suggested pronunciation of selected plural endings that are frequently encountered in the field of medicine:

PLURAL ENDINGS	EXAMPLES
-a /-ə/	**inoculum,** *pl.* **inocula** /inok'yoolə/
-ae /-ē/	**vertebra,** *pl.* **vertebrae** /vur'təbrē/
-ces /-sēz/	**thorax,** *pl.* **thoraces** /thôr'əsēz/
	apex, *pl.* **apices** /ā'pisēz/
-era /-ərə/	**genus,** *pl.* **genera** /jen'ərə/
-ges /-jēz/	**meninx,** *pl.* **meninges** /minin'jēz/
-i /-ī/	**calculus,** *pl.* **calculi** /kal'kyəlī/
	coccus, *pl.* **cocci** /kok'sī/
-ia /-ē·ə/	**criterion,** *pl.* **criteria** /krītir'ē·ə/
-ides /-idēz/	**epulis,** *pl.* **epulides** /ipyoo'lidēz/
-ina /-ənə/	**foramen,** *pl.* **foramina** /fəram'ənə/
-ines /-ənēz/	**lentigo,** *pl.* **lentigines** /lentij'ənēz/
-omata /-ō'mətə/	**hematoma,** *pl.* **hematomata** /hē'mətō'mətə/
-ones /-ō'nēz/	**comedo,** *pl.* **comedones** /kom'ədō'nēz/
-ora /-ərə/	**corpus,** *pl.* **corpora** /kôr'pərə/
	femur, *pl.* **femora** /fem'ərə/
-ses /-sēz/	**analysis,** *pl.* **analyses** /ənal'əsēz/
-udes /-oo'dēz/	**incus,** *pl.* **incudes** /inkoo'dēz/
-us /-oos/	**ductus** (/duk'təs/), *pl.* **ductus** /duk'toos/

NOTE: Notwithstanding the listing of Latin and Greek plurals in this dictionary, and notwithstanding the foregoing examples, in most instances it is acceptable or even preferable to pluralize Latin and Greek words according to the rules of English words. (For certain kinds of entries, both the English and the foreign plurals are given in this dictionary, usually showing the English form first, as, for example, in nearly all **-oma** nouns: **hematoma,** *pl.* **hematomas, hematomata.**)

W.D.G.

I. ETYMOLOGIES AND EPONYMS

The word roots, or etymologies, of the headwords in this dictionary are shown in square brackets following the pronounciations of the headwords. Meanings are given in roman typeface and represent the original connotation of the word from which the medical term is derived. In compound medical terms formed from two or more elements, a plus sign (+) is used to indicate an element has been translated in a previous headword, as in [L *acidus* + Gk *philein* to love]. A semicolon (;) is used to separate word elements having more than one origin, as in [L *abdomen;* Gk *skopein* to view]. Word fragments representing etymologic elements, such as prefixes, are separated from the rest of the word root by a comma (,), as in [Gk *a, basis* not step]. A comma is also used to separate the abbreviation for the language of origin and its translation when the English-language equivalent for the word is the same, as in the term **ala** [L, wing].

The following abbreviations are used to identify language sources:

Afr	African	Jpn	Japanese
Ar	Arabic	L	Latin
AS	Anglo-Saxon	ME	Middle English
Dan	Danish	OE	Old English
D	Dutch	OFr	Old French
Fr	French	ONorse	Old Norse
Ger	German	Port	Portuguese
Gk	Greek	Scand	Scandinavian
Heb	Hebrew	Sp	Spanish
It	Italian	Swe	Swedish
		Turk	Turkish

Some other languages sources, such as Singhalese or Welsh, may be indicated without abbreviations.

Eponymous entries, in which the surname of an individual is incorporated in the headword, are also treated in square brackets with brief biographic details, as in **Alcock's canal** [Joseph Alcock, English surgeon, b. 1784]. When an eponym contains two or more surnames, a semicolon (;) is used to separate the identities of the individuals. Medical terms derived from other proper nouns, such as geographic sites, are presented in a similar manner, as **calabar swelling** [Calabar, a Nigerian seaport], or **ytterbium (Yb)** [Ytterby, Sweden].

K.N.A.

PRONUNCIATION KEY

Vowels

SYMBOLS	KEY WORDS
/a/	hat
/ä/	father
/ā/	fate
/e/	flesh
/ē/	she
/er/	**air, ferry**
/i/	sit
/ī/	**eye**
/ir/	**ear**
/o/	proper
/ō/	nose
/ô/	saw
/oi/	**boy**
/o͞o/	move
/o͝o/	book
/ou/	**out**
/u/	cup, love
/ur/	**fur, first**
/ə/	(the neutral vowel, always unstressed, as in) **ago**, foc**u**s
/ər/	teach**er**, doct**or**

Consonants

SYMBOLS	KEY WORDS
/b/	book
/ch/	chew
/d/	day
/f/	fast
/g/	good
/h/	happy
/j/	gem
/k/	keep
/l/	late
/m/	make
/n/	no
/ng/	sing, drink
/ng·g/	finger
/p/	pair
/r/	ring
/s/	set
/sh/	shoe, lotion
/t/	tone
/th/	thin
/th/	than
/v/	very
/w/	work
/y/	yes
/z/	zeal
/zh/	azure, vision

For /œ/, /Y/, /kh/, /kh/, /N/, and /nyə/, see FOREIGN SOUNDS, p. xxxi.

COLOR ATLAS
OF HUMAN ANATOMY

SKELETAL SYSTEM

ANTERIOR VIEW OF SKELETON
Axial skeleton is shown in blue. Appendicular system is bone colored.

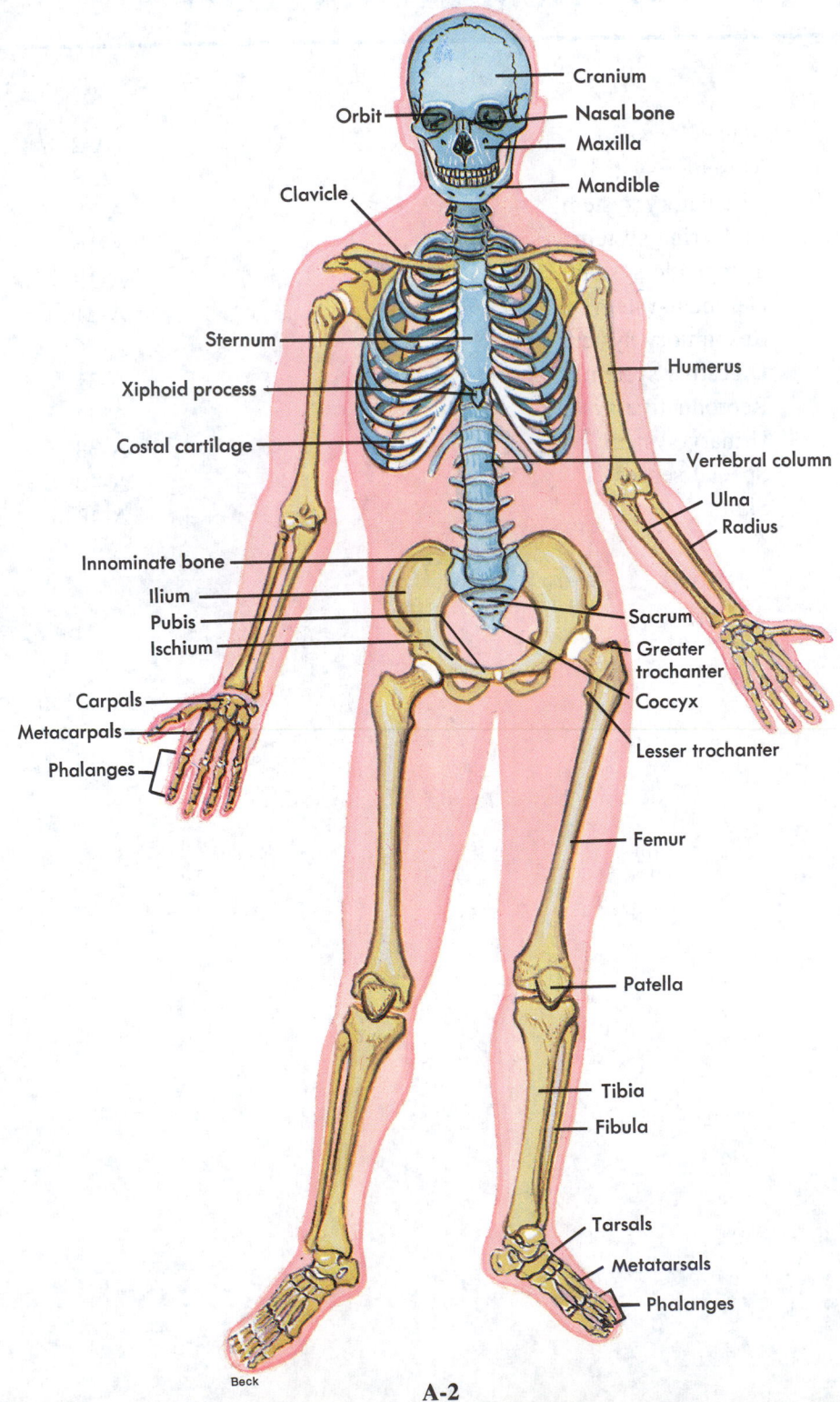

Cranium

Orbit

Nasal bone

Maxilla

Mandible

Clavicle

Sternum

Humerus

Xiphoid process

Costal cartilage

Vertebral column

Ulna

Radius

Innominate bone

Ilium

Pubis

Sacrum

Ischium

Greater trochanter

Coccyx

Carpals

Metacarpals

Lesser trochanter

Phalanges

Femur

Patella

Tibia

Fibula

Tarsals

Metatarsals

Phalanges

Beck

A-2

POSTERIOR VIEW OF SKELETON
Axial skeleton is shown in blue. Appendicular system is
bone colored.

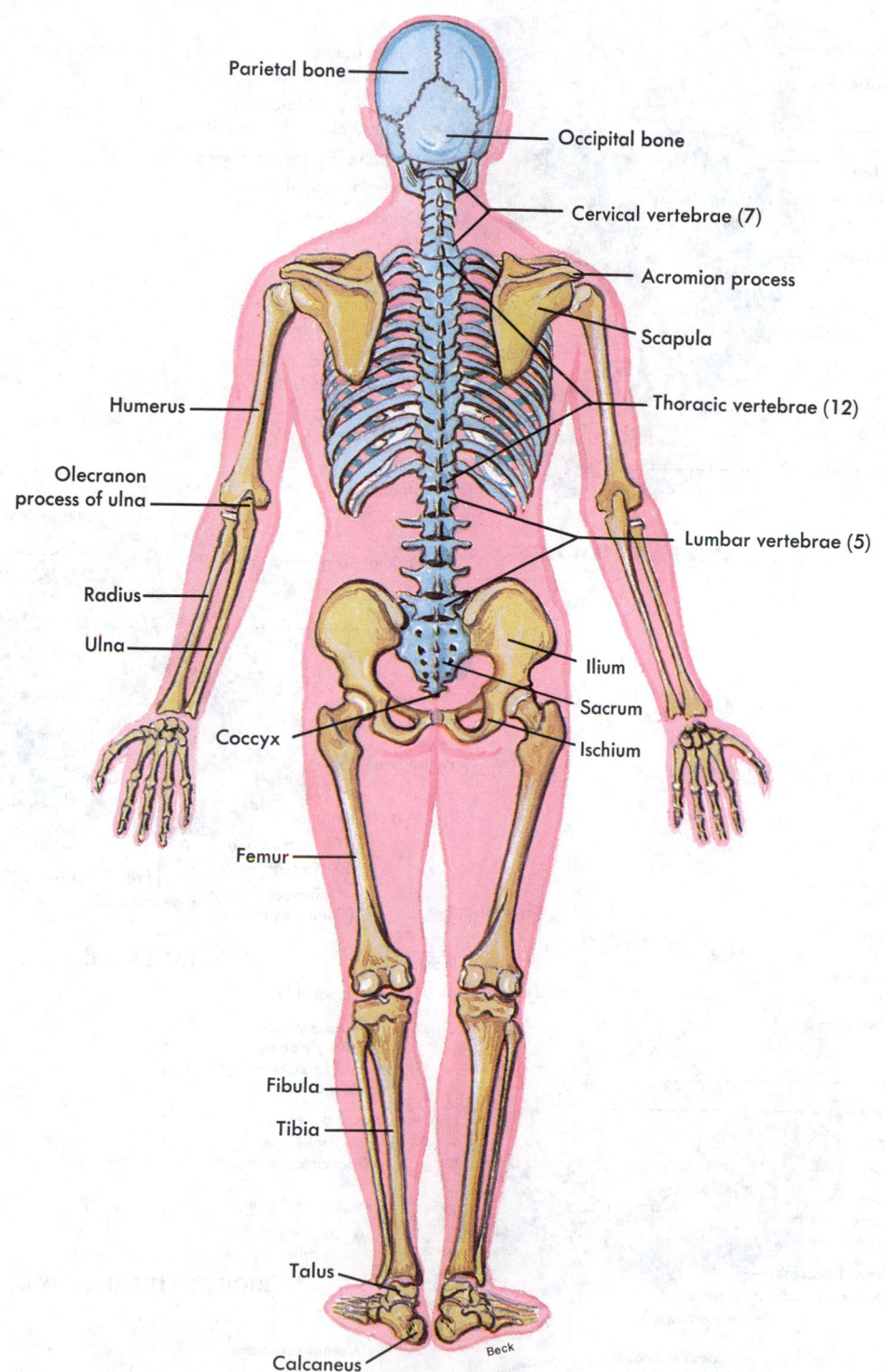

Parietal bone

Occipital bone

Cervical vertebrae (7)

Acromion process

Scapula

Humerus

Thoracic vertebrae (12)

Olecranon
process of ulna

Radius

Lumbar vertebrae (5)

Ulna

Ilium

Sacrum

Coccyx

Ischium

Femur

Fibula

Tibia

Talus

Calcaneus

Beck

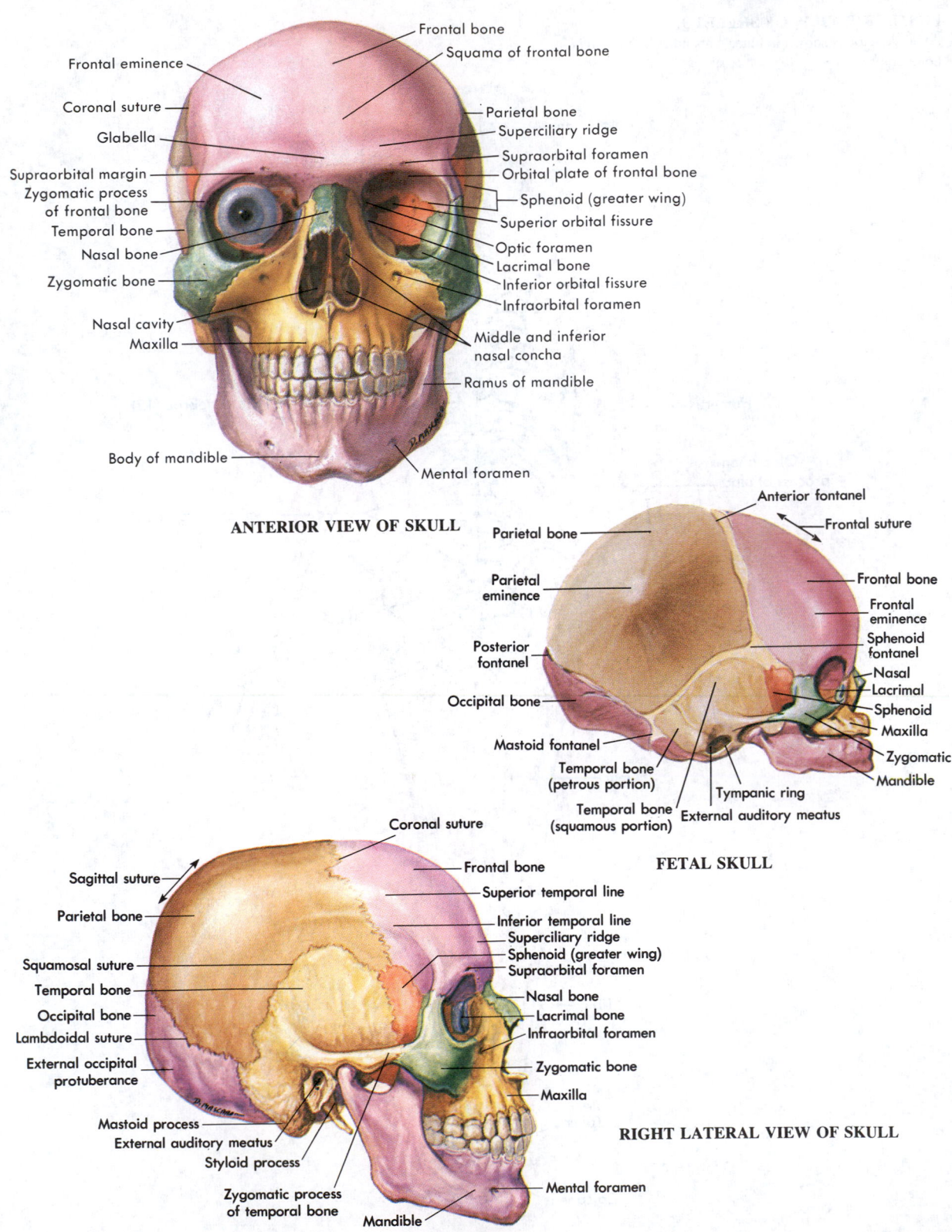

Frontal bone
Squama of frontal bone
Frontal eminence
Coronal suture
Glabella
Parietal bone
Superciliary ridge
Supraorbital foramen
Supraorbital margin
Orbital plate of frontal bone
Zygomatic process
of frontal bone
Sphenoid (greater wing)
Temporal bone
Superior orbital fissure
Nasal bone
Optic foramen
Zygomatic bone
Lacrimal bone
Inferior orbital fissure
Infraorbital foramen
Nasal cavity
Maxilla
Middle and inferior
nasal concha
Ramus of mandible
Body of mandible
Mental foramen

ANTERIOR VIEW OF SKULL

Anterior fontanel
Parietal bone
Frontal suture
Parietal
eminence
Frontal bone
Frontal
eminence
Sphenoid
fontanel
Posterior
fontanel
Nasal
Lacrimal
Occipital bone
Sphenoid
Maxilla
Mastoid fontanel
Zygomatic
Temporal bone
(petrous portion)
Mandible
Tympanic ring
Temporal bone
(squamous portion)
External auditory meatus

FETAL SKULL

Coronal suture
Sagittal suture
Frontal bone
Superior temporal line
Parietal bone
Inferior temporal line
Superciliary ridge
Sphenoid (greater wing)
Squamosal suture
Supraorbital foramen
Temporal bone
Nasal bone
Occipital bone
Lacrimal bone
Lambdoidal suture
Infraorbital foramen
External occipital
protuberance
Zygomatic bone
Maxilla
Mastoid process
External auditory meatus
Styloid process
Zygomatic process
of temporal bone
Mental foramen
Mandible

RIGHT LATERAL VIEW OF SKULL

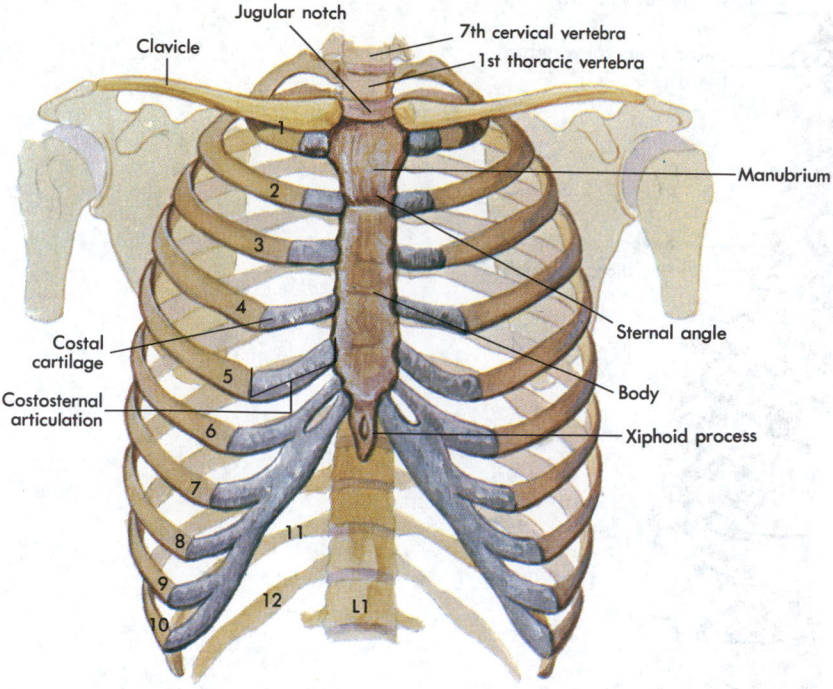

THORAX AND RIBS

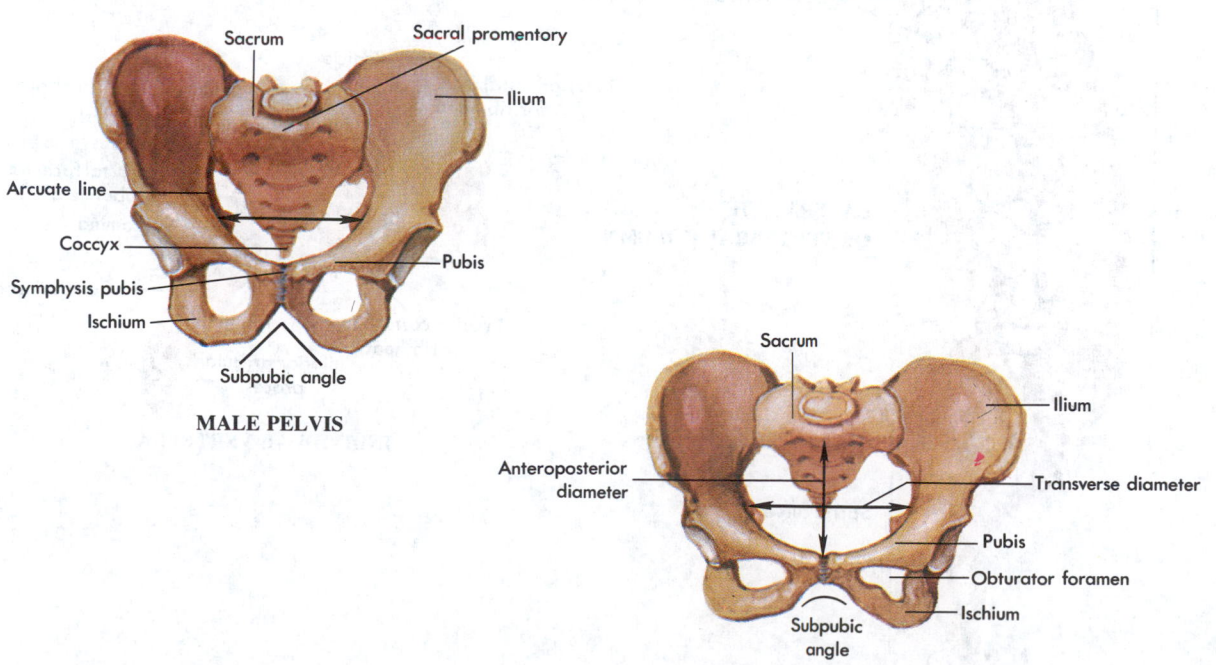

MALE PELVIS

FEMALE PELVIS

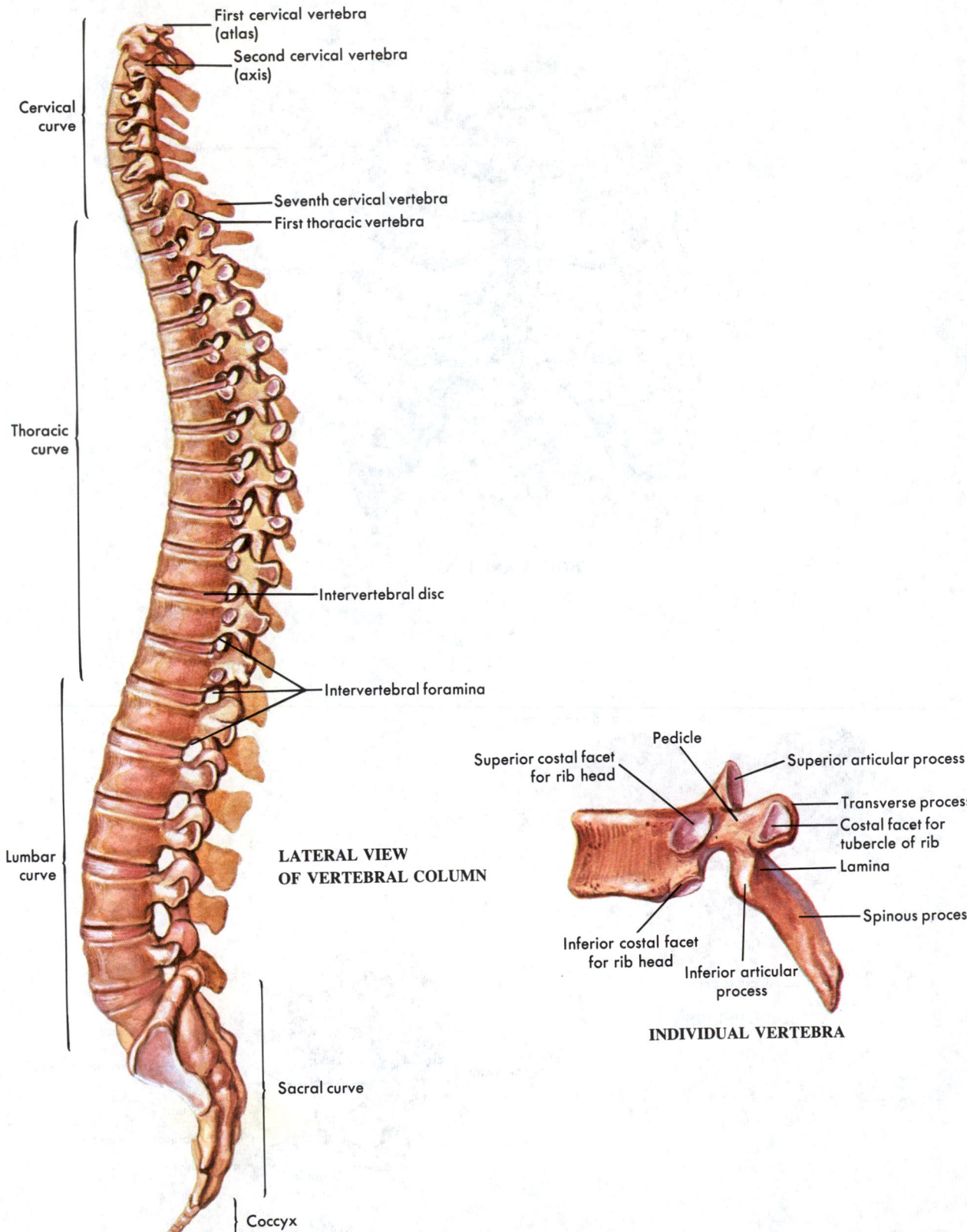

First cervical vertebra
(atlas)

Second cervical vertebra
(axis)

Cervical
curve

Seventh cervical vertebra

First thoracic vertebra

Thoracic
curve

Intervertebral disc

Intervertebral foramina

Lumbar
curve

**LATERAL VIEW
OF VERTEBRAL COLUMN**

Sacral curve

Coccyx

Pedicle

Superior costal facet
for rib head

Superior articular process

Transverse process

Costal facet for
tubercle of rib

Lamina

Spinous process

Inferior costal facet
for rib head

Inferior articular
process

INDIVIDUAL VERTEBRA

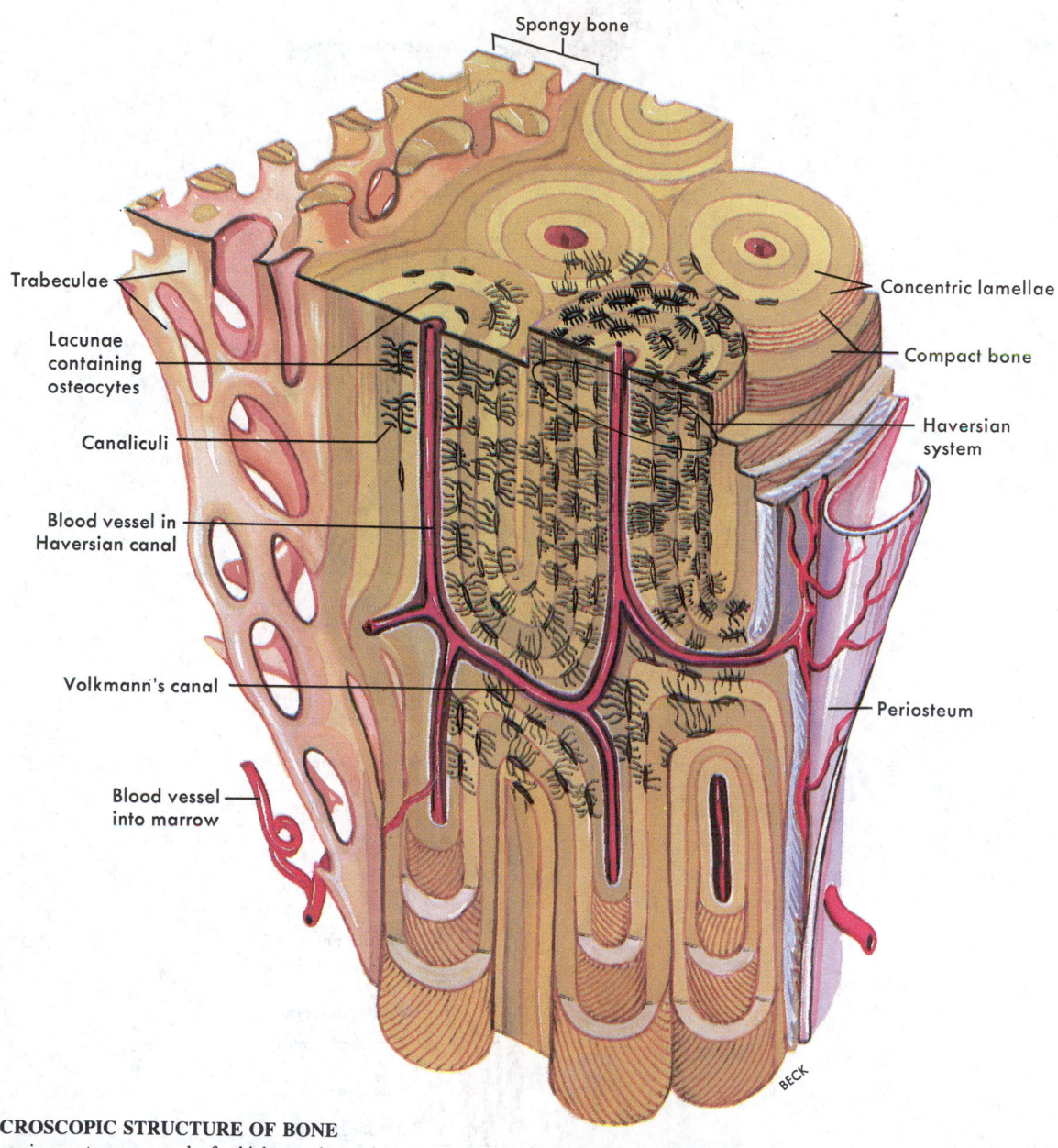

Spongy bone

Trabeculae

Lacunae
containing
osteocytes

Canaliculi

Blood vessel in
Haversian canal

Volkmann's canal

Blood vessel
into marrow

Concentric lamellae

Compact bone

Haversian
system

Periosteum

BECK

MICROSCOPIC STRUCTURE OF BONE

Haversian systems, several of which are shown here,
compose compact bone. Note the structures that make
up one haversian system: concentric lamellae, lacunae,
canaliculi, and a haversian canal. Shown bordering the
compact bone on the left is spongy bone, a name
descriptive of the many open spaces that characterize
it.

MUSCULAR SYSTEM

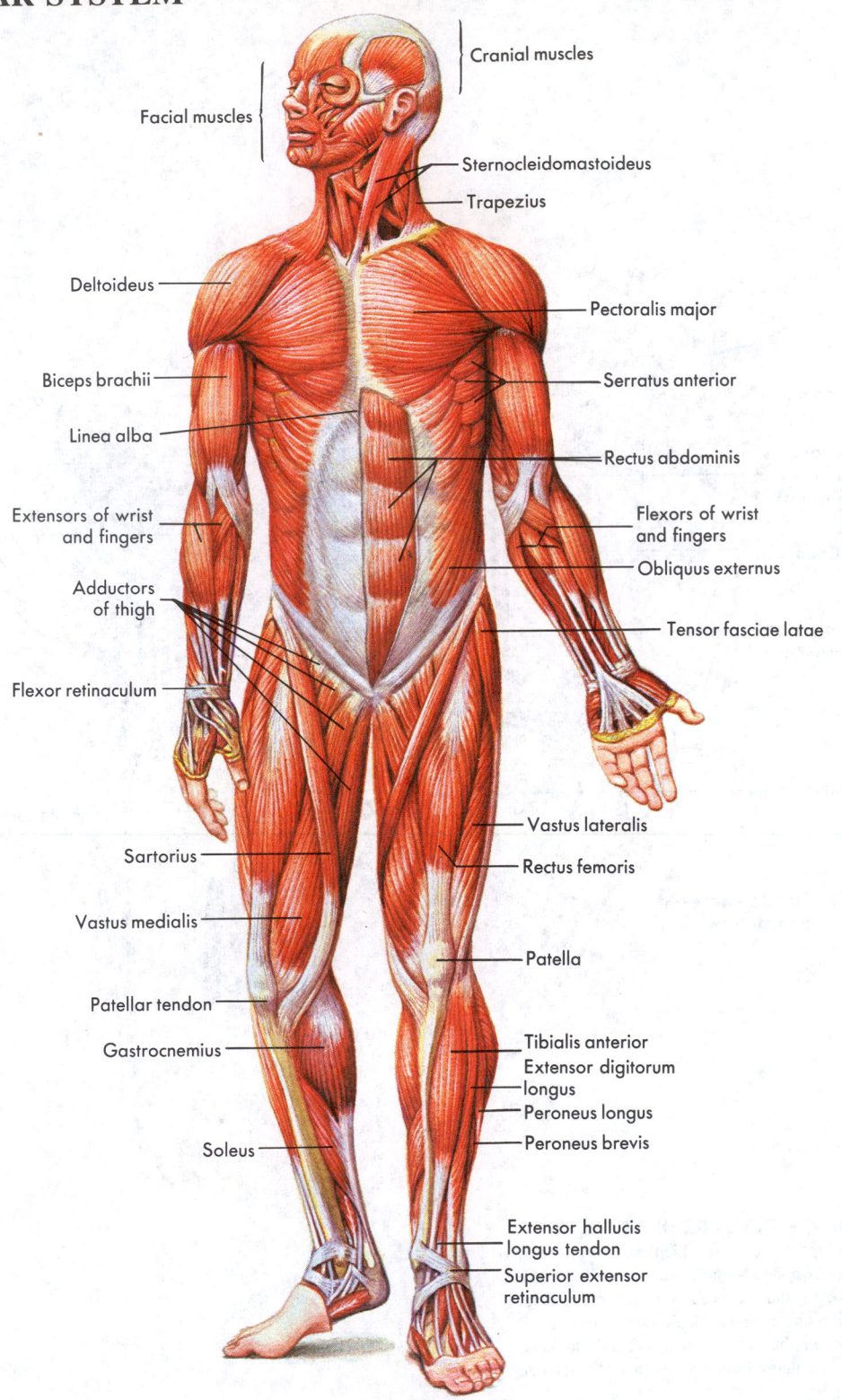

Cranial muscles

Facial muscles

Sternocleidomastoideus

Trapezius

Deltoideus

Pectoralis major

Biceps brachii

Serratus anterior

Linea alba

Rectus abdominis

Extensors of wrist
and fingers

Flexors of wrist
and fingers

Obliquus externus

Adductors
of thigh

Tensor fasciae latae

Flexor retinaculum

Vastus lateralis

Sartorius

Rectus femoris

Vastus medialis

Patella

Patellar tendon

Tibialis anterior

Gastrocnemius

Extensor digitorum
longus

Peroneus longus

Peroneus brevis

Soleus

Extensor hallucis
longus tendon

Superior extensor
retinaculum

ANTERIOR VIEW

A-8

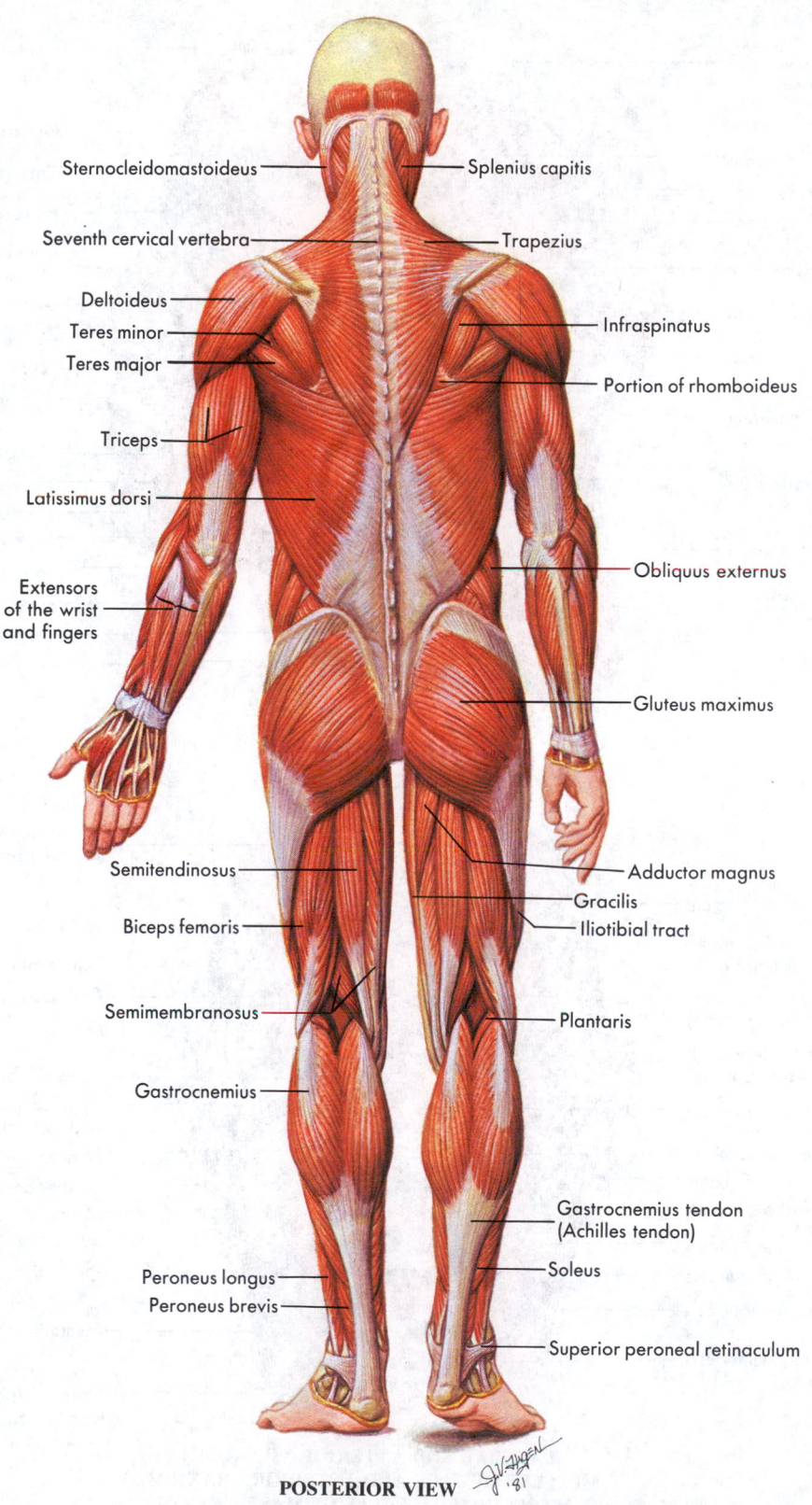

Sternocleidomastoideus — Splenius capitis

Seventh cervical vertebra — Trapezius

Deltoideus

Teres minor

Teres major

Triceps

Latissimus dorsi

Extensors
of the wrist
and fingers

Infraspinatus

Portion of rhomboideus

Obliquus externus

Gluteus maximus

Semitendinosus — Adductor magnus

Biceps femoris — Gracilis

Iliotibial tract

Semimembranosus — Plantaris

Gastrocnemius

Gastrocnemius tendon
(Achilles tendon)

Peroneus longus — Soleus
Peroneus brevis

Superior peroneal retinaculum

POSTERIOR VIEW

A-9

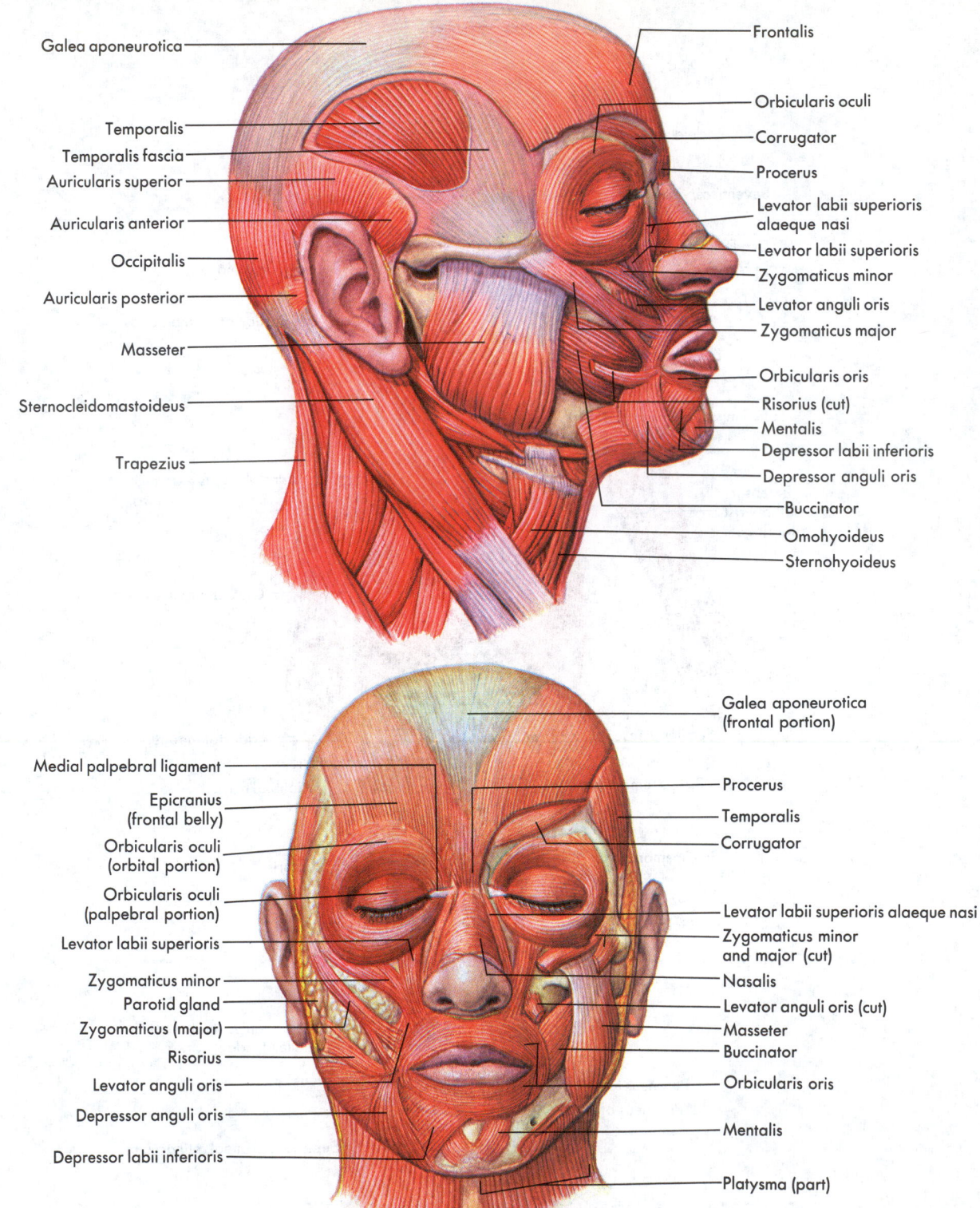

Galea aponeurotica

Temporalis

Temporalis fascia

Auricularis superior

Auricularis anterior

Occipitalis

Auricularis posterior

Masseter

Sternocleidomastoideus

Trapezius

Frontalis

Orbicularis oculi

Corrugator

Procerus

Levator labii superioris
alaeque nasi

Levator labii superioris

Zygomaticus minor

Levator anguli oris

Zygomaticus major

Orbicularis oris

Risorius (cut)

Mentalis

Depressor labii inferioris

Depressor anguli oris

Buccinator

Omohyoideus

Sternohyoideus

Galea aponeurotica
(frontal portion)

Medial palpebral ligament

Epicranius
(frontal belly)

Orbicularis oculi
(orbital portion)

Orbicularis oculi
(palpebral portion)

Levator labii superioris

Zygomaticus minor

Parotid gland

Zygomaticus (major)

Risorius

Levator anguli oris

Depressor anguli oris

Depressor labii inferioris

Procerus

Temporalis

Corrugator

Levator labii superioris alaeque nasi

Zygomaticus minor
and major (cut)

Nasalis

Levator anguli oris (cut)

Masseter

Buccinator

Orbicularis oris

Mentalis

Platysma (part)

**LATERAL AND ANTERIOR VIEWS OF
MUSCLES OF FACE AND ANTERIOR CRANIUM
AND SEVERAL MUSCLES OF MASTICATION**

A-10

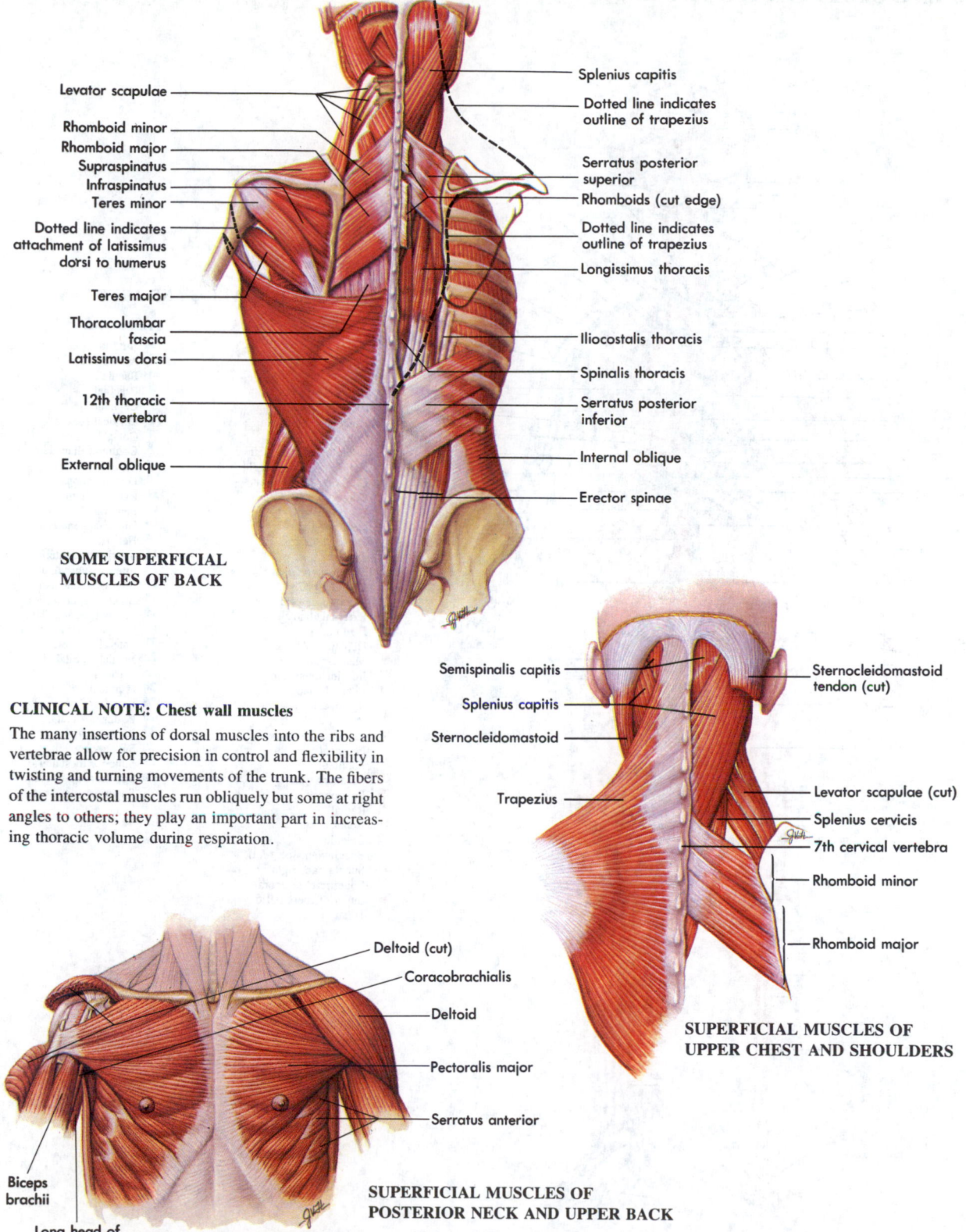

Levator scapulae

Rhomboid minor

Rhomboid major

Supraspinatus

Infraspinatus

Teres minor

Dotted line indicates attachment of latissimus dorsi to humerus

Teres major

Thoracolumbar fascia

Latissimus dorsi

12th thoracic vertebra

External oblique

Splenius capitis

Dotted line indicates outline of trapezius

Serratus posterior superior

Rhomboids (cut edge)

Dotted line indicates outline of trapezius

Longissimus thoracis

Iliocostalis thoracis

Spinalis thoracis

Serratus posterior inferior

Internal oblique

Erector spinae

SOME SUPERFICIAL MUSCLES OF BACK

CLINICAL NOTE: Chest wall muscles

The many insertions of dorsal muscles into the ribs and vertebrae allow for precision in control and flexibility in twisting and turning movements of the trunk. The fibers of the intercostal muscles run obliquely but some at right angles to others; they play an important part in increasing thoracic volume during respiration.

Semispinalis capitis

Splenius capitis

Sternocleidomastoid

Trapezius

Sternocleidomastoid tendon (cut)

Levator scapulae (cut)

Splenius cervicis

7th cervical vertebra

Rhomboid minor

Rhomboid major

SUPERFICIAL MUSCLES OF UPPER CHEST AND SHOULDERS

Deltoid (cut)

Coracobrachialis

Deltoid

Pectoralis major

Serratus anterior

Biceps brachii

Long head of the triceps

SUPERFICIAL MUSCLES OF POSTERIOR NECK AND UPPER BACK

CIRCULATORY SYSTEM

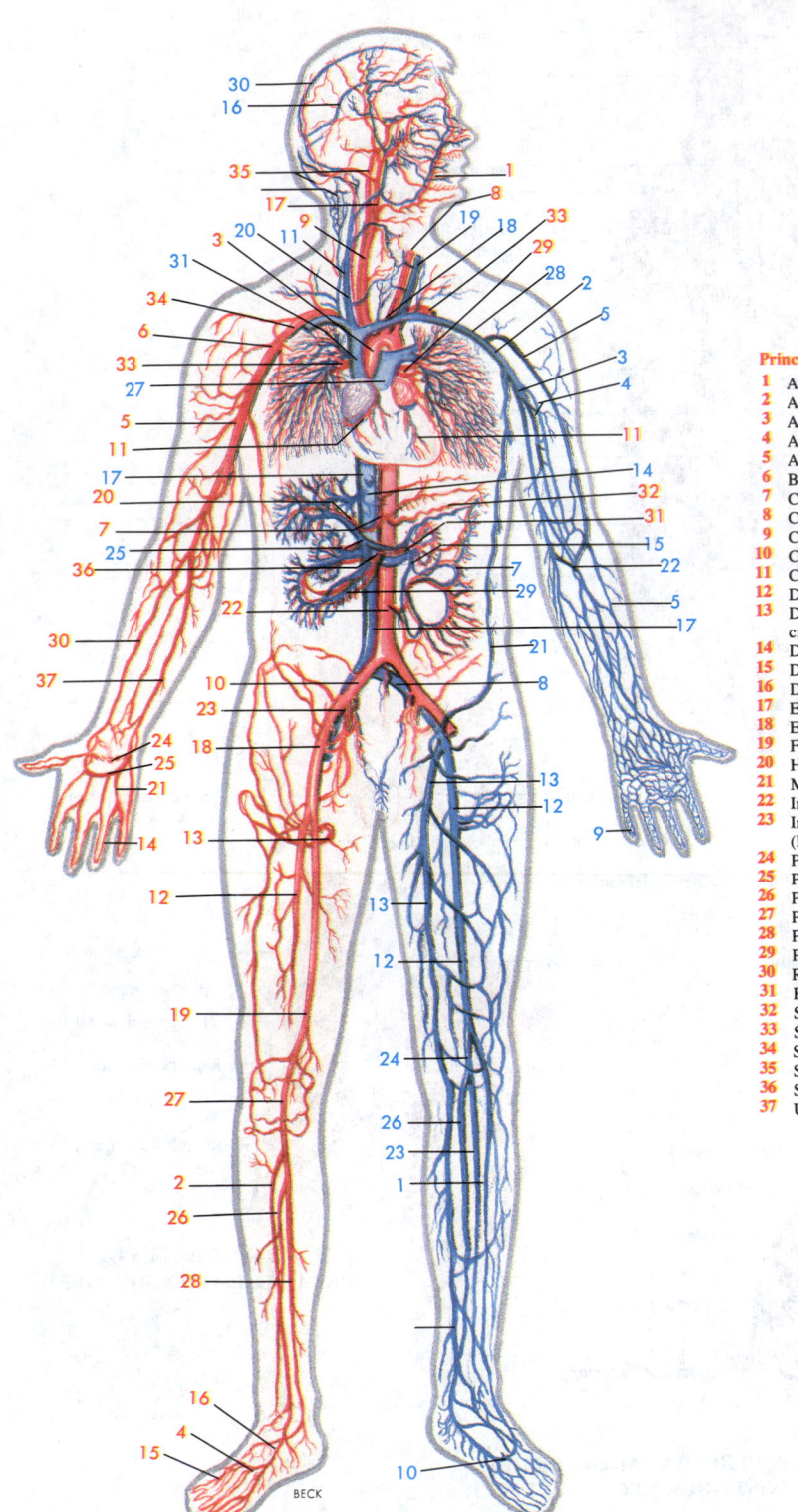

PRINCIPAL VEINS AND ARTERIES

Principal arteries

1 Angular
2 Anterior tibial
3 Aorta
4 Arcuate
5 Axillary
6 Brachial
7 Celiac
8 Common carotid, left
9 Common carotid, right
10 Common iliac, right
11 Coronary, left
12 Deep femoral
13 Deep medial
    circumflex femoral
14 Digital
15 Dorsal metatarsal
16 Dorsalis pedis
17 External carotid
18 External iliac
19 Femoral
20 Hepatic
21 Metacarpal
22 Inferior mesenteric
23 Internal iliac
    (hypogastric)
24 Palmar arch, deep
25 Palmar arch, superficial
26 Peroneal
27 Popliteal
28 Posterior tibial
29 Pulmonary
30 Radial
31 Renal
32 Splenic
33 Subclavian, left (cut)
34 Subclavian, right
35 Superficial temporal
36 Superior mesenteric
37 Ulnar

Principal veins

1 Anterior tibial
2 Axillary
3 Basilic
4 Brachial
5 Cephalic
6 Cervical plexus
7 Colic
8 Common iliac, left
9 Digital
10 Dorsal venous arch
11 External jugular
12 Femoral
13 Great saphenous
14 Hepatic
15 Inferior mesenteric
16 Inferior sagittal sinus
17 Inferior vena cava
18 Brachiocephalic, left
19 Internal jugular, left
20 Internal jugular, right
21 Lateral thoracic
22 Median cubital
23 Peroneal
24 Popliteal
25 Portal
26 Posterior tibial
27 Pulmonary
28 Subclavian, left
29 Superior mesenteric
30 Superior sagittal sinus
31 Superior vena cava

BECK

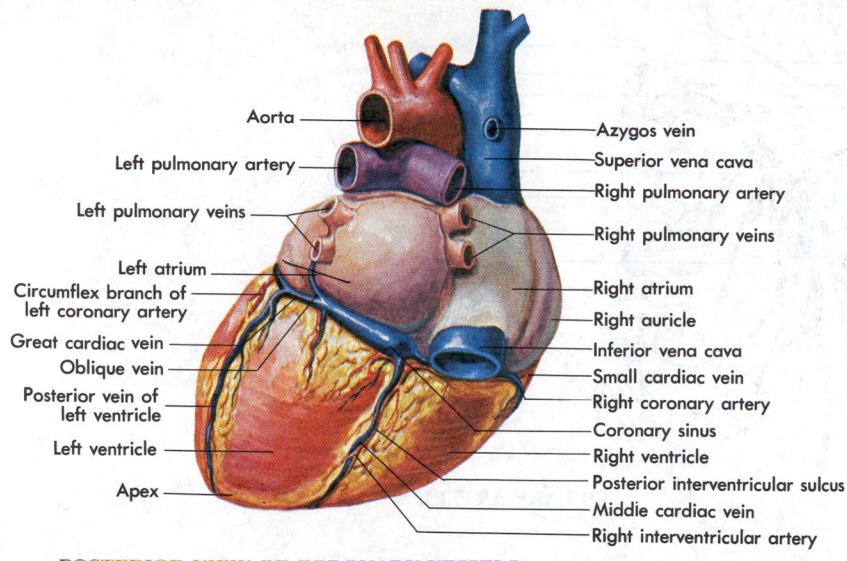

POSTERIOR VIEW OF CORONARY VESSELS

Aorta
Left pulmonary artery
Left pulmonary veins
Left atrium
Circumflex branch of left coronary artery
Great cardiac vein
Oblique vein
Posterior vein of left ventricle
Left ventricle
Apex

Azygos vein
Superior vena cava
Right pulmonary artery
Right pulmonary veins
Right atrium
Right auricle
Inferior vena cava
Small cardiac vein
Right coronary artery
Coronary sinus
Right ventricle
Posterior interventricular sulcus
Middle cardiac vein
Right interventricular artery

Brachiocephalic artery
Left common carotid artery

Right common carotid artery
Right internal jugular vein
Right subclavian vein
Superior vena cava
Right pulmonary arteries
Right pulmonary veins
Right atrium
Aortic valve (dotted lines)
Section of right ventricle intact
Tricuspid valve
Right ventricle
Inferior vena cava
Papillary muscle

Left subclavian artery
Aortic arch
Ligamentum arteriosus
Pulmonary trunk
Left pulmonary arteries
Left pulmonary veins
Pulmonary valve leaflet
Left atrium and mitral valve
Chordae tendineae
Papillary muscle
Left ventricle
Interventricular septum
Myocardium

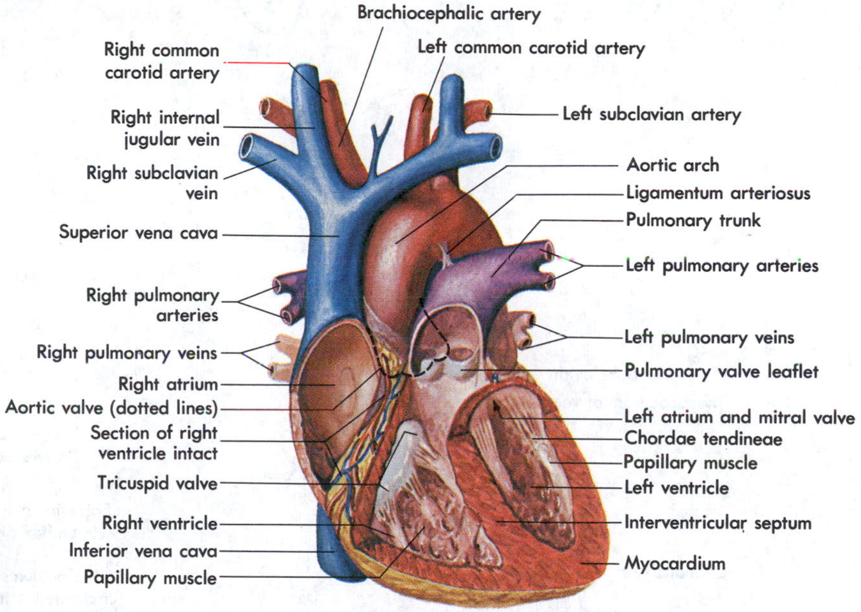

HUMAN HEART IN FRONTAL SECTION

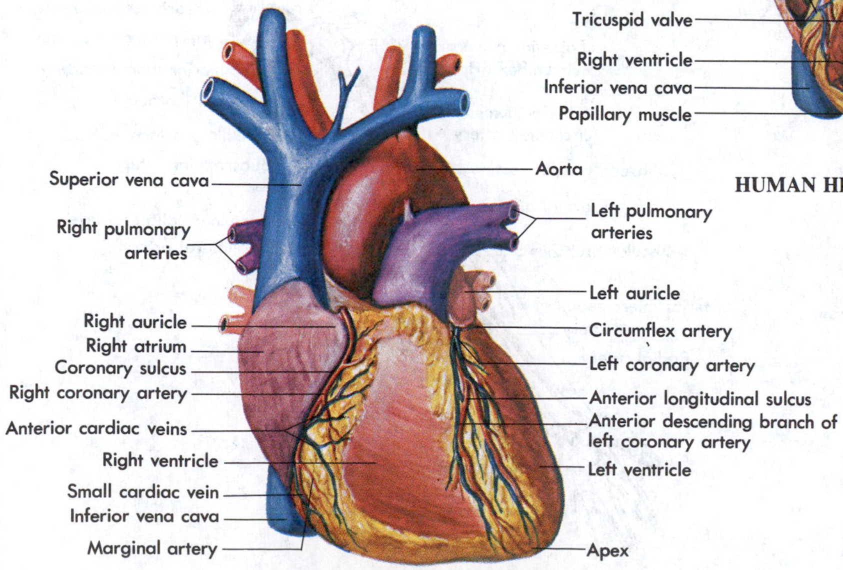

Superior vena cava
Right pulmonary arteries
Right auricle
Right atrium
Coronary sulcus
Right coronary artery
Anterior cardiac veins
Right ventricle
Small cardiac vein
Inferior vena cava
Marginal artery

Aorta
Left pulmonary arteries
Left auricle
Circumflex artery
Left coronary artery
Anterior longitudinal sulcus
Anterior descending branch of left coronary artery
Left ventricle
Apex

ANTERIOR VIEW OF CORONARY VESSELS

Circulatory system

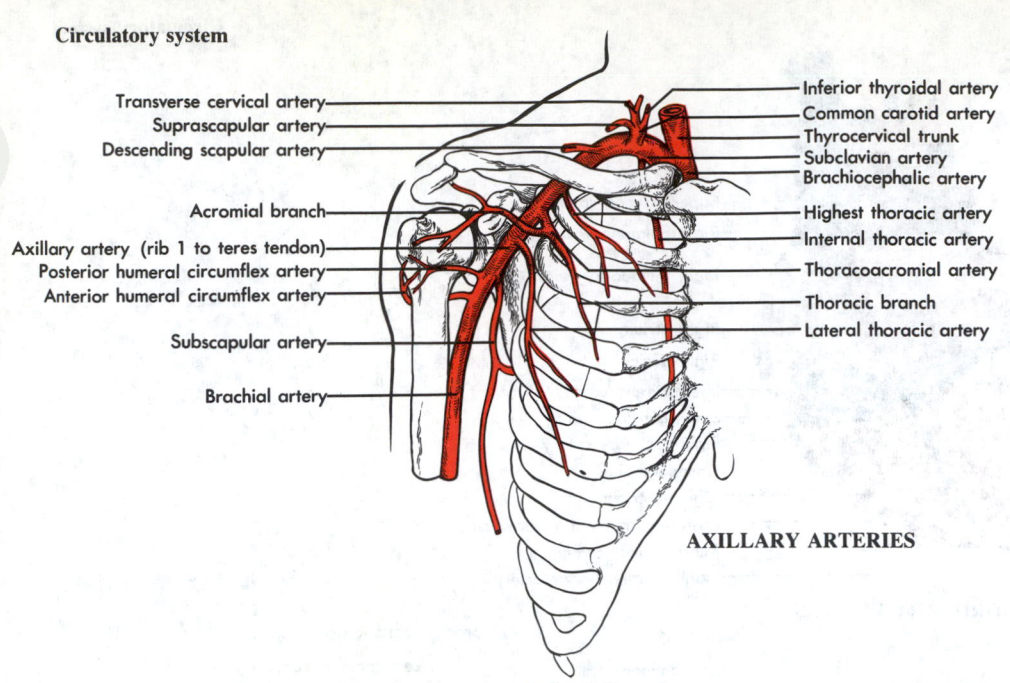

Transverse cervical artery
Suprascapular artery
Descending scapular artery

Inferior thyroidal artery
Common carotid artery
Thyrocervical trunk
Subclavian artery
Brachiocephalic artery

Acromial branch

Highest thoracic artery
Internal thoracic artery

Axillary artery (rib 1 to teres tendon)
Posterior humeral circumflex artery
Anterior humeral circumflex artery

Thoracoacromial artery

Thoracic branch
Lateral thoracic artery

Subscapular artery

Brachial artery

AXILLARY ARTERIES

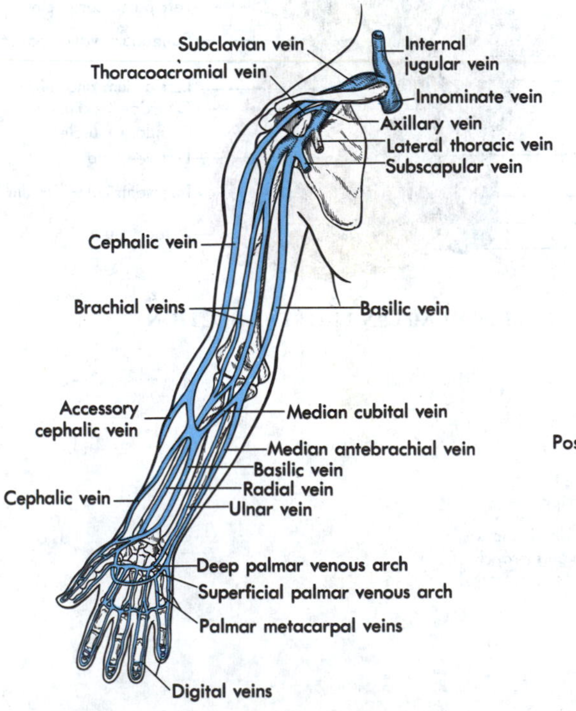

Subclavian vein
Thoracoacromial vein

Internal jugular vein
Innominate vein
Axillary vein
Lateral thoracic vein
Subscapular vein

Cephalic vein

Brachial veins

Basilic vein

Accessory cephalic vein

Median cubital vein
Median antebrachial vein
Basilic vein
Radial vein
Ulnar vein

Cephalic vein

Deep palmar venous arch
Superficial palmar venous arch
Palmar metacarpal veins

Digital veins

MAJOR VEINS OF UPPER APPENDAGES

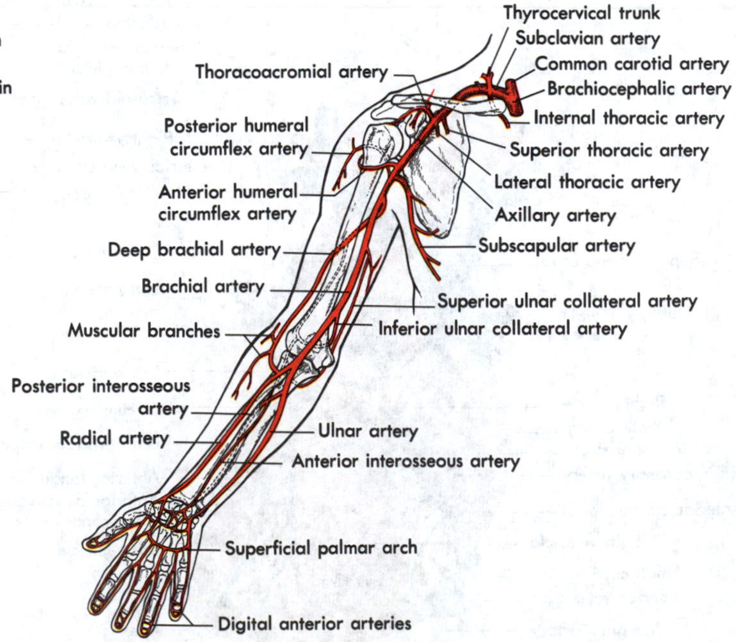

Thoracoacromial artery

Thyrocervical trunk
Subclavian artery
Common carotid artery
Brachiocephalic artery
Internal thoracic artery
Superior thoracic artery
Lateral thoracic artery
Axillary artery
Subscapular artery

Posterior humeral circumflex artery

Anterior humeral circumflex artery

Deep brachial artery

Brachial artery

Muscular branches

Superior ulnar collateral artery
Inferior ulnar collateral artery

Posterior interosseous artery

Radial artery

Ulnar artery
Anterior interosseous artery

Superficial palmar arch

Digital anterior arteries

MAJOR ARTERIES OF UPPER APPENDAGES

A-14

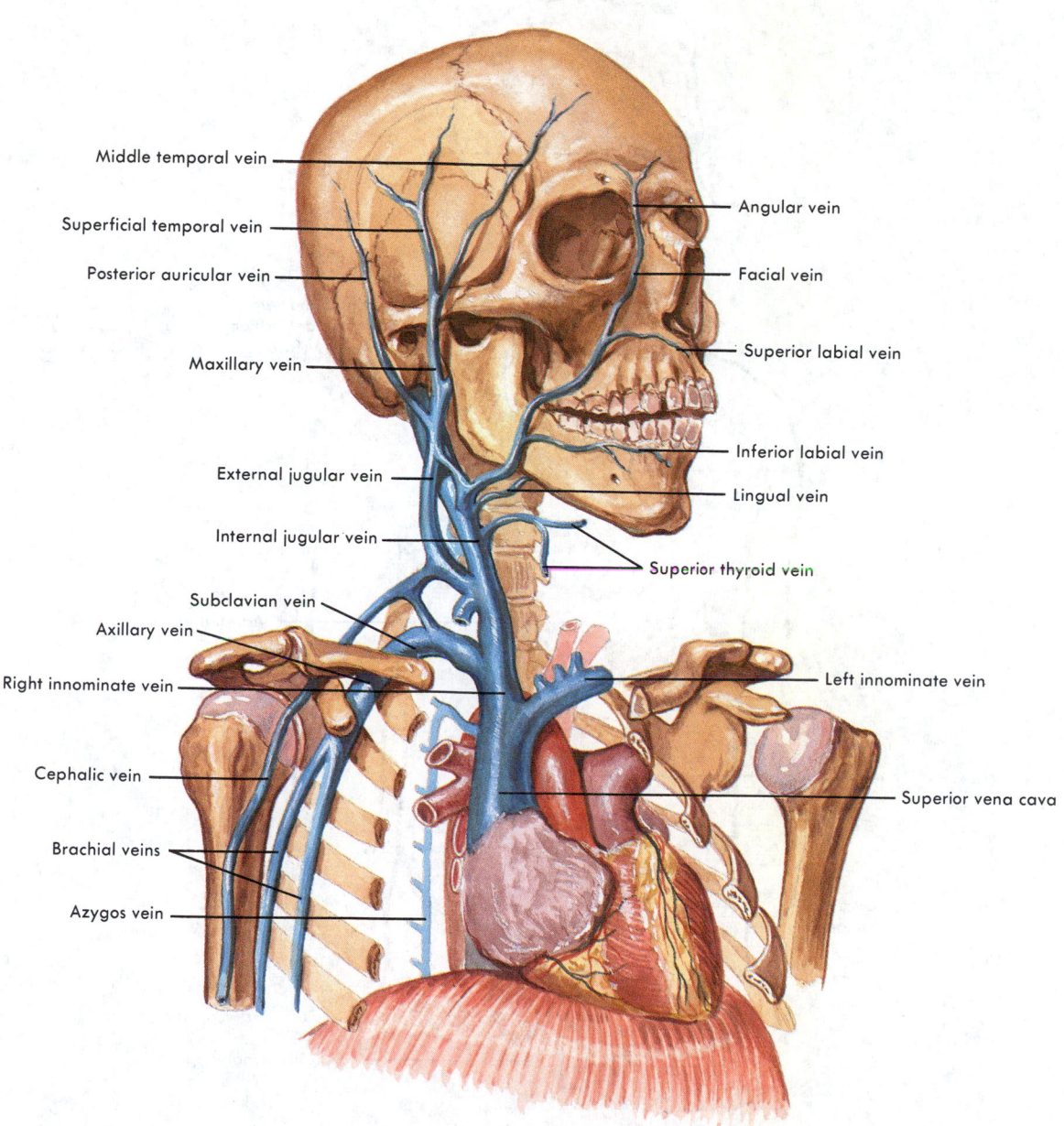

Middle temporal vein

Superficial temporal vein

Posterior auricular vein

Maxillary vein

External jugular vein

Internal jugular vein

Subclavian vein

Axillary vein

Right innominate vein

Cephalic vein

Brachial veins

Azygos vein

Angular vein

Facial vein

Superior labial vein

Inferior labial vein

Lingual vein

Superior thyroid vein

Left innominate vein

Superior vena cava

VEINS FORMING SUPERIOR VENA CAVA

ENDOCRINE SYSTEM

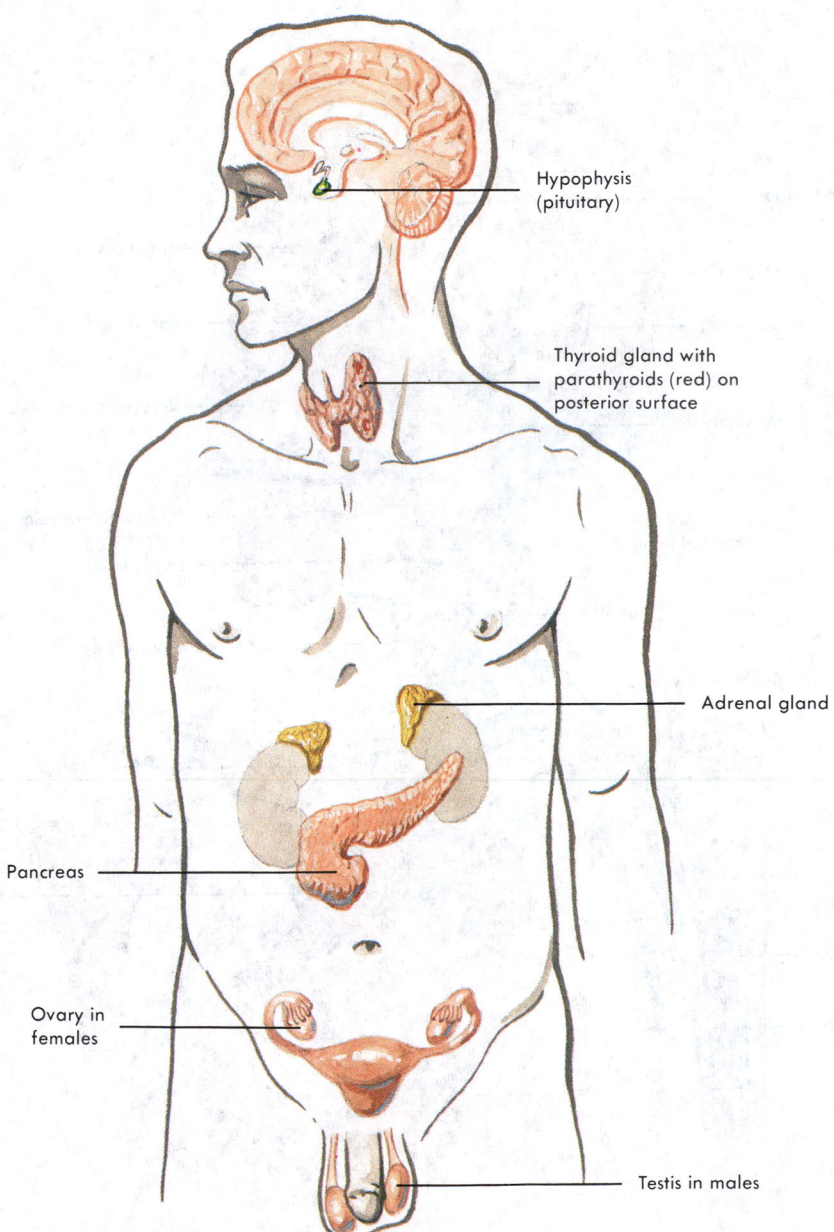

Hypophysis
(pituitary)

Thyroid gland with
parathyroids (red) on
posterior surface

Adrenal gland

Pancreas

Ovary in
females

Testis in males

ENDOCRINE SYSTEM

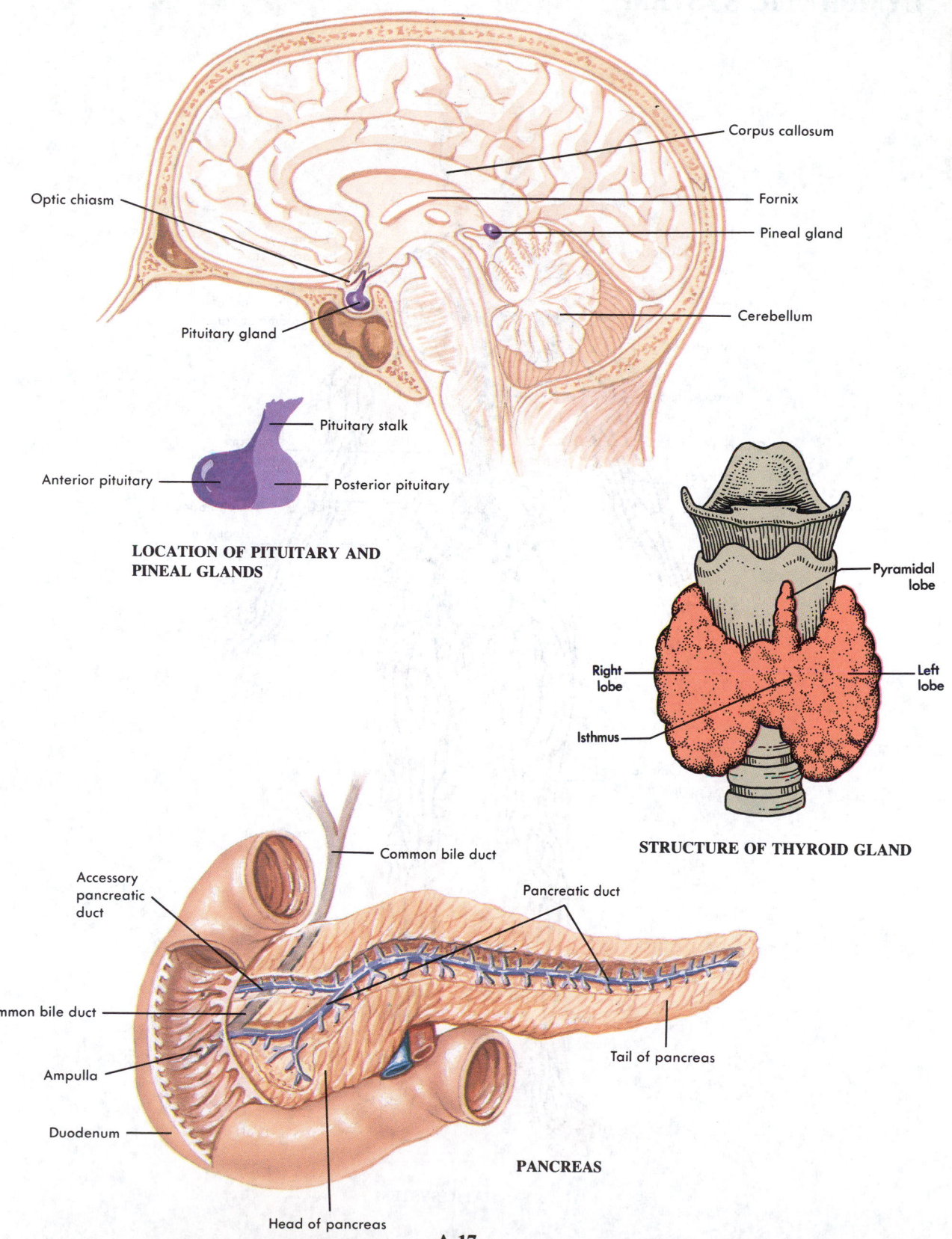

Corpus callosum

Optic chiasm

Fornix

Pineal gland

Cerebellum

Pituitary gland

Pituitary stalk

Anterior pituitary

Posterior pituitary

LOCATION OF PITUITARY AND PINEAL GLANDS

Pyramidal lobe

Right lobe

Left lobe

Isthmus

STRUCTURE OF THYROID GLAND

Common bile duct

Accessory pancreatic duct

Pancreatic duct

Common bile duct

Ampulla

Duodenum

Tail of pancreas

PANCREAS

Head of pancreas

A-17

LYMPHATIC SYSTEM

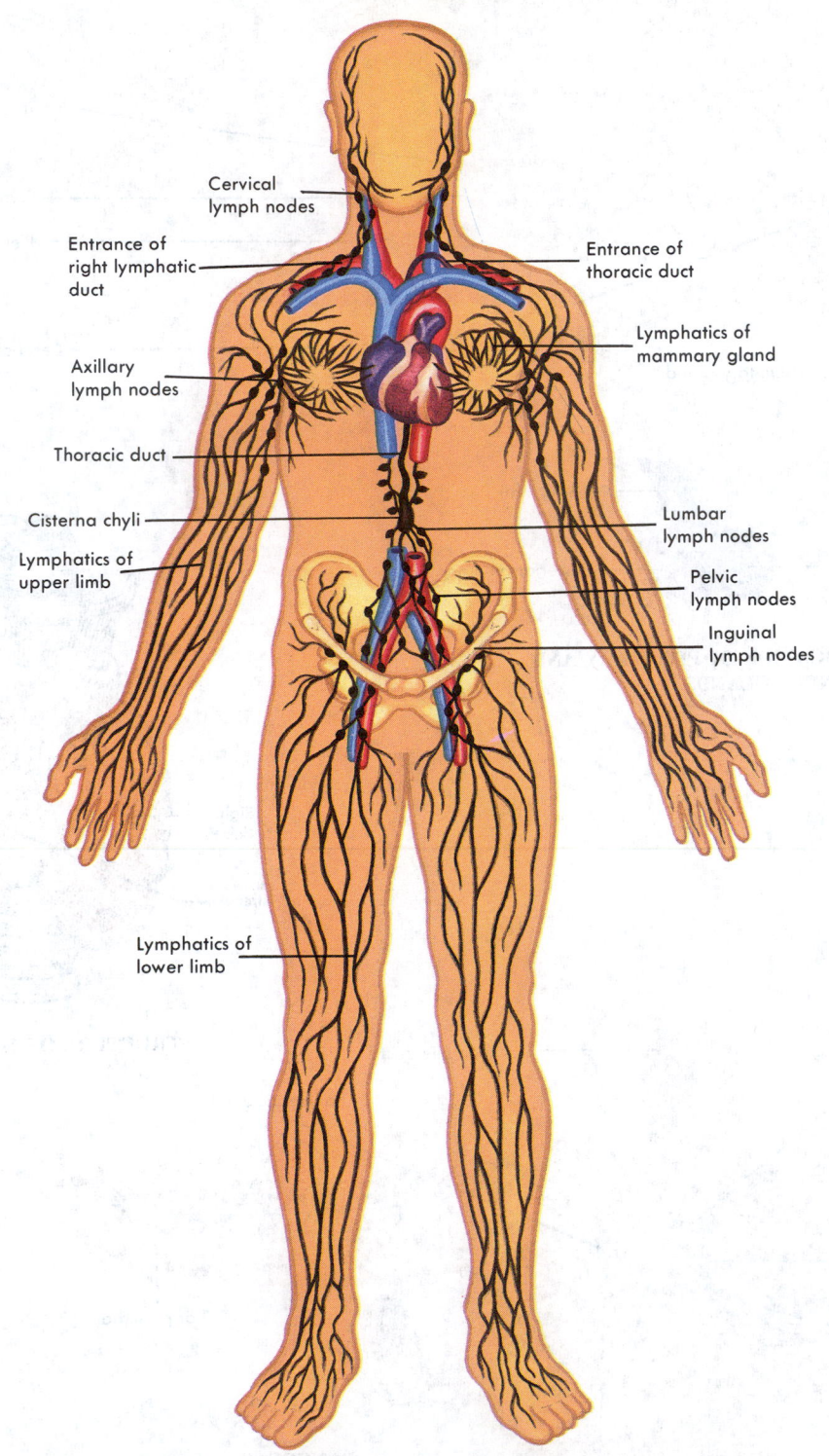

Cervical
lymph nodes

Entrance of
right lymphatic
duct

Entrance of
thoracic duct

Axillary
lymph nodes

Lymphatics of
mammary gland

Thoracic duct

Cisterna chyli

Lumbar
lymph nodes

Lymphatics of
upper limb

Pelvic
lymph nodes

Inguinal
lymph nodes

Lymphatics of
lower limb

LYMPHATIC SYSTEM

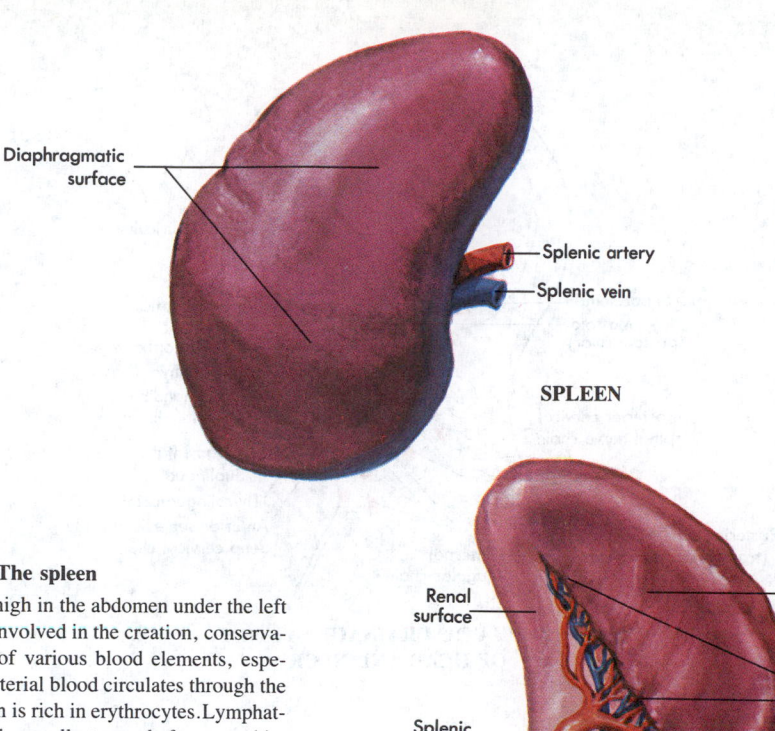

Diaphragmatic surface

Splenic artery

Splenic vein

SPLEEN

Renal surface

Gastric surface

Hilus

Splenic artery

Splenic vein

CLINICAL NOTE: The spleen

The spleen is located high in the abdomen under the left hemidiaphragm. It is involved in the creation, conservation, and destruction of various blood elements, especially erythrocytes. Arterial blood circulates through the red splenic pulp, which is rich in erythrocytes. Lymphatic tissue surrounding the smallest vessels forms a white pulp material.

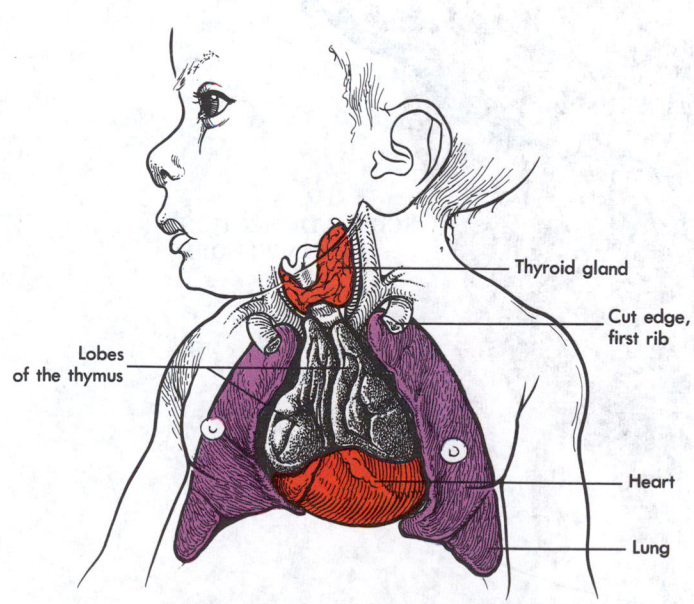

Thyroid gland

Cut edge, first rib

Lobes of the thymus

Heart

Lung

LOCATION AND GROSS ANATOMY OF THYMUS

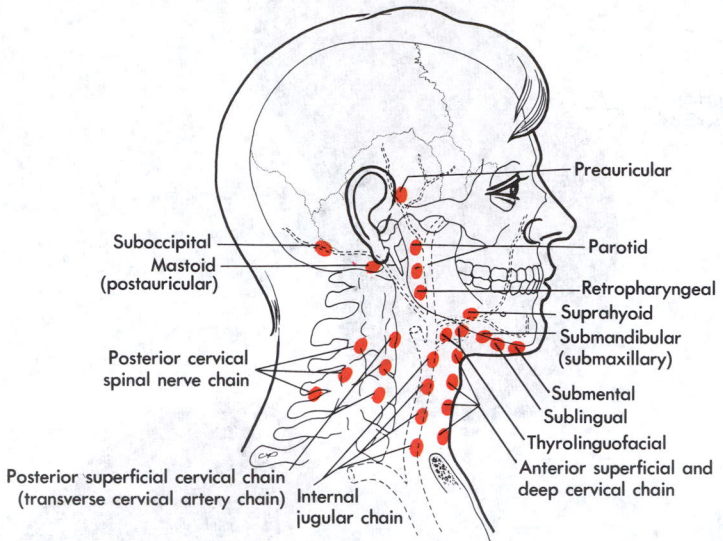

Preauricular

Suboccipital

Mastoid
(postauricular)

Parotid

Retropharyngeal

Suprahyoid

Submandibular
(submaxillary)

Posterior cervical
spinal nerve chain

Submental

Sublingual

Thyrolinguofacial

Anterior superficial and
deep cervical chain

Posterior superficial cervical chain
(transverse cervical artery chain)

Internal
jugular chain

**LYMPHATIC DRAINAGE SYSTEM
OF HEAD AND NECK**

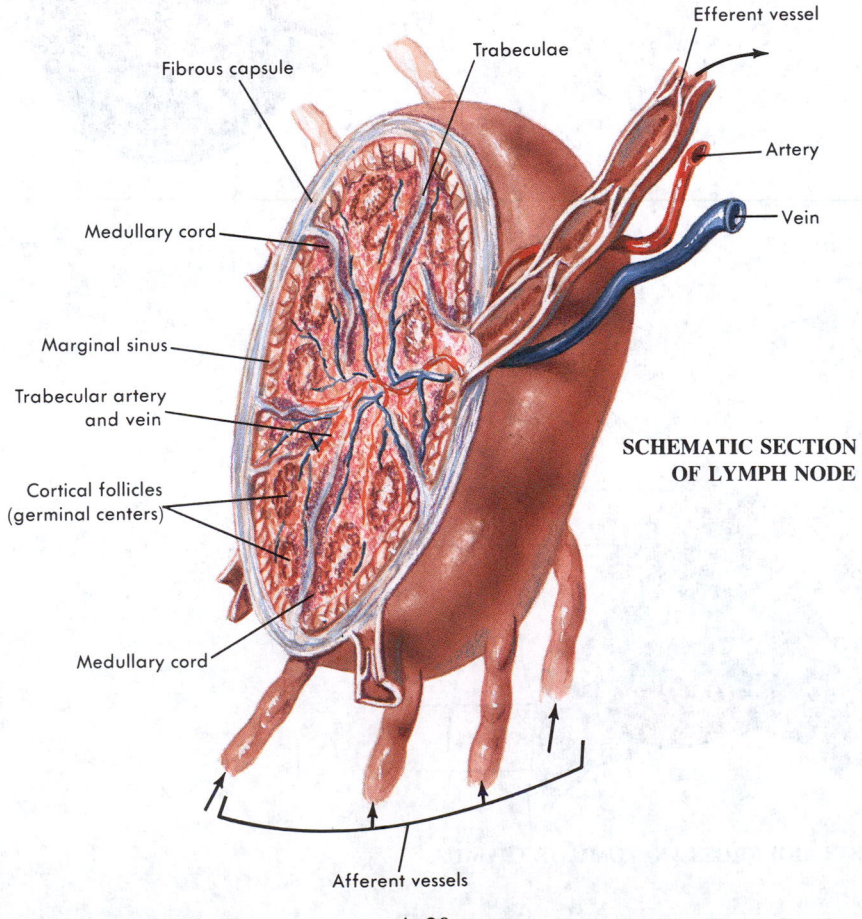

Efferent vessel

Fibrous capsule

Trabeculae

Artery

Vein

Medullary cord

Marginal sinus

Trabecular artery
and vein

**SCHEMATIC SECTION
OF LYMPH NODE**

Cortical follicles
(germinal centers)

Medullary cord

Afferent vessels

A-20

NERVOUS SYSTEM

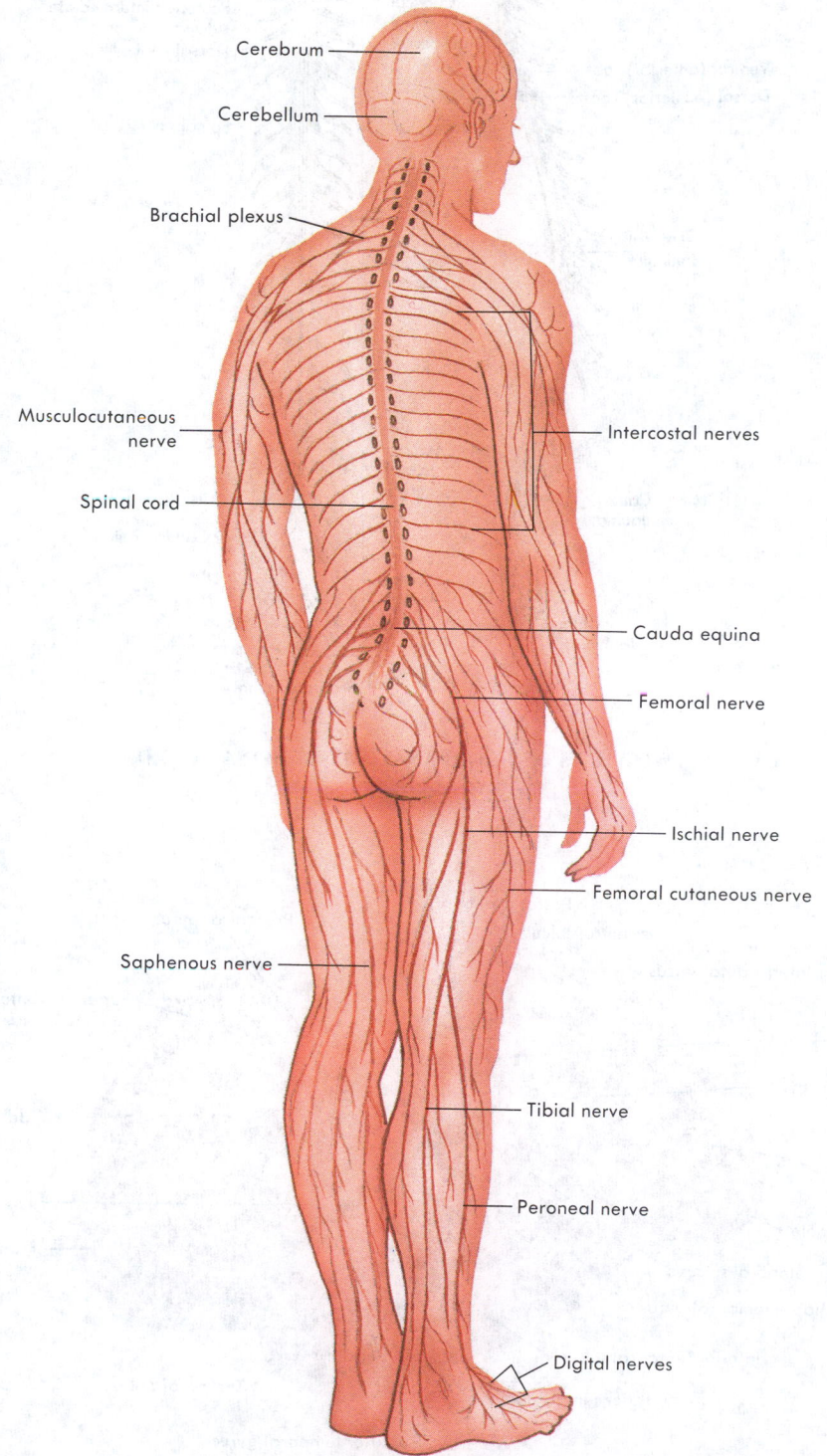

Cerebrum

Cerebellum

Brachial plexus

Musculocutaneous nerve

Spinal cord

Intercostal nerves

Cauda equina

Femoral nerve

Ischial nerve

Femoral cutaneous nerve

Saphenous nerve

Tibial nerve

Peroneal nerve

Digital nerves

SIMPLIFIED VIEW OF NERVOUS SYSTEM

A-21

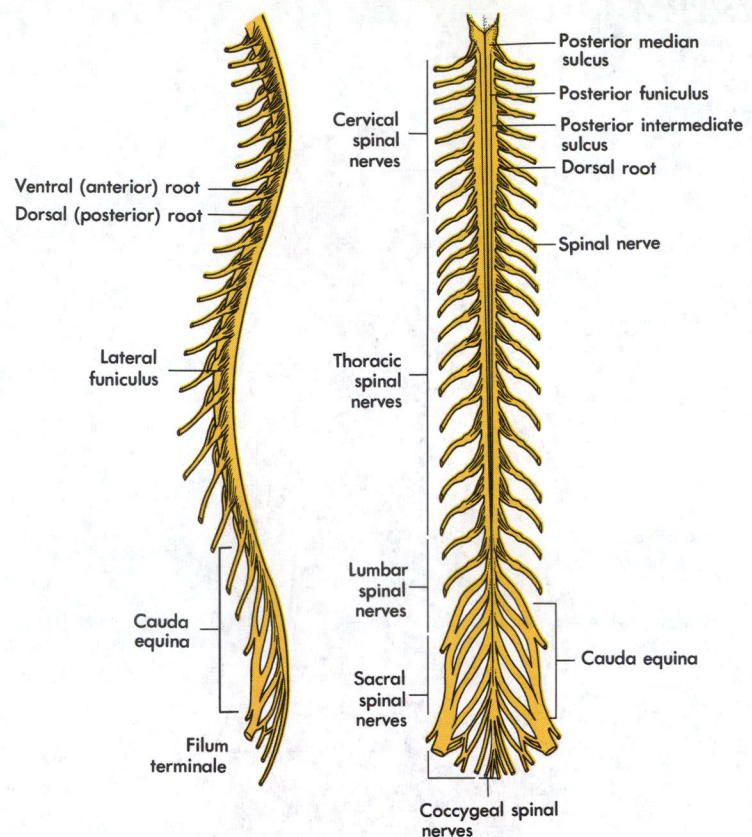

Posterior median sulcus

Posterior funiculus

Posterior intermediate sulcus

Dorsal root

Cervical spinal nerves

Ventral (anterior) root

Dorsal (posterior) root

Spinal nerve

Lateral funiculus

Thoracic spinal nerves

Lumbar spinal nerves

Cauda equina

Cauda equina

Sacral spinal nerves

Filum terminale

Coccygeal spinal nerves

TWO VIEWS OF GROSS ANATOMY OF SPINAL CORD

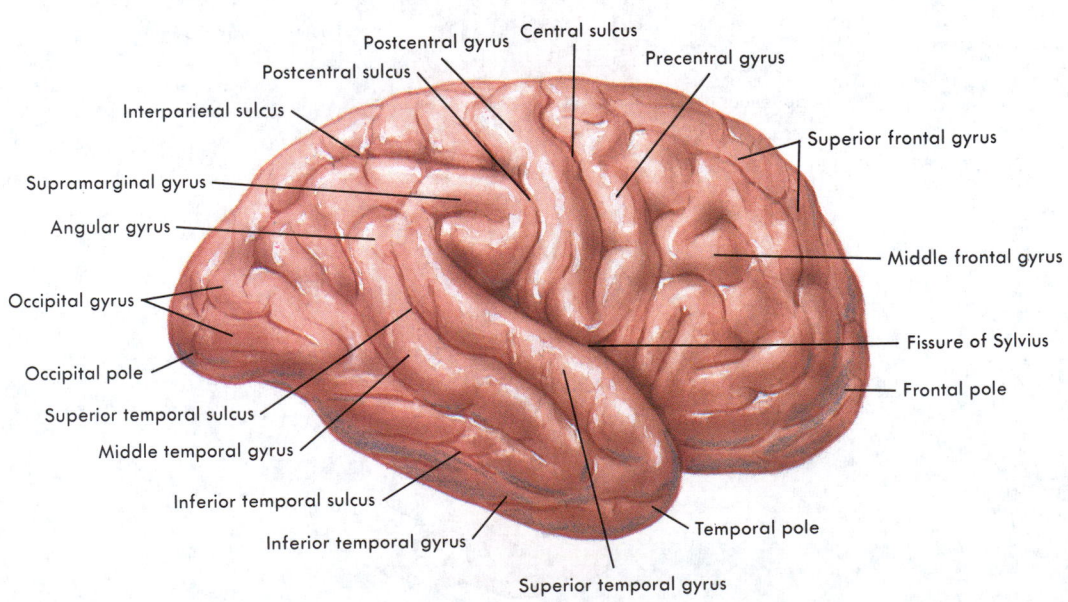

Postcentral gyrus **Central sulcus**

Postcentral sulcus **Precentral gyrus**

Interparietal sulcus

Superior frontal gyrus

Supramarginal gyrus

Angular gyrus

Middle frontal gyrus

Occipital gyrus

Occipital pole **Fissure of Sylvius**

Superior temporal sulcus **Frontal pole**

Middle temporal gyrus

Inferior temporal sulcus

Inferior temporal gyrus **Temporal pole**

Superior temporal gyrus

SURFACE ANATOMY OF CEREBRAL CORTEX

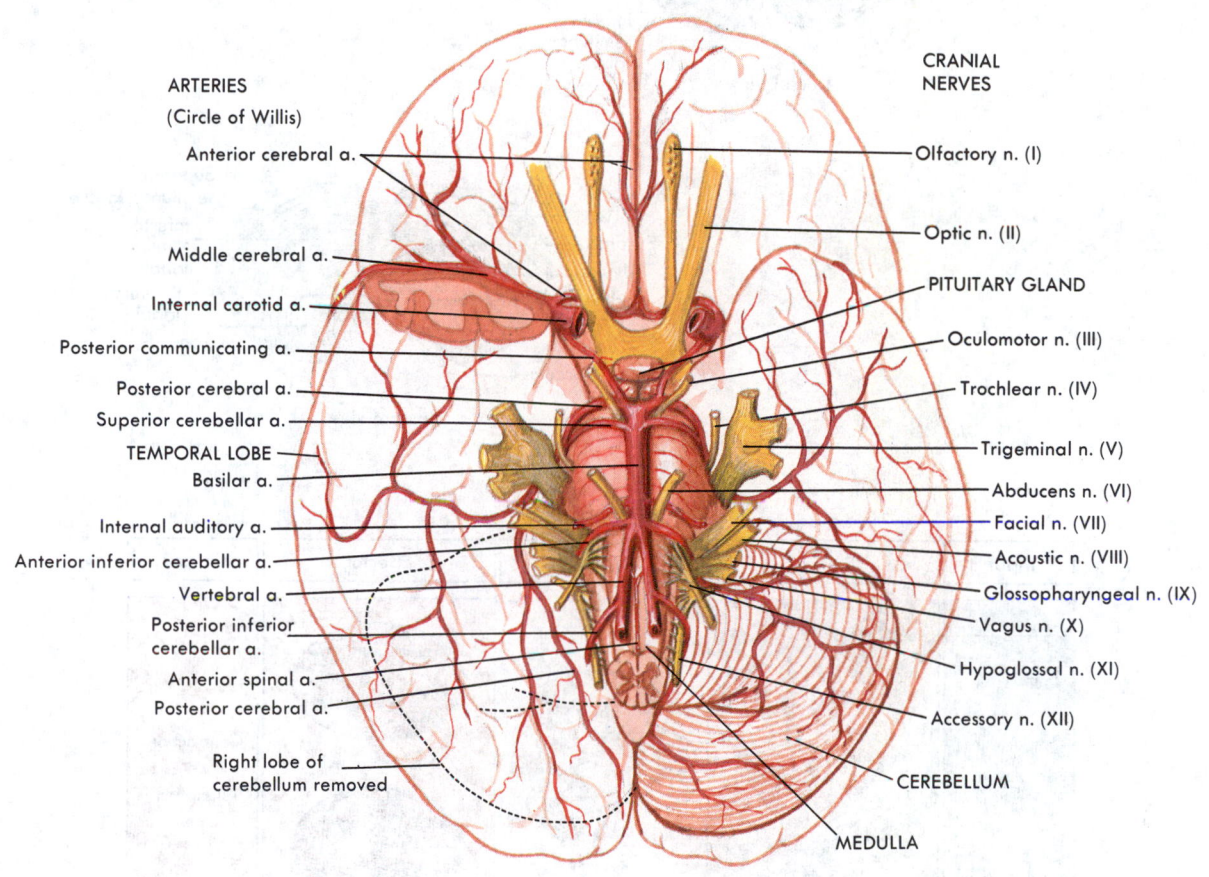

ARTERIES
(Circle of Willis)
Anterior cerebral a.
Middle cerebral a.
Internal carotid a.
Posterior communicating a.
Posterior cerebral a.
Superior cerebellar a.
TEMPORAL LOBE
Basilar a.
Internal auditory a.
Anterior inferior cerebellar a.
Vertebral a.
Posterior inferior cerebellar a.
Anterior spinal a.
Posterior cerebral a.
Right lobe of cerebellum removed

CRANIAL
NERVES
Olfactory n. (I)
Optic n. (II)
PITUITARY GLAND
Oculomotor n. (III)
Trochlear n. (IV)
Trigeminal n. (V)
Abducens n. (VI)
Facial n. (VII)
Acoustic n. (VIII)
Glossopharyngeal n. (IX)
Vagus n. (X)
Hypoglossal n. (XI)
Accessory n. (XII)
CEREBELLUM
MEDULLA

BASE OF BRAIN

ANATOMY OF CEREBELLUM

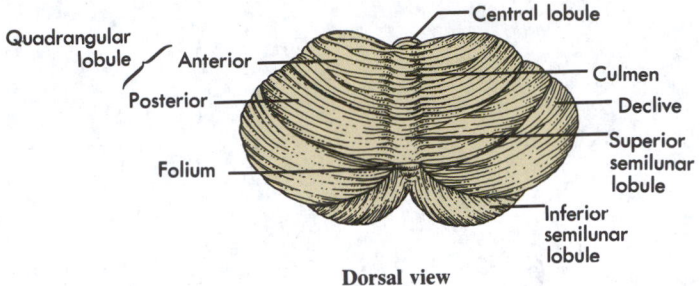

Quadrangular lobule
Anterior
Posterior
Folium
Central lobule
Culmen
Declive
Superior semilunar lobule
Inferior semilunar lobule

Dorsal view

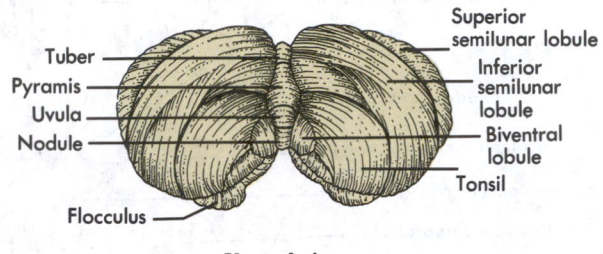

Tuber
Pyramis
Uvula
Nodule
Flocculus
Superior semilunar lobule
Inferior semilunar lobule
Biventral lobule
Tonsil

Ventral view

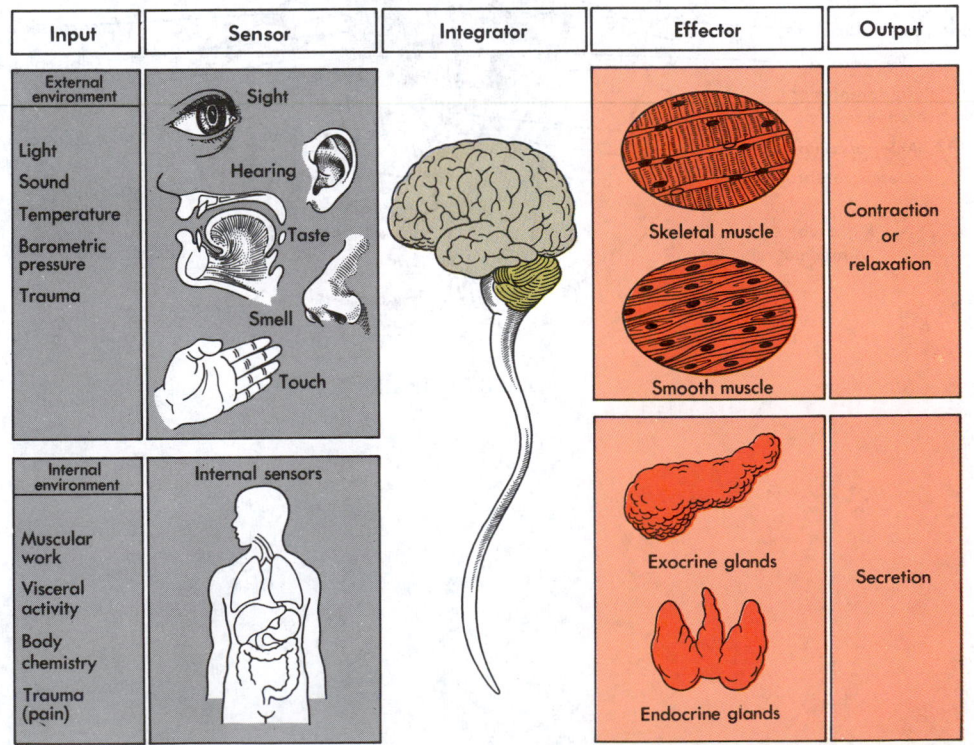

Input	Sensor	Integrator	Effector	Output
External environment Light Sound Temperature Barometric pressure Trauma	Sight Hearing Taste Smell Touch		Skeletal muscle Smooth muscle	Contraction or relaxation
Internal environment Muscular work Visceral activity Body chemistry Trauma (pain)	Internal sensors		Exocrine glands Endocrine glands	Secretion

COMPONENTS OF NERVOUS SYSTEM

A-24

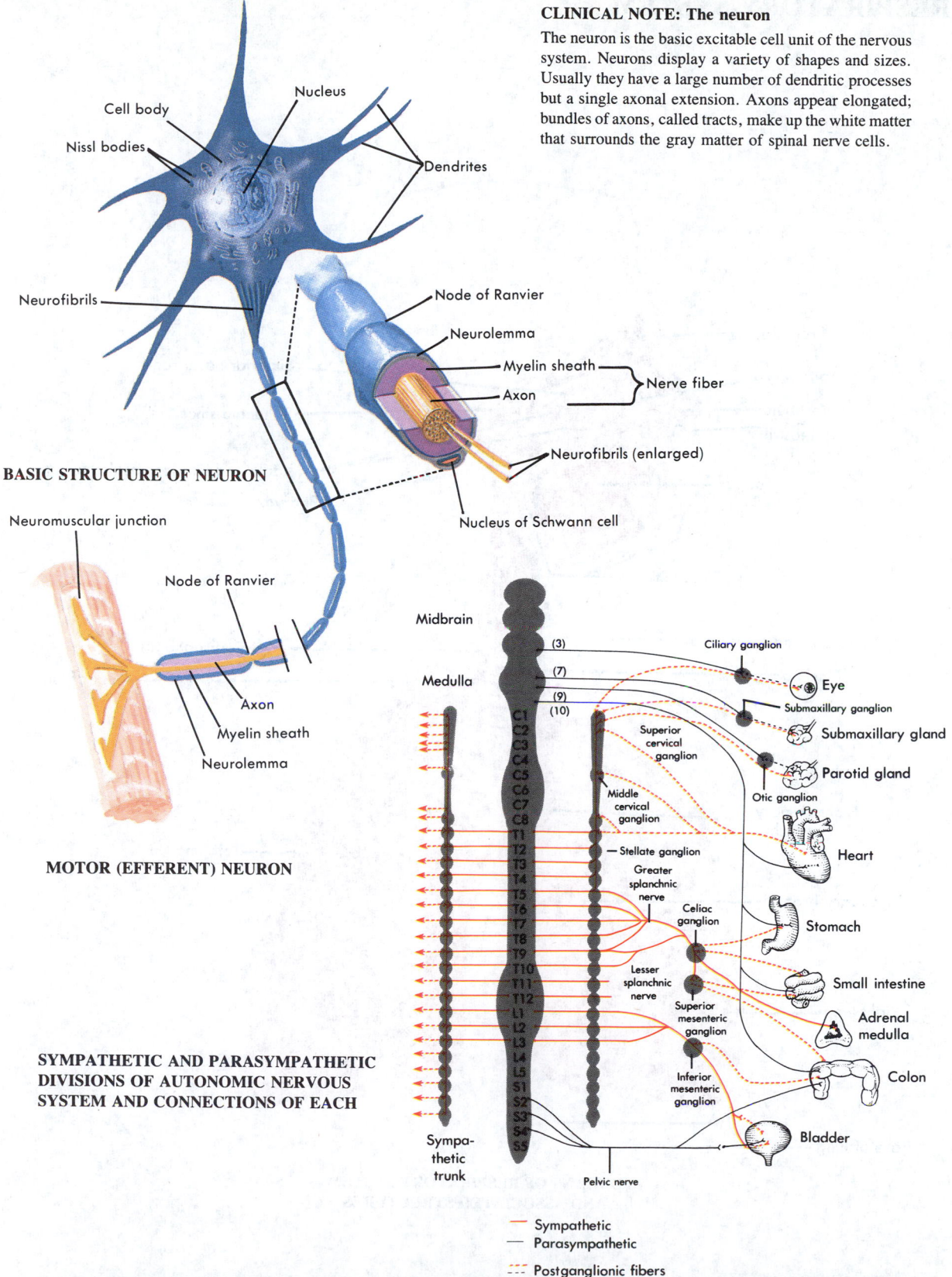

CLINICAL NOTE: The neuron

The neuron is the basic excitable cell unit of the nervous system. Neurons display a variety of shapes and sizes. Usually they have a large number of dendritic processes but a single axonal extension. Axons appear elongated; bundles of axons, called tracts, make up the white matter that surrounds the gray matter of spinal nerve cells.

Cell body

Nucleus

Nissl bodies

Dendrites

Neurofibrils

Node of Ranvier

Neurolemma

Myelin sheath

Axon

Nerve fiber

Neurofibrils (enlarged)

BASIC STRUCTURE OF NEURON

Nucleus of Schwann cell

Neuromuscular junction

Node of Ranvier

Axon

Myelin sheath

Neurolemma

MOTOR (EFFERENT) NEURON

Midbrain

Medulla

Ciliary ganglion

(3)

(7)

(9)

(10)

Eye

Submaxillary ganglion

Submaxillary gland

Superior cervical ganglion

Parotid gland

Middle cervical ganglion

Otic ganglion

Stellate ganglion

Heart

Greater splanchnic nerve

Celiac ganglion

Stomach

Lesser splanchnic nerve

Small intestine

Superior mesenteric ganglion

Adrenal medulla

Inferior mesenteric ganglion

Colon

Bladder

Sympathetic trunk

Pelvic nerve

C1 C2 C3 C4 C5 C6 C7 C8 T1 T2 T3 T4 T5 T6 T7 T8 T9 T10 T11 T12 L1 L2 L3 L4 L5 S1 S2 S3 S4 S5

SYMPATHETIC AND PARASYMPATHETIC DIVISIONS OF AUTONOMIC NERVOUS SYSTEM AND CONNECTIONS OF EACH

Sympathetic

Parasympathetic

Postganglionic fibers

RESPIRATORY SYSTEM

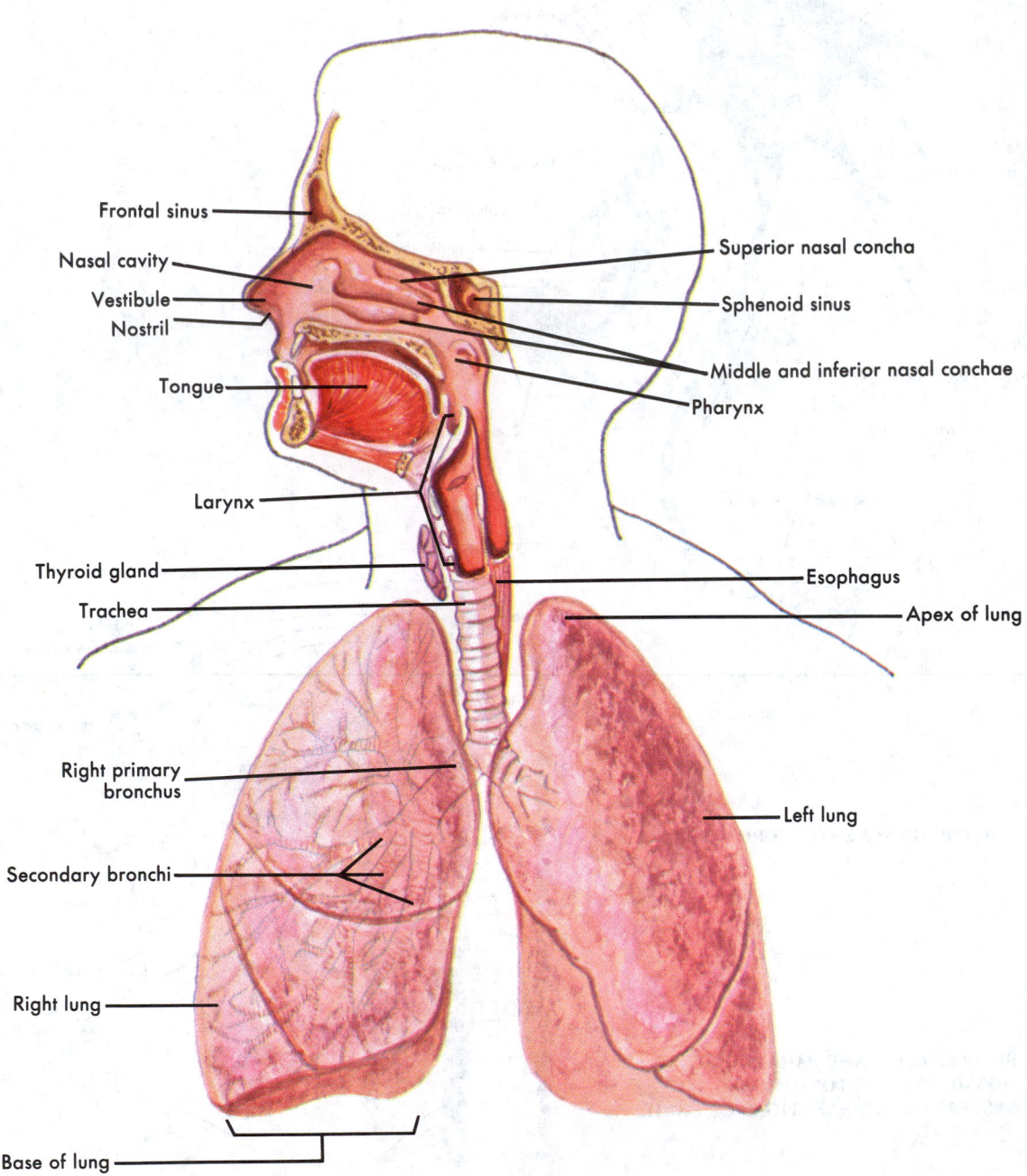

Frontal sinus

Nasal cavity

Vestibule

Nostril

Tongue

Larynx

Thyroid gland

Trachea

Right primary bronchus

Secondary bronchi

Right lung

Base of lung

Superior nasal concha

Sphenoid sinus

Middle and inferior nasal conchae

Pharynx

Esophagus

Apex of lung

Left lung

**ORGANS OF RESPIRATORY SYSTEM
AND ASSOCIATED STRUCTURES**

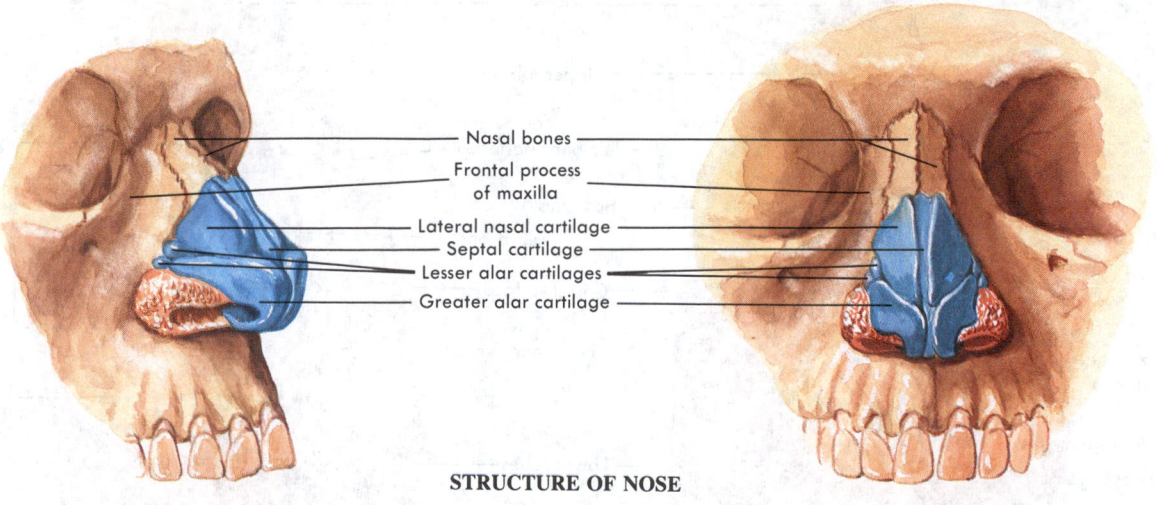

Nasal bones

Frontal process
of maxilla

Lateral nasal cartilage

Septal cartilage

Lesser alar cartilages

Greater alar cartilage

STRUCTURE OF NOSE

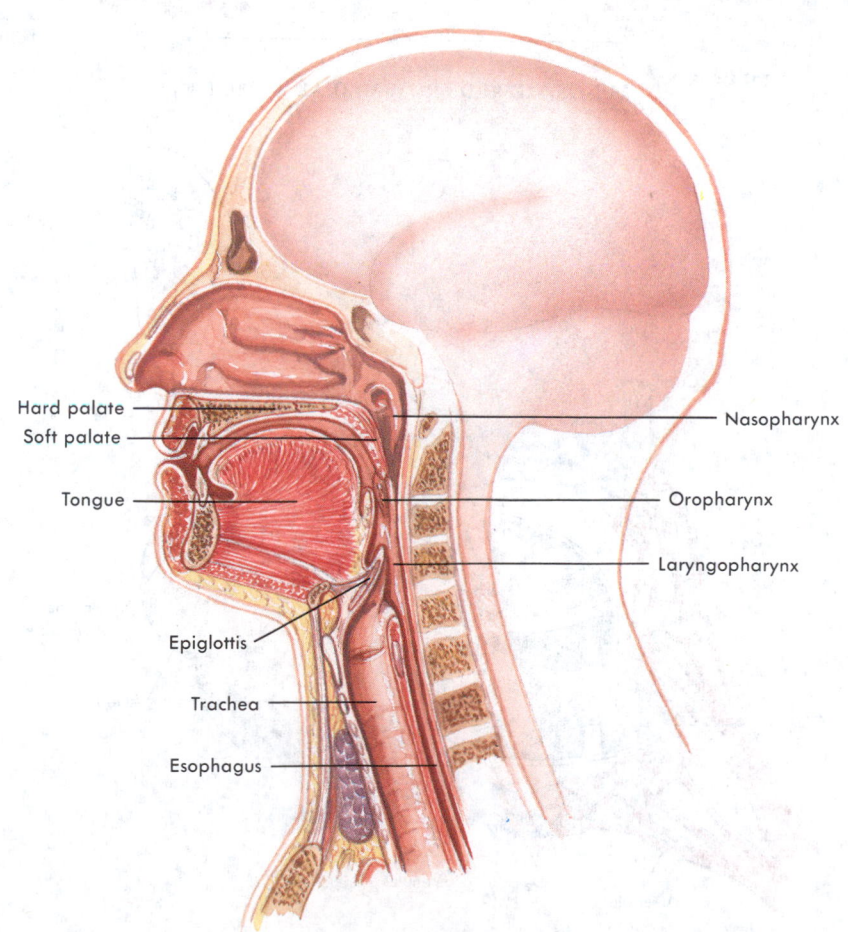

Hard palate

Soft palate

Tongue

Epiglottis

Trachea

Esophagus

Nasopharynx

Oropharynx

Laryngopharynx

STRUCTURES OF NASAL PASSAGES AND THROAT

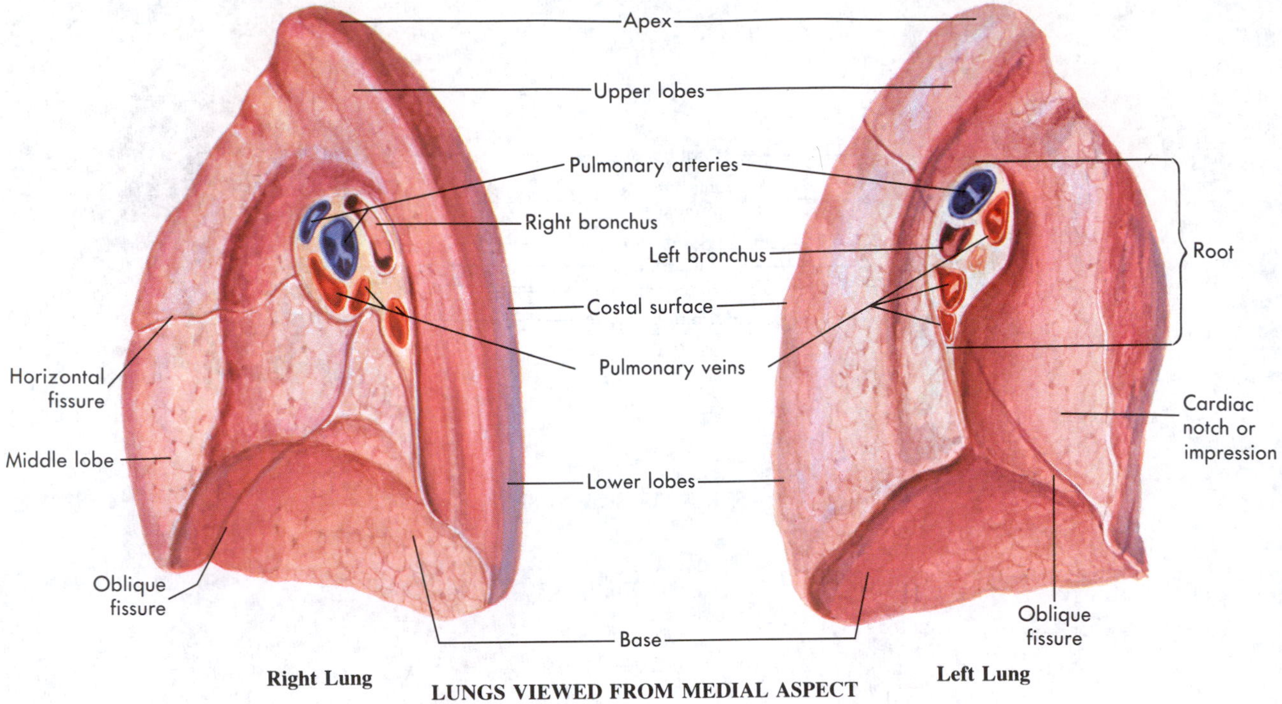

Apex

Upper lobes

Pulmonary arteries

Right bronchus

Left bronchus

Costal surface

Pulmonary veins

Root

Horizontal
fissure

Middle lobe

Cardiac
notch or
impression

Oblique
fissure

Lower lobes

Oblique
fissure

Base

Right Lung

Left Lung

LUNGS VIEWED FROM MEDIAL ASPECT

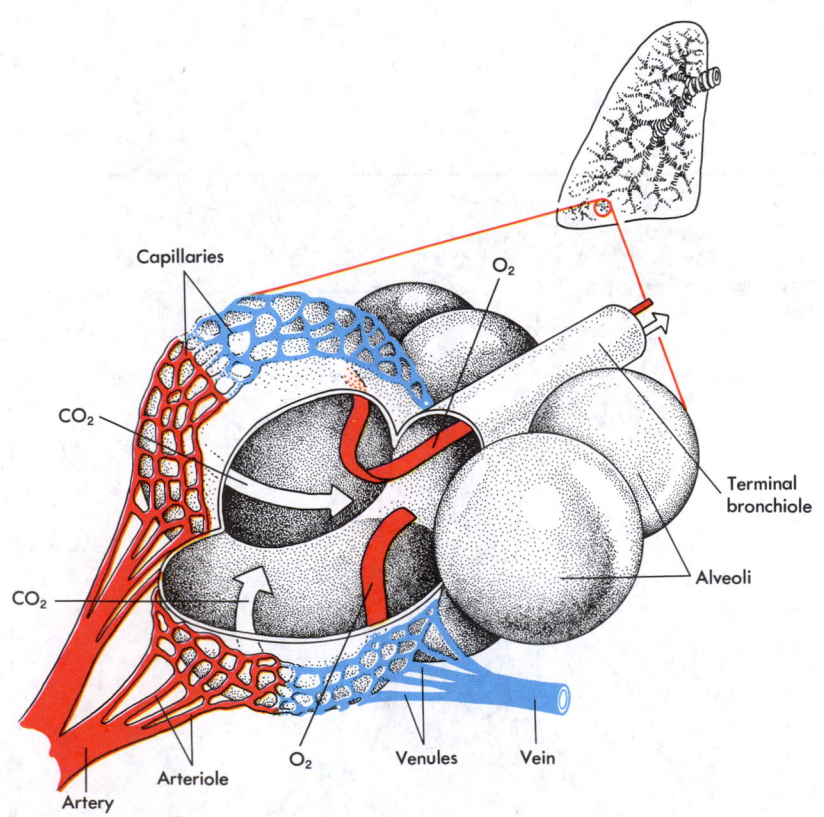

Capillaries

O_2

CO_2

Terminal
bronchiole

CO_2

Alveoli

O_2

Venules

Vein

Arteriole

Artery

ANATOMY OF AIR-EXCHANGING SURFACE OF LUNGS

CLINICAL NOTE: Respiratory muscles

Unlike cardiac muscle, respiratory muscles are skeletal and striated and possess no inherent rhythm. The periodic nature of respiratory movements results instead from the activity of certain pontine and medullary cells belonging to the reticular formation. Some stimulate breathing movements, others the opposite (inspiratory and expiratory centers).

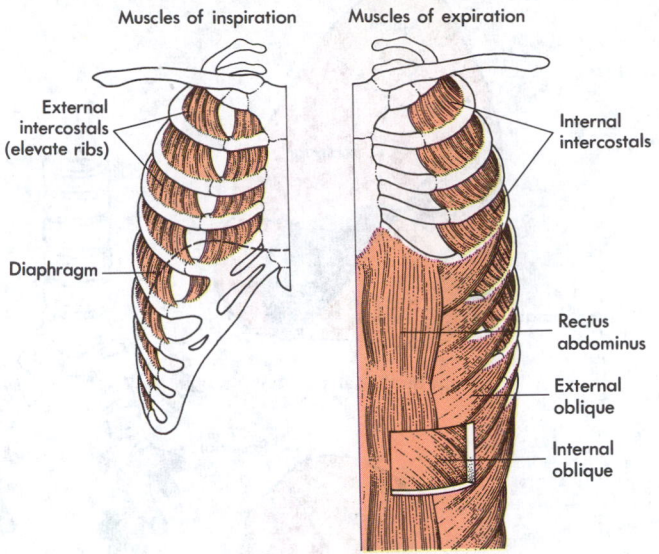

Muscles of inspiration   Muscles of expiration

External intercostals (elevate ribs)
Diaphragm
Internal intercostals
Rectus abdominus
External oblique
Internal oblique

MECHANICS OF RESPIRATION:
Muscles required for inspiration and expiration

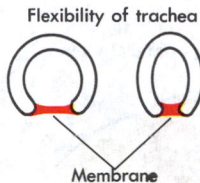

Flexibility of trachea

Membrane

FLEXIBILITY OF TRACHEA

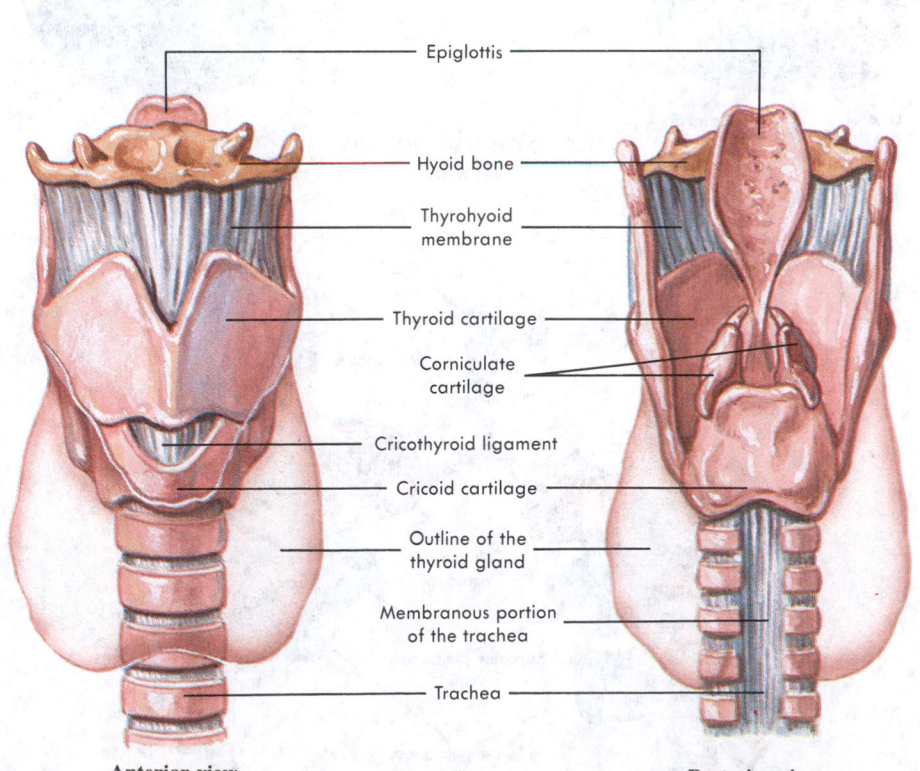

Epiglottis

Hyoid bone

Thyrohyoid membrane

Thyroid cartilage

Corniculate cartilage

Cricothyroid ligament

Cricoid cartilage

Outline of the thyroid gland

Membranous portion of the trachea

Trachea

Anterior view   Posterior view

CARTILAGINOUS STRUCTURE OF LARYNX AND UPPER TRACHEA

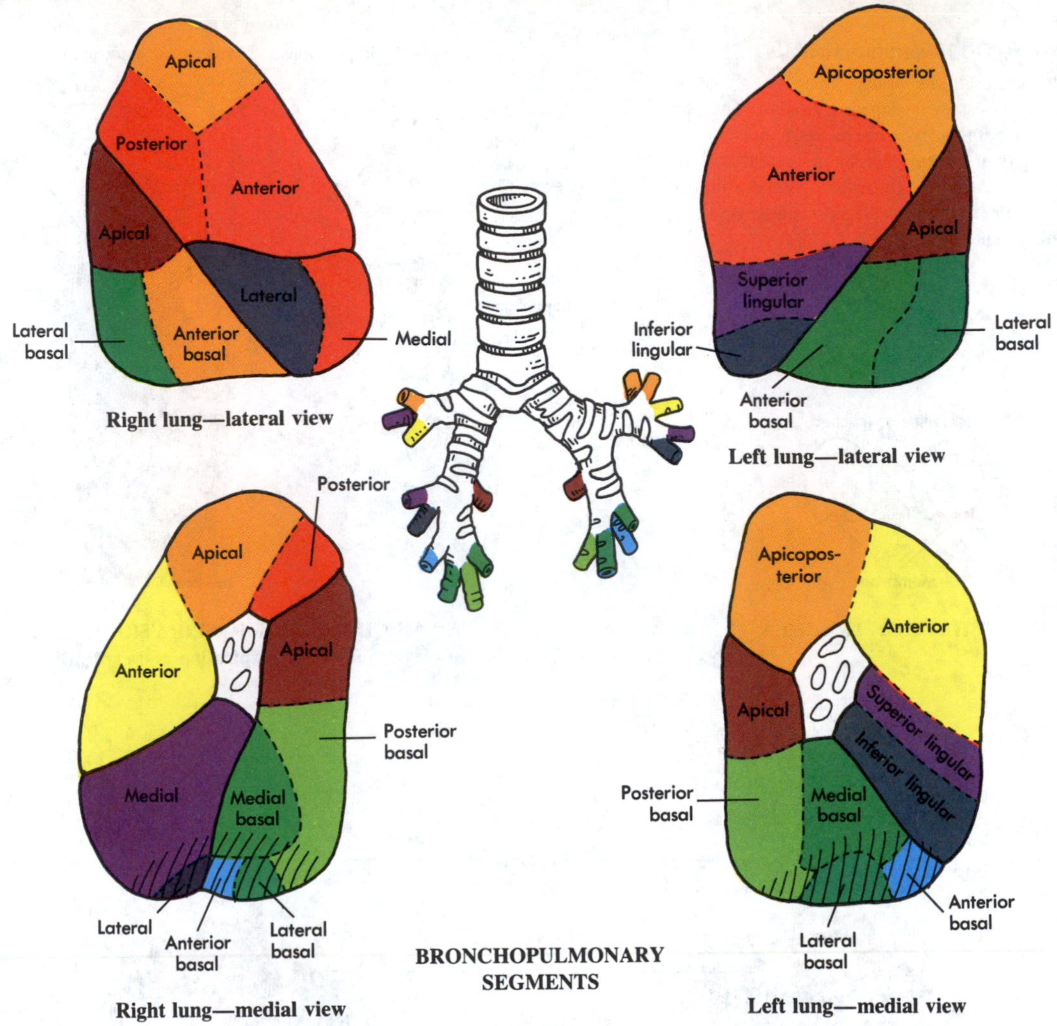

Apical

Posterior

Anterior

Apical

Lateral

Lateral basal

Anterior basal

Medial

Right lung—lateral view

Apicoposterior

Anterior

Apical

Superior lingular

Inferior lingular

Lateral basal

Anterior basal

Left lung—lateral view

Apical

Posterior

Anterior

Apical

Posterior basal

Medial

Medial basal

Lateral

Anterior basal

Lateral basal

Right lung—medial view

Apicoposterior

Anterior

Apical

Superior lingular

Inferior lingular

Posterior basal

Medial basal

Lateral basal

Anterior basal

Left lung—medial view

BRONCHOPULMONARY SEGMENTS

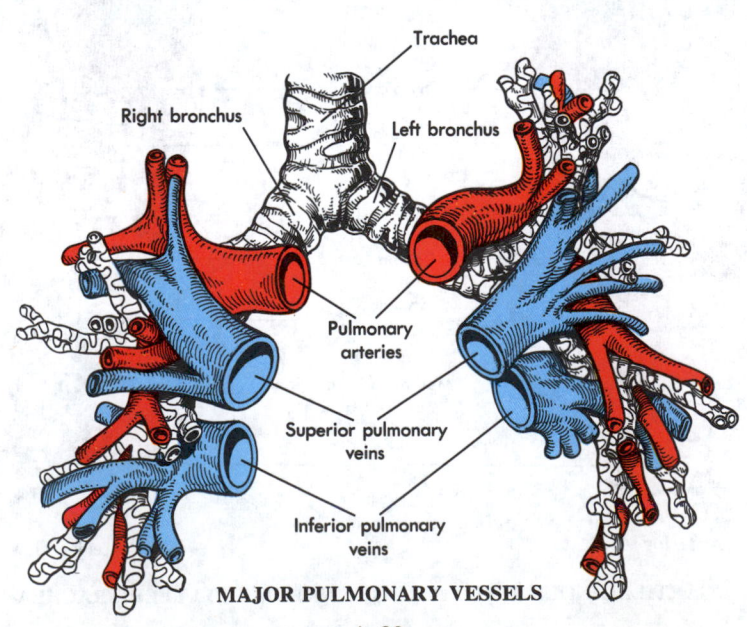

Trachea

Right bronchus

Left bronchus

Pulmonary arteries

Superior pulmonary veins

Inferior pulmonary veins

MAJOR PULMONARY VESSELS

A-30

DIGESTIVE SYSTEM

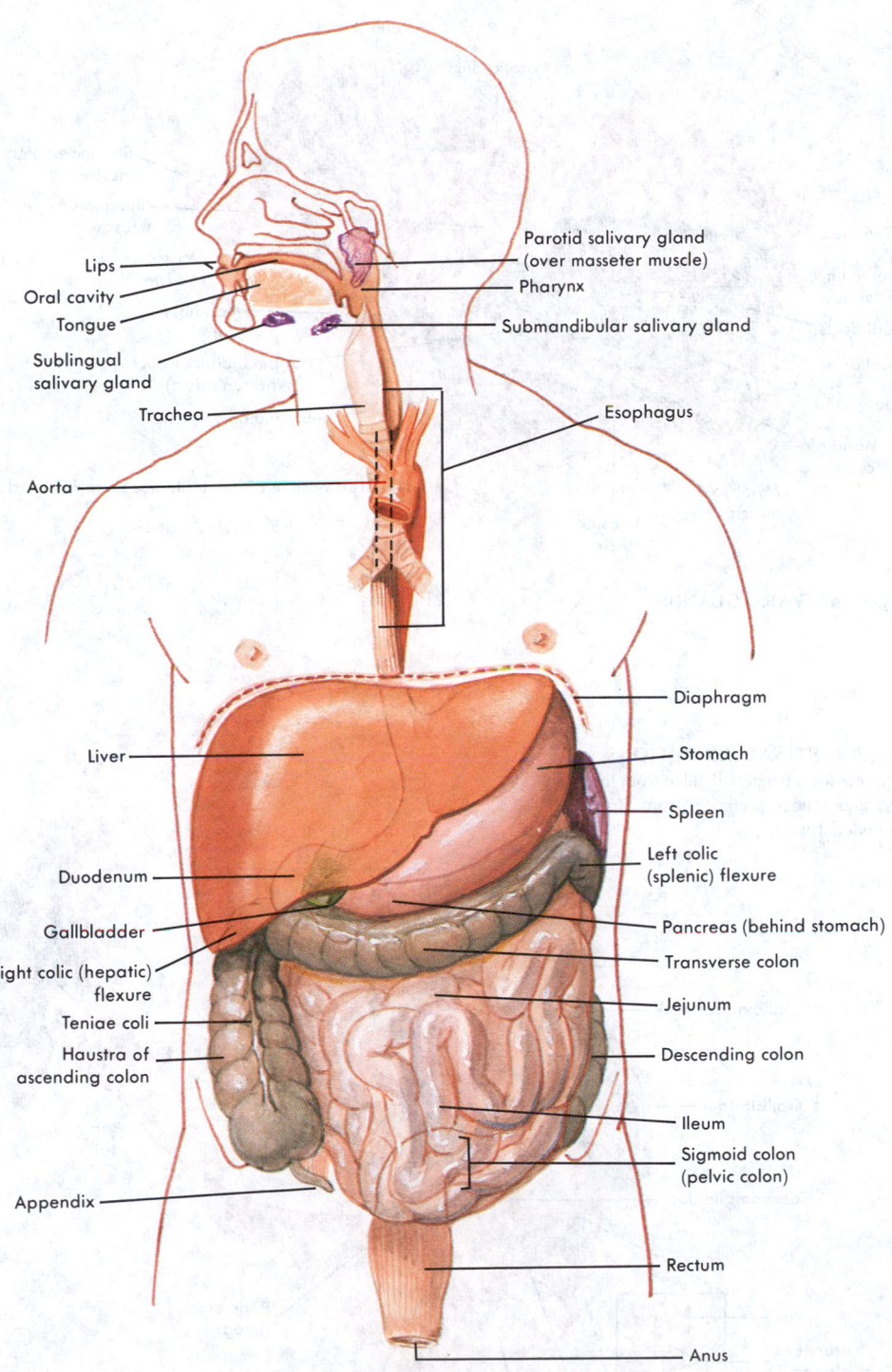

Lips

Oral cavity

Tongue

Sublingual
salivary gland

Trachea

Aorta

Parotid salivary gland
(over masseter muscle)

Pharynx

Submandibular salivary gland

Esophagus

Liver

Duodenum

Gallbladder

Right colic (hepatic)
flexure

Teniae coli

Haustra of
ascending colon

Appendix

Diaphragm

Stomach

Spleen

Left colic
(splenic) flexure

Pancreas (behind stomach)

Transverse colon

Jejunum

Descending colon

Ileum

Sigmoid colon
(pelvic colon)

Rectum

Anus

**ORGANS OF DIGESTIVE SYSTEM AND
SOME ASSOCIATED STRUCTURES**

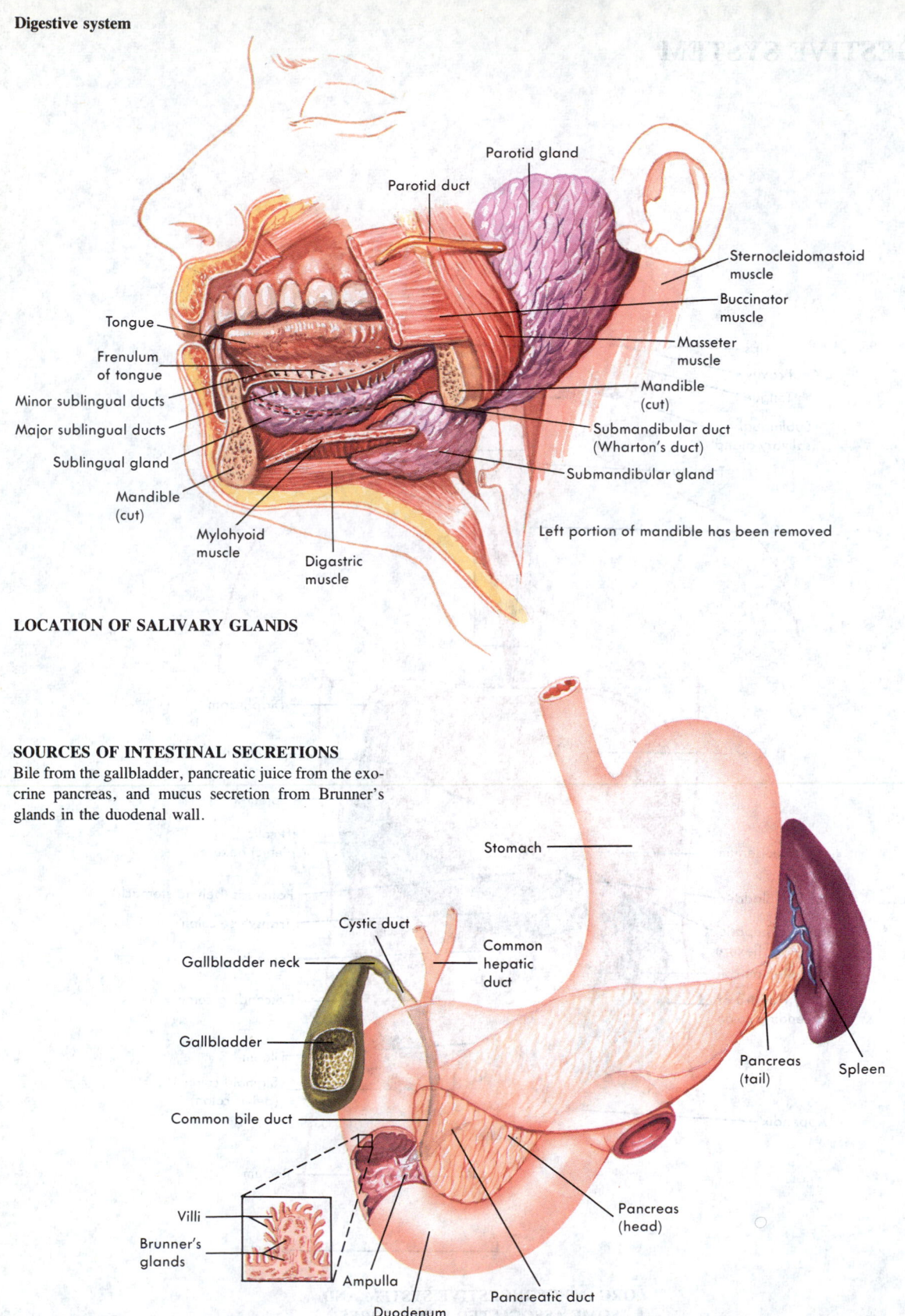

Parotid gland

Parotid duct

Sternocleidomastoid muscle

Buccinator muscle

Masseter muscle

Tongue

Frenulum of tongue

Minor sublingual ducts

Major sublingual ducts

Sublingual gland

Mandible (cut)

Mandible (cut)

Submandibular duct (Wharton's duct)

Submandibular gland

Mylohyoid muscle

Digastric muscle

Left portion of mandible has been removed

LOCATION OF SALIVARY GLANDS

SOURCES OF INTESTINAL SECRETIONS

Bile from the gallbladder, pancreatic juice from the exocrine pancreas, and mucus secretion from Brunner's glands in the duodenal wall.

Stomach

Cystic duct

Common hepatic duct

Gallbladder neck

Gallbladder

Pancreas (tail)

Spleen

Common bile duct

Villi

Brunner's glands

Ampulla

Duodenum

Pancreatic duct

Pancreas (head)

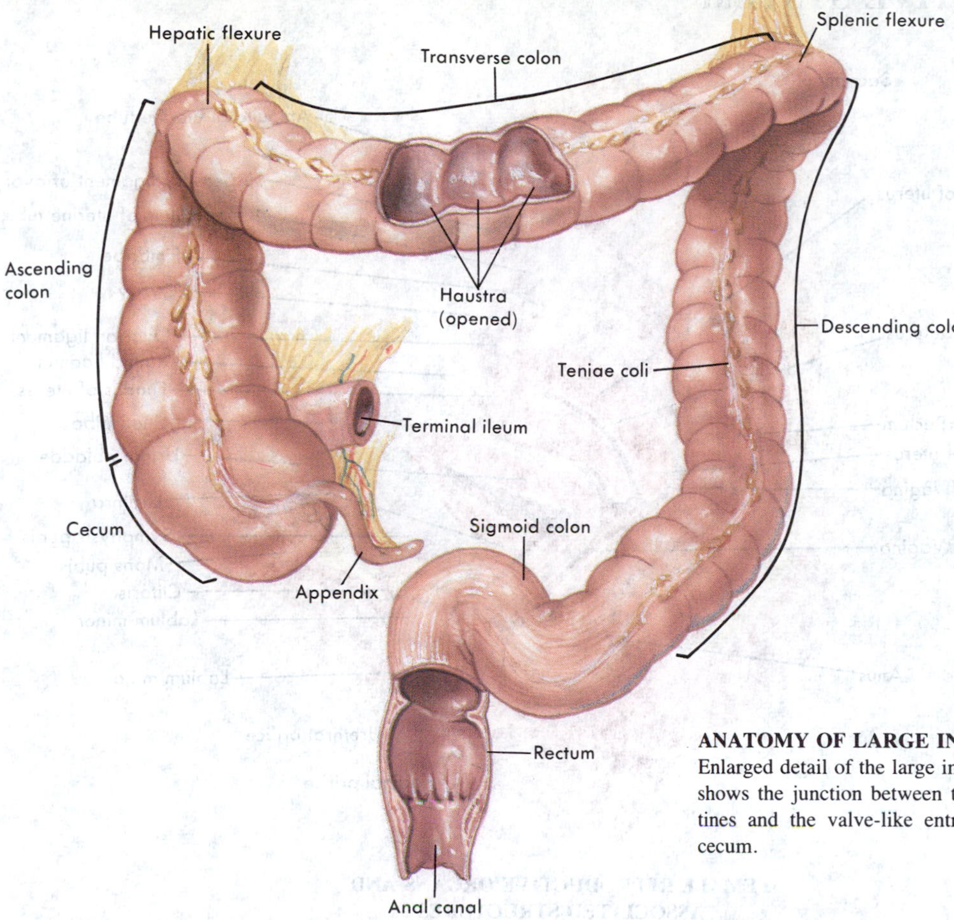

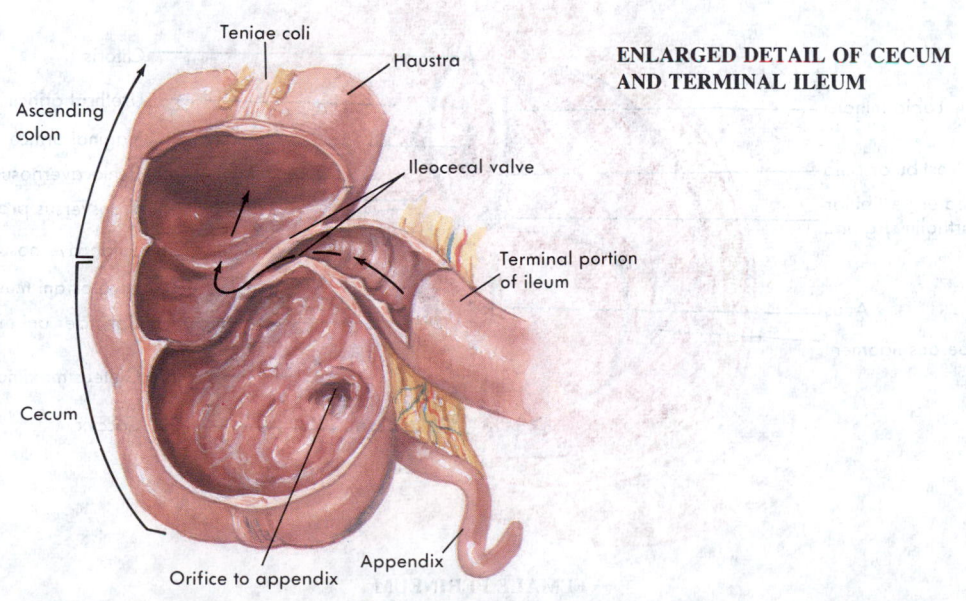

Hepatic flexure

Transverse colon

Splenic flexure

Ascending colon

Haustra (opened)

Descending colon

Teniae coli

Terminal ileum

Cecum

Sigmoid colon

Appendix

Rectum

Anal canal

ANATOMY OF LARGE INTESTINE

Enlarged detail of the large intestine, rectum, and anus shows the junction between the large and small intestines and the valve-like entry of the ileum into the cecum.

Teniae coli

Haustra

ENLARGED DETAIL OF CECUM AND TERMINAL ILEUM

Ascending colon

Ileocecal valve

Terminal portion of ileum

Cecum

Orifice to appendix

Appendix

REPRODUCTIVE SYSTEM

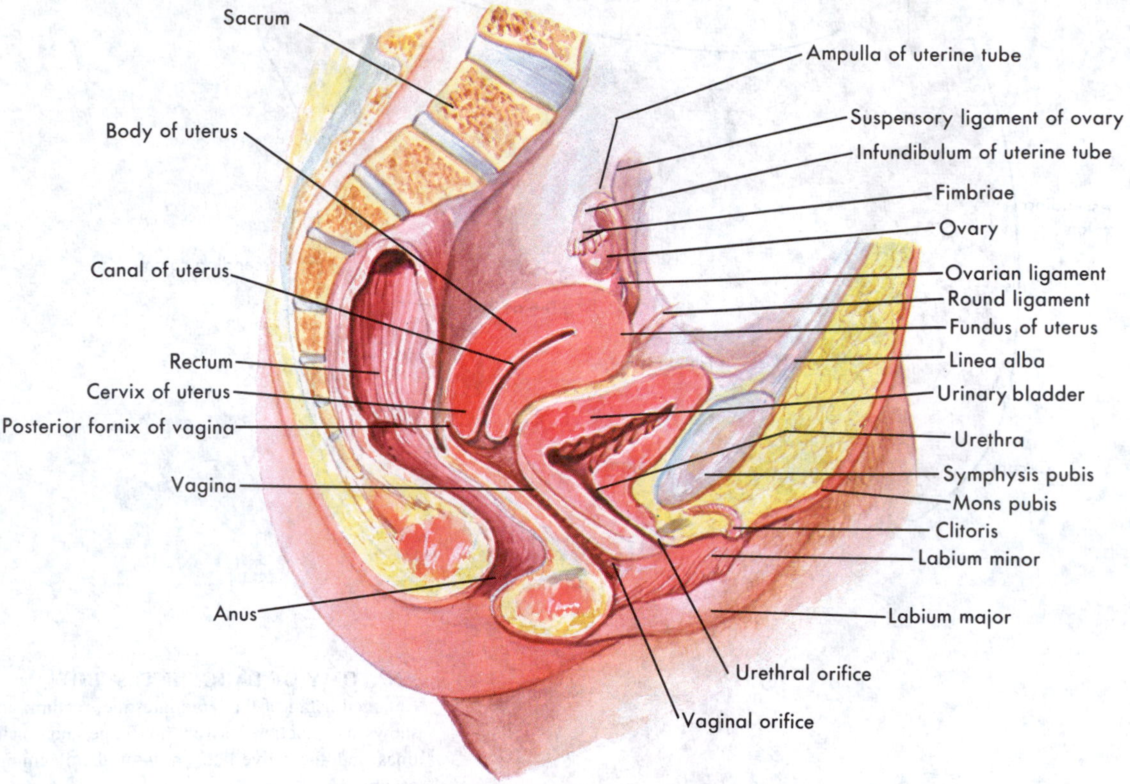

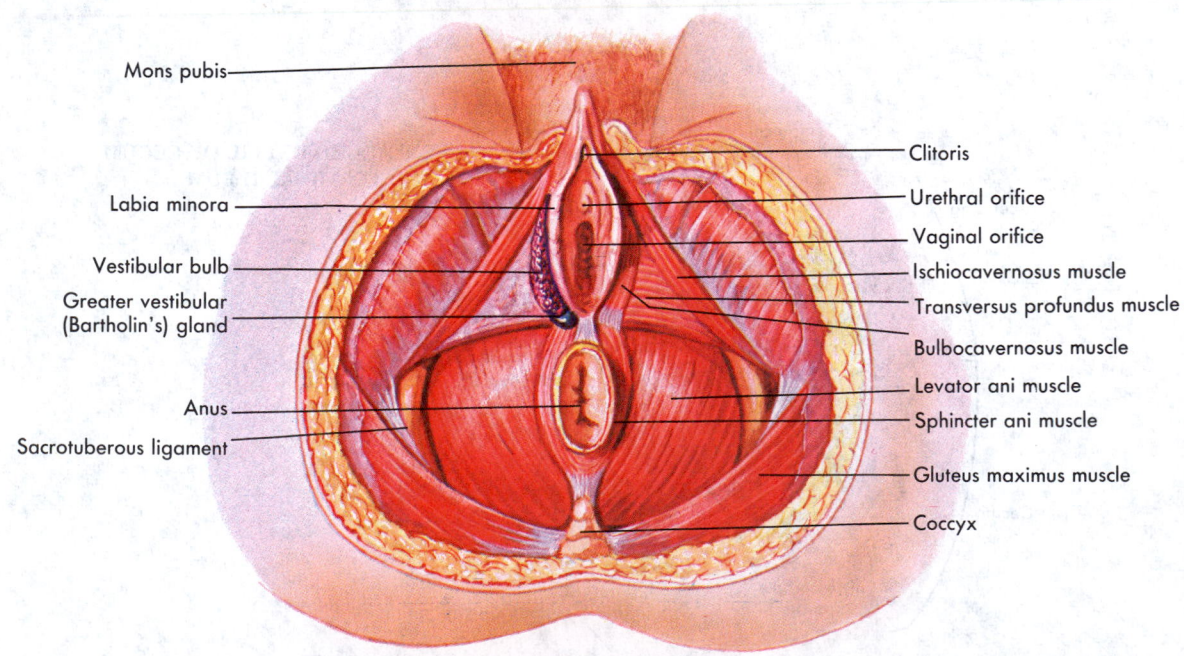

Sacrum

Body of uterus

Canal of uterus

Rectum

Cervix of uterus

Posterior fornix of vagina

Vagina

Anus

Ampulla of uterine tube

Suspensory ligament of ovary

Infundibulum of uterine tube

Fimbriae

Ovary

Ovarian ligament

Round ligament

Fundus of uterus

Linea alba

Urinary bladder

Urethra

Symphysis pubis

Mons pubis

Clitoris

Labium minor

Labium major

Urethral orifice

Vaginal orifice

**FEMALE REPRODUCTIVE ORGANS AND
ASSOCIATED STRUCTURES**

Mons pubis

Labia minora

Vestibular bulb

Greater vestibular
(Bartholin's) gland

Anus

Sacrotuberous ligament

Clitoris

Urethral orifice

Vaginal orifice

Ischiocavernosus muscle

Transversus profundus muscle

Bulbocavernosus muscle

Levator ani muscle

Sphincter ani muscle

Gluteus maximus muscle

Coccyx

FEMALE PERINEUM

A-34

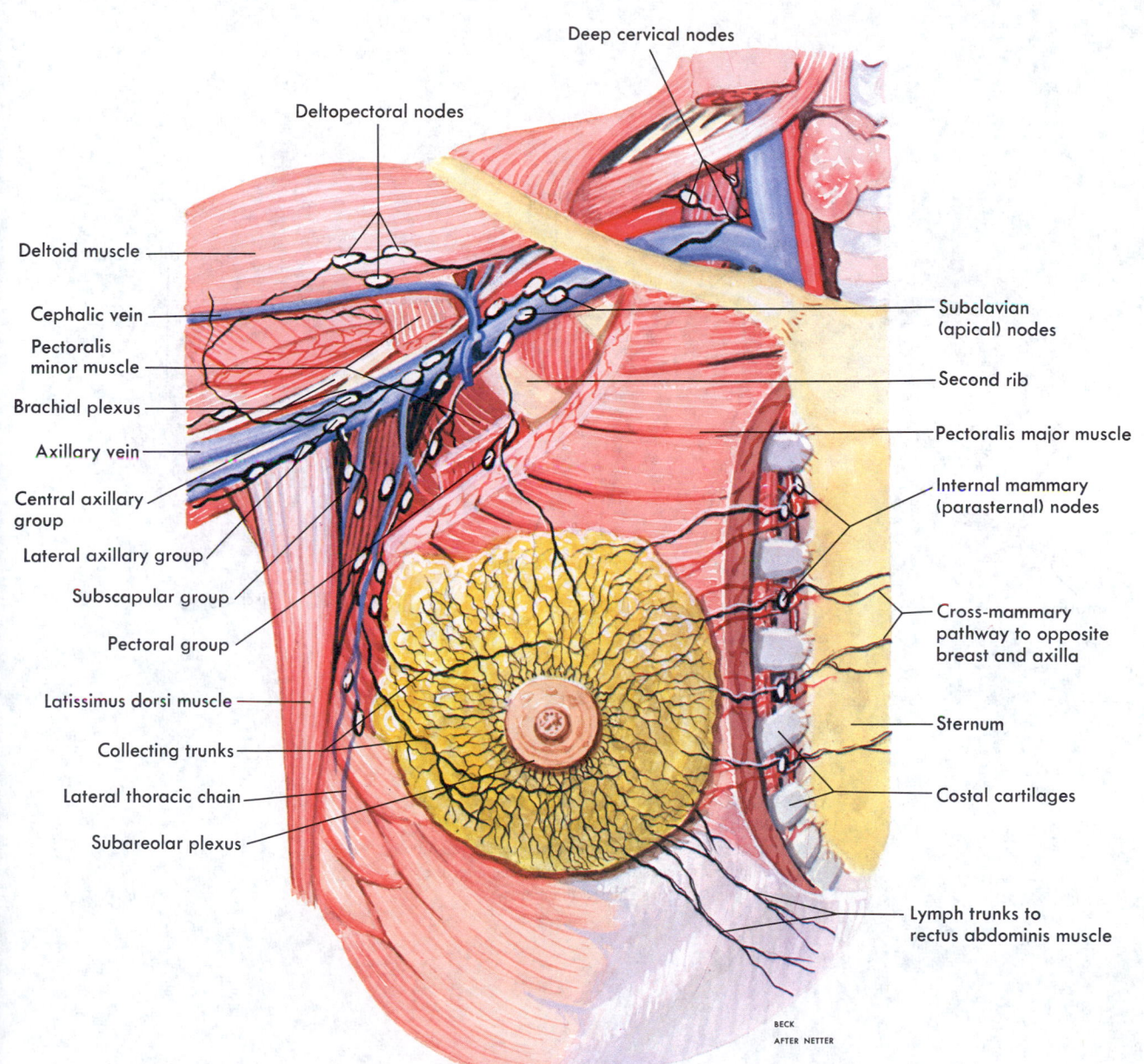

Deep cervical nodes

Deltopectoral nodes

Deltoid muscle

Cephalic vein

Pectoralis minor muscle

Brachial plexus

Axillary vein

Central axillary group

Lateral axillary group

Subscapular group

Pectoral group

Latissimus dorsi muscle

Collecting trunks

Lateral thoracic chain

Subareolar plexus

Subclavian (apical) nodes

Second rib

Pectoralis major muscle

Internal mammary (parasternal) nodes

Cross-mammary pathway to opposite breast and axilla

Sternum

Costal cartilages

Lymph trunks to rectus abdominis muscle

BECK
AFTER NETTER

LYMPHATIC AND RETICULOENDOTHELIAL SYSTEM

CLINICAL NOTE: Female reproductive system
Immense structural changes occur within the uterus during pregnancy. However, if fertilization does not take place, then the endometrial lining is shed cyclically under hormonal control in the phenomenon of menstruation.

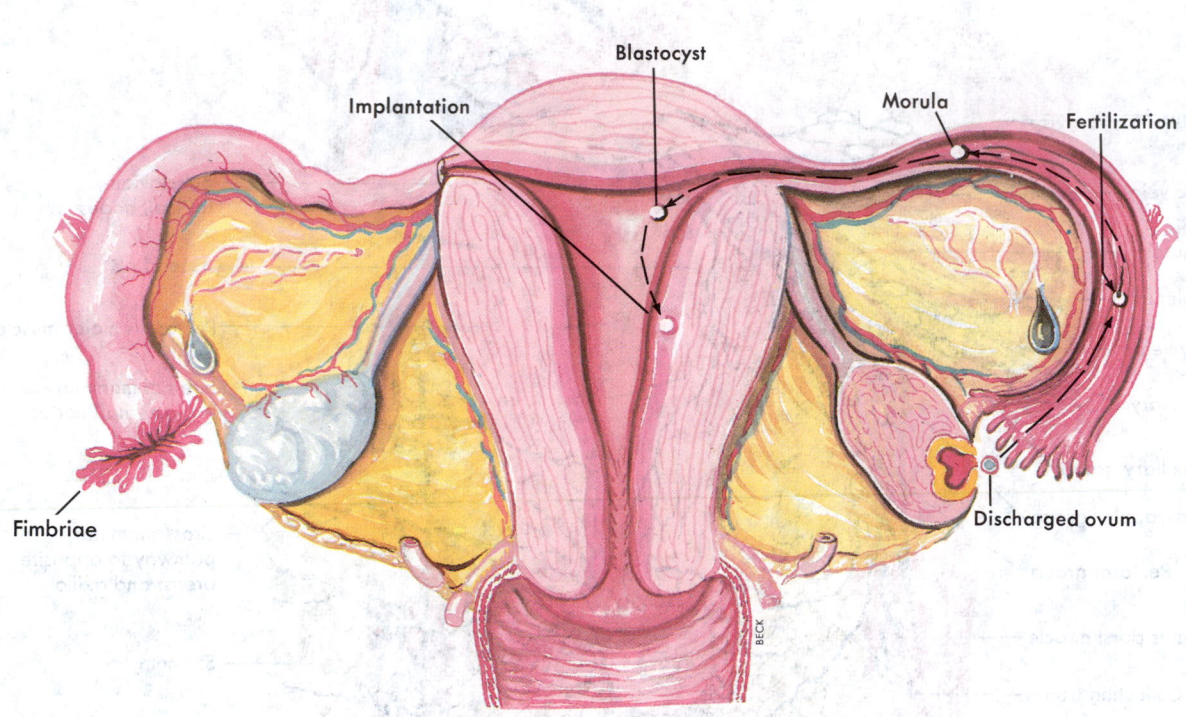

APPEARANCE OF UTERUS AND UTERINE TUBES FROM FERTILIZATION TO IMPLANTATION
Fertilization occurs in the outer third of the uterine tube. Development reaches the blastocyst stage after the embryo has entered the uterus.

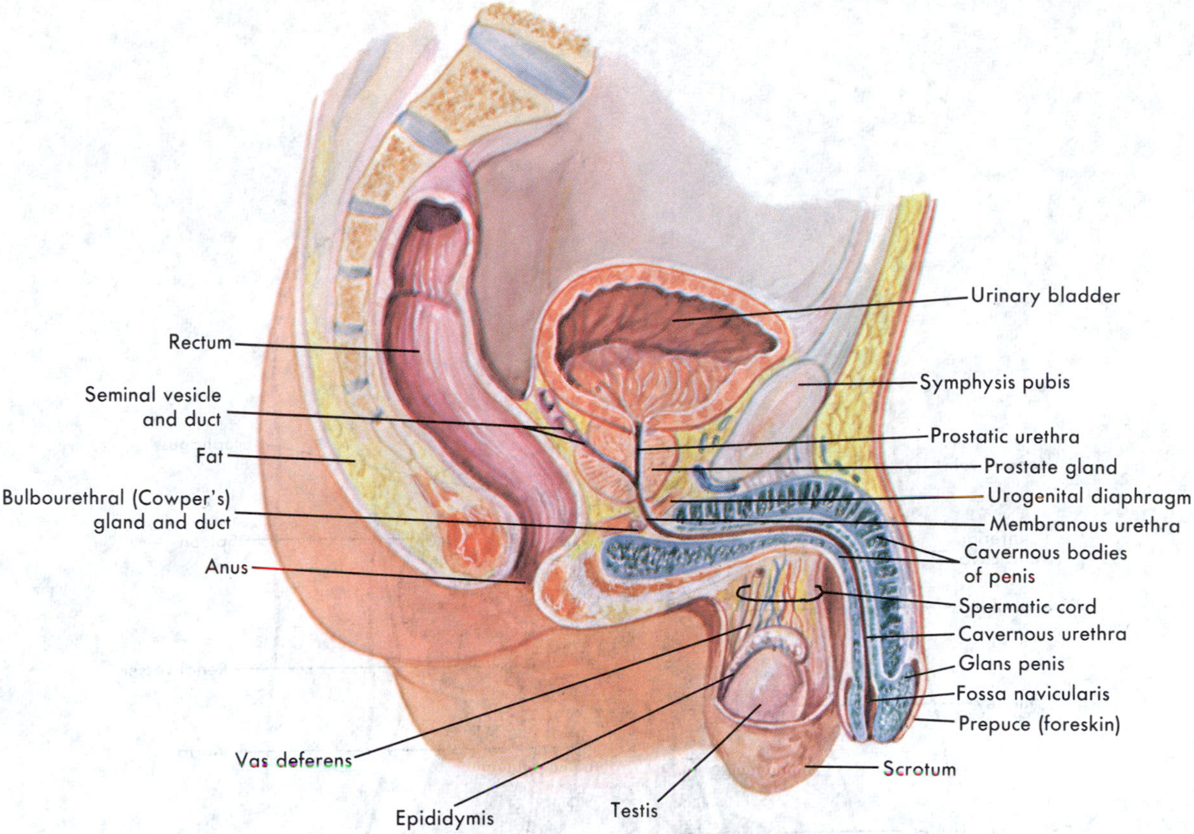

Rectum

Seminal vesicle
and duct

Fat

Bulbourethral (Cowper's)
gland and duct

Anus

Urinary bladder

Symphysis pubis

Prostatic urethra

Prostate gland

Urogenital diaphragm

Membranous urethra

Cavernous bodies
of penis

Spermatic cord

Cavernous urethra

Glans penis

Fossa navicularis

Prepuce (foreskin)

Scrotum

Vas deferens

Epididymis

Testis

**MALE REPRODUCTIVE ORGANS AND
ASSOCIATED STRUCTURES**

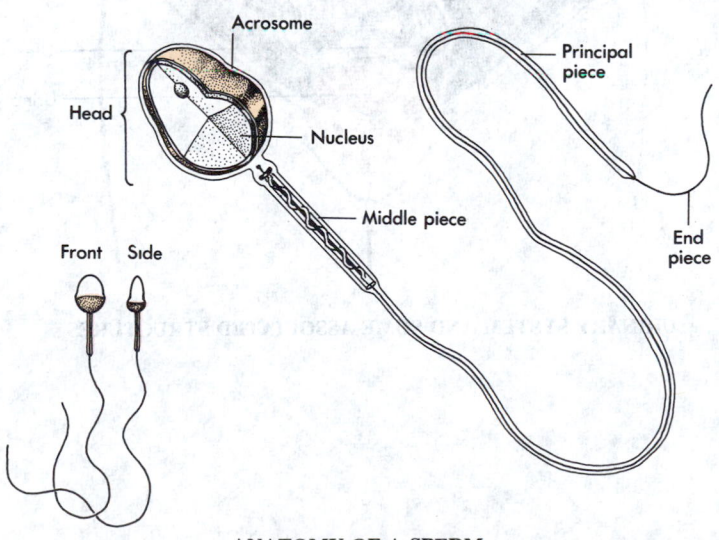

Acrosome

Head

Nucleus

Middle piece

Principal
piece

End
piece

Front   Side

ANATOMY OF A SPERM

URINARY SYSTEM

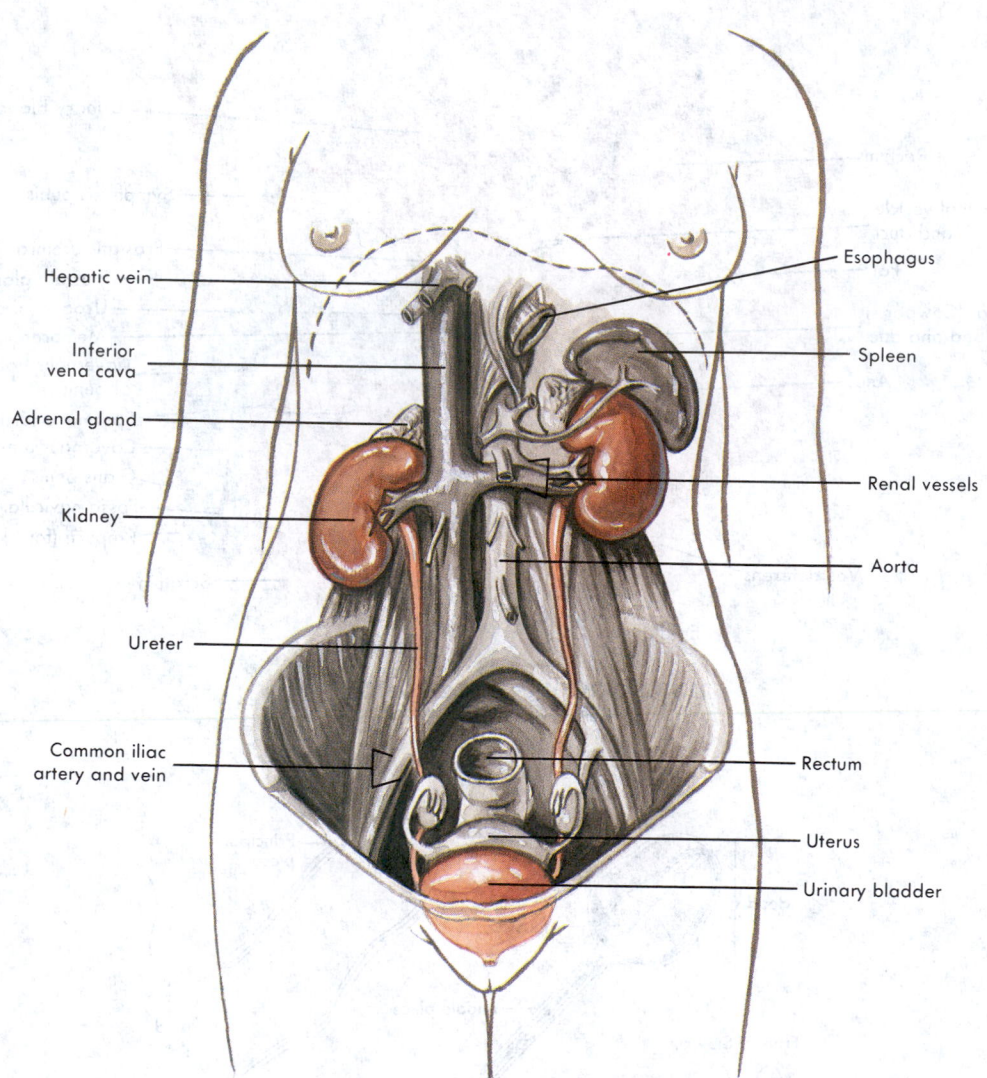

Hepatic vein

Inferior vena cava

Adrenal gland

Kidney

Ureter

Common iliac artery and vein

Esophagus

Spleen

Renal vessels

Aorta

Rectum

Uterus

Urinary bladder

URINARY SYSTEM AND SOME ASSOCIATED STRUCTURES

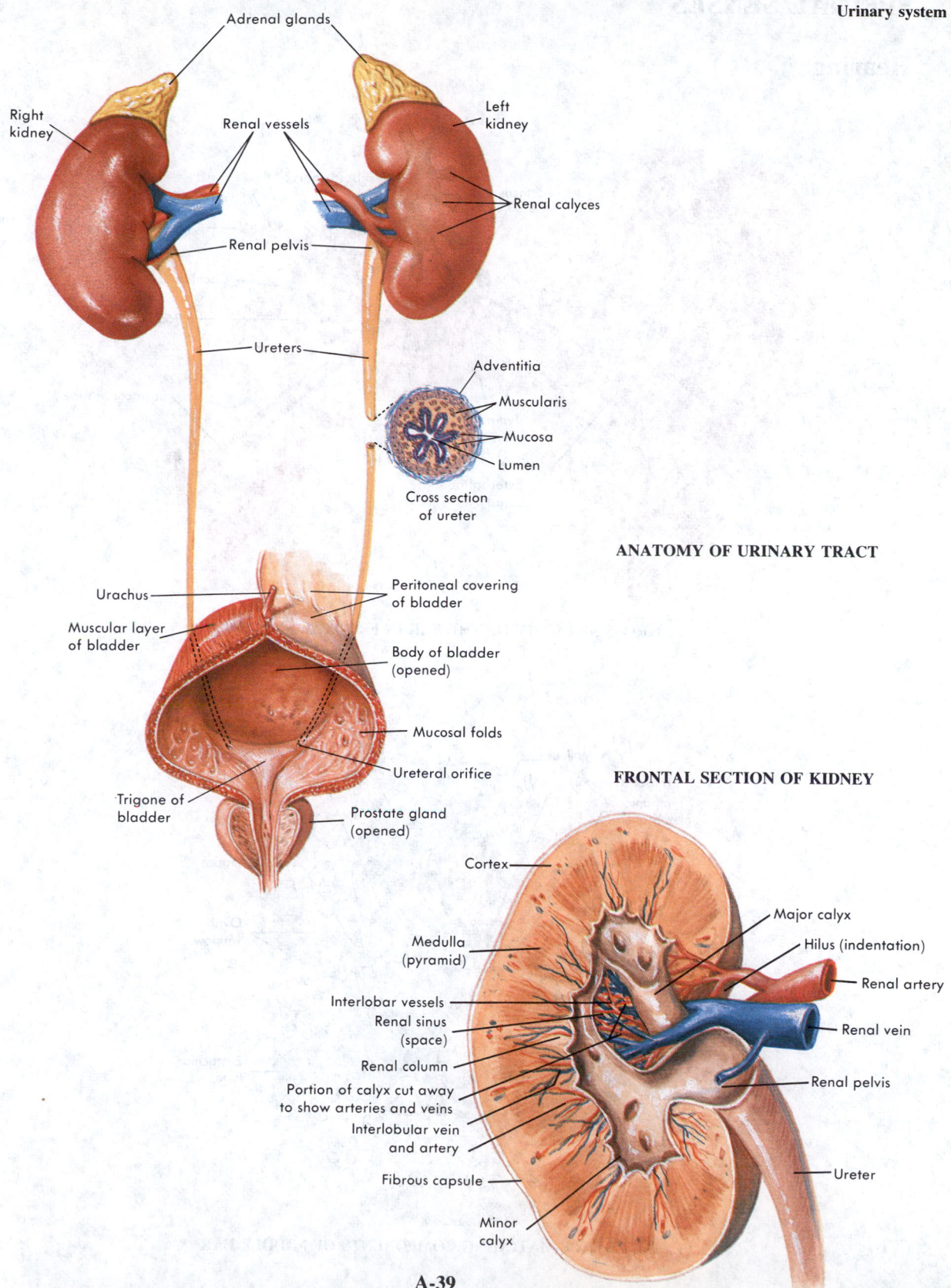

Adrenal glands

Right
kidney

Renal vessels

Left
kidney

Renal calyces

Renal pelvis

Ureters

Adventitia

Muscularis

Mucosa

Lumen

Cross section
of ureter

ANATOMY OF URINARY TRACT

Urachus

Peritoneal covering
of bladder

Muscular layer
of bladder

Body of bladder
(opened)

Mucosal folds

Ureteral orifice

FRONTAL SECTION OF KIDNEY

Trigone of
bladder

Prostate gland
(opened)

Cortex

Major calyx

Medulla
(pyramid)

Hilus (indentation)

Renal artery

Interlobar vessels

Renal sinus
(space)

Renal vein

Renal column

Renal pelvis

Portion of calyx cut away
to show arteries and veins

Interlobular vein
and artery

Ureter

Fibrous capsule

Minor
calyx

A-39

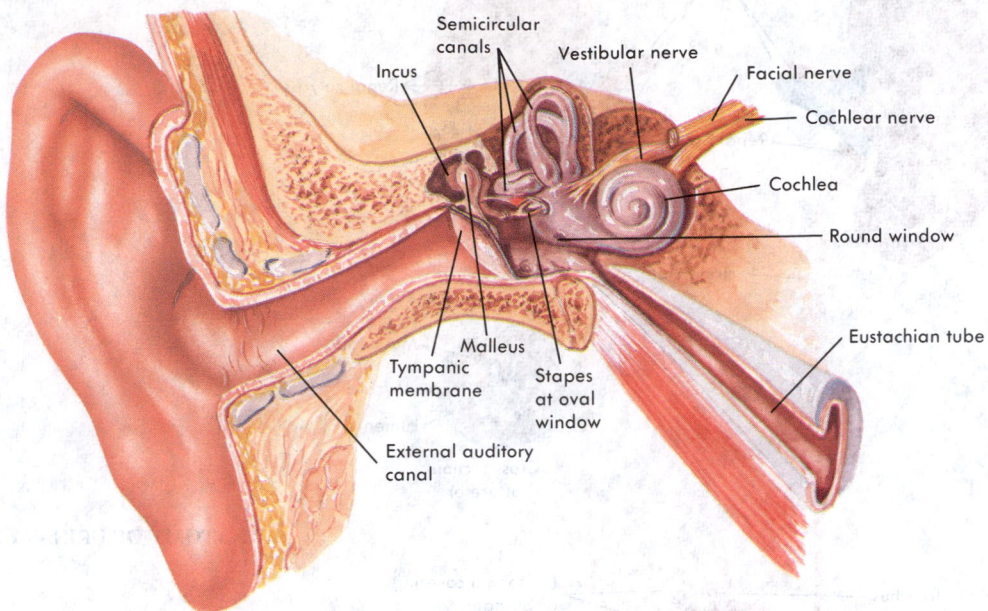

GROSS ANATOMY OF THE EAR IN FRONTAL SECTION

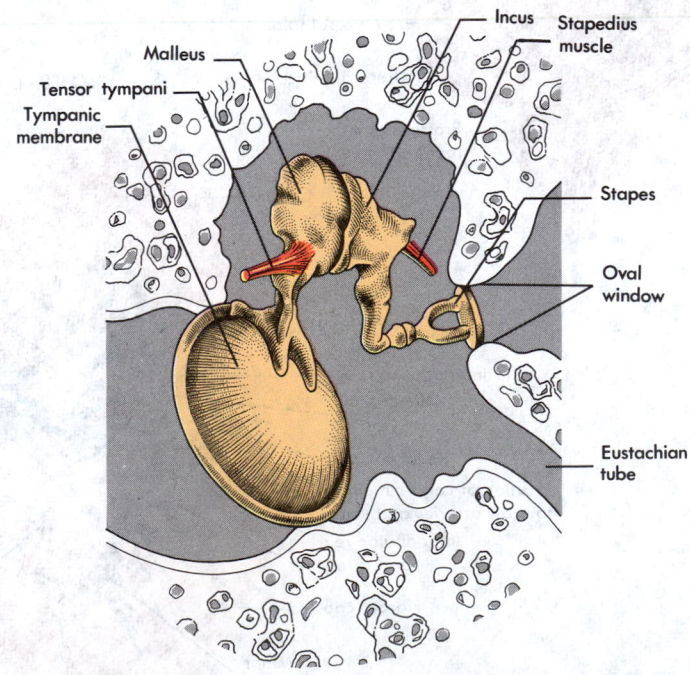

IMPEDENCE-MATCHING COMPONENTS OF MIDDLE EAR

Sight

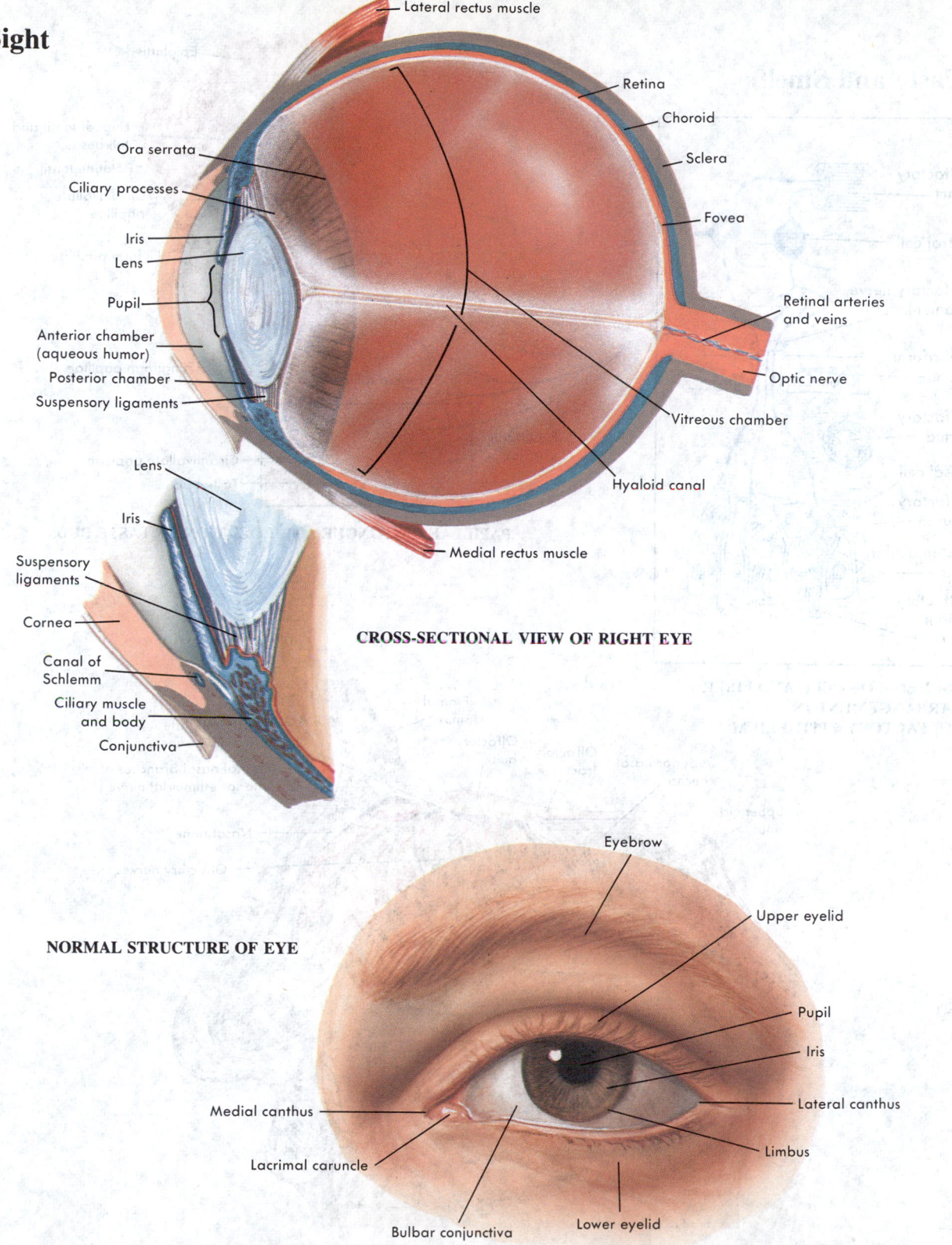

Lateral rectus muscle

Retina

Choroid

Sclera

Fovea

Ora serrata

Ciliary processes

Iris

Lens

Pupil

Anterior chamber (aqueous humor)

Posterior chamber

Suspensory ligaments

Retinal arteries and veins

Optic nerve

Vitreous chamber

Hyaloid canal

Medial rectus muscle

CROSS-SECTIONAL VIEW OF RIGHT EYE

Lens

Iris

Suspensory ligaments

Cornea

Canal of Schlemm

Ciliary muscle and body

Conjunctiva

NORMAL STRUCTURE OF EYE

Eyebrow

Upper eyelid

Pupil

Iris

Lateral canthus

Limbus

Medial canthus

Lacrimal caruncle

Bulbar conjunctiva

Lower eyelid

A-41

Taste and Smell

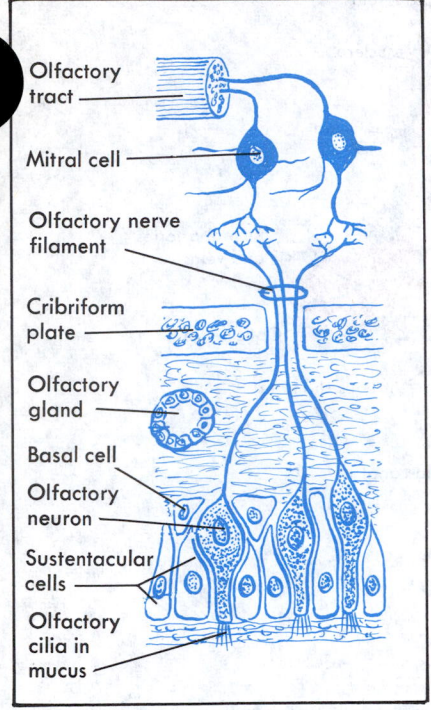

Olfactory tract

Mitral cell

Olfactory nerve filament

Cribriform plate

Olfactory gland

Basal cell

Olfactory neuron

Sustentacular cells

Olfactory cilia in mucus

SCHEME OF CELL AND FIBER ARRANGEMENT IN OLFACTORY EPITHELIUM

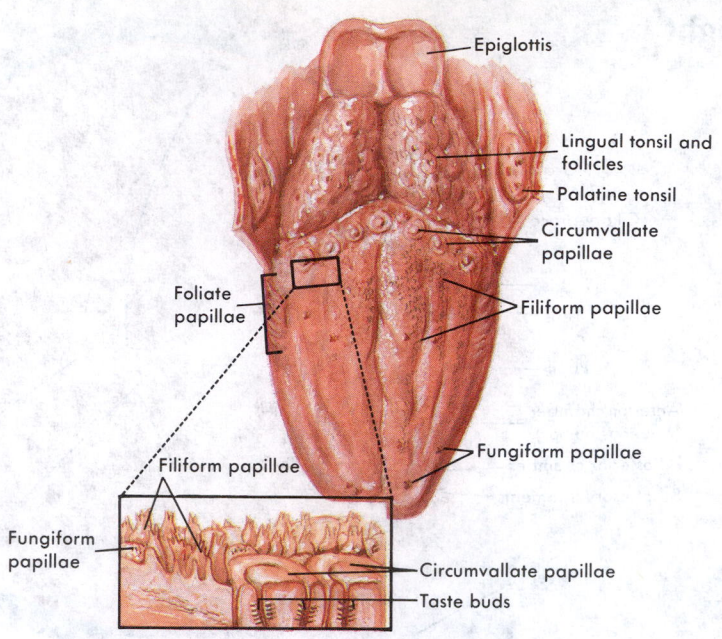

Epiglottis

Lingual tonsil and follicles

Palatine tonsil

Circumvallate papillae

Filiform papillae

Foliate papillae

Fungiform papillae

Filiform papillae

Fungiform papillae

Circumvallate papillae

Taste buds

PAPILLAE ON TONGUE AND LOCATION OF TASTE BUDS

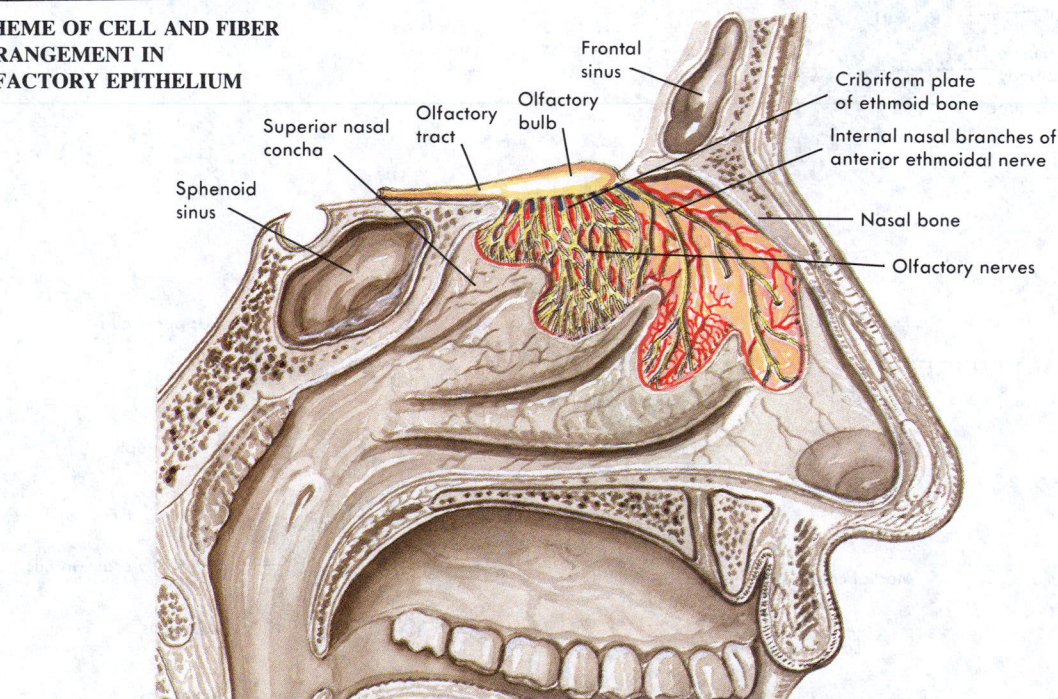

Frontal sinus

Superior nasal concha

Olfactory tract

Olfactory bulb

Cribriform plate of ethmoid bone

Internal nasal branches of anterior ethmoidal nerve

Sphenoid sinus

Nasal bone

Olfactory nerves

OLFACTORY NERVE DISTRIBUTION TO MUCOSA OF NASAL CAVITY

A-42

SKIN

Protection and Touch

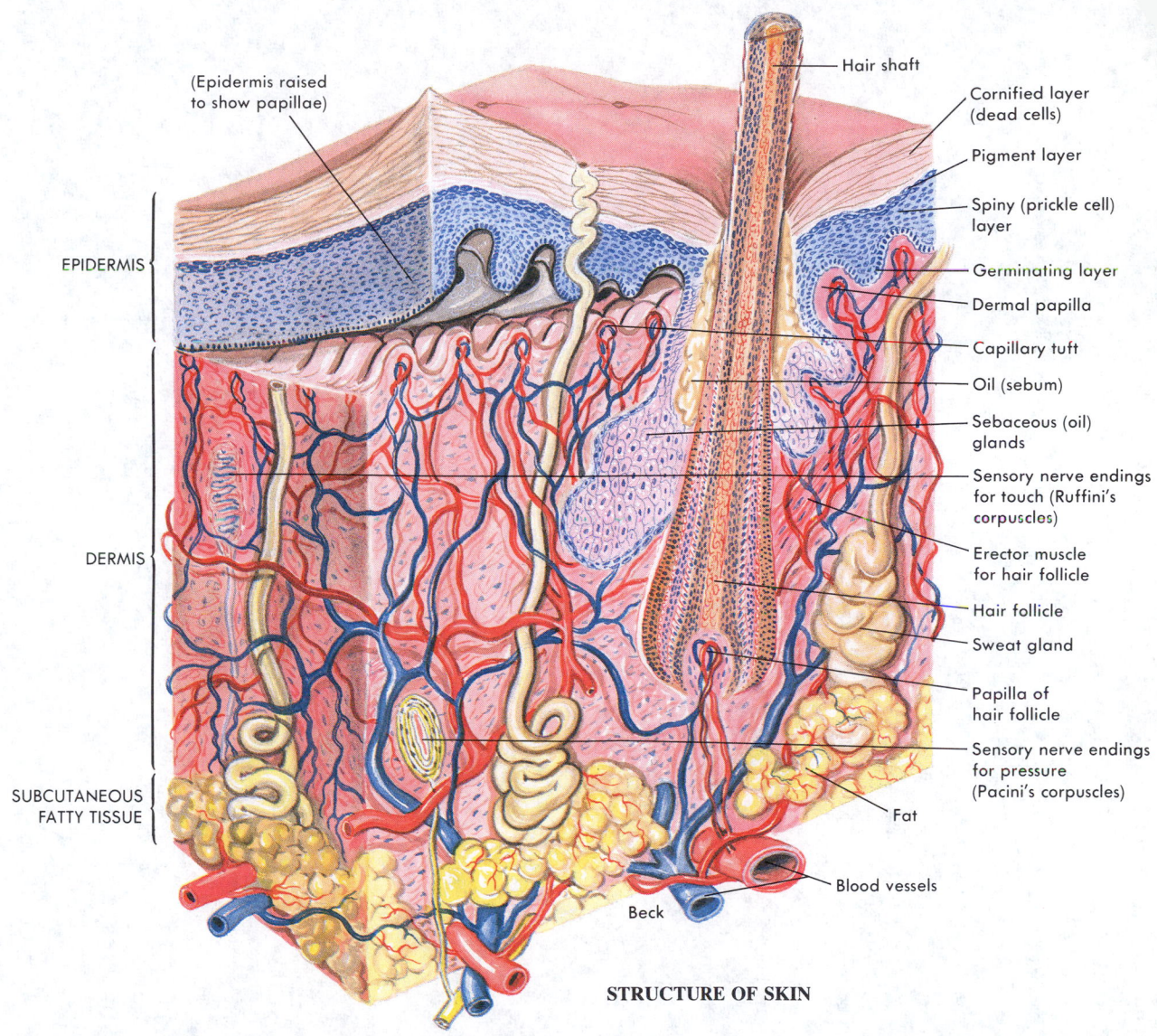

(Epidermis raised to show papillae)

EPIDERMIS

DERMIS

SUBCUTANEOUS FATTY TISSUE

Hair shaft

Cornified layer (dead cells)

Pigment layer

Spiny (prickle cell) layer

Germinating layer

Dermal papilla

Capillary tuft

Oil (sebum)

Sebaceous (oil) glands

Sensory nerve endings for touch (Ruffini's corpuscles)

Erector muscle for hair follicle

Hair follicle

Sweat gland

Papilla of hair follicle

Sensory nerve endings for pressure (Pacini's corpuscles)

Fat

Blood vessels

Beck

STRUCTURE OF SKIN

a, symbol for **arterial blood.**

A, **1.** abbreviation for **accommodation. 2.** symbol for alveolar gas. **3.** abbreviation for **ampere. 4.** abbreviation for **anterior. 5.** abbreviation for **atomic weight. 6.** abbreviation for **axial. 7.** symbol for **mass number.**

A68, symbol for a protein found in the brain tissue of Alzheimer's disease patients. It is also found in the developing normal brains of fetuses and infants but begins to disappear by the age of 2 years.

Å, symbol for **angstrom.**

a-, a prefix meaning 'without, not, lack of': *abacterial, abasia, anemia.*

AA, **1.** abbreviation for **achievement age. 2.** abbreviation for **Alcoholics Anonymous. 3.** abbreviation for **amplitude of accommodation. 4.** abbreviation for **anesthesiologist's assistant.**

āa, āā, ĀĀ, (in prescriptions) abbreviation for *ana,* indicating an equal amount of each ingredient to be compounded.

AAAI, abbreviation for **American Academy of Allergy and Immunology.**

AACN, **1.** abbreviation for **American Association of Colleges of Nursing. 2.** abbreviation for **American Association of Critical Care Nurses.**

AAFP, abbreviation for *American Academy of Family Practice.*

AAGP, abbreviation for *American Academy of General Practice.* Now called *American Academy of Family Practice.*

AAIN, abbreviation for **American Association of Industrial Nurses.**

AAMC, abbreviation for **American Association of Medical Colleges.**

AAMI, abbreviation for **Association for the Advancement of Medical Instrumentation.**

AAN, abbreviation for **American Academy of Nursing.**

AANA, abbreviation for **American Association of Nurse Anesthetists.**

AANN, **1.** abbreviation for **American Association of Neuroscience Nurses. 2.** abbreviation for **American Association of Neurological Nurses.**

AANNT, abbreviation for **American Association of Nephrology Nurses and Technicians.**

AAOHN, abbreviation for *American Association of Occupational Health Nurses.*

AAOMS, abbreviation for *American Association of Oral and Maxillofacial Surgeons.*

AAPA, abbreviation for **American Academy of Physicians' Assistants.**

AAPB, abbreviation for **American Association of Pathologists and Bacteriologists.**

AAPMR, abbreviation for **American Academy of Physical Medicine and Rehabilitation.**

AARP, abbreviation for *American Association of Retired Persons.*

AART, abbreviation for *American Association for Respiratory Therapy.*

AAUP, abbreviation for **American Association of University Professors.**

AAV, abbreviation for **adenoassociated virus.**

Ab, abbreviation for **antibody.**

ab-, abs-, a prefix meaning 'from, off, away from': *abstract, abduction.*

abacterial /ab′aktir′ē·əl/, any atmosphere or condition free of bacteria; literally, without bacteria.

abaissement /ä′bāsmäN′ [Fr, a lowering]/, a falling or depressing; in ophthalmology, the displacement of a lens.

abalienation /abāl′yənā′shən/, **1.** a state of physical deterioration or mental decay. **2.** a state of insanity. **—abalienate,** *v.,* **abalienated,** *adj.*

A band, the area between two I bands of a sarcomere, marked by partial overlapping of actin and myosin filaments.

abandonment of care /əban′dənment/, (in law) wrongful cessation of the provision of care to a patient, usually by a physician.

abarticular /ab′ärtik′yo͞olər/, **1.** of or pertaining to a condition that does not affect a joint. **2.** of or pertaining to a site or structure remote from a joint.

abarticulation /ab′ärtik′yəlā′shən/, **1.** dislocation of a joint. **2.** a synovial joint.

abasia /əbā′zhə/ [Gk, *a, basis,* not step], the inability to walk, caused by lack of motor coordination. **—abasic, abatic,** *adj.*

abasia-astasia. See **astasia-abasia.**

abate /əbāt′/ [ME, *abaten,* to beat down], to decrease or reduce in severity or degree.

abaxial /abak′sē·əl/ [L, *ab, axis* from axle], **1.** of or pertaining to a position outside the axis of a body or structure. **2.** of or pertaining to a position at the opposite extremity of a structure.

-abatic. See **abasia.**

Abbé-Estlander operation /ab′ē·est′/ [Robert Abbé, American surgeon, b. 1851; Jakob A. Estlander, Finnish surgeon, b. 1831], a surgical procedure that transfers a full-thickness section of one oral lip to the other lip, using an arterial pedicle for ensuring survival of a graft.

Abbé-Zeiss apparatus /äbā′tsīs′/, [Abbé; Carl Zeiss, German optician, b. 1816], an apparatus for calculating the number of blood cells in a measured amount of blood. See also **hemocytometer.**

Abbokinase, a trademark for a plasminogen activator (urokinase).

Abbott pump /ab′ət/, a small portable pump that can be adjusted and finely calibrated to deliver precise amounts of medication in solution through an intravenous infusion set.

1

It is similar to a Harvard pump, but the flow rate may be increased or decreased by smaller increments.

ABC, abbreviation for **aspiration biopsy cytology.**

abdomen /ab'dəmən, abdō'mən/ [L, belly], the portion of the body between the thorax and the pelvis. The abdominal cavity contains the lower portion of the esophagus, the stomach, the intestines, the liver, the spleen, the pancreas, and other visceral organs. The walls of the abdominal cavity are lined with the parietal layer of the peritoneum, a serous membrane. The covering, or outermost layer of each organ, is formed by the visceral layer of the peritoneum. A small amount of serous fluid in the space between the membranous layers allows the organs to slide freely, as in the normal process of digestion, evacuation, and breathing. Also called (*informal*) **belly.** See also **abdominal regions. –abdominal** /abdom'-/, *adj.*

abdominal actinomycosis. See **actinomycosis.**

abdominal adhesion, the binding together of tissue surfaces of abdominal organs, usually involving the intestines and causing obstruction. The condition may be the result of trauma or inflammation and may form after abdominal surgery. The patient experiences pain, nausea, vomiting, and increased pulse rate. Surgery may be required.

abdominal aorta, the portion of the descending aorta that passes from the aortic hiatus of the diaphragm into the abdomen, descending ventral to the vertebral column, and ending at the fourth lumbar vertebra, where it divides into the two common iliac arteries. It supplies many different parts of the body, such as the testes, ovaries, kidneys, and stomach. Its branches are the celiac, superior mesenteric, inferior mesenteric, middle suprarenal, renal, testicular, ovarian, inferior phrenic, lumbar, middle sacral, and common iliac arteries. See also **descending aorta.** Compare **thoracic aorta.**

abdominal aortography, the process of producing a radiograph of the abdominal aorta using a radiopaque contrast medium.

abdominal aponeurosis, the conjoined tendons of the oblique and transverse muscles of the abdomen.

abdominal bandage, a broad supportive bandage commonly used after abdominal surgery.

abdominal binder, a bandage or elasticized wrap that is applied around the lower part of the torso to support the abdomen. An abdominal binder is sometimes applied after abdominal surgery to decrease discomfort, thereby increasing a patient's ability to begin ambulatory activities and accelerate convalescence. A kind of abdominal binder is the **scultetus binder.**

abdominal breathing, breathing in which the majority of ventilatory work is done by the diaphragm and abdominal muscles. It is sometimes used to treat respiratory deficiencies; the patient is trained to strengthen the contractile force of the abdominal wall muscles so as to elevate the diaphragm and empty the lungs. The patient places a hand on the epigastrium during training to focus attention on that portion of the body.

abdominal cavity, the space within the abdominal walls between the diaphragm and the pelvic area, containing the liver, stomach, intestines, spleen, kidneys, and associated tissues and vessels.

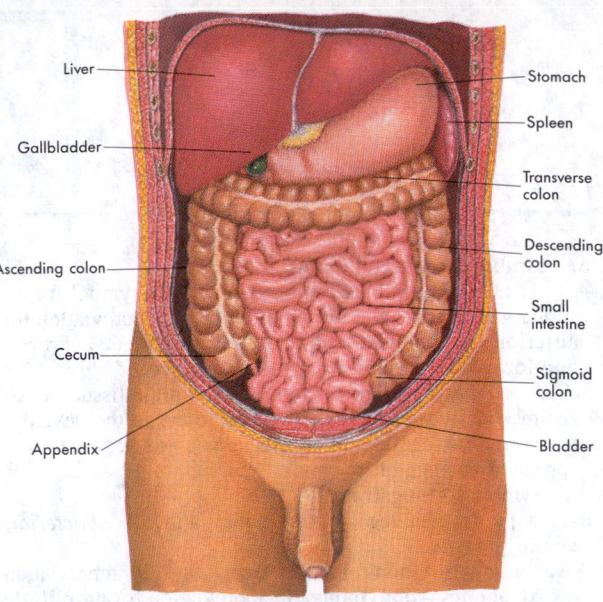

Abdominal cavity (Seidel, 1991)

abdominal delivery, the delivery of a child through a surgical incision in the abdomen. See **cesarean section.**

abdominal fistula, an abnormal passage from an abdominal organ to the surface of the abdomen. In a colostomy, a passage from the bowel to an opening on the surface of the abdomen is created surgically.

abdominal gestation, the implantation of a fertilized ovum outside the uterus but within the peritoneal cavity. See also **ectopic pregnancy.**

abdominalgia /abdom'ənal'jə/, [L, *abdomen*, belly; Gk, *algos*, pain], a pain in the abdomen.

abdominal girth, the circumference of the abdomen, usually measured at the umbilicus.

abdominal hernia, a hernia in which a loop of bowel protrudes through the abdominal musculature, often through the site of an old surgical scar which has stretched and thinned. Also called **ventral hernia.** See also **hernia.**

abdominal hysterectomy, the excision of the uterus through the abdominal wall. Also called **abdominohysterectomy.**

abdominal nephrectomy [L, *abdominis*, belly; Gk, *nephr*, kidney, *ektome*, cutting out], the surgical removal of a kidney through an incision into the abdomen.

abdominal pain, acute or chronic localized or diffuse pain in the abdominal cavity. Abdominal pain is a significant symptom because its cause may require immediate surgical or medical intervention. The most common causes of severe abdominal pain are inflammation, perforation of an intraabdominal structure, circulatory obstruction, intestinal or ureteral obstruction, or rupture of an organ located within the abdomen. Specific conditions include appendicitis, perforated gastric ulcer, strangulated hernia, superior mesenteric arterial thrombosis, and small and large bowel obstruction. The differential diagnosis of the cause of acute abdominal pain requires localization and characterization of the pain by means of light and deep percussion, auscultation and palpation and by abdominal, rectal, or pelvic examination. Direct physical examination may be supplemented by various laboratory and radiologic examinations. Aspiration of peritoneal fluid for bacteriologic and chemical evaluation is sometimes indicated. Conditions producing acute abdominal pain that may require surgery include appendicitis, acute or severe and chronic diverticulitis, acute and chronic cholecystitis, cholelithiasis, acute pancreatitis, perforation of a peptic ulcer, various intestinal obstructions, abdominal aortic aneurysms, and trauma affecting any of the abdominal organs. Gynecologic causes of acute abdominal pain that may require surgery include acute pelvic inflammatory disease, ruptured ovarian cyst, and ectopic pregnancy. Abdominal pain associated with pregnancy may be caused by the weight of the enlarged uterus; rotation, stretching, or compression of the round ligament; or squeezing or displacement of the bowel. In addition, uterine contractions associated with premature labor may produce severe abdominal pain. Chronic abdominal pain may be functional or the result of overeating or aerophagia. When the symptoms are recurrent, an organic cause is considered. Organic sources of abdominal pain include peptic ulcer, hiatus hernia, gastritis, chronic cholecystitis and cholelithiasis, chronic pancreatitis, pancreatic carcinoma, chronic diverticulitis, intermittent low-grade intestinal obstruction, and functional indigestion. Some systemic conditions may be responsible for abdominal pain. Examples include systemic lupus erythematosus, lead poisoning, hypercalcemia, sickle cell anemia, diabetic acidosis, porphyria, tabes dorsalis, and black widow spider poisoning.

abdominal paracentesis [L, *abdominis,* belly; Gk, *para,* near, *kentesis,* puncturing], the surgical puncturing of the abdominal cavity in order to remove fluid for diagnosis or treatment.

abdominal pregnancy, an extrauterine pregnancy in which the conceptus develops in the abdominal cavity after being extruded from the fimbriated end of the fallopian tube or through a defect in the tube or uterus. The placenta may implant on the abdominal or visceral peritoneum. Abdominal pregnancy may be suspected when the abdomen has enlarged but the uterus has remained small for the length of gestation. Abdominal pregnancies constitute approximately 2% of ectopic pregnancies and approximately 0.01% of all pregnancies. The condition results in perinatal death of the fetus in most cases, maternal death in approximately 6%. Because of its rarity, the condition may be unsuspected, and diagnosis is often delayed. Ultrasound or x-ray visualization showing gas in the maternal bowel below the fetus is diagnostic of the condition. Surgical removal of the placenta, sac, and embryo or fetus is necessary, but the procedure is often complicated by massive bleeding, and, because the placenta tends to adhere firmly to the peritoneum and to the bowel, complete removal is seldom possible. Postoperative sequelae may include necrotization of retained placental tissue, infection, continued bleeding, and sterility.

abdominal pulse, the pulse of the abdominal aorta.

abdominal quadrant, any of four topographic areas of the abdomen divided by two imaginary vertical and horizontal lines intersecting at the umbilicus. The divisions are the left upper quadrant (LUQ), the left lower quadrant (LLQ), the right upper quadrant (RUQ), and the right lower quadrant (RLQ).

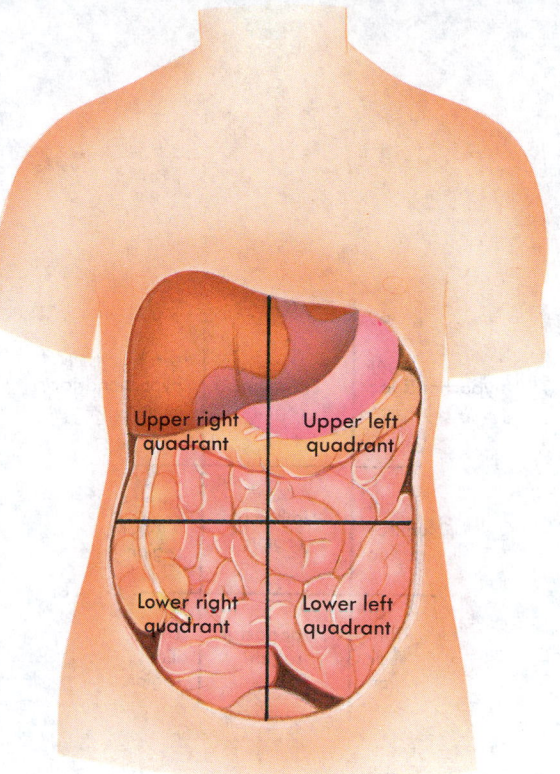

Abdominal quadrants (Seeley, 1992/Nadine Sokol)

abdominal reflex, a superficial neurologic reflex obtained by firmly stroking the skin of the abdomen, normally resulting in a brisk contraction of abdominal muscles in which the umbilicus moves toward the site of the stimulus. This reflex is lost in diseases of the pyramidal tract. See also **superficial reflex.**

abdominal regions, the nine topographic subdivisions of the abdomen, determined by four imaginary lines, in a tic-tac-toe pattern, imposed over the anterior surface. The upper horizontal line passes along the level of the cartilages of the nine ribs; the lower along the iliac crests. The two vertical lines extend on each side of the body from the cartilage of the eighth rib to the center of the inguinal ligament. The lines, which are drawn straight or curved in an alternate formation, divide the abdomen into three upper, three middle, and three lower zones: right hypochondriac, epigastric, and left hypochondriac regions (upper zones); right lateral, umbilical, and left lateral regions (middle zones); right inguinal, pubic, and left inguinal regions (lower zones). (See Fig. p. 4.)

abdominal splinting, a rigid contraction of the muscles of the abdominal wall. It usually occurs as an involuntary reaction to the pain of a visceral disease or disorder or postoperative discomfort. Abdominal splinting, in turn, may result in hypoventilation and respiratory complications.

abdominal sponge [L, *abdomen,* belly; Gk, *spongia,* sponge], a thin flat surgical sponge used as packing, absorbent, and covering for the viscera. See also **sponge.**

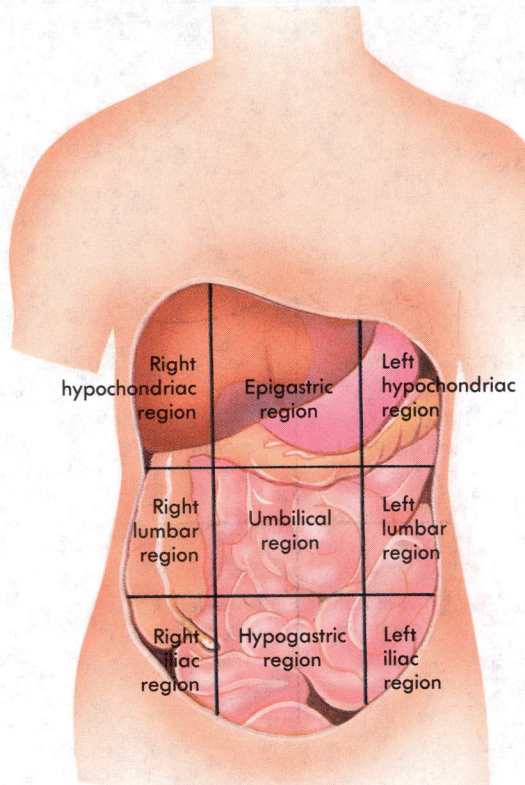

Abdominal regions *(Seeley, 1992/Nadine Sokol)*

abdominal surgery,   any operation that involves an incision into the abdomen. Before surgery a complete blood count and a urinalysis are done. An enema may be given. The skin is shaved and cleansed from the nipple line to the pubis. Food and fluids by mouth are withheld for 8 hours prior to surgery. Postoperatively, the nurse ensures that the airway is open, checks tubes and catheters, connects drainage tubes to collection containers, and checks the dressing for excessive bleeding or drainage. Close observation of vital signs is essential. A careful record is kept of fluid intake and output. The patient is turned and is helped to cough and breathe deeply every hour. Medication is given as needed for relief from pain. Some kinds of abdominal surgery are **appendectomy, cholecystectomy, colostomy, gastrectomy, herniorrhaphy,** and **laparotomy.** See also **acute abdomen, laparotomy.**

abdominal tenaculum.   See **tenaculum.**

abdomino- /abdom′inō-/,   a combining form meaning 'pertaining to the abdomen': *abdominocentesis, abdominoscopy, abdominothoracic.*

abdominocentesis.   See **paracentesis.**

abdominocyesis /abdom′inōsī·ē′sis/,   an abdominal pregnancy.

abdominohysterectomy.   See **abdominal hysterectomy.**

abdominohysterotomy   /-his′tərot′əmē/,   hysterotomy through an abdominal incision. See **hysterotomy.**

abdominopelvic cavity /-pel′vik/,   the space between the diaphragm and the groin. There is no structurally distinct separation between the abdomen and pelvic regions.

abdominoperineal /-per′inē′əl/,   pertaining to the abdomen and the perineum, including the pelvic area, female vulva and anus and the male anus and scrotum.

abdominoplasty /abdom′ənōplas′tē/,   plastic surgery involving the abdominal tissues.

abdominoscopy /abdom′inos′kəpē/ [L, *abdomen;* Gk, *skopein,* to view],   a procedure for examining the contents of the peritoneum in which an electrically illuminated tubular device is passed through a trocar into the abdominal cavity. Also called **peritomeoscopy.** See also **endoscopy, laparoscopy.**

abducens /abdo͞o′sənz/ [L, drawing away],   pertaining to a movement away from the median line of the body.

abducens muscle,   the extraocular lateral rectus muscle that moves the eyeball outward.

abducens nerve [L, *abducere,* to take away],   the sixth cranial nerve. It arises in the pons, near the fourth ventricle, leaves the brainstem between the medulla oblongata and pons, and passes through the cavernous sinus and the superior orbital fissure. It controls the lateral rectus muscle, turning the eye outward. Also called **abducent nerve, nervus abducens.**

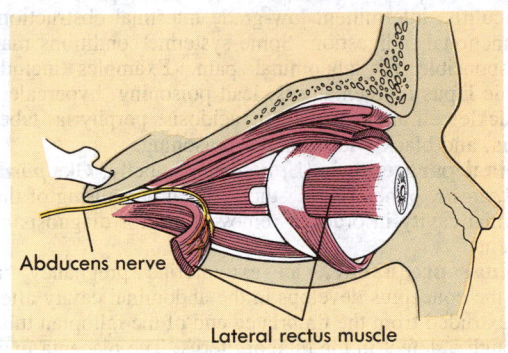

Abducens nerve *(Seeley, 1992/Michael Schenk)*

abduct /abdukt′/,   to move away from the median plane of the body.

abduction [L, *abducere,* to take away],   movement of a limb away from the body. Compare **adduction.**

abduction boots,   a pair of orthopedic casts for the lower extremities, available in both short-leg and long-leg configurations, with a bar incorporated at ankle level to provide hip abduction. Abduction boots are used for postoperative positioning and immobilization after hip adductor releases and to promote proper positioning during healing after surgery to repair structures in the lower extremities.

abductor /abduk′tər/ [L, *abducere*],   a muscle that draws a body part away from the midline, or one part from another. Compare **adductor.**

Abernethy's sarcoma. /ab′ərnē′thēz/,   a malignant neoplasm of fat cells, usually occurring on the trunk.

aberrancy.   See **aberrant ventricular conduction.**

aberrant /aber′ənt/ [L, *aberrare,* to wander],   **1.** of or pertaining to a wandering from the usual or expected course, such as various ducts, nerves, and vessels in the body. **2.** (in botany and zoology) of or pertaining to an abnormal individual, such as certain atypical members of a species.

aberrant goiter, an enlargement of a supernumerary or ectopic thyroid gland.

aberrant ventricular conduction (AVC), the temporary abnormal intraventricular conduction of a supraventricular impulse, usually associated with a change in cycle length. This conduction pattern is fairly common after a very premature impulse with the QRS complex most often conducted with a right bundle branch block. Also called **aberrancy, ventricular aberration.**

aberration /ab′ərā′shən/ [L, *aberrare*, to wander], **1.** any departure from the usual course or normal condition. **2.** abnormal growth or development. **3.** (in psychology) an illogical and unreasonable thought or belief, often leading to an unsound mental state. **4.** (in genetics) any change in the number or structure of the chromosomes. See also **chromosomal aberration. 5.** (in optics) any imperfect image formation caused by unequal refraction or focalization of light rays through a lens.

abetalipoproteinemia /əbā′təlip′ōprō′tinē′mē·ə/ [Gk, *a, beta,* not beta, *lipos,* fat, *proteios,* first rank, *haima,* blood], a rare inherited disorder of fat metabolism, characterized by acanthocytosis, low or absent serum betalipoproteins, and hypocholesterolemia. In severe cases steatorrhea, ataxia, nystagmus, motor incoordination, and retinitis pigmentosa occur. Also called **Bassen-Kornzweig syndrome** /-kôrn′zwīg/.

ABG, abbreviation for **arterial blood gas.**

abient /ab′ē·ənt/ [L, *abire,* to go away], characterized by a tendency to move away from stimuli. Compare **adient. –abience,** *n.*

ability /əbil′itē/, the capacity to act in a specified way because of the possession of appropriate skills and mental or physical fitness.

abiogenesis /ab′ē·ōjen′əsis/ [Gk, *a, bios,* not life, *genein,* to produce], spontaneous generation; the theory that organic life can originate from inanimate matter. Compare **biogenesis. –abiogenetic,** *adj.*

abiosis /ab′ē·ō′sis/ [Gk, *a, bios* not life], a nonviable condition or a situation that is incompatible with life. **–abiotic,** *adj.*

abiotrophy /ab′ē·ot′rəfē/ [Gk, *a, bios* + *trophe* nutrition], a premature depletion of vitality or the deterioration of certain cells and tissues, especially those involved in genetic degenerative diseases. **–abiotrophic** /ab′ē·ətrō′fik/, *adj.*

ablate ablāt′ [L, *ab, latus,* caried away], to cut away or remove.

ablation /ablā′shən/ [L, *ab, latus,* carried away], an amputation, an excision of any part of the body, or a removal of a growth or harmful substance.

ablatio placentae. See **abruptio placentae.**

-able, -ible, a suffix indicating ability or capacity: *intractable, flexible.*

ablepsia /əblep′sē·ə/ [Gk, *a, blepein,* not to see], the condition of being blind. Also called **ablepsy.**

ABMS, abbreviation for *American Board of Medical Specialties.*

abnerval current /abnur′vəl/ [L, *ab,* from; Gk, *neuron,* nerve], an electric current that passes from a nerve to and through muscle.

abnormal behavior /abnôr′məl/ [L, *ab, norma,* away from rule], maladaptive acts or activities detrimental to the individual or to society. The acts range from the brief inability to cope with a stressful situation to persistent bizarre or destructive behavior or total disorientation and withdrawal from the realities of everyday life. See also **behavior disorder.**

abnormality /ab′nôrmal′itē/ [L, *ab,* away from; *norma,* the rule], a condition that differs from the usual physical or mental state.

abnormal psychology, the study of mental disorders and maladaptive behavior and of normal phenomena that are not completely understood, such as dreams and altered states of consciousness.

ABO blood groups, A system for classifying human blood based on the antigenic components of red blood cells and their corresponding antibodies. The ABO blood group is identified by the presence or absence of two different antigens, A and B, on the surface of the red blood cell. The four blood types in this grouping, A, B, AB, and O, are determined by and named for these antigens. Type AB indicates the presence of both antigens; type O the absence of both. Corresponding antibodies, anti-A and anti-B agglutinins, can be found in the plasma of type O blood. The plasma components of type A and type B blood are, respectively, devoid of anti-A and anti-B agglutinins; both agglutinins are absent from type AB blood plasma. In addition to its significant role in transfusion therapy and transplantation, the ABO blood grouping contributes to forensic medicine, to genetics, and, together with the less important blood groups, to anthropology and legal medicine. See also **blood group, Rh factor, transfusion.**

aboiement /ä′bô·ämäN′/, an involuntary making of abnormal, animal-like sounds, such as barking. Aboiement may be a clinical sign of Gilles de la Tourette's syndrome.

abort /əbôrt′/ [L, *ab,* away from, *oriri,* to be born], **1.** to deliver a nonviable fetus; to miscarry. See also **spontaneous abortion. 2.** to terminate a pregnancy before the fetus has developed enough to live ex utero. See also **induced abortion. 3.** to terminate in the early stages or to discontinue before completion, as to arrest the usual course of a disease, to stop growth and development, or to halt a project.

aborted systole, a contraction of the heart that is usually weak and is not associated with a radial pulse.

abortifacient /əbôr′tifā′shənt/, **1.** producing abortion. **2.** an agent that causes abortion.

abortion /əbor′shən/ [L, *ab* + *oriri*], the spontaneous or induced termination of pregnancy before the fetus has developed to the stage of viability. Kinds of abortion include **habitual abortion, infected abortion, septic abortion, threatened abortion,** and **voluntary abortion.** See also **complete abortion, criminal abortion, elective abortion, incomplete abortion, induced abortion, medical abortion, missed abortion, spontaneous abortion, therapeutic abortion.**

abortion on demand, a concept promoted by prochoice health advocates that it is the right of a pregnant woman to have an abortion performed at her request. That right may be limited by time of gestation, or it may pertain to any period of gestation.

abortive infection /əbôr′tiv/, an infection in which some or all viral components have been synthesized, but no infective virus is produced. The situation may result from an infection with defective viruses or because the host cell is nonpermissive and prohibits replication of the particular virus.

abortus /əbôr′təs/, any incompletely developed fetus that results from an abortion, particularly one weighing less than 500 g.

abortus fever, a form of brucellosis, the only one .UL ONendemic to North America. It is caused by *Brucella abortus,* an organism so named because it causes abortion in cows. Infection in humans results from the ingestion of contaminated milk from cows infected with *B. abortus,* from handling infected meat, or from skin contact with the excreta of living infected animals. Streptomycin and tetracycline are usually prescribed together as treatment. Also called **Rio Grande fever.** See also **brucellosis.**

abouchementä′bo͞oshmäN′/ [Fr, a tube connection], the junction of a small blood vessel with a large blood vessel.

aboulia. See **abulia.**

ABP, abbreviation for **arterial blood pressure.**

ABPM, abbreviation for **ambulatory blood pressure monitoring**.

abrachia /əbrā′kē·ə/ [Gk, *a, brachion* not arm], the absence of arms. **−abrachial,** *adj.*

abrade /əbrād′/ to remove the epidermis or other skin layers, usually by scraping or rubbing.

abrasion /əbrā′zhən/ [L, *abradere,* to scrape off], a scraping, or rubbing away of a surface of skin by friction. Abrasion may be the result of trauma, such as a skinned knee; of therapy, as in dermabrasion of the skin for removal of scar tissue; or of normal function, such as the wearing down of a tooth by mastication. Compare **laceration.** See also **bruxism, friction burn. −abrade,** *v.,* **abrasive,** *adj.*

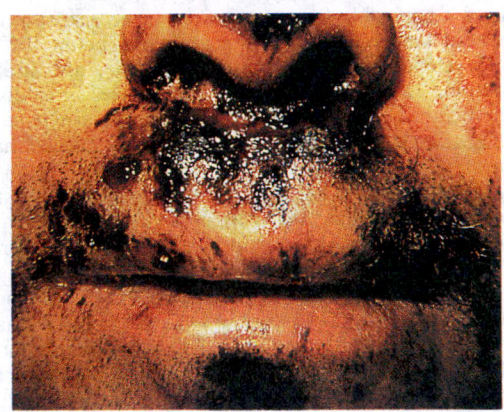

Abrasions of the nose and lips *(Grossman, 1993)*

abreaction /ab′rē·ak′shən/ [L, *ab,* from, *re,* again, *agere,* to act], an emotional release resulting from mentally reliving or from bringing into consciousness, through the process of catharsis, a long-repressed, painful experience. See also **catharsis.**

abrosia /əbrō′zhə/ [Gk, fasting], a condition caused by fasting or abstaining from food. See also **anoxia.**

abruptio placentae [L, *ab,* away from, *rumpere,* to rupture], separation of the placenta implanted in normal position in a pregnancy of 20 weeks or more or during labor before delivery of the fetus. It occurs approximately once in 200 births, and, because it often results in severe hemorrhage, it is a significant cause of maternal and fetal mor-

tality. Hypertension and preeclampsia are associated with increased rates of occurrence, but in many cases there is no explanation. Complete separation brings about immediate death of the fetus. Bleeding from the site of separation causes abdominal pain, uterine tenderness, and tetanic uterine contraction. Bleeding may be concealed within the uterus or may be evident externally, sometimes as sudden massive hemorrhage. In severe cases, shock and death can come in minutes. Cesarean section must be performed immediately and rapidly. Extensive extravasation of blood within the wall of the uterus may deplete fibrinogen, prolong clotting time, bring about intractable bleeding, lead to DIC, and, by damaging the musculature of the uterus, prevent the uterus from contracting well after delivery. Hysterectomy may be necessary to prevent exsanguination. Partial separation may cause little bleeding and may not interfere with fetal oxygenation. If the pregnancy is near term, labor may be permitted or induced by amniotomy. A premature pregnancy may be allowed to continue under close observation of the mother at bed rest. The nurse must be alert to the possibility that bleeding is present but concealed internally and that if all the blood can escape, there may be little pain. Also called **ablatio placentae, accidental hemorrhage.** Compare **placenta previa.** See also **Couvelaire uterus.**

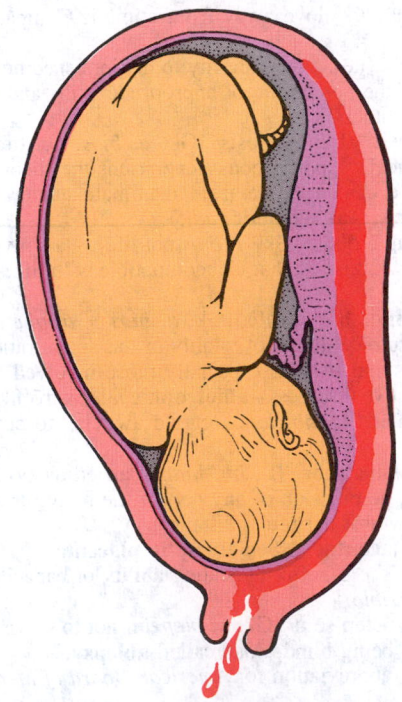

Abruptio placentae *(Thibodeau, 1993/Marcia Williams)*

abscess /ab′səs/ [L, *abscedere,* to go away], **1.** a cavity containing pus and surrounded by inflamed tissue, formed as a result of suppuration in a localized infection (characteristically, a staphylococcal infection). Healing usually occurs when an abscess drains or is incised. If an abscess is deep in tissue, drainage is made by means of a sinus tract that connects it to the surface. In a sterile abscess, the contents are not the result of pyogenic bacteria. **2. dental abscess,** an abscess that develops anywhere along the root length of a tooth. It is usually characterized by pain due to the pressure of pus against the nerve tissue, redness because of blood accumulation, and swelling due to the suppuration.

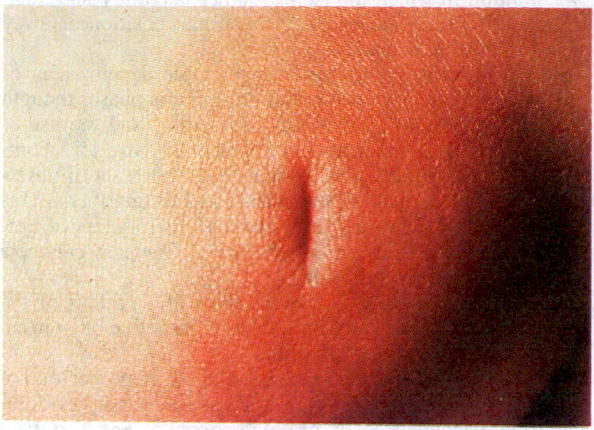

Breast abscess (Zitelli, 1992)

abscess of liver [L, *abscedere,* to go away; AS, *lifer*], an abscess in the liver cells, usually caused by an amebic infection, bacterial infections, or trauma, characteriazed by sweats and chills, pain, nausea and vomiting.

abscissa /absis′ə/ [L, *ab,* away; *scindere,* to cut], a point on a horizontal Cartesian coordinate plane measured from the y-axis running perpendicular to the plane.

absence seizure, an epileptic seizure characterized by a sudden, momentary loss of consciousness occasionally accompanied by minor myoclonus of the neck or upper extremities, slight symmetric twitching of the face, or a loss of muscle tone. The seizures usually occur many times a day without a warning aura and are most frequent in children and adolescents, especially at the time of puberty. The patient experiencing a typical seizure has a vacant facial expression and ceases all voluntary motor activity; with the rapid return of consciousness, the patient may resume conversation at the point of interruption without realizing what occurred. During and between seizures, the patient's electroencephalogram shows three cycle-per-second spike and wave discharges. Anticonvulsant drugs used to prevent absence seizures include ethosuximide and valproic acid. Also called **petit mal seizure.** See also **epilepsy.**

absenteeism /ab′səntē′izəm/, (for health or related reasons) absence from work. Absenteeism varies according to job assignments, with professional and managerial personnel taking an average annual sick leave of 4 days while unskilled workers claim an average of 18 days sick leave during the year. Surveys also indicate that fewer than 10% of workers account for nearly 50% of all absenteeism. The most common causes of absenteeism include influenza and occupationally related skin diseases.

absentia epileptica /absen′shə/ [L, *absens,* not present; Gk, *epilepsia,* seizure], a brief loss of consciousness. It usually occurs without convulsions but may be accompanied

by minor involuntary muscle contractions. Formerly called **petit mal seizures.**

absent without leave (AWOL) /ā′wôl/ [L, *absentia*], describing a patient who leaves a psychiatric facility without authorization.

absolute agraphia [L, *absolutus,* set loose; Gk, *a,* not, *graphein,* to write], a complete inability to write caused by a central nervous system lesion. The person is unable to write even the letters of the alphabet. See also **agraphia.**

absolute alcohol. See **dehydrated alcohol.**

absolute cephalopelvic disproportion. See **cephalopelvic disproportion.**

absolute discharge /ab′səloot/ [L, *absolutus,* set free], a final and complete termination of the patient's relationship with a care-giving agency.

absolute growth, the total increase in size of an organism or a particular organ or part, such as the limbs, head, or trunk.

absolute humidity, the actual weight or content of water in a measured volume of air. It is usually expressed in grams per cubic meter or pounds per cubic foot or cubic yard.

absolute refractory period. See **refractory period.**

absolute temperature, temperature that is measured from a base of absolute zero on the Kelvin scale or the Rankine scale.

absolute threshold, [L, *absolutus,* set loose; AS, *therscold*], the lowest point at which a stimulus can be perceived.

absolute zero, the temperature at which all molecular activity ceases. It is a theoretical value derived by calculations and projections from experiments with the behavior of gases at extremely low temperatures. On the Kelvin scale, absolute zero is estimated to be equal to −273° C. On the Rankine scale, the equivalent temperature is calculated at −460° F.

absolutum glaucoma /ab′səloo′təm/ [L, *abolutus;* Gk, *cataract*], complete blindness in which vision is permanently lost and intraocular pressure is increased. The optic disc is white and deeply excavated, and the pupil is usually widely dilated and immobile. Also called **glaucoma consummatum.**

absorb /absôrb′, əbzôrb′/ [L, *absorbere,* to swallow], **1.** the act of drinking in, wholly engulfing, assimilating, or taking up various substances; for example, the tissues of the intestines absorb fluids. **2.** the energy transferred to tissues by radiation, such as an absorbed dose of radioactivity.

absorbable gauze /əbsôr′bəbəl/, a gauzelike material, produced from oxidized cellulose, that can be absorbed. It is applied directly to bleeding tissue for hemostasis.

absorbable surgical suture, [L, *absorbere,* to suck up; Gk, *cheirourgos,* surgery; L, *sutura*], a suture made from material that can be completely removed by the body's phagocytes.

absorbance /əbsôr′bəns/, the degree of absorption of light or other radiant energy by a medium through which the radiant energy passes. It is expressed as the logarithm of the ratio of energy transmitted through a pure solvent to the intensity of energy transmitted through the medium. Absorbance varies with such factors as wavelength, the solution, concentration, and path length.

absorbed dose, (in radiotherapy) the energy imparted by ionizing radiation per unit mass of irradiated material at the place of interest. The SI unit of absorbed dose is the gray, which is 1 joule/kg and equals 100 rad.

absorbent /absôr′bənt/ [L, *absorbere,* to suck up], **1.** capable of attracting and absorbing substances into itself. **2.** a product or substance that can absorb liquids or gases.

absorbent dressing, a dressing of any material applied to a wound or incision to absorb secretions.

absorbent gauze, a gauze for absorbing fluids. The form, weight, and use vary. Gauze may be a fine fabric in rolled single layers for spiral bandages, or it may be a thick, many-layered pad for a sterile pressure dressing.

absorbifacient /absôr′bifā′shənt/ [L, *absorbere* + *facere,* to make], **1.** any agent that promotes or enhances absorption. **2.** causing or enhancing absorption.

absorption /absôrp′shən/ [L, *absorbere*], **1.** the incorporation of matter by other matter through chemical, molecular, or physical action, such as the dissolving of a gas in a liquid or the taking up of a liquid by a porous solid. **2.** (in physiology) the passage of substances across and into tissues, such as the passage of digested food molecules into intestinal cells or the passage of liquids into kidney tubules. Kinds of absorption are **agglutinin absorption, cutaneous absorption, external absorption, intestinal absorption, parenteral absorption,** and **pathologic absorption. 3.** (in radiology) the process of absorbing radiant energy by living or nonliving matter with which the radiation intereacts.

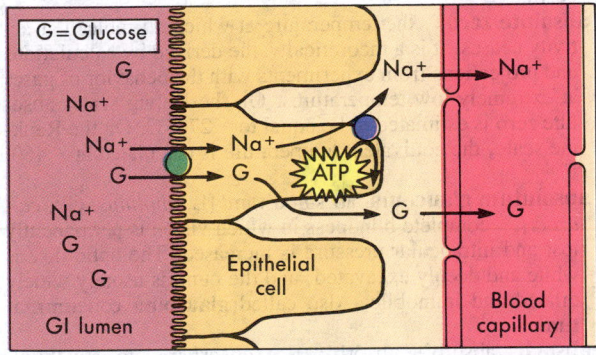

Absorption of sodium, glucose, and amino acids
(Thibodeau, 1993/Rolin Graphics)

absorption coefficient, (in radiology) the fractional loss in intensity of electromagnetic energy as it interacts with an absorbing material. It is usually expressed per unit of thickness or per unit mass.

absorption rate constant, a value describing how much drug is absorbed per unit of time.

absorption spectrum, the range of electromagnetic energy that is used for spectroanalysis, including both visible light and ultraviolet radiation; also, a graph of spectrum for a specific compound.

absorptivity /ab′sôrptiv′itē/, absorbance divided by the product of the concentration of a substance and the sample path length.

abstinence /ab′stinəns/, voluntary avoidance of a substance or the performance of an act for which the person has an appetite.

abstinence syndrome [L, *abstinere,* to hold back; Gk, *syn,* together, *dromos,* course], the withdrawal symptoms experienced by a chemically dependent person who is suddenly deprived of a regular intake of alcohol or other drugs.

abstract /ab′strakt, abstrakt′/, a condensed summary of a scientific article, literary piece, or address.

abstraction /abstrak′shən/ [L, *abstrahere,* to drag away], a condition in which the teeth or other maxillary and mandibular structures are below their normal position or away from the occlusal plane.

abstract thinking, the final stage in the development of the cognitive thought processes. During this phase, thought is characterized by adaptability, flexibility, and the use of concepts and generalizations. Problem solving is accomplished by drawing logical conclusions from a set of observations, such as making hypotheses and testing them. This type of thinking appears from about 12 to 15 years of age, usually after some degree of education. Compare **concrete thinking, syncretic thinking.**

abulia /əboo′lyə/ [Gk, *a, boule,* not will], a loss of the ability or a reduced capacity to exhibit initiative or to make decisions. Also spelled **aboulia.**

abuse /əbyoos′/ [L, *abuti,* to waste], **1.** improper use of equipment, a substance, or a service, such as a drug or program, either intentionally or unintentionally. See also **drug abuse. 2.** to physically or verbally attack or injure. A kind of abuse is **child abuse.**

abuse of the elderly, physical, psychologic, or material abuse, as well as violation of the rights of safety, security, and adequate health care of older adults. The victim of such abuse is generally an older woman with physical or mental impairment who lives with an adult child or another relative. Abusers are often middle-aged women, related or unrelated caretakers, who are themselves under stress. Contributing factors may include economics, interpersonal conflicts, health, and dependency. Often the abused person denies that abusive acts occur, leading to a climate of helplessness and resignation to abuse. The condition is often corrected by placing the abused adult in a protected setting away from the family, by vacations that provide respite for the family and older adult, and by sharing of caretaking responsibilities among children.

abutment /əbut′mənt/ [Fr, *abouter* to place end to end], a tooth, root, or implant which serves to support and retention of a fixed or movable prosthesis.

abutment tooth, a tooth selected to support a prosthesis.

ABVD, an anticancer drug combination of doxorubicin, bleomycin, vinblastine, and dacarbazine.

Ac, symbol for the element **actinium.**

AC, 1. abbreviation for **alternating current. 2.** abbreviation for *accommodative convergence.* See **AC/A ratio.**

ac-. See **ad-.**

a.c., (in prescriptions) abbreviation for *ante cibum,* a Latin phrase meaning 'before meals.' The times of administration are commonly 7 AM, 11 AM, and 5 PM.

A-C, abbreviation for *alveolar-capillary.*

acacia gum, a dried, gummy exudate of the acacia tree *(Acacia senegal)* used as a suspending or emulsifying agent in medicines.

academic ladder /ak′ədem′ik/ [Gk, *akademeia,* school], the hierarchy of faculty appointments in a university through which a faculty member must advance from the rank of instructor to assistant professor, to associate professor, and, finally, to professor.

acalculia /a'kalkoo'lyə/ [Gk, *a*, not; L, *calculare*, to reckon], a type of aphasia characterized by the inability to solve simple mathematic calculations.

acampsia /əkamp'sē·ə/ [Gk, *a, kampsein*, not to bend], a condition in which a joint becomes rigid. See also **ankylosis.**

acantha /əkan'thə/ [Gk, *akantha*, thorn], a spine or a spinous projection. **–acanthoid,** *adj.*

acanthiomeatal line /əkan'thē·ō'mē·ā'təl/, a hypothetical line extending from the external auditory meatus to the acanthion. In dentistry, a full maxillary denture is constructed so that its occlusal plane is parallel with this line.

acanthion, a point at the center of the base of the anterior nasal spine.

acantho-, a combining form meaning 'thorny or spiny': *acanthesthesia, acanthoid, acantholysis.*

Acanthocheilonema perstans /akan'thōkī'lənē'mə/, a threadworm usually found in Africa. It commonly infects wild and domestic animals and occasionally invades the bloodstream of humans, causing a skin rash, muscle and joint pains, various neurologic disorders, and nodules in the subcutaneous tissues. The larvae are also found in the cerebrospinal fluid of affected patients.

acanthocyte /əkan'thəsīt'/ [Gk, *akantha + kytos*, cell], an abnormal red blood cell with spurlike projections. Large numbers are present in abetalipoproteinemia; fewer occur in cirrhosis and in certain malabsorption syndromes. Compare **burr cell.** See also **abetalipoproteinemia, acanthocytosis.**

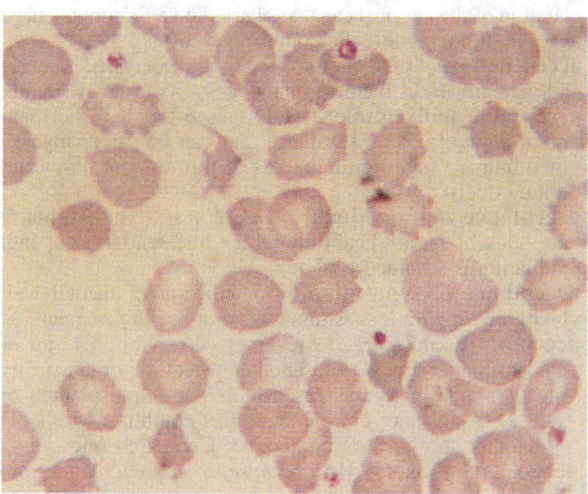

Acanthocytes *(Bain, 1989)*

acanthocytosis /akan'thōsītō'sis/ [Gk, *akantha, kytos + osis,* condition], the abnormal presence of acanthocytes in the circulating blood, most commonly associated with abetalipoproteinemia, in which as many as 80% of the erythrocytes are acanthocytes. See also **abetalipoproteinemia, elliptocytosis.**

acanthoid. See **acantha.**

acanthoma /ak'anthō'mə/ [Gk, *akantha + oma,* tumor], any localized benign or malignant tumor arising from the prickle-cell layer of the epidermis.

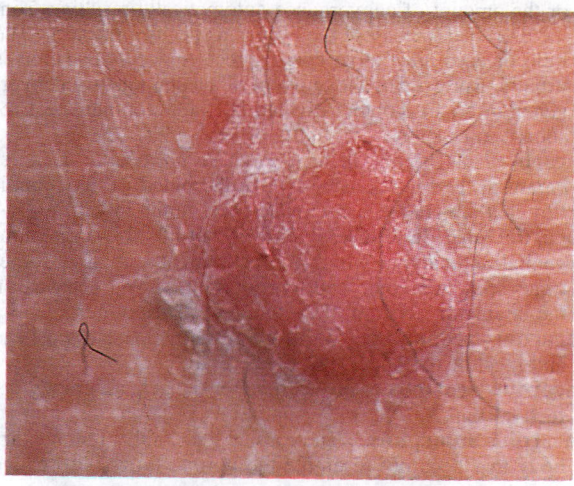

Clear cell acanthoma of Degas
(du Vivier, 1993/Courtesy The Institute of Dermatology, London)

acanthoma adenoides cysticum. See **trichoepithelioma.**

acanthoma verrucosa seborrheica. See **seborrheic keratosis.**

acanthosis /ak'ənthō'sis/ [Gk, *akantha + osis,* condition], an abnormal, diffuse thickening of the prickle-cell layer of the skin, as in eczema and psoriasis. See also **acanthosis nigricans, epidermis. –acanthotic,** *adj.*

acanthosis nigricans /nē'grikanz'/, a skin disease characterized by hyperpigmented, warty lesions of the axillae and perianal body folds. There are benign and malignant forms, the latter associated with cancers of the GI tract. See also **acanthosis.**

-acanthosis. See **acanthosis.**

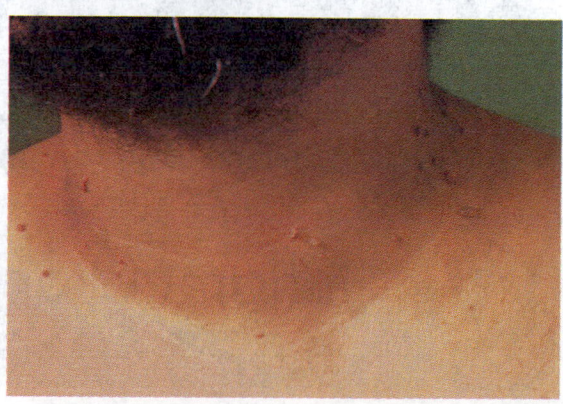

Acanthosis nigricans *(McKee, 1993)*

acapnia /akap'nē·ə/, a deficiency of carbon dioxide in the blood. The condition is usually the result of hyperventilation.

AC/A ratio, in ophthalmology, the proportion between accommodative convergence (AC) and accommodation (A), or the amount of convergence automatically resulting from the dioptric focusing of the eyes at a specified distance. The ratio of accommodative convergence to accommodation is usually expressed as the quotient of accommodative convergence in prism diopters divided by the accommodative response in diopters.

acarbia /akär'bē·ə/ [Gk, *a*, not; L, *carbo*, coal], **1.** a decrease in the bicarbonate level in the blood. **2.** any condition that lowers the bicarbonate level in the blood.

acardia /akär'dē·ə/ [Gk, *a, kardia*, not heart], a rare congenital anomaly in which the heart is absent. It is sometimes seen in a conjoined twin whose survival depends on the circulatory system of its twin. **–acardiac,** *adj*.

acardius acephalus, an acardiac fetus that lacks a head and most of the upper part of the body.

acardius acormus, an acardiac fetus that has a grossly defective trunk.

acardius amorphus, an acardiac fetus with a rudimentary body that does not resemble the normal form. Also called **acardius anceps.**

acariasis /ak'ərī'əsis/ [Gk, *akari*, mite, *osis*, condition], any disease caused by an acarid, such as scrub typhus, which is transmitted by trombiculid mites.

acarid /ak'ərid/, one of the many mites that are members of the order Acarina, which includes a great number of parasitic and free-living organisms. Most are yet undescribed, but several types are of medical interest because they infect humans. The kinds associated with disease are those acting as intermediate hosts of pathogenic agents, those that directly cause skin or tissue damage, and those that cause loss of blood or tissue fluids. Important as vectors of scrub typhus and other rickettsial agents are the six-legged larvae of trombiculid mites, which are parasitic of humans, many other mammals, and birds. See also **chigger, scabies.**

acaro-, a combining form meaning 'pertaining to mites': *acarodermatitis, acaroid, acarophobia*.

acc, Acc, abbreviation for **accommodation.**

accelerated hypertension See **malignant hypertension.**

accelerated idiojunctional rhythm /aksel'ərā'tid id'ē·ō-/, an automatic junctional rhythm at a rate exceeding the normal firing rate of the junction but slower than 100 per minute (60 to 99 per minute) and without retrograde conduction to the atria.

accelerated idioventricular rhythm (AIVR), an automatic ectopic ventricular rhythm, faster than the normal rate of the His-Purkinje system but slower than 100 per minute (50 to 99 per minute) and without retrograde conduction to the atria. In acute myocardial infarction, an AIVR is a sign of reperfusion, spontaneous or as a result of thrombolytic therapy.

accelerated junctional rhythm, an ectopic junctional heart rhythm with a rate that exceeds the normal firing rate of junctional tissue, with or without retrograde atrial conduction.

acceleration /aksel'ərā'shən/ [L, *accelerare*, to quicken], an increase in the speed or velocity of an object or reaction. Compare **deceleration. –accelerator,** *n*.

acceleration phase, (in obstetrics) the first period of active labor, Stage I, characterized by an increased rate of dilatation of the cervical canal as charted on a Friedman curve.

accelerator urinae. See bulbocavernosus.

accentuation /aksen'choo·ā'shən/, [L, *accentus*, accent], an increase in distinctness or loudness, as in heart sounds.

acceptable daily intake (ADI) /aksep'təbəl/, the maximum amount of any substance that can be safely ingested by a human. Ingestion in excess of this amount may cause toxic effects.

acceptance of individuality /aksep'təns/, (in psychiatry) an index of family health by which differentiation or individuation is a valued goal.

acceptance of separation, an indicator of mental well-being in which a loss is mourned in a healthy manner.

acceptor [L, *accipere*, to receive] /aksep'tər/, **1.** an organism that receives from another person or organism living tissue, such as transfused blood or a transplanted organ. **2.** a substance or compound that combines with a part of another substance or compound. Compare **donor.**

access cavity /ak'ses/ [L, *accedere*, to approach], a coronal opening in a tooth, required for effective cleaning, shaping, and filling of the pulp canal and chamber during endodontic or root canal therapy.

accessory /akses'ərē/ [L, *accessonis*, appendage], **1.** a supplement employed chiefly for convenience or for safety, such as the electric elevator mechanisms for hospital beds. **2.** a structure that serves one of the main anatomic systems, such as the accessory sex organs in men and women; the accessory organs of the skin; the hair; the nails; and the skin glands. **3.** one who aids in perpetrating a crime.

accessory chromosome, an unpaired X or Y sex chromosome. Also called **monosome.**

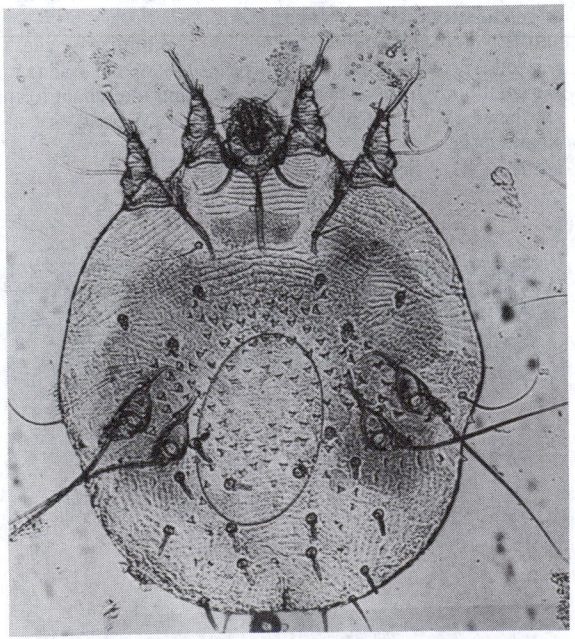

Acarid (Stone, 1989)

accessory diaphragm, a congenital defect in which a second diaphragm or portion of a diaphragm develops in the chest. It is usually found on the right side and is oriented upward and backward to the posterior chest wall. It may be separated from the true diaphragm by a lobe of a lung.

accessory ligament, [L, *accessionis,* a thing added, *ligare,* to bind], a ligament that helps strengthen a union between two bones, even though it is not part of a joint capsule.

accessory movements, joint movements that are necessary for a full range of motion, but that are not under direct voluntary control of the individual. Examples include rotation and gliding motions.

accessory muscle, a relatively rare anatomic duplication of a muscle that may appear anywhere in the muscular system. The most common sign associated with an accessory muscle is the appearance of a soft-tissue mass. Differential diagnosis without surgical intervention and exploration is difficult because of the similar appearance of some tumors or soft-tissue masses, such as ganglia. The appearance of the soft-tissue mass associated with an accessory muscle may be transient, or it may be constant, depending on the location of the accessory muscle in relation to motion. In many individuals with accessory muscles, specific treatment is not indicated unless the accessory muscle interferes with normal function.

accessory muscles of respiration [L, *supplementary*], additional or reinforcing muscles, such as muscles of the neck, back, and abdomen, that may play a more prominent role in respiration during a breathing disorder or during exercise.

accessory nasal sinuses [L, *accessus,* extra + nasus, nose + *sinus,* hollow], the paranasal sinuses that occur as hollows within the skull but open into the nasal cavity and are lined with a mucous membrane that is continuous with the nasal mucous membrane.

accessory nerve, either of a pair of cranial nerves essential for speech, swallowing, and certain movements of the head and shoulders. Each nerve has a cranial and a spinal portion, communicates with certain cervical nerves, and connects to the nucleus ambiguus of the brain. Also called **eleventh nerve, nervus accessorius, spinal accessory nerve.**

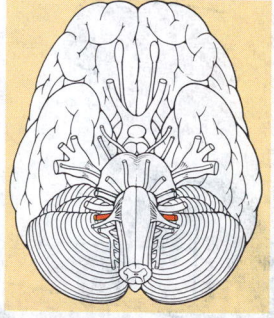

Accessory nerve
(Seeley, 1992/David J Mascaro & Associates)

accessory pancreas [L, *accessionis,* a thing added, Gk, *pan,* all, *kreas,* flesh], small clusters of pancreas cells detached from the pancreas and sometimes found in the wall of the stomach or intestines.

accessory pancreatic duct, a small duct opening into the pancreatic duct or duodenum near the mouth of the common bile duct.

accessory pathway, an abnormal muscle connection between the atria and ventricles that is outside the conduction system. Ventricular activation via this pathway causes initial ventricular forces to slow, producing preexcitation and the delta wave of Wolff-Parkinson-White syndrome. Because of the delta wave, the PR interval is short and the QRS broad. Patients have a tendency to develop paroxysmal supraventricular tachycardia due to AV reentry and a broad QRS, irregular tachycardia due to atrial fibrillation with conduction over the accessory pathway. Patients may be cured by transvenous radio frequency ablation of the accessory pathway.

accessory phrenic nerve, the nerve that joins the phrenic nerve at the root of the neck or in the thorax, forming a loop around the subclavian vein. It may arise from the nerve to the subclavius or from the fifth cervical nerve. Resection of the phrenic nerve to immobilize the diaphragm may be only partially successful if the accessory phrenic nerve is not also resected. Compare **phrenic nerve.**

accessory placenta [L, *accessionis,* a thing added, *placenta,* flat cake], a small placenta that may develop attached to the main placenta by umbilical blood vessels. Also called **succenturiate placenta.**

accessory root canal, a lateral branching of the pulp canal in a tooth, usually occurring in the apical third of the root.

accessory sinus of the nose. See **paranasal sinus.**

accessory spleen [L, *accessus,* extra; Gk, *splen*], small nodules of spleen tissue that may occur in the gastrosplenic ligament, greater omentum, or other visceral sites.

accessory thymus [L, *accessus,* extra; Gk, *thymos,* thymelike], a nodule of thymus issue that is isolated from the gland.

accessory tooth, a supernumerary tooth that does not resemble a normal tooth in size, shape, or position.

access time, the amount of time required for a computer to retrieve a word from its memory or from its disk drive.

ACCH, abbreviation for **Association for the Care of Children's Health.**

accident /ak′sidənt/ [L, *accidere,* to happen], any unexpected or unplanned event that may result in death, injury, property damage, or a combination of serious effects. The victim may or may not be directly involved in the cause of the accident. Accidents frequently are the result of both physical and mental factors that can result in unsafe operating systems at work, home, or other sites.

accidental hemorrhage. See **abruptio placentae.**

acclimate /əklī′mit, ak′limāt/ [L, *ad,* toward; Gk, *klima,* region], to adjust physiologically to a different climate or environment, or to changes in altitude or temperature. Also **acclimatize** /əklī′mətīz′/. –**acclimation, acclimatization,** *n.*

accommodation (A, acc, Acc) /əkom′ədā′shən/ [L, *acommodatio,* adjustment], **1.** the state or process of adapting or adjusting one thing or set of things to another. **2.** the continuous process or effort of the individual to adapt or adjust to surroundings to maintain a state of homeostasis, both physiologically and psychologically. **3.** the adjustment of the eye to variations in distance. See also **accommodation**

reflex. **4.** (in sociology) the reciprocal reconciliation of conflicts between individuals or groups concerning habits and customs, usually through a process of compromise, arbitration, or negotiation. Also called **adjustment.** Compare **adaptation.**

accommodation reflex, an adjustment of the eyes for near vision, consisting of pupillary constriction, convergence of the eyes, and increased convexity of the lens. Also called **ciliary reflex.** See also **light reflex.**

accommodative strabismus /əkom'ədā'tiv/ [L, *accommodatio,* adjustment; Gk, *strabismos,* squint], **1.** strabismus resulting from abnormal demand on accommodation, such as convergent strabismus, uncorrected hypermetropia or divergent strabismus uncorrected myopia. **2.** strabismus resulting from the act of accommodating in association with a high AC/A ratio.

accomplishment quotient /əkom'plishmənt/, a numerical evaluation of a person's achievement age compared with mental age, expressed as a ratio multiplied by 100. See also **achievement quotient, intelligence quotient.**

accountability /əkoun'təbil'itē/, being accountable or responsible for the moral and legal requirements of proper patient care.

accreditation /əkred'itā'shən/, a process whereby a professional association or nongovernmental agency grants recognition to a school or institution for demonstrated ability to meet predetermined criteria, such as the accreditation of hospitals by the Joint Commission on Accreditation of Hospitals or of nursing schools by the National League for Nursing. Compare **certification, licensure.**

accrementition /ak'rəmentish'ən/, growth or increase of size by the addition of similar tissue or material, as in cellular division, simple fission, budding, or gemmation.

-accrete. See **accretion.**

accretio cordis /əkrē'shē·ō/ [L, *accrescere,* to increase; *cordis,* heart], an abnormal condition in which there is an adhesion of the pericardium to a structure around the heart.

accretion /əkrē'shən/ [L, *accrescere,* to increase], **1.** growth or increase by the addition of material of the same nature that is already present. **2.** the adherence or growing together of parts that are normally separated. **3.** the accumulation of foreign material, especially within a cavity. **–accrete,** *v.,* **accretive,** *adj.*

acculturation /əkul'chərā'shən/, the process of adopting the cultural traits or social patterns of another population group.

accumulated dose equivalent /əkyoo'myəlā'tid/, an estimated lifetime maximum permissible dose (MPD) of radiation for persons working with radioactive materials or x-rays. It is 5 rems per year.

accumulator /əkyoo'myəlā'tər/, the 'scratch pad' of a computer's central processing unit (CPU). Data written there can be accessed and processed very rapidly.

accuracy /ak'yərəsē'/, the extent to which a measurement is close to the true value.

accurate empathy /ak'yərit/, a communication technique used by a nurse to convey an understanding of the patient's feelings and experiences.

Accurbron, a trademark for a bronchodilator (theophylline).

Accutane, a trademark for an antiacne agent (isotretinoin).

ACE, abbreviation for **angiotensin-converting enzyme.**

Ace bandage, trademark for a woven elastic bandage.

acebutolol /as'əboo'təlol/, a beta-adrenergic blocking agent. Also called **butanamide.**

■ INDICATIONS: It is prescribed in the treatment of hypertension, angina pectoris, cardiac arrhythmias, and other cardiovascular disorders.

■ CONTRAINDICATIONS: The drug should not be given to patients with asthma, heart failure, or peripheral vascular disease.

■ ADVERSE EFFECTS: The side effects most often reported include bradycardia, flatulence, leg pains, nausea, headache, skin rashes, dizziness, and drowsiness.

acedia /əsē'dē·ə/ [Gk, *akedia,* apathy], a condition of listlessness and a form of melancholy, marked by indifference and sluggish mental processes.

acelius /āsē'lē·əs/, an individual without a body cavity.

acentric /āsen'trik/ [Gk, *a, kentron,* not center], **1.** having no center. **2.** (in genetics) describing a chromosome fragment that has no centromere.

acentric occlusion. See **eccentric occlusion.**

-aceous /-ā'shəs/, a suffix meaning 'having the appearance of' or 'like' something specified: *coriaceous, foliaceous, testaceous.*

acephalia. See **acephaly.**

acephalism. See **acephaly.**

acephalo-, a combining form meaning 'having no head': *acephalobrachia, acephalus, acephaly.*

acephalobrachia /asef'əlōbrā'kē·ə/ [Gk, *a, kephale* + *brachion,* arm], a congenital anomaly in which a fetus lacks both arms and a head.

acephaly /əsef'əlē/ [Gk, *a, kephale,* not head], a congenital defect in which the head is absent or not properly developed. Also called **acephalia** /as'əfā'lē·ə/, **acephalism** /əsef'əliz'əm/. **–acephalic,** *adj.*

acet, abbreviation for an acetate carboxylate anion.

acet-, a combining form meaning 'vinegar': *acetify, acetoin, acetyl.*

acetabula. See **acetabulum.**

acetabular /as'ətab'yələr/ [L, *acetabulum,* little saucer], pertaining to the acetabulum, or cup-shaped hip socket into which the head of the femur is set.

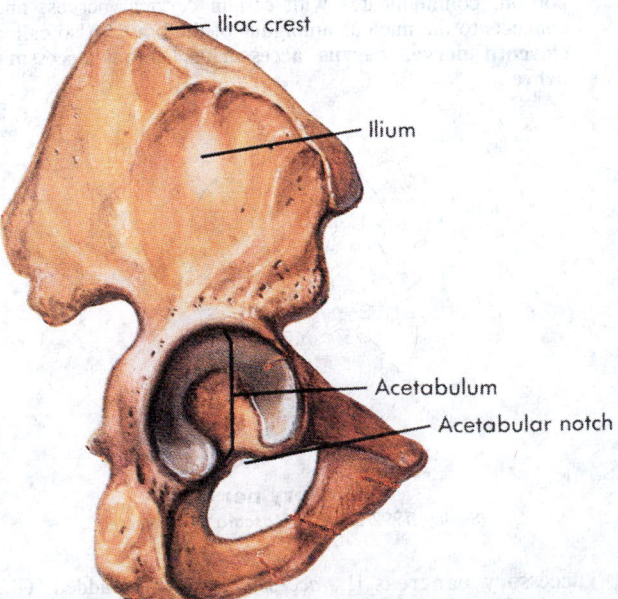

Acetabulum at the junction of the ilium, ischium, and pubus (Seeley, 1992/David J Mascaro & Associates)

acetabulum /as′ətab′yələm/, *pl.* **acetabula** [L, vinegar cup], the large, cup-shaped, articular cavity at the juncture of the ilium, the ischium, and the pubis, containing the ball-shaped head of the femur.

acetaldehyde /as′ətəldē′hīd/, a colorless, volatile liquid with a pungent odor produced by the oxidation of ethyl alcohol. In the human body, acetaldehyde is produced in the liver by the action of alcohol dehydrogenase and other enzymes. It is used commercially in the manufacture of acetic acid and various aromas and flavors. Exposure to high levels of acetaldehyde can result in headache, corneal injury, rhinitis, and respiratory disorders.

acetaminophen /əset′əmin′əfin/, an analgesic and antipyretic drug used in many nonprescription pain relievers. It has no anti-inflammatory properties.
■ INDICATIONS: It is often prescribed for mild to moderate pain and fever.
■ CONTRAINDICATION: Known hypersensitivity to acetaminophen prohibits its use.
■ ADVERSE EFFECTS: Among the most serious adverse reactions are anaphylaxis and hemolytic anemia. Overdosage can result in fatal hepatic necrosis.

acetaminophen poisoning, a toxic reaction to the ingestion of excessive doses of acetaminophen. In adults dosages exceeding 10 to 15 g can produce liver failure, and doses above 25 g can be fatal. Large amounts of acetaminophen metabolites can overwhelm the glutathione-detoxifying mechanism of the liver, resulting in progressive necrosis of the liver within 5 days. The onset of symptoms may be marked by nausea and vomiting, profuse sweating, pallor, and oliguria. The nausea and vomiting increase, accompanied by jaundice and pain in the upper abdomen, hypoglycemia, encephalopathy, and kidney failure. Treatment requires emesis and gastric lavage. Acetylcysteine may prevent extensive liver damage if given soon after ingestion (via nasogastric tube).

acetanilide /as′ətan′ilīd/, an analgesic drug with antipyretic and antirheumatic properties, derived from aniline. Because the use of acetanilide has been associated with an increased risk of methemoglobinemia, it has been generally replaced by acetaminophen. See also **acetaminophen.**

acetate /as′itāt/, a salt of acetic acid.

acetate kinase, an enzyme that catalyzes the transfer of a phosphate group from adenosine triphosphate to acetate. Also called **acetokinase** /as′ətōkī′nās, əsē′tō-/.

acetazolamide /as′ətəzō′ləmīd/, a carbonic anhydrase inhibitor.
■ INDICATIONS: It is prescribed for edema, glaucoma, and epilepsy (primarily petit mal).
■ CONTRAINDICATIONS: Hyponatremia, hypocalcemia, severe liver or kidney disease or dysfunction, Addison's disease, or known hypersensitivity to this drug prohibits its use.
■ ADVERSE EFFECTS: Among the most serious adverse reactions are anorexia and depression, particularly in the elderly; acidosis; hyperuricemia; and crystalluria. GI disturbances and lethargy are common.

Acetest, a trademark for a product used to test for the presence of abnormal quantities of acetone in the urine of patients with diabetes mellitus or other metabolic disorders. A large quantity of acetone causes a rapid change in the color of the Acetest tablet. See also **acidosis, ketone bodies.**

acetic /əsē′tik, əset′ik/ [L, *acetum,* vinegar], pertaining to substances having the sour properties of vinegar or acetic acid; also, chemical compounds possessing the radical, CH3CO—.

acetic acid a clear, colorless, pungent liquid that is miscible with water, alcohol, glycerin, and ether and that constitutes 3% to 5% of vinegar. Acetic acid is produced commercially by the destructive distillation of wood or from methyl alcohol, or it may be converted from ethyl alcohol by the action of many aerobic bacteria. Various concentrations of acetic acid are used in the manufacture of plastics, dyes, insecticides, cellulose acetate, photographic chemicals, and pharmaceutic preparations, including vaginal jellies and antimicrobial solutions for the treatment of superficial infections of the external auditory canal. Also called **ethanoic acid.**

acetic acid test. See **albumin test.**

acetic fermentation, the production of acetic acid or vinegar from a weak alcoholic solution.

acetoacetic acid /as′ətō·əsē′tik, əsē′tō-/, a colorless, oily keto acid produced by the metabolism of lipids and pyruvates. It is excreted in trace amounts in normal urine and in elevated levels in diabetes mellitus, especially in ketoacidosis. Acetoacetic acid is also increased during starvation as a result of incomplete oxidation of fatty acids. Soluble in water, alcohol, and ether, acetoacetic acid decomposes at temperatures below 100° C to acetone and carbon dioxide. Also called **acetone carboxylic acid** /kär′boksil′ik/, **acetylacetic acid** /əsē′tiləsē′tik, as′ətil-/, **beta-ketobutyric acid** /bet′əkē′tōbyŏŏtir′ik/, **diacetic acid** /dī·əsē′tik/.

acetohexamide /-hek′səmīd/, a sulfonylurea oral antidiabetic.
■ INDICATION: It is prescribed in the treatment of Type II, non-insulin-dependent diabetes mellitus (NIDDM).
■ CONTRAINDICATIONS: Diabetes, severe liver or kidney dysfunction, or known hypersensitivity to this drug or to other sulfonylureas prohibits its use.
■ ADVERSE EFFECTS: Among the most serious adverse reactions are blood dyscrasias, hypoglycemia, and allergic reactions. GI disturbances are common.

acetokinase. See **acetate kinase.**

acetol kinase, an enzyme that catalyzes the transfer of a phosphate group from adenosine triphosphate to hydroxyacetone.

acetone /as′ətōn/, a colorless, aromatic, volatile liquid ketone body found in small amounts in normal urine and in larger quantities in the urine of diabetics experiencing ketoacidosis or starvation. Commercially prepared acetone is used to clean the skin before injections, but prolonged exposure to the compound can be irritating. It also has many varied industrial uses.

acetone bodies. See **ketone bodies.**

acetone carboxylic acid. See **acetoacetic acid.**

acetone in urine test, a test for the presence of dimethylketone in the urine of patients, used as a laboratory indication of ketosis and the severity of diabetes. The test consists of exposing chemically treated test paper strips or sticks to urine. If acetone is present in the urine as the result of incomplete breakdown of fatty and amino acids in the body, the test strips change color. A similar test uses a compound added directly to a urine sample.

acetonide grouping, an acetone-based ketal present in some corticosteroid drugs, such as flucinolone acetonide.

acetonuria /as′ətōnŏŏr′ē·ə/, the presence of acetone and diacetic bodies in the urine. See also **ketoaciduria.**

acetophenetidin. See **phenacetin.**

acetpyrogall /as′ətpī′rəgal/, a topical irritant used as a caustic and keratolytic agent. Also called **pyrogallol triacetate.**

acetyl-CoA. See **acetylcoenzyme A.**

acetylacetic acid. See **acetoacetic acid.**

acetylcholine (ACh) /as′ətilkō′lēn, əsē′til-/, a neurotransmitter substance widely distributed in body tissues, with a primary function of mediating synaptic activity of the nervous system and skeletal muscles. Its active phase is transient because it is rapidly destroyed by acetylcholinesterase. Acetylcholine activity also can be blocked by atropine at junctions of nerve fibers with glands and smooth muscle tissue. It is a stimulant of the vagus and parasympathetic nervous system and functions as a vasodilator and cardiac depressant. Acetylcholine is used therapeutically as an adjunct to eye surgery and has limited benefits in certain circulatory disorders due to its short half-life.

acetylcholinesterase /-kō′lines′tərās/ **(AChE),** an enzyme present at endings of voluntary nerves and parasympathetic involuntary nerves. It inactivates and prevents accumulation of the neurotransmitter acetylcholine released during nerve impulse transmission by hydrolyzing the substance to choline and acetate. The action reduces or prevents excessive firing of neurons at neuromuscular junctions. However, acetylcholinesterase activity can be blocked by many chemicals, including morphine and organophosphate pesticides.

acetylcoenzyme A /əsē′til-kō·en′zīm, as′ətil-/, a 2-carbon molecule that is formed in the course of several important metabolic processes. The formation of acetylcoenzyme A is the critical intermediate step between anaerobic glycolysis and the citric acid cycle. Also called **acetyl-CoA.** See also **Krebs' cycle, tricarboxylic acid cycle.**

acetylcysteine /-sis′tēn/, a mucolytic.
- INDICATIONS: It is prescribed in the treatment of chronic pulmonary disease, acute bronchopulmonary disease, atelectasis resulting from mucous obstruction, and acetaminophen poisoning.
- CONTRAINDICATION: Known sensitivity to this drug prohibits its use.
- ADVERSE EFFECTS: Among the most serious adverse reactions are stomatitis, nausea, rhinorrhea, and bronchospasm.

acetylsalicylic acid. See **aspirin.**

acetylsalicylic acid poisoning /əsē′təlsal′isil′ik, as′itəl-/, the toxic effects of overdosage of the commonly used antipyretic and analgesic drug, aspirin. Early symptoms of overdosage include dizziness, ringing in the ears, changes in body temperature, gastrointestinal discomfort, and hyperventilation. Severe poisoning is marked by respiratory alkalosis, which may lead to metabolic acidosis. Children are particularly vulnerable to the potential toxic effects of salicylates. See also **Reye's syndrome, salicylate poisoning.**

acetyltransferase /-trans′fərās/, any of several enzymes that transfer acetyl groups from one compound to another. See also **acetylcoenzyme A.**

ACG, abbreviation for *apexcardiography.*

ACh, abbreviation for **acetylcholine.**

ACH, abbreviation for **adrenocortical hormone.**

achalasia /ak′əlā′zhə/ [Gk, *a, chalasis* not relaxation], an abnormal condition characterized by the inability of a muscle to relax, particularly the cardiac sphincter of the stomach. Compare **corkscrew esophagus.** See also **dysphagia.**

Achard-Thiers syndrome /ash′ärtērz′/ [Émile C. Achard, French physician, b. 1860; Joseph Thiers, French physician, b. 1873], a hormonal disorder seen in postmenopausal women with diabetes, characterized by growth of body hair in a masculine distribution. Treatment includes mechanical removal or bleaching of excess hair and hormonal therapy to correct endocrine imbalances related to systemic disease. See also **hirsutism.**

ache /āk/ [OE, *acan,* to hurt], **1.** a pain characterized by persistence, dullness, and, usually, moderate intensity. An ache may be localized, as a stomachache, headache, or bone ache, or general, as the myalgia that accompanies a viral infection or a persistent fever. **2.** to suffer from a dull, persistent pain of moderate intensity.

AChE, abbreviation for **acetylcholinesterase.**

achievement age /əchēv′mənt/, the level of a person's educational development as measured by an achievement test and compared with the normal score for chronologic age. Compare **mental age.** See also **developmental age.**

achievement quotient (AQ), a numeric expression of a person's achievement age, determined by various achievement tests, divided by the chronologic age and expressed as a multiple of 100. Compare **intelligence quotient.** See also **accomplishment quotient.**

achievement test, a standardized test for the measurement and comparison of knowledge or proficiency in various fields of vocational or academic study. Compare **aptitude test, intelligence test, personality test, psychologic test.**

Achilles tendon /əkil′ēz/ [Achilles, Greek mythologic hero], the common tendon of the soleus and gastrocnemius muscles. It is the thickest and strongest tendon in the body and begins near the middle of the posterior part of the leg. In an adult it is about 15 cm long. The tendon becomes contracted about 4 cm above the heel and flares out again to insert into the calcaneus. Also called **tendo calcaneus.**

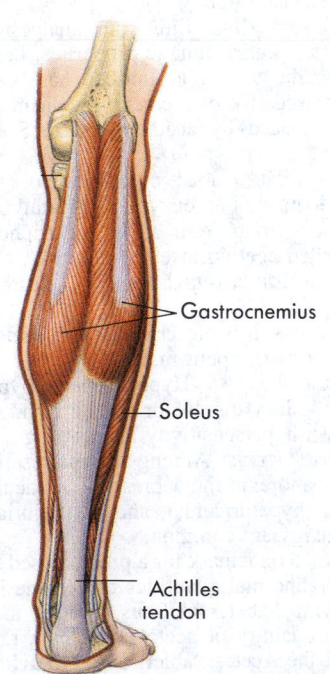

Gastrocnemius

Soleus

Achilles tendon

Achilles tendon *(Thibodeau, 1993/John V Hagen)*

Achilles tendon reflex, a deep tendon reflex consisting of plantar flexion of the foot when a sharp tap is given directly to the tendon of the gastrocnemius muscle at the back of the ankle. This reflex is often absent in diabetics and people with peripheral neuropathies. A sluggish return of the flexed foot may be seen in patients with hypothyroidism. A hyperactive reflex may be caused by hyperthyroidism or by pyramidal tract disease. Also called **ankle reflex. See also deep tendon reflex.**

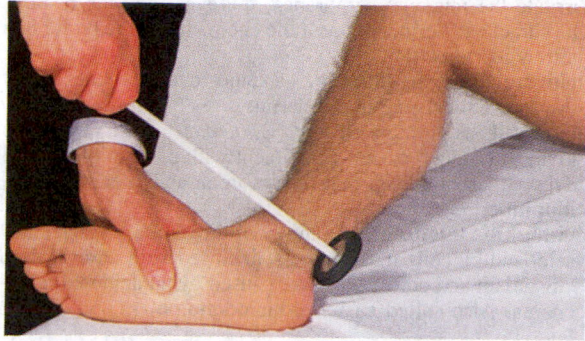

Elicitation of the Achilles tendon reflex *(Epstein, 1992)*

achlorhydria /āˈklôrhīˈdrē·ə/ [Gk, *a, chloros,* not green, *hydor* water], an abnormal condition characterized by the absence of hydrochloric acid in the gastric juice. Achlorhydria occurs most commonly in atrophy of the gastric mucosa, gastric carcinoma, and pernicious anemia involving metabolism and absorption of intrinsic and extrinsic factors. It is also found in severe iron deficiency anemia. Achlorhydria in a patient with symptoms of gastric ulcer almost always indicates that the lesion is malignant. Protein digestion is severely impaired in patients with achlorhydria, but overall digestion in the alimentary tract is relatively normal, because trypsin and other enzymes of the pancreas and small intestine are not affected. See also **achylia, pernicious anemia. –achlorhydric,** *adj.*

acholia /akōˈlē·ə/ [Gk, *a, chole,* not bile], **1.** the absence or decrease of bile secretion. **2.** any condition that suppresses the flow of bile into the small intestine. **–acholic,** *adj.*

acholuria /akˈəlŏŏrˈē·ə/ [Gk, *a, chole + ouron,* urine], the absence or lack of bile pigments in the urine.

achondrogenesis /ākonˈdrōjenˈəsis/, a form of dwarfism characterized by gross limb shortening and hydropic head and trunk. It is transmitted by an autosomal recessive gene.

achondroplasia /ākonˈdrōplāˈzhə/ [Gk, *a, chondros,* not cartilage, *plassein,* to form], a disorder of the growth of cartilage in the epiphyses of the long bones and skull that results in premature ossification, permanent limitation of skeletal development, and dwarfism typified by protruding forehead and short, thick arms and legs on a normal trunk. Onset is in fetal life. Familial achondroplasia is inherited as an autosomal dominant gene; the chance is 50% that an offspring of an affected parent will be affected. The majority of affected individuals die during gestation or the first year of life. The minority that survive have relatively normal longevity. There is no treatment other than orthopedic

surgery. Antenatal diagnosis is possible. Also called **chondrodystrophy, fetal rickets.**

achondroplastic dwarf /-plasˈtik/, the most common type of dwarf, characterized by disproportionately short limbs, a normal-sized trunk, large head with a depressed nasal bridge and small face, stubby hands, and lordosis. The condition results from an inherited defect in bone-forming tissue and is often associated with other defects or abnormalities, although there is usually no involvement of the central nervous system and intelligence is normal. See also **achondroplasia.**

achromatic lens /akˈrəmatˈik/, [Gk, *a,* without, *chroma,* color; L, *lentil*], a lens in which the focal lengths for red and blue colors of the spectrum are the same, refracting light without decomposing it into its component colors.

achromatic vision. See **color blindness.**

achromatocyte. See **achromocyte.**

achromia /akrōˈmēə/ [Gk, *a, chroma,* not color], the absence or loss of normal skin pigment. The condition may be the result of a disease such as psoriasis.

achromocyte /ākrōˈməsīt/, a sickle-shaped, hypochromic erythrocyte. Also called **achromatocyte** /āˈkrōmatˈəsīt/.

Achromycin V, a trademark for an antibiotic (tetracycline hydrochloride).

achylia /ākīˈlē·ə/ [Gk, *a, chylos,* not juice], an absence or severe deficiency of hydrochloric acid and pepsinogen (pepsin) in the stomach. This condition may also occur in the pancreas when the exocrine portion of that gland fails to produce digestive enzymes. Also called **achylosis.** See also **achlorhydria.**

achylous /ākīˈləs/, **1.** of or pertaining to a lack of gastric juice or other digestive secretions. **2.** of or pertaining to a lack of chyle.

acicular /əsikˈyələr/ [L, *aciculus,* little needle], needle-shaped, such as certain leaves and crystals.

acid /asˈid/ [L *acidus* sour], **1.** a compound that yields hydrogen ions when dissociated in solution. Acids turn blue litmus red, have a sour taste, and react with bases to form salts. Acids have chemical properties essentially opposite to those of bases. See also **alkali. 2.** *slang.* lysergic acid diethylamide (LSD). See also **lysergide.**

acid-, a prefix meaning 'sour, bitter, acid': *acidemia, acidophil.*

-acid, 1. a suffix meanning an 'acid': *sulfacid.* **2.** a combining form meaning 'pertaining to acid': *subacid, semiacid, superacid.*

acid-base balance, a condition existing when the net rate at which the body produces acids or bases equals the net rate at which acids or bases are excreted. The result of acid-base balance is a stable concentration of hydrogen ions in body fluids. See also **acid, base.**

acid-base metabolism, the metabolic processes that maintain the balance of acids and bases essential in regulating the composition of body fluids. Acids release hydrogen ions, and bases accept them; the number of hydrogen ions present in a solution governs whether it is acid, alkali, or neutral. Hydrogen ions are measured on a pH scale of 1 to 14, with a reading of 7 being neutral. Above 7, the solution is alkaline; below 7, it is acid. Blood is slightly alkaline, ranging from 7.35 to 7.45. Metabolic buffer systems within the body maintain this ratio, and, when it is upset, either acidosis or alkalosis results. Acidosis may be caused by diarrhea, vomiting, uremia, diabetes mellitus, and the action of certain drugs. Alkalosis may be caused by overingestion of alkaline drugs, loss of chloride in gastric vomitus, and the action of certain diuretic drugs. See also **acid-base balance, acidosis, alkalosis, pH.**

acid bath, a bath taken in water containing a mineral acid to help reduce excessive sweating.

acid burn, damage to tissue caused by exposure to an acid. The severity of the burn is determined by the strength of the acid and the duration and extent of exposure. Emergency treatment includes washing the affected area with large amounts of water. Compare **alkali burn.**

acid dust, an accumulation of highly acidic particles of dust. Such substances accumulate in the atmosphere and account for much of the smog hanging over large metropolitan areas. Many respiratory illnesses, such as lung cancer and asthma, may be aggravated or caused by such dust. See also **acid rain.**

-acidemia /-as′idē′mē·ə/, a suffix meaning an 'increased hydrogen-ion concentration in the blood' or 'abnormal acidity in the blood': *lactacidemia, lipacidemia.*

acid-fast bacillus (AFB), a type of bacillus that resists decolorizing by acid after accepting a stain. Examples include *Mycobacterium tuberculosis* and *M. leprae.*

acid-fast stain, a method of staining used in bacteriology in which a smear on a slide is treated with carbol-fuchsin stain, decolorized with acid alcohol, and counterstained with methylene blue to identify acid-fast bacteria. Acid-fast organisms resist decolorization and appear red or yellow against a dark background when viewed under a microscope. The stain may be performed on any clinical specimen but is most commonly used in examining sputum for *Mycobacterium tuberculosis,* an acid-fast bacillus. See also **Ziehl-Neelsen test.**

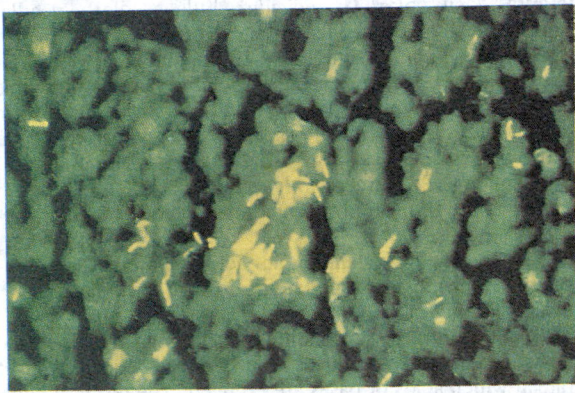

Acid-fast stain of *mycobacterium tuberculosis*
(Murray, 1990)

acid flush, a runoff of precipitation with a high acid content, as may occur during thaws in various parts of the world. Acid flushes may pollute rivers and reservoirs, killing fish and endangering the natural balance of the ecosystem. See also **acid rain.**

acidify /asid′əfī/, **1.** to make a substance acid, as through the addition of an acid. **2.** to become acid. Compare **alkalinize.**

acidity /asid′itē/ [L, *acidus,* sour], the degree of sourness, sharpness of taste, or ability of a chemical to yield hydrogen ions in an aqueous solution.

acidity of the stomach, the degree of gastric acid in the stomach. The acidity varies during any 24-hour period but averages in the range of pH 0.9 to pH 1.5. The main source of stomach acidity is hydrochloric acid secreted by gastric glands of the stomach.

acid mist, mist containing a high concentration of acid or particles of any toxic chemical, such as carbon tetrachloride or silicon tetrachloride. Such chemicals are often used by industry and stored in tanks that may leak their contents into residential areas, becoming especially dangerous if the toxic substance mixes with fog. Inhalation of acid mists may irritate the mucous membranes, the eyes, and the respiratory tract and seriously upset the chemistry of the body. See also **acid rain.**

acid mucopolysaccharide, a major chemical constituent of ground substance in the dermis.

acidophil /as′idōfil, əsid′əfil/ [L, *acidus* + Gk, *philein,* to love], **1.** a cell or cell constituent with an affinity for acid dyes. **2.** an organism that thrives in an acid medium. **—acidophilic,** *adj.*

acidophilic adenoma, a tumor of the pituitary gland characterized by cells that can be stained red with an acid dye. Gigantism and acromegaly are caused by an acidophilic adenoma. Also called **eosinophilic adenoma.**

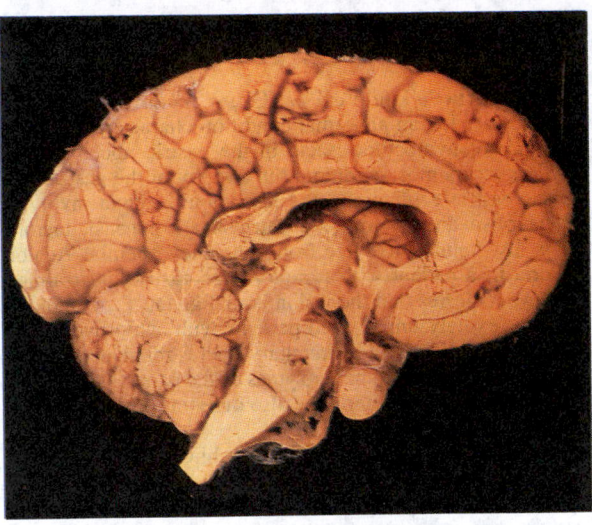

Acidophilic adenoma *(Skarin, 1991)*

acidophilus milk /as′idof′ələs/, milk inoculated with cultures of *Lactobacillus acidophilus,* used in various enteric disorders to change the bacterial flora of the GI tract.

acidosis /as′idō′sis/ [L, *acidus* + Gk, *osis,* condition], an abnormal increase in hydrogen ion concentration in the body resulting from an accumulation of an acid or the loss of a base. It is indicated by a blood pH below 7.4. The various forms of acidosis are named for the cause of the condition; for example, renal tubular acidosis results from failure of the kidney to secrete hydrogen ions or reabsorb bicarbonate ions, respiratory acidosis results from respiratory retention of CO_2, and diabetic acidosis results from an accumulation of ketones associated with poorly controlled diabetes mellitus. Treatment depends on diagnosis of the underlying pathology and concurrent correction of the acid-base imbalance. Compare **alkalosis.** –**acidotic,** *adj.*

acidosis dialysis, a type of metabolic acidosis that may develop when contaminating bacteria alter the pH of the dialysis bath. The condition is most likely to occur after prolonged hemodialysis.

acidotic, pertaining to acidosis, either depletion of base or accumulation of acid.

acid-perfusion test, a test to demonstrate sensitivity of the esophagus to acid, a condition suggestive of reflux esophagitis. A weak hydrochloric acid solution and normal saline are dripped alternately into the esophagus via a nasal-esophageal tube without telling the patient which solution is being infused. A positive response is pain with acid but not with saline. An alternative method is to compare acid barium swallows with neutral barium swallows. If acid sensitivity is present, diffuse spasm of the esophagus may be seen by fluoroscopy when acid barium is infused and no spasm with neutral barium. Also called **Bernstein test.**

acid phosphatase, an enzyme found in the kidneys, serum, semen, and prostate gland. It is elevated in serum in cancers of the prostate and in trauma. Normal concentrations in serum are 0 to 1.1 Bodansky units/ml. See also **alkaline phosphatase.**

acid poisoning, a toxic condition caused by the ingestion of a toxic acid agent such as hydrochloric, nitric, phosphoric, or sulfuric acids, some of which are ingredients in common household cleaning compounds. Emergency treatment includes giving copious amounts of water, milk, or beaten eggs to dilute the acid. Vomiting is not induced, and mild solutions of alkali are not given. The victim is transported immediately to the hospital for observation of any corrosive damage to the esophagus or stomach, for metabolic abnormality, and for mechanical removal of the acid by gastric lavage. Compare **alkali poisoning.**

acid rain, the precipitation of moisture, as rain, with high acidity caused by release into the atmosphere of pollutants from industry, motor vehicle exhausts, and other sources. Acid precipitation with a pH of 5.6 or less is blamed by various authorities for numerous human health problems, fish kills, and the destruction of timber. Also called **acid precipitation, acid snow.**

acid rebound, a condition of hypersecretion of gastric acid that may occur after the initial buffering effect of an antacid. It occurs most noticeably when antacids containing calcium carbonate are used.

acid salt, a salt that is formed from only partial replacement of hydrogen ions from the related acid, leaving some degree of acidity in the salt. An example is sodium bicarbonate, which is also identified as sodium acid carbonate.

acid snow. See **acid rain.**

acid therapy, a method for removing warts, which employs plaster patches impregnated with acid, such as 40% salicylic acid, or with acid drops, such as 5% to 16.7% salicylic and lactic acids in flexible collodion. The application is made every 12 to 24 hours for 2 to 4 weeks. Acid therapy is not usually recommended for body areas that perspire heavily or that are likely to become wet or for exposed body parts where the patches would detract from the patient's appearance.

acidulous /əsid′yələs/, slightly acidic or sour.

aciduria [L, *acidus* + Gk, *ouron* urine, the presence of acid in the urine. The condition may be caused by a diet rich in meat proteins or certain fruits, the introduction of a

medication for the treatment of a urinary tract disorder, an inborn error of metabolism, or ketoacidosis.

acinar adenocarcinoma. See **acinic cell adenocarcinoma.**

acinar cell /as′inər/ [L, *acinus,* grape], a cell of the tiny lobules of a compound gland or similar saclike structure such as an alveolus.

Acinetobacter /as′inē′təbak′tər/, a genus of nonmotile, aerobic bacteria of the family Neisseriaceae that often occurs in clinical specimens. The *Acinetobacter* contains gram-negative or gram-variable cocci and does not produce spores. This bacterium grows on regular media without serum and is oxidase negative and catalase positive.

acini. See **acinus.**

acinic cell adenocarcinoma /asin′ik/ [L, *acinus,* grape], an uncommon, low-grade malignant neoplasm that develops in the secreting cells of racemose glands, especially the salivary glands. The tumor consists of cells with clear or slightly granular cytoplasm and small eccentric dark nuclei. Also called **acinar adenocarcinoma, acinous adenocarcinoma** /as′inəs/.

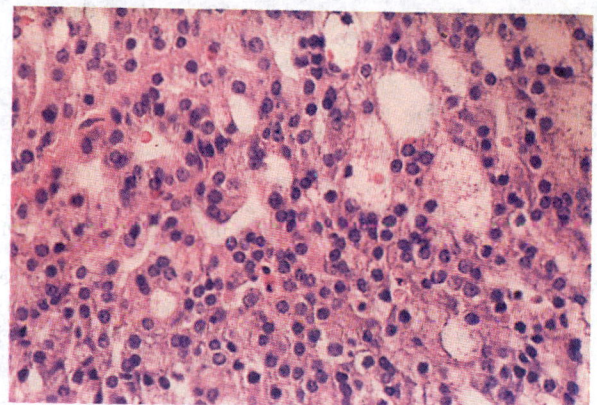

Acinic cell adenocarcinoma (Skarin, 1991)

acinitis /as′inī′tis/, any inflammation of the tiny, grape-shaped portions of certain glands.

acinous adenocarcinoma. See **acinic cell adenocarcinoma.**

acinus /as′inəs/, *pl.* **acini** [L, grape], **1.** any small saclike structure, particularly one found in a gland. **2.** a subdivision of the lung consisting of the tissue distal to a terminal bronchiole. Also called **alveolus.**

A.C. joint, abbreviation for *acromioclavicular joint.* See **acromioclavicular articulation.**

Aclovate, a trademark for a topical corticosteroid (alclometasone dipropionate).

ACLS, abbreviation for **advanced cardiac life support.**

ACMC, abbreviation for **Association of Canadian Medical Colleges.**

acme /ak′mē/, the peak or highest point, such as the peak of intensity of a uterine contraction during labor.

acne /ak′nē/ /ak′nē/ [Gk, *akme,* point], an inflammatory, papulopustular skin eruption occurring usually in or near the sebaceous glands on the face, neck, shoulders, and upper back. Its cause is unknown but involves bacterial breakdown of sebum into fatty acids irritating to surrounding subcutaneous tissue. Treatment includes topical and oral antibiotics, topical vitamin A derivatives, benzyl benzoate, and dermabrasion. Kinds of acne include **acne conglobata, acne vulgaris, chloracne,** and **rosacea.** See also **comedo.**

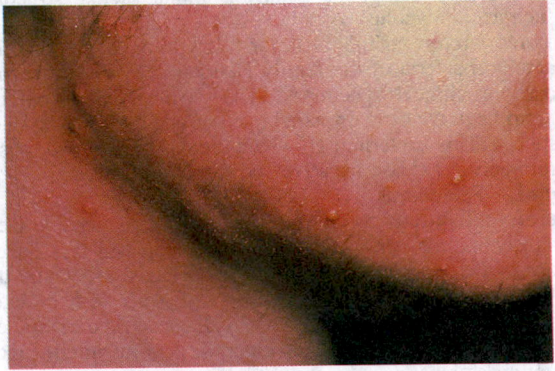

Moderate acne
(Goldstein, 1992/Courtesy Department of Dermatology, University of North Carolina at Chapel Hill)

acne artificialis, an eruption in the skin caused by an external irritant, such as tar, or ingestion of halogen compounds.

acne cachecticorum, an eruption or irritation of the skin that may occur in patients who are very weak and debilitated. It is characterized by soft, mildly infiltrated pustular lesions.

acne conglobata /kong′glōbā′tə/, a severe form of acne with abscess, cyst, scar, and keloid formation. Acne conglobata may affect the lower back, buttocks, and thighs, as well as the face and chest. Also called **cystic acne.**

Acne conglobata *(Zitelli, 1992)*

acneform /ak′nifôrm/, resembling acne. Also **acneiform** /aknē′əfôrm/.

acneform drug eruption, any one of various skin reactions to a drug that is characterized by papules and pustules erupting in acne, with or without comedones.

acnegenic /ak′nijen′ik/ [Gk, *akme* + *genein,* to produce], causing or producing acne.

acneiform. See **acneform.**

acne indurata, a pathologic skin condition characterized by hard, deep-seated lesions that are secondary to fibroblastic proliferation and formation of new tissue. Also called **chronic acne vulgaris.**

acne keloid, [Gk, *akme,* point, *kelis,* spot, *eidos,* form], a cellular overgrowth at the site of an acne lesion.

acne keratosa, a skin condition characterized by hard conic plugs that usually appear at the corners of the mouth and inflame surrounding tissue.

acne necrotica miliaris, a rare, chronic type of folliculitis of the scalp, occurring mostly in adults and characterized by tiny pustules, probably a pyoderma or tuberculid. Also called **acne varioliformis.**

acne neonatorum, a skin condition of newborns caused by sebaceous gland hyperplasia and characterized by the formation of grouped comedones on the nose, cheeks, and forehead.

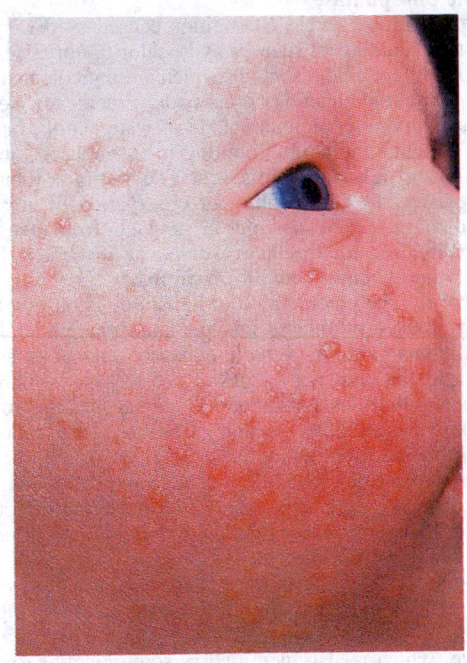

Acne neonatorum *(Zitelli, 1992)*

acne papulosa, a common skin condition that develops small papular lesions. It is considered a papular form of acne vulgaris.

acne rosacea. See **rosacea.**

acne varioliformis. See **acne necrotica miliaris.**

acne vulgaris, a common form of acne seen predominantly in adolescents and young adults. Acne vulgaris, characterized by comedones with black centers, papules, pustules, and miliary sebaceous cysts, or whiteheads, is probably an effect of androgenic hormones (which stimulate the production of sebum) and *Propionibacterium acnes* in the hair follicle.

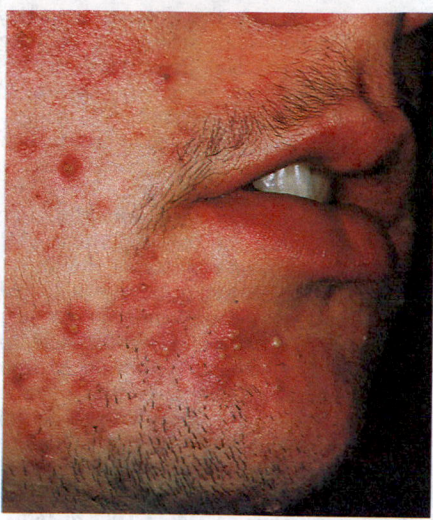

Acne vulgaris (Habif, 1990)

ACNM, abbreviation for *American College of Nurse-Midwives.*

ACOG, abbreviation for **American College of Obstetricians and Gynecologists.**

acognosia /ak′og·nō′zhə/, a knowledge of remedies.

acoria /akôr′ē·ə/ [Gk, *a, koros,* not satiety], a condition characterized by constant hunger and eating, even when the appetite is small.

acorn-tipped catheter, a flexible catheter with an acorn-shaped tip used in various diagnostic procedures, especially in urology.

acous-, acus-, acust/o-, a combining form meaning 'pertaining to hearing': *acoustic, acousma.*

-acousia, -acusia, -acusis, -akusis, a suffix meaning a '(specified) condition of the hearing'.

acousma /əkooz′mə/, *pl.* **acousmas, acousmata** [Gk, *akousma,* something heard], a hallucinatory impression of strange sounds.

acoustic/əkoos′tik/ [Gk *akouein* to hear], of or pertaining to sound or hearing. Also **acoustical.**

-acoustic, -acoustical, 1. a suffix meaning 'pertaining to the hearing organs': *entacoustic, otacoustic.* **2.** a suffix meaning 'pertaining to amplified sound waves': *micracoustic, microcoustic, stethacoustic.*

acoustic cavitation, a potential biologic effect of ultrasonography, marked by large-amplitude oscillations of microscopic gas bubbles. As normally used, ultrasound pulses are too short to cause acoustic cavitation in human tissues.

acoustic center, the portion of the brain, in the temporal lobe of the cerebrum, in which the sense of hearing is located.

acoustic hair cell. See **auditory hair.**

acoustic impedance, the effect of interference with the passage of sound waves, such as those generated by ultrasound equipment, by objects in the path of the sound wave. It is calculated as the product of the velocity of sound in a medium and the density of the medium. The impedance increases if either the speed of the sound waves or the density of the medium increases. The acoustic impedance of bone may be nearly five times as great as that of blood. Test-

ing of middle ear impedance is part of audiologic test batteries to detect middle ear problems.

acoustic meatus [Gk, *akoustikos,* hearing; L, *meatus,* a passage], either the external or the internal canal of the ear.

acoustic microscope, a microscope in which the object being viewed is scanned with sound waves and its image reconstructed with light waves. Acoustic microscopes produce excellent resolution of the objects being studied and allow very close examination of cells and tissues without staining or damaging the specimen.

acoustic nerve, either of a pair of cranial nerves composed of fibers from the cochlear nerve and the vestibular nerve in the inner ear, conveying impulses of both the sense of hearing and the sense of balance. Also called **eighth cranial nerve.**

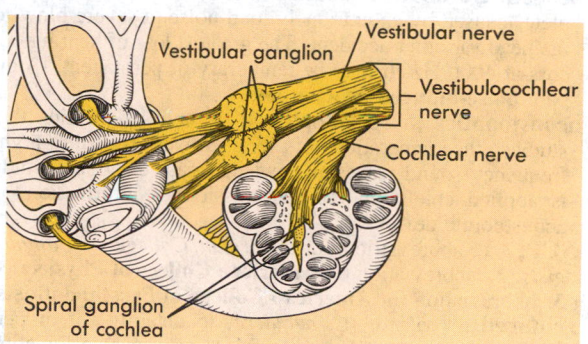

Acoustic nerve (Seeley, 1992)

acoustic neuroma, a benign unilateral or bilateral tumor that develops from the eighth cranial (auditory) nerve and grows within the auditory canal. Depending on the location and size of the lesion, tinnitus, progressive hearing loss, headache, facial numbness, papilledema, dizziness, and an unsteady gait may result. Paresis and difficulty in speaking and swallowing may occur in the later stage. Also called **acoustic neurilemoma, acoustic neurinoma, acoustic neurofibroma.**

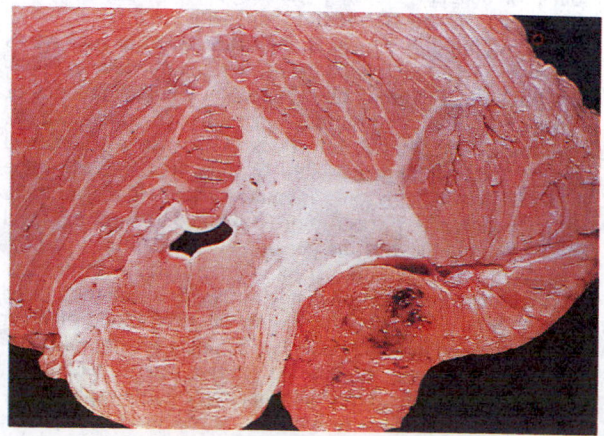

Acoustic neuroma seen in horizontal section
(Okazaki, 1988/by permission of Mayo Foundation)

acoustic reflex, contraction of the stapedius muscle in the middle ear in response to a loud sound. The muscle contraction pulls the stapes out of the oval window and thus protects the inner ear from damage resulting from loud noise. The **acoustic reflex threshold** is the lowest level of sound that will elicit an acoustic reflex and is in the range of 85 to 90 dB HL in individuals with normal hearing. Acoustic reflexes are usually elevated or absent in cases of conductive or neural hearing loss and present at normal or lower levels in the case of cochlear (inner ear) hearing loss.

acoustics /əkoos'tiks/ [Gk, *akoustikos,* hearing], the perception of sound.

acoustic shadow, an ultrasound image produced by the presence of dense material, such as calculi, in a scan of soft tissue. It is often used to detect gallstones.

acoustic trauma, a sudden loss of hearing, partial or complete, caused by an extremely loud noise, a severe blow to the head, or other accident. The greatest loss of hearing occurs at 4000 Hz. It may be temporary or permanent. Compare **noise-induced hearing loss.**

acoustooptics /əkoos'tō·op'tiks/, a field of physics that studies the generation of light waves by ultra-high-frequency sound waves. Knowledge gained by such study is applied chiefly in the transmission of information by acoustooptic devices.

ACP, **1.** abbreviation for *American College of Pathologists.* **2.** abbreviation for **American College of Physicians. 3.** abbreviation for **American College of Prosthodontists.**

acquired /əkwī'ərd/ [L, *acquiere,* to obtain], of or pertaining to a characteristic, condition, or disease originating after birth, not caused by hereditary or developmental factors but by a reaction to environmental influences outside of the organism. Compare **congenital, familial, hereditary.**

acquired hypogammaglobulinemia [L, *acquirere,* to obtain; Gk, *hypo,* a deficiency, *gamma,* third letter of Greek alphabet; L, *globulus,* small globe; Gk, *haima,* blood], an acquired deficiency of the gamma globulin blood fraction. See also **hypogammaglobulinemia.**

acquired immunodeficiency syndrome (AIDS) /ādz/, a disease involving a defect in cell-mediated immunity that has a long incubation period, follows a protracted and debilitating course, is manifested by various opportunistic infections, and has a poor prognosis. The disorder originally was found in homosexual men and intravenous drug users but now occurs increasingly among female sex partners of bisexual men and children of those with the disease.

■ OBSERVATIONS: A patient is characterized as having AIDS if he or she has contracted the human immunodeficiency virus (HIV) and exhibits one or more of 23 specific signs or symptoms, including various types of pneumonia, cancer, and fungal and parasitic infections. AIDS also is determined by the level of the patient's T4 lymphocytes, indicating the efficiency of the person's immune system. If that number drops below 200-500 per mm³, compared to a normal level of 1000 lymphocytes, the person may be identified as having AIDS. The causative agent is a retrovirus, identified as HIV (human immunodeficiency virus), transmitted through sexual contact or exposure to contaminated blood or other body fluids of infected patients, including breast milk. Initial symptoms include extreme fatigue, intermittent fever, night sweats, chills, lymphadenopathy, enlarged spleen, anorexia and consequent weight loss, severe diarrhea, apathy, and depression. As the disease progresses, there is a general failure to thrive, anergy, and any number and kind of recurring opportunistic infections, most commonly *Pneumocystis carinii* pneumonia, meningitis, or encephalitis caused by aspergillosis, candidiasis, crytococcosis, cytomegalovirus, toxoplasmosis, or herpes simplex. Most patients with the disorder are susceptible to malignant neoplasms, especially Kaposi's sarcoma, Burkitt's lymphoma, and non-Hodgkin's lymphoma, that cause as well as result from immunodeficiency.

■ INTERVENTIONS: Treatment consists primarily of combined chemotherapy to counteract the opportunistic diseases. Although there is no known cure for an HIV infection, the antiviral drug zidovudine has been shown to reduce the progress of the disease and prolong the lives of patients. Alternative antiviral drugs include didanosine (ddi) and zalcitabine (ddc); vaccines may be developed from glycoproteins gp120 or gp160. Interferon and other immunomodulators have been used, with little success, to correct the underlying immune defect. The fatality rate is 90% in those diagnosed more than 2 years. See also **AIDS-dementia complex, AIDS-wasting syndrome, human immunodeficiency virus, CD4, CD8, gp160, retrovirus.**

■ NURSING CONSIDERATIONS: Nursing care of the patient with AIDS varies with the patient's symptoms. Intervention is directed at providing education to prevent the spread of disease, preventing infections, modifying alterations in body temperature, promoting self-care, promoting optimal nutrition, and providing emotional support for patients and their families.

acquired immunity, any form of immunity that is not innate and is obtained during life. It may be natural or artificial and actively or passively induced. **Naturally acquired immunity** is obtained by the development of antibodies resulting from an attack of infectious disease or by the transmission of antibodies from the mother through the placenta to the fetus or to the infant through the colostrum. **Artificially acquired immunity** is obtained by vaccination or by the injection of antiserum. Compare **natural immunity.** See also **active immunity, passive immunity.**

acquired reflex. See **conditioned reflex.**

acquired sterility [L, *acquiere,* to obtain + *sterilis,* barren], the failure to conceive after once bearing a child. Also called **one-child sterility.**

acquired trait [L, *acquiere,* to obtain + *trahere,* to draw], a physical characteristic that is not inherited, but which may be an effect of the environment or a mutation.

ACR, abbreviation for **American College of Radiology.**

acrid /ak'rid/, sharp or pungent, bitter and unpleasant to the smell or taste.

acridine /ak'ridēn/, a dibenzopyridine compound used in the synthesis of dyes and drugs. Its derivatives include fluorescent yellow dyes and the antiseptic agents acriflavine hydrochloride, acriflavine base, and proflavine.

acrimony /ak'rəmō'nē/ [L, *acrimonia,* pungency], a quality of bitterness, harshness, or sharpness.

acro-, a prefix meaning 'pertaining to the extremities': *acroataxia, acrocyanosis.*

acrocentric /ak'rōsen'trik/ [Gk, *akron,* extremity, *kentron,* center], pertaining to a chromosome in which the centromere is located near one of the ends so that the arms of the chromatids are extremely uneven. Compare **metacentric, submetacentric, telocentric.**

acrocephalosyndactylism. See **Apert's syndrome.**

acrocephaly. See **oxycephaly.**

acrochordon /ak′rōkôr′don/, a benign, pedunculated skin tag commonly occurring on the eyelids or neck or in the axilla or groin.

acrocyanosis /ak′rōsī′ənō′sis/ [Gk, *akron* + *kyanos* blue], a condition characterized by cyanotic discoloration, coldness, and sweating of the extremities, especially the hands, caused by arterial spasm that is usually precipitated by cold or by emotional stress. Acrocyanosis may be treated with antiadrenergic drugs, and attacks may be prevented by not smoking and by avoiding exposure to cold. Another kind of acrocyanosis is **peripheral acrocyanosis of the newborn.** Acrocyanosis is also called **Raynaud's phenomenon, Raynaud's sign.**

acrodermatitis /-dur′mətī′tis/ [Gk, *akron* + *derma*, skin, *itis* inflammation], any eruption of the skin of the hands and feet caused by a parasitic mite belonging to the order Acarina.

acrodermatitis enteropathica /en′tərōpath′ikə/, a rare, chronic disease of infants characterized by vesicles and bullae of the skin and mucous membranes, alopecia, diarrhea, and failure to thrive. An autosomal recessive disorder of zinc malabsorption, the disease may be lethal if not treated. Zinc sulfate is usually prescribed.

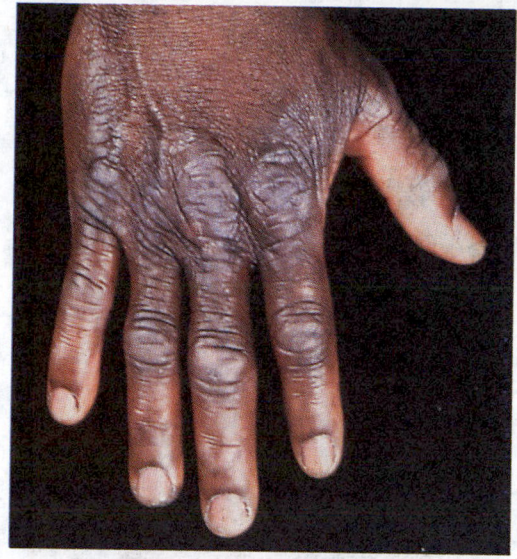

Acrokeratosis verruciformis (du Vivier, 1993)

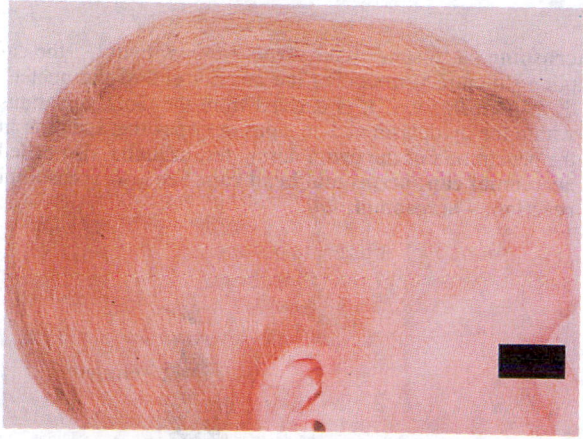

Acrodermatitis enteropathica on the scalp
(Baran, 1991)

acrodynia /ak′rōdin′ē·ə/ [Gk, *akron* + *odyne*, pain], a disease that occurs in infants and young children. Symptoms include edema, pruritus, generalized skin rash, with pink coloration of the extremities and scarlet coloration of the cheeks and nose, profuse sweating, digestive disturbances, photophobia, polyneuritis, extreme irritability alternating with periods of listlessness and apathy, and failure to thrive. The cause is unknown, although the condition is usually associated with ingestion of or contact with mercury and often with inflammatory changes of obscure origin in the central nervous system. Also called **erythredema polyneuropathy, Feer's disease, pink disease, Swift's disease.**

acrokeratosis verruciformis /ak′rōker′ətō′sis/, a skin disorder characterized by the appearance of wartlike lesions on the dorsum of the hands and feet and occasionally on the wrists, forearms, and knees. It is an inherited disease, transmitted as a dominant trait.

acrokinesis /-kīnē′sis/ [Gk, *akron*, extremity, + *kinesis*, motion], a state in which there is an abnormally wide range of motion of the limbs.

acromegalia. See **acromegaly.**

acromegalic eunuchoidism, /-məgal′ik/ a rare disorder characterized by genital atrophy and the development of female secondary sex characteristics, occurring in men with advanced acromegaly caused by a tumor in the anterior pituitary gland. Initially, the gonadal function of the anterior lobe may be stimulated, but with the growth of the tumor the patient may become impotent; lose facial, axillary, and pubic hair; and develop a soft skin and a feminine distribution of fat. Also called **retrograde infantilism.**

acromegaly /ak′rəmeg′əlē/ [Gk, *akron* + *megas*, great], a chronic metabolic condition characterized by a gradual, marked enlargement and elongation of the bones of the face, jaw, and extremities. The condition, which afflicts middle-aged and older persons, is caused by the overproduction of growth hormone and is treated by x-ray or surgery, often involving partial resection of the pituitary gland. Also called **acromegalia.** Compare **gigantism.** See also **adenohypophysis, growth hormone—acromegalic,** *adj*. (See Fig. p. 22.)

-acromial. See **acromion.**

acromial process /əkrō′mēəl/ [Gk, *akron*, extremity, + *omos,* shoulder], a flat triangular plate at the end of the scapula.

acromicria /ak′rəmik′rē·ə/, an anomaly characterized by abnormally small hands and feet. The person may also possess unusually small facial features, such as nose and ears.

acromioclavicular articulation /-mī′ōklavik′yələr/, the gliding joint between the acromial end of the clavicle and the medial margin of the acromion of the scapula. The joint has six ligaments.

acromiocoracoid /-kôr′əkoid/, pertaining to the acromion and coracoid process.

acromiohumeral /-hyōō′mərəl/, pertaining to the acromion and the humerus.

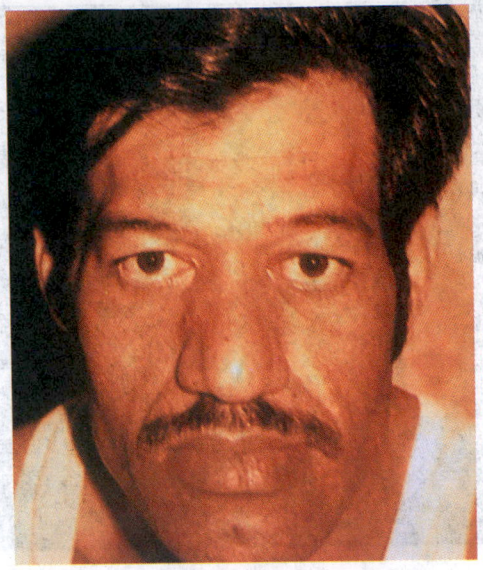

Acromegaly
(Seidel, 1991/Courtesy Paul W Ladenson, MD, The Johns Hopkins University and Hospital, Baltimore)

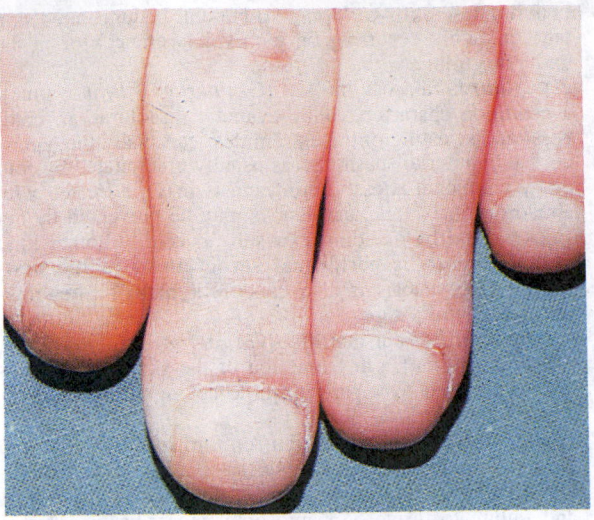

Acroosteolysis in PVC disease
(Baran, 1991/Courtesy Prof. G. Moulin)

acromion /əkrō'mē·ən/ [Gk, *akron* + *omos*, shoulder], the lateral extension of the spine of the scapula, forming the highest point of the shoulder and connecting with the clavicle at a small oval surface in the middle of the spine. It gives attachment to the deltoideus and trapezius. Also called **acromion process.** Compare **coracoid process. – acromial,** *adj.*

acromioscapular /-skap'yələr/, pertaining to the acromion process and the scapula.

acroosteolysis /ak'rō·os'tē·ol'isis/, an occupational disease that mainly affects people who work with polyvinylchloride (PVC) plastic materials. It is characterized by Raynaud's phenomenon, loss of bone tissue in the hands, and sensitivity to cold temperatures. A nonoccupational form of the disease is believed to be inherited.

acroparesthesia /ak'rōpar'isthē'zhə/ [Gk, *akron* + *para,* near, *aisthesis*, feeling], **1.** an extreme sensitivity at the tips of the extremities of the body, caused by compression of the nerves in the affected area or by polyneuritis. **2.** a disease characterized by tingling, numbness, and stiffness in the extremities, especially in the fingers, the hands, and the forearms. It sometimes produces pain, skin pallor, or mild cyanosis. The disease occurs in a simple form, which may produce acrocyanosis, and in an angiospastic form, which may produce gangrene.

acrophobia [Gk, *akron* + *phobos*, fear], a pathologic fear or dread of high places that results in extreme anxiety. Therapy attempts to overcome or eliminate the phobic reaction. See also **obsession, phobia.**

-acrosomal. See **acrosome.**

acrosomal cap, acrosomal head cap See **acrosome.**

acrosomal reaction /ak'rəsō'məl/, the pattern of various chemical changes that occur in the anterior of the head of the spermatozoon in response to contact with the ovum and that lead to the penetration by the sperm and fertilization of the ovum.

acrosome /ak'rəsōm'/ [Gk, *akron* + *soma*, body], the caplike structure surrounding the anterior end of the nucleus of a spermatozoon. It is derived from the Golgi apparatus within the cytoplasm and contains enzymes that function in the penetration of the ovum during fertilization. Also called **acrosomal cap, acrosomal head cap.** See also **acrosomal reaction. – acrosomal,** *adj.*

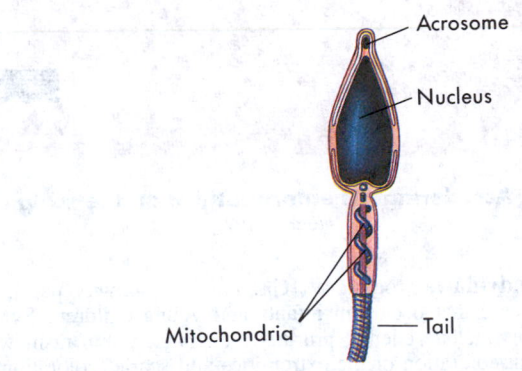

Acrosome

Nucleus

Mitochondria

Tail

Acrosome at the tip of a human sperm
(Thibodeau, 1993/Bill Ober)

acrotic /əkrot'ik/ [Gk, *a, krotos*, not beating], **1.** of or pertaining to the surface or to the skin glands. **2.** of or pertaining to the absence or the weakness of a pulse.

acrylic resin base /əkril'ik/, (in dentistry) a denture base made of acrylic resin. Compare **denture base.**

acrylic resin dental cement, a dental cement for restoring or repairing damaged teeth. In powder form it contains polymethyl methacrylate, which acts as filler, plasticizer, and polymerization initiator. In liquid form it contains methyl methacrylate with an inhibitor and an activator.

acryl(o)-, a prefix for terms relating to acrylic compounds.

ACS, 1. abbreviation for *American Cancer Society*. **2.** abbreviation for *American Chemical Society*. **3.** abbreviation for **American College of Surgeons. 4.** abbreviation for *anodal closing sound*.

ACSM, abbreviation for *American College of Sports Medicine*.

act-, a prefix meaning 'to do, drive, act': *action, activate, actor*.

ACTH, abbreviation for **adrenocorticotropic hormone.**

Acthar, a trademark for adrenocorticotropic hormone (corticotropin).

-actide, a combining form designating a synthetic corticotropin.

Actidil, a trademark for an antihistamine (triprolidine hydrochloride), used for the symptomatic relief of allergic conditions.

Actifed, a trademark for a fixed-combination drug containing an adrenergic vasoconstrictor (pseudoephedrine hydrochloride) and an antihistamine (triprolidine hydrochloride).

actigraph /ak'tigraf'/, any instrument that records changes in the activity of a substance or an organism and produces a graphic record of the process, such as an electrocardiograph machine, which produces a record of cardiac activity.

actin, a protein found in muscle fibers that acts with myosin to bring about contraction and relaxation. Also called **actinin. See also myosin.**

actin-. See **actino-.**

acting out, the expression of intrapsychic conflict or painful emotion through overt behavior that is usually neurotic, defensive, and unconscious and that may be destructive or dangerous. In controlled situations, like psychodrama, Gestalt therapy, or play therapy, such behavior may be therapeutic in itself and may also serve to reveal to the patient the underlying conflict governing his behavior. See also **transference.**

actinic /aktin'ik/ [Gk, *aktis*, ray], of or pertaining to radiation, such as sunlight or x-rays.

actinic conjunctivitis [Gk, *actis*, ray, + L, *conjunctivus*, connecting, + Gk, *itis*, inflammation], an eye inflammation caused by exposure to the ultraviolet radiation of sunlight or other UV sources, such as acetylene torches, therapeutic lamps (sun lamps), and klieg lights. Also called **actinic ophthalmia.**

actinic dermatitis, a skin inflammation or rash resulting from exposure to sunlight, x-ray, or atomic particle radiation. Chronic or recurrent actinic dermatitis can predispose to skin cancer. See also **actinic keratosis.**

actinic keratosis, a slowly developing, localized thickening of the outer layers of the skin as a result of chronic, prolonged exposure to the sun. Treatment of this potentially malignant lesion includes surgical excision, cryotherapy, and topical chemotherapy. Also called **senile keratosis, senile wart, solar keratosis.**

actinin. See **actin.**

Actinic ophthalmia. See **actinic conjunctivitis.**

actinium (Ac), a rare, radioactive metallic element. Its atomic number is 89; its atomic weight is 227. It occurs in some ores of uranium.

actino-, actin-, a prefix meaning 'pertaining to a ray or to radiation': *actinocardiogram, actinocutitis, actinogen*.

Actinomyces /ak'tinōmī'sēz/ [Gk, *aktis*, ray, *mykes*, fungus], a genus of anaerobic or facultative anaerobic, gram-positive bacteria. Species that may cause disease in humans,

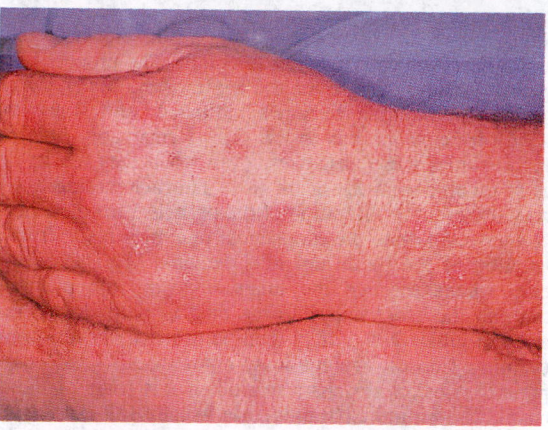

Actinic keratosis
(Greenberger, 1993/Courtesy Dr. Loren H. Amundson, University of South Dakota, Sioux Falls)

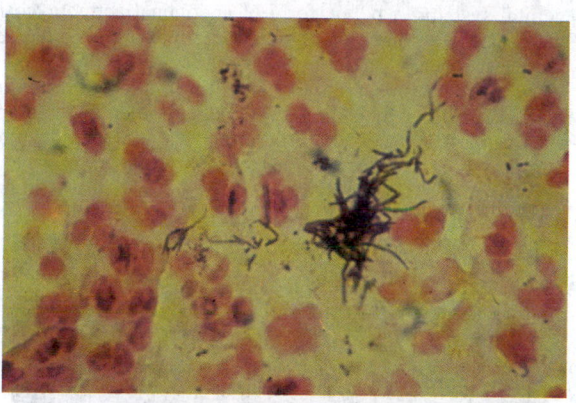

Actinomyces israelii *(Baron, 1990)*

such as *Actinomyces israelii*, are normally present in the mouth and throat. See also **actinomycosis.**

actinomycin A /-mī'sin/, the first of a group of chromopeptide antibiotic agents derived from soil bacteria. Most are derivatives of phenoxazine and contain actinocin. They are generally active against gram-positive bacteria, fungi, and neoplasms. See **dactinomycin.**

actinomycin B, an antibiotic agent derived from *Actinomyces antibioticus*.

actinomycin D. See **dactinomycin.**

actinomycosis /ak'tinōmīkō'sis/, a chronic, systemic disease characterized by deep, lumpy abscesses that extrude a thin, granular pus through multiple sinuses. The disease occurs worldwide but is seen most frequently in those who live in rural areas. It is not spread from person to person or from animal to humans. The most common causative organism in humans is *A. israelii*, a normal inhabitant of the bowel and mouth. Disease occurs after tissue damage, usually in the presence of another infectious organism. It can be diagnosed by microscopic identification of sulfur granules, pathognomonic of *Actinomyces*, in the exudate. There are four principal forms of actinomycosis. **Cervicofacial**

actinomycosis occurs with the spread of the bacterium into the subcutaneous tissues of the mouth, throat, and neck, as a result of dental or tonsillar infection. The process begins with a hard swelling over the angle of the lower jaw and neck. The swelling becomes indurated, and sinus tracts form, draining the pus to the skin. Remarkably little pain accompanies these abscesses, even when they are so deep as to involve the bone of the jaw. **Thoracic actinomycosis** may represent proliferation of the organism from cervicofacial abscesses into the esophagus, or it may result from inhalation of the bacterium into the bronchi. The infection may spread through the lungs, reaching the pleura, or through the esophagus into the mediastinum. Ribs, heart, and the great vessels may then be affected. Fever, cough, draining sinuses, weight loss, night sweats, and, rarely, pleural effusion are characteristic of this form of the disease. **Abdominal actinomycosis** usually follows an acute inflammatory process in the stomach or intestines, such as appendicitis, diverticulum of the large bowel, or a perforation of the stomach. A large mass may be palpated, and sinus tracts may be found in the groin or other area that drains exudate from abscesses deep in the abdomen. **Generalized actinomycosis** may involve the skin, brain, liver, and urogenital system. A pelvic form of abdominal actinomycosis may occur after insertion of an intrauterine contraceptive device. All forms of actinomycosis are treated with at least 6 weeks of daily injections of penicillin in large doses. Surgical excision or incision and drainage of deep or large abscesses may be necessary. Abdominal actinomycosis can be cured in 40% of cases, thoracic actinomycosis in 80%, and cervicofacial actinomycosis in 90%.

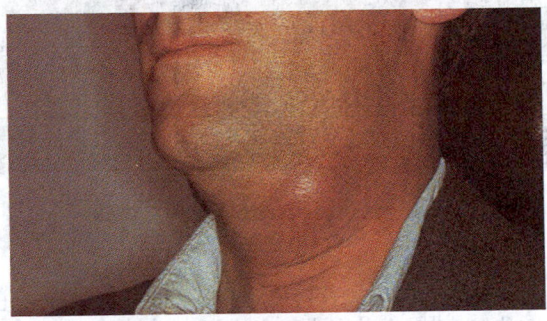

Cervicofacial actinomycosis (Lamey, 1988)

action current. See **action potential.**

action level, the level of concentration at which an undesirable or toxic component of a food is considered dangerous enough to public health to warrant government prohibition of the sale of that food. The United States Food and Drug Administration tests foods for action levels.

action potential, an electric impulse consisting of a self-propagating series of polarizations and depolarizations, transmitted across the cell membranes of a nerve fiber during the transmission of a nerve impulse and across the cell membranes of a muscle cell during contraction or other activity of the cell. Also called **action current.**

action tremor, [L, *agere,* to do + *tremor,* shaking], a tremor that occurs or is evident during voluntary movements. Also called **intention tremor.**

Activase, a trademark for a commercial form of tissue plasminogen activator (t-PA).

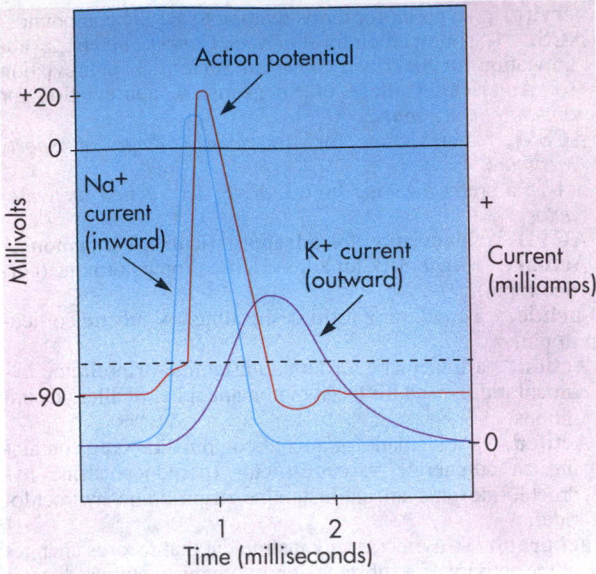

Action potential (Potter, 1993)

activate /ak′təvāt/, [L, *activus,* active], to induce or prolong an activity or render optimal action.

activated charcoal, a general-purpose antidote and a powerful pharmaceutic adsorbent.

- INDICATIONS: It is prescribed in the treatment of acute poisoning and to control flatulence.
- CONTRAINDICATIONS: There are no known contraindications, but activated charcoal is ineffective in poisoning caused by a strong acid or alkali or by cyanide. It should not be administered to unconscious persons.
- ADVERSE EFFECTS: There are no known adverse effects.

activated 7-dehydrocholesterol. See **vitamin D₃.**

activated partial thromboplastin time (APTT), a timed blood test that determines the efficacy of various clotting factors used in the diagnosis of coagulation disorders. The normal value in venous blood is 32 to 51 seconds.

activating enzyme, an enzyme that promotes or sustains an activity, such as an enzyme that catalyzes the combining of amino acids to form peptides or proteins.

activation energy /ak′tivā′shən/ [L, *activus,* active], the energy required to convert reactants to transition-state species that will spontaneously proceed to products.

activation factor. See **factor XII.**

activator /ak′tivā′tər/, 1. a substance, force, or device that stimulates activity in another substance or structure, especially a substance that activates an enzyme. 2. a substance that stimulates the development of an anatomic structure in the embryo. 3. an internal secretion of the pancreas. 4. an apparatus for making substances radioactive, such as a cyclotron or neutron generator. 5. (in dentistry) a removable orthodontic appliance that functions as a passive transmitter and stimulator of the perioral muscles.

active algolagnia. See **sadism.**

active anaphylaxis [Gk, *ana,* up, *phylaxis,* protection], a condition of hypersensitivity caused by the reaction of the body's immune system to injection of a foreign protein. See also **anaphylaxis.**

active assisted exercise [L, *activus*], the movement of the body or any of its parts primarily through the individual's own efforts but accompanied by the aid of a therapist or some device, such as an exercise machine. See also **exercise, passive exercise.**

active carrier [OFr, *carier*], a person without signs or symptoms of an infectious disease who carries the causal micro-organisms.

active electrode [Gk, *elektron*, amber, *hodos*, way], an electrode that is applied at a specific point to produce stimulation in a concentrated area in electrotherapy.

active euthanasia. See **euthanasia.**

active exercise, repetitive movement of a part of the body as a result of voluntary contraction and relaxation of the controlling muscles. Compare **passive exercise.** See also **aerobic exercise, anaerobic exercise.**

active expiration [L, *expirare*, to breathe out], forced exhalation, using the muscles of the abdominal wall and rib cage, in addition to the diaphragm and recoil of elastic tissues.

active hyperemia [L, *activus*, Gk, *hyper*, excessive, *haima*, blood], the increased flow of blood into a particular body part.

active immunity, a form of long-term, acquired immunity that protects the body against a new infection as the result of antibodies that develop naturally after an initial infection or artificially after a vaccination. Compare **passive immunity.** See also **immune response.**

active labor [L, *activus*, active, *labor*, work], the normal progress of the birth process, including uterine contractions, dilatation of the cervix, and descent of the fetus into the birth canal.

active listening, an attitude of alert hearing and of showing an interest in what a person has to say.

active movement, muscular action at a joint as a result of voluntary effort without outside help. Compare **passive movement.**

active-passive, (in psychiatry) a concept that characterizes persons as either actively involved in shaping events or passively reacting to events.

active play, any activity from which one derives amusement, entertainment, enjoyment, or satisfaction by taking a participatory rather than a passive role. Children of all age groups engage in various forms of active play, from the exploration of objects and toys by the infant and toddler to the formal games, sports, and hobbies of the older child. Compare **passive play.**

active range of motion, (AROM), the range of movement through which a joint can be moved without assistance.

active resistance exercise, the movement or exertion of the body or any of its parts performed totally through the individual's own efforts against a resisting force. See also **progressive resistance exercise.**

active resistance training (ART), a conditioning or rehabilitation program designed to enhance a patient's muscular strength, power, and endurance through progressive active resistance exercises and muscle overloading.

active sensitization [L, *agere*, to do + *sentire*, to feel], the condition that results when a specific antigen is injected into a person known to be susceptible. See also **sensitization.**

active site, the place on the surface of an enzyme where its catalytic action occurs.

active specific immunotherapy, a therapy in which a cancer patient is injected with irradiated tumor cells. The injected cells stimulate the production of antibodies that resist the tumor cells.

active transport, the movement of materials across the

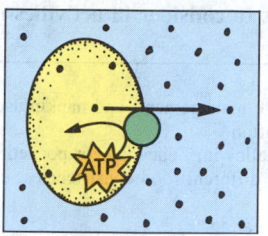

Active transport *(Potter, 1993)*

membrane of a cell by means of chemical activity that allows the cell to admit larger molecules than would otherwise be able to enter. Expediting active transport are carrier molecules within the cell that bind themselves to incoming molecules, rotate around them, and disconnect, setting the incoming molecule free inside the cell wall. The entry of large molecules in the process of active transport disturbs the equilibrium of the internal environment of the cell, which compensates for the imbalance by releasing materials through its membrane. Active transport is the means by which the cell absorbs glucose and other substances needed to sustain life and health. Certain enzymes play a role in active transport, providing a chemical 'pump' that helps move substances through the cell membrane. Compare **osmosis, passive transport.**

activities of daily living (ADL) /aktiv′itēz/, the activities usually performed in the course of a normal day in the person's life, such as eating, toileting, dressing, washing, or brushing the teeth. The ability to perform the activities of daily living may be compromised by a variety of causes, including chronic illnesses and accidents. The limitation imposed may be temporary or permanent; rehabilitation may involve relearning the skills or learning new ways to accomplish an activity. Health care professionals have significant roles in helping a person to maintain or regain his or her ability to perform the necessary activities of daily living, thus remaining independent to the greatest degree possible. An ADL checklist is often used before discharge from a hospital. If any activities cannot be adequately performed, arrangements are made with an outside agency, such as a visiting nurse service, or with family members to provide the necessary assistance. Follow-up with physical therapy or other health care professions such as occupational therapy on an outpatient basis may be useful in maintaining or increasing the person's ability to perform the activities. See also **Barthel Index.** (See Table p. 26.)

activity, the action of an enzyme on an amount of substrate that is converted to product per unit time under defined conditions.

activity coefficient, a proportionality constant, γ, relating activity, α, to concentration, expressed in the equation, $\alpha = \gamma c$.

activity intolerance, a nursing diagnosis accepted by the Fifth National Conference on the Classification of Nursing Diagnoses. Activity intolerance is a state in which an individual has insufficient physiologic or psychologic energy to endure or complete required or desired daily activities. The cause of the condition may be generalized weakness, a sedentary life-style, imbalance between oxygen supply and demand, or bed rest or immobility. The defining characteristics of the condition include verbal report of fatigue or weakness, abnormal heart rate or blood pressure response to

Specific elements to consider in activities of daily living training

Feeding:
- Utensil, cup, plate management, and napkin use.
- Tidiness/organization.
- Awareness of swallowing, chewing, or pocketing problems.
- Ability to handle different food consistencies, e.g., finger foods versus soups.
- Mouth care after eating.

Bathing:
- Assembling of items and appropriate equipment.
- Management of caps, lids, sprays, etc.
- Facial cleansers and cosmetic application.
- Shaving foam or soap application versus electric razor.
- Shaving face, underarms, and/or legs.
- Hair care.
- Deodorant application.
- Tooth/denture care.
- Nail care.
- Replacement of care items.
- Location of bath facilities in hospital and home.
- Transfer ability to bathtub or shower.

Dressing:
- Selection of clothing.
- Assembling of clothing.
- Application of underwear.
- Management of fasteners.
- Application of trousers/slacks, belt, or suspenders.
- Management of pullover tops.
- Application of shirt, jacket, dress (front opening), or tie.
- Management of buttons.
- Application of socks or stockings.
- Application of shoes and tying laces.
- Location of dressing activities: bed, sitting or standing.
- Ability to care for and apply glasses, contact lenses, or hearing aid.

Toileting and elimination management:
- Transfer ability.
- Clothing management.
- Cognitive function.
- Bowel and bladder control.
- External devices: assembly, application, removal, and care of equipment.
- Suppository insertion (include preparation of suppository and cleaning of insertion device if used).
- Post-toileting hygiene.
- Timing of bowel program (morning or evening).
- Employment/school/home/environment considerations.
- Colostomy or ileal conduit care.
- Performance of bladder management programs.
- Accident management.

Adapted from Mumma CM, editor: *Rehabilitation nursing concepts and practice: a core curriculum*, ed 2, Skokie, IL, 1987, Rehabilitation Nursing Foundation.

activity, exertional discomfort or dyspnea, and electrocardiographic changes reflecting arrhythmias or ischemia. See also **nursing diagnosis.**

activity intolerance, high risk for, a nursing diagnosis accepted by the Seventh National Conference on the Classification of Nursing Diagnoses. Activity intolerance is a state in which an individual is at risk of experiencing insufficient physiologic or psychologic energy to endure or complete required or desired daily activities. Risk factors are a history of previous intolerance, deconditioned status, presence of circulatory or respiratory problems, and inexperience with activity. See also **nursing diagnosis.**

activity theory, a concept proposed by Robert J. Havighurst, an American educator and gerontologist, that activity promotes well-being and satisfaction in aging. Thus older adults who are actively involved in social situations, and establish new roles and relationships, are more likely to age with a sense of satisfaction.

activity tolerance, the type and amount of exercise a patient may be able to perform without undue exertion or possible injury.

actual cautery /ak′chōō·əl/ [L, *actus*, act], the application of heat, rather than a chemical substance, in the destruction of tissue.

actual charge, the amount actually charged or billed by a medical practitioner for a service. The actual charge may not be the same as that paid for the service by an insurance plan.

actual damages. See **damages.**

actualize /ak′chōō·əlīz′/, the act of fulfilling a potential, as by a person who may develop capabilities through experience and education.

acu-, a combining form meaning 'pertaining to a needle': *acuclosure, aculeate, acupressure.*

acuity /əkyōō′itē/, the clearness or sharpness of perception, such as visual acuity.

acuminate wart. See **genital wart.**

acupressure /ak′yəpresh′ər/ [L, *acus*, needle, *pressura*, pressure], a therapeutic technique of applying digital pressure in a specified way on designated points on the body to relieve pain, produce anesthesia, or regulate a body function.

acupuncture /ak′yəpunk′tshər/ [L, *acus* + *punctura*, puncture], a method of producing analgesia or altering the function of a system of the body by inserting fine, wire-thin needles into the skin at specific sites on the body along a series of lines, or channels, called meridians. The needles are twirled or energized electrically or warmed. Acupuncture originated in the Far East and has gained increasing attention in the West since the early 1970s. Research seeks to determine the usefulness of acupuncture and to understand the mechanisms by which it produces analgesia or alters sensory function. Some studies indicate that the analgesic effect of this technique is reversed by naloxone, suggesting that the release of enkephalin is significantly involved. See also **moxibustion.** –**acupuncturist,** *n.*

acupuncture point, one of many discrete points on the skin along the several meridians, or chains of points of the body. Stimulation of any of the various points may induce an increase or decrease in function or sensation in an area or system of the body. The meridians are named and the points numbered to allow specific location of the points to be stimulated in acupuncture, acupressure, or moxibustion.

-acusis. See **-acousia.**

acute /əkyōōt′/ [L, *acutus*, sharp], **1.** (of a disease or disease symptoms) beginning abruptly with marked intensity or sharpness, then subsiding after a relatively short period of time. **2.** sharp or severe. Compare **chronic.**

acute abdomen, an abnormal condition characterized by the acute onset of severe pain within the abdominal cavity. An acute abdomen requires immediate evaluation and diagnosis because it may indicate a condition that calls for surgical intervention. Information about the onset, duration, character, location, and symptoms associated with the pain is critical in making an accurate diagnosis. The patient is asked what decreases or increases the pain; constant, increasing pain is associated with appendicitis and diverticulitis, whereas intermittent pain is more likely indicative of a bowel obstruction, ureteral calculi, or gallstones. Appendicitis may often be differentiated from a perforated ulcer by the slower onset or development of pain. Although sometimes misleading because of referral, radiation, or reflection of pain, the patient's report of the location of the pain may serve to identify a specific organ or system. Factors in the patient's history that are useful in the diagnosis and management of an acute abdomen include changes in bowel habits, weight loss, bloody stool, diarrhea, menses in females, vomiting, and clay-colored stool. Also called **surgical abdomen.** See also **abdominal pain.**

acute abscess, [L, *acutus,* sharp, *abscedere,* to go away], a collection of pus in a body cavity accompanied by localized inflammation, pain, pyrexia, and swelling.

acute air trapping, a condition of bronchiolar collapse that may occur without warning. The patient's respiratory system becomes immobilized in a position of partial exhalation. The individual is unable to inhale or exhale. The patient may panic and become cyanotic. The episode can usually be treated by a series of sharp, forceful lateral squeezes to the sides of the thorax that overcome the pressure of bronchiolar collapse and empty the lungs. Persons prone to episodes of acute air trapping often learn to control exhalations through pursed-lip breathing.

acute alcoholism, drunkenness or intoxication resulting from excessive consumption of alcoholic beverages. The syndrome is temporary and is characterized by depression of the higher nerve centers causing impaired motor control, stupor, lack of coordination, and often nausea, dehydration, headache, and other physical symptoms. Compare **chronic alcoholism.** See also **alcoholism.**

acute angle, [L, *acutus,* + *angulus*], any angle of less than 90 degrees.

acute anicteric hepatitis [Gk, *a,* without, *ikteros,* jaundice, *hepar,* liver, *itis,* inflammation], an acute hepatitis that is not accompanied by jaundice.

acute articular rheumatism [L, *articulare,* to divide into joints; Gk, *rheumatismos,* that which flows], a common form of adult rheumatism, possibly associated with a pyogenic infection in the joints. Symptoms include fever and arthritis.

acute ascending myelitis [L, *ascendere,* to go up; Gk, *myelos,* marrow, *itis,* inflammation], an inflammation of the spinal cord that extends progressively upward with corresponding interference in nerve functions. See also **myelitis.**

acute ascending spinal paralysis, a progressive spinal paralysis that spreads upward toward the brain.

acute atrophic paralysis [Gk, *a,* without, *trophe,* nourishment, *paralyein,* to have palsy], an acute poliomyelitis involving the anterior horns of the spinal cord and resulting in flaccid paralysis of involved muscle groups and later by atrophy.

acute bacterial arthritis. See **septic arthritis.**

acute bronchitis. See **bronchitis.**

acute care, a pattern of health care in which a patient is treated for an acute episode of illness, for the sequelae of an accident or other trauma, or during recovery from surgery. Acute care is usually given in a hospital by specialized personnel using complex and sophisticated technical equipment and materials, and it may involve intensive care or emergency care. This pattern of care is often necessary for only a short time, unlike chronic care.

acute catarrhal sinusitis [Gk, *kata* + *rhoia,* flow; L, *sinus,* hollow], an inflammation that involves the nose and the sinuses.

acute cervicitis. See **cervicitis.**

acute childhood leukemia, a progressive, malignant disease of the blood-forming tissues that is characterized by the uncontrolled proliferation of immature leukocytes and their precursors, particularly in the bone marrow, spleen, and lymph nodes. It is the most frequent cancer in children, with a peak onset occurring between 2 and 5 years of age.

■ OBSERVATIONS: Acute leukemia is classified according to cell type: **acute lymphoid leukemia (ALL)** includes lymphatic, lymphocytic, lymphoblastic, and lymphoblastoid types; **acute nonlymphoid leukemia (ANLL)** includes granulocytic, myelocytic, monocytic, myelogenous, monoblastic, and monomyeloblastic types (the myelocytic and monocytic series are abbreviated **AML**). ALL is predominantly a disease of childhood, whereas AML and ANLL occur in all age groups. The traditional classification of leukemia into chronic and acute types is based on duration or expected course of the illness and the relative maturity of the leukemic cells. The exact cause of the disease is unknown, although various factors are implicated, including genetic defects, immune deficiency, viruses, and carcinogenic environmental factors, primarily ionizing radiation. In acute leukemia, large immature leukocytes accumulate rapidly and infiltrate other tissues of the body, especially the reticuloendothelial system, causing decreased production of erythrocytes and platelets. Neutropenia, anemia, an increased susceptibility to infection and hemorrhage, and weakening of the bones with a tendency to fracture also occur. Initial symptoms of the disease include fever, pallor, fatigue, anorexia, secondary infections (usually of the mouth, throat, or lungs), bone, joint, and abdominal pain, subdermal or submucosal hemorrhage, and enlargement of the spleen, liver, and lymph nodes. Onset may be abrupt or follow a gradual, progressive course. Involvement of the central nervous system may lead to leukemic meningitis. Characteristically, a peripheral blood smear reveals many immature leukocytes. The diagnosis is confirmed by bone marrow aspiration or biopsy and examination, which show a highly elevated number of lymphoblasts with almost complete absence of erythrocytes, granulocytes, and megakaryocytes. The prognosis is poor in untreated cases, and death occurs usually within 6 months after the onset of symptoms. Survival rates have dramatically increased in recent years with the use of antileukemic agents in combination regimens. Remission of 5 years or longer occurs in 50% to 70% of children with ALL, with 20% to 30% achieving complete remission. For children with AML, the prognosis is poorer, and the remission rate is far less.

■ INTERVENTIONS: Treatment of acute leukemia consists of a three-stage process involving the use of chemotherapeutic agents and irradiation. In the first phase (remission induction), complete destruction of all leukemic cells is achieved within a 4- to 6-week period using a combination drug-therapy regimen. The main drugs used in ALL are the corticosteroids, usually three daily oral doses of prednisone; vincristine, administered intravenously once a week; and l-asparaginase, given intramuscularly three times a week for a total of nine doses. Allopurinol, a xanthine-oxidase inhibitor, is usually administered to inhibit uric acid production. Other drugs used in various combination regimens in sequential cycles include methotrexate, 6-mercaptopurine, cyclophosphamide, cytosine arabinoside, hydroxyurea, daunorubicin, and doxorubicin. In children with AML the primary drugs for induction remission are 6-thioguanine, daunomycin, cytosine arabinoside, 5-azacytidine, vincristine, and prednisone. The child is usually hospitalized for part or all of the treatment because of the many side effects of the drugs and the high risk of complications, especially infection and hemorrhage. If severe hemorrhaging occurs and does not respond to local treatment, platelet transfusions may be necessary, and in cases of severe anemia, especially during induction therapy, whole blood or packed red cells may be needed to raise hemoglobin levels. The second stage of treatment involves prophylactic maintenance to prevent leukemic infiltration of the central nervous system. Because chemotherapy drugs do not cross the blood-brain barrier, therapy usually consists of daily high-dose cranial irradiation for about 2 weeks after induction remission and weekly or twice-weekly doses of intrathecal methotrexate, for a total of five or six injections, although in some cases only the drug is given. In small children the irradiation is limited to the cranium to prevent retardation of linear growth, but older children may receive craniospinal radiation. Therapy to maintain remission usually begins after the child is discharged from the hospital and consists of various regimens of drugs in combination. A common schedule includes daily oral doses of 6-mercaptopurine and weekly doses of oral methotrexate, intermittent short-term therapy with prednisone and vincristine, and periodic doses of intrathecal methotrexate for prophylaxis against spread to the central nervous system. Complete blood counts are done weekly or monthly, and bone marrow examinations are performed every 3 to 4 months to detect myelosuppression and drug toxicity. Maintenance therapy is discontinued after a period of 2 to 3 years if initial remission is maintained. Continuous treatment beyond 3 years is not advised, as the adverse affects of the medications increase with prolonged use. Relapse occurs in as many as 20% of treated children. If relapse occurs, the child begins the treatment cycle again, usually with prednisone, vincristine, and a combination of other drugs not previously tried. With each relapse the prognosis becomes poorer. Other treatments for prolonging remission include immunotherapy using periodic inoculation with BCG vaccine or bone marrow transplant, which has been successful in inducing long-term remissions in about 10% to 20% of the cases, especially those with AML or severe, terminal ALL.

■ NURSING CONSIDERATIONS: Nursing care for the child with acute leukemia involves intensive physical and emotional support during all phases of the disease, its diagnosis, and treatment. Foremost is the preparation of the child and parents for the various diagnostic and therapeutic procedures, including venipuncture, bone-marrow aspiration or biopsy, lumbar puncture, and x-ray treatment. Specific medical and nursing management depends on the particular regimen of drug therapy, although most of the chemotherapeutic agents used in treatment cause myelosuppression that may lead to secondary complications of infection, hemorrhage, and anemia. Overwhelming infection is a major problem and one of the most frequent causes of death. Severe neutropenia indicates increased risk of infection. It may occur during immunosuppressive therapy or after prolonged antibiotic therapy. The most common infectious organisms are viruses, especially varicella, herpes zoster, herpes simplex, measles, mumps, rubella, and poliomyelitis, both gram-positive and gram-negative bacteria, including *Staphylo-*

coccus aureus, S. epidermidis, group-A [Grk b]-hemolytic *Streptococcus, Pseudomonas aeruginosa, Escherichia coli, Proteus,* and *Klebsiella,* and various parasites and fungi, especially *Pneumocystis carinii* and *Candida albicans.* To prevent infection, the nurse isolates the child as much as possible, screens visitors for active infection, institutes strict aseptic procedures, monitors temperature closely, evaluates possible sites of infection (such as needle punctures), encourages adequate nutrition, helps the child to avoid exertion or fatigue, and, at discharge, teaches the child and parents the necessity for avoiding all known sources of infection, primarily the common childhood communicable diseases. Preventive measures to control infection also help decrease the tendency toward hemorrhage. Special attention is given to skin care, oral hygiene, cleanliness of the perineal area, and restriction of activities that could result in accidental injury. A major nursing consideration is the management of the many side effects resulting from drug toxicity and irradiation, including nausea and vomiting, anorexia, oral and rectal ulceration, alopecia, hemorrhagic cystitis, and peripheral neuropathy, including weakness and numbing of the extremities and severe jaw pain. Although corticosteroid treatment usually increases the appetite and produces a euphoric sense of well-being in the child, it also causes moon face, which is reversed with cessation of the steroid therapy. During maintenance therapy, the nurse continues to provide emotional support and guidance, specifically teaching parents which side effects are normal reactions to drugs and which indicate toxicity and require medical attention. In terminal stages of the disease, relief of discomfort and pain become the primary focus. Effective measures include careful physical handling of the child, frequent position changes, avoidance of pressure on painful areas, and control of annoying environmental factors, such as excessive light and noise. Nonsalicylate analgesics are used as needed, depending on the severity of pain. See also **acute lymphocytic leukemia, acute myelocytic leukemia, leukemia.**

acute cholecystitis.   See **cholecystitis.**

acute circulatory failure /sur′kyələtôr′ē/,   a drop in heart output resulting from cardiac or noncardiac causes and leading to tissue hypoxia. Acute circulatory failure usually happens so rapidly that the body does not have time to adjust to the changes. If not controlled immediately, the condition usually progresses to one of shock syndrome.

acute circumscribed edema [L, *circum,* around, *scribere,* to draw; Gk, *oidema,* swelling],   a localized edema, often associated with an inflammatory lesion or process.

acute confusional state,   a form of central nervous system dysfunction caused by interference with the metabolic or other biochemical processes essential for normal brain functioning. Symptoms may include disturbances in cognition, levels of awareness, memory, and orientation, accompanied by restlessness, apprehension, irritability, and apathy. The condition may be associated with delirium, toxic psychosis, or acute brain syndrome.

acute decubitus [L, *decumbere,* to lie down],   an ulceration that may develop secondary to increased pressure.

acute delirium,   an episode of delirium that is sudden, severe, and transient. See also **delirium.**

acute diarrhea [Gk, *dia, rhein,* to flow],   a sudden severe attack of diarrhea.

acute diffuse peritonitis [L, *diffundere,* to pour out; Gk, *peri,* near, *tenein,* to stretch, *itis,* inflammation],   an acute widespread attack of peritonitis affecting most of the peritoneum and usually caused by a perforation of the stomach or appendix. Also called **generalized peritonitis.**

acute disease, a disease characterized by a relatively short duration of symptoms that are usually severe. An episode of acute disease results in recovery to a state comparable to the patient's state of health and activity before the disease, in passage into a chronic phase, or in death. Examples are adenoviral pharyngitis, caisson disease, mountain sickness. See also **chronic disease.**

acute endarteritis [Gk, *endon,* within, *arteria,* windpipe, *itis,* inflammation], an inflamed condition of the cells lining an artery. It may be caused by an infection or the proliferation of fibrous tissue inside the wall of a large artery.

acute epiglottitis, a severe, rapidly progressing bacterial infection of the upper respiratory tract that occurs in young children, primarily between 2 and 7 years of age. It is characterized by sore throat, croupy stridor, and an inflamed epiglottis, which may cause sudden respiratory obstruction and be quickly fatal. The infection is generally caused by *Haemophilus influenzae,* type B, although streptococci may occasionally be the causative agent. Transmission occurs by infection with airborne particles or contact with infected secretions. The diagnosis is made by bacteriologic identification of *H. influenzae,* type B, in a specimen taken from the upper respiratory tract or in the blood. An x-ray film of the neck from the side shows an enlarged epiglottis and distention of the hypopharynx, which distinguishes the condition from croup. Direct visualization of the inflamed, cherry-red epiglottis by depression of the tongue or indirect laryngoscopy is also diagnostic but may produce total acute obstruction and should be attempted only by trained personnel with equipment to establish an airway or to provide respiratory resuscitation, if necessary. Compare **croup.**

■ OBSERVATIONS: The onset of the infection is abrupt, and it progresses rapidly. The first signs—sore throat, hoarseness, fever, and dysphagia—may be followed by an inability to swallow, drooling, varying degrees of dyspnea, inspiratory stridor, marked irritability and apprehension, and a tendency to sit upright and hyperextend the neck in order to breathe. Difficulty in breathing may progress to severe respiratory distress in minutes or hours. Suprasternal, supraclavicular, intercostal, and subcostal inspiratory retractions may be visible. The hypoxic child appears frightened and anxious; the color of the skin ranges from pallor to cyanosis.

■ INTERVENTIONS: Establishment of an airway is urgent, either by endotracheal intubation or by tracheostomy. Humidity and oxygen are provided, and airway secretions are drained or suctioned. Intravenous fluids are usually required, and antibiotic therapy is initiated immediately, usually with penicillin, ampicillin, or chloramphenicol. Sedatives are contraindicated because of their depressant effect on the respiratory system, and steroids, antihistamines, and adrenergic drugs are not usually of any therapeutic value.

■ NURSING CONSIDERATIONS: The nurse may assist with intubation or tracheostomy once the diagnosis is confirmed. Intensive nursing care is required for a child with acute epiglottitis. The most acute phase of the condition passes within 24 to 48 hours, and intubation is rarely needed beyond 3 to 4 days. As the child responds to therapy, breathing becomes easier, and there is usually rapid recovery so that bed rest and quiet activity to relieve boredom become primary nursing concerns. The infection may spread, causing such complications as otitis media, pneumonia, and bronchiolitis. Complications of the tracheostomy may also

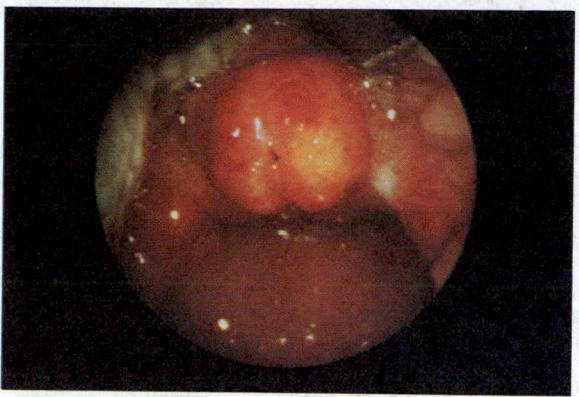

Acute epiglottitis *(Bingham, 1992/Courtesy Dr. Bruce Benjamin)*

develop, including infection, atelectasis, cannula occlusion, tracheal bleeding, granulation, stenosis, and delayed healing of the stoma. Also called **acute epiglottiditis.**

acute febrile polyneuritis. See **Guillain-Barré syndrome.**

acute fibrinous pericarditis [L, *fibra,* fibrous; Gk, *peri,* near, *kardia,* heart, *itis,* inflammation], an acute inflammation of the pericardium with fibers extending into the pericardial sac. The endothelial cells of the pericardium become inflamed.

acute gastritis. See **gastritis.**

acute glaucoma. See **glaucoma.**

acute glomerulonephritis. See **postinfectious glomerulonephritis.**

acute goiter, [L, *guttur,* throat], a condition of sudden enlargement of the thyroid gland.

acute granulocytic leukemia (AGL). See **acute myelocytic leukemia (AML).**

acute hallucinatory paranoia, a form of psychosis in which hallucinations are combined with the systematized delusions.

acute hallucinosis. See **alcoholic hallucinosis.**

acute hemorrhagic conjunctivitis, a highly contagious eye disease usually caused by enterovirus type 70. The disease is found primarily in densely populated humid areas, particularly the developing countries or places with a large immigrant population. Clinical features include sudden onset of ocular pain, itching, redness, photophobia, edema of the eyelid, and profuse watery discharge. Spontaneous improvement occurs within 2 to 4 days and is complete by 7 to 10 days. Treatment consists of hygienic measures and ophthalmic preparations.

acute hemorrhagic leukoencephalitis. See **acute necrotizing hemorrhagic encephalopathy.**

acute hemorrhagic pancreatitis [Gk, *haima,* blood, *rhegnynei,* to gush, *pan,* all, *kreas,* flesh], a potentially fatal inflammation of the pancreas characterized by bleeding, tissue necrosis, and digestive tract paralysis.

acute hydrocele [Gk, *hydor,* water, *kele,* hernia], a benign fluid accumulation within the tunica vaginalis that causes swelling of the scrotum. It is a frequent, minor disorder in infant boys, as well as adults. Surgery eliminates the condition.

acute hypoxia, a sudden or rapid depletion in available oxygen at the tissue level, as may result from asphyxia, airway obstruction, acute hemorrhage, blockage of the alveoli by edema or infectious exudate, or abrupt cardiorespiratory failure. Clinical signs may include hypoventilation or hyperventilation to the point of air hunger and neurologic deficits ranging from headache and confusion to loss of consciousness.

acute idiopathic polyneuritis. See **Guillain-Barré syndrome.**

acute idiopathic thrombocytopenic purpura. See **idiopathic thrombocytopenic purpura.**

acute illness, any illness characterized by signs and symptoms that are of a short duration, are usually severe, and impair the normal functioning of the patient.

acute immune disease. See **autoimmunity.**

acute infectious paralysis [L, *inficere,* to stain; Gk, *paralyein,* to be palsied], **1.** an alternative term for acute anterior poliomyelitis. **2.** infectious polyneuritis.

acute intermittent porphyria (AIP), a genetically transmitted metabolic disorder characterized by acute attacks of neurologic dysfunction that can be started by environmental or endogenous factors. Women are affected more frequently than men, and attacks often are precipitated by starvation or crash dieting, alcohol ingestion, bacterial or viral infections, and a wide range of pharmaceutic products. Any part of the nervous system can be affected, and a common effect is mild to severe abdominal pain associated with autonomic neuropathy. Other effects can include peripheral neuropathy, hyponatremia, and organic brain dysfunction marked by seizures, coma, hallucinations, and respiratory paralysis. A frequent diagnostic factor is a high level of porphyrin precursors in the urine, which usually increase during periods of acute attacks. Treatment is generally symptomatic, with emphasis on pain control and education of the patient about environmental factors, particularly medications, that are known to cause an onset of symptoms. A high-carbohydrate diet is reported to reduce the risk of acute attacks because glucose tends to block the induction of hepatic gamma-aminolevulinic acid (ALA) synthetase, an enzyme involved in the porphyrias. See also **porphyria.**

acute interstitial nephritis. See **interstitial nephritis.**

acute laryngotracheobronchitis. See **croup.**

acute lymphoblastic leukemia. See **acute lymphocytic leukemia.**

acute lymphocytic leukemia (ALL), a progressive, malignant disease characterized by large numbers of immature cells, resembling lymphoblasts in the bone marrow, circulating blood, lymph nodes, spleen, liver, and other organs. The number of normal blood cells is reduced. More than three-fourths of the cases in the United States occur in children, with the greatest number diagnosed between 2 and 5 years of age. The risk of the disease is increased for people with Down syndrome and for siblings of leukemia patients. The disease has a sudden onset and rapid progression marked by fever, pallor, anorexia, fatigue, anemia, hemorrhage, bone pain, splenomegaly, and recurrent infection. Blood and bone marrow studies are used for diagnosis and for determining the type of proliferating lymphocyte, which may be B cells, T cells (which usually respond poorly to therapy), or null cells (as are found in most cases). Treatment includes intensive combination chemotherapy, therapy for secondary infections and hyperuricemia, irradiation, and intrathecal methotrexate.

acute lymphoid leukemia (ALL). See **acute childhood leukemia.**

acute mastitis. See **mastitis.**

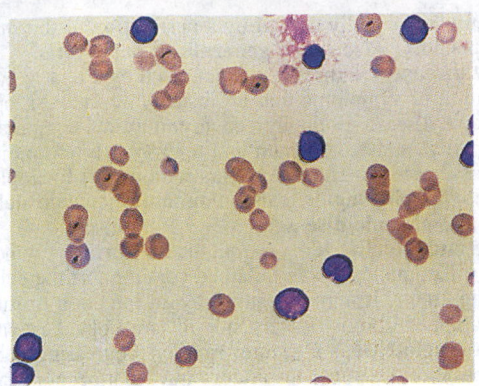

Peripheral blood smear of acute lymphocytic leukemia
(Zitelli, 1992)

acute mountain sickness. See **altitude sickness.**

acute myelitis, a sudden, severe inflammation of the spinal cord. See also **acute transverse myelitis, myelitis.**

acute myelocytic leukemia (AML), a malignant neoplasm of blood-forming tissues characterized by the uncontrolled proliferation of immature granular leukocytes that usually have azurophilic Auer rods in their cytoplasm. Symptoms that appear gradually are spongy bleeding gums, anemia, fatigue, fever, dyspnea, moderate splenomegaly, joint and bone pains, and repeated infections. AML occurs most frequently in adolescents and young adults. The risk of the disease is increased among people who have been exposed to massive doses of radiation and who have certain blood dyscrasias, such as polycythemia vera, primary thrombocytopenia, and refractory anemia. Variants of AML, in which only one cell line proliferates, are erythroid, eosinophilic, basophilic, monocytic, and megakaryocytic leukemias. The diagnosis is based on blood counts and bone marrow biopsies. Radiotherapy, biotherapy, and bone marrow transplantation are used, but long remissions resulting from any form of treatment are rare. Also called **acute granulocytic leukemia (AGL), acute myelogenous leukemia, acute nonlymphocytic leukemia (ANLL), myeloid leukemia, splenomedullary leukemia, splenomyelogenous leukemia.** See also **acute childhood leukemia, chronic myelocytic leukemia.**

acute myocardial infarction (AMI) [L, *acutus,* + Gk, *mys,* muscle, *kardia,* heart; L, *infarcire,* to stuff], the early critical stage of mycardial infarction, characterized by elevated ST segments in the reflecting leads. See **myocardial infarction.**

acute necrotizing hemorrhagic encephalopathy, a degenerative disease of the brain, characterized by marked edema, numerous minute hemorrhages, necrosis of blood vessel walls, especially those of small veins, demyelination of nerve fibers, and infiltration of the meninges with neutrophils, lymphocytes, and histiocytes. Typical signs are severe headache, fever, and vomiting; convulsions may occur, and the patient may rapidly lose consciousness. Treatment consists of decompression by withdrawing cerebrospinal fluids. Also called **acute hemorrhagic leukoencephalitis.**

acute necrotizing ulcerative gingivitis (ANUG), a distinct, recurring periodontal disease that primarily affects the

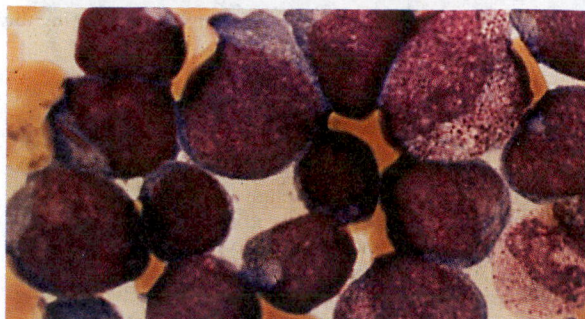

Peripheral blood smear in acute myelocytic leukemia
(Zitelli, 1992)

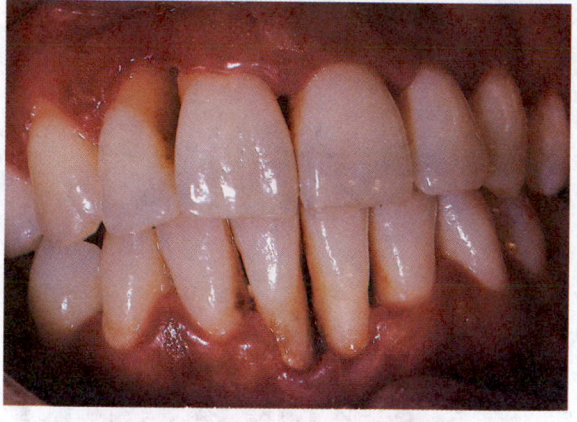

Acute necrotizing ulcerative gingivitis (Murray, 1990)

interdental papillae, causing necrosis and ulceration of the gums and throat, fever, and enlarged lymph nodes in the neck. It is usually associated with poor oral hygiene and is most common in conditions in which there is crowding and malnutrition. Treatment includes peroxide mouthwashes, antibiotics, analgesics, and dental care. Also called **trench mouth, Vincent's angina, Vincent's infection.**

acute nephritis, a sudden inflammation of the kidney, characterized by albuminuria and hematuria, but without edema or urine retention. It affects children most commonly and usually involves only a few glomeruli. See also **nephritis.**

acute nicotine poisoning [L, *Nicotiana, potio,* drink], a toxic effect produced by nicotine, usually in the insecticide form. Characteristics include burning sensation in the mouth, nausea and vomiting, diarrhea, palpitations, pulmonary edema, and convulsions that may lead to death.

acute nongonorrheal vulvitis [L, *non,* not; Gk, *gone,* seed + *rhoia,* flow; L, *vulva,* wrapper; Gk, *itis,* inflammation], an inflammation of the vulva resulting from chafing, accumulation of sebaceous material, or other causes that are nonvenereal.

acute nonlymphocytic leukemia. See **acute myelocytic leukemia.**

acute nonspecific pericarditis [Gk, *peri,* around, *kardia,* heart, *itis,* inflammation], an inflammation of the pericardium, with or without effusion. It often is associated with myocarditis but usually resolves without complications. See also **pericarditis.**

acute pain, severe pain, as may follow surgery or trauma or accompany myocardial infarction or other conditions and diseases. Acute pain occurring in the first 24 to 48 hours after surgery is often difficult to relieve, even with drugs. Some studies show that patients over 50 years of age need less analgesia to relieve acute pain than do younger patients. Another study indicates that 23% of surgical patients, except for orthopedic patients, do not require analgesia. Acute pain in individuals with orthopedic problems originates from the periosteum, the joint surfaces, and the arterial walls. Muscle pain associated with bone surgery results from muscle ischemia rather than muscle tension. Acute abdominal pain often causes the individual involved to lie on one side and draw up the legs in the fetal position. Compare **chronic pain.** See also **pain intervention.**

acute pancreatitis [Gk, *pan,* all, *kreas,* flesh, *itis,* inflam-

mation], a sudden inflammation of the pancreas marked by symptoms of acute abdomen and escape of pancreatic enzymes into the pancreas tissues. The condition is associated with biliary disease or alcoholism. See also **pancreatitis.**

acute paranoid disorder, a psychopathologic condition characterized by a persecutory delusional system of rapid onset, quick development, and short duration, usually lasting less than 6 months. The disorder, which rarely becomes chronic, is most commonly seen in persons who have experienced drastic changes in their environment, such as immigrants, refugees, prisoners, military inductees, and, in a less severe form, those leaving home for the first time.

acute pharyngitis, a sudden, severe inflammation of the pharynx. See also **pharyngitis.**

acute pleurisy, an inflammation of the pleura, often secondary to a disease of the lung. It is characterized by irritation without recognizable effusion and is localized. See also **pleurisy.**

acute primary myocarditis, **1.** an inflammation of the heart muscle caused by a bacterial infection initiated locally or carried through the bloodstream. **2.** a severe inflammation of the heart muscle associated with degeneration in the muscle fibers with the release of leukocytes into the interstitial tissues. See also **myocarditis.**

acute promyelocytic leukemia, a malignancy of the blood-forming tissues, characterized by the proliferation of promyelocytes and blast cells with distinctive Auer rods. Symptoms include severe bleeding, bruises, and low fibrinogen level and platelet count. Management of the disease requires replacement of coagulation factors and the administration of cytotoxic drugs. See **leukemia.** (See Fig. p. 32.)

acute prostatitis [L, *acutus,* sharp; Gk, *prostates,* one standing before, *itis,* inflammation], a sudden, severe inflammation of the prostate gland. See also **prostate, prostatitis.**

acute psychosis, one of a group of disorders in which the ego disintegrates and functioning is either impaired or inhibited. The ability to process information is diminished and disordered. The cause of the particular disorder may be a known physiologic abnormality. In other cases the physiologic abnormality may not be recognized, but the defect in function is clearly present.

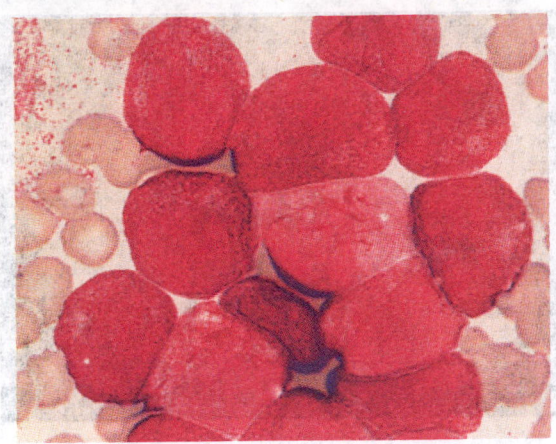

Acute promyelocytic leukemia (Hayhoe, 1992)

acute pyelonephritis.   See **pyelonephritis.**

acute pyogenic arthritis,   an acute bacterial infection of one or more joints, caused by trauma or a penetrating wound and occurring most frequently in children. Typical signs are pain, redness, and swelling in the affected joint, muscular spasms in the area, chills, fever, diaphoresis, and leukocytosis. Treatment consists of immobilization of the joint, the intravenous administration of an antibiotic, analgesia, and sedation. If required, the joint may be irrigated with normal saline and an antibiotic. Hospitalization is usually required.

acute radial nerve palsy,   a type of mononeuropathy characterized by damage to the radial nerve and consequent weakening of the muscles of the forearm. It may be caused by excessive compression of the radial nerve against a hard surface in individuals insensitized by the intake of alcohol or sedatives. It may also be caused by the repeated compression of the nerve by various weights, such as the weight of the head of a bed partner. Time and the withdrawal of causative compression usually ensure full recovery.

acute radiation exposure,   exposure of short duration to intense ionizing radiation, usually occurring as the result of an accident. Exposure of the whole body to approximately 10,000 rad (100 gray) causes neurologic and cardiovascular breakdown and is fatal within 24 hours. A dose between 500 and 1200 rad (5 and 12 gray) destroys GI mucosa, produces bloody diarrhea, and may cause death in several days. Death may occur weeks after exposure to a dose of 200 to 500 rad (2 to 5 gray) because of the destructive effect on blood-forming organs, but 600 rad (6 gray) is generally considered the fatal dose. See also **radiation exposure.**

acute rejection [L, *rejicere,* to throw back],   the rapid reaction against allograph or xenograph tissue that is incompatible after about a week's delay, during which the immune response increases in intensity.

acute respiratory distress syndrome.   See **adult respiratory distress syndrome.**

acute respiratory failure (ARF) [L, *acutus,* + *respirare,* respiratory, *fallere,* to deceive],   a sudden inability of the lungs to maintain normal respiratory function. It may be caused by an obstruction in the airways or failure of the lungs to exchange gases in the alveoli.

acute rheumatic arthritis,   arthritis that occurs during the acute phase of rheumatic fever.

acute rhinitis.   See **rhinitis.**

acute schizophrenia,   a form of psychosis that is characterized by the sudden onset of personality disorganization with symptoms that include disturbances in thought, mood, and behavior. Episodes appear suddenly in persons whose previous behavior has been relatively normal and are usually of short duration. Recurrent episodes are common, and in some instances a more chronic type of the disorder may develop. Also called **undifferentiated schizophrenia.** See also **schizophrenia, schizophreniform disorder.**

acute secondary myocarditis,   a sudden severe inflammation of the heart muscle, secondary to a disease of the endocardium or the pericardium, or a generalized infection. See also **myocarditis.**

acute septic myocarditis [Gk, *septikos,* putrid, *mys,* muscle, *kardia,* heart, *itis,* inflammation],   a severe inflammation of the myocardium associated with pus formation, necrosis, and abscess formation. See also **myocarditis.**

acute suppurative sinusitis [L, *acutus,* sharp + *suppurare,* to form pus + *sinus,* hollow; Gk, *itis,* inflammation],   a purulent infection of the sinuses. Symptoms are pain over the inflamed area, headache, chills, and fever.

acute tonsillitis [L, *acutus,* sharp + *tonsilla;* Gk, *itis,* inflammation],   an inflammation of tonsil(s) associated with a catarrhal exudate over the tonsil or the discharge of caseous or suppurative material from the tonsil crypts.

acute toxicity,   the harmful effect of a toxic agent that manifests itself in seconds, minutes, hours, or days after entering the patient.

acute transverse myelitis,   an inflammation of the entire thickness of the spinal cord, affecting both the sensory and the motor nerves. It can develop rapidly, accompanied by necrosis and neurologic deficit that commonly persist after recovery. Patients who develop spastic reflexes soon after the onset of this disease are more likely to recover. This disorder may develop from a variety of causes, such as acute multiple sclerosis, measles, pneumonia, and the ingestion of certain toxic agents, such as carbon monoxide, lead, and arsenic. Such poisonous substances can destroy the entire circumference of the spinal cord, including the myelin sheaths, the axis cylinders, and the neurons, and can also cause hemorrhage and necrosis. There is no effective treatment, and the prognosis for complete recovery is poor. Nursing care includes frequent assessment of vital signs, vigilance for signs of spinal shock, maintenance of Foley catheters, and proper skin care.

acute tubular necrosis (ATN) [L, *tubulus,* tubule; Gk, *nekros,* dead, *osis,* condition],   sudden failure of the kidney tubules. The condition is commonly caused by an interruption of the blood supply to the tubules, resulting in ischemia.

acute urethral syndrome [Gk, *ourethra,* urethra, *syn,* together, *dromos,* course],   a group of pelvic area symptoms experienced by women, including dysuria, urinary frequency, urinary tenesmus, lower back pain, and suprapubic aching and cramping. However, clinical evidence of a pathogen or other factor to account for the symptoms is usually absent.

acyanotic /ā′sī·ənot′ik/ [Gk, *a,* not, *kyanos,* blue],   pertaining to the absence of the blue appearance of the skin and mucous membranes. See also **cyanosis.**

acyanotic congenital defect /āsī′ənot′ik/ [Gk, *a, kyanos,* not blue], a congenital heart defect that does not produce cyanosis under normal circumstances. However, the condition does increase the load on the pulmonary circulation, and cyanosis, right ventricular failure, or other complications may result from physical exertion.

acyclovir /əsī′klōvir/, an antiviral (acycloguanosine).
■ INDICATIONS: It is prescribed topically in an ointment for the treatment of herpes simplex keratitis and both topically and systemically in other types of herpes infections, including genital herpes. Acyclovir appears to act selectively by inhibiting the functions of herpesvirus DNA molecules, but the drug has no demonstrated activity against other types of viral infections.
■ CONTRAINDICATION: Known sensitivity to this drug prohibits its use.
■ ADVERSE EFFECTS: After topical use, irritation or pruritus may occur; after systemic use, diaphoresis, headache, and nausea may occur. When it is administered intravenously in the treatment of immunosuppressed patients, there may be pain at the site of the injection.

acyesis /ā′sī·ē′sis/, **1.** the absence of pregnancy. **2.** a condition of sterility in women.

acylation /as′ilā′shən/, the incorporation into a molecule of an organic compound of an acyl group.

a.d., abbreviation for **auris dextra,** or right ear.

ad-, ac-, af-, ag-, ap-, as-, at-, a prefix meaning 'to, toward, addition to, or intensification': *adneural, adoral, adrenal.*

-ad, a suffix meaning 'toward (a specified terminus)': *cephalad.*

A/D, abbreviation for **analog-to-digital.**

ADA, 1. abbreviation for *American Dental Association.* **2.** abbreviation for *American Diabetes Association.* **3.** abbreviation for *American Dietetic Association.* **4.** abbreviation for **adenosine deaminase.**

adactyly /ādak′tilē/ [Gk, *a, daktylos,* not finger or toe], a congenital defect in which one or more digits of the hand or foot are missing.

Adalat, a trademark for a calcium channel blocker (nifedipine).

adamantinoma, adamantoblastoma. See **ameloblastoma.**

ADAMHA, abbreviation for United States *Alcohol, Drug Abuse, and Mental Health Administration.*

Adam's apple, *informal.* the bulge at the front of the neck produced by the thyroid cartilage of the larynx. Also called **laryngeal prominence.**

Adams-Stokes syndrome [Robert Adams, Dublin surgeon, b. 1791; William Stokes, Dublin physician, b. 1804], a condition characterized by sudden recurrent episodes of loss of consciousness because of incomplete heart block. Seizures may accompany the episodes. Also called **Stokes-Adams syndrome.** See also **infranodal block.**

adaptation /ad′aptā′shən/ [L, *adaptatio,* act of adapting], a change or response to stress of any kind, such as inflammation of the nasal mucosa in infectious rhinitis or an increase in crying in a frightened child. Adaptation may be normal, self-protective, and developmental, such as a child learning to talk; it may be all encompassing, creating further stress, such as polycythemia, which occurs naturally at high altitudes to provide more oxygen-carrying red blood cells, but which may also lead to thrombosis, venous congestion, or edema. The degree and nature of adaptation shown by a patient is evaluated regularly by the nurse. It is a measure of the effectiveness of nursing care, the course of the disease, and the ability of the patient to cope with stress. Compare **accommodation.**

adaptation model, (in nursing) a conceptual framework that focuses on the patient as an adaptive system, one in which nursing intervention is required when a deficit develops in the patient's ability to cope with the internal and external demands of the environment. These demands are classified in four groups: physiologic needs, the need for a positive self-concept, the need to perform social roles, and the need to balance dependence and independence. The nurse assesses the patient's maladaptive response and identifies the kind of demand that is causing the problem. Nursing care is planned to promote adaptive responses to cope successfully with the current stress on the patient's well-being. This model, first proposed by Sister Callista Roy, is frequently used as a conceptual framework for programs of nursing education.

adaptation syndrome. See **general adaptation syndrome.**

adapted clothing, clothing that has been modified, as with Velcro fasteners, to permit disabled persons to dress themselves with a minimum of difficulty.

adaptive device /adap′tiv/ [L, *adaptatio,* process of adapting; OFr, *devise*], any structure, design, instrument, contrivance, or equipment that enables a person with a disability to function independently. Also called **self-help device.**

adaptive hypertrophy [L, *adaptatio,* process of adapting; Gk, *hyper,* excessive, *trophe,* nourishment], an increase in amount of tissue that compensates for a loss of the same or similar tissue so that function is not impaired.

adaptive response, an appropriate reaction to an environmental demand.

adaptor RNA. See **transfer RNA.**

ADC, abbreviation for **AIDS-dementia complex.**

Addams, Jane (1860–1935), an American social reformer. In 1889 she founded Hull House in Chicago, one of the first social settlements in the United States, where volunteers from many disciplines, including nursing, lived and continued working in their professions. She was at the center of most of the social reforms of her time and was an inspiration to those in the nursing profession who were striving to establish high educational standards and better working conditions. She was corecipient of the Nobel peace prize in 1931.

addict /ad′ikt/ [L, *addicere,* to devote], a person who has become physiologically or psychologically dependent upon a chemical, such as alcohol or other drugs, so that normal social, occupational, and other responsible life functions are disrupted.

addiction /ədik′shən/ [L, *addictere,* to devote], compulsive, uncontrollable dependence on a substance, habit, or practice to such a degree that cessation causes severe emotional, mental, or physiologic reactions. Compare **habituation.**

addictive personality /ədik′tiv/, a personality marked by traits of compulsive and habitual use of a substance or practice to cope with psychic pain engendered by conflict and anxiety.

Addis count, a method for counting red blood cells, white blood cells, epithelial cells, casts, and protein content in a sedimented 12-hour urine sample. Results are expressed as the number of each formed element excreted per 24 hours. The count is useful for diagnosing and managing kidney disease, because there should be none or nearly none of these components in the urine.

addisonian anemia.   See **pernicious anemia.**

addisonian crisis, Addison's crisis.   See **adrenal crisis.**

addisonism, [Thomas Addison, London physician, b.1793], a condition characterized by the physical signs of Addison's disease, although loss of adrenocortical functions is not involved. The signs include increased pigmentation of the skin and mucous membranes, general debility, and a tendency to develop tubercular infections.

Addison's disease [Thomas Addison, London physician, b. 1793], a life-threatening condition caused by partial or complete failure of adrenocortical function, often resulting from autoimmune processes, infection (especially tubercular or fungal), neoplasm, or hemorrhage in the gland. All three general functions of the adrenal cortex are lost: glucocorticoid, mineralocorticoid, and androgenic. Also called **addisonism, Addison's syndrome.** See also **adrenal crisis.**
■ OBSERVATIONS: The disease is characterized by weakness, decreased endurance, increased pigmentation of the skin and mucous membranes, described as bronzing, anorexia, dehydration, weight loss, GI disturbances, anxiety, depression, and other emotional distress, and decreased tolerance to cold. The onset is usually gradual, occurring over a period of weeks or months. Laboratory tests show abnormally low blood concentrations of sodium and glucose, a greater than normal level of serum potassium, and a decreased urinary output of certain steroids. The diagnosis is established if, after stimulation with adrenocorticosteroids, the amount of cortisol in the plasma and steroid in the urine fails to increase.
■ INTERVENTIONS: Treatment includes replacement therapy with glucocorticoid and mineralocorticoid drugs, an adequate intake of fluids, control of sodium and potassium balance, and a diet high in complex carbohydrate and protein. The person's requirements for glucocorticoid, mineralocorticoid, and salt are increased by stress, as in infection, trauma, and surgical procedures. Follow-up care includes frequent monitoring of sugar in the blood or urine, urinary acetone, and continued administration of corticoid drugs.
■ NURSING CONSIDERATIONS: The complications of Addison's disease include high fever, psychotic behavior, and adrenal crisis (addisonian crisis). Under careful management, the patient's resistance to infection, capacity for work, and general well-being may be maintained. Nurses administer steroid and other drugs, observe the patient for signs of abnormal sodium and potassium levels, monitor body weight and fluid intake and output, and encourage an adequate intake of nutrients. The patient needs protection against stress while in the hospital and instruction in the importance of avoiding stress at home. The significance of emotional distress, the value of wearing a medical-alert bracelet or tag, the signs of impending crisis, the use of a prepared kit for emergencies, and the importance of scrupulous attention to drug and diet regimens are emphasized before discharge. Discharge teaching also emphasizes the need to take cortisone after meals or with milk to avoid gastric irritation and the development of ulcers.

Addison's keloid.   See **morphea.**

Addison's syndrome.   See **Addison's disease.**

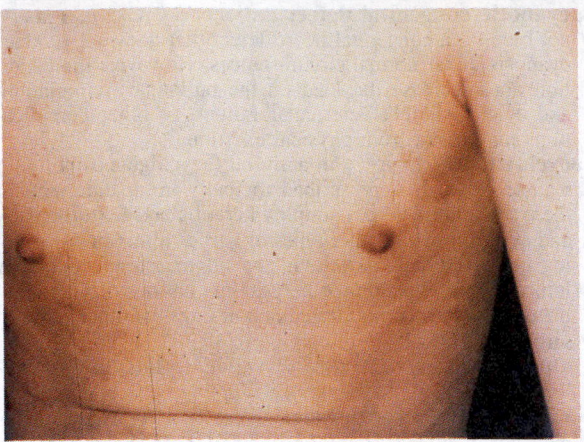

Hyperpigmentation of Addison's disease
(Zitelli, 1992/Courtesy Dr. M. New)

addition [L, *additio*, something added], a chemical reaction in which two complete molecules combine to form a new product, usually by attachment to carbon atoms at a double or triple bond of one of the molecules.

additive effect /ad'itiv/ [L, *additio*, something added, *effectus*], the combined effect of drugs that when used in combination produce an enhanced effect that is no greater than the sum of their separately measured individual effects.

adduct /ədukt'/ [L, *adducere*, to bring to], to move toward the median line or axis of the body.

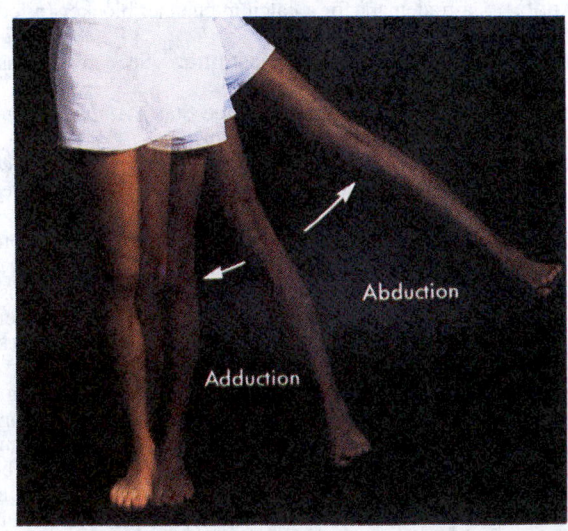

Adduction (Thibodeau, 1993)

adduction /əduk'shən/ [L, *adducere,* to bring to], movement of a limb toward the axis of the body. Compare **abduction.**

adductor /əduk'tər/, a muscle that acts to draw a part toward the axis or midline of the body. Compare **abductor, tensor.**

adductor brevis, a somewhat triangular muscle in the thigh and one of the five medial femoral muscles. Arising from the inferior ramus of the pubis between the gracilis and the obturator externus, it passes downward, backward, and to the side to insert into the line leading from the lesser trochanter to the linea aspera of the femur. It is innervated by a branch of the obturator nerve, which contains fibers from the third and fourth lumbar nerves, and it acts to adduct and rotate the thigh medially and to flex the leg. Compare **adductor longus, adductor magnus, gracilis, pectineus.**

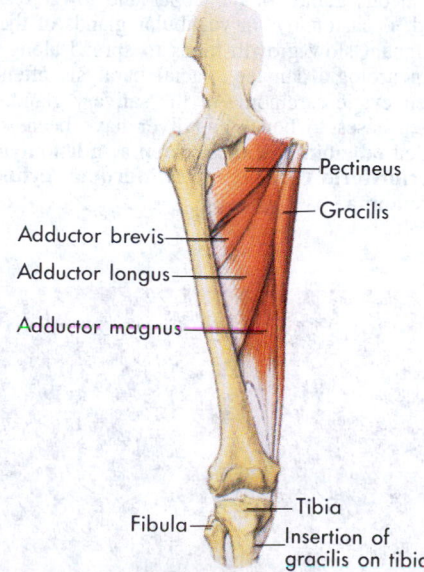

Adductor brevis, adductor longus, and adductor mangus muscles of the anterior thigh
(Thibodeau, 1993/John V. Hagen)

adductor canal, a triangular channel beneath the sartorius muscle and between the adductor longus and vastus medialis through which the femoral vessels and the saphenous nerve pass. Also called **Hunter's canal, subsartorial canal.**

adductor longus, the most superficial of the three adductor muscles of the thigh and one of five medial femoral muscles. A triangular muscle that arises from the anterior surface of the pubis, it spreads to form a broad fleshy belly, passing downward, backward, and to the side to insert into the linea aspera of the femur, between the vastus medialis and the adductor magnus. It is innervated by a branch of the obturator nerve, which contains fibers from the third and

fourth lumbar nerves, and it functions to adduct and flex the thigh. Compare **adductor brevis, adductor magnus, gracilis, pectineus.**

adductor magnus, the long, heavy triangular muscle of the medial aspect of the thigh. It arises from the inferior rami of the ischium and pubis and the inferior margin of the ischial tuberosity. The fibers of the muscle insert into the rough surface of the greater trochanter, into the linea aspera via a broad aponeurosis, and into the distal third of the femur via a rounded, thick tendon. The muscle is innervated by the obturator nerve, which contains fibers of the third and fourth lumbar nerves, and by a branch of the sciatic nerve. The adductor magnus acts to adduct the thigh. The proximal portion acts to rotate the thigh medially and to flex it on the hip; the distal portion acts to extend the thigh and rotate it laterally.

aden-. See **adeno-.**

adenalgia /ad'ənal'jə/ [Gk, *aden,* gland, *algos,* pain], a pain in any of the glands. Also called **adenodynia** /ad'ənōdin'ē·ə/.

adenectomy /ad'ənek'təmē/ [Gk, *aden* + *ektome,* excision], the surgical removal of any gland.

Aden fever. See **dengue fever.**

-adenia, a suffix meaning '(condition of the) glands': *anadenia, heteradenia.*

adenine /ad'ənin/, a purine-base component of the nucleic acids, DNA and RNA, and a constituent of cyclic AMP and the adenosine portion of AMP, ADP, and ATP. See **ATP, DNA, RNA.**

adenine arabinoside. See **vidarabine.**

adenine-D-ribose. See **adenosine.**

adenitis /ad'ənī'tis/, an inflammatory condition of a lymph node or gland. Acute adenitis of the cervical lymph nodes manifests itself as a sore throat and stiff neck, simulating mumps if severe. It is usually a sign of secondary infection related to an oral, pharyngeal, or ear infection. Scarlet fever may cause an acute suppurative cervical adenitis, as may infectious mononucleosis. Swelling of the lymph nodes in the back of the neck is often the result of a scalp infection,

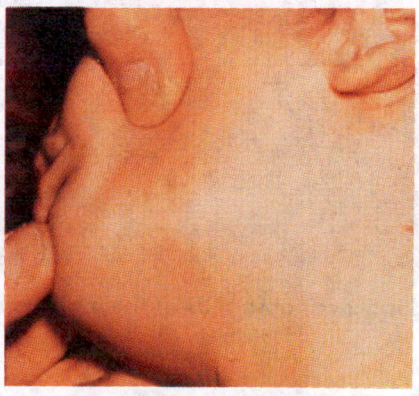

Myobacterial adenitis
(Zitelli, 1992/Courtesy Dr. Michael Sherlock)

insect bite, or infestation by head lice. Inflammation of the lymph nodes of the mesenteric portion of the peritoneum often produces pain and other symptoms similar to those of appendicitis. Mesenteric adenitis may be mistaken for appendicitis, but, characteristically, mesenteric adenitis is preceded by a respiratory infection, the pain is less localized and less constant than in appendicitis, and it does not increase in severity. Generalized adenitis is a secondary symptom of syphilis. Therapy requires treatment of the primary infection by the administration of antimicrobial agents, application of warm compresses, and, in rare cases, incision and drainage. Also called **lymphadenitis.** Compare **acinitis.**

adeno-, aden-, a prefix meaning 'pertaining to a gland': *adenocarcinoma, adenocellulitis, adenofibrosis.*

adenoacanthoma /ad'ənō·ak'anthō'mə/ [Gk, *aden* + *akantha*, thorn, *oma*, tumor], a neoplasm that may be malignant or benign, derived from glandular tissue with squamous differentiation shown by some of the cells.

adenoameloblastoma /ad'ənō·amel'ōblastō'mə/, *pl.* **adenoameloblastomas, adenoameloblastomata,** a benign tumor of the maxilla composed of ducts lined with columnar or cuboidal epithelial cells. It develops in tissue that normally gives rise to the teeth, and it is most often seen in young people.

adenoassociated virus (AAV) /ad'ənō-/, a defective virus that can reproduce only in the presence of adenoviruses. It is not yet known what role, if any, these organisms have in causing disease.

adenocarcinoma /ad'ənōkärsinō'mə/, *pl.* **adenocarcinomas, adenocarcinomata** [Gk, *aden* + *karkinos*, crab, *oma*], any one of a large group of malignant, epithelial cell tumors of the glands. Specific tumors are diagnosed and named by cytologic identification of the tissue affected; for example, an adenocarcinoma of the uterine cervix is characterized by tumor cells resembling the glandular epithelium of the cervix. **—adenocarcinomatous,** *adj.*

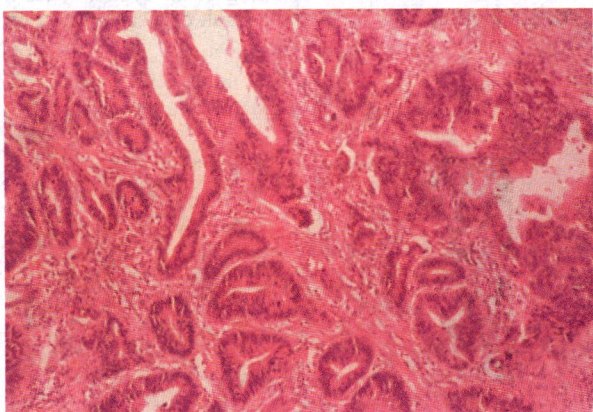

Adenocarcinoma cells of the intestines
(Misiewicz, 1985)

adenocarcinoma in situ, a localized growth of abnormal glandular tissue that may become malignant. However, the abnormal cells have not extended beyond the basement membrane. It is most common in the endometrium and in the large intestine.

adenocarcinoma of the kidney. See **renal cell carcinoma.**

adenocarcinomata. See **adenocarcinoma.**

adenocarcinomatous. See **adenocarcinoma.**

adenocele /ad'ənōsēl'/, a cystic, glandular tumor.

adenochondroma /ad'ənōkondrō'mə/, *pl.* **adenochondromas, adenochondromata** [Gk, *aden* + *chondros*, cartilage, *oma*], a neoplasm of cells derived from glandular and cartilaginous tissues, as a mixed tumor of the salivary glands. Also called **chondroadenoma.**

adenocyst /ad'ənōsist'/ [Gk, *aden* + *kytis*, bag], a benign tumor in which the cells form cysts. Also called **adenocystoma.** A kind of adenocyst is **papillary adenocystoma lymphomatosum.**

adenocystic carcinoma, a malignant neoplasm composed of cords of uniform small epithelial cells arranged in a sievelike pattern around cystic spaces that often contain mucus. The tumor occurs most frequently in the salivary glands, breast, mucous glands of the upper and lower respiratory tract, and, occasionally, in vestibular glands of the vulva. The malignant slow growth tends to spread along nerves, causing neurologic damage. Facial paralysis often results from adenocystic carcinoma of the salivary gland. Bloodborne metastases to bones and liver have been reported. Also called **adenoid cystic carcinoma, adenomyoepithelioma, cribriform carcinoma, cylindroma, cylindromatous carcinoma.**

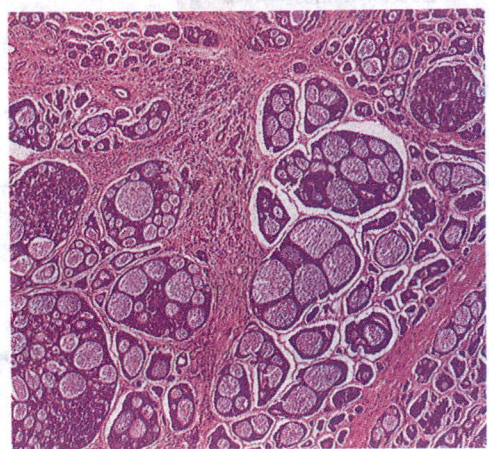

Adenocystic carcinoma cells *(Cawson, 1987)*

adenocystoma. See **adenocyst.**

adenodynia. See **adenalgia.**

adenoepithelioma /ad'ənō·ep'ithē'lē·ō'mə/, *pl.* **adenoepitheliomas, adenoepitheliomata** [Gk, *aden* + *epi*, on, *thele* nipple, *oma*], a neoplasm consisting of glandular and epithelial components.

adenofibroma /ad'ənōfībrō'mə/, *pl.* **adenofibromas, adenofibromata** [Gk, *aden* + L, *fibra*, fiber, *oma*], a tumor of the connective tissues that contains glandular elements.

adenofibroma edematodes, a neoplasm consisting of glandular elements and connective tissue in which marked edema is present.

adenofibromata. See **adenofibroma.**

adenohypophysis /ad'ənō'hīpof'isis/ [Gk, *aden* + *hypo,* beneath, *phyein,* to grow], the anterior lobe of the pituitary gland. It secretes growth hormone, thyrotropin, adrenocorticotropic hormone, melanocyte stimulating hormone, follicle stimulating hormone, luteinizing hormone, prolactin, beta lipotropin molecules, and endorphins. Releasing hormones from the hypothalamus regulate secretions. Also called **anterior pituitary.**

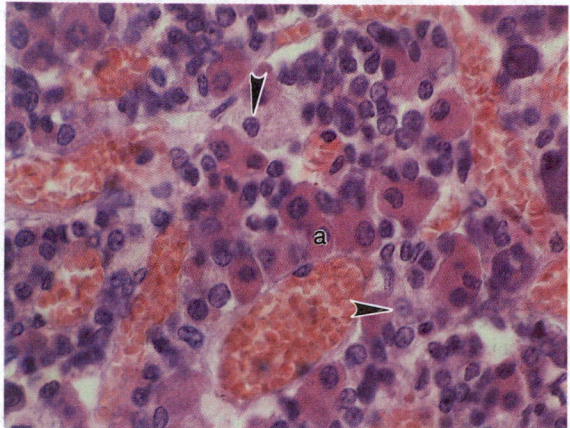

Histology of the adenohypophysis *(Erlandsen, 1992)*

adenoid /ad'ənoid/ [Gk, *aden* + *eidos,* form], **1.** having a glandular appearance, particularly lymphoid. **2.** adenoids, hypertrophy of the pharyngeal tonsil. —**adenoidal,** *adj.*

adenoidal speech, an abnormal manner of speaking caused by hypertrophy of the adenoidal tissue that normally exists in the nasopharynx of children. It is often characterized by a muted, nasal quality and may be corrected by a natural reduction of the swollen tissues or by surgical excision of the adenoids.

adenoid cystic carcinoma. See **adenocystic carcinoma.**

adenoidectomy /ad'ənoidek'təmē/ [Gk, *aden* + *eidos,* form, *ektome,* excision], removal of the lymphoid tissue in the nasopharynx. The surgical procedure may be performed because the adenoids are enlarged, causing obstruction, or chronically infected. Normal adenoids may be excised as a prophylactic measure during tonsillectomy. Preoperative procedures include a partial thromboplastin time test and for black patients a sickle cell preparation test. The operation is performed under general anesthesia in children, but local anesthesia may be used in adults. After removal of the adenoids, bleeding is stemmed with pressure; in some cases vessels may be ligated with sutures, or an electrocoagulation current may be used. Postoperatively, the patient is observed for signs of hemorrhage, and the pulse is checked every 15 minutes for the first hour and every 30 minutes for several hours thereafter. See also **tonsillectomy.**

adenoid hyperplasia, a condition in which enlarged adenoid glands cause partial respiratory obstruction, especially in children. Enlarged adenoids, often in association with enlarged tonsils, are a frequent cause of recurrent otitis media, sinusitis, and conduction deafness. Severe nasopharyngeal obstruction can result in alveolar hypoventilation and pulmonary hypertension with congestive heart failure. Treatment is usually surgical removal of the adenoids.

adenoid hypertrophy [Gk, *aden,* gland, *eidos,* form, *hyper,* excessive, *trophe,* nourishment], an enlargement of the pharyngeal tonsil.

adenoids, small masses of lymphoid tissue forming the pharyngeal tonsils on the posterior wall of the nasopharynx. Also called **pharyngeal tonsils.**

adenoid tissue, the lymphoid tissue that forms the pharyngeal tonsils.

adenoleiomyofibroma /ad'ənōlī'ōmī'ōfibrō'mə/, *pl.* **adenoleiomyofibromas, adenoleiomyofibromata** [Gk, *aden* + *leios,* smooth, *mys,* muscle; L, *fibra,* fiber; Gk, *oma*], a glandular tumor with smooth muscle, connective tissue, and epithelial elements.

adenolipoma /ad'ənōlipō'mə/, *pl.* **adenolipomas, adenolipomata** [Gk, *aden* + *lipos,* fat, *oma*], a neoplasm consisting of elements of glandular and fatty tissue.

adenolipomatosis /ad'ənōlipōmətō'sis/, a condition characterized by the growth of adenolipomas in the groin, axilla, and neck.

adenolymphoma. See **papillary adenocystoma lymphomatosum.**

adenoma /ad'ənō'mə/, *pl.* **adenomas, adenomata** [Gk, *aden* + *oma*], a tumor of glandular epithelium in which the cells of the tumor are arranged in a recognizable glandular structure. An adenoma may cause excess secretion by the affected gland, such as acidophilic pituitary adenoma resulting in an excess of growth hormone. Kinds of adenomas include **acidophilic adenoma, basophilic adenoma, fibroadenoma,** and **insulinoma.** —**adenomatous,** *adj.*

-adenoma, a suffix meaning a 'tumor composed of glandular tissue or glandlike in structure': *sarcoadenoma, splenadenoma.*

adenoma sebaceum /sebā'sē·əm/, an abnormal skin condition consisting of multiple, wartlike, yellowish red, waxy papules on the face that are true adenomas composed chiefly of fibrovascular tissue. The lesions are usually benign. See also **tuberous sclerosis.**

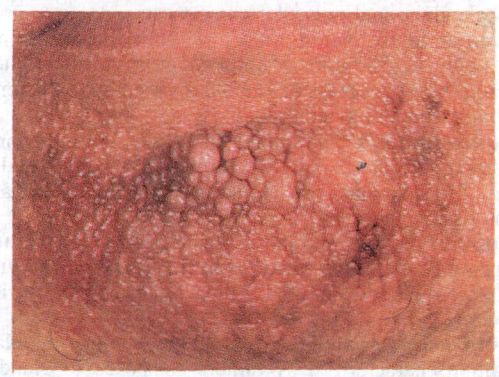

Adenoma sebaceum *(duVivier, 1993)*

adenomata. See **adenoma.**

adenomatoid /ad'ənō'mətoid/ [Gk, *aden, oma* + *eidos,* form], resembling a glandular tumor.

adenomatosis /ad'ənōmətō'sis/, an abnormal condition in which hyperplasia or tumor development affects two or more glands, usually the thyroid, adrenals, or pituitary.
-adenomatous. See **adenoma.**

adenomatous goiter /ad'ənō'mətəs/, an enlargement of the thyroid gland because of an adenoma or numerous colloid nodules.

adenomatous polyp [Gk, *aden*, gland, *oma*, tumor, *polys*, many, *pous*, foot], a tumor that develops in glandular tissue.

adenomatous polyposis coli (APC), a gene associated with **familial adenomatous polyposis,** an inherited disorder characterized by the development of myriad polyps in the colon beginning in late adolescence or early adulthood. Untreated, the condition may lead to colon cancer. The gene is located on chromosome 5.

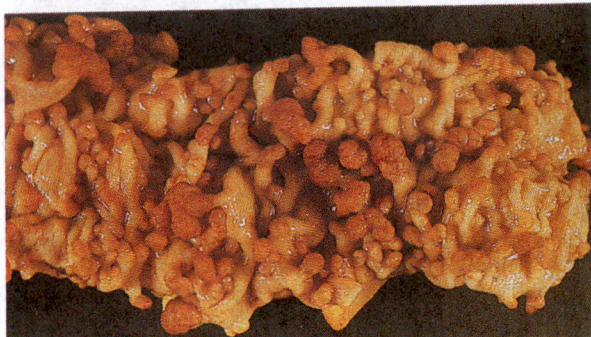

Familial adenomatous polyposis (Fletcher, 1987)

adenomyoepithelioma. See **adenocystic carcinoma.**

adenomyofibroma /ad'ənōmī'ōfībrō'mə/, *pl.* **adenomyofibromas, adenomyofibromata** [Gk, *aden* + *mys*, muscle; L, *fibra*, fiber; Gk, *oma*], a fibrous tumor that contains glandular and muscular components.

adenomyoma /ad'ənōmī'ō'mə/, *pl.* **adenomyomas, adenomyomata,** a tumor of the endometrium of the uterus characterized by a mass of smooth muscle containing endometrial tissue and glands.

adenomyomatosis /ad'ənōmī'ōmətō'sis/, an abnormal condition characterized by the formation of benign nodules resembling adenomyomas, found in the uterus or in parauterine tissue.

adenomyosarcoma /ad'ənōmī'ōsärkō'mə/, *pl.* **adenomyosarcomas, adenomyosarcomata,** a malignant tumor of soft tissue containing glandular elements and striated muscle.

adenomyosis /ad'ənōmī·ō'sis/, **1.** a benign neoplastic condition characterized by tumors composed of glandular tissue and smooth muscle cells. **2.** a malignant neoplastic condition characterized by the invasive growth of uterine mucosa in the uterus, pelvis, colon, or oviducts.

adenopathy /ad'ənop'əthē/ [Gk, *aden* + *pathos*, suffering], an enlargement of any gland. **—adenopathic,** *adj.*

adenosarcoma /ad'ənōsärkō'mə/, *pl.* **adenosarcomas, adenosarcomata** [Gk, *aden* + *sarx*, flesh, *oma*], a malignant glandular tumor of the soft tissues of the body.

adenosarcorhabdomyoma /ad'ənōsär'kōrab'dōmīō'mə/, *pl.* **adenosarcorhabdomyomas, adenosarcorhabdomyomata,** a tumor composed of glandular, connective tissue, and striated muscle elements.

adenosine /əden'əsin, -sēn/, a compound derived from nucleic acid, composed of adenine and a sugar, D-ribose. Adenosine is the major molecular component of the nucleotides adenosine monophosphate, adenosine diphosphate, and adenosine triphosphate and of the nucleic acids deoxyribonucleic acid and ribonucleic acid. Also called **adenine-D-ribose.** See also **adenosine phosphate.**

adenosine deaminase (ADA) /dē·am'inās/, an enzyme that catalyzes the conversion of adenosine to the nucleoside inosine through the removal of an amino group. A deficiency of ADA can lead to **severe combined immunodeficiency syndrome (SCIDS).** See also **adenosine.**

adenosine diphosphate, a product of the hydrolysis of adenosine triphosphate.

adenosine hydrolase, an enzyme that catalyzes the conversion of adenosine into adenine and ribose.

adenosine kinase, an enzyme in the liver and kidney that catalyzes the transfer of a phosphate group from adenosine triphosphate to produce adenosine phosphate.

adenosine monophosphate (AMP), an ester, composed of adenine, D-ribose, and phosphoric acid, that affects energy release in work done by a muscle. Also called **adenylic acid.**

adenosine phosphate, a compound consisting of the nucleotide adenosine attached through its ribose group to one, two, or three phosphoric acid molecules. Kinds of adenosine phosphate, all of which are interconvertible, are **adenosine diphosphate, adenosine monophosphate,** and **adenosine triphosphate.**

adenosine 3':5'-cyclic phosphate. See **cyclic adenosine monophosphate.**

adenosine triphosphatase (ATPase), an enzyme in skeletal muscle that catalyzes the hydrolysis of adenosine triphosphate to adenosine diphosphate and inorganic phosphate. Among various enzymes in this group associated with cell membranes and intracellular structures, mitochondrial ATPase is involved in obtaining energy for cellular metabolism, and myosin ATPase is involved in muscle contraction.

adenosine triphosphate (ATP), a compound consisting of the nucleotide adenosine attached through its ribose group to three phosphoric acid molecules. It serves to store energy in muscles, which is released when it is hydrolized to adenosine diphosphate.

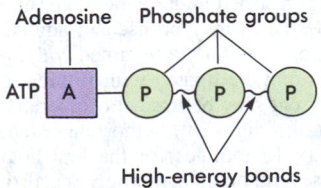

Structure of ATP (Thibodeau, 1993/Rolin Graphics)

adenosis /ad'ənō'sis/, **1.** any disease of the glands, especially a lymphatic gland. **2.** an abnormal development or enlargement of glandular tissue.

adenovirus /ad′ənōvī′rəs/ [Gk, *aden* + L, *virus*, poison], any one of the 33 medium-sized viruses of the Adenoviridae family, pathogenic to humans, that cause conjunctivitis, upper respiratory infection, or GI infection. After the acute and symptomatic period of illness, the virus may persist in a latent stage in the tonsils, adenoids, and other lymphoid tissue. Compare **rhinovirus. – adenoviral,** *adj.*

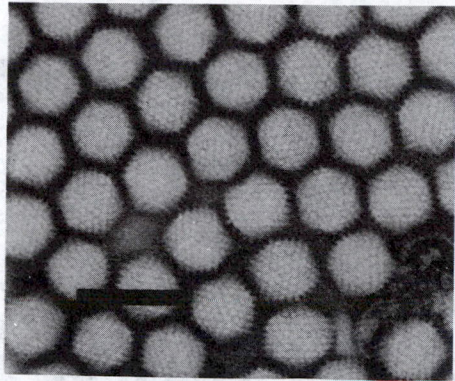

Adenovirus seen in feces (Baron, 1990)

adenylate /əden′ilāt/, a salt or ester of adenylic acid.

adenylate cyclase, an enzyme that initiates the conversion of adenosine triphosphate (ATP) to cyclic adenosine monophosphate (cAMP), a mediator of many physiologic activities.

adenylate kinase, an enzyme in skeletal muscle that makes possible the reaction ATP + AMP = 2ADP. Also called **myokinase.**

adenylic acid. See **adenosine monophosphate.**

adequate and well-controlled studies, clinical and laboratory studies that the sponsors of a new drug are required by law to conduct to demonstrate the truth of the claims made for its effectiveness.

adermia /ədur′mē·ə/ [Gk, *a, derma,* not skin], a congenital or acquired skin defect or the absence of skin.

ADH, abbreviation for **antidiuretic hormone.**

ADHA, abbreviation for the **American Dental Hygienists' Association.**

adhere /adhir′/, to stick together or become fastened together, as two surfaces.

adherence /adhir′əns/, **1.** the quality of clinging or being closely attached. **2.** the process in which a person follows rules, guidelines, or standards, especially as a patient follows prescription and recommendations for a regimen of care.

adherent /adhir′ənt/, [L, *adhaerens,* sticking to], having the tendency to cling as one substance to the surface of another substance.

adherent placenta [L, *adhesio,* sticking to, *placenta,* flat cake], a placenta that remains attached to the uterine wall beyond the normal time after delivery of the fetus.

adhesion /adhē′zhən/ [L, *adhesio,* clinging to], a band of scar tissue that binds together two anatomic surfaces that are normally separate from each other. Adhesions are most commonly found in the abdomen, where they form after abdominal surgery, inflammation, or injury. A loop of intestine may adhere to unhealed areas and cause an intestinal

obstruction if scar tissue develops and constricts the lumen of the bowel, blocking the intestinal flow. The condition is characterized by abdominal pain, nausea and vomiting, and distention. Nasogastric intubation and suction may relieve the symptoms. If the blockage does not resolve spontaneously, surgery may be necessary. See also **adhesiotomy, intestinal obstruction.**

adhesiotomy /adhē′sē·ot′əmē/ [L, *adhesio* + Gk, *temnein* to cut], the surgical dividing or separating of adhesions, usually performed to relieve an intestinal obstruction. See also **abdominal surgery.**

adhesive /adhē′siv/ [L, *adhesio,* clinging to], a quality of a substance that enables it to become attached to another substance.

adhesive absorbent dressing, an absorbent dressing on an adhesive backing.

adhesive pericarditis, a condition characterized by adhesions between the visceral and the parietal layers of the pericardium or by adhesions between the pericardium and the mediastinum, diaphragm, or chest wall. Adhesions between the pericardial layers may completely obstruct the pericardial cavity. Adhesive pericarditis may seriously impair normal movements of the heart.

adhesive peritonitis, an inflammation of the peritoneum, characterized by adhesions between adjacent serous surfaces. This condition may be marked by exudations of serum, fibrin, cells, and pus, accompanied by abdominal pain and tenderness, vomiting, constipation, and fever.

adhesive phlebitis, See **obliterative phlebitis.**

adhesive plaster, a strong fabric material covered on one side with an adhesive. Often water-repellent, it may be used to hold bandages and dressings in place, to immobilize a part, or to exert pressure. Also called **adhesive tape.**

adhesive pleurisy, inflammation of the pleura with exudation, causing obliteration of the pleural space through the fusion of the visceral pleural layer covering the lungs and the parietal layer lining the walls of the thoracic cavity.

adhesive skin traction, one of two kinds of skin traction in which the therapeutic pull of traction weights is applied with adhesive straps that stick to the skin over the body structure involved, especially a fractured bone. Adhesive skin traction is used only when continuous traction is desired and skin care for the affected area is easily maintained. The adhesive straps spread the pull over a wide plot of skin, decreasing the vulnerability of the patient to skin breakdown. Compare **nonadhesive skin traction.**

adhesive tape, a strong fabric material covered on one side with an adhesive. Often water-repellent, it may be used to hold bandages and dressings in place, to immobilize a part, or to exert pressure. Also called **adhesive plaster.**

ADI, abbreviation for **acceptable daily intake.**

adiadochokinesia /ā′dē·ad′əkōkinē′sis, ədī′ədō′kō-/, an inability to perform rapidly alternating movements, such as pronation and supination, or elbow flexion and extension. The exercise is commonly done as part of a neurologic examination.

adiastole /ā′dī·as′təlē/ [Gk, *a,* not, *dia,* across, *stellein,* to set], absence or imperceptibility of the diastolic stage of the cardiac cycle. See also **diastole.**

adiathermance /a′dī·əthur′məns/ [Gk, *a, dia,* not through, *therme,* heat], the quality of being unaffected by radiated heat.

adient /ad′ē·ənt/ [L, *adire,* moving toward], characterized by a tendency to move toward rather than away from stimuli. Compare **abient. – adience,** *n.*

Adie's pupil /ā´dēz/ [William J. Adie, London physician, b. 1816], an abnormal condition of the eyes marked by one pupil that reacts much more slowly to light changes or accommodation or convergence than the pupil of the other eye. There is no specific therapy for the condition, which is considered a pupillary muscle problem. Also called **tonic pupil.**

Adie's syndrome, the condition of Adie's pupil accompanied by depressed or absent tendon reflexes, particularly the ankle and knee-jerk reflexes. See **Adie's pupil.**

adip-. See **adipo-.**

adipectomy. See **lipectomy.**

adiphenine hydrochloride /ədif´ənin/, an anticholinergic with smooth muscle relaxant properties that has been used for spastic disorders of the GI and genitourinary tract.

adipic /ədip´ik/ [L, *adeps*, fat], of or pertaining to fatty tissue.

adipo-, adip-, a combining form meaning 'pertaining to fat': *adipocele, adipogenesis.*

adipocele /ad´ipōsēl´/ [L, *adeps* + Gk, *kele*, hernia], a hernia containing fat or fatty tissue. Also called **lipocele.**

adipocyte /ad´ipōsīt´/, a fat cell.

adipofibroma /ad´ipōfībrō´mə/, *pl.* **adipofibromas, adipofibromata** [L, *adeps* + *fibra*, fiber; Gk, *oma*], a fibrous neoplasm of the connective tissue with fatty components.

adipokinesis /ad´ipō´kinē´sis/, the mobilization of fat or fatty acids in lipid metabolism.

adiponecrosis /ad´ipōnikrō´sis/ [L, *adeps* + Gk, *nekros*, dead, *osis* condition], a necrosis of fatty tissue in the body. The condition may be associated with hemorrhagic pancreatitis. **–adiponecrotic,** *adj.*

adiponecrosis subcutanea neonatorum, an abnormal dermatologic condition of the newborn characterized by patchy areas of hardened subcutaneous fatty tissue and a bluish red discoloration of the overlying skin. The lesions,

often a result of manipulation during delivery, spontaneously resolve within a period of days to several weeks without scarring. Also called **pseudosclerema, subcutaneous fat necrosis.**

-adiponecrotic. See **adiponecrosis.**

adipose /ad´ipōs/, fatty. Adipose tissue is composed of fat cells arranged in lobules. See also **fat, fatty acid, lipoma.**

adipose degeneration. See **fatty degeneration.**

adipose tissue [L, *adeps*, fat, OFr, *tissu*], a collection of fat cells. See also **fatty tissue.**

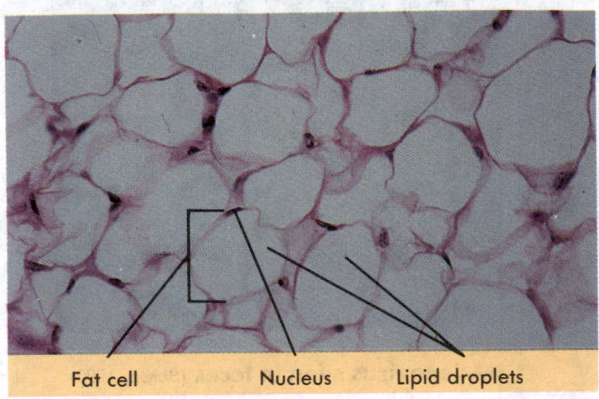

Fat cell   Nucleus   Lipid droplets

Adipose tissue *(Seeley, 1992/Ed Reschke)*

adipose tumor. See **lipoma.**

adiposogenital dystrophy /ad´ipō´sōjen´itəl/ [L, *adeps* + *genitalis*, generation], a disorder occurring in adolescent boys, characterized by genital hypoplasia and feminine secondary sex characteristics, including female distribution of fat. It is caused by hypothalamic malfunction or by a tumor in the anterior pituitary gland. A subnormal body temperature, low blood pressure, and reduced blood glucose are frequently associated with the disorder. Diabetes insipidus often occurs because of hyposecretion of antidiuretic hormone, and involvement of the hypothalamic satiety center may induce overeating and result in pronounced obesity. If a tumor is present, there may be drowsiness and symptoms of increased intracranial pressure. Treatment may include the administration of testosterone and a weight reduction program, excision or radiologic ablation of a tumor, and replacement of hormones, as necessary. Also called **adiposogenital syndrome, Fröhlich's syndrome.**

adipsia /ādip´sē·ə/ [Gk, *a, dipsa*, not thirst], absence of thirst.

aditus /ad´itəs/ [L, going to], an approach or an entry.

adjunct /ad´jungkt/ [L, *adjungere* to join], (in health care) an additional substance, treatment, or procedure used for increasing the efficacy or safety of the primary substance, treatment, or procedure or to facilitate its performance. **–adjunctive,** *adj.*

adjunctive group /adjungk´tiv/, a group with specific activities and focuses, such as socialization, perceptual stimulation, sensory stimulation, or reality orientation.

adjunctive psychotherapy, a form of psychotherapy that concentrates on improving a person's general mental and physical outlook without trying to resolve basic emotional problems. Some kinds of adjunctive psychotherapy are **music therapy, occupational therapy, physical therapy,** and **recreational therapy.**

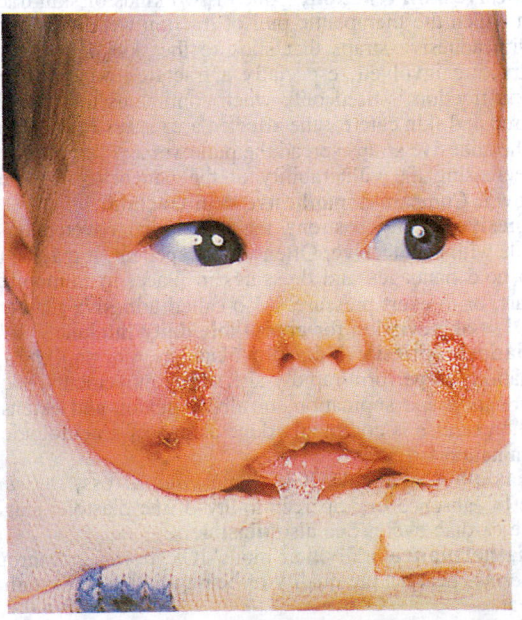

Adiponecrosis subcutanea neonatorum
(McKee, 1993/Courtesy Institute of Dermatology, London)

adjunct to anesthesia, one of a number of drugs of five different classes. Each class of drug has a use in anesthetic procedures, as well as a therapeutic indication in other aspects of health care. Adjuncts to anesthesia are used as premedications, as intravenous supplements to hypnotic or analgesic medications, and as neuromuscular blocking agents, analeptics, and therapeutic gases. Premedications are given to reduce anxiety, sedate the patient, reduce salivation and secretions of the respiratory passages, and prevent bradycardia. Strong analgesics, sedatives and hypnotics, phenothiazines, anticholinergics, and antianxiety agents are also sometimes prescribed as premedications. Intravenous hypnotic and analgesic supplements given to augment the effects of nitrous oxide include morphine, meperidine, diazepam, fentanyl, and droperidol. Neuromuscular blocking agents are given to produce and sustain relaxation of the skeletal muscles during the surgical procedure. These agents are of two kinds: depolarizing or nondepolarizing. Depolarizing agents (including succinylcholine) act by depolarizing the postsynaptic membranes, rendering them refractory to stimulation and producing muscle paralysis. Nondepolarizing agents (including tubocurarine, metocurine, gallamine, and pancuronium) act by competing with acetylcholine for receptor sites on the postjunctional receptor sites, producing paralysis of the muscles. The use of these agents usually requires assisted or controlled respiration by an anesthetist or anesthesiologist and a careful evaluation of the recovery of neuromuscular transmission in the postoperative period. Analeptics may be administered to stimulate the function of the central nervous system in ventilatory insufficiency caused by drug overdose, drowning, electric shock, carbon monoxide poisoning, or other conditions resulting in hypoxemia. The effects of these agents are transitory and may paradoxically result in further depression; therefore, they are not usually recommended. Therapeutic gases include carbon dioxide and oxygen and various general anesthetics. Carbon dioxide and oxygen are given to maintain normal respiratory metabolism and function and as vehicles to carry anesthetic gases.

adjustable orthodontic band /adjus′təbəl/, a thin metal ring, usually made of stainless steel, equipped with an adjusting screw to allow alteration in size, fitted to a tooth and serving for the attachment of orthodontic appliances. See also **orthodontic band.**

adjusted death rate. See **standardized death rate.**

adjustment. See **accommodation.**

adjustment, impaired, a nursing diagnosis accepted by the Seventh National Conference on the Classification of Nursing Diagnoses. Impaired adjustment is a state in which the individual is unable to modify his or her life-style behavior in a manner consistent with a change in health status. The major defining characteristics of the condition are verbalization of nonacceptance of health status change and nonexistent or unsuccessful ability to be involved in problem solving or goal setting. Minor defining characteristics are lack of movement toward independence, lack of future-oriented thinking, and extended period of shock, disbelief, or anger regarding health status change. Related factors include a disability requiring a change in life-style, inadequate support systems, impaired cognition, sensory overload, an assault to self-esteem, altered locus of control, or incomplete grieving. See also **nursing diagnosis.**

adjustment reaction, [L, *adjuxtare,* to bring together], a temporary disorder of varying severity that occurs as an acute reaction to overwhelming stress in persons of any age who have no apparent underlying mental disorders. Symptoms include anxiety, withdrawal, depression, brooding, temper outbursts, crying spells, attention-getting behavior, enuresis, loss of appetite, aches, pains, and muscle spasms. It can result from such situations as separation of an infant from its mother, the birth of a sibling, loss or change of a job, death of a loved one, or forced retirement. Symptoms usually recede and eventually disappear as stress diminishes. See also **neurotic disorder.**

adjuvant /ad′jəvənt/ [L, *ad, juvare,* to help], **1.** a substance, especially a drug, added to a prescription to assist in the action of the main ingredient. **2.** in immunology, a substance added to an antigen that enhances or modifies the antibody response to the antigen.

adjuvant chemotherapy, the use of anticancer drugs in the absence of any detectable residual cancer, as after apparently complete surgical removal of a cancer. The method is employed when there is a significant risk that undetectable cancer cells may still be present. Adjuvant chemotherapy is most commonly used in treating breast cancers.

adjuvant therapy, the treatment of a disease with substances that enhance the action of drugs, especially drugs that promote the production of antibodies.

ADL, abbreviation for **activities of daily living.**

ad lib, an abbreviation of the Latin phrase *ad libitum,* meaning to be taken as desired and sometimes used in pharmaceutic prescriptions.

administration of parenteral fluids /admin′istrā′shən/, the intravenous infusion of various solutions to maintain adequate hydration, restore fluid volume, reestablish lost electrolytes, or provide partial nutrition. See **parenteral.**

■ METHOD: Fluid is administered parenterally through a closed system consisting of a bottle or sterile bag of sterile solution, tubing, and an attached intracatheter or scalp vein needle that is inserted into a peripheral vein and securely taped to the patient's arm, leg, or scalp. The fluid is infused slowly. Five percent dextrose in distilled water may be used to maintain volume or restore blood volume; ascorbic acid and B vitamins are often added to the solution. Five percent dextrose in saline solution plus potassium chloride may be infused to reestablish electrolyte balance, but potassium is contraindicated in renal failure and untreated adrenal insufficiency. A one-sixth molar lactate solution may be administered if sodium is deficient, and an ammonium chloride solution may be administered when replacement of chloride is required. Distilled water containing 10% to 20% glucose or fructose may be used to supply carbohydrate, but, because these solutions are hypertonic, additional hydration is needed for proper excretion. Low molecular weight dextran is frequently used as a plasma volume expander in treating shock, but it increases bleeding time and is contraindicated in pregnancy and severe renal disease. During parenteral fluid administration, the venipuncture site is observed every 1 to 2 hours for signs of redness, swelling, warmth, and leakage; for the security and comfort of the tape; and for the position of the patient's extremity. The flow rate, level, color, and clarity of the fluid, the label, and the patency of the tubing are checked, and the patient is monitored for signs of dehydration, fever, and signs of circulatory overload, such as headache, tachycardia, elevated blood pressure, dyspnea, engorged neck veins, and pulmonary edema.

■ NURSING INTERVENTION: Depending on the service, the nurse may select the necessary equipment, prepare the venipuncture site, check the labels of fluid bottles for content, and perform the venipuncture. During the administration of fluid, the nurse keeps the system closed, watches the flow rate, records the amount of solution given, and observes the venipuncture site and the patient's general condition. If there are any signs of increased blood volume, the nurse reduces the flow of the infusion until further orders are obtained. The nurse changes the dressing daily and ensures that the patient understands the importance of keeping the extremity still, of not disturbing the tubing, and of reporting pain or swelling.

■ OUTCOME CRITERIA: Parenteral fluid therapy is usually uneventful, but infants, elderly patients with circulatory or renal impairment, and burn patients, whose plasma may shift suddenly from interstitial tissue, causing increased blood volume, require special attention.

Administration On Aging (AOA), the principal agency designated to carry out the provisions of the Older Americans Act of 1965. The AOA advises the Secretary of the Department of Health and Human Services and other federal departments and agencies on the characteristics and needs of older people and develops programs designed to promote their welfare.

ADN, abbreviation for **Associate Degree in Nursing.**

ad nauseam [L, *ad*, to + Gk, *nausia*, seasickness], to the extent of inducing nausea and vomiting.

adnexa /adnek′sə/, *sing.* **adnexus** [L, *adnectere*, to tie together], tissue or structures in the body that are next to or near another, related structure. The ovaries and the uterine tubes are adnexa of the uterus. –**adnexal,** *adj.*

adnexal [L, *adnectere*, to tie to], pertaining to accessory organs or tissues, as in the relationship of the fallopian tubes and uterus.

adnexitis /ad′neksī′tis/, an inflammation of the adnexal organs of the uterus, such as the ovaries or the fallopian tubes.

-adol, a combining form designating an analgesic.

adnexus. See **adnexa.**

adolescence /ad′əles′əns/ [L, *adolescere*, to grow up], **1.** the period in development between the onset of puberty and adulthood. It usually begins between 11 and 13 years of age, with the appearance of secondary sex characteristics, and spans the teen years, terminating at 18 to 20 years of age with the acquisition of completely developed adult form. During this period the individual undergoes extensive physical, psychologic, emotional, and personality changes. **2.** the state or quality of being adolescent or youthful. See also **postpuberty, prepuberty, psychosexual development, psychosocial development, pubarche.**

adolescent, **1.** of, pertaining to, or characteristic of adolescence. **2.** one in the state or process of adolescence; a teenager.

adolescent vertebral epiphysitis. See **Scheuermann's disease.**

adoption /ədop′shən/ [L, *adoptere*, to choose], a selection and bringing into a previously established relationship.

ADP, abbreviation for **adenosine diphosphate.**

adrenal /ədrē′nəl/ [L, *ad*, to, *ren*, kidney], pertaining to the adrenal or suprarenal glands that are located atop the kidneys.

adrenal cortex [L *ad*, *ren* to kidney], the outer and greater portion of the adrenal or suprarenal gland, fused with the gland's medulla and producing mineralocorticoids, androgens, and glucocorticoids, hormones essential to homeostasis. The outer cortex is normally a deep yellow; the inner part, dark red or brown. It is recognizable in the embryo

during the sixth week as a groove in the coelom at the base of the mesentery near the cranial end of the mesonephros.

adrenal cortical carcinoma, a malignant neoplasm of the adrenal cortex that may cause adrenogenital syndrome or Cushing's syndrome. Such tumors vary in size, occur at any age, and are more common in females than in males. Metastases frequently spread the cancer to the lungs, liver, and other organs. See also **adrenal virilism, Cushing's syndrome.**

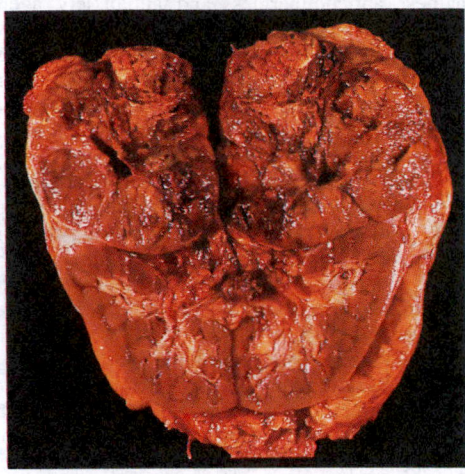

Adrenal cortical carcinoma compressing the upper pole of the kidney
(Skarin, 1991)

adrenal crisis, an acute, life-threatening state of profound adrenocortical insufficiency in which immediate therapy is required. It is characterized by glucocorticoid deficiency, a drop in extracellular fluid volume, and hyperkalemia. Also called **addisonian crisis, adrenergic crisis.** See also **Addison's disease, adrenal cortex.**

■ OBSERVATIONS: Typically, the patient appears to be in shock or coma with a low blood pressure, severe prostration, and loss of vasomotor tone. The person's medical history may include Addison's disease or reveal symptoms indicating its presence. Laboratory tests show hyperkalemia and hyponatremia.

■ INTERVENTIONS: An intravenous isotonic solution of sodium chloride containing a water-soluble glucocorticoid is administered rapidly. Vasopressor agents may be necessary to combat hypotension. If the patient is vomiting, a nasogastric tube is usually inserted. Total bed rest and the monitoring of blood pressure, temperature, and other vital signs are mandatory. After the first critical hours, the patient is followed as for Addison's disease, and steroid dosage is tapered to maintenance levels. In all cases the precipitating cause is sought. Infection and a failure to increase the maintenance dose are common causes of crisis in people who have Addison's disease.

■ NURSING CONSIDERATIONS: Nursing care during adrenal crisis includes eliminating all forms of stimuli, especially loud noises or bright lights. The patient is not moved unless absolutely necessary and is not allowed to perform self-care activities. If the condition is identified and treated promptly, the prognosis is good. Discharge instructions include a reminder to the patient to seek medical attention in any stressful situation, whether physiologic or psychologic, to prevent a recurrence of the crisis.

adrenalectomy /ədrē′nəlek′təmē/ [L, *ad, ren* + Gk, *ek-tome,* excision], the surgical removal of one or both adrenal glands or the resection of a portion of one or both glands, performed to reduce the excessive secretion of adrenal hormones when an adrenal tumor or a malignancy of the breast or prostate is present. The incision is made under the twelfth rib in the rear flank area with the patient under a general anesthetic. Preoperative laboratory tests include electrolytes, fasting blood glucose, and glucose tolerance. Corticosteroid drugs are given, and frequent blood pressure measurements are recorded. Before surgery a nasogastric tube is inserted and a venous cutdown is done. Postoperative care focuses on monitoring vital signs and maintaining blood pressure with an IV solution containing a vasopressor and corticosteroids. An abrupt drop in blood pressure, increasing weakness, and a rise in temperature are signs of acute corticosteroid insufficiency. Blood electrolyte levels are checked frequently, and fluid intake and output are carefully recorded. Steroids are given by mouth a few days after surgery. When oral steroids can be tolerated, the dosage is tapered to a maintenance level; if both glands are removed, the maintenance dosage continues for life. Stress and fatigue must be avoided. See also **Addison's disease, Cushing's syndrome.**

adrenal gland, either of two secretory organs perched atop the kidneys and surrounded by the protective fat capsule of the kidneys. Each consists of two parts having independent functions: the cortex and the medulla. The adrenal cortex, in response to adrenocorticotropic hormone secreted by the anterior pituitary, secretes cortisol and androgens. Adrenal androgens serve as precursors that are converted by the liver to testosterone and estrogens. Renin

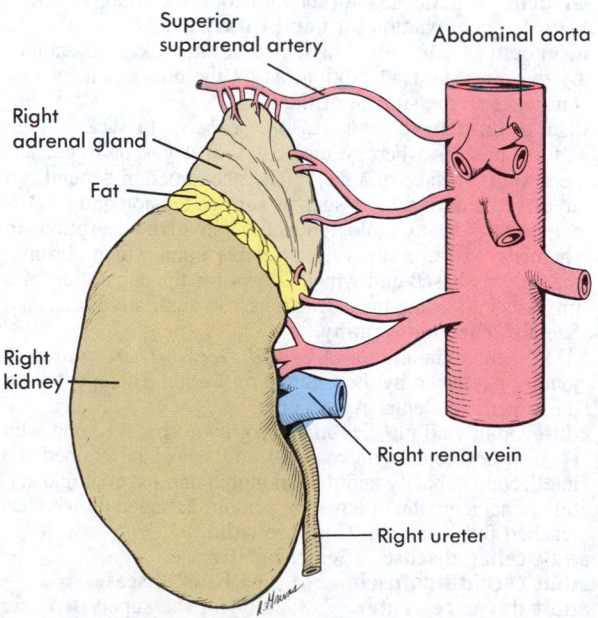

Superior suprarenal artery

Abdominal aorta

Right adrenal gland

Fat

Right kidney

Right renal vein

Right ureter

Adrenal gland *(Seeley, 1992/Andrew Grivas)*

from the kidney controls adrenal cortical production of aldosterone. The adrenal medulla manufactures the catecholamines epinephrine and norepinephrine.

Adrenalin, a trademark for an adrenergic (epinephrine).

adrenaline. See **epinephrine.**

adrenal insufficiency [L, *ad,* to, *ren,* kidney, *in,* not, *sufficere,* to suffice], a condition in which the adrenal gland is unable to function adequately. See also **Addison's disease.**

adrenalize /ədrē′nəlīz/, to stimulate or excite.

adrenal medulla, the inner portion of the adrenal gland. Adrenal medulla cells secrete epinephrine and norepinephrine. See **adrenal cortex.**

adrenal virilism, a condition characterized by hypersecretion of adrenocortical androgens, resulting in somatic masculinization. Excessive production of the hormone may be caused by a virilizing adrenal tumor, congenital adrenal hyperplasia, or an inborn deficiency of enzymes required to transform endogenous androgenic steroids to glucocorticoids. Girls born with adrenogenitalism may be pseudohermaphroditic with clitoral enlargement and labial fusion in infancy and later hirsutism, low vocal pitch, acne, amenorrhea, and masculine distribution of hair and development of muscles. Boys with congenital adrenogenitalism show precocious development of the penis and prostate and of pubic and axillary hair, but their testes remain small and immature because negative feedback from the high level of adrenal androgens prevents the normal pubertal increase in pituitary gonadotropin. Children with the disorder are unusually tall, but their epiphyses close prematurely, and as adults they are abnormally short. Virilizing tumors are more common or more frequently diagnosed in women. They usually occur between 30 and 40 years of age but may arise later, after the menopause. Signs of the tumor in women include hirsutism, amenorrhea, oily skin, ovarian changes, muscular hypertrophy, and atrophy of the uterus and breasts. Treatment may involve tumor resection, administration of cortisol, and plastic surgical procedures. Electrolytic epilation may be indicated. Also called **adrenogenital syndrome.** See also **congenital adrenal hyperplasia, pseudohermaphroditism, virilization.**

adrenarche /ad′rinär′kē/ [L, *ad, ren* + Gk, *arche,* beginning], the intensified activity in the adrenal cortex that occurs at about 8 years of age and increases the elaboration of various hormones, especially androgens.

adrenergic /ad′rinur′jik/ [L, *ad, ren* + Gk, *ergon,* work], of or pertaining to sympathetic nerve fibers of the autonomic nervous system that use as neurotransmitters epinephrine or epinephrine-like substances. Compare **cholinergic.** See **sympathomimetic.**

adrenergic blocking agent. See **antiadrenergic.**

adrenergic bronchodilator, a drug that acts on the sympathetic nervous system receptors to relax bronchial smooth muscle cells. Examples include drugs that contain epinephrine, ephedrine, isoproterenol, or albuterol.

adrenergic crisis. See **adrenal crisis.**

adrenergic drug. See **sympathomimetic.**

adrenergic fibers, nerve fibers of the autonomic nervous system that release the neurotransmitter norepinephrine and, in some areas, dopamine. Most postganglionic sympathetic fibers are of this type.

adrenergic nerve [L, *ad,* to, *ren,* kidney; Gk, *ergon,* work, L, *nervus*], a nerve of the autonomic system that controls the release of norepinephrine at its synapses.

adrenergic receptor [L, *ad, ren,* kidney; Gk, *ergon,* work; L, *recipere,* to receive], a site in a sympathetic effector cell that reacts to adrenergic stimulation. Two types of adrenergic receptors are recognized: **alpha-adrenergic,** which act in response to sympathomimetic stimuli, and **beta-adrenergic,** which block sympathomimetic activity. In general, stimulation of alpha receptors is excitatory of the function of the host organ or tissue, and stimulation of the beta-receptors is inhibitory.

-adrenia, a combining form meaning '(degree or condition of) adrenal activity': *anadrenia, dysadrenia, hypadrenia.*

adrenocortical /-kôr′tikəl/ [L, *ad,ren,* + *cortex,* bark], pertaining to the outer or superficial portion of the adrenal gland.

adrenocortical hormone (ACH) [L, *ad,* to, *ren,* kidney, *cortex,* bark; Gk, *hormaein,* to set in motion], any of the hormones secreted by the cortex of the adrenal gland, including the glucocorticoids, mineralocorticoids, and sex hormones.

adrenocorticotrophic hormone. See **adrenocorticotropic hormone.**

adrenocorticotropic /ədrē′nōkôr′tikōtrop′ik/ [L, *ad, ren* + *cortex,* rind; Gk, *trope,* a turning], of or pertaining to stimulation of the adrenal cortex. Also **adrenocorticotrophic** /-trof′ik/.

adrenocorticotropic hormone (ACTH), a hormone of the anterior pituitary gland that stimulates the growth of the adrenal gland cortex and the secretion of corticosteroids. ACTH secretion, regulated by corticotropin releasing factor (CRF) from the hypothalamus, increases in response to a low level of circulating cortisol and to stress, fever, acute

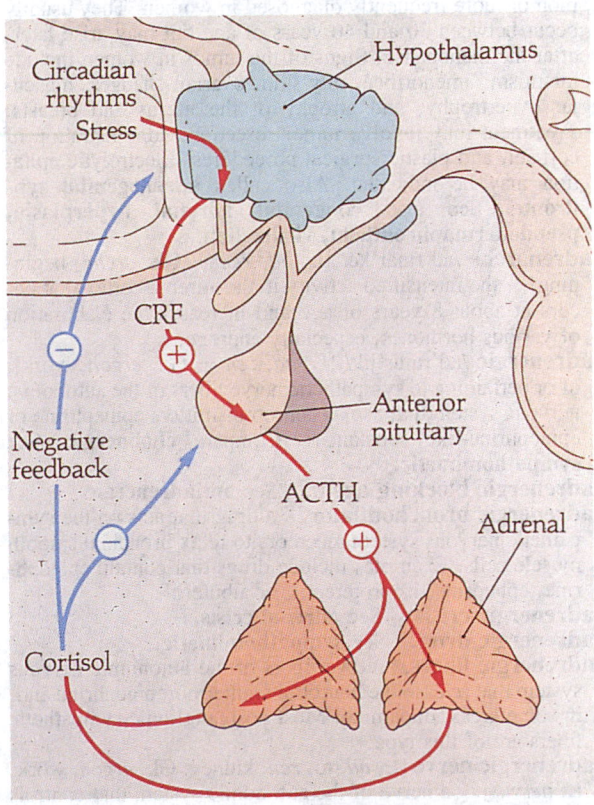

Feedback regulation of ACTH *(Zitelli, 1992)*

hypoglycemia, and major surgery. Under normal conditions there is a diurnal rhythm in ACTH secretion with an increase beginning after the first few hours of sleep and reaching a peak at the time a person awakens. ACTH stimulates the formation of cyclic adenosine monophosphate (AMP), which is thought to activate the enzyme system that catalyzes the conversion of cholesterol to pregnenolone, the precursor of all steroidal hormones. A purified preparation of ACTH in gelatin is widely used in the treatment of rheumatoid arthritis, acquired hemolytic anemia, intractable allergic states, various dermatologic diseases, and many other disorders. Normal findings range from 15-100 pg/ml or 10-80 ng/L am to less than 50 pg/ml or 50 ng/L pm. Also called **adrenocorticotrophic hormone, corticotropin.**

adrenocorticotropin /-trop′in/, the adrenocorticotropic hormone **(ACTH)** secreted by the anterior pituitary gland that stimulates secretion of other hormones by the adrenal cortex.

adrenodoxin /ədrē′nōdok′sin/, a protein, produced by the adrenal glands, that participates in the transfer of electrons within animal cells.

adrenogenital syndrome. See **adrenal virilism.**

adrenoleukodystrophy (ALD), a rare, hereditary childhood metabolic disease that is transmitted as a recessive sex-linked trait and that affects only boys. It is characterized by adrenal atrophy and widespread cerebral demyelination, producing progressive mental deterioration, aphasia, apraxia, and eventual blindness. Prognosis is poor, with death occurring usually in 1 to 5 years. ALD was formerly classified under Schilder's disease.

adrenomegaly /-meg′əlē [L, *ad,ren,* + Gk, *megaly,* large], an abnormal enlargement of one or both adrenal glands.

Adriamycin RDF, a trademark for a cytotoxic agent (doxorubicin hydrochloride).

adromia /ədrō′mē·ə/ [Gk, *a, dromos,* not course], the absence of the conductive capacity of any nerve that normally innervates a muscle.

Adrucil, a trademark for an antineoplastic (fluorouracil).

ADRV, abbreviation for **adult rotavirus.**

adsorbent /adsôr′bənt/, a substance that takes up another by the process of adsorption, as by the attachment of one substance to the surface of the other.

adsorption /adsôrp′shən/ [L, *ad, sorbere,* to suck in], a natural process whereby molecules of a gas or liquid adhere to the surface of a solid. The phenomenon depends on an assortment of factors such as surface tension and electrical charges. Many biologic reactions involve adsorption. In chemistry, adsorption is the principle upon which chromatography is based and which allows for the separation of a mixture into component fractions for qualitative analysis. See also **chromatography.**

ADT, abbreviation for *Accepted Dental Therapeutics,* a journal published by the Council on Dental Therapeutics of the American Dental Association.

adult /ədult′, ad′ult/ [L, *adultus,* grown up], **1.** one who is fully developed and matured and who has attained the intellectual capacity and the emotional and psychologic stability characteristic of a mature person. **2.** a person who has reached full legal age. Compare **child.**

adult celiac disease. See **celiac disease.**

adult ceroid-lipofuscinosis. See **Kufs' disease.**

adult day-care center, a facility for the supervised care of older adults, providing such activities as meals and socialization during specified day hours, with the participants returning to their homes each evening.

adult ego state, in psychiatry, a part of the self that analyzes and solves problems, using information received from the parent ego and child ego states. It is assumed to be fully developed in a normal individual at the age of 12.

adulteration /ədul′tərā′shən/ [L, *adulterare,* to defile], the debasement or dilution of the purity of any substance, process, or activity by the addition of extraneous material.

adult hemoglobin. See **hemoglobin A.**

adulthood, the phase of development characterized by physical and mental maturity.

adult nurse practitioner, a registered nurse who has received additional education in the primary health care of adults. The additional education may be obtained through a master's degree program or a nondegree continuing education certificate program.

adult-onset diabetes. See **non-insulin-dependent diabetes mellitus.**

adult polycystic disease. See **polycystic kidney disease.**

adult respiratory distress syndrome (ARDS), a respiratory syndrome characterized by respiratory insufficiency and hypoxemia. Triggers include aspiration of a foreign body, cardiopulmonary bypass surgery, gram-negative sepsis, multiple blood transfusions, oxygen toxicity, trauma, pneumonia, or other respiratory infection. Also called **acute respiratory distress syndrome, congestive atelectasis, pump lung, shock lung, wet lung.** See also **chronic obstructive pulmonary disease.**

■ OBSERVATIONS: The symptoms and signs of ARDS include shortness of breath, rapid breathing, inadequate oxygenation of the arterial blood, and decreased lung compliance. The changes that occur within the lungs include damage to the membranes of the capillaries, hemorrhage, capillary leaking, interstitial edema, impairment in gas exchange, and ventilation-perfusion abnormalities. These sequelae lead to decreased lung compliance and increased dyspnea.

■ INTERVENTIONS: The patient with ARDS usually requires mechanical ventilation, often using positive end-expiratory pressure (PEEP). Treatment is directed toward establishing an airway, administering oxygen, improving the underlying condition, and removing the cause. Also used in management are suctioning of the respiratory passages as necessary, postural drainage, and cupping and vibration. When ventilation cannot be maintained and there is evidence of a rising Pco_2, mechanical ventilation with a ventilator is necessary. Positive end-expiratory pressure is widely used in the treatment of ARDS.

■ NURSING CONSIDERATIONS: The patient with ARDS requires constant and meticulous care, reassurance, and observation for changes in respiratory function and adequacy including signs of hypercapnia, hypoxemia, especially confusion, skin flushing, and behavior changes that include agitation and restiveness. Increasing hypoxia may be recognized by tachycardia, elevated blood pressure, and increased peripheral resistance; fulminant respiratory failure is accompanied by falling blood pressure and cyanosis. If PEEP is being used, one is careful to observe for a sudden disappearance of breath sounds accompanied by signs of respiratory distress—an indication that pneumothorax may be present. Care is taken when weaning patients from the ventilator, and intermittent mandatory ventilation (IMV) and pressure ventilation (PSV) may be used. Adequate humidification, respiratory therapy, sterile suction techniques, and position changes are continued as necessary. Weight is taken frequently, x-ray films of the chest are taken and evaluated, and input and bacteriologic cultures of secretions are ana-

lyzed in the laboratory. Throughout treatment, ventilation is carefully monitored using blood gas studies and spirometry.

adult rickets, a disease affecting adults that resembles rickets. See also **osteomalacia, rickets.**

adult rotavirus (ADRV), a form of rotavirus that causes severe diarrhea in adults. The virus resembles the usual rotavirus and its genome, but it is not antigenically related and does not react against rotavirus antibodies. ADRV antibodies have been found in adults in China and Australia. See also **rotavirus.**

advance /advans′/ [Fr, *avancer,* to move forward], a surgical technique in which a muscle or tendon is brought forward.

advanced cardiac life support (ACLS), emergency medical procedures in which basic life support efforts of cardiopulmonary resuscitation are augmented by establishment of an intravenous fluid line, drug administration, control of cardiac arrhythmias, and ventilation equipment. The procedures usually require direct or indirect supervision by a physician.

advance declaration. See **advance directive, living will.**

advance directive [Fr, *avancer,* to move forward; L, *dirigere,* to direct], **1.** an advance declaration by a patient adjudged to be hopelessly and terminally ill that the person does not want to be connected to life support equipment. The document, signed and witnessed, may generally serve as a "Living Will," depending upon current state laws. **2.** a Durable Power of Attorney for Health Care, in which a terminally ill person assigns to someone else the power to make health care decisions if the patient is no longer able to make such decisions. The document directs the surrogate person to function as "attorney-in-fact" and make the final decision regarding cessation of treatment. Also called **advance declaration.**

advanced life support. See **Emergency Medical Technician-Advanced Life Support.**

adventitia /ad′ventish′ə/ [L, *adventitius,* coming from abroad], the outermost layer, composed of connective tissue with elastic and collagenous fibers, of an artery or other structure.

adventitious [L, *adventitius, from outside sources*], of or pertaining to an accidental condition or an arbitrary action.

adventitious bursa, an abnormal bursa that develops as a response to friction or pressure.

adventitious crisis, an accidental, uncommon, and unexpected tragedy that may affect an entire community or population, such as an earthquake, flood, or airplane crash. In addition to injuries, loss of life, and property damage, an adventitious crisis often results in psychologic effects that require long-term crisis intervention.

adventitious sounds, breath sounds that are not normally heard, such as crackles and rhonchi. They may be superimposed on normal breath sounds.

adverse drug effect /advurs′, ad′vers/, a harmful, unintended reaction to a drug administered at normal dosage.

adverse reaction, any harmful or unintended effect of a medication, diagnostic test, or therapeutic intervention.

advocacy /ad′vəkas′ē/, **1.** a process whereby a nurse provides a patient with the information to make certain decisions. **2.** a method by which patients, their families, attorneys, health professionals, and citizen groups can work together to develop programs that ensure the availability of high-quality health care for a community.

adynamia /ad′inā′mē·ə/ [Gk, *a, dynamis,* not strength], lack of physical strength due to a pathologic condition. See also **asthenia.** **–adynamic,** *adj.*

adynamia episodica hereditaria, a condition seen in infancy, characterized by muscle weakness and episodes of flaccid paralysis. It is inherited as an autosomal dominant trait. Also called **hyperkalemic periodic paralysis.**

adynamic. See **adynamia.**

adynamic fever, an elevated temperature with a feeble pulse, nervous depression, and a cool, moist, skin. Also called **asthenic fever.**

adynamic ileus. See **ileus.**

AE amputation, the amputation of the arm above the elbow. A short AE amputation (near the shoulder) results in the loss of shoulder rotation. After a long AE amputation (just above the elbow) the patient should retain good shoulder function.

Aedes /ā·ē′dēz/ [Gk, *aedes,* unpleasant], a genus of mosquito, prevalent in tropical and subtropical regions. Several species are capable of transmitting pathogenic organisms to humans, including dengue, equine encephalitis, St. Louis encephalitis, tularemia, and yellow fever.

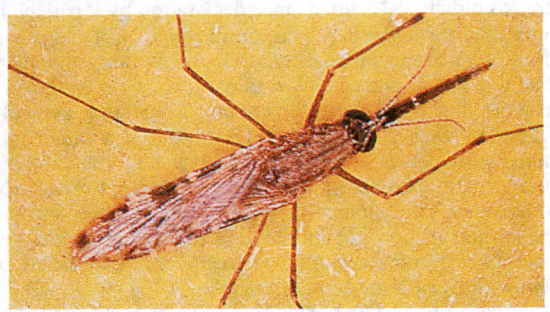

Female aedes mosquito
(Muller, 1990/Courtesy Prof. WW MacDonald)

aer-. See **aero-.**

aerate /er′āt/ [Gk, *aer,* air], to charge a substance or a structure with air, carbon dioxide, or oxygen.

aeration [Gk, *aer,* air], **1.** exchange of carbon dioxide for oxygen by blood in the lungs. **2.** a process of exposing a tissue or fluid to the air, or artificially charging it with oxygen or another gas, such as carbon dioxide.

aero-, aer-, a combining form meaning 'pertaining to air or to gas': *aerobe, aerocystography, aerodontalgia.*

Aerobacter aerogenes. See **Enterobacter cloacae.**

aerobe /er′ōb/ [Gk, *aer* + *bios,* life], a microorganism that lives and grows in the presence of free oxygen. Aerobes may be **facultative** or **obligate aerobes.** Compare **anaerobe, microaerophile.**

aerobic /erō′bik/, **1.** of or pertaining to the presence of air or oxygen. **2.** able to live and function in the presence of free oxygen. **3.** requiring oxygen for the maintenance of life. **4.** of or pertaining to aerobic exercise.

aerobic exercise, any physical exercise that requires additional effort by the heart and lungs to meet the increased demand by the skeletal muscles for oxygen. The exercise generally requires heavier breathing than passive muscular activity and results in increased heart and lung efficiency

with a minimum of wasted energy. Examples of aerobic exercise include running, jogging, swimming, and vigorous dancing or cycling. Also called **aerobics.** See also **active exercise, passive exercise.**

aerobic glycolysis. See **glycolysis.**

aerobics. See **aerobic exercise.**

aerobic training, physical exercises designed to require an increased intake and distribution of oxygen. Such exercises involve depletion of the body's normal tissue stores of oxygen by comparatively strenuous exertion and replacement of the oxygen through deep breathing. This training can be accomplished by biking, walking, jogging or other similar activities for at least 20 minutes, 3 times per week. Also called **aerobics.**

aerodontalgia /er′ōdontal′jə/ [Gk, *aer* + *odous,* tooth, *algos,* pain], a painful sensation in the teeth because of a change in atmospheric pressure, as may occur at high altitudes.

aeroembolism. See **embolism.**

aerophagy /erof′əjē/ [Gk, *aer* + *phagein,* to eat], the swallowing of air, usually followed by belching, gastric distress, and flatulence. Also called **aerophagia** /er′ōfā′jē·ə/.

aerosinusitis /er′ōsī′nəsī′tis/ [Gk, *aer* + L, *sinus,* curve; Gk, *itis*], inflammation, edema, or hemorrhage of the frontal sinuses, caused by expansion of air within the sinuses when barometric pressure is decreased, as in aircraft at high altitudes. Also called **barosinusitis.**

aerosol /er′əsol′/ [Gk, *aer* + *hydor,* water; L, *solutus,* dissolved], **1.** nebulized particles suspended in a gas or air. **2.** a pressurized gas containing a finely nebulized medication for inhalation therapy. **3.** a pressurized gas containing a nebulized chemical agent for sterilizing the air of a room.

aerosol bronchodilator therapy, the use of drugs that provide relaxation of the respiratory tract smooth muscle tissue when administered as tiny droplets or a mist to be inhaled.

aerospace medicine /er′ōspās/, a branch of medicine concerned with the physiologic and psychologic effects of living and working in an artificial environment beyond the atmospheric and gravitational forces of the earth. The stress of extraterrestrial travel requiring long periods of weightlessness is a major concern. See also **aviation medicine.**

Aerosporin, a trademark for an antibiotic (polymyxin B sulfate).

aerotitis /er′ətī′tis/ [Gk, *aer* + *otikos,* ear, *itis*], an inflammation of the ear caused by changes in atmospheric pressure. Also called **barotitis.**

aerotitis media, inflammation or bleeding in the middle ear caused by a difference between the air pressure in the middle ear and that of the atmosphere, as occurs in sudden changes in altitude, in diving, or in hyperbaric chambers. Symptoms are pain, tinnitus, diminished hearing, and vertigo. Also called **barotitis media.**

Æsculapius /es′kyoŏlā′pē·əs/, the ancient Greek god of medicine. According to legend, Æsculapius, the son of Apollo, was trained by the centaur Chiron in the art of healing, becoming so proficient that he not only cured sick patients but also brought the dead back to life. Because Zeus feared that Æsculapius could help humans escape death altogether, he killed the healer with a bolt of lightning. Later, Æsculapius was raised to the stature of a god and was worshiped also by the Romans, who believed he could prevent pestilence. Serpents were regarded as sacred by

Æsculapius, and he is symbolized in modern medicine by a staff with a serpent entwined about it. See **staff of Æsculapius.**

-aesthesia, -esthesia, a suffix meaning '(condition of) feeling, perception, or sensation': *allaesthesia, cinaesthesia, hypercrysaesthesia.*

-aesthetic. See **-esthetic.**

Aesthetics. See **esthetics**.

AF, abbreviation for **atrial fibrillation.**

af-. See **ad-.**

AFB, abbreviation for **acid-fast bacillus.**

afebrile /āfē'bril, āfeb'ril/ [Gk, *a, febris,* not fever], without fever.

affect /əfekt'/ [L *affectus* influence], an outward manifestation of a person's feelings or emotions. −**affective,** *adj.*

affection /əfek'shən/ [L, *affectare,* to be influenced], **1.** an emotional state expressed by a warm or caring feeling toward another individual. **2.** a morbid process affecting all or a part of the human body.

affective /əfek'tiv/ [L, *affectus*], pertaining to emotion, mood, or feeling.

affective disorder. See **major affective disorder.**

affective intimacy, a measure of well-being in a family group in which members feel close to one another but do not lose their individuality.

affective learning, the acquisition of behaviors involved in expressing feelings in attitudes, appreciations, and values.

affective psychosis, a psychologic reaction in which the ego is disintegrated and the primary clinical feature is a severe disorder of mood or emotions.

affect memory, a particular emotional feeling that recurs whenever a significant experience is recalled.

afferent /af'ərənt/ [L, *ad, ferre,* to carry], proceeding toward a center, as applied to arteries, veins, lymphatics, and nerves. Compare **efferent.**

afferent nerves [L, *ad, ferre,* to bear, + *nervus*], nerve fibers that transmit impulses from the periphery toward the central nervous system.

afferent pathway [L, *ad,* to, *ferre,* to bear, AS, *paeth, weg*], the course or route taken, usually by a linkage of neurons, from the periphery of the body toward the center.

afferent tract [L, *ad, ferre,* to bear + *tractus*], a pathway for nerve impulses traveling inward or toward the brain, the center of an organ, or other body structure. Also called **ascending tract.**

affidavit /af'idā'vit/ [L, he has pledged] a written statement that is sworn to before a notary public or an officer of the court.

affiliated hospital /əfil'ē·ā'tid/ [L, *ad, filius,* to son], a hospital that is associated to some degree with a medical school or health program.

affinity /əfin'itē/ [L, *affinis,* related], the measure of the binding strength of the antibody-antigen reaction.

affirmative defense /əfur'mətiv/ [L, *affirmare,* to make firm], (in law) a denial of guilt or wrongdoing based on new evidence rather than on simple denial of a charge, as a plea of immunity according to a good samaritan law. The defendant bears the burden of proof in an affirmative defense.

afibrinogenemia /afī'brinōjenē'mē·ə/ [Gk, *a,* not; L, *fibra,* fiber; Gk, *genein,* to produce, *haima,* blood], a relative lack or absence of fibrinogen in the blood. It may be the result of a primary, congenital blood dyscrasia or acquired, as in disseminated intravascular coagulation.

aflatoxins /af'lātok'sins/ [Gk, *a,* not; L, *flavus,* yellow; Gk, *toxikon* poison], a group of carcinogenic and toxic factors produced by *Aspergillus flavus* food molds. The mucotoxins have been found to cause liver necrosis and liver cancer in laboratory animals and are believed to be responsible for a high incidence of liver cancer among people in tropic regions of Africa and Asia who may consume moldy grains, peanuts, or other *Aspergillus*-contaminated foods. See *Aspergillus*.

AFO, abbreviation for **ankle-foot orthosis.**

AFP, abbreviation for **alpha fetoprotein.**

African lymphoma. See **Burkitt's lymphoma.**

African sleeping sickness. See **African trypanosomiasis.**

African tick fever. See **relapsing fever.**

African tick typhus, a rickettsial infection transmitted by ixodid ticks and characterized by fever, maculopapular rash, and swollen lymph nodes. At the onset of the infection, a local lesion called tache noire, a buttonlike ulcer with a black center, appears. The rash usually begins on the forearms and spreads over the rest of the body. The fever may persist into the second week, but death or complications are rare.

African trypanosomiasis, a disease caused by the parasite *Trypanosoma brucei gambiense* or *Trypanosoma brucei rhodesiense,* transmitted to humans by the bite of the tsetse fly. African trypanosomiasis occurs only in the tropical areas of Africa, where tsetse flies are found. The disease progresses through three phases: localized, at the site of invasion of the organism; systemic, marked by fever, chills, headache, anemia, edema of the hands and feet, and enlargement of the lymph glands; and neurologic, marked by symptoms of central nervous system involvement, including lethargy, sleepiness, headache, convulsions, and coma. The disease is fatal unless treated, though it may be years before the patient reaches the neurologic phase. Antimicrobial medication specific for the treatment of trypanosomiasis is available in the United States only from the Centers for Disease Control. Kinds of African trypanosomiasis are **Gambian trypanosomiasis** and **Rhodesian trypanosomiasis.** Also called **African sleeping sickness, sleeping sickness.** See also **trypanosomiasis, tsetse fly.**

Afrin, a trademark for an adrenergic vasoconstrictor (oxymetazoline hydrochloride) used as a decongestant.

afterbirth [AS, *aefter;* ME, *burth*], the placenta, the amnion, the chorion, and some amniotic fluid, blood, and blood clots expelled from the uterus after childbirth.

aftercare [AS, *aefter, caru*], health care offered a patient after discharge from a hospital or other health care facility. The patient may require a certain amount of medical or nursing attention for a health problem that no longer demands inpatient status.

afterdepolarization /dēpō'lərizā'shən/, a second depolarization that follows an action potential. It is thought to be responsible for atrial and ventricular ectopic beats, especially in the setting of digitalis toxicity. Also called **afterpotential.**

afterload [AS, *aefter;* ME, *lod*], the load, or resistance, against which the left ventricle must eject its volume of blood during contraction. The resistance is produced by the volume of blood already in the vascular system and the vessel walls.

afterloading, (in radiotherapy) a technique in which an unloaded applicator or needle is placed within the patient at the time of an operative procedure and subsequently loaded with the radioactive source under controlled conditions in which health care personnel are protected against exposure to radiation. A kind of afterloading is **remote afterloading.**

aftermovement, an involuntary muscle contraction that causes a continued movement of a limb after a strong exertion against resistance has stopped. It is often demonstrated in abduction of the arm. Also called **Kohnstamm's phenomenon.**

afterpains [AS, *aefter;* Gk, *poine,* penalty], contractions of the uterus common during the first days postpartum. They tend to be strongest in nursing mothers during breastfeeding and multiparas, large babies, overdistended uterus, resolve spontaneously, and may require analgesia. The nurse may reassure the mother that afterpains are normal and prove that the uterus is contracting as it should.

afterpotential. See **afterdepolarization.**

afterpotential wave /-pəten′shəl/, either of two smaller waves, positive or negative, that follow the main spike potential wave of a nerve impulse, as recorded on an oscillograph tracing of an action potential that propagates along a nerve fiber.

Ag, symbol for the element **silver.**

ag-. See **ad-.**

AGA, abbreviation for **appropriate for gestational age.**

against medical advice (ama), a phrase pertaining to a client's decision to discontinue a therapy despite the advice of medical professionals.

agalactia /ā′gəlak′shə/ [Gk *a, gala* not milk], the inability of the mother to secrete enough milk to breast-feed an infant after childbirth.

agamete /āgam′ēt/ [Gk *a, gamos* not marriage], **1.** any of the unicellular organisms that reproduce asexually by multiple fission, such as bacteria and protozoa. **2.** any asexual reproductive cell, such as a spore or merozoite, that forms a new organism without fusion with another cell.

agametic /āgəmē′tik,/ asexual; without recognizable sex organs or gametes. Also **agamous** /ag′əməs/.

agamic /āgam′ik/, reproducing asexually, without the union of gametes; asexual.

agammaglobulinemia /agam′əglob′yoolinē′mē·ə/ [Gk *a, gamma* not gamma (third letter of Greek alphabet); L *globulus* small sphere; Gk *haima* blood], the absence of the serum immunoglobulin, gamma globulin, associated with an increased susceptibility to infection. The condition may be transient, congenital, or acquired. The transient form is common in infancy before 6 weeks of age, when the infant becomes able to synthesize the immunoglobulin. The congenital form is rare, sex-linked, and results in decreased production of antibodies. The acquired form usually occurs in malignant diseases such as leukemia, myeloma, or lymphoma. See also **Bruton's agammaglobulinemia, immune gamma globulin.**

agamogenesis /əgam′ōjen′əsis/ [Gk, *a, gamos,* not marriage, *genein,* to produce], asexual reproduction, as by budding or simple fission of cells; parthenogenesis. Also called **agamocytogeny** /əgam′ōsītoj′ənē/, **agamogony** /ag′əmog′ənē/. **–agamocytogenic, agamogenetic, agamogenic, agamogonic,** *adj.*

agamont. See **schizont.**

agamous. See **agametic.**

aganglionic megacolon. See **Hirschsprung's disease.**

agar-agar /a′gära′gär/ [Malay], a dried hydrophilic, colloidal product obtained from certain species of red algae. Because it is unaffected by bacterial enzymes, it is widely used as the basic ingredient in solid culture media in bacteriology. Agar-agar is also used as a suspending medium, as an emulsifying agent, and as a bulk laxative. Also called **agar.**

agarose /ag′ärōs/, an essentially neutral fraction of agar used as a medium in electrophoresis, particularly for separation of serum proteins, hemoglobin variants, and lipoprotein fractions.

agastric /āgas′trik/ [Gk, *a,* not, *gaster,* stomach], a condition of lacking a stomach or digestive tract.

age [L, *aetus*], a stage of development at which the body has arrived, as compared by physical and laboratory examinations to what is normal for a man or woman of the same chronologic span of life.

aged /ājd/, a state of having grown older or more mature than others of the population group.

ageism /ā′jizəm/ [L, *aetas,* lifetime], an attitude that discriminates, separates, stigmatizes, or otherwise disadvantages older adults on the basis of chronologic age.

agency [L, *agere,* to do], (in law) a relationship between two parties in which one authorizes the other to act in his or her behalf as agent. It usually implies a contractual arrangement between two parties managed by a third party, the agent.

agenesia. See **agenesis.**

agenesia corticalis /ā′jenē′zhə/ [Gk, *a, genein,* not to produce; L, cortex], the failure of the cortical cells of the brain, especially the pyramidal cells, to develop in the embryo, resulting in infantile cerebral paralysis and severe mental retardation.

agenesis /ājen′əsis/ [Gk, *a, genein,* not to produce], **1.** congenital absence of an organ or part, usually caused by a lack of primordial tissue and failure of development in the embryo. **2.** impotence or sterility. Also called **agenesia** /ā′jinē′zhə/. Compare **dysgenesis. –agenic,** *adj.*

agenetic fracture /ā′jenet′ik/, a spontaneous fracture caused by an imperfect osteogenesis.

-agenic. See **agenesis.**

ageniocephaly /ājen′ē·ōsef′əlē/ [Gk, *a, genein,* not to produce, *kephale,* head], a form of otocephaly in which the brain, cranial vault, and sense organs are intact but the lower jaw is malformed. Also called **ageniocephalia** /ājen′ē·ōsəfā′lē·ə. –ageniocephalic, ageniocephalous,** *adj.*

agenitalism /ājen′itəliz′əm/, a condition caused by the lack of sex hormones and the absence or malfunction of the ovaries or testes.

agenosomia /əjen′əsō′mē·ə/, a congenital malformation characterized by the absence or defective formation of the genitals and protrusion of the intestines through an incompletely developed abdominal wall.

agenosomus /əjen′əsō′məs/ [Gk, *a, genein,* not to produce, *soma,* body], a fetus with agenosomia.

agent [L, *agere,* to do], (in law) a party authorized to act on behalf of another and to give the other an account of such actions.

Agent Orange, a U.S. military code name for a mixture of two herbicides, 2,4-D and 2,4,5-T, used as a defoliant in Southeast Asia during the 1960s war in Vietnam. The herbicides were unintentionally contaminated with the highly toxic chemical dioxin, a cause of cancer and birth defects in animals and of chloracne and porphyria cutanea tarda in humans. See **dioxin.**

age of majority, the age at which a person is considered to be an adult in the eyes of the law.

age 30 transition, in psychiatry, a period between the ages of 28 and 33 when an individual may reevaluate the choices made in his or her twenties.

ageusia /əgyōō′sē·ə/ [Gk, *a*, not, *geusis*, taste], a loss or impairment of the sense of taste. The degree and cause may vary. Also called **ageustia.**

agglutinant /əglōō′tənənt/ [L, *agglutinare*, to glue], something that causes adhesion, such as an antibody produced in the blood that is stimulated by the presence of an antigen to adhere to it.

agglutination /əglōō′tinā′shən/ [L, *agglutinare*, to glue], the clumping together of cells as a result of interaction with specific antibodies called agglutinins. Agglutinins are used in blood typing and in identifying or estimating the strength of immunoglobulins or immune sera. See also **agglutinin, blood typing, precipitin.**

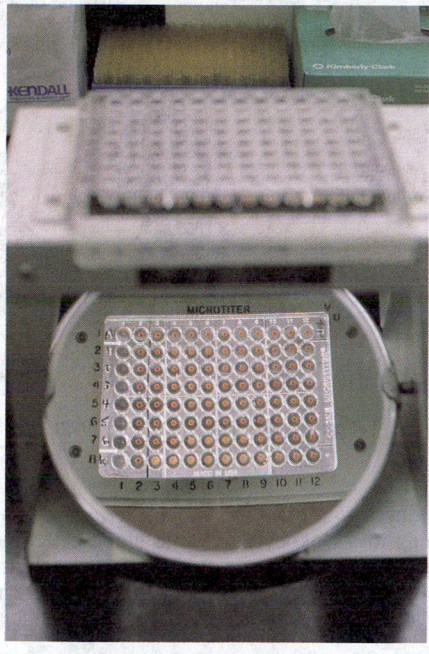

Agglutination assay (Mudge-Grout, 1992)

agglutination-inhibition test, a serologic technique useful in testing for certain unknown soluble antigens. The unknown antigen is mixed with a known agglutinin. If there is a reaction, the agglutinin can no longer adhere to the cells or particles that carry its corresponding antigen, and the unknown antigen is thus identified. One type of pregnancy test is based on agglutination inhibition.

agglutinin /əglōō′tinin/, an antibody that interacts with antigens, resulting in agglutination. Usually multivalent, ag-

glutinins act on insoluble antigens in stable suspension to form a cross-linking lattice that may clump or precipitate. Compare **precipitin.** See also **agglutination, blood typing, hemagglutination.**

agglutinin absorption, the removal from immune serum of antibody by treatment with homologous antigen, followed by centrifugation and separation of the antigen-antibody complex.

agglutinogen /ag′lōōtin′əjin/ [L, *agglutinare* + Gk, *genein*, to produce], any antigenic substance that causes agglutination by the production of agglutinin.

aggregate /ag′rəgāt/ [L, *ad, gregare*, to gather together], the total of a group of substances or components making up a mass or complex.

aggregate anaphylaxis, an exaggerated reaction of hypersensitivity rapidly induced by the injection of an antigen that forms a soluble antigen-antibody complex.

aggregation /ag′rəgā′shən [L, *ad, gregare,* to form a flock], an accumulation of substances, objects, or individuals, as in the clumping of blood cells or the clustering of clients with the same disorder.

aggression /əgresh′ən/ [L, *aggressio,* to attack], a forceful, action or attitude that is expressed physically, verbally, or symbolically. It may arise from innate drives or occur as a defensive mechanism and is manifested by either constructive or destructive acts directed toward oneself or against others. Kinds of aggression are **constructive aggression, destructive aggression,** and **inward aggression.**

aggressive personality /əgres′iv/, a personality with behavior patterns characterized by irritability, tantrums, destructiveness, or violence in response to frustration.

aggressive-radical therapy, (in psychiatry) a form of therapy that introduces the political and social viewpoints of the therapist into the therapeutic process. Proponents of this technique believe that by making all values explicit, sometimes through actual didactic input, the patient will view the solution of an emotional conflict and the raising of political consciousness as one and the same.

aging [L, *aetas,* lifetime], the process of growing old, resulting in part from a failure of body cells to function normally or to produce new body cells to replace those that are dead or malfunctioning. Normal cell function may be lost through infectious disease, malnutrition, exposure to environmental hazards, or genetic influences. Among body cells that exhibit early signs of aging are those that normally cease dividing after reaching maturity. See also **assessment of the aging patient, senile.**

agitated /aj′ətā′təd [L, *agitare,* to shake], describing a condition of psychomotor excitement characterized by purposeless, restless activity. Pacing, crying, and laughing, sometimes without apparent cause, are often seen and may serve to release nervous tension associated with anxiety, fear, or other mental stress. **–agitate,** *v.,* **agitation,** *n.*

agitated depression, a form of depression characterized by severe anxiety accompanied by continuous physical restlessness. See also **depression.**

agitation, a state of chronic restlessness, generally observed as a psychomotor expression of emotional tension.

agitographia /aj′itōgraf′ē·ə/ [L, *agitare* + Gk, *graphein,* to write], a condition characterized by abnormally rapid writing in which words or parts of words are unconsciously omitted. The condition is commonly associated with agitophasia.

agitophasia /aj'itōfā'zhə/ [L, *agitare* + Gk, *phasis*, speech], a condition characterized by abnormally rapid speech in which words, sounds, or syllables are unconsciously omitted, slurred, or distorted. The condition is commonly associated with agitographia. Also called **agitolalia.**

aglycemia /ā'glīsē'mē·ə/ [Gk, *a, glykis,* not sweet, *haima,* blood], an absence of blood sugar.

agnathia /ag·nath'ē·ə/ [Gk, *a, gnathos,* not jaw], a developmental defect characterized by total or partial absence of the lower jaw. It is usually accompanied by the union or approximation of the ears. Also called **agnathy** /ag'nəthē/. Compare **synotia.** See also **otocephaly. –agnathous,** *adj.*

agnathocephalia. See **agnathocephaly.**

-agnathocephalic. See **agnathocephaly.**

-agnathocephalous. See **agnathocephaly.**

agnathocephalus /ag·nath'əsef'ələs/, a fetus with agnathocephaly.

agnathocephaly /ag·nath'əsef'əlē/ [Gk, *a, gnathos* + *kephale,* head], a congenital malformation characterized by the absence of the lower jaw, defective formation of the mouth, and placement of the eyes low on the face with fusion or approximation of the zygomas and the ears. Also called **agnathocephalia.** See also **otocephaly. –agnathocephalic, agnathocephalous,** *adj.*

agnathus /ag·nath'əs/ [Gk, *a, gnathos,* not jaw], a fetus with agnathia.

agnathy. See **agnathia.**

agnogenic myeloid metaplasia. See **myeloid metaplasia.**

agnosia /ag·nō'zhə/ [Gk, *a, gnosis,* not knowledge], total or partial loss of the ability to recognize familiar objects or persons through sensory stimuli as a result of organic brain damage. The condition may affect any of the senses and is classified accordingly as auditory, visual, olfactory, gustatory, or tactile agnosia. Also called **agnosis.** See also **autotopagnosia.**

-agnosia, -agnosis, a suffix meaning '(condition of the) loss of the faculty to perceive': *autotopagnosia, paragnosia.*

-agogue, -agog, a suffix meaning an 'agent promoting the expulsion of a (specified) substance': **lymphagogue, succagogue, uragogue.**

agonal /ag'ənəl/ [Gk, *agon,* struggle], pertaining to death and dying.

agonal respiration [Gk, *agon,* struggle], a type of breathing that usually follows a pattern of gasping succeeded by apnea. It generally indicates the onset of respiratory arrest or the breathing pattern of a dying individual.

agonal thrombus, an aggregation of blood platelets, fibrin, clotting factors, and cellular elements that forms in the heart in the process of dying.

agonist /ag'ənist/ [Gk, *agon,* struggle], **1.** a contracting muscle whose contraction is opposed by another muscle (an antagonist). **2.** a drug or other substance having a specific cellular affinity that produces a predictable response.

agony /ag'ənē/ [Gk, *agon*], severe physical or emotional anguish or distress, as in pain.

agoraphobia /ag'ərə-/ [Gk, *agora,* marketplace, *phobos,* fear], an anxiety disorder characterized by a fear of being in an open, crowded, or public place, such as a field, tunnel, bridge, congested street, or busy department store, where escape may be difficult or help not available in case of sudden incapacitation. This phenomenon is observed more often in women than in men and generally can be

traced to some sudden loss or separation. Treatment consists of antianxiety medication and psychotherapy to uncover the cause of the phobic reaction and of behavior therapy, specifically systemic desensitization and flooding techniques for reducing the anxiety and altering the behavioral response. If untreated, fear and avoidance behavior dominate life, and the person refuses to leave home.

-agra, a suffix meaning a 'pain or painful seizure': **cardiagra, podagra, trachelagra.**

agranular endoplasmic reticulum. See **endoplasmic reticulum.**

agranulocyte /āgran'yoolōsīt'/ [Gk, *a,* not; L, *granulum,* small grain; Gk, *kytos,* cell], any leukocyte that does not contain predominant cytoplasmic granules, such as a monocyte or lymphocyte. Compare **granulocyte.** See also **leukocyte.**

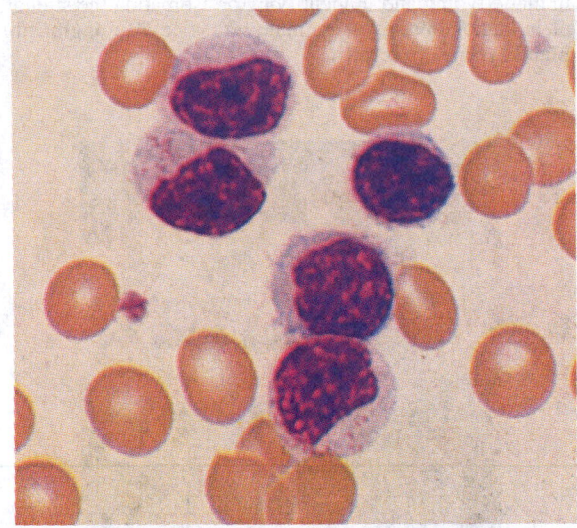

Agranulocytes *(Hayhoe, 1992)*

agranulocytic /-si'tik/ [Gk, *a,* not, *granule, kytos,* cell], pertaining to a leukocyte or white blood cell which, upon being stained, shows no granules in the cytoplasm.

agranulocytosis /āgran'yoolōsītō'sis/, a severe reduction in the number of granulocytes (basophils, eosinophils, and

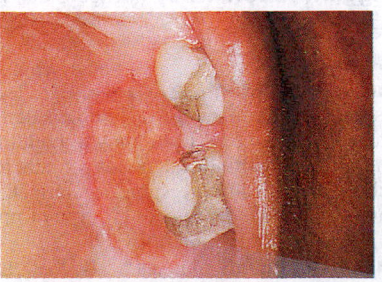

Agranulocytosis in the oral cavity *(Lamey, 1988)*

neutrophils). Fever, prostration, and bleeding ulcers of the rectum, mouth, and vagina may be present. The acute disease may be an adverse reaction to a medication or the result of radiation therapy.

agraphia /āgraf′ē·ə/ [Gk, *a, graphein*, not to write], an abnormal neurologic condition characterized by loss of the ability to write, resulting from injury to the language center in the cerebral cortex. Compare **dysgraphia**. –**agraphic**, *adj*.

A:G ratio, the ratio of protein albumin to globulin in the blood serum. On the basis of differential solubility with neutral salt solution the normal values are 3.5 to 5 g/dl for albumin and 2.5 to 4 g/dl for globulin.

agrypnia. See **insomnia.**

agrypnocoma /agrip′nōkō′mə/ [Gk, *agrypnos*, sleepless], a coma in which there is some degree of wakefulness. The condition may be manifested by extreme lethargy or drowsiness accompanied by delirium.

agrypnotic /ag′ripnot′ik/, **1.** insomniac. **2.** a drug or other substance that prevents sleep.

agyria /əjī′rē·ə/, **1.** an abnormal condition caused by excessive absorption and tissue deposition of silver salts. It is marked by a slate-gray coloration of the skin and mucous membranes. **2.** a cerebral cortex abnormality in which the gyri are poorly developed. The cortical tissue is reduced, leading to severe mental retardation.

AHA, abbreviation for **American Hospital Association.**

"aha" reaction /ähä′/, (in psychology) a sudden realization or inspiration, experienced especially during creative thinking. Some psychologists associate great scientific discoveries and artistic inspirations with this reaction, which is not necessarily related to intelligence. The term has apparently replaced **"aha" experience,** formerly used by psychologists, especially those of the Gestalt school, to label experiences in which an individual utters "Aha!" during a moment of revelation.

AHF, abbreviation for **antihemophilic factor.**

AHH, abbreviation for **aryl hydrocarbon hydroxylase.**

Ahumada-del Castillo syndrome /ä′hoomä′dädel′ kästē′yō/, a form of secondary amenorrhea that may be associated with a pituitary gland tumor. It is characterized by both galactorrhea and amenorrhea in the absence of a pregnancy.

AI, abbreviation for **artificial intelligence;** abbreviation for **artificial insemination.**

aid, assistance given a person who is ill, injured, or otherwise unable to cope with normal demands of life.

AID, abbreviation for **artificial insemination-donor.**

AIDS /ādz/, abbreviation for **acquired immunodeficiency syndrome.**

AIDS-dementia complex (ADC), a neurologic effect of encephalitis or brain inflammation experienced by nearly one-third of all AIDS patients. The condition is characterized by memory loss and other forms of dementia. A suggested cause is that the AIDS virus may destroy neurons without actually entering the brain cells. Autopsies indicate the neuron density in AIDS patients may be 40% lower than in the brains of persons who have not experienced AIDS. Also called **AIDS-related dementia.**

AIDS-wasting syndrome, a category of acquired immunodeficiency syndrome (AIDS). Signs and symptoms may include weight loss, fever, malaise, lethargy, oral thrush, and immunologic abnormalities characteristic of AIDS. Previously called **AIDS-related complex (ARC).**

AIH, abbreviation for **artificial insemination-husband.**

ailment [OE, *eglan*], any disease or physical disorder or complaint, generally of a chronic, acute, or mild nature.

ainhum. See **autoamputation.**

air [Gk *aer*], the colorless, odorless gaseous mixture constituting the earth's atmosphere. It consists of 78% nitrogen, 21% oxygen, almost 1% argon, small amounts of carbon dioxide, hydrogen, and ozone, traces of helium, krypton, neon, and xenon, and varying amounts of water vapor.

air bath, the exposure of the naked body to warm air for therapeutic purposes. Also called **balneum pneumaticum** /bal′nē·əm noomat′ikəm/.

airborne contaminants, materials in the atmosphere that can affect the health of persons in the same or nearby environments. Particularly vulnerable are tissues of the upper respiratory tract and lungs, including the terminal bronchioles and alveoli. The effects depend in part on the solubility of the inhaled matter. Inhaled contaminants may cause tissue damage, tissue reaction, disease, or physical obstruction. Some airborne contaminants, such as carbon monoxide gas, may have little or no direct effect on the lungs but can be absorbed into the bloodstream and carried to other organs or damage the blood itself. Biologically inert gases may dilute the atmospheric oxygen below the normal blood saturation value, thereby disturbing cellular respiration.

air compressor, a contrivance that compresses air for storage and use in handpieces and other air-driven medical and dental tools.

air embolism, the abnormal presence of air in the cardiovascular system, resulting in obstruction of the flow of blood through the vessel. Air may be inadvertently introduced by injection, during intravenous therapy or surgery, or traumatically, as by a puncture wound. See also **decompression sickness, embolus, gas embolism.**

air encephalography. See **encephalography.**

air entrainment, the movement of room air into the chamber of a jet nebulizer used to treat respiratory diseases. Air entrainment increases the rate of nebulization and the amount of liquid administered per unit of time.

airflow pattern, the pattern of movement of respiratory gases through the respiratory tract, such as laminar, turbulent, or tracheobronchial. The pattern is affected by such factors as gas density and viscosity.

air fluidization, the process of blowing warm air through a collection of microspheres to create a fluidlike environment. The technique is used in special mattresses designed to reduce pressure against a patient's skin. See also **air-fluidized bed.**

air-fluidized bed, a bed with body support provided by thousands of tiny soda-lime glass beads suspended by pressurized warm air. The patient rests on a polyester filter sheet that covers the beads. The special bed is designed for use by patients with posterior pressure sores or posterior grafts, burns, or donor areas. Pressure against the skin surface of the patient is less than capillary filling pressure. The improved capillary blood flow to the skin speeds the growth of granulation tissue. The temperature of the bed can be controlled.

air hunger, a form of respiratory distress characterized by gasping, labored breathing, or dyspnea.

airplane splint, a splint used for immobilizing a fractured humerus during healing. The splint holds the arm in an abducted position at shoulder level, with the elbow bent. It extends to the waist and may be made of wire or leather, or it may be supported by a plaster body.

air pump, a pump that forces air in or out of a cavity or chamber.

air sickness. See **motion sickness.**

air spaces, the alveolar ducts, alveolar sacs, and alveoli of the respiratory system.

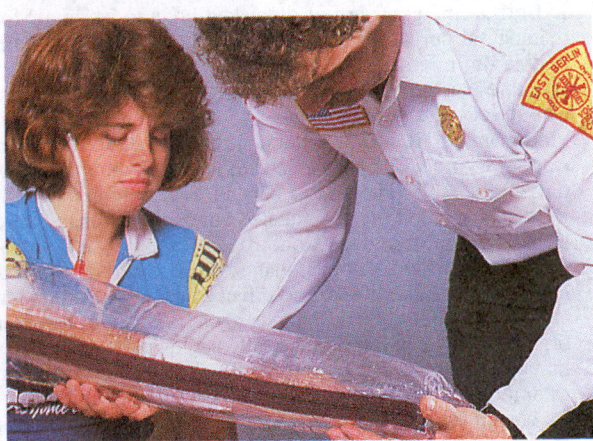

Air splint *(Judd, 1988)*

air splint, a device for temporarily immobilizing fractured or otherwise injured extremities. It consists of an inflatable cylinder that can be closed at both ends and becomes rigid when filled with air under pressure.

air thermometer, a thermometer using air as its expansible medium. See also **thermometer.**

airway [Gk, *aer* + AS, *weg*, way], any tubular passage for the movement of air into and out of the lungs, such as the trachea and bronchi; a respiratory anesthesia device; or an oropharyngeal tube used for mouth-to-mouth resuscitation. An airway with a diameter greater than 2 mm is defined as a large, or central, airway; one smaller than 2 mm is called a small, or peripheral, airway.

airway clearance, ineffective, a nursing diagnosis accepted by the Fourth National Conference on the Classification of Nursing Diagnoses. It is a state in which an individual is unable to clear secretions or obstructions from the respiratory tract to maintain airway patency. The defining characteristics of the condition include abnormal breath sounds, change in the rate or depth of respiration, tachypnea, cough, cyanosis, and dyspnea. Related factors include decreased energy or fatigue, infection, obstruction, or secretions of the tracheobronchial tree, perceptual or cognitive impairment, or trauma. See also **nursing diagnosis.**

airway conductance, the instantaneous volumetric gas flow rate in the airway per unit of pressure difference between the mouth, nose, or other airway opening and the alveoli. It is also the reciprocal of airway resistance. It is indicated by the symbol G_{aw}.

airway division, one of the 18 segments of the bronchopulmonary system. The segments are usually numbered from 1 to 10 for both the right and left lungs, although there are usually only two lobes in the left lung, compared with three lobes in the right lung, resulting in two fewer bronchial branches on the left side.

airway obstruction, an abnormal condition of the respiratory system characterized by a mechanical impediment to the delivery or to the absorption of oxygen in the lungs, as in bronchospasm, choking, croup, laryngospasm, chronic obstructive lung disease, goiter, tumor, or pneumothorax.

■ OBSERVATIONS: If the obstruction is minor, as in sinusitis or pharyngitis, the person is able to breathe, but not normally. If the obstruction is acute, the person may grasp the neck, gasp, become cyanotic, and lose consciousness.

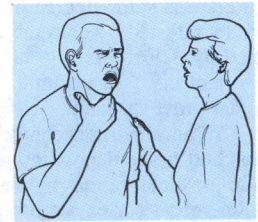

Airway obstruction: Victim gives international choking sign; rescuer asks if victim can speak

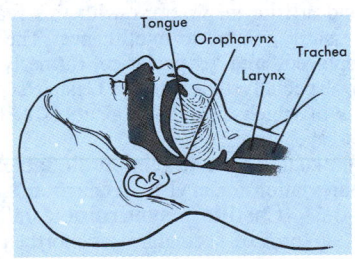

Airway obstruction by tongue

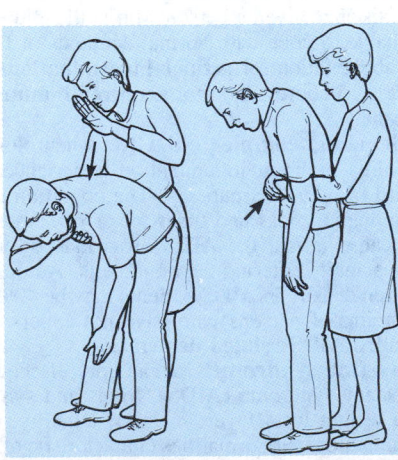

Airway obstruction: back blows and chest thrusts

■ INTERVENTIONS: Acute airway obstruction requires rapid intervention to save the person's life. A bolus of food, a collection of mucus, or a foreign body may be removed manually, by suction, or with the Heimlich maneuver. Obstruction of the airway caused by inflammatory or allergic reaction may be treated with bronchodilating drugs, corticosteroids, intubation, and the administration of oxygen. An emergency tracheotomy may be required if the obstruction cannot be mechanically removed or pharmacologically reduced within a few minutes.

■ NURSING CONSIDERATIONS: The patient is usually very apprehensive and may physically resist assistance. The cause of the obstruction is identified, if possible. Medical assistance is summoned, and the most highly trained person available begins emergency care, including removing the obstruction, if possible; administering oxygen; and performing cardiopulmonary resuscitation, if necessary. See also **aspiration, cardiopulmonary resuscitation, Heimlich maneuver.**

airway resistance, the ratio of pressure difference between the mouth, nose, or other airway opening and the alveoli to the simultaneously measured resulting volumetric gas flow rate. It is the reciprocal of airway conductance and is indicated by the symbol R_{aw}.

AK, abbreviation for *above the knee,* a term referring to amputations, amputees, prostheses, and orthoses.

akathisia /ak'əthē'zhə/ [Gk, *a, kathizein,* not to sit], a pathologic condition characterized by restlessness and agitation, such as an inability to sit still. −**akathisiac,** *adj.*

akinesia /ā'kinē'zhə, ā'kīnē'zhə/ [Gk, *a, kinesis,* not movement], an abnormal state of motor and psychic hypoactivity or muscular paralysis. −*akinetic* /ā'kinet'ik/, *adj.*

akinetic, /ā'kinet'ik/ [Gk, *a,kinesis],* without movement], pertaining to a loss of ability to move a part or all of the body.

akinetic apraxia, the inability to perform a spontaneous movement. See also **apraxia.**

akinetic mutism, a state in which a person is unable or refuses to move or to make sounds, resulting from neurologic or psychologic disturbance.

akinetic seizure, a type of seizure disorder observed in children. It is a brief, generalized seizure in which the child suddenly falls to the ground.

Akineton, a trademark for an anticholinergic (biperiden hydrochloride or biperiden lactate), used as an antiparkinsonian.

-akusis. See -acousia.

Al, symbol for the element **aluminum.**

-al, a suffix designating a compound containing a member of the aldehyde group: **benzal, chloral, ethanal.**

-al, -ale, a suffix meaning 'pertaining to or characterized by': **appendiceal, calyceal, meningeal.**

ala /ā'lə/, *pl.* **alae** [L, wing], **1.** any winglike structure. **2.** the axilla.

Ala, abbreviation for **alanine.**

ALA, abbreviation for **aminolevulinic acid.**

ala auris, the auricle of the ear.

ala cerebelli /ser'əbel'ī/, the ala of the central lobule of the cerebellum.

ala cinerea /sinir'ē·ə/, the triangular area on the floor of the fourth ventricle of the brain from which the autonomic fibers of the vagus nerve arise.

alactasia. See **lactase deficiency.**

ala nasi /nā'sī/, the outer flaring cartilaginous wall of each nostril.

alanine (Ala) /al'ənin/, a nonessential amino acid found in many food protein sources as well as in the body. It is degraded in the liver to produce pyruvate and glutamate. See also **amino acid, protein.**

Chemical structure of alanine (Seeley, 1992)

alanine aminotransferase (ALT), an enzyme normally present in the serum and tissues of the body, especially the tissues of the liver. This enzyme catalyzes the transfer of an amino group from l-alanine to alpha-ketoglutarate, forming pyruvate and L-glutamate. The reaction is reversible. The enzyme is released into the serum because of tissue injury and may increase in persons with acute liver damage. Normal findings are 5-35 IU/L. Also called **glutamic-pyruvic transaminase.** Compare **aspartate aminotransferase.**

Al-Anon, an international organization that offers guidance, counseling, and support for the relatives, friends, and associates of alcoholics. See also **Alcoholics Anonymous.**

ala of the ethmoid, a small projection on each side of the crista galli of the ethmoid bone. Each ala fits into a corresponding depression of the frontal bone.

ala of the ilium, the upper flaring portion of the iliac bone.

ala of the sacrum, the flat extension of bone on each side of the sacrum.

alar /ā'lär/ [L, *ala,* wing], pertaining to a winglike structure, such as the shoulder.

alar lamina [L, *ala,* wing, *lamina,* thin plate], the posterolateral area of the embryonic neural tube through which sensory nerves enter.

alar ligament, one of a pair of ligaments that connects the axis to the occipital bone and limits rotation of the cranium. Also called **check ligament, odontoid ligament.** Compare **membrana tectoria.**

alar process [L, *ala,* wing, *processus],* a projection of the cribriform plate of the ethmoid bone articulating with the frontal bone.

alarm reaction, the first stage of the general adaptation syndrome, characterized by the mobilization of the various defense mechanisms of the body or the mind to cope with a stressful situation of a physical or emotional nature. See also **stress.**

alastrim /al'əstrim/ [Port, *alastrar,* to spread], a mild form of smallpox, thought to be caused by a weak strain of *Poxvirus variolae.* Unlike smallpox, alastrim is rarely fatal. Also called **Cuban itch, milkpox, variola minor.** See also **smallpox.**

Alateen, an international organization that offers guidance, counseling, and support for the children of alcoholics. See also **Alcoholics Anonymous.**

ala vomeris /vō'məris/, an extension of bone on each side of the upper border of the vomer.

alb-, a prefix meaning 'white': *albumin*.

alba /al'bə/, literally, 'white,' as in *linea alba*.

Albers-Schönberg disease /-shœn'burg, -shōn'-/ [Heinrich E. Albers-Schönberg, Hamburg radiologist, b. 1865], a form of osteopetrosis characterized by marblelike calcification of bones. The condition is often discovered by chance during x-ray examination. The disease is transmitted as an autosomal dominant trait. See also **osteopetrosis.**

Albert's disease, an inflammation of the bursa that lies between the Achilles tendon and the calcaneus. It is most frequently caused by injury but may also result from the wearing of poorly fitted shoes, increased strain on the tendon, or rheumatoid arthritis. If treatment is delayed, the inflammation may cause erosion of the calcaneus. Also called **anterior Achilles bursitis.**

albicans /al'bikənz/ [L, *albus,* white], pertaining to the whitish yellow scar tissue of the **corpus albicans** of the ovary. The scar tissue forms following rupture of the ovarian follicle after ovulation. The scar decreases in size and eventually disappears over time. See also **corpus luteum.**

albinism /al'biniz'əm/, a congenital condition characterized by partial or total lack of melanin pigment in the body. Total albinos have pale skin that does not tan, white hair, pink eyes, nystagmus, astigmatism, and photophobia. Albinos are prone to severe sunburn, actinic dermatitis, and skin cancer. Compare **piebald, vitiligo.**

albino /albī'nō/ [L, *albus*] white], an individual with a marked deficiency of pigment in the eyes, hair, and skin. Because of a lack of eye pigment, the choroid is vulnerable to adverse effects of sunlight frequently resulting in photophobia, astigmatism, and other visual disorders. Lack of skin pigment predisposes the individual to skin cancer.

Albright's syndrome /ôl'brīts/ [Fuller Albright, Boston physician, b. 1900], a disorder characterized by fibrous dysplasia of bone, isolated brown macules on the skin, and endocrine dysfunction. It causes precocious puberty in girls but not in boys. The osseous lesions are reddish gray, gritty fibromas containing areas of coarse fiber that may be confined to one bone or occur in several, frequently causing deformities. Hyperthyroidism is present in some cases. Treatment may involve osteotomy, curettage, and bone grafts. Also called **Albright-McCune-Sternberg syndrome, osteitis fibrosa disseminata.** See **pseudohypoparathyroidism.**

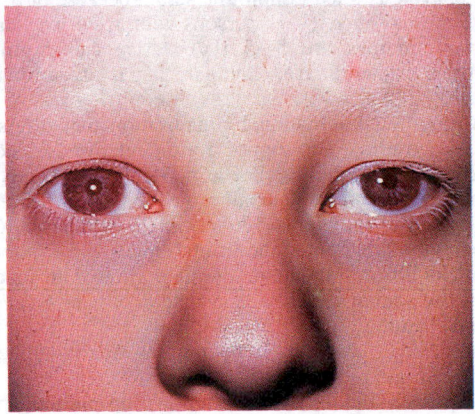

Pale fundus of albinism *(Zitelli, 1992)*

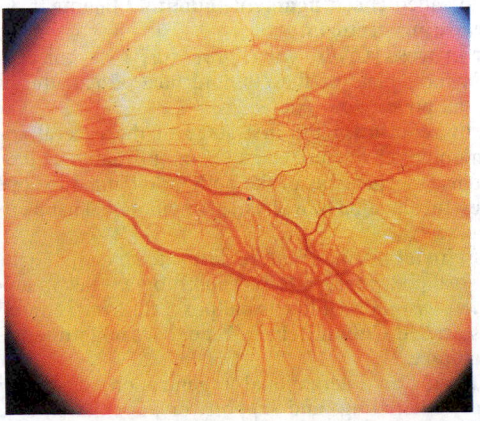

White hair and pale skin of albinism *(Zitelli, 1992)*

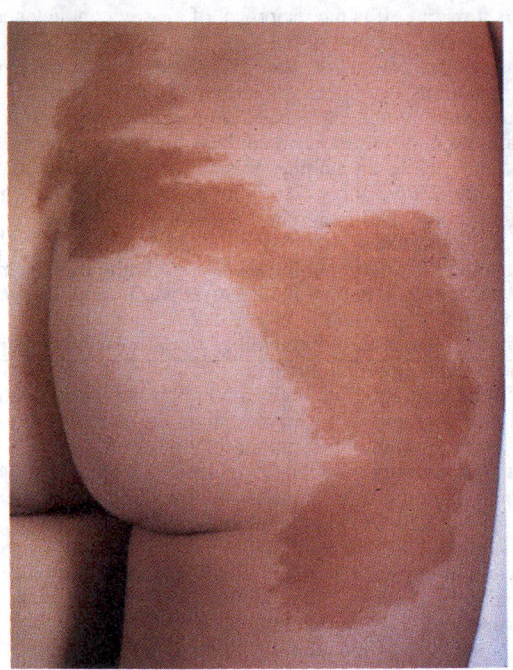

Albright's syndrome
(du Vivier, 1993/Courtesy Dr. David Atherton)

albumin /albyoo'min/ [L, *albus,* white], a water-soluble, heat-coagulable protein. Various albumins are found in practically all animal tissues and in many plant tissues. Determination of the levels and kinds of albumin in urine, blood, and other body tissues is the basis of a number of laboratory diagnostic tests.

albumin A, a blood serum constituent that gathers in cancer cells but is deficient in circulation in cancer patients.

albumin (human), a plasma-volume expander.

■ INDICATIONS: It is prescribed in the treatment of hypoproteinemia, hyperbilirubinemia, and hypovolemic shock.

■ CONTRAINDICATIONS: Severe anemia or cardiac failure prohibits its use.

■ ADVERSE EFFECTS: Among the most serious adverse reactions are chills, hypotension, fever, and urticaria.

albuminous liver. See **amyloid liver.**

albumin test [L, *albus,* white], any of several tests for the presence of albumin, a class of simple proteins, in the urine, a common sign of renal or functional disorders. One type of albumin test depends upon the change in color of a chemically treated strip of paper in the presence of albumin. The **Heller's test** involves the addition of a thin layer of urine on a small amount of concentrated nitric acid and is regarded as positive if an opaque line forms at the junction of the two fluids. In an **acetic acid test,** a test tube of urine is heated until a cloudiness develops. The test is considered positive if the cloudiness increases when three drops of acetic acid are added.

albuminuria. See **proteinuria.**

-albuminuria, a suffix meaning a '(specified) condition characterized by excess serum proteins in the urine': *noctalbuminuria, pseudalbuminuria.*

albuterol, an adrenergic used as a bronchodilator.

■ INDICATION: It is prescribed in the treatment of bronchospasm in patients with reversible obstructive airway disease.

■ CONTRAINDICATION: Known sensitivity to this drug prohibits its use.

■ ADVERSE EFFECTS: Among the most serious adverse reactions are tachycardia, insomnia, dizziness, and hypertension.

alcalase, a protein enzyme contained in concentrations of about 60 ppm in certain laundry detergents. It is a cause of enzymatic detergent asthma.

alclometasone dipropionate, a topical corticosteroid.

■ INDICATIONS: It is prescribed for the relief of symptoms of inflammation and pruritus of corticosteroid-responsive dermatoses.

■ CONTRAINDICATIONS: Children may absorb proportionally greater amounts of the drug per area of skin surface and should be treated with the smallest amount of the drug needed.

■ ADVERSE EFFECTS: Among adverse reactions reported are burning, stinging, and itching.

Alcock's canal [Joseph Alcock, English surgeon, b. 1784], a canal formed by the obturator internus muscle and the obturator fascia through which the pudendal nerve and vessels pass. Also called **pudendal canal.**

alcohol /al′kəhôl/ [Ar *alkohl* subtle essence], **1.** (USP) a preparation containing at least 92.3% and not more than 93.8% by weight of ethyl alcohol, used as a topical antiseptic and solvent. **2.** a clear, colorless, volatile liquid that is miscible with water, chloroform, or ether, obtained by the fermentation of carbohydrates with yeast. **3.** a compound derived from a hydrocarbon by replacing one or more hydrogen atoms with an equal number of hydroxyl (OH) groups. Depending on the number of hydroxyl radicals, alcohols are classified as monohydric, dihydric, trihydric. Some kinds of alcohol are **rubbing alcohol, sugar alcohol,** and **unsaturated alcohol.**

alcohol bath, a procedure for decreasing an elevated body temperature. A tepid solution of 25% to 50% alcohol in water is sponged lightly on each limb, then on the trunk, turning the person only once from supine to prone position and then back again. Some sources recommend the placement of a hot-water bottle at the feet and a cold compress on the head to accelerate heat loss through vasodilatation, to promote the comfort of the patient during the procedure, and to reduce the temperature of the circulation to the brain. As the alcohol evaporates quickly, the bed is less likely to get wet, the patient does not need to be dried, and, for an equal result, the solution does not need to be as cold as a plain bath with cold water.

Alcohol, Drug Abuse, and Mental Health Administration (ADAMHA), an agency of the U.S. Department of Health and Human Services with three components—the National Institute on Alcohol Abuse and Alcoholism, the National Institute on Drug Abuse, and the National Institute of Mental Health. It conducts and supports research on the biologic, psychologic, epidemiologic, and behaviorial aspects of alcoholism, drug abuse, and mental health and illness.

alcoholic ataxia [Ar, *alkohl,* essence, + Gk, *ataxia,* disorder], a loss of control of voluntary movements associated with peripheral neuritis secondary to alcoholism. A similar form of ataxia may occur with neuritis resulting from other toxic agents.

alcoholic cardiomyopathy [Ar, *alkohl,* essence, + Gk, *kardia,* heart, *mys,* muscle, *pathos,* disease], a cardiac disease associated with alcohol abuse. It is characterized by an enlarged heart and low cardiac output.

alcoholic cirrhosis. See **Laënnec's cirrhosis.**

alcoholic coma [Ar, *alkohl,* + Gk, *koma,* deep sleep], a state of unconsciousness that results from severe alcoholic intoxication.

alcoholic dementia [Ar, *alkohl,* + L, *de,* away, *mens,* mind], a deterioration of normal cognitive and intellectual functions associated with long-term alcohol abuse.

alcoholic fermentation, the conversion of carbohydrates to ethyl alcohol.

alcoholic hallucinosis, a form of alcoholic psychosis characterized primarily by auditory hallucinations, abject fear, and delusions of persecution. The condition develops in acute alcoholism as withdrawal symptoms shortly after stopping or reducing the intake of alcohol. Also called **acute hallucinosis.** See also **alcoholic psychosis, hallucinosis.**

alcoholic hepatitis, acute toxic liver injury associated with excess ethanol consumption. This is characterized by necrosis, polymorphonuclear inflammation, and in many instances Mallory bodies.

alcoholic ketoacidosis, the fall in blood pH (acidosis) sometimes seen in alcoholics and associated with a rise in serum ketone bodies (acetone, beta-hydroxybutyric acid, and acetoacetic acid).

alcoholic neuropathy. See **alcoholic paralysis.**

alcoholic-nutritional cerebellar degeneration, a sudden, severe incoordination in the lower extremity, characteristic of poorly nourished alcoholics. The patient walks, if at all, with an ataxic or wide-based gait. Cerebellar tumors, multiple sclerosis, and other neurologic disorders have similar motor impairments. Treatment consists of improved nutrition, abstinence from alcohol, and physical therapy. See also **alcoholism.**

alcoholic paralysis [Ar, *alkohl,* essence; Gk, *paralyein,* to be palsied], a paralysis affecting the peripheral nerves as a result of alcohol consumption. Also called **alcoholic neuropathy.**

alcoholic psychosis, any of a group of severe mental disorders, such as pathologic intoxication, delirium tremens,

Korsakoff's psychosis, and acute hallucinosis, characterized by brain damage or dysfunction that results from the excessive use of alcohol.

Alcoholics Anonymous (AA), an international nonprofit organization, founded in 1935, consisting of abstinent alcoholics whose purpose is to help other alcoholics stop drinking and maintain sobriety through group support, shared experiences, and faith in a power greater than themselves. The AA program, which emphasizes both medical and religious resources for help in overcoming alcoholism, consists of attending meetings and coping with abstinence "one day at a time." Meetings are held at convenient times in factories, schools, churches, hospitals, and many other institutions and community buildings. Similar groups who work with the children, relatives, friends, and associates of alcoholics are **Al-Anon** and **Alateen.**

alcoholic trance, a state of automatism resulting from ethanol intoxication.

alcoholism /al′kəhôliz′əm/, the extreme dependence on excessive amounts of alcohol, associated with a cumulative pattern of deviant behaviors. Alcoholism is a chronic illness with a slow, insidious onset, which may occur at any age. The cause is unknown, but cultural and psychosocial factors are suspect, and families of alcoholics have a higher incidence of alcoholism. Frequent intoxication has cumulative destructive effects on an individual's family and social life, working life, and physical health. The most frequent medical consequences of alcoholism are central nervous system depression and cirrhosis of the liver. The severity of each of these is possibly increased in the absence of food intake. Alcoholic patients also may suffer from alcoholic gastritis, peripheral neuropathies, auditory hallucinations, and cardiac problems. Abrupt withdrawal of alcohol in addiction causes weakness, sweating, and hyperreflexia. The severe form of alcohol withdrawal is called delirium tremens. Extreme caution should be used in administering drugs to the alcoholic patient because of the possibility of additive central nervous system depression. The treatment of alcoholism consists of psychotherapy (especially group therapy, by organizations like Alcoholics Anonymous), electroshock treatments, or drugs such as disulfiram that cause an aversion to alcohol. See also **acute alcoholism, chronic alcoholism, delirium tremens.**

alcohol poisoning, poisoning caused by the ingestion of any of several alcohols, of which ethyl, isopropyl, and methyl are the most common. Ethyl alcohol (grain alcohol) is found in whiskies, brandy, gin, and other beverages. Ordinarily, it is lethal only if large quantities are ingested in a brief period. Isopropyl alcohol is more toxic: Ingestion of 8 ounces may result in respiratory or circulatory failure. Methyl alcohol (wood alcohol) is extremely poisonous: in addition to nausea, vomiting, and abdominal pain, it may cause blindness, and death may follow the consumption of only 2 ounces. Treatment for alcohol poisoning may include gastric lavage and other supportive intervention.

alcohol withdrawal syndrome, the clinical symptoms associated with cessation of alcohol consumption. These may include tremor, hallucinations, autonomic nervous system dysfunction, and seizures.

ALD, abbreviation for **adrenoleukodystrophy.**

Aldactazide, a trademark for a fixed-combination drug containing two diuretics (hydrochlorothiazide and spironolactone).

Aldactone, a trademark for a potassium-sparing diuretic (spironolactone).

aldehyde /al′dəhīd′/ [Ar, alkohl + L, dehydrogenatum, dehydrogenated], any of a large category of organic compounds derived from a corresponding alcohol by the removal of two hydrogen atoms, as in the conversion of ethyl alcohol to acetaldehyde. Each aldehyde is characterized by a carbonyl (-CHO) group in its empiric formula and can be converted into a corresponding acid by the addition of one oxygen atom, as in the conversion of acetaldehyde to acetic acid.

Aldoclor, a trademark for a fixed-combination antihypertensive drug containing chlorothiazide and methyldopa.

aldolase /al′dəlās/, an enzyme found in muscle tissue that catalyzes the step in anaerobic glycolysis involving the breakdown of fructose 1,6-diphosphate to glyceraldehyde 3-phosphate. The enzyme can also catalyze the reverse reaction. Normal adult findings are 3.0-8.2 Sibley-Lehninger U/dl or 22-59 mU at 37 degrees C. See also **glycolysis.**

Aldomet, a trademark for an antihypertensive (methyldopa).

Aldoril, a trademark for a fixed-combination drug containing a diuretic (hydrochlorothiazide) and an antihypertensive (methyldopa).

aldose /al′dōs/, the chemical form of monosaccharides in which the carbonyl group is an aldehyde.

aldosterone /al′dōstərōn′, aldos′tərōn/, a mineral corticoid steroid hormone produced by the adrenal cortex with action in the renal tubule to regulate sodium and potassium balance in the blood.

aldosteronism /al′dōstərō′nizəm, aldos′-/, a condition characterized by hypersecretion of aldosterone, occurring as a primary disease of the adrenal cortex or, more often, as a secondary disorder in response to various extraadrenal pathologic processes. Primary aldosteronism, also called **Conn's syndrome,** may be caused by adrenal hyperplasia or by an aldosterone-secreting tumor. Secondary aldosteronism is associated with increased plasma renin activity and may be induced by the nephrotic syndrome, hepatic cirrhosis, idiopathic edema, congestive heart failure, trauma, burns, or other kinds of stress. Hypersecretion of aldosterone promotes sodium retention and potassium excretion, leading to increased blood volume and blood pressure, alkalosis, muscular weakness, tetany, paresthesias, nephropathy, ventricular arrhythmias, and other cardiac abnormalities. The electrolyte imbalance in aldosteronism usually causes polydipsia and polyuria. Treatment of primary aldosteronism caused by a tumor may include surgical resection and chemotherapy with the adrenal cytotoxic agent mitotane. Spironolactone, an aldosterone antagonist, is frequently used to treat symptoms of aldosteronism. Also called **hyperaldosteronism.**

aldosteronoma /al′dōstir′ənō′mə/, pl. **aldosteronomas, aldosteronomata,** an aldosterone-secreting adenoma of the adrenal cortex that is usually small and occurs more frequently in the left than the right adrenal gland. Hyperaldosteronism with salt retention, expansion of the extracellular fluid volume, and increased blood pressure may occur.

-aldrate, a suffix designating an antacid aluminum salt.

Aleppo boil. See **oriental sore.**

alertness [Fr, alerte], a condition of being quick, active, and keenly aware of the environment.

aleukemic leukemia /ā′lōōkē′mik/, a type of leukemia in

which the total leukocyte count remains within normal limits and few abnormal forms appear in the peripheral blood. Diagnosis requires bone marrow biopsy. Also called **subleukemic leukemia.** See also **leukemia.**

aleukemic myelosis.   See **myeloid metaplasia.**

aleukia /āloo̅'kē·ə/ [Gk, *a, leukos,* not white],   a marked reduction in or the complete absence of white blood cells or blood platelets. Compare **leukopenia, thrombocytopenia.** See also **aplastic anemia.**

aleukocythemic leukemia.   See **aleukemic leukemia.**

Alexander technique,   a body-focused alternative mental health therapy introduced by Frederick Alexander. It focuses on individual variations in body musculature, posture, and the breathing process and the correction of defects to avoid stress, tension, and possible dysfunction.

alexia /əlek'sē·ə/ [Gk, *a, lexis,* not speech],   an inability to comprehend written words. Also called **word blindness.** Compare **dyslexia. –alexic,** *adj.*

alexic /əlek'sik/ [Gk, *a,* without, *lexis,* speech],   pertaining to a condition of alexia.

alexithymia /əlek'sithī'mē·ə, -thim'ē·ə/,   an inability to consciously experience and communicate feelings.

alfa.   See **alpha.**

alg-.   See **algesi-.**

alga /al'gə/, *pl.* **algae** /al'jī, al'jē/ [L, seaweed],   any of a large group of nonmotile, or motile, marine plants containing chlorophyll. Many genera and species of algae are found worldwide in fresh water, in salt water, and on land. All belong to the phylum Thallophyta. **–algal,** *adj.*

algesi-, alg-, alge-, algo-,   a prefix meaning 'pertaining to pain': *algesia.*

-algesia,   a suffix meaning '(condition of) sensitivity to pain': *asphalgesia, haphalgesia, hyperthermalgesia.*

-algesic,   a suffix meaning 'pertaining to sensitivity to pain': *analgesic, hypalgesic, paralgesic.*

-algia, -algy,   a suffix meaning 'pain, painful condition': *epigastralgia, sacralgia, uteralgia.*

-algic,   a suffix meaning 'related to pain': *cardialgic, ophthalmalgic, tibialgic.*

algid malaria /al'jid/ [L, *algere,* to be cold],   a stage of malaria caused by the protozoan *Plasmodium falciparum,* characterized by coldness of the skin, profound weakness, and severe diarrhea. See also **falciparum malaria, malaria.**

algo-.   See **algesi-.**

algodystrophy /al'gōdis'trəfē/,   a painful wasting of the muscles of the hands, often accompanied by tenderness and a loss of bone calcium. The condition may begin in the hand or in the shoulder and spread over the entire limb, causing contractures, edema, and cyanosis of the skin. It may be associated with injury, heart disease, stroke, or a viral infection.

ALGOL /al'gôl/,   abbreviation for *algorithmic language,* a type of computer language.

algolagnia /al'gōlag'nē·ə/ [Gk, *algos,* pain, *lagneia,* lust],   a form of sexual perversion characterized by sadism or masochism. See also **sadism, sadomasochism.**

algologist /algol'əjist/,   **1.** a person who specializes in the study of or the treatment of pain. **2.** also called **phycologist.** a person who specializes in the study of algae.

algology,   **1.** the branch of medicine that is concerned with the study of pain. **2.** also called **phycology.** the branch of science that is concerned with algae.

algophobia [Gk, *algos,* pain, *phobos,* fear],   an anxiety disorder characterized by an abnormal, pervasive fear of experiencing pain or of witnessing pain in others.

algorithm /al'gərith'əm/,   **1.** a step-by-step procedure for the solution of a problem by computer, using specific mathematic or logical operations. Compare **heuristic. 2.** an explicit protocol with well-defined rules to be followed in solving a health care problem.

algor mortis,   the reduction in body temperature and accompanying loss of skin elasticity that occur after death. Also called **death chill.**

alien /āl'yən/ [L, *alienare,* to estrange],   strange, unusual, or foreign.

alienate /al'yənāt/ [L, *alienare*],   to cause a withdrawal or transference of affection, or detachment.

alienation /āl'yənā'shən/ [L, *alienare,* to estrange],   the act or state of being estranged or isolated. See also **depersonalization.**

alignment /əlīn'mənt/,   **1.** the arrangement of a group of points or objects along a line. **2.** the placing or maintaining of body structures in their proper anatomic positions, such as straightening the teeth or repairing a fractured bone. Also spelled **alinement.**

alimentary /al'əmen'tərē/ [L, *alimentum,* nourishment],   pertaining to food or nourishment and to the digestive organs.

alimentary bolus.   See **bolus,** def. 1.

alimentary canal.   See **digestive tract.**

alimentary system [L, *alimentum,* nourishment; Gk, *systema*],   the digestive system.

alimentary tract.   See **digestive tract.**

alimentation.   nourishment. See also **feeding.**

alinement.   See **alignment.**

aliphatic /al'ifat'ik/ [Gk, *aleiphar,* oil],   pertaining to fat or oil, specifically to those hydrocarbon compounds that are open chains of carbon atoms, such as the fatty acids, rather than ring structures.

aliphatic acid,   an acid of a nonaromatic hydrocarbon.

aliphatic alcohol,   an alcohol that contains an open chain or fatty series of hydrocarbons. Examples include ethyl alcohol and isopropyl alcohol, both of which have fat-solvent properties as well as bactericidal effects.

-alis,   a suffix meaning 'pertaining to' something specified.

alkalemia [Ar, *al, galiy,* wood ash; Gk, *haima,* blood],   a condition of increased pH of the blood, above the normal range of 7.38 to 7.42.

alkali /al'kəlī/ [Ar, *al, galiy,* wood ash],   a compound with the chemical characteristics of a base. Alkalis combine with fatty acids to form soaps, turn red litmus blue, and enter into reactions that form water-soluble carbonates. See also **acid, base. alkaline,** *adj.* **alkalinity,** *n.*

alkali burn,   damage to tissue caused by exposure to an alkaline compound like lye. Treatment includes washing the area with copious amounts of water to remove the chemical. The victim should be immediately taken to a medical facility if the tissue damage is more than slight and superficial. Compare **acid burn.**

-alkaline,   a suffix meaning 'of or referring to alkali': **subalkaline.**

alkaline-ash /al'kəlīn/,   residue in the urine having a pH of higher than 7.

alkaline-ash-producing foods,   foods that may be ingested in order to produce an alkaline pH in the urine, thereby reducing the incidence of acidic urinary calculi, or that may be avoided in order to reduce the incidence of alkaline calculi. Some of the foods that result in alkaline ash are milk, cream, buttermilk, fruit (except prunes, plums, and cranberries), vegetables (except corn and lentils), almonds, chestnuts, coconuts, and olives.

alkaline bath, a bath taken in water containing sodium bicarbonate, used especially for skin disorders.

alkaline phosphatase, an enzyme present in bone, the kidneys, the intestine, plasma, and teeth. It may be elevated in the serum in some diseases of the bone and liver and in some other illnesses. The normal concentrations of this enzyme in the serum of adults are 1.5 to 4.5 Bodansky units; in children, 5 to 14 Bodansky units. See **Bodansky units.**

alkaline reserve, an additional amount of sodium bicarbonate the body produces to maintain an arterial blood pH of 7.40 when the carbon dioxide level increases as a result of hypoventilation. The alkaline reserve is maintained by the kidneys, which control excretion of bicarbonate ions in the urine.

alkalinity /al'kəlin'itē/, pertaining to the acid-base relationship of any solution that has fewer hydrogen ions or more hydroxyl ions than pure water, which is an arbitrarily neutral standard with a pH of 7.

alkalinize /al'kəlinīz/, **1.** to make a substance alkaline, as through the addition of a base. **2.** to become alkaline. Also **alkalize** /al'kəlīz/. Compare **acidify.**

alkali poisoning, a toxic condition caused by the ingestion of an alkaline agent like liquid ammonia, lye, and some detergent powders. Emergency treatment includes giving copious amounts of water or milk to dilute the alkali. Vomiting is not induced, and mild acids are not administered. The victim is transported immediately to the hospital for observation of any corrosive damage to the esophagus or of any metabolic abnormality and for mechanical removal of the alkali by gastric lavage. Compare **acid poisoning.**

alkali reserves [Ar, *al, galiy,* the wood ashes, + L, *reservare,* to save], the volume of carbon dioxide or carbonates at standard temperature and pressure held by 100 ml of blood plasma to be neutralized by lactic or other acids. The principal buffer in blood is bicarbonate, which essentially represents the alkali reserve. Hemoglobin phosphates and additional bases also act as buffers. If the alkali reserve is low, a state of acidosis exists; if the alkali reserve is high, alkalosis exists.

alkalize. See **alkalinize.**

alkaloid /al'kəloid/ [Ar, *al, galiy* + Gk, *eidos,* form], any of a large group of nitrogen-containing organic compounds produced by plants, including many pharmacologically active substances, such as atropine, caffeine, cocaine, morphine, nicotine, and quinine. The term also may be applied to synthetic chemicals, such as procaine, that are similar to the alkaloid substances found in leaves, stems, seeds, or other plant parts.

alkalosis /al'kəlō'sis/ [Ar, *al, galiy* + Gk, *osis,* condition], an abnormal condition of body fluids, characterized by a tendency toward a pH level greater than 7.44, as from an excess of alkaline bicarbonate or a deficiency of acid. Respiratory alkalosis may be caused by hyperventilation, resulting in an excess loss of carbon dioxide and a carbonic acid deficit. Metabolic alkalosis may result from an excess intake or retention of bicarbonate, loss of gastric acid in

vomiting, potassium depletion, or any stimulus that increases the rate of sodium-hydrogen exchange. Alkalosis is said to be compensated if an adaptive mechanism, such as a buffer system, carbon dioxide retention, or bicarbonate excretion, prevents a shift in pH. Treatment of uncompensated alkalosis involves correction of dehydration and various ionic deficits to restore the normal acid-base balance in which the ratio of carbonic acid to bicarbonate is 20:1. Compare **acidosis.**

alkaptonuria /alkap'tōnoor'ē·ə/ [Ar, *al, galiy* + Gk, *haptein* to possess, *ouron* urine], a rare inherited disorder resulting from the incomplete metabolism of tyrosine, an amino acid, in which abnormal amounts of glycosuric acid are excreted, staining the urine dark. In this disorder, which is transmitted by an autosomal recessive gene, a key metabolic enzyme is absent from the body. Usually, the condition does not cause symptoms until middle age, at which point ochronosis, a type of arthritis, may develop. The condition also can be caused by chronic phenol poisoning. See also **ochronosis. –alkaptonuric,** *adj.*

alkene /al'kēn/, an unsaturated aliphatic hydrocarbon containing one double bond in the carbon chain, such as ethylene. Also called **olefin.**

Alkeran, a trademark for an antineoplastic (melphalan).

alkyl /al'kil/, a hydrocarbon fragment derived from alkane by the removal of one of the hydrogen atoms.

alkylamine /al'kiləmīn'/, an amine in which an alkyl group replaces one to three of the hydrogen atoms that are attached to the nitrogen atom, such as methylamine.

alkylating agent /al'kilā'ting/, any substance that contains an alkyl radical and is capable of replacing a free hydrogen atom in an organic compound. This type of chemical reaction results in interference with mitosis and cell division, especially in rapidly proliferating tissue. The agents are useful in the treatment of cancer. Agents include cyclophosphamide. Adverse effects include nausea, vomiting, alopecia, and anemia.

alkylation, a chemical reaction in which an alkyl group is transferred from an alkylating agent. When such organic reactions occur with a biologically significant cellular constituent, such as DNA, they result in interference with mitosis and cell division.

ALL, abbreviation for **acute lymphocytic leukemia.** See also **acute childhood leukemia.**

all-. See **allo-.**

allanto-, a combining form meaning 'pertaining to the allantois': *allantotoxicon.*

-allantoic. See **allantois.**

allantoidoangiopagus /al'əntoi'dō·an'jē·op'əgəs/ [Gk, *allantoeides,* sausagelike, *aggeion,* vessel, *pagos,* fixed], conjoined monozygotic twin fetuses of unequal size that are united by the vessels of the umbilical cord. Also called **omphaloangiopagus.** See also **omphalosite. –allantoidoangiopagous,** *adj.*

allantoin /əlan'tō·in/, a chemical compound (5-ureidohydantoin), $C_4H_6N_4O_3$, that occurs as a white crystallizable substance found in many plants and in the allantoic and amniotic fluids and fetal urine of primates. It is also present in the urine of mammals other than the primates as a product of purine metabolism. The substance, which can be produced synthetically by the oxidation of uric acid, was once used to promote tissue growth in the treatment of suppurating wounds and ulcers.

allantois /əlan'tois/ [Gk, *allas,* sausage, *eidos,* form], a tubular extension of the endoderm of the yolk sac that extends with the allantoic vessels into the body stalk of the embryo. In human embryos, allantoic vessels become the umbilical vessels and the chorionic villi. See also **body stalk, umbilical cord.** –**allantoic** /al'əntō'ik/, *adj.*

allele /əlēl'/, **1.** one of two or more alternative forms of a gene that occupy corresponding loci on homologous chromosomes. **2.** Also called **allelomorph** /əlēl'əmôrf'/. one of two or more contrasting characteristics transmitted by alternative genes.

allelo-, a combining form meaning 'pertaining to another': *allelocatalysis, allelomorph, allelotaxis.*

allelomorph. See **allele.**

Allen correction, multichromatic analysis of reaction to correct for background absorbance.

Allen-Doisy test [Edgar Allen, American anatomist, b. 1892; Edward Doisy, American physiologist, b. 1893], a bioassay test for estrogen and gonadotropins by injecting ovariectomized mice with an estrogenic substance. The appearance of cornified cells on vaginal smears is regarded as positive.

Allen test, a test for the patency of the radial artery after insertion of an indwelling monitoring catheter. The patient's hand is formed into a fist while the nurse compresses the ulnar artery. Compression of the ulnar artery is continued while the fist is opened. If blood perfusion through the radial artery is adequate, the hand should flush and resume normal pinkish coloration.

allergen /al'ərjin/ [Gk, *allos*, other, *ergein*, to work, *genein*, to produce], a substance that can produce a hypersensitive reaction in the body but is not necessarily intrinsically harmful. Some common allergens are pollen, animal dander, house dust, feathers, and various foods. Some studies indicate that one of every six Americans is hypersensitive to one or more allergens. The bodies of normal individuals develop a natural or acquired immunity to allergens, but in less fortunate individuals the immune system may be overly sensitive to foreign substances and to others produced naturally by the body. The body normally protects itself against allergens or antigens by the complex chemical reactions of the humoral immune and the cell-mediated immune systems. Methods to identify specific allergens affecting individuals continue to improve. The most common method involves a skin test in which several allergens can be examined simultaneously. –**allergenic,** *adj.*

allergenic extract /al'ərjen'ik/, an extract of the protein of a substance to which a person may be sensitive. The extract, which may be prepared from a wide variety of substances from food to fungi, can be used for diagnosis or for desensitization therapy.

allergic /əlur'jik/, **1.** of or pertaining to allergy. **2.** having an allergy.

allergic alveolitis. See **diffuse hypersensitivity pneumonia.**

allergic asthma, a form of asthma caused by the exposure of the bronchial mucosa to an inhaled airborne antigen. This allergen causes the production of antibodies that bind to mast cells in the bronchial tree. The mast cells then release histamine, which stimulates contraction of bronchial smooth muscle and causes mucosal edema. Psychologic factors may provoke asthma attacks in bronchi already sensitized by allergens. Hyposensitization treatments are more effective for pollen sensitivity than for house dust, animal hair, molds, and insects. Often, a diurnal pattern of hista-

mine release is seen, causing variable degrees of bronchospasm at different times of the day. See also **asthma, asthma in children, asthmatic eosinophilia, status asthmaticus.**

allergic bronchopulmonary aspergillosis, a form of aspergillosis that occurs in asthmatics when the fungus *Aspergillus fumigatus,* growing within the bronchial lumen, causes a type I or type III hypersensitivity reaction. The characteristics of the condition are similar to those of asthma, including dyspnea and wheezing. Chest examination and pulmonary function tests may reveal airway obstruction. Serologic tests usually reveal precipitating antibodies to *A. fumigatus.* Bacteriologic and microscopic examination of sputum may reveal *A. fumigatus* in addition to Charcot-Leyden crystals. Eosinophilia is usually also present. Compare **aspergillosis.**

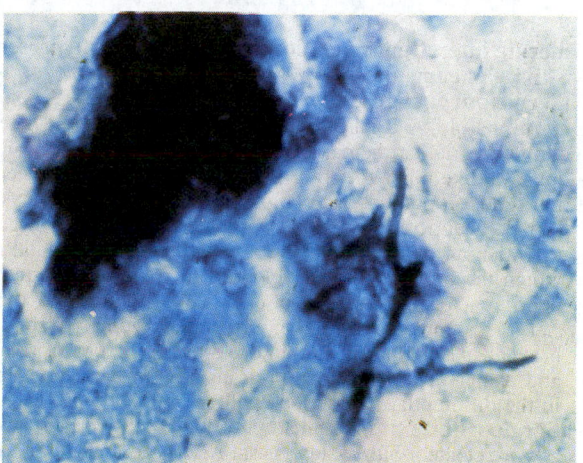

Allergic bronchopulmonary aspergillosis—sputum smear
(Zitelli, 1992/Borrowed from Slavin RG, Laird TS, Cherry JD: Allergic bronchopulmonary aspergillosis in a child. Pediatr 1970; 76:416-421)

allergic conjunctivitis, hyperemia of the conjunctiva caused by an allergy. Common allergens that cause this condition are pollen, grass, topical medications, air pollutants, occupational irritants, and smoke. It is bilateral and usually starts before puberty and lasts about 10 years, commonly recurring in a seasonal pattern.
- OBSERVATIONS: The common signs of allergic conjunctivitis are excessive tearing and pain. Eosinophils predominate in stained blood smears, and diagnosis is commonly based on cultures and sensitivity tests to identify the causative allergen.
- INTERVENTIONS: Treatment commonly includes the administration of vasoconstrictor eyedrops, such as epinephrine, and oral antihistamines.
- NURSING CONSIDERATIONS: Cold compresses may be administered.

allergic coryza, acute rhinitis caused by exposure to any allergen to which the person is hypersensitive.

allergic dermatitis [Ger, *allergie*, reaction, + Gk, *derma*, skin, *itis*, inflammation], an acute inflammatory condition of the skin after exposure of a body area to an allergen to which the patient is hypersensitive. (See Fig. p. 60.)

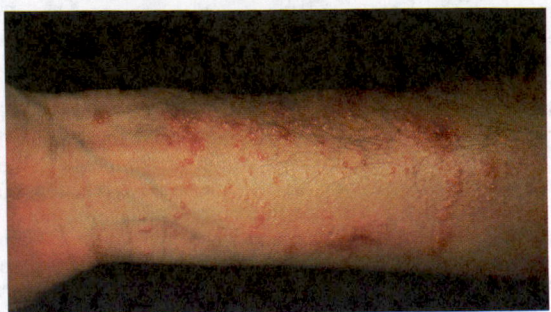

Allergic dermatitis resulting from contact with poison ivy
(Goldstein, 1992)

allergic interstitial pneumonitis.   See **diffuse hypersensitivity pneumonia.**

allergic purpura [Gk, *allos,* other, *ergein,* to work; L, *purpura,* purple], a chronic disorder of the skin associated with urticaria, erythema, asthma, and rheumatic joint swellings. Unlike other forms of purpura, platelet count, bleeding time, and blood coagulation are normal.

allergic reaction, a hypersensitive response to an allergen to which an organism has previously been exposed and to which the organism has developed antibodies. Subsequent exposure causes the release of chemical mediators and a variety of symptoms including urticaria, eczema, dyspnea, bronchospasm, diarrhea, rhinitis, sinusitis, laryngospasm, and anaphylaxis. Eosinophilia is usually present, revealed in the differential white blood cell count.

allergic rhinitis, inflammation of the nasal passages, usually associated with watery nasal discharge and itching of the nose and eyes caused by a localized sensitivity reaction to house dust, animal dander, or an antigen, commonly pol-

len. The condition may be seasonal, as in hay fever, or perennial, as in allergy to dust or animals. Treatment may include the local, systemic, or topical administration of antihistamines, avoidance of the antigen, and hyposensitization by injections of diluted antigen in gradually increasing amounts.

allergic vasculitis, an inflammatory condition of the blood vessels that is induced by an allergen. Disseminated intravascular inflammation sometimes occurs in patients treated with iodides, penicillin, sulfonamides, and thioureas. Allergic cutaneous vasculitis is characterized by itching, malaise, and a slight fever and by the presence of papules, vesicles, urticarial wheals, or small ulcers on the skin.

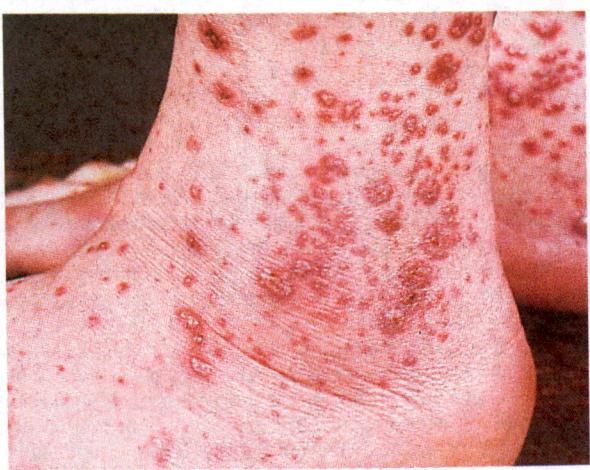

allergic vasculitis in the foot
(du Vivier, 1993/Courtesy St. Mary's Hospital)

allergist /al'ərjist/, a physician who specializes in the diagnosis and treatment of allergic disorders.

allergy /al'ərjē/ [Gk, *allos,* other, *ergein,* to work], a hypersensitive reaction to intrinsically harmless antigens, most of which are environmental. Studies show that one of every six Americans has a severe allergy and that more than 20 million Americans have allergic reactions to airborne or inhaled allergens, such as cigarette smoke, house dust, and pollens. Allergic rhinitis, which is associated with airborne allergens, affects predominantly young children and adolescents but occurs in all age groups. Allergies are divided into those that produce immediate or antibody-mediated reactions and those that produce delayed or cell-mediated reactions. Immediate allergic reactions release certain substances into the circulation, such as histamine, bradykinin, acetylcholine, immunoglobulin IgG, and leukotaxine. Delayed allergic reactions are caused by antigens but do not seem to depend on antibodies. Depending on the type of hypersensitivity involved, some common symptoms of allergy are bronchial congestion, conjunctivitis, edema, fever, urticaria, and vomiting. Severe allergic reactions such as anaphylaxis can cause systemic shock and death. Symptoms of limited duration, such as those associated with hay fever, serum sickness, bee stings, and urticaria, can be suppressed by glucocorticoids administered as supplements to primary therapy. Severe allergic reactions such as anaphylaxis and angioneurotic edema of the glottis commonly re-

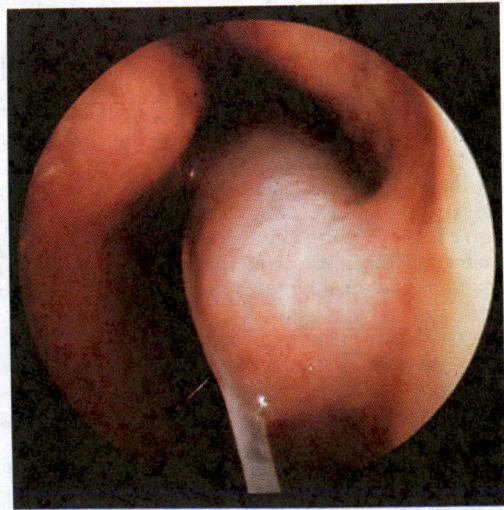

Allergic rhinitis as seen through fiberoptic rhinoscope
(Zitelli, 1992)

quire immediate therapy with epinephrine administered subcutaneously. When allergic reactions are life threatening, steroids, such as dexamethasone sodium phosphate, may be administered intravenously. For milder diseases, such as serum sickness and hay fever, antihistamines are usually administered. See also **allergy testing, immunoglobulins.**

allergy testing, any one of the various procedures used in identifying the specific allergens that afflict a patient. Such tests are helpful in prescribing treatment to prevent allergic reactions or to reduce their severity. The most common is skin testing, which exposes the patient to small quantities of the suspected allergens. Positive reactions usually occur within 20 minutes as varying degrees of erythema. Factors considered in performing allergy tests include the medical history of the patient, the allergy history, the environment, and the diet. Individuals to be tested are usually instructed to discontinue the use of any antihistamines at least 24 hours before the test, because these drugs can interfere with normal test responses. The most common kinds of allergy testing include the intradermal, scratch, patch, conjunctival, and use tests.

all fours position, the sixth stage in the Rood system of ontogenetic motor patterns. In this stage, the lower trunk and lower extremities are brought into a cocontraction pattern while stretching of the trunk and limb girdles develops cocontractions of the trunk flexors and extensors.

allied health personnel. See **paramedical personnel.**

alligator forceps, 1. a forceps with heavy teeth and a double clamp, employed in orthopedic surgery. **2.** a forceps with long, thin, angular handles and interlocking teeth.

allo-, all-, a prefix meaning 'differing from the normal, reversal, or referring to another': *allobiosis, allochezia, allopathy.*

allodiploid /al'ōdip'loid/ [Gk, *allos,* other, *diploos,* double, *eidos,* form], **1.** also **allodiploidic.** of or pertaining to an individual, organism, strain, or cell that has two genetically distinct sets of chromosomes derived from different ancestral species, as occurs in hybridization. **2.** such an individual, organism, strain, or cell. See also **autopolyploid.**

allodiploidy /al'ōdip'loidē/, the state or condition of having two genetically distinct sets of chromosomes derived from different ancestral species.

alloeroticism, alloerotism. See **heteroeroticism.**

alloesthesia /al'ō·esthē'zhə/, a referred pain or other sensation that may be perceived on the same or opposite side of the body but not at the site stimulated.

allogamy. See **cross fertilization.**

allogenic /al'ōjen'ik/ [Gk, *allos* + *genein,* to produce], **1.** (in genetics) denoting an individual or cell type that is from the same species but genetically distinct. **2.** (in transplantation biology) denoting tissues that are from the same species but antigenically distinct; homologous. Compare **syngeneic, xenogeneic.**

allograft /al'əgraft/ [Gk, *allos,* other + *graphion,* stylus], the transfer of tissue between two genetically dissimilar individuals of the same species, such as a tissue transplant between two humans who are not identical twins. Also called **homograft.** Compare **autograft, isograft, xenograft.** See also **graft.**

allohexaploid, allohexaploidic. See **allopolyploid.**

-allometric. See **allometry.**

allometric growth, the increase in size of different organs or parts of an organism at various rates. Also called **heterauxesis** /het'ərôksē'sis/. Compare **isometric growth.** See also **allometry.**

allometron /əlom'itron/, a quantitative change in the proportional relationship of the parts of an organism as a result of the evolutionary process.

allometry /əlom'itrē/ [Gk, *allos* + *metron,* measure], the measurement and study of the changes in proportions of the various parts of an organism in relation to the growth of the whole or within a series of related organisms. See also **allometric growth. –allometric,** *adj.*

allomorphism /al'ōmôr'fizəm/ [Gk, *allos,* other, *morphe,* form], **1.** a change in crystalline form without a change in chemical composition. **2.** a change in the shape of a group of cells due to pressure or other physical factors.

allopathic physician /al'ōpath'ik/, a physician who treats disease and injury with active interventions, such as medical and surgical treatment, intended to bring about effects opposite from those produced by the disease or injury. Almost all practicing physicians in the United States are allopathic. Compare **chiropractic, homeopathy.**

allopathy /əlop'əthē/ [Gk, *allos* + *pathos,* suffering], a system of medical therapy in which a disease or an abnormal condition is treated by creating an environment that is antagonistic to the disease or condition; for example, an antibiotic toxic to a pathogenic organism is given in an infection, or an iron supplement may be given to increase the synthesis of hemoglobin in iron deficiency anemia.

allopentaploid, allopentaploidic. See **allopolyploid.**

alloplastic maneuver [Gk, *allos* + *plassein,* to form], (in psychology) a process that is part of adaptation, involving an adjustment or change in the external environment. Compare **autoplastic maneuver.**

alloploid, alloploidic. See **allodiploid, allopolyploid.**

alloploidy. See **allodiploidy, allopolyploidy.**

allopolyploid /al'əpol'iploid/ [Gk, *allos* + *polyplous,* many times, *eidos* form], **1.** also **allopolyploidic.** of or pertaining to an individual, organism, strain, or cell that has more than two genetically distinct sets of chromosomes derived from two or more different ancestral species, as occurs in hybridization. They are referred to as allotriploid, allotetraploid, allopentaploid, allohexaploid, and so on, depending on the number of multiples of haploid sets of chromosomes they contain. **2.** such an individual, organism, strain, or cell. See also **mosaic.** Compare **autopolyploid.**

allopolyploidy /al'əpol'iploi'dē/, the state or condition of having more than two genetically distinct sets of chromosomes from two or more ancestral species. See **mosaic.** Compare **autopolyploidy.**

allopurinol /al'əpyoor'ənôl/, a xanthine oxidase inhibitor.
■ INDICATIONS: It is prescribed in the treatment of gout and other hyperuricemic conditions.
■ CONTRAINDICATIONS: It is not prescribed for children (except those with hyperuricemia secondary to malignancy), for lactating mothers, or for people suffering an acute attack of gout. Known hypersensitivity to this drug prohibits its use.
■ ADVERSE EFFECTS: Among the most serious adverse reactions to this drug are blood dyscrasias and severe rashes and other allergic reactions. GI and ophthalmologic disturbances also may occur.

all-or-none law, 1. the principle in neurophysiology that if a stimulus is strong enough to trigger a nerve impulse, the entire impulse is discharged. A weak stimulus will not produce a weak reaction. **2.** the principle that the heart muscle, under any stimulus above a threshold level, will respond either with a maximal strength contraction or not at all. Also called **Bowditch's law.**

allosteric sites /al'ōster'ik/ [Gk, *allos* + *stereos,* solid], the sites, other than the active site or sites, of an enzyme that bind regulatory molecules.

allotetraploid, allotetraploidic. See **allopolyploid.**

allotrio-, a prefix meaning 'strange or foreign': *allotriodontia.*

allotriploid, allotriploidic. See **allopolyploid.**

allowable charge /əlou′əbəl/, the maximum amount that a third party, usually an insurance company, will pay to reimburse a provider for a specific service.

allowable costs, components of an institution's costs that are reimbursable as determined by a payment formula. In general, costs of services not considered to be reasonable or necessary to the proper provision of health services are excluded from allowable costs.

allowable dose. See **maximum permissible dose.**

allowable error, the amount of error that can be tolerated without invalidating the medical usefulness of the analytic result. Allowable error is defined as having a 95% limit of analytic error; only 1 sample in 20 can have an error greater than this limit.

alloxan /əlok′san/, an oxidation product of uric acid that is found in the human intestine in diarrhea. Because it can destroy the insulin-secreting islet cells of the pancreas, alloxan may cause diabetes.

alloy /al′oi/ [Fr, *aloyer*, to combine metals], a mixture of two or more metals or of substances with metallic properties. Most alloys are formed by mixing molten metals that dissolve in each other. A number of alloys have medical applications, such as those used for prostheses and in dental amalgams. See **amalgam.**

aloe /al′ō/ [Gk], the inspissated juice of various species of *Aloe* plants, formerly used as a cathartic but generally discontinued because it often causes severe intestinal cramps. It is a component of many topical preparations.

alopecia /al′əpē′shə/ [Gk, *alopex*, fox (mange)], partial or complete lack of hair resulting from normal aging, endocrine disorder, drug reaction, anticancer medication, or skin disease. Kinds of alopecia include **alopecia areata, alopecia totalis,** and **alopecia universalis.**

alopecia areata /er′ē·ā′tə/, a disease of unknown cause in which well-defined bald patches occur. The bald areas are usually round or oval and located on the head and other hairy parts of the body. The condition is usually self-limited and clears completely within 6 to 12 months without treatment. Recurrences are common. Compare **alopecia totalis, alopecia universalis.**

alopecia totalis, an uncommon condition characterized by the loss of all the hair on the scalp. The cause is unknown, and the baldness is usually permanent. No treatment is known. Compare **alopecia areata, alopecia universalis.**

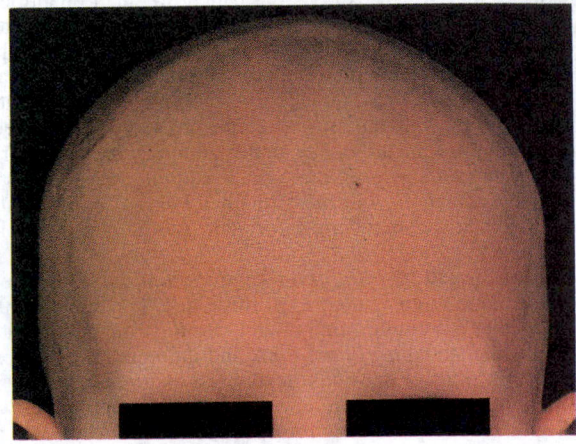

Alopecia totalis (Baran, 1992)

alopecia universalis, a total loss of hair on all parts of the body. The condition is occasionally an extension of alopecia areata. Compare **alopecia areata, alopecia totalis.**

alpha /al′fə/, A, α, the first letter of the Greek alphabet. It is often used in chemical nomenclature to distinguish one variation in a chemical compound from others. Also spelled **alfa.**

alpha-$_1$ antitrypsin [Gk, *anti*, against, + trypsin], a plasma protein produced in the liver that inhibits the action of proteolytic enzymes such as trypsin. Deficiencis are associated with hepatitis in children and panacinar emphysema in adults. The latter is an inherited condition.

alpha-adrenergic. See **adrenergic receptor.**

alpha-adrenergic blocking agent. See **antiadrenergic.**

alpha-adrenergic receptor. See **alpha receptor.**

alpha alcoholism, a mild form of alcoholism in which the dependence is psychologic rather than physical. The person may consume alcohol in excessive amounts to relieve physical pain or psychologic distress but is usually able to retain control and can cease use of alcohol voluntarily.

alpha-aminoisovalerianic acid. See **valine.**

alpha-antitrypsin. See **anti-trypsin.**

alpha cells [Gk, *alpha*, first letter of the Greek alphabet, + L, *cella*, storeroom], cells located in the anterior lobe of the pituitary gland or in the pancreatic islets. In the pancreas, they produce glucagon.

alpha fetoprotein (AFP), a protein normally synthesized by the liver, yolk sac, and GI tract of a human fetus, but which may be found elevated in the sera of adults having certain malignancies. AFP measurements in amniotic fluid are used for early diagnosis of fetal neural tube defects, such as spina bifida and anencephaly. Elevated serum levels may be present in ataxia-telangiectasia, hereditary tyrosinemia, cirrhosis, alcoholic hepatitis, and viral hepatitis. Although

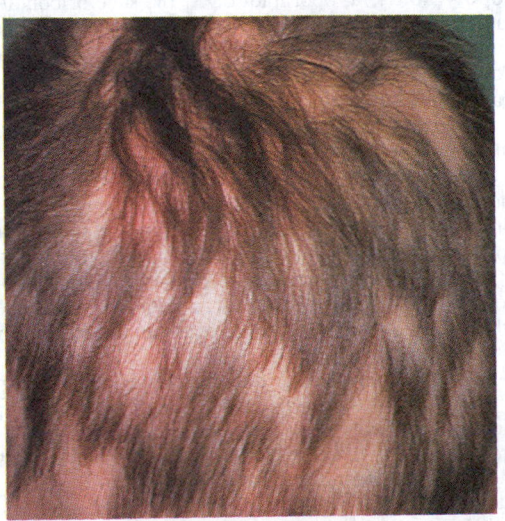

Alopecia areata (Baran, 1992)

not a specific marker for malignancies, AFP may be used to monitor effectiveness of surgical and chemotherapeutic management of hepatomas and germ cell neoplasms. Normal adult findings are less than 40 ng/ml or 40 µg/L.

alpha-galactosidase, an enzyme that catalyzes the conversion of alpha-D-galactoside to D-galactose.

alpha hemolysis, the development of a greenish zone around a bacterial colony growing on blood-agar medium, characteristic of pneumococci and certain streptococci and caused by the partial decomposition of hemoglobin. Compare **beta hemolysis.**

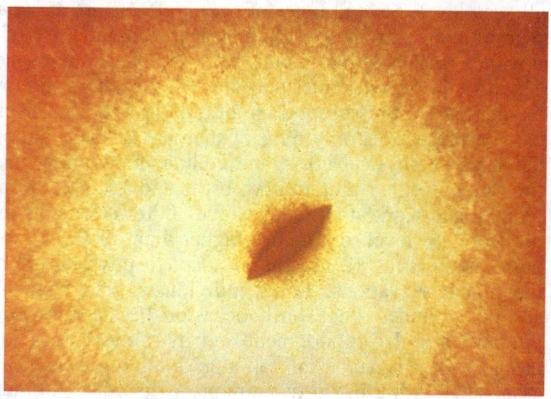

Alpha hemolysis *(Baron, 1990)*

alpha-hydroxypropionic acid. See **lactic acid.**

alpha$_2$-interferon /in'tərfir'on/, a protein molecule found effective in controlling the spread of common colds caused by rhinoviruses. It is administered as a nasal spray.

alpha-methyldopa. See **methyldopa.**

alphanumeric, pertaining to a system of characters in which information is coded in combinations of letters and numerals. The characters, which also may include punctuation, are used commonly in computer programing to code signals or data.

alpha particle, a particle emitted from an atom during one kind of radioactive decay. It consists of two protons and two neutrons, the equivalent of a helium nucleus. Ordinarily, alpha particles are a weak form of radiation with a short range and are not considered hazardous unless inhaled or ingested.

alpha receptor, any one of the postulated adrenergic components of receptor tissues that responds to norepinephrine and to various blocking agents. The activation of the alpha receptors causes such physiologic responses as increased peripheral vascular resistance, dilatation of the pupils, and contraction of pilomotor muscles. Also called **alpha-adrenergic receptor.** Compare **beta receptor.**

alpha redistribution phase, a period after intravenous administration of a drug when the blood level begins to fall from its peak. It is caused primarily by redistribution of the drug throughout the body.

alpha rhythm. See **alpha wave.**

alpha state, a condition of relaxed, peaceful wakefulness devoid of concentration and sensory stimulation. It is characterized by the alpha rhythm of brain wave activity, as recorded by an electroencephalograph, and is accompanied by feelings of tranquillity and a lack of tension and anxiety. Biofeedback training and meditation techniques are used to achieve this state.

Alpha Tau Delta /al'fə tou' del'tə/, a national fraternity for professional nurses.

alpha-tocopherol. See **vitamin E.**

alphavirus /al'favī'rəs/, any of a group of very small togaviruses consisting of a single molecule of single-stranded DNA within a lipoprotein capsule. Many alphaviruses multiply in the cytoplasm of cells of arthropods and are transmitted to humans through insect bites, such as equine encephalitis. See also **encephalitis, togaviruses.**

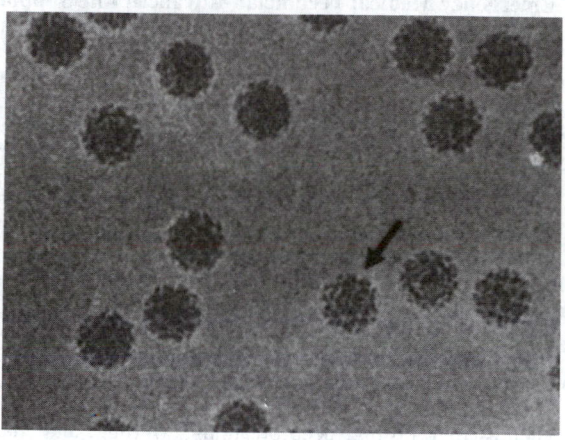

Alphavirus
(Murray, 1990/Borrowed from Fuller SD; Cell 48:923, 1987)

alpha wave, one of the four types of brain waves, characterized by a relatively high voltage or amplitude and a frequency of 8 to 13 Hz. Alpha waves are the "relaxed waves" of the brain and constitute the majority of waves recorded by electroencephalograms registering the activity of the parietal and the occipital lobes and the posterior parts of the temporal lobes when the individual is awake but nonattentive and relaxed, with the eyes closed. Opening and closing the eyes affects the patterns of the alpha waves and the beta waves. Also called **alpha rhythm, Berger wave.** Compare **beta wave, delta wave, theta wave.**

Alport's syndrome, a form of hereditary nephritis with symptoms of glomerulonephritis, hematuria, progressive sensorineural hearing loss, and occasional ocular disorders such as cataracts, drusen, and lenticonus. The trait is transmitted most often through females, although symptoms have a higher frequency and tend to be more severe in males. Females are often asymptomatic. Males tend to develop kidney impairment in their third decade and die of renal complications in middle age. Treatment is directed toward relief of uremia or other kidney disorders. Kidney transplants are sometimes successful.

alprazolam /al'praz'ələm/ a benzodiazepine antianxiety agent.

■ INDICATIONS: It is prescribed in the treatment of anxiety disorders or the short-term relief of the symptoms of anxiety.

■ CONTRAINDICATIONS: Acute narrow-angle glaucoma or known sensitivity to this drug or other benzodiazepines prohibits its use.

■ ADVERSE EFFECTS: Among the most serious adverse reactions are drowsiness and lightheadedness.

alprostadil, a proprietary form of prostaglandin E$_1$ used to maintain the patency of the ductus arteriosus in certain neonates.

■ INDICATIONS: It is recommended as a palliative therapy for neonates awaiting surgery to correct congenital heart defects, such as tetralogy of Fallot and tricuspid atresia.

■ CONTRAINDICATIONS: There are no contraindications.

■ ADVERSE EFFECTS: The most common adverse effects include apnea, fever, seizures, cerebral bleeding, and flushing.

ALS, 1. abbreviation for **advanced life support.** See **Emergency Medical Technician-Advanced Life Support.** 2. abbreviation for **amyotrophic lateral sclerosis.** 3. abbreviation for **antilymphocyte serum.**

Älstrom's syndrome /äl'strəmz/, an inherited disease characterized by multiple end organ resistance to hormones. Clinical features include retinal degeneration leading to childhood blindness, vasopressin-resistant diabetes insipidus, baldness, hyperuricemia, and hypertryglyceridemia. Males are also likely to have high plasma gonadotropin levels and hypogonadism. The condition is transmitted through an autosomal recessive gene.

ALT, abbreviation for **alanine aminotransferase.**

altered state of consciousness (ASC) [Gk, *alterare,* to change], any state of awareness that differs from the normal awareness of a conscious person. Altered states of consciousness have been achieved, especially in Eastern cultures, by many individuals using various techniques, such as long fasting, deep breathing, whirling, and chanting. Researchers now recognize that such practices can affect the chemistry of the body and help induce the desired state. Experiments suggest that telepathy, mystical experiences, clairvoyance, and other altered states of consciousness may be subconscious capabilities in most individuals and can be used to improve health and help fight disease.

alternans /ôl'tərnənz/ [L, *alternare,* to alternate], a regular rhythm of the heart where the pulse alternates between strong beats and weak beats (pulsus alternans).

alternate generation /ôl'tərnit/ [L, *alter,* other of two], a type of reproduction in which a sexual generation alternates with one or more asexual generations, as in many plants and lower animals. Also called **alternation of generations.**

alternating current (AC) /ôl'tərnā'ting/, an electric current that reverses direction, according to a consistent sinusoidal pattern. Compare **direct current.** See also **current.**

alternating mydriasis, a visual disorder in which there is abnormal dilatation of the pupils of the eyes that affects the left and right eyes alternately. See also **mydriasis.**

alternating pulse, See **pulsus alternans.**

alternation of generations. See **alternate generation.**

alternation rules, (in psychology) the sociolinguistic rules that establish options available to a person when he or she is speaking to someone else. The rules are influenced by social categories, such as kinship, sex, status, age, and the type of interpersonal relationship.

alternative inheritance /ôltur'nətiv/, the acquisition of all genetic traits and conditions from one parent, as in self-pollinating plants and self-fertilizing animals.

alternative pathway of complement activation, a process of antigen-antibody interaction in which activation of the C3 step occurs without prior activation of C1, C4, and C2. The initiating substance may be endotoxin, yeast cell wall, bacterial capsule, or IgA. Also called **properidin system.**

alternobaric vertigo, a condition of dysequilibrium caused by unequalized pressure differences in the middle ear, as may be experienced by divers during ascent. The pressure difference exerts its effect on the oval window of the inner ear.

alt.h., abbreviation for the Latin prescription term *alternis horis,* meaning 'every other hour'.

altitude /ôl'tityōod/ [L, *altitudo,* height], any location on earth with reference to a fixed surface point, which is usually sea level. Several types of health effects are associated with altitude extremes, including a greater intensity of ultraviolet radiation that results from a thinner atmosphere. There are fewer molecules per liter of atmosphere and lower oxygen partial pressure. At an altitude of 5500 m, inspired oxygen pressure is only 50% of that at sea level, although demands of physical effort and cellular respiration remain the same at either altitude. An estimated 25,000,000 people live and work at altitudes above 3000 m. Persons moving from sea level to altitudes higher than 3000 m may require as much as 12 months to adapt to physical effort at the higher elevations. Some individuals who have lived at high altitudes since birth occasionally develop an intolerance for the environment and must move to a lower altitude to survive. High altitude intolerance is usually associated with a blood or pulmonary disorder. As mining is a common occupation in mountainous regions, altitude intolerance is frequently associated with silicosis, which usually produces symptoms earlier and progresses more rapidly than at lower altitudes. See also **altitude sickness.**

altitude anoxia [L, *altus,* high, + Gk, *a,* without, *oxys,* sharp, *genein,* to produce], oxygen deprivation in a high altitude atmosphere.

altitude sickness, a syndrome associated with the relatively low partial pressure (reduced barometric pressure) of oxygen in the atmosphere at altitudes encountered during mountain climbing or travel in unpressurized aircraft. The acute symptoms may include dizziness, headache, irritability, breathlessness, and euphoria. Older people and those affected by pulmonary or cardiac disorders may suffer pulmonary edema, heart failure, or prostration, requiring emergency treatment and removal to lower altitudes. A chronic form of altitude sickness is characterized by an increased production of red blood cells, resulting in blood that is thick and difficult to move through the circulatory system. Also called **acute mountain sickness, Monge's disease.** See also **polycythemia.**

altruism /al'trōo·iz'əm/, a sense of concern for the welfare of others. It may be expressed at the level of the individual or the larger social system.

alum /al'əm/ [L, *alumen*], a topical astringent, used primarily in lotions and douches. Common potassium is applied topically as a 0.5% to 5% solution.

alum bath, a bath taken in water containing the mineral salt alum, used primarily for skin disorders.

aluminum (Al) /əlōo'minəm/ [L, *alumen* alum], a widely used metallic element and the third most abundant of all the elements. Its atomic number is 13; its atomic weight is 26.97. It occurs in the ores feldspar, mica, and kaolin but most abundantly in bauxite. Aluminum is commonly obtained by purifying bauxite to produce alumina, which is reduced to aluminum. It is light and durable and used extensively in the manufacture of aircraft components, prosthetic devices, and dental appliances. It is also a component of many antacids, antiseptics, astringents, and styptics. Aluminum salts, such as aluminum hydroxychloride, can cause allergic reactions in susceptible individuals. Aluminum hydroxychloride is the most commonly used agent in antiperspirants and is also effective as a deodorant.

aluminum acetate solution. See **Burow's solution.**

aluminum attenuator, an aluminum filter used to control the hardness of an x-ray beam. The attenuator removes low-energy x-ray photons before they can reach the patient and be absorbed.

aluminum hydroxide gel [L, *alumen,* alum, + Gk, *hydor,* water, *oxys,* sharp, + L, *gelare,* to congeal], an antacid that works by chemical neutralization and also by adsorption of hydrochloric acid, gases, and toxins.

Alupent, a trademark for a beta-adrenergic bronchodilator (metaproterenol sulfate).

Alurate Elixir, a trademark for a sedative-hypnotic (aprobarbital).

Alu sequences, a family of repeated sequences in the human genome.

alve-, a prefix meaning 'trough, channel, cavity': *alveolate, alveolus.*

alveobronchitis [L, *alveolus,* little hollow + Gk, *bronchos,* windpipe, *itis,* inflammation], inflammation of the alveoli and bronchioles. Also called **alveobronchiolitis. See** also **bronchopneumonia.**

alveolar /alvē′ələr/[L, *alveolus,* little hollow], pertaining to an alveolus.

alveolar adenocarcinoma [L, *alveolus,* small hollow], a neoplasm in which the tumor cells form alveoli.

alveolar air, the respiratory gases in an alveolus, or air sac, of the lung. Alveolar air can be analyzed for its content of oxygen, carbon dioxide, or other gaseous components by collecting the last portion of air expelled by maximum exhalation.

alveolar air equation, a method of calculating the approximate alveolar oxygen tension from the arterial partial pressure of carbon dioxide, fractional inspired oxygen, and the ratio of carbon dioxide production to oxygen consumption.

alveolar-arterial end-capillary gas pressure difference, the gas pressure difference that exists between alveolar gas and pulmonary capillary blood as the latter leaves the alveolus. It is measured in torr units or mm Hg.

alveolar-arterial gas pressure difference, the difference between the measured or calculated mean partial pressure of a gas, such as CO_2, in the alveoli and the simultaneously measured partial pressure of that gas in systemic arterial blood. The difference may indicate ventilation-perfusion mismatching. A negative difference indicates that the partial pressure of the gas is higher in systemic arterial blood than it is in alveolar gas. It is measured in torr units.

alveolar bone. See alveolar process.

alveolar canal, any of the canals of the maxilla through which the posterior superior alveolar blood vessels and the nerves to the upper teeth pass. Also called **dental canal.**

alveolar-capillary membrane, a lung tissue structure, varying in thickness from 0.4 to 2.0 μm, through which diffusion of oxygen and carbon dioxide molecules occurs during the respiration process. It consists of an alveolar cell

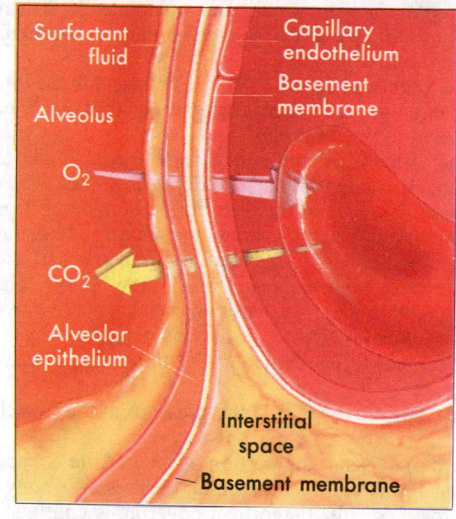

Alveolar-capillary membrane (Thibodeau, 1993)

separated from a capillary cell by an interstitial space and is essentially a fluid barrier.

alveolar cell carcinoma, a malignant pulmonary neoplasm that arises in a bronchiole and spreads along alveolar surfaces. The tumor consists of cuboidal or nonciliated columnar epithelial cells with abundant eosinophilic cytoplasm that may contain droplets of mucus. This form of lung cancer is characterized by a severe cough and copious sputum. Also called **bronchiolar carcinoma.**

alveolar cleft, a form of cleft palate in which the fusion failure extends forward to include the alveolar ridge.

alveolar dead space. See dead space.

alveolar distending pressure, the pressure difference between the alveolus and the intrapleural space.

alveolar duct, any of the air passages in the lung that branch out from the respiratory bronchioles. From the ducts arise the alveolar sacs.

alveolar edema, an accumulation of fluid within the alveoli. The cause is usually the movement of blood components through the pulmonary capillary walls resulting from a change in osmotic pressure, increased permeability of the walls, or related factors.

alveolar fiber, any one of the many white collagenous fibers of the periodontal ligament that extend from the alveolar bone to the intermediate plexus, where their terminations mix with those of the cemental fibers.

alveolar fistula. See dental fistula.

alveolar gas, the gas mixture within the gas-exchange regions of the lungs, reflecting the combined effects of alveolar ventilation and respiratory gas exchange or the expired gas that has come from the alveoli and gas exchange regions. Alveolar gas composition is influenced by technical problems of gas sampling, the discontinuous nature of pulmonary ventilation, regional variations in inspired gas distribution, and imperfect matching of the different aspects of lung function. Alveolar gas is assumed to be saturated with water vapor at 37° C.

alveolar gas volume, the aggregate volume of gas in the lung regions within which respiratory gas exchange occurs. It is indicated by the symbol V_A.

alveolar gingiva, gingiva that covers the alveolar bone and process in the maxilla and mandible. It is firmly attached to the bone and to the cementum of the teeth. Also called **attached gingiva.**

alveolar macrophages, defense cells within the lungs that act by engulfing and digesting foreign substances that may be inhaled into the alveoli.

alveolar microlithiasis, a disease characterized by the presence of calcium phosphate deposits in the alveolar sacs and ducts. Because of the distribution of mineral deposits in the lung tissue, the entire lung may appear radiopaque, with fine sandlike deposits. It is familial in about half of cases.

alveolar periosteum [L, *alveolus,* little hollow; Gk, *peri,* near, *osteon,* bone], a dense layer of connective tissue that lines the alveolar cavities of the upper and lower jaws, joining the bones to the cementum of the teeth. See also **periosteum.**

alveolar pressure (P$_A$), the pressure in the alveoli of the lungs.

alveolar process, the portion of the maxilla or the mandible that forms the dental arch and serves as a bony investment for the teeth. Its cortical covering is continuous with the compact bone of the body of the maxilla or the mandible and is continuous with the spongy bone of the body of the jaws. Also called **alveolar bone.** See also **alveolar ridge.**

alveolar proteinosis, a disorder marked by the accumulation of plasma proteins, lipoproteins, and other blood components in the alveoli of the lungs. The disease tends to affect previously healthy young adults, with a higher incidence among males than females. The cause is unknown and clinical signs vary, although only the lungs are affected. Some patients are asymptomatic, whereas others show dyspnea and an unproductive cough. The condition may be treated with bronchopulmonary lavage. There is a risk of secondary infections.

alveolar ridge, the bony ridge of the maxilla or the mandible that contains the alveoli of the teeth. See also **alveolar process.**

alveolar sac [L, *alveolus,* little hollow; Gk, *sakkos*], an air sac at one of the terminal cavities of lung tissue.

alveolar socket [L, *alveolus,* little hollow; OFr, *soket*], a cavity in the alveolar bone of the maxilla and mandible that accommodates a tooth.

alveolar soft part sarcoma, a tumor in subcutaneous or fibromuscular tissue, consisting of numerous large round or polygonal cells in a netlike matrix of connective tissue.

alveolar ventilation, the volume of air that ventilates all the perfused alveoli, measured as minute volume in liters. The figure is also the difference between total ventilation and dead space ventilation. The normal average is between 4 and 5 liters per minute.

alveolectomy /al′vē·əlek′təmē/ [L, *alveolus* + Gk, *ektome,* excision], the excision of a portion of the alveolar process for aiding the extraction of a tooth or teeth, the modification of the alveolar contour after tooth extraction, or the preparation of the mouth for dentures.

alveoli /alvē′əlī/, small outpouchings of walls of alveolar space through which gas exchange takes place between alveolar air and pulmonary capillary blood.

alveolitis /al′vē·əlī′tis/, an allergic pulmonary reaction to the inhalation of antigenic substances characterized by acute episodes of dyspnea, cough, sweating, fever, weakness, and pain in the joints and muscles lasting from 12 to 18 hours. Recurrent episodes may lead to chronic obstructive lung disease with weight loss, increasing exertional dyspnea, and interstitial fibrosis. Radiologic films of the lungs may show cellular thickening of alveolar septa and ill-defined generalized infiltrates. Kinds of alveolitis include **bagassosis, farmer's lung,** and **pigeon breeder's disease.**

alveolo-, a combining form meaning 'pertaining to an alveolus': *alveoloplasty.*

alveolus /alvē′ələs/, *pl.* **alveoli** [L, small hollow], a small saclike structure. Often used interchangeably with **acinus.** See also **alveoli, dental alveolus, pulmonary alveolus.** **–alveolar,** *adj.*

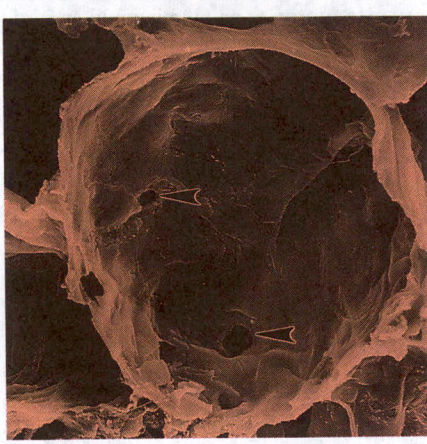

Alveolus—scanning electron microscope view
(Erlandsen, 1992)

alvine constipation. See **obstructive constipation.**

alymphocytosis /alim′fōsītō′sis/ [Gk, *a,* not; L, *lympha,* water; Gk, *kytos,* cell, *osis,* condition], a severe reduction in the total number of circulating lymphocytes in the blood. Compare **aplastic anemia, lymphocytopenia.** See also **leukocyte, lymphocyte.**

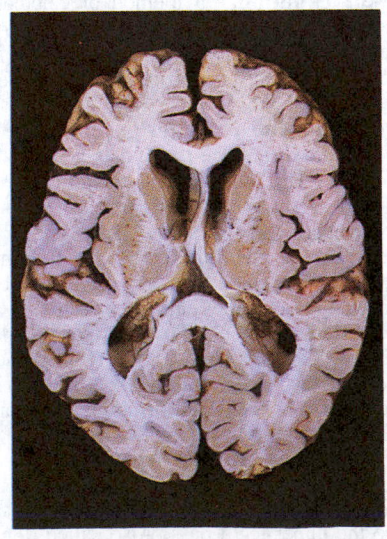

Axial section of brain exhibiting Alzheimer's disease
(Okazaki, 1988/by permission of Mayo Foundation)

Alzheimer's disease /ôl'zīmərz/ [Alois Alzheimer, German neurologist, b. 1864], presenile dementia, characterized by confusion, memory failure, disorientation, restlessness, agnosia, speech disturbances, inability to carry out purposeful movements, and hallucinosis. The patient may become hypomanic, refuse food, and lose sphincter control without focal impairment. The disease usually begins in later middle life with slight defects in memory and behavior and occurs with equal frequency in men and women. Typical pathologic features are miliary plaques in the cortex and fibrillary degeneration within pyramidal ganglion cells. Treatment can only be palliative. Nursing care is concerned primarily with preventing injury, promoting activity, promoting sleep, and preventing agitation and violence. Also called **senile dementia-Alzheimer type (SDAT).**

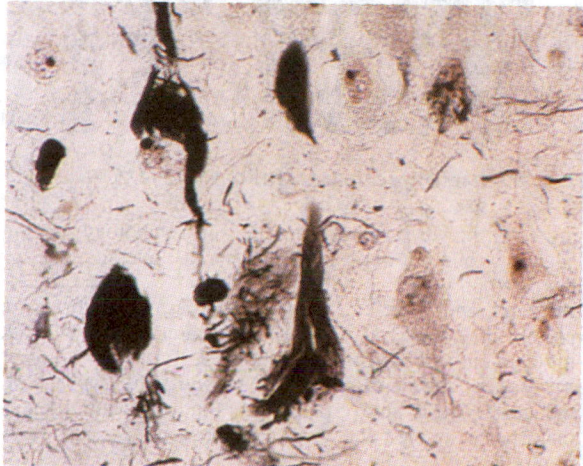

Neurofibrillary tangles common in Alzheimer's disease
(Okazaki, 1988/by permission of Mayo Foundation)

Alzheimer's sclerosis [Alois Alzheimer; Gk, *sklerosis,* hardening], the degeneration of small cerebral blood vessels resulting in mental changes.

am, abbreviation for an *ammonium cation.*

Am, symbol for the element **americium.**

ama, abbreviation for **against medical advice.**

AMA, abbreviation for **American Medical Association.**

amalgam /əmal'gəm/ [Gk, *malagma,* soft mass], **1.** a mixture or combination. **2.** an alloy of mercury and another metal or metals.

amalgam carrier, (in dentistry) an instrument for carrying plastic amalgam for inserting into a prepared tooth cavity (cavity prep) or mold.

amalgam carver, a dental instrument for shaping plastic amalgam restoration used in some tooth cavity fillings.

amalgam condenser, (in dentistry) an instrument used for compacting plastic amalgam in filling teeth.

amalgam core, a rigid base for the retention of a cast crown restoration, used in the replacement of a damaged tooth crown. The core may be retained by undercuts, slots, pins, or the pulp chamber of an endodontically treated tooth. Compare **cast core, composite core.** See also **core.**

amalgam tattoo, a discoloration of the gingiva or buccal membrane caused by particles of silver amalgam filling material that became embedded under the surface. The condition causes no symptoms and is left in situ.

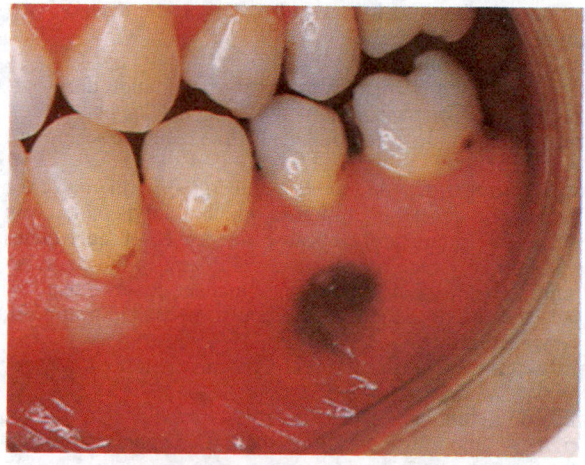

Amalgam tatoo *(Lamey, 1988)*

Amanita [Gk, *amanitai,* fungus], a genus of mushrooms. Some species, such as *Amanita phalloides,* are poisonous, causing hallucinations, GI upset, and pain that may be followed by liver, kidney, and central nervous system damage.

amantadine hydrochloride /əman'tədēn/, an antiviral and antiparkinsonian drug.

■ INDICATIONS: It is prescribed in the prophylaxis and early treatment of influenza virus A_2, and for symptomatic treatment of parkinsonian symptoms.

■ CONTRAINDICATIONS: It is used with caution in patients with congestive heart failure and during pregnancy and lactation. Known hypersensitivity to this drug prohibits its use.

■ ADVERSE EFFECTS: Among the most serious adverse reactions are central nervous system effects and livedo reticularis. Nervousness, blurred vision, and slurred speech also may occur.

amastia /əmas'tē·ə/ [Gk, *a, mastos,* not breast], absence of the breasts in women caused by a congenital defect, an endocrine disorder resulting in faulty development, lack of development of secondary sex characteristics, or a bilateral mastectomy. Also called **amazia.**

amaurosis /am'ôrō'sis/ [Gk, *amauroein,* to darken], blindness, especially lack of vision resulting from an extraocular cause, such as disease of the optic nerve or brain, diabetes, renal disease, or systemic poisoning produced by excessive use of alcohol or tobacco, rather than from damage to the eye itself. Unilateral or, more rarely, bilateral amaurosis may follow an emotional shock and may continue for days or months. Amaurosis may accompany an attack of acute gastritis. One kind of congenital amaurosis is transmitted as an autosomal recessive trait. —**amaurotic,** *adj.*

amaurosis fugax /foo'gaks/, transient episodic blindness due to decreased blood flow to the retina. Compare **amaurosis.**

amaurosis partialis fugax, transitory partial blindness, usually caused by vascular insufficiency of the retina or optic nerve as a result of carotid artery disease. Other related symptoms include dizziness, nausea, and vomiting.

amaurotic. See **amaurosis.**

amaurotic familial idiocy. See **Tay-Sachs disease.**

amazia. See **amastia.**

amb-. See **ambi-.**

Ambenyl, a trademark for a fixed-combination drug containing a narcotic analgesic-antitussive (codeine phosphate), an antihistamine (bromodiphenhydramine hydrochloride), and alcohol.

amber mutation [Ar, *anbar,* ambergris], (in molecular genetics) a genetic alteration in which a polypeptide chain terminates prematurely because the triplet of nucleotides that normally code for the next amino acid in the chain becomes UAG, the uracil-adenine-guanine sequence that signals the end of the chain. Also called **nonsense mutation, ochre mutation.**

ambi-, ambo-, amb-, a prefix meaning 'on both sides' or 'both': *ambidexterity, ambilateral.*

ambidextrous /am'bēdek'strəs/ [L, *ambo,* both, *dexter,* right], able to use use either the left or right hand to perform a task.

ambient /am'bē·ənt/ [L, *ambire,* on both sides], pertaining to the surrounding area or atmosphere, usually a defined area such as a room or other large enclosed space.

ambient air standard, the maximum tolerable concentration of any air pollutant, such as lead, nitrogen dioxide, sodium hydroxide, or sulfuric dioxide. Federal authorities in the United States have indicated that Los Angeles, Chicago, Salt Lake City, and metropolitan New York City may not meet the ambient air standard for nitrogen dioxide and that those cities and many others throughout the world have an atmosphere polluted by various toxic chemicals that are dangerous to breathe. Research and medical evidence show the strong correlation between many diseases and toxic chemicals, but little is known about the precise effects and movement of airborne pollutants.

ambient noise [L, *ambiens,* around + ME, clamor], the total noise in a given environment.

ambient pressure, the atmospheric pressure, or pressure in the environment or surrounding area. It is given a reference value of zero (0) cm H_2O.

ambient temperature [L, *ambi,* around + *temperatura*], the temperature of the enviroment.

ambiguous genitalia [L, *ambigere,* to go around], external genitalia that are not normal and morphologically typical of either sex, as occurs in pseudohermaphroditism.

ambilateral. See **ambi.**

ambilhar. See **niridazole.**

ambiopia. See **diplopia.**

ambivalence /ambiv'ələns/ [L, *ambo,* both, *valentia,* strength], 1. a state in which a person experiences conflicting feelings, attitudes, drives, desires, or emotions, such as love and hate, tenderness and cruelty, pleasure and pain toward the same person, place, or object. To some degree, ambivalence is normal. Treatment in severe, debilitating cases consists of psychotherapy appropriate to the underlying cause. 2. uncertainty and fluctuation caused by an inability to make a choice between opposites. 3. a continuous oscillation or fluctuation. –**ambivalent,** *adj.*

ambivalent [L, *ambo,* both, *valentia,* strength], 1. hav-

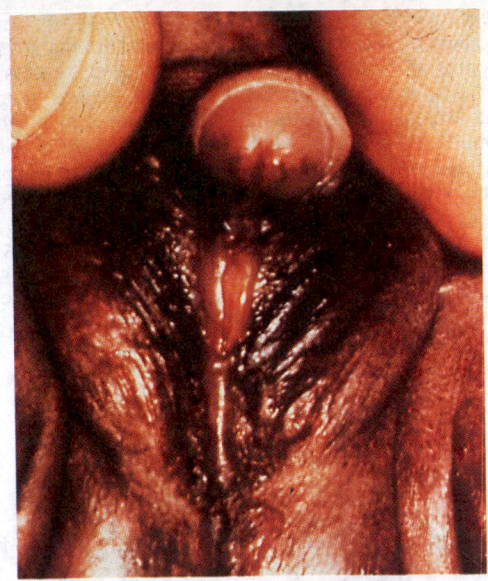

Ambiguous genitalia (*Zitelli,* 1992)

ing equal power on both sides. 2. in psychology, having equally strong but opposing emotions, as love and hate for the same person.

ambivert /am'bivurt'/ [L, *ambo,* both, *vertere,* to turn], a person who possesses some of the characteristics of both introversion and extroversion.

amblyopia /am'blē·ō'pē·ə/ [Gk, *amblys,* dull, *ops,* eye], reduced vision in an eye that appears to be structurally normal when examined with an ophthalmoscope. See also **toxic amblyopia.**

amblyopia cruciata. See **crossed amblyopia.**

ambo-. See **ambi-.**

Ambu-bag, a trademark for a breathing bag used to assist respiratory ventilation. (See Fig. p. 69.)

ambulance /am'byələns/ an emergency vehicle usually used for the transport of patients to a medical facility in cases of accident, trauma, or sudden, severe illness.

ambulatory /am'byələtôr'ē/ [L, *ambulare,* to walk about], able to walk, hence describing a patient who is not confined to bed or designating a health service for people who are not hospitalized.

ambulatory automatism, aimless wandering or moving about or performance of mechanical acts without conscious awareness of the behavior. See also **fugue, poriomania.**

ambulatory blood pressure monitoring (ABPM), a device that permits recording of a patient's blood pressure under normal living and working conditions.

ambulatory care, health services provided on an outpatient basis to those who visit a hospital or other health care facility and depart after treatment on the same day.

ambulatory electrocardiograph. See **Holter monitor.**

ambulatory schizophrenia, a mild form of psychosis, characterized mainly by a tendency to respond to questions with vague and irrelevant answers. The person also may seem somewhat eccentric and wander aimlessly.

ambulatory splint. See **functional splint.**

ambulatory surgery center, a medical facility designed and equipped to handle relatively minor surgery cases, such

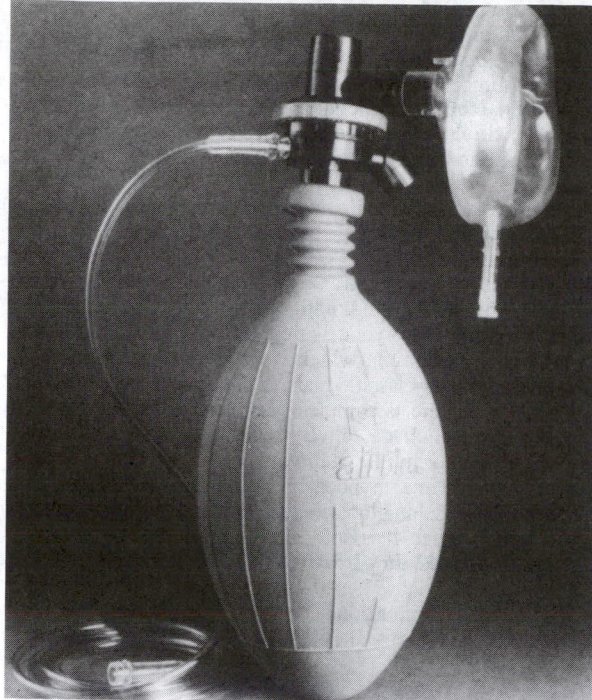

Ambu bag

as cataracts, herniorrhaphy, and meniscectomy, that do not require overnight hospitalization. Only patients who are in good health, usually children, are admitted for treatment at ambulatory surgery centers. The centers may be part of a community general hospital or independent medical facilities with prearranged hospital backup. The centers are staffed with the same health professionals as conventional surgery departments of general hospitals.

AM care, routine hygienic care that is given patients before breakfast or early in the morning.

amcinonide /amsin′ōnīd/, a topical corticosteroid.
- INDICATION: It is used as an antiinflammatory agent.
- CONTRAINDICATIONS: Viral and fungal diseases of the skin, circulation impairment, or known hypersensitivity to steroids prohibits its use.
- ADVERSE EFFECTS: Among the most serious adverse reactions are various skin eruptions. Systemic side effects may occur from prolonged or excessive application.

amdinocillin /am′dinōsil′in/, a penicillin derivative that is used as a parenteral antibiotic.
- INDICATIONS: It is prescribed for the treatment of urinary infections caused by susceptible strains of *Escherichia coli* and various species of *Klebsiella* and *Enterobacter*.
- CONTRAINDICATIONS: It is contraindicated in patients allergic to penicillin.
- ADVERSE EFFECTS: Among the most serious adverse effects reported are eosinophilia, thrombocytosis, elevated serum aspartate aminotransferase and serum alkaline phosphatase, skin rash, thrombophlebitis, diarrhea, nausea, dizziness, and various blood disorders.

ameba /əmē′bə/ [Gk, *amoibe*, change], a microscopic, single-celled, parasitic organism. Several species may be parasitic in humans, including *Entamoeba coli* and *E. histolytica*. Also spelled **amoeba**. See also **amebiasis. —amebic,** *adj.*

-ameba, -amoeba, a suffix meaning a '(specified) protozoan': *caudameba, Dientamoeba, Entamoeba*.

amebiasis /am′ēbī′əsis/, an infection of the intestine or liver by species of pathogenic amebas, particularly *Entamoeba histolytica*, acquired by ingesting food or water contaminated with infected feces. Mild amebiasis may be asymptomatic; severe infection may cause profuse diarrhea, acute abdominal pain, jaundice, anorexia, and weight loss. It is most serious in infants, the elderly, and debilitated people. Metronidazole is often effective in curing the infection. Also spelled **amoebiasis.** See also **ameba, amebic abscess, amebic dysentery, hepatic amebiasis.**

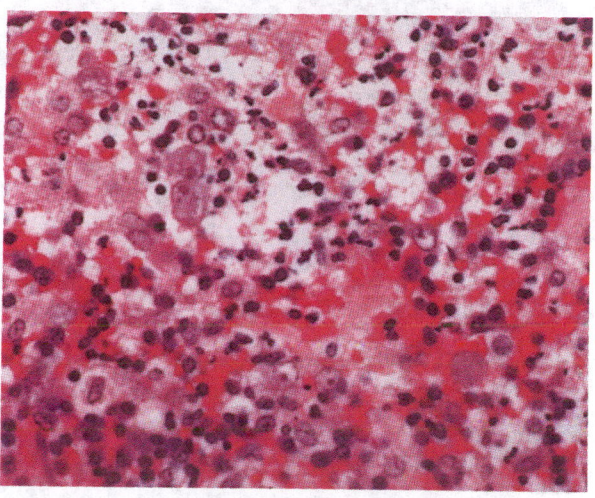

Amebiasis *(Mitros, 1988)*

amebic. See **ameba.**

amebic abscess, a collection of pus formed by disintegrated tissue in a cavity, usually in the liver, caused by the protozoan parasite *Entamoeba histolytica*. Cysts of the organism, ingested in fecally contaminated food or water, pass into the intestine, where active trophozoites of the parasite are released. The trophozoites enter the intestinal mucosa, causing ulceration, nausea, vomiting, abdominal pain, and severe diarrhea, and they may invade the liver and produce an abscess. Oral metronidazole and chloroquine hydrochloride administered orally or intramuscularly are used in treating hepatic amebic abscesses. See also **amebiasis.**

amebic carrier state, a condition in which a patient may be a carrier of amebic organisms without showing signs or symptoms of an amebic infection. A **precocious carrier** may appear healthy but subsequently develop the amebic infection.

amebic dysentery, an inflammation of the intestine caused by infestation with *Entamoeba histolytica* and characterized by frequent, loose stools flecked with blood and mucus. Intestinal amebiasis may be accompanied by symptoms of liver involvement. Also called **intestinal amebiasis.** See also **amebiasis, hepatic amebiasis.**

amebicide /əmē'bəsīd/, a drug or other agent that is destructive to amebas.

ameboid movement /əmē'boid/ [Gk, *amoibe,* ameba, *eidos,* form + L, *movere,* to move], the amebalike movement of certain types of body cells that can migrate through tissues. The movement generally consists of extension of a portion of the cell wall through a small opening between other tissue cells, which allows the cytoplasmic contents to follow.

amelanic melanoma /am'ilan'ik/, a melanoma that lacks melanin.

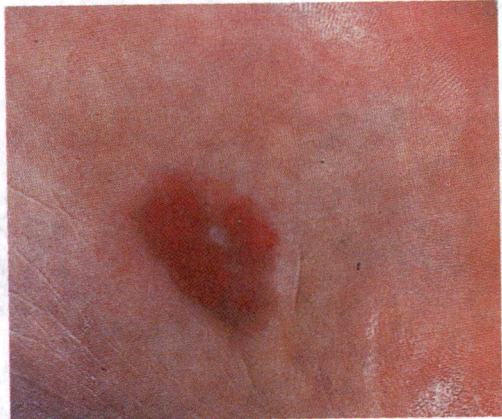

Amelanotic malignant melanoma *(du Vivier, 1993)*

amelanotic /am'ilənot'ik/ [Gk, *a, melas,* not black], of or pertaining to tissue that is unpigmented because it lacks melanin.

amelia /əmē'lyə/ [Gk, *a, melos,* not limb], **1.** a birth defect, marked by the absence of one or more limbs. The term may be modified to indicate the number of legs or arms missing at birth, such as **tetramelia** for the absence of all four limbs. **2.** a psychologic trait of apathy or indifference associated with certain forms of psychosis.

amelification /əmel'ifikā'shən/ [OFr, *amel,* enamel; L, *facere,* to make], the differentiation of ameloblasts, or enamel cells, into the enamel of the teeth.

amelioration [L, *ad,* to, *melior,* better], an improvement in conditions.

ameloblast /am'ilōblast'/ [OFr, *amel* + Gk, *blastos,* germ], an epithelial cell from which tooth enamel is formed.

ameloblastic /-blas'tik/, *adj.*

ameloblastic fibroma, an odontogenic neoplasm in which simultaneous proliferation of mesenchymal and epithelial tissues occurs without the formation of dentin or enamel.

ameloblastic hemangioma, a highly vascular tumor of cells covering the dental papilla. See also **hemangioma.**

ameloblastic odontoma, an odontogenic tumor characterized by an ameloblastoma within an odontoma. See also **composite odontoma.**

ameloblastic sarcoma, a malignant odontogenic tumor, characterized by the proliferation of epithelial and mesen-

chymal tissue without the formation of dentin or enamel.

ameloblastoma /am'əlōblastō'mə/ [OFr, *amel* + Gk, *blastos,* germ, *oma*], a highly destructive, malignant, rapidly growing tumor of the jaw. Also called **adamantinoma, adamantoblastoma, epithelioma adamantinum.**

amelodentinal /am'əlōden'tinəl/ [OFr, *amel* + L, *dens,* tooth], pertaining to both the enamel and the dentin of the teeth.

amelogenesis /am'əlōjen'əsis/ [OFr, *amel* + Gk, *genein,* to produce], the formation of the enamel of the teeth. **—amelogenic,** *adj.*

amelogenesis imperfecta, a hereditary dental defect characterized by a brown coloration of the teeth and resulting from either severe hypocalcification or hypoplasia of the enamel. The condition, which is inherited as an autosomal dominant trait, is classified according to severity as agenesis, in which there is complete lack of enamel; enamel hypoplasia, in which defective matrix formation causes the enamel to be normal in quality of hardness but deficient in quantity; or enamel hypocalcification, in which defective maturation of the ameloblasts results in the normal quantity of enamel, though it is soft and undercalcified in context. Also called **hereditary brown enamel, hereditary enamel hypoplasia.** Compare **dentinogenesis imperfecta.** See also **enamel hypocalcification, enamel hypoplasia.**

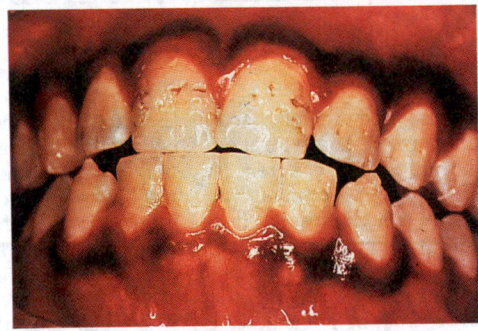

Amelogenesis imperfecta, hypoplastic type
(Zitelli, 1992)

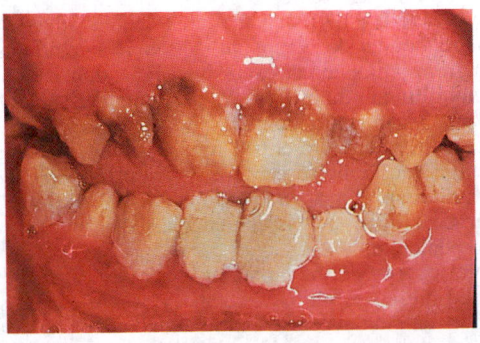

Amelogenesis imperfecta, hypocalcified type
(Zitelli, 1992)

amenorrhea /ā′menərē ′ə/ [Gk, *a, men,* not month, *rhoia,* to flow], the absence of menstruation. Amenorrhea is normal before sexual maturity, during pregnancy, after menopause, and during the intermenstrual phase of the monthly hormonal cycle but is otherwise caused by dysfunction of the hypothalamus, pituitary gland, ovary, or uterus, by the congenital absence or surgical removal of both ovaries or the uterus, or by medication. **Primary amenorrhea** is the failure of menstrual cycles to begin. **Secondary amenorrhea** is the cessation of menstrual cycles once established. See also **hypothalamic amenorrhea, postpill amenorrhea.** –**amenorrheic.** *adj.*

amentia /āmen′shə/ [Gk, *a,* not; L, *mens,* mind], **1.** an obsolete term for congenital mental retardation. See **mental retardation. 2.** also called **confusional insanity.** a state of mind characterized by apathy and disorientation, bordering on stupor, as in Stearns' alcoholic amentia.

American Academy of Allergy and Immunology (AAAI), a national organization of physicians specializing in the diagnosis and treatment of allergies and immune system disorders.

American Academy of Nursing (AAN), the honorary organization of the American Nurses' Association, created to recognize superior achievement in nursing in order to promote advances and excellence in nursing practice and education. A person who is elected to membership is given the title of Fellow of the American Academy of Nursing and may use the abbreviation FAAN as an honorific.

American Academy of Physical Medicine and Rehabilitation (AAPMR), a national association of professional health care workers concerned with the diagnosis of physical impairment and the development of therapies and devices to improve physical function.

American Academy of Physicians' Assistants (AAPA), a national organization of physicians' assistants or associates.

American Association for Respiratory Therapy (AART), a national organization of nurses and other health workers in the field of respiratory therapy.

American Association of Colleges of Nursing (AACN), a national organization of baccalaureate and higher degree programs in nursing that was established to address issues in nursing education.

American Association of Critical Care Nurses (AACN), a national organization of nurses who work in critical care units.

American Association of Industrial Nurses (AAIN), a national professional association of nurses working in industry and concerned with issues in occupational health.

American Association of Medical Colleges (AAMC), a national organization of faculty members and deans of medical schools and colleges that was established to address issues in medical education.

American Association of Nephrology Nurses and Technicians (AANNT), an organization of nurses and technicians working in the fields of dialysis and renal diseases.

American Association of Neurological Nurses (AANN), a national organization of nurses working in the field of neurology.

American Association of Neuroscience Nurses (AANN), a national organization of nurses working with neurologically impaired patients. The organization is affili-

ated with the American Association of Neurological Surgeons.

American Association of Nurse Anesthetists (AANA), a professional association of certified registered nurse anesthetists. See also **nurse anesthetist.**

American Association of Pathologists and Bacteriologists (AAPB), a national professional organization of specialists in pathology and bacteriology.

American Association of Retired Persons (AARP), a voluntary US organization of older persons, who may or may not be retired, with the goal of improving the welfare of persons over the age of 50. The AARP claims a membership of 30,000,000 and advises members of congress and state legislatures regarding legislation affecting older individuals.

American Association of University Professors (AAUP), a national organization of faculty members of institutions of higher learning. The AAUP represents faculty in matters of academic freedom, appointment policies, and procedures and serves as the bargaining agent for the faculties of some universities.

American College of Obstetricians and Gynecologists (ACOG), the national organization of obstetricians and gynecologists. It is concerned with the education of physicians in the specialty standards of practice, the continued education and well-being of its members, and the board certification of eligible members as fellows of the organization.

American College of Physicians (ACP), a national professional organization of physicians.

American College of Prosthodontists, an organization of dentists who specialize in restoration of dental or oral structures, such as dentures, crowns, and bridges, and in the diagnosis and treatment of temporomandibular joint and maxillofacial disorders.

American College of Radiology (ACR), a national professional organization of physicians who specialize in radiology.

American College of Surgeons (ACS), a national professional organization of physcians who specialize in surgery.

American Dental Hygienists' Association (ADHA), a national organization, a tripartite group, composed of constituent or state, local (city), and regional associations. National headquarters are in Chicago, Illinois.

American Hospital Association (AHA), a national organization of individuals, institutions, and organizations that works to improve health services for all people. The AHA publishes several journals and newsletters.

American Journal of Nursing, the professional journal of the American Nurses' Association (ANA). It contains articles of general and specialized clinical interest to nurses and is an important resource regarding the profession in the United States.

American leishmaniasis, a group of mucocutaneous infections caused by various species of *Leishmania,* characterized by disfiguring ulcerative lesions of the nose, mouth, and throat. These infections are most prevalent in forested areas of southern Mexico and in Central and South America. Illness may be prolonged, rendering patients susceptible to serious secondary infections. Kinds of American leishmaniasis are **chiclero's ulcer, espundia, forest yaws,** and **uta.** Also called **mucocutaneous leishmaniasis, New World leishmaniasis.** See also **leishmaniasis.**

American Medical Association (AMA), a professional association whose membership is made up of approximately half of the total licensed physicians in the United States, including practitioners in all recognized medical specialties, as well as general primary care physicians. The AMA is governed by a Board of Trustees and House of Delegates who represent various state and local medical associations and government agencies such as the Public Health Service and medical departments of the Army, Navy, and Air Force. The AMA maintains directories of all qualified physicians (including nonmembers) in the United States, including graduates of foreign medical colleges, evaluates prescription and nonprescription drugs, advises congressional and state legislators regarding proposed health care laws, and publishes a variety of journals that report on scientific and socioeconomic developments in the field of medicine. See also **British Medical Association (BMA).**

American mountain fever. See **Colorado tick fever.**

American National Standards Institute (ANSI), a private, nonprofit organization that coordinates voluntary developments of standards for medical and other devices in the United States and represents the United States in areas of international standardization.

American Nurses' Association (ANA), the national professional association of registered nurses in the United States. It was founded in 1896 to improve standards of health and the availability of health care given in order to foster high standards for nursing, to promote the professional development of nurses, and to advance the economic and general welfare of nurses. The ANA is made up of 53 constituent associations from 50 states, the District of Columbia, Guam, and the Virgin Islands, representing more than 900 district associations. National conventions are held biennially in even-numbered years. Members may join one or more of the five Divisions on Nursing Practice: Community Health, Gerontological, Maternal and Child Health, Medical-Surgical, and Psychiatric and Mental Health Nursing. These Divisions are coordinated by the Congress for Nursing Practice. The Congress evaluates changes in the scope of practice, monitors scientific and educational developments, encourages research, and develops statements that describe ANA policies regarding legislation affecting nursing practice. Other commissions within the Association include the Commission on Nursing Education, the Commission on Nursing Services, and the Commission on Nursing Research. In addition, the ANA is politically active on the federal level in all issues relevant to nursing. Statistical services enable the Association to fulfill its role as the most authoritative source of data on nursing in the United States. The publications of the ANA include the *American Nurse,* the *Publications List,* and *The American Journal of Nursing.*

American Psychiatric Association (APA), a national professional psychiatric society concerned with the development of standards for psychiatric facilities, the formulation of mental health programs, the dissemination of data, and the promotion of psychiatric education and research. It publishes the *Diagnostic and Statistical Manual of Mental Disorders.*

American Red Cross, one of more than 120 national organizations that seek to reduce human suffering through various health, safety, and disaster relief programs in affiliation with the International Committee of the Red Cross. The Committee and all Red Cross organizations evolved from the Geneva Convention of 1864, following the example and urging of Swiss humanitarian Jean Henri Dunant, who aided wounded French and Austrian soldiers at the Battle of Solferino in 1859. The American Red Cross has more than 130 million members in about 3100 chapters throughout the United States. Volunteers comprise the entire staffs of about 1700 chapters. Other chapters maintain small paid staffs and some professionals but depend largely on volunteers. The American Red Cross blood program collects and distributes more blood than any other single agency in the United States and coordinates distribution of blood and blood products to the U.S. Defense Department on request or during national emergencies. The organization annually collects about 4 million blood donations and gives blood to more than 4000 hospitals. American Red Cross nursing and health programs include courses in the home on parenthood, prenatal and postnatal care, hygiene, and venereal disease. Nursing students are enrolled for service in American Red Cross community programs and during disasters. Four area offices at Alexandria, Virginia, Atlanta, Georgia, St. Louis, Missouri, and San Francisco, California, supervise and assist 70 divisions of the American Red Cross and direct field staff members assigned to military installations. National headquarters of the organization is at 17th and D Streets, NW, Washington, DC 20006. The President of the United States is honorary chairman of the organization, for which a 50-member board of governors, all volunteers, develops policy. The symbol of the American Red Cross, like that of most other Red Cross societies throughout the world, is a red cross on a field of white; in Switzerland it is a white cross on a red field, in Muslim countries, a red crescent, and in Israel, a red star of David.

American Registry of Radiologic Technologists (ARRT), a national professional organization of technicians specializing in radiology.

American Society of Parenteral and Enteral Nutrition, an organization that provides education, support, and accreditation to persons who specialize in nutrition that is provided through intravenous, enteral, or related types of feeding.

American Speech, Language, and Hearing Association (ASHA), the professional association that certifies audiologists and speech-language pathologists.

American Type Culture Collection (ATCC), a nonprofit, nongovernmental organization that is concerned with the preservation of specimens of cellular and microbiologic cultures and with the distribution of the cultures to research centers and laboratories in the academic, scientific, and medical communities.

americium (Am) /am′ərish′ē·əm/, a synthetic radioactive element of the actinide group. Its atomic number is 95; its atomic weight is 243.

Ameslan /am′islan/, abbreviation for *American Sign Language,* a method of manual communication used by some deaf people in which the position, shape, and motion of the hands and fingers convey concepts and messages. Ameslan is considered to be a true language, with a unique grammatical structure different from that of English. See also **sign language.**

Ames test /āmz/, a method for testing substances for possible carcinogenicity by exposing a strain of *Salmonella* bacteria to a sample of the substance. The rate of mutations observed is interpreted as an indication of the carcinogenic potential of the substance tested. Also called **mutagenicity test.**

amethopterin. See **methotrexate.**

ametropia /am′itrō′pē·ə/ [Gk, *ametros,* irregular, *opsis,* sight], a condition characterized by an optic defect involving an error of refraction, such as astigmatism, hyperopia, or myopia. –**ametropic,** *adj.*

AMI, 1. abbreviation for *anterior myocardial infarction.* **2.** abbreviation for **acute myocardial infarction.**

Amicar, a trademark for a hemostatic (aminocaproic acid).

Amici's disk. See **Z disk.**

amide-compound local anesthetic, any of more than two dozen compounds that are safe, versatile, and effective local anesthetics. If hypersensitivity to a drug in this group precludes its use, one of the ester-compound local anesthetics may provide analgesia without adverse effect. Some kinds of amide-compound local anesthetics are **bupivacaine, dibucaine, etiodocaine, lidocaine, mepivacaine,** and **prilocaine.**

amido-, prefix meaning 'the presence of the radical NH_2 along with the radical CO': *amidoacetal, amidobenzene, amidopyrine.*

amidobenzene. See **aniline.**

Amigo, a trademark for a battery-operated scooterlike vehicle that gives mobility to some patients who cannot walk.

amikacin sulfate /am′ikā′sin/, an aminoglycoside antibiotic.

■ INDICATIONS: It is prescribed in the treatment of various severe infections that are resistant to other antibiotics.

■ CONTRAINDICATIONS: Concurrent use of certain diuretics or known hypersensitivity to this or other aminoglycosides prohibits its use. The drug is used with caution in patients who have impaired renal function or myasthenia gravis or patients under the influence of neuromuscular blockers or other nephrotoxins.

■ ADVERSE EFFECTS: Among the more serious adverse reactions are nephrotoxicity, auditory and vestibular ototoxicity, and neuromuscular blockade. GI disturbances, pain at the site of injection, and hypersensitivity reactions may occur.

Amikin, a trademark for an antibiotic (amikacin sulfate).

amiloride hydrochloride /am′ilôr′id/, a potassium-sparing diuretic and antihypertensive agent.

■ INDICATIONS: It is prescribed as adjunctive therapy in the treatment of congestive heart failure or hypertension. It is often given with a thiazide medication.

■ CONTRAINDICATIONS: Concurrent use of potassium-conserving agents, hyperkalemia, impaired renal function, or known hypersensitivity to this drug prohibits its use.

■ ADVERSE EFFECTS: Among the most serious adverse reactions are headache, diarrhea, nausea and vomiting, anorexia, hyperkalemia, dizziness, encephalopathy, impotence, muscle cramps, photosensitivity, irregular heart rhythm, mental confusion, and paresthesia.

amine /am′in, əmēn′/ [L, *ammonia*], (in chemistry) a type of organic compound that contains nitrogen.

amine pump, *informal.* an active transport system in the presynaptic nerve endings that takes up released amine neurotransmitters. Adverse reactions to some drugs, notably tricyclic antidepressants, block this function, resulting in a high concentration of norepinephrine in cardiac tissue and resultant tachycardia and arrhythmia. See also **monoamine oxidase inhibitor (MAO).**

aminoacetic acid. See **glycine.**

amino acid /əmē′nō/, an organic chemical compound composed of one or more basic amino groups and one or more acidic carboxyl groups. Twenty of the more than 100 amino acids that occur in nature are the building blocks of peptides, polypeptides, and proteins. The eight essential amino acids are isoleucine, leucine, lysine, methionine, phenylalanine, threonine, tryptophan, and valine. Arginine and histidine are essential in infants. Cysteine and tyrosine are quasiessential because they may be synthesized from methionine and phenylalanine, respectively. The main nonessential amino acids are alanine, asparagine, aspartic acid, glutamine, glutamic acid, glycine, proline, and serine. From their structures, the amino acids can be classified as neutral, basic, or acidic, each group being transported across cell membranes by different carrier mechanisms. Arginine, histidine, and lysine are basic amino acids, aspartic acid and glutamic acid are acidic, and the remainder are neutral.

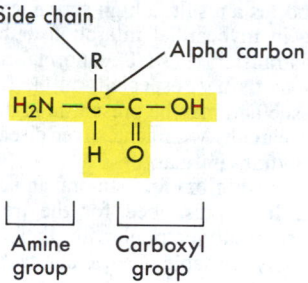

Basic structural formula for an amino acid
(Thibodeau, 1993)

amino acid group, a category of organic chemicals containing the monovalent amine radical NH_2, an acid or COOH, and a group idiosyncratic to that particular amino acid group.

aminoaciduria /əmē′nō·as′idoÖor′ē·ə/, the abnormal presence of amino acids in the urine that usually indicates an inborn metabolic defect, as in cystinuria. Also called **acidaminuria.**

aminobenzene. See **aniline.**

aminobenzoic acid /-benzō′ik/, a metabolic product of the catabolism of the amino acid tryptophan. Also called **anthranilic acid.** See also **para-aminobenzoic acid (PABA).**

aminocaproic acid /əmē′nōkəprō′ik, am′inō-/, a hemostatic.

■ INDICATION: It is prescribed to stop excessive bleeding that results from hyperfibrinolysis.

■ CONTRAINDICATION: Active intravascular coagulation prohibits its use.

■ ADVERSE EFFECTS: Among the most serious adverse reactions are thrombosis and hypotension. Inhibition of ejaculation, nasal congestion, diarrhea, and various allergic reactions also may occur.

aminoglycoside antibiotic. See **antibiotic.**

aminolevulinic acid (ALA) /am′inōlev′oÖolin′ik/, the aliphatic precursor of heme. It is formed in the body from the condensation of glycine and succinyl coenzyme A and undergoes further condensation to form porphobilinogen.

Aminolevulinic acid may be detected in the urine of some patients with porphyria, liver disease, and lead poisoning.

aminophylline /am'ənōfil'in, əmē'nō-/, a bronchodilator.

■ INDICATIONS: It is prescribed in the treatment of bronchial asthma, emphysema, and bronchitis.

■ CONTRAINDICATIONS: Known hypersensitivity to this drug or other xanthine medication prohibits its use. It is used with caution in patients who have peptic ulcer and those in whom cardiac stimulation would be harmful.

■ ADVERSE EFFECTS: Among the more serious adverse reactions are GI disturbances, central nervous system stimulation, palpitations, tachycardia, nervousness, and seizures.

aminosalicylic acid. See **paraaminosalicylic acid.**

aminosuccinic acid. See **aspartic acid.**

aminotransferase /-trans'fərās/, an enzyme that catalyzes the transfer of an amino group from an alpha-amino acid to an alpha-keto acid, with pyridoxal phosphate and pyridoxamine phosphate acting as coenzymes. Aspartate amino transferase (AST), normally present in serum and various tissues, especially in the heart and liver, is released by damaged cells and, as a result, a high serum level of AST may be diagnostic in myocardial infarction or hepatic disease. Alanine aminotransferase (ALT), a normal constituent of serum and various tissues, especially in the liver, is released by injured tissue and may be present in high concentrations in the sera of patients with acute liver disease. Also called **transaminase** /transam'inās/.

amiodarone hydrochloride, an oral antiarrhythmic drug.

■ INDICATIONS: It is prescribed for the treatment of life-threatening, recurrent ventricular fibrillation and recurrent, hemodynamically unstable ventricular tachycardia refractory to other drugs.

■ CONTRAINDICATIONS: This drug should not be given to patients with severe sinus-node dysfunction, second- and third-degree atrioventricular block, and when episodes of bradycardia have resulted in syncope, except when used in conjunction with a pacemaker.

■ ADVERSE EFFECTS: Among the most serious adverse effects reported are pulmonary toxicity, liver dysfunction, nausea, vomiting, constipation, anorexia, malaise, fatigue, tremor, involuntary movements, visual disorders, bradycardia, cyanosis, and congestive heart failure.

Amipaque, a trademark for an intrathecal and intravascular diagnostic drug (metrizamide).

amitosis /am'ətō'sis/ [Gr, *a, mitos,* not thread], direct cell division in which there is simple fission of the nucleus and cytoplasm. It does not involve the complex stages of chromatin separation of the chromosomes that occur in mitosis. –**amitotic,** *adj.*

amitriptyline /am'itrip'tilin/, a tricyclic antidepressant.

■ INDICATION: It is prescribed in the treatment of depression.

■ CONTRAINDICATIONS: Concomitant administration of monoamine oxidase inhibitors, recent myocardial infarction, or known hypersensitivity to this drug or to other tricyclic medication prohibits its use. It is used with caution in patients having a seizure disorder or in those with cardiovascular disease.

■ ADVERSE EFFECTS: Among the more serious adverse reactions are sedation and a variety of GI, cardiovascular, and neurologic reactions. This drug interacts with many other drugs.

AML, abbreviation for **acute myelocytic leukemia.**

ammoni-, a prefix meaning 'pertaining to ammonium': *ammoniemia, ammonirrhea, ammoniuria.*

ammonia /amō'nē·a/ [Gk, *ammoniakos,* salt of Ammon, Egyptian god], a colorless pungent gas consisting of nitrogen and hydrogen, produced by the decomposition of nitrogenous organic matter. Some of its many uses are as an aromatic stimulant, a detergent, and an emulsifier.

ammoniacal fermentation /am'ənī'əkəl/, the production of ammonia and carbon dioxide from urea by the enzyme urease.

ammonium ion, an $NH_4 +$ ion formed by the reaction of ammonia (NH_3) with a hydrogen ion ($H+$). The ammonium ion is highly soluble in water but does not pass easily through cell membranes, as does the ammonia molecule, and its rate of excretion is influenced in part by the acidity of urine. The lower the pH, the greater the proportion of ammonium ions present, assuming a constant level of ammonia production from amino acid metabolism.

Ammon's horn. See **hippocampus.**

amnesia /amnē'zhə/ [Gk, *a, mnemonic,* not memory], a loss of memory caused by brain damage or by severe emotional trauma. Kinds of amnesia are **anterograde amnesia, posttraumatic amnesia,** and **retrograde amnesia.**

amnesic /amnē'sik/ [Gk, *amnesia,* forgetfulness], in a state of forgetfulness or showing signs of memory loss or impairment.

amnesic aphasia [Gk, *amnesia, + a, phasis,* without speech], an inability to remember spoken words or to use words for names of objects, circumstances, or characteristics.

amnestic apraxia /amnes'tik/, the inability to carry out a movement in response to a request because of a lack of ability to remember the request rather than to a loss of motor function. See also **apraxia.**

amnio-, a prefix meaning 'pertaining to the amnion': *amniogenesis, amnioma, amniorrhexis.*

amniocentesis /am'nē·ōsentē'sis/ [Gk, *amnos,* lamb's caul, *kentesis* pricking], an obstetric procedure in which a small amount of amniotic fluid is removed for laboratory analysis. It is usually performed between the sixteenth and twentieth weeks of gestation to aid in the diagnosis of fetal abnormalities.

■ METHOD: With the use of ultrasound scanning techniques the position of the fetus and the location of the placenta are determined. The skin on the mother's abdomen is aseptically prepared, and a local anesthetic is usually injected. A needle attached to a syringe is introduced into a part of the uterus where there is the least chance of perforating the placenta or scratching the fetus. Between 20 and 25 ml of amniotic fluid is aspirated. Amniocentesis is performed to diagnose various genetic defects, including chromosomal abnormalities, neural tube defects, and Tay-Sachs disease. It is also performed to discover the sex of the fetus if certain sex-linked genetic defects are suspected. Later in pregnancy, amniocentesis may be performed to assess fetal lung maturity by testing the lecithin-sphingomyelin (L/S) ratio and the presence of phosphatidyl-glycerol (PG) in the laboratory before elective delivery. The fluid may be tested for the concentration of creatinine, another indicator of fetal maturity. When postmaturity is suspected, amniocentesis is performed to examine the amniotic fluid for meconium.

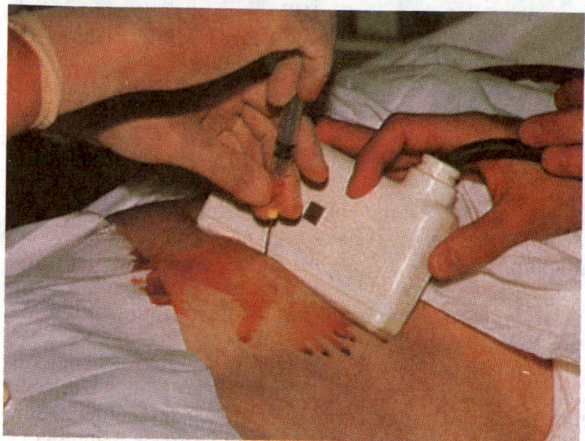

Amniocentesis—placement of needle through abdomen
(Al-Azzawi, 1991)

■ NURSING INTERVENTION: Proof of informed consent is required to be signed by the woman before amniocentesis. Specifically stated in the consent form are the reasons for performing the procedure and the facts that fluid is to be removed after needle puncture of the uterus, that ultrasound imaging techniques are usual adjuncts, that the procedure may fail to give the results intended, and that spontaneous abortion, nausea, abdominal pain, or fetal injury may occur. The woman is reassured that complications and failure are rare; she is given emotional support before, during, and after the procedure. In testing for genetic abnormalities 3 or more weeks is usually necessary for tissue culture before a diagnosis may be made; this waiting period is extremely stressful for the mother. The woman is warned to report any signs of infection or of the onset of labor. Rh immune globulin should be given to pregnant women who are Rh negative.

■ OUTCOME CRITERIA: Spontaneous abortion occurs in approximately 1% of women undergoing amniocentesis. Perforation of the placenta or a blood vessel in the umbilical cord or placenta may cause hemorrhage or isoimmunization and hemolytic disease of the fetus, possibly leading to fetal death. Maternal and fetal infection with attendant morbidity or mortality may occur, but it is rare. Premature rupture of the membranes, premature labor, or trauma to the fetus or umbilical cord may occur. The procedure is not usually performed for genetic diagnosis unless the mother plans to terminate the pregnancy if the procedure indicates the presence of a genetic disease or abnormality.

amniography /am′nē·og′rəfē/, a procedure used to detect placement of the placenta by x-ray examination with injection of a radiopaque contrast medium into the amniotic fluid. It is seldom used, having been largely supplanted by ultrasonography.

amnion /am′nē·on/ [Gk, *amnos,* lamb's caul], a membrane, continuous with and covering the fetal side of the placenta, that forms the outer surface of the umbilical cord and becomes the outermost layer of the skin of the developing fetus. Compare **chorion.**

amnionitis /am′nē·ōnī′tis/, an inflammation of the amnion. The condition may develop after early rupture of the fetal membranes.

amnioscopy /am′nē·os′kəpē/, direct visual examination of the fetus and amniotic fluid with an endoscope that is inserted into the amniotic cavity through the uterine cervix or an incision in the abdominal wall.

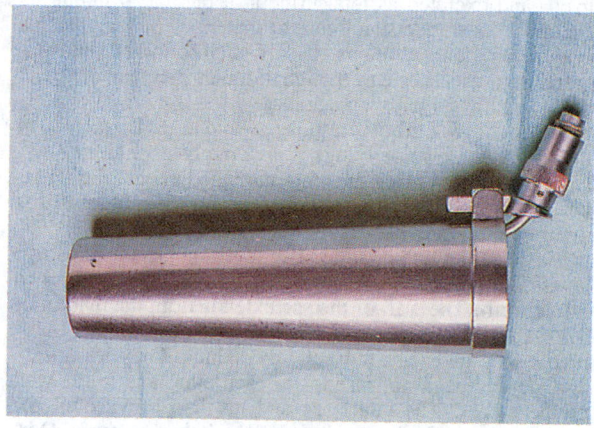

Amnioscope *(Al-Azzawi, 1991)*

amniotic /am′nē·ot′ik/, pertaining to the amnion.

amniotic band syndrome, an abnormal condition of fetal development characterized by the development of fibrous bands within the uterus that entangle the fetus, leading to deformities in structure and function. The syndrome is associated with a variety of congenital defects, including clubbed feet, amputated limbs, simian creases, and skull and visceral defects.

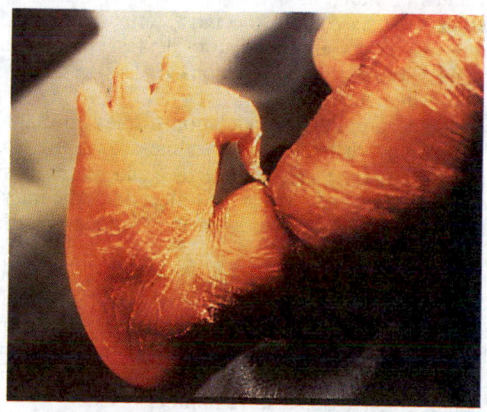

Amniotic bands *(Zitelli, 1992)*

amniotic cavity, [Gk, *amnion,* fetal membrane + L, *cavum*], the fluid-filled cavity of the amniotic sac surrounding the fetus.

amniotic fluid, a liquid produced by the fetal membranes and the fetus. It surrounds the fetus throughout pregnancy, protecting it from trauma, temperature variations, provides freedom of fetal movements, and helps maintain the fetal oxygen supply. The volume totals about 1000 ml at term. In addition to providing the fetus with physical protection, the amniotic fluid is a medium of active chemical exchange. It is secreted and resorbed by cells lining the amniotic sac at a rate of 500 ml/hr at term, and is swallowed, metabolized, and excreted as fetal urine at a rate of 50 ml/hr. Its chemical constituents are those of maternal and fetal plasma in different concentrations. Its pH is close to neutral. Amniotic fluid itself is clear, though desquamated fetal cells and lipids give it a cloudy appearance.

amniotic fluid embolism [Gk, *amnion,* + L, *fluere,* to flow, + Gk, *embolos,* plug], an embolism resulting from amniotic fluid entering the maternal blood system during labor and/or delivery. It is usually fatal for the mother if it is a pulmonary embolism.

amniotic sac, a thin-walled bag that contains the fetus and amniotic fluid during pregnancy, having a capacity of 4 to 5 L at term. The wall of the sac extends from the margin of the placenta. The amnion, chorion, and decidua that make up the wall are each a few cell layers thick. They are closely applied—though not fused—to each other and to the wall of the uterus. The intact sac and its fluid provide for the equilibration of hydrostatic pressure within the uterus. During labor, the sac effects the uniform transmission of the force of uterine contractions to the cervix for dilatation. See also **amnion, chorion, decidua.**

amniotomy /am′nē·ot′əmē/ the artificial rupture of the fetal membranes (ARM). It is usually performed to stimulate or accelerate the onset of labor. The procedure is painless.

amobarbital /am′ōbär′bətal/, a barbiturate sedative-hypnotic.
- INDICATIONS: It is prescribed for the relief of anxiety and insomnia and as an anticonvulsant.
- CONTRAINDICATIONS: Porphyria or known hypersensitivity to barbiturates prohibits its use.
- ADVERSE EFFECTS: Among the most serious adverse reactions are respiratory and circulatory depression, drug hangover, and various allergic reactions. It is also involved in many drug interactions.

A-mode, the amplitude modulation display in diagnostic ultrasonography. It represents the time taken for the ultrasound beam to strike a tissue interface and return its signal to the transducer. The greater the reflection at the interface, the larger the signal amplitude on the A-mode screen. See also **B-mode, M-mode.**

A-mode ultrasound [L, *ultra,* beyond + *sonus,* sound], a display of ultrasonic echoes in which the horizontal axis of the cathode ray tube display represents the time required for the return of the echo and the vertical oscilloscope trace represents the strength of the echo. The mode is used in echoencephalography. See also **A-mode.**

amoeba. See ameba.

-amoeba. See -ameba.

amoebiasis. See amebiasis.

amoebic dysentery. See amebic dysentery.

amok [Malay, *amoq,* furious], a psychotic frenzy with a desire to kill anybody encountered. The murderous episodes may follow periods of severe depression.

amorph /ā′môrf, əmôrf′/ [Gk, *a, morphe*f, not shape], **1.** inactive gene; a mutant allele that has little or no effect on the expression of a trait. Compare **antimorph, hypermorph, hypomorph. 2.** abbreviation for *amorphous,* such as amorph IZS (amorphous insulin zinc suspension).

amorphic, (in genetics) of or pertaining to a gene that is inactive or nearly inactive so that it has no determinable effect.

amorphous crystals /əmôr′fəs/, shapeless, ill-defined crystals, usually phosphates.

amoxapine /əmok′sepin/, an antidepressant similar to the tricyclics.
- INDICATION: It is prescribed in the treatment of mental depression.
- CONTRAINDICATIONS: It is used with caution in conditions where anticholinergics are contraindicated, in seizure disorders, and in patients with cardiovascular disorders. Concomitant administration of monoamine oxidase inhibitors, recent myocardial infarction, or known hypersensitivity to this drug prohibits its use.
- ADVERSE EFFECTS: Among the most serious adverse reactions are sedation and anticholinergic side effects. A variety of GI, cardiovascular, and neurologic reactions may also occur. It is involved in many potential drug interactions.

amoxicillin /əmok′səsil′in/, a semisynthetic oral penicillin antibiotic similar to ampicillin.
- INDICATIONS: It is prescribed in the treatment of several infections that are caused by a susceptible gram-negative or gram-positive organism.
- CONTRAINDICATION: Known hypersensitivity to any penicillin prohibits its use.
- ADVERSE EFFECTS: Among the most serious adverse reactions are anaphylaxis, nausea, and diarrhea. Various allergic reactions and rashes are common.

Amoxil, a trademark for an antibiotic (amoxicillin).

AMP, abbreviation for **adenosine monophosphate.**

ampere (A) /am′pēr/ [André M. Ampere, French physicist, b. 1775], a unit of measurement of the amount of electric current. An ampere, according to the meter-kilogram-second (MKS) system, is the amount of current passed through a resistance of 1 ohm by an electrical potential of 1 volt. The standard international ampere is the amount of current that deposits 0.001118 g of silver per second when passed, according to certain specifications, through a silver nitrate solution. See also **ohm, volt, watt.**

amperometry /am′parom′ətrē/, the measurement of current at a single applied potential.

amph-. See amphi-.

amphetamines /amfet′əmēnz/, a group of nervous system stimulants, including amphetamine and its chemical congeners dextroamphetamine and methamphetamine, that are subject to abuse because of their ability to produce wakefulness and euphoria. Abuse leads to compulsive behavior, paranoia, hallucinations, and suicidal tendencies. They have many street names, such as **black beauties, lid poppers, pep pills, speed,** an injectable form, and **ice,** a crystalline form of methamphetamine that is smoked. See also **dextroamphetamine sulfate, methamphetamine hydrochloride.**

amphetamine poisoning, toxic effects of overdosage of amphetamines. Symptoms usually include excitement, tremors, tachycardia, hallucinations, delirium, convulsions, and circulatory collapse. Emergency first aid requires gastric lavage with tap water and charcoal or induced emesis.

amphi-, amph-, a prefix meaning 'on both sides': *amphiarthrosis, amphibious.*

amphiarthrosis. See **cartilaginous joint.**

amphigenesis. See **amphigony.**

amphigenetic /am′fijənet′ik/ [Gk, *amphi,* both sides, *genein,* to produce], **1.** produced by the union of gametes from both sexes. **2.** bisexual; having both testicular and ovarian tissue. Compare **hermaphroditism, pseudohermaphroditism.**

amphigenous inheritance /amfij′ənəs/, the acquisition of genetic traits and conditions from both parents. Also called **biparental inheritance, duplex inheritance.**

amphigonadism /am′figō′nədiz′əm/, true hermaphroditism; having both testicular and ovarian tissue. −**amphigonadic,** *adj.*

amphigony /amfig′ənē/ [Gk, *amphi* + *gonos,* generation], sexual reproduction. Also called **amphigenesis.** −**amphigonic** /am′figon′ik/, *adj.*

amphikaryon /am′fiker′ē·on/ [Gk, *amphi* + *karyon,* nucleus], a nucleus containing the diploid number of chromosomes. −**amphikaryotic,** *adj.*

amphimixis /am′fimik′sis/ [Gk, *amphi* + *mixis,* mingling], **1.** the union of germ cells in reproduction so that both maternal and paternal hereditary characteristics are derived; interbreeding. **2.** (in psychoanalysis) the union and integration of oral, anal, and genital libidinal impulses in the development of heterosexuality.

amphipathic /-path′ik/ [Gk, *amphi* + *pathos,* suffering], pertaining to a molecule having two sides with characteristically different properties, such as a detergent, which has both a polar (hydrophilic) end and a nonpolar (hydrophobic) end but is long enough so that each end demonstrates its own solubility characteristics.

ampho-, a prefix meaning 'around, both, doubly': *amphochromophil, amphodiplopia, amphogenic.*

amphoric breath sound /amfôr′ik/ [Gk, *amphoreus,* jug], an abnormal, resonant, hollow blowing sound heard with a stethoscope. It indicates a cavity opening into the bronchus or a pneumothorax.

amphoteric /am′fōter′ik/ [Gk, *amphoteros,* pertaining to both], a substance that can have a positive, zero, or negative charge, depending on conditions.

amphotericin B /am′fəter′əsin/, an antifungal medication.

■ INDICATIONS: It is prescribed for topical or systemic use in the treatment of fungal infections.

■ CONTRAINDICATION: Known hypersensitivity to this drug prohibits its use.

■ ADVERSE EFFECTS: Among the most serious adverse reactions are, when used systemically, thrombophlebitis, blood dyscrasias, nephrotoxicity, nausea, and fever; chills and shaking may occur on administration. With topical use, local hypersensitivity reactions are the most common adverse reactions.

amphotericin methyl ester (AME), an antiviral drug used in experimental treatment of HIV infections.

amphoterism /-ter′izəm/ [Gk, *amphoteros,* both], a quality of a chemical compound that permits it to act as an acid or a base.

ampicillin /am′pəsil′in/, a semisynthetic penicillin.

■ INDICATIONS: It is prescribed in the treatment of a variety

of infections caused by a broad spectrum of sensitive gram-negative and gram-positive organisms.

■ CONTRAINDICATION: Known hypersensitivity to any penicillin prohibits its use.

■ ADVERSE EFFECTS: Among the most serious adverse reactions are anaphylaxis, nausea, and diarrhea. Fever, rashes, other allergic reactions, and suprainfection also may occur.

amplification /am′plifikā′shən/ [L, *amplificare,* to make wider], **1.** (in molecular genetics) a process in which the amount of plasmid DNA is increased in proportion to the amount of bacterial DNA by treatment with certain substances, including chloramphenicol. **2.** the replication in bulk of an entire gene library. −**amplify,** *v.*

amplitude /am′plityōōd/ [L, *amplus,* wide], width or breadth of range or extent, such as amplitude of accommodation or amplitude of convergence.

amplitude of accommodation (AA), the total accommodative power of the eye, determined by the difference between the refractive power for farthest vision and that for nearest vision.

amplitude of convergence, the difference in the power needed to turn the eyes from their far point to their near point of convergence. Also called **fusional amplitude, vergence ability.**

ampule /am′pyōōl/ [Fr, *ampoule,* phial], a small, sterile glass or plastic container that usually contains a single dose of a solution to be administered parenterally. Also spelled **ampoule.**

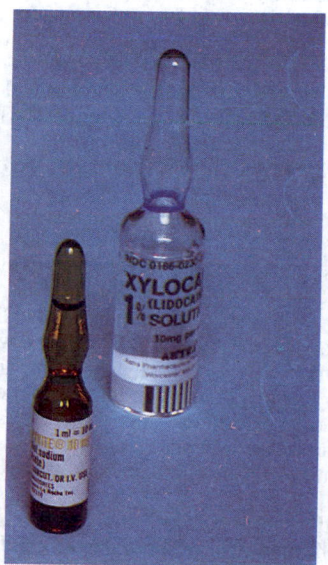

Ampule *(Potter, 1993)*

ampulla /ampōōl′ə/ [L, flasklike bottle], a rounded, saclike dilatation of a duct, canal, or any tubular structure, such as the lacrimal duct, semicircular canal, uterine tube, rectum, or vas deferens.

ampulla of Vater. See **hepatopancreatic ampulla.**

ampullary aneurysm. See **saccular aneurysm.**

ampullary tubal pregnancy /ampo͞o'lərē/, am'pəler'ē/, a kind of tubal pregnancy in which implantation occurs in the ampulla of one of the fallopian tubes. See also **tubal pregnancy.**

amputation /am'pyo͞otā'shən/ [L, *amputare*, to excise], the surgical removal of a part of the body or a limb or part of a limb, performed to treat recurrent infections or gangrene in peripheral vascular disease, to remove malignant tumors, and in severe trauma. With the patient under anesthesia, the part is removed and a shaped flap is cut from muscular and cutaneous tissue to cover the end of the bone. A section may be left open for drainage if infection is present. Preoperative care includes an assessment of circulation in the affected part and the shaving and cleansing of the area. Postoperatively, the stump is elevated on a pillow, and, if necessary, protected with plastic from urinary and fecal contamination. Vital signs are monitored carefully. If a soft dressing is used, it is watched for excessive bleeding. The stump is moved frequently to prevent circulatory complications and tissue necrosis. If the dressing is rigid (a cast), it must remain in place for 8 to 14 days. Should the cast come off inadvertently, the stump must be wrapped tightly at once with elastic compression bandage and plans must be made to replace the cast. With the cast on, the patient who has had part of a leg removed can stand briefly after 24 hours and bear some weight on the prosthesis. Medication may relieve incisional and phantom limb pain. Kinds of amputation include **closed amputation, congenital amputation, open amputation, primary amputation,** and **secondary amputation.**

amputation neuroma, a form of traumatic neuroma that may develop near the stump after the amputation of an extremity.

amputee /am'pyətē'/, a person who has had one or more extremities traumatically, congenitally, or surgically removed. See also **congenital amputation.**

A.M.R.A, abbreviation for *American Medical Records Association.*

amrinone lactate /am'rinōn/, an intravenous cardiac inotropic drug.

■ INDICATIONS: It is prescribed in the short-term management of congestive heart failure in patients who do not respond to therapy with digitalis, diuretics, and vasodilators.

■ CONTRAINDICATIONS: The drug may interact with other cardiovascular medications, particularly disopyramide, and any combination therapy should be closely monitored.

■ ADVERSE EFFECTS: Among more serious adverse reactions are thrombocytopenia, dysrhythmias, hypotension, nausea, vomiting, liver impairment, and hypersensitivity effects.

Amsler grid [Marc Amsler, Swiss ophthalmologist, b. 1891], a checkerboard grid of intersecting dark horizontal and vertical lines with one dark spot in the middle. To discover a visual field defect, the person simply covers or closes one eye and looks at the spot with the other. A visual field defect is perceived as a defect, distortion, blank, or other fault in the grid. The person may record the defects directly on a paper copy of the grid that may be kept as a permanent record.

A.M.T, abbreviation for *American Medical Technologists.*

amu, abbreviation for **atomic mass unit.**

amusia /əmyo͞o'sē·ə/, a form of agnosia characterized by a loss of the ability to recognize melodies. The neurologic defect may follow a stroke or other damage to the parietal lobe of the brain.

amyelinic neuroma /amī'əlin'ik/ [Gk, *a, myelos*, not marrow, *neuron*, nerve, *oma*], a tumor that contains only nonmyelinated nerve fibers.

amygdala /amig'dələ/ [Gk, *amygdale*, almond], **1.** an almond-shaped mass of gray matter in the front portion of the temporal lobe of the brain. **2.** an obsolete term for the tonsil.

amygdalin /əmig'dəlin/ [Gk, *amygdale*, almond], a naturally occurring cyanogenic glycoside obtained from bitter almonds and apricot pits. It has been promoted as a potential cancer remedy under the trademark of Laetrile. Also called **vitamin B$_{17}$.**

amygdaloid /-dəloid/, resembling a tonsil.

amygdaloid fossa [Gk, *amylon, eidos,* starchlike + L, *fossa,* ditch], a space in the wall of the oropharynx, between the pillars of the fauces, that is occupied by the palatine tonsil. Also called **tonsillar fossa.**

amygdaloid nucleus [Gk, *amygdale,* almond, *eidos,* form; L, *nucleus,* nut], one of the basal nuclei, found in the inferior horn of the lateral ventricle.

amyl-. See **amylo-.**

amyl alcohol /am'il/ [Gk, *amylon,* starch], a colorless, oily liquid that is only slightly soluble in water but can be mixed with ethyl alcohol, chloroform, or ether.

amyl alcohol tertiary. See **amylene hydrate.**

amylase /am'ilās/ [Gk, *amylon,* starch], an enzyme that catalyzes the hydrolysis of starch into smaller carbohydrate molecules. Alpha-amylase, found in saliva, pancreatic juice, malt, certain bacteria, and molds, catalyzes the hydrolysis of starches to dextrins, maltose, and maltotriose. Beta-amylase, found in grains, vegetables, and malt, is involved in the hydrolysis of starch to maltose. Normal blood findings are 56-190 IU/L. See also **enzyme.**

amylene hydrate /am'əlēn/, a clear, colorless liquid with a camphorlike odor, miscible with alcohol, chloroform, ether, or glycerin and used as a solvent and a hypnotic.

amylic fermentation /əmil'ik/, the formation of amyl alcohol from sugar.

amyl nitrite, a vasodilator.

■ INDICATION: It is prescribed to relieve the vasospasm of angina pectoris.

■ CONTRAINDICATIONS: Known hypersensitivity to this drug or to other nitrites prohibits its use.

■ ADVERSE EFFECTS: Among the more serious adverse reactions are hypotension, allergic reactions, nausea, headache, and dizziness.

amylo-, amyl-, a prefix meaning 'pertaining to starch': *amyloclast, amylodextrin, amyloid.*

amylobarbitone. See **amobarbital.**

amyloid /am'iloid/ [Gk, *amylon,* starch + *eidos,* form], **1.** pertaining to or resembling starch. **2.** a starchlike protein-carbohydrate complex that is deposited abnormally in some tissues during certain chronic disease states, such as amyloidosis, rheumatoid arthritis, and tuberculosis.

amyloid disease. See **amyloidosis.**

amyloid liver [Gk, *amylon,* starch, *eidos,* form; AS, *lifer*], liver in which the cells have been infiltrated with amyloid deposits. Also called **albuminous liver.**

amyloidosis /am'iloidō'sis/ [Gk, *amylon* + *eidos,* form, *osis,* condition], a disease in which a waxy, starchlike, glycoprotein (amyloid) accumulates in tissues and organs,

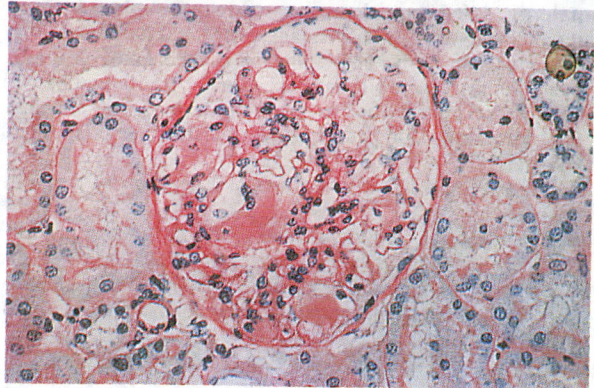

Amyloid deposits in the kidney (Shipley, 1993)

impairing their function. There are two major forms of the condition. **Primary amyloidosis** usually occurs with multiple myeloma. Patients with **secondary amyloidosis** usually suffer from another chronic infectious or inflammatory disease, such as tuberculosis, osteomyelitis, rheumatoid arthritis, or Crohn's disease. The cause of both types of amyloidosis is unknown. Almost all organs are affected, most often the heart, lungs, tongue, and intestines in primary amyloidosis, and the kidneys, liver, and spleen in the secondary type. Elderly patients tend to experience cardiac effects of the disease. Diagnosis is made through biopsy of the suspected organ. There is no known cure for amyloidosis, and treatment in the secondary type is aimed at alleviating the underlying chronic disease. Patients with renal amyloidosis are frequently candidates for kidney dialysis and transplantation.

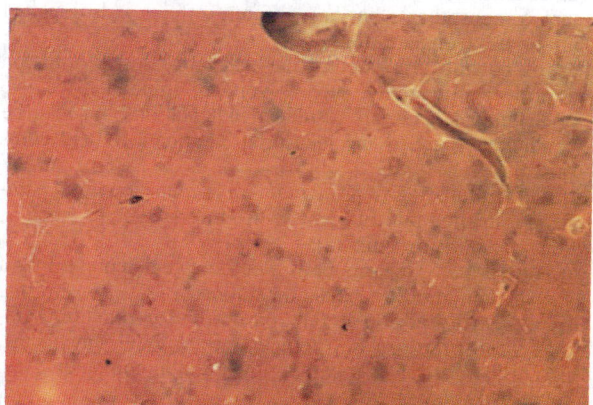

Amyloidosis involving the spleen (Fletcher, 1987)

amylopectinosis.   See **Andersen's disease.**
amyoplasia congenita.   See **arthrogryposis multiplex congenita.**
amyotonia /ā′mī·ōtō′nē·ə/ [Gk, *a, mys,* not muscle, *tonos,*

tone],   an abnormal condition of skeletal muscle, characterized by a lack of tone, weakness, and wasting, usually the result of motor neuron disease. —**amyotonic,** *adj.*
amyotrophic lateral sclerosis (ALS) /ā′mī·ōtrof′ik/ [Gk, *a, mys + trophe,* nourishment],   a degenerative disease of the motor neurons, characterized by weakness and atrophy of the muscles of the hands, forearms, and legs, spreading to involve most of the body and face. It results from degeneration of the motor neurons of the anterior horns and corticospinal tracts, beginning in middle age and progressing rapidly, causing death within 2 to 5 years. There is no known treatment. Also called **Lou Gehrig's disease.** See also **Aran-Duchenne muscular atrophy.**
an-, ana-,   a prefix meaning 'not, without': *anoxia, anosmic, analgesia.*
-an, -ian,   a suffix meaning 'belonging to, characteristic of, similar to': *amphibian, protozoan, salpingian.*
ana (āa, āā, ĀĀ),   (in prescriptions) 'so much of each,' indication of the amount of each ingredient to be compounded. Usually written as an abbreviation.
ANA,   1. abbreviation for **American Nurses' Association.** 2. abbreviation for **antinuclear antibody.**
ana-.   See **an-.**
anabolic.   See **anabolism.**
anabolic steroid /an′əbol′ik/ [Gk, *anaballein,* to build up],   any one of several compounds derived from testosterone or prepared synthetically to promote general body growth, to oppose the effects of endogenous estrogen, or to promote masculinizing effects. All such compounds cause a mixed androgenic-anabolic effect. Anabolic steroids are prescribed in the treatment of aplastic anemia, red-cell aplasia, and hemolytic anemia and in anemias associated with renal failure, myeloid metaplasia, and leukemia. Some common compounds used in such therapies are calusterone, methandriol, and nandrolone. Anabolic steroids used in the palliation of carcinoma of the breast in women carry the risk of causing masculinization. The earliest symptoms of such undesirable effects are acne, the growth of facial hair, and the hoarsening or deepening of the voice. Continued use of these compounds in women may also produce prominent musculature, excessive body hair, and hypertrophy of the clitoris.
anabolism /ənab′əliz′əm/ [Gk, anaballein, to build up],   constructive metabolism characterized by the conversion of simple substances into the more complex compounds of living matter. Compare **catabolism.** —**anabolic** /an′əbol′ik/, *adj.*
anacatadidymus /an′əkat′ədid′iməs/ [Gk, *ana,* up, again *kata,* down, *didymos,* twin],   conjoined twins that are fused in the middle but separated above and below.
anaclisis /an′əklī′sis/ [Gk, *ana + klisis,* leaning],   1. a condition, normal in childhood but pathologic in adulthood, in which a person is emotionally dependent on other people. 2. a condition in which a person consciously or unconsciously chooses a love object because of a resemblance to the mother, father, or other person who was an important source of comfort and protection in infancy. —**anaclitic** /an′əklit′ik/, *adj.*
anaclitic depression /an′əklit′ik/,   a syndrome occurring in infants, usually after sudden separation from the mothering person. Symptoms include apprehension, withdrawal, incessant crying, refusal to eat, sleep disturbances, and, eventually, stupor leading to severe impairment of the infant's physical, social, and intellectual development. If the

mothering figure or a substitute is made available within 1 to 3 months, the infant recovers quickly with no long-term effects. See also **hospitalism.**

anacrotic pulse /an'əkrot'ik/ [Gk, *ana* + *krotos,* stroke], (on a sphygmographic tracing) a pulse characterized by one transient drop in amplitude on the curve of the primary elevation. It is seen in valvular aortic stenosis.

anacusis /an'əkoo'sis/ [Gk, *a, akouein,* not to hear], a total loss of hearing.

anadicrotic pulse /an'ədīkrot'ik/ [Gk, *ana* + *dis,* twice, *krotos,* stroke], (on a sphygmographic tracing) a pulse characterized by two transient drops in amplitude on the curve of primary elevation.

anadidymus /an'ədid'iməs/ [Gk, *ana* + *dydymos,* twin], conjoined twins that are united at the pelvis and lower extremities but are separated in the upper half. Also called **duplicatus anterior.**

anadipsia /an'ədip'sē·ə/ [Gk, *ana* + *dipsa,* thirst], extreme thirst, often occurring in the manic phase of bipolar mood disorder. The condition is the result of dehydration caused by the excessive perspiration, continuous urination, and relentless physical activity produced by the intense excitement characteristic of the manic phase.

Anadrol-50, a trademark for an androgen (oxymetholone), used as an anabolic agent.

anaerobe /aner'ōb/ [Gk, *a, aer,* not air, *bios,* life], a microorganism that grows and lives in the complete or almost complete absence of oxygen. An example is *Clostridium botulinum.* Anaerobes are widely distributed in nature and in the body. Some kinds of anaerobes are **facultative anaerobe** and **obligate anaerobe.** Compare **aerobe, microaerophile.** See also **anaerobic infection.**

anaerobic /an'ərō'bik/, **1.** pertaining to the absence of air or oxygen. **2.** able to grow and function without air or oxygen.

anaerobic catabolism, the breakdown of complex chemical substances into simpler compounds, with the release of energy, in the absence of oxygen.

anaerobic exercise, muscular exertion sufficient to result in metabolic acidosis because of accumulation of lactic acid as a product of muscle metabolism. Compare **aerobic exercise.** See also **active exercise, passive exercise.**

anaerobic glycolysis. See **glycolysis.**

anaerobic infection, an infection caused by an anaerobic organism, usually occurring in deep puncture wounds that exclude air or in tissue that has diminished oxygen-reduction potential as a result of trauma, necrosis, or overgrowth of bacteria. Kinds of anaerobic infection are **gangrene** and **tetanus.** See also *Clostridium.*

anaerobic myositis. See **gas gangrene.**

Ana-Kit, a trademark for an insect sting treatment kit containing epinephrine in a sterile 1 ml syringe.

anal /ā'nəl/ [L, *anus*], of or pertaining to the anus.

anal agenesis. See **imperforate anus.**

anal canal, the final portion of the alimentary tract, about 4 cm long, between the rectal ampulla and the anus.

anal character, (in psychoanalysis) a kind of personality exhibiting patterns of behavior originating in the anal phase of infancy, characterized by extreme orderliness, obstinacy, perfectionism, cleanliness, punctuality, and miserliness, or their extreme opposites. See also **anal eroticism, anal stage, psychosexual development.**

anal crypt, the depression between rectal columns that encloses networks of veins that, when inflamed and swollen, are called hemorrhoids.

analeptic See **central nervous system stimulant.**

anal eroticism, (in psychoanalysis) libidinal fixation at or regression to the anal stage of psychosexual development, often reflected in such personality traits as miserliness, stubbornness, and overscrupulousness. Also called **anal erotism.** Compare **oral eroticism.** See also **anal character.**

anal fissure, a linear ulceration or laceration of the skin of the anus.

anal fistula, an abnormal opening on the cutaneous surface near the anus, usually resulting from a local crypt abscess and also common in Crohn's disease. A perianal fistula may or may not communicate with the rectum. Also called **fistula-in-ano.**

analgesia /an'əljē'zē·ə/ [Gk, *a, algos,* not pain], a decreased or absent sensation of pain.

analgesia algera. See **anesthesia dolorosa.**

analgesic /an'əljē'zik/, **1.** relieving pain. **2.** a drug that relieves pain. The narcotic analgesics act on the central nervous system and alter the patient's perception; they are more often used for severe pain. The nonnarcotic analgesics act at the site of the pain, do not produce tolerance or dependence, and do not alter the patient's perception; they are used for mild to moderate pain. Compare **anodyne.** See also **pain intervention.**

analgesic nephropathy [Gk, *a,* without, *algos,* pain + *nephros,* kidney, *pathos,* disease], a condition of kidney damage resulting from the consuming of excessive amounts of aspirin or similar analgesic pills.

analgia [Gk, *a,* without, *algos,* pain], an absence of pain.

anal incontinence [L, *anus, incontinentia,* an inability to retain], the lack of voluntary control over fecal discharge.

anal membrane. See **cloacal membrane.**

anal membrane atresia. See **imperforate anus.**

analog /an'əlog/ [Gk, *analogos,* proportionate], **1.** a substance, tissue, or organ that is similar in appearance or function to another but differing in origin or development, such as the eye of a fly and the eye of a human. **2.** a drug or other chemical compound that resembles another in structure or constituents but has different effects. Also spelled **analogue.** Compare **homolog.**

analog computer, a computer that processes information as a physical quantity, such as voltage, amperage, weight, or length and presents results of calculations that can be continuously varied and measured. Compare **hybrid computer.**

analogous /ənal'əgəs/ [Gk, *analogos,* proportionate], similar in function but different in origin or structure, such as wings of birds and flies.

analog signal, a continuous electric signal representing a specific condition, such as temperature or ECG waveforms.

analog-to-digital converter, a device for converting analog information, such as temperature or ECG waveforms, into digital form for processing by a digital computer. Also called A/D converter.

analogue. See **analog.**

analogy /ənal'əjē/ [Gk, *analogos*], similar to a degree in function or form but different structurally or in origin.

anal phase. See **anal stage.**

anal reflex, a superficial neurologic reflex obtained by stroking the skin or mucosa of the region around the anus, which normally results in a contraction of the external anal sphincter. This reflex may be lost in disease of the pyramidal tract above the upper lumbar spine level (S3-4). See also **superficial reflex.**

anal sadism, (in psychoanalysis) a sadistic form of anal eroticism, manifested by such behavior as aggressiveness and selfishness. Compare **oral sadism.**

anal stage, (in psychoanalysis) the pregenital period in psychosexual development, occurring between 1 and 3 years of age, when preoccupation with the function of the bowel and the sensations associated with the anus are the predominant source of pleasurable stimulation. It is regarded as an important determinant of ultimate personality type. Adult patterns of behavior associated with fixation on this stage include extreme neatness, orderliness, cleanliness, perfectionism, and punctuality or their extreme opposites. Also called **anal phase.** See also **anal character, psychosexual development.**

anal stenosis. See **imperforate anus.**

anal verge [L, *anus* + *vergere,* to bend], the area between the anal canal and the perianal skin.

analysand /ənal′isand′/, a person undergoing psychoanalysis.

analysis /ənal′əsis/ [Gk, *ana* + *lyein,,* to loosen], the separation of substances into their constituent parts and the determination of the nature, properties, and composition of compounds. In chemistry, **qualitative analysis** is the determination of the elements present in a substance; **quantitative analysis** is the determination of how much of each element is present in a substance. Analysis is also an informal term for **psychoanalysis. –analytic,** *adj.* **analyze,** *v.*

analysis of variance (ANOVA), a series of statistical procedures for determining whether the differences among two or more groups of scores are attributable to chance alone.

analyst /an′əlist/, **1.** a psychoanalyst. **2.** a person who analyzes the chemical, physical, or other properties of a substance or product.

analyte /an′əlīt/, any substance that is measured. The term is usually applied to a component of blood or other body fluid.

analytic. See **analysis.**

analytic psychology /an′əlit′ik/, **1.** the system in which phenomena such as sensations and feelings are analyzed and classified by introspective rather than by experimental methods. Compare **experimental psychology. 2.** also called **Jungian psychology,** a system of analyzing the psyche according to the concepts developed by Carl Gustav Jung. It differs from the psychoanalysis of Sigmund Freud in stressing a "collective unconscious" and a mystic, religious factor in the development of the personal unconscious while minimizing the role of sexual influence on early emotional and psychologic development.

analyze. See **analysis.**

analyzing /an′əlī′zing/, (in five-step nursing process) a category of nursing behavior in which the health care needs of the client are identified and the goals of care are defined. The nurse interprets data; identifies problems involving the client, the client's family, and significant others; defines goals and establishes priorities; integrates the information; and projects the expected outcomes of nursing activities. Although analyzing follows assessing and precedes planning in the five steps of the nursing process, in practice, analyzing is integral to effective nursing practice at all steps of the process. See also **assessing, evaluating, implementing, nursing process, planning.**

anamnesis /an′amnē′sis/ [Gk, *anamimneskein,* to recall],

1. remembrance of the past. **2.** the accumulated data concerning a medical or psychiatric patient and the patient's background, including family, previous environment, experiences, and, particularly, recollections, for use in analyzing his or her condition. Compare **catamnesis.**

anaphase /an′əfāz/ [Gk, *ana* + *phainein,* to appear], the third of four stages of nuclear division in mitosis and in each of the two divisions of meiosis. In mitosis and the second meiotic division the centromeres divide, and the two chromatids, which are arranged along the equatorial plane of the spindle, separate and move to the opposite poles of the cell, forming daughter chromosomes. In the first meiotic division the pairs of homologous chromosomes separate from each other and move intact to the opposite poles of the spindle. See also **interphase, meiosis, metaphase, mitosis, prophase, telophase.**

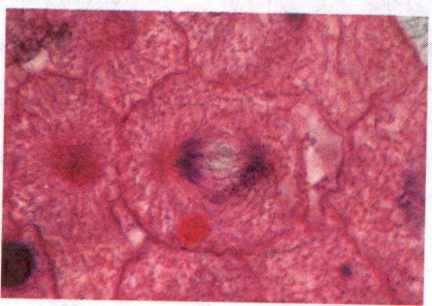

Anaphase
(Seeley, 1992/Ed Reschke/Michael Abbey, Science Source)

anaphia /ənā′fē·ə/, an inability to perceive tactile stimuli.

anaphylactic /an′əfilak′tik/ [Gk, *ana,* up, *phylaxis,* protection], pertaining to anaphylaxis.

anaphylactic hypersensitivity an IgE- or IgG-, dependent, immediate-acting humoral hypersensitivity response to an exogenous antigen. An intradermal skin test produces a wheal and flare reaction and edema within 30 minutes. Histamine, kinins, and other substances are released from mast cells, causing vasodilatation and muscle contraction. Systemic anaphylaxis, atopic allergies, hay fever, and insect-sting reactions are all anaphylactic hypersensitivity reactions. Also called **type I hypersensitivity.** Compare **cell-mediated immune response, cytotoxic hypersensitivity, immune complex hypersensitivity.** See also **anaphylactic shock, immunoglobulin.**

anaphylactic reactions [Gk, *ana, phylaxis,* protection; L, *re, agere,* to act], a hypersensitive condition induced by contact with certain antigens. The second contact with the same antigen may result in dyspnea, severe convulsions, shock, and, in some cases, death. The reaction is particularly severe if the antigen contact is by injection.

anaphylactic shock, a severe and sometimes fatal systemic hypersensitivity reaction to a sensitizing substance, such as a drug, vaccine, certain food, serum, allergen extract, insect venom, or chemical. This condition may occur within seconds from the time of exposure to the sensitizing factor and is commonly marked by respiratory distress and vascular collapse. The more quickly any systemic atopic reaction occurs in the individual after exposure, the more severe the associated shock is likely to be. The involved al-

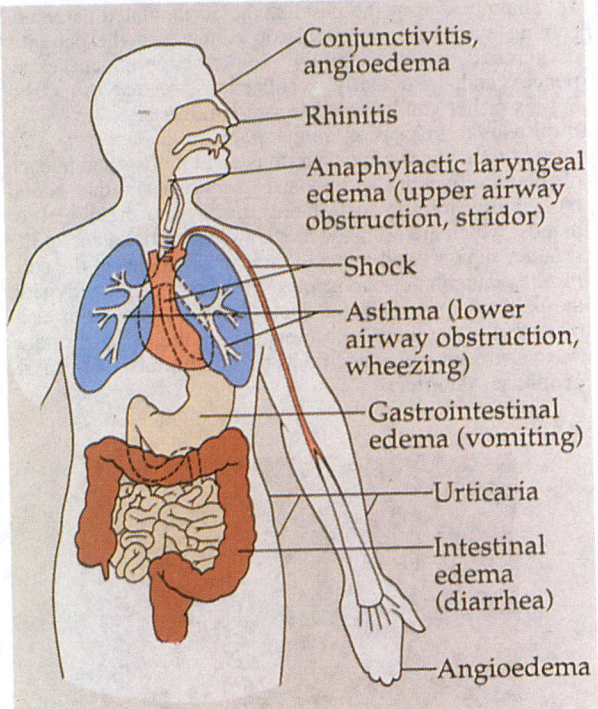

**Systemic manifestations of
anaphylactic hypersensitivity**
(Zitelli, 1992)

Labels on figure:
Conjunctivitis, angioedema
Rhinitis
Anaphylactic laryngeal edema (upper airway obstruction, stridor)
Shock
Asthma (lower airway obstruction, wheezing)
Gastrointestinal edema (vomiting)
Urticaria
Intestinal edema (diarrhea)
Angioedema

lergen enters the systemic circulation and triggers an incomplete humoral response that allows the allergen to combine with IgE and cause the release of histamine. Also entering into the reaction are IgG and IgM, which cause the release of complement fractions, further stimulating histamine action.

■ OBSERVATIONS: Anaphylactic shock can occur within seconds or minutes after exposure to an allergen. The first symptoms are intense anxiety, weakness, sweating, and shortness of breath. Other symptoms may include hypotension, shock, arrhythmia, respiratory congestion, laryngeal edema, nausea, and diarrhea.

■ INTERVENTIONS: If the patient is conscious and normotensive, treatment requires the immediate injection of epinephrine intramuscularly or subcutaneously with vigorous massage of the injection site to ensure faster distribution of the drug. If the patient is unconscious, epinephrine is administered intravenously. The airway is maintained, and the patient is carefully monitored for signs of laryngeal edema, which may require the insertion of an endotracheal tube or a tracheotomy and oxygen therapy. The signs of laryngeal edema include stridor, hoarseness, and dyspnea. Cardiopulmonary resuscitation may be required for cardiac arrest; it often involves closed-chest heart massage, assisted ventilation, and the administration of sodium bicarbonate.

■ NURSING CONSIDERATIONS: Nursing care of patients experiencing anaphylactic shock requires the performance of appropriate emergency treatment and the close monitoring of the patient for hypotension and decreased circulatory volume; volume expanders, as plasma, saline, and albumin, are often ordered. After the emergency, other medications, such

as subcutaneous epinephrine, corticosteroids, and diphenhydramine IV, are administered as prescribed; blood pressure, central venous pressure, and urinary output are monitored. Patients with food allergies that produce anaphylactic shock are instructed to avoid offending allergens; patients with insect sting allergies are instructed to carry emergency anaphylactic kits when outdoors. Such kits contain epinephrine, antihistamine, and tourniquets.

anaphylactoid purpura See **Henoch-Schönlein purpura.**

anaphylatoxin /an'əfī'lətok'sin/, a polypeptide derived from complement. It mediates changes in mast cells leading to the release of histamine and other pharmacologically active substances.

anaphylaxis /an'əfilak'sis/ [Gk, *ana* + *phylaxis*, protection], an exaggerated, life-threatening hypersensitivity reaction to a previously encountered antigen. The response, which is mediated by antibodies of the IgE class of immunoglobulins, causes the release of chemical mediators from the mast cells. The reaction may be a localized wheal and flare of generalized itching, hyperemia, angioneurotic edema, and in severe cases vascular collapse, bronchospasm, and shock. The severity of symptoms depends on the original sensitizing dose of the antigen, the amount and distribution of antibodies, the route of entry and size of the dose of antigen producing anaphylaxis. Insect stings, contrast media containing iodide, aspirin, antitoxins prepared with animal serum, and allergens used in testing and desensitizing patients who are hypersensitive produce anaphylaxis in some individuals. Penicillin injection is the most common cause of anaphylactic shock. Kinds of anaphylaxis are **aggregate anaphylaxis, antiserum anaphylaxis, cutaneous anaphylaxis, cytotoxic anaphylaxis, indirect anaphylaxis,** and **inverse anaphylaxis. –anaphylactic,** *adj.*

anaplasia /an'əplā'zhə/ [Gk, *ana* + *plassein*, to shape], a change in the structure and orientation of cells, characterized by a loss of differentiation and reversion to a more primitive form. Anaplasia is characteristic of malignancy. Compare **metastasis. –anaplastic** /an'əplas'tik/, *adj.*

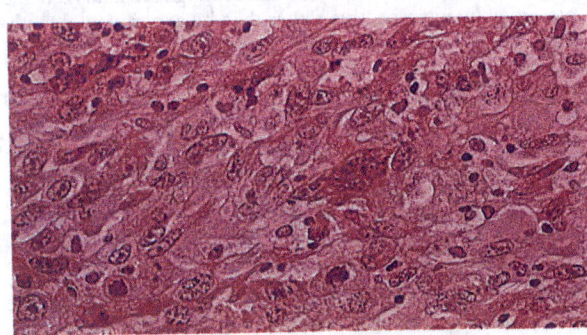

Anaplastic carcinoma *(Besser, 1987)*

anaplastic [Gk, *ana*, backward, *plassein*, to mold], pertaining to anaplasia.

anaplastic astrocytoma. See **glioblastoma multiforme.**

Anaprox, a trademark for a nonsteroidal antiinflammatory drug (naproxen sodium).

anarthria /anär'thrē·ə/ [Gk, *a, arthron*, not joint], a loss of control of the muscles of speech, resulting in the inability to utter words. The condition is usually caused by damage to a central or peripheral motor nerve.

anasarca /anʹəsärʹkə/ [Gk, *ana* + *sarx*, flesh], generalized, massive edema. Anasarca is often observed in edema associated with renal disease when fluid retention continues for an extended period of time. See also **edema. –anasarcous,** *adj.*

anastomose /ənasʹtəmōs/ [Gk, *anastomoein,* to provide a mouth], to open a channel or passage between two vessels or cavities that are normally separate.

anastomosis /ənasʹtōmōʹsis/ *pl.* **anastomoses** [Gk, *anastomoien,* to provide a mouth], a surgical joining of two ducts, blood vessels, or bowel segments to allow flow from one to the other. A vascular anastomosis may be performed to bypass an aneurysm or a vascular or arterial occlusion. With the patient under anesthesia, a section of the saphenous vein or a synthetic prosthesis is grafted to the prepared vessels. Postoperative nursing care includes preventing tissue injury and wound infection by the use of a bed cradle over the incision and padded rails. An adequate airway is maintained, oxygen is given if necessary, and vital signs are closely monitored. The systolic blood pressure is kept at about 20 mm Hg above normal to maintain blood flow through the graft. Lack of blood flow may allow the graft to close, a major complication that requires exploratory surgery and sometimes amputation. Pulses distal to the anastomosis are evaluated and their locations marked. Capillary filling time and the color and temperature of the skin are checked. Prophylactic antibiotic therapy may be started. Urinary output is monitored. The patient is turned and frequently encouraged to cough and breathe deeply. Kinds of anastomoses are **end-to-end anastomosis, side-to-side anastomosis.** See also **aneurysm, bypass.**

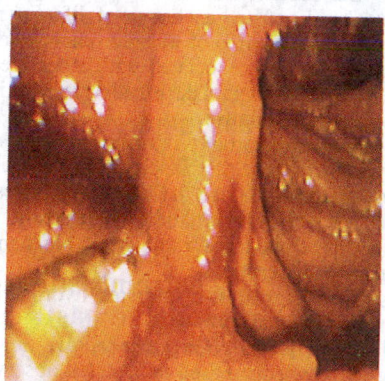

Anastomosis, seen postoperatively
(Winawer, 1992/Courtesy Dr. Jerome D. Waye)

anastomosis at elbow joint, a convergence of blood vessels at the elbow joint, consisting of various veins and portions of the brachial and deep brachial arteries and their branches.

anastomotic /ənasʹtəmotʹik/, pertaining to or resembling an anastomosis.

anatomic [Gk, *ana, temnein,* to cut], pertaining to the structure of the body.

anatomical age, the estimated age of an individual based on the stage of development or deterioration of the body as compared to other persons of the same chronologic age.

anatomical neck of the humerus [Gk, *ana,* up, *temnein,* to cut; AS, *hnecca;* L, *humerus,* shoulder], the portion of the humerus where there is a slight constriction adjoining the head.

anatomical topography [Gk, *ana, temnein,* to cut + *topos,* place, + *graphein,* to write], a system of identification of a body part in terms of the region in which it is located and its nearby structures.

anatomic crown, the portion of the dentin of a tooth, covered by enamel. See also **artificial crown, clinical crown, partial crown.**

anatomic curve, the curvature of the different segments of the vertebral column. In the lateral contour of the back, the cervical curve appears concave, the thoracic curve appears convex, and the lumbar curve appears concave.

anatomic dead space. See **dead space.**

anatomic height of contour, an imaginary line that encircles and designates the greatest convexity of a tooth. Also called **surveyed height of contour.** See also **height of contour.**

anatomic impotence. See **impotence.**

anatomic pathology [Gk, *ana,* up, *temnein,* to cut + *pathos,* disease, *logos,* science], the study of the effects of disease on the structure of the body.

anatomic position, a position of the body in which a person stands erect, facing directly forward, feet pointed for-

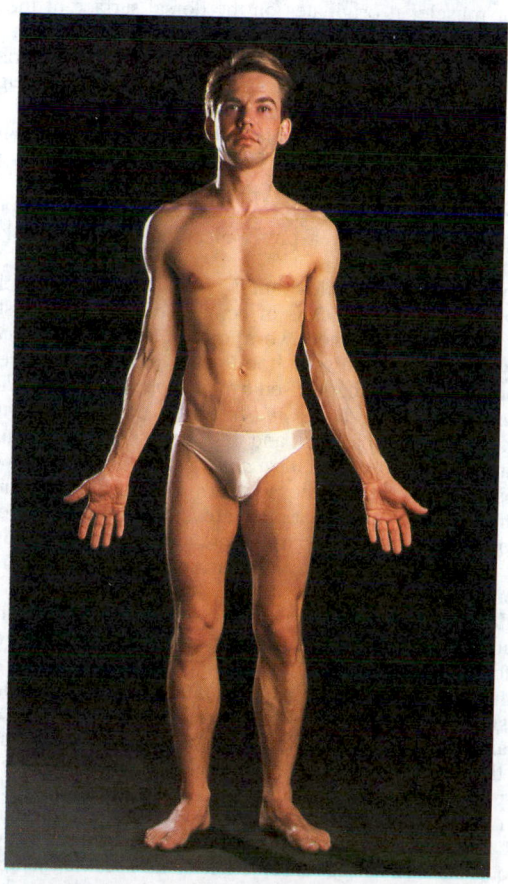

Anatomic position
(Seeley, 1992/Terry Cockerham, Synapse Media Production)

ward slightly apart, arms hanging down at the sides with palms facing forward. This is the standard neutral position of reference used to describe sites or motions of various parts of the body.

anatomic snuffbox, a small, cuplike depression on the back of the hand near the wrist formed by the tendons reaching toward the thumb and index finger as the thumb is abducted, the wrist flexed, and the digits extended.

anatomic zero joint position, the beginning point of a joint range of motion.

anatomy /ənat′əmē/ [Gk, *ana + temnein,* to cut], **1.** the study, classification, and description of structures and organs of the body. Kinds of anatomy are **applied, comparative, descriptive, gross, microscopic,** and **surface. 2.** the structure of an organism. **3.** a text on anatomy. **4.** *archaic.* dissection of a body. Compare **physiology.**

Anavar, a trademark for an androgen (oxandrolone), used as an anabolic agent.

A.N.C., abbreviation for **Army Nurse Corps.**

-ance. See **-ency.**

Ancef, a trademark for a semisynthetic cephalosporin (cefazolin sodium).

ancillary /an′səler′ē/, pertaining to something that is subordinate, auxiliary, or supplementary.

Ancobon, a trademark for an antifungal (flucytosine).

anconeus /angkō′nē·əs/ [Gk, *agkon,* elbow], one of seven superficial muscles of the posterior forearm. A small triangular muscle, it originates on the dorsal surface of the lateral condyle of the humerus and inserts in the olecranon process of the ulna. It is innervated by a branch of the radial nerve, which contains fibers from the seventh and eighth cervical nerves, and it functions to extend the forearm.

ancrod /ang′krod/, the venom of the Malayan pit viper, used to remove fibrinogen from the circulation, thus preventing clotting of the blood.

-ancy. See **-ency.**

ancylo-, anchylo-, a prefix meaning 'bent or crooked': *ancylostoma.*

Ancylostoma /ang′kilos′təmə/ [Gk, *agkylos,* crooked, *stoma,* mouth], a genus of nematode that is an intestinal parasite and causes hookworm disease. See also *Necator.*

ancylostomiasis /an′səlos′təmī′əsis/, hookworm disease, more specifically that caused by *Ancylostoma duodenale, A. braziliense,* or *A. caninum.* Infection by *A. duodenale* is generally more harmful and less responsive to treatment than that by *Necator americanus,* which is the hookworm most often found in the southern United States. Clinical manifestations and treatment are similar for all types of hookworms. Infection may be prevented by eliminating fecal pollution of soil and by wearing shoes. See also **hookworm.**

Andersen's disease [Dorothy H. Andersen, American pediatrician, b. 1901], a rare glycogen storage disease characterized by a genetic deficiency of branching enzyme (amylo-1:4, 1:6 transglucosidase), causing the deposition in tissues of abnormal glycogen with long inner and outer chains. Infants with the disease are normal at birth but fail to thrive and soon show hepatomegaly, splenomegaly, and hypotonic muscles, associated with the progressive development of liver cirrhosis or heart failure of unknown mechanisms. Diagnosis is by enzyme assays of white blood cells and fibroblasts. There is no specific therapy for the disease, which is usually fatal in the first few years of life. Also called **amylopectinosis, glycogen storage disease type IV.**

andr-. See **andro-.**

-andr-, a combining form designating an androgen.

andreioma, andreoblastoma. See **arrhenoblastoma.**

andro-, andr-, a prefix meaning 'pertaining to man or to the male': *androcyte, androgen, androgone.*

androgamone /an′drōgam′ōn/ [Gk, *andros,* man, *gamos,* marriage], a gamone secreted by the male gamete.

androgen /an′drəjin/ [Gk, *andros + genein,* to produce], any steroid hormone that increases male characteristics. Natural hormones, such as testosterone and its esters and analogs, are primarily used as substitutional therapy during the male climacteric. Androgens may be administered orally or parenterally. —**androgenic** /an′drōjen′ik/, *adj.*

androgenic [Gk, *ander,* man, *genein,* to produce], pertaining to the production or development of masculine characteristics.

androgynous /androj′inəs/, **1.** (of a man or woman) having some characteristics of both sexes. Social role, behavior, personality, and appearance are reflections of individuality and are not determined by gender. **2.** hermaphroditic. Compare **gynandrous.** —**androgyny** /-droj′ənē/, *n.*

android [Gk, *andros + eidos,* form], pertaining to something that is typically masculine, or manlike, such as an android pelvis.

android pelvis, a type of pelvis in which the structure is characteristic of the male. It is not uncommon in women. The bones are thick and heavy, and the inlet is heart-shaped. The sacrum inclines anteriorly, the side walls are convergent, and the pubic arch is small. The diameters of the midplane and the outlet are smaller than in the normal gynecoid pelvis. Vaginal delivery is likely to be difficult unless the overall pelvis is large and the fetus small. See **pelvis.**

androma. See **arrhenoblastoma.**

andropause /an′drəpôs/, a change of life for males that may be expressed in terms of a career change, divorce, or reordering of life. It is associated with a decline in androgen levels that occurs in men during their late forties or early fifties. See also **menopause.**

androsterone /andros′tərōn/ [Gk, *andros + stereos,* solid], originally believed to be the principal male sex hormone, it is used less frequently since the discovery of testosterone. The greater potency of several other male sex hormones has relegated androsterone largely to historic biochemical interest. See also **testosterone.**

-ane, a suffix designating a saturated hydrocarbon of the methane series: *butane, propane.*

anecdotal /an′əkdot′əl/ [Gk, *anekdotos,* unpublished], pertaining to knowledge based on isolated observations and not yet verified by controlled scientific studies.

anechoic /an′ekō′ik/, (in ultrasonography) free of echoes or without echoes.

Anectine, a trademark for a skeletal muscle relaxant (succinylcholine chloride), used as an adjunct to anesthesia.

anemia /ənē′mē·ə/ [Gk, *a, haima,* not blood], a decrease in hemoglobin in the blood to levels below the normal range of 4.2 million/mm^3 to 6.1 million/mm^3. Anemia may be caused by a decrease in red cell production, increased red cell destruction, or blood loss. A morphologic classification system describes anemia by the hemoglobin content of the red cells (normochromic or hypochromic) and by differences in red cell size (macrocytic, normocytic, or microcytic). See also **hemolytic anemia, hypoplastic anemia, iron deficiency anemia, iron metabolism.**

■ OBSERVATIONS: Depending on severity, anemia may be accompanied by clinical findings that stem from the diminished oxygen-carrying capacity of the blood. Signs include fatigue, exertional dyspnea, dizziness, headache, insomnia, and pallor. Anorexia, dyspepsia, palpitations, tachycardia, cardiac dilatation, and systolic murmurs also may occur. Iron deficiency is the most common etiology factor. Additional laboratory studies may be required to establish the less common forms of anemia.

■ INTERVENTIONS: The therapeutic response to anemia is variable and depends on the causative factors. Moderate to severe anemia, with hemoglobin levels that are below 7 to 8 g/dl, may require transfusion of one or more units of blood especially if the condition is acute and specific clinical signs are present. Depending on the kind of anemia, treatment includes providing supplements of the deficient component, eliminating the cause of the blood loss, or alleviating the hemolytic component. The latter may involve the administration of adrenal corticosteroids or splenectomy. Appropriate laboratory tests are repeated at intervals to monitor the response and need for continued therapy.

-anemia, -anaemia, -nemia a suffix meaning '(condition of) red blood cell deficiency or its remedy': *achylanemia, melanemia, sulfanemia.*

anemia of pregnancy, a condition of pregnancy characterized by a reduction in the concentration of hemoglobin in the blood. It may be physiologic or pathologic. In physiologic anemia of pregnancy, the reduction in concentration results from dilution because the plasma volume expands more than the red blood cell volume. The hematocrit in pregnancy normally drops several points below the level it was before pregnancy. In pathologic anemia of pregnancy, the oxygen-carrying capacity of the blood is deficient because of disordered erythrocyte production or excessive loss of erythrocytes through destruction or bleeding. Pathologic anemia is a common complication of pregnancy occurring in approximately one half of all pregnancies. Disordered production of erythrocytes may result from nutritional deficiency of iron, folic acid, or vitamin B_{12}, or from sickle cell or other chronic disease, malignancy, chronic malnutrition, or exposure to toxins. Destruction of erythrocytes may result from inflammation, chronic infection, sepsis, autoimmune disorders, microangiopathy, or a hematologic disease in which the red cells are abnormal. Excessive loss of erythrocytes through bleeding may result from abortion, bleeding hemorrhoids, intestinal parasites such as hookworm, placental abnormalities such as placenta previa and premature separation, or postpartum uterine atony.

anemic /ənē′mik/ [Gk, *a*, without, *haima*, blood], pertaining to anemia.

anemic anoxia, a condition characterized by a deficiency of oxygen in body tissues, resulting from a decrease in the number of erythrocytes in the blood or in the amount of hemoglobin.

anemo-, a prefix meaning 'pertaining to the wind': *anemophobia.*

anencephaly /an′ensef′əlē/ [Gk, *a*, *egkephalos*, not brain], congenital absence of the brain and spinal cord in which the cranium does not close and the vertebral canal remains a groove. Transmitted genetically, anencephaly is not compatible with life. It can be detected early in gestation by amniocentesis and analysis or by ultrasonography. See also **neural tube defect.**

anephrogenesis /anef′rōjen′əsis/ [Gk, *a*, without, *nephros*, kidney, *genein*, to produce], to be born without kidneys.

anergic. See **anergy.**

anergic stupor /ənur′jik/, a kind of dementia characterized by quietness, listlessness, and nonresistance.

anergy /an′ərjē/ [Gk *a*, ergon not work], **1.** lack of activity. **2.** an immunodeficient condition characterized by a lack of or diminished reaction to an antigen or group of antigens. This state may be seen in advanced tuberculosis and other serious infections, acquired immune deficiency syndrome, and some malignancies. **–anergic,** *adj.*

aneroid /an′əroid/, not containing a liquid, used especially to describe a device in contrast to one performing a similar function that does contain liquid, such as aneroid sphygmomanometer, which does not contain a column of liquid mercury.

aneroid barometer, a device consisting of a flexible spring in a sealed, evacuated metal box that is used to measure atmospheric pressure. It is less accurate than a mercury barometer and is generally used for nonscientific work.

Anestacon, a trademark for an endourethral local anesthetic solution (2% lidocaine hydrochloride).

anesthesia /an′esthē′zhə/ [Gk, *anaisthesia*, lack of feeling], the absence of normal sensation, especially sensitivity to pain, as induced by an anesthetic substance or by hypnosis or as occurs with traumatic or pathophysiologic damage to nerve tissue. Anesthesia induced for medical or surgical purposes may be topical, local, regional, or general and is named for the anesthetic agent used, the method or procedure followed, the area or organ anesthetized, or the age or class of patient served. See also **general anesthesia, Guedel's signs, local anesthesia, regional anesthesia, topical anesthesia,** and see specific anesthetic agents. (See Fig. p. 86.)

anesthesia dolorosa, a severe tactile or spontaneous, paradoxical pain in an anesthetized area. Also called **analgesia algera.**

anesthesia machine, an apparatus for administering inhalant anesthetic agents. Although there are many different models, all have the following features: an accommodation for a source of gas; a meter to measure the flow of gas; vessels for volatilizing and mixing the anesthetic agents and the carrier gases; and a system for delivering the gas to the patient.

anesthesia paralysis [Gk, *anaisthesia*, lack of feeling + *paralyein*, to be palsied], paralysis that may develop after administration of a general anesthetic.

anesthesia patients, classification of, the system by which the American Society of Anesthesiologists classifies anesthesia patients in five categories by anesthetic risk factors. Class I includes patients who are generally healthy, without serious organic, physiologic, biochemical, or psychiatric problems, and for whom anesthesia is required only for a local condition, such as an inguinal hernia or fibroid uterus. Class II includes patients who have mild to moderate systemic problems, whether involving or extraneous to the condition requiring anesthesia, such as anemia, mild diabetes, essential hypertension, extreme obesity, or chronic bronchitis. Class III includes patients who have severe systemic disturbances or disease, whether or not related to the procedure requiring surgical anesthesia. Class IV includes patients who are suffering from a life-threatening, but not necessarily terminal, condition that may or may not be related to the intended surgical procedure. Class V includes the moribund patient who has little chance of survival, such as a person in shock with a burst abdominal aneurysm or a massive pulmonary embolus. The letter E is added to the roman numeral to indicate an emergency procedure, such

Common postanesthesia problems

Apnea, Hypoventilation, and Hypoxia
Contributing factors
   Airway obstruction
   Respiratory depressant drugs
   Residual effects of muscle relaxants
   Pain
   Constrictive abdominal or thoracic dressings
Treatment
   Airway maintenance
   Oxygen administration
   Reversal of anesthetic agents by narcotic antagonists and
      anticholinesterases
   Respiratory stimulants
   Wake-up regimen
   Pain relief

Hypotension
Contributing factors
   Hypovolemia (blood loss; fluid deficit)
   Cutaneous vasodilation with rewarming
   Loss of sympathetic tone
   Myocardial dysfunction
   Drugs
   Technical problems
Treatment
   Determine cause
   Replace volume deficits
   Place patient in Trendelenburg position
   Administer vasopressors

Hypertension
Contributing factors
   Pain
   Delirium and agitation
   Hypoxia
   Hypercarbia
   Excess fluid administration
   Moderate hypothermia
   Gastric or bladder distention
   Preoperative hypertension
Treatment
   Determine cause
   Drug therapy (analgesics; sedation)

From Beare PG, Myers JL: *Principles and practice of adult health nursing,*
St Louis, 1990, Mosby.

as a patient scheduled for an elective herniorrhaphy who becomes an emergency case when his hernia becomes an obstruction.

anesthesia screen, a metal inverted U-shaped frame that attaches to the sides of an operating table, 12 to 18 inches above a patient's upper chest. It is covered with a sheet to prevent contamination of an operative site on the chest or abdomen by airborne infection from the patient or the anesthetist and to provide a wide sterile field for the surgeon.

anesthesia shock, [Gk, *anaisthesia;* Fr, *choc*], a condition of shock produced by an overdose of anesthetic.

anesthesiologist /anʹəsthēʹzē·olʹəjist/, a physician trained in the administration of anesthetics and in the provision of respiratory and cardiovascular support during anesthetic procedures. Compare **nurse anesthetist.**

anesthesiologist's assistant (AA), an allied health professional who assists the anesthesiologist in collecting preoperative data, such as taking an accurate health history and

performing an appropriate physical examination; in performing various preoperative tasks, such as the insertion of intravenous and arterial lines, central venous pressure monitors, special catheters; in airway management and drug administration for induction and maintenance of anesthesia; in administering supportive therapy, such as intravenous fluids and vasodilators; in providing recovery room care and in performing other functions and tasks relating to care in an intensive care unit or pain clinic; in providing anesthesia monitoring services; and in performing administrative functions and tasks, such as staff education.

anesthesiology /-olʹəjē/, the branch of medicine that is concerned with the relief of pain and with the administration of medication to relieve pain during surgery. It is a specialty requiring competency in general medicine, a broad understanding of surgical procedures, a wide knowledge of clinical pharmacology, biochemistry, cardiology, and respiratory physiology. See also **anesthesiologist, nurse anesthetist.**

anesthetic /anʹesthetʹik/, a drug or agent that is capable of producing a complete or partial loss of feeling (anesthesia).

anesthetist /anesʹthətist/, **1.** a person who administers anesthesia. **2.** an anesthesiologist. See also **nurse anesthetist.**

anesthetize /anesʹthətīz/ [Gk, *anaisthesia,* lack of feeling], to induce a state of anesthesia.

anetoderma /anʹətōdurʹmə/ [Gk, *anetos,* relaxed, *derma,* skin], an idiopathic, patchy atrophy and looseness of skin for which there is no known effective treatment.

aneuploid /anʹyo͞oploid/ [Gk, *a, eu,* not good, *ploos,* fold, *eidos,* form], **1.** of or pertaining to an individual, organism, strain, or cell that has a chromosome number that is not an exact multiple of the normal, basic haploid number characteristic of the species. **2.** such an individual, organism, strain, or cell. Also **aneuploidic** /-ploiʹdik/. Compare **euploid.** See also **monosomy, trisomy.**

aneuploidy /anʹyo͞oploiʹdē/, any variation in chromosome number that involves individual chromosomes rather than entire sets. There may be fewer chromosomes, as in Turner's syndrome, or more chromosomes, as in Down's syndrome. Such individuals have various abnormal physiologic and morphologic traits. Compare **euploidy.** See also **monosomy, trisomy.**

aneurysm /anʹyo͞orizʹəm/ [Gk, *aneurysma,* widening], a localized dilatation of the wall of a blood vessel, usually caused by atherosclerosis and hypertension, or, less frequently, by trauma, infection, or a congenital weakness in the vessel wall. Aneurysms are common in the aorta but also occur in peripheral vessels and are fairly common in the lower extremities of older people, especially in the pop-

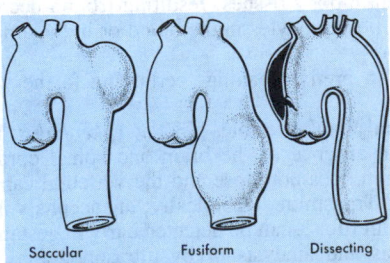

Saccular   Fusiform   Dissecting

Types of aneurysms: saccular, fusiform, dissecting

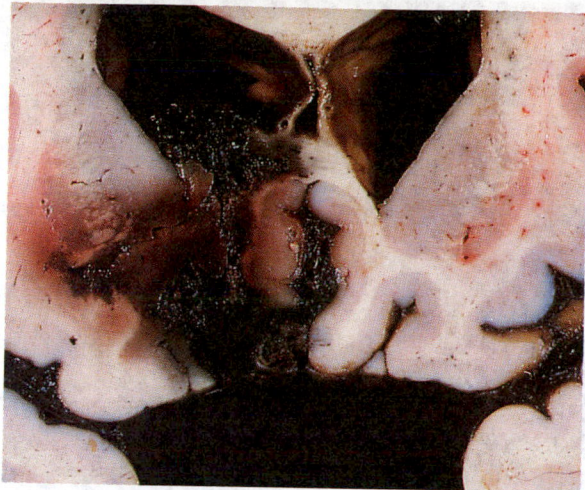

Cerebral aneurysm seen in postmortem section
(Okazaki, 1988/by permission of Mayo Foundation)

liteal arteries. A sign of an arterial aneurysm is a pulsating swelling that produces a blowing murmur on auscultation. An aneurysm may rupture, causing hemorrhage, or thrombi may form in the dilated pouch and give rise to emboli that may obstruct smaller vessels. Kinds of aneurysms include **aortic, bacterial, berry, cerebral, compound, dissecting, fusiform, mycotic, racemose, Rasmussen's, saccular, varicose** and **ventricular aneurysm.** –**aneurysmal** /an'yooriz'məl/, *adj*.

aneurysmal bone cyst, a cystic bone lesion that tends to develop in the metaphyseal region of long bones but may occur in any bone, including the vertebrae. It produces pain and swelling and generally increases in size gradually. It is usually removed surgically, but radiation may be used in cases when the tumor is not easily accessible.

aneurysmal varix [Gk, *aneurysma*, a widening; L, *varix*, a dilated vein], a varicose vein in which the enlargement is of aneurysmal proportions. Also called **aneurysmoid varix.**

aneurysmectomy. See **ventricular aneurysm.**

aneurysm needle, a needle equipped with a handle, used to ligate aneurysms.

aneurysmoid varix. See **aneurysmal varix.**

ANF, abbreviation for *American Nurses Foundation; Australian Nursing Federation.*

angel dust. See **phencyclidine hydrochloride (PCP).**

anger [L *angere* to hurt], an emotional reaction characterized by extreme displeasure, rage, indignation, or hostility. It is considered to be of pathologic origin when such a response does not realistically reflect a person's actual circumstances. However, expressions of anger vary widely from individual to individual and culture to culture.

angi-. See **angio-.**

angiitis /anjē·ī'tis/ [Gk, *aggeion*, vessel, *itis*], an inflammatory condition of a vessel, chiefly a blood or lymph vessel. See also **vasculitis.**

angina /anjī'nə, an'jinə/ [L, *angor*, quinsy (strangling)], **1.** a spasmodic, cramplike choking feeling. **2.** a term now used primarily to denote angina pectoris, the paroxysmal chest pain caused by anoxia of the myocardium. **3.** a de-scriptive feature of various diseases characterized by a feeling of choking, suffocation, or crushing pressure and pain. Kinds of angina are **intestinal, Ludwig's, Prinzmetal's, stable, unstable,** and **streptococcal angina.** –**anginal,** *adj*.

-angina, a suffix meaning 'severe ulceration, usually of the mouth or throat.'

angina acuta [L, *angina*, quinsy, *acutus*, sharp], an old term for a simple sore throat.

angina decubitus, a condition characterized by periodic attacks of angina pectoris that occur when the person is lying down.

anginal, pertaining to angina.

angina pectoris, a paroxysmal thoracic pain caused most often by myocardial anoxia as a result of atherosclerosis of the coronary arteries. The pain usually radiates down the inner aspect of the left arm and is frequently accompanied by a feeling of suffocation and impending death. Attacks of angina pectoris are often related to exertion, emotional stress, and exposure to intense cold. The pain may be relieved by rest and vasodilatation of the coronary arteries by medication, as with nitroglycerin.

angina sine dolore /sē'nə dolôr'ə, sī'nē/, a painless episode of coronary insufficiency.

angina trachealis. See **croup.**

angio-, angei-, angi-, a combining form meaning 'pertaining to a vessel, usually a blood vessel': *angioblastic, angiochondroma, angioglioma.*

angioblastic meningioma /an'jē·ōblas'tik/, a tumor of the blood vessels of the meninges covering the spinal cord or the brain.

angioblastoma /an'jē·ōblastō'mə/, *pl.* **angioblastomas, angioblastomata** [Gk, *aggeion*, vessel, *blastos*, germ, *oma*], a tumor of blood vessels in the brain. Kinds of angioblastomas are **angioblastic meningioma** and **cerebellar angioblastoma.**

angiocardiography /an'jē·ōkär'dē·ōgram'/ [Gk, *aggeion* + *kardia*, heart, *graphein* to record], the process of producing a radiograph of the heart and great vessels of the heart. A radiopaque contrast medium is injected directly into the heart by a catheter introduced through the antecubital veins. X-ray films are taken as the contrast medium passes through the heart and great vessels. See also **angiography.**

angiocardiopathy /-kär'dē·op'əthē/ [Gk, *aggeion*, vessel, *kardia*, heart, *pathos*, disease], a disease of the blood vessels of the heart.

angiocatheter /an'jē·ōkath'ətər/, a hollow, flexible tube inserted into a blood vessel to withdraw or instill fluids.

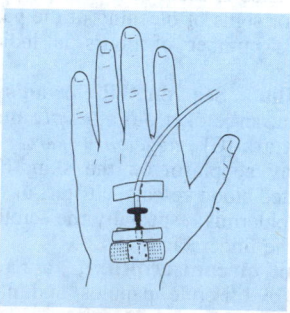

Angiocatheter securing method

angiochondroma /an′jē·ōkondrō′mə/, *pl.* **angiochondromas, angiochondromata** [Gk, *aggeion* + *chondros,* cartilage, *oma*], a cartilaginous tumor characterized by an excessive formation of blood vessels.

angioedema. See **angioneurotic edema.**

angioendothelioma. See **hemangioendothelioma.**

angiofibroma /an′jē·ōfibrō′mə/, *pl.* **angiofibromas, angiofibromata** [Gk, *aggeion* + L, *fibra,* fiber; Gk, *oma*], an angioma containing fibrous tissue. Also called **fibroangioma, telangiectatic fibroma.**

angiogenesis /an′jē·ōjen′əsis/ [Gk, *aggeion* + *genesis,* origin], the ability to evoke blood vessel formation, a common property of malignant tissue. The presence of angiogenesis in breast tissue is regarded as a precursor of histologic evidence of breast cancer.

angiogenin /an′jē·ōjen′in/, a protein that mediates the formation of blood vessels. A single-chain basic protein cloned from molecules of the tumor angiogenesis factor (TAF) in human colon cancer cells. Angiogenin does not bind to heparin and does not induce proliferation or migration of tissue-cultured endothelial cells. Angiogenin is used experimentally to stimulate the development of new blood vessels in wound healing, stroke, or coronary heart disease. See also **tumor angiogenesis factor.**

angioglioma /an′jē·ōglē·ō′mə/, *pl.* **angiogliomas, angiogliomata** [Gk, *aggeion* + *glia,* glue, *oma*], a highly vascular tumor composed of neuroglia.

angiogram /an′jē·əgram/ [Gk, *aggeion,* vessel, *gramma,* writing], a radiographic image of a blood vessel after the injection of a contrast medium. Also called **arteriogram.**

angiograph /an′jē·əgraf/ [Gk, *aggeion,* vessel, *graphein,* to record], a sphygmographic device that records the patterns of pulse waves.

angiography /an′jē·og′rəfē/ [Gk, *aggeion* + *graphein,* to record], the x-ray visualization of the internal anatomy of the heart and blood vessels after the intravascular introduction of radiopaque contrast medium. The procedure is used as a diagnostic aid in myocardial infarction, vascular occlusion, calcified atherosclerotic plaques, cerebrovascular accident, portal hypertension, renal neoplasms, renal artery stenosis as a causative factor in hypertension, pulmonary emboli, and congenital and acquired lesions of pulmonary vessels. The contrast medium may be injected into an artery or vein or introduced into a catheter inserted in a peripheral artery and threaded through the vessel to a visceral site. Because the iodine in the contrast medium may result in a marked allergic reaction in some patients, testing for hypersensitivity is indicated before the radiopaque substance is used. After the procedure the patient is monitored for signs of bleeding at the puncture site, and bed rest for a number of hours is indicated. **–angiographic,** *adj.*

angiohemophilia. See **von Willebrand's disease.**

angiokeratoma /an′jē·ōker′ətō′mə/, *pl.* **angiokeratomas, angiokeratomata** [Gk, *aggeion* + *keras,* horn, *oma*], a vascular, horny neoplasm on the skin, characterized by clumps of dilated blood vessels, clusters of warts, and thickening of the epidermis, especially the scrotum and the dorsal aspect of the fingers and toes.

angiokeratoma circumscriptum, a rare skin disorder characterized by discrete papules and nodules in small patches on the legs or on the trunk.

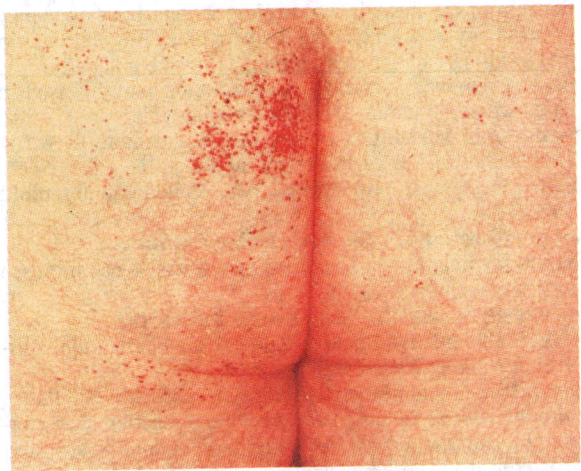

Angiokeratoma *(du Vivier, 1993)*

angiokeratoma corporis diffusum, an uncommon familial disease in which phospholipids are stored in many parts of the body, especially the blood vessels, causing vasomotor, urinary, and cutaneous disorders and, in some cases, muscular abnormalities. Characteristic signs of the disease are edema, hypertension, and cardiomegaly, especially enlargement of the left ventricle; diffuse nodularity of the skin; albumin, erythrocytes, leukocytes, and casts in the urine; and vacuoles in muscle bundles. Also called **Fabry's disease, Fabry's syndrome.**

Angiokeratoma corporis diffusum seen on the buttocks
(McKee, 1993)

angiokeratomata. See **angiokeratoma.**

angiolipoma /an′jē·ōlipō′mə/, *pl.* **angiolipomas, angiolipomata** [Gk, *aggeion* + *lipos,* fat, *oma*], a benign neoplasm containing blood vessels and tissue. Also called **lipoma cavernosum, telangiectatic lipoma.**

angioma /an′jē·ō′mə/, *pl.* **angiomas, angiomata** [Gk *aggeion* vessel, *oma* tumor], any benign tumor with blood vessels (hemangioma) or lymph vessels (lymphangioma). Most angiomas are congenital; some, like cavernous hemangiomas, may disappear spontaneously.

-angioma, a suffix meaning a 'tumor composed chiefly of blood and lymph vessels': *fibroangioma, glomangioma.*

angioma arteriale racemosum /ärtir′ē·ā′lē ras′əmō′səm/ [Gk *aggeion, oma* + L *arteria* airpipe, *racemus* grape], a vascular neoplasm characterized by the intertwining of many small, newly formed, dilated blood vessels. Normal blood vessels become affected.

angioma cavernosum. See **cavernous hemangioma.**

angioma cutis, a nevus composed of a network of dilated blood vessels.

angioma lymphaticum. See **lymphangioma.**

angioma serpiginosum /sərpij′inō′səm/ [Gk *aggeion, oma* + L *serpere* to creep], a cutaneous disease characterized by rings of tiny vascular points appearing as red dots. Also called **Hutchinson's disease.**

angiomatosis /an′jē·ōmətō′sis/, a condition characterized by the presence of numerous vascular tumors.

angiomyoma, *pl.* **angiomyomas, angiomyomata** [Gk *aggeion* + *mys* muscle, *oma*], a tumor composed of vascular and muscular tissue elements.

angiomyoneuroma. See **glomangioma.**

angiomyosarcoma /an′jē·ōmī′ōsärkō′mə/, *pl.* **angiomyosarcomas, angiomyosarcomata** [Gk *aggeion* + *mys* muscle, *sarx* flesh, *oma*], a tumor containing vascular, muscular, and connective tissue elements.

angioneuroma. See **glomangioma.**

angioneurotic anuria /-nŏorot′ik ənyŏor′ē·ə/ [Gk *aggeion* + *neuron* nerve; *a, ouron* not urine], an abnormal condition characterized by an almost complete absence of urination caused by destruction of tissue in the renal cortex.

angioneurotic edema [Gk *aggeion* + *neuron* nerve; *oidema* swelling], an acute, painless, dermal, subcutaneous or submucosal swelling of short duration involving the face, neck, lips, larynx, hands, feet, genitalia, or viscera. It may result from food or drug allergy, infection, or emotional stress, or it may be hereditary. Treatment depends on the cause. For severe forms, subcutaneous injections of epinephrine, intubation, or tracheotomy may be necessary to

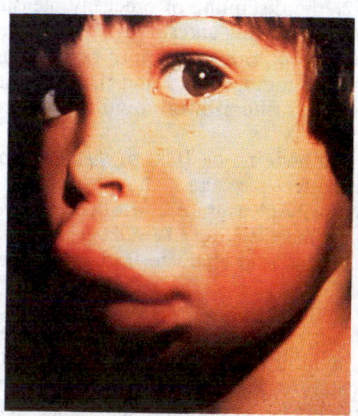

Angioneurotic edema (Zitelli, 1992)

prevent respiratory obstruction. Prevention depends on the identification and avoidance of causative factors. Also called **angioedema** /an′jē·ōdē′mə/. See also **anaphylaxis, serum sickness, urticaria.**

angioneurotic gangrene, [Gk, *aggeion, neuron,* nerve, *gaggraina*], the death and putrefaction of tissue due to an interruption of the blood supply resulting from thrombotic arteries or veins.

angiopathy /an′jē·op′əthē/ [Gk, *aggeion,* vessel, *pathos,* disease], a disease of the blood vessels.

angioplasty /an′jēōplas′tē/ [Gk, *aggeion,* vessel, *plassein,* to mold], the reconstruction of blood vessels damaged by disease or injury.

angiorraphy /an′jē·ôr′əfē/ [Gk, *aggeion,* vessel, *rhaphe,* suture], the repair by suture of any blood vessel.

angiosarcoma /an′jē·ōsärkō′mə/, a rare, malignant tumor consisting of endothelial and fibroblastic tissue that proliferates and eventually surrounds vascular channels. The condition usually occurs in older persons. Angiosarcoma has been associated with exposure to vinyl chloride and arsenic. Also called **hemangiosarcoma, malignant hemangioendothelioma.** Compare **angioma.**

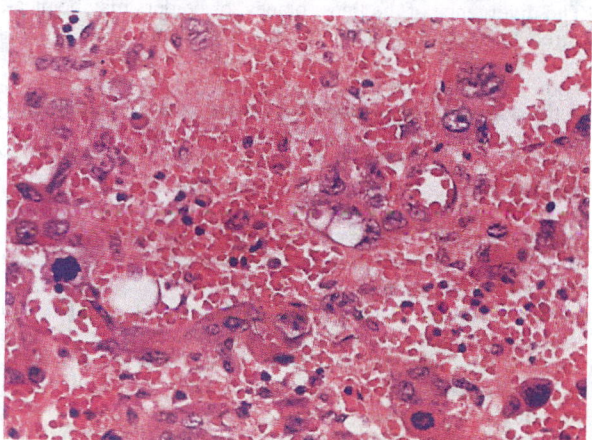

Angiosarcoma (Cawson, 1987)

angiosclerosis /-sklerō′sis/ [Gk, *aggeion,* vessel + *skleros,* hard; *osis,* condition], a thickening and hardening of the walls of the blood vessels. See also **atherosclerosis.**

angiospasm /an′jē·ōspaz′əm/, a sudden, transient constriction of a blood vessel. Also called **vasospasm.** See also **vasoconstriction.**

angiotensin /an′jē·ōten′sin/ [Gk, *aggeion* + L, *tendere,* to stretch], a polypeptide occurring in the blood causing vasoconstriction, increased blood pressure, and the release of aldosterone from the adrenal cortex. Angiotensin is formed by the action of renin on angiotensinogen, an alpha-2-globulin that is produced in the liver and constantly circulates in the blood. Renin, elaborated by juxtaglomerular cells in the kidney in response to decreased blood volume and serum sodium, acts as an enzyme in the conversion of angiotensinogen to angiotensin I, which is rapidly hydrolyzed to form the active compound angiotensin II. The vasoconstrictive action of angiotensin II decreases the glomerular filtration rate, and the concomitant action of aldosterone promotes sodium retention, with the result that blood volume and sodium reabsorption increase. Plasma angiotensin increases during the luteal phase of the menstrual cycle and is probably responsible for an elevated level of aldosterone during that period. Angiotensin is inactivated by peptidases, called angiotensinases, in plasma and tissues.

angiotensin-converting enzyme (ACE), a protein (dipeptidyl carboxypeptidase) that catalyzes the conversion of angiotensin I to angiotensin II by splitting two terminal amino acids. ACE-inhibiting agents are used in hypertension control.

angiotensinogen /-tensin'əjən/, a serum globulin produced in the liver that is the precursor of angiotensin.

angiotensin sensitivity test (AST), a test for sensitivity to angiotensin II by infusion of angiotensin-II-amide into the right cubital vein. Angiotensin is metered in doses that increase by 1 ng/kg/min at 5-minute intervals. A positive AST result is an effective pressor dose, or one that causes a 20 mm Hg rise in diastolic blood pressure at an infusion rate of less than 10 ng/kg/min.

angle /ang'gəl/ [L, *angulus*], **1.** the space or the shape formed at the intersection of two lines, planes, or borders. The divergence of the lines, planes, or borders may be measured in degrees of a circle. **2.** (in anatomy and physiology) the geometric relationships between the surfaces of body structures and the positions affected by movement.

angle board, (in dentistry) a device used for facilitating the establishment of reproducible angular relationships between a patient's head, the x-ray beam, and the x-ray film.

angle-closure glaucoma. See **glaucoma.**

angle former, (in dentistry) one of a series of paired cutting instruments having cutting edges at an angle other than a right angle in relation to the axis of the blade. Also called **bayonet angle former.**

angle of incidence, the angle at which an ultrasound beam hits the interface between two different types of tissues, such as the facing surfaces of bone and muscle. The angle is also affected by the difference in acoustic impedance of the different tissues.

angle of Louis, the sternal angle between the manubrium and the body of the sternum.

angle of mandible, the angular relationship between the body and the ramus of the mandible. Also called **gonial angle.**

angle of refraction [L, *angulus* + *refringere*, to break apart], the angle between a refracted ray and the normal to the surface of the refracting medium. Also called **refracting angle.**

angle of Treitz /trīts/, a sharp curve or flexure at the junction of the duodenum and jejunum.

Angle's Classification of Malocclusion, a classification of the various types of malocclusion, established by Edward Hartley Angle, American orthodontist (1855–1930). This system has since been modified and includes three main classes of occlusion, each class having several types or division. Classification is based on the relation of different teeth in the upper and lower jaws, such as the maxillary and the mandibular molars. See also **classification of malocclusion.**

angstrom (Å) /ang'strəm/ [Anders J. Angström, Swedish physicist, b. 1814], a unit of measure of length equal to 0.1 millimicron (1/10,000,000 meter), or 10^{-10} meter. Also called **angstrom unit, a.u.**

angstrom unit, see **angstrom (Å).**

angular gyrus /ang'gyələr/ [L, *angulus,* + Gk, *gyros*], a folded convolution in the inferior parietal lobe where it unites with the temporal lobe of the cerebral cortex.

angular movement [L, *angularis,* sharply bent], one of the four basic kinds of movement allowed by the various joints of the skeleton in which the angle between two adjoining bones is decreased, as in flexion, or increased, as in extension. Compare **circumduction, gliding, rotation.**

angular spinal curvature [L, *agulus* + *spina,* backbone + *curvatura,* bend], a sharp bending or sloping of the vertebral column.

angular stomatitis, inflammation at the corner of the mouth.

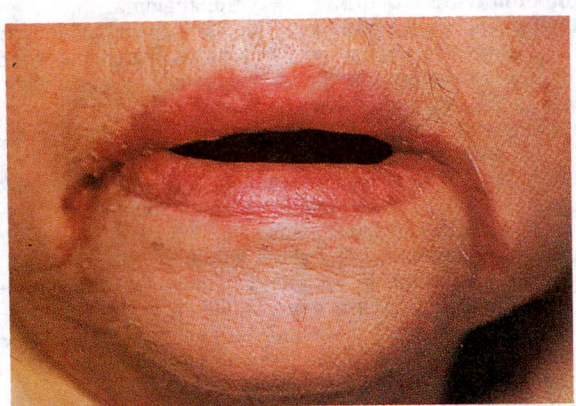

Angular stomatitis *(Kamal, 1992)*

angular vein, one of a pair of veins of the face, formed by the junction of the frontal and the supraorbital veins. At the root of the nose each angular vein receives the flow of venous blood from the infraorbital, the superior palpebral, the inferior palpebral, and the external nasal veins, becoming the first part of one of the two facial veins.

angulated fracture /ang'gyələ'tid/, a fracture in which the fragments of bone are at angles.

angulation [L, *angulatus,* bent], **1.** an angular shape or formation. **2.** the discipline of precisely measuring angles, as in mechanical drafting and surveying. **3.** (in radiography) the direction of the primary beam of radiation in relation to the object being radiographed and the film used to record its image. See also **horizontal angulation, vertical angulation.**

anhedonia /an'hēdō'nē·ə/ [Gk *a, hedone* not pleasure], the inability to feel pleasure or happiness from experiences that are ordinarily pleasurable. **–anhedonic,** *adj.*

anhidrosis /an'hidrō'sis, an'hī-/ [Gk, *a, hidros,* not sweat], an abnormal condition characterized by inadequate perspiration.

anhidrotic /an'hidrot'ik, an'hī-/, **1.** of or pertaining to anhidrosis. **2.** an agent that reduces or suppresses sweating.

anhydrase /anhī'drās/ [Gk, *a,* not, *hydor,* water], an enzyme that catalyzes the elimination of water molecules from certain compounds, as carbonic anhydrase dehydrates carbonic acid, thereby controlling the amount of carbon dioxide in the blood and lungs.

anhydride /anhī'drīd/ [Gk, *a, hydor,* not water], a chemical compound, especially an acid, derived by the removal of water from a substance.

anhydrous /anhī′drəs/ [Gk, *a*, without, *hydor*, water], an absence of water.

anicteric /an′ikter′ik/ [Gk, *a*, *icterus*, not jaundice], pertaining to the absence of jaundice.

anicteric hepatitis, a mild form of hepatitis in which there is no jaundice (icterus). Symptoms include anorexia, GI disturbances, and slight fever. AST and ALT are elevated. The infection may be mistaken for flu or go unnoticed. Compare **hepatitis.** See also **jaundice.**

anidean /anid′ē·ən/ [Gk, *a*, *eidos*, not form], formless; shapeless; denoting an undifferentiated mass, such as an anideus. Also **anidian, anidous** /an′idəs/.

anideus /anid′ē·əs/, an anomalous, rudimentary embryo consisting of a simple rounded mass with little indication of the body parts. A kind of anideus is **embryonic anideus.** Also called **fetus anideus.**

anidian. See **anidean.**

anidous. See **anidean.**

aniline /an′ilēn/ [Ar, *alnil*, indigo], an oily, colorless poisonous liquid with a strong odor and burning taste, formerly extracted from the indigo plant and now made synthetically using nitrobenzene in the manufacture of aniline dyes. Industrial workers exposed to aniline are at risk of developing methemoglobinemia and bone marrow depression. Also called **amidobenzene, aminobenzene.**

anilism [Ar, *alnil*, indigo, + Gk, *ismos*, state], a condition of poisoning from exposure to aniline compounds. Symptoms generally include cyanosis, weakness, cold sweats, irregular pulse, breathing difficulty, coma, convulsions, and possible sudden heart failure. Treatment includes gastric lavage and induction of emesis. Also called **anilinism.** See also **aniline.**

anilinparasulfonic acid. See **sulfanilic acid.**

anima /an′imə/ [L, soul], **1.** the soul or life. **2.** the active ingredient in a drug. **3.** (in Jungian psychology) a person's true, inner, unconscious being or personality, as distinguished from overt personality, or persona. **4.** (in analytic psychology) the female component of the male personality. Compare **animus.**

animal pole [L, *anima*], the active, formative part of the ovum protoplasm that contains the nucleus and bulk of the cytoplasm and where the polar bodies form. In mammals it is also the site where the inner cell mass gives rise to the ectoderm. Also called **germinal pole.** Compare **vegetal pole.**

animal starch. See **glycogen.**

animus /an′iməs/ [L, spirit], **1.** the active or rational soul; the animating principle of life. **2.** the male component of the female personality. **3.** (in psychiatry) a deep-seated antagonism that is usually controlled but may erupt with virulence under stress. Compare **anima.**

anion /an′ī·ən/ [Gk, *ana*, *ion*, backward going], **1.** a negatively charged ion that is attracted to the positive electrode (anode) in electrolysis. **2.** a negatively charged atom, molecule, or radical. Compare **cation.**

anion exchange resin, any one of the simple organic polymers with high molecular weights that exchange anions with other ions in solution. Anion exchange resins are used as antacids in treating ulcers. Compare **cation exchange resin.**

anion gap, the difference between the concentrations of serum cations and anions, determined by measuring the concentrations of sodium cations and chloride and bicarbonate anions. It is helpful in the diagnosis and treatment of acidosis, and it is estimated by subtracting the sum of sodium and bicarbonate concentrations in the plasma from that of sodium. It is normally about 8 to 14 mEq/L and represents the negative charges contributed to plasma by unmeasured ions or ions other than those of chloride and bicarbonate, mainly phosphate, sulfate, organic acids, and plasma proteins. Anions other than chloride and bicarbonate normally constitute about 12 mEq/L of the total anion concentration in plasma. Acidosis can develop with or without an associated anion increase. An increase in the anion gap often suggests diabetic ketoacidosis, drug poisoning, renal failure, or lactic acidosis and usually warrants further laboratory tests.

anionic /an′ī·on′ik/ [Gk, *ana*, not, *ion*, going], pertaining to an anion.

anise /an′is/, the fruit of the *Pimpinella anisum* plant. Extract of anise is used in the preparation of carminatives and expectorants.

aniseikonia /an′īsīkō′nē·ə/ [Gk, *anisos*, unequal, *eikon*, image], an abnormal ocular condition in which each eye perceives the same image as being of a different form and size.

aniso- /anī′sō-/, a prefix meaning 'unequal, asymmetric, or dissimilar': *anisochromia, anisognathous.*

anisocytosis /anī′sōsītō′sis/ [Gk, *anisos* + *kytos*, cell], an abnormal condition of the blood characterized by red blood cells of variable and abnormal size. Compare **poikilocytosis.** See also **macrocytosis, microcytosis.**

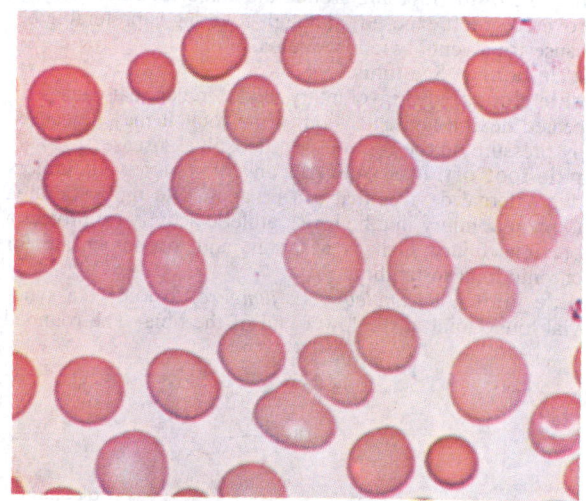

Anisocytosis *(Hayhoe, 1992)*

anisogamete /-gam′ēt/ [Gk, *anisos* + *gamos*, marriage], a gamete that differs considerably in size and structure from the one with which it unites, as the macrogamete and microgamete of certain sporozoa. Compare **heterogamete, isogamete.** –**anisogametic,** *adj.*

anisogamy /an′īsog′əmē/, sexual conjugation of gametes that are of unequal size and structure, as in certain thallophytes and sporozoa. Compare **heterogamy, isogamy.** –**anisogamous,** *adj.*

anisognathic, /an′īsōnath′ik/ [Gk, *anisos* + *gnathos*, jaw], of or pertaining to an abnormal condition in which the maxillary and the mandibular arches or jaws are of significantly different sizes in the same individual.

anisokaryosis /anī′sōker′ē·ō′sis/, significant variation in the size of the nucleus of cells of the same general type. **-anisokaryotic,** *adj.*

anisomastia /anī′sōmas′tē·ə/, a condition in which one female breast is much larger than the other.

anisometropia /anī′sōmetrō′pē·ə/ [Gk, *anisos* + *metron* measure, *ops*, eye], an abnormal ocular condition characterized by a difference in the refractive powers of the eyes.

anisopia /an′īsō′pē·ə/, a condition in which the visual power of one eye is greater than that of the other.

anisotropine methylbromide, an anticholinergic drug.

■ INDICATION: It is prescribed as adjunctive therapy in the treatment of peptic ulcer.

■ CONTRAINDICATIONS: Glaucoma, obstructive uropathy, obstructive conditions of the GI tract, paralytic ileus, intestinal atony, unstable cardiovascular status in acute hemorrhage, severe ulcerative colitis or toxic megacolon complicating ulcerative colitis, or myasthenia gravis prohibits its use.

■ ADVERSE EFFECTS: Among the most serious adverse reactions are blurred vision, tachycardia, mydriasis, cycloplegia, impotence, mental confusion, urinary retention, constipation, allergic reactions, and urticaria.

ankle [AS, *ancleow*], **1.** the joint of the tibia, the talus, and the fibula. **2.** the part of the leg where this joint is located.

ankle bandage, a figure-of-eight bandage looped under the sole of the foot and around the ankle. The heel may be covered or left exposed, although covering is preferable because it prevents 'window edema.'

ankle bone. See **talus.**

ankle clonus, an involuntary tendon reflex that causes repeated flexion and extension of the foot. It may be caused by pressure on the foot or a corticospinal disease.

ankle-foot orthosis (AFO), any of a variety of protective external devices that can be applied to the ankle area to prevent injury in a high-risk athletic activity, to protect a previous injury such as a sprain, and to compensate for chronic joint instability.

ankle joint [AS, *ancleow*, L, *jumgere*, to join], a synovial hinge joint at the lower end of the tibia. The rounded

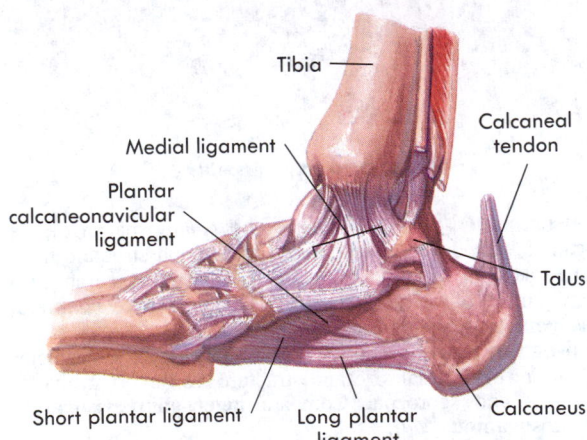

Ankle joint of the right foot—medial view
(Seeley, 1992/David J Mascaro & Associates)

malleous prominences on either side of the joint form a mortise for the upper surface of the talus.

ankle reflex. See **Achilles tendon reflex.**

ankylo-. a prefix meaning 'fusion, stiffness, crooked, bent': *ankylosis.*

ankyloglossia /ang′kilōglos′ē·ə/ [Gk, *agkylos*, crooked, *glossa* tongue], an oral defect, characterized by an abnormally short lingual frenum that limits tongue movement and impairs the speech. It may be surgically corrected by a frenotomy. Also called **tongue-tie.**

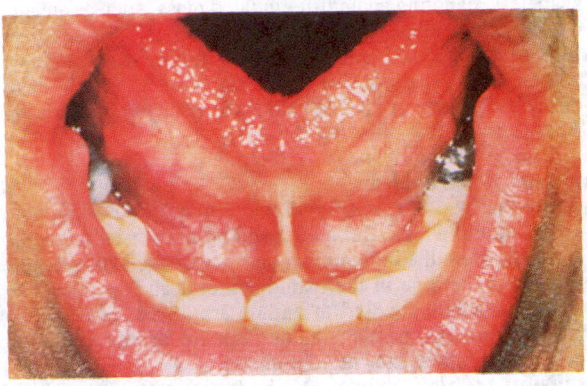

Ankyloglossia (Lamey, 1988)

ankylosed /ang′kilōst/, pertaining to the immobility of a joint resulting from pathologic changes in the joint or in adjacent tissues.

ankylosing spondylitis /ang′kilō′sing/, a chronic inflammatory disease of unknown origin, first affecting the spine and adjacent structures and commonly progressing to eventual fusion (ankylosis) of the involved joints. In extreme cases the patient develops a forward flexion of the spine, called a "poker spine" or "bamboo spine." The disease affects primarily males under 30 years of age, and generally burns itself out after a course of 20 years. There is a strong hereditary tendency. In addition to the spine, the joints of the hip, shoulder, neck, ribs, and jaw are often involved. When the costovertebral joints are involved, the patient may have difficulty in expanding the rib cage while breathing. Ankylosing spondylitis is a systemic disease, often affecting the eyes and the heart. Many patients with the disease also have inflammatory bowel disease. The aim of treatment is to reduce pain and inflammation in the involved joints, usually with nonsteroidal antiinflammatory drugs. Physical therapy aids in keeping the spine as erect as possible to prevent flexion contractures. In advanced cases surgery may be performed to straighten a badly deformed spine. Compare **rheumatoid arthritis.** See also **ankylosis.** Also called **Marie-Strümpell disease.**

ankylosis /ang′kilō′sis/ [Gk, *agkylosis*, bent condition], **1.** fixation of a joint, often in an abnormal position, usually resulting from destruction of articular cartilage and subchondral bone, as occurs in rheumatoid arthritis. **2.** also called arthrodesis, **fusion.** Surgically induced fixation of a joint to relieve pain or provide support.

anlage /on′lägə/ [Ger, *Anlage,* disposition, aptitude], (in embryology) the undifferentiated layer of cells from which

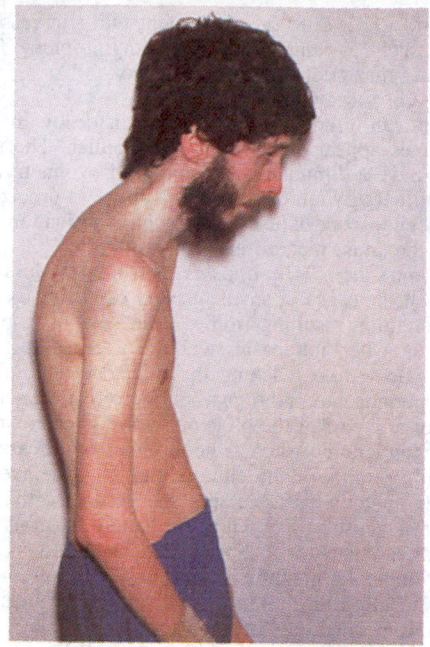

Posture typical of ankylosing spondylitis
(Shipley, 1993)

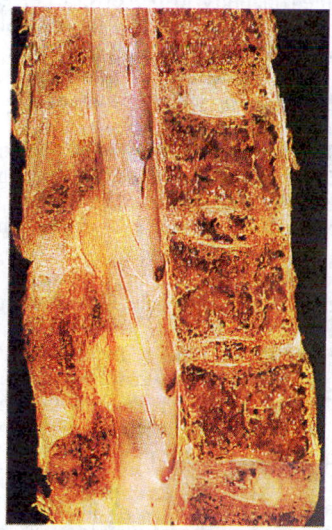

Ankylosing spondylitis, seen in lumbar vertebrae
(Fletcher, 1987/Courtesy Prof. PG Bullough, Cornell University Medical College, New York)

a particular organ, tissue, or structure develops; primordium rudiment. See also **blastema**.

ANLL, abbreviation for **acute nonlymphocytic leukemia**. See **acute myelocytic leukemia**.

annihilation /ənī′ələ′shən/, the total transformation of matter into energy, as when an antimatter positron collides with an electron. Two photons are created, each equaling the rest mass of the individual particles.

annular. See **anular**.

annular ligament. See **anular ligament**.

annulus /an′yələs/ [L, a ring], any ring-shaped structure, such as the outer edge of an intervertebral disc.

anodic stripping voltammetry /ənō′dik/, /anod′ik/, a process of electroanalytic chemistry used to detect trace metals. It involves the use of a metal-exchange reagent that releases lead or other metals from macromolecular binding sites.

anodmia. See **anosmia**.

anodontia /an′ōdon′tē·ə/ [Gk, *a*, not, *odous*, tooth], a congenital defect in which some or all of the teeth are missing. The term is generally applied to cases in which most teeth are missing and there are no tooth follicles present.

anodyne /an′ədīn/ [Gk *a, odyne* not pain], a drug that relieves or lessens pain. Compare **analgesic**.

anomalo-, a combining form meaning 'uneven, deviation from normal, or irregular': *anomalopia, anomaloscope*.

anomaly /ənom′əlē/ [Gk, *anomalos*, irregular], **1.** deviation from what is regarded as normal. **2.** congenital malformation, such as the absence of a limb or the presence of an extra finger. **–anomalous,** *adj*.

anomia /ənō′mē·ə/ [Gk, *a, onoma*, not name], a form of aphasia characterized by the inability to name objects, caused by a lesion in the temporal lobe of the brain.

anomie /an′əmē/, a state of apathy, alienation, anxiety, personal disorientation, and distress, resulting from the loss of social norms and goals previously valued. Also spelled **anomy**.

anoopsia /an′ō·op′sē·ə/ [Gk, *ana*, up, *ops*, eye], a strabismus in which one or both eyes are deviated upward. Also called **hypertropia**.

Anopheles /ənof′əlēz/ [Gk, *anopheles*, harmful], a genus of mosquito, many species of which transmit malaria-causing parasites to humans. See also **malaria**, *Plasmodium*.

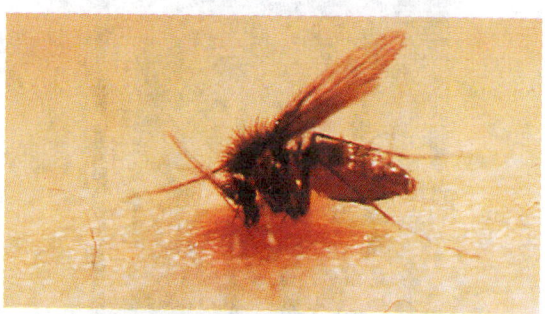

Female *Anopheles* mosquito *(Muller, 1990)*

anopia /anō′pē·ə/ [Gk, *a, ops*, not eye], blindness resulting from a defect in or the absence of one or both eyes.

-anopia, -anopsia, 1. a suffix meaning '(condition involving) nonuse or arrested development of the eye': *hemianopia, quadrantanopsia*. **2.** a suffix meaning '(condition of) defective color vision': *cyanopia, deuteranopia, tritanopia*.

anoplasty /an′ōplas′tē/ [L, *anus;* Gk, *plassein,* to shape], a restorative operation on the anus.

-anopsia. See **-anopia.**

anorchia /anôr′kē·ə/ [Gk, *a, orchis,* not testis], congenital absence of one or both testes. Also called **anorchism.**

anorectal /an′ōrek′təl/, ā′nō- [L, *anus* + *rectus,* straight], of or pertaining to the anal and rectal portions of the large intestine.

anorectal abscess [L, *anus* + *rectus,* straight, *abscedere,* to go away], an abscess in the area of the anus and rectum. See also **abscess.**

anorectal stricture [L, *anus* + *rectus,* straight + *strictura,* compression], a narrowing of the anorectal canal, sometimes congenital but also the result of surgery to correct a fissure or to remove hemorrhoids.

anorectic /an′ōrek′tik/, **1.** of or pertaining to anorexia. **2.** lacking appetite. **3.** causing a loss of appetite, as an anorexiant drug. Also **anorectous, anorexiant, anorexic.**

anorexia /an′ōrek′sē·ə/ [Gk, *a, orexis,* not appetite], lack or loss of appetite, resulting in the inability to eat. The condition may result from poorly prepared or unattractive food or surroundings, unfavorable company, or various physical and psychologic causes. Compare **pseudoanorexia.** See also **anorexia nervosa.**

anorexia nervosa, a disorder characterized by a prolonged refusal to eat, resulting in emaciation, amenorrhea, emotional disturbance concerning body image, and an abnormal fear of becoming obese. The condition is seen primarily in adolescents, predominantly in girls, and is usually associated with emotional stress or conflict, such as anxiety, irritation, anger, and fear, which may accompany a major change in the person's life. Treatment consists of measures to improve nourishment, followed by therapy to overcome the underlying emotional conflicts.

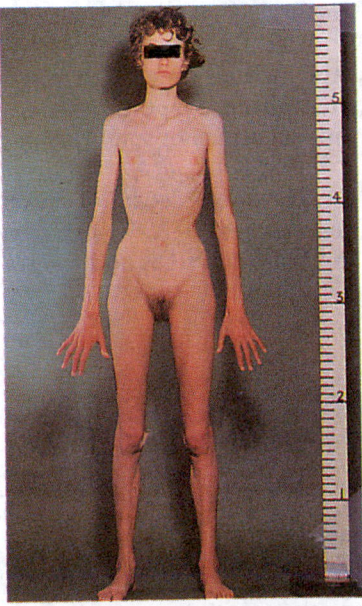

Anorexia nervosa in 20-year-old woman
(Forbes, 1993)

anorexiant, 1. a drug or other agent that suppresses the appetite, such as amphetamine, diethylpropion, fenfluramine, and mazindol. **2.** See **anorectic.**

anorexic. See **anorectic.**

anorthopia /an′ôrthō′pē·ə/, a visual distortion in which straight lines appear to be curved or angular. The person also may have a diminished perception of symmetry.

anosigmoidoscopy /an′ōsig′moidos′kəpē/, a procedure in which an endoscope is used for direct examination of the lining of the anus, rectum, and colon.

anosmia /anoz′mē·ə/ [Gk, *a, osme,* not smell], loss or impairment of the sense of smell, usually occurring as a temporary condition resulting from a head cold or respiratory infection or when intranasal swelling or other obstruction prevents odors from reaching the olfactory region. It becomes a permanent condition when the olfactory neuroepithelium or any part of the olfactory nerve is destroyed as a result of intracranial trauma, neoplasms, or disease, such as atrophic rhinitis or the chronic rhinitis associated with the granulomatous diseases. In some instances, the condition may be caused by psychologic factors, such as a phobia or fear associated with a particular smell. Kinds of anosmia are **anosmia gustatoria** and **preferential anosmia.** Also called **anodmia, anosphrasia, olfactory anesthesia.** Compare **hyperosmia.** –**anosmatic, anosmic,** *adj.*

anosmia gustatoria, the inability to smell foods.

anosmic [Gk, *a,* without, *osme,* smell], pertaining to a loss of the sense of smell.

anosognosia /an′əsog·nō′zhə/ [Gk, *a, nosos,* not disease, *gnosis* knowing], an abnormal condition characterized by a real or feigned inability to perceive a defect, especially paralysis, on one side of the body, possibly attributable to a lesion in the right parietal lobe of the brain.

anosphrasia, anosphresia. See **anosmia.**

anotia /anō′tē·ə/ [Gk, *a,* without, *ous,* ear], a congenital absence of one or both ears.

ANOVA, abbreviation for **analysis of variance.**

anovaginal /ā′nōvaj′inəl/ [L, *anus, vagina,* sheath], pertaining to the perineal region of the anus and vagina.

anovesical /-ves′ikəl/ [L, *anus* + *vesicula,* small bladder], pertaining to the anus and bladder.

anovular /anov′yələr/ [Gk, *a,* not, *ovulum*], pertaining to a menstrual discharge not associated with the production or release of an ovum.

anovular menstruation [Gk, *a, ovulum,* not egg], menstrual bleeding that occurs even though ovulation has not taken place. The ovum either remains within the follicle and undergoes degeneration or in rare cases becomes impregnated, resulting in an ovarian pregnancy.

anovulation /an′ovyələ̄′shən/, failure of the ovaries to produce, mature, or release eggs as a result of ovarian immaturity or postmaturity; of altered ovarian function, as in pregnancy and lactation; of primary ovarian dysfunction, as in ovarian dysgenesis; or of disturbance of the interaction of the hypothalamus, pituitary gland, and ovary, caused by stress or disease. Hormonal contraceptives prevent conception by suppressing ovulation. Anovulation may be an adverse side effect of medications prescribed in the treatment of other disorders. –**anovulatory** /anov′yələtôr′ē/, *adj.*

anoxemia /an′oksē′mē·ə/, a deficiency of oxygen in the blood.

anoxia /anok′sē·ə/ [Gk, *a, oxys,* not sharp], an abnormal condition characterized by a lack of oxygen. Anoxia may be local or systemic and may be the result of an inadequate supply of oxygen to the respiratorysystem or of an inability of the blood to carry oxygen to the tissues, as in anemic anoxia, or of the tissues to absorb the oxygen from the circulation, as in histotoxic anoxia. Kinds of anoxia include **cerebral anoxia** and **stagnant anoxia.** See also **hypoxemia, hypoxia. −anoxic,** *adj.*

-ans, a suffix meaning '-ing': *aberrans, penetrans, proliferans*.

ansa /an′sə/, *pl.* **ansae** [L, handle], (in anatomy) a looplike structure resembling a curved handle of a vase.

ansa cervicalis, one of three loops of nerves in the cervical plexus, branches of which innervate the infrahyoid muscles. It has a superior root, which connects with the hypoglossal nerve and contains fibers of the first and the second cervical nerves, and an inferior root, which connects with the second and the third cervical nerves. Also called **ansa hypoglossi.**

-anserin, a suffix designating a serotonin antagonist.

ANSI, abbreviation for **American National Standards Institute.**

ant-. See **anti-.**

Antabuse, a trademark for an alcohol abuse deterrent (disulfiram).

antacid /antas′id/ [Gk, *anti*, against, *acidus*, sour], **1.** opposing acidity. **2.** a drug or dietary substance that buffers, neutralizes, or absorbs hydrochloric acid in the stomach. Most antacids are not absorbed systemically. Antacids containing aluminum and calcium are constipating; those containing magnesium have a laxative effect.

antagonism /antag′əniz′əm/ [Gk, *antagonisma*, struggle], an inhibiting action between physiologic processes, such as muscle actions. Also, opposing actions of drugs.

antagonist /antaga′nist/, [Gk, *antagonisma*, struggle], **1.** one who contends with or is opposed to another. **2.** (in physiology) any agent, such as a drug or muscle, that exerts an opposite action to that of another or competes for the same receptor sites. Kinds of antagonists include **antimetabolite, associated antagonist, direct antagonist,** and **narcotic antagonist.** Compare **agonist. 3.** (in dentistry) a tooth in the upper jaw that articulates during mastication or occlusion with a tooth in the lower jaw. **−antagonistic,** *adj.,* **antagonize,** *v.*

antagonistic reflexes [Gk, *antagonisma;* L, *reflectere,* to bend back], two or more reflexes initiated at the same time that produce opposite effects. The most adaptive or persistent response occurs.

antagonize. See **antagonist.**

ante-, a prefix meaning 'before in time or in place': *anteflexion, antenatal, antepartal.*

antecardium. See **epigastric region.**

antecubital /-kyoo′bitəl/ [L, *ante*, before, *cubitum*, elbow], in front of the elbow; at the bend of the elbow.

antecubital fossa [L, *ante*, before, *cubitum*, elbow, *fossa*, ditch], a depression at the bend of the elbow.

Acid-neutralizing capacity of antacids

Antacids	Ingredients	Acid-neutralizing capacity	Dose to neutralize 80 mEq HCl
Liquid preparations		*mEq/ml*	*ml needed*
Aludrox	AlOH, MgOH	2.8	28
Amphojel	AlOH	2	40
Gelusil		2.4	33
Gelusil-II	AlOH, MgOH, simethicone	4.8	16.6
Gelusil-M		3	26.6
Maalox		2.7	29.6
Maalox Plus	AlOH, MgOH (plus:	2.7	29.6
Maalox TC	simethicone)	5.7	14
Mylanta	AlOH, MgOH, simethicone	2.5	32
Mylanta-II		5.1	15.6
Phosphalgel	AlPO$_4$	0.4	200
Tablet preparations		*mEq per tablet*	*Tablets needed*
Gelusil Chewable		11	7.3
Gelusil-II Chewable	AlOH, MgOH, simethicone	21	3.8
Maalox No. 1 Chewable		8.5	9.4
Maalox No. 2 Chewable	AlOH, MgOH	18	4.4
Maalox Plus Chewable		11.4	7
Mylanta Chewable		11.5	7
Mylanta II Chewable	AlOh, MgOH, simethicone	23	3.5
Riopan Tablet		13.5	5.9
Riopan Chewable Tablet	magaldrate (plus:	13.5	5.9
Riopan Plus Chewable Tablet	simethicone)	13.5	5.9
Rolaids	Dihydroxyaluminum sodium carbonate	8	10
Titralac Tablet	Calcium carbonate, glycine	7.5	10.7

Adapted from Zaenger P. *Fa J Hosp Pharm* 1(1):1, 1981; and Kutsop JJ: *Am Pharmacy* N524(12):778, 1984; USP-DI, 1990.
From McKenry L, Salerno E: *Mosby's pharmacology in nursing,* ed. 18, St Louis, 1992, Mosby.

antefebrile.   See **antipyretic.**

anteflexion /-flek′shən/ [L, *ante* + *flectare*, bend],   an abnormal position of an organ in which the organ is tilted acutely forward, folded over on itself.

antegonial notch /-gō′nē·əl/ [L, *ante* + *gonia*, angle],   a depression or concavity commonly present at the junction of the ramus and the mandible, near the attachment of the anterior margin of the masseter.

antegrade /an′təgrād/ [L, *ante*, before, *gredi*, to go],   moving forward, or proceeding toward the front. Also called **anterograde.**

-antel,   a combining form designating an anthelmintic.

ante mortem [L, *ante*, before, *mors*, death],   before death.

antenatal.   See **prenatal.**

antenatal diagnosis.   See **prenatal diagnosis.**

antepartal /an′təpär′təl/ [L, *ante* + *parturire*, to have labor pains],   pertaining to the period spanning conception and labor.

antepartal care,   care of a pregnant woman during the time in the maternity cycle that begins with conception and ends with the onset of labor. See also **intrapartal care, postpartal care.**

■ METHOD: A medical, surgical, gynecologic, obstetric, social, and family history is taken with particular emphasis on the discovery of familial or transmissable diseases. A physical examination is performed, including observation and evaluation of the skin, thyroid gland, heart, breasts, abdomen, lungs, and pelvic organs. The vaginal part of the pelvic examination may include estimation of the size of the pelvis, a Pap smear and tests for *Neisseria gonorrhoeae, Candida albicans, Chlamydia,* and *Trichomonas vaginalis.* Blood pressure, weight, urinalysis for glucose and protein, measurement of the height of the fundus and auscultation of the fetal heart are routinely performed at monthly intervals or even more frequently. Laboratory tests are performed to determine blood type and Rh factor, rubella antibody titers, hematocrit, and hemoglobin. A serologic test for syphilis is performed, and various diagnostic studies may be done to discover *Chlamydia,* genital herpes, or other viral infections. Amniocentesis may be performed if certain fetal abnormalities are suspected.

antepartum hemorrhage [Gk, *ante,* before; L, *parturire,* to have labor pains; Gk, *haima,* blood, *rhegnynei,* to gush],   bleeding from the uterus during a pregancy in which the placenta appears to be normally situated, particularly after the 28th week.

antepyretic /-pīret′ik/ [L, *ante,* before + Gk, *pyretos,* fever],   before the onset of fever. Also called **antefebrile.**

anterior (A) /antir′ē·ər/ [L, *ante, prior,* foremost],   **1.** the front of a structure. **2.** of or pertaining to a surface or part situated toward the front or facing forward. Compare **posterior.** See also **ventral.**

anterior Achilles bursitis.   See **Albert's disease.**

anterior asynclitism.   See **asynclitism.**

anterior atlantoaxial ligament /atlan′tō·ak′sē·əl/,   one of five ligaments connecting the atlas to the axis. It is fixed to the inferior border of the anterior arch of the atlas and to the ventral surface of the body of the axis. Compare **posterior atlantoaxial ligament.**

anterior atlantooccipital membrane,   one of two broad, densely woven fibrous sheets that form part of the atlantooccipital joint between the atlas and the occipital bone. It is continuous with two articular capsules and strengthened ventrally by a strong, rounded cord connecting the base of the occipital bone to the anterior arch of the atlas. Also called **anterior atlantooccipital ligament.** Compare **posterior atlantooccipital membrane.**

anterior cardiac vein,   one of several small vessels that return deoxygenated blood from the ventral portion of the myocardium of the right ventricle to the right atrium. In some individuals, the right marginal vein opens into the right atrium and in those instances is regarded as one of the anterior cardiac veins. See also **coronary sinus.**

anterior cerebral commissure [L, *anterior,* foremost, *cerebrum,* brain, *commissura,* ajoining],   a bundle of fibers in the anterior wall of the forebrain connecting the olfactory bulb and cortex on one side with the similar structures on the other side.

anterior chamber [L, *anterior,* foremost + Gk, *kamara,* an arched cover],   the part of the anterior cavity of the eye in front of the iris. It contains the aqueous humor.

anterior common ligament.   See **anterior longitudinal ligament.**

anterior crural nerve.   See **femoral nerve.**

anterior cutaneous nerve,   one of a pair of cutaneous branches of the cervical plexus. It arises from the second and the third cervical nerves, bends around the middle of the sternocleidomastoideus, crosses the muscle obliquely, passes beneath the platysma, and divides into the ascending and the descending branches. The ascending branches pass upward, pierce the platysma, and are distributed to the cranial, the ventral, and the lateral parts of the neck. The descending branches are distributed to the skin of the ventral and the lateral parts of the neck as far down as the sternum.

anterior determinants of cusp,   (in dentistry) the characteristics of the anterior teeth that determine the cusp elevations and the fossa depressions in restoration of the postcanine teeth. Some such determinants are occlusion, alignment overlaps, and the capacity to disocclude conjointly with condylar trajectories.

anterior elastic lamina.   See **Bowman's lamina.**

anterior fontanel,   a diamond-shaped area between the frontal and two parietal bones just above the baby's forehead at the junction of the coronal and sagittal sutures. See also **fontanel.**

anterior guide,   (in dentistry) the portion of an articulator that is contacted by the incisal guide pin to maintain the selected separation of the upper and lower members of the articulator. The guide influences the changing relationships of mounted casts in eccentric movements. Compare **condylar guide, incisal guide.**

anterior horn cell,   a large nerve cell, as seen in cross-section, of the anterior column of the spinal cord. It is the axon of a somatic efferent nerve.

anterior horn of the spinal cord [L, *anterius,* foremost, *cornu,* horn, *spina,* spine; Gk, *chorde,* string],   one of the hornlike projections of gray matter into the white matter of the spinal cord. The anterior, or ventral horn, contains efferent fibers innervating muscle tissue.

anterior longitudinal ligament,   the broad, strong ligament attached to the ventral surfaces of the vertebral bodies. It extends from the occipital bone and the anterior tubercle of the atlas to the sacrum. Also called **anterior common ligament.** Compare **posterior longitudinal ligament.**

anterior mediastinal node,   a node in one of the three groups of thoracic visceral nodes of the lymphatic system that drains lymph from the nodes of the thymus, the pericardium, and the sternum. They are located ventral to the brachiocephalic veins and to the arterial trunks from the aortic arch. The efferents of the nodes form the right and the left bronchomediastinal trunks. Compare **posterior mediastinal node.** See also **lymph, lymphatic system, lymph node.**

anterior mediastinum, a caudal portion of the mediastinum in the middle of the thorax, bounded ventrally by the body of the sternum and parts of the fourth through the seventh ribs and dorsally by the parietal pericardium, extending downward as far as the diaphragm. It contains a few lymph nodes and a few vessels and a thin layer of subserous fascia, which is separated from the endothoracic fascia by a fascial cleft. Compare **middle mediastinum, posterior mediastinum, superior mediastinum.**

anterior nares, the ends of the nostrils that open anteriorly into the nasal cavity and allow the inhalation and the exhalation of air. Each is an oval opening that measures about 1.5 cm anteroposteriorly and about 1 cm in diameter. The anterior nares connect with the nasal fossae. Also called **nostrils.** Compare **posterior nares.**

anterior neuropore, the opening of the embryonic neural tube in the anterior portion of the forebrain. It closes at the 20 somite stage, which indicates the end of horizon XI in the numerical anatomic charting of human embryonic development. Compare **posterior neuropore.** See also **horizon.**

anterior pituitary. See **adenohypophysis.**

anterior rhizotomy [L, *anterior,* foremost; Gk, *rhiza,* root + *temnein,* to cut], the surgical cutting of the ventral root of a spinal nerve, usually to relieve peristent spasm or involuntary movement.

anterior tibial artery, one of the two divisions of the popliteal artery, arising in back of the knee, dividing into six branches, and supplying various muscles of the leg and foot. Its six branches are the posterior tibial recurrent, fibular, anterior tibial recurrent, muscular, anterior medial malleolar, and anterior lateral malleolar. Compare **posterior tibial artery.**

anterior tibial node, one of the small lymph glands of the lower limb, lying on the interosseous membrane near the proximal portion of the anterior tibial vessels. Compare **inguinal node, popliteal node.**

anterior tooth, any of the incisors or canine cuspid teeth. Compare **posterior tooth.**

antero- /an′tərō-/, a prefix denoting front.

anterocclusion /an′tərōkloō′shən/ [L, *ante* + *occludere,* to shut], (in dentistry) a malocclusion in which the mandibular teeth are anterior to their normal position relative to the teeth in the maxillary arch. Compare **anteversion.**

anterograde. See **antegrade.**

anterograde amnesia [L, *ante, prior,* foremost, *gredi,* to go], the inability to recall events of long ago with normal recall of recent events. Compare **anterograde memory, retrograde amnesia.**

anterograde memory, the ability to recall events of long ago but not those of recent occurrence. Compare **anterograde amnesia.** Also called **senile memory.**

anterolateral /-lat′ərəl/, in front and on either side of another structure or object.

anterolateral thoracotomy a chest surgery technique in which entry to the chest is made with an incision below the breast but above the costal margins. The incision involves the pectoralis, serratus anterior, and intercostal muscles.

Compare **median sternotomy, posterolateral thoracotomy.** See also **thoracotomy.**

anteroposterior (A.P.) /an′tərōpostir′ē·ər/ [L, *ante, prior,* foremost, *posterus,* coming after], from the front to the back of the body, commonly associated with the direction of the x-ray beam.

anteroposterior vaginal repair, a surgical procedure in which the upper and lower walls of the vagina are reconstructed to correct relaxed tissue.

anteversion /-vur′shən/ [L, *ante* + *versio,* turning], **1.** an abnormal position of an organ in which the organ is tilted forward on its axis, away from the midline. **2.** (in dentistry) the tipping or the tilting of teeth or other mandibular structures more anteriorly than normal. Compare **anterocclusion. 3.** the angulation created in the transverse plane between the neck and shaft of the femur. The normal angle is between 15 and 20 degrees. –**anteverted,** *adj.*

anthelmintic /ant′helmin′tik/ [Gk, *anti, helmins,* against worms], **1.** of or pertaining to a substance that destroys or prevents the development of parasitic worms, such as filariae, flukes, hookworms, pinworms, roundworms, schistosomes, tapeworms, trichinae, and whipworms. **2.** an anthelmintic drug. An anthelmintic may interfere with the parasites' carbohydrate metabolism, inhibit their respiratory enzymes, block their neuromuscular action, or render them susceptible to destruction by the host's macrophages. Among a number of drugs used in treating specific helmintic infections are piperazine, pyrantel pamoate, pyrvinium pamoate, mebendazole, nic[001e]losamide, hexylresorcinol, diethylcarbamazine, and thiabendazole.

-anthema, a suffix meaning a '(specified) type of skin eruption or rash': *eisanthema, enanthema, exanthema.*

anthraco-, a combining form meaning 'pertaining to a carbuncle or to coal': *anthracoid, anthraconecrosis, anthracosis.*

anthracosis /an′thrəkō′sis/ [Gk, *anthrax,* coal, *osis,* condition], a chronic lung disease occurring in coal miners, characterized by the deposit of coal dust in the lungs and the formation of black nodules on the bronchioles and resulting in focal emphysema. The condition is aggravated by cigarette smoking. There is no specific treatment; most cases are asymptomatic, and the progress of the condition may

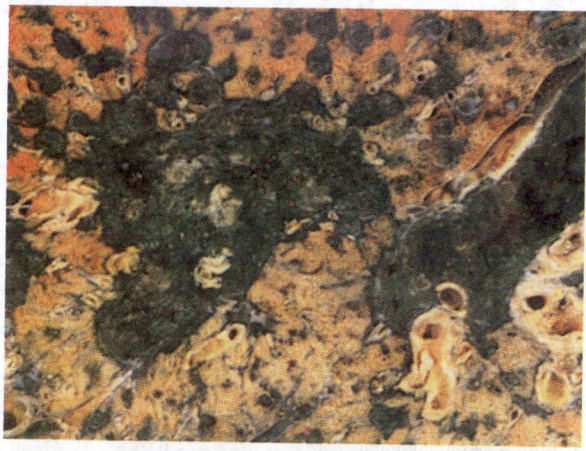

Anthracosis *(Fletcher, 1987)*

be halted by the prevention of further exposure to coal dust. Also called **black lung disease, coal worker's pneumoconiosis, miner's pneumoconiosis.** See also **inorganic dust.**

anthracosis linguae. See **parasitic glossitis.**

anthralin /an'thrəlin/, a topical antipsoriatic.

■ INDICATIONS: It is prescribed in the treatment of psoriasis and chronic dermatitis.

■ CONTRAINDICATIONS: Renal dysfunction or known hypersensitivity to this drug prohibits its use. It is not applied to acute psoriatic eruptions or near the eyes.

■ ADVERSE EFFECTS: The most serious adverse reaction is nephrotoxicity resulting from systemic absorption.

anthranilic acid. See **aminobenzoic acid.**

anthrax /an'thraks/ [Gk, coal, carbuncle], a disease affecting primarily farm animals (cattle, goats, pigs, sheep, and horses), caused by the bacterium *Bacillus anthracis*. Anthrax in animals is usually fatal. Humans most often acquire it when a break in the skin comes into direct contact with infected animals and their hides, but they may also contract a pulmonary form of anthrax by inhaling the spores of the bacterium. The cutaneous form begins with a reddish brown lesion that ulcerates and then forms a dark scab. The signs and symptoms that follow include internal hemorrhage, muscle pain, headache, fever, nausea, and vomiting. The pulmonary form, called woolsorter's disease, is often fatal unless treated early. Treatment for both forms is penicillin G or tetracycline. A vaccine is available for veterinarians and for others for whom anthrax is an occupational hazard. Also called **malignant pustule.**

anthropo-, a prefix meaning 'pertaining to man or to a human being': *anthropocentric, anthropocracy, anthropoid.*

anthropoid /an'thrəpoid/ [Gk, *anthropos*, human, *eidos*, form], a noun or adjective generally applied to humanlike apes or other primates; also used to describe a certain kind of pelvis in gynecology and obstetrics.

anthropoid pelvis [Gk, *anthropos*, human, *eidos*, form], a type of pelvis in which the inlet is oval; the anteroposterior diameter is much greater than the transverse, and, because of the posterior inclination of the sacrum, the posterior portion of the space in the true pelvis is much greater than the anterior portion. The side walls are somewhat convergent, and the ischial spines are prominent. If the pelvis is large, vaginal delivery is not compromised, but the occiput posterior position of the fetus is favored. This type of pelvis is present in 40% of nonwhite women and in more than 25% of white women. See **pelvis.**

anthropology [Gk, *anthropos*, human, *logos*, science], the science of human beings, from animal-like characteristics to social and environmental aspects.

anthropometry /an'thrəpom'ətrē/ [Gk, *anthropos* + *metron*, measure], the science of measuring the human body

Anthropometric measurements

Test	Gender	Normal values	Values showing malnutrition
Triceps skinfold (TSF)	Male	11-12.5 mm	7.5-11 mm
	Female	15-16.5 mm	10-15 mm
Mid upper arm circumference (MUAC)	Male	26-29 cm	20-26 cm
	Female	26-28.5 cm	20-26 cm
Arm muscle circumference (AMC)	Male	23-25 cm	16-23 cm
	Female	20-23 cm	14-20 cm

AMC = MUAC − 0.314 = TSF

as to height, weight, and size of component parts, including measurement of skinfolds, to study and compare the relative proportions under normal and abnormal conditions. Also called **anthropometric measurement. –anthropometric,** *adj.*

anti-, ant-, a prefix meaning 'against or over against': *antialexin, antibiosis, antichlorotic.*

antiadrenergic /an'ti·ad'rənur'jik, an'tī-/ [Gk, *anti* + L, *ad, ren*, to kidney], **1.** of or pertaining to the blocking of the effects of impulses transmitted by the adrenergic postganglionic fibers of the sympathetic nervous system. **2.** an antiadrenergic agent. Drugs that block the response to norepinephrine bound to alpha-adrenergic receptors reduce the tone of smooth muscle in peripheral blood vessels, causing increased peripheral circulation and decreased blood pressure. Alpha-blocking agents include ergotamine derivatives, used in treating migraine; phenoxybenzamine and phentolamine, administered for Raynaud's disease, pheochromocytoma, and diabetic gangrene; and tolazoline hydrochloride, administered to patients with spastic vascular disease. Agents that block beta-adrenergic receptors decrease the rate and force of heart contractions among other effects. Propranolol and its congeners are beta-blocking agents and are administered for hypertension, angina, and arrhythmias. Also called **sympatholytic.** Compare **adrenergic.**

antiagglutinin /-əgloo'tinin/ [Gk, *anti*, against + L, *agglutinare*, to glue], a specific antibody that counteracts the effects of an agglutinin.

antianabolic /-an'əbol'ik/, pertaining to drugs or other agents that inhibit or retard anabolic processes, such as cell division or the creation of new tissue by protein synthesis.

antianaphylaxis /-an'əfilak'sis/ [Gk, *anti*, against, *ana*, back, *phylaxis*, protection], a procedure to prevent anaphylactic reactions by injecting a patient with small desensitizing doses of the antigen.

antianemic /-ənē'mik/ [Gk, *anti* + *a, haima*, without blood], **1.** of or pertaining to a substance or procedure that counteracts or prevents a deficiency of erythrocytes. **2.** an agent used to treat or to prevent anemia. Whole blood is transfused in the treatment of anemia resulting from acute blood loss, and packed red cells are usually administered when the deficiency is caused by chronic blood loss. Transfusions of blood components are used in the treatment of aplastic anemia. Iron deficiency anemia, the most common form of anemia, is usually treated with oral preparations of ferrous sulfate, fumarate, or gluconate, but a parenteral preparation is indicated for people who are unable to absorb iron from the GI tract or for those who develop nausea and diarrhea when taking iron orally. Cyanocobalamin is administered parenterally in the treatment of pernicious anemia. Folic acid is prescribed to correct a deficiency of that vitamin in the anemias accompanying general malnutrition or alcoholic cirrhosis and to treat the common anemia of infants who are on a milk diet exclusively. A combination of folic acid and vitamin B_{12} is prescribed for people who are anemic as a result of an inadequate dietary intake of both vitamins.

antianginal drug /-anji'nəl/, any medication that increases oxygen supplies to the coronary arteries, thereby improving the blood flow to the myocardium to prevent symptoms of angina pectoris.

antiantibody /an'ti·an'tibodē/ [Gk, *anti, anti* + AS, *bodig*], an immunoglobulin formed as the result of the administration of an antibody that acts as an immunogen. The antiantibody then interacts with the antibody. See also **antibody, immune gamma globulin.**

antiantitoxin /-tok'sin/ [Gk, *anti, anti, toxikon,* poison], an antibody that may form in the body during immunization, inhibiting or counteracting the effect of the antitoxin administered. See also **antiantibody.**

antianxiety agent. See **sedative-hypnotic.**

antiarrhythmic /-ərith'mik/ [Gk, *anti* + *rhythmos,* rhythm], **1.** of or pertaining to a procedure or substance that prevents, alleviates, or corrects an abnormal cardiac rhythm. **2.** an agent used to treat a cardiac arrhythmia. A defibrillator that delivers a precordial electric shock is often used to restore a normal rhythm to rapid, irregular atrial or ventricular contractions. A pacemaker may be implanted in a patient with an extremely slow heart rate or other arrhythmia. The electrode catheter of an external pacemaker may be threaded through a vein to the heart in cases of ventricular standstill or complete heart block. Two of the major antiarrhythmic drugs are lidocaine, which increases the threshhold of electric stimulation in the ventricles during diastole, and a combination of disopyramide, procainamide, and quinidine, which decreases the excitability of the myocardium and prolongs the refractory period. The beta-adrenergic blocking agent propranolol may be used in treating arrhythmias. Isoproterenol is indicated for complete heart block and ventricular arrhythmias requiring an increased force of cardiac contractions to establish a normal rhythm. Atropine may be used in the treatment of bradycardia, a sedative in the treatment of tachycardia, and digitalis in the treatment of atrial fibrillation. Verapamil and other calcium blockers control arrhythmias by inhibiting calcium ion influx across the cell membrane of cardiac muscle, thus slowing atrioventricular conduction and prolonging the effective refractory period within the atrioventricular node. See also **arrhythmia.**

antiarthritic /-ärthrit'ik/ [Gk, *anti,* against, *arthron,* joint, *itis,* inflammation], pertaining to a therapy that relieves symptoms of arthritis.

antibacterial /-baktir'ē·əl/ [Gk, *anti* + *bakterion,* small staff], **1.** of or pertaining to a substance that kills bacteria or inhibits their growth or replication. **2.** an antibacterial agent. Antibiotics synthesized chemically or derived from various microorganisms exert their bactericidal or bacteriostatic effect by interfering with the production of the bacterial cell wall, by interfering with protein synthesis, nucleic acid synthesis, or cell membrane integrity, or by inhibiting critical biosynthetic pathways in the bacteria.

antiberiberi factor. See **thiamine.**

antibiotic /-bī·ot'ik/ [Gk, *anti* + *bios,* life], **1.** of or pertaining to the ability to destroy or interfere with the development of a living organism. **2.** an antimicrobial agent, derived from cultures of a microorganism or produced semisynthetically, used to treat infections. The penicillins, derived from species of the fungus *Penicillium* or manufactured semisynthetically, consist of a thiazolidine ring fused to a beta-lactam ring connected to side chains; these agents exert their action by inhibiting mucopeptide synthesis in bacterial cell walls during multiplication of the organisms. Penicillin G and V are widely used in treating many gram-positive coccal infections but are inactivated by the enzyme penicillinase produced by strains of staphylococci; cloxacillin, dicloxacillin, methicillin, nafcillin, and oxacillin are penicillinase-resistant penicillins. Broad-spectrum penicillins effective against gram-negative organisms are ampicillin, carbenicillin, and hetacillin. Hypersen-

sitivity reactions, such as rash, fever, bronchospasm, vasculitis, and anaphylaxis, are relatively common side effects of penicillin therapy. Aminoglycoside antibiotics, composed of amino sugars in glycoside linkage, interfere with the synthesis of bacterial proteins and are used primarily for the treatment of infections caused by gram-negative organisms. The aminoglycosides include gentamicin derived from *Micromonospora,* semisynthetic amikacin, kanamycin, neomycin, streptomycin, and tobramycin. These agents commonly cause nephrotoxic and ototoxic reactions as well as GI disturbances. Macrolide antibiotics, consisting of a large lactone ring and deoxamino sugar, interfere in protein synthesis of susceptible bacteria during multiplication without affecting nucleic acid synthesis. Oleandomycin, which is added to feed to improve the growth of poultry and swine, and broad-spectrum erythromycin, used to treat various gram-positive and gram-negative infections and intestinal amebiasis, are macrolides derived from species of *Streptomyces.* Erythromycin may cause mild allergic reactions and GI discomfort, but nausea, vomiting, and diarrhea occur infrequently with the usual oral dose. Polypeptide antibiotics derived from species of *Streptomyces* or certain soil bacilli vary in their spectra; most of these agents are nephrotoxic and ototoxic. Bacitracin and vancomycin are polypeptides used to treat severe staphylococcal infections; capreomycin and vancomycin are antituberculosis agents; and gramicidin is included in ointments for topical infections. Among polypeptide antibiotics effective against gram-negative organisms, colistin and neomycin are administered for diarrhea caused by enteropathogenic *Escherichia coli.* The tetracyclines, including the prototype derived from *Streptomyces,* chlortetracycline, demeclocycline, doxycycline, minocycline, and oxytetracycline, are active against a wide range of gram-positive and gram-negative organisms and some rickettsiae. Antibiotics in this group are primarily bacteriostatic and are thought to exert their effect by inhibiting protein synthesis in the organisms. Tetracycline therapy may cause GI irritation, photosensitivity, renal toxicity, and hepatic toxicity, and administration of a drug of this group during the last half of pregnancy, during infancy, or before 8 years of age may result in permanent discoloration of the teeth. The cephalosporins, derived from the soil fungus *Cephalosporium* or produced semisynthetically, inhibit bacterial cell wall synthesis, resist the action of penicillinase,

Mode of action of antibiotics

Mode of action	Representative antibiotics
Inhibition of bacterial cell wall synthesis	Penicillins
	Cephalosporins
	Bacitracins
Alteration of membrane permeability	Polymyxin B
	Amphotericin B
	Nystatin
Inhibition of microbial DNA translation and transcription	Erythromycin
	Tetracyclines
	Streptomycin
	Lincomycin
	Kanamycin
	Chloramphenicol
Inhibition of essential metabolite synthesis	Paraaminosalicylic acid
	Sulfonamides

and are used in treating infections of the respiratory tract, urinary tract, middle ear, and bones, as well as septicemia caused by a wide range of gram-positive and gram-negative organisms. The group includes cefadroxil, cefamandole, cefazolin, cephalexin, cephaloglycin, cephaloridine, cephalothin, cephapirin, and cephradine. Treatment with a cephalosporin may cause nausea, vomiting, diarrhea, enterocolitis, or an allergic reaction, such as rash, angioneurotic edema, or exfoliative dermatitis; use of antibiotics in this group is contraindicated in patients who have shown hypersensitivity to a penicillin. Chloramphenicol, a broad-spectrum antibiotic initially derived from *Streptomyces venezuelae*, inhibits protein synthesis in bacteria. Because the drug may cause life-threatening blood dyscrasias, its use is reserved for the treatment of acute typhoid fever, serious gram-negative infections (including *Haemophilus influenzae* meningitis), and rickettsial diseases.

antibiotic anticancer agents, drugs that may have both antibiotic and anticancer activity. Examples include bleomycin, dactinomycin, daunorubicin, and mitomycin.

antibiotic sensitivity tests, a laboratory method for determining the susceptibility of bacterial infections to therapy with antibiotics. After the infecting organism has been recovered from a clinical specimen, it is cultured and tested against several antibiotic drugs, often in two groups, gram-positive and gram-negative. If the growth of the organism is inhibited by the action of the drug, it is reported as sensitive to that antibiotic. If the organism is not susceptible to the antibiotic in question, it is reported as resistant to that drug. See also **Gram's stain.**

antibody (Ab) /an'tibod'ē/ [Gk, *anti* + AS, *bodig*], an immunoglobulin produced by lymphocytes in response to bacteria, viruses, or other antigenic substances. An antibody is specific to an antigen. Each class of antibody is named for its action. Antibodies include agglutinins, bacteriolysins, opsonins, and precipitin. See also **antiantibody, antigen determinant, plasma protein, T cell.**

antibody absorption, the process of removing or tying up undesired antibodies in an antiserum reagent by allowing them to react with undesired antigens.

antibody instructive theory, a theory that each antigenic contact in the life of an individual develops a new antibody, as when a B cell comes in contact with an antigen and subsequently produces plasma cells and memory cells. The theory maintains that the random contact of B cells with antigens induces the reticuloendothelial system to instruct memory cells to produce antibodies against antigens at any time. Compare **antibody specific theory.**

antibody specific theory, (in immunology) a theory of antibody formation proposed by F.M. Burnet, stating that preprogramed, or precommitted, clones of lymphoid cells that are produced in the fetus are capable of interacting with a limited number of antigenic determinants with which the host may come in contact. Any precommitted immunocompetent cells that encounter the specific antigen in utero are destroyed or suppressed so that entire clones are eliminated or inactivated. This in effect removes the cells programmed to become endogenous autoantigens and prevents the development of autoimmune diseases, leaving intact those cells capable of reacting with exogenous antigens. The theory holds that the body contains an enormous number of diverse clones of cells, each genetically programmed to synthesize a different antibody. This theory further maintains that any antigen entering the body selects the specific clone pro-

grammed to synthesize the antibody for that antigen and stimulates the cells of the clone to proliferate and produce more of the same antibody. Also called **clonal selection theory.** Compare **antibody instructive theory.** See also **autoimmunity.**

antibromic. See **deodorant.**

anticancer diet /-kan'sər/, a diet, based on recommendations of the American Cancer Society (ACS), National Cancer Institute (NCI), and National Academy of Sciences, to reduce cancer risk factors associated with eating habits. A fat intake of not more that 30% of total calories, adequate daily intake of high-fiber foods, intake of foods rich in vitamins A and C, and cruciferous vegetables (broccoli, cabbage, cauliflower), and moderation in the consumption of alcohol and salt-cured, smoked, or nitrite-cured foods are recommended. The diet is based on data from various epidemiologic studies.

anticarcinogenic /-kär'sinəjen'ik/ [Gk, *anti,* against, *karkinos,* crab, *oma,* tumor, *genein,* to produce], pertaining to a substance or device that neutralizes the effects of a carcinogen.

anticholinergic /-kō'lənur'jik/ [Gk, *anti* + *chole,* bile, *ergein,* to work], **1.** of or pertaining to a blockade of acetylcholine receptors that results in the inhibition of the transmission of parasympathetic nerve impulses. **2.** an anticholinergic agent that functions by competing with the neurotransmitter acetylcholine for its receptor sites at synaptic junctions. Anticholinergic drugs reduce spasms of smooth muscle in the bladder, bronchi, and intestine; relax the iris sphincter; decrease gastric, bronchial, and salivary secretions; decrease perspiration; and accelerate impulse conduction through the myocardium by blocking vagal impulses. Many anticholinergic agents reduce parkinsonian symptoms; atropine in large doses stimulates the central nervous system and in small doses acts as a depressant. Among numerous cholinergic blocking agents are anisotropine methylbromide, belladonna, glycopyrrolate, hyoscyamine sulfate, methixene hydrochloride, and scopolamine. Various members of the group are used to treat spastic disorders of the GI tract, to reduce salivary and bronchial secretions preoperatively, or to dilate the pupil. Also called **parasympatholytic.** Compare **cholinergic.**

anticholinergic agent. See **anticholinergic.**

anticholinesterase /an'tikol'ənes'tərās/, a drug that inhibits or inactivates the action of acetylcholinesterase. Drugs of this class cause acetylcholine to accumulate at the junctions of various cholinergic nerve fibers and their effector sites or organs, allowing potentially continuous stimulation of cholinergic fibers throughout the central and peripheral nervous systems. Anticholinesterase drugs include neostigmine, edrophonium, and pyridostigmine. Neostigmine and pyridostigmine are prescribed in the treatment of myasthenia gravis; edrophonium in the diagnosis of myasthenia gravis and the treatment of overdosage of curariform drugs. Many agricultural insecticides have been developed from anticholinesterases; these are the highly toxic chemicals called organophosphates. Nerve gases developed as potential chemical warfare agents contain potent, irreversible forms of anticholinesterase.

anticipatory adaptation /antis'əpətôr'ē/ [L, *anticipare,* to receive before], the act of adapting to a potentially distressing situation before actually confronting the problem, as when a person tries to relax before learning the results of a medical examination.

anticipatory grief, feelings of grief that develop before, rather than after, a loss.

anticipatory guidance, the psychologic preparation of a person to help relieve fear and anxiety of an event expected to be stressful, such as the preparation of a child for surgery by explaining what will happen and what it will feel like and the showing of equipment or the part of the hospital where the child will be. It is also used to prepare parents for normal growth and development.

anticoagulant /-kō·ag′yəlent/ [Gk, *anti* + *coagulare,* curdle], **1.** of or pertaining to a substance that prevents or delays coagulation of the blood. **2.** an anticoagulant drug. Heparin, obtained from the liver and lungs of domestic animals, is a potent anticoagulant that interferes with the formation of thromboplastin, with the conversion of prothrombin to thrombin, and with the formation of fibrin from fibrinogen. Synthetic coumarin and phenindione derivatives administered orally are vitamin K antagonists that prevent coagulation by inhibiting the formation of vitamin K-dependent clotting factors.

anticoagulant therapy [Gk, *anti,* L, *coagulare,* to curdle; Gk, *therapeia*], the administration of drugs that reduce the tendency of blood to coagulate, thereby reducing the risk of thrombosis.

anticodon /an′tikō′don/ [Gk, *anti* + *caudex,* book], (in genetics) a sequence of three nucleotides in transfer RNA that pairs complementarily with a specific codon of messenger RNA during protein synthesis to specify a particular amino acid in the polypeptide chain. See also **genetic code, transcription, translation.**

anticonvulsant /-kənvul′sənt/ [Gk, *anti* + L, *convellere,* to shake], **1.** of or pertaining to a substance or procedure that prevents or reduces the severity of epileptic or other convulsive seizures. **2.** an anticonvulsant drug. Hydantoin derivatives, especially phenytoin, apparently exert their anticonvulsant effect by stabilizing the cell membrane and decreasing intracellular sodium, with the result that the excitability of the epileptogenic focus is reduced. Phenytoin prevents the spread of excessive discharges in cerebral motor areas and suppresses dysrhythmias originating in the thalamus, frontal lobes, and other brain areas. Phenacemide and primidone are also used in treating grand mal epilepsy, and succinic acid derivatives, valproic acid, paramethadione, and various barbiturates are among the drugs prescribed to limit or prevent petit mal seizures. Many of these agents have a potential for producing fetal malformations when administered to pregnant women.

antideformity positioning and splinting /-dəfôr′mitē/, the use of splints, braces, or similar devices to prevent or control contractures or other musculoskeletal deformities that may result from disuse, burns, or other injuries. Examples include the application of axillary or airplane splints to prevent adduction contracture of the shoulder and a neck conformer splint to prevent flexion contractures of the neck.

antidepressant /-dəpres′ənt/, **1.** of or pertaining to a substance or a measure that prevents or relieves depression. **2.** an antidepressant agent. Tricyclic antidepressant agents, such as amitryptyline and imipramine hydrochloride, block reuptake of amine neurotransmitters, but the exact mechanism of the antidepressant action of these drugs is unknown. Monoamine oxidase (MAO) inhibitors, such as isocarboxazid, pargyline hydrochloride, phenelzine sulfate, and tranylcypromine, increase the concentration of epinephrine, norepinephrine, and serotonin in storage sites in the nervous system, and it is theorized that this increased level of monoamines in the brainstem is responsible for the drugs' antidepressant effect. MAO inhibitors also have antihypertensive action. See also **antipsychotic.**

antidiarrheal /-dī′ərē′əl/, a drug or other agent that relieves the symptoms of diarrhea. Antidiarrheals work by absorbing water from the digestive tract, by altering intestinal motility, by altering electrolyte transport, or by adsorption of toxins or microorganisms.

antidiuretic /-dī′əret′ik/ [Gk, *anti* + *dia,* through, *ourein,* to urinate], **1.** of or pertaining to the suppression of urine formation. **2.** an antidiuretic agent. Antidiuretic hormone (vasopressin), produced in hypothalamic nuclei and stored in the posterior lobe of the pituitary gland, suppresses urine formation by stimulating the resorption of water in distal tubules and collecting ducts in the kidneys. **–antidiuresis,** *n.*

antidiuretic hormone (ADH), a hormone that decreases the production of urine by increasing the reabsorption of water by the renal tubules. ADH is secreted by cells of the hypothalamus and stored in the posterior lobe of the pituitary gland. It is released in response to a decrease in blood volume or an increased concentration of sodium or other substances in plasma, or by pain, stress, or the action of certain drugs. ADH can cause contraction of smooth muscle in the digestive tract and blood vessels, especially capillaries, arterioles, and venules. Acetylcholine, methacholine, nicotine, large doses of barbiturates, anesthetics, epinephrine, and norepinephrine stimulate ADH release; ethanol and phenytoin inhibit production of the hormone. Increased intracranial pressure promotes inappropriate increases and decreases in ADH. Synthetic ADH is used in the treatment of diabetes insipidus. Normal values are 1-5 pg/ml or less than 1.5 ngL. Also called **vasopressin.**

antidotal /-dō′təl/ [Gk, *anti,* against, *dotos,* that which is given], a substance that renders a poison or drug ineffective.

antidote /an′tidōt/ [Gk, *anti* + *dotos,* that which is given], a drug or other substance that opposes the action of a poison. An antidote may be mechanical, acting to coat the stomach and prevent absorption; or chemical, acting to make the toxin inert; or physiologic, acting to oppose the action of the poison, as when a sedative is given to a person who has ingested a large amount of a stimulant, or when a receptor blocker is administered to a person who has taken a large dose of the receptor agonist.

antidromic conduction /an′tidrom′ik/ [Gk, *anti* + *dromos,* course], the conduction of a neural impulse backward from a receptor in the midportion of an axon. It is an unnatural phenomenon and may be produced experimentally. Because synaptic junctions allow conduction in one direction only, any backward, antidromic impulses that occur fail to pass the synapse, dying at that point. Compare **orthodromic conduction.**

antiembolism hose /-em′bəliz′əm/ [Gk, *anti* + *embolos,* plug], elasticized stockings worn to prevent the formation of emboli and thrombi, especially in patients after surgery or those restricted to bed. Return flow of the venous circulation is promoted, preventing venous stasis and dilatation of the veins, conditions that predispose to varicosities and thromboembolic disorders.

antiemetic /-imet′ik/ [Gk, *anti* + *emesis,* vomiting], **1.** of or pertaining to a substance or procedure that prevents or alleviates nausea and vomiting. **2.** an antiemetic drug or agent. Belladonna derivatives, bromides, barbiturates and other sedatives, and substances that protect the stomach lining, such as lime water or mild gastric astringents, have weak antiemetic properties. Chlorpromazine and other phenothiazines are sometimes effective antiemetic agents. In motion sickness scopolamine and antihistamines provide relief. Marijuana may alleviate the nausea induced by certain antineoplastic drugs in cancer patients.

antiepileptic. See **anticonvulsant.**

antiestrogen drug /-es′trəjən/, any of a group of hormone-based products used predominantly in cancer chemotherapy. The group includes tamoxifen. They are used mainly in treating estrogen-dependent tumors, such as breast cancer.

antifebrile. See **antipyretic.**

antifungal /-fung′gəl/, **1.** of or pertaining to a substance that kills fungi or inhibits their growth or reproduction. **2.** an antifungal, antibiotic drug. Amphotericin B and ketoconazole, both effective against a broad spectrum of fungi, probably act by binding to sterols in the fungal cell membrane and changing the membrane's permeability. Griseofulvin, another broad-spectrum antifungal agent, binds to the host's new keratin and renders it resistant to further fungal invasion. Miconazole inhibits the growth of common dermatophytes, including yeastlike *Candida albicans,* and nystatin is effective against yeast and yeastlike fungi. Also called **antimycotic.**

antigalactic /-gəlak′tik/, pertaining to a drug or other agent that prevents or reduces milk secretion in some mothers of newborns.

anti-GBM disease, an immunologically mediated kidney disorder involving the glomerular basement membrane (GBM), which is damaged in the antigen-antibody reaction. The kidney itself may serve as the antigenic target in the reaction.

antigen /an′tijən/ [Gk, *anti* + *genein,* to produce], a substance, usually a protein, that causes the formation of an antibody and reacts specifically with that antibody.

antigen-antibody reaction, a process of the immune system in which immunoglobulin-coated B cells recognize an intruder or antigen and stimulate antibody production. The T cells assist in the antigen-antibody reaction, but the B cells play the key role. Antigen-antibody reactions activate the complement system of the body, amplifying the humoral immunity response of the B cells and causing lysis of the antigenic cells. Antigen-antibody reactions involve the binding of antigens to antibodies to form antigen-antibody complexes that may render the toxic antigen harmless, agglutinize antigens on the surface of microorganisms, or activate the complement system by exposing the complement-binding sites on the antibody molecule. Complement protein immediately binds to these sites and triggers the activity of the other complement proteins to produce cytolysis of the antigen cells. The antigen-antibody reaction may start immediately with antigen contact, or it may start as much as 48 hours later. Antigen-antibody reactions are essential to the immune response of the body and are precipitated by contact of antigenic protein molecules with antibody protein molecules. The antigen-antibody reactions occur and antigen-antibody complexes are formed when unique areas on the surfaces of antigen molecules fit precisely into appropriate concave combining sites on the surfaces of antibody molecules. Various amounts of IgM, IgG, IgA, IgE, and IgD are normally present during any antigenic chal-

lenge. Antigen-antibody reactions normally produce immunity, but they can also produce allergy, autoimmunity, and fetomaternal hematologic incompatibility. Antigen-antibody reaction in the immediate allergic response activates certain enzymes and causes an imbalance between these enzymes and their inhibitors. Simultaneously released into the circulation are certain pharmacologically active substances, such as acetylcholine, bradykinin, histamine, IgG, and leukotaxine. Autoimmunity occurs when the immune system seeks to distinguish between self and a foreign substance. There are several theories that seek to explain why the body reacts to autoimmune diseases by producing antibodies that attack not only the invading organisms but the cells of the body as well. They are the forbidden clone theory, the sequestered antigens theory, and the immune complex activity theory. The antigen-antibody reactions associated with autoimmunity are still not well understood. In erythroblastosis fetalis, an antigen-antibody reaction stems from the incompatibility of the fetal and the maternal blood and produces a maternal antibody that acts against fetal red cells. See also **serum sickness.**

antigen determinant, a small area on the surface of an antigen molecule that fits a combining site of an antibody molecule and binds the antigen in the formation of an antigen-antibody complex. Antigen determinants commonly consist of a sequence of amino acids that decrees the shape of these reactive areas. Also called **epitope.** See also **antibody.**

antigenic drift /-jen′ik/ [Gk, *anti,* against, *genein,* to produce + AS, *drifan,* drift], the tendency of a virus or other microorganism to alter its genetic makeup, periodically resulting in a mutant antigen requiring new antibodies and vaccines to combat its effects.

antigenicity /an′tijənis′ətē/, the ability to cause the production of antibodies. The degree of antigenicity depends on the kind and amount of the particular substance, the condition of the host, and the degree to which the host is sensitive to the antigen and able to produce antibodies.

antigerminal pole. See **vegetal pole.**

antiglobulin /an′tiglob′yŏŏlin/ [Gk, *anti* + L *globulus,* small globe], an antibody occurring naturally or prepared in laboratory animals against human globulin. Specific antiglobulins are used in the detection of specific antibodies, as in blood typing. See also **antiglobulin test, Coombs' test, precipitin.**

antiglobulin test, a test for the presence of antibodies that coat and damage red blood cells as a result of any of several diseases or conditions. The test can detect Rh antibodies in maternal blood and is used to anticipate hemolytic disease of the newborn. It is also used to diagnose and screen for autoimmune hemolytic anemias and to determine the compatibility of blood types. When exposed to a sample of the patient's serum, the antiglobulin serum will cause agglutination if human globulin antibody or its complement is present. Also called **Coombs' test.** See also **autoimmune disease, erythroblastosis fetalis.**

antigravity muscles /-grav′itē/, the muscle groups involved with stabilization of joints or other body parts by opposing the effects of gravity on the body. Examples include the muscles of the jaw that automatically keep the mandible raised and the mouth closed.

anti-G suit. See **military antishock trousers.**

antihemophilic C factor. See **factor XI.**

antihemophilic factor (AHF) /-hē′mōfil′ik/, blood factor VIII, a systemic hemostatic.

■ INDICATION: It is prescribed in the treatment of hemophilia A, a deficiency of factor VIII.

■ CONTRAINDICATION: There are no known contraindications.

■ ADVERSE EFFECTS: The most serious adverse reaction is hepatitis, because the factor is obtained from pools of human plasma. Various allergic reactions may also occur.

antihemophilic factor plasma [Gk, *anti,* against, *haima,* blood, *philein,* to love; L, *facere,* to make; Gk, *plassein,* to mold], blood plasma that contains the antihemophilic factor VIII.

antihemorrhagic /-hē′môraj′ik/, any drug or agent used to prevent or control bleeding, such as thromboplastin or thrombin, either of which mediates the blood clotting process.

antihidrotic /-hidrot′ik/ [Gk, *anti,* + *hidros,* sweat], an agent that inhibits or prevents the production of sweat.

antihistamine /-his′təmin/ [Gk, *anti* + *histos,* tissue, amine (ammonia compound)], any substance capable of reducing the physiologic and pharmacologic effects of histamine, including a wide variety of drugs that block histamine receptors. Many such drugs are readily available as nonprescription medicines for the management of allergies. Toxicity resulting from the overuse of antihistamines and their accidental ingestion by children is common and sometimes fatal. These substances do not stop the release of histamine, and the ways in which they act on the central nervous system (CNS) are not completely understood. The antihistamines are divided into H_1 and H_2 blockers depending on the responses to histamine they prevent. The H_1 blocking drugs, such as the alkylamines, ethanolamines, ethylenediamines, and piperazines, are effective in the symptomatic treatment of acute exudative allergies, such as pollinosis and urticaria. The H_2 blocking drugs, such as cimetidine, are effective in the control of gastric secretions and are often used in the treatment of duodenal ulcers. Antihistamines can both stimulate and depress the CNS. The side effects of H_1 blockers may include sedation, nausea, constipation, and dryness of the throat and respiratory tract. About 25% of the individuals who use antihistamines experience some bothersome reaction.

antihistaminic [Gk, *anti* + *histos,* tissue, amine], pertaining to a substance that counteracts the effects of histamine.

antihypercholesterolemic /-hī′pərkō′lestərōlē′mik/, a drug that prevents or controls an increase of cholesterol in the blood. Examples include clofibrate, lovastatin, and colestipol.

antihypertensive /-hī·pərten′siv/, **1.** of or pertaining to a substance or procedure that reduces high blood pressure. **2.** an antihypertensive agent. Various drugs achieve their antihypertensive effect by depleting tissue stores of catecholamines in peripheral sites, by stimulating pressor receptors in the carotid sinus and heart, by blocking autonomic nerve impulses that constrict blood vessels, by stimulating central inhibitory alpha-adrenergic receptors, or by direct vasodilatation. Thiazides and other diuretic agents reduce blood pressure by decreasing blood volume. Among the numerous drugs used to treat hypertension are reserpine, captopril, verapamil, diazoxide, guanethidine, methyldopa, pargyline hydrochloride, and trimethaphan camsylate.

antiimmune /an′ti·imyŌŌn′/ [Gk, *anti* + L, *immunis,* free from], pertaining to the prevention or inhibition of immunity. See **immune response.**

antiinfection vitamin. See **vitamin A.**

antiinfectious /-infek′shəs/ [Gk, *anti* + L, *inficere,* to stain], pertaining to an agent that prevents or treats infection.

antiinflammatory /-inflam′ətor′ē/ [Gk, *anti* + L, *inflammare,* to set afire], **1.** of or pertaining to a substance or procedure that counteracts or reduces inflammation. **2.** an antiinflammatory drug or agent. Betamethasone, prednisolone, prednisone, and other synthetic glucocorticoids are used extensively in treating inflammation. The basis of the antiinflammatory effect of salicylates and nonsteroidal antiinflammatory agents, such as phenylbutazone and indomethacin, appears to involve inhibition of prostaglandin biosynthesis.

antiinitiator /-inish′ē·ātər/, a substance that is a potential cocarcinogen but that may protect cells against cancer development if given before exposure to an initiator. An example is the food additive BHT. An antiinitiator given after exposure to an initiator may also act as a promoter and encourage rather than block cancer development.

antileprotic /-leprot′ik/, a drug or other agent that is effective in treating leprosy.

antilipidemic /an′tilip′idē′mik/ [Gk, *anti* + *lipos,* fat, *haima,* blood], **1.** of or pertaining to a regimen, diet, or agent that reduces the amount of lipids in the serum. **2.** a drug used to reduce the amount of lipids in the serum. Antilipidemic diets and drugs are prescribed to reduce the risk of atherosclerotic cardiovascular disease (ACVD) based on two facts: Atheromatous plaques contain free cholesterol, and lower serum cholesterol levels and less coronary heart disease are found in populations consuming a low-fat diet than in those on a high-fat diet. Although it has not been proven that food intake affects the development of ACVD, a prudent low-fat diet with polyunsaturates replacing saturated fats is considered a valuable preventive measure by many cardiologists. A number of pharmacologic agents are used to reduce serum lipids, but it is not established whether drug-induced lowering of serum cholesterol or triglyceride levels has a beneficial effect, no effect, or a detrimental effect on ACVD morbidity or mortality. Clofibrate reduces very low density lipoproteins in serum; the drug may reduce the risk of a second, nonfatal myocardial infarction, but it increases the risk of cholelithiasis, cardiac arrhythmias, intermittent claudication, and thromboembolism. Cholestyramine and colestipol exert their antilipidemic action by combining with bile acids in the intestine to form an insoluble complex that is excreted in the feces; it may reduce serum cholesterol markedly, but it prevents the absorption of essential fat-soluble vitamins and may be associated with several serious side effects. Colestipol also binds and removes bile acids from the intestine; sitosterol may interfere with intestinal absorption of cholesterol, but the exact mechanism of its action and that of antilipidemic probucol are unknown. Lovastatin interferes with the biosynthesis of cholesterol. See also **hyperlipidemia.**

Antilirium, a trademark for an acetylcholinesterase drug inhibitor (physostigmine salicylate).

antilymphocyte serum (ALS) /-lim′fəsīt/, a serum prescribed as an immunosuppressive agent for the reduction of rejection reactions in organ transplant and as an adjunct in chemotherapy for malignant neoplasms. Its effects have been promising in some cases of leukemia and in kidney transplant. It is associated with some adverse effects, such as serious serum sickness, generalized infection, anaphylaxis, and antigen-antibody-induced glomerulonephritis.

antimalarial /-məler′ē·əl/, **1.** of or pertaining to a substance that destroys or suppresses the development of malaria plasmodia or to a procedure that exterminates the mosquito vectors of the disease, such as spraying insecticides or draining swamps. **2.** an antimalarial drug that destroys or prevents the development of plasmodia in human hosts. Chloroquine hydrochloride and hydroxychloroquine sulfate are effective against *Plasmodium vivax, P. malariae,* and certain strains of *P. falciparum.* Patients with drug-resistant *P. falciparum* are often treated with a combination of quinine, pyrimethamine, and sulfadoxine. See also **malaria.**

antimessage, a strand of RNA that cannot act as mRNA because of its negative coding sequence. It must be converted to a positive-strand sequence by a viral transcriptase before it can function as a messenger.

antimetabolite /-mətab′əlīt/ [Gk, *anti + metabole,* change], a drug or other substance that is an antagonist or that resembles a normal human metabolite and interferes with its function in the body, usually by competing for the metabolite's receptors or enzymes. Among the antimetabolites used as antineoplastic agents are the folic acid analog methotrexate and the pyrimidine analogs fluorouracil and floxuridine. Antineoplastic mercaptopurine, an analog of the nucleotide adenine and the purine base hypoxanthine, is a metabolic antagonist of both compounds. Thioguanine, another member of a large series of purine analogs, interferes with nucleic acid synthesis. Cytarabine, used in the treatment of acute myelocytic leukemia, is a synthetic nucleoside that resembles cytidine and kills cells actively synthesizing DNA, apparently by inhibiting the enzyme DNA polymerase.

antimicrobial /-mīkrō′bē·əl/ [Gk, *anti + mikros,* small, *bios,* life], **1.** of or pertaining to a substance that kills microorganisms or inhibits their growth or replication. **2.** an agent that kills or inhibits the growth or replication of microorganisms. See also **antibiotic.**

antimicrobial drugs [Gk, *anti + mikros,* small, *bios,* life, Fr, *drogue*], drugs that destroy or inhibit the growth of microorganisms.

Antiminth, a trademark for an anthelmintic (pyrantel pamoate).

antimitochondrial antibody /-mī′tōkon′drē·əl/, an antibody that acts specifically against mitochondria. These antibodies are not normally present in the blood of healthy people. A laboratory test for the presence of the antibodies in the blood is a valuable diagnostic aid in liver disease. Low titers may occur in chronic hepatitis, drug-induced hepatotoxicity, and various other diseases. High titers are virtually diagnostic of primary biliary cirrhosis.

antimitotic /-mītot′ik/, pertaining to the inhibition of cell division.

antimony /an′təmō′nē/ [L *antimonium*], a bluish, crystalline metallic element occurring in nature, both free and as salts. Various antimony compounds are used in the treatment of filariasis, leishmaniasis, lymphogranuloma, schistosomiasis, and trypanosomiasis and as an emetic.

antimony poisoning, poisoning caused by the ingestion or inhalation of antimony or antimony compounds, characterized by vomiting, sweating, diarrhea, and a metallic taste in the mouth. Irritation of the skin or mucous membrane may result from external exposure. Severe poisoning resembles arsenic poisoning. Dimercaprol is used for chelation. Antimony and antimony compounds are common ingredients of many substances used in medicine and industry.

antimorph /an′təmôrf/ [Gk, *anti + morphe,* form], a mutant gene that inhibits or antagonizes the normal influence of its allele in the expression of a trait. Compare **amorph, hypermorph, hypomorph.**

antimuscarinic /-mus′kərin′ik/ [Gk, *anti + L, musca,* fly], inhibiting the stimulation of the postganglionic parasympathetic receptor.

antimutagen /-myoo′təjən/ [Gk, *anti + L, mutare,* to change; Gk *genein* to produce], **1.** any substance that reduces the rate of spontaneous mutations or counteracts or reverses the action of a mutagen. **2.** any technique that protects cells against the effects of mutagenic agents. **- antimutagenic,** *adj.*

antimycotic. See **antifungal.**

antineoplastic /-nē′ōplas′tik/ [Gk, *anti + neos,* new, *plasma,* something formed], **1.** of or pertaining to a substance, procedure, or measure that prevents the proliferation of malignant cells. **2.** a chemotherapeutic agent that controls or kills cancer cells. Drugs used in the treatment of cancer are cytotoxic but are generally more damaging to dividing cells than to resting cells. Cycle-specific antineoplastic agents are more effective in killing proliferating cells than in killing resting cells, and phase-specific agents are most active during a specific phase of the cell cycle. Most anticancer drugs prevent the proliferation of cells by inhibiting the synthesis of DNA by various mechanisms. Alkylating agents, such as nitrogen mustard derivatives, ethylenimine derivatives, and alkyl sulfonates, interfere with DNA replication by causing cross-linking of DNA strands and abnormal pairing of nucleotides. Antimetabolites exert their action by interfering with the formation of compounds required for cell division. The folic acid analog and 5-fluorouracil, a pyrimidine analog, inhibit enzymes required for the formation of the essential DNA constituent thymidine. Hypoxanthine analog 6-mercaptopurine and 6-thioguanine, an analog of guanine, interfere with the biosynthesis of purine. Vinblastine and vincristine, alkaloids derived from the periwinkle plant, disrupt cell division by interfering with the formation of the mitotic spindle. Antineoplastic antibiotics, such as doxorubicin, daunomycin, and mitomycin, block or inhibit DNA synthesis, while dactinomycin and mithramycin interfere with RNA synthesis. Cytotoxic chemotherapeutic agents may be administered orally, intravenously, or by infusion. All have untoward and unpleasant side effects and are potentially immunosuppressive and dangerous. Estrogens and androgens, although not considered antineoplastic agents, frequently cause tumor regression when administered in high doses to patients with hormone-dependent cancers. See also **alkylating agent, antimetabolite.**

antineoplastic antibiotic, a chemical substance derived from a microorganism or a synthetic analog of the substance, used in cancer chemotherapy. Dactinomycin, employed in the treatment of Wilms' tumor, testicular carcinoma, choriocarcinoma, rhabdomyosarcoma, and some other sarcomas, exerts its antineoplastic effect by interfering with RNA synthesis. Mithramycin, with a similar mechanism of action, is also administered for testicular cancer and for trophoblastic neoplasms. Doxorubicin, a broadspectrum agent that is especially useful in treating breast carcinoma, lymphomas, sarcomas, and acute leukemia, and closely related daunomycin, which is also effective in acute leukemias, block the biosynthesis of RNA. Mitomycin C, prescribed for gastric, breast, cervical, and head and neck carcinomas, cross links strands of DNA. Bleomycin, used in the treatment of squamous cell carcinomas of the head and neck, testicular carcinoma, and lymphomas, damages DNA and prevents its repair. Antineoplastic antibiotics depress bone marrow and usually cause nausea and vomiting; several cause alopecia. Doxorubicin and daunomycin may be cardiotoxic, and mitomycin and bleomycin may produce pulmonary changes.

antineoplastic hormone, a chemical substance produced by an endocrine gland or a synthetic analog of the naturally occurring compound, used to control certain disseminated cancers. Hormonal therapy is designed to counteract the effect of an endogenous hormone required for the growth of the tumor. The estrogens diethylstilbestrol (DES) and ethinyl estradiol are employed in palliative treatment of a prostatic carcinoma that is nonresectable or unresponsive to radiotherapy. An androgen, such as testosterone propionate, testolactone, or fluoxymesterone, may be administered postoperatively to control disseminated breast cancer in women whose tumors are estrogen-dependent. The antiestrogen tamoxifen produces responses in many patients with advanced estrogen-dependent breast cancer. Paradoxically, large doses of estrogen, frequently used to control disseminated breast cancer in postmenopausal women, apparently check the growth of tumors by inhibiting the secretion of estrogen by the adrenal gland. Some progestins produce a favorable response in women with disseminated endometrial carcinoma and, occasionally, in patients with prostatic or renal cancers. These progestins include megestrol acetate, medroxyprogesterone acetate, and 17-alphahydroxyprogesterone caproate.

antineuritic vitamin. See **thiamine.**

antinuclear antibody (ANA) /-nōō′klē·ər/, an autoantibody that reacts with nuclear material. Antinuclear antibodies are found in the blood serum of patients with rheumatoid arthritis, systemic lupus erythematosus, Sjögren's syndrome, polymyositis, and a number of nonrheumatic disorders ranging from lymphomas and leukemias to adverse drug ractions. The antibodies are detected with an immunofluorescent assay technique.

antioxidant /-ok′sidənt/, a chemical or other agent that inhibits or retards oxidation of a substance to which it is added. Examples include butylated hydroxyanisole (BHA) and butylated hydroxytoluene (BHT). These substances are added to foods containing fats or oils to prevent oxygen from combining with the fatty molecules, thereby causing them to become rancid.

antiparallel /-per′ələl/ [Gk, anti + parallelos, side-by-side], (in molecular genetics) the condition in which molecules, such as strands of DNA, are parallel but point in opposite directions.

antiparasitic /-per′əsit′ik/ [Gk, anti + parasitos, guest], **1.** of or pertaining to a substance or procedure that kills parasites or inhibits their growth or reproduction. **2.** an antiparasitic drug including amebicides, anthelmintics, antimalarials, schistosomicides, trichomonacides, and trypanosomicides.

antiparkinsonian /-pär′kənsəniz′əm/, of or pertaining to a substance or procedure used to treat parkinsonism. Drugs for this neurologic disorder are of two kinds: those that compensate for the lack of dopamine in the corpus striatum of parkinsonism patients, and anticholinergic agents that counteract the activity of the abundant acetylcholine in the striatum. Synthetic levodopa, a dopamine precursor that crosses the blood-brain barrier, is administered to patients to reduce the rigidity, sluggishness, dysphagia, drooling, and instability characteristic of the disease, but the drug does not alter the relentless course of the disorder. Centrally active cholinergic blockers, notably benztropine, biperiden, procyclidine, and trihexyphenidyl, may relieve tremors and rigidity and improve mobility. The antiviral agent amantadine is often effective in the treatment of parkinsonism; the mechanism of its action is not established, but it apparently increases release of dopamine in the brain. Therapeutic approaches to the relief of the symptoms of parkinsonism include alcohol injection, cautery, cryosurgery, and surgical excision performed to destroy the globus pallidus (reducing rigidity) and parts of the thalamus (reducing tremor). Extrapyramidal symptoms similar to idiopathic parkinsonism are frequently induced by antipsychotic drugs. See also **tardive dyskinesia.**

antipathy /antip′əthē/ [Gk, anti + pathos, suffering], a strong feeling of aversion or antagonism to particular objects or individuals.

antiperistaltic /-per′əstal′tik/ [Gk, anti + peristellein, to wrap around], **1.** of or pertaining to a substance that inhibits or diminishes peristalsis. **2.** an antiperistaltic agent. Narcotics, such as paregoric, diphenoxylate, and loperamide hydrochloride, are antiperistaltic agents used to provide symptomatic relief in diarrhea. Anticholinergic (parasympatholytic) drugs reduce spasms of intestinal smooth muscle and are frequently prescribed to decrease excessive GI motility.

antipernicious anemia factor. See **cyanocobalamin.**

antiprotoplasmatic /-prō′təplasmat′ik/, pertaining to agents that damage the protoplasm of cells.

antipruritic /-prōōrit′ik/ [Gk, anti + L, prurire, to itch], **1.** of or pertaining to a substance or procedure that tends to relieve or prevent itching. **2.** an antipruritic drug. Topical

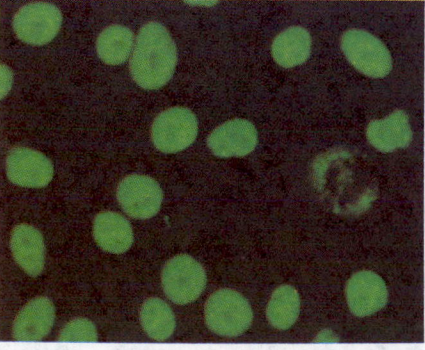

Immunofluorescence of antinuclear antibodies
(Shipley, 1993)

anesthetics, corticosteroids, and antihistamines are used as antipruritic agents.

antipsoriatic /an′tisôr′ē·at′ik/ [Gk, *anti* + *psora,* itch], pertaining to an agent that relieves the symptoms of psoriasis.

antipsychotic /-sīkot′ik/ [Gk, *anti* + *psyche,* mind, *osis,* condition], **1.** of or pertaining to a substance or procedure that counteracts or diminishes symptoms of a psychosis. **2.** an antipsychotic drug. Phenothiazine derivatives are the most frequently prescribed antipsychotics for use in the treatment of schizophrenia and other major affective disorders. They apparently act by enhancing the filtering mechanisms of the reticular formation in the brainstem and by blocking central dopamine receptors. Common side effects of phenothiazines are a dry mouth, blurred vision, and extrapyramidal reactions requiring treatment with antiparkinsonian agents. See also **antidepressant, neuroleptic, tranquilizer.**

antipyresis /-pīrē′sis/ [Gk, *anti* + *pyretos,* fever], treatment to reduce and ameliorate fever.

antipyretic /-pīret′ik/ [Gk, *anti* + *pyretos,* fever], **1.** of or pertaining to a substance or procedure that reduces fever. **2.** an antipyretic agent. Such drugs usually lower the thermodetection set point of the hypothalamic heat regulatory center, with resulting vasodilatation and sweating. Widely used antipyretic agents are acetaminophen, administered orally or through rectal suppositories, aspirin, and other salicylates. A tepid alcohol sponge bath or lukewarm tub bath may decrease an elevated temperature, and hypothermia produced by a cooling blanket is sometimes used for patients with a prolonged, high fever. Also called **antifebrile, antithermic, febrifuge.**

antipyretic bath, a bath in which tepid water is used to reduce the temperature of the body.

antipyrotic /-pīrot′ik/ [Gk, *anti* + *pyr,* fire], pertaining to the treatment of burns or scalds.

antirachitic /-rəkit′ik/, pertaining to an agent used to treat rickets.

antirheumatic /-roōmat′ik/ [Gk, *anti* + *rheumatismos,* that which flows], pertaining to the relief of symptoms of any painful or immobilizing disorder of the musculoskeletal system.

antiscorbutic vitamin. See **ascorbic acid.**

antiseborrheic /-seb′ərē′ik/, pertaining to a drug or agent that is applied to the skin to control seborrhea or seborrheic dermatitis. Antiseborrheic preparations usually contain salicylic acid, resorcinol, sulfur, selenium sulfide, pyrithione zinc, or benzalkonium chloride.

antisense /an′tēsens/, (molecular genetics) an RNA molecule that is complementary to the mRNA (sense) molecule produced by transcription of a given gene. The antisense strands of many genes have been synthesized in the laboratory and are useful because they hybridize with the mRNA sense strand and block their translation into amino acids and proteins.

antisepsis /-sep′sis/ [Gk, *anti* + *sepein,* putrefaction], destruction of microorganisms to prevent infection.

antiseptic /-sep′tik/, **1.** tending to inhibit the growth and reproduction of microorganisms. **2.** a substance that tends to inhibit the growth and reproduction of microorganisms.

antiseptic dressing, a dressing treated with an antiseptic, germicide, or bacteriostat, applied to a wound or an incision to prevent or treat infection.

antiseptic gauze, gauze permeated with an antiseptic solution, sometimes packaged in individual, sealed packets.

antiserum /an′tisir′əm/, *pl.* **antisera, antiserums** [Gk, *anti* + L, whey], serum of an animal or human containing antibodies against a specific disease, used to confer passive immunity to that disease. Antisera do not provoke the production of antibodies. There are two types of antiserum. Antitoxin is an antiserum that neutralizes the toxin produced by specific bacteria, but it does not kill the bacteria. Antimicrobial serum acts to destroy bacteria by making them more susceptible to the leukocytic action. Polyvalent antiserum acts on more than one strain of bacteria; univalent antiserum acts on only one strain. Antibiotic drugs have largely replaced antimicrobial antisera. Caution is always to be used in giving antiserum of any kind, as hepatitis or hypersensitivity reactions can occur. Also called **immune serum.** Compare **vaccine.**

antiserum anaphylaxis, an exaggerated reaction of hypersensitivity in a normal person caused by the injection of serum from a sensitized individual. Also called **passive anaphylaxis.**

antiserums. See **antiseptic gauze.**

antisialogogue /-sī·al′əgōg′/ [Gk, *anti* + *sialon,* saliva + *agogos,* leading], a drug that reduces saliva secretion.

antisocial personality /-sō′shəl/ [Gk, *anti* + L, *socius,* companion], a person who exhibits attitudes and overt behavior contrary to the customs, standards, and moral principles accepted by society. Also called **psychopathic personality, sociopathic personality.** See also **antisocial personality disorder.**

antisocial personality disorder, a condition characterized by repetitive behavioral patterns that lack moral and ethical standards and bring a person into continuous conflict with society. Symptoms include aggressiveness, callousness, impulsiveness, irresponsibility, hostility, a low frustration level, a marked emotional immaturity, and poor judgment. A person who has this disorder neglects the rights of others, is incapable of loyalty to others or to social values, is unable to feel guilt or to learn from experience, is impervious to punishment, and tends to rationalize his behavior or to blame it on others. Also called **antisocial reaction.** See also **psychopathic.**

antisocial reaction. See **antisocial personality disorder.**

antispasmodic /-spazmod′ik/, a drug or other agent that prevents smooth muscle spasms, as in the uterus, digestive system, or urinary tract. Belladonna and dicyclomine hydrochloride are among drugs used in antispasmodic preparations.

antistreptolysin-O test (ASOT, ASLT) /an′tistrep′təli′sinō′/, a streptococcal antibody test for finding and measuring serum antibodies to streptolysin-O, an exotoxin produced by most group A and some group C and G streptococci. The test is often used as an aid in the diagnosis of rheumatic fever and glomerulonephritis. A low titer of antistreptolysin-O antibody is present in most people, since streptococcal infection is common. Elevated or increasing titers indicate a recent infection. The normal findings for adults are equal to or less than 160 Todd units/ml. See also **Lancefield's classification.**

antithermic. See **antipyretic.**

antithymocyte globulin (ATG) /an′tithī′məsīt/, a gamma globulin fraction rendered immune to T lymphocytes.

antithyroid drug /-thī′roid/, any one of several preparations that can inhibit the synthesis of thyroid hormones and are commonly used in the treatment of hyperthyroidism. The major antithyroid drugs are thioamides, such as propylthiouracil, and methimazole.In the body such substances interfere with the incorporation of iodine into the tyrosyl residues of thyroglobulin required for the production of the hormones thyroxine and triiodothyronine. These drugs are often used to control hyperthyroidism during an anticipated remission and before a thyroidectomy. Such substances cross the placenta, can cause fetal hypothyroidism and goiter, and are contraindicated for mothers who breast-feed their children.

antitoxin /-tok′sin/ [Gk, *anti* + *toxikon*, poison], a subgroup of antisera usually prepared from the serum of horses immunized against a particular toxin-producing organism, such as botulism antitoxin given therapeutically in botulism and tetanus and diphtheria antitoxin given prophylactically to prevent those infections.

antitrust /-trust′/, (in law) against the operation, establishment, or maintenance of a monopoly in the manufacture, production, or sale of a commodity, providing of a service, or practice of a profession.

antitrypsin /-trip′sin/, a protein, produced in the liver, that blocks the action of trypsin and other proteolytic enzymes. A deficiency of antitrypsin is associated with emphysema, in which the basic lesion is believed to result from effects of proteolytic enzymes on the walls of the alveoli. Also called **alpha-antitrypsin.**

antitubercular /-tōōbur′kyələr/, any agent or any of a group of drugs used to treat tuberculosis. At least two drugs, and usually three, are required in various combinations in pulmonary tuberculosis therapy. They include isoniazid (INH), ethambutol (EMB), streptomycin (SM), and rifampin (RMP). Supplements of pyridoxine (vitamin B$_6$) also may be needed to relieve the symptoms of peripheral neuritis that can occur as an INH side effect.

antitussive /an′titus′iv/ [Gk, *anti* + L, *tussive*, cough], **1.** against a cough. **2.** any of a large group of narcotic and nonnarcotic drugs that act on the central and peripheral nervous systems to suppress the cough reflex. Because the cough reflex is necessary for clearing the upper respiratory tract of obstructive secretions, antitussives should not be used with a productive cough. Codeine and hydrocodone are potent narcotic antitussives. Dextromethorphan is an equally effective antitussive with no dependence liability. Antitussives are administered orally, usually in a syrup with a mucolytic or expectorant and alcohol, or, sometimes, in a capsule with an antihistaminic and a mild analgesic.

antivenin /an′tiven′in/ [Gk, *anti* + L, *venenum*, poison], a suspension of venom-neutralizing antibodies prepared from the serum of immunized horses. Antivenin confers passive immunity and is given as a part of emergency first aid for various snake and insect bites. Also called **antivenom.**

Antivert, a trademark for an antihistamine (meclizine hydrochloride).

antiviral, destructive to viruses.

antivitamin [Gk, *anti* + L, *vita*, life, amine], a substance that inactivates a vitamin.

antixerophthalmic vitamin See **vitamin A.**

Anton's syndrome, a form of anosognosia in which a person with partial or total blindness denies being visually impaired, despite medical evidence to the contrary. The patient typically contrives excuses for the inability to see, suggesting, for example, that the light is inadequate.

antr-. See **antro-.**

antral gastritis [Gk, *antron*, cave], an abnormal narrowing of the antrum, or distal portion of the stomach. The narrowing is not a true gastritis, but a radiographic finding that may represent gastric ulcer or tumor.

antro-, antr-, a prefix meaning 'pertaining to an antrum or sinus': *antrocele, antrodynia, antrophore*.

antrum cardiacum /an′trəm/, a constricted passage from the esophagus to the stomach, lying just inside the opening formed by the cardiac sphincter.

antrum of Highmore. See **maxillary sinus.**

Anturane, a trademark for a uricosuric (sulfinpyrazone).

ANUG, abbreviation for **acute necrotizing ulcerative gingivitis.**

anular /an′yələr/ [L, *annulus*, ring], describing a ring-shaped lesion surrounding a clear, normal, unaffected disk of skin.

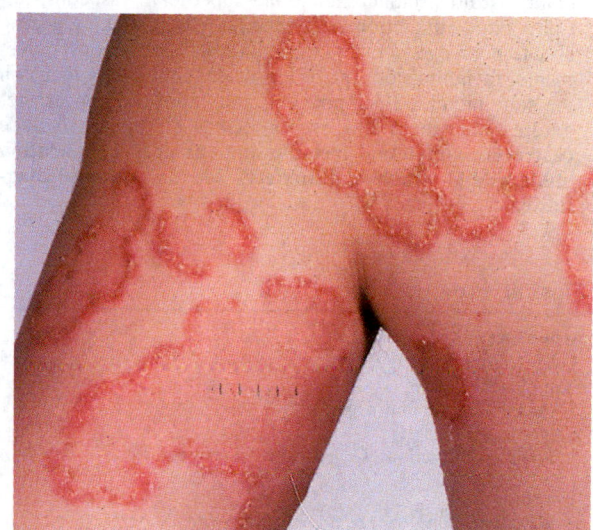

Anular psoriasis (du Vivier, 1993)

anular ligament, a ligament that encircles the head of the radius and holds it in the radial notch of the ulna. Distal to the notch, the anular ligament forms a complete fibrous ring.

anulus /an′yələs/, a ring of circular tissue, such as the whitish tympanic anulus around the perimeter of the tympanic membrane.

anuresis. See **anuria.**

anuria /ənōōr′ē·ə/ [Gk, *a, ouron*, not urine], the cessation of urine production, or a urinary output of less than 100 ml per day. Anuria may be caused by kidney failure or dysfunction, a decline in blood pressure below that required to maintain filtration pressure in the kidney, or an obstruction in the urinary passages. A rapid decline in urinary output, leading ultimately to anuria and uremia, occurs in acute renal failure. Kinds of anuria include **angioneurotic anuria, calculus anuria, obstructive anuria, postrenal anuria, prerenal anuria,** and **renal anuria.** Also called **anuresis** /an′yōōrē′sis/. **–anuric, anuretic,** *adj*. Compare **oliguria.**

anus /ā′nəs/, the opening at the terminal end of the anal canal.

anxietas /angzī′ətas/ [L, anxiety], a state of anxiety, nervous restlessness, or apprehension, often accompanied by a feeling of oppression in the epigastrium. Kinds of anxietas are **anxietas presenilis** and **restless legs syndrome.**

anxietas presenilis [L, *anxietas; prae,* before, *senex,* aged], a state of extreme anxiety associated with the climacteric period of life.

anxietas tibiarum.   See **restless legs syndrome.**

anxiety /angzī′ətē/ [L *anxietas*], a nursing diagnosis accepted by the Fifth National Conference on the Classification of Nursing Diagnoses. Anxiety is defined as a vague, uneasy feeling, the source of which is often nonspecific or unknown to the individual. The defining characteristics of the condition may be subjective or objective. The subjective characteristics include increased tension, apprehension, painful and persistent increased helplessness, feelings of uncertainty and inadequacy, fear, feelings of overexcitedness, distress, jitteriness, and worry. Objective characteristics include cardiovascular excitation, superficial vasoconstriction, pupil dilatation, restlessness, insomnia, glancing about, poor eye contact, trembling and extraneous movements, facial tension, quivering voice, continuous focus on the self, increased perspiration, and expressed concern regarding change in life events. Kinds of anxiety include **castration anxiety, free-floating anxiety, separation anxiety,** and **situational anxiety.** See also **nursing diagnosis.**

Signs of anxiety

Appearance
↑ Muscle tension (rigidity)
Skin blanches, pales
↑ Perspiration, clammy skin
Fatigue
↑ Small motor activity (e.g., restlessness, tremor)

Behavior
↓ Attention span
↓ Ability to follow directions
↑ Acting out
↑ Somatizing
↑ Immobility

Conversation
↑ Number of questions
Constantly seeks of reassurance
Frequently shifts topics of conversation
Describes fears with sense of helplessness
Avoids focusing on feelings
Focuses on equipment or procedures

Physiologic signs mediated through autonomic nervous system
↑ Heart rate
↑ Rate or depth of respirations
Rapid extreme shifts in body temperature, blood pressure, menstrual flow
Diarrhea
Urinary urgency
Dryness of mouth
↓ Appetite
↑ Perspiration
Dilation of pupils

Signs of anxiety are dependent on the degree of anxiety. Mild anxiety heightens the use of capacities, whereas severe and panic states severely paralyze or overwork capacities.

anxiety attack. an acute, psychobiologic reaction manifested by intense anxiety and panic. Symptoms vary according to the individual and the intensity of the attack but typically include palpitations, shortness of breath, dizziness, faintness, profuse sweating, pallor of the face and extremities, GI discomfort, and a vague feeling of imminent death. Attacks usually occur suddenly, last from a few seconds to an hour or longer, and vary in frequency from several times a day to once a month. Treatment consists of reassurance, administration of a sedative, if necessary, and appropriate psychotherapy to identify the stresses perceived as threatening. See also **anxiety.**

anxiety complex.   See **castration anxiety.**

anxiety disorders, disorders characterized by persistent worry. The symptoms range from mild, chronic tenseness, with feelings of timidity, fatigue, apprehension, and indecisiveness, to more intense states of restlessness and irritability that may lead to aggressive acts or indecisiveness. In extreme cases, the overwhelming emotional discomfort is accompanied by physical reactions, including tremor, sustained muscle tension, tachycardia, dyspnea, hypertension, increased respiration, and profuse perspiration. Other physical signs include changes in skin color, nausea, vomiting, diarrhea, restlessness, immobilization, insomnia, and changes in appetite, all occurring without underlying organic cause. The symptoms of anxiety may be controlled with medication, such as tranquilizers, but psychotherapy is the preferred treatment. See also **anxiety reaction, anxiety state.** See also **anxiety, anxiety attack.**

anxiety dream, a dream that occurs during rapid-eye-movement (REM) sleep and is accompanied by restlessness and a gradual increase in pulse rate. Anxiety dreams tend to occur in children, who usually recall the content clearly.

anxiety hysteria [L, *anxietas;* Gk, *hystera,* womb], a disorder characterized by symptoms of both anxiety and hysteria. See also **anxiety, hysteria.**

anxiety neurosis, a neurotic disorder characterized by persistent anxiety. The symptoms range from mild, chronic tenseness, with feelings of timidity, fatigue, apprehension, and indecisiveness, to more intense states of restlessness and irritability that may lead to aggressive acts or indecisiveness. In extreme cases, the overwhelming emotional discomfort is accompanied by physical reactions, including tremor, sustained muscle tension, tachycardia, dyspnea, hypertension, increased respiration, and profuse perspiration. Other physical signs include changes in skin color, nausea, vomiting, diarrhea, restlessness, immobilization, insomnia, and changes in appetite, all occurring without underlying organic cause. The symptoms of anxiety may be controlled with medication, such as tranquilizers, but psychotherapy is the preferred treatment and sometimes cures the neurosis. Also called **anxiety reaction, anxiety state.** See also **anxiety, anxiety attack.**

anxiety reaction [L, *anxietas* + *re, agere,* to act], any of a group of disorders in which anxiety is the predominant characteristic, or is experienced by a person facing a dreaded situation to the extent that the individual's functioning is impaired. The reaction may be expressed as a panic disorder, a phobia, or a compulsion.

anxiety state [L, *anxietas* + *state*], a mental reaction characterized by apprehension, uncertainty, and fear. Anxiety states may be accompanied by physiologic changes as sweating and tremors.

anxiolytic /angk′sē·ōlit′ik/,   a sedative or minor tranquilizer used primarily to treat episodes of anxiety. Kinds of anxiolytics include barbiturates, benzodiazepines, chlormezanone, hydroxyzine, meprobamate, and tybamate.

AOA,   abbreviation for **Administration On Aging.**

AORN,   abbreviation for **Association of Operating Room Nurses.**

aorta /ā·ôr′tə/ [Gk, *aerein,* to raise],   the main trunk of the systemic arterial circulation, comprising four parts: the ascending aorta, the arch of the aorta, the thoracic portion of the descending aorta, and the abdominal portion of the descending aorta. It starts at the aortic opening of the left ventricle, where it has a diameter of about 3 cm, rises a short distance toward the neck, bends to the left and dorsally over the root of the left lung, descends within the thorax on the left side of the vertebral column, and passes through the aortic hiatus of the diaphragm into the abdominal cavity. Opposite the caudal border of the fourth lumbar vertebra, it narrows to about 1.75 cm in diameter and branches into the two common iliac arteries.

aortic /ā·ôr′tik/ [Gk, *aerein,* to raise],   pertaining to the aorta.

aortic aneurysm,   a localized dilatation of the wall of the aorta caused by atherosclerosis, hypertension, or, less frequently, syphilis. The lesion may be a saccular distention, a fusiform or cylindroid swelling of a length of the vessel, or a longitudinal dissection between the outer and middle layers of the vessel wall. Syphilitic aneurysms almost always occur in the thoracic aorta and usually involve the aortic arch, while more common atherosclerotic aneurysms are usually in the abdominal section of the great vessel below the renal arteries and above the bifurcation of the aorta. These lesions often contain atheromatous ulcers covered by thrombi that may discharge emboli, causing obstruction of smaller vessels. See also **dissecting aneurysm.**

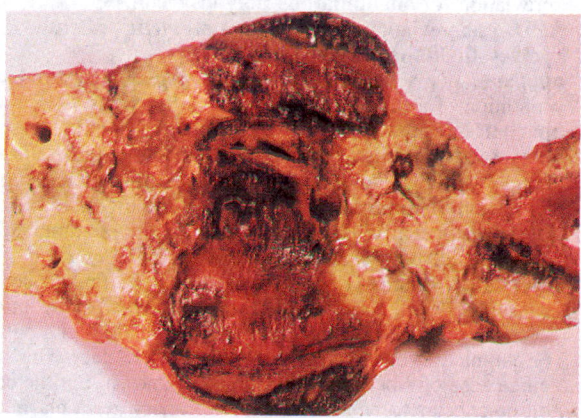

Aortic aneurysm *(McLaren, 1992/Courtesy Dr. HM Gilmore)*

aortic arch   See **arch of the aorta.**

aortic arch syndrome,   any of a group of occlusive conditions of the aortic arch producing a variety of symptoms related to obstruction of the large branch arteries, including the innominate, left common carotid, or left subclavian. Such conditions as atherosclerosis, Takayasu's arteritis, and syphilis may cause aortic arch syndrome. The symptoms include syncope, temporary blindness, hemiplegia, aphasia, and memory loss.

aortic atresia [Gk, *aerein + a, tresis,* a boring],   a congenital anomaly in which the left side of the heart is defective and there is an imperforation of the aortic valve.

aortic balloon pump.   See **intraaortic balloon pump.**

aortic body.   See **carotid body.**

aortic body reflex,   See **carotid body reflex.**

aortic insufficiency,   See **aortic regurgitation.**

aortic notch [Gk, *arein,* to raise; OFr, enochier],   the dicrotic notch on the descending limb of an arterial pulse sphygmogram. It marks the closure of the aortic valve and immediately precedes a dicrotic wave.

aortic regurgitant murmur [Gk, *arein,* to raise; L, *re,* again, *gurgitare,* to flow + *murmur,* humming],   a heart murmur that is a sign of aortic incompetence. A failure of the aortic valves to close completely during ventricular diastole allows some blood to flow back into the left ventricle.

aortic regurgitation,   the flow of blood during systole from the aorta back into the left ventricle. Also called **aortic insufficiency.**

aortic sinus [Gk, *aerein,* to rise; L, *sinus,* little hollow],   any of three dilatations, one anterior and two posterior, between the aortic wall and the semilunar cusps of the aortic valve. Also called **Petit's sinuses, sinuses of Morgagni, Sinuses of Valsalva.**

aortic stenosis (AS) [Gk, *aerein + stenos,* narrow, *osis,* condition],   a cardiac anomaly characterized by a narrowing or stricture of the aortic valve secondary to congenital malformation or of fusion of the cusps, as may result from rheumatic fever. Aortic stenosis obstructs the flow of blood from the left ventricle into the aorta, causing decreased cardiac output and pulmonary vascular congestion. Clinical manifestations include faint peripheral pulses, exercise intolerance, anginal pain, and a systolic murmur. Diagnosis is confirmed by cardiac catheterization and echocardiography. Surgical repair is usually indicated, followed by frequent examinations because recurrence of the stenosis and bacterial endocarditis are relatively common sequelae. Children with aortic stenosis are usually restricted from strenuous, competitive sports activities. See also **congenital cardiac anomaly, valvular heart disease.**

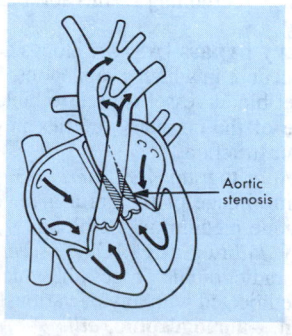

Aortic stenosis

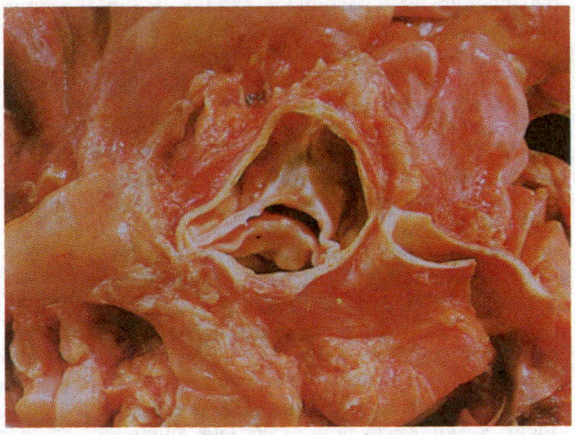

Aortic stenosis as seen from above (Fletcher, 1987)

aortic thrill [Gk, *aerein*, to rise; AS, *thyrlian*], a palpable chest vibration caused by stenosis of the aortic valve, or by an aortic aneurysm. It is usually felt or palpated in the second intercostal space to the right of the sternum in systole, by using the flat of the hand or the fingertips.

aortic valve, a valve in the heart between the left ventricle and the aorta. It is composed of three semilunar cusps that close in diastole to prevent blood from flowing back into the left ventricle from the aorta. The three cusps are separated by sinuses that resemble tiny buckets when they are filled with blood. These cup-shaped flaps grow from the lining of the aorta and, in systole, open to allow oxygenated blood to flow from the left ventricle into the aorta and on to the peripheral circulation. The right coronary artery arises from the sinus between the right posterior cusp of the valve and the aortic wall; the left coronary artery arises from the sinus of the left posterior cusp. The anterior cusp is the third flap of the valve. Compare **mitral valve, pulmonary valve, tricuspid valve.**

aortic valvular stenosis. See **subaortic stenosis.**

aortitis /ā′ôrtī′tis/, an inflammatory condition of the aorta, occurring most frequently in tertiary syphilis and occasionally in rheumatic fever. Kinds of aortitis are **rheumatic aortitis** and **syphilitic aortitis.**

aortocoronary /ā·ôr′tōkôr′əner′ē/ [Gk, *aerein* + L, *corona*, crown], pertaining to the aorta and coronary arteries.

aortocoronary bypass [AS, *bi*, alongside; Fr, *passer*], a surgical procedure in which a saphenous vein, mammary artery, or other blood vessel is used to build a shunt from the aorta to one of the coronary arteries in order to bypass a circulatory obstruction.

aortogram /ā·ôr′təgram/ [Gk, *aerein* + *gramma*, record], a radiographic image of the aorta made after the injection of a radiopaque medium in the blood.

aortography /ā·ôrtog′rəfē/ [Gk, *aerein* + *graphein*, to record], a radiographic process in which the aorta and its branches are injected with any of various contrast media for visualization. –**aortographic,** *adj.*

aortopulmonary fenestration /ā·ôr′tōpul′mənər′ē/ [Gk, *aerein* + L, *pulmoneus*, lung; *fenestra*, window], a congenital anomaly characterized by an abnormal fenestration in the ascending aorta and the pulmonary artery cephalad to the semilunar valve, allowing oxygenated and unoxygenated blood to mix, resulting in a decrease in the oxygen available in the peripheral circulation.

aosmic. See **anosmia.**

AOTA, abbreviation for **American Occupational Therapy Association.**

A.O.T.F., abbreviation for *American Occupational Therapy Foundation*.

ap-apo-. a prefix meaning 'separation or derivation from': *apeidosis, apenteric.*

A.P., abbreviation for **anteroposterior.**

APA, 1. abbreviation for **American Psychiatric Association.** 2. abbreviation for *American Psychological Association*.

apareunia /ā′pəro͞o′nē·ə/, an inability to perform sexual intercourse because of a physical or psychologic sexual dysfunction.

apathetic. See **apathy.**

apathetic hyperthyroidism /ap′əthet′ik/, a form of thyrotoxicosis that tends to affect mainly older adults who have stereotyped "senile" physical features and are apathetic and inactive rather than hyperkinetic in behavior. Medical treatment not only restores normal behavioral activity but also results in a loss of wrinkles and a younger physical appearance. Untreated, the patient is likely to succumb to the effects of stress or acute illness.

apathy /ap′əthē/ [Gk, *a, pathos*, not suffering], an absence or suppression of emotion, feeling, concern, or passion; an indifference to things found generally to be exciting or moving. The condition is commonly seen in patients with neurasthenic neurosis and schizophrenia. –**apathetic,** *adj.*

apatite /ap′ətīt/ [Gk, *apate*, deceit], an inorganic mineral composed of calcium and phosphate that is found in the bones and teeth.

APC, 1. abbreviation for **aspirin, phenacetin, caffeine.** 2. abbreviation for *atrial premature contraction*. 3. abbreviation for **adenomatous polyposis coli.**

APD, abbreviation for **adult polycystic disease.** See **polycystic kidney disease.**

apepsia /āpep′sē·ə/ [Gk, *a*, without, *pepsis*, digestion], a condition of a failure of the digestive functions.

aperient /əpir′ē·ənt/ [L, *aperire*, to open], a mild laxative.

aperistalsis /āper′istal′sis/ [Gk, *a*, without, *peristellein*, to clasp], a failure of the normal waves of contraction and relaxation that move contents through the digestive tract.

aperitive /əper′itiv/ [L, *aperere*, to open], a stimulant of the appetite. Also called **aperitif** /əper′itif/.

Apert's syndrome /operz′/ [Eugene Apert, French pediatrician, b. 1868], a rare condition characterized by an abnormal craniofacial appearance in combination with partial or complete syndactyly of the hands and the feet. The specific cause of Apert's syndrome is not known, but the condition appears to be the result of a primary germ plasm defect. Characteristic features of this condition include premature synostosis of the cranial bones, with resultant growth disturbances. Some signs of Apert's syndrome are a peaked and vertically elongated head, widespread and bulging eyes, and a high, arched posterior palate with bony defects of the maxilla and the mandible. The degree of syndactyly varies greatly and may be complete, with the apparent fusion of all the digits externally. The treatment of Apert's syndrome usually includes an osteotomy of the cranial bones to prevent increased intracranial pressure. The syndactyly may be surgically corrected, the specific procedure depending on the severity of the deformity. Also called **acrocephalosyndactylism.**

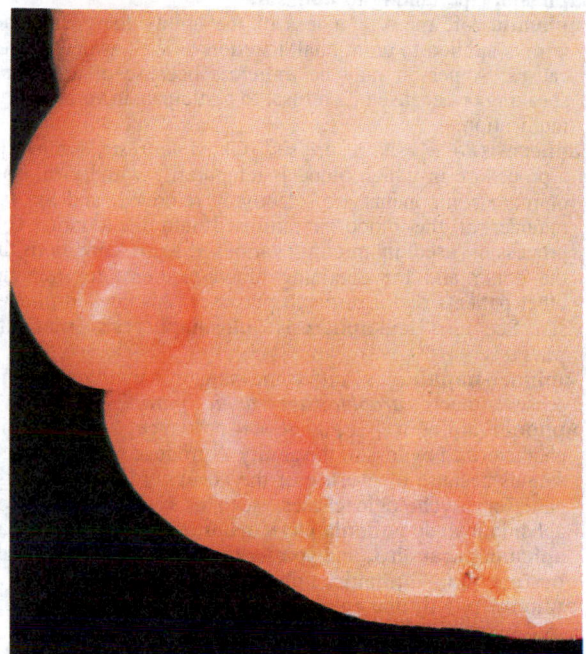

Syndactyly of the foot in Apert's syndrome
(Baran, 1991)

aperture /ap'ərchər/ [L, *apertura,* an opening], an opening or hole in an object or anatomic structure. See specific apertures.

aperture of frontal sinus, an external opening of the frontal sinus into the nasal cavity.

aperture of glottis, an opening between the true vocal cords and the arytenoid cartilages.

aperture of larynx, an opening between the pharynx and larynx.

aperture of sphenoid sinus, a round opening between the sphenoid sinus and nasal cavity, situated just above the superior nasal concha.

apex /ā'peks/, *pl.* **apices** /ā'pisēz/ [L, tip], the top, the end, or the tip of a structure, such as the apex of the heart or the apices of the teeth.

apex beat, a pulsation of the left ventricle of the heart, palpable and sometimes visible at the fifth intercostal space, approximately 9 cm to the left of the midline.

apexcardiogram /-kär'dē·əgram'/, a graphic representation of the pulsations of the chest over the heart in the region of the cardiac apex.

apex cordis [L, *apex + cordis,* of the heart], the pointed lower border of the heart. It is directed downward, forward, to the left, and usually located at the level of the fifth intercostal space.

apexification /-if'ikā'shən/ [L, *apex + facere,* to make], (in dentistry) the process of induced tooth root development, or apical closure of the root by the deposit of hard tissue.

apexigraph /āpek'sigraf'/, (in denistry) a device used for determining the position of the apex of a tooth root.

apex murmur [L, *apex,* summit + *murmur,* humming], a murmur heard best at the apex of the heart. Also called **apical murmur.**

apex pneumonia [L, *apex,* summit; Gk, *pnemon,* lung], pneumonia in which consolidation is limited to the upper lobe of one lung. Also called **apical pneumonia.**

apex pulmonis /pəlmō'nis/ [L, *apex + pulmoneus,* lung], the rounded upper border of each lung, projecting above the clavicle into the root of the neck.

Apgar score /ap'gär/ [Virginia Apgar, American anesthesiologist, b. 1909], the evaluation of an infant's physical condition, usually performed 1 minute and again 5 minutes after birth, based on a rating of five factors that reflect the infant's ability to adjust to extrauterine life. Virginia Apgar, M.D., developed the system for the rapid identification of infants requiring immediate intervention or transfer to an intensive care nursery.
■ METHOD: The infant's heart rate, respiratory effort, muscle tone, reflex irritability, and color are scored from a low value of 0 to a normal value of 2. The five scores are combined, and the totals at 1 minute and 5 minutes are noted; for example, Apgar 9/10 is a score of 9 at 1 minute and 10 at 5 minutes. See table below.
■ NURSING CONSIDERATIONS: A low 1-minute score requires immediate intervention, including the administration of oxygen, the clearing of the nasopharynx, and usually transfer to an intensive care nursery. A baby with a low score that persists at 5 minutes requires expert care, which may include assisted ventilation, umbilical catheterization, cardiac massage, blood gas evaluation, correction of acid-base deficit, or medication to reverse the effects of maternal medication.
■ OUTCOME CRITERIA: A score of 0 to 3 represents severe distress, a score of 4 to 7 indicates moderate distress, and a score of 7 to 10 indicates an absence of difficulty in adjusting to extrauterine life. The 5-minute total score is normally higher than the 1-minute score. Because a normal, vigor-

Infant evaluation at birth—Apgar scoring system

Sign	0	1	2
Heart rate	Absent	Slow, <100	>100
Respiratory effort	Absent	Weak cry, hyperventilates	Good, strong cry
Muscle tone	Limp	Some flexion of extremities	Well flexed
Reflex irritability (response to skin stimulation of feet)	No response	Some motion	Cry, sneeze
Color	Blue, pale	Body pink, extremities blue	Completely pink

From Wong, DL: Whaley and Wong's *Essentials of pediatric nursing,* ed 4, St Louis, 1993, Mosby.

ous, healthy newborn almost always has bluish hands and feet at 1 minute, the first score will include a 1 rather than a perfect 2; but at 5 minutes the blueness may have passed, and a score of 2 may be given. A 5-minute score of 0 to 1 correlates with a 50% neonatal mortality rate; infants who survive exhibit three times as many neurologic abnormalities at 1 year of age as do children with a 5-minute score of 7 or more.

APHA, abbreviation for *American Public Health Association.*

aphacia. See **aphakia.**

-aphacic. See **aphakia.**

aphagia /əfā′jē·ə/ [Gk, *a, phagein,* not to eat], a condition characterized by the loss of the ability to swallow as a result of organic or psychologic causes. A kind of aphagia is **aphagia algera.** See also **dysphagia.**

aphagia algera, a condition characterized by the refusal to eat or swallow because doing so causes pain.

aphakia /əfā′kē·ə/ [Gk, *a, phakos,* not lens], (in ophthalmology) a condition in which part or all of the crystalline lens of the eye is absent, usually because it has been surgically removed, as in the treatment of cataracts. Also called **aphacia** /əfā′shə/. −**aphakic, aphacic,** *adj.*

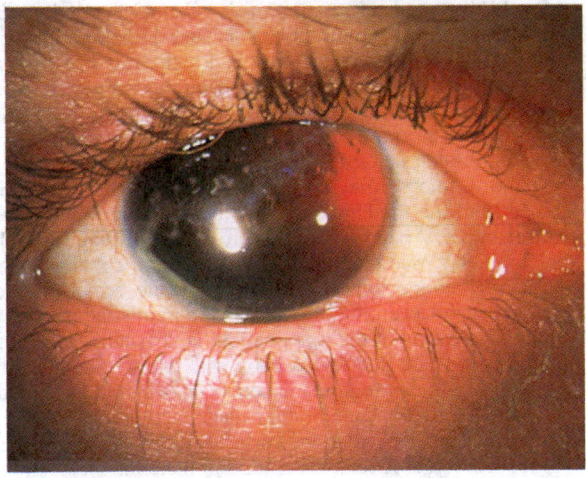

Aphakia (Eagling, 1986)

aphakic /əfākik/ [Gk, *a,* without, *phakos,* lens], pertaining to a condition in which the lens of the eye is absent because of congenital or surgical events.

aphasia /əfā′zhə/ [Gk, *a, phasis,* not speech], an abnormal neurologic condition in which language function is defective or absent because of an injury to certain areas of the cerebral cortex. The deficiency may be sensory or receptive, in which language is not understood, or expressive or motor, in which words cannot be formed or expressed. Sensory aphasia may be complete or partial, affecting specific language functions, as in dyslexia or alexia. Expressive aphasia may be complete, as in dysphasia, in which speech is impaired, or as in agraphia, in which writing is affected, or it may be partial, diminishing either or both functions. Most commonly, the condition is a mixture of incomplete expressive and receptive aphasia. It may occur after severe head trauma, prolonged hypoxia, or cardiovascular accident. It is sometimes transient, as when the swelling in the brain that follows a stroke or injury subsides and language returns. See also **Broca's area, Wernicke's aphasia.**

aphasic, pertaining to **aphasia.**

aphemia /əfē′mē·ə/, a loss of the ability to speak. The term is applied to emotional disorders as well as neurologic causes. A person may be **aphemic** because of a fear of speaking or because of a refusal to participate in verbal communication.

apheresis /əfer′əsis, af′ərē′sis/ [Gk, *aphairesis,* removal], a procedure in which blood is temporarily withdrawn, one or more components are selectively removed, and the remainder of the blood is reinfused into the donor. The process is used in treating various disease conditions in the donor and for obtaining blood elements for treating other patients or for research purposes. Also called **pheresis.** See also **leukapheresis, plasmapheresis, plateletpheresis.**

-aphia, -haphia, a suffix meaning a 'condition of the sense of touch': *araphia, hyperaphia, paraphia.*

aphonia /āfō′nē·ə/ [Gk, *a, phone,* not voice], a condition characterized by loss of the ability to produce normal speech sounds because of overuse of the vocal cords, organic disease, or psychologic causes, such as hysteria. Kinds of aphonia include **aphonia clericorum, aphonia paralytica, aphonia paranoica,** and **spastic aphonia.** See also **speech dysfunction.** −**aphonic, aphonous,** *adj.*

aphonia paralytica /par′əlit′ikə/, a condition characterized by a loss of the voice because of paralysis or disease of the laryngeal nerves.

aphonia paranoica, an inability to speak that lacks an organic basis and that is characteristic of some forms of mental illness.

-aphonic. See **aphonia.**

aphonic speech /āfon′ik/, abnormal speech in which vocalizations are whispered.

-aphonous. See **aphonia.**

aphoria /əfôr′ē·ə/, a condition in which physical weakness is not improved as a result of exercise.

aphrasia /əfā′zhə/, a form of aphasia in which a person may be able to speak single words or understand single words but is not able to communicate with words that are arranged in meaningful phrases or sentences.

-aphrodisia, a suffix meaning a '(specified) condition of sexual arousal': *anaphrodisia, hypaphrodisia.*

aphronia /əfrō′nē·ə/ [Gk, *a, phronein,* not to understand], (in psychiatry) a condition characterized by an impaired ability to make common-sense decisions. −**aphronic,** *n., adj.*

aphthae /af′thē/ [Gk, *aphtha,* eruption], a condition of shallow, painful ulcerations that usually affect the oral mucosa. Aphthae occasionally may affect other body tissues, including the GI tract and the external genitalia. See also **aphthous stomatitis, foot-and-mouth disease.**

aphthous [Gk, *aphtha,* eruption], pertaining to aphthae.

aphthous fever. See **foot-and-mouth disease.**

aphthous stomatitis /af′thəs/ [Gk, *aptha,* eruption; *stoma,* mouth, *itis* inflammation], a recurring condition characterized by the eruption of painful ulcers (commonly called canker sores) on the mucous membranes of the mouth. The cause is unknown, but there is evidence to suggest that aphthous stomatitis is an immune reaction. See also **canker sore.**

APIC, abbreviation for **Association for Practitioners of Infection Control.**

apical /ap'ikəl, ā'pi-/ [L, *apex*, tip], **1.** of or pertaining to the summit or apex. **2.** of or pertaining to the end of a tooth root.

apical curettage [L, *apex;* Fr, scraping], (in dentistry) debridement of the apical surface of a tooth and removal of diseased soft tissues in the surrounding bony crypt. Compare **apicoectomy, root curettage, subgingival curettage.**

apical fiber, any one of the many fibers of the periodontal ligament that radiate around the apex of the tooth.

apical lordotic view /lôrdot'ik/, a radiograph made by positioning the patient leaning backward at an angle of approximately 45 degrees to visualize the apices of the lung under the clavicle.

apical murmur. See **apex murmur.**

apical odontoid ligament /ōdon'toid/, a ligament connecting the axis to the occipital bone. It extends from the process of the axis to the anterior margin of the foramen magnum and lies between the two alar ligaments, blending with the anterior atlantooccipital membrane. It is considered a rudimentary intervertebral disk and contains traces of the embryonic notochord.

apical periodontitis [L, *apex*, summit; Gk, *peri*, near, *odous*, tooth, *itis*, inflammation], an inflammation around the apex of the root of a tooth.

apical pneumonia. See **apex pneumonia.**

apical pulse, the heart rate as auscultated with a stethoscope placed on the chest wall adjacent to the cardiac apex.

apicectomy /ap'isek'təmē/ [L, *apex* + Gk, *ektome* excision], the surgical removal of the apex or the apical portion of a tooth root, usually in conjunction with apical curettage or root canal therapy. Also called **root amputation, root resection.**

apices, plural of **apex.**

apituitarism /ā'pityo̅o̅'itəriz'əm/ [Gk, *a*, without + L, *pituita*, phlegm + Gk, *ismos*, a state], an absence or loss of function of the pituitary gland.

APKD, abbreviation for *adult polycystic kidney disease.* See also **polycystic kidney disease.**

aplasia /əplā'zhə/ [Gk *a, plassein* not to form], **1.** a developmental failure resulting in the absence of an organ or tissue. **2.** in hematology, a failure of the normal process of cell generation and development. See also **aplastic anemia, hyperplasia.**

aplasia cutis congenita [Gk, *a, plassein;* L, *cutis,* skin; *congenitus* born with], the congenital absence of a localized area of skin. The defect occurs predominantly on the scalp, less frequently on the limbs and trunk, and is usually covered by a thin, translucent membrane or scar tissue, or it may be raw and ulcerated. The condition is genetically transmitted, although the mode of inheritance is not known.

aplastic /āplas'tik/ [Gk *a, plassein* not to form], **1.** pertaining to the absence or defective development of a tissue or organ. **2.** failure of a tissue to produce normal daughter cells by mitosis. See also **aplastic anemia.**

aplastic anemia, a deficiency of all of the formed elements of the blood, representing a failure of the cell-generating capacity of the bone marrow. Neoplastic disease of the bone marrow, destruction of the bone marrow by exposure to toxic chemicals, ionizing radiation, or some antibiotics or other medications are common etiologies. An id-

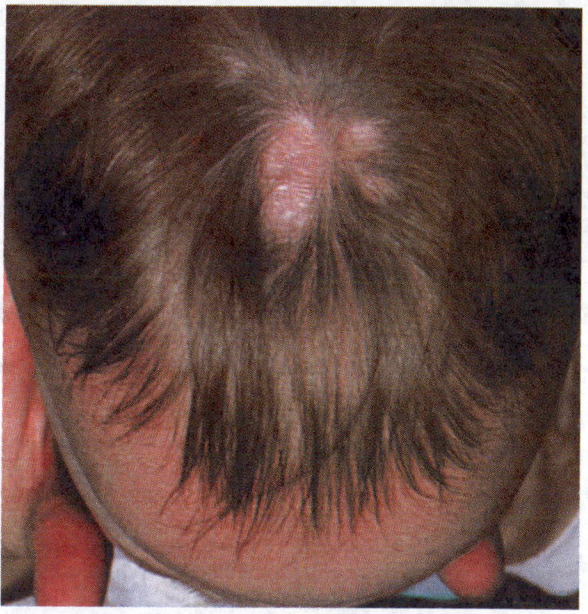

Aplasia cutis congentia *(Baran, 1991)*

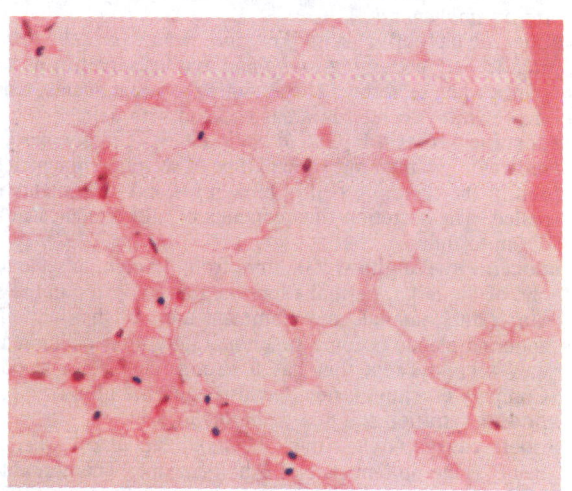

Aplastic anemia *(Hayhoe, 1992)*

iopathic form of the disease occurs rarely. Compare **alymphocytosis, hemolytic anemia, hypoplastic anemia.** See also **aleukia, leukopenia.**

Aplisol, a trademark for a tuberculin protein derivative used in the diagnosis of tuberculosis.

Aplitest, a trademark for a tuberculin protein derivative used in the diagnosis of tuberculosis.

APMA, abbreviation for *American Podiatric Medical Society.*

AP mobile projection. See **AP portable chest radiograph.**

apnea /apnē'ə, ap'nē·ə/ [Gk, *a, pnein,* not to breath], an absence of spontaneous respiration. Types of apnea include **cardiac apnea, deglutition apnea, periodic apnea of the**

newborn, primary apnea, reflex apnea, secondary apnea, and **sleep apnea. −apneic,** *adj.*

apnea alarm mattress [Gk, *a, pnein*, to breathe], a mattress for infants, designed to sound an alarm if the child stops breathing for a given period of time.

apnea monitoring, the act of closely observing the respiratory activity of individuals, particularly infants. The procedure may involve the use of electronic devices that detect changes in thoracic or abdominal movements and heart rate. Apneic detection devices may include an alarm that sounds if breathing stops. See also **apnea alarm mattress.**

-apneic. See **apnea.**

apneic oxygenation /apnē′ik/ [Gk, *a, pnein*, to breathe; *oxys*, sharp + *genein*, to produce], the maintenance of oxygen flow to the upper airway of patients with breathing difficulty.

apneustic breathing /apnoo′stik/ [Gk, *a, pneusis*, not breathing], a pattern of respirations characterized by a prolonged inspiratory phase followed by expiration apnea. The rate of apneustic breathing is usually around 1.5 cycles per minute.

apneustic center, an area of nerve tissue in the lower portion of the pons that controls the inspiratory phase of respiration. Disorders affecting the pons can result in abnormal stimulation of the apneustic center, marked by a gasping type of ventilation with maximum inspirations. Also called **pontine center.**

apo-, ap-, a prefix meaning 'separation or derivation from': *aponeurosis*.

apocrine /ap′əkrīn, -krin/ [Gk, *apo*, from + *krinein*, to separate], **1.** pertaining to a gland that loses part of its substance when secreting. **2.** pertaining to sweat glands, which are generally located in areas covered with hair.

apocrine secretion [Gk, *apo* + *krinein*; L, *secernere*, to separate], a mammary gland type of secretion in which the end of the secreting cell is broken off and its contents expelled. The secretion thus contains cellular granules in addition to fluid.

apocrine sweat gland [Gk, *apo*, from, *krinein*, to separate], one of the large, dermal exocrine glands located in the axillary, anal, genital, and mammary areas of the body. The apocrine glands become functional only after puberty, and they secrete sweat that has a strong, characteristic odor. Compare **eccrine gland.** See also **exocrine gland.**

apodial symmelia. See *sirenomelia*.

apoenzyme /ap′ō·en′zīm/ [Gk, *apo* + *en*, into, *zyme*, ferment], the protein part of a holoenzyme. The nonprotein part is the prosthetic group, which is usually permantly attached to the apoenzyme.

apogee /ap′əjē/ [Gk, *apo* + *ge*, earth], the climax of a disease or the period of greatest severity of signs and symptoms, usually followed by a crisis.

apolipoprotein /ap′ōlip′ōprō′tēn/ [Gk, *apo* + *lipos*, fat, *protos*, first], the protein component of lipoprotein complexes.

aponeurosis /ap′ōnoo̅ro̅′sis/, *pl.* **aponeuroses** [Gk, *apo* + *neuron*, nerve, sinew], a strong sheet of fibrous connective tissue that serves as a tendon to attach muscles to bone or as fascia to bind muscles together.

aponeurosis of the obliquus externus abdominis, the strong membrane that covers the entire ventral surface of the abdomen and lies superficial to the rectus abdominis. Fibers from both sides of the aponeurosis interlace in the midline to form the linea alba. The upper part of the apo-

neurosis serves as the inferior origin of the pectoralis major; the lower part ends in the inguinal ligament.

aponeurotic fascia /-noo̅rot′ik/ [Gk, *apo*, from + *neuron*, tendon], a thickened layer of connective tissue that provides attachment to a muscle.

apophyseal /ap′əfiz′ē·əl/, pertaining to an apophysis.

apophyseal fracture, a fracture that separates a projection of a bone from the main osseous tissue at a point of strong tendinous attachment.

apophysis /əpof′isis/ [Gk, a growing away], any small projection, process, or outgrowth, usually on a bone. Examples include the zygomatic apophysis of the temporal bone and the basilar apophysis of the occipital bone.

apophysitis /əpof′əsī′tis/, a condition characterized by the inflammation of an outgrowth or swelling, especially a bony outgrowth that is not separated from the bone. Apophysitis occurs most frequently as a disorder of the foot caused by disease of the epiphysis of the quadrangular bone at the back of the tarsus.

apoplexy /ap′əplek′sē/ [Gk, *apoplexia*, stroke], *obsolete.* a cerebrovascular accident, resulting in paralysis. **−apoplectic,** *adj.*

apoprotein /ap′ōprō′tēn/, a polypeptide chain not yet complexed to its specific prosthetic group.

apothecaries' measure /əpoth′əker′ēz/ [Gk, *apotheke*, a store], a system of graduated liquid volumes originally based on the minim, formerly equal to one drop of water but now standardized to 0.06 ml; 60 minims equals 1 fluid dram, 8 fluid drams equals 1 fluid ounce, 16 fluid ounces equals 1 pint, 2 pints equals 1 quart, 4 quarts equals 1 gallon. See also **apothecaries' weight, metric system.**

apothecaries' weight, a system of graduated amounts arranged in order of heaviness and based upon the grain, formerly equal to the weight of a plump grain of wheat but now standardized to 65 mg; 20 grains equals one scruple, 3 scruples equals 1 dram, 8 drams equals 1 ounce, 12 ounces equals 1 pound. Compare **avoirdupois weight.** See also **apothecaries' measure, metric system.**

apothecary /əpoth′əker′ē/ [Gk, *apotheke*, store], a pharmacist. See also **apothecaries' measure, apothecaries' weight.**

apparatus /ap′ərat′əs/ [L, *ad*, toward, *parare*, to make ready], a device or a system composed of different parts that act together to perform some special function.

apparent death. See **death.**

appendage /əpen′dij/ [L, *appendere*, to add something], an accessory structure attached to another part or organ. Also called **appendix.**

appendectomy /ap′əndek′təmē/ [L, *appendere* + Gk, *ektome*, excision], the surgical removal of the vermiform appendix through an incision in the right lower quadrant of the abdomen. The operation is performed in acute appendicitis to remove an inflamed appendix before it ruptures and prophylactically at the time of other abdominal surgery. Unless the appendix has perforated and peritonitis is present or suspected, postoperative care and nursing considerations are the same as for any other abdominal operation. If the appendix has perforated, a drain may be left in the incision, dressing changes are more frequent, and appropriate antibiotics are prescribed; ileus may be present and pain may be acute. Intravenous fluids, electrolytes, and analgesics are usually given. See also **abdominal surgery, peritonitis.**

appendiceal /ap′endish′əl/, of or pertaining to the vermiform appendix. Also **appendicial, appendical** /əpen′dikəl/.

appendiceal abscess. See **appendicular abscess.**

appendicial. See **appendiceal.**

appendices. See **appendix.**

appendices epiploicae. See **appendix epiploica.**

appendicitis /əpen′disī′tis/ [L, *appendere* + Gk, *itis*], inflammation of the vermiform appendix, usually acute, which if undiagnosed leads rapidly to perforation and peritonitis. The most common symptom is constant pain in the right lower quadrant of the abdomen around McBurney's point, which the patient describes as having begun as intermittent pain in midabdomen. To decrease the pain, the patient keeps knees bent to avoid tension of abdominal muscles. Appendicitis is characterized by vomiting, a low-grade fever of 99° to 102°, an elevated white blood count, rebound tenderness, a rigid abdomen, and decreased or absent bowel sounds. The inflammation is caused by an obstruction such as a hard mass of feces or a foreign body in the lumen of the appendix, fibrous disease of the bowel wall, an adhesion, or a parasitic infestation. Treatment is appendectomy, within 24 to 48 hours of the first symptoms because delay usually results in rupture and peritonitis as fecal matter is released into the peritoneal cavity. The fever rises sharply once peritonitis begins, and the patient may have sudden relief from pain followed by increased, diffuse pain. The nurse is alert to the other indications of peritonitis: increasing abdominal distention, tachycardia, rapid shallow breathing, and restlessness. If peritonitis is suspected, intravenous antibiotic therapy, fluids, and electrolytes are given. Appendicitis is most apt to occur in teenagers and young adults and is more frequent in males. A kind of appendicitis is **chronic appendicitis.** See also **McBurney's point, peritonitis.**

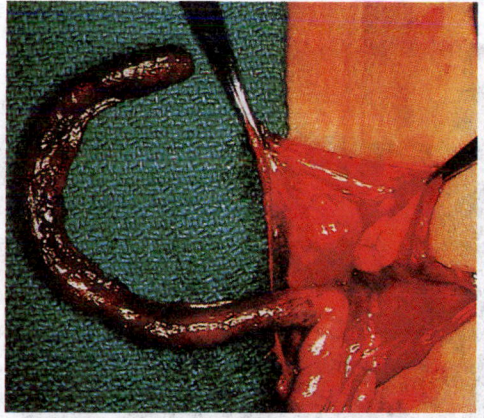

Acute appendicitis (*Zitelli, 1992*)

appendicitis pain [L, *appendere*, to hang upon + *poena*, penalty], severe general abdominal pain that develops rapidly and usually becomes localized in the lower right quadrant. It is accompanied by extreme tenderness over the right rectus muscle with rebound pain at McBurney's point. Occasionally, the pain is on the left side.

appendicular /ap′ǝndik′yǝlǝr/, **1.** pertaining to the vermiform appendix. **2.** pertaining to the limbs of the skeleton.

appendicular abscess, **1.** an abscess on a limb. **2.** an abscess of the vermiform appendix. Also called **appendiceal abscess.**

appendicular skeleton, the bones of the limbs and their girdles, attached to the axial skeleton. See also **axial skeleton.**

appendix /əpen′diks/, *pl.* **appendixes, appendices, 1.** an accessory part of a main structure. Also called **appendage. 2.** See **vermiform appendix.**

appendix dyspepsia [L, *appendere* + Gk, *dys,* difficult, *peptein,* to digest], an abnormal condition characterized by the impairment of the digestive function associated with chronic appendicitis. See also **dyspepsia.**

appendix epididymidis /ep′ididim′idis/, a cystic structure sometimes found on the head of the epididymis. It represents a remnant of the mesonephros.

appendix epiploica /əp′iplô′ikə/, *pl.* **appendices epiploicae** [L, *appendere* + Gk, *epiploon,* caul], one of the fat pads, 2 to 10 cm long, scattered through the peritoneum along the colon and the upper part of the rectum, especially along the transverse and the sigmoid parts of the colon.

appendixes. See **appendix.**

appendix vermiformis. See **vermiform appendix.**

apperception /ap′ərsep′shən/ [L, *ad,* toward, *percipere,* to perceive], **1.** mental perception or recognition. **2.** (in psychology) a conscious process of understanding or perceiving in terms of a person's previous knowledge, experiences, emotions, and memories. **–apperceptive,** *adj.*

appetite /ap′ətīt/ [L, *appetere,* to long for], a natural or instinctive desire, such as for food.

appliance /əplī′əns/ [L, *applicare,* to apply], a device or instrument designed for a specific purpose, such as a dental orthodontic appliance.

application /ap′likā′shən/, a computer procedure or problem to be processed, such as payroll, inventory, data about patients, scheduling of procedures and activities, pharmacy requisition and control, recording of nursing notes, or care planning.

applied. See **anatomy.**

applied anatomy /əplīd′/, the study of the structure and morphology of the organs of the body as it relates to the diagnosis and treatment of disease. Kinds of applied anatomy are **pathologic anatomy, radiologic anatomy,** and **surgical anatomy.** Also called **practical anatomy.** See also **comparative anatomy.**

applied chemistry, the application of the study of chemical elements and compounds to industry and the arts.

applied psychology, **1.** the interpretation of historical, literary, medical, or other data according to psychologic principles. **2.** any branch of psychology that emphasizes practical rather than theoretic approaches and objectives, such as clinical psychology, child psychology, industrial psychology, and educational psychology.

applied science. See **science.**

AP portable chest radiograph, a radiographic examination of the chest performed in the room of an immobilized patient with a portable x-ray machine. The film holder is placed behind the patient with the x-ray tube in front. The patient is positioned as upright as possible to allow for visualization of fluid levels in the lungs. Also called **AP mobile projection.**

apposition /ap′əsish′ən/ [L, *apponere,* to put to], the placing of objects in close proximity, as in the layering of tissue cells or juxtapositioning of facing surfaces side-by-side.

appositional growth, an increase in size by the addition of new tissue or similar material at the periphery of a particular part or structure, as in the addition of new layers in bone and tooth formation. Compare **interstitial growth.**

approach-approach conflict [L, *ad, propiare,* to draw near], a conflict resulting from the simultaneous presence of two or more incompatible impulses, desires, or goals, each of which is desirable. Also called **double-approach conflict.** See also **conflict.**

approach-avoidance conflict, a conflict resulting from the presence of a single goal or desire that is both desirable and undesirable. See also **conflict.**

appropriate for gestational age (AGA) infant /əprō′prē·it/ [L, *ad,* toward, *proprius,* ownership], a newborn infant whose size, growth, and maturation are normal for gestational age, whether delivered prematurely, at term, or later than term. Such infants, if born at term, fall within the average range of size and weight on intrauterine growth curves, measuring from 48 to 53 cm in length and weighing between 2700 and 4000 g.

approximate /əprok′simit/ [L, *ad, proximare,* to come near], to bring two tissue surfaces close together, as in the repair of a wound or to bring the bones of a joint together, as in physical therapy.

approximator /əprok′səmā′tər/, a medical instrument used to draw together the edges of divided tissues, as in closing a wound or in repairing a fractured rib.

apraxia /əprak′sē·ə/ [Gk, *a, pressein,* not to act], an impairment in the ability to perform purposeful acts or to manipulate objects. **Ideational apraxia** is characterized by impairment caused by a loss of the perception of the use of an object. **Motor apraxia** is characterized by an inability to use an object or perform a task without any loss of perception of the use of the object or the goal of the task. **Amnestic apraxia** is characterized by an inability to perform the function because of an inability to remember the command to perform it. **Apraxia of speech** is an articulatory disorder caused by brain damage and resulting in an inability to program the position of speech muscles and the sequence of muscle movements necessary to produce understandable speech. **–apraxic,** *adj.*

Apresoline Hydrochloride a trademark for an antihypertensive (hydralazine hydrochloride).

aprobarbital /ap′rōbär′bital/, an intermediate-acting barbiturate.
■ INDICATIONS: It is prescribed as a sedative-hypnotic for sedation and induction of sleep on a short-term basis.
■ CONTRAINDICATIONS: The drug is contraindicated for patients with a known sensitivity to barbiturates or with a history of porphyria.
■ ADVERSE EFFECTS: The most commonly reported adverse effects include nausea, vomiting, dizziness, nervousness, headache, skin rash, and purpura.

aprosody /āpros′odē/ [Gk, *a, prosodia,* not modulated voice], a speech defect characterized by the absence of the normal variations in pitch, intonation, and rhythm of word formation.

aprosopia /ā′prəsō′pē·ə/ [Gk, *aprosopos,* faceless], a congenital anomaly characterized by the absence of part or all of the facial structures. The condition is usually associated with other malformations.

APTA, abbreviation for *American Physical Therapy Association.*

aptitude /ap′tətyōōd/ [L, *aptitudo,* ability], a natural ability, tendency, talent, or capability to learn, understand, or acquire a particular skill; mental alertness.

aptitude test, any of a variety of standardized tests for measuring an individual's ability to learn certain skills. Compare **achievement test, intelligence test, personality test, psychologic test.**

apyretic /ā′pīret′ik/ [Gk, *a,* without, *pyretos,* fever], an afebrile condition.

apyrexia /ā′pīrek′sē·ə/ [Gk, *a,* without, *pyrexis,* fever], an absence or remission of fever.

aq. See **aqua.**

AQ, abbreviation for **achievement quotient.**

aqua (aq) /ā′kwə/, the Latin word for water.

aqua amnii. See **amniotic fluid.**

AquaMEPHYTON, a trademark for vitamin K (phytonadione).

aquaphobia /ā′kwəfō′bē·ə/ [L, *aqua,* water + Gk, *phobos,* fear], fear of water.

aquapuncture /-pungk′chər/ [L, *aqua,* water, *punctura,* puncture], the injection of water under the skin or spraying of a fine jet of water on the surface of the skin to relieve a mild irritation.

aquathermia pad, /-thur′ mē·ə/ a waterproof plastic or rubber pad that can be applied to areas of muscle sprain, edema, or mild inflamation. The pad contains channels through which heated or cooled water flows. The device is connected by hoses to a bedside control unit that contains a temperature regulator, a motor for circulating the water, and a reservoir of distilled water. Although generally safer than a conventional heating pad, the aquathermia pad should be checked periodically to avoid the risk of accidental burns. Also called **water flow pad.**

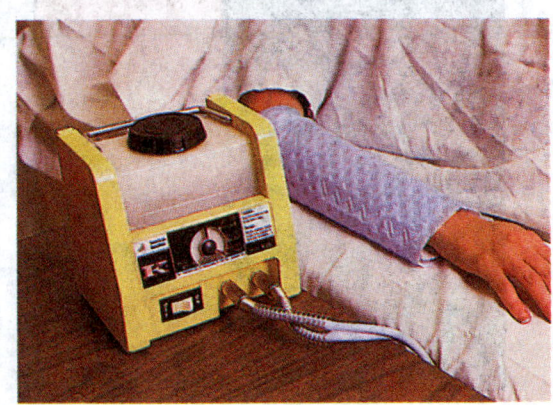

Aquathermia pad (Potter, 1993)

aqueduct /-dukt/ [L, *aqua,* water, *ductus,* act of leading], any canal, channel, or passage through or between body parts, as the aqueduct of Sylvius in the brain.

aqueduct of Sylvius. See **cerebral aqueduct.**

aqueductus /ak′wəduk′təs/, the Latin word for canal.

aqueous /ā′kwē·əs, ak′wē·əs/ [L, *aqua*], **1.** watery or waterlike. **2.** a medication prepared with water. See also **aqueous humor.**

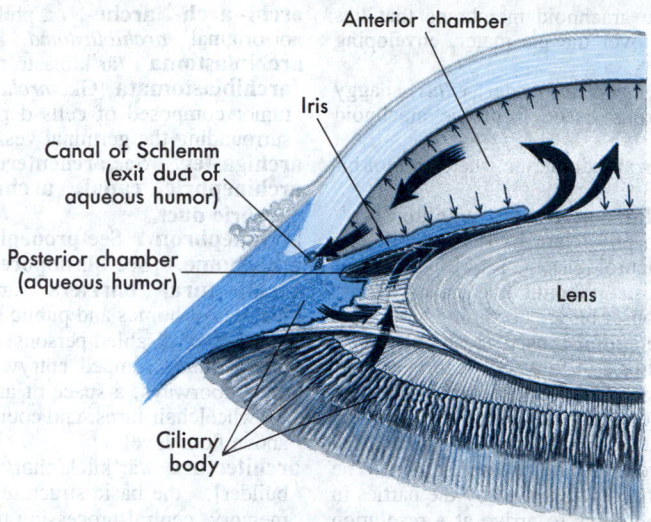

Anterior chamber

Iris

Canal of Schlemm (exit duct of aqueous humor)

Posterior chamber (aqueous humor)

Lens

Ciliary body

Aqueous chambers (Thibodeau, 1993/Ernest W Beck)

aqueous chambers [L, *aqua*, water + Gk, *kamara*, something with an arched cover], the anterior and posterior chambers of the eye, containing the aqueous humor.

aqueous humor, the clear, watery fluid circulating in the anterior and posterior chambers of the eye. It is produced by the ciliary processes and is reabsorbed into the venous system at the iridocorneal angle by means of the sinus venosus, or canal of Schlemm.

aqueous solution [L, *aqua*, water + *solutus*, dissolved], a homogenous liquid preparation of any substance dissolved in water.

Ar, symbol for the element **argon.**

AR, abbreviation for *assisted respiration*.

arabinosylcytosine. See **cytarabine.**

arachidonic acid /ar'əkidon'ik/ [L, *arachos*, a legume], an essential fatty acid that is a component of lecithin and a basic material for the biosynthesis of some prostaglandins.

arachnid [Gk, *arachne*, spider], pertaining to the animal class of Arachnida, which includes spiders, scorpions, mites, and ticks.

arachno-, arachn-, a combining form meaning 'pertaining to the arachnoid membrane or to a spider': *arachnoidal, arachnoidea.*

arachnodactyly /ərak'nōdak'tilē/ [Gk, *arachne*, spider, *dactylos,* finger], a congenital condition of having long, thin, spiderlike fingers and toes, which is seen in Marfan's syndrome.

arachnoid /ərak'noid/ [Gk, *arachne* + *eidos,* form], a delicate, fibrous structure resembling a cobweb or spiderweb, such as the arachnoid membrane. See also **arachnoid membrane. –arachnoidal,** *adj.*

arachnoidea encephali /ar'aknoi'dē·ə ensef'əlē/ [Gk, spiderweb; *enkephalos,* brain], the arachnoid membrane surrounding the brain. Also called **arachnoid of the brain, cranial arachnoid.**

arachnoidea spinalis [Gk, spiderweb; L *spina,* spine], a continuation of the arachnoid membrane of the brain, extending along the spinal cord as far as the cauda equina with sheaths that cover the various spinal nerves as they pass out-

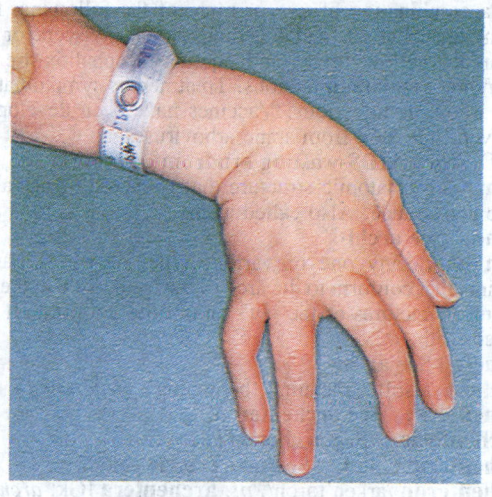

Arachnodactyly, as seen in Marfan's syndrome
(Zitelli, 1992)

ward to the intervertebral foramina. Also called **arachnoid of the spinal cord, spinal arachnoid.**

arachnoidism /ərak'noidiz'əm/ [Gk, *arachne*, spider, *eidos*, form], the condition produced by the bite of a venomous spider.

arachnoid membrane, a thin, delicate membrane enclosing the brain and the spinal cord, interposed between the pia mater and the dura mater. The subarachnoid space lies between the arachnoid membrane and the pia, and the subdural space lies between the arachnoid and the dura mater.

arachnoid of the brain. See **arachnoidea encephali.**

arachnoid of the spinal cord. See **arachnoidea spinalis.**

arachnoid sheath [Gk, *arachne*, spider + *eidos*, form; AS, *scaeth*], pertaining to the arachnoid membrane that lies under the dura mater and over the pia mater, enveloping the brain and spinal cord.

arachnoid villi /vil′ī/ [Gk, *arachne*, spider, *villus*, shaggy hair], projections of fibrous tissue from the arachnoid membrane.

Aramine, a trademark for an adrenergic (metaraminol bitartrate).

Aran-Duchenne muscular atrophy /aran′dōōshen′/ [François A. Aran, French physician, b. 1817; Guillaume B. A. Duchenne, French neurologist, b. 1806], a form of amyotrophic lateral sclerosis affecting the hands, arms, shoulders, and legs at the onset before becoming more generalized. Also **progressive spinal muscular atrophy.**

arbitrary inference /är′bitrer′ē in′fərəns/, a form of cognitive distortion in which a judgment based on insufficient evidence leads to an erroneous conclusion.

arbitrator /är′bətrā′tər/ [L, *arbiter*, umpire], an impartial person appointed to resolve a dispute between parties. The arbiter listens to the evidence as presented by the parties in an informal hearing and attempts to arrive at a resolution acceptable to both parties. –**arbitration,** *n*.

arborization test. See **ferning test.**

arbovirus /är′bōvī′rəs/, any one of more than 300 arthropod-borne viruses that cause infections characterized by a combination of two or more of the following: fever, rash, encephalitis, and bleeding into the viscera or skin. Dengue, yellow fever, and equine encephalitis are three common arboviral infections. Treatment is symptomatic for all arbovirus infections. Vaccines have been developed to prevent infection from some arboviruses.

ARC. See **AIDS-wasting syndrome.**

arch, any anatomic structure that is curved or has a bow-like appearance. Also called **arcus.**

arch-. See **archi-.**

arch bar, any one of various types of wires, bars, or splints that conform to the arch of the teeth, used in the treatment of fractures of the jaws and in the stabilization of injured teeth.

arche-. See **archi-.**

-arche, a suffix meaning 'beginning': *menarche*.

archentera. See **archenteron.**

-archenteric. See **archenteron.**

archenteric canal. See **neurenteric canal.**

archenteron /arken′təron/, *pl*. **archentera** [Gk, *arche*, beginning, *enteron*, intestine], the primitive digestive cavity formed by the invagination into the gastrula in the embryonic development of many animals. It corresponds to the tubular cavity in the vertebrates that connects the amniotic cavity with the yolk sac. Also called **archigaster, coelenteron, gastrocoele, primitive gut.** See also **gastrula.** –**archenteric,** *adj*.

arches of the foot [L, *arcus*, bow + AS, *fot*], the bony arches of the instep, including the longitudinal, or anteroposterior, and the transverse arches.

archeocortex. See **olfactory cortex.**

archetype /är′kətīp′/ [Gk, *arche* + *typos*, type], **1.** an original model or pattern from which a thing or group of things is made or evolves. **2.** (in analytic psychology) an inherited primordial idea or mode of thought derived from the experiences of the human race and present in the unconscious of the individual in the form of drives, moods, and concepts. See also **anima.** –**archetypal, archetypic, archetypical,** *adj*.

archi- arch-, arche-, a prefix meaning 'first, beginning, or original': *archiblastoma*.

archiblastoma /är′kiblastō′mə/, *pl*. **archiblastomas, archiblastomata** [Gk, *arche* + *blastos*, germ, *oma*], a tumor composed of cells derived from the layer of tissue surrounding the germinal vesicle.

archigaster. See **archenteron.**

archinephric canal, archinephric duct. See **pronephric duct.**

archinephron. See **pronephros.**

archistome. See **blastopore.**

architectural barriers /är′kətek′chərəl/, architectural features of homes and public buildings that limit access and mobility of disabled persons. Wheelchair access, for example, requires ramped entryways, a minimum of 32-inch-wide doorways, a space of at least 60 inches by 60 inches for wheelchair turns, and counters no more than 26.5 inches above floor level.

architecture /är′kitek′chər/ [Gk, *architekton*, master builder], the basic structure of a computer, including the memory, central processing unit, and input/output units.

architis /ärkī′tis/ [Gk, *archos*, anus, *itis*, inflammation], an inflammation of the anus. Also called **proctitis.**

arch length /ärch/, the length of a dental arch, usually measured through the points of contact between adjoining teeth. See also **available arch length.**

arch length deficiency, the difference in any dental arch between the required length to accommodate all the natural teeth and the actual space available.

archo-, a prefix meaning 'pertaining to the rectum or anus': *archocele, archoptoma, archostenosis*.

arch of the aorta, one of the four portions of the aorta, giving rise to three arterial branches called the innominate (brachiocephalic), left common carotid, and left subclavian arteries. The arch rises at the level of the cranial border of the second sternocostal articulation of the right side, passes to the left in front of the trachea, bends dorsally, and becomes part of the descending aorta. Also called **aortic arch.**

arch width, the width of a dental arch, which varies in all diameters between the left and right opposite teeth and is determined by direct measurement between the canines, the first molars, and the second premolars. The intercanine, interpremolar, and intermolar distances may be cited as the arch width.

arch wire, an orthodontic wire fastened to two or more teeth through fixed attachments, used to cause or guide tooth movement. See also **full-arch wire, sectional arch wire.**

arcing spring contraceptive diaphragm /är′king/, a kind of contraceptive diaphragm in which the flexible metal spring that forms the rim is a combination of a flexible coil spring and a flat band spring made of stainless steel. The rubber dome is approximately 4 cm deep, and the diameter of the rubber-covered rim is between 5.5 and 10 cm. Ten sizes, in increments of 0.5 cm, allow the clinician to fit the diaphragm to each individual woman. The kind of spring and the size of the rim in millimeters are stamped on the rim, for example, 75 mm arcing spring. This kind of diaphragm is prescribed for a woman whose vaginal musculature is relaxed and does not afford strong support, as in first-degree cystocele, rectocele, or uterine prolapse. Compare **coil-spring contraceptive diaphragm, flat spring contraceptive diaphragm.** See also **contraceptive diaphragm fitting.**

arcuate /är'kyoo·at/ [L, *arcuare, to bow*], an arch or bow shape.

arcuate scotoma [L *arcuatus* bowed; Gk, *skotoma*, darkness], an arc-shaped blind area that may develop in the field of vision of a person with glaucoma. It is caused by damage to nerve fibers in the retina.

arcus. See **arch.**

arcus senilis /senē'lis/ [L, bow, aged], an opaque ring, gray to white in color, that surrounds the periphery of the cornea. The condition is caused by deposits of fat granules in the cornea or hyaline degeneration and occurs primarily in older persons. Also called **gerontoxon.**

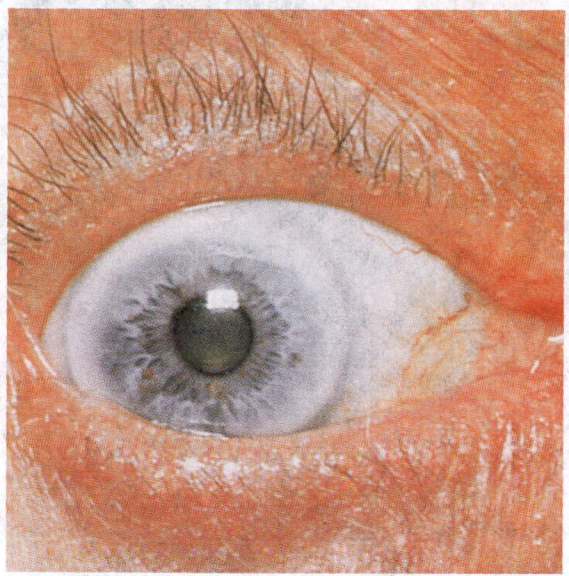

Arcus senilis (Kamal, 1991)

ARDS, abbreviation for **acute respiratory distress syndrome.**

area /er'ē·ə/ [L, space], (in anatomy) a limited anatomic space that contains a specific structure of the body or within which certain physiologic functions predominate, such as the aortic area and the association areas of the cerebral cortex.

area under the concentration curve (AUC), a method of measurement of the bioavailability of a drug based on a plot of blood concentrations sampled at frequent intervals. It is directly proportional to the total amount of unaltered drug in the patient's blood.

areflexia /ā'rēflek'sē·ə/, the absence of the reflexes.

Arenavirus /er'inəvī'rəs/, a genus of viruses usually transmitted to humans by oral or cutaneous contact with the excreta of wild rodents. Individual arenaviruses are identified with specific geographic areas, such as **Bolivian hemorrhagic fever** in one river valley in Bolivia, **Lassa fever** in Nigeria, Liberia, and Sierra Leone, and **Argentine hemorrhagic fever** in two agricultural provinces in Argentina. Arenavirus infections are characterized by slow onset, fever, muscle pain, rash, petechiae, hemorrhage, delirium, hypotension, and ulcers of the mouth. Treatment is supportive; there is no specific antimicrobial agent or vaccine. Fluid

and electrolyte balance, rest, and adequate nutrition are the goals of treatment.

areola /erē'ōlə/, *pl.* **areolae, 1.** a small space or a cavity within a tissue. **2.** a circular area of a different color surrounding a central feature, such as the discoloration about a pustule or vesicle. **3.** the part of the iris around the pupil.

areola mammae /mam'ē/, the pigmented, circular area surrounding the nipple of each breast. Also called **areola papillaris.**

areolar /erē'ələr/ [L, *areola*, little space], pertaining to areola.

areolar gland one of the large sebaceous glands in the areolae encircling the nipples on the breasts of women. The areolar glands secrete a lipoid fluid that lubricates and protects the nipple during nursing and contain smooth muscle bundles that cause the nipples to become erect when stimulated. Also called **gland of Montgomery.**

areolar tissue, a kind of connective tissue having little tensile strength and consisting of loosely woven fibers and areolae. Also called **fibroareolar tissue.** Compare **fibrous tissue.**

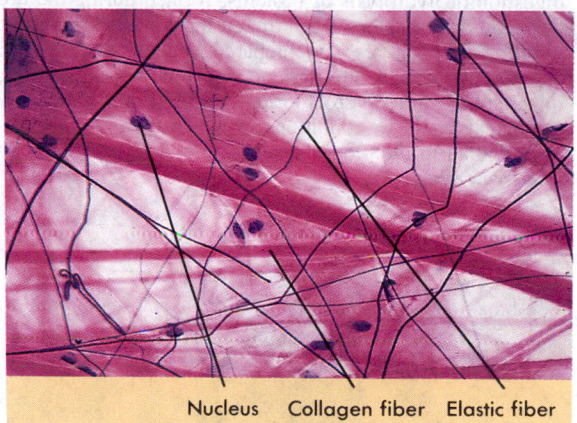

Nucleus   Collagen fiber   Elastic fiber

Areolar tissue (Seeley, 1992/Ed Reschke)

ARF, abbreviation for **acute respiratory failure.**

Arfonad, a trademark for a ganglion blocking agent antihypertensive (trimethaphan camsylate).

Arg, abbreviation for **arginine.**

argentaffin cell /är'jentaf'in/ [L, *argentum*, silver, *affinitas*, affinity], a cell containing serotonin-secreting granules that stain readily with silver and chromium parts. Such cells occur in most regions of the GI tract and are especially abundant in the crypts of Lieberkühn. Also called **enterochromaffin cell, Kulchitsky's cell.** See also **carcinoid, carcinoid syndrome.**

argentaffinoma /är'jentaf'inō'mə/, *pl.* **argentaffinomas, argentaffinomata,** a carcinoid tumor arising most often from argentaffin cells in epithelium of the crypts of Lieberkühn in the digestive tract. The neoplasm, which occurs primarily in middle-aged or elderly persons, may be a nodule or plaque in the early stage and a growth encircling the bowel in the later stage. Highly vascular tumors formed of silver-staining argentaffin cells may also develop in the bronchi.

argentaffinomata. See **argentaffinoma.**

argentaffinoma syndrome. See **carcinoid syndrome.**

Argentine hemorrhagic fever, an infectious disease caused by an arenavirus transmitted to humans by the ingestion of food contaminated by the excreta of infected rodents and by personal contact. Initially, it is characterized by chills, fever, headache, myalgia, anorexia, nausea, vomiting, and a general feeling of malaise. As the disease progresses, the victim may develop a high fever, dehydration, hypotension, flushed skin, abnormally slow heartbeat, bleeding from the gums and internal tissues, hematuria, and hematemesis. There may be involvement of the central nervous system, shock, and pulmonary edema. There is no specific treatment for the disease other than hydration, rest, warmth, and adequate nutrition. Rarely, intravenous fluids and dialysis are necessary. Usually, the prognosis is complete recovery. See also **Arenavirus, Bolivian hemorrhagic fever, Lassa fever.**

arginase /är′ginās/, an enzyme that catalyzes the hydrolysis of arginine during the urea cycle, producing urea and ornithine. The enzyme is found primarily in the liver but also occurs in the mammary gland, testes, and kidney.

arginine (Arg) /är′ginin/, an amino acid produced by the digestion or hydrolysis of proteins, formed during the urea cycle by the transfer of a nitrogen atom from aspartate to citrulline. It can also be prepared synthetically. Certain compounds made from arginine, especially arginine glutamate and arginine hydrochloride, are used intravenously in the management of conditions in which there is an excess of ammonia in the blood because of liver dysfunction. See also **urea cycle.**

Chemical structure of arginine (Seeley, 1992)

argininemia /är′jininē′mē·ə/, an autosomal recessive disorder characterized by an increased amount of arginine in the blood caused by a deficiency of arginase. Without arginase, ammonia cannot be metabolized into urea. Partial deficiency may result in hyperammonemia, metabolic alkalosis, convulsions, hepatomegaly, mental retardation, and growth failure; total deficiency is fatal.

argininosuccinic acidemia /är′jin′inō′suksin′ik/, an inherited amino acid metabolism disorder in which the lack of an enzyme, argininosuccinase, results in an excess of argininosuccinic acid in the blood. The condition is characterized by seizures and mental retardation. Treatment involves mainly a low-protein diet containing essential amino acids or amino acid analogs.

argon (Ar) /är′gon/ [Gk, *argos,* inactive], a colorless, odorless, chemically inactive gas and one of the six rare gases in the atmosphere. Its atomic weight is 39.95; its atomic number is 18. It forms no compounds.

Argyll Robertson pupil [Douglas M. C. L. Argyll Robertson, Scottish physician, b. 1837], a pupil that constricts on accommodation but not in response to light. It is most often seen with miosis and in advanced neurosyphilis.

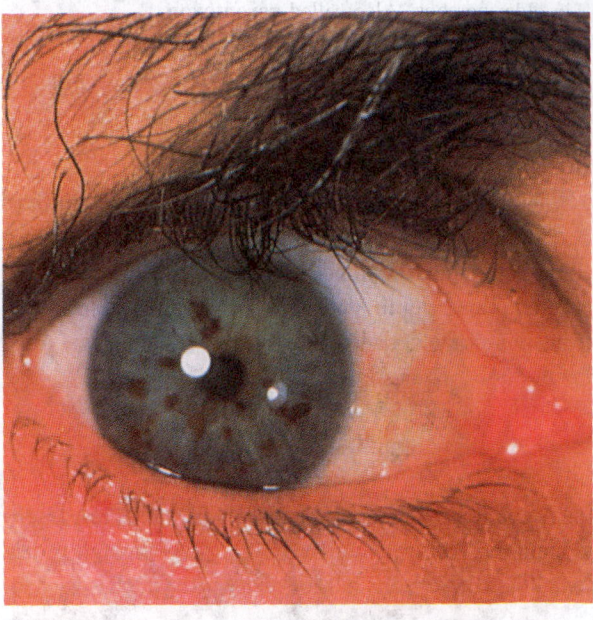

Argyll Robertson pupil (Epstein, 1992)

argyrophil /ärjī′rəfil/ [Gk, *argyros,* silver, *philein,* to love], a cell or other object that is easily stained or impregnated with silver.

arhythmia. See **arrhythmia.**

ariboflavinosis /ārī′bōflā′vinō′sis/ [Gk, a, not, ribose; L, *flavus,* yellow; Gk, *osis*], a condition caused by deficiency of vitamin B2 [0E] (riboflavin) in the diet and characterized by lesions at the corners of the mouth, on the lips, and around the nose and eyes, by seborrheic dermatitis, and by various visual disorders. See also **riboflavin.**

Arica therapy, an alternative mental health treatment introduced by Oscar Ichazo that focuses on altered states of consciousness with a goal of increasing the powers of the mind. It requires a 40-day training program of physical exercise and meditation, climaxed by a mild form of sensory deprivation during which the patient practices self-observation.

Aristocort, a trademark for a glucocorticoid (triamcinolone).

-arit, a combining form designating an antirheumatic drug.

arithmetic mean. See **mean.**

Arkansas stone /är′kənsô/, a fine-grained stone of novaculite, used for making hones with which surgical instruments may be sharpened.

Arlidin, a trademark for a peripheral vasodilator (nylidrin hydrochloride).

arm [L *armus*], **1.** a portion of the upper limb of the body between the shoulder and the elbow. The bone of the arm is the humerus. The muscles of the arm are the coracobrachialis, the biceps brachii, the brachialis, and the triceps brachii. Investing these structures is the brachial fascia. The arm is innervated by various nerves, such as the musculocutaneous nerve and the radial nerve, and is nourished by various arteries, such as the brachial artery and the radial collateral artery. **2.** *nontechnical.* the arm and the forearm. See also **shoulder joint.**

ARM, abbreviation for *artificial rupture of the (fetal) membranes.* Also spelled **AROM.** See also **amniotomy.**

armamentarium /är′məmenter′ē·əm/ [L, *armamentum*, implement], the total therapeutic assets of a physician or medical facility, including medicines and equipment.

arm board, 1. a board used to position the affected arm of a hemiplegic person. It fastens to the arm rest of a wheelchair, supporting the arm in correct position for subluxtion of the shoulder and flaccid arm, and to prevent edema. **2.** a board used to keep the arm still to permit the drawing of blood or for starting an intravenous needle.

arm bone. See **humerus.**

arm cylinder cast, an orthopedic device of plaster of paris or fiberglass, used for immobilizing the upper limb from the wrist to the upper arm. It is most often applied to aid the healing of a dislocated elbow, for postoperative immobilization or positioning of the elbow, or in the correction or the maintenance of a correction of a deformity of the elbow.

armpit. See **axilla.**

Army Nurse Corps (A.N.C.), a branch of the U.S. Army, founded February 2, 1901, with headquarters in Falls Church, Virginia.

Arnold-Chiari malformation /är′nəldkē·är′ē/ [Julius Arnold, German pathologist, b. 1835; Hans Chiari, French pathologist, b. 1851], a congenital herniation of the brainstem and lower cerebellum through the foramen magnum into the cervical vertebral canal, often associated with meningocele and spina bifida. See also **neural tube defect.**

-arol, a combining form designating a dicoumarol-type anticoagulant.

AROM, abbreviation for **active range of motion.**

aroma [Gk, spice], any agreeable odor or pleasing fragrance, especially of food, drink. spices, or medication.

aromatic /er′ōmat′ik/ [Gk, *aroma*, spice], **1.** pertaining to a strong but agreeable odor such as a spicy odor. **2.** a stimulant or spicy medicine.

aromatic alcohol, a fatty alcohol in which part of the hydrogen of the alcohol radical is replaced by a phenyl hydrocarbon.

aromatic ammonia spirit [Gk, *aroma, Ammon temple*, ancient source of ammonium chloride salt, *spiritus*, breath], a strongly fragrant solution of ammonium carbonate in dilute liquid ammonia, oils, alcohol, and water. It is used as a reflex stimulus, antacid, and carminitive. Also called **aromatic spirit of ammonia.**

aromatic bath, a medicated bath in which aromatic substances or essential oils are added to the water.

aromatic compounds, organic compounds that contain a benzene, naphthalene, or analogous ring. Many of these compounds have agreeable odors, which accounts for the origin of this term for such compounds.

aromatic hydrocarbon [Gk, *aroma*, spice; *hydor*, water; L, *carbo*, coal], an organic compound that has a benzene or quinoid ring, as distinguished from open-chain aliphatic compounds.

aromatic spirit of ammonia. See **aromatic ammonia spirit.**

arousal [OE, to rise], to awaken from sleep, to excite, or to evoke action or response to sensory stimuli.

arrest [L, *ad, resistare*, to withstand], to inhibit, restrain, or stop, as to arrest the course of a disease. See also **cardiac arrest.**

arrested dental caries, dental caries in which the area of decay has stopped progressing and infection is not present but in which the demineralized area in the tooth remains as a cavity. Also called **eburnation of dentin.**

arrested development, the cessation of one or more phases of the developmental process in utero before normal completion, resulting in congenital anomalies. Also called **developmental arrest.**

arrested labor [L, *ad, restare*, to withstand + *labor*, work], an interruption in the labor process that may be caused by an obstruction in the pelvis or lack of uterine contractions.

arrheno-, a prefix meaning 'male': *arrhenoblastoma, arrhenogenic, arrhenoplasm.*

arrhenoblastoma /erē′nōblastō′mə/ [Gk, *arrhen*, male, *blastos*, germ, *oma*, tumor], an ovarian neoplasm whose cells mimic those in testicular tubules and secrete male sex hormone, causing virilization in females. Also called **andreioma, andreoblastoma, androma, arrhenoma, Sertoli-Leydig cell tumor.**

arrhenogenic /erē′nōjen′ik/, producing only male offspring.

arrhenokaryon /erē′nōker′ē·on/ [Gk, *arrhen*, male, *karyon*, nucleus], an organism that is produced from an egg that has only paternal chromosomes.

arrhenoma. See **arrhenoblastoma.**

arrhythmia /ərith′mē·ə, ərith′mē·ə/ [Gk, *a, rhythmos*, not rhythm], any deviation from the normal pattern of the heartbeat. Kinds of arrhythmias include **atrial fibrillation, atrial flutter, heart block, premature atrial contraction,** and **sinus arrhythmia.** Also spelled **arhythmia.** Compare **dysrhythmia. –arrhythmic, arrhythmical,** *adj.*

arrhythmic [Gk, *a*, without, *rhythmos*, rhythm], pertaining to an absence or irregularity of normal rhythm.

ARRT, abbreviation for **American Registry of Radiologic Technologists.**

arsenic (As) /är′sənik/ [Gk, *arsen*, strong], an element that occurs throughout the earth's crust in metal arsenides, arsenious sulfides, and arsenious oxides. Its atomic number is 33; its atomic weight is 74.91. The arsenic atom occurs in the elemental form and in trivalent and pentavalent oxidation states. This element has been used for centuries as a therapeutic agent and as a poison and continues to have limited use in some trypanocidal drugs, as melarsoprol and tryparsamide. The introduction of nonarsenic trypanosomicides with less dangerous side effects in the treatment of trypanosomiasis has greatly reduced its use. Arsenic is usually not mined in raw form but recovered as a by-product from the smelting of copper, lead, zinc, and other ores. Such processes release arsenic into the environment, as does the leaching of large amounts of the element from the soil by mineral springs and the effluent from geothermal power plants. It is a component of coal, released during combustion. The environmental distribution of arsenic ensures its concentration in the food chain. The average concentration in the human adult is about 20 mg, an amount stored mainly in the liver, the kidney, the GI tract, and the lungs. The mechanisms for the biotransformation of arsenics in humans are not well understood. Most arsenics are slowly excreted in the urine and feces, which accounts for the toxicity of the element. **–arsenic** /ärsen′ik/, *adj.*

arsenic poisoning, poisoning caused by the ingestion or inhalation of arsenic or a substance containing arsenic, an ingredient in some pesticides, herbicides, dyes, and medicinal solutions. Small amounts absorbed over a period of time may result in chronic poisoning, producing nausea, headache, coloration and scaling of the skin, hyperkeratoses, anorexia, and white lines across the fingernails. Ingestion of large amounts of arsenic results in severe GI pain, diarrhea, vomiting, and swelling of the extremities. Renal failure and shock may occur, and death may result. Determination of the presence of arsenic in the urine, hair, or fingernails is diagnostic. Treatment may includes gastric lavage with water and administration of dimercaprol, intravenous fluid therapy, and other supportive treatment as indicated for anemia, renal failure, or shock.

arsenic stomatitis [Gk, *arsen,* strong; *stoma,* mouth, *itis,* inflammation], an abnormal oral condition associated with arsenic poisoning, characterized by dry, red, and painful oral mucosa, ulceration, purpura, and mobility of teeth. Compare **Atabrine stomatitis, bismuth stomatitis.** See also **arsenic poisoning.**

ART, abbreviation for **active resistance training.**

Artane, a trademark for an anticholinergic (trihexyphenidyl hydrochloride).

artefact, See **artifact.**

arteri-. See **arterio-.**

arteria alveolaris inferior. See **inferior alveolar artery.**

arterial /ärtir′ē·əl/ [Gk *arteria* airpipe], of or pertaining to an artery.

arterial bleeding [Gk, *arteria,* windpipe, ME, *blod*], loss of blood from an artery, an event usually characterized by blood that is bright red and spurting.

arterial blood gas (ABG), the oxygen and carbon dioxide in arterial blood, measured by various methods to assess the adequacy of ventilation and oxygenation and the acid-base status. Oxygen saturation of hemoglobin is normally 95% or higher. The partial pressure of oxygen (PaO_2[0E]), normally 80 to 100 mm Hg, is increased in hy-

Arterial blood gases

Respiratory function	Measurements	Normal value
Acid-base balance	pH-hydrogen ion concentration	7.35-7.45
Oxygenation	PaO_2: partial pressure of dissolved O_2 in blood	80-100 mm Hg
	SaO_2: percentage of O_2 bound to hemoglobin	95%-98%
Ventilation	$PaCO_2$: partial pressure of CO_2 dissolved in blood	38-45 mm Hg

From Phipps WF, Long BC, Woods NF, Cassmeyer VL: *Medical surgical nursing: concepts and clinical practice,* ed 4, St Louis, 1991, Mosby.

perventilation and decreased in cardiac decompensation, chronic obstructive pulmonary disease, and certain neuromuscular disorders. The carbon dioxide content, normally 46%, is increased in emphysema and aldosteronism and by severe vomiting; it is decreased in starvation, acute renal failure, diabetic acidosis, and severe diarrhea. Partial pressure of carbon dioxide ($PaCO_2$[0E]), normally 38 to 45 mm Hg, may be higher in emphysema, obstructive lung disease, and reduced function of the respiratory center and lower in pregnancy and in the presence of pulmonary emboli and anxiety. The normal pH of arterial blood is 7.4.

arterial blood pressure (ABP), the pressure of the blood in the arterial system, which depends upon the pumping pressure of the heart, the resistance of the arterial walls, the amount of blood, and its viscosity.

arterial capillaries, microscopic blood vessels (capillaries) extending beyond the terminal ends of arterioles.

arterial catheter [Gk, *arteria,* windpipe, *katheter,* a thing lowered into], a catheter that can be inserted into an artery either to draw blood or to measure blood pressure directly.

arterial circle of Willis. See **circle of Willis.**

arterial circulation [Gk, *arteria* + L, *circulare,* to go around], the movement of blood through the arteries directed away from the heart, as opposed to venous circulation.

arterial insufficiency, inadequate blood flow in arteries caused by occlusive atherosclerotic plaques or emboli, by damaged, diseased, or intrinsically weak vessels, by arteriovenous fistulas, by aneurysms, by hypercoagulability states, or by heavy use of tobacco. Signs of arterial inadequacy include pale, cyanotic, or mottled skin over the affected area, absent or decreased sensations, tingling, diminished sense of temperature, muscle pains, reduced or absent peripheral pulses, and, in advanced disease, atrophy of muscles of the involved extremity. Arterial insufficiency may be diagnosed by checking and comparing peripheral pulses in contralateral extremities, by angiography, by ultrasound using a Doppler device, and by skin temperature tests. Treatment of arterial insufficiency may include a diet low in saturated fats, moderate exercise, sleeping on a firm mattress, the use of a vasodilator, and, if indicated, surgical repair of an aneurysm or arteriovenous fistula. Smoking, prolonged standing, and sitting with the knees bent are discouraged.

arterial insufficiency of lower extremities, a condition characterized by hardening, thickening, and loss of elasticity of the walls of peripheral arteries causing decreased circulation, sensation, and function. Symptoms include sharp, cramping pain during exercise or rest at night, numbness, skin changes ranging from pallor to ulceration, and loss of hair on the legs. Pedal and popliteal pulses may be diminished or absent. Laboratory studies usually show elevated plasma lipids.

arterial line, an arterial blood monitoring system consisting of a catheter inserted into an artery and connected to pressure tubing and a transducer. The device permits continuous direct blood pressure readings as well as access to the blood supply when samples are needed for analysis.

arterial nephrosclerosis [Gk, *arteria,* windpipe + *nephros,* kidney, *sklera,* hard, *osis,* condition], arteriosclerosis of the kidney arteries, leading to deprivation of oxygenated blood to the kidney tissues and their destruction.

arterial network. See **rete arteriosum.**

arterial palpitation [Gk, *arteria,* windpipe; L, *palpitare,* to flutter], a palpitation felt in an artery.

arterial pH, the hydrogen ion concentration of arterial blood. Normal range is 7.35 to 7.45. The figure respresents a ratio of 20:1 between bicarbonate ions and carbon dioxide dissolved in the blood.

arterial pressure, the stress exerted by the circulating blood on the walls of the arteries. It is the product of the cardiac output and the systemic vascular resistance. A number of extrinsic and intrinsic factors regulate and maintain a reasonably constant arterial pressure. Extrinsic factors include neurologic stimulation, catecholamines, and prostaglandins and other hormones. Intrinsic factors include chemoreceptors and pressure-sensitive receptors in the arterial walls that cause vasoconstriction or vasodilatation. Arterial blood pressure is commonly measured with a sphygmomanometer and stethoscope. Stress, hypervolemia, hypovolemia, and various drugs may alter the arterial pressure.

arterial rete /rē′tē/ [Gk, *arteria,* windpipe; L, *rete,* net], a network of arteries and arterioles.

arterial sclerosis [Gk, *arteria,* windpipe + *sklerosis,* hardening], a thickening of the arteries. See **atherosclerosis.**

arterial tension, the pressure on artery walls caused by the force of blood being squeezed into the systemic circulation by contraction of the heart's left ventricle.

arterial wall, the fibrous muscular enclosure of the many vessels that carry oxygenated blood from the heart to structures throughout the body, and of the pulmonary arteries that carry venous blood from the heart to the lungs. The arteries, like the veins, are cylindric tubes enclosed by layers of different kinds of tissue. The inner layer is composed of a membrane of endothelium, a subendothelial layer of delicate connective tissue, and an internal elastic membrane. The endothelium of the inner layer is composed of a single layer of simple squamous cells and is continuous with the endothelium of the capillaries and the endocardium of the heart. The middle layer of tissue around each artery comprises most of the arterial wall and is composed of circular sheets of smooth muscle cells and elastic tissue. The outer layer consists of areolar connective tissue with a fine network of collagenous and elastic fibers. Most of the arteries in the body are of medium size, with a diameter of about 4 mm. The muscular coat is well developed, and nerves from the sympathetic system control the flow of blood into the areas served by the artery. The middle layer in smaller arteries is almost entirely muscular and in larger arteries is more elastic. The thickness of the outer layer varies with the location of the artery. In protected areas, such as the abdominal and cranial cavities, the outer layer of associated arteries is very thin, but in more exposed locations, as in the limbs, it is much thicker. Larger arteries have a thick inner layer, which in older people may contain atherosclerotic plaques of cholesterol and calcium salts or other pathologic deposits.

arteriectomy /ärtir′ē·ek′təmē/ [Gk, *arteria* + *ektome,* cutting out], the surgical removal of a portion of an artery.

arteries. See **blood vessel.**

arterio-, arteri-, a prefix meaning 'pertaining to an artery': *arteriosclerosis, arteriovenous, arteritis.*

arteriogram /ärtir′ē·əgram′/, an x-ray film of an artery injected with a radiopaque medium. See also **arteriography.**

arteriography /ärtir′ē·og′rəfē/ [Gk, *arteria,* airpipe, *graphein,* to record], a method of radiologic visualization of arteries performed after a radiopaque contrast medium is introduced into the bloodstream or into a specific vessel by injection or through a catheter. See also **angiography. – arteriographic,** *adj.*

arteriole /ärtir′ē·ōl/ [L, *arteriola,* little artery], the smallest vascular branch of the arterial circulation. Blood flowing from the heart is pumped through the arteries to the arterioles to the capillaries into the veins and returned to the heart. The muscular wall of the arterioles constricts and dilates in response to neurochemical stimuli; thus, arterioles play a significant role in peripheral vascular resistance and in regulation of blood pressure. Also called **arteriola.** See also **artery.**

arteriopathy /ärtir′ē·op′əthē/ [Gk, *arteria* + *pathos,* suffering], a disease of an artery.

arterioplasty /ärtir′ē·əplas′tē/ [Gk, *arteria* + *plassein,* to mold], plastic surgery of an artery. The procedure is often performed to correct an aneurysm.

arteriosclerosis /ärtir′ē·ō′sklərō′sis/ [Gk, *arteria* + *sklerosis,* hardening], a common arterial disorder characterized by thickening, loss of elasticity, and calcification of arterial walls, resulting in a decreased blood supply, especially to the cerebrum and lower extremities. The condition often develops with aging and in hypertension, nephrosclerosis, scleroderma, diabetes, and hyperlipidemia. Typical signs and symptoms include intermittent claudication, changes in skin temperature and color, altered peripheral pulses, bruits over an involved artery, headache, dizziness, and memory defects. Vasodilators and exercise may relieve symptoms, but there is no specific treatment for the disorder. Preventive measures include therapy of predisposing diseases, adequate rest and exercise, and avoidance of stress. Kinds of arteriosclerosis are **atherosclerosis** and **Mönckeberg's arteriosclerosis.**

arteriosclerosis obliterans [Gk, *arteria, skleros,* + L, *obliterare,* efface], a gradual narrowing of the arteries with degeneration of the intima and thrombosis. The condition may lead to complete occlusion of the artery and subsequent gangrene.

arteriosclerotic /-sklərot′ik/ [Gk, *arteria* + *skleros,* hard], pertaining to a thickening and hardening of the arterial wall.

arteriosclerotic heart disease (ASHD), a thickening and hardening of the walls of the coronary arteries.

arteriosclerotic retinopathy [Gk, *arteria,* windpipe + *sklerosis,* hardening; L, *rete,* net; Gk, *pathos,* disease], a disorder of the retina associated with hardening and thickening of the arteries supplying that part of the eye. The condition often accompanies hypertension.

arteriospasm /ärtir′ē·ōspaz′əm/ [Gk, *arteria* + *spasmos,* spasm], a spasm of an artery.

arteriovenous /-vē′nəs/ [Gk, *arteria* + L, *vena,* vein], of or pertaining to arteries and veins.

arteriovenous anastomosis [Gk, *arteria* + L, *vena;* Gk, *anastomoein,* to form a mouth], a communication between an artery and a vein, either as a congenital anomaly or a surgically produced link between vessels.

arteriovenous aneurysm, an aneurysm affecting both an artery and a vein, often as an abnormal linkage between a vein and artery.

arteriovenous angioma of the brain, a congenital tumor consisting of a tangle of coiled, usually dilated arteries and veins, islets of sclerosed brain tissue, and, occasionally, cartilaginous cells. The lesion, which may be distinguished by an intracranial bruit, generally arises in the vascular system of the pia mater and may grow to project deeply into the brain, causing seizures and progressive hemiparesis.

arteriovenous fistula, an abnormal communication between an artery and vein occurring congenitally or resulting from trauma, infection, arterial aneurysm, or a malignancy. A continuous murmur and palpable thrill may be detected over the fistula and may be obliterated by compressing the feeding artery; this maneuver may slow the heart beat (Branham's sign). Chronic arteriovenous fistulas may cause varicosities, cutaneous ulcers, and cardiac enlargement. A congenital fistula may result in a cavernous hemangioma. If an arteriovenous fistula is limited in size and is accessible, it can be treated by surgical excision. An arteriovenous fistula is often created surgically to provide vascular access for hemodialysis.

arteriovenous oxygen (a-vo₂) difference, the arterial oxygen content minus the central venous oxygen content.

arteriovenous shunt, a passageway, artificial or natural, that allows blood to flow from an artery to a vein without going through a capillary network.

arteritis /är′tərī′tis/ [Gk, *arteria + itis*], an inflammatory condition of the inner layers or the outer coat of one or more arteries, occurring as a clinical entity or accompanying another disorder, such as rheumatoid arthritis, rheumatic fever, polymyositis, or systemic lupus erythematosus. Kinds of arteritis include **infantile arteritis, rheumatic arteritis, Takayasu's arteritis,** and **temporal arteritis.** See also **endarteritis, periarteritis.**

arteritis obliterans. See **Friedländer's disease.**

arteritis umbilicalis, a septic inflammation of the umbilical artery in newborn infants, usually by the bacteria of the species *Clostridium tetani.*

artery /är′tərē/ [Gk, *arteria,* airpipe], one of the large blood vessels carrying blood in a direction away from the heart. The wall of an artery has three layers: the **tunica adventitia,** the outer coat; the **tunica media,** the middle coat; and the **tunica intima,** the inner coat. See also **arteriole.**

artery forceps, any forceps used for grasping, compressing, and holding the end of an artery during ligation. Generally self-locking, its handles are scissorlike. Also called **hemostatic forceps.**

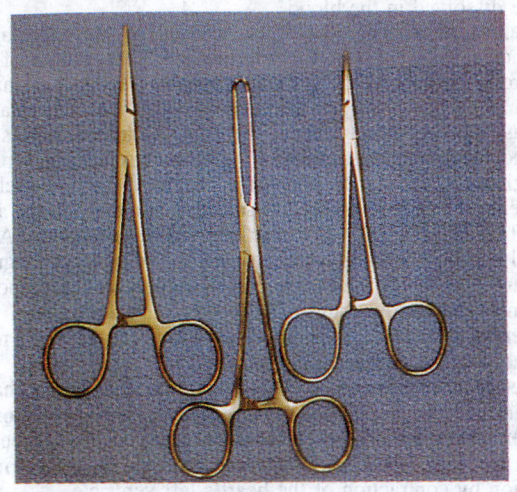

Artery forceps (*Grossman, 1993*)

arthr-, arthro-, a combining form meaning 'pertaining to a joint': *arthralgia, arthrocentesis.*

arthralgia /ärthral′jə/ [Gk, *arthron,* joint, *algos,* pain], joint pain. —**arthralgic,** *adj.*

-arthria, a suffix meaning a '(specified) condition involving the ability to articulate': *anarthria, dysarthria, pararthria.*

-arthritic, -arthritical, a suffix meaning 'pertaining to an arthritic condition': *antarthritic, antiarthritic, postarthritic.*

arthritis /ärthrī′tis/ [Gk, *arthron,* joint, *itis*], any inflammatory condition of the joints, characterized by pain and swelling. See also osteoarthritis, rheumatoid arthritis.

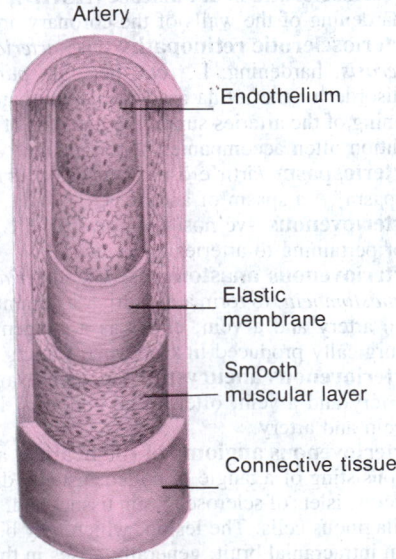

Artery

— Endothelium

— Elastic membrane

— Smooth muscular layer

— Connective tissue

Cross-section of an artery (*Cannobio, 1990*)

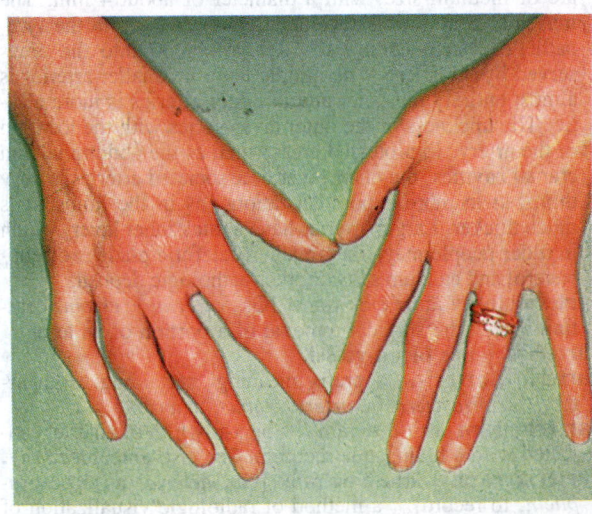

Hand involvement in arthritis (*Shipley, 1993*)

arthritis deformans.   See **rheumatoid arthritis.**

arthro- [Gk, *arthron,* joint],   a combining form relating to joints, articulations.

arthrocentesis /är′thrōsintē′sis/ [Gk, *arthron* + *kentesis,* pricking],   the puncture of a joint with a needle and the withdrawal of fluid, performed to obtain samples of synovial fluid for diagnostic purposes. A local anesthetic is usually administered; surgical asepsis is observed in the procedure. Normal synovial fluid is a clear, straw-colored, slightly viscous liquid that forms a white, viscous clot when mixed with glacial acetic acid; but if inflammation is present, as in rheumatoid arthritis, the fluid is watery and turbid, and its mixture with glacial acetic acid results in a flocculent, easily broken clot. The number of leukocytes, especially polymorphonuclear cells, and the protein content are increased and the glucose level is decreased if inflammation is present. Synovial fluid samples are also cultured and examined microscopically to diagnose a septic process, such as bacterial arthritis.

arthrodesis.   See **ankylosis,** def. 2.

arthrodia.   See **gliding joint.**

arthrogram /är′thrəgram/,   a radiogram of a joint after injection of a contrast medium.

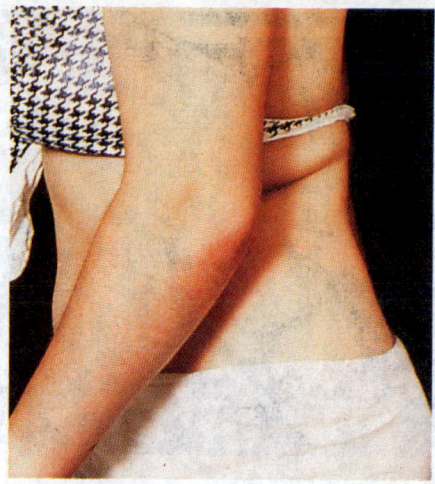

Limited motion of the elbow in arthrogryposis multiplex congenita (Zitelli, 1992)

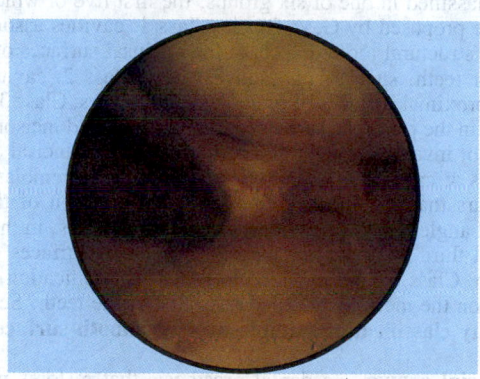

Arthrogram of knee (Johnson, 1981)

arthrography [Gk, *arthron,* joint, *graphein,* to record],   a method of radiographically visualizing the inside of a joint by injecting air or a contrast medium.

arthrogryposis multiplex congenita [Gk, *arthron, gryposis,* joint curve; L, *multus,* many, *plica,* fold; *congenitus,* born with],   fibrous stiffness of one or more joints, present at birth, often associated with incomplete development of the muscles that move the involved joints and degenerative changes of the motor neurons that innervate those muscles. The cause of the condition, which is uncommon, is unknown. Physiotherapy to loosen the joints is the only treatment. Also called **amyoplasia congenita** /əmī′ō-plä′zhə/.

arthrokinematic /är′thrəkin′əmat′ik/,   pertaining to the movement of joint surfaces.

arthron /är′thron [Gk]/,   a joint, including its various components of bones, cartilaginous inserts, all soft tissue structures intervening between the rigid skeletal parts, and the adjacent muscular elements.

arthropathy /ärthrop′əthē/ [Gk, *arthron* + *pathos,* suffering],   any disease or abnormal condition affecting a joint. **—arthropathic,** *adj.*

arthroplasty /är′thrəplast′ē/ [Gk, *arthron* + *plassein,* to shape],   the surgical reconstruction or replacement of a painful, degenerated joint, to restore mobility to a joint in osteoarthritis or rheumatoid arthritis or to correct a congenital deformity. Either the bones of the joint are reshaped and soft tissue or a metal disk is placed between the reshaped ends, or all or part of the joint is replaced with a metal or plastic prosthesis. Preoperative care may include the typing and crossmatching of blood. Postoperatively, the patient may be placed in traction to immobilize the affected limb. Exercise to increase muscle strength and range of motion is allowed in a slow, progressive schedule. Frequent checks of distal circulation are made and the nurse watches for signs of surgical shock, thrombophlebitis, pulmonary embolism, or fat embolism. Antibiotics are usually given to prevent infection, which is the most common cause of failure of the surgery. See also **osteoarthritis.**

arthropod /är′thrəpod′/ [Gk, *arthron* + *pous,* foot],   a member of the Arthropoda, a large phylum of animal life that includes crabs and lobsters as well as mites, ticks, spiders, and insects. Arthropods generally are distinguished by a jointed exoskeleton (shell) and paired, jointed legs; they bite, sting, cause allergic reactions, and carry viruses and other disease agents.

arthroscope /-skōp′/ [Gk, *arthron* + *skopein,* to watch],   a type of endoscope used to examine joints.

arthroscopy /ärthros′kəpē/ [Gk, *arthron* + *skopein* to watch],   the examination of the interior of a joint, performed by inserting a specially designed endoscope through a small incision. The procedure, used chiefly in knee problems, permits biopsy of cartilage or synovium, the diagnosis of a torn meniscus, and, in some instances, the removal of loose bodies in the joint space. **—arthroscopic,** *adj.* (See Fig. p. 126.)

arthrous /är′thrəs/ [Gk, *arthron*],   **1.** pertaining to joints or articulation of bones. **2.** pertaining to a disease of a joint.

Arthus reaction /ärtoos′/ [Nicholas M. Arthus, French

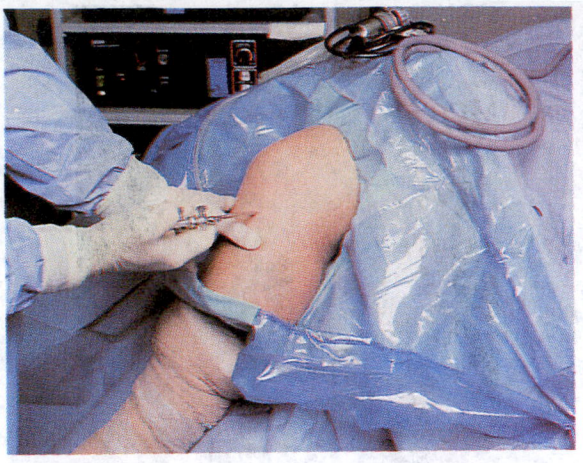

Arthroscopy of the knee (Mourad, 1991)

physiologist, b. 1862], a rare, severe, immediate hypersensitivity reaction to injection of a foreign substance, which is usually not irritating but in certain individuals is antigenic. An acute local inflammatory reaction, marked by edema, hemorrhage, and necrosis, occurs at the site of injection. A sterile abscess may form that is slow to heal and may become secondarily infected. Also called **Arthus phenomenon.** See also **serum sickness.**

articul-, a combining form meaning 'pertaining to a joint, structure and function': *articular, articulatio.*

articular /ärtik'yələr/ [L, *articulare*, to divide into joints], relating to a joint or the involvement of joints.

articular capsule [L, *articulare*, to divide into joints], an envelope of tissue that surrounds a freely moving joint, composed of an external layer of white fibrous tissue and an internal synovial membrane. See also **fibrous capsule.**

articular cartilage [L, *articulare* + *cartilago*], a type of hyaline connective tissue that covers the articulating surfaces of bases within synovial joints. See also **cartilage.**

articular disk, the platelike end of certain bones in movable joints, developed from unabsorbed mesoderm and sometimes closely associated with surrounding muscles or with cartilage.

articular fracture, a fracture involving the articular surfaces of a joint.

articulated partial denture. See **partial denture.**

articulatio cubiti. See **elbow joint.**

articulatio ellipsoidea. See **condyloid joint.**

articulatio genus. See **knee joint.**

articulation. See **joint.**

articulation of the pelvis /ärtik'yəlā'shən/, any one of the connections between the bones of the pelvis, involving four groups of ligaments. The first group connects the sacrum and the ilium; the second, the sacrum and the ischium; the third, the sacrum and the coccyx; and the fourth, the two pubic bones.

articulatio plana. See **gliding joint.**

articulatio sellaris. See **saddle joint.**

articulator /ärtik'yəlā'tər/ [L, *articulare*, to divide into joints], (in dentistry) a mechanical device used in the fabrication and testing of dentures. It represents the temporo-

mandibular joints and jaw members to which maxillary and mandibular casts may be attached. Some articulators are adjustable, allowing movement of attached casts into various eccentric relationships.

artifact /är'təfakt/ [L, *ars*, skill, *facere*, to make], anything extraneous, irrelevant, or unwanted, such as a substance, structure, or piece of data or information. In radiologic imaging, spurious electronic signals may appear as an artifact in an image with as much strength as the signals produced by the real objects, thereby confusing the radiologist and the results of any examination.

artifactual modification /är'təfak'chōō·əl/, a change in protein structure caused by in vitro manipulation.

artificial airway /är'tifish'əl/ [L, *artificiosum*, skillfully made], a plastic or rubber device that can be inserted into the upper or lower respiratory tract to facilitate ventilation or the removal of secretions.

artificial alimentation, See **parenteral nutrition.**

artificial assists, any prosthetic devices or contrivances that may enable a physically challenged person to function. Examples include heart pacemakers, crutches, and artificial limbs.

artificial blood. See **perfluorocarbons.**

artificial classification of cavities, any cavity that may be classified in one of six groups, the first five of which are those proposed by G.V. Black. Class 1: cavities associated with structural tooth defects in the occlusal surfaces of posterior teeth, such as pits and fissures; Class 2: cavities in the proximal surfaces of premolars and molars; Class 3: cavities in the proximal surfaces of the canines and incisors that do not involve removal and restoration of the incisal angle; Class 4: cavities in the proximal surfaces of premolars and molars that require the removal and restoration of the incisal angle; Class 5: cavities, except pit cavities, in the gingival third of the labial, buccal, or lingual surfaces of the teeth; Class 6: (not included in Black's classification) cavities on the incisal edges and cusp tips of the teeth. See also **cavity classification, simple cavity, smooth surface cavity.**

artificial crown, a dental prosthesis that restores part or all of the coronal portion of a natural tooth. Compare **anatomic crown, clinical crown, partial crown.**

artificial fever, an elevated body temperature produced by artificial means, such as the injection of malarial parasites or of a vaccine known to produce fever symptoms, or by applying heat to the body. An artificial fever may be prescribed for a patient to arrest a disease that is sensitive to elevated body temperatures. Also called **fever therapy.**

artificial heart, a mechanical device of molded polyurethane, consisting of two ventricles implanted in the body and powered by an air compressor located outside the body. The first artificial heart for humans was implanted in December 1982 at the University of Utah Medical Center in Salt Lake City. The mechanical heart was attached to the atria and major blood vessels of the native heart with Dacron fittings. The first artificial heart for humans kept the patient alive for 112 days. See also **Jarvik-7.**

artificial insemination (AI), the introduction of semen into the vagina or uterus by mechanical or instrumental means rather than by sexual intercourse. The procedure is planned to coincide with the expected time of ovulation so that fertilization can occur. Kinds of artificial insemination are **artificial insemination-donor** and **artificial insemination-husband.** Also called **artificial impregnation.** See also **menstrual cycle.**

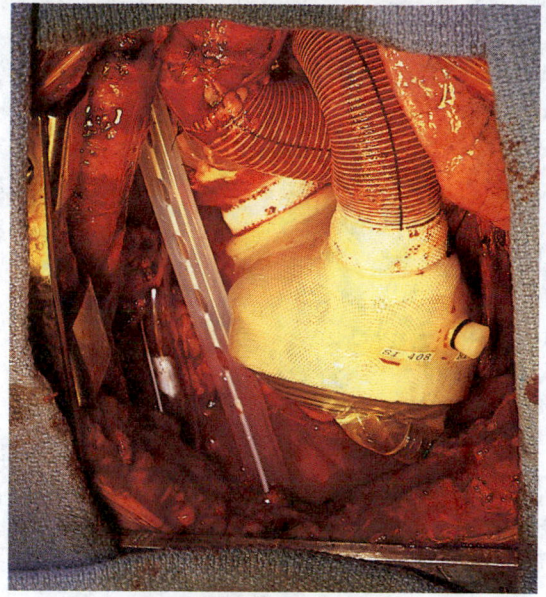

Jarvik-7 artificial heart
(Seeley, 1992/Courtesy the University Medical Center,
Tucson, Arizona)

artificial insemination-donor (AID), artificial insemination in which the semen specimen is provided by an anonymous donor. The procedure is used primarily in cases where the husband is sterile. Also called **heterologous insemination.** Compare **artificial insemination-husband.**

artificial insemination-husband (AIH), artificial insemination in which the semen specimen is provided by the husband. The procedure is used primarily in cases of impotency, low sperm count, a vaginal disorder, or when the husband is incapable of sexual intercourse because of some physical disability. Also called **artificial homologous insemination.** Compare **artificial insemination-donor.**

artificial intelligence (AI), a system that makes it possible for a machine to perform functions similar to human intelligence, such as learning, reasoning, self-correcting, and adapting. Computer technology produces many instruments and systems that mimic and surpass some human capabilities, as speed of counting, correlating, sensing, and deducing.

artificial kidney, a device used to rid blood, circulated outside of the body, of substances commonly excreted in urine. It usually consists of a set of tubes or catheters which pass the blood through a dialysate solution where wastes are removed by osmosis and diffusion. Also called **kidney machine.** See also **hemodialysis, peritoneal dialysis.**

artificial labor [L, *artificiosus,* artificial + *labor,* work], induced labor, as when started with drugs or mechanical devices.

artificial limb. See **prosthesis.**

artificial lung. See **Drinker respirator.**

artificially acquired immunity. See **acquired immunity.**

artificial menopause [L, *artificiosus,* artificial + *mensis,* month; Gk, *pauein,* to cease], the termination of menstrual periods by surgery, radiation, or other methods.

artificial pacemaker. See **pacemaker.**

artificial pneumothorax. See **therapeutic pneumothorax.**

artificial respiration. See **artificial ventilation.**

artificial rupture of membranes (AROM). See amniotomy.

artificial saliva [L, *artificialis,* artifice + *saliva,* spittle], a mixture of carboxymethylcellulose, sorbitol, sodium and potassium chloride in an aqueous solution. It is available in a spray container for the treatment of xerostomia, or drymouth.

artificial selection, the process by which the genotypes of successive plant and animal generations are determined through controlled breeding. Compare **natural selection.**

artificial stone, a calcined gypsum derivative similar to but stronger than plaster of paris, used for making dental casts and dies.

artificial ventilation, the process of supporting respiration by manual or mechanical means when normal breathing is inefficient or has stopped. Effective ventilation of the lungs may fail because of bronchial obstruction by swelling, a foreign body, increased secretions, neuromuscular weakness, status asthmaticus, exhaustion, pharmacologic depression, or trauma to the chest wall. Before an attempt to administer artificial ventilation, the airway is tested and any obstruction removed. See also **cardiopulmonary resuscitation (CPR), resuscitation, ventilator.** Also called **artificial respiration.** (See Fig. p. 128.)

art therapy, a type of mental health treatment in which the patient is encouraged to express his or her feelings through various forms of artwork.

aryepiglottic folds /er′ē·ep′iglot′ik/, folds of mucous membrane that extend around the margins of the larynx from a junction with the epiglottis. They function as a sphincter during swallowing.

aryl- /er′il/ [*aromatic* + *yl*], an alkyl univalent radical derived from an aromatic hydrocarbon and used to denote aromatic groups.

aryl hydrocarbon hydroxylase (AHH), an enzyme that converts carcinogenic chemicals in tobacco smoke and in polluted air into active carcinogens within the lungs. Aryl hydrocarbon hydroxylase is the subject of numerous studies to determine why some smokers develop cancer and others do not. Experimental blood tests indicate that the level of aryl hydrocarbon hydroxylase may be a factor in hereditary predisposition of a cigarette smoker to cancer.

As, symbol for the element **arsenic.**

AS, abbreviation for **aortic stenosis.**

as-. See **ad-.**

a.s., abbreviation for **auris sinistra.**

ASA, **1.** abbreviation for *American Society of Anesthesiologists.* **2.** abbreviation for **aspirin** (acetylsalicylic acid).

ASAHP, abbreviation for *American Society of Allied Health Professionals.*

ASAP, abbreviation for *as soon as possible.*

asbestos /asbes′təs/ [Gk, *asbestos,* unquenchable], a group of fibrous impure magnesium silicate minerals. Inhalation of the fibers can lead to pulmonary fibrosis if the fibers accumulate in terminal bronchioles. Continued exposure to asbestos fibers can result in lung cancer.

asbestosis [Gk, *asbestos,* inextinguishable, *osis,* condition], a chronic lung disease caused by the inhalation of asbestos fibers that results in the development of alveolar, interstitial, and pleural fibrosis. Asbestos miners and workers are most frequently affected, but the disease sometimes occurs

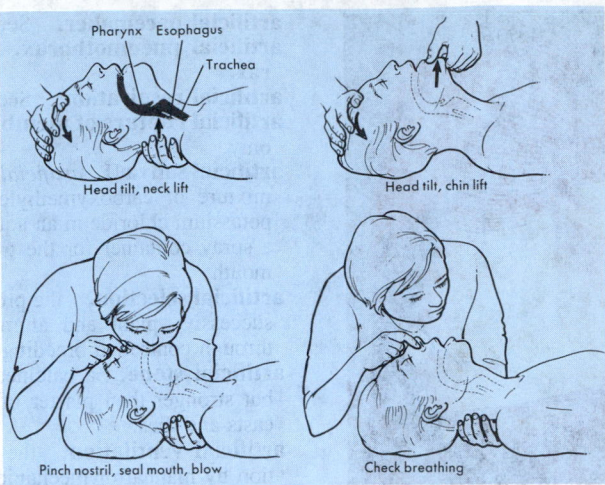

Artificial ventilation

in other people who have been exposed to asbestos building materials. Chest x-ray films show the characteristic small linear opacities distributed throughout the lungs. The disease is progressive: Shortness of breath develops eventually into respiratory failure. Cigarette smoking and continuous exposure to asbestos aggravate the condition. Fatal mesothelial tumors sometimes occur. There is no treatment. See also **chronic obstructive pulmonary disease, inorganic dust.**

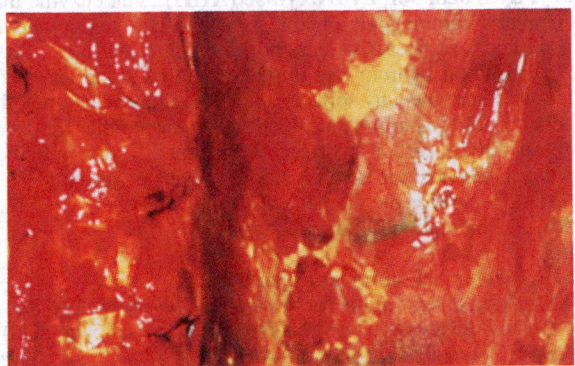

Asbestosis—lung biopsy specimen
(Fletcher, 1987)

ASC, abbreviation for **altered state of consciousness.**
ascariasis /as′kərī′əsis/ [Gk, askaris, intestinal worm, osis, condition], an infection caused by a parasitic worm, Ascaris lumbricoides, that migrates through the lungs in its larval stage. The eggs are passed in human feces, contaminating the soil and allowing transmission to the mouths of others through hands, water, or food. After hatching in the small intestine, the larvae travel through the wall of the intestine, whence they are carried by the lymphatics and blood to the lungs. Early respiratory symptoms of coughing, wheezing, and fever are caused by the passage through the respiratory tract. The larvae are swallowed, they mature in the jejunum, where they release eggs, and the cycle is repeated. Intestinal infection may result in abdominal cramps and obstruction. In children, migration of the adult worms into the liver, gallbladder, or peritoneal cavity may cause death. The infective eggs are readily identified in the feces. Piperazine citrate, pyrantel pamoate, and mebendazole are effective treatments. The disease can be prevented by educating people, especially children, about good sanitation habits such as handwashing.

Ascaris /as′kəris/, a genus of large parasitic intestinal roundworms, such as *Ascaris lumbricoides,* a cause of ascariasis, found throughout temperate and tropic regions.

ascending aorta /asen′ding/ [L, ascendere, to climb], one of the four main sections of the aorta, branching into the right and left coronary arteries, rising from the semilunar valve of the left ventricle, curving to the right near the cranial border of the second right costal cartilage, and lying about 6 cm deep to the dorsal surface of the sternum. It is about 5 cm long and has three small aortic sinuses at its origin, opposite the aortic valve.

ascending colon, the segment of the colon that extends from the cecum in the lower right side of the abdomen to the transverse colon at the hepatic flexure on the right side, usually at the level of the umbilicus.

ascending current. See **centripetal current.**

ascending neuritis [L, ascendere, to rise; Gk, neuron, nerve, itis, inflammation], a nerve inflammation that begins on the periphery and moves upward along a nerve trunk.

ascending neuropathy, a disease of the nervous system that begins at a lower place in the body and spreads upward.

ascending oblique muscle. See **obliquus internus abdominis.**

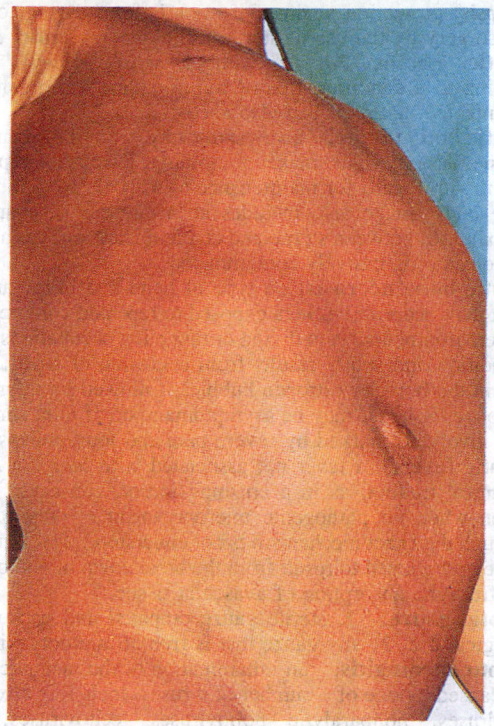

Intestinal obstruction due to infestation by
ascaris lumbricoides
(Zitelli, 1992)

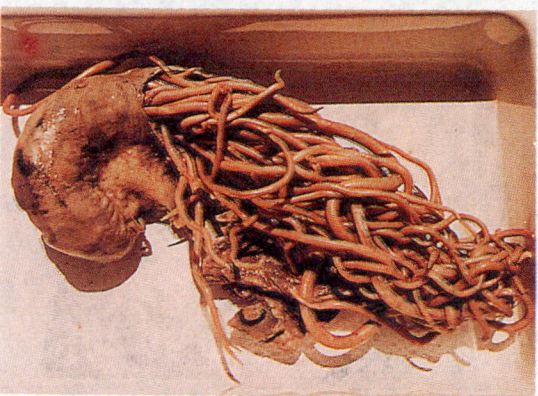

Portion of small intestine blocked by *ascaris*
(Muller, 1990/Courtesy Prof. RB Holliman)

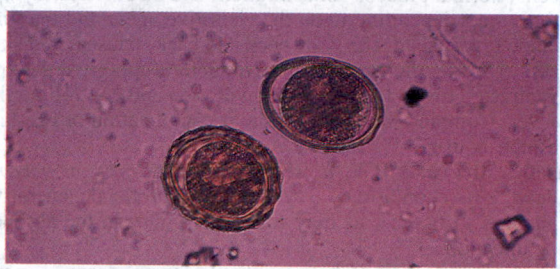

Ascaris lumbricoides eggs (Murray, 1990)

ascending paralysis, a condition in which there is successive flaccid paralysis of the legs, then the trunk and arms, and finally the muscles of respiration. Causes may include poliomyelitis, infectious polyneuritis, or exposure to toxic chemicals.

ascending pharyngeal artery, one of the smallest arteries that branch from the external carotid artery, deep in the neck, supplying various organs and muscles of the head, such as the tympanic cavity, the longus capitis, and the longus colli. It divides into five branches, the pharyngeal, palatine, prevertebral, inferior tympanic, and posterior meningeal.

ascending poliomyelitis [L, *ascendere,* to rise; Gk, *polios,* gray, *myelos,* marrow, *itis,* inflammation], poliomyelitis that begins in the legs and spreads upward to involve the trunk and respiratory muscles. See also **ascending paralysis.**

ascending tract [L, *tractus*], a nervous system pathway found in the spinal cord that carries impulses toward the brain. Also called **afferent tract.**

ascending urography. See **urography.**

asceticism /aset′isiz′əm/ [Gk, *askein,* to exercise], (in psychiatry) a defense mechanism that involves repudiation of all instinctual impulses. The concept is derived from the religious doctrine that material things are evil and only spiritual things are good.

Aschheim-Zondek (AZ) test /ash′hīmtson′dek/, an obsolete biologic test for pregnancy.

Aschoff bodies [Karl Albert Ludwig Aschoff, German pathologist, b. 1866; AS, *bodig*], tiny rounded or spindle-shaped nodules containing multinucleated giant cells, fibroblasts, and basophilic cells found in joints, tendons, the pleura, and the cardiovascular system of rheumatic fever patients.

ascites /əsī′tēz/ [Gk, *askos,* bag], an abnormal intraperitoneal accumulation of a fluid containing large amounts of protein and electrolytes. Ascites may be detectable when more than 500 ml of fluid has accumulated. The condition may be accompanied by general abdominal swelling, hemodilution, edema, or a decrease in urinary output. Identification of ascites is made through auscultation, percussion, and palpation. Ascites is a complication of cirrhosis, congestive heart failure, nephrosis, malignant neoplastic disease, peritonitis, or various fungal and parasitic diseases. Ascites is treated with dietary therapy and diuretic drugs; abdominal paracentesis may be performed to relieve pain and improve respiratory and visceral function by relieving the pressure of the accumulated fluid. By lowering pressure within the portal system, paracentesis is therapeutic in ascites accompanied by bleeding. See also **paracentesis. –ascitic,** *adj.* (See Fig. p. 130.)

ascites adiposus. See **chylous ascites.**

ascites praecox /prē′koks/ [Gk, *askos* + L, premature], an abnormal accumulation of fluid within the peritoneal cavity preceding the development of generalized edema associated with pericarditis. See also **ascites.**

ascitic fluid /əsit′ik/ [Gk, *askos,* bag], a watery fluid containing albumin, glucose, and electrolytes that accumulates in the peritoneal cavity in association with certain disease conditions, such as liver disease or congestive heart failure.

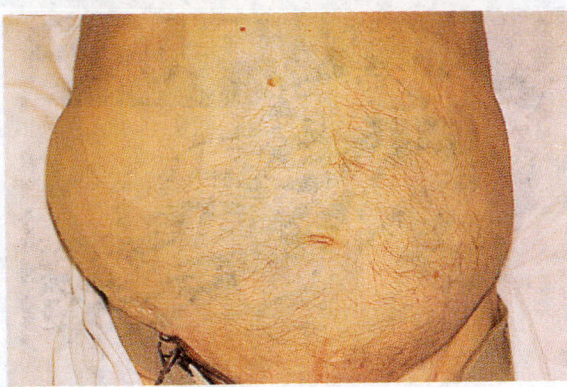

Abdominal distension caused by ascites
(Kamal, 1991)

The fluid occurs as leakage from the veins and lymphatics into extravascular spaces.

ascorbemia /as'kôrbē'mē·ə/ [Gk, *a*, not; AS, *scurf*, scurvy; Gk, *haima*, blood], the presence of ascorbic acid in the blood in amounts greater than normal, usually reflecting only an excess of ascorbic acid intake. The condition is usually due to the use of ascorbic acid supplements.

ascorbic acid /əskôr'bik/ [Gk, *a*, not; AS, *scurf*, scurvy], a water-soluble, white crystalline vitamin present in citrus fruits, tomatoes, berries, potatoes, and fresh, green, leafy vegetables, such as broccoli, brussels sprouts, collards, turnip greens, parsley, sweet peppers, and cabbage. It is essential for the formation of collagen and fibrous tissue for normal intercellular matrices in teeth, bone, cartilage, connective tissue, and skin, and for the structural integrity of capillary walls. It also aids in fighting bacterial infections and interacts with other nutrients. Signs of deficiency are bleeding gums, tendency to bruising, swollen or painful joints, nosebleeds, anemia, lowered resistance to infections, and slow healing of wounds and fractures. Severe deficiency results in scurvy. An excess of ascorbic acid may cause a burning sensation during urination, diarrhea, skin rash, and nausea and may disturb the absorption and metabolism of cyanocobalamin. Tests for glycosuria, uric acid, and iron may be inaccurate when large amounts of the vitamin are being administered. Also called **antiscorbutic vitamin, cevitamic acid, vitamin C.** See also **ascorbemia, bioflavonoid, infantile scurvy, scurvy.**

ascorburia /as'kôrbyŏŏr'ē·ə/ [Gk, *a*, not; AS, *scurf*, scurvy; Gk, *ouron*, urine], the presence of ascorbic acid in the urine in amounts greater than normal, usually reflecting only an excess of ascorbic acid intake. It is usually caused by the use of ascorbic acid supplements.

ascribed role /əskrībd'/, an assigned role in society, based on age, sex, or other factors about which the individual has no choice. See also **assumed role.**

ASD, abbreviation for **atrial septal defect.**

-ase, a suffix used in naming enzymes: *lipase, oxidase, protease.*

Asendin, a trademark for an antidepressant (amoxapine).

asepsis /āsep'sis/ [Gk, *a, sepsis,* not decay], **1.** the absence of germs. **2. medical asepsis,** the removal or destruction of disease organisms or infected material. **3. surgical**

asepsis, protection against infection before, during, or after surgery by the use of sterile technique. **–aseptic,** *adj.*

aseptic /āsep'tik/ [Gk, *a,* without, *sepsis,* decay], pertaining to a condition free of living pathogenic organisms or infected material. See also **asepsis.**

aseptic body image, an awareness by operating room personnel of body, hair, makeup, clothing, jewelry, and placement with regard for maintenance of a sterile environment. The body image also includes an awareness of changing proximities between sterile and contaminated areas as a field becomes progressively contaminated.

aseptic bone necrosis, a type of bone and joint damage that may occur in workers exposed to repeated compressed-air environments, as in diving or tunneling occupations. The condition apparently results from occlusion of small arteries in the bone by nitrogen bubbles, followed by infarction of bone tissue. It may be asymptomatic or, if joint surfaces are involved, marked by severe pain and joint collapse.

aseptic fever, a fever not associated with infection. Mechanical trauma, as in a crushing injury, can cause fever even when no pathogenic microorganism is present. Although the exact mechanism is not understood, fever in such cases is believed to result from the breakdown of leukocytes or from the absorption of avascular tissue.

aseptic gauze, 1. sterile gauze prepared and packed for surgical use. **2.** any gauze that is free of microorganisms.

aseptic meningitis, an inflammation of the meninges that is caused by one of a number of viruses, including coxsackieviruses, nonparalytic polioviruses, echoviruses, and mumps. The disease is especially common in children during the late summer and early fall. In about one third of the cases no pathogen can be demonstrated, but analysis of cerebrospinal fluid reveals increased numbers of white blood cells, normal glucose concentration, and no bacteria. Symptoms vary depending upon the causative agent and may include fever, headache, stiff neck and back, nausea, and skin rash. No specific treatment is available. Supportive therapy is directed toward maintaining hydration and controlling the fever. Complete recovery, without complication or residual effect, is usual.

aseptic necrosis [Gk, *a, sepsis,* without decay + *nekros,* dead, *osis,* condition], cystic and sclerotic degenerative changes in tissues, as may follow an injury in the absence of infection.

aseptic peritonitis [Gk, *a,* without, *sepsis,* decay + *peri,* near, *teinein,* to stretch, *itis,* inflammation], peritonitis in which inflammation of the peritoneum is caused by chemicals, radiation, or injury, rather than by an infectious agent.

aseptic surgery [Gk, *a, sepsis,* decay + *cheirourgos,* surgeon], the avoidance of contamination during surgical procedures.

aseptic technique, any health care procedure in which added precautions are used to prevent contamination of a person, object, or area by microorganisms.

Asepto syringe, a trademark for a bulb-fitted, blunt-tipped syringe used primarily for irrigation of wounds.

asexual /āsek'shoo·əl/ [Gk, *a,* not; L *sexus* male or female], **1.** not sexual. **2.** of or pertaining to an organism that has no sexual organs. **3.** of or pertaining to a process that is not sexual. **–asexuality,** *n.*

asexual dwarf, an adult dwarf whose genital organs are underdeveloped.

asexual generation, any type of reproduction that occurs without the union of male and female gametes, such as fission, budding, sporulation, or parthenogenesis. Also called **direct generation, nonsexual generation.**

-asexuality. See **asexual.**

asexualization /āsek′shōō·əlīzā′shən/, the process of making one incapable of reproduction; sterilization of an individual or animal by castration, vasectomy, removal of the ovaries, or used of chemicals.

asexual reproduction, a type of reproduction found in plants and lower animals in which new organisms are formed without the union of gametes, as occurs in budding, fission, and spore formation. Compare **sexual generation.**

ASHA, abbreviation for **American Speech, Language, and Hearing Association.**

ASHD, abbreviation for **arteriosclerotic heart disease.**

Asherman syndrome, secondary amenorrhea in a hormonally normal woman, caused by obliteration of the endometrial cavity by adhesions that form as a result of curettage or infection.

asialorrhea. See **hyposalivation.**

Asian flu. See **influenza.**

asiderosis /ā′sidərō′sis/, an iron deficiency and a cause of anemia.

-asis, a suffix meaning an 'action, process, or result of': *basis, metabasis, oxydasis.*

ASLT, abbreviation for **antistreptolysin-O test.**

A.S.M.T., abbreviation for *American Society for Medical Technology.*

Asn, abbreviation for **asparagine.**

asocial /āsō′shəl/ [Gk, *a*, without; L, *socius*, companion], withdrawn or disengaged from normal contacts with other individuals.

ASOT, abbreviation for **antistreptolysin-O test.**

asparaginase /aspar′əjinās/ [Gk, *asparagos*, asparagus], an enzyme that catalyzes the hydrolysis of asparagine to asparaginic acid and ammonia. Asparaginase is used as a chemotherapeutic agent in the treatment of acute lymphoblastic leukemia.

asparagine (Asn) /aspar′əjin/, a nonessential amino acid found in many proteins in the body. It is easily hydrolyzed to aspartic acid and has diuretic properties. See also **amino acid, protein.**

Chemical structure of asparagine (Seeley, 1992)

aspartame /aspär′tām, as′pərtām/, a white, almost odorless crystalline powder with an intensely sweet taste that is used as an artificial sweetener. It is approximately 180 times as sweet as the same amount of sucrose and is used to enhance the flavor of cold or uncooked foods. Aspartame tends to lose its sweetness in the presence of heat, moisture, and alkaline media. Excessive use of aspartame should be avoided by patients with phenylketonuria (PKU) because the substance hydrolyzes to form aspartylphenylalanine.

aspartate aminotransferase (AST) /aspär′tāt/, an enzyme normally present in body serum and in certain body tissues, especially those of the heart and liver. This enzyme affects the intermolecular transfer of an amino group from aspartic acid to alpha-ketoglutaric acid, forming glutamic acid and oxaloacetic acid. The reaction is reversible. The enzyme is released into the serum because of tissue injury and thus may increase as a result of myocardial infarction and liver damage. Normal findings for adults are 8-20 U/L or 5-40 IU/L. Also called **glutamic-oxaloacetic transaminase, serum glutamic oxaloacetic transaminase.** Compare **alanine aminotransferase.**

aspartate kinase, an enzyme that catalyzes the transfer of a phosphate group from adenosine triphosphate to aspartate to produce phosphoaspartate.

aspartate transaminase. See **aspartate aminotransferase.**

aspartic acid (Asp) /aspär′tik/, a nonessential amino acid present in sugar cane, beet molasses, and the breakdown products of many proteins. Pure aspartic acid is a water-soluble, colorless crystalline substance. In the Krebs' cycle, aspartic acid and oxaloacetic acid are interconvertible. Aspartic acid is used in culture media, dietary supplements, detergents, fungicides, and germicides. Also called **aminosuccinic acid.** See also **amino acid, protein.**

Chemical structure of aspartic acid (Seeley, 1992)

ASPEN, abbreviation for **American Society of Parenteral and Enteral Nutrition.**

aspergillic acid /as′pərjil′ik/, an antibiotic substance derived from *Aspergillus flavus*, an aflatoxin-producing mold found on corn, grain, and peanuts. See **aflatoxins.**

aspergillosis /as′pərjilō′sis/ [L, *aspergere*, to sprinkle; Gk, *osis*, condition], an infection caused by a fungus of the genus *Aspergillus*, most commonly affecting the ear but capable of causing inflammatory, granulomatous lesions on or in any organ. The infection is relatively uncommon and typically occurs in a person already weakened by some other disorder. Topical fungicides can be used on the skin; amphotericin B is used to treat systemic aspergillosis, especially if it has spread to the lungs. The prognosis, as for most systemic fungal infections, is poor. Compare **allergic bronchopulmonary aspergillosis.**

Aspergillus /as′pərjil′əs/ [L, *aspereger*, to sprinkle], a genus of fungi that is a common contaminant in the laboratory and a cause of nosocomial infection. The fungus has hyphae and spores, lives in the soil, is ubiquitous, and proliferates rapidly. Inhalation of the spores of the two pathogenic species, *Aspergillus fumigatus* and *A. flavus*, is common, but infection is rare.

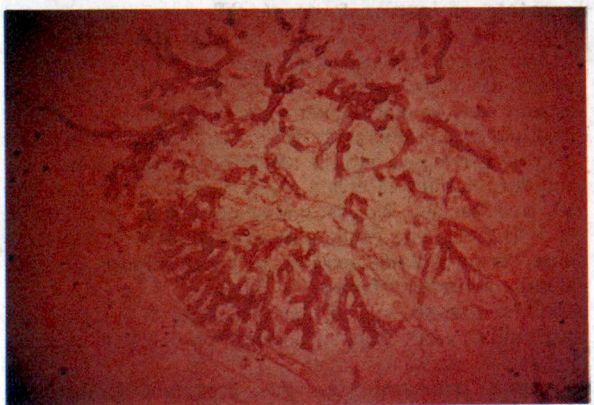

Aspergillus fumigatus *(Murray, 1990)*

aspermia /āspur′mē·ə/ [Gk, *a, sperma,* not seed], lack of formation or ejaculation of semen.

asphyxia /asfik′sē·ə/ [Gk, *a, sphyxis,* not pulse], severe hypoxia leading to hypoxemia and hypercapnia, loss of consciousness, and, if not corrected, death. Some of the more common causes of asphyxia are drowning, electric shock, aspiration of vomitus, lodging of a foreign body in the respiratory tract, inhalation of toxic gas or smoke, and poisoning. Artificial ventilation and oxygen are promptly administered to avoid damage to the brain. The underlying cause is then treated. See **artificial ventilation. –asphyxiate,** *v.,* **asphyxiated,** *adj.*

asphyxia livida /liv′ədə/, an abnormal condition in which a newborn infant's skin is cyanotic, the pulse is weak and slow, and the reflexes are slow or absent. Also called **blue asphyxia.**

asphyxia neonatorum, a condition in which a newborn does not breath spontaneously. The asphyxia may develop before or during labor or immediately after delivery. The condition may involve placental or neonatal pulmonary dysfunction with underlying causes that can include abruptio placentae, umbilical compression, or uterine tetany. Other factors may include congenital defects, such as a diaphragmatic hernia, or adverse effects of anesthetics or analgesics administered to the mother. Immediate resuscitation is required to prevent death or brain damage. Also called **perinatal asphyxia.** See also **asphyxia livida, asphyxia pallida.**

asphyxia pallida /pal′ədə/, an abnormal condition in which a newborn infant appears pale and limp, shows signs of apnea, and suffers from bradycardia as marked by a heartbeat of 80 beats per minute or less.

asphyxiate /asfik′sē·āt/ [Gk, *a,* without, *sphyxis,* pulse], to induce an inability to breathe. Causes may include circulatory congestion, chemical poisoning, electrical shock, or physical suffocation.

asphyxiated. See **asphyxia.**

asphyxiating thoracic dysplasia. See **Jeune's syndrome.**

asphyxiation [Gk, *a,* without, *sphyxis,* pulse], a state of asphyxia or inability to breathe.

aspirant /as′pirənt/, the fluid, gas, or solid particles that are withdrawn from the body by aspiration methods.

aspirant maneuver, a procedure used in making x-ray films of the laryngopharyngeal area. The patient exhales completely, then slowly inhales while making a harsh, high-pitched sound. The maneuver adducts the vocal cords so the ventricle of the larynx is clearly visible in the x-ray.

aspirate /-rāt/ [L, *aspirare,* to breathe upon], to withdraw fluid or air from a cavity. The process is usually aided by the use of a syringe or a suction device. See **paracentesis, thoracentesis.**

aspirating needle, a long hollow needle used to remove fluid from a cavity, vessel, or structure of the body.

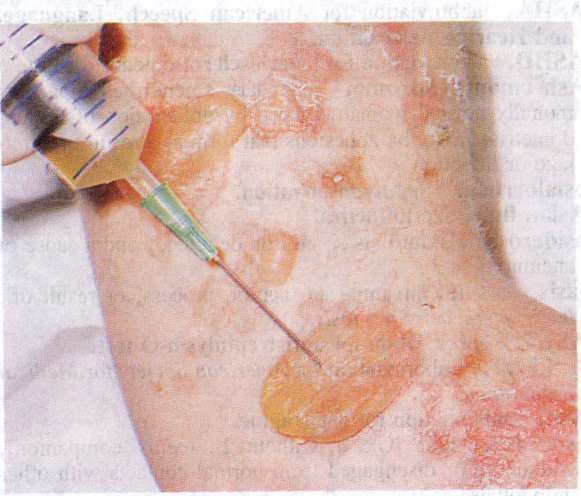

Aspirating needle *(Stone, 1989)*

aspirating syringe /-rā′ting/, (in dentistry) a hypodermic syringe used in the injection of local anesthetics. It can be checked by aspirating to ensure that the anesthetic solution is not being deposited in a blood vessel.

aspiration /as′pirā′shən/, **1.** the act of taking a breath, inhaling. **2.** the act of withdrawing a fluid, such as mucus or serum, from the body by a suction device. See also **aspiration pneumonia. –aspirate,** *n.*

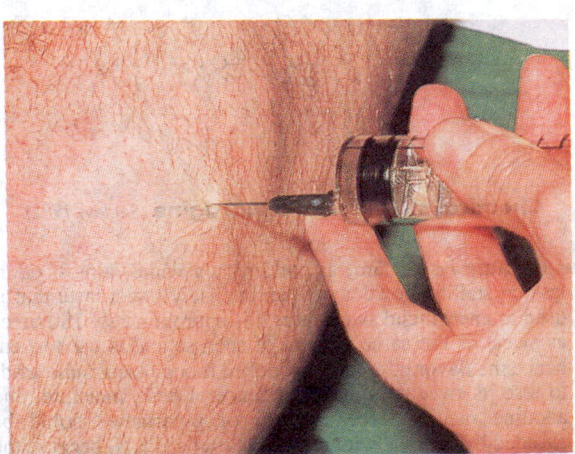

Aspiration of fluid from the knee joint *(Shipley, 1993)*

aspiration biopsy, the removal of living tissue for microscopic examination by suction through a fine needle attached to a syringe. The procedure is used primarily to obtain cells from a lesion containing fluid or when fluid is formed in a serous cavity. See also **cytology, needle biopsy.**

aspiration biopsy cytology (ABC), a microscopic examination of cells obtained directly from living body tissue by aspiration through a fine needle. It is used primarily as a diagnostic procedure, generally as a technique for detecting nuclear and cytoplasmic changes in cancerous tissue. Compare **exfoliative cytology.**

aspiration, high risk for, a nursing diagnosis accepted by the Eighth National Conference on the Classification of Nursing Diagnoses. Potential for aspiration is a state in which an individual is at risk for entry of gastric secretions, oropharyngeal secretions, or exogenous food or fluids into tracheobronchial passages caused by dysfunction or absence of normal protective mechanisms. The defining characteristics are the presence of risk factors including reduced level of consciousness, depressed cough and gag reflexes, the presence of a tracheostomy or endotracheal tube, an overinflated tracheostomy or endotracheal tube cuff, inadequate inflation of a tracheostomy or endotracheal tube cuff, gastrointestinal tubes, and bolus tube feedings or medication administration. Other risk factors are situations hindering elevation of the upper body, increased intragastric pressure, increased gastric residual, decreased gastrointestinal motility, delaying gastric emptying, impaired swallowing, wired jaws, and facial, oral, or neck surgery or trauma. See also **nursing diagnosis.**

aspiration drug abuse, the inhalation of a liquid, solid, or gaseous chemical into the respiratory system for nontherapeutic purposes. Examples include glue sniffing and cocaine snorting.

aspiration of vomitus, the inhalation of regurgitated gastric contents into the pulmonary system. See also **aspiration, aspiration pneumonia.**

aspiration pneumonia, an inflammatory condition of the lungs and bronchi caused by the inhalation of foreign material or vomitus containing acid gastric contents. Compare **bronchopneumonia.** See also **pneumonia.**

■ OBSERVATIONS: Aspiration pneumonia may occur during anesthesia or recovery from anesthesia or during a seizure of acute alcoholic intoxication or other condition characterized by vomiting and a decreased level of consciousness.

■ INTERVENTIONS: Treatment requires prompt suctioning of the bronchi and the administration of 100% oxygen. Continued artificial ventilation may be required. Corticosteroids may be given to diminish inflammation. The sputum is cultured regularly, and any bacterial infection thus diagnosed is treated with an appropriate antibiotic. As long as oxygen is required, frequent analyses of the levels of gases in the blood may be indicated.

■ NURSING CONSIDERATIONS: The pulse rate and quality of respirations, level of consciousness, and the color of the skin are carefully monitored. Infection and respiratory failure are frequent complications. Aspiration pneumonia may be avoided by correctly positioning unconscious patients with the head slightly elevated (15 to 30 degrees) and turned to the side and by paying careful attention to the maintenance of an adequate airway. An oral airway is left in place until the patient's condition improves, and secretions are removed by suction as necessary.

aspirator /as'pirā'tər/ [L, *aspirare*, to breathe upon], any instrument that removes a substance from body cavities by suction, such as a bulb syringe, piston pump, or hypodermic syringe.

aspirin (ASA) /as'pirin/, an analgesic, antipyretic, and antirheumatic. Also called **acetylsalicylic acid** /əsē'təlsal'isil'ik, as'itəl-/.

■ INDICATIONS: It is prescribed to reduce fever and for the relief of pain and inflammation.

■ CONTRAINDICATIONS: Bleeding disorders, peptic ulcer, pregnancy, the concomitant use of anticoagulants, or known hypersensitivity to salicylates prohibits its use.

■ ADVERSE EFFECTS: Among the most serious adverse reactions are GI effects (ulcers, occult bleeding). Sustained treatment with large doses can cause clotting defects, liver toxicity, and renal toxicities. Reye's syndrome has been associated with aspirin use in children. An asthmatic-like and other allergic reactions are occasionally seen. Tinnitus and dyspepsia are the most common adverse effects.

aspirin poisoning. See **salicylate poisoning.**

asplenia /āsplē'nē·ə/ [Gk, *a*, without, *spleen*], absence of a spleen. The condition may be congenital or the result of surgical removal.

A.S.R.T., abbreviation for *American Society of Radiologic Technologists.*

Assam fever. See **kala-azar.**

assault /əsôlt'/ [L, *assilirere*, to leap upon], **1.** an unlawful act that places another person, without that person's consent, in fear of immediate bodily harm or battery. The act must be apparently possible, thus causing well-founded apprehension in the victim of the assault. **2.** the act of committing an assault. **3.** to threaten a person with bodily harm or injury.

assay /asā', as'ā/ [Fr, *essayer*, to try], the analysis of the purity or effectiveness of drugs and other biologic substances, including laboratory and clinical observations.

assertion training. See **assertive training.**

assertiveness /əsur'tivnes/, a form of behavior that is directed toward claiming one's rights without denying the rights of others.

assertive training /əsur'tiv/ [L, *asserere*, to join to oneself], a technique used in behavior therapy to help individuals become more self-assertive and self-confident in interpersonal relationships. It focuses on the direct, honest statement of feelings and beliefs, both positive and negative. The technique is learned by role playing in a therapeutic setting, usually in a group, followed by practice in actual situations. Also called **assertion training.**

-assess. See **assessment.**

assessing /əses'ing/ [L, *assidere*, to sit beside], (in five-step nursing process) a category of nursing behavior that includes the gathering, verifying, and communicating of information relative to the client. The nurse collects information from verbal interactions with the patient, the patient's family and significant others; examines standard data sources for information; systematically checks for symptoms and signs; determines the patient's ability to perform self-care activities; assesses the patient's environment; and identifies reactions of the staff (including the nurse who is performing the assessment) to the patient and to the patient's family and significant others. To verify the data, the nurse confirms the observations and perceptions by gathering additional information; discusses the orders and decisions made by other members of the staff with them, when indicated; and personally evaluates and checks the patient's condition. The nurse reports the information that has been gathered and verified. Although assessing is the first of the five steps of the nursing process, preceding analyzing, in practice assessing is integral to effective nursing practice at all steps of the process. See also **analyzing, evaluating, implementing, nursing process, planning.**

assessment /əses′mənt/ [L, *assidere*, to sit beside], (in medicine and nursing) **1.** an evaluation or appraisal of a condition. **2.** the process of making such an evaluation. **3.** (in a problem oriented medical record) an examiner's evaluation of the disease or condition based on the patient's subjective report of the symptoms and course of the illness or condition and the examiner's objective findings, including data obtained through laboratory tests, physical examination, and medical history. See also **nursing assessment, problem oriented medical record. –assess,** *v.*

assessment of the aging patient, an evaluation of the changes characteristic of advancing years exhibited by an elderly person.

■ METHOD: The patient is measured, weighed, examined, observed, and questioned about physical, functional, and behavioral changes; height normally diminishes 1-2 inches with aging, and weight steadily decreases in men over 65 years of age but increases in women. The skin is examined for dryness, wrinkles, sagging, thinning over the back of the hands, areas of vitiligo, keratoses, warts, skin tags, and senile telangiectases, and the hair for depigmentation, lack of luster, and thinning or loss on the scalp and in the axillary and the pubic areas. Observations are made of enlargement of the nose and ears relative to face size, dryness of the eyes, discoloration of the sclera and iris, an opaque ring near the edge of the cornea (arcus senilis), decreased size of the pupil, and diminished peripheral vision. Tests are performed to determine if there is hearing loss, especially of high-frequency tones, decreased tidal volume, diminished peripheral perfusion, or deviation of the trachea, especially if scoliosis is present. Examination may reveal gum recession, loss of teeth and taste perception, diminished salivation, a decreased resting heart rate and cardiac output, and an easily palpable arterial pulse. The elderly patient may show decreased muscle mass, osteoarthritic joints, Heberden's or Bouchard's nodes at finger joints, contracture of lateral fingers, osteoporosis, a broad-based stance, and slow voluntary movements. The sense of position, of smell, and of touch and the sensitivity to heat and cold may be diminished, and deep tendon reflexes may be decreased. Signs of aging that may be found in women are pendulous, flaccid breasts; vaginal narrowing and shortening and diminished lubrication, causing painful coitus; and effects of long-term estrogen therapy, such as uterine bleeding, mastalgia, weight gain, fluid retention, and hypertension. Signs of aging in men include decrease in the size and firmness of the testes and in the amount and viscosity of seminal fluid, an increased diameter of the penis, and prostatic hypertrophy; libido and a sense of satisfaction usually do not diminish.

■ NURSING CONSIDERATIONS: The nurse faces the patient during the evaluation, establishes eye contact, repeats questions if necessary, avoids shouting, and addresses the person by name. If the patient's visual perception and tactile sense are diminished, the nurse uses color contrasts and items of marked textural differences in the assessment.

■ OUTCOME CRITERIA: Aging does not progress at a uniform rate, and its effects may vary widely from one individual to the next, but, in many cases, changes considered normal in elderly patients are disease processes that may respond to treatment. A careful assessment distinguishes the effects of pathology from those of aging and elucidates the care needed by the patient.

assimilate /əsim′əlāt/ [L, *assimilare*, to make alike], to absorb nutritive substances from the digestive tract to the circulatory system and consequently convert into living tissues.

assimilation [L, *assimulare*, to make alike], **1.** the process of incorporating nutritive material into living tissue; the end stage of the nutrition process, after digestion and absorption or occurring simultaneously with absorption. **2.** (in psychology) the incorporation of new experiences into a person's pattern of consciousness. Compare **apperception. 3.** (in sociology) the process in which a person or a group of people of a different ethnic background become absorbed into a new culture. **–assimilate,** *v.*

assist-control mode, a system of mechanical ventilation in which the patient is allowed to initiate breathing, although the ventilator delivers a set volume with each breath. The machine can also be programmed to take over at a backup rate if the patient's breathing slows beyond a certain point or stops altogether.

assisted breech [L, *assistere*, to stand by], an obstetric operation in which a baby being born feet or buttocks first is permitted to deliver spontaneously as far as its umbilicus and is then extracted. Also called **partial breech extraction.** Compare **breech extraction.**

assisted circulation [L, *assistere*, to stand, *circulare*, to go around], a method of treating patients with severe circulatory deficiencies by introducing a mechanical pumping system to aid the blood flow.

assisted death, a form of euthanasia in which an individual expressing a wish to die prematurely is helped to accomplish that goal by another person, either by counseling and/or by providing a poison or other lethal instrument. The assisted death may be regarded as a homicide or suicide by local authorities, and the person giving assistance may be held responsible for the death. In most cases, the deceased was a terminally ill patient.

assisted suicide, a form of euthanasia in which a person wishes to commit suicide but feels unable to perform the act alone because of a physical disability or lack of knowledge about the most effective means. An individual who assists a suicide victim in accomplishing that goal may or may not be held responsible for the death, depending on local laws.

assisted ventilation, the use of mechanical or other devices to help maintain respiration, usually by delivering air or oxygen under positive pressure. See also **IPPB.**

Associate Degree in Nursing (ADN) /əsō′shē·āt/ [L, *associare*, to unite], an academic degree awarded upon satisfactory completion of a 2-year course of study, usually at a community or junior college. The recipient is eligible to take the national licensing examination to become a registered nurse. An associate degree in nursing is not available in Canada.

associate nurse *U.S.,* **1.** (in primary nursing) a nurse who is responsible for implementing a primary nurse's care plans. **2.** in some states, a registered nurse who holds a diploma from a hospital school of nursing or an associate degree.

associated antagonist, one of a pair of muscles or group of muscles that pull in opposite directions but whose combined action results in moving a part in one direction.

association /əsō'shē·ā'shən/ [L, *associare*, to unite], **1.** a connection, union, joining, or combination of things. **2.** (in psychology) the connection of remembered feelings, emotions, sensations, thoughts, or perceptions with particular persons, things, or ideas. Kinds of association are **association of ideas, clang association, controlled association, dream association,** and **free association.**

association area, any part of the cerebral cortex involved in the integration of sensory information. Also called **association cortex.**

Association for Practitioners of Infection Control (APIC), a national professional organization of nurses who work in the field of infection control.

Association for the Advancement of Medical Instrumentation (AAMI), a nonprofit organization involved ineducation and standards relating to biomedical engineering.

Association for the Care of Children's Health (ACCH), an international, interdisciplinary organization concerned with the psychosocial needs of children and their families in health care settings. A quarterly journal and a bimonthly newsletter are available to members. There are affiliate organizations throughout the United States and Canada.

Association of Canadian Medical Colleges (ACMC), a Canadian organization of the deans and faculty members of the nation's 16 medical schools. It is concerned with all aspects of the education of physicians and acts as the liaison between the member schools and other professional organizations and governmental agencies. The official languages of the ACMC are English and French.

associationist model of learning /əsō'shē·ā'shənist/, a theory that defines learning as behavioral change that is a result of reinforced practice. If the response has not been reinforced repeatedly, an alternative behavior may be substituted.

association of ideas, a mental connection established between similar or simultaneously occurring ideas, feelings, or perceptions.

Association of Operating Room Nurses (AORN), a national organization of operating room nurses.

association test, a technique used in psychiatric diagnosis and in educational and psychologic evaluation in which a person is asked to respond to a stimulus word with the first word that comes to mind. The time taken to respond and the associations offered are compared with pretested responses and are classified and enumerated for diagnostic significance. Also called **word association test.**

association paralysis, a motor neuron disease in which wasting, weakness, and fasciculation of the tongue, facial muscles, pharynx, and larynx occur. Also called **progressive bulbar paralysis.**

associative looseness /əsō'shətiv/, a form of thought disorder in which the patient is unable to maintain consistent thought for more than a few minutes and jumps from thought to thought in the same conversation.

associative play, a form of play in which a group of children participate in similar or identical activities without formal organization, group direction, group interaction, or a definite goal. The children may borrow or lend toys or pieces of play equipment, and they may imitate others in the group, but each child acts independently, as on a playground or among a group riding tricycles or bicycles. Compare **cooperative play.** See also **parallel play, solitary play.**

assortive mating, the matching of males and females for reproduction in a manner that avoids random selection.

assumed role /əs(y)ōomd'/, a role in life that an individual usually selects or achieves by choice, such as one's role in marriage or employment. See also **ascribed role.**

-ast, a combining form designating an antiasthmatic or antiallergic drug not acting primarily as an antihistamine.

AST, 1. abbreviation for **angiotensin sensitivity test. 2.** abbreviation for **aspartate aminotransferase.**

astasia /astā'zhə/, a motor nerve disorder marked by an inability to stand or sit without assistance.

astasia-abasia [Gk, *a, stasis,* not stand + *a, basis,* not step], a form of ataxia in which the patient is unable to stand or walk because of lack of motor coordination although able to carry out natural leg movements when sitting or lying down. Also called **abasia-astasia.**

astatine (At) [Gk, *astasis,* unsteady], a very unstable, radioactive element that occurs naturally in tiny amounts. Its atomic number is 85; its atomic weight is 210.

asteatosis /as'tē·ətō'sis/ [Gk, *a, stear,* not tallow, *osis,* condition], a dry skin condition caused by a deficiency of sebaceous gland secretions. There may be scales and fissures as a result of the dryness. The condition is treated with creams and ointments that replace the missing skin oils.

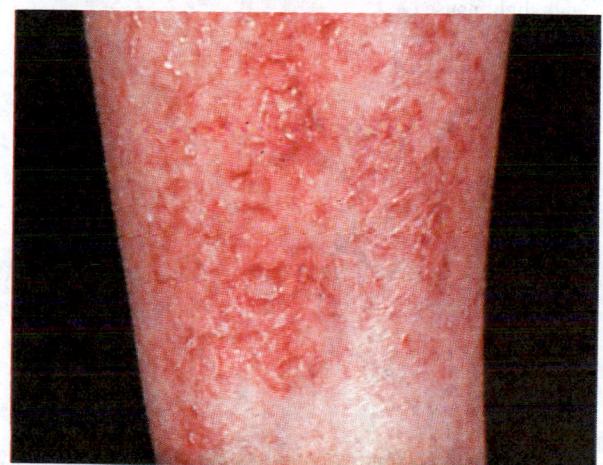

Asteatotic eczema *(du Vivier, 1993)*

-aster, a suffix meaning 'star-shaped': *cytaster, diaster, oleaster.*

astereognosis /əstir'ē·og·nō'sis/ [Gk, *a, stereos,* not solid, *gnosis,* knowledge], an inability to identify objects by touch.

asterixis /as'tərik'sis/ [Gk, *a, sterixis,* not fixed position], a hand-flapping tremor, often accompanying metabolic disorders. The tremor is usually induced by extending the arm and dorsiflexing the wrist. Asterixis is seen frequently in hepatic encephalopathy. Also called **flapping tremor, liver flap.**

asteroid body [Gk, *aster,* star, *eidos,* form], an irregular star-shaped structure that develops in the giant cells in certain diseases, including sarcoidosis, actinomycosis, and nocardiosis.

asthenia /asthē′nē·ə/ [Gk, *a, sthenos,* not strength], **1.** the lack or loss of strength or energy; weakness; debility. **2.** (in psychiatry) lack of dynamic force in the personality. Kinds of asthenia include **myalgic asthenia** and **neurocirculatory asthenia.** See also **adynamia.** –**asthenic,** *adj.*

-asthenia, a suffix meaning '(condition of) debility, loss of stength and energy, depleted vitality': *gangliasthenia, neurasthenia, phlebasthenia.*

asthenic /asthen′ik/ [Gk, *a,* without, *sthenos,* strength], pertaining to a condition of weakness, feebleness, or loss of vitality.

asthenic habitus [Gk, *a, sthenos,* not strength; L *habere* to have], a body structure characterized by a slender build with long limbs, an angular profile, and prominent muscles or bones. Compare **athletic habitus, pyknic.** See also **ectomorph.**

asthenic personality, a personality characterized by low energy, lack of enthusiasm, depressed emotions, and oversensitivity to physical and emotional strain. A person who has this kind of personality may be easily fatigued and self-pitying and may place the burden of physical and emotional difficulties on others.

asthenopia /as′thənō′pē·ə/ [Gk, *a, sthenos* + *ops,* eye], a condition in which the eyes tire easily because of weakness of the ocular or ciliary muscles. Symptoms include pain in or around the eyes, headache, dimness of vision, dizziness, and slight nausea.

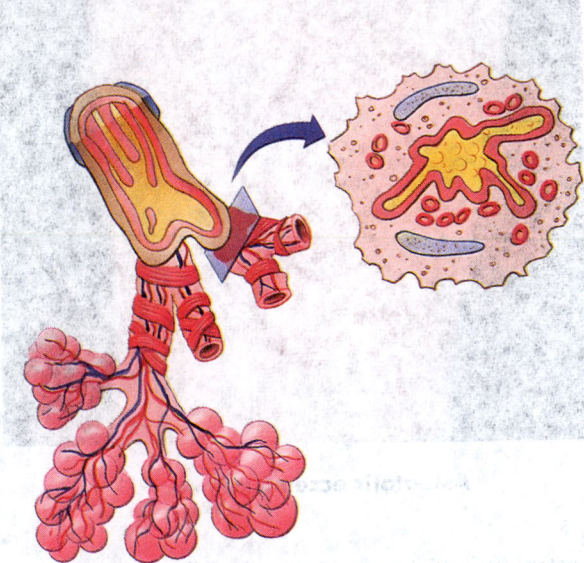

Asthma—obstruction of airways by excessive mucous production and edeman of respiratory mucosa
(Thibodeau, 1993/Rolin Graphics)

asthma /az′mə/ [Gk, panting], a respiratory disorder characterized by recurring episodes of paroxysmal dyspnea, wheezing on expiration/inspiration due to constriction of the bronchi, coughing, and viscous mucoid bronchial secretions. The episodes may be precipitated by inhalation of allergens or pollutants, infection, cold air, vigorous exercise, or emotional stress. Treatment may include elimination of the causative agent, hyposensitization, aerosol or oral bronchodilators, beta-adrenergic drugs, methylxanthines, and short-term use of corticosteroids. Sedatives and cough suppressants may be contraindicated. Also called **bronchial asthma.** See also **allergic asthma, asthma in children, exercise-induced asthma, intrinsic asthma, organic dust, status asthmaticus.**

-asthma, a suffix meaning '(condition of) labored breathing'.

asthma crystal. See **Charcot-Leyden crystal.**

asthma in children, an obstructive respiratory condition characterized by recurring attacks of paroxysmal dyspnea, wheezing, prolonged expiration, and an irritative cough that is a common, chronic illness in childhood. Onset usually occurs between 3 and 8 years of age. Asthmatic attacks are caused by constriction of the large and small airways, resulting from bronchial smooth muscle spasm, edema or inflammation of the bronchial wall, or excessive production of mucus. It is a complex disorder involving biochemical, immunologic, infectious, endocrinologic, and psychologic factors. Asthma in children is usually extrinsic, that is, most attacks are associated with an allergenic hypersensitivity to a foreign substance, such as airborne pollen, mold, house dust, certain foods, animal hair and skin, feathers, insects, smoke, and various chemicals or drugs. In infants, especially those born into a family with a history of allergic reactions, food allergy is a common precipitating factor. In some instances, episodes are triggered by nonallergenic factors, such as infection or inflammation, bronchial compression from external pressure, obstruction by a foreign body, physical stress resulting from fatigue or exercise, exposure to cold air, or psychologic stress. Such cases are classified as nonallergic, or intrinsic, asthma. A few cases may be caused by an inherited or acquired defect of adrenergic and cholinergic control of airway diameter. There is a strong hereditary factor associated with the disease. As many as 75%

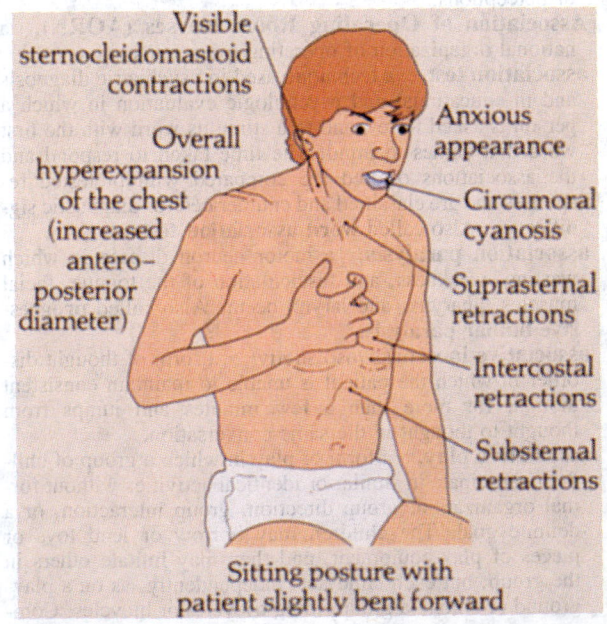

Visible sternocleidomastoid contractions

Overall hyperexpansion of the chest (increased antero-posterior diameter)

Anxious appearance

Circumoral cyanosis

Suprasternal retractions

Intercostal retractions

Substernal retractions

Sitting posture with patient slightly bent forward

Asthma in children—physical findings *(Zitelli, 1992)*

of children with asthma have a family history of the disorder, and the child usually has other allergic manifestations, such as hay fever, eczema, or urticaria. The disease occurs twice as often in boys as in girls before puberty, but boys and girls are affected equally during adolescence.

■ OBSERVATIONS: The condition is often confused with acute middle and lower respiratory tract infections, congenital stridor, obstruction of the bronchi or trachea, bronchial or tracheal compression, and cystic fibrosis. The diagnosis is generally determined by observation during a physical examination, a medical history confirming a presence of allergic reactions and familial allergic disease, and, to a lesser degree, laboratory tests and x-ray studies, which primarily eliminate identification of other diseases. A unique diagnostic feature is the presence of large numbers of eosinophils and their crystalloid degenerative fragments, called Charcot-Leyden crystals, in the sputum. Pulmonary function tests are valuable for assessing the degree of airway obstruction and the volume of gas exchange. Asthmatic episodes vary greatly in frequency, duration, and degree of symptoms, ranging from occasional periods of wheezing, mild coughing, and slight dypsnea to severe attacks that can lead to total airway obstruction and respiratory tract failure (status asthmaticus). An attack may begin gradually or abruptly and is often preceded by an upper respiratory infection. In general, episodes caused by infection have a gradual onset and are of long duration, whereas those resulting from allergenic factors are acute and subside quickly if the causative agent is removed. Typically, an attack begins with signs of air hunger, yawning, sighing, shortness of breath, paroxysms of wheezing, and a hacking, nonproductive cough. As secretions increase, the expiratory phase becomes prolonged, the cough gets deeper and more rattling, and a large quantity of thick, tenacious, mucoid sputum is produced as the attack subsides. The child appears apprehensive, speaks in a panting manner, and may assume a bent-over position to facilitate breathing. The prolonged expiratory phase is not as noticeable in infants and young children. In severe spasm or obstruction the respirations become shallow and irregular. A sudden increase in the rate of respiration, repeated hacking, and nonproductive coughing are indicative of lack of air movement with impending ventilatory failure and asphyxia. Children with chronic asthma develop a barrel chest from the continuous hyperventilated state and usually carry their shoulders in an elevated position to make better use of the accessory muscles of respiration.

■ INTERVENTIONS: An acute asthmatic attack is a medical emergency and requires immediate relief of bronchial obstruction with bronchodilating drugs, reduction of mucosal edema, and removal of excess bronchial secretions. The major drugs used to relieve bronchospasm are the beta-adrenergic agents, including epinephrine, isoproterenol, ephedrine, isoetharine, metaproterenol, terbutaline, and salbutamol; the methylxanthines, including theophylline and aminophylline; corticosteroids; expectorants; and antibiotics for cases in which infection is the triggering mechanism. Rarely, an acute attack does not respond to any of these measures, resulting in status asthmaticus. Hospitalization is required. The child is usually in a state of dehydration and acidosis with hypoxia and hypercapnia. Management consists of intravenous fluids; humidified oxygen given by tent, face mask, or cannula; administration of sodium bicarbonate or tromethamine to keep pH at acceptable levels; and use of bronchodilators to alleviate bronchospasm and of an-

tibiotics to reduce risk of infection. Children with mild, intermittent episodes of asthma are treated with bronchodilators in aerosol sprays, which provide quick relief and are effective in controlling an attack at the outset; oral administration is preferred for younger children. Those with persistent chronic asthma receive daily oral doses of a bronchodilator, often theophylline, usually in combination with an expectorant and corticosteroids. Bronchospasm induced by exercise can be treated prophylactically with cromolyn sodium, which inhibits the release of histamine in the lungs. Long-range management and treatment consist of physical training and exercises to induce physical and mental relaxation, improve posture, strengthen respiratory musculature, and develop better breathing patterns. Hyposensitization is recommended when an allergen is known and cannot be avoided. Prognosis for children with asthma varies considerably; many children lose their symptoms at puberty but the symptoms reaapear in their 40's. Prognosis depends on the number and severity of symptoms, emotional factors, and the family history of allergy.

■ NURSING CONSIDERATIONS: The primary focus of nursing care for children with acute asthma is to relieve symptoms of respiratory distress by initiating intravenous infusion and oxygen therapy, correcting acidosis, and administering bronchodilators and corticosteroids. The nurse implements measures to promote physical comfort, induce rest, and reduce fatigue and anxiety. It is especially important to reassure the child and parents concerning procedures, equipment, and prognosis. The nurse also plays an important role in the long-term support of children with chronic asthma, primarily in teaching the child and parents about the disease and how to cope with the condition. Once an allergen is determined, the home environment may be modified to reduce contact with the causative agents. The nurse teaches the child and parents how to use prescribed medications, especially nebulizers and aerosol devices, how to detect early signs of an attack so that it can be controlled with medication, how to determine any adverse effects of the drugs, especially the dangers of overuse, and how to implement physical exercise and play activities as therapeutic measures, especially those that promote proper breathing techniques. Children with emotional problems require special attention; psychologic stresses often trigger asthmatic attacks, and psychotherapy or behavior therapy is often necessary.

-asthmatic, a suffix meaning 'pertaining to asthma, its symptoms, or its treatment': *antiasthmatic, nonasthmatic, postasthmatic.*

asthmatic breathing /azmat'ik/ [Gk, *asthma,* panting, AS, *braeth*], breathing marked by prolonged wheezing upon exhalation because of spasmodic contractions of the bronchi.

asthmatic cough [Gk, *asthma,* AS, *cohhetan*], a wheezing cough accompanied by signs of breathing difficulty.

asthmatic eosinophilia, a form of eosinophilic pneumonia, characterized by allergic bronchospasm, by expectoration of bronchial casts containing eosinophils and mycelium, and by cough and fever. The condition usually occurs in the fourth or fifth decade of life, and is twice as common in women as in men. It is a result of hypersensitivity to *Aspergillus fumigatus* or *Candida albicans.* Untreated, the condition may result in pleural effusion, pericarditis, ascites, encephalitis, hepatomegaly, and respiratory failure. Treatment is similar to that for asthma and includes administration of corticosteroids and antibiotics.

Desensitization to the allergen is not usually effective. See also **allergic asthma, eosinophilic pneumonia.**

Astiban, a trademark for an investigational parasiticide (sodium stibocaptate), available only from the Centers for Disease Control.

astigmatic /as′tigmat′ik/ [Gk, *a*, without, *stigma*, point], pertaining to astigmatism, or an error of refraction in which a ray of light is not sharply focused on the retinal tissue, but is spread over a more diffuse area. Astigmatism is due to differences in curvature in the various meridians of the cornea and lens of the eye.

astigmatism /əstig′mətiz′əm/ [Gk, *a, stigma*, not point], an abnormal condition of the eye in which the light rays cannot be focused clearly in a point on the retina because the spheric curve of the cornea is not equal in all meridians. Vision is blurred, and use of the eyes causes discomfort. The person cannot accommodate to correct the problem. The condition usually may be corrected with contact lenses or with eye glasses ground to neutralize the defect.

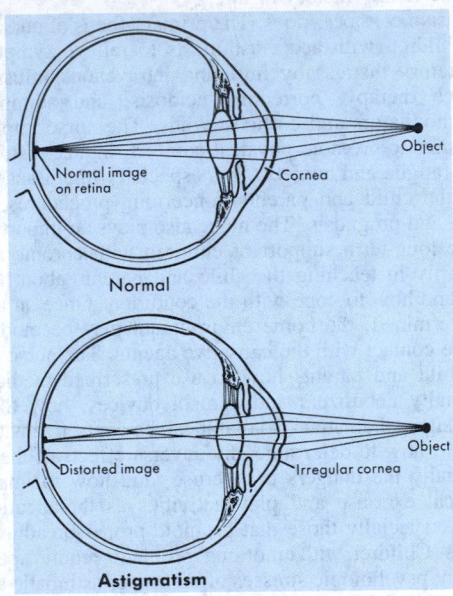

Astigmatism

-astine, a combining form designating an antihistaminic.

astragalus. See **talus.**

astringent /əstrin′jənt/ [Gk, *astringere*, to tighten], **1.** a substance that causes contraction of tissues upon application, usually used locally. **2.** having the quality of an astringent. **−astringency,** *n.*

astringent bath, a bath in which alum, tannic acid, or another astringent is added to the water.

astro-, a prefix meaning 'pertaining to a star, or star-shaped': *astroblastoma, astrocytoma, astrophorous.*

astroblastoma /as′trōblastō′mə/, *pl.* **astroblastomas, astroblastomata** [Gk, *aster*, star, *blastos*, germ, *oma*, tumor], a malignant neoplasm of the brain and spinal cord. Cells of an astroblastoma lie around blood vessels or around connective tissue septa.

astrocyte /as′trōsīt′/ [Gk, *aster* + *kytos*, cell], a large, star-shaped cell found in certain tissues of the nervous system.

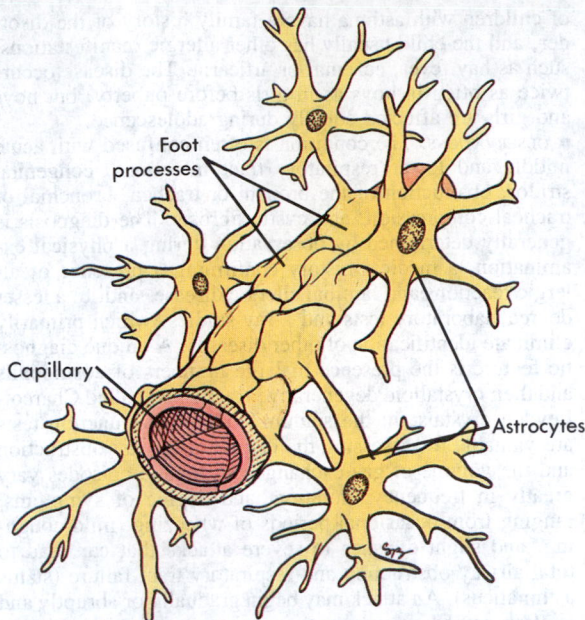

Astrocytes *(Seeley, 1992/Scott Bodell)*

astrocytoma /as′trōsītō′mə/, *pl.* **astrocytomas, astrocytomata** [Gk, *aster, kytos* + *oma*], a primary tumor of the brain composed of astrocytes and characterized by slow growth, cyst formation, invasion of surrounding structures, and the development of a highly malignant glioblastoma within the tumor mass. Complete surgical resection of an astrocytoma may be possible early in the development of the tumor. Also called **astrocytic glioma.**

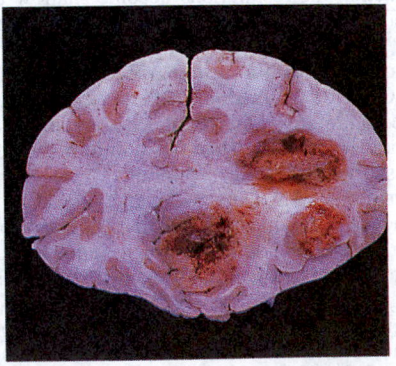

Astrocytoma
(Okazaki, 1988/by permission of Mayo Foundation)

astrocytosis /as′trōsītō′sis/ [Gk, *aster, kytos* + *osis*, condition], an increase in the number of neuroglial cells with fibrous or protoplasmic processes frequently observed in an irregular area adjacent to degenerative lesions, such as abscesses, certain brain neoplasms, and encephalomalacia.

Astrocytosis represents a reparative process, and in some cases may be diffuse in a large region.

asymmetric /āˈsimetˈrik, asˈimetˈrik/ [Gk, *a, symmetria,* not proportion], (of the body or parts of the body) unequal in size or shape; different in placement or arrangement about an axis. Also **asymmetrical.** Compare **symmetric.** −**asymmetry** /āsimˈitrē, asimˈ-/, *n.*

asymmetric tonic neck reflex. See **tonic neck reflex.**

-asymmetry. See **asymmetric.**

asymptomatic /āsimpˈtəmatˈik/ [Gk, *a,* without, *symptom*], without symptoms.

asymptomatic neurosyphilis [Gk, *a,* without, *symptoma* + *neuron,* nerve; Fr, *syphilide*], a form of neurosyphilis that shows pathologic changes in the cerebrospinal fluid, although there are no symptoms of nervous system damage. Asymptomatic neurosyphilis may occur many years before actual nervous system damage is noticeable.

asynchronous /āsingˈkrənəs/ [Gk, *a, synchronos,* not simultaneous], (of an event or device) a computer operation in which the next command is performed in response to a signal that the previous command has been completed. One operation is completed before the next is initiated.

asynclitism /āsingˈklitizˈəm/ [Gk, *a, syn,* not together, *kleisis,* to lean], presentation of a parietal aspect of the fetal head to the maternal pelvic inlet in labor, the sagittal suture being parallel to the transverse diameter of the pelvis but anterior or posterior to it. In normal labor, the fetal head usually engages with some degree of asynclitism. **Anterior asynclitism,** in which the anterior part presents, is called Nägele's obliquity. **Posterior asynclitism** is called Litzmann's obliquity. See also **cardinal movements of labor, engagement.**

asyndesis /əsinˈdəsis/, a mental disorder marked by an inability to assemble related ideas or thoughts into one coherent concept.

asynergy /āsinˈərjē/ [Gk, *a, syn* + *ergein,* to work], **1.** a condition characterized by faulty coordination among groups of organs or muscles that normally function harmoniously. **2.** the state of muscle antagonism found in cerebellar disease. See also **ataxia, cerebellum.**

asyntaxia /āˈsintakˈsē·ə/ [Gk, *a, syn* + *taxis,* arrangement], any interference with the orderly sequence of growth and differentiation of the fetus during embryonic development, resulting in one or more congenital anomalies. A kind of asyntaxia is **asyntaxia dorsalis.** See also **developmental anomaly.**

asyntaxia dorsalis, failure of the neural tube to close during embryonic development. See also **neural tube defect.**

asystole /āsisˈtəlē/ [Gk, *a, systole,* not contraction], a life-threatening cardiac condition characterized by the absence of electrical and mechanical activity in the heart. Clinical signs include absent pulse and breathing. Without cardiac monitoring, asystole cannot be distinguished from ventricular fibrillation. −**asystolic** /āˈsistolˈik/, *adj.*

At, symbol for the element **astatine.**

at-. See **ad-.**

Atabrine Hydrochloride, a trademark for an antimalarial (quinacrine hydrochloride).

Atabrine stomatitis, an abnormal oral condition that may be associated with the use of Atabrine, characterized by oral changes simulating lichen planus. Compare **arsenic stomatitis, bismuth stomatitis.**

ataractic /atˈərakˈtik/ [Gk, *ataraktos,* quiet], pertaining to a drug or other agent that has a tranquilizing or sedating effect.

Atarax, a trademark for an antianxiety, antiemetic, and anticholinergic (hydroxyzine hydrochloride).

atavism /atˈəvizˈəm/ [L, *atavus,* ancestor], the appearance in an individual of traits or characteristics more like those of a grandparent or earlier ancestor than of the parents. Atavistic data may offer clues to an examining physician of genetic or familial health factors. −**atavistic,** *adj.*

atavistic [L, *atavus,* ancestor], the tendency for a genetic trait of a remote ancestor to be expressed in an individual due to chance recombination of genes.

ataxia /ətakˈsē·ə/ [Gk, disorder], an abnormal condition characterized by impaired ability to coordinate movement. A staggering gait and postural imbalance are caused by a lesion in the spinal cord or cerebellum, which might be the sequela of birth trauma, congenital disorder, infection, degenerative disorder, neoplasm, toxic substance, or head injury. See also **hereditary ataxia.** −**ataxial, ataxic,** *adj.*

ataxial. [Gk, *ataxia,* without order], pertaining to ataxia.

ataxia-telangiectasia [Gk, *ataxia* + *telos,* end, *aggeion,* vessel, *ektasis,* expansion], a rare genetic disease involving immunoglobulin metabolism that is transmitted as an autosomal recessive trait. The onset usually occurs in infancy and progresses slowly with increasing cerebellar degeneration and recurrent infections. Telangiectasias are most prominent on the ears, facial skin, and bulbar conjunctiva. There is an increased risk of malignancy, especially lymphoma. Also called **Louis-Bar syndrome.**

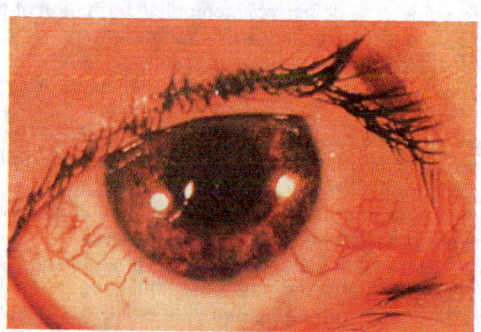

Bulbar telangiectasia typical of ataxia-telangiectasia
(Zitelli, 1992)

ataxic. See **ataxia.**

ataxic aphasia. See **motor aphasia.**

ataxic breathing, a type of breathing associated with a lesion in the medullary respiratory centers and characterized by a series of inspirations and expirations.

ataxic gait. See **cerebellar gait.**

ataxic speech, abnormal speech characterized by faulty formation of the sounds because of neuromuscular dysfunction.

ATCC, abbreviation for **American Type Culture Collection.**

-ate, 1. a suffix meaning 'acted upon or being in a (specified) state': *degenerate, disparate, enucleate.* **2.** a suffix meaning 'possessing': *caudate, cuspidate, longipedate.* **3.** a suffix meaning a 'chemical compound derived from a (specified) source': *silicate, sulfate, opiate.* **4.** a suffix meaning an 'acid compound': *acetate, oxalate, phosphate.*

atelectasis /at'ilek'təsis/ [Gk, *ateles,* incomplete, *ektasis,* expansion], an abnormal condition characterized by the collapse of lung tissue, preventing the respiratory exchange of carbon dioxide and oxygen. Symptoms may include diminished breath sounds, a mediastinal shift toward the side of the collapse, fever, and increasing dyspnea. The condition may be caused by obstruction of the major airways and bronchioles, by pressure on the lung from fluid or air in the pleural space, or by pressure from a tumor outside the lung. As the remaining portions of the lung eventually hyperinflate, oxygen saturation of the blood is often nearly normal. Loss of functional lung tissue may secondarily cause increased heart rate, blood pressure, and respiratory rate. The retained secretions are rich in nutrients for the growth of bacteria, a condition often leading to stasis pneumonia in critically ill patients. See also **postoperative atelectasis, primary atelectasis.**

atelectatic rale /at'iləktat'ik/ [Gk, *ateles, ektasis* + Fr, *rale,* rattle], an abnormal intermittent crackling sound heard during auscultation of the chest. It usually disappears after the individual being examined coughs or breathes deeply several times.

ateliotic dwarf /at'əlē·ot'ik/, a dwarf whose skeleton is incompletely formed, resulting from the nonunion of the epiphyses and diaphyses during bone development.

atelo-, a prefix meaning 'imperfect or incomplete': *atelocardia, ateloglossia, atelopodia.*

atelorachidia /at'əlôr'əkid'ē·ə/ [Gk, *ateles,* incomplete, *rhachis,* spine], a defective, incomplete formation of the spinal column. Also spelled **atelorhachidia.**

atenolol /aten'əlôl/, a beta-1 blocker.
- INDICATION: It is prescribed for the treatment of hypertension.
- CONTRAINDICATIONS: Sinus bradycardia, second- or third-degree atrioventricular block, cardiogenic shock, or cardiac failure prohibits its use.
- ADVERSE EFFECTS: Among the more serious adverse reactions are bradycardia, dizziness, and nausea.

ATG, abbreviation for **antithymocyte globulin.**

atherectomy catheter /ath'ərek'təmē/, a specially designed catheter for cutting away atheromatous plaque from the lining of an artery. A tiny metal cone at the tip of the catheter has cutting edges for loosening the plaque and has openings through which the plaque fragments can be aspirated. The catheter is positioned and monitored by fluoroscopy.

atheroembolic renal disease /ath'ərō·embol'ik/, a condition of gradual or rapid kidney failure resulting from obstruction of the renal arteries by atheromas and emboli. It is associated with atherosclerosis and hypertension and occurs most frequently in persons over 60 years of age. The patient is usually azotemic and also experiences emboli in other body areas.

atherogenesis [Gk, *athere,* porridge, *oma,* tumor, *genein,* to produce], the formation of subintimal plaques in the lining of arteries.

atheroma /ath'ərō'mə/, *pl.* **atheromas, atheromata** [Gk, *athere,* meal, *oma,* tumor], an abnormal mass of fat or lipids, as in a sebaceous cyst or in deposits in an arterial wall. **–atheromatous,** *adj.*

atheromatosis /ath'ərōmətō'sis/, the development of many atheromas.

atheromatous [Gk, *athere,* porridge, *oma,* tumor], pertaining to atheroma.

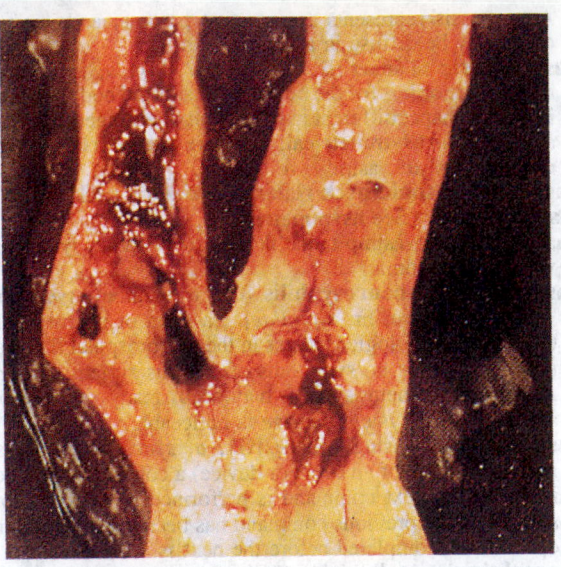

Atheroma in patient with prolonged hypertension
(Kamal, 1991/Courtesy Dr. Pauline Sambrook & Ciba-Geigy)

atheromatous plaque, a yellowish raised area on the lining of an artery formed by fatty deposits.

atherosclerosis /ath'ərōsklərō'sis/ [Gk, *athere,* meal, *sklerosis,* hardening], a common arterial disorder characterized by yellowish plaques of cholesterol, lipids, and cellular debris in the inner layers of the walls of large and medium-sized arteries. The vessel walls become thick, fibrotic, and calcified, and the lumen narrows, resulting in reduced blood flow to organs normally supplied by the artery. Atheromatous lesions are major causes of coronary heart disease, angina pectoris, myocardial infarction, and other cardiac disorders. The pathogenesis of atherosclerosis is not clear; it may be induced by injury to arterial endothelium, the proliferation of smooth muscle in vessel walls, or the accumulation of lipids in hyperlipidemia. Atherosclerosis usually occurs with aging and is often associated with obesity, hypertension, and diabetes. Segments of arteries obstructed or severely damaged by atheromatous lesions may be replaced by patch grafts or bypassed, as in coronary bypass surgery, or the lesion may be removed from the vessel via endarterectomy. Antilipidemic agents do not reverse atherosclerosis, but a diet low in cholesterol, calories, and saturated fats, adequate exercise, and the avoidance of smoking and stress may help prevent the disorder. Also called **arterial sclerosis, intimal sclerosis.** See also **arteriosclerosis.**

atherosclerotic aneurysm /-ot'ik/ [Gk, *athere, skleros,* hard, *aneurysma,* a widening], an aneurysm that develops as a result of atherosclerotic weakening of an arterial wall.

athetoid /ath'ətoid/, pertaining to athetosis, as in the involuntary, purposeless weaving motions of the body or its extremities.

athetosis /ath'ətō'sis/ [Gk, *athetos,* not fixed], a neuromuscular condition characterized by slow, writhing, continuous, and involuntary movement of the extremities, as seen in some forms of cerebral palsy and in motor disorders re-

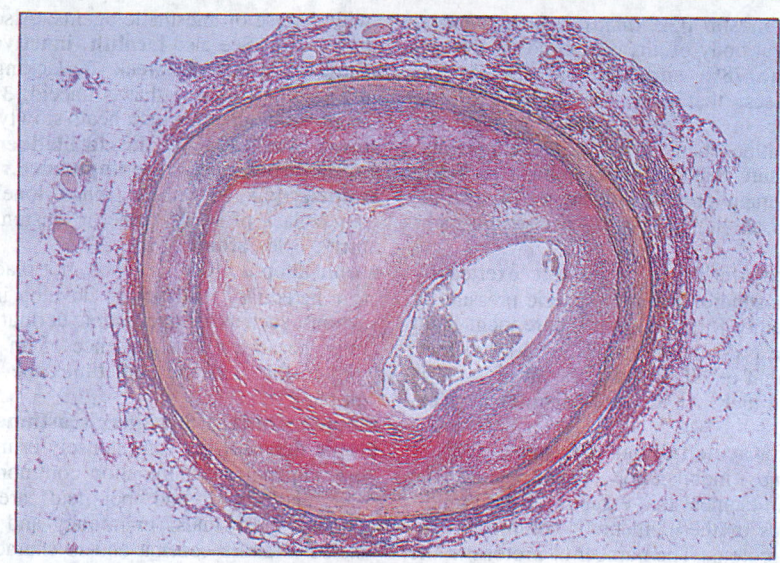

Athersclerotic plaque in an artery
(Seeley, 1992/Ronald J Ervin)

sulting from lesions in the basal ganglia, tabes dorsalis, or other conditions.

athiaminosis /əthī'əminō'sis/, a condition resulting from lack of thiamine in the diet. See also **beriberi, thiamine.**

athlete's foot. See **tinea pedis.**

athlete's heart /ath'lēts/, the typical normal but enlarged heart of an athlete trained for endurance, characterized by a slow heart rate, an increased pumping capacity, and greater than average ability to deliver oxygen to skeletal muscles. Also called **athletic heart syndrome (AHS).**

athletic habitus /athlet'ik/, a physique characterized by a well-proportioned, muscular body with broad shoulders, thick neck, deep chest, and flat abdomen. Compare **asthenic habitus, pyknic.** See also **mesomorph.**

athletic heart syndrome. See **athlete's heart.**

athletic trainer, an allied health professional who, with the consultation and supervision of attending physicians, is an integral part of the health care system associated with sports. Through preparation in both academic and practical experience, the athletic trainer provides a variety of services including injury prevention and recognition, immediate care, treatment, and rehabilitation of athletic trauma. Standards for recognition of athletic training as an allied health occupation were approved by the American Medical Association in 1990.

Athrombin-K, a trademark for an anticoagulant (warfarin).

Ativan, a trademark for an antianxiety agent (lorazepam), a benzodiazepine used as an adjunct to anesthesia.

atlantal /ətlan'təl/, pertaining to the atlas, the first cervical vertebra.

atlantoaxial /ətlan'tō·ak'sē·ə/[Gk, *atlas*, to bear + *axis*, pivot], pertaining to the first two cervical vertebrae.

atlantooccipital joint /-oksip'itəl/ [Gk, *Atlas, theni*, to bear; L, *ob*, against, *caput*, head], one of a pair of condyloid joints formed by the articulation of the atlas of the vertebral column with the occipital bone of the skull. It in-

cludes two articular capsules, two membranes, and two lateral ligaments. The atlantooccipital joint permits nodding and lateral movements of the head.

atlas [Gk, *Atlas*, a mythical king-giant], the first cervical vertebra, articulating with the occipital bone and the axis.

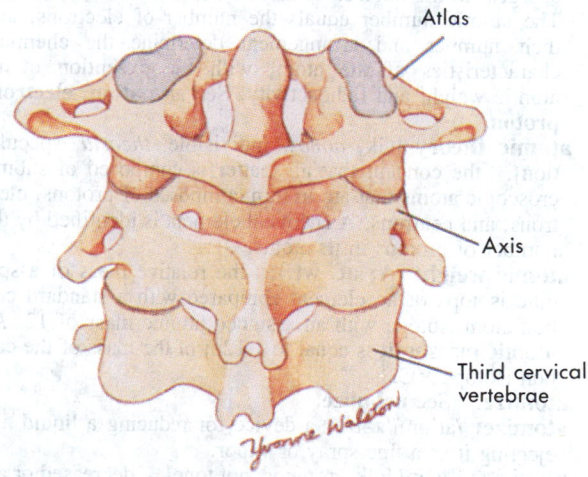

Atlas
Axis
Third cervical
vertebrae

Atlas (Thibodeau, 1993)

atm, **1.** abbreviation for **atmosphere. 2.** abbreviation for **atmospheric.**

atman /ät'män/, (in psychiatry) a concept derived from Eastern Indian philosophy that the highest value is to know one's true self. The atman represents the most inward reality, the innermost spirit, and the highest controlling power of a person.

atmo-, a prefix meaning 'pertaining to steam or vapor': *atmocausis, atmolysis, atmotherapy.*

atmosphere (atm) /at′məsfir/ [Gk, *atmos*, vapor, *sphaira*, sphere],   **1.** the natural body of air, composed of approximately 20% oxygen, 78% nitrogen, and 2% carbon dioxide and other gases, that covers the surface of the earth. **2.** an envelope of gas, which may or may not duplicate the natural atmosphere in chemical components. **3.** a unit of gas pressure that is usually defined as being equivalent to the average pressure of the earth's atmosphere at sea level, or about 14.7 pounds per square inch. **–atmospheric,** *adj.*

atmospheric pressure /-fer′ik/,   the pressure exerted by the weight of the atmosphere. The atmospheric pressure at sea level is approximately 15 pounds per square inch. With increasing altitude the pressure decreases: At 30,000 feet, approximately the height of Mt. Everest, the air pressure is 4.3 pounds per square inch. Also called **barometric pressure.**

ATN,   abbreviation for **acute tubular necrosis.**

atom /at′əm/ [Gk, *atmos*, indivisible],   **1.** (in physics) the smallest division of an element that exhibits all the properties and characteristics of the element. It comprises neutrons, electrons, and protons. The number of protons in the nucleus of every atom of any given element is the same and is called its atomic number. **2.** *nontechnical.* the amount of any substance that is so small further division is not possible. **3.** *informal.* a minute amount of any substance. **–atomic,** *adj.*

atomic mass unit (amu) /ətom′ik/,   the mass of a neutral atom of an element, expressed as 1/12 of the mass of carbon, which has an arbitrarily assigned value of 12. The energy equivalent of 1 amu is 931.2 MeV. The mass equivalent of 1 amu is $1.66(10^{-24}$ gm).

atomic number,   the number of protons, or positive charges, in the nucleus of an atom of a particular element. The atomic number equals the number of electrons, and their number and arrangement determine the chemical characteristics of the atom, with the exception of its atomic weight and radioactivity. See also **atom, electron, proton.**

atomic theory [Gk, *atmos,* indivisible, *theoria,* speculation],   the concept that all matter is composed of submicroscopic atoms that are in turn composed of protons, electrons, and neutrons. A chemical element is identified by the number of protons in its atoms.

atomic weight (A, at. wt.),   the relative mass of a specific isotope of an element compared with a standard carbon atom isotope with an assigned atomic mass of 12. An **atomic mass unit** is equal to 1/12th of the mass of the carbon isotope ^{12}C.

atomize.   See **nebulize.**

atomizer /at′əmī′zər/,   a device for reducing a liquid and ejecting it as a fine spray or vapor.

atonia /ātō′nē·ə/ [Gk, *a, tonos,* not tone],   decreased or absent muscle tone.

atonia constipation,   constipation caused by the failure of the colon to respond to the normal stimuli for evacuation due to loss of muscle tone. It may occur in elderly or bedridden patients or after prolonged dependence on laxatives. To prevent fecal impaction in the colon and rectum, a moderately irritant oral laxative or a mild suppository may be recommended. Patients are encouraged to develop regular, unhurried bowel habits and may be given a diet rich in fruits and vegetables. If fecal impaction develops, it may be removed by means of a mild enema or manual disimpaction,

with the use of anesthetic agents. Also called **colon stasis, lazy colon.** See also **fecalith, inactive colon.**

atonic /əton′ik/,   **1.** weak. **2.** lacking normal tone, as in the case of a muscle that is flaccid. **3.** lacking vigor, such as an atonic ulcer, which heals slowly. **–atony** /at′onē/, *n.*

atonic bladder.   See **flaccid bladder.**

atonic impotence.   See **impotence.**

atonicity [Gk, *a,* without, *tonos,* tone],   a condition of atony or lack of muscle tone or tension.

atony.   See **atonic.**

atopic /ātop′ik/ [Gk, *a, topos,* not place],   of or pertaining to a hereditary tendency to develop immediate allergic reactions, such as asthma, atopic dermatitis, or vasomotor rhinitis, because of the presence of an antibody (atopic reagin) in the skin and sometimes the bloodstream. **–atopy** /at′opē/, *n.*

atopic asthma.   See **allergic asthma.**

atopic dermatitis,   an intensely pruritic, often excoriated, maculopapular inflammation commonly found on the face and antecubital and popliteal areas of allergy-prone (atopic) individuals. In infancy and early childhood it is called infantile eczema and is characterized by erythema, oozing, and crusting. In adults the disease manifests itself with crusting and excoriation. Treatment includes identification and avoidance of allergens and administration of topical and parenteral corticosteroids, tar ointments, antihistamines, and wet compresses of Burow's solution. Also called **atopic eczema.** Compare **contact dermatitis.** See also **atopic.**

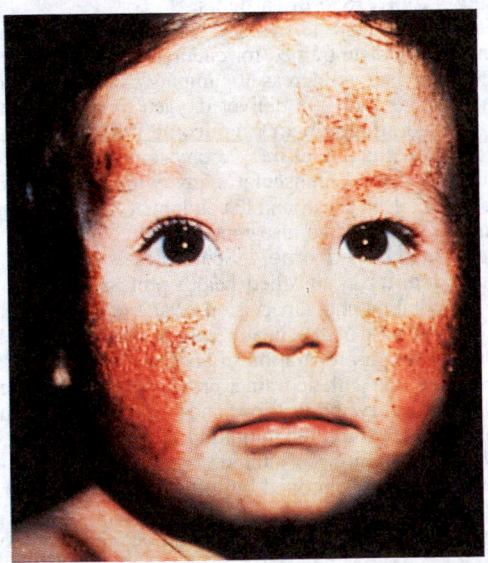

Infantile atopic dermatitis (*Zitelli, 1992*)

atopic reagin.   See **reagin.**

atopognosia /ātop′əgnō′zhə/ [Gk, *a, topos,* not place, *gnosis,* knowledge],   a form of corporeal agnosia in which a person is unable to locate a sensation properly.

atopy.   See **atopic.**

atoxic.   See **nontoxic.**

ATP, abbreviation for **adenosine triphosphate.**

ATPase, abbreviation for **adenosine triphosphatase.**

ATPD, abbreviation for *ambient temperature, ambient pressure, dry.*

ATPS, abbreviation for *ambient temperature, ambient pressure, saturated* (with water vapor). See also **volume (ATPS).**

atransferrinemic anemia /ā′transfer′inē′mik/, an iron-transport deficiency disease characterized by a failure of iron to move from the liver or other storage sites to tissues in which erthyrocytes develop. The condition is believed to be caused by a transferrin molecule defect, iron-binding protein. In addition to anemia, the patient usually suffers from hemosiderosis.

atraumatic /ā′trômat′ik/ [Gk, *a*, without, *trauma*], pertaining to therapies or therapeutic instruments and devices that are unlikely to cause tissue damage.

atresia /ətrē′zhə/ [Gk, *a, tresis*, not perforation], the absence of a normal body opening, duct, or canal, such as the anus, vagina, or external ear canal. —**atresic, atretic,** *adj.*

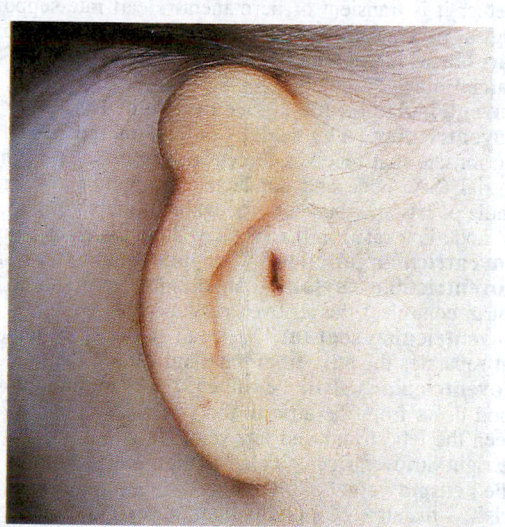

Atresia of the right external ear *(Zitelli, 1992)*

-atresia, a suffix meaning a 'condition of abnormal occlusion': *gynatresia, hedratresia, urethratresia.*

atresic teratism /ətrē′sik/ [Gk, *a, tresis* + *tera*, monster], a congenital anomaly in which any of the normal openings of the body, such as the mouth, nares, anus, or vagina, fail to form.

-atretic. See **atresia.**

atreto-, a prefix meaning 'closed, or lacking an opening': *atretoblepharia, atretolemia, atretorrhinia.*

atria. See **atrium.**

atrial. See **pacing.**

atrial appendix. See **auricle.**

atrial fibrillation (AF) /ā′trē·əl/, a cardiac dysrhythmia characterized by disorganized electrical activity in the atria accompanied by a rapid, irregular ventricular response. The atria quiver instead of pumping in an organized fashion, resulting in compromised ventricular filling and reduced

stroke volume. Stasis of flow increases the risk of embolic events. Atrial fibrillation is associated with rheumatic heart diseases, mitral stenosis, heart failure, and heart surgery. Treatment includes digitalis, antidysrhythmic drugs, electrical cardioversion, and surgical interruption of impulse transmission.

atrial flutter, a type of atrial tachycardia with rates from 230 to 380/min. Two types (I and II) have been identified and are distinguished from each other by their rates. In Type I the atrial rate is 290-310/min, but can range between 230 and 350/min. In Type II the atrial rate is 360-380/min but can range between 340 and 430/min. Type I can be interrupted with rapid atrial pacing; Type II cannot be terminated in this way and often requires aggressive pharmacologic treatment. Compare **atrial fibrillation.**

atrial gallop, an abnormal cardiac rhythm in which a low-pitched, extra sound is heard late in diastole, just before the S_1, on auscultation of the heart. It indicates increased resistance to ventricular filling and is frequently heard in hypertensive cardiovascular disease, coronary artery disease, and aortic stenosis. Also called S_4. See also **gallop, heart sound.**

atrial myxoma, a benign, pedunculated, gelatinous tumor that originates in the interatrial septum of the heart. The tumor is characterized by palpitations, disseminated neuritis, nausea, weight loss, fatigue, dyspnea, fever, and, occasionally, sudden loss of consciousness. It is treated by surgical removal of the tumor.

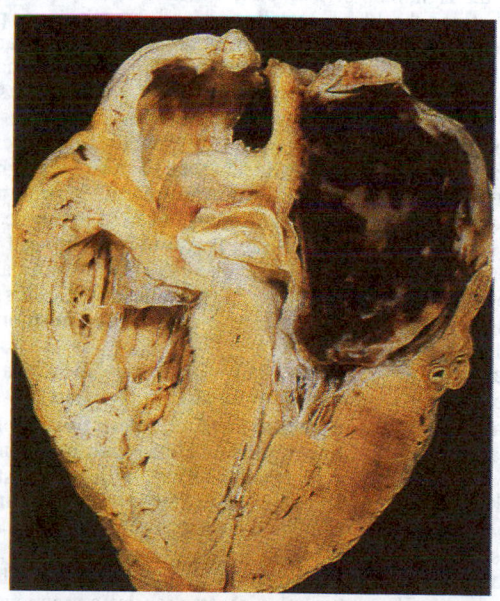

Left atrial myxoma *(Anderson, 1986)*

atrial pacing. See **pacing.**

atrial septal defect (ASD), a congenital cardiac anomaly characterized by an abnormal opening between the atria. The severity of the condition depends on the size and location of the defect, which depend on the stage at which em-

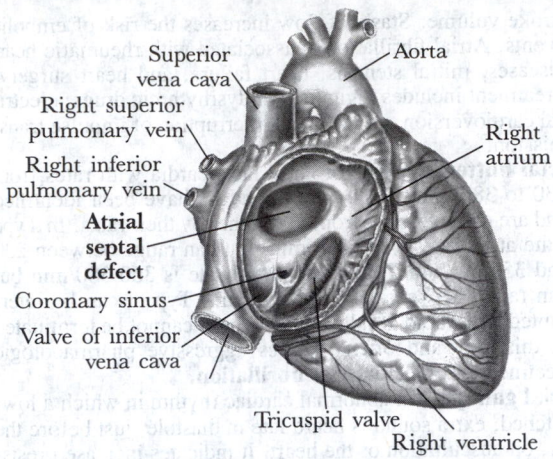

Superior vena cava

Aorta

Right superior pulmonary vein

Right inferior pulmonary vein

Right atrium

Atrial septal defect

Coronary sinus

Valve of inferior vena cava

Tricuspid valve

Right ventricle

Atrial septal defect (Cannobio, 1989)

bryonic development of the septum was arrested. The defects are classified as ostium secundum defect, in which the aperture in the septum secundum, or second septum, of the fetal heart fails to close; ostium primum defect, in which there is inadequate development of the endocardial cushions of the first septum of the heart; and sinus venosus defect, in which the superior portion of the atrium fails to develop. Atrial septal defects increase the flow of oxygenated blood into the right side of the heart, which is usually well tolerated, since the blood is delivered under much lower pressure than in ventricular septal defect. Clinical manifestations include right atrial and ventricular enlargement, a characteristic harsh, scratchy systolic murmur, and a fixed splitting of the second heart sound, which does not vary with respiration. X-ray films and electrocardiograms generally show right atrial and ventricular enlargement, although definitive diagnosis is made by cardiac catheterization or echocardiogram. Surgical closure is indicated in most cases, but unless the defect is severe, it is usually postponed until later childhood to prevent complications during early adulthood, such as atrial arrhythmias, bacterial endocarditis, and congestive heart failure. See also **endocardial cushion defect.**

atrial septum [L, *atrium,* hall + *saeptum,* fence], a partition between the left and right atria of the heart.

atrial standstill, a condition of complete failure of the atria to contract. Generally, a junctional pacemaker maintains continuation of ventricular activity during atrial standstill. P waves are absent in all ECG surface leads and A waves are absent in the jugular venous pulse and right atrial pressure tracings.

atrial systole, the contraction of the atria of the heart, which precedes ventricular contraction by a fraction of a second.

atrial tachycardia [L, *atrium,* hall; Gk, *tachys,* quick + *kardia,* heart], rapid contraction of the atria because of an ectopic focus that may increase the rate to more than 200 beats min. The ventricles usually respond to each atrial contraction. When an attack begins or ends suddenly it is referred to as **paroxysmal atrial tachycardia (PAT)** and may be influenced by impulses from the vagus nerve. Attacks are often terminated by stimulation of the vagus nerve. Also called **auricular tachycardia.**

atrichosis /ā'trikō'sis/ [Gk, *a, trichia* without hair + *osis,* condition], a congenital absence of hair.

atrio-, a prefix meaning 'pertaining to the atrium of the heart': *atriocommissuropexy, atrionector, atrioseptopexy.*

atrioventricular (AV) /ā'trē·ōventrik'yələr/ [L, *atrium,* hall, *ventriculum*], pertaining to an atrium and a ventricle.

atrioventricular (AV) block (AVB) [L, *atrium* + *ventriculus,* little belly], a disorder of cardiac impulse transmission that reflects prolonged, intermittent, or absent conduction of the impulse between the atria and ventricles. It commonly occurs at the AV node or within the bundle branch system. Treatment depends on the location of the block and whether it is transient or permanent. Heart rate-supporting drugs or pacemaker insertion are common options. See also **heart block, intraatrial block, intraventricular block, sinoatrial block.**

atrioventricular bundle. See **bundle of His.**

atrioventricular (AV) node, an area of specialized cardiac muscle that receives the cardiac impulse from the sinoatrial (SA) node and conducts it to the atrioventricular bundle of His and thence to the walls of the ventricles. The AV node is located in the septal wall of the right atrium.

atrioventricular junction. See **junctional extrasystole.**

atrioventricular rhythm, an obsolete term for a heart beat in control of the atrioventricular node.

atrioventricular septum, a small portion of membrane that separates the atria from the ventricles of the heart.

atrioventricular valve, a valve in the heart through which blood flows from the atria to the ventricles. The valve between the left atrium and left ventricle is the mitral valve; the right atrioventricular valve is the tricuspid valve. Also called **cuspid valve.**

at risk, the state of an individual or population being vulnerable to a particular disease or injury. The factors determining risk may be environmental or physiologic. An example of an environmental factor is exposure to harmful substances or organisms. An example of a physiologic factor is genetic predisposition to a disease.

atrium /ā'trē·əm/, *pl.* **atria** [L, hall], a chamber or cavity, such as the right and left atria of the heart or the nasal cavity.

atrium of the heart, one of the two upper chambers of the heart. The right atrium receives deoxygenated blood from the superior vena cava, the inferior vena cava, and the coronary sinus. The left atrium receives oxygenated blood

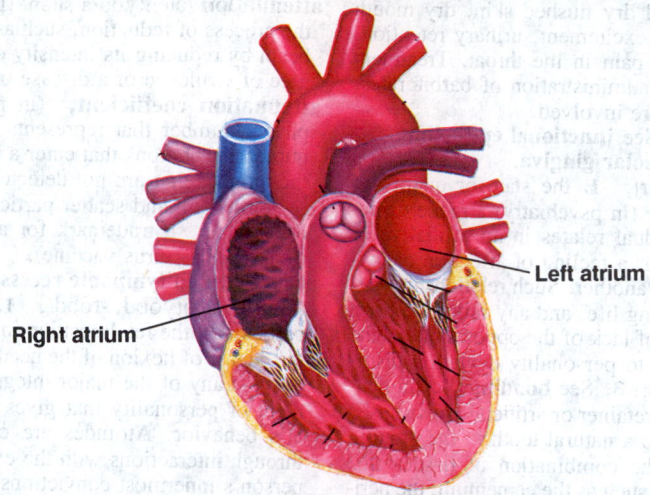

Atria of the heart (Cannobio, 1989)

from the pulmonary veins. Blood is emptied into the ventricles from the atria during diastole.

Atromid-S, a trademark for an antihyperlipidemic (clofibrate).

-atrophia, -trophy, 1. a suffix meaning a 'condition of malnutrition': *metatrophia, metratrophia, pantatrophia.* **2.** a combining form meaning a 'progressive decline of a body part': *dermatrophia, neuratrophia, splenatrophia.*

atrophic /ātrof′ik/ [Gk, *a*, without, *trophe*, nourishment], characterized by a wasting of tissues, usually associated with general malnutrition or a specific disease state.

atrophic arthritis. See rheumatoid arthritis.

atrophic catarrh [Gk, *a, trophe*, not nourishment; *kata*, down, *rhoia* flow], an abnormal condition characterized by inflammation and discharge from the mucous membranes of the nose, accompanied by the loss of mucosal and submucosal tissue. Compare **hypertrophic catarrh.** See also **catarrh.**

atrophic cirrhosis [Gk, *a,trophe*, atrophy, *kirrhos*, yellowish coloration], a form of advanced portal cirrhosis with massive shrinkage of the liver.

atrophic fracture, a spontaneous fracture caused by atrophy, as in the bones of an elderly person.

atrophic gastritis, a chronic inflammation of the stomach, associated with degeneration of the gastric mucosa. Seen in elderly patients and in persons with pernicious anemia, atrophic gastritis rarely causes epigastric pain. See also **pernicious anemia.**

atrophic glossitis, a pathologic condition in which the various papillae are lost from the dorsum of the tongue resulting in a very sore and highly sensitive surface that makes eating difficult. See also **glossitis.**

atrophic rhinitis [Gk, *a, trophe,* nourishment, *rhis,* nose + *itis,* inflammation], a nasal condition in which there is atrophy of the mucous membrane of the nose, resulting in failure of the ciliary function and drying and crusting of the lining of the nasal passages. This may alter olfactory sensation.

atrophic vaginitis [Gk, *a, trophe,* nourishment; L, *vagina,* sheath; Gk, *itis,* inflammation], a condition of degeneration of the vaginal mucous membrane after menopause.

atrophied /at′rōfīd/ [Gk, *a, trophe*], decreased in size as an organ, tissue, or body part because of disuse or disease.

atrophoderma /at′rōfədur′mə/ [Gk, *a, trophe* + *derma,* skin], the wasting away or decrease in size of the skin. The atrophy may affect the entire body surface or only localized areas. The condition is often associated with aging and may occur as a primary or secondary symptom of various diseases.

atrophy /at′rəfē/ [Gk, *a, trophe,* not nourishment], a wasting or diminution of size or physiologic activity of a part of the body because of disease or other influences. A skeletal muscle may undergo atrophy because of lack of physical exercise or as a result of neurologic or musculoskeletal disease. Cells of the brain and central nervous system may atrophy in old age because of restricted blood flow to those areas. See also **aging.** –**atrophic,** *adj.,* **atrophy,** *v.*

atrophy of disuse [Gk, *a, trophe,* L, *dis,* opposite of, *usus*], a shrinkage of tissues resulting from immobility or lack of exercise.

atropine /at′rōpin/ [Gk, *Atropos,* one of the three Fates], an alkaloid from *Atropa belladonna* and *Datura stramonium* plants. It is related to other drugs, such as scopolamine and hyoscyamine, and has a similar action of blocking parasympathetic stimuli by raising the threshold of response of effector cells to acetylcholine.

atropine sulfate, an antispasmodic and anticholinergic.
■ INDICATIONS: It is prescribed in the treatment of GI hypermotility, inflammation of the iris or the uvea, cardiac dysrhythmias, parkinsonism, and certain kinds of poisoning and as an adjunct to anesthesia.
■ CONTRAINDICATIONS: GI obstruction, glaucoma, hepatitis, liver or kidney dysfunction, porphyria, or known hypersensitivity to this drug or other anticholinergics prohibits its use.
■ ADVERSE EFFECTS: Among the more serious adverse reactions are tachycardia, angina, loss of taste, nausea, diarrhea, skin rash, blurred vision, and eye pain. Dry mouth and constipation are common effects.

atropine sulfate poisoning [Gk, *Atropos,* fate; L, *sulphur; potio,* drink], toxic effects of an overdose of a drug sometimes used as an adjunct to general anesthesia. Symptoms include tachycardia, hot and dry flushed skin, dry mouth with thirst, restlessness and excitement, urinary retention, constipation, and a burning pain in the throat. Treatment includes gastric lavage and administration of barbiturates, and pilocarpine if the eyes are involved.

attached epithelial cuff.   See **junctional epithelium.**

attached gingiva.   See **alveolar gingiva.**

attachment [Fr, *attachement*],   **1.** the state or quality of being affixed or attached. **2.** (in psychiatry) a mode of behavior in which one individual relates in an affiliative or dependent manner to another; a feeling of affection or loyalty that binds one person to another. Such relationships develop at critical periods during life, and any failure to form these attachments, because of lack of the opportunity or the inability to relate, can lead to personality deviation disorders or maladaptive behavior. **3.** See **bonding. 4.** (in dentistry) any device, such as a retainer or artificial crown, used to secure a partial denture to a natural tooth in the mouth.

attachment apparatus,   the combination of tissues that invest and support the teeth, such as the cementum, the periodontal ligament, and the alveolar bone. See also **masticatory system.**

attending physician [L, *attendere* to, stretch],   the physician who is responsible for a particular, usually private, patient. In a university setting, an attending physician often also has teaching responsibilities and holds a faculty appointment. Also called (*informal*) **attending.**

attention [L, *attendere*, to stretch],   the element of cognitive functioning in which the mental focus is maintained on a specific issue, object, or activity.

attention deficit disorder,   a syndrome affecting children, adolescents, and, rarely, adults characterized by learning and behavior disabilities. The symptoms may be mild or severe and are associated with functional deviations of the central nervous system without signs of major neurologic or psychiatric disturbance. The people affected are usually of normal or above average intelligence. Symptoms include impairment in perception, conceptualization, language, memory, and motor skills, decreased attention span, increased impulsivity and emotional lability, and usually, but not always, hyperactivity. The condition is 10 times more prevalent in boys than in girls and may result from genetic factors, biochemical irregularities, or perinatal or postnatal injury or disease. There is no known cure, and symptoms often subside or disappear with time. Medication with methylphenidate, pemoline, or the dextroamphetamines is frequently prescribed for children with hyperactive symptoms, and some form of psychotherapeutic counseling is often recommended. Some treatments include abstinence from certain foods and food additives. Also called **hyperactivity, hyperkinesis, minimal brain dysfunction.** See also **learning disability.**

attention-deficit disorder with hyperactivity.   See **hyperactive child syndrome.**

attenuated /əten′yo͞o·ā′tid/ [L, *attenure*, to make thinner], pertaining to the dilution of a solution or the reduction in virulence or toxicity of a microorganism or a drug by weakening it.

attenuated virus [L, *attenuare*, to make thin + *virus*, poison],   a strain of virus whose virulence has been lowered by physical or chemical processes, or by repeated passage through the cells of another species. Vaccines made by attenuated strains are used to prevent tuberculosis, small pox, measles, mumps, rubella, polio, and yellow fever.

attenuation /əten′yo͞o·ā′shən/ [L, *attenuare*, to make thin], the process of reduction, such as the attenuation of an x-ray beam by reducing its intensity or the weakening of the degree of virulence of a disease organism.

attenuation coefficient,   (in positron emission tomography) a number that represents the difference between the number of photons that enter a body part being studied and the number that are not detected. The difference is caused by absorption and scatter particles within the body tissues.

Attenuvax,   a trademark for an active immunizing agent (live measles virus vaccine).

attic.   See **epitympanic recess.**

attitude /at′əto͞od, -to͞od/,   **1.** a body position or posture, particularly the fetal position in the uterus as determined by the degree of flexion of the head and extremities. **2.** (in psychiatry) any of the major integrative forces in the development of personality that gives consistency to an individual's behavior. Attitudes are cognitive in nature, formed through interactions with the environment. They reflect the person's innermost convictions about good or bad, right or wrong, desirable or undesirable.

attitudinal isolation /at′əto͞o′dənəl/ [L, *attitudo*, posture], a type of social isolation that results from a person's own cultural or personal values.

attitudinal reflex,   any reflex initiated by a change in position of the head or by a change in position of the head with respect to the position of the body. Kinds of attitudinal reflexes include **tonic neck reflex** and **tonic labyrinthine reflex.** Also called **statotonic reflex.**

attraction [L, *attrahere*, to draw to],   a tendency of the teeth or other maxillary or mandibular structures to elevate above their normal position.

attrition /ətrish′ən/ [L, *atterere*, to wear away],   the process of wearing away or wearing down by friction.

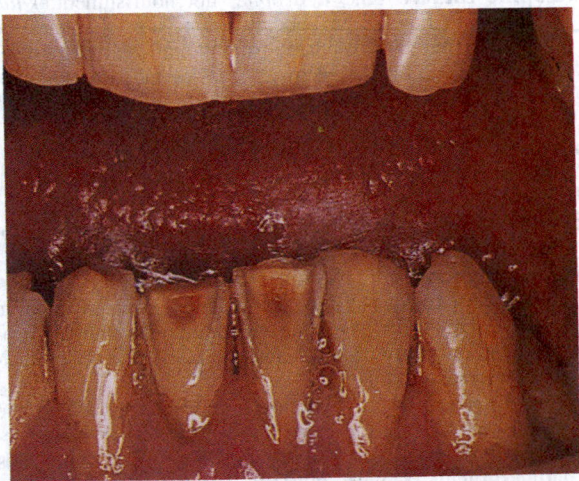

Attrition of the teeth (Lamey, 1988)

-ature,   a noun-forming combining form: *armature, ligature, tubulature.*

at. wt.,   abbreviation for **atomic weight.**

atypia /ātip′ēə/ [Gk, *a, typos*, not type],   a condition of being irregular or not standard.

atypical /ātip′əkəl/ [Gk, *a*, not, *typos*, type], a condition or object that is not of a usual or standard type.

atypical measles syndrome (AMS), a form of measles (rubeola) that tends to infect persons previously immunized by killed measles vaccine or live, attenuated measles vaccine that may have been stored improperly. Symptoms vary somewhat from typical measles, beginning with a sudden high fever, headache, abdominal pain, and coughing. The measles rash may appear only 1 or 2 days later, usually starting on the hands and feet rather than the head and neck. The infection may be complicated by edema of the extremities and pneumonia.

atypical *Mycobacterium* [Gk, *a*, not, *typos*, type, *mykes*, fungus, *bakterion*, small staff], a group of mycobacteria, including pathogenic and nonpathogenic forms, that are classified according to their ability to produce pigments, growth characteristics, and reactions to chemical tests.

atypical pneumonia [Gk, *a*, not, *typos*, type, *peumon*, lung, *ia*, condition], a group of relatively mild symptoms of chills, headache, muscular pains, moderate fever, and coughing, but without evidence of a bacterial infection. Chest x-ray film may show mottling at the bases. Eaton's agent, or *Mycoplasma pneumoniae*, may be the cause of the symptoms.

atypical somatoform disorder, an abnormal condition marked by physical symptoms and complaints that appear related to a preoccupation with an imagined defect in one's personal appearance or ability.

Au, symbol for the element **gold.**

audible /ô′dəbəl/ [L, *audire*, to hear], capable of being heard. Some animals are able to hear sounds of higher or lower frequencies and different intensities than those audible to most humans.

audio-, a combining form meaning 'hearing': *audiology.*

audioanalgesia /ô·dē·ō·an′əliē″sē·a/ [L, *audire*, to hear; Gk, *a*, *algos*, not pain], the use of music to enhance relaxation and to distract a patient's mind from pain, as during dentistry. The procedure has also been tried experimentally during labor.

audiogram /ô′dē·əgram′/ [Gk, *audire* + Gk, *gramma* record], a chart showing the faintest sounds an individual is able to hear and to distinguish different speech sounds. See also **audiometry.**

-audiologic. See **audiology.**

audiologist /-ol′əjist/ [L, *audire*, to hear + Gk, *logos*, science], a health professional with at least a master's degree who studies the sense of hearing, detects and diagnoses hearing loss, and works to rehabilitate individuals with hearing loss.

audiology /-ol′əjē/ [L, *audire* + Gk, *logos*, science], a field of research devoted to the study of hearing, especially impaired hearing that cannot be corrected by medical means. **–audiologic,** *adj.*

audiometer /ô′dē·om′ətər/ [L, *audire* + Gk, *metron*, measure], an electric device for testing the hearing. Earphones are placed over the ears; the ear being tested is stimulated by a series of tones, from very low to very high frequencies at various decibels of intensity. The patient signals when a tone is heard, and the lowest level at which the tone is heard is noted on an audiogram.

audiometry /ô′dē·om′ətrē/, the testing of the sensitivity of the sense of hearing. Various audiometric tests determine the lowest intensity of sound at which an individual can perceive an auditory stimulus (hearing threshold), hear differ-

ent frequencies, and distinguish different speech sounds. Pure tone audiometry assesses the person's ability to hear frequencies, usually ranging from 125 to 8000 hertz (Hz), and can indicate if a hearing loss is caused by an outer or middle ear problem or by one in the inner ear or the acoustic nerve. In this test the subject sits in a soundproof booth and signals when sounds are first heard through earphones. The operator slowly decreases the decibel level until it can no longer be heard. Speech audiometry tests the ability to repeat selected words. Impedance audiometry is an objective method of assessing the resistance or compliance of the conducting mechanism of the middle ear with a probe inserted in the ear canal. Cortical audiometry indicates auditory activity by measuring and averaging electric potentials evoked from the cortex of the brain by pure tones. Localization audiometry is a method for measuring the individual's ability to locate the source of a sound tone received binaurally in a sound field. **–audiometric,** *adj.*

audit /ô′dit/, a review and evaluation of health care procedures.

auditory /ô′dətôr′ē/ [L, *auditorius*, hearing], pertaining to the sense of hearing and the hearing organs involved.

auditory amnesia, [L, *auditorius*, hearing, Gk, *amnesia*, forgetfulness], a loss of memory for the meaning of sounds. Also called **word deafness.**

auditory canal, one of two passageways for sound impulses passing through the ear. One leads from the outer ear to the tympanic membranes. The other, located in the temporal bone, contains the auditory nerve, which transmits impulses from the inner ear to the brain. Compare **eustachian tube (auditory tube).**

auditory hair [L, *audire*, to hear, AS, *haer*], one of the cells with hairlike processes in the spiral organ of Corti. The hairs, or cilia, function as sensory receptors. Also called **acoustic hair cell, cell of Corti.**

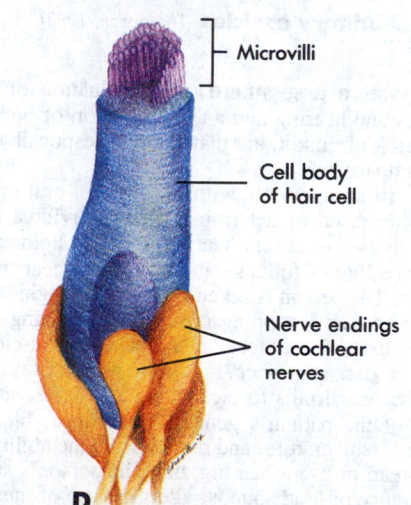

Auditory hair cell (Seeley, 1992/Lisa Chuck/Michael Schenk)

auditory hallucination [L, *audire*, to hear, *alucinari*, a wandering mind], a subjective experience of hearing voices or other sounds despite the absence of a real-world stimulus to account for the phenomenon.

auditory meatus [L, *audire*, to hear; *meatus*, passage], **1.** the external auditory meatus, a tubelike channel of the external ear extending from the auricle to the tympanum of the middle ear. **2.** the internal auditory meatus, a short channel extending from the petrous part of the temporal bone to the fundus near the vestibule. It contains the eighth cranial nerve.

auditory nerve,   See **acoustic nerve.**

auditory ossicles [L, *audire* + *ossiculum*, little bone], the incus, the malleus, and the stapes, small bones in the middle ear that articulate with each other and the tympanic membrane. Sound waves are transmitted through them as the tympanic membrane vibrates.

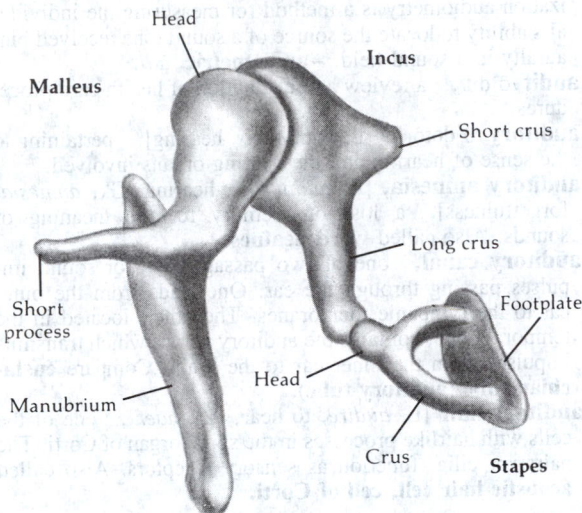

Auditory ossicles *(Thompson, 1993)*

auditory system assessment, an evaluation of the patient's ears and hearing and an investigation of present and past diseases or conditions that may be responsible for an auditory impairment.

■ METHOD: In an interview with the patient, oral or written questions are used to determine if the individual has earaches, decreased or absent hearing in one or both ears, vertigo, or a feeling of fullness, itching, or the heart pulsating in the ears. The person is asked if there is a ringing or buzzing in the ears or a popping noise when yawning or swallowing, if the voice echoes, if the ears drain a clear, yellow, red, or dark substance, and if the person uses oils, cotton swabs, or hairpins to clean the ears. Observations are recorded of the patient's general appearance, blood pressure, pulse, temperature, and respirations, the ability to hear or to lip-read or use a hearing aid. The person's startle reflex, tolerance of loud sounds, allergies, use of medication, especially of eardrops, streptomycin, salicylates, and quinine, and the color, character, and amount of ear drainage are carefully noted. The presence of otitis media, otosclerosis, acoustic nerve tumor, labyrinthitis, Méniére's disease, diabetes mellitus, arteriosclerosis, hypertension, mastoiditis, or a cerebral tumor, head contusion, or skull fracture is investigated. It is determined if the patient previously underwent stapes mobilization, suffered from otitis media, head trauma, or syphilis, or if the person is exposed to a high decibel level on the job or to recreational ear hazards, as in swimming. Diagnos tic procedures indicated by the history may include an audiogram, audiometric test, a mastoid x-ray film, otologic examination, Rinne and Weber tuning-fork tests, and microbiologic studies for potential pathogens in smears of ear drainage.

■ NURSING CONSIDERATIONS: The nurse conducts the interview, makes the observations, and collects the pertinent background information and the results of the diagnostic procedures.

■ OUTCOME CRITERIA: A thorough assessment of the patient's auditory system is essential in establishing the diagnosis of an ear disorder.

auditory threshold [L, *audire*, to hear; AS, *therscold*], the lowest intensity at which a sound may be heard.

auditory tube.   See **eustachian tube.**

auditory vertigo [L, *audire*, to hear + *vertigo*, dizziness], a form of vertigo that is associated with ear disease, characterized by sensations of gyration and, when severe, with prostration and vomiting.

Auerbach's plexus [Leopold Auerbach, Polish anatomist, b. 1828; L, *plexus*, plaited], the myenteric plexus, a group of autonomic nerve fibers and ganglia located in the muscle tissue of the intestinal tract.

Auer rod /ou′ər/ [John Auer, American physiologist, b. 1875], an abnormal, needle-shaped or round, pink-staining inclusion in the cytoplasm of myeloblasts and promyelocytes in acute myelogenous or myelomonocytic leukemia. These inclusions contain enzymes such as acid phosphatase, peroxidase, and esterase and may represent abnormal derivatives of cytoplasmic granules. The finding of Auer rods in stained blood smears helps to differentiate acute myelogenous leukemia from acute lymphoblastic leukemia. Also called **Auer body.**

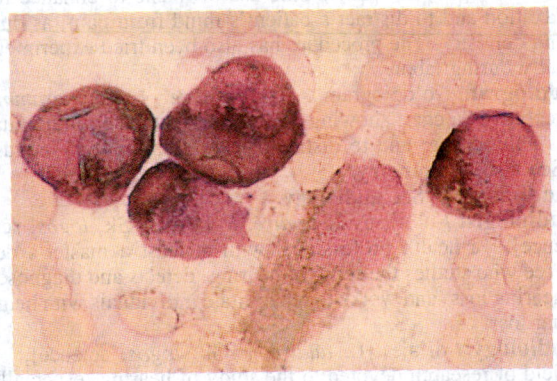

Auer rods *(Hayhoe, 1992)*

augmentation /ôg′məntā′shən/ [L, *augmentare*, to increase], a process in which a substance or mechanism can stimulate an increased rate of biologic activity, such as faster cell division or heart beat.

aur-, a prefix meaning 'pertaining to the ear': *auralgan, auricle, auricular.*

aura /ôr′ə/ [L, breath], **1.** *pl.* **aurae** /ôr′ē/, a sensation, as of light or warmth, that may precede an attack of migraine or an epileptic seizure. **2.** *pl.* **auras,** an emanation of light or color surrounding a person as seen in Kirlian photography and studied in current nursing research in healing techniques.

aural[1] /ôr′əl/,   of or pertaining to the ear or hearing. **−aurally**, *adv.*

aural[2],   of or pertaining to an aura.

aural forceps,   a dressing forceps with fine, bent tips, used in surgery.

aurally.   See **aural.**

aural rehabilitation,   a form of therapy in which hearing-impaired individuals are taught to improve their ability to communicate. Methods taught include, but are not limited to, speech-reading, auditory training, use of hearing aids, and use of assistive listening devices such as telephone amplifiers.

auramine /ôr′əmēn/,   a yellow aniline dye used in the manufacture of paints, textiles, and rubber products. The experimental carcinogen in animals has been identified as a cause of bladder cancer in humans. Also called **dimethyl aniline.**

auranofin /ôr′ənof′in/,   an oral antiarthritic drug.

■ INDICATIONS: It is prescribed for the treatment of rheumatoid arthritis.

■ CONTRAINDICATIONS: Auranofin is contraindicated for patients who have disorders that are caused by or aggravated by medicines containing gold.

■ ADVERSE EFFECTS: Among the most severe adverse reactions reported are diarrhea, loose stools, abdominal pain, nausea, vomiting, rash, pruritus, stomatitis, anemia, leukopenia, thrombocytopenia, eosinophilia, proteinemia, hematuria, and elevated liver enzyme levels.

aurantiasis cutis /ôr′əntī′əsis/ [L, *aurantium*, orange; Gk, *osis*, condition; L, *cutis*, skin],   a yellowish skin pigmen-

tation that results from eating excessive amounts of foods containing carotene, such as carrots.

auras.   See **aura.**

Aureomycin,   a trademark for a tetracycline antibiotic (chlortetracycline hydrochloride).

auricle /ôr′ikəl/ [L, *auricula*, little ear],   **1.** also called

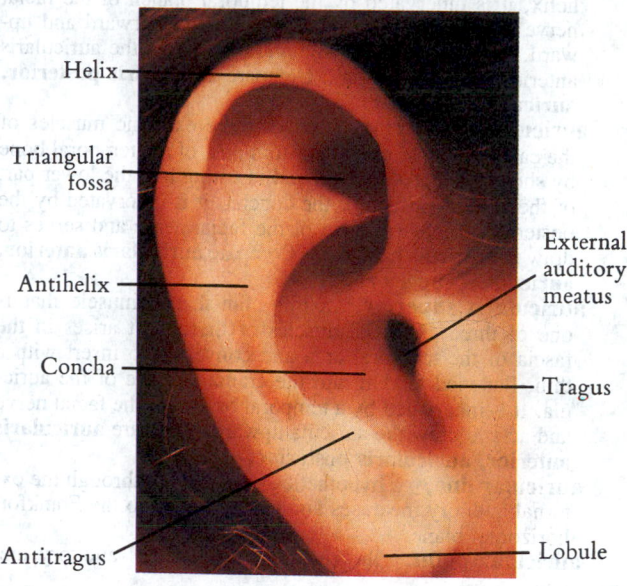

Auricle *(Seidel, (1991)*

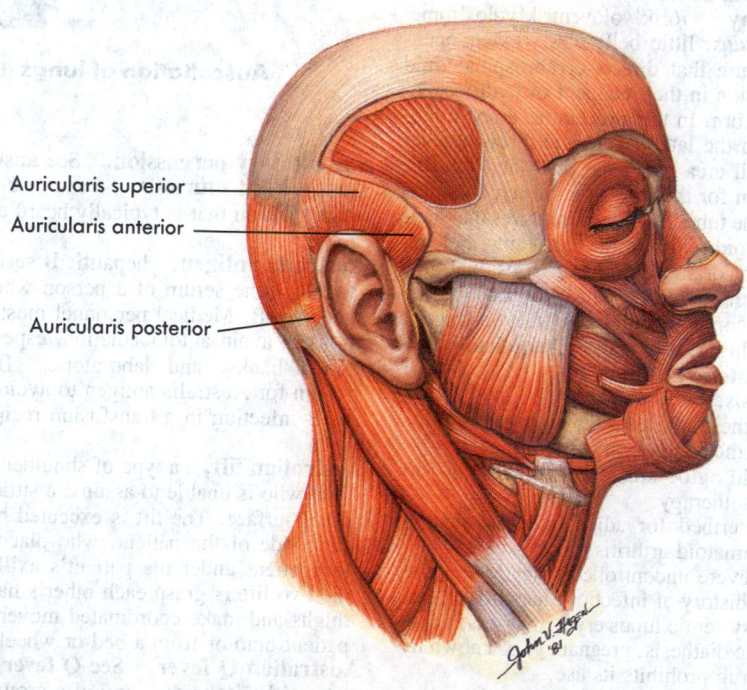

Extrinsic muscles of the ear: auricularis anterior, auricularis posterior, and auricularis superior
(Seeley, 1992/John V Hagen)

pinna. the external ear. **2.** the left or right cardiac atrium, so named because of its earlike shape.

auricular /ôrik′yələr/, **1.** of or pertaining to the auricle of the ear. **2.** otic.

auricularis anterior, one of three extrinsic muscles of the ear. Arising from the anterior portion of the fascia in the temporal area and inserting into a projection in front of the helix, it is innervated by the temporal branch of the facial nerve and functions to move the auricula forward and upward. Some people can voluntarily contract the auricularis anterior to move the ears. Compare **auricularis posterior, auricularis superior.**

auricularis posterior, one of three extrinsic muscles of the ear. Arising from the mastoid area of the temporal bone by short aponeurotic fibers and inserting into the lower part of the cranial surface of the concha, it is innervated by the posterior auricular branch of the facial nerve and serves to draw the auricula backward. Compare **auricularis anterior, auricularis superior.**

auricularis superior, a thin, fan-shaped muscle that is one of three extrinsic muscles of the ear. It arises in the fascia of the temporal area and converges to insert with a thin, flattened tendon into the cranial surface of the auricula. It is innervated by a temporal branch of the facial nerve and acts to draw the auricula upward. Compare **auricularis anterior, auricularis posterior.**

auricular line, a hypothetical line passing through the external auditory meatuses and perpendicular to the Frankfort horizontal plane.

auricular point, the center of the external auditory meatus.

auricular tachycardia. See **atrial tachycardia.**

auriculin /ôrik′yəlin/, a hormonelike substance with diuretic activity produced in the atria of the heart.

auriculoventriculostomy /ôrik′yəlōventrik′yəlos′təmē/ [L, *auricula* + *ventriculus,* little belly; Gk, *stoma,* opening], a surgical procedure that directs cerebrospinal fluid into the general circulation in the treatment of hydrocephalus, usually in the newborn. In this procedure, a polyethylene tube is passed from the lateral ventricle through a bur hole in the parietal skull area under the scalp and into the jugular vein or abdomen for the discharge of cerebrospinal fluid. The insertion of the tube into these structures that have one-way valves is to avoid reflux of the blood into the ventricles and to continue the drain of excess cerebrospinal fluid when ventricular pressure increases. This procedure is performed to correct the communicating and the obstructive forms of hydrocephalus. Also called **ventriculoatrial shunt, ventriculoatriostomy.**

auriosis. See **chrysiasis.**

auris dextra (a.d.), the Latin term for right ear.

auris sinistra (a.s.), the Latin term for left ear.

aurothioglucose /ôr′ōthī′ōglōō′kōs/, an organic gold antiarthritic used in chrysotherapy.

■ INDICATION: It is prescribed for adjunctive treatment of adult and juvenile rheumatoid arthritis.

■ CONTRAINDICATIONS: Severe uncontrolled diabetes, renal or hepatic dysfunction, a history of infectious hepatitis, hypertension, heart failure, systemic lupus erythematosus, agranulocytosis, hemorrhagic diathesis, pregnancy, or known hypersensitivity to this drug prohibits its use.

■ ADVERSE EFFECTS: Among the most serious adverse effects are kidney and liver damage and various allergic reactions. Dermatitis and lesions of mucous membranes are common.

auscultation /ôs′kəltā′shən/ [L, *auscultare,* to listen], the act of listening for sounds within the body to evaluate the condition of the heart, blood vessels, lungs, pleura, intestines, or other organs or to detect the fetal heart sound. Auscultation may be performed directly, but most commonly a stethoscope is used to determine the frequency, intensity, duration, and quality of the sounds. During auscultation of the lungs the patient usually sits upright and is instructed to breathe slowly and deeply through the mouth. The anterior and posterior surfaces of the thorax are auscultated from apex to base with comparisons made between the right and left sides; when the posterior chest is examined, the patient is asked to bring the shoulders forward so that a greater surface of the lung can be auscultated. The heart and abdomen may be auscultated with the patient supine or sitting upright. **–auscultate,** *v.,* **auscultatory** /ôskul′tətôr′ē/, *adj.*

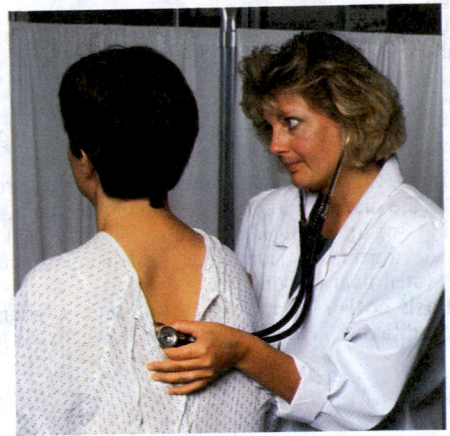

Auscultation of lungs *(Belcher, 1992)*

auscultatory percussion. See **auscultation, percussion.**

Austin Flint murmur, a murmur characteristic of aortic regurgitation that is typically heard during ventricular diastole.

Australia antigen, hepatitis B surface antigen (HBsAG), found in the serum of a person who has acute or chronic hepatitis B. Medical personnel must take adequate precautions to avoid autoinoculation, especially in dialysis units, blood banks, and laboratories. Blood banks routinely screen for Australia antigen to avoid causing active hepatitis B infection in a transfusion recipient. See also **hepatitis.**

Australian lift, a type of shoulder lift used to move a patient who is unable to assume a sitting position on a bed or other surface. The lift is executed by two persons, one on each side of the patient, who place their shoulder nearest the patient under the patient's axillae. At the same time, the two lifters grasp each other's hands under the patient's thighs and make coordinated movements needed to lift the patient onto or from a bed or wheelchair.

Australian Q fever. See **Q fever.**

autacoid /ô′təkoid/, any of a group of substances, as hormones, that are produced in one organ and are transported via blood or lymph as a means to control a physiologic process in another part of the body.

authenticity /ô′thəntis′itē/, (in psychiatry) emotional and behavioral openess; a quality of being genuine and trustworthy.

authoritarian personality, a group of behavioral traits characteristic of one who advocates obedience and strict adherence to the rules.

authority /ôthôr′ətē/, a relationship between two or more persons or groups characterized by the influence one may exercise over the other through ideas, commands, suggestions, or instructions.

authority figure, a person who by virtue of status, strength, knowledge, or other recognized superiority exerts influence over others.

autism [Gk *autos* self], a mental disorder characterized by extreme withdrawal and an abnormal absorption in fantasy, accompanied by delusion, hallucination, and an inability to communicate verbally or to otherwise relate to people. Schizophrenic children are often autistic. See also **infantile autism. –autistic,** *adj.*

autistic disorder /ôtis′tik/ [Gk, *autos*, self], a severe pervasive developmental disorder with onset in infancy or childhood, characterized by impaired social interaction, impaired communication, and a remarkably restricted repertoire of activities and interests. See also **infantile autism. –autistic,** *adj.*

autistic phase, a period of preoedipal development, according to Mahler's system of personality stages. It lasts from birth to around 1 month and is considered normal. Children then become aware that they cannot satisfy their body needs by themselves.

autistic thought, a form of thinking in which the ideas have a private meaning to the individual. In autistic thinking, fantasy life may be interpreted as reality.

auto- /ô′tō-/, a prefix meaning 'pertaining to self': *autoblast, autocatharsis, autoclasis.*

autoactivation /-ak′tivā′shən/[Gk, *autos*, self + *activus*, active], a process of self-activation, as when a gland is stimulated by its own secretions.

autoagglutination /-əglōō′tənā′shən/ [Gk, *autos*, self + L, *agglutinare*, to glue], **1.** the agglutination or clumping of red blood cells by the serum of the same individual. Also called **autohemagglutination. 2.** the agglutination or clumping together of certain antigens such as bacteria.

autoamputation /-amp′yōōtā′shən/, the spontaneous detachment of a body part, usually the fourth or fifth toe, as occurs among the males of some African peoples. A depression develops across the digitoplantar fold of the toe and gradually progresses until the toe falls off. The condition is usually painless and has no other symptoms. Also called **ainhum** /ān′hōōm, īnyoon′/.

autoantibody /ô′tō·an′tibod′ē/ [Gk, *autos* + *anti*, against; AS, *bodig*, body], an immunoglobulin that reacts against a normal constituent in a person's body, such as nuclear material in the patient with systemic lupus erythematosus. There are several mechanisms that may trigger the production of autoantibodies. An antigen formed during fetal development and then sequestered may be released as a result of infection or trauma and elicit the synthesis of autoantibodies, as occurs in autoimmune thyroiditis, sympathetic uveitis, and aspermia. Antibodies produced against certain streptococcal antigens during infection may cross-react with myocardial tissue, causing rheumatic heart disease, or with glomerular basement membrane, causing glomerulonephritis. Normal body proteins may be converted to autoantigens by chemicals, infectious organisms, or therapeutic drugs.

Autoantibodies are found against gastric parietal cells in pernicious anemia, against platelets in autoimmune thrombocytopenia, and against antigens on the surface of erythrocytes in autoimmune hemolytic anemia.

autoantigen /ô′tō·an′tijin/ [Gk, *autos* + *anti*, against, *genein*, to produce], an endogenous body constituent that stimulates the production of autoantibody and a resulting autoimmune reaction against one or more tissues of the person in whom the abnormal reaction occurs. An autoantigen associated with **Addison's disease** has been identified as an enzyme molecule, 17α-hydroxylase. See also **autoantibody, autoimmune disease.**

autochthonous idea /ôtok′thənəs/ [Gk, *autos*, + *chthon*, earth], an idea that originates in the unconscious and arises spontaneously in the mind, independent of the conscious train of thought.

autoclave /ô′təklāv/, an appliance used to sterilize medical instruments or other objects with steam under pressure.

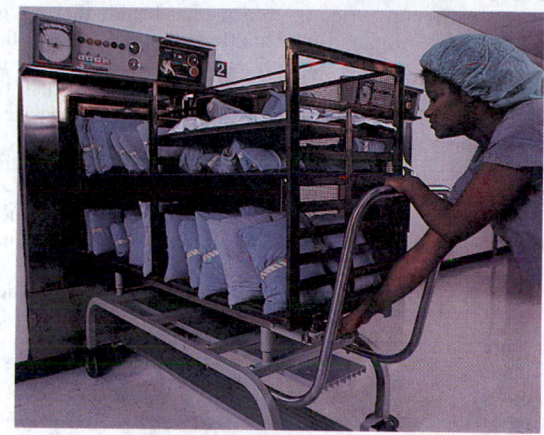

Autoclave *(Sorrentino, 1992)*

autodermic graft. See **autograft.**

autodiploid /ô′tōdip′loid/ [Gk, *autos* + *diploos*, double, *eidos*, form], **1.** also **autodiploidic.** of or pertaining to an individual, organism, strain, or cell containing two genetically identical or nearly identical chromosome sets that are derived from the same ancestral species and result from the duplication of the haploid set. **2.** such an individual, organism, strain, or cell. Compare **allodiploid.** See also **autopolyploid.**

autodiploidy /ô′tōdip′loidē/, the state or condition of having two genetically identical or nearly identical chromosome sets from the same ancestral species. Such a state enables cell division to occur in a normal manner. Compare **allodiploidy.**

autoeroticism /-irot′əsiz′əm/ [Gk, *autos* +*eros*, love], **1.** sensual, usually sexual, gratification of the self, usually obtained through the stimulus of one's own body without the participation of another person and derived from such acts as stroking, masturbation, and fantasy, or from other oral, anal, or visual sources of stimulation. **2.** sexual feeling or desire occurring without any external stimulus. **3.** (in Freudian psychoanalytic theory) an early phase of psychosexual development, occurring in the oral and the anal stages. Also called **autoerotism.** Compare **heteroeroticism. –autoerotic,** *adj*.

autoerythrocyte sensitization /ô′tō·ərith′rəsīt/ [Gk, *autos* + *erythros*, red, *kytos*, cell], an unusual disorder characterized by the spontaneous appearance of painful, hemorrhagic spots on the anterior aspects of the arms and legs, resulting from hypersensitivity to the patient's own red blood cells. Autoimmune hemolytic anemia, an extreme example of hypersensitivity to antigens on the surface of the patient's erythrocytes, may cause fulminant hemolysis, fever, abdominal pain, hyperbilirubinemia, thrombosis, and shock. Psychoneurotic disorders may be associated with the disorder. Also called **Gardner-Diamond syndrome.**

autoerythrocyte sensitization syndrome. See **Gardner-Diamond syndrome.**

autogenesis /ô′tōjen′əsis/ [Gk, *autos* + *genein*, to produce], **1.** abiogenesis. **2.** self-produced condition; a condition originating from within the organism. Also called **autogeny** /ôtoj′ənē/. Compare **heterogenesis, homogenesis. –autogenetic, autogenic,** *adj*.

autogenic therapy /-jen′ik/, a mental health therapy introduced by Wolfgang Luthe and based on the concept that natural forces in the brain are able to remove disturbing influences so that functional harmony can be restored in the mind and body. It was developed from research on sleep and hypnosis and involves biofeedback exercises.

autogenous /ôtoj′ənəs/, **1.** self-generating. **2.** originating from within the organism, as a toxin or vaccine.

autogenous graft [Gk, *autos*. self, *genein*, to produce, *graphion*, stylus], a self-produced skin graft transplanted from one site to another in the same individual.

autogenous vaccine [Gk, *autos*, self + *genein*, to produce; L, *vaccinus*, cow], a vaccine prepared from cultures of the microorganism taken from a lesion of the patient to be treated.

autogeny. See **autogenesis.**

autograft /ô′təgraft′/ [Gk, *autos* + *graphion*, stylus], surgical transplantation of any tissue from one part of the body to another location in the same individual. Autografts are commonly used to replace skin lost in severe burns and several forms of plastic surgery. An obsolete term is **autodermic graft.** Compare **allograft, isograft, xenograft.** See also **graft.**

autographism. See **dermatographia.**

autohemagglutination. See **autoagglutination.**

autohemolysis /-hēmol′isis/ [Gk, *autos*, self + *haima*, blood, *lysein*, to loosen], the destruction of erythrocytes by hemolytic agents found in the blood serum of the individual.

autohexaploid, autohexaploidic. See **autopolyploid.**

autohypnosis [Gk, *autos* + *hypnos,* sleep], the self-induction of hypnois by an individual who concentrates on one subject to attain an altered state of consciousness. It may also occur in a person who has become sensitized to the process by undergoing hypnosis a number of times.

autoimmune /-imyōōn′/ [Gk, *autos* + L, *immunus*, exempt], pertaining to the development of an immune response (autoantibodies or cellular immune response) to one's own tissues.

autoimmune disease, one of a large group of diseases characterized by the subversion or alteration of the function of the immune system of the body. Antigens normally present in the internal cells stimulate the development of an-

tibodies, and the antibodies, unable to distinguish antigens of the internal cells from external antigens, act against the internal cell to cause localized and systemic reactions. These reactions affect the epithelial and the connective tissues of the body, causing a variety of diseases that can be divided into two general categories: the collagen diseases (including systemic lupus erythematosus, dermatomyositis, periarteritis nodosa, scleroderma, and rheumatoid arthritis) and the autoimmune hemolytic disorders (including idiopathic thrombocytopenic purpura, acquired hemolytic anemia, and autoimmune leukopenia). The precise pathophysiologic processes and the origin of these diseases are unknown.

■ OBSERVATIONS: The manifestations and clinical characteristics depend on the specific disease and on the organ or systems affected. See specific diseases.

■ INTERVENTIONS: Therapy includes corticosteroid, antiinflammatory, and immunosuppressive drugs. The symptoms are treated specifically, such as a transfusion for hemorrhage, analgesics for pain, and physical therapy for the prevention of contracture. Diet may be regulated for specific needs; for example, iron might be increased to treat anemia in a person with thrombocytopenic purpura, or calories might be reduced in a weight-loss diet for a person with rheumatoid arthritis. Surgical treatment may be corrective or preventive, such as a hip replacement in rheumatoid arthritis or a splenectomy in thrombocytopenic purpura.

■ NURSING CONSIDERATIONS: Many of these diseases are characterized by periods of crisis and periods of remission. During a crisis, the patient may be hospitalized and require extensive nursing care, with relief from pain, applications of heat or cold, range of motion exercises, or assistance in movement and ambulation. The nurse observes for signs of hemorrhage, puts side rails or a trapeze in place if necessary, protects the person from infection, and prevents chilling or overheating. Because the patient is in particular need of emotional support, the nurse helps the person verbalize feelings of anger and frustration, recognize limitations, focus on strengths, set realistic goals, and understand the disease process. It is important also to teach the patient and the family the side effects of the drugs being prescribed and how the drugs are to be taken.

autoimmune polyglandular syndromes. See **polyendocrine deficiency syndromes.**

autoimmunity /-imyōō′nitē/, an abnormal characteristic or condition in which the body reacts against constituents of its own tissues. Autoimmunity may result in hypersensitivity and autoimmune disease. It is not yet fully understood, but there are several common theories to explain autoimmunity, such as the forbidden clone theory and the sequestered antigens theory. See also **acute immune disease, antibody specific theory, autoantibody, autoantigen.**

autoimmunization /-im′yəniza′shən/, the process whereby an individual's immune system develops antibodies against one or more of the person's own tissues. See also **autoimmune disease, autoimmunity.**

autoinoculation /-inok′yəla′shən/ [Gk, *autos* + L, *inoculare*, to graft], the inoculation of a microorganism obtained by contact with a lesion on one's own body, producing a secondary infection.

autointoxication /-intok′sika′shən/ [Gk, *autos* + L, *in;* Gk, *toxikon*, poison], a condition of poisoning by substances generated by one's own body, such as toxins resulting from a metabolic disorder.

autolet /ô′tōlet/, a small, sharp instrument, as a lancet, that is used to obtain a capillary blood specimen.

autologous /ôtol′əgəs/ [Gk, *autos* + *logos*, ratio], pertaining to a tissue or structure occurring naturally and derived from the same individual.

autologous blood. See **bank blood.**

autologous graft [Gk, *autos, logos, graphion,* stylus], the transfer of tissue from one site to another on the same body.

autologous transfusion a procedure in which blood is removed from a donor and stored for a variable period before it is returned to the donor's own circulation.

automatic behavior. See **automatism.**

automatic bladder. See **spastic bladder.**

automatic infiltration detector /ô′təmat′ik/ [Gk, *automatismos,* self-action] a temperature-sensitive device that activates an alarm and automatically stops an intravenous infusion when infiltration of the intravenous fluid occurs. The device detects any cooling of the skin at the intravenous site, a common sign of infiltration. The detector is usually secured to the skin with tape and attaches by a small cable to the fluid-monitoring circuit of an intravenous pump.

automaticity /ô′tōmətis′itē/, a property of specialized excitable tissue that allows self-activation through spontaneous development of an action potential, as in the pacemaker cells of the heart.

automatic mallet condenser. See **mechanical condenser.**

automatic speech, speech composed of or containing words or phrases spoken without voluntary control, often consisting of expletives, profanities, and greetings.

automatic document entry. See optical character recognition.

automation /ô′təmā′shən/, use of a machine designed to follow repeatedly and automatically a predetermined sequence of individual operations.

automatism /ôtom′ətiz′əm/ [Gk, *automatismos,* self-action], **1.** (in physiology) involuntary function of an organ system independent of apparent external stimuli, such as the beating of the heart, or dependent on external stimuli but not consciously controlled, such as the dilatation of the pupil of the eye. **2.** (in philosophy) the theory that the body acts as a machine and that the mind, whose processes depend solely on brain activity, is a noncontrolling adjunct of the body. **3.** (in psychology) mechanical, repetitive, and undirected behavior that is not consciously controlled, as seen in psychomotor epilepsy, hysterical states, and such acts as sleepwalking. Kinds of automatism include **ambulatory automatism, command automatism,** and **immediate posttraumatic automatism.** Also called **automatic behavior.**

autonomic /ô′tənom′ik/ [Gk, *autos* + *nomos,* law], **1.** having the ability to function independently without outside influence. **2.** of or pertaining to the autonomic nervous system.

autonomic-active bronchodilators, a category of drugs with actions that dilate bronchiolar smooth muscle tissue by acting on the autonomic nervous system. Examples include adrenergic drugs, such as epinephrine, and anticholinergic products, such as atropine sulfate.

autonomic drug, any of a large group of drugs that mimic or modify the function of the autonomic nervous system.

autonomic dysreflexia, a dysreflexia that is the result of impaired function of the autonomic nervous system caused by simultaneous sympathetic and parasympathetic activity.

It occurs in quadriplegics and some paraplegics, with symptoms of hypertension, bradycardia, severe headaches, pallor below and flushing above the cord lesions, and convulsions. A cerebrovascular accident and death may occur during an attack. See also **autonomic hyperreflexia.**

autonomic ganglion [Gk, *autos,* self + *nomos,* law; *gagglion,* knot], a group of autonomic neuron cell bodies with a common function.

autonomic hyperreflexia, a neurologic disorder characterized by a discharge of sympathetic nervous system impulses as a result of stimulation of the bladder, large intestine, or other visceral organs. It occurs in persons with certain spinal cord injuries. Symptoms may include bradycardia, profuse sweating, headache, and hypertension.

autonomic imbalance [Gk, *autos,* self, *nomos,* law; L, *in,* not, *bilanx,* having two scales], a disruption of a segment of the autonomic nervous system, as in autonomic ataxia.

autonomic nerve [Gk, *autos,* self, *nomos,* law, *neuron,* nerve], a nerve of the autonomic nervous system, which includes both the sympathetic and parasympathetic nervous systems, with the ability to function independently and spontaneously as needed to maintain optimum status of bodily activities.

autonomic nervous system, the part of the nervous system that regulates involuntary vital function, including the activity of the cardiac muscle, smooth muscles, and glands. It has two divisions: The **sympathetic nervous system** accelerates heart rate, constricts blood vessels, and raises blood pressure; the **parasympathetic nervous system** slows heart rate, increases intestinal peristalsis and gland activity, and relaxes sphincters.

autonomic neuropathy, self-controlling, functionally independent disturbances in the peripheral nervous system.

autonomic reflex, any of a large number of normal reflexes governing and regulating the functions of the viscera. Autonomic reflexes control such activities of the body as blood pressure, heart rate, peristalsis, sweating, and urination.

autonomous /ôton′əməs/ [Gk, *autos,* self + *nomos,* law], being functionally independent.

autonomous bladder. See **flaccid bladder.**

autonomy /ôton′əmē/ [Gk, *autos*+ *nomos,* law], the quality of having the ability or tendency to function independently. **–autonomous,** *adj.*

autonomy drive, a behavioral trait characterized by the attempt of an individual to master the environment and to impose the person's purposes on it.

autopentaploid, autopentaploidic. See **autopolyploid.**

autoplastic maneuver /-plas′tik/, (in psychology) a process that is part of adaptation, involving an adjustment within the self. Compare **alloplastic maneuver.**

autoplasty /ô′təplas′tē/ [Gk, *autos* + *plassein,* to shape], a plastic surgery procedure in which autografts, or parts of the patient's own tissues, are used to replace or repair body areas damaged by disease or injury.

autopolyploid /ô′tōpol′iploid/ [Gk, *autos* + *polyploos,* many times, *eidos* form], **1.** also **autopolyploidic.** of or pertaining to an individual, organism, strain, or cell that has more than two genetically identical or nearly identical sets of chromosomes that are derived from the same ancestral species. They result from the duplication of the haploid chromosome set and are referred to as autotriploid, autotetraploid, autopentaploid, autohexaploid, and so on, depending on the number of multiples of the haploid chromosomes they contain. **2.** such an individual, organism, strain, or cell. Compare **allopolyploid.** See also **allodiploid.**

autopolyploidy /ô′tōpol′iploi′dē/, the state or condition of having more than two identical or nearly identical sets of chromosomes. Compare **allopolyploid.**

autopsy /ô′topsē/ [Gk, *autos* + *opsis*, view], a postmortem examination performed to confirm or determine the cause of death. Also called **necropsy** /nek′ropsē/, **thanatopsy** /than′ətop′sē./ −**autopsic, autopsical,** *adj.,* **autopsist,** *n.*

autopsy pathology, the study of disease by the examination of the body after death by a pathologist. The organs and tissues are first described by their appearance at the time of dissection, then by their appearance in the microscopic examination or laboratory analysis of small representative samples of tissue taken for their diagnostic value.

autoregulation [Gk, *autos,* self + L, *regula,* rule], an intrinsic capacity of tissues to regulate their own blood flow thanks to the self-excitable contractile process of smooth muscle that acts to constrict and dilate vessels. It allows organ systems to maintain constant blood flow despite variations in systemic arterial pressure and is an essential mechanism to meet the metabolic needs of an organ.

autoserous treatment /ô′təsir′əs/ [Gk, *autos* + L, *serum* whey], therapy of an infectious disease by inoculating the patient with the patient's own serum.

autosensitization /-sen′sətīzā′shən/ [Gk, *autos,* self + L, *sentire,* to feel], the sensitization of an individual by humoral antibodies or a delayed cellular reaction to substances in his or her own body tissues.

autosite /ô′təsīt/ [Gk, *autos* + *sitos,* food], the larger, more normally formed member of unequal or asymmetric conjoined twins on whom the other smaller fetus depends for various physiologic functions and for nutrition and growth. Compare **parasitic fetus.** −**autositic.** *adj.*

autosomal /ô′təsō′məl/ [Gk, *autos* + *soma,* body], **1.** pertaining to or characteristic of an autosome. **2.** pertaining to any condition transmitted by an autosome.

autosomal dominant inheritance, a pattern of inheritance in which the transmission of a dominant gene on an autosome causes a characteristic to be expressed. Males and females are affected with equal frequency. Affected individuals have an affected parent unless the condition is the result of a fresh mutation. Each child of a heterozygous affected parent has a 50% chance of being affected. Each child of a heterozygous affected parent has a 25% chance of being normal, 25% chance of being homozygous affected, and 50% chance of being heterozygous affected. All of the children of a homozygous affected parent are affected. Normal children of an affected parent do not carry the trait. Traits can be traced vertically through previous generations. A family history may be illustrated by drawing a pedigree. The first case, the propositus, appears suddenly in the pedigree, usually as a mutation. Achondroplasia, osteogenesis imperfecta, polydactyly, and Marfan's syndrome are autosomal dominant disorders. Compare **autosomal recessive inheritance.** See also **dominance.**

autosomal inheritance, a pattern of inheritance in which the transmission of traits depends on the presence or absence of certain genes on the autosomes. The pattern may be dominant or recessive, and males and females are affected with equal frequency. The majority of hereditary disorders are the result of a defective gene on an autosome. Kinds of autosomal inheritance are **autosomal dominant inheritance**

and **autosomal recessive inheritance.** See **inheritance.**

autosomal recessive inheritance, a pattern of inheritance in which the transmission of a recessive gene on an autosome results in a carrier state if the person is heterozygous for the trait and in the affected state if the person is homozygous for the trait. Males and females are affected with equal frequency. Affected individuals have unaffected parents who are heterozygous for the trait. One fourth of the children of two unaffected heterozygous parents are affected. All of the children of two homozygous affected parents are affected. The children of a couple in which one parent has the trait and the other does not are all carriers who show no effect of the trait. There is usually no family history of the trait; it becomes manifest when two unaffected parents who are heterozygous for a particular recessive gene have a child who is homozygous for the trait. Cystic fibrosis, phenylketonuria, and galactosemia are examples of autosomal recessive inheritance. Compare **autosomal dominant inheritance.** See also **recessive.**

autosome /ô′təsōm/, any chromosome that is not a sex chromosome and that appears as a homologous pair in the somatic cell. Humans have 22 pairs of autosomes, which are involved in transmitting all genetic traits and conditions other than those that are sex-linked. Also called **euchromosome** /yoo′krəsōm/. Compare **sex chromosome.**

autosplenectomy /ô′tōsplinek′təmē/ [Gk, *autos* + *splen,* spleen, *ektome,* excision], a progressive shrinking of the spleen that may occur in sickle cell anemia. The spleen is replaced by fibrous tissue and becomes nonfunctional.

autosuggestion [Gk, *autos* + L, *suggerere,* to suggest], an idea, thought, attitude, or belief suggested to oneself, often as a formula or incantation, as a means of controlling one's behavior. Compare **suggestion.**

autotetraploid, autotetraploidic. See **autopolyploid.**

autotopagnosia /ô′tōtop′əg·nō′zhə/ [Gk, *autos* + *topos,* place, *a, gnosis,* not knowledge], the inability to recognize or localize the various parts of the body because of organic brain damage. It is associated generally with lesions of the dominant hemisphere of the patient and may be an effect of some cases of cerebrovascular accident (CVA). It is also characterized by a loss of the patient's ability to distinguish left from right, manifested during a neurologic examination when the patient is unable to perform a task such as touching the right ear with the left thumb. Retraining involves touching various parts of the patient's body and asking the patient to identify the area touched and by having the patient assemble human figure puzzles. Also called **body-image agnosia, body-scheme disorder.** See also **agnosia, proprioception.**

autotransfusion /-transfyoo′zhən/, the collection, anticoagulation, filtration, and reinfusion of blood from an active bleeding site. It may be used in cases of major trauma or in major surgery when blood can be collected from a sterile site.

autotriploid, autotriploidic. See **autopolyploid.**

autumn fever. See **leptospirosis.**

auxanology /ôks′ənol′əjē/ [Gk, *auxein,* to grow, *logos,* science], the scientific study of growth and development. −**auxanologic,** *adj.*

auxesis /ôksē′sis/, *pl.* **auxeses** [Gk, *auxein* + *osis,* condition], an increase in size or volume because of cell expansion rather than of an increase in the number of cells or tissue elements; hypertrophy. Also called **auxetic growth.** Compare **merisis.** −**auxetic,** *adj., n.*

auxiliary /ôksil′yərē/ [L, *auxilium,* aid], an individual or group serving in helpful, supporting, or complementary tasks in a clinical setting.

auxiliary enzyme [L, *auxilium,* assist], in a coupled assay system, an enzyme that links the enzyme being measured with an indicator enzyme.

auxiliary storage, a storage device for adding to the main storage of the computer, employing such media as floppy disks, hard disks, cassette tapes, magnetic tapes, or cartridge tapes.

auxo-, a prefix meaning 'pertaining to growth, to acceleration, or to stimulation': *auxochrome, auxocyte, auxotonic.*

AV, abbreviation for *arteriovenous, atrioventricular, auriculoventricular.*

available arch length /əvā′ləbəl/ [ME, *availen,* to be of use], the length or space in a dental arch that is available for all the natural teeth of an individual. See also **arch length, arch length deficiency, arch width.**

avalvular /āvalv′yələr/ [Gk, *a,* without + L, *valva,* valve], an absence of one or more valves.

avantin. See **isopropyl alcohol.**

avascular /āvas′kyələr/ [Gk, *a,* not; L, *vasculum,* vessel], **1.** (of a tissue area) not receiving a sufficient supply of blood. The reduced flow may be the result of blockage by a blood clot or the deliberate stoppage of flow during surgery or of measures taken to control a hemorrhage. **2.** (of a kind of tissue) not having blood vessels.

avascular graft [Gk, *a,* without + L, *vasculum,* vessel; Gk, *graphion,* stylus], a tissue graft in which there is no infiltration of blood vessels.

avascularization [Gk, *a,* without, L, *vasculum,* vessel], pertaining to a diversion of blood flow away from tissues

AVB, abbreviation for **atrioventricular block.**

aversion therapy /əvur′zhən/ [L, *aversus,* a turning away], a form of behavior therapy in which punishment or unpleasant or painful stimuli, such as electric shock or drugs that induce nausea, are used to suppress undesirable behavior. The procedure is used in treating such conditions as drug abuse, alcoholism, gambling, overeating, smoking, and various sexual deviations. Also called **aversive conditioning.** See also **behavior therapy.**

aversive stimulus /əvur′siv/, a stimulus, as electric shock, that causes psychic or physical pain. See also **aversion therapy.**

aviation medicine /āv′ē·ā′shən/, a branch of medicine that is concerned with the health effects of travel by aircraft, including such aspects as jetlag, restricted body movement for long periods, and reaction to violent aircraft movement in turbulent weather. Also called **aerospace medicine.** See also **aviation physiology.**

aviation physiology, a branch of physiology that is concerned with the effects on humans and animals exposed for long periods in pressurized cabins, radiation hazards at high altitudes, weightlessness, disturbances of biologic rhythms, acceleration, and mental functions under stressful flying conditions.

avidin, a glycoprotein in raw egg white that interacts with biotin to render it unavailable to the body.

avidity /avid′itē/ [L, *avidus,* eager], a measure of the binding strength of antibodies to multiple antigenic determinants on natural antigens.

A-V interval [L, *intervallum,* space between ramparts], the time or space that separates an atrial systole and a ventricular systole in producing an electrocardiogram.

avirulent /āvir′yələnt/ [Gk, *a,* not; L, *virus,* poison], not virulent; not pathogenic.

avitaminosis /āvī′təminō′sis/ [Gk, *a,* not; L, *vita,* life, amine, *osis* condition], a condition resulting from a deficiency of or the lack of absorption or use of one or more vitamins in the diet. Also called **hypovitaminosis.** Compare **hypervitaminosis.** See also specific vitamins.

AV nicking, a vascular abnormality on the retina of the eye, visible on ophthalmologic examination, in which a vein is compressed by an arteriovenous crossing. The vein appears "nicked," because of constriction or spasm. It is a sign of hypertension, arteriosclerosis, and other vascular conditions.

Avogadro's law /av′ōgad′rōz/ [Count Amedeo Avogadro, Italian physicist, b. 1776], a law in physics stating that equal volumes of all gases at a given temperature and pressure contain the identical number of molecules.

Avogadro's number, the number of atoms in exactly 12 g of the isotope of carbon C_{12}, or 6.02×10^{23}. One mole of any monoatomic element contains this number of atoms and one mole of any polyatomic element or molecule contains this number of molecules. The mass of a mole of any element or compound is a mass in grams numerically equal to the relative atomic mass of the atoms or molecules.

avoidance [ME *avoiden* to empty], (in psychiatry) a conscious or unconscious defense mechanism, physical or psychologic, by which an individual tries to avoid or escape from unpleasant stimuli, conflicts, or feelings, such as anxiety, fear, pain, or danger.

avoidance-avoidance conflict, a conflict resulting from the confrontation of two or more alternative goals or desires that are equally aversive and undesirable. Also called **double-avoidant conflict.** See also **conflict.**

avoidance conditioning, the establishment of certain patterns of behavior to avoid unpleasant or painful stimuli.

avoidant personality, a personality disorder characterized by hypersensitivity to rejection and a reluctance to start a relationship because of a fear of not being accepted uncritically. The person has a strong desire for affection and acceptance and may be distressed by an inability to relate comfortably with others.

avoirdupois weight /av′ərdəpoiz′/ [OF, *avoir de pois,* property of weight], the English system of weights in which there are 7000 grains, 256 drams, or 16 ounces to 1 pound. One ounce in this system equals 28.35 g, and 1 pound equals 453.59 g. Compare **apothecaries' weight.** See also **metric system.**

-avulse. See **avulsion.**

avulsed teeth /əvulst/ [L, *avulsio,* a pulling away], teeth that have been forcibly displaced from their normal position. In some cases, if attended to early, they can be surgically reimplanted. Also spelled **evulsed teeth.** See also **avulsion.** (See Fig. p. 156.)

avulsion /əvul′shən/ [L, *avulsio,* a pulling away], the separation, by tearing, of any part of the body from the whole, such as an umbilical cord torn in the process of delivering the placenta. **–avulse,** *v.* (See Fig. p. 156.)

avulsion fracture, a fracture caused by the tearing away of a fragment of bone where a strong ligamentous or tendinous attachment forcibly pulls the fragment away from osseous tissue.

awake anesthesia [ME, *awakenen*], an anesthetic procedure in which analgesia and anesthesia are accomplished without loss of consciousness. Dental procedures, surgery

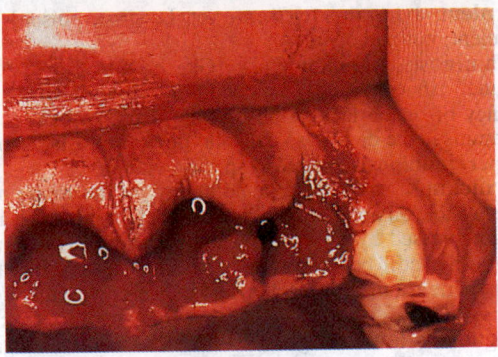

Avulsed teeth (Zitelli, 1992)

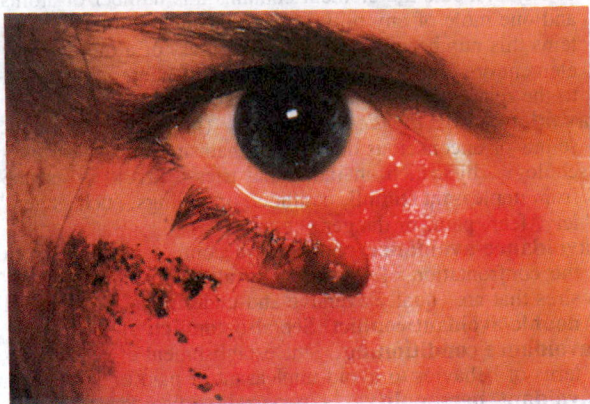

Avulsion of the lower eyelid (Shingleton, 1991)

on a limb or an extremity, scopic examinations, and certain kinds of head surgery are ordinarily performed using awake anesthesia. Awake anesthesia is not as complete as general anesthesia, and muscle relaxation is not required. Various combinations of sedatives, tranquilizers, and low concentrations of anesthetic gas may be used. Also called **conscious sedation.**

AWOL /āʹwôl/, abbreviation for **absent without leave.**

ax-, axio-, axo-, axon-, a prefix meaning 'pertaining to an axis': *axial, axofugal, axon.*

axetil, a contraction for *L-acetoxyethyl.*

axial (A) /akʹsē·əl/ [Gk, *axon*, axle], **1.** pertaining to or situated on the axis of a structure or part of the body. **2.** (in dentistry) relating to the long axis of a tooth.

axial current, the central part of the blood current.

axial gradient, 1. the variation in metabolic rate in different parts of the body. **2.** the development toward the body axis or its parts in relation to the metabolic rate in the various parts.

axial illumination. See **illumination.**

axial neuritis. See **parenchymatous neuritis.**

axial skeleton [L, *axis*, axle, Gk, *skeletos*, dried up], the bones forming the axis of the skeleton, including the skull,

vertebrae, ribs, and sternum. See also **appendicular skeleton.**

axial spillway, a groove that crosses a cusp ridge or a marginal ridge and extends onto an axial surface of a tooth. Compare **interdental spillway, occlusal spillway.**

axilla /aksilʹə/, *pl.* **axillae** [L, wing], a pyramid-shaped space forming the underside of the shoulder between the upper part of the arm and the side of the chest. Also called **armpit. –axillary,** *adj.*

axillary /akʹsilerʹē/ [L, *axilla,* wing], pertaining to the armpit.

axillary abscess [L, *axilla,* wing, *abscedere,* to go away], an abscess in the armpit.

axillary anesthesia. See **brachial plexus anesthesia.**

axillary artery /akʹsələrʹē/ [L, *axilla,* wing], one of a pair of continuations of the subclavian arteries that starts at the outer border of the first rib and ends at the distal border of the teres major, where it becomes the brachial artery. It has three parts and six branches, supplying various chest and arm muscles, such as the pectoral, deltoid, and subclavius. The six branches are the highest thoracic, thoracoacromial, lateral thoracic, subscapular, posterior humeral circumflex, and anterior humeral circumflex.

axillary nerve, one of the last two branches of the posterior cord of the brachial plexus before the posterior cord becomes the radial nerve. The axillary nerve passes over the insertion of the subscapularis, crosses the teres minor, and leaves the axilla, accompanied by the posterior humeral circumflex artery. It passes through the quadrilateral space bounded by the neck of the humerus, the two teres muscles, and the long head of the triceps and divides into a posterior branch and an anterior branch. The posterior branch innervates the teres minor, part of the deltoideus, and part of the skin overlying the deltoideus; the anterior branch winds around the neck of the humerus and innervates the deltoideus. Some fibers of the nerve also supply the capsule of the shoulder joint.

axillary node, one of the lymph glands of the axilla that helps fight infections in the chest, armpit, neck, and arm and drains lymph from those areas. The 20 to 30 axillary nodes are divided into the lateral group, the anterior group, the posterior group, the central group, and the medial group. The lateral group is associated with lymphatic vessels that drain the whole arm, the anterior group with vessels that drain the thoracic muscles, the posterior group with vessels that drain the dorsal muscles of the neck and the muscles of the thoracic wall, the central group with vessels that drain the lymph from the nodes of the three preceding groups, and the medial group with afferent vessels that drain lymph from the breast and efferent vessels that form the subclavian lymphatic trunk. See also **lymphatic system, lymph node.**

axillary temperature [L, *axilla,* wing + *temperatura*], the body temperature as recorded by a thermometer placed in the armpit. The reading is generally 0.5 to 1.0 degree less than the oral temperature.

axillary vein, one of a pair of veins of the upper limb that begins at the junction of the basilic and the brachial veins near the distal border of the teres major and becomes the subclavian vein at the outer border of the first rib. It receives deoxygenated blood from the venous tributaries that correspond to the branches of the axillary artery and near its termination, from the cephalic vein. It contains a pair of valves at the distal border of the subscapularis. Compare **subclavian vein.**

axio-.   See **ax-.**

axis, *pl.* **axes** /ak'sēz/ [Gk, *axon*, axle],   **1.** (in anatomy) a line that passes through the center of the body, or a part of the body, such as the frontal axis, binauricular axis, and basifacial axis. **2.** the second cervical vertebra about which the atlas rotates, allowing the head to be turned, extended, and flexed. Also called **epistropheus, odontoid vertebra.**

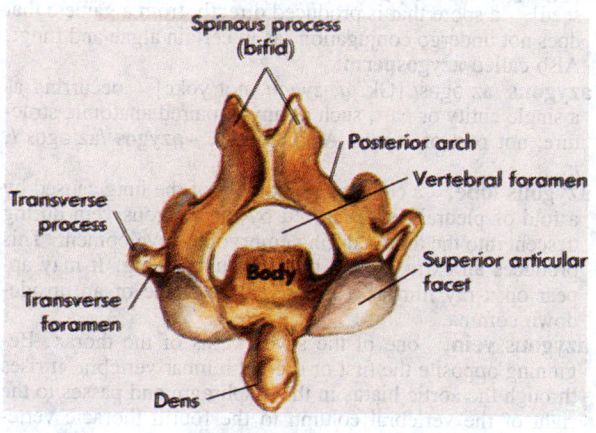

Spinous process (bifid)

Posterior arch

Vertebral foramen

Transverse process

Body

Superior articular facet

Transverse foramen

Dens

Axis *(Seeley, 1991)*

axis artery,   one of a pair of extensions of the subclavian arteries, running into and supplying the upper limb, continuing into the forearm as the palmar interosseous artery. Each artery is divided into subclavian, axillary, and brachial portions, developing radial and ulnar arteries from the brachial section.

axis cylinder.   See **axon.**

axis traction,   **1.** the process of pulling a baby's head with obstetric forceps in a direction in line with the path of least resistance, following the curve of Carus through the mother's birth canal. **2.** *informal.* any mechanical device attached to obstetric forceps to facilitate pulling in the proper direction.

axo-.   See **ax-.**

axoaxonic synapse /ak'sō·akson'ik/ [Gk, *axon*, axle (to) *axon* axle],   a type of synapse in which the axon of one neuron comes in contact with the axon of another neuron.

axodendrite /-den'trīt/ [Gk, *axon,* axle, *dendron,* tree],   a nonmedullated fibril appendage of the main axon of a nerve cell.

axodendritic synapse /-dendrit'ik/ [Gk, *axon* + *dendron,* tree],   a type of synapse in which the axon of one neuron comes in contact with the dendrites of another neuron.

axodendrosomatic synapse /-den'drōsōmat'ik/,   a type of synapse in which the axon of one neuron comes in contact with both the dendrites and the cell body of another neuron.

axon /ak'son [Gk, axle]/,   the cylindric extension of a nerve cell that conducts impulses away from the neuron cell body. Axons may be bare or sheathed in myelin. Also called **axone** /ak'sōn/, **axis cylinder.** Compare **dendrite.**

axon-.   See **ax-.**

axon flare,   vasodilatation, reddening, and increased sensitivity of skin surrounding an injured area, caused by an axon reflex. Axon flare or reflex is considered part of a triple response in which injury or stroking of the skin results in local reddening, the release of histamine or a histamine-like substance, a surrounding flare, and wheal formation. A pinprick in the involved area causes more intense pain than a similar stimulus before injury.

axonotmesis /ak'sənotmē'sis/ [Gk, *axon* + *temnein*, to cut],   an interruption of the axon with subsequent wallerian degeneration of the distal nerve segment. Connective tissue of the nerve, including the Schwann cell basement membranes, may remain intact.

axon reflex [Gk, *axon*, axle],   a neuron reflex in which an afferent impulse travels along a nerve fiber away from the cell body until it reaches a branching, where it is diverted to an end organ without entering the cell body. It does not involve a complete reflex arc, and therefore it is not a true reflex (vasodilation that occurs when the skin is stimulated).

axon sheath [Gk, *axle*, AS, *scaeth*],   a laminated myelin sheath that is interrupted at intervals by nodes of Ranvier.

axoplasmic flow /ak'sōplaz'mik/ [Gk, *axon* + *plassein*, to shape],   the continuous pulsing, undulating movement of the cytoplasm between the cell body of a neuron, where protein synthesis occurs, and the axon fiber to supply it with the substances vital for the maintenance of activity and for repair. The nerve fiber depends totally on the cell body for metabolites, and any interruption in the axoplasmic flow caused by disease or trauma results in the degeneration of the unsupplied areas of the axon.

axosomatic synapse /ak'sōsōmat'ik/ [Gk, *axon* + *soma*, body],   a type of synapse in which the axon of one neuron comes in contact with the cell body of another neuron.

Aygestin,   a trademark for an oral progestin drug (norethindrone acetate).

azatadine maleate /azat'ədēn/,   an antihistamine with antiserotonin, anticholinergic, and sedative effects.

- INDICATIONS: It is used in the treatment of allergic rhinitis and chronic urticaria.

- CONTRAINDICATIONS: It is contraindicated in patients hypersensitive to this drug or similar antihistamines and should not be given to patients also taking monoamine oxidase inhibitors or those with asthma or lower respiratory tract symptoms.

- ADVERSE EFFECTS: The most commonly reported adverse effects are drowsiness, urticaria, drug rash, anaphylactic shock, photosensitivity, chills, dry mouth, and diaphoresis.

azathioprine /az'əthī'ōprēn/,   an immunosuppressive.

- INDICATIONS: It is prescribed to prevent organ rejection after transplantation and in the treatment of lupus erythematosus and other systemic inflammatory diseases.

- CONTRAINDICATION: Known hypersensitivity to this drug prohibits its use.

- ADVERSE EFFECTS: Among the most serious adverse reactions are bone marrow depression and hepatotoxicity. Nausea and fever are common.

-azepam,   a combining form designating a diazepam-type antianxiety agent.

azidothymidine.   See **zidovudine.**

Azlin,   a trademark for an antibiotic (azlocillin).

azlocillin sodium /az'lōsil'in/,   a semisynthetic penicillin antibiotic.

- INDICATIONS: It is prescribed for lower respiratory tract, urinary tract, skin, and bone and joint infections and bacterial septicemia caused by susceptible strains of microorganisms, mainly *Pseudomonas aeruginosa.*

■ CONTRAINDICATION: Hypersensitivity to any of the penicillins prohibits its use.

■ ADVERSE EFFECTS: The most serious adverse reactions are anaphylactic reactions, convulsive seizures, epigastric pain, reduction in blood elements, and elevation in hepatic and renal parameters.

azo-, a prefix meaning 'containing nitrogen': *azotenesis, azotemin.*

-azocine, a combining form designating a narcotic agonist or antagonist.

azo compounds /ā′zō/ [Fr, *azote,* nitrogen], one of many organic aromatic compounds containing the divalent chromophore, -N=N-. They are produced by the alkaline reduction of nitro compounds.

azo dye a type of nitrogen-containing compound used in commercial coloring materials. Some forms of the chemical are potential carcinogens.

-azoline, a combining form designating an antihistaminic or local vasoconstrictor.

azoospermia /āzō′əspur′mē·ə/ [Gk, *a, zoon,* not animal, *sperma* seed], lack of spermatozoa in the semen. It may be caused by testicular dysfunction or by blockage of the tubules of the epididymis, or it may be induced by vasectomy. Infertility but not impotence is associated with azoospermia. Compare **oligospermia.**

-azosin, a combining form designating a prazosin-type antihypertensive agent.

azotemia /az′ōtē′mē·ə/ [Fr, *azote,* nitrogen; Gk, *haima,* blood], retention of excessive amounts of nitrogenous compounds in the blood. This toxic condition is caused by failure of the kidneys to remove urea from the blood and is characteristic of uremia. See also **uremia. –azotemic,** *adj.*

azoturia /az′ōtŌŌr′ēə/ [Fr, *azote,* nitrogen + Gk, *ouron,* urine], an excess of nitrogenous compounds including urea in the urine.

AZT, a trademark for an HIV virus inhibitor (Zidovudine). Also called Retrovir.

AZ test. See **Aschheim-Zondek test.**

azul, azula. See **pinta.**

Azulfidine, a trademark for an antibacterial (sulfasalazine).

azygos. See **azygous.**

azygospore /az′igəspô′r/ [Gk, *a, zygon,* not yoke, *sporos,* seed], a spore that is produced directly from a gamete that does not undergo conjugation, as in certain algae and fungi. Also called **azygosperm.**

azygous /az′əgəs/ [Gk, *a, zygon,* not yoke], occurring as a single entity or part, such as any unpaired anatomic structure; not part of a pair. Also **azygos. –azygos** /az′əgos′/, *n.*

azygous lobe, a congenital anomaly of the lung caused by a fold of pleural tissue carried by the azygous vein during descent into the thorax during embryonic development. This produces an extra lobe in the right upper lung. It may appear on x-ray film as a fissure in the shape of an upside-down comma.

azygous vein, one of the seven veins of the thorax. Beginning opposite the first or second lumbar vertebra, it rises through the aortic hiatus in the diaphragm and passes to the right of the vertebral column to the fourth thoracic vertebra, then arches ventrally over the root of the right lung, and ends in the superior vena cava. It receives numerous veins, such as the hemiazygous veins, several esophageal veins, and the right bronchial vein. Compare **internal thoracic vein, left brachiocephalic vein, right brachiocephalic vein.**

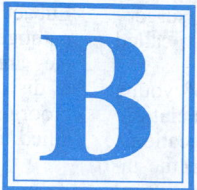

B, symbol for the element **boron.**

Ba, symbol for the element **barium.**

BA, abbreviation for *Bachelor of Arts.*

babbling, a stage in speech development characterized by the production of strings of speech sounds in vocal play.

Babcock's operation [William W. Babcock, American surgeon, b. 1872], the extirpation of a varicosed saphenous vein by inserting an acorn-tipped sound, tying the vein to the sound, and drawing it out. Also called **subcutaneous stripping.**

babesiosis /bəbē′sē·ō′sis/ [Victor Babés, Romanian bacteriologist, b. 1854], an infection caused by protozoa of the genus *Babesia.* The parasite is introduced into the host through the bite of ticks of the species *Ixodes dammini* and infects red blood cells. Incidence of the disease is highest in the U.S. in the northeast and north-central regions. Symptoms include headache, fever, nausea and vomiting, myalgia, and hemolysis. Also called **babesiasis** /bab′əsī′əsis/.

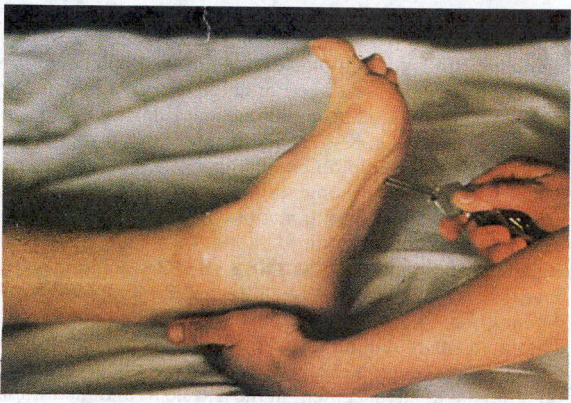

Babinski's reflex in an older adult *(Kamal, 1991)*

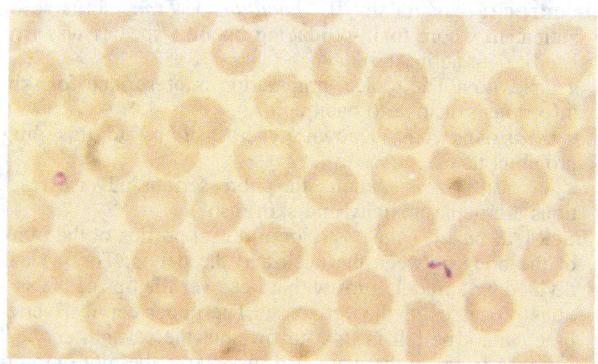

Red blood cells exhibiting babesiosis *(Bain, 1989)*

Babinski's reflex /bəbin′skēz/ [Josef F.F. Babinski, French neurologist, b. 1857], dorsiflexion of the big toe with extension and fanning of the other toes elicited by firmly stroking the lateral aspect of the sole of the foot. The reflex is normal in newborn infants and abnormal in children and adults, in whom it may indicate a lesion in the pyramidal tract.

baby [ME *babe*], **1.** an infant or young child, especially one who is not yet able to walk or talk. **2.** to treat gently or with special care.

Baby bottle tooth decay, a dental condition that occurs in children between 12 months and 3 years of age as a result of being given a bottle at bedtime, resulting in prolonged exposure of the teeth to milk or juice. Caries are formed because pools of milk or juice in the mouth break down to lactic acid and other decay-causing substances. Preventive measures include elimination of the bedtime feeding or substitution of water for milk or juice in the nighttime bottle. Formerly called **nursing bottle caries.**

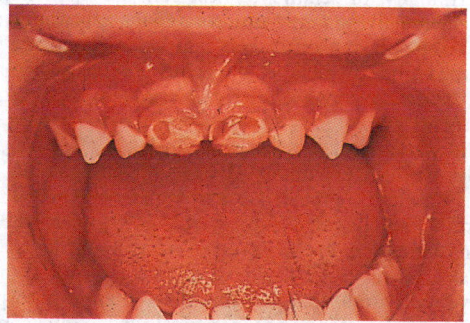

Baby bottle tooth decay
(Seidel, 1991/Courtesy Drs. Abelson and Cameron, Lutherville, MD)

Baby Jane Doe regulations, rules established in 1984 by the U.S. Health and Human Services Department requiring state governments to investigate complaints about parental decisions involving the treatment of handicapped infants. The rules also allowed the federal government to have access to children's medical records and required hospitals to post notices urging doctors and nurses to report any suspected cases of infants denied proper medical care. The controversial regulations have been held illegal by a federal court. The popular name for the federal rules was taken from the name "Jane Doe" given to an infant born in New York with an open spinal column and other defects and who became the object of a campaign to force lifesaving surgery for the child over the objections of the parents. Also called **Baby Doe rules.**

baby talk, **1.** the speech patterns and sounds of young children learning to talk, characterized by mispronunciation, imperfect syntax, repetition, and phonetic modifications, such as lisping or stuttering. See also **lallation. 2.** the intentionally oversimplified manner of speech, imitative of young children learning to talk, used by adults in addressing children or pets. **3.** the speech patterns characteristic of regressive stages of various mental disorders, especially schizophrenia.

bacampicillin hydrochloride, a semisynthetic penicillin.
■ INDICATIONS: It is prescribed in the treatment of respiratory tract, urinary tract, skin, and gonococcal infections.
■ CONTRAINDICATIONS: Known sensitivity to this drug or other penicillin antibiotics prohibits its use.
■ ADVERSE EFFECTS: Among the most serious adverse reactions are hypersensitivity reactions, gastritis, enterocolitis, and transient blood disorders.

Bachelor of Science in Nursing (BSN) /bach′ələr/, an academic degree awarded on satisfactory completion of a 4-year course of study in an institution of higher learning. The recipient is eligible to take the national certifying examination to become a registered nurse. A BSN degree is prerequisite to advancement in most systems and institutions that employ nurses. Compare **associate degree in nursing, diploma program in nursing.**

bacill-, a combining form meaning 'pertaining to any rod-shaped bacterium': **bacillemia, bacillosis.**

Bacillaceae /bas′əlā′si·ē/ [L, *bacillum,* small rod], a family of *Schizomycetes* of the order *Eubacteriales,* consisting of gram-positive, rod-shaped cells that can produce cylindric, ellipsoid, or spheric endospores situated terminally, subterminally, or centrally. These cells are chemoheterotropic and mostly saprophytic, commonly appearing in soil. Some are parasitic on insects and animals and are pathogenic. The family includes the genus *Bacillus,* which is aerobic, and the genus *Clostridium,* which is facultatively anaerobic.

bacillary dysentery. See **shigellosis.**

bacille Calmette-Guérin (BCG) /kalmet′gāraN′/ [Léon C.A. Calmette, French bacteriologist, b. 1863; Camille Guérin, French bacteriologist, b. 1872], an attenuated strain of tubercle bacilli, used in many countries as a vaccine against tuberculosis, most often administered intradermally, with a multiple-puncture disk. It appears to prevent the more serious forms of tuberculosis and to give some protection to persons living in areas where tuberculosis is prevalent. BCG is also administered to stimulate the immune response in people who have certain kinds of malignancy. It induces a positive tuberculin reaction and may mask early, active infection by removing the diagnostic sign of conversion from the negative to the positive skin reaction. See also **tuberculin test, tuberculosis.**

bacillemia. See **bacill.**

bacilli /bəsil′ī/, *sing.* **bacillum** [L, *bacillum,* small rod], any rod-shaped bacteria. See **Bacillus.**

bacilliform /bəsil′ifôrm/, rod-shaped, like a bacillus.

bacillosis. See **bacill.**

bacillum. See **bacill.**

bacilluria /bas′əloŏr′ē·ə/ [L, *bacillum* + Gk, *ouron,* urine], the presence of bacilli in the urine.

Bacillus /bəsil′əs/, a genus of aerobic, gram-positive spore-producing bacteria in the family Bacillaceae, order

Eubacteriales, including 33 species, three of which are pathogenic and the rest saprophytic soil forms. Some species are nonpathogenic, but others cause of a wide variety of diseases, ranging from anthrax to tuberculosis. Many microorganisms formerly classified as *Bacillus* are now classified in other genera. See also **Bacillaceae.**

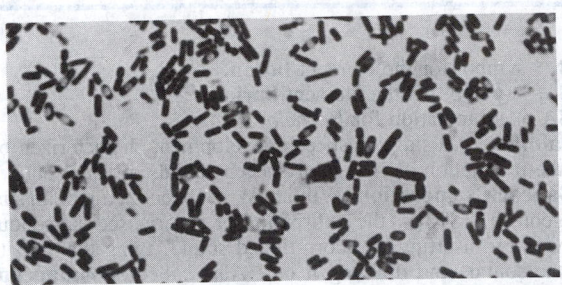
Bacillus *(Baron, 1990)*

Bacillus anthracis, a species of gram-positive, facultative anaerobe that causes anthrax, a disease primarily of cattle and sheep. The spores of this organism, if inhaled, can cause a pulmonary form of anthrax; spores can live for many years in animal products, such as hides and wool, and in soil. See also **anthrax, wool-sorter's disease.**

bacillus Calmette-Guérin vaccine. See **BCG vaccine.**

bacitracin /bas′itrā′sin/ [L, *bacillum* + *Tracy* surname of patient in whom toxin-producing bacillus species was isolated], an antibacterial.
■ INDICATION: The topical preparation is prescribed for skin infections sensitive to bacitracin.
■ CONTRAINDICATION: Known hypersensitivity to this drug prohibits its use.
■ ADVERSE EFFECTS: Among the more serious adverse reactions are nephrotoxicity and skin rash.

back [AS *baec*], the posterior or dorsal portion of the trunk of the body between the neck and the pelvis. The back is divided by a middle furrow that lies over the tips of the spinous processes of the vertebrae. The upper cervical vertebrae cannot be felt in this furrow, but the seventh cervical vertebra is easily distinguished just above the more prominent first thoracic vertebra. The skeletal portion of the back includes the thoracic and the lumbar vertebrae and both scapulae. The root of the spine of the scapula is on a level in the back with the spine of the third thoracic vertebra, and the inferior angle of the scapula is on a level with the spine of the seventh thoracic vertebra. The superficial muscles of the back are large and include the trapezius, the rhomboideus major, and the latissimus. The deep muscles of the back are the erector spinae iliocostalis, interspinales, intertransversarii, longissimus, multifidi, rotatores, splenius, semispinales, spinales, transversocostal, and transversospinal. The nerves that innervate the various muscles of the back include some branches of the dorsal primary divisions of the spinal nerves, the lateral branches of the dorsal primary division of the middle and the lower cervical nerves, some branches of the primary division of the spinal nerves, and some branches of the ventral primary divisions of the spinal nerves.

backache /bak′āk/ [AS, *baec* + ME, *aken*], a pain in the lumbar, lumbosacral, or cervical regions of the back, varying in sharpness and intensity. Causes may include muscle strain or other muscular disorders or pressure on the root of a nerve, such as the sciatic nerve, caused in turn by a variety of factors, including a herniated vertebral disk. Treatment may include heat, ultrasound, and devices to provide support for the affected area while in bed or while standing or sitting, bed rest, surgical intervention, and medications to relieve pain and relax spasm of the muscle of the affected area.

back-action condenser, (in dentistry) an instrument for compacting amalgams that has a U-shaped shank to develop the condensing force from a pulling motion rather than the more common pushing motions.

backcross [AS, *baec + cruc,* cross], **1.** (in genetics) the cross of a first filial generation hybrid with one of the parents or with a genotype that is identical to the parental strain. **2.** the organism or strain produced by such a cross.

back knee. See **genu recurvatum.**

background radiation [AS, *baec* + OE, *grund* ground], naturally occurring radiation emitted by materials in the soil, groundwater, and building material, radioactive substances in the body, especially potassium 40 (40K), and cosmic rays from outer space. Each year the average person is exposed to 44 millirads (mrad) of cosmic radiation, 44 mrads from external terrestrial radiation, and 18 mrads from naturally occurring internal radioactive sources. Background radiation levels may vary in different locales.

back pressure [AS, *baec;* L, *premere,* to press], pressure that builds in a vessel or a cavity as fluid is accumulated. The pressure increases and extends backward if the normal mechanism for egress or passage of the fluid is not restored.

backscatter radiation. See **scattered radiation.**

backup, a duplicate computer, data file, equipment, or procedure for use in the event of equipment failure.

baclofen, an antispastic agent.
■ INDICATION: It is prescribed for the alleviation of spasticity.
■ CONTRAINDICATION: Known hypersensitivity to this drug prohibits its use.
■ ADVERSE EFFECTS: Among the more serious adverse reactions are confusion, hypotension, dyspnea, impotence, nausea, and transient drowsiness.

-bactam, a combining form designating a beta-lactamase inhibitor.

bacter-. See **bacterio-.**

bacteremia /bak'tirē'mē·ə/ [Gk, *bakterion* small, staff, *haima,* blood], the presence of bacteria in the blood. Undocumented bacteremias occur frequently and usually abate spontaneously. Bacteremia is demonstrated by blood culture. Antibiotic treatment, if given, is specific for the organism found and appropriate to the locus of infection. Compare **septicemia.** See also **septic shock.** **–bacteremic,** *adj.*

bacteremic shock. See **septic shock.**

bacteria /baktir'ē·ə/, *sing.* **bacterium** [Gk, *bakterion,* small staff], any of the small unicellular microorganisms of the class Schizomycetes. The genera vary morphologically, being spheric (cocci), rod-shaped (bacilli), spiral (spirochetes), or comma-shaped (vibrios). The nature, severity, and outcome of any infection caused by a bacterium are characteristic of that species.

-bacteria, a suffix meaning 'genus of microscopic plants forming the class Schizomycetes': *lysobacteria, nitrobacteria, streptobacteria.*

bacterial aneurysm /baktir'ē·əl/, a localized dilatation in the wall of a blood vessel caused by the growth of bacteria, often following septicemia or bacteremia and usually occurring in peripheral vessels. See also **mycotic aneurysm.**

bacterial count. See **count.**

bacterial endocarditis, an acute or subacute bacterial infection of the endocardium or the heart valves or both. The condition is characterized by heart murmur, prolonged fever, bacteremia, splenomegaly, and embolic phenomena. The acute variety progresses rapidly and is usually caused by staphylococci. The subacute variety is usually caused by lodging of *Streptococcus viridans* in valves of the heart damaged by rheumatic fever. Prompt treatment of both types with antibiotics, such as penicillin, cephalosporin, or gentamicin given intravenously, is essential to prevent destruction of the valves and cardiac failure. See also **endocarditis, subacute bacterial endocarditis.**

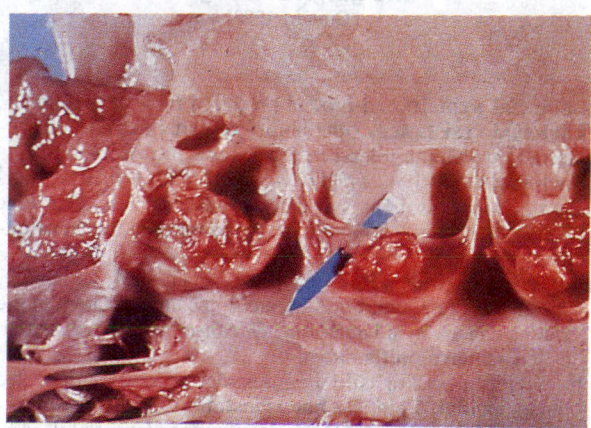

Bacterial endocarditis *(Farrar, 1992)*

bacterial food poisoning, a toxic condition resulting from the ingestion of food contaminated by certain bacteria. Acute infectious gastroenteritis caused by various species of *Salmonella* is characterized by fever, chills, nausea, vomiting, diarrhea, and general discomfort beginning 8 to 48 hours after ingestion and continuing for several days. Similar symptoms caused by *Staphylococcus,* usually *S. aureus,* appear much sooner and rarely last more than a few hours. Food poisoning caused by the neurotoxin of *Clostridium botulinum* is characterized by GI symptoms, disturbances of vision, weakness or paralysis of muscles, and, in severe cases, respiratory failure. See also **botulism.**

bacterial inflammation [L, *bacterium, inflammare,* to set afire], any inflammation that is part of a body's response to a bacterial infection.

bacterial kinase, **1.** a kinase of bacterial origin. **2.** a bacterial enzyme that activates plasminogen, the precursor of plasmin.

bacterial meningitis. See **meningitis.**

bacterial plaque, a film comprised of microorganisms that attaches with acquired pellicle to the teeth and causes caries and infections of the gingival tissue. Mucin secreted by the salivary glands is also a component of plaque; it varies in thickness and consistency, depending on individual metabolism, dental hygiene, diet, and environmental factors. Also called **dental plaque.** (See Fig. p. 162.)

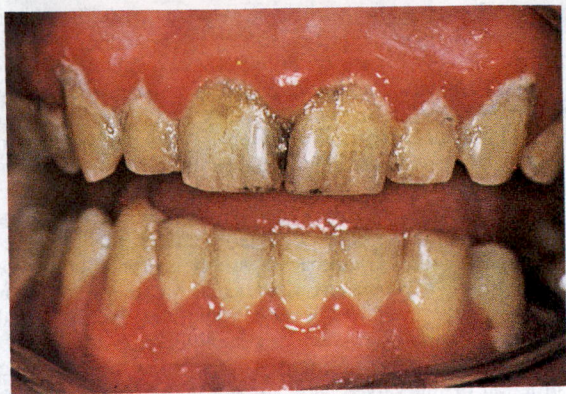

Gross bacterial plaque deposits near the gingival margin
(Grundy, 1992)

bacterial protein, a protein produced by a bacterium.

bacterial resistance, the ability of certain strains of bacteria to develop a tolerance toward specific antibiotics.

bacterial toxin [Gk, *bakterion*, small staff + *toxikon*, poison], any poisonous substance produced by a bacterium. Kinds of bacterial toxins include **endotoxins** and **exotoxins**.

bacterial vaginosis [Gk, *bakterion*, small staff; L, *vagina*, sheath; Gk, *osis*, condition], a chronic inflammation of the vagina caused by a bacterium, *Gardnerella vaginalis*. Also called **vulvovaginitis**.

bactericidal /baktir′isī′dəl/, destructive to bacteria. Also **bacteriocidal**. Compare **bacteriostatic**.

bactericidal antibiotic [L, *bacterium*, *caedere*, to kill, Gk, *anti*, against, *bios*, life], an antibiotic drug that kills bacteria.

bactericide /baktir′əsīd/ [GK, *bakterion*; L, *caedere*, to kill], any drug or other agent that kills bacteria.

bactericidin [Gk, *bakterion* + L, *caedere*, to kill], an antibody that kills bacteria in the presence of complement.

bacterio-, bacter-, a combining form meaning 'pertaining to any bacterial microorganism': *bacteriogenic, bacteriophytoma, bacteriosis*.

bacteriocidal. See **bactericidal**.

bacteriocidal antibiotic, See **bactericidal antibiotic**.

bacterioidal. See **bacteroid**.

bacteriologic /baktir′ē·əloj′ik/ [L, *bacterium*], pertaining to **bacteriology**. Also **bacteriological**.

bacteriologic sputum examination, a laboratory procedure to determine the presence or absence of bacteria in a specimen of a patient's sputum. Part of the specimen is stained and examined microscopically on a glass slide, and part is mixed with culture media and allowed to incubate for more specific examination later.

bacteriologist /baktir′ē·ol′əjist/, a specialist in bacteriology.

bacteriology /-ol′əjē/ [Gk, *bakterion* + *logos*, science], the scientific study of bacteria.

bacteriolysin /baktir′ē·əlī′sin/ [Gk, *bakterion* + *lyein*, to loosen], an antibody that causes the breakdown of a particular species of bacterial cell. Complement is usually also necessary for this reaction. See also **bacteriolysis**.

bacteriolysis /baktir′ē·ol′əsis/, the breakdown of bacteria intracellularly or extracellularly. See also **bacteriolysin**. —**bacteriolytic**, *adj*.

bacteriophage /baktir′ē·əfāj′/ [Gk, *bakterion* + *phagein*, to eat], any virus that causes lysis of host bacteria, including the blue-green "algae." Bacteriophages resemble other viruses in that each is composed of either ribonucleic acid(RNA) or deoxyribonucleic acid(DNA). They vary in structure from simple fibrous bodies to complex forms with contractile "tails." Bacteriophages associated with temperate bacteria may be genetically intimate with the host and are named after the bacterial strain for which they are specific, such as coliphage and corynebacteriophage. —**bacteriophagic**, *adj.*, **bacteriophagy** /-of′əjē/, *n*.

bacteriophage typing, the process of identifying a species of bacteria according to the type of virus that attacks it.

-bacteriophagic. See **bacteriophage**.

-bacteriophagy See **bacteriophage**.

bacteriostasis /baktir′ē·os′təsis/ [L, *bacterium*, Gk, *stasis*, standing still], a state of suspended growth and/or reproduction of bacteria.

bacteriostatic /baktir′ē·əstat′ik/ [Gk, *bakterion* + *statikos*, standing], tending to restrain the development or the reproduction of bacteria. Compare **bactericidal**.

bacterium. See **bacteria**.

bacteriuria /baktir′ēyŏŏr′ē·ə/, the presence of bacteria in the urine. The presence of more than 100,000 pathogenic bacteria per milliliter of urine is usually considered significant and diagnostic of urinary tract infection. See also **urinary tract infection**.

bacteroid /bak′təroid/, **1.** of, pertaining to, or resembling bacteria. **2.** a structure that resembles a bacterium. Also **bacterioid** /baktir′ē·oid/. —**bacteroidal, bacterioidal,** *adj*.

Bacteroides /bak′təroi′dēz/ [Gk, *bakterion*, small staff, *eidos*, form], a genus of obligate anaerobic bacilli normally found in the colon, mouth, genital tract, and upper respiratory system. Severe infection may result from the invasion of the bacillus through a break in the mucous membrane into the venous circulation, where thrombosis and bacteremia may occur. Foul-smelling abcesses, gas, and putrefaction are characteristic of infection with this organism. Of the 30 species, *Bacteroides fragilis* is the most common and most virulent.

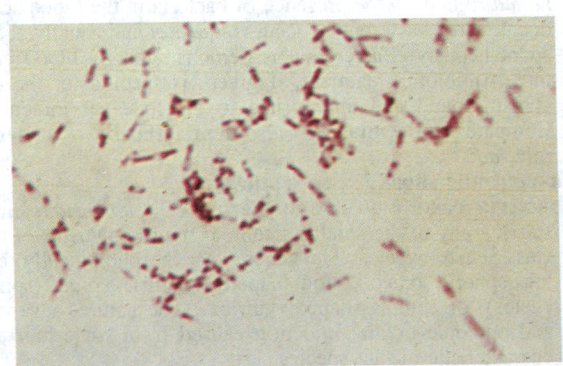

Bacteroides fragilis *(Baron, 1990)*

Bactrim, a trademark for a fixed-combination drug containing two antibacterials (sulfamethoxazole and trimethoprim).

BAEP, abbreviation for **brainstem auditory-evoked potential.**

baffling, the process of removing large water particles from suspension in a jet nebulizer so that the particles entering the patient's airways are of a uniform therapeutic size. The function may be performed in part by a perforated plate against which liquid particles impinge, fracture, and are reflected into the vapor chamber of the nebulizer.

bag [AS *baelg*], a flexible or dilatable sac or pouch designed to contain gas, fluid, or semisolid material such as crushed ice. An Ambu bag or breathing bag is used to control the flow of respiratory gases entering the lungs of a patient. Several types of bags are used in medical or surgical procedures to dilate the anus, vagina, or other body openings.

bagasse /bəgas′/ [Fr, cane trash], the crushed fibers or the residue of sugar cane, a source of the thermophilic actinomycetes antigen that is a cause of bagassosis hypersensitivity pneumonitis.

bagassosis /bag′əsō′sis/, a self-limited lung disease caused by an allergic response to bagasse, the fungi-laden, dusty debris left after the syrup has been extracted from sugar cane. It is characterized by fever, dyspnea, and malaise.

bagging, *informal.* the artificial respiration performed with a ventilator or respirator bag, such as an Ambu bag or Hope resuscitator. The bag is squeezed to deliver air to the patient's lungs as the mask is held over the mouth. During general anesthesia the anesthetist may also use this technique to correct the respiratory pattern of an unconscious patient.

bag of waters. the membranous sac of amniotic fluid surrounding the fetus in the uterus of a pregnant woman. See **amnion.**

bag-valve-mask resuscitator, a device consisting of a manually compressible container with a plastic bag of oxygen at one end and at the other a one-way valve and mask that fit over the mouth and nose of the person to be resuscitated. See also **Ambu bag.**

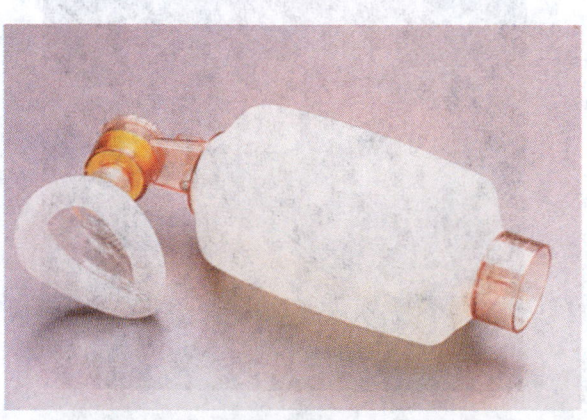

Bag valve mask *(Judd, 1988)*

Bain Breathing Circuit, a continuous-flow anesthetic system that does not require a soda-lime absorber.

Bainbridge reflex [Francis A. Bainbridge, English physiologist, b. 1874], a cardiac reflex consisting of an increased pulse rate, resulting from stimulation of stretch receptors in the wall of the left atrium. It may be produced by the infusion of large amounts of intravenous fluids.

Baker's cyst, a synovial cyst that forms at the back of the knee. It is often associated with rheumatoid arthritis and may appear only when the leg is straightened.

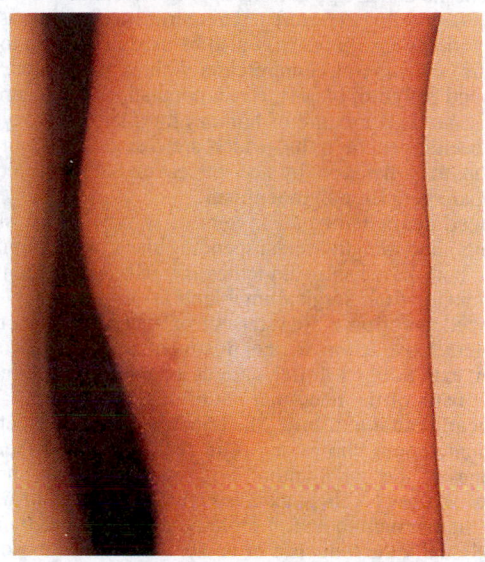

Baker's cyst *(Zitelli, 1992/Courtesy Dr. M Sherlock)*

baker's itch [AS, *giccan*, to bake], a rash that may develop on the hands and forearms of bakery workers, probably as an allergic reaction to flours or other ingredients in bakery products.

BAL, abbreviation for **British antilewisite.** See **dimercaprol.**

balance [L, *bilanx*, having two scales], **1.** an instrument for weighing. **2.** a normal state of physiologic equilibrium. **3.** a state of mental or emotional equilibrium. **4.** to bring into equilibrium.

balanced anesthesia, *informal,* one of a number of variable techniques of general anesthesia in which no single anesthetic agent or preset proportion of the combination of agents is used; rather, an individualized mixture of anesthetics is prescribed according to the needs of a particular patient for a particular operation. One type of balanced anesthesia may combine a local or regional anesthetic with general anesthetic agents; another may combine a muscle relaxant, an analgesic, oxygen, an anesthetic gas, and a sedative.

balanced articulation, the simultaneous contacting of the upper and lower teeth as they glide over each other when the mandible is moved from centric relation to various eccentric relations. See also **balanced occlusion.**

balanced diet, a diet containing all of the essential nutrients that cannot be synthesized in adequate quantities by the body, in amounts adequate for growth, energy needs, nitrogen equilibrium, repair of wear, and maintenance of normal health.

balanced occlusion, 1. an occlusion of the teeth that presents a harmonious relation of the occluding surfaces in centric and eccentric positions within the functional range of mandibular positions and tooth size. **2.** the simultaneous contacting of the upper and lower teeth on both sides and in the anterior and posterior occlusal areas of the jaws. An appropriate dental prosthesis develops such an occlusion to prevent the denture base from tipping or rotating in relation to the supporting structures. This term is primarily associated with the mouth but may also be used in relation to testing the occlusion of denture casts with an articulator.

balanced polymorphism, in a population, the recurrence of an equalized mixture of homozygotes and heterozygotes for specific genetic traits, which are maintained from generation to generation by the forces of natural selection. Compare **genetic polymorphism.**

balanced suspension, a system of splints, ropes, slings, pulleys, and weights for suspending the lower extremities of the body, used as an aid to healing and recuperation from fractures or from surgical intervention.

balanced traction, a system of balanced suspension that supplements traction in the treatment of fractures of the lower extremities or after various operations affecting the lower parts of the body that require traction.

balanced translocation, the transfer of segments between nonhomologous chromosomes in such a way that there are changes in the configuration and total number of chromosomes, but each cell or gamete contains no more or no less than the normal amount of diploid or haploid genetic material. Usually the long arm of an acrocentric chromosome is transferred to another chromosome, and the small fragment containing the centromere is lost, leaving only 45 chromosomes. A person with balanced translocation is phenotypically normal but may produce children with trisomies. Compare **reciprocal translocation, robertsonian translocation.**

balancing side, (in dentistry) the side of the mouth opposite the working side of a dentition or denture.

balanic /bəlan'ik/ [Gk, *balanos*, acorn], of or pertaining to the glans penis or the glans clitoridis.

balanitis /bal'ənī'tis/ [Gk, *balanos* + *itis*], inflammation of the glans penis.

balanitis xerotica obliterans /zirot'ikə oblit'ərans/ [Gk, *balanos, itis; xeros,* dry, *tokos,* labor; L *obliterare* to efface], a chronic skin disease of the penis, characterized by a white indurated area surrounding the meatus. Local antibacterial and antiinflammatory agents are used to treat it.

balano-, a combining form meaning 'pertaining to the glans penis': *balanocele, balanoplasty, balanoposthitis.*

balanoplasty /bal'ənōplas'tē/ [Gk, *balanos* + *plassein,* to shape], an operation involving plastic surgery of the glans penis.

balanoposthitis /bal'ənōposthī'tis/ [Gk, *balanos* + *posthe,* penis, foreskin, *itis*], a generalized inflammation of the glans penis and prepuce, characterized by soreness, irritation, and discharge, occurring as a complication of bacterial or fungal infection. Smear and culture can determine the causative agent—often a common venereal disease—

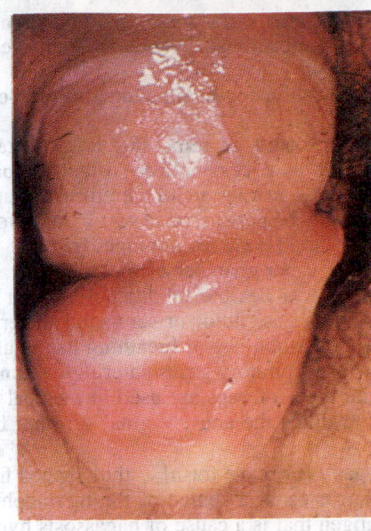

Balanitis *(Shipley, 1993)*

whereupon specific antimicrobial therapy can be instituted. Circumcision may be considered in severe cases. To relieve discomfort, the inflamed area can be irrigated with a warm saline solution several times a day.

balanopreputial /bal'ənōpripyoo'shəl/ [Gk, *balanos* + L, *praeputium,* foreskin], of or pertaining to the glans penis and the prepuce.

balanorrhagia /bal'ənōrā'jē·ə/ [Gk, *balanos* + *thegnynai,* to gush], balanitis in which pus is discharged copiously from the penis.

balantidiasis /bal'əntidī'əsis/, an infection caused by ingestion of cysts of the protozoan *Balantidium coli.* In some cases the organism is a harmless inhabitant of the large intestine, but infection with *B. coli* usually causes diarrhea. Infrequently the infection progresses, and the protozoan invades the intestinal wall and produces ulcers or abscesses,

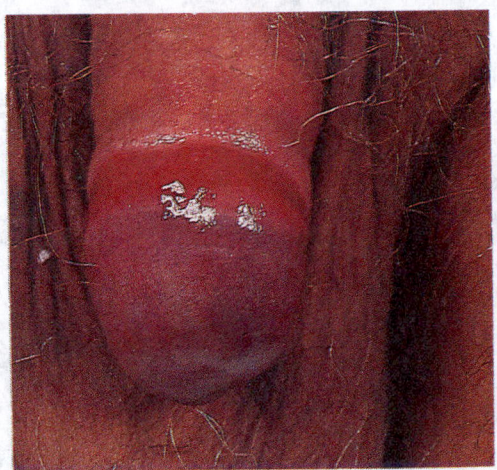

balanitis xerotica obliterans *(duVivier, 1993)*

which may cause dysentery and death. The diagnosis is made by the identification of cysts and trophozoites in the stool or in the exudate from intestinal ulcers. Metronidazole is usually prescribed to treat the infection.

Balantidium coli /bal'əntid'ē·əm/ [Gk, *balantidion*, little bag; *kolon*, colon], the largest and the only ciliated protozoan species that is pathogenic to humans, causing balantidiasis. The organism is seen in two life stages: the motile trophozoite and the encysted cercaria. It is a normal inhabitant of the domestic hog and is transmitted to humans by the ingestion of cysts excreted in the feces of the hog.

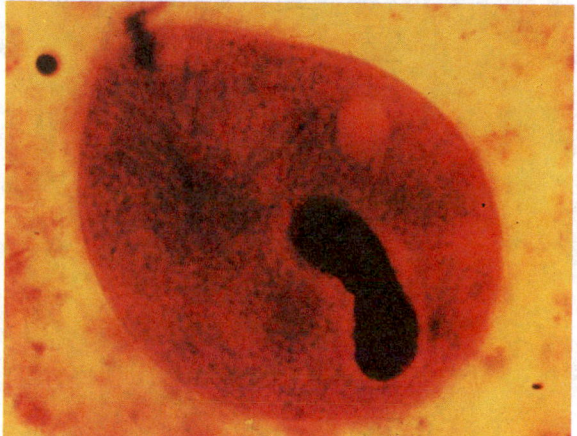

Balantidium coli (Baron, 1990)

baldness [ME, *balled*], absence of hair, especially from the scalp. See also **alopecia.**

BAL in Oil, a trademark for a heavy metal antagonist (dimercaprol).

Balkan traction frame, an overhead rectangular frame, attached to the bed of an orthopedic patient, for attaching splints, suspending or changing the position of immobilized limbs, and providing continuous traction with weights and pulleys.

Balkan tubulointerstitial nephritis /tōo'byəlō·in'tərstish'əl/, a chronic kidney disorder marked by renal insufficiency, proteinuria, tubulointerstitial nephritis, and anemia. The onset is gradual, but end-stage disease occurs within 5 years after the first signs. About one third of the patients also suffer from urinary tract cancers. The disease is endemic in the Balkans but is not hereditary.

ball [ME *bal*], a relatively spheric mass, such as one of the chondrin balls embedded in hyaline cartilage.

ball-and-socket joint, a synovial joint in which the globular (ball-shaped) head of an articulating bone is received into a cuplike cavity, allowing the distal bone to move around an indefinite number of axes with a common center, such as in hip and shoulder joints. Also called **enarthrosis, spheroidea.** Compare **condyloid joint, pivot joint, saddle joint.**

ball-catcher position, a position of the hands for the purpose of making a radiograph to diagnose rheumatoid arthritis. The hands are held with the palms upward and the fingers cupped, as if to catch a ball.

ballism /bôl'izəm/ [Gk, *ballismo*, dancing], an abnormal neuromuscular condition characterized by uncoordinated swinging of the limbs and jerky movements. Ballism is associated with extrapyramidal disorders, such as Sydenham's chorea. The condition may occur in a unilateral form as hemiballismus. Also called **ballismus.**

ballistic movement /bəlis'tik/, a high-velocity musculoskeletal movement, such as a tennis serve or boxing punch, requiring reciprocal organization of agonistic and antagonistic synergies.

ballistics /bəlis'tiks/ [Gk, *ballein*, to throw], the study of the motion, trajectory, and impact of projectiles, including bullets and rockets.

ballistocardiogram /bəlis'tōkär''dē·əgram'/ [Gk, *ballein*, to throw, *kardia*, heart, *graphein*, to record], a record of the motion of the body—toward the head and toward the feet—caused by the thrust of the heart during systolic ejection of the blood into the aorta and the pulmonary arteries. The patient is placed on a special table, a **ballistocardiograph**, that is so delicately balanced that vibrations of the body can be recorded by a machine attached to the table. The ballistocardiogram is a sensitive tool that is useful in measuring cardiac output and the force of contraction of the heart.

ball of the foot, the part of the foot composed of the distal heads of the metatarsals and their surrounding fatty fibrous tissue pad.

balloon angioplasty /bəlōon'/, a method of dilating or opening an obstructed blood vessel by threading a small balloon-tipped catheter into the vessel. The balloon is inflated to widen the blood vessel by compressing the foreign material against the walls, leaving a larger lumen through which blood can pass.

balloon bezoar [Fr, *ballon*, a large ball, Ar, *bazahr*, counterpoison], a balloon that is inserted into the stomach and inflated to create a sensation of fullness, used as a therapy for obesity.

balloon septostomy. See **Rashkind procedure.**

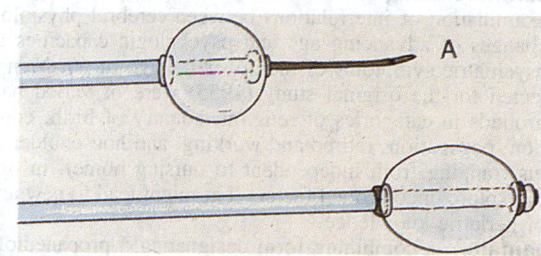

Double-lumen balloon-tip catheter (Geenen, 1992)

balloon-tip catheter, a catheter bearing a nonporous inflatable sac around its distal end. After insertion of the catheter the sac can be inflated with air or sterile water, introduced via injection into a special port at the proximal end of the catheter. The inflated sac secures the catheter in the correct position. Kinds of balloon-tip catheters include **Foley catheter, and Swan-Ganz catheter.**

ballottable /bəlot'əbəl/ [Fr, *balloter*, a shaking about], pertaining to a use of palpation to detect the movement of objects suspended in fluid, such as the body of a fetus in its amniotic fluid. See **ballottement**.

ballottable head [Fr, *ballotage,* shaking up], a fetal head that has not descended and has not become fixed in the maternal bony pelvis.

ballottement /bä'lôtmäN', bəlot'ment/ [Fr, tossing], a technique of palpating an organ or floating structure by bouncing it gently and feeling it rebound. Ballottement of a fetus within a uterus is a probable objective sign of pregnancy. In late pregnancy a fetal head that can be ballotted is said to be **floating** or **unengaged,** as differentiated from a fixed or an engaged head, which cannot be easily dislodged from the pelvis.

ball thrombus, a relatively round, coagulated mass of blood, containing platelets, fibrin, and cellular fragments, that may obstruct a blood vessel or an orifice, usually the mitral valve of the heart.

ball-valve action, the intermittent opening and closing of an orifice by a buoyant, ball-shaped mass, which acts as a valve. Some kinds of objects that may act in this manner are kidney stones, gallstones, and blood clots.

balm /bäm/ [Gk, *balsamon,* balsam], **1.** also called **balsam.** a healing or a soothing substance, such as any of various medicinal ointments. **2.** an aromatic plant of the genus *Melissa* that relieves pain.

balneology /bal'nē·ol'əjē/ [L, *balneum,* bath; Gk, *logos,* science], a field of medicine that deals with the chemical compositions of various mineral waters and their healing characteristics, especially in baths. **–balneologic,** *adj.*

balneotherapy /bal'nē·ōther'əpē/ [L, *balneum* + Gk, *therapeia,* treatment], a use of baths in the treatment of many diseases and conditions.

balneum pneumaticum. See **air bath.**

balsam[1] /bôl'səm/ [Gk *balsamon*], any of a variety of resinous saps, generally from evergreens, usually containing benzoic or cinnamic acid. Balsam is sometimes used in rectal suppositories and dermatologic agents as a counterirritant.

balsam[2]. See **balm.**

Baltimore Longitudinal Study of Aging, a long-range examination of interrelations between cerebral physiologic changes of advancing age and psychologic capacities and psychiatric symptoms of men over the age of 65. Men selected for the original study (1955) were of varied backgrounds in categories of religion, country of birth, education, occupation, retired and working, and householder status (ranging from independent to nursing home), in order to explore uncontrolled factors that might lead to new areas of geriatric knowledge.

-bamate, a combining form designating a propanediol or pentanediol derivative.

bamboo spine /bambōō'/ [Malay, *bambu*], the characteristically rigid spine of advanced ankylosing spondylitis. Also called **poker spine.** See also **ankylosing spondylitis.**

band [ME *bande* strip], **1.** (in anatomy) a bundle of fibers, as seen in striated muscle, that encircles a structure or binds one part of the body to another. **2.** (in dentistry) a strip of metal that fits around a tooth and serves as an attachment for orthodontic components. **3.** also called **stab form.** *informal.* the immature form of a segmented granulocyte characterized by a sausage-shaped nucleus. It is the only immature leukocyte normally found in the peripheral circulation. Bands represent 3% to 5% of the total white cell volume.

An increase in the relative number of bands indicates bacterial infection or acute stress to the bone marrow.

band adapter, an instrument for aiding in the fitting of a circumferential orthodontic band to a tooth.

bandage /ban'dij/ [ME, *bande,* strip], **1.** a strip or roll of cloth or other material that may be wound around a part of the body in a variety of ways to secure a dressing, maintain pressure over a compress, or immobilize a limb or other part of the body. **2.** to apply a bandage.

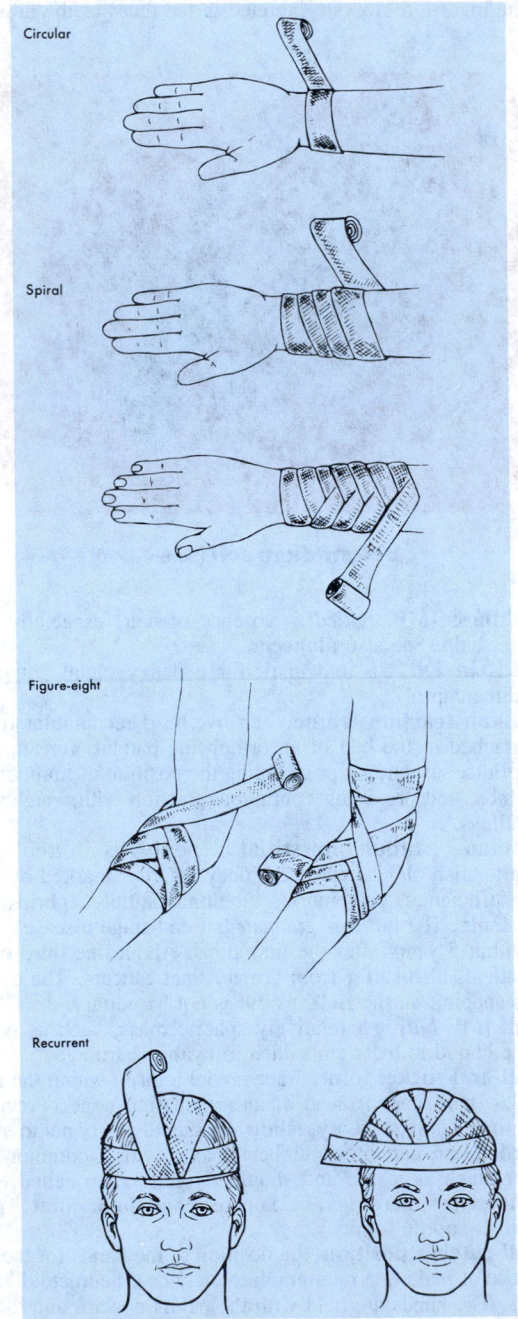

Types of bandage turns *(Potter, 1993)*

bandage shears, a sturdy pair of scissors used to cut through bandages. The blades of most bandage shears are angled to the shaft of the instrument, and the lower blade has a rounded blunt protuberance to facilitate insertion under the bandage without harming the patient's skin.

band cell, a developing granular leukocyte in circulating blood, characterized by a curved or indented nucleus. Band cells are intermediate leukocytic forms between metamyelocytes and adult leukocytes with segmented nuclei.

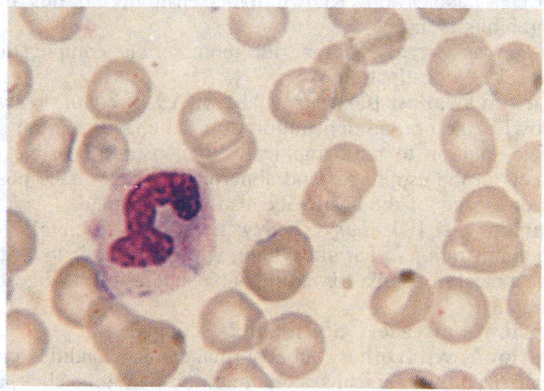

Band cell (Bain, 1989)

banding [ME, *bande,* strip], (in genetics) any of several techniques of staining chromosomes with fluorescent stains or chemical dyes that produce a series of lateral light and dark areas whose intensity and position are characteristic for each chromosome. Banding patterns are identified according to the staining technique used, as C-banding, G-banding, Q-banding, and R-banding. Also called **chromosome banding.**

Bandl's ring. See **pathologic retraction ring.** Compare **constriction ring.**

bandpass, (in radiology) a measure of the number of times per second an electron beam can be modulated. It is a factor that influences horizontal resolution on a cathode-ray tube. The higher the bandpass, the greater the horizontal resolution. Also called **bandwidth.**

band pusher, an instrument used for adapting metal circumferential orthodontic bands to the teeth.

band remover, an instrument used for removing circumferential orthodontic bands from the teeth.

bandwidth. See **bandpass.**

bang. See **bhang.**

Bangkok hemorrhagic fever. See **dengue fever.**

bank blood [It, *banca,* bench; AS, *blod*], anticoagulated, preserved blood collected from donors usually in units of 500 ml and stored under refrigeration for future use. Dated and identified as to blood type, it is stored for a usual maximum period of 21 days. Bank blood may be used directly after cross matching against the recipient's blood or for the extraction and preparation of any of its components. See also **autologous blood, frozen blood, packed cells, pooled plasma, whole blood.**

Banthine, a trademark for an anticholinergic (methantheline bromide) used as an antispasmodic.

Banti's syndrome /ban'tēz/ [Guido Banti, Italian patholo-

gist, b. 1852], a serious, progressive disorder involving several organ systems, characterized by portal hypertension, splenomegaly, anemia, leukopenia, GI tract bleeding, and cirrhosis of the liver. Obstruction of the blood vessels that lie between the intestines and the liver leads to venous congestion, an enlarged spleen, and abnormal destruction of red and white blood cells. Early symptoms are weakness, fatigue, and anemia. Surgical removal of the spleen and creation of a portacaval shunt to improve portal circulation are sometimes necessary. Since the syndrome is often a complication of alcoholic cirrhosis of the liver, medical treatment includes prescribing improved nutrition, vitamins, abstinence from alcohol, and rest. Also called **Banti's disease.** See also **congestive splenomegalia, cirrhosis, portacaval shunt, portal hypertension.**

BAO, abbreviation for **basal acid output.**

bar-. See **baro-.**

bar, a measure of air pressure. It is equal to 1000 millibars, or 106 dynes/cm^2, or approximately 1 standard atmosphere (1 atm).

baralyme (BL) /ber'əlīm/ [Gk, *barys,* heavy; AS *lim* lime], a mixture of calcium and barium compounds used to absorb exhaled carbon dioxide in an anesthesia rebreathing system.

Bárány's test. See **caloric test.**

-barb, a combining form designating a barbituric acid derivative.

barber's itch. See **sycosis barbae.**

barbiturate /bärbichŏōrāt, -ərit/ [Saint Barbara, drug discovered on day of the saint, 1864], a derivative of barbituric acid that acts as a sedative or hypnotic. These derivatives are in widespread use and act by depressing the respiratory rate, blood pressure, temperature, and central nervous system. They may have addiction potential. Some barbiturates are used in anesthesia and for seizures. Among the more common derivatives are amobarbital, butabarbital, pentobarbital, phenobarbital, secobarbital, and thiopental.

barbiturate coma [Ger, Saint Barbara's Day, Gk, *koma,* deep sleep], an effect of barbituric acid or its derivatives, which may be rapid-acting sedatives, hypnotics, and respiratory depressants. Death may result from intentional or accidental overdosage.

-barbituric, a combining form given to compounds derived from barbituric acid: *dibromobarbituric, isobarbituric, phenylethylbarbituric.*

barbiturism /bärbich'əriz'əm/, **1.** acute or chronic poisoning by any of the derivatives of barbituric acid. Ingestion of such preparations in excess of therapeutic quantities may be fatal or may produce physiologic, pathologic, and psychologic changes, such as depressed respiration, cyanosis, disorientation, and coma. **2.** addiction to a barbiturate.

Bardeleben's bone. See **ostrigonum.**

Bard-Pic syndrome /bärd'pik'/ [Louis Bard, French anatomist, b. 1857; Adrian Pic, French physician, b. 1863], a condition characterized by progressive jaundice, enlarged gallbladder, and cachexia, associated with advanced pancreatic cancer.

Bard's sign [Louis Bard, French anatomist, b. 1857], the increased oscillations of the eyeball in organic nystagmus when the patient tries to visually follow a target moved from side to side across the line of sight. Such oscillations usually cease during the same test if the patient has congenital nystagmus.

bar graph [OF, *barre*], a graph in which frequencies are represented by bars extending from the ordinate or the abscissa, allowing the distribution of the entire sample to be seen at once.

bariatrics /ber′ē·at′riks/ [Gk, *baros*, weight, *iatros*, physician], the field of medicine that focuses on the treatment and control of obesity and diseases associated with obesity.

baritosis /ber′ətō′sis/, a benign form of pneumoconiosis caused by an accumulation of barium dust in the lungs. Barium is an inert mineral, does not cause fibrosis, and is not a common cause of functional impairment. The condition is most likely to affect persons involved in the mining and processing of barite, a barium product used in the manufacture of paints.

barium (Ba) /ber′ē·əm/ [Gk, *barys,* heavy], a pale yellow, metallic element classified with the alkaline earths. Its atomic number is 56; its atomic weight is 137.36. The acid-soluble salts of barium are poisonous. Barium carbonate, formerly used in medicine, is now used to prepare the cardiac stimulant, barium chloride; fine, milky barium sulfate is used as a contrast medium in radiographic imaging of the digestive tract.

barium enema, a rectal infusion of barium sulfate, a radiopaque contrast medium, which is retained in the lower intestinal tract during roentgenographic studies for diagnosing obstruction, tumors, or other abnormalities, such as ulcerative colitis. For the procedure to be most effective, the colon must be free of all fecal material, accomplished by a minimum residue diet for 2 days, a cathartic the night before, and a cleansing enema or suppository on the morning of the study. The patient takes only liquids the previous night and has no breakfast before the examination. After the x-ray studies are made, the barium is removed by a cleansing enema. The procedure is used therapeutically in children to reduce nonstrangulated intussusception. Also called **contrast enema.**

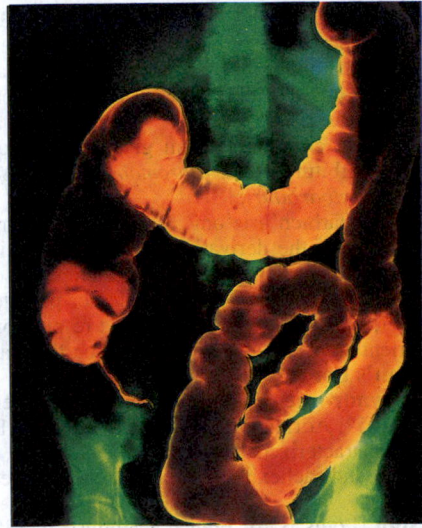

Barium enema *(Thibodeau, 1993/Ernest W Beck)*

barium meal, the ingestion of barium sulfate, a radiopaque contrast medium, for the radiographic examina-

tion of the esophagus, stomach, and intestinal tract in the diagnosis of such conditions as dysphagia, peptic ulcer, and fistulas. The movement of the barium through the GI tract is followed by fluoroscopy, x-ray studies, or both. Before the test, the patient receives nothing by mouth for at least 8 hours. See also **barium swallow.**

barium sulfate, a radiopaque medium used as a diagnostic aid in roentgenology.

■ INDICATION: It is prescribed for x-ray examination of the GI tract.

■ CONTRAINDICATION: Known hypersensitivity to this drug prohibits its use.

■ ADVERSE EFFECTS: Among the more serious complications is severe constipation.

barium swallow [Gk, *barys,* heavy, AS, *swelgan,* to swallow], the oral administration of a radiopaque barium sulfate solution to radiographically demonstrate possible defects in the esophagô and abnormal borders of the posterior aspects of the heart. See also **barium meal.**

barium test [Gk, *barys,* heavy; L, *testum,* crucible], the administration of barium sulfate, which is opaque to x-rays, as a meal or enema for radiographic studies of the digestive tract.

Barlow's disease. See **infantile scurvy.**

Barlow's syndrome, an abnormal cardiac condition characterized by an apical systolic murmur, a systolic click, and an electrocardiogram indicating inferior ischemia. These signs are associated with mitral regurgitation caused by prolapse of the mitral valve. Also called **electrocardiographic-auscultatory syndrome, mitral valve prolapse.**

baro-, bar-, a combining form meaning 'pertaining to pressure, heaviness': *baresthesia, barognosis, barospirator.*

barognosis /ber′əgnō′sis/, *pl.* **barognoses** [Gk, *baros* weight, *gnosis,* knowledge], the ability to perceive and evaluate weight, especially that held in the hand.

barograph /ber′əgraf′/ [Gk, *baros* + *graphein,* to record], an instrument that continuously monitors barometric pressure and provides a record on paper of pressure changes.

barometer /bərom′ətər/ [Gk, *baros* + *metron,* measure, an instrument for measuring atmospheric pressure, commonly consisting of a slender tube filled with mercury, sealed at one end, and inverted into a reservoir of mercury. At sea level the normal height of mercury in the tube is 760 mm. At higher elevations the mercury column height (barometric pressure) is less. Fluctuations in barometric pressure may occur preceding major changes in the weather, making a barometer useful in weather forecasting. **–barometric,** *adj.*

barometric pressure. See **atmospheric pressure.**

baroreceptor /ber′ōrisep′tər/ [Gk, *baros* + L, *recipcre,* to receive], one of the pressure-sensitive nerve endings in the walls of the atria of the heart, the vena cava, the aortic arch, and the carotid sinus. Baroreceptors stimulate central reflex mechanisms that allow physiologic adjustment and adaptation to changes in blood pressure via vasodilatation or vasoconstriction. Baroreceptors are essential for homeostasis.

barosinusitis. See **aerosinusitis.**

Barosperse, a trademark for a radiopaque medium (barium sulfate).

barotitis. See **aerotitis.**

barotitis media. See **aerotitis media.**

barotrauma /ber′ōtrô′mə, -trou′mə/ [Gk, *baros* + *trauma,* wound], physical injury sustained as a result of exposure to increased environmental pressure, such as barotitis media or rupture of the lungs or paranasal sinuses, as may occur among deep-sea divers or caisson workers. Compare **decompression sickness.**

Barr body. See **sex chromatin.**

barrel chest, a large, rounded thorax, considered normal in some stocky individuals and certain others who live in high-altitude areas and consequently develop increased vital capacities. Barrel chest, however, may also be a sign of pulmonary emphysema.

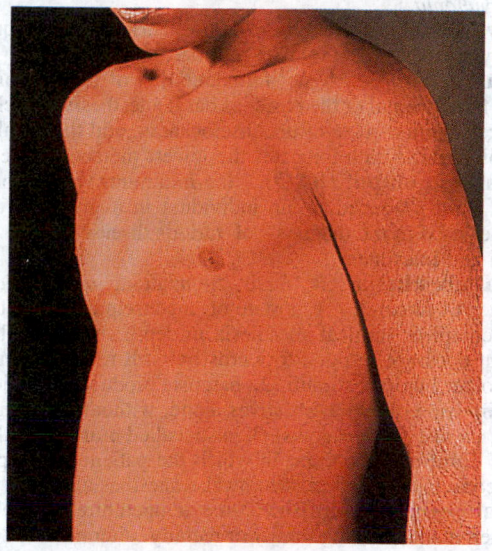

Barrel chest (Zitelli, 1992/Courtesy of Dr. Meyer B Marks)

Barr-Epstein virus. See **Epstein-Barr virus.**

Barré's pyramidal sign /bäräz'/ [Jean A. Barré, French neurologist, b. 1880], a diagnostic sign of a prefrontal brain lesion observed as a phenomenon in which the lateral or vertical movement of one leg of a recumbent patient is followed by a similar movement of the other leg.

Barrett's syndrome [Norman R. Barrett, English surgeon, b. 1903], a disorder of the lower esophagus marked by a benign ulcerlike lesion in columnar epithelium, resulting most often from chronic irritation of the esophagus by gas-

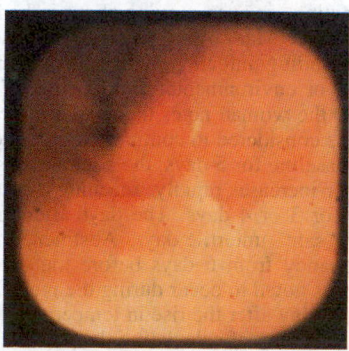

Endoscopic view of Barret's syndrome (Mitros, 1988)

tric reflux of acidic digestive juices. Major symptoms include dysphagia and heartburn. Symptoms may be relieved by eating frequent small meals, avoiding foods that produce gas, taking antacid medication, and elevating the head of the bed to prevent passive reflux when lying down. Also called **Barrett's esophagus, Barrett's ulcer.**

barrier /ber'ē·ər/ [ME, barrere], **1.** a wall or other obstacle that can restrain or block the passage of substances. Barrier methods of contraception, such as the condom or cervical diaphragm, prevent the passage of spermatazoa into the uterus. Membranes and cell walls of body tissues function as screenlike barriers to permit the movement of water or certain other molecules from one side to the other while preventing the passage of other substances. Barriers in kidney tissues adjust automatically to regulate the retention or excretion of water and other substances according to the needs of organ systems elsewhere in the body. **2.** something nonphysical that obstructs or separates, such as barriers to communication or compliance. **3.** (in radiography) any device that intercepts beams of x-rays. A primary barrier is one that blocks the passage of the useful x-ray beam, such as the walls and floor. A secondary barrier is one that intercepts only leakage and scattered x-ray emissions. An example is the ceiling.

barrier creams, ointments, lotions, and similar preparations applied to exposed areas of the skin to protect skin cells from exposure to various allergens, irritants, and carcinogens, including sunlight.

barrier-free design [ME, barrere; AS, freo, barreres; L, designare, to mark out], the design of homes, workplaces, and public buildings so that physically challenged individuals can make regular use of such structures.

Barsony-Koppenstein method, a procedure for making x-ray images of the cervical intervertebral foramina.

Barthel Index (BI), a disability profile scale developed by D.W. Barthel in 1965 to evaluate a patient's self-care abilities in 10 areas, including bowel and bladder control. The patient is scored from 0 to 15 points in various self-care categories, depending on his or her need for help, such as in feeding, bathing, dressing, and walking. A person who is continent, does not require help in feeding, dressing, bathing, ascending or descending stairs, and is able to walk at least a block may score 100 points on the BI scale. However, that person may still require help in such activities of daily living as cooking, keeping house, and functioning normally in public.

Bartholinian abscess. See **Bartholin's abscess.**

bartholinitis /bär'təlinī'tis/ [Caspar Bartholin; Gk itis], an inflammatory condition of one or both Bartholin's glands, caused by bacterial infection. Usually, the causative microorganism is a species of Streptococcus or Staphylococcus or a strain of gonococci. The condition is characterized by swelling of one or both glands, pain, and the development of an abscess in the infected gland. A fistula may develop from the gland to the vagina, anus, or perineum. Treatment includes local application of heat, often by soaking in hot water, antibiotics, or, if necessary, incision of the gland and drainage of the purulent material or excision of the entire gland and its duct.

Bartholin's abscess /bär'təlinz/ [Caspar T. Bartholin, Danish anatomist, b. 1655; L, abscedere, to go away], an abscess of the greater vestibular gland of the vagina. Also called **Bartholinian abscess.**

Bartholin's cyst a cyst that arises from one of the vestibular glands or from its ducts, filling with clear fluid that replaces the suppurative exudate characteristic of chronic inflammation.

Bartholin's duct, the major duct of the sublingual salivary gland.

Bartholin's gland, one of two small, mucus-secreting glands located on the posterior and lateral aspect of the vestibule of the vagina. Also called **greater vestibular glands.**

Barton, Clara (1821–1912), an American philanthropist, humanitarian, and founder of the American National Red Cross. During the Civil War, she was a volunteer nurse, often on the battlefield, and at its end she organized a bureau of records to help in the search for missing men. When the Franco-Prussian War erupted, she assisted in the organization of military hospitals in Europe in association with the International Red Cross. This experience led to her advocacy of an American Red Cross organization, of which she became the first president.

Bartonella /bär′tənel′ə/ [Alberto Barton, Peruvian bacteriologist, b. 1871], a genus of small, gram-negative flagellated pleomorphic coccobacilli. Members of the genus are intracellular parasites that infect red blood cells and the epithelial cells of the lymph nodes, liver, and spleen. They are transmitted at night by the bite of a sandfly of the genus *Phlebotomus*. The only known species of *Bartonella* is *B. bacilliformis*, the organism that causes bartonellosis. Because of its distinctive appearance, it is easily identified on microscopic examination of a smear of blood stained with Wright's stain.

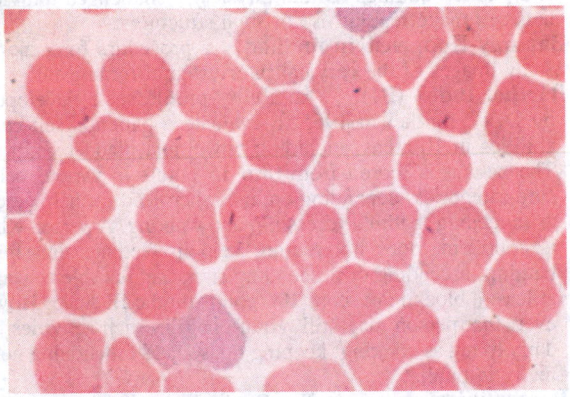

Blood smear infected with *Bartonella bacilliformis*
(Hayhoe, 1992)

bartonellosis /bär′tənəlō′sis/, an acute infection caused by *Bartonella bacilliformis*, transmitted by the bite of a sandfly. It is characterized by fever, severe anemia, bone pain, and, several weeks after the first symptoms are observed, by multiple nodular or verrucose skin lesions. The disease is endemic in the valleys of the Andes in Peru, Colombia, and Ecuador. The treatment usually includes chloramphenicol, penicillin, streptomycin, or tetracycline. Untreated, the infection is often fatal. Also called **Carrión's disease, Oroya fever, verruga peruana.**

Barton forceps. See **obstetric forceps.**

Barton's fracture [John R. Barton, American surgeon, b. 1794], a fracture of the distal articular surface of the ra-

dius, which may be accompanied by the dorsal dislocation of the carpus on the radius.

Bartter's syndrome /bär′tərz/ [Frederick C. Bartter, American physiologist, b. 1914], a rare hereditary disorder, characterized by hyperplasia of the juxtaglomerular apparatus and secondary hyperaldosteronism. Renin and angiotensin levels may be elevated, but blood pressure usually remains normal. Early signs in childhood are abnormal physical growth and mental retardation, often accompanied by chronic hypokalemia and alkalosis.

bary-, a combining form meaning 'heavy or difficult': *baryphonia.*

barye /ber′ē/, a measure of atmospheric pressure equal to 1 dyne/cm², or 1/1000 of a millibar.

basal /bā′səl/ [Gk, *basis*, foundation], of or pertaining to the fundamental or the basic, as basal anesthesia, which produces the first stage of unconsciousness, and the basal metabolic rate, which indicates the lowest metabolic rate.

basal acid output (BAO), the minimum volume of gastric fluid produced by an individual in a given period of time, used in the diagnosis of various diseases of the stomach and intestines.

basal anesthesia [Gk, *basis*, foundation; *anaisthesia*, absence of feeling], **1.** a state of unconsciousness just short of complete surgical anesthesia in depth, in which the patient does not respond to words but still reacts to pinprick or other noxious stimuli. **2.** narcosis produced by injection or infusion of potent sedatives alone, without added narcotics or anesthetic agents. **3.** also called **narcoanesthesia.** any form of anesthesia, in which the patient is completely unconscious, in contrast to awake anesthesia.

basal body temperature, the temperature of the body taken in the morning, orally or rectally, after at least 8 hours of sleep and before doing anything else, including getting out of bed, smoking a cigarette, moving around, talking, eating, or drinking.

basal-body-temperature method of family planning, a natural method of family planning that relies on the identification of the fertile period of the menstrual cycle by noting the progesterone-mediated rise in basal body temperature of 0.5° to 1° F that occurs with ovulation. The rate and pattern of the increase vary greatly from woman to woman, and somewhat from cycle to cycle in any one woman. Several cycles are observed, and careful records are kept in which the woman takes her temperature at the same time every morning, before getting out of bed or doing anything else. It may be taken orally or rectally but should be done the same way every day. Talk ing, getting up, smoking a cigarette, eating, or even moving about in bed may change the temperature. Many other factors may also change the reading, including infection, stress, a bad night's sleep, medication, or environmental temperature. If any of these are present, the woman notes them on her record. The fertile period is considered to continue until the temperature is above the baseline for 5 days; the rise occurs slowly during all 5 days or increases rapidly, reaching a plateau at which it remains for 3 or 4 days. The days after that period are considered "safe" unfertile days. Abstinence is required to avoid pregnancy from 6 days before the earliest day that ovulation was noted to occur during the preceding 6 months until the fifth day after the rise in temperature in the current cycle. Another way of calculating the possible beginning of the fertile days is to subtract 19 days from the shortest complete menstrual cycle of the preceding 6 months. The basal body temperature method is more effective when used with the ovulation method than is either method used alone. The combination of these methods is called the symptothermal method of family planning. Compare **calendar method of family planning, ovulation method of family planning.**

basal bone, **1.** (in prosthodontics) the osseous tissue of the mandible and the maxillae, except for the rami and the processes, which provides support for artificial dentures. **2.** (in orthodontics) the fixed osseous structure that limits the movement of teeth in the creation of a stable occlusion.

basal cell, any one of the cells in the deepest layer of stratified epithelium.

basal cell acanthoma. See **basal cell papilloma.**

basal cell carcinoma [Gk, *basis* + L, *cella* storeroom; Gk, *karkinos,* crab, *oma,* tumor], a malignant, epithelial cell tumor that begins as a papule and enlarges peripherally, developing a central crater that erodes, crusts, and bleeds. Metastasis is rare, but local invasion destroys underlying and adjacent tissue. In 90% of cases the lesion is seen between the hairline and the upper lip. The primary cause of the cancer is excessive exposure to the sun or to x-rays. Treatment is eradication of the lesion, often by electrodesiccation or cryotherapy. Also called **basal cell epithelioma, basaloma, basiloma, carcinoma basocellulare, hair matrix carcinoma.** See also **rodent ulcer.**

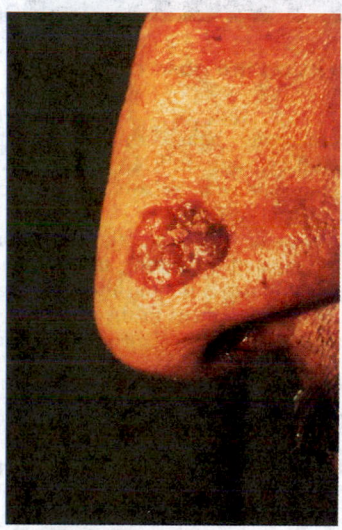

Basal cell carcinoma (Belcher, 1992)

basal cell papilloma [Gk, *basis* + L, *cella,* storeroom, *papilla,* nipple; Gk, *oma,* tumor], a benign, epidermal neoplasm characterized by multiple yellow or brown raised oval lesions that usually develop in middle age. Also called **basal cell acanthoma, seborrheic keratosis, seborrheic wart.**

basal ganglia [Gk, *basis* + *ganglion,* knot], the islands of gray matter within each cerebral hemisphere, the most important being the caudate nucleus, the putamen, and the pallidum. The basal ganglia are surrounded by the rings of the limbic system and lie between the thalamus of the diencephalon and the white matter of the hemisphere.

Basaljel, a trademark for an antacid (aluminum carbonate gel).

basal lamina [Gk, *basis* + L, thin, plate], a thin, noncellular layer of ground substance lying just under epithelial surfaces. Constituting the uppermost layer of the basement membrane, it can be examined with an electron microscope. Also called **basement lamina.**

basal layer. See **stratum basale.**

basal membrane, a sheet of tissue that forms the outer layer of the choroid and lies just under the pigmented layer of the retina. It is composed of elastic fibers and a thin homogenous layer.

basal metabolic rate (BMR), the amount of energy used in a unit of time by a fasting, resting subject to maintain vital functions. The rate, determined by the amount of oxygen used, is expressed in calories consumed per hour per square meter of body surface area or per kilogram of body weight.

basal metabolism [Gk, *basis* + *metabole,* change], the amount of energy needed to maintain essential basic body functions, such as respiration, circulation, temperature, peristalsis, and muscle tone. Basal metabolism is measured when the subject is awake and at complete rest, has not eaten for 14 to 18 hours, and is in a comfortable, warm environment. It is expressed as a basal metabolic rate, according to large calories per hour per square meter of body surface.

basal narcosis [Gk, *basis,* foundation, *narkosis,* a benumbing], a complete unconsciousness that is induced in a surgical patient before general anesthetic is administered. The state of induced unconsciousness is less profound than that of general anesthesia. The patient is unresponsive to verbal stimuli but may respond to noxious stimuli. Also called **basis narcosis.**

basaloid carcinoma /bā′səloid/ [Gk, *basis* + *eidos,* form; *karkinos* crab, *oma* tumor], a rare, malignant neoplasm of the anal canal containing areas that resemble basal cell carcinoma of the skin. Basaloid carcinoma is rapidly invasive. Tumor may spread to the skin of the perineum.

basaloma. See **basal cell carcinoma.**

basal seat, (in dentistry) the oral tissues and structures that support a denture. See also **basal seat outline.**

basal seat area, the portion of the oral structures that is available to support a denture. Also called **denture-bearing area, stress-bearing area.**

basal seat outline, (in dentistry) a profile on the mucous membrane or on a cast of the entire oral area to be covered by a denture. See also **basal seat.**

basal temperature. See **basal body temperature.**

basal temperature chart [Gk, *basis,* foundation; L, *temperatura;* + *charta,* paper], a daily temperature chart, usually including the temperature on awakening. A basal temperature chart is sometimes used by women to establish a date of ovulation, when the temperature may show a sudden increase. *basal tidal volume,* the tidal volume of a healthy person at complete rest, with all bodily functions at a minimal level of activity, adjusted for age, weight, and sex. The reported basal tidal volume figures would not apply to persons whose physiology is altered by such factors as illness or surgery.

base [Gk, *basis,* foundation], **1.** a chemical compound that combines with an acid to form a salt. Compare *alkali.* **2.** a molecule or radical that takes up or accepts protons. **3.** the major ingredient of a compounded material, particularly one that is used as a medication. Petroleum jelly is frequently used as a base for ointments. **4.** (in radiology) the rigid but flexible foundation of a sheet of x-ray film. The base is essentially transparent but is given a bluish tint during manufacture to reduce eyestrain for the radiologist viewing x-ray films.

base analogue [Gk, *basis* + *analogos*, proportionate], an analogue of one of the purine or the pyrimidine bases normally found in ribonucleic acid or deoxyribonucleic acid.

Basedow's goiter /bä′sədōz/ [Karl A. von Basedow, German physician, b. 1799], an enlargement of the thyroid gland, characterized by the hypersecretion of thyroid hormone after iodine therapy.

base excess, a measure of metabolic alkalosis or metabolic acidosis (negative value of base excess) expressed as the amount of acid or alkali needed to titrate 1 L of fully oxygenated blood to a pH of 7.40, the temperature being held at a constant 37° C and the P_{CO_2} at 40 torr.

base-forming food, a food that increases the pH of the urine. Base-forming foods include mainly fruits, vegetables, and dairy products, which are sources of sodium and potassium. Some foods that are acidic in their natural state may be converted to alkaline metabolites.

baseline /bās′līn/ [Gk, *basis* + L, *linea*], **1.** a known value or quantity with which an unknown is compared when measured or assessed. **2.** (in radiology) any of several basic anatomic planes or locations used for positioning purposes. They include the orbitomeatal, infraorbitomeatal, acanthomeatal, and glabellomeatal lines.

baseline behavior, a specified frequency and form of a particular behavior during preexperimental or pretherapeutic conditions.

baseline condition, an environmental condition during which a particular behavior reflects a stable rate of response before the introduction of experimental or therapeutic conditions.

baseline fetal heart rate, the fetal heart rate pattern between uterine contractions. An electronic fetal monitor is used to detect abnormally rapid or slow rates (less than 110 or more than 160 per minute) at term.

basement lamina. See **basal lamina.**

basement membrane [Fr, *soubassement*, under base], the fragile, noncellular layer of tissue that secures the overlying layers of stratified epithelium. It is the deepest layer, may contain reticular fibers, and can be selectively stained with silver stains.

base of the heart, the portion of the heart opposite the apex, directed to the right side of the body. It forms the upper border of the heart, lies just below the second rib, and involves primarily the left atrium, part of the right atrium, and the proximal portions of the great vessels. Passing between the base of the heart and the bodies of the fifth to the eighth thoracic vertebrae are the descending aorta, the esophagus, and the thoracic duct.

base of the skull, the floor of the skull, containing the anterior, middle, and posterior cranial fossae and numerous foramina, such as the optic foramen, foramen ovale, foramen lacerum, and foramen magnum.

base pair, a pair of nucleotides in a nucleic acid. One of the pair must be a purine, the other a pyrimidine. Base pairing finds guanine paired with cytosine and adenine paired with thymine.

base pairing, (in molecular genetics) the association in nucleic acids of the purine bases adenine and guanine with the pyrimidine bases cytosine, thymine, and uracil. In

Zygomatic arch — Zygomatic process of maxilla — Incisive foramen — Palatine process of maxilla — Hard palate — Horizontal plate of palatine bone — Vomer — Medial pterygoid lamina of sphenoid — Foramen ovale — Foramen spinosum — Foramen lacerum — Mandibular fossa — Stylomastoid foramen — Jugular foramen — Parietal bone — Temporal bone — Occipital condyle — Foramen magnum — Occipital bone

Landmarks on the base of the skull *(Vidik, 1984)*

DNA, adenine always pairs with thymine, and guanine always pairs with cytosine. In RNA, adenine invariably pairs with uracil, and guanine invariably pairs with cytosine. Thymine is not present in RNA.

baseplate [Gk, *basis* + ME, *plate*], a temporary form that represents the base of a denture, used for making records of maxillomandibular relationships, arranging artificial teeth, or for trial placement in the mouth to ensure a precise fit of a denture. Also called **record base, temporary base.**

base ratio, the ratio of molar quantities of the bases in ribonucleic and deoxyribonucleic acids.

bas-fond /bäfôN′/ [Fr, bottom], the bottom or fundus of any structure, especially the fundus of the urinary bladder.

basi-, basio-, a prefix meaning 'pertaining to a foundation or a base': *basicranial, basilaris, basiotribe.*

-basia /bā′zhə/, a suffix meaning 'ability to walk': *abasia, brachybasia, dysbasia.*

BASIC /bā′sik/, abbreviation for *b*eginner's *a*ll-purpose *s*ymbolic *i*nstruction *c*ode, a computer programing language considered the easiest form of programing language to learn.

-basic, a suffix meaning 'relating to or containing alkaline compounds': *ammonobasic, polybasic, tribasic.*

basic amino acid, an amino acid that has a positive electric charge in solution at a pH of 7. The basic amino acids are arginine, histidine, and lysine.

basic group identity, (in psychiatry) the shared social characteristics, such as world view, language, and value and ideologic system, that evolve from membership in an ethnic group.

basic health services, the minimum degree of health care considered to be necessary to maintain adequate health and protection from disease.

basic human needs, the things required for survival and normal mental and physical health, such as food, water, shelter, protection from environmental threats, and love.

basic life support (BLS) [Gk, *basis*, foundation; AS, *lif*, L, *supportare*, to bring up to], the role of cardiopulmonary resuscitation (CPR) and emergency cardiac care (ECC) in reinstituting either circulatory or respiratory function, or both, in the emergency treatment of a victim of cardiac or respiratory arrest.

basic salt, a salt that contains an unreplaced hydroxide ion from the base generating it, such as Ca(OH)Cl.

basifacial /bā′sifā′shəl/ [Gk, *basis* + L, *facies* face], pertaining to the lower portion of the face.

basilar /bas′ilər/ [Gk *basis* foundation], of or pertaining to a base or a basal area.

basilar artery, the single posterior arterial trunk formed by the junction of the two vertebral arteries at the base of the skull, extending from the inferior to the superior border of the pons, dividing into the left and right cerebral arteries, and supplying the internal ear and parts of the brain through the five branches of each artery. The branches are the pontine, labyrinthine, anterior inferior cerebellar, superior cerebellar, and posterior cerebral.

basilar artery insufficiency syndrome, the composite of clinical indicators associated with insufficient blood flow through the basilar artery, a condition that may be caused by arterial occlusion. Some of the common signs of this syndrome are dizziness, blindness, numbness, depression, dysarthria, dysphagia, and weakness on one side of the body.

basilar artery occlusion, an obstruction of the basilar artery, resulting in dysfunction involving cranial nerves III through XII, cerebellar dysfunction, hemiplegia or quadriplegia, and loss of proprioception.

basilar membrane, the cellular structure that forms the floor of the cochlear duct and is supported by bony and fibrous projections from the cochlear wall. It provides a fibrous base for the spiral organ of Corti.

basilar plexus [Gk, *basis* + L, braided], the venous network interlaced between the layers of the dura mater over the basilar portion of the occipital bone. It connects the two petrosal sinuses and communicates with the anterior vertebral venous plexus.

basilar sulcus [Gk, *basis* + L, furrow], the sulcus that cradles the basilar artery in the midline of the pons.

basilic vein /bəsil′ik/, one of the four superficial veins of the arm, beginning in the ulnar part of the dorsal venous network and running proximally on the posterior surface of the ulnar side of the forearm. It veers toward the anterior surface of the forearm distal to the elbow and is joined by the median cubital vein, then ascends obliquely between the biceps brachii and the pronator teres and crosses the brachial artery. It then runs proximally along the medial border of the biceps brachii, pierces the deep fascia, and ascends to join the brachial vein to form the axillary vein. Compare **dorsal digital vein, median antebrachial vein.**

basiloma /bas′ilō′mə/, *pl.* **basilomas, basilomata** See **basal cell carcinoma**

basiloma terebrans /ter′əbrənz/ [Gk, *basis, oma* + L, *terebare*, to bore], an invasive basal cell epithelioma.

basio-. See **basil-.**

basioccipital /bā′si·oksip′ətəl/ [Gk, *basis* + L, *occiput*, back of the head], of or pertaining to the basilar process of the occipital bone.

basion /bā′sē·on/ [Gk, *basis*, foundation], the midpoint on the anterior margin of the foramen magnum of the occipital

bone, opposite the opisthion in the middle of the posterior margin.

basis narcosis. See **basal narcosis.**

basis pedunculi cerebri. See **crus cerebri.**

basket cell [L, *bascauda*, dishpan], a cerebral cotex cell with a horizontal axon that sends out branches. Each branch breaks up into a basketlike mesh that surrounds a Purkinje cell.

Basle Nomina Anatomica (BNA), an international system of anatomic terminology adopted at Basel, Switzerland.

basophil /bā′səfil/ [Gk, *basis* + *philein* to love], a granulocytic white blood cell characterized by cytoplasmic granules that stain blue when exposed to a basic dye. Basophils represent 1% or less of the total white blood cell count. The relative number of basophils increases in myeloproliferative diseases and decreases in severe allergic reactions. Compare **eosinophil, neutrophil.** See also **agranulocyte, differential white blood cell count, granulocyte, leukocyte, polymorphonuclear leukocyte.**

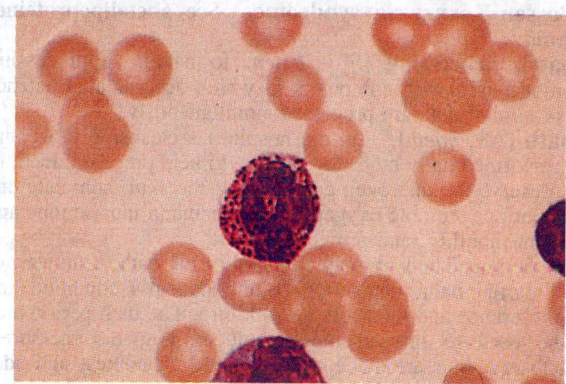

Basophil *(Hayhoe, 1992)*

basophilic adenoma [Gk, *basis* + *philein*, to love, *aden* gland, *oma*], a tumor of the pituitary gland composed of cells that can be stained with basic dyes. Compare **acidophilic adenoma, chromophobic adenoma.**

basophilic erythrocyte [Gk, *basis*, foundation, *philein*, to love, *erythros*, red, *kytos*, cell], a red blood cell that contains basophilic material resulting in the appearance of blue stippling in the erythrocyte. The effect can be a sign of lead poisoning.

basophilic leukemia [Gk, *basis* + *philein,* to love, *leukos* white, *haima*, blood], an acute or chronic malignant neoplasm of blood-forming tissues, characterized by large numbers of immature basophilic granulocytes in peripheral circulation and in tissues. See also **acute myelocytic leukemia.**

basophilic stippling [Gk, *basis* + *philein*, to love; D, *stippen* to prick], the presence of punctate, blue nucleic acid remnants in red blood cells, observed under the microscope on a Wright-Giemsa-Gram-stained blood smear. Stippling is characteristic of lead poisoning. See also **basophil, lead poisoning.**

basosquamous cell carcinoma /bā′sōskwā′məs/ [Gk, *basis* + L, *squamosus*, scaly], a malignant epidermal tumor composed of basal and squamous cells.

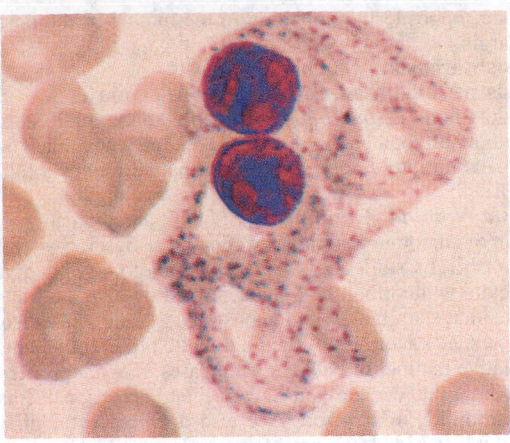

Basophilic stippling (Hayhoe, 1992)

Bassen-Kornzweig syndrome. See **abetalipoproteine-mia.**

batch processing [ME, *baten,* to bake], a processing mode used with computers in which accumulated batches of similar data are processed simultaneously.

bath [AS, *baeth*], (in the hospital) a cleansing procedure performed daily by or for patients to help prevent infection, preserve the unbroken condition of the skin, stimulate circulation, promote oxygen intake, maintain muscle tone and joint mobility, and provide comfort.

■ METHOD: The bath may be a bed or tub bath, a shower, or a partial bath, depending on the patient's condition and preference and the room temperature. The bath period may be used to instruct the patient on hygienic measures. Observations are made of the general cleanliness and odor of the patient's body, the color, dryness, turgor, and elasticity of the skin, the condition of the hair, hands, feet, fingernails, and toenails. Any discoloration, abrasion, rash, discharge, perineal or rectal irritation, clubbing of the digits, hair loss, or evidence of lice is carefully noted. Mild soap and water are used for the bath, and a lanolin-based lotion is used for the afterbath massage. The patient's hair is combed daily and shampooed as desired; fingernails and toenails are cleaned and trimmed whenever required. Petroleum jelly or other suitable lubricant and a thin layer of cornstarch are applied to the perineal and perianal areas if indicated.

■ NURSING INTERVENTION: The nurse gives the bed bath in a setting that provides privacy for the patient. Firm, gentle strokes are used to wash, dry, and massage the person; vigorous rubbing is avoided. The partial bath is given with the patient seated in or on the side of the bed or in a chair. Self-help is encouraged, and the procedure is completed as soon as possible to avoid chilling. In preparation for a tub bath, the nurse checks the safety strips in the bottom of the tub and the temperature of the water and assists the patient into the tub. Precautions are taken to avoid chilling, and on completion of the bath the nurse may help the patient out of the tub. In preparation for a shower, the nurse explains the operation of the dials regulating the water temperature, provides a bath mat, and cautions the patient not to become chilled.

■ OUTCOME CRITERIA: A daily bath helps prevent decubiti, provides an opportunity to assess external signs of disease and effects of therapy, and improves the patient's sense of well-being and self-esteem.

bath blanket, a thin, lightweight blanket used to cover a patient during a bath. It absorbs moisture while keeping the patient warm. See also **blanket bath.**

bathesthesia /bath′əsthē′zhə/ [Gk, *bathys,* deep, *anaisthesia,* loss of feeling], a loss of deep feeling, such as that associated with organs or structures beneath the surface of the body, or muscles and joints. Also called **bathyesthesia** /bath′ē·əsthē′zhə/.

bathmic evolution. See **orthogenic evolution.**

bathy-, batho-, a prefix meaning 'pertaining to depth, deep': *bathycentesis, bathypnea, bathomorphic.*

bathyesthesia. See **bathesthesia.**

Batten's disease [Frederick E. Batten, English neurologist, b. 1865], a progressive childhood encephalopathy with disturbed metabolism of polyunsaturated fatty acids.

battered baby. See **child abuse.**

battered woman syndrome (BWS), repeated episodes of physical assault on a woman by the man with whom she lives, often resulting in serious physical and psychologic damage to the woman. Such violence tends to follow a predictable pattern. The violent episodes usually follow verbal argument and accusation and are accompanied by verbal abuse. Almost any subject—housekeeping, money, childrearing—may begin the episode. Over time, the violent episodes escalate in frequency and severity. Once a month becomes once a week; a shove becomes a punch. Most battered women report that they thought that the assaults would stop; but, unfortunately, study shows that the longer the women stay in the relationship the more likely they are to be seriously injured. Less and less provocation seems to be enough to trigger an attack once the syndrome has begun. The use of alcohol increases the severity of the assault; a man who usually shoves or slaps his partner is more likely to punch or kick her if he is drunk. Other drugs do not have this effect. The man is more likely to be abusive as the drug is wearing off. Battering occurs in cycles of violence. The first phase is characterized by the man acting increasingly irritable, edgy, and tense. Verbal abuse, insults, and criticism increase, and shoves or slaps begin. The second phase is the time of the acute, violent activity. As the tension mounts, the woman becomes unable to placate the man, and she may argue or defend herself. The man uses this as the justification for his anger and assaults her, often saying that he is "teaching her a lesson." The third stage is characterized by apology and remorse on the part of the man, with promises of change. The calm continues until tension builds again. The battered woman syndrome occurs at all socioeconomic levels, and one half to three quarters of female assault victims are the victims of an attack by a lover or husband. It is estimated that in the United States between 1 and 2 million women a year are beaten by their husbands. Men who grew up in homes in which the father abused the mother are more likely to beat their wives than are men who lived in nonviolent homes. Personal and cultural attitudes also affect the incidence of wife battering. Aggressive behavior is a normal part of male socialization in most cultures; physical aggression may be condoned as a means of resolving a conflict. A personality profile obtained by psychologic testing reveals the typical battered woman to be reserved, withdrawn, depressed, and anxious, with low self-esteem, a poorly integrated self-image, and a general inability to cope with life's demands. The parents of such women encouraged compliance, were not physically affectionate, and socially restricted their daughters' independence, preventing the widening of social contact that normally occurs in adolescence. Victims of the battered woman syndrome are often afraid to leave the man and the situation; change, loneliness, and the unknown are perceived as more painful than the beatings. Nurses are in an excellent position to offer assistance to battered women in several ways, because encouraging a woman to talk about the battering and the injuries may help her to admit what she may have been too embarrassed to reveal even to her parents. A realistic appraisal of the situation is then possible; the woman wants to hear that the nurse thinks the battering will not recur, but the nurse can tell her only that the usual pattern is for the abuse to continue and to become more severe. The woman may be referred to the social service department or given directions for contacting special community agencies, such as a battered women's shelter or a hotline to a counseling service. Caring for and counseling a battered woman often require great patience because she is usually ambivalent about her situation and may be confused to the point of believing that she deserves the assaults she has suffered. Records are maintained to document the extent of the problem, including the form of abuse reported, the injuries sustained, and a summary of similar incidents and previous admissions.

battery [Fr, *batterie*], **1.** a complex of two or more electrolytic cells connected together to form a single source providing direct current or voltage. **2.** a series or a combination of tests to determine the cause of a particular illness or the degree of proficiency in a particular skill or discipline. **3.** the unlawful use of force on a person. See **assault.**

Battey bacillus /bat′ē/ [Battey Hospital, in Rome, Georgia, where bacteria strain first isolated], any of a group of atypical mycobacteria, including *Mycobacteria aviu* and *M. intracellulare,* that cause a chronic pulmonary disease resembling tuberculosis. These organisms are resistant to most of the common bacteriostatic and antibiotic medications but may be treated with multiple drug regimens. Surgical resection of involved lung tissue may be necessary and may improve the outcome in serious cases. Rest, good nutrition, and general supportive care are usually recommended. Compare **tuberculosis.**

battledore placenta /bat′əldôr′/ [ME, *batyldoure,* a beating instrument; L, flat cake], a placenta to which the umbilical cord is attached at the periphery. It rarely occurs and does not affect placental functioning.

Battle's sign [William H. Battle, English surgeon, b. 1855], a small hemorrhagic spot behind the ear that appears in cases may indicate a fracture of a bone of the lower skull.

batyl alcohol /bat″əl/ an alcohol found in fish liver oil that is used to treat bracken poisoning in cattle.

baud /bôd/ [J.M.E. Baudot, French inventor, b. 1845], binary units or bits per second, used as a measure of data flow or the speed with which a computer device transmits information.

Baudelocque's diameter. See **external conjugate.**

Baudelocque's method /bô′dəlok′s/ [Jean L. Baudelocque, French obstetrician, b. 1746], (in obstetrics) a maneuver used to convert a face presentation to a vertex presentation. The operator flexes the fetal head vaginally and applies counterpressure to the back of the head abdominally while an assistant rotates the fetus in the direction of flexion until the vertex is fixed in the pelvis.

Bayley Scales of Infant Development, a three-part scale

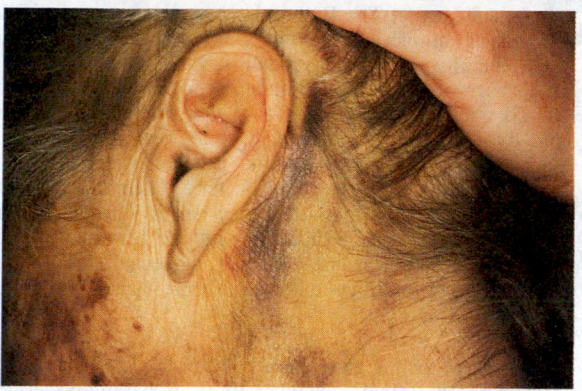

Battle's sign *(Bingham, 1992)*

for assessing the development of children between the ages of 2 months and 2½ years. Infants are tested for perception, memory, and vocalization on the mental scale; sitting, stairclimbing, and manual manipulation on the motor scale; and attention span, social behavior, and persistence on the behavioral scale.

Baynton's bandage /bān′tənz/ [Thomas Baynton, English surgeon, b. 1761], a spiral adhesive wrap applied to the leg over a dressing, used in the treatment of indolent ulcers of the leg.

bayonet angle former /bā′ənit/ [Fr, *baionette,* a steel blade], a hoe-shaped paired cutting instrument for accenting angles in a Class 3 tooth cavity. The cutting edge of this device is at an angle to the axis of the blade that is parallel to the axis of the shaft. Also called **angle former.**

bayonet condenser [Fr, *baionette*], (in dentistry) an instrument for compacting restorative material. It has an offset nib device and a shank with right angle bends for varying the line of force, used primarily in condensing direct filling gold. There are many variations in angles, length, and nib diameter.

BBB, 1. abbreviation for **blood-brain barrier.** 2. abbreviation for **bundle branch block.**

B cell, a type of lymphocyte that originates in the bone marrow. A precursor of the plasma cell, it is one of the two lymphocytes that play a major role in the body's immune response. Compare **T cell.** See also **plasma cell.**

BCG, abbreviation for **bacille Calmette-Guérin.**

BCG vaccine, an active immunizing agent prepared from bacille Calmette-Guérin.

■ INDICATION: It is prescribed most commonly for immunization against tuberculosis.

■ CONTRAINDICATIONS: Hypogammaglobulinemia, immunosuppression, or concomitant use of corticosteroids or isoniazid prohibits its use. It is not given after a vaccination for smallpox, nor is it given to patients with a positive tuberculin reaction or a burn.

■ ADVERSE EFFECTS: Among the most serious adverse reactions are anaphylaxis and disseminated pulmonary tuberculosis. Pain, inflammation, and granuloma may develop at site of injection.

BCNU. See **carmustine.**

B complex vitamins, a large group of water-soluble substances that includes **vitamin B$_1$** (thiamine), **vitamin B$_{12}$** (cyanocobalamin), **biotin, folic acid, vitamin B$_3$** (niacin), **B$_6$** (pyridoxal, pyridoxine, pyridoxamine, riboflavin, and pantothenic acid.) The B complex vitamins are essential in converting simple carbohydrates like glucose into energy, for metabolism of fats and proteins, for normal functioning of the nervous system, for maintenance of muscle tone in the GI tract, and for the health of skin, hair, eyes, mouth, and liver. They are found in brewer's yeast, liver, whole grain cereals, nuts, eggs, meats, fish, and vegetables and are produced by the intestinal bacteria. Maintaining milk-free diets or taking antibiotics may destroy these bacteria. Symptoms of vitamin B deficiency include nervousness, depression, insomnia, neuritis, anemia, alopecia, acne or other skin disorders, and hypercholesterolemia. See also specific vitamins.

b.d. See **b.i.d.**

Be, symbol for the element **beryllium.**

beaded /bē′did/ [ME, *bede*], **1.** of or having a resemblance to a row of beads. **2.** of or pertaining to bacterial colonies that develop along the inoculation line in various stab cultures. **3.** of or pertaining to stained bacteria that develop more deeply stained beadlike granules.

beaker cell. See **goblet cell.**

beam [ME, *beem*, tree], **1.** a bedframe fitting for pulleys and weights, used in the treatment of patients requiring weight traction. See **Balkan frame.** **2.** in radiology, the primary beam of radiation emitted from the x-ray tube.

BEAM /bēm, bē′ē′ā′em′/, abbreviation for **brain electric activity map.**

beam alignment, the process of locating the radiographic tube head so it is aligned properly with the x-ray film.

beam collimation, the restriction of x-radiation to only the area being examined or treated by confining the beam with collimators or metal diaphragms or shutters with high radiation absorption power. In addition to protecting the patient and others from scatter radiation, beam collimation reduces fogging of the film.

beam hardening, the process of increasing the energy level of the x-ray beam spectrum by filtering out the low-energy photons.

BE amputation, an amputation of the arm below the elbow.

beam quality, (in radiology) the energy of the x-ray beam.

beam restrictors, devices that reduce scatter radiation from x-ray equipment. Three basic types of restrictors are variable-aperture collimators, cones or cylinders, and aperture diaphragms.

beam-splitting mirror, a device that allows a radiologist to view a fluoroscopic examination of a patient while the same view is being recorded on film. The mirror can be adjusted to reflect from 10% to 90% of the x-ray beam to the cathode-ray screen while the rest is directed to the film in the camera.

bean [ME *bene*], the pod-enclosed flattened seed of numerous leguminous plants. Beans used in pharmacologic preparations are alphabetized by specific name.

bearing down /ber′ing/ [OE, *beran*, to bear, *adune*, down], a voluntary effort by a woman in in the second stage of labor to aid in the expulsion of a fetus. By applying the Valsalva maneuver, the mother increases intra-abdominal pressure.

bearing down pains [OE, *beran*, to bear, *adune*, down; L, *poena*, penalty], the pains experienced by a woman during the second stage of labor while performing the Valsava maneuver to help expel the fetus.

beat, the contraction of the heart muscle, which may be detected and recorded as the pulse.

Beck depression inventory (BDI). See **Beck's Diagnostic Inventory (BDI).**

Becker's muscular dystrophy, a chronic degenerative disease of the muscles, characterized by progressive weakness. It occurs in childhood between 8 and 20 years of age. It occurs less frequently, progresses more slowly, and has a better prognosis than the more common pseudohypertrophic form of muscular dystrophy. The pathophysiology of the disease is not understood; it is transmitted genetically as an autosomal recessive trait. Also called **benign pseudohypertrophic muscular dystrophy.** Compare **Duchenne's muscular dystrophy.**

Beck operation, [Claude S. Beck, American surgeon, b. 1894] a now obsolete surgical procedure to provide collateral circulation to the heart.

Beck's Diagnostic Inventory (BDI), a system of classifying a total of 18 criteria of depressive illness. It was developed by A.T. Beck in the 1970s as a diagnostic and therapeutic tool for the treatment of childhood affective disorders. The BDI is similar to the 21-criteria DSM-III diagnostic system of the 1980s except that the DSM-III scale includes loss of interest, restlessness, and sulkiness, which are missing from the BDI, while the Beck inventory lists somatic complaints and loneliness, which are criteria not included in the DSM-III inventory. Also called **Beck depression inventory (BDI).** See also **DSM.**

Beck's triad, a combination of three symptoms that characterize cardiac tamponade: high venous pressure, low arterial pressure, and a small, quiet heart.

Beckwith's syndrome [John B. Beckwith, American pathologist, b. 1933], an hereditary disorder of unknown cause associated with neonatal hypoglycemia and hyperinsulinism. Clinical manifestations include gigantism, macroglossia, omphalocele or umbilical hernia, visceromegaly, hyperplasia of the kidney and pancreas, extreme enlargement of the cells of the adrenal cortex, and often various other abnormalities. Treatment consists of adequate glucose, diazoxide, and glucocorticoid therapy. Subtotal pancreatectomy is often necessary in cases of beta cell hyperplasia, nesidioblastosis, or beta cell tumor of the pancreas.

Beckwith-Wiedemann syndrome. See **EMG syndrome.**

beclomethasone dipropionate, a glucocorticoid.

■ INDICATION: It is prescribed in an inhaler in the treatment of bronchial asthma.

■ CONTRAINDICATIONS: Status asthmaticus, acute asthma, or known hypersensitivity to this drug prohibits its use.

■ ADVERSE EFFECTS: Among the more serious adverse reactions of systemic administration are the symptoms of adrenal insufficiency. Hoarseness, sore throat, and fungal infections of the oropharynx and larynx may occur.

becquerel (Bq) /bekrel′, bek′ərel′/ [Antoine H. Becquerel, French physicist, b. 1852], the SI unit of radioactivity, equal to one radioactive decay per second. See **curie.**

bed [AS *bedd*], (in anatomy) a supporting matrix of tissue, such as the nail beds of modified epidermis over which the fingernails and the toenails move as they grow.

bedbug [AS, *bedd* + ME *bugge*, hobgoblin], a blood-sucking arthropod of the species *Cimex lectularius* or the species *C. hemipterus* that feeds on humans and other animals. The bedbug can be removed after covering it with petrolatum. The bite, which causes itching, pain, and redness, can be treated with a lotion or cream containing a corticosteroid or other topical antiinflammatory or analgesic preparation.

Bedford finger stall, a removable finger splint that holds the injured finger in a brace or cast along with the adjacent finger. It can be worn for prolonged periods of time.

Bednar's aphthae /bed′närz/ [Alois Bednar, Austrian pediatrician, b. 1816], the small, yellowish, slightly elevated ulcerated patches that occur on the posterior portion of the hard palate of infants who place infected objects in their mouths. It is also associated with marasmus. Compare **Epstein's pearls, thrush.**

bed pan, a vessel, usually made of metal, used to collect feces and urine of bedridden patients.

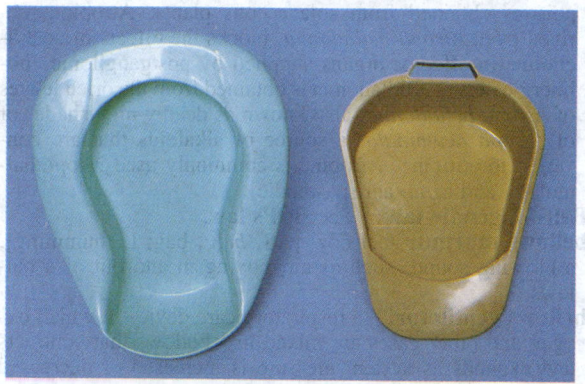

Bed pans: fracture and regular *(Potter, 1993)*

bed rest, the restriction of a patient to bed for therapeutic reasons for a prescribed period.

bedside manner, the behavior of a nurse or doctor as perceived by a patient.

bedside thermometer. See **clinical thermometer.**

bedsore. See **decubitus ulcer.**

bedwetting. See **enuresis.**

Bee cell pessary. See **pessary.**

beef tapeworm. See *Taenia saginata.*

beef tapeworm infection [OF, *buef,* cow; AS, *taeppe, wyrm*], an infection caused by the tapeworm *Taenia saginata,* transmitted to humans when they eat contaminated beef. The adult worm can live for years in the intestine of humans without causing any symptoms. The infection is rarely found in North America and Western Europe, where beef is carefully inspected before being made available and is often thoroughly cooked before eating, but it is commonly found in other parts of the world. See **tapeworm infection.**

bee sting [AS, *beo, stingan*], an injury caused by the venom of bees, usually accompanied by pain and swelling. The stinger of the honeybee usually remains implanted and should be removed. Pain may be alleviated by application of an ice pack or a paste of sodium bicarbonate and water. Serious reactions may result from multiple stings, stings on some areas of the head, or the injection of venom directly into the circulatory system. In a hypersensitive person, a single bee sting may result in death because of anaphylactic shock and bronchospasm. Hypersensitive individuals are encouraged to carry emergency treatment supplies with them when the possibility of bee sting exists. Compare **wasp.**

behavior /bihā′vyər/ [ME, *behaven*], **1.** the manner in which a person acts or performs. **2.** any or all of the activities of a person, including physical actions, which are observed directly, and mental activity, which is inferred and interpreted. Kinds of behavior include **abnormal behavior, automatic behavior, invariable behavior,** and **variable behavior.**

behavioral isolation /behā′vyərəl/, social isolation that occurs because of a person's socially unacceptable behavior.

behavioral objective, a goal in therapy or research that concerns an act or a specific behavior or pattern of behaviors.

behavioral science, any of the various interrelated disciplines, such as psychiatry, psychology, sociology, and anthropology, that observes and studies human activity, including psychologic and emotional development, interpersonal relationships, values, and mores.

behavior disorder, any of a group of antisocial behavior patterns occurring primarily in children and adolescents, such as overaggressiveness, overactivity, destructiveness, cruelty, truancy, lying, disobedience, perverse sexual activity, criminality, alcoholism, and drug addiction. Treatment may include psychotherapy, milieu therapy, medication, and family counseling. See also **antisocial personality disorder.**

behaviorism, a school of psychology founded by John B. Watson that studies and interprets behavior by observing measurable responses to stimuli without reference to consciousness, mental states, or subjective phenomena, such as ideas and emotions. See also **neobehaviorism.**

behaviorist, a disciple of the school of behaviorism.

behavioristic psychology. See **behaviorism.**

behavior modification. See **behavior therapy.**

behavior reflex. See **conditioned response.**

behavior systems model, a conceptual framework describing factors that may affect the stability of a person's behavior. The model examines systems of behavior, not the behavior of an individual at any particular time. In one model, behavior is defined as an integrated response to stimuli. Several subsystems of behavior form the eight human microsystems, which are: ingestion, elimination, dependency, sex, achievement, affiliation, aggression, and restoration. Each subsystem comprises several structural components called 'imperatives,' which are goal, set, choice, action, and support. The goal of nursing care is to attain, maintain, or restore balance of the subsystems of behavior for the stability of the patient.

behavior therapy, a kind of psychotherapy that attempts to modify observable, maladjusted patterns of behavior by the substitution of a new response or set of responses to a given stimulus. The treatment techniques involve the methods, concepts, and procedures derived from experimental psychology and include assertiveness training, aversion therapy, contingency management, flooding, modeling, operant conditioning, and systemic desensitization. Also called **behavior modification.** See also **biofeedback.**

Behçet's disease /bā′sets/ [Hulusi Behçet, Turkish dermatologist, b. 1889], a rare and severe illness of unknown cause, mostly affecting young males and characterized by severe uveitis and retinal vasculitis. Some other signs are optic atrophy and aphthous lesions of the mouth and the gen-

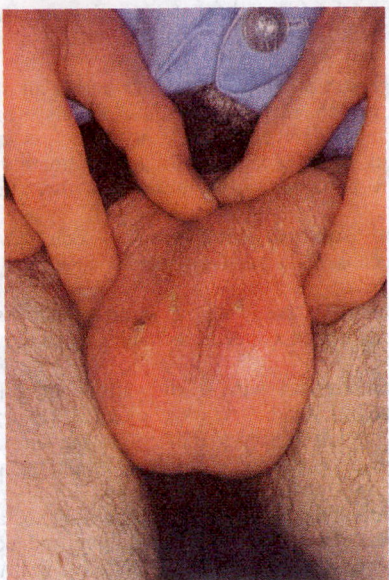

Behcet's disease (Shipley, 1993)

itals, indicating diffuse vasculitis. Also called **Behçet's syndrome.**

Behla's bodies. See **Plimmer's bodies.**

BEI, abbreviation for **butanol-extractable iodine.**

BEIR-III Report, a report, *The Biological Effects of Low Doses of Ionizing Radiation*, by the National Academy of Sciences; it estimates the risk of cancer deaths from exposure to radiation at various dose levels.

bejel /bej′əl/ [Ar, *bajal*], a nonvenereal form of syphilis prevalent among children in the Middle East and North Africa, caused by the spirochete *Treponema pallidum II*. It is transmitted by person-to-person contact and by the sharing of drinking and eating utensils. The primary lesion is usually on or near the mouth, appearing as a mucous patch, followed by the development of pimplelike sores on the trunk, arms, and legs. Chronic ulceration of the nose and soft palate occurs in the advanced stages of the infection. Destructive changes in the tissues of the heart, central nervous system, and mouth, often associated with the venereal form of syphilis, rarely develop. Intramuscular injection of penicillin is effective in curing the infection, but if extensive tissue destruction has occurred, scar tissue forms and may be permanently disfiguring.

Békésy audiometry /bek′əsē/ [George von Békésy, Hungarian-American physicist, b. 1899], a type of hearing test in which the subject controls the intensity of the stimulus by pressing a button while listening to a pure tone whose frequency slowly moves through the entire audible range. The intensity diminishes as long as the button is pressed. When the intensity is too low for the subject to hear the tone, the button is released and the intensity begins to increase. When the subject again hears the tone, the button is again pressed, yielding a zig-zag tracing. Continuous and interrupted tones are used, and the tracings of the two are compared. The test may be used to differentiate between hearing losses of cochlear and neural origins.

bel [Alexander G. Bell, Canadian inventor, b. 1847], a unit that expresses intensity of sound. It is the logarithm (to the

base 10) of the ratio of the power of any specific sound to the power of a reference sound. The most common reference sound has a power of 10^{-16} watts per cm^2, or the approximate minimum intensity of sound at 1000 cycles per second that is perceptible to the human ear. An increase of 1 bel approximately doubles the intensity or loudness of most sounds.

belching. See **eructation.**

belladonna /bel′ədon′ə, belädôn′ä/ [It, fair lady], the dried leaves, roots, and flowering or fruiting tops of *Atropa belladonna*, a common perennial called deadly nightshade, containing the alkaloids hyoscine and hyoscyamine. Hyoscyamine is a source of atropine with anticholinergic properties.

belladonna and atropine poisons [It, *belladonna*, fair lady; Gk, *Atropos*, fate; L, *potio*, drink], two powerful poisons obtained from solanaceous plants. Atropine, derived from *Atropa belladonna*, blocks the effects of acetylcholine in effector organs supplied by postganglionic cholinergic nerves. Belladonna is obtained from the dried leaves of *Atropa belladonna*, also known as deadly nightshade, or of *Atropa acuminata*, a source of alkaloids that are converted to atropine. Atropine is commonly used in ophthalmology and as an antispasmodic.

Bell-Magendie law. See **Bell's law.**

bellows murmur /bel′ōōz/ [AS, *belg*, bag; L, humming], a blowing sound, such as air moving in and out of a bellows.

bellows ventilator, a respiratory care device in which oxygen and other gases are mixed in a bellows that contracts and expands as system pressure is increased or decreased in the chamber surrounding the bellows. As system pressure pushes the bellows upward, the gases in the bellows are moved into the patient circuit. As the patient exhales, the bellows falls and fills again with gases from air and oxygen intakes.

Bell's law [Charles Bell, Scottish surgeon, b. 1774], an axiom stating that the ventral spinal roots are motor and the dorsal spinal roots are sensory. Also called **Bell-Magendie law, Magendie's law.**

Bell's mania [Luther V. Bell, American physician, b. 1806], *obsolete*. a mood disorder characterized by acute delirium. See also **delirium, mania.**

Bell's palsy [Charles Bell, Scottish surgeon, b. 1774], a paralysis of the facial nerve, resulting from trauma to the nerve, compression of the nerve by a tumor, or, possibly, an unknown infection. Any or all branches of the nerve may be affected. The person may not be able to close an eye or control salivation on the affected side. The condition is usually unilateral and can be transient or permanent.

Bell's phenomenon, a sign of peripheral facial paralysis, manifested by the upward and outward rolling of the eyeball when the affected individual tries to close the eyelid.

belly. See **abdomen.**

belly button. See **umbilicus.**

belonephobia /bel′ənəfō′bē·ə/ [Gk, *belone*, needle, *phobos*, fear], a morbid fear of sharp-pointed objects, especially needles and pins.

belt restraint, a device used to secure a patient on a stretcher or in a chair.

Benadryl, a trademark for an antihistaminic (diphenhydramine hydrochloride).

Benassi method /bənas′ē/, a positioning procedure for producing x-ray images of the liver. With the patient in a

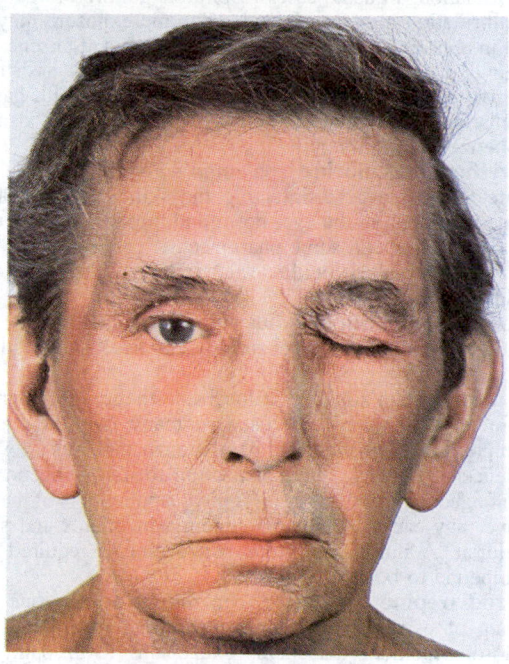

Bell's palsy *(Perkin, 1986)*

prone position so that the liver is closer to the x-ray film, two radiographs are made from the angles of 25 degrees caudad and 10 degrees cephalad.

Bence Jones protein /bens/ [Henry Bence Jones, English physician, b. 1813], a protein found almost exclusively in the urine of patients with multiple myeloma. The protein constitutes the light chain component of myeloma globulin; it coagulates at temperatures of 45° to 55° C and redissolves completely or partially on boiling. See also **multiple myeloma, protein.**

bench research *informal.* (in medicine) any research done in a controlled laboratory setting using other than human subjects.

-bendazole /ben'dəzōl/ a combining form designating a tibendazole-type anthelmintic.

Bender's Visual Motor Gestalt test [Lauretta Bender, American psychiatrist, b. 1897; L, *visus,* vision, *movere,* to move; Ger, *Gestalt,* form; L, *testum,* crucible], a standard psychological test in which the subject copies a series of patterns.

bending fracture, a fracture indirectly caused by the bending of an extremity, such as the foot or the big toe.

bendrofluazide. See **bendroflumethiazide.**

bendroflumethiazide /ben'drōflōō'məthī'əzīd/, a diuretic and antihypertensive.

■ INDICATIONS: It is prescribed in the treatment of hypertension and edema.

■ CONTRAINDICATIONS: Anuria or known hypersensitivity to this drug, to other thiazide medication, or to sulfonamide derivatives prohibit its use.

■ ADVERSE EFFECTS: Among the more serious adverse reactions are hypokalemia, hyperglycemia, hyperuricemia, and various hypersensitivity reactions.

bends. See **decompression sickness.**

Benedict's qualitative test [Stanley R. Benedict, American biochemist, b. 1884], a test for sugar in the urine based on the reduction by glucose of cupric ions. Formation of an orange or red precipitate indicates more than 2% sugar (called 4+), yellow indicates 1% to 2% sugar (called 3+), olive green indicates 0.5% to 1% sugar (called 2+), and green indicates less than 0.5% sugar (called 1+). Also called **Benedict's method.**

Benemid, a trademark for a uricosuric (probenecid).

benign /binīn'/ [L *benignus,* well], (of a tumor) noncancerous and therefore not an immediate threat, even though treatment eventually may be required for health or cosmetic reasons. See **benign neoplasm.** Compare **malignant.**

benign familial chronic pemphigus [L, *benedicere,* to bless, *familia,* household; Gk, *pemphix,* bubble], a hereditary condition of the skin characterized in the early stages by blisters which break, leaving red, eroded areas followed by crusts. Also called **Hailey-Hailey disease.**

benign hypertension, a misnomer implying an innocent elevation of blood pressure. Because any sustained elevation of blood pressure may adversely affect health, it is incorrect to refer to the condition as "benign." See also **essential hypertension.**

benign intracranial hypertension. See **pseudotumor cerebri.**

benign juvenile melanoma, a benign, pink or fuchsia raised papule with a scaly surface, usually on a cheek. Occurring most commonly in children between 9 and 13 years of age, it may be mistaken for a malignant melanoma. Also called **compound melanocytoma, spindle cell nevus, Spitz nevus.**

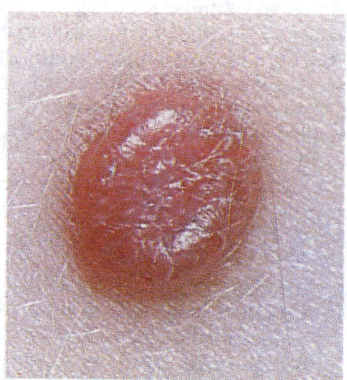

Benign juvenile melanoma *(Zitelli, 1992)*

benign lymphocytic meningitis. See **sterile meningitis.**

benign lymphoreticulosis. See **cat scratch fever.**

benign mesenchymoma [L, *benignare* + Gk, *meso,* middle, *egchyma,* infusion, *oma,* tumor], a benign neoplasm that has two or more definitely recognizable mesenchymal elements in addition to fibrous tissue.

benign myalgic encephalomyelitis. See **postviral fatigue syndrome.**

benign neoplasm [L, *benignare* +Gk, *neos,* new, *plasma,* formation], a localized tumor that has a fibrous capsule, limited potential for growth, a regular shape, and cells that are well differentiated. A benign neoplasm does not invade surrounding tissue or metastasize to distant sites. Some kinds of benign neoplasms are **adenoma, fibroma, hemangioma,** *and* **lipoma.** See also **malignant neoplasm.**

benign nephrosclerosis, a renal disorder marked by arteriolosclerotic lesions in the kidney. It is associated with hypertension.

benign prostatic hypertrophy, enlargement of the prostate gland, common among men after the age of 50. The condition is not malignant or inflammatory but is usually progressive and may lead to obstruction of the urethra and to interference with the flow of urine, possibly causing frequency of urination, the need to urinate during the night, pain, and urinary tract infections. Treatment may consist of nonsurgical measures, such as localized application of heat, medication, and balloon dilatation. Surgical resection of the enlarged prostate is sometimes necessary. Compare *prostatitis.* See also *prostatectomy.*

benign pseudohypertrophic muscular dystrophy. See **Becker's muscular dystrophy.**

benign stupor, a state of apathy or lethargy, such as occurs in severe depression.

benign thrombocytosis. See **thrombocytosis.**

benign tumor [L, *benignare,* to bless; L, swelling], a neoplasm that does not invade other tissues or metastasize to other sites. A benign tumor is usually encapsulated, and its cells exhibit less anaplasia than those of a malignant growth.

Bennet's small corpuscle. See **Drysdale's corpuscle.**

Bennett angle [Norman G. Bennett, English dentist, b. 1870], (in dentistry) the angle formed by the sagittal plane and the path of the advancing condyle during lateral mandibular movement, as viewed in the horizontal plane.

Bennett hand tool test, a test used in occupational therapy and prevocational testing to measure hand function and coordination and speed in performance.

Bennett's fracture [Edward H. Bennett, Irish surgeon, b. 1837], a fracture that runs obliquely through the base of the first metacarpal bone and into the carpometacarpal joint, detaching the greater part of the articular facet. Bennett's fracture may be associated with dorsal subluxation or with dislocation of the first metacarpal.

Benoquin, a trademark for a depigmenting agent (monobenzone).

bent fracture [ME, *benden*], an incomplete greenstick fracture.

bentonite [Fort Benton, Montana], colloidal, hydrated aluminum silicate, that, when added to water, swells to approximately 12 times its dry size. It is used as a bulk laxative and as a base for skin care preparations. Also called **mineral soap.**

bentonite test, a flocculation test for the presence of rheumatoid factor in patient blood samples. After sensitized bentonite particles are added to the serum, the test is considered positive for rheumatoid arthritis if adsorption has occurred with 50% of the particles.

Bentyl, a trademark for an anticholinergic antispasmodic (dicyclomine hydrochloride).

benz, abbreviation for a *benzoate carboxylate anion.*

benzalkonium chloride, a disinfectant and fungicide prepared in an aqueous solution in various strengths.

benzathine penicillin G. See **penicillin G benzathine.**

benzene poisoning /ben′zēn/, a toxic condition caused by ingestion of benzene, the inhalation of benzene fumes, or exposure to benzene-related products such as toluene or xylene, characterized by nausea, headache, dizziness, and in-

coordination. In acute cases respiratory failure or ventricular fibrillation may cause death. Chronic exposure may result in aplastic anemia or a form of leukemia. Benzene poisoning by inhalation is treated with ventilatory assistance and oxygen; poisoning by ingestion is treated with gastric intubation, removal of the poison, and lavage. See also **nitrobenzene poisoning.**

benzethonium chloride /ben′zəthō′nē·əm/, a topical antiinfective used for disinfecting the skin and for treating some infections of the eye, nose, and throat. It is also used as a preservative in some pharmaceutic preparations.

benzhexol hydrochloride. See **trihexyphenidyl hydrochloride.**

benzo(a)pyrene dihydrodiol epoxide (BPDE-I), a carcinogenic derivative of benzo(a)pyrene associated with tobacco smoke.

benzocaine /ben′zəkān/, a local anesthetic agent derived from aminobenzoic acid, used in many over-the-counter compounds for pruritus and pain. Benzocaine has a low incidence of toxicity, but sensitization to it may occur with prolonged or frequent use. Topical application of benzocaine may cause methemoglobinemia in infants and small children. A minimum of 5% benzocaine is required in a compound to be effective.

benzodiazepine derivative /ben′zōdī·az′əpin/, one of a group of psychotropic agents, including the tranquilizers chlordiazepoxide, diazepam, oxazepam, lovazepam, and chlorazepate, prescribed to alleviate anxiety, and the hypnotics flurazepam and nitrazepam, prescribed in the treatment of insomnia. Some of the drugs have further clinical application: Diazepam is often prescribed to relieve spasm of the muscles and to increase the seizure threshold. Tolerance and physical dependence occur with prolonged high dosage. Withdrawal symptoms, including seizures and acute psychosis, may follow abrupt discontinuation. Adverse reactions to the benzodiazepines include drowsiness, ataxia, and a paradoxical increase in aggression and hostility; these reactions are not commonly seen in association with the usual recommended dosage.

benzoic acid /benzō′ik/, a keratolytic agent, usually used with salicylic acid as an ointment in the treatment of athlete's foot and ringworm of the scalp. It has little antifungal action but makes deep infections accessible to more potent preparation. Mild irritation may occur at the site of application.

benzonatate /benzō′nətāt/, a nonopiate antitussive.
- INDICATION: It is prescribed to suppress the cough reflex.
- CONTRAINDICATION: Known hypersensitivity to this drug prohibits its use.
- ADVERSE EFFECTS: A serious reaction may be convulsions. Vertigo, headache, constipation, and hypersensitivity reactions, usually mild, sometimes occur.

benzoyl peroxide /benzō′il/, an antibacterial, keratolytic, drying agent.
- INDICATION: It is prescribed in the treatment of acne.
- CONTRAINDICATIONS: Known hypersensitivity to this drug prohibits its use. It is not used in the eye, on inflamed skin, or on mucous membranes.
- ADVERSE EFFECTS: Among the more serious adverse reactions are excessive drying and allergic contact sensitization.

benzphetamine hydrochloride /benzfet′əmēn/, a sympathomimetic used as an anorexic agent.
- INDICATIONS: It is prescribed to decrease the appetite in the treatment of obesity.

- CONTRAINDICATIONS: Arteriosclerosis, cardiovascular disease, hypertension, glaucoma, hyperthyroidism, or known hypersensitivity to this or other sympathomimetic drugs prohibits its use.
- ADVERSE EFFECTS: Among the more serious adverse reactions are restlessness, insomnia, tachycardia, increased blood pressure, and dry mouth.

benzquinamide /benzkwin′əmīd/, an antiemetic.
- INDICATIONS: It is prescribed in the treatment of postoperative nausea and vomiting.
- CONTRAINDICATIONS: Severe hypertension, severe cardiovascular disease, or known hypersensitivity to this drug prohibits its use. It is not usually administered to children or to pregnant women.
- ADVERSE EFFECTS: Among the most serious adverse reactions are sudden increase in blood pressure and cardiac arrhythmia. Drowsiness, chills, and shivering are commonly noted.

benzthiazide /benzthī′əzid/, a diuretic and antihypertensive.
- INDICATIONS: It is prescribed in the treatment of hypertension and edema.
- CONTRAINDICATIONS: Anuria or known hypersensitivity to this drug, to other thiazide medication, or to sulfonamide derivatives prohibits its use.
- ADVERSE EFFECTS: Among the more serious adverse effects are hypokalemia, hyperglycemia, hyperuricemia, and hypersensitivity reactions.

benztropine mesylate /benztrō′pēn/, an anticholinergic and antihistaminic agent.
- INDICATIONS: It is prescribed as adjunctive therapy in the treatment of all forms of parkinsonism.
- CONTRAINDICATIONS: Known sensitivity to this drug prohibits its use, and it is not administered to children under 3 years of age.
- ADVERSE EFFECTS: Among the most serious adverse reactions are blurred vision, xerostoma, nausea and vomiting, constipation, depression, and skin rash.

benzyl alcohol /ben′zil/, a clear, colorless, oily liquid, derived from certain balsams, used as a topical anesthetic and as a bacteriostatic agent in solutions for injection. Also called **phenyl carbinol, phenyl methanol.**

benzyl benzoate /benzō′āt/, a clear, oily liquid with a pleasant, aromatic odor. It is used as an agent to destroy lice and scabies, as a solvent, and as a flavor for gum.

benzyl carbonol. See **phenylethyl alcohol.**

benzylpenicillin. See **penicillin G.**

bereavement /bərēv′mənt/ [ME, *bereven* to rob], a form of depression with anxiety symptoms that is a common reaction to the loss of a loved one. It may be accompanied by insomnia, hyperactivity, and other effects. Although bereavement does not necessarily lead to depressive illness, it may be a triggering factor in a person who is otherwise vulnerable to depression. See also **grief, mourning.**

Berger's disease, a kidney disorder characterized by recurrent episodes of macroscopic hematuria, proteinuria, and a granular deposition of IgA from the glomerular mesangium. The condition may or may not progress to renal failure over a period of many years. A spontaneous remission occurs in some cases. The onset of disease is usually in childhood or early adulthood, and males are affected twice as often as females. Treatment is similar to that of other renal diseases. Also called **mesangial IgA nephropathy** /mesan′jē·əl/.

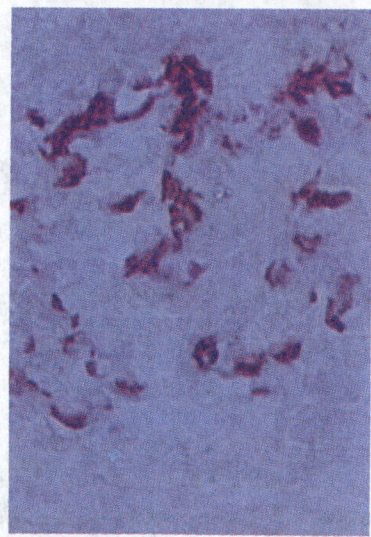

**Renal biopsy taken from patient
with Berger's disease**
(Swales, 1991)

Berger's paresthesia [Oskar Berger, German neurologist, b. 1844; Gk, *para*, near, *aisthesia*, sensation], a condition of tingling, prickliness, or weakness and a loss of feeling in the legs without evidence of organic disease. The condition affects young people.

Berger wave. See **alpha wave.**

Bergonié-Tribondeau law /ber′gônē′trä′bônō′/ [Jean A. Bergonié, French radiologist, b. 1857; Louis Frédéric A. Tribondeau, French physician, b. 1872], (in radiotherapy) a rule stating that the radiosensitivity of tissue depends on the number of undifferentiated cells, their mitotic activity, and the length of time they are actively proliferating.

beriberi /ber′ēber′ē/ [Singhalese, *beri*, weakness], a disease of the peripheral nerves caused by a deficiency of or an inability to assimilate thiamine. It is frequently the result of a diet limited to polished white rice, and it occurs in endemic form in eastern and southern Asia. Rare cases in the United States are associated with stressful conditions, such as hypothyroidism, infections, pregnancy, lactation, and chronic alcoholism. Symptoms are fatigue, diarrhea, appetite and weight loss, disturbed nerve function causing paralysis and wasting of limbs, edema, and heart failure. Kinds of beriberi include alcoholic beriberi, atrophic beriberi, cardiac beriberi, and cerebral beriberi. Administration of thiamine prevents and cures most cases of the disease. Also called **athiaminosis, kakke disease.** See also **thiamine.** (See Fig. p. 182.)

berkelium (Bk) /burk′lē·əm/ [Berkeley, California], an artificial radioactive transuranic element. Its atomic number is 97; its atomic weight is 247.

berlock dermatitis [Fr, *breloque*, bracelet charm], a a temporary skin condition, characterized by hyperpigmentation and skin lesions, caused by a unique reaction to psoralen-type photosynthesizers, which are commonly used in perfumes, colognes, and pomades, such as oil of bergamot. This condition affects mostly women and children and may result from the use of products containing psoralens

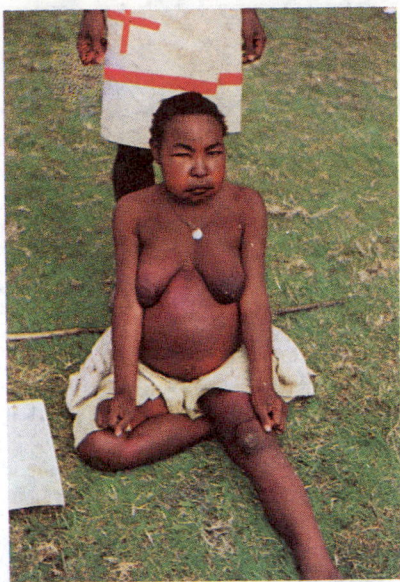

Cardiac beriberi
(McLaren, 1992/Courtesy Prof. AJ Radford)

and from exposure to ultraviolet light. Also spelled **berloque dermatitis.**

■ OBSERVATIONS: Berlock dermatitis commonly produces an acute erythematous reaction, similar to that associated with sunburn. The area affected becomes hyperpigmented and surrounded by darker pigmentation. Areas of the neck where perfume containing oil of bergamot is applied often become affected by pendantlike lesions. Diagnosis is based on the appearance of such signs and on patient history, which may include recent exposure to psoralens.

■ INTERVENTION: Treatment seeks to identify and eliminate the cause of the condition. Topical steroids may be administered to relieve discomfort.

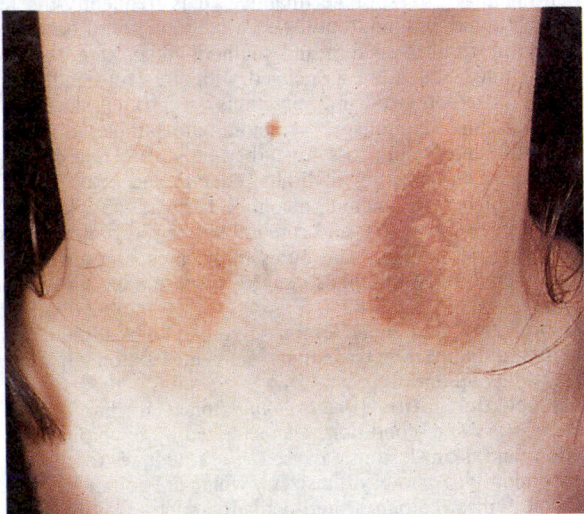

Berlock dermatitis *(duVivier, 1993)*

■ NURSING CONSIDERATIONS: Patients benefit from advice about the complications of prolonged exposure to sunlight and ultraviolet light. They also appreciate the reassurance that the lesions will vanish within a few months.

Bernard-Soulier syndrome /bernär'so͞olyā'/, a coagulation disorder characterized by an absence of or a deficiency in the ability of the platelets to aggregate because of the relative lack of an essential glycoprotein in the membranes of the platelets. On microscopic examination the platelets appear large and dispersed. The use of aspirin may provoke hemorrhage in people who have this condition. After trauma and surgery, loss of blood may be greater than normal and transfusion may be required.

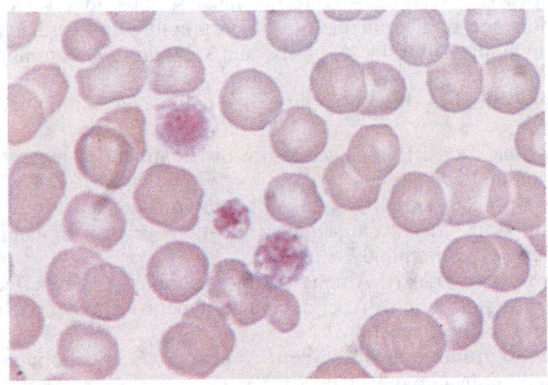

Bernard-Soulier syndrome *(Bain, 1989)*

Bernoulli's principle /bərno͞o'lēz/ [Daniel Bernoulli, Swiss scientist, b. 1700], (in physics) the principle stating that the sum of the velocity and the kinetic energy of a fluid flowing through a tube is constant. The greater the velocity, the less the lateral pressure on the wall of the tube. Thus, if an artery is narrowed by an atherosclerotic plaque, the flow of blood through the constriction increases in velocity and decreases in lateral pressure. Also called **Bernoulli's law.**

Bernstein test. See **acid-perfusion test.**

berry aneurysm [ME, *berye;* Gk, *aneurysma,* widening], a small, saccular dilatation of the wall of a cerebral artery, occurring most frequently at the junctures of vessels in the circle of Willis. A berry aneurysm may be the result of a congenital developmental defect and may rupture without warning, causing intracranial hemorrhage.

Bertel method /bur'təl/, a positioning procedure for producing x-ray images of the inferior orbital fissures. The central beam is directed through the nasion at an angle of 20 to 25 degrees cephalad.

berylliosis /bəril'ē·ō'sis/, poisoning that results from the inhalation of dusts or vapors containing beryllium or beryllium compounds. The substance also may enter the body through or under the skin. It is characterized by granulomas throughout the body and by diffuse pulmonary fibrosis, resulting in a dry cough, shortness of breath, and chest pain. Symptoms may not appear for several years after exposure. See also **inorganic dust.**

beryllium (Be), a steel-gray, lightweight metallic element. Its atomic number is 4; its atomic weight is 9.012. Beryllium occurs naturally as beryl and is used in metallic alloys and in fluorescent powders. Inhalation of beryllium fumes or particles may cause the formation of granulomas in the lungs, skin, and subcutaneous tissues. See also **berylliosis.**

bestiality /bes'chē·al'itē/, [L, *bestia*, beast], **1.** a brutal or animal-like character or nature. **2.** conduct or behavior characterized by beastlike appetites or instincts. **3.** also called **zooerastia** /zoo·əras'tē·ə/. sexual relations between a human being and an animal. **4.** sodomy. See also **zoophilia.**

besylate, a contraction for benzenesulfonate.

beta /bē'tə, bā'tə/, B, β, the second letter of the Greek alphabet, employed as a combining form with chemical names to distinguish one of two or more isomers or to indicate the position of substituted atoms in certain compounds.

beta-adrenergic blocking agent. See **antiadrenergic.**

beta-adrenergic receptor. See **beta receptor.**

beta-adrenergic stimulating agent. See **adrenergic.**

beta-alaninemia /-al'əninē'mē·ə/, an inherited metabolic disorder marked by a deficiency of an enzyme, beta-alanine-alpha-ketoglutarate amino transferase. The clinical signs include seizures, somnolence, and, if uncorrected, death. The condition is sometimes treated with vitamin B$_6$ (pyridoxine).

beta-carotene [Gk, beta; L, *carota*, carrot], an ultraviolet screening agent.

■ INDICATION: It is prescribed to ameliorate photosensitivity in patients with erythropoetic protoporphyria.

■ CONTRAINDICATIONS: It is used with caution in patients with impaired renal or hepatic function. Known hypersensitivity to this drug prohibits its use.

■ ADVERSE EFFECTS: No serious adverse reactions have been observed. Diarrhea may occur.

beta cells, **1.** insulin-producing cells situated in the islets of Langerhans. They contain granules that are soluble in alcohol and tend to be concentrated in the central portion of each islet. The insulin-producing function of the beta cells tends to accelerate the movement of glucose, amino acids, and fatty acids out of the blood and into the cellular cytoplasm, countering glucagon function of alpha cells. **2.** the basophilic cells of the anterior lobe of the pituitary gland.

beta decay, a type of radioactivity that results in the emission of beta particles, such as electrons or positrons. See **beta particle.**

Betadine, a trademark for a topical antiinfective (povidone-iodine).

beta fetoprotein, a protein found in fetal liver and in some adults with liver disease. It is now known to be identical with normal liver ferritin. See also **alpha fetoprotein, ferritin, fetoprotein.**

beta-galactosidase. See **lactase.**

Betagan, a trademark for a topical ophthalmic drug for glaucoma (levobunolol hydrochloride).

beta hemolysis, the development of a clear zone around a bacterial colony growing on blood agar medium, characteristic of certain pathogenic bacteria. Compare **alpha hemolysis.**

beta-hemolytic streptococci, the pyogenic streptococci of groups A, B, C, E, F, G, H, K, L, M, and O that cause hemolysis of red blood cells in blood agar in the laboratory. These organisms cause most of the acute streptococcal infections seen in humans, including rheumatic fever, scarlet fever, many cases of pneumonia and sepsis syn-

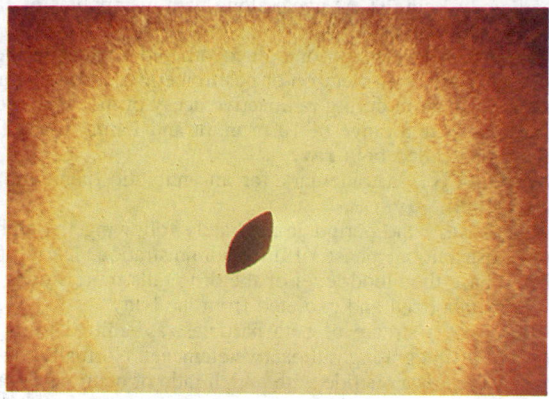

Beta hemolysis *(Baron, 1990)*

drome, and streptococcal sore throat. Penicillin is usually prescribed to treat these infections when they are suspected, even before the results of the bacteriologic culture are available, because it is known that these organisms as a group are usually sensitive to the effects of penicillin, and because the sequelae of untreated streptococcal infection may include glomerulonephritis and rheumatic fever.

beta-hydroxyisovaleric aciduria, an inherited metabolic disease caused by a deficiency of an enzyme needed to metabolize the amino acid leucine. The condition results in an accumulation of leucine in the tissues, causing an unpleasant urine odor, retardation, and muscle atrophy. See also **maple syrup urine disease.**

beta$_2$-interferon. See IL-6.

beta-ketobutyric acid. See **acetoacetic acid.**

beta-lactamase /-lak'təmāz/ [*lactam*, a cyclic amide, *ase*, enzyme], an enzyme that catalyzes the hydrolysis of the beta-lactam ring of some penicillins and cephalosporins, producing penicilloic acid and rendering the antibiotic ineffective. Also called **cephalosporinase, penicillinase.**

beta-lactamase resistance. See **beta-lactamase-resistant antibiotics**.

beta-lactamase-resistant antibiotics, antibiotcs that are resistant to the enzymatic effects of **beta-lactamase**.

beta-lactamase-resistant penicillin, See **beta-lactamase-resistant antibiotics**.

betamethasone. a glucocorticoid.

■ INDICATION: It is prescribed as a topical antiinflammatory agent.

■ CONTRAINDICATIONS: Systemic fungal infections, dermatologic viral and fungal infections, impaired circulation, or known hypersensitivity to this drug prohibits its use.

■ ADVERSE EFFECTS: Among the more serious adverse reactions associated with prolonged use of the drug are GI, endocrine, neurologic, and fluid and electrolyte disturbances.

beta-naphthylamine /-nafthil'əmēn/, an aromatic amine used in aniline dyes and a cause of bladder cancer in humans.

beta-oxidation, a catabolic process in which fatty acids are used by the body as a source of energy. The fatty acid molecules are converted through a series of intermediates into acetylcoenzyme A molecules, which then enter the tricarboxylic acid (TCA) cycle along with metabolites of carbohydrates and proteins.

Betapar, a trademark for a glucocorticoid (meprednisone).

beta particle, an electron or positron emitted from the nucleus of an atom during radioactive decay of the atom. Beta particles have a range of 10 m in air and 1 mm in soft tissue. Also called **beta ray.**

Betapen-VK, a trademark for an antibiotic (penicillin V potassium).

beta phase, the period immediately following the alpha, or redistribution, phase of drug administration. During the beta phase the blood level of the drug falls more slowly as it is metabolized and excreted from the body.

beta rays a stream of beta particles, as emitted from atoms of disintegrating radioactive elements. Normally, when the element is a nuclide with a high ratio of neutrons to protons, the beta particle is an electron; when the nuclide has a higher proportion of protons to neutrons, the beta particle is a positron.

beta receptor, any one of the postulated adrenergic components of receptor tissues that responds to epinephrine and such blocking agents as propranolol. Activation of beta receptors causes various physiologic reactions, such as relaxation of the bronchial muscles and an increase in the rate and force of cardiac contraction. Also called **beta-adrenergic receptor.** Compare **alpha receptor.**

beta rhythm. See **beta wave.**

betatron /bā′tətron/, a cyclic accelerator that produces high-energy electrons for radiotherapy treatment. The magnetic field of the betatron deflects electrons into a circular orbit, and an increasing magnetic orbital flux produces an induced circumferential electric field that accelerates the electrons.

beta wave, one of the four types of brain waves, characterized by relatively low voltage and a frequency of more than 13 Hz. Beta waves are the "busy waves" of the brain, recorded by electroencephalograph from the frontal and the central areas of the cerebrum when the patient is awake and alert with eyes open. Also called **beta rhythm.** Compare **alpha wave, delta wave, theta wave.**

betaxolol hydrochloride /betak′sələl/, a topical drug for open-angle glaucoma.
- INDICATIONS: This drug is prescibed for the relief of ocular hypertension and chronic open-angle glaucoma.
- CONTRAINDICATIONS: Betaxolol hydrochloride is contraindicated in patients with sinus bradycardia, greater than first-degree atrioventricular block, cardiogenic shock, overt heart failure. Caution is advised in use of the product by patients who are also receiving oral beta-blocker drugs.
- ADVERSE EFFECTS: Reported adverse reactions include stinging and tearing of the eyes. Systemic effects are rare.

bethanechol chloride /bethan′əkol/, a cholinergic.
- INDICATIONS: It is prescribed in the treatment of fecal and urinary retention and neurogenic atony of the bladder.
- CONTRAINDICATIONS: Uncertain strength of the bladder, obstruction of the GI or urinary tract, hyperthyroidism, peptic ulcer, bronchial asthma, cardiovascular disease, epilepsy, Parkinson's disease, hypotension, or known hypersensitivity to this drug prohibits its use. It is not given during pregnancy.
- ADVERSE EFFECTS: Among the more serious adverse reactions are flushing, headache, GI distress, diarrhea, excessive salivation, sweating, and hypotension.

Betopic, a trademark for a topical glaucoma medication (betaxolol hydrochloride).

Betz cells [Vladimir Aleksandrovich Betz, Russian anatomist, b. 1834; L, *cella,* storeroom], large pyramidal neurons of the motor cortex with axons that form part of the pyramidal tract associated with voluntary movements.

bevel /bev′əl/ [OFr, *baif,* open mouth angle], **1.** any angle, other than a right angle, between two planes or surfaces. **2.** (in dentistry) any angle other than 90 degrees between a tooth cut and a cavity wall in the preparation of a tooth cavity. Compare **cavosurface bevel, contra bevel.**

bezoar /bē′zôr/ [Ar, *bazahr,* protection against poison], a hard ball of hair or vegetable fiber that may develop within the stomach of humans. More often it is found in the stomachs of ruminants. In some societies it was formerly considered a useful medicine and possessed of certain magical properties. It is apparently still used as a therapeutic and mystical device by some, especially in the Far East.

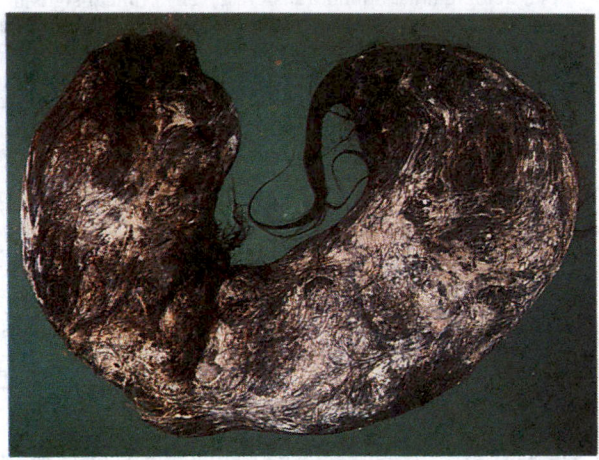

Bezoar *(Mitros, 1988/Courtesy Dr. TH Kent)*

B/F, a symbol for *black female,* often used in the initial identifying statement in a patient record.

β-galactosidase. See **lactase.**

bhang /bang/ [Hindi, *bag*], an Asian Indian hallucinogenic, composed of dried leaves and the young stems of uncultivated *Cannabis sativa.* It is usually ingested as a boiled mixture with milk, sugar, or water; it produces euphoria. It also may be smoked or chewed. Also spelled **bang.** See also **cannabis.**

Bi, symbol for the element **bismuth.**

bi-, a prefix meaning 'twice, two': *biarticular, bicapsular, bicaudal.* See also **bio-, bis-.**

BIA, abbreviation for **bioelectric impedance analysis.**

-bia, a suffix meaning 'creature possessing a mode of life': *aerobia.*

bias /bī′əs/ [MFr, *biais*], **1.** an oblique or a diagonal line. **2.** a prejudiced or subjective attitude. **3.** (in statistics) the systematic distortion of a statistic caused by a particular sampling process. **4.** (in electronics) a voltage applied to an electronic device, such as a vacuum tube or a transistor, to control operating limits.

biased sample /bī′əst/ [OFr, *biais*, slant; L, *exemplum*, sample], (in research), a sample of a group in which all factors or particpants were not equally balanced or objectively represented.

biasing /bī′əsing/, a method of treating neuromuscular dysfunction by contracting a muscle against resistance, causing the muscle spindles to readjust to the shorter length. It results in the muscle tissue being more responsive and sensitive to stretching.

Biavax, a trademark for a rubella and mumps vaccine.

bibliotherapy, a type of group therapy in which books, poems, and newspaper articles are read in the group to help stimulate thinking about events in the real world and to foster relations between group members.

bicarbonate /bīkär′bənāt/ [L, *bis*, two, *carbo*, coal], any salt of carbonic acid in which only one of the hydrogen atoms has been replaced by a metal or radical, as sodium bicarbonate (NaHCO₃).

bicarbonate of soda. See **sodium bicarbonate.**

bicarbonate precursor, an injection of sodium lactate used in the treatment of metabolic acidosis. It is metabolized in the body to sodium bicarbonate.

bicarbonate therapy, a procedure to increase a patient's stores of bicarbonate when there are signs of severe acidosis. It is usually performed only in certain cases and as a stopgap measure to partially neutralize the acidosis when the patient's blood pH has fallen to levels that may be a hazard to survival of vital tissues.

bicarbonate transport, the route by which most of the carbon dioxide is carried in the bloodstream. Once dissolved in the blood plasma, carbon dioxide combines with water to form carbonic acid, which immediately ionizes into hydrogen and bicarbonate ions. The bicarbonate ions serve as part of the alkaline reserve.

biceps brachii /bī′seps brā′kē·ī/ [L, *bis*, twice, *caput*, head; *bracchii* arm], the long fusiform muscle of the upper arm on the anterior surface of the humerus, arising in two heads from the scapula. The short head arises in a thick, flat tendon from the coracoid process, the long head arises in the glenoid cavity. Both parts of the muscle converge in a flattened tendon that inserts into the radius of the forearm. The biceps brachii is innervated by branches of the musculocutaneous nerve, containing fibers from the fifth and the sixth cervical nerves. It flexes the arm and the forearm and supinates the hand. The long head draws the humerus toward the glenoid fossa, strengthening the shoulder joint. Also called **biceps, biceps flexor cubiti.** Compare **brachialis, triceps brachii.**

biceps femoris [L, *bis,* twice, *caput*, head; thigh], one of the posterior femoral muscles. It has two heads at its origin. The long head arises from the tuberosity of the ischium and from the inferior part of the sacrotuberous ligament; the short head arises from the linea aspera and from the lateral intermuscular septum. The fibers passing from both heads join in a tendon that inserts into the lateral side of the fibula and, by a few fibers, into the lateral condyle of the tibia. The tendon of insertion forms the lateral hamstring. The long head of the muscle is innervated by branches of the sciatic nerve containing fibers from the first three sacral nerves. The short head is innervated by a branch of the peroneal nerve containing fibers from the fifth lumbar and first two sacral nerves. The biceps femoris flexes the leg and rotates it laterally and extends the thigh, rotating it laterally. Also called **hamstring muscle.**

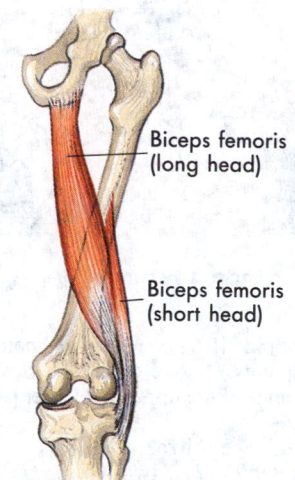

Biceps femoris *(Thibodeau, 1993/Ernest W Beck)*

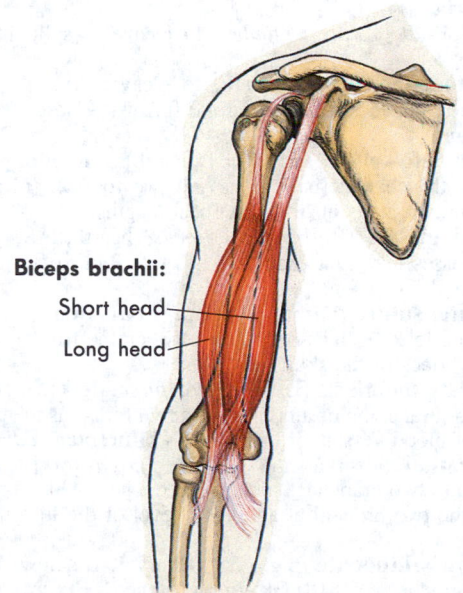

Biceps brachii *(Thibodeau, 1993/Ernest W Beck)*

biceps flexor cubiti. See **biceps brachii.**

biceps reflex, a contraction of a biceps muscle produced when the tendon is tapped with a percussor in testing deep tendon reflexes. See also **deep tendon reflex.**

bicipital groove /bīsip′ətəl/ [L, *bis*, two, *caput*, heads; D, *groeve*], a groove between the greater and lesser tubercles

of the humerus for passage of the tendon of the long head
of the biceps muscle.

Bickerdyke /bik'ərdīk/, **Mary Ann** (1817–1901), an
American nurse who, after taking a short course in homeopathy, cared for the sick and wounded on the battlefields
during the Civil War. She insisted on cleanliness, good
food, and the best of medical care for her patients. At night
she searched the battlefield with a lantern looking for survivors.

biclor /bī'klôr/, abbreviation for a *bichloride noncarboxylate anion*.

biconcave /bīkon'kāv/ [L, *bis*, twice, *concavare*, to make
hollow], concave on both sides, especially as applied to a
lens. **–biconcavity,** *n*.

biconvex /bīkon'veks/ [L, *bis* + *convexus*, vaulted],
convex on both sides, especially as applied to a lens.
–biconvexity, *n*.

bicornate /bīkôr'nāt/ [L, *bis* + *cornu*, horn], having two
horns or processes.

bicornate uterus, an abnormal uterus that may be either
a single or a double organ with two horns, or branches. The
anomaly is believed to result from an embryonic development error and is associated with a high incidence of premature labor, spontaneous abortion, and infertility.

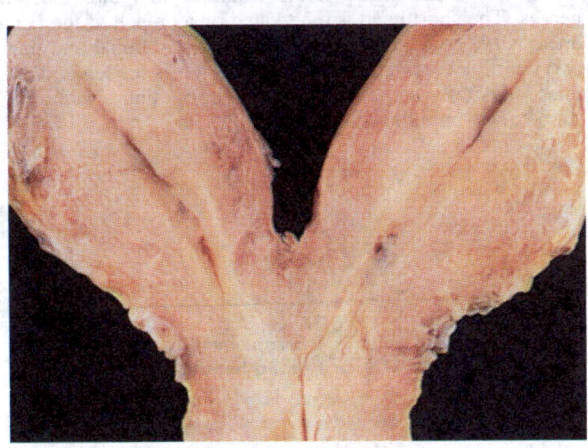

Bicornate uterus (Fletcher, 1987)

bicuspid /bīkus'pid/ [L, *bis* + *cuspis*, point], **1.** having
two cusps or points. **2.** one of the two teeth between the
molars and canines of the upper and lower jaws. Also called
premolar.

bicuspid valve. See **mitral valve.**

bicycle ergometer [L, *bis*, two; Gk, *kyklos*, circle, *ergon*,
work, *metron*, measure], a stationary bicycle dynamometer that measures the power of the contraction of the muscles of an individual.

b.i.d., (in prescriptions) abbreviation for *bis in die* /dē'ā/,
a Latin phrase meaning 'twice a day.' The times of administration are commonly 9 AM and 7 PM.

bidactyly /bīdak'tilē/ [L, *bis* + Gk, *daktylos*, finger], an
abnormal condition in which the second, third, and fourth
digits on the same hand are missing and only the first and
fifth are represented. Also called **lobster claw deformity. –bidactylous,** *adj*.

bidermoma /bī'dər'mō'mə/, *pl.* **bidermomas, bidermo-**

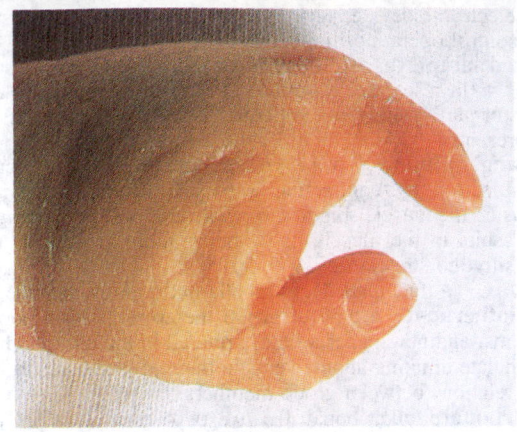

Bidactyly
(Zitelli, 1992/Courtesy Dr. Christine L Williams, New York
Medical College)

mata [L, *bis* + Gk, *derma*, skin, *oma*, tumor], a teratoid
neoplasm composed of cells and tissues originating in two
germ layers.

bidet /bidā'/ [Fr, pony], a fixture resembling a toilet bowl,
with a rim to sit on and usually equipped with plumbing
implements for cleaning the genital and rectal areas of the
body.

biduotertian fever /bī'dŏŏ·ətur'shən/ [L, *bis* + *dies*, day,
tertius three], a form of malaria characterized by overlapping paroxysms of chills, fever, and other symptoms,
caused by infection with two strains of *Plasmodium,* each
having its own cycle of symptoms, such as in quartan and
tertian malaria. Compare **double quartan fever.** See also
malaria.

bifid /bī'fid/ [L, *bis* + *findere* to cleave], split into two
parts.

bifid tongue [L, *bis, findere*, to cleave; AS, *tunge*], a
tongue divided by a longitudinal furrow. Also called **cleft
tongue.**

bifocal /bīfō'kəl/ [L, *bis* + *focus* hearth], **1.** of or pertaining to the characteristic of having two foci. **2.** (of a lens)
having two areas of different focal lengths.

bifocal glasses [L, *bis*, two, *focus*, hearth; AS, *glaes*],
eyeglasses in which each lens has two foci to permit both
near and far vision.

bifrontal suture /bīfron'təl/ [L, *bi, frons*, front + *sutura*],
the interlocking lines of fusion between the frontal and parietal bones of the skull.

bifurcate /bīfur'kāt/ [L, *bis*, two, *furca*, fork], the division or branching of an object into two forks, as the branching of blood vessels or bronchi. **–bifurcated,** *adj*.

bifurcation /bī'fərkā'shən/ [L, *bis* + *furca*, fork], a splitting into two branches, such as the trachea, which branches
into the two bronchi at about the level of the fifth thoracic
vertebra.

Bigelow's lithotrite /big'əlōz/ [Henry J. Bigelow, American surgeon, b. 1818; Gk, *lithos*, stone; L, *terere*, to rub],
a long-jawed lithotrite, passed through the urethra, for
crushing a calculus in the bladder.

-bigeminal. See **bigeminy.**

bigeminal pulse /bījem′inəl/, an abnormal pulse in which two beats in close succession are followed by a pause during which no pulse is felt. See also **trigeminal pulse, trigeminy.**

bigeminal rhythm [L, *bis, geminus,* twins; Gk, *rhythmos*], a coupled heart beat with ventricular or atrial ectopic beats alternating with sinus beats or ventricular ectopics occurring in pairs, such as ventricular tachycardia with 3:2 exit block. Also called **coupled rhythm.**

bigeminy /bījem′inē/ [L, *bis + geminus,* twin], **1.** an association in pairs. **2.** a cardiac arrhythmia characterized by pairs of beats in which each normal beat is followed by an abnormal or ectopic beat in a repeating manner. **–bigeminal,** *adj.*

bilabe /bī′lāb/ [L, *bis,* + *labium,* lip], a narrow forceps used to remove small calculi from the bladder.

bilaminar /bīlam′ənər/ [L, *bis,* + *lamina,* thin plate], pertaining to or having two layers, such as the basal lamina and the reticular lamina that constitute the basement membrane of the epithelium.

bilaminar blastoderm, the stage of embryonic development before mesoderm formation in which only the ectoderm and entoderm primary germ layers have formed. Compare **trilaminar blastoderm.**

bilateral /bilat′ərəl/ [L, *bis + lateralis,* side], **1.** having two sides. **2.** occurring or appearing on two sides. A patient with bilateral hearing loss may have partial or total deafness in both ears. **3.** having two layers.

bilateral carotid [L, *bis,* two, *latus,* side; Gk, *karos,* heavy sleep], a main artery to the head and neck that divides into left and right branches and again into external and internal branches.

bilateral lithotomy [L, *bis,* two, *latus,* side; Gk, *lithos,* stone, *temnein,* to cut], a surgical procedure for removing urinary tract stones from the bladder by making transverse perineal incisions through the lateral lobes of the prostate.

bilateral long-leg spica cast, an orthopedic device of plaster of paris, fiberglass, or other casting material that encases and immobilizes the trunk cranially as far as the nipple line and both legs caudally as far as the toes. A horizontal crossbar to improve immobilization connects the parts of the cast encasing both legs at ankle level. It is used to aid the healing of fractures of the hip, the femur, the acetabulum, or the pelvis and to correct or maintain the correction of a hip deformity. Compare **one-and-a-half spica cast, unilateral long-leg spica cast.**

bilateral strabismus [L, *bis, latus,* side; Gk, *strabismos*], an eye disorder, characterized by bilateral squint, in which the condition is caused by a failure of ocular accommodation.

bilateral symmetry [L, *bis, latus,* side; Gk, *syn,* together + *metron,* measure], the symmetry of the halves of an organism.

Bilbao tube /bilbō′ə/, a long, thin, flexible tube that is used to inject barium into the small intestine. The tube is guided with a stiff wire to the end of the duodenum under fluoroscopic control.

bile /bīl/ [L, *bilis*], a bitter, yellow-green secretion of the liver. Stored in the gallbladder, bile receives its color from the presence of bile pigments such as bilirubin. Bile passes from the gallbladder through the common bile duct in response to the presence of a fatty meal in the duodenum. Bile emulsifies these fats, preparing them for further digestion and absorption in the small intestine. Any interference in the flow of bile will result in the presence of unabsorbed fat in the feces and in jaundice. Also called **gall.** See also **biliary obstruction, jaundice. –biliary,** *adj.*

bile acid, a steroid acid of the bile, produced during the metabolism of cholesterol. On hydrolysis bile acid yields glycine and cholic acid.

bile duct. See **biliary duct.**

bile pigments, a group of substances that contribute to the colors of bile, which may range from a yellowish-green to brown. A common bile pigment is bilirubin, which contains a reddish iron pigment derived from the breakdown of old red blood cells.

bile salts [L, *bilis,* bile; AS, *sealt*], a mixture of sodium salts of the bile acids and cholic and chendoxychoic acids synthesized in the liver as a derivative of cholesterol. Their low surface tension contributes to the emulsification of fats in the intestine.

bile solubility test, a bacteriologic test used in the differential diagnosis of pneumococcal and streptococcal infection. A broth culture of each organism is placed into two tubes. Ox bile is added to one and salt to the other. Pneumococci dissolve in ox bile, resulting in a clear solution; streptococci do not dissolve, resulting in a cloudy solution. The tube with salt is used for comparative purposes.

Bilharzia. See *Schistosoma.*

bilharziasis. See **schistosomiasis.**

bili-, a prefix meaning 'pertaining to the bile': *biliary, bilidigestive, bilifuscin.*

biliary /bil′ē·er′ē/, of or pertaining to bile or to the gallbladder and bile ducts, which transport bile. These are often called the **biliary tract** or the biliary system. Also **bilious.** See also **bile, biliary calculus.**

biliary atresia, congenital absence or underdevelopment of one or more of the biliary structures, causing jaundice and early liver damage. As the condition worsens, the child may show retarded growth and develop portal hypertension. Surgery can correct the defective ducts in only a small percentage of cases. Most infants die in early childhood from biliary cirrhosis. It is essential to distinguish between this condition and neonatal hepatitis, which is treatable. See also **biliary cirrhosis.**

biliary calculus [L, *bilis,* bile, *calculus,* pebble], a stone formed in the biliary tract, consisting of cholesterol or bile pigments and calcium salts. Biliary calculi may cause jaun-

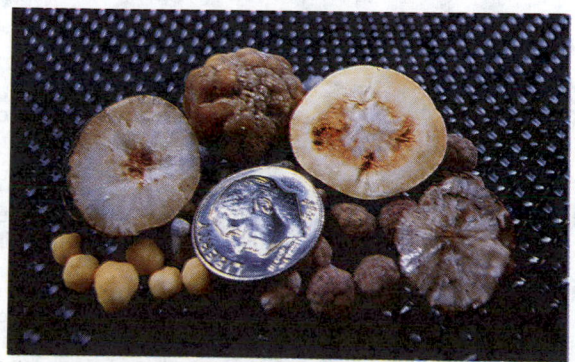

Biliary calculus
(Seeley, 1992/SIU Biomedical Communications/Science Source/Photoresearchers, Inc)

dice, right upper quadrant pain, obstruction, and inflammation of the gallbladder. If stones cannot pass spontaneously into the duodenum, cholangiography or similar processes will reveal their location, and they can be removed. Also called **choledocholithiasis, gallstones.** See also **cholangitis, cholecystitis, cholelithiasis.**

biliary cirrhosis [L, *bilis* + *kirrhos,* yellow, *osis* condition], an inflammatory condition in which the flow of bile through the ductules of the liver is obstructed. Primary biliary cirrhosis most commonly affects women in their middle years, and its cause is unknown. It is characterized by itching, jaundice, steatorrhea, and enlargement of the liver and spleen. The disease is slowly progressive. There is no specific medical or surgical treatment. Care must be taken to rule out secondary biliary cirrhosis due to obstruction of the biliary structures outside the liver, because the latter condition can be treated successfully. Compare **biliary calculus, biliary obstruction.**

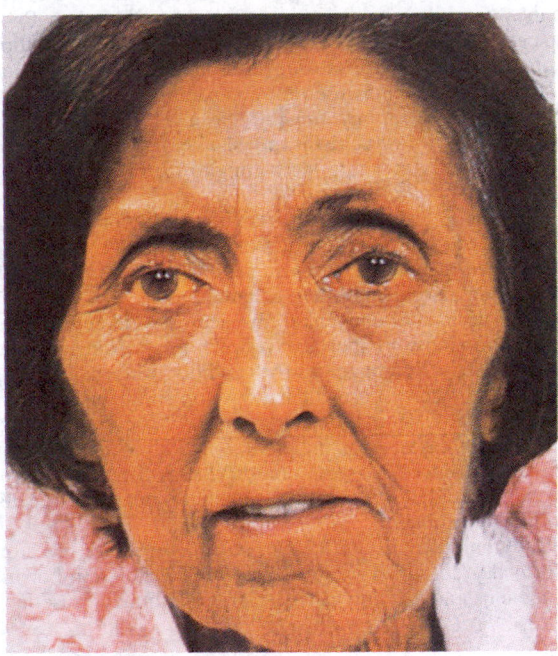

Biliary cirrhosis *(Kamal, 1991)*

biliary colic [L, *bilis* + *kolikos,* colon pain], a type of smooth muscle or visceral pain specifically associated with the passing of stones through the bile ducts. Also called **cholecystalgia.** See also **biliary calculus.**

biliary duct, a muscular duct through which bile passes from the liver to the duodenum. Also called **common bile duct.**

biliary fistula, an abnormal passage from the gallbladder, a bile duct, or the liver to an internal organ or the surface of the body. Biliary fistulae into the duodenum may complicate cholelithiasis; a gallstone may become impacted, usually in the ileocecal valve, and cause intestinal obstruction.

biliary obstruction, blockage of the common or cystic bile duct, usually caused by one or more gallstones. It impedes bile drainage and produces an inflammatory reaction. Uncommon causes of biliary obstruction include choledochal cysts, pancreatic and duodenal tumors, Crohn's disease, pancreatitis, echinococcosis, ascariasis, and sclerosing cholangitis. Stones, consisting chiefly of cholesterol, bile pigment, and calcium, may form in the gallbladder and in the hepatic duct in persons of either sex at any age but are more common in middle-aged women. Increased amounts of serum cholesterol in the blood, such as occurs in obesity, diabetes, hypothyroidism, biliary stasis, and inflammation of the biliary system, promote the formation of gallstones. Cholelithiasis may be asymptomatic until a stone lodges in a biliary duct, but the patient usually has a history of indigestion and discomfort after eating fatty foods.

■ OBSERVATIONS: Biliary obstruction is characterized by severe epigastric pain, often radiating to the back and shoulder, nausea, vomiting, and profuse diaphoresis. The dehydrated patient may have chills, fever, jaundice, clay-colored stools, dark, concentrated urine, an electrolyte imbalance, and a tendency to bleed because the absence of bile prevents the synthesis and absorption of fat-soluble vitamin K.

■ INTERVENTIONS: The patient is placed in bed in a semi-Fowler's position and is usually administered intermittent nasogastric suctioning, parenteral fluids with electrolytes and fat-soluble vitamins, and medication for pain. Antibiotics, anticholinergic and antispasmodic drugs, and a cholecystogram or ultrasound scan may be ordered. The blood pressure, temperature, pulse, and respirations are noted, and the patient is helped to turn, cough, and deep breathe every 2 to 4 hours. The intake and output of fluids are measured, and the color and character of urine and stools are noted. When the nasogastric tube is removed, the patient initially receives a low-fat liquid diet and progresses to a soft or normal diet, as tolerated; up to 2500 ml of fluids a day are forced, unless contraindicated. Cholecystectomy is usually the definitive treatment, but in most cases surgery is delayed until the patient's condition is stabilized and any prothrombin deficiency (caused by vitamin K malabsorption) is corrected.

biliary system. See **biliary.**

biliary tract [L, *bilis,* bile + *tractus*], the pathway for bile flow from the canaliculi in the liver to the opening of the bile duct into the duodenum.

biliary tract cancer, a rare adenocarcinoma in an extrahepatic bile duct, occurring more often in men than in women, characterized by progressive jaundice, pruritus, weight loss, and, severe pain. Transhepatic cholangiography and x-ray examination are used to identify and determine the site of the lesion. Results of laboratory studies indicative of extrahepatic biliary obstruction include greater than normal levels of serum alkaline phosphatase and bilirubin in the blood. If the tumor is in the ampulla of Vater, occult blood may be found in the stool. The lesion may be papillary or flat and ulcerated. The tumor is generally inoperable if located in the hepatic or common bile duct. Periampullary lesions may be treated by pancreatoduodenectomy. Preoperative, postoperative, and palliative irradiation may be given. With the exception of a rare remission induced by 5-fluorouracil, chemotherapy is not effective in treating these lesions.

bilingulate /bīling′gyəlit/ [L, *bis,* twice, *lingula,* little tongue], having two tongues or two tonguelike structures.

bilious /bil′yəs/ [L, *bilis*, bile], **1.** of or pertaining to bile. **2.** characterized by an excessive secretion of bile. **3.** characterized by a disorder affecting the bile.

bilirubin /bil′ir o͞o′bin/ [L, *bilis* + *ruber*, red], the orange-yellow pigment of bile, formed principally by the breakdown of hemoglobin in red blood cells after termination of their normal lifespan. Water-insoluble, unconjugated bilirubin normally travels in the bloodstream to the liver, where it is converted to a water-soluble, conjugated form and excreted into the bile. In a healthy person about 250 mg of bilirubin are produced daily. The majority of bilirubin is excreted in the stool. The characteristic yellow pallor of jaundice is caused by the accumulation of bilirubin in the blood and in the tissues of the skin. Testing for bilirubin in the blood provides information for diagnosis and evaluation of liver disease, biliary obstruction, and hemolytic anemia. Normal levels of total bilirubin are 0.1 to 1.0 mg/dl or 5.1-17.0 μmol/L. See also **jaundice, van den Bergh test.**

bilirubinemia /-ē′mē·ə/ [L, *bilis*, bile, *ruber*, red; Gk, *haima*, blood], the presence of biirubin in the blood.

bilirubinuria /-o͞or′ē·ə/, the presence of bilirubin in urine.

biliuria /bil′iyo͞or′ē·ə/ [L, *bilis* + Gk, *ouron*, urine], the presence of bile in the urine.

biliverdin /bil′ivur′din/ [L, *bilis* + *virdis*, green], a greenish bile pigment formed in the breakdown of hemoglobin and converted to bilirubin. See also **bile, bilirubin.**

billing limit. See **limiting charge.**

Billings method, a way of estimating ovulation time by changes in the cervical mucus that occur during the menstrual cycle.

Billroth's operation I [Christian A. Billroth, Austrian surgeon, b. 1829], the surgical removal of the pylorus in the treatment of gastric cancer. The proximal end of the duodenum is anastomosed to the stomach.

Billroth's operation II, the surgical removal of the pylorus and duodenum. The cut end of the stomach is anastomosed to the jejunum through the transverse mesocolon.

bilobate /bīlō′bāt/ [L, *bis*, twice, *lobus*, lobe], having two lobes.

bilobate placenta [L, *bis*, two, *lobus*, lobe, *placenta*, a flat cake], a placenta with two connected lobes. Also called **bilobed placenta, placenta bipartitia.**

bilobulate /bīlob′yəlāt/, having two lobules. Also **bilobular.**

bilocular /bīlok′yələr/ [L, *bis* + *loculus*, compartment], **1.** divided into two cells. **2.** containing two cells. Also **biloculate.**

Biltricide, a trademark for a trematocide (praziquantel).

bimanual /bīman′yo͞o·əl/ [L, *bis* + *manus*, hand], of or pertaining to the functioning of both hands.

bimanual palpation, the examination of a woman's pelvic organs conducted by the examiner placing one hand on the abdomen and one or two fingers of the other hand in the vagina.

bimanual percussion [L, *bis*, two, *manus*, hand, *percutere*, to strike through], a diagnostic technique of producing sound vibrations in body cavities by the use of two hands, one serving as the plexor and the other as the pleximeter.

bimaxillary /bīmak′siler′ē/ [L, *bis* + *maxilla*, jawbone], of or pertaining to the right and left maxilla.

bimodal distribution /bīmo′dəl/ [L, *bis* + *modus*, measure], the distribution of quantitative data around two separate modes. It is suggestive of two separate normally distributed populations from which the data are drawn.

bimolecular reaction (E2) /bī′molek′yələr/, an elimination reaction in which more than one kind of molecule is involved. Enzyme-catalyzed reactions usually consist of a series of bimolecular reactions. It may follow first-order, second-order, or more complicated chemical kinetics.

binangle /bin′ang·gəl/ [L, *bini*, twofold, *angulus*, angle], a surgical or operative instrument that has a shank with two offsetting angles to keep the cutting edge of the instrument within 3 mm of the shaft axis.

binary fission /bī′nərē/ [L, *bini*, twofold; *fissionis*, splitting], direct division of a cell or nucleus into two equal parts. It is the common form of asexual reproduction of bacteria, protozoa, and other lower forms of life. Also called **simple fission.** Compare **multiple fission.**

binary number, a number represented in the binary system, and represented by 0s and 1s. See **binary system.**

binary system, a number system based on the number two, used in digital computers. Each digit, represented by a zero or one, represents a power of two. Thus the decimal number 47 (actually representing $4 \times 10^1 + 7 \times 10^0$) is expressed in binary notation as 101111 (that is, $1 \times 2^5 + 0 \times 2^4 + 1 \times 2^3 + 1 \times 2^2 + 1 \times 2^1 + 1 \times 2^0$).

binaural stethoscope /bīnôr′əl/ [L, *bini* + *auris*, ear], a stethoscope having two earpieces.

bind [AS, *binden*], **1.** to bandage or wrap in a band. **2.** to join together with a band or with a ligature. **3.** (in chemistry) to combine or unite molecules by employing reactive groups within the molecules or by using a binding chemical. Binding is especially associated with chemical bonds that are fairly easily broken, such as in the bonds between toxins and antitoxins.

binder, a bandage made of a large piece of material to fit and support a specific body part.

binding energy, the amount of energy required to remove a particle from the orbit or nucleus of an atom.

binding site [ME, *binden*, L, *situs*], the location on the surface of a cell or a molecule where other cell fragments or molecules attach to initiate a chemical or physiologic action.

Binet age /binā′/ [Alfred Binet, French psychologist, b. 1857], the mental age of an individual, especially a child, as determined by the Binet-Simon tests, which are evaluated on the basis of tested intelligence of the 'normal' individual at any given age. The Binet age corresponding to 'profoundly retarded' is 1 to 2 years; to 'severely retarded,' 3 to 7 years; and to 'mildly retarded,' 8 to 12 years.

binocular /binok′yələr, bin-/ [L, *bini* + *oculus*, eye], **1.** pertaining to both eyes, especially regarding vision. **2.** a microscope, telescope, or field glass that can accommodate viewing by both eyes.

binocular fixation, the process of having both eyes directed at the same object at the same time, which is essential to having good depth perception.

binocular ophthalmoscope, an ophthalmoscope having two eyepieces through which stereoscopic examination of the eye may be made.

binocular parallax /per′əlaks/ [L, *bini, oculus;* Gk, *parallax*, in turn], the difference in the angles formed by the sight lines to two objects situated at different distances from the eyes. Binocular parallax is a major factor in depth perception. Also called **stereoscopic parallax.**

binocular perception, the visual ability to judge depth or distance by virtue of having two eyes.

binocular vision, the use of both eyes simultaneously so that the images perceived by each eye are combined to appear as a single image. Compare **diplopia.**

binomial /bīnō'mē·əl/, containing two names or terms.

binomial nomenclature [L, *bis,* two; Gk, *nomos,* law; L, *nomenclatio,* calling by name], a system of classification of animals and plants by assigning Latinized genus and species names to each, such as *Homo sapiens* for humans.

binovular /bīnov'yələr/ [L, *bini + ovum,* egg], developing from two distinct ova, as in dizygotic twins. Also **diovular.** Compare **uniovular.**

binovular twins. See **dizygotic twins.**

binuclear /bīnoo'klē·ər/ [L, *bis,* two; *nucleus,* nut], having two nuclei, as in the example of a heteroakryon or binucleate hybrid cell. Also **binucleate** /bīnoo'klē·āt/.

bio-, /bī'ō-/ a prefix meaning 'pertaining to life': *bioassay, biogenesis, biolysis.*

bioactive [**Gk,** *bios,* life; L, *activus,* with energy], of or pertaining to a substance that has an effect on or causes a reaction in living tissue.

bioactivity /-aktiv'itē/, any response from or reaction in living tissue.

bioassay /bī'ō·as'ā, -əsā'/ [Gk, *bios + Fr, assayer,* to try], the laboratory determination of the concentration of a drug or other substance in a specimen by comparing its effect on an organism, an animal, or an isolated tissue with that of a standard preparation. Also called **biologic assay.**

bioavailability /-əvā'libil'itē/ [Gk, *bios + ME, availen,* to serve], the degree of activity or amount of an administered drug or other substance that becomes available for activity in the target tissue.

biochemical genetics. See **molecular genetics.**

biochemical marker /-kem'ikəl/ [Gk, *bios + chemeia,* alchemy], any hormone, enzyme, antibody, or other substance that is detected in the urine or other body fluids or tissues that may serve as a sign of a disease or other abnormality. An example is the Bence Jones protein that appears in the urine of multiple myeloma patients.

biochemistry /-kem'istrē/, the chemistry of living organisms and life processes. Also called **biologic chemistry, physiologic chemistry.**

biochromatic analysis /-krōmat'ik/ [Gk, *bios + chroma,* color], the spectrophotometric monitoring of a reaction at two wavelengths. It is used to correct for background color.

biodegradable /-digrā'dəbəl/ [Gk, *bios,* life; L, *de,* away, *gradus,* step], the natural ability of a chemical substance to be broken down into less complex compounds or compounds having fewer carbon atoms by bacteria or other microrganisms.

bioelectric impedance analysis (BIA) /-ilek'trik/, a method of measuring the fat composition of the body, compared to other tissues, by its resistance to electricity. Fat tissue does not conduct electricity; muscle and bone are poor conductors. The method is reported to be 95% accurate, with some variations due to body water content, which may fluctuate with exercise, diet, sweating, and use of alcohol or drugs. See also **total body electric conductivity (TOBEC).**

bioelectricity /-ilektris'itē/ [Gk, *bios + elektron,* amber], electric current that is generated by living tissues, such as nerves and muscles. The electric potentials of human tissues, recorded by electrocardiograph, electroencephalograph, and similar sensitive devices, are used in diagnosing the condition of various vital organs.

bioenergetics /-en'ərjet'iks/ [Gk, *bios + energein,* to be active], a system of exercises based on the concept that natural healing will be enhanced by bringing into harmony the patient's body rhythms and the natural environment.

bioequivalent /bī'ō·ikwiv'ələnt/ [Gk, *bios + L, aequus,* equal, *valere,* to be strong], **1.** (in pharmacology) of or pertaining to a drug that has the same effect on the body as another drug, usually one nearly identical in its chemical formulation. **2.** a bioequivalent drug. –**bioequivalence,** *n.*

biofeedback /-fēd'bak/ [Gk, *bios + AS, faedan,* food, *baec,* back], a process providing a person with visual or auditory information about the autonomic physiologic functions of his or her body, such as blood pressure, muscle tension, and brain wave activity, usually through use of instrumentation. By trial and error, the person learns to consciously control these processes, which were previously regarded as involuntary. Biofeedback may be used clinically to treat many conditions, such as hypertension, insomnia, and migraine headache.

bioflavonoid /bī'ōflā'vənoid/ [Gk, *bios + L, flavus,* yellow; Gk, *eidos,* form], a generic term for any of a group of colored flavones found in many fruits and essential for the absorption and metabolism of ascorbic acid. The bioflavonoids are needed for the maintenance of collagen and of the capillary walls and may aid in protection against infection. The components are citrin, hesperidin, rutin, flavones, and flavonoids. Rich sources include lemons, grapes, plums, grapefruit, black currants, apricots, buckwheat, cherries, and blackberries. Deficiency can result in a tendency to bleed or bruise easily. The bioflavonoids are completely nontoxic. See also **ascorbic acid.**

biogenesis /bī'ōjen'əsis/ [Gk, *bios + genein,* to produce], **1.** also called **biogeny** /bī·oj'ənē/. the doctrine that living material can originate only from preexisting life and not from inanimate matter. **2.** the origin of life and living organisms; ontogeny and phylogeny. –**biogenetic,** *adj.*

biogenetic law. See **recapitulation theory.**

biogenic /bī'ōjen'ik/, **1.** produced by the action of a living organism, such as fermentation. **2.** essential to life and the maintenance of health, such as food, water, and proper rest.

biogenic amine, one of a large group of naturally occurring biologically active compounds most of which act as neurotransmitters. The most dominant, norepinephrine, is involved in such physiologic functions as emotional reactions, memory, sleep, and arousal from sleep. Other biochemicals of the group include three catecholamines: histamine, serotonin, and dopamine. These substances are active in regulating blood pressure, elimination, body temperature, and many other centrally mediated body functions.

biogenous /bī·oj'ənəs/, **1.** biogenetic. **2.** biogenic.

biogeny. See **biogenesis.**

biohazard /-haz'ərd/ [Gk, *bios,* life; OFr, *hasard*], anything that is a risk to living organisms, such as exposure to ionizing radiation.

biokinetics /-kinet'iks/ [Gk, *bios,* life, *kinetikos,* moving], a branch of science that deals with movements within developing organisms.

biologic /-loj'ik/ [Gk, *bios + logos* science], **1.** pertaining to living organisms and their products. **2.** any preparation made from living organisms or the products of living organisms and used as diagnostic, preventive, or therapeutic agents. Kinds of biologics are **antigens, antitoxins, serums,** and **vaccines.** Also called **biological.**

biologic activity, the inherent capacity of a substance, such as a drug or toxin, to alter one or more of the chemical or physiologic functions of a cell. The capacity has relationships not only to the physical and chemical nature of the substance but also to its concentration and the duration of cellular exposure to the substance. Theoretically, biologic activity may have a "domino effect" in that alteration of one function may disrupt the normal activity of one or more chemical reactions within a cell with the possible events being equivalent to a factorial (N!) of the total number of reactions within the cell.

biologic armature, the connective-tissue-rich aggregate of larger ducts, vessels, and autonomic nerves that in many mammalian exocrine glands serve as an internal framework whose function of support, and often anchorage, resembles that of the armature within a clay sculpture.

biologic assay. See **bioassay.**

biologic chemistry. See **biochemistry.**

biologic half-life, the time required for the body to eliminate one half of an administered dose of any substance by regular physiologic processes. The time required is approximately the same for both the stable and radioactive isotopes of a specific element. Also called **metabolic half-life.** See also **effective half-life, half-life.**

biologic monitoring, **1.** a process of measuring the levels of various physiologic substances, drugs, or metabolites within a patient during diagnosis or therapy. **2.** the measurement of toxic substances in the environment and the identification of health risks to the population. Biologic monitoring often uses indirect methods of identifying and measuring substances by analysis of samples of blood, urine, feces, hair, nails, sweat, saliva, or exhaled air and by extrapolating from metabolic effects.

biologic plausibility, a method of reasoning used to establish a cause and effect relationship between a biologic factor and a particular disease.

biologic psychiatry, a school of psychiatric thought that stresses the physical, chemical, and neurologic causes of and treatments for mental and emotional disorders.

biologic rhythm [Gk, *bios*, life + *logos*, science + *rhythmos*], the periodic recurrence of certain biologic phenomena, such as circadian rhythms.

biologic vector. See **vector.**

biologist /bī·ol′əjist/ [Gk, *bios*, life, *logos*, science], a person who studies the science of life.

biology /bī·ol′əje/, the scientific study of plants and animals. Some branches of biology are **biometry, ecology, molecular biology,** and **paleontology.**

biome /bī′ōm/ [Gk, *bios* + *oma*, tumor, mass], the total group of biologic communities existing in and characteristic of a given geographic region, such as a desert, woodland, or marsh. A biome includes all plants, animals, and microorganisms of a particular region.

-biomechanic. See **biomechanics.**

biomechanic adaptation /-məkan′ic/, a process in the use of orthotic treatment to enable a disabled person to resume normal function of a body part with the aid of a device, such as an ankle-foot brace or a patellar-tendon bearing prosthesis. The process of adaptation includes the central nervous system input received during therapeutic exercises with the orthotic appliance.

biomechanics [Gk, *bios* + *mechane*, machine], the study of mechanical laws and their application to living organisms, especially the human body and its locomotor system. **–biomechanic, biomechanical,** *adj.*

biomedical engineering /-med′ikəl/ [Gk, *bios* + L, *medicare*, to heal], a system of techniques in which knowledge of biologic processes is applied to solve practical medical problems and to answer questions in biomedical research.

biometry. See **biology.**

bionics /bī·on′iks/, the science of applying electronic principles and devices, such as computers and solid state miniaturized circuitry, to medical problems, such as artificial pacemakers used to correct abnormal heart rhythms. **–bionic,** *adj.*

biophore /bī′əfôr′/ [Gk, *bios* + *phora*, bearer], according to German biologist A.F.L. Weismann, the basic hereditary unit contained in the germ plasm from which all living cells develop and all inherited characteristics are transmitted. Compare **gemmule.**

biopotentials /-pəten′shəlz/, electric charges produced by various tissues of the body, particularly muscle tissue during contractions. Electrocardiography depends on measurement of changing potentials in heart muscle contractions, and electromyography functions similarly in diagnosis of neuromuscular problems.

biopsy /bī′opsē/ [Gk, *bios* + *opsis*, view], **1.** the removal of a small piece of living tissue from an organ or other part of the body for microscopic examination to confirm or establish a diagnosis, estimate prognosis, or follow the course of a disease. **2.** the tissue excised for examination. **3.** *informal,* to excise tissue for examination. Kinds of biopsy include **aspiration biopsy, needle biopsy, punch biopsy,** and **surface biopsy.** **–bioptic** /bī·op′tik/, *adj.*

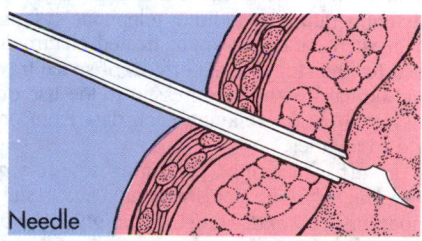

Aspiration biopsy *(Belcher, 1992)*

biopsychic /bī′ōsī′kik/ [Gk, *bios* + *psyche*, mind], of or pertaining to psychic factors as they relate to living organisms.

biopsychology. See **psychobiology.**

biopsychosocial /bī′ōsī′kōsō′shəl/ [Gk, *bios* + *psyche*, mind; L, *socius,* companion], of or pertaining to the complex of biologic, psychologic, and social aspects of life.

-bioptic. See **biopsy.**

bioptome tip catheter /bī·op′tōm/, a catheter with a special tip designed for obtaining endomyocardial biopsy samples. It is advanced under fluroscopy through a guiding catheter to the right ventricle, where it snips small tissue samples from the septal wall for pathologic examination. The bioptome tip device is used to monitor heart transplant patients for early signs of tissue rejection.

biorhythm /bī′ōrithm/ [Gk, *bios* + *rhythmos* rhythm], any cyclic, biologic event or phenomenon, such as the sleep cycle, the menstrual cycle, or the respiratory cycle. —**bio-rhythmic,** *adj.*

-biosis, a suffix meaning 'life': *macrobiosis, necrobiosis, otobiosis.*

biostatistics /-stətis′tiks/, numeric data on births, deaths, diseases, injuries, and other factors affecting the general health and condition of human populations. Also called **vital statistics.**

biosynthesis /-sin′thəsis/ [Gk, *bios* + *synthesis,* putting together], any one of thousands of chemical reactions continually occurring throughout the body in which molecules form more complex biomolecules, especially the carbohydrates, the lipids, the proteins, the nucleotides, and the nucleic acids. Biosynthetic reactions constitute the anabolism of the body. —**biosynthetic,** *adj.*

biotaxis /bī′ōtak′sis/ [Gk, *bios* + *taxis,* arrangement], the ability of living cells to develop into certain forms and arrangements. See also **cytoclesis.** —**biotactic,** *adj.*

biotaxy /bī′ōtak′sē/, **1.** biotaxis. **2.** the systematic classification of living organisms according to their anatomic characteristics; taxonomy.

biotechnology /-teknol′əjē/ [Gk, *bios* + *techne,* art, *logos,* science], **1.** the study of the relationships between humans or other living organisms and machinery, such as the health effects of computer equipment on office workers or the ability of airplane pilots to perform tasks when traveling at supersonic speeds. **2.** the industrial application of the results of biologic research, particularly in fields such as recombinant DNA or gene splicing, which permits the production of synthetic hormones or enzymes by combining genetic material from different species. See **recombinant DNA.**

biotelemetry /-təlem′ətrē/, the transmission of physiologic data, such as ECG and EEG recordings, heart rate, and body temperature by radio or telephone systems. Transmission of such data uses sophisticated electronic devices developed for the study of the effects of space travel on animals and humans; it has progressed to the use of communications satellites for relaying such data from one part of the world to another.

-biotic, a suffix meaning 'pertaining to life': *anabiotic, catabiotic, microbiotic;* also, meaning 'possessing a (specified) mode of life': *endobiotic, parabiotic, photobiotic.*

biotic potential /bī·ot′ik/, the possible growth rate of a population of organisms under ideal conditions, including absence of predators and maximum nutrients and space for expansion.

biotin /bī′ətin/ [Gk, *bios,* life], a colorless, crystalline, water-soluble B complex vitamin that acts as a coenzyme in fatty acid production and in the oxidation of fatty acids and carbohydrates. It also aids in the use of protein, folic acid, pantothenic acid, and vitamin B_{12}. Rich sources are egg yolk, beef liver, kidney, unpolished rice, brewer's yeast, peanuts, cauliflower, and mushrooms. Also called **vitamin H.** See also **avidin.**

biotin deficiency syndrome, an abnormal condition caused by a deficiency of biotin, characterized by dermatitis, hyperesthesia, muscle pain, anorexia, slight anemia, and changes in electrocardiographic activity of the heart. The average daily requirement of biotin for an adult is 100 to 200 [mu]g; the average American diet provides 100 to 300 [mu]g of the vitamin. Because biotin is synthesized by intestinal bacteria, naturally occurring deficiency disease is unknown, although it can be induced by large quantities of raw egg whites in the diet. Symptoms include scaly dermatitis, grayish pallor, extreme lassitude, anorexia, muscle pains, insomnia, some precordial distress, and slight anemia. Some authorities consider seborrheic dermatitis in infants a form of biotin deficiency.

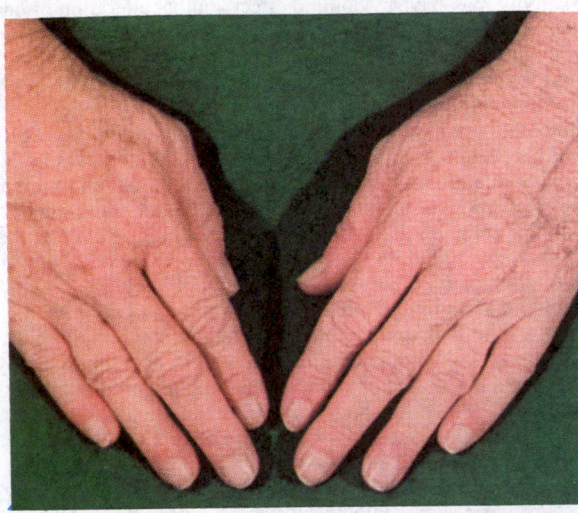

Scaly dermatitis resulting from biotin deficiency
(McLaren, 1992/Courtesy Dr. CE Butterworth Jr)

biotope /bī′ətōp/ [Gk, *bios* + *topos,* place], a specific biologic habitat or site.

biotransformation /-trans′fôrmā′shən/ [Gk, *bios* + L, *trans* across, *formare,* to form], the chemical changes a substance undergoes in the body, such as by the action of enzymes. See also **metabolic.**

Biot's respiration /bē·ōz′/ [Camille Biot, French physician, b. 1878], an abnormal respiratory pattern, characterized by irregular breathing with periods of apnea. The breathing may be slow and deep or rapid and shallow and is often accompanied by sighing. Biot's respiration is symptomatic of meningitis or increased intracranial pressure.

biovular twins. See **dizygotic twins.**

bipara /bip′ərə/, a woman who has given birth twice in separate pregnancies.

biparental inheritance. See **amphigenous inheritance.**

biparietal /bīpərī′ətəl/ [L, *bis,* twice, *paries,* wall], of or pertaining to the two parietal bones of the head, such as the biparietal diameter.

biparietal diameter, the distance between the protuberances of the two parietal bones of the skull.

biparietal suture [L, *bis, paries,* wall + *sutura*], the interlocking lines of fusion between two parietal bones of the skull.

biparous [L, *bis,* twice, *parere* to produce], pertaining to the birth of two infants in separate pregnancies.

bipartite /bīpär′tīt/, having two parts.

biped /bī′ped/, **1.** having two feet. **2.** any animal with only two feet.

bipedal /bīpē′əl, -ped′əl/ [L, *bis,* twice, *pes,* foot], capable of locomotion on two feet.

bipenniform /bīpen′ifôrm′/ [L, *bis* + *penna,* feather, *forma,* form], (of bodily structure) having the bilateral symmetry of a feather, such as the pattern formed by the fasciculi that converge on both sides of a muscle tendon in the rectus femoris. Compare **multipenniform, penniform, radiate.**

biperiden /bīper′idən/, a synthetic anticholinergic agent.
■ INDICATIONS: It is prescribed in the treatment of Parkinson's disease and drug-induced extrapyramidal disorders. Biperiden hydrochloride is administered orally, and biperiden lactate is administered intramuscularly or intravenously.
■ CONTRAINDICATIONS: Narrow-angle glaucoma, asthma, obstruction of the genitourinary or GI tract, or known hypersensitivity to this drug prohibits its use.
■ ADVERSE EFFECTS: Among the more serious adverse reactions are blurred vision, central nervous system effects, tachycardia, dry mouth, decreased sweating, and hypersensitivity reactions.

biphasic /bīfā′zik/ [L, *bis* + Gk, *phasis*, appearance], having two phases, parts, aspects, or stages.

bipolar /bīpō′lər/ [L, *bis* + *polus*, pole], **1.** having two poles, such as in certain electrotherapeutic treatments using two poles or in certain bacterial staining that affects only the two poles of the microorganism under study. **2.** (of a nerve cell) having an afferent and an efferent process.

bipolar disorder, a major psychologic disorder characterized by episodes of mania, depression, or mixed mood. One or the other phase may be predominant at any given time, one phase may appear alternately with the other, or elements of both phases may be present simultaneously. Characteristics of the manic phase are excessive emotional displays, excitement, euphoria, hyperactivity accompanied by elation, boisterousness, impaired ability to concentrate, decreased need for sleep, and seemingly unbounded energy, often accompanied by delusions of grandeur. In the depressive phase, marked apathy and underactivity are accompanied by feelings of profound sadness, loneliness, guilt, and lowered self-esteem. Causes of the disorder are multiple and complex, often involving biologic, psychologic, interpersonal, and social and cultural factors. Treatment includes lithium, carbamezapine, valproic acid, antipsychotic medication, antidepressants, tranquilizers and antianxiety drugs, or the use of electroconvulsive therapy for persons who present an immediate and serious risk of suicide, followed by long-term psychotherapy. Careful nursing observation is important during depression, particularly during the recovery from depression, because of the possibility of suicide. See also **major depressive disorder.**

bipolar lead /lēd/, **1.** an electrocardiographic conductor having two electrodes placed on different body regions, with each electrode contributing significantly to the record. **2.** *informal.* a tracing produced by such a lead on an electrocardiograph.

bipotentiality /bī′pəten′shē·al′itē/ [L, *bis* + *potentia*, power], the characteristic of acting or reacting according to either of two potentials.

bird breeder's lung. See **pigeon breeder's lung.**

bird face retrognathism, an abnormal facial profile with an underdeveloped mandible, which may be caused by interference of condylar growth associated with trauma or condylar infection. See also **prognathism.**

bird headed dwarf, a person affected with Seckel's syndrome, a congenital disorder characterized by a proportionate shortness of stature; a proportionally small head with hypoplasia of the jaws, large eyes, and a beaklike protru-

sion of the nose; mental retardation; and various other skeletal, cutaneous, and genital defects. Also called **nanocephalic dwarf.**

birth [ME, *burth*], **1.** the event of being born, the coming of a new person out of its mother into the world. Kinds of birth are **breech birth, live birth,** and **stillbirth.** See also **effacement, labor. 2.** the child-bearing event, the bringing forth by a mother of a baby. **3.** a medical event, the delivery of a fetus by an obstetric attendant.

birth canal, *informal.* the passage that extends from the inlet of the true pelvis to the vaginal orifice through which an infant passes during vaginal birth. See also **clinical pelvimetry.**

birth control. See **contraception.**

birth defect. See **congenital anomaly.**

birthing chair, a chair used in labor and delivery to promote the comfort of the mother and the efficiency of parturition. The chair may be specially designed, having many technical features, or it may be a simple three-legged stool with a high, slanted back and a circular seat with a large central hole in it. The newer birthing chairs allow woman to sit straight up or to recline. The chair has a lower section that may be removed or folded out of the way. Lights, mirrors, and basins may be attached for the attendant's convenience. The upright position appears to shorten the time in labor, particularly the second or expulsive stage of labor, probably because of gravity and increased participation of the mother. The chair is not suitable for use with anesthesia.

birth injury, trauma suffered by a baby while being born. Some kinds of birth injury are **Bell's palsy, cerebral palsy,** and **Erb's palsy.**

birthmark. See **nevus.**

birth mother, The biologic mother or woman who bears a child. The child may have been conceived in a surrogate mother with sperm of the biologic father.

birth palsy [ME, *burth;* Gk, *paralyein,* to be palsied], a loss of motor or sensory nerve function in some part of the body because of a nerve injury during the birth process.

birth paralysis [ME, *burth;* Gk, *paralyein,* to be palsied], paralysis, usually of an arm, caused by a brachial plexus injury during the birth process.

birth parents, the biologic parents, or the combined source of the entire genetic information of a child.

birth rate, the proportion of the number of births in a specific area during a given period to the total population of that area, usually expressed as the number of births per 1000 of population. Compare **crude birth rate, refined birth rate, true birth rate.**

birth trauma, 1. any physical injury suffered by an infant during the process of delivery. **2.** the supposed psychic shock, according to some psychiatric theories, that an infant suffers during delivery.

birth weight, the measured heaviness of a baby when born, usually about 3500 g (7.5 pounds). In the United States, 97% of newborns weigh between 2500 g (5.5 pounds) and 4500 g (10 pounds). Babies weighing less than 2500 g at term are considered **small for gestational age.** Babies weighing more than 4500 g are considered **large for gestational age** and are often infants of mothers with diabetes.

bis-, a prefix meaning 'twice, two': *bisacromial, bisaxillary, bisferious.* See also *bi-.*

bisacodyl /bisak′ōdil/, a cathartic.

■ INDICATIONS: It is prescribed in the treatment of acute or chronic constipation, to empty the bowel pre- or postoperatively or before diagnostic radiographic procedures.

■ CONTRAINDICATIONS: Abdominal pain, nausea, vomiting, rectal fissures, ulcerated hemorrhoids, or known hypersensitivity to this drug prohibits its use.

■ ADVERSE EFFECTS: Among the more serious adverse reactions are colic, abdominal pain, and diarrhea.

bisect /bīsekt′/ [L, bis + secare, to cut], to divide into two equal lengths or parts.

bisexual /bīsek′shoo·əl/ [L, bis + sexus, male or female], **1.** hermaphroditic; having gonads of both sexes. **2.** possessing physical or psychologic characteristics of both sexes. **3.** engaging in both heterosexual and homosexual activity. **4.** desiring sexual contact with persons of both sexes.

bisexual libido, (in psychoanalysis) the tendency in a person to seek sexual gratification with people of either sex.

bisferial pulse /bisfer′ē·əs/ [L, bis + ferire, to beat], an arterial pulse that has two palpable peaks, the second of which is slightly weaker than the first. It may be detected in cases of aortic regurgitation and obstructive cardiomyopathy. Compare **dicrotic pulse.**

bishydroxycoumarin. See **dicumarol.**

bis in die (b.d., b.i.d.) /dē′ā/, a Latin phrase, used in prescriptions, meaning twice a day. It is more commonly used in its abbreviated form.

bismuth (Bi) /biz′məth, bis′-/ [Ger, wismut, white mass], a reddish, crystalline, trivalent metallic element. Its atomic number is 83; its atomic weight is 209. It is combined with various other elements, such as oxygen, to produce numerous salts used in the manufacture of many pharmaceutic substances.

bismuth gingivitis, a symptom of metallic poisoning caused by bismuth administered in the treatment of systemic disease. It is characterized by a dark bluish line along the gingival margin. See also **bismuth stomatitis, gingivitis.**

bismuth stomatitis, an abnormal oral condition caused by systemic use of bismuth compounds over prolonged periods, characterized by a blue-black line on the inner aspect of the gingival sulcus or pigmentation of the buccal mucosa, a sore tongue, metallic taste, and a burning sensation in the mouth. Compare **arsenic stomatitis, Atabrine stomatitis.**

bit /bit/, abbreviation for binary digit, a single digit of a binary number. See also **byte.**

bitart, abbreviation for a bitartrate carboxylate anion.

bite [AS, bitan], **1.** the act of cutting, tearing, holding, or gripping with the teeth. **2.** the lingual portion of an artificial tooth between its shoulder and incisal edge. **3.** an occlusal record or relationship of upper and lower teeth or jaws. Compare **closed bite, open bite.**

bite block. See **occlusion rim.**

bitegage /bīt′gāj′/ [AS, bitan + OFr, gauge measure], a prosthetic dental device that helps attain proper occlusion of the teeth rooted in the maxilla and the mandible.

biteguard [AS, bitan + OFr, garder, to defend], a resin appliance that covers the occlusal and incisal surfaces of the teeth. It is designed to stabilize the teeth and provide a platform for the excursive glides of the mandible. Also called **biteplane, night guard.**

biteguard splint, a device, usually made of resin, for covering the occlusal and incisal surfaces of the teeth and for protecting them from traumatic occlusal forces during immobilization and stabilization processes. See also **Gunning's splint.**

bitelock /bīt′lok′/, a dental device for retaining the occlusion rims in the same relation outside the mouth as inside the mouth.

bitemporal /bītem′pərəl/ [L, bis, twice, tempora, temples], of or pertaining to both temples or both temporal bones.

bitemporal hemianopia [L, bis, two, tempora, temples; Gk, hemi, half, opsis, vision], a loss of the temporal half of the vision in each eye, usually resulting from a lesion in the chiasmal area, such as pituitary tumors.

biteplane /bīt′plān/, **1.** a plane formed by the biting surfaces of the teeth. See **occlusal plane. 2.** a metal sheet laid across the biting surfaces of mandibular or maxillary teeth to determine the relationship of the teeth to this predetermined plane. **3.** an orthodontic appliance of acrylic resin worn over the maxillary occlusal surfaces and used to treat pain of the temporomandibular joint and adjacent muscles. Although removable, the device is kept in place by labial wires and wrought wire clasps.

biteplate /bīt′plāt/, a device used in dentistry as a diagnostic or a therapeutic aid for prosthodontics or for orthodontics. It is fabricated of wire and plastic and worn in the palate. It may also be used to correct temperomandibular joint problems or as a splint in restoring the full mouth.

bite reflex, a swift, involuntary biting action that may be triggered by stimulation of the oral cavity. The bite can be difficult to release in some cases, such as when a spoon or tongue depressor is placed in a patient's mouth.

bite wing film [AS, bitan + ME, winge], a type of dental x-ray film that has a central tab or wing on which the teeth close to maintain film position during radiographic examination. Also called **interproximal film.**

bite wing radiograph, a kind of dental radiograph that reveals approximately the coronal portions of maxillary and mandibular teeth and portions of the interdental septa on the same film. See also **occlusal radiograph.**

bithionol (TBP) /bithī′ənôl/, a pale gray powder, soluble in acetone, alcohol, or ether, used as a local antiseptic and administered orally in the treatment of infestations of the giant liver fluke (Fasciola gigantica hepatica) and of the lung fluke (Paragonimus westermani), which cause parasitic hemoptysis in Asiatic countries.

Bithynia /bəthin′ē·ə/, a genus of snails, species of which act as intermediate hosts to *Opisthorchis*.

biting in childhood, a natural behavior trait and reflex action in infants, acquired at about 5 to 6 months of age in response to the introduction of solid foods in the diet and the beginning of the teething process. The activity represents a significant modality in the psychosocial development of the child, because it is the first aggressive action the infant learns, and through it the infant learns to control the environment. The behavior also confronts the infant with one of the first inner conflicts, because biting can produce both pleasing and displeasing results. Biting during breast-feeding causes withdrawal of the nipple and anxiety in the mother, yet it also serves as a means of soothing teething discomfort. Infants continue to use biting as a mechanism for exploring their surroundings. Toddlers and older children often use biting for expressing aggression toward their parents and other children, especially during play or as a means of gaining attention. Most children normally outgrow the tendency unless severe maladaptive or emotional problems are present. See also **psychosexual development, psychosocial development.**

bitolterol mesylate /bitol′tərol mes′ilāt/, an orally inhaled bronchodilator.

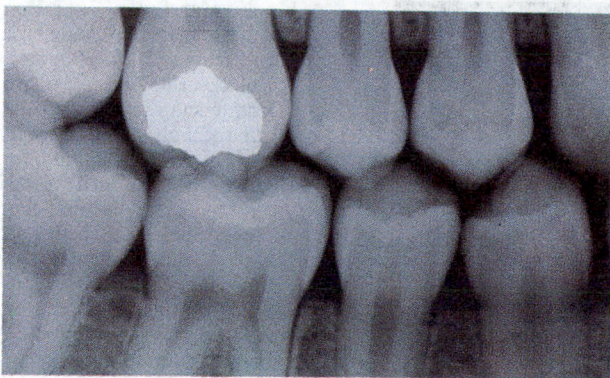

Bite wing radiograph (Jordan, 1993)

■ INDICATIONS: It is used in the treatment of bronchial asthma and reversible bronchospasm.

■ CONTRAINDICATIONS: This product is contraindicated in patients who are sensitive to bitolterol mesylate.

■ ADVERSE EFFECTS: Among adverse reactions reported are tremor, nervousness, headache, dizziness, palpitations, chest discomfort, tachycardia, coughing, and throat irritation.

Bitot's spots /bitōz'/ [Pierre Bitot, French surgeon, b. 1822], white or gray triangular deposits on the bulbar conjunctiva adjacent to the lateral margin of the cornea, a clinical sign of vitamin A deficiency. Also called **Bitot's patches.**

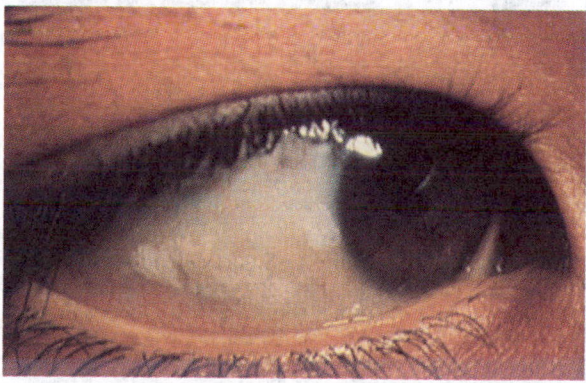

Bitot's spots (McLaren, 1992)

bitrochanteric lipodystrophy /bī'trōkənter'ik/ [L, *bis* + Gk, *trochanter*, runner; *lipos*, fat, *dys*, bad, *trophe*, nourishment], an abnormal and excessive deposition of fat on the buttocks and the outer aspect of the upper thighs, occurring most commonly in women. See also **lipodystrophy.**

biuret test /bī'yŏŏret/ [L, *bis* + Gk, *ouron*, urine], a method for detecting urea and other soluble proteins in serum. In alkaline solution, copper sulfate ions react with the peptide bonds of proteins to produce a purple color, called the biuret reaction. The amount of serum protein in a sample solution is estimated by comparing its color with that of a standard solution whose protein concentration is known.

bivalent /bīvā'lənt/ [L, *bis* + *valere*, to be powerful], 1. also **divalent.** (in genetics) a pair of synapsed homologous chromosomes that are attached to each other by chiasmata during the early first meiotic prophase of gametogenesis. The structure serves as the basis for the tetrads from which gametes are produced during the two meiotic divisions. 2. See **valence,** def. 1. – **bivalence,** *n.*

bivalent chromosome, a pair of synapsed homologous chromosomes during the early stages of gametogenesis. See also **bivalent.**

bivalve cast [L, *bis* + *valva*, valve], an orthopedic cast used for immobilizing a section of the body for the healing of one or more broken bones or for correcting or maintaining correction of an orthopedic deformity. The cast is cut in half to detect or relieve pressure under the cast, especially with a patient who has decreased sensation or who has no sensation in the portion of the body surrounded by the cast. If dangerous pressure areas are detected, "windows" are often cut out of the cast over the pressure areas to relieve the problem.

bizarre leiomyoma. See **epithelioid leiomyoma.**

BK, abbreviation for *below the knee,* a term referring to amputations, amputees, prostheses, and orthoses.

Bk, symbol for the element **berkelium.**

BL, abbreviation for **baralyme.**

black beauties, *slang,* amphetamines.

black damp. See **damp.**

black death. See **bubonic plague.**

Blackett-Healy method, a procedure for positioning a patient for making radiographs of the subscapularis area. It involves placing the patient in a supine position with the affected shoulder joint centered to the midline of the film, the arm abducted, and the elbow flexed. The opposite shoulder is raised about 15 degrees and supported with a sandbag.

black eye, an eyelid contusion with bruising, discoloration, and swelling. It is usually treated for the first 24 hours with ice packs to reduce swelling, then treated with hot compresses to aid in resorption of blood from the hematoma. (See Fig. p. 196.)

black fever. See **kala-azar.**

black hairy tongue [AS, *blac* + *haer* + *tunge*], a black or brown patch on the back of the tongue accompanied by filiform papillae. The condition is associated with heavy smoking or the use of broad-spectrum antibiotics. See also **parasitic glossitis.** (See Fig. p. 196.)

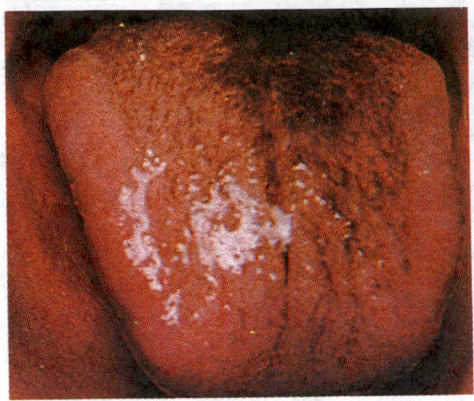

Black hairy tongue *(Bingham, 1992)*

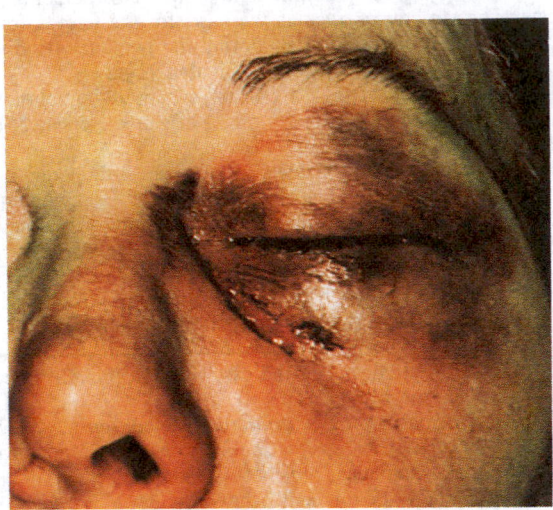

Black eye *(Bedford, 1986)*

blackhead. See **comedo.**

black light. See **Wood's light.**

black lung disease. See **anthracosis, pneumoconiosis.**

black measles [AS, *blac*; OHG, *masala*], hemorrhagic measles characterized by a darkened rash caused by bleeding into the skin and mucous membranes. Also called **hemorrhagic measles.**

blackout, informal. a temporary loss of vision or consciousness.

black plague. See **bubonic plague.**

Black's Classification of Caries. See **classification of caries.**

black spots film fault, a defect in a radiograph, seen as dark spots throughout the image area. It is caused by dust particles or developer on the x-ray film before development or by outdated film.

black tongue. See **parasitic glossitis.**

blackwater fever, a serious complication of chronic falciparum malaria, characterized by jaundice, hemoglobinuria, acute renal failure, and the passage of bloody dark red or black urine because of massive intravascular hemolysis. Death occurs in 20% to 30% of all cases; mortality is particularly high among Europeans. See also **falciparum malaria, malaria,** *Plasmodium.*

Blackwell, Elizabeth (1821–1910), a British-born American physician, the first woman to be awarded a medical degree. She established the New York Infirmary, a 40-bed hospital staffed entirely by women, in which she trained nurses in a 4-month course. Her influence helped others establish nursing schools to improve patient care.

black widow spider [AS, *blac, widewe*], a poisonous arachnid found in many parts of the world. The venom injected with its bite causes perspiration, abdominal cramps, nausea, headaches, and dizziness of various levels of intensity. Small children, old people, or persons with heart conditions are most severely affected and may require hospitalization and the administration of an antivenin.

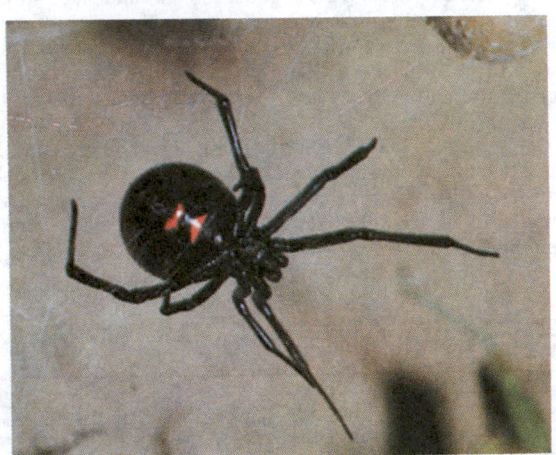

Black widow spider *(Judd, 1988)*

black widow spider bite [AS, *blac + widewe*; ME, *spithre;* AS, *bitan*], the bite of the spider species *Lactrodectus mactans,* causing generalized spastic contractions and localized tissue necrosis. Black widow venom contains some enzymatic proteins, including a peptide that affects neuromuscular transmission. The bite is perceived as a sharp pinprick pain, followed by a dull pain in the area of the bite, muscular rigidity in the shoulders, back, and abdomen, restlessness, anxiety, sweating, weakness, and drooping eyelids.

black widow spider antivenin, a passive immunizing agent.

■ INDICATION: It is prescribed in the treatment of black widow spider bite.

■ CONTRAINDICATIONS: Known hypersensitivity to this drug or to horse serum prohibits its use.

■ ADVERSE EFFECTS: Among the more serious adverse effects are allergic reactions.

bladder [AS, *blaedre*], **1.** a membranous sac serving as a receptacle for secretions. **2.** the urinary bladder.

bladder cancer, the most common malignancy of the urinary tract, characterized by multiple growths that tend to recur in a more aggressive form. Bladder cancer occurs 2.3 times more often in men than in women, is more prevalent in urban than in rural areas. The risk of bladder cancer is increased with cigarette smoking and exposure to aniline dyes, beta-naphthylamine, mixtures of aromatic hydrocarbons, or benzidine and its salts, used in chemical, paint, plastics, rubber, textile, petroleum, wood industries, and in medical laboratories. Other predisposing factors are chronic urinary tract infections, calculous disease, and schistosomiasis. Early symptoms of bladder cancer include hematuria, frequent urination, dysuria, and cystitis. Urinalysis, excretory urography, cystoscopy, or transurethral biopsy are performed for diagnosis. The majority of bladder malignancies are transitional cell carcinomas; a small percentage are squamous cell carcinomas or adenocarcinomas. Superficial or multiple lesions may be treated by fulguration or open loop resection. A segmental resection is usually performed if the tumor is at the dome or in a lateral wall of the bladder. Total cystectomy may be performed for an invasive lesion of the trigone. In patients requiring cystectomy, a conduit is constructed to divert urine to the colon, to a rectal bladder, or to an abdominal stoma. External radiation may be administered preoperatively or as palliation for inoperable lesions. Internal radiation, the introduction of radioisotopes via a balloon of a catheter, or the implantation of radon seeds may be used in treating small localized tumors on the bladder wall. Medications that are often used as palliatives are BCG, 5-fluorouracil, and adriamycin. See also **cystectomy.**

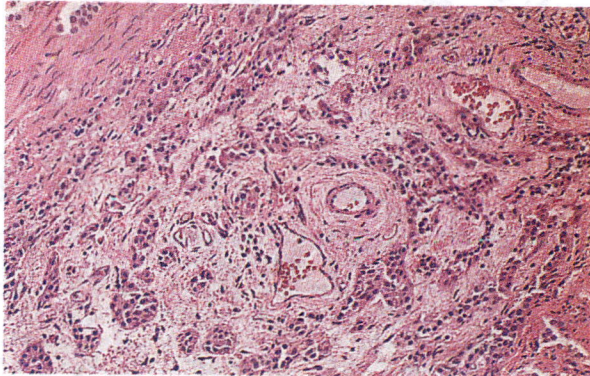

Transitional cell carcinoma, common in bladder cancer
(Weiss, 1988)

bladder flap, *informal.* the vesicouterine fold of peritoneum that is incised during low cervical cesarean section so that the bladder can be separated from the uterus to expose the lower uterine segment for incision. The flap is reapproximated with sutures during closure to cover the uterine incision. See also **cesarean section.**

bladder irrigation [AS, *blaedre*; L, *irrigare,* to conduct water], the washing out of the bladder by a continuous or intermittent flow of water or a medicated solution. The bladder also may be irrigated by an oral intake of fluid.

bladder retraining [AS, *blaedre*; L, *trahere,* to draw], a system of therapy for incontinence in which a patient, in a hospital setting, practices withholding urine for intervals that begin with 1 hour and increase over a period of 10 days while maintaining a normal intake of fluid. The patient also learns to recognize and react to the urge to void.

bladder sphincter [AS, *blaedre*; Gk, *sphigkter,* one that binds], a circular muscle surrounding the opening of the urinary bladder into the urethra.

bladder stone. See **vesicle calculus.**

Blakemore-Sengstaken tube. See **Sengstaken-Blakemore tube.**

Blalock-Taussig procedure /blā′loktô′sig/ [Alfred Blalock, American surgeon, b. 1899; Helen B. Taussig, American physician, b. 1898], surgical construction of a shunt as a temporary measure to overcome congenital pulmonary stenosis and atrial septal defect, as in an infant born with tetralogy of Fallot. Preoperatively, a cardiac catheterization is done to identify the defect or defects, and the levels of arterial blood gases are analyzed. Hypothermia anesthesia and a cardiac bypass machine are used. The subclavian artery is joined end to end with the pulmonary artery, directing blood from the systemic circulation to the lungs. Thrombosis of the shunt is the major postoperative complication. Nursing care includes giving humidified oxygen, monitoring fluids and electrolytes, maintaining the IV, and giving nasogastric feedings. Restlessness may signal a lack of oxygen or a low cardiac output. Permanent surgical correction is performed in early childhood. See also **heart surgery.**

blame placing, the process of placing responsibility for one's behavior on others.

blanch /blanch, blänch/ [Fr, *blanchir,* to become white], **1.** to cause to become pale, as a spider angiomata may be blanched using digital pressure. **2.** to whiten or bleach a surface or substance. **3.** to become white or pale, as from vasoconstriction accompanying fear or anger.

blanch test [Fr, *blanchir,* to become white; L, *testum,* crucible], a test of blood circulation in the fingers or toes. Pressure is applied to the nail over a finger or toe until normal color is lost. The pressure is then removed, and, if the circulation is normal, color will return within about five seconds. Also called **blanching test, capillary refill.**

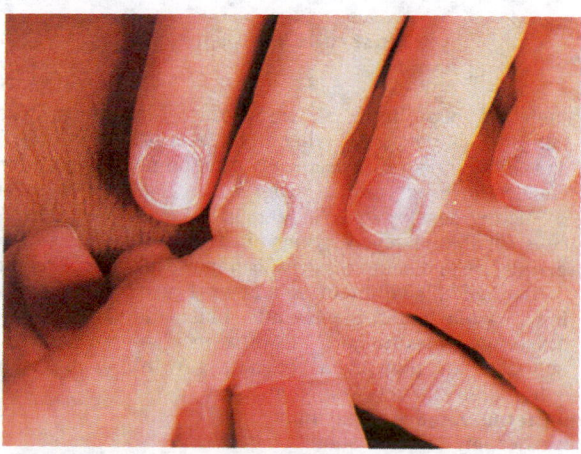

Blanch test *(Judd, 1988)*

bland [L *blandus*],   mild or having a soothing effect.

bland aerosols,   aerosols that consist of water, saline solutions, or similar substances that lack important pharmacologic action. They are primarily used for humidification and liquefaction of secretions.

bland diet,   a diet that is mechanically, chemically, physiologically, and sometimes thermally nonirritating. It is often prescribed in the treatment of peptic ulcer, ulcerative colitis, gallbladder disease, diverticulitis, gastritis, idiopathic spastic constipation, and mucous colitis and after abdominal surgery. The diet may include eggs, meat, poultry, fish, and enriched fine cereals; milk is usually an important ingredient. A bland diet may be planned that includes or excludes any specific foods. Spicy or highly seasoned foods, carbonated beverages, raw fruits and vegetables, and rich desserts are avoided.

blanket bath [OFr, *blanchet*, a white garment],   the procedure of wrapping the patient in a wet pack and then in blankets.

-blast,   a suffix meaning an 'embryonic state of development': *leucoblast, megaloblast, osteoblast.*

blast cell [Gk *blastos* germ],   any immature cell, such as an erythroblast, a lymphoblast, or a neuroblast.

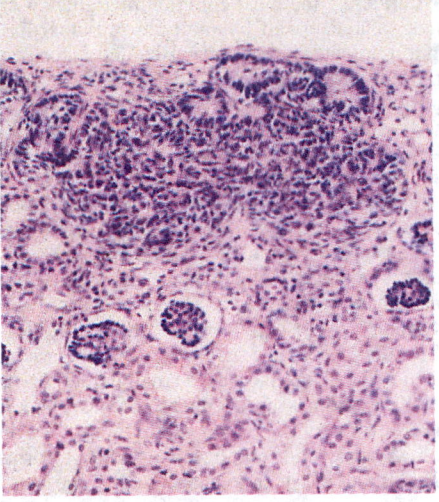

Renal blastema (*Weiss, 1988*)

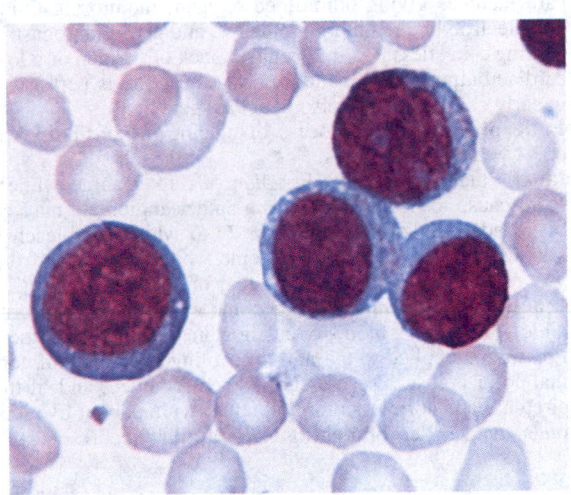

Blast cells (*Hayhoe, 1992*)

blastema /blastē′mə/, *pl.* **blastemas, blastemata** [Gk, bud],   **1.** any mass of living protoplasm capable of growth and differentiation, specifically the primordial undifferentiated cellular material from which a particular organ or tissue develops. **2.** in certain animals, a group of cells capable of regenerating a lost or damaged part or of giving rise to a complete organism in asexual reproduction. **3.** the budding or sprouting area of a plant. See also **anlage. –blastemal, blastematic, blastemic,** *adj.*

-blastema /-blas′rtəmə/,   a suffix meaning a 'beginning substance or foundation for new growth': *epiblastema, scleroblastema, scytoblastema.*

blastemata. See **blastema.**

-blastemal. See **blastema.**

-blastematic. See **blastema.**

-blastemic. See **blastema.**

blastic transformation,   a late stage in the progress of chronic granulocytic leukemia; the leukemic cells become more undifferentiated and morphologically and genetically more abnormal, with more aggressive growth patterns. There are signs of anemia and blood platelet deficiency, and half of the blood cells in the bone marrow are immature forms. Blastic transformation indicates that the patient has developed resistance to therapy and has entered a terminal stage of leukemia.

blastid /blas′tid/ [Gk, *blastos*, germ],   the site in the fertilized ovum where the pronuclei fuse and the nucleus forms. Also called **blastide.**

blastin /blas′tin/ [Gk, *blastanein*, to grow],   any substance that provides nourishment for or stimulates the growth or proliferation of cells, such as allantoin.

blasto-,   a combining form meaning 'pertaining to an early embryonic or developing stage': *blastocele, blastocytoma, blastomatosis.*

blastocoele /blas′təsēl′/ [Gk, *blastos*, germ, *koilos*, hollow],   the fluid-filled cavity of the blastocyst in mammals and the blastula or discoblastula of lower animals. The cavity increases the surface area of the developing embryo for better absorption of nutrients and oxygen. Also spelled **blastocoel, blastocele.** Also called **cleavage cavity, segmentation cavity, subgerminal cavity.**

blastocyst /blas′təsist/ [Gk, *blastos* + *kystis*, bag],   the embryonic form that follows the morula in human development. It is a spheric mass of cells having a central, fluid-filled cavity (blastocele) surrounded by two layers of cells. The outer layer (trophoblast) later forms the placenta; the inner layer (embryoblast) later forms the embryo. Implantation in the wall of the uterus usually occurs at this stage, on approximately the eighth day after fertilization.

blastocyte /blas′təsīt/ [Gk, *blastos* + *kytos*, cell],   an undifferentiated embryonic cell before germ layer formation. **–blastocytic,** *adj.*

blastocytoma. See **blastoma.**

blastoderm /blas′tədurm′/ [Gk, *blastos* + *derma*, skin],   the layer of cells forming the wall of the blastocyst in mammals and the blastula in lower animals during the early stages of embryonic development. It is produced by the

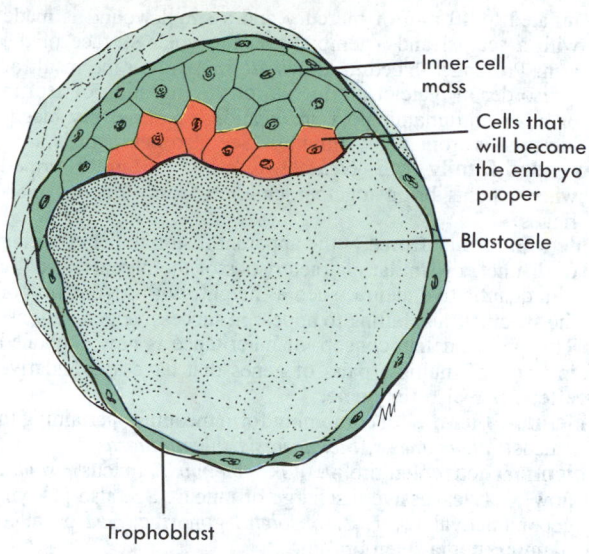

Blastocyst (Seeley, 1992)

Inner cell mass

Cells that will become the embryo proper

Blastocele

Trophoblast

cleavage of the fertilized ovum and gives rise to the primary germ layers, the ectoderm, mesoderm, and endoderm from which the embryo and all of its membranes are derived. In animals in which the ovum contains a large amount of yolk and undergoes partial cleavage, the cells form a small caplike structure, or cellular disk, above the yolk mass. Kinds of blastoderm are **bilaminar blastoderm, embryonic blastoderm, extraembryonic blastoderm,** and **trilaminar blastoderm.** Also called **germinal membrane.** –**blastodermal, blastodermic,** *adj.*

blastodisk /blas'tədisk/, the disklike nonyolk area of the protoplasm surrounding the animal pole where cleavage occurs in a fertilized ovum containing a large amount of yolk, as in birds and reptiles. As cleavage continues, the blastomeres form a convex structure, the blastula, which eventually develops into the embryo. Also spelled **blastodisc.**

blastogenesis /blas'tōjen'əsis/ [Gk, *blastos* + *genein*, to produce], **1.** asexual reproduction by budding. **2.** the theory of the transmission of hereditary characteristics by the germ plasm, as opposed to the theory of pangenesis. **3.** the early development of the embryo during cleavage and formation of the germ layers. **4.** the process of transforming small lymphocytes in tissue culture into large blastlike cells by exposure to phytohemagglutin or other substances, often for the purpose of inducing mitosis. –**blastogenetic,** *adj.*

blastogenic /-jen'ik/, **1.** originating in the germ plasm. **2.** initiating tissue proliferation. **3.** relating to or characterized by blastogenesis.

blastogeny /blastoj'ənē/, the early stages in ontogeny; the germ plasm history of an organism or species, which traces the history of the inherited characteristics.

blastokinin /blas'təkī'nin/ [Gk, *blastos* + *kinein,* to move], a globulin, secreted by the uterus in many mammals, that may stimulate and regulate the implantation process of the blastocyst in the uterine wall. Also called **uteroglobulin.**

blastolysis /blastol'isis/ [Gk, *blastos* + *lysis,* loosening], destruction of a germ cell or blastoderm. –**blastolytic,** *adj.*

blastoma /blastō'mə/, *pl.* **blastomas, blastomata** [Gk, *blastos* + *oma,* tumor], a neoplasm of embryonic tissue developing from the blastema of an organ or tissue. A blastoma derived from a number of scattered cells is pluricentric, and one arising from a single cell or group of cells is unicentric. Also called **blastocytoma.** –**blastomatous** /blastom'ətəs/, *adj.*

blastomatosis /blast'tōmətō'sis/ [Gk, *blastos* + *oma,* tumor, *osis* condition], the development of many tumors derived from embryonic tissue.

–blastomatous. See **blastoma.**

blastomere /blas'təmēr/ [Gk, *blastos* + *meros,* part], one of a pair of cells that develops in the first mitotic division of the segmentation nucleus of a fertilized ovum. The two blastomeres divide and subdivide to form the morula in the first several days of pregnancy. –**blastomeric,** *adj.*

blastomerotomy /-merot'əmē/ [Gk, *blastos* + *meros,* part, *tome* cut], the destruction or the separation of blastomeres, either caused naturally or induced artificially. Also called **blastotomy** /blastot'əmē/. –**blastomerotomic,** *adj.*

Blastomyces /blas'tōmī'sēz/ [Gk, *blastos* + *mykes,* fungus], a genus of yeastlike fungus, usually including the species *Blastomyces dermatitidis,* which causes North American blastomycosis, and *Paracoccidioides brasiliensis,* which causes South American blastomycosis.

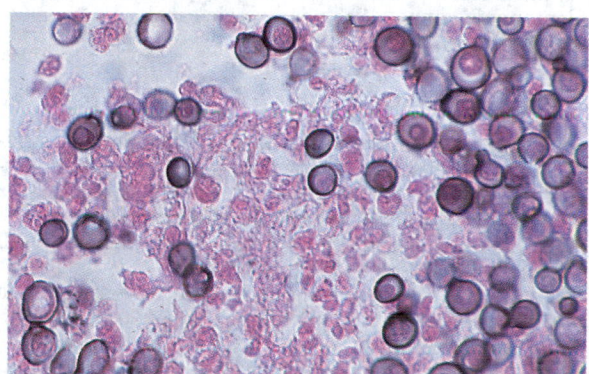

Blastomyces dermatitides (Baron, 1990)

blastomycosis /blas'tōmīkō'sis/ [Gk, *blastos* + *mykes,* fungus, *osis,* condition], an infectious disease caused by a yeastlike fungus, *Blastomyces dermatitidis,* that usually affects only the skin but may invade the lungs, kidneys, central nervous system, and bones. The disease is most common in young men living in North America, particularly the southeastern United States, but outbreaks have occurred in Africa and Latin America. Skin infections are almost always a result of hematogenous seeding from a primary infection and often begin as small papules on the hand, face, neck, or other exposed areas where there has been a cut, bruise, or other injury. The infection may spread gradually and irregularly into surrounding areas. When the lungs are involved, x-ray films of the chest show tumors resembling cancer. The person usually has a cough, dyspnea, chest pain, chills, and a fever with heavy sweating. Diagnosis is made by identification of the disease organism in a culture of specimens from lesions. Treatment usually involves the administration of amphotericin B in pulmonary disease or

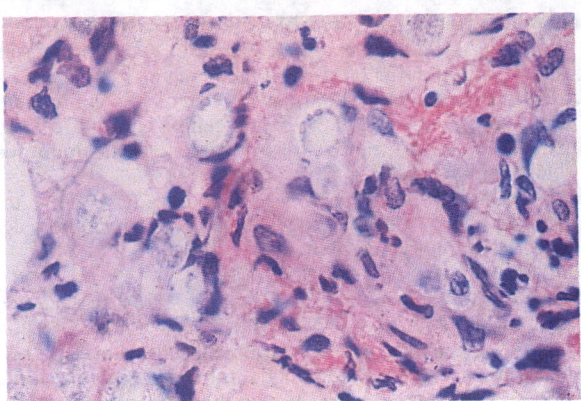

Blastomycosis (Ioachim, 1989)

ketoconazole or one of the newer triazole compounds, fluconazole or intraconazole. Recovery usually begins within the first week of treatment. Also called **Gilchrist's disease.** See also **fungus, mycosis.**

blastopore /blas′təpôr/ [Gk, *blastos* + *poros*, opening], (in embryology) the invagination into a blastula that occurs in the process of the blastula becoming a gastrula.

blastoporic canal. See **neurenteric canal.**

blastosphere. See **blastula.**

blastotomy. See **blastomerotomy.**

blastula /blas′tyələ/ [Gk, *blastos,* germ], an early stage of the process through which a zygote develops into an embryo, characterized by a fluid-filled sphere formed by a single layer of cells. The spheric layer of cells is called a blastoderm, and the fluid-filled cavity is the blastocoele. The blastula develops from the morula stage and is usually the form in which the embryo becomes implanted in the wall of the uterus. Also called **blastosphere.**

-blastula, a suffix meaning an 'early embryonic stage in the development of a fertilized egg': *coeloblastula, diblastula, steroblastula.*

blastulation, the transformation of the morula into a blastocyst or blastula by the development of a central cavity, the blastocoele.

BLB mask, abbreviation for **Boothby-Lovelace-Bulbulian mask.**

bleb /bleb/ [ME, blob], an accumulation of fluid under the skin.

bleed [AS, *blod*, blood], **1.** to lose blood from the blood vessels of the body. The blood may flow externally through an orifice or a break in the skin or flow internally into a cavity, into an organ, or between tissues. The color, quantity, and source of blood are noted. **2.** to cause blood to flow from a vein or an artery.

bleeder, *informal.* **1.** a person who has hemophilia or any other vascular or hematologic condition associated with a tendency to hemorrhage. **2.** blood vessel that bleeds, especially one cut during a surgical procedure.

bleeding, the release of blood from the vascular system as a result of damage to a blood vessel. See also **blood clotting.**

bleeding diasthesis, a predisposition to abnormal blood clotting.

bleeding time, the time required for blood to stop flowing from a tiny wound. A test of bleeding time is the Ivy method, in which a blood pressure cuff on the upper arm is inflated to 40 mm of mercury and a small wound is made with a scalpel and a template on the volar surface of the arm. Prolonged bleeding times are most often the result of a disorder of platelet production or the ingestion of aspirin or other antiinflammatory medications. Normal Ivy bleeding time is from 1 to 9 minutes. See also **hemostasis.**

blended family [ME, *blenden,* to mix], a family formed when parents bring together children from previous marriages.

blending inheritance, the apparent fusion in the offspring of distinct, dissimilar characteristics of the parents, usually of a quantitative nature, such as height, with segregation of the specific traits failing to appear in successive generations. This premendelian concept of inheritance is now explained in terms of multiple pairs of genes that have a cumulative effect. See also **polygene.**

blenno-, blenn-, a combining form meaning 'pertaining to mucus': *blennemesis, blennostasis, blennothorax.*

blennorrhea /blen′ərē′ə/ [Gk, *blennos,* mucus, *rhoia,* flow], **1.** excessive discharge of mucus. See also pharyngoconjunctival fever. **2.** *obsolete.* gonorrhea. Also called **blennorrhagia** /blen′ôrā′jē·ə/.

Blenoxane, a trademark for an antineoplastic (bleomycin sulfate).

bleomycin sulfate /blē·əmī′sin/, an antineoplastic antibiotic.

■ INDICATIONS: It is prescribed in the treatment of a variety of neoplasms.

■ CONTRAINDICATION: Hypersensitivity to this drug prohibits its use.

■ ADVERSE EFFECTS: Among the most serious adverse reactions are pneumonitis, pulmonary fibrosis, and a syndrome of hyperpyrexia and circulatory collapse. Rashes and skin reactions commonly occur.

blephar-. See **blepharo-.**

blepharal /blef′ərəl/ [Gk, *blepharon,* eyelid], of or pertaining to the eyelids.

-blepharia, a suffix meaning '(condition of the) eyelid': *ablepharia, atretoblepharia, macroblepharia.*

blepharitis /blef′ərī′tis/ [Gk, *blepharon* + *itis*], an inflammatory condition of the lash follicles and meibomian glands of the eyelids, characterized by swelling, redness, and crusts of dried mucus on the lids. **Ulcerative blepharitis** is caused

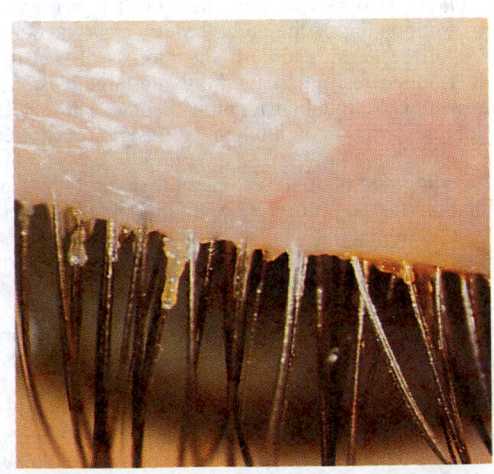

Blepharitis (Zitelli, 1992)

by bacterial infection. **Nonulcerative blepharitis** may be caused by psoriasis, seborrhea, or an allergic response.

blepharo-, blephar- /blef'ərō-/, a combining form meaning 'pertaining to the eyelid or eyelash': *blepharochalasis, blepharal, blepharelosis.*

blepharoadenoma /-ad'inō'mə/, *pl.* **blepharoadenomas, blepharoadenomata,** a glandular epithelial tumor of the eyelid.

blepharoatheroma /-ath'ərō'mə/, *pl.* **blepharoatheromas, blepharoatheromata,** a tumor of the eyelid.

blepharoncus /blef'ərōn'kəs/ [Gk, *blepharon* + *onkos* swelling], a tumor of the eyelid.

blepharoplasty /blef'əroplas'tē/ [Gk, *blepharon,* eyelid, *plassein,* to mold], the use of plastic surgery to restore or repair the eyelid and eyebrow.

blepharoplegia /-plē'jē·ə/ [Gk, *blepharon* + *plege,* stroke], paralysis of the eyelid.

blepharospasm /blef'ərōspaz'əm/ [Gk, *blepharon,* eyelid, *spasmos,* spasm], the involuntary contraction of eyelid muscles. The condition may be caused by a local lesion of the eye, a neurologic irritation, or psychologic stress.

blight, any disease of plants caused by fungus.

blighted ovum /blī'tid/, a fertilized ovum that fails to develop. On x-ray or ultrasonic visualization it appears to be a fluid-filled cyst attached to the wall of the uterus. It may be empty, or it may contain amorphous parts. Many first trimester spontaneous abortions represent the expulsion of a blighted ovum. Suction curettage may be necessary if the blighted ovum is retained.

blind [AS, *blind*], the absence of sight. The term may indicate a total loss of vision or may be applied in a modified manner to describe certain visual limitation, as in yellow color blindness (tritanopia) or word blindness (dyslexia).

blind fistula [AS, *blind;* L, pipe], an abnormal passage with only one open end; the opening may be on the body surface or on or within an internal organ or structure. Also called **incomplete fistula.**

blindgut. See **cecum.**

blind intubation. See **intubation.**

blind loop [AS, *blind;* ME, *loupe*], a redundant segment of intestine. Bacterial overgrowth occurs and may lead to malabsorption, obstruction, and necrosis. Blind loops may be created inadvertently by surgical procedures, such as side to side ileotransverse colostomy. See also **blind spot.**

blindness See **blind.**

blind spot, **1.** a normal gap in the visual field occurring when an image is focused on the space in the retina occupied by the optic disc. **2.** an abnormal gap in the visual field because of a lesion on the retina, or in the optic pathways, or because of hemorrhage or choroiditis, often perceived as light spots or flashes.

blink reflex [ME, *blenken;* L, *reflectere,* to bend back], the automatic closure of the eyelid when an object is perceived to be approaching the eye rapidly.

blister, a vesicle or bulla.

bloat [ME, *blout*], a swelling or filling with gas, such as the distention of the abdomen from swallowing air or from intestinal gas. The stomach on auscultation will have a tympany sound.

Blocadren, a trademark for a beta-adrenergic receptor blocking agent (timolol maleate).

blockade /blokād'/, an agent that interferes with or prevents a specific action in an organ or tissue, such as a cholinergic blockade that inhibits transmission of acetylcholine-stimulated nerve impulses along fibers of the autonomic nervous system.

block anesthesia. See **conduction anesthesia.**

blocked communication, a situation in which communication with a patient is difficult because of incongruent verbal and nonverbal messages and messages that contain discrepancies and inconsistencies. To clarify blocked communication, therapists may record meetings with patients on videotapes that can be studied for eye contact and other clues to the patient's thinking processes.

blocking [ME, *blok*], **1.** preventing the transmission of an impulse, such as by an antiadrenergic agent or by the injection of an anesthetic. **2.** interrupting an intracellular biosynthetic process, such as by the injection of actinomycin D or the action of an antivitamin. **3.** being unable to remember or involuntarily interrupting a train of thought or speech, usually because of emotional or mental conflict. **4.** repressing an idea or emotion to keep it from obtruding into the consciousness.

blocking antibody, an antibody that fails to cross-link and cause agglutination. When such antibodies are present in high concentration, they interfere with the action of other antibodies by occupying all the antigenic sites. See also **antigen-antibody reaction, hapten.**

blood [AS, *blod*], the liquid pumped by the heart through all the arteries, veins, and capillaries. The blood is composed of a clear yellow fluid, called plasma, and the formed elements, and a series of cell types with different functions. The major function of the blood is to transport oxygen and nutrients to the cells and to remove from the cells carbon dioxide and other waste products for detoxification and elimination. Adults normally have a total blood volume of 7% to 8% of body weight, or 70 mL/kg of body weight for men and about 65 mL/kg for women. Blood is pumped through the body at a speed of about 30 cm/second, with a complete circulation time of 20 seconds. Compare **lymph.** See also **blood cell, erythrocyte, leukocyte, plasma, platelet.**

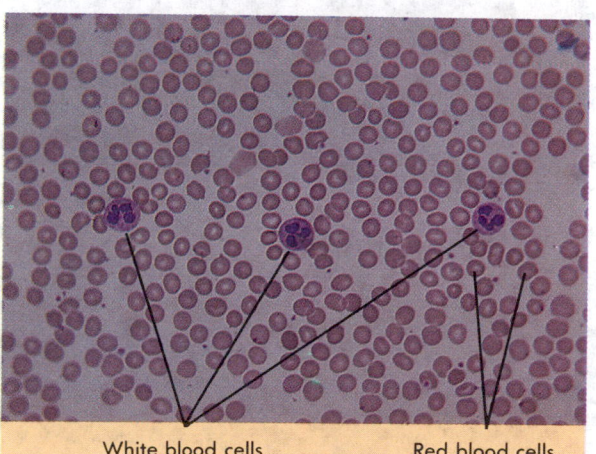

White blood cells   Red blood cells

Blood *(Seeley, 1992)*

blood agar, a culture medium consisting of blood and nutrient agar, used in bacteriology to cultivate certain microorganisms, including *Staphylococcus epidermidis, Diplococcus pneumoniae,* and *Clostridium perfringens.*

blood albumin [AS, *blod;* L, *albus*], the albumin circulating in blood serum. Also called **serum albumin.**

blood bank, an organizational unit responsible for collecting, processing, and storing blood for transfusion and other purposes. The blood bank is usually a subdivision of a laboratory in a hospital and is often charged with the responsibility for serologic testing. See also **bank blood, component therapy, transfusion.**

blood bank technology specialist an allied health professional who performs both routine and specialized tests in blood bank immunohematology in technical areas of the modern blood bank and who performs transfusion services using methodology that conforms to the *Standards for Blood Banks and Transfusion Services* of the American Association of Blood Banks. The individual may be responsible for testing for blood group antigens, compatibility, and antibody identification; investigating abnormalities such as hemolytic diseases of the newborn, hemolytic anemias, and adverse responses to transfusions; supporting physicians in transfusion therapy, including patients for homologous organ transplant; blood collection and processing, including selecting donors, drawing and typing blood, and performing pretransfusion tests to ensure the safety of the patient.

Blood borne pathogens pathogenic microorganisms that are present in human blood and cause disease in humans. They include, but are not limited to, Hepatitis B virus (HBV) and Human Immunodeficiency Virus (HIV).

blood-brain barrier (BBB) [AS, *blod; bragen;* ME *barrere*], an anatomic-physiologic feature of the brain thought to consist of walls of capillaries in the central nervous system and surrounding glial membranes. The barrier separates the parenchyma of the central nervous system from blood. The blood-brain barrier prevents or slows the passage of some drugs and other chemical compounds, radioactive ions, and disease-causing organisms such as viruses from the blood into the central nervous system.

oxide and bicarbonate ions, that functions in maintaining the proper pH of the blood. See also **buffer, pH.**

blood capillaries [AS, *blod;* L, *capillaris,* hairlike], the hairlike vessels that convey blood between the arterioles and the venules. The capillary wall generally has a thickness of one cell; occasional tiny openings permit the distribution of oxygen and nutrients to the tissues supplied by the capillary network and the collection of waste products released by the cells.

blood cell, any of the formed elements of the blood, including red cells (erythrocytes), white cells (leukocytes), and platelets (thrombocytes). Blood cells constitute about 50% of the total volume of the blood. See also **erythrocyte, leukocyte, platelet.**

blood cell casts [AS, *blod;* L, *cella,* storeroom, ONorse, *kasta*], a mass of blood debris released from a diseased body surface or excreted in the urine.

blood circulation [AS, *blod;* L, *circulare,* to go around], the circuit of blood through the body, from the heart through the arteries, arterioles, capillaries, venules, and veins and back to the heart.

blood clot [AS, *blod; clott,* lump], a semisolid, gelatinous mass, the end result of the clotting process in blood. Red cells, white cells, and platelets are enmeshed in an insoluble fibrin network of the blood clot. Compare **embolus, thrombus.** See also **blood clotting, fibrinogen.**

blood clotting, the conversion of blood from a free-flowing liquid to a semisolid gel. Although clotting can occur within an intact blood vessel, the process usually starts with tissue damage. Within seconds of injury to the vessel wall, platelets clump at the site. If normal amounts of calcium, platelets, and tissue factors are present, prothrombin will be converted to thrombin. Thrombin acts as a catalyst for the conversion of fibrinogen to a mesh of insoluble fibrin, in which all the formed elements are immobilized. Also called **blood coagulation.** Compare **hemostasis.** See also **anticoagulant, coagulation.**

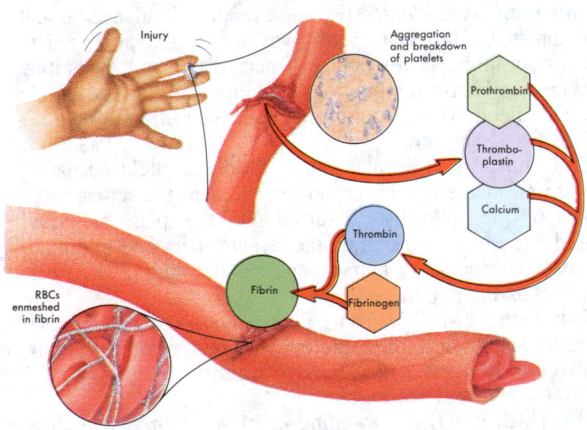

Blood clotting (Thibodeau, 1993)

Blood-brain barrier (Raven, 1992/Nadine Sokol)

blood buffers [AS, *blod;* ME, *buffe,* to cushion], a system of buffers, composed primarily of dissolved carbon di-

blood corpuscle [AS, *blod;* L, *corpusculum,* little body], a blood cell, either an erythrocyte or a leukocyte.

blood count. See **complete blood count.**

blood culture medium, a liquid enrichment medium for the growth of bacteria in the diagnosis of blood infections. It contains a suspension of brain tissue in meat broth with dextrose, peptone, and citrate and has a pH of 7.4.

blood donor, anyone who donates his or her blood. See also **blood bank, transfusion.**

blood dyscrasia [AS, *blod;* Gk, *dys,* bad, *krasis,* mingling], a pathologic condition in which any of the constituents of the blood are abnormal in structure, function, or quality, as in leukemia or hemophilia.

blood fluke, a parasitic flatworm of the class Trematoda, genus *Schistosoma,* including the species *S. haematobium, S. japonicum,* and *S. mansoni.* See also *Schistosoma,* **schistosomiasis.**

blood gas, gas dissolved in the liquid part of the blood. Blood gases include oxygen, carbon dioxide, and nitrogen.

	pH	CARBONIC ACID	BICARBONATE
ACIDOSIS	Low	Increase	Decrease
ALKALOSIS	High	Decrease	Increase

Acid-base balance is normally maintained by three different body systems: the respiratory system, the renal system, and the buffer system.

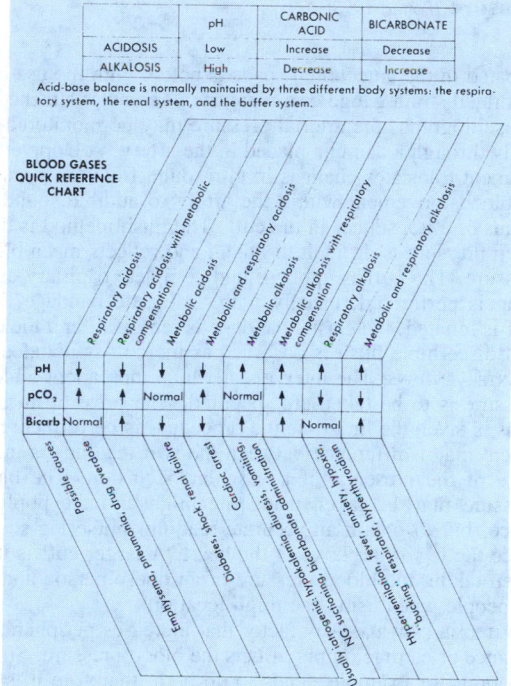

Blood gases

blood gas determination, an analysis of the pH of the blood and the concentration and pressure of oxygen, carbon dioxide, and hydrogen ion in the blood. It can be performed rapidly as an emergency procedure to assess acid base balance and ventilatory status. Blood gas determination is often important in the evaluation of cardiac failure, hemorrhage, kidney failure, drug overdose, shock, uncontrolled diabetes mellitus, or any other condition of severe stress. The blood for examination is drawn from a vein or artery as ordered in a heparinized syringe, placed in ice, and immediately transported for analysis. Normal arterial blood gas values are: pH 7.35-7.45; Pco_2 35-45 mm Hg; HCO^-_3 21-28 mEq/L; Po_2 80-100 mm Hg; O_2 saturation 95%-100%. See also **acid base balance, acidosis, alkalosis, oxygenation,** PCO_2, pH, PO_2.

blood gas tension, the partial pressure of a gas in the blood.

blood glucose. See **blood sugar.**

blood group, the classification of blood based on the presence or absence of genetically determined antigens on the surface of the red cell. Several different grouping systems have been described. These include ABO, Duffy, high-frequency antigens, I, Kell, Kidd, Lewis, low-frequency antigens, Lutheran, MNS, P, Rh, and Xg. Their relative importance depends on their clinical significance in transfusion therapy, organ transplantation, maternal-fetal compatibility, and genetic studies. See also **ABO blood groups.**

blood island, one of the clusters of mesodermal cells that proliferate on the outer surface of the embryonic yolk sac and give it a lumpy appearance. The outermost cells flatten into primitive endothelium; the inner cells develop primitive blood plasma and elaborate hemoglobin within their cytoplasm.

blood lactate, lactic acid that appears in the blood as a result of anaerobic metabolism when oxygen delivery to the tissues is insufficient to support normal metabolic demands.

blood lavage [AS, *blod;* L, *lavere,* to wash], the removal of toxic elements from the blood by the injection of serum into the veins.

bloodless phlebotomy [AS, *blod;* ME, *les;* Gk, *phleps,* vein, *tomos,* cutting], a technique of trapping blood in a body region by the application of tourniquet pressure that is less than needed to interrupt arterial blood flow.

blood level, the concentration of a drug or other substance in a measured amount of plasma, serum, or whole blood.

blood level of glucose [AS, *blod;* OFr, *livel;* Gk, *glykys,* sweet], the amount of glucose found in the bloodstream, normally about 80 to 120 mg/dl. Concentrations higher or lower than normal can be a sign of a variety of diseases, such as diabetes mellitus or pancreatic cancer.

blood osmolality [AS, *blod;* Gk, *osmos,* impulsion], the osmotic pressure of blood. The normal values in serum are 280 to 295 mOsm/L. See also **osmolality.**

blood patch. See **epidural blood patch.**

blood pH, the hydrogen ion concentration of the blood, a measure of blood acidity or alkalinity. The normal pH values for arterial whole blood are 7.38 to 7.44; for venous whole blood, 7.36 to 7.41; for venous serum or plasma, 7.35 to 7.45.

blood plasma [AS, *blod;* Gk, *plassein,* to mold], the liquid portion of the blood, free of its formed elements and particles. Plasma represents approximately 50% of the total volume of blood and contains glucose, proteins, amino acids, and other nutritive materials, urea, other excretory products, as well as hormones, enzymes, vitamins, and minerals. Compare **serum.** See also **blood, plasma protein, pooled plasma.**

blood platelet. See **platelet, thrombocyte.**

blood poisoning. See **septicemia.**

blood pressure (BP) [AS, *blod;* L, *premere,* to press], the pressure exerted by the circulating volume of blood on the walls of the arteries, the veins, and the chambers of the heart. Overall blood pressure is maintained by the complex interaction of the homeostatic mechanisms of the body, moderated by the volume of the blood, the lumen of the arteries and arterioles, and the force of the cardiac contraction. The pressure in the aorta and the large arteries of a healthy young adult is approximately 120 mm Hg during systole and 70 mm Hg in diastole. The pulse pressure is approximately 50 mm Hg. See also **hypertension, hypotension.**

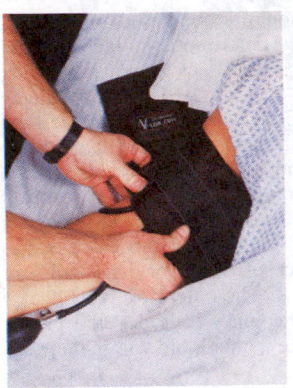 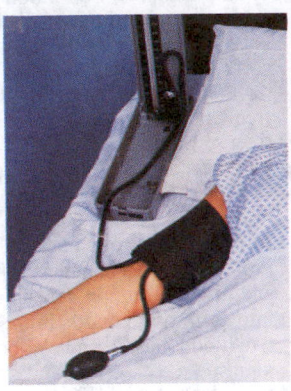 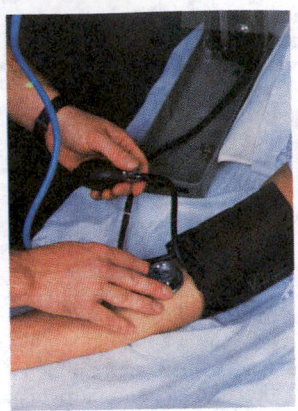 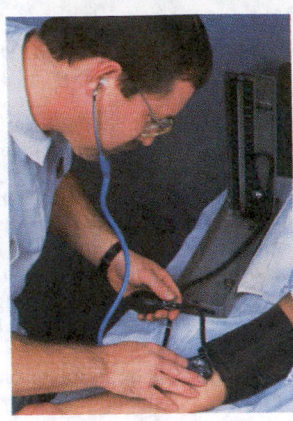

Measurement of blood pressure (Potter, 1993)

■ METHOD: The blood pressure is most often measured by auscultation, using an aneroid or mercury sphygmomanometer, a stethoscope, and a blood pressure cuff. The cuff is placed around the upper arm and inflated to a pressure greater than the systolic pressure, occluding the artery. The diaphragm of the stethoscope is placed over the brachial artery in the antecubital space, and the pressure in the cuff is slowly released. No sound is heard until the cuff pressure falls to less than the systolic pressure in the artery; at that point a pulse is heard. As the cuff pressure continues to fall slowly, the pulse continues; first becoming louder, then dull and muffled. These sounds, called the sounds of Korotkoff, are produced by turbulence of the blood flowing through a vessel that is partially occluded as the arterial pressure falls to the low pressure of diastole. When the cuff pressure is less than the diastolic pressure, no pulse is heard. Thus the cuff pressure at which the first sound is heard is the systolic blood pressure indicative of the pressure in the large arteries during systole; the cuff pressure at which the sounds stop is the diastolic blood pressure, indicative of the pressure on the arteries during diastole. Other methods include the use of palpation in place of auscultation to determine the systolic pressure: The pressure at which a pulse is first palpated in the antecubital space is noted; with the use of a calibrated strain gauge or a mercury manometer attached to an oscillograph, the arterial pressure may be monitored directly through a cannula placed in the artery. A Doppler instrument translates changes in ultrasound frequency caused by blood movement within the artery to audible sound by means of a transducer in the cuff. The flush method is used when pressure is difficult to obtain and reflects mean blood pressure. The cuff is applied, and complete capillary emptying is performed, usually with an elastic bandage. The cuff is inflated, the elastic bandage is removed, and the earliest discernible flush is observed as the cuff is deflated.

■ INTERVENTIONS: The intervals at which the patient's blood pressure is to be taken are specified. The pressure in both arms is taken the first time the procedure is performed; persistent major difference between the two readings is indicative of the presence of a vascular occlusion. The blood pressure may be taken using the thigh and the popliteal space, but to obtain an accurate reading, nurse leg should place the leg at the level of the heart. A larger cuff is used when taking the blood pressure of an obese person and for all people when using the thigh location.

■ OUTCOME CRITERIA: Any factor that increases peripheral resistance or cardiac output affects the blood pressure. Strong emotion, for example, tends to do both; therefore it is important to try to secure a blood pressure reading when the person is at rest. Increased peripheral resistance usually increases the diastolic pressure, and increased cardiac output tends to increase the systolic pressure. Blood pressure increases with age, primarily because of the decreased distensibility of the veins. As a person grows older, an increase in systolic pressure precedes an increase in diastolic pressure.

blood pressure monitor [AS, *blod;* L, *premere,* to press, *monere,* to warn], a device that automatically measures blood pressure and records the information continuously. Automatic monitorng of blood pressure may be required in surgery or in an intensive care unit.

blood proteins [AS, *blod;* Gk, *proteios,* of first rank], the proteins normally in the blood, such as albumin, globulin, hemoglobin, proteins bound to hormones or other compounds.

blood pump, **1.** a pump for regulating the flow of blood into a blood vessel during transfusion. **2.** a component of a heart-lung machine that pumps the blood through the ma-

Classification of blood pressure

Range*	Category
Diastolic	
<85	Normal blood pressure
85-89	High normal blood pressure
90-104	Mild hypertension
105-114	Moderate hypertension
≥115	Severe hypertension
Systolic, when diastolic BP is <90	
<140	Normal blood pressure
140-159	Borderline isolated systolic hypertension
≥160	Isolated systolic hypertension

*In mm Hg.
From The Joint National Committee on Detection, Evaluation, and Treatment of High Blood Pressure: The 1988 report of the Joint National Committee on Detection, Evaluation, and Treatment of High Blood Pressure, *Arch Intern Med* 148:1023, 1988.

chine for oxygenation and then through the peripheral circulatory system of the body. Also called **mechanical heart-lung.** See also **oxygenation.**

blood serum. See **serum.**

bloodshot, a reddening of the conjunctiva or sclera of the eye caused by dilation of blood vessels in the tissues.

blood smear, a small specimen of blood that is smeared or spread onto a glass microscope slide for examination.

blood substitute, a substance used for a replacement or volume expansion for circulating blood. Plasma, human serum albumin, packed red cells, platelets, leukocytes, and concentrates of clotting factors are often administered in place of whole blood transfusions in the treatment of various disorders. Substances that are sometimes used to expand blood volume include dextran, hetastarch, albumin solutions, or plasma protein fraction. Perfluorocarbon emulsions, although potentially toxic, have been tested as blood substitutes; they are able to carry oxygen to tissues, have a long shelf life without refrigeration, and do not induce antigen-antibody reactions.

blood sugar, 1. one of a group of closely related substances, such as glucose, fructose, and galactose, that are normal constituents of the blood and are essential for cellular metabolism. 2. *nontechnical.* the concentration of glucose in the blood, represented in milligrams of glucose per deciliter of blood. Also called **blood glucose.** See also **hyperglycemia, hypoglycemia.**

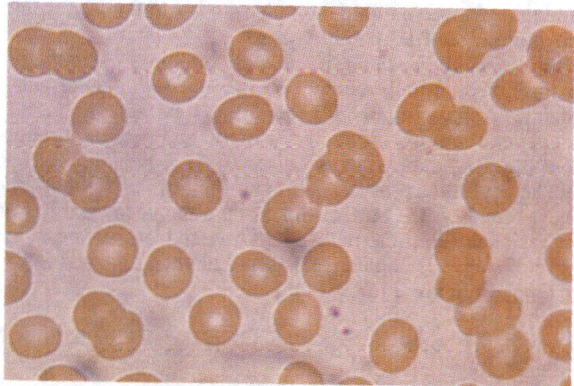

Blood smear *(Zitelli, 1992)*

blood test, 1. any test that determines something about the characteristics or properties of the blood.

blood transfusion [AS, *blod;* L *transfundere* to pour through], the administration of whole blood or a component, such as packed red cells, to replace blood lost through trauma, surgery, or disease.

■ METHOD: Blood for transfusion is obtained from a healthy donor or donors whose ABO blood group and antigenic subgroups match those of the recipient and who have an adequate hemoglobin level (above 13.5 g/100 ml for men and above 12.5 g/100 ml for women). Each 500 ml of blood collected from a donor is stored in a plastic bag containing citrate-dextrose or citrate-phosphate. A unit can be stored under refrigeration for only 3 weeks; at that time the leukocytes, platelets, and 20% to 30% of the red cells are nonviable, and the levels of clotting factors V and VIII are low.

The blood is removed from the refrigerator no more than 30 minutes before transfusion and is checked according to hospital policy. The necessary equipment is assembled, the blood tubing is flushed with normal saline solution, and the patient's venipuncture site is prepared. During transfusion the position of the extremity is checked, and the venipuncture site is observed for signs of erythema, swelling, or leakage. The procedure is stopped if there is evidence of a systemic reaction. An acute hemolytic reaction, characterized by chills, fever, headache, back pain, decreased blood pressure, hematuria, and nausea, may occur if the recipient's and donor's blood groups are not exactly matched. Circulatory overload may cause shortness of breath, lung congestion, and frothy sputum. A pyrogenic reaction caused by bacteria or an antigen on the leukocytes or platelets of the transfused blood may result in fever, chills, and palpitations. An allergic reaction to serum protein in transfused blood may be characterized by urticaria, laryngeal edema, and asthmatic wheezing. After a transfusion has been completed, pressure is applied to the venipuncture site and a bandage or dressing is applied. The patient is observed at 30-minute intervals to make certain that a reaction does not occur.

■ NURSING INTERVENTION: The nurse prepares the required equipment and venipuncture site, observes the patient during and after transfusion, and instructs the patient to report any symptoms associated with the procedure.

■ OUTCOME CRITERIA: All possible measures are taken to prevent the reactions that occur in an estimated 2% to 3% of transfused patients. Acute hemolytic reactions can be fatal; delayed hemolysis, characterized by jaundice and anemia, may occur weeks or months after transfusion. Air embolism may occur if blood is administered under air pressure after hemorrhaging; massive replacement may cause hyperkalemia, thrombocytopenia, ammonia, and citrate toxicity. Viral hepatitis, cytomegalovirus disease, and other dis-

Blood products and their uses

Blood product	Uses
Red blood cells	Acute or chronic anemia, aplastic anemia, bone marrow failure, congestive heart failure, chronic renal failure, hepatic coma
Whole blood	Acute massive blood loss, hypovolemic shock
Platelets	Thrombocytopenia, platelet function abnormality
Fresh frozen plasma	Hypovolemia combined with hemorrhage because of deficiencies
Cryoprecipitate	Hemophilia, von Willebrand's disease, hypofibrinogenemia, factor XIII deficiency
Albumin	Shock caused by burns; maintains blood volume in patients with hypovolemia; hypoproteinemia
Leukocyte-poor red blood cells	Repeated febrile reaction; reaction from leukocyte antibodies and patients who are candidates for organ transplants

Adapted from Sheehy SB: *Emergency nursing principles and practice,* ed 3, St Louis, 1992, Mosby. Data courtesy Eastern Maine Medical Center, Bangor, Maine.

eases may be transmitted by transfused blood. But in most cases transfusion is an uneventful procedure.

blood typing, identification of genetically determined antigens on the surface of the red blood cell used to determine blood groups. Usually a blood bank procedure, typing is the first step in testing blood to be used in transfusion and is followed by cross-matching. See also **ABO blood groups, blood group, Rh factor, transfusion reaction.**

blood urea nitrogen (BUN) [AS, *blod;* Gk, *ouron,* urine + *nitron,* soda + *genein,* to produce], nitrogen in the blood in the form of urea. The urea is formed in the liver as the end product of protein metabolism and is deposited in the blood to be excreted through the kidney. The BUN, determined by a blood test, is directly related to the metabolic function of the liver and the excretory function of the kidney. Normal findings are: adult, 10-20 mg/dl or 3.6-7.1 mm/L; elderly, may be slightly higher than normal adult levels; children, 5-18 mg/dl; infants, 5-18 mg/dl; newborn, 3-12 mg/dl; cord, 21-40 mg/dl. A value w 100 mg/dl indicates serious impairment of renal function. Also called **urea nitrogen, serum urea nitrogen.** See also **azotemia.**

blood vessel, any one of the network of muscular tubes that carry blood. Kinds of blood vessels are **arteries, arterioles, capillaries, veins,** and **venules.**

blood warming coil, a device constructed of coiled plastic tubing used for the warming of reserve blood before massive transfusions, such as those often required for patients who develop extensive GI bleeding. Administration of cold blood in such transfusions may cause the patient to go into shock. The blood warming coil is a prepackaged, sterile single-use device. Aseptic technique is used to remove the coil from its wrapper. The coil is immersed in water warmed to 99° F (37.6° C), and blood from the transfusion bag is allowed to flow through the coil until warm enough to administer. The coil is equipped with clamps for control of the blood flow to the primary transfusion line. During prolonged transfusions the blood warming coil is replaced every 24 hours. Compare **electric blood warmer.**

bloody show. See **vaginal bleeding.**

bloody sputum [AS, *blod;* L, *sputum,* spittle], blood-tinged material expelled from the respiratory passages. The amount and color of blood in sputum expelled by coughing or clearing the throat may indicate the cause and location of the bleeding.

Bloom's syndrome [David Bloom, American physician, b. 1892], a rare genetic disease occurring mainly in Ashkenazi Jews. It is transmitted as an autosomal recessive trait and is characterized by growth retardation, telangiectatic erythema of the face and arms, sensitivity to sunlight, and an increased risk of leukemia.

blow bottles, a device used in respiratory care to provide resistance to expiration. The bottles are partially filled with water, and the patient is encouraged to blow the water from one bottle to another, a practice that requires deep inspiration and lung expansion to develop increased lung pressure.

blow-out fracture, a fracture of the floor of the orbit caused by a blow that suddenly increases the intraocular pressure.

BLS, abbreviation for **basic life support.**

blue asphyxia. See **asphyxia livida.**

blue baby [OFr, *blou;* ME, *babe*], an infant born with cyanosis caused by a congenital heart lesion, such as transposition of the great vessels, tetralogy of Fallot, or incomplete

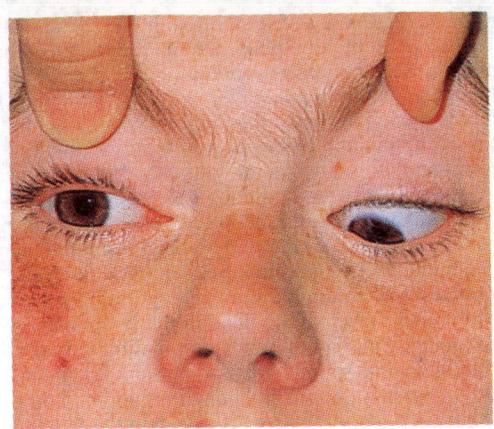

Blow-out fracture (*Zitelli, 1992*)

expansion of the lungs (congenital atelectasis). Tetralogy of Fallot is the most common congenital cyanotic cardiac lesion. Congenital cyanotic heart lesions are diagnosed by cardiac catheterization, angiography, or echocardiography and are corrected surgically, preferably in early childhood. See also **congenital cardiac anomaly, tetralogy of Fallot, transposition of the great vessels.**

blue fever, *informal.* Rocky Mountain spotted fever, so named for the dark cyanotic discoloration of the skin after the initial rickettsial infection. See also **rickettsiosis, Rocky Mountain spotted fever, typhus.**

blue nevus [OFr, *blou;* L, *naevus,* mole], a sharply circumscribed, usually benign, steel blue skin nodule with a diameter between 2 and 7 mm. It is found on the face or upper extremities, grows very slowly, and persists throughout life. The dark color is caused by large, densely packed melanocytes deep in the dermis of the nevus. Nodular blue nevi found on the buttocks or in the sacrococcygeal region occasionally become malignant. Any sudden change in the size of such a lesion demands surgical attention and biopsy. Compare **melanoma.**

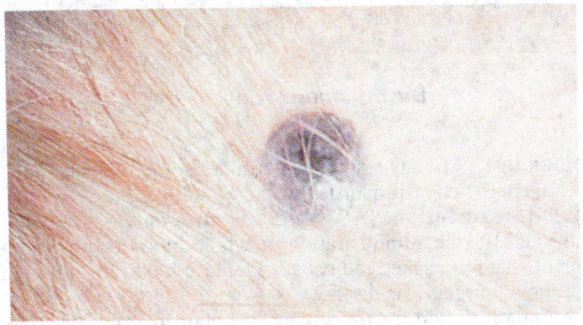

Blue nevus (*Baran, 1991*)

blue phlebitis. See **phlegmasia cerulea dolens.**

blue spot, **1.** also called **macula cerulea** /seroo'lē·ə/. one of a number of small grayish blue spots that may appear near the armpits or around the groins of individuals infested with lice, such as in pediculosis corporis and pediculosis pubis. These spots are usually less than 1 cm in diameter and are caused by a substance in the saliva of lice that converts bilirubin to biliverdin. **2.** one of a number of dark blue round or oval spots that may appear as a congenital condition in the sacral regions of certain children under 4 or 5 years of age. They usually disappear spontaneously as the affected individual matures. Also called **mongolian spot.**

blunt dissection [ME, *blunt*; L, *dissecare*, to cut apart], a dissection performed by separating tissues along natural lines of cleavage without cutting.

blunthook /blunt'hŏŏk/ [ME, *blunt* + AS, *hoc*], **1.** a sturdy hook-shaped bar used in obstetrics for traction between the abdomen and the thigh in cases of difficult breech deliveries. **2.** a hook-shaped device with a blunt end used in embryotomy.

blunting, a decrease in the intensity of emotional expression from the level one would normally expect as a reaction to a specific situation. It is the opposite of overreaction and may be marked by apathy, minimal response, or indifference.

blurred film fault /blurd'/, a defect in a photograph or radiograph that appears as an indistinct or blurred image. It is caused by film movement during exposure, bent film during exposure, double exposure, or film emulsion flow during processing in excessively warm solutions.

blush [ME, *blusshen*, to redden], a brief, diffuse erythema of the face and neck, commonly the result of dilatation of superficial small blood vessels in response to heat or sudden emotion.

B lymphocyte. See **B cell.**

B/M, symbol for black male, often used in the initial identifying statement in a patient record.

BMA, abbreviation for **British Medical Association.**

BMD, abbreviation for **Bureau of Medical Devices.**

B-mode, brightness modulation, an imaging technique used in ultrasound scanning in which bright dots on an oscilloscope screen represent echoes and the intensity of the brightness indicates the strength of the echo.

BMR, abbreviation for **basal metabolic rate.**

BNA, abbreviation for *Basle Nomina Anatomica.*

BOA, abbreviation for **born out of asepsis.**

board. See **custodial care.**

board certification, a process by which physicians are certified in a given medical specialty or subspecialty. Certification is provided by the 23-member boards of the American Board of Medical Specialties and is given on completion of accredited training and examinations, as well as fulfilling individual requirements of the particular board.

board certified, denoting a physician who has completed the certification requirements established by a medical specialty board and has been certified as a specialist in a particular field of medicine.

board eligible, denoting a physician who has completed all of the requirements for admission to a medical specialty board.

boarder baby, an infant abandoned to a hospital because the mother is unable to care for him or her. Many boarder babies are infants born with AIDS or delivered to mothers who are drug users.

board of health, an administrative body acting on a municipal, county, state, provincial, or national level. The functions, powers, and responsibilities of boards of health vary with the locales. Each board is generally concerned with the recognition of the health needs of the people and

the coordination of projects and resources to meet and identify these needs. Among the tasks of most boards of health are prevention of disease, health education, and implementation of laws pertaining to health.

Boas' test /bō'az/ [Ismar I. Boas, German physician, b. 1858], **1.** also called **resorcinol** /risôr'sinol/ **test.** a test for hydrochloric acid in the contents of the stomach in which a glass rod dipped in a specially prepared reagent is touched to a drop of filtered stomach liquid. A scarlet streak forms along the rod in the presence of hydrochloric acid. **2.** a test for free hydrochloric acid in the contents of the stomach in which filtered stomach fluid is boiled with a special reagent. Free hydrochloric acid produces a transient rosy mirror. **3.** a test for lactic acid in a sample of gastric juice that depends on the oxidation of the lactic acid to aldehyde and formic acid by sulfuric acid and manganese. **4.** also called **chlorophyll test.** a test for gastric motility in which a fasting patient drinks 400 ml of water that has been tinted green by the addition of 20 drops of chlorophyll solution. After 30 minutes, the contents of the stomach are aspirated and the amount of tinted water that has passed through the stomach is determined.

Bodansky unit [Aaron Bodansky, American biochemist, b. 1887], the quantity of phosphatase in 100 ml of serum needed to liberate 1 mg of phosphorous as phosphate ion from sodium betaglycerophosphate in 1 hour at 37° C. It is used to express the measure of certain enzymes, such as acid phosphatase, in the body.

body [AS, *bodig*], **1.** the whole structure of an individual with all the organs. **2.** a cadaver or a corpse. **3.** the largest or the main part of any organ, such as the body of the tibia or the body of the vastus lateralis. Also called **corpus, soma.**

body cast [AS, *bodig,* body; ONorse, *kasta*], a molded cast that may extend from the chest to the groin to immobilize the spine.

body cavity, any of the spaces in the chest and abdomen that contain body organs. One major cavity, the thoracic cavity, is subdivided into a pericardial and two pleural cav-

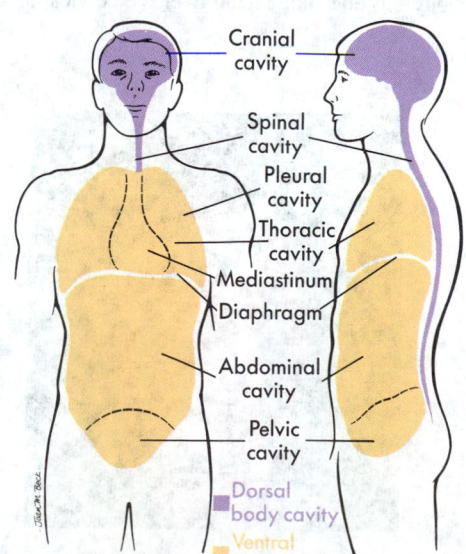

Major body cavities (Thibodeau, 1993/Joan M Beck)

ities. The abdominal cavity has no intervening partition, but the lower portion is known as the pelvic cavity.

body fluid [AS, *bodig;* L, *fluere,* to flow], a fluid contained in the three fluid compartments of the body: the blood plasma of the circulating blood, the interstitial fluid between the cells, and the cell fluid within the cells. Blood plasma and interstitial fluid make up the extracellular fluid; the cell fluid is the intracellular fluid. The chemical constituents of the fluids vary greatly; for example, sodium is present in large amounts in both compartments of the extracellular fluid but is nearly absent in the intracellular fluid; protein is present in the blood plasma and cell fluid but not in the interstitial fluid.

body image [AS, *bodig;* L, *imago,* likeness], a person's subjective concept of his or her physical appearance. The mental representation, which may be realistic or unrealistic, is constructed from self-observation, the reactions of others, and a complex interaction of attitudes, emotions, memories, fantasies, and experiences, both conscious and unconscious. A marked inability to conceptualize one's personal body characteristics may be caused by organic brain damage, as in autotopagnosia, by a physical disability, such as the loss of a limb, or by psychologic and emotional disturbances, as in anorexia nervosa.

body image agnosia. See **autotopagnosia.**

body image disturbance, a nursing diagnosis accepted by the Seventh National Conference on the Classification of Nursing Diagnoses. The condition is defined as a disruption in the way one perceives one's body image. The cause of a disturbance in body image may be a biophysical, cognitive, perceptual, psychosocial, cultural, or spiritual factor. The defining characteristics of the deficit include verbal or nonverbal responses to a real or perceived change in structure or function, a missing body part, personalization of the missing part by giving it a name, refusal by the client to look at a part of the body, negative feelings about the body, trauma to a nonfunctioning part, a change in general social involvement or life-style, and a fear of rejection by others. See also **nursing diagnosis.**

body jacket, an orthopedic cast that encases the trunk of the body but does not extend over the cervical area; it may be equipped with shoulder straps. It is used to help immobilize the trunk for the healing of spinal injuries and scoliosis and for postoperative positioning and immobilization after spinal surgery. Compare **Risser cast.**

body language [AS, *bodig;* L, *lingua,* tongue], a set of nonverbal signals, including body movements, postures, gestures, spatial positions, facial expressions, and bodily adornment, that give expression to various physical, mental, and emotional states. See also **kinesics.**

body louse. See **lice, pediculus humanus corporis.**

body mechanics, the field of physiology that studies muscular actions and the function of muscles in maintaining the posture of the body.

body movement, motion of all or part of the body, especially at a joint or joints. Some kinds of body movements are **abduction, adduction, extension, flexion,** and **rotation.**

body odor, a fetid smell associated with stale perspiration. Freshly secreted perspiration is odorless, but after exposure to the atmosphere and bacterial activity at the surface of the skin, chemical changes occur to produce the odor. Common body odor usually can be eliminated by bathing with soap and water. Body odors also can be the result of discharges from a variety of skin conditions, including cancer, fungus, hemorrhoids, leukemia, and ulcers. See also **bromhidrosis.**

body of Retzius /ret′sē·əs/ [Magnus G. Retzius, Swedish anatomist, b. 1842], any one of the masses of protoplasm containing pigment granules at the lower end of a hair cell of the organ of Corti in the internal ear.

body plethysmograph [AS, *bodig;* Gk, *plethynein,* to increase, *graphein* to record], a device for studying alveolar pressures, lung volumes, and airway resistance. The patient sits or reclines in an airtight compartment and breathes normally. The pressure changes in the alveoli are reciprocated in the compartment and are recorded automatically.

body position, attitude or posture of the body. Some kinds of body position are **anatomic position, decubitus, Fowler's position, prone, supine,** and **Trendelenburg position.**

body righting reflex [AS, *bodig;* L, *rectus,* straight; *reflectere* to bend back], any one of the neuromuscular responses to restore the body to its normal upright position when it has been displaced. The righting reflexes involve complicated mechanisms and processes associated with the structures of the internal ear, such as the utricle, the saccule, the macula, and the semicircular canals. Also involved in the righting mechanism are receptors for the vestibular branch of the eighth cranial nerve. Any change in the position of the head produces a change in the pressure on the gelatinous membrane of the macula and causes tiny otoliths within the membrane to pull on hair cells, stimulating adjacent receptors of the vestibular nerve. The fibers of the nerve transmit impulses to the brain, producing a sense of position of the head by a sensation of change in the gravitational pull, activating muscles that tend to restore the body to its optimum position. Also activating righting reflexes are proprioceptors in muscles and tendons and visual nerve impulses. Interruption of the impulses associated with body righting reflexes may disturb equilibrium and cause nausea and vomiting.

body scheme, a Piagetian term for a cognitive structure that develops in infants in the sensorimotor period during

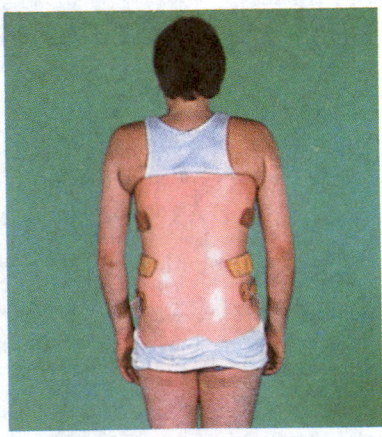

Body jacket *(Houghton, 1989)*

the first 2 years of life as they learn to differentiate between themselves and the world around them.

body-scheme disorder. See **autotopagnosia.**

body-section radiography, a radiographic technique employed to produce a more distinct image of a selected body plane by moving the film and x-ray tube in opposite directions. The process has the effect of blurring adjacent body structures during exposure. Also called **tomography.**

body stalk, the elongated part of the embryo that is connected to the chorion. The stalk first extends from the posterior end of the embryo to the chorion but later moves to the midventral region and forms the lengthening umbilical cord. As the embryo develops and the amnion expands, the umbilical cord comes to enclose the body stalk and the yolk sac. See also **allantois.**

body surface area. See **surface area.**

body systems model, (in nursing education) a conceptual framework in which illness is studied in relation to the functional systems of the body, such as the circulatory, nervous, GI, and reproductive. In this model, nursing care is directed toward manipulating the patient's environment in such a way that the signs and symptoms of the health problem are alleviated. As the body systems model focuses on the disease rather than the patient, current educational programs tend to integrate it with other concepts that allow the nurse to approach the patient in a more holistic framework, recognizing the complexity of the external and internal agents that contribute to illness and to health. Also called **medical model.**

body temperature, the level of heat produced and sustained by the body processes. Variations and changes in body temperature are major indicators of disease and other abnormalities. Heat is generated within the body through metabolism of food and lost from the body surface through radiation, convection, and evaporation of perspiration. Heat production and loss are regulated and controlled in the hypothalamus and brainstem. Fever is usually a function of an increase in the generation of heat, but some abnormal conditions, such as congestive heart failure, produce slight elevations of body temperature through impairment of the heat loss function. Contributing to the failure to dissipate heat are reduced activity of the heart, lower rate of blood flow to the skin, and the insulating effect of edema. Diseases of the hypothalamus or interference with the other regulatory centers may produce abnormally low body temperatures. Normal adult body temperature, as measured orally, is 98.6° F. Oral temperatures ranging from 96.5° F to 99° F are consistent with good health, depending on the physical activity of the person, the ambient temperature, and the particular normal body temperature for that person. Axillary temperature is usually 1° F lower than the oral temperature. Rectal temperatures may be 0.5° to 1° F higher than oral readings. Body temperature appears to vary 1° to 2° F throughout the day, with lows recorded early in the morning and peaks between 6 PM and 10 PM. This diurnal variation may increase in range during a fever. While adult body temperature, normal and abnormal, tends to vary within a relatively narrow range, the temperatures of children respond more dramatically and rapidly to disease, changes in ambient temperature, and levels of physical activity.

body temperature, altered, high risk for, a nursing diagnosis accepted by the Seventh National Conference on the Classification of Nursing Diagnoses. The condition is a state in which the individual is at risk for failure to maintain body temperature within normal range. Risk factors are extremes of age; extremes of weight; exposure to cool-to-cold or warm-to-hot environments; dehydration; inactivity or vigorous activity; medications causing vasoconstriction or vasodilation; altered metabolic rate; sedation; inappropriate clothing for environmental temperature; and illness or trauma affecting temperature regulations. See also **nursing diagnosis.**

body type, the general physical appearance of an individual human body. Three commonly used terms for body types are ectomorph, describing a thin, fragile physique; endomorph, denoting a round, soft body; and mesomorph, indicating a muscular, athletic body of average size. See also **asthenic habitus, athletic habitus, ectomorph, endomorph, mesomorph, pyknic.**

Boeck's sarcoid. See **sarcoidosis.**

Boerhaave's syndrome /bôr′hävz/ [Hermann Boerhaave, Dutch physician, b. 1668], a condition marked by spontaneous rupture of the esophagus, leading to mediastinitis and pleural effusion. Emergency care with surgery and drainage is needed to save the life of the patient.

Bohr effect [Christian Bohr, Danish physiologist, b. 1855], the effect of CO_2 and H+ on the affinity of hemoglobin for molecular O_2. Increasing P_{CO_2} and H+ decrease oxyhemoglobin saturation, whereas decreasing concentrations have the opposite effect. In humans a decrease of pH from 7.4 to 7.3 at 40 torr P_{O_2} decreases oxyhemoglobin saturation by 6%. The Bohr effect is particularly significant in the capillaries of working muscles and the myocardium and in maternal and fetal exchange vessels of the placenta.

boil [AS, *byle*, sore], a skin abscess. See **furuncle.**

boiling point [ME, *boilen*, to make bubbles; L, *pungere*, to prick], the temperature at which a substance passes from the liquid to the gaseous state at a particular atmospheric pressure. See also **evaporation.**

-bol, a combining form designating an anabolic steroid.

bole /bōl/, any of a variety of soft, friable clays of various colors, although usually red from iron oxide. They consist of hydrous silicate of aluminum, are used as pigments, and were once commonly used as absorbents and astringents.

Bolivian hemorrhagic fever /bəliv′ē·ən/, an infectious disease caused by an arenavirus, generally transmitted from infected rodents to humans through contamination of food by rodent urine. After an incubation period of from 1 to 2 weeks, the patient experiences chills, fever, headache, muscle ache, anorexia, nausea, and vomiting. As the disease progresses, hypotension, dehydration, bradycardia, pulmonary edema, and internal hemorrhages may occur. The mortality rate may reach 30%; pulmonary edema is the most common cause of death. There is no specific therapy. Peritoneal dialysis is sometimes performed. Also called **Machupo.** See also **Arenavirus, Argentine hemorrhagic fever, Lassa fever.**

bolus /bō′ləs/ [Gk, *bolos*, lump], **1.** also called **alimentary bolus.** a round mass, specifically a masticated lump of food ready to be swallowed. **2.** a large round preparation of medicinal material for oral ingestion, usually soft and not prepackaged. **3.** a dose of a medication or a contrast material, radioactive isotope, or other pharmaceutic preparation injected all at once intravenously. **4.** in radiotherapy, material used to fill in irregular body surfaces in order to get a better dose distribution for hyperthermia or to increase the dose to the skin when high-energy photon beams are used.

Bombay phenotype /bombā'/, a rare genetic trait involving the phenotypic expression of the ABO blood groups. The gene for the H antigen, which in the usual dominant form of HH or Hh is responsible for the precursor necessary for the production of the A and B antigens, is homozygous recessive in individuals with this trait so that the expression of the A, B, and H antigens is suppressed. Cells of such individuals are phenotypically of blood type O, and the serum contains anti-A, anti-B, and anti-H antigens. In such cases the offspring from two phenotypic O blood type parents may be blood type AB. The phenomenon is an example of the intricate interaction of linked genes in which one gene on a chromosome controls the expression or suppression of another gene that is not its allele. The trait is named for the city in which it was first reported. See also **ABO blood groups.**

bonding[1] [ME, *band*, to bind], the attachment process that occurs between an infant and the parents, especially the mother, and is significant in the formation of affectionate ties that later influence both the physical and psychologic development of the child. The process is reciprocal and is usually initiated immediately after birth by placing the nude infant on the mother's abdomen so that both the parents and child can see and touch one another and begin to interact. The newborn is in an alert, reactive state for about 30 minutes to 1 hour after birth and displays such behavior as crying, sucking, clinging, grasping, and following with the eyes, which in turn stimulates the expression of the parenting instincts. By about the second to third week of life, there is a definite reciprocal pattern of interacting behavior, involving an attention and nonattention cycle, during each encounter of parents and child. At the peak of the attention phase, the infant reaches out toward the parent and is very attentive. This is followed in a short time by deceleration of excitement in the infant and a turning away from the parent. This nonattentive phase prevents the infant from being overwhelmed by excessive stimuli, and no amount of visual or verbal attempt will regain his attention. Recognition of these cycles and especially the fact that the nonattention phase is not a form of rejection help the mother and father to develop competence in parenting. Assessment of the attachment process is an important function of the nurse and requires skill in terms of observation and interviewing. The nurse observes the mother's reactions, especially while feeding, bathing, and comforting her infant, for potential signs of inadequate or delayed mothering. Perhaps the most important actions for forming positive parent-child attachment are eye contact in the en face position and embracing the infant close to the body. Many variables determine the development of attachment and parenting, including the parents' fantasies about the child, the conditions surrounding the pregnancy, what arrangements have been made concerning changes in life-style with the addition of a dependent family member, and what type of parenting the mother and father received as children. Although bonding is considered primarily an emotional response, it is theorized that there may be some biochemical and hormonal interaction in the mother that may stimulate the response, but studies are still inconclusive. Also called **maternal-child attachment.** See also **maternal deprivation syndrome, maternal-infant bonding.**

bonding[2], (in dentistry) a technique of joining orthodontic brackets or other attachments directly to the enamel surface of a tooth, using orthodontic adhesives.

bond specificity, the nature of enzyme action that causes the disruption of only certain bonds between atoms.

bone [AS, *ban*], **1.** the dense, hard, and slightly elastic connective tissue comprising the 206 bones of the human skeleton. It is composed of compact osseous tissue surrounding spongy cancellous tissue permeated by many blood vessels and nerves and enclosed in membranous periosteum. Long bones contain yellow marrow in longitudinal cavities and red marrow in their articular ends. Red marrow also fills the cavities of the flat and the short bones, the bodies of the vertebrae, the cranial diploe, the sternum, and the ribs. Blood cells are produced in active red marrow. Osteocytes form bone tissue in concentric rings around an intricate haversian system of interconnecting canals that accommodates blood vessels, lymphatic vessels, and nerve fibers. **2.** any single element of the skeleton, such as a rib, the sternum, or the femur. Also called *(Latin)* **os** /os/. See also **connective tissue.**

bone age [AS, *ban*; L, *aetas*], the stage of development or decline of the skeleton or its segments, as seen in radio-

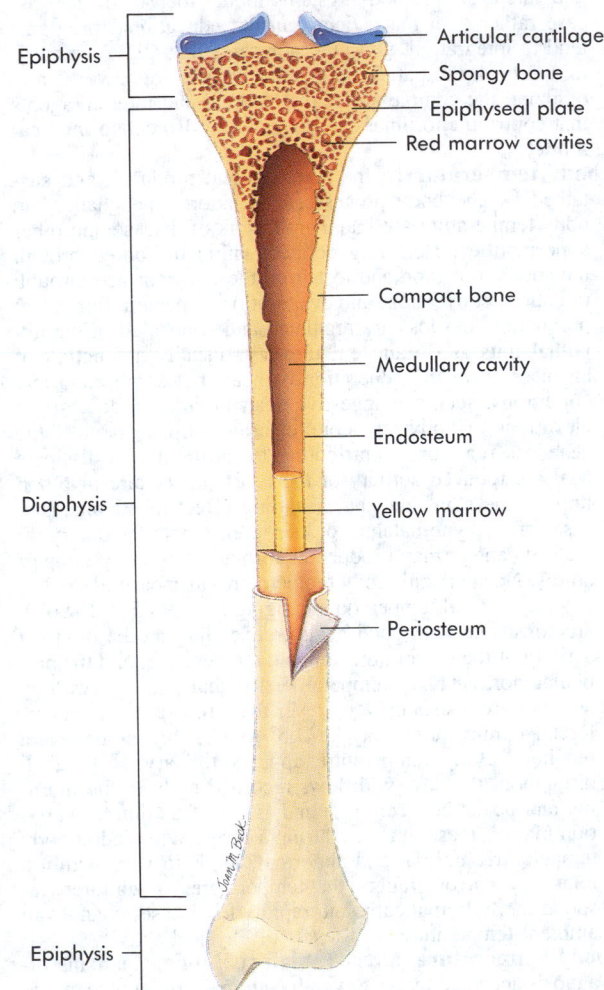

Long bone *(Thibodeau, 1993/Joan M Beck)*

Epiphysis — Articular cartilage, Spongy bone, Epiphyseal plate, Red marrow cavities
Compact bone
Medullary cavity
Endosteum
Diaphysis — Yellow marrow
Periosteum
Epiphysis

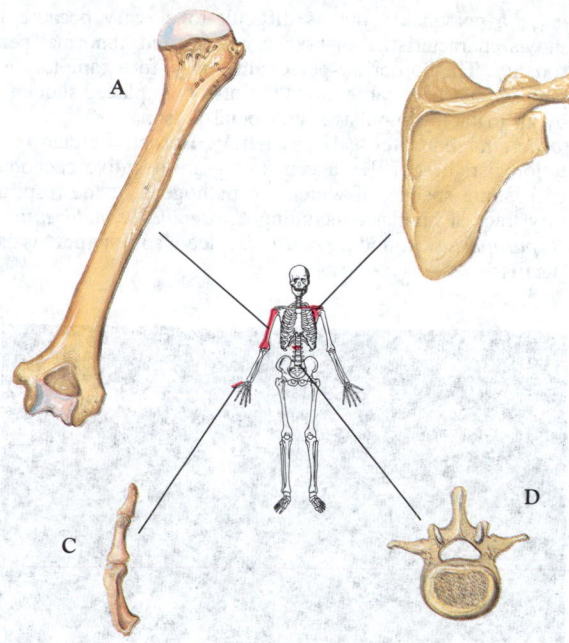

Types of bones: Long (A), flat (B), short (C), and irrecular (D).
(Thibodeau, 1993/Ernest W Beck)

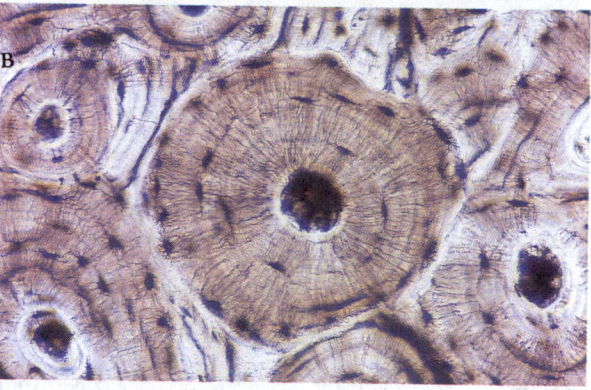

Bone tissue *(Thibodeau, 1993/Carolina Biological Supply)*

graphic examination, when compared with x-ray views of the bone structures of other individuals of the same chronologic age.

bone cancer [AS, *ban;* Gk, *karkinos,* crab], a skeletal malignancy occurring primarily as a sarcoma in an area of rapid growth or, secondarily, as metastasis from cancer elsewhere in the body. Primary bone tumors are rare; the incidence peaks during adolescence, decreases, and then rises slowly after the age of 35. In adults, bone cancer is linked to exposure to ionizing radiation. Paget's disease, hyperparathyroidism, chronic osteomyelitis, old bone infarcts, and fracture callosities increase the risk of many bone tumors. Most osseous malignancies are metastatic lesions found most often in the spine or pelvis and less often in sites away from the trunk. Bone cancers progress rapidly but are often difficult to detect. Bone pain that increases at night may be the only symptom. X-ray films, radioisotopic scans, arteriography, and biopsies are diagnostic; alkaline phosphatase levels are elevated in osteoblastic tumors, and serum calcium and urinary calcium are increased in highly destructive lesions. The most common osseous malignancies are osteosarcomas, followed by chondrosarcomas, fibrosarcomas, and Ewing's sarcoma. Surgical treatment consists of local resection of slow-growing tumors or amputation, including the joint above the tumor, if the lesion is aggressive. Radiotherapy may be given preoperatively or as the primary form of treatment of radiosensitive tumors, such as Ewing's sarcoma, reticulum cell sarcoma, and multiple myeloma.

bone cell [AS, *ban;* L, *cella,* storeroom], an osteocyte, a cell resembling a melon seed, but with myriad spidery processes.

bone cutting forceps, a kind of forceps that has long handles, single or double joints, and heavy blades.

bone cyst [AS, *ban;* Gk, *kytis,* cyst], **1.** an aneurysmal vascular bone cyst, usually eccentrically placed. **2.** osteitis fibrosa cystica, a parathyroid disorder characterized by cyst formation and replacement of bone by fibrous tissue.

bone graft, the transplantation of a piece of bone from one part of the body to another to repair a skeletal defect.

bone lamella [AS, *ban,* bone, *lamella,* small plate], a thin plate of bone matrix, a basic structural unit of mature bone.

bone marrow [AS, *ban;* ME, *marowe*], specialized, soft tissue filling the spaces in cancellous bone of the epiphyses. Fatty, **yellow marrow** is found in the compact bone of most adult epiphyses. **Red marrow** is found in many bones of infants and children and in the spongy bone of the proximal epiphyses of the humerus and femur and in the sternum, ribs, and vertebral bodies of adults. It is composed of myeloid tissue and is essential in the manufacture and maturation of red blood cells.

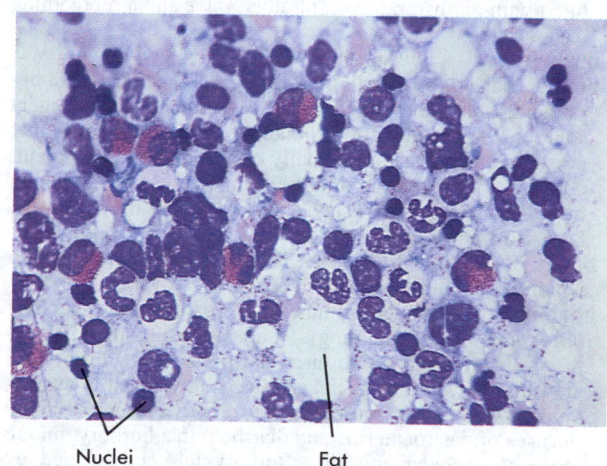

Nuclei   Fat

Bone marrow *(Seeley, 1992/Ed Reschke)*

bone marrow transplant, the transplantation of bone marrow from healthy donors to stimulate production of formed blood cells. It is used in treatment of hematopoietic or lymphoreticular diseases, such as aplastic anemia, leukemia, immune deficiency syndromes, and acute radiation syndrome. The bone marrow is removed from the donor by aspiration and infused intravenously into the recipient.

bone plate [AS, *ban*, bone; OFr, *plate*], a metal plate used to reconstruct a bone that has been fractured. The plate is designed to hold fragments in apposition.

bone recession [AS, *ban*; L, *recedere*, to recede], apical progression of the level of the alveolar crest, associated with inflammatory or dystrophic periodontal disease and resulting in decreased bone support for the teeth.

bone tissue [AS, *ban*; OFr, *tissu*], a hard form of connective tissue composed of osteocytes and a calcified collogenous intercellular substanc arranged in thin plates. Also called **bony tissue.**

Bonine, a trademark for an antiemetic (meclizine hydrochloride).

Bonnevie-Ullrich syndrome. See **Turner's syndrome.**

Bonwill's triangle [William G. A. Bonwill, American dentist, b. 1833], an equilateral triangle with 4 inch (10 cm) sides formed by lines from the contact points of the lower central incisors (or the median line of the residual ridge of the mandible) to the condyle on either side and from one condyle to the other. Compare **Tweed triangle.**

bony landmark [AS, *ban*; AS, *land, meark*], a groove or prominence on a bone that serves as a guide to the location of other body structures.

bony palate. See **hard palate.**

bony thorax [AS, *ban*; Gk, *thorax*, chest], the skeletal part of the chest, including the thoracic vertebrae, ribs, and sternum.

bony tissue. See **bone tissue.**

booster injection, the administration of an antigen, such as a vaccine or toxoid, usually in a smaller amount than the original immunization. It is given to maintain the immune response at an appropriate level.

Boothby-Lovelace-Bulbulian (BLB) mask, an apparatus for the administration of oxygen consisting of a mask fitted with an inspiratory-expiratory valve and a rebreathing bag.

boracic acid. See **boric acid.**

borate /bôr′āt/, any salt of boric acid. Borate salts and boric acid, although formerly used as mild antiseptic irrigant solutions, especially for ophthalmic conditions, are highly poisonous when taken internally or absorbed through a cut, abrasion, or other wound in the skin. Because of the potential for fatal poisoning, such solutions are rarely used now. See also **boric acid.**

borax bath [Ar, *bauraq*; AS, *baeth*], a medicated bath in which borax and glycerin are added to the water.

borborygmos /bôr′bərig′məs/, *pl.* **borborygmi** [Gk, *borborygmos*, bowel rumbling], an audible abdominal sound produced by hyperactive intestinal peristalsis. Borborygmi are rumbling, gurgling, and tinkling noises heard in auscultation. Although increased intestinal activity may be noted in cases of gastroenteritis and diarrhea, true borborygmi are more intense and episodic. Borborygmi accompanied by vomiting, distension, and intestinal cramps suggest a mechanical obstruction of the small intestine.

borderline [OFr, *bordure*; L, *linea*], pertaining to a state of health in which the patient has some of the signs and symptoms of a disease but not enough to justify a definite diagnosis.

borderline personality [OFr, *bordure*; L, *linea, persona-*

lis], a personality that is difficult to classify because it shows characteristics of both a normal and abnormal personality. The borderline personality may, for example, display a consistent stable mood but also be replaced suddenly by an irritable, impulsive, antisocial persona.

Bordetella /bôr′ditel′ə/ [Jules J.B.V. Bordet, Belgian bacteriologist, b. 1870], a genus of gram-negative coccobacilli, some species of which are pathogens of the respiratory tract of humans, including *Bordetella bronchiseptica*, *B. parapertussis*, and *B. pertussis*. See also **parapertussis, pertussis.**

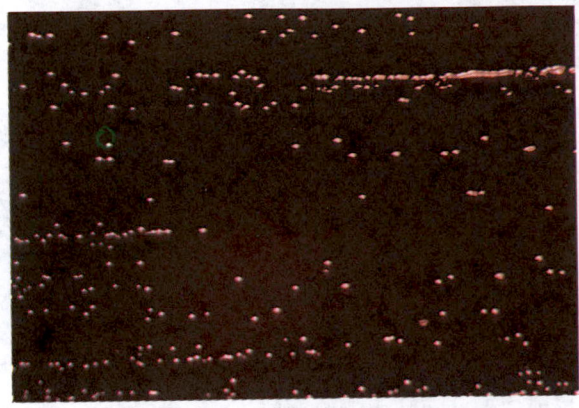

Bordetella pertussis (Baron, 1990)

boric acid /bôr′ik/, a white, odorless powder or crystalline substance used as a buffer and formerly employed as a topical antiseptic and eye wash. Also called **boracic acid** /bôras′ik/, **orthoboric acid** /ôr′thə-/.

Bornholm disease. See **epidemic pleurodynia.**

born out of asepsis (BOA), (in a hospital) denoting a newborn infant who was not delivered in the usual place in an obstetric unit. Depending on the policy of the institution, a BOA-designated infant may have been born on the way to the hospital or in the hospital, on the way to the delivery suite, or in a labor room.

■ OBSERVATIONS: Initial assessment on the admitting unit includes evaluation of respiration, quality of cry, skin color, apical pulse rate, muscle tone, reflexes, temperature, condition of umbilical cord or cord stump, ability to suck, presence of meconium, congenital defect, skin eruption, or signs of sepsis, including jaundice, anorexia, vomiting, diarrhea, irritability or lethargy, high-pitched cry, and hypothermia or hyperthermia.

■ INTERVENTIONS: The usual steps in caring for a newborn are performed. Head and chest circumferences are measured, weight is taken, the baby is placed in a warmer until the axillary temperature is 36.5° C. Vitamin K and silver nitrate are usually given, and a bath is given when the body temperature is over 36.5° C and stable. In many hospitals BOA infants are placed in a special nursery and isolated from other infants to prevent contagion if the BOA baby is infected.

■ NURSING CONSIDERATIONS: Daily care for the newborn BOA is the same as that given to other newborns, but, in addition, close observation for signs of sepsis is made. The parents are involved in the care of the infant as soon as is possible, and the usual instructions are given for care of the baby at home after discharge.

boron (B) /bôr'on/, a nonmetallic element, similar to aluminum. Its atomic number is 5; its atomic weight is 10.8. Elemental boron occurs in the form of dark crystals and as a greenish yellow amorphous mass. Certain concentrations of this element are toxic to plant and animal life, but plants need traces of boron for normal growth. It is the characteristic element of boric acid, which is used chiefly as a dusting powder and ointment for minor skin disorders. Boric acid in solution was formerly extensively employed as an antiinfective and eyewash, but the high incidence of toxic reactions and fatalities associated with these preparations has greatly reduced their use.

Borrelia /bərel'ē·ə/ [Amédée Borrel, French bacteriologist, b. 1867], a genus of coarse, unevenly coiled, helical spirochetes, several species of which cause tickborne and louseborne relapsing fever. The organism is spread to offspring from generation to generation. This does not occur in lice. Many animals serve as reservoirs and hosts for *Borrelia*. The spirochete may be identified by microscopic examination of a smear of blood stained with Wright's stain; it is also easily inoculated onto culture media for bacterial culture and identification.

Borrelia burgdorferi /burg'dôrfer'ī/, the etiologic agent in Lyme disease. The organism is transmitted to humans by tick vectors, primarily *Ixodes dammini*.In the United States the disease is found primarily in the northeast, north-central, and northwest regions.

boss [ME, *boce*], a swelling, eminence, or protuberance on an organ, such as a tumor or overgrowth on a bone surface. For example, on the forehead it is often a sign of rickets.

Boston exanthem [Boston; Gk, *ex* out, *anthema*, blossoming], an epidemic disease characterized by scattered, pale red maculopapules on the face, chest, and back, occasionally accompanied by small ulcerations on the tonsils and soft palate. There is little or no adenopathy, and the rash disappears spontaneously in 2 or 3 weeks. It is caused by echovirus 16 and requires no treatment. Compare **herpangina.**

bottle feeding [OFr, *bouteille*; AS, *faeden*], feeding an infant or young child from a bottle with a rubber nipple on the end as a substitute for or supplement to breastfeeding.
■ METHOD: The infant is held on one arm close to the body of the mother or nurse during feeding. The bottle is held at an angle to ensure that the nipple is always filled with liquid so that the infant does not ingest air while feeding. For a newborn infant, rest periods may be given every several minutes. At least once in the course of the feeding and again at the end the infant is encouraged to burp by being held upright on the mother's or nurse's shoulder or on its stomach on the feeder's lap. Gentle rubbing or patting on the back and pressure on the stomach often helps to induce burping.
■ NURSING INTERVENTION: The formula contains protein, fats, carbohydrates, vitamins, and minerals in amounts similar to those in breast milk. The formula may be warmed before feeding by immersing the bottle in warm water for several minutes (although this is not necessary if the formula is kept at room temperature), and the size of the nipple hole is adjusted to the needs of the infant. Smaller infants need larger nipple holes, which require less sucking. Premature or weak infants may be fed using a special, long soft nipple through which it is very easy for the infant to feed.

■ OUTCOME CRITERIA: Bottle feeding is used as a substitute for breastfeeding when the mother is unable to breastfeed or chooses not to. Bottle feeding can also be substituted for breastfeeding occasionally, once lactation has been established. Bottle feeding is recommended if the mother has active tuberculosis or other active, acute contagious disease, if she has a serious chronic disease, such as cancer or cardiac disease, or if she has recently undergone extensive surgery. Severe mastitis, narcotic addiction, or concurrent use of medication that is secreted in the breast milk usually requires the mother to bottle-feed.

botulinus toxin /boch'əlī'nəs/ [L, *botulus*, sausage; Gk, *toxikon*, poison], any of a group of potent bacterial toxins produced by different strains of *Clostridium botulinum*. The strains are sometimes identified by letters of the alphabet, such as A, B, or C, Also called **botulinum toxin.**

botulism /boch'əliz'əm/ [L, *botulus*, sausage], an often fatal form of food poisoning caused by an endotoxin produced by the bacillus *Clostridium botulinum*. The toxin is ingested in food contaminated by *C. botulinum*, although it is not necessary for the live bacillus to be present if the toxin has been produced. In rare instances the toxin may be introduced into the human body through a wound contaminated by the organism. Botulism differs from most other types of food poisoning in that it develops without gastric distress and may not occur for from 18 hours up to 1 week after the contaminated food has been ingested. Botulism is characterized by a period of lassitude and fatigue followed by visual disturbances, such as double vision, difficulty in focusing the eyes, and loss of ability of the pupil to accommodate to light. Muscles may become weak, and the victim often develops dysphagia. Nausea and vomiting occur in less than half the cases. Hospitalization is required, and antitoxins are administered. Sedatives are given, mainly to relieve anxiety. Approximately two thirds of the cases of botulism are fatal, usually as a result of delayed diagnosis and respiratory complications. For those who survive, recovery is slow. Most botulism occurs after eating improperly canned or cooked foods. See also *Clostridium*.

bouba. See **yaws.**

Bouchard's node /bo͞oshärz'/ [Charles J. Bouchard, French physician, b. 1837], an abnormal cartilaginous or bony enlargement of a proximal interphalangeal joint of a finger, usually occurring in degenerative diseases of the joints. Compare **Heberden's node.**

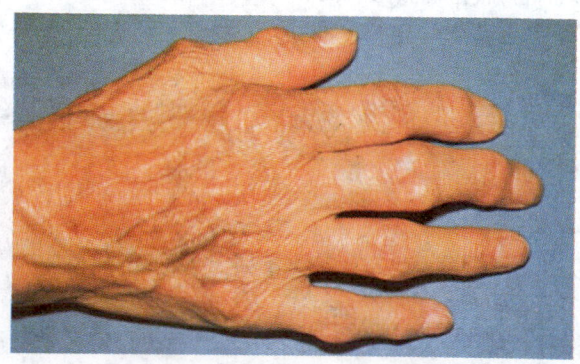

Bouchard's nodes (Kamal, 1991)

bougie /boō'zhē, boōzhē'/ [Fr, candle],   a thin, cylindric instrument made of rubber, waxed silk, or other flexible material for insertion into canals of the body in order to dilate, examine, or measure them.

-boulia. See **-bulia.**

boulimia. See **bulimia.**

boundary /bound'dərē/   ,(in psychology) an aspect of family health in which the generations are clearly defined and issues dealt with by the appropriate generation. There are also limits between the family "turf" and the larger society.

boundary lubrication,   a coating of a thin layer of molecules on each weight-bearing surface of a joint to facilitate a sliding action by the opposing bone surfaces.

boundary maintenance mechanisms,   (in psychology) behavior and practices that exclude members of some groups from the customs and values of another group.

bound carbon dioxide,   carbon dioxide that is transported in the bloodstream as part of a sodium bicarbonate molecule, as distinguished from dissolved carbon dioxide or bicarbonate ion.

bounding pulse [OFr, *bondir*, to leap; L, *pulsare*, to beat],   a pulse that, on palpation, feels full and springlike because of an increased thrust of cardiac contraction or an increased volume of circulating blood within the elastic structures of the vascular system.

bouquet fever. See **dengue fever.**

Bourdon regulator,   a commonly used adjustable regulator with an attached pressure gauge for cylinders of oxygen or other medical gases.

Bourneville's disease. See **tuberous sclerosis.**

boutonneuse fever /boō'tənoōz'/ [Fr, *bouton*, pustule; L, *febris*],   an infectious disease caused by *Rickettsia conorii*, transmitted to humans through the bite of a tick. The onset of the disease is characterized by a lesion called a tache noire /täshnô·är'/, or black spot, at the site of the infection, fever lasting from a few days to 2 weeks, and a papular erythematous rash that spreads over the body to include the skin of the palms and soles. Treatment usually involves administration of antibiotics. There is no prophylactic medication available, and prevention depends primarily on avoiding ticks. The disease is similar to Rocky Mountain spotted fever and to other rickettsial diseases. It is prevalent in parts of Europe, Asia, Africa, and the Middle East. See also **rickettsiosis, Rocky Mountain spotted fever.**

boutonnière deformity /boō'tônyer'/ [Fr, buttonhole],   an abnormality of a finger marked by the fixed flexion of the proximal interphalangeal joint and the hyperextension of the distal interphalangeal joint.

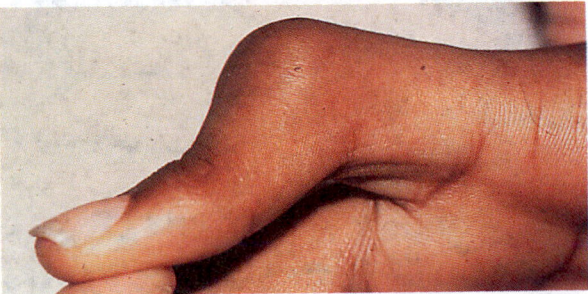

Boutonnière deformity *(Zitelli, 1992)*

bovine tuberculosis /bō'vīn/ [L, *bos*, ox + *tuber*, swelling, Gk, *osis*, condition],   a form of tuberculosis caused by *Mycobacterium tuberculosis* that primarily affects cattle. Mastitis and pulmonary symptoms can occur.

Bowditch's law. See **all-or-none law.**

bowel. See **intestine.**

bowel training /bou'əl/ [OFr, *boel*],   a method of establishing regular evacuation by reflex conditioning used in the treatment of fecal incontinence, impaction, chronic diarrhea, and autonomic hyperreflexia. In patients with autonomic hyperreflexia, distention of the rectum and bladder causes paroxysmal hypertension, restlessness, chills, diaphoresis, headache, elevated temperature, and bradycardia.

■ METHOD: The patient's previous bowel habits are ascertained, and the necessity of developing a program to induce an evacuation at the same time each day or every other day is explained. Exercises to strengthen abdominal muscles, such as pushing up, bearing down, and contracting the musculature, are demonstrated. A bedside commode is provided, and privacy is ensured. The patient is instructed to recognize and respond promptly to signals indicating a full bowel, such as goose pimples, perspiration, piloerection on arms or legs, and to develop cues to stimulate the urge to defecate, such as drinking coffee, massaging the abdomen, pressing the inner thigh, or stroking the anus. Fluids to 3000 ml daily are encouraged; prune juice, orange juice, and coffee are included in the daily diet, and the importance of having well-balanced meals that include bulk and roughage and of avoiding constipating or gas-producing foods, such as bananas, beans, and cabbage, is discussed. Depending on the patient and the problem, the training program may involve drinking 4 to 10 ounces of prune juice each night or 12 hours before the time set for evacuation, drinking warm water, coffee, or milk 30 minutes before the set time, and inserting a lubricated glycerine suppository before the set time. The patient is told that no formed stools for 3 days, semiliquid feces, restlessness, and discomfort are signs of impending impaction and that the condition may be treated with a laxative suppository or with a tap water or oil retention enema. The importance of reporting symptoms of autonomic hyperreflexia to the physician is stressed. The possibility that emotional stress or illness may cause accidental incontinence after the program has been established is discussed.

■ NURSING INTERVENTION: The nurse provides instruction and encourages the patient to establish a program of regular evacuation.

■ OUTCOME CRITERIA: Reflex conditioning is often an effective method of developing regular bowel habits in incontinent patients, especially those who are highly motivated and are given good instruction and understanding support. Young persons with spinal cord lesions are able to develop automatic defecation when adequately trained, but some elderly incontinent people may not be able to learn the program.

Bowen's disease, Bowen's precancerous dermatosis. See **intraepidermal carcinoma.**

bowleg. See **genu varum.**

Bowman's capsule /bō'mənz/ [Sir William Bowman, English surgeon, b. 1816],   the cup-shaped end of a renal tubule containing a glomerulus. Also called **glomerular capsule.**

Bowman's glands [William Bowman, English surgeon, b. 1816; L, *glans*, acorn],   glands in the mucous membrane of the mouth.

Bowman's lamina [William Bowman; L, *lamina*, thin plate], a tough membrane beneath the corneal epithelium. Also called **anterior elastic lamina, Bowman's layer, Bowman's membrane**.

bowtie filter /bō´tī/, (in radiology) a special bowtie-shaped filter that may be used in computed tomography procedures to compensate for the shape of the patient's head or body. It is used with fan-shaped x-ray beams to equalize the amount of radiation reaching the film.

box bath. See **cabinet bath.**

boxer's fracture [Dan, *bask*, a blow; L, *fractura*, break], a fracture of one or more metacarpal bones, usually the fourth or the fifth, caused by punching a hard object. Such a fracture is often distal, angulated, and impacted.

boxing, (in dentistry) the forming of vertical walls, most commonly made of wax, to produce the desired shape and size of the base of a cast.

Boyle's law /boilz/ [Robert Boyle, English scientist, b. 1627], (in physics) the law stating that the product of the volume and pressure of a gas contained at a constant temperature remains constant.

BP, abbreviation for **blood pressure.**

BPDE-I, abbreviation for **benzo(a)pyrene dihydrodiol epoxide.**

Br, symbol for the element **bromine.**

brace [OFr, *bracier*, to embrace], an orthotic device, sometimes jointed, to support and hold any part of the body in the correct position to allow function, such as a leg brace that permits walking and standing. Compare **splint.**

brachi- /brā´kē-/ , a prefix meaning 'pertaining to the arm': *brachialgia, brachiation, brachiocyllosis*.

-brachia /-brā´kē·ə/, a suffix meaning an 'anatomic condition involving an arm': *acephalobrachia, diantebrachia, monobrachia*.

brachial /brā´kē·əl/ [Gk, *brachion*, arm], of or pertaining to the arm.

brachial artery, the principal artery of the upper arm that is the continuation of the axillary artery. It has three branches and terminates at the bifurcation of its main trunk into the radial artery and the ulnar artery.

brachialgia /-al´jē·ə/ [L, *brachium*, arm; Gk, *algos*, pain], a severe pain in the arm, often related to a disorder involving the brachial plexus.

brachialis /brā´kē·al´is/ [Gk, *brachion*, arm], a muscle of the upper arm, covering the anterior part of the elbow joint and the distal half of the humerus. It arises from the anterior surface of the humerus and inserts by a thick tendon into the tuberosity of the coronoid process of the ulna. It is innervated by a branch of the musculocutaneous nerve, containing fibers from the fifth and the sixth cervical nerves, and functions to flex the forearm. Compare **biceps brachii, triceps brachii.**

brachial paralysis [L, *brachium*, arm; Gk, *paralyein*, to be palsied], paralysis of an arm or a hand.

brachial plexus [Gk, *brachion*; L, braided], a network of nerves in the neck, passing under the clavicle and into the axilla, originating in the fifth, sixth, seventh, and eighth cervical and first two thoracic spinal nerves and innervating the muscles and skin of the chest, shoulders, and arms.

brachial plexus anesthesia, an anesthetic block of the region innervated by the anterior divisions of the last four cervical and first two thoracic nerves. The plexus extends from the transverse processes to the apex of the axilla, where the terminal nerves are formed. Because of the anatomy of the

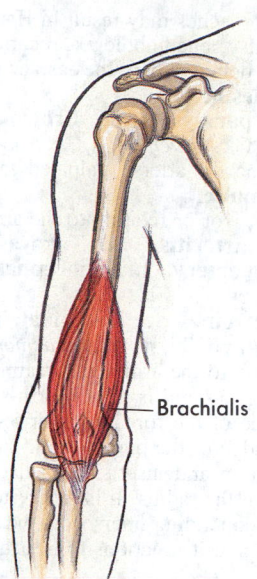

Brachialis *(Thibodeau, 1993/Ernest W Beck)*

area, many approaches are possible, the axillary being most common; supraclavicular and interscalene are also used. Perivascular axillary block has the least incidence of complications, it being limited to minimal extravasation of

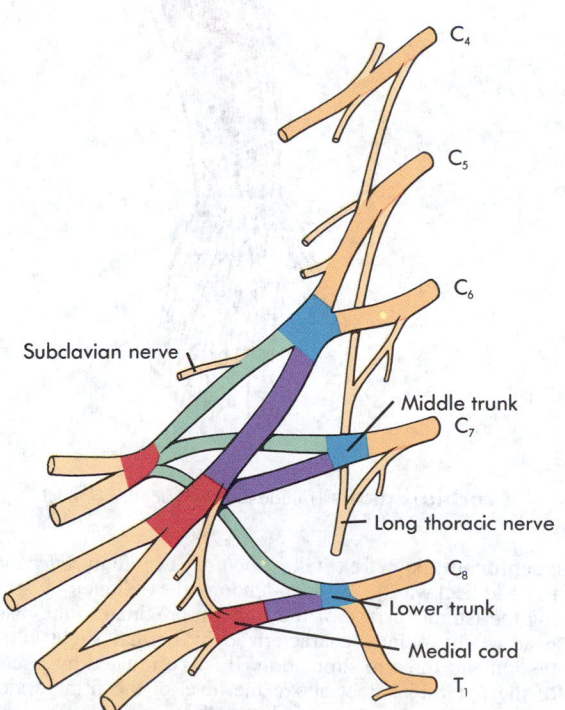

Brachial plexus *(Seeley, 1992/Michael Schenk)*

blood. Other approaches may result in Horner's syndrome, phrenic nerve palsy, pneumothorax, recurrent laryngeal paralysis, sensory deficits, paresthesias, or hematomas. See also **regional anesthesia.**

brachial plexus paralysis. See **Erb's palsy.**

brachial pulse [Gk, *brachion;* L, *pulsare,* to beat], the pulse of the brachial artery, palpated in the antecubital space. See also **pulse.**

brachiocephalic, of or relating to the arm and head.

brachiocephalic arteritis. See **Takayasu's arteritis.**

brachiocephalic artery, brachiocephalic trunk. See **innominate artery.**

brachiocephalic vein. See **innominate vein.**

brachiocubital /-kyōo′bitəl/ [Gk, *brachion;* L, *cubitus,* elbow], pertaining to the arm and forearm.

brachioradialis /-rā′dē·al′is/, the most superficial muscle on the radial side of the forearm. It arises from the lateral supracondylar ridge of the humerus and from the lateral intermuscular septum and inserts, by a flat tendon, into the styloid process of the radius. It is innervated by a branch of the radial nerve containing fibers from the fifth and the sixth cervical nerves, and it functions to flex the forearm.

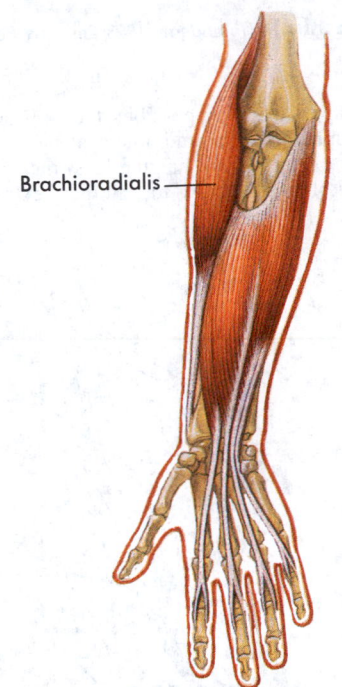

Brachioradialis

Brachioradialis *(Thibodeau, 1993/John V Hagen)*

brachioradialis reflex [Gk, *brachion;* L, *radial; reflectare,* to bend backward], a deep tendon reflex elicited by striking the lateral surface of the forearm proximal to the distal head of the radius, characterized by normal slight elbow flexion and forearm supination. It is accentuated by disease of the pyramidal tract above the level of the fifth cervical vertebra. See also **deep tendon reflex.**

-brachium /-brā′kē·əm/, **1.** a suffix meaning 'the upper arm from shoulder to elbow'. **2.** 'a suffix meaning an arm

or armlike growth': *antibrachium, prebrachium, pontibrachium.*

brachy- /brak′ē-/, a prefix meaning 'short': *brachycheilia, brachygnathia, brachyskelous.*

brachycardia /-kär′dē·ə/ [Gk, *brachys,* short, *kardia,* heart], slowness of the heart. See **bradycardia.**

brachycephaly /-sef′əlē/ [Gk, *brachys,* short, *kephale,* head], a congenital malformation of the skull in which premature closure of the coronal suture results in excessive lateral growth of the head, giving it a short, broad appearance with a cephalic index of between 81 and 85. Also called **brachycephalia** /-səfā′lē·ə/, **brachycephalism** /-sef′əlizəm/. See also **craniostenosis.** −**brachycephalic** /-səfal′ik/, **brachycephalous** /-sef′ələs/, *adj.*

brachydactyly /-dak′təlē/, a condition of abnormally short fingers or toes.

brachytherapy [Gk, *brachys* + *therapeia,* treatment], the placement of radioactive sources in contact with or implanted into the tissues to be treated. Compare **teletherapy.**

Bradford frame [Edward H. Bradford, American surgeon, b. 1848], a rectangular orthopedic frame made of pipes to which heavy movable straps of canvas are attached, running from side to side to support a patient in a prone or supine position. The straps can be removed to permit the patient to urinate or defecate while remaining immobile.

Bradford solid frame, a rectangular orthopedic device of metal covered with canvas to aid in immobilization, especially of children in traction. The Bradford solid frame provides support for the entire body and is especially appropriate for patients who are under 5 years of age, hyperactive, or mentally retarded. The main purpose of the device is to assist in maintaining proper immobilization, positioning, and alignment by controlling movement. To facilitate nursing care, the Bradford solid frame is not placed directly on a bed but elevated at both ends by plywood blocks or by other suitable devices. It is most often used with Bryant traction but never with balanced suspension traction, cervical traction, cervical tongs, or certain other kinds of traction.

Bradford split frame, a rectangular orthopedic device of metal covered with two separate pieces of canvas fastened at both ends of the frame. Used especially in pediatrics to aid in the immobilization of children in traction, it is divided in the middle by a large opening designed to accommodate the excretory functions of an incontinent patient in a hip spica cast. The division also allows for the upper and lower extremities of the patient to be elevated separately and for the maintenance of a clean and dry cast.

Bradley method, a method of psychophysical preparation for childbirth developed by Robert Bradley, M.D., comprising education about the physiology of childbirth, exercise and nutrition during pregnancy, and techniques of breathing and relaxation for control and comfort during labor and delivery. The father is extensively involved in the classes and acts as the mother's "coach" during labor. Among the advantages of the method are its simplicity, the involvement of the father, and the realistic approach to the efforts and discomfort of labor. Also called **husband-coached childbirth.** Compare **Lamaze method, Read method.**

brady- /brad′ē-/, a prefix meaning 'slow, dull': *bradyacusia, bradydiastalsis, bradyphagia.*

bradyarrhythmia /-ərith′mē·ə/ [Gk, *bradys,* slow, *a, rhythmos,* rhythm], an abnormally slow heart rhythm.

bradycardia /-kär′dē·ə/ [Gk, *bradys,* slow, *kardia,* heart], a circulatory condition in which the myocardium contracts steadily but at a rate of less than 60 contractions a minute. The heart normally slows during sleep, and in some physically fit people the pulse may be quite slow. Pathologic bradycardia may be symptomatic of a brain tumor, digitalis toxicity, or vagotonus. Cardiac output is decreased, causing faintness, dizziness, chest pain, and eventually syncope and circulatory collapse. Treatment may include administration of atropine, implantation of a pacemaker, or change in medical treatment

bradycardia-tachycardia syndrome [Gk, *bradys, kardia,* + *tachys,* fast, *kardia; syn,* together, *dromos,* course], a heart disorder characterized by a heart rate that alternates between abnormally slow and abnormally rapid rhythms. Also called **sick sinus syndrome.**

bradydiastole /-dī·as′tǝlē/ [Gk, *bradys,* slow, *dia,* through, *stellein,* to set], a diastolic phase that is abnormally long. It is associated with myocardial infarction.

bradyesthesia /-esthē′zhǝ/ [Gk, *bradys,* slow, *aisthesis,* feeling], a slowness in perception.

bradykinesia /-kinē′zhǝ,-kīnē′zhǝ/ [Gk, *bradys* + *kinesis,* motion], an abnormal condition characterized by slowness of all voluntary movement and speech, such as caused by parkinsonism, other extrapyramidal disorders, and certain tranquilizers.

bradykinin /-kī′nin/ [Gk, *bradys* + *kinein,* to move], a peptide of nonprotein origin containing nine amino acid residues. It is produced from α_2-globulin by kallikrein, and it is a potent vasodilator.

bradypnea /-pnē′ǝ/ [Gk, *bradys* + *pnein,* to breath], an abnormally slow rate of breathing. Compare **hypopnea.** See also **respiratory rate.**

bradytachycardia [Gk, *bradys,* slow, *tachy,* fast, *kardia,* heart], a heart rate that alternates between abnormally slow and abnormally fast, as in *sick sinus syndrome.*

Bragg curve [Sir William H. Bragg, English physicist, b. 1862], in radiation therapy, the path followed by ionizing particles used in a treatment. Because certain particles reach a peak of potential near the end of their path, the Bragg curve can be used to direct the radiation so that it reaches deep seated tumors while significantly sparing the normal overlying tissues.

Braille /brāl, brä′yǝ/ [Louis Braille, French teacher of blind, b. 1809], a system of printing for the blind consisting of raised dots or points that can be read by touch.

brain [AS, *bragen*], the portion of the central nervous system contained within the cranium. It consists of the cerebrum, cerebellum, pons, medulla, and midbrain. Specialized cells in its mass of convoluted, soft, gray or white tissue coordinate and regulate the functions of the central nervous system.

brain abscess [AS, *bragen;* L, *abscedere,* to go away], a pocket of infection in a part of the brain, usually as a result of the spread of an infection from another source, such as the skull, sinuses, or other structures in the head. The infection also may be secondary to a disease in the bones, the nervous system outside the brain, or the heart. Also called **cerebral abscess, intracranial abscess.**

brain compression. See **cerebral compression.**

brain concussion [AS, *bragen;* L, *concussus,* a shaking], a violent jarring or shaking or other blunt, nonpenetrating injury to the brain caused by a sudden change in momentum of the head. Characteristically, after a mild concussion there may be a transient loss of consciousness followed, on

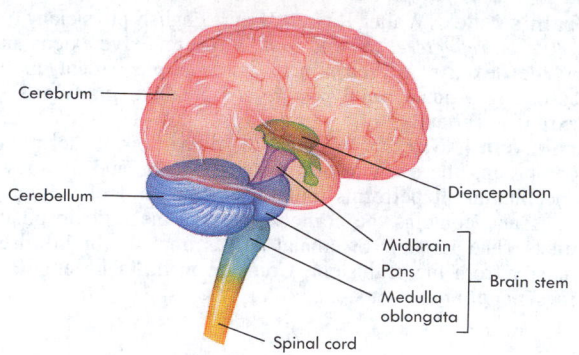

Adult brain *(Seeley, 1992/Barbara Cousins)*

Cerebrum
Cerebellum
Diencephalon
Midbrain
Pons
Medulla oblongata
Brain stem
Spinal cord

awakening, by a headache. Severe concussion may cause prolonged unconsciousness and disruption of certain vital functions of the brainstem, such as respiration and vasomotor stability. The treatment for a person recovering from a concussion consists principally of observation for signs of intracranial bleeding and increased ICP. Also called **concussion.**

brain death [AS, *bragen, death*], an irreversible form of unconsciousness characterized by a complete loss of brain function while the heart continues to beat. The legal definition of this condition varies from state to state. The usual clinical criteria for brain death include the absence of reflex activity, movements, and spontaneous respiration. The pupils are dilated and fixed. Because hypothermia, anesthesia, poisoning, or drug intoxication may cause deep physiologic depression that resembles brain death, a diagnosis of brain death may require evaluating and demonstrating that electric activity of the brain is absent on two electroencephalograms performed 12 to 24 hours apart. Also called **irreversible coma.** Compare **coma, sleep, stupor.**

brain edema. See **cerebral edema.**

brain electric activity map (BEAM), a topographic map of the brain created by a computer that is able to respond to the electric potentials evoked in the brain by a flash of light. Potentials recorded at 4-msec intervals are converted into a many-colored map of the brain, showing them to be positive or negative. The waves may be observed traveling through the brain. If the wave is disordered, blocked, too small, or too large, there may be a tumor or other lesion causing the abnormal pattern.

brain fever, *informal.* any inflammation of the brain or meninges. See also **encephalitis.**

brain scan [AS, *bragen;* L, *scandere,* to climb], a diagnostic procedure employing radioisotope imaging techniques to localize and identify intracranial masses, lesions, tumors, or infarcts. Radioisotopes are injected intravenously to circulate to the brain, where they accumulate in abnormal tissue. The radioisotopes are traced and photographed by a scintillator or scanner, and the size and location of the abnormality are determined. The nature and rate of accumulation of radioisotopes in pathologic tissue in some cases are diagnostic of a particular lesion. A brain scan, which is painless, requires only injection of the isotopes and an explanation of the procedure to the patient. Compare **CT.** See also **isotope, radioisotope.**

Brain's reflex [Walter Russell Brain, English physician, b. 1895; L, *reflectere,* to bend back], the reflexive extension of the flexed paralyzed arm of a hemiplegia patient upon assuming a quadripedal posture. Also called **quadripedal extensor reflex.**

brainstem [AS, *bragen, stemm*], the portion of the brain comprising the medulla oblongata, the pons, and the mesencephalon. It performs motor, sensory, and reflex functions and contains the corticospinal and the reticulospinal tracts. The 12 pairs of cranial nerves from the brain arise mostly from the brainstem. Compare **medulla oblongata, mesencephalon, pons.**

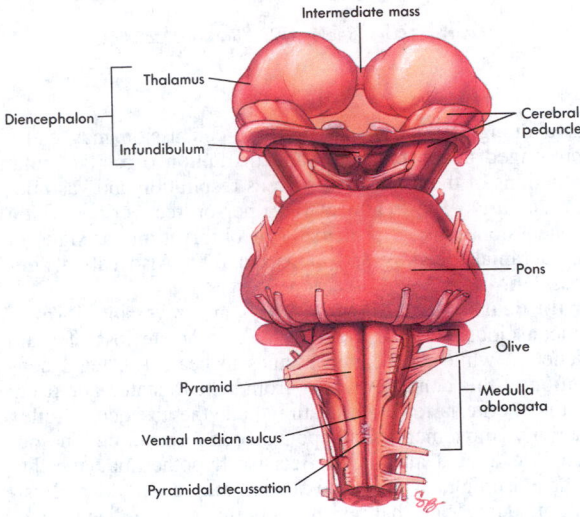

Brainstem, anterior view *(Seeley, 1992/Scott Bodell)*

brainstem auditory evoked potential (BAEP), the electric activity that may be recorded from the brainstem in the first 10 msec following presentation of an auditory stimulus. In a subject with normal brainstem functioning, seven peaks are observed. A delayed, normally shaped waveform may indicate a hearing loss caused by middle or inner ear pathology, while one or more missing peaks may indicate neural pathology.

brain swelling, See **cerebral edema.**

brain syndrome, a group of symptoms resulting from impaired function of the brain. It may be acute and reversible or chronic and irreversible. Organic mental disorder designates a particular organic mental syndrome in which the etiology is known or presumed. Organic mental syndrome (OMS) indicates a temporary or permanent brain dysfunction without reference to etiology.

brain tumor, an invasive neoplasm of the intracranial portion of the central nervous system. Brain tumors cause significant morbidity and mortality, but are treated successfully. Intracranial tumors in children are usually the result of a developmental defect. In adults 20% to 40% of malignancies in the brain are metastatic lesions from cancers in the breast, lung, GI tract, kidney, or any site of a malignant melanoma. The origin of primary brain tumors is not known, but the risk is increased in individuals exposed to

vinyl chloride, in the siblings of cancer patients, and in recipients of renal transplant being treated with immunosuppressant medication. Symptoms of a brain tumor are often those of increased intracranial pressure, such as headache, nausea, vomiting, papilledema, lethargy, and disorientation. Localizing signs, such as loss of vision on the side of an occipital neoplasm may occur. Diagnostic measures include visual field and funduscopic examinations, skull x-ray examinations, electroencephalography, cerebral angiography, brain scanning, computerized axial tomography, and spinal fluid studies. Gliomas, chiefly astrocytomas, are the most common malignancies. Medulloblastomas occur often in children. Surgery is the initial treatment for most primary tumors of the brain. Radiotherapy is indicated for inoperable lesions, medulloblastomas, and tumors with multiple foci, and as postoperative treatment of residual tumor tissue. Beams of neutrons and high energy pi-mesons currently show promise in the treatment of highly malignant brain tumors. The blood-brain barrier impedes the effect of some antineoplastic agents, but responses are obtained in some cases treated with procarbazine and various nitrosoureas administered alone or with vincristine. Compare **spinal cord tumor.**

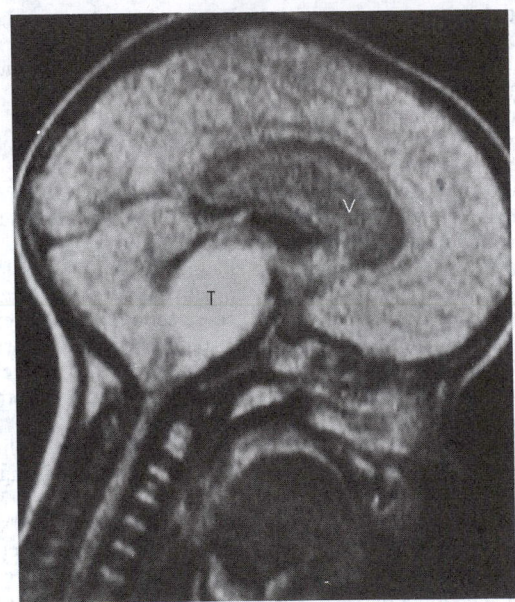

Brain tumor *(Ballinger, 1991, Vol 3)*

brain wave [AS, *bragen* + *wafian*], any of a number of patterns of rhythmic electric impulses produced in different parts of the brain. Most patterns, identified by the Greek letters alpha, beta, delta, gamma, kappa, and theta, are similar for all normal persons and are relatively stable for each individual. Alpha waves are produced when the person is awake but resting, beta waves signal an active phase of cerebral function, and delta waves are emitted during deep sleep. Brain waves also help in the diagnosis of certain neurologic disorders, such as epilepsy or brain tumors.

bran bath [OFr, *bren;* AS, *baeth*], a bath in which bran has been boiled in the water. It is used for the relief of skin irritation.

branched chain ketoaciduria. See **maple syrup urine disease.**

branched tubular gland [OFr, *branche*], one of the many multicellular glands with one excretory duct from two or more tube-shaped secretory branches, such as some of the gastric glands.

branchial /brang′kē·əl/ [Gk, *branchia*, gills], pertaining to body structures of the neck and throat area, particularly the muscles.

branchial arches [Gk, *brachia*, gills; L, *arcus,* bow], arched structures in the embryonic pharynx. In aquatic vertebrates, the arches develop into gills.

branchial cleft [Gk, *brachial*, gills; ME, *clift*], a linear depression in the pharynx of the early embryo opposite a branchial, or pharyngeal, pouch.

branchial cyst [Gk, *brachia*, gills, *kystis*, bag], a cyst derived from a branchial remnant in the neck.

branchial fistula, a congenital, abnormal passage from the pharynx to the external surface of the neck, resulting from the failure of a branchial cleft to close during fetal development. Introduction of a sound into a branchial fistula may cause pallor and arrhythmic pounding of the heart. Also called **cervical fistula.**

branching canal. See **collateral pulp canal.**

branchiogenic /brang′kē·ōjen′ik/ [Gk, *brachia,* gills, *genein,* to produce], pertaining to any tissues originating in the branchial cleft or arch. Also **branchiogenous** /-kē·oj′ənes/.

brand name. See **trademark.**

Brandt-Andrews maneuver [M.L. Brandt, American obstetrician, b. 1894; C.J. Andrews, American surgeon], a method of expressing the placenta from the uterus in the third stage of labor. One hand grasps the umbilical cord while the other is placed on the mother's abdomen with the fingers over the anterior surface of the uterus. While the hand on the abdomen is pressed backward and slightly upward, the other applies gentle traction on the cord.

brassfounder's ague. See **metal fume fever.**

brassy cough [AS, *brase,* brassy, *cohhetan,* to cough], a high-pitched cough caused by irritation of the recurrent pharyngeal nerve or by pressure on the trachea.

brassy eye. See **chalkitis.**

Braun's canal. See **neurenteric canal.**

Braxton Hicks contraction /brak′stənhiks′/ [John Braxton Hicks, English physician, b. 1823], irregular tightening of the pregnant uterus that begins in the first trimester and increases in frequency, duration, and intensity as pregnancy progresses. Contractility of uterine muscle increases in pregnancy. Near term, strong Braxton Hicks contractions are often difficult to distinguish from the contractions of true labor. Also called **Braxton Hicks sign, false labor.**

Braxton Hicks version, one of several types of maneuvers sometimes used to turn the fetus from an undesirable position to one that is more likely to facilitate delivery. See also **version.**

Brazelton assessment, a system for assessing the interactional behavior of newborns with a series of 27 reaction tests, including response to inanimate objects, to a pinprick, to light, and to the sound of a rattle or bell.

Brazilian trypanosomiasis. See **Chagas' disease.**

breach of contract, the failure to perform as promised or agreed in a contract. The breach may be complete or partial and may occur by repudiation, by failure to recognize the contract, or by prevention or hindrance of performance.

breach of duty, 1. the failure to perform an act required by law. 2. the performance of an act in an unlawful way.

breakbone fever. See **dengue fever.**

break test, a test of muscle strength of a patient by applying resistance after the patient has reached the end of a range of motion. Resistance is applied gradually in a direction opposite to the line of pull of the muscle or muscle group being tested. The resistance is released immediately if there is a sign of pain or discomfort.

breakthrough bleeding [AS, *brecan;* ME, *thurh,* across], the escape of uterine blood between menstrual periods, a side effect experienced by some women using oral contraceptives.

breast [AS, *breast*], 1. the anterior aspect of the surface of the chest. 2. a mammary gland. (See Fig. p. 220.)

breast cancer, a malignant neoplastic disease of breast tissue, the most common malignancy in women in the United States. The incidence increases exponentially with age from the third to the fifth decade and reaches a second peak at age 65, suggesting that breast cancer in premenopausal women may be related to ovarian hormonal function and in postmenopausal patients to adrenal function. Based on the great prevalence of breast cancer in affluent countries, especially in high socioeconomic groups, it is thought that a high-fat diet may be a causative factor, but the relationship is unproven and the origin is unknown. Risk factors include a family history of breast cancer, nulliparity, exposure to ionizing radiation, early menarche, late menopause, obesity, diabetes, hypertension, chronic cystic disease of the breast, and, possibly, postmenopausal estrogen therapy. Women who are over 40 years of age when they bear their first child and patients with malignancies in other body sites also have an increased risk of developing breast cancer. Initial symptoms, detected in most cases by self-examination, include a small painless lump, thick or dimpled skin, or nipple retraction. As the lesion progresses, there may be nipple discharge, pain, ulceration, and enlarged axillary glands. The diagnosis may be established by a careful physical examination, mammography, and cytologic examination of tumor cells obtained by biopsy. Infiltrating ductal carcinomas are found in about 75% of cases, and infiltrating lobular, infiltrating medullary, colloid, comedo, or papillary carcinomas in the others. Tumors are more common in the left than in the right breast and in the upper and outer quadrant than in the other quadrants. Metastasis through the lymphatic system to axillary lymph nodes and to bone, lung, brain, and liver is common, but there is evidence that primary carcinomas of the breast may exist in multiple sites and that tumor cells may enter the bloodstream directly without passing through lymph nodes. Surgical treatment, depending on the assessment of the tumor, may be a radical, modified radical, or simple mastectomy, with dissection of axillary nodes, or a lumpectomy. Postoperative radiotherapy, chemotherapy, or both are usually prescribed. Chemotherapeutic agents frequently administered in various combinations are cyclophosphamide, methotrexate, 5-fluorouracil, phenylalanine mustard (L-PAM), thio-TEPA, doxorubicin, vincristine, methotrexate, and prednisone. The presence of estrogen receptors in breast tumors is considered an indication for ovarian ablation, adrenalectomy, or hypophysectomy or for the administration of androgens or antiestrogens in order to reduce the amount of

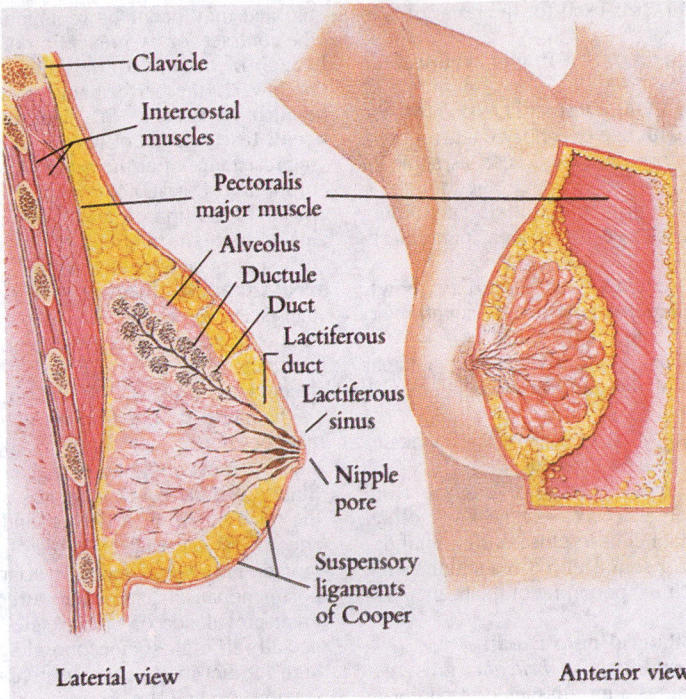

Female breast (Seidel, 1991)

endogenous estrogen. Implantation of a prosthesis after mastectomy is gaining currency but is painful initially and is not universally approved. Less than 1% of breast cancers occur in men, but those with Klinefelter's syndrome are at 60 times greater risk. In men, the tumor may be successfully treated with surgical excision and with combination chemotherapy, orchiectomy, adrenalectomy, or hypophysectomy. The prognosis is generally less favorable in women. See also **lumpectomy, mastectomy, scirrhous carcinoma.**

breast examination, a process in which the breasts and their accessory structures are observed and palpated in as-

sessing the presence of changes or abnormalities that could indicate malignant disease. See also **self-breast examination.**

■ METHOD: The breasts are observed with the patient sitting with her arms at her sides, sitting with her arms over her head, back straight, then leaning forward, and, finally, sitting upright as she contracts the pectoral muscles. The breasts are observed for symmetry of shape and size and for surface characteristics, including moles or nevi, hyperpigmentation, retraction or dimpling, edema, abnormal distribution of hair, focal vascularity, or lesions. With the patient still sitting, the axillary nodes and the supraclavicular and subclavicular areas are palpated. With the patient lying down on her back, each breast is shifted medially, and the glandular area in each is palpated with the flat of the fingers of a hand in concentric circles or in a pattern like the spokes of a wheel, from the periphery inward. The areolar areas, the nipples, and the axillary tail of Spence in the upper outer quadrant extending toward the axilla are then palpated.

■ NURSING INTERVENTION: The patient should be taught how to perform a self-breast examination and encouraged to do it monthly. Many women find it helpful to check their breasts every time they shower for the first few months after being taught the procedure to practice and to become very familiar with their own breasts.

■ OUTCOME CRITERIA: Early diagnosis greatly improves the rate of cure in cancer of the breast. The breast examination thoroughly performed serves as a valuable means of screening women to discover those who require further diagnostic examination by xeroradiography, mammography, biopsy, or, less frequently, thermoradiography.

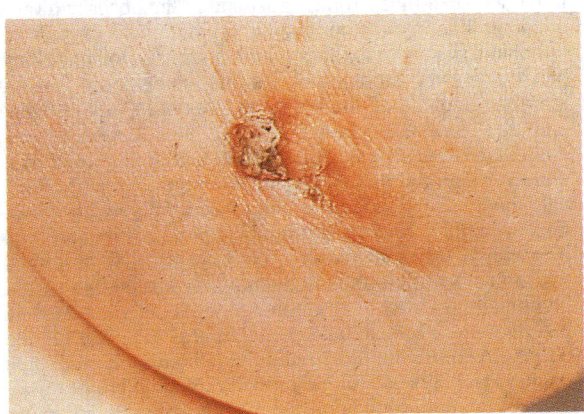

Breast cancer (Skarin, 1991)

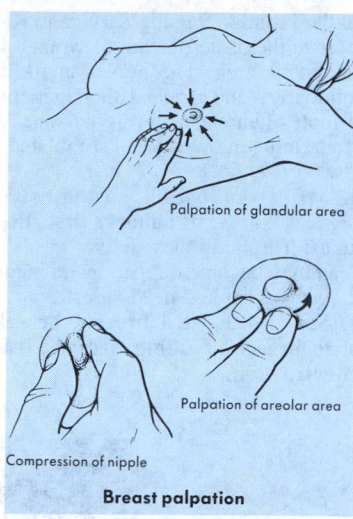

Palpation of glandular area

Palpation of areolar area

Compression of nipple

Breast palpation

Breast examination

breastfeeding [AS, braest; ME *feden*], **1.** suckling or nursing, such as giving a baby milk from the breast. Breast-feeding encourages postpartum uterine involution and slows the natural return of the menses. **2.** taking milk from the breast. See also **breast milk, lactation.**

breastfeeding, effective, a nursing diagnosis accepted by the Ninth National Conference on the Classification of Nursing Diagnoses. Effective breastfeeding is a state in which a mother-infant dyad/family exhibits adequate proficiency and satisfaction with the breastfeeding process. The defining characteristics are the mother's ability to position the infant at the breast to promote a successful latch-on response, regular and sustained suckling/swallowing at the breast, infant content after feeding, appropriate infant weight patterns for age, effective mother-infant communication patterns, signs and/or symptoms of oxytocin release, adequate infant elimination patterns for age, eagerness of the infant to nurse, and maternal verbalization of satisfaction with the breast-feeding process. Related factors include basic breastfeeding knowledge, normal breast structure, normal infant oral structure, infant gestational age greater than 34 weeks, support sources, and maternal confidence.

breastfeeding, ineffective, a nursing diagnosis accepted by the Eighth National Conference on the Classification of Nursing Diagnoses. Ineffective breastfeeding is a state in which a mother, infant, and/or family experiences dissatisfaction or difficulty with the breastfeeding process. The major defining characteristic is the unsatisfactory breastfeeding process. Other characteristics include an actual or perceived inadequate milk supply, no observable signs of oxytocin release, persistence of sore nipples beyond the infant's first week of life, and maternal reluctance to put the infant to breast as necessary. The infant may be unable to attach to the maternal nipple correctly or may resist latching on with arching and crying at the breast. Within the first hour after breastfeeding the infant may exhibit fussiness or crying and be unresponsive to other comfort measures. There may also be observable signs of an inadequate infant intake, nonsustained suckling at the breast, suckling at only one breast per feeding, and nursing less than 7 times in 24 hours.

Related factors in the diagnosis of ineffective breastfeeding are prematurity; infant anomaly; maternal breast anomaly; previous breast surgery; previous history of breastfeeding failure; infant receiving supplemental feedings with an artificial nipple; poor infant sucking reflex; nonsupportive partner or family; knowledge deficit; and interruption in breast-feeding. See also **nursing diagnosis.**

breastfeeding, interrupted, a nursing diagnosis accepted by the Tenth National Conference on the Classification of Nursing Diagnoses. Interrupted breastfeeding is a break in the continuity of the breastfeeding process as a result of inability or inadvisability to put the baby to the breast for feeding. The defining characteristics include the infant not receiving nourishment at the breast for some or all feedings, a maternal desire to maintain lactation and provide her breast milk for her infant's nutritional needs, separation of mother and infant, and lack of knowledge about expression and storage of breast milk. Related factors include maternal or infant illness, prematurity, maternal employment, contraindications to breastfeeding (e.g., drugs, true breast mild jaundice), or a need to abruptly wean the infant.

breast milk [AS, *braest; meoluc*], human milk. The nurse should counsel mothers that it is easily digested, clean, and warm, that it confers some immunities (bronchiolitis and gastroenteritis are rare in breastfed babies). Infants fed breast milk are less likely to become obese or to develop dental malocclusions. See also **breastfeeding.**

breast milk jaundice, jaundice and hyperbilirubinemia in breastfed infants that occur in the first weeks of life as a result of a metabolite in the mother's milk that inhibits the infant's ability to conjugate bilirubin to protein for excretion. See also **hyperbilirubinemia of the newborn.**

■ OBSERVATIONS: Breast milk jaundice usually occurs after the fifth day of life and peaks toward the end of the second or third week. Serum bilirubin levels usually exceed 5 mg/100 ml but rarely reach dangerous levels of 20 mg/100 ml, at which point kernicterus may develop. The infant seems normal and healthy, but the skin, the whites of the eyes, and the serum are jaundiced.

■ INTERVENTIONS: If serum bilirubin exceeds acceptable levels, breastfeeding may be interrupted until there is a decrease to the normal range, usually a period of 1 to 3 days. During this interval, the infant is bottle-fed with a supplemental formula and the mother uses a breast pump or manual devices to maintain lactation without becoming engorged. Phototherapy may be used to accelerate excretion of bilirubin through the skin.

■ NURSING CONSIDERATIONS: The primary concern of the nurse is to observe for signs of increasing jaundice, to monitor serum bilirubin levels, and usually to reassure the mother that her child is well and that the jaundice resolves slowly but completely in time.

breast pump, a device for withdrawing milk from the breast.

breast self-examination. See **self-breast examination.**

breast shadows, artifacts on chest radiographs of women caused by breast tissue. The shadows accentuate the underlying tissue and may cause the appearance of an interstitial disease process. Breast nipples may also appear on the radiograph as 'coin lesions,' requiring a second radiograph to be made with special markers attached to the nipples so the two films can be compared.

breast transillumination [AS, *braest;* L *trans,* through, *illuminare,* to light up], a method of examining the inner structures of the breast by directing light through the outer wall. See also **diaphanography.**

Breathalyzer /breth'əlī'zər/, a trademark for a device that analyzes exhaled air. It is commonly used to test for blood alcohol levels, based on a relationship between alcohol in the breath and alcohol in the blood circulating through the lungs. Also spelled **Breathalyser.**

breath-holding /breth-/ [AS, *braeth;* ME, *holden*], a form of voluntary apnea that is usually, but not necessarily, performed with a closed glottis. Although breath-holding may be prolonged for several minutes, it is invariably terminated by an involuntary breaking point.

breathing. See **respiration.**

breathing cycle /brē'thing/, a ventilatory cycle consisting of an inspiration followed by the expiration of a volume of gas called the tidal volume. The duration or total cycle time of a breathing cycle is the breathing or ventilatory period.

breathing frequency (f), the number of breathing cycles per a given unit of time.

breathing nomogram [AS, *braeth;* Gk, *nomos,* law, *gramma,* a record], a chart that presents scales of data for body weight, breathing frequency, and predicted basal tidal volume arranged in a pattern. It allows calculation of an unknown value on one scale by drawing a line that connects known values on two other scales.

breathing pattern, ineffective, a nursing diagnosis accepted by the Fourth National Conference on the Classification of Nursing Diagnoses. An ineffective breathing pattern is the state in which an inhalation and/or exhalation pattern does not enable adequate pulmonary inflation or emptying. The cause of the condition includes neuromuscular impairment, pain, musculoskeletal impairment, impairment of perception or cognition, anxiety, decreased energy, and fatigue. The defining characteristics of the problem include dyspnea, shortness of breath, tachypnea, fremitus, abnormal arterial blood gases, cyanosis, cough, nasal flaring, change in depth of respiration, pursed lip breathing or prolonged expiratory phase, increased anteroposterior diameter of the chest, use of accessory muscles of breathing, and altered excursion of the chest wall with respiration. See also **nursing diagnosis.**

breathing tube, a device inserted into the trachea through the mouth or nose to ensure a patent airway for adequate respiration during artificial or assisted ventilation. See also **extubation, intubation.**

breathing work, the energy required for breathing movements. It is the cumulative product of instantaneous pressure developed by the respiratory muscles and the volume of air moved during a breathing cycle.

breathlessness. See **dyspnea.**

breath odor /breth/, an odor usually produced by substances or diseases in the lungs or mouth. Certain specific odors are associated with some diseases, such as diabetes, liver failure, uremia, or a lung abscess. In the absence of eructation, breath odors usually do not originate in the digestive tract because the esophagus is normally collapsed.

breath sound [AS, *braeth;* L, *sonus*], the sound of air passing in and out of the lungs as heard with a stethoscope. Vesicular, bronchovesicular, and tracheal breath sounds are normal. Decreased breath sounds may indicate an obstruction of an airway, collapse of a portion or all of a lung, thickening of the pleurae of the lungs, emphysema, or other chronic obstructive lung disease.

Breckinridge, Mary (1881–1965), an American nurse who founded the Frontier Nursing Service in Kentucky, designed to improve the obstetric care of women living in the remote mountainous area. The nurses in the Service had training in midwifery and reached their patients on horseback and on foot, often encountering personal danger. The Service began training midwives and stimulated the increase of other midwifery schools.

breech birth [ME, *brech, burth*], parturition in which the baby emerges feet, knees, or buttocks first. Breech birth is often hazardous: The body may deliver easily, but the aftercoming head may become trapped by an incompletely dilated cervix because babies' heads are usually larger than their bodies. See also **assisted breech, breech presentation, complete breech, footling breech, frank breech, version and extraction.**

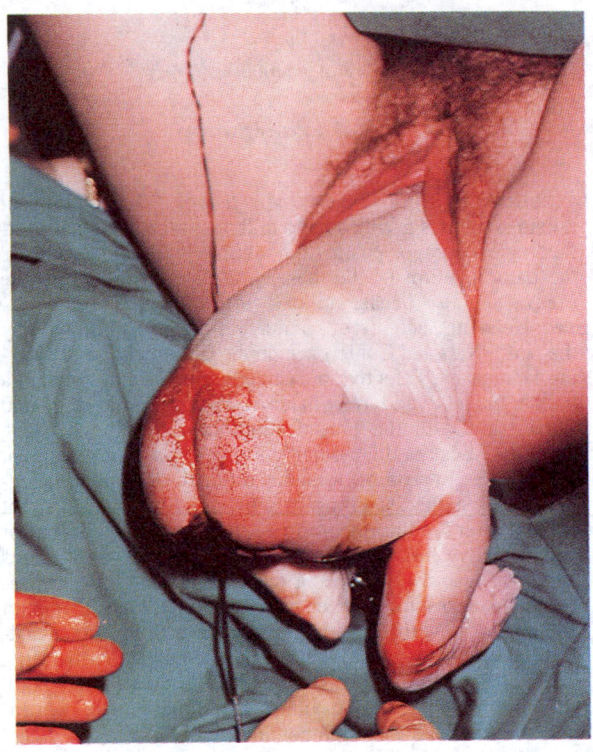

Breech birth *(Al-Azzawi, 1991)*

breech extraction [ME, *brech;* L, *ex,* out, *trahere,* to pull], an obstetric operation in which a baby being born feet or buttocks first is grasped before any part of the trunk is born and delivered by traction. Compare **assisted breech.**

breech presentation [ME, *brech;* L, *praesentare,* to show], intrauterine position of the fetus in which the buttocks or feet present, occurring in approximately 3% of labors. Kinds of breech presentation are **complete breech, footling breech,** and **frank breech.** Compare **vertex presentation.** See also **breech birth.**

bregma /breg'mə/ [Gk, the front of the head], the junction of the coronal and sagittal sutures on the top of the skull. **–bregmatic,** *adj.*

bremsstrahlung radiation /brems'shträ'lŏŏng/ [Ger, braking radiation], a type of x-ray in which there is a loss of kinetic energy from interaction with the nucleus of a target atom, resulting in an x-ray photon.

Brenner tumor [Fritz Brenner, German pathologist, b. 1877], an uncommon, benign ovarian neoplasm consisting of nests or cords of epithelial cells containing glycogen that are enclosed in fibrous connective tissue. The tumor may be solid or cystic and is sometimes difficult to distinguish from certain granulosa-theca cell neoplasms.

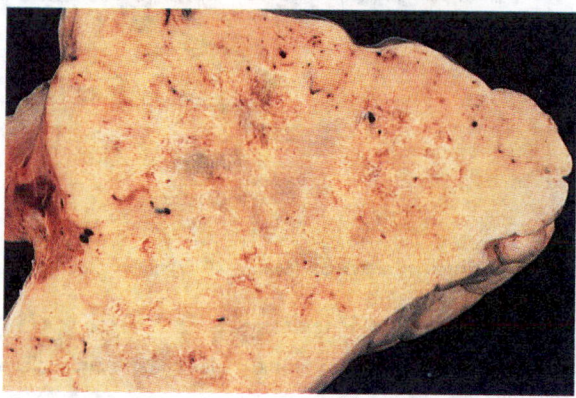

Brenner tumor *(Fletcher, 1987)*

Brethine, a trademark for a beta agonist bronchodilator (terbutaline sulfate).

bretylium tosylate /britil′ē·əm/, an antiarrhythmic agent.
■ INDICATION: It is prescribed in the treatment of life-threatening ventricular arrhythmias when other measures have not been effective.
■ CONTRAINDICATION: Known hypersensitivity to this drug prohibits its use.
■ ADVERSE EFFECTS: Among the more serious adverse reactions are hypotension, nausea and vomiting, anginal pain, and nasal stuffiness.

Bretylol, a trademark for an adrenergic blocking agent (bretylium tosylate) used as an antiarrhythmic agent.

brevi- /brev′ē-/, a prefix meaning 'short': *brevicollis, brevi-flexor, breviradiate*.

Brevicon, a trademark for a norethidrone-ethinyl estradiol oral contraceptive.

Brevital Sodium, a trademark for a barbiturate (methohexital sodium) used as a general anesthetic.

brewer's yeast /broo′ərz/ [ME, *brewen*, to boil, *yest*, foam], a preparation containing the dried pulverized cells of a yeast, such as *Saccharomyces cerevisiae*, that is used as a leavening agent and as a dietary supplement. It is one of the best sources of the B complex vitamins and of many minerals and is also a high grade of protein. Brewer's yeast may protect against toxicity of large doses of vitamin D, is used to prevent constipation, and is a good source of enzyme-producing agent.

Bricanyl, a trademark for a beta-adrenergic drug (terbutaline sulfate).

brick dust urine, a sign of precipitated urates in acidic urine in a urinalysis sample.

bridge of Varolius. See **pons.**

bridgework, a fixed prosthetic appliance which is cemented permanently to abutment teeth.

bridging [AS, *brycg*], **1.** a nursing technique of positioning a patient so that bony prominences are free of pressure on the mattress by using pads, bolsters of foam rubber, or pillows to distribute body weight over a larger surface. **2.** a nursing technique for supporting a part of the body, such as the testicles in treating orchitis using a Bellevue bridge made of a towel or other material.

brief psychotherapy, (in psychiatry) treatment directed toward the active resolution of personality or behavioral problems rather than toward the speculative analysis of the unconscious. It usually concentrates on a specific problem or symptom and is limited to a specified number of sessions with the therapist.

brief reactive psychosis, a short episode, usually less than 2 weeks, of psychotic behavior that occurs in response to a significant psychosocial stressor.

brightness gain /brīt′nes/, (in radiology) the ability of an image intensifier to increase the illumination level of an image. It is calculated as the product of the minification gain and the flux gain, which is the ratio of the number of photons at the output phosphor to the number at the input phosphor.

Brill-Symmers disease. See **giant follicular lymphoma.**

Brill-Zinsser disease /bril′zin′sər/ [Nathan E. Brill, American physician, b. 1860; Hans Zinsser, American bacteriologist, b. 1878], a mild form of typhus that recurs in a person who appears to have completely recovered from a severe case of the disease. Some rickettsiae remain in the body after the symptoms of the disease abate, causing the recurrence of symptoms, especially when stress, illness, or malnutrition weaken the person. Treatment with antibiotics may eradicate the organism. See also **epidemic typhus, murine typhus, rickettsiosis, typhus.**

brim, the edge of the upper border of the true pelvis, or the pelvic inlet. See also **pelvis.**

Brinnell hardness test, a means of determining the surface hardness of a material by measuring the amount of resistance to the impact of a steel ball. The test result is recorded as the Brinnell hardness number (BHN); the higher the number, the harder the material. The BHN is generally indicative of abrasion resistance, and the associated test is commonly used to measure this quality in various materials used in dental restorations, such as amalgams, cements, and porcelains. Compare **Knoop hardness test.**

Briquet's syndrome. See **somatization disorder.**

Brissaud's dwarf /brisōz′/ [Edouard Brissaud, French physician, b. 1852], a person affected with infantile myxedema in which short stature is associated with hypothyroidism.

British antilewisite. See **dimercaprol.**

British Medical Association (BMA), a national professional organization of physicians in the United Kingdom.

British Pharmacopoeia (BP), the official British reference work setting forth standards of strength and purity of medications and containing directions for their preparation to ensure that the same prescription written by different doctors and filled by different pharmacists will contain exactly the same ingredients in the same proportions. The first *British Pharmacopoeia* was published in 1864 by the General Medical Council; it superseded the *London Pharmacopoeia,* which had been published since 1618. See also

British Medical Association, *United States Pharmacopeia (USP).*

British thermal unit (BTU),　a unit of heat energy. The amount of thermal energy that must by absorbed by 1 lb of water to raise its temperature by one degree Fahrenheit at 39.2°F. It is also equivalent to 1055 joules or 252 calories.

brittle bones.　See **osteogenesis imperfecta.**

brittle diabetes.　See **insulin-dependent diabetes mellitus.**

broach,　an elongated, tapering dental instrument used for shaping and enlarging holes, particularly in removing pulp or cleansing of a root canal.

broad beta disease,　a familial type of hyperlipoproteinemia in which a lipoprotein, high in cholesterol and triglycerides, accumulates in the blood. The condition, which affects males in their 20s and females in their 30s and 40s, is characterized by yellowish nodules (xanthomas) on the elbows and knees, peripheral vascular disease, and elevated serum cholesterol levels. Persons with this disease are at risk of developing early coronary disease. Therapy includes dietary measures to reduce weight and serum lipids. Also called **dysbetalipoproteine mia** /disbet′əlip′ōprō′tēnē′mē·ə/, **hyperlipidemia type III.** See also **hyperlipidemia, hyperlipoproteinemia.**

broad ligament [ME, *brood;* L, *ligare,* to tie], a folded sheet of peritoneum draped over the uterine tubes, the uterus, and the ovaries. It extends from the sides of the uterus to the sidewalls of the pelvis, dividing the pelvis from side to side and creating the vesicouterine fossa and pouch in front of the uterus and the rectouterine fossa and pouch behind it. Also called **ligamentum latum uteri.** See also **cardinal ligament.**

broad ligament of liver [ME, *brod;* L, *ligare,* to bind; AS, *lifer*], a crescent-shaped fold of peritoneum attached to the lower surface of the diaphragm, connecting with the liver and the anterior abdominal wall. Also called **falciform ligament of the liver, ligamentum falciforme hepatis.**

broad-spectrum antibiotic,　an antibiotic that is effective against a wide range of infectious microorganisms.

Broca's area /brō′kəz/ [Pierre P. Broca, French surgeon, b. 1824], an area, involved in speech production, situated on the inferior frontal gyrus of the brain. See also **aphasia.**

Broca's plane [Pierre P. Broca], a plane that extends from the tip of the interalveolar septum between the upper central incisors to the lowest point of the occipital condyle.

Brodie's abscess [Sir Benjamin Brodie, English surgeon, b. 1783], a form of osteomyelitis consisting of an indolent staphylococcal infection of bone, usually in the metaphysis of a long bone of a child, characterized by a necrotic cavity surrounded by dense granulation tissue. See also **osteomyelitis.** Also called **circumscribed abscess of bone.**

Brodmann's areas /brod′manz, brōt′mons/ [Korbinian Brodmann, German anatomist, b. 1868], the 47 different areas of the cerebral cortex that are associated with specific neurologic functions and distinguished by different cellular components. Compare **motor area.** See also **cerebral cortex.**

brom,　abbreviation for a *bromide noncarboxylate anion.*

brom-, bromo-,　a prefix pertaining to a compound containing bromine or meaning 'odor, stench': *bromacetone, bromhidrosis, bromoacetophenon.*

Bromfed,　a trademark for a fixed combination deconges-

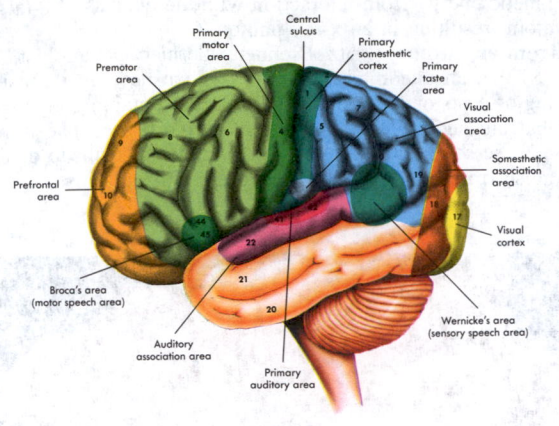

Brodmann's areas *(Seeley, 1992/William Ober)*

tant containing brompheniramine maleate and pseudoephedrine maleate.

bromhidrosis /brō′midrō′sis/ [Gk, *bromos,* stench, *hidros,* sweat], an abnormal condition in which the apocrine sweat has an unpleasant odor. The odor is usually caused by bacterial decomposition of perspiration on the skin. Treatment includes frequent bathing, changing of socks and underclothes, and the use of deodorants, antibacterial soaps, and dusting powders. Also called **body odor.**

bromide /brō′mīd/ [Gk, *bromos,* stench], a compound in which the negative element is bromine, especially a salt of hydrobromic acid. Bromides, once widely prescribed as sedatives, are now seldom used for that purpose because they may cause serious mental disturbances as side effects.

bromine (Br) /brō′mēn/, a toxic, red-brown, liquid element of the halogen group. Its atomic number is 35; its atomic weight is 79.909. Bromine is used in industry, in photography, in the manufacture of organic chemicals and fuels, and in medications. Bromine gives off a red vapor that is extremely irritating to the eyes and the respiratory tract. Liquid bromine is irritating to the skin; bromates used as neutralizers in cold wave products are toxic if ingested. Bromides are binary compounds of bromine; they have been used as sedatives, hypnotics, and analgesics and are still used in some nonprescription, over-the-counter preparations. Prolonged use of these products may cause brominism, a toxic condition characterized by acneiform eruptions, headache, loss of libido, drowsiness, and fatigue. See also **bromide.**

bromo-.　See **brom-.**

bromocriptine mesylate /brō′mōkrip′tēn/, a dopamine receptor agonist.

■ INDICATIONS: It is prescribed for the treatment of amenorrhea and galactorrhea associated with hyperprolactinemia, female infertility, and Parkinson's disease.

■ CONTRAINDICATION: Sensitivity to any ergot alkaloid prohibits its use.

■ ADVERSE EFFECTS: Among the more severe adverse reactions are palpitations, hypotension, bradycardia, hallucinations, syncope, nausea, ataxia, dyspnea, dysphagia, and confusion.

bromoderma /brō′mōdur′mə/ [Gk, *bromos,* stench, *derma* skin], an acneiform, bullous, or nodular skin rash, occurring as a hypersensitivity reaction to ingested bromides.

brompheniramine maleate /brom′fənir′əmin/, an antihistamine.

■ INDICATIONS: It is prescribed in the treatment of a variety of hypersensitivity reactions, including rhinitis, skin reactions, and itching.

■ CONTRAINDICATIONS: Asthma or known hypersensitivity to this drug prohibits its use. It is not given to newborn infants, lactating mothers, or other people for whom anticholinergic medications are contraindicated.

■ ADVERSE EFFECTS: Drowsiness, skin rash, hypersensitivity reactions, dry mouth, and tachycardia commonly occur.

Brompton's cocktail, an analgesic solution containing alcohol, morphine or heroin, cocaine, and, in some cases, a phenothiazine. Formulations vary, and recently cocaine has generally been eliminated from the mixture. The cocktail is administered in the control of pain in the terminally ill patient. Given frequently at the lowest effective dose, it may relieve pain for many months. It was developed at the Brompton Hospital in England. Also called **Brompton's mixture.**

Bromsulphalein (BSP) test /bromsul′falin/, a trademark for sulfobromophthalein, a dye prepared for use in a highly sensitive, nonspecific test that measures the ability of liver cells to remove the sulfobromophthalein from the blood. The test is rarely indicated in current clinical practice because it may cause severe allergic reactions and because it cannot indicate a specific dysfunction of the liver. See also **sulfobromophthalein.**

bronch-, a combining form meaning 'pertaining to the bronchus': *bronchiectasis, bronchiotetany, bronchodilatation.*

bronchial /brong′kē·əl/ [Gk, *bronchos,* windpipe], pertaining to the bronchi or bronchioles.

bronchial asthma. See **asthma.**

bronchial breath sound [Gk, *bronchos,* windpipe], an abnormal sound heard with a stethoscope over the lungs, indicating consolidation because of pneumonia or compression. Expiration and inspiration produce loud, high-pitched sounds of equal duration.

bronchial drainage. See **postural drainage.**

bronchial fremitus, a vibration that can be palpated or auscultated on the chest wall over a bronchus congested by secretions that rattle as the air passes during respiration. See also **fremitus.**

bronchial hyperreactivity [Gk, *bronchos; hyper,* excess; L, *re,* again, *agere,* to act], an abnormal respiratory condition characterized by reflex bronchospasm in response to histamine or a cholinergic drug. It is a universal feature of asthma and is used in the differential diagnosis of asthma and heart disease. An asthmatic person experiences episodes of bronchospasm in response to the cholinergic effect of endogenous histamine and to exposure via inhalation of histamine or a cholinergic drug such as methacholine in testing for asthma.

bronchial pneumonia. See **bronchopneumonia.**

bronchial secretion, a substance produced in the bronchial tree that consists of mucus secreted by the goblet cells and mucous glands of the bronchi, protein salts released from disintegrating cells, plasma fluid, and proteins, including fibrinogen, escaping from pulmonary capillaries.

bronchial spasm, an excessive and prolonged contraction of the involuntary muscle fibers in the walls of the bronchi and bronchioles. The contractions may be localized or general and may be caused by irritation or injury to the respiratory mucosa, infections, or allergies. Also called **bronchiospasm, bronchospasm.**

bronchial toilet, special care that is given patients with tracheostomies and respiratory disorders, including stimulation of coughing, deep breathing, and the suctioning of the respiratory tract with a tracheobronchial aspiration pump.

bronchial tree, an anatomic complex of the bronchi and the bronchial tubes. The bronchi branch from the trachea, and the bronchial tubes branch from the bronchi. The right bronchus is wider and shorter than the left bronchus, and it diverges less abruptly from the trachea. The right bronchus branches into three secondary bronchi, one passing to each of the three lobes that comprise the right lung. The left bronchus is smaller in diameter but about twice as long as the right bronchus and passes inferior to the pulmonary artery before branching into the secondary bronchi for the inferior and the superior lobes of the left lung.

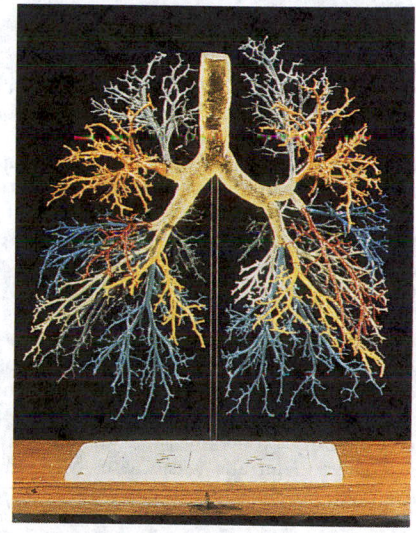

Cast of the bronchial tree (Turner-Warwick, 1989)

bronchial washing [Gk, *bronchos,* windpipe; ME, *wasshen,* to wash], the irrigation of the bronchi and bronchioles to cleanse them and to collect specimens for laboratory examination.

bronchiectasis /brong′kē·ek′təsis/ [Gk, *bronchos* + *ektasis,* stretching], an abnormal condition of the bronchial tree, characterized by irreversible dilatation and destruction of the bronchial walls. The condition is sometimes congenital but is more often a result of bronchial infection or of obstruction by a tumor or an aspirated foreign body. Symptoms of bronchiectasis include a constant cough productive of copious purulent sputum, hemoptysis, chronic sinusitis, clubbing of fingers, and persistent moist, coarse rales. Some of the complications of bronchiectasis are pneumonia, lung abscess, empyema, brain abscess, and amyloidosis. Treatment includes frequent postural drainage, antibiotics, and, rarely, surgical resection of the affected part of the lungs.

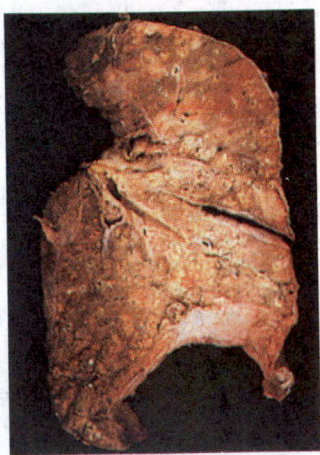

Bronchiectasis *(Fletcher, 1987)*

bronchiolar. See **bronchiole.**

bronchiolar carcinoma. See **alveolar cell carcinoma.**

bronchiolar collapse /brong′kyələr/ [L, *bronchiolus*, little windpipe; *conlabi*, to fall], a condition in which bronchioles, pliable soft-walled tubes without cartilage support, become compressed by the pressure of surrounding structures and the lack of inflowing air needed to keep them inflated. The condition occurs in such disorders as emphysema, cystic disease, and bronchiectasis.

bronchiole /brong′kē·ōl/ [L, *bronchiolus*, little windpipe], a small airway of the respiratory system extending from the bronchi into the lobes of the lung. There are two divisions of bronchioles: The terminal bronchioles pass inspired air from the bronchi to the respiratory bronchioles and expired waste gases from the respiratory bronchioles to the bronchi. The respiratory bronchioles function similarly, allowing the exchange of air and waste gases between the alveolar ducts and the terminal bronchioles. **–bronchiolar** /brongkē′ələr/, *adj.*

bronchiolitis /brong′kē·ōlī′tis/ [L, *bronchiolus*, little windpipe + Gk, *itis*, inflammation], an acute viral infection of the lower respiratory tract that occurs primarily in infants under 18 months of age, characterized by expiratory wheezing, respiratory distress, inflammation, and obstruction at the level of the bronchioles. The most common causative agents are the respiratory syncytial viruses (RSV) and the parainfluenza viruses. *Mycoplasma pneumoniae,* the rhinoviruses, enteroviruses, and measles virus are less common causative agents. Transmission occurs by infection with airborne particles or by contact with infected secretions. The diagnosis consists of evidence of hyperinflation of the lungs through percussion or chest x-ray examination.

■ OBSERVATIONS: The condition typically begins as an upper respiratory tract infection with serous nasal discharge and, often, low-grade fever. Increasing respiratory distress follows, characterized by tachypnea, tachycardia, intercostal and subcostal retractions, a paroxysmal cough, an expiratory wheeze, and, often, an elevated temperature. The chest may appear barrel-shaped; x-ray films show hyperinflated lungs and a depressed diaphragm. Respiration becomes more shallow, causing increased alveolar oxygen tension and leading to respiratory acidosis. Complete obstruction and absorption of trapped air may lead to atelectasis and respiratory failure. Blood gas determinations indicate the degree of carbon dioxide retention.

■ INTERVENTIONS: Routine treatment includes humidity and oxygen via a mist tent, vaporizer, or Croupette, generally combined with oxygen; an adequate fluid intake, usually given intravenously because of tachypnea, weakness, and fatigue; suctioning of the airways to remove secretions; and rest. Endotracheal intubation is indicated when carbon dioxide retention occurs, when bronchial secretions do not loosen and clear, or when oxygen therapy does not alleviate hypoxia. Such medications as antibiotics, bronchodilators, corticosteroids, cough suppressants, and expectorants are not routinely used. Sedatives are contraindicated because of their suppressant effect on the respiratory tract. The infection typically runs its course in 7 to 10 days, with good prognosis. A major complication is bacterial infection, most commonly after prolonged use of a mist tent. The disorder is often confused with asthma: A family history of allergy, the presence of other allergic manifestations, and improvement with epinephrine injection is usually indicative of asthma, not bronchiolitis. Cystic fibrosis, pertussis, the bronchopneumonias, and foreign body obstruction of the trachea are other disorders that may be confused with bronchiolitis.

■ NURSING CONSIDERATIONS: The focus of nursing care is to promote rest and to conserve the child's energy by reducing anxiety and apprehension; to increase the ease of breathing with humidity and oxygen as needed; to aid in changing position for comfort; and to induce drainage of secretions or to suction when necessary. Fever is usually controlled by the cool atmosphere of the mist tent and by administering antipyretics as needed. Frequent changing of clothing and bed linen is often necessary in a mist environment to reduce chilling. Vital signs and chest and breath sounds are continuously monitored to detect early signs of respiratory distress.

bronchiospasm. See **bronchial spasm.**

bronchitis /brongkī′tis/ [Gk, *bronchos*, windpipe + *itis*, inflammation], an acute or chronic inflammation of the mucous membranes of the tracheobronchial tree. **Acute bronchitis** is characterized by a productive cough, fever, hypertrophy of mucus-secreting structures, and back pain. Caused by the spread of upper respiratory viral infections to the bronchi, it is often observed with or after childhood infections like measles, whooping cough, diphtheria, and typhoid fever. Treatment includes bed rest, aspirin, expectorants, and appropriate antibiotic therapy. **Chronic bronchitis** is distinguished by an excessive secretion of mucus in the bronchi with a productive cough for at least 3 consecutive months in at least 2 successive years. Additional symptoms are frequent chest infections, cyanosis, hypoxemia, hypercapnia, and a marked tendency for the development of cor pulmonale and respiratory failure. Predisposing factors for chronic bronchitis include cigarette smoking, chronic infections, and abnormal physical development of the bronchi that distorts the structures sufficiently to interfere with bronchial drainage. Most common in adults, it is often a com-

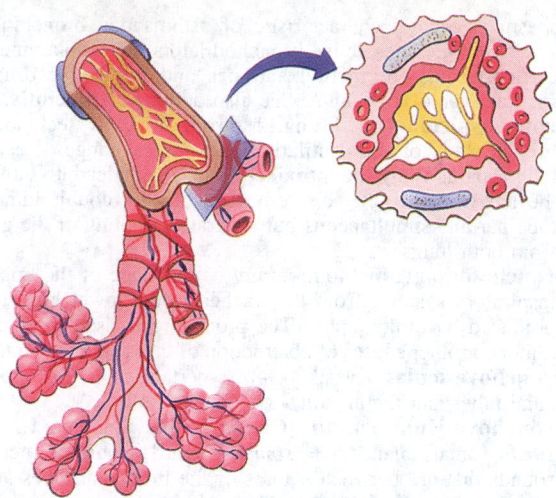

Chronic bronchitis *(Thibodeau, 1993/Rolin Graphics)*

plication of cystic fibrosis in children. Treatment includes the cessation of cigarette smoking, avoidance of airway irritants, the use of expectorants, and postural drainage. Currently, prophylactic antibiotics, steroids, and desensitization therapy are not recommended. See also **chronic obstructive pulmonary disease (COPD), respiratory syncytial virus.**

bronchoalveolar /-alvē′ələr/ [Gk, *bronchos,* windpipe; L, *alveolus,* little hollow],   pertaining to the terminal air sacs at the ends of the bronchioles.

bronchoconstriction [Gk, *bronchos,* windpipe; L, *constringere,* to draw tight],   a constriction of the bronchi, resulting in a narrowing of the airway lumen.

bronchodilatation /-dil′ətā′shən/ [Gk, *bronchos,* windpipe; L, *dilatare,* to widen],   an increase in the diameter or lumen of the bronchi, allowing increased airflow to and from the lungs.

bronchodilator /-dilā′tər/,   a substance, especially a drug, that relaxes contractions of the smooth muscle of the bronchioles to improve ventilation to the lungs. Pharmacologic bronchodilators are prescribed to improve aeration in asthma, bronchiectasis, bronchitis, and emphysema. Commonly used bronchodilators include corticosteroids, ephedrine, isoproterenol hydrochloride, theophylline, and various derivatives and combinations of these drugs. Beclomethasone dipropionate and triamcinolone are available in aerosol form. The adverse effects vary, depending on the particular class of the bronchodilating drug. In general, bronchodilators are given with caution to people with impaired cardiac function. Nervousness, irritability, gastritis, or palpitations of the heart may occur.

bronchofibroscopy.   See **fiberoptic bronchoscopy.**

bronchogenic /-jen′ik/ [Gk, *bronchos* + *genein,* to produce],   originating in the bronchi.

bronchogenic carcinoma,   one of the more than 90% of malignant lung tumors that originate in bronchi. Lesions, usually associated with cigarette smoking, may cause coughing and wheezing, fatigue, chest tightness, and aching joints. In the late stages, bloody sputum, clubbing of the fingers, weight loss, and pleural effusion may be present. Diagnosis is made by bronchoscopy, sputum cytology, lymph node biopsy, radioisotope scanning procedures, or exploratory surgery. About 45% of the tumors are squamous cell or epidermoid carcinomas, 33% are oat cell carcinomas, and 15% to 20% are adenocarcinomas. Surgery is the most effective treatment, but approximately 50% of cases are advanced and inoperable when first seen. Palliative treatment includes radiotherapy and chemotherapy.

bronchography /brongkog′rəfē/,   an x-ray examination of the bronchi after they have been coated with a radiopaque substance.

bronchomotor tone,   the state of contraction or relaxation of smooth muscle in the bronchial walls that regulates the caliber of the airways.

bronchophony /brongkof′ənē/ [Gk, *bronchos* + *phone,* voice],   an increase in intensity and clarity of vocal resonance that may result from an increase in lung tissue density, such as in the consolidation of pneumonia.

bronchopneumonia [Gk, *bronchos* + *pneumon,* lung],   an acute inflammation of the lungs and bronchioles, characterized by chills, fever, high pulse and respiratory rates, bronchial breathing, cough with purulent bloody sputum, severe chest pain, and abdominal distension. The disease is usually a result of the spread of bacterial infection from the upper respiratory tract to the lower respiratory tract, caused by *Mycoplasma pneumoniae, Staphylococcus pyogenes,* or *Streptococcus pneumoniae.* Atypical forms of bronchopneumonia may occur in viral and rickettsial infections. The most common cause in infancy is the respiratory syncytial virus (RSV). The condition results in pleural effusion, empyema, lung abscess, peripheral thrombophlebitis, respiratory failure, congestive heart failure, and jaundice. Treatment includes an antibiotic, often penicillin or ampicillin, oxygen therapy, supportive measures to keep the bronchi clear of secretions, and relief of pleural pain. Also called **bronchial pneumonia.** Compare **aspiration pneumonia, eosinophilic pneumonia, interstitial pneumonia.** See also **lobar pneumonia, respiratory syncytial virus.**

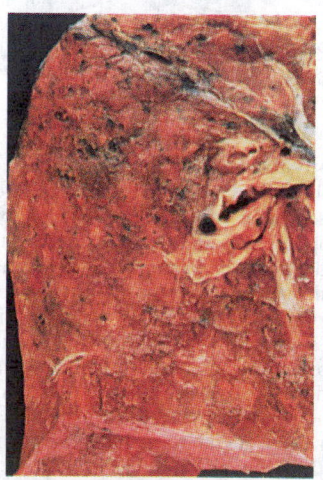

Bronchopneumonia *(Fletcher, 1987)*

bronchopulmonary /-pul'mōner'ē/ [Gk, *bronchos* + L, *pulmonis*, lung], of or pertaining to the bronchi and the lungs of the respiratory system.

bronchopulmonary hygiene, the care and cleanliness of the respiratory tract, including ventilatory/respiratory therapy equipment and natural air passages. Hygienic care also allows for complete assessment of the patient's respiratory condition and of any equipment or devices used to support his or her breathing. The patient may need assistance in performing postural drainage and controlled coughing techniques or may require percussion, vibration, or rib shaking. Respiratory care equipment is a potential source and reservoir of infectious organisms and must be cleaned and sterilized periodically.

bronchopulmonary lavage [Gk, *bronchos*, windpipe; L, *pulmonis*, lung; Fr, *lavage*, washing out], the irrigation or washing out of the bronchi and bronchioles to remove pulmonary secretions.

bronchoscope /brong'kəskōp'/, a curved, flexible tube for visual examination of the bronchi. It contains fibers that carry light down the tube and project an enlarged image up the tube to the viewer. The bronchoscope is used to examine the bronchi, to secure a specimen for biopsy or culture, or to aspirate a foreign body from the respiratory tract. See also **fiberoptic bronchoscopy.** –**bronchoscopic,** *adj.*

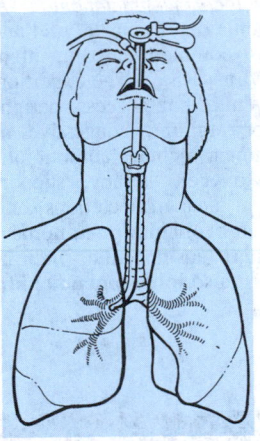

Bronchoscope

bronchoscopy /brongkos'kəpē/, the visual examination of the tracheobronchial tree, using the standard rigid, tubular metal bronchoscope or the narrower, flexible fiberoptic bronchoscope. The patient is in a fasting state and is usually sedated before the examination, which is routinely performed under topical anesthesia. In addition to visualization, the procedure can be used for suctioning, for obtaining a biopsy and fluid or sputum for examination, for removal of foreign bodies, and for diagnosing such conditions as localized atelectasis, bronchial obstruction, lung abscess, and tracheal extubation. See also **bronchoscope.**

bronchospasm, an abnormal contraction of the smooth muscle of the bronchi, resulting in an acute narrowing and obstruction of the respiratory airway. A cough with generalized wheezing usually indicates this condition. Broncho-

spasm is a chief characteristic of asthma and bronchitis. Treatment includes active bronchodilators, catecholamines, corticosteroids, or methylxanthines and preventive drugs such as cromolyn sodium. See also **asthma, bronchitis.**

bronchospirometry /brong'kōspīrom'ətrē/, a technique for the study of the ventilation and gas exchange of each lung separately by the introduction of a catheter into either the left or the right mainstem bronchus. A double-lumen tube permits simultaneous but separate sampling of the gas from both lungs.

bronchotomogram /-tom'əgram/, an image of the upper respiratory system, from the trachea to the lower bronchi, produced by tomography. The procedure is used to detect tumors or other causes of obstruction of the respiratory tract.

bronchovesicular /-vesik'yələr/, pertaining to the bronchial tubes and the alveoli.

bronchovesicular sounds [Gk, *bronchos*, windpipe; L, *vesicula*, small bladder + *sonus*, sound], normal breath sounds that are between sounds of the bronchial tubes and those of the alveoli, or a combination of the two sounds.

bronchus /brong'kəs/, *pl.* **bronchi** /-kī/ [L; Gk, *bronchos*, windpipe], any one of several large air passages in the lungs through which pass inspired air and exhaled waste gases. Each bronchus has a wall consisting of three layers. The outermost is made of dense fibrous tissue, reinforced with cartilage. The middle layer is a network of smooth muscle. The innermost layer consists of ciliated mucous membrane. Kinds of bronchi are **lobar bronchus, primary bronchus, secondary bronchus,** and **segmental bronchus.** See also **arteriole, bronchiole.** –**bronchial,** *adj.*

Bronkephrine, a trademark for a sympathomimetic bronchodilator (ethylnorepinephrine hydrochloride).

Bronkodyl, a trademark for a smooth muscle relaxant (theophylline).

Bronkosol, a trademark for a bronchodilator (isoetharine hydrochloride) used for temporary relief of bronchial asthma, acute paroxysms, and bronchial spasms of bronchitis and emphysema.

Brönsted-Lowry base, any chemical compound that accepts a proton. It may or may not be a hydroxide.

bronze diabetes. See **exogenous hemochromatosis.**

bronzed diabetes. See **hepatic siderosis.**

broth, **1.** a fluid culture medium, such as a solution of lactose or thioglycollate, used to support the growth of bacteria for laboratory analysis. **2.** a beverage or other fluid made with meat extract and water, such as chicken bouillon.

brow, the forehead, particularly the eyebrow or ridge above the eye.

brown fat [ME, *broun;* AS, *faett,* filled], a type of fat present in newborn infants and rarely found in adults. Brown fat is a unique source of heat energy for the infant because it has greater thermogenic activity than ordinary fat. Brown fat deposits occur around the kidneys, neck, and upper chest area.

brownian movement /brou'nyən/ [Robert Brown, Scottish botanist, b. 1773], a random movement of microscopic particles suspended in a liquid or gas, such as the continuing erratic behavior of dust particles in still water. The movement is produced by the natural kinetic activity of molecules of the fluid striking the foreign particles.

brown recluse spider bite [L, *recludere,* to shut off; ME, *spithre;* AS, *bitan*], the bite of the brown or violin spider, *Loxosceles reclusa,* producing a characteristic necrotic lesion. There is little or no initial pain but localized pain

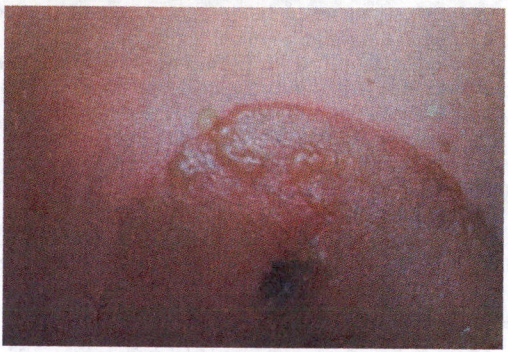

Brown recluse spider bite *(Weston, 1991)*

develops about an hour later. A bleb forms, sometimes in a target or bull's eye pattern. The blood-filled bleb increases in size and eventually ruptures, leaving a black scar. The patient may also experience systemic symptoms.

Brown-Séquard's treatment. See **organotherapy.**

Brown-Séquard syndrome /broun'säkär'/ [Charles E. Brown-Séquard, French physiologist, b. 1817], a traumatic neurologic disorder resulting from compression of one side of the spinal cord, above the tenth thoracic vertebrae, characterized by spastic paralysis on the injured side of the body, loss of postural sense, and loss of the senses of pain and heat on the other side of the body.

brown spider, a poisonous insect, also known as the brown recluse or violin spider, found in both North and South America. The venom from its bite usually creates a blister surrounded by concentric white and red circles. This so-called 'bull's eye' appearance is helpful in distinguishing it from other spider bites. The wound ordinarily ulcerates and sometimes becomes infected. Pain, nausea, fever, and chills are common, but the reaction is usually self-limited. Antivenin is not available in the United States, but corticosteroids may be administered.

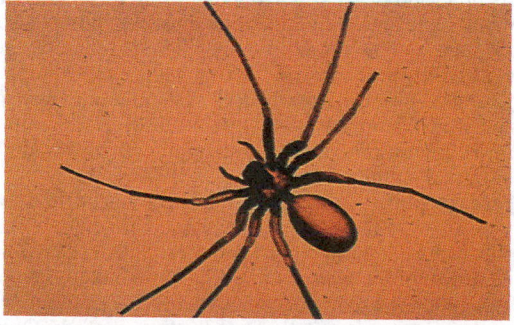

Brown recluse spider *(Habif, 1990)*

brow presentation, an obstetric situation in which the brow, or forehead, of the fetus is the first part of the body to enter the birth canal. Because the diameter of the fetal head at this angle may be greater than the mother's pelvic outlet, a cesarean section may be recommended. However, the fetus usually converts to a face presentation.

Brucella abortus. See **abortus fever.**

brucellosis /broo'səlō'sis/ [Sir David Bruce, English pathologist, b. 1855], a disease caused by any of several species of the gram-negative coccobacillus *Brucella*. Brucellosis is most prevalent in rural areas among farmers, veterinarians, meat packers, slaughterhouse workers, and livestock producers. It is primarily a disease of animals (including cattle, pigs, and goats), and humans usually acquire it by ingesting contaminated milk or milk products or through a break in the skin. It is characterized by fever, chills, sweating, malaise, and weakness. The fever often comes in waves, rising in the evening and subsiding during the day, occurring at intervals separated by periods of remission. Other signs and symptoms may include anorexia and weight loss, headache, muscle and joint pain, and an enlarged spleen. In some victims the disease is acute; more often it is chronic, recurring over a period of months or years. Although brucellosis itself is rarely fatal, treatment is important because serious complications such as pneumonia, meningitis, and encephalitis can develop. Tetracycline plus streptomycin is the treatment of choice; bed rest is also important. Also called **Cyprus fever, Gibraltar fever, Malta fever, Mediterranean fever, rock fever, undulant fever.** See also **abortus fever.**

Bruch's disease. See **Marseilles fever.**

Brudzinski's sign /broodzin'skēz/ [Josef Brudzinski, Polish physician, b. 1874], an involuntary flexion of the arm, hip, and knee when the neck is passively flexed, seen in patients with meningitis.

bruise. See **contusion, ecchymosis.**

bruit /broo'ē/ [Fr, noise], an abnormal sound or murmur heard while auscultating a carotid artery, organ or gland, such as the liver or thyroid. The specific character of the bruit, its location, and the time of its occurrence in a cycle of other sounds are all of diagnostic importance.

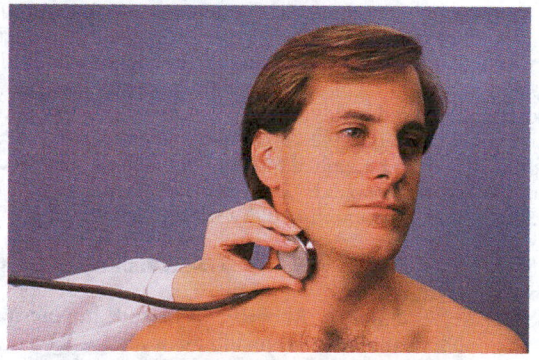

Auscultation for bruits *(Canobbio, 1990)*

Brunnstrom hemiplegia classification, an evaluation procedure that assesses muscle tone and voluntary control of movement patterns in a stroke patient. Results indicate the patient's progress through stages of recovery.

brush border, microvilli on the free surfaces of certain epithelial cells, particularly the absorptive surfaces of the intestine and the proximal convoluted tubules of the kidney. The tiny cylindric processes increase the surface area of the tissues.

Brushfield's spots [Thomas Brushfield, English physician, b. 1858; ME *spotte* stain], pinpoint, white or light yellow spots on the iris of a child with Down's syndrome. Occasionally, they are seen in normal infants.

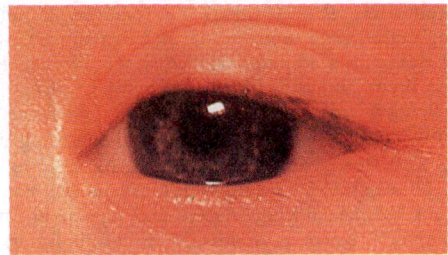

Brushfield spots (Zitelli, 1992)

Bruton's agammaglobulinemia [Ogden C. Bruton, American physician, b. 1908], a sex-linked, inherited condition characterized by the absence of gamma globulin in the blood. Patients (usually children) with this syndrome are deficient in antibodies and susceptible to repeated infections. Compare **agammaglobulinemia.**

bruxism /bruk′sizəm/ [Gk, *brychein*, to gnash the teeth], the compulsive, unconscious grinding of the teeth, especially during sleep or as a mechanism for the release of tension during periods of extreme stress in the waking hours. Also called **bruxomania.**

bry-, a prefix meaning 'tree moss': *bryocyte, bryocytole, bryocytic.*

Bryant's traction /brī′ənts/ [Sir Thomas Bryant, English physician, b. 1828; L, *trahere*, to pull], an orthopedic mechanism used only with infants to immobilize both lower extremities in the treatment of a fractured femur or in the correction of the congenital dislocation of the hip. This mechanism consists of a traction frame supporting weights, connected by ropes that run through pulleys to traction foot plates worn by the infant. The traction pull elevates the lower extremities to a vertical position with the patient supine, the trunk and the lower extremities forming a right angle. The weight applied to the traction mechanism is usually less than 35 pounds. Compare **Buck's traction.**

BSA, 1. abbreviation for **body surface area.** See **surface area.** 2. abbreviation for *bovine serum albumin.*

BSE, abbreviation for **breast self-examination.** See **self-breast examination.**

BSN, abbreviation for **Bachelor of Science in Nursing.**

BSP, abbreviation for **Bromsulphalein.**

BT, abbreviation for **bleeding time.**

BTPD, abbreviation for *body temperature, ambient pressure, dry.*

BTPS, abbreviation for *body temperature, ambient pressure, saturated* (with water vapor). See also **volume (BTPS).**

BTU, abbreviation for **British Thermal Unit.**

buba See **yaws.**

bubbling rale [ME, *bubblen*, to make bubbles; Fr, *ralement*, a rattling], an abnormal chest sound characteristic of moisture moving in the lungs. Compare **amphoric breath sound, atelectatic rale, dry rale.**

bubble-diffusion humidifier, a device that provides hu-

midified oxygen or other therapeutic gases by allowing the gas to bubble through a reservoir of water.

bubble oxygenator, a heart-lung device that oxygenates the blood while it is diverted outside the patient's body.

bubo /byoo′bō/, *pl.* **buboes** [Gk, *boubon*, groin], a greatly enlarged, inflamed lymph node usually in the axilla or groin that is associated with diseases such as chancroid, lymphogranuloma venereum, bubonic plague, and syphilis. Treatment includes specific antibiotic therapy, application of moist heat, and, sometimes, incision and drainage.

bubonic plague /byoobon′ik/ [Gk, *boubon*, groin; L, *plaga*, stroke], the most common form of plague. It is characterized by painful buboes in the axilla, groin, or neck, fever often rising to 106° F (41.11°C), prostration with a rapid, thready pulse, hypotension, delirium, and bleeding into the skin from the superficial blood vessels. The symptoms are caused by an endotoxin released by a bacillus, *Yersinia pestis,* usually introduced into the body by the bite of a rat flea that has bitten an infected rat. Inoculation with plague vaccine confers partial immunity; infection provides lifetime immunity. Treatment includes antibiotics, supportive nursing care, surgical drainage of buboes, isolation, and stringent precautions against spread of the disease. Conditions favor a plague epidemic when a large infected rodent population lives with a large nonimmune human population in a damp, warm climate. Improved sanitary conditions and the eradication of rats and other rodent reservoirs of *Y. pestis* may prevent outbreaks of the disease. Killing the infected rodents, which may include squirrels and rabbits, and not the fleas allows a continued threat of human infection. Also called (*informal*) **black death, black plague.** Compare **pneumonic plague, septicemic plague.** See also **bubo,** plague, *Yersinia pestis.*

bucca-. See **bucco-.**

buccal /buk′əl/ [L, *bucca*, cheek], of or pertaining to the inside of the cheek, the surface of a tooth, or the gum next to the cheek.

buccal administration of medication, oral administration of a drug, usually in the form of a tablet, by placing it between the cheek and the teeth or gum until it dissolves.

buccal bar, a portion of an orthodontic appliance that consists of a rigid metal wire extending from the buccal side of a molar band anteriorly. See also **arch bar, labial bar, lingual bar.**

buccal contour [L, *bucca; cum*, together with, *tornare*, to turn], the shape of the buccal side of a posterior tooth, usually characterized by a slight occlusocervical convexity with its largest prominence at the gingival third of the clinical buccal surface.

buccal fat pad, a fat pad in the cheek under the subcutaneous layer of the skin, over the buccinator. It is particularly prominent in infants and is often called a sucking pad.

buccal flange [L, *bucca;* OFr, *flanche*, flank], the portion of a denture base that occupies the buccal vestibule of the mouth and extends distally from the buccal notch. Compare **labial flange, lingual flange.** See also **flange.**

buccal glands [L, *bucca*, cheek, *glans*, acorn], small salivary glands located between the buccinator muscle and the mucous membrane in the vestibule of the mouth.

buccal notch, a depression in a denture flange that accommodates the buccal frenum. See also **labial notch.**

buccal smear, a sample of cells removed from the buccal mucosa for purposes of obtaining a karyotype to determine the genetic sex of an individual.

buccal splint, any material, usually plaster, placed on the buccal surfaces of fixed partial denture units to hold the units in position for assembly.

bucci-. See **bucco-.**

buccinator /buk′sinā′tər/ [L, *buccina*, trumpet], the main muscle of the cheek, one of the 12 muscles of the mouth. It arises from the maxilla above and the mandible below, inserting in the lips; its superficial surface is covered by the buccopharyngeal fascia and the buccal fat pad. Its deep part is pierced by the duct of the parotid gland opposite the second molar tooth. The buccinator, innervated by buccal branches of the facial nerve, compresses the cheek, acting as an important accessory muscle of mastication by holding food under the teeth.

bucco-, bucca-, bucci-, a combining form meaning 'pertaining to the cheek': *buccocervical, buccodistal, buccogingival.*

buccogingival /buk′ōjinjī′vəl/, pertaining to the internal mouth structures, particularly the cheeks and gums.

buccolinguomasticatory triad /buk′ōling′wōmas′təkətôr′e/ [L *bucca* cheek, *lingua* tongue, *masticare* to gnash the teeth], a complex of involuntary lip, tongue, jaw, and head movements seen in tardive dyskinesia.

buccopharyngeal /buk′ōfərin′jē·əl/, of or pertaining to the cheek and the pharynx or to the mouth and the pharynx.

bucket. See **socket.**

bucket handle fracture [OFr, *buket*, tub; ME, *handel*, part grasped; L, *fractura*, break], a fracture that produces a tear in a semilunar cartilage along the medial side of the knee joint.

bucking, *informal.* **1.** gagging on an endotracheal tube. **2.** involuntarily resisting insufflation by a positive pressure respirator.

buck knife, a periodontal surgical knife with a spear-shaped cutting point, used for interdental incision associated with a gingivectomy.

Buck's skin traction, an orthopedic procedure that applies traction to the lower extremity with the hips and the knees extended. It is used in the treatment of hip and knee contractures, in postoperative positioning and immobilization, and in disease processes of the hip and the knee. This type of traction may be unilateral, involving one leg, or bilateral, involving both legs.

Buck's traction [Gurdon Buck, American surgeon, b. 1807; L, *trahere*, to pull], one of the most common orthopedic mechanisms by which pull is exerted on the lower extremity with a system of ropes, weights, and pulleys. Buck's traction, which may be unilateral or bilateral, is used to immobilize, position, and align the lower extremity in the treatment of contractures and diseases of the hip and knee. The mechanism commonly consists of a metal bar extending from a frame at the foot of the patient's bed, supporting traction weights connected by a rope passing through a pulley to a cast or a splint around the affected body structure. Compare **Bryant's traction.**

Bucky diaphragm [Gustav P. Bucky, American radiologist, b. 1880; Gk, *diaphragma*, partition], (in radiology) a device consisting of a moving grid that limits the amount of scattered radiation reaching the film and thus obtains finer x-ray film contrast and detail. Also called **Bucky grid.**

buclizine hydrochloride /bōō′kləzēn/, an antiemetic drug derived from piperazine but with antihistamine properties. It is also used to treat allergies and vertigo.

Budd-Chiari syndrome /bud′kē·ãr′ē/ [George Budd, English physician, b. 1880; Hans Chiari, Czech-French pathologist, b. 1851], a disorder of hepatic circulation, marked by venous obstruction, that leads to liver enlargement, ascites, extensive development of collateral vessels, and severe portal hypertension. Also called **Chiari's syndrome, Rokitansky's disease.**

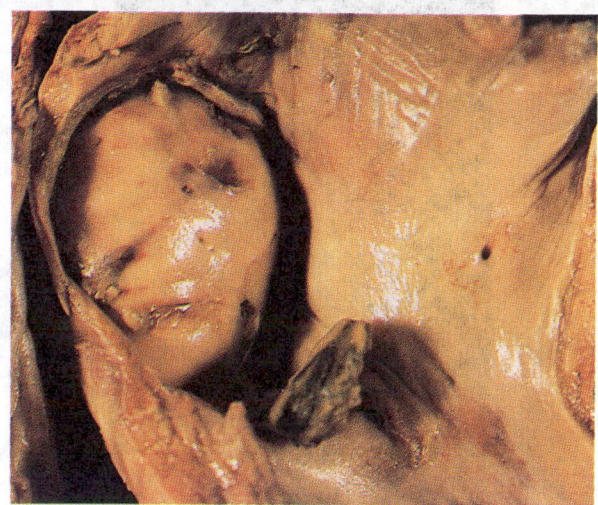

Budd-Chiari syndrome (Fletcher, 1987)

budding [ME *budde*], a type of asexual reproduction in which the cell produces a budlike projection containing chromatin that eventually separates from the parent and develops into an independent organism. It is a common form of reproduction in the lower animals and plants, such as sponges, yeasts, and molds.

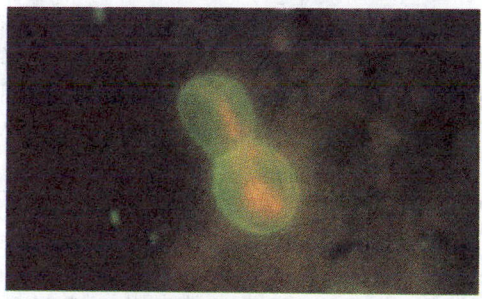

Budding (Baron, 1990)

buddy splint, a splinting technique commonly used after a finger injury requiring immobilization. The injured finger and the adjacent finger are typically taped together to limit the range of motion of the affected finger.

Buerger's disease. See **thromboangiitis obliterans.**

Buerger's postural exercises [Leo Buerger, American physician, b. 1879; L, *ponere*, to place, *exercere*, to continue working], a set of special exercises designed to maintain circulation in a limb.

buffalo hump, an accumulation of fat on the back of the neck associated with the prolonged use of large doses of glucocorticoids or the hypersecretion of cortisol caused by Cushing's syndrome.

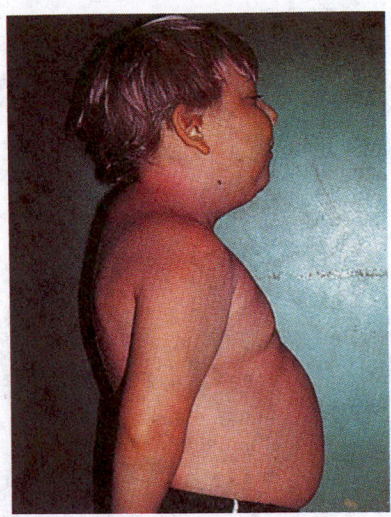

Buffalo hump (Zitelli, 1992)

buffer [ME, *buffe,* to cushion], a substance or group of substances that tends to control the hydrogen ion concentration in a solution by absorbing hydrogen ions when an acid is added to the system and releasing hydrogen ions upon the addition of a base. Buffers minimize significant changes of pH in a chemical system. Among the functions carried out by buffer systems in the body are maintenance of the acid-base balance of the blood and maintenance of the proper pH in kidney tubules. See also **blood buffers, pH.**

buffer anions, the negatively charged bicarbonate, protein, and phosphate ions that comprise the buffer systems of the body.

buffer cations, the positively charged ions of the body's electrolytes, including sodium, calcium, potassium, and magnesium.

buffer solution [ME, *buffet;* L, *solutus,* dissolved], a solution that will maintain or will a given pH value despite dilution or the addition of a small amount of base or acid.

buffy coat [ME, *buffet;* Fr, *cote*], a grayish-white layer of white blood cells and platelets, mixed with some red blood cells, that accumulates on the surface of sedimented erythrocytes when blood plasma is allowed to stand.

buffy coat transfusion. See **granulocyte transfusion.**

bug, an error in a computer program (software bug) or a design flaw in computer hardware (hardware bug), usually resulting in the inability to make a computer process data correctly.

bulb [L, *bulbus,* swollen root], any rounded structure, such as the eyeball, hair roots, and certain sensory nerve endings.

bulbar /bul'bər/ [L, *bulbus*], **1.** pertaining to a bulb. **2.** pertaining to the medulla oblongata of the brain and the cranial nerves.

bulbar ataxia [L, *bulbus,* a swollen root; Gk, *ataxia,* lack of order], a loss of motor coordination caused by a lesion in the medulla oblongata or pons.

bulbar conjunctiva. See **conjunctiva.**

bulbar myelitis [L, *bulbus,* swollen root; Gk, *myelos,* marrow, *itis,* inflammation], an inflammation of the central nervous system involving the medulla oblongata.

bulbar palsy [L, *bulbus,* swollen root; Gk, *paralyein,* to be palsied], a form of paralysis resulting from a defect in the motor centers of the medulla oblongata. See also **bulbar poliomyelitis.**

bulbar paralysis, a degenerative neurologic condition characterized by progressive paralysis of cranial nerves and involving the lips, tongue, mouth, pharynx, and larynx. The condition occurs most commonly in people over 50 years of age, in multiple sclerosis, and in amyotrophic lateral sclerosis.

bulbar poliomyelitis [L, *bulbus,* swollen root; Gk, *polios,* gray, *myelos,* marrow, *itis,* inflammation], a form of poliomyelitis that involves the medulla oblongata and gradually progresses to bulbar paralysis, with respiratory and circulatory failure.

bulbocavernosus /bul'bōkav'ərnō'səs/ [L, *bulbus,* swollen root, *cavernosum,* full of hollows], a muscle that covers the bulb of the penis in the male and the bulbus vestibuli in the female. Also called **accelerator urinae, ejaculator urinae,** *(in females)* **sphincter virginae.**

bulbourethral gland /-yŏŏrē'thrəl/, one of two small glands located on each side of the prostate, draining to the urethra. Bulbourethral glands secrete a fluid component of the seminal fluid. Also called **Cowper's gland.**

bulbous [L, *bulbus,* swollen root], pertaining to a structure that resembles a bulb or that originates in a bulb.

bulb syringe, a blunt-tipped, flexible syringe usually made of rubber or plastic. Bulb syringes are used primarily for irrigating external orifices, such as the auditory canal.

bulbus oculi. See **eye.**

-bulia, -boulia, a suffix meaning '(condition of the) will': *abulia, parabulia, hyperbulia.*

bulimia /byŏŏlim'ē·ə/ [Gk, *bous,* ox, *limos,* hunger], an insatiable craving for food, often resulting in episodes of continuous eating, and often followed by purging, depression, and self-deprivation. Also spelled **boulimia.** See also **anorexia nervosa.** –**bulemic,** *n., adj.*

bulk. See **dietary fiber.**

bulk cathartic [ME, *bulke,* heap; Gk, *kathartikos,* evacuation of bowels], a cathartic that acts by softening and increasing the mass of fecal material in the bowel. Bulk cathartics contain a hydrophilic agent such as methylcellulose or psyllium seed.

bulla /bŏŏl'ə, bul'ə/, *pl.* **bullae** [L, bubble], a thin-walled blister of the skin or mucous membranes greater than 1 cm in diameter containing clear, serous fluid. Compare **vesicle.** –**bullous,** *adj.*

bulldog forceps, short, spring forceps for clamping an artery or vein for hemostasis. The jaws may be padded to avoid injury to vascular tissue.

bullet forceps, a kind of forceps that has thin, curved, serrated blades that are designed for extracting a foreign object, such as a bullet, from the base of a puncture wound.

-bullous. See **bulla.**

bullous disease /bŏŏl'əs/, any disease marked by erup-

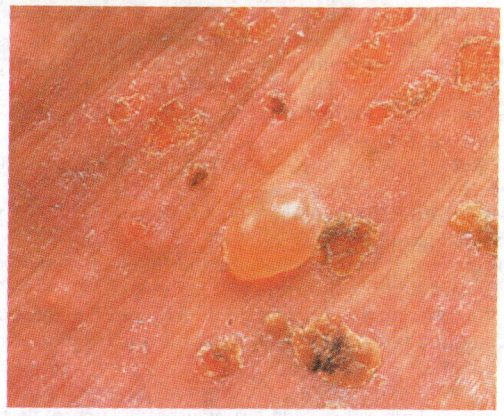

Bulla (duVivier, 1993)

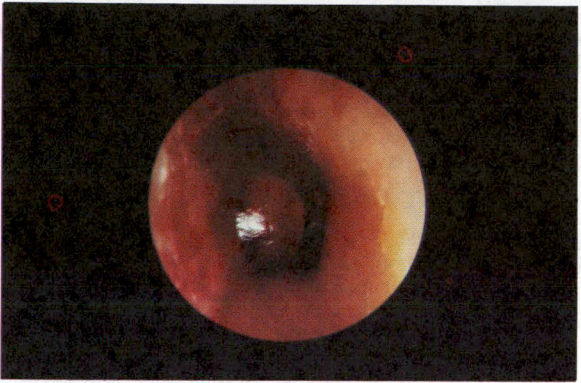

bullous myringitis (Bingham, 1992)

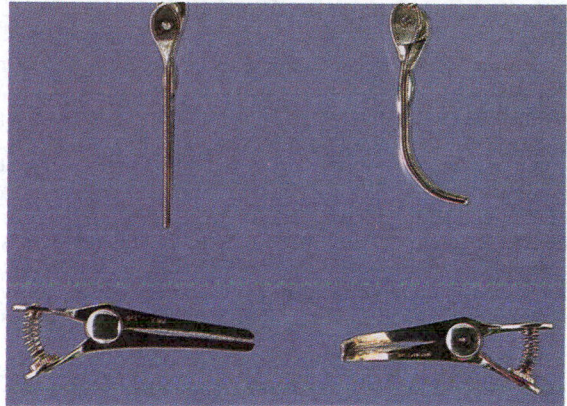

Bulldog forceps (Brooks-Tighe, 1989)

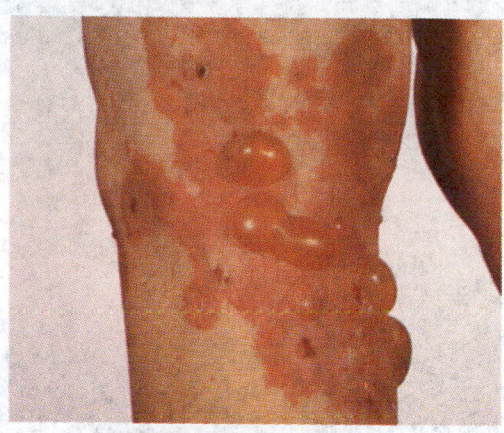

Bullous pemphigoid, seen on the back of the leg
(duVivier, 1993)

tions of blisters, or bullae, filled with fluid, or bullae, on the skin or mucous membranes. An example is pemphigus.

bullous myringitis [L, *bulla; myringa,* eardrum], an inflammatory condition of the ear, characterized by fluidfilled vesicles on the tympanic membrane and the sudden onset of severe pain in the ear. The condition often occurs with bacterial otitis media. Treatment includes the administration of antibiotics, analgesics, and surgical draining of the vesicles. See also **otitis media.**

bullous pemphigoid [L, *bulla,* bubble; Gk, *pemphix,* bubble, *eidos,* form], a condition characterized by chronic eruptions of skin blisters over multiple body areas.

bumetanide /bo͞omet′ənīd/, a loop diuretic related to furosemide.

■ INDICATIONS: It is prescribed for edema caused by cardiac, hepatic, or renal disease.

■ CONTRAINDICATIONS: Anuria, electrolyte depletion, or known sensitivity to this drug prohibits its use.

■ ADVERSE EFFECTS: Among the most serious adverse reactions are hypokalemia, hyperuricemia, azotemia.

Bumex, a trademark for a diuretic (bumetanide).

Buminate, a trademark for a blood volume expander (human albumin).

BUN, abbreviation for **blood urea nitrogen.**

-bund, a suffix meaning 'prone to' something specified: *furibund, moribund.*

bundle branch [Dan *bondel;* Fr *branche*], a segment of a network of specialized conducting fibers that transmit electrical impulses within the ventricles. It is a continuation of the bundle of His, extending from the upper part of the intraventricular septum of the heart. The AV bundle divides into a left and a right branch, each going to its respective ventricle by passing down the septum and beneath the endocardium. Within the ventricles the bundle branches and terminates in the Purkinje fibers.

bundle branch block (BBB), an abnormal conduction of the cardiac impulse within the ventricles, resulting in an abnormally shaped QRS complex. BBB is commonly caused by ischemia or necrosis of the bundle bracnhes, trauma (as in surgical manipulation), or mechanical compression of the branches by a tumor. Pacemaker insertion may be performed if further deterioration in conduction is anticipated. Also called **infranodal block, intraventricular block.**

bundle of His /his/ [Dan, *bondel;* Wilhelm His, German physician, b. 1863], a band of atypical cardiac muscle fibers with few contractile units. It arises from the distal portion of the AV node and extends across the AV groove to the top of the intraventricular septum, where it divides into the bundle branches. Also called **atrioventricular bundle, His bundle.**

bunion /bun′yən/ [Gk, *bounion,* turnip], an abnormal enlargement of the joint at the base of the great toe. It is caused by inflammation of the bursa, usually as a result of chronic irritation and pressure from poorly fitted shoes. It is characterized by soreness, swelling, thickening of the skin, and lateral displacement of the great toe.

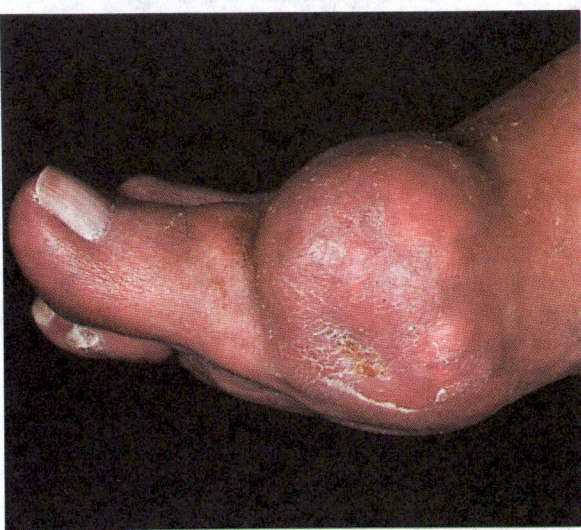

Bunion (duVivier, 1993)

bunionectomy /bun′yənek′təmē/, excision of a bunion.

bunionette /bun′yənet′/, an abnormal enlargement and inflammation of the joint at the base of the small toe. Also called **tailor's bunion.**

Bunnell block, a small wooden block used in exercise of the fingers after surgery. The exercises with the block allow each joint to be exercised individually with full tendon excursion while the other joints are held extended.

Bunyamwera arbovirus /bun′yəmwir′ə/, one of a group of arthropod-borne viruses that infect humans, carried by mosquitoes from rodent hosts causing California encephalitis, Rift Valley fever, and other diseases characterized by headache, weakness, low-grade fever, myalgia, and a rash. Convalescence is prolonged. Outbreaks have occurred in North America, South America, Africa, and Europe.

buphthalmos. See **congenital glaucoma.**

bupivacaine hydrochloride /byōōpiv′əkān/, a local anesthetic.

■ INDICATIONS: It is prescribed for caudal, epidural, peripheral, or sympathetic anesthetic block.

■ CONTRAINDICATIONS: Known hypersensitivity to this drug or to any of the amide class of local anesthetics prohibits its use.

■ ADVERSE EFFECTS: Among the more serious adverse reactions are central nervous system disturbances, cardiovascular depression, respiratory arrest, cardiac arrest, and hypersensitivity reactions. The adverse effects vary depending on the condition of the patient, the dosage, and the route of administration.

Buprenex, a trademark for a parenteral analgesic (buprenorphine hydrochloride).

buprenorphine hydrochloride /bōō′prənôr′fēn/, a parenteral analgesic.

■ INDICATIONS: It is prescribed for the relief of moderate to severe pain.

■ CONTRAINDICATIONS: This Schedule V controlled substance is contraindicated for patients who may be narcotic-dependent.

■ ADVERSE EFFECTS: Among the reported adverse effects are respiratory depression, sedation, nausea, dizziness, vertigo, headache, vomiting, miosis, diaphoresis, and hypotension.

Bureau of Medical Devices (BMD), an agency of the Food and Drug Administration organized in 1976 with the responsibility of providing standards for and regulation of the manufacture and uses of medical devices.

buret /byōōret′/ [Fr, small jug], a laboratory utensil used to deliver a wide range of volumes accurately. Also spelled **burette.**

buried suture [L, *sutura*], a suture that is inserted to bring together soft tissues between the viscus and the skin.

Burkitt's lymphoma /bur′kits/ [Denis P. Burkitt, English physician, b. 1911], a malignant neoplasm composed of undifferentiated lymphoreticular cells that form a large osteolytic lesion in the jaw or, in children, an abdominal mass. The tumor, which is seen chiefly in Central Africa, is characteristically a gray-white mass with a branlike consistency, sometimes containing areas of hemorrhage and necrosis. Central nervous system involvement often occurs, and other organs may be affected. The Epstein-Barr virus (EBV), a herpesvirus, is associated with this lymphoma. Chemotherapy usually results in rapid shrinking of the osteolytic lesion and complete cure of the disease. Also called **African lymphoma, Burkitt's tumor.**

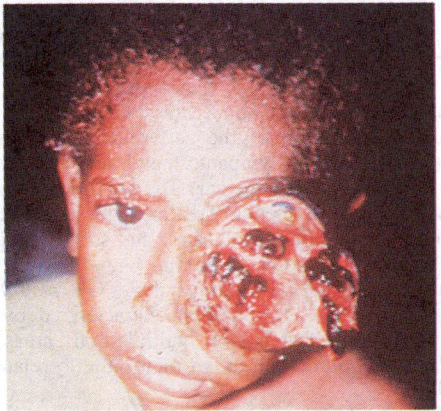

Burkitt's lymphoma (Hart, 1992)

burn [AS, *baernan*], any injury to tissues of the body caused by heat, electricity, chemicals, radiation, or gases in which the extent of the injury is determined by the amount of exposure of the cell to the agent and to the nature of the agent. The treatment of burns includes pain relief, careful asepsis, prevention of infection, maintenance of the balance in the body of fluids and electrolytes, and good nutrition. Severe burns of any origin may cause shock, which is treated before the wound. See also **chemical burn, electrocution, thermal burn.**

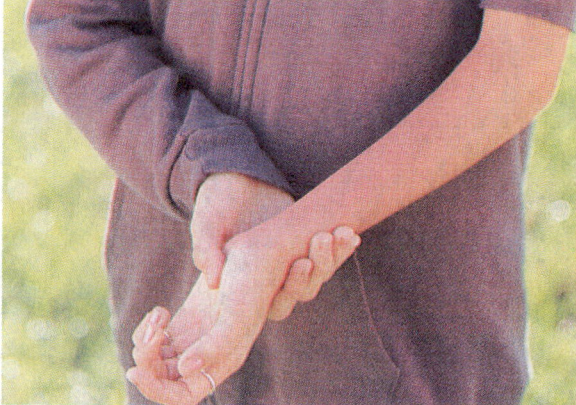

First degree burn

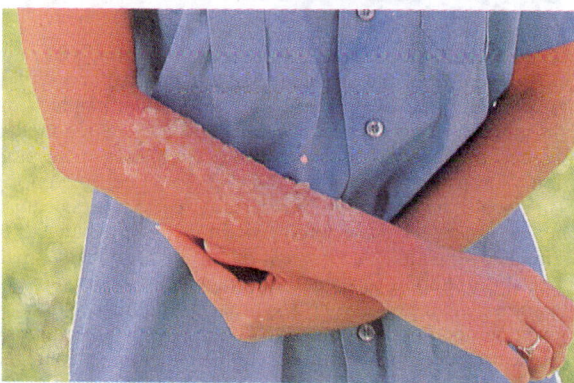

Second degree burn

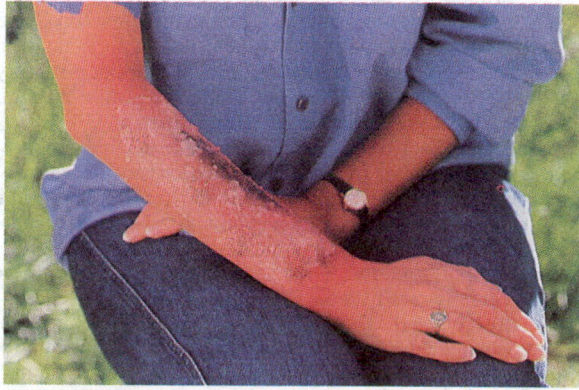

Third degree burn *(Judd, 1988)*

burn center, a health care facility that is designed to care for patients who have been severely burned. A network of burn centers has been established throughout the United States and Canada to provide sophisticated advanced techniques of care for burn victims.

burning feet syndrome, a neurologic disorder characterized by symptoms of a burning sensation in the sole of the foot. The burning tends to be more intense at night and may also involve the hands. Possible causes include causalgia from injury to the sciatic nerve, degeneration of the spinal cord, and acute polyneuropathy. The condition is also associated with diabetes mellitus, kidney disease, and a B-vitamin deficiency.

burning pain [AS, *baernan,* to burn; L, *poena,* penalty], the pain experienced as a result of a thermal burn.

burnisher /bur'nishər/ [ME, *burnischen,* to make brown], a noncutting dental instrument with one end shaped as a beveled nib, used to smooth out rough edges of restorations.

burnout, a popular term for the condition of having mental or physical energy depletion after a period of chronic, unrelieved job-related stress characterized sometimes by physical illness. The health professional loses concern or respect for patients and often develops cynical, dehumanized perceptions of people, labeling them in a derogatory manner. Causes of burnout peculiar to the nursing profession often include stressful, even dangerous, work environments; lack of support; lack of respectful relationships within the health care team; low pay scales compared with physicians' salaries; shift changes and long work hours; understaffing of hospitals; pressure from the responsibility of providing continuous high levels of care over long periods of time; and frustration and disillusionment resulting from the difference between job realities and job expectations.

burn therapy, the management of a patient burned by flames, hot liquids, explosives, chemicals, or electric current. Partial thickness burns may be first degree, involving only the epidermis, or second degree, involving the epidermis and corium, whereas full thickness or third degree burns involve all skin layers. Second degree burns covering more than 30% of the body and third degree burns on the face and extremities, or more than 10% of the body surface, are critical. In the first 48 hours of a severe burn, vascular fluid, sodium chloride, and protein rapidly pass into the affected area causing local edema, blister formation, hypovolemia, hypoproteinemia, hyponatremia, hyperkalemia, hypotension, and oliguria. The initial hypovolemic stage is followed by a shift of fluid in the opposite direction resulting in diuresis, increased blood volume, and decreased serum electrolytes. Potential complications in serious burns include circulatory collapse, renal damage, gastric atony, paralytic ileus, infections, septic shock, pneumonia, and stress ulcer (Curling's ulcer), characterized by hematemesis and peritonitis.

■ METHOD: The extent of the burn, its cause, and time of occurrence and the patient's age, weight, allergies, and any preexisting illness are recorded. If respiratory distress is present, endotracheal intubation or tracheostomy may be performed. Specimens are obtained for urinalysis, blood type, blood urea nitrogen level, hematocrit, prothrombin time, electrolyte levels, blood gases, and cultures of nasal, throat, wound, and stool organisms. Parenteral fluids and electrolytes, antibiotics, tetanus prophylaxis, and pain medication are administered as ordered; large doses of analgesics and sedatives are avoided when possible to prevent depressing respiration and the masking of symptoms. An in-

	Depth of burn / Detailed classification	Pain and pinprick sensitivity	Appearance	Healing time	End result of healing	Treatment
1°	Erythema only, no loss of epidermis	Hyperalgesia	Erythema		Normal skin	Allow to heal by natural processes / Protect from further injury and infection
2° Partial skin loss	Superficial, no loss of dermis	Hyperalgesia or normal		6-10 days	Normal skin	
	Intermediate, healing from hair follicles	Normal to hypo- algesia	Erythema to opaque, white blisters are characteristic	7-14 days	Normal to slightly pitted and/or poorly pigmented	
	Deep, healing from sweat glands	Hypoalgesia to analgesia		14-21 days	Hairless and depigmented / Texture normal to pitted or flat and shiny	Elective skin grafting may save time and give better end result
3° Whole skin loss	Deep dermal, occassionally heal from scattered epithelium	Analgesia	White opaque to charred, coagulated; subcutaneous veins may be visible	More than 21 days	Poor texture / Hypertrophic / Scar frequent	
	Whole skin loss, healing from edges only			Never if area is large	Hypertrophic scar and chronic granulations unless grafted	Skin grafting mandatory
4° Deep tissue loss	Deep structure loss	May be some algesia				

Burn classification

dwelling urinary catheter is inserted, and a nasogastric tube and catheter for monitoring central venous pressure may be indicated. Local treatment of the burn may be by the closed method or the more frequently used open method in which the injured area is cleaned and exposed to air and the patient is kept warm by a blanket or linen over a bed cradle or by a heater or lamp. In the closed method, a germicidal or bacteriostatic cream, ointment, or solution is applied to the burn, and the wound is covered with a dressing. A porcine heterograft may be used to cover the wound temporarily; this technique prevents loss of fluid and reduces the risk of infection, but the graft dries in 1 or 2 days and may pull and cause pain. Newly developed artificial skin holds great promise for treating severe burns. During the acute stage of a burn, the patient's blood pressure, pulse, respiration, and cerebrovascular pressure are checked every 30 to 60 minutes, and the rectal temperature every 2 to 4 hours. Oral hygiene, assistance in turning, coughing, and deep breathing are provided every 2 hours, and the patient's sensorium is evaluated hourly. If oral fluids are ordered, juices and carbonated drinks are offered, but plain water and ice chips are avoided. Fluid intake and output are measured hourly; if a child excretes less than 1 ml/kg of urine or an adult less than 0.5 ml/kg, a diuretic or an increase in intravenous infusion of fluid may be necessary. Blood transfusions, steroid therapy, and antipyretics may be ordered; aspirin is contraindicated. Excessive chilling and exposure to upper respiratory and wound infections are carefully avoided. Burned extremities are elevated, and contractures are prevented by using firm supports to keep affected areas properly aligned, such as by using a footboard to keep the feet at a 90 degree angle to the ankles in burns of the lower extremities or by having the patient grasp a ball when the back of the hand is burned. In burns of the arm, axilla, or chest, the arm of the affected side is supported at a 90 degree angle to the body slightly above shoulder height. Linear incision of the eschar on the wound may be required if the constricting crust interferes with circulation or respiration. The patient is weighed daily at the same time on the same scale, and, after the initial acute period, an adequate intake of a high-calorie, high-protein diet is encouraged; to stimulate appetite, the patient is offered frequent small meals of preferred foods and beverages that are high in potassium. Vitamins may be required. Tranquilizers may be given before wound care, but narcotics for pain usually are not needed after the acute phase. The patient is encouraged to stand for a few minutes every hour or every second hour and is generally able to walk in 7 to 10 days, but convalescence may be prolonged. Burned patients often are frightened, withdrawn, and disoriented initially, but after a few days they may become angry, depressed, or rebellious and in need of emotional support to help them cooperate with their treatment and rehabilitation. Extensive plastic surgery and repeated skin grafts may be required to restore function and the physical appearance of burn patients.

■ NURSING INTERVENTION: The burned patient requires intensive, prolonged care to avoid complications and prevent disfiguring contractures. The nurse administers parenteral fluids, medication, and implements wound care, closely monitors the patient, limits physical discomfort, provides emotional support and diversion, and encourages the family to visit regularly and become involved in the patient's care.

■ OUTCOME CRITERIA: The outcome for the severely burned patient depends greatly on the detailed, near-constant care required during the acute phase of treatment. Scarring may cause residual dysfunction and discouragement. Encourage ment to participate fully in physical therapy and to continue treatments may be helpful. Although protection from infection is essential, the nurse does not isolate the patient unless necessary.

Burow's solution /byo͞or′ōz/ [Karl A. von Burow, German physician, b. 1809], a liquid preparation containing aluminum sulfate, acetic acid, precipitated calcium carbonate, and water, used as a topical astringent, antiseptic, and antipyretic for a wide variety of skin disorders. Also called **aluminum acetate solution.**

burp, *informal*. **1.** to belch, or eructate. **2.** a belch, or eructation.

burr cell [ME, *burre;* L, *cella,* storeroom], a form of mature erythrocyte in which the cells or cell fragments have spicules, or tiny projections, on the surface.

burrowing flea. See **chigoe.**

bursa /bur′sə/, *pl.* **bursae** [Gk, *byrsa,* wineskin], **1.** a fibrous sac between certain tendons and the bones beneath them. Lined with a synovial membrane that secretes synovial fluid, the bursa acts as a small cushion that allows the tendon to move over the bone as it contracts and relaxes. See also **adventitious bursa, bursa of Achilles, olecranon bursa, prepatellar bursa. 2.** a sac or closed cavity. See also **omental bursa, pharyngeal bursa.**

bursa of Achilles, bursa separating the tendon of Achilles and the calcaneus.

bursectomy /bərsek′təmē/ [Gk, *byrsa,* wine skin, *ektome,* cutting out], the excision of a bursa.

bursitis /bərsī′tis/, an inflammation of the bursa, the connective tissue structure surrounding a joint. Bursitis may be precipitated by arthritis, infection, injury, or excessive or traumatic exercise or effort. The chief symptom is severe pain of the affected joint, particularly on movement. The goals of treatment for bursitis include the control of pain and the maintenance of joint motion. A frequent measure used for the relief of acute pain is an intrabursal injection of an adrenocorticosteroid. Other commonly used treatments are analgesics, antiinflammatory agents, cold, and immobilization of the inflamed site. After the inflammatory process has subsided, heat may be helpful. In chronic cases surgery may be required to remove calcium deposits. Some

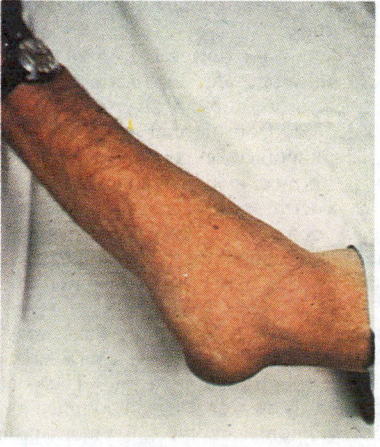

Bursitis (Shipley, 1993)

kinds of bursitis are **housemaid's knee, miner's elbow,** and **weaver's bottom.** See also **rheumatism.**

bursting fracture [ME, *bersten;* L, *fractura,* break], any fracture that disperses multiple bone fragments, usually at or near the end of a bone.

bus, a group of wires, a circuit, or a group of circuits in a computer in which each separate wire carries the electric current representing one bit. Buses interconnect the parts of the computer that communicate with each other.

Buschke's disease. See **cryptococcosis.**

BuSpar, a trademark for an oral antianxiety drug (buspirone hydrochloride)

buspirone hydrochloride /bo͞ospir′ōn/, an oral antianxiety drug.
- INDICATIONS: It is prescribed for anxiety disorders and the short-term relief of anxiety symptoms.
- CONTRAINDICATIONS: This drug is contraindicated in patients with severe hepatic or renal impairment. Patients taking a benzodiazepine drug should be gradually withdrawn from that medication before starting therapy with buspirone.
- ADVERSE EFFECTS: Among adverse reactions reported are dizziness, headache, lightheadedness, excitement, and nausea.

busulfan /bo͞osul′fən/, an alkylating agent.
- INDICATION: It is prescribed in the treatment of chronic myelocytic leukemia.
- CONTRAINDICATIONS: Radiation, depressed neutrophil or platelet counts, concurrent administration of neoplastic medication, or known hypersensitivity to this drug prohibits its use.
- ADVERSE REACTIONS: Among the more serious adverse reactions are alveolar hyperplasia (busulfan lung), depression of the bone marrow, and severe nausea and diarrhea. Amenorrhea commonly occurs.

butabarbital sodium /byo͞o′təbär′bitôl/, a sedative.
- INDICATIONS: It is prescribed for the relief of anxiety, nervous tension, and insomnia.
- CONTRAINDICATIONS: Porphyria, seizure disorders, or known hypersensitivity to this drug prohibits its use.
- ADVERSE EFFECTS: Among the more serious adverse reactions are jaundice, skin rash, and paradoxical excitement.

butaconazole nitrate /byo͞o′təkō′nəzōl/, an intravaginal antifungal cream.
- INDICATIONS: This drug is prescribed for the treatment of vulvovaginal fungal infections caused by *Candida* species.
- CONTRAINDICATIONS: Its use is contraindicated during the first trimester of a pregnancy.
- ADVERSE EFFECTS: Adverse reactions reported include vulvar and vaginal burning and itching.

butamben picrate /byo͞otam′bən pik′rāt/, a topical local anesthetic for the temporary relief of pain from minor burns.

butanamide. See **acebutolol.**

butanoic acid. See **butyric acid.**

butanol. See **butyl alcohol.**

butanol-extractable iodine (BEI) /byo͞o′tənôl/, iodine that can be separated from plasma proteins by a solvent, as butanol, and measured for analyzing thyroid function. The normal concentrations of butanol-extractable iodine in serum are 3.5 to 6.5 [Grk m]g/dl. Concentration values are inaccurate if the patient has ingested any iodine compound just before a butanol-extractable iodine test.

butaperazine maleate /byo͞o′təper′əzēn mal′ē·āt/, an antipsychotic.

■ INDICATIONS: It is prescribed in the treatment of schizophrenia and chronic brain syndrome.

■ CONTRAINDICATIONS: Bone marrow depression, the concomitant use of an antiadrenergic, or known hypersensitivity to this drug or to other phenothiazines prohibits its use. It is not given to children under 12 years of age.

■ ADVERSE EFFECTS: Among the more serious adverse reactions are skin rash, leukopenia, tardive dyskinesia, and jaundice.

Butazolidin, a trademark for an antirheumatic (phenylbutazone).

Butesin Picrate, a trademark for a local anesthetic (butamben picrate).

Butisol Sodium, a trademark for a sedative (butabarbital sodium).

butorphanol tartrate /byōōtôr′fənôl/, a parenteral agonist/antagonist narcotic of the phenanthrene family, given for surgical premedication and as an analgesic component of balanced anesthesia. Because it provides almost immediate relief from pain when given intravenously and begins to take effect within 10 minutes when given intramuscularly (with peak analgesic activity within 30 to 60 minutes), it is useful for the relief of moderate to severe pain associated with surgical procedures. Butorphanol tartrate is not given to patients known to be sensitive to phenanthrenes or to persons dependent on narcotics because it may provoke withdrawal symptoms. Toxicity may result from the use of butorphanol with other narcotics.

butterfly bandage [AS, *buttorfleoge*], a narrow adhesive strip with broader winglike ends used to approximate the edges of a superficial wound and to hold the sides together as they heal. It is used in place of a suture in certain cases. Also called **butterfly.**

butterfly fracture, a bone break in which the center fragment contained by two cracks forms a triangle.

butterfly rash, an erythematous, scaling eruption of both cheeks joined by a narrow band of rash across the nose. It may be seen in lupus erythematosus, rosacea, and seborrheic dermatitis.

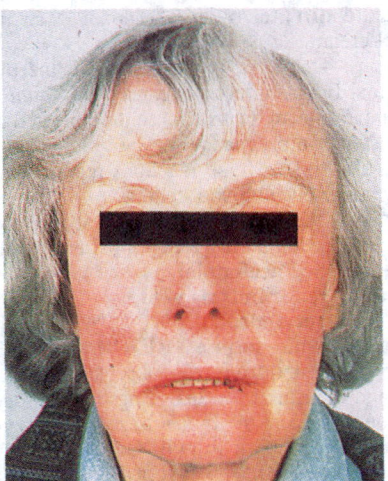

Butterfly rash *(Shipley, 1993)*

buttermilk [Gk, *boutyron*, butter; AS, *meoluc*], **1.** the slightly sour tasting liquid residue remaining after the solids in cream have been churned into butter. It is nearly fat free and is nutritionally comparable to whole milk. **2.** cultured milk made by the addition of certain organisms to fat-free milk.

buttock. See **nates.**

buttonhole [OFr, *boton;* AS, *hol*], a small slitlike hole in the wall of a structure or a cavity of the body.

buttonhole fracture, any fracture caused by the perforation of a bone by a bullet.

buttonhook, any of a variety of devices designed to help patients with limited finger range of motion or amputations to fasten clothing.

button suture, a technique in suturing in which the ends of the suture material are passed through buttons on the surface of the skin and tied. It is used to prevent the suture from cutting through the skin.

butyl /byōō′til/ [Gk, *boutyron*, butter, *hyle,* matter], a hydrocarbon radical (C_4H_9), the compounds of which are obtained from petroleum. Butyl compounds, some of which are toxic and irritating, are used in a variety of industrial and medical applications, including anesthesia.

butyl alcohol, a clear, toxic liquid used as an organic solvent. It is one of four isomers, the others being isobutyl, secondary butyl, and tertiary butyl alcohol. Also called **butanol.**

butyr-, a combining form meaning 'pertaining to butter': *butyraceous, butyric, butyrinase.*

butyric acid /byōōtir′ik/, a fatty acid occurring in rancid butter, feces, urine, perspiration, and, in trace amounts, in the spleen and blood. Butyric acid is used in the preparation of flavorings, emulsifying agents, and pharmaceutics. Also called **butanoic acid** /byōō′tənō′ik/, **propylformic acid.**

butyric fermentation, the conversion of carbohydrates to butyric acid.

butyrophenone /byōō′tərōfē′nōn/, one of a small group of major tranquilizers used in treating psychosis to decrease the choreic symptoms of Huntington's chorea and the tics and coprolalia of Gilles de la Tourette's syndrome and as an adjunct in neuroleptanesthesia. Principal butyrophenones are pimozide, fluspirilene, haloperidol, and droperidol. Butyrophenones are pharmacologically and clinically similar to the phenothiazines.

BWS, abbreviation for **battered woman syndrome.**

bypass [AS, *bi,* alongside; Fr, *passer*], **1.** any one of various surgical procedures to divert the flow of blood or other natural fluids from normal anatomic courses. A bypass may be temporary or permanent. Bypass surgery is commonly performed in the treatment of cardiac and GI disorders. **2.** a term used by some hospitals to signal that its emergency department lacks the personnel and equipment to handle additional cases, thereby advising that ambulances transporting new cases be diverted to other hospitals.

byssinosis /bis′inō′sis/ [Gk, *byssos,* flax, *osis,* condition], an occupational respiratory disease characterized by shortness of breath, cough, and wheezing. The condition is an allergic reaction to dust or fungi in cotton, flax, and hemp fibers. The symptoms are typically more pronounced on Mondays when the workers return after a weekend break.

They are reversible in the early stages, but prolonged exposure results in chronic airway obstruction, bronchitis, and emphysema with fibrosis, leading to respiratory failure, pulmonary hypertension, and cor pulmonale. Treatment is symptomatic for the irreversible changes of emphysema and chronic bronchitis. Compare **pneumoconiosis.** See also **organic dust.**

byte /bīt/, the number of bits required to encode one character of information (letter, number, or symbol) in a computer system. See also **bit.**

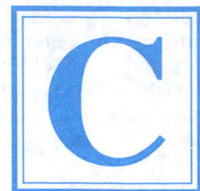

c, 1. symbol for *capillary blood*. 2. abbreviation for **cu-rie**.

C, 1. symbol for **compliance** in respiratory physiology. 2. symbol for *concentration of gas in the blood*. 3. symbol for the element **carbon**.

Ca, symbol for the element **calcium**.

CABG, abbreviation for *coronary artery bypass graft*.

cabinet bath [ME, *cabane*, cabin], a bath in which the patient is enclosed in a cabinet, except for the head, heated by hot air or radiant heat. Also called **box bath.**

Cabot rings /kab′ot/ [Richard C. Cabot, American physician, b. 1868], threadlike figures, often appearing as loops or rings, observed in red blood cells of patients with severe anemia. The inclusions are seen after blood smears are stained with Wright stain. Also called **Cabot bodies.**

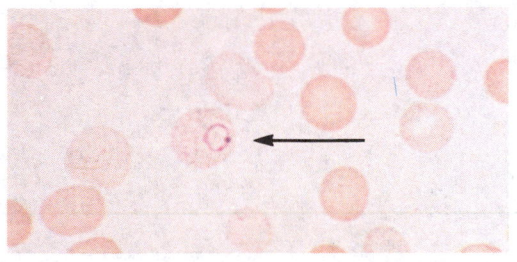

Cabot rings *(Hayhoe, 1992)*

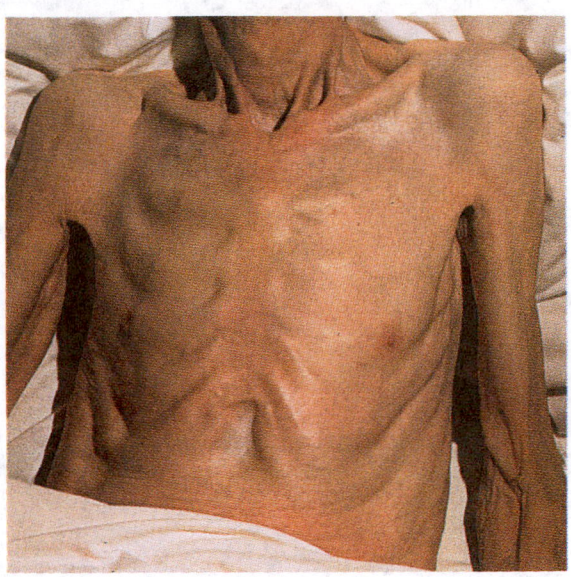

Cachexia *(Kamal, 1991)*

Cabot's splint [Arthur T. Cabot, American surgeon, b. 1852], a metal splint worn behind the thigh and leg for support.

cac-. See caco-.

cacao [/kəkā′ō/ *caca*], 1. cocoa. 2. the substance *Theobroma cacao*. 3. the seeds of *Theobroma cacao*.

cacesthesia /kak′əsthē′zhə/ [Gk, *kakos*, bad, *aisthesis*, feeling], any morbid feeling or disordered sensibility. −cacesthetic, *adj*.

cache /kash/ (in computer technology) a fast storage buffer in the CPU. Also called **cache memory.**

cachectic /kəkek′tik/ [Gk, *kakos*, bad, *hexis*, state], pertaining to a state of generally poor health and malnutrition.

cachet /käshā′/ [Fr, tablet], any lenticular edible capsule that encloses a dose of medicine.

cachexia /kəkek′sē·ə/ [Gk, *kakos*, bad, *hexis*, state], general ill health and malnutrition, marked by weakness and emaciation, usually associated with serious disease, as tuberculosis or cancer. Also called **cachexy** /kəkek′sē/. −cachectic, *adj*.

cachinnation /kak′ənā′shən/ [L, *cachinnare*, to laugh aloud], an excessive laughter for no apparent reason, often part of the behavioral pattern in schizophrenia. −cachinnate, *v*.

caco-, cac-, a prefix meaning 'ill, unpleasant, or bad': *cacodontia, cacogeusia, cacosmia*.

cacodemonomania /kak′ōdē′mənōmā′nē·ə/ [Gk, *kakos* + *daimon*, spirit, *mania*, madness], an abnormal mental condition in which the patient claims to be possessed by an evil spirit.

cacophony /kəkof′ənē/, *pl*. cacophonies [Gk, *kakos* + *phone*, voice], a harsh or discordant sound or a mixture of confused, different sounds. −cacophonic, cacophonous, *adj*.

cacosmia /kakoz′mē·ə/ [Gk, *kakos* + *osme*, odor], the perception of foul odors or stench when none exists. In most instances the condition results from psychologic factors, as in olfactory hallucinations that occur during certain psychoses, although it may be caused by a brain lesion. Also spelled **kakosmia.**

CAD, 1. abbreviation for **coronary artery disease**. 2. abbreviation for *computer assisted design*.

cadaver /kədä′vər/ [L, dead body], a dead body used for dissection and study.

cadaver graft, the transfer of tissue from the body of a dead individual to repair a defect in a living body. Also called **postmortem graft.**

cadaveric /kad'äver'ik/, pertaining to or resembling a cadaver.

cadence /kā'dəns/ [L, *cadere*, to fall], a rhythm as in voice, music, or movement.

cadmium /kad'mē·əm/ (Cd) [Gk, *kadmeia*, zinc ore], a metallic, bluish-white element that resembles tin. Its atomic number is 48; its atomic weight is 112.40. Cadmium has many uses in industry and was formerly used in medications. Such medications have been replaced by less toxic drugs. Cadmium bromide, used in engraving, lithography, and photography, can cause severe GI symptoms if swallowed. Cadmium may also cause poisoning by inhalation of fumes from metal-plating processes or by the ingestion of acidic foods prepared and stored in cadmium-lined containers, as lemonade in certain metal cans.

cadmium poisoning, poisoning resulting from the inhalation of cadmium in fumes created by welding, smelting, or other industrial processes involving solder. The effects may include vomiting, dyspnea, headache, prostration, pulmonary edema, and, possibly, years later, cancer. Treatment for acute poisoning includes intravenous fluids and hyperbaric oxygen.

caduceus /kədōō'sē·əs/ [L; Gk, *karykeion,* herald], the wand of the god Hermes or Mercury, used as the symbol for the U.S. Army Medical Corps. It is represented as a staff with two serpents coiled around it and is often confused with the staff of Æsculapius, a rod with one snake entwined about it.

caecal. See **cecal.**

caenogenesis. See **cenogenesis.**

caenogenetic. See **cenogenesis.**

cade oil. See **juniper tar.**

Caesarean hysterectomy. See **cesarean hysterectomy.**

Caesarean section. See **cesarean section.**

café-au-lait spot /kaf'ā·ōlā'/ [Fr, coffee with milk], a pale tan macule the color of coffee with milk. Several café-au-lait spots developing simultaneously are associated with neurofibromatosis, but occasional café-au-lait spots occur normally. See also **neurofibromatosis.**

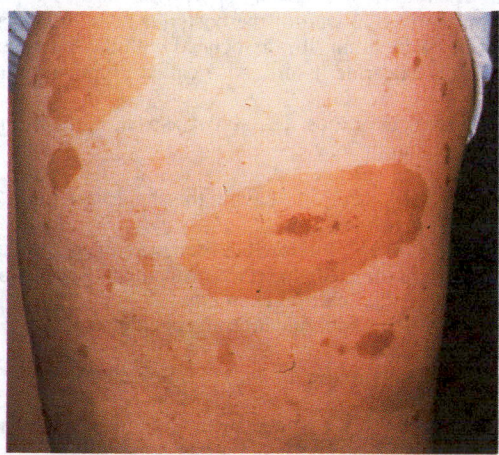

Café-au-lait patches in neurofibromatosis
(Epstein, 1992)

Cafergot, a trademark for a fixed-combination drug containing caffeine and ergotamine, commonly administered in the treatment of migraine headaches.

caffeine /kafēn', kaf'ē·in/ [Ar, *gahwah,* coffee], a central nervous system stimulant.

■ INDICATIONS: It is prescribed to counteract migraine, drowsiness, and mental fatigue.

■ CONTRAINDICATIONS: It is used with caution in patients with heart disease and peptic ulcer. Known hypersensitivity to this drug prohibits its use.

■ ADVERSE EFFECTS: Among the most serious adverse reactions are tachycardia and diuresis. GI distress, restlessness, and insomnia are common.

caffeine poisoning [Ar, *qahwah,* coffee, L, *potio,* drink], a toxic condition caused by the chronic ingestion of excessive amounts of caffeine, which is found in coffee, tea, cola beverages, or certain stimulant drugs. Symptoms include restlessness, anxiety, general depression, tachycardia, tremors, nausea, diuresis, and insomnia. In cases of caffeine poisoning, death may occur from cardiovascular and respiratory collapse. Also called **caffeinism** /kafē'niz'əm/, **caffeism** /kaf'ē·izm/. See also **xanthine derivative.**

Caffey's disease. See **infantile cortical hyperostosis.**

Caffey's syndrome, the battered baby syndrome, first described by American pediatrician John Caffey in 1946. See also **child abuse.**

CAH, **1.** abbreviation for *chronic active hepatitis.* **2.** Abbreviation for **congenital adrenal hyperplasia.**

C.A.H.E.A., abbreviation for **Committee on Allied Health Education and Accreditation.**

CAI, abbreviation for **computer-assisted instruction.**

-caine, a combining form usually indicating a synthetic alkaloid anesthetic: *cocaine, isocaine, lidocaine, metycaine, neurocaine.*

caisson disease. See **decompression sickness.**

cajeputol. See **eucalyptol.**

caked /kākt/ [ONorse, *kaka*], formed into a compact mass or crust, as the scab of coagulated blood on a healing wound.

caked breast, an accumulation of milk in the secreting ducts of the breast after child delivery, causing all or a part of the breast to become hardened and the tissues to become engorged. Also called **lactation mastitis.**

cal, **1.** abbreviation for **small calorie.** **2.** abbreviation for a *calcium cation.*

Cal, abbreviation for **large calorie.**

calabar swelling /kal'əbär/ [Calabar, a Nigerian seaport], an abnormal condition characterized by fugitive, swollen lumps of subcutaneous tissue caused by a parasitic, filarial worm endemic to central and west Africa. The swollen areas migrate with the worm through the body at a speed of about 1 cm per minute and may become as large as a small egg. At times the worm may move under the conjunctiva of the eye and may live in the anterior chamber of the eye. Treatment includes the oral administration of diethylcarbamazine, which destroys the adult worms and their offspring. Antihistamines and other medications may be given. A kind of calabar swelling is *Loa loa.* See also **loiasis.** (See Fig. p. 242.)

Caladryl, a trademark for a topical, fixed-combination drug containing a protectant (calamine) and an antihistaminic (diphenhydramine hydrochloride).

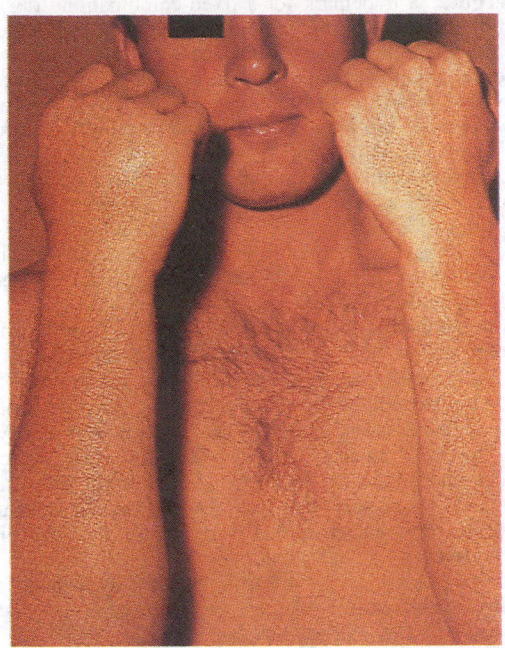

Calabar swellings (du Vivier, 1993)

calamine /kal′əmīn/ [Gk, *kadmeia*, zinc ore], a pink, odorless, powdered concoction used as a protectant or as an astringent and sometimes prepared as a lotion. It is composed of zinc oxide with 0.5% ferric oxide.

Calan, a trademark for a slow calcium channel blocker. (verapamil).

calc-, calci-, **1.** a combining form meaning 'pertaining to lime or limestone': *calcarea, calcariuria, calciosis.* **2.** a combining form meaning 'pertaining to the heel': *calcaneum, calcaneocavus, calcanodynia.*

-calcaneal. See **calcaneus.**

calcaneal /kalkā′nē·əl/ [L, *calcaneum*, heel], of or pertaining to the calcaneus at the back of the tarsus.

calcaneal epiphysitis, a painful disorder involving the calcaneus at its epiphysis. The condition tends to affect mainly children who are physically active and whose heel bones are still divided by a layer of cartilage. The stress of jumping and other athletic activities may break the union of the bone segments at the cartilage layer. Treatment may require immobilization of the foot in a cast. Also called **Sever's disease.**

calcaneal spurs, abnormal, often painful, bony outgrowths on the lower surface of the calcaneus, resulting from chronic traumatic pressure on the heel.

calcaneal tendon. See **Achilles tendon.**

calcaneal tuberosity, a transverse elevation on the plantar surface of the calcaneus to which are attached the abductor digiti minimi, the long plantar ligament, and various other muscles, including the abductor hallucis and the flexor digitorum brevis.

calcanean. See **calcaneus.**

calcaneodynia /kalkā′nē·ōdin′ē·ə/ [L, *calcaneum;* Gk, *odyne* pain], a painful condition of the heel.

calcaneovalgus. See **clubfoot.**

calcaneovarus. See **clubfoot.**

calcaneum. See **calcaneus.**

calcaneus /kalkā′nē·əs/ [L, *calcaneum,* heel], the heel bone. The largest of the tarsal bones, it articulates proximally with the talus and distally with the cuboid. **–calcaneal, calcanean,** *adj.*

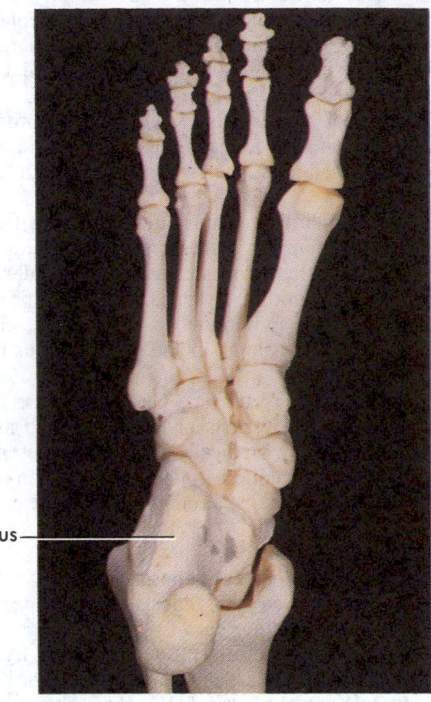

Calcaneus—

Calcaneus bone (Vidic, 1984)

calcar /kal′kär/, *pl.* **calcaria,** a spur or a structure that resembles a spur.

calcar avis /ā′vis/ [L, *calcar,* spur; *avis,* bird], a projection on the medial wall of the posterior horn of the lateral ventricle of the brain. It is associated with the lateral extension of the calcarine fissure. Also called **hippocampus minor.**

calcareous /kalker′ē·əs/ [L, *calcar,* spur], of or pertaining to calcium or lime.

calcaria. See **calcar.**

calcarine /kal′kərīn/, **1.** having the shape of a spur. **2.** of or pertaining to the calcar.

calcarine fissure, a fissure between the cuneus and the lingual gyrus on the medial surface of the occipital lobe of the brain. Also called **calcarine sulcus.**

calcemia. See **hypercalcemia, hypocalcemia.**

calci-. See **calc-.**

calcifediol /kal′sife′dē·ol/, a physiologic form of vitamin D.

■ INDICATION: It is prescribed in the treatment of metabolic bone disease associated with chronic renal failure.

■ CONTRAINDICATIONS: Hypercalcemia, vitamin D toxicity, or known hypersensitivity to this drug prohibits its use.

■ ADVERSE EFFECTS: Among the most serious adverse reactions are renal toxicity and those reactions associated with hypercalcemia, as soft tissue calcification and GI and central nervous system disturbances.

calciferol /kalsif′ərôl/ [L, *calx*, lime, *ferre*, to bear], a fat-soluble, crystalline, unsaturated alcohol produced by ultraviolet irradiation of ergosterol and used as a dietary supplement in the prophylaxis and treatment of rickets, osteomalacia, and other hypocalcemic disorders. It occurs naturally in milk and fish-liver oils. Also called **ergocalciferol, oleovitamin D₂**, vitamin D₂. See also **rickets, viosterol.**

calcific /kalsif′ik/ [L, *calx*, lime, *facere*, to make], pertaining to the formation of chalk, lime, or calcium.

calcific aortic disease [L, *calx*, lime], an abnormal condition characterized by small deposits of calcium in the aorta.

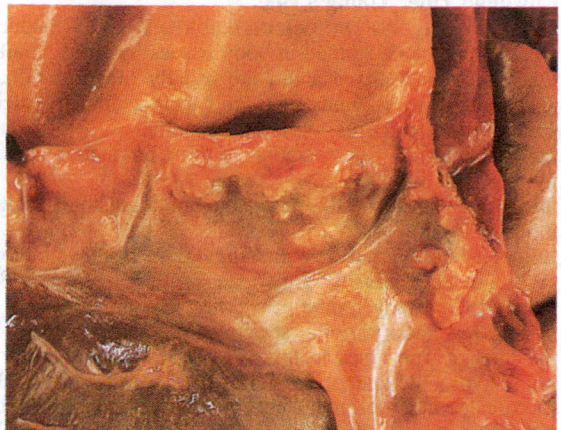

Calcific aortic disease *(Fletcher, 1987)*

calcification [L, *calx* + *facere*, to make], the accumulation of calcium salts in tissues. Normally, about 99% of all the calcium entering the human body is deposited in the bones and teeth; the remaining 1% is dissolved in body fluids such as the blood. Disorders affecting the delicate balance between calcium and other minerals, parathyroid hormone, and vitamin D can result in calcium deposits in arteries, kidneys, lung alveoli, and other tissues, interfering

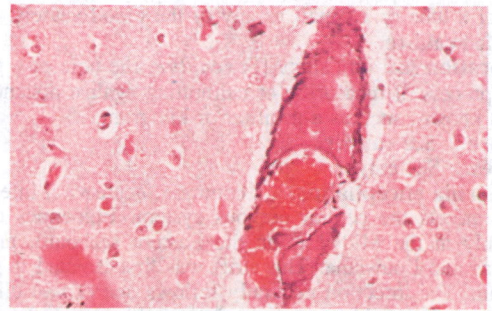

Calcification of a blood vessel wall *(Trotot, 1991)*

with usual organ functions. See also **calcitonin, calcium, calculus.**

calcific tendinitis [L, *calx*, lime, *facere*, to make, *tendo*, tendon; Gk, *itis*, inflammation], a chronic inflammation of a tendon as a result of an accumulation of calcium deposits in the tissue.

calcified fetus. See **lithopedion.**

Calcimar, a trademark for calcitonin.

calcination /kal′sinā′shən/ [L, *calcinare*, to burn lime], (in dentistry) a process of removing water by heat, used in the manufacture of plaster and stone from gypsum. Compare **calcification.**

calcinosis /kal′sənō′sis/, a condition characterized by abnormal deposits of calcium salts in various tissues of the body. The deposits appear as nodules or plaques and may occur in the skin, connective tissue, muscles, or intervertebral disks. Usually the nodules occur secondary to a preexisting inflammatory degenerative or neoplastic dermatosis, primarily scleroderma, and dermatomyositis.

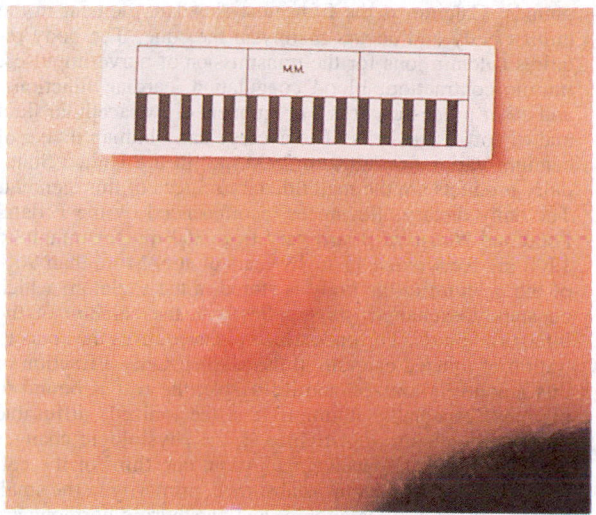

Nodule on knee caused by calcinosis *(Ansell, 1992)*

calcitonin /kal′sitō′nin/ [L, *calx* + Gk, *tonos*, tone], a hormone produced in parafollicular cells of the thyroid that participates in regulating the blood level of calcium and stimulates bone mineralization. A synthetic preparation of the hormone is used in the treatment of certain bone disorders. Calcitonin acts to reduce the blood level of calcium and to inhibit bone resorption, whereas parathyroid hormone acts to increase blood calcium and bone resorption. Calcitonin has a short-term effect in enhancing bone formation and causes transient decreases in the volume and acidity of gastric juice and in the volume of amylase and trypsin in pancreatic juice. The hormone also promotes the excretion of phosphate, sodium, and calcium by decreasing their reabsorption in kidney tubules. The secretion of calcitonin is regulated by the amount of calcium in plasma, and an infusion of calcium may increase the concentration of the circulating hormone two- to threefold. Men usually have a higher level of plasma calcitonin than women.

calcitriol /kalsit′rē·ôl/, the active form of vitamin D, a regulator of calcium metabolism.

- INDICATION: It is prescribed in the management of hypocalcemia occurring in patients undergoing chronic renal dialysis.
- CONTRAINDICATIONS: Hypercalcemia, evidence of vitamin D toxicity, or known sensitivity to this drug prohibits its use.
- ADVERSE EFFECTS: Among the more serious adverse reactions are renal toxicity and those associated with hypercalcemia, such as soft tissue calcification, and GI and central nervous system disturbances.

calcium (Ca) /kal′sē·əm/ [L, *calx*, lime], an alkaline earth metal element. Its atomic number is 20; its atomic weight is 40. Its metallic form is a white, flammable solid, somewhat harder than lead. Calcium is commonly produced by the electrolysis or by the thermal dissociation of calcium chloride. Calcium carbonate is the most common calcium compound, which, when treated with hydrochloric acid, forms calcium chloride. Calcium also occurs as a component of the natural compound gypsum, which forms plaster of paris when heated. It is also a component of calcium cyanamid, a fertilizer and progenitor of other nitrogen compounds. Calcium is the fifth most abundant element in the human body and occurs mainly in the bone. The body requires calcium ions for the transmission of nerve impulses, muscle contraction, blood coagulation, cardiac functions, and other processes. It is a component of extracellular fluid and of soft tissue cells. The average daily human intake of calcium varies from 200 to 2500 mg. In the United States dairy products are the major dietary sources of this element. The daily dietary allowances recommended by the Federal Food and Nutrition Board vary from 360 mg for infants to 1200 mg for women 15 to 18 years of age. More than 90% of the calcium in the body is stored in the skeleton, which constantly exchanges its supplies with the calcium of the interstitial fluids. The endocrine system controls the concentration of ionized calcium in the plasma. Only a fraction of this amount is ionized and diffusable; the rest is bound to proteins, especially albumin. It is the ionized, diffusable portion of calcium that figures in the physiologic changes associated with hypocalcemia. About one third of the calcium ingested by humans is absorbed, primarily in the small bowel. Vitamin D, calcitonin, and parathyroid hormone are essential in the metabolism of calcium. The degree of cell permeability varies inversely with calcium ion concentration. Abnormally high levels of ionized calcium in the extracellular fluid can produce muscle weakness, lethargy, and coma. A relatively small decrease from the normal level of this element can produce tetanic seizures. Normal blood levels of calcium are 9.0-10.5 mg/dl or 2.25-2.75 nmol/L.

calcium channel blocker, a drug that inhibits the flow of calcium ions across the membranes of smooth muscle cells. By reducing the calcium flow, smooth muscle tone is relaxed and the risk of muscle spasms is diminished. Calcium channel blockers are used primarily in the treatment of heart diseases marked by coronary artery spasms. Also called **calcium antagonist, calcium blocker.**

calcium chloride, a concentrated solution of the chloride salt of calcium used to replenish calcium in the blood.

- INDICATIONS: It is prescribed for hypocalcemic tetany and as an antidote for magnesium poisoning or an overdose of magnesium sulfate.
- CONTRAINDICATIONS: Renal insufficiency, ventricular fibrillation, hypercalcemia, or known hypersensitivity to this drug prohibits its use.

- ADVERSE EFFECTS: Among the more serious adverse reactions is hypercalcemia.
- CAUTION: Calcium chloride is never injected into tissue.

calcium gluconate ($C_{12}H_{22}CaO_{14}$), a white, odorless, tasteless powder or granules administered orally or intravenously to replenish the body's calcium stores, as after a transfusion.

calcium phosphate [$Ca_3(PO_4)_2$], an odorless, tasteless white powder used as a calcium supplement, laxative, and antacid.

calcium pump, a theoretical, energy-requiring mechanism for transmitting calcium ions across a cell membrane from a region of low calcium ion concentration to one of higher concentration. Compare **sodium pump.**

calciuria /kal′sinŏŏr′ē·ə/ [L, *calx*, lime; Gk, *ouron*, urine], the presence of calcium in the urine.

calculation for children dosage. See **Clark's rule, Cowling's rule, Young's rule.**

calculus /kal′kyələs/, *pl.* **calculi** /kal′kyəlī/ [L, little stone], an abnormal stone formed in body tissues by an accumulation of mineral salts. Calculi are usually found in biliary and urinary tracts. Kinds of calculi include **biliary calculus** and **renal calculus.** Also called **stone.**

calculus anuria, the cessation of urine production caused by renal calculi.

Calderol, a trademark for a calcium regulator (calcifediol).

Caldwell-Moloy pelvic classification /kôl′dwelməloi′/ [William E. Caldwell, American obstetrician, b. 1880; Howard C. Moloy, American gynecologist, b. 1903], a system for classifying the structure of the bony pelvis of the female. The types in this system are android, anthropoid, gynecoid, and platypelloid. The sacrum, sidewalls, sacrosciatic notch, ischial spines, pubic arch, and ischial tuberosities are the anatomic points of reference used to determine pelvic type. The classification system requires that a mixed pelvis be named for the character of its posterior section with the name of the type characterized by the anterior portion following a hyphen, as in a gynecoid-android pelvis. See also **pelvic classification.**

calefacient /kal′əfā′shənt/ [L, *calare*, to be warm, *facere*, to make], **1.** making or tending to make anything warm or hot. **2.** an agent that imparts a sense of warmth when applied, such as a hot-water bottle or a hot compress.

calendar method of family planning. See **natural family planning.**

calf, *pl.* **calves** [ONorse, *kalfi*], the fleshy mass at the back of the leg below the knee, composed chiefly of the gastrocnemius muscle.

calf bone. See **fibula.**

caliber /kal′ibər/ [Fr, *calibre*, bore of a gun], the diameter of a tube or a canal, as any of the blood vessels. Also spelled **calibre.**

calibration /kal′ibrā′shən/ [Fr, *calibre*, the bore of a gun], the process of measuring or calibrating against a standardized known, such as a deciliter or kilogram.

calibre. See **caliber.**

calices. See **calyx.**

California encephalitis, a common, acute viral infection that affects the central nervous system. Epidemics occur mainly in the Midwest, on the Eastern seaboard, and in Texas and Louisiana. The virus was first isolated in California. The infection generally follows one of two clinical courses. The mild form is characterized by headache, malaise, GI symptoms, and a fever that may reach 104° F. The more severe form may be marked by a sudden onset of fever, vomiting, headaches, lethargy, and signs of neurologic involvement such as loss of reflexes, disorientation, seizure, loss of consciousness, and flaccid paralysis. Recovery usually begins in 1 week. Mortality is very low, but a significant number of patients have neurologic sequelae for 1 year or more. Treatment usually involves administration of anticonvulsant and sedative medications. See also **arbovirus, encephalitis.**

californium (Cf) [State of California], an artificial element in the actinide group. Its atomic number is 98; its atomic weight is 251. Californium 252 isotope is a potent source of neutrons.

calipers /kal′ipərz/ [Fr, *calibre,* bore of a gun], an instrument with two hinged, adjustable, curved legs, used to measure the thickness or the diameter of a convex or solid body.

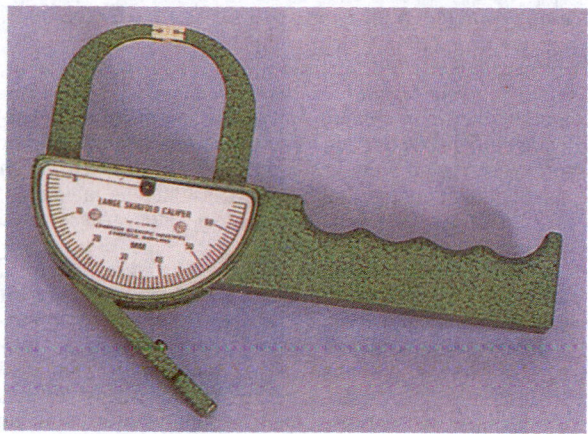

Triceps skinfold calipers
(Seidel, 1991)

calosum. See **corpus callosum.**

callous. See **callus.**

callous ulcer /kal′əs/ [L, *callosus,* hard + *ulcus,* ulcer], an ulcer with a hard, indurated base and thick inelastic margins. It lacks a blood supply and is frequently associated with edema of the legs.

callus /kal′əs/ [L, hard skin], **1.** also called **callosity.** a common, usually painless thickening of the epidermis at locations of external pressure or friction. Compare **corn. 2.** bony deposit formed between and around the broken ends of a fractured bone during healing. –**callous,** *adj.*

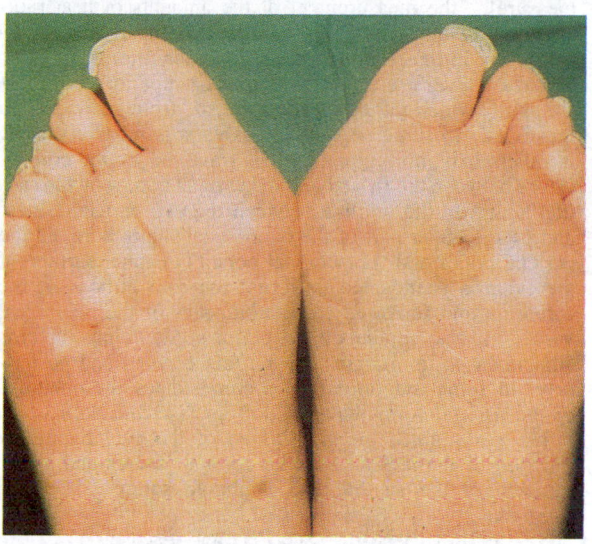

Callus *(Shipley, 1993)*

caliper splint, a splint for the leg consisting of two metal rods running from the back of a band around the thigh or from a cushioned ring around the lower portion of the pelvis. The rods are attached to a metal plate under the shoe below the arch of the foot.

calix. See **calyx.**

Calliphoridae /kal′əfôr′ədē/ [Gk, *kallos,* beauty, *pherein,* to bear], a family of medium-sized to large flies that belong to the order Diptera, serve as pathogenic vectors, and may cause intestinal or nasopharyngeal myiasis in humans. These flies include the genera *Auchmeromyia, Calliphora, Cordylobia, Cochliomyia, Chrysomyia, Lucilia, Phaenicia,* and *Phormia.*

callomania /kal′ōmā′nē·ə/ [Gk, *kallos,* beauty, *mania,* madness], an abnormal psychologic condition characterized by delusions of personal beauty.

callosal fissure /kəlos′əl/ [L, *callosus,* hard; *fissura,* cleft], a groove following the convex aspect of the corpus callosum.

callosity. See **callus.**

callosomarginal fissure /kəlō′sōmär′jənəl/, a long, irregular groove on the medial surface of a cerebral hemisphere. It divides the cingulate gyrus from the medial frontal gyrus and from the paracentral lobule. Also called **cingulate sulcus** /sin′gyəlit/.

calmodulin /kalmod′yəlin/, a calcium-binding protein that mediates a variety of biochemical and physiologic processes, including the contraction of muscles and the release of norepinephrine. Depending on its form and function, calmodulin may act independently of, in concert with, or antagonistically to reactions involving cyclic adenosinemonophosphate.

calor /kal′ôr/ [L, warmth], heat, as that generated by inflammation of tissues or that from the normal metabolic processes of the body.

calor-, a prefix meaning 'pertaining to heat': *calorie, calorifacient, calorization.*

caloric /kalôr′ik/, of or pertaining to heat or calories.

caloric test, a procedure in which the ears are alternately irrigated with warm water or air and cold water or air. The warm irrigation produces a rotatory nystagmus toward the irrigated side. Cold irrigation produces a rotatory nystagamus away from the irrigated side. If the ear is normal, all irrigations will produce nystagmus that is approximately equal in intensity. If the ear is diseased, irrigation may produce less nystagmus than the normal ear. Also called **Bárány's test.**

calorie /kal′ôrē/ [L, *calor,* warmth], **1.** also called **gram calorie, small calorie (cal.).** the amount of heat required to raise 1 g of water 1° C at atmospheric pressure. **2.** also called **great calorie, kilocalorie, kilogram calorie, large**

calorie (Cal.). a quantity of heat equal to 1000 small calories. **3.** a unit, equal to the large calorie, used to denote the heat expenditure of an organism and the fuel or energy value of food. **–caloric,** *adj.*

calorific /kal'ərif'ik/, pertaining to the production of heat.

calorigenic /kəlôr'ijen'ik/ [L, *calor,* warmth; Gk, *genein,* to produce], of or pertaining to a substance or process that produces heat or energy or that increases the consumption of oxygen.

calorimeter /kal'ərim'ətər/, a device used for measuring quantities of heat generated by friction, by chemical reaction, or by the human body. **–calorimetric,** *adj.*

calorimetry /kal'ərim'ətrē/ [L, *calor,* warmth; Gk, *metron,* measure], the measurement of the amounts of heat radiated and the amounts of heat absorbed. Compare **direct calorimetry, indirect calorimetry. –calorimetric,** *adj.*

calvaria /kalver'ē·ə/, the skull cap or superior portion of the skull, which varies greatly in shape from individual to individual. In some persons the calvaria is relatively oval, in others it is more circular. It is traversed by the coronal suture between the frontal and the parietal bones, by the sagittal suture in the midline between the two parietal bones, and by the upper part of the lambdoidal suture between the parietal bones and the occipital bone. The inner surface of the calvaria is indented to accept the convolutions of the cerebrum and furrowed for the branches of the meningeal vessels. It also contains the superior sagittal sinus, affords attachment at its margins for the falx cerebri, and posteriorly, in some individuals, it accommodates the openings of the parietal foramina. The soft spots in the skull of an infant are situated on the surface of the calvaria at the junction of the sagittal and the coronal sutures and at the junction of the sagittal and lambdoid sutures. See also **bregma.**

Calve-Perthes disease, See **Perthes' disease**.

calvous. See **calvities.**

calvities /kalvish'i·ēz/ [L, *calvus,* without hair], baldness. **–calvous,** *adj.*

calyx /kā'liks/, *pl.* **calyces** /kal'isēz/, calyxes [Gk, *kalyx,* shell], **1.** a cup-shaped organ. **2.** a renal calyx. **3.** the wall of an ovarian follicle after expulsion of the ovum at ovulation. Also spelled **calix.**

cambium layer [L, *cambire,* to exchange], **1.** the loose, inner cellular layer of the periosteum that develops during ossification. **2.** a cellular layer of formative tissue that lies between the wood and the bark in plants.

camera /kam'ərə/ [L, vaulted chamber], (in anatomy) any cavity or chamber, as those of the eye or the heart.

camisole restraint. See **straitjacket.**

cAMP, abbreviation for **cyclic adenosine monophosphate.**

camphor /kam'fər/ [L, *camphora*], a colorless or white crystalline substance with a penetrating odor and pungent taste, occurring naturally in certain plants, especially *Cinnamomum camphora.* Also called **camphora, gum camphor.**

camphorated oil /kam'fərā'tid/ [Malay, *kapur,* chalk; L, *oleum,* oil], a colorless to yellowish liquid with the penetrating, pungent odor of camphor. It is derived from a combination of a dozen organic chemicals, including terpenes, safrole, and acetaldhehyde obtained from the camphor laurel plant. It is used mainly as a liniment, counterirritant, and rubefacient.

camphor bath, an air bath in which the air is filled with camphor vapor.

camphor poisoning, a severe toxic condition resulting from the accidental ingestion of camphorated oils. Symptoms may include headache, hallucinations, nausea, vomiting, diarrhea, convulsions, and kidney failure. Treatment may require ipecac emesis, gastric lavage, and, in some cases, dialysis. Diazepam may be administered to control convulsions.

camphor salicylate, a crystalline substance formed by the fusion of 84 parts of camphor and 65 parts of salicylic acid, previously used in skin ointments and administered internally for diarrhea.

camptodactyly /kamp'tədak'təlē/ [Gk, *kamptos,* bent, *daktylos,* finger], the permanent flexion of one or more fingers. **–campodactylic,** *adj.*

camptomelia /kamp'təmē'lyə/ [Gk, *kamptos,* bent, *melos,* arm], a congenital anomaly characterized by bending of one or more limbs, causing permanent bowing or curving of the affected area. **–camptomelic,** *adj.*

Campylobacter [Gk, *campylos,* curved, *bacterion,* rod], a genus of bacteria found in the family Spirillaceae. The organisms consist of gram-negative, non-spore-forming, spirally curved, motile rods that have a single polar flagellum at either or both ends of the cell and move in a characteristic coil-like motion. The organisms require little or no oxygen for growth. The type species is *C. fetus,* which consists of several subspecies that cause human infections, as well as abortion and infertility in cattle. Also called *Vibrio fetus.*

camsylate, shortened word form for *camphorsulfonate.*

Camurati-Engelmann disease, an inherited disorder of bone development marked by an onset of symptoms of muscular pain, weakness, and wasting, mainly in the legs, during childhood. The symptoms vary individually from mild to disabling. Radiographic examination usually reveals thickening of the periosteal and medullary surfaces of the diaphyseal edges of the long bones. In some cases there may be compression of nerve tissue. The symptoms usually subside during early adulthood. Also called **diaphyseal dysplasia.**

Canadian Association of Occupational Therapists. See **CAOT.**

Canadian Association of University Schools of Nursing (CAUSN), a national organization of baccalaureate and higher degree programs in nursing in Canada. It includes an accreditation system established in 1987.

Canadian Association of University Teachers (CAUT), a national Canadian organization representing the interests of all who teach in the universities of the provinces and territories of Canada. The official languages of the CAUT are English and French.

Canadian crutch, a wooden or a metal device that helps a disabled patient stand or walk. It consists of two uprights with a crosspiece to accommodate the hand and a concave crosspiece that fits the armpit for support.

Canadian Journal of Public Health (CJPH), the official publication of the Canadian Public Health Association.

Canadian Medical Association Journal (CMAJ), the official publication of the Canadian Medical Association.

Canadian Nurses Association (CNA), the official national organization for the professional registered nurses of Canada who are members of the 10 provincial nurses' associations and the Northwest Territory's association. The CNA, a federation of these 11 associations, is supported by contributions of the members of the associations. The chief objective of the CNA is to promote conditions conducive to the good health of Canadians and to good patient care. It is concerned with the quality and quantity of nurses available, the standards of education for nurses, social and economic welfare of nurses, advancement of competence and expertise within the profession, promotion of unity and understanding among the members, and the representation of the organized profession of nurses nationally and internationally. A board of elected volunteers and a permanent staff working at CNA House in Ottawa manage the affairs of the organization. Among the services provided are a research and advisory unit that studies trends in nursing and health and prepares briefs, when necessary; a library containing reference works, the archives of the CNA, and up-to-date lists of educational programs in nursing; an information service that collects and disseminates information about nursing and publishes *The Canadian Nurse* and *L'Infirmie*[ac]re Canadienne; a labor relations service; a certification program; a testing service; a governmental liaison service; and an international service that facilitates a working relationship with various organizations such as the World Health Organization and the Pan American Health Organization. All services are provided in the two official languages of Canada, English and French.

Canadian Nurses' Association Testing Service (CNATS), the organizational affiliate of the Canadian Nurses' Association that is concerned with testing the graduates of approved schools of nursing to qualify them as registered nurses.

Canadian Nurses Foundation (CNF), a national Canadian foundation organized to support scholarship in nursing. The CNF awards financial support to nurses undertaking baccalaureate and graduate studies in nursing and to nurses conducting research in nursing.

Canadian Nurses' Respiratory Society (CNRS), an organization of nurses working with or interested in alleviating the problems of respiratory disease. The CNRS is an affiliate of the Canadian Nurses' Association, and it is a section of the Canadian Lung Association.

Canadian Orthopedic Nurses' Association (CONA), a national Canadian organization concerned with the nursing care of orthopedic patients and the continuing education of nurses working in orthopedics. Membership includes orthopedic nurses and other professionals concerned with orthopedics.

Canadian Public Health Association (CPHA), a national Canadian organization concerned with issues in public health and epidemiology. Membership is open to professionals and to others interested in these issues.

canal /kənal'/ [L, *canalis*, channel], **1.** (in anatomy) a narrow tube or channel. Some kinds of canals are **adductor canal, Alcock's canal,** and **alveolar canal. 2.** (in dentistry) one of the accessory root canals and collateral pulp canals in the teeth.

canal debridement. See **epithelial debridement.**

canaliculus /kan'əlik'yələs/, *pl.* **canaliculi** [L, little channel], a very small tube or channel, like the tiny haversian canaliculi throughout bone tissue.

canalization /kan'əlīzā'shən/, the formation of canals or of passages through any tissue.

canal of Schlemm /shlem/ [Friedrich Schlemm, German anatomist, b. 1795], a tiny vein at the angle of the anterior chamber of the eye that connects with the pectinate villi, draining the aqueous humor and funneling it into the bloodstream. Also called **Schlemm's canal.**

canavanine /kan'əvan'in/, an amino acid antagonist present in alfalfa sprouts in concentrations of about 15,000 ppm, or 1.5% by weight. Canavanine can displace arginine in cellular proteins, thereby rendering them inactive. In laboratory experiments canavanine fed to monkeys produces a severe toxic syndrome similar to human lupus erythematosus.

cancellous /kan'siləs/ [L, *cancellus,* lattice], (of tissue) latticelike, porous, spongy. Cancellous tissue is normally present in the interior of many bones, where the spaces are usually filled with marrow.

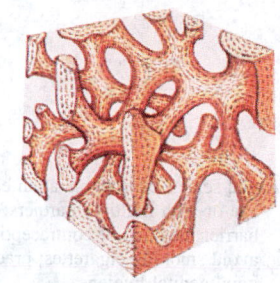

Cancellous bone (Mourad, 1991)

cancer /kan'sər/ [L, crab], **1.** a neoplasm characterized by the uncontrolled growth of anaplastic cells that tend to invade surrounding tissue and to metastasize to distant body sites. **2.** any of a large group of malignant neoplastic diseases characterized by the presence of malignant cells. Each cancer is distinguished by the nature, site, or clinical course of the lesion. The basic origin of cancer is undetermined, but many potential causes are recognized. More than 80% of cases of cancer are attributed to cigarette smoking, exposure to carcinogenic chemicals, ionizing radiation, and ultraviolet rays; overexposure to the sun is the major cause of skin cancer. Many viruses induce malignant tumors in animals, and viral particles are detected in some human tumors; but with possible exception of HIV and EB viral links, there is no clear evidence that any microorganism causes human cancer. The high incidence of various kinds of cancer in certain families suggests that genetic susceptibility is an important factor. An excess rate of malignant tumors in organ transplant recipients after immunosuppressive therapy indicates that the immune system plays a major role in controlling the proliferation of anaplastic cells. The basic defect may be a biochemical anomaly that triggers abnormal cell growth and glucose metabolism and in which certain vital proteins and respiratory enzymes are reduced. The incidence of different kinds of cancer varies markedly with sex, age,

Cancer's seven warning signals

- Change in bowel or bladder habits
- A sore that will not heal
- Unusual bleeding or discharge
- Thickening or lump in breast or elsewhere
- Indigestion or difficulty swallowing
- Obvious change in a wart or mole
- Nagging cough or hoarseness

From Cancer facts and figures 1990, Atlanta, 1990, American Cancer Society.

Prevention, screening, and early detection guidelines

Site	Prevention and risk reduction	Warning signals	Early detection screening for asymptomatic persons
Breast	Follow nutrition guidelines to maintain normal weight and reduce the daily intake of fats	Mass or thickening in breast or axilla Skin dimpling, puckering, or nipple retraction Nipple discharge or scaliness Edema (peau d'orange) Erythema, ulceration Change in size, contour, shape of the breast	Breast self-exam every month beginning at age 20 Breast physical examination every 3 years between ages 20 and 40, then yearly Mammography between ages 35 and 39 for a baseline Mammography every 1-2 years between ages 40 and 49; yearly at age 50 and over; with a positive family history, it may be recommended to begin regular mammograms 5 years earlier than the age at which the relative was diagnosed
Cervix	Avoid sexual intercourse at an early age or with multiple partners; use barrier methods of contraception; avoid smoking cigarettes; practice good genital hygiene	Abnormal vaginal bleeding Persistent postcoital spotting	Annual Pap test and pelvic examination for women who are sexually active or age 18 or older; after three or more consecutive normal annual examinations, the Pap test can be done less frequently at discretion of physician
Colon/Rectum	Removal of colorectal polyp(s); follow nutrition guidelines	Rectal bleeding Change in bowel habits Abdominal pain Decreased diameter of stool Rectal pressure	Annual digital rectal examination beginning at age 40 Annual stool blood test at age 50 and over Sigmoidoscopy beginning at age 50 every year until two normal examinations 1 year apart, then every 3-5 years; more frequent, earlier, and extensive exams in persons with familial polyposis syndrome or a family history of colon cancer
Endometrium	Follow nutrition guidelines; in considering estrogen replacement therapy, discuss the benefits and risks with the patients and individualize therapy based on latest medical research	Abnormal vaginal bleeding or spotting Abdominal or pelvic pain or mass	Pelvic examination. At menopause, an endometrial biopsy is done in high-risk women (history of infertility, failure to ovulate, abnormal uterine bleeding, estrogen therapy use, or obesity)
Head and neck	Avoid tobacco in all forms Drink alcohol only in moderation Good oral hygiene Practice occupational safety to reduce exposure to carcinogens	Color change in mouth Painless lesions in mucosal areas of head and neck Difficulty chewing Earache Persistent sore throat Immobility of tongue Hoarseness Problems opening mouth Neck mass Loss of ability to smell Difficulty breathing	Monthly oral self-examination Annual examination by a health professional
Lung	Stop smoking or using other tobacco products Follow workplace safety practices to reduce exposure to carcinogens	Persistent, nagging cough Dull pain in chest Persistent respiratory cold Wheezing, dyspnea Hemoptysis Change in volume or odor of sputum	None
Prostate	None	Difficulty urinating Painful, frequent urination Blood in urine	Annual digital rectal examination after age 40

From Otto S: *Oncology nursing*, St. Louis, 1991, Mosby.

Prevention, screening, and early detection guidelines—cont'd

Site	Prevention and risk reduction	Warning signals	Early detection screening for asymptomatic persons
Skin	Protect against overexposure to sun by using sunscreen with a protective factor of at least 15 Wear protective clothing when in the sun Limit sun exposure during the hours of 10 AM to 2 PM Avoid suntanning parlors Excise suspicious looking lesions	Change in a wart or mole Sore that does not heal	Annual physical examination Monthly self-examination of skin, especially moles, scars, and birthmarks People with dysplastic nevus syndrome should be carefully monitored
Testicle	None (surgical transfer of the undescended testicle does not decrease the risk but facilitates testicular palpation for screening)	Testicular mass or nodule "Heavy" sensation in the scrotum Painless swelling of the testicle Gynecomastia	Annual physical examination Monthly testicular self-examination (beginning in adolescence)

ethnic group, and geographic location. The age-adjusted death rate for oral cancer is almost 10 times higher in Hong Kong than in Denmark, and that for prostate cancer is more than 10 times greater in Sweden than in Japan, but leukemia mortality is similar throughout the world. In the United States, cancer is second only to heart disease as a cause of mortality and is a leading cause of death in children between 3 and 14 years of age. The most common sites for the development of malignant tumors are the lung, breast, colon, uterus, oral cavity, and bone marrow. Surgery remains the major form of treatment, but irradiation is widely used as preoperative, postoperative, or primary therapy; chemotherapy, with single or multiple antineoplastic agents, is often highly effective. Many malignant lesions are curable if detected in the early stage. Depending on the site, the warning signal may be a change in bowel or bladder habits, a nonhealing sore, unusual bleeding or discharge, a thickening or lump in the breast or elsewhere, indigestion or dysphagia, an obvious change in a wart or mole, or a nagging cough or persistent hoarseness.

cancer bodies. See **Russell's bodies.**

cancericidal /kan′sərisī′dəl/ [L, crab, *caedere,* to kill], of or pertaining to a substance or procedure capable of destroying cancer cells.

cancer in situ. See **carcinoma in situ.**

cancer of the small intestine, a neoplastic disease of the duodenum, jejunum, or ileum. Its characteristics vary, depending on the kind of tumor and the site, but may include abdominal pain, vomiting, weight loss, diarrhea, intermittent bowel obstruction, GI bleeding, or a mass deep in the right abdomen. Diagnosis is made with barium x-ray examination, but such studies may be inconclusive until lesions are large. Adenocarcinomas, the most common tumors, occur more frequently in the duodenum or upper jejunum and form polypoid or constricting napkin-ring growths. Lymphomas, found most often in the lower small intestine, may impair bowel motility by invading nerves and in some cases are associated with a malabsorption syndrome. Less common tumors of the small intestine are carcinoids, usually found in the ileum, and sarcomas, including Kaposi's sarcoma, usually seen in the jejunum and ileum. A leiomyosarcoma may sometimes form a large extraluminal mass but does not metastasize, unlike other cancers of the small intestine. Surgery, including a wide resection of mesenteric lymph nodes, is indicated for adenocarcinomas. Irradiation is not effective in ablation of these tumors but is recommended postoperatively for lymphomas to treat metastatic lesions in mesenteric lymph nodes, the liver, and spleen. Resection of carcinoids is advised to prevent bowel obstruction even if metastatic disease is present, and some patients with these lesions may respond to chemotherapeutic agents, such as cyclophosphamide, 5-fluorouracil, methotrexate, and streptozocin. Cancer of the small intestine, which is uncommon considering the great length and surface area of that organ, occurs slightly more often in men than in women.

cancerigenic. See **carcinogenic.**

cancerous /kan′sərəs/ [L, crab, *oma,* tumor], pertaining to or resembling a cancer.

cancer staging, a system for describing the size and extent of spread of a malignant tumor, used to plan treatment and predict prognosis. Staging may involve a physical examination, diagnostic procedures, surgical exploration, and histologic examination. The system developed by the American Joint Committee for Cancer Staging and End Results Reporting uses the letter T to represent the tumor, N for the regional lymph node involvement, M for distant metastases, and numeric subscripts in each category to indicate the degree of dissemination. According to this system $T_1N_0M_0$ designates a small, localized tumor; $T_2N_1M_0$ is a larger primary tumor that has extended to regional nodes; and $T_4N_3M_3$ is a very large lesion involving regional nodes and distant sites. Other systems may be used for staging breast carcinoma, colorectal cancer, and cutaneous melanoma.

cancr-, chancr-, a combining form meaning 'pertaining to or resembling cancer': *cancriform, cancroid, cancrology.*

cancriform /kang′krifôrm′/ [L, crab, *forma,* form], of or pertaining to a lesion resembling a cancer.

cancroid [L, crab; Gk, *eidos,* form], **1.** of or pertaining to a lesion resembling a cancer. **2.** a moderately malignant skin cancer.

candela. See **candle.**

Candida /kan′didə/ [L, *candidus,* white], a genus of yeastlike fungi including the common pathogen, *Candida albicans.*

Candida albicans /al′bəkanz/, a common, budding, yeastlike, microscopic fungal organism normally present in the mucous membranes of the mouth, intestinal tract, and vagina and on the skin of healthy people. Under certain circumstances, it may cause superficial infections of the mouth or vagina and, in persons with AIDS, infection of the esoph-

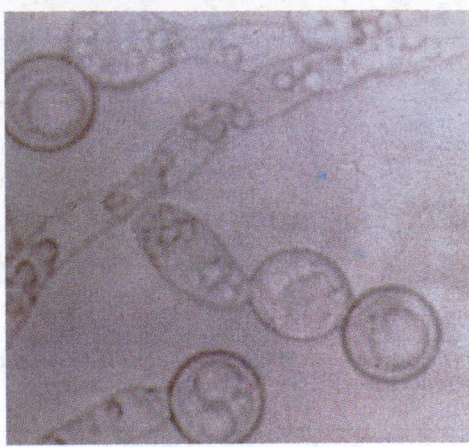

Candida albicans
(Zitelli, 1992/Courtesy Dr. Ellen Wald, Children's Hospital of Pittsburgh)

agus, and serious invasive systemic infections. See also **candidiasis.**

Candida vaginitis. See **candidiasis.**

candidiasis /kan′didī′əsis/ [L, *candidus* + Gk, *osis,* condition], any infection caused by a species of *Candida,* usually *Candida albicans,* characterized by pruritus, a white exudate, peeling, and easy bleeding. Diaper rash, intertrigo, vaginitis, and thrush are common topical manifestations of candidiasis. Endocarditis and infection of the kidney, spleen, liver, and lungs sometimes occur in debilitated patients. Treatment includes the oral and topical administration of antifungal drugs, as nystatin, clotrimazole, and for more severe infections, amphotericin B or fluconazole. Oral candidiasis without a history of recent antibiotic therapy, chemotherapy, cortcosteroid therapy, radiation therapy to the head and neck or other immunosuppressive disorder may indicate the possibility of HIV infection. Also called **candidosis.**

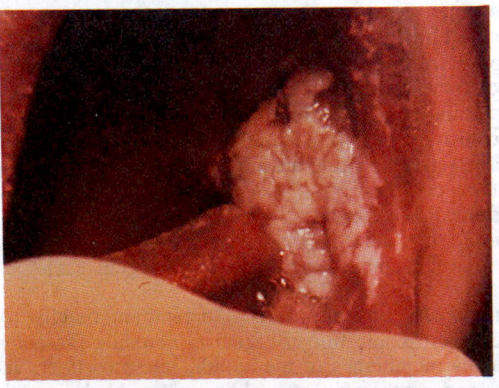

Oral candidiasis *(Zitelli, 1992)*

Candiru fever /kan′dirōō′/, an arbovirus infection transmitted to humans by the bite of a sandfly, characterized by an acute fever, headache, and muscle aches. Recovery occurs, without treatment, within a few days. It occurs mainly in the forests of Brazil. See also **arbovirus, phlebotomus fever.**

candle [L, *candela,* light], (in optics) the basic unit of measurement for luminous intensity, equal to ¹⁄₆₀ of the luminous intensity of a square centimeter of a black body heated to 1773.5° C or the solidification temperature of platinum, adopted in 1948 as the international standard of luminous intensity. Also called **candela** /kandē′lə/.

candle power. See **CP.**

candy-striper, *informal.* a hospital volunteer, named for the striped pink and white uniforms traditionally worn by the young people who perform this service.

cane [Ar, *qanah,* reed], a sturdy wooden or metal shaft, or walking stick, used to give support and mobility to an ambulatory but partially disabled person. A cane should be of an appropriate length to allow a patient with an injured leg to walk with the cane held on the side of the sound leg. In walking, the person may rest his or her weight on the cane and the impaired leg while moving the unaffected leg forward. To take the next step, the weight is placed on the sound leg while the impaired leg and cane are moved forward. The cane should allow 25 degrees of elbow flexion.

cane-cutter's cramp. See **heat cramp.**

canefield fever. See **field fever.**

canine fossa /kā′nīn/ [L, *canis,* dog; L, ditch], (in dentistry) either of the wide depressions on the external surface of each maxilla, superolateral to the canine tooth socket. It is the origin of the levator anguli oris muscle. Also called **maxillary fossa.**

canine tooth, any one of the four teeth, two in each jaw, situated immediately lateral to the incisor teeth in the human dental arches. The canine teeth are larger and stronger than the incisors, have both anterior and posterior tooth characteristics, and they project beyond the level of the other teeth in both arches. Their roots sink deeply into the bones, causing marked prominences on the alveolar arch. The upper canine teeth, or eye teeth, are larger and longer than the lower ones and have a distinct basal ridge. The lower canine teeth, or stomach teeth, are situated nearer the middle line than the upper ones, and their summits correspond to the intervals between the upper canines and the incisors. The crowns of the canines are very large and conic and taper to blunted points or cusps. The canines erupt as deciduous teeth about 16 to 20 months after birth. The eruption of the permanent canines occurs during the eleventh or the twelfth year of life.

canker /kang′kər/ [L, *cancer,* crab], an ulcer or sore in the mouth or genitals. Also called **aphthous stomatitis, chancre.**

canker sore, an ulcerous lesion of the mouth, characteristic of aphthous stomatitis. See also **aphthous stomatitis.**

cannabis /kan′əbis/ [Gk, *kannabis,* hemp], a psychoactive herb derived from the flowering tops of hemp plants. It has no currently acceptable clinical use in the United States but has been employed in the treatment of glaucoma and as an antiemetic in some cancer patients to counter the nausea and vomiting associated with chemotherapy. Cannabis is controlled under Schedule I of the Comprehensive Drug Abuse Prevention and Control Act of 1970. The common hemp from which cannabis is obtained is an herbaceous annual of which *Cannabis sativa* is the sole species. All parts of the plant contain psychoactive substances or cannabinoids, the highest concentrations of which are in the resin of the flowering tops of the plant. Cannabinoids synthesized by the hemp plant include cannabinol, cannabidiol, cannabinolic acid, cannabigerol, cannabicyclol, and several isomers of tetrahydrocannabinol (THC). THC is believed to cause the most characteristic psychologic effects, which include alterations of mood, memory, motor coordination, cognitive ability, and self-perception. Low doses of cannabis seldom impair the ability to perform simple motor tasks but commonly hinder more complex actions, as driving and flying, which involve complex sensory perception, concentration, and information processing. Cannabis may also enhance the nondominant senses of touch, taste, and smell. Higher doses in some persons can produce delusions, paranoid feelings, anxiety, and panic. This drug also increases the heart rate and systolic blood pressure. Pharmacologic effects of smoking marijuana occur within minutes after smoking begins and produce peak plasma concentrations of THC within 10 to 30 minutes. The effects of one cigarette rarely last more than 2 or 3 hours. Marijuana is about three times more powerful when smoked than when taken orally. Studies indicate that it is used by many individuals in all socioeconomic and ethnic groups. Research indicates that some cannabinoids may be therapeutic as anticonvulsants and helpful in reducing intraocular pressure associated with glaucoma. Also called **bhang, ganja, grass, hashish, marijuana, pot, reefer, tea, weed.**

cannabism /kan'əbiz'əm/, a condition associated with excessive or extended use of cannabis drugs. It is characterized by anxiety, disorientation, hallucinations, memory defects, and paranoia.

cannon wave [L, *cane*, tube; *AS, wafian*], a powerful "a" wave in the jugular venous pulse, characteristic of a complete heart block and of premature ventricular beats. Cannon waves are caused by the contraction of the right atrium against a closed tricuspid valve.

cannula /kan'yələ/, *pl.* **cannulas, cannulae** [L, small tube], a flexible tube containing a stiff, pointed trocar that may be inserted into the body, guided by the trocar. As the trocar is removed, a body fluid may be passed through the cannula to the outside. **–cannular, cannulate,** *adj.*

cannulation /kan'yəlā'shən/, the insertion of a cannula into a body duct or cavity, as into the trachea, bladder, or a blood vessel. Also called cannulization. **–cannulate, cannulize,** *v.*

cantharides. See **cantharis.**

cantering rhythm [*Canterbury gallop*; Gk, *rhythmos*, beat], a pattern of three heart sounds in each cardiac cycle, resembling the canter of a horse. Also called **gallop rhythm.**

cantharis /kan'thäris/, *pl.* **cantharides** /kanther'idēz/ [Gk, *kantharis*, beetle], the dried insect *Cantharis vesicatoria* containing cantharidin, formerly used as a topical vesicant. Also called **Spanish fly.**

canthi. See **canthus.**

canthic. See **canthus.**

cantho-, a combining form meaning 'pertaining to the canthus': *cantholysis, canthorraphy, canthotomy.*

canthus /kan'thəs/, *pl.* **canthi** [Gk, *kanthus*, corner of the eye], the angle at the medial and the lateral margins of the eyelids. The medial canthus opens into a small space

containing the opening to a lacrimal duct. Also called **palpebral commissure. –canthic,** *adj.*

Cantil, a trademark for an anticholinergic antispasmodic (mepenzolate bromide).

C.A.O.T., abbreviation for **Canadian Association of Occupational Therapists.**

cap, abbreviation for Latin *capiat,* 'let him or her take,' used in prescriptions.

CAP, 1. abbreviation for **College of American Pathologists. 2.** (in molecular genetics) abbreviation for **catabolic activator protein.** CAP participates in initiating the transcription of RNA in organisms without a true nucleus, as bacteria.

capacitance vessels /kəpas'ətəns/ [L, *capacitas*, capacity], **1.** the blood vessels that hold the major portion of the intravascular blood volume. **2.** the veins.

capacitation /kəpas'itā'shən/, the process in which the spermatozoon, after it reaches the ampulla of the fallopian tube, undergoes a series of changes that lead to its ability to fertilize an ovum.

capacity factor /kəpas'itē/ [L, *capacitas; factum*, to make], the ratio of the elution volume of a substance to the void volume in the column.

Capastat, a trademark for an antibiotic (capreomycin).

CAPD, abbreviation for **continuous ambulatory peritoneal dialysis.**

capeline bandage /kap'əlin/ [Fr, hooded cape], a caplike covering used for protecting the head, shoulder, or a stump. Also called **Hippocrates' bandage.**

capillaries. See **blood vessel.**

capillaritis /kap'ilərī'tis/ [L, *capillaris*, hairlike; Gk, *itis*, inflammation], an abnormal condition characterized by a progressive pigmentary disorder of the skin and dilatation of the capillaries without inflammation. It does not involve any systemic problems and runs a benign self-limiting course.

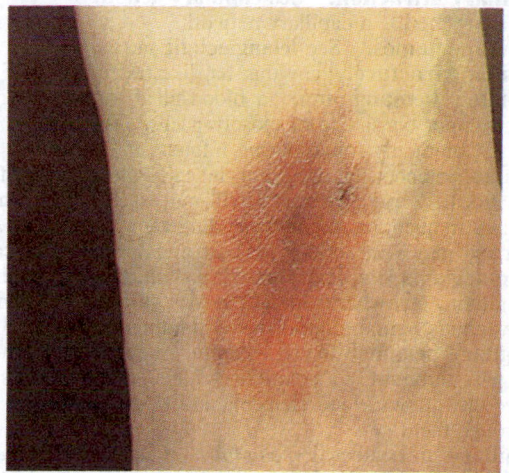

Capillaritis *(du Vivier, 1993)*

capillarity. See **capillary action.**

capillary /kap'iler'ē/ [L, *capillaris*, hairlike], one of the tiny blood vessels (about 0.008 mm in diameter) joining arterioles and venules. Through their walls, which consist of

a single layer of endothelial cells, specialized squamous epithelial cells, blood and tissue cells exchange various substances.

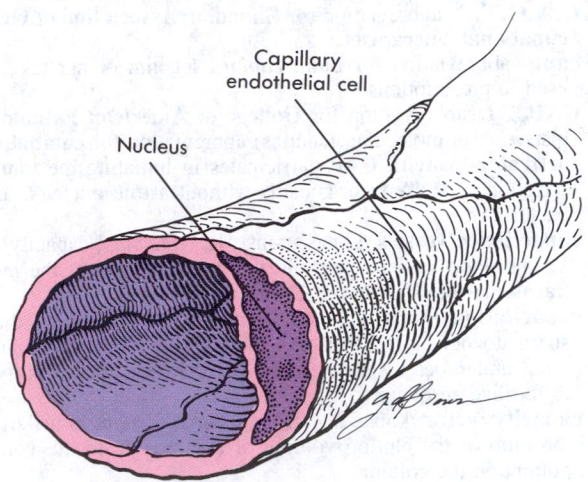

Capillary *(Seeley, 1992/Ronald J Ervin)*

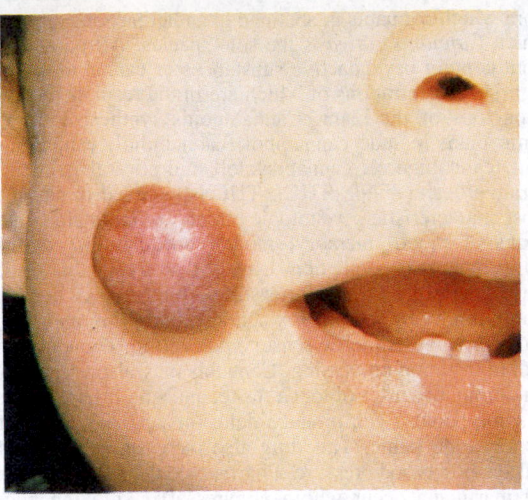

Capillary hemanogioma *(Zacarian, 1985)*

capillary action,   the action involving molecular adhesion
by which the surface of a liquid in a tube is either elevated
or depressed, depending on the cohesiveness of the liquid
molecules. The more cohesive the molecules the more elevated will be the surface of the liquid. Less cohesive liquid
molecules will adhere to the surfaces of the tube in which
they are contained and depress the surface of the liquid.
Also called **capillary attraction, capillarity.**

capillary angioma.   See **cherry angioma.**

capillary attraction.   See **capillary action.**

capillary bed,   a capillary network.

capillary flames.   See **telangiectatic nevus.**

capillary fracture,   any thin hairlike fracture.

capillary hemangioma,   a blood-filled birthmark or benign tumor consisting of closely packed, small blood vessels. Commonly found during infancy, it first grows, then
may spontaneously disappear in early childhood without
treatment. Surgical removal will not usually be attempted
unless frequent trauma and bleeding are present. However,
surgery may be used later for cosmetic reasons. Also called
**hemangioma simplex, port-wine stain, strawberry hem-
angioma, strawberry mark, nevus vascularis.** Compare
cavernous hemangioma, nevus flammeus.

capillary permeability [L, *capillaris*, hairlike, *permeare*,
to pass through],   a condition of the capillary wall structure that allows blood elements and waste products to pass
through them.

capillary pressure [L, *capillaris*, hairlike, *premere*, to
press],   the blood pressure within a capillary.

capillary pulse.   See **Quincke's pulse.**

capillary refill.   See **blanch test.**

capillary refilling,   the process of blood returning to a portion of the capillary system after being interrupted briefly.
When cardiac output is reduced and digital perfusion is
poor, capillary refill is slow. It is tested by pressing firmly
for 5 seconds on a fingernail and estimating the speed at
which blood returns after pressure is released. In a normal

person with good cardiac output and digital perfusion, capillary refilling should take less than 3 seconds. A capillary
refill of more than 3 seconds is considered a sign of sluggish digital circulation, and a time of 5 seconds is regarded
as abnormal.

capillary tufting,   an abnormal condition in which pulmonary capillaries project as tufts, or small masses, into the
alveoli.

capillus /kəpil′əs/, *pl.* **capilli** [L, filament],   one of the
hairs of the body, especially one of the hairs of the scalp.

capit-,   a combining form meaning 'pertaining to the head':
capitate, capitopedal, capitular.

capita.   See **caput.**

capitate /kap′itāt/,   having the shape of a head.

capitate bone [L, *caput*, head; AS, *ban*],   one of the
largest carpal bones, located at the center of the wrist and
having a rounded head that fits the concavity of the scaphoid and the lunate bones. Various ligaments are attached to
the rough dorsal and palmar surfaces. The capitate articulates with the scaphoid and lunate proximally, the second,
third, and fourth metacarpals distally, the trapezoid on the
radial side, and the hamate on the ulnar side. Also called
os capitatum, os magnum.

capitation fee /kap′ita′shən/ [L, *caput*, head; ME, *fief*, pay-
ment],   a method of paying a physician for annual services
based on a fee per patient.

capitatum.   See **capitate bone.**

capitulum /kəpich′ələm/, *pl.* **capitula** [L, small head],   a
small, rounded prominence on a bone where it articulates
with another bone.

capitulum humeri /hyo͞o′mərī, ho͞o′mərē/ [L, small head;
humerus, shoulder],   a rounded eminence at the distal end
of the humerus. It articulates with the radius.

-capnia,   a suffix meaning '(condition of) carbon dioxide
content in the blood': *acapnia, eucapnia, hypocapnia.*

capnograph /kap′nəgraf′/ [Gk, *kapnos*, smoke, *graphein*,
to record],   an instrument used in anesthesia, respiratory
physiology, and respiratory therapy to produce a tracing, or
capnogram, which shows the proportion of carbon dioxide
in expired air.

capnometry /kapnom′ətrē/,   the measurement of carbon

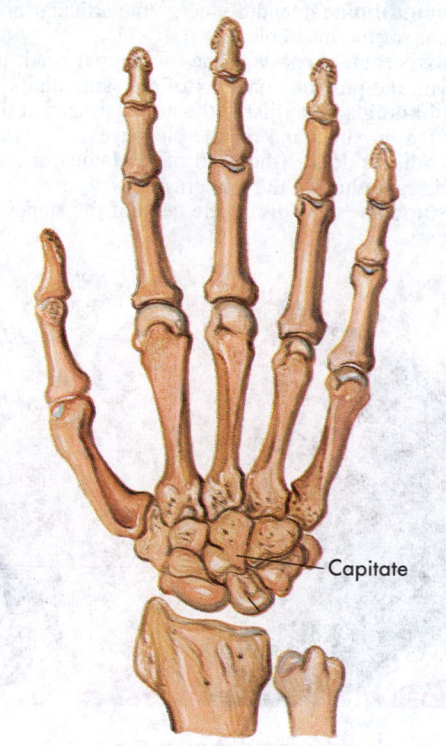

Capitate bone (Thibodeau, 1993/Ernest W Beck)

dioxide in a volume of gas, usually by methods of infrared absorption or mass spectrometry. The most common monitoring units use the infrared absorption technique in which infrared light is absorbed by carbon dioxide and water vapor but not oxygen, nitrogen, and some of the rare gases in the atmosphere. Also **end-tidal CO_2 monitor-ing.**

Capoten, a trademark for an angiotensin-converting enzyme (captopril).

capotement /käpōtmäN′, kəpōt′mənt/, a splashing sound made by fluid movements in a dilated stomach.

capreomycin /kap′rē·ōmī′sin/, an antibiotic.

■ INDICATIONS: It is prescribed in the treatment of pulmonary infections caused by capreomycin-susceptible strains of *Mycobacterium tuberculosis* when the primary agents are ineffective or cannot be used.

■ CONTRAINDICATIONS: Known sensitivity to this drug prohibits its use. It must be used with caution in patients with preexisting renal or auditory impairment.

■ ADVERSE EFFECTS: Among the most serious adverse reactions are nephrotoxicity, hearing loss, tinnitus, vertigo, leukocytosis, leukopenia, urticaria, and skin rash.

capric acid /kap′rik/ [L, *caper*, goat], a white, crystalline substance with a rancid odor, occurring as a glyceride in natural oils. Capric acid is used in the production of perfumes, flavors, wetting agents, and food additives. Also called **decanoic acid, decoic acid.**

caproic acid /kaprō′ik/, a fatty acid that occurs in milk fat and some plant oils. It is used in the production of artificial flavors. Also called **hexanoic acid.**

caps-, kaps-, a prefix meaning 'capsule or container': *capsitis, capsulation, capsuloplasty.*

capsid /kap′sid/ [L, *capsa*, box], the layer of protein enveloping a virion. A capsid is composed of structural units, called capsomeres, and its symmetry may be cubic or helical.

capsomere /kap′səmir/, one of the building blocks of a viral capsid. It consists of groups of identical protein molecules and is visible in an electron microscope.

capsula. See **capsule.**

capsular /kap′sələr/ [L, *capsula*, little box], pertaining to or resembling a small container.

capsular cataract [L, *capsula*; Gk, *katarrhaktes*, waterfall], a visual opacity caused by a thickening of the epithelial cells lining the capsule. The condition is frequently the result of the aging process or a disease that involves surrounding eye tissues.

capsular pattern, a series of limitations of joint movement when the joint capsule is a limiting structure. An example is the range in glenohumeral joints from flexion as the least limited movement to external rotation as the most limited movement. It occurs only in synovial joints that are controlled by muscles and not in joints, such as the sacroiliac, that depend primarily on ligamentous stability.

capsular swelling test. See **quellung reaction.**

capsule /kap′syəl, kap′səl/ [L, *capsula*, little box], **1.** a small, soluble container, usually made of gelatin, used for enclosing a dose of medication for swallowing. Compare **tablet. 2.** a membranous shell surrounding certain microorganisms, such as the pneumococcus bacterium. **3.** a well-defined anatomic structure that encloses an organ or part, such as the capsule of the adrenal gland. Also called **capsula** (*pl.* capsuli).

capsulectomy /kap′sələk′təmē/, the surgical excision of a capsule, usually the capsule of a joint or the capsule of the lens of the eye.

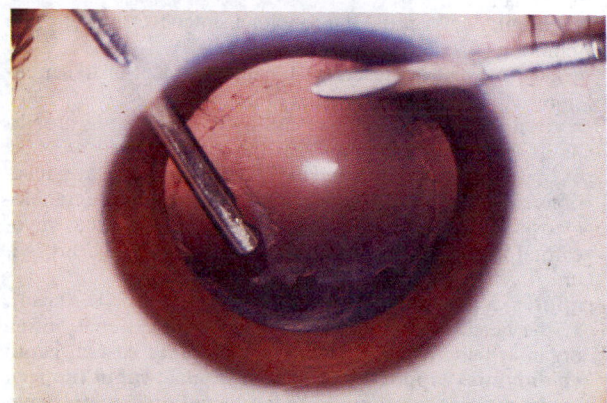

Capsulectomy of the eye (Jaffe, 1990)

capsule of Tenon. See **fascia bulbi.**

capsule of the kidney, the fatty enclosure of the kidney, consisting of adipose tissue continuous at the hilus with the fat of the renal sinus. This investment of perirenal fat covers the fibrous capsule and helps protect the organ from bumps and shocks. It also encloses the adrenal glands. Compare **Bowman's capsule.**

capsule of the lens. See **lens capsule.**

capsuli. See **capsule.**

capsulitis /-ī'tis/ [L, *capsula*, little box; Gk, *itis*, inflamation], an inflammation involving any anatomic capsule.

capsuloma /kap'səlō'mə/, *pl.* capsulomas, capsulomata [L, *capsula* + Gk, *oma*, tumor], a neoplasm of the capsule or the subcapsular area of the kidney.

capsulotomy /kap'səlot'əmē/ [L, *capsula* + Gk, *temnein*, to cut], an incision into a capsule, such as in an operation to remove a cataract.

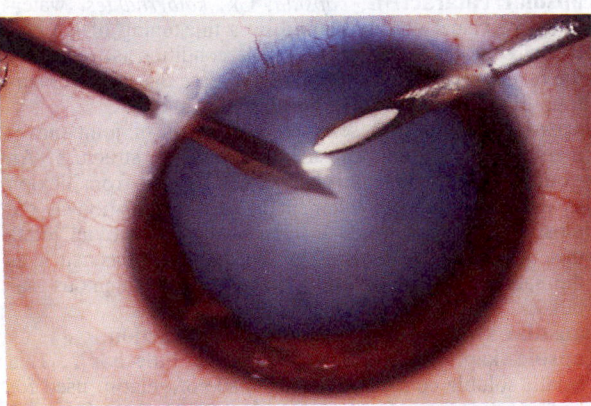

Capsulotomy of the eye (Jaffe, 1990)

captain-of-the-ship doctrine, the medicolegal principle that the physician is ultimately responsible for all patient-care activities and thus may be held accountable and may be sued for negligence or malpractice when the act at issue is performed by an employee or other person under the physician's control, even if not ordered by the physician.

captopril /kap'tōpril/, an angiotensin-converting enzyme inhibitor.

■ INDICATION: It is prescribed for the treatment of hypertension.

■ CONTRAINDICATION: Known sensitivity to this drug prohibits its use.

■ ADVERSE EFFECTS: Among the most serious adverse reactions are proteinurea, renal failure, neutropenia, agranulocytosis, angioneurotic edema, hypotension, angina, myocardial infarction, Raynaud's disease, congestive heart failure.

caput /kā'pət, kap'ət/, *pl.* capita /cap'itə/ [L, head], **1.** the head. **2.** the enlarged or prominent extremity of an organ or part. Kinds of capita include **caput costae, caput epididymis, caput femoris, caput fibulae, caput humeri, caput mallei, caput mandibulae, caput ossis metacarpalis, caput phalangis, caput radii, caput stapedis,** and **caput succedaneum.**

caput costae /kos'tē/ [L, head; *costa*, rib], the head of a rib; it articulates with a vertebral body.

caput epididymidis, the head of the epididymis.

caput femoris /fem'əris/, the head of the femur; it fits into the acetabulum.

caput fibulae /fib'yəlē/, the head of the fibula; it articulates with the lateral condyle of the tibia.

caput humeri /hyoo'mərī/, the head of the humerus; it fits into the glenoid cavity of the scapula.

caput mallei /mal'ē·ī/, the head of the malleus.

caput mandibulae /mandib'yəlē/, the articular process of the ramus of the mandible.

caput ossis metacarpalis, the metacarpal head; it articulates with the proximal phalanx of the same digit.

caput phalangis /falan'jis/, the articular head at the distal end of the proximal and middle phalanges.

caput radii /rā'dē·ī/, the head of the radius; it articulates with the capitulum of the humerus.

caput stapedis /stapē'dis/, the head of the stapes.

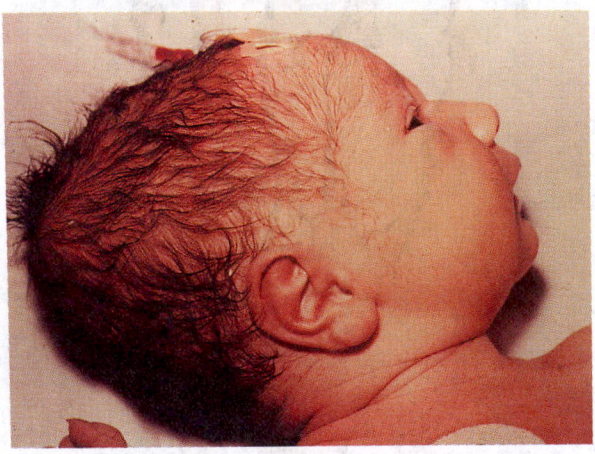

Caput succedaneum (Zitelli, 1992)

caput succedaneum /suk'sədənē'əm/ [L, head; *succeder*, to replace], a localized pitting edema in the scalp of a fetus that may overlie sutures of the skull. It is usually formed during labor as a result of the circular pressure of the cervix on the fetal occiput. On vaginal examination the swelling may be mistaken for unruptured membranes. If the caput enlarges appreciably during labor, it may give an erroneous impression of fetal descent on successive examinations. At birth the baby's head may appear markedly deformed, but the swelling begins to resolve immediately and is usually gone in a few days. Compare **cephalhematoma, molding.**

Carafate, a trademark for a peptic ulcer medication (sucralfate).

caramiphen edisylate /kəram'ifən'ēdis'ilāt/, an antitussive.

■ INDICATION: It is prescribed in the treatment of coughs.

■ CONTRAINDICATION: Known sensitivity to this drug prohibits its use.

■ ADVERSE EFFECTS: Among the most serious adverse reactions are dizziness, GI upset, nausea, and drowsiness.

carapace /kar'əpās/ [Sp, *carapacho*, hard shell], a horny shield or shell covering the dorsal surface of an animal, such as a turtle.

carate. See **pinta.**

carb, abbreviation for a *carbonate noncarboxylate anion.*

carbam, abbreviation for a *carbamate carboxylate anion.*

carbamate /kär'bəmāt/, any of a group of anticholinesterase enzymes that cause reversible inhibition of cholinesterase. They are used in certain medications and insecticides. Some carbamates are toxic and may cause convulsions and death through ingestion or skin contact. Atropine is a commonly recommended antidote.

carbamate kinase, a liver enzyme that catalyzes the transfer of a phosphate group from adenosine triphosphate, associated with ammonia and carbon dioxide, to form adenosine diphosphate and carbamoylphosphate.

carbamazepine /kär′bəmaz′əpin/, an anticonvulsant and specific analgesic for trigeminal neuralgia.
■ INDICATIONS: It is prescribed in the treatment of trigeminal neuralgia and certain seizure disorders.
■ CONTRAINDICATIONS: Concomitant use of monoamine oxidase inhibitors, a history of bone marrow depression, or known hypersensitivity to this drug or to any of the tricyclic antidepressants prohibits its use.
■ ADVERSE EFFECTS: Among the more serious adverse reactions are life-threatening blood dyscrasias, drowsiness, dizziness, ataxia, and nausea. Dermatologic and hypersensitivity reactions may occur.

carbamide peroxide /kär′bəmīd/, a topical antiinfective and ceruminolytic.
■ INDICATIONS: It is prescribed in the treatment of canker sores and other minor inflammatory conditions of the gums and mouth and to soften impacted earwax.
■ CONTRAINDICATION: Perforated eardrum prohibits its use.
■ ADVERSE EFFECTS: The most serious adverse reaction is local irritation.

carbamino compound /kärbam′inō/, a chemical complex formed by the binding of carbon dioxide molecules to plasma proteins. A small fraction of carbon dioxide binds with protein as it leaves a tissue cell.

carbamino-hemoglobin, a chemical complex formed by carbon dioxide and hemoglobin after the release of oxygen by the hemoglobin to a tissue cell. The action is similar to that of the formation of a carbamino compound. It accounts for nearly 25% of the carbon dioxide released in the lung.

carbenicillin disodium /kär′bənəsil′in/, a semisynthetic penicillin antibiotic.
■ INDICATIONS: It is prescribed in the treatment of certain infections.
■ CONTRAINDICATIONS: Known hypersensitivity to this drug or to other penicillins prohibits its use.
■ ADVERSE EFFECTS: Among the more serious adverse effects are hypersensitivity reactions, neurologic disturbances, and clotting defects. The high sodium content (5.5-6.5 mEq/g) may aggravate fluid and electrolyte imbalance in people affected with kidney, heart, or liver disease.

carbidopa /kär′bidō′pə/, a DOPA decarboxylase inhibitor.
■ INDICATION: It is prescribed in combination with levodopa in the treatment of idiopathic Parkinson's disease because it inhibits the degradation of levadopa.
■ CONTRAINDICATIONS: Glaucoma, hypertension, the use of a monoamine oxidase inhibitor within the past 14 days, or known hypersensitivity to this drug prohibits its use.
■ ADVERSE EFFECTS: Among the most serious adverse reactions are GI bleeding, cardiac irregularity, hemolytic anemia, tardive dyskinesia, mental depression, blurred vision, and activation of malignant melanoma.

carbinoxamine maleate /kär′bənok′səmēn/, an antihistamine.
■ INDICATIONS: It is prescribed in the treatment of a variety of hypersensitivity reactions, including rhinitis, skin reactions, and itching.
■ CONTRAINDICATIONS: Asthma or known hypersensitivity to this drug prohibits its use. It should not be administered to newborn infants or lactating mothers.

■ ADVERSE EFFECTS: Among the more serious adverse reactions are tachycardia and other side effects of anticholinergic medications. Drowsiness, skin rash, hypersensitivity reactions, and dry mouth commonly occur.

carbo-, carbon-, a combining form meaning 'carbon, carbonic acid, or charcoal': *carbonate, carboneol, carbonometry.*

Carbocaine Hydrochloride, a trademark for a local anesthetic (mepivacaine hydrochloride).

carbocyclic. See **closed-chain.**

carbohydrate /kär′bōhī′drit/ [L, *carbo,* coal; Gk, *hydor,* water], any of a group of organic compounds, the most important being the saccharides, starch, cellulose, and gum. They are classified according to molecular structure as mono-, di-, tri-, poly-, and heterosaccharides. Carbohydrates constitute the main source of energy for all body functions, particularly brain functions, and are necessary for the metabolism of other nutrients. They are synthesized by all green plants and in the body are either absorbed immediately or stored in the form of glycogen. Cereals, vegetables, fruits, rice, potatoes, legumes, and flour products are the major sources of carbohydrates. They can also be manufactured in the body from some amino acids and the glycerol component of fats. Symptoms of deficiency include fatigue, depression, breakdown of essential body protein, and electrolyte imbalance. Muscle protein-sparing amounts of food carbohydrates have been estimated to be 50 to 100 grams per day for most people. Excessive consumption of carbohydrates is associated with tooth decay, obesity, diabetes mellitus, and cardiovascular disease.

Summary of carbohydrate classes

Chemical class name	Class members	Sources
Polysaccharides Multiple sugars, complex carbohydrates	Starch	Grains and grain products Cereal, bread, crackers, and other baked goods Pasta Rice, corn, bulgur Legumes Potatoes and other vegetables
	Glycogen	Animal tissues, liver and muscle meats
	Dietary fiber	Whole grains Fruits Vegetables Seeds, nuts, skins
Disaccharides Double sugars, simple carbohydrates	Sucrose	"Table" sugar: sugar cane, sugar beets Molasses
	Lactose	Milk
	Maltose	Starch digestion, intermediate Sweetener in food products Starch digestion, final
Monosaccharides Single sugars, simple carbohydrates	Glucose (dextrose)	Corn syrup (large use in processed foods)
	Fructose	Fruits, honey
	Galactose	Lactose (milk)

From Williams SW: *Basic nutrition and diet therapy,* ed 9, St Louis, 1992, Mosby.

carbohydrate loading, a dietary practice of some endurance atheletes, such as marathon runners, intended to increase glycogen stores in the muscle tissue. It begins with a period of several days of carbohydrate abstinence designed to deplete stored glycogen. During the period of carbohydrate abstinence, the individual eats mainly a high-protein, high-fat diet with only enough carbohydrates to prevent ketosis. The athlete ends the glycogen-depletion phase by consuming a diet high in complex carbohydrates for 3 days before the event. Other approaches simply involve a high carbohydrate diet (about 70% of total food calories) sustained five to seven days before competition. The practice is controversial and not universally practiced.

carbohydrate metabolism, the sum of the anabolic and catabolic processes of the body involved in the synthesis and breakdown of carbohydrates, principally galactose, fructose, and glucose. Some of the processes are glycogenesis, glyconeogenesis, and glycolysis. Energy-rich phosphate bonds are produced in many metabolic reactions requiring carbohydrates.

carbolated camphor /kär′bōlā′tid/ [L, *carbo,* coal; *camphora*], a mixture of 1.5 parts camphor with 1 part each of alcohol and phenol, used as an antiseptic dressing for wounds.

carbol-fuchsin solution /kär′bolfŏok′sin/ [L, *carbo,* coal; Leonard Fuchs, German botanist, b. 1501], a preparation used in the treatment of superficial fungal infections. It contains boric acid, phenol, resorcinol, fuchsin, acetone, and alcohol in water. Also called **Castellani's paint.**

carbol-fuchsin stain, a solution of dilute phenol and basic fuchsin used on microorganisms and cell nuclei for microscopic examination. Also called **Ziehl's stain.**

carbolic acid /kärbol′ik/ [L, *carbo,* coal; *acidus,* sour], a poisonous, colorless to pale pink crystalline compound obtained from coal tar distillation and converted to a clear liquid with a strong odor and burning taste by the addition of 10% water. Low concentrations of carbolic acid are used in antiseptic preparations. Also called **hydroxybenzene, oxybenzene, phenic acid, phenol, phenylic acid, phenylic alcohol.**

carbolic acid poisoning. See **phenol poisoning.**

carbon /kär′bən/ (C) [L, *carbo,* coal], a nonmetallic, chiefly tetravalent element. Its atomic number is 6; its atomic weight is 12.011. Carbon occurs in pure form in diamonds, graphite, and fullerenes and is a component of all living tissue. Most of the study of organic chemistry focuses on the vast number of carbon compounds. Carbon occurs in impure form in charcoal, coke, and soot, and in the atmosphere as carbon dioxide. Carbon is essential to the chemistry of the body, participating in many metabolic processes and acting as a component of carbohydrates, amino acids, triglycerides, deoxyribonucleic and ribonucleic acids, and many other compounds. Carbon dioxide produced in glycolysis is important in the acid-base balance of the body and in controlling respiration. Carbon is a component of carbon monoxide, which can be lethal if inhaled, and of many hydrocarbons, the fumes of which can cause death from respiratory failure. Brief incidental exposures to low concentrations of solvent vapors that contain carbon, such as gasoline, lighter fluids, aerosol sprays, and spot removers, may be relatively harmless, but exposures to concentrations of hydrocarbon vapors often found in the home and in manufacturing environments may be dangerous. Many occupational pulmonary diseases, such as coal worker's pneumoconiosis, black lung disease, and byssinosis, are caused by chronic inhalation of dusts containing carbon compounds. See also **carbon 11, carbon 14.**

carbon-. See **carbo-.**

carbon 11, a radioisotope of carbon with a half-life of 20 minutes. It is produced by a cyclotron and emits positrons. Compare **carbon 14.**

carbon 14, a beta-emitter with a half-life of 5760 years. It occurs naturally, arising from cosmic rays, and is used as a tracer in studying various aspects of metabolism and in dating relics that contain natural carbonaceous materials. Compare **carbon 11.**

carbon arc lamp, an electric lamp producing a strong white light of adjustable intensity from an arc of current between carbon electrodes.

carbonate /kär′bənāt/, a CO_3^- anion. Carbonates are in equilibrium with bicarbonates in water and frequently occur in compounds as insoluble salts, such as calcium carbonate.

carbon cycle, the steps by which carbon in the form of carbon dioxide is extracted from and returned to the atmosphere by living organisms, especially human beings. The process starts with the photosynthetic production of carbohydrates by plants, progresses through the consumption of carbohydrates by animals and human beings, and ends with the exhalation of carbon dioxide by those same animals and human beings, and also with the release of carbon dioxide during the decomposition of dead plants and animals. Various chemical processes intervene between the ingestion of carbohydrates and the release of carbon dioxide. Carbohydrate metabolism starts with the movement of glucose through cell membranes and subsequently involves glycolysis, the processes of the citric acid cycle, electron transport, and oxidative phosphorylation. See also **Krebs' cycle, tricarboxylic acid cycle.**

carbon damp. See **damp.**

carbon dioxide (CO$_2$) [L, *carbo;* Gk, *dis,* twice, *oxys,* sharp], a colorless, odorless gas produced by the oxidation of carbon. Carbon dioxide, as a product of cell respiration, is carried by the blood to the lungs and is exhaled. The acid-base balance of body fluids and tissues is affected by the level of carbon dioxide and its carbonate compounds. Solid carbon dioxide (dry ice) is used in the treatment of some skin conditions. Normal adult blood levels of carbon dioxide are 23-30 mEq/L or 23-30 mmol/L (SI units).

carbon dioxide acidosis. See **respiratory acidosis.**

carbon dioxide bath, a bath taken in water that is saturated with carbon dioxide. See also **Nauheim bath.**

carbon dioxide narcosis, a condition of severe hypercapnia, with symptoms of confusion, tremors, convulsions, and possible coma, that may occur if blood levels of carbon dioxide are increased to 70 mm Hg or higher. Generally, carbon dioxide is near 40 mm Hg when ventilation is sufficient to maintain normal levels of oxygen partial pressure in the arteries. See also **carbon dioxide poisoning.**

carbon dioxide poisoning, toxic effects of inhaling excessive amounts of carbon dioxide. Carbon dioxide is a respiratory stimulant, but it is also an asphyxiant. Concentrations of 10% or greater can cause unconsciousness and death from ventilatory failure. Particularly vulnerable are persons who work in confined spaces with poor air circulation, such as mine shafts, silos, or holds of ships. See also **carbon dioxide narcosis.**

carbon dioxide pressure. See **carbon dioxide tension.**

carbon dioxide retention, any increased partial pressure and body stores of carbon dioxide resulting from impaired carbon dioxide elimination in conditions such as alveolar hypoventilation, strangulation, apnea, and bronchopulmonary conditions associated with ventilation-perfusion abnormalities. Respiratory acidosis may result from carbon dioxide retention.

carbon dioxide response, the ventilatory reaction to increased concentrations of carbon dioxide gas. Ventilation normally increases linearly up to a concentration of 8% to 10%. The carbon dioxide response curve flattens slightly near the peak and falls off at concentrations of about 20%. At concentrations around 25%, the person is conscious but is unable to perform simple tasks. At concentrations of 30%, carbon dioxide is an anesthetic.

carbon dioxide stores, the volume of carbon dioxide contained in the body as a gas and also in the form of carbonic acid, carbonate, bicarbonate, and carbamino-hemoglobin. During a steady state of ventilation and aerobic respiration, the carbon dioxide output rate equals the production rate, and the quantity of carbon dioxide stores remains constant.

carbon dioxide tension, the partial pressure of carbon dioxide gas, expressed as Pco_2, which is proportional to its percentage or relative concentration in the blood or lungs. It is expressed quantitatively in millimeters (mm) of mercury. Alveolar Pco_2 directly reflects adequate pulmonary gas exchange in relation to blood flow. A high rate of ventilation causes a lower alveolar Pco_2; a lower rate of breathing leads to higher amounts of alveolar and blood carbon dioxide. Normal values for arterial and alveolar carbon dioxide tension are between 37 and 43 mm Hg. Higher levels occur in conditions of slow blood flow, slow ventilatory rate. Below-normal values are caused by hyperventilation, respiratory alkalosis. Also called **carbon dioxide pressure.** See also **carbon dioxide, hypercapnia, hyperventilation, hypoventilation.**

carbon dioxide therapy, the therapeutic inhalation of a low concentration of carbon dioxide gas. Such therapy may be used to dilate the blood vessels, stimulate the cardiovascular brain centers and the central nervous system, overcome hyperventilation, assist in developing a productive cough needed to remove mucous secretions, and control hiccups.

carbon dioxide titration curve, a line plotted on a graph showing the blood pH and total carbon dioxide concentration changes that result from the addition or removal of carbon dioxide.

carbon fiber, a material consisting of graphite fibers in a plastic matrix used in radiologic devices to reduce patient exposure to x-rays.

carbonate dehydratase. See **carbonic anhydrase.**

carbonic acid (H_2CO_3) /kärbon'ik/ [L, *carbo*, coal, *acidus*, acid], an unstable acid formed by dissolving carbon dioxide in water. It is the basis of carbonated beverages and is related to the carbonate group of compounds.

carbonic anhydrase /anhī'drās/, a zinc-containing enzyme in red blood cells that assists in the hydration of carbon dioxide to carbonic acid in the red blood cell so it can be transported from the tissue cell to the lungs. Also called **carbonate dehydratase.**

carbonic anhydrase inhibitor, a substance that decreases the rate of carbonic acid and H+ production in the kidney, thereby increasing the excretion of solutes and the rate of urinary output. An example of a carbonic anhydrase inhibitor is acetazolamide. Some carbonic anhydrase inhibitors are used as diuretics, others in the treatment of glaucoma.

carbon monoxide [L, *carbo;* Gk, *monos*, single, *oxys*, sharp], a colorless, odorless, poisonous gas produced by the combustion of carbon or organic fuels in a limited oxygen supply, as in the cylinders of an internal combustion engine. Carbon monoxide combines irreversibly with hemoglobin, preventing the formation of oxyhemoglobin and reducing the oxygen supply to the tissues. Prolonged exposure to high levels of carbon monoxide results in asphyxiation.

carbon monoxide poisoning, a toxic condition in which carbon monoxide gas has been inhaled and absorbed by erythrocytes in the pulmonary circulation, displacing oxygen from the red blood cells and decreasing the capacity of the blood to carry oxygen to the cells of the body. Characteristically, headache, dyspnea, drowsiness, confusion, cherry-pink skin, unconsciousness, and apnea occur in sequence as the level of carbon monoxide in the blood increases. The most common source of carbon monoxide in cases of poisoning is exhaust fumes from an automobile. Treatment includes removal of the victim from the toxic environment, cardiac resuscitation, as necessary, administration of high-flow oxygen, monitoring of carboxyhemoglobin levels and potential hyperbaric oxygen therapy.

carbon tetrachloride [L, *carbo;* Gk, *tetra*, four, *chloros*, greenish], a colorless, volatile, toxic liquid used as a solvent and in fire extinguishers. Ingestion of the liquid or inhalation of the fumes usually results in headaches, nausea, CNS depression, abdominal pain, and convulsions. In poisoning by inhalation, ventilatory assistance and oxygen may be necessary. In poisoning by ingestion, removal of the poison and gastric lavage are the usual treatments. Carbon tetrachloride is particularly toxic to the kidneys and liver; permanent damage to these organs may result.

carbon tetrachloride poisoning [L, *carbo*, coal; Gk, *tetra*, four, *chloros*, greenish; L, *potio*, drink], toxic effects of exposure to carbon tetrachloride, a colorless commercial dry cleaning fluid also used in fire extinguishers and industrial solvents. It may attack both liver and kidneys. Symptoms include persistent headache, nausea, vomiting, diarrhea, uremia, lethargy, confusion from CNS depression, and degeneration of the liver and kidneys.

carboxyfluoroquinolone /kärbok'sēflōō'ərōkwī'nəlōn/, any of a group of oral quinolone antibiotics that is generally effective against Enterobacteriaceae and shows varying activity against *Pseudomonas* and other species. The drugs differ in their oral absorption. Examples include ofloxacin and perfloxacin.

carboxyhemoglobin /kärbok'sēhē'məglō'bin, -hem'-/ [L, *carbo* + Gk, *oxys*, sharp, *haima*, blood; L, *globus*, ball], a compound produced by the exposure of hemoglobin to carbon monoxide. Carbon monoxide from the environment is inhaled into the lungs, absorbed through the alveoli, and bound to hemoglobin in the blood, blocking the sites for oxygen transport. Oxygen levels decrease, hypoxia and anoxia may result. See also **carbon monoxide poisoning, oxyhemoglobin.**

carboxyl /kärbok'sil/, a monovalent radical COOH characteristic of organic acids. The hydrogen of the radical can be replaced by metals to form salts.

carboxylation /-lā'shən/, a chemical process in which a carboxyl group (-COOH) replaces a hydrogen atom.

carbuncle /kär'bungkəl/ [L, *carbunculus*, little coal], a large staphylococcal infection containing purulent matter in deep, interconnecting, subcutaneous pockets. Pus eventually discharges to the skin surface through openings. Common sites for carbuncles are the back of the neck and the buttocks. Treatment may include the use of antibiotics, hot compresses, and surgical drainage. Compare **furuncle.**

carbunculosis /karbung′kyəlō′sis/, an abnormal condition characterized by a cluster of deep painful abscesses that drain through multiple openings onto the skin surface, usually around hair follicles. Carbunculosis is a form of folliculitis, most commonly caused by the coagulase-positive *Staphylococcus aureus.* The lesions caused by this condition may result in fever and malaise.
■ OBSERVATIONS: Carbunculosis commonly follows persistent *S. aureus* infection and furunculosis. Diagnosis is based on obvious skin lesions, a patient history of previous furunculosis, and *S. aureus* in wound culture.
■ INTERVENTIONS: Treatment of carbunculosis requires the administration of systemic antibiotics. The prognosis depends on the severity of the infection and the physical condition of the patient.
■ NURSING CONSIDERATIONS: Nursing care for this disorder is mainly supportive and educative to impress the patient with the importance of meticulous personal and family hygiene. The nurse explains that reducing the intake of sugars and fats is important and cautions the patient never to squeeze a carbuncle or furuncle because it may rupture into the surrounding area. The patient is also instructed not to share towels and washcloths with other family members because this may spread the bacteria. Also stressed is the importance of boiling towels and washcloths before reusing them and the need for daily changes of boiled clothes and bedsheets. The patient is additionally encouraged to change dressings frequently and to discard them in paper bags. Because carbunculosis often follows furunculosis, a disorder associated with diabetes, the patient should have a thorough physical examination.

carcin-, a combining form meaning 'pertaining to cancer': *carcinelcosis, carcinogen, carcinolytic.*

carcinoembryonic antigen (CEA) /kär′sənō·em′brē-on′ik/ [Gk, *karkinos*, crab, *en*, into, *bryein*, to grow; *anti* against, *genein*, to produce], an antigen present in very small quantities in adult tissue. A greater than normal amount is suggestive of cancer. Presence of CEA aids in evaluating recurrent or disseminated disease, and in monitoring treatment effectiveness. Normal CEA findings are less than 5 ng/ml or 0-2.5 micrograms/L.

carcinogen /kärsin′əjin/ [Gk, *karkinos* + *genein*, to produce], a substance or agent that causes the development or increases the incidence of cancer.

carcinogenesis /kär′sinəjen′əsis/, the process of initiating and promoting cancer. Compare **oncogenesis, sarcomagenesis, tumorigenesis.**

carcinogenic /kär′sinəjen′ik/, of or pertaining to the ability to cause the development of a cancer. Also called **cancerigenic, cancerogenic.**

carcinoid /kär′sinoid/ [Gk, *karkinos* + *eidos*, form], a small yellow tumor derived from argentaffin cells in the gastrointestinal mucosa that secrete serotonin and other catecholamines. Carcinoid tumors spread slowly locally but may metastasize widely. Also called **argentaffinoma, Kulchitsky-cell carcinoma.** See also **argentaffin cell, carcinoid syndrome.**

carcinoid syndrome, the systemic effects of serotonin-secreting carcinoid tumors manifested by flushing, diarrhea, cramps, skin lesions resembling pellagra, labored breathing, palpitations, and valvular heart disease, especially of the pulmonary valve. Treatment includes surgical excision of

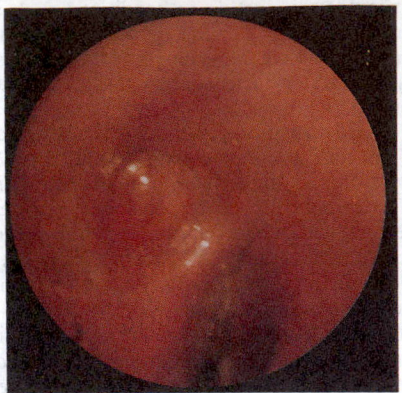

Carcinoid tumor (du Bois, 1987)

the tumor, if feasible, administration of alpha-adrenergic blocking agents to produce vasodilatation, and medication to counteract bronchospasm. Also called **argentaffinoma syndrome.** See also **carcinoid.**

carcinolysis /kär′sinol′isis/ [Gk, *karkinos* + *lysis*, loosening], the destruction of cancer cells. –**carcinolytic,** *adj.*

carcinoma /kär′sinō′mə/, *pl.* **carcinomas, carcinomata** [Gk, *karkinos* + *oma*, tumor], a malignant epithelial neoplasm that tends to invade surrounding tissue and to metastasize to distant regions of the body. Carcinomas develop most frequently in the skin, large intestine, lungs, stomach, prostate gland, cervix, or breast. The tumor is firm, irregular, nodular, with a well-defined border. Microscopically, the cells are characterized by anaplasia, abnormal size and shape, disproportionately large nuclei, and clumps of nuclear chromatin. –**carcinomatous,** *adj.*

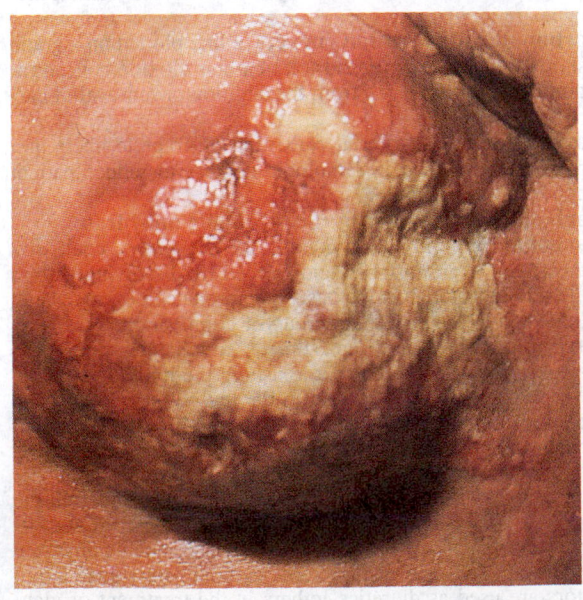

Carcinoma of the breast (Kamal, 1991)

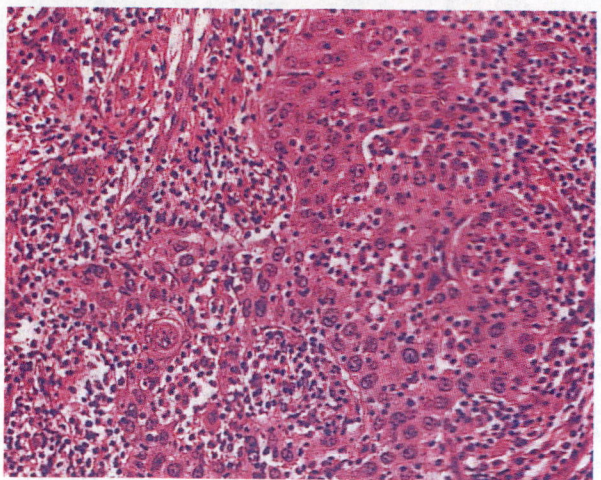

Microscopic changes in a carcinoma *(Weiss, 1988)*

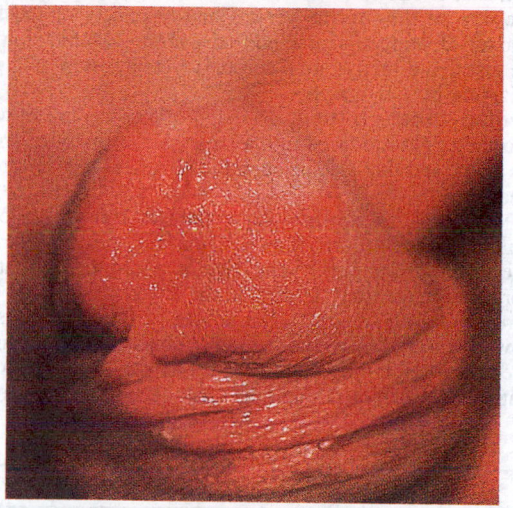

Carcinoma in situ
(Weiss, 1988/Courtesy K.R. Greer, MD, Charlottesville, VA)

-carcinoma, a suffix meaning a 'malignant tumor composed of epithelial cells, with a tendency to metastasize': *ophthalmocarcinoma, osteocarcinoma, phlebocarcinoma.*

carcinoma basocellulare. See **basal cell carcinoma.**

carcinoma cutaneum. See **basal cell carcinoma, squamous cell carcinoma.**

carcinoma en cuirasse /äN'kērās'/ [Gk, *karkinos, oma;* Fr, breastplate], a rare neoplasm accompanying advanced breast cancer and characterized by progressive extensive fibrosis and rigidity of the skin of the chest, neck, back, and, abdomen.

carcinoma fibrosum. See **scirrhous carcinoma.**

carcinoma gigantocellulare. See **giant cell carcinoma.**

carcinoma in situ /insit'ōō, insī'tōō [Gk, *karkinos, oma;* L, in position], a premalignant neoplasm that has not invaded the basement membrane but shows cytologic characteristics of cancer. Such neoplastic changes in stratified squamous or glandular epithelium are frequently seen on the uterine cervix, and in the anus, bronchi, buccal mucosa, esophagus, eye, lip, penis, uterine endometrium, and vagina. Also called **cancer in situ, intraepithelial carcinoma, preinvasive carcinoma.** See also **erythroplasia of Queyrat.**

carcinoma lenticulare /len'tikōōlär'ə/ [Gk, karkinos, oma; L, lens], a form of carcinoma tuberosum or scirrhous skin cancer characterized by the development of many small, flat nodules that coalesce to form larger areas resembling a fungous infection.

carcinoma medullare, carcinoma molle. See **medullary carcinoma.**

carcinoma mucocellulare. See **Krukenberg's tumor.**

carcinoma scroti /skrō'tī/, an epithelial cell carcinoma of the scrotum.

carcinoma spongiosum /spon'jē·ō'səm/, a soft and spongy carcinoma with small and large cavities. See also **medullary carcinoma.**

carcinomata. See **carcinoma.**

carcinoma telangiectaticum /telan'jē·ektat'ikəm/ [Gk, *karkinos, oma; telos,* end, *aggeion,* vessel, *ektasis,* dilatation], a neoplasm of the capillaries of the skin causing dilatation of the vessels and red spots on the skin that blanch with pressure.

carcinomatoid /kär'sinō'mətoid/, resembling a carcinoma.

carcinomatosis. See **carcinosis.**

carcinomatous /-om'ətəs/, pertaining to carcinoma. Also **carcinous.**

carcinomatous pericarditis. See **neoplastic pericarditis.**

carcinoma tuberosum. See **tuberous carcinoma.**

carcinoma villosum. See **villous carcinoma.**

carcinophilia /kär'sinō'fil'yə/ [Gk, *karkinos + philein,* to love], the property in which there is an affinity for carcinomatous tissue. **—carcinophilic,** *adj.*

carcinosarcoma /kär'sinōsärkō'mə/, *pl.* **carcinosarcomas, carsinosarcomata** [Gk, *karkinos + sarx,* flesh, *oma,* tumor], a malignant neoplasm composed of carcinomatous and sarcomatous cells. Tumors of this type may occur in the esophagus, thyroid gland, and uterus.

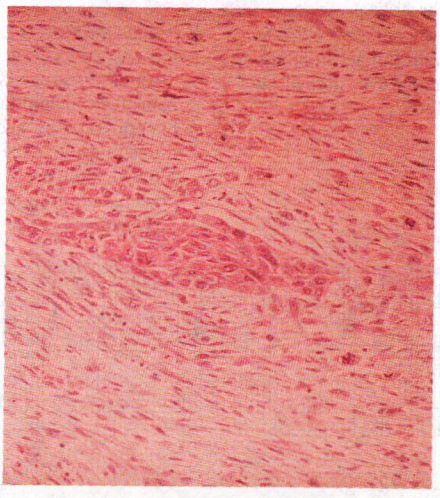

Carcinosarcoma *(Mitros, 1988/Courtesy FH Straus, MD)*

carcinosis /kär'sinō'sis/, *pl.* carcinoses, a condition characterized by the development of many carcinomas throughout the body. Kinds of carcinoses are **carcinosis pleurae, miliary carcinosis, pulmonary carcinosis.** Also called **carcinomatosis.**

carcinosis pleurae /plŏŏ'rē/, a secondary malignancy of the pleura in which nodules develop throughout the membranes.

carcinostatic /kär'sinōstat'ik/ [Gk, *karkinos* + *statikos,* causing to stand], of or pertaining to the tendency to slow or halt the growth of a carcinoma.

carcinous See **carcinomatous**

card-, cardio-, a combining form meaning 'heart': *cardioclasis, cardiography, cardiomegaly.*

cardia /kär'dē·ə/ [Gk, *kardia,* heart], **1.** the opening between the esophagus and the cardiac portion of the stomach. **2.** the portion of the stomach surrounding the esophagogastric connection, characterized by the absence of acid cells. **3.** an obsolete term formerly and vaguely used to describe the heart and the region around the heart. **–cardiac,** *adj.*

cardia-. See **cardio-.**

-cardia, a suffix meaning a 'type of heart action or location': *araiocardia, brachycardia, miocardia.*

cardiac [Gk *kardia* heart], **1.** of or pertaining to the heart. **2.** pertaining to a person with heart disease. **3.** of or pertaining to the proximal part of the stomach.

-cardiac, 1. a suffix meaning 'to characterize types and locations of heart ailments': *gravidocardiac, intracardiac, precardiac.* **2.** a suffix meaning 'to identify heart ailment patients': *diplocardiac, hemicardiac, phrenopericardiac.*

cardiac aneurysm. See **ventricular aneurysm.**

cardiac angiography [Gk, *kardia,* heart, *aggeion,* vessel, *graphein,* to record], the radiographic study of the heart and coronary vessels after injection with medium.

cardiac aneurysm. See **ventricular aneurysm.**

cardiac apnea [Gk, *kardia* + *a, pnein,* not to breathe], abnormal, temporary absence of ventilation, as in Cheyne-Stokes respiration.

cardiac arrest [Gk, *kardia* + L, *ad, restare,* to withstand], a sudden cessation of cardiac output and effective circulation, usually precipitated by ventricular fibrillation or ventricular asystole. When cardiac arrest occurs, delivery of oxygen and removal of carbon dioxide stop, tissue cell metabolism becomes anaerobic, and metabolic and repiratory acidosis ensue. Immediate initiation of cardiopulmonary resuscitation is required to prevent heart, lung, kidney, and brain damage. Also called **cardiopulmonary arrest.** See also **cardiac standstill, cardiopulmonary resuscitation.**

cardiac arrhythmia [Gk, *kardia* + *a, rhythmos,* not rhythm], an abnormal cardiac rate or rhythm. The condition may be caused by a defect in the node to maintain its pacemaker function, or by a failure of the electrical conduction system. Kinds of arrhythmia include **bradycardia, tachycardia, extrasystole, and heart block.**

cardiac asthma, an attack of asthma associated with heart disease, such as left ventricular failure, and characterized by predominant pulmonary congestion with some bronchoconstriction.

cardiac catheter, a long, fine catheter designed to be passed into the heart through a blood vessel. Used for diagnosis, it allows the determination of blood pressure and the rate of flow in the vessels and chambers of the heart and the identification of abnormal anatomy. Medication may be instilled directly into a coronary vessel, often with visualization by tomography.

cardiac catheterization, a diagnostic procedure in which a catheter is introduced into a large vein, usually of an arm or a leg, and threaded through the circulatory system to the heart.

■ METHOD: A sterile radiopaque catheter 100 to 125 cm in length is passed through an incision into the vein, through the vein to the superior vena cava, and into the right atrium (or through an artery leading to the left ventricle) and other structures to be studied. The course of the catheter is followed with fluoroscopy, and radiographs may be taken. An electrocardiogram is monitored on an oscilloscope. As the catheter tip passes through the chambers and vessels of the

Common basic cardiac arrhythmias

Rhythm characteristics	Etiology	Clinical significance	Management
Sinus tachycardia			
Regular rhythm, rate 100-180 beats/min (higher in infants), normal P-wave, normal QRS complex	Rate increase may be normal response to exercise, emotion, or stressors such as pain, fever, pump failure, hyperthyroidism, and certain drugs (e.g., caffeine, nitrates, atropine, epinephrine, isoproterenol, nicotine)	May have hemodynamic consequences in client with damaged heart that is unable to sustain increased workloads (increased myocardial oxygen consumption) brought on by persistent increases in heart rate	Correct underlying factors, remove offending drugs

Adapted from Canobbio MM: *Cardiovascular disorders,* St Louis, 1990, Mosby, pp. 64-67; from Potter P, Perry AG: *Fundamentals of nursing: concepts, process, & practice,* ed 3, St Louis, 1992, Mosby.

Common basic cardiac arrhythmias—cont'd

Rhythm characteristics	Etiology	Clinical significance	Management
Sinus bradycardia Regular rhythm, rate less than 60 beats/min, normal P-wave, normal PR interval, normal QRS complex	Rate decrease may be normal response to sleep or in well-conditioned athlete; abnormal drops in rate may be caused by diminished blood flow to SA node, vagal stimulation, hypothyroidism, increased intracranial pressure, or pharmacological agents (e.g., digoxin, propranolol, quinidine, procainamide)	No clinical significance unless associated with signs of impaired cardiac output and symptoms of dizziness, syncope, chest pain	Correct underlying causes, administer atropine 0.5-1.0 mg IV, implant transvenous pacemaker

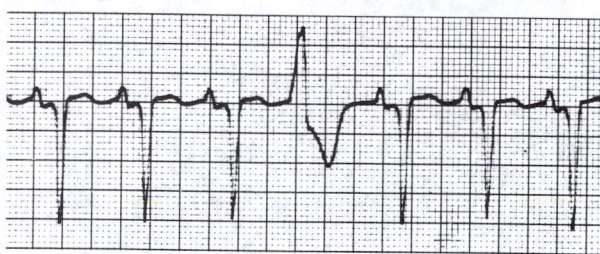

Sinus dysrhythmia Irregular rhythm; possibly phasic with respiration, slowing during inspiration and increasing with expiration; rate of 60-100 beats/min; normal P-wave; normal PR interval; normal QRS complex	Sinus rhythm with cyclic variation caused by vagal impulses that influence rhythm during respiration; occurs commonly in children, young adults, and older adults; usually disappears as heart rate increases	No clinical significance unless heart rate decreases and symptoms of dizziness with decreased rate	None indicated unless heart rate decreases and symptoms occur

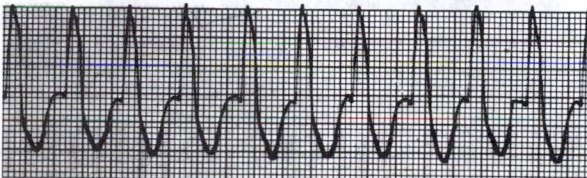

Supraventricular tachycardia (SVT) Sudden, rapid onset of tachycardia with stimulus originating above AV node; regular rhythm; rate 150-250 beats/min; P-wave uniform, possibly buried in preceding T-wave; PR interval variable, often difficult to measure; normal QRS complex	May begin and end spontaneously or be precipitated by excitement, fatigue, or caffeine, smoking, or alcohol use	Usually no significant impairment; client complains of palpitations and shortness of breath; if persistent or occurring in client with preexisting organic heart disease, may cause decrease in cardiac output and/or blood pressure resulting in pump failure or shock	Perform vagal stimulation with carotid sinus massage; decrease ventricular response with medication to block AV conduction: verapamil 5-10 mg IV push, propranolol slowly IV in 1 mg increments up to 4 mg [contraindicated in clients with heart failure], edrophonium, test dose 1 mg followed by 10 mg IV; perform cardioversion if resistant to preceding measures

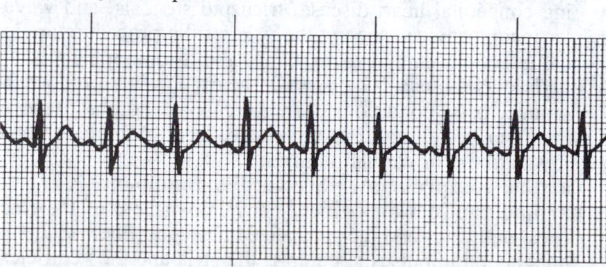

Continued.

Common basic cardiac arrhythmias—cont'd

Rhythm characteristics	Etiology	Clinical significance	Management
Premature ventricular contractions (PVCs) Irregular rhythm with ectopic beats followed by full compensatory pause; rate normal or increased depending on number of ectopic beats; P-wave absent in ectopic beat; PR interval absent; QRS complex widened and distorted; T-wave in opposition to R-wave	Caused by irritable focus within ventricle, commonly associated with myocardial infarction; other causes include hypoxia, hypocalcemia, acidosis	PVCs occurring frequently (more than 6/min) or in pairs indicating increased ventricular irritability	Try to suppress PVCs; if PVCs frequent, administer IV bolus of lidocaine (50-100 mg) followed by continuous IV infusion; administer additional antiarrhythmic agents as needed

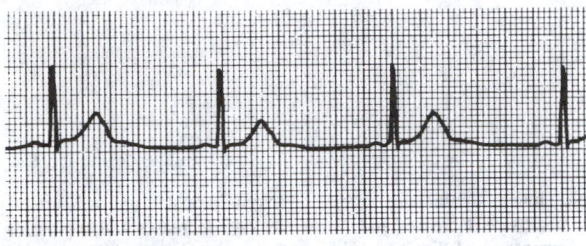

Ventricular tachycardia Rhythm slightly irregular, rate 100-200 beats/min, P-wave absent, PR interval absent, QRS complex wide and bizarre, >0.12 second	Caused by irritable ventricular foci firing repetitively, commonly caused by myocardial infarction	Often a forerunner of ventricular fibrillation; if condition persistent and rapid, causes decreased cardiac output because of decreased ventricular filling time	Most episodes terminate abruptly without treatment; administer lidocaine bolus 75-100 mg IV followed by continuous intravenous drip; perform defibrillation

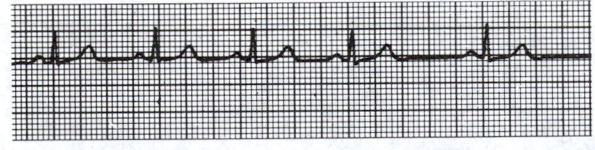

Adapted from Canobbio MM: *Cardiovascular disorders,* St Louis, 1990, Mosby, pp. 64-67; from Potter P, Perry AG: *Fundamentals of nursing: concepts, process, & practice,* ed 3, St Louis, 1992, Mosby.

heart, the pressure of the flow of blood is monitored, and samples of the blood are taken to study the oxygen content. ■ NURSING INTERVENTION: Cardiac catheterization takes from 1 to 3 hours, and the patient has to lie still during the entire procedure. It is not painful, but, because it is anxiety producing, the patient needs explanation and emotional support. A young child may need a sedative in order to lie still. An antibiotic is often given the day before. The pulse on the operative side and the blood pressure on the other side of the body are monitored every 15 minutes for 1 hour and every half hour thereafter. In left heart catheterization, peripheral pulses are also monitored. The temperature may be elevated for several hours, and there may be pain at the site of the incision. The nurse observes the site for bleeding and for signs of infection, thrombophlebitis, and cardiac arrhythmia. Cardiac catheterization is often performed by a special team in a special laboratory. By offering information and counseling, a member of the team may be of great help to the patient and the nursing staff before and after the procedure. ■ OUTCOME CRITERIA: Many conditions may be accurately identified and assessed using cardiac catheterization, including congenital heart disease, tricuspid stenosis, and valvular incompetence. Among the risks of the procedure are local infection, cardiac arrhythmia, and thrombophlebitis.

cardiac cirrhosis [Gk, *kardia,* heart, *kirrhos,* yellowish-orange, *osis,* condition], an increase of fibrous tissue in the liver resulting from congestive heart failure, chronic myocarditis, or cardiac fibrosis.

cardiac compression. See **cardiac tamponade.**

cardiac conduction defect, any impairment of the electrical pathways and the specialized muscular fibers that conduct action impulses to contract the atria and the ventricles. Conduction defects may develop in the sinus node, the atrioventricular node, the bundle of His, the left or the right fiber bundle branches. Defective transmission of cardiac impulses

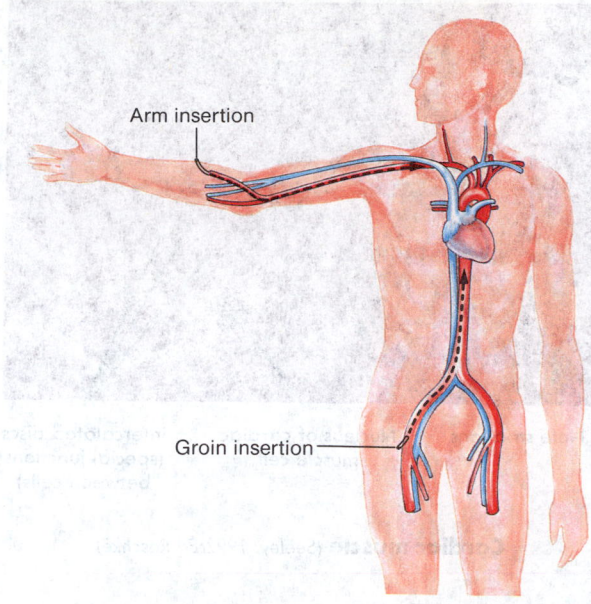

Insertion sites for cardiac catheterization
(Canobbio, 1990)

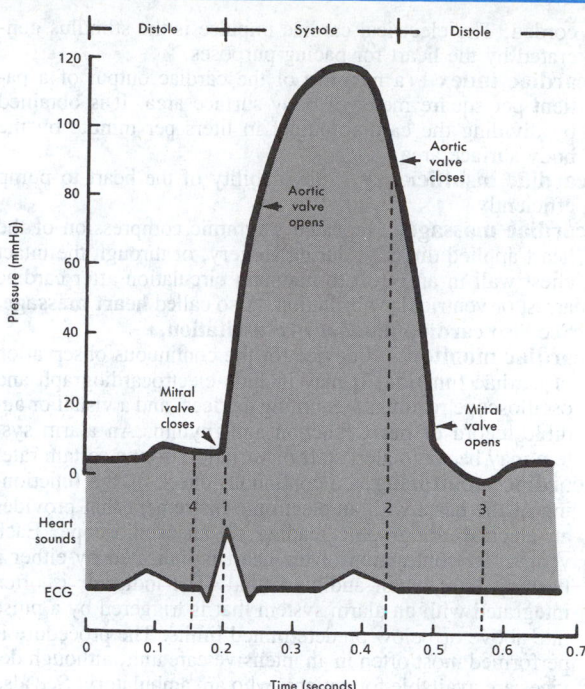

Cardiac cycle *(Thompson, 1993)*

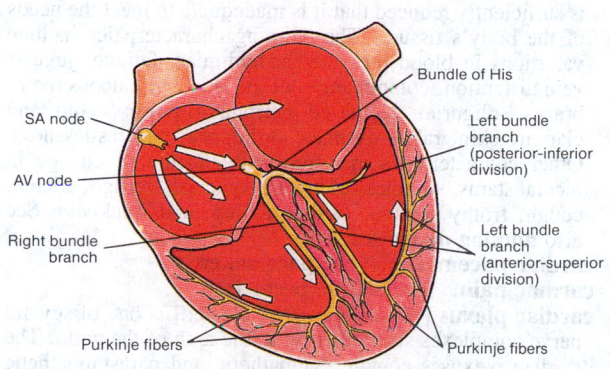

Cardiac conduction *(Canobbio, 1990)*

along the conduction routes may be caused by ischemia, necrosis, drug effects, electrolyte disturbances, or trauma. See also **heart block.**

cardiac cycle [Gk, *kardia* + *kyklos*, circle], the cycle of events during which an electrical impulse is conducted through special fibers over the myocardium, from the sinoatrial (SA) node to the atrioventricular (AV) node, to the bundle of His and the bundle branches, and to the Purkinje fibers, causing contraction of the atria followed by contraction of the ventricles. Contraction occurs following depolarization of the muscle fibers. Deoxygenated blood enters the right atrium of the heart from the inferior and superior venae cavae and is pumped through the tricuspid valve into the right ventricle. From the right ventricle, blood is pumped through the pulmonary valve into the pulmonary artery and the lungs for oxygenation. Oxygen-rich blood is returned to the heart through the branches of the pulmonary veins to the left atrium and pumped through the mitral valve

into the left ventricle. The blood is pumped through the aortic valve into the aorta for peripheral circulation. The contractions of the left and the right atria are nearly simultaneous; they precede the nearly simultaneous contractions of the ventricles. Structural, chemical, or electric abnormalities may cause a large variety of anomalies in electric conduction, muscular contraction, and blood flow in the heart.

cardiac decompensation, a condition of heart failure in which the heart is unable to fulfill its normal function of ensuring adequate cellular perfusion to all parts of the body without assistance. Causes may include myocardial infarction, increased work load, infection, toxins, or defective heart valves.

cardiac depressant [L, *deprimere*, to press down], an agent that decreases the heart rate and contractility. See also **antiadrenergic, calcium channel blocker.**

cardiac dyspnea [Gk, *dys*, difficult, *pnoia*, breath], breathing distress that is caused by heart disease, most commonly the result of pulmonary venous congestion.

cardiac edema [Gk, *oidema*, swelling], an accumulation of serum fluid from blood plasma in the interstitial tissues as a result of congestive heart failure. In severe cases, the fluid may also accumulate in serous cavities.

cardiac electric axis, the angle the mean cardiac vector in the frontal plane makes with a horizontal plane drawn through the center of Einthoven's triangle and left hip.

cardiac failure. See **heart failure.**

cardiac hypertrophy, an abnormal enlargement of the heart muscle.

cardiac impulse [Gk, *kardia* + L, *impellere*, to set in motion], the mechanical movement of the thorax, caused by the beating of the heart. It is readily palpable and easily recorded. The electrical cardiac impulse is the stimulus generated by the heart for pacing purposes.

cardiac index, a measure of the cardiac output of a patient per square meter of body surface area. It is obtained by dividing the cardiac output in liters per minute by the body surface area.

cardiac insufficiency, the inability of the heart to pump efficiently.

cardiac massage, repeated, rhythmic compression of the heart applied directly, during surgery, or through the intact chest wall in an effort to maintain circulation after cardiac arrest or ventricular fibrillation. Also called **heart massage.** See also **cardiopulmonary resuscitation.**

cardiac monitor, a device for the continuous observation of cardiac function. It may include electrocardiograph and oscilloscope readings, recording devices, and a visual or audible record of heart function and rhythm. An alarm system may be set to alert staff of variation from a certain rate.

cardiac monitoring, a continuous check on the functioning of the heart with an electronic instrument that provides an electrocardiographic reading on an oscilloscope. Each ventricular contraction of the heart is indicated by either a flashing light or an audible sound. The indicator is often integrated with an alarm system that is triggered by a pulse rate above or below predetermined limits. The procedure is performed most often in an intensive care unit, although devices are available for patients who are ambulatory. See also **electrocardiograph.**

cardiac murmur, an abnormal sound heard during auscultatory examination of the heart, caused by altered blood flow into a chamber or through a valve. A murmur is classified by the time of its occurrence during the cardiac cycle, the duration, and the intensity of the sound on a scale of I to V. Also noted is the part of the heart over which the murmur is heard and any parts to which it radiates. In general, many systolic murmurs are benign and of no significance, but some signal cardiac pathophysiology. Most diastolic murmurs are pathologic. Also called **heart murmur.**

cardiac muscle, a special striated muscle of the myocardium, containing dark intercalated disks at the junctions of abutting fibers. Cardiac muscle is an exception among involuntary muscles, which are characteristically smooth. Its contractile fibers resemble those of skeletal muscle but are only one third as large in diameter, are richer in sarcoplasm, and contain centrally located instead of peripheral nuclei. Studies with the electron microscope indicate that the intercalated disks in cardiac muscle represent cell boundaries. The connective tissue of cardiac muscle is sparser than that of skeletal muscle.

cardiac output, the volume of blood expelled by the ventricles of the heart, equal to the amount of blood ejected at each beat (the stroke output) multiplied by the heart rate per minute · number of beats in the period of time used in the computation. Cardiac output is commonly measured by the thermodilution technique in which a catheter with a thermistor at the tip is inserted in the pulmonary artery, and a solution is injected through the lumen of the catheter into the right atrium. The thermistor measures the temperature of the solution when it flows past the thermistorreaches the pulmonary artery, and the output is calculated on the basis of the temperature change; the increase in the temperature of the solution is inversely related to the functioning of the heart. A normal heart in a resting adult ejects from 4 to 8 L of blood per minute.

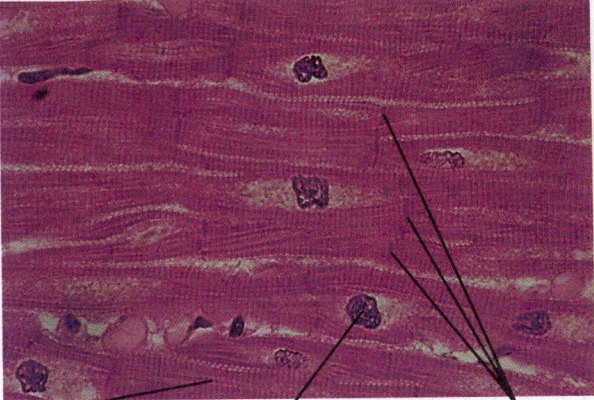

Note striations   Nucleus of cardiac   Intercalated discs
                 muscle cell   (special junctions
                                    between cells)

Cardiac muscle *(Seeley, 1992/Ed Reschke)*

cardiac output, decreased, a nursing diagnosis accepted by the Fourth National Conference on the Classification of Nursing Diagnoses. Decreased cardiac output is a state in which the amount of blood pumped by an individual's heart is sufficiently reduced that it is inadequate to meet the needs of the body's tissues. The defining characteristics include variations in blood pressure, arrhythmias, fatigue, jugular vein distention, color changes of the skin and mucous membranes, oliguria, decreased peripheral pulses, cold and clammy skin, rales, dyspnea, orthopnea, and restlessness. Other characteristics that frequently occur are change in mental status, shortness of breath, syncope, vertigo, edema, cough, frothy sputum, cardiac gallop, and weakness. See also **nursing diagnosis.**

cardiac pacemaker. See **pacemaker.**

cardiac pain. See **angina pectoris**.

cardiac plexus [Gk, *kardia* + L, pleated], one of several nerve complexes situated close to the arch of the aorta. The cardiac plexuses contain sympathetic and parasympathetic nerve fibers that leave the plexuses, accompany the right and the left coronary arteries, and enter the heart. Some of the fibers from the plexuses terminate in the sinoatrial node; others terminate in the atrioventricular node and in the atrial myocardium.

cardiac radionuclide imaging [Gk, *kardi* + L, *radiare*, to shine, *nucleus* kernel; *imago* image], the noninvasive examination of the heart, using a radiopharmaceutical, such as thallium 201, and a detection device, such as a gamma camera, positron camera, or rectilinear scanner. The main clinical applications of cardiac radionuclide imaging are the gated cardiac blood pool scan, myocardial imaging, and the detection of myocardial necrosis.

cardiac reflex [L, *reflectere*, to bend back], reaction to a pair of stimuli that automatically increases or reduces the heart rate. Stimulation of vagus fibers in the right side of the heart by increased venous return accelerates the heart rate, whereas increased arterial blood pressure stimulates nerve endings in the carotid sinus to slow the heart rate.

cardiac regurgitation [Gk, *kardia*, heart; L, *re*, *gurgitare*, to flow], a backward flow of blood through one or more defective heart valves.

cardiac rehabilitation [Gk, *kardia*, heart; L, *re*, *habilitas*, ability], a supervised program of progressive exercise, psychologic support, and education or training to enable a myocardial infarction patient to resume the activities of daily living on an independent basis. Special training may be needed to adapt the patient to a new occupation and lifestyle.

cardiac reserve, the potential capacity of the heart to function well beyond its basal level, responding to alterations in physiologic demands.

cardiac rhythm [Gk, *kardia*, heart + *rhythmos*], the recurring beat of the heart.

cardiac souffle [Gk, *kardia*, heart; Fr, puff], a heart murmur.

cardiac sphincter [Gk, *kardia* + *sphigkter*, binder], a ring of muscle fibers at the juncture of the esophagus and stomach.

cardiac standstill, the complete cessation of ventricular contractions and ejection of blood by the heart. Cardiac standstill requires immediate cardiopulmonary resuscitation. See also **cardiac arrest.**

cardiac stenosis [Gk, *kardia*, heart; Gk, *stenos*, narrow + *osis*, condition], an obstruction of blood flow through any of the chambers of the heart that is not valvular in origin. The cause may be a thrombosis or tumor.

cardiac stimulant, a pharmacologic agent that increases the action of the heart. Cardiac glycosides, such as digitalis, digitoxin, digoxin, deslanoside, lanatoside, acetyldigitoxin, and ouabain, increase the force of myocardial contractions and decrease the heart rate and conduction velocity, allowing more time for the ventricles to relax and become filled with blood. These glycosides, which are composed of a steroid nucleus, a lactone ring, and a sugar, are used in the treatment of congestive heart failure, atrial flutter and fibrillation, paroxysmal atrial tachycardia, and cardiogenic shock. Toxic signs and symptoms, resulting from an overdose or the cumulative effect of slowly eliminated digitalis preparations, include anorexia, nausea, vomiting, diarrhea, abdominal pain, headache, muscle weakness, confusion, drowsiness, irritability, visual disturbances, bradycardia or tachycardia, ectopic heart beats, bigeminy, and a pulse deficit. Epinephrine, a potent vasopressor and cardiac stimulant, is sometimes used to restore heart rhythm in cardiac arrest but is not employed in treating heart failure or cardiogenic shock. Isoproterenol hydrochloride, which is related to epinephrine, may be used in treating heart block. Amrinone, dobutamine hydrochloride, and dopamine are employed in the short-term treatment of cardiac decompensation resulting from depressed contractility.

cardiac syncope [Gk, *kardia*, heart + *syncope*, fainting], a temporary loss of consciousness caused by inadequate cerebral blood flow resulting, in turn, from a sudden failure in cardiac output for any reason.

cardiac tamponade, compression of the heart produced by the accumulation of blood in the pericardial sac resulting from the rupture of the wall of the heart, as by a penetrating wound. Also called **cardiac compression.**

■ OBSERVATIONS: Signs of cardiac tamponade may include distended neck veins, hypotension, decreased heart sounds, tachypnea, peripheral pulses that are weak or absent or that fall sharply during inspiration (pulsus paradoxus), reduced left atrial pressure, and a pericardial friction rub. The patient, who is usually anxious and restless, may sit upright or lean forward, and the skin may be pale, dusky, or cya-

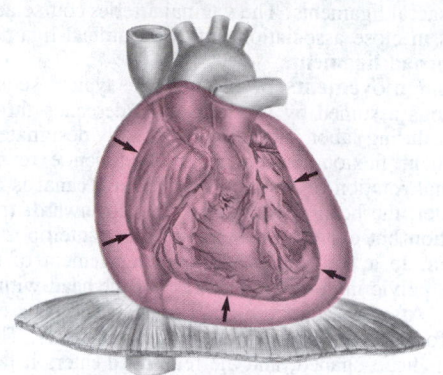

Hemopericardium and tamponade
Cardiac tamponade (Canobbio, 1990)

notic. The electrocardiogram generally shows decreased cardiac voltage, and the chest x-ray film may reveal an enlarged heart shadow ('water bottle' heart).

■ INTERVENTIONS: The patient is maintained on bed rest; the head of the bed is elevated 45 degrees, and a defibrillator and emergency drugs are kept at the bedside. Blood pressure, respiration, apical pulse, and atrial and pulmonary wedge pressures are checked every 15 to 30 minutes. Auscultation for pulsus paradoxus is performed, and peripheral pulses are checked every 30 minutes. A 12-lead electrocardiogram is usually ordered, and, when possible, the patient is placed on a cardiac monitor and the rhythm strip is checked every hour. Cardiotonic and antiarrhythmic drugs and measures for controlling pain are administered as ordered. Aspiration of the fluid or blood in the pericardial sac (pericardiocentesis) is performed for diagnosis and for therapy. If surgery is indicated, the patient is prepared for the procedure, and the bleeding vessel or vessels are ligated.

cardiac thrombosis [Gk, *kardia*, heart + *thrombos*, lump + *osis*, condition], a blood clot located at a heart valve or in one of the heart chambers. A left ventricular thrombosis may follow a large infarct.

cardiac valve. See **heart valve.**

cardiasthenia [Gk, *kardia*, heart, *a*, without, *sthenos*, strength], a form of neurasthenia in which cardiovascular symptoms are prominent.

Cardilate, a trademark for an antianginal (erythrityl tetranitrate).

cardinal /kär′dənal/ [L, *cardo*, hinge], so fundamental that other things hinge on it, such as a cardinal trait that influences one's total behavior.

cardinal frontal plane [L, *cardo*, hinge; *frons*, forehead; *planum*, level ground], the plane that divides the body into front and back portions. Also called **vertical plane.**

cardinal horizontal plane. See **transverse plane.**

cardinal ligament [L, *cardo*, hinge; *ligare*, to bind], a sheet of subserous fascia extending across the female pelvic floor as a continuation of the broad ligament. It is embedded in the adipose tissue on each side of the vagina and is formed by the fasciae of the vagina and the cervix converging at the lateral borders of these organs. The ligament forms ventral and dorsal extensions at the lateral portion of the pelvic diaphragm. The ventral extension joins the tissue supporting the bladder. The dorsal extension blends with the uterosacral ligaments. The vaginal arteries course across the pelvis in close association with the cardinal ligament. See also **broad ligament.**

cardinal movements of labor, the typical sequence of positions assumed by the fetus as it descends through the pelvis during labor and delivery, usually designated as engagement, flexion, descent, internal rotation, extension, and external rotation or restitution. The birth canal is a curved cylinder; the head must enter it in a downward, transverse direction but exit it in a more forward, anteroposterior direction. In a vertex presentation, engagement of the head in the pelvic inlet requires flexion of the head with chin on chest. After descent, the head must undergo extension to turn forward and be born under the symphysis. The pelvic inlet is heart-shaped, and the fetal head enters it facing obliquely; however, the pelvic outlet is diamond-shaped, and the head usually exits it facing posteriorly and must undergo internal rotation to do so. After delivery of the head, the shoulders remain for a time in the oblique plane and the head undergoes external rotation or restitution to allow the widest diameter of the shoulders to be delivered from the longer anteroposterior diameter of the pelvic outlet. See illustration at **labor.**

cardinal position of gaze, (in ophthalmology) one of six positions to which the normal eye may be turned. Each position requires the function of a specific ocular muscle and a cranial nerve. The positions and the corresponding muscles and nerves are as follows:
1. Straight nasal: medial rectus and the third cranial nerve
2. Up nasal: inferior oblique and the third cranial nerve
3. Down nasal: superior oblique and the fourth cranial nerve
4. Straight temporal: lateral rectus and the sixth cranial nerve
5. Up temporal: superior rectus and the third cranial nerve
6. Down temporal: inferior rectus and the third cranial nerve

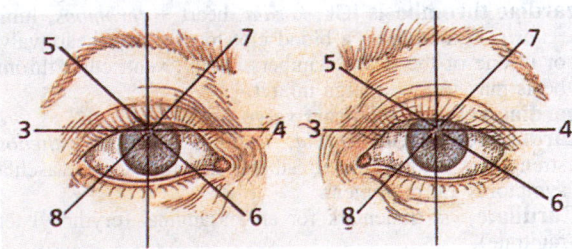

Cardinal positions of gaze (Potter, 1993)

cardinal sagittal plane. See **median plane.**
cardinal symptom. See **symptom.**
cardio-, cardia-, a combining form meaning 'pertaining to the heart': *cardiocele, cardiocirrhosis, cardiodynia.*
cardioangiography, See **cardiac angiography.**
cardiocatheterization /kär′dē·ō·kath′ərīzā′shən/ [Gk, *kardia,* heart, *katheter,* a thing lowered into], the introduction of a flexible radio-opaque catheter through a saphenous or median basilic vein and the superior vena cava to the heart chambers. It may be used to collect samples of blood in the heart and to measure blood pressure in various heart chambers, as well as to illuminate the coronary arteries.

cardiocirculatory /kär′dē·ō·sur′kyŏŏlətôr′ē/ [Gk, *kardia* heart; L, *circulare,* to go around], of or pertaining to the heart and the circulation.
cardioesophageal reflux /-əsof′əjē′əl/ [Gk, *kardia,* heart, *oisophagos,* gullet; L, *refluere,* to flow back], a backward flow or regurgitation of stomach contents into the esophagus. Repeated episodes of reflux can lead to esophagitis. Among factors contributing to the condition are stomach pressure greater than pressure in the esophagus, hiatus hernia, and incompetence of the lower esophageal sphincter.
cardiogenic shock /kär′dē·ō·jen′ik/ [Gk, *kardia* + *genein,* to produce; Fr, *choc*], an abnormal condition characterized by critically low cardiac output in association with acute myocardial infarction and congestive heart failure. Although low cardiac output is a common sign of this disorder, cardiogenic shock may also occur in association with normal output. Cardiogenic shock is fatal in about 80% of cases, and immediate therapy is necessary. Depending on the signs, therapy may include diuretics, vasoactive drugs, and the application of various devices. Compare **hypovolemic shock.** See also **electric shock, shock.**
cardiogram /kär′dē·əgram′/, an electronically recorded tracing of cardiac activity.
cardiograph. See **electrocardiogram, electrocardiograph.**
cardiography /kär′dē·og′rəfē/, the technique of graphically recording the movements of the heart by means of a cardiograph.
cardiologist /-ol′əjist/, a physician specializing in the diagnosis and treatment of disorders of the heart.
cardiology /-ol′əjē/ [Gk, *kardia* + *logos,* science], the study of the anatomy, normal functions, and disorders of the heart.
cardiolysis /kär′dē·ol′isis/ [Gk, *kardia* + *lysein,* to loosen], an operation that separates the heart and the pericardium from the sternal periosteum in a procedure to correct adhesive mediastinopericarditis. The operation resects the ribs and the sternum over the pericardium.
cardiomegaly /kär′dē·ō·meg′əlē/ [Gk, *kardia* + *megas,* large], enlargement of the heart caused hypertrophy (thickening) of the walls of the heart. In athletes an enlarged, well-functioning heart is a normal finding. See also **athlete's heart.**
cardiomyopathy /kär′dē·ō·mī·op′əthē/ [Gk, *kardia* + *mys,* muscle, *pathos,* disease], any disease that affects the structure and function of the heart.
cardiomyopexy /kär′dē·omī′əpek′sē/ [Gk, *kardia* + *mys,* muscle, *pexis,* fixation], a surgical procedure in which the blood supply from the nearby pectoral muscles of the chest is diverted directly to the coronary arteries of the heart.
cardiopathy /kär′dē·op′əthē/ [Gk, *kardia,* heart, *pathos,* disease], a disease of the heart.
cardioplasty /kär′dē·ōplas′tē/, a surgical procedure to correct a defect in the cardiac sphincter of the esophagus that frequently leads to cardiospasm. Cardiospasm is caused by failure of the sphincter to relax so that food can enter the stomach.
cardioplegia /kär′dē·ōplē′jə/ [Gk, *kardia* + *plege,* stroke], 1. paralysis of the heart. 2. the arrest of myocardial contractions by injection of chemicals, hypothermia, or electrical stimuli for the purpose of performing surgery on the heart. See also **cardiac standstill.**
cardiopulmonary /-pul′məner′ē/ [Gk, *kardia* + L, *pulmoneus* lungs], of or pertaining to the heart and the lungs.

cardiopulmonary arrest. See **cardiac arrest.**

cardiopulmonary bypass, a procedure used in heart surgery in which the blood is diverted from the heart and lungs by means of a pump oxygenator and returned directly to the aorta.

cardiopulmonary murmur [Gk, *kardia*, heart; L, *pulmo*, lung, *murmur*, humming], a sound heard over the heart during breathing and during the heart beat. It is caused by vibrations resulting from the heart striking the lung tissue with every beat. Also called **cardiorespiratory murmur.**

cardiopulmonary resuscitation (CPR), a basic emergency procedure for life support, consisting of artificial respiration and manual external cardiac massage. It is used in cases of cardiac arrest to establish effective circulation and ventilation in order to prevent irreversible cerebral damage resulting from anoxia. External cardiac massage compresses the heart between the lower sternum and the thoracic vertebral column. During compressions, blood is forced into systemic and pulmonary circulation, and venous blood refills the heart when the compression is released. Mouth-to-mouth breathing or a mechanical form of ventilation is used concomitantly with CPR to oxygenate the blood being pumped through the circulatory system. (Table, pages 268-269)

■ METHOD: Basic cardiopulmonary resuscitation requires no adjunctive equipment, although mechanical devices can be used. It can be done by one or two rescuers and involves three interrelated actions: opening the airway, restoring breathing, and restoring circulation. For an adult, the procedure is performed in the following manner:

1. The victim is placed on a hard flat surface, such as a CPR board, a backboard, or, if necessary, the floor. Resuscitation efforts are not delayed while the rescuer is waiting for such a support.

2. The victim is examined closely. If unresponsive, the victim is tapped on the shoulder, or the ear is pinched. The rescuer asks loudly, "Can you hear me? Are you all right?" If there is no response, it is assumed the victim is unconscious.

3. The rescuer establishes and maintains an open airway. In the supine position, relaxed muscles allow the tongue to drop back in the throat, blocking the airway. This can be easily relieved by tilting the head. One hand is placed on the forehead of the victim and the other is used to lift the lower jaw or chin, placing the fingers and thumb on top of the jaw. The head is held in this position. This extends the neck and lifts the tongue from the back of the throat. In a case of suspected cervical spine injury, the neck is not hyperextended. Instead, the lower jaw is lifted by placing the fingers behind the angles of the victim's jaw in front of the earlobes and displacing it upward. If available, an oropharyngeal airway is inserted; if not, the head is held in position, either tilted back or with jaw lifted, throughout the resuscitation procedure.

4. The rescuer evaluates the need for artificial respiration by looking, listening, and feeling for signs of air exchange or respiratory effort. If there is no spontaneous exchange and if there is no stoma (artificial airway device) over the larynx, regular artificial respiration is begun immediately. If there is a stoma, mouth-to-stoma respiration is initiated.

5. To begin artificial respiration, the rescuer rotates the hand that has been placed on the victim's forehead and, using the thumb and index finger of this hand, pinches the nostrils closed. A tight seal is made with the rescuer's mouth around the mouth of the victim, and four breaths, each

of increasing strength and volume, are given. The rescuer's mouth is removed, and the victim is allowed to exhale passively. The rescuer watches the chest fall and then breathes in another series of breaths. The cycle is repeated every 5 seconds as long as respiratory deficiency exists. If indicated, mouth-to-nose respiration may be used. If the chest does not expand, the head is repositioned and ventilation is again attempted. A second unsuccessful attempt indicates an obstructed airway. See also **Heimlich maneuver.**

6. The rescuer takes the carotid pulse and checks for cardiac arrest. If the pulse is absent or inadequate, the carotid artery is palpated for 5 seconds immediately after the two initial breaths are given. Absence or questionable pressure of the pulse at that time indicates the need to begin external cardiac compression.

7. To start external massage, the rescuer takes a position facing the side of the victim. To find the correct location for the hands (the landmark position), the chest is uncovered and the xiphoid process is identified. With the middle finger on the notch and the index finger next to it, the heel of the other hand is placed on the sternum, directly adjacent to the fingers marking the xiphoid. With the fingers extended upward and away from the ribs, the first hand is placed on top of the second and the fingers are interlocked. With arms straight, the rescuer rocks back and forth from the hip joints, exerting sufficient downward pressure with the forward swing of the body to depress the victim's sternum from 1.5 to 2 inches. It is extremely important to be positioned properly to avoid depressing the xiphoid process and the possibility of causing severe internal injury. After each compression, a rest is allowed for a time equal to the time of compression, but the hands are not moved from their position on the chest. The cycle is repeated using a ratio of 15 compressions to two breaths at the rate of 80 compressions a minute. The proper rhythm may be achieved by counting 'one and two and three,' up to 15. If two rescuers are available, CPR is performed with one rescuer giving compressions and the other giving breaths, at a 5:1 ratio at a rate of 60 compressions a minute. The proper rhythm can be determined by counting 'one-one thousand, two-one thousand,' up to 'five-one thousand.' Effectiveness of CPR is checked frequently by palpating the carotid artery for the return of a spontaneous heartbeat and by watching for 'pinking' of the skin, con striction of the pupils, and a return of respiration. If the rescuer doing compressions becomes tired, a switch may be made by changing the counting rhythm to 'switch-one thousand, two-one thousand,' up to 'five-one thousand.' At the end of that cycle, the rescuer giving compressions moves to the victim's head and checks the pulse. The rescuer who has been at the head, after giving a breath, moves to the victim's side, and checks the pulse for 5 seconds. If the pulse is absent or its pressure is inadequate, the rescuer at the head says, 'No pulse. Continue CPR.'

The technique for infants up to 1 year of age and for children up to 8 years of age is like that for adults, with the following exceptions. In infants, the neck is not hyperextended because soft cartilage and neck tissues may occlude the airway if the head is tilted too far; placing a hand beneath the shoulders of an infant provides adequate tilt. The rescuer's mouth covers the infant's mouth and nose, and the infant's pulse is checked on the brachial artery. For a small infant, both thumbs are placed on the midsternum while joining the fingers behind the infant's back. It is best ap-

Emergency cardiopulmonary resuscitation (CPR)

Findings	CPR basic sequence	ABCD's of action	
1. No response	1. Call for help Stimulate or arouse		
2. Abscence of respirations Cyanosis Dilated pupils Limp extremities	2. Open airway using head tilt–chin lift maneuver	A - Open airway	
3. Respirations still absent	3. Initiate artificial respiration a. Pinch nostrils and make a seal with rescuer's mouth; two quick breaths ($\frac{1}{2}$ sec per breath)	B - Restore breathing	
4. Pulse—not palpable	4. a. Palpate brachial artery in infants, carotid artery in children and adults b. Initiate external cardiac compressions and continue rescue breathing	C - Restore circulation	

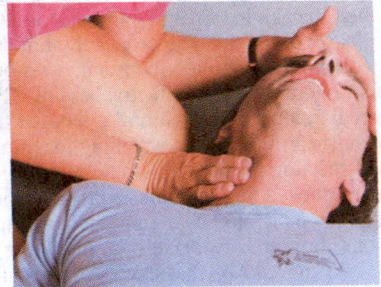
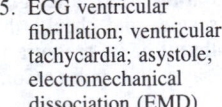
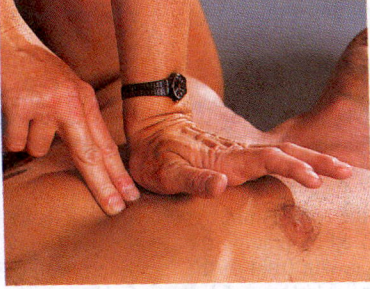
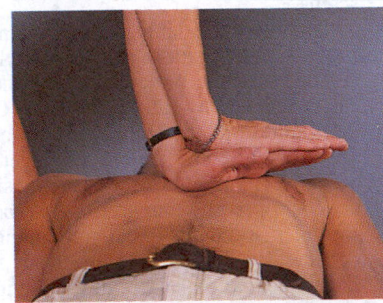

5. ECG ventricular fibrillation; ventricular tachycardia; asystole; electromechanical dissociation (EMD)	5. Drug therapy; defibrillation	D - Provide definitive treatment	

Victim *must* be supported on hard surface; gastric emptying (decompression) is recommended only if the abdomen is so tense that ventilation is ineffective; effective CPR is accompanied by improvement in skin color, pupillary constriction, spontaneous movement, and some grasping respirations; effectiveness should be evaluated after 1 minute, and periodically thereafter (every 1 to 3 minutes)

Adapted from Emergency Cardiac Care Committee and Subcommittees, American Heart Association. Guidelines for cardiopulmonary resuscitation and emergency cardiac care. Parts I and II, *JAMA* 268:2172-2198, 1992.
Illustrations from Judd, RL and Ponsell, DD *Mosby's First Responder,* ed. 2. St. Louis, 1988, The CV Mosby Company.

Age	Consideration	Procedures	
Infants (less than 1 year)	Breathing point	Mouth *and* nose	
	Pressure point	Midsternum—on line with nipples	
	Hands	Tips of 2 or 3 fingers	
	Compression distance	½ to 1 inch (1.3 to 2.5 cm)	
	Compression/ventilation C/V ratio	5/1 100C/20V/minute; use only slight hyperextension of neck; mouth or mask covers nose and mouth; use only small breaths from cheeks	
Children (1 through 8 years)	Breathing point	Mouth	
	Pressure point	Slightly below midsternum	
	Hands	Heel of one hand	
	Compression distance	1 to 1½ inches (2.5 to 3.8 cm)	
	Compression/ventilation C/V ratio	5/1 80-100C/15-20V/minute	
Older children and adults	Breathing point	Mouth	
	Pressure point	Lower half of sternum	
	Hands	Both	
	Compression distance	1½ to 2 inches (4 to 5 cm)	
	Compression/ventilation	Alone—15/2 2 Rescuers—5/1 80-100 C/150-20V/ minute	

plied from the superior direction with the operator at the infant's head. For an older infant, pressure is applied with two fingers on the midsternum, exerting a sharp downward thrust. For children older than 5 years, the heel of one hand is used. Because the ventricles of the heart in infants and small children lie higher in the chest cavity than they do in adults, external pressure is applied midsternum and only to a depth of 0.5 to 0.75 inches for infants, 0.75 to 1 inch for young children, and 1.5 to 2 inches for older children. The rate of cardiac compression for infants is 100 a minute, with breaths interposed as quickly as possible after each five compressions—approximately one every 3 seconds. The rate of compression for children is 80 a minute, with ventilations delivered once every 4 seconds. Less air is necessary for a child than for an adult. For an infant, only the air held in the cheeks is puffed in.

■ OUTCOME CRITERIA: To provide adequate basic life support, these rules for correct performance should be followed:

1. CPR should not be interrupted for more than 5 seconds, except for endotracheal intubation or for moving a victim. In these cases, the interruption should not exceed 15 seconds.

2. Compressions should be smooth, regular, and uninterrupted.

3. The victim should be stabilized before transportation to a more convenient site.

4. The pressure on the chest should be completely released after each compression, although the palm of the hand remains in contact with the chest wall.

5. The shoulders of the rescuer should be placed directly above the victim's sternum to provide the most effective thrusts.

6. The sternum should be depressed to the correct degree according to the size and age of the victim.

7. The xiphoid process should not be compressed because of the danger of lacerating the liver.

8. Gastric distension should not be relieved unless it becomes so severe that it interferes with ventilation.

CPR is used only in cases of sudden cardiac arrest. Even if CPR is initiated as soon as possible and all steps are performed correctly, there are some cases, such as with severe emphysema or crushing chest injuries, in which it is not successful. Even properly performed, CPR may cause rib fractures in some victims. Other complications include fracture of the sternum, separation of costochondral cartilage, hepatic hematoma, lung contusions, and fat embolism. The danger of complications is minimized by correct performance. Properly performed, external cardiac massage can produce a systolic blood pressure peaking at more than 100 mm Hg in the carotid arteries. With no heartbeat the diastolic pressure is 0; thus the mean pressure with CPR is usually about 40 mm Hg, and the flow of arterial blood is approximately 25% to 35% of the normal flow. These figures point out the need for immediate action and for continuous effort to effect a rescue; they also indicate that CPR can be effective and can save lives if properly given in a carefully monitored fashion. CPR is an interim measure used until advanced life support action and definitive measures can be taken. Once initiated, it is continued until one of the following occurs: Spontaneous circulation and respiration are restored; resuscitation efforts are transferred to someone who can continue life-support procedures, either basic or advanced; a physician assumes responsibility for the victim; the victim is handed over to the care of a medical facility; or the rescuer is physically unable to continue.

■ INTERVENTIONS: Cardiopulmonary resuscitation is considered an emergency procedure, and knowledge of the principles, procedures, requirements, and complications of this maneuver is essential. In the hospital, there are additional tasks to perform to implement CPR. Primarily, the nurse evaluates the extent of the emergency and the indications for initiating lifesaving measures. The nurse is also prepared to undertake immediate action should it be necessary to do so before the medical team arrives. If not immediately involved in performing CPR, the nurse prepares for the initiation of definitive therapy by readying equipment, including an electrocardiograph, a defibrillator, a tracheostomy set, oxygen, and a suction machine. Epinephrine for direct injection into the heart, sodium bicarbonate to combat acidosis, and calcium chloride to stimulate cardiac contraction are also prepared for injection and properly labeled. While resuscitation proceeds, efforts are made to start an intravenous infusion, and ECG electrodes are applied to the patient. In the hospital, mouth-to-mask ventilation is recommended to protect health-care workers from making direct contact with oral secretions of the patient. The decision to terminate resuscitation efforts is made by a physician.

cardiorespiratory murmur. See **cardiopulmonary murmur.**

cardiorrhaphy /kär′dē·ôr′əfē/ [Gk, *kardia + rhaphe*, suture], an operation in which the heart muscle is sutured.

cardioscope /kär′dē·əskōp′/, an obsolete device for inspecting and manipulating the internal structures of the heart.

cardiospasm /kär′dē·əspaz′əm/ [Gk, *kardia + spasmos*, pull], a form of achalasia characterized by a failure of the cardia at the distal end of the esophagus to relax, causing dysphagia and regurgitation, and sometimes requiring surgical division of the muscle.

cardiotachometer /kär′dē·ō′təkom′ətər/ [Gk, *kardia + tachos*, speed, *metron*, measure], an instrument that continuously monitors and records the heartbeat.

cardiotomy /kär′dē·ot′əmē/ [Gk, *kardia + temnein*, to cut], 1. an operation in which the heart is incised. 2. an operation in which the cardiac end of the stomach or cardiac orifice is incised.

cardiotonic /kär′dē·ōton′ik/ [Gk, *kardia + tonos*, tone], 1. of or pertaining to a substance that tends to increase the efficiency of contractions of the heart muscle. 2. a pharmacologic agent that increases the force of myocardial contractions. Cardiac glycosides, derived from certain plant alkaloids, exert a tonic effect by altering the transport of electrolytes across the myocardial membrane, causing an increased influx of sodium and calcium and an increased efflux of potassium. Digitalis, digitoxin, and digoxin, widely used cardiac glycosides obtained from leaves of a species of foxglove, increase the force of myocardial contractions, extend the refractory period of the atrioventricular node, and, to a lesser degree, affect the sinoatrial node and the heart's conduction system. Other cardiac glycosides are ouabain and strophanthin, obtained from species of *Strophanthus;* scillaridin, derived from squill; and bufotalin, obtained from the skin and saliva of a European toad.

cardiotoxic /-tok′sik/ [Gk, *kardia + toxikon*, poison], having a toxic or injurious effect on the heart.

cardiovascular /kär′dē·ōvas′kyələr/ [Gk, *kardia + L, vasculum* small vessel], of or pertaining to the heart and blood vessels.

cardiovascular assessment, an evaluation of the condition, function, and abnormalities of the heart and circulatory system.

■ METHOD: The patient is asked to describe the onset, duration, location, and characteristics of any pain present and the occurrence of weakness, fatigue, shortness of breath, fever, coughing, wheezing, and palpitations. Questions are asked regarding episodes of fainting, indigestion, nausea, edema of extremities, cyanosis, and changes in vision, and whether the hands and feet ever feel numb or cold. The person's general appearance, color, assumed position, rate and rhythm of all arterial pulses, the presence of pulsus paradoxus or pulsus alternans, and the distention, pulsation, and pressure of neck veins are observed. Blood pressure, temperature, rate, and character of respirations are checked, and the precordium is examined for the point of maximal impulse, symmetry, the cardiac border, pulsations, and evidence of lifts or bulges. Auscultation of the chest is performed to determine the intensity, pitch, duration, timbre, origin, and frequency of heart sounds and murmurs and to identify the location and character of breath sounds, including rales, rhonchi, and rubs. Color, temperature, turgor, and dryness or sweating of the skin are noted, and the appearance of the extremities, capillary filling time, nails, and lesions are described. The patient's level of consciousness, reflexes, neurologic signs, and responses to pain are recorded, along with data on concurrent hypertension, obesity, diabetes, and any pulmonary and renal conditions. Information is obtained on any previous cardiovascular surgery and illnesses, such as rheumatic fever, myocardial infarction, angina, congenital heart disease, occlusive vascular disease, and lung and kidney disorders. Pertinent background data include the patient's response to stress, methods of coping, relationships, occupation, environment, sleep pattern, exercise levels, leisure activities, and use of alcohol and tobacco. Other factors considered in the evaluation are the patient's family history, the patient's history of medication with digitalis preparations, antihypertensives, diuretics, aspirin, sleeping pills, and over-the-counter cold and influenza remedies and family history of heart disease, hypertension, diabetes, obesity, vascular disorders, stroke, and renal disease. Diagnostic aids used are electrocardiogram, chest x-ray film, echocardiogram, radionuclide imaging, coronary arteriogram, cardiac catheterization, and arterial and pulmonary wedge pressure readings. Appropriate laboratory studies include a complete blood count, hemoglobin and hematocrit determinations, electrolyte and clotting profiles, and assays of serum cholesterol, triglycerides, serum glutamic oxaloacetic transaminase (SGOT), serum glutamic pyruvic transaminase (SGPT), creatine phosphokinase (CP), and lactic acid dehydrogenase (LAD).

■ NURSING INTERVENTION: The nurse usually obtains the patient's history, records the external observations, checks the blood pressure, temperature, respiration, and pulse, auscultates the chest, and assembles the pertinent background information and the reports on diagnostic tests. In a coronary care unit the nurse may have a greatly expanded role, interpreting the data on an electrocardiographic tracing and adjusting medications.

■ OUTCOME CRITERIA: An accurate and complete assessment of cardiovascular function is an essential adjunct to a complete physical examination and is vital to the diagnosis and proper continuing care of a patient who has cardiovascular disease.

cardiovascular disease, any abnormal condition characterized by dysfunction of the heart and blood vessels. Some common kinds of cardiovascular disease are **atherosclerosis, cardiomyopathy, rheumatic heart disease, syphilitic heart disease,** and **systemic hypertension.** In the United States cardiovascular disease is the leading cause of death.

cardiovascular shunt [Gk, *kardia,* heart; L, *vasculum,* little vessel; ME, *shunten*], any abnormal passage between chambers of the heart or between systemic and pulmonary circulatory systems.

cardiovascular system, the network of anatomical structures, including the heart and the blood vessels, that pump blood throughout the body. The system includes thousands of miles of vessels to deliver nutrients and other essential materials to the fluids surrounding the cells and to remove waste products, which are conveyed to excretory organs.

cardiovascular technologist, an allied health professional who performs diagnostic examinations at the request or direction of a physician in one or more of the following three areas: (1) invasive cardiology; (2) noninvasive cardiology; and (3) massive peripheral vascular study. Through subjective sampling and/or recording, the technologist creates an easily definable foundation of data from which a correct anatomic and physiologic diagnosis may be established for each patient.

cardioversion /-vur′zhən/ [Gk, *kardia* + L, *vertere,* to turn], the restoration of the heart's normal sinus rhythm by delivery of a synchronized electric shock through two

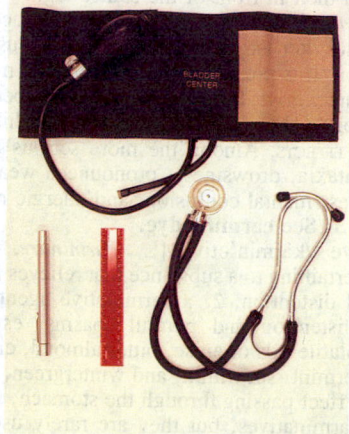

Equipment for cardiovascular assessment
(Canobbio, 1990)

Multiple risk factors in cardiovascular disease

Personal characteristics (no control)	Learned behaviors (intervene and change)	Background conditions (screen-treat)
Sex	Stress/coping	Hypertension
Age	Smoking cigarettes	Diabetes mellitus
Family history	Sedentary life	Hyperlipidemia (especially
	Obesity	hypercholesterolemia)
	Food habits	
	Excess fat	
	Excess sugar	
	Excess salt	

From Williams SR: *Basic nutrition and diet therapy,* ed 9, St Louis, 1992, Mosby.

metal paddles placed on the patient's chest. Cardioversion is used to slow the heart rate or to restore the heart's normal sinus rhythm when drug therapy is ineffective.

carditis /kärdī′tis/, an inflammatory condition of the muscles of the heart, usually resulting from infection. In most cases more than one layer of muscles is involved. Chest pain, cardiac arrhythmia, circulatory failure, and damage to the structures of the heart may occur. Kinds of carditis are **endocarditis, myocarditis,** and **pericarditis.**

Cardizem, a trademark for a slow calcium channel blocker or calcium antagonist (diltiazem).

career ladder, (in nursing education) a pathway for upward mobility that begins with a course of study in practical nursing or a program that grants an associate degree in nursing. Upon completion of this basic level, the candidate may continue up the ladder, to earn a baccalaureate degree in nursing, and then to the graduate level to earn a master's degree and a doctoral degree in nursing.

caregiver, one who contributes the benefits of medical, social, economic, or environmental resources to a dependent or partially dependent individual, such as a critically ill person.

caregiver role strain, a nursing diagnosis accepted by the Tenth National Conference on the Classification of Nursing Diagnoses. Caregiver role strain is a state in which a caregiver perceives difficulty in performing the family caregiver role. Defining characteristics include the caregiver's report of difficulty in providing specific caregiving activities, inadequate resources to provide required care, worry about the care receiver, the feeling that caregiving interferes with other important roles in the caregiver's life, feeling of loss, family conflict, stress, and depression. Related factors may be pathophysiological/physiological, developmental, psychosocial, or situational. Pathophysiological/physiological factors include severity of the care receiver's illness, addiction or codependency, premature birth or congenital defect, discharge of a family member with significant home health needs, caregiver health impairment, unpredictable illness course or instability in the care receivers health, or gender of the caregiver (female). Developmental factors include a developmental inability to fulfill the caregiver role and developmental delay or retardation of the care receiver or caregiver. Psychosocial factors include psychological or cognitive problems in the care receiver, marginal family adaptation or dysfunction before caregiving became necessary, marginal coping patterns of the caregiver, history of a poor relationship with the care receiver, spousal relationship to care receiver, and deviant, bizarre behavior exhibited by the care receiver. Situational factors include the presence of abuse or violence, presence of normal situational stressors, duration of caregiving required, inadequate physical environment for providing care, isolation, lack of respite and recreation, inexperience with caregiving, competing role commitments, and complexity and number of caregiving tasks. See also **nursing diagnosis.**

caregiver role strain, high risk for, a nursing diagnosis accepted by the Tenth National Conference on the Classification of Nursing Diagnoses. High risk for caregiver role strain is a state of vulnerability for feeling difficulty in performing the family caregiver role. Risk factors may be physiological, developmental, psychosocial, or situational. Physiological factors include severity of the care receiver's illness, addiction or codependency, premature birth or congenital defect, discharge of a family member with significant home health needs, caregiver health impairment, un-

predictable illness course or instability in the care receivers health, or gender of the caregiver (female). Developmental factors include a developmental inability to fulfill the caregiver role and developmental delay or retardation of the care receiver or caregiver. Psychosocial factors include psychological or cognitive problems in the care receiver, marginal family adaptation or dysfunction before caregiving became necessary, marginal coping patterns of the caregiver, history of a poor relationship with the care receiver, spousal relationship to care receiver, and deviant, bizarre behavior exhibited by the care receiver. Situational factors include the presence of abuse or violence, presence of normal situational stressors, duration of caregiving required, inadequate physical environment for providing care, isolation, lack of respite and recreational, inexperience with caregiving, competing role commitments, and complexity and number of caregiving tasks. See also **nursing diagnosis.**

care of the chronically ill, a pattern of medical and nursing care that focuses on long-term care of people with chronic diseases or conditions, either at home or in a medical facility. It includes care specific to the problem, as well as other measures to encourage self-care, to promote health, and to prevent loss of function.

care of the sick, (in public health nursing) the care of sick patients in their homes, as distinguished from health supervision. Public health nursing agencies are reimbursed for the nursing services rendered by the nurses according to the kind of service rendered, such as a sick visit or a health supervision visit. Compare **health supervision.**

care plan. See **nursing care plan.**

C.A.R.F., abbreviation for *Commission on Accreditation of Rehabilitation Facilities.*

caries /ker′ēz/ [L, decay], an abnormal condition of a tooth or a bone characterized by decay, disintegration, and destruction of the structure. Kinds of caries include **dental caries, radiation caries,** and **spinal caries.**

carina /kərē′nə/, *pl.* *carinae* [L, keel], any structure shaped like a ridge or keel, such as the carina of the trachea, that projects from the lowest tracheal cartilage.

caring behaviors, behaviors associated with concern for the well-being of a patient, such as sensitivity, comforting, attentive listening, and honesty.

cariocas /kär′ē·ō′kəs/, a form of lateral movement in a gait cycle in which the side-stepping leg is brought successively behind and then in front of the stance leg.

cariogenic /ker′ē·ōjen′ik/, tending to produce caries.

carisoprodol /ker′isōprō′dol/, a skeletal muscle relaxant.
■ INDICATION: It is prescribed for the relief of muscle spasm.
■ CONTRAINDICATIONS: Porphyria or known hypersensitivity to this drug or to chemically similar drugs prohibits its use.
■ ADVERSE EFFECTS: Among the more serious adverse reactions are ataxia, drowsiness, pronounced weakness, visual disturbances, mental confusion, and allergic reactions.

carmalum. See **carmine dye.**

carminative /kärmin′ətiv/ [L, *carminare,* to cleanse], **1.** of or pertaining to a substance that relieves flatulence and abdominal distention. **2.** a carminative agent that relieves gaseous distention and painful spasms, especially after meals. Volatile oils of anise, bitter almond, cinnamon, fennel, peppermint, spearmint, and wintergreen, which have a soothing effect passing through the stomach, were formerly used as carminatives, but they are rarely used in modern medicine except as flavoring agents.

carmine dye /kär′min/ [AR, *qirmize;* AS, *deag*], a red coloring substance, produced by the addition of alum to an extract of cochineal, used for staining specimens in histology. Also called **carmalum.**

carmustine /kärmus'tin/, a lipid-soluble nitrosourea, 1,3-bis(2-chloroethyl)-1-nitrosourea, used as a single antineoplastic agent or with other approved chemotherapeutic agents in the treatment of brain tumors, multiple myeloma, Hodgkin's disease, and non-Hodgkin's lymphomas. Also called **BCNU.**

carnal /kär'nəl/ [L, *caro*, flesh], pertaining to the flesh or body, or worldly things, as distinguished from spiritual.

carneous /kär'nē·əs/, having the quality of flesh.

carnitine /kär'nitin/, a substance found in skeletal and cardiac muscle and certain other tissues that functions as a carrier of fatty acids across the membranes of the mitochondria. It is used therapeutically in treating angina and certain deficiency diseases, particularly endocardial fibroelastosis and as an antithyroid agent. It has actions that closely resemble those of amino acids and B vitamins.

Carnitor, a trademark for a carnitine-deficiency drug (L-carnitine).

carnivore /kär'nivôr/ [L, *caro*, flesh, *vorare*, to devour], an animal belonging to the order *Carnivora*, classified as a flesheater, with appropriate teeth and a characteristically simple stomach and a short intestine for such a diet. — **carnivorous** /kärniv'ərəs/, *adj.*

carotene /kar'ətin/ [L, *carota*, carrot], a red or orange hydrocarbon found in carrots, sweet potatoes, milk fat, egg yolk, and leafy vegetables, as beet greens, spinach, and broccoli. Beta-carotene is a provitamin and in the body is converted into vitamin A. An inability to utilize carotene results in vitamin A deficiency. Also spelled **carotin, carrotene, carrotine.** See also **vitamin A.**

carotenemia /kar'ətinē'mē·ə/, the presence of high levels of carotene in the blood resulting in an abnormal yellow appearance of the plasma and skin. The conjunctivae are not discolored. Also called **pseudojaundice, xanthemia** /zanthē'mē·ə/. See also jaundice.

carotenoid /kərot'ənoid/, any of a group of red, yellow, or orange highly unsaturated pigments that are found in some animal tissue and in foods, such as carrots, sweet potatoes, and leafy green vegetables. Many of these substances, such as carotene, are necessary for the formation of vitamin A in the body, whereas others, including lycopene and xanthophyll, show no vitamin A activity. Also spelled **carotinoid.**

carotenosis. See **carotenemia.**

carotid /kərot'id/ [Gk, *karos*, heavy sleep], of or pertaining to the carotid artery. See also **carotid body, carotid sinus, common carotid artery.**

carotid arch [Gk, *karos*, heavy sleep; L, *arcus*, bow], the third arch of the aorta, the source of the common carotid arteries.

carotid body [Gk, *karos;* AS, *bodig*], a small structure containing neural tissue at the bifurcation of the carotid arteries. It monitors the oxygen content of the blood and assists in regulating respiration.

carotid-body reflex [Gk, *karos* + AS, *bodig;* L, *reflecere,* to bend backward], a normal chemical reflex initiated by a decrease in oxygen concentration in the blood and, to a lesser degree, by increased carbon dioxide and hydrogen ion concentrations that act on chemoreceptors at the bifurcation of the common carotid arteries. The resulting nerve impulses cause the respiratory center in the medulla to increase respiratory activity. See also **aortic-body reflex.**

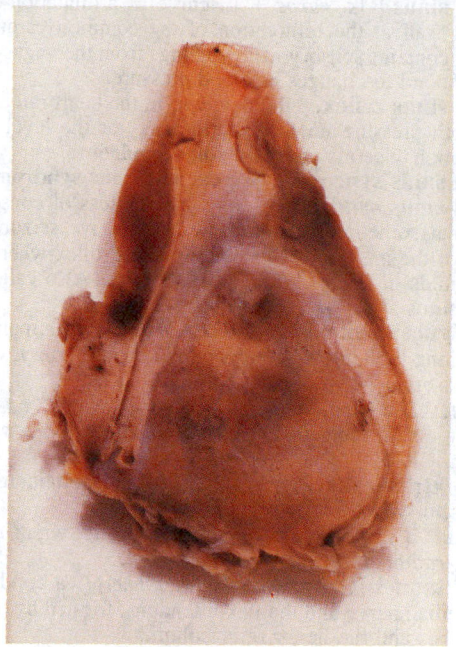

Carotid body tumor *(Skarin, 1991)*

carotid-body tumor, a benign, round, firm growth that develops at the bifurcation of the common carotid artery. The tumor may cause dizziness, nausea, and vomiting, if it impedes the flow of blood and pressure is increased in the vascular system. Surgical excision may be used for treatment in some cases.

carotid plexus [Gk, *karos* + L, pleated], any one of three nerve plexuses associated with the carotid arteries. Compare **common carotid plexus, external carotid plexus, internal carotid plexus.**

carotid pulse, the pulse of the carotid artery, palpated by gently pressing a finger in the groove between the larynx and the sternocleidomastoid muscle in the neck. See also **pulse.**

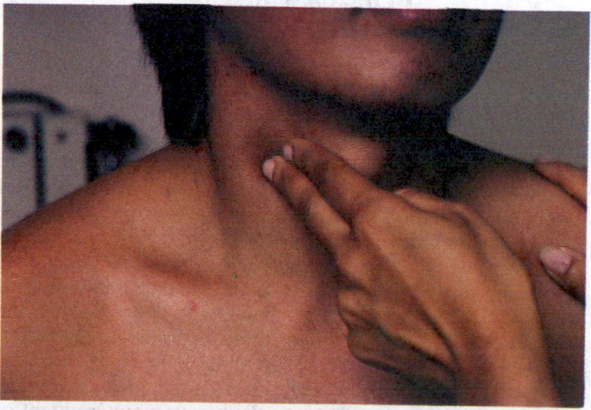

Measurement of carotid pulse *(Canobbio, 1990)*

carotid sinus [Gk, *karos* + L, curve], a dilatation of the arterial wall at the bifurcation of the common carotid artery. It contains sensory nerve endings from the vagus nerve that respond to changes in blood pressure.

carotid sinus reflex, the decrease in the heart rate resulting from pressure on the carotid artery at the level of its bifurcation. See also **carotid sinus syndrome.**

carotid sinus syncope, See **carotid sinus syndrome.**

carotid sinus syndrome, a temporary loss of consciousness that sometimes accompanies convulsive seizures because of the intensity of the carotid sinus reflex when pressure builds in one or both carotid sinuses. Also called **carotid sinus syncope.**

carotidynia /kərot′ōdin′ē·ə/ [Gk, *karos* + *odyne*, pain], a pain along the length of the common carotid artery, caused by pressure.

carotin. See **carotene.**

-carp, a suffix meaning 'fruit': *archicarp, ascocarp, pericarp.*

carpal /kär′pəl/ [Gk, *karpos*, wrist], of or pertaining to the carpus, or wrist.

-carpal, a combining form referring to the wrist: *extracarpal, radiocarpal, trapeziometacarpal.*

carpal tunnel [Gk, *karpos* + Fr, *tonnel*], a conduit for the median nerve and the flexor tendons, formed by the carpal bones and the flexor retinaculum.

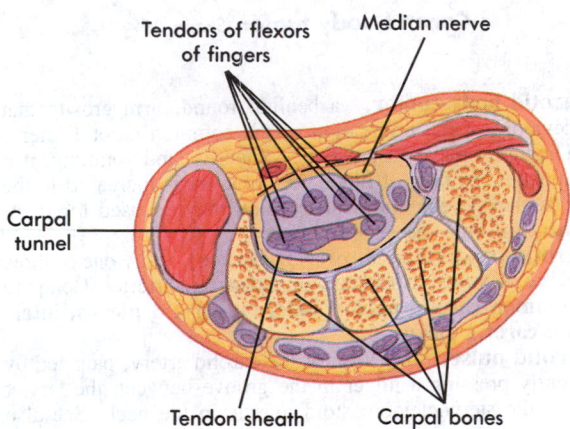

Carpal tunnel syndrome—compression of the median nerve
(Thibodeau, 1993/Rolin Graphics)

carpal tunnel syndrome, a common painful disorder of the wrist and hand, induced by compression on the median nerve between the inelastic carpal ligament and other structures within the carpal tunnel. The syndrome is seen more often in women, especially in pregnant and in menopausal women. Symptoms may result from trauma, synovitis, or tumor, or may develop with rheumatoid arthritis, amyloidosis, acromegaly, or diabetes. The median nerve innervates the palm and the radial side of the hand; compression of the nerve causes weakness, pain with opposition of the thumb, and burning, tingling, or aching, sometimes radiating to the forearm and to the shoulder joint. Weakness and atrophy of muscles may increase from lack of use, impairing thumb and finger dexterity. Pain may be intermittent or constant and is often most intense at night. Symptomatic

treatment usually relieves mild symptoms of recent onset, but if the pain becomes disabling, the injection of corticosteroids often brings dramatic relief. Surgical division of the volar carpal ligament to relieve nerve pressure is usually curative. Nursing treatment includes emotional support, nocturnal splinting of the hand and forearm, elevation of the arm to relieve the swelling of soft tissue, and encouragement of mild wrist and finger movements to prevent atrophy of muscles.

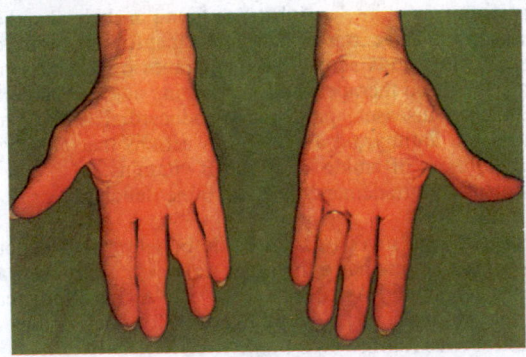

Carpal tunnel syndrome—atrophy and weakness of the hand
(Shipley, 1993)

carpo- /kär′pō-/ [Gk, *karpos*, wrist], a combining form meaning 'wrist.'

carpometacarpal /-met′əkär′pəl/ (CMC) joint [Gk, *karpos*, wrist, *meta*, next, *karpos*], any of the joints formed by the distal row of carpal bones and the bases of the metacarpals. The joints are essential for prehensile patterns.

carpopedal spasm /-ped′əl/ [Gk, *karpos* + L, *pes*, foot], a spasm of the hand, thumbs, foot, or toes that sometimes accompanies tetany.

carpus /kär′pəs/ [L; Gk, *karpos*], the wrist, made up of eight bones arranged in two rows. The proximal row consists of the scaphoid, lunate, triangular, and pisiform. The distal row consists of the trapezium, trapezoid, capitate, and hamate.

Carrel-Lindbergh pump. See **Lindbergh pump.**

carrier /ker′ē·ər/ [OFr, *carier*], **1.** a person or animal who harbors and spreads an organism causing disease in others but who does not become ill. **2.** one whose chromosomes carry a recessive gene.

Carrión's disease. See **bartonellosis.**

Carroll Quantitative Test of Upper Extremity Function, a six-part test of the ability of the patient to grasp and lift objects of different shapes and sizes. It is designed to measure the ability to perform general arm and hand movements required for the activities of daily living.

carrotene. See **carotene.**

carrotine. See **carotene.**

carrying angle, the angle at which the humerus and radius articulate.

carry-over [L, *carrus*, wagon; AS *ofer*], contamination of a specimen by the previous one.

car sickness [L, *carrus*, wagon; AS, *seoc*], nausea and vomiting due to the motion of the vehicle. See also **motion sickness.**

cartilage /kär'tilij/ [L, *cartilago*], a nonvascular support-ing connective tissue composed of various cells and fibers, found chiefly in the joints, the thorax, and various rigid tubes, such as the larynx, trachea, nose, and ear. Tempo-rary cartilage, such as that comprising most of the fetal skel-eton at an early stage, is later replaced by bone. Permanent cartilage remains unossified, except in certain diseases and, sometimes, in advanced age. Kinds of permanent cartilage are **hyaline cartilage, white fibrocartilage,** and **yellow cartilage.** –**cartilaginous** /kär'tilaj'inəs/, *adj.*

cartilage capped exostosis. See **exostosis cartilagines.**

cartilage graft, the transplantation of cartilage. It is used to correct congenital ear and nose defects in children and to treat severe injuries in adults. Because chondrocytes can be allografted without the risk of an immune reaction, cadaver cartilage can be used for tissue grafts.

cartilage-hair hypoplasia [L, *cartilago* + AS, *haer;* Gk, *hypo,* under, *plasis,* forming], a genetic disorder, inher-ited as an autosomal recessive trait, characterized by dwarf-ism caused by hypoplasia of the cartilage, multiple skeletal abnormalities, and excessively sparse, short, fine, brittle hair that is usually light colored. The condition is found pri-marily among Amish people in the United States and Can-ada.

cartilaginous [L, *cartilago,* cartilage], pertaining to carti-lage.

cartilaginous joint [L, *cartilago* + *junger,* to join], a slightly movable joint in which cartilage unites bony sur-faces. Two types of articulation involving cartilaginous joints are synchondrosis and symphysis. Also called **am-phiarthrosis, junctura cartilaginea.** Compare **fibrous joint, synovial joint.**

cartilagenous skeleton [L, *cartilago;* Gk, *skeletos,* dried up], the parts of the skeleton that are formed by cartilage.

CARTOS /kär'tos/, abbreviation for *computer-aided re-construction by tracing of serial sections,* a technique in which serial, hand-drawn copies of electron micrographs are programed on a computer for display on a television screen. The image can be manipulated for study of all dimensions of the structure.

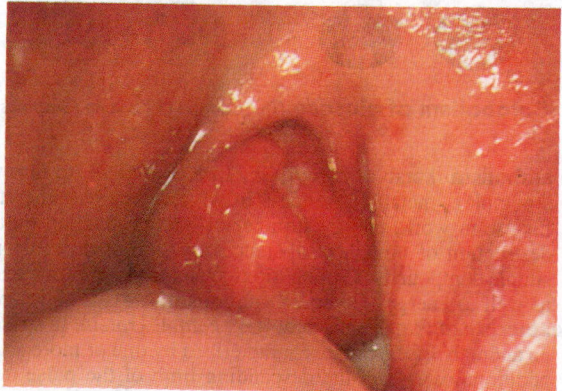

Caruncle *(Kamal, 1991)*

caruncle /kär'ungkəl/ [L, *caruncula,* small piece of flesh], a small, fleshy projection, as one of the lacrimal caruncles at the inner canthus of the eye or the hymenal caruncles that are the hymenal remnants. Also called **caruncula.**

carunculae hymenales [L, *caruncula* + Gk, *hymen,* mem-brane], remnants of a ruptured hymen that appear as ir-regular projections of normal skin around the introitus to the vagina. Also called **hymenal tags.**

caryo-, karyo-, a combining form meaning 'pertaining to a nucleus': *caryokinesis, caryophyllus.*

cascade /kaskād'/ [L, *cadere,* to fall], any process that de-velops in stages, with each stage dependent on the preced-ing one, often producing a cumulative effect.

cascade humidifier, a bubbling respiratory care device in which gases travel down a tower and pass through a grid into a chamber of heated water. As water is displaced, it rises above the grid, forming a liquid film that is converted to a froth as the gas also rises from the chamber through the grid. The process results in an air flow that can have a relative humidity of up to 100 percent.

cascara sagrada /kasker'ə səgrä'də/ [Sp, sacred bark], a stimulant cathartic prepared from the bark of the *Rhamnus purshianus* tree.

■ INDICATION: It is prescribed for constipation.

■ CONTRAINDICATIONS: Symptoms of appendicitis, intestinal obstruction or perforation, fecal impaction, or known hy-persensitivity to this drug prohibits its use. It is not given to lactating mothers.

■ ADVERSE EFFECTS: Among the more serious adverse reac-tions are rectal bleeding, muscle cramps, dizziness, and lax-ative dependence.

case [L, *causus,* a happening], **1.** an episode of illness or injury. **2.** a container.

caseation /kā'sē·ā'shən/ [L, *caseus,* cheese], a form of tis-sue necrosis in which there is loss of cellular outline and the appearance is that of crumbly cheese. It is typical of tuberculosis. See also **caseous.** –**caseate,** *v.*

caseation necrosis [L, *caseus,* cheese; Gk, *nekros,* dead, *osis* condition], necrosis that transforms tissue into a dry cheeselike mass.It occurs primarily in tuberculosis.

case-control study, an investigation employing an epide-miologic approach in which previously existing cases of the condition are used in lieu of gathering new information from a randomized population.A group of patients with a partic-ular disease or disorder, such as myocardial infarction, is compared with a control group of persons who have not de-veloped that medical problem. The two groups, matched for age, sex, and other personal data, are examined to deter-mine what possible factor (cigarette smoking, coffee drink-ing, etc.) might account for the increased disease incidence in the case group.

case fatality rate [L, *causus,* a happening, *fatum,* fate, *(pro) rata*], the number of registered deaths caused by any specific disease, expressed as a percentage of the total num-ber of reported cases of a specific disease.

casefinding, the act of locating individuals with a disease.

case history [L, *causus, historia*], a complete medical record of a patient prior to a current illness or injury. The history will include any infectious diseases experienced by the person, all immunizations, hospitalizations or therapies, information relating to deaths or illnesses of parents and other close family members, allergies, and congenital or ac-quired physical defects.

case management, the assignment of a health care pro-vider to assist a patient in assessing health and social ser-vice systems and to assure that all required services are ob-tained.

case nursing [L, *casus,* a happening, *nutrix,* nourish], an organizational mode for assigning nursing staff in which one nurse is assigned to provide total nursing care to one or more patients.

caseous /kā′sē·əs/, cheeselike; describing the mixture of fat and protein that appears in some body tissues undergoing necrosis.

caseous abscess. See **cheesy abscess.**

caseous fermentation [L, *caseus,* cheese; *fermentum,* yeast], the coagulation of soluble casein through the action of rennin.

cassette /kaset′/ [Fr, little box], a device used in radiography for holding a sheet of x-ray film and a set of screens. A cassette also may have a grid to absorb scattered radiation.

cast [ONorse, *kasta*], **1.** a stiff, solid dressing formed with plaster of Paris or other material around a limb or other body part to immobilize it during healing. **2.** a mold of a part or all of a patient's teeth and internal jaw area for fitting prostheses or dentures. **3.** a tiny structure formed by deposits of mineral or other substances on the walls of renal tubules, bronchioles, or other organs. Casts often appear in samples of urine or blood collected for laboratory examination. **4.** the deviation of an eye from the normal parallel lines of vision, such as in strabismus.

cast brace, a combination of a brace within a cast at a joint.

cast core [ONorse, *kasta;* L, *cor,* heart], a metal casting, shaped like a stump of a tooth and incorporating a post in the root canal for retaining an artificial tooth crown. Compare **amalgam core, composite core.** See also **core.**

Castellani's paint. See **carbol-fuchsin solution.**

casting, 1. the act of encasing a body part in a cast. **2.** (in dentistry) the process by which crowns, inlays, and other metallic restorations are produced.

casting tape, an adhesive or resin-impregnated tape used for shaping lightweight casts.

castor oil /kas′tər/ [L, beaver, *oleum* olive oil], an oil derived from *Ricinus communis,* used as a stimulant cathartic.
■ INDICATIONS: It is prescribed for constipation and for a cleansing preparation of the bowel or colon before examination.
■ CONTRAINDICATIONS: Symptoms of appendicitis, intestinal obstruction or perforation, and fecal impaction prohibit its use. It is not to be used during menstruation or pregnancy.
■ ADVERSE EFFECTS: Among the most serious adverse reactions are rectal bleeding and laxative dependence. Nausea, abdominal cramps, and dizziness also may occur.

castration /kastrā′shən/ [L, *castrare,* to castrate], the surgical excision of one or both testicles or ovaries, performed most frequently to reduce the production and secretion of certain hormones that may stimulate the proliferation of malignant cells in women with breast cancer or in men with cancer of the prostate. The patient must be informed that bilateral excision of the gonads causes sterility. See also **oophorectomy, orchidectomy.**

castration anxiety, 1. the fantasized fear of injury or loss of the genital organs, often as the reaction to a repressed feeling of punishment for forbidden sexual desires. It may also be caused by some apparently threatening everyday occurrence, such as a humiliating experience, loss of a job, or loss of authority. **2.** a general threat to the masculinity or femininity of a person or an unrealistic fear of bodily injury or loss of power. Also called **anxiety complex.** See also **anxiety neurosis.**

castration complex. See **castration anxiety.**

cast saw, a saw used to cut through a plaster cast.

cast shoe, a shoe worn over a foot that is encased in a plaster cast.

cast stabilization, the use of rods, pins, broom handles, or other devices to lend stability to a cast.

casuistics /kazh′əwis′tiks/ [L, *casus,* a happening], the recording and the study of the cases of any disease.

CAT /kat/, abbreviation for **computerized axial tomography.** See **computed tomography**

cata-, cat-, kata-, a combining form meaning 'down, under, against, lower, with': *catabasis, catabolic, catacausis.*

catabasis /kətab′əsis/, *pl.* **catabases** [Gk, *kata,* down, *bainein,* to go], the phase in which a disease declines. **–catabatic** /kat′əbat′ik/, *adj.*

catabiosis /kat′əbī·ō′sis/, the normal aging of cells. **–catabiotic,** *adj.*

catabolic. See **catabolism.**

catabolic activator protein. See **CAP.**

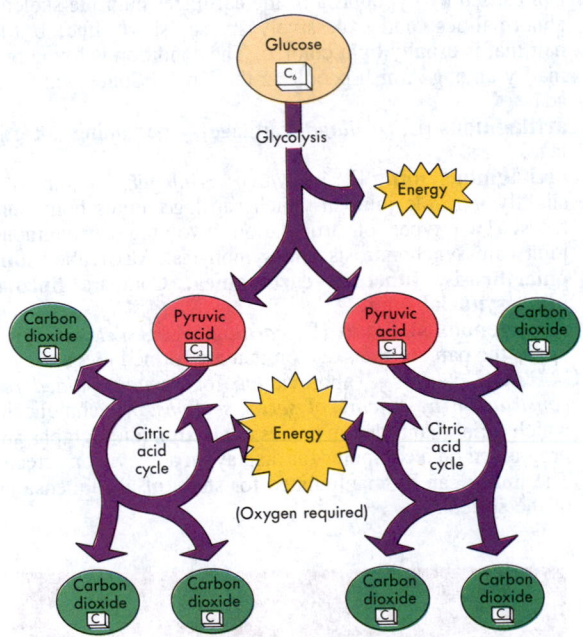

Catabolism of glucose (Thibodeau, 1993/Rolin Graphics)

catabolism /kətab′əliz′əm/ [Gk, *kata* + *ballein,* to throw], a complex, metabolic process in which energy is liberated for use in work, energy storage, or heat production by the destruction of complex substances by living cells to form simple compounds. Carbon dioxide and water are produced, as well as energy. Compare **anabolism.** **–catabolic,** *adj.*

catacrotism /kətak′rətiz′əm/ [Gk, *kata* + *krotein,* to strike], an anomaly of the pulse, characterized by one or more small additional waves in the descending limb of the pulse tracing. **–catacrotic,** *adj.*

catagen. See **hair.**

catagenesis /kat′əjen′əsis/ [Gk, *kata,* down, *genein,* to produce], a form of evolution that is retrogressive.

catalase /kat′əlās/ [Gk, *katalein,* to dissolve], a heme enzyme, found in almost all biologic cells, that catalyzes the decomposition of hydrogen peroxide to water and oxygen.

catalepsy /kat′ələp′sē/ [Gk, *kata* + *lambanein*, to seize], an abnormal state characterized by a trancelike level of consciousness and postural rigidity. It occurs in hypnosis and in certain organic and psychologic disorders, such as schizophrenia, epilepsy, and hysteria.

catalysis /kətal′əsis/ [Gk, *katalein*, to dissolve], an increase in the rate of a chemical reaction that is caused by a substance that is neither permanently altered or consumed by the reaction. Compare **negative catalysis.** See also **catalyst.** −**catalytic,** *adj.*

catalyst /kat′əlist/ [Gk, *katalein*, to dissolve], a substance that influences the rate of a chemical reaction without being permanently altered or consumed by the process. Most catalysts, including enzymes in living organisms, accelerate chemical reactions; negative catalysts retard such reactions. See also **enzyme.**

-catalytic, -catalytical, a suffix meaning 'pertaining to a chemical reaction caused by an agent unchanged by the reaction': *allelocatalytic, autocatalytic, photocatalytic.*

catamenia. See **menses.**

catamnesis /kat′amnē′sis/ [Gk, *kata* + *men,* month], the medical history of a patient from the onset of an illness. Compare **anamnesis.**

cataphylaxis /kat′əfəlak′sis/ [Gk, kata + *phylax,* guard], **1.** the migration of leukocytes and antibodies to the site of an infection. **2.** the deterioration of the natural defense system of the body. cataphylactic, *adj.*

cataplexy /kat′əplek′sē/ [Gk, *kata* + *plexis,* stroke], a condition characterized by sudden muscular weakness and hypotonia, caused by emotions, such as anger, fear or surprise, often associated with narcolepsy. −**cataplectic,** *adj.*

Catapres, a trademark for an antihypertensive (clonidine hydrochloride).

cataract /kat′ərakt/ [Gk, *katarrhakies,* waterfall], an abnormal progressive condition of the lens of the eye, characterized by loss of transparency. A gray-white opacity can be seen within the lens, behind the pupil. Most cataracts are caused by degenerative changes, occurring most often after 50 years of age. The tendency to develop cataracts is inherited. Trauma, such as a puncture wound, may result in cataract formation; less often, exposure to such poisons as dinitrophenol or naphthalene causes them. **Congenital cataracts** are usually hereditary but may be caused by viral infection during the first trimester of gestation. If cataracts are untreated, sight is eventually lost. At onset vision is blurred; then, bright lights glare diffusely, and distortion and double vision may develop. Uncomplicated cataracts of old age (**senile cataracts**) are usually treated with excision of the lens and prescription of special contact lenses or glasses. The soft cataracts of children and young adults may either be incised and drained or fragmented by ultrasound, followed by irrigation and aspiration of the fragments through a minute incision.

catarrh /kətär′/ [Gk, *kata* + *rhoia,* flow], *obsolete.* inflammation of the mucous membranes with discharge, especially inflammation of the air passages of the nose and the trachea. −**catarrhal, catarrhous,** *adj.*

catarrhal /kətär′əl/ [Gk, *kata,* down, *rhoia,* flow], pertaining to catarrh or discharge from an inflamed mucous membrane.

catarrhal conjunctivitis [Gk, *kata, rhoia;* L, *conjunctivus,* connecting; Gk, *itis,* inflammation], a simple form of inflammation of the conjunctiva, usually associated with an

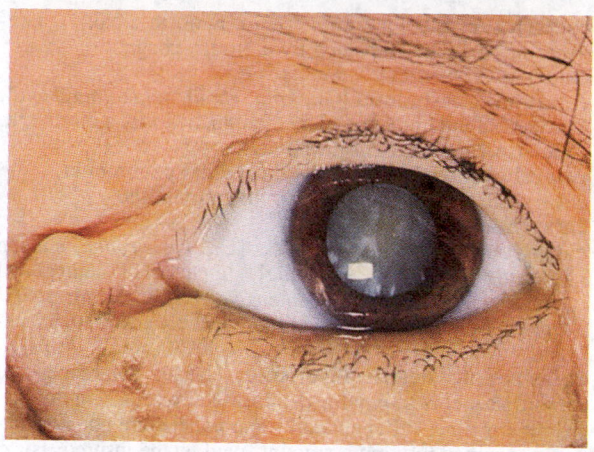

Appearance of eye with cataract *(Bedford, 1986)*

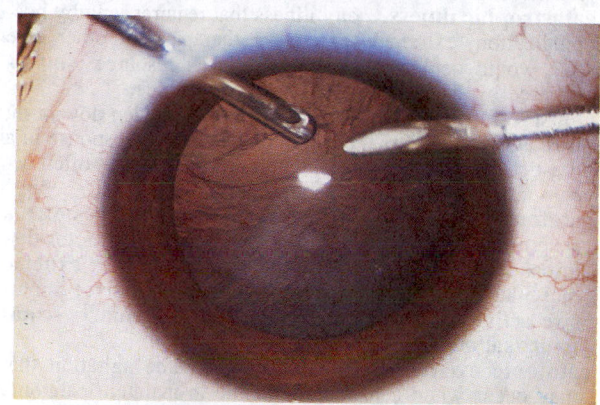

Cataract removal by aspiration *(Jaffe, 1990)*

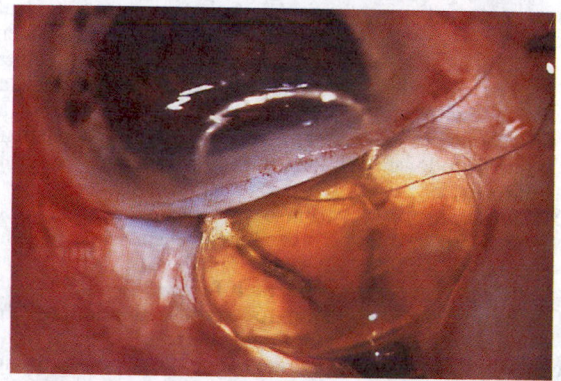

Cataract removal by excision *(Jaffe, 1990)*

infection, allergy, exposure to pollution, or physical irritation as by an eyelash in the eye and accompanied by a discharge.

catarrhal croup [Gk, *kata, rhoia*; Scot, to croak], a severe laryngitis acompanied by a croupy cough.

catarrhal dysentery. See **sprue.**

catarrhal ophthalmia [Gk, *kata, rhoia, ophthalmos*, eye], a catarrhal inflammation of the conjunctiva with a discharge. See also **catarrhal conjunctivitis.**

catarrhal pneumonia. See **bronchial pneumonia.**

catarrhal stomatitis. See **simple stomatitis.**

catarrhous. See **catarrh.**

catastrophic care /kat'əstrof'ik/ [Gk, *katastrophe*, sudden downturn; L, *garrire*, to babble], a pattern of medical and nursing care that involves intensive, highly technical life-support care of an acutely ill or severely traumatized patient.

catastrophic health insurance, health insurance that awards benefits to pay for the cost of severe or lengthy disability or illness. Benefits on some policies are not paid until a specified minimum amount, paid by the insured, is exceeded. Most policies have a limit in total benefits paid, and payment for certain kinds of services may be precluded or limited to a maximum indemnity.

catastrophic illness, any illness that requires lengthy hospitalization, extremely expensive therapies, or other care that would deplete a family's financial resources, unless covered by special medical insurance policies.

catastrophic reaction [Gk, *katastrophe*, sudden downturn; L *re* again, *agere* to act], the uncoordinated response to a drastic shock or a sudden threatening condition, as often occurs in the victims of car crashes and disasters.

catatonia /kat'ətō'nē·ə/ [Gk, *kata* + *tonos*, tension], a state or condition characterized by conspicuous motor disturbance, manifested usually as immobility with extreme muscular rigidity or, less commonly, as excessive, impulsive activity. See also **catatonic schizophrenia. –catatonic** /kat'əton'ik/, *adj.*

catatonic excitement, a state of extreme agitation that may occur when a patient is unable to maintain catatonic immobility.

catatonic schizophrenia [Gk, *kata, tonos* + *schizein*, to split, *phren*, mind], a form of schizophrenia characterized by alternating periods of extreme withdrawal and extreme excitement. During the withdrawal stage stupor, muscular rigidity, mutism, blocking, negativism, and catalepsy (cerea flexibilitas) may be seen; during the period of excitement, purposeless and impulsive activity may range from mild agitation to violence. Treatment may include tranquilizers, antipsychotic, or antianxiety medication or electroconvulsive therapy, followed by long-term psychotherapy. See also **catatonia.**

catatonic stupor, a form of catatonia marked by a lack of response; it may be related to a patient's fear of losing the ability to control his or her impulses.

cat-bite fever. See **cat-scratch fever.**

CAT-CAM, abbreviation for **contoured adducted trochanteric controlled alignment method.**

catchment area [L, *capere*, to take; *area*, space], the specific geographic area for which a particular institution, especially a mental health center, is responsible.

catch-up growth [L, *capere* + As, *uf, gruowan*], an acceleration of the growth rate following a period of growth retardation caused by a secondary deficiency, such as acute malnutrition or severe illness. The phenomenon, which is routinely seen in premature infants, involves rapid increase in weight, length, and head circumference and continues until the normal individual growth pattern is resumed. The se-

verity, duration, and the developmental timing at which the deficiency occurs may result in some growth inadequacy or permanent deficit, especially in such tissue as the brain.

cat-cry syndrome [L, *catta,* cat, *quiritare,* to cry out; Gk, *syndromos,* course], a rare, congenital disorder recognized at birth by a kittenlike cry caused by a laryngeal anomaly. The condition is associated with a defect in chromosome 5. Other characteristics include low birth weight, microcephaly, 'moon face,' wide-set eyes, strabismus, and low-set misshaped ears. Infants are hypotonic; heart defects and mental and physical retardation are common. Also called **cri-du-chat syndrome** /crēdōōshä'/, **chromosome 5p–syndrome.**

catecholamine /kat'əkələm'in/, any one of a group of sympathomimetic compounds composed of a catechol molecule and the aliphatic portion of an amine. Some catecholamines are produced naturally by the body and function as key neurologic chemicals. Catecholamines are also synthesized as drugs used in the treatment of various disorders, such as anaphylaxis, asthma, cardiac failure, and hypertension. Some important endogenous catecholamines are dopamine, epinephrine, and norepinephrine. Norepinephrine mediates a host of physiologic and metabolic responses that follow the stimulation of the sympathetic nerves. In response to stress, the adrenal medulla is stimulated, causing the elevation of epinephrine and norepinephrine concentrations in the circulation. Epinephrine dilates blood vessels to the skeletal muscles. Norepinephrine slightly constricts these blood vessels. Both compounds stimulate the myocardium. Dopamine is found primarily in the basal ganglia of the central nervous system (CNS), but dopaminergic nerve endings and specific receptors for this compound have been found in other CNS areas. The major functions of catecholamines and drugs that mimic their actions include the peripheral excitation of certain muscles, peripheral inhibition of certain muscles, cardiac excitation, metabolic actions, endocrine actions, and CNS actions. Differences in the actions of the catecholamines depend on alpha and beta receptors in nerve terminals throughout the body. The brain contains separate neuronal systems that use dopamine, epinephrine, and norepinephrine. More than half of the catecholamine content of the CNS is dopamine, large quantities of which are found in the basal ganglia, the central nucleus of the amygdala, the median eminence, the olfactory tubercle, and the restricted fields of the frontal cortex. The hypothalamus and certain zones of the limbic system contain relatively large amounts of norepinephrine, which is also found in lesser amounts in other brain areas. Neurons in the CNS that contain epinephrine are situated primarily in the medullary reticular formation. Norepinephrine is converted to epinephrine in the adrenal medulla. Catecholamines act directly on sympathetic effector cells by binding to receptors in cellular plasma membranes. Sympathomimetic drugs influence biochemical reactions and functional responses in all the tissues they affect.

catechol-o-methyl transferase (COMT) /kat'əkol'ōmeth'il/, an enzyme that deactivates the catecholamines epinephrine and norepinephrine.

cat-eye syndrome [L, *catta* + AS, *eage*; Gk, *syndromos* course], a rare, congenital autosomal anomaly, marked by the presence of an extra, small chromosome 22 and pupils that resemble the vertical pupils of a cat. Anal atresia, heart abnormalities, and severe mental retardation are common.

categoric data /kat′əgôr′ik/ [Gk, *kategorikos,* affirmation; L, *datus,* giving], (in research) any data that are classified by name rather than by number, such as race, religion, ethnicity, or marital status.

catgut [L, *catta* + AS, *guttas*], a nonabsorbable suture material, prepared from the intestines of sheep, used to close surgical wounds.

catharsis /kəthär′sis/, **1.** a cleansing or purging. **–cathartic,** *n.* **2.** the therapeutic release of pent-up feelings and emotions by open discussion of ideas and thoughts. **3.** also called **psychocatharsis.** the process of bringing repressed ideas and feelings into the consciousness by the technique of free association, often in conjunction with hypnosis and the use of hypnotic drugs. See also **abreaction.**

cathartic /kəthär′tik/ [Gk, *katharsis,* cleansing], **1.** of or pertaining to a substance that causes evacuation of the bowel. **2.** also called **coprogogue** /kop′rəgōg/. a cathartic agent that promotes bowel evacuation by stimulating peristalsis, increasing the fluidity or bulk of intestinal contents, softening the feces, or lubricating the intestinal wall. The term *cathartic* implies a fluid evacuation; this is in contrast to *laxative,* which implies the elimination of a soft, formed stool. Cathartics that increase peristalsis, usually by irritating intestinal mucosa, include certain plant substances, such as aloe, colocynth, croton oil, podophyllum senna, phenolphthalein, bisacodyl, and dehydrocholic acid. Saline cathartics, such as sodium sulfate, magnesium sulfate, and magnesium hydroxide, dilute the intestinal contents by retaining water through osmotic forces. Suppositories containing sodium biphosphate, sodium acid pyrophosphate, and sodium bicarbonate induce defecation when the salts react to form carbon dioxide and the expanding gas stimulates peristalsis. See also **laxative.** **–catharsis,** *n.*

-cathartic, a suffix meaning 'pertaining to cleaning': *cephalocathartic, emetocathartic, hematocathartic.*

cathetic. See **cathexis.**

catheter /kath′ətər/ [Gk, *katheter,* something lowered], a hollow, flexible tube that can be inserted into a vessel or cavity of the body to withdraw or to instill fluids. Most catheters are made of soft plastic or rubber and may be used for treatment or diagnosis. Kinds of catheters include **acorn-tipped catheter, Foley catheter,** and **intrauterine catheter.**

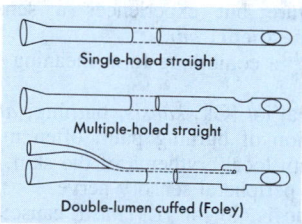

Single-holed straight

Multiple-holed straight

Double-lumen cuffed (Foley)

Catheters

catheter hub, a threaded plastic connection at the end of an intravenous catheter.

catheterization /kath′əturī′zā′shən/, the introduction of a catheter into a body cavity or organ to inject or remove a fluid. The most common procedure is the insertion of a catheter into the bladder through the urethra for the relief of urinary retention and for emptying the bladder completely before surgery. It is also used when a urine specimen may oth-

erwise be contaminated, such as when a woman is menstruating. Self-catheterization is taught to those patients with neurogenic bladder. Sterile, aseptic techniques are necessary to prevent infection; trauma is also to be avoided, particularly to the male urethra and when the procedure is performed on children, who are frightened by the technique and cannot cooperate. For indwelling catheters, attention is given to maintaining continuous free drainage and to the increased possibility of infection. Frequent washing of the area surrounding the urinary meatus reduces the risk of infection and eliminates unpleasant odors and irritation. Kinds of catheterization are **cardiac catheterization, hepatic vein catheterization,** and **laryngeal catheterization.** See also **female catheterization, Foley catheter, male catheterization.** **–catheterize** /kath′ətərīz/, *v.*

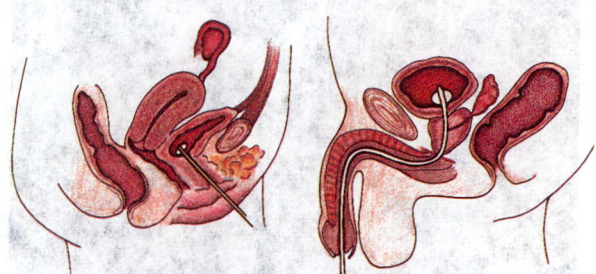

Female catheterization   Male catheterization

Catheterization
(Potter, 1993)

cathexis /kəthek′sis/ [Gk, *kathexis,* retention], the conscious or unconscious attachment of emotional feeling and importance to a specific idea, person, or object. **–cathectic,** *adj.*

cathode /kath′ōd/ [Gk, *kata,* down, *hodos,* way], **1.** the electrode at which reduction occurs. **2.** the negative side of the x-ray tube which consists of the focusing cup and the filament.

cathode ray, a stream of electrons emitted by the negative electrode of a gaseous discharge device when the cathode is bombarded by positive ions, such as in a cathode ray tube, an oscilloscope, or a television picture tube. The ray itself is usually focused by a series of electromagnets that control its direction and position on a screen coated with a phosphor to create a visible pattern.

cathode ray oscilloscope [Gk, *kata, hodos;* L, *radius; ocillare,* to swing; Gk, *skopein,* to view], an instrument that produces a visual representation of electric variations by means of the fluorescent screen of a cathode ray tube. Oscilloscopes have many applications in medicine and in nursing, such as the displaying of patients' brain waves and heart beats for monitoring and diagnostic purposes.

cathode ray tube (CRT), a vacuum tube that focuses a beam of electrons onto a spot on a screen coated with a phosphor, creating a visible image of information on the face of the tube. The CRT provides a means for graphically representing data processed by a computer.

cation /kat′ī·on/ [Gk, *kata,* down, *ion,* going], a positively charged ion that in solution is attracted to the negative electrode. Compare **anion.**

cation-exchange resin, any one of various insoluble organic polymers with high molecular weights that exchange their cations for other ions in solution. Cation-exchange resins are used especially to restrict intestinal sodium absorption in patients with edema. Compare **anion-exchange resin.**

catling, a long, sharp, double-edged knife used in amputation. Also called **catlin.**

catoptric /kətop′trik/ [Gk, *katoptron*, mirror], of or pertaining to a reflected image or reflected light, such as from a mirror.

CAT scan. See **computed tomography.**

cat scratch disease, See **cat scratch fever.**

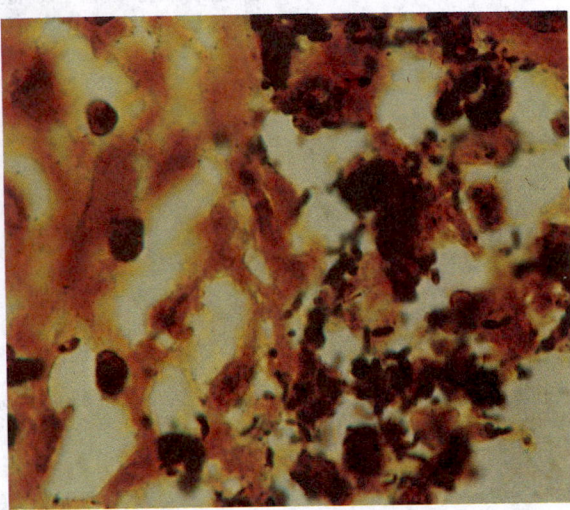

Cat scratch fever bacillus in lymph node tissue
(Baron, 1990/Courtesy Dr. Ellen Kahn, North Shore University Hospital, Manhasset, NY)

cat scratch fever, a disease that results from the scratch or bite of a healthy cat. Inflammation and pustules are found on the scratched skin, and lymph nodes in the neck, head, groin, or axilla swell 2 weeks later. Although patients are seldom seriously ill, fever, headache, and malaise may occur and symptoms can persist for months. Tetracycline may aid rapid recovery. The cat scratch skin test is available to help in the diagnosis. There may be spontaneous remission of symptoms in about two weeks. Also called **cat scratch disease, benign lymphoreticulosis.**

cat's eye amaurosis [L, *catta;* AS, *aege;* Gk, *amauroin,* to darken], a monocular blindness, with a bright reflection from the pupil caused by a white mass in the vitreous humor resulting from inflammation or a malignant lesion.

Caucasian, pertaining to a person whose ancestors were believed to have in ancient times inhabited the geographic region of the Caucasus, in Southeastern Europe, or whose ancestors were members of the hypothetical Indo-European cultures identified with the Caucuses.

caud-, a combining form meaning 'pertaining to a tail': *caudal, caudalward, caudocephalad.*

caudad /kô′dad/ [L, *cauda,* tail], toward the tail or end of the body, away from the head. Compare **cephalad.**

cauda equina [L, *cauda* + *equus,* horse], the lower end of the spinal cord at the first lumbar vertebra and the bundle of lumbar, sacral, and coccygeal nerve roots that emerge from the spinal cord and descend through the spinal canal of the sacrum and coccyx before reaching the intervertebral foramina of their particular vertebrae. The cauda equina looks like a horse's tail.

caudal /kô′dəl/, signifying a position toward the distal end of the body.

caudal anesthesia, the injection of a local anesthetic agent into the caudal portion of the spinal canal through the sacrum. It is performed in labor and in such procedures as culdoscopy and anorectal and genitourinary surgery. Complications of caudal anesthesia include infection, a high (5% to 10%) rate of failure, frequent neurologic complications, arterial hypotension, and, in obstetrics, reduced force of labor. See also **regional anesthesia.**

caudate /kô′dāt/, having a tail.

caudate lobe of the liver [L, *cauda,* tail; Gk, *lobos,* lobe; AS, *lifer*], a part of the right lobe of the liver that lies near the vena cava.

caudate nucleus [L, *cauda,* tail, *nucleus,* nut], a crescent-shaped mass of gray matter lateral to the thalamus in the floor of the anterior horn and body of the lateral ventricle.

caudate process [L, *cauda* + *processus,* projection], a small elevation of tissue that extends obliquely from the lower extremity of the caudate lobe of the liver to the visceral surface of the right lobe. It separates the fossa for the gallbladder from the beginning of the fossa for the inferior vena cava.

caudocephalad /kô′dōsef′əlad/ [L, *cauda,* tail; Gk, *kephale,* head; L, *ad,* toward], movement from the tail toward the head.

caul /kôl/ [ME, *cawel,* basket], the intact amniotic sac surrounding the fetus at birth. The sac usually ruptures or is ruptured during the course of labor or delivery; when it remains intact, it must be torn or cut to allow the baby to breathe. In the past, pieces of the caul were sold to sailors as a good luck token that would protect the bearer from death by drowning.

cauliflower ear [L, *caulis,* cabbage, *fiore,* flower; AS, *eare*], a thickened, deformed ear caused by repeated trauma, such as that suffered by boxers. Plastic surgery may be a means of restoring the normal appearance of the ear.

caumesthesia /kô′məsthē′zhə/ [Gk, *kauma,* heat, *aisthesis,* feeling], an abnormal condition in which a patient has a low temperature but experiences a sense of intense heat. **–caumesthetic,** *adj.*

caus-, caut-, a combining form meaning 'burn': *causalgia, cautery.*

causalgia /kôzal′jə/ [Gk, *kausis,* burning, *algos,* pain], a severe sensation of burning pain, often in an extremity, sometimes with local erythema of the skin. It is the result of injury to a peripheral sensory nerve.

causal hypothesis /kô′səl/ [L, *causa,* cause; Gk, *hypotithenia,* foundation], (in research) a hypothesis that predicts a cause-and-effect relationship among the variables to be studied.

causal hypothesis testing study, (in nursing research) an experimental design used in testing a hypothesis that predicts a cause-and-effect relationship within the data to be studied.

causality /kôsal′itē/, (in research) a relationship between one phenomenon or event (A) and another (B) in which A precedes and causes B and the direction of influence and the nature of the effect are predictable and reproducible and may be empirically observed. Causality is difficult to prove;

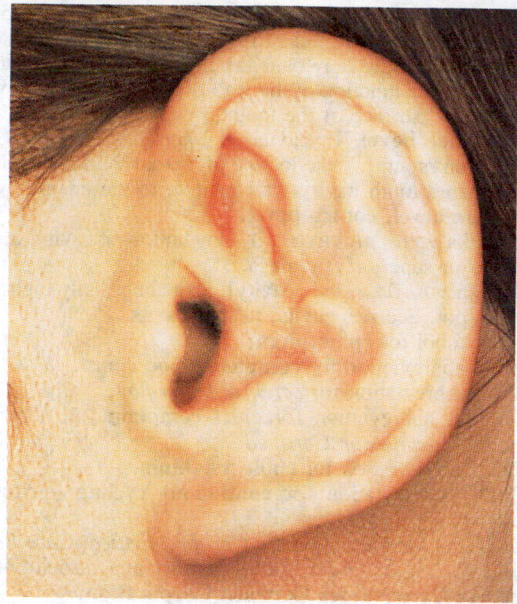

Cauliflower ear
*(Bingham, 1992/Courtesy Mouth Clinic, Sunnybrook Medical
Centre, Toronto)*

some social scientists contend that it is impossible to prove a causal relationship.

causal treatment. See **treatment.**

causation /kôsā'shən/ [L, *causa*], (in law) the existence of a reasonable connection between the misfeasance, malfeasance, or nonfeasance of the defendant and the injury or damage suffered by the plaintiff. In a lawsuit in which negligence is alleged, the harm suffered by the plaintiff must be proved to result directly from the negligence of the defendant; causation must be demonstrated.

cause [L, *causa*], any process, substance, or organism that produces an effect or condition.

CAUSN, abbreviation for **Canadian Association of University Schools of Nursing.**

caustic /kôs'tik/ [Gk, *kaustikos*, burning], **1.** any substance that is destructive to living tissue, such as silver nitrate, nitric acid, or sulfuric acid. **2.** exerting a burning or corrosive effect.

caustic poisoning, the accidental ingestion of strong acids or alkalis, resulting in burns and tissue damage to the mouth, esophagus, and stomach. The victim experiences immediate pain, swelling, and edema. The pulse may be weak and rapid. Respirations become shallow, and edema may close the airway. Complications of circulatory shock, perforation of the esophagus, and pharyngeal edema leading to asphyxia can be fatal. The victim should be hospitalized or seen by a physician immediately. Recommended first aid is dilution of the acid or alkali with copious amounts of water and removal of any clothing contaminated by the chemical. Administration of 'neutralizing' substances is not recommended because of the risk of a heat-producing chemical reaction. See also **acid burn, alkali burn.**

CAUT, abbreviation for **Canadian Association of University Teachers.**

cauterization /kô'tərīzā'shən/ [Gk, *kauterion*, branding

iron], the process of burning a part of the body by cautery.

cauterize /kô'tərīz/ [Gk, *kauterion*, branding iron], to burn tissues by thermal heat, including steam, hot metal, or solar radiation, or electricity or other agent, including dry ice, usually with the objective of destroying damaged or diseased tissues.

cautery /kô'tərē/ [Gk, *kauterion*, branding iron], **1.** a device or agent that scars and burns the skin, such as in the coagulation of tissue by heat or caustic substances. **2.** a destructive effect produced by a cauterizing agent.

cautery knife, a surgical knife that cuts tissue and cauterizes it to prevent bleeding. The knife is connected to an electric source that generates the heat necessary for cauterization.

cav-, a combining form meaning 'hollow': *cavascope, cavernome, cavity.*

cava. See **cavum.**

cavalry bone. See **rider's bone.**

Cavell Edith /kəvel'/, (1865–1915), an English nurse who trained at London Hospital. In 1907 she became the head of a nurses' training school in Brussels, with the task of raising nursing standards to match those of Britain. By 1912, the school offered a 3-year intensive course and was associated with four hospitals in Brussels. After the Germans occupied Belgium in World War I, she nursed or sheltered more than 200 fleeing soldiers and helped them reach Holland; to her, this was an extension of her nursing: helping those in need. She was arrested by the Germans, tried, and shot on October 12, 1915. Her execution, which she met with courage and fortitude, brought her widespread fame.

cavernoma. See **cavernous hemangioma.**

cavernous /kav'ərnəs/ [L, *caverna*, hollow place], containing cavities or hollow spaces. See also **cavernous hemangioma.**

cavernous angioma. See **cavernous hemangioma.**

cavernous body of the clitoris, cavernous body of the penis. See **corpus cavernosum.**

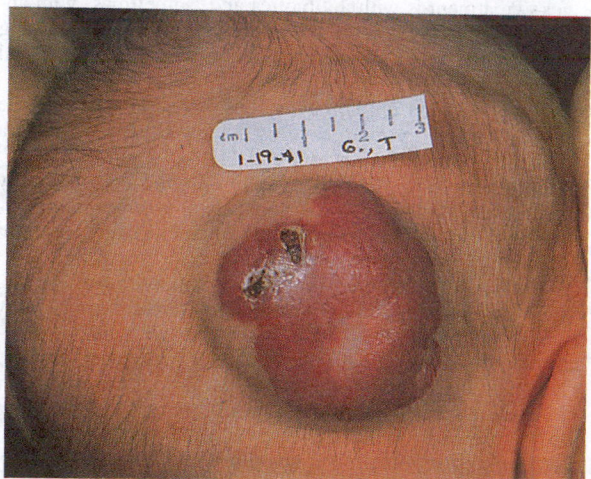

Cavernous hemangioma *(Baran, 1991)*

cavernous hemangioma [L, *caverna*, hollow place; Gk *haima*, blood, *oma*, tumor], a benign, congenital tumor consisting of large, blood-filled, cystic spaces. The scalp, face, and neck are the most common sites, but these tumors have been found in the liver and other organs. Superficial cavernous hemangiomas are friable and easily infected if the skin is broken. Treatment includes observation, irradiation, sclerosing solutions, and surgery. Also called **angioma cavernosum, cavernoma.** Compare **capillary hemangioma, nevus flammeus.**

cavernous lymphangioma. See **lymphangioma cavernosum.**

cavernous rale [L, *caverna* + Fr, rattle], an abnormal hollow, metallic sound heard during auscultation of the thorax. It is caused by contraction and expansion of a pulmonary cavity during respiration and indicates a pathologic condition.

cavernous sinus [L, *caverna* + *sinus,* curve], one of a pair of irregularly shaped, bilateral venous channels between the sphenoid bone of the skull and the dura mater. It is one of the five anterior inferior venous sinuses that drain the blood from the dura mater into the internal jugular vein. Like the other anterior inferior sinuses, the cavernous sinus has no valves. Coursing through the sinus are the oculomotor nerve, the trochlear nerve, the abducent nerve, the ophthalmic and the maxillary divisions of the trigeminal nerve, and the internal carotid artery. The cavernous sinus receives the superior and the inferior ophthalmic veins, some of the cerebral veins, and the sphenoparietal sinus, and joins the cavernous sinus from the opposite side through the intercavernous sinuses. The cavernous sinus drains into the inferior petrosal sinus, thence into the internal jugular vein.

cavernous sinus syndrome, an abnormal condition characterized by edema of the conjunctiva, the upper eyelid, and the root of the nose and by paralysis of the third, the fourth, and the sixth nerves. It is caused by a thrombosis of the cavernous sinus.

cavernous sinus thrombosis, a syndrome, usually secondary to infections near the eye or nose, characterized by orbital edema, venous congestion of the eye, and palsy of the nerves supplying the extraocular muscles. The infection may spread to involve the cerebrospinal fluid and meninges. Treatment is with antibiotics and, sometimes, with anticoagulants. Prevention includes avoidance of squeezing pimples and other skin lesions in the area of the nose and central face.

cavitary /kav′iter′ē/ [L, *cavus,* hollow], **1.** denoting the presence of one or more cavities. **2.** any entozoon having a body cavity or an alimentary canal.

cavitate /kav′itāt/ [L, *cavus,* hollow], the act of rapidly forming and collapsing vapor pockets or bubbles in a flowing fluid with low pressure areas, often causing damage to surrounding structures.

cavitation, 1. the formation of cavities within the body, such as those formed in the lung by tuberculosis. **2.** any cavity within the body, such as the pleural cavities.

cavity /kav′itē/ [L, *cavus*], **1.** a hollow space within a larger structure, such as the peritoneal cavity or the oral cavity. See also **body cavity. 2.** *nontechnical.* a space in a tooth formed by dental caries.

cavity classification, the taxonomy of carious lesions according to the tooth surfaces on which they occur, such as labial, buccal, or occlusal; type of surface, such as pitted or smooth; numeric designation of cavity type according to the classification proposed by G.V. Black. See also **artificial classification cavity.**

cavogram /kav′əgram′/ [L, *cavus* + Gk, *gramma,* record], an angiogram of the inferior or superior vena cava.

cavosurface angle /kāv′ōsur′fəs/, (in dentistry) the angle formed by the junction of the wall of a prepared cavity with the external surface of the tooth.

cavosurface bevel [L, cavus + *superficies,* surface; OFr, *baif,* open mouth], the incline of the cavosurface angle of a pre pared tooth cavity wall relative to the enamel wall. Compare **bevel, contra bevel.**

cavum /kā′vəm/, *pl.* **cava, 1.** any hollow or cavity. **2.** the inferior or superior vena cava.

cavus /kā′vəs/ [L, *cavus,* cavity], an abnormally high arch of the foot. See **pes cavus, talipes cavus.**

Cb, symbol for **columbium.**

CBC, abbreviation for **complete blood count.**

CBF, abbreviation for *cerebral blood flow.*

C.C., 1. abbreviation for **chief complaint. 2.** abbreviation for *Commission Certified.*

CCK, abbreviation for **cholecystokinin.**

CCPD, abbreviation for **continuous cycling peritoneal dialysis.**

CCRN, 1. abbreviation for *Certified Critical Care Registered Nurse;* **2.** trademark of **American Association of Critical-Care Nurses Certified Corporation.**

CCU, abbreviation for **coronary care unit.**

Cd, symbol for the element **cadmium.**

CD, abbreviation for **compact disk.**

CDC, abbreviation for **Centers for Disease Control and Prevention.**

CDE, 1. the major symbols used in one system for the nomenclature of the Rh system, in which D is the same as RhO, the major determining factor of Rh positivity. **2.** abbreviation for **common duct exploration.**

CD4, symbol for a glycoprotein expressed on the surface of most thymocytes and some lymphocytes, including Helper T cells. Human CD4 is the receptor that serves as a docking site for HIV viruses on certain lymphocyte cells. Binding of the viral glycoprotein gp120 to CD4 is the first step in viral entry, leading to the fusion of viral and cell membranes.

CD4 cell count, a method of analyzing the prognosis of HIV-infected patients. As the virus binds to CD4 and kills T cells bearing this antigen, the level of CD4 helper T cells in the blood is an indicator of the progress of the infection. The CD4 cell count helps measure effectiveness of clinical trials of HIV antiviral drugs and the CD4 count in a patient can be reinforced by administering doses of the antigen.

CD8, symbol for peripheral lymphocyte T cells that secrete large amounts of gamma-interferon, a lymphokine involved in the body's defense against viruses. Whereas CD4 T cells produce mainly lymphokine interleukin 2 (IL2), an autocrine and paracrine T-cell growth factor, preactivated or memory CD4 T cells secrete a much larger array of lymphokines upon restimulation. CD4 and CD8 lymphocytes carry out different functions during immune reactions partly because of distinct patterns of lymphokines secreted upon stimulation. Also called **cytotoxic T cells.**

CD/ROM, abbreviation for **compact disk/read only memory.**

Ce, symbol for the element **cerium.**

CEA, abbreviation for **carcinoembryonic antigen.**

ceasmic /sē·az′mik/ [Gk *keazein* to split], pertaining to or characterized by a persistent embryonic fissure or abnormal cleavage of parts.

ceasmic teratism [Gk, *keazein* + *teras*, monster], a congenital anomaly, caused by developmental arrest, in which parts of the body that should be fused remain in their fissured embryonic state, such as in cleft palate.

cec-, a combining form meaning 'pertaining to a cecum': *cecitis, cecectomy, cecoplication.*

cecal /sē′kəl/ [L, *caecus*, blind (gut)], **1.** of or pertaining to the cecum. **2.** of or pertaining to the optic disc or the blind spot in the retina. Also spelled **caecal.**

cecal appendix. See **vermiform appendix.**

Ceclor, a trademark for a cephalosporin antibiotic (cefaclor).

cecocolostomy /sē′kōkəlos′təmē/ [L, *caecus*, blind (gut); Gk, *kolon*, colon, *stoma*, mouth], **1.** a surgical operation that creates an anastomosis between the cecum and the colon. **2.** the anastomosis produced by this operation.

cecofixation. See **cecopexy.**

cecoileostomy /-il′ē·os′təmē/ [L, *caecus* + *ilia*, intestine, *stoma*, mouth], a surgical operation that connects the ileum with the cecum. Also called **ileocecostomy** /il′ē·ōsēkos′təmē/.

cecopexy /sē′kōpek′sē/ [L, caecus + Gk, *pexis*, fix], a surgical operation that fixes or suspends the cecum to correct its excessive mobility. Also called **cecofixation.**

cecostomy /sēkos′təmē/ [L, *caecus* + Gk, *stoma*, mouth], the surgical construction of an opening into the cecum, performed as a temporary measure to relieve intestinal obstruction in a patient who cannot tolerate major surgery. Twenty-four hours before surgery, if time permits, a low residue diet is given, with only clear liquids allowed. Cleansing enemas and antibiotics are prescribed to reduce the number of bacteria in the bowel. IV fluids and electrolytes are given, and a nasointestinal tube is inserted. With the patient under local anesthesia, a tube is inserted into the cecum to allow drainage of feces. The procedure may also be done to decompress the large bowel and prevent distention until peristalsis is restored after intestinal surgery. Postoperatively, the tube is connected to a drainage bottle. The nurse irrigates the cecostomy tube with saline solution as necessary, allowing the solution to flow in and out by gravity, if possible. Frequent changes of dressings are needed to keep the skin clean and dry. An ileostomy bag may be used. When edema and inflammation have subsided, the obstruction (usually cancer) is resected, the healthy sections of bowel reconnected, and the cecostomy closed. See also **abdominal surgery, intestinal obstruction.**

cecum /sē′kəm/ [L, *caecus*, blind (gut)], a cul-de-sac constituting the first part of the large intestine. It joins the ileum, the last segment of the small intestine.

CED, abbreviation for *Certified Diabetes Educator.*

Cedilanid-D, a trademark for a cardiac glycoside (deslanoside).

CeeNU, a trademark for an antineoplastic (lomustine).

cef-, a combining form designating a cephalosporin.

cefaclor /sē′fəklôr/, a cephalosporin antibiotic.

■ INDICATIONS: It is prescribed in the treatment of certain infections.

■ CONTRAINDICATIONS: Known hypersensitivity to cephalosporins prohibits its use. It is administered with caution to patients who have a history of allergy to penicillin.

■ ADVERSE EFFECTS: Among the most serious adverse reactions are hypersensitivity reactions and severe diarrhea, nausea, and vomiting.

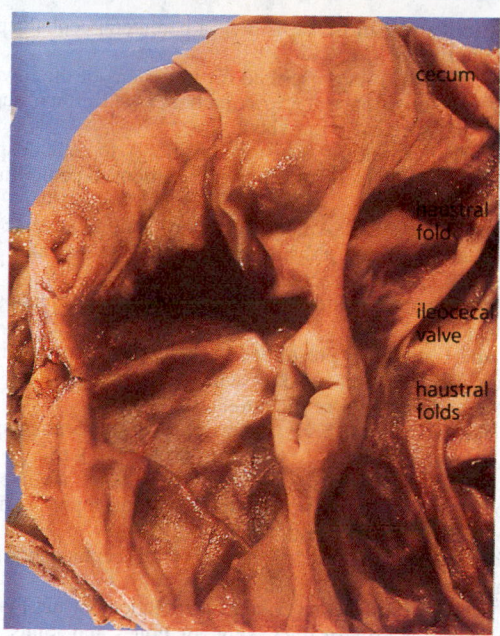

Cecum *(Mitros, 1988)*

cefadroxil monohydrate /sē′fədrok′sil/, a cephalosporin antibiotic.

■ INDICATIONS: It is prescribed in the treatment of certain bacterial infections.

■ CONTRAINDICATIONS: Known hypersensitivity to cephalosporins prohibits its use. It is administered with caution to patients with a history of allergy to penicillins.

■ ADVERSE EFFECTS: Among the most serious adverse reactions are hypersensitivity reactions and severe diarrhea, nausea, and vomiting.

Cefadyl, a trademark for an antibiotic (cephapirin).

cefamandole nafate /sēfəman′dōlnaf′āt/, a cephalosporin antibiotic.

■ INDICATIONS: It is prescribed in the treatment of certain bacterial infections.

■ CONTRAINDICATIONS: Known hypersensitivity to cephalosporins prohibits its use. It is administered with caution to patients who have a history of allergy to penicillin.

■ ADVERSE EFFECTS: Among the most serious adverse reactions are various hypersensitivity reactions, phlebitis, suprainfection, and pain on intramuscular injection.

cefazolin sodium /sēfaz′olin/, a cephalosporin antibacterial.

■ INDICATIONS: It is prescribed in the treatment of a variety of infections.

■ CONTRAINDICATIONS: Known hypersensitivity to this drug or to any cephalosporin medication prohibits its use. It is used with caution in patients who are allergic to penicillin.

■ ADVERSE EFFECTS: Among the more serious adverse reactions are pain at the site of injection and hypersensitivity reactions.

Cefizox, a trademark for a cephalosporin antibiotic (ceftizoxime).

Cefobid, a trademark for a cephalosporin antibiotic (cefoperazone).

cefonicid sodium /sēfon′isid/,   a parenteral cephalosporin-type antibiotic.
■ INDICATIONS: It is prescribed for infections of the lower respiratory or urinary tract, skin, bones and joints, septicemia, and surgical prophylaxis.
■ CONTRAINDICATIONS: A history of allergy to cephalosporins or acute anaphylactic or urticarial reactions to penicillin prohibits its use.
■ ADVERSE EFFECTS: Among the more serious adverse reactions are pain and phlebitis at the injection site and, occasionally, allergic reactions and GI effects.

cefoperazone sodium /sē′fōper′əzōn/,   a cephalosporin antibiotic.
■ INDICATIONS: It is prescribed in the treatment of respiratory tract, intraabdominal, skin, and female genital tract infections and bacterial septicemia.
■ CONTRAINDICATIONS: Hypersensitvity to the cephalosporins or known sensitivity to this drug prohibits its use.
■ ADVERSE EFFECTS: Among the most serious adverse reactions are pruritus, urticaria, transient eosinophilia, neutropenia, and injection site reactions.

ceforanide /sefôr′ənīd/,   a parenteral cephalosporin-type antibiotic.
■ INDICATIONS: It is prescribed for infections of the lower respiratory or urinary tract, skin, or bones and joints, septicemia, endocarditis, and surgical prophylaxis.
■ CONTRAINDICATIONS: A history of allergy to cephalosporins or acute anaphylactic or urticarial reactions to penicillin prohibit its use.
■ ADVERSE EFFECTS: Among the more serious adverse reactions are allergic reactions and GI effects.

cefotaxime sodium /sēfōtak′zēm/,   a cephalosporin antibiotic.
■ INDICATIONS: It is prescribed for lower respiratory tract, genitourinary, gynecologic, intraabdominal, skin, bone and joint, and central nervous system infections caused by susceptible strains of microorganisms.
■ CONTRAINDICATIONS: Hypersensitivity to the cephalosporins or known hypersensitivity to this drug prohibits its use.
■ ADVERSE EFFECTS: The most serious adverse reactions are pruritus, colitis, fungal infections, and injection site reactions.

cefotetan disodium /sē′fōtet′ən/,   a cephalosporin antibiotic for parenteral administration.
■ INDICATIONS: It is prescribed for infections of the lower respiratory tract, urinary tract, skin, abdomen, bones or joints, reproductive organs, or surgical prophylaxis.
■ CONTRAINDICATIONS: This drug is contraindicated for patients who are hypersensitive to cefotetan or to other cephalosporin antibiotics.
■ ADVERSE EFFECTS: Among adverse reactions reported are skin rash, diarrhea, eosinophillia, positive Coombs test results, and elevated liver enzyme levels.

Cefotan,   a trademark for a cephalosporin antibiotic (cefotetan disodium).

cefoxitin sodium /sēfok′sitin/,   a cephalosporin antibiotic.
■ INDICATIONS: It is prescribed in the treatment of certain bacterial infections.
■ CONTRAINDICATIONS: Known hypersensitivity to cephalosporins prohibits its use. It is administered with caution to patients who have a history of allergy to penicillin.
■ ADVERSE EFFECTS: Among the most serious adverse reactions are various hypersensitivity reactions, phlebitis, suprainfection, and pain on intramuscular injection.

ceftazidime /seftaz′idēm/,   a cephalosporin-type parenteral antibiotic.
■ INDICATIONS: It is prescribed for treatment of infections of the lower respiratory tract, urinary tract, skin, abdomen, blood, bones and joints, and central nervous system.
■ CONTRAINDICATIONS: This drug is contraindicated in pa tients who are hypersensitive to this product or to other cephalosporin antibiotics.
■ ADVERSE EFFECTS: Among adverse reactions reported are pruritis, fever, skin rash, diarrhea, eosinophilia, thrombocytosis, phlebitis, discomfort at the site of injection, and positive Coombs test result.

ceftizoxime sodium /sef′tizok′zēm/,   a cephalosporin antibiotic.
■ INDICATIONS: It is prescribed in the treatment of several bacterial infections.
■ CONTRAINDICATIONS: Known sensitivity to this drug prohibits its use. It is administered with caution to patients who are allergic to penicillin.
■ ADVERSE EFFECTS: Among the most serious adverse reactions are hypersensitivity reactions, neutropenia, leukopenia, thrombocytopenia, and pain at the injection site.

ceftriaxone sodium /sef′trī·ak′sōn/,   a cephalosporin-type parenteral antibiotic.
■ INDICATIONS: It is prescribed for infections of the lower respiratory tract, urinary tract, skin, abdomen, bones, and joints. It is also used to treat gonorrhea, septicemia, and meningitis, and for surgical prophylaxis, particularly in coronary bypass operations.
■ CONTRAINDICATIONS: Ceftriaxone sodium is contraindicated in patients who are hypersensitive to this product or to other cephalosporin antibiotics.
■ ADVERSE EFFECTS: Among reported adverse reactions are skin rash, diarrhea, eosinophilia, thrombocytosis, leukopenia, increased liver enzyme and blood urea nitrogen levels, and pain and tenderness at the site of injection.

cefuroxime sodium /sef′ōōrok′zēm/,   a cephalosporin antibiotic.
■ INDICATIONS: It is prescribed in the treatment of lower respiratory tract, urinary tract, skin, and gonococcal infections, bacterial septicemia, meningitis, and for the prevention of postoperative infections.
■ CONTRAINDICATIONS: Hypersensitivity to the cephalosporins or known sensitivity to this drug prohibits its use.
■ ADVERSE EFFECTS: Among the most serious adverse reactions are pruritus, urticaria, transient eosinophilia, neutropenia, leukopenia, and injection site reactions.

cel-, coel-,   1. a combining form meaning 'a cavity of the body': *celarium, celoschisis, celozoic.* 2. a combining form meaning 'a swelling or tumor, hernia': *celectome, celology, celosomia.*

-cele,   a suffix meaning 'relating to a hernia or swelling': *rectocele, cystocele.*

cele 2.   See **coel.**

-cele, -coel, -coele   a combining form meaning a 'cavity': *paracele, orchidocele, syringocele.*

Celestone,   a trademark for a glucocorticoid (betamethasone).

celiac /sē′lē·ak/ [Gk, *koilia,* belly],   pertaining to the abdominal cavity.

celiac artery [Gk, *koilia,* belly; *arteria,* air pipe],   a thick visceral branch of the abdominal aorta, arising caudal to the diaphragm, usually dividing into the left gastric, the common hepatic, and the splenic arteries.

celiac disease [Gk, *koilia* + L, *dis,* opposite of; Fr, *aise,* ease],   an inborn error of metabolism characterized by the inability to hydrolyze peptides contained in gluten. The disease affects adults and young children, who suffer from abdominal distention, vomiting, diarrhea, muscle wasting, and extreme lethargy. A characteristic sign is a pale, foul-smelling stool that floats on water because of its high fat content. There may be a secondary lactose intolerance, and it may become necessary to eliminate all milk products from the diet. Most patients respond well to a high-protein, high-calorie, gluten-free diet. Rice and corn are good substitutes for wheat, and any vitamin or mineral deficiencies can be corrected with oral preparations. Prognosis for full recovery is excellent. Failure to respond generally indicates misdiagnosis. Also called **celiac sprue, gluten-induced enteropathy, nontropical sprue.** Compare **malabsorption syndrome.**

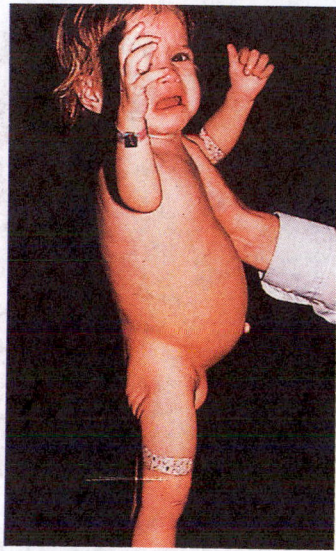

Celiac disease *(Zitelli, 1992)*

celiac plexus. See **solar plexus.**
celiac rickets [Gk, *koilia* + *rhachis,* spine, *itis,* inflammation],   arrested growth and osseous deformities resulting from malabsorption of fat and calcium. See also **celiac disease, rickets.**
celiac sprue. See **celiac disease.**
celio-,   a prefix meaning 'pertaining to the abdomen': *celioma, celiopathy, celiorrhaphy.*
celio-, -celo, cel-, coel-,   a combining form meaning 'pertaining to the belly or abdominal area': *celioscope, celiac, coelom,* relating to hernias or hollow structures.
celiocolpotomy /sē′lē·ōkəlpot′əmē/ [Gk, *koilia* + *kolpos,* vagina, *temnein,* to cut],   an incision into the abdomen through the vagina.
celioma /sē′lē·ō′mə/, *pl.* **celiomas, celiomata** [Gk, *koilia* + *oma,* tumor],   an abdominal neoplasm, especially a mesothelial tumor of the peritoneum.
celioscope. See **laparoscope.**
celiothelioma /sē′lē·ōthē′lē·ō′mə/, *pl.* **celiotheliomas, celiotheliomata,**   a mesothelioma of the abdomen.

cell [L *cella* storeroom],   the fundamental unit of all living tissue. Eukaryotic cells consist of a nucleus, cytoplasm, and organelles surrounded by a cytoplasmic membrane. Within the nucleus are the nucleolus (containing RNA) and chromatin granules (containing protein and DNA) that develop into chromosomes, the determinants of hereditary characteristics. Organelles within the cytoplasm include the endoplasmic reticulum, ribosomes, the Golgi complex, mitochondria, lysosomes, and the centrosome. Prokaryotic cells are similar but lack a nucleus. The specialized nature of body tissue reflects the specialized structure and function of its constituent cells. See also **cell theory.**

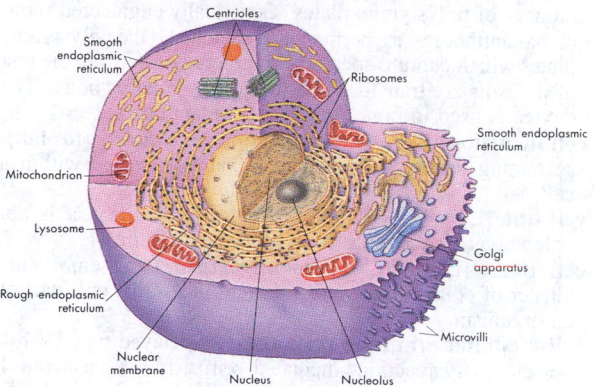

Cell *(Thibodeau, 1993/William Ober)*

cella /sel′ə/, *pl.* cellae [L, storeroom,   an enclosed space.
cell biology,   the science that deals with the structures, living processes, and functions of cells, especially human cells.
cell body [L, *cella* + AS, *bodig*],   the part of a cell that contains the nucleus and surrounding cytoplasm exclusive of any projections or processes, such as the axon and dendrites of a neuron or the tail of a spermatozoon. This enlarged area is concerned more with the metabolism of the cell than with a specific function.
cell culture [L, *cella,*   storeroom, *colere,* to cultivate], living cells that are maintained in vitro in artificial media of serum and nutrients for the study and growth of certain strains or for experiments in controlling diseases, such as cancer.
cell cycle,   the sequence of events that occurs during the growth and division of tissue cells.
cell death,   1. terminal failure of a cell to maintain the essential life functions. **2.** the point in the process of dying at which vital functions have ceased at the cellular level.
cell division,   the continuous process by which a cell divides in four stages; prophase, metaphase, anaphase, and telophase. Preliminary to prophase, the centrosome of the cell divides into two parts, which become oriented at opposite poles of the nucleus. During the prophase, previously dispersed chromatin condenses into chromomeres strung along a threadlike chromonema composed of deoxyribonucleic acid. The chromonema then condenses into compact chromosomes. During metaphase, the chromosomes become oriented in the equatorial plane with a clear area directed toward the two centrosomes. Each chromosome meanwhile has doubled into chromatids attached to each

other at the centromere. Each centromere divides during late metaphase and early anaphase. In telophase, the chromosomes form a compact mass, lose their individuality, and disperse into the chromatin of the intermitotic nucleus. Cell division does not occur in discrete steps; each phase is part of a continuous process that may require hours to complete. The cycle of cell division includes an interphase period during which new DNA, RNA, and protein molecules are synthesized before the start of the next prophase. Also called **mitosis.** Compare **meiosis.**

cellae.   See **cella.**

Cellector,   trademark for a device that modifies human blood cells by circulating them through a box containing a number of polystyrene plates. Genetically engineered monclonal antibodies are permanently attached o the polystyrene plates which capture specifically targeted cells while the rest of the cells are transfused back into the patient's body. The device is used in bone marrow transplant cases.

cell inclusion [L, *cella,* storeroom + *in, claudere,* to shut], pertaining to any foreign matter that is enclosed within a cell.

cell line [L, *cella + linea*],   a colony of animal cells developed as a subculture from a primary culture.

cell mass [L, *cella,* storeroom, *massa*],   the embryonic cluster of cells that develops into an individual or a part of an organism.

cell-mediated immune response,   a delayed type IV hypersensitivity reaction, mediated primarily by sensitized T cell lymphocytes as opposed to antibodies. Cell-mediated immune reactions are responsible for defense against certain bacterial, fungal, and viral pathogens, malignant cells, and other foreign protein or tissue. Also called **cellular hypersensitivity reaction, type IV hypersensitivity.** Compare **anaphylactic hypersensitivity, immune complex hypersensitivity.**

cell-mediated immunity.   See **cellular immunity.**

cell membrane,   the outer covering of a cell, often having projecting microvilli and containing the cellular cytoplasm. The cell membrane is so thin and delicate that it is barely visible with a light microscope and can be studied in detail only with an electron microscope. The membrane controls the exchange of materials between the cell and its environment by various processes, such as osmosis, phagocytosis, pinocytosis, and secretion. Also called **plasma membrane.**

cell of Corti.   See **auditory hair.**

cell organelle [L, *cella,* storeroom; Gk, *organon,* instrument],   any of a number of membrane-bound structures within a cell that have specific functions, such as reproduction or metabolism. Examples include mitochondria and Golgi bodies.

cells of Paneth /pä′nət, pan′əth/ [Josef Paneth, Austrian physiologist, b. 1857],   large granular epithelial cells found in intestinal glands. They secrete digestive enzymes. Also called **Davidoff's cells.**

cell theory,   the proposition that cells are the basic units of all living substance and that cellular function is the essential process of life.

cellular /sel′yələr/ [L, *cella,* storeroom],   pertaining to or consisting of cells.

cellular hypersensitivity reaction.   See **cell-mediated immune response.**

cellular immunity [L, *cellula,* little cell; *immunis,* exempt], the mechanism of acquired immunity characterized by the dominant role of small T cell lymphocytes. Cellular immunity is involved in resistance to infectious diseases caused by viruses and some bacteria, in delayed hypersensitivity reactions, some aspects of resistance to cancer, certain autoimmune diseases, graft rejection, and certain allergies. Also called **cell-mediated immunity.** Compare **humoral immunity.**

cellular infiltration,   the migration and grouping of cells within tissues throughout the body.

cellulitis /sel′yəlī′tis/ [L, *cellula,* little cell; Gk, *itis,* inflammation],   a diffuse, acute infection of the skin and subcutaneous tissue characterized most commonly by local heat, redness, pain, and swelling, and occasionally by fever, malaise, chills, and headache. Abscess and tissue destruction usually follow if antibiotics are not taken. The infection is more likely to develop in the presence of damaged skin, poor circulation, or diabetes mellitus. In addition to appropriate antibiotics, treatment includes warm soaks, elevation, and avoidance of pressure to the affected areas.

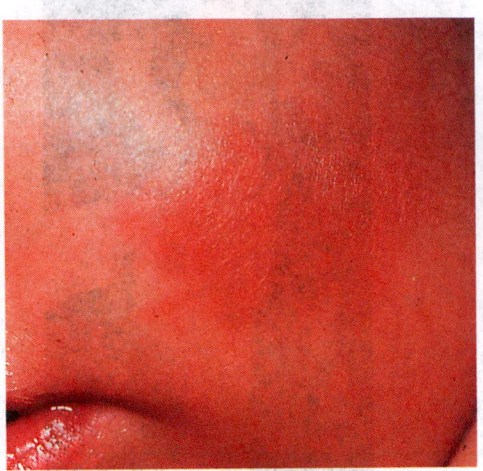

Cellulitis *(Zitelli, 1992)*

cellulose /sel′yōōlōs/ [L, *cellula,* little cell],   a colorless, insoluble, nondigestible, transparent solid carbohydrate that is the primary constituent of the skeletal substances of the cell walls of plants. In the diet it provides the bulk necessary for proper digestive tract functioning. Rich sources are fruits, such as apples and bananas, and legumes, bran, and green vegetables, especially celery. See also **dietary fiber.**

cell wall,   the structure that covers and protects the cell membrane in some kinds of cells, such as certain bacteria and all plant cells. The cell walls of plant cells are composed of cellulose.

celom.   See **coelom.**

celomic.   See **coelom.**

Celontin,   a trademark for an anticonvulsant (methsuximide).

celosomia /sē′ləsō′mē·ə/ [Gk, *kele,* hernia, *soma,* body], a congenital malformation characterized by a fissure or absence of the sternum and ribs and protrusion of the viscera.

celosomus /sē′ləsō′məs/,   a fetus with celosomia.

celothelioma.   See **mesothelioma.**

Celsius (C) /sel′sē·əs/ [Anders Celsius, Swedish scientist, b. 1701],   denoting a temperature scale in which 0° is the freezing point of water and 100° is the boiling point of water at sea level. Also called **centigrade.** Compare **Fahrenheit.**

Celsius thermometer. See **Celsius.**

cement /siment'/ [L, *caementum,* rough stone], **1.** a sticky or mucilaginous substance that helps neighboring tissue cells stick together. **2.** any of a variety of dental materials used to fill cavities or to hold bridgework or other dental prostheses in place. **3.** a material used in the fixation of a prosthetic joint in adjacent bone, such as methyl methacrylate.

cemental fiber /simen'təl/ [L, *caementum,* rough stone; *fibra*], any one of the many fibers of the periodontal membrane that extend from the cementum to the intermediate plexus, where their terminations are mixed with those of the alveolar fibers.

cement base, (in dentistry) a layer of insulated dental cement, sometimes medicated, pressed into the bottom of a prepared cavity to protect the pulp, to reduce the bulk of metallic restoration, or eliminate undercuts in a tapered preparation.

cementifying fibroma /-ifī'ing/ [L, *caementum* + *facere,* to make; *fibra,* fiber; Gk, *oma,* tumor], **1.** an intrabony lesion composed of fibrous connective tissue enclosing foci of calcified material resembling cementum. **2.** a rare odontogenic tumor composed of vary ing amounts of fibrous connective tissue resembling cementum. **3.** central jaw lesion.

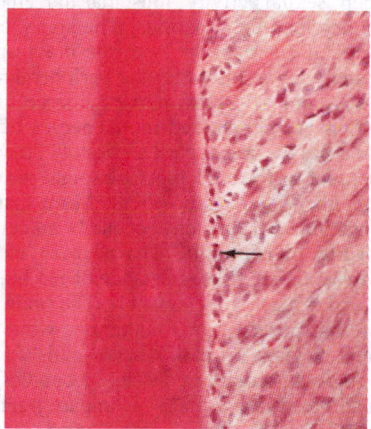

Layer of cementoblasts (arrows) lining the cementum *(Berkovitz, 1992)*

cementoblast /simen'təblast/, (in dentistry), a large squamous or cuboidal cell that is responsible for the formation of cementum on the root dentin of a developing tooth.

cementoblastoma /simen'tōblastō'mə/, *pl.* cementoblastomas, cementoblastomata [L, *caementum* + Gk, *blastos,* germ, *oma,* tumor], an odontogenic fibrous tumor consisting of cells developing into cementoblasts but containing only a small amount of calcified tissue.

cementoma /sē'mentō'mə/, *pl.* **cementomas, cementomata** [L, *caementum* + Gk, *oma,* tumor], an accumulation of cementum existing free at the apex of a tooth, probably caused by trauma rather than neoplastic growth.

cementopathia /-ōpath'ē·ə/ [L, *caementum* + Gk, *pathos,* disease], an abnormal condition of the teeth caused by necrotic cementum and insufficient cementogenesis. Cementopathia is implicated in periodontitis and periodontosis.

cementum /simen'təm/, the bonelike connective tissue that covers the roots of the teeth and helps to support them in the alveolar bone.

cen, abbreviation for **centromere.**

cen-, a combining form meaning 'common': *cenadelphus, cenesthesia, cenesthopathia.*

CEN, abbreviation for *Certified Emergency Nurse.*

cenesthesia /sē'nesthē'zhə/ [Gk, *kenos,* empty, *aisthesis,* feeling], the general sense of existing, derived as the aggregate of all the various stimuli and reactions throughout the body at any specific moment to produce a feeling of health or of illness. Also called **cenesthesis, coenesthesis.**

ceno-, a combining form meaning 'new': *cenogenesis, cenophobia, cenopsychic.*

cenogenesis /sē'nōjen'əsis/ [Gk, *kenos,* empty, *genein,* to produce], the development of structural characteristics that are absent in earlier forms of a species, as an adaptive response to environmental conditions. Also spelled **coenogenesis, caenogenesis, kenogenesis.** Compare **palingenesis. –cenogenetic, coenogenetic, caenogenetic,** *adj.*

ceno-, a prefix meaning 'new, empty, or having a common feature': *cenogenesis, cenagonous.*

cenophobia. See **kenophobia.**

censor [L, *censere,* to assess], **1.** a person who monitors or evaluates books, newspapers, plays, works of art, speech, or other means of expression in order to suppress certain kinds of information. **2.** (in psychoanalysis) a psychic suppression that allows unconscious thoughts to rise to consciousness only if they are heavily disguised.

cente-, a combining form meaning 'puncture': *centesis.*

center [Gk, *kentron*], **1.** the middle point of the body or geometric entity, equidistant from points on the periphery. **2.** a group of neurons with a common function, such as the accelerating center in the brain that controls the heartbeat.

center of gravity, the midpoint or center of the weight of a body or object. In the standing adult human the center of gravity is in the midpelvic cavity, between the symphysis pubis and the umbilicus.

Centers for Disease Control and Prevention (CDC), a federal agency of the U.S. government that provides facilities and services for the investigation, identification, prevention, and control of disease. It is concerned with all aspects of the epidemiology and the laboratory diagnosis of disease. Immunization programs, quarantine regulations and programs, laboratory standards, and community surveillance for disease are among the activities of the CDC, which is located in Atlanta. Many state and local health workers and scientists receive training in specific techniques there. Originally, the Communicable Disease Center, it was concerned only with communicable diseases; today its interests include environmental health, smoking, malnutrition, poisoning, and issues in occupational health. The name was changed again in 1992 when 'and Prevention' was added.

centesis /sentē'sis/ [Gk, *kentesis,* pricking], a perforation or a puncture of a cavity, such as paracentesis, abdominocentesis, or thoracocentesis.

centi-, a combining form meaning 'a hundred or a hundredth': *centibar, centiliter, centipoise.*

centigrade. See **Celsius.**

centimeter (cm) /sen'timē'tər/ [L, *centum,* hundred; Gk, *metron,* measure], the metric unit of measurement equal to one hundredth of a meter, or 0.3937 inches.

centimeter-gram-second system (cgs, CGS), the internationally accepted scientific system of expressing length, mass, and time in basic units of centimeters, grams, and seconds. The CGS system is gradually being replaced by the Systeme International d'Unités (SI) or the International System of Units, based on the meter, kilogram, and second.

centipede bite /sen'təpēd/ [L, *centum*, hundred, *pes,* foot], a wound produced by the poison claws and the first body segment of a centipede, an elongate arthropod with many pairs of legs. The bite of a few species, including *Scolopendra morsitans* in the southern United States, may cause painful local inflammation, fever, headache, vomiting, and dizziness.

centipoise /sen'təpois/ [Jean L. M. Poiseuille, French physiologist, b. 1799], a measure of the viscosity of a liquid, equal to one hundredth of a poise. The centipoise of glycerine is 1490 centipoise, compared with 1.005 centipoise for water.

central [Gk, *kentron*, center], pertaining to or situated at a center.

central amaurosis [Gk, *kentron; amauroein,* to darken], blindness caused by a disease of the central nervous system.

central auditory processing disorder (CAPD), difficulty in processing and interpreting auditory stimuli in the absence of a peripheral hearing loss, usually resulting from a problem in the brainstem or cerebral cortex. Children with CAPD often have difficulty reading and may exhibit other learning disabilities as well.

central canal of spinal cord [Gk, *kentron; L, canalis,* channel], the conduit that runs the entire length of the spinal cord and contains most of the 140 ml of cerebrospinal fluid in the body of the average individual. The central canal of the spinal cord lies in the center of the cord between the ventral and the dorsal gray commissures and extends cranialward into the medulla oblongata, where it opens into the fourth ventricle of the brain. Caudalward, the canal runs into the filum terminale after forming a triangular, fusiform dilatation about 10 mm long in the conus medullaris. Cerebrospinal fluid flows into the canal from the fourth ventricle of the brain, into the subarachnoid space around the spinal cord, and into the subarachnoid space around the brain. Subarachnoid hemorrhage may form blood clots that block drainage of the cerebrospinal fluid from the subarachnoid space. Lumbar puncture, often performed to obtain samples of cerebrospinal fluid for diagnostic purposes, draws fluid from the subarachnoid space around the spinal cord and not from the central canal. See also **lumbar puncture.**

central catheter [Gk, *kentron,* central, *katheter,* a thing lowered into], a catheter inserted into either a central artery or a central vein for diagnostic or therapeutic procedures.

central chemoreceptor, any of the sensory nerve cells or chemical receptors that are located in the medulla of the brain. Also called **medullary chemoreceptor.**

central chondrosarcoma [Gk, *kentron; chondros,* cartilage, *sarx* flesh, *oma* tumor], a malignant cartilaginous tumor that forms inside a bone. Also called **enchondrosarcoma.**

central deafness. See **central auditory processing disorder.**

central electrode, a key part of a radiation detection instrument. It consists of a positively charged rigid wire in the center of a gas-filled cylinder. The electrode attracts electrons liberated by ionization effects of radiation and converts them into an electric current.

central fissure. See **central sulcus.**

central implantation. See **superficial implantation.**

central line, an intravenous line inserted for continuous access to a central vein for administering fluids and medicines and for obtaining diagnostic information. Keeping the central line in place ensures accessibility to the venous system in case the veins collapse.

central lobe, one of the lobes constituting each of the cerebral hemispheres, lying hidden in the depths of the lateral sulcus. The central lobe can be seen only if the lips of the sulcus are parted or cut away. The lips of the lateral sulcus are parts of the frontal, the parietal, and the temporal lobes and are separated by the rami of the lateral sulcus, thus constituting the frontal, the parietal, and the temporal opercula. With the opercula cut away, the insula appears as a triangular area with the limen insulae as the apex. Also called **island of Reil.** Compare **frontal lobe, occipital lobe, parietal lobe, temporal lobe.**

central necrosis [Gk, *kentron,* central, *nekros,* dead, *osis,* condition], death of the central part of a tissue or organ.

central nervous system (CNS) [Gk, *kentron; L, nervus,* nerve; Gk, *systema*], one of the two main divisions of the nervous system of the body, consisting of the brain and the spinal cord. The central nervous system processes information to and from the peripheral nervous system and is the main network of coordination and control for the entire body. The brain controls many functions and sensations, such as sleep, sexual activity, muscular movement, hunger, thirst, memory, and the emotions. The spinal cord extends various types of nerve fibers from the brain and acts as a switching and relay terminal for the peripheral nervous system. The 12 pairs of cranial nerves emerge directly from the brain. Sensory nerves and motor nerves of the peripheral system leave the spinal cord separately between the vertebrae but unite to form 31 pairs of spinal nerves containing sensory fibers and motor fibers. More than 10 billion neurons constitute but one tenth of the brain cells, the other cells consisting of neuroglia. The neurons and the neuroglia form the soft, jellylike substance of the brain, which is supported and protected by the skull. The brain and the spinal cord are composed of gray matter and white matter. The gray matter contains primarily nerve cells and associated processes; the white matter consists of bundles of predominantly myelinated nerve fibers. Compare **peripheral nervous system.** See also **brain, spinal cord.**

central nervous system depressant, any drug that decreases the function of the central nervous system, such as alcohol, barbiturates, and hypnotics. Such drugs can produce tolerance, physical dependence, and compulsive drug use. The compulsive use of barbiturates, benzodiazepines, and related drugs varies greatly and is believed to exceed that of the opiates. Depressants, especially the benzodiazepines, are the most widely prescribed drugs throughout the world. These substances depress excitable tissue throughout the central nervous system by stabilizing neuronal membranes, decreasing the amount of transmitter released by the nerve impulse, and generally depressing postsynaptic responsiveness and ion movement. The central nervous system is more affected by alcohol than any other body system, with effects generally proportional to the concentration of alcohol in the blood. Central nervous system depressants elevate the seizure threshold and can produce physical dependence in a relatively short period of time. All depressants are subject to abuse, particularly through the use of

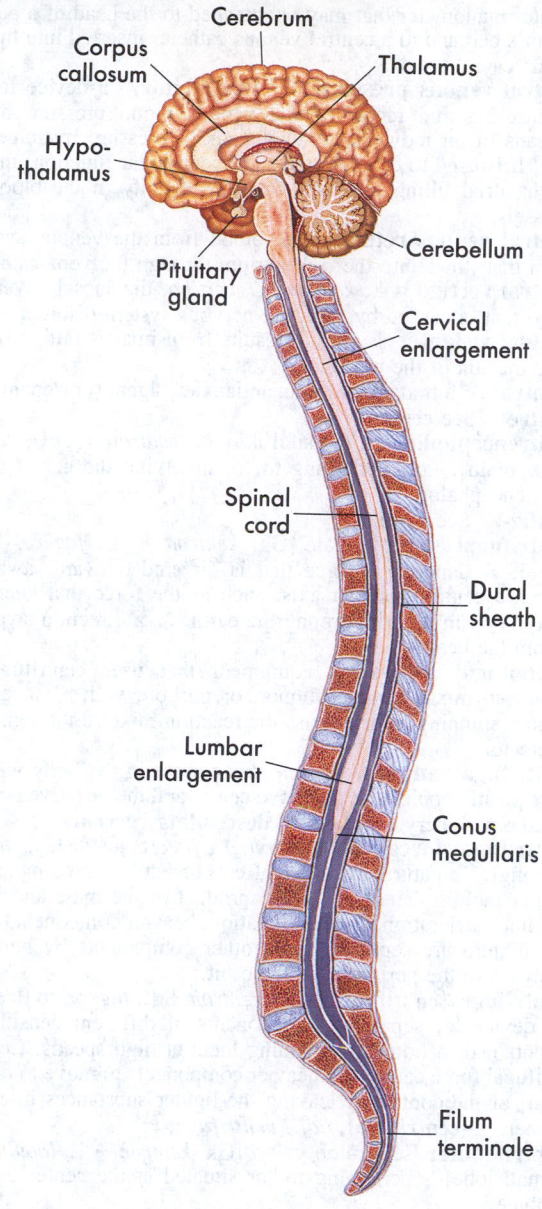

Central nervous system (Chipps, 1992)

illicitly procured depressants. The most abused depressants are the short-acting barbiturates, especially pentobarbital, secobarbital, glutethimide, methyprylon, and methaqualone. These substances have popular street names on the illicit market, such as 'reds' (secobarbital) and 'yellows' (pentobarbital). Sudden withdrawal of general central nervous system depressants that have been used in high doses for prolonged periods can be fatal to some individuals. Withdrawal treatment commonly involves the substitution of pentobarbital or diazepam administered orally to produce a stabilization level followed by gradual reduction in dosage for a period of 10 days to 3 weeks.

central nervous system stimulant, a substance that quickens the activity of the central nervous system by increasing the rate of neuronal discharge or by blocking an inhibitory neurotransmitter. Many natural and synthetic compounds stimulate the central nervous system, but only a few are used therapeutically. Caffeine, a potent central nervous system stimulant, is used to help restore mental alertness and overcome respiratory depression, but it may cause nausea, nervousness, tinnitus, tremor, tachycardia, extra systoles, diuresis, and visual disturbances. Amphetamines, sympathomimetic amines with central nervous system stimulating activity, are employed in treating narcolepsy and obesity, but these drugs have a high potential for abuse and may cause dizziness, restlessness, tachycardia, increased blood pressure, headache, mouth dryness, an unpleasant taste, GI symptoms, and urticaria. Various amphetamines, especially methylphenidate, and deanol acetamidobenzoate, a precursor of acetylcholine, are prescribed for the hyperkinetic child syndrome because central nervous system stimulants may act as depressants on children. Doxapram, ethamivan, and nikethamide are used to stimulate the respiratory center and restore consciousness after anesthesia or in the treatment of acute sedative-hypnotic intoxication. Flurothyl is employed in convulsive therapy in psychiatry. Also called **analeptic.**

central nervous system syndrome (CNS syndrome), a constellation of neurologic and emotional signs and symptoms that results from a massive whole-body dosage of radiation. The syndrome includes hysteria and disorientation, increasing during the last 24 to 48 hours before death.

central nervous system tumor, a neoplasm of the brain or spinal cord that characteristically does not spread beyond the cerebrospinal axis, although it may be highly invasive locally and have widespread effects on body functions. Intracranial neoplasms are about four times more common than those arising in the spinal cord. From 20% to 40% of brain tumors are metastatic lesions from primary cancer in the breast, lung, GI tract, kidney, or a site of melanoma. See also **brain tumor, spinal cord tumor.**

central neurogenic hyperventilation (CNHV) [Gk, *kentron; neuron*, nerve, *genein*, to produce], a pattern of breathing marked by rapid and regular ventilations at a rate of about 25 per minute. Increasing regularity, rather than rate, is an important diagnostic sign because it indicates an increasing depth of coma.

central pain [Gk, *kentron*; L, *poena*, penalty], pain caused by a lesion in centrally located nerve tissue.

central paralysis [Gk, *kentron, paralyein*, to be palsied], paralysis caused by a lesion in the central nervous system.

central placenta previa [Gk, *kentron*; L, flat cake; *praevius*, preceding], placenta previa in which the placenta is implanted in the lower segment of the uterus and completely covers the internal os of the uterine cervix. In labor, as the cervix dilates, the placenta is gradually separated from the underlying blood vessels in the uterine lining, resulting in bleeding that usually begins slowly, is painless, and progresses to hemorrhage that is life-threatening to the mother and the baby. Cesarean section is usually performed to save the mother and the baby. The condition may be discovered by ultrasound visualization before any bleeding occurs or by digital palpation in the normal course of prenatal care. Also called **complete previa.** See also **placenta previa.**

central processing unit (cpu, CPU), a component of a computer that controls the encoding and execution of instructions, consisting mainly of an arithmetic unit, which performs arithmetic functions, and an internal memory, which controls the sequencing of operations. Also called **processor.**

central ray (CR), the portion of the x-ray beam that is directed toward the center of the film or of the object being radiographed.

central scotoma [Gk, *kentron; skotos,* darkness, *oma,* tumor], an area of blindness or site of depressed vision involving the macula of the retina.

central sleep apnea, a form of sleep apnea resulting from a decreased respiratory center output. It may involve primary brainstem medullary depression resulting from a tumor of the posterior fossa, poliomyelitis, or idiopathic central hypoventilation.

central stimulant. See **central nervous system stimulant.**

central sulcus [Gk, *kentron;* L, furrow], a cleft separating the frontal from the parietal lobes of brain. Also called **central fissure, fissure of Rolando.**

central tendon, a broad connective tissue sheet that forms the diaphragm. It is composed of interlacing fibers that arise from the lumbar vertebrae, the costal margin, and the xiphoid process of the sternum.

central venous catheter, a catheter that is threaded through the internal jugular, antecubital, or subclavian vein, usually with the tip resting in the superior vena cava or the right atrium.

central venous oxygen saturation (CVSo$_2$), the oxygen saturation in the vena cava. The CVSo$_2$ is measured through a central venous catheter and is useful in measuring cardiac output. A reading of less than 55% usually indicates a falling cardiac output and probable cardiac failure.

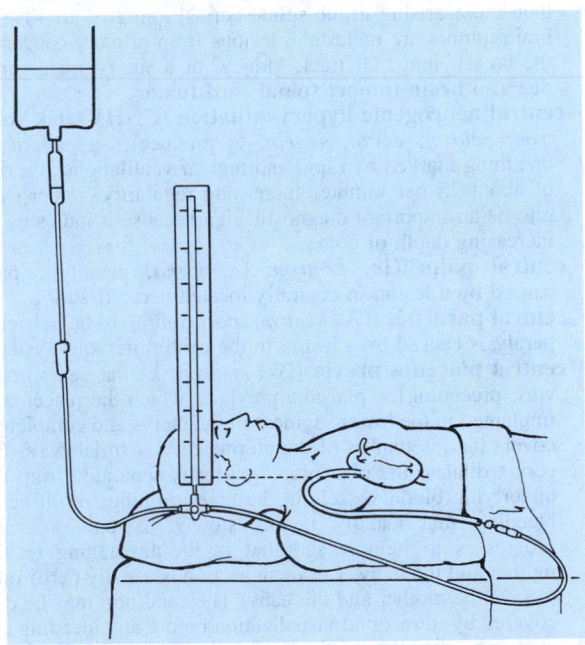

Measurement of central venous pressure

central venous pressure (CVP), the blood pressure in the large veins of the body, as distinguished from peripheral venous pressure in an extremity. It is measured with a water manometer that may be attached to the head of a patient's bed and to a central venous catheter inserted into the vena cava.

central venous pressure (CVP) monitor, a device for measuring and recording the venous blood pressure by means of an indwelling catheter and a pressure manometer. It is used to evaluate the right ventricular function, the right atrial filling pressure, and the capacity of the blood vessels.

central venous return, the blood from the venous system that flows into the right atrium through the vena cava.

central vertigo [Gk, *kentron;* L, *vertigo,* dizziness], vertigo that is caused by a central nervous system disorder.

central vision, vision that results from images falling on the macula of the retina.

Centrax, a trademark for an antianxiety agent (prazepam).

centre. See **center.**

centrencephalic /sen'trensifal'ik/ [Gk, *kentron* + *enkephalos,* brain], of, pertaining to, or involving the center of the encephalon.

centri-. See **centro-.**

centrifugal /sentrif'ŏŏgəl/ [Gk, *kentron* + L, *fugere,* to flee], **1.** denoting a force that is directed outward, away from a central point or axis, such as the force that keeps the moon in its orbit around the earth. **2.** a direction away from the head.

centrifugal analyzer, equipment that uses centrifugal force to mix a sample aliquot, or portion, with a reagent and a spinning rotor to pass the reaction mixture through a detector.

centrifugal current, an electric current in the body with the positive pole near the nerve center and the negative pole at the periphery. Also called **descending current.**

centrifugal force [Gk, *kentron;* L, *fugere,* to flee, *fortis,* strong], a natural force that affects objects undergoing circular motion. The force is the product of the mass and its radial acceleration. In centrifugation, heavier components of a mixture are separated from other components by being thrown to the periphery of the orbit.

centrifuge /sen'trifyŏŏj'/ [Gk, *kentron* + L, *fugere,* to flee], a device for separating components of different densities contained in liquid by spinning them at high speeds. Centrifugal force causes the heavier components to move to one part of the container, leaving the lighter substances in another. —**centrifugal,** *adj., ***centrifuge,** *v.*

centrilobular /sen'trəlob'yələr/ [Gk, *kentron* + L, *lobulus,* small lobe], pertaining to, or situated at the center of a lobule.

centriole /sen'trē·ōl'/ [Gk, *kentron*], an intracellular organelle, usually as a component of the centrosome. Often occurring in pairs, centrioles are associated with cell division and can be closely studied only with an electron microscope; under a light microscope the centrioles appear as tiny dots. They are actually tiny cylinders positioned at right angles to each other, with walls consisting of nine bundles of fine tubules, three tubules to a bundle. The centriole measures approximately 150 nm by 300 nm to 500 nm. Numerous centrioles occur in some large cells, such as the giant cells in bone marrow. The precise function of centrioles is still a mystery, but they appear to aid in the formation of the spindle that develops during mitosis.

centripetal /sentrip'ətəl/ [Gk, *kentron* + L, *petere,* to seek], **1.** denoting an afferent direction, such as that of a sensory nerve impulse traveling toward the brain. **2.** denoting the direction of a force pulling an object toward an axis of rotation or constraining an object to a specific curved path.

centripetal current, an electric current passing through the body from a peripheral positive electrode to a negative pole near the nerve center. Also called **ascending current.**

centripetal force, (in radiology) a 'center-seeking' electrical force that holds electrons in their orbits about the nucleus of an atom. The centripetal force exactly balances the electron velocity so that electrons normally maintain a constant distance from the nucleus.

centro-, centri-, a combining form meaning 'center, central, to the center': *centrocecal, centrocinesia, centrosclerosis.*

centromere /sen′trəmir/ [Gk, *kentron* + *meros,* part], the specialized, constricted region of the chromosome that joins the two chromatids to each other and attaches to the spindle fiber in mitosis and meiosis. During cell division the centromeres split longitudinally, half going to each of the new daughter chromosomes. The position of the centromere is constant for a specific chromosome and is identified accordingly as acrocentric, metacentric, submetacentric, or telocentric. Also called **kinetochore, kinomere, primary constriction. –centromeric,** *adj.*

centrosome [Gk, *kentron* + *soma,* body], a self-propagating cytoplasmic organelle present in animal cells and in those of some lower plants. The structure, which consists of the centrosphere and the centrioles, is located near the nucleus and functions as the dynamic center of the cell, especially during mitosis. Also called **cytocentrum, microcentrum, paranuclear body.**

centrosphere [Gk, *kentron* + *sphaira,* ball], the differentiated, condensed area of cytoplasm surrounding the centrioles in the centrosome of the cell.

centrum, *pl.* centra [L; Gk, *kentron*], any kind of center, especially one related to a structure of the body, as the centrum semiovale of a cerebral hemisphere.

CEO, C.E.O., abbreviation for **Chief Executive Officer.**

cephal-. See **cephalo.**

cephalad /sef′əlad/ [Gk, *kephale,* head], toward the head, away from the ends, or tail. Compare **caudad.**

cephalalgia /sef′əlal′jə/ [Gk, *kephale,* head, *algos,* pain], headache, often combined with another word to indicate a specific type of headache, such as histamine cephalalgia. Also called **cephalgia.** See also **histamine headache.**

cephalexin /sef′əlek′sin/, a cephalosporin antibacterial.

■ INDICATIONS: It is prescribed orally in the treatment of certain infections.

■ CONTRAINDICATIONS: Known hypersensitivity to this drug or to any cephalosporin medication prohibits its use. It is used with caution in patients who are allergic to penicillin.

■ ADVERSE EFFECTS: Nausea, diarrhea, and hypersensitivity reactions may occur.

cephalgia. See **cephalalgia, headache.**

cephalhematoma /sef′əlhē′mətō′mə, -hem′ətō′mə/, swelling caused by subcutaneous bleeding and accumulation of blood. It may begin to form in the scalp of a fetus during labor and enlarge slowly in the first few days after birth. It is usually a result of trauma, often from forceps. Large cephalhematomas may become infected, require surgical drainage, and take several months to resolve. Compare **caput succedaneum, molding.**

-cephalia, -cephaly, a suffixm meaning a specified '(condition of the) head': *hemicephalia, megacephalia, notancephalia.*

cephalic /sifal′ik/, of or pertaining to the head.

-cephalic, a suffix meaning 'relating to the head': *holocephalic, megalocephalic, postcephalic.*

cephalic index [Gk, *kephale,* head, *index,* pointer], a ratio between the breadth and length of the head. It is calculated as 100 times the maximum breadth of the head measured at the greatest diameter of the cranial vault above the supramastoid crest divided by the maximum length measured from the most prominent point on the glabella to the opisthocranion.

cephalic presentation, a classification of fetal position in which the head of the fetus is at the uterine cervix. Cephalic presentation is usually further qualified by an indication of the part of the head presenting, such as the occiput, bregma, or mentum.

cephalic vein, one of the four superficial veins of the upper limb. It begins in the dorsal venous network of the hand and winds upward to end in the axillary vein just caudal to the clavicle. It receives deoxygenated blood from the dorsal and the palmar surfaces of the forearm. Just distal to the antecubital fossa, it has a wide anastomosis with the median cubital vein. In the proximal third of the arm it passes between the pectoralis major and the deltoideus where it is accompanied by the thoracoacromial artery. Compare **basilic vein, dorsal digital vein, median antebrachial vein.**

cephalo-, cephal-, a combining form meaning 'pertaining to the head': *cephalocaudal, cephalocentesis, cephalogenesis.*

cephalocaudal /sef′əlōkô′dəl/ [Gk, *kephale* + L, *cauda,* tail], pertaining to the long axis of the body, or the relationship between the head and the base of the spine. Also called **cephalocercal** /sef′əlōsur′kəl/.

cephalomelus /sef′əlom′ələs/ [Gk, *kephale* + *melos,* limb], a deformed individual with a structure resembling an arm or a leg protruding from the head.

cephalometry /-ətrē/, scientific measurement of the head, such as that performed in dentistry to determine appropriate orthodontic procedures for correcting malocclusions and other abnormal conditions. **–cephalometric,** *adj.*

cephalopagus. See **craniopagus.**

cephalopelvic /-pel′vik/, pertaining to a relationship between the fetal head and the maternal pelvis.

cephalopelvic disproportion (CPD) [Gk, *kephale* + L, *pelvis,* basin; *dis,* opposite of, *proportio,* similarity], an obstetric condition in which a baby's head is too large or a mother's birth canal too small to permit normal labor or birth. In **relative CPD,** the size of the baby's head is within normal limits but larger than average or the size of the mother's birth canal is within normal limits but smaller than average, or both; relative CPD is often overcome by molding of the head, the forces of labor, or by the use of forceps to effect delivery. In **absolute CPD,** the baby's head is markedly or abnormally enlarged or the mother's birth canal is markedly or abnormally contracted, making vaginal delivery impossible. See also **clinical pelvimetry, x-ray pelvimetry.**

cephaloridine /sef′əlôr′idēn/, a cephalosporin antibiotic.

■ INDICATIONS: It is prescribed in the treatment of a variety of infections.

■ CONTRAINDICATIONS: Concurrent administration of medications causing nephrotoxicity or known hypersensitivity to this drug or to cephalosporin medication prohibits its use. It is used with caution in patients who are allergic to penicillin.

■ ADVERSE EFFECTS: Among the more serious adverse reac-

tions are nephrotoxicity, pain at the site of injection, and hypersensitivity reactions.

cephalosporin /sef′əlōspôr′in/ [Gk, *kephale* + *sporos*, seed], a semisynthetic derivative of an antibiotic originally derived from the microorganism *Cephalosporium acremonium.* Cephalosporins are similar in structure to penicillins except for a beta-lactam-dihydrothiazine ring in place of beta-lactam-thiazolidin in penicillin.

cephalosporinase. See **beta-lactamase.**

cephalothin sodium /sef′əlō′thin/, a cephalosporin antibacterial.

■ INDICATIONS: It is prescribed in the treatment of a variety of infections.

■ CONTRAINDICATIONS: Known hypersensitivity to this drug or to any cephalosporin medication prohibits its use. It is used with caution in patients who are allergic to penicillin.

■ ADVERSE EFFECTS: Among the more serious adverse reactions are pain at the site of injection and hypersensitivity reactions.

cephalothoracoiliopagus. See **synadelphus.**

cephalothoracopagus /sef′əlōthôr′əkop′əgəs/ [Gk, *kephale,* + *thorax,* chest, *pagos,* joined], a conjoined twin fetal monster united at the head, neck, and thorax.

-cephaly, -cephalia, a combining form meaning a '(specified) condition of the head': *macrencephaly, platycephaly, trochocephaly.*

cephapirin /sef′əprin/, an antibiotic.

■ INDICATIONS: It is prescribed in the treatment of infections caused by cephapirin-susceptible strains of a wide variety of microorganisms causing septicemia, endocarditis, osteomyelitis, and infections of the respiratory tract, urinary tract, and skin.

■ CONTRAINDICATION: Known sensitivity to cephalosporin antibiotics prohibits its use.

■ ADVERSE EFFECTS: Among the most serious adverse reactions are neutropenia, leukopenia, anemia, and allergic reactions.

cephradine /sef′rədēn/, a cephalosporin antibacterial.

■ INDICATIONS: It is prescribed in the treatment of certain bacterial infections.

■ CONTRAINDICATIONS: Known hypersensitivity to this drug or to any cephalosporin medication prohibits its use. It is used with caution in patients who are allergic to penicillin.

■ ADVERSE EFFECTS: Nausea, diarrhea, and hypersensitivity reactions may occur.

cer-, a combining form meaning 'wax': *ceraceous, cerate, cerumen.*

ceramics /səram′iks/, (in dentistry) the technology of making dental restorations from fused porcelain and other glasses.

cerato-, kerato-, a combining form meaning 'pertaining to the cornea or to horny tissue': *ceratocricoid, ceratohyal, ceratopharyngeus.*

cercaria /sərker′ē·ə/, pl. **cercariae** [Gk, *kerkos,* tail], a minute, wormlike early developmental form of trematode. It develops in a freshwater snail, is released into the water, and swims toward the sun, rising to the surface of the water in the warmest part of the day. Cercariae enter the body of the next host by ingestion, by direct invasion through the skin, or through a cut or other break in the skin. Some cercariae of the genera *Schistosoma, Chlonorchis, Paragonimus, Fasciolopsis,* and *Fasciola* are known to infect humans. They encyst and complete their development in various organs of the body. Each species tends to migrate to

one organ, such as *Fasciola hepatica,* which grows to become a liver fluke. See also **fluke, schistosomiasis.**

cerclage /serkläzh′/ [Fr, cask hooping], **1.** an orthopedic procedure in which the ends of an oblique bone fracture or the chips of a broken patella are bound together with a wire loop or a metal band to hold the bone fragments in position until healed. **2.** a procedure in which a taut silicone band is applied around the sclera to restore contact between the retina and the choroid when the retina is detached. **3.** an obstetric procedure in which a nonabsorbable suture is used for holding the cervix closed to prevent spontaneous abortion in a woman who has an incompetent cervix. The band is usually released when the pregnancy is at full term to allow labor to begin. See also **incompetent cervix.**

cerea flexibilitas /sirē′ə flek′sibil′itas/ [L, waxlike flexibility], a cataleptic state, frequently observed in catatonic schizophrenia, in which the limbs retain for an indefinite period of time the positions in which they are placed. Also called **flexibilitas cerea, waxy flexibility.** See **catalepsy.**

cerebella. See **cerebellum.**

cerebellar /ser′əbel′ər/ [L, *cerebellum,* small brain], of or pertaining to the cerebellum.

cerebellar angioblastoma [L, *cerebellum;* Gk, *aggeion,* vessel, *blastos,* germ, *oma*], a cystic tumor in the cerebellum composed of a mass of blood vessels. It is frequently associated with von Hippel-Lindau disease.

cerebellar artery occlusion, an obstruction of one of the arteries supplying the cerebellum. It can result in ipsilateral ataxia, facial analgesia, contralateral hemiparesis, and loss of temperature and pain sensations.

cerebellar ataxia [L, *cerebellum,* small brain; Gk, *ataxia,* lack of order], a loss of muscle coordination caused by a lesion in the cerebellum.

cerebellar atrophy [L, *cerebellum;* Gk, *a, trophe,* not nourishment], deterioration and wasting of tissues of the cerebellum. Causes of the condition include nutritional/metabolic factors, such as alcohol abuse, or degenerative disease. See also **spinocerebellar disorder.**

cerebellar cortex, the superficial gray matter of the cerebellum covering the white substance in the medullary core and consisting of two layers, an external molecular layer and an internal granule cell layer. The layers are separated by an incomplete stratum of Purkinje cells. Also called **cortical substance of cerebellum.**

cerebellar gait [L, *cerebellum,* small brain, ONorse, *geta,* a way], a staggering gait in which the person walks with a wide base and has difficulty turning. The feet are thrown outward and the person comes down first on the heel and then on the toes. The condition is caused by a lesion in the cerebellum or cerebellar pathways. Also called **ataxic gait.**

cerebellar inferior peduncle [L, *cerebellum,* small brain, *inferior,* lower, *pes,* foot], a band of nerve fibers that forms the lateral boundary of the bottom part of the fourth ventricle and carries afferent fibers into the cerebellum.

cerebellar middle peduncle [L, *cerebellum,* small brain, *medius, pes,* foot], a lateral extension of the transverse nerve fibers of the pons. It consists mainly of fibers from the pontine nuclei to the neocerebellum.

cerebellar speech [L, *cerebellum;* AS, *spaec*], abnormal speech seen in diseases of the cerebellum. It is characterized by slow, jerky, and slurred articulation that may be intermittent and explosive or monotonous and unvaried in pitch. Also called **ataxic speech.**

cerebellar superior peduncle [L, *cerebellum*, small brain, *superior*, *pes*, foot], a band of nerve fibers that pass from the cerebellum on either side of the superior medullary velum. It includes nerve tracts linking the dentate nucleus to the red nucleus of the midbrain and to the thalamus.

cerebellar tremor [L, *cerebellum*, small brain + *tremor*, shaking], an intention tremor or trembling during voluntary movements, due to lesions in the cerebellum. Also called **Hunt's tremor**.

cerebellopontine /ser′əbel′ōpon′tīn/ [L, *cerebellum* + *pons*, bridge], leading from the cerebellum to the pons varolii.

cerebellospinal /ser′əbel′ōspī′nəl/ [L, *cerebellum* + *spina*, backbone], leading from the cerebellum to the spinal cord.

cerebellum /ser′əbel′əm/, *pl.* **cerebellums, cerebella** [L, small brain], the part of the brain located in the posterior cranial fossa behind the brainstem. It consists of two lateral cerebellar hemispheres, or lobes, and a middle section called the vermis. Three pairs of peduncles link it with the brain stem. Its functions are concerned with coordinating voluntary muscular activity.

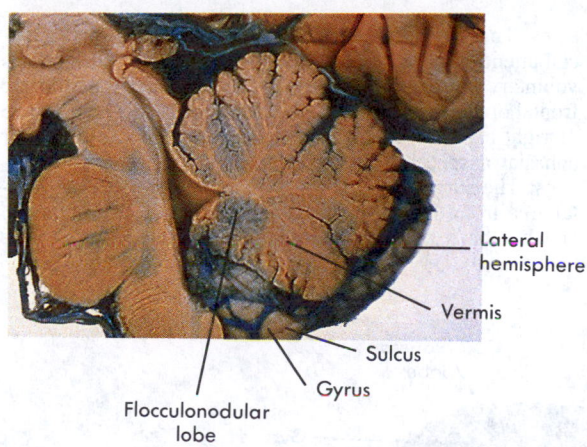

Lateral hemisphere

Vermis

Sulcus

Gyrus

Flocculonodular lobe

Cerebellum *(Seeley, 1992/RT Hutchings)*

cerebr-, prefix meaning 'pertaining to the cerebrum': *cerebralgia, cerebrocardiac, cerebropathy*.

cerebra. See **cerebrum**.

cerebral /ser′əbrəl, sərē′brəl/, of or pertaining to the cerebrum.

-cerebral, a suffix referring to the brain: *craniocerebral, medicerebral, postcerebral*.

cerebral abscess. See **brain abscess**.

cerebral aneurysm [L, *cerebrum*, brain; Gk, *aneurysma*, widening], an abnormal localized dilatation of a cerebral artery, most commonly the result of congenital weakness of the media or muscle layer of the vessel wall. Cerebral aneurysms may also be caused by infection, such as subacute bacterial endocarditis or syphilis, and by neoplasms, arteriosclerosis, and trauma. The most frequent sites are the middle cerebral, internal carotid, basilar, and anterior cerebral arteries, especially at bifurcations of vessels. Cerebral aneurysms may occur in infancy or old age and may be fusiform dilatations of the entire circumference of an artery or saccular outcroppings of the side of a vessel, which may be as small as a pinhead or as large as an orange but are usually the size of a pea.

■ OBSERVATIONS: Depending on its size and site, a cerebral aneurysm may cause headache, drowsiness, confusion, vertigo, facial weakness and pain, tinnitus, visual impairment, neck stiffness, and monoplegia or hemiplegia. Because a cerebral aneurysm may rupture, the patient is closely monitored for signs of subarachnoid hemorrhage and increased intracranial pressure. Few aneurysms rupture that are less than 1 cm in diameter.

■ INTERVENTIONS: The patient is placed in a bed, in which the head is raised at a 45-degree angle, and is maintained in a quiet, darkened environment. Antifibrinolytic, analgesic, anticonvulsant, antiemetic, or antihypertensive medication, steroids, and parenteral fluids may be administered as ordered. The pulse, blood pressure, respiration, and neurologic status of the patient are checked frequently. Any sudden change in blood pressure or pupillary response is reported promptly. An ice bag may be applied to relieve headache, and hypothermia or cooling measures may be indicated to reduce blood flow to the brain and decrease the risk of rupture of the aneurysm. The patient is turned gently every 2 to 4 hours and may need to be fed. Passive range of motion exercises to the extremities are performed to maintain function. A lumbar puncture, which can reveal rupture of the aneurysm if there is blood in the cerebrospinal fluid, and an angiogram, to show the site of the lesion, may be ordered; the contrast medium for angiography can be injected into the carotid artery, but placement in a femoral artery is preferred because there is less risk of dislodging a carotid plaque. Surgery, if indicated, involves a craniotomy and the application of a silver clip to the neck of the aneurysm or the use of an electric current to produce thrombosis. If the base of the aneurysm is too large to be ligated, a coating containing methyl methacrylate may be applied to support the weakened artery. When craniotomy is contraindicated, the neurosurgeon may apply a special clamp to a common carotid artery to reduce blood flow to the site of the aneurysm if collateral vessels can supply enough blood to maintain vital brain functions.

■ NURSING CONSIDERATIONS: The patient with a cerebral aneurysm requires intensive care and as little stress as possible. The nurse limits the number of visitors and the length of visits but involves the family in the patient's care and instructions. The patient is almost certain to be anxious about the possibility of rupture of the aneurysm and resultant neu-

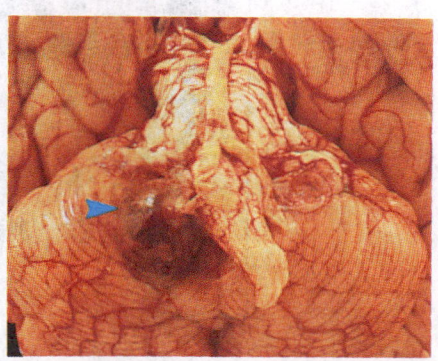

Cerebral aneurysm *(Fletcher, 1987)*

rologic problems. This concern may be anticipated by the nurse in order to help the patient express the fear and adapt to the situation.

cerebral angiography [L, *cerebrum*, brain; Gk, *angeion*, vessel + *graphein*, to record], an radiographic procedure used to visualize the vascular system of the brain after injection of a radiopaque contrast medium. **cerebral anoxia,** a condition in which oxygen is deficient in brain tissue. This state, which is caused by circulatory failure, can exist for no more than 4 to 6 minutes before the onset of irreversible brain damage.

cerebral aqueduct [L, *cerebrum; aqueductus,* water canal], the narrow conduit, between the third and the fourth ventricles in the midbrain, that conveys the cerebrospinal fluid. Also called **aqueduct of Sylvius.**

cerebral compression [L, *cerebrum*, brain, *comprimere*, to press together], any abnormal condition, such as hemorrhage, abscess, or tumor, that increases intracranial pressure. If untreated, the compression destroys the brain tissues and causes herniation of the brain. Also called **brain compression.**

cerebral cortex [L, *cerebrum; cortex,* bark], a thin layer of gray matter on the surface of the cerebral hemisphere, folded into gyri with about two thirds of its area buried in fissures. It integrates higher mental functions, general movement, visceral functions, perception, and behavioral reactions. It has been classified many different ways, with reference according to supposed phylogenetic and ontogenetic differences, structure, cell, and fiber layers, and function areas. Research has described more than 200 areas on the basis of differences in myelinated fiber patterns and has defined 47 separate function areas with different cell de-

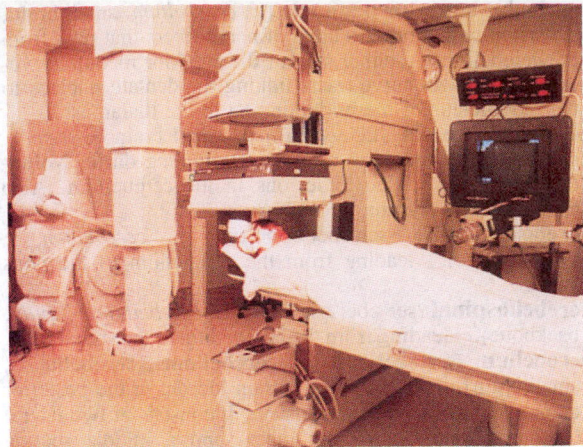

Positioning of patient for cerebral angiography
(Chipps, 1992)

signs. The precentral cortex or motor area has received special attention because its stimulation with electrodes causes voluntary muscle contractions. A motor speech area in the frontal operculum is better developed in the left hemisphere of right-handed persons, and its destruction causes motor aphasia or speech defects despite healthy, intact vocal organs. The surgical operation of lobotomy isolates the frontal area from the rest of the brain, especially the thalamus, and has been used in the treatment of severe psychoses.

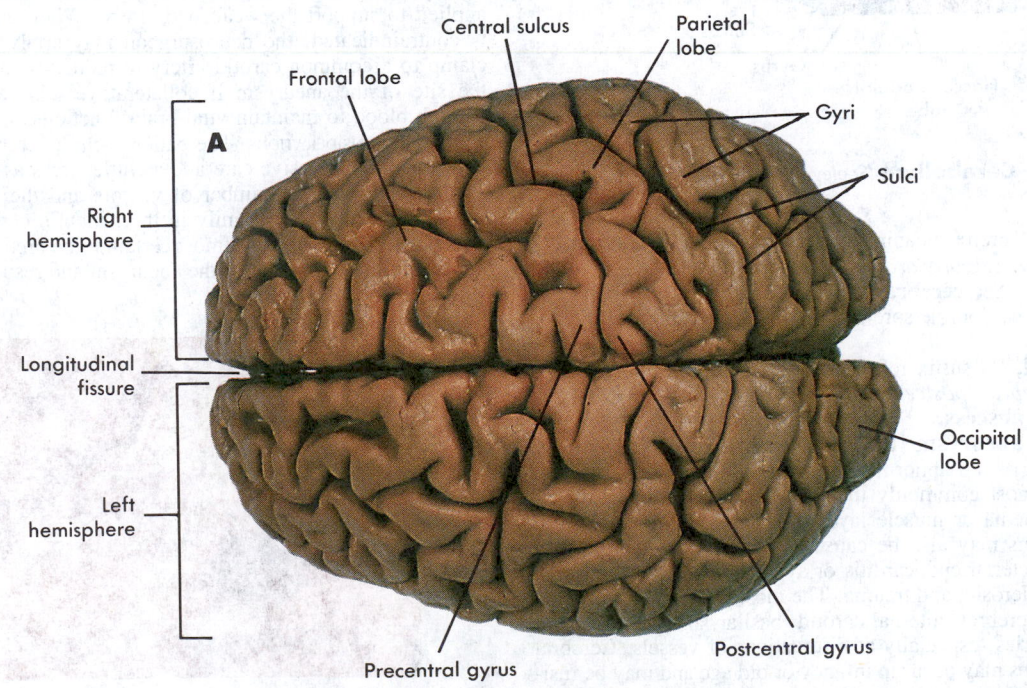

Cerebral cortex, superior view *(Seeley, 1992/RT Hutchings)*

Stimulation of the frontal area affects circulation, respiration, pupillary reaction, and other visceral activity. Also called **pallium.**

cerebral deafness. See **central auditory processing disorder.**

cerebral depressant [L, *cerebrum*, brain, *deprimere*, to press down], a drug or other agent that has a sedating effect on the brain, reducing activity and alertness, and, in some instances, causing a loss of consciousness.

cerebral dominance, the specialization of each of the two cerebral hemispheres in the integration and control of different functions. In 90% of the population, the left cerebral hemisphere specializes in or dominates the ability to speak and write and the ability to understand spoken and written words. The areas that control these activities are situated in the frontal, parietal, and temporal lobes of the left hemisphere. In the other 10% of the population, either the right hemisphere or both hemispheres dominate the speech and writing abilities. The right cerebral hemisphere dominates the integration of certain sounds other than those associated with speaking, such as sounds of coughing, laughter, crying, and melodies. The right cerebral hemisphere perceives tactual stimuli and visual spatial relationships better than the left cerebral hemisphere. See also **Brodmann's areas.**

cerebral edema [L, *cerebrum*; Gk, *oidema*, swelling], an accumulation of fluid in the brain tissues. Causes can include an infection, tumor, trauma, or exposure to certain toxins. Because the skull cannot expand to accommodate the fluid pressure, brain tissues are compressed. Early symptoms are changes in level of consciousness; sluggish, then dilated pupils, and a gradual loss of consciousness. Cerebral edema can be fatal.

cerebral embolism [L, *cerebrum*; *embolos*, plug], an embolus that blocks the flow of blood through the vessels of the cerebrum, resulting in tissue ischemia distal to the occlusion. See also **cerebrovascular accident.**

cerebral gigantism [L, *cerebrum*; Gk, *gigas*, giant], an abnormal condition characterized by excessive weight and size at birth, accelerated growth during the first 4 or 5 years after birth without any increase in the level of growth hormone, and then reversion to normal growth. Some typical signs of this condition are prognathism, antimongoloid slant, dolichocephalic skull, moderate mental retardation, and impaired coordination. Also called **Sotos' syndrome.**

cerebral hemiplegia [L, *cerebrum*; Gk, *hemi*, half, *plege*, stroke], paralysis of one side of the body caused by a lesion in the brain.

cerebral hemisphere [L, *cerebrum*; Gk, *hemi*, half, *sphaira*, ball], one of the halves of the cerebrum. The two cerebral hemispheres are divided by a deep longitudinal fissure and are connected medially at the bottom of the fissure by the corpus callosum. Prominent grooves, subdividing each hemisphere into four major lobes, are the central sulcus, the lateral fissure, and the parietooccipital fissure. Each hemisphere also has a fifth major lobe deep in the brain. The central fissure separates the frontal lobe from the parietal lobe. The lateral fissure separates the temporal lobe, which lies below the fissure, from the frontal and parietal lobes, which lie above it. The parietooccipital fissure separates the occipital lobe from the two parietal lobes. The hemispheres consist of external gray substance, internal white substance, and internal gray substance and are covered by cerebral cortexes at the surface.

cerebral hemorrhage [L, *cerebrum*; Gk, *haima*, blood,

rhegnynei, to gush], a hemorrhage from a blood vessel in the brain. Three criteria used to classify cerebral hemorrhages are location (subarachnoid, extradural, subdural), the kind of vessel involved (arterial, venous, capillary), and origin (traumatic, degenerative). Each kind of cerebral hemorrhage has its own clinical characteristics. Most cerebral hemorrhages occur in the region of the basal ganglia and are caused by the rupture of a sclerotic artery as a result of hypertension. Other causes of rupture include congenital aneurysm, cerebrovascular thrombosis, and head trauma.

■ OBSERVATIONS: Bleeding may lead to displacement or destruction of brain tissue. Extensive hemorrhage is usually fatal. Depending on the extent and the location of the damaged tissue, residual effects may include aphasia, diminished mental function, or disturbance of the function of a special sense.

■ INTERVENTIONS: Lumbar puncture may reveal blood in the spinal fluid. A CT scan may be performed to locate the lesion and to differentiate the hemorrhage from an embolus or thrombus, or cerebral angiography may be utilized for these purposes. Surgery is often necessary to stop the bleeding and to prevent death from greatly increased intracranial pressure. The person is kept immobile, with the body in a position that assures adequate blood flow to and from the head. Physical therapy and speech therapy may be necessary during convalescence.

cerebral infarction [L, *cerebrum*, brain, *infarcire*, to stuff], an area of brain tissue that undergoes necrosis secondary to an interruption of the blood supply, with or without hemorrhage. An infarct may be the result of thrombosis, an embolism, or vasospasm.

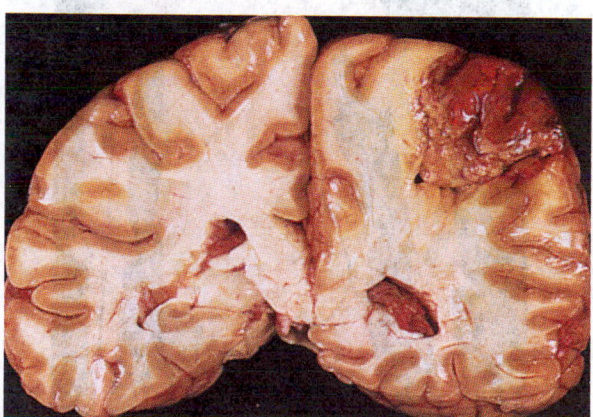

Cerebral infarction (Fletcher, 1987)

cerebral localization, 1. the determination of various areas in the cerebral cortex associated with specific functions, such as the 47 areas of Brodmann. 2. the diagnosis of a cerebral condition, such as a brain lesion, by determining the area of the brain affected, a determination made by analysis of the signs manifested by the patient.

cerebral nerve. See **cranial nerve.**

cerebral palsy [L, *cerebrum*; Gk, *para*, beyond, *lysis*, loosening], a motor function disorder caused by a permanent, nonprogressive brain defect or lesion present at birth or shortly thereafter. The neurologic deficit may result in spastic hemiplegia, monoplegia, diplegia, or quadriplegia, athetosis or ataxia, seizures, paresthesia, varying degrees of mental retardation, and impaired speech, vision, and hearing. The disorder is usually associated with premature or abnormal birth and intrapartum asphyxia, causing damage to the nervous system. Abnormalities in breathing, sucking, swallowing, and responsiveness are usually apparent soon after birth, but the characteristic stiff, awkward movements of the infant's limbs may be overlooked for several months. Walking is usually delayed, and, when attempted, the child manifests a typical scissors gait. The arms may be affected only slightly, but the fingers are often spastic. Deep-tendon reflexes are exaggerated, and there may be slurred speech, delay in acquiring sphincter control, and athetotic movements of the face and hands. Early identification of the disorder facilitates the handling of infants with cerebral palsy and the initiation of an exercise and training program. Treatment is individualized and may include the use of braces, surgical correction of deformities, speech therapy, and various indicated drugs, such as muscle relaxants and anticonvulsants. Also called **congenital cerebral diplegia, Little's disease.**

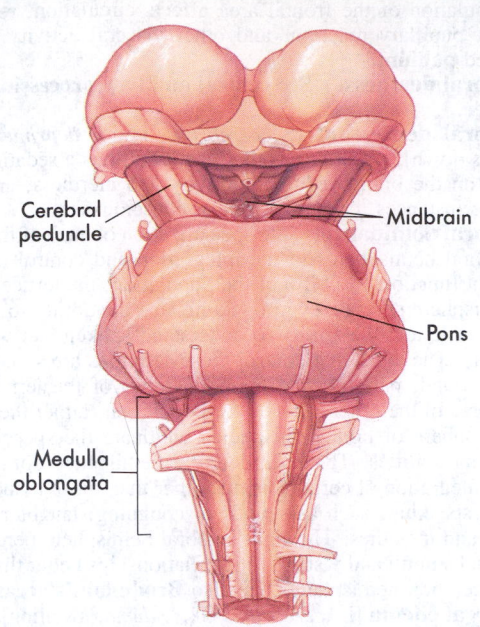

Cerebral peduncle (Thibodeau, 1993/Scott Bodell)

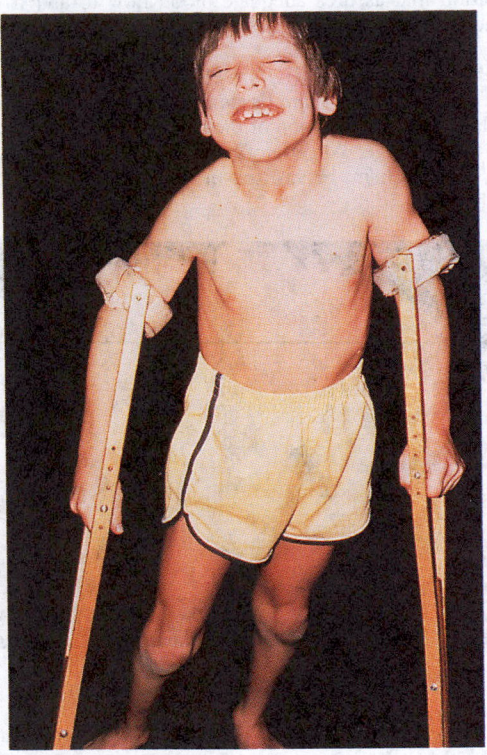

Cerebral palsy (Zitelli, 1992)

cerebral peduncle [L, *cerebrum*, brain, *pes*, foot], a pair of cylindrical masses of nerve fibers at the upper border of the pons which disappears into the left and right hemispheres. It includes corticopointine and pyramidal-tract fibers.

cerebral perfusion pressure (CPP), a measure of the amount of blood flow to the brain. It is calculated by subtracting the intracranial pressure from the mean systemic arterial blood pressure.

cerebral thrombosis [L, *cerebrum;* Gk, *thrombos,* lump, *osis,* condition], a clotting of blood in any cerebral vessel, such as the middle cerebral artery or the ascending parietal artery.

cerebral vertigo [L, *cerebrum,* brain + *vertigo,* dizziness], vertigo that is caused by organic brain disease.

cerebriform carcinoma. See **medullary carcinoma.**

cerebritis /ser′əbrī′tis/, *obsolete.* **1.** any inflammation of the cerebrum or brain. **2.** bacterial meningitis.

cerebrocerebellar atrophy /ser′əbrōser′əbel′ər/ [L, *cerebrum,* brain, *cerebellum,* small brain; Gk, *a, trophe,* without nourishment], a deterioration of the cerebellum caused by certain abiotrophic diseases.

cerebroid /ser′əbroid/ [L, *cerebrum* + Gk, *eidos,* form], resembling the substance of the brain.

cerebroma /ser′əbrō′mə/, *pl.* **cerebromas, cerebromata,** any unusual mass of brain tissue.

cerebromedullary tube. See **neural tube.**

cerebropathia psychia toxemia. See **Korsakoff's psychosis.**

cerebroretinal angiomatosis /ser′əbrōret′ənəl, sərē′brō-/ [L, *cerebrum* + *rete,* net; Gk, *aggeion,* vessel, *oma,* tumor, *osis* condition], a hereditary disease characterized by congenital, tumorlike vascular nodules in the retina and cerebellum. Similar spinal cord lesions, cysts of the pancreas, kidneys, and other viscera, seizures, and mental retardation may be present. Also called **Lindau-von Hippel disease, retinocerebral angiomatosis, von Hippel-Lindau disease.**

cerebroside /ser′əbrōsīd′/, any of a group of glycolipids found in the brain and other tissue of the nervous system, especially the myelin sheath.

cerebroside sulfatase [L, *cerebrum,* brain, *sulfur,* brimstone, *ase,* enzyme], an enzyme of the hydrolase class that catalyzes the reaction of cerebroside 3-sulfate + H_2O. A deficiency of the enzyme, which is transmitted as an autosomal recessive gene, is a cause of metachromatic leukodystrophy.

cerebrospinal /ser′əbrōspī′nəl, sərē′brō-/, pertaining to or involving the brain and the spinal cord.

cerebrospinal axis [L, *cerebrum*, brain, *spina*, spine, *axle*], a line formed by the brain and spinal cord about which the body turns.

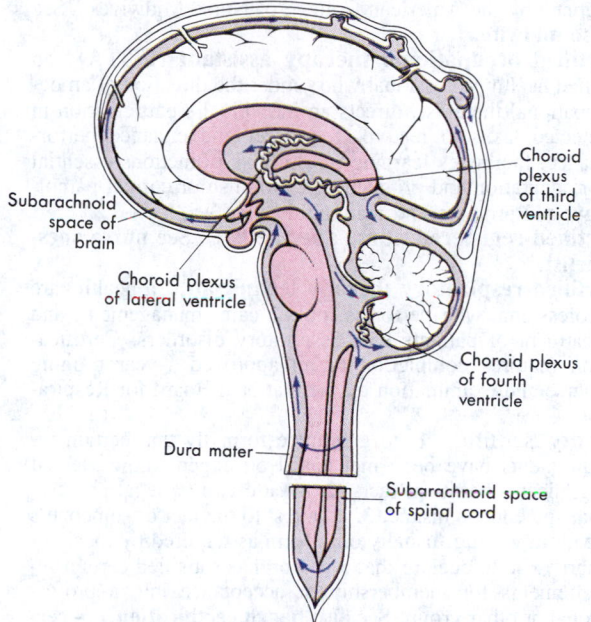

Cerebrospinal fluid circulation (Seeley, 1989)

Subarachnoid space of brain
Choroid plexus of lateral ventricle
Dura mater
Choroid plexus of third ventricle
Choroid plexus of fourth ventricle
Subarachnoid space of spinal cord

cerebrospinal fluid (CSF), the fluid that flows through and protects the four ventricles of the brain, the subarachnoid space, and the spinal canal. It is composed mainly of secretions of the choroid plexi in the lateral ventricles and in the third and the fourth ventricles of the brain. Openings in the roof of the fourth ventricle allow the fluid to flow into the subarachnoid spaces around the brain and the spinal cord. The flow of fluid is from the blood in the choroid plexi, through the ventricles, the central canal, the subarachnoid spaces, and back into the blood. The volume of CSF in the average adult is about 140 ml, including about 23 ml in the ventricles and 117 ml in the subarachnoid spaces of the brain and the spinal cord. Changes in the carbon dioxide content of CSF affect the respiratory center in the medulla, helping to control breathing. A brain tumor may press against the cerebral aqueduct and shut off the flow of the fluid from the third to the fourth ventricle, resulting in an accumulation of fluid in the lateral and the third ventricles, called internal hydrocephalus. Other blockages of the flow of CSF, such as those caused by blood clots, result in serious complications. Certain illnesses and various diagnoses may require microscopic examination and chemical analysis of CSF. Samples of the fluid may be removed by lumbar puncture between the third and the fourth lumbar vertebrae.

cerebrospinal nerves, the 12 pairs of cranial nerves and 31 pairs of spinal nerves that originate in the brain and spinal cord.

cerebrospinal pressure [L, *cerebrum*, *spina*, *premere*, to press], the pressure of cerebrospinal fluid in the central nervous system. It usually measures between 100 and 150 mm of water and is measured by a manometer attached to the end of a needle after it has been inserted into the subarachnoid space.

cerebrospinal rhinorrhea [L, *cerebrum*, brain + *spina*, backbone; Gk, *rhis*, nose + *rhoia*, flow], a discharge of cerebrospinal fluid from the nose.

cerebrotendinous xanthomatosis. See **van Bogaert's disease.**

cerebrovascular /ser′əbrōvas′kyələr, sərē′brō-/ [L, *cerebrum* + *vasculum*, little vessel], of or pertaining to the vascular system and blood supply of the brain.

cerebrovascular accident (CVA), an abnormal condition of the blood vessels of the brain characterized by occlusion by an embolus, a thrombus, or cerebrovascular hemorrhage, resulting in ischemia of the brain tissues normally perfused by the damaged vessels. The sequelae of a cerebrovascular accident depend on the location and extent of ischemia. Paralysis, weakness, sensory change, speech defect, aphasia, or death may occur. Symptoms remit somewhat after the first few days as brain swelling subsides.

cerebrum /ser′əbrəm, sərē′brəm/, *pl.* **cerebrums, cerebra** [L, brain], the largest and uppermost section of the brain, divided by a central sulcus into the left and the right cerebral hemispheres. At the bottom of the groove, the hemispheres are connected by the corpus callosum. The internal structures of the hemispheres merge with those of the diencephalon and further communicate with the brain stem through the cerebral peduncles. Each cerebral hemisphere is composed of the extensive outer cerebral cortex with its gray substance, the underlying semiovale with its white substance, the internal basal ganglia, and certain centrally and medially located structures comprising the rhinencephalon. The surface of the cerebrum is convoluted and lobed, each lobe bearing the name of the bone under which it lies. The cerebrum performs sensory functions, motor functions, and less easily defined integration functions associated with various mental activities. It generates a variety of electric waves that may be recorded on an electroencephalogram to localize areas of brain dysfunction, to identify altered states of consciousness, or to establish brain death. Some of the other processes that are controlled or affected by the cerebrum are memory, speech, writing, and emotional response. See also **cerebral cortex.** –**cerebral,** *adj.*

cerium (Ce) /sir′ē·əm/ [L, *Ceres*, Roman goddess of agriculture], a ductile, gray rare-earth element. Its atomic number is 58; its atomic weight is 140.13. A compound of cerium, cerium oxalate, is used as a sedative, an antiemetic, and an antitussive.

cerium nitrate, a topical antiseptic used to control bacterial and fungal infections in the treatment of burns.

ceroid /sir′oid/ [L, *cera*, wax; Gk, *eidos*, form], a golden, waxy pigment appearing in the cirrhotic livers of some individuals, in the GI tract, in the nervous system, and in the muscles. It is an insoluble, acid-fast, sudanophilic pigment.

ceroma /sirō′mə/, *pl.* **ceromas, ceromata** [L, *cera,* wax; Gk, *oma,* tumor], a neoplasm that has undergone waxy degeneration.

certifiable /sur′tifī′əbəl/ [L, *certus,* certain, *facere,* to make], **1.** a legal term pertaining to a patient with a mental illness who has been found incompetent and requires care by a guardian or in a hospital. **2.** pertaining to infectious diseases or dangerous conditions that must be reported to local health authorities.

certificate-of-need or -necessity, a statement or certificate issued by a governmental agency to the effect that a proposed construction or modification of a health facility will be needed at the time of its completion. The certificate is issued to the individual or group intending to build or modify the facility.

certification [L, *certus,* certain, *facere,* to make], **1.** a process in which an individual, an institution, or an educational program is evaluated and recognized as meeting certain predetermined standards. Certification is usually made by a nongovernmental agency. The purpose of certification is to assure that the standards met are those necessary for safe and ethical practice of the profession or service. **2.** (in nursing) a process in which the professional organization or association verifies the fact that a person who is licensed to practice has met the standards for specialty practice specified by the profession. The purpose of certification is to assure other professionals and the public that the person has mastered the skills necessary to practice a particular specialty and has acquired the standard body of knowledge common to that specialty.

certification for excellence, (in nursing) certification that recognizes professional achievement, advanced education, and superior performance in a special or subspecial field of practice.

certification in nursing, one of two processes in which a professional organization formally recognizes the competence of a nurse to practice a subspecialty of nursing. One process, certification for excellence, bases recognition on professional achievement, advanced education, and superior performance. The second process, entry level certification, bases recognition on advanced education in a program approved by the certifying organization. Criteria vary according to the particular requirements of the professional organization but always require current licensure as a registered nurse and usually include an examination and certain educational or practice requirements. Submission and evaluation of documented clinical practice and a statement of a philosophy of practice may also be required by some professional organizations.

certified dental assistant /sur′tifīd/, a person who has successfully completed the education, training, and testing of the Certification Examination. A dental assisstant may also become certified without receiving a formal education by working two years as a fulltime chairside dental assistant before taking the Certification Examination.

certified medical transcriptionist. See **medical transcriptionist.**

certified milk, raw milk that is obtained, handled, and marketed in compliance with state health laws. The milk must be produced by disease-free cows, which are regularly inspected by a veterinarian and are milked by sterilized equipment in hygienic surroundings, contain less than a specified low bacterial count, and be not older than 36 hours when delivered.

certified nurse-midwife (CNM), (according to the American College of Nurse-Midwives) 'an individual educated in the two disciplines of nursing and midwifery, who possesses evidence of certification according to the requirements of the American College of Nurse-Midwives. Nurse-midwifery practice is the independent management of care of essentially normal newborns and women, antepartally, intrapartally, postpartally, and/or gynecologically, occurring within a health care system which provides for medical consultation, collaborative management, or referral and is in accord with the qualifications, standards, and functions for the practice of nurse-midwifery as defined by the American College of Nurse-Midwives.' See also **midwife.**

certified occupational therapy assistant (COTA) an allied health professional who, under the direction of an occupational therapist, directs an individual's participation in selected tasks to restore, reinforce, and enhance performance; facilitates learning of skills and functions essential for adaptation and productivity; diminish or correct pathology; and promote and maintain health.

certified registered nurse anesthetist. See **nurse anesthetist.**

certified respiratory therapy technician, a health care professional who performs routine care, management, and treatment of patients with respiratory disorders. Certification requires completion of an approved 1-year training course and examination by the National Board for Respiratory Care.

certify /sur′tifī/, **1.** to guarantee formally that certain requirements have been met based on expert knowledge of significant, pertinent facts. **2.** to attest, by a legal process, that someone is insane. **3.** to attest to the fact of someone's death in writing, usually on a form as required by local authority. **4.** to declare that a person has satisified certain requirements for membership or acceptance into a professional or other group. See also **board certification.** −**certification,** *n.,* **certifiable,** *adj.*

Cerubidine, a trademark for an antineoplastic (daunorubicin hydrochloride).

cerulean /sirŏŏ′lē·ən/ [L, *caelum,* sky], sky-blue in color.

ceruloplasmin /sirŏŏ′lōplaz′min/ [L, *caelum,* sky; Gk, *plassein,* to shape], a glycoprotein in plasma that transports 96% of the plasma copper.

cerumen /sirŏŏ′mən/ [L, *cera,* wax], a yellowish or brownish waxy secretion produced by vestigial apocrine sweat glands in the external ear canal. Also called **earwax.**

ceruminolytic /sirŏŏ′mənōlit′ik/, pertaining to a drug or other agent that dissolves cerumen.

ceruminolytic agent [L, *cera,* wax; Gk, *lysis,* a loosening; L, *agere,* to do], a medication that dissolves or loosens cerumen (earwax) to allow for removal.

ceruminosis /sirŏŏ′minō′sis/, excessive buildup of cerumen or earwax in the external auditory canal. It can cause discomfort, symptoms of hearing loss, and irritation leading to the development of infection. Removal of excess cerumen is accomplished by the local use of a wax softening agent followed by careful flushing with an ear syringe. A cerumen spoon is sometimes used to scoop out hard collections of old wax.

ceruminous gland /sirŏŏ′minəs/, one of a number of tiny structures in the external ear canal, believed to be modified sweat glands. They secrete a waxy cerumen instead of watery sweat.

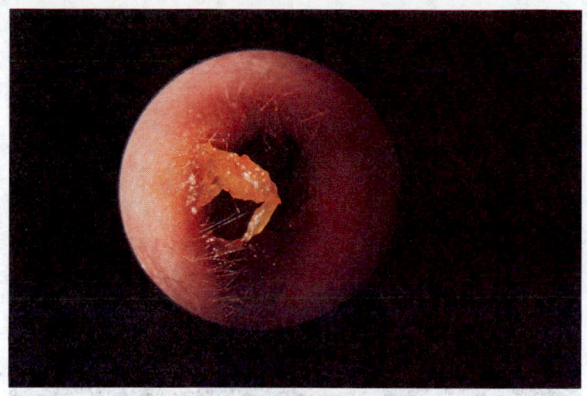

Cerumen in the external auditory meatus
(Bingham, 1992/Courtesy Dr. Arnold Noyek)

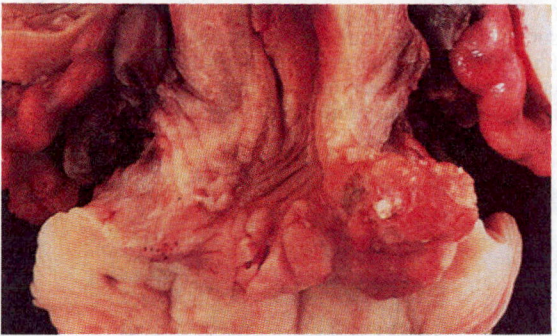

Cervical cancer *(Fletcher, 1987)*

cervic-, a combining form meaning 'pertaining to the neck': *cervicectomy, cervicitis, cervicobrachial.*

cervical /sur′vikəl/ [L, *cervix,* neck], **1.** of or pertaining to the neck or the region of the neck. **2.** of or pertaining to the constricted area of a necklike structure, such as the neck of a tooth or the cervix of the uterus.

cervical abortion [L, *cervix; ab,* away, from, *oriri,* to be born], spontaneous expulsion of a cervical pregnancy.

cervical adenitis [L, *cervix;* Gk, *aden,* gland, *itis,* inflammation], an abnormal condition characterized by enlarged, tender lymph nodes of the neck. It often occurs in association with acute infections of the throat.

cervical amputation, the removal of the neck of the uterus.

cervical canal, the canal within the uterine cervix, which protrudes into the vagina. The uterine end of the canal is closed at the internal os and, in the nullipara, at the distal end by the external os. The canal is a passageway through which the menstrual flow escapes and, vastly dilated and effaced by labor, through which the infant must come to be delivered vaginally. Various diagnostic and therapeutic procedures require dilatation of the muscular cervix surrounding the canal, including endometrial biopsy, suction or surgical curettage, or radium implantation. Pelvic inflammatory disease is the result of the entry of pathogenic bacteria into the uterus through the cervical canal. Sperm must travel upward through the canal to reach the uterus and fallopian tubes. The mucus that is secreted by endocervical glands changes in appearance and consistency through the menstrual cycle. For the first few days after menstruation little mucus is secreted. As ovulation approaches, increasing amounts of sticky, cloudy-white or yellowish secretions are seen. Around the time of ovulation, the volume of mucus increases, and it becomes clear, slippery, and elastic, resembling the uncooked white of an egg. After ovulation the mucus becomes cloudy, thick, sticky, and progressively less profuse until menstruation supervenes to begin the cycle again.

cervical cancer, a neoplasm of the uterine cervix that can be detected in the early, curable stage by the Papanicolaou (Pap) test. Factors associated with the development of cervical cancer are coitus at an early age, many sexual partners, genital herpesvirus infections, multiparity, and poor obstetric and gynecologic care. Early cervical neoplasia is usually asymptomatic, but there may be a watery vaginal discharge or occasional spotting of blood; advanced lesions may cause a dark, foul-smelling vaginal discharge, leakage from bladder or rectal fistulas, anorexia, weight loss, and back and leg pains. Pap smears of cervical cells are highly important in screening, but definitive diagnoses are based on colposcopic examination and cytologic study of specimens obtained by biopsy. Suitable sites for biopsy may be indicated by applying 3% acetic acid to the cervix to accentuate characteristic changes in neoplastic epithelium or by using Schiller's test in which an iodine solution stains normal cervical cells dark brown and does not stain the nonglycogen-producing cells of malignant epithelium. Cervical dysplasia may regress, persist, or progress to clinical disease, but carcinoma in situ is considered to be a precursor of invasive carcinoma. About 90% of cervical tumors are squamous cell carcinomas, fewer than 10% are adenocarcinomas, and others are mixtures of these kinds, or, in rare cases, sarcomas. Tumors on the surface of the cervix may be huge, polypoid masses whereas endophytic lesions tend to be small and hard; ulcerative lesions may cause extensive erosion. Cervical cancer invades the tissues of adjacent organs and may metastasize through lymphatic channels to distant sites, including the lungs, bone, liver, brain, and paraaortic nodes. Treatment depends on the kind and the extent of the malignancy, the age of the woman, and her general health. Also considered are her wishes in regard to maintaining her reproductive function. Carcinoma in situ may be treated by excisional conization or cryosurgery. Invasive tumors may be treated with radium implants or with radiotherapy or vaginal or abdominal hysterectomy.

cervical cap, a contraceptive device consisting of a small rubber cup fitted over the uterine cervix to prevent spermatozoa from entering the cervical canal. In some studies, its contraceptive effectiveness equals or exceeds that of the diaphragm. It may be more comfortable than the diaphragm and may be left safely on the cervix for days or weeks and remain effective.

cervical cauterization, the destruction, usually by heat or electric current, of the superficial tissues of the cervix.

cervical conization, the excision of a cone-shaped section of tissue from the endocervix. See also **cone biopsy.**

cervical cyst [L, *cervix,* neck; Gk, *kystis,* bag], a mucus cyst of the uterine cervix. Also called **Nabothian cyst.**

cervical dilatation /dil′ətā′shən/ [L, *dilatare,* to widen], the diameter of the opening of the cervix in labor as measured on vaginal examination, expressed in centimeters or finger breadths, one finger breadth being approximately 2 cm. At full dilatation the diameter of the cervical opening is 10 cm. See also **dilatation.**

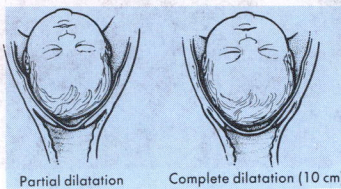

Partial dilatation   Complete dilatation (10 cm)

Cervical dilatation

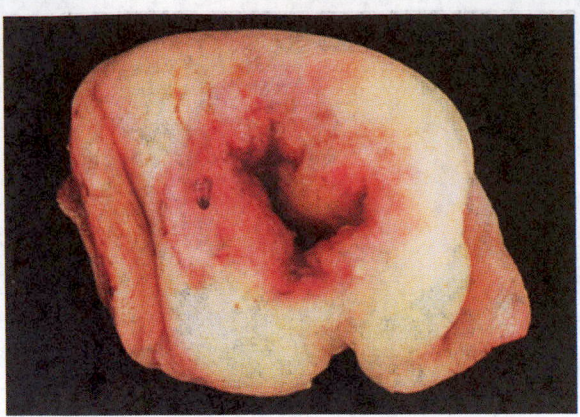

Cervical erosion (Fletcher, 1987)

cervical disk syndrome, an abnormal condition characterized by compression or irritation of the cervical nerve roots in or near the intervertebral foramina before the roots divide into the anterior and the posterior rami. Cervical disk syndrome may be caused by ruptured intervertebral disks, degenerative cervical disk disease, or cervical injuries. The form caused by ruptured cervical intervertebral disks or by degenerative disease may produce varying degrees of malalignment, causing nerve root compression. Most cervical disk syndromes are caused by injuries that involve hyperextension, which results in compression of the anatomic structures. Flexion injuries in the cervical area do not result in nerve compression. Edema usually occurs in all cases of cervical disk syndrome. Pain, the most common symptom, usually emanates from the cervical area but may radiate down the arm to the fingers and increase with cervical motion. The pain may increase sharply with coughing, sneezing, or any radical movement. Other signs and symptoms associated with cervical disk syndrome may be paresthesia, headache, blurred vision, decreased skeletal function, and weakened hand grip. Physical examination may reveal varying degrees of muscular atrophy, sensory abnormalities, muscular weakness, and decreased reflexes. Radiographic examination may show a loss of normal lordosis associated with the cervical vertebrae and may also reveal some minor malalignment of the vertebrae. Nonsurgical intervention, which is usually a successful treatment, may include immobilization of the cervical vertebrae to decrease irritation and to provide rest for the traumatized area. Other treatment may include special exercises, heat therapy, and intermittent traction. Mild analgesics are usually successful in controlling the pain associated with cervical disk syndrome, especially when employed with immobilization. Surgery is usually recommended only when signs and symptoms persist despite nonsurgical treatment. The prognosis for this condition is usually good, but recurrence of symptoms is common. Also called **cervical root syndrome.** See also **herniated disk, whiplash injury.**

cervical endometritis, an inflammation of the inner lining of the cervix uteri. See also **endometritis.**

cervical erosion [L, *cervix; erodere,* to consume], a condition in which the squamous epithelium of the cervix is abraded as a result of irritation caused by infection or trauma, such as childbirth, and is replaced by columnar epithelium. Early treatment is desirable to avoid possible malignancy later and consists of cryosurgery, cauterization, and douches.

cervical fistula, an abnormal passage from the cervix to the vagina or bladder that may be caused by a malignant lesion, radiotherapy, surgical trauma, or injury during childbirth. A cervical fistula communicating with the bladder permits leakage of urine, causing irritation, odor, and embarrassment. See also **branchial fistula.**

cervical mucus, a secretion of the columnar epithelium lining the upper portion of the cervical canal of the uterus. See **mucous plug.**

cervical mucus method of family planning. See **ovulation method of family planning.**

cervical nerves [L, *cervix,* neck, *nervus,* nerve], the eight pairs of spinal nerves that arise from the neck area of the spinal cord, from above the atlas to below the seventh vertebra. The first four supply the head and neck and the other four mainly innervate the upper limbs, scalp, and back. See also **cervical plexus.**

cervical os. See **external cervical os, internal cervical os.**

cervical plexus, the network of nerves formed by the ventral primary divisions of the first four cervical nerves. Each nerve, except the first, divides into the superior branch and the inferior branch, and both branches unite to form three loops. The plexus is located opposite the cranial aspect of the first four cervical vertebrae, ventrolateral to the levator scapulae and the scalenus medius, and deep to the sternocleidomastoideus. It communicates with certain cranial nerves and numerous muscular and cutaneous branches.

cervical plexus anesthesia, nerve block at any point below the mastoid process from C_2 or the second cervical vertebra transverse process to the sixth cervical vertebra. This method is used for operations on the area between the jaw and clavicle. Complications may include Horner's syndrome, inadvertent stellate ganglion or brachial plexus block, vertebral artery bleeding, subarachnoid or peridural penetration, phrenic nerve block or palsy, or laryngeal nerve block, manifested by sudden hoarseness.

cervical polyp [L, *cervix;* Gk, *polys,* mean, *pous,* foot], an outgrowth of columnar epithelial tissue of the endocervical canal, usually attached to the wall of the canal by a slender pedicle. Often there are no symptoms, but multiple

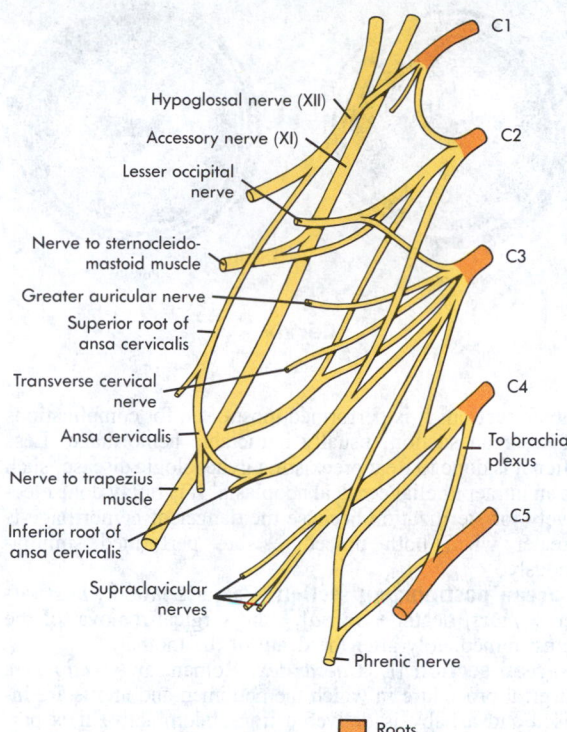

Cervical plexus *(Seeley, 1992/Michael Schenk)*

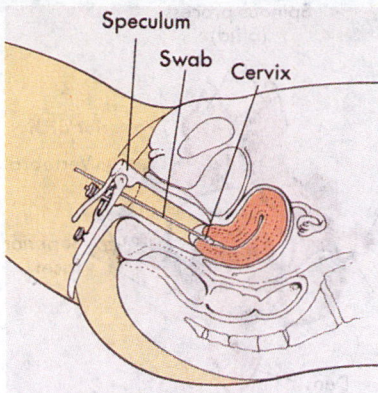

Obtaining a cervical smear *(Grimes, 1991)*

or abraded polyps may cause bleeding, especially with contact during coitus. Polyps are most common in women over 40 years of age. The cause is not known. Treatment of a symptomatic polyp is removal by simple torsion, turning the polyp on its stalk while pulling gently until it tears off. Scant bleeding and prompt healing usually follow.

cervical root syndrome. See **cervical disk syndrome.**

cervical smear [L, *cervix;* AS, *smero,* grease], a small amount of the secretions and superficial cells of the cervix, secured from the external os of the cervix with a sterile applicator or special small wooden or plastic spatula. For a Pap smear, it is obtained from the squamocolumnar junction of the uterine cervix and from the vaginal vault and endocervical canal. The specimen is spread on a specially labeled glass slide and sent for cytologic examination by a special laboratory. For bacteriologic culture and identification, only the applicator is used; the specimen is spread on a glass slide and stained and examined under a microscope or placed in or on a culture medium and sent to a bacteriologic laboratory for culture and identification.

cervical spondylosis [L, *cervix;* Gk, *spondylos,* vertebra, *osis,* condition], a form of degenerative joint and disk disease affecting the cervical vertebrae and resulting in compression of the associated nerve roots. Symptoms include pain or loss of feeling in the affected arm and shoulder and stiffness of the cervical spine.

cervical stenosis [L, *cervix;* Gk, *stenos,* narrow, *osis,* condition], a narrowing of the canal between the body of the uterus and the cervical os.

cervical tenaculum. See **tenaculum.**

cervical triangle, one of two triangular areas formed in the neck by the oblique course of the sternocleidomastoideus. The anterior triangle is bounded by the midline of the throat anteriorly, the sternocleidomastoideus laterally, and the body of the mandible superiorly. The posterior triangle is bounded by the clavicle inferiorly and by the borders of the sternocleidomastoideus and the trapezius superiorly.

cervical vertebra, one of the first seven segments of the vertebral column. They differ from the thoracic and the lumbar vertebrae by the presence of a foramen in each transverse process. The first, second, and seventh cervical vertebrae present exceptional features. The bodies of the four remaining cervical vertebrae are small, oval, and broader than the other three in transverse diameter and contain large, triangular foramina within their transverse processes. Their spinous processes are short and bifid. The first cervical vertebra has no body, supports the head, and contains a smooth, oval facet for articulation with the dens of the second cervical vertebra. The dens extends from the cranial portion of the body of the second cervical vertebra, which has a very large, strong spinous process with a bifid extremity. The seventh cervical vertebra has a very long, prominent spinous process that is nearly horizontal in direction and is often used as a palpable reference for locating the other cervical spines. Compare **coccygeal vertebra, lumbar vertebra, sacral vertebra, thoracic vertebra.** See also **vertebra.** (See Fig. p. 302.)

cervicitis /sur′visi′tis/, acute or chronic inflammation of the uterine cervix. **Acute cervicitis** is infection of the cervix marked by redness, edema, and bleeding on contact. Symptoms do not always occur but may include any or all of the following: copious, foul-smelling discharge from the vagina, pelvic pressure or pain, scant bleeding with intercourse, and itching or burning of the external genitalia. The principal causative organisms are: *Trichomonas vaginalis, Candida albicans,* and *Haemophilus vaginalis.* Diagnosis is by microscopic examination, confirmed in some cases by culture and Pap smear. Specific antimicrobial medication may be effective. Acute cervicitis tends to be a recurrent problem because of reexposure to the germ, undertreatment, or predisposing factors such as HIV infection, multiple sexual partners or poor nutritional status. **Chronic cervicitis** is a persistent inflammation of the cervix usually occurring

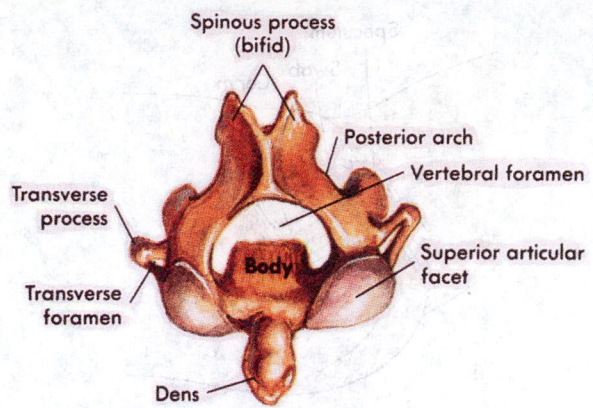

Cervical vertebra
(Seeley, 1992/David J Mascaro and Associates)

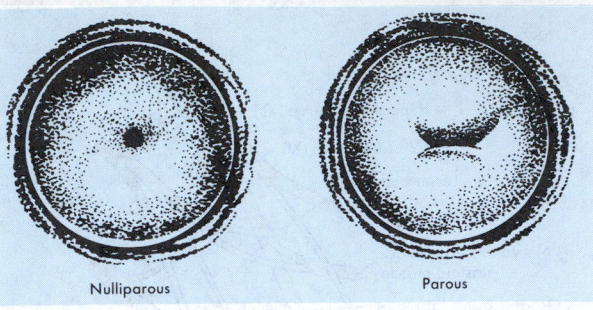

Nulliparous   Parous

Cervix

among women in their reproductive years. Symptoms include a thick, irritating, malodorous discharge that may in severe cases be accompanied by significant pelvic pain. The cervix looks congested and enlarged, nabothian cysts are often present, and there are signs of eversion of the cervix and often old lacerations from childbirth. A Pap smear should be performed before treatment. The most effective treatments are hot or cold cautery. See also **Candida albicans, cautery, cervical cancer, cervical polyp, condylomatum acuminatum, nabothian cyst.**

cervico-, a combining form meaning 'neck': *cervicodynia, cervicolabial, cervicotomy.*

cervicodynia /sur'vikōdin'ē·ə/, pain in the neck. Also called **trachelodynia.**

cervicofacial actinomycosis. See **actinomycosis.**

cervicolabial /sur'vikōlā'bē·əl/ [L, *cervix* + *labium*, lip], pertaining to or situated in the labial area of the neck of an incisor or a canine tooth.

cervicouterine /sur'vikōyōō'tərin/, pertaining to or situated at the cervix of the uterus.

cervicovaginitis /-vaj'inītis/, an inflammation of the cervix and vagina.

cervicovesical /sur'vikōves'ikəl/ [L, *cervix* + *vesica*, bladder], of or pertaining to the cervix of the uterus and the bladder.

cervix /sur'viks/ [L, neck], the part of the uterus that protrudes into the cavity of the vagina. The cervix is divided into the supravaginal portion and the vaginal portion. The supravaginal portion is separated ventrally from the bladder by the parametrium, which attaches to the sides of the cervix and contains the uterine arteries. The vaginal portion of the cervix projects into the cavity of the vagina and contains the cervical canal and the internal and external os of the canal. The mucous membrane lining the endocervix is broken by numerous oblique ridges, deep glandular follicles, little cysts, and papillae. See also **effacement.**

ceryl alcohol /sē'ril/ [L, *cera*, wax; Ar, *alkohl*, essence], a fatty alcohol present in many waxes. Also called **hexacosanol.**

cesarean hysterectomy /sizer'ē·ən/ [L, *Caesar lex*, Roman law; Gk, *hys tera*, womb, *ektome*, excision], a surgical operation in which the uterus is removed at the time of ce-

sarean section. It is performed most often for complications of cesarean section, usually intractable hemorrhage. Less often it is done to treat preexisting gynecologic disease, such as an intraepithelial cervical neoplasia. It is rarely done electively for sterilization because the danger of hemorrhage is greater when both procedures are performed simultaneously.

cesarean postmortem section [Caesar's law; L, *post*, after + *mors*, death + *sectio*], the surgical removal of the fetus immediately after the death of the mother.

cesarean section [L, *Caesar lex*, Roman law, *sectio*], a surgical procedure in which the abdomen and uterus are incised and a baby is delivered transabdominally. It is performed when abnormal maternal or fetal conditions exist that are judged likely to make vaginal delivery hazardous. Approximately 25% to 30% of births in the United States are by cesarean section; the operation is performed less frequently in other countries. Maternal indications for the operation include placenta previa or abruptio placenta, and dysfunctional labor. Prior delivery by cesarean section is no longer considered an absolute indication for repeating it in future deliveries. Cesarean birth is less traumatic for babies than difficult midforceps delivery. Fetal indications for the operation include fetal distress, cephalopelvic disproportion, and abnormal presentation, such as breech and transverse lie. The incision in the skin of the abdomen may be horizontal or vertical, regardless of the kind of internal incision into the uterus. Because she must begin mothering while she is recovering from major surgery, the mother requires special care that provides for both her postoperative medical needs and her need to nurture her new baby, who may also be ill or recovering during the crucial neonatal period. See also **classic cesarean section, extraperitoneal cesarean section, low cervical cesarean section.**

cesium (Cs) /sē'zē·əm/ [L, *caesius*, sky blue], an alkali metal element. Its atomic number is 55; its atomic weight is 132.9. Like other alkali metals cesium emits electrons when exposed to visible light and is used in photoelectric cells and in television cameras.

cesium 137, a radioactive material with a half-life of 30.2 years that is used in radiotherapy as a sealed source of gamma rays intended for application to various malignancies that are treated by brachytherapy. Cesium has replaced radium for such applications. See also **brachytherapy.**

cesspool fever, *informal.* typhoid fever.

cestode. See **tapeworm.**

cestode infection, cestodiasis. See **tapeworm infection.**

cestodiasis. See **tapeworm infection.**

cestoid /ses'toid/ [Gk, *kestos*, girdle, *eidos*, form], **1.** cestodlike, or resembling a tapeworm. **2.** a tapeworm of the Cestoda subclass.

CET, abbreviation for *Certified Enterostomal Therapist.*

Cetacaine, a trademark for a fixed-combination, anesthetic spray, containing several local anesthetics (benzocaine, butyl aminobenzoate, tetracaine), applied to mucous membranes.

cetyl alcohol /sē'til/ [L, *cetus*, whale; Ar, *alkohl,* essence], a fatty alcohol, derived from spermaceti, used as an emulsifier and stiffening agent in creams and ointments. Also called **hexadecanol, palmityl alcohol.**

cetylpyridinium chloride /sē'təlpī'ridin'ē·əm/, an antiinfective used as a preservative in pharmaceutical preparations and as a topical cleanser.

■ INDICATIONS: It is prescribed prophylactically to prevent infection of the skin or mucous membranes.

■ CONTRAINDICATIONS: Known hypersensitivity to this drug is the only contraindication.

■ NOTE: It is inactivated by soap, serum, and tissue fluids; therefore the surface of the skin must be clean and well rinsed.

CEU, abbreviation for **continuing education unit.**

Ce-Vi-Sol, a trademark for vitamin C (ascorbic acid).

cevitamic acid. See **ascorbic acid.**

Cf, symbol for the element **californium.**

CF test, abbreviation for **complement-fixation test.**

CGC, abbreviation for *Certified Gastrointestinal Clinician.*

cGMP, abbreviation for **cyclic guanosine monophosphate.**

cgs, CGS, abbreviation for **centimeter-gram-second system.**

Ch1, symbol for **Christchurch chromosome.**

CHB, abbreviation for **complete heart block.**

Chaddock reflex [Charles G. Chaddock, American neurologist, b. 1861], an abnormal reflex, induced by firmly stroking the ulnar surface of the forearm, characterized by flexion of the wrist and extension of the fingers in fanlike position. It is seen on the affected side iun hemiplegia. Compare **Gordon's reflex, Oppenheim reflex.** See also **Babinski's reflex.**

Chaddock's sign [Charles G. Chaddock, American neurologist, b. 1861], a variation of Babinski's reflex, elicited by firmly stroking the side of the foot just distal to the lateral malleolus, characterized by extension of the great toe and fanning of the other toes. It is seen in pyramidal tract disease. See **Babinski reflex.**

Chadwick's sign /chad'wiks/ [James R. Chadwick, American gynecologist, b. 1844], the bluish coloration of the vulva and vagina that develops after the sixth week of pregnancy as a normal result of local venous congestion. It is an early sign of pregnancy.

chafe [L *calefacere* to make warm], an irritation of the skin by friction, such as when rough material rubs against an unprotected area of the body.

chafing, superficial irritation of the skin by friction.

Chagas' disease /chag'əs/ [Carlos Chagas, Brazilian physician, b. 1879], a parasitic disease caused by *Trypanosoma cruzi* transmitted to humans by the bite of bloodsucking insects. It may occur in acute or chronic form. The acute form, which is common in children and rare in adults, is marked by a lesion at the site of the bite, fever, weakness, enlarged spleen and lymph nodes, edema of the face and legs, and tachycardia. This form resolves within 4 months unless complications, such as encephalitis, develop. The chronic form may be manifested by cardiomyopathy or by dilatation of the esophagus or colon. Often, infections are asymptomatic. Also called **Brazilian trypanosomiasis, Chagas-Cruz disease, Cruz trypanosomiasis, South American trypanosomiasis.** See also **trypanosomiasis.**

Chagres fever /chag'ris/ [Chagres River, Panama; L, *febris*], a phlebotomus arbovirus infection transmitted to humans through the bite of a sandfly. The disease is rarely fatal and is characterized by fever, headache, and muscle pains of the chest or abdomen. There may be nausea and vomiting, giddiness, weakness, photophobia, and pain on moving the eyes. The infection subsides within a week. Supportive treatment includes analgesics, bed rest, and adequate fluid intake. The disease is most common in Central America. Also called **Panama fever.**

chain [L, *catena*], **1.** a length of several units linked together in a linear pattern, such as a polypeptide chain of amino acids or a chain of atoms forming a chemical molecule. **2.** a group of individual bacteria linked together, such as streptococci formed by a chain of cocci. **3.** the serial relationship of certain structures essential to function, such as the chain of ossicles in the middle ear. Each of the small bones moves successively in response to vibration of the tympanic membrane, thus transmitting the auditory stimulus to the oval window. See also **chain ligature.**

chain ligature [L, *catena; ligare,* to bind], an interlocking ligature that ties off a pedicle at several places by passing a long thread through the pedicle at different points.

chain reaction, **1.** (in chemistry) a reaction that produces a compound needed for the reaction to continue, such as each product that is produced in the chain reaction of glycolysis that is essential for each succeeding reaction and the total catabolism of glucose. **2.** (in physics) a reaction that perpetuates itself by the proliferating fission of nuclei and the release of atomic particles that cause more nuclear fissions.

chain reflex, a series of reflexes, each stimulated by the preceding one.

chain-stitch suture, a continuous surgical stitch in which each loop of the suture is secured by the next loop.

chalasia /kəlā'zhə/ [Gk, *chalasis,* relaxation], abnormal relaxation or incompetence of the cardiac sphincter of the stomach, resulting in reflux of the gastric contents into the esophagus with subsequent regurgitation. Conservative treatment in infancy includes feeding several small meals a day to avoid distention of the stomach and holding the baby upright while giving the feeding. The symptoms and treatment are similar to those of a hiatal hernia. See also **gastroesophageal reflux.**

chalazion /kəlā'zion/ [Gk, hailstone], a small, localized swelling of the eyelid resulting from obstruction and retained secretions of the meibomian glands. It is a nonmalignant condition that often requires surgery for correction. Compare **hordeolum, sty.** (See Fig. p. 304.)

chalice cell. See **goblet cell.**

chalicosis /kal'ikō'sis/, a type of fibrosis that results from the inhalation of calcium dusts. Pure calcium dusts are soluble and are absorbed. Calcium dusts from marble, limestone, or Portland cement usually do not cause fibrosis. Re-

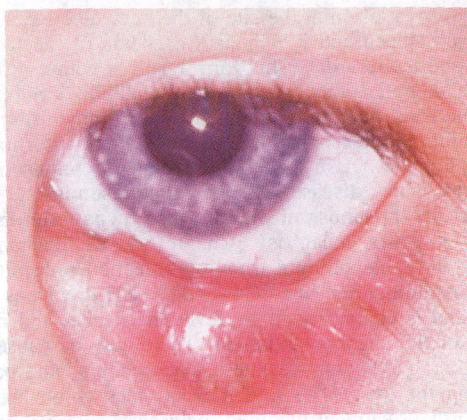

Chalazion (Zitelli, 1992)

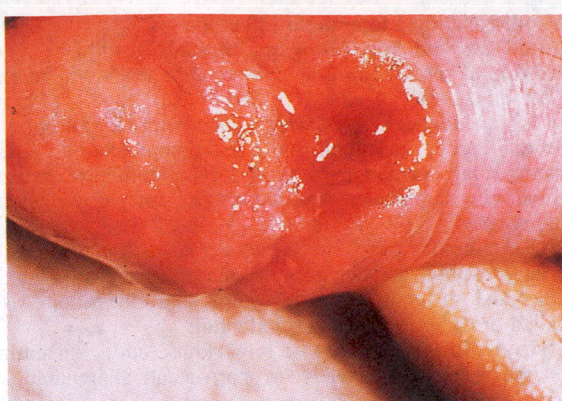

Primary chancre of syphilis (Epstein, 1992)

spiratory impairment is generally caused by the presence of free silica in the calcium dust.

chalkitis /kalkī′tis/ [Gk, *chalkos,* brass, *itis,* inflammation], an abnormal condition characterized by inflammation of the eyes, caused by rubbing the eyes with the hands after touching or handling brass. Also called **brassy eye.**

challenge, a method of testing the sensitivity of an individual to a hormone, allergen, or other substance by administering a sample. To challenge the person's sensitivity to a particular antigen, a small amount may be injected to determine whether the immune system will react by producing appropriate antibodies.

chalone /kā′lōn/ [Gk, *chalan,* to relax], any one of numerous polypeptide inhibitors that is elaborated by a tissue and functions like a hormone on specific target organs.

chamaeprosopy /kam′əpros′əpē/ [Gk, *chamai,* low, *prosopon,* face], a facial appearance characterized by a low brow and a broad face with a facial index of 90 or less. **–chamaeprosopic,** *adj.*

chamber [Gk, *kamara,* vaulted enclosure], **1.** a hollow but not necessarily empty space or cavity in an organ, as in the anterior and posterior chambers of the eye or the atrial and ventricular chambers of the heart. **2.** a room or closed space used for research or therapeutic purposes, such as a decompression chamber or hyperbaric oxygen chamber.

Chamberlain's line [W. E. Chamberlain, American radiologist, b. 1891], a line that extends from the posterior of the hard palate to the dorsum of the foramen magnum.

Chamberlen forceps [Peter Chamberlen, English obstetrician, b. 1560], one of the earliest kinds of obstetric forceps, introduced in the seventeenth century.

CHAMPUS, abbreviation for **Civilian Health and Medical Programs for Uniformed Services.**

chancr-. See **cancr-.**

chancre /shang′kər/ [Fr, canker], **1.** also called **venereal sore.** a skin lesion, usually of primary syphilis, that begins at the site of infection as a papule and develops into a red, bloodless, painless ulcer with a scooped-out appearance. It heals without treatment and leaves no scar. Two or more chancres may develop at the same time, occurring usually in the genital area but sometimes on the hands, face, or other body surface. The chancre teems with *Treponema pallidum* spirochetes and is highly contagious. **2.** a papular lesion or ulcerated area of the skin that marks the point of infection of a nonsyphilitic disease, such as tuberculosis. Compare **chancroid.** See also **syphilis.**

chancroid /shang′kroid/ [Fr, *chancre,* canker; Gk, *eidos,* form], a highly contagious, sexually transmitted disease caused by infection with a bacillus, *Haemophilus ducreyi.* It characteristically begins as a papule, usually on the skin of the external genitalia; it then grows and ulcerates, other papules form, and, if untreated, the bacillus spreads, causing buboes in the groin. An intradermal skin test is more reliable than smear and culture techniques in diagnosing this condition. Erythromycin or ceftriaxone are prescribed to treat chancroid. Because the lesion resembles syphilis and lymphogranuloma venereum, the diagnosis must be made before treatment to avoid obscuring simultaneous infections. Symptoms may not appear until 10 days after infection. Compare **chancre.**

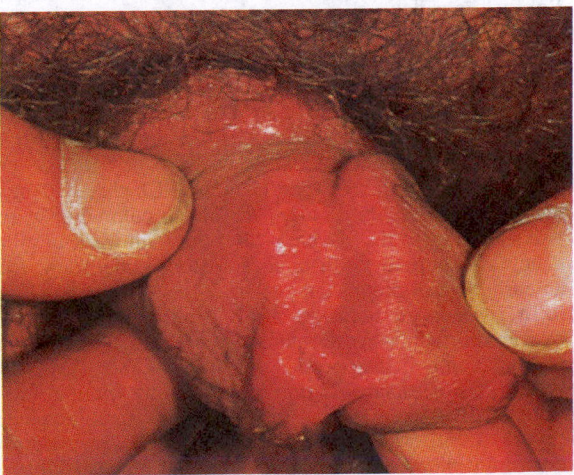

Chancroid (Habif, 1990)

change agent, a role in which communication skills, education, and other resources are applied to help a client adjust to changes caused by illness or disability.

change of life, *informal.* the female climacteric; menopause.

channel [L, *canalis,* pipe], a passageway or groove that conveys fluid, such as the central channels that connect the arterioles with the venules.

channel ulcer [L, *canalis,* pipe, *ulcus,* sore], a rare type of peptic ulcer found in the pyloric canal between the stomach and the duodenum. See also **peptic ulcer.**

chaotic atrial tachycardia /kā·ot′ik/, an atrial rhythm of more than 100 beats per minute due to multifocal atrial activity with at least three different shapes of P′ waves on the electrocardiogram. The condition is often associated with chronic obstructive lung disease.

chapped /chapt/ [ME, *chappen,* cracked], pertaining to skin that is roughened, cracked, or reddened by exposure to cold or excessive moisture evaporation. Stinging or burning sensations often accompany the disorder. Prevention is by protection against exposure to cold and wind. Treatment includes the avoidance of frequent washing, the replacement of soaps and detergents with superfatted soaps, and the application of emollients. Compare **frostbite. –chap,** *v.*

character [Gk, *charassein,* to engrave], **1.** the integrated composite of traits and behavioral tendencies that enable a person to react in a relatively consistent way to the customs and mores of society. Character, as contrasted with personality, implies volition and morality. Compare **personality. 2.** any letter, number, symbol, or punctuation mark, usually composed of eight bits or one byte, that can be transmitted as output by a computer. See also **bit.**

character analysis, a systematic investigation of the personality of an individual with special attention to psychologic defenses and motivations, usually undertaken to improve behavior.

character disorder, a chronic, habitual, maladaptive, and socially unacceptable pattern of behavior and emotional response. The condition is usually accompanied by minimal feelings of anxiety. Also called **character neurosis.** See also **antisocial personality disorder.**

characteristic curve /ker′əktəris′tik/, (in radiology) the pattern of a plot on a graph representing the relationship between the density, or degree of blackness of an x-ray film, and the exposure.

characteristic radiation, radiation produced when a projectile electron interacts with an inner-shell electron of a target atom, causing total removal of the electron. It is one of the principles of x-ray production.

character neurosis. See **character disorder.**

character printer, a printer for computers that prints a fully formed character, such as a letter, number, or symbol, with each impression stroke. Compare **dot-matrix printer.**

charcoal. See **activated charcoal.**

Charcot-Bouchard aneurysm /shärkō′bōōshär′/ [Jean M. Charcot, French neurologist, b. 1825; Charles J. Bouchard, French physician, b. 1837], a small, round aneurysm of a small artery of the cerebral cortex or basal ganglia. Charcot-Bouchard aneurysms often occur in individuals with very high blood pressure.

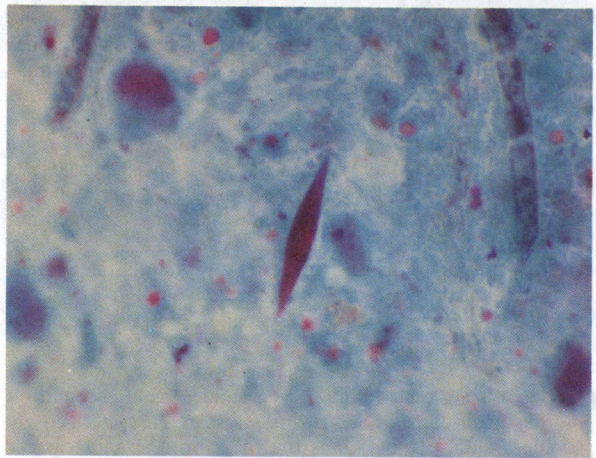

Charcot-Leyden crystals *(Baron, 1990)*

Charcot-Leyden crystal /shärkō′lī′dən/ [Jean M. Charcot; Ernst V. von Leyden, German physician, b. 1832], any one of the crystalline structures shaped like narrow, double pyramids found in the sputum of individuals suffering from bronchial asthma. They are also found in the feces of dysentery patients. The Charcot-Leyden crystals are protein compounds and occur in association with the fragmentation of eosinophils. Also called **asthma crystal, leukocytic crystal.**

Charcot-Marie-Tooth disease /shärkō′mərē′tōōth′/ [Jean M. Charcot; Pierre Marie, French neurologist, b. 1853; Howard H. Tooth, English neurologist, b. 1856], a progressive hereditary disorder characterized by degeneration of the peroneal muscles of the fibula, resulting in clubfoot, foot drop, and ataxia. Progressive arm weakness can also be present as distal muscles atrophy.

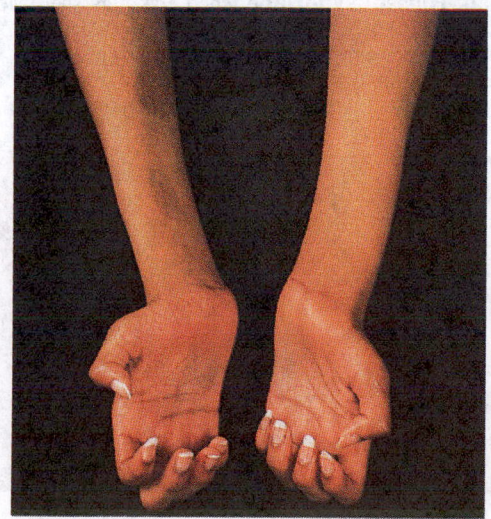

Charcot-Marie-Tooth atrophy *(Zitelli, 1992)*

Charcot's fever /shärkōz′/ [Jean M. Charcot], a syndrome characterized by a recurrent fever, jaundice, and abdominal pain in the right upper quadrant occurring with inflammation of the bile ducts. It is caused by the intermittent impaction of a stone in the ducts.

Charcot's joint, See **neuropathic joint disease.**

Charcot's triad [Jean Martin Charcot, French neurologist, b. 1825; Gk, *trias,* three], a set of three signs of brainstem involvement in multiple sclerosis. They are intention tremor, nystagmus, and scanning speech.

charlatan /shär′lətən/ [Fr, imposter], a totally unqualified individual posing as an expert, especially an individual pretending to be a physician. Also called **quack.** –**charlatanical,** *adj.*

Charles' law. See **Gay-Lussac's law.**

charley horse /chär′lē hôrs′/, a sudden painful condition of the quadriceps or hamstring muscles characterized by soreness and stiffness. It is the result of a strain, tear, or bruise of the muscle, is aggravated by movement, and is often associated with athletic activity. Treatment includes rest and massage. Compare **cramp.**

chart /chärt/ [L, *charta,* paper], **1.** *informal.* a patient record. **2.** to note data in a patient record, usually at prescribed intervals.

charta /kär′tə/, *pl.* **chartae** [L, paper], a piece of paper, especially one treated with medicine, as for external application, or with a chemical for a special purpose, such as litmus paper.

chauffeur's fracture /shō′fərz/ [Fr, stoker; L, *fractura* break], any fracture of the radial styloid, produced by a twisting or a snapping type injury.

Chaussier's areola /shôsyāz′/ [François Chaussier, French anatomist, b. 1746; L, little space], an areola of indurated tissue surrounding a malignant pustule.

CHB, abbreviation for **complete heart block.**

CHC, abbreviation for *community health center.*

CHD, abbreviation for **coronary heart disease.**

check ligament. See **alar ligament.**

check-up [Fr, *eschec* acquire; AS, *uf*], a thorough study or examination of the health of an individual.

Chediak-Higashi syndrome /ched′ē·ak·higä′shē/ [Moises Chediak, twentieth century French physician; Ototaka Higa shi, twentieth century Japanese physician], a congenital, autosomal disorder, characterized by partial albinism, photophobia, massive leukocytic inclusions, psychomotor abnormalities, recurrent infections, and early death. Antenatal diagnosis can be made by amniocentesis and tissue culture. Treatment includes antibiotics and transfusions.

cheek [AS, *ceace*], a fleshy prominence, especially the fleshy protuberances on both sides of the face between the eye and the jaw and the ear and the nose and mouth. Also called **bucca.**

cheekbone. See **zygomatic bone.**

cheesy abscess [AS, *cese*; L, *abscedere,* to go away], an abscess that contains a yellowish semisolid, cheeselike, material. It is found in tuberculous abscesses. Also called **caseous abscess.**

cheil-. See **cheilo-.**

-cheilia, -chilia, a suffix meaning '(condition of the) lips': *atelocheilia, dicheilia, xerocheilia.*

cheilitis /kīlī′tis/ [Gk, *cheilos,* lip, *itis,* inflammation], an abnormal condition of the lips characterized by inflammation and cracking of the skin. There are several forms, including those caused by excessive exposure to sunlight, allergic sensitivity to cosmetics, and vitamin deficiency. Compare **cheilosis.**

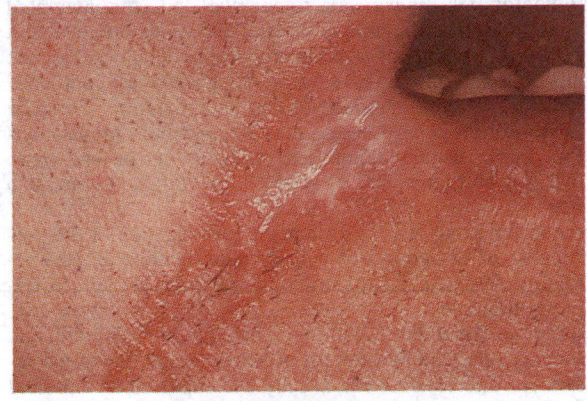

Angular cheilitis
(Lamey, 1988)

cheilo-, cheil-, a combining form meaning 'pertaining to the lip': *cheiloangioscopy, cheilocarcinoma, cheiloplasty.*

cheilocarcinoma /kī′lōkär′sinō′mə/, *pl.* **cheilocarcinomas, cheilocarcinomata,** a malignant epithelial tumor of the lip.

cheiloplasty /kī′ləplas′tē/ [Gk, *cheilos,* lip, *plassein,* to mold], surgical correction of a defect of the lip.

cheilorrhaphy /kīlôr′əfē/ [Gk, *cheilos,* lip, *raphe,* suture], a surgical procedure that sutures the lip, such as in the repair of a congenitally cleft lip or a lacerated lip.

cheilosis /kīlō′sis/, a disorder of the lips and mouth characterized by scales and fissures, resulting from a deficiency of riboflavin in the diet.

cheir-. See **cheiro-.**

cheiragra. See **cheiro.**

cheiralgia /kəral′jə/ [Gk, *cheir* + *algos,* pain], a pain in the hand, especially the pain associated with arthritis. –**cheiralgic,** *adj.*

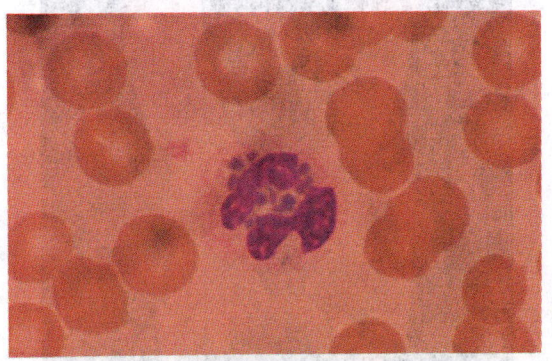

Chediak-Higashi syndrome
(Zitelli, 1992/Courtesy Dr. William Zinkham)

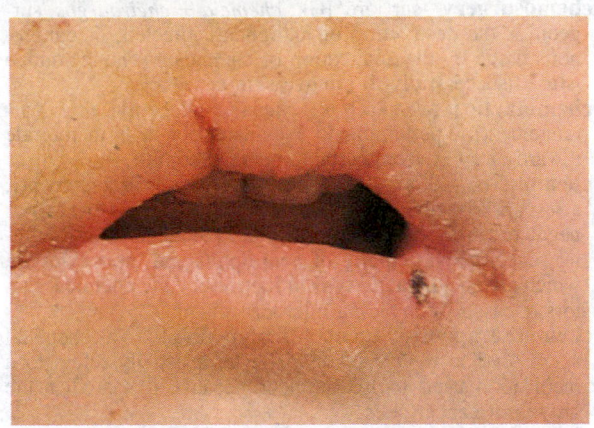

Cheilosis *(McLaren, 1992)*

-cheiria. See **-chiria.**

cheiro-, cheir-, chir-, chiro-, a combining form meaning 'pertaining to the hand': *cheiragra, cheiromegaly, cheiroplasty.*

cheiromegaly /kī′rōmeg′əlē/ [Gk, *cheir* + *megas,* large], an abnormal condition characterized by excessively large hands. **–cheiromegalic,** *adj.*

cheiroplasty /kī′rōplas′tē/, an operation involving plastic surgery of the hand. **–cheiroplastic,** *adj.*

chelate /kē′lāt/ [Gk, *chele,* claw], **1.** (of a metal ion and two or more polar groups of a single molecule) to form a bond, thus creating a ringlike complex. **2.** (in medicine) any coordination compound composed of a central metal ion and an organic molecule with multiple bonds, arranged in ring formations, used especially in chemotherapeutic treatments for metal poisoning. **3.** of or pertaining to chelation.

chelating agent /kē′lāting/, a substance that promotes chelation. Chelating agents are used in the treatment of metal poisoning. See also **chelation.**

chelation /kēlā′shən/, a chemical reaction in which there is a combination with a metal to form a ring-shaped molecular complex in which the metal is firmly bound and sequestered. See also **chelating agent.**

cheloid. See **keloid.**

cheloidal. See **keloid.**

cheloidosis. See **keloidosis.**

chemabrasion /kem′əbrā′zhən/ [Gk, *chemeia,* alchemy; L, *ab, radere,* to scrape off], a method of treating scars, chromatosis, or other skin disorders by applying chemicals that remove the surface layers of skin cells. See also **chemical cauterization, chemosurgery.**

chemical /kem′əkəl/ [Gk, *chemeia,* alchemy], **1.** a substance composed of chemical elements or a substance produced by or used in chemical processes. **2.** pertaining to chemistry.

chemical action, any process in which natural elements and compounds react with each other to produce a chemical change or a different compound; for example, hydrogen and oxygen combine to produce water.

chemical affinity [Gk, *chemeia,* alchemy; L, *affinis,* re-lated], an attraction that results in the formation of molecules from atoms.

chemical agent, any chemical power, active principle, or substance that can produce an effect in the body by interacting with various body substances, such as aspirin, which produces an analgesic effect.

chemical antidote [Gk, *chemeia; anti,* against, *dotos,* that which is given], any substance that reacts chemically with a poison to form a compound that is harmless. There are few true antidotes, and treatment of poisoning depends largely on eliminating the toxic agent before it can be absorbed by the body.

chemical burn, tissue damage caused by exposure to a strong acid or alkali, such as phenol, creosol, mustard gas, or phosphorus. Emergency treatment includes washing the surface with copious amounts of water to remove the chemical and, if the damage is more than slight and superficial, immediate transport to a medical facility. See also **acid burn, acid poisoning, alkali burn, alkali poisoning.**

chemical carcinogen [Gk, *chemeia,* alchemy, *karkinos,* crab, *oma,* tumor, *genein,* to produce], any chemical agent that can induce the development of cancer in living tissue.

chemical cauterization [Gk, *chemeia; kauterion,* branding iron], the corroding or burning of living tissue by a caustic chemical substance, such as potassium hydroxide. Also called **chemocautery.**

chemical diabetes. See **impaired glucose tolerance.**

chemical energy. See **energy.**

chemical equivalent, a drug or chemical containing similar amounts of the same ingredients as another drug or chemical.

chemical fog, a curtain effect on x-ray film resulting in the loss of image quality. It appears as a dull gray discoloration and is usually caused by chemical contamination of the developer used.

chemical gastritis, inflammation of the stomach caused by the ingestion of a chemical compound. Treatment is determined by the substance ingested. Gastric lavage is often advisable, but neither lavage nor emetics should be administered in cases involving the most corrosive poisons. Compare **corrosive gastritis, erosive gastritis.**

chemical indicator, a commercially prepared device that monitors all or part of the physical conditions of the sterilization cycle. It usually consists of a sensitive ink dye that changes colors under certain conditions.

chemical mediator, a neurotransmitter chemical, such as acetylcholine.

chemical name, the exact designation of the chemical structure of a drug as determined by the rules of accepted systems of chemical nomenclature. For example, N,N-bis-(2-chloroethyl)-N′-(3-hydroxypropyl) phosphordiamidic acid cyclic acid monohydrate is the chemical name of cyclophosphamide, a drug used in cancer chemotherapy.

chemical peritonitis [Gk, *chemeia,* alchemy, *peri,* near, *teinein,* to stretch, *itis,* inflammation], an inflammation of the peritoneum resulting from chemicals, including digestive substances, in the peritoneum.

chemical shift, (in nuclear magnetic response spectometry) the position of a resonance in the substance of interest relative to the position of the resonance of a standard. Non equivalent atoms of a molecule will have different chemical shifts.

chemical warfare, the waging of war with poisonous chemicals and gases.

cheminosis /kem'ənō'sis/ [Gk, *chemeia* + *osis,* condition], any disease caused by a chemical substance.

chemistry /kem'istrē/ [Gk, *chemeia,* alchemy], the science dealing with the elements, their compounds, and the molecular structure and interactions of matter. Kinds of chemistry include **inorganic chemistry** and **organic chemistry.**

chemistry, normal values, the amounts of various substances in the normal human body, determined by testing a large sample of people presumed to be healthy. Normal values are expressed in ranges of numbers, and ranges vary from laboratory to laboratory. For example, a normal concentration of a substance in the blood might be expressed as 5 to 20 mg/dl. Although variations from normal values may be highly significant tools in the diagnoses of certain diseases, in all cases an abnormal result must be cautiously interpreted. See also specific tests.

chemo- /kem'ō-/, kē'mō-/, a combining form meaning 'by chemical reaction' or'pertaining to a chemical or to chemistry': *chemoantigen, chemobiotic, chemokinesis.*

chemocautery. See **chemical cauterization.**

chemodifferentiation /-dif'əren'shē·ā'shən/, a stage in embryonic development that precedes and controls specialization and differentiation of the cells into rudimentary organs.

chemonucleolysis /-nōō'klē·ol'isis-/ [Gk, *chemeia* + L, *nucleus,* kernel; Gk, *lysein,* to loosen], a method of dissolving the nucleus pulposus of an intervertebral disk by the injection of a chemolytic agent, such as the enzyme chymopapain. The procedure is used primarily in the treatment of a herniated disk and other intervertebral disk lesions.

chemoprophylaxis /-prō'filak'sis/ [Gk, *chemeia* + *prophylax,* advance guard], the use of antimicrobial drugs to prevent the acquisition of pathogens in an endemic area or to prevent their spread from one body area to another.

chemoreceptor /-risep'tər/ [Gk, *chemeia* + L, *recipere,* to receive], a sensory nerve cell activated by chemical stimuli, such as a chemoreceptor in the carotid artery that is sensitive to the P_{CO_2} in the blood, signaling the respiratory center in the brain to increase or decrease respiration.

chemoreflex /-rē'fleks/, any reflex initiated by the stimulation of chemical receptors, such as the carotid and aortic bodies, which respond to changes in carbon dioxide, hydrogen ion, and oxygen concentrations in the blood. See also **chemoreceptor.**

chemosis /kimō'sis/ [Gk, *cheme,* cockle, *osis,* condition], an abnormal edematous swelling of the mucous membrane covering the eyeball and lining the eyelids that is usually the result of local trauma or infection. Chemosis may also occur in acute conjunctivitis. An obstruction of normal lymph flow, such as might occur from growth of a tumor within the eye socket, may less commonly be found to be the cause of chemosis. Systemic disorders, such as angioneurotic edema, anemia, and Bright's disease, may also cause the condition. Also called **conjunctival edema.**

chemostat /kē'məstat'/, a device that assures a steady rate of cell division in bacterial populations by maintaining a constant environment.

chemosurgery /-sur'jərē/ [Gk, *chemeia* + *cheirourgos,* surgeon], the destruction of malignant, infected, or gangrenous tissue by the application of chemicals. The technique is used successfully to remove skin cancers.

chemotactic /-tak'tik/ [Gk, *chemeia,* alchemy, *taxis,* arrangement], pertaining to a tendency of cells to migrate toward or away from certain chemical stimuli.

chemotaxis /-tak'sis/ [Gk, *chemeia* + *taxis,* arrangement], a response involving movement that is positive (toward) or negative (away from) to a chemical stimulus. It is a cellular function, particularly of neutrophils and monocytes, in which phagocytic activity is influenced by the chemical factors released by invading microorganisms.

chemotherapeutic agent /-ther'əpyōō'tik/, a chemical agent used to treat diseases. The term usually refers to a medication used to treat cancer because it can alter the growth of cancer cells.

chemotherapy /-ther'əpē/, the treatment of infections and other diseases with chemical agents. The term has been applied over the centuries to a variety of therapies, including the treatment of malaria with herbs and the use of mercury for syphilis. In modern usage, chemotherapy usually refers to the use of chemicals to destroy cancer cells on a selective basis. The cytotoxic agents used in cancer treatments generally function in the same manner as ionizing radiation; they do not kill the cancer cells directly but instead impair their ability to replicate. Most of the nearly 40 anticancer drugs commonly used act by interfering with DNA and RNA activities associated with cell division. Chemotherapeutic agents are often used in combination with radiation treatments for their synergistic effect. A cytotoxic agent, for example, may be used to render a tumor cell more sensitive to the effects of radiation. Thus, by making the cancer cell more vulnerable to the effects of ionizing radiation, the cancer can be controlled with smaller doses of radiation than would be possible with radiation alone.

chemotherapy (unsealed radioactive), the oral or parenteral administration of a radioisotope, such as iodine 131 (^{131}I) for the treatment of hyperthyroidism or thyroid cancer, phosphorus 32 (^{32}P) for leukemia or polycythemia vera, or peritoneal ascites resulting from widely disseminated carcinoma.

■ METHOD: Before unsealed radioactive chemotherapy is administered, the patient receives an explanation of the procedure and of the need for isolation during the half-life of the radioisotope (8.1 days for ^{131}I, 14 days for ^{32}P, and 2.7 days for ^{198}Au). The room in which the patient is isolated adjoins a private bathroom and is equipped with convenient furniture, a freshly made bed placed next to the building's outer wall, a functioning phone and television set, adequate lighting, reading and hobby materials, and containers for contaminated linen, dressings, and excreta. Radioactive tags are posted on the door. The patient's chart is kept at the door, and individual radioactive badges are worn by each staff member entering the room to record the amount of radiation exposure; pregnant staff members are not assigned to the patient's care. Urine excreted by a patient treated with ^{131}I is collected directly or via an indwelling catheter, in a lead-lined container, which is sent to the laboratory for assay of the radioisotope. Feces, sputum, and vomitus are placed in the toilet and decontaminated with a dropperful of a saturated solution of potassium iodide before the bowl is flushed. If excreta spills on the skin, the area is rinsed in running water for 2 minutes and washed in soap and water for an additional 3 minutes. If the bed or another surface in the room is contaminated with excreta, the radiation control officer is notified and the area is monitored before being cleaned. Dressings and bed linen are handled with rubber or plastic gloves; contaminated linens are placed in a hamper and trash in plastic bags, and they are not removed from the room until monitored with a Geiger-Müller counter. The staff member limits exposure by repositioning the debilitated patient with a turn sheet, by bathing only the soiled body areas, and by preparing and cutting food on the diet tray before entering the room. The patient treated with ^{131}I is observed for evidence of neck tenderness, changes in exophthalmia, a transient productive cough, hypoparathyroidism, hypothyroidism, and hyperthyroidism. Special precautions are required in caring for the patient treated with radioactive gold, which emits gamma and beta rays. After purple liquid ^{198}Au is injected into the body cavity, the patient is turned with a sheet every 15 minutes for 2 hours so that the radionuclide can spread. Dressings and cleansing tissues contaminated by the purple seepage from wounds are burned immediately; linen in contact with wounds is placed in special containers. The patient injected with ^{198}Au is usually terminally ill, and, if death occurs, a tag is placed on the body to alert the mortician to the presence of the radionuclide.

■ NURSING INTERVENTION: The nurse wears a radiation badge when entering the patient's room and limits exposure by performing planned procedures efficiently. Routine nursing functions are kept to a minimum, especially if the patient is ambulatory, but emotional support is provided in brief hourly visits at the door and via the intercommunication system. The nurse anticipates and fulfills the isolated patient's requests as promptly as possible, arranges diversional activities, and assures the patient that when a certain period of time has passed the patient will no longer be a source of radioactivity.

■ OUTCOME CRITERIA: Radioactive iodine usually counteracts hyperthyroidism and is frequently used in conjunction with surgery in the treatment of thyroid cancer. Radioactive phosphorus often controls polycythemia vera, but other agents are generally more effective in leukemia therapy. Radioactive gold is usually administered as a last resort in advanced lung cancer or peritoneal ascites resulting from malignant disease.

chenodeoxycholic acid /kē′nōdē·ok′sikō′lik/, a secondary bile acid. It is used in vivo to dissolve cholesterol gallstones, particularly in the elderly and poor-risk patients. See also **ursodeoxycholic acid.**

cherry angioma [L, *cerasus; aggeion,* vessel, *oma,* tumor], a small, bright red, clearly circumscribed vascular tumor on the skin. It occurs most often on the trunk but may be found anywhere on the body. The lesion is very common; more than 85% of people over 45 years of age have several cherry angiomas. Also called **capillary angioma, capillary hemangioma, De Morgan's spots, senile angioma.**

cherry red spot, an abnormal red circular area of the choroid, seen through the fovea centralis of the eye and surrounded by a contrasting white edema. It is associated with cases of infantile cerebral sphingolipidosis and sometimes appears in the late infantile form of amaurotic familial idiocy. Also called **Tay's spot.**

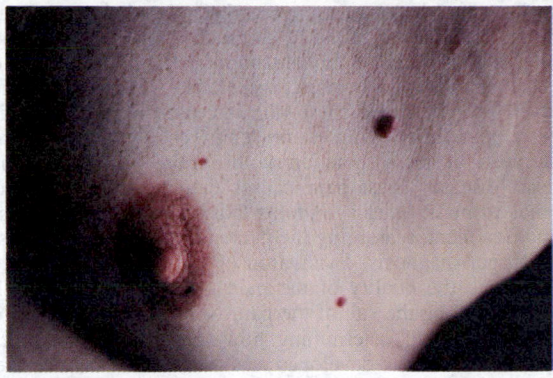

Cherry angioma *(Christiansen, 1993)*

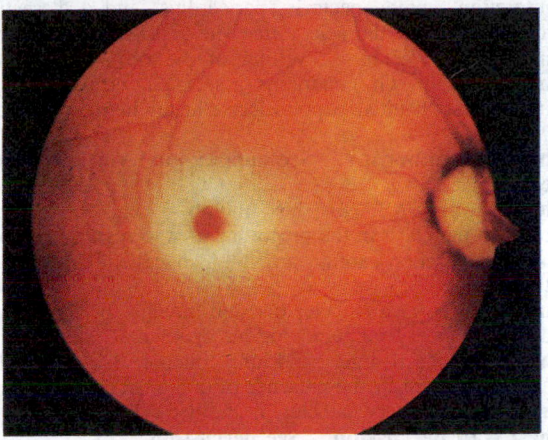

Cherry red spot *(Apple, 1991)*

cherubism /cher′əbiz′əm/ [Heb, *kerubh*], an abnormal hereditary condition characterized by progressive bilateral swelling at the angle of the mandible, especially in children. In some cases of cherubism, the entire jaw swells and the eyes turn up, enhancing the cherubic facial appearance. The condition tends to regress during adult life.

chest. See **thorax.**

chest cavity. See **body cavity.**

chest lead /lēd/, **1.** an electrocardiographic conductor in which the exploring electrode is placed on the chest or precordium. The indifferent electrode is placed on the patient's back for a CB (chest back) lead, on the front of the chest for a CF (chest front) lead, on the left arm for a CL (chest left) lead, and on the right arm for a CR (chest right) lead. **2.** *informal.* the tracing produced by such a lead on an electrocardiograph.

chest pain [AS, *cest,* box; L, *poena,* punishment], a physical complaint that requires immediate diagnosis and evaluation. Chest pain may be symptomatic of cardiac disease, such as angina pectoris, myocardial infarction, or pericarditis, or of disease of the lungs, such as pleurisy, pneumonia, or pulmonary embolism or infarction. The source of chest pain may also be musculoskeletal, GI, or psychogenic. Over 90% of severe chest pain is caused by coronary disease, spinal root compression, or psychologic disturbance. Because of its association with serious, life-threatening heart disease, chest pain causes extreme anxiety, which tends to mask other symptoms that would aid in diagnosis and treatment; reassuring the person being examined assists in proper diagnosis. Evaluation of chest pain requires determining the quality of the pain—dull, sharp, or crushing—locating the site of the pain—in the center or side of the chest—and determining how long the pain has persisted, how it has developed, and whether it has occurred in the past. The patient is asked to describe the spread of pain to other parts of the body and to identify such factors as exertion, emotional distress, movement, or deep breathing, that aggravate or relieve the pain. Specific cardiovascular conditions associated with chest pain are myocardial infarction, angina pectoris, pericarditis, and a dissecting aneurysm of the thoracic aorta. Musculoskeletal conditions include rib fractures, swelling of the rib cartilage, and muscle strain. GI conditions associated with chest pain include esophagitis, peptic ulcers, hiatus hernia, and pancreatitis.

chest physiotherapy. See **cupping and vibrating, percussion.**

chest thump [AS, *cest*, box; thump = echoic], a sharp blow to the chest in the precordial area to restore a normal heart beat after cardiac arrest. Also called **precordianl thump**.

chest tube, 1. a catheter inserted through the thorax into the chest cavity for removing air or fluid. It is commonly used after chest surgery and lung collapse. 2. radiographic artifacts caused by the presence of oral or tracheal tubes, or a pulmonary artery catheter, in the body of a patient.

chest wall percussion. See **percussion.**

chewing gum diarrhea. See **osmotic diarrhea.**

chewing reflex, a pathologic sign in brain-damaged adults, characterized by repetitive chewing motions when the mouth is stimulated.

Cheyne-Stokes respiration (CSR) /chān'stōks'/ [John Cheyne, Scottish physician, b. 1777; William Stokes, Irish physician, b. 1804; L *respirare* to breathe], an abnormal pattern of respiration, characterized by alternating periods of apnea and deep, rapid breathing. The respiratory cycle begins with slow, shallow breaths that gradually increase to abnormal depth and rapidity. Respiration gradually subsides as breathing slows and becomes shallower, climaxing in a 10- to 20-second period without respiration before the cycle is repeated. Each cyclic episode may last from 45 seconds to 3 minutes. The immediate cause of CSR is a complex alteration in the functioning of the respiratory center in the brain, caused by dysfunction of the diencephalon or by bilateral hemispheric lesions. Changes in blood gases, especially an increase in carbon dioxide, may be the proximal cause. Alternatively, a direct reduction in the sensitivity of the respiratory center may occur in the presence of normal concentrations of blood gases, such as seen in cerebral vascular disease, in tumors of the brainstem, or as a result of severe head injury. The most common cause of an alteration in the blood

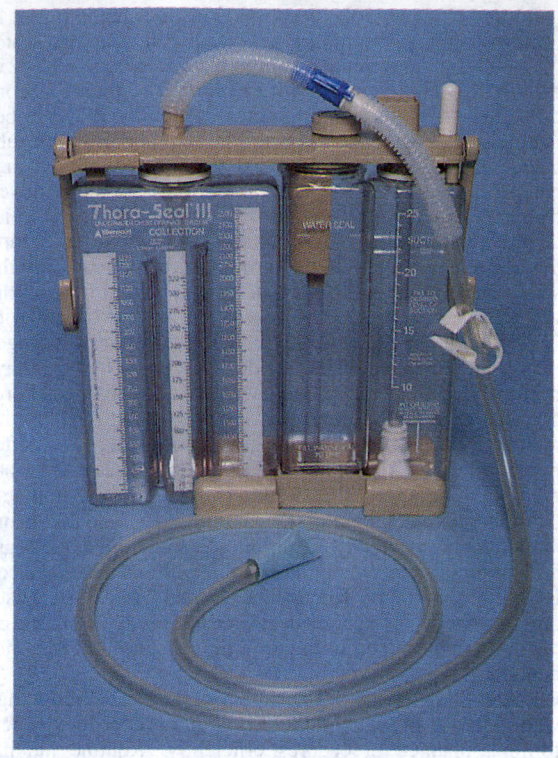

Commercial chest drainage system (Potter, 1993)

chemistry that might induce CSR is congestive heart failure, especially in elderly patients with degenerative arterial disease. Bronchopneumonia or other respiratory diseases in elderly people may likewise induce Cheyne-Stokes breathing, and CSR may occur in an otherwise healthy person through hyperventilation or exposure to high altitudes. This pattern of breathing may also be induced by an overdose of a narcotic or hypnotic drug, and it occurs more frequently during sleep. Compare **Biot's respiration.**

-chezia, -chesia, a suffix meaning '(condition of) defecation, especially involving the discharge of foreign substances': *dyschezia, hematochezia, pyochezia.*

CHF, abbreviation for **congestive heart failure.**

ch'i, a Chinese concept of a fundamental life energy that flows in orderly ways along meridians, or channels, in the body. See also **acupuncture.**

Chiari-Frommel syndrome /kē·är'ēfrom'əl/ [Johann B. Chiari, German physician, b. 1817; Richard Frommel, German gynecologist, b. 1854], a hormonal disorder that occurs after a pregnancy in which weaning does not spontaneously end lactation. The syndrome is usually the result of a decrease in pituitary gonadotropins and an excess of pituitary prolactin and may be accompanied by amenorrhea. Treatment includes observation, hormonal therapy, and investigation to confirm or rule out pituitary tumor.

Chiari's syndrome. See **Budd-Chiari syndrome.**

chiasm /kī'azəm/ [Gk, *chiasma*, lines that cross], 1. the crossing of two lines or tracts, as the crossing of the optic

Differentiating characteristics of chest pain

Precipitating factors	Character	Relief
Cardiovascular		
Effort angina		
Exercise, emotion, extreme temperatures, eating heavy meals	Constricting, squeezing, pressure; usually lasting more than 2 minutes and less than 15 minutes	Rest or nitroglycerin
Rest angina		
Spontaneous; possible daily cycle	Like effort angina	Nitroglycerin
Acute myocardial infarction		
Spontaneous	Like angina but more severe, crushing; usually lasting longer than 20 minutes	Narcotic analgesics, rest or glycerin not effective
Pericarditis		
Deep breath, lying down	Sharp, stabbing; continuous	Antiinflammatories, analgesics sitting up, leaning forward
Hypertrophic cardiomyopathy		
Exercise, stress	Anginal pain associated with lightheadedness, dizziness, syncope	Rest, β-blockers
Mitral valve prolapse		
Spontaneous	Variable in character, possibly migratory	Time
Acute dissecting aortic aneurysm		
Spontaneous	Sudden, severe, tearing pain in center of chest, radiating to back or abdomen	Large doses of analgesics
Pulmonary		
Pulmonary embolism		
Spontaneous; accentuated by dyspnea and pleuritic respiration	Sharp, stabbing, knifelike; continuous	Time
Pleurisy		
History of recent respiratory illness; worse with respiratory movement	Sharp, burning, ache or "catch" on one side of the chest	Time
Musculoskeletal		
Coughing, deep breath, movement	Sharp, stabbing, tenderness, localized; fleeting or lasting for days	Antiinflammatories, analgesics
Gastrointestinal		
Gastric or duodenal ulcer		
Empty stomach	Burning in epigastrium 60 to 90 minutes after eating	Milk or antacids
Esophageal spasm or irritation		
Spontaneous	Buring deep in throat; accompanying weight loss, dysphagia, regurgitation	Nitroglycerin
Other		
Emotional stress		
Stress stimulus	Tightness, aching; if accompanied by hyperventilation, possible ST-segment and T-wave changes	Stimulus removal
Mediastinitis or mediastinal tumors		
Spontaneous	Pleuritic, constriction	Time Removal of mass
Tissue rupture or tear		
Blunt injury	Abrupt, sharp	Time, repair

From Guzzetta C, Dossey B: *Cardiovascular nursing: holistic practice*, St Louis, 1992, Mosby, p 230.

nerves at the optic chiasm. **2.** (in genetics) the crossing of two chromatids in the prophase of meiosis. **–chiasmal, chiasmic,** *adj.*

chiasma /kī·az′mə/, *pl.* ***chiasmata*** [Gk, lines that cross], (in genetics), the visible point of connection between homologous chromosomes during the first meiotic division in gametogenesis. The X-shaped configurations form during the late prophase stage and provide the means by which exchange of genetic material occurs. See also **crossing over. –chiasmatic, chiasmic.** *adj.*

chiasmal. See **chiasm.**

chiasmatypy. See **crossing over.**

chiasmic. See **chiasm, chiasma.**

chickenpox /chik′ənpoks′/ [AS, *cicen;* ME, *pokke*], an acute, highly contagious viral disease caused by a herpesvirus, varicella zoster virus (VZV). It occurs primarily in young children and is characterized by crops of pruritic vesicular eruptions on the skin. The disease is transmitted by direct contact with skin lesions or, more commonly, by droplets spread from the respiratory tract of infected persons, usually in the prodromal period or the early stages of the rash. The vesicular fluid and the scabs are infectious until entirely dry. Indirect transmission through uninfected persons or objects is rare. The diagnosis is usually made by physical examination and by the characteristic appearance of the disease. The virus may be identified by culture of the vesicle fluid. Also called **varicella.**
■ OBSERVATIONS: The incubation period averages 2 to 3 weeks, followed by slight fever, mild headache, malaise, and anorexia occurring about 24 to 36 hours before the rash begins. The prodromal period is usually mild in children but may be severe in adults. The rash, which is highly pruritic, begins as macules and progresses in 1 or 2 days to papules and, finally, to vesicles surrounding an erythematous base and containing clear fluid. Within 24 to 48 hours the vesicles turn cloudy and become umbilicated, are easily broken, and become encrusted. The lesions, which erupt in crops so that all three stages are present simultaneously, appear first on the back and chest and then spread to the face, neck, and limbs; they occur only rarely on the soles and palms. In severe cases, laryngeal or tracheal vesicles in the pharynx, larynx, and trachea may cause dyspnea and dysphagia. Prolonged fever, lymphadenopathy, and extreme irritability from pruritus are other symptoms. The symptoms last from a few days to 2 weeks.

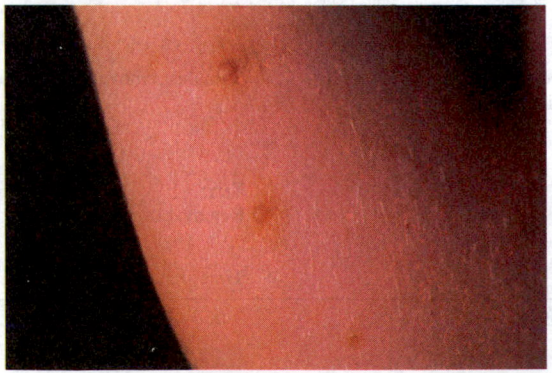

Chicken pox *(Goldstein, 1992/Courtesy John Cook MD)*

■ INTERVENTIONS: Routine treatment consists of bed rest; antipyretics to reduce fever; applications of topical antipruritics, such as wet compresses, calamine lotion, or a paste made from baking soda and water; or oral antihistamines, given for the relief of itching. Infected vesicles may be treated with neomycin-bacitracin, and systemic antibiotics may be given if the secondary bacterial infection is extensive. People who are susceptible and at risk for severe disease when exposed to the infection may be passively protected with zoster immune globulin (ZIG), varicella-zoster immune globulin (VZIG), immune serum globulin (ISG), or zoster immune plasma (ZIP). A preparation of the virus for active immunization is not yet available. Babies born to women who develop chickenpox within 5 days of delivery are especially likely to get a severe case of the disease. One attack of the disease confers permanent immunity, although recurring episodes of herpes zoster occur, especially in elderly or debilitated people, resulting from reactivation of the virus. Herpes zoster virus (HZV), like all herpesviruses, lies dormant in certain sensory nerve roots after primary infection.
■ NURSING CONSIDERATIONS: Chickenpox in childhood is usually benign. Few cases require hospitalization. It may be serious or fatal in immunocompromised people, such as those receiving chemotherapy or radiotherapy for malignant disease, in those who have undergone organ transplantation, in those with congenital or acquired defects in cell-mediated immunity, or in those receiving high doses of steroids. Common complications are secondary bacterial infections, such as abscesses, cellulitis, pneumonia, and sepsis, and hemorrhagic varicella (tiny hemorrhages that may occur in the vesicles or surrounding skin). Less common complications are encephalitis, Reye's syndrome (associated with the use of aspirin by patients), thrombocytopenia, and hepatitis.

chiclero's ulcer /chikler′ōz/ [Mex, *tzictli,* chicle; L, *ulcus*], a kind of American leishmaniasis caused by *Leishmania mexicana*. It is endemic among the workers in the Yucatan and Central America who harvest chicle from the forest. The disease is characterized by cutaneous ulcers on the head that usually heal spontaneously by 6 months, except for those on the pinna of the ear, which may last for years and cause scarring and deformities. See also **American leishmaniasis, leishmaniasis.**

chief cell [Fr, *chef;* L, *cella,* storeroom], **1.** also called **zymogenic cell.** any one of the columnar epithelial cells or the cuboidal epithelial cells that line the gastric glands and secrete pepsinogen and intrinsic factor, which is needed for the absorption of vitamin B_{12} and the normal development of red blood cells. Anemia is caused by the absence of intrinsic factor. **2.** any one of the epithelioid cells with pale-staining cytoplasm and a large nucleus containing a prominent nucleolus. Cords of such cells form the main substance of the pineal body. **3.** also called **principal cell.** any one of the polyhedral epithelial cells, within the parathyroid glands, which contain pale, clear cytoplasm and a vesicular nucleus.

chief complaint (C.C.), a subjective statement made by a patient describing the patient's most significant or serious symptoms or signs of illness or dysfunction.

Chief Executive Officer (CEO, C.E.O.), the most senior official of an organization or institution.

chief resident, a senior resident physician who acts temporarily as the clinical and administrative director of the

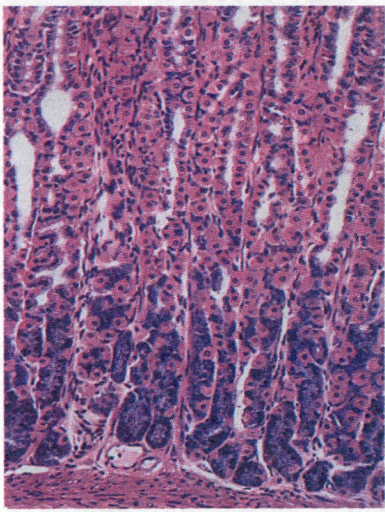

Chief cells (Mitros, 1988)

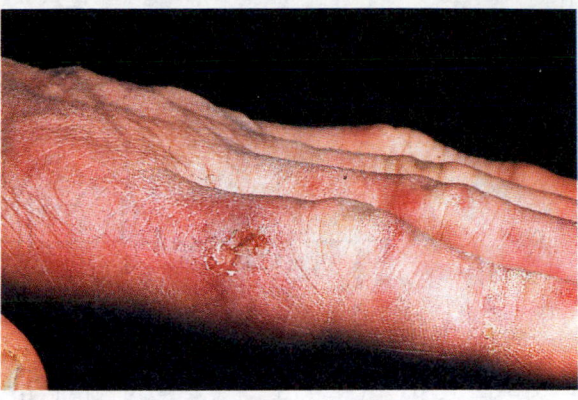

Chilblains (du Vivier, 1993)

house staff in a department of the hospital. The period of duty varies depending on the size of the department, the length of the residency, and the number of house staff members.

chief surgeon, a surgeon appointed or elected head of the surgeons on the staff of a health care facility.

chigger /chig′ər/ [Fr, *chique*], the larva of *Trombicula* mites found in tall grass and weeds. It sticks to the skin and causes irritation and severe itching. Also called **harvest mite, red mite.**

chigoe /chig′ō/, a flea found in tropical and subtropical America and Africa. The pregnant female flea burrows into the skin of the feet, causing an inflammatory condition that may lead to spontaneous amputation of a toe. Also called **burrowing flea, jigger, sand flea.** See also **chigger.**

chikungunya encephalitis /chik′ən·gun′yə/ [Bantu, to bend upward; Gk, *enkephalos*, brain, *itis*, inflammation], an arbovirus infection characterized by a high fever that begins abruptly, muscle aches, a rash, and pain in the joints. It is transmitted by the bite of a mosquito and occurs mainly in Africa, Asia, and on some of the Pacific islands, including Guam. The fever may last for a week, then rise again after a remission of several days. Pain in the joints may continue after other symptoms have ceased. Supportive nursing care and symptomatic relief are the only treatments.

chilblain /chil′blān/ [AS, *cele*, cold, *bleyn*, blister], redness and swelling of the skin because of excessive exposure to cold. Burning, itching, blistering, and ulceration that are similar to a thermal burn, may occur. Treatment includes protection against cold and injury, gentle warming, and avoidance of tobacco. Also called **pernio.** Compare **frostbite.**

child [AS, *cild*], **1.** a person of either sex between the time of birth and adolescence. **2.** an unborn or recently born human being; fetus, neonate, infant. **3.** an offspring or descendant; a son or daughter or a member of a particular tribe or clan. **4.** one who is like a child or immature.

child abuse, the physical, sexual, or emotional maltreatment of a child. It may be overt or covert and often results

Warning signs of child abuse

Physical evidence of abuse and/or neglect, including previous injuries

Conflicting stories about the "accident" or injury from the parents or others

Cause of injury blamed on sibling or other party

An injury inconsistent with the history, such as a concussion and broken arm from falling off a bed

History inconsistent with child's developmental level, such as a 6-month-old turning on the hot water

A complaint other than the one associated with signs of abuse (e.g., a chief complaint of a cold when there is evidence of first- and second-degree burns)

Inappropriate response of caregiver, such as an exaggerated or absent emotional response; refusal to sign for additional tests or agree to necessary treatment; excessive delay in seeking treatment; absence of the parents for questioning

Inappropriate response of child, such as little or no response to pain; fear of being touched; excessive or lack of separation anxiety; indiscriminate friendliness to strangers

Child's report of physical or sexual abuse

Previous reports of abuse in the family

Repeated visits to emergency facilities with injuries

From Wong DL, *Whaley & Wong's essentials of pediatric nursing*, ed 4, St Lous, 1993, Mosby, p 411.

in permanent physical or psychiatric injury, mental impairment, or sometimes death. Child abuse occurs predominantly with children less than 3 years of age and is the result of multiple and complex factors involving both the parents and the child, compounded by various stressful environmental circumstances, such as poor socioeconomic conditions, inadequate physical and emotional support within the family, and any major life change or crisis, especially those crises arising from marital strife. Parents at high risk for abuse are characterized as having unsatisfied needs, difficulty in forming adequate interpersonal relationships, unrealistic expectations of the child, and a lack of nurturing experience, often involving neglect or abuse in their own childhoods. Predisposing factors among children include the temperament, per sonality, and activity level of

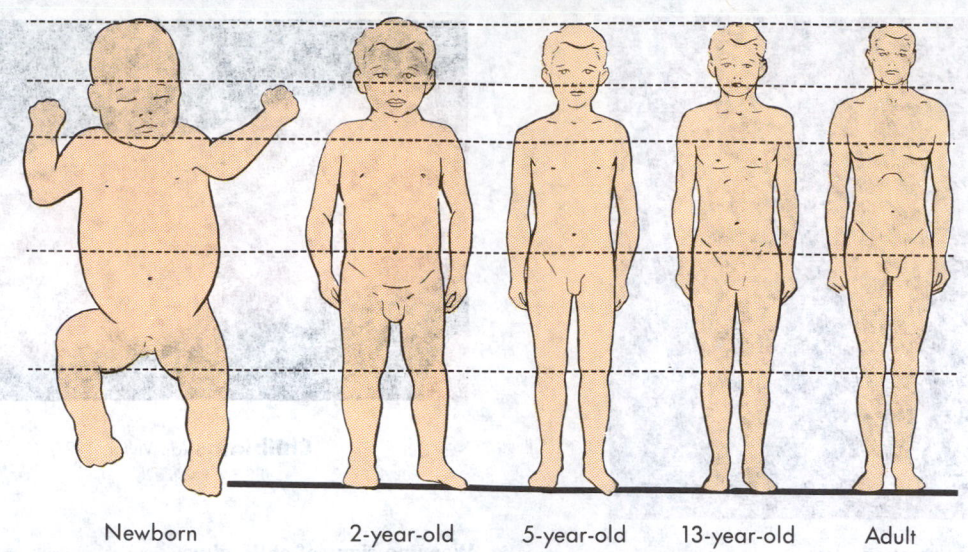

Newborn   2-year-old   5-year-old   13-year-old   Adult

Child development and proportion

the child, order of birth in the family, sensitivity to parental needs, and a need for special physical or emotional care resulting from illness, premature birth, or congenital or genetic abnormalities. Identification of abused children or potential child abusers is a major concern for all health care workers. Obvious physical marks on a child's body, as burns, welts, or bruises, and signs of emotional distress, including symptoms of failure to thrive, are common indications of some degree of neglect or abuse. Often, x-ray film to detect healed or new fractures of the extremities or diagnostic tests to identify sexual molestation are necessary. If abuse is suspected, the nurse is required to make the necessary report. Special counseling services or support groups, such as Parents Anonymous, exist to help families in which a child is abused. The nurse can play a significant role in preventing abuse by promoting a positive parent-child relationship, especially in the neonatal period, by teaching parents proper child care and disciplinary techniques, and by explaining normal child development and behavior so that parents can formulate realistic guidelines for discipline. Compare **child neglect.**

childbearing period [AS, *cild + beran,* to bear; Gk, *peri,* around, *hodos,* way], the reproductive period in a woman's life, from puberty to menopause. It is the time during which she is physiologically able to conceive children.

childbed fever. See **puerperal fever.**

childbirth. See **birth.**

childbirth center, a health facility where prenatal care and delivery services are made available to low-risk pregnant women by a team of nurse-midwives, obstetricians, pediatricians, and ancillary health professionals.

child development, the various stages of physical, social, and psychologic growth that occur from birth through adulthood. See also **adolescence, development, growth, infant, neonatal period, psychosexual development, psychosocial development, toddler.**

childhood, 1. the period in human development that extends from birth until the onset of puberty. 2. the state or quality of being a child. See also **development, growth.**

childhood aphasia, an inability to process language because of a brain dysfunction in childhood.

childhood myxedema [AS, *cildhad;* Gk, *myxa,* mucus, *oidema,* swelling], a juvenile form of hypothyroidism characterized by atrophy of the thyroid gland following a severe infection of the gland. Also called **juvenile myxedema.**

childhood-onset pervasive developmental disorders, disturbances in thought, affect, social relatedness, and behavior that emerge between the ages of 30 months and 12 years.

childhood polycystic disease. See **polycystic kidney disease.**

childhood triad, three types of behavior—fire setting, bedwetting, and cruelty to animals—that may predict emerging sociopathy when they occur consistently and in combination.

child neglect, the failure by parents or guardians to provide for the basic needs of a child by physical or emotional deprivation that interferes with normal growth and development or that places the child in jeopardy. Compare **child abuse.** See also **failure to thrive, maternal deprivation syndrome.**

child psychology, the study of the mental, emotional, and behavioral development of infants and children.

child welfare, any service sponsored by the community or special organizations that provide for the physical, social, or psychologic care of children in need of it.

-chilia. See **-cheilia.**

chill [AS, *cele*], 1. the sensation of cold caused by exposure to a cold environment. 2. an attack of shivering with pallor and a feeling of coldness, often occurring at the beginning of an infection and accompanied by a rapid rise in temperature.

chilo-, cheilo- [Gr, *cheilos,* lip], a prefix for medical terms relating to the lips.

Chilomastix /kī'lōmas'tiks/, a genus of flagellate protozoa, as *Chilomastix mesnili,* a nonpathogenic intestinal parasite of humans.

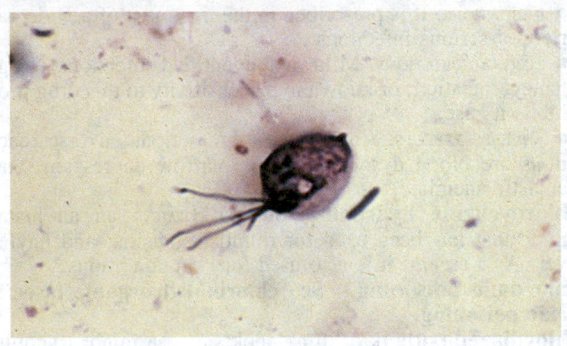

Chilomastix mesnili **trophozoite** *(Baron, 1990)*

chimera /kimir′ə, kīmir′ə/ [Gk, *khimaros,* fire-breathing monster], an organism carrying cell populations derived from two or more different zygotes of the same or of different species. It may be a natural phenomenon, such as in a bone marrow graft. Compare **mosaic.**

chimerism /kimir′izəm/, a state in bone marrow transplantation in which bone marrow and host cells exist compatibly without signs of graft-versus-host rejection disease.

chimney-sweeps′ cancer. See **scrotal cancer.**

chin, the raised triangular portion of the mandible below the lower lip. It is formed by the mental protuberance.

Chinese restaurant syndrome, a syndrome consisting of tingling and burning sensations of the skin, facial pressure, headache, and chest pain that occurs immediately after eating food containing monosodium glutamate, frequently used in Chinese cooking.

chin reflex, chin-jerk reflex. See **mandibular reflex.**

chip [AS, *kippen,* to slice], **1.** a relatively small piece of a bone or tooth. **2.** to break off or cut away a small piece. **3.** a semiconductor in which an integrated circuit is embedded.

chip fracture, any small fragmental fracture, usually one involving a bony process near a joint.

chir-. See **cheiro-.**

chiralgia /kəral′jə/, a pain in the hand, particularly one that does not result from a nerve injury or disease.

chirality. See **handedness.**

-chiria, -cheiria, 1. a suffix meaning a '(specified) condition involving hands': *acephalochiria, atelochiria, dichiria.* **2.** a suffix meaning a '(specified) condition involving stimulus and its perception': *allochiria, dyschiria, synchiria.*

chiro-. See **cheiro-.**

chiroplasty /kir′əplas′tē/ a surgical procedure to restore an injured or congenitally deformed hand to normal use.

chiropodist /kirop′ədist, shir-/, *obsolete* a health professional trained to diagnose and treat diseases and other disorders of the feet. See **podiatrist.**

chiropody /kirop′ədē, shir-/ [Gk, *cheir,* hand, *pous,* foot], *obsolete* the study of minor disorders of the feet and the practice of treating these disorders.

chiropractic /kī′rōprak′tik/ [Gk, *cheir,* hand, *practikos,* efficient], a system of therapy based on the theory that the state of a person's health is determined in general by the condition of his nervous system. In most cases treatment provided by chiropractors involves the mechanical manipulation of the spinal column. Some practitioners employ radiology for diagnosis and use physiotherapy and diet in addition to spinal manipulation. Chiropractic does not employ drugs or surgery, the primary basis of treatment used by medical physicians. A chiropractor is awarded the degree of Doctor of Chiropractic, or D.C., after completing at least 2 years of premedical studies followed by 4 years of training in an approved chiropractic school. Compare **allopathic physician.**

chiropractor /-prak′tər/, a practitioner of **chiropractic.**

chirospasm. See **writer's cramp.**

-chirurgia. See **-surgery.**

chisel fracture, any fracture in which there is oblique detachment of a bone fragment from the head of the radius.

chi square (χ^2) /kī/, (in statistics) a statistic test for an association between observed data and expected data represented by frequencies. The test yields a statement of the probability of the obtained distribution having occurred by chance alone.

Chlamydia /kləmid′ē·ə/ [Gk, *chlamys,* cloak], **1.** a microorganism of the genus *Chlamydia.* **2.** a genus of microorganisms that live as intracellular parasites, have a number of properties in common with gram-negative bacteria, and are currently classified as specialized bacteria. Three species of *Chlamydia* have been recognized; all are pathogenic to humans. *Chlamydia trachomatis,* an organism that lives in the conjunctiva of the eye and the epithelium of the urethra and cervix, is responsible for inclusion conjunctivitis, lymphogranuloma venereum, pelvic inflammatory disease (PID), and trachoma. It is one of the most common sexually transmitted diseases in North America and a frequent cause of sterility. *Chlamydia psittaci* is an organism that infects birds and causes a type of pneumonia in humans. *Chlamydia pneumoniae* is the causative organism of TWAR, which is responsible for both upper and lower respiratory tract infections and commonly causes community acquired pneumonias. See also **psittacosis.** **–chlamydial,** *adj.*

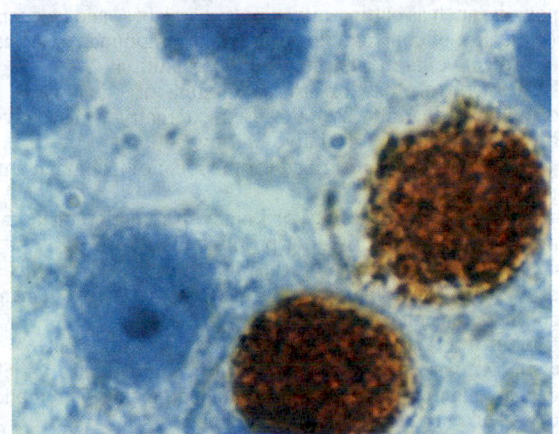

Chlamydia trachomatis *(Tilton, 1992)*

chloasma /klō·az′mə/ [Gk, *chloazein,* to be green], tan or brown pigmentation, particularly of the forehead, cheeks, and nose, commonly associated with pregnancy or the use of oral contraceptives. The hyperpigmentation may be permanent or may disappear only to recur with subsequent

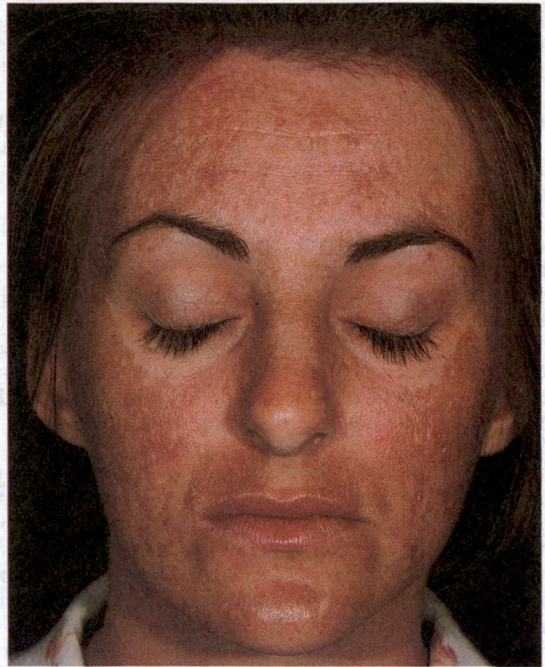

Chloasma (Habif, 1990)

pregnancies or use of oral contraceptives. Also called **mask of pregnancy, melasma.**

chlor-, a combining form meaning 'green': *chloremia, chlorephidrosis, chlorine.*

chloracne /klôrak′nē/ [Gk, *chloros,* green, *akme,* point], a skin condition characterized by small, black follicular plugs and papules on exposed surfaces, especially on the arms, face, and neck of workers in contact with chlorinated compounds, such as cutting oils, paints, varnishes, and lacquers. Avoidance of contact with chlorinated compounds or the use of protective garments prevents the condition.

chloral camphor /klôr′əl/, a mixture of equal parts of camphor and chloral hydrate, used externally as a sedative.

chloral hydrate, a sedative and hypnotic.
- INDICATIONS: It is prescribed for the relief of insomnia, anxiety, or tension.
- CONTRAINDICATIONS: Liver or kidney dysfunction or known hypersensitivity to this drug prohibits its use.
- ADVERSE EFFECTS: Among the more serious adverse reactions are GI disturbances, skin rash, paradoxic excitement, and hypotension.

chlorambucil /klôr′ambōō′sil/, an alkylating agent.
- INDICATIONS: It is prescribed in the treatment of a variety of malignant neoplastic diseases, including chronic lymphocytic leukemia and Hodgkin's disease.
- CONTRAINDICATIONS: Bone marrow depression or known hypersensitivity to this drug prohibits its use. It is not given during the first trimester of pregnancy or within 28 days of chemotherapy or radiation therapy.
- ADVERSE EFFECTS: Among the more serious adverse reactions are bone marrow depression, GI disturbance, skin rash, and hepatotoxicity.

chloramphenicol /-amfē′nikol/, an antibacterial and antirickettsial.

- INDICATIONS: It is prescribed in the treatment of a wide variety of serious infections.
- CONTRAINDICATIONS: Mild or unidentified infections, pregnancy, lactation, or known hypersensitivity to this drug prohibits its use.
- ADVERSE EFFECTS: Among the more serious adverse reactions are blood dyscrasias, bone marrow depression, and aplastic anemia.

chlorcyclizine hydrochloride /-sī′klizin/, an antihistamine that has been used for rhinitis, sinusitis, and hayfever. As a cream, it is also used for skin conditions.

chlordane poisoning. See **chlorinated organic insecticide poisoning.**

chlordiazepoxide /klôr′dī·az′əpok′sīd/, a minor tranquilizer.
- INDICATIONS: It is prescribed in the treatment of anxiety and nervous tension and alcohol withdrawal symptoms.
- CONTRAINDICATIONS: Psychosis, acute narrow-angle glaucoma, or known hypersensitivity to this drug prohibits its use.
- ADVERSE EFFECTS: Among the more serious adverse reactions are withdrawal symptoms occurring on discontinuation of treatment. Drowsiness and fatigue commonly occur.

chlorhexidine /-hek′sidēn/, an antimicrobial agent used as a surgical scrub, hand rinse, and topical antiseptic.

chlorhydria /-hī′drē·ə/, an excessive level of hydrochloric acid in the stomach.

-chloric, a suffix meaning 'referring to or containing chlorine': *hydrochloric, hyperchloric, perchloric.*

chloride /klôr′īd/ [Gk, *chloros,* green], a compound in which the negative element is chlorine. Chlorides are salts of hydrochloric acid, the most common being sodium chloride (table salt).

chloride shift, an exchange of chloride ions in red blood cells in peripheral tissues in response to P_{CO_2} of blood. The shift reverses in the lungs.

chloriduria, an excessive level of chlorides in the urine.

chlorinated /klôr′ənā′tid/ [Gk, *chloros,* greenish], pertaining to material that contains or has been treated with chlorine.

chlorinated organic insecticide poisoning, poisoning resulting from the inhalation, ingestion, or absorption of DDT and other insecticides containing chlorophenothane, as heptachlor, dieldrin, and chlordane. It is characterized by vomiting, weakness, malaise, convulsions, tremors, ventricular fibrillation, respiratory failure, and pulmonary edema. Treatment includes control of the neurologic and neuromuscular symptoms and supportive therapy as indicated by monitoring vital functions. Also called **DDT poisoning.**

chlorination [Gk, *chloros,* green], the disinfection or treatment of water or other substances with free chlorine.

chlorine (Cl) /klôr′ēn/, a yellowish-green, gaseous element of the halogen group. Its atomic number is 17; its atomic weight is 35.453. It has a strong, distinctive odor, is irritating to the respiratory tract, and is poisonous if ingested or inhaled. It occurs in nature chiefly as a component of sodium chloride in sea water and in salt deposits. It is used as a bleach and as a disinfectant to purify water for drinking or for use in swimming pools. Chlorine compounds in general use include many solvents, cleaning fluids, and chloroform. Most of the solvents and cleaning fluids containing chlorine are toxic when inhaled or ingested. Chloroform was formerly in general use as an anesthetic.

chlormezanone /-mez′ənōn/, an antianxiety agent.

■ INDICATIONS: It is prescribed for mild anxiety and for nervous tension.

■ CONTRAINDICATION: Known hypersensitivity to this drug prohibits its use.

■ ADVERSE EFFECTS: Among the most serious adverse reactions are hypersensitivity and sedation. Dizziness, nausea, and rashes often occur.

chloroform /klôr'əfôrm'/ [Gk, *chloros* + L, *formica,* ant], a nonflammable, volatile liquid that was the first inhalation anesthetic to be discovered. Chloroform is a dangerous anesthetic drug: A difference of only 10% in drug-plasma levels can result in hypotension, myocardial and respiratory depression, cardiogenic shock, ventricular fibrillation, coma, and death. Delayed poisoning, even weeks after apparently complete recovery, can occur, and serious ocular damage is frequently reported.

chloroformism /-iz'əm/, **1.** the habit of inhaling chloroform for its narcotic effect. **2.** the anesthetic effect of chloroform.

chloroleukemia /klôr'ōloōokē'mē·ə/ [GK, *chloros,* green, *leukos,* white, *haima,* blood], a kind of myelogenous leukemia in which specific tumor masses are not seen at autopsy but body fluids and organs are green. See also **myelogenous leukemia.**

chlorolymphosarcoma /-lim'fōsärkō'mə/, *pl.* **chlorolymphosarcomas, chlorolymphosarcomata** [Gk, *chloros* + L, *lympha,* water; Gk, *sarx,* flesh, *oma,* tumor], a greenish neoplasm of myeloid tissue occurring in patients with myelogenous leukemia. The mononuclear cells in the peripheral blood are believed to be lymphocytes rather than myeloblasts, such as found with chloroma.

chloroma /klôrō'mə/, *pl.* **chloromas, chloromata,** a malignant, greenish neoplasm of myeloid tissue occurring anywhere in the body in patients with myelogenous leukemia. The green pigment, primarily myeloperoxidase (verdoperoxidase), has no definite metabolic function. The tumor tissue fluoresces bright red under ultraviolet light. Also called **granulocytic sarcoma, green cancer.**

Chloromycetin, a trademark for an antibacterial and antirickettsial (chloramphenicol).

chloromyeloma. See **chloroma.**

chlorophyll /klôr'əfil/ [Gk, *chloros* + *phyllon,* leaf], a plant pigment capable of absorbing light and converting it to energy for the oxidation and reduction involved in photosynthesis of carbohydrates. Chlorophylls a and b are found in green plants; chlorophyll c occurs in brown algae, and chlorophyll d occurs in red algae. See **photosynthesis.**

chlorophyll test. See **Boas' test.**

chloroprocaine /-prō'kān/, a local anesthetic with a chemical structure similar to procaine.

chloroquine /klôr'əkwīn'/, an antimalarial.

■ INDICATIONS: It is prescribed in the treatment of malaria, extraintestinal amebiasis, rheumatoid arthritis, some forms of lupus erythematosus, and photoallergic reactions.

■ CONTRAINDICATIONS: Retinal or visual field changes, porphyria, or known hypersensitivity to this drug prohibits its use.

■ ADVERSE EFFECTS: Among the more serious adverse reactions are GI disturbances, headache, visual disturbances resulting from retinal damage., and pruritus.

chlorosis /klôrō'sis/, *obsolete.* an iron deficiency anemia of young women characterized by hypochromic, microcytic erythrocytes, and a small reduction in the total number of erythrocytes. See also **anemia.**

chlorothiazide /-thī'əzīd/, a diuretic and antihypertensive.

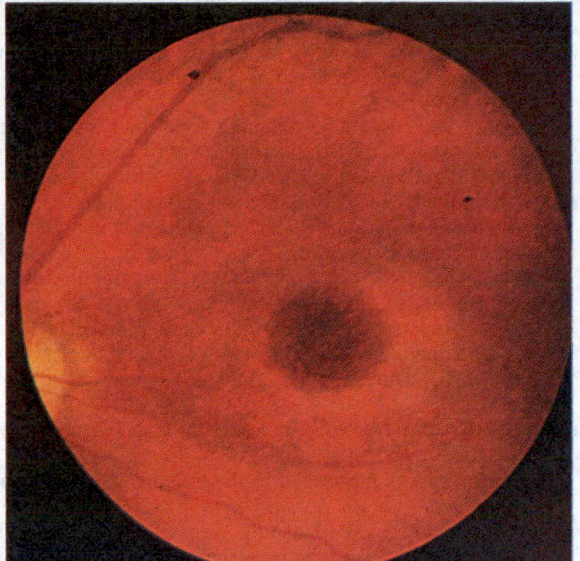

Retinal damage caused by chloroquine
(Shipley, 1993)

■ INDICATIONS: It is prescribed in the treatment of hypertension and edema.

■ CONTRAINDICATIONS: Anuria or known hypersensitivity to thiazide medication or to sulfonamide derivatives prohibits its use.

■ ADVERSE EFFECTS: Among the more serious adverse reactions are hypokalemia, hyperglycemia, and hyperuricemia. Hypersensitivity reactions may occur.

chlorotrianisene /-trī·an'isēn/, an estrogen.

■ INDICATIONS: It is prescribed in the treatment of postpartum breast engorgement, menopausal symptoms, and prostatic cancer.

■ CONTRAINDICATIONS: Liver dysfunction, thromboembolic disorders, unusual vaginal bleeding, known or suspected pregnancy, suspected estrogen-dependent neoplastic disease, or known hypersensitivity to this drug prohibits its use.

■ ADVERSE EFFECTS: Among the more serious adverse reactions are GI distress, breakthrough bleeding, and, in men, gynecomastia, decreased libido, and impotence.

chlorpheniramine maleate /-fenir'əmēn/, an antihistamine.

■ INDICATIONS: It is prescribed in the treatment of a variety of hypersensitivity reactions, including rhinitis, skin rash, and pruritus.

■ CONTRAINDICATIONS: Asthma or known hypersensitivity to this drug prohibits its use. It is not given to newborn infants or nursing mothers.

■ ADVERSE EFFECTS: Among the more serious adverse reactions are skin rash, hypersensitivity reactions, and tachycardia. Drowsiness and dry mouth commonly occur.

chlorpromazine /-prō'məzēn/, a phenothiazine tranquilizer and antiemetic.

■ INDICATIONS: It is prescribed in the treatment of psychotic disorders, severe nausea and vomiting, and intractable hiccups.

■ CONTRAINDICATIONS: Parkinson's disease, concurrent administration of central nervous system depressants, liver or renal dysfunction, severe hypotension, or known hypersensitivity to this drug or to other phenothiazine medication prohibits its use.

■ ADVERSE EFFECTS: Among the more serious adverse effects are hypotension, liver toxicity, a variety of extrapyramidal reactions, blood dyscrasias, and hypersensitivity reactions.

chlorpropamide /-prō′pəmīd/, an oral antidiabetic.

■ INDICATION: It is prescribed in the treatment of non-insulin-dependent diabetes mellitus.

■ CONTRAINDICATIONS: Liver or kidney dysfunction or known hypersensitivity to this drug prohibits its use.

■ ADVERSE EFFECTS: Among the most serious adverse reactions are hematologic derangements and jaundice. Hypoglycemia, GI distress, and rashes are common adverse effects.

chlorprothixene /-prōthik′sēn/, a thioxanthene antipsychotic agent.

■ INDICATIONS: It is prescribed in the treatment of psychotic disorders.

■ CONTRAINDICATIONS: Parkinson's disease, concurrent administration of central nervous system depressants, liver or renal dysfunction, severe hypotension, or known hypersensitivity to this drug prohibits its use.

■ ADVERSE EFFECTS: Among the more serious adverse effects are hypotension, liver toxicity, a variety of extrapyramidal reactions, blood dyscrasias, and hypersensitivity reactions.

chlortetracycline hydrochloride /-tet′rəsī′klēn/, an antibiotic.

■ INDICATIONS: It is prescribed in the treatment of a variety of infections.

■ CONTRAINDICATIONS: Renal or liver dysfunction, pregnancy, early childhood, or known hypersensitivity to this drug or to other tetracycline medication prohibits its use.

■ ADVERSE EFFECTS: Among the more serious adverse effects are GI disturbances, phototoxicity, potentially serious suprainfections, and hypersensitivity reactions. Discoloration of teeth may occur in children exposed to this drug in utero or before 8 years of age.

chlorthalidone /-thal′idōn/, a diuretic and antihypertensive.

■ INDICATIONS: It is prescribed in the treatment of high blood pressure and edema.

■ CONTRAINDICATIONS: Anuria or known hypersensitivity to this drug, to other thiazide medication, or to sulfonamide derivatives prohibits its use.

■ ADVERSE EFFECTS: Among the more serious adverse reactions are hypokalemia, hyperglycemia, hyperuricemia, and hypersensitivity reactions.

Chlor-Trimeton, a trademark for an antihistamine (chlorpheniramine maleate).

chlorzoxazone /-zok′səzōn/, a skeletal muscle relaxant.

■ INDICATION: It is prescribed for the relief of muscle spasm.

■ CONTRAINDICATION: Known hypersensitivity to this drug is the only contraindication.

■ ADVERSE EFFECTS: Among the more serious adverse reactions are jaundice and GI bleeding.

CHN, abbreviation for *Certified Hemodialysis Nurse.*

choana /kō′ənə/, *pl.* **choanae, 1.** a funnel-shaped channel. **2.** See **posterior nares.**

choanal atresia /kō′ənəl/ [Gk, *choane,* funnel, *a, tresis,* not hole], a congenital anomaly in which a bony or membranous occlusion blocks the passageway between the nose and pharynx. The condition, which is caused by the failure of the nasopharyngeal septum to rupture during embryonic development, can result in serious ventilation problems in the neonate, and providing an oral airway or endotracheal intubation may be necessary. The defect is usually repaired surgically shortly after birth.

chocolate cyst [Mex, *chocolatl;* Gk, *kystis,* bag], a darkly pigmented cyst sometimes found in the endometrium.

choke [ME, *choken*], to interrupt breathing by compression or obstruction of larynx or trachea.

choke damp. See **damp.**

choked disc. *informal.* papilledema; edema of the optic disc.

chokes, a respiratory condition, occurring in decompression sickness, characterized by shortness of breath, substernal pain, and a nonproductive paroxysmal cough caused by bubbles of gas in the blood vessels of the lungs.

choking, the condition in which a respiratory passage is blocked by constriction of the neck, an obstruction in the trachea, or swelling of the larynx. It is characterized by sudden coughing and a red face that rapidly becomes cyanotic. The person cannot breathe and clutches his throat. Emergency treatment requires removal of the obstruction and resuscitation if necessary. See also **Heimlich maneuver.**

chol-. See **chole-.**

cholangeostomy /kōlan′jē·os′təmē/ [Gk, *chloe,* bile, *aggeion,* small vessel, *stoma,* mouth], a surgical operation to form an opening in a bile duct.

cholangiocarcinoma /-okär′sinō′mə/, a cancer of the biliary epithelium in the liver that occurs mainly in patients who have had ulcerative colitis or an infestation of liver flukes. Diagnosis is based on histological evaluation, and the prognosis is poor.

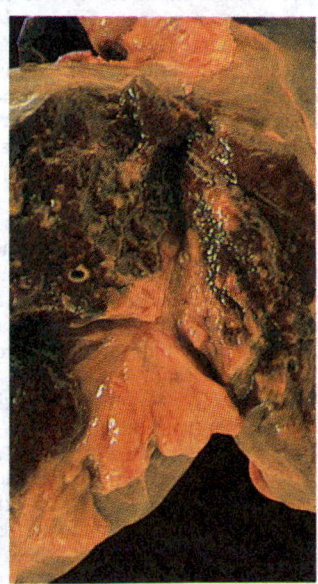

Cholangiocarcinoma *(Fletcher, 1987)*

cholangiogram /kōlan′jē·əgram′/, an x-ray film of the bile ducts produced after injection of a radiopaque contrast medium. A cholangiogram is routinely performed as a part of biliary tract surgery, before or after the procedure. A postoperative radiogram may be made after injecting an iodinated contrast medium through an indwelling T-tube. The medium also may be introduced directly into the biliary system or intravenously. See also **cholangiography, cholecystography.**

cholangiography /kōlan′jē·og′rəfē/, a special roentgenographic test procedure for outlining the major bile ducts by the intravenous injection or the direct instillation of a radiopaque contrast material.

■ METHOD: For intravenous cholangiography the contrast agent is given slowly by vein, and x-ray films are taken of the region of the gallbladder. Operative and postoperative cholangiography employ the injection of contrast material into the common bile duct via a drainage T-tube inserted during surgery, the purpose being to discover any small, residual gallstones. In percutaneous transhepatic cholangiography the contrast material is injected through a long needle or needle-catheter, which is introduced directly through the skin into the substance of the liver. Endoscopic retrograde cholangiography is accomplished by cannulating the ampulla of Vater through a flexible fiberoptic duodenoscope and instilling radiopaque material directly into the common bile duct.

■ NURSING INTERVENTION: Intravenous cholangiography cannot be used in the presence of severe liver disease or jaundice, because the dye will not be concentrated and excreted into the bile. The patient fasts, and fluids are restricted overnight. An early morning cleansing enema is given, usually followed by a sedative. The patient is warned about a brief period of a burning sensation that occurs as the dye is injected. For percutaneous transhepatic cholangiography, sedative premedication is often ordered and a local anesthetic injected at the site of needle puncture. Appropriate evaluation for bleeding tendencies must be carried out before percutaneous transhepatic cholangiography. Bile peritonitis is occasionally a complication of T-tube or percutaneous cholangiography, and close nursing observation is essential after the test is completed. For endoscopic retrograde cholangiography, nothing is given by mouth after midnight, an explanation is given to the patient, dentures are removed, and, to permit administration of medications, intravenous infusion is begun. The endoscope is passed with the patient in the left lateral position; then the patient is turned to the prone position, the ampulla is cannulated, the dye is injected, and films are taken. Vital signs are observed and the patient is given a light meal 2 to 4 hours after the procedure.

■ OUTCOME CRITERIA: The resulting cholangiograms from any of these procedures are examined for unobstructed outlining of the biliary system. Calculi may be noted as shadows within the opaque medium. See also **cholecystography.**

cholangiohepatoma /kōlan′jē·ōhep′ətō′mə/, *pl.* **cholangiohepatomas, cholangiohepatomata,** a neoplasm in which an abnormal mixture of liver cord cells and bile ducts exists.

cholangiolitis /-lī′tis/, an abnormal condition characterized by inflammation of the fine tubules of the bile duct system, which may cause cholangiolitic cirrhosis. **–cholangiolitic,** *adj.*

cholangioma /kōlan′jē·ō′mə/, *pl.* **cholangiomas, cholangiomata,** a neoplasm of the bile ducts.

cholangitis /kō′lanjī′tis/, inflammation of the bile ducts, caused either by bacterial invasion or by obstruction of the ducts by calculi or a tumor. The condition is characterized by severe right upper quadrant pain, jaundice (if an obstruction is present), and intermittent fever. Blood tests reveal

an elevated level of serum bilirubin. Diagnosis is made by ultrasounds and cholangiography. Treatment is with antibiotics for infection and with surgery for acute obstruction. See also **biliary calculus.**

chole-, chol-, cholo-, a combining form meaning 'pertaining to the bile': *cholecystectomy, cholelithotomy, cholesterase.*

cholecalciferol. See **vitamin D₃.**

cholecystalgia. See **biliary colic.**

cholecystectomy /kō′lisistek′təmē/ [Gk, *chole + kystis,* bag, *ektome* excision], the surgical removal of the gallbladder, performed to treat cholelithiasis and cholecystitis. Surgery may be delayed while the acute inflammation is treated. Before surgery, an electrocardiogram and tests of hepatic function may be ordered. Under general anesthesia, the gallbladder is excised and the cystic duct ligated; the common duct is searched, and any stones found are removed. The most common complication is a disruption of the hepatic or other ducts of the biliary system, requiring surgical correction. Wound infection, hemorrhage, bile leakage, and jaundice may also occur. See also **cholecystitis, cholelithiasis.**

cholecystitis /kō′lisistī′tis/ [Gk, chole + *kystis,* bag, *itis,* inflammation], acute or chronic inflammation of the gallbladder. **Acute cholecystitis** is usually caused by a gallstone that cannot pass through the cystic duct. Pain is felt in the right upper quadrant of the abdomen, accompanied by nausea, vomiting, eructation, and flatulence. Diagnosis is usually made with ultrasound. Surgery is the preferred mode of treatment. **Chronic cholecystitis,** the more common type, has an insidious onset. Pain, often felt at night, may follow a fatty meal. Complications include biliary calculi, pancreatitis, and carcinoma of the gallbladder. Again, surgery is the preferred treatment. See also **biliary calculus, cholecystectomy, cholelithiasis.**

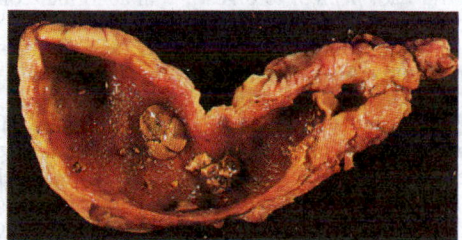

Chronic cholecystitis (Fletcher, 1987)

cholecystogram /kō′lisis′təgram′/, an x-ray film of the gallbladder, made after the ingestion or injection of a radiopaque substance, usually a contrast material containing iodine.

cholecystography /kō′lisistog′rəfē/, an x-ray examination of the gallbladder. At least 12 hours before the study the patient has a fat-free meal and ingests a contrast material containing iodine, usually in the form of tablets; it may also be given intravenously. The iodine, which is opaque to x-rays, is excreted by the liver into the bile in the gallbladder. After the procedure, the patient consumes a fatty meal or cholecystokinin, which stimulates the gallbladder to contract, expelling bile and contrast material into the bile duct.

Additional x-ray films are taken about 1 hour later. The test is useful in the diagnosis of cholecystitis, cholelithiasis, tumors, and the differential diagnosis of a mass in the upper right quadrant of the stomach.

cholecystoileostomy /kō'lisis'tō·il'ē·os'təmē/ [Gk, *chole*, bile, *kystis*, bag, *eilein*, to twist, *stoma*, mouth], a surgical procedure performed to connect the gall bladder to the ileum.

cholecystokinin /-kī'nin/ [Gk, *chole* + *kystis*, bag, *kinein*, to move], a hormone, produced by the mucosa of the upper intestine, that stimulates contraction of the gallbladder and the secretion of pancreatic enzymes.

choledochal /-dok'əl/ [Gk, *chole*, bile, *dochus*, containing], pertaining to the common bile duct.

choledochojejunostomy /-dok'ōjē'jōōnos'təmē/ [Gk, *chole*, bile, *dochus*, containing; L, *jejunus*, empty; Gk, *stoma*, mouth], a surgical procedure in which the bile duct is connected to the jejunum.

choledocholithiasis. See **biliary calculus.**

choledocholithotomy /-lithot'əmē/ [Gk, *chole* + *dochus*, containing, *lithos*, stone, *temnein*, to cut], a surgical operation to make an incision in the common bile duct to remove a stone.

Choledyl, a trademark for a theophylline derivative (oxtriphylline), used as a bronchodilator.

cholelithiasis /-lithī'əsis/ [Gk, *chole* + *lithos*, stone, *osis*, condition], the presence of gallstones in the gallbladder. The condition affects about 20% of the population over 40 years of age and is more prevalent in women and in persons with cirrhosis of the liver. Many patients complain of unlocalized abdominal discomfort, eructation, and intolerance to certain foods. Other patients will have no symptoms at all. In patients with severe attacks of biliary pain associated with cholelithiasis, cholecystectomy is recommended to prevent such complications as cholecystitis, cholangitis, and pancreatitis. See also **biliary calculus, cholecystitis.**

cholelithic dyspepsia /kō'lilith'ik/ [Gk, *chole* + *lithos*, stone; *dys* bad, *peptein* to digest], an abnormal condition characterized by sudden attacks of indigestion associated with the dysfunction of the gallbladder. See **dyspepsia.**

cholelithotomy /-lithot'əmē/, a surgical operation to remove gallstones through an incision in the gallbladder.

cholera /kol'ərə/ [Gk, *chole* + *rhein*, to flow], an acute bacterial infection of the small intestine, characterized by severe diarrhea and vomiting, muscular cramps, dehydration, and depletion of electrolytes. The disease is spread by water and food that have been contaminated by feces of persons previously infected. The symptoms are caused by toxic substances produced by the infecting organism, *Vibrio cholerae*. The profuse, watery diarrhea, as much as a liter an hour, depletes the body of fluids and minerals. Complications include circulatory collapse, cyanosis, destruction of kidney tissue, and metabolic acidosis. Mortality is as high as 50% if the infection remains untreated. Treatment includes the administration of antibiotics that destroy the infecting bacteria and the restoration of normal amounts of fluids and electrolytes with intravenous solutions. A cholera vaccine is available for people traveling to areas where the infection is endemic, but is of questionable benefit in protection from the disease. Other preventive measures include drinking only boiled or bottled water decontaminated as by iodine, and eating only cooked foods. See also *Vibrio cholerae, Vibrio gastroenteritis.*

choleragen /kol'ərəjin/, an exotoxin, produced by the cholera vibrio, that stimulates the secretion of electrolyte and water into the small intestine in Asiatic cholera, draining body fluids and weakening the patient.

cholera vaccine, an active immunizing agent.
- INDICATION: It is prescribed as an immunization against cholera.
- CONTRAINDICATIONS: Immunosuppression, acute infection, concomitant administration of corticosteroids, or known hypersensitivity to this drug prohibits its use.
- ADVERSE EFFECTS: The most serious adverse reaction is anaphylaxis.

choleretic /kō'ləret'ik/ [Gk, *chole* + *eresis*, removal], **1.** stimulating the production of bile in the liver either by cholepoiesis or by hydrocholeresis. **2.** a choleretic agent.

choleric /kol'ərik, kəler'ik/, having a hot temper or an irritable nature.

cholestasis /-stā'sis/ [Gk, *chole* + *stasis*, standing still], interruption in the flow of bile through any part of the biliary system, from liver to duodenum. It is essential for the physician to discover whether the cause is within the liver (intrahepatic) or outside it (extrahepatic). Intrahepatic causes include hepatitis, drug and alcohol use, metastatic carcinoma, and pregnancy. Extrahepatic causes may be an obstructing calculus or tumor in the common bile duct or carcinoma of the pancreas. Symptoms of both types of cholestasis include jaundice, pale and fatty stools, dark urine, and intense itching over the skin. If liver disease is suspected, liver biopsy can confirm the suspicion, and attempts can be made to treat the underlying disorder. Extrahepatic cholestasis usually requires surgery. See also **cholestatic hepatitis, hyperbilirubinemia of the newborn.** −**cholestatic,** *adj.*

cholestatic hepatitis /-stat'ik/, a variant of viral hepatitis. Signs are persistent jaundice, itching, and elevated alkaline phosphatase. These signs usually abate when the hepatitis remits. See also **cholestasis, hepatitis.**

cholesteatoma /kōles'tē·ətō'mə/ [Gk, *chole* + *stear*, fat, *oma*, tumor], a cystic mass composed of epithelial cells and cho lesterol that is found in the middle ear and occurs as a congenital defect or as a serious complication of chronic otitis media. The mass may occlude the middle ear, or enzymes produced by it may destroy the adjacent bones, including the ossicles. Surgery is required to remove a cholesteatoma. See also **otitis media.**

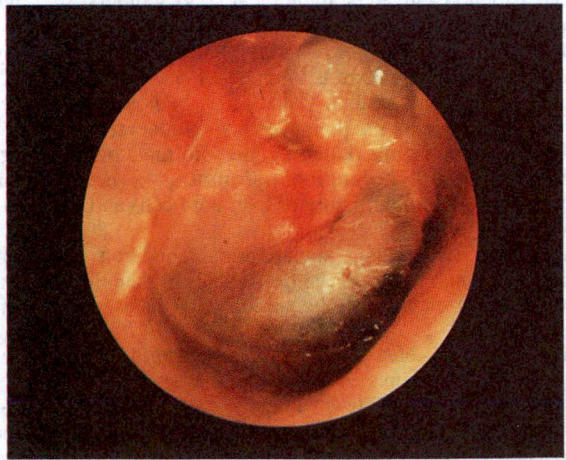

Cholesteatoma (Epstein, 1992)

cholesterase /kəles′tərās′/ [Gk, *chole* + *aither*, air; Ger, *Saure,* acid; *ase,* enzyme suffix], an enzyme in the blood and other tissues that forms cholesterol and fatty acids by hydrolyzing cholesterol esters.

cholesteremia. See **cholesterolemia.**

cholesterol /kəles′tərôl/ [Gk, *chole* + *steros,* solid], a fat-soluble crystalline steroid alcohol found in animal fats and oils, and egg yolk, and widely distributed in the body, especially in the bile, blood, brain tissue, liver, kidneys, adrenal glands, and myelin sheaths of nerve fibers. It facilitates the absorption and transport of fatty acids and acts as the precursor for the synthesis of vitamin D at the surface of the skin, as well as for the synthesis of the various steroid hormones, including cortisol, cortisone, and aldosterone in the adrenal glands and of the sex hormones progesterone, estrogen, and testosterone. It sometimes crystallizes in the gallbladder to form gallstones. Cholesterol is found almost exclusively in foods of animal origin and is continuously synthesized in the body, primarily in the liver and

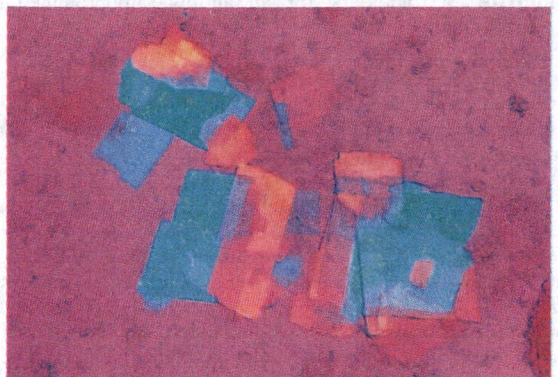

Cholesterol crystals *(Schumacher, 1988)*

$$CH_3$$
$$CH-CH_2CH_2CH_2 CH$$
$$CH_3 \qquad CH_3$$
$$CH_3$$
$$HO$$

Cholesterol

Chemical structure of cholesterol *(Thibodeau, 1993)*

Serum cholesterol levels identifying persons at moderate and high risk who require treatment (diet therapy and weight control; drug therapy only after careful maximal diet therapy)

Age (years)	Moderate risk	High risk
	Greater than:	Greater than:
2-19	170 mg/dl	185 mg/dl
20-29	200 mg/dl	220 mg/dl
30-39	220 mg/dl	240 mg/dl
40 and older	240 mg/dl	260 mg/dl

From National Institutes of Health: *Nutr Today* 20(1):13, 1985.

the adrenal cortex. Increased levels of LDL cholesterol may be associated with the pathogenesis of atherosclerosis while higher levels of HDL cholesterol appear to lower the person's risk for heart disease. Normal adult levels of blood cholesterol are 150-200 mg/dl or 3.90-6.50 mmol/L (SI units). Also called **cholesterin.** See also **high-density lipoprotein, low-density lipoprotein, vitamin D.**

cholesterolemia /-ē′mē·ə/, **1.** the presence of excessive amounts of cholesterol in the blood. **2.** the abnormal condition of having excessive amounts of cholesterol in the blood. Also called **cholesteremia.**

cholesteroleresis /-er′isis/ /kəles′tərôler′isis/ [Gk, *chole, steros* + *eresis,* removal], the increased elimination of cholesterol in the bile.

cholesterol metabolism, the sum of the anabolic and catabolic processes in the synthesis and degradation of cholesterol in the body. Ingested cholesterol is quickly absorbed. It is also synthesized in the liver and can be synthesized by most other tissues of the body. As more cholesterol is ingested, less is synthesized. Cholesterol is removed from the body by conversion in the liver and excretion in the bile.

cholesterolopoiesis /kəles′tərō′lōpō·ē′sis/ [Gk, *chole, steros* + *poiesis,* producing], the elaboration of cholesterol by the liver.

cholesterolosis /kəles′tərəlō′sis/, an abnormal condition, found in about 5% of patients with chronic cholecystitis, in which there are deposits of cholesterol within large macrophages in the submucosa of the gallbladder. This produces a spotty appearance, sometimes referred to as a strawberry gallbladder. Cholesterolosis is often associated with gallstones and may be asymptomatic or accompanied by biliary colic. See also **cholecystitis.**

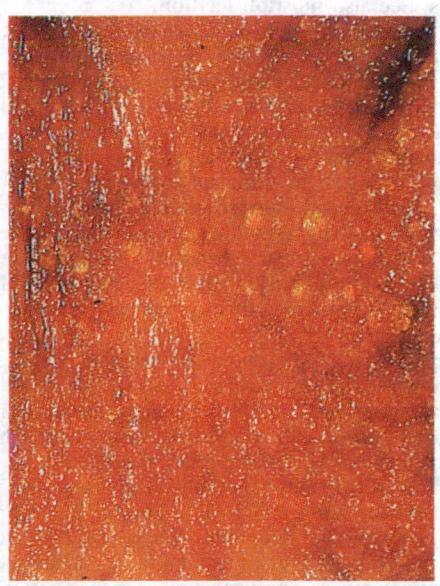

Cholesterolosis *(Fletcher, 1987)*

cholesteryl ester storage disease /kōles′təril/, an inherited disorder in which there is an accumulation of neutral lipids, such as cholesterol esters and glycerides, in body tissues. The disease may be asymptomatic or be characterized by hepatosplenomegaly, steatorrhea, and adrenal calcification. The cause is a deficiency of the enzyme cholesterol ester hydrolase. There is no specific treatment. A form of the disorder affecting infants, with symptoms in the first weeks after birth, is Wolman's disease.

cholestyramine /-tir′əmēn/, a substance that acts on the liver's bile acids, interrupting the bile-acid cycle and increasing the function of LDL receptors, thereby increasing cellular cholesterol uptake and lowering blood cholesterol levels.

cholestyramine resin, an ion-exchange resin and antihyperlipoproteinemic agent.

■ INDICATIONS: It is prescribed for hyperlipoproteinemia and for pruritus resulting from partial biliary obstruction.

■ CONTRAINDICATIONS: Complete biliary obstruction or known hypersensitivity to this drug prohibits its use.

■ ADVERSE EFFECTS: Among the more serious adverse reactions are fecal impaction, GI disturbances, and depletion of vitamins A, D, and K. Constipation is common.

-cholia, -choly, a suffix meaning '(condition of the) bile': *albuminocholia, syncholia, uricocholia.*

choline /kō′lēn/ [Gk, *chole,* bile], a lipotropic substance sometimes included in the vitamin B complex as essential for the metabolism of fats in the body. Found in most animal tissues, choline is a primary component of acetylcholine, the neurotransmitter, and functions with inositol as a basic constituent of lecithin. It prevents the deposition of fats in the liver and facilitates the movement of fats into the cells. The richest sources of choline are liver, kidneys, brains, wheat germ, brewer's yeast, and egg yolk. Deficiency leads to hepatic cirrhosis, resulting in bleeding stomach ulcers and impaired kidney function, hypertension, high blood levels of cholesterol, and atherosclerosis and arteriosclerosis. See also **inositol, lecithin.**

choline esters, a group of cholinergic drugs that act in body sites where acetylcholine is the neurotransmitter. Examples include bethanechol, carbachol, and methacholine.

cholinergic /-ur′jik/ [Gk, *chole* + *ergon,* to work], **1.** of or pertaining to nerve fibers that elaborate acetylcholine at the myoneural junctions. **2.** the tendency to transmit or to be stimulated by or to stimulate the elaboration of acetylcholine. Compare **adrenergic, anticholinergic.**

cholinergic blocking agent, any agent that blocks the action of acetylcholine and substances similar to acetylcholine. Such agents, in effect, block the action of cholinergic nerves that transmit impulses by the release of acetylcholine at their synapses.

cholinergic crisis, a pronounced muscular weakness and respiratory paralysis caused by excessive acetylcholine, often apparent in patients suffering from myasthenia gravis as a result of overmedication with anticholinesterase drugs.

cholinergic fibers [Gr, *chole,* bile, *ergon,* work; L, *fibra*], nerve fibers of the autonomic nervous system that release the neurotransmitter acetylcholine. They include all preganglionic fibers, all postganglionic sympathetic fibers to sweat glands and efferent fibers innervating skeletal muscle.

cholinergic nerve, a nerve that releases the neurotransmitter acetylcholine at its synapse. The cholinergic nerves include all the preganglionic sympathetic and the preganglionic parasympathetic nerves, the postganglionic parasympathetic nerves, the somatic motor nerves to skeletal muscles, and some nerves to sweat glands and to certain blood vessels.

cholinergic receptor [Gk, *chole,* bile + *ergein,* to work; L, *recipere,* to receive], a specialized sensory nerve ending that responds to the stimulation of acetylcholine.

cholinergic stimulant. See **cholinergic.**

cholinergic urticaria [Gk, *chole* + *ergon,* to work; L, *urtica,* nettle], an abnormal and usually temporary vascular reaction of the skin, often associated with sweating in susceptible individuals subjected to stress, strong exertion, or hot weather. The condition is characterized by small, pale, itchy papules surrounded by reddish areas; it is caused by the action of acetylcholine on mast cells.

cholinesterase /kō′lines′tərās/, an enzyme that acts as a catalyst in the hydrolysis of acetylcholine to choline and acetate.

choliopancreatography /kō′lē·ōpan′krē·ātog′rəfē/ [Gk, *chole* + *pan,* all, *kreas,* flesh, *graphein,* to record], the x-ray visualization of the bile and pancreatic ducts.

cholo-. See **chole-.**

Cholografin, a trademark for a diagnostic dye (iodipamide), used in radiology.

Choloxin, a trademark for an antihyperlipoproteinemic (dextrothyroxine sodium).

-choly. See **-cholia.**

chondr-. See **chondro-.**

chondral /kon′drəl/, of or pertaining to cartilage.

chondrectomy /kondrek′təmē/, the surgical excision of a cartilage.

chondri-. See **chondro-.**

-chondria, **1.** a suffix meaning a 'condition involving granules in cell composition': *lipochondria, mitochondria, plastochondria.* **2.** a combining form meaning an 'abnormal preoccupation with worry about disease': *hypochondria.*

chondrial bone [Gk, *chondros,* cartilage; AS, *ban,* bone], pertaining to bone that forms under the periostial membrane. Also called **perichondrial bone.**

chondriocont /kon′drē·ōkont′/, a threadlike or rod-shaped mitochondrion.

chondriome /kon′drē·ōm/ [Gk, *chondros,* cartilage], the total mitochondria content of a cell, taken as a unit. Also called **chondrioma.**

chondriomite /kon′drē·ōmīt′/ [Gk, *chondros* + *mitos,* thread], a single granular mitochondrion or a group of such organelles appearing in a chain formation.

chondriosome. See **mitochondrion.**

chondritis /kondrī′tis/, any inflammatory condition affecting the cartilage.

chondro-, chondr-, chondri-, a combining form meaning 'pertaining to cartilage': *chondroblast, chondroclast, chondrocostal.*

chondroadenoma. See **adenochondroma.**

chondroangioma /kon′drō·an′jē·ō′mə/, *pl.* **chondroangiomas, chondroangiomata** [Gk, *chondros* + *aggeion,* little vessel, *oma* tumor], a benign, mesenchymal tumor containing vascular and cartilaginous elements.

chondroblast /kon′drōblast/ [Gk, *chondros* + *blastos,* germ], any one of the cells that develops from the mesenchyma and forms cartilage. Also called **chondroplast.**

chondroblastoma /kon′drōblastō′mə/, *pl.* **chondroblastomas, chondroblastomata,** a benign tumor, derived from precursors of cartilage cells, that develops most frequently in epiphyses of the femur and humerus, especially in young men. The lesions may contain scattered areas of calcification and necrosis. Also called **Codman's tumor.**

chondrocalcinosis /kon′drōkal′sinō′sis/ [Gk, *chondros* + L, *calyx*, lime; Gk, *osis*, condition], an arthritic disease in which calcium deposits are found in the peripheral joints. It resembles gout and is often found in patients over 50 years of age who have osteoarthritis or diabetes mellitus. It most commonly invades the knee joint. Aspiration of synovial fluid from the affected joints reveals crystals of calcium salts, especially calcium pyrophosphate dihydrate (CPPD). Inflammation and pain may be relieved by intraarticular injections of hydrocortisone and by antiinflammatory medications. Also called **pseudogout.** Compare **gout, gouty arthritis.**

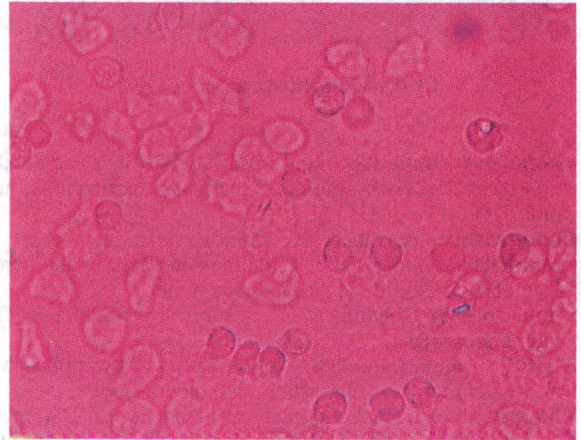

Chondrocalcinosis *(Shipley, 1993)*

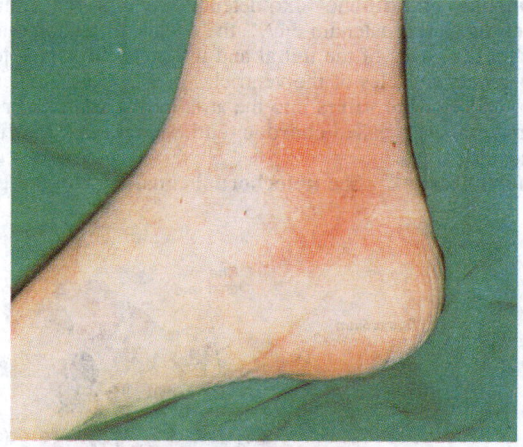

Acute pseudogout of the ankle *(Shipley, 1993)*

chondrocarcinoma /kon′drōkär′sinō′mə/, *pl.* **chondrocarcinoma, chondrocarcinomata** [Gk, *chondros* + *karkinos*, crab, *oma*, tumor], a malignant epithelial tumor in which cartilaginous metaplasia is present.
chondroclast /kon′drōklast′/ [Gk, *chondros* + *klasis,*

breaking], a giant multinucleated cell associated with the resorption of cartilage. **—chondroclastic,** *adj.*
chondrocostal /kon′drōkos′təl/ [Gk, *chondros* + L, *costa*, rib], of or pertaining to the ribs and the costal cartilages.
chondrocyte /kon′drəsīt/ [Gk, *chondros* + *kytos*, cell], any one of the polymorphic cells that form the cartilage of the body. Each contains a nucleus, a relatively large amount of clear cytoplasm, and the common organelles. **—chondrocytic,** *adj.*

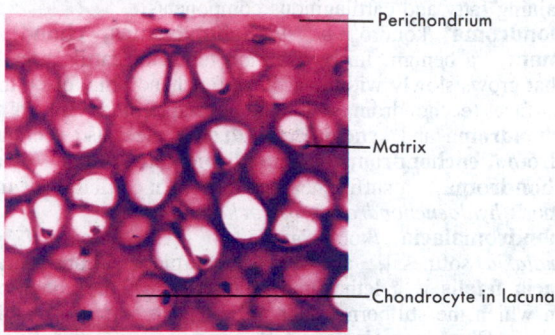

— Perichondrium

— Matrix

—Chondrocyte in lacuna

Chondrocyte in lacuna *(Thibodeau, 1993)*

chondrodysplasia /kon′drōdisplā′zhə/ [Gk, *chondros* + *dys*, bad, *plassein* to form], an inherited disease characterized by abnormal growth at the ends of bones, particularly the long bones of the arms and legs. Bones of the hands and feet may be similarly affected.
chondrodysplasia punctata, an inherited form of dwarfism characterized by skin lesions, radiographic epiphyseal stippling, and a pug nose. There are two types of the anomaly, a benign Conradi-Hunermann form marked by mild asymmetric limb shortening, and a lethal rhizomelic form with marked proximal limb shortening. The Conradi-Hunermann form of the disorder is transmitted by an autosomal dominant gene and the rhizomelic form by an autosomal recessive gene.
chondrodystrophia calcificans congenita /-distrō′fē·ə/ [Gk, *chondros* + *dys*, bad, *trophe*, nourishment; L, *calyx*, lime; *congenitus* born with], an inherited defect characterized by many small opacities in the epiphyses of the long bones. This sign is present on x-ray films of the newborn. Dwarfism, contractures, cataracts, mental retardation, and short stubby fingers develop as the infant grows into childhood. Also called **chondrodystrophia fetalis calcificans, Conradi's disease.**
chondrodystrophy /kon′drōdis′trəfē/ [Gk, *chondros* + *dys*, bad, *trophe*, nourishment], a group of disorders in which there is abnormal conversion of cartilage to bone, particularly in the epiphyses of the long bones. Patients are dwarfed, with normal trunks and shortened extremities. See also **achondroplasia.**
chondroectodermal dysplasia /kon′drō·ek′tədur′məl/, an inherited form of dwarfism marked by distal limb shortening, postaxial polydactyly, and cardiovascular abnormalities. It is transmitted by an autosomal recessive gene. Also called **Ellis-van Creveld syndrome.**
chondroendothelioma /kon′drō·en′dōthē′lē·ō′mə/, *pl.* **chondroendotheliomas, chondroendotheliomata** [Gk, *chondros* + *endon*, within, *thele*, nipple, *oma*, tumor], a

benign mesenchymal tumor containing cartilaginous and endothelial components.

chondrofibroma /kon'drōfībrō'mə/, *pl.* **chondrofibromas, chondrofibromata,** a fibrous tumor containing cartilaginous components.

chondrogenesis /kon'drōjen'əsis/, the development of cartilage. –**chondrogenetic,** *adj*.

chondroid /kon'droid/, resembling cartilage.

chondrolipoma /kon'drōlipō'mə/, *pl.* **chondrolipomas, chondrolipomata,** a benign mesenchymal tumor containing fatty and cartilaginous components.

chondroma /kondrō'mə/, *pl.* **chondromas, chondromata,** a benign, fairly common tumor of cartilage cells that grows slowly within cartilage (enchondroma) or on the surface (ecchondroma). Kinds of chondromas are **joint chondroma** and **synovial chondroma.** See also **ecchondroma, enchondroma.** –**chondromatous,** *adj*.

-chondroma, a suffix meaning a 'benign cartilaginous tumor': *hyaloenchondroma, osteochondroma.*

chondromalacia /kon'drōmələ'shə/ [Gk, *chondros* + *malakia,* softness], a softening of cartilage. **Chondromalacia fetalis** is a lethal congenital form of the condition in which the stillborn infant is born with soft and pliable limbs. **Chondromalacia patellae** occurs in young adults after knee injury and is characterized by swelling, pain, and degenerative changes, which are revealed on examination by x-ray.

chondroma sarcomatosum. See **chondrosarcoma.**

chondromatosis /kon'drōmətō'sis/, a condition characterized by the presence of many cartilaginous tumors. A kind of chondromatosis is **synovial chondromatosis.**

chondromatous. See **chondroma.**

chondromere /kon'drōmir/ [Gk, *chondros* + *meros,* part], a cartilaginous, embryonic vertebra and its costal component.

chondromyoma /kon'drōmī·ō'mə/, *pl.* **chondromyomas, chondromyomata** [Gk, *chondros* + *mys,* muscle, *oma,* tumor], a benign mesenchymal tumor containing myomatous and cartilaginous tissue.

chondromyxofibroma /kon'drōmik'sōfībrō'mə/ [Gk, *chondros* + *myxa,* mucus; L, *fibra,* fiber; *oma,* tumor], a benign tumor that develops from cartilage-forming connective tissue. The lesion, typically a firm, grayish-white, somewhat mass, tends to occur in the knee and small bones of the foot and may be confused with chondrosarcoma. Also called **chondromyxoid fibroma.**

chondromyxoid /kon'drōmik'soid/ [Gk, *chondros* + *myxa,* mucus, *eidos,* form], composed of cartilaginous and myxoid elements.

chondromyxoid fibroma. See **chondromyxofibroma.**

chondrophyte /kon'drōfīt'/ [Gk, *chondros* + *phyton,* growth], an abnormal mass of cartilage. –**chondrophytic,** *adj*.

chondroplasia /-plā'zhə/ [Gk, *chondros,* cartilage, *plassein,* to form], the formation of cartilage.

chondroplast. See **chondroblast.**

chondroplasty /kon'drōplas'tē/ [Gk, *chondros* + *plassein,* to form], the surgical repair of cartilage.

chondrosarcoma /kon'drōsärkō'mə/, *pl.* **chondrosarcomas, chondrosarcomata** [Gk, *chondros* + *sarx,* flesh, *oma,* tumor], a malignant neoplasm of cartilaginous cells or their precursors that occurs most frequently in long bones, the pelvic girdle, and the scapula. The tumor is a large, smooth, lobulated growth composed of nodules of hyaline cartilage that may show slight to marked calcification.

Also called **chondroma sarcomatosum.** –**chondrosarcomatous,** *adj*.

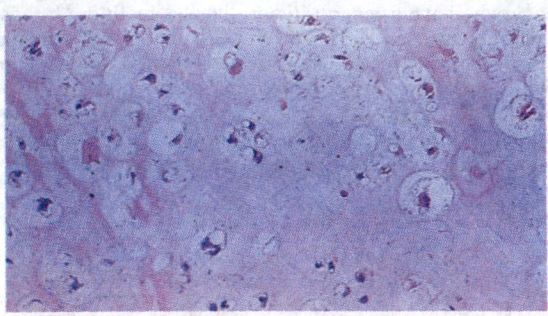

Chondrosarcoma (Lewis, 1988)

chondrosarcomatosis /kon'drōsär'kōmətō'sis/, a condition characterized by multiple, malignant cartilaginous tumors.

chondrosarcomatous. See **chondrosarcoma.**

chondrosis /kondrō'sis/, **1.** the development of the cartilage of the body. **2.** a cartilaginous tumor.

chondrotomy /kondrot'əmē/, a surgical procedure for dividing a cartilage.

CHOP, an anticancer drug combination of cyclophosphamide, doxorubicin, vincristine, and prednisone.

chopping, a therapeutic exercise to improve the strength and coordination of upper trunk nerves and muscles by lifting the arms overhead and bringing them down in a chopping or slashing movement.

chord-, a combining form meaning 'string, cord': *chordoblastoma, chordoma, chordotomy.*

chordae tendineae /kô'dētendin'i·ē/, *sing.* **chorda tendinea** /kô'dätendin'ē·ä/, the strands of tendon that anchor the cusps of the mitral and the tricuspid valves to the papillary muscles of the ventricles of the heart, preventing prolapse of the valves into the atria during ventricular contraction. Also called **chordae tendineae cordis, tendinous cords.**

chordal canal. See **notochordal canal.**

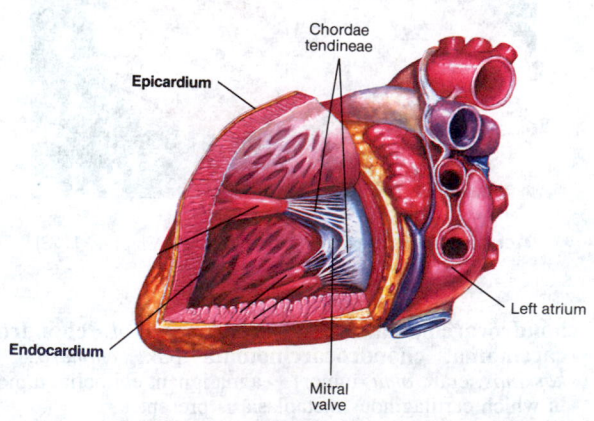

Chordae tendineae (Canobbio, 1990)

chorda spinalis.   See **spinal cord.**

chorda umbilicalis.   See **umbilical cord.**

chordee /kôr′dē, kôr′dā/ [Gk, *chorde*, cord],   a congenital defect of the genitourinary tract resulting in a ventral curvature of the penis, caused by a fibrous band of tissue instead of normal skin along the corpus spongiosum. The condition is often associated with hypospadias and is surgically corrected in early childhood. The goals of surgery are to improve the appearance of the genitalia cosmetically for psychologic reasons, to construct an organ that allows the boy to void in a standing position, and to produce a sexually adequate organ.

chordencephalon /kôrd′ensef′əlon/ [Gk, *chorde* + *enkephalos*, brain],   the portion of the central nervous system that develops in the early weeks of pregnancy from the neural tube and includes the mesencephalon, the rhombencephalon, and the spinal cord. The chordencephalon is segmented and divided into the alar and the basal plates. The alar plate becomes the sensory portion of the gray substance of the spinal cord; the basal plate becomes the motor portion of the gray substance. *chordencephalic, adj.*

chorditis /kôrdī′tis/,   **1.** inflammation of a spermatic cord. **2.** inflammation of the vocal cords or of the vocal folds.

chordoid /kôr′doid/ [Gk, *chorde* + *eidos*, form],   resembling the notocord or notochordal tissue.

chordoma /kôrdō′mə/, *pl.* **chordomas, chordomata,**   a rare, congenital tumor of the brain developing from the fetal notochord. It is usually located in the midline, behind the sella, slow growing, but highly invasive.

chordotomy /kôrdot′əmē/ [Gk, *chorde* + *temnein*, to cut],   an operation in which the anterolateral tracts of the spinal cord are surgically divided to relieve pain.

chorea /kôrē′ə/ [Gk, *choreia*, dance],   a condition characterized by involuntary, purposeless, rapid motions, as flexing and extending the fingers, raising and lowering the shoulders, or grimacing. In some forms, the person is also irritable, emotionally unstable, weak, restless, and fretful. See also **chorea gravidarum, Huntington's chorea, Sydenham's chorea.** −**choreic** /kôrā′ik/, *adj.*

-chorea,   a suffix meaning a '(specified) nervous disorder characterized by involuntary muscle twitching': *hemichorea, monochorea, orthochorea.*

chorea gravidarum /kôr′ē·əgrav′idär′əm/,   a form of chorea occurring during a first pregnancy subsequent to an episode of Sydenham's chorea in childhood. Similar symptoms may develop in a woman taking oral contraceptives.

chorea minor.   See **Sydenham's chorea.**

choreic.   See **chorea.**

choreic ataxia /kôrē′ik/ [Gk, *choreia*, dance, *ataxia*, lack of order],   a form of ataxia in which patients lack muscular coordination and movements are marked by involuntary twitchng and abrupt jerking.

choreiform /kərē′əfôrm′/,   resembling the rapid jerky movements associated with chorea.

choreiform spasm [Gk, *chorea*, dance; L, *forma;* Gk, *spasmos*],   a condition of involuntary muscle contractions that result in dancing motions. One type of dancing spasm involves powerful contractions of the leg muscles, resulting in a leaping, jumping action. It can also involve arm, shoulder and neck muscles.

choreoathetoid cerebral palsy /kôr′ē·ō·ath′ətoid/,   a form of cerebral palsy characterized by choreiform (jerky, ticlike twitching) and athetoid (slow, writhing) movements.

chorio-,   a combining form meaning 'pertaining to the pro-

tective fetal membrane': *chorioblastosis, choriocele, chorioma.*

chorioadenoma /kərē′ō·ad′inō′mə/, *pl.* **chorioadenomas, chorioadenomata** [Gk, *chorion*, skin, *aden*, gland, *oma*, tumor],   an epithelial cell tumor of the outermost fetal membrane that is intermediate in the malignant development of a hydatid mole to invasive choriocarcinoma.

chorioadenoma destruens /-ad′ənō′mədes′troo′ əns/[Gk, *chorion, aden, oma* + L, *destruere,* to pull down],   an invasive hydatidiform mole in which the chorionic villi of the mole penetrate into the myometrium and parametrium of the uterus and metastasize to distant parts of the body, most commonly to the lungs. Also called **metastasizing mole.**

chorioallantoic graft /-əlan′toid/ [Gk, *chorion* + *allas*, sausage, *eidos*, form; *graphion*, stylus],   the grafting of tissue onto the chorioallantoic membrane of the egg of a hen to improve the environment for embryonic growth.

chorioamnionic /-am′nē·ot′ik/,   of or pertaining to the chorion and the amnion.

chorioamnionitis /-am′nē·ōtī′tis/ [Gk, *chorion* + *amnion*, fetal membrane, *itis*, inflammation],   an inflammatory reaction in the amniotic membranes caused by bacteriaor viruses in the amniotic fluid. The membranes become infiltrated with polymorphonuclear leukocytes.

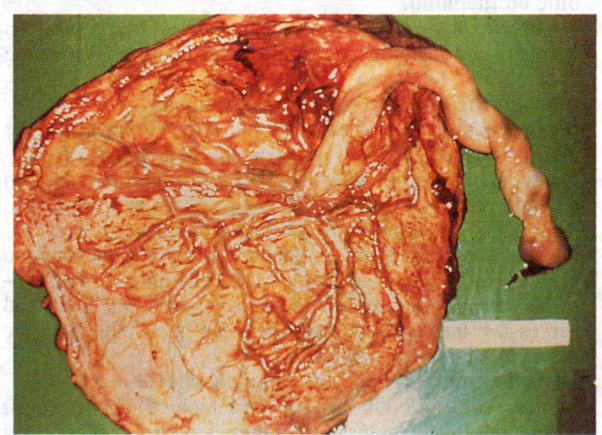

Chorioamnionitis (Zitelli, 1992)

choriocarcinoma /kôr′ē·ōkär′sinō′mə/, *pl.* **choriocarcinomas, choriocarcinomata,**   an epithelial malignancy of fetal origin that develops from the chorionic portion of the products of conception, usually from a hydatidiform mole. The primary tumor usually appears in the uterus as a soft, dark red, crumbling mass, may invade and destroy the uterine wall, and metastasize through lymph or blood vessels, forming secondary hemorrhagic and necrotic tumors in the vaginal wall, vulva, lymph nodes, lungs, liver, and brain. The urine often contains much more chorionic gonadotropin than is expected in pregnancy. The hormone level returns to normal when the tumor is completely removed. This form of cancer, which is more common in older than in younger women, responds to chemotherapy with cytotoxic drugs, such as methotrexate. Rarely, a choriocarcinoma may arise in a teratoma of the testis, mediastinum, or pineal gland, and chemotherapy is usually not ef-

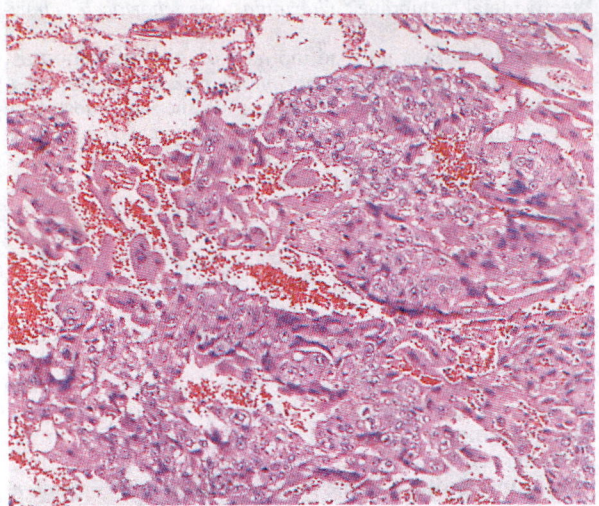

Choriocarcinoma
(Okazaki, 1988/by permission of Mayo Foundation)

fective in treating these tumors. Also called **chorioblastoma, chorioepithelioma, chorionic carcinoma, chorionic epithelioma.**

choriocele /kôr′ē·əsēl′/ [Gk, *chorion* + *kele*, hernia], a hernia or protrusion of the tissue of the choroid layer of the eye.

chorioepithelioma. See **choriocarcinoma.**

choriogenesis /kôr′ē·ōjen′əsis/, the development of the chorion, which is first evident in the first month of pregnancy, after the trophoblast anchors to the uterine tissue and extends primary villi into the intervillous space. The chorion at first contains fluid and loose filaments of extraembryonic mesoderm. As pregnancy proceeds, the amnion grows into the chorionic space and obliterates it. The chorion continues to expand to accommodate the fetus and serves as the outer barrier between the fetus and the uterus. **–choriogenetic,** *adj.*

choriomeningitis. See **lymphocytic choriomeningitis.**

chorion /kôr′ē·on/ [Gk, a skin], (in biology) the outermost extraembryonic membrane composed of trophoblast lined with mesoderm. It develops villi about 2 weeks after fertilization and is vascularized by allantoic vessels 1 week later. It gives rise to the placenta and persists until birth as the outer of the two layers of membrane containing the amniotic fluid and the fetus. Compare **amnion.** See also **amniotic sac.**

-chorion, a suffix meaning a 'membrane': *allantochorion, omphalochorion, prochorion.*

chorionic carcinoma, chorionic epithelioma. See **choriocarcinoma.**

chorionic gonadotropin (CG) /kôr′ē·on′ikgon′ədōtrop′in/ [Gk, *chorion; gone,* seed, *trophe,* nutrition], a chemical component of the urine of pregnant women or pregnant mares. This glycoprotein hormone is secreted by the placental trophoblastic cells. It is composed of two subunits, alpha and beta human chorionic gonadotropin. The alpha subunit is nearly identical to similar subunits of the follicle-stimulating, luteinizing, and thyroid-stimulating hormones. The specific hormonal effects of chorionic gonadotropin are activated by the beta portion. They include stimulation of the corpus luteum to secrete estrogen and progesterone and to decrease lymphocyte activation, both important factors in preparing the uterus to accept the fetus immunologically. Chorionic gonadotropin is also administered in the treatment of some cases of cryptorchidism and male hypogonadism, and to induce ovulation in some infertile women. Also called **human chorionic gonadotropin (HCG).** See also **gonadotropin.**

chorionic plate [Gk, *chorion; platys,* flat], the part of the fetal placenta that gives rise to chorionic villi, which attach to the uterus during the early stage of formation of the placenta.

chorionic sac [Gk, *chorion,* a skin + *sakkos,* sack], the saclike membrane that develops from the blastocyst wall to envelop the embryo.

chorionic villi [Gk, *chorion;* L, *villus,* shaggy hair], tiny vascular fibrils on the surface of the chorion that infiltrate the maternal blood sinuses of the endometrium and help form the placenta.

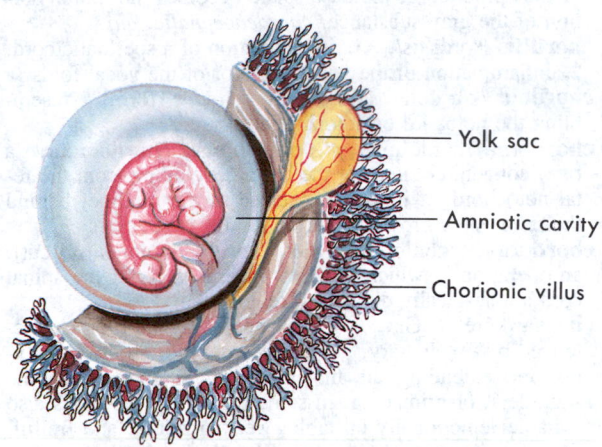

Yolk sac

Amniotic cavity

Chorionic villus

Chorionic villus *(Thibodeau, 1993/Ernest W Beck)*

chorionic villi sampling [Gk, *chorion,* skin; L, *villus,* shaggy hair, *exemplum,* sample], a procedure for obtaining prenatal evaluation data early in a pregnancy by withdrawing a chorionic villi sample from the fetal membranes. The sample is obtained through a catheter inserted into the uterus. See also **amniocentesis.**

chorioretinitis /kôr′ē·ōret′inī′tis/, an inflammatory condition of the choroid and retina of the eye, usually as a result

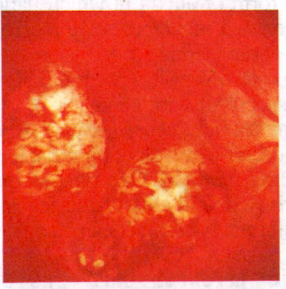

Chorioretinitis *(Stein, 1988)*

of parasitic or bacterial infection. It is characterized by blurred vision, photophobia, and distorted images.

chorioretinopathy /kôr′ē·ōret′ənop′əthē/ [Gk, *chorion* + L, *rete* net; Gk, *pathos,* disease], a noninflammatory process caused by disease that involves the choroid and the retina. Also called **choroidoretinitis.**

choroid /kôr′oid/ [Gk, *chorion* + *eidos,* form], a thin, highly vascular membrane covering the posterior five sixths of the eye between the retina and sclera.

choroidal malignant melanoma /kôroi′dəl/ [Gk, *chorion, eidos* + L, *malignus,* ill-disposed; Gk, *melas,* black, *oma,* tumor], a tumor of the choroid coat that grows into the vitreous humor, causing detachment and degeneration of the overlying retina. Typically mound shaped or mushroom shaped, the neoplasm may break through the sclera and present under the conjunctiva.

choroiditis /kôr′oidī′tis/, an inflammatory condition of the choroid membrane of the eye. See also **chorioretinitis.**

choroidocyclitis /kôroi′dōsiklī′tis/ [Gk, *chorion, eidos* + *kyklos,* circle, *itis,* inflammation], an abnormal condition characterized by inflammation of the choroid and the ciliary processes.

choroidoretinitis. See **chorioretinopathy.**

choroid plexectomy /pleksek′təmē/ [Gk, *chorion, eidos*; L, *plexus,* pleated; Gk, *ektome,* excision], a surgical procedure for the reduction of cerebrospinal fluid production in the ventricles of the brain in hydrocephalus, usually in the newborn. The procedure involves transcortical entry of the lateral ventricles to coagulate or to excise the choroid plexuses and seeks to correct a communicating type of hydrocephalus.

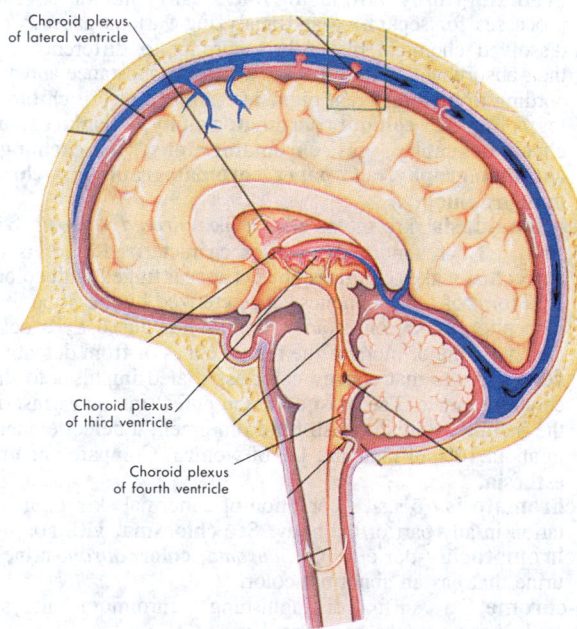

Choroid plexus of lateral ventricle

Choroid plexus of third ventricle

Choroid plexus of fourth ventricle

Choroid plexus *(Thibodeau, 1993/Barbara Cousins)*

choroid plexus [Gk, *chorion, eidos*; L, pleated], any one of the tangled masses of tiny blood vessels contained within the third, the lateral, and the fourth ventricles of the brain.

The choroid plexus of the third ventricle is part of the roof of the anterior commissure of the third ventricle, lying above the interventricular foramen. The choroid plexus of the lateral ventricle is continuous with the choroid plexus of the third ventricle, extending from the interventricular foramen, through the body of the ventricle, to the rostral end of the inferior horn. The choroid plexus of the fourth ventricle, on each side, is an elongated tuft of blood vessels extending through the roof of the ventricle.

Christchurch chromosome (Ch1) [Christchurch, city on South Island of New Zealand], an abnormally small acrocentric chromosome of the G group, involving any members of chromosome pairs 21 or 22, in which the short arms are missing or partially deleted. The aberration is associated with chronic lymphocytic leukemia but has also been found in patients with various other defects. See also **Philadelphia chromosome.**

Christian-Weber disease [Henry Asbury Christian, American physician, b. 1876; Frederick Parkes Weber, English physician, b. 1863], a rare form of panniculitis characterized by nodular formations in the subcutaneous tissues and prolonged intermittent relapsing fever.

Christmas disease. See **hemophilia B.**

Christmas factor. See **factor IX.**

-chroia, a suffix meaning '(condition of) skin coloration': *cacochroia, cyanochroia, xanthochroia.*

chrom-. See **chromo-.**

chromaffin /krō′məfin/ [Gk, *chroma,* color; L, *affin,* affinity], having an affinity for strong staining with chromium salts, especially strong staining of the cells of the adrenal, the coccygeal, and the carotid glands, certain cells of the adrenal medulla, and the cells of the paraganglions. Also **chromaphil** /krō′məfil/.

chromaffin body. See **paraganglion.**

chromaffin cell, any one of the special cells comprising the paraganglia and connected to the ganglia of the celiac, the renal, the suprarenal, the aortic, and the hypogastric plexuses. Chromaffin cells are also sometimes found in association with other sympathetic plexuses. The chromaffin cells of the adrenal medulla secrete two catecholamines, epinephrine and norepinephrine, which affect smooth muscle, cardiac muscle, and glands in the same way as sympathetic stimulation, increasing and prolonging sympathetic effects. The chromaffin cells of the adrenal medulla are especially active in response to stress and the associated reception of nerve impulses from the hypothalamus. These impulses synapse with the chromaffin cells in the adrenal medulla and stimulate them to increase hormonal production, about 80% of which is epinephrine, the rest being norepinephrine.

chromaffinoma. See **pheochromocytoma.**

chromaphil. See **chromaffin.**

-chromasia, **1.** a suffix meaning '(condition of) color (as of cells, skin)': *allochromasia, hyperchromasia, oligochromasia.* **2.** a suffix meaning '(condition of the) stainability of tissues': *amblychromasia, anisochromasia, anochromasia.*

chromatic /krōmat′ik/ [Gk, *chroma,* color], **1.** of or pertaining to color. **2.** stainable by a dye. **3.** of or pertaining to chromatin. Also **chromatinic.**

-chromatic. See **-chromic.**

chromatic asymmetry of iris [Gk, *chroma,* color, *a, symmetria,* commensurability, *iris,* rainbow], a difference in color of the two irides.

chromatic dispersion [Gk, *chroma* + L, *dis,* apart, *spar-*

gere, to scatter], the splitting of light into its various component wavelengths or frequencies, such as with a prism, to separate and study the different colors.

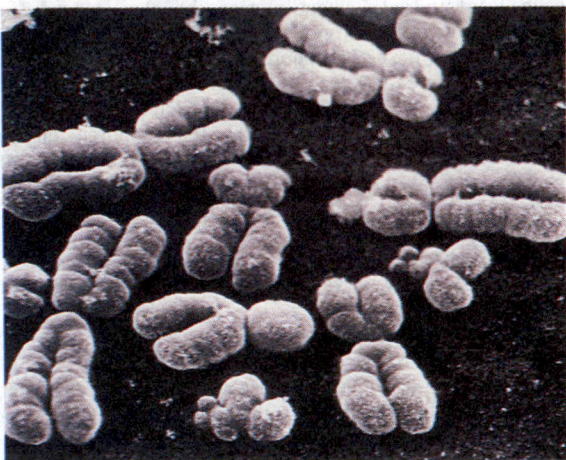

Chromatids
(Raven, 1992/Biophoto Associates/Photo Researchers)

chromatid /krō′mətid/ [Gk, *chroma,* color], one of the two identical threadlike filaments of a chromosome. It results from the self-replication of the chromosome during interphase, is held together by a common centromere, and, during anaphase of mitosis and meiosis, divides longitudinally to form daughter chromosomes.

chromatid deletion, the breakage of a chromatid. The breakage may be caused by a single-hit effect produced by radiation. If the hit occurs in the G_1 phase of a cell cycle, before DNA synthesis, both the deletion and the remaining portion of the damaged chromosome will be replicated as the two sister chromatids with material missing and two acentric fragments. The fragments are isochromatids.

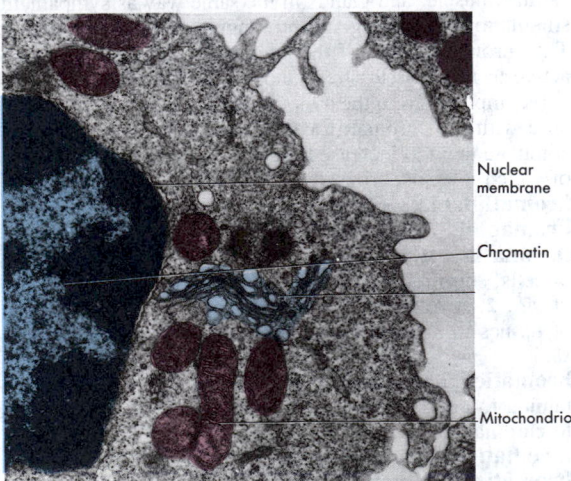

Nuclear membrane

Chromatin

Mitochondrion

Portion of a cell showing location of chromatin
(Thibodeau, 1993/KG Murti)

chromatin /krō′mətin/ [Gk, *chroma,* color], the material within the cell nucleus from which the chromosomes are formed. It consists of fine, threadlike strands of deoxyribonucleic acid attached to a protein base, usually histone; it is readily stained with basic dyes; and it occurs in two different forms, euchromatin and heterochromatin, which are distinguishable during the phases of the cell cycle by variant degrees of staining depending on the amount of dispersion or coiling that occurs. During cell division, portions of the chromatin condense and coil to form the chromosomes. A kind of chromatin is **sex chromatin.** Chromatin is also called **chromoplasm, karyotin.** See also **chromatid, euchromatin, heterochromatin.** —**chromatinic,** *adj.*

chromatinic. See **chromatic.**

chromatin-negative, pertaining to or descriptive of the nuclei of cells that lack sex chromatin, specifically characteristic of the normal male, but also occurring in certain chromosomal abnormalities.

chromatin nucleolus. See **karyosome.**

chromatin-positive, pertaining to or descriptive of the nuclei of cells that contain sex chromatin, specifically characteristic of the normal female, but occurring also in certain chromosomal abnormalities.

chromatism /krō′mətiz′əm/, **1.** an abnormal condition characterized by hallucinations in which the affected individual sees colored lights. **2.** abnormal pigmentation.

chromatogram /krōmat′əgram′/, **1.** the record produced by the separation of gaseous substances or dissolved chemical substances moving through a column of absorbent material that filters out the various absorbates in different layers. **2.** any graphic record produced by any chromatographic method.

chromatography /krō′mətog′rəfē/, any one of several processes for separating and analyzing various gaseous or dissolved chemical materials according to differences in their absorbency with respect to a specific substance and according to their different pigments. Some kinds of chromatography are **column chromatography, displacement chromatography, gas chromatography, ion-exchange chromatography,** and **paper chromatography.** —**chromatographic,** *adj.*

chromatopsia /krō′mətop′sē·ə/ [Gk, *chroma* + *opsis,* vision], **1.** an abnormal condition characterized by a visual defect that makes colorless objects appear tinged with color. **2.** a form of color blindness characterized by the imperfect perception of various colors. It may be caused by a deficiency in one or more of the retinal cones or from defective nerve circuits that convey color-associated impulses to the cerebral cortex. The most common defect in color sense is the inability to distinguish red from green, a defect evident in about 10% of men and 1% of women. Compare **chromesthesia.**

chromatosis /-ō′sis/, condition of abnormal skin pigmentation in any part of the body. See **chloasma, vitiligo.**

chromaturia /-ŏŏr′ē·ə/ [Gk, *chroma,* color, *ouron,* urine], urine that has an abnormal color.

-chrome, a suffix distinguishing 'chromium alloys': *hallachrome, nichrome, nicochrome.*

-chromemia, a suffix meaning '(condition of the) hemoglobin in the blood': *hyperchromemia, lipochromemia, polychromemia.*

chromesthesia /krō′misthē′zhə/ [Gk, *chroma* + *aisthesis,* feeling], **1.** the color sense that depends on the mixture of wavelengths in the light that enters the eye and the response of the different types of retinal cones associated with color vision. According to one theory of color vision, one type of cone responds to green light, a second type to red light, and a third to blue light. The human eye can distinguish hundreds of different colors that are combinations of the basic light wavelengths for red, green, and blue. Some of the retinal cones can be stimulated by the whole visual spectrum, and variable stimulation of all the cones can produce all the color sensations known to humans. Changes in the pigments with in the cones affect color vision, and defects in the cones cause various kinds of color blindness. **2.** an abnormal condition characterized by the confusion of other senses, such as taste and smell, with imagined sensations of color. Compare **chromatopsia.**

chromhidrosis /krō'midrō'sis/ [Gk, *chroma* + *hidros*, sweat], a rare, functional disorder in which apocrine sweat glands secrete colored sweat. The sweat may be yellow, blue, green, or black and often also fluoresces. A known cause is occupational exposure to copper, catechols, or ferrous oxide. Industrial nurses should be aware of this benign condition.

-chromia, a suffix meaning a 'state or condition of pigmentation': *metachromia, normochromia, orthochromia.*

-chromic, -chromatic, 1. a suffix meaning the '(specified) number of colors seen by the eye': *bichromic, hexachromic, tetrachromic.* **2.** a suffix meaning a '(specified) color of the blood indicating the hemoglobin content': *hypochromic, normochromic.* **3.** a suffix meaning the 'staining ability of bacteria and tissues': *bathochromic, hemochromic, perchromic.* **4.** a suffix meaning a '(specified) skin color as indicative of disease': *heterochromic, pleiochromic, xanthochromic.* **5.** a suffix meaning a 'coloring substance within a cell or chemical compound: *cytachrome, hemochrome, serochrome.*

chromic catgut /krō'mik/ [Gk, *chroma*, color; L, *catta*; AS, *guttas*], surgical catgut that has been treated with chromium trioxide to strengthen it.

chromic myopia, a kind of color blindness characterized by the ability to distinguish colors only of those objects that are close to the eye.

chromium (Cr) /krō'mē·əm/ [Gk, *chroma*, color], a hard, brittle, metallic element. Its atomic number is 24; its atomic weight is 51.9. It does not occur naturally in pure form but exists in combination with iron and oxygen in chromite, a mineral found chiefly in Africa, Albania, Russia, and Turkey. Chromium strongly resists corrosion and is used extensively to plate other metals and harden steel and, in combination with other elements, to form colored compounds. Stainless steels are more than 10% chromium and strongly resist rusting. Traces of chromium occur in plants and animals, and there is evidence this element may be important in human nutrition, especially in carbohydrate metabolism. Some experts estimate that the safe and adequate daily intake of chromium ranges from 0.1 to 0.2 mg, depending on the age of the individual. Workers in chromite mines are susceptible to pneumoconiosis caused by the inhalation of chromite dust particles that lodge in the lung. Chromium 51 isotope is used in blood studies.

chromium alum, a chemical commonly used to fix, or harden, the emulsion of an x-ray film during manual processing.

chromo-, chrom-, chromat-, chromato-, a combining form meaning 'pertaining to color': *chromocrinia, chromocyte, chromotrichia.*

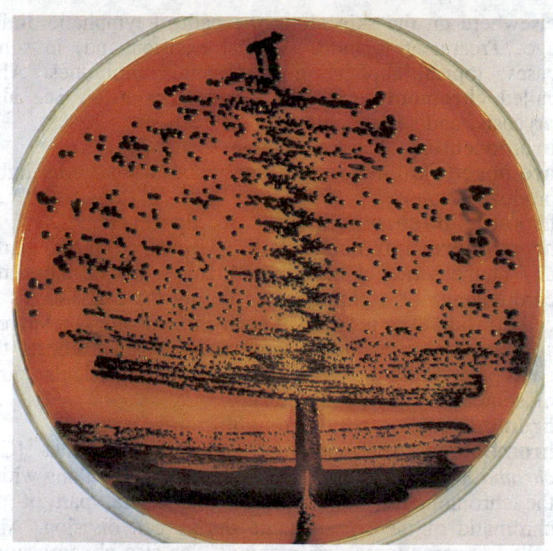

Chromobacterium violaceum (Baron, 1990)

chromobacteriosis /krō'məbaktir'ē·ō'sis/, an extremely rare, usually fatal systemic infection caused by a gramnegative bacillus *Chromobacterium violaceum,* found in fresh water in tropic and subtropic regions, which enters the body through a break in the skin. The disease is characterized by sepsis, multiple liver abscesses, and severe prostration. Early diagnosis, surgical drainage of abscesses, and the administration of chloramphenicol markedly improve the chance of survival.

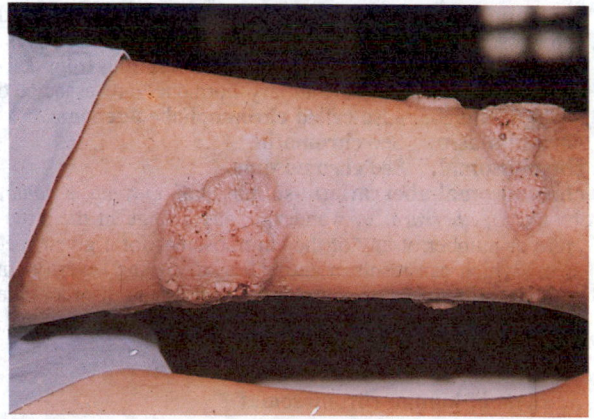

Chromoblastomycosis (Murray, 1990)

chromoblastomycosis /krō'mōblas'tōmīkō'sis/ [Gk, *chroma,* + *blastos,* germ, *mykes,* fungus, *osis,* condition], a chronic infectious skin disease caused by any of a variety of fungi and characterized by the appearance of pruritic, warty nodules that develop in a cut or other break in the skin. What may first appear as a small dull-red lesion gradually develops into a large ulcerated growth. Over a period of weeks or months, additional warty growths may appear elsewhere on the skin along the path of lymphatic drainage. Treatment includes surgical excision and, in some cases, topical application of systemic antibiotics. Also called **chromomycosis, verrucous dermatitis.** See also **mycosis,** and see specific fungal infections.

chromocenter. See **karyosome.**

chromogen /krō'mōjən/, a substance that absorbs light, producing color.

chromolipid, chromolipoid. See **lipochrome.**

chromomere /krō'məmir/ [Gk, *chroma + meros,* part], any of the series of beadlike structures that lie along the chromonema of a chromosome during the early stages of cell division. The position of each chromomere is relatively constant for each chromosome and probably reflects the coiling pattern of the DNA molecule for the particular chromosome. Also called **idiomere.**

chromomycosis. See **chromoblastomycosis.**

chromonema /krō'mənē'mə/, *pl.* chromonemata [Gk, *chroma + nema,* thread], the coiled filament along which the chromomeres lie that forms the central part of the chromatid of the chromosome during cell division. Also called **chromoneme** /krō'mənēm/. See also **chromosome.** –**chromonemal, chromonematic, chromonemic,** *adj.*

chromophilic /krō'məfil'ik/ [Gk, *chroma + philein,* to love], denoting a cell, tissue, or microorganism that is easily stained, particularly certain leukocytes. Compare **chromophobic.**

chromophobe adenoma. See **chromophobic adenoma.**

chromophobia /krō'mə-/ [Gk, *chroma + phobos,* fear], **1.** the resistance of certain cells and tissues to stains. **2.** a morbid aversion to colors. –**chromophobe,** *n.*

chromophobe. See **chromophobia.**

chromophobic /krō'məfō'bik/, denoting a cell, tissue, or microorganism that is not easily stained, particularly certain cells of the anterior lobe of the pituitary gland. Compare **chromophilic.**

chromophobic adenoma, a tumor of the pituitary gland composed of cells that do not stain with acid or basic dyes. Diabetes insipidus and other conditions resulting from deficiency of one or more pituitary hormones are associated with this tumor. Also called **chromophobe adenoma.**

chromoplasm. See **chromatin.**

chromosomal. See **chromosome.**

chromosomal aberration /-sō'məl/ [Gk, *chroma + soma,* body; L, *aberrare,* to wander], any change in the structure or number of any of the chromosomes for a given species, which can result in anomalies of varying severity. In humans, a number of physical disabilities and disorders are directly associated with chromosomal defects of both the autosomes and the sex chromosomes, including Down's syndrome, Turner's syndrome, and Kleinfelter's syndrome. The incidence for most of the chromosomal disorders is significantly higher than that for the single gene disorders. See also specific trisomy syndromes.

chromosomal nomenclature, a standard nomenclature that serves to identify the complement of chromosomes in an individual according to the number of chromosomes, sex, and the deletion or addition of a specific chromosome or part of a chromosome. Complement in a normal female is recorded as 46,XX, and for a normal male, 46,XY. The morphologically paired autosomes are separated into 7 groups and numbered from 1 to 22, with 1 through 3 being designated group A; 4 and 5, group B; 6 through 12, group C; 13 through 15, group D; 16 through 18, group E; 19 and 20, group F; and 21 and 22, group G. The chromosomes are arranged according to decreasing length, followed by the sex chromosome complement, in the usual karyotype representation. Chromosomal aberrations are designated by indicating the total chromosomal number, sex complement, and the group or specific chromosome in which the addition or deletion occurs. For example, 47,XY,G+ indicates a male with an extra chromosome in the G group; 47,XX,21+ shows a female with an extra chromosome 21, or Down's syndrome. The short arm of a chromosome is designated "p," the long arm is "q," and a translocation is "t".

chromosomal sex [Gk, *chroma,* color + *soma,* body; L, *sexus,* male or female], in mammals, the sex of an individual as determined by the presence or absence of the Y chromosome.

chromosome /krō'məsōm/ [Gk, *chroma + soma,* body, any one of the threadlike structures in the nucleus of a cell that function in the transmission of genetic information. Each consists of a double strand of the nucleoprotein deoxyribonucleic acid (DNA), which is coiled in a helix formation and attached to a protein base, usually a histone. The genes, which contain the genetic material that controls the inheritance of traits, are arranged in a linear pattern along the entire length of each DNA strand. Chromosomes are readily stainable with basic dyes and can be seen easily during cell division when they are compactly coiled and in their most condensed state. During interphase, the chromosomes disperse into chromatin and undergo self-replication, forming identical chromatids that separate during mitosis so that each new cell receives a full set of chromosomes. Each species has a characteristic number of chromosomes in the somatic cell, which in humans is 46 and includes 22 homologous pairs of autosomes and one pair of sex chromo-

Analysis of human chromosomes

Description of chromosomes		Group	Autosomes	Sex chromosomes	Number of chromosomes in all body (somatic) cells	
Size	Position of centromere				Male	Female
Large	Metacentric or submetacentric	A	1, 2, 3		6	6
Large	Submetacentric	B	4, 5		4	4
Medium	Metacentric and submetacentric	C	6, 7, 8, 9, 10, 11, 12	X	15	16
Medium	Acrocentric (subterminal)	D	13, 14, 15		6	6
Small	Metacentric and submetacentric	E	16, 17, 18		6	6
Smallest	Metacentric	F	19, 20			
Small	Acrocentric (subterminal)	G	21, 22	Y	5	4
				TOTAL	46	46

somes, with one member of each pair being derived from each parent. Kinds of chromosomes include **accessory chromosome, Christchurch chromosome, daughter chromosome, gametic chromosome, giant chromosome, homologous chromosomes, Philadelphia chromosome, sex chromosome, somatic chromosome, W chromosome,** and **Z chromosome.** See also **centromere, chromatid, chromatin, Denver classification, gene, karyotype, mitosis. –chromosomal,** *adj.*

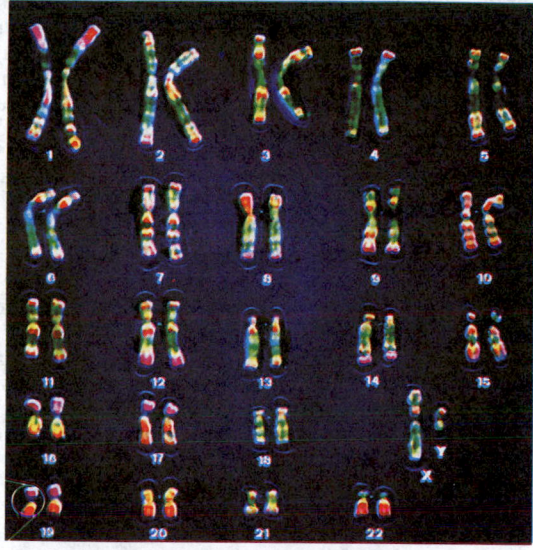

Human chromosomes
(Thibodeau, 1993/CNRI/Science Photo Library)

chromosome banding. See **banding.**

chromosome coil, the spiral formed by the coiling of two or more chromonemata of the chromatid within the chromosome.

chromosome complement, the normal number of chromosomes found in the somatic cell of any given species. In humans it is 46, consisting of 22 pairs of homologous autosomes and one pair of sex chromosomes.

chromosome 5p–syndrome. See **cat-cry syndrome.**

chromosome mapping. See **mapping.**

chromosome puff, a band of accumulated chromatic material located at a specific site on a giant chromosome. It is indicative of gene activity, specifically DNA and RNA synthesis, for the particular locus. Such bands appear at certain chromosomal locations within a given tissue at specific developmental stages in insects and are significant for studying the mode of genetic transmission.

chromosome walking, the process by which overlapping molecular clones that span large chromosomal intervals are isolated.

chromotrope /krō'mətrōp/ [Gk, *chroma* + *trepein,* to turn], **1.** a component of tissue that stains metachromatically with metachromatic dyes. **2.** any one of several dyes differentiated by numeric suffixes. **–chromotropic,** *adj.*

chron-. See **chrono-.**

chronaxie /krō'naksē/ [Gk, *chronos,* time, *axia,* value], (in electroneuromyography) a measure of the shortest dura-

tion of an electric stimulus needed to excite nerve or muscle tissue.

-chronia, -chrone, 1. a suffix meaning '(condition of) processes with respect to time': *isochronia, heterochronia, synchronia.* **2.** a suffix meaning '(condition of) chronaxy between muscle and nerve': *isochronia.* **3.** a suffix meaning the 'time of formation of a part or tissue': *heterochronia, synchronia.*

chronic /kron'ik/ [Gk, *chronos,* time], (of a disease or disorder) developing slowly and persisting for a long period of time, often for the remainder of the lifetime of the individual. Glaucoma is an example of a disease that may develop gradually and insidiously, although it may also occur as an acute disorder marked by sudden severe pain, requiring emergency treatment. Compare **acute.**

chronic abscess [Gk, *chronos,* time; L, *abscedere,* to go away], a slowly developing abscess that produces pus but shows little or no inflammation, redness, or pain. It is usually a tuberculous abscess. Also called **cold abscess.**

chronic airway obstruction, a type of pulmonary disorder in which the patient, when at rest, breathes at a normal rate and may have prolongation of the expiratory phase with pursed-lip breathing. The patient may be barrel chested and have large supraclavicular fossae. The intercostal spaces retract during inspiration, and accessory muscles are used during inspiration. The clinical signs are seen in cases of emphysema and chronic bronchitis.

chronic alcoholic delirium. See also **Korsakoff's psychosis.**

chronic alcoholism, a pathologic condition resulting from the habitual use of alcohol in excessive amounts. The syndrome involves complex cultural, psychologic, social, and physiologic factors and usually impairs an individual's health and ability to function normally in society. Symptoms of the disease include anorexia, diarrhea, weight loss, neurologic and psychiatric disturbances (most notably depression), and fatty deterioration of the liver, sometimes leading to cirrhosis. Treatment depends on the severity of the disease and its resulting complications; hospitalization may be necessary. Nutritional therapy, use of tranquilizers in the detoxification process, use of disulfiram as an aid to continued abstinence, and psychotherapy are all methods of treatment. Alcoholism often goes unrecognized in patients admitted to the hospital for care after an accident or for esophagitis, gastritis, peripheral neuropathy, anemia, or depression, all of which are secondary effects of their alcoholism. If alcoholism is not diagnosed and treated, the patient may not recover. The nurse usually spends more time with a patient than the physician does and is in a better position to discover the condition and to observe signs of withdrawal; the nurse should inform the physician responsible so that detoxification, sedation, and other treatment can be instituted. If the patient is to undergo an operation, it is imperative that the anesthesiologist be notified of the alcoholism, which can affect sensitivity to anesthetics. Alcoholism is a family disease, and the nurse can be instrumental in guiding the patient's family to seek treatment. Long-term support for the alcoholic and his family is offered by such organizations as Alcoholics Anonymous, Al-Anon, and Alateen, and rehabilitation facilities for alcoholism. Compare **acute alcoholism.** See also **alcoholism.**

chronic appendicitis, 1. a type of appendicitis characterized by thickening or scarring of the vermiform appendix, caused by previous inflammation. **2.** an obsolete term for chronic pain in the appendiceal area without any evidence of inflammation.

chronic brain syndrome, an obsolete term for **dementia.**

chronic bronchitis, a very common debilitating pulmonary disease, characterized by greatly increased production of mucus by the glands of the trachea and bronchi and resulting in a cough with expectoration for at least 3 months of the year for more than 2 consecutive years.

■ OBSERVATIONS: The condition has a strong association with smoking. Formerly seen almost exclusively in males, the disease is becoming more common in women who smoke. Productive cough, often with wheezing, is a universal feature, followed by progressive dyspnea on exertion, repeated purulent respiratory infections, airway narrowing and obstruction, and often respiratory failure. Cor pulmonale with right ventricular heart failure is a common result. Some patients develop secondary polycythemia caused by chronic hypoxemia. Acute attacks of respiratory distress with rapid, labored respirations, prolonged expiratory phase, prominent cough, and cyanosis have resulted in these patients being called 'blue bloaters.' Common laboratory findings include elevated hematocrit, with or without respiratory acidosis, abnormal liver function caused by right-sided heart failure and hepatic congestion, pathogenic bacteria in the sputum, abnormal pulmonary function tests, and often chest x-ray signs of increased bronchial markings and emphysema.

■ INTERVENTIONS: Broad-spectrum antibiotics, as ampicillin or erythromycin, are usually prescribed during acute exacerbations of symptoms. Bronchodilators, as theophylline or albuterol, as well as sympathomimetic drugs, such as terbutaline and metaproterenol, are prescribed to prevent worsening of the condition. Heart failure is managed with sodium restriction, diuretics, and sometimes digitalis.

■ NURSING CONSIDERATIONS: A major effort should be made to have the patient discontinue smoking and avoid exposure to toxic inhalants, such as hair sprays, aerosol insecticides, and occupational irritants and poisons. Patients with chronic bronchitis should be immunized against influenza and pneumococcal infections. The use of low-flow oxygen in the home may require patient education and monitoring. Exercise, especially walking, chest physiotherapy, and postural drainage are often indicated, and nurses may give instruction to patients and their families in these therapeutic programs. See also **asthma, chronic obstructive pulmonary disease, cor pulmonale, emphysema, respiratory failure.**

chronic care. See **care of the chronically ill.**

chronic carrier, an individual who acts as host to pathogenic organisms for an extended period of time without displaying any signs of disease.

chronic cervicitis. See **cervicitis.**

chronic cholecystitis. See **cholecystitis.**

chronic chorea. See **Huntington's chorea.**

chronic cystic mastitis. See **fibrocystic disease.**

chronic delirium [Gk, *chronos,* time; L, *delirare,* to rave], a form of delirium in which the patient shows signs of psychosis but is afebrile. The condition is sometimes associated with exhaustion, malnutrition, and wasting.

chronic disease, a disease that persists over a long period of time as compared with the course of an acute disease. The symptoms of chronic disease are usually less severe than those of the acute phase of the same disease. Chronic disease may result in complete or partial disability.

chronic endoarteritis [Gk, *chronos,* time, *endon,* within, *arteria,* windpipe, *itis,* inflammation], an inflammatory condition of the tunica intima lining of an artery wall. It may be accompanied by fatty degeneration of arterial tissue

and calcium deposits. Also called **endarteritis deformans.**

chronic endocarditis [Gk, *chronos,* time, *endon,* within, *kardia,* heart, *itis,* inflammation], an inflammatory condition of the endocardium lining the heart, usually following an attack of acute endocarditis, syphilis, or an atheroma. It frequently involves the cardiac valves, making them incompetent.

chronic fatigue syndrome (CFS), a condition characterized by the onset of disabling fatigue after an initial viral-like illness. The fatigue is accompanied by a constellation of symptoms including myalgias, arthralgias without frank arthritis, low-grade fevers, painful cervical adenopathy, sore throat, headache, memory deficits, and sleep disturbances. The diagnosis is one of exclusion; the cause remaining obscure. Therapy is directed toward the relief of symptoms. Psychiatric intervention is frequently helpful in support of depression which frequently accompanies the condition. The disorder usually resolve spontaneously. Also called **chronic fatigue and immune dysfunction syndrome (CFIDS).**

chronic gastritis. See **gastritis.**

chronic glaucoma. See **glaucoma.**

chronic glomerulonephritis, a noninfectious disease of the glomerulus of the kidney characterized by proteinuria, hematuria, edema, and decreased production of urine. Of unknown cause, it is asymptomatic for years: The symptoms develop slowly, but the disease progresses to kidney failure. Transplantation and dialysis are the only treatments available. See also **postinfectious glomerulonephritis, subacute glomerulonephritis, uremia.**

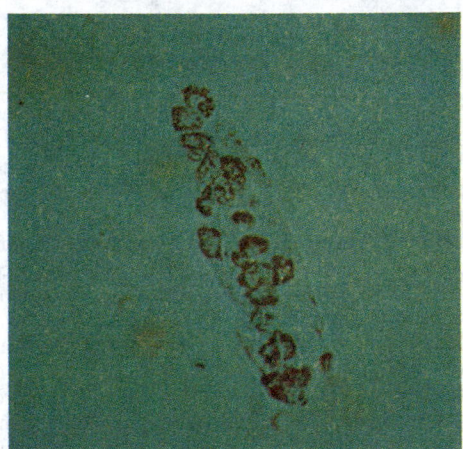

White blood cell cast from patient with chronic glomerulonephritis
(Zitelli, 1992)

chronic gout [Gk, *chronos,* time; L, *gutta,* drop], a persistent condition of purine metabolism, characterized by abnormally high levels of serum uric acid and attacks of arthritis, with deposits of urates in the joints. The disorder may be familial and if untreated can lead to renal failure.

chronic hepatitis [Gk, *chronos,* time, *hepar,* liver, *itis,* inflammation], a state in which the symptoms continue for several months and may increase in severity. In some cases of hepatitis B, the patient may become a lifelong carrier of the antigen and may show prolonged evidence of the infection.

chronic hyperplastic rhinitis [Gk, *chronos,* time + *hyper,* excess + *plassein,* to form + *rhis,* nose + *itis,* inflammation], chronic inflammation of the mucous membranes of the nose, with polyp formation.

chronic hyperplastic sinusitis [Gk, *chronos,* time + *hyper,* excess + *plassein,* to form; L, *sinus,* hollow; Gk, *itis,* inflammation], chronic sinus inflammation, with polyp formation in the nose and sinuses.

chronic hypertrophic rhinitis [Gk, *chronos,* time + *hyper,* excess + *trophe,* nourishment + *rhis,* nose + *itis,* inflammation], a condition of chronic inflammation of the nasal mucosa associated with enlargement of the mucous membrane.

chronic hypoxia, a usually slow, insidious reduction in tissue oxygenation resulting from gradually destructive or fibrotic lung diseases, congenital or acquired heart disorders, or chronic blood loss. There is usually an absence of acute symptoms, but the person develops persistent mental and physical fatigue, shows sluggish mental responses, and complains of a loss of ability to perform physical tasks. Unless treated, the condition may lead to cyanosis and disability, although there may be some physiologic adjustment to the lack of oxygen as occurs in individuals who move from sea level to mountainous areas where oxygen pressures are reduced.

chronic idiopathic thrombocytopenic purpura. See **idiopathic thrombocytopenic purpura.**

chronic illness, any illness that persists over a long period of time and affects physical, emotional, intellectual, social, or spiritual functioning.

chronic intestinal ischemia. See **intestinal angina.**

chronic interstitial nephritis. See **interstitial nephritis.**

chronic intractable pain [Gk, *chronos,* time; L, *intractabilis* + *poena,* penalty], persistent pain that fails to respond to nonnarcotic analgesics and other treatment measures.

chronicity /krōnis′itē/, a state of being chronic.

chronic leg ulcer [Gk, *chronos,* time; ONorse, *leggr*; L, *ulcus,* ulcer], a slow-healing ulcer of the leg, usually associated with varicose veins or a similar circulatory obstacle.

chronic lingual papillitis [Gk, *chronos* + L, *lingua,* tongue; *papilla,* nipple; Gk, *itis*], an inflammatory disorder of the tongue, sometimes extending to the buccal mucosa and palate. It is characterized by irregularly scattered red patches, thinning of the lingual papillae, severe burning pain, and shedding of epidermal tissue. The disorder affects middle-aged individuals, especially women, and occurs in attacks alternating with remissions lasting weeks or months. Also called **Moeller's glossitis.**

chronic lymphocytic leukemia (CLL) [Gk, *chronos* + L, *lympha,* water; Gk, *kytos,* cell; *leukos,* white, *haima,* blood], a neoplasm of blood-forming tissues, characterized by a proliferation of small, long-lived lymphocytes, chiefly B cells, in bone marrow, blood liver, and lymphoid organs. CLL is rare under 35 years of age, increases in frequency with age, and is more common in men than in women. The disease has an insidious onset and progresses to cause malaise, easy fatigability, anorexia, weight loss,

nocturnal sweating, lymphadenopathy, and hepatosplenomegaly. Most patients can continue normal activities for years; 25% die of unrelated diseases. No treatment is curative, but remissions may be induced by chemotherapy, busulfan and cytoxan, with chlorambucil and glucocorticoids or by thymic, splenic, or total body irradiation.

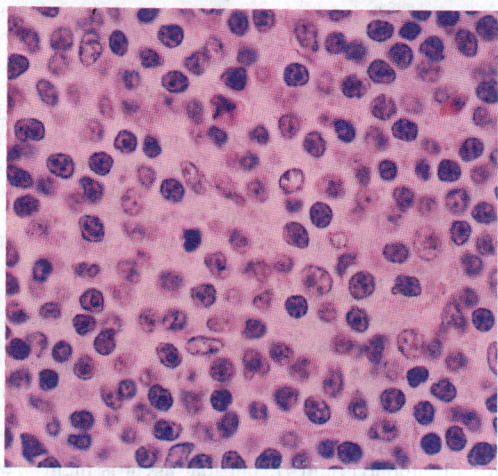

Chronic lymphocytic leukemia— lymph node biopsy
(Skarin, 1991)

chronic mastitis. See **mastitis.**

chronic mountain sickness [Gk, *chronos,* time; L, *montana*; AS, *soec*], a form of altitude sickness in which the increased production of red cells results in polycythemia. Some symptoms of mountain sickness such as headache, weakness, and limb aches occasionally develop in indigenous mountain dwellers as well as persons who had become acclimatized to the higher altitudes. See also **altitude sickness.**

chronic mucocutaneous candidiasis, an abnormal condition and rare form of candidiasis, characterized by candidal infection lesions of the skin, mucous membranes, gastrointestinal tract, and respiratory tract. This disease usually occurs during the first year of life but can develop any time. It affects both men and women and may be associated with an inherited defect of the cell-mediated immune system which can allow autoantibodies to develop against target organs. The humoral immune system functions normally in this disease. The onset of infections associated with the disease may precede endocrinopathy.

■ OBSERVATIONS: Chronic mucocutaneous candidiasis may affect the skin, the mucous membranes, the nails, and the vagina, usually causing large, circular lesions. Associated viral infections may lead to endocrinopathy and hepatitis. Infections of the mouth, nose, and palate may cause problems with speech and eating. Tetany and hypocalcemia are the most common symptoms associated with the endocrinopathy and are usually confined to the involved organ. Other complications associated with chronic mucocutaneous candidiasis may include diabetes, Addison's disease, hypothyroidism, and pernicious anemia. Some patients also develop psychiatric problems because of disfigurements and extensive endocrinal disorders. Diagnosis of this disease usually includes laboratory tests, which commonly show a normal T-cell count and normal immunologic responses to antigens other than *Candida albicans*. The endocrinopathy associated with this disease may include nonimmunologic aberrations, such as hypocalcemia, abnormal hepatic function, hyperglycemia, iron deficiency, and abnormal vitamin B_{12} absorption. Other immunodeficiency diseases associated with chronic *Candida* infection must be excluded by diagnosis. Such immunodeficiency diseases as DiGeorge's syndrome, ataxia-telangiectasia, and severe combined immunodeficiency disease all cause serious immunologic defects. Required after diagnosis of chronic mucocutaneous candidiasis are evaluations of numerous functions of the patient, such as adrenal, gonadal, pancreatic, parathyroid, pituitary, and thyroid functions. Chronic mucocutaneous candidiasis is progressive and usually leads to endocrinopathy.

■ INTERVENTIONS: Chronic mucocutaneous candidiasis resists treatment with topical antifungal agents, miconazole, and nystatin. Endocrinopathies associated with the disease must be treated individually by hormone replacement; some success in this regard has been reported with experimental injections of thymosin and levamisole. Most success in treating severe cases has been with transfer factor from a *Candida*-positive donor, with intravenous amphotericin B. Some success may also be possible against systemic infection with amphotericin B, but that agent is highly nephrotoxic. Some patients respond fairly well to fetal thymus transplants. Plastic surgery may also be part of the treatment to aid patients in coping with disfigurements caused by the disease. Treatment may also include iron replacement orally or intramuscularly.

■ NURSING CONSIDERATIONS: Patients with chronic mucocutaneous candidiasis must be closely monitored for signs of other associated diseases, as Addison's disease, diabetes, hepatitis, and pernicious anemia. Patients suffering psychologically from disfigurements associated with the disease often respond positively to the counsel, encouragement, and kindness of the nursing staff. If amphotericin B is involved in the treatment, the patient must be carefully monitored for renal function, because amphotericin B is nephrotoxic. Patients benefit from calm explanations about the progressive manifestations of the disease and the importance of regular endocrinologic checkups.

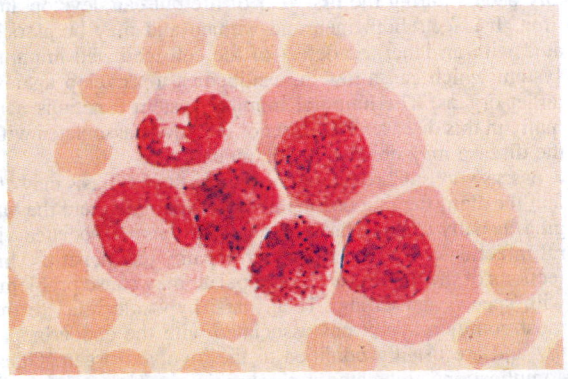

Chronic myelocytic leukemia *(Hayhoe, 1992)*

chronic myelocytic leukemia (CML), a malignant neoplasm of blood-forming tissues, characterized by a proliferation of granular leukocytes and, often, of megakaryocytes. The disease occurs most frequently in mature adults and begins insidiously. Its progress is marked by malaise, fatigue, heat intolerance, bleeding gums, purpura, skin lesions, weight loss, hyperuricemia, abdominal discomfort, and massive splenomegaly. Differential blood count and bone-marrow biopsies are performed to aid in the diagnosis. The alkaline phosphatase activity of the leukocytes is low, and the Philadelphia chromosome is present in myeloblasts in most patients with CML. Therapy with an oral alkylating agent is usual, but advanced CML is refractory to chemotherapy. Also called **chronic granulocytic leukemia (CGL), chronic myelogenous leukemia (CML), chronic myeloid leukemia, splenomedullary leukemia, splenomyelogenous leukemia.**

chronic myocarditis [Gk, *chronos,* time, *mys,* muscle, *kardia,* heart, *itis,* inflammation], an inflammatory condition of the myocardium that persists after an acute bacterial attack. Chronic myocarditis is characterized by degeneration of muscle tissue and fibrosis or infiltration of interstitial tissues.

chronic nephritis [Gk, *chronos,* time, *nephros,* kidney, *itis,* inflammation], a form of kidney inflammation usually secondary to another disease, such as chronic pyelonephritis. In chronic interstitial nephritis, the kidney becomes small and granular with thickening of arteries and arterioles and proliferation of interstitial tissue. There may be functional abnormalities, such as urea retention, hematuria, and casts.

chronic nephropathy, a kidney disorder characterized by generalized or local damage to the tubulointerstitial areas of the kidney. The condition frequently results from more than a single cause, such as diabetes and a bacterial infection. Toxins, in the form of drugs or heavy metals, including cadmium or lead, are common causes, as are gout, cystinosis, and other metabolic disorders. Sickle cell disease is one of several inherited factors that may contribute to chronic nephropathy, but the condition can also develop from no known cause. Symptoms include polyuria, renal acidosis, edema, proteinuria, and blood in the urine. Treatment varies with correction of underlying causal factors. See also **kidney disease.**

chronic obstructive pulmonary disease (COPD), a progressive and irreversible condition characterized by diminished inspiratory and expiratory capacity of the lungs. The person complains of dyspnea with physical exertion, of difficulty in inhaling or exhaling deeply, and sometimes of a chronic cough. The condition includes chronic bronchitis, pulmonary emphysema, asthma, or chronic bronchiectasis and is aggravated by cigarette smoking and air pollution. Also called **chronic obstructive lung disease.**

chronic (open-angle) glaucoma. See **glaucoma.**

chronic pain, pain that continues or recurs over a prolonged period, caused by various diseases or abnormal conditions, such as rheumatoid arthritis. Chronic pain is often less intense than the acute pain. The person with chronic pain does not display increased pulse and rapid respiration because these autonomic reactions to pain cannot be sustained for long periods. Others with chronic pain may withdraw from their environment and concentrate solely on their affliction, totally ignoring their family, their friends, and external stimuli. Some of the factors that can complicate the treatment of persons with chronic pain are scarring, continuing psychologic stress, and medication. Compare **acute pain.** See also **pain intervention, pain mechanism.**

chronic pancreatitis [Gk, *chronos*, time + *pan*, all + *kreas*, flesh + *itis*, inflammation], chronic inflammation of the pancreas with fibrosis and calcification of the gland. It may follow repeated acute attacks and can lead to diabetes.

chronic peritonitis [Gk, *chronos*, time, *peri*, near, *tenein*, to stretch, *itis*, inflammation], a form of peritonitis in which the peritoneum thickens and ascites develop. The condition is usually associated with another disorder, such as pericarditis or polyserositis.

chronic pharyngitis [Gk, *chronos*, time, *pharynx*, throat, *itis*, inflammation], a form of throat inflammation that may be associated with the lymphoid granules in the pharyngeal mucosa.

chronic prostatitis [Gk, *chronos*, time, *prostates*, one standing before, *itis*, inflammation], a persistent inflammatory condition of the prostate gland characterized by a dull, aching pain in the lower back or perineal area, dysuria, fever, and discharge from the penis.

chronic purulent synovitis. See **chronic synovitis.**

chronic pyelonephritis. See **pyelonephritis.**

chronic rheumatism [Gk, *chronos*, time + *rheumatismos*, that which flows], a chronic nonspecific painful condition of the musculoskeletal tissues, including non-articular forms of arthritis.

chronic synovitis [Gk, *chronos*, time + *syn*, together; L, *ovum*, egg(white); Gk, *itis*, inflammation], chronic inflammation of the synovial membrane of a joint. Kinds of chronic synovitis include: **chronic purulent synovitis; chronic serous synovitis.**

chronic tetanus [Gk, *chronos*, time + *tetanos*, convulsive tension], **1.** a form of tetanus with a delayed onset, slow progress of the disease, and milder than usual symptoms. **2.** a reactivated tetanus infection in a healed wound.

chronic tuberculous mastitis, a rare infection of the breast resulting from extension of tuberculosis of underlying ribs. The condition is also characterized by multiple sinus tracts and the presence of tuberculosis elsewhere in the body.

chronic undifferentiated schizophrenia, a condition marked by the symptoms of more than one of the classic types of schizophrenia—simple, paranoid, catatonic, or hebephrenic. See also **acute schizophrenia.**

chrono-, chron-, a combining form meaning 'pertaining to time': *chronognosis, chronophobia, chronotropism.*

chronograph /kron'əgraf/ [Gk, *chronos* + *graphein*, to record], a device that records small intervals of time, such as a stopwatch. **—chronographic,** *adj.*

chronologic /kron'əloj'ik/ [Gk, *chronos* + *logos*, reason], **1.** arranged in time sequence. **2.** of or pertaining to chronology. Also **chronological.**

chronologic age, the age of an individual expressed as a period of time that has elapsed since birth, as the age of an infant, which is expressed in hours, days, or months, and the age of children and adults, expressed in years.

chronopsychophysiology /kron'ōsī'kofis'ē·ol'əjē/, the science of physiologic cyclic processes in the body.

chronotropism /krənot'rəpiz'əm/ [Gk, *chronos* + *trepein*, to turn], the act or process of affecting the regularity of a periodic function, especially interference with the rate of heartbeat. **—chronotropic,** *adj.*

chrys- a combining form meaning 'pertaining to gold': *chrysotherapy, chrysoderma.*

chrysarobin /kris'ərō'bin/, a substance obtained from the wood of araboa trees and used as an irritant in the treatment of parasitic skin diseases and psoriasis.

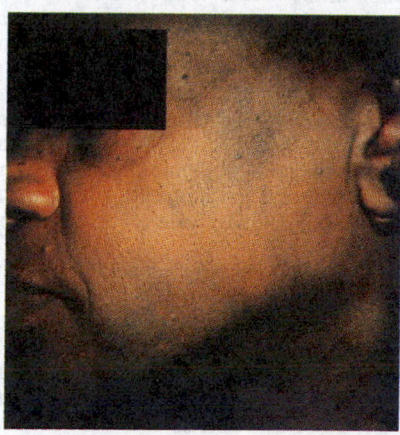

Chrysiasis (Schumacher, 1988)

chrysiasis /krəsī'əsis/ [Gk, *chrysos*, gold, *osis*, condition], an abnormal condition characterized by the deposition of gold in the tissues of the body. Also called **auriosis.**

chrysotherapy /kris'ōther'əpē/ [Gk, *chrysos* + *therapeia*, treatment], the treatment of any disease with gold salts. **—chrysotherapeutic,** *adj.*

Chua K'a, a holistic counseling system of muscle tension release that emphasizes clarification and cleansing of the mind and emotions.

Churg-Strauss syndrome /churg'strous'/, an allergic disorder marked by granulomatosis, usually of the lungs, and often involving the circulatory system.

Chvostek's sign /khvôsh'teks/ [Franz Chvostek, Austrian surgeon, b. 1835], an abnormal spasm of the facial muscles elicited by light taps on the facial nerve in patients who are hypocalcemic. It is a sign of tetany.

Chvostek-Weiss sign. See **Chvostek's sign.**

chyl-. See **chylo-.**

chyle /kīl/ [Gk, *chylos*, juice], the cloudy liquid products of digestion taken up by the small intestine. Consisting mainly of emulsified fats, chyle passes through fingerlike projections in the small intestine, called lacteals, and into the lymphatic system for transport to the venous circulation at the thoracic duct in the neck. Also called **chylus. —chylous,** *adj.*

chyli-. See **chylo-.**

-chylia, a suffix meaning '(condition of the) digestive juices, or chyle': *dyschylia, euchylia, polychylia.*

chyliform ascites. See **chylous ascites.**

chylo-, chyl-, chyli-, a combining form meaning 'pertaining to chyle': *chylocyst, chylophonic, chylosis.*

chyloid /kī'loid/, resembling the chyle that fills the lacteals of the small intestine during the digestion of fatty foods.

chylomediastinum /kī'lōmē'dē·astī'nəm/ [Gk, *chylos*, juice; L, *mediastinus*, midway], the presence of chyle in the mediastinum.

chylomicron /kī'lōmī'kron/ [Gk, *chylos* + *mikros*, small], minute droplets of the lipoproteins measuring less than 0.5

μm in diameter. Chylomicrons consist of about 90% triglycerides with small amounts of cholesterol, phospholipids, and protein. They are synthesized in the GI tract and carry dietary glycerides from the intestinal mucosa via the thoracic lymphatic duct into the plasma and ultimately to sites of utilization in the tissues. The remnant chylomicron particles are removed by the liver and converted into high and low density lipoproteins seen later in the circulation.

chylosus ascites. See **chylous ascites.**

chylothorax /kī'lōthôr'aks/ [Gk, *chylos* + *thorax,* chest], a condition marked by the effusion of chyle from the thoracic duct into the pleural space. The cause is usually a traumatic injury to the neck or a tumor that invades the thoracic duct. Treatment is directed at repairing damage to the duct.

chylous /kī'ləs/ [Gk, *chylos,* juice], pertaining to or resembling chyle.

chylous ascites, an abnormal condition characterized by an accumulation of chyle in the peritoneal cavity. Chylous ascites results from an obstruction of the thoracic duct that may be caused by a tumor or by a destructive lesion, resulting in rupture of a lymph vessel. Also called **ascites adiposus, chylosus ascites, chyliform ascites, fatty ascites, milky ascites.** See also **ascites.**

chyluria /kīlŏŏr'ē·ə/ [Gk, *chylos* + *ouron,* urine], a condition characterized by the milky appearance of the urine because of the presence of chyle.

chylus. See **chyle.**

chyme /kīm/ [Gk, *chymos,* juice], the viscous, semifluid contents of the stomach present during digestion of a meal. Chyme then passes through the pylorus into the duodenum, where further digestion occurs.

-chymia, -chymy, a combining form meaning '(condition of) partly digested food in the duodenum': *achymia, ischochymia, oligochymia.*

chymopapain /kī'mōpəpā'ēn/ [Gk, *chymos* + Sp, *papaya*], a proteolytic enzyme isolated from the fruit of *Carica papaya* and related to papain. It is used in the treatment of prolapsed intervertebral or herniated disks.

chymosin. See **rennin.**

chymotrypsin /kī'mōtrip'sin/ [Gk, *chymos* + *tryein,* to rub, *pepsin* digestion], **1.** a proteolytic enzyme, produced by the pancreas, that catalyzes the hydrolysis of casein and gelatin. **2.** a yellow crystalline powder prepared from an extract of ox pancreas, used in treating digestive disorders in which the enzyme is present in less than normal amounts or is totally lacking.

chymotrypsinogen /kī'mōtripsin'əjən/, a substance, produced in the pancreas, that is the zymogen precursor to the enzyme chymotrypsin. It is converted to chymotrypsin by trypsin.

-chymy. See **-chymia.**

Ci, abbreviation for **curie.**

C.I., abbreviation for **color index.**

C.I., abbreviation for **Colour Index.**

cibophobia /sē'bə-/ [L, *cibus,* food; Gk, *phobos,* fear], an abnormal or morbid aversion to food or to eating.

CIC, abbreviation for *Certified Infection Control.*

cicatrices. See **cicatrix.**

cicatricial entropion. See **cicatrix, entropion.**

cicatrical scar [L, *cicatrix,* scar; Gk, *eschara,* scab], a fibrous scar that remains after a wound has healed.

cicatricial stenosis [L, *cicatrix,* scar; Gk, *stenos,* narrow, *osis,* condition], the narrowing of a duct or tube because of the formation of scar tissue.

cicatrix /sik'ətriks, sikā'triks/, *pl.* **cicatrices** /sik'ətrī'sēz/ [L, scar], scar tissue that is avascular, pale, contracted, and firm after the earlier phase of skin healing characterized by redness and softness. **–cicatricial** /sik'ətrish'əl/, *adj.* **–cicatrize,** *v.*

cicatrize /sik'ətrīz/ [L, *cicatrix,* scar], to heal so as to form a scar.

ciclopirox /sī'kləpī'roks/, an antifungal agent.

■ INDICATIONS: It is prescribed in the treatment of tinea and candidiasis.

■ CONTRAINDICATION: Known sensitivity to this drug prohibits its use.

■ ADVERSE EFFECTS: Among the most serious adverse reactions are hypersensitivity of the skin.

ciclosporin. See **cyclosporine.**

cicutism /sik'yŏŏtiz'əm/ [L, *Cicuta,* hemlock; Gk, *ismos,* process], poisoning caused by water hemlock, resulting in cyanosis, dilated pupils, convulsions, and coma.

CID, abbreviation for **cytomegalic inclusion disease.**

-cide, -cid, a suffix meaning 'killing': *amebicide, herbicide, protozoacide.*

-cidin, a combining form designating a natural antibiotic.

cigarette drain [Sp, *cigarro;* AS, *dranen*], a surgical drain fashioned from a section of gauze or surgical sponge drawn into a tube of gutta-percha.

cigarette smoking, the inhalation of the gases and hydrocarbon vapors generated by slowly burning tobacco in cigarettes. The practice stems partly from the effect on the nervous system of the nicotine contained in the smoke. In addition to nicotine, nearly 1000 other chemicals have been identified in cigarette smoke, including carcinogenic polycyclic aromatic alcohols, cocarcinogenic phenols and fatty acids, carbon monoxide, hydrogen sulfide, hydrocyanic acid, nitrogen oxides, and various irritants that suppress protease inhibition and impair alveolar macrophage function. Cigarette smoke is considered more dangerous than pipe or cigar smoke because it is less irritating and more likely to be inhaled. See also **lung cancer, nicotine.**

ciguatera poisoning /sē'gwəter'ə/ [Sp, *cigua,* sea snail; L, *potio,* drink], a nonbacterial food poisoning that results from eating fish contaminated with the ciguatera toxin. Any of over 300 varieties of fish from the Caribbean or South Pacific have been implicated. The toxin is believed to block acetylcholinesterase activity. Characteristics of ciguatera poisoning are vomiting, diarrhea, tingling or numbness of extremities and the skin around the mouth, itching, muscle weakness, pain, and respiratory paralysis. Cold liquids feel hot to the surfaces of the mouth and throat. No specific treatment has been developed.

cili-, **1.** a combining form meaning 'pertaining to an eyelid': *ciliectomy, cilioretinal, cilioscleral.* **2.** a combining form meaning 'pertaining to an eyelash': *ciliary, cilium.* **3.** a combining form meaning 'pertaining to a minute vibratile': *ciliated, ciliogenesis.*

cilia /sil'ē·ə/, *sing.* **cilium** [L, eyelids], **1.** the eyelids or eyelashes. **2.** small, hairlike processes on the outer surfaces of some cells, aiding metabolism by producing motion, eddies, or current in a fluid. **–ciliary,** *adj.*

ciliary /sil'ē·er'ē/ [L, *cilium,* eyelash], pertaining to the eyelashes or eyelids.

ciliary body [L, *cilium,* eyelid], the thickened part of the vascular tunic of the eye that joins the iris with the anterior portion of the choroid. It is composed of the ciliary crown,

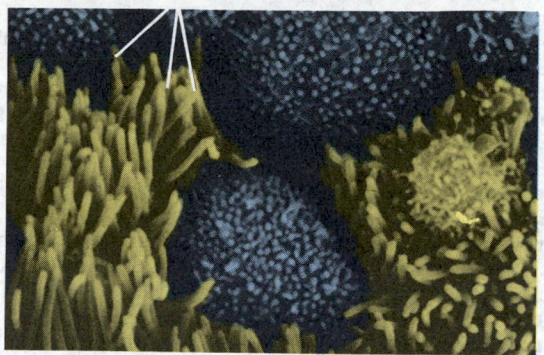

Cilia *(Thibodeau, 1993/Andrew P Evan)*

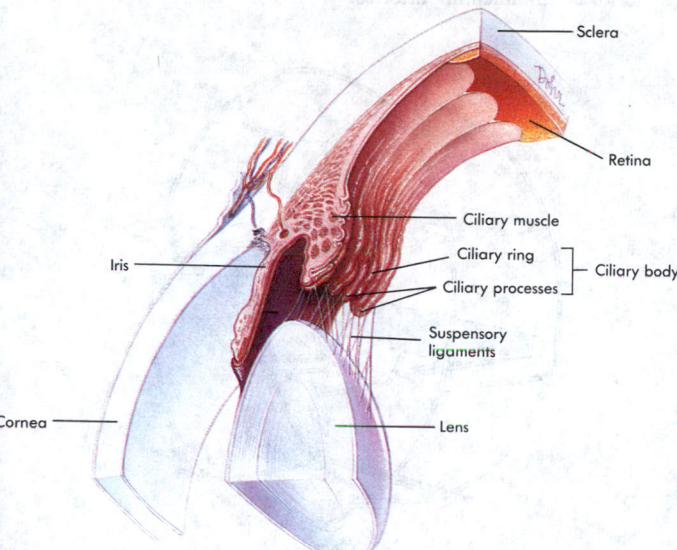

Ciliary body *(Thibodeau, 1993/Marsha J Dohrmann)*

ciliary processes and folds, ciliary orbiculus, ciliary muscle, and a basal lamina.

ciliary canal, the spaces of the iridocorneal angle.

ciliary gland, one of the numerous tiny, modified sweat glands arranged in several rows near the free margins of the eyelids. The apertures of the glands lie near the attachments of the eyelashes. Acute localized bacterial infection of one or more of the ciliary glands causes external sties. Also called **gland of Zeiss.** Compare **tarsal gland.**

ciliary margin, the peripheral border of the iris, continuous with the ciliary body.

ciliary movement, the waving motion of the hairlike processes projecting from the epithelium of the respiratory tract and from certain microorganisms.

ciliary mucus transport, the movement of particles from the upper respiratory tract by means other than exhalation, particularly through the constant wave motion of microscopic cilia lining the tract from the bronchioles to the trachea and the mucous layer that carries trapped particles upward to the lower pharynx.

ciliary muscle, a semitransparent, circular band of smooth muscle fibers attached to the choroid of the eye, the chief agent in adjusting the eye to view near objects. It draws the ciliary process centripetally, relaxing the suspensory ligament of the crystalline lens and allowing the lens to become more convex. It consists of meridional fibers and circular fibers and is thickest anteriorly. The circular fibers close to the circumference of the iris are well developed in hypermetropic eyes but are rudimentary or absent in myopic eyes.

ciliary process, any one of about 80 tiny fleshy projections on the posterior surface of the iris, forming a frill around the margin of the crystalline lens of the eye. The larger ciliary processes are about 2.5 mm long and are more regularly arranged than the smaller ones. The processes comprise one of the two zones of the ciliary body of the eye and are formed by infolding of the various layers of the choroid. They are attached anteriorly to the orbicularis ciliaris and posteriorly to the suspensory ligament of the crystalline lens. See also **ciliary body.**

ciliary reflex. See **accommodation reflex.**

ciliary ring, a small grooved band of tissue, about 4 mm wide, that forms the posterior part of the ciliary body of the eye. It extends from the ora serrata of the retina to the ciliary processes and is thicker near the ciliary processes, because of the thickness of the ciliary muscle.

ciliary zone, an outer circular area on the anterior surface of the iris, separated from the inner circular area by the angular line. The ciliary zone contains the stroma of the iris. Also called **zonula ciliaris.**

Ciliata /sil'ē·ā'tə/, a class of protozoa of the subphylum Ciliophora, characterized by cilia throughout the life cycle. The class includes the subclasses Euciliata and Protociliata. The only significant ciliate in humans is the intestinal parasite *Balantidium coli,* which causes dysentery.

ciliate /sil'ē·it/, of or having cilia, as certain epithelial cells of the body or protozoa of the class Ciliata.

ciliated epithelium /sil'ē·ā'tid/ [L, *cilium,* eyelid; Gk, *epi,* upon, *thele,* nipple], any epithelial tissue that projects cilia from its surface, such as portions of the epithelium in the respiratory tract.

ciliophora. See **protozoa.**

ciliospinal reflex /sil'ē·ōspī'nəl/ [L, *cilium* + *spina,* backbone, *reflectere,* to bend backward], a normal brainstem reflex initiated by scratching or pinching the skin of the back of the neck, resulting in dilatation of the pupil. Also called **pupillary skin reflex.**

cilium. See **cilia.**

-cillin, a suffix designating a penicillin.

cimetidine /simet'idēn/, a histamine H_2-receptor antagonist.

■ INDICATIONS: It is prescribed to inhibit the production and secretion of acid in the stomach in the treatment of duodenal ulcer, pancreatitis, and hypersecretory conditions.

■ CONTRAINDICATION: Known hypersensitivity to this drug prohibits its use.

■ ADVERSE EFFECTS: Among the more serious adverse reactions are diarrhea, dizziness, rash, confusion (usually in elderly patients given large doses), and gynecomastia.

Cimex lectularius. See **bedbug.**

cinchona /singkō'nə, chinchō'nə/ [Countess of Chinchon, Peru], the dried bark of the stem or root of species of *Cinchona,* containing the alkaloids quinine and quinidine.

cinchonism /sin′kōniz′əm/, a condition resulting from excessive ingestion of cinchona bark or its alkaloid derivatives. Cinchonism is characterized by deafness, headache, ringing in the ears, and signs of cerebral congestion. See also **quinine.**

cine-, kine-, kinesio-, a prefix meaning 'pertaining to movement': *cineangiogram, cinefluorography, cineradiography.*

cineangiocardiogram /sin′ē·an′jē·ōkär′dē·əgram′/, a radiograph of the cardiovascular system obtained by special instruments that employ a combination of x-ray, fluoroscopic, and motion-picture techniques.

cineangiocardiography /sin′ē·an′jē·ōkär′dē·og′rəfē/ [Gk, *kinesis,* movement, *aggeion,* vessel, *kardia,* heart, *graphein,* to record], the filming of fluorescent images of the cardiovascular system combining use of fluoroscopic, x-ray, and motion-picture techniques. See also **cineradiography.**

cineangiogram /sin′ē·an′jē·əgram′/, a movie film record of a blood vessel or of a portion of the cardiovascular system, obtained by injecting a patient with a nontoxic radiopaque medium and filming the action of the vessels through which it courses.

cineangiograph /sin′ē·an′jē·əgraf′/, a special movie camera for recording fluorescent images of the cardiovascular system.

cine film /sin′ē/, a special type of motion picture film used in cineradiography, usually in cardiac catheterization or GI studies.

cinefluorography. See **cineradiography.**

cinematics. See **kinematics.**

cineradiography /sin′irā′dē·og′rəfē/ [Gk, *kinesis,* movement; L, *radiere,* to shine; Gk, *graphein,* to record], the filming with a movie camera of the images that appear on a fluorescent screen, especially those images of body structures that have been injected with a nontoxic, radiopaque medium, for diagnostic purposes. Cineradiography incorporates the techniques of cinematography, fluoroscopy, and radiography as a diagnostic technique. Also called **cinefluorography, cineroentgenofluorography.** See also **cineangiocardiography.**

-cinesis, -cinesia, See **-kinesis.**

cingulate /sing′gyəlit/ [L, *cingulum,* girdle], **1.** having a zone or a girdle, usually with transverse markings. **2.** of or pertaining to a cingulum.

cingulate sulcus. See **callosomarginal fissure.**

cingulectomy /sing′gyo͞olek′təmē/ [L, *cingulum* + Gk, *ektome,* excision], the surgical excision of a portion of the cingulate gyrus in the frontal lobe of the brain and the immediately surrounding tissue.

cingulotomy /sing′gyo͞olot′əmē/ [L, *cingulum* + temnein, to cut], a procedure in brain surgery to alleviate intractable pain by producing lesions in the tissue of the cingulate gyrus of the frontal lobe. The operation interrupts the fibers of the white matter in the gyrus by the stereotactic application of heat or cold.

cinnamon /sin′ə mən/ [Gk, *kinnamomon*], the aromatic inner bark of several species of *Cinnamomum,* a tree native to the East Indies and China. Saigon cinnamon is commonly used as a carminative, an aromatic stimulant, or a spice. **–cinnamic,** *adj.*

CIPM, abbreviation for **Comité International des Poids et Mesures.**

circadian dysrhythmia /sərkā′dē·ən, sur′kədē′ən/ [L *circa,* about, *dies,* day; Gk, *dys,* bad, rhythmos], the biologic and psychologic stress effects of jet lag, or rapid travel through several time zones. In addition to a shift in normal eating and sleeping patterns, medication schedules and other therapies may be disrupted.

circadian rhythm [L, *circa* about, *dies,* day; Gk, rhythmos], a pattern based on a 24-hour cycle, especially the repetition of certain physiologic phenomena, as sleeping and eating.

circinate /sur′sināt/ [L, *circinare,* to make round], having a ring-shaped outline or formation; annular.

circle [L, *circulus*], (in anatomy) a circular or nearly circular structure of the body, as the circle of Willis and circle of Zinn. **–circular,** *adj.*

circle of Carus. See **curve of Carus.**

circle of Willis [Thomas Willis, English physician, b. 1621], a vascular network at the base of the brain, formed by the interconnection of the internal carotid, anterior cerebral, posterior cerebral, anterior communicating, and posterior communicating arteries.

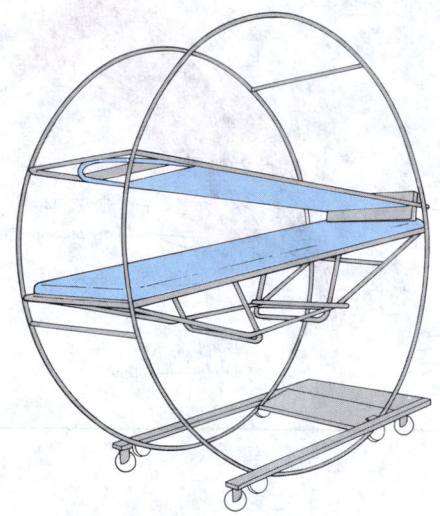

CircOlectric bed (Sorrentino, 1992)

CircOlectric (COL) bed, a trademark for an electronically controlled bed that can be vertically rotated 210 degrees and permits vertical alteration of the position of the patient from prone to supine. This bed is used especially in orthopedics and in the treatment of patients with severe burns. The bed consists of a strong aluminum circular frame supporting an anterior and a posterior straight frame within the exterior aluminum circle. The patient is "sandwiched" and secured between the two straight frames during rotation. Additionally, some advantages of the COL bed are its versatility in changing bed-patient position, the accommodation for patient transfer to walkers, and the capability for gradually orienting the cardiovascular patient to a vertical position before walking. The COL bed also permits greater patient comfort during position changes essential to postoperative treatment for orthopedic surgery, controlled weight-bearing for patients after hip surgery, and easy mobilization of elderly patients who may be at lesser risk in a COL bed than they would be with 5 to 7 days of bed rest in a regular hospital bed. Disadvantages of the COL bed include the development of "CircOlectric feet"; a patient without protective sensations may get decubiti from the pressure of the footboard against the feet and from the posterior mattress resting on the heels when the patient is prone. An additional hazard of the COL bed is the height of the frame and the absence of any high-low electric adjustment mechanism. Patients that are elderly, postanesthesia, or heavily sedated may be injured by falling from the bed unless they are properly secured with safety belts. Many orthopedists caution about the use of the COL bed for patients with unstable spines. Compare **Foster bed, hyperextension bed, Stryker wedge frame.**

circuit /sur'kit/ [L, *circuitus*, going around], a course or pathway, particularly one through which an electric current passes. Current passes through a closed or continuous circuit and stops if the circuit is open, interrupted, or broken. See also **volt.**

circuit training, a method of physcial exercise in which activities are arranged in sets so that the participant moves quickly from one activity to another with a minimum of rest between sets.

circular. See **circle.**

circular bandage /sur'kyələr/ [L, *circularis*, round], a bandage wrapped around an injured part, usually a limb.

circular fiber, any one of the many fibers in the free gingiva that encircle the teeth. Compare **alveolar fiber, apical fiber.**

circular fold, one of the numerous annular projections in the small intestine. They vary in size and frequency in the duodenum, the jejunum, and the ileum, and are formed by mucous and submucous tissue. Most of the folds make less than a full turn around the inside circumference of the intestine, but others spiral through the lumen, making as manyas three turns. Also called **plica circularis, valve of Kerkring.**

circulation /sur'kyəlā'shən/ [L, *circulatio,* to follow a circuit], movement of an object or substance through a circular course so that it returns to its starting point, such as the circulation of blood through the circuitous network of arteries and veins.

circulation rate [L, *circulare,* to go around, *ratum,* calculation], the velocity of blood flow, usually measured in the

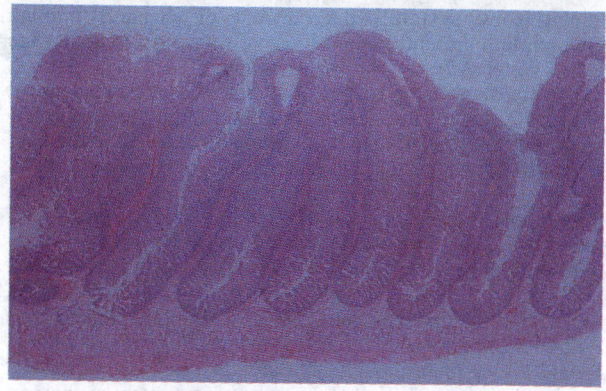
Circular folds (*Mitros, 1988*)

amount of blood pumped through the heart per minute. The rate varies with such factors as blood volume and cardiac contractility.

circulation time, normal, the time required for blood to flow from one part of the body to another. Timing a particle of blood involves injecting a traceable dye or radioisotope into a vein and timing its reappearance in an artery at the point of injection. Alternatively, a tastable substance such as saccharin can be injected, and the time it takes to travel to the tongue can be noted.

circulatory failure /sur'kyələtôr'ē/ [L, *circulatio* + *fallere,* to deceive], failure of the cardiovascular system to supply the cells with enough oxygenated blood to meet metabolic demands. The condition results from abnormal cardiac function as in myocardial infarction; from an inadequate circulating volume of blood, as with hemorrhage; or from collapse of the peripheral vascular system, as in Gram-negative septicemia. See also **shock.**

circulatory fluid. See **blood, lymph.**

circulatory overload [L, *circulare,* to go around; AS, *ofer*; ME, *lod*], an effect of increased blood volume, as by transfusion, that raises the blood pressure. The condition can lead to heart failure or pulmonary edema.

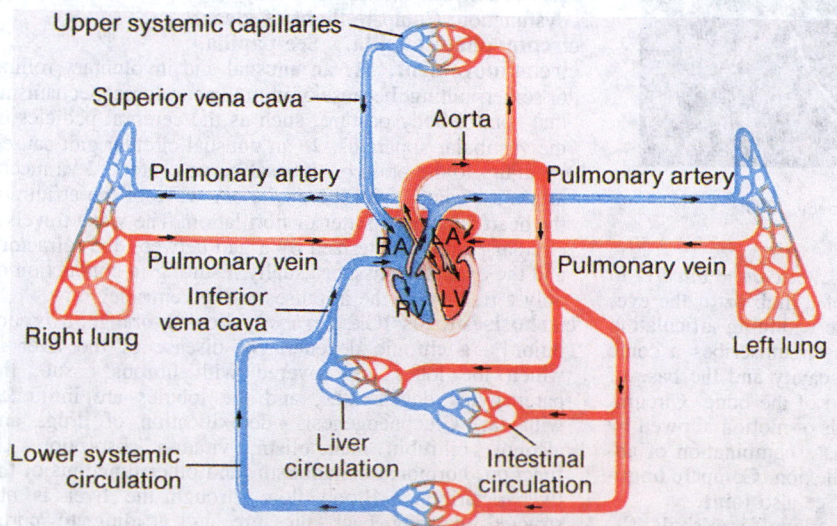

The right chamber receives oxygen-depleted blood from the circulation. Blood is pumped out of the RV, routed through the lungs, where the oxygen is replenished, and returned to the left side of the heart. From the LV, blood is propelled into the systemic circulation.

Circulatory system (*Canobbio, 1990*)

circulatory system, the network of channels through which the nutrient fluids (blood) of the body circulate. See also Color Atlas of Human Anatomy.

circulus arteriosus minor [L, circle; Gk *arteria* air pipe; L, less], the small artery encircling the outer circumference of the iris. Also called **circulus arteriosis iridus.**

circum- /sur′kəm-/, a prefix meaning 'around': *circumanal, circumgemmal, circumvascular.*

circumanal /sur′kəmā′nəl/ [L, *circum,* around, *anus*], of or pertaining to the area surrounding the anus.

circumcision /-sizh′ən/ [L, *circum,* around, *cadere,* to cut], a surgical procedure in which the prepuce of the penis or, rarely, the prepuce of the clitoris is excised. Circumcision is widely performed on newborn boys despite the demonstrable lack of medical benefit and the small but significant risk of serious or lethal complications, such as hemorrhage, urethral injury, or postoperative infection. The operation is performed on newborns with penile block anesthesia, using one of several kinds of clamp. Circumcision is sometimes performed on adult males in the treatment of phymosis and balanitis. Ritual circumcision is required by the religions of approximately one sixth of the population of the world.

circumcorneal /-kôr′nē·əl/, pertaining to the area of the eye surrounding the cornea.

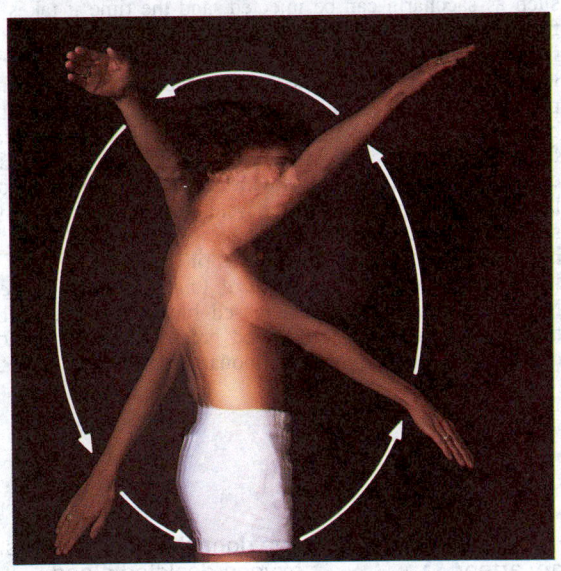

Circumduction (Thibodeau, 1993)

circumduction /sur′kəmduk′shən/ [L, *circum* + *ducere,* to lead], **1.** the circular movement of a limb or of the eye. **2.** the motion of the head of a bone within an articulating cavity, as the hip joint. The bone circumscribes a conic space, the apex of which is in the cavity and the base of which is described by the distal end of the bone. Circumduction is one of the four basic kinds of motion allowed by various joints of the skeleton and is a combination of abduction, adduction, extension, and flexion. Compare **angular movement, gliding, rotation.** See also **joint.**

circumferential fibrocartilage /sərkum′fəren′shəl/ [L, *circum* + *ferre,* to bring; *fibra,* fiber, *cartilago*], a structure made of fibrocartilage, in which fibrocartilaginous rims surround the margins of various articular cavities, as the glenoid labra of the hip and the shoulder. The rims deepen such cavities and protect their edges. Compare **connecting fibrocartilage, interarticular fibrocartilage, stratiform cartilage.**

circumferential implantation. See **superficial implantation.**

circumflex /sur′kəmfleks/ [L, *circum,* around, *flexcere,* to bend], pertaining to blood vessels or nerves that wind around other body structures.

circumlocution /-lōkōō′shən/, the use of pantomime or nonverbal communication or word substitution by a patient to avoid revealing that a word has been forgotten.

circumoral /sur′kəmôr′əl/ [L, *circum* + *os,* mouth], of or pertaining to the area of the face around the mouth.

circumoral pallor [L, *circum,* around, *os,* mouth, *pallor,* paleness], a pale skin area around the mouth, a possible sign of scarlet fever.

circumscribed /-skrībd′/ [L, *circum,* around, *scribere,* to draw], within a well-defined area, or in one with definite boundaries or limits.

circumscribed abscess [L, *circum,* around, *scribere,* to draw, *abscedere,* to go away], an abscess separated from surrounding tissues by a wall of fibroblasts.

circumscribed abscess of bone. See **Brodie's abscess.**

circumscribed scleroderma. See **morphea.**

circum-speech [L, *circum* + AS, *spaec*], (in psychiatry) behavioral characteristics associated with conversation. The characteristics include body language, maintenance of personal space between individuals, handsweeps, head nods, and task-oriented activities such as walking or knitting while carrying on a conversation.

circumstantiality /-stan′shē·al′itē/ [L, *circum* + *stare,* to stand], (in psychiatry) a speech pattern in which a patient has difficulty in separating relevant from irrelevant information while describing an event. The patient may not only include every detail but present the details in a sequential order with the result that the main thread of thought becomes lost as one association leads to another. Very often the person may need to have questions repeated because the main point of answers become lost in the confusion of unnecessary detail. Circumstantiality may be a sign of chronic brain dysfunction. Compare **flight of ideas.**

circumvallate papilla. See **papilla.**

circus movement, **1.** an unusual and involuntary rolling or somersaulting, because of injured neurologic mechanisms that control body posture, such as the cerebral pedicles or the vestibular apparatus. **2.** an unusual circular gait caused by injury to the brain or to basal nerve centers. **3.** a mechanism associated with the excitatory wave of the atrium of the heart and atrial flutter or fibrillation. The wave travels a circular path characterized by a gap between the refractory and the excitatory tissue, usually resulting in conduction of only a fraction of the impulses to the ventricle.

cirrhosis /sirō′sis/ [Gk, *kirrhos,* yellowish-orange, *osis* condition], a chronic degenerative disease of the liver in which the lobes are covered with fibrous tissue, the parenchyma degenerates, and the lobules are infiltrated with fat. Gluconeogenesis, detoxification of drugs and alcohol, bilirubin metabolism, vitamin absorption, GI function, hormonal metabolism, and other functions of the liver deteriorate. Blood flow through the liver is obstructed, causing back pressure and leading to portal hypertension and esophageal varices. Unless the cause of the disease is removed, hepatic coma, GI hemorrhage, and kidney failure may occur. Cirrhosis is most commonly the result of chronic alcohol abuse and sometimes nutritional deprivation, hepatitis, or other causes. The symptoms of cirrhosis are the same regardless of the cause: nausea, fatigue, anorexia, weight loss, ascites, varicosities, and spider angiomas. Diagnosis is made definitively by biopsy, but x-ray and physical examinations and several blood tests of liver function are serially performed to monitor the course of the disease. Treatment depends on the etiology. The liver has remarkable ability to regenerate, but recovery may be very slow.

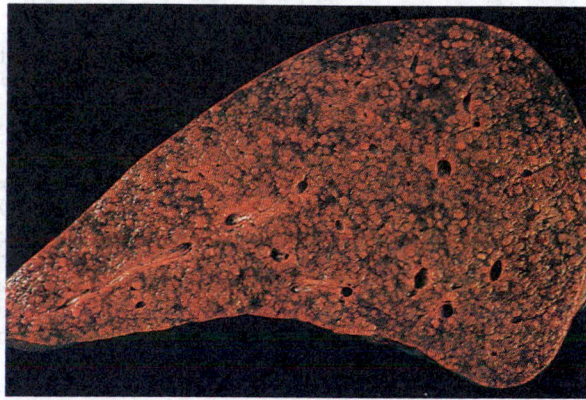

Cirrhosis (Fletcher, 1987)

cirsoid aneurysm. See **racemose aneurysm.**

cis configuration /sis/, **1.** the presence of the dominant alleles of two or more pairs of genes on one chromosome and the recessive alleles on the homologous chromosome. **2.** the presence of the mutant genes of a pair of pseudoalleles on one chromosome and the wild-type genes on the homologous chromosome. Compare **coupling, transconfiguration. 3.** (in chemistry) a form of isomerism in which two substituent groups are on the same side of a double bond. Also called **cis arrangement, cis position.**

cisplatin /sisplat′in/, an antineoplastic.
- INDICATIONS: It is prescribed in the treatment of a wide variety of neoplasms, as metastatic testicular, prostatic, and ovarian tumors.
- CONTRAINDICATIONS: Preexisting renal dysfunction, myelosuppression, hearing impairment, or known hypersensitivity to this drug or other drugs containing platinum prohibits its use.
- ADVERSE EFFECTS: Among the most serious adverse reactions are nephrotoxicity, ototoxicity, myelosuppression, severe nausea, anorexia, vomiting, and allergic reactions.

cistern /sis′tərn/ [L, *cisterna*, a vessel], a storage reservoir for fluids.

cis position. See **cis configuration.**

cisterna /sistur′nə/, *pl.* **cisternae** [L, a vessel], a cavity that serves as a reservoir for lymph or other body fluids. Kinds of cisternae include **cisterna chyli** and **cisterna subarachnoidea.**

cisterna chyli [L, vessel; *chylos*, juice], a dilatation at the beginning of the thoracic duct, situated ventral to the body

of the second lumbar vertebra, on the right side of and dorsal to the aorta. It receives the two lumbar lymphatic trunks and the intestinal lymphatic trunk.

cisternal puncture /sistur′nəl/ [L, vessel; *punctura*, a piercing], the insertion of a needle into the cerebellomedullary cistern to withdraw cerebrospinal fluid for examination. The puncture is made between the atlas and the occipital bone.

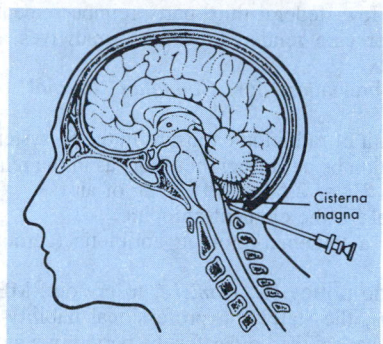

Cisternal puncture

cisterna subarachnoidea [L, vessel; *sub*, under; Gk, *arachne*, spider, *eidos*, form], any one of many small subarachnoid spaces that serve as reservoirs for cerebrospinal fluid.

cistron /sis′tron/ [L, *cis*, this side, *trans*, across], a fragment or portion of DNA that codes for a specific polypeptide. It is the smallest unit functioning as a transmitter of genetic information. In modern molecular genetics the cistron is essentially synonymous with the gene. **–cistronic,** *adj.*

cisvestitism /sisves′titiz′əm/ [L, *cis*, this side, *vestis*, garment], the practice of wearing attire appropriate to the sex of the individual involved but not suitable to the age, occupation, or status of the wearer, as when a male bookkeeper impersonates a male police officer by wearing a police uniform.

cit, abbreviation for a *citrate carboxylate anion.*

Citanest Hydrochloride, a trademark for a local anesthetic (prilocaine hydrochloride).

citrate /sit′rāt, sī′trāt/ [L, *kitron*, citron], **1.** any salt or ester of citric acid. **2.** the act of treating with a citrate or citric acid. **–citration,** *n.*

citric acid /sit′rik/ [Gk, *kitron*, citron; L, *acidus*, sour], a white, crystalline, organic acid soluble in water and alcohol. It is extracted from citrus fruits, especially lemons and limes, or obtained by fermentation of sugars and is used as a flavoring agent in foods, carbonated beverages, and certain pharmaceutic products, especially laxatives. Compare **ascorbic acid.**

citric acid cycle. See **Kreb's cycle.**

citrin /sit′rin/ [Gk, *kitron*, citron], a crystalline flavonoid concentrate that is used as a source of bioflavonoid.

citrovorum factor. See **folinic acid.**

citrulline /sitrul′ēn/ [*Citrullus*, watermelon], an amino acid that is produced from ornithine during the urea cycle and is subsequently transformed to arginine by the transfer of a nitrogen atom from aspartate.

citrullinemia /-ē′mē·ə/, a disorder of amino acid metabolism caused by a deficiency of an enzyme, argininosuccinic acid synthetase. The clinical features include vomiting, convulsions, and coma. It is treated with a low-protein diet providing an essential amino acid mixture, ketoacid analogs of amino acids, and arginine.

Civilian Health and Medical Programs for Uniformed Services (CHAMPUS), a health care insurance system for military dependents and members of the military services when certain kinds of care are not available through the usual military medical service. CHAMPUS is the first, and one of the few, federal third-party reimbursement systems that pay for care rendered by nurse-midwives and nurse practitioners.

CJPH, abbreviation for *Canadian Journal of Public Health.*

C/kg, a unit of radiation exposure in the SI system. It represents coulombs per kilogram of air, as in the relationship, 1 roentgen (R) = 2.58×10^{-4} C/kg of air.

Cl, symbol for the element **chlorine.**

Claforan, a trademark for an antibiotic (cefotaxime sodium).

claims-made policy [L, *clamere,* to cry out; ME, *maken;* L, *politicus,* the state], a professional liability-insurance policy that covers the holder for the period in which a claim of malpractice is made. The alleged act of malpractice may have occurred at some previous time, but the policy insures the holder when the claim is made. Compare **occurrence policy.**

clairvoyance /klervoi'əns/, the alleged power or ability to perceive or to be aware of objects or events without the use of the physical senses. Also called **clairsentience.** See also **extrasensory perception, parapsychology, telepathy.**

clam poisoning. See **shellfish poisoning.**

clamp [AS, *clam,* to hold together], an instrument with serrated tips and locking handles, used for gripping, holding, joining, supporting, or compressing an organ or vessel. In surgery, clamps generally are used for hemostasis.

clamp forceps. See **pedicle clamp.**

clang association /klang/ [L, *clangere,* to resound; *associare* to unite], the mental connection between dissociated ideas made because of similarity in the sounds of the words used to describe the ideas. The phenomenon occurs frequently in the manic phase of bipolar disorder. Also spelled *(German)* **klang association.**

clapping [AS, *cloeppan,* to beat], (in massage) the procedure of making percussive movements on the body, usually on the chest wall, of a patient by lowering the cupped palms alternately in a series of rapid, stimulating blows. In this procedure the movement of the hands is from the wrist. Clapping stimulates the circulation and refreshes the skin and is often done to improve the comfort of bedridden patients, especially during the administration of a bed bath. Also called **percussion.**

clarification /kler'ifikā'shən/ [L, *clarus,* clear, *facere,* to make], (in psychology) an intervention technique designed to guide the patient in focusing on and recognizing gaps and inconsistencies in his or her statements.

clarify /kler'əfī/, (in chemistry) to clear a turbid liquid by allowing any suspended matter to settle, by adding a substance that precipitates any suspended matter, or by heating. –**clarification,** *n.*

Clark's rule [Cecil Clark, 20th century English chemist; L *regula* model], a method of calculating the approximate pediatric dosage of a drug for a child using this formula: weight in pounds/150 [ti] adult dose. See also **pediatric dosage.**

clas-, a combining form meaning 'a piece broken off, or

fragmentation': *clasmatocyte, clasmatodendrosis, clasmatosis.*

-clasia, a suffix meaning a '(specified) condition involving crushing or breaking up': *aortoclasia, colloidoclasia, osteoclasia.*

clasp [ME, *clippen,* to embrace], **1.** (in dentistry) a sleeve-like fitting that is fastened over a tooth to hold a partial denture in place. **2.** (in surgery) any device for holding tissues together, especially bones.

clasp-knife reflex, an abnormal sign in which a spastic limb resists passive motion and then suddenly gives way, similar to the blade of a jackknife. It is an indication of damage to the pyramidal tract.

clasp torsion, the twisting of a dental retentive clasp arm on its long axis.

Class II biologic safety cabinet, a vertical or other container that recirculates air through a high-efficiency filter. It is usually located in a hospital pharmacy and is used to prepare chemotherapeutic agents in an environment that protects personnel from exposure to potentially hazardous materials.

classic cesarean section [L, *classicus,* first-class, *Caesar lex,* Roman law; *sectio,* a cutting], a method for surgically delivering a baby through a vertical midline incision of the upper segment of the uterus. For many practitioners this is the fastest method of cesarean delivery, but it results in a weaker scar, and because the upper segment is thicker and more vascular, there is more bleeding during surgery than from the low cervical cesarean section. Compare **extraperitoneal cesarean section.** See also **cesarean section.**

classic conditioning, a form of learning in which a previously neutral stimulus comes to elicit a given response through associative training. Also called **respondent conditioning.** See also **conditioned reflex.**

classical conditioning. See **conditioned response.**

classic tomography [L, *classicus* + Gk, *tome,* section, *greaphein,* to record], a method that moves the x-ray source and the x-ray plate during an exposure to produce an image in which all but a particular plane is blurred out. This enables an approximate isolation of the image of a detail, which might otherwise be obscured by overlying or underlying structures. See also **computed tomography.**

classic typhus. See **epidemic typhus.**

classification /klas'ifikā'shən/ [L, *classis,* collection, *facere,* to make], (in research) a process in data analysis in which data are grouped according to previously determined characteristics. –**classify,** *v.*

classification of caries [L, *classis,* class, *facere,* to make, *caries,* decay], a system of defining dental caries according to the part of the tooth. The system, devised by G.V. Black, defines Class I caries as pits and fissures in the occlusal surfaces of molars and premolars (bicuspids), in facial and lingual surfaces of molars and in the lingual surfaces of maxillary incisors; Class II, proximal surfaces of premolars and molars, not broken through from proximal to occlusal; Class III, proximal surfaces of incisors and canines not including the incisal angles; Class IV, proximal surfaces of incisors and canines which include the incisal angles; and Class V, cervical one-third of facial or lingual surfaces, not pits and fissures.

classification of malocclusion [L, *classis,* collection, *mallus,* bad, *occludere,* to close up], a system developed by E. H. Angle for defining malposition and contact of the maxillary and mandibular teeth. The system: Class I (neutroclusion), a normal anteroposterior relationship of the jaws, but with crowding of maxillary or mandibular teeth; protruded or retruded maxillary incisors; anterior and/or posterior crossbite, and mesial drift of molars in cases of premature loss of teeth. Class II (distocclusion), the buccal groove of the first mandibular molar is distal to the mesiobuccal cusp of the maxillary first permanent molar by at least the width of a premolar. Class III (mesiocclusion), the lower arch is anterior to the upper in one or both lateral segments, and the lower first molar is mesial to the upper first molar, and Class IV, the occlusal relations of the dental arches present the peculiar condition of being in distal occlusion upon one lateral half and in mesial occlusion upon the other half of the mouth.

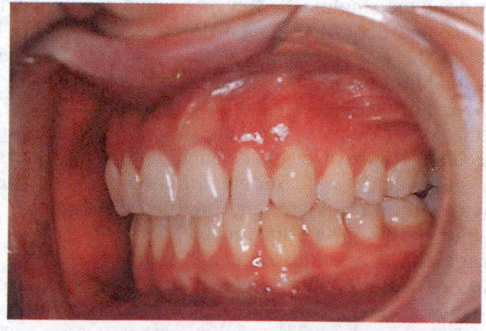

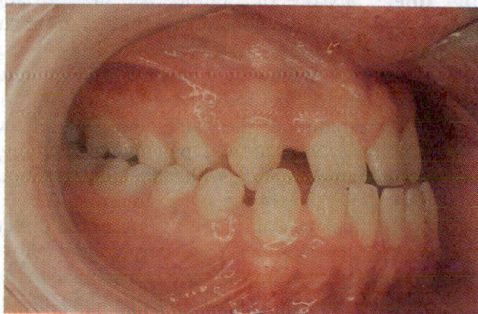

Classification of malocclusion
Class I malocclusion
Class III malocclusion
(Seidel, 1991/Courtesy Drs. Abelson and Cameron, Lutherville, MD)

classification schemes, systems of organizing data or information, usually involving categories of items with similar characteristics. An example is the *International Classification of Diseases (ICD)* compiled by the World Health Organization (WHO), in which basic disease categories are assigned a three-digit code with optional digits for specific disease entities. An example is candidiasis, which is assigned the basic three-digit code 112. Candidiasis of the mouth is 112.0, of the skin and nails, 112.3. A fifth digit is assigned to specified sites, such as 112.81 for candidal endocarditis and 112.82 for candidal otitis externa. Other classification schemes include that of the North American Nursing Diagnoses Association (NANDA) and the *Diagnostic and Statistical Manual of Mental Disorders (DSM)*, prepared by the American Psychiatric Association. See also **nursing diagnosis.**

classify. See **classification.**

-clast, a suffix meaning 'something that breaks': *angioclast, cranioclast, myeloclast.*

-clastic, a suffix meaning 'causing disintegration': *hemoclastic, histoclastic, lipoclastic.*

claudication /klô′dikā′shən/ [L, *claudicatio,* a limping], cramplike pains in the calves caused by poor circulation of the blood to the leg muscles. The condition is commonly associated with atherosclerosis. Intermittent claudication is a form of the disorder that is manifested only at certain times, usually after an extended period of walking, and is relieved by rest.

claustra. See **claustrom.**

claustrophobia /klôs′trə-/ [L, *claustrum,* a closing; Gk, *phobos,* fear], a morbid fear of being in or becoming trapped in enclosed or narrow places. The phenomenon is observed more often in women than in men and can generally be traced to some traumatic situation involving enclosed spaces, usually occurring in childhood. Treatment consists of psychotherapy to uncover the cause of the phobic reaction, followed by behavior therapy, specifically systematic desensitization or flooding technique.

claustrum /klôs′trəm/, *pl.* **claustra** [L, a closing], **1.** a barrier, as a membrane that partially closes an aperture. **2.** a thin sheet of gray matter, composed chiefly of spindle cells, situated lateral to the external capsule of the brain and separating the internal capsule from white matter of the insula. Also called **claustrum of insula.**

clavicle /klav′ikəl/ [L, *clavicula,* little key], a long, curved, horizontal bone just above the first rib, forming the ventral portion of the shoulder girdle. It articulates medially with the sternum and laterally with the acromion of the scapula and accommodates the attachment of numerous muscles. It starts to ossify before any other bone in the body and does not totally unite with the sternum until about the twenty-fifth year. It is shorter, thinner, less curved, and smoother in the female than in the male and is thicker, more curved, and more prominently ridged for muscle attachment in persons performing consistent, strenuous manual labor.

clavicular notch /kləvik′yələr/ [L, *clavicula* + OFr, *enochier*], one of a pair of oval depressions at the superior end of the sternum. Each clavicular notch is situated on one side of the sternum and articulates with the clavicle from the same side.

clavus. See **corn.**

clawfoot. See **pes cavus.**

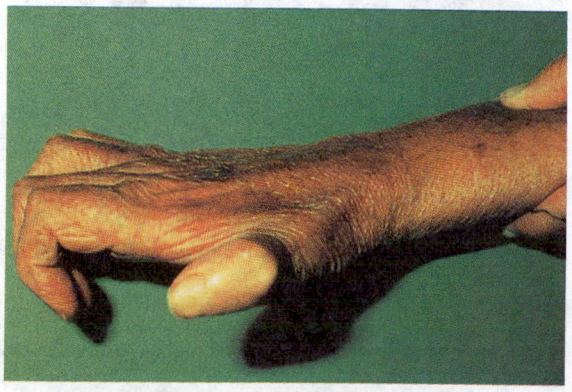

Clawhand *(Kamal, 1991)*

clawhand [AS, *clawu, hand*], an abnormal condition of the hand characterized by extreme flexion of the middle and distal phalanges and hyperextension of the metacarpophalangeal joints. It is caused by atrophy of the interosseous muscles. Also called **main en griffe** /menäNgrif'/.

claw-type traction frame, an orthopedic apparatus that holds various pieces of traction equipment, such as the pulleys, the ropes, and the weights by which traction is applied to various parts of the body or by which various parts of the body are suspended. It consists of two metal uprights, one at the head of the bed and the other at the foot. Both the uprights are secured by claw-type attachments and support an overhead metal bar secured by metal clamps. Compare **Balkan frame, IV-type traction frame.**

clean-catch specimen, a urine specimen that is as free from bacterial contamination as possible without the use of a catheter.

cleansing enema, an enema, usually composed of soapsuds, administered to remove all formed fecal material from the colon.

clearance /klir'əns/ [L, *clarus*, clear], the removal of a substance from the blood via the kidneys. Kidney function can be tested by measuring the amount of a specific substance excreted in the urine in a given length of time.

clear cell [L, *clarus + cella*, storeroom], **1.** a type of cell found in the parathyroid gland that does not take on a color with the ordinary tissue stains used for microscopic examination. **2.** the principal cell of most renal cell carcinomas and, occasionally, of ovarian and parathyroid tumors. **3.** a specific type of epidermal cell, probably of neural origin, that has a dark-staining nucleus but clear cytoplasm with hematoxylin and eosin stain.

clear cell carcinoma, 1. a malignant tumor of the tubular epithelium of the kidney. Characteristically the malignant cells contain abundant clear cytoplasm. See also **renal cell carcinoma. 2.** an uncommon ovarian neoplasm characterized by cells with clear cytoplasm.

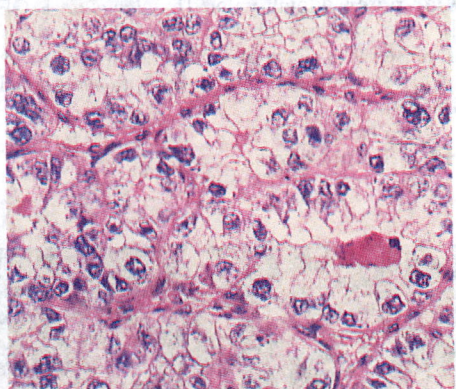

Clear cell carcinoma (Skarin, 1991)

clear cell carcinoma of the kidney. See **renal cell carcinoma.**

clearing agent, a chemical, such as ammonium thiosulfate, used in the processing of exposed x-ray film to remove unexposed and undeveloped silver halide from the emulsion.

clearing test, a range of motion test that moves the joint to its limits, stretching the capsule and other soft tissues in an attempt to reproduce symptoms. If the range of motion is normal and no symptoms are produced, the joint is cleared as a cause of a musculoskeletal disorder.

clear-liquid diet [L, *clarus + liquere*, to flow], a diet that supplies fluids and provides minimal residue. It consists primarily of dissolved sugar and flavored liquids, such as ginger ale, sweetened tea or coffee, fat-free broth, plain gelatin desserts, and strained fruit juices. The diet is nutritionally inadequate and is usually prescribed for a limited amount of time, such as 1 day, postoperatively.

cleavage /klē'vij/ [AS, *cleofan*, to split], **1.** the series of repeated mitotic cell divisions occurring in the ovum immediately after fertilization to form a mass of cells that transforms the single-celled zygote into a multicellular embryo capable of growth and differentiation. At this initial stage, as the zygote remains uniform in size, the cleavage cells, or blastomeres, become smaller with each division. **2.** the act or process of cleaving or splitting, primarily the splitting of a complex molecule into two or more simpler molecules. Kinds of cleavage include **determinate cleavage, equal cleavage, indeterminate cleavage, partial cleavage, total cleavage,** and **unequal cleavage.**

cleavage cavity. See **blastocoele.**

cleavage cell. See **blastomere.**

cleavage fracture, any fracture that splits cartilage with the avulsion of a small piece of bone from the distal portion of the lateral condyle of the humerus.

cleavage line, any one of a number of linear striations in the skin that delineate the general structural pattern and tension of the subcutaneous fibrous tissue. They correspond closely to the crease lines on the surface of the skin and are present in all areas of the body but are visible only in certain sites, as the palms of the hands and soles of the feet. The lines follow a characteristic pattern for each region of the body, although they vary with body configuration; they are consistent in persons of the same build regardless of age. In general, the lines run obliquely, lying in the direction in which the skin stretches the least, perpendicular to the direction of the greatest stretch. Incisions made parallel to these lines heal with much less scarring than those made perpendicular to them. To a certain degree, cleavage lines determine the direction and arrangement of lesions in skin diseases. Also called **Langer's line.**

cleavage nucleus. See **segmentation nucleus.**

cleavage plane, 1. the area in a fertilized ovum where cleavage takes place; the axis along which any cell division occurs. **2.** any plane within the body where organs or structures can be separated with minimal damage to surrounding tissue.

cleave /klēv/ [AS, *cleofan*], segmentation or division, as in cell division or the splitting of a complex molecule into simpler molecules.

cleft [ME, *clift*], **1.** divided. **2.** a fissure, especially one that originates in the embryo, as the branchial cleft or the facial cleft.

cleft foot, an abnormal condition in which the division between third and fourth toes extends into the metatarsus of the foot.

cleft lip, a congenital anomaly consisting of one or more clefts in the upper lip resulting from the failure in the embryo of the maxillary and median nasal processes to close. Treatment is surgical repair in infancy. Also called **harelip.** See also **cleft palate.**

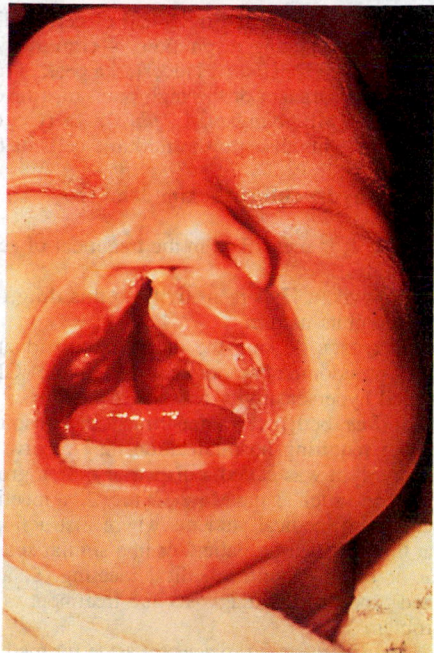

Cleft lip and palate
(Zitelli, 1992/Courtesy Dr. Michael Sherlock)

cleft-lip repair, the surgical correction of a unilateral or bilateral congenital interruption of the upper lip, usually resulting from the embryologic failure of the median nasal and maxillary processes to unite.
■ METHOD: A cleft lip may sometimes be repaired during the infant's first 48 hours of life, but some surgeons follow a "rule of 10s" and perform the operation when the child is 10 weeks old, weighs 10 or more pounds, and has a hemoglobin of at least 10 g per 100 ml. Preoperatively, elbow restraints, used to prevent the infant from touching the incision, are prepared in the proper size and are sent to the operating room with the patient. Postoperatively, the infant is maintained with ventilatory support as necessary until respirations are normal and is observed for respiratory stridor or obstruction, excessive bleeding, separation of the incision, and redness under the elbow restraints. The wire bow applied to the infant's upper lip and taped to the cheeks to prevent tension on the sutures is kept in place; if it becomes loose, it is reapplied with tincture of benzoin. The infant is given clear liquids and juices through an Asepto syringe or special feeding unit; parenteral fluids are administered until the oral intake is adequate; milk products, solids, and a nipple or pacifier are not allowed. The diet and manner of feeding may vary, but the infant is fed while held with the head up or is placed in a cardiac chair and burped after the intake of each ounce of food. The intake and output of fluids are measured. The elbow restraints are worn at all times except when range-of-motion exercises are performed, one arm at a time, while skin care is administered to that limb.
■ NURSING INTERVENTION: The nurse administers preoperative and postoperative care and prepares for the infant's discharge by ensuring that the parents understand the proper diet and feeding schedule and technique. The nurse emphasizes the importance of using elbow restraints, of maintaining motion and skin integrity of the arms, of avoiding injury to the surgical area, and of reporting symptoms of infection, including separation of the incision, excessive swelling, redness, bleeding, and drainage.
■ OUTCOME CRITERIA: Modern surgical techniques permit remarkable repair of cleft lips, but in some cases a second operation is required to eliminate the scar.

cleft palate, a congenital defect characterized by a fissure in the midline of the palate, resulting from the failure of the two sides to fuse during embryonic development. The fissure may be complete, extending through both the hard and soft palates into the nasal cavities, or it may show any degree of incomplete or partial cleft. The condition, which occurs approximately once in every 2500 live births and affects females more than males, is often associated with a cleft in the upper lip. Together, these abnormalities are the most common of the craniofacial malformations, accounting for half of the total number of defects. Feeding is best accomplished with special feeding devices. Surgical repair of the defect is usually not begun until the first or second year of life and is usually performed in steps. Care of the child requires a team approach that includes a plastic surgeon, orthodontist, dentist, nurse, speech and hearing therapists, and social workers. Long-term postoperative problems, including speech impairment and hearing loss, improper tooth development and alignment, chronic respiratory and ear infections, and varying levels of emotional and social maladjustment, may be largely prevented by modern techniques and reconstructive surgery. See also **cleft lip.**

cleft-palate repair, the surgical correction of a congenital fissure in the midline of the partition separating the oral and nasal cavities. Palatine clefts range from a simple separation in the uvula to an extensive fissure involving the soft and hard palate and extending forward unilaterally or bilaterally through the alveolar ridge. A cleft lip often accompanies a cleft palate. Repair of a cleft palate is usually undertaken in the child's second year.
■ METHOD: Before surgery, properly sized elbow restraints to prevent the child from touching the mouth are prepared and sent to the operating room with the patient. Postoperatively, the youngster is kept in a moist oxygen-rich environment using a Croupette or other tent device until respirations are normal, and the child is observed for signs of airway obstruction or excessive bleeding. Parenteral fluids are administered until the oral intake is adequate. Clear liquids and juices are given by cup only; straws, nipples, pacifiers, utensils, or toys may not be put in the mouth. Milk products and solids are contraindicated, but the kind of feeding ordered may vary. The child is fed in a high chair when possible, and a bib is used to accommodate drooling. Only circumoral mouth care is administered; the teeth are not brushed. The intake and output of fluids are measured. The elbow restraints are worn continuously, except when daily range-of-motion exercises are performed and skin care is administered, to one arm at a time. With improvement, the child is permitted to walk as tolerated.
■ NURSING INTERVENTION: Before discharge, the nurse ensures that the parents understand the required diet and the need to feed by cup only, to use elbow restraints, to maintain the motion and skin integrity of the arms, and to avoid injury to the mouth. The nurse reminds the parents to administer the required medication in the proper dosage and on schedule and to report symptoms of incision infection, such as drainage, mouth odor, or bleeding.

■ OUTCOME CRITERIA: Depending on the extent and nature of a cleft palate, it may be repaired in one or in several operations. Some experts believe that early repair of a defect in the bony palate can lead to structural malrelations and advise delaying the operation until the child is between 5 and 7 years of age and has achieved more bone growth. Successful repair often greatly improves the child's oronasopharyngeal physiology, speech, and appearance.

cleft tongue [ME, *clift*; AS, *tunge*], a tongue divided by a longitudinal fissure. Also called **bifid tongue**.

cleft uvula, an abnormal congenital condition in which the uvula is split into halves because of the failure of the posterior palatine folds to unite.

cleido-, cleid-, a combining form meaning 'pertaining to the clavicle': *cleidocostal, cleidocranial, cleidomastoid.*

cleidocranial dysostosis /klē'dōkrā'nē·əl/ [Gk, *kleis,* key, *kranion,* skull; *dys,* bad, *osteon,* bone], a rare, abnormal hereditary condition characterized by defective ossification of the cranial bones and by the complete or partial absence of the clavicles. It is transmitted as an autosomal dominant trait. The defective ossification of the cranial bones delays the closing of the cranial sutures and results in large fontanels. The complete or partial absence of the clavicles allows the shoulders to be brought together. This condition also involves dental and vertebral anomalies. Also called **cleidocranial dysplasia.** See also **dysostosis.**

cleidocranial dystrophia. See also **cleidocranial dysostosis.**

clemastine /klemas'tēn/, an antihistaminic agent.

■ INDICATIONS: It is prescribed in the treatment of symptoms of allergic rhinitis, as sneezing, rhinorrhea, pruritus, or lacrimation.

■ CONTRAINDICATIONS: Use by nursing mothers or those undergoing monamine oxidase inhibitor therapy or having known sensitivity to this drug or other antihistamines is contraindicated.

■ ADVERSE EFFECTS: Among the most serious adverse reactions are hypersensitivity reactions, skin rash, and tachycardia. Transient drowsiness commonly occurs.

Cleocin, a trademark for an antibacterial (clindamycin).

cleptomania. See **kleptomania.**

click [Fr, *cliquer,* to clash], (in cardiology) an extra heart sound that occurs during systole. See also **ejection click, systolic click.**

client /klī'ənt/ [L, *clinare,* to lean], 1. a person who is recipient of a professional service. 2. a recipient of health care regardless of the state of health. 3. a recipient of health care who is not ill or hospitalized. 4. a patient.

client-centered therapy, a nondirective method of group or individual psychotherapy, originated by Carl Rogers, in which the role of the therapist is to listen to and then reflect or restate without judgment or interpretation the words of the client. The goal of the therapy is personal growth achieved by the client's increased awareness and understanding of his attitudes, feelings, and behavior.

client interview. See **patient interview.**

climacteric. See **menopause.**

climacteric melancholia. See **involutional melancholia.**

climate /klī'mit/ [Gk, *klima,* inclination], a composite of the prevailing weather conditions that characterizes any particular geographic region. Various phenomena constitute climate, such as air pressure, temperature, precipitation, sunshine, and humidity. These health factors must be con-

sidered in the diagnosis and treatment of certain illnesses, especially those affecting respiration. —**climatic,** *adj.*

climax /klī'maks/ [Gk, *klimax,* ladder], a peak of intensity, such as a sexual orgasm or the high point of a fever.

climbing fiber [ME, *climben;* L, *fibra*], a type of nerve fiber that carries impulses to the Purkinje cells of the cerebellar cortex.

clindamycin hydrochloride /klin'dəmī'sin/, an antibacterial.

■ INDICATIONS: It is prescribed in the treatment of certain serious infections.

■ CONTRAINDICATION: Hypersensitivity to this drug or to lincomycin prohibits its use.

■ ADVERSE EFFECTS: Among the more serious adverse reactions are pseudomembranous colitis, severe GI disturbances, and hypersensitivity reactions.

clinic [Gk, *kline,* bed], 1. a department in a hospital where persons not requiring hospitalization may receive medical care. Formerly it was called a dispensary. 2. a group practice of doctors, such as the Mayo Clinic. 3. a meeting place for doctors and medical students where instruction can be given at the bedside of a patient or in a similar setting. 4. a seminar or other scientific medical meeting. 5. a detailed published report of the diagnosis and treatment of a health care problem.

-clinic, a suffix meaning 'places set aside for medical treatment': *policlinic, polyclinic, psychoclinic.*

clinical /klin'ikəl/ [Gk, *kline,* bed], 1. of or pertaining to a clinic. 2. of or pertaining to direct, bedside medical care. 3. of or pertaining to materials or equipment used in the care of a sick person.

clinical crown, 1. the portion of a tooth that is covered by enamel and visible in the mouth. 2. the portion of a tooth that is occlusal to the deepest part of the gingival crevice. Compare **anatomic crown, artificial crown, partial crown.**

clinical-crown/clinical-root ratio, the proportion between the length of the portion of the teeth lying coronal to the epithelial attachment and the length of the portion of the root lying apical to the epithelial attachment. The clinical-crown/clinical-root ratio is useful in the diagnosis and prognosis of periodontal disease.

clinical cytogenetics, the branch of genetics that studies the relationship between chromosomal abnormalities and pathologic conditions.

clinical diagnosis, a diagnosis made on the basis of knowledge obtained by medical history and physical examination alone, without benefit of laboratory tests or x-rays films.

clinical disease, a stage in the history of a pathologic condition that begins with anatomic or physiologic changes that are sufficient to produce recognizable signs and symptoms of a disease.

clinical genetics, a branch of genetics that studies inherited disorders and investigates the possible genetic factors that may influence the occurrence of any pathologic condition. Also called **medical genetics.**

clinical horizon, the imaginary line above which detectable signs and symptoms of a disease first begin to appear. Compare **subclinical.**

clinical humidity therapy, respiratory therapy in which water is added to the therapeutic gases to make them more comfortable to breathe.

clinical laboratory, a laboratory in which tests directly related to the care of patients are performed. Such laboratories use material obtained from patients for testing, as compared with research laboratories, where animal and other sources of test material are also used.

clinical nurse specialist (CNS), a registered nurse who holds a master's degree in nursing and who has acquired advanced knowledge and clinical skills in a specific area of nursing practice. The CNS, as a practitioner, assumes a leadership role in the distribution of clinical care to a specific patient population while interacting within the total health care system. The unique functions of the CNS are based on clinical expertise and judgment and include caring for patients, delegating responsibility, teaching other staff members, and influencing and effecting change with respect to the needs of the patient and family and the total health care system.

clinical-pathologic conference, a teaching conference in which a case is presented to a clinician who then demonstrates the process of reasoning that leads to his diagnosis. A pathologist then presents an anatomic diagnosis, based on the study of tissue removed at surgery or obtained in autopsy. Often the students will have been asked to suggest a diagnosis based on the same information presented to the clinician. A discussion usually follows that serves to demonstrate the origin of errors present in any of the diagnoses offered. The pathologist's diagnosis is usually the definitive one. The clinical-pathologic conference is the model for the long series called 'case-reports' in the *New England Journal of Medicine* and is a part of the curricula of most medical schools.

clinical pathology, the laboratory study of disease by a pathologist using techniques appropriate to the specimen being studied. Among the many branches of clinical pathology are hematology, bacteriology, chemistry, and serology.

clinical pelvimetry, a process used to assess the size of the birth canal by means of the systematic vaginal palpation of specific bony landmarks in the pelvis and an estimation of the distances between them. Internal pelvic diameters are not accessible to direct measurement; they must be inferred. Clinical pelvimetry is usually performed by a midwife or an obstetrician during the first prenatal examination of a pregnant woman. Findings are commonly recorded in terms such as 'adequate,' 'borderline,' or 'inadequate,' rather than in centimeters or inches. Compare **x-ray pelvimetry.** See also **birth canal, cephalopelvic disproportion, contraction, dystocia.**

clinical psychology, the branch of psychology concerned with the diagnosis, treatment, and prevention of personality and behavioral disorders.

clinical research center, an organization, often associated with a medical school or a teaching hospital, that studies, analyzes, correlates, and describes medical cases. Such centers usually have extensive laboratory facilities and specialized staffs of physicians and medical technicians. Clinical research centers often offer free or very inexpensive diagnoses and treatment for patients participating in various research programs and often produce significant new medical information distributed through articles, journals, reports, seminars, and lectures. Funding for such facilities may come from minimal fees for various medical services and from grants.

clinical specialist, a physician or nurse having advanced training in a particular field of practice, as a nurse-midwife, pediatrician, or radiologist.

clinical thermometer [Gk, *kline*, bedside + *therme*, heat + *metron*, measure], a thermometer designed for measuring the body temperature of patients. Also called **bedside thermometer.**

clinical thermometry, a method for determining temperature in heated tissue.

clinical trials, organized studies to provide large bodies of clinical data for statistically valid evaluation of treatment.

Clinitest, a trademark for reagent tablets used to test for the presence of reducing sugars, such as glucose, in the urine. The tablets contain copper sulfate, and the procedure is a modified version of Benedict's test.

Clinitron bed, a special bed containing an air-fluidization mattress that conforms to the body shape of the patient. It reduces pressure exerted against the skin and soft tissues.

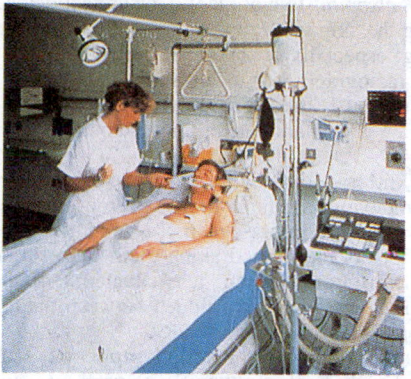

Clinitron bed
(Morison, 1992/Courtesy Support Systems International)

clino-, a combining form meaning 'to bend or make lie down': *clinodactyl, clinostatic, clinostatism.*

clinocephaly /klī′nōsef′əlē/ [Gk, *klinein*, to bend, *kephale*, head], a congenital anomaly of the head in which the upper surface of the skull is saddle-shaped or concave. Also called **clinocephalism.** –**clinocephalic, clinocephalous,** *adj.*

clinodactyly /klī′nōdak′təlē/ [Gk, *klinein* + *daktylos*, finger], a congenital anomaly characterized by abnormal lateral or medial bending of one or more fingers or toes. Also called **clinodactylism.** —**clinodactylic, clinodactylous,** *adj.* (See Fig. p. 349.)

clinoid processes /klī′noid/ [Gk, *kline*, bed, *eidos*, form; L, *processus*], the anterior, middle, and posterior processes of the sphenoid bone at the base of the skull.

clinometer /klīnom′ətər/, an instrument used to measure angular convergence of the eyes or the degree of paralysis of extraocular muscles. Also called **clinoscope.**

Clinoril, a trademark for an antiinflammatory (sulindac).

clinoscope. See **clinometer.**

clioquinol. See **iodochlorhydroxyquin.**

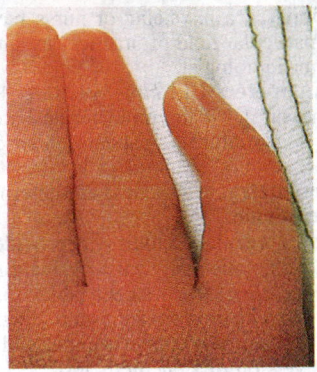

Clinodactyly
(Zitelli, 1992/Courtesy Dr. Christine L Williams, New York
Medical College)

clip [AS, *clyppan,* to embrace], a surgical device used for grasping the skin to align the edges of a wound and to stop bleeding, especially of the smaller blood vessels. It is also used in radiography for localization.

clipped speech. See **scamping speech.**

Clistin, a trademark for an antihistamine (carbinoxamine maleate).

clitoris /klit'əris/ [Gk, *kleitoris*], the vaginal erectile structure homologous to the corpora cavernosa of the penis. It consists of two corpora cavernosa within a dense layer of fibrous membrane, joined along their inner surfaces by an incomplete fibrous septum. It is situated beneath the anterior commissure, partially hidden between the anterior extremities of the labia minora.

CLL, abbreviation for **chronic lymphocytic leukemia.**

cloaca /klō·ā'kə/, *pl.* **cloacae** [L, sewer], **1.** (in embryology) the end of the hindgut before the developmental division into the rectum, the bladder, and the primitive genital structures. **2.** (in pathology) an opening into the sheath of tissue around a necrotic bone.

cloacal membrane /klō·ā'kəl/, a thin sheath that separates the internal and external portions of the cloaca in the developing embryo. It is formed from endoderm and ectoderm and closes the fetal anus during early prenatal development; it later ruptures and is absorbed so that the anal canal becomes continuous with the rectum. Also called **anal membrane.**

cloacal septum. See **urorectal septum.**

clobetasol propionate /klōbet'əsol prō'pyōnāt/, a topical corticosteroid.
■ INDICATIONS: It is prescribed for the short-term treatment of inflammation and pruritus associated with certain moderate to severe types of dermatitis.
■ CONTRAINDICATIONS: Its use is contraindicated for prolonged use, for applications to large areas of poor skin integrity, and with the use of occlusive dressing.
■ ADVERSE EFFECTS: Possible adverse effects may include hyperglycemia, glycosuria, Cushing's syndrome, and suppression of hypothalamic-pituitary-adrenal functions. Because of the greater ratio of skin surface to body weight in children, they are at risk of absorbing a greater proportion of topical steroid.

clocortolone pivalate /klōkôr'təlōn piv'əlāt/, a topical corticosteroid.
■ INDICATION: It is used topically as an antiinflammatory agent.
■ CONTRAINDICATIONS: Viral and fungal diseases of the skin or local impairment of circulation prohibits its use.
■ ADVERSE REACTIONS: Among the more serious adverse reactions are various systemic side effects that may occur from prolonged or excessive application. Local irritation of the skin may occur.

clofibrate /klō'fəbrāt/, an antihyperlipoproteinemic.
■ INDICATIONS: It is prescribed in the treatment of high blood levels of cholesterol, triglycerides, or both.
■ CONTRAINDICATIONS: Liver or kidney dysfunction, pregnancy, lactation, biliary cirrhosis, or known hypersensitivity to this drug prohibits its use.
■ ADVERSE EFFECTS: Among the more serious adverse reactions are nausea, diarrhea, weight gain, and a syndrome resembling influenza. This drug interacts with many other drugs.

Clomid, a trademark for a nonsteroidal fertility drug (clomiphene citrate).

clomiphene citrate /klō'məfēn/, a nonsteroidal antiestrogen that acts to stimulate ovulation.
■ INDICATIONS: It is prescribed principally in the treatment of anovulation and oligoovulation in women.
■ CONTRAINDICATIONS: Abnormal vaginal bleeding, liver dysfunction, or known hypersensitivity to this drug prohibits its use.
■ ADVERSE EFFECTS: Among the more serious adverse reactions are enlargement of the ovaries, blurred vision, gastric upset, rashes, and abdominal pain.

clomiphene stimulation test, a test used to evaluate gonadal function in males who show signs of abnormal pubertal development. Clomiphene, a nonsteroidal analog of estrogen, stimulates the hypothalamic-pituitary system to raise FSH and LH levels of the blood. Failure to respond to clomiphene indicates hypothalamic-pituitary disease, possibly a pituitary tumor. See also **clomiphene citrate, gonadotropins.**

clonal selection theory. See **antibody specific theory.**

clonazepam /klōnaz'əpam/, a benzodiazepine anticonvulsant.
■ INDICATIONS: It is prescribed in the prevention of seizures in petit mal epilepsy and other convulsive disorders.
■ CONTRAINDICATIONS: Liver disease, acute narrow-angle glaucoma, or known hypersensitivity to this drug or to other benzodiazepine drugs prohibits its use. It is not given during lactation.
■ ADVERSE EFFECTS: Among the more serious adverse reactions are anemia, coma, palpitations, mental and respiratory depression, muscle weakness, and shortness of breath.

clone [Gk, *klon,* a plant cutting], a group of genetically identical cells or organisms derived from a single common cell or organism through mitosis.

-clonia, a suffix meaning '(condition involving) spasms': *logoclonia, myoclonia, polyclonia.*

clonic /klon'ik/ [Gk, *klonos,* tumult], pertaining to increased reflex activity, as in upper motor neuron lesions when repetitive muscular contractions and relaxations in rapid succession are induced by stretching.

clonic convulsion [Gk, *klonos,* tumult; L, *convulsio,* cramp], a form of convulsion characterized by rhythmic alternate involuntary contraction and relaxation of muscle groups.

clonic spasm [Gk, *klonos,* tumult, *spasmos*], involuntary alternate contractions and relaxations of muscles.

clonidine hydrochloride /klōˈnədēn/, an antihypertensive.

■ INDICATIONS: It is prescribed for the reduction of high blood pressure.

■ CONTRAINDICATIONS: Known hypersensitivity to this drug prohibits its use.

■ ADVERSE EFFECTS: Among the more serious adverse reactions are a withdrawal syndrome occurring on discontinuation of the medication, characterized by tachycardia, a rapid increase in blood pressure, and anxiety. Drowsiness, sexual dysfunction, and dry mouth commonly occur.

clonorchiasis /klōˈnôrkīˈəsis/, an infestation of liver flukes. See also **Clonorchis sinensis, schistosomiasis.**

Clonorchis sinensis /klōnôrˈkis sinenˈsis/, the Chinese or Oriental liver fluke, a form of tapeworm that is acquired by humans who eat raw or imperfectly cooked fish that is the intermediate host of the parasite. The fluke exists in a dormant stage as a cercaria, encysted in the skin of a fish and unable to continue its life cycle until ingested by a warmblooded animal in which the larvae mature and produce eggs. The eggs are excreted in the feces of the host to enter water where the new generation evolves first in aquatic snails and then in fish. In human hosts, the liver fluke lives in the bile ducts and gallbladder, causing chronic liver disease with enlargement of the liver, diarrhea, edema, and, eventually, death. Also called **Opisthorchis sinensis.**

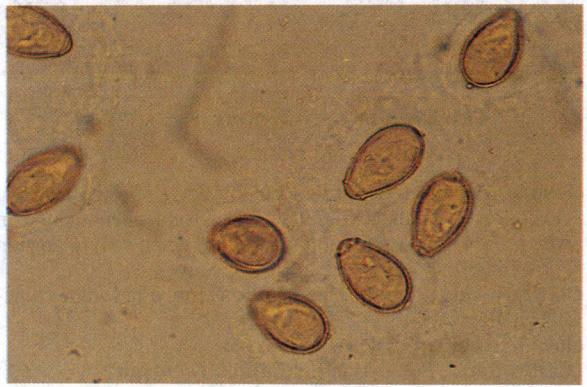

***Clonorchis sinesis* egg** (Murray, 1990)

clonus /klōˈnəs/ [Gk, *klonos,* tumult], an abnormal pattern of neuromuscular activity, characterized by rapidly alternating involuntary contraction and relaxation of skeletal muscle. Compare **tonus.** –**clonic,** *adj.*

C-loop, a surgically formed loop of bowel with a C-shape.

Clogquet's hernia. See **crural hernia.**

clor, abbreviation for a *chloride noncarboxylate anion.*

clorazepate dipotassium /klôrazˈəpāt dī-/, a benzodiaepine tranquilizer.

■ INDICATIONS: It is prescribed in the treatment of anxiety, nervous tension, and alcohol withdrawal.

■ CONTRAINDICATIONS: Psychosis, acute narrow-angle glaucoma, or known hypersensitivity to this drug prohibits its use.

■ ADVERSE EFFECTS: Among the more serious adverse reactions are withdrawal symptoms occurring on discontinuation of treatment. Drowsiness and fatigue commonly occur.

closed amputation [L, *claudere,* to shut; *amputare,* to cut away], a kind of amputation in which one or two broad flaps of muscular and cutaneous tissue are retained to form a cover over the end of the bone. It is performed only when no infection is present. Compare **open amputation.**

closed-angle glaucoma. See **glaucoma.**

closed bite [L, *claudere* + AS, *bitan*], **1.** an abnormal overbite. **2.** a decrease in the occlusal vertical dimension produced by various factors, such as tooth abrasion and insufficient eruption of supportive posterior teeth. Compare **open bite.**

closed-chain, (in organic chemistry) of or pertaining to a compound in which the carbon atoms are bonded together to form a closed ring. Also called **carbocyclic.**

closed-circuit breathing, any breathing system in which a contained gas mixture is rebreathed, either directly or after recirculation through a water or carbon dioxide absorbing unit. An example is a spirometer.

closed-circuit helium dilution, a technique for measuring residual lung volume and functional residual capacity by having a patient breathe through a spirometer containing a known concentration of helium.

closed dislocation [L, *claudere,* to close, *dis,* apart, *locare,* to place], a dislocation that is not accompanied by a skin break at the joint.

closed drainage. See **drainage.**

closed fracture [L, *claudere,* to close, *fractura*], a bone fracture that is not accompanied by a break in the skin.

closed group, a group in which all members are admitted at the same time and vacancies that occur in the membership are unfilled.

closed reduction of fractures [L, *claudere,* to close + *reducere,* to lead back + *fractura*], the manual reduction of a fracture without incision.

closed system, a system that does not interact with its environment.

closed-system helium dilution method, a technique for measuring functional residual capacity and residual volume. It is based on the principle that if a known volume and concentration of helium are added to a patient's respiratory system, the helium will be diluted in proportion to the lung volume to which it is added. Helium, an inert gas, is not significantly absorbed from the lungs by the blood.

closed-wound suction, any one of several techniques for draining potentially harmful fluids, such as blood, pus, serosanguineous fluid, and tissue secretions from surgical wounds. Such fluids interfere with the healing of wounds and often promote infection. Postoperative drainage aids the healing process by removing dead spaces where extravascular fluids collect and helps draw healing tissues together. Many surgical authorities prefer closed-wound suction to other wound-drainage methods, such as pressure bandages and wicks, because it minimizes danger of infection. Closed-wound suction is often an important part of postoperative treatment and may be accomplished with a variety of reliable devices that create a gentle negative pressure to drain away undesirable exudates. The uses of closed-wound suction are as varied as the different surgical procedures. The technique is used as an aid to many operations, such as mastectomies, augmentations, plastic and reconstructive procedures, and urologic and urogenital procedures. Closed-wound suction devices usually consist of disposable transparent containers attached to suction tubes and portable suction pumps. After thoroughly irrigating the wound to remove blood clots and debris, the surgeon inserts the perforated wound tubing into the wound and brings it out through healthy tissue, approximately 5 cm from the incision line. When silicone tubing is used, the tube is passed through a stab wound made adjacent to the surgical wound. With the drainage tubing brought out away from the incision line, the closed-wound suction system remains completely closed. Air cannot infiltrate the wound and cause contamination. When the suction tube has been inserted, the wound is closed and a light dressing is applied. Since the tubing drains most fluids, the dressing usually does not require frequent changing. Closed-wound suction usually continues postoperatively for 2 or 3 days or until the wound stops exuding fluid. The surgeon then removes the suction tubing, and all drainage components of the suction device are discarded. The transparent tubing and reservoir are checked regularly while the suction is functioning as a precaution against clogging and to monitor the volume of exudate drawn from the wound. In some individuals closed-wound suction systems can also accommodate antibiotic drips, which are connected to accessory tubing placed within the wound beside the suction tube. Closed-wound suction also allows irrigation of the wound with special flow controls to permit a periodic change in the flow direction of solutions.

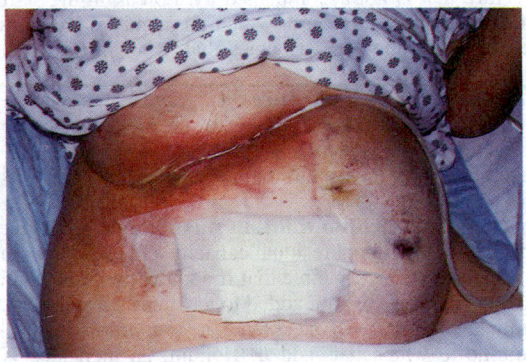

Closed wound suction
(Bryant, 1992/Courtesy Abbott Northwestern Hospital, Minneapolis)

closing capacity (CC), (in respiratory therapy) the sum of the closing volume and the residual volume of gas in the lungs.

closing volume (CV), the volume of gas remaining in the lungs when the small airways begin to close during a controlled maximum exhalation.

clostridial /klostrid′ē·əl/ [Gk, *kloster,* spindle], of or pertaining to anaerobic spore-forming bacteria of the genus *Clostridium.*

clostridial myonecrosis. See **myonecrosis.**

Clostridium /-ē·əm/ [Gk, *kloster,* spindle], a genus of spore-forming, anaerobic bacteria of the Bacillaceae family: *Clostridium novyi, C. septicum,* and *C. bifermentans* are involved in gas gangrene; *C. botulinum* causes botulism; *C. perfringens* causes food poisoning, cellulitis, and wound infections; *C. tetani* is the cause of tetanus.

Clostridium botulinum [Gk, *kloster,* spindle], a species of anaerobic bacteria that cause botulism in humans and botulismlike diseases in other animals. Botulinus food poisoning results from ingesting food containing preformed toxins produced by the species. It is a proteolytic pathogen commonly present in soil, where its endospores can survive for years. Their resistance to heat makes the spores an impoprtant cause of poisoning in improperly cooked or canned foods.

Clostridium perfringens [Gk, *kloster,* spindle], a species of anaerobic Gram-positive bacteria capable of causing gas gangrene in humans and various digestive and urinary tract disease in livestock. The oval spores of the bacteria are found in the soil and in the intestinal tracts of humans and animals. Also called ***Clostridium welchii.***

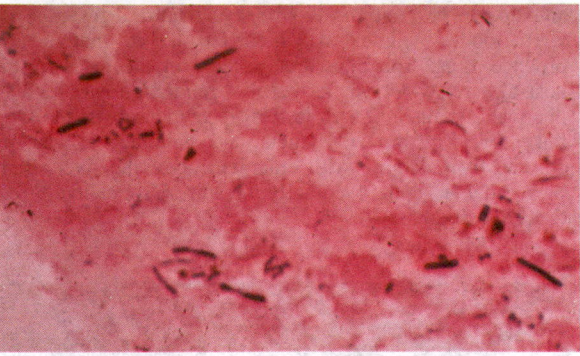

Clostridium perfringens *(Baron, 1990)*

closure /klō′zhər/ [L, *claudere,* to shut], **1.** the surgical closing of a wound by suture. **2.** a visual phenomenon in which the mind "sees" an entire figure when only a portion is actually visible. **See also flask closure**

closylate /klos′ilāt/, a contraction for *p*-chlorobenzenesulfonate.

clot. See **blood clot.**

clothes lice. See **pediculus humanus corporis.**

clotrimazole /klōtrim′əzōl/, a broad spectrum antifungal agent of the imidazole group used in topical applications to treat fungal and yeast infections.

■ INDICATIONS: It is prescribed in the treatment of a variety of superficial fungal infections and for candidal vulvovaginitis.

■ CONTRAINDICATIONS: Known hypersensitivity to this drug prohibits its use. It is not prescribed for ophthalmic use; contact with eyes is avoided.

■ ADVERSE EFFECTS: The most serious adverse reactions are severe hypersensitivity reactions of the skin.

clotting. See **blood clotting.**

clotting time [AS, *clott*], the time required for blood to form a clot, tested by collecting 4 ml of blood in a glass tube and examining it for clot formation. The first appearance of a clot is noted and timed. This simple test has been used to diagnose hemophilias, but it does not detect mild coagulation disorders. Its chief application is in monitoring anticoagulant therapy. Also called **coagulation time.**

cloud baby [AS, *clud; babe*],   a newborn who appears well and healthy but is a carrier of infectious bacterial or viral organisms. The infant may contaminate the surrounding environment with airborne droplets from the respiratory tract forming clouds of the organisms. A cloud baby may be the source of a nursery epidemic, especially one caused by a staphylococcal organism.

clouding of consciousness,   a mental state in which a patient is confused about or is not fully aware of the immediate surroundings.

clove /klōv/ [L, *clavus,* nail],   the dried flower bud of *Eugenia caryophyllata.* It contains the lactone caryophyllin and a volatile oil used as a dental analgesic, a germicide, and a salve. Clove is also used as a spice and a carminative against nausea, vomiting, and flatulence.

cloverleaf nail /klō'vərlēf'/ [AS, *clafre, leaf; nagel*],   a surgical nail shaped in cross section like a cloverleaf, used especially in the repair of fractures of the femur.

cloverleaf skull deformity,   a congenital defect characterized by a trilobed skull resulting from the premature closure of multiple cranial sutures during embryonic development. The condition is associated with hydrocephalus, facial anomalies, and skeletal deformities. Also called **kleeblattschädel deformity syndrome** /klä'blochä'dəl/.

cloxacillin sodium /klok'səsil'in/,   an antibacterial.

■ INDICATIONS: It is prescribed in the treatment of certain serious infections, primarily those caused by penicillin-resistant strains of staphylococci.

■ CONTRAINDICATION: Known hypersensitivity to this drug or to any penicillin prohibits its use.

■ ADVERSE EFFECTS: Among the more serious adverse reactions are GI discomfort, rash, and hypersensitivity reactions.

clubbed penis, [ME, *clubbe*; L, *penis*],   a penis that is curved or twisted, or both. The abnormality may be accompanied by epispadias or hypospadias.

clubbing [ME, *clubbe*],   an abnormal enlargement of the distal phalanges, usually associated with cyanotic heart disease or advanced chronic pulmonary disease but sometimes occurring with biliary cirrhosis, colitis, chronic dysentery, and thyrotoxicosis. The mechanism whereby diminished ox-

ygen tension in the blood causes clubbing is not understood. Clubbing occurs in all the digits but is most easily seen in the fingers. Advanced clubbing is obvious, but early clubbing is difficult to diagnose. Clubbing is present if the transverse diameter of the base of the fingernail is greater than the transverse diameter of the most distal joint of the digit. The affected phalanx is full, fleshy, and quite vascular; the skin may be excoriated.

clubfoot [ME, *clubbe;* AS, *fot*],   a congenital deformity of the foot, sometimes resulting from intrauterine constriction and characterized by unilateral or bilateral deviation of the metatarsal bones of the forefoot. Ninety-five percent of clubfoot deformities are **equinovarus,** characterized by medial deviation and plantar flexion of the forefoot, but a few are **calcaneovalgus,** or **calcaneovarus,** characterized by lateral deviation and dorsiflexion either outward from or inward toward the midline of the body. Treatment depends on the extent and rigidity of the deformity. Splints and casts in infancy may produce complete correction; surgery in several steps may be necessary to achieve normal function. See also **Denis Browne splint, talipes.**

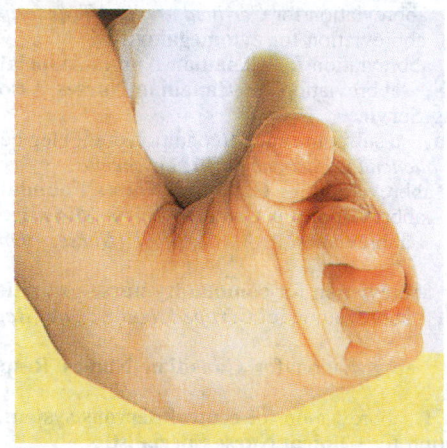

Clubfoot
(Zitelli, 1992/Courtesy Dr. Christine L Williams, New York Medical College).

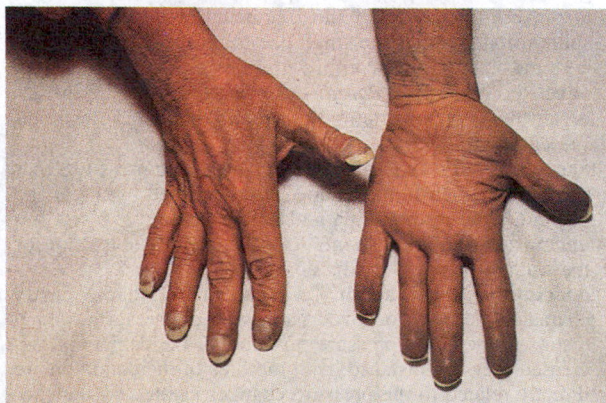

Clubbing *(Wilson, 1990)*

club hair,   a hair in the resting, or final, stage of the growth cycle. See also **hair.**

clubhand,   a congenital disorder in which the hand develops abnormally as a widened stump at the end of the wrist with stunted fingers.

cluster analysis [AS, *clyster,* growing together; Gk, *analyein,* to loosen],   (in statistics) a complex technique of data analysis of numeric scale scores that produces clusters of variables related to one another. The technique is performed with a computer.

cluster breathing,   a breathing pattern in which a closely grouped series of respirations is followed by apnea. The activity is associated with a lesion in the lower pontine region of the brainstem.

cluster headache.   See **histamine headache.**

cluttering [ME, *clotter*],   a speech defect characterized by a rapid, confused, nervous delivery with uneven rhythmic patterns and the omission or transposition of various letters or syllables. The condition is commonly associated with other language disorders, such as difficulty in learning to speak, read, and spell, and with various personality and behavior problems.

clysis /klī'sis/ [Gk, *klyster,* washout], the administration of an enema.

cm, symbol for **centimeter.**

cm², symbol for **square centimeter.**

cm³, symbol for **cubic centimeter.**

Cm, symbol for the element **curium.**

CMA, abbreviation for *Canadian Medical Association.*

CMAJ, abbreviation for *Canadian Medical Association Journal.*

CMC, abbreviation for **carpometacarpal.**

CMF, an anticancer drug combination of cyclophosphamide, methotrexate, and fluorouracil.

CMHC, abbreviation for **community mental health center.**

CMI, abbreviation for **computer-managed instruction.**

CML, abbreviation for **chronic myelocytic leukemia.**

CMRNG, abbreviation for *chromosomally mediated resistant Neisseria gonorrhea.*

CMT, abbreviation for *Certified Medical Transcriptionist.*

CMV, abbreviation for **cytomegalovirus.**

CNA, abbreviation for **Canadian Nurses Association.**

CNATS, abbreviation for **Canadian Nurses Association Testing Service.**

-cnemia, a suffix meaning '(condition of the) leg below the knee': *bucnemia, cacocnemia, microcnemia.*

CNF, abbreviation for **Canadian Nurses Foundation.**

CNM, abbreviation for **Certified Nurse-Midwife.**

CNOR, abbreviation for *Certified Nurse, Operating Room.*

CNP, abbreviation for **community nurse practitioner.**

CNRN, abbreviation for *Certified Neuroscience Registered Nurse.*

CNRS, abbreviation for **Canadian Nurses Respiratory Society.**

CNS, 1. abbreviation for **central nervous system.** 2. abbreviation for **Clinical Nurse Specialist.**

CNSN, abbreviation for *Certified Nutrition Support Nurse.*

CNS sympathomimetic, a drug, such as cocaine or amphetamine, whose effects mimic those of sympathetic nervous system stimulation.

CNS syndrome. See **central nervous system syndrome.**

Co, symbol for the element **cobalt.**

CO, 1. symbol for **carbon monoxide.** 2. abbreviation for **cardiac output.**

co-, col-, com-, con-, cor-, a combining form meaning 'together, with': *coadaptation, coagulate, coarctate.*

CO₂, symbol for **carbon dioxide.**

CoA, abbreviation for **coenzyme A.**

Coactin, a trademark for an antibiotic (amdinocillin).

coagglutination /kō'əgloo'tənā'shən/ [L, *cum, agglutinare,* to glue], a clumping of red blood cells by mixtures of protein antigens and their antisera.

coaguability /kō·ag'yəlbil'itē/ [L, *coagulare,* to curdle], the state of being able to coagulate or form blood clots.

coagulant /kō·ag'yələnt/ [L, *coagulare,* to curdle], an agent that causes a coagulum, or blood clot, to form.

coagulase /kō·ag'yəlās/ [L, *coagulare,* to curdle], an enzyme produced by bacteria, particularly the *Staphylococcus aureus,* that promotes the formation of thrombi.

coagulation /kō·ag'yəlā'shən/ [L, *coagulare,* to curdle], 1. the process of transforming a liquid into a solid, especially of the blood. See also **blood clotting.** 2. (in colloid chemistry) the transforming of the liquid dispersion medium into a gelatinous mass. 3. the hardening of tissue by some physical means, as by electrocoagulation or photocoagulation.

coagulation current, an electric current delivered by a needle ball or other variously shaped points that coagulates tissue. See also **electrocautery, electrocoagulation.**

coagulation factor, one of 13 factors in the blood, the interactions of which are responsible for the process of blood clotting. The factors, using standardized numeric nomenclature, are factor I, fibrinogen; factor II, prothrombin; factor III, tissue thromboplastin; factor IV, calcium ions; factors V and VI, proaccelerin or labile factors; factor VII, proconvertin or stable factor; factor VIII, antihemophilic globulin; factor IX, plasma thromboplastin component (PTC); factor X, Stuart factor; factor XI, plasma thromboplastin antecedent (PTA); factor XII, Hageman factor or glass factor; factor XIII, fibrin stabilizing factor or Laki-Lorand factor. See also **blood clotting, coagulation, fibrinogen, hemophilia A, hemophilia B, hemophilia C, prothrombin, thromboplastin,** and see **factor IV** through **factor XIII.**

coagulation necrosis. See **necrosis.**

coagulation time. See **clotting time.**

coagulopathy /kō·ag'yəlop'əthē/, a pathologic condition affecting the ability of the blood to coagulate.

coalesce /kō'əles'/ [L, *coalescere,* to grow together], to grow together.

coal tar, a topical antieczematic.

■ INDICATIONS: It is prescribed in the treatment of chronic skin diseases, as eczema and psoriasis.

■ CONTRAINDICATIONS: Known hypersensitivity to this drug prohibits its use.

■ ADVERSE EFFECTS: Among the most serious adverse effects are skin irritation and local hypersensitivity reactions.

coal worker's pneumoconiosis. See **anthracosis.**

Coanda effect, a phenomenon of fluid movement similar to the Bernoulli effect in which passage of a stream of gas next to a wall results in a pocket of turbulence between the wall and the gas flow. The turbulence forms a low-pressure bubble that makes the gas stream adhere to the wall. The principle is used in fluidic ventilators.

coaptation splint /kō'aptā'shən/ [L, *coaptare,* to fit together; ME *splinte*], a small splint fitted to a fractured limb to prevent overriding of the fragments of bone. A longer splint usually covers the small one to provide for more support and fixation of the entire limb.

coarct /kō·ärkt'/ [L, *coarctare,* to press together], the act of narrowing or constricting, especially the lumen of a blood vessel.

coarctate retina /kō·ärk'tāt/ [L, *coartare,* to press together + *rete,* net], a funnel-shaped retina caused by a leakage of fluid between the retina and the choroid.

coarctation /kō'ärktā'shən/, a stricture or contraction of the walls of a vessel as the aorta.

coarctation of the aorta, a congenital cardiac anomaly characterized by a localized narrowing of the aorta, which results in increased pressure proximal to the defect and decreased pressure distal to it. Symptoms of the condition are directly related to the pressure changes created by the constriction. The most common site of coarctation is just beyond the origin of the left subclavian artery from the aorta, resulting in high blood pressure in the upper extremities and head and low blood pressure in the lower extremities. Clinical manifestations include dizziness, headaches, fainting, epistaxis, reduced or absent femoral pulses, and muscle cramps in the legs from tissue anoxia during increased exercise. Diagnosis is based on characteristic pressure changes in the upper and lower body and specific radiologic findings, including notching of the lower ribs, left ventricular hypertrophy, and dilatation of the aorta proximal to the stricture. A murmur may or may not be present. Surgical repair is recommended for minor defects because of the high incidence of untreated complications, including aortic rupture, hypertension, infective endocarditis, subarachnoid hemorrhage, and congestive heart failure.

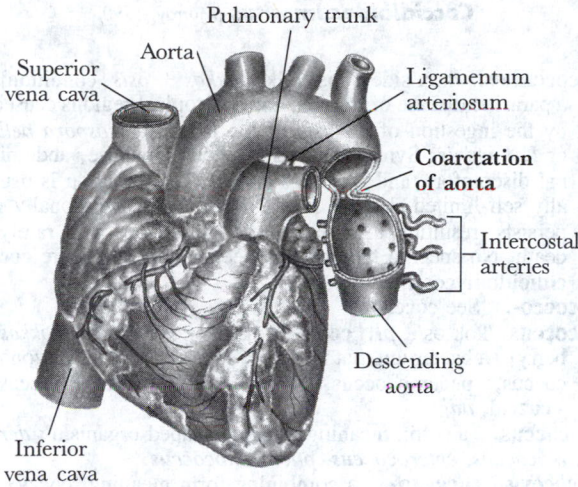

Pulmonary trunk

Aorta

Superior vena cava

Ligamentum arteriosum

Coarctation of aorta

Intercostal arteries

Descending aorta

Inferior vena cava

Coarctation of the aorta *(Canobbio, 1990)*

coarse /kôrs/ [ME, *cors,* common], (in physiology) involving a wide range of movements, such as those associated with tremors and other involuntary movements of the skeletal muscle.

coarse fremitus, a rough, loud, tremulous vibration of the chest wall noted on palpation of the chest during a physical examination as the person inhales and exhales. It is most common in pulmonary conditions characterized by consolidation.

coarse râle [of course (ordinary); Fr, *rale,* rattle], an abnormal breathing sound caused by air moving through an excessive amount of fluid present in an airway, as in pulmonary edema.

coarse tremor [of course (ordinary); L, *tremor,* shaking], a tremor in which the movements are relatively slow and may involve larger muscle groups.

coat [ME *cote*], **1.** a membrane that covers the outside of an organ or part. **2.** one of the layers of a wall of an organ or part, especially a canal or a vessel.

coated tablet [OFr, *cote*; Fr, *tablette*], a solid disc of one or more pharmaceutical agents coated with sugar or a flavoring to mask the taste or by a substance that resists dissolution in the stomach but allows release of the medication in the intestine.

coated tongue [OFr, *cote*; AS, *tunge*], a tongue with a white, yellow, or brown furred surface, representing a possible accumulation of mycelia, bacteria, food debris, or desquamated epithelial cells. There are many possible causes, ranging from a fungal infection to sleeping with the mouth open.

cobalamin /kōbôl′əmin/ [Ger, *kobold,* mine goblin], a generic term for a chemical portion of the vitamin B_{12} group. See also **cyanocobalamin.**

cobalt (Co) /kō′bôlt/ [Ger, *kobold,* mine goblin], a metallic element that occurs in the minerals cobaltite, smaltite, and linnaeite. Its atomic number is 27; its atomic weight is 58.9. Extensive deposits of cobalt minerals are found in Ontario, Canada. Pure cobalt is obtained by reducing the oxide with aluminum or with carbon. It is used in special alloys, such as Alnico. Cobalt is a component of vitamin B_{12}, is found in most common foods, and is readily absorbed by the GI tract. Research has established that this element is common in the human diet, but the precise daily intake requirement is not known, and cobalt deficiency in humans is not known. The administration of cobalt in the form of cobaltous chloride has been successful in some patients with certain types of anemia because of the capacity of cobalt to produce polycythemia. Accidental intoxication by cobaltous chloride, especially in children, may produce cyanosis, coma, and death. Certain amounts of cobalt stimulate the production of erythropoietin, but the exact mechanisms of this process are not completely understood. Large doses of cobalt depress erythrocyte production. It is believed that in stimulating the production of erythropoietin cobalt inhibits enzymes involved in oxidative metabolism and that erythropoietin increases as the result of tissue hypoxia. The only disease for which some experts still advocate the use of cobalt is normochromic, normocytic anemia associated with renal failure. The radioisotope ^{60}Co emits gamma rays and is often used as an encapsulated radiation source in the treatment of cancer.

cobalt 60 (^{60}Co), (in radiotherapy) a radioactive isotope of the silver-white metallic element cobalt with a mass number of 60 and a half-life of 5.2 years. ^{60}Co emits high-energy gamma rays and is the most frequently used radioisotope in radiotherapy. In ^{60}Co machines, the high-energy radioactive source is stored in a position well shielded by lead or uranium.

Coban, a trademark for an elastic pressure wrap applied to reduce edema in an injured finger.

COBOL /kō′bol/, abbreviation for *common business oriented language,* a high-level compiler computer language for programing.

cobra venom solution [L, *colubra,* snake, *venenum,* venom, *solutus,* dissolved], a sterile physiological salt solution containing minute amounts of cobralysin, the hemolytic substance in cobra venom.

coca, a species of South American shrubs, native to Bolivia and Peru and cultivated in Indonesia. The leaves are dried and then chewed for their stimulant effect by some of the people of the region. It is a natural source of cocaine.

cocaine babies /kōkān′/, infants with birth defects caused by exposure to cocaine in utero. Contributing causes may include poor sperm quality of a male cocaine user, poor nutritional habits and/or alcohol or tobacco abuse by the mother while pregnant, and direct effect of the drug itself, which can cross the placental barrier.

cocaine hydrochloride, a white crystalline powder used as a local anesthetic. It was originally derived from coca leaves but can also be prepared synthetically.

■ INDICATIONS: In solution the drug is an effective topical anesthetic commonly used in the examination and treatment of the eye, ear, nose, and throat. The vasoconstrictive action of the drug slows bleeding and limits absorption. Prolonged or frequent use may damage the mucous membranes.

■ CONTRAINDICATIONS: Cocaine is incompatible with all alkaloid precipitants, mercurials, and silver nitrate. Central nervous system overstimulation may result from use with monoamine oxidase inhibitors, amphetamines, or guanethidine. Combination with epinephrine or norepinephrine can lead to cardiac arrhythmias or ventricular fibrillation. Cocaine is not given to patients with severe cardiovascular disease, thyrotoxicosis, hypotension, or hypertension.

■ ADVERSE REACTIONS: Among the most serious adverse reactions are excitement, depression, euphoria, restlessness, tremors, vertigo, nausea, vomiting, hypotension, hypertension, abdominal cramps, exophthalmia, mydriasis, peripheral vascular collapse, tachypnea, tachycardia, chills, fever, coma, or death from respiratory failure.

■ NOTE: Cocaine hydrochloride solution should be freshly made; it deteriorates rapidly on standing and cannot be heat-sterilized. Cocaine is a Schedule II drug under the Controlled Substances Act. A crystalline form of cocaine with the street names of **crack** or **crack cocaine** is smoked.

cocaine hydrochloride poisoning [Sp, *coca, HCl*; L, *potio,* drink], toxic effects of exposure to the colorless crystalline alkaloid derived from coca leaves. Although used as a local analgesic for a century, cocaine is highly toxic with moderate vasoconstrictor activity and serious psychotropic effects. Symptoms include nervous excitement, restlessness, incoherent speech, fever, hypertension, cardiac arrythmias, leading to convulsions, collapse, respiratory arrested, and death. The euphoric effect of cocaine lasts about 30 minutes.

cocarcinogen /kōkär′sənəjən/ [L, *cum,* together with; Gk, *karkinos,* crab, *genein,* to produce], an agent that, alone, does not transform a normal cell into a cancerous state but in concert with another agent can effect the transformation.

cocci-, cocco-, a combining form meaning 'seed or berry; pertaining to a spherical bacterial cell': *coccobacillus, coccogenous, coccoid.*

coccidioidomycosis /koksid′ē·oi′dōmīkō′sis/ [Gk, *kokkos,* berry, *eidos,* form, *mykes,* fungus, *osis,* condition], an infectious fungal disease caused by the inhalation of spores of the bacterium *Coccidioides immitis,* which is carried on windborne dust particles. The disease is endemic in hot, dry regions of the southwestern United States and Central and South America and is an opportunistic disease associated with AIDS. Primary infection is characterized by symptoms resembling those of the common cold or influenza. Secondary infection, occurring after a period of remission and lasting from weeks to years, is marked by low-grade fever, anorexia and weight loss, cyanosis, dyspnea, hemoptysis, focal skin lesions resembling erythema nodosum, and arthritic pain in the bones and joints. The diagnosis is made by learning that the patient was living in or visiting an endemic area and by identifying *C. immitis* in sputum, exudate, or tissue. Treatment usually consists of bed rest and the administration of antibiotics, such as Amphotericin B or fluconazole. Also called **desert fever, desert rheumatism, San Joaquin fever, valleyfever.**

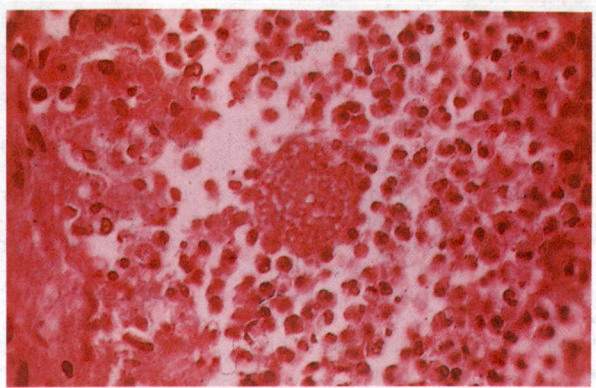

Coccidioides immitus (Murray, 1990)

coccidiosis /kok′sidē·ō′sis/ [Gk, *kokkos* + *osis,* condition], a parasitic disease of tropical and subtropical regions caused by the ingestion of oocysts of the protozoa *Isospora belli* or *I. hominis.* Symptoms include fever, malaise, abdominal discomfort, and watery diarrhea. The infection is usually self-limited, lasting 1 to 2 weeks, but occasionally it persists, resulting in malabsorption syndrome and, rarely, death. No specific therapy has been found. Compare **coccidioidomycosis.**

cocco-. See **cocci-.**

coccus /kok′əs/, *pl.* **cocci** /kok′sī, kok′ī/ [Gk, *kokkos,* berry], a bacterium that is round, spheric, or oval, as gonococcus, pneumococcus, staphylococcus, streptococcus. **–coccal,** *adj.*

-coccus, a suffix meaning a 'berry-shaped organism': *dermococcus, enterococcus, pneumonococcus.*

coccyg-, coccygo-, a combining form meaning 'coccyx': *coccygeal, coccygectomy, coccygodynia.*

coccygeal. See **coccyx.**

coccygeal body /koksid′ē·əl/ [Gk, *kokkyx,* cuckoo; AS, *bodig,* the coccyx.

coccygeal vertebra, one of the four segments of the vertebral column that fuse to form the adult coccyx. They are considered rudimentary vertebrae and have no pedicles, laminae, or spinous processes. Compare **cervical vertebra, lumbar vertebra, sacral vertebra, thoracic vertebra.** See also **coccyx, vertebra.**

coccyges. See **coccyx.**

coccygeus /koksij′ē·əs/ [Gk, *kokkyx,* cuckoo's beak], one of two muscles in the pelvic diaphragm. Stretching across the pelvic cavity like a hammock, it is a triangular sheet of muscle and tendinous fibers, dorsal to the levator ani, arising from the spine of the ischium and from the sacrospinous ligament. It inserts into the coccyx and into the sacrum, it is innervated by branches of the pudendal plexus, which contain fibers from the fourth and the fifth sacral nerves, and it acts to draw the coccyx ventrally, helping to support the pelvic floor. Compare **levator ani.**

coccygodynia /kok′sigōdin′ē·ə/, a pain in the coccygeal area of the body.

coccyx /kok′siks/, *pl.* **coccyges** /koksī′jēz, kok′sijēz/ [Gk, *kokkyx,* cuckoo's beak], the beaklike bone joined to the sacrum by a disk of fibrocartilage at the base of the vertebral column. It is formed by the union of three to five rudimentary vertebrae. The pieces of the coccyx fuse together in men at an earlier period in life than in women. In men and in women, the coccyx becomes fused with the sacrum by the sixth decade of life. The coccyx is freely movable on the sacrum during pregnancy.　**–coccygeal** /koksij'ē·əl/, *adj.*

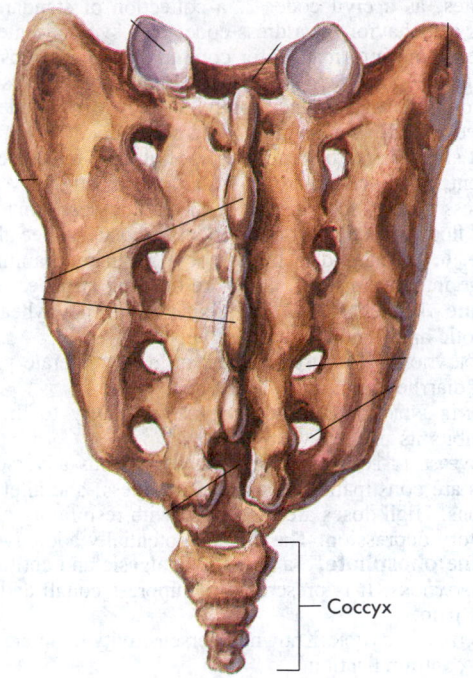

Coccyx—posterior view
(Seeley, 1992/David J Mascaro & Associates)

cochineal /koch'inēl'/ [L, *coccineus,* bright red], a red dye prepared from the dried female insects of the species *Coccus cacti* containing young larvae. During the preparation of the dye the larvae are extracted with an aqueous solution of alum, and the resulting dye has been used in coloring medicines.

cochlea /kok'lē·ə/ [L, snail shell], a conic bony structure of the inner ear, perforated by numerous apertures for passage of the cochlear division of the acoustic nerve. Part of a complex tubular network called the osseous labyrinth, it is a spiral tunnel about 30 mm long with two full and three quarter-turns, resembling a tiny snail shell. **–cochlear,** *adj.*

cochlear canal /kok'lē·ər/, [L *cochlea + canalis* channel], a bony spiral tunnel within the cochlea of the internal ear. It narrows gradually in diameter as it rises to the apex of the cochlea. It contains one opening that communicates with the tympanic cavity, a second that connects with the vestibule, and a third that leads to a tiny canal opening on the inferior surface of the temporal bone.

cochlear duct. See **cochlear canal.**

cochlear implant, an electronic device that is surgically implanted into the cochlea of a deaf individual. A transmitter placed outside the scalp sends signals to a receiver under the scalp, which in turn transmits an electrical code to the auditory nerve. While the implant does not transmit speech clearly, it allows the individual to be aware of sounds that would not otherwise be heard and to use those sounds along with other environmental cues to improve communication.

cochlear nerve [L, *cochlea,* snail shell, *nervus,* nerve], one of the main divisions of the eighth cranial nerve, with fibers that arise in spiral ganglion cells and terminate in the dorsal and ventral cochlear nuclei of the brainstem. Also called **acoustic nerve.**

cochlear toxicity, toxic effects of drugs that may result in hearing disorders, such as sensorineural hearing loss and tinnitus.

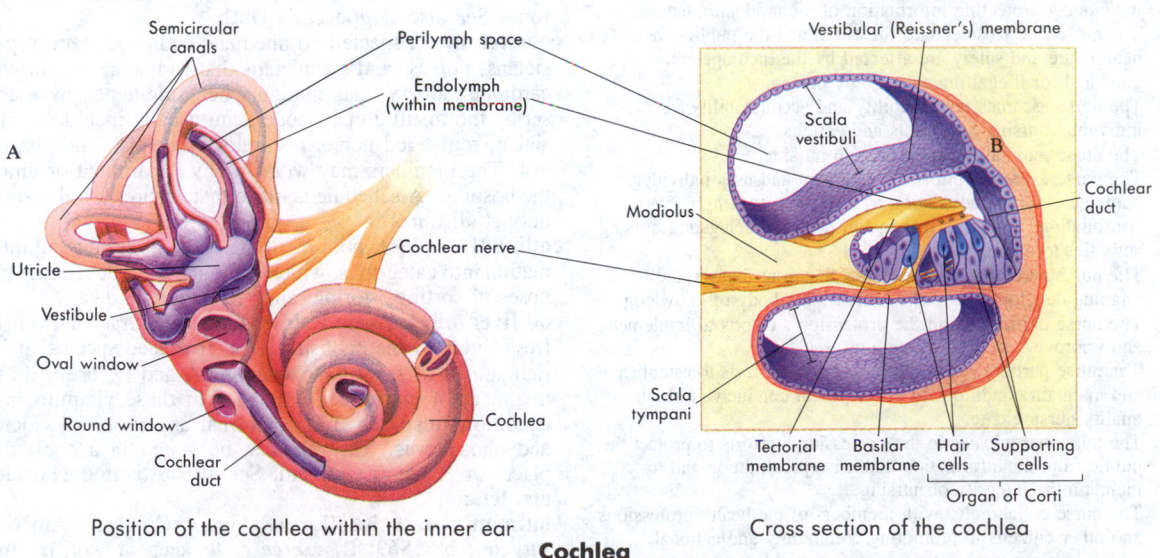

Position of the cochlea within the inner ear　　　Cross section of the cochlea

Cochlea
(Thibodeau, 1993/Rolin Graphics)

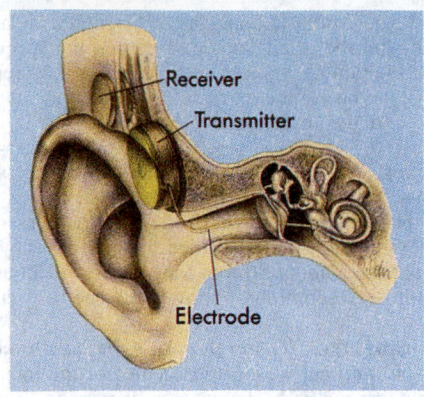

Cochlear implant *(Thibodeau, 1993/Rolin Graphics)*

cochlear window. See **round window.**

cockroach, the common name of members of the Blattidae family of insects that infest homes, workplaces, and other areas inhabited by humans. Cockroaches transmit a number of disease agents, including bacteria, protozoa, and eggs of parasitic worms.

cockscomb papilloma /kok'skōm/ [AS, *cocc, camb;* L, *papilla,* nipple; Gk, *oma,* tumor], a benign, small red lesion that may project from the uterine cervix during pregnancy; it regresses after delivery.

cocktail [AS, *cocc, toegel*], *informal.* an unofficial mixture of drugs, usually in solution, combined to achieve a

Code for nurses

1. The nurse provides services with respect for human dignity and the uniqueness of the client unrestricted by considerations of social or economic status, personal attributes, or the nature of health problems.
2. The nurse safeguards the client's right to privacy by judiciously protecting information of a confidential nature.
3. The nurse acts to safeguard the client and the public when health care and safety are affected by the incompetent, unethical, or illegal practice of any person.
4. The nurse assumes responsibility and accountability for individual nursing judgments and actions.
5. The nurse maintains competence in nursing.
6. The nurse exercises informed judgment and uses individual competence and qualification as criteria in seeking consultation, accepting responsibilities, and delegating nursing activities to others.
7. The nurse participates in activities that contribute to the ongoing development of the profession's body of knowledge.
8. The nurse participates in the profession's efforts to implement and improve standards of nursing.
9. The nurse participates in the profession's efforts to establish and maintain conditions of employment conducive to high quality nursing care.
10. The nurse participates in the profession's efforts to protect the public from misinformation and misrepresentation and to maintain the integrity of nursing.
11. The nurse collaborates with members of the health professions and other citizens in promoting community and national efforts to meet the health needs of the public.

From American Nurses' Association: *Code for nurses with interpretive statements,* Kansas City, MO, 1985, The Association.

specific purpose. See also **Brompton's cocktail.**

cockup splint, a splint used to immobilize the wrist and leave the fingers free.

cocontraction /kō'kəntrak'shən/, the simultaneous contraction of agonist and antagonist muscles around a joint to hold a position. Also called **coinnervation.**

code [L, *caudex,* book], **1.** (in law) a published body of statutes, as a civil code. **2.** a collection of standards and rules of behavior, as a dress code. **3.** a symbolic means of representing information for communication or transfer, as a genetic code. **4.** a system of notation that allows information to be transmitted rapidly, such as Morse code, or in secrecy, such as a cryptographic code. **5.** *informal.* a discreet signal used to summon a special team to resuscitate a patient, as in "code zero, 3 west" announced over a public address system to bring the team to the west wing of the third floor without alarming patients or visitors. See also **nocode. 6.** to enter data by use of a given programing language into a computer. Compare **decode, encode.**

codeine /kō'dēn, kō'dē·in/ [Gk, *kodeia,* poppyhead], a narcotic analgesic and antitussive.

■ INDICATIONS: It is used to treat mild to moderate pain, to treat diarrhea, and as an antitussive.

■ CONTRAINDICATIONS: Known hypersensitivity to this drug prohibits its use.

■ ADVERSE EFFECTS: Among the most serious adverse reactions are constipation, nausea, drowsiness, and allergic reactions. High doses are associated with respiratory and circulatory depression. The drug is potentially addictive.

codeine phosphate, a narcotic analgesic and antitussive.

■ INDICATIONS: It is prescribed to suppress cough and to relieve pain.

■ CONTRAINDICATION: Known hypersensitivity to opiates is the only contraindication.

■ ADVERSE EFFECTS: Among the more serious adverse reactions are depression of the central nervous system, paradoxical excitement, and drug dependence.

code of ethics, a statement encompassing the set of rules by which practitioners of a profession are expected to conform. See also **Hippocratic Oath.**

code team, a specially trained and equipped team of physicians, nurses, and technicians that is available to provide cardiopulmonary resuscitation when summoned by a code set by the institution. A code team usually includes a physician, registered nurse, respiratory therapist, and pharmacist. The members may work in any department or unit of the hospital. A schedule is made that ensures a full team on duty at all times.

coding [L, *caudex,* book], the process of organizing information into categories, which are assigned codes for the purposes of sorting, storing, and retrieving the data.

cod-liver oil, a pale-yellow, fatty oil extracted from the fresh livers of the codfish and other related species. It is a rich source of fat-soluble vitamins A and D, useful in the treatment of nutritional deficiency of those vitamins or of conditions resulting from abnormal absorption of calcium and phosphorus. The oil must be stored in a cool, dark place, or it becomes rancid. See also **osteomalacia, rickets, tetany.**

Codman's exercise [Ernest Amory Codman, American surgeon, b. 1869; L, *exercere,* to keep at work], mild exercises for restoring range of motion and function in the arms after immobilization of the limbs. The patient flexes the trunk over a surface to create a pendulum. The arm then hangs free and can be moved through the motions of the trunk without active contraction of the shoulder muscle.

Codman's tumor. See **chondroblastoma.**

codominant /kōdom′ənənt/ [L, *cum*, together with, *dominari*, to rule], of or pertaining to the equal degree of dominance of two alleles or traits fully expressed in a phenotype, as when a person inherits both the A and B genes of the ABO blood group and has AB type blood. **–codominance,** *n.*

codominant inheritance, the transmission of a trait or condition in which both alleles of a pair are given full expression in a heterozygote, such as in the AB or MNS blood group antigens and the leukocyte antigens.

codon /kō′don/, a unit of three adjacent nucleotides along a DNA or messenger RNA molecule that designates a specific amino acid in the polypeptide chain during protein synthesis. Each codon consists of a specific section of the DNA molecule so that the order of the codons along the molecule determines the sequence of the amino acids in each protein. See also **genetic code.**

coefficient /kō′efish′ənt/ [L, *cum*, together with, *efficere*, to effect], a mathematic relationship between factors that can be used to measure or evaluate a characteristic under specified conditions. Examples include Henry's law, which measures **solubility coefficient;** Graham's law, which calculates **diffusion coefficient;** and the **oxygen-utilization coefficient,** which measures the amount of oxygen in a patient's venous blood in terms of the proportion of oxygen in his or her arterial blood.

coel-, a combining form meaning 'pertaining to the colon': *colalgia, colauxe, colectasia.* See also **cel-.**

-coel, -coele. See **-cele2.**

coelentera. See **coelenteron.**

Coelenterates /sēlen′tɨrā′tēz/, a phylum of marine animals that includes jellyfish, sea anemones, hydroids, and corals.

coelenteron /sēlen′təron/, *pl.* **coelentera** [Gk, *koilos*, hollow, *enteron*, intestine], the digestive cavity of those animals having only two germ layers, such as the hydra and jellyfish. See also **archenteron.**

coelom /sē′ləm/ [Gk, *koilos*, hollow], the body cavity of the developing embryo. It is situated between the layers of mesoderm and in mammals gives rise to the pericardial, pleural, and peritoneal cavities. A kind of coelom is **extraembryonic coelom.** Also spelled **coelome, celom.** Also called **coeloma** (*pl.* **coelomata**), **somatic cavity. –coelomic, celomic,** *adj.*

coelosomy /sē′ləsō′mē/ [Gk, *koilos* + *soma*, body], a congenital anomaly characterized by the protrusion of the viscera from the body cavity.

coenesthesia, coenesthesis, coenogenesis. See **cenesthesia.**

coenogenetic. See **cenogenesis.**

coenzyme /kō·en′zīm/ [L, *cum*, together with, *en*, in, *zyme*, ferment], a nonprotein substance that combines with an apoenzyme to form a complete enzyme or holoenzyme. Coenzymes include some of the vitamins, such as B_1 and B_2, and have smaller molecules than enzymes. Coenzymes are dialyzable and heat-stable and usually dissociate easily from the protein portions of the enzymes with which they combine. See also **acetylcoenzyme A.**

coenzyme A (CoA) [L, *cum, en*, into, *zyme*, ferment], an important metabolite in the citric acid cycle. Although not a true enzyme, it plays a significant role in the transfer of acetyl groups and the metabolism of acids and amino acids.

coffee [Ar, *qahwah*], the dried and roasted ripe seeds of *Coffea arabica, C. liberica,* and *C. robusta* trees that may have originated in Africa but now grow in almost all tropical areas. Coffee contains the alkaloid caffeine and is the basis for a stimulating drink that has been used in treating the common headache, chronic asthma, and narcotic poisoning.

coffee-ground vomitus, dark brown vomitus the color and consistency of coffee grounds, composed of gastric juices and old blood and indicative of slow upper GI bleeding. Compare **hematemesis.**

Cogentin, a trademark for an antiparkinsonian (benztropine mesylate).

cognition /kognish′ən/ [L, *cognoscere*, to know], the mental process characterized by knowing, thinking, learning, and judging. Compare **conation.** *cognitive, adj.*

cognitive /kog′nitiv/, pertaining to the mental processes of comprehension, judgment, memory, and reasoning, as contrasted with emotional and volitional processes.

cognitive development, the developmental process by which an infant becomes an intelligent person, acquiring, with growth, knowledge and the ability to think, learn, reason, and abstract. Jean Piaget demonstrated the orderly sequence of this process from early infancy through childhood. See also **psychosexual development, psychosocial development.**

cognitive dissonance [L, *cognoscere*, to know, *dis*, opposite of, *sonare*, to sound], a state of tension resulting from a discrepancy in a person's emotional and intellectual frame of reference for interpreting and coping with his or her environment. It usually occurs when new information contradicts existing assumptions or knowledge.

cognitive function, an intellectual process by which one becomes aware of, perceives, or comprehends ideas. It involves all aspects of perception, thinking, reasoning, and remembering. Compare **conation.**

cognitive learning, 1. learning that is concerned with acquisition of problem-solving abilities and with intelligence and conscious thought. **2.** a theory that defines learning as behavioral change based on the acquisition of information about the environment.

cognitive psychology, the study of the development of thought, language, and intelligence in infants and children.

cognitive restoration, an intervention technique designed to restore cognitive functioning.

cognitive restructuring, a change in attitudes, values, or beliefs that limit a person's self-expression; it occurs as a result of insight or behavioral achievement.

cognitive structuring, the process of reviewing with a patient the changes that have occurred in the patient's thinking to show a sense of change and a sense of playing an active role in bringing about that change.

cognitive therapy, any of the various methods of treating mental and emotional disorders that help a person change attitudes, perceptions, and patterns of thinking. Therapeutic approaches include behavior therapy, existential therapy, Gestalt therapy, and transactional analysis.

cogwheel rigidity [ME, *cugge*, tooth on a gear; AS, *hweol*; L, *rigiditas*, unbending], an abnormal rigor in muscle tissue, characterized by jerky movements when the muscle is passively stretched. Some authorities believe cogwheel rigidity masks a muscular tremor that is not evident until the affected muscle is manipulated. The condition is often found in cases of Parkinson's disease.

cohabitate /kōhab'itāt/, to live together in a heterosexual relationship when not married.

cohere /kōhir'/ [L, *cohaerere*, to cling together], to stick together, as similar molecules of a common substance.

coherence /kōhir'əns/, 1. the property of sticking together, as the molecules within a common substance. 2. (in psychology) the logical pattern of expression and thought evident in the speech of a normal, stable individual. –**coherent**, *adj*.

cohesiveness /kōhē'sivnəs/ [L, *cohaerere*, to cling together], 1. (in psychiatry) a force that attracts members to a group and causes them to remain in the group. 2. (in dentistry) a property of annealed pure gold that allows it to be used as a filling material.

cohesive termini /kōhē'siv/, (in molecular genetics) the complementary single-stranded ends projecting from a double-stranded DNA segment that can be joined to introduced fragments. Also called **sticky ends**.

COHN, abbreviation for *Certified Occupational Health Nurse*.

cohort /kō'hôrt/ [L, *cohortem*, large group], (in statistics) a collection or sampling of individuals who share a common characteristic, such as members of the same age or the same sex.

cohort study, (in research) a study concerning a specific subpopulation, such as the children born between December and May in 1975 and the children born in the same months in 1955. See also **prospective study**.

coil. See **intrauterine device**.

coiled tubular gland [L, *colligere*, to gather together; *tubulus*, small tube; *glans*, acorn], one of the many multicellular glands that contain a coiled, tube-shaped secretory portion, such as the sweat glands.

coil-spring contraceptive diaphragm, a kind of contraceptive diaphragm in which the flexible metal spring that forms the rim is a coiled, circular spring. The rubber dome of the diaphragm is approximately 3.8 cm deep, and the diameter of the rubber-covered rim is from 5.5 to 10 cm. Ten sizes, in increments of 0.5 cm, allow the clinician to fit the diaphragm to the individual woman. This kind of diaphragm is prescribed for a woman whose vaginal musculature offers good support, whose uterus is not acutely retroflexed or anteflexed, and whose vagina, neither very long nor very short, has a deeper than usual arch behind the symphysis pubis.

coincidence counting /kō·in'sidəns/ [L, *coincidere*, to occur together], (in radiotherapy) the detection of two photons that arrive at separate counters simultaneously as the result of annihilation of a positron (created during a radioactive decay) and an electron. As an imaging technique, the coincidence counting of two photons greatly reduces the significance of any background radiation.

coinnervation. See **cocontraction**.

coitus /kō'itəs/ [L, *coire*, to come together], the sexual union of two people of opposite sex in which the penis is introduced into the vagina, typically resulting in mutual excitation and usually orgasm. Also called **coition, copulation, sexual intercourse.** –**coital**, *adj*.

coitus interruptus. See **withdrawal method**.

col-, a combining form meaning 'pertaining to the colon': *colalgia, colauxe, colectasia*. See also **co-**.

Colace, a trademark for a stool softener (docusate sodium sulfosuccinate).

colation /kōlā'shən/ [L, *colare*, to strain], the act of filtering or straining, as urine is often strained for medical examination.

COL bed. See **CircOlectric bed**.

ColBENEMID, a trademark for an antigout medication (probenecid-colchicine).

colchicine /kol'chəsēn/ [Gk, *kolchikon*], a gout suppressant.

■ INDICATIONS: It is prescribed in the treatment of acute gout and prophylaxis of recurrent gouty arthritis.

■ CONTRAINDICATIONS: Ulcer, ulcerative colitis, or known hypersensitivity to this drug prohibits its use. The drug is highly toxic and is not given to elderly, debilitated patients or to those people who have chronic renal, hepatic, cardiovascular, or GI disease.

■ ADVERSE EFFECTS: Among the most serious adverse reactions are severe GI distress including diarrhea with blood, bone marrow depression, peripheral neuritis, liver dysfunction, and alopecia.

cold [AS, *kald*], 1. the absence of heat. 2. also called **common cold.** a contagious viral infection of the upper respiratory tract, usually caused by a strain of rhinovirus. It is characterized by rhinitis, tearing, low-grade fever, and malaise and is treated symptomatically with rest, mild analgesia, decongestants, and an increased intake of fluids.

cold abscess, a site of infection that does not show common signs of heat, redness, and swelling.

cold agglutinin, a nonspecific antibody, found on the surface of red blood cells in certain diseases, that may cause clumping of the cells at temperatures below 4° C and may cause hemolysis. The phenomenon does not occur at body temperature. Mycoplasma pneumonia, infectious mononucleosis, and many lymphoproliferative disorders are associated with cold agglutinins.

cold agglutinin disease [AS, *kald*; L, *agglutinare*, to glue, *dis*, without; Fr, *aise*, ease], a disorder characterized by circulating antibodies that can agglutinate red cells at less than normal body temperatures. They occur in the sera of patients with atypical pneumonia and blood diseases, particularly hemolytic anemia. The disease also tends to affect elderly patients.

cold bath, a bath in which the water temperature is approximately 50° F (10° C) to 65° F (18° C), used primarily to reduce body temperature.

cold-blooded, unable to regulate body heat, as fishes, reptiles, and amphibians that have internal temperatures that are close to the temperatures of the environments in which they live. Also called **poikilothermic.** Compare **warm-blooded**.

cold cautery. See **cryocautery**.

cold caloric irrigation, a procedure for testing the integrity of brainstem function. It is carried out by irrigating the external auditory canal of the patient with a cold saline solution while the head is flexed at approximately 30 degrees, after checking the patency of the ear canal. The stimulus results in jerky but regular eye movements in a normal patient. Absence of the reaction may be a sign of a lesion at the pontine level of the brainstem.

cold compress [AS, *kald*; L, *comprimere*, to press together], a pad of damp, thickly folded, soft absorbent cloth, dipped in cold water, wrung out, and applied to a body part for the relief of pain or reduction of inflammation.

cold environment, a human environment arbitrarily designated as one in which the temperature is below 10° C (50° F). Nearly two thirds of the world population, including most of North America, Europe, and Asia north of the Indian subcontinent, lives in a naturally cold environment for at least a part of each year. The human body generally begins to experience some functional impairment when unprotected in temperatures below 15° C (59° F). The hands and fingers lose sensitivity, and the risk of errors and accidents increases. The body's hemostatic mechanism reacts with vasoconstriction, reducing heat loss to the environment but cooling the skin with a resultant chilling of the extremities. When vasoconstriction no longer eases the thermal strain between the skin and the environment, muscular hypertonus and shivering become mechanisms for maintaining body temperature.

cold hemoglobinuria. See **hemoglobinuria.**

cold injury, any of several abnormal and often serious physical conditions caused by exposure to cold temperatures. See also **chilblain, frostbite, hypothermia, immersion foot.**

cold pack [AS, *kald*; ME, *pakke*], a method, now generally obsolete, of lowering body temperature by wrapping the patient in a blanket or sheet that has been dipped in cold water and wrung out.

cold-pressor test, a test for the tendency to develop essential hypertension. One hand of the individual is immersed in ice water for about 60 seconds. An excessive rise in the blood pressure or an unusual delay in the return of normal blood pressure when the hand is removed from the water is believed to indicate that the individual is at risk for hypertension.

cold-sensitive mutation, a genetic alteration resulting in a gene that functions at a high temperature and not at a low temperature.

cold sore. See **herpes simplex (HSV-I).**

cold stress. See **hypothermia.**

cold urticaria [AS, *kald*; L, *urtica,* nettle], wheals caused by exposure to cold temperatures.

cold-wet-sheet pack, a form of somatic therapy for agitated patients. The patient is swathed in cold, wet sheets, which are then warmed by body heat. The warmth and immobilization are reported to be soothing to very agitated patients.

colectomy /kəlek′təmē/ [Gk, *kolon,* colon, *ektome,* excision], surgical excision of part or all of the colon, performed to treat cancer of the colon or severe chronic ulcerative colitis. For several days before surgery, a low-residue diet is prescribed. Antibiotics and cleansing enemas are given to reduce the number of bacteria in the bowel. Parenteral fluids and electrolytes are given, and a nasointestinal tube is passed. The nurse gives postoperative care as for any abdominal surgery. The nasointestinal tube is connected to suction and remains in place until bowel sounds are heard. See **abdominal surgery.**

Colestid, a trademark for an antihyperlipoproteinemic (colestipol hydrochloride).

colestipol hydrochloride /kōles′tipol/, an antihyperlipoproteinemic that acts by sequestering bile acids in the intestine, thus reducing plasma levels of cholesterol.

■ INDICATIONS: It is prescribed in the treatment of hypercholesterolemia and xanthoma.

■ CONTRAINDICATIONS: Biliary obstruction or known hypersensitivity to this drug prohibits its use.

■ ADVERSE EFFECTS: Among the more serious adverse reactions are skin rash, fecal impaction, and a deficiency of vitamins A, D, and K.

colic /kol′ik/ [Gk, *kolikos,* colon pain], **1.** sharp visceral pain resulting from torsion, obstruction, or smooth muscle spasm of a hollow or tubular organ, such as a ureter or the intestines. Kinds of colic include **biliary colic, infantile colic,** and **renal colic. 2.** of or pertaining to the colon. – **colicky,** *adj.*

colicinogen /kol′isin′əjən/ [(E.) *coli* + L, *caedere,* to kill; Gk, *genein,* to produce], an episome in some strains of *Escherichia coli* that induces secretion of a colicin, a protein lethal to other strains of the bacterium. Specific colicins attach to specific receptors on the cell membrane and impair the synthesis of macromolecules or the production of energy. Also called **colicinogenic factor.**

colicky. See **colic.**

coliform /kol′ifôrm/ [(E.) *coli* + L, *forma,* form], **1.** of or pertaining to the colon-acrogenes group, or the *Escherichia coli* species of microorganisms, constituting most of the intestinal flora in humans and other animals. **2.** having the characteristic of a sieve or cribriform structure, such as some of the porous bones of the skull.

colistimethate sodium /kō′listim′əthāt/, an antibacterial. Also called **colistin sulfomethate sodium.**

■ INDICATIONS: It is prescribed in the treatment of GI infections caused by certain gram-negative microorganisms and as a topical medication.

■ CONTRAINDICATIONS: Known hypersensitivity to this drug or to polymyxin B prohibits its use.

■ ADVERSE EFFECTS: Among the more serious adverse reactions are nephrotoxicity and neurotoxicity, including neuromuscular blockade.

colistin sulfate /kōlis′tin/, an antibacterial.

■ INDICATIONS: It is prescribed topically in the treatment of infections of the outer ear and systemically for serious gram-negative infections and for the treatment of gastroenteritis caused by *Escherichia coli* infections.

■ CONTRAINDICATION: Known hypersensitivity to this drug prohibits its use.

■ ADVERSE EFFECTS: Among the more serious systemic reactions are respiratory arrest, renal toxicity, and neuromuscular blockade.

colistin sulfomethate sodium. See **colistimethate sodium.**

colitis /kōlī′tis/, an inflammatory condition of the large intestine. Inflammatory bowel disease is characterized by severe diarrhea, bleeding, and ulceration of the mucosa of the intestine. Weight loss and pain are significant. Steroids, fluids, electrolytes, antibiotics, and careful attention to diet are the usual modes of therapy. Most of the diseases of this group are of unknown origin. Kinds of inflammatory bowel disease include **Crohn's disease** and **ulcerative colitis.** – **colitic,** *adj.*

collaborative power structure /kəlab′ərətiv′/, an arrangement whereby adult family members of a functional family make major decisions and are in agreement about power distribution.

collagen /kol′əjən/ [Gk, *kolla,* glue, *genein,* to produce], a protein consisting of bundles of tiny reticular fibrils, which combine to form the white glistening inelastic fibers of the tendons, the ligaments, and the fascia. – **collagenous** /kəlaj′ənəs/, *adj.*

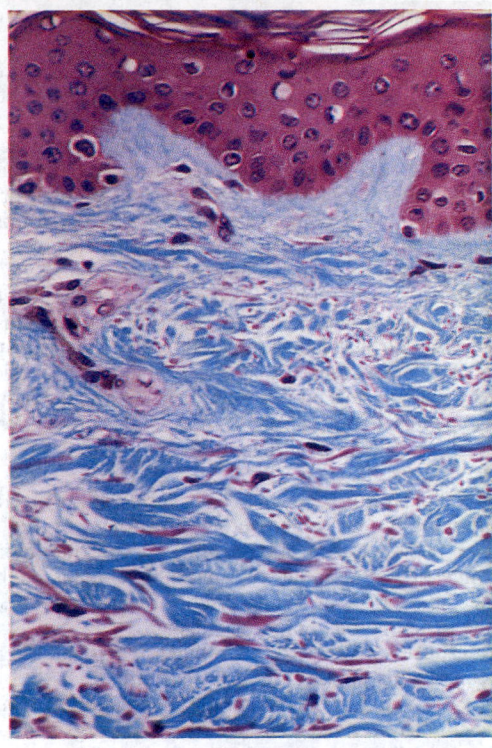

Collagen (du Vivier, 1993)

collagenase ointment /kəlaj′ənās/, a medication used in the treatment of decubitus ulcers, burns, and other epidermal lesions. It is an enzyme preparation derived from the fermentation of *Clostridium histolyticum.*

collagen disease, an abnormal condition characterized by extensive disruption of the connective tissue, such as inflammation and fibrinoid degeneration. Some collagen diseases are polyarteritis nodosa, systemic lupus erythematosus, rheumatic fever, rheumatoid arthritis. Such disorders may also cause coronary problems, which are often controlled with glucocorticoids.

collagenoblast /kəlaj′ənōblast′/ [Gk, *kolla, genein* + *blastos,* germ], a cell that differentiates from a fibroblast and functions in the formation of collagen. It can also transform into cartilage and bone tissue by metaplasia.

collagenous. See **collagen.**

collagenous fiber /kəlaj′ənəs/, any one of the tough, white fibers that constitute much of the intercellular substance and the connective tissue of the body. Collagenous fibers contain collagen; they are often arranged in bundles that strengthen the tissues in which they are imbedded.

collagen vascular disease, any of a group of acquired disorders that have in common diffuse immunologic and inflammatory changes in small blood vessels and connective tissue. The cause of most of these diseases is unknown. Hereditary factors and deficiencies, environmental antigens, infections, allergies, and antigen-antibody complexes in various combinations are probably involved. Common features of most of these entities include arthritis, skin lesions, iritis and episcleritis, pericarditis, pleuritis, subcutaneous nodules, myocarditis, vasculitis, and nephritis. Often associated are also Coombs test-positive hemolytic anemia, thrombocytopenia, leukopenia, B and T cell abnormalities, antinuclear antibodies, cryoglobulins, rheumatoid factors, false-positive serologic tests for syphilis, alterations in serum complement, and immunologic abnormalities. The diseases usually included in this category are mixed connective tissue disease, necrotizing vasculitis, and other vasculopathies, polymyositis, relapsing polychondritis, rheumatic fever, rheumatoid arthritis, scleroderma, and systemic lupus erythematosus. Also called **connective tissue disease.**

collapse /kəlaps′/ [L, *collabi,* to fall], **1.** *nontechnical.* a state of extreme depression or a condition of complete exhaustion because of physical or psychosomatic problems. **2.** an abnormal condition characterized by shock. **3.** the abnormal sagging of an organ or the obliteration of its cavity.

collapse of the lung [L, *collabi,* to fall together; AS, *lungen*], a reduction in the volume of the lung and the amount of air in it as a result of increased intrapleural pressure from accumulating air or fluid in the pleural cavity or because of a loss of internal pressure and elastic recoil of the lung. See also **atelectasis, hemothorax, pneumothorax.**

collar [L *collum* neck], any structure that encircles another, usually around its neck, such as the periosteal bone collars that form around the diaphyses of young bones.

collarbone. See **clavicle.**

collateral /kōlat′ərəl/ [L, *cum,* together with, *lateralis,* side], **1.** secondary or accessory. **2.** (in anatomy) a small branch, such as any one of the arterioles or venules in the body.

collateral circulation [L, *cum, latus,* side, *circulare,* to go around], a redundant blood pathway developed through enlargement of secondary vessels following obstruction of a main channel.

collateral fissure, a fissure separating the subcalcarine and the subcollateral gyri of the cerebral hemisphere.

collateral pulp canal, (in dentistry) a branch of the pulp canal that emerges from the root at a place other than the apex. Also called **branching canal.** Compare **accessory root canal.**

collateral ventilation, the ventilation of pulmonary air spaces (alveoli) through indirect pathways, such as Kohn's pores in alveolar septa or anastomosing bronchioles.

collateral vessel [L, *cum, latus,* side + *vascellum,* small vase], a branch of an artery or vein used as an accessory to the blood vessel from which it arose.

collecting tubule [L, *colligere,* to gather; *tubulus,* small tube], any one of the many relatively large straight tubules of the kidney that funnel urine into the renal pelvis. The collecting tubules drain the urine from the distal convoluted tubules in the renal cortex and descend into the renal medulla before connecting with each other at various intervals along the path to the renal pelvis. The collecting tubules play an important role in maintaining the fluid balance of the body by allowing water to osmose through their membranes into the interstitial fluid in the renal medulla. Antidiuretic hormone in the blood makes the collecting tubules permeable to water. If no antidiuretic hormone is present in the blood, membranes of the collecting tubules are practically impermeable to water. See **Bowman's capsule, kidney.**

collective bargaining /kəlek′tiv/, the use of collective action by employees in negotiating working conditions and economic issues with their employer.

collective hysteria. See **major hysteria.**

collective unconscious [L, *colligere,* to gather; AS, *un,* not; L, *conscious,* aware], (in analytic psychology) that portion of the unconscious common to all mankind. Also called **racial unconscious.** See also **analytic psychology.**

collector, (in medicine) a device with various modifications, used for collecting secretions from the bronchi and esophagus for bacteriologic and cytologic examination.

college [L, *collegium,* society], **1.** an organization of individuals with common professional training and interests, as the American College of Nurse-Midwives, the American College of Cardiology, or the American College of Surgeons. **2.** an institution of higher learning.

College of American Pathologists (CAP), a national professional organization of physicians who specialize in pathology.

Colles' fascia /kol′ēz/ [Abraham Colles, Irish surgeon, b. 1773; L, band], the deep layer of the subcutaneous fascia of the perineum, constituting a distinctive structure in the urogenital region of the body. It is a strong, smooth sheet of tissue containing elastic fibers that give it a characteristic yellow tint. Ventrally, it is continuous with the deep layer of the subcutaneous abdominal fascia and fills a groove between the scrotum and the thigh or between the labium and the thigh; medially, it joins the superficial layer of the subcutaneous perineal fascia to form the dartos tunic of the scrotum or to form the thick fascial sheath of the labium; later ally, it firmly adheres to the ischiopubic ramus; and dorsally, it dips toward the ischiorectal fossa and attaches firmly to deep perineal fascia. In the anal region of the perineum, Colles' fascia adheres to both the superficial layer and the deep layer of the subcutaneous fascia.

Colles' fracture [Abraham Colles], a fracture of the radius at the epiphysis within 1 inch of the joint of the wrist, easily recognized by the dorsal and lateral position of the hand that it causes.

colligative /kol′igā′tiv/ [L, *colligere,* to gather], (in physical chemistry) of or pertaining to those properties of matter that depend on the concentration of particles, such as molecules and ions, rather than the chemical properties of any substance. One such colligative property is the pressure of a specific volume of gas.

collimator /kol′imā′tər/ [L, *collinare,* to bring into alignment], a device for limiting particles of radiation to parallel paths, used to restrict the beam of a radiotherapy machine to a specified area.

colliquation /kol′ikwā′shən/ [L, *cum,* together with, *liquifacere,* to make liquid], the degeneration of a tissue of the body to a liquid state, usually associated with necrotic tissue.

colliquative /kol′ikwā′tiv/, characterized by the profuse discharge of fluid, as in suppurating wounds and structures of the body that are infected.

collision tumor /kəlizh′ən/ [L, *cum,* together with, *laedere,* to strike], a tumor formed as two separate growths, developing close to each other, join. See also **carcinoma.**

collodion /kəlō′dē·ən/ [Gk, *kolla,* glue, *eidos,* form], a clear or a slightly opaque, highly inflammable liquid composed of pyroxylin, ether, and alcohol. It dries to a strong, transparent film that is used as a surgical dressing.

collodion baby, an infant whose skin at birth is covered with a scaly, parchmentlike membrane. See also **harlequin fetus, lamellar exfoliation of the newborn.**

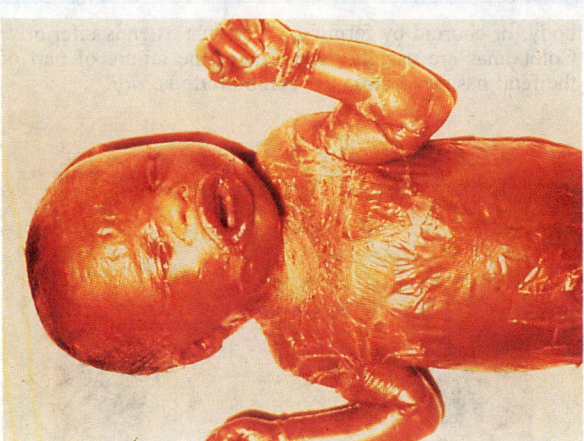

Collodion baby (*Zitelli, 1992*)

colloid /kol′oid/ [Gk, *kolla,* glue, *eidos,* form], a state or division of matter in which large molecules or aggregates of molecules that do not precipitate, and that measure between 1 and 100 nm, are dispersed in another medium. In a suspension colloid the particles are insoluble and the medium may be solid, liquid, or gas. In an emulsion colloid the particles are usually water, and the medium is any of several complex hydrophilic, organic substances that become evenly dispersed among the particles of water. Compare **solution, suspension.**

colloidal solution /koloi′dəl/ [Gk, *kolla,* glue + *eidos,* form; L, *solutus,* dissolved], a solution in which small particles, such as large polymeric molecules, are homogenously dispersed through a liquid medium. See also **colloid.**

colloidal sulfur, a form of very finely divided sulfur that is used in the treatment of acne and other skin disorders.

colloid bath, a bath taken in water that contains such substances as bran, gelatin, and starch, used to relieve irritation and inflammation. See also **emollient bath.**

colloid carcinoma, a former term for mucinous carcinoma.

colloid chemistry, the science dealing with the composition and nature of chemical colloids.

colloid cyst [Gk, *kolla,* glue, *eidos,* form, *kystis,* bag], **1.** a thyroid gland follicle distended with thyroid secretion. **2.** a cyst in the third ventricle, leading to hydrocephalus.

colloid goiter, a greatly enlarged, soft thyroid gland in which the follicles are distended with colloid.

colloid osmotic pressure, an abnormal condition of the kidney caused by the pressure of concentrations of large particles, such as protein molecules, that will pass through a membrane. Also called **oncotic pressure.**

colloid suspension [Gk, *kolla,* glue, *eidos,* form; L, *suspendere,* to hang], a system of solids dispersed in a liquid medium, with particles generally smaller than 100 nm.

collyrium /kolir′ē·əm/, an ophthalmic liquid containing medications to be instilled into the eye.

colo-, colon-, colonic- a combining form meaning 'pertaining to the colon': *colocolic, colodyspepsia, cololysis.*

coloboma /kol′əbō′mə/, *pl.* **colobomas, colobomata** [Gk *koloboma* defect], a congenital or pathologic defect in the ocular tissue of the body, usually affecting the iris, ciliary body, or choroid by forming a cleft that extends inferiorly. Colobomas are usually the result of the failure of part of the fetal fissure to close. **—colobomatous,** *adj.*

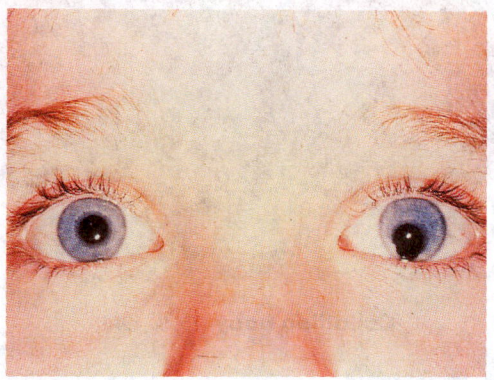

Coloboma (*Zitelli, 1992*)

-coloboma, a suffix meaning the 'absence or defect of an ocular tissue affecting function, especially of the iris': *blepharocoloboma, iridocoloboma, pseudocoloboma.*

coloenteritis. See **enterocolitis.**

colon /kō'lən/ [Gk, *kolon*], the portion of the large intestine extending from the cecum to the rectum. It has four segments: ascending colon, transverse colon, descending colon, and sigmoid colon. **—colonic** /kəlon'ik/, *adj.*

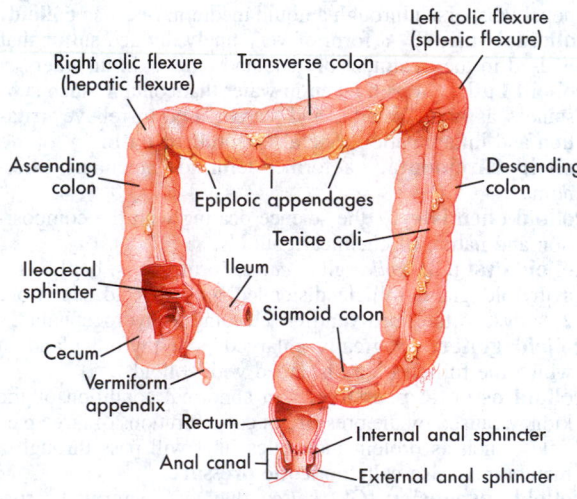

Colon (*Seeley, 1992*)

colon-. See **colo-.**

-colon, a suffix meaning the 'part of the large intestine between the cecum and rectum': *cecocolon, megacolon, paracolon.*

colonic. See **colon.**

-colonic /kolon'ik/, a suffix meaning 'relating to the colon': *pericolonic, rectocolonic, vesicocolonic.*

colonic fistula [Gk, *kolon*; L, pipe], an abnormal passage from the colon to the surface of the body or an internal organ or structure. In regional enteritis, chronic inflammation may lead to the formation of a fistula between two adjacent loops of bowel. An external opening from the colon to the surface of the abdomen may be created surgically after the removal of a malignant or severely ulcerated segment of the bowel. See also **colostomy.**

colonic irrigation, a procedure for washing the inner wall of the colon by filling it with water, then draining it. It is not considered an enema, but rather a technique for removing any material that may be present high in the colon.

colonization /kol'ənīzā'shən/, the presence and multiplication of microorganisms without tissue invasion or damage.

colonoscope /kō'lənōskōp'/ [Gk, *kolon, skopein,* to watch], a long instrument with a light and lens that permits examination of the interior of the colon.

colonoscopy /kō'lənos'kəpē/, the examination of the mucosal lining of the colon using a colonoscope, an elongated endoscope.

colon stasis. See **atonia constipation.**

colony /kol'ənē/ [L, *colonia*], **1.** (in bacteriology) a mass of microorganisms in a culture that originates from a single cell. Some kinds of colonies, according to different configurations, are smooth colonies, rough colonies, and dwarf colonies. **2.** (in cell biology) a mass of cells in a culture or in certain experimental tissues, such as a spleen colony.

colony counter, a device used for counting colonies of bacteria growing in a culture and usually consisting of an illuminated, transparent plate divided into sections of known area. Petri dishes containing colonies of bacteria are placed over the plate, and the colonies are counted according to the number within the areas viewed.

coloproctitis /kō'ləproktī'tis/, an inflammation of both the colon and rectum. Also called **colorectitis, rectocolitis.**

coloptosis /kō'lopto'sis/ [Gk, *kolon* + *ptosis,* fall], the prolapse or downward displacement of the colon.

-color, a combining form meaning 'hue or hues': *cuticolor, tricolor, versicolor.*

Colorado tick fever, a relatively mild, self-limited arbovirus infection transmitted to humans by the bite of a tick. It is most prevalent in the spring and summer months throughout the Rocky Mountains, particularly in Colorado. Symptoms, occurring in two phases separated by a period of remission, include chills, fever, headache, pain in the eyes, legs, and back, and sensitivity to light. Treatment is supportive; analgesics can be given for headache and other pains. Also called **American mountain fever, mountain fever, mountain tick fever.** Compare **Rocky Mountain spotted fever.**

color blindness [L, color; AS *blint*], an abnormal condition characterized by an inability to clearly distinguish colors of the spectrum. In most cases, it is not a blindness but a weakness in perceiving colors distinctly. There are two forms of color blindness. **Daltonism,** the most common form, is characterized by an inability to distinguish reds from greens. It is an inherited, sex-linked disorder. **Total color blindness, or achromatic vision,** is characterized by an inability to perceive any color at all. Only white, gray, and black are seen. It may be the result of a defect in or the absence of the cones in the retina.

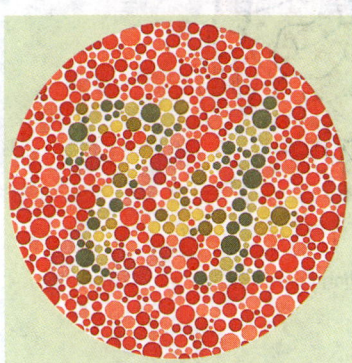

Color blindness chart
(Seeley, 1992/S Ishihara, Tokyo, Japan; Courtesy Washington University Department of Ophthalmology)

color dysnomia /disnō′mē·ə/ [L, color; Gk *dys,* difficult, *onoma,* name],   an inability to name colors despite an ability to match and distinguish them. It may be caused by expressive dysphasis.

colorectal cancer /kō′lərek′təl/ [Gk, *kolon,* colon; L, *rectus* straight],   a malignant neoplastic disease of the large intestine, characterized by a change in bowel habits and the passing of blood (melena). Malignant tumors of the large bowel usually occur after the age of 50, are slightly more frequent in women than in men, and are almost as common as lung cancer in the United States. The high incidence of colorectal cancer in the western world, as contrasted with the low incidence in Japan and rural Africa, suggests that a diet high in refined carbohydrates and beef and low in roughage may be a causative factor. The risk of large bowel cancer is increased in chronic ulcerative colitis, in diverticulosis, in villous adenomas, and especially in familial polyposis of the colon. People who have inhaled asbestos fibers or who have been irradiated are more likely than others to develop colorectal cancer. In the vermiform appendix, carcinoid is the most common tumor. Most lesions of the large bowel are adenocarcinomas; one half arise in the rectum, one fifth in the sigmoid colon, approximately one sixth in the cecum and ascending colon, and the rest in other sites. Rectal tumors may cause pain, bleeding, and a feeling of incomplete evacuation; they may metastasize slowly through lymphatic channels and veins, and occasionally prolapse through the anus. Typical napkin ring tumors in the sigmoid and descending colon constrict the intestinal lumen, causing partial obstruction and the production of flat or pencil-shaped stools. Malignant lesions in the ascending colon are usually large growths that may be palpable on physical examination; they generally cause severe anemia, nausea, and alternating constipation and diarrhea. The diagnosis of colorectal cancer is based on digital rectal examination, testing for blood in the stool, proctosigmoidoscopic examination of the sigmoid, and x-ray studies of the GI tract

after a barium enema. Suspicious polyps may be removed for histologic study, often through a sigmoidoscope or colonoscope or by a laparotomy. Surgical treatment of colorectal cancer may involve a wide resection of the lesion, the surrounding colon, and the attached tissues, with an end-to-end anastomosis of the remaining intestinal segments whenever possible. Tumors of the lower two thirds of the rectum usually require removal of the entire rectum by abdominoperineal resection and the creation of a permanent colostomy. Transanal electric coagulation is currently being studied and tried in the treatment of certain rectal cancers. Irradiation may be administered preoperatively and postoperatively as palliative therapy for inoperable tumors. Chemotherapy with 5-fluorouracil infused intraluminally in the bowel at surgery and intravenously after surgery may be used as adjunctive treatment.

colorectitis.   See **coloproctitis.**

colorimetry /kol′ərim′ətrē/,   **1.** measurement of the intensity of color in a fluid or substance. See also **spectrophotometry. 2.** measurement of color in the blood by use of a colorimeter to determine hemoglobin concentration. The technique is useful only for gross screening purposes, because it is not exact and interpretation is subjective.   **—colorimetric,** *adj.*

color index (C.I.),   the ratio between the concentration of hemoglobin and the number of red blood cells in any given sample of blood. The color index is computed by dividing the concentration of hemoglobin, expressed as a percentage of normal concentration, by the approximate number of red blood cells, expressed as a percentage of a normal concentration of 5 million red cells per cubic millimeter. The average color index is about 0.85. Compare *Colour Index.*

color vision,   a recognition of color as the result of changes in the pigments of the cones in the retina that react to varying intensities of red, green, and blue light. The exact mechanisms of color vision are not completely understood, but some experts believe they depend on three specialized types of cones, each type responding to red, green, or blue light. Some retinal cones respond to the entire visual spectrum. See also **color blindness.**

colosigmoidoscopy /kō′ləsig′moidos′kəpē/ [Gk, *kolon* + *sigma,* S-shaped, *eidos,* form, *skopein,* to look],   the direct examination of the sigmoid portion of the colon with a sigmoidscope.

colostomate /kəlos′təmāt/ [Gk, *kolon* + *stoma,* mouth; L, *atum,* one acted upon],   a person who has undergone a colostomy.

colostomy /kəlos′təmē/ [Gk, *kolon* + *stoma,* mouth],   surgical creation of an artificial anus on the abdominal wall by incising the colon and bringing it out to the surface, performed for cancer of the colon and benign obstructive tumors, and severe abdominal wounds. A colostomy may be single-barreled, with one opening, or double-barreled, with distal and proximal loops open onto the abdomen. The latter is performed when the lower bowel is completely blocked or in paraplegia to simplify daily management. A temporary colostomy may be done to divert feces, after surgery, as in the repair of Hirschsprung's disease, from an inflamed area; it is repaired when the colon has healed or the inflammation subsides. Preoperative nursing care focuses on teaching the patient what to expect after surgery. A high-calorie, low-residue diet is given; an antibiotic, usu-

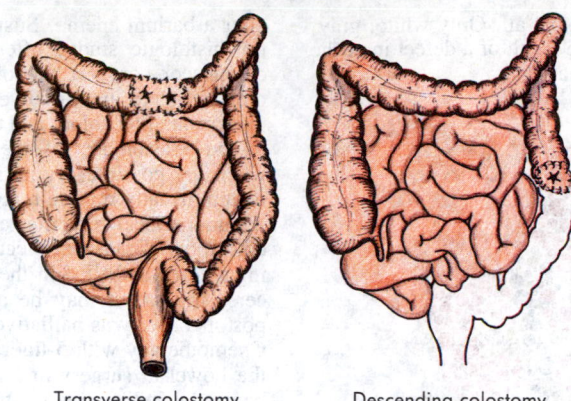

Transverse colostomy   Descending colostomy

Colostomies *(Potter, 1993)*

ally neomycin, is prescribed to reduce the bacterial count in the bowel, and enemas are given until returns are clear. Immediate postoperative care is the same as for abdominal surgery. The color of the stoma is checked: a dark blue-black color (rather than bright red) indicates a circulation block, and the surgeon is notified. Saline irrigations are begun on the fourth or fifth day. A type of colostomy is **loop colostomy.** Compare **enterostomy.**

colostomy irrigation, a procedure used by colostomates to clear the bowel of fecal matter and to help establish an evacuation schedule.

■ METHOD: Daily irrigation may be ordered beginning 7 to 10 days after the operation, and the patient is involved in assisting in the procedure as soon as possible. In preparation for self-care, the technique is explained in a step-by-step manner and irrigation is carried out with the equipment the patient will use at home. In the hospital the procedure is performed as the patient sits in bed in a semi- or high-Fowler's position or on a commode, if ambulatory; at home the individual will probably find a toilet more convenient. A catheter, lubricated with petroleum jelly, is gently inserted in the stoma to a depth of about 3 inches; the catheter tip is advanced only as far as it will go easily and is never forced. If it is not accepted, the stoma is usually dilated by gently inserting and rotating a gloved, lubricated finger approximating the size of the opening. An irrigating bag containing 500 to 1000 ml of warm solution is held 12 to 18 inches above the stoma, and the fluid is allowed to flow slowly into the colon. If the patient complains of cramps, the catheter is clamped for a few minutes before the flow is resumed. The fluid is retained for several minutes and then drained through outlet tubing into a basin or commode. From 30 to 45 minutes is allowed for draining; if the return is slow, the patient is asked to lean forward or move from side to side; the abdomen may be massaged. The character and amount of the return flow is noted. A dehydrated patient may retain some fluid.

■ NURSING INTERVENTION: The nurse performs and teaches colostomy irrigation and ensures that the patient knows how to carry out the procedure correctly and where to

purchase the necessary equipment. The person is urged to report any symptoms of obstruction or prolapse of the stoma. A home nurse is available in many areas for home visits if help is needed.

■ OUTCOME CRITERIA: Many colostomates establish a regular schedule of evacuation with irrigation, but the procedure may be unsatisfactory for patients with a liquid or semisoft fecal stream, for patients who, before the operation, had a tendency to develop diarrhea under stress, or for patients with irregular bowel habits.

colostrum /kəlos'trəm/ [L, first milk after delivery], the fluid secreted by the breast during pregnancy and the first days postpartum before lactation begins, consisting of immunologically active substances (maternal antibodies) and white blood cells, water, protein, fat, minerals, vitamins, and carbohydrate in a thin, yellow, serous fluid.

colotomy /kōlot'əmē/, a surgical incision into the colon, usually performed through the abdominal wall.

Colour Index (C.I.), a publication of dyers, colorists, and textile chemists that specifies all the standard industrial pigments and stains according to five-digit numbers associated with chemical coloring materials. For example, methylene blue is assigned number 52015. Compare **color index.**

colovaginal /kō'lōvaj'inəl/ [Gk, *kolon,* colon; L, *vagina,* sheath], pertaining to the colon and vagina, or to a communication between the two structures.

colp-. See **colpo-.**

colpalgia /kolpal'jə/, a pain in the vagina.

colpectomy /kolpek'təmē/, the surgical excision of the vagina.

colpitis /kolpī'tis/, a vaginal inflammation.

colpo-, colp-, kolpo-, kysth-, kystho-, a combining form meaning 'pertaining to the vagina': *colpocele, colpocystitis, colpodynia.*

colpocystitis /kol'pōsistī'tis/, an inflammation of the vagina and urinary bladder.

colpocystocele /kol'pəsis'təsēl/ the prolapse of the urinary bladder into the vagina, usually through the anterior vaginal wall.

colpohysterectomy /-his'tərek'təmē/ [Gk, *kolpos* vagina, *hystera,* womb, *ektome,* excision],   vaginal hysterectomy. See also **hysterectomy.**

colporrhaphy /kolpôr'əfē/ [Gk, *kolpos* + *raphe,* suture], a surgical procedure in which the vagina is sutured, as for the purpose of narrowing the vagina.

colposcope /kol'pəskōp/,   a lighted instrument with lenses for direct examination of the surfaces of the vagina and cervix.

colposcopy /kolpos'kəpē/ [Gk, *kolpos* + *skopein,* to watch], an examination of the vagina and cervix with a colposcope.

colpotomy /kolpot'əmē/ [Gk, *kolpos* + *temnein,* to cut], any surgical incision into the wall of the vagina.

columbium,   former name for **niobium.**

columna posterior.   See **posterior column.**

columnar cell /kəlum'nər/ [L, *columna,* column, *cella,* storeroom],   an epithelial cell that appears long and narrow when sectioned along its long axis.

columnar epithelium [L, *columna,* column; Gk, *epi,* upon, *thele,* nipple],   a type of epithelial cell that resembles a hexagonal prism and approximately rectangular when sectioned along its long axis.

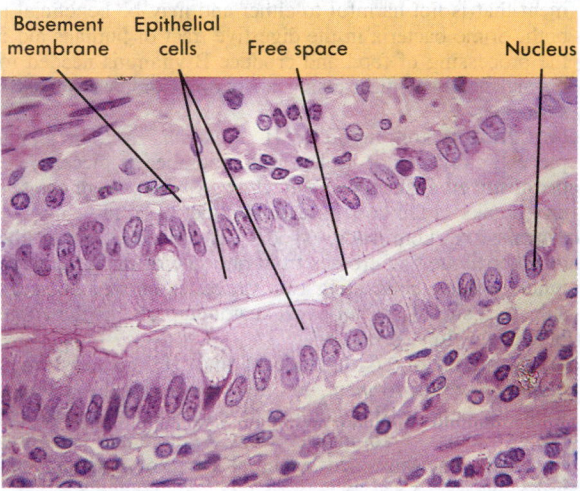

Simple columnar epithelium *(Seeley, 1992/Trent Stephens)*

columnar layer [L, *columna,* column; AS, *lecgan*],   the layer of rods and cones in the retina.

column chromatography [L, *columna;* Gk, *chroma,* color, *graphein* to record],   the process of separating and analyzing a group of substances according to the differences in their absorption affinities for a given absorbent as evidenced by pigments deposited during filtration through the same absorbent contained in a glass cylinder or tube. The substances are dissolved in a liquid that is passed through the absorbent. The absorbates move down the column at different rates and leave behind a band of pigments that is subsequently washed with a pure solvent to "develop" discrete pigmented bands that constitute a chromatograph. The cylinder of absorbent is then pushed from the tube, and the individual bands are either separated with a knife or further diluted with the pure solvent and collected in the bottom of the tube for analysis. Effective column chromatography depends on the selection of the appropriate absorbent and solvent and a flow rate that is slow enough to allow complete diffusion of the absorbates from the solvent to the absorbent and the retardation of the absorbates according to their different affinities for the absorbent. Compare **gas chromatography, ion-exchange chromatography.**

Coly-Mycin M,   a trademark for a parenteral antibacterial (colistimethate sodium).

Coly-Mycin S,   a trademark for an oral antibacterial (colistin sulfate).

com-.   See **co-.**

coma /kō'mə/ [Gk, *koma,* deep sleep],   a state of profound unconsciousness, characterized by the absence of spontaneous eye openings, response to painful stimuli, and vocalization. The person cannot be aroused. Coma may be the result of trauma, space-occupying brain tumor, hematoma, toxic metabolic condition, acute infectious disease with encephalitis, vascular disease, or brain ischemia. See also **Glasgow Coma Scale, unconscious.**

-coma,   **1.** a suffix meaning '(condition of) profound unconsciousness': *narcoma, semicoma.* **2.** a combining form meaning '(condition of) torpor': *agrypnocoma.*

comatose /kō'mətōs/,   pertaining to a state of coma, or abnormally deep sleep, caused by illness or injury.

combat fatigue [L, *com,* together, *battuere,* to beat; *fatigare,* to tire],   any of a variety of psychoneurotic disorders, usually temporary but sometimes leading to permanent neurosis, resulting from exhaustion, the stress of combat, or the cumulative emotions and psychologic strain of warfare or similar situations. It is characterized by anxiety, depression, irritability, memory and sleep disorders, and various related symptoms. Also called **combat neurosis, war neurosis.** See also **posttraumatic stress disorder, shell shock.**

combination chemotherapy /kom'binā'shən/,   the use of two or more anticancer drugs at the same time.

combined anesthesia.   See **balanced anesthesia.**

combined carbon dioxide [L, *com,* together, *bini,* twofold],   the portion of the total carbon dioxide that is contained in blood carbonate and can be calculated as the difference between the total and dissolved carbon dioxide.

combined cycling ventilator,   a mechanical ventilator that has more than one cycling mechanism, such as equipment that may have time cycling or pressure cycling as a backup to a volume cycling control device.

combined modality treatment,   the use of chemotherapy in combination with surgery or radiation or both in the treatment of cancer.

combined oxygen,   the oxygen that is physically bound to hemoglobin as oxyhemoglobin (Hb_{O_2}) One gram-molecular weight of oxygen can combine with 16,700 g of hemoglobin, and each gram of hemoglobin can bind with and carry 1.34 ml of oxygen.

combined patterns,   a method of evaluating the neuromuscular functions of a patient through tests that reveal the degree of coordination between movement patterns of the trunk and the extremities.

combined system disease,   a disorder of the nervous system caused by a deficiency of vitamin B_{12} that results in pernicious anemia and degeneration of the spinal cord and peripheral nerves, marked by increased difficulty in walking, a feeling of vibration in the legs, and a loss of sense of position. Also known as **subacute combined degeneration of the spinal cord.** See also **pernicious anemia, vitamin B₁₂.**

combining sites, **1.** concave features on antibody molecules that serve as locations for binding antigens. Because of possible variations in antibody amino acid sequences and molecule configurations, each kind of antibody can provide combining sites for a specific antigen. **2.** locations on protein molecules where drugs or other substances may become bound by electrochemical attraction.

combustion /kəmbus′chen/, the process of burning or oxidation, which may be accompanied by light and heat. Oxygen itself does not burn, but oxygen supports combustion. The rate of combustion is influenced by both oxygen concentration and its partial pressure.

comedo /kom′idō/, *pl.* **comedones** /komidō′nēz/ [L, *comedere,* to consume], blackhead, the basic lesion of acne vulgaris, caused by an accumulation of keratin and sebum within the opening of a hair follicle. It is dark because of the effect of oxygen on sebum, not because of the presence of dirt. Compare **milium.**

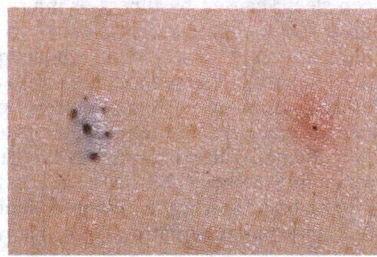

Comedo *(Stone, 1989)*

comedocarcinoma /kom′idōkär′sinō′mə/, *pl.* **comedocarcinomas, comedocarcinomata** [L, *comedere,* to consume; Gk, *karkinos,* crab, *oma,* tumor], a malignant intraductal neoplasm of the breast, in which the central cells degenerate and may be easily expressed from the cut surface of the tumor. Growth confined in the mammary ducts carries a better prognosis than do cases of invasive breast lesions.

comedogenicity /kom′idōjənis′itē/, the ability of certain drugs or agents, such as anabolic steroids, to produce acne comedones.

comedone. See **comedo.**

COMDU, abbreviation for *cardiac monitor and diagnostic unit.*

comfort measure [L, *com,* together, *fortis,* strong], any action taken to promote comfort of the patient, as a back rub, a change in position, or the prewarming of a stethoscope or a bedpan.

comfort zone [ME, *comforten*; Gk, *zone,* belt], the boundaries of temperature, humidity, wind velocity, and solar radiation within which a person dressed in a specified manner can perform certain tasks without discomfort.

Comité International des Poids et Mesures (CIPM) /kômitā′ aNternäsyōnäl′ dä pô·ä′ ä mesYr′/, a group of scientists that meets periodically to define the international (SI) units of physical quantities, as the volume of a liter, the length of a meter, or the precise amount of time in a minute. See also **SI units.**

-comma, a combining form meaning a 'piece of a structure or to cut off a piece': *inocomma, myocomma, osteocomma.*

command [L, *commendare,* protection of anyone], an order given to the computer to execute a specific instruction, as a code that evokes a particular program or performs a particular function.

command automatism, a condition characterized by an abnormal mechanical responsiveness to commands, usually followed without critical judgment, such as may be seen in hypnosis and certain psychotic states.

command hallucination, a psychotic condition in which the patient hears and obeys voices that command him or her to perform certain acts. The hallucinations may influence the individual to engage in behavior that is dangerous to himself or to others.

commensal /kəmen′səl/ [L, *com,* together, *imensa,* table], (of two different organisms) living together in an arrangement that is not harmful to either and may be beneficial to both. Some bacteria in the digestive tract of humans aid in the processing of food and produce B vitamins needed for normal health while causing no harm. Compare **parasite, synergist.**

comminuted /kom′inyōo′tid/ [L, *comminuere,* to break into pieces], crushed or broken into a number of pieces.

comminuted fracture, a fracture in which there are several breaks in the bone, creating numerous fragments.

commissure /kom′isŏor, -syŏor/ **1.** a band of nerve fiber or other tissue that crosses from one side of the body to the other, usually connecting two structures or masses of tissue. **2.** a site of union of two anatomic parts, as the corner of the eye, lips, or labia.

commissurotomy /kom′ishŏorot′əmē/ [L, *commissura,* a connection; Gk, *temnein,* to cut], the surgical division of a fibrous band or ring connecting corresponding parts of a body structure. A commissurotomy is commonly performed to separate the thickened, adherent leaves of a stenosed mitral valve.

commitment [L, *committere,* to entrust], **1.** the placement or confinement of an individual in a specialized hospital or other institutional facility. See also **institutionalize. 2.** the legal procedure of admitting a mentally ill person to an institution for psychiatric treatment. The process varies from state to state but usually involves judicial or court action based on medical evidence certifying that the person is mentally ill. See also **certification. 3.** a pledge or contract to fulfill some obligation or agreement, used especially in some forms of psychotherapy or marriage counseling.

common bile duct [L, *communis,* common, *bilis,* bile, *ducere* to lead], the duct formed by the juncture of the cystic duct and hepatic duct.

common carotid artery [L, *communis* + Gk, *karos,* heavy sleep, *arteria* air pipe], one of the major arteries supplying blood to the head and neck. The left common carotid is a branch of the brachiocephalic trunk. Each divides into an external common carotid and an internal common carotid.

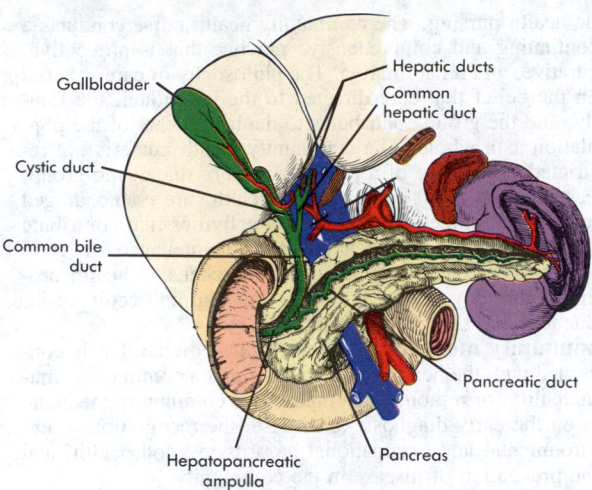

Common bile duct
(Seeley, 1992/David J Mascaro & Associates)

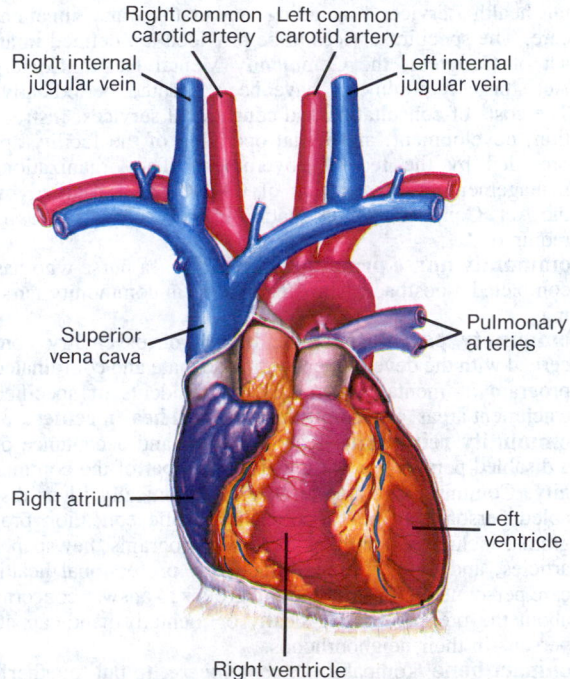

Common carotid artery *(Canobbio, 1990)*

Branches of the external carotid supply the face, scalp, and most of the neck and throat tissues. The internal common carotids supply the brain and other tissues generally accessible from within the skull, as the eyes.

common carotid plexus, a network of nerves on the common carotid artery, supplying sympathetic fibers to the head and the neck, with branches that accompany the cranial blood vessels. The common carotid plexus is formed by the internal and external carotid plexuses and by the cervical ganglia of the sympathetic system.

common cold. See **cold.**

common duct exploration. See **CDE.**

common hepatic artery, the visceral branch of the celiac trunk of the abdominal aorta, passing to the pylorus and dividing into five branches, the gastroduodenal, right gastric, right hepatic, left hepatic, and middle hepatic.

common iliac artery, a division of the abdominal aorta, starting to the left of the fourth lumbar vertebra, passing caudally about 5 cm, and dividing into external and internal iliac arteries. The right common iliac artery is somewhat longer than the left.

common iliac node, a node in one of the seven groups of parietal lymph nodes serving the abdomen and the pelvis. The nodes are arranged in clusters of about five nodes lying along the dorsal aspect of the common iliac artery. They drain the internal and the external iliac nodes and pass their materials to the lateral aortic nodes. Compare **external iliac node, internal iliac node, iliac circumflex node.** See also **lymph, lymphatic system, lymph node.**

common iliac vein, one of the two veins that are the sources of the inferior vena cava, formed by the union of the internal and the external iliac veins, ventral to the sacroiliac articulation. The right common iliac vein runs almost vertically, ascends dorsally and laterally to its corresponding artery, and is shorter than the left common iliac vein. The left common iliac vein ascends more obliquely, at first to the medial side of the corresponding artery and then dorsal to the right common iliac vein. Each common iliac vein receives the iliolumbar and, in some individuals, the lateral sacral veins. The left common iliac vein also receives the middle sacral vein. Neither of the common iliacs contains valves. Compare **external iliac vein, internal iliac vein.**

communicability period /kəmyo͞o′nəkəbil′itē/, the usual time span during which contact with an infected person is most likely to result in spread of the infection. For measles the communicability period ranges from 4 days before the appearance of a rash until 5 days after the onset of symptoms.

communicable /kəmyo͞o′nəkəbəl/ [L, *communis,* common], contagious; transmissible by direct or indirect means, as a communicable disease.

communicable disease, any disease transmitted from one person or animal to another directly, by contact with excreta or other discharges from the body; or indirectly, via substances or inanimate objects, such as contaminated drinking glasses, toys, or water; or via vectors, as flies, mosquitoes, ticks, or other insects. To control a communicable disease, it is important to identify the organism, prevent its spread to the environment, protect others against contamination, and treat the infected person. Many communicable diseases, by law, must be reported to the local health department. Kinds of communicable diseases include those caused by bacteria, chlamydia, fungi, parasites, rickettsiae, and viruses. Also called **contagious disease.**

Communicable Disease Center, former name of the **Centers for Disease Control and Prevention.**

communicating hydrocephalus /kəmyo͞o′nikā′ting/ [L, *communicans;* Gk, *hydor,* water, *kephale,* head], a form of hydrocephalus in which there is an increase in cerebrospinal fluid that involves the entire ventricle system and the subarachnoid space because of an abnormality in the ability to absorb fluid in the subarachnoid space.

communication /kəmyoō′nikā′shən/ [L, *communis,* common], any process in which a message containing information is transferred, especially from one person to another, via any of a number of media. Communication may be verbal or nonverbal; it may occur directly, such as in a face-to-face conversation or with the observation of a gesture; or it may occur remotely, spanning space and time, such as in writing and reading or in making or playing back a recording. Communication is basic to all nursing and contributes to the development of all therapeutic relationships. See also **kinesics.**

communication channels, (in communication theory) any gesture, action, sound, written word, or visual image used in transmitting messages.

communication, impaired verbal, a nursing diagnosis accepted by the Fourth National Conference on the Classification of Nursing Diagnoses. Impaired verbal communication is defined as the state in which an individual experiences a decreased or absent ability to use of understand language in human interaction. The origin of the condition includes decreased circulation to the brain; a physical barrier to speech, as a brain tumor, laryngectomy, tracheostomy, or intubation; an anatomic deficit, as a cleft palate; a psychologic barrier, as a psychosis or lack of stimuli; a cultural difference; or a developmental or age-related factor. The defining characteristics of the condition include slurring, stuttering, difficulty in forming words or sentences, difficulty in expressing thoughts verbally, inappropriate verbalization, dyspnea, and disorientation. The critical defining characteristics, one of which must be present for the diagnosis to be made, are an inability to speak the dominant language of the culture, a difficulty in speaking or verbalizing, or the absence of speech. See also **nursing diagnosis.**

communication theme, (in psychiatry) a recurrent concept or idea that ties together components of communication. Kinds of communication themes include **content theme,** in which a single concept links varied topics of discussion; **mood theme,** in which the underlying idea is the emotion communicated by the individual; and **interaction theme,** in which a particular idea best describes the dynamics between communicating participants.

communication theory, a theory that describes a model of a system of communication consisting of a source of information (the sender), a transmitter, a communication channel, a source of noise (interference), a receiver, and a purpose for the message.

community /kəmyoō′nitē/ [L, *communis,* common], a group of species who reside in a designated geographical area and who share common interests or bonds.

community-acquired infection, an infection acquired from the environment, including infections acquired indirectly from the use of medications. Community-acquired infections are distinguished from nosocomial, or hospital-acquired, diseases by the types of organisms that affect patients who are recovering from a disease or injury. Community-acquired respiratory infections commonly involve strains of *Haemophilus influenzae* or *Streptococcus pneumoniae* and are usually more antibiotic sensitive.

community health nursing, a field of nursing that is a blend of primary health care and nursing practice with pub-

lic health nursing. The community health nurse conducts a continuing and comprehensive practice that is preventive, curative, and rehabilitative. The philosophy of care is based on the belief that care directed to the individual, the family, and the group contributes to the health care of the population as a whole. The community health nurse is not restricted to the care of a particular age or diagnostic group. Participation of all consumers of health care is encouraged in the development of community activities that contribute to the promotion, education, and maintenance of good health. These activities require comprehensive health programs that pay special attention to social and ecologic influences and specific populations at risk.

community medicine, a branch of medicine that is concerned with the health of the members of a community, municipality, or region. The emphasis in community medicine is on the early diagnosis of disease, the recognition of environmental and occupational hazards to good health, and the prevention of disease in the community.

community mental health, a treatment philosophy based on the social model of psychiatric care that advocates a comprehensive range of mental health services to be made readily available to all members of the community.

community mental health center (CMHC), a community-based center that provides comprehensive mental health services, including ambulatory and inpatient care. The specific services to be provided are defined in an act of Congress, the Community Mental Health Centers Act; these requirements have been updated periodically. The costs of consultation and educational services, instruction, development, and initial operation of the facility are provided by the federal government. The organization, management, and operation of CMHCs are specified by the Act. Consumer representation in each of these areas is required.

community nurse practitioner (CNP), a nurse who has completed a postbaccalaureate program in community nursing.

community psychiatry, the branch of psychiatry concerned with the development of an adequate and coordinated program of mental health care for residents of specified catchment areas. See **community mental health center.**

community reintegration, the return and acceptance of a disabled person as a participating member of the community. Community reintegration of a chronically ill or disabled person may be supported by public education programs, including radio and television programs, newspaper articles, and by public appearances by professional health care personnel before community groups to answer concerns about the presence of physically or mentally handicapped persons in their neighborhoods.

compact bone /kompakt/ [L, *compingere,* to put together], hard, dense bone that is usually found at the surface of skeletal structures, as distinguished from spongy cancellous bone.

compact disc (CD) an optical disk on which computer data are encoded. A CD may also contain recorded music.

compact disc/read only memory. See **CD/ROM.**

companionship /kəmpan′yənship′/ [L, *com,* together, *panis,* food], (in psychiatric nursing) the assignment of a staff member or of another patient to stay with a disturbed patient to provide support and to protect the patient from self-harm or the harming of others. In constant companionship, the disturbed patient is accompanied in all activities

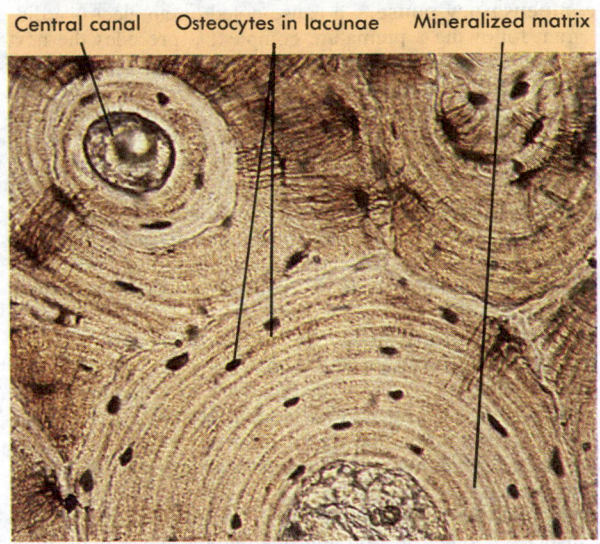

Central canal   Osteocytes in lacunae   Mineralized matrix

Compact bone *(Seeley, 1992/Trent Stephens)*

until the companion is convinced the patient has regained control.

comparative anatomy /kəmper′ətiv/ [L, *com + par,* equal], the study of the morphology and function of all living animals. A comparison of the forms indicates a progression on a scale from the simplest to the most highly specialized animals. The adult stage of animals that are lower in the scale resembles the immature stages of many animals that are higher in the scale. See also **applied anatomy, ontogeny, phylogeny.**

comparative embryology, the study of the similarities and differences among various organisms during the embryologic period of development.

comparative method, the analytic method to which the test method is compared in the comparison-of-methods experiment. This term makes no inference about the quality of the comparative method.

comparative physiology, the study of the similarities and differences of the vital processes found in various species of living organisms to determine fundamental physiologic relationships between members of the animal and plant kingdoms.

comparative psychology, **1.** the study of human behavior as it relates to or differs from animal behavior. **2.** the study of the psychologic and behavioral differences among various peoples.

compartment model /kəmpärt′mənt/, a mathematical representation of the body or an area of the body created to study physiologic or pharmacologic kinetics. A compartment model can simulate all of the biologic processes involved in the kinetic behavior of a drug after it has been introduced into the body, leading to a better understanding of the drug's pharmacodynamic effects. Studies most frequently employ one- or two-compartment models. In a one-compartment model the body assumes the characteristics of a homogenous unit in which an administered drug diffuses instantaneously in the volume of body fluid. In a two-compartment model the body is represented as two definite

compartments, a central and a peripheral compartment, with two separate fluid volumes.

compartment syndrome [L, *com + partiri,* to share], a pathologic condition caused by the progressive development of arterial compression and reduced blood supply. It can result in a permanent contracture deformity of the hand or foot, with or without a fracture. See also **Volkmann's contracture.**

compatibility /kəmpat′əbil′itē/ [L, *compatibilis,* agreeable], **1.** the quality or state of existing together in harmony; congruity. **2.** the orderly, efficient integration of the elements of one system with those of another. **3.** the formation of a stable chemical or biochemical system, specifically in medication, so that two or more drugs can be administered at the same time without producing undesired side effects or without canceling or changing the therapeutic effects of the others. **4.** (in immunology) the degree to which the body's defense system will tolerate the presence of foreign material, such as transfused blood, grafted tissue, or transplanted organs, without an immune reaction. Usually, complete compatibility exists between identical twins. **5.** (in blood grouping or crossmatching) the lack of reaction between blood groups so that there is no agglutination when the red blood cells of one sample are mixed with the serum of another sample; no reaction from transfused blood. **–compatible,** *adj.*

Compazine, a trademark for a phenothiazine (prochlorperazine), used as an antiemetic and antipsychotic.

compendium /kəmpen′dē·əm/, *pl.* **compendia** [L, *compendere,* to weigh together], a collected body of information on the standards of strength, purity, and quality of drugs. The official compendia in the United States are the *United States Pharmacopoeia,* the *Homeopathic Pharmacopoeia of the United States,* and their supplements. See also **formulary.**

compensated acidosis /kom′pənsā′tid/ [L, *compensare,* to weigh together, *acidus,* sour; Gk, *osis,* condition], a condition in which the pH of the blood is maintained within normal limits although the blood bicarbonate level is below normal.

compensated alkalosis, a condition in which the blood bicarbonate is increased but buffering keeps the blood pH within the normal range.

compensated flow meter [L, *compensare,* to balance], a gas therapy device with a scale that is calibrated against a constant pressure of 50 psi instead of the atmosphere. Because it is equipped with a valve distal to the gauge, the flow to the patient is recorded accurately, whereas an uncompensated flow meter, with a valve proximal to the gauge, may record less than the actual output.

compensated gluteal gait, one of the more common abnormal gaits associated with a weakness of the gluteus medius. It is a variation of the Trendelenburg gait and involves the dropping of the pelvis on the unaffected side of the body during the walking cycle between the moment of heelstrike on the affected side and the moment of heelstrike on the unaffected side. The compensated gluteal gait is also characterized by the dropping of the entire trunk downward and sideways over the affected hip and a short step on the unaffected side. In a compensated gait, the trunk is forcibly thrown laterally during the weight-bearing or stance phase in the movement of the affected lower limb. This lateral movement is the result of an attempt to shift a significant portion of body weight above and outside the center of rotation of the affected hip. During this movement, the erector spinae and the quadratus lumborum of the involved side function to lift the whole weight of the pelvis and the opposite lower extremity off the ground to allow the uninvolved leg to clear during its swing phase. Also called **gluteal gait.**

compensated heart failure, an abnormal cardiac condition in which heart failure is compensated for by such mechanisms as increased sympathetic adrenergic stimulation of the heart, fluid retention with increased venous return, increased end-diastolic ventricular volume and fiber length, and hypertrophy. Compensation may be aided by the administration of digitalis glycosides, with associated improved myocardial function, or by diuresis. However, diuretics may relieve only the symptoms of pulmonary and peripheral congestion, whereas the ventricular function remains severely abnormal. See also **heart failure.**

compensating current /kom′pənsā′ting/, an electric current that neutralizes the intensity of a muscle current.

compensating curve, the curvature of alignment of the occlusal surfaces of the teeth, developed to compensate for the paths of the condyles as the mandible moves from centric to eccentric positions. It is used to maintain posterior tooth contacts on the molar teeth and to provide balancing contacts on dentures associated with a protruding mandible. The compensating curve corresponds to the curve of Spee of natural teeth.

compensating filter, (in radiology) a device, such as a wedge fashioned from aluminum or plastic, that is positioned over a body area to compensate for differences in radiopacity. An example is the placement of a wedge of material over a foot with the thick portion shadowing the toes and the thin edge toward the heel to compensate for the range of thickness of the foot. See also **bowtie filter.**

compensation /kom′pənsā′shən/ [L, compensare, to balance], **1.** the process of counterbalancing any defect in bodily structure or function. **2.** (in cardiology) the process of maintaining an adequate blood flow through such normal cardiac and circulatory mechanisms as tachycardia, fluid retention with increased venous return, and hypertrophy. Failure of the heart to compensate and to provide the required cardiac output indicates a diseased heart muscle. See also **compensated heart failure. 3.** (in psychiatry) a complex defense mechanism that allows one to avoid the unpleasant or painful emotional stimuli that result from a feeling of inferiority or inadequacy. Examples include making an extraordinary effort to overcome a handicap, scorning the quality lacking ("sour grapes"), and substituting hard work and excellent performance in one field for a lack of ability in another. See also **overcompensation.**

compensation neurosis, an unconscious process by which one prolongs the symptoms resulting from an injury or disease in order to receive secondary gains, especially money. Compare **malingering.**

compensator /kom′pənsā′tər/, a device used in radiotherapy to correct for irregularities in body surfaces by providing a differential attenuation of the beam before it reaches the patient. The result is a more uniform distribution of radiation dose in the tumor. Compensators are generally mounted on the collimator system of a teletherapy unit.

compensatory hypertrophy /kəmpen′sətôr′ē/ [L, compensare, to balance], an increase in the size or the function of an organ or part to counteract a structural or functional defect. See also **compensated heart failure.**

compensatory pause, a pause noted on an electrocardiogram following a premature complex; it precedes the next normal complex.

competence /kom′pətəns/ [L, competentia, capable], **1.** (in embryology) the total capacity of an embryonic cell to react to determinative stimuli in various ways of differentiation. **2.** the ability of bacteria to take up donor DNA molecules.

competent community /kom′pətənt/, a population that is aware of resources and alternatives, can make reasoned decisions about issues facing the group, and can cope adaptively with problems. It parallels the concept of positive mental health.

competitive antagonist. See **antimetabolite.**

competitive-binding assay /kompet′itiv/ [L, competere, to come together], an analytic procedure based on the reversible binding of a ligand to a binding protein. In proportion to its concentration, the ligand competes with a labeled derivative for binding to the limited number of available binding sites.

competitive displacement, the tendency of one drug to displace another at a protein-binding site when both drugs are taken at the same time. The bound drug becomes less pharmacologically active than the free drug. An example is phenylbutazone, which has a greater affinity for binding sites than warfarin. As a result, if both drugs are taken at the same time, fewer binding sites are available for warfarin, which remains active in the body, increasing its anticoagulant action.

competitive identification, the unconscious modeling of one's personality on that of another as a means of outdoing or bettering the other person. See also **identification.**

competitive inhibitor, an inhibitor of an enzyme reaction that competes with the substrate by binding at the active site.

complaint [L, complangere, to beat the breast], **1.** (in law) a pleading by a plaintiff made under oath to initiate a suit. It is a statement of the formal charge and the cause for action against the defendant. For a minor offense, the defendant is tried on the basis of the complaint. A more serious felony prosecution requires an indictment with evidence presented by a state's attorney. **2.** informal. any ailment, problem, or symptom identified by the client, patient, member of the person's family, or other knowledgeable person. The chief complaint is often the reason that the person seeks health care.

complement /kom′pləmənt/ [L, complementum, that which completes], one of 11 complex, enzymatic serum proteins. In an antigen-antibody reaction, complement causes lysis. Complement is also involved in other physiologic reactions, including anaphylaxis and phagocytosis. Normal findings of total complement are 41-90 hemolytic U. See also **antibody, antigen, antigen-antibody reaction, immune gamma globulin.**

complement abnormality, an unusual condition characterized by deficiencies or by dysfunctions of any of the nine functional components of the enzymatic proteins of blood serum. The components are labeled C1 through C9. Intensive research currently seeks to determine the relationship between complement abnormalities or deficiencies and numerous disorders. Theoretically, any of the nine complement components may be lacking. The most common abnormalities are C2 and C3 deficiencies and C5 familial dysfunction. Patients with complement deficiencies or with complement dysfunctions may be more susceptible to infections and to collagen vascular diseases. Some patients with lupus erythematosus or dermatomyositis have displayed complement abnormalities. Studies indicate that primary complement deficiencies may be inherited. Secondary complementary deficiencies may stem from immunologic reactions, such as drug-induced serum disease, which depletes complement. Complement deficiencies may be associated with other illnesses, such as acute streptococcal glomerulonephritis and acute systemic lupus erythematosus.

■ OBSERVATIONS: Increased susceptibility to systemic bacterial infection is associated with C2 and C3 deficiencies and with C5 familial dysfunction. Chronic renal failure and lupus erythematosus may also be associated with C2 deficiency. Signs of C5 dysfunction are malaise, diarrhea, and seborrheic dermatitis. It is difficult and often expensive to diagnose complement abnormalities, but some indications are ECG conduction abnormalities, detection of complement and immunoglobulin in the walls of blood vessels in glomerulonephritis, cerebrospinal fluid pleocytosis, increased erythrocyte sedimentation rate, and the presence in urine of RBCs, RBC casts, and protein.

■ INTERVENTIONS: Replacement of complement-fixing antibodies and the control of infection and associated illnesses are part of the standard treatment of complement abnormalities. The patient with complement deficiency or dysfunction commonly receives transfusions of fresh plasma to replace antibodies. Bone marrow transplants and injections of gamma globulin may also be employed, but bone marrow transplant carries the risk of a fatal graft-versus-host reaction. Complement abnormalities may usually be temporarily corrected by replacement therapy, but no permanent cure is yet available.

■ NURSING CONSIDERATIONS: Authorities recommend careful monitoring of patients with complement abnormalities, especially patients who receive gamma globulin injections. The gamma globulin is injected into a large muscle mass and massaged well after each injection. More than one site is usually selected if the dosage is more than 1.5 ml. If frequent doses are ordered, the injection sites are rotated. With plasma infusions, careful matching of leukocytes for HLA cell types is important to prevent graft-versus-host reaction and other undesirable responses. Bone marrow transplants require close monitoring for transfusion reactions and are usually followed by instructions to the patient for scrupulous hygiene, prompt treatment of the smallest wound, and avoidance of crowds or persons with active infections. Renal infections require meticulous monitoring of intake and output, tests for serum electrolytes and acid-base balance, and observation for symptoms of renal failure. Neurologic damage resulting from infection is cause for special alertness to detect early signs of ataxia or slight changes in mental activity.

complemental inheritance /kom′pləmen′təl/, the acquisition or expression of a trait or condition from the presence of two independent pairs of nonallelic genes. Both of the genes must be present for the characteristic to appear in the phenotype.

complementarity /kom′pləmənter′itē/, a relationship in which differences are maximal.

complementary feeding /kom′pləmen′tərē/ [L, complementum, that which completes], a supplemental feeding given an infant that is still hungry after breast feeding.

complementary gene, either member of two or more non-allelic gene pairs that interact to produce an effect not expressed in the absence of any of the pairs. Also called **reciprocal gene.**

complement cascade, a biochemical process involving the C1 to C9 complement components in which one complement interacts with another in a specific sequence called a complement pathway. The reaction sequence is C1, 4, 2, 3, 5, 6, 7, 8, 9 (the first complements being out of numerical sequence for historical reasons). The cascade effect leads to an accumulation of fluid in a cell and finally lysis of the membrane, causing the cell to rupture.

complement fixation, an immunologic reaction in which an antigen combines with an antibody and its complement, causing the complement factor to become inactive or "fixed." The complement-fixation reaction can be tested in the laboratory by exposing the patient's serum to antigen, complement, and specially sensitized red blood cells. Complement-fixation tests are widely used to detect antibodies for infectious diseases, especially syphilis and viral illnesses. See also **complement, immune system, immunity, Wassermann blood test.**

complement-fixation test (C-F test), any serologic test in which complement fixation is detected, indicating the presence of a particular antigen. Specific C-F tests are used to aid in the diagnosis of amebiasis, Rocky Mountain spotted fever, trypanosomiasis, and typhus. The Wassermann test is a C-F test for syphilis.

complement protein molecule [L, complementum, proteios, first rank], any of the proteins molecules that are chief humoral mediators of antigen-antibody reactions in the immune system. Nine are involved in the "classical pathway" cascade resulting in the lysis of antibody-coated bacteria. They are designated C_1 to C_9.

complete abortion [L, complere, to fill up], termination of pregnancy in which the conceptus is expelled or removed in its entirety. Because no products of conception remain in the uterus, surgical evacuation is not necessary. Compare **incomplete abortion.**

complete bed bath, a bath in which the entire body of a patient is washed while the person is in bed. See also **blanket bath.**

complete blood count (CBC), a determination of the number of red and white blood cells per cubic millimeter of blood. A complete blood count is one of the most routinely performed tests in a clinical laboratory and one of the most valuable screening and diagnostic techniques. The count can be performed manually by staining a smear of blood on a slide and counting the different types of cells under a microscope. Most laboratories use an electronic counter for reporting numbers of red and white blood cells. Platelets are more difficult to count automatically, and many laboratories continue to do this manually. Examining a stained slide of blood yields useful information about red-cell morphology. Each type of white cell can be represented as a percentage of the total number of white cells observed. This is called a differential count. Many electronic blood counters also automatically determine hemoglobin or hematocrit and include this value in the complete blood count. See also **differential white blood cell count, erythrocyte, hematocrit, hemoglobin, leukocyte.**

complete breech, a fetal presentation in which the nates present with the legs folded on the thighs and the thighs on the abdomen. The position of the fetus is the same as in a normal vertex presentation but upside down. Compare **frank breech.** See also **breech birth.**

complete dislocation [L, *complere,* to fill up, *dis,* apart, *locare,* to place], a dislocation in which the articular surfaces of the joint are completely separated.

complete fistula, an abnormal passage from an internal organ or structure to the surface of the body or to another internal organ or structure.

complete fracture, a bone break that completely disrupts the continuity of osseous tissue across the entire width of the bone involved.

complete health history, a health history that includes a history of the present illness, a health history, social history, occupational history, sexual history, and a family health history. See also **functional health history, health history.**

complete heart block (CHB) [L, *complere,* to fill up; Gk, *kardia,* heart; OFr, *bloc*], a condition of complete failure of the conduction of all impulses from the atria to the ventricles so they beat independently.

complete hernia [L, *complere,* to fill up, *hernia,* rupture], a hernia characterized by protrusion of the hernial sac and abdominal contents through the abdominal wall.

complete paralysis [L, *complere,* to fill up; Gk, *paralyein,* to be palsied], paralysis characterized by a complete loss of motor function.

complete previa. See **central placenta previa.**

complete rachischisis, a rare congenital fissure of the entire vertebral column and spinal cord, resulting from the failure of the embryonic neural tube to close. The condition is characterized by flaccid paralysis and impaired sensations. It is often accompanied by other birth defects, such as cleft palate, cleft lip, and hydrocephalus, and is frequently fatal. Also called **rachischisis totalis, holorachischisis.** See also **spina bifida.**

complete response (CR), (in oncology) the total disappearance of a tumor.

complex /kom'pleks, kəmpleks'/ [L, *complexus,* an embrace], **1.** a group of items, as chemical molecules, that are related in structure or function as are the iron and protein portions of hemoglobin or the cobalt and protein portions of vitamin B_{12}. **2.** a combination of signs and symptoms of disease that forms a syndrome. **3.** (in psychology) a group of associated ideas with strong emotional overtones affecting a person's attitudes.

complex carbohydrate, a polysaccharide, such as a carbohydrate that is composed of a large number of glucose molecules, so called to distinguish it from simple sugars.

complex cavity, a cavity that involves more than one surface of a tooth. Compare **gingival cavity.**

complex ectopic beat [L, *complexus,* an embrace; Gk, *ektos,* outside, *topos,* place], a heart contraction impulse that originates from a point other than the sinoatrial node.

complex fracture, a closed fracture in which the soft tissue surrounding the bone is severely damaged.

complex odontoma. See **composite odontoma.**

complex protein, a protein that contains a simple protein and at least one molecule of another substance, as a glycoprotein, nucleoprotein, or hemoglobin.

complex spatial relations, the perceptual relationship of one figure or part of a figure to another.

complex sugars, sugar molecules that can be hydrolyzed or digested to yield two molecules of the same or different simple sugars, as sucrose, lactose, and maltose. Also called **disaccharides.**

compliance /kəmpli'əns/ [L, *complere,* to complete], **1.** fulfillment by the patient of the care-giver's prescribed course of treatment. **2. (C)** (in respiratory physiology) a measure of distensibility of the lung volume produced by a unit pressure change.

compliance factor, a measure of the amount of trapped tidal volume in a mechanical ventilating system associated with expansion of the flexible tubing when pressure is applied.

complicated dislocation [L, *complicare,* to fold together, *dis,* apart, *locare,* place], a dislocation complicated by damage to other tissues.

complicated labor [L, *complicare,* to fold together, *labor,* work], any labor that is complicated by a deviation from the normal procedure.

complication [L, *com + plicare,* to fold], a disease or injury that develops during the treatment of an earlier disorder. An example is a bacterial infection that is acquired by a person weakened by a viral infection. The complication frequently alters the prognosis.

component /kəmpō'nənt/ [L, *componere,* to assemble], a significant part of a larger unit.

component drip set, a device used for delivering intravenous fluids, especially whole blood. It includes plastic tubing and a combination drip-chamber and filter. Compare **component syringe set, microaggregate recipient set, straight-line blood set, Y-set.**

component syringe set, a device used for delivering intravenous fluids. It includes plastic tubing, two slide clamps, a Y-connector, and a syringe. The component syringe set may be used in various procedures, as in the transfusion of platelets and in the transfusion of cryoprecipitates. In such transfusions the component syringe set is used primarily to avoid clogging the intravenous line. Compare **component drip set, microaggregate recipient set, straight-line blood set, Y-set.**

component therapy, a transfusion of specific blood components instead of whole blood. Packed red cells or platelet-rich plasma suspensions may be transfused in larger quantities than would be possible if whole blood were used. More sophisticated processing provides fibrinogen or antihemophilic globulin solutions for administration in therapeutic amounts in excess of what might be given with conventional blood transfusion therapy. Compare **plasmapheresis.** See also **packed cells, pooled plasma.**

composite core /kəmpos'it/ [L, *componere,* to assemble], a buildup of composite resin, designed and installed to retain an artificial tooth crown. See also **core.** Compare **amalgam core, cast core.**

composite odontoma, an odontogenic tumor composed of abnormally arranged calcified enamel and dentin. Also called **complex odontoma.**

compos mentis /kom'pōs men'tis/, the quality of having a sound mind. Compare **non compos mentis.**

compound [L, *componere,* to assemble], **1.** /kom'pound/ (in chemistry) a substance composed of two or more different elements, chemically combined in definite proportions, that cannot be separated by physical means. **2.** /kom'pound/ any substance composed of two or more different ingredients. **3.** /kəmpound'/ to make a substance by combining ingredients, such as a pharmaceutic. **4.** denoting an injury characterized by multiple factors, such as a compound fracture.

compound aneurysm, a localized dilatation of an arterial wall in which some of the layers are distended and others are ruptured or dissected.

compound dislocation [L, *componere,* to put together, *dis,* apart, *locare,* to place], a dislocation in which there is a break in the skin associated with the affected joint.

compound fracture, a fracture in which the broken end or ends of the bone have torn through the skin. Also called **open fracture.**

compound joint [L, *componere,* to put together, *jungere,* to join], any joint that involves more than two bones.

compound melanocytoma. See **benign juvenile melanoma.**

compound microscope [L, *componere,* to put together; Gk, *mikros,* small, *skopein,* to view], a microscope with two or more simple or complex lens systems.

compound monster, a fetus in which some of the parts or organs are duplicated but not fully developed.

compound tubuloalveolar gland /too'byəlo'alve'ələr/, one of the many multicellular glands with more than one secretory duct that contains both tube-shaped and sac-shaped portions, as the salivary glands.

comprehensive care. See **holistic health care.**

Comprehensive Health Manpower Act of 1971, legislation passed by the U.S. Congress providing educational funding for nurse-practitioner (NP) and physician-assistant (PA) programs.

Comprehensive Health Planning (CHP) and Public Health Services Amendments, legislation passed by the U.S. Congress in 1966 that emphasized regional planning and established for the first time the concept that each person has a "right to health care."

compress /kom'pres/ [L, *comprimere,* to press together], a soft pad, usually made of cloth, used to apply heat, cold, or medications to the surface of a body area. A compress also may be applied over a wound to help control bleeding. Compare **dressing.**

compressed air hazards. See **decompression sickness.**

compressibility factor /kəmpres'ibil'itē/, a measure of the amount of tidal volume that may be trapped in a mechanical ventilator system in relation to the water pressure applied. It is expressed in milliliters of gas per centimeter of water pressure.

compressible volume /kəmpres'əbəl/, a part of the tidal volume of gas produced by a mechanical ventilator that does not reach the patient because of compression of the gas and expansion of the flexible tubing in the equipment.

compression /kəmpresh'ən/ [L, *comprimere,* to press together], the act of pressing, squeezing, or otherwise applying pressure to an organ, tissue, or body area. An intracranial tumor or hemorrhage may cause compression of brain tissue. Kinds of pathologic compression include **compression fracture,** in which bone surfaces are forced against each other, causing a break, and **compression paralysis,** marked by paralysis of a body area caused by pressure on a nerve.

compression fracture, a bone break, especially in a short bone, that disrupts osseous tissue and collapses the affected bone. The bodies of vertebrae are often sites of compression fractures.

compression neuropathy, any of several disorders involving damage to sensory nerve roots or peripheral nerves,

caused by mechanical pressure or localized trauma and characterized by paresthesia, weakness, or paralysis. The carpal, peroneal, radial, and ulnar nerves are most commonly involved. Compare **neuritis.** See also **paresthesia.**

compression paralysis [L, *comprimere,* to press together; Gk, *paralyein,* to be palsied], a paralysis that is caused by sustained pressure on a peripheral nerve. The condition can be temporary or permament, depending on the duration and intensity of the pressure.

compressive atelectasis /kəmpres'iv/, a loss of the ability of the lung to move air in and out of the atelectatic region because of intrathoracic pressures that compress the alveoli. The condition may result from a pulmonary embolism. The embolism releases chemicals that cause vasoconstriction and bronchospasm, leading to compression of the alveoli in the affected area into a dense, airless mass of tissue.

compressor naris /kompres'ôr nät'is/, the transverse part of the nasalis muscle that serves to depress the cartilage of the nose and to draw the ala toward the septum. Compare **dilatator naris.**

compromise /kom'prəmīs/ [L, *com,* together, *promittere,* to promise], an action that may involve a change in a person's behavior, as in substituting goals or delaying satisfaction of needs in one area to reduce stress in another.

compromise body image, a new body image acquired by a patient as part of his or her adjustment to a physical dysfunction. It may harbor important emotional factors for the individual. A compromise body image incorporates and modifies unacceptable features of the condition through psychologic defense mechanisms as denial, sublimation, repression, and overcompensation.

compromised host, a person who is less-than-normally able to resist infection, because of immunosuppressive therapy, immunologic defect, severe anemia, or concurrent disease or condition, including AIDS, metastatic malignancy, cachexia, or severe malnutrition.

Compton scatter [Arthur H. Compton, American physicist, b. 1892], the principal interaction process of photons with tissue in the diagnostic and therapeutic radiology energy range. In this process, the incoming photon transfers energy to an electron in the material and is deflected with reduced energy into a path that generally leads to additional interactions.

compulsion [L, *compellere,* to urge], an irresistible, repetitive, irrational impulse to perform an act that is usually contrary to one's ordinary judgments or standards yet results in overt anxiety if it is not completed. The impulse is usually the result of an obsession. A kind of compulsion is **repetition compulsion.** Compare **phobia.** See also **obsession.** –**compulsive,** *adj.*

compulsion need [L, *compellere,* to urge; Gk, *neuron,* nerve, *osis,* condition], a need characterized by a compulsion to perform certain acts repeatedly in spite of conscious recognition that it is abnormal behavior. The compulsive act may have symbolic significance to the patient.

compulsive /kəmpul'siv/ [L, *compellere,* to urge], pertaining to an act repeatedly performed under the stress of compulsion.

compulsive idea [L, *compellere,* to urge], a recurring, irrational idea that persists in the mind, usually resulting in an irresistible urge to perform some inappropriate act. Also called **imperative idea.**

compulsive personality, a type of character structure in which there is a pattern of chronic and obsessive adherence to rigid standards of conduct. The person is usually excessively conscientious and inhibited, is extremely inflexible, has an extraordinary capacity for work, and lacks a normal ability to relax and to relate to other people. The compulsive person is likely to follow repetitive patterns of behavior, such as snapping the fingers, crossing the legs, tapping the foot, or refusing to walk on cracks in the sidewalk, and often leads an impoverished emotional life, being dominated by a need for order, cleanliness, punctuality, rules, and systems. See also **compulsive personality disorder.**

compulsive personality disorder, a condition in which an irrational preoccupation with order, rules, ritual, and detail interferes with everyday functioning and normal behavior. The disorder is characterized by an excessive devotion to work, a pathologic adherence to a definite set of rules or system of behavior, and a persistent, compulsive following of specific rituals. The person cannot make decisions when faced with unexpected situations and cannot take pleasure in the normal activities of daily life. Psychotherapy is the usual treatment and may include behavior therapy with desensitization and flooding in order to reduce maladaptive anxiety. See also **compulsive personality.**

compulsive polydipsia, a compelling urge to drink excessive amounts of liquid. The condition is psychogenic; it is not caused by any organic dysfunction or physical deprivation. Extreme cases can result in death from water intoxication and electrolyte imbalance. See also **polydipsia.**

compulsive ritual, a series of acts a person feels must be carried out even though he recognizes the behavior to be useless and inappropriate. Failure to complete the acts results in extreme tension or anxiety.

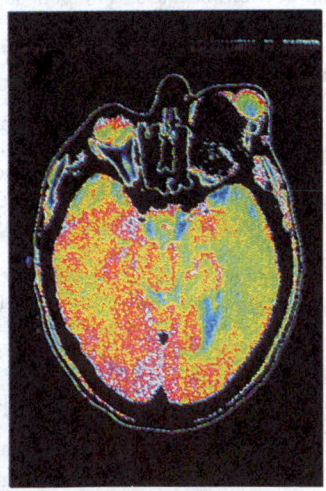

CT scan *(Seeley, 1992/Howard Sochurek)*

computed tomography (CT) /kəmpyōō′tid/, an x-ray technique that produces a film representing a detailed cross section of tissue structure. The procedure is painless, noninvasive, and requires no special preparation. Computed tomography employs a narrowly collimated beam of x-rays that rotates in a continuous 360-degree motion around the patient to image the body in cross-sectional slices. An ar-

ray of detectors, positioned at several angles, records those x-rays that pass through the body. The image is created by computer using multiple attenuation readings taken around the periphery of the body part. The computer calculates tissue absorption, displays a printout of the numeric values, and produces a visualization of the tissues that demonstrates the densities of the various structures. Tumor masses, infractions, bone displacement, and accumulations of fluid may be detected. Formerly called **computerized axial tomography.**

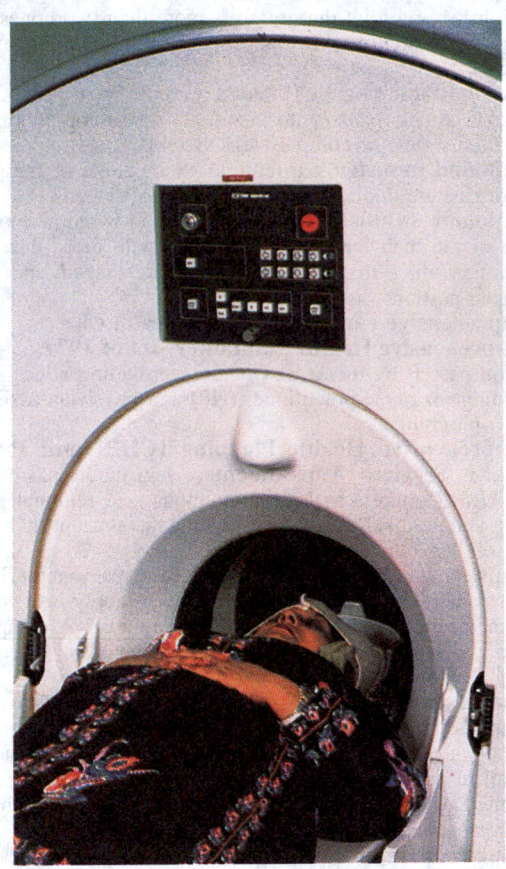

Positioning of patient for computed tomography
(Perkin, 1986)

computer [L *computare* to calculate], an electronic device for processing and storing large amounts of information very quickly. See also **analog computer. main-frame computer, microcomputer, minicomputer.**

computer-assisted instruction (CAI), a teaching process employing a computer in the presentation of instructional materials, often in such a way as to require the student to interact with it. Also called **computer-assisted learning (CAL).**

computerized axial tomography (CAT). See **computed tomography.**

computer-managed instruction (CMI), a system in which a computer is employed to manage several or many aspects of instruction including lerarning assessment through administration of pre- and post-tests, design and preapation of learning prescriptions, and calculation, analysis, and storage of student scores.

con-. See **co-.**

CONA, abbreviation for **Canadian Orthopedic Nurses Association.**

conation /kōnā′shən/ [L, *conari,* to attempt], the mental process characterized by desire, impulse, volition, and striving. Compare **cognition.** –**conative,** *adj.*

-conazole, a suffix designating a miconazole-type systemic antifungal agent.

concanavalin A /kon′kənav′əlin/, a hemagglutinin, isolated from the meal of the jack bean, that reacts with polyglucosans in the blood of mammals causing agglutination. It has been used in immunology to stimulate T cell production.

concatenates /kənkat′ənāts/, long molecules formed by continuous repeating of the same molecular subunit.

concave-convex joint relationship /kon′kāv, konkāv′/, the relative shape of each component of a joint's articulating surfaces. One surface is usually concave and the other convex.

concave spherical lens [L, *concavare,* to make hollow; Gk, *sphaira,* ball; L, *lentil*], a lens that has curved, depressed surfaces to diverge the rays of light. It is used for the management of myopia.

concavity /kən′kav′itē/, a deep depression or inward curving surface of an organ or body structure.

concealed accessory pathway /kənsēld/ [L, *con,* together, *celare,* to hide], (in cardiology) a condition in which an accessory pathway is present but is cpable of retrograde conduction only. The electrocardiogram is normal during sinus rhythm (no delta wave) but the patient is prone to paraoxysmal supraventricular tachycardia due to orthodontic circus movement tachycardia. During atrial fibrillation conduction into the ventricles is normal since the accessory pathway does not conduct anterogradely.

concealed junctional extrasystole, a junctional impulse that arises in and discharges the atrioventricular junction but fails to reach either atria or ventricles.

conceive /kənsēv′/ [L, *concipere,* to take together], to become pregnant.

concentrate /kon′səntrāt/ [L, *con* + *centrum,* center], **1.** to decrease the bulk of a liquid and increase its strength per unit of volume by the removal of inactive ingredients through evaporation or other means. **2.** a substance, particularly a liquid, that has been strengthened and reduced in volume through such means.

concentration gradient, a gradient that exists across a membrane separating a high concentration of a particular ion from a low concentration of the same ion.

concentric /kənsen′trik/ [L, *con* + *centrum,* center], describing two or more circles that have a common center.

concentric contraction, a common form of muscle contraction that occurs in rhythmic activities when the muscle fibers shorten as tension develops. See also **isotonic exercise.**

concentric fibroma, a fibrous tumor surrounding the uterine cavity.

concentric hypertrophy [L, *cum,* together, *centrum,* center; Gk, *hyper,* excessive, *trophe,* nourishment], a type of tissue overgrowth in which the walls of an organ continue to increase but the exterior size remains the same but the internal size is diminished.

concept [L, *concipere,* to take together], a construct or abstract idea or thought that originates and is held within the mind. –**conceptual,** *adj.*

conception /kənsep′shən/ [L, *concipere,* to take together], **1.** the beginning of pregnancy, usually taken to be the instant that a spermatozoon enters an ovum and forms a viable zygote. **2.** the act or process of fertilization. **3.** the act or process of creating an idea or notion. **4.** the idea or notion created; a general impression resulting from the interpretation of a symbol or set of symbols.

conceptional age, in fetal development, the number of weeks since conception. Because the exact time of conception is difficult to determine, conceptional age is assumed to be 2 weeks less than gestational age.

conception control. See **contraception.**

conceptive /kənsep′tiv/ [L, *concipere,* to take together], **1.** able to become pregnant. **2.** pertaining to or characteristic of the mental process of forming ideas or impressions.

conceptual. See **concept.**

conceptual disorder /kənsep′chōō·əl/ [L, *concipere,* to take together], a disturbance in thought processes, in cognitive activities, or in the ability to formulate concepts.

conceptual framework, a group of concepts that are broadly defined and systematically organized to provide a focus, a rationale, and a tool for the integration and interpretation of information. Usually expressed abstractly using word models, a conceptual framework is the conceptual basis for many theories, as communication theory and general systems theory.

conceptus /kənsep′təs/ [L, *concipere,* to take together], the product of conception; the fertilized ovum and its enclosing membranes at all stages of intrauterine development, from implantation to birth. See also **embryo, fetus.**

concha /kong′kə/, a body structure that is shell shaped, as the cavity in the external ear that surrounds the external auditory canal meatus.

concoction /kənkok′shən/ [L, *con* + *coquere,* to cook], a remedy prepared from a mixture of two or more drugs or substances that have been heated.

concomitant /konkom′itənt/ [L, *con* + *comitari,* to accompany], designating one or more of two or more things, occurring simultaneously, that may or may not be interrelated or produced as a result of the others; accompanying.

concomitant symptom, any symptom that accompanies a primary symptom.

concordance /kənkôr′dəns/ [L, *concordare,* to agree], (in genetics) the expression of one or more specific traits in both members of a pair of twins. Compare **discordance.** –**concordant,** *adj.*

concreteness /kənkrēt′nes/ [L, *concrescere,* to be formed], the content of a communication that is not vague, but which includes specific feelings, behaviors, and experiences or situations.

concrete operation /kon′krēt, konkrēt′/, a thought process based on concrete rather than abstract points of reference.

concrete thinking, a stage in the development of the cognitive thought processes in the child. During this phase, thought becomes increasingly logical and coherent so that the child is able to classify, sort, order, and organize facts while still being incapable of generalizing or dealing in abstractions. Problem solving is accomplished in a concrete, systematic fashion based on what is perceived, keeping to the literal meaning of words, as the word 'horse' applying to a particular animal and not to horses in general. In Piaget's classification, this stage occurs between 7 and 11 years of age, is preceded by syncretic thinking, and is followed by abstract thinking.

concretion. See **calculus.**

concurrent disinfection /kənkur′ənt/ [L, *concurrere,* to meet at one place; *dis,* opposite of, *inficere,* to taint], the daily handling and disposal of contaminated material or equipment.

concurrent infection [L, *concurrere,* to run together, *inficere,* to stain], a condition during which a person has two or more infections at the same time.

concurrent nursing audit. See **nursing audit.**

concurrent sterilization, a method of preparing an infant-feeding formula in which all ingredients and equipment are sterilized before mixing the formula.

concurrent validity, validity of a test or a measurement tool that is established by concurrently applying a previously validated tool or test to the same phenomena, or data base, and comparing the results. Concurrent validity is achieved if the results are the same or similar at a statistically significant level. See also **validity.**

concussion /konkush′ən/ [L, *concutere,* to shake violently], **1.** a violent jarring or shaking, as caused by a blow or an explosion. **2.** *informal.* **brain concussion.**

condensation /kon′dənsā′shən/ [L, *condensare,* to make denser], **1.** a reduction to a denser form, such as from water vapor to a liquid. **2.** (in psychology) a process often present in dreams in which two or more concepts are fused so that a single symbol represents the multiple components. In some cases of schizophrenia condensation, several thoughts and feelings fuse into a single verbal or nonverbal message and may be seen in repetitive statements or gestures that can have a variety of meanings.

condensation nuclei, neutral particles, such as dust, in the atmosphere that are able to absorb or adsorb water and grow in size. At relatively high humidities, they form fogs or hazes. Condensation nuclei consisting of sulfuric or nitric acid vapors or nitrogen oxides may be a source of respiratory irritants.

condensed milk, a thick liquid prepared by the evaporation of half of the water content of cow's milk.

condenser, (in dentistry) an instrument for compacting restorative material into a prepared tooth cavity. It has a working end, or nib, with a flat or serrated face.

condition /kəndish′ən/ [L, *condicere,* to make arrangements], **1.** a state of being, specifically in reference to physical and mental health or well-being. **2.** anything that is essential for or that restricts or modifies the appearance or occurrence of something else. **3.** to train the body or mind, usually through specific exercises and repeated exposure to a particular state or thing. **4.** (in psychology) to subject a person or animal to conditioning or associative learning so that a specific stimulus will always elicit a particular response. See also **classic conditioning.**

conditional discharge /kəndish′ənəl/, a specified leave of absence or liberty from a psychiatric hospital in which certain behaviors are expected from the patient and the original commitment order remains in effect.

conditioned avoidance response, a learned reaction that is performed either consciously or unconsciously to avoid an unpleasant or painful stimulus or to prevent such stimuli from occurring.

conditioned escape response, a learned reaction that is performed either consciously or unconsciously to stop or to escape from an aversive stimulus.

conditioned orientation response (COR), the desired response in an audiometry technique used in hearing tests for children under the age of 2 years. A toy mounted on a loudspeaker moves or lights up after presentation of a test tone. If later test sounds are audible to the child, he or she will look toward the toy after hearing a tone.

conditioned reflex, a reflex developed gradually by training in association with a specific, repeated external stimulus. An example of a conditioned reflex is Pavlov's experiment in which a dog salivates at the ringing of a bell if over a period of time every feeding is preceded by the bell-ringing stimulus.

conditioned response, an automatic reaction to a stimulus that does not normally elicit such response but which has been learned through training. Such responses can be physical or psychologic and are produced by repeated association of some physiologic function or behavioral pattern with an unrelated stimulus or event. In Pavlov's classic experiments, dogs learned to associate the sound of a ringing bell with feeding time so that they would salivate at the sound of the bell regardless of whether or not food was given to them. Also called **acquired reflex, behavior reflex, conditioned reflex, trained reflex.** Compare **unconditioned response.** See also **classical conditioning.**

conditioned stimulus [L, *conditio* + *stimulus,* goad], any stimulus to which a reflex response has become conditioned by previous training or experience.

conditioning /kəndish′əning/ [L, *condicere,* to make arrangements], a form of learning based on the development of a response or set of responses to a stimulus or series of stimuli. Kinds of conditioning are **classical conditioning, instrumental conditioning,** and **operant conditioning.**

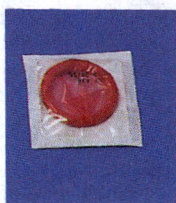

Condom *(Edge, 1994)*

condom /kon′dəm/, a soft, flexible sheath that covers the penis and prevents semen from entering the vagina in sexual intercourse, and is used to avoid the transmittal of an infection and to prevent conception. Condoms are made of plastic, rubber, or skin. Also called **prophylactic,** *(informal)* **rubber.**

conduct disorder /kon′dukt/, (in psychiatry) behavior in an adolescent or child that is unacceptable in the social environment and could be considered criminal in an adult.

conduction /kənduk'shən/ [L, *conducere*, to lead], **1.** (in physics) a process in which heat is transferred from one substance to another because of a difference in temperature; a process in which energy is transmitted through a conductor. **2.** (in physiology) the process by which a nerve impulse is transmitted.

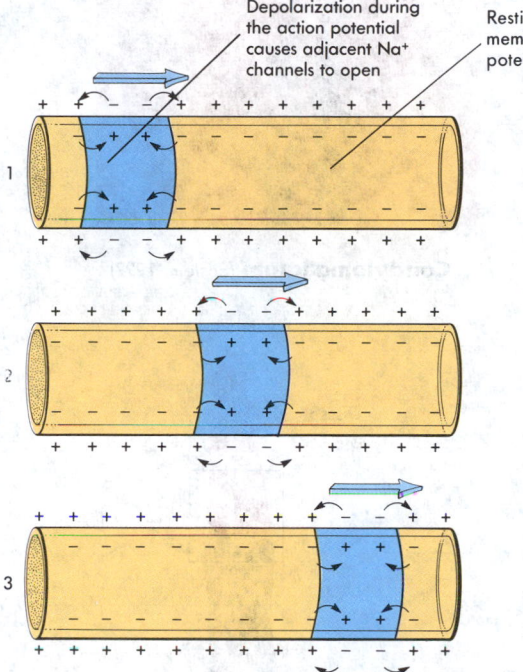

Conduction of an action potential
(Thibodeau, 1993/Joan M Beck)

conduction anesthesia, a loss of sensation, especially pain, in a region of the body, produced by injecting a local anesthetic along the course of a nerve or nerves to inhibit the conduction of impulses to and from the area supplied by that nerve or nerves. Also called **block anesthesia, nerve block anesthesia.**

conduction aphasia, a dissociative speech phenomenon in which there is no difficulty in comprehending words seen or heard and in which there is no dysarthria, yet the patient has problems in self-expression. The patient may substitute words similar in sound or meaning for the correct ones but is unable to repeat from dictation, to spell, and to read aloud. The patient is alert and aware of the deficit. A common cause is an embolus in a branch of the middle cerebral artery. The nurse should try to reduce tension and frustration in the patient, encourage socialization, find the best means of communication for the patient, use simple language and direct questions requiring simple answers, and help the family to understand the problem and deal with it. See also **aphasia.**

conduction deafness. See **conductive hearing loss.**

conduction system, specialized tissue that carries electrical impulses, such as bundle branches and Purkinje fibers.

conduction system of the heart, the network of nervous tissue that transmits the electrical impulses needed for a heart beat. It includes the sinoatrial and atrioventricular nodes, the bundle of His, the Purkinje fibers, and the left and right bundle branches.

conduction velocity, the speed with which an electrical impulse can be transmitted through excitable tissue, as in the movement of a action potential through His-Purkinje fibers of the heart.

conductive hearing loss /kənduk'tiv/ [L, *conducere*, to lead], a form of hearing loss in which sound is inadequately conducted through the external or middle ear to the sensorineural apparatus of the inner ear. Sensitivity to sound is diminished, but clarity (interpretation of the sound) is not changed. Compare **sensorineural hearing loss.**

conductor, **1.** any substance through which electrons flow easily. **2.** (in psychiatry) a family therapist who uses his or her own personality to give direction to a family in therapy.

conduit /kon'dit, kon'doo·it/, **1.** an artificial channel or passage that connects two organs or different parts of the same organ. **2.** a tube or other device for conveying water or other fluids from one region to another.

condylar fracture /kon'dilər/ [Gk, *kondylos*, knuckle], any fracture of the round end of a hinge joint, usually occurring at the distal end of the humerus or at the distal end of the femur, frequently detaching a small bone fragment that includes the condyle.

condylar guide, a mechanical device on a dental articulator, designed to guide articular movement similar to that produced by the paths of the condyles in the temporomandibular joints. Compare **anterior guide, incisal guide.**

condyle /kon'dīl/ [Gk, *kondylos*, knuckle], a rounded projection at the end of a bone that anchors muscle ligaments and articulates with adjacent bones.

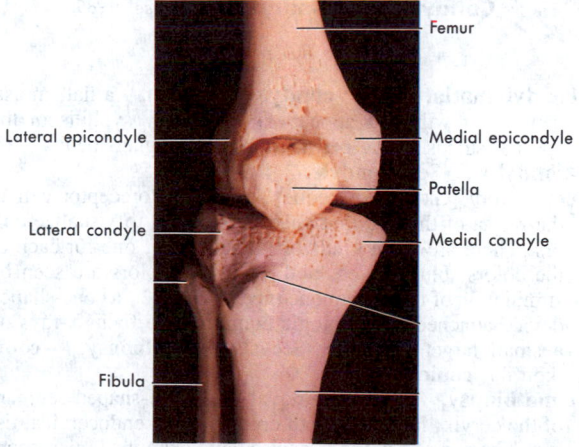

Condyles of the knee *(Vidic, 1984)*

-condyle, -condylus, a suffix meaning a 'knucklelike projection on a bone': *entepicondyle, epicondyle, entocondyle.*

condyloid /kon′diloid/ [Gk, *kondylos,* knuckle], resembling a knuckle.

condyloid joint [L, *kondylos + eidos,* form], a synovial joint in which a condyle is received into an elliptic cavity, as the wrist joint. A condyloid joint permits no axial rotation but allows flexion, extension, adduction, abduction, and circumduction. Also called **articulatio ellipsoidea.** Compare **ball-and-socket joint, pivot joint, saddle joint.**

condyloma /kon′dilō′mə/, *pl.* **condylomas,** [Gk, *kondyloma,* a knob], a wartlike growth on the anus, vulva, or glans penis, usually sexually transmitted.

condyloma acuminatum, *pl.* **condylomata acuminata,** a soft, wartlike or papillomatous growth common on warm and moist skin and the mucous membrane of the genitalia. It is caused by a virus and is transmitted by sexual contact. Also called **acuminate wart, venereal wart.**

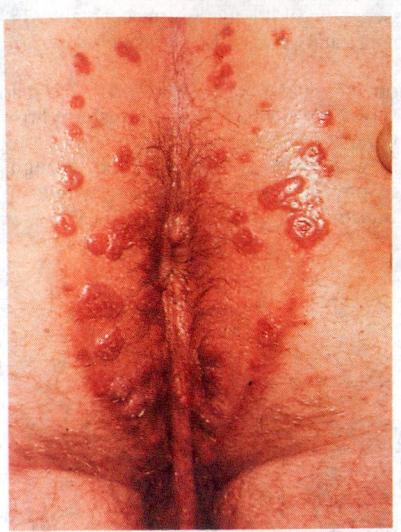

Condyloma latum *(Epstein, 1992)*

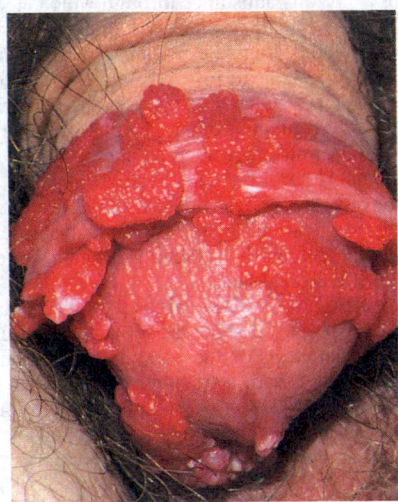

Condyloma acuminatum *(Chessel, 1985)*

condyloma latum, *pl.* **condylomata lata,** a flat, moist, papular growth that appears in secondary syphilis in the coronal sulcus of the perineum or on the glans penis.

-condylus. See **-condyle.**

cone /kōn/ [Gk, *konos,* cone], **1.** a photoreceptor cell in the retina of the eye that enables a person to visualize colors. There are three kinds of retinal cones, one for each of the colors, blue, green, and red; other colors are seen by stimulation of more than one type of cone. **2.** a cone-shaped device attached to radiologic equipment to focus x-rays on a small target of tissue. See also **cone biopsy.** **–conic** /kon′ik/, **conical,** *adj.*

cone biopsy, surgical removal of a cone-shaped segment of the cervix, including both epithelial and endocervical tissue. The cone of tissue is excised and examined microscopically to establish a precise diagnosis, usually to confirm or evaluate a positive Papanicolaou test. Postoperatively, hemorrhage sometimes occurs. If bleeding occurs 7 to 10 days later, suturing may be required. See also **biopsy, cone.**

cone cutting, the interference by a radiographic cone with an x-ray beam caused by misalignment of the tube, cone,

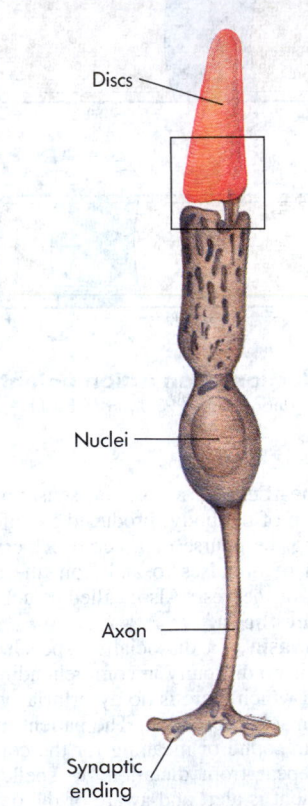

Cone cell of the retina
(Seeley, 1992/Lisa Chuck, Michael Schenk)

and film. It may result in the loss of one portion of the x-ray image.

cone of light, **1.** a triangular reflection observed during an ear examination when the light of an otoscope is focused on the image of the malleus. **2.** the group of light rays entering the pupil of the eye and forming an image on the retina.

confabulation /kənfab′yəlā′shən/ [L, *con* + *fabulari*, to speak], the fabrication of experiences or situations, often recounted in a detailed and plausible way to fill in and cover up gaps in the memory. The phenomenon occurs principally as a defense mechanism and is most commonly seen in alcoholics, especially those who have Korsakoff's psychosis, and persons with head injuries, dementia, or lead poisoning. Also called **fabrication.**

confession /kənfesh′ən/, an act of seeking expiation through another from guilt for a real or imagined transgression.

confidentiality, /kon′fiden′shē·al′itē/ the nondisclosure of certain information except to another authorized person.

configuration /kənfig′yərā′shən/ [L, *configuare*, to form from], the hardware, software, and peripherals assembled to work as a computer unit in a specific situation.

configurationism. See **Gestalt psychology.**

confinement /kənfīn′mənt/ [L, *confinis*, common boundary], **1.** a state of being held or restrained within a specific place in order to hinder or minimize activity. **2.** the final phase of pregnancy during which labor and childbirth occur; parturition. See also **puerperium.**

confinement deprivation, an emotional disorder that may result when an individual is separated from familiar surroundings or denied contact with familiar persons or objects. It may occur when one is confined to a single room.

conflict /kon′flikt/ [L, *conflictere,* to strike together], **1.** a mental struggle, either conscious or unconscious, resulting from the simultaneous presence of opposing or incompatible thoughts, ideas, goals, or emotional forces, such as impulses, desires, or drives. **2.** a painful state of consciousness caused by the arousal of such opposing forces and the inability to resolve them; a kind of stress found to a certain degree in every person. **3.** (in psychoanalysis) the unconscious emotional struggle between the demands of the id and those of the ego and superego or between the demands of the ego and the restrictions imposed by society. Kinds of conflict include **approach-approach conflict, approach-avoidance conflict, avoidance-avoidance conflict, extrapsychic conflict,** and **intrapsychic conflict.**

confluence of the sinuses /kon′floo·əns/ [L, *confluere,* to flow together], the wide junction of the superior sagittal, the straight, and the occipital sinuses with the two large transverse sinuses of the dura mater. The right transverse sinus usually receives most of the blood from the superior sagittal sinus, and the left transverse sinus receives the blood from the straight sinus. The confluence is one of six posterior superior sinuses of the dura matter, draining blood from the section and an inner bulging granular section.

confluent /kon′floo·ənt/ [L, *confluere,* to flow together], running together, such as the sinuses of the dura mater, or skin eruptions that are confluent.

confrontation test /kon′frəntā′shən/ [L, *con* + *frons,* forehead], a method of assessing the visual field of a patient by moving an object into the periphery of each of the visual quadrants. The test is conducted while one eye is covered and the vision of the other is fixed on a point straight ahead. The patient reports when the moving object, which may be the examiner's finger, is first detected at the edge of the visual field.

confusion /kənfyoo′shən/ [L, *confundere,* to mingle], a mental state characterized by disorientation regarding time, place, or person, causing bewilderment, perplexity, lack of orderly thought, and inability to choose or act decisively, and perform the activities of daily living. It is usually symptomatic of an organic mental disorder, but it may accompany severe emotional stress and various psychologic disorders. **—confusional,** *adj.*

confusional insanity. See **amentia.**

confusional state, a mild form of delirium that may be experienced by an elderly person or a patient with preexisting brain disease. The confusional state may be triggered by a sudden or unexpected change in the person's environment. The confusion may be characterized by failure to perform activities of daily living, memory deficits, disruptive behavior, and inappropriate speech.

congener /kon′jənər/ [L, *con* + *genus,* origin], one of two or more things that are similar or closely related in structure, function, or origin. Examples of congeners are muscles that function identically, chemical compounds similar in composition and effect, or species from the same genus of plants or animals. **—congenerous** /kənjen′ərəs/, *adj.*

congenital /kənjen′itəl/ [L, *congenitus,* born with], present at birth, as a congenital anomaly or defect.

congenital absence of sacrum and lumbar vertebrae, an abnormal condition present at birth and characterized by varying degrees of deformity, ranging from the absence of the lower segment of the coccyx to the absence of the entire sacrum and all lumbar vertebrae. Congenital absence of the sacrum and the lumbar vertebrae is relatively rare. Lesser degrees of this anomaly may present so few signs that marked deformities are not present, and the condition may not be diagnosed unless accidentally found on radiographic examination. More severe forms display gross deformities and neurologic deficits. Signs and symptoms of the more severe kinds include short stature, flattened buttocks, muscle paralysis to varying degrees, muscle atrophy in the lower extremities, foot deformities, contractures of the hips and the knees, and varying degrees of loss of sensation, especially sensation distal to the knees. The treatment varies greatly for the congenital absence of the sacrum and the lumbar vertebrae and depends on severity. Surgical intervention may be reconstructive or may involve disarticulation procedures at various spinal levels and subsequent fusion of the remaining vertebrae. Depending on the severity, many patients with this anomaly may be surgically provided with enough stability to sit and to walk with assistance. The most severe forms are usually fatal.

congenital adrenal hyperplasia, a group of disorders that have in common an enzyme defect resulting in low levels of cortisol and increased secretion of ACTH. The net effect is adrenal gland overgrowth and increased production of cortisol precursors and androgens. During intrauterine life, the disorder leads to pseudohermaphroditism in female infants and macrogenitosomia in male infants. Treatment involves hydrocortisone therapy and reconstructive surgery. See also **adrenal virilism, macrogenitosomia, pseudohermaphroditism.**

congenital amputation, the absence of a fetal limb or part at birth, previously attributed to amputation by constricting bands in utero but now regarded as a developmental defect. See also **amputee.**

congenital anomaly, any abnormality present at birth, particularly a structural one, which may be inherited genetically, acquired during gestation, or inflicted during parturition. Also called **birth defect.**

congenital aspiration pneumonia [L, *congenitus,* born with, *aspirare,* to breathe upon; Gk, *pneumon,* lung], a neonatal lung inflammation caused by the aspiration of fluid or meconium during labor.

congenital cataracts. See **cataract.**

congenital cardiac anomaly, any structural or functional abnormality or defect of the heart or great vessels existing from birth. Congenital heart disease is a major cause of neonatal distress and is the most common cause of death in the newborn other than problems related to prematurity. Approximately 90% of all deaths from congenital heart disease occur during the first year of life. Congenital heart defects may result from genetic causes or from environmental factors, such as maternal infection or exposure to radiation or noxious substances during pregnancy. Most defects are probably caused by some interaction between genetic and environmental factors that results in arrested embryonic development. Congenital heart anomalies are classified broadly according to the resulting alteration in circulation as acyanotic, in which no unoxygenated blood mixes in the circulatory system, or cyanotic, in which unoxygenated blood enters the system. The general effects of cardiac malformations on cardiovascular functioning are increased cardiac workload, increased pulmonary vascular resistance, inadequate cardiac output, and decreased oxygen saturation from the shunting of unoxygenated blood directly into the circulatory system. The general physical symptoms of these pathophysiologic alterations are growth retardation, decreased exercise tolerance, recurrent respiratory infections, dyspnea, tachypnea, tachycardia, cyanosis, tissue hypoxia, and murmurs, all of which vary in severity depending on the type and degree of the defect. Kinds of congenital cardiac anomalies include **atrial septal defect, coarctation of the aorta, tetralogy of Fallot, transposition of the great vessels, tricuspid atresia,** and **ventricular septal defect.** See also **aortic stenosis, patent ductus arteriosus, pulmonic stenosis, valvular stenosis.**

congenital cerebral diplegia. See **cerebral palsy.**

congenital cloaca. See **persistent cloaca.**

congenital cyanosis [L, *congenitus,* born with; Gk, *kyanos,* blue, *osis,* condition], cyanosis present at birth because of a congenital heart disease or atelectasis of the lungs. See also **blue baby.**

congenital cyst [L, *congenitus,* born with; Gk, *kystis,* bag], a cyst present at birth, as a dermoid cyst resulting from an embryonic defect in the skin or midline structures.

congenital cytomegalovirus (CMV) disease. See **cytomegalic inclusion disease.**

congenital dermal sinus, a channel present at birth, extending from the surface of the body and passing between the bodies of two adjacent lumbar vertebrae to the spinal canal.

congenital dislocation of the hip, a congenital orthopedic defect in which the head of the femur does not articulate with the acetabulum, because of an abnormal shallowness of the acetabulum. Treatment consists of maintaining continuous abduction of the thigh so that the head of the femur presses into the center of the shallow cavity, causing it to deepen. Also called **congenital dysplasia of the hip, congenital subluxation of the hip.** See also **Frejka splint.**

congenital erythropoietic porphyria [L, *congenitus,* born with; Gk, *erythros,* red, *poein,* to make, *porphyros,* purple], a rare autosomal recessive trait caused by a defect in hemoglobin synthesis in erythrocytes and release of porphyrin from normoblasts in the bone marrow. The porphyrin is excreted in the urine. Symptoms may include dermatitis, enlarged spleen, and hemolytic anemia.

congenital facial diplegia. See **Möbius' syndrome.**

congenital glaucoma, a rare form of glaucoma affecting infants and young children, resulting from a congenital closure of the iridocorneal angle by a membrane that obstructs the flow of aqueous humor and increases the intraorbital pressure. The condition is progressive, usually bilateral, and may damage the optic nerve. It may be corrected surgically. Also called **buphthalmos, hydrophthalmos.**

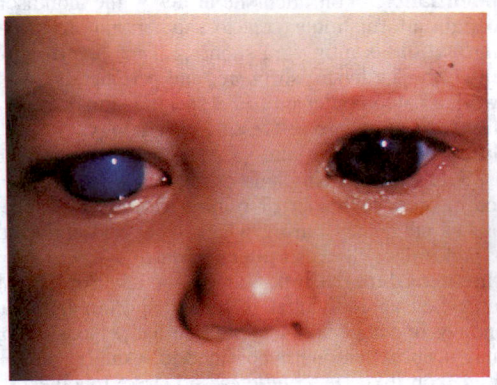

Congenital glaucoma *(Zitelli, 1992)*

congenital goiter, an enlargement of the thyroid gland at birth. It may be caused by a deficiency of enzymes or iodine required for the production of thyroxine.

congenital heart disease. See **congenital cardiac anomaly.**

congenital hernia [L, *congenitus,* born with, *hernia,* rupture], a hernia caused by a defect present at birth, as with an umbilical hernia.

congenital hypogammaglobulinemia [L, *congenitus,* born with; Gk, *hypo,* deficiency, *gamma,* third letter of Greek alphabet; L, *globus,* small globe, *haima,* blood], a genetic disease characterized by a deficiency of gamma globulin and antibody in the serum. The cause may be a genetic defect leading to a failure to develop a normal β-lymphocyte system and immune responses.

congenital hypoplastic anemia. See **Diamond-Blackfan syndrome.**

congenital immunity [L, *congenitus,* born with, *immunis,* free from], the immunity one has at birth that is acquired from the mother's antibodies as they pass through the placenta.

congenital jaundice [L, *congenitus,* born with; Fr, *jaune,* yellow], jaundice found at birth or during the first 24 hours of life. It is usually caused by poorly developed bile ducts.

congenital laryngeal stridor [L, *congenitus,* born with; Gk, *larynx,* L, *stridens,* a grating noise], a harsh respiratory sound that some infants make the first weeks after birth.

congenital megacolon. See **Hirschsprung's disease.**

congenital nonspherocytic hemolytic anemia, a group of blood disorders made up of a number of similar inherited diseases, each with a deficiency of one of the enzymes of red-cell glycolysis. Most are associated with varying degrees of hemolysis, but all are less severe than and are to be differentiated from the more serious disorder associated with spherocytosis. Compare **hemolytic anemia, spherocytic anemia.** See also **elliptocystosis, heme, sickle cell anemia.**

congenital oculofacial paralysis. See **Möbius' syndrome.**

congenital polycystic disease. See **polycystic kidney disease.**

congenital pulmonary arteriovenous fistula, a direct connection between the arterial and venous systems of the lung present at birth that results in a right-to-left shunt and permits unoxygenated blood to enter the systemic circulation. The anomaly is probably caused by faulty development of the network of vessels covering the embryonic lungs and is often accompanied by hereditary hemorrhagic telangiectasis (Rendu-Osler-Weber disease). The fistula may be single or multiple and may occur in any part of the lung; if it is in an accessible site, surgical correction is the method of treatment.

congenital scoliosis, an abnormal condition present at birth, characterized by a lateral curvature of the spine, resulting from specific congenital rib and vertebral anomalies. The etiologic and the pathologic characteristics of congenital scoliosis are divided into six categories. Category I is associated with partial unilateral failure of the formation of a vertebra. Category II is associated with complete unilateral failure of the formation of a vertebra. Category III is associated with bilateral failure of segmentation with the absence of disk space. Category IV is associated with the unilateral failure of segmentation with the unsegmented bar. Category V is associated with the fusion of ribs. Category VI is associated with any condition not covered in the other categories. Category IV scoliosis seems to progress more rapidly and cause the greatest degree of deformity. The degree of obvious deformity caused by congenital scoliosis depends on the cause of the disease. The deformity increases with growth and age, usually progressing slowly during periods of slow growth of the trunk of the body. Diagnosis of the specific congenital anomaly may be confirmed by radiographic examination. The specific rate of progression of many congenital curvatures cannot be predicted. There may be little correlation between the rate of progression and the severity of the curvature at the time of diagnosis. Treatment of congenital scoliosis may be surgical or nonsurgical. Some kinds of nonsurgical treatment techniques are exercise programs and the use of orthotic devices, such as scoliosis splints, a Milwaukee brace, a Risser localizer, or a turnbuckle cast. Surgical intervention in this disease may involve an anterior or a posterior spinal fusion. In a few individuals with this disease, additional procedures, such as spinal osteotomy, Harrington rod, or halo traction, may be required. See also **scoliosis.**

congenital short neck syndrome, a rare congenital malformation of the cervical spine in which the cervical vertebrae are fused, usually in pairs, into one mass of bone, resulting in decreased neck motion and decreased cervical length, sometimes with neurologic involvement. The posterior portion of the laminar arches in the cervical area is not fully developed, resulting in spina bifida in the cervical region, usually involving the lower cervical vertebrae and, in some cases, one or more of the upper thoracic vertebrae. Congenital short neck syndrome is often associated with a cervical rib or with hemivertebrae. Neurologic complica-

tions, such as nerve-root compression and peripheral nerve symptoms, are secondary to deformities of the vertebral bodies. The extreme shortness of the neck is the most common sign of this deformity, which allows only limited motion, lateral bending, and rotation. When the deformity involves nerve-root compression, symptoms of peripheral nerve involvement, as pain or a burning sensation, may be evident, accompanied by paralysis, hyperesthesia, or paresthesia. Involvement of the spinal cord may present signs of abnormalities of lower extremities with associated signs of an upper motor lesion. Congenital short neck syndrome may require no treatment. Mild associated symptoms may be alleviated with traction, cast application, or cervical collars. Surgery may be required to relieve neurologic manifestations. Also called **Klippel-Feil syndrome** /klipel′fel′, klip′əlfil′/.

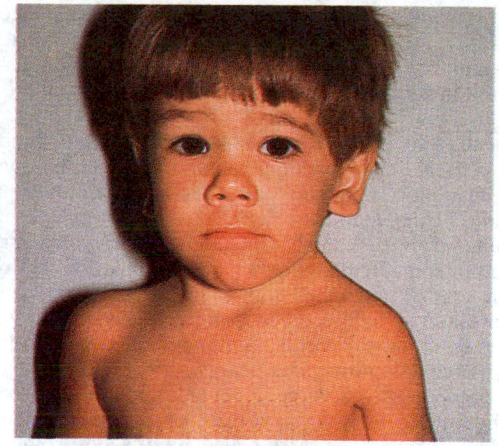

Congenital short neck syndrome (Zitelli, 1992)

congenital subluxation of the hip. See **congenital dislocation of the hip.**

congenital syphilis [L, *congenitus*, born with; Gk, *syn*, together + *philein*, to love], a form of syphilis acquired *in utero* and generally characterized by osteitis, rashes, coryza, and wasting in the first months of life. Later childhood signs of the infection include interstitial keratitis, deafness, and notches in the incisor teeth. Some infected infants may appear disease-free at birth but develop typical signs of the disease in adolescence. Infants are treated with penicillin; all infected infants require an ophthalmic examination. If left untreated, the infection may result in deafness, blindness, crippling or death.

congestion /kənjes′chən/ [L, *congerere*, to accumulate], abnormal accumulation of fluid in an organ or body area. The fluid is often blood, but it may be bile or mucus.

congestive atelectasis /kənjes′tiv/ [L, *congerere* + Gk, *ateles*, incomplete, *ektasis*, stretching], severe pulmonary congestion characterized by diffuse injury to alveolar-capillary membranes, resulting in hemorrhagic edema, stiffness of the lungs, difficult ventilation, and respiratory failure. Fulminating sepsis, especially when gram-negative organisms are involved, is the most common cause, but congestive atelectasis may occur after trauma, near drowning, aspiration of gastric acid, paraquat ingestion, inhalation of corrosive chemicals, such as chlorine, ammonia, or phosgene, or the use of certain drugs, including barbiturates, chlordiazepoxide, heroin, methadone, propoxyphene, and salicylates. This serious pulmonary disorder may also be caused by diabetic ketoacidosis, fungal infections, high altitudes, pancreatitis, tuberculosis, and uremia. Management of congestive atelectasis consists of treatment of the underlying cause, frequent changes of the patient's position to promote drainage, careful dehydration, assistance with ventilation, and the use of bronchodilators and steroids. Also called **adult respiratory distress syndrome, hemorrhagic lung, pump lung, stiff lung, wet lung.**

congestive cardiomyopathy [L, *congerere,* to heap together; Gk, *kardia,* heart, *mys,* muscle, *pathos,* disease], a heart muscle disease characterized by heart failure and enlargement.

congestive dysmenorrhea [L, *congerere,* to heap together; Gk, *dys,* difficult, *mens,* month, *rhein,* to flow], a form of secondary dysmenorrhea caused by pelvic congestion, arising in turn from an increased blood supply in the area due to a pelvic disease.

congestive heart failure (CHF), an abnormal condition that reflects impaired cardiac pumping, caused by myocardial infarction, ischemic heart disease, or cardiomyopathy. Failure of the ventricle to eject blood efficiently results in volume overload, chamber dilatation, and elevated intracardiac pressure. Retrograde transmission of increased hydrostatic pressure from the left heart causes pulmonary congestion; elevated right heart pressure causes systemic venous congestion and peripheral edema. See also **heart failure.**

congestive splenomegalia [L, *congerere,* to heap together; Gk, *splen* + *megas,* large], an enlarged spleen associated with gastric hemorrhages, anemia, portal hypertension, and cirrhosis of the liver. Also called **Banti's syndrome, congestive splenomegaly, hepatolienal fibrosis.**

conglomerate silicosis /kənglom′ərit/ [L, *con* + *glomerare,* to wind into a ball], a severe form of silicosis marked by conglomerate masses of mineral dust in the lungs, causing acute shortness of breath, coughing, and production of sputum. The conglomerates may encroach on the pulmonary circulation, causing pulmonary hypertension, right ventricular hypertrophy, and complete disability. The patient usually develops cor pulmonale.

Congolese red fever. See **murine typhus.**

Congress for Nursing Practice, a unit of the American Nurses Association whose activities concern the scope of nursing practice, legal aspects of nursing practice, public recognition of the significance of nursing practice in health care, and implications of health care trends for nursing practice.

congruent communication /kong′grōō·ənt/, a communication pattern in which the person sends the same message on both verbal and nonverbal levels.

-conia, a suffix meaning 'small particles in the (specified) fluid or part of the body': *chondroconia, otoconia, statoconia.*

conic. See **cone.**

conical. See **cone.**

conic papilla. See **papilla.**

conization /kon′īzā′shən/, the removal of a cone-shaped sample of tissue, as in a cone biopsy.

conjoined manipulation /kənjoind′/ [L, *con* + *jungere,* to join], the use of both hands in obstetric and gynecologic procedures, with one positioned in the vagina and the other on the abdomen.

conjoined tendon. See **inguinal falx.**

conjoined twins, two fetuses developed from the same ovum who are physically united at birth. The defect ranges from a superficial anatomic union of varying extent between equally or nearly equally formed fetuses to one in which only a part of the body is duplicated or in which a small, incompletely developed fetus, or parasite, is attached to a more fully formed one, the autosite. Conjoined twins result when separation of the blastomeres in early embryonic development does not occur until a late cleavage phase and is incomplete, causing the fused condition. Viability depends on the extent of the fusion and the degree of development of the fetuses. See also **Siamese twins.**

conjoint family therapy, /kənjoint/ a form of psychotherapy in which a single nuclear family is seen, and the issues and problems raised by family members are addressed by the therapist.

conjugate /kon′jəgit/ [L, *con* + *jungere,* to join], (in pelvimetry) the measurement of the female pelvis to determine whether the presenting part of a fetus can enter the birth canal. See also **diagonal conjugate, true conjugate.**

conjugated estrogen /kon′jəgā′tid/, a mixture of sodium salts of estrogen sulfates, chiefly those of estrone, equilin, and 17-alpha-dihydroequilin, blended to approximate the average composition of estrogenic substances in the urine of pregnant mares. Conjugated estrogens may be prescribed to relieve postmenopausal vasomotor symptoms, as hot flushes, for the treatment of atrophic vaginitis, female hypogonadism, primary ovarian failure, and palliation in advanced prostatic carcinoma and metastatic breast cancer in selected patients. The drug, in conjunction with other therapeutic measures, may also retard the progress of postmenopausal osteoporosis. Continued use of estrogens increases the risk of endometrial carcinoma, gallbladder disease, and thromboembolic disorders; because of the danger of damage to the fetus, all female sex hormones are contraindicated during pregnancy. Among the adverse effects of conjugated estrogens are breakthrough bleeding, breast tenderness, nausea, headache, water retention, and acneiform skin eruptions.

conjugate deviation [L, *conjugere,* to yoke together, *deviare,* to turn aside], pertaining to movements of the two eyes in which their visual axes function in parallel. The cause is a dysfunction of the ocular muscles, allowing the eyes to diverge to the same side when at rest.

conjugated protein, a compound that contains a protein molecule united to a nonprotein substance.

conjugate paralysis [L, *conjugere,* to yoke together; Gk, *paralyein,* to be palsied], a condition of paralysis of the conjugate movements of the two eyes, up or down, or to the right or left. There is no diplopia. The cause is a cranial nerve lesion.

conjugation /kon′jəgā′shən/, (in genetics) a form of sexual reproduction in unicellular organisms in which the gametes temporarily fuse so that genetic material can transfer from the donor male to the recipient female, where it is incorporated, recombined, and then passed on to the progeny through replication.

conjugon /kon′jōōgon/, an episome that induces bacterial conjugation.

conjunctiva /kon′jungktī′və/ [L, *conjunctivus,* connecting], the mucous membrane lining the inner surfaces of the eyelids and anterior part of the sclera. The **palpebral conjunctiva** lines the inner surface of the eyelids and is thick, opaque, and highly vascular. The **bulbar conjunctiva** is loosely connected, thin, and transparent, covering the sclera of the anterior third of the eye.

conjunctival burns /-ī·vəl/, chemical burns of the conjunctiva. Emergency treatment involves irrigating the eye with copious amounts of water for as long as 30 minutes or until the chemical has been neutralized, as indicated by paper pH indicators. An anesthetic may be instilled to relieve pain. The injured eye should be examined and treated by an ophthalmologist to prevent complications.

conjunctival edema. See **chemosis.**

conjunctival fornix. See **inferior conjunctival fornix, superior conjunctival fornix.**

conjunctival reflex, a protective mechanism for the eye in which the eyelids close whenever the conjunctiva is touched. Compare **corneal reflex.**

conjunctival sac [L, *conjunctivus,* connecting; Gk, *sakkos*], the space enclosed by the conjunctiva and the eyelids.

conjunctival test, a procedure used to identify offending allergens by instilling the eye with a dilute solution of the allergenic extract. A positive reaction in the allergic patient causes tearing and redness of the conjunctiva within 5 to 15 minutes. See also **allergy testing.**

conjunctivitis /kənjungk′tivī′tis/, inflammation of the conjunctiva, caused by bacterial or viral infection, allergy, or environmental factors. Red eyes, a thick discharge, sticky eyelids in the morning, and inflammation without pain are characteristic. The cause may be found by microscopic examination or bacteriologic culture of a specimen of the discharge. Choice of treatment depends on the causative agent and may include antibacterial agents, antibiotics, or corticosteroids. Also called **pinkeye.** See also **choroiditis, uveitis.**

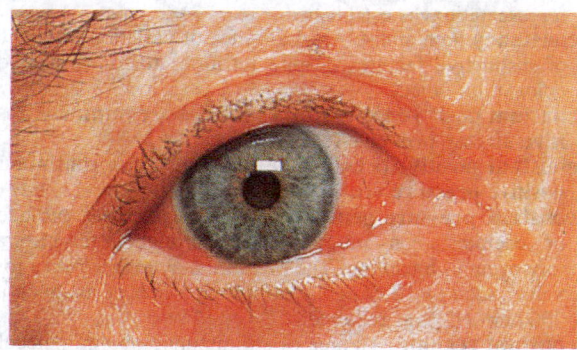

Conjunctivitis *(Kamal, 1991)*

conjunctivitis of newborn [L, *conjunctivus,* connecting; *itis,* inflammation; ME, *newe, borne*], a condition characterized by a purulent discharge from the eyes of an infant during the first three weeks of life. A frequent cause is a gonococcal infection, which may lead to blindness if untreated. Also called **ophthalmia neonatorum.**

connecting fibrocartilage [L, *con + nectere,* to bind], a disk of fibrocartilage found between many joints, especially those with limited mobility, such as the spinal vertebrae. Each disk is composed of concentric rings of fibrous tissue

separated by cartilaginous laminae. The disk swells outward if it is compressed by the vertebrae above or below. Compare **circumferential fibrocartilage, interarticular fibrocartilage, stratiform fibrocartilage.**

connective /kənek′tiv/ [L, *cum,* with, *nectere,* to bind], pertaining to a binding or connection.

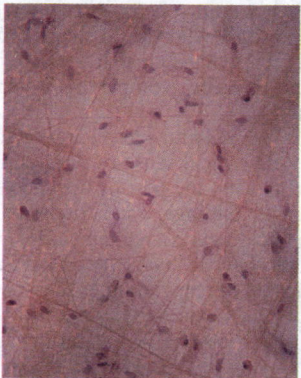

Loose connective tissue
(Raven, 1992/Trent Stephens)

connective tissue, tissue that supports and binds other body tissue and parts. It derives from the mesoderm of the embryo and is dense, containing large numbers of cells and large amounts of intercellular material. The intercellular material is composed of fibers in a matrix or ground substance that may be liquid, gelatinous, or solid, such as in bone and cartilage. Connective tissue fibers may be collagenous or elastic. The matrix or ground material surrounding fibers and cells is a dynamic substance, susceptible to its own special diseases. Kinds of connective tissue are **bone, cartilage, fibrous,** and loose **connective tissue.**

connective tissue disease. See **collagen vascular disease.**

Conn's syndrome [Jerome W. Conn, American physician, b. 1907, Gk, *syn,* together, *dromos,* course], primary hyperaldosteronism, characterized by excessive secretion of aldosterone with symptoms of headache, fatigue, nocturia,

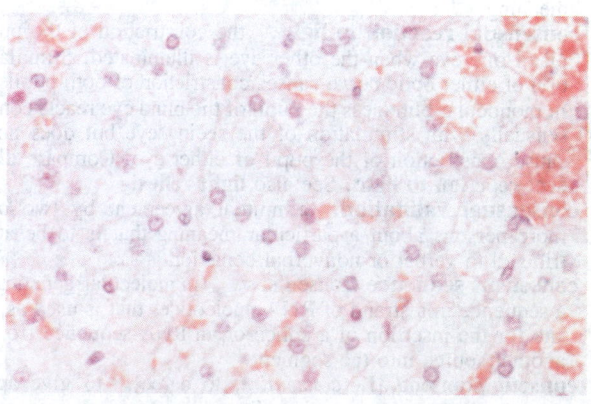

Conn's syndrome *(Swales, 1991)*

and polyuria. The patient may also experience hypertension, hypokalemic alkalosis potassium depletion, and hypervolemia.

Conor's disease. See **Marseilles fever.**

Conradi's disease. See **chondrodystrophia calcificans congenita.**

consanguinity /kon'sang·gwin'itē/ [L, *con* + *sanguis,* blood], a hereditary or "blood" relationship between persons, by having a common parent or ancestor. In unions between first cousins, who would share 12.5% of the same genes, it has been calculated that the risk of an abnormal offspring is less than 3%, compared with about 2% for unrelated parents.

conscience [L, *conscientia,* to be privy to information], **1.** the moral, self-critical sense of what is right and wrong. **2.** (in psychoanalysis) the part of the superego system that monitors thoughts, feelings, and actions and measures them against internalized values and standards.

conscious /kon'shəs/ [L, *conscire,* to be aware], **1.** (in neurology) capable of responding to sensory stimuli; awake, alert; aware of one's external environment. **2.** (in psychiatry) that part of the psyche or mental functioning in which thoughts, ideas, emotions, and other mental content are in complete awareness. Compare **preconscious, unconscious.**

consciousness /kon'shəsnes/, a clear state of awareness of self and the environment in which attention is focused on immediate matters, as distinguished from mental activity of an unconscious or subconscious nature.

conscious proprioception, the conscious awareness of body position and movement of bodily segments. It is regulated by the lemniscal system through pathways that begin in joint receptors and end in the parietal lobe of the cerebral cortex; it enables the cortex to refine voluntary movements.

conscious sedation. See **awake anesthesia.**

consensual /konsen'choo·əl/ [L, *con* + *sentire,* to feel], pertaining to a reflex action in which stimulation of one part of the body results in a response in another part.

consensual light reflex, a normally present crossed reflex in which light directed at one eye causes the opposite pupil to contract. In monocular blindness the pupil of the blind eye reacts consensually with stimulation of the seeing eye but does not cause constriction of the pupil of either eye. Also called **consensual reaction to light.** See also **light reflex.** Compare **direct reaction to light.**

consensually validated symbols, symbols that are accepted by enough people that they have an agreed-upon meaning.

consensual reaction to light, the constriction of the pupil of one eye when the other eye is illuminated. Stimulation of either optic nerve causes constriction of both pupils. In monocular blindness the pupil of the blind eye reacts consensually with stimulation of the seeing eye but does not cause constriction of the pupil of either eye. Compare **direct reaction to light.** See also **light reflex.**

consensual validation, a mutual agreement by two or more persons about a particular meaning that is to be attributed to verbal or nonverbal behavior.

consensus sequence /kənsen'səs/, (in molecular genetics) a sequence in a strand of RNA nucleotides that is used as a site for the insertion of a splice of an RNA sequence from another source into the segment.

consent /kənsent/ [L, *consentire,* to agree], to give approval, assent, or permission. See also **informed consent.**

consenting adult, an adult who willingly agrees to participate in an activity with one or more other adults. The term is usually applied to sexual activity.

consequences /kon'səkwen'səs/, stimulus events following a behavior that strengthen or weaken the behavior. They may be either reinforcers or punishers.

conservation of energy /kon'sərvā'shən/ [L, *conservare,* to preserve], (in physics) a law stating that in any closed system the total amount of energy is constant.

conservation of matter, (in physics) a law stating that matter can neither be created nor destroyed and that the amount of matter in the universe is finite. Also called **conservation of mass.** See also **conservation of energy.**

conservation principles of nursing, a conceptual framework for nursing that is directed toward maintaining the wholeness or integrity of the patient when the normal ability to cope is disturbed or exceeded by stress. Nursing intervention is determined by the patient's need to conserve energy and to maintain structural, personal, and social integrity. The patient is perceived as a person whose wholeness is threatened by stress. Subjective and objective indicators of stress are assessed by the nurse, the stimuli for the stress are identified, and the level of integrity in each area is evaluated. The nurse acts as a "conservationist."

conservative treatment. See **treatment.**

consolidation /kənsol'idā'shən/ [L, *consolidare,* to make solid], **1.** the combining of separate parts into a single whole. **2.** a state of solidification. **3.** (in medicine) the process of becoming solid, as when the lungs become firm and inelastic in pneumonia.

consolidation of individuality and emotional constancy, (in psychiatry) the fourth and final subphase in Mahler's system of the separation-individuation phase of preoedipal development. It begins toward the end of the second year and is seen as open ended. A degree of object constancy is accomplished, and separation of self and object representations is established.

constancy /kon'stənsē/, an absence of variation in quality of distinctive features despite location, rotation, size, or color of an object.

constant positive airway pressure. See **continuous positive airway pressure (CPAP).**

constant positive pressure ventilation. See **continuous positive pressure ventilation (CPPV).**

constant pressure generator, a generator that provides or generates a constant gas pressure throughout the inspiratory cycle of breathing. The pressure may range from a low value, such as 12 cm H_2O, to a high value of as much as 3500 cm H_2O, as required.

constant region, an area of an immunoglobulin molecule in which the amino acid sequence is relatively constant. See also **variable region.**

constant touch, a technique to diagnose the sensibility of an injured body part, such as a hand, by pressing the eraser end of a pencil or another object in various areas to determine the ability of the person to detect the pressure.

constipation /kon'stipā'shən/ [L, *constipare,* to crowd together], **1.** difficulty in passing stools or an incomplete or infrequent passage of hard stools. There are many causes, both organic and functional. Among the organic causes are intestinal obstruction, diverticulitis, and tumors. Functional impairment of the colon may occur in elderly or bedridden patients who fail to respond to the urge to defecate. For constipation that is not organically caused, the nurse can encourage a liberal diet of fruits, vegetables, and plenty of water. The patient should be encouraged to exercise moderately, if possible, and to develop regular, unhurried bowel habits. **2.** a nursing diagnosis accepted by the Fourth National Conference on the Classification of Nursing Diagnoses. The cause of the condition, developed at the Fifth National Conference, is less than adequate intake and bulk, less than adequate physical activity, a side effect of medications, chronic use of medications and enemas, GI obstructive lesions, neuromuscular or musculoskeletal impairment, weak abdominal musculature, pain on defecation, diagnostic procedures, lack of privacy for personal habits, pregnancy, or emotional stature. The defining characteristics include decreased frequency of elimination; a hard, formed stool; a palpable rectal mass; straining at stool; decreased bowel sounds; reported feeling of abdominal or rectal fullness or pressure; less than useful amount of stool; and nausea. Abdominal pain, appetite impairment, back pain, headache, and interference with daily living may also be present. See also **atonia constipation, nursing diagnosis. —constipated,** *adj.*

constipation, colonic, a nursing diagnosis accepted by the Eighth National Conference on the Classification of Nursing Diagnoses. Colonic constipation is a state in which an individual's pattern of elimination is characterized by hard, dry stool that results from a delay in passage of food residue. Major defining characteristics are decreased frequency, hard dry stool, straining at stool, painful defecation, abdominal distention, and a palpable mass. Minor characteristics are rectal pressure, headache, appetite impairment, and abdominal pain. Related factors are less than adequate fluid intake or dietary intake; less than adequate fiber; less than adequate physical activity; immobility; lack of privacy; emotional disturbance; chronic use of medication and enemas; stress; change in daily routine; and metabolic problems, such as hypothyroidism, hypocalcemia, and hypokalemia. See also **nursing diagnosis.**

constipation, perceived, a nursing diagnosis accepted by the Eighth National Conference on the Classification of Nursing Diagnoses. Perceived constipation is a state in which an individual makes a self-diagnosis of constipation and ensures a daily bowel movment through use of laxatives, enemas, and suppositories. The defining characteristic is an expectation of a daily bowel movment, which may be expected at the same time every day, with the resulting overuse of laxatives, enemas, and suppositories. Related factors are cultural and family health beliefs, faulty appraisal, and impaired thought processes. See also **nursing diagnosis.**

constipation, rectal, a nursing diagnosis accepted by the Eighth National Conference on the Classification of Nursing Diagnoses. Rectal constipation is a state in which an individual's pattern of elimination is characterized by stool retention, normal stool consistency, and delayed elimination that results from biopsychosocial disruptions. There is also abdominal discomfort, rectal fullness, and a change in flatus. Related factors are weak plevis floor muscles; painful anorectal lesions; self-care deficits; environmental constraints; altered mobility; low or no social support; impaired communication; altered awareness; and emotional disturbances. See also **nursing diagnosis.**

constitutional delay /kon′stityōō′shənəl/ [L, *constituere,* to establish], a period in the development of a child during which growth may be interrupted. In some cases constitutional delay may be associated with an illness or stressful event, and growth resumes later. The lost growth may or may not be regained. A form of constitutional delay is associated with some types of dwarfism.

constitutional disease [L, *constituere,* to set up; Gk, *dis,* without; Fr, *aise,* ease], any disease associated with the inborn physical condition of the client, such as a hereditary susceptibility.

constitutional psychology, the study of the relationship of individual psychologic makeup to body morphology and organic functioning.

constitutional symptom. See **symptom.**

constitutive resistance /kənstich′ōōtiv/, the bacterial resistance to antibiotics that is contained in the DNA molecules of the organism. The trait can be passed on to daughter cells through cell division, but it cannot be transmitted to other species of bacteria.

constriction /kənstrik′shən/ [L, *constringere,* to draw tight], an abnormal closing or reduction in the size of an opening or passage of the body, as in vasoconstriction of a blood vessel. See also **stenosis.**

constriction ring, a band of contracted uterine muscle that forms a stricture around part of the fetus during labor, usually after premature rupture of the membranes and sometimes impeding labor. The uterine wall is thickened in the zone of the ring and is not prone to rupture. Compare **pathologic retraction ring.**

constrictive cardiomyopathy /kənstrik′tiv/ [L, *constringere,* to draw tight; Gk, *kardia,* heart, *mys,* muscle, *pathos,* disease], a heart disorder in which there is decreased diastolic compliance of the ventricles, imitating constrictive pericarditis. Also called **restrictive cardiomyopathy.**

constrictive pericarditis, a fibrous thickening of the pericardium caused by gradual scarring or fibrosis of the membrane, which may also undergo calcification. The pericardium gradually becomes a rigid membrane that resists the normal dilation of the heart chambers during the blood-filling phases of the cardiac cycle.

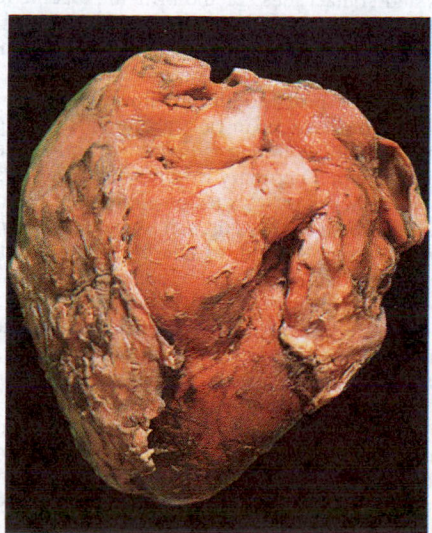

Constrictive pericarditis (Fletcher, 1987)

constrictor /kənstrik'tər/, a muscle that causes a narrowing of an opening, as the ciliary body fibers that control the size of the pupil.

constructional apraxia /kənstruk'shənəl/ [L, *construere,* to build], a form of apraxia characterized by the inability to copy drawings or to manipulate objects to form patterns or designs. It is caused by a right hemisphere lesion. The deficit is tested by asking the patient to copy two-dimensional geometric patterns, such as circles, squares, diamonds, and hexagons, and to copy three-dimensional structures constructed of 1-inch building blocks.

constructive aggression /kənstruk'tiv/, an act of self-assertiveness in response to a threatening action for purposes of self-protection and preservation. See also **aggression.**

constructive interference, (in ultrasonography) an increase in amplitude of sound waves that results when multiple waves of equal frequency are transmitted precisely in phase.

construct validity /kon'strakt/, validity of a test or a measurement tool that is established by demonstrating its ability to identify the variables that it proposes to identify. See also **validity.**

consultant /kənsul'tənt/ [L, *consultare,* to deliberate], a person who by training and experience has acquired a special knowledge in a subject area which has been recognized by a peer group.

consultation /kon'səltā'shən/ [L, *consultare,* to deliberate], a process in which the help of a specialist is sought to identify ways to handle problems in patient management or in the planning and implementation of health care programs.

consultee-centered communication /kon'sultē'/, expert advice or guidance that is given a consultee (health care worker) to improve the consultee's capacity to function more effectively in working with patients.

consumption, an obsolete term for tuberculosis.

consumption coagulopathy. See **disseminated intravascular coagulation (DIC).**

contact [L, *contingere,* to touch], **1.** the touching or bringing together of two surfaces, as those of upper and lower teeth. The term is often used attributively, as in contact dermatitis and contact lens. **2.** the bringing together either directly or indirectly, as through the handling of food or clothing, of two individuals so as to allow the transmission of an infectious organism from one to the other. **3.** a person who has been exposed to an infectious disease.

contact dermatitis, skin rash resulting from exposure to a primary irritant or to a sensitizing antigen. In the first, or nonallergic, type, a primary irritant, such as an alkaline detergent or an acid, causes a lesion similar to a thermal burn. Emergency treatment is to drench liberally and immediately with water. In the second, or allergic, type, sensitizing antigens result in an immunologic change in certain lymphocytes. Subsequent exposure to the antigen causes the lymphocytes to release irritating chemicals leading to inflammation, edema, and vesiculation. Poison ivy and nickel dermatitis are common examples of this delayed hypersensitivity reaction. The diagnosis can be aided by patch testing with suspected antigens. Treatment includes avoidance of the irritant or sensitizer, administration of topical corticosteroid preparations, and soothing or drying lotions. In severe cases, systemic corticosteroids may be used. Also called **dermatitis venenata.** Compare **atopic dermatitis.** See also **hypersensitivity reaction.**

contact factor. See **factor XII.**

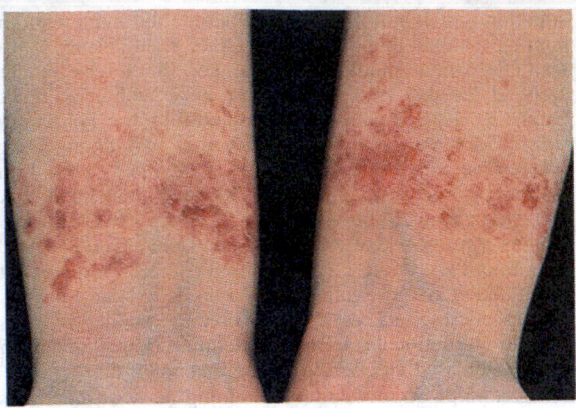

Contact dermatitis (Cerio, 1992)

contact lens, a small, curved, glass or plastic lens shaped to fit the person's eye and to correct refraction. Contact lenses float on the precorneal tear film and must be inserted, removed, cleaned, and stored as directed to avoid damage or infection to the eyes.

contactor /kəntak'tər/, a switching device that is part of the timer for the control of voltage across an x-ray tube.

contact shield, a protective device constructed of metal or other material that is positioned directly over the eyes or gonads of a patient to be exposed to an x-ray beam.

contagion /kəntā'jən/ [L, *contingere,* to touch], the transmission of a disease by direct contact with a person who has the disease or by indirect contact through handling of clothing, bedding, dishes, or other objects the person has used.

contagious /kəntā'jəs/ [L, *contingere,* to touch], communicable, such as a disease that may be transmitted by direct or indirect contact. **–contagion,** *n.*

contagious disease. See **communicable disease.**

contagious pustular dermatitis [L, *contingere,* to touch, *pustula,* pustules; Gk, *derma,* skin, *itis,* inflammation], a skin disease normally affecting sheep but transmitted to humans who handle infected animals. It is caused by a pox virus and results in lesions on the hands, and occasionally on the face. The lesions resolve spontaneously, but slowly. Also called **orf.**

contaminant /kəntaminənt/ [L, *contaminare,* to bring in contact], an agent that causes contamination, pollution, or spoilage, such as a mold spore making food unsafe to eat.

contamination /-ā'shən/ [L, *contaminare,* to pollute], a condition of being soiled, stained, touched, or otherwise exposed to harmful agents, such as by entry of infectious or toxic materials into a previously clean or sterile environment, making an object potentially unsafe for use as intended or without barrier techniques.

content theme. See **communication theme.**

content validity, validity of a test or a measurement as a result of the use of previously tested items or concepts within the tool. See also **validity.**

context [L, *contexere,* to weave together], (in communications theory) the setting, meaning, and language of a message. If a message is interpreted without strict regard for these limits, it will be taken out of context.

continence /kon'tinəns/ [L, *continere,* to contain], **1.** the ability to control bladder or bowel function. **2.** the use of self-restraint, particularly in regard to sexual intercourse.

continent ileostomy /kon′tinənt/, an ileostomy that drains into a surgically created pouch or reservoir in the abdomen. Involuntary discharge of intestinal contents is prevented by a nipple valve created from the ileum.

■ METHOD: After surgery, the pouch is kept relatively empty by means of a catheter placed in it at surgery. It is removed a week or two afterward, depending on the status of intestinal function and wound healing. Once the indwelling catheter is removed, the pouch is drained by periodically inserting a catheter through the stoma into the pouch through the valve. The length of time allowed to elapse between catheterizations is gradually lengthened as the capacity of the pouch increases to between 500 and 1000 ml. Six months after surgery, drainage may be necessary only 3 or 4 times a day. The patient learns to recognize a feeling of fullness that indicates the need for drainage. When the patient is seated on the toilet, the dressing over the stoma is removed, and the tip of a French size 28 to 32 catheter is lubricated and inserted into the stoma. The distal end of the catheter is in a receptacle or in the toilet, at least 30 cm below the stoma. The lubricated tip of the catheter is advanced carefully through the stoma. Resistance is usually felt at a depth of about 5 cm where the valve covers the opening to the pouch. Flow usually begins when the tip of the catheter has passed the valve, at a distance of approximately 7.5 cm from the stoma. Drainage may take up to 15 minutes to complete.

■ INTERVENTIONS: After surgery, the patient is usually instructed to add foods one at a time. High-fiber foods and those that cause gas formation are particularly likely to be problematic. Thick secretions may be thinned by the injection of a little water into the pouch through the catheter. The stoma may be covered with a 3-inch square cut from a disposable diaper. It is important to teach the patient to avoid irritation of the skin around the stoma. Nonallergenic tape may be used to hold the pad in place. After healing, if there is no danger of a blow to the abdomen, a pad is often not necessary. After surgery, activity is resumed as the patient is able. There is no reason for activity to be curtailed once healing is complete and the person feels well.

■ OUTCOME CRITERIA: The patient may expect to be able to care for the stoma and to manage the drainage of the pouch before discharge from the hospital. A continent ileostomy has several advantages, including the avoidance of unpleasant odors, and the convenience of not having to use a colostomy or ileostomy bag.

continua. See **continuum.**

contingency contracting /kəntin′jənsē/ [L, *contingere,* to touch], a formal agreement between a psychotherapist and a patient undergoing behavior therapy regarding the consequences of certain actions by both parties.

contingency management, any of a group of techniques used in behavior therapy that attempts to modify a behavioral response by controlling the consequences of that response. Kinds of contingency management include **contingency contracting, shaping,** and **token economy.**

continuing care nurse /kəntin′yo͞o·ing/, [L, *continuare,* to unite], a nurse specializing in coordination of the overall needs of the patient with the potential health care resources of the community. Much of the emphasis is on discharge planning and assessment of the availability of participation in the patient's care after discharge by members of the fam-

ily or other parties. Continuing care nursing responsibilities and discharge planning ideally begin at the time a patient is admitted to a hospital.

continuing education, (in nursing) formal, organized, educational programs designed to promote the knowledge, skills, and professional attitudes of nurses. The programs are usually short-term and specific; a certificate may be offered for completion of a course, and a number of continuing education units (CEUs) may be conferred. Continuing education is required for relicensure in many states. It is not to be confused with academic, degree-granting programs, such as advanced education or graduate education.

continuing education unit (CEU), a point awarded to a professional person by a professional organization for having attended an educational program relevant to the goals of the organization. A value is established for the course and that number of points is given. Many states require professionals in the various fields of medicine and nursing to obtain a specific number of CEUs annually for relicensure.

continuity theory /kon′tinyo͞o′itē/, a concept that an individual's personality does not change as the person ages, with the result that his or her behavior becomes more predictable.

continuous ambulatory peritoneal dialysis (CAPD) /kəntin′yo͞o·əs/ [L, *continuare,* to join on, *ambulare,* to walk about; Gk, *peri,* near, *tenein,* to stretch, *dia,* through, *lysis,* loosening], a maintenance system of peritoneal dialysis in which an indwelling catheter permits fluid to drain into and out of the peritoneal cavity by gravity.

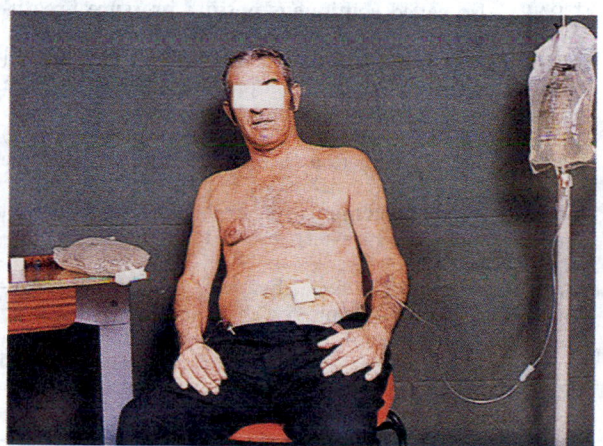

Continuous ambulatory peritoneal dialysis
(Bodansky, 1989/Courtesy Dr. EJ Will, Leeds)

continuous anesthesia [L, *continuare,* to unite], a method for maintaining regional nerve block in anesthesia for surgical operations or labor in which an anesthetic solution drips either at intervals or at a low rate of flow. The procedure is named according to the area infiltrated: continuous spinal, caudal, epidural, peridural, or lumbar. Also called **fractional anesthesia.**

continuous bath. See **continuous tub bath.**

continuous cycling peritoneal dialysis (CCPD), a type of dialysis in which the patient is attached to an automatic cycler for short exchanges while sleeping at night. Mobility is not feasible because of the cumbersome equipment.

During waking hours, the patient receives long dialysis exchanges but has ambulatory freedom.

continuous fever, a fever that persists steadily for a prolonged period of time. Compare **intermittent fever.**

continuous murmur [L, *continuare*, to join on, *murmur*, humming], a heart or venous murmur that characteristically begins in systole and spills into diastole. The cause may be a patent ductus arteriosus.

continuous negative chest wall pressure, a negative pressure (below ambient pressure) that is applied to the chest wall during the entire respiratory cycle, thus providing increased transpulmonary pressure.

continuous passive motion (CPM), a technique for maintaining or increasing the amount of movement in a joint with the use of a mechanical device that applies force to bring about motion in a joint without normal musle function.

continuous phase [L, *continuare*, to join on, Gk, *phasis*, appearance], the phase of a colloidal solution corresponding to that of the solvent of a true solution. Also called **external phase, dispersion medium.**

continuous positive airway pressure (CPAP), (in respiratory therapy) ventilation assisted by a flow of air delivered at a constant pressure throughout the respiratory cycle. It is performed for patients who can initiate their own respirations but who are not able to maintain adequate arterial oxygen levels without assistance. CPAP may be given through a ventilator and endotracheal tube, through a nasal cannula, or into a hood over the patient's head. Respiratory distress syndrome in the newborn is often treated with CPAP. Also called **continuous positive pressure breathing (CPPB).** Compare **positive end expiratory pressure.**

continuous positive pressure ventilation (CPPV), a positive pressure above ambient pressure maintained at the upper airway throughout the breathing cycle. The term is usually applied to positive end expiratory pressure (PEEP) and mechanical ventilation. See also **continuous positive airway pressure.**

continuous reinforcement, a schedule of reinforcement in which omission of a response is followed by the reinforcer.

continuous tremor, fine, rhythmic, purposeless movements that persist during rest but sometimes disappear briefly during voluntary movements. The pill-rolling movements and trembling seen in Parkinson's disease are typical of continuous tremors. Also called **resting tremor.** Compare **intention tremor.** See also **tremor.**

continuous tub bath, a therapeutic bath, usually prescribed in the treatment of some dermatologic conditions, in which the patient lies supported in a medicated solution of tepid water.
■ METHOD: The bath is prepared as for a medicated tub bath. The patient is immersed in the water, and a towel saturated with the solution is placed over the torso. The patient may wear a loin cloth, and a harness is fitted comfortably around the chest and under the shoulders and head to hold the head safely out of the water as the patient sleeps or dozes. A pillow or folded towel is placed over the wide supporting straps under the head and neck to add to the patient's comfort. A board is placed on top of the tub from the patient's shoulders to the end of the tub, and a sheet is draped over it. A bell for calling for assistance, a container of drinking water with a flexible straw, and any other materials that may be needed are placed on the board.

■ NURSING INTERVENTION: The method and the reason for the treatment are explained to the patient. Privacy is maintained; close supervision by a nurse is available throughout the treatment. The procedure is psychologically trying and may be physically unpleasant for the patient. Psychosocial support and attention to making the patient as comfortable as possible improves the patient's tolerance for the procedure.
■ OUTCOME CRITERIA: The patient is observed for any febrile reaction, rapid or weak pulse, faintness, or increased severity of symptoms, as itching, burning, or pain. The solution is changed completely every 4 hours, the linen is changed twice a day, and the harness is changed once a day.

continuum /kəntin′yoo·əm/, *pl.* **continua,** 1. a continuous series or whole. 2. (in mathematics) a system of real numbers.

contoured adducted trochanteric controlled alignment method /kon′tŏord/ **(CAT-CAM),** a design for an artificial lower limb for persons who have undergone above the knee (AK) amputations.

contra-, a prefix meaning 'against': *contraception, contralateral, contraparetic.*

contra bevel [L, *contra*, against; OFr, *baif*, open mouth], 1. also called **reverse bevel.** (in dentistry) the angle between a cutting blade and the base of the periodontal pocket when the blade is held so that it separates the sulcular epithelium from the external epithelium of the gingiva. 2. (in dentistry) an external bevel of a tooth preparation extending onto a buccal or lingual cusp from an intracoronal restoration.

contraception /kon′trəsep′shən/ [L, *contra + concipere*, to take in], a process or technique for the prevention of pregnancy by means of a medication, device, or method that blocks or alters one or more of the processes of reproduction in such a way that sexual union can occur without impregnation. Kinds of contraception include **cervical cap, condom, contraceptive diaphragm, intrauterine device, natural family-planning method, oral contraceptive, spermicide,** and **sterilization.** Also called **birth control, conception control, family planning.** See also **basal-body-temperature method of family planning; Norplant; planned parenthood.**

contraceptive /kon′trəsep′tiv/, [L, *contra + concipere*, to take in], any device or technique that prevents conception. (Table pp. 389-390) See also **contraception.**

contraceptive diaphragm a contraceptive device consisting of a hemisphere of thin rubber bonded to a flexible ring, inserted in the vagina together with spermicidal jelly or cream up to 2 hours before coitus. Fitted between the pubic symphysis and the posterior fornix of the vagina, the diaphragm cups the cervix in a pool of spermacide so that spermatozoa cannot enter the uterus, thus preventing conception. The rate of failure of the diaphragm method of contraception is approximately 5 to 10 unplanned pregnancies in 100 women using the method properly for 1 year. The principal advantage of the diaphragm are that it has no systemic effects. The most often reported disadvantages are that it is messy, that it is uncomfortable for some people, and that insertion may interfere with spontaneity or continuity in making love. Diaphragms are manufactured in seven standard sizes from 60 mm to 90 mm in diameter. Kinds of diaphragms are **arcing spring, coil spring,** and **flat spring.** Also called **diaphragm.**

contraceptive diaphragm fitting, a procedure, performed in an office or clinic, in which a contraceptive dia-

Methods of contraception*

Device/method	Action	Failure rates	Advantages	Disadvantages
Intrauterine devices (Paragard Copper T380A, Progestasert)	Small plastic or metal devices placed in the uterus that somehow prevent fertilization or implantation; some contain copper, others release hormones	1-5	Convenient, highly effective, need to be replaced infrequently	Can cause excess menstrual bleeding and pain; danger of perforation, infection, and expulsion; not recommended for those who are childless or not monogamous, risk of pelvic inflammatory disease or infertility; dangerous in pregnancy
Oral contraceptives	Hormones, either in combination or progestin only, that primarily prevent release of egg	1-5, depending on type	Convenient and highly effective; provide significant noncontraceptive health benefits, such as protection against ovarian and endometrial cancers	Pills must be taken regularly; possible minor side effects, which new formulations have reduced; not for women with cardiovascular risks, mostly those over 35 who smoke
Condom	Thin penis sheath (usually made of latex) collects semen	3-15	Easy to use, effective, and inexpensive; protects against sexually transmitted diseases	Requires male cooperation; may diminish spontaneity; may deteriorate on the shelf
Diaphragm	Soft rubber cup that covers entrance to uterus, prevents sperm from reaching egg, and holds spermicide	4-25	No dangerous side effects; reliable if used properly; provides some protection against sexually transmitted diseases and cervical cancer	Requires careful fitting; some inconvenience associated with insertion and removal; may be dislodged during sex
Cervical cap	Miniature diaphragm that covers cervix closely, prevents sperm from reaching egg, and holds spermicide	Probably comparable to diaphragm	No dangerous side effects; fairly effective; can remain in place longer than diaphragm	Problems with fitting and insertion; comes in limited number of sizes
Foams, creams, jellies, vaginal suppositories	Chemical spermicides inserted in vagina before intercourse that also prevent sperm from entering uterus	10-25	Can be used by anyone who is not allergic; protect against some sexually transmitted diseases; no known side effects	Relatively unreliable, sometimes messy; must be used 5 to 10 minutes before each act of intercourse
Sponge	Acts as sperm barrier and releases spermicide	15-30	Safe; easy to insert; provides some protection against sexually transmitted diseases; can be left in place for 24 hours; needs no fitting	Relatively unreliable; comes in only one size; some sensitivity and removal problems; cannot be used during menstruation
Implant (Norplant)	Capsules surgically implanted under skin that slowly release a hormone that blocks release of eggs	0.3	Very safe, convenient, and effective; very long-lasting (5 years); may have nonreproductive health benefits like those of oral contraceptives	Irregular or absent periods; necessity of minor surgical procedure to insert and remove
Injectable contraceptive (DepoProvera) Unavailable in U.S.	Injection every 3 months of a hormone slowly released from the muscle that prevents ovulation	1	Convenient and highly effective; no serious side effects other than occasional heavy menstrual bleeding	Animal studies suggest that it may cause cancer, though new studies of women are mostly encouraging

Adapted from Raven P, Johnson G: *Biology,* ed 3. St Louis, 1992, Mosby. Data from American College of Obstetricians and Gynecologists: Benefits, Risks, and Effectiveness of Contraception, Washington, D.C., ACOG, Bobak IM, Jensen MD: *Maternity and gynecologic care: the nurse and the family,* ed 5, St Louis, 1993, Mosby and Denney NW, Quadagno D: *Human sexuality,* ed 2, St Louis, 1992, Mosby.
*Approximate effectiveness of these reversible methods of birth control is measured in pregnancies per 100 actual users per year.

Continued.

Methods of contraception—cont'd

Device/method	Action	Failure rates	Advantages	Disadvantages
Periodic abstinence				
Calendar method	Determine fertile period by (1) subtracting 18 days from length of shortest menstrual cycle to determine first "unsafe" day; (2) subtract 11 days from length of longest menstrual cycle to determine last "unsafe" day; abstinence during fertile periods	9-23%	No side effects; acceptable to members of religions that prohibit use of contraceptives	Length of menstrual cycle may be unpredictable; requires abstinence for long periods of time
Basal body temperature (BBT)	time of ovulation determined by drop and subsequent rise in BBT; abstinence during fertile periods	7-21%	No side effects; acceptable to members of religions that prohibit use of contraceptives; increased understanding and appreciation of own body	BBT may fluctuate because of fatigue, inadequate sleep, infection, or anxiety; success requires motivation and commitment
Cervical mucus	Time of ovulation determined by observation of changes in characteristics of cervical mucus	3-15%	No side effects; acceptable to members of religions that prohibit use of contraceptives; increased understanding and appreciation of own body	Woman may be uncomfortable touching her genitals; mucus can be affected by douches, medications, semen, or discharge from vaginal infections; success requires motivation and commitment
Symptothermal	Combination of BBT and cervical mucus methods; abstinence on fertile days	3-27%	More reliable than other calendar methods; couple often report improvement in sexual relationships	Same disadvantages as for BBT and cervical mucus methods

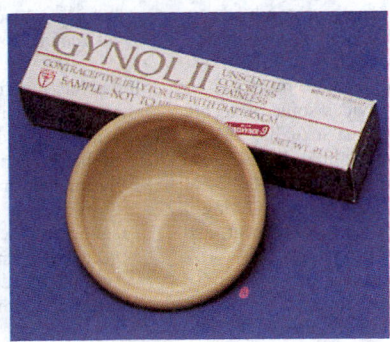

Contraceptive diaphragm
(Edge, 1994)

phragm is selected according to the clinical assessment of certain anatomic factors specific to the woman being fitted, including the size of the vagina, the position of the uterus, the depth of the arch behind the symphysis pubis, and the degree of support afforded by the muscles surrounding the vagina. See also **arcing-spring contraceptive diaphragm, coil-spring contraceptive diaphragm, flat-spring contraceptive diaphragm.**

contraceptive effectiveness, the effectiveness of a method of contraception in preventing pregnancy. For clinical purposes, it combines the theoretic effectiveness of the device, medication, or method and the use effectiveness. It is sometimes represented as a percentage but more accurately as the number of pregnancies per 100 woman-years. The average pregnancy rate for a couple that is sexually active without the use of contraceptives is equivalent to 90 pregnancies per 100 woman-years. A contraceptive method that results in a pregnancy rate of less than 10 pregnancies per 100 woman-years is considered highly effective. See also **pregnancy rate, woman-year.**

contraceptive jelly [L, *contra,* opposed, *concipere,* to take in, *gelare,* to congeal], a gelatinous preparation containing a spermicide for introduction into the vagina to prevent conception.

contraceptive method, any act, device, or medication for avoiding conception or a viable pregnancy. See also **cervical cap, condom, diaphragm, intrauterine device, natural family-planning method, oral contraceptive, spermatocide, sterilization.**

contract [L, *con + trahere,* to draw], /kon'trakt/ **1.** an agreement or a promise that meets certain legal requirements, including competence of both or all parties to the contract, proper lawful subject matter, mutuality of agreement, mutuality of obligation, and consideration (the giving of something of value in payment for the obligation undertaken). **2.** /kəntrakt'/, to make such an agreement or promise. **–contractual** /kəntrak'chōō·əl/, *adj.*

contractile /kəntrak'tĭl/ [L, *cum*, with, *trahere*, to draw], capable of becoming reduced in size or length or of being drawn together in response to some stimulus.

contractile ring dysphagia [L, *con* + *trahere*, to draw; AS, *hring*], an abnormal condition characterized by difficulty in swallowing because of an overreactive interior esophageal sphincteric mechanism that induces painful sticking sensations under the lower sternum. Compare **dysphagia lusoria, vallecular dysphagia.**

contractility /kon'traktĭl'ĭtē/, (in cardiology) a property of muscle tissue, particuarly cardiac muscle, that reflects its ability to contract, or shorten.

contraction /kəntrak'shən/ [L, *con* + *trahere*, to draw], **1.** a reduction in size, especially of muscle fibers. **2.** an abnormal shrinkage. **3.** (in labor) a rhythmic tightening of the musculature of the upper uterine segment that begins mildly and becomes very strong late in labor, occurring as frequently as every 2 minutes, and lasting over 1 minute. Contractions decrease the size of the uterus and squeeze the fetus through the birth canal. **4.** abnormal smallness of the birth canal or part of it, a cause of dystocia. **Inlet contraction** exists if the anteroposterior diameter is 10 cm or less or if the transverse diameter is 11.5 cm or less. **Midpelvic contraction** exists if the sum of the measurements in centimeters of the interspinous diameter (normally 10.5 cm) and the posterior sagittal diameter (normally 5 cm) is 13.5 cm or less. **Outlet contraction** exists if the intertuberous diameter is 8 cm or less. See also **clinical pelvimetry, concentric contraction, dystocia, eccentric contraction, x-ray pelvimetry.**

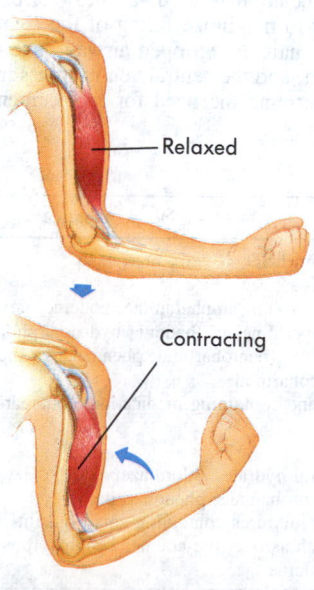

Isotonic muscle contraction
(Tibodeau, 1993/Rolin Graphics)

contractual. See **contract.**

contracture /kəntrak'chər/ [L, *contractura,* a pulling together], an abnormal, usually permanent condition of a joint, characterized by flexion and fixation and caused by atrophy and shortening of muscle fibers or by loss of the normal elasticity of the skin, such as from the formation of extensive scar tissue over a joint. See also **Volkmann's contracture.**

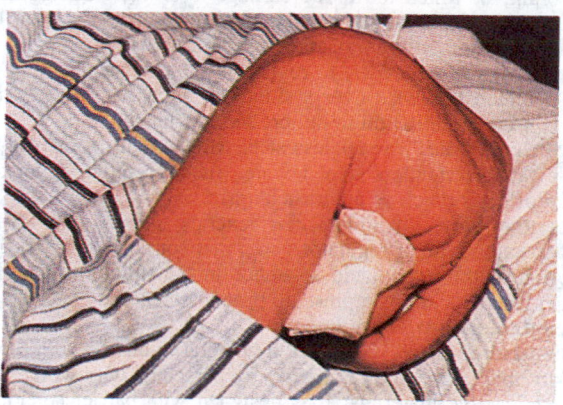

Contracture *(Forbes, 1993)*

contraindicate /kon'trə·in'dikāt/ [L, *contra,* opposed, *indicare,* to make known], to report the presence of a disease or physical condition that makes it impossible or undesirable to treat a particular client in the usual manner or to prescribe medicines that might otherwise be suitable.

contraindication /'in'dikā'shən/ [L, *contra,* against, *indicare,* to make known], a factor that prohibits the administration of a drug or the performance of an act or procedure in the care of a specific patient; for example, pregnancy is a contraindication for the prescription of tetracycline, immunosuppression is a contraindication for vaccination, and complete placenta previa is a contraindication for vaginal delivery.

contralateral /'-lat'ərəl/ [L, *contra* + *lateralis,* side], affecting or originating in the opposite side of a point or reference, such as a point on a body.

contralateral reflexes [L, *contra,* opposed, *latus,* side, *reflectere,* to bend back], an overflow phenomenon of the nervous system in which a reflex is elicited on one side of the body by a stimulus to the opposite side.

contrast /kon'trast/ [L, *contra* + *stare,* to stand], a measure of the differences between two adjacent areas in an image. Contrast may be based on differences in optic density or differences in radiation transmission, or other parameters. Contrast plays an important role in the ability of a radiologist to perceive image detail.

contrast bath, a bath in which the patient alternately immerses a part of the body, usually the hands or feet, in hot and cold water for a specified period of time. The procedure is used to increase the blood flow to a particular area.

contrast enema. See **barium enema.**

contrast examination, the use of radiopaque materials to make internal organs visible on x-ray film. Because of their high atomic numbers, substances such as iodine and barium have an x-ray photoelectric interaction that is nearly 400 times that of soft tissue, resulting in the increased visibility of internal organs or cavities oulined by contrast materials.

contrast medium, a radiopaque substance injected into the body to facilitate radiographic imaging of internal structures that otherwise are difficult to visualize on x-ray films.

contrecoup. See **coup.**

contrecoup injury /kôntrekōō′/ [L, *contra,* opposed; Fr, *coup,* blow; L, *injuria*], an injury, usually involving the brain, in which the tissue damage is on the side opposite the site of the trauma, as when a blow to the left side of the head results in brain damage on the right side.

control [Fr, *contrôler,* to register], to exercise restraint or maintain influence over a situation, as in self-control, the conscious limitation or suppression of impulses.

control cable, a stainless steel wire, usually contained in a flexible stainless steel housing, used to move or lock a prosthesis, such as an artificial arm.

control gene, (in molecular genetics) a gene, such as the operator gene or regulator gene, that controls the transcription of the amino-acid sequence in the structural gene by either inducing or repressing protein synthesis.

control group. See **group.**

controlled area, a part of a hospital or other health facility that is occupied primarily by personnel who work with radioactive materials. It is designed with barrier shielding to confine the radiation exposure rate in the area to less than 100 milliroentgen per week (mR/wk).

controlled association, **1.** a direct connection of relevant ideas as the result of a specific stimulus. **2.** a process of bringing repressed ideas into the consciousness in response to words spoken by a psychoanalyst. Also called **word association.**

controlled hypotension. See **deliberate hypotension.**

controlled oxygen therapy, the administration of oxygen to a patient on a dose-response basis in which oxygen is regarded as a drug and only the smallest amount of gas is used to obtain a desired therapeutic effect.

controlled substance [Fr, *contrôle,* check; L, *substantia,* essence], any drug as defined in the five categories of the federal **Controlled Substances Act of 1970.** The categories, or schedules, cover opium and its derivatives, hallucinogens, depressants, and stimulants.

Controlled Substances Act, a U.S. law enacted in 1970 that regulates the prescribing and dispensing of psychoactive drugs, including stimulants, depressants, and hallucinogens. The Act lists five categories of restricted drugs, depending upon their medical acceptance, abuse potential, and ability to produce dependence.

controlled ventilation, the use of an intermittent positive pressure breathing unit or other respirator that has an automatic cycling device that replaces spontaneous respiration. Some units measure expired volume, nebulize medication or fluids in the air, exert negative pressure at the end of the expiration, or have a variety of alarms.

control of hemorrhage, the limitation of the flow of blood from a break in the wall of a blood vessel.

■ METHOD: Some of the methods for controlling hemorrhage are direct pressure, use of a tourniquet, or application of pressure on pressure points proximal to the wound. Direct pressure with a thick compress is applied in such a way that the edges of the wound are brought together. A tourniquet is applied proximal to the site of bleeding only in the most drastic emergency, for the limb may then have to be sacrificed because of tissue anoxia stemming from the use of the tourniquet. Pressure is applied to a pressure point by using firm manual pressure over the main artery supplying the wound. Points used to obtain the pulse may be used as pressure points to stop hemorrhage. See also **tourniquet.**

■ NURSING INTERVENTION: The flow of blood to an area is limited by restricting activity, elevating the part, and applying pressure. Specific treatment depends on the cause of the hemorrhage and the condition of the patient. In addition to intravenous infusion equipment and fluids, the nurse may anticipate the need for vasopressor drugs, ventilatory assistance, central venous pressure monitoring equipment, and materials for obtaining and recording the blood pressure and urinary output. If signs of shock are present, the patient may be placed supine at a 45-degree angle to the pelvis, with the knees straight and the pelvis slightly higher than the chest. The head may be supported with a pillow. If Trendelenburg's position is used, a pillow is placed under the left shoulder to maximize filling of the right atrium of the heart and to maintain an open airway. The person may be given oxygen, and the central venous pressure may be measured to determine the need for replacement of fluid vol-

Classification of controlled substances

Classification	Description	Specific substances
Schedule I (Schedule H*)	Drugs that have high potential for abuse and no accepted medical use. Containers are marked C-1	Heroin, LSD, peyote, marijuana
Schedule II (Schedule F*)	Drugs that have high potential for abuse but have accepted medical use. Dependence may include strong physical and psychologic dependence. Containers are marked C-II.	Amobarbital, amphetamine, codeine, dextroamphetamine, meperidine, methadone, hydromorphone, morphine, opium, pentobarbital, phenazocine, methylphenidate, secobarbital
Schedule III (Schedule F*)	Medically accepted drugs that may cause dependence but are less prone to abuse than drugs in Schedules I and II. Containers are marked C-III	Codeine-containing medications, butabarbital, paregoric
Schedule IV (Schedule F*)	Medically accepted drugs that may cause mild physical or psychologic dependence. Containers are marked C-IV	Chloral hydrate, chlordiazepoxide, diazepam, meprobamate, phenobarbital
Schedule V	Medically accepted drugs with very limited potential for causing mild physical or psychologic dependence. Containers are marked C-V	Drug mixtures containing small quantities of narcotics, such as over-the-counter cough syrups containing codeine

*Canadian classification.
Adapted from Clark JF, Queerer SF, Karb VB: *Pharmacologic basis of nursing practice,* ed 4, St Louis, 1993, Mosby.

ume. Sudden, severe hemorrhage with signs of shock usually is treated with intravenous infusion of fluids and a transfusion of blood. The application of additional warmth to the skin is not recommended, because heat increases the metabolism and the need for oxygen.

■ OUTCOME CRITERIA: Signs of continued bleeding, tachycardia, cold sweat, decreasing blood pressure, and anxiety on the part of the patient alert the nurse to the probability that bleeding has begun again or that replacement fluids administered after the hemorrhage are not adequate. The person is kept calm and quiet; if the fluid balance is promptly restored, recovery is usual. Excessive loss of blood leads to hypoxia of all the tissues of the body, including the brain and vital organs, and causes death.

control process, a system of establishing standards, objectives, and methods, and measuring actual performance, comparing results, reinforcing strengths, and taking necessary corrective action.

contusion /kənt(y) o͞o′zhən/ [L, *contundere*, to bruise], an injury that does not disrupt the integrity of the skin, caused by a blow to the body and characterized by swelling, discoloration, and pain. The immediate application of cold may limit the development of a contusion. Also called **bruise.** Compare **ecchymosis.**

convalescence /kon′vəles′əns/ [L, *convalescere*, to grow strong], the period of recovery after an illness, injury, or surgery.

convalescent home. See **extended care facility.**

convection /kənvek′shən/ [L, *convehere*, to bring together], (in physics) the transfer of heat through a gas or liquid by the circulation of heated particles.

convergence /kənvur′jəns/ [L, *convegere*, to bend together], the movement of two objects toward a common point, such as the turning of the eyes inward to see an object close to the face.

convergent evolution, the development of similar structures or functions within widely differing phylogenetic species in response to similar environmental conditions.

convergent squint [L, *convergere*, to incline together; ME, *squint*], a visual disorder in which a deviating eye looks inward toward the nose.

convergent strabismus. See **esotropia.**

conversion /kənvur′zhən/ [L, *convertere*, to turn around], **1.** changing from one form to another, transmutation. **2.** (in obstetrics) the correction of a fetal position during labor. **3.** (in psychiatry) an unconscious defense mechanism by which emotional conflicts ordinarily resulting in anxiety are repressed and transformed into symbolic physical symptoms having no organic basis. Loss of sensation, paralysis, pain, or other dysfunction of the nervous system are the most common somatic expressions of conversion.

conversion disorder, a disorder in which repressed emotional conflicts are converted into sensory, motor, or visceral symptoms having no underlying organic cause, such as blindness, anesthesia, hypesthesia, hyperesthesia, paresthesia, involuntary muscular movements (for example, tics or tremors), paralysis, aphonia, mutism, hallucinations, catalepsy, choking sensations, and respiratory difficulties. The person who has conversion disorder is usually indifferent to the symptoms yet firmly believes the condition exists. Causal factors include a conscious or unconscious desire to escape from or avoid some unpleasant situation or responsibility or to obtain sympathy or some other secondary gain. Treatment usually consists of psychotherapy. Also called

conversion hysteria, conversion reaction, somatoform disorder.

conversion reaction, an ego defense mechanism whereby intrapsychic conflict is expressed symbolically through physical symptoms.

convulsion. See **seizure.**

convoluted kidney tubules /kon′vəlo͞o′tid/[L, *convolvere*, to roll together; ME, *kidenei*; L, *tubulus*], pertaining to the convoluted portion of the nephron that leads from the glomerulus to the connecting ducts. The proximal and distal sections are convoluted while the ascending and descending limbs of the loop of Henle are relatively straight.

convoluted seminiferous tubules, the long, threadlike tubes in the aerolar tissue of the testes. The testes also contain straight segments of seminiferous tubules.

convulsive seizure /kənvul′siv/ [L, *convulsio*, cramp; OFr, *seisir*], a sudden onset of a disease characterized by convulsions, palpitations, and other symptoms. The term is sometimes applied to an attack of an epileptic disorder.

convulsive syncope. See **vasovagal.**

convulsive tic, a disorder of the facial nerve, causing involuntary spasmodic contractions of the facial muscles supplied by that nerve. Also called **hemifacial spasm.** See also **Gilles de la Tourette's syndrome.**

Cooley's anemia. See **thalassemia.**

Coolidge tube, a basic type of hot-cathode x-ray tube that, with modern refinements, has been used by radiologists since it was invented in 1913.

cooling [AS, *colian*, cool], reducing body temperature by the application of a hypothermia blanket, cold moist dressings, ice packs, or an alcohol bath. Subnormal body temperature may be induced to reduce metabolic function before some kinds of surgery. Very high fevers of any origin may be treated in part by reduction of the fever with cooling techniques. See also **alcohol bath, hypothermia, hypothermia blanket.**

cooling rate, the rate at which temperature decreases with time (°C/minute) immediately after the completion of hyperthermia treatment.

Coombs' positive hemolytic anemia /ko͞omz/ [Robin R. A. Coombs, British immunologist, b. 1921], a form of anemia resulting from premature destruction of circulating red blood cells. See also **antiglobulin test.**

Coombs' test. See **antiglobulin test.** (See Fig. p. 394.)

cooperative play /kō·op′erətiv′/, any organized play among a group of children in which activities are planned for the purpose of achieving some goal. It usually occurs among older children. Compare **associative play, parallel play, solitary play.**

coordinated reflex /kō·ôr′dinā′tid/ [L, *coordinare*, to arrange], a sequence of muscular actions occurring in a purposeful, orderly progression, such as the act of swallowing.

COPD, abbreviation for **chronic obstructive pulmonary disease.**

coping [Gk, *kolaphos*, buffet], a process by which a person deals with stress, solves problems, and makes decisions. The process has two components, cognitive and noncognitive. The cognitive component includes the thought and learning necessary to identify the source of the stress. The noncognitive components are automatic and focus on relieving the discomfort. Many defense mechanisms fall into this category. Although sometimes useful, noncognitive measures may fail to relieve the stress because the response may

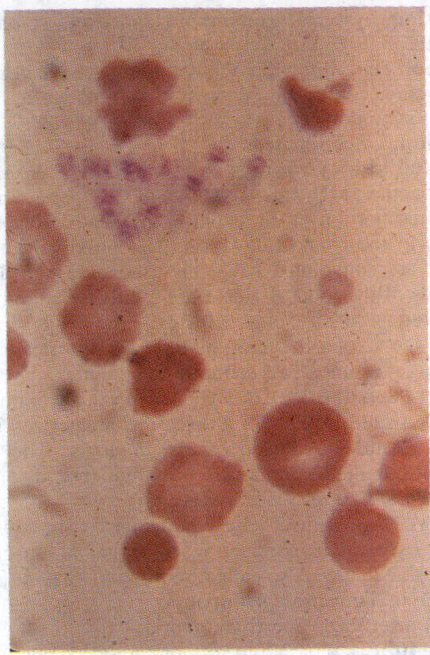

Coombs—positive hemolytic anemia (*Zitelli, 1992*)

be inappropriate, may have the wrong effect, and, as it replaces cognitive coping measures, may prevent the person from learning more about the cause and a better solution for the problem.

coping, defensive, a nursing diagnosis accepted by the Eighth National Conference on the Classification of Nursing Diagnoses. Defensive coping is a state in which an individual experiences falsely positive self-evaluation based on a self-protective pattern that defends against undelying perceived threats to positive self-regard. Major defining characteristics are denial of obvious problems or weaknesses, projection of blame or responsibility, rationalization of failures, defensiveness and hypersensitivity to slight or criticism and grandiosity. Minor characteristics are a superior attitude toward others, difficulty in establishing or maintaining relationships, hostile laughter or ridicule of others, difficulty in reality testing perceptions, and lack of follow through or participation in treatment or therapy. See also **nursing diagnosis.**

coping, family: potential for growth, a nursing diagnosis accepted by the Fourth National Conference on the Classification of Nursing Diagnoses. The condition is defined as effective managing of adaptive tasks by the family member involved with the patient's health challenge, who now is exhibiting desire and readiness for enhanced health and grown in regard to self and in relation to the client. The defining characteristics of the family's potential for growth in this area are the family's expressed wish to discuss the impact of the situation on the client's own life and values, interest in meeting with others in similar situations, and choice of healthful options available to the client. See also **nursing diagnosis.**

coping, ineffective family: compromised, a nursing diagnosis accepted by the Fourth National Conference on the Classification of Nursing Diagnoses. The diagnosis refers to a lack or absence of emotional and psychologic support for the client that is usually available from a family member or other supportive person, a deficiency that causes further difficulty for the client in coping with the current health problem. The cause of the situation may be inadequate or faulty understanding of the health problem by the supportive person, or it may result from temporary preoccupation with emotional conflicts on the part of the supportive person. Illness or health problems may cause changes in roles, resulting in temporary disorganization of the network of family and friends, who may become exhausted by the demands of filling the needs of the client. Many situational crises may interrupt or prevent adequate expression of support for the client, and the client may be able to give little support in return. The defining characteristics of ineffective compromised family coping include expression by the client that support is lacking or expression by the supportive person that fear, anticipatory grief, anxiety, or other reaction is interfering with the ability to give support to the client. A frank statement of an inadequate understanding of the health problem from the client or supportive person may be made. Objectively, the nurse may observe that the support given is inadequate, that the communication between the parties is limited and unsatisfactory, or that the supportive person offers help that is disproportionate to the need. See also **nursing diagnosis.**

coping, ineffective family: disabling, a nursing diagnosis accepted by the Fourth National Conference on the Classification of Nursing Diagnoses. The diagnosis refers to the detrimental attitudes and behavior of a family, a family member, or other person who is important to the client. The cause of the problem is often the disablement of the significant person by grief, anxiety, guilt, hostility, or despair. The defining characteristics of this kind of ineffective family coping include neglect in the care of the client, intolerance, rejection or abandonment, adoption of the symptoms of the client, disregard of the client's needs, and marked distortion of reality in regard to the client's health problem. See also **nursing diagnosis.**

coping, ineffective individual, a nursing diagnosis accepted by the Fourth National Conference on the Classification of Nursing Diagnoses. The cause of the problem includes situational crises, maturational or developmental crises, or personal vulnerability. The defining characteristics include an inability to meet the expectations of a role, an inability to meet one's basic needs, or an alteration in ability to participate in society. The critical defining characteristics, one of which must be present for the diagnosis to be made, are an inability to ask for help, an inability to solve problems, and verbalization of the inability to cope. Other characteristics that may be present are destructive behavior, inappropriate or excessive use of defense mechanisms, a change in patterns of communication, verbal manipulation, and a greater-than-expected incidence of accidents and illness. See also **nursing diagnosis.**

coping mechanism, any effort directed toward stress management, including task-oriented and ego-defense mechanisms; the factors that enable an individual to regain emotional equilibrium after a stressful experience.

coping resources, the characteristics of a person, group, or environment that are helpful in assisting individuals in adapting to stress.

coping style, the cognitive, affective, or behavioral responses of a person to problematic or traumatic life events.

COPP, an anticancer drug combination of cyclophosphamide, procarbazine, and prednisone.

copper (Cu) [L, *cuprum*], a malleable, reddish-brown, metallic element. Its atomic number is 29; its atomic weight is 63.54. Copper occurs in a pure state in nature and in many ores. It is a component of several important enzymes in the body and is essential to good health. Copper deficiency in the body is rare because only 2 to 5 mg daily, easily obtained from a variety of foods, is sufficient for a proper balance. Copper accumulates in individuals with Wilson's disease, primary biliary cirrhosis, and, occasionally, chronic extrahepatic biliary tract obstruction. Copper is an excellent conductor of heat and electricity and a valuable component of numerous alloys, and it may be compounded with arsenic to form insecticides. Copper-sulfate solution was previously used to test for reducing agents, such as glucose, in the urine. See also **ceruloplasmin, hepatolenticular degeneration.**

copperhead /kop'ərhed'/ [L, *cuprum* + ME, *hed*], a poisonous pit viper found mainly in the southeastern United States. A similar snake of a different genus is found in Australia. The reddish-brown, darkly banded snake is responsible for nearly 40% of the snake bites in the United States; few bites are fatal. Pain, swelling, fang marks, and a bruise are usually present. Immediate treatment includes placing a constricting band above the bite that is tight enough to prevent lymphatic and superficial venous flow from the wound to the general circulation but that is not tight enough to stop deep arterial and venous flow to the limb. The fang marks are incised, the venom is drained, and free bleeding is allowed. The victim should be taken to a medical facility and given antivenin if necessary. See also **coral snake, cottonmouth, rattlesnake.**

Copper Kettle, a trademark for a kind of vaporizer used in the circuits of an anesthesia machine to mix the carrier gas and the volatile anesthetic liquid to form an anesthetizing vapor.

Copper T, a trademark for a T-shaped plastic intrauterine device (IUD). It is recommended only for women over 25 who have been pregnant, have a monogamous relationship, and have not had pelvic inflammatory disease.

copro-, copr-, kopr-, kopra-, a combining form meaning 'pertaining to feces': *coprolalia, coprolith.*

coprogogue. See **cathartic.**

coprolalia /kop'rōlā'lyə/ [Gk, *kopros*, dung, *lalein*, to babble], the excessive use of obscene language.

coprology. See **scatology.**

coproporphyria /kop'rōpôrfir'ē·ə/ [Gk, *kopros* + *porphyros*, purple], a rare, hereditary, metabolic disorder in which large quantities of nitrogenous substances, called porphyrins, are excreted in the feces. Attacks, with varying GI and neurologic symptoms, may be precipitated by certain drugs, including barbiturates, sulfonamides, and steroids. Patients are often helped by a high-carbohydrate diet. See also **acute intermittent porphyria, coproporphyrin, porphyria.**

coproporphyrin /kop'rōpôr'firin/ [Gk, *kopros* + *porphyros*, purple], any of the nitrogenous organic substances normally excreted in the feces that are products of the breakdown of bilirubin from hemoglobin decomposition.

copulation. See **coitus.**

cor /kôr/, **1.** the heart. **2.** relating to the heart.

cor-. See **co-.**

coracobrachialis /kôr'əkōbrā'kē·al'is/, a muscle with its origin on the scapula and its insertion on the inner side of the humerus. It is innervated by the musculocutaneous nerve and functions by adducting the shoulder.

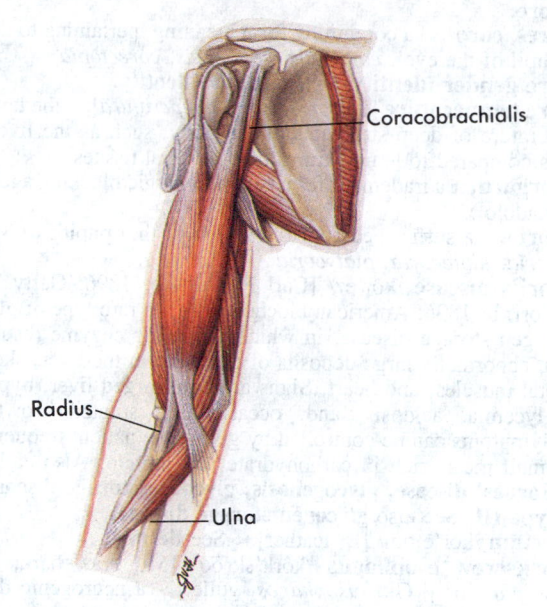

Corachobrachialis muscle
(Thibodeau, 1993/John V Hagen)

coracoid process /kôr'əkoid/ [Gk, *korax*, crow, *eidos*, form; L, *processus*], the thick, curved extension of the superior border of the scapula, to which the pectoralis minor is attached. Compare **acromion.**

coral calculus. See **dendritic calculus.**

coral snake, a poisonous snake with transverse red, black, and yellow bands that is native to the southern United States. Bites are rare; pain is not always present, but neuromuscular and respiratory effects may be severe. Coral snake antivenin and oxygen are the usual emergency treatments.

Coramine, a trademark for a respiratory stimulant (nikethamide).

cord [Gk, *chorde*, string], any long, rounded, flexible structure. The body contains many different cords, such as the spermatic, vocal, spinal, nerve, umbilical, and hepatic cords. Cords serve many different purposes, depending on location, kind of enclosed cells, and body parts or tissue involved. —**cordal,** *adj.*

Cordarone, a trademark for an oral antiarrhythmic drug (amiodarone hydrochloride).

corditis /kôrdī'tis/ [Gk, *chorde* + *itis*, inflammation], an abnormal inflammation of the spermatic cord, accompanied by pain in the testis, often caused by an infection originating in the urethra or by tumor, hydrocele, or varicocele. Injury to the groin often causes hematoma of the cord. Inflammatory conditions of the testis may lead to swelling and tenderness.

Cordran, a trademark for a glucocorticoid (flurandrenolide).

core [L, *cor*, heart], **1.** a kind of main computer memory. **2.** (in dentistry) a section of a mold, usually of plaster, made over assembled parts of a dental restoration to record and maintain their relationships so that the parts can be reassembled in their original position. Also called **laboratory core.**

core-, coro-, a combining form meaning 'pertaining to the pupil of the eye': *coreclisis, corectasis, corectopia.*

core gender identity. See **gender identity.**

core temperature [L, *cor*, heart + *temperatura*], the temperature of deep structures of the body, such as the liver, as compared to temperatures of peripheral tissues.

Corgard, a trademark for a beta-adrenergic blocking agent (nadolol).

-coria, a suffix meaning '(condition of the) pupil': *anisocoria, diplocoria, platycoria.*

Cori's disease /kôr′ēz/ [Carl F. Cori, b. 1896; Gerty T. Cori, b. 1896; American biochemists], a rare type of glycogen storage disease, in which a missing enzyme results in abnormally large deposits of glycogen in the liver, skeletal muscles, and heart. Signs are an enlarged liver, hypoglycemia, acidosis, and, occasionally, stunted growth. Symptoms can be controlled by giving the patient frequent, small meals rich in carbohydrate and protein. Also called **Forbes' disease, glycogenosis, glycogen storage disease, type III.** See also **glycogen storage disease.**

corium /kôr′ē·əm/ [L, leather]. See **dermis.**

corkscrew esophagus /kôrk′skrōō/ [ME *cork* bark; L, *scrofa*, sow]; Gk, *oisophagos*, gullet], a neurogenic disorder in which normal peristaltic contractions of the esophagus are replaced by spastic movements occurring spontaneously or with swallowing or gastric acid reflux. Difficulty in swallowing, weight loss, severe pain over the upper chest, and a characteristic corkscrew image on x-ray pictures are the symptoms usually present. Management may include the use of antispasmodic drugs, avoidance of cold fluids, surgical dilatation, or myotomy. Compare **achalasia.** See also **dysphagia.**

-cormia, -cormy, a suffix meaning an 'abnormal development of the trunk of the body': *camptocormia, nanocormia, schistocormia.*

corn [L, *cornu*, horn], a horny mass of condensed epithelial cells overlying a bony prominence. Corns result from chronic friction and pressure. The conic shape of the corn compresses the underlying dermis, making it thin and tender. Corns can become soft and macerated by perspiration. Treatment includes relief of the mechanical pressure and surgical paring or chemical peeling of the excess keratin. Also called **clavus.** Compare **callus.**

cornea /kôr′nē·ə/ [L, *corneus*, horny], the convex, transparent, anterior part of the eye, comprising one sixth of the outermost tunic of the eye bulb. It allows light to pass through it to the lens. The cornea is a fibrous structure with five layers: the anterior corneal epithelium, continuous with that of the conjunctiva; the anterior limiting layer (Bowman's membrane); the substantia propria; the posterior limiting layer (Descemet's membrane); and the endothelium of the anterior chamber (keratoderma). It is dense, uniform in thickness, and nonvascular, and it projects like a dome beyond the sclera, which forms the other five sixths of the eye's outermost tunic. The degree of corneal curvature varies in different individuals and in the same person at differ-

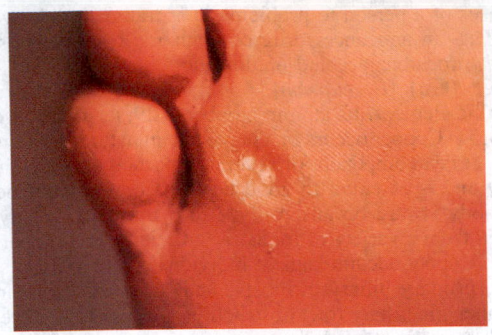

Corn *(Weston, 1991)*

ent ages, the curvature being more pronounced in youth than in advanced age.

-cornea, a suffix meaning 'condition of the cornea': *entocornea, mesocornea, microcornea.*

corneal abrasion /kôr′nē·əl/ [L, *corneus* horny; *abrasio* scraping], the rubbing off of the outer layers of the cornea.

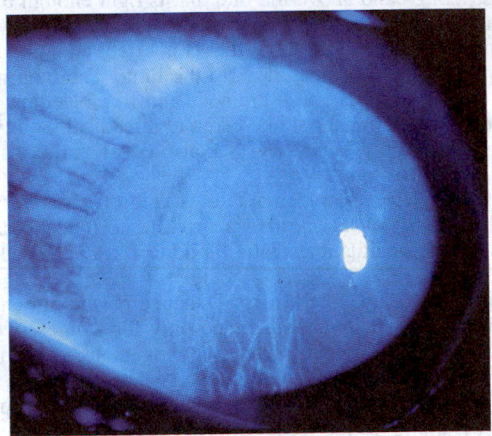

Corneal abrasion *(Zitelli, 1992)*

corneal grafting, transplantation of corneal tissue from one human eye to another, performed to improve vision in corneal scarring or distortion or to remove a perforating ulcer. Preoperative preparation includes constricting the pupil with a miotic drug, such as pilocarpine. Under local anesthesia the affected area is excised; an identical section of clear cornea is cut from the donor eye and sutured in place, using an operating microscope. Cataract surgery may be performed at the same time. Postoperatively, the eye is covered with a protective metal shield. The patient is cautioned to avoid coughing, sneezing, sudden movement, or lifting. The dressing is changed daily, and antibiotics are instilled. A complication that may occur after several weeks is a clouding over of the graft, because of the body's rejection of foreign tissue. Corticosteroid drugs administered immediately postoperatively may prevent the reaction. Healing is slow, and the sutures are usually left in place for 1 year. Also called **keratoplasty.**

corneal loupe, (in ophthalmology) a magnifying lens designed especially for examining the cornea.

corneal reflex, a protective mechanism for the eye in which the eyelids close when the cornea is touched. This reflex is mediated by the ophthalmic division of the fifth cranial nerve (sensory)and seventh cranial nerve (motor) may be used as a test of integrity of those nerves. People who wear contact lenses may have a diminished or absent corneal reflex. Compare **conjunctival reflex.**

corneal transplant. See **corneal grafting.**

corneus layer. See **stratum corneum.**

cornification /kôr′nifikā′shən/, the conversion of cells into the horny layer of the skin. Also called **keratinization.**

corn pad, a device that helps relieve the pressure and the pain of a corn by transferring the pressure to surrounding, unaffected areas. Corn pads are constructed of pliable fabric and fashioned in various ways to accommodate different conditions. Some common kinds of corn pads are the foam toe cap, the foam toe sleeve, the soft corn shield, and the hard corn shield.

cornual pregnancy /kôr′nyo͞o·əl/ [L, *cornu,* horn; *praegnans,* child bearing], an ectopic pregnancy in one of the straight or curved extensions of the body of the uterus. The signs include a uterus that is asymmetric and tender, and cramping and spotting occur. The cornu of the uterus usually ruptures between 12 and 16 weeks of the pregnancy unless the condition is treated surgically to remove the products of conception. In most cases the uterus can be repaired. Also called **interstitial pregnancy.** See also **ectopic pregnancy.**

cornu posterioris. See **dorsal horn, posterior horn.**

coro-. See **core-.**

corona /kərō′nə/ [L, crown], **1.** a crown. **2.** a crownlike projection or encircling structure, such as a process extending from a bone. **—coronal, coronoid,** *adj.*

coronal plane. See **frontal plane.**

coronal section [L, *corona,* crown + *sectio*], a section of the body cut in the plane of the coronal suture, or parallel to it.

coronal suture, the serrated transverse suture between the frontal bone and the parietal bone on each side of the skull.

corona radiata, *pl.* **coronae radiatae** [L, crown; *radiare* to emit rays], **1.** a network of fibers that weaves through the internal capsule of the cerebral cortex and intermingles with the fibers of the corpus callosum. **2.** an aggregate of cells that surrounds the zona pellucida of the ovum.

coronary /kôr′əner′ē/ [L, *corona,* crown], **1.** (in anatomy) of or pertaining to encircling structures, such as the coronary arteries; of or pertaining to the heart. **2.** *nontechnical.* myocardial infarction or occlusion.

coronary arteriovenous fistula, an unusual congenital abnormality characterized by a direct communication between a coronary artery, usually the right, and the right atrium or ventricle, the coronary sinus, or the vena cava. There may be a left-to-right shunt of small magnitude causing no symptoms, but a large shunt may result in growth failure, limited exercise tolerance, dyspnea, and anginal pain. Possible complications with a large shunt are bacte-

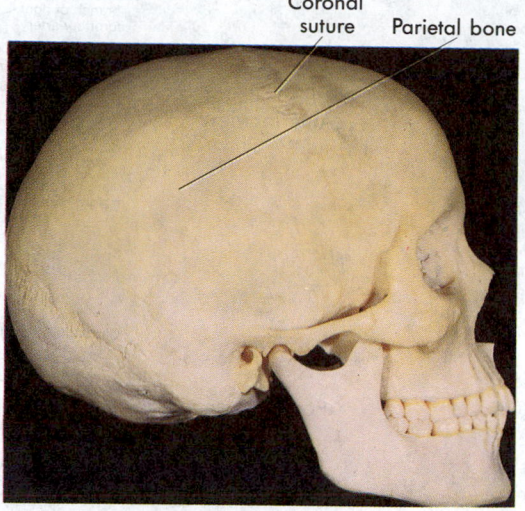

Coronal suture Parietal bone

Coronal suture (*Thibodeau, 1993*)

rial endocarditis, rupture of an aneurysmal fistula, thrombus formation causing occlusion or distal embolization, and, in rare cases, pulmonary hypertension and congestive heart failure. A loud continuous murmur heard at the lower or midsternal border of the heart suggests a coronary arteriovenous fistula; the diagnosis may be confirmed by coronary arteriography or aortography. Closure of the fistulous tract is a safe surgical procedure with excellent long-term results.

coronary artery, one of a pair of arteries that branch from the aorta, including the left and the right coronary arteries. Because these vessels and their branches supply the heart, any dysfunction or disease that affects them can cause serious, sometimes fatal complications. Coronary arterial anastomoses occur throughout the heart and are especially numerous within the interventricular and interatrial septums, at the apex of the heart, at the crux, over the anterior surface of the right ventricle, and between the sinus-node artery and the other atrial arteries. These anastomoses are more numerous and larger in the epicardium than in the endocardium, and they provide important collateral circulation in the recovery of patients who suffer coronary occlusions. The branches of the coronary arteries are affected by many different disorders, such as embolic, neoplastic, inflammatory, and noninflammatory diseases.

coronary artery disease, any one of the abnormal conditions that may affect the arteries of the heart and produce various pathologic effects, especially the reduced flow of oxygen and nutrients to the myocardium. Any of the coronary artery diseases, such as coronary atherosclerosis, coronary arteritis, or fibromuscular hyperplasia of the coronary arteries, may produce the common characteristic symptom of angina pectoris. The most common kind of coronary artery disease is coronary atherosclerosis, now the leading cause of death in the Western world. The disease is not necessarily part of the aging process. It affects more men than women and occurs more often in whites, the middle-aged

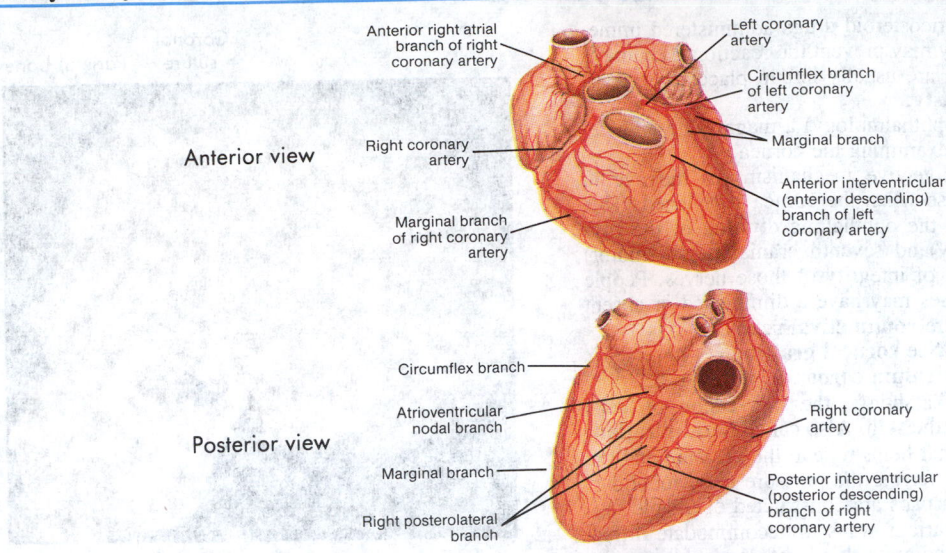

Anterior view

Anterior right atrial branch of right coronary artery

Right coronary artery

Marginal branch of right coronary artery

Left coronary artery

Circumflex branch of left coronary artery

Marginal branch

Anterior interventricular (anterior descending) branch of left coronary artery

Posterior view

Circumflex branch

Atrioventricular nodal branch

Marginal branch

Right posterolateral branch

Right coronary artery

Posterior interventricular (posterior descending) branch of right coronary artery

Coronary artery circulation (Canobbio, 1990)

or elderly, and individuals from affluent countries. Studies over the last 30 years confirm that coronary atherosclerosis occurs most frequently in populations with regular diets high in calories, total fat, saturated fat, cholesterol, and refined carbohydrates. Other risk factors include cigarette smoking, hypertension, serum cholesterol levels, coffee intake, alcohol intake, deficiencies of vitamins C and E, water hardness, hypoxia, carbon monoxide, social overcrowding, heredity, climate, and viruses. Atherosclerosis develops with the formation of fatty fibrous plaques that narrow the lumen of the coronary arteries and may lead to thrombosis and myocardial infarction. Although no single cause of atherosclerosis has been found, the development of the disease is closely associated with the plasma lipids and the lipoproteins that transport the plasma lipids from one tissue to another.

■ OBSERVATIONS: Angina pectoris, the classic symptom of coronary artery disease, results from myocardial ischemia. Angina is usually described as a substernal pain that radiates to the left arm, neck, jaw, or shoulder blade. In affected individuals, angina commonly follows physical exertion, emotional excitement, or exposure to cold. Diagnosis of coronary artery disease is usually based on patient history and the use of tests such as exercise stress tests, ECG, coronary angiography, and myocardial perfusion imaging.

■ INTERVENTION: Treatment of the patient with coronary artery disease concentrates on reducing myocardial oxygen demand or on increasing oxygen supply. Therapy commonly includes the administration of nitrates, such as nitroglycerin, isosorbide dinitrate, or propranolol, a beta-adrenergic blocker. Coronary-artery-bypass surgery may use vein grafts to obviate obstructive lesions. Angioplasty to relieve occlusion by compressing fatty deposits in coronary arteries with no calcification may also be performed. The prevalence of coronary artery disease highlights the importance of preventive measures, such as the reduction of

caloric intake for the obese patient; reduction of salt, fats, and cholesterol; regular exercise; abstention from smoking; and reduction of stress.

■ NURSING CONSIDERATIONS: Nursing care of the patient with coronary artery disease involves monitoring of blood pressure and heart rate, taking of ECGs during anginal episodes, and administration of nitrates, such as nitroglycerin. Nurses are especially alert to signs of ischemia and arrhythmias and, before the patient is discharged, stress the importance of following the prescribed regimens of diet, medication, and exercise.

coronary artery fistula, a congenital anomaly characterized by an abnormal communication between a coronary artery and the right side of the heart or the pulmonary artery.

coronary bypass, open-heart surgery in which a prosthesis or a section of a blood vessel is grafted onto one of the coronary arteries, bypassing a narrowing or blockage in a coronary artery. The operation is performed in coronary artery disease to improve the blood supply to the heart muscle, and to relieve anginal pain. Coronary arteriography pinpoints the areas of obstruction preoperatively. Under general anesthesia and with the use of a cardiopulmonary bypass machine, one end of a 15 to 20 cm prosthesis or a segment of saphenous vein from the patient's leg is grafted to the ascending aorta. The other end is sutured to the clogged coronary artery at a point distal to the stoppage. The internal mammary artery may also be used as graft tissue. Usually, double or triple grafts are done for multiple areas of blockage. Postoperatively, close observation in a coronary intensive care unit or surgical recovery unit is essential to ensure adequate ventilation and cardiac output. The systolic blood pressure is not allowed to drop more than 10 mm Hg below the preoperative baseline, nor is it allowed to rise significantly, because hypertension can rupture a graft site. Arrhythmias occur frequently and are treated with lidocaine, procainamide, or digitalis, given intravenously, or by electrical cardioversion. The patient is usually dis-

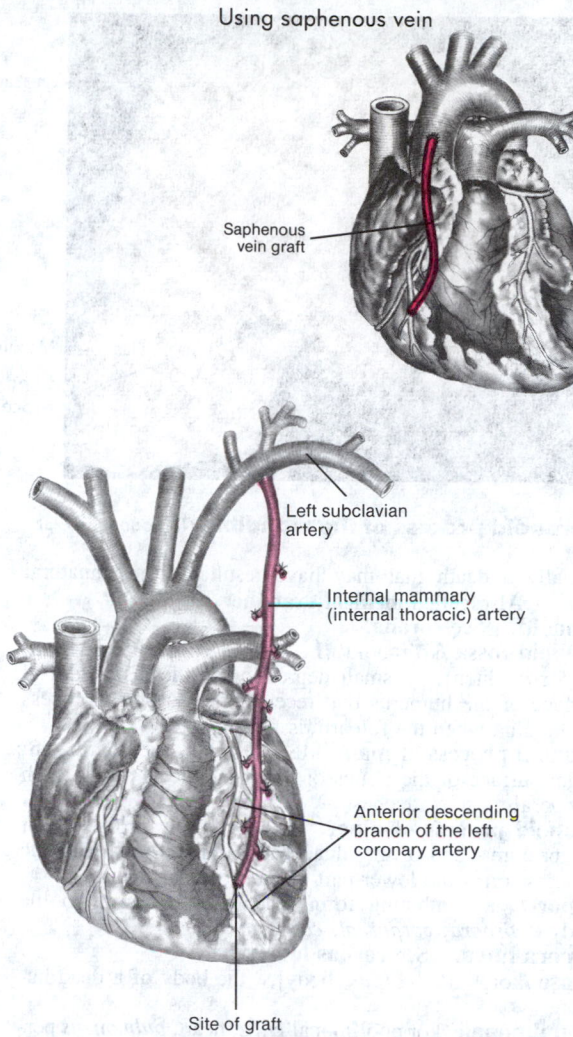

Using saphenous vein

Saphenous vein graft

Left subclavian artery

Internal mammary (internal thoracic) artery

Anterior descending branch of the left coronary artery

Site of graft

Using internal mammary artery

Coronary bypass (Thelan, 1989/George Wassilchenko)

charged within 10 to 14 days. Nearly 20% of cases are associated with thrombosis within the first year after surgery, making the surgery controversial.

coronary care nursing, the nursing care provided in a hospital in a coronary care unit. Nursing in this setting requires technical knowledge, judgment, and skills, as well as an ability to give emotional support to patients and their families during the acute stage of cardiac dysfunction.

coronary care unit (CCU), a specially equipped hospital area designed for the treatment of patients with sudden, life-threatening cardiac conditions, as myocardial infarction. Such units contain resuscitation and monitoring equipment and are staffed by personnel especially trained and skilled in recognizing and immediately responding to cardiac emergencies. See also **intensive care unit.**

coronary collateralization, the spontaneous development of new blood vessels in or around areas of restricted blood flow to the heart.

coronary heart disease. See **CHD.**

coronary occlusion, an obstruction of any one of the coronary arteries, usually caused by progressive atherosclerosis and often complicated by thrombosis. Obstruction of a coronary artery develops gradually from the accumulation of fatty, fibrous plaques that narrow the arterial lumen, reducing blood flow to the heart muscle. In certain heart diseases arterial spasms may narrow the lumen of a coronary artery, blocking blood flow. Occlusions that lead to myocardial infarction are common, and mortality is high when treatment is delayed. Almost half the sudden deaths caused by myocardial infarction occur before the affected individual is hospitalized. If treatment begins immediately after the onset of symptoms, the prognosis significantly improves. Treatment of coronary occlusion and associated myocardial infarction often includes the administration of lidocaine or other antiarrhythmic drugs, vasodilators, nitroglycerin to relieve pain, oxygen, and bed rest. See also **coronary artery disease.**

coronary plexus, [L, *corona,* crown, *plexus,* plaited], a network of autonomic nerve fibers located near the base of the heart.

coronary sinus, the wide venous channel, about 2.25 cm long, situated in the coronary sulcus and covered by muscular fibers from the left atrium. It drains five coronary veins through a single semilunar valve. They are the great cardiac vein, the small cardiac vein, the middle cardiac vein, theposterior vein of the left ventricle, and the oblique vein of the left atrium.

coronary thrombosis, a development of a thrombus that blocks a coronary artery, often causing myocardial infarction and death. Coronary thromboses commonly develop in segments of arteries with atherosclerotic lesions.

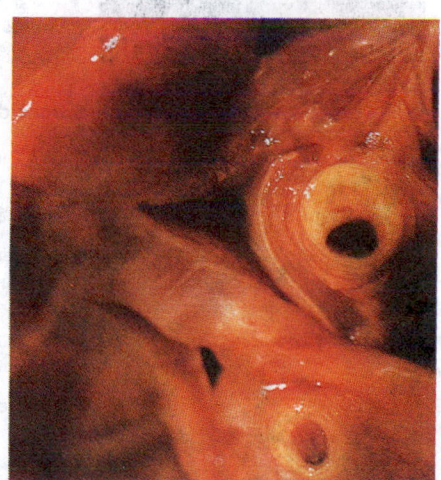

Coronary thrombosis (Fletcher, 1987)

coronary valve [L, *corona,* crown + *valva,* leaf of a door], the valve of the coronary sinus, a semicircular fold of endocardium, leading into the right atrium.

coronary vein, one of the veins of the heart that drains blood from the capillary beds of the myocardium through the coronary sinus into the right atrium. A few small coronary veins that collect blood from a small area in the right ventricle drain directly into the right atrium.

coronavirus /kôr′ənəvī′rəs/ [L, *corona* + *virus*, poison], a member of a family of viruses that includes several types capable of causing acute respiratory illnesses.

coroner /kôr′ənər/ [L, *corona*, crown], a public official who investigates the causes and circumstances of a death occurring within a specific legal jurisdiction or territory, es-

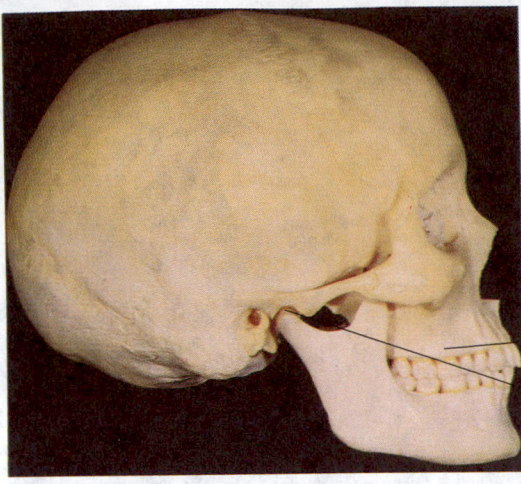

Coronoid process of the mandible (*Thibodeau, 1993*)

pecially a death that may have resulted from unnatural causes. Also called **medical examiner.**

coronoid. See **corona.**

coronoid fossa /kô′rənoid/ [L, *corona* + Gk, *eidos*, form; L, *fossa*, ditch], a small depression in the distal, dorsal surface of the humerus that receives the coronoid process of the ulna when the forearm is flexed.

coronoid process of mandible, a prominence on the anterior surface of the ramus of the mandible to which each temporal muscle attaches.

coronoid process of ulna, a wide, flaring projection of the proximal end of the ulna. The proximal surface of the process forms the lower part of the trochlear notch.

corpor-, a combining form meaning 'pertaining to the body': *corpora, corporeal, corporic.*

corpora lutea. See **corpus luteum.**

corpse /kôrps/ [L, *corpus*, body], the body of a dead human.

cor pulmonale /kôr pōōl′mənal′ē/ [L, heart; *pulmoneus* pertaining to the lungs], an abnormal cardiac condition characterized by hypertrophy of the right ventricle of the heart as a result of hypertension of the pulmonary circulation. Pulmonary hypertension associated with this condition is caused by some disorder of the pulmonary parenchyma or of the pulmonary vascular system between the origin of the left pulmonary artery and the entry of the pulmonary veins into the left atrium. Chronic cor pulmonale commonly increases the size of the right ventricle of the heart, because the right ventricle cannot accommodate an increase in pressure as easily as the left ventricle. In some patients, however, the disease also increases the size of the left ventricle. Some of the diseases associated with cor pulmonale include cystic fibrosis, myasthenia gravis, myopathies, and pulmonary arteritis.

corpus. See **body.**

corpus albicans /kôr′pəs/ a pale white spot on the surface of the ovary which arises from the corpus leuteum if conception does not occur. Compare **corpus luteum.**

corpus callosum. See **callosum.**

corpus cavernosum [L, body; *caverna* hollow place], a type of spongy erectile tissue within the penis or clitoris. The tissue becomes engorged with blood during sexual excitement.

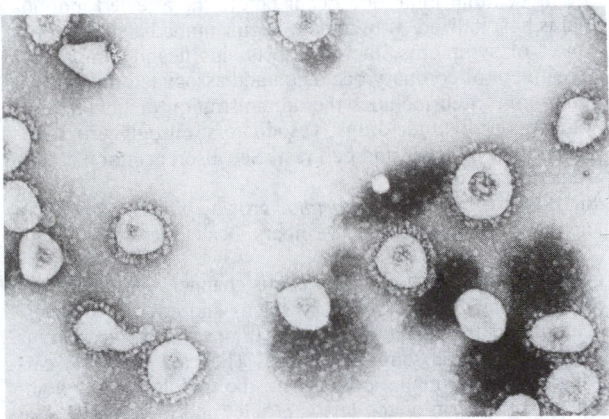

Coronavirus
(*Murray, 1990/Courtesy Center for Disease Control, Atlanta, Georgia*)

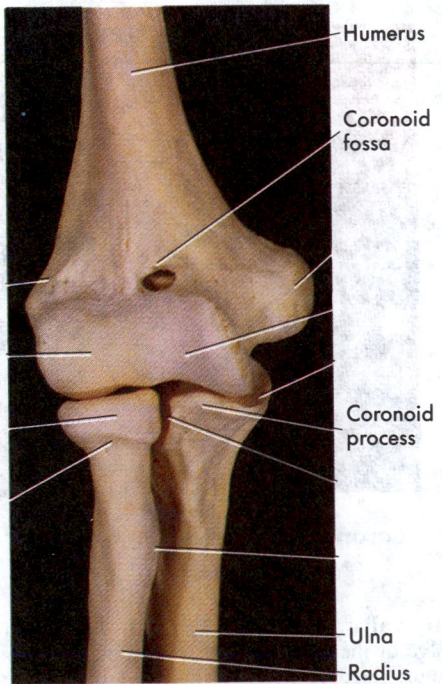

Coronoid fossa and coronoid process of the elbow
(*Thibodeau, 1993*)

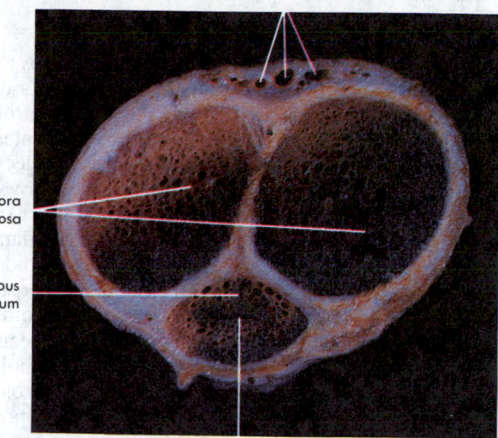

Dorsal blood vessels of penis

Corpora
cavernosa

Corpus
spongiosum

Urethra

Cross-section of the penis showing the corpus cavernosum and corpus spongiosum
(Thibodeau, 1993)

corpuscle /kôr′pəsəl/ [L, *corpusculum,* little body], **1.** any cell of the body. **2.** a red or white blood cell. Also called **corpuscule.** –corpuscular, *adj.*

corpuscular radiation /kôrpus′kyələr/ [L, *corpusculum; radiare,* to emit rays], the radiation associated with subatomic particles, such as electrons, protons, neutrons, or alpha particles, that travel in streams at various velocities. All these particles have definite masses and have radiation properties very different from electromagnetic radiations, which have no mass and travel in wave forms at the speed of light. See also **background radiation, leakage radiation, scattered radiation.**

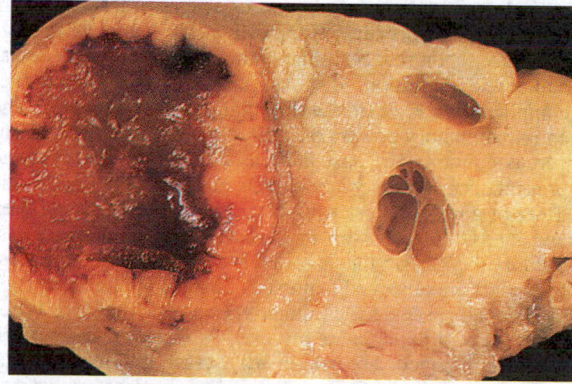

Corpus luteum *(Fletcher, 1987)*

corpus luteum /kôr′pəs lōo′tē·əm/, *pl.* **corpora lutea** [L, body; *luteus,* yellow], an anatomic structure on the surface of the ovary, consisting of a spheroid of yellowish tissue 1 to 2 cm in diameter that grows within the ruptured ovarian follicle after ovulation. The pleated wall of the collapsed follicle is made up of several layers of granulosa cells that grow toward the center of the cavity to form the struc-

ture. During the reproductive years of a woman's life, a corpus luteum forms after every ovulation. It acts as a short-lived endocrine organ that secretes progesterone, which serves to maintain the decidual layer of the endometrium in the richly vascular state necessary for implantation and pregnancy. If conception occurs, the corpus luteum grows and secretes increasing amounts of progesterone. It reaches its maximum function and size (2 to 3 cm) at 10 to 12 weeks of gestation. It persists, slowly diminishing in size and function, until 6 months after the onset of gestation. During the 2 weeks before menstruation, the corpus luteum secretes progesterone in decreasing amounts, atrophies, undergoes fibrotic degeneration, and becomes a pale spot on the surface of the ovary. Compare **corpus albicans.**

corpus spongiosum /spon′jē·ō′səm/, one of the cylinders of spongy tissue that, with the corpora cavernosa, form the penis.

corpus vitreum. See **vitreous humor.**

corrected pressure [L, *corrigere,* to make straight], a method of applying Boyle's law of gas pressures to adjust simultaneously for changes in both pressure and humidity.

corrective emotional experience /kərek′tiv/, a process by which a patient gives up old patterns of behavior and learns or relearns new patterns by reexperiencing early unresolved feelings and needs.

corrective exercise. See **therapeutic exercise.**

correlation /kôr′əlā′shən/ [L, *com + relatio,* a carrying back], (in statistics) a relationship between variables that may be negative (inverse), positive, or curvilinear. Correlation is measured and expressed using numeric scales.

correlative differentiation /kərel′ətiv/, (in embryology) specialization or diversification of cells or tissues caused by an inductor or other external factor. Also called **dependent differentiation.**

Corrigan's pulse [Dominic J. Corrigan, Irish physician, b. 1802], a bounding pulse in which a great surge is felt followed by a sudden and complete absence of force or fullness in the artery. This kind of pulse occurs in excited emotional states, in various abnormal cardiac conditions, including patent ductus arteriosus, and as a result of systemic arteriosclerosis.

corrode. See **corrosive.**

corrosion. See **corrosive.**

corrosion of surgical instruments /kərō′zhen/ [L, *corrodere,* to gnaw away], the rusting of surgical instruments or the gradual wearing away of their polished surfaces because of oxidation and the action of contaminants. Though minimized by the use of stainless steel alloys in the fabrication of the instruments, corrosion persists as a problem, even when cleaning procedures seem more than adequate. It usually occurs because of inadequate cleaning and drying of surgical instruments after use, the use of sterilizing solutions that eat into the surface, overexposure to such solutions, or a faulty autoclave. Cleanliness is the single most important factor in preventing corrosion. Any foreign material, either organic or inorganic, on the surface of stainless steel is likely to promote corrosion, and microscopic examinations often reveal foreign material and chlorides from cleaning solutions scattered over the surface of cleaned and sterilized instruments. The more chromium in the stainless steel alloys of which surgical instruments are made, the more resistant the instruments are to corrosion. Carbon, which hardens such alloys, also reduces their resistance to corrosion. Most corrosion of surgical instruments is superficial and may be removed by soaking in a solution of ammonia and alcohol or by repolishing by the manufacturer.

corrosive /kərō'siv/ [L, *corrodere*, to gnaw away], **1.** eating away a substance or tissue, especially by chemical action. **2.** an agent or substance that eats away a substance or tissue. **−corrode,** *v.,* **corrosion,** *n.*

corrosive gastritis, an acute inflammatory condition of the stomach caused by the ingestion of an acid, alkali, or other corrosive chemical in which the lining of the stomach is eaten away by the corrosive substance. The amount of tissue destruction and recommended treatment depend on the nature of the corrosive agent and the extent of exposure. Compare **chemical gastritis, erosive gastritis.** See also **acid poisoning, alkali poisoning.**

corrugator supercilii /kôr'əgā'tər sōo'pərsil'ē·ī/ [L, *corrugare*, to wrinkle; *super*, above, *cilium*, eyelash], one of the three muscles of the eyelid. Arising from the medial end of the supercilliary arch and inserting into the skin above the orbital arch, it is innervated by temporal and zygomatic branches of the facial nerve and functions to draw the eyebrow downward and inward, as if to frown. Also called **corrugator.** Compare **levator palpebrae superioris, orbicularis oculi.**

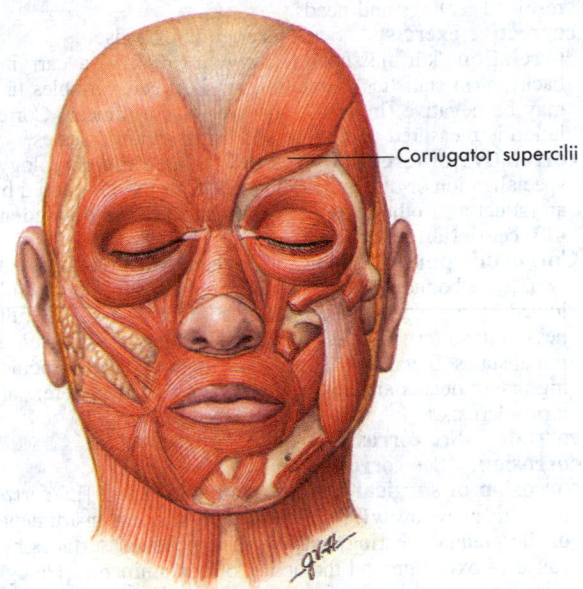

Corrugator supercilii

Corrugator supercilli muscle
(Thibodeau, 1983/John V Hagen)

-cort-, a suffix designating a cortisone derivative.

cortex, *pl.* **cortices** /kôr'tisēz/ [L, bark], the outer layer of a body organ or other structure, as distinguished from the internal substance.

cortic-, a combining form meaning 'pertaining to the cortex or bark': *corticipetal, corticobulbar, corticothalamic.*

cortical audiometry. See **audiometry.**

cortical blindness /kôr'tikəl/ [L, *cortex* + AS, *blind*], blindness that results from a lesion in the visual center of the cerebral cortex of the brain.

cortical bone, bone that is 70% to 90% mineralized.

cortical fracture [L, *cortex* + *fractura*, break], any fracture that involves the cortex of the bone.

cortical substance of cerebellum. See **cerebellar cortex.**

cortices. See **cortex.**

corticosteroid /kôr'tikōstir'oid/ [L, *cortex* + *steros*, solid], any one of the natural or the synthetic hormones associated with the adrenal cortex, which influences or controls key processes of the body, such as carbohydrate and protein metabolism, maintenance of serum glucose levels, electrolyte and water balance, and the functions of the cardiovascular system, the skeletal muscle, the kidneys, and other organs. The corticosteroids synthesized by the adrenal glands include the glucocorticoids and the mineralocorticoids. The principal glucocorticoids are cortisol and corticosterone. The only physiologically important mineralocorticoid in humans is aldosterone. The glucocorticoids tend to cause the cells of the body to shift from carbohydrate catabolism to fat catabolism, to accelerate the breakdown of proteins to amino acids, and to help maintain normal blood pressure. The secretion of these hormones increases during stress, especially that produced by anxiety and severe injury. Chronic overproduction of these substances is associated with various disorders, such as Cushing's syndrome. A high blood level of glucocorticoids markedly increases the number of eosinophils and decreases the size of lymphatic tissues, especially the thymus and the lymph nodes. The decrease in lymphocytes retards antibody formation and affects the immune system of the body. Aldosterone is the most powerful of the natural mineralocorticoids in the regulation of electrolyte balance, especially in the balance of sodium and potassium. Cortisol induces sodium retention and potassium excretion but not as effectively as aldosterone. The effects of the corticosteroids on the cardiovascular system, which are not precisely understood, are most evident in hypocorticism when the reduction in blood volume, accompanied by increased viscosity, may cause hypotension and cardiovascular collapse. The absence of corticosteroids increases capillary permeability, decreases the vasomotor response of the small vessels, and reduces cardiac size and output. The skeletal muscles require adequate amounts of the corticosteroids to function normally; excessive amounts cause them to function abnormally. Cortisol and its synthetic analogs can prevent or reduce inflammation by inhibiting edema, leukocytic migration, disposition of collagen, and other complications associated with inflammatory processes. The antiinflammatory powers of synthetic hormones can be dangerous, however, because they mask the disease process and prevent accurate observation of its progress. Pharmacologic doses of glucocorticosteroids retard bone growth of children and inhibit cell division in various developing structures, such as the gastric mucosa, liver, lung, and brain. Glucocorticoids are absorbed from sites of local application, such as synovial spaces, the conjunctival sac, and the skin. When large areas of the skin are involved or when the administration is prolonged, absorption may cause systemic effects, including adrenocortical suppression. Corticosteroids may be administered orally, parenterally, or topically. Toxic effects may result from the too rapid withdrawal of such drugs after prolonged therapy or from the continued use of large doses. Toxic effects associated with prolonged corticosteroid therapy include fluid and electrolyte imbalance, hyperglycemia and glycosuria, increased susceptibility to infections, myopathy, arrested growth, ecchymoses, Cushing's syndrome, acne, and behavioral disturbances. The increased susceptibility to infection associated with corticosteroids is not specific for any particular pathogen, and those patients who develop infections while undergoing corticosteroid therapy are usually treated concomitantly with appropriate antibacterial agents. Peptic ulceration occurs in some patients undergoing corticosteroid therapy, and some patients receiving large doses of these drugs develop myopathy, characterized by weakness of the proximal musculature of the arms and the legs and of associated shoulder and pelvic muscles. Corticosteroid therapy may also produce behavioral changes, such as schizophrenia, suicidal tendencies, nervousness, and insomnia. See also **adrenal crisis.**

corticosteroid-binding globulin. See **transcortin.**

corticotropin. See **adrenocorticotropic hormone.**

corticotropin-releasing factor (CRF) /kôr′tikōtrop′in/, a polypeptide secreted by the hypothalamus into the bloodstream. It triggers the release of ACTH from the pituitary gland.

cortisol /kôr′təsôl/, a steroid hormone occurring naturally in the body and produced synthetically for pharmacologic use. Also called **hydrocortisone.**
- INDICATION: It is prescribed as an antiinflammatory agent.
- CONTRAINDICATIONS: Fungal infections or known hypersensitivity to this drug prohibits its systemic use. Viral or fungal infections of the skin, impaired circulation, or known hypersensitivity to this drug prohibits its topical use.
- ADVERSE EFFECTS: Among the more serious adverse reactions to the systemic administration of this drug are GI, endocrine, neurologic, fluid, and electrolyte disturbances. A variety of hypersensitivity reactions may occur from topical administration of this drug.

cortisone /kôr′təsōn/, a glucocorticoid produced in the liver and also made synthetically.
- INDICATION: It is prescribed as an antiinflammatory agent.
- CONTRAINDICATIONS: Fungal infections or known hypersensitivity to this drug prohibits its systemic use. Viral or fungal infections of the skin, impaired circulation, or known hypersensitivity to this drug prohibits its topical use.
- ADVERSE EFFECTS: Among the more serious adverse reactions to the systemic administration of the drug are GI, endocrine, neurologic, fluid, and electrolyte disturbances. A variety of skin reactions may occur from topical administration of this drug.

Corti's organ. See **organ of Corti.**

Cortisporin, a trademark for a topical fixed-combination drug containing a glucocorticoid (hydrocortisone) and three antibacterials (neomycin sulfate, polymyxin B sulfate, and bacitracin zinc).

Corynebacterium /kôr′inē′baktir′ē·əm/ [Gk, *koryne,* club, *bakterion,* small staff], a common genus of rod-shaped, curved bacilli having many species. The most common pathogenic species are *Corynebacterium acnes,* commonly found in acne lesions, and *C. diphtheriae,* the cause of diphtheria. See also *Propionibacterium.*

coryza. See **rhinitis.**

coryza spasmodica. See **hay fever.**

Corzide, a trademark for a combination antihypertensive medication (nadolol and bendroflumethiazide).

Cosmegen, a trademark for an antineoplastic (dactinomycin).

cosmetic surgery /kosmet′ik/ [Gk, *kosmesis,* adornment], reconstruction of cutaneous or underlying tissues, performed to improve and correct a structural defect or to remove a scar, birthmark, or some normal evidence of aging. A local anesthetic is usually sufficient. Kinds of cosmetic surgery include **blepharoplasty, rhinoplasty, rhytidoplasty.** Compare **plastic surgery.**

cosmic radiation /kos′mik/, high-energy particles with great penetrating power originating in outer space and reaching the earth as normal background radiation. The rays consist partly of high-energy atomic nuclei.

cost-. See **costi-.**

costal /kos′təl/ [L, *costa,* rib], **1.** of or pertaining to a rib. **2.** situated near a rib or on a side close to a rib.

costal arch [L, *costa* + *arcus,* bow], an arch formed by the shafts of the ribs.

costal cartilage, the cartilage at the anterior end of each rib.

costalgia /kostal′jē·ə/[L, *costa,* rib; Gk, *algos,* pain], a pain in the ribs.

cost analysis [L *costare* to stand firm; Gk, *ana,* again, *lyein,* to loosen], an analysis of the disbursements of a given activity, agency, department, or program.

COSTAR /kō′stär/, abbreviation for *COmputer STored Ambulatory Record* system, an on-line interactive computerized information system, accessible via a minicomputer, for the public health field.

cost-benefit ratio, a ratio that represents the relationship of the cost of an activity to the benefit of its outcome or product.

cost cap, *informal.* a limit on the amount of money that an agency, department, or institution may spend.

cost center, a department, division, or other subunit of an institution established within its accounting system so that the income and expenses of the subunit can be separated from the income or expenses of other centers and monitored for cost and benefit.

cost control, the process of monitoring and regulating of the expenditure of funds by an agency or institution. Budgets, reports, and cost-accounting procedures are performed to achieve cost control.

cost effectiveness, the extent to which an activity is thought to be as valuable as it is expensive, such as a public-assistance program that gives vouchers for nutritious foods in pregnancy being cost-effective if it were to prevent the costly incidence of perinatal morbidity.

Costen's syndrome. See **temporomandibular joint pain-dysfunction syndrome.**

costi-, cost-, costo-, a prefix meaning 'pertaining to a rib': *costicartillage, costicervical, costifluous.*

costocervical /kos′tōsur′vikəl/ [L, *costa,* rib, *cervix,* neck], pertaining to or involving the ribs and the neck.

costochondral /kos′təkon′drəl/ [L, *costa* + Gk, *chondros,* cartilage], of or pertaining to a rib and its cartilage.

costoclavicular /-klavik′yələr/ [L, *costa* + *clavicula,* little key], pertaining to or involving the ribs and the clavicle.

costophrenic (CP) angle /-fren′ik/ [L, *costa* + *phrenicus,* diaphragm], the angle at the bottom of the lung where the diaphragm and chest wall meet.

costosternal /-stur′nəl/, pertaining to or involving the ribs and the sternum.

costotransverse articulation /-transvurs′/ [L, *costa* + *transversus,* a cross direction], any one of 20 gliding joints between the ribs and associated vertebrae, except for the eleventh and twelfth ribs. The five ligaments that associate with each costotransverse joint are the articular capsule, the superior costotransverse ligament, the posterior costotransverse ligament, the ligament of the neck of the rib, and the ligament of the tubercle of the rib.

costovertebral /-vur′təbrəl/, of or relating to a rib and the vertebral column.

costovertebral angle (CVA), one of two angles that outline a space over the kidneys. The angle is formed by the lateral and downward curve of the lowest rib and the vertical column of the spine itself. CVA tenderness to percussion is a common finding in pyelonephritis and other infections of the kidney and adjacent structures.

cosyntropin /kō′sintrop′in/, a synthetic form of ACTH that is used in the diagnosis and treatment of adrenal hypofunction disorders, such as Addison's disease.

C.O.T.A., abbreviation for **Certified Occupational Therapy Assistant.**

Cotazym, a trademark for an enzyme (pancrelipase).

cot death. See **sudden infant death syndrome.**

cotton-mill fever. See **byssinosis.**

cottonmouth, a poisonous pit viper commonly found near water and swamps of the southeastern part of the United States. The symptoms of the bite of a cottonmouth are rapid swelling, severe pain, skin discoloration at bite marks, and weakness. Antivenin and oxygen are the usual treatments. Also called **water moccasin.**

Cotton's fracture, a trimalleolar fracture involving medial, lateral, and posterior malleoli.

cotton-wool exudate [Ar, *qutun;* AS, *wull,* ME, *spot*], a soft-white exudate seen on the retina of patients with certain systemic conditions, such as AIDS, hypertension, and lupus. Thry can also be observed in retinal infections. Also called **cotton-wool spot, cotton-wool patch.**

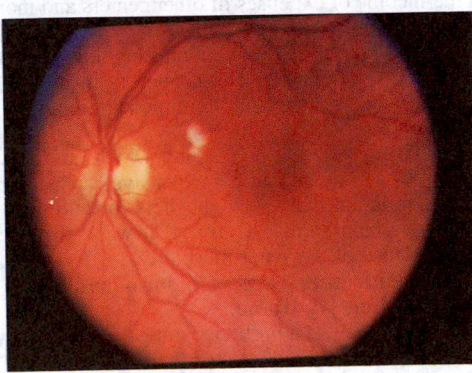

Cotton-wool exudate (Zitelli, 1992)

cotyledon /kot′ilē′don/ [Gk, *kotyledon,* cup-shaped], one of the visible segments on the maternal surface of the placenta. A typical placenta may have 15 to 28 cotyledons, each consisting of fetal vessels, chorionic villi, and intervillous space.

cotyloid cavity. See **acetabulum.**

cough /kôf/ [AS, *cohhetan*], a sudden, audible expulsion of air from the lungs. Coughing is preceded by inspiration, the glottis is partially closed, and the accessory muscles of expiration contract to expel the air forcibly from the respiratory passages. Coughing is an essential protective response that serves to clear the lungs, bronchi, or trachea of irritants and secretions or to prevent aspiration of foreign material into the lungs. It is a common symptom of diseases of the chest and larynx. Chronic coughing may be indica-

tive of tuberculosis, lung cancer, bronchiectasis, or bronchitis. Otitis media, subdiaphragmatic irritation, congestive heart failure, and mitral valve disease may be associated with episodes of severe chronic coughing. Coughing is a reflex action that may be induced voluntarily and, to some extent, voluntarily inhibited. The cough-reflex center is located in the medulla of the brain. It responds to stimulation transmitted by the glossopharyngeal or vagus nerve. The reflex is initiated by chemical or mechanical irritation of the pharynx, larynx, or tracheobronchial tree. Because the function of coughing is to clear the respiratory tract of secretions, it is important that the cough bring out accumulated debris. Where it does not, because of weakness or inhibition of the force of the cough caused by pain, instruction and assistance in effective coughing and deep-breathing exercises are required. Persons with chronic coughs may obtain symptomatic relief through environmental controls that reduce irritants in the air and provide humidification. Medication may be supplied to dilate the bronchi, liquefy secretions, and increase expectoration. Rest, increased fluid intake, and adequate nutrition are necessary. Antitussive medications are sometimes prescribed in the treatment of a cough in the absence of mucus or congestion.

cough fracture, any fracture of a rib, usually the fifth or the seventh rib, caused by violent coughing.

cough syncope [AS, *cohhetan;* Gk, *syncope,* fainting], a temporary loss of consciousness due to an interruption in cerebral blood flow during coughing. The coughing spell increases the intrathoracic pressure enough to impede venous return, thereby interfering with normal blood flow to the brain.

coulomb /kōō′lōm/ [Charles A. de Coulomb, French physicist, b. 1736], the SI unit of electricity equal to the quantity of charge transferred in 1 second across a conductor in which there is a constant current of 1 ampere, or 1 ampere-second.

Coulomb's law, (in physics) a law stating that the force of attraction or repulsion between two electrically charged bodies is directly proportional to the strength of the electric charges and inversely proportional to the square of the distance between them.

coulometry /kōōlom′ətrē/, a type of electroanalytic chemistry in which a reagent generated at the surface of an electrode reacts with a substance to be measured. The substance, usually a metal ion, is measured in terms of the coulombs required for the reaction.

Coulter counter /kōl′tər/ [W. H. Coulter, 20th century American engineer], a trademark for an electric device that rapidly identifies, sorts, and counts the various kinds of cells present in a small specimen of blood.

Coumadin, a trademark for an anticoagulant (warfarin sodium).

coumarin /kōō′mərin/, an anticoagulant.

■ INDICATIONS: It is prescribed for prophylaxis and treatment of thrombosis and embolism.

■ CONTRAINDICATIONS: Known hypersensitivity to the drug prohibits its use. It is not used in situations where there is a risk of hemorrhage.

■ ADVERSE EFFECTS: The most serious adverse reaction is hemorrhage. Many other drugs interact with this drug to increase or decrease its effect.

counseling [L, *consulere,* to consult], the act of providing advice and guidance to a patient or the patient's family. It is a therapeutic technique that helps the patient recognize and manage stress and that facilitates interpersonal relationships between the patient and the family, significant others, or the health care team. See also **genetic counseling.**

count [L, *computere*, to calculate], a computation of the number of objects or elements present per unit of measurement. Kinds of counts include **Addis count, bacteria count, blood count,** and **platelet count.**

counterclaim [L, *contra* + *clamere*, to cry out], (in law) a claim made by a defendant establishing a cause for action in his favor against the plaintiff. The purpose of a counterclaim is to oppose or detract from the plaintiff's claim or complaint.

counterconditioning, a process used in behavioral therapy in which a learned response is replaced by an alternative response that is less disruptive.

countercurrent, a change in the direction of the flow of a fluid, as occurs in the ascending branch of a kidney tubule where osmolality undergoes a reversal after a gradual change in sodium chloride concentrations.

counterinjunction /-injungk'shən/, (in transactional analysis) an overt message from the parent ego state of the mother or father that may be difficult to follow if the message conflicts with earlier parental instructions. For example, the person may obey an earlier injunction to avoid close relationships, then be instructed later to "grow up and get married."

counterphobic behavior /-fō'bik/, an expression of reaction to a phobia by a patient who actively seeks exposure to the type of situation that precipitates phobic symptoms.

counterpulsation /-pulsā'shən/ [L, *contra* + *pulsare*, to beat], **1.** the action of a circulatory-assist pumping device synchronized counter to the normal action of the heart. **2.** the process of increasing the intraaortic pressure in diastole by inflation of an intraaortic balloon and deflation of the balloon immediately preceding the next systole.

countershock [L, *contra* + Fr, *choc*], (in cardiology) a high-intensity, short-duration electric shock applied to the area of the heart, resulting in total cardiac depolarization. See also **cardioversion, defibrillation.**

countertraction /-trak'shən/ [L, *contra* + *trahere*, to pull], a force that counteracts the pull of traction, especially in orthopedics, such as the force of body weight resulting from the pull of gravity. Orthopedic countertraction may also be obtained by altering the angle of the body force in relation to the pull of traction, such as by elevating the foot of the bed with shock blocks to attain Trendelenburg's position. The magnitude of countertraction depends on the amount of force needed to counteract the pull of the traction and is usually developed gradually by methodically changing the position of a patient and by adding or by removing weights from weight hangers.

countertransference /-transfur'əns/, the conscious or unconscious emotional response of a psychotherapist or psychoanalyst to a patient. The response is inappropriate to the content and context of the therapeutic relationship. See also **transference.**

countertransport /-trans'pôrt/ [L, *contra* + *trans,* across, *portare*, carry], the simultaneous transport of two different substances across the same membrane, each in the opposite direction.

counting cell hemocytometer [OFr, *conter;* L, *cella,* storeroom; Gk, *haima,* blood, *metron,* measure], a device for counting the number of cells in a volume of blood or other fluid. It consists of a microscope slide with a counting chamber. The chamber has a known volume and the slide has a ruled area to help count the cells.

coup /ko̅o̅/ [Fr, blow], any blow or stroke or the effects of such a blow or stroke to the body, usually used with a French word identifying a type of stroke: **1. coup de sabre** /ko̅o̅dəsäb'r(ə)/, a wound resembling a sword cut. **2. coup de soleil.** See **sunstroke. 3. coup sur coup** /ko̅o̅sYrko̅o̅'/, administration of a drug in small amounts over a short period of time rather than in a single larger dose. **4. contre coup** /kôNtrəko̅o̅'/, an injury most often associated with a blow to the skull in which the force of the impact is transmitted through the skull bones to the opposite side of the head where the bruise, fracture, or other sign of injury appears.

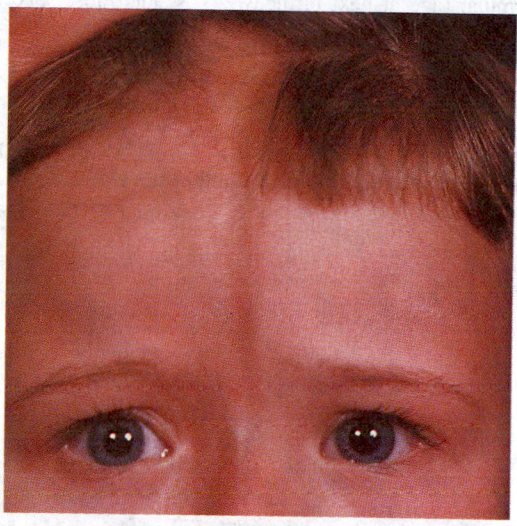

Coup de sabre (du Vivier, 1993)

coupled. See **pacing.**

coupled pacing. See **pacing.**

coupled rhythm. See **bigeminal rhythm.**

couples therapy, psychotherapy in which couples, who may be married or unmarried but living together, undergo therapy together.

coupling /kup'ling/ [L, *copula,* bonding], **1.** the act of coming together, joining, or pairing. **2.** (in genetics) the situation in linked inheritance in which the nonalleles of two or more mutant genes are located on the same chromosome and are close enough so that they are likely to be inherited together. **3.** (in radiation therapy) the efficiency of transfer of power from an applicator to the treatment site. Compare **repulsion.** See also **cis configuration.**

coupling interval, the interval between the dominant heartbeat and a linked ectopic beat, measured from the beginning of a normal QRS complex to the beginning of the ectopic QRS complex that follows it.

coup sur coup. See **coup.**

courseware /kôrs'wer/, software programs for use in instruction.

Courvoisier's law /ko̅o̅rvô·ä·zē·āz'/ [Ludwig Courvoisier, Swiss surgeon, b. 1843], a statement that the gallbladder is smaller than usual if a gallstone blocks the common bile duct but is dilated if the common bile duct is blocked as a result of a cause other than a gallstone, such as cancer of the pancreas.

couvade /ko͞ovä´d´/, a custom in some non-Western cultures whereby the husband goes through mock labor while his wife is giving birth.

Couvelaire uterus /ko͞ovəler´/ [Alexandre Couvelaire, French obstetrician, b. 1873], a hemorrhagic process in uterine musculature that may accompany severe abruptio placenta. Extravasated blood effuses between the muscle fibrils and under the uterine peritoneum. The uterus takes on a purplish color and does not contract well. Also called **uteroplacental apoplexy.** See also **abruptio placenta.**

Cowling's rule /Kou´lings/, a method of calculating the approximate pediatric dosage of a drug for a child using this formula: (age at next birthday/24) × adult dose. See also **pediatric dosage.**

Cowper's gland /kou´pərz/ [William Cowper, English surgeon, b. 1666], either of two round, pea-sized glands embedded in the urethral sphincter of the male. Normally yellow in color, they consist of several lobes with ducts that join and form a single excretory duct. Also called **bulbourethral gland.** Compare **Bartholin's gland.**

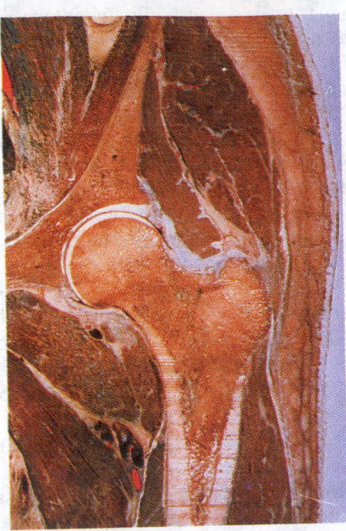

Coaxl articulation (Seeley, 1992/RT Hutchings)

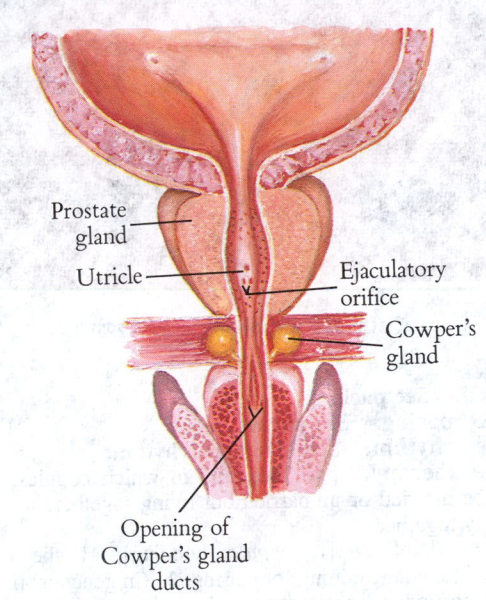

Prostate gland

Utricle

Ejaculatory orifice

Cowper's gland

Opening of Cowper's gland ducts

Cowper's gland (Seidel, 1991)

cowpox /kou´poks/ [AS, cu; ME, pokkes], a mild infectious disease characterized by a pustular rash, caused by the vaccinia virus transmitted to humans from infected cattle. Cowpox infection usually confers immunity to smallpox, because of the similarity of the variola and vaccinia viruses. See also **smallpox, vaccinia.**

coxa /kok´sə/, pl. **coxae** [L, hip], the hip joint; the head of the femur and the acetabulum of the innominate bone.

coxa adducta, coxa flexa. See **coxa vara.**

coxal articulation /kok´səl/ [L, coxa + articularis, relating to the joints], the ball-and-socket joint of the hip, formed by the articulation of the head of the femur into the cup-shaped cavity of the acetabulum. It involves seven ligaments and permits very extensive movements, such as flexion, extension, adduction, abduction, circumduction, and rotation. Also called **hip joint.** Compare **shoulder joint.**

coxa magna, an abnormal widening of the head and neck of the femur.

coxa plana. See **Perthes' disease.**

coxa valga, a hip deformity in which the angle formed by the axis of the head and neck of the femur and the axis of its shaft is significantly increased.

coxa vara, a hip deformity in which the angle formed by the axis of the head and neck of the femur and the axis of its shaft is decreased. Also called **coxa adducta, coxa flexa.**

coxa vara luxans, a fissure or crack in the neck of the femur with dislocation of the head, caused by coxa vara.

coxsackievirus /koksak´ē-/ [Coxsackie, New York; L, virus, poison], any of 30 serologically different enteroviruses associated with a variety of symptoms and primarily affecting children during warm weather. The coxsackieviruses resemble the virus responsible for poliomyelitis, particularly in size; both are picornaviruses. Among the diseases associated with coxsackievirus infections are herpangina, hand, foot, and mouth disease, epidemic pleurodynia, myocarditis, pericarditis, aseptic meninigitis, and several exanthems. There is no known preventive measure except isolation of infected persons, and the treatment is generally directed toward relief of symptoms. See also **viral infection.**

C.P., 1. abbreviation for **candle power.** 2. abbreviation for **cerebral palsy.** 3. abbreviation for **chemically pure.**

CPAN, abbreviation for *Certified Post-Anesthesia Nurse.*

CPAP, abbreviation for **continuous positive airway pressure.**

CPD, 1. abbreviation for **cephalopelvic disproportion.** 2. abbreviation for **childhood polycystic disease.** See **polycystic kidney disease.** 3. abbreviation for **congenital polycystic disease.** See **polycystic kidney disease.**

C-peptide, a biologically inactive residue of insulin for mation in the beta cells of the pancreas. When proinsulin is converted to insulin, an equal amount of C-peptide, a chain of amino acids, is also secreted into the blood stream. Beta cell secretory function can be determined by measuring the C-peptide in a blood sample.

CPHA, abbreviation for the **Canadian Public Health Association.**

CPK, abbreviation for *creatine phosphokinase.* See **creatine kinase.**

CPK isoenzyme fraction, one of several blood-borne enzymes that are released after myocardial necrosis. The isoenzyme of CPK (creatine phosphokinase) is identified as MB isomer, or MB-CPK, and is a diagnostic clue to heart damage. See also **lactate dehydrogenase (LDH), serum glutamic oxaloacetic transaminase (SGOT).**

CPNP/A, abbreviation for *Certified Pediatric Nurse Practitioner/Associate.*

CPPB, abbreviation for **continuous positive pressure breathing.**

CPPD, abbreviation for *calcium pyrophosphate dihydrate.* See *chondrocalcinosis.*

CPPV, abbreviation for **continuous positive pressure ventilation.**

CPR, abbreviation for **cardiopulmonary resuscitation.**

CPRAM, abbreviation for *controlled partial rebreathing anesthesia method.*

CPT, abbreviation for **current procedural terminology.**

cpu, CPU, abbreviation for **central processing unit** of a computer.

Cr, symbol for the element **chromium.**

CR, abbreviation for *controlled respiration.*

crab louse [AS, *crabba, lus*], a species of body louse, *Phthirus pubis,* that infests the hairs of the genital area and is often transmitted between persons by venereal contact. Also called *Pediculus pubis, (informal)* **crab.** See also **pediculosis.**

crack [ME, *craken*], a street drug made by chemically converting cocaine hydrochloride to a form that can be smoked. Smoking crack is a faster, more direct way of getting cocaine molecules into the brain. Because larger amounts of the drug reach the brain more quickly, the effects are more intense than when cocaine, in the white-powder form, is injected, ingested, or inhaled. Also called **crack cocaine, freebase.**

crack baby, an infant who was exposed to effects of cocaine in utero by a mother who used the "crack" form of the drug while pregnant.

crack cocaine. See **cocaine hydrochloride, crack.**

cracked-pot sound [ME, *craken, pott;* L, *sonus,* sound], a sound sometimes heard on percussion over a cavity with an opening to a bronchus.

crackle, a common abnormal respiratory sound heard on auscultation of the chest during inspiration, characterized by discontinuous bubbling noises. Fine crackles have a crackling sound produced by air entering distal bronchioles or alveoli that contain serous secretions, as in congestive heart failure, pneumonia, or early tuberculosis. Coarse sounds may originate in the larger bronchi or trachea and have a lower pitch. Also called *(obsolete)* **rale.** Compare **rhonchus, wheeze.**

crackling rale /râle/ [AS, *cracian;* Fr, rattle], an abnormal breathing sound produced by fluid in the bronchioles during inspiration.

cradle cap [AS, *cradel, caeppe*], a common seborrheic dermatitis of infants consisting of thick, yellow, greasy scales on the scalp. Treatment includes oil or ointment to soften the scales and frequent shampoos. Also called **seborrhea capitis.**

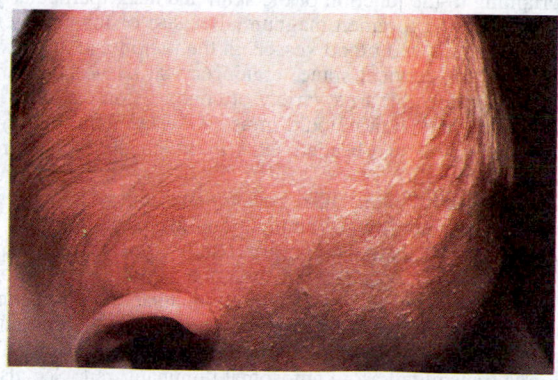

Cradle cap
(Goldstein, 1992/Courtesy Department of Dermatology, University of North Carolina at Chapel Hill)

cramp [AS, *crammian,* to fill], **1.** a spasmodic and often painful contraction of one or more muscles. **2.** a pain resembling a muscular cramp. Kinds of cramps include **cane-cutter's cramp, fireman's cramp, miner's cramp, stoker's cramp,** and **writer's cramp.** See also **charley horse, dysmenorrhea, heat cramp, wryneck.**

-crania, a suffix meaning '(condition of the) skull or head': *diastematocrania, hemicrania, platycrania.*

cranial. See **cranium.**

cranial arachnoid. See **arachnoidea encephali.**

cranial arteritis. See **temporal arteritis.**

cranial bones /krā′nē·əl/ [Gk, *kranion,* cranium; AS, *ban*], the bones of the skull, particularly the part of the cranium that encloses the brain.

cranial nerves [Gk, *kranion,* skull; L, *nervus*], the 12 pairs of nerves emerging from the cranial cavity through various openings in the skull. Beginning with the most anterior, they are designated by Roman numerals and named (I) olfactory, (II) optic, (III) oculomotor, (IV) trochlear, (V) trigeminal, (VI) abducens, (VII) facial, (VIII) acoustic or auditory, (IX) glossopharyngeal, (X) vagal, (XI) accessory, (XII) hypoglossal. The cranial nerves originate in the base of the brain and carry impulses for such functions as smell, vision, ocular move ment, pupil contraction, muscular sensibility, general sensibility, mastication, facial expression, glandular secretion, taste, cutaneous sensibility, hearing, equilibrium, swallowing, phonation, tongue movement, head movement, and shoulder movement. Certain cranial nerves, particularly V, VII, and VIII, contain two or more distinct functional components considered as independent nerves by some authorities. In this category the masticatory nerve would be separated from the trigeminal (V), the glossopalatine from the facial (VII), and the equilibrium from the acoustic (VIII), making 15 pairs in all. Some anatomists also classify the terminal nerve as the first cranial. Also called **cerebral nerves.** See also the specific nerves.

craniectomy /krā′nē·ek′təmē/ [Gk, *kranion,* cranium, *ektome,* cutting out], the surgical removal of a portion of the cranium.

cranio- /krā′nē·ō-/, a prefix meaning 'pertaining to the skull or cranium': *craniobuccal, craniognomy, craniosacral.*

craniocele. See **encephalocele.**

craniocervical /-sur′vikəl/ [Gk, *kranion* + L, *cervix*, neck], pertaining to the junction of the skull and neck, particularly the area of the foramen magnum. Because of the complex of nerve fibers and blood vessels in the region and the flexibility of the cervical spine, craniocervical tissues are particularly vulnerable to a variety of compression disorders.

craniodidymus /krā′nē·ōdid′iməs/ [Gk, *kranion* + *didymos*, twin], a two-headed fetus in which the bodies are fused.

craniofacial /-fā′shəl/ [Gk, *kranion*, cranium, L, *facies*, face], pertaining to the cranium and the face.

craniofacial dysostosis [Gk, *kranion* + L, *facies*, face; Gk, *dys*, bad, *osteon*, bone], an abnormal hereditary condition characterized by acrocephaly, exophthalmos, hypertelorism, strabismus, parrot-beaked nose, and hypoplastic maxilla with relative mandibular prognathism. This condition is transmitted as an autosomal dominant trait. See also **dysostosis.**

craniohypophyseal xanthoma /krā′nē·ōhī′pōfiz′ē·əl/ [Gk, *kranion* + *hypo*, deficient, *phyein*, to grow; *xanthos*, yellow, *oma*, tumor], a condition in which cholesterol deposits are formed around the hypophyses of the bones, as in Hand-Schüller-Christian disease.

craniometaphyseal dysplasia /-met′əfiz′ē·əl/, an inherited bone disorder characterized by paranasal overgrowth, thickening of the skull and jaw, and entrapment of cranial nerves. The long bones have widened, club-shaped metaphyses. The patient may experience nasorespiratory infections, associated with bone overgrowth at the sinuses, and malocclusion of the jaws.

craniopagus /krā′nē·op′əgəs/ [Gk, *kranion* + *pagos*, fixed], conjoined twins united at the heads. Fusion can occur at the frontal, occipital, or parietal regions. Also called **cephalopagus.**

craniopharyngeal /krā′nē·ōfərin′jē·əl/ [Gk, *kranion* + *pharynx*, throat], of or pertaining to the cranium and the pharynx.

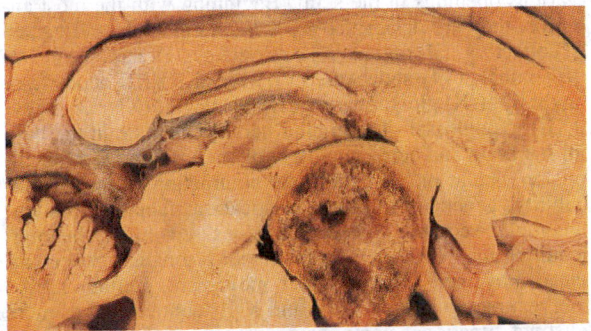

Craniopharyngioma *(Fletcher, 1987)*

craniopharyngioma /krā′nē·ōfərin′jē·ō′mə/, *pl.* **craniopharyngiomas, craniopharyngiomata,** a congenital pituitary tumor, appearing most often in children and adolescents, that arises in cells derived from Rathke's pouch or the hypophyseal stalk. The lesion, a solid or cystic body ranging in size from 1 to 8 cm, may expand into the third ventricle or the temporal lobe, frequently becoming calcified. The tumor may interfere with pituitary function, damage the optic chiasm, disrupt hypothalamic control of the autonomic nervous system, and result in hydrocephalus. Increased intracranial pressure, severe headaches, vomiting, stunted growth, defective vision, irritability, somnolence, and infantile genitalia are often associated with the lesion in children. Development of the tumor after puberty usually results in amenorrhea in women and loss of libido and potency in men. Also called **ameloblastoma, craniopharyngeal duct tumor, pituitary adamantinoma, Rathke's pouch tumor.**

craniostenosis /krā′nē·ō′stənō′sis/ [Gk, *kranion* + *stenos*, narrow, *osis*, condition], a congenital deformity of the skull resulting from premature closure of the sutures between the cranial bones. The severity of the malformation depends on which sutures close, the point in the developmental process the closure occurred, and the success or failure of the other sutures to compensate by expansion. Impaired brain growth may or may not be involved. The most common form of the condition is permanent closure of the sagittal suture with anteroposterior elongation of the skull. Surgery is generally indicated when multiple sutures are fused to relieve cerebral pressure and may be performed for cosmetic reasons. See also **brachycephaly, oxycephaly, plagiocephaly, scaphocephaly. –craniostenotic,** *adj.*

craniostosis /krā′nē·ostō′sis/ [Gk, *kranion* + *osteon*, bone, *osis*, condition], premature ossification of the sutures of the skull, often associated with other skeletal defects. The sutures close before or soon after birth. If no surgical correction is made, the growth of the skull is inhibited, the head is deformed, and the eyes and brain are often damaged. Also called **craniosynostosis.**

craniotabes /krā′nē·ōtā′bēz/ [Gk, *kranion* + L, *tabes*, wasting], benign, congenital thinness of the top and back of the skull of a newborn, common because the rate of brain growth exceeds the rate of calcification of the skull during the last month of gestation. The bones feel brittle when pressed by an examiner's fingers. The condition disappears with normal nutrition and growth but may persist in infants who develop rickets.

craniotomy /kran′ē·ot′əmē/ [Gk, *kranion*, skull, *temnein*, to cut], any surgical opening into the skull, performed to relieve intracranial pressure, to control bleeding, or to remove a tumor. X-ray films of the skull are taken preoperatively, and a CT scan or an electroencephalogram is done to establish the diagnosis. The operative site is shaved and cleansed. Parenteral corticosteroids are given to reduce cerebral edema; mannitol and urea are administered to decrease intracranial pressure. Neuroleptic drugs that sedate but do not narcotize the patient may be combined with local anesthesia, or general anesthesia may be given. A semicircular skin incision is made just above the hairline, a series of burr holes are made and connected with a cut, and the flap of bone is removed. The meninges are incised, and the brain is exposed. The flap may be replaced after surgery or left off temporarily to prevent the buildup of pressure from the cerebral edema. Postoperatively, if the cerebral area is involved, the head of the patient's bed is elevated to 45 degrees to reduce the risk of hemorrhage and edema; if the cerebellum or brainstem is affected, the patient is kept flat. The dressing is checked frequently for yellowish drainage of cerebrospinal fluid. Any moist areas are reinforced with sterile materials to avoid infection. Frequent observation of neurologic signs, including the level of consciousness, speech, and strength, is essential.

craniotubular /-tŏŏb′yələr/, pertaining to a bossing, or overgrowth, of bone that results in an abnormal contour and increased bone density. An example of a craniotubular disorder is craniometaphyseal dysplasia.

cranium /krā′nē·əm/ [Gk, kranion, skull], the bony skull that holds the brain. It is composed of eight bones: frontal, occipital, sphenoid, and ethmoid bones, and paired temporal and parietal bones. **–cranial,** adj.

-cranium, a suffix meaning 'referring to the skull': chondrocranium, desmocranium, endocranium.

crankcase-spool catheter /krangk′kās/, a special, elastic catheter stored within a plastic spool to facilitate its insertion, especially for hyperalimentation. Most experts recommend the indirect method of venipuncture for insertion of this kind of catheter, usually into a peripheral vein that connects with the subclavian vein. When fully inserted, the crankcase-spool catheter is usually lodged in the subclavian vein. The catheter is highly flexible, and each revolution of the crankcase spool feeds about 5 inches of the catheter into the vein involved. When the crankcase-spool catheter is fully inserted, an x-ray exposure is made of the insertion area to confirm its correct placement. The venipuncture site for insertion is prepared, dressed, and taped in the same manner as any other venipuncture site. The crankcase-spool catheter is less irritating than a regular catheter, allows greater limb movement, and minimizes the risk of thrombosis. It may, however, cause complications, such as occlusion, phlebitis, infection, and catheter sensitivity. Occlusion of the vein, a common risk, is usually countered by flushing the vein with dilute streptokinase. If the patient develops phlebitis and receives proper treatment, the catheter may be left in place. Infection, usually evidenced by purulent drainage at the insertion site, is accompanied by an elevated white blood cell count. In cases of such infection the attending physician may order an antibiotic or the removal of the catheter. Catheter sensitivity, evidenced by fever and phlebitis, may require removal of the catheter.

crash [ME, crasschen, to break violently], a malfunction of computer hardware or software. A crash in a hard disk drive occurs when the read/write head impacts on the disk surface.

crash cart, a cart carrying emergency equipment, such as analgesics, antiseptics, suction devices, sutures, scalpels, surgical needles, sponges, swabs, retractors, hemostats, forceps, trachea tubes, and often a defibrillator. Hospital emergency rooms and intensive care units usually have several crash carts equipped according to prescribed specifications. Efficient, effective emergency care often depends on the careful provisioning of crash carts and the precise knowledge of their layouts.

-crasia, **1.** a suffix meaning '(condition of a) mixture, good or bad': eucrasia, orthocrasia, spermacrasia. **2.** a combining form meaning a '(specified) condition involving loss of control': copracrasia, uracrasia.

-cratia, a suffix meaning '(condition of) incontinence': scatacratia, scoracratia, uracratia.

cravat bandage /krəvat′/ [Fr, cravate, scarf; bande, strip], a triangular bandage, folded lengthwise. It may be used as a circular, figure-of-eight, or spiral bandage to control bleeding or to tie splints in place.

crawling reflex. See **symmetric tonic neck reflex.**

C-reactive protein (CRP) /-rē·ak′tiv/, a protein not nor-mally detected in the serum but present in many acute inflammatory conditions and with necrosis. CRP appears in the serum before the erythrocyte-sedimentation rate begins to rise, often within 24 to 48 hours of the onset of inflammation. After a myocardial infarction, it is present in 24 hours, begins to fall 3 days later, and is absent after 2 weeks. Acute rheumatic fever is monitored with serial estimations of CRP, because the serum level of the protein is the most sensitive indicator of rheumatic activity. Bacterial infections and widespread neoplastic disease are also associated with C-reactive protein in the serum. CRP disappears when an inflammatory process is suppressed by salicylates steroids, or both. Also called **serum C-reactive protein.**

cream [Gk, chrima, oil], **1.** the portion of milk rich in butterfat. **2.** any fluid mixture of thick consistency. Creams are often used as a method of applying medication to the surface of the body. Compare **ointment.**

crease [ME, creste, crest], an indentation or margin formed by a doubling back of tissue, such as the folds or creases on the palm of the hand and sole of the foot.

creat-, a combining form meaning 'pertaining to flesh': creaton, creatorrhea, creatotoxism.

creatine /krē′ətēn, -tin/ [Gk, kreas, flesh], an important nitrogenous compound produced by metabolic processes in the body. Combined with phosphorus, it forms high-energy phosphate. In normal metabolic reactions the phosphorus is yielded to combine with a molecule of adenosine diphosphate to produce a molecule of the very-high-energy molecule adenosine triphosphate. See also **creatinine.**

creatine kinase, an enzyme in muscle, brain, and other tissues that catalyzes the transfer of a phosphate group from adenosine triphosphate to creatine, producing adenosine diphosphate and phosphocreatine. Also called **creatine phosphokinase (CPK).** See also **Duchenne's muscular dystrophy.**

creatine phosphate [Gk, kreas, flesh; Du, potasschen], an enzyme that increases in blood levels when there has been muscle damage, as in pseudohypertrophic muscular dystrophy.

creatine phosphokinase. See **creatine kinase.**

creatinine /krē·at′inēn, -nin/, a substance formed from the metabolism of creatine, commonly found in blood, urine, and muscle tissue. It is measured in blood and urine tests as a clue to kidney function. Normal adult blood levels of creatinine are 0.5-1.1 mg/dl for females and 0.6-1.2 mg/dl for males; the numbers decrease in elderly patients because of a smaller muscle mass. See also **creatine.**

creatinine clearance test, a diagnostic test for kidney function, as a measure of the filtration rate of creatinine, the end product of muscle metabolism. It is calculated on the basis of a urine volume in milliliters per minute times the amount of milligrams per liter of urinary creatinine excreted in 24 hours. The resulting figure is divided by the amount of serum creatinine in milligrams per deciliter.

creatinine height index (CHI), a measurement of a 24-hour urinary excretion of creatinine, which is generally related to the patient's muscle mass and an indicator of malnutrition, particularly in young males.

credentials /kriden′shelz/, a predetermined set of standards, such as licensure or certification, establishing that a person or institution has achieved professional recognition in a specific field of health care.

Credé's method /kredāz′/ [Karl S. Credé, German physician, b. 1819], a technique for promoting the expulsion of urine by manual compression of the bladder through pressure on the lower abdominal wall.

Credé's prophylaxis [Karl S. Credé], the instillation of a 1% silver-nitrate solution into the conjunctiva of newborn infants to prevent ophthalmia neonatorum.

creep, a rheologic effect of metals and other solid materials that may become elongated or deformed as a result of a load being applied for a long period of time. For example, creep can occur in silver amalgam fillings that have been in place for some time.

creeping eruption [AS, *creopan,* bent; L *erumpere* to burst forth], a skin lesion characterized by irregular, wandering red lines on the foot made by the burrowing larvae of hookworms and certain roundworms. Infestation occurs when people walk barefoot where these parasites are present. Antiparasitic treatment is specific to the organism. Also called **larva migrans.**

cremaster /krimas'tər/ [Gk, *kremastos,* hanging], a thin, muscular layer spreading out over the spermatic cord in a series of loops. It is a continuation of the obliquus internus. The muscle arises from the inguinal ligament and inserts into the crest of the pubis and into the sheath of the rectus abdominis. It is innervated by the genital branch of the genitofemoral nerve and functions to draw the testis up toward the superficial inguinal ring in response to cold or to stimulation of the nerve.

cremasteric reflex /krē'məster'ik/, a superficial neural reflex elicited by stroking the skin of the upper inner aspect of the thigh in a male. This normally results in a brisk retraction of the testis on the side of the stimulus. The reflex is lost in diseases of the pyramidal tract above the level of the first lumbar vertebra. See also **superficial reflex.**

crenation /krinā'shən/ [L, *crena,* notch], the formation of notches or leaflike, scalloped edges on an object. Red blood cells exposed to a hypertonic saline solution acquire a notched, shriveled surface because of the osmotic effect of the solution. They are then called crenated red blood cells. *crenate, crenated, adj.*

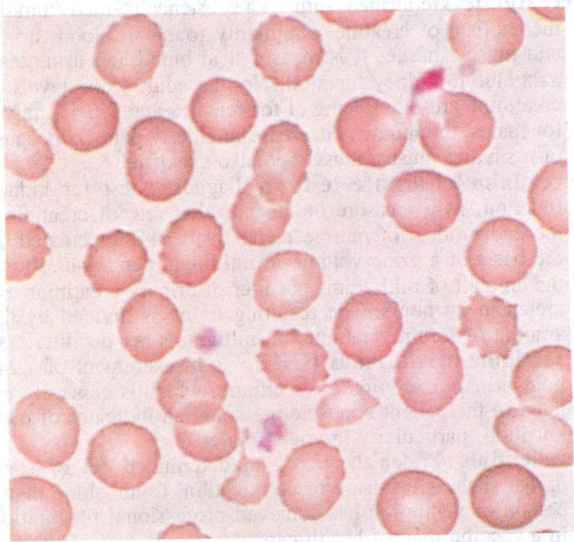

Crenated red blood cells *(Hayhoe, 1992)*

creosol /krē'əsol/, an oily liquid that is one of the active constituents (phenol) of creosote. It should not be confused with cresol.

creosote /krē'əsōt/, a flammable, oily liquid with a smoky odor that is used primarily as a wood preservative. It can be a cause of a wide variety of health problems, ranging from cancer and corneal damage to convulsions, dermatitis, and vertigo. Persons who work with treated wood are usually at the greatest risk of exposure. See also **phenol poisoning.**

crepitant /krep'itənt/ [L, *crepitans,* crackling], pertaining to a sound of crackling or rattling, or of rough surfaces being rubbed together.

crepitation. See **crepitus.**

crepitant rale [L, *crepitans,* crackling; Fr, rattle], an abnormal breathing sound produced at the end of inspiration and caused by air entering collapsed alveoli that contain fibrous exudate. It is heard in cases of pneumonia, tuberculosis, and pulmonary edema.

crepitus /krep'itəs/ [L, crackling], **1.** flatulence or the noisy discharge of fetid gas from the intestine through the anus. **2.** a sound that resembles the crackling noise heard when rubbing hair between the fingers or throwing salt on an open fire. Crepitus is associated with gas gangrene, the rubbing of bone fragments, or the rales of a consolidated area of the lung in pneumonia. Also called **crepitation.**

cresc-, a combining form meaning 'to grow': *crescograph.*

crescendo angina /krishen'dō/ [L, *crescere,* to increase], a form of anginal discomfort associated with ischemic electrocardiographic changes, marked by increased frequency, provocation, intensity, or character.

crescendo murmur [L, *crescere,* to increase, *murmur,* humming], a murmur of steadily increasing intensity to a sudden termination.

cresol /krē'sol/, a mixture of three isomers in a liquid with a phenolic odor. It is derived from coal tar and used in synthetic resins and disinfectants. Cresol is a potentially lethal protoplasmic poison that can be absorbed through the skin. Symptoms of chronic poisoning include skin eruptions, digestive disorders, uremia, jaundice, nervous disorders, vertigo, and mental changes. Acute poisoning by oral intake of 8 g or more can cause circulatory collapse and death. See also **phenol poisoning.**

CREST syndrome /krest/, abbreviation for *calcinosis, Raynaud's phenomenon, esophageal dysfunction, sclerodactyly, and telangiectasis,* which may occur for varying periods of time in patients with scleroderma.

cretin. See **cretinism.**

cretin dwarf /krē'tən/, a person in whom short stature is caused by infantile hypothyroidism and severe deficiency of thyroid hormone. Also called **hypothyroid dwarf.** See also **cretinism.**

cretinism /krē'təniz'əm/ [Fr, *cretin,* idiot], a condition characterized by severe congenital hypothyroidism and often associated with other endocrine abnormalities. Typical signs of cretinism include dwarfism, mental deficiency, puffy facial features, dry skin, a large tongue, umbilical hernia, and muscular incoordination. The disorder occurs usually in areas where the diet is deficient in iodine and where goiter is endemic. Early treatment with thyroid hormone generally promotes normal physical growth but may not prevent mental retardation. The use of iodized salt dramatically reduces the incidence of cretinism in a population. The con-

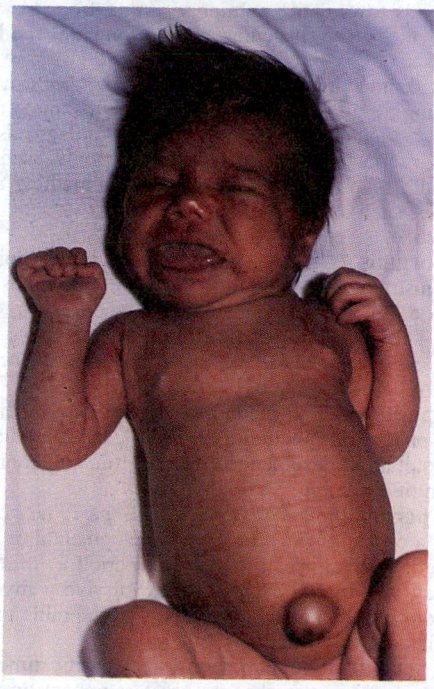

Cretinism *(Zitelli, 1992/Courtesy Dr. TP Foley, Jr)*

dition is rare in the United States, but in some areas, including parts of Ecuador, the Himalayas, and Zaire, more than 5% of the people are cretins. See also **familial cretinism.** **–cretinoid, cretinous,** *adj.,* **cretin,** *n.*

Creutzfeldt-Jakob disease /kroits′feltyä′kôp/ [Hans G. Creutzfeldt, German neurologist, b. 1885; Alfons M. Jakob, German neurologist, b. 1884], a rare, fatal encephalopathy caused by an as yet unidentified slow virus. The disease occurs in middle age, and symptoms are progressive dementia, dysarthria, muscle wasting, and various involuntary movements, such as myoclonus and athetosis. Deterioration is obvious week to week. Death ensues, usually within a year. Transmission between humans is unusual, but the disease has been observed years after exposure to needles, instruments, and electrodes previously used in the treatment of a patient with the disease. Isolation is not necessary. Special care in disposal or sterilization of potentially infective items is always necessary. Also called **Jakob-Creutzfeldt disease, spastic pseudoparalysis, spastic pseudosclerosis.**

CRF, abbreviation for **corticotropin-releasing factor.**

crib death. See **sudden infant death syndrome.**

cribriform carcinoma. See **adenocystic carcinoma.**

crico-, a combining form meaning 'ring': *cricoderma, cricoid, cricoidectomy.*

cricoid /krī′koid/ [Gk, *krikos,* ring, *eidos,* form], **1.** having a ring shape. **2.** a ring-shaped cartilage connected to the thyroid cartilage by the cricothyroid ligament at the level of the sixth cervical vertebra.

cricoid cartilage, a ringshaped cartilage of the larynx, consisting of a narrow anterior arch and a wide quadrilateral lamina posteriorly.

cricoidectomy /-ek′təmē/ [Gk, *krikos* + *eidos* + *ektome,*

cutting out], a surgical procedure for removing the cricoid cartilage.

cricoid pressure, a technique to reduce the risk of the aspiration of stomach contents during induction of general anesthesia. The cricoid cartilage is pushed against the esophagus to prevent passive regurgitation. The technique cannot, however, stop vomiting that has begun. Cricoid pressure is applied before intubation, immediately after injection of the anesthetic drug or muscle relaxant. Also called **Sellick's maneuver.**

cricopharyngeal /krī′kōfərin′jē·əl/ [Gk, *krikos* + *pharynx,* throat], of or pertaining to the cricoid cartilage and the pharynx.

cricopharyngeal incoordination, a defect in the normal swallowing reflex. The cricopharyngeus muscle ordinarily serves as a sphincter to keep the top of the esophagus closed except when the person is swallowing, vomiting, or belching. The trachea remains open for breathing, but air normally does not enter the esophagus during respiration. In swallowing, the reverse effect occurs and the larynx is closed while food slides past it into the esophagus, which is located immediately behind the larynx. When the somewhat complex series of neuromuscular actions is not properly coordinated as a result of disease or injury, the patient may choke, swallow air, regurgitate fluid into the nose, or experience discomfort in swallowing food. See also **dysphagia.**

cricothyroid membrane /-thī′roid/, a fibroelastic membrane including the cricothyroid ligament that connects the cricoid and thyroid cartilages. Also called **elastic membrane.**

cricothyrotomy /krī′kōthīrot′əmē/ [Gk, *krikos* + *thyreos,* shield, *eidos* form, *temnein* to cut], an emergency incision into the larynx, performed to open the airway in a person who is choking. A small vertical midline cut is made just below the Adam's apple and above the cricoid cartilage. The incision is opened further with a transverse cut through the cricothyroid membrane, and the wound is spread open with a knife handle or other dilator. The new opening must be held open with a tube that is open at both ends to allow air to move in and out. The cartridge end of a ballpoint pen will suffice until a tracheostomy can be done. Compare **tracheostomy.**

cri-du-chat syndrome. See **cat-cry syndrome.**

Crigler-Najjar syndrome /krig′lərnaj′är/ [John F. Crigler, Jr., American pediatrician, b. 1919; Victor A. Najjar, American pediatrician, b. 1914], a congenital, familial, autosomal anomaly, in which glucuronyl transferase, an enzyme, is deficient or absent. The condition is characterized by nonhemolytic jaundice, an accumulation of unconjugated bilirubin in the blood, and severe disorders of the central nervous system. See also **hyperbilirubinemia of the newborn.**

crime [L, *crimen*], any act that violates a law and may include criminal intent.

Crimean-Congo hemorrhagic fever /krīmē′ən/, an arbovirus infection transmitted to humans through the bite of a tick, characterized by fever, dizziness, muscle ache, vomiting, headache, and other neurologic symptoms. After several days, in severe cases, bleeding from the skin and mucous membranes, particularly from the mouth and nose, bloody sputum or vomit, and blood-tinged feces may be seen. Transfusion may be necessary to replace lost blood; otherwise, treatment is symptomatic and supportive. There is no specific medication or therapy available for prevention or cure. It occurs mainly in the U.S.S.R., Asia, and Africa; agricultural workers are most often afflicted. See also **hemorrhagic fever, Omsk hemorrhagic fever.**

criminal abortion /krim'inəl/, the intentional termination of pregnancy under any condition prohibited by law. See also **induced abortion.**

criminal psychology, the study of the mental processes, motivational patterns, and behavior of criminals.

crin-, a combining form meaning 'to separate or secrete': *crinin, crinogenic.*

-crinat, a suffix designating an ethacrynic acid –derived diuretic.

-crine, a suffix designating an acridine derivative.

-crine, -crinia, a suffix meaning '(condition of) endocrine secretion': *hemocrinia, hypercrinia, neurocrinia.*

-crisia, **1.** a suffix meaning a 'diagnosis or to judge': *acrisia, urocrisia.* **2.** a combining form meaning a '(specified) condition of endocrine secretion': *hypercrisia, hyperendocrisia, hypocrisia.*

crisis /krī'sis/ [Gk, *krisis,* turning point], **1.** a turning point for better or worse in the course of a disease, usually indicated by a marked change in the intensity of signs and symptoms. A crisis may be celiac, marked by an attack of watery diarrhea and vomiting leading, in turn, to dehydration; hepatic, characterized by intense pain in the region of the liver; or ocular, manifested by eye pain, a flow of tears, and sensitivity to light. **2.** a turning point in events affecting the emotional state of a person, such as death or divorce. **3.** a characteristically self-limiting period of from 4 to 6 weeks that constitutes a transitional phase representing both the danger of increased psychological vulnerability and an opportunity for personal growth. See also **crisis intervention.**

crisis intervention, (in psychiatry) a therapeutic goal of psychological resolution of the patient's immediate crisis and restoration to at least a level of functioning that existed before the crisis period. A maximum goal is improvement of functioning above the precrisis level. The goal is to restore in the person the level of functioning that existed before the current crisis.

crisis-intervention unit, a group trained in emergency medical treatment and in various methods for rendering psychiatric therapeutic assistance to a person or group of persons during a period of crisis, especially instances involving suicide attempts or drug abuse. Such networks are found within community hospitals, health care centers, or as specialized self-contained units, such as suicide-prevention centers, and operate 24 hours a day. The primary objective of such crisis assistance is to help the person cope with the immediate problem and to offer guidance and support for long-term therapy.

crisis resolution, (in psychiatry) the development of effective adaptive and coping devices to resolve a crisis.

crisis theory, a conceptual framework for defining and explaining the phenomena that occur when a person faces a problem that appears to be insoluble. The theory is the basis of crisis therapy.

crisscross inheritance [*Christ cross*; L, *in, hereditas,* in heredity], the acquisition of genetic characteristics or conditions from the parent of the opposite sex.

crista supraventricularis /kris'tə sŏŏ'prəven'trik'yəler'is/ [L, *crista,* ridge; *supra,* above, *ventriculum,* belly], the muscular ridge on the interior dorsal wall of the right ventricle of the heart. It defines the limit of the arterial cone

and extends toward the pulmonary trunk from the ventral cusp of the atrioventricular ring. Compare **moderator band.**

criterion /krītir'ē·ən/, *pl.* **criteria** [Gk, *kriterion,* a means for judging], a standard or rule by which something may be judged, such as a health condition, or a diagnosis established. Criteria (the plural form is commonly used) are a set of rules or principles against which something may be measured, such as health care practices.

critical care. See **intensive care.**

critical organs /krit'ikəl/ [Gk, *krisis,* turning point; *organon,* instrument], tissues that are the most sensitive to irradiation, such as the gonads, lymphoid organs, and intestine. The skin, cornea, oral cavity, esophagus, vagina, cervix, and optic lens are the next most sensitive organs to irradiation.

critical pathway, a schedule of critical care medical and nursing procedures, including diagnostic tests, medications, and consultations designed to effect an efficient, coordinated program of treatment.

critical period [Gk, *kritikos,* critical, *peri,* near, *hodos,* way], a period of time during a developmental or rehabilitation crisis. Examples are the brief period in which a zygote may be formed, a patient may survive a myocardial infarction, or when an embryo is most vulnerable to effects of medications used by the mother.

critical period of development, a specific time during which the environment has its greatest impact on an individual's development.

critical point, the temperature and pressure at which, in a sealed system, the densities of the liquid and gas forms of a substance will be equal and the two are not visibly separated.

critical pressure, the pressure exerted by a vapor in a closed system at the critical temperature.

critical temperature, the highest temperature at which a substance can exist as a liquid outside a sealed system.

CRNA, abbreviation for *certified registered nurse anesthetist.* See also **Nurse Anesthetist.**

CRNI, abbreviation for *certified registered nurse, intravenous.*

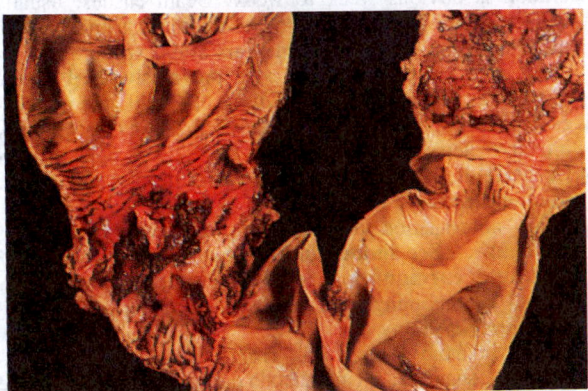

Crohn's disease *(Fletcher, 1987)*

Crohn's disease /krōnz/ [Burrill B. Crohn, American physician, b. 1884], a chronic inflammatory bowel disease of unknown origin, usually affecting the ileum, the colon, or

Comparison of ulcerative colitis and Crohn's disease

	Ulcerative colitis	Crohn's disease
Usual area affected	Left colon, rectum	Distal ileum, right colon
Extent of involvement	Diffuse areas, contiguous	Segmental areas, noncontiguous
Inflammation	Mostly mucosal	Transmural
Mucosal appearance	Ulcerations	Cobblestone effect, granulomas
Character of stools	Blood present	No blood present
	No fat	Steatorrhea
	Frequent liquid stools	Three to five semisoft stools per day
Abdominal pain	May occur, mild	Right lower quadrant pain, cramping
Abdominal mass	No	Common in right lower quadrant
Complications	Toxic megacolon	Fistulas
	Pseudopolyps	Perianal disease
	Hemorrhoids	Strictures
	Hemorrhage	Abscesses
		Perforation
Extraintestinal manifestations	Anemia	Anemia
	Erythema nodosum	Malabsorption of fat and fat-soluble vitamins
	Pyoderma gangrenosa	Arthritis
	Arthritis	Hepatobiliary disease
	Liver disease	Iritis, conjunctivitis
	Iritis, conjunctivitis	Renal stones, obstructive uropathy
	Stomatitis	
	Thrombophlebitis	
Reasons for surgery	Poor response to medical therapy	Presence of complications
	Complications	
Response to surgery	Curative	Noncurative, high recurrence rate

From Phipps WJ, Long BC, Woods NF, Cassmeyer VL: *Medical surgical nursing concepts and clinical practice*, ed 4, St Louis, 1991, Mosby, p 1310.

both structures. Diseased segments may be separated by normal bowel segments. Also called **regional enteritis.** Compare **ulcerative colitis.** See also **colitis, ileitis.**
- OBSERVATIONS: Crohn's disease is characterized by frequent attacks of diarrhea, severe abdominal pain, nausea, fever, chills, weakness, anorexia, and weight loss. Children with the disease often suffer retarded physical growth. The diagnosis of Crohn's disease is based on clinical signs, x-ray studies using a contrast medium, and endoscopy. The disease is easily confused with ulcerative colitis, which is also an inflammatory bowel disease affecting the colon and rectum.
- INTERVENTIONS: Corticosteroids, antibiotics, and antiinflammatory agents are used to control symptoms and to attempt to induce remission. In patients who are malnourished because of the disease, intravenous hyperalimentation is used to ensure adequate intake of nutrients and to rest the bowel. Surgical removal of the diseased segment of the bowel provides some relief, but recurrence after surgery is likely.
- NURSING CONSIDERATIONS: In many cases the inflammation extends to other areas of the bowel or to the stomach, duodenum, or mouth. Other complications are arthritis, ankylosing spondylitis, kidney and liver disease, and skin and eye disorders. The formation of fistulas from the diseased bowel to the anus, vagina, skin surface, or to other loops of bowel are common. Persons with Crohn's disease are hospitalized frequently and often become depressed because of the relentless, painful character of the disease. Continued support and encouragement are essential in helping the patient maintain a hopeful outlook.

-cromil, a suffix designating a cromoglicic acid –type antiallergic agent.

cromoglicic acid. See **cromolyn sodium.**

cromolyn sodium /krom′əlin/, an antiasthmatic that acts by decreasing allergic bronchospasm resulting from an inhaled allergen.
- INDICATION: It is prophylactically prescribed in the treatment of bronchial asthma. The drug has no effect after an attack has begun.
- CONTRAINDICATION: Known hypersensitivity to this drug prohibits its use.
- ADVERSE EFFECTS: Bronchospasm, wheezing, nasal congestion, pharyngeal irritation, and other hypersensitivity reactions may occur.

Cronkhite-Canada syndrome /krong′kīt/ [Leonard W. Cronkhite, American physician, b. 1919; Wilma J. Canada, American radiologist], an abnormal familial condition characterized by GI polyposis accompanied by ectodermal defects, such as nail atrophy, alopecia, and excessive skin pigmentation. In some individuals it is also accompanied by protein-losing enteropathy, malabsorption, and deficiency of blood calcium, potassium, and magnesium.

cross [L, *crux*], (in genetics) any method of crossbreeding or any individual, organism, or strain produced from crossbreeding. Kinds of crosses include **dihybrid cross, monohybrid cross, polyhybrid cross,** and **trihybrid cross.**

cross-bite tooth [L, *crux* + AS, *bitan, toth*], any of the posterior teeth that allow the modified buccal cusps of the upper teeth to be positioned in the central fossae of the lower teeth, instead of having those cusps buccal to the lower teeth.

crossbreeding [L, *crux* + *bredan*], the production of offspring by the mating of plants and animals from different varieties, strains, or species; hybridization. See also **inbreeding. –crossbred,** *adj.*

crossed amblyopia [L, *crux,* cross; Gk, *amblys,* dull, *ops,* eyes], a visual disorder in which the patient is unable to see on one side of the visual field, associated with hemianesthesia of the opposite side of the body. Also called **amblyopia cruciata.**

crossed extension reflex, one of the spinal-mediated reflexes normally present in the first 2 months of life. It is demonstrated by the flexion, adduction, and extension of one leg when the foot of the other leg is stimulated.

crossed grid, (in radiography) an assembly of two parallel x-ray grids that are rotated at right angles to each other so that it cleans up scattered radiation from more than one direction. Also called **crosshatch grid.** See also **grid.**

crossed reflex, any neural reflex in which stimulation of one side of the body results in a response on the other side, such as the consensual light reflex.

cross-eye. See **esophoria.**

cross fertilization, 1. (in zoology), the union of gametes from different species or varieties to form hybrids. 2. (in botany) the fertilization of the flower of one plant by the pollen from a different plant, as opposed to self-fertilization. Also called **allogamy.**

crosshatch grid. See **crossed grid.**

cross infection [L, *crux*, cross, *inficere*, to stain], the transmittal of an infection from one patient in a hospital or health care setting to another patient in the same environment.

crossing over, the exchange of sections of chromatids between homologous pairs of chromosomes during the prophase stage of the first meiotic division. The process occurs through the formation of chiasmata and results in the recombination of genes. Also called **chiasmatypy.**

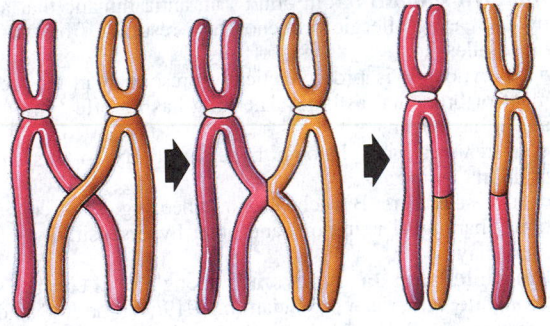

Crossing over (Thibodeau, 1993/Kevin A Sommerville)

crossmatching of blood [L, *crux* + AS, *gemaecca*, matching], a procedure used to determine compatibility of a donor's blood with that of a recipient after the specimens have been matched for major blood type. Serum from the donor's blood is mixed with red cells from the recipient's blood, and cells from the donor are mixed with serum from the recipient. If agglutination occurs, an antigenic substance is present and the bloods are not compatible. If no agglutination occurs, the donor's blood may safely be transfused to the recipient. Compare **blood typing.** See also **ABO blood groups, Rh factor, transfusion, transfusion reaction.**

crossover /kros'ovər/ [L, *crux* + AS, *ofer*], the result of the recombination of genes on homologous pairs of chromosomes during meiosis. See also **crossing over.**

cross-reacting antibody [L, *crux*, cross, *re, agere,* to act; Gk, *anti;* AS, *bodig,* body], an antibody that reacts with antigens that are similar but different than the specific antigens with which it originally reacted.

cross resistance, the resistance to a particular antibiotic that also results in resistance against a different antibiotic, usually from a similar chemical class, to which the bacteria may not have been exposed. Cross resistance can occur between colistin and polymyxin B or clindamycin and lincomycin.

cross-sectional [L, *crux* + *secare,* to cut], (in statistics) pertaining to the comparative data of two groups of persons at one point in time.

cross-sectional anatomy, the study of the relationship of the structures of the body by the examination of cross sections of the tissue or organ. Compare **surface anatomy.**

cross sensitivity, a sensitivity to one substance that predisposes an individual to sensitivity to other substances that are related in chemical structure. Cross sensitivity with allergic reactions may develop between antibiotics of similar chemical structures.

cross-sequential /-sikwen'shəl/ [L, *crux* + *sequi,* to follow], (in statistics) pertaining to data that compare several cohorts at different points in time.

cross tolerance, a tolerance to other drugs that develops after exposure to only one agent. An example is the cross tolerance that develops between alcohol and barbiturates.

crotamiton /krōtam'iton/, a scabicide.

■ INDICATIONS: It is prescribed in treating scabies and other pruritic skin diseases.

■ CONTRAINDICATIONS: Known hypersensitivity to this drug prohibits its use. It is not applied near the eyes or on the mouth or raw skin.

■ ADVERSE EFFECTS: Among the most serious adverse reactions are irritation and allergic reactions of the skin.

croup /krōop/ [Scot, to croak], an acute viral infection of the upper and lower respiratory tract that occurs primarily in infants and young children 3 months to 3 years of age after an upper respiratory tract infection. It is characterized by hoarseness, fever, a distinctive harsh, brassy cough, persistent stridor during inspiration, and varying degrees of respiratory distress resulting from obstruction of the larynx. The most common causative agents are the parainfluenza viruses, especially type 1, followed by the respiratory syncytial viruses (RSV) and influenza A and B viruses. Also called **angina trachealis, exudative angina, laryngostasis.** Compare **acute epiglottitis.** —**croupous, croupy,** *adj.*

■ OBSERVATIONS: Transmission occurs by infection with airborne particles or with infected secretions. Leukocytosis with an increased proportion of polymorphonuclear cells may be present at first, followed by leukopenia and lymphocytosis. A lateral neck x-ray film shows subepiglottic narrowing and a normal-sized epiglottis, which differentiate the condition from acute epiglottitis. Onset of the acute stage is rapid, usually occurs at night, and may be preciptated by exposure to cold air. The child becomes irritable, develops stridor, dyspnea, tachypnea, the characteristic barking cough, and, in severe cases, cyanosis or pallor. The child's condition often improves in the morning, but it may worsen at night.

■ INTERVENTIONS: Routine treatment consists of bed rest, adequate fluid intake, and the alleviation of airway obstruction to ensure adequate respiratory exchange. Children with mild infections are usually managed at home with supportive measures, such as vaporizers, humidifiers, or steam from hot running water in an enclosed bathroom to reduce the spasm of the laryngeal muscles and to free secretions. Hospitalization is indicated for children with high temperatures, progressive stridor and respiratory distress, and hypoxia, cyanosis, or pallor. Endotracheal intubation and tracheostomy may be necessary. Humidity and oxygen are usually prescribed. The vital signs are continuously monitored; a change in pulse and respiration may be early signs of hypoxia and impending airway obstruction. Fluids are often given intravenously to reduce physical exertion and the possibility of vomiting, with its attendant increased risk of aspiration. Corticosteroids or other drugs, such as expectorants, bronchodilators, and antihistamines, are rarely used, and sedatives are contraindicated, because they exert a depressant effect on the respiratory tract.

■ NURSING CONSIDERATIONS: The primary focus of nursing care is to ease breathing by providing humidity and to maintain continuous monitoring and surveillance for signs of respiratory distress and impending airway obstruction, with intubation and tracheostomy equipment kept readily available. To conserve the child's energy and to reduce apprehension, the nurse encourages rest, disturbs the child as little as possible, remains in constant attendance, provides comfort with a familiar toy or other device, and encourages parental involvement whenever possible. Fever is usually reduced by the cool atmosphere of the mist tent; antipyretics are given as needed. To prevent chilling, frequent changes of clothing and bed linen are often necessary in the humid environment. The nurse also explains the condition to the parents and discusses appropriate care after discharge, including continued use of humidity and ensurance of adequate hydration and proper nutrition. In most children the condition is relatively mild and runs its course in 3 to 7 days. The infection may spread to other areas of the respiratory tract and may cause complications, such as bronchiolitis, pneumonia, and otitis media. The most serious complication is laryngeal obstruction, which may cause death. If a tracheostomy is required, as may happen with a small percentage of children, other complications, such as infection, atelectasis, cannula occlusion, tracheal bleeding, granulation, stenosis, and delayed healing of the stoma, may develop.

Croupette /kro͞opet′/, a trademark for a device that provides cool humidification with the administration of oxygen or of compressed air, used especially in the treatment of pediatric patients. The Croupette consists of a nebulizer with attached tubing that connects with a canopy to enclose the patient and contain the humidifying mist. The environment of the patient may be cooled by adding ice to the ice compartment or by using a Croupette with its own refrigeration unit. This device is especially used with pediatric patients from 1 month to 10 years of age to relieve hypoxia, liquefy secretions, and cool the environment of the patient. It is also often used in the treatment of the croup, bronchiolitis, cystic fibrosis, asthma, laryngitis, postoperative dehydration, and hyperpyrexia. The oxygen concentration obtainable is approximately 21% to 60%. Nursing care associated with this device usually involves assembling the unit, ensuring proper water level in the nebulizer, and adjusting the oxygen flow rate. The flow rate may be adjusted from 6 L to 10 L per minute or according to equipment specifications. Explaining the equipment and the humidifying treatment also helps reassure the patient. Precautions in using the Croupette with a patient receiving periodic therapy involve ensuring that the flow of oxygen or compressed air is turned on when the canopy is placed over the patient and that the patient is carefully monitored throughout the therapy period.

Some of the advantages of the Croupette are its capability for providing a cool, moist environment, its adaptability for the delivery of oxygen or the delivery of compressed air, and the ease of canopy installation. Croupette canopies are disposable. Some of the limitations associated with the device are that some Croupette units have awkward, bulky frames; nebulizer water reservoirs are usually small and require constant refilling; periodic refills of ice are required; and excess humidity may wet the bed linen and the patient.

croupous. See **croup.**

croupy. See **croup.**

Crouzon's disease /kro͞ozonz′/ [Octave Crouzon, French neurologist, b. 1874; L, *dis;* Fr, *aise,* ease], a familial disease characterized by a malformed skull and various ocular disorders, including exophthalmos, divergent squint, and optic atrophy.

crowing inspiration /krō′ing/ [ME, *crouen*; L, *inspirare,* to breathe in], a harsh noise heard on inhalation caused by an acute obstruction in the larynx. Also called **laryngismus stridulus, spasmodic croup.**

crown [L, *corona*], **1.** the upper part of an organ or structure, such as the top of the head. **2.** the portion of a human tooth that is covered by enamel.

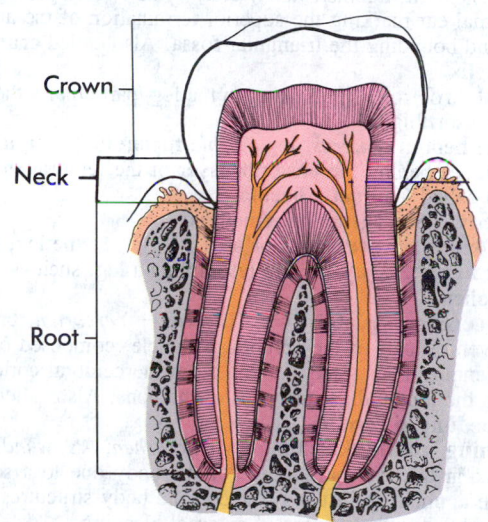

Crown *(Potter, 1993)*

crown-heel length [L, *corona* + AS, *hela, lengthu*], the length of an embryo, fetus, or newborn as measured from the crown of the head to the heel. It is compared to the standing height of an older individual.

crowning [L, *corona*], (in obstetrics) the phase at the end of labor in which the fetal head is seen at the introitus of the vagina. The labia are stretched in a crown around the head just before delivery.

crown/root ratio, the relation of the clinical crown to the clinical root of a tooth.

crown-rump length, the length of an embryo, fetus, or newborn as measured from the crown of the head to the prominence of the buttocks.

crown static, an x-ray film artifact caused by a buildup of electrons in the film emulsion. It is most likely to occur during periods of low environmental humidity.

CRP, abbreviation for **C-reactive protein.**

CRRN, abbreviation for *Certified Rehabilitation Registered Nurse.*

CRT, abbreviation for **cathode-ray tube.**

CRTT, abbreviation for **Certified Respiratory Therapy Technician.**

crucial anastomosis /krōō'shəl/ [L, *crux*, cross; Gk, *anastomoein*, to provide a mouth], an anastomosis in the upper part of the thigh, formed between the first perforating branch of the profunda femoris artery, the inferior gluteal artery, and the lateral and medial circumflex arteries.

crucial bandage. See **T bandage.**

cruciate ligament of the atlas [L, *crux*, cross; *ligare*, to bind], a crosslike ligament attaching the atlas to the base of the occipital bone above and the posterior surface of the body of the axis below.

crude birth rate [L, *crudus*, raw; ME, *burth*; L, *reri*, to reckon], the number of births per 1000 people in a population during 1 year. Compare **birth rate, refined birth rate, true birth rate.**

crur-, a suffix meaning 'pertaining to the leg or thigh': *crura, crural, crureus.*

crura. See **crus.**

crura anthelicis /krōōr'ə anthel'isis, ant·hē'lisis/ [L, *crus*, leg; Gk, *anti*, against, *helix*, coil], the two ridges on the external ear marking the superior termination of the anthelix and bounding the triangular fossa. Also called **crura of anthelix.**

crural /krōō'rəl/, pertaining to the leg, particularly the upper leg or thigh.

crural hernia [L, *crus*, leg, *hernia* rupture], a hernia that protrudes behind the posterior layer of the femoral sheath. Also called **Cloquet's hernia.**

crureus. See **vastus intermedius.**

crus /krus/, *pl.* **crura** /krōōr'ə/ [L, *leg*], **1.** the leg, from knee to foot. **2.** a structure resembling a leg, such as crura anthelicis.

crus cerebri /ser'əbrī, -brē/ [L, *crus* + *cerebrum*, brain], the ventral part of the cerebral peduncle, composed of the descending fiber tracts passing from the cerebral cortex to form the longitudinal fascicles of the pons. Also called **basis pedunculi cerebri.**

crushing wound /krush'ing/ [ME, *crushen*; AS, *wund*], a break in the external surface of the body due to a severe force applied against the tissues. The body structures may be crushed without signs of external bleeding.

crush syndrome [OFr, *cruisir*, to crush], **1.** a severe, life-threatening condition caused by extensive crushing trauma, characterized by destruction of muscle and bone tissue, hemorrhage, and fluid loss resulting in hypovolemic shock, hematuria, renal failure, and coma. Massive supportive therapy, with fluids, electrolytes, antibiotics, analgesia, oxygen, and intensive care with close monitoring of all vital functions are usually necessary. **2.** a severe complication of heroin-induced coma characterized by edema, vascular occlusion, and lymphatic obstruction.

crust [L, *crusta*, shell], a solidified, hard outer layer formed by the drying of a bodily exudate, common in dermatologic conditions such as eczema, impetigo, seborrhea, and favus and during the healing of burns and lesions; a scab.

crutch [AS, *cryce*], a wooden or metal staff, the most common kind of which reaches from the ground almost to the axilla, to aid a person in walking. A padded, curved

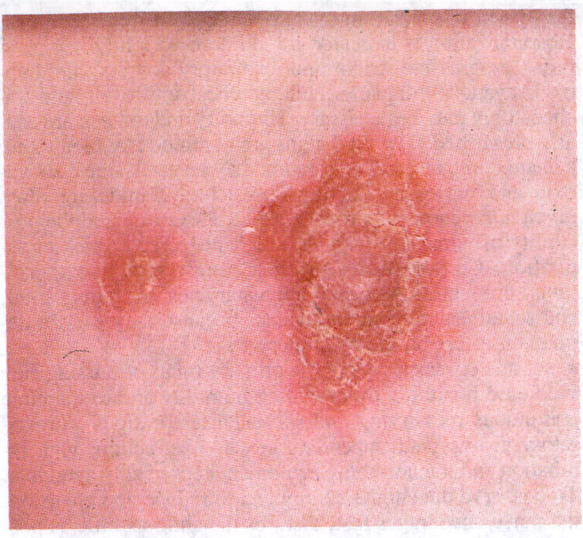

Crust (du Vivier, 1993)

surface at the top fits under the arm; a grip in the form of a crossbar is held in the hand at the level of the palms to support the body. It is important that the person be taught how to use the crutches safely and how to achieve a stable and acceptable gait. Kinds of crutches include *axillary crutches, forearm crutches.*

Crutchfield tongs [W. Gayle Crutchfield, American surgeon, b. 1900; ME, *tonges*], an instrument inserted into the skull to hyperextend the head and neck of patients with fractured cervical vertebrae.

■ METHOD: The tongs are inserted into small bur holes drilled in each parietal region of the skull; the surrounding skin is sutured and covered with a collodion dressing. A weight of from 10 to 20 pounds is suspended from a rope extending from the center of the tongs, over a pulley attached to head of the bed allowing the weights to hang freely. The insertion sites of the tongs are inspected and cleaned every 1 to 2 hours; any formed crusts are removed with hydrogen peroxide twice a day or as required. The patient is turned and assisted in deep breathing every other hour and is given scalp and skin care every 2 to 4 hours. The bed linen is kept dry and smooth, an air mattress or sheepskin is used, and back rubs are administered to prevent decubiti, especially of the scapulae, coccyx, and heels. Passive range-of-motion exercises of all extremities are performed. Sandbags may be used to prevent the patient from sliding to the head of the bed, and the call bell is placed within easy reach. The immobilized patient receives food that is easy to swallow and is fed with care to prevent aspiration; suction apparatus is kept at the bedside as an emergency measure.

■ NURSING INTERVENTION: The nurse maintains the patient's body alignment, checks the weight and traction apparatus, administers meticulous skin care, feeds the patient, and provides for other care as necessary.

■ OUTCOME CRITERIA: A patient may be immobilized by Crutchfield tongs for weeks before surgery is performed; during an operation on the cervical spine and cord, the tongs may be left in place for proper alignment.

crutch gait, a gait achieved by a person on crutches by alternately bearing weight on one or both legs and on the

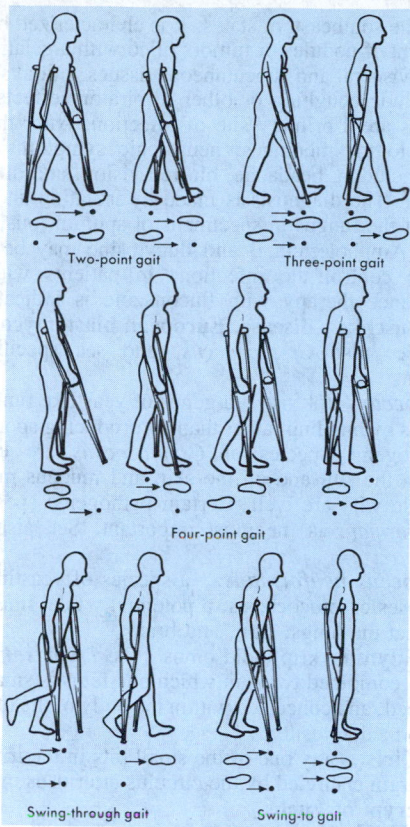

Two-point gait   Three-point gait

Four-point gait

Swing-through gait   Swing-to gait

Crutch gaits

crutches. The gait selected and learned is determined by physical and functional abilities of the patient and on the diagnosis. In a three-point gait, weight is borne on the non-involved leg, then on both crutches, then on the noninvolved leg. Touchdown and progression to full-weight bearing on the involved leg are usual. Four-point gait gives stability but requires bearing weight on both legs. Each leg is used alternately with each crutch. Two-point gait characteristically uses each crutch with the opposing leg. The swing-to and swing-through gaits are often used by paraplegic patients with weight-supporting braces on the legs. Weight is borne on the supported legs; the crutches are placed one stride in front of the person who then swings to that point or through the crutches to a spot in front of them.

crutch palsy, the temporary or permanent loss of sensation or muscle control resulting from pressure on the radial nerve by a crutch. The radial nerve passes under the axillary area superficially. Pressure, often caused by mismatching the height of the patient and the crutch, can lead to paralysis of the elbow and wrist extensors.

Cruz trypanosomiasis. See **Chagas' disease.**

cry [OFr, *crier*], **1.** a sudden, loud, voluntary, or automatic vocalization in response to pain, fear, or a startle reflex. **2.** weeping, because of pain or as an emotional response to depression or grief. **3.** See **cri-du-chat syndrome.**

crying vital capacity (CVC), a measurement of the tidal volume while an infant is crying. The CVC may be valu-

able in monitoring infants with lung diseases that cause changes in functional residual capacity.

cryo-, cry-, crymo-, a prefix meaning 'pertaining to cold': *cryocautery, cryophilia, cryotolerant.*

cryoanesthesia /krī′ō·an′isthē′zhə/ [Gk, *kryos,* cold, *aisthesis,* feeling], the freezing of a part to achieve adequate deadening of neural sensitivity to pain during brief minor surgical procedures.

cryocautery /krī′ōkô′tərē/ [Gk, *kryos* + *kauterion,* branding iron], the application of any substance, such as solid carbon dioxide, that destroys tissue by freezing. Also called **cold cautery.**

cryogen /krī′əjən/ [Gk, *kryos* + *genein,* to produce], **1.** a chemical that induces freezing, used to destroy diseased tissue without injury to adjacent structures. Cell death is caused by dehydration after cell membranes rupture. **2.** (in magnetic resonance imaging) a chemical used to cool the MRI electromagnet so that higher energies can be achieved. Kinds of cryogens include **carbon dioxide, liquid nitrogen,** and **nitrous oxide. −cryogenic,** *adj.*

cryoglobulin /krī′ōglob′yoŏlin/ [Gk, *kryos* + L, *globulus,* small sphere], an abnormal plasma protein that precipitates and coalesces at low temperatures and dissolves and disperses at body temperature.

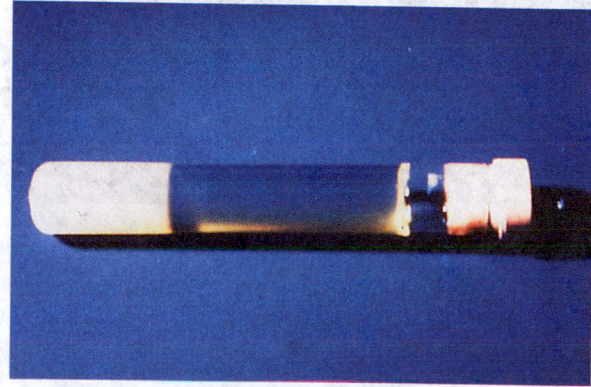

Cryoglobulin *(Skarin, 1991)*

cryoglobulinemia /krī′ōglob′yoŏlinē′mē·ə/ [Gk, *kryos* + L, *globulus,* small sphere; Gk, *haima,* blood], the presence of cryoglobulins in the blood. Cryoglobulins may be found associated with Waldenström's macroglobulinemia.

cryonics /krī·on′iks/ [Gk, *kryos,* cold], the techniques in which cold is applied for a variety of therapeutic goals, including brief local anesthesia, destruction of superficial skin lesions, and preservation of cells, tissue, organs, or the entire body. **−cryonic,** *adj.*

cryoprecipitate /-prisip′itāt/. **1.** any precipitate formed upon cooling a solution. **2.** a preparation rich in factor VIII needed to restore normal coagulation in hemophilia. It is collected from fresh human plasma that has been frozen and thawed.

cryostat /krī′ōstat/ [Gk, *kryos* + *statos,* standing], a device used in surgical pathology that consists of a special microtome used for freezing and slicing sections of tissue for study by a surgical pathologist.

cryosurgery /-sur′jərē/ [Gk, *kryos* + *cheirourgos*], use of subfreezing temperature to destroy tissue. Cryosurgery is performed in the destruction of the ganglion of nerve cells in the thalamus in the treatment of Parkinson's disease, in the destruction of the pituitary gland to halt the progress of some kinds of metastatic cancer, and in the treatment of various cancers and lesions of the skin. The process is also used in ophthalmology to cause the edges of a detached retina to heal and to remove cataracts. The coolant is circulated through a metal probe, chilling it to as low as −160° C, depending on the chemical used. The moist tissues adhere to the cold metal of the probe and freeze. Cells are dehydrated as their membranes burst; they are eventually discarded or absorbed by the body. No specific postoperative nursing care is required.

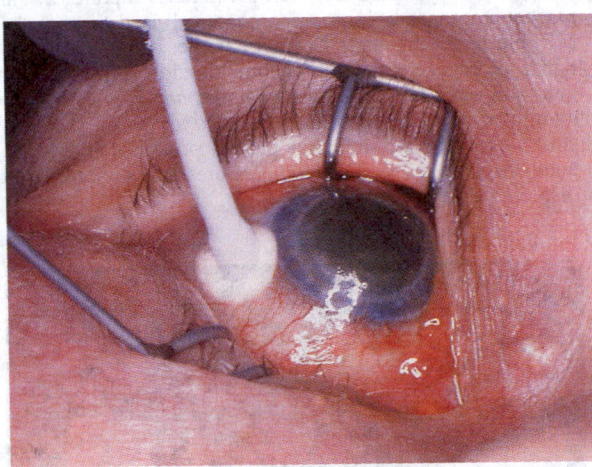

Cryosurgery *(Jaffe, 1990)*

cryotherapy /krī'ōther'əpē/ [Gk, *kryos* + *therapeia*], a treatment using cold as a destructive medium. Cutaneous tags, warts, condylomata acuminatum, actinic keratosis, and dermatofibromas are some of the common skin disorders responsive to cryotherapy. Solid carbon dioxide or liquid nitrogen is applied briefly with a sterile cotton-tipped applicator. A blister forms, followed by necrosis. The procedure may be repeated.

crypt /kript/ [Gk, *kryptos*, hidden], a blind pit or tube on a free surface. Some kinds of crypts are **anal crypt, dental crypt,** and **synovial crypt.**

crypt-. See **crypto-.**

cryptic /krip'tik/ [Gk, *kryptos*, hidden], pertaining to something concealed.

crypto-, crypt-, krypto-, a prefix meaning 'hidden': *cryptocephalus, cryptocrystalline, cryptodidymus.*

cryptocephalus /krip'tōsef'ələs/ [Gk, *kryptos* + *kephale*, head], a malformed fetus that has a small, underdeveloped head. **–cryptocephalic, cryptocephalous,** *adj.*, **cryptocephaly,** *n.*

cryptococcosis /krip'tōkokō'sis/, an infectious disease caused by a fungus, *Cryptococcus neoformans,* which spreads from the lungs to the brain and central nervous system, skin, skeletal system, and urinary tract. The disease occurs in all parts of the world, but in North America it is most likely to afflict persons with AIDS and middle-aged

men in the southeastern states. It is characterized by the development of nodules or tumors filled with a gelatinous material in visceral and subcutaneous tissues. Initial symptoms may include coughing or other respiratory effects because the lungs are a primary site of infection. After the fungus spreads to the meninges, neurologic symptoms may develop, including headache, blurred vision, and difficulty in speaking. The diagnosis is made by isolation and identification of the fungus in specimens of sputum, pus, or tissue biopsy. Amphotericin B and flucytosine may be administered to control the infection. In patients with AIDS, maintenance therapy with fluconazole is indicated. Also called **Buschke's disease, European blastomycosis, torulosis.** See also *Cryptococcus,* and see specific fungal infections.

Cryptococcus /-kok'əs/, a genus of yeastlike fungi that reproduces by budding rather than by producing spores. Many nonpathogenic species of *Cryptococcus* are commonly found in the soil and on the skin and mucous membranes of people who are well. Certain pathogenic species exist; *C. neoformans* is the most important. See also **fungus, yeast.**

Cryptococcus neoformans, a species of yeastlike fungus that causes cryptococcosis, a potentially fatal infection that can affect the lungs, skin, and brain.

cryptodidymus /krip'tōdid'əməs/ [Gk, *kryptos* + *didymos*, twin], conjoined twins in which one fetus is small, underdeveloped, and concealed within the body of the other, more fully formed autosite.

crypt of iris, any one of the small pits in the iris along its free margin encircled by the circulus arteriosus minor. Also called **crypt of Fuchs.**

crypt of Lieberkuhn. See **Lieberkuhn's glands.**

cryptogenic /-jen'ik/ [Gk, *kryptos,* hidden, *genein,* to produce], **1.** pertaining to a disease of unknown etiology. **2.** a parasitic organism living within another organism.

cryptomenorrhea /krip'tōmenôrē'ə/ [Gk, *kryptos* + L, *mensis,* month; Gk, *rhoia,* flow], an abnormal condition in which the products of menstruation are retained within the vagina because of an imperforate hymen, or, less often, within the uterus because of an occlusion of the cervical canal. Cryptomenorrhea is usually accompanied by subjective symptoms of menstruation with scant or absent flow and sometimes by severe pain. If the flow is completely obstructed, uterotubal reflux of menstrual flow into the pelvic cavity may cause peritonitis, pain, adhesions, and endometriosis. **–cryptomenorrheal,** *adj.*

cryptophthalmos /krip'təfthal'məs/ [Gk, *kryptos* + *ophthalmos,* eye], a developmental anomaly characterized by complete fusion of the eyelids, usually with defective formation or lack of the eyes.

cryptorchid /kriptôr'kid/[Gk, *kryptos,* hidden, *orchis,* testis], a developmental defect characterized by failure of the testicles to descend into the scrotum. They are retained in the abdomen or inguinal canal.

cryptorchidism /kriptôr'kidiz'əm/ [Gk, *kryptos* + *orchis,* testis], failure of one or both of the testicles to descend into the scrotum. If spontaneous descent does not occur by the age of 1 year, hormonal injections may be given. If not successful, surgery, called orchiopexy, will likely be performed before the boy is 5 years of age. Also called **undescended testis.**

cryptorchis. See **cryptorchid, cryptorchidism.**

cry reflex, a normal infantile reaction to pain, hunger, or

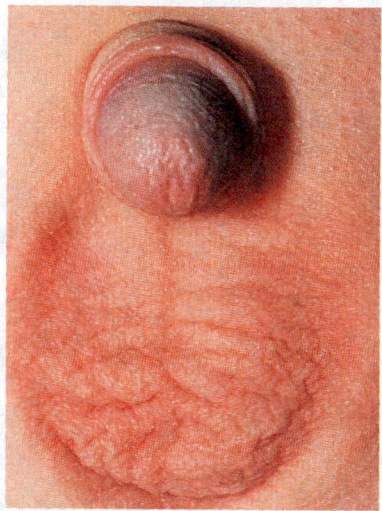

Cryptorchidism *(Zitelli, 1992)*

need for attention. The reflex may be absent in an infant born prematurely or one in poor health.

crystal /kris'təl/ [Gk, *krystallos*], a solid inorganic substance, the atoms or molecules of which are arranged in a regular, repeating three-dimensional pattern, which determines the shape of a crystal. **—crystalline,** *adj.*

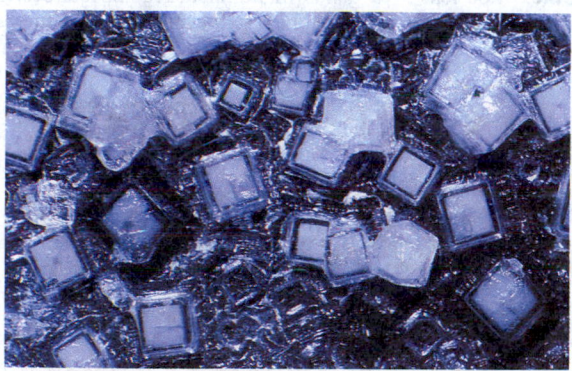

Sodium chloride crystals
(Seeley, 1992/Michael Godomski/Tom Stack & Associates)

crystalline lens /kris'təlin, -līn/ [Gk, *krystallos;* L, lentil], a transparent structure of the eye, enclosed in a capsule, situated between the iris and the vitreous humor, and slightly overlapped at its margin by the ciliary processes. It refracts light to focus images on the retina. The capsule of the lens is a transparent, elastic membrane that touches the free border of the iris anteriorly and is secured by the suspensory ligament of the lens. The circumference of the capsule recedes from the iris to form the posterior chamber of the eye. The lens is a transparent biconvex structure with the posterior surface more convex than the anterior. It is composed of a soft, cortical material, a firm nucleus, and concentric laminae and is covered anteriorly by transparent epithelium. In the fetus the lens is very soft and has a slightly reddish tint; in the adult it is colorless and firm; in old age it becomes flattened, more dense, slightly opaque, and amber-tinted. See also **eye.**

crystallization /kris'təlīzā'shən/ [Gk, *krystallos,* rock crystal], the production of crystals, either by cooling a liquid or gas to a solid state or by cooling a solution until the solute precipitates as a crystalline deposit.

crystalloid /kris'təloid/ [Gk, *krystallos + eidos,* form], a substance in a solution that can be diffused through a semipermeable membrane. Compare **colloid.**

crystalluria /kris'təlŏŏr'ē·ə/, the presence of crystals in the urine. The condition may be a source of urinary tract irritation.

Crystodigin, a trademark for a cardiac glycoside (digitoxin).

Cs, symbol for the element **cesium.**

CS, abbreviation for **cesarean section.**

c-section, see **cesarean section.**

CSF, abbreviation for **cerebrospinal fluid.**

CSN, abbreviation for *certified school nurse.*

CSR, abbreviation for **Cheyne-Stokes respiration.**

CT, abbreviation for **computed tomography.**

C3 nephritic factor, a C3 complement protein molecule that may be deposited in glomerular capillary walls and mesangial tissues, precipitating or contributing to local immune inflammatory injury and kidney damage.

Cu, symbol for the element **copper.**

Cuban itch. See **alastrim.**

cubic centimeter (cm³) [Gk, *kybos;* L, *centum,* hundred; Gk, *metron,* measure], a theoretical cube or its equivalent, each edge of which is 1 centimeter long. One cubic centimeter is equivalent to 1 milliliter (ml).

cubital /kyōō'bitəl/, pertaining to the elbow or the forearm.

cuboidal epithelium /kyōōboi'dəl/ [Gk, *kybos,* cube, *eidos,* form, *epi,* above, *thele,* nipple], simple epithelial cells that are generally cubeshaped and one layer in thickness.

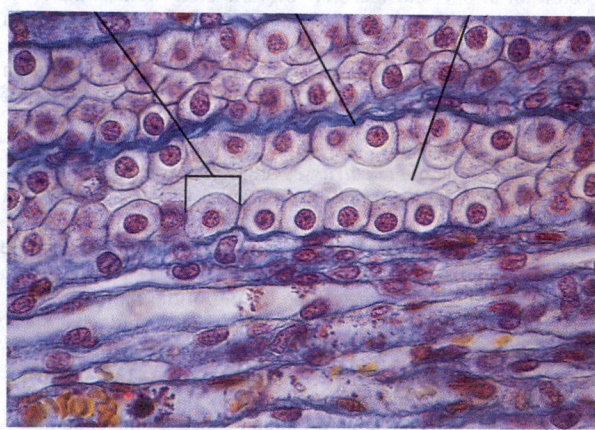

Simple cuboidal epithelium *(Seeley, 1992/Ed Reschke)*

cuboid bone /kyoo'boid/ [Gk, *kybos*, cube, *eidos*, form], the cuboidal tarsal bone on the lateral side of the foot, proximal to the fourth and fifth metatarsal bones. It articulates with the calcaneus, lateral cuneiform, and fourth and fifth metatarsal bones, and, occasionally, the navicular. Also called **os cuboideum.**

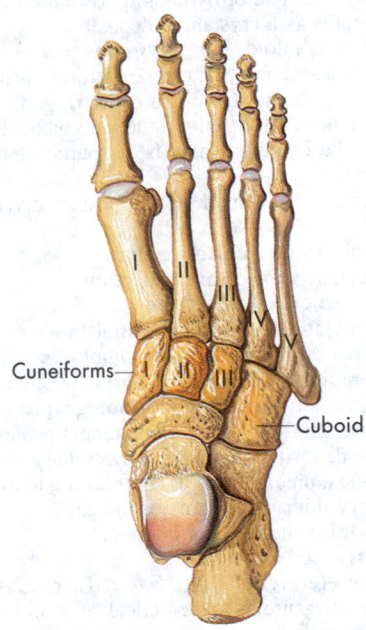

Cuneiforms

Cuboid

Cuboid bone *(Thibodeau, 1993)*

cu.cm., abbreviation for **cubic centimeter.**

cue /kyoo/, a stimulus that determines or may prompt the nature of a person's response.

cuff [ME], an inflatable elastic tube that is placed about the upper arm and expanded with air to restrict arterial circulation during blood pressure examination. See also **cuffed endotracheal tube, Dacron cuff.**

cuffed endotracheal tube, an endotracheal tube with a balloon at one end that may be inflated to tighten the fit of the tube in the lumen of the airway. The balloon forms a cuff that prevents gastric contents from passing into the lungs and gas from leaking back from the lungs. Both high pressure and low pressure cuffs are in use. Overinflation of the cuff can cause contusion, hemorrhage, mucosal sloughing, or stenosis may develop.

cuirass /kwiras'/ [Fr, *cuirasse,* breastplate], **1.** a negative-pressure full body respirator. It consists of a rigid shell that conforms to the surfaces of the body from the neck to the hips. Ventilating pressure is delivered through a flexible hose attached to the top of the device. An electric-driven pump is adjusted to match the timing of the patient's spontaneous breathing. **2.** a tightly fitted chest bandage.

cul-de-sac /kul'dəsak, kYdesok'/, *pl.* **culs-de-sac, cul-de-sacs** [F, bottom of the bag], a blind pouch or cecum, such as the conjunctival cul-de-sac and the dural cul-de-sac.

cul-de-sac of Douglas, a pouch formed by the caudal portion of the parietal peritoneum. Also called **pouch of Douglas, rectouterine excavation, rectouterine pouch.**

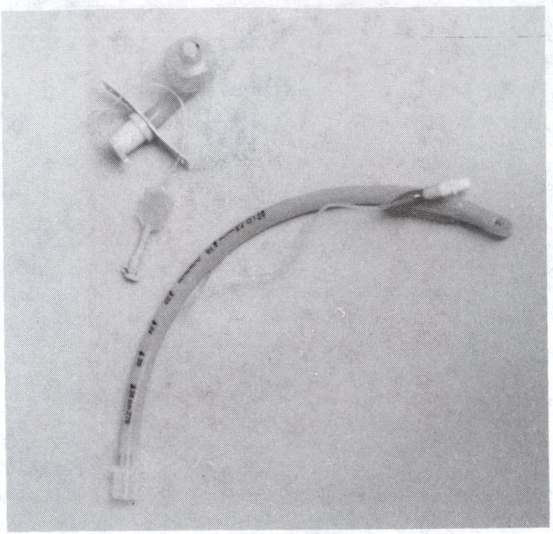

Cuffed tracheostomy tube and cuffed endotracheal tube
(Wilson, 1990)

culdocentesis /kul'dōsentē'sis/, the use of needle puncture or incision through the vagina to remove intraperitoneal fluid, including purulent material.

culdotomy /kuldot'əmē/, incision or needle puncture of the cul-de-sac of Douglas by way of the vagina.

Culex /koo'leks/, a genus of humpbacked mosquitoes. It includes species that transmit viral encephalitis and filariasis.

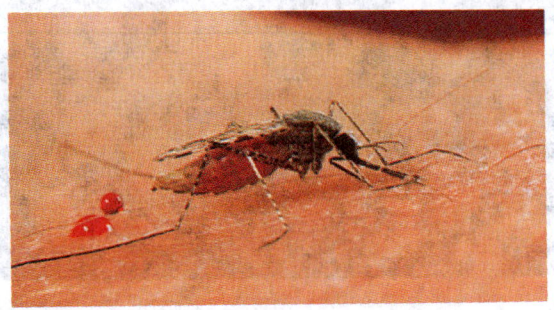

Female Culex mosquito *(Muller, 1990)*

Cullen's sign [Thomas S. Cullen, American gynecologist, b. 1868], the appearance of faint, irregularly formed hemorrhagic patches on the skin around the umbilicus. The discolored skin is blue-black and becomes greenish-brown or yellow. Cullen's sign may appear 1 to 2 days after the onset of anorexia and the severe, poorly localized abdominal pains that are characteristic of acute pancreatitis. Cullen's sign is also present in massive upper GI hemorrhage and ruptured ectopic pregnancy. Compare **Grey Turner's sign.** See also **pancreatitis.**

culs-de-sac. See **cul-de-sac.**

cult, a specific complex of beliefs, rites, and ceremonies maintained by a social group in association with some particular person or object. A cult is often considered as having magical significance.

cultural assimilation /kul′chərəl/, a process by which members of an ethnic minority group lose cultural characteristics that distinguish them from the dominant cultural group.

cultural event, a communication of meaning that takes place each time one member of a society interacts with another member.

cultural healer, a member of an ethnic or cultural group who uses traditional methods of healing rather than modern scientific methods to provide health care for other members of the group or members of another ethnic minority group.

cultural relativism, a concept that health and normality emerge within a social context, and that the content and form of mental health will vary greatly from one culture to another. Differences may be due to variations in stressors, symbolic interpretation, acceptance of expression and repression, and cohesion of social groups and their tolerance of deviation.

culturally relativistic perspective, an ability to understand the behavior of transcultural patients (those who move from one culture to another) within the context of their own culture. See also **transcultural nursing.**

culture /kul′chər/ [L, *colere*, to cultivate], **1.** (in microbiology) a laboratory test involving the cultivation of microorganisms or cells in a special growth medium. See also **medium. 2.** (in psychology) a set of learned values, beliefs, customs, and behavior that is shared by a group of interacting individuals.

culture-bound, pertaining to a health condition that is specific to a particular culture, such as a belief in the effects of certain kinds prayer or the "evil eye."

culture medium. See **medium.**

culture procedure, (in bacteriology) any of several techniques for growing colonies of microorganisms to identify a pathogen and to determine its sensitivity to various antibiotics. Usually, a specimen is secured and a small amount is placed in or on one or more culture media, because different organisms are nourished by different nutrients and grow best at specific but different pH levels. The environment in which the media are held during observation is maintained at body temperature, and the ambient oxygen level is adjusted to achieve an aerobic or anaerobic state. All procedures are aseptic and all equipment is sterile to avoid accidental contamination of the media. As colonies appear in or on the media, small amounts of each (there are often several) are spread on other media to allow examination of a pure specimen of the microorganisms.

culture shock, the psychologic effect of a drastic change in the cultural environment of an individual. The person may exhibit feelings of helplessness, discomfort, and disorientation in attempting to adapt to a different cultural group with dissimilar practices, values, and beliefs.

cu.mm., abbreviation for *cubic millimeter.*

cumulative /kyōo′myəlā′tiv/ [L, *cumulare*, to pile on], increasing by incremental steps with an eventual total that may exceed the expected result.

cumulative action, 1. the increased activity of a therapeutic measure or agent when administered repeatedly, as the cumulative action of a regular exercise program. **2.** the increased activity demonstrated by a drug when repeated doses accumulate in the body and exert a greater biologic effect than the initial dose.

cumulative dose, the total dose that accumulates from repeated exposure to radiation or a radiopharmaceutic product.

cumulative gene. See **polygene.**

cune-, a combining form meaning 'pertaining to a wedge': *cuneate, cuneiform, cuneus.*

cuneate /kyōo′ne·āt/ [L, *cuneus*, wedge], (of tissue) wedge-shaped, used especially in describing cells of the nervous system.

cuneiform /kyōone′əfôrm′/ [L, *cuneus*, wedge, *forma*], (of bone and cartilage) wedge-shaped.

cuneiform bone. See **triangular bone.**

cuneiform cartilage [L, *cuneus*, wedgeshaped, *forma, cartilago*], an elongated elastic laryngeal cartilage at the edge of the aryepiglottic fold, above and anterior to the corniculate cartilage.

-cuneo, cuneo- [L, *cuneus*, wedgeshaped], a combining form 'pertaining to wedgeshaped structures': *cunneus, cuneiform.*

cunnilingus /kun′əling′gəs/, the oral stimulation of the female genitalia.

cup arthroplasty of the hip joint [L, *cupa*, cask; Gk, *arthron*, joint, *plassein*, to form], the surgical replacement of the head of the femur by a metal or plastic mold to relieve pain and increase motion in arthritis or to correct a deformity. The damaged or diseased bone is removed, and the acetabulum and the head of the femur are reshaped. A cup is inserted between the two and becomes the articulating surface of the femur. Postoperatively, the patient's leg is suspended in traction to hold it in a position of abduction and internal rotation to keep the disk in place in the acetabulum. Continued abduction may be necessary for 6 weeks. Possible complications include infection, thrombophlebitis, pulmonary embolism, and fat embolism. The patient receives extensive physical therapy; crutches are necessary to avoid bearing of full weight for 6 months, and an exercise program must be followed for several years. Compare **hip replacement.** See also **arthroplasty, knee replacement, osteoarthritis, plastic surgery.**

cupping, a counterirritant technique of applying a suction device to the skin to draw blood to the surface of the body.

cupping and vibrating, the procedures to help remove mucus and fluid from the lungs by the use of the techniques of manual percussion and vibration to dislodge and mobilize the secretions.

■ METHOD: Cupping is performed by the rhythmic percussion of the affected segments of the lungs or bronchi by the practitioner's cupped hands. Cupping is begun gently and is increased in forcefulness as the patient tolerates increased percussion. Vibration is done by placing the practitioner's hands over the affected area and tensing and contracting the muscles of the hand, arm, and, mainly, shoulder, as if having a shaking chill during the exhalation. The movements are transmitted to the patient's chest, which increases the turbulence and velocity of exhaled air in the small bronchi. See also **postural drainage.**

■ NURSING INTERVENTION: Cupping is never performed over breast tissue, over the spine, or below the ribs because it causes discomfort and can cause damage to soft tissue. After head-down postural drainage with cupping and vibrating, the patient is helped to a position favorable for effective coughing and asked to breathe deeply at least three times and to cough at least twice.

■ OUTCOME CRITERIA: Thick, tenacious mucus is difficult to

evacuate from the bronchi, the bronchioles, and the alveoli. As an adjunct to postural drainage, cupping and vibrating may greatly facilitate the clearing of the passages. The patient can breathe more deeply and with less effort, and the potential of pneumonia or atelectasis is reduced.

cupric /kyoo′prik/ [L, *cuprum,* copper], of or pertaining to copper in its divalent form, as cupric sulfate.

Cuprid, a trademark for a copper chelating agent (trientine hydrochloride).

Cuprimine, a trademark for a chelating agent (D-penicillamine), used in treating poisoning by heavy metals.

cupulolithiasis /kyoo′pyoolōlithī′əsis/ [L, *cupula,* little cup; Gk, *lithos,* stone], a severe, long-lasting vertigo brought on by movement of the head to certain positions. There are many possible causes, among them otitis media, ear surgery, or injury to the inner ear. In addition to extreme dizziness, signs are nausea, vomiting, and ataxia. There is no treatment except avoidance of the offending head positions. Also called **postural vertigo.**

curare /kyoorä′rē/ [S.Am. Indian, *ourari*], a substance derived from tropic plants of the genus *Strychnos.* It is a potent neuromuscular blocker that acts by preventing transmission of neural impulses across the myoneural junctions. Large dosage can cause complete paralysis, but action is usually reversible with anticholinergics. Pharmacologic preparations of the substance are used as adjuncts to general anesthesia. The use of curare or other neuromuscular blocking agents requires respiratory and ventilatory assistance by a qualified anesthetist or anesthesiologist. See also **tubocurarine chloride.**

curariform /kyoorä′rifôrm′/ [*curare* + L, *forma*], **1.** chemically similar to curare. **2.** having the effect of curare.

curative treatment. See **treatment.**

cure /kyoor/ [L, *cura*], **1.** restoration to health of a person afflicted with a disease or other disorder. **2.** the favorable outcome of the treatment of a disease or other disorder. **3.** a course of therapy, a medication, a therapeutic measure, or another remedy used in treatment of a medical problem, as faith healing, fasting, rest cure, or work cure.

curet /kyooret′/ [Fr, *curette,* scoop], **1.** a surgical instrument shaped like a spoon or scoop for scraping and removing material or tissue from an organ, cavity, or surface. A curet may be blunt or sharp and is designed in a shape and size appropriate to its use. **2.** to remove tissue or debris with such a device. Kinds of curets include **Hartmann's curet.**

curettage /kyoor′ətäzh′/ [Fr, *curette,* scoop], scraping of material from the wall of a cavity or other surface, performed to remove tumors or other abnormal tissue or to obtain tissue for microscopic examination. Curettage also refers to clearing unwanted material from fistulas and areas of chronic infection. It may be performed with a blunt or a sharp curet or by suction.

curie (c, Ci) /kyoor′ē/ [Marie S. Curie, Polish-born chemist, b. 1867; Pierre Curie, French scientist, b. 1859], a unit of radioactivity used before adoption of the becquerel (Bq) as the SI unit. It is equal to 3.70×10^{10} Bq.

curium (Cm) /kyoo′rē·əm/ [Marie S. Curie; Pierre Curie], a radioactive metallic element. Its atomic number is 96; its atomic weight is 247. Curium is an artificial element produced by bombarding plutonium with helium ions in a cyclotron. Numerous isotopes of curium are produced by bombarding lighter transuranium elements. Curium is so radioactive that it glows in the dark.

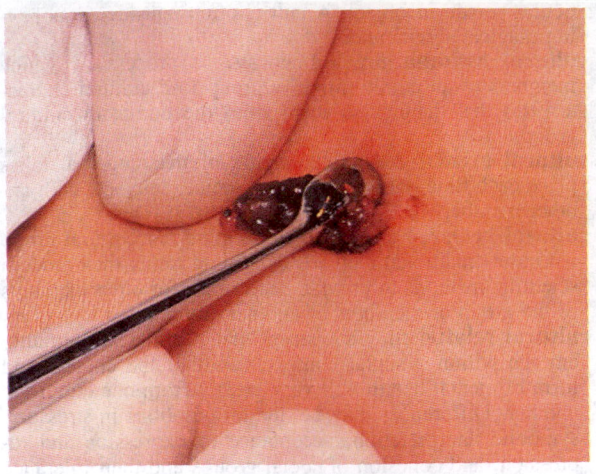

Curettage *(Stone, 1989)*

-curium, a suffix designating a neuromuscular blocking agent.

Curling's ulcer [Thomas B. Curling, English surgeon, b. 1811], a duodenal ulcer that develops in people who have severe burns on the surface of the body. Also called **Curling's stress ulcer.** See also **milk therapy.**

CURN, abbreviation for *Certified Urological Registered Nurse.*

-curonium, a suffix designating a neuromuscular blocking agent.

currant jelly clot /kur′ənt/ [ME, *corauns;* L, *gelare,* to congeal; AS, *clott*], a red, jellylike blood clot that is rich in hemoglobin from erythrocytes in the clot.

current /kur′ənt/ [L, *currere,* to run], **1.** a flowing or streaming movement. **2.** a flow of electrons along a conductor in a closed circuit; an electric current. **3.** certain physiologic electric activity and characteristics of blood circulation. Physiologic currents include abnerval current, action current, axial current, centrifugal current, centripetal current, compensating current, demarcation current, and electrotonic current. See also **alternating current, direct current, volt, watt.**

-current, a suffix meaning 'running, flowing, happening': *concurrent, excurrent, intercurrent.*

current of injury. an abnormal current flow to and from injured myocardium resulting from reduced membrane potential in the injured area conpared to that of the normal fibers. See **demarcation current.**

Current Procedural Terminology (CPT), a system developed by the American Medical Association for standardizing the terminology and coding used to describe medical services and procedures.

current validity. See **validity.**

curriculum vitae (CV) /kərik′ələm wē′tī, vē′tē/, *pl.* **curricula vitae** [L, *curriculum,* course; *vita,* life], a summary of educational and professional experiences, including activities and honors, to be used in seeking employment, for biographic citations on professional meeting programs, or for related purposes. Also called **résumé, resume** /rā′zəmā/.

Curschmann spiral /koorsh′mon/ [Heinrich Curschmann, German physician, b. 1846; Gk, *speira,* coil], one of the coiled fibrils of mucus occasionally found in the sputum of persons with bronchial asthma.

cursor /kur′sər/   a movable indicator light on a computer CRT that shows the position for entering, modifying, or deleting data.

curtain effect /kur′tən/,   (in radiology) an x-ray film artifact caused by chemical processing stains that were not properly squeezed from the film during development.

curvature myopia /kur′vəchər/,   a type of nearsightedness caused by refractive errors associated with an excessive curvature of the cornea.

curve [L, *curvare,* to bend],   (in statistics) a straight or curved line used as a graphic method of demonstrating the distribution of data collected in a study or survey.

curve of Carus [Karl G. Carus, German physician, b. 1789],   the normal axis of the pelvic outlet. Also called **circle of Carus.**

curve of occlusion,   **1.** a curved occlusal surface that simultaneously contacts the major portion of the incisal and occlusal prominences of the existing teeth. **2.** the curve of dentition on which lie the occlusal surfaces of the teeth. See also **reverse curve.**

curve of Spee /shpā, spē/ [Ferdinand Graf von Spee, German embryologist, b. 1855],   **1.** the anatomic curvature of the occlusal alignment of the teeth, beginning at the tip of the lower canine, following the buccal cusps of the natural premolars and molars, and continuing to the anterior border of the ramus. **2.** the curve of the occlusal surfaces of the arches in vertical dimension, produced by a downward dipping of the mandibular premolars, with a corresponding adjustment of the upper premolars.

curvilinear /kur′vilin′ē·ər/ [L, *curvus,* bent, *linea,* line], pertaining to a curved line.

curvilinear trend [L, *curvus,* bent, *linea,* line; AS, *trendan,* to turn],   (in statistics) a trend in which a graphic representation of the data yields a curved line. The value of the independent variable may be expressed as a polynomial coefficient, by a more complete mathematic expression, such as a logistic curve, or by a smoothing process, as a moving average.

cushingoid /kōōsh′ingoid/ [Harvey W. Cushing, American surgeon, b. 1869; Gk, *eidos,* form],   having the habitus and facies characteristic of Cushing's disease: fat pads on the upper back and face, striae on the limbs and trunk, and excess hair on the face.

Cushing's disease /kōōsh′ingz/ [Harvey W. Cushing],   a metabolic disorder characterized by the abnormally increased secretion of adrenocortical steroids caused by increased amounts of adrenocorticotropic hormone (ACTH) secreted by the pituitary, such as by a pituitary adenoma. Excess adrenocortical hormones result in accumulations of fat on the chest, upper back, and face and the occurrence of edema, hyperglycemia, increased gluconeogenesis, muscle weakness, purplish striae on the skin, decreased immunity to infection, osteoporosis with susceptibility to fracture of bones, acne, and facial hirsutism. Hyperglycemia resulting from Cushing's disease does not usually respond to treatment; diabetes mellitus may become a chronic condition. Therapy is aimed at removal or destruction of ACTH secreting tissue, most commonly by surgical or radiologic procedures. If this is not possible, the adrenal glands are totally or subtotally removed and pharmacologic preparations of adrenal steroids are administered. Also called **hyperadrenalism.** Compare **Cushing's syndrome.**

Cushing's syndrome [Harvey W. Cushing],   a metabolic disorder resulting from the chronic and excessive production of cortisol by the adrenal cortex or by the administration of glucocorticoids in large doses for several weeks or longer. When occurring spontaneously, the syndrome represents a failure in the body's ability to regulate the secretion of cortisol or adrenocorticotropic hormone (ACTH). (Normally cortisol is produced only in response to ACTH, and ACTH is not secreted in the presence of high levels of cortisol.) The most common cause of the syndrome is a pituitary tumor that causes an increased secretion of ACTH. It can be caused by idiopathic hyperplasia of adrenal tissue functioning outside the control of the negative feedback system. Also called **hyperadrenocorticism.** See also **Addison's disease, Cushing's disease, Nelson's syndrome.**

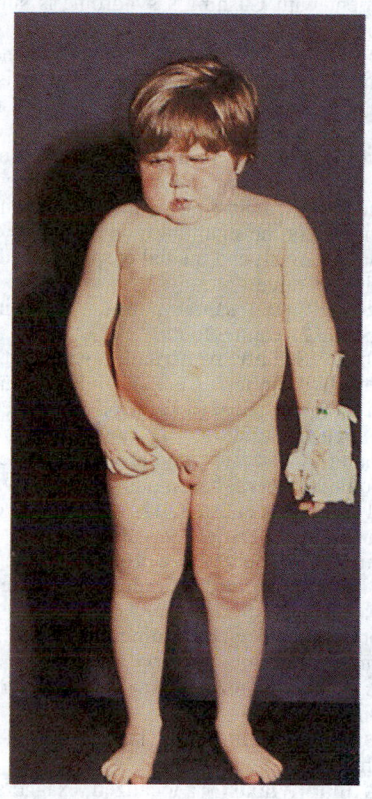

Cushing's syndrome *(Zitelli, 1992)*

■ OBSERVATIONS: Characteristically, the patient with Cushing's syndrome has a decreased glucose tolerance, central obesity, round "moon" face, supraclavicular fat pads, a pendulous, striae-covered pad of fat on the chest and abdomen, oligomenorrhea or decreased testosterone levels, muscular atrophy, edema, hypokalemia, and some degree of emotional change. The skin may be abnormally pigmented and fragile; minor infections may become systemic and long-lasting. Children with the disorder may stop growing. Occasionally, hypertension, kidney stones, and psychosis occur.

■ INTERVENTIONS: The objective of all treatment is reduction of the secretion of cortisol. The source of the excess ACTH is discovered by a series of tests that challenge the function of the adrenal and pituitary glands. Once known, the cause is treated. If the excess ACTH is caused by an adenoma of the anterior pituitary, x-ray irradiation or surgical excision of the tumor corrects the condition. If the condition is the result of medication, decreasing or changing the medication may alleviate the symptoms.

■ NURSING CONSIDERATIONS: In caring for children, the nurse normally observes height and weight, because rapidly developing obesity and failure to grow are suggestive of Cushing's syndrome. The patient with the syndrome may usually be reassured that treatment is largely successful and that the appearance may be expected to return to normal. Some of the medications used for some forms of the condition may cause nausea and anorexia, somnolence, and lethargy, and the patient is informed of this. Nursing care of the hospitalized patient with Cushing's syndrome is similar to that of Addison's disease, Cushing's disease, and other endocrinologic disorders; weight and electrolyte and fluid balance are monitored, an adequate, balanced diet is urged, and emotional changes are observed with a goal of maintaining emotional equilibrium.

cusp [L, *cuspis,* point], **1.** a sharp projection or a rounded eminence that rises from the chewing surface of a tooth, such as the two pyramidal cusps that arise from the premolars. **2.** any one of the small flaps on the valves of the heart, as the ventral, dorsal, and medial cusps attached to the right atrioventricular valve.

cuspid /kus′pid/ [L, *cuspis,* point], **1.** having but one cusp, or point. **2.** canine tooth.

cuspid valve. See **atrioventricular valve.**

cuspless tooth /kusp′les/, a tooth without cuspal prominences on its masticatory surface, possibly due to attriton.

custodial care /kəstō′dē·əl/ [L, *custodia,* guarding; *garrire,* to chatter], services and care of a nonmedical nature provided on a long-term basis, usually for convalescent and chronically ill individuals. Kinds of custodial care include **board, room,** and **personal assistance.**

cut, (in molecular genetics) a fissure or split in a double strand of DNA in contrast to a nick in a single strand. See also **nick.**

cut-, a prefix meaning 'pertaining to the skin': *cutaneous, cuticle, cuticularization.*

cutaneous /kyo͞otā′nē·əs/ [L, *cutis,* skin], of or pertaining to the skin.

cutaneous absorption, the taking up of substances through the skin.

cutaneous anaphylaxis, a localized, exaggerated reaction of hypersensitivity in the form of a wheal and flare caused by an antigen injected into the skin of a sensitized individual, generally used as a test of sensitivity to various allergens. Passive cutaneous anaphylaxis, the response to an intradermally injected antibody, is used in studies of antibodies that induce immediate reactions of hypersensitivity.

cutaneous horn, a hard, skin-colored projection of the epidermis, usually on the head or face.

cutaneous larva migrans, a skin condition caused by a hookworm, *Ancylostoma braziliense,* a parasite of cats and dogs. Its ova are deposited in the ground with the feces of infected animals, develop into larvae, and invade the skin of people, particularly bare feet, but any skin may be involved. The larvae rarely develop into adult hookworms in the human body, but as the larvae migrate through the epidermis, a trail of inflammation follows the burrow, causing severe pruritus. Secondary infections often occur if the skin has been broken by scratching. Topical application of a so-

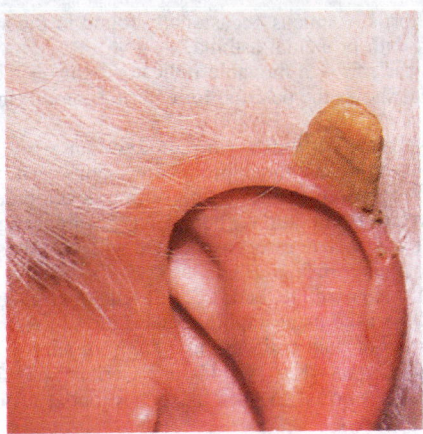

Cutaneous horn
(duVivier, 1993/Courtesy St. Mary's Hospital)

lution of thiabendazole usually eradicates the larvae. Also called **creeping eruption.**

cutaneous leishmaniasis. See **Oriental sore.**

cutaneous lupus erythematosus. See **discoid lupus erythematosus.**

cutaneous membrane. See **skin.**

cutaneous nerve, a nerve that enters the skin.

cutaneous nevus [L, *cutis,* skin, *naevus,* a mole on the body], a congenital discoloration of a skin area, such as a strawberry birthmark.

cutaneous papilloma, a small brown or flesh-colored outgrowth of skin, occurring most frequently on the neck of an older person. Also called **cutaneous tag, skin tag.**

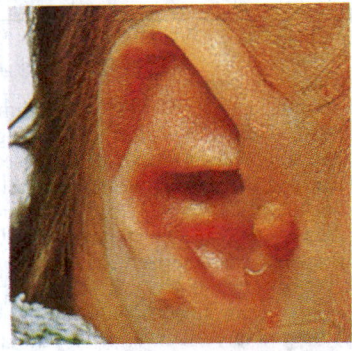

Cutaneous papilloma
(Zitelli, 1992/Courtesy Dr. Christine L Williams, New York Medical College)

cutaneous sensation [L, *cutis,* skin + *sentire,* to feel], a sensation experienced in or arising from receptors of the skin.

cutaneous tag. See **cutaneous papilloma.**

cutdown [ME, *cutten, doun*], an incision into a vein with the insertion of a catheter for intravenous infusion. It is performed when an infusion cannot be started by venipuncture and in hyperalimentation therapy, when highly concentrated solutions are given via catheter into the superior vena cava. The skin is cleansed before the procedure; the incision is sutured, and a sterile dressing is applied at its conclusion. See also **hyperalimentation, venipuncture.**

cuticle /kyōō′təkəl/ [L, *cuticula*, little skin],   **1.** epidermis. **2.** the sheath of a hair follicle. **3.** the thin edge of cornified epithelium at the base of a nail.

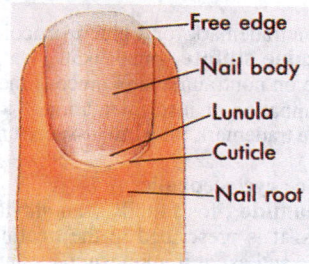

Cuticle *(Thibodeau, 1993/Joan M Beck)*

cutis.   See **skin.**
cutis laxa /kyōō′təs/ [L, skin; *laxus*, loose],   abnormally loose, relaxed skin resulting from an absence of elastic fibers in the body, usually a hereditary condition.
cutis marmorata.   skin that has a "marbled" appearance due to conspicuous veining and dilatation of small vessels. See **livedo.**
cutting oil dermatitis,   a skin disorder that affects machinists and others who use cutting oils as coolants and lubricants. Exposure to the oil obstructs hair follicles, sweat ducts, and sebaceous glands, leading to development of comedones and folliculitis; sometimes there are secondary infections complicated by minute metal particles in the oil.
cuvette /kyōōvet′/ [Fr, *cuva*, tub],   a small transparent tube or container with specific optical properties that is used in laboratory research and analyses, such as photometric evaluations, colorimetric determinations, and turbidity studies. The chemical composition of the container determines the vessel's use, such as Pyrex glass for examining materials in the visible spectrum and one containing silica for those in the ultraviolet range.
CVA,   **1.** abbreviation for **cerebrovascular accident. 2.** abbreviation for **costovertebral angle.**
CVP,   **1.** abbreviation for **central venous pressure. 2.** an anticancer drug combination of cyclophosphamide, vincristine, and prednisone.
CVP monitor.   See **central venous pressure monitor.**
cyan-.   See **cyano-.**
cyanide poisoning /sī′ənid, -nīd/ [Gk, *kyanos*, blue],   poisoning resulting from the ingestion or inhalation of cyanide from such substances as bitter almond oil, wild cherry syrup, prussic acid, hydrocyanic acid, or potassium or sodium cyanide. Characterized by tachycardia, drowsiness, convulsion, and headache, cyanide poisoning may result in death within 1 to 15 minutes. Treatment may include gastric lavage, amyl-nitrite inhalation, oxygen, and sodium thiosulfate.
cyano-, cyan-,   a combining form meaning 'blue': *cyanochroia, cyanocrystallin, cyanodermia.*
cyanocobalamin /sī′ənōkōbal′əmin/ [Gk, *kyanos* + Ger, *kobald*, mine goblin],   a red, crystalline, water-soluble

substance with activity similar to that of vitamin B_{12}. It is involved in the metabolism of protein, fats, and carbohydrates, normal blood formation, and neural function. It is the first substance containing cobalt that is found to be vital to life. It cannot be produced synthetically but can be obtained from cultures of *Streptomyces griseus*. Rich dietary sources are liver, kidney, meats, fish, and dairy products. Deficiency is usually caused by the absence of intrinsic factor, which is necessary for the absorption of cyanocobalamin from the GI tract and which results in pernicious anemia and brain damage. Deficiency can also occur in persons whose diet is strictly vegetarian thereby excluding meat and dairy sources of the nutrient. Symptoms of deficiency include nervousness, neuritis, numbness and tingling in the hands and feet, poor muscular coordination, unpleasant body odor, and menstrual disturbances. Cyanocobalamin is used in the prophylaxis and treatment of pernicious anemia, tropical and nontropical sprue, and other macrocytic and megaloblastic anemias. It is nontoxic, even when administered in amounts greater than those recommended for therapeutic purposes. Also called **antipernicious anemia factor, extrinsic factor, LLD factor, vitamin B_{12}. See also intrinsic factor, pernicious anemia.**
cyanogenetic glycosides /sī′ənōjənet′ik/,   chemical compounds contained in foods that release hydrogen cyanide when chewed or digested. The act of chewing or digestion disrupts the structure of the substances, causing cyanide to be released. Cyanogenetic glycosides are present in apples, apricots, cherries, peaches, plums, and quinces, particularly in the seeds of such fruits. The chemicals are also found in almonds, sorghum, lima beans, cassava, corn, yams, chickpeas, cashews, and kirsch. Although human poisoning from cyanogenetic glycosides is rare, cases have been reported of cyanide poisoning from certain varieties of lima beans, cassava, and bitter almonds.
cyanomethemoglobin /sī′ənō′met·hē′məglō′bin/ [Gk, *kyanos* + *meta*, together with, *haima*, blood; L, *globus*, ball],   a hemoglobin derivative formed during nitrite therapy for cyanide poisoning.
cyanosis /sī′ənō′sis/ [Gk, *kyanos*, blue, *osis*, condition],   bluish discoloration of the skin and mucous membranes caused by an excess of deoxygenated hemoglobin in the blood or a structural defect in the hemoglobin molecule, such as in methemoglobin.   –**cyanotic,** *adj.*

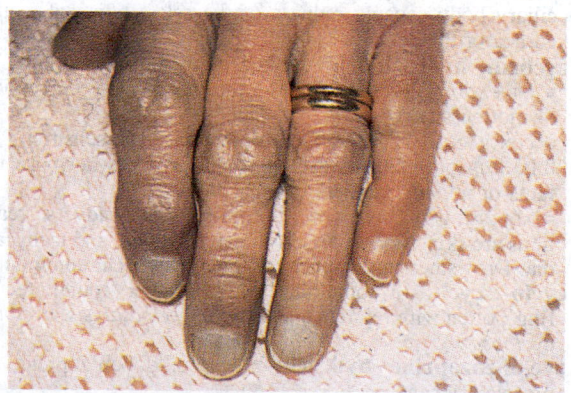

Peripheral cyanosis *(Kamal, 1991)*

cyanotic congenital defect /sī'ənot'ik/, a congenital heart defect that allows the mixing of unsaturated (venous) blood with saturated (arterial) blood to produce cyanosis.

cycl-. See **cyclo-**.

cyclacillin /sī'kləsī'lin/, a penicillin antibiotic.

■ INDICATIONS: It is prescribed in the treatment of certain bacterial infections.

■ CONTRAINDICATION: Known hypersensitivity to penicillins prohibits its use.

■ ADVERSE EFFECTS: Among the most serious adverse reactions are hypersensitivity reactions and severe diarrhea and nausea. Skin rash may also occur.

cyclamate /sī'kləmāt/, an artificial, nonnutritive sweetener formerly used in the form of calcium or sodium salt.

cyclandelate /sīklan'dəlāt/, a vasodilator.

■ INDICATIONS: It is prescribed in the treatment of muscular ischemia and peripheral vascular obstruction or spasm.

■ CONTRAINDICATIONS: Pregnancy or known hypersensitivity to this drug prohibits its use.

■ ADVERSE EFFECTS: Tachycardia, GI distress, and flushing may occur.

Cyclapen-W, a trademark for a penicillin antibiotic (cyclacillin).

cyclencephaly /sīk'lənsef'əlē/ [Gk, *kyklos*, circle, *enkephalos*, brain], a developmental anomaly characterized by the fusion of the two cerebral hemispheres. **–cyclencephalic, cyclencephalous,** *adj.*, **cyclencephalus,** *n.*

cyclic adenosine monophosphate (cAMP) /sik'lik, sī'k-lik/, a cyclic nucleotide formed from adenosine triphosphate by the action of adenyl cyclase. This cyclic compound, known as the "second messenger," participates in the action of catecholamines, vasopressin, adrenocorticotropic hormone, and many other hormones. Also called **cyclic AMP, adenosine 3':5'-cyclic phosphate.**

cyclic guanosine monophosphate (cGMP), a substance that mediates the action of certain hormones in a manner similar to that of cyclic adenosine monophosphate (cAMP). In response to the stimulation of cholinergic receptors in a parasympathetic nerve, guanylate cyclase triggers the conversion of guanosine triphosphate (GTP) to cGMP with the release of various enzymes. Atropine, an anticholinergic drug, can block cholinergic stimulation by means of this process.

cyclic phosphate. See **cyclic adenosine monophosphate.**

-cycline, a suffix designating a tetracycline –derivative antibiotic.

cyclitis /sīklī'tis/ [Gk, *kyklos* + *itis*], inflammation of the ciliary body causing redness of the sclera adjacent to the cornea of the eye.

cyclizine hydrochloride /sī'klizēn/, an antihistamine.

■ INDICATION: It is prescribed in the treatment or prevention of motion sickness.

■ CONTRAINDICATIONS: Asthma or known hypersensitivity to this drug prohibits its use. It is not given to newborn infants or nursing mothers.

■ ADVERSE EFFECTS: Among the more serious adverse reactions are skin rash, hypersensitivity reactions, and tachycardia. Drowsiness and dryness of the mouth occur commonly.

cyclo-, cycl-, a combining form meaning 'round, recurring'; often with reference to the eye: *cyclodialysis, cycloid, cyclops.*

cyclobenzaprine hydrochloride, /sī'kləben'zəprēn/, a muscle relaxant.

■ INDICATION: It is prescribed in the short-term treatment of muscle spasm.

■ CONTRAINDICATIONS: Hyperthyroidism, cardiac arrhythmia, cardiac failure, concomitant use of a monoamine oxidase inhibitor, or known hypersensitivity to this drug prohibits its use. It is used with caution in conditions in which anticholinergics are contraindicated.

■ ADVERSE EFFECTS: The most serious adverse effects are hypersensitivity reactions. Drowsiness, dry mouth, and dizziness commonly occur.

cyclocephalic, cyclocephalous, cyclocephaly. See **cyclopia.**

Cyclocort, a trademark for a glucocorticoid (amcinonide).

cyclomethycaine sulfate /-meth'ikān/, a local anesthetic agent for use on nontraumatized mucous membranes before clinical examination or instrumentation.

Cyclopar, a trademark for a broad-spectrum antibiotic (tetracycline).

cyclopia. See **cyclocephalic.**

cyclophosphamide /-fos'fəmīd/, an alkylating agent.

■ INDICATIONS: It is prescribed in the treatment of a variety of neoplasms and as an immunosuppressant in organ transplants.

■ CONTRAINDICATIONS: This drug is teratogenic in animals. It is not used during pregnancy; adequate methods of contraception should be considered for both males and females taking the drug. It is used with caution with impaired renal or hepatic function or with various blood disorders.

■ ADVERSE EFFECTS: Among the more serious adverse reactions are anorexia, vomiting, alopecia, leukopenia, and potentially serious hemorrhagic cystitis.

cyclopia /sīklō'pē·ə/ [Gk, *Cyclops*, mythic one-eyed giant], a developmental anomaly characterized by fusion of the orbits into a single cavity containing one eye. The condition is usually combined with various other head and facial defects. Also called **cyclocephaly** (*adj.* **cyclocephalic, cyclocephalous**), **synophthalmia.** **–cyclops,** *n.*

cycloplegia /sī'kləplē'jə/ [Gk, *kyklos* + *plege*, stroke], paralysis of the ciliary muscles, as induced by certain ophthalmic drugs to allow examination of the eye. See also **cycloplegic.**

cycloplegic /sī'kləplē'jik/, **1.** of or pertaining to a drug or treatment that causes paralysis of the ciliary muscles of the eye. **2.** one of a group of anticholinergic drugs used to paralyze the ciliary muscles of the eye for ophthalmologic examination or surgery. Any of the cycloplegics may cause adverse effects in persons sensitive to anticholinergics.

cyclopropane /sī'klōprō'pān/, a highly flammable and explosive potent anesthetic gas that gives good analgesia and skeletal muscle relaxation, with low toxicity, minimal adverse effects, and rapid induction and emergence. It has been replaced by the nonflammable halogenated hydrocarbons and is no longer used because of its high flammability and explosion potential. Also called **trimethylene.**

cyclops. See **cyclopia.**

cycloserine /sī'klōser'ēn/, an antibiotic.

■ INDICATIONS: It is prescribed in the treatment of active pulmonary and extrapulmonary tuberculosis.

■ CONTRAINDICATIONS: Epilepsy, depression, severe anxiety, psychosis, severe renal insufficiency, excessive concurrent use of alcohol, or known hypersensitivity to this drug prohibits its use.

■ ADVERSE EFFECTS: Among the most serious reactions are central nervous system toxicity, including tremor, drowsiness, convulsions, and psychotic changes.

Cyclospasmol, a trademark for a vasodilator (cyclandelate).

cyclosporin /-spôr′in/, any of a group of biologically active metabolites of *Tolypocladium inflatum Gams* and certain other fungi. The major forms are cyclosporin A and C, which are cyclic oligopeptides with immunosuppressive, antifungal, and antipyretic effects. As immunosuppressants, cyclosporins affect primarily the T cell lymphocytes. Seven other metabolites have been identified as cyclosporin B and cyclosporins D through I. Also spelled **ciclosporin.**

cyclosporine /-spôr′ēn/, an alternative term for cyclosporin A.

cyclothymic disorder /-thĭm′ik/ [Gk, *kyklos* + *thymos,* mind], a disorder of mood, whereby the essential feature is a chronic mood disturbance of at least two years' duration, involving numerous periods of depression and hypomania, but not of sufficient severity and duration to meet the criteria for a major depressive or manic episode. See also **bipolar disorder, depression, dysthymic disorder.**

cyclothymic personality, a personality characterized by extreme swings in mood from elation to depression.

cyclotomy /sīklot′əmē/, a surgical procedure for the correction of a defect in the ciliary muscle of the eye.

cyclotron /sī′klətron/ [Gk, *kyklos* + *electron,* amber], a device used to accelerate charged particles or ions. The particles bombard special targets where they create radioactive species to be used as radiopharmaceuticals or to make neutrons that can be used for radiotherapy.

cyesis [Gk, *kyesis,* pregnancy], pregnancy.

Cylert, a trademark for a central nervous system stimulant (pemoline).

cylindrical grasp /silin′drikəl/, the normal position of the hand and fingers when holding cylindrical objects, such as a glass tumbler, railing, or pot handle. The fingers close and flex around the object, which is stabilized against the palm of the hand. It occurs as a reflex action in infants and later is developed into a voluntary gross grasp.

cylindroma /sil′indrō′mə/, *pl.* **cylindromas, cylindromata** [Gk, *kylindros,* cylinder], **1.** See **adenocystic carcinoma. 2.** also called **cylindromatous spiradenoma, trichobasalioma hyalinicum.** a benign neoplasm of the skin, usually of the scalp or face, developing from a hair follicle or sweat gland.

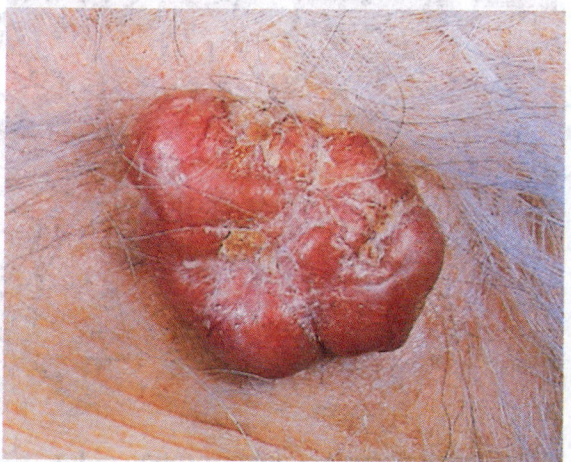

Cylindroma (du Vivier, 1986)

cylindromatous carcinoma. See **adenocystic carcinoma.**

cylindromatous spiradenoma. See **cylindroma.**

cyma line /sī′mə/, an S-shaped line seen on radiographs at the articulation of the talonavicular and calcaneocuboid bones of the foot. An abnormality in the joint, including pronation or supination of the talar head, will show as a broken cyma line on radiographs.

cyno-, cyn-, a combining form meaning 'pertaining to dogs, doglike': *cynobax, cynocephalic, cynophobia.*

cyproheptadine hydrochloride /sī′prōhep′tədēn/, an antihistamine.

■ INDICATIONS: It is prescribed in the treatment of a variety of hypersensitivity reactions, including rhinitis, skin rash, and pruritus.

■ CONTRAINDICATIONS: Asthma or known hypersensitivity to this drug prohibits its use. It is not given to newborn infants or lactating mothers.

■ ADVERSE EFFECTS: Among the more serious adverse reactions are skin rash, hypersensitivity reactions, and tachycardia. Drowsiness and dry mouth commonly occur.

cypionate /sī′pyōnāt/, a contraction for cyclopentanepropionate.

Cyprus fever. See **brucellosis.**

Cys, abbreviation for **cysteine.**

cyst /sist/ [Gk, *kystis,* bag], a closed sac in or under the skin lined with epithelium and containing fluid or semisolid material, as a **sebaceous cyst.**

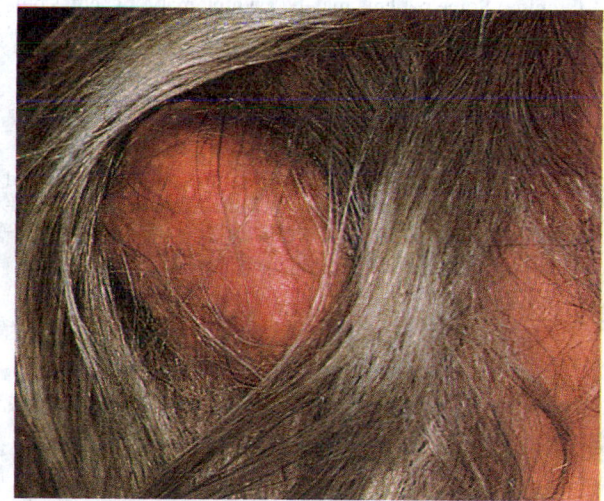

Sebaceous cyst (Kamal, 1991)

cyst-. See **cysto-.**

-cyst, -cystis, a suffix meaning a 'pouch or bladder': *enterocyst, microcyst, zoocyst.*

cystadenocarcinoma /sis′tədē′nəkär′sinō′mə/, a type of pancreatic tumor that evolves from a mucus cystadenoma. Clinical features include epigastric pain and a palpable abdominal mass that may also be seen by ultrasonography or CT scan. It is treated by surgical removal of the tumor or total pancreatectomy.

cystadenoma /sis′tədinō′mə/, *pl.* **cystadenomas, cystadenomata** [Gk, *kystis* + *aden,* gland, *oma,* tumor], **1.** an adenoma associated with a cystoma. **2.** an adenoma containing multiple cystic structures. The cysts may be serous, containing serum, or pseudomucinous, containing clear serous fluid or thick, viscid fluid.

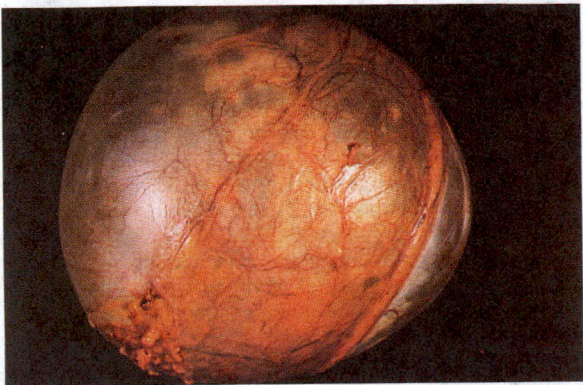

Serous cystadenoma *(Fletcher, 1987)*

cystathioninemia /sis′təthī′əninē′mē·ə/, an inherited metabolic disorder caused by a deficiency of the enzyme cystathionase. It results in an excess of the amino acid methionine. Some patients may be asymptomatic, whereas others show signs of mental retardation. It is treated with large doses of vitamin B_6 (pyridoxine).

cystectomy /sistek′təmē/ [Gk, *kystis* + *ektome,* excision], a surgical procedure in which all or a part of the bladder is removed, as may be required in treating cancer of the bladder.

cysteine (Cys) /sis′tēn/, a nonessential amino acid found in many proteins in the body, including keratin. It is a metabolic precursor of cystine and an important source of sulfur for various body functions.

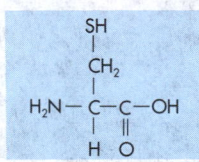

Chemical structure of cysteine *(Seeley, 1992)*

cysti-. See **cysto-.**

cystic /sis′tik/ [Gk, *kystis,* bag], **1.** pertaining to a cyst. **2.** pertaining to a fluid-filled sac, such as the gall bladder or urinary bladder.

cystic acne. See **acne conglobata.**

cystic carcinoma, a malignant neoplasm containing cysts or cystlike spaces. These tumors may occur in the breast and ovary.

cystic duct, the duct through which bile from the gallbladder passes into the common bile duct.

cysticercosis /sis′tisərkō′sis/ [Gk, *kystis* + *kerkos,* tail, *osis,* condition], an infection and infestation by the larval stage of the pork tapeworm *Taenia solium* or the beef tapeworm *T. saginata.* The eggs are ingested and hatch in the intestine; the larvae invade the subcutaneous tissue, brain, eye, muscle, heart, liver, lung, and peritoneum. They attach themselves with two rows of hooklets, grow, mature, and become covered with a dense, fibrous capsule. The invasive, early phase of the infection is characterized by fever, malaise, muscle pain, and eosinophilia. Years later, epilepsy and personality change may appear if the brain is affected, and calcification and destruction of local structures are apparent in other infested areas of the body. Prophylaxis depends on avoiding ingestion of inadequately cooked, infected pork or beef.

cysticercus /sis′tisur′kəs/, a larval form of tapeworm. It consists of a single scolex enclosed in a bladderlike cyst.

cystic fibroma, a fibrous tumor in which cystic degeneration has occurred.

cystic fibrosis, an inherited disorder of the exocrine glands, causing those glands to produce abnormally thick secretions of mucus, elevation of sweat electrolytes, increased organic and enzymatic constituents of saliva, and overactivity of the autonomic nervous system. The glands most affected are those in the pancreas, the respiratory system, and the sweat glands. Cystic fibrosis is usually recognized in infancy or early childhood, occurring chiefly among whites. The earliest manifestation is meconium ileus, an obstruction of the small bowel by viscid stool. Other early signs are a chronic cough, frequent, foul-smelling stools, and persistent upper respiratory infections. The most reliable diagnostic tool is the sweat test, which shows elevations of both sodium and chloride. Because there is no known cure, treatment is directed at the prevention of respiratory infections, which are the most frequent cause of death. Mucolytic agents and bronchodilators are used to help liquefy the thick, tenacious mucus. Physical therapy measures, such as postural drainage and breathing exercises,

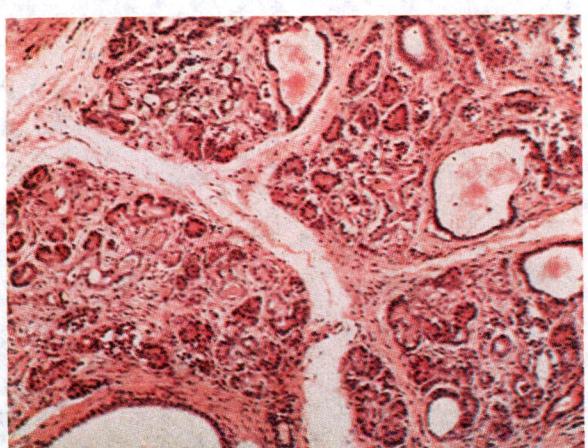

Cystic fibrosis—malabsorption of fat
(McLaren, 1992/Courtesy Professor CM Anderson)

can also dislodge secretions. Broad spectrum antibiotics may be used prophylactically. The nurse's role is vital in instructing the family in health promotion and in all the aspects of care needed by the child. Particular attention is paid to teaching the child and family the use of pancreatic enzymes, equipment, food selection, prevention of infection, and techniques of expectorating sputum. The nurse can provide emotional support for the family and counsel them on community resources. Life expectancy in cystic fibrosis has improved markedly over the past several decades, and with early diagnosis and treatment, most patients can be expected to reach adulthood. Also called **fibrocystic disease of the pancreas, mucoviscidosis.**

cystic goiter, an enlargement of the thyroid gland containing cysts resulting from mucoid or colloid degeneration, or liquifaction.

cystic hygroma. See **cystic lymphangioma.**

cystic kidney [Gk, *kystis,* bag; ME, *kidenei*], pertaining to any of several cystic disorders of the kidney, including congenital polycystic disease, solitary renal cysts, or cortical cysts associated with nephroslcerosis.

cystic lymphangioma, a cystic growth formed by lymph vessels, usually congenital and occurring most frequently in the neck, axilla, or groin of children. Also called **cystic hygroma, lymphangioma cysticum.**

cystic mastitis, a form of mammary dysplasia with inflammation and the formation of nodular cysts in the breast tissue. The cysts contain a turbid fluid. Symptoms may vary with individual breast changes that occur during the menstrual cycle.

cystic mole. See **hydatid mole.**

cystic myxoma, a tumor of the connective tissue that has undergone cystic degeneration.

cystic neuroma, a neoplasm of nerve tissue that has degenerated and become cystic. Also called **false neuroma.**

cystic tumor, a tumor with cavities or sacs containing a semisolid or a liquid material.

cystido-. See **cysto-.**

cystine /sis'tin/, a nonessential amino acid found in many proteins in the body, including keratin and insulin. Cystine is a product of the oxidation of two cysteine molecules.

cystinosis /sis'tinō'sis/ [*cystine* + Gk, *osis,* condition], a congenital disease characterized by glucosuria, proteinuria, cystine deposits in the liver, spleen, bone marrow, and cornea, rickets, excessive amounts of phosphates in the urine, and retardation of growth. Also called **cystine storage disease, Fanconi's syndrome.** See also **cystine.**

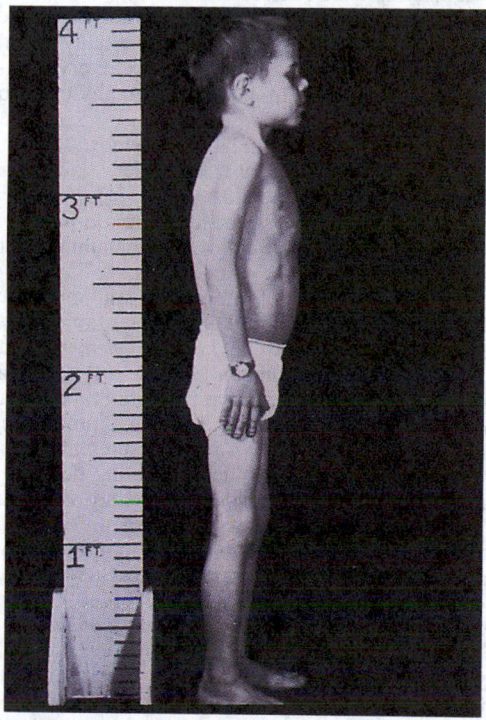

Cystic fibrosis—poor nutritional status (*Zitelli, 1992*)

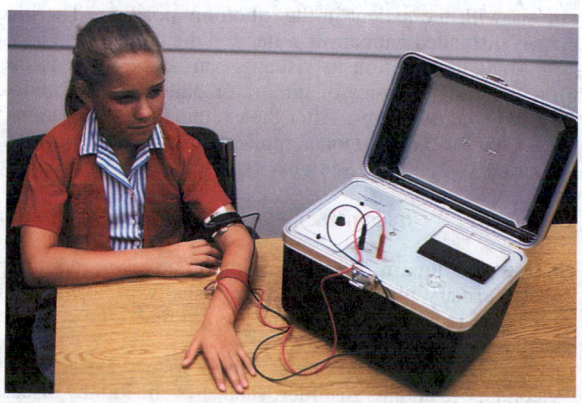

Sweat test for cystic fibrosis (*Wilson, 1990*)

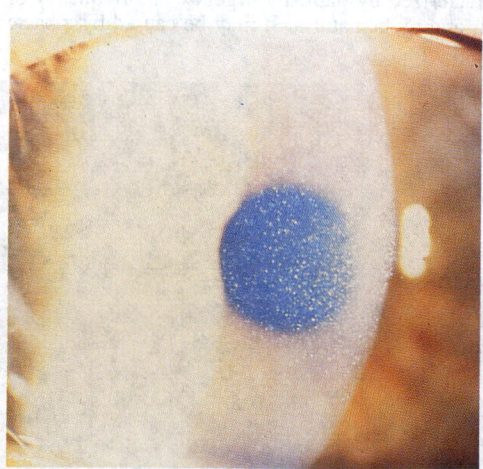

Cystinosis—deposits of cystine crystals on the cornea
(*Zitelli, 1992*)

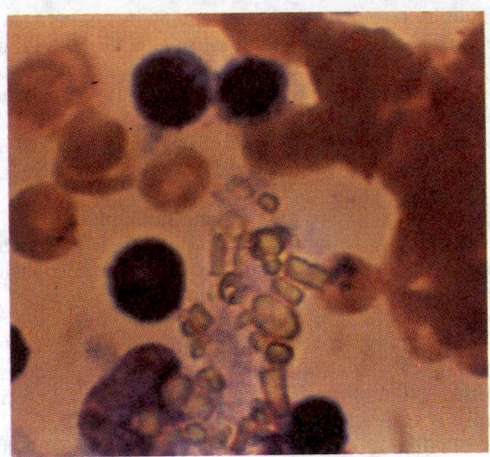

Cystinosis—deposits of cystine crystals in the bone marrow
(Zitelli, 1992)

cystinuria /sis′tinŏŏr′ē·ə/ [*cystine* + Gk, *ouron*, urine],
1. abnormal presence of the amino acid cystine in the urine.
2. an inherited defect of the renal tubules, characterized by excessive urinary excretion of cystine and several other amino acids. The disorder is caused by an autosomal recessive trait that impairs cystine reabsorption by the kidney tubules. In high concentration, cystine tends to precipitate in the urinary tract and form kidney or bladder stones. Treatment attempts to prevent the formation of stones or to dissolve them by increasing the volume of urine flow, decreasing the pH of the urine, and increasing the solubility of cystine. In addition to a large fluid intake, sodium bicarbonate, acetazolamide, and, in refractory cases, D-penicillamine are sometimes prescribed.

-cystis. See **-cyst.**

cystitis /sistī′tis/ [Gk, *kystis* + *itis,* inflammation], an inflammatory condition of the urinary bladder and ureters, characterized by pain, by urgency and frequency of urination, and by hematuria. It may be caused by a bacterial in-

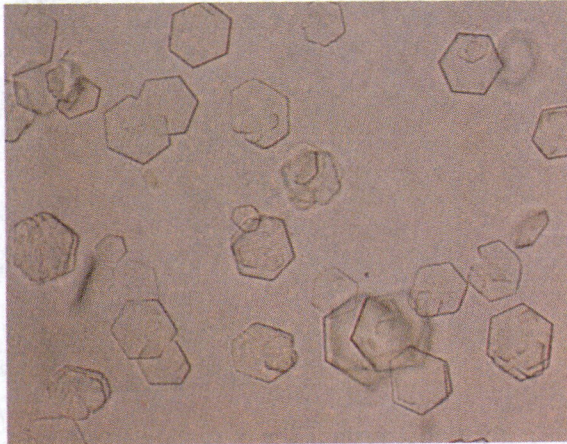

Cystinuria *(Weiss, 1988)*

fection, calculus, or tumor. Depending on the diagnosis, treatment may include antibiotics, increased fluid intake, bed rest, medications to control bladder wall spasms, and, when necessary, surgery.

-cystitis, a combining form meaning an 'inflammation of the bladder or cyst': *epicystitis, gonecystitis, pericystitis.*

cysto-, cyst-, cysti-, cystido-, a prefix meaning 'pertaining to the bladder, or to a cyst or sac': *cystocele, cystodynia, cystomyoma.*

cystocele /sis′təsēl′/ [Gk, *kystis* + *kele*, hernia], a herniation or protrusion of the urinary bladder through the wall of the vagina. Compare **rectocele.**

cystogram /sis′təgram′/ [Gk, *kystis* + *gramma*, record], a graphic record of the urinary bladder, usually a series of x-ray films, obtained as a part of any excretory urographic procedure, such as in retrograde pyelography or retrograde cystoscopy.

cystoid /sis′toid/ [Gk, *kystis*, bag + *eidos*, form], pertaining to or resembling a cyst or bladder.

cystolith. See **vesicle calculus.**

cystoma /sistō′mə/, *pl.* **cystomas, cystomata** [Gk, *kystis* + *oma*, tumor], any tumor or growth containing cysts, especially one in or near the ovary.

-cystoma, a combining form meaning a 'cystic tumor': *enterocystoma, hydrocystoma, inocystoma.*

cystometry /sistom′ətrē/ [Gk, *kystis* + *metron*, measure], the study of bladder function by use of a **cystometer** /sistom′ətər/, an instrument that measures capacity in relation to changing pressure. The urologic procedure, **cystometography** /sis′tōmətog′rəfē/, measures the amount of pressure exerted on the bladder at varying degrees of capacity. The results of the measurements are traced graphically on a **cystometogram** /sis′tōmet′əgram′/.

cystosarcoma phyllodes /sis′tōsärkō′məfilō′dēs/, a benign breast tumor that grows rapidly and tends to recur if not adequately excised.

cystoscope /sis′təskōp′/ [Gk, *kystis* + *skopein,* to look], an instrument for examining and treating lesions of the urinary bladder, ureter, and kidney. It consists of an outer sheath with a lighting system, a viewing obturator, and a passage for catheters and operative devices.

cystoscopic. See **cystoscopy.**

cystoscopic urography. See **retrograde cystoscopy.**

cystoscopy /sistos′kəpē/, the direct visualization of the urinary tract by means of a cystoscope inserted in the urethra. The procedure is usually performed under sedation or anesthesia with the patient in the lithotomy position. The bladder is distended with air or water and the patient is in a fasting state. In addition to visualization, cystoscopy is used for obtaining biopsies of tumors or other growths and for the removal of polyps. After the examination, the patient is observed for the common complications of trauma and signs of urinary infection. See also **cystoscope.** −**cystoscopic,** *adj.*

Cystospaz, a trademark for an anticholinergic (hyoscyamine).

cystourethrogram /sis′tə·yŏŏrē′thrəgram′/, a radiograph of the urinary bladder and urethra usually performed with use of an iodinated contrast medium to make the structures visible.

cysts of liver, small, single, simple watery cysts, usually secondary to another disorder, such as cystic kidney disease.

cyt-, cyto-, a prefix meaning 'cell or cytoplasm': *cytochrome, cytogenesis, cytosome.*

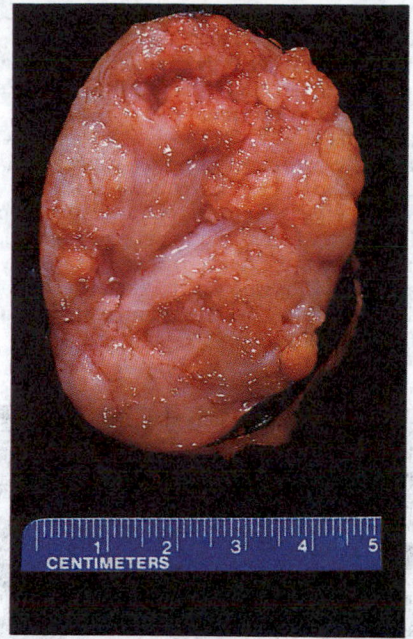

Cystosarcoma phylloides
(Skarin, 1991/Courtesy N Weidner, MD, Brigham and Women's Hospital, Boston, MA)

Cytadren, a trademark for an inhibitor of adrenocortico-steroid biosynthesis (aminoglutethimide).

cytarabine /siter′əbēn/, an antineoplastic agent. Also called **arabinosylcytosine, cytosine arabinoside.**

■ INDICATIONS: It is prescribed in the treatment of acute and chronic myelocytic leukemia, acute lymphocytic leukemia, and erythroleukemia.

■ CONTRAINDICATION: Known hypersensitivity to this drug prohibits its use.

■ ADVERSE EFFECTS: The most serious adverse reactions are bone marrow depression, stomatitis, phlebitis, liver toxicity, and fever. GI disturbances may occur.

-cyte, a suffix meaning a 'cell' of a specified type: *gliacyte, hemacyte, plasmacyte.*

-cythemia, -cythaemia, a combining form meaning a 'condition involving cells in the blood': *achroiocythemia, rhestocythemia, thrombocythemia.*

cyto-. See **cyt-.**

cytoarchitectonic /sī′tō·är′kitekton′ik/ /sī′tō-/ [Gk, *kytos,* cell; L, *architectura,* architecture], pertaining to the cellular arrangement within a tissue or structure.

cytoarchitecture /-är′kitek′chər/, the typical pattern of cellular arrangement within a particular tissue or organ, as in the cerebral cortex. **−cytoarchitectural,** *adj.*

cytobiotactic. See **cytoclesis.**

cytobiotaxis. See **cytoclesis.**

cytoblast /sī′təblast′/, *obsolete.* the nucleus of a cell.

cytocentrum. See **centrosome.**

cytocerastic. See **cytokerastic.**

cytochemism /sī′tōkem′izəm/ [Gk, *kytos* + *chemeia,* alchemy], the chemical activity within the living cell, specifically the various reactions to and affinity for chemical substances.

cytochemistry /-kem′istrē/, the study of the various chemicals within a living cell and their actions and functions.

cytochrome /si′tōkrōm/ [Gk, *kytos,* cell, *chroma,* color], **1.** a class of hemoproteins whose function is electron transport. These proteins have the ability to reverse the valence of heme-iron compounds, alternating between ferrous and ferric states. **2.** proteins involved in mitochondrial exudative electron transport systems associated with ATP production.

cytochrome P-450 [Gk, *kytos,* cell, *chroma,* color], a cytochrome protein involved with extramitochondrial electron transport in the liver and in drug detoxification.

cytocide [Gk, *kytos* + L, *caedere,* to kill], any substance that is destructive to cells. **−cytocidal,** *adj.*

cytoclesis /sī′tōklē′sis/ [Gk, *kytos* + *klesis,* calling for], the influence exerted by one cell on the action of other cells; the vital principle of all living tissue. Also called **cytobiotaxis.** **−cytocletic, cytobiotactic,** *adj.*

cytoctony /sītok′tənē/ [Gk, *kytos* + *ktonos,* killing], the destruction of cells, specifically the killing of cells in culture by viruses.

cytode /sī′tōd/ [Gk, *kytos* + *eidos,* form], the simplest type of cell, consisting of a protoplasmic mass without a nucleus, such as a bacterium.

cytodieresis /sī′tōdī·er′isis/, *pl.* **cytodiereses** [Gk, *kytos* + *diairesis,* separation], cell division, especially the phenomena involving the division of the cytoplasm. See also **meiosis, mitosis.** **−cytodieretic,** *adj.*

cytodifferentiation /-dif′ərən·shē·ā′shən/ [Gk, *kytos* + L, *differentia,* difference], **1.** a process by which embryonic cells acquire biochemical and morphologic properties essential for specialization and diversification. **2.** the total and gradual transformation from an undifferentiated to a fully differentiated state.

cytofluorograph /-flôr′əgraf/, a diagnostic instrument used to measure the level of CD4 T lymphocytes in HIV-positive patients. The lymphocytes are stained with specific monclonal antibodies. The normal value of the CD4 count is 800 per mm^3. Antiretroviral therapy may begin when the CD4 level drops below 500 per mm^3.

cytogene /sī′təjēn/ [Gk, *kytos* + *genein,* to produce], a particle within the cytoplasm of a cell that is self-replicating, derived from the genes in the nucleus, and capable of transmitting hereditary information.

cytogenesis /sī′tōjen′əsis/ [Gk, *kytos* + *genein,* to produce], the origin, development, and differentiation of cells. **−cytogenetic, cytogenic,** *adj.*

cytogeneticist /sī′tōjənet′isist/, one who specializes in cytogenetics.

cytogenetics /sī′tōjənet′iks/, the branch of genetics that studies the cellular constituents concerned with heredity, primarily the structure, function, and origin of the chromosomes. One kind of cytogenetics is **clinical cytogenetics.** Also called **cytogenics.** **−cytogenetic,** *adj.*

cytogenic /-jen′ik/, pertaining to the formation of cells.

cytogenic gland, a glandular organ that secretes living cells, specifically the testes and ovary.

cytogenic reproduction, the formation of a new organism from a unicellular germ cell, either sexually through the fusion of gametes to form a zygote or asexually by means of spores.

cytogenics. See **cytogenetics.**

cytogeny /sītoj′ənē/, **1.** cytogenetics. **2.** the origin and development of the cell. **−cytogenic, cytogenous,** *adj.*

cytogony /sītog′ənē/,   cytogenic reproduction.

cytohistogenesis /sī′tōhis′tōjen′əsis/ [Gk, *kytos* + *histos,* tissue, *genein,* to produce],   the structural development and formation of cells.   **−cytohistogenetic,** *adj.*

cytohyaloplasm.   See **hyaloplasm.**

cytoid /sī′toid/ [Gk, *kytos* + *eidos,* form],   like a cell.

cytoid body,   a small white spot on the retina of each eye that is seen by using an ophthalmoscope in examining the eyes of a patient affected with systemic lupus erythematosus.

cytokerastic /sī′tōkəras′tik/ [Gk, *kytos* + *kerastos,* mixed], pertaining to or characteristic of cellular development from a lower to a higher form or from a simple to more complex arrangement. Also **cytocerastic** /-səras′tik/.

cytokinesis /sī′tōkinē′sis, -kīnē′sis/ [Gk, *kytos* + *kinesis,* movement],   the division of the cytoplasm, exclusive of nuclear division, that occurs during the final stages of mitosis and meiosis to form daughter cells; the total of all the changes that occur in the cytoplasm during mitosis, meiosis, and fertilization.   **−cytokinetic,** *adj.*

cytologic.   See **cytology.**

cytological.   See **cytology.**

cytologic map [Gk, *kytos* + *logos,* science; L, *mappa,* table napkin],   the graphic representation of the location of genes on a chromosome, based on correlating genetic recombination test-crossing results with the structural analysis of chromosomes that have undergone such changes as deletions or translocations as detected by banding techniques.

cytologic sputum examination,   a microscopic examination of a specimen of bronchial secretions, including a search for cells that may be cancerous or otherwise abnormal.

cytologist /sītol′əjist/,   one who specializes in the study of cells, specifically one who uses cytologic techniques in the differential diagnosis of neoplasms.

cytology /sītol′əjē/ [Gk, *kytos* + *logos,* science],   the study of cells, including their formation, origin, structure, function, biochemical activities, and pathology. Kinds of cytology are **aspiration biopsy cytology** and **exfoliative cytology.   −cytologic, cytological,** *adj.*

cytolymph.   See **hyaloplasm.**

cytolyses.   See **cytolysis.**

cytolysin /sītol′isin/ [Gk, *kytos* + *lyein,* to loosen],   an antibody that dissolves antigenic cells. Kinds of cytolysin are **bacteriolysin** and **hemolysin.**

cytolysis /sītol′isis/, *pl.* **cytolyses** [Gk, *kytos* + *lyein,* to loosen],   the destruction or breakdown of the living cell, primarily by the disintegration of the outer membrane. A kind of cytolysis is **immune cytolysis. −cytolytic,** *adj.*

cytomegalic inclusion disease (CID) /sī′tōmegal′ik/ [Gk, *kytos* + *megas,* large; L, *in, claudere,* in enclosure],   a viral infection caused by the cytomegalovirus (CMV), a virus of the herpesviruses family, characterized by malaise, fever, lymphadenopathy, pneumonia, hepatosplenomegaly, and superinfection with various bacteria and fungi as a result of the depression of immune response characteristic of herpesviruses. It is primarily a congenitally acquired disease of newborn infants, transmitted in utero from the mother to the fetus. Results may range from spontaneous abortion or fatal neonatal illness to birth of a normal infant, depending on such factors as the virulence of the viral strain, fetal age when infected, and whether the mother's infection was pri-

mary or recurrent. About 10% of newborns with congenital CMV show clinical signs, such as microcephaly, retarded growth, hepatosplenomegaly, hemolytic anemia, and pathologic fracture of long bones. There is no specific treatment. See also **TORCH syndrome.**

cytomegalovirus (CMV) /sī′tōmeg′əlōvī′rəs/ [Gk, *kytos* + *megas,* large; L, *virus,* poison],   a member of a group of large species-specific herpes-type viruses with a wide variety of disease effects. It causes serious illness in persons with AIDS, in newborns, and in people being treated with immunosuppressive drugs and therapy, especially after an organ transplant. The virus usually results in a retinal or gastrointestinal infection. See also **cytomegalic inclusion disease, TORCH syndrome.**

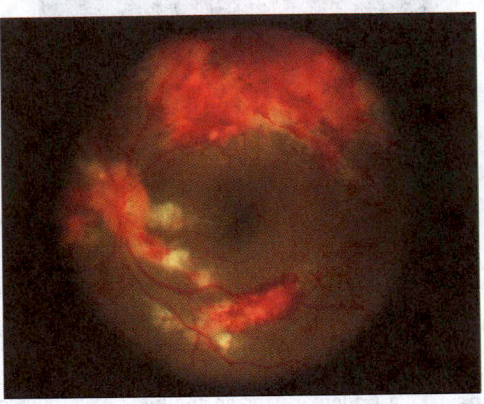

Cytomegalovirus retinitis
(Seidel, 1991/Courtesy Douglas A Jabs, MD, The Wilmer Ophthalmological Institute, The Johns Hopkins University and Hospital, Baltimore)

cytomegalovirus (CMV) disease.   See **cytomegalic inclusion disease.**

Cytomel,   a trademark for a thyroid hormone (liothyronine sodium).

cytometer /sītom′ətər/ [Gk, *kytos* + *metron,* measure],   a device for counting and measuring the number of cells within a given amount of fluid, as blood, urine, or cerebrospinal fluid.

cytometry /sītom′ətrē/,   the counting and measuring of cells, specifically blood cells.   **−cytometric,** *adj.*

cytomitome /sī′təmī′tōm/ [Gk, *kytos* + *mitos,* thread],   the fibrillary network within the cytoplasm of a cell, as contrasted with that in the nucleoplasm. See also **karyomitome.**

cytomorphology /-môrfol′əjē/ [Gk, *kytos* + *morphe,* shape, *logos,* science],   the study of the various forms of cells and the structures contained within them.   **−cytomorphologic, cytomorphological,** *adj.,* **cytomorphologist,** *n.*

cytomorphosis /sī′tōmôr′fəsis/, *pl.* **cytomorphoses** [Gk, *kytos* + *morphosis,* shaping],   the various changes that occur within a cell during the course of its life cycle, from the earliest undifferentiated stage until destruction.

cyton /sī′ton/ [Gk, *kytos,* cell],   the cell body of a neuron or that portion containing the nucleus and its surrounding cytoplasm from which the axon and dendrites are formed. Also called **cytone** /sī′tōn/.

cytopenia /-pē'nē·ə/, [Gk, *kytos* + *penes,* poor], a deficiency of cells in the blood.

cytopheresis /sī'tōfer'əsis/ [Gk, *kytos* + *aphairesis,* withdrawal], **1.** a therapeutic technique to remove red or white blood cells or platelets from patients with certain blood disorders. **2.** a laboratory procedure for separating specific components, such as white blood cells or platelets, from donor blood by centrifugation.

cytophotometer /sī'tōfətom'ətər/ [Gk, *kytos* + *phos,* light, *metron,* measure], an instrument for measuring light density through stained portions of cytoplasm, used for locating and identifying chemical substances within cells.

cytophotometry /sī'tōfətom'ətrē/, the identification of chemical substances within cells, using a cytophotometer. Also called **microfluorometry.** **−cytophotometric,** *adj.*

cytophysiology /-fis'ē·ol'əjē/ [Gk, *kytos* + *physis,* nature, *logos* science], the study of the biochemical processes involved in the functioning of an individual cell, as contrasted with the functioning of organs or tissues. **−cytophysiologic, cytophysiological,** *adj.,* **cytophysiologist,** *n.*

cytoplasm /sī'təplaz'əm/ [Gk, *kytos* + *plassein,* to mold], all of the substance of a cell other than the nucleus. See also **cell, nucleus.**

cytoplasmic bridge. See **intercellular bridge.**

cytoplasmic inheritance /sī'tōplaz'mik/, the acquisition of traits or conditions controlled by self-replicating substances within the cytoplasm, such as mitochondria or chloroplasts, rather than by the genes on the chromosomes in the nucleus. The phenomenon occurs in plants and lower animals but has not yet been demonstrated in humans.

Cytosar-U, a trademark for an antineoplastic (cytarabine).

cytoscopy /sītos'kəpē/ [Gk, *kytos* + *skopein,* to watch], the diagnostic study of cells obtained from patient specimens with the aid of microscopes and other laboratory equipment.

cytosine /sī'təsin/, a major pyrimidine base found in nucleotides and a fundamental constituent of DNA and RNA. In free or uncombined form it occurs in trace amounts in most cells, usually as products of the enzymatic hydrolysis of nucleic acids and nucleotides. Upon hydrolysis, it is converted to urea and ammonia. See also **thymine, uracil.**

cytosine arabinoside. See **cytarabine.**

cytoskeleton /-skel'ətən/ [Gk, *kytos* + *skeletos,* dried body], the cytoplasmic elements, including the tonofibrils, keratin, and other microfibrils, that function as a supportive system within a cell, especially an epithelial cell.

cytosome /sī'təsōm/, a multilayered membrane-bound lamellar body found in type II pneumocytes. It is a precursor of pulmonary surfactant.

cytotechnologist /-teknol'əjist/, an allied health professional who specializes in the study of the structure and function of cells. Cytotechnologists prepare cellular samples for study under the microscope and assist in the diagnosis of disease by the examination of the samples. Cell specimens may be obtained from various body sites, such as the female reproductive tract, the oral cavity, the lung, or any body cavity shedding cells. Using the findings of the cytotechnologist, the physician is able to detect cancer and other diseases at a very early stage.

cytotoxic /tok'sik/ [Gk, *kytos* + *toxikon,* poison], pertaining to a pharmacologic compound or other agent that destroys or damages tissue cells.

cytotoxic anaphylaxis, an exaggerated reaction of hyper-

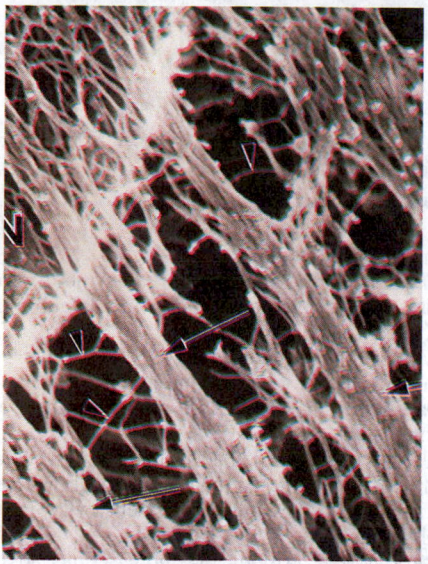

Cytoskeleton (Thibodeau, 1993/Klaus Weber, Mary Osborn)

sensitivity to an injection of antibodies specific for antigenic substances that occur normally on surfaces of body cells.

cytotoxic drug, any pharmacologic compound that inhibits the proliferation of cells within the body. Such compounds as the alkylating agents and the antimetabolites are designed to destroy abnormal cells selectively, while sparing as many normal cells as possible; they are commonly used in chemotherapy. Cytotoxic agents have a potential for producing teratogenesis, mutagenesis, and carcinogenesis.

cytotoxic hypersensitivity [Gk, *kytos* + *toxikon,* poison; *hyper,* above; L, *sentire,* to feel], an IgG or an IgM complement-dependent, immediate-acting hypersensitive humoral response to foreign cells or to alterations of surface antigens on the cells. Direct and immediate destruction of cells occurs, as seen in hemolytic disease of the newborn and in severe transfusion reactions. Also called **type II hypersensitivity.** Compare **anaphylactic hypersensitivity, immune complex hypersensitivity.** See also **immune gamma globulin.**

cytotoxic T cells. See **CD8.**

cytotoxin /sī'tōtok'sin/ [Gk, *kytos* + *toxikon,* poison], a substance that has a toxic effect on certain cells. An antibody may act as a cytotoxin. **−cytotoxic,** *adj.*

cytotrophoblast /sī'tōtrof'əblast'/ [Gk, *kytos* + *trophe,* nutrition, *blastos,* germ], the inner layer of cells of the trophoblast of the early mammalian embryo that gives rise to the outer surface and villi of the chorion. Also called **Langhans' layer.** Compare **syncytiotrophoblast.** **−cytotrophoblastic,** *adj.*

Cytovene, trademark for a brand of ganciclovir, an antiviral drug active against the retinitis of cytomegalovirus.

Cytoxan, a trademark for an antineoplastic (cyclophosphamide).

CY-VA-DIC, an anticancer drug combination of cyclophosphamide, vincristine, doxorubicin, and dacarbazine.

d, symbol for one tenth.

D, 1. symbol for *dead space gas*. **2.** symbol for **diffusing capacity. 3.** abbreviation for *diopter*. **4.** abbreviation for *dexter*, meaning 'right.'

da, symbol for the multiple 10.

DA, abbreviation for **developmental age.**

dacarbazine /dekär′bəzēn/, an alkylating agent used as an antineoplastic.

■ INDICATIONS: It is prescribed primarily in the treatment of malignant melanoma, sarcoma, and Hodgkin's disease

■ CONTRAINDICATION: Known hypersensitivity to this drug prohibits its use.

■ ADVERSE EFFECTS: Among the more serious adverse reactions are bone marrow depression, GI symptoms, kidney and liver impairment, alopecia, and fever.

D/A converter. See **digital-to-analog converter.**

Dacron cuff, a sheath of Dacron surrounding an atrial or venous catheter to prevent ascending infections and accidental displacement of the catheter.

dacryadenitis. See **dacryoadenitis.**

dacryo-, dacry-, a combining form meaning 'pertaining to tears': *dacryocele, dacryolin, dacryorrhea.*

dacryoadenitis /dak′rē·ō·ad′ənī′tis/, an inflammation of the lacrimal gland. The condition may be seen in mumps infection that involves a lacrimal gland. Also called **dacry-adenitis** /-ad′ənī′tis/.

dacryocyst /dak′re·ōsist′/ [Gk, *dakryon*, tear, *kytis*, bag], a lacrimal sac at the medial angle of the eye, a normal anatomic feature.

dacryocystectomy /dak′rē·ōsistek′təmē/ [Gk, *dakryon* + *kytis*, bag, *ektome*, excision], partial or total excision of the lacrimal sac.

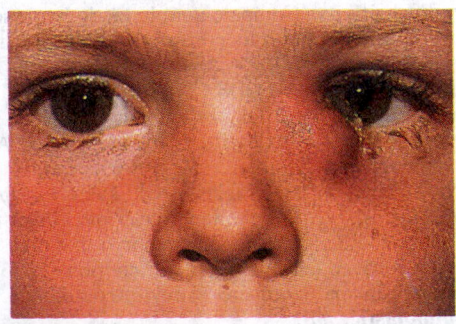

Dacryocystitis *(Zitelli, 1992)*

dacryocystitis /dak′rē·ōsistī′tis/, an infection of the lacrimal sac caused by obstruction of the nasolacrimal duct, characterized by tearing and discharge from the eye. In the acute phase, the sac becomes inflamed and painful. The disorder is nearly always unilateral and usually occurs in infants. Systemic administration of antibiotics is usual; local, topical treatment is seldom effective; and, rarely, a dacryocystorhinostomy may be required. Compare **dacryostenosis.**

dacryocystorhinostomy /dak′rē·ōsis′tôrīnos′təmē/ [Gk *dakryon* + *kytis*, bag, *rhis*, nose, *stoma*, mouth], a surgical procedure for restoring drainage into the nose from the lacrimal sac when the nasolacrimal duct is obstructed.

dacryon. See **tears.**

dacryostenosis /dak′rē·ōstinō′sis/ [Gk, *dakryon* + *stenos*, narrow, *osis*, condition], an abnormal stricture of the nasolacrimal duct, occurring either as a congenital condition or as a result of infection or trauma. Dacryocystorhinostomy may be required to correct this condition. Compare **dacryocystitis.**

dactinomycin /dak′tinōmī′sin/, an antibiotic used as an antineoplastic agent.

■ INDICATIONS: It is prescribed in the treatment of a variety of malignant neoplastic diseases, including Wilms' tumor and rhabdomyosarcoma in children.

■ CONTRAINDICATIONS: Herpes zoster infection or known hypersensitivity to this drug prohibits its use.

■ ADVERSE EFFECTS: Among the more serious adverse reactions are bone marrow depression, severe GI disturbances, proctitis, alopecia, and ulcers of the mouth.

dactyl /dak′til/ [Gk, *dactylos*, finger], a digit (finger or toe). –**dactylic** /daktil′ik/, *adj.*

dactyl-. See **dactylo-.**

-dactyl, a suffix meaning 'digit (finger or toe)': *hermodactyl, pachydactyl, pentadactyl.*

-dactylia, -dactyly, a suffix meaning '(condition of the) fingers or toes': *ankylodactylia, heptadactylia, oligodactylia.*

-dactylic See **dactyl.**

dactylitis /dak′tīlī′tis/, a painful inflammation of the fingers or toes, usually associated with sickle cell anemia or certain infectious diseases, particularly syphilis or tuberculosis.

dactylo-, dactyl-, a combining form meaning 'pertaining to a finger or toe': *dactylophasia, dactylospasm, dactylosymphysis.*

-dactyly. See **-dactylia.**

daily adjusted progressive resistance exercise (DAPRE), a program of isotonic exercises that allows for individual differences in the rate at which a patient regains strength in an injured or diseased body part.

daisy-wheel printer, a character printer for computers in which the character dies are on a number of narrow, flexible "fingers" projecting from a central hub, resembling a daisy. The wheel spins in front of the position for printing, and as the desired character appears, it is struck by a hammer and the pattern is impressed on the paper through an inked ribbon. Compare **dot-matrix printer, laser printer.**

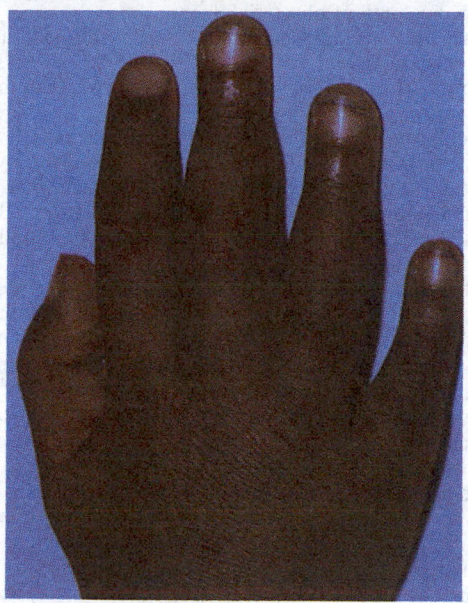

Dactylitis (Zitelli, 1992)

Dakin's solution [Henry D. Dakin, American biochemist, b. 1880; L *solutus* dissolved], an antiseptic solution containing boric acid and 0.4% to 0.5% of sodium hypochlorite.

Dalmane, a trademark for a benzodiazepine sedative-hypnotic (flurazepam hydrochloride).

dalton [John Dalton, English chemist, b. 1766], an obsolete unit of atomic mass, based on 1/16 of the mass of the oxygen atom. See **atomic weight**.

daltonism /dôl′təniz′əm/ [John Dalton, English chemist, b. 1766], *informal*. a form of red-green color blindness. It is genetically transmitted as a sex-linked autosomal recessive trait.

Dalton's law of partial pressures /dôl′tənz/ [John Dalton], (in physics) a law stating that the total pressure exerted by a mixture of gases is equal to the sum of the pressures that could be exerted by the gases if they were present alone in the container. See also **Avogadro's law, Boyle's law, Gay-Lussac's law.**

damages /dam′ijəs/ [L, *damnum*, loss], (in law) a sum of money awarded to a plaintiff by a court as compensation for any loss, detriment, or injury to the plaintiff's person, property, or rights caused by the malfeasance or negligence of the defendant. **Actual damages** are awarded to reimburse the plaintiff for the loss or injury sustained. **Nominal damages** are awarded to show that a legal wrong has been committed although no recoverable loss can be determined. **Punitive damages** exceed the actual cost of injury or damage and are awarded when the defendant has acted maliciously or in reckless disregard of the plaintiff's rights.

damp [AS, vapor], a potentially lethal atmosphere in caves and mines. **Black damp** or **choke damp** is caused by absorption of the available oxygen by coal seams. **Fire damp** is composed of methane and other explosive hydrocarbon gases. **White damp** is another name for carbon monoxide.

damping [AS, vapor], (in cardiology) a diminishing of the amplitude of a series of waves or oscillations, as in damping of the arterial pressure wave form.

danazol /dan′əzol/, a synthetic androgen that acts to suppress the output of gonadotropins from the pituitary.
■ INDICATION: It is prescribed in the treatment of endometriosis.
■ CONTRAINDICATIONS: Genital bleeding, cardiac, liver, or kidney dysfunction, or known hypersensitivity to this drug prohibits its use. It is not used during pregnancy or lactation.
■ ADVERSE EFFECTS: Among the most serious adverse reactions are muscle spasms, nausea, weight gain, acne, edema, oily skin, voice changes, and other androgenic effects.

dance reflex [ME, *dauncen;* L, *reflectere,* to look backward], a normal response in the neonate to simulate walking by a reciprocal flexion and extension of the legs when held in an erect position with the soles touching a hard surface. The reflex disappears by about 3 to 4 weeks of age and is replaced by controlled, deliberate movement. Also called **step reflex, stepping reflex.**

dance therapy, (in psychology) the use of rhythmic body movements or dance to release expression of feelings.

dander, dry scales shed from the scalp.

dandruff /dan′druf/, an excessive amount of scaly material composed of dead, keratinized epithelium shed from the scalp that may be a mild form of seborrheic dermatitis. Treatment with a keratolytic shampoo is usually recommended to soften and remove the scales.

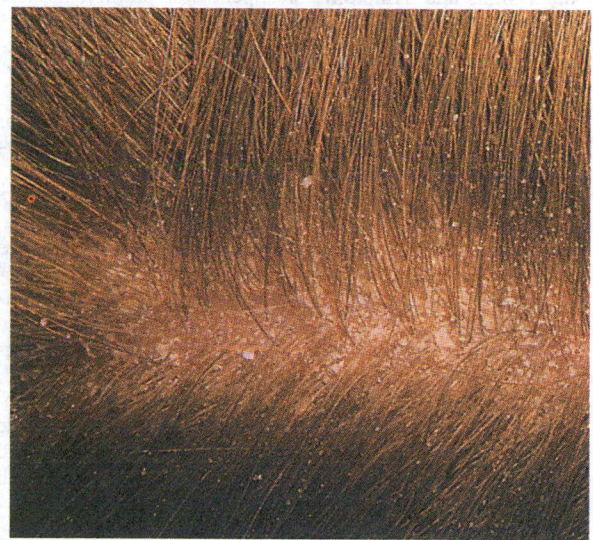

Dandruff (Baran, 1991)

dandy fever. See **dengue fever.**

Dandy-Walker cyst [Walter E. Dandy, American neurosurgeon, b. 1886; Arthur E. Walker, American surgeon, b. 1907], a cystic malformation of the fourth ventricle of the brain, resulting from hydrocephalus. Diagnosis of the defect is made with CT scan, with x-ray films, and less commonly with a ventriculogram. See also **hydrocephalus, shunt.** (See Fig. p. 436.)

Danocrine, a trademark for an anterior pituitary suppressant (danazol).

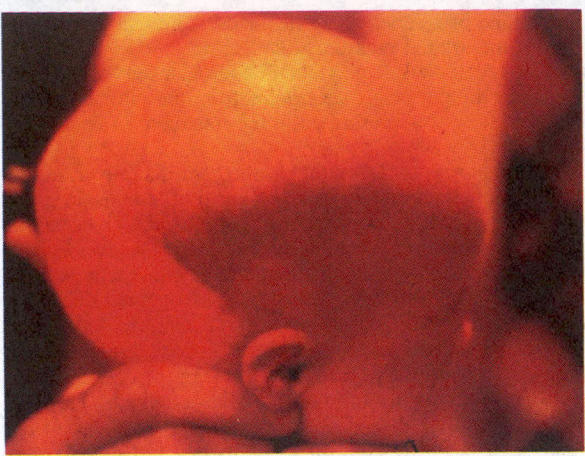

Dandy-Walker cyst
(Zitelli, 1992/Courtesy Dr. Michael J Painter)

danthron /dan′thron/, a stimulant laxative.

■ INDICATIONS: It is prescribed in the treatment of constipation or for bowel evacuation before radiologic or surgical procedures.

■ CONTRAINDICATIONS: Abdominal pain, nausea, vomiting, or other signs and symptoms of appendicitis prohibit its use. It is not recommended for nursing mothers.

■ ADVERSE EFFECTS: Among the most serious adverse reactions are dizziness, palpitations, stomach cramps, and excessive bowel activity.

Dantrium, a trademark for a skeletal muscle relaxant (dantrolene sodium), used in the treatment of malignant hyperthermia or hyperpyrexia.

dantrolene sodium /dan′trəlēn/, a skeletal muscle relaxant.

■ INDICATIONS: It is prescribed in the treatment of muscle spasticity resulting from injury to the spinal cord or cerebrum. It is not indicated in treatment of spasm from rheumatic disorders.

■ CONTRAINDICATIONS: Liver dysfunction or known hypersensitivity to this drug prohibits its use.

■ ADVERSE EFFECTS: The most serious adverse reaction is potentially fatal hepatotoxicity. Common reactions include confusion, drowsiness, diarrhea, dizziness, fatigue, and muscular weakness. Side effects may continue for several days.

DAP, abbreviation for **Draw-A-Person Test.**

DAPRE, abbreviation for **daily adjusted progressive resistance exercise.**

dapsone (DADPS) /dap′sōn/, a bacteriostatic sulfone derivative.

■ INDICATIONS: It is prescribed in the treatment of lepromatous leprosy and dermatitis herpetiformis.

■ CONTRAINDICATIONS: Pregnancy or known hypersensitivity to this drug prohibits its use.

■ ADVERSE EFFECTS: Among the more serious adverse reactions are hemolysis (particularly in people who have glucose-6-phosphate dehydrogenase deficiency), lepra reactions, methemoglobinemia, neuropathy, nausea, anorexia, and skin rash.

-dapsone, a suffix designating a diaminodiphenylsulfone-

derivative antimycobacterial agent.

Daraprim, a trademark for an antimalarial (pyrimethamine).

Darbid, a trademark for an anticholinergic (isopropamide iodide).

Darier's disease. See **keratosis follicularis.**

dark adaptation, a normal increase in sensitivity of the retinal rod cells of the eye to detect any light that may be available for vision in a dimly lighted environment. The process is accompanied by an adjustment of the pupils to allow more light to enter the eyes.

darkfield microscopy [AS, *deorc,* hidden, *feld,* field; Gk, *mikros,* small, *skopein,* to look], examination with a darkfield microscope, in which the specimen is illuminated by a peripheral light source. Organisms in specimens that have been prepared for use with a darkfield microscope appear to glow against a dark background. The technique is used primarily to identify the syphilis spirochete. Also called **darkfield illumination, ultramicroscopy.**

dark-film fault [AS, *deorc,* hidden, *filmen,* skin; L, *fallere,* to disappoint], a defect in a photograph or radiograph, which appears as an excessively darkened image and image area. It is caused by overexposure of the film to light or radiation, film fog from excessive development, accidental exposure to light, or an unsafe darkroom light.

darkroom, a room in a hospital or similar facility for the storage and processing of light-sensitive materials, such as x-ray film.

Darvocet-N, a trademark for a fixed-combination drug containing an analgesic-antipyretic (acetaminophen) and an analgesic (propoxyphene napsylate).

Darvon, a trademark for an analgesic (propoxyphene hydrochloride).

Darvon Compound, a trademark for a fixed-combination drug containing an analgesic (propoxyphene hydrochloride) and APC (aspirin, phenacetin, and caffeine).

Darvon-N, a trademark for an analgesic (propoxyphene napsylate).

darwinian. See **darwinian theory.**

darwinian reflex. See **grasp reflex.**

darwinian theory /därwin′ē·ən/ [Charles R. Darwin, English naturalist, b. 1809], the theory postulated by Charles Darwin that organic evolution results from the process of natural selection of those variants of plants and animals best suited to survive in their environmental surroundings. Also called **darwinism.** Compare **lamarckism. –darwinian,** *adj., n.*

DAS, abbreviation for **data acquisition system.**

DASE, abbreviation for **Denver Articulation Screening Examination.**

data /dā′tə, dat′ə, dä′tə/, *sing.* **datum** [L, *datum,* giving], **1.** pieces of information, especially those that are part of a collection of information to be used in an analysis of a problem, such as the diagnosis of a health problem. **2.** information stored and processed by a computer.

data acquisition system (DAS), a radiation detection system that measures the amount of radiation passing through a patient.

data analysis, (in research) the phase of a study that includes classifying, coding, and tabulating information needed to perform quantitative or qualitative analyses according to the research design and appropriate to the data. Data analysis follows data collection and precedes interpretation or application of the data.

data base, a large store or bank of information, especially in a form that can be processed by computer.

data clustering, the grouping of related information from the patient's health history, physical examination, and laboratory results as part of the process of making a diagnosis.

data collection, (in research) the phase of a study that includes the gathering of information and identification of sampling units as directed by the research design. Data collection precedes data analysis.

data processing, the techniques and practices involved in the manipulation of information by a computer.

data retrieval, the recovery of information from an organized filing system, such as a computer data base, index card file, or color-coded record folders.

dataset /dā′təset/, **1.** a modem. **2.** a collection of similar and related data for processing by computer.

data source, the origin of information relevant to a patient's level of wellness and health patterns.

data validation, the process of determining if information gathered during the process of data collection is complete and accurate.

date/acquaintance rape, a sexual assault or rape by a person known to the victim, such as a date, employer, friend, or casual acquaintance. See also **rape.**

datum. See **data.**

daughter cell [ME, *doughter*; L, *cella*, storeroom], one of the cells produced by the division of a parent cell.

daughter chromosome [AS, *tohter*, female, child; Gk, *chroma*, color, *soma*, body], either of the paired chromatids that during the anaphase stage of mitosis separate and migrate to opposite ends of the cell before division. Each contains the complete genetic information of the original chromosome and was formed during interphase by the duplication of the DNA molecule.

daughter element, an element that results from the radioactive decay of a parent element. An example is technetium 99, which is the daughter element created by the decay of an atom of molybdenum 99.

daughter product. See **decay product.**

daunorubicin hydrochloride /dô′nōrōō′bisin/, an anthracycline antibiotic antineoplastic agent.

■ INDICATIONS: It is prescribed in the treatment of cancer, particularly the leukemias and neuroblastoma.

■ CONTRAINDICATIONS: Preexisting drug-induced bone marrow depression or known hypersensitivity to this drug prohibits its use. It is not given to patients who have previously received a complete course of treatment with daunorubicin or doxorubicin.

■ ADVERSE EFFECTS: Among the most serious adverse reactions are bone marrow depression and cardiotoxicity. GI disturbances, stomatitis, and alopecia are common.

Davidoff's cells [M. Davidoff, German histologist, d. 1904], See **cells of Paneth.**

Davidson regimen [Edward C. Davidson, American physician, b. 1894; L, direction], a method of treating chronic constipation in children, of developing regular bowel habits, and of identifying those with functional bowel disease or obstructive disorders. If necessary, the fecal impactions are removed by a series of enemas. The child is then given mineral oil in increasing doses, until four or five loose bowel movements occur daily. The condition usually subsides within 2 to 3 weeks unless Hirschsprung's disease or another obstructive disorder is present. Some children, especially those under 2 years of age, require supplemental, fat-

soluble vitamins to maintain proper nutrition. The regimen may be continued in children older than 3 years as a training procedure for developing regular bowel habits. The child is placed on a potty-chair at a specific time each day for 5 to 15 minutes, and, as regular habits develop, the mineral oil is gradually withdrawn over a period of several weeks. See also **toilet training.**

dawn phenomenon [ME, *daunen*; Gk, *phainomenon*, anything seen], a tendency for patients with insulin-dependent diabetes mellitus to require an increased insulin dose in the early morning hours because of an increase in plasma glucose concentration. Compare **Somogyi phenomenon.**

day blindness. See **hemeralopia.**

day care [OE, *doeg*; L, *garrire*, to chatter], a specialized program or facility that provides care for preschool children, usually within a group framework, either as a substitute for or extension of home care, particularly for single parents or for parents who are both employed outside the home. Day care groups vary in size and function and range from casual neighborhood parent-supervised play groups to formal nursery schools or organized centers run by trained personnel. Most day care programs incorporate a daily schedule of quiet play, outdoor activities, group games and projects, creative or educational play, and snack and rest periods.

daydream, a usually nonpathologic reverie that occurs while a person is awake. The content is usually the fulfillment of wishes that are not disguised, and fulfillment is imagined as direct.

day health care services, the provision of hospitals, nursing homes, or other facilities for health-related services to adult patients who are ambulatory or can be transported and who regularly use such services for a certain number of daytime hours but do not require continuous inpatient care.

day hospital [OE, *doeg*; L, *hospes*, guest], a psychiatric facility that offers a therapeutic program during daytime hours for patients.

day patient. See **inpatient.**

day sight. See **nyctalopia.**

dB, abbreviation for **decibel.**

DBMS, abbreviation for *data base management system.*

DC, abbreviation for **direct current.**

d/c abbreviation for *discontinue.*

D & C, abbreviation for **dilatation and curettage.**

D&E, abbreviation for **dilation and evacuation.**

DD, abbreviation for **developmental disability.**

DDAVP, a trademark for an antidiuretic (desmopressin acetate).

ddC, symbol for 2′3-dideoxycytidine, an antiretroviral drug used in the treatment of AIDS. It is related chemically to DDI.

DDI, **1.** abbreviation for 2′,3′-dideoxyinosine, an antiretroviral medication. Also called **didanosine. 2.** abbreviation for **dideoxyinose.**

D.D.S., abbreviation for *Doctor of Dental Surgery.*

DDST, abbreviation for **Denver Developmental Screening Test.**

DDT (dichlorodiphenyltrichloroethane), a nondegradable water-insoluble chlorinated hydrocarbon once used worldwide as a major insecticide, especially in agriculture. In recent years, knowledge of its adverse impact on the environment has led to restrictions in its use. In addition, because tolerance in formerly susceptible organisms develops rapidly, DDT has been largely replaced by organophosphate insecticides in the United States, where DDT was banned by the FDA in 1971. It is still used as a pediculocide where epidemic-scale delousing is justified, as in barracks and refugee camps. Its value as a scabicide is marginal, since scabies and crab lice quickly become resistant to it. See also **scabicide.**

DDT poisoning. See **chlorinated organic insecticide poisoning.**

DE, abbreviation for **dose equivalent.**

de-, a prefix meaning 'to do the opposite, away, off of, to remove entirely, down or from': *deaquation, decartation, dedentition.*

DEA, 1. abbreviation for *Drug Enforcement Administration.* 2. abbreviation for **Drug Enforcement Agency.**

deactivation /dē·ak′tivā′shən/ [L, *de,* from, *activus,* active], the process of becoming or making something inactive or inoperable.

dead-end host [AS, *dead, ende;* L, *hospes,* guest], any animal from which a parasite cannot escape to continue its life cycle. Humans are dead-end hosts for trichinosis, because the larvae encyst in muscle and human flesh is unlikely to be a source of food for other animals susceptible to this parasite. Compare **definitive host, intermediate host, reservoir host.**

dead fetus syndrome, a condition in which the fetus has died but has remained in the uterus for more than 6 weeks. The condition leads to a blood coagulation disorder, DIC, and the eventual delivery is usually accompanied by massive bleeding. See also **disseminated intravascular coagulation.**

dead pulp. See **nonvital pulp**.

dead space [AS; L, *spatium*], 1. a cavity that remainsafter the incomplete closure of a surgical or traumatic wound, leaving an area in which blood can collect and delay healing. 2. the amount of lung in contact with ventilating gases but not in contact with pulmonary blood flow. **Alveolar dead space** refers to alveoli that are ventilated by the pulmonary circulation but are not perfused. The condition may exist when pulmonary circulation is obstructed, as by a thromboembolus. **Anatomic dead space** is an area in the trachea, bronchi, and air passages containing air that does not reach the alveoli during respiration. As a general rule, the volume of air in the anatomic dead space in milliliters is approximately equal to the weight in pounds of the involved individual. Certain lung disorders, such as emphysema, increase the amount of anatomic dead space. **Physiologic dead space** is an area in the respiratory system that includes the anatomic dead space together with the space in the alveoli occupied by air that does not contribute to the oxygen-carbon dioxide exchange.

dead space effect, any of several potential adverse effects of dead space resulting from mechanical ventilation, particularly when there is alveolar dead space. In hospitalized patients it can be responsible for producing hypoxemia and hypercarbia. A pulmonary embolism can also produce a dead space effect; blood flow in the pulmonary arteries is reduced without impeding ventilation.

deaf [AS], 1. unable to hear; hard of hearing. 2. people who are unable to hear or who suffer hearing impairment. **–deafness,** *n.*

deafferentation /dē·af′ərəntā′shən/ [L, *de,* from, *ad, ferre,* to bear], an interruption in an afferent nerve system.

deaf-mute, an obsolete term for a person who is unable to hear or to speak.

deaf-mutism [AS, *déaf;* L, *mutus*], an obsolete term for a state of being both unable to hear and unable to speak.

deafness, a condition characterized by a partial or complete loss of hearing. In assessing deafness, the patient's ears are examined for drainage, crusts, accumulation of cerumen, or structural abnormality. It is determined if the deafness is conductive or sensory, temporary or permanent, and congenital or acquired in childhood, adolescence, or adulthood. The effect of aging, when applicable, is evaluated, and a psychosocial assessment is conducted to ascertain if the individual is well adjusted to deafness or reacts to the handicap with fear, anxiety, frustration, depression, anger, or hostility. In all cases the degree of loss and the kind of impairment causing the loss are determined. See also **conductive hearing loss, sensorineural hearing loss.**

■ OBSERVATIONS: Many conditions and diseases may result in deafness. More than 6 million people in the United States have some degree of bilateral hearing loss, and more than 50% of those people are over 65 years old. The person with a slight hearing loss may be initially unaware of the problem. Recognition, diagnosis, and early treatment may help prevent further impairment and prevent frustration, embarrassment, and danger for the person. An older person with a hearing impairment usually has a sensorineural loss. High sounds are hard to hear, and discernment of such letter sounds as /s/ and /f/ becomes difficult. Speaking clearly and slowly, allowing the person to speech-read, is helpful, as are visual cues clear with enunciation; shouting is not. A severe or sudden hearing loss usually drives the person to seek help. If the loss is sudden, confusion, fear, and even panic are common. The person's speech becomes loud and slurred. There is new danger because the person cannot hear horns, whistles, or sirens and has not developed a way to cope with the impairment safely. The congenitally deaf person needs special speech and language training before reaching school age.

■ INTERVENTIONS: The treatment of deafness depends on the cause. Merely removing impacted cerumen from the external auditory canal may significantly improve hearing. Hearing aids, amplification of sound, or speech reading may be useful. Speech therapy is useful in teaching a person to speak or helping a person to retain the ability to speak.

■ NURSING CONSIDERATIONS: Caring for a deaf person who is hospitalized for treatment of another problem requires certain adjustments in communication between nurse and patient. To communicate with the deaf patient who speech-reads, staff members speak slowly, enunciate distinctly, use simple phrases, and rephrase any statements that are not understood; the speaker avoids shouting, chewing gum, or covering or obscuring the mouth in other ways while speaking. If the patient uses a hearing aid, its placement and operation are checked before the speaker begins to talk; the voice is modulated to a level that is comfortable for the patient, and the speaker stands or sits where the lips are visible to the deaf individual. If the patient uses sign language, an interpreter or another means of communication is sought; when a pad and pencil are used, a frequent practice with the newly deaf, the messages are written clearly in short, simple phrases, and adequate time is allowed for the patient to understand and answer. Because hospitalization increases the stress imposed by deafness and because persons with impaired hearing are acutely aware of movement and changes in light, the patient is maintained in a calm, nonstressful, and safe environment. The bed is located so that the patient can see the door.

deaminase /dē·am′ĭnās/ [L, *de*, away, *amine*, ammonia; Fr, *diastase*, enzyme], an enzyme that catalyses the hydrolysis of the NH_2 bond in amino compounds. The enzymes are usually named according to the substrate, such as **adenosine deaminase, guanine deaminase,** or **guanosine deaminase.**

deamination /dē′amĭnā′shən/, the removal, usually by hydrolysis, of the NH_2 radical from an amino compound. Also called **deaminization.**

dean [L *decanus* chief of ten], chief executive and educational officer of a unit of a university, school, or college.

Deaner, a trademark for a psychostimulant (deanol).

deanol /dē′ənol/, a psychostimulant.
- INDICATIONS: It is prescribed in the treatment of learning problems and hyperkinetic-behavior problems.
- CONTRAINDICATIONS: There are no known absolute contraindications, but it should be used with caution in patients with grand mal epilepsy.
- ADVERSE EFFECTS: Among the most serious adverse reactions are insomnia, mild overstimulation, and pruritus.

death [AS], **1. apparent death,** the cessation of life as indicated by the absence of heartbeat or respiration. **2. legal death,** the total absence of activity in the brain and central nervous system, the cardiovascular system, and the respiratory system as observed and declared by a physician. See also **cell death, emotional care of the dying patient, stages of dying, sudden infant death syndrome.**

death chill. See **algor mortis.**

death instinct, instinctive behavior that tends to be self-destructive.

death mask [AS, *déath*, Fr, *masque*], a mask made from a plaster of paris cast of the face of a dead person.

death rate, the number of deaths occuring within a specified population during a particular time period, usually expressed in terms of deaths per 1000 persons per year.

death rattle, a sound produced by air moving through mucus that has accumulated in the throat of a dying person after loss of the cough reflex, often accompanied by agonal respiration.

death trance, a state in which a person appears to be dead.

"death with dignity" [AS, *déath*; L, *dignus*, worthy], the philosophical concept that a terminally ill client should be allowed to die naturally, rather than experience a comatose, vegetative life prolonged needlessly by mechanical support systems.

debilitating /dibil′itā′ting/, pertaining to a disease or injury that enfeebles, weakens, or otherwise disables a person.

debility /dibil′itē/, feebleness, weakness, or loss of strength. See also **asthenia.**

debride /dibrēd′/ [Fr, *debridle*, remove], to remove dirt, foreign objects, damaged tissue, and cellular debris from a wound or a burn to prevent infection and to promote healing. In treating a wound, debridement is the first step in cleansing it; debridement also allows thorough examination of the extent of the injury. In treating a burn, debridement of the eschar may be performed in a hydrotherapy bath. **–debridement** /debrēdmäN′/, *n.*

debris /dəbrē′/, the dead, diseased, or damaged tissue and any foreign material that is to be removed from a wound or other area being treated.

Debrox, a trademark for a topical antiinfective (carbamide peroxide).

debug /dibug′, dē′bug/ [L, *de*, Welsh; *bwg*, hobgoblin to find and correct errors in a computer program or hardware.

dec-, 1. a prefix meaning 'ten': *decagram, decaliter, decipara.* **2.** a combining form meaning 'tenth': *decigram, deciliter, decinormal.*

Decadron, a trademark for a glucocorticoid (dexamethasone).

Deca-Durabolin, a trademark for an androgen (nandrolone decanoate), used as an anabolic agent.

decalcification /dēkal′sifikā′shən/ [L, *de* + *calyx*, lime, *facere*, to make], loss of calcium salts from the teeth and bones caused by malnutrition, malabsorption, or other dietary or physiologic factors. It may result, particularly in older people, from a diet that lacks adequate calcium. Malabsorption may be caused by a lack of vitamin D necessary for the absorption of calcium from the intestine, by an excess of dietary fats that can combine with calcium to form an indigestible soaplike compound, by the presence of oxalic acid that can combine with calcium to form a relatively insoluble calcium oxalate salt, or by a relative lack of acid in the digestive tract that can decrease the solubility of calcium. Other factors include the parathyroid hormone control of the calcium level in the bloodstream, the ratio of calcium to phosphorus in the blood, and the relative activity of osteoblast cells that form calcium deposits in the bones and teeth and osteoclast cells that absorb calcium from bones and teeth. Bone tissue tends to be maintained in quantities no greater than needed to meet current physical stress. Therefore inactive and, particularly, bedridden people lose calcium from their bones; osteoclastic activity exceeds osteoblastic activity, and decalcification occurs. See also **calcium, mineral.**

decannulation /dēkan′yəlā′shən/ [L, *de*, from, *cannula*, small reed], the removal of a cannula or tube that may have been inserted during a surgical procedure.

decanoic acid. See **capric acid.**

decay product /dikā′/ [L, *de* + *cadere*, to fall; *producere*, to produce], (in radiology) a stable or radioactive nuclide formed directly from the radioactive disintegration of a radionuclide or as a result of successive transformation in a radioactive series. Also called **daughter product.**

deceleration /dēsel′ərā′shən/ [L, *de* + *accelerare*, to hasten], a decrease in the speed or velocity of an object or reaction. Compare **acceleration.**

deceleration phase, (in obstetrics) the latter part of active labor characterized by a decreased rate of dilatation of the cervical os on a Friedman curve.

decerebrate posture /dēser′əbrat/ [L, *de* + *cerebrum*, brain; *ponere* to place], the position of a patient, who is usually comatose, in which the arms are extended and internally rotated and the legs are extended with the feet in forced plantar flexion. The posture is usually observed in patients afflicted by compression of the brainstem at a low level. Also called **decerebrate rigidity.**

decerebration /-brā′shən/ [L, *de*, from, *cerebrum*,], the process of removing the brain or of cutting the brain stem above the level of the red nucleus, thus eliminating cerebral function.

deci-, a combining form indicating one tenth.

decibel (dB) /des′əbəl/ [L, *decimus*, one tenth, *bel*, Alexander G. Bell], a unit of measure of the intensity of sound.

A decibel is one tenth of 1 bel; an increase of 1 bel is perceived as a tenfold increase in loudness, based on a sound-pressure reference level of 0.0002 dyn/cc.

decidua /disij′ōō·ə/ [L, *decidere*, to fall off], the epithelial tissue of the endometrium lining the uterus. It envelops the conceptus during gestation and is shed in the puerperium. It is also shed periodically during menstruation. Kinds of decidua are **decidua basalis, decidua capsularis,** and **decidua vera.** See also **amniotic sac.**

decidua basalis, the decidua of the endometrium in the uterus that lies beneath the implanted ovum. Also called **decidua serotina.**

decidua capsularis, the decidua of the endometrium of the uterus covering the implanted ovum. Also called **decidua reflexa.**

decidual endometritis /disij′ōō·əl/, an inflammation or infection of any portion of the decidua during pregnancy. See also **endometritis.**

decidua menstrualis, the endometrium shed during menstruation.

decidua parietalis. See **decidua vera.**

decidua reflexa. See **decidua capsularis.**

decidua serotina. See **decidua basalis.**

decidua vera, the decidua of the endometrium lining the uterus except for those areas beneath and above the implanted and developing ovum called, respectively, the decidua basalis and the decidua capsularis. Also called **decidua parietalis.**

deciduoma /disij′ōō·ō′mə/, a benign or malignant tumor of endometrial tissue. A deciduoma may develop after a pregnancy, regardless of the outcome of the pregnancy. It may be detected on a Pap smear.

deciduous dentition /disij′ōō·əs/, the teeth in proximal arrangement in the maxilla and mandible that appear in the mouth first. Also called **primary dentition.** See **deciduous tooth.**

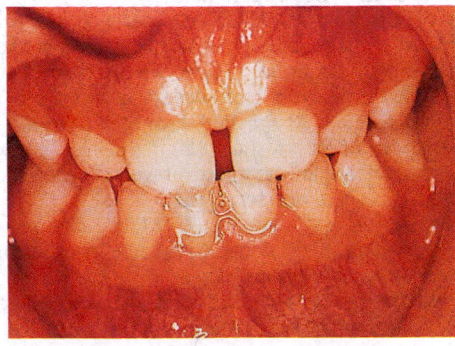

Deciduous dentition (*Zitelli, 1992*)

deciduous tooth [L, *decidere*, to fall off; AS, *toth*], any one of the set of 20 teeth that appear normally during infancy, consisting of four incisors, two canines, and four molars in each jaw. Deciduous teeth start developing at about the sixth week of fetal life as a thickening of the epithelium along the line of the future jaw. During the seventh week, the epithelium splits longitudinally into the labial strand and the lingual strand. The labial strand forms the labiodental

lamina. The lingual strand becomes the dental lamina, which develops ten enlargements in each jaw. The enlargements appear about the ninth week and correspond to the future deciduous teeth. In most individuals the first deciduous tooth erupts through the gum about 6 months after birth. Thereafter, one or more deciduous teeth erupt about every month until all 20 have appeared. The deciduous teeth are usually shed between the ages of 6 and 13, although the timing varies greatly from person to person. Also called **milk tooth, deciduous dentition, first dentition, primary dentition.** Compare **permanent tooth.** See also **predeciduous dentition, teething, tooth.**

decisional conflict, a nursing diagnosis accepted by the Eighth National Conference on the Classification of Nursing Diagnoses. The condition is a state of uncertainty about the course of action to be taken when choice among competing actions involves risk, loss, or challenge to personal life values. The focus of conflict is to be specified, such as choices regarding health, family relationships, career, or finances. Major defining characteristics include a verbalized feeling of distress related to uncertainty about choices, verbalization of undesired consequences of alternative actions being considered, vacillation between alternative choices, and delayed decision making. Minor characteristics include self-focusing, questioning personal values and beliefs while attempting a decision, and physical signs of distress or tension, such as increased heart rate, increased muscle tension, and restlessness. Related factors are unclear personal values or beliefs; perceived threat to his or her value system; lack of experience or interference with decision making; lack of relevant information; and a support system deficit. See also **nursing diagnosis.**

Declomycin, a trademark for an antibacterial (demeclocycline hydrochloride).

decoction /dikok′shən/ [L, *de* + *coquere,* to cook], a liquid medicine made from an extract of water-soluble substances, usually with the aid of boiling water. Herbal remedies are usually decoctions. See also **concoction.**

decode /dikōd′/, to interpret coded information into a form usable by people.

decoded message, (in communication theory) a message as translated by a receiver. If it is correctly interpreted within the context of the message as sent by the sender, the decoded message is the same as the encoded message; if it is not understood and interpreted as sent, it is not the same as the encoded message.

decoic acid. See **capric acid.**

decompensation /kē′kəmpənsā′shən/ [L, *de* + *compensare,* to weigh together], the failure of a system, as cardiac decompensation in heart failure.

decomposition /dī′kəmpəsish′ən/ [L, *de* + *componere,* to put together], the dissolution of a substance into simpler chemical forms.

decompression /dē′kəmpresh′ən/ [L, *de* + *comprimere,* to press together], **1.** a technique used to readapt an individual to normal atmospheric pressure after exposure to higher pressures, as in diving. **2.** the removal of pressure caused by gas or fluid in a body cavity, as the stomach or intestinal tract.

decompression sickness, a painful, sometimes fatal syndrome caused by the formation of nitrogen bubbles in the tissues of divers, caisson workers, and aviators who move too rapidly from environments of higher to those of lower atmospheric pressures. Nitrogen breathed in air under pressure dissolves in tissue fluids. When ambient pressure is reduced too rapidly, nitrogen comes out of solution faster than it can be circulated to the lungs for expiration. Gaseous nitrogen then accumulates in the joint spaces and peripheral circulation, impairing tissue oxygenation. Disorientation, severe pain, and syncope follow. Treatment is by rapid return of the patient to an environment of higher pressure followed by gradual decompression. Death is more often caused by accident during syncope rather than by decompression sickness itself. Also called **bends, caisson disease** /kā'sän/. Compare **barotrauma.**

decongestant [L, *de + congerere,* to pile up], **1.** of or pertaining to a substance or procedure that eliminates or reduces congestion or swelling. **2.** a decongestant drug. Adrenergic drugs (α-1 stimulants), such as ephedrine, pseudoephedrine, and phenylpropanolamine hydrochloride, that cause vasoconstriction of nasal mucosa are used as decongestants.

decontamination /dā'kəntam'inā'shən/, the process of making a person, object, or environment free of microorganisms, radioactivity, or other contaminants.

decorticate posture /dēkôr'tikāt/ [L, *de + cortex,* bark; *ponere,* to place], the position of a comatose patient in which the upper extremities are rigidly flexed at the elbows and at the wrists. The legs also may be flexed. The decorticate posture indicates a lesion in a mesencephalic region of the brain. In some instances the posture may be produced by application of a painful stimulus to a comatose patient. Also called **decorticate rigidity.**

decortication /dēkôr'tikā'shən/ [L, *de + cortex,* bark], (in medicine) the removal of the cortical tissue of an organ or structure, such as the kidney, the brain, and the lung. —**decorticate,** *v., adj.*

decrement /dek'rəmənt/ [L, *de + crescere,* to grow], a decrease or stage of decline, as of a uterine contraction.

decremental conduction /dek'rəmen'təl/, (in cardiology) conduction that slows progressively as the effectiveness of the propagating impulse gradually decreases.

decrudescence /dē'krōōdes'əns/ [L, *de,* from, *crudescere,* to become bad], a decrease in the severity of symptoms.

decubital /dikyōō'bitəl/ [L, *decumbere,* to lie down], pertaining to bedsores.

decubitus /dikyōō'bitəs/ [L, *decumbere,* to lie down], a recumbent or horizontal position, as lateral decubitus, which

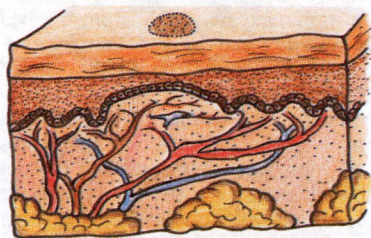

Stage I

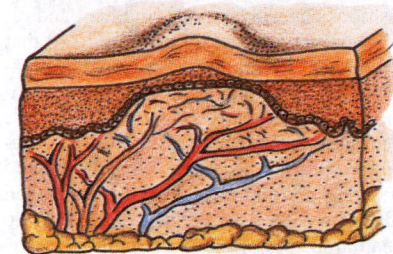

Stage II

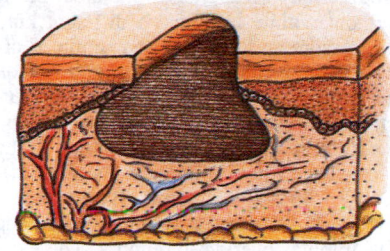

Stage III

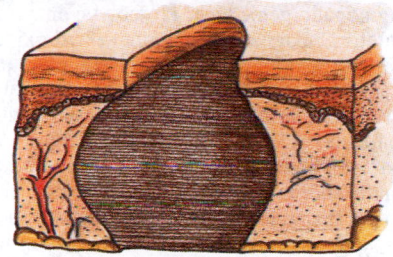

Stage IV

Stages of decubitus ulcers
(Potter, 1993)

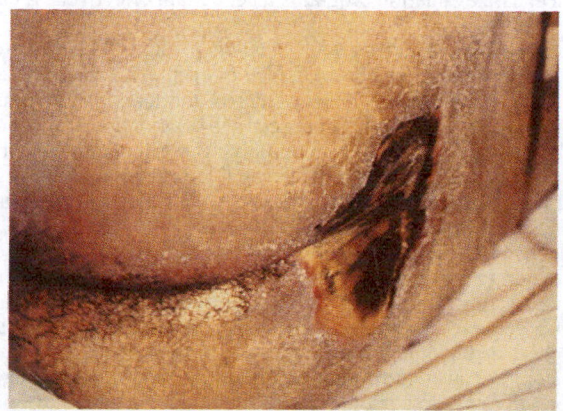

Decubitus ulcer *(Baron, 1990)*

is lying on one side. See also **decubitus care, decubitus ulcer.**

decubitus care, the management and prevention of decubitus ulcers that occur most frequently on the sacrum, elbows, heels, outer ankles, inner knees, hips, shoulder blades, and ear rims of immobilized patients, especially those who are obese, elderly, or suffering from infections, injuries, or a poor nutritional state.

■ METHOD: Decubiti may be prevented by repositioning the immobile patient every 2 hours, keeping the skin dry, and inspecting pressure areas every 4 to 6 hours for signs of redness. Bed linen is kept dry and wrinkle-free; a sheet is used to lift the patient, who is moved frequently from the bed but is not allowed to sit in one place for more than 30 minutes. A high-protein diet, vitamins, and iron may be ordered for vulnerable patients, and a prophylactic measure is daily skin care, in which all areas are washed, rinsed, and dried thoroughly and lotion is gently rubbed on bony prominences. A thin layer of cornstarch or a noncaking powder is applied to areas showing excessive perspiration, and the perineal and perianal areas are washed with soap and water after each defecation and urination. Preventive devices include air mattresses, flotation mattresses, sheepskins, silicone pads, foam cushions for wheelchairs, and heel and elbow guards. Stage I decubiti, characterized by redness that is not relieved by circulatory stimulation or removal of pressure, and Stage II lesions, involving excoriation, vesiculation, or breaks in the skin, are treated similarly. The area is cleaned every 8 hours as indicated with mild soap and water, dilute hydrogen peroxide, or normal saline solution and is blotted dry. To increase circulation, the area is massaged gently and exposed every 2 to 4 hours for 15 minutes to air, sunlight, or a heat lamp. Magnesium aluminum hydroxide gel, karaya powder, A & D ointment, tincture of benzoin, or povidone-iodine may be applied to the area, but if there is no improvement within 48 hours, a different kind of dressing is tried. Pressure and irritation to excoriated areas are avoided at all times. Stage III decubiti, in which there is full-thickness skin loss, and Stage IV pressure ulcers, which characteristically invade fascia, connective tissue, muscle, or bone, require more extensive treatment. The patient is turned every 1 to 2 hours, and the lesion is irrigated with water every 6 to 8 hours. The affected area is exposed to air for 15 to 30 minutes every 2 to 4 hours and to a heat lamp for 15 minutes every 4 to 6 hours. The ulcer may be incised, debrided, and covered with a nonadhering dressing secured by nonallergenic tape. Proteolytic enzyme preparations, antibiotics, magnesium aluminum hydroxide gel, gold-leaf flakes, or povidone-iodine may be applied to the wound, and granulated sugar dressings may be used after removal of necrotic tissue, although they are contraindicated in diabetic patients.

■ NURSING INTERVENTION: The nurse plays a major role in the prevention of decubiti and in their treatment if they occur, turning the patient at frequent intervals, applying the ordered medications and dressings to the lesions, and, in the administration of daily skin care, avoiding vigorous rubbing. The nurse conducts active or passive exercises with massage to the patient's extremities and, when indicated, prepares for incision and debridement of advanced ulcers.

■ OUTCOME CRITERIA: Decubiti are often resistant to treatment, and large areas of ulceration can be life-threatening, especially in a debilitated patient. Prompt and continued care of early lesions can prevent invasion of underlying tissue and promote healing. The nurse may elicit the cooperation and participation of the patient in a nursing care plan that includes all preventive measures. The importance of frequent change of position, dryness, cleanliness, and good nutrition are emphasized.

decubitus position [L, *decumbere*, to lie down, *positio*], the position gradually assumed by a person who is bedridden over a long period.

decubitus posture, the position acquired by a bedridden patient to rest on his or her side to relieve the pressure of body weight on the sacrum, heels, or other body areas vulnerable to decubitus ulcers.

decubitus projection, (in radiology) a position for producing a radiograph of the chest or abdomen of a patient who is lying down, with the central ray parallel to the horizon. Variations of the position include left and right AP oblique, dorsal decubitus, ventral decubitus, and left and right lateral decubitus.

decubitus ulcer, an inflammation, sore, or ulcer in the skin over a bony prominence. It results from ischemic hypoxia of the tissues because of prolonged pressure on the part. Decubitus ulcers are most often seen in aged, debilitated, immobilized, or cachectic patients. The sores are graded by stages of severity. Stage I: The skin is red; the color of the skin does not return to normal. Stage II: The skin is blistered, peeling, or cracked, although damage is still superficial. Stage III: The skin is broken; a full thickness of skin is lost, subcutaneous tissue may also be damaged, and a serous or bloody drainage may be seen. Stage IV: A deep, craterlike ulcer has formed. The full thickness of skin and the subcutaneous tissues are destroyed. Fascia, connective tissue, bone, or muscle underlying the ulcer are exposed and may be damaged. Prevention of decubitus ulcers is a cardinal aspect of nursing care; treatment is planned specific to the location and the extent of the condition. Also called **bedsore, pressure necrosis, pressure ulcer.**

decussate /dəcus′āt/ [L, *decussis*, intersection], to cross in the form of an "X," as certain nerve fibers from the retina cross at the optic chiasm. −**decussation,** *n*.

decussation /di′kusā′shən/ [L, *decussare*, to make a cross], a crossing of central nervous system fibers in the brain, with some fibers on the left side crossing to the right side and vice versa.

decussation of pyramids [L, *decussare*, to make a cross; Gk, *pyramis*], the crossing of nerve fibers of the corticospinal motor tract at the ventral side on the lower portion of the medulla oblongata.

deduction [L, *deducere*, to lead], a system of reasoning that leads from a known principle to an unknown, or from the general to the specific. Deductive reasoning is used to test diagnostic hypotheses.

deemed status /dēmd/ [AS, *deman*, to judge; L, a standing], a status conferred on a hospital by a professional standards review organization (PSRO) in formal recognition that the hospital's review, continued-stay review, and medical care evaluation programs meet certain effectiveness criteria.

deep brachial artery [As, *dyppan*, to dip; Gk, *brachion*, arm; *arteria* air pipe], a branch of each of the brachial arteries, arising at the distal border of the teres major, passing deeply into the arm between the long and lateral heads of the triceps brachii, and supplying the humerus and the muscles of the upper arm. It has five branches: ascending, radial collateral, middle collateral, muscular, and nutrient. Also called **superior profunda artery.**

deep breathing and coughing exercises, the exercises taught to a person to improve aeration or to maintain respiratory function, especially after prolonged inactivity or after general anesthesia. Incisional pain after surgery in the chest or abdomen often inhibits normal respiratory excursion. See also **cupping and vibrating, postural drainage.**

■ METHOD: The person is assisted to a comfortable position, supine or sitting up. An analgesic may be indicated before

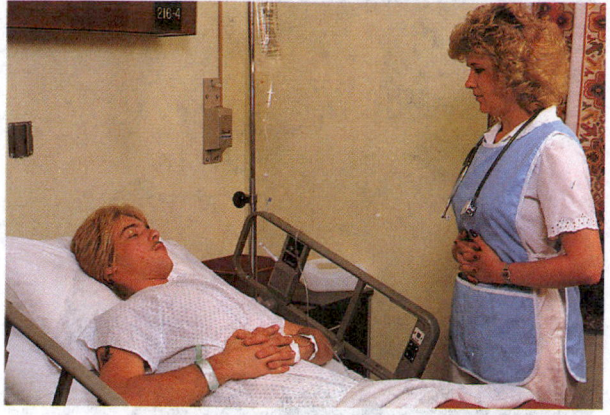

Hands placed over rib cage for deep breathing

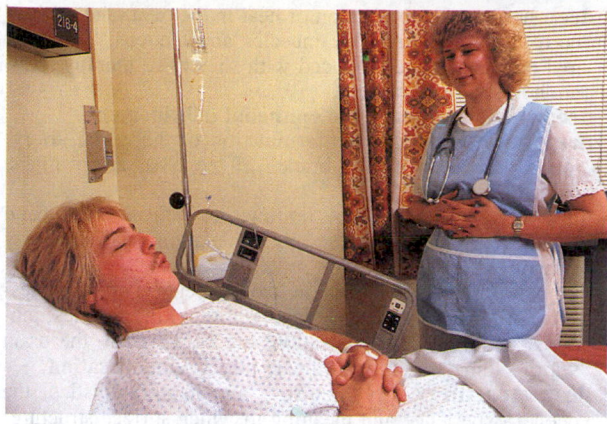

Exhaling through pursed lips

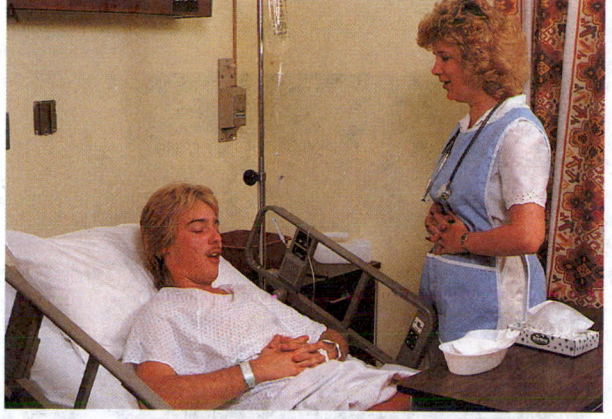

Supporting the incision with a small pillow

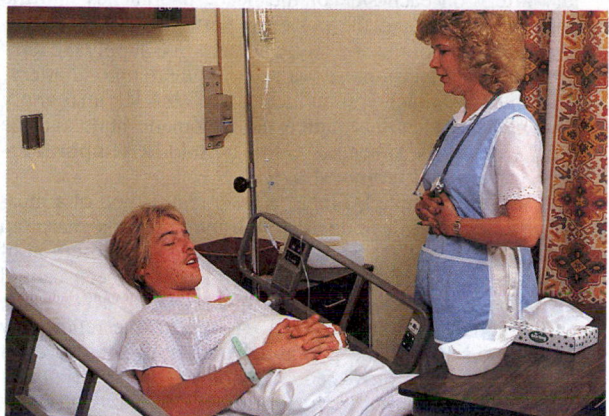

Supporting the incision with fingers interlaced

Deep breathing and coughing exercises *(Sorrentino, 1992)*

the exercises if pain is present. Inhalation through the nose and exhalation through the mouth are encouraged. With the incision supported, the patient is asked to cough after a deep inhalation. If pain prevents the person from producing a deep, effective cough, a series of short barklike coughs may be encouraged.

■ NURSING INTERVENTION: The use of simple techniques and encouragement significantly improve the effectiveness of the exercises. Positioning increases comfort, allows the abdominal contents to fall away from the diaphragm, and encourages full expansion of the chest wall on inspiration. If an incision is present, it may be supported with the hands or with a book or pillow held against the abdomen. The person is often reluctant to breathe deeply or to cough; adequate analgesia, encouragement, and a patient explanation to the person of the benefits may overcome that resistance. Various devices are available for use in respiratory exercises, as those used in atelectasis to strengthen the muscles used in expiration and to empty the air sacs of retained gas.

Postural drainage is commonly performed concurrently with coughing and deep-breathing exercises.

■ OUTCOME CRITERIA: When shallow breathing has replaced deep breathing, secretions tend to dry in the airway, causing damage to the mucous membranes lining the passages. Coughing and deep breathing serve to clear the dried or thick and viscid mucus, to allow moisturized air to enter the bronchi, bronchioles, and alveoli, and to expand the lungs and increase the exchange of gases, thereby improving ventilation.

deep fascia, the most extensive of three kinds of fascia comprising an intricate series of connective sheets and bands that hold the muscles and other structures in place throughout the body, wrapping the muscles in gray, feltlike membranes. The deep fasciae comprise a continuous system, splitting and fusing in an elaborate network attached to the skeleton and divided into the outer investing layer, the internal investing layer, and the intermediate membranes. Compare **subcutaneous fascia, subserous fascia.**

deep heat, the application of heat in the treatment of deep body tissues, particularly muscles and tendons. The thermal effects may be produced with shortwave therapy, phonophoresis, or ultrasound.

deepithelialization. See **epithelial debridement.**

deep palmar arch, the termination of the radial artery, joining the deep palmar branch of the ulnar artery in the palm of the hand.

deep reflexes [ME, *dep*, hollow; L, *reflectere*, to bend back], any reflexes caused by stimulation of a deep body structure, such as a tendon reflex.

deep sensation, the awareness or perception of pain, pressure, or tension in the deep layers of the skin, muscles, tendons, or joints. Such sensations are conveyed to the brain via the spinal column. Compare **superficial sensation.**

deep structure, (in linguistics and neurolinguistics) the deeper experience and meaning to which surface structures in a communication may refer.

deep temporal artery, one of the branches of the maxillary artery on each side of the head. It branches into the anterior portion and the posterior portion, both rising between the temporalis and the pericranium to supply the temporalis and to anastomose with the middle temporal artery. The anterior branch communicates with the lacrimal artery by small branches that pierce the zygomatic bone and the great wing of the sphenoid. Compare **middle temporal artery, superficial temporal artery.**

deep tendon reflex (DTR), a brisk contraction of a muscle in response to a sudden stretch induced by a sharp tap by a finger or rubber hammer on the tendon of insertion of the muscle. Absence of the reflex may have been caused by damage to the muscle, the peripheral nerve, nerve roots, or the spinal cord at that level. A hyperactive reflex may indicate disease of the pyramidal tract above the level of the reflex arc being tested. Generalized hyperactivity of DTRs may be caused by hyperthyroidism. Kinds of DTRs include **Achilles tendon reflex, biceps reflex, brachioradialis reflex, patellar reflex,** and **triceps reflex.** Also called **myotatic reflex, tendon reflex.**

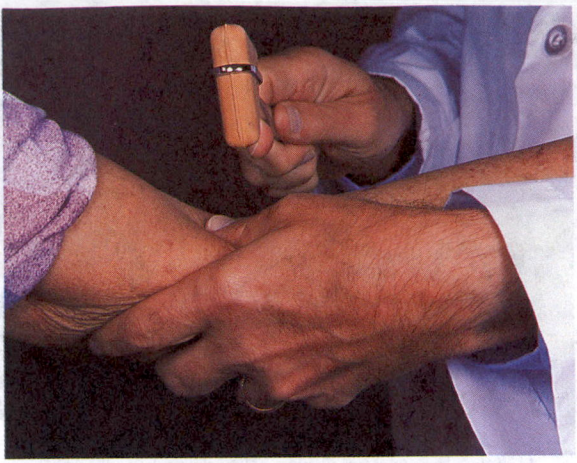

Biceps reflex *(Seidel, 1991)*

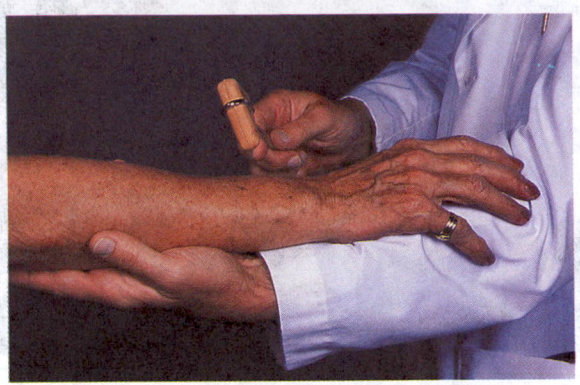

Brachioradial reflex *(Seidel, 1991)*

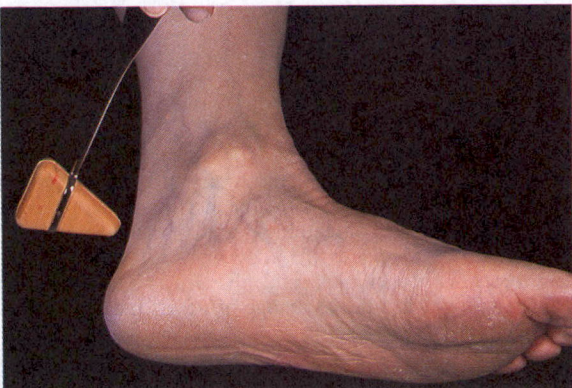

Achilles reflex *(Seidel, 1991)*

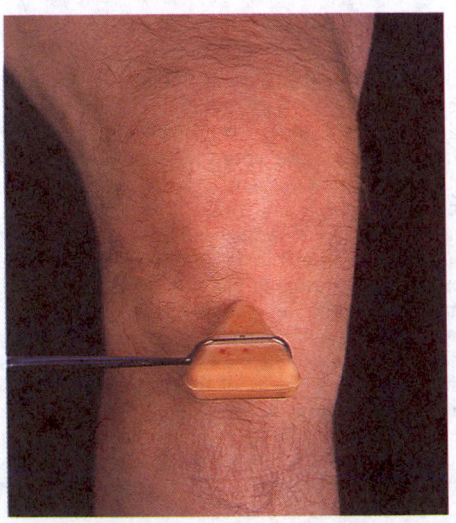

Patellar reflex *(Seidel, 1991)*

deep vein, one of the many systemic veins that accompanies the arteries, usually enclosed in a sheath that wraps both the vein and the associated artery. The larger arteries, such as the axillary, femoral, popliteal, and subclavian, are usu-

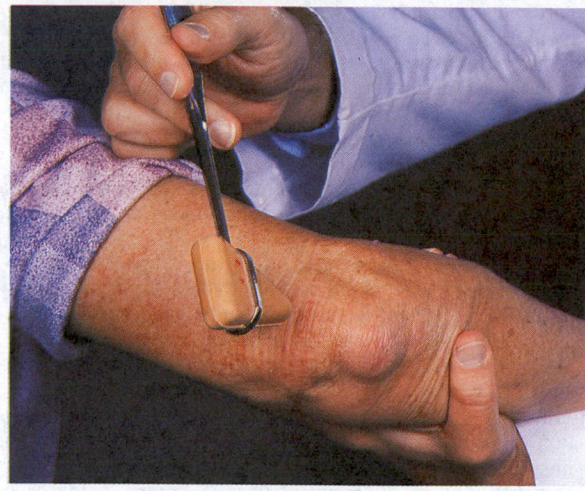

Triceps reflex *(Seidel, 1991)*

ally accompanied by only one deep vein. The deep veins accompanying the smaller arteries, such as the brachial, peroneal, and radial, occur usually in pairs, one vein on each side of the artery. Various structures, such as the skull, vertebral column, and liver, are served by less closely associated arteries and veins. Compare **superficial vein.**

deep vein thrombosis, a disorder involving a thrombus in one of the deep veins of the body. Among deep veins most commonly affected are the iliac and femoral veins. Symptoms include tenderness, pain, swelling, warmth, and discoloration of the skin. A deep vein thrombus is potentially life threatening, and treatment, including bed rest and anticoagulant drugs, is directed toward prevention of movement of the thrombus toward the lungs.

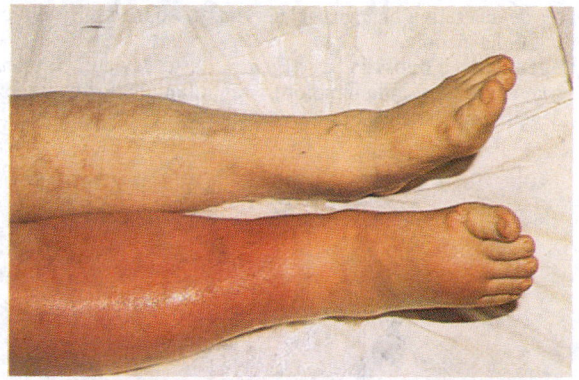

Deep vein thrombosis *(Kamal, 1991)*

deep x-ray therapy, the treatment of internal neoplasms, such as Wilms' tumor of the kidney, Hodgkin's disease, and other cancers, with ionizing radiation from an external source. The dose delivered is determined according to the radiosensitivity, size, pathologic grade and differentiation of the tumor, the tolerance of normal surrounding tissue to irradiation, and the condition of the patient. Deep x-ray therapy frequently causes nausea, malaise, diarrhea, and skin reactions, such as blanching, erythema, itching, burning, oozing, or desquamation, but with modern techniques the ray is beamed directly to the site, reducing side scatter, and the skin can be spared. Because tumor cells are hypoxic and are more effectively eradicated when they are well oxygenated, the patient may breathe hyperbaric oxygen or atmospheric oxygen with 5% carbon dioxide during deep x-ray therapy.

deerfly fever. See **tularemia.**

defamation /def′əmā′shən/ [L, *diffamare,* to discredit], any communication, written or spoken, that is untrue and that injures the good name or reputation of another or that in any way brings that person into disrepute.

default judgment /difôlt′/ [L, *defallere,* to lack; *judicare,* to decide], (in law) a judgment rendered against a defendant because of the defendant's failure to appear in court or to answer the plaintiff's claim within the proper time.

defecation /def′ikā′shən/ [L, *defaecare,* to clean], the elimination of feces from the digestive tract through the rectum. See also **constipation, diarrhea, feces.** –**defecate** /def′ikāt/, *v.*

defecation reflex. See **rectal reflex.**

defecography /def′əkog′rəfē/, a radiographic procedure for evaluating the rectum and anal canal of children with fecal incontinence. The child is examined while sitting on a radiolucent toilet seat or potty. Barium is injected through an enema tube that is left in place until the child indicates a desire to defecate. The fluoroscopic view of the bowel movement may be recorded on videotape for review and study.

defective /difek′tiv/ [L, *defectus,* a failing], pertaining to something that is imperfect, or, as in an outdated term, to an individual who may be suffering from a any disorder.

defendant /difen′dənt/, (in law) the party that is named in a plaintiff's complaint and against whom the plaintiff's allegations are made. The defendant must respond to the allegations.

defense mechanism [L, *defendere,* to repulse; *mechanicus,* machine], an unconscious, intrapsychic reaction that offers protection to the self from a stressful situation. Defense mechanisms can be separated into two categories: those that diminish anxiety and are used by an individual to integrate more fully into society, and those that do not reduce anxiety but simply postpone the effects of feeling it. Anxiety-reducing defenses include compensation, identification, imitation, introjection, some forms of repression, substitution, and sublimation. Defenses that postpone full expression of anxiety include denial, displacement, isolation, projection, reaction formation, rationalization, regression, repression, suppression, and undoing.

defensin /difen′sin/, a peptide with natural antibiotic activity found within human neutrophils. Three types of defensins have been identified, each consisting of a chain of about 30 amino acids. Similar molecules occur in white blood cells of other animal species. They show activity toward viruses and fungi, in addition to bacteria.

defensive radical therapy /difen′siv/, (in psychology) a view of the therapeutic process in which as a survival tactic the therapist begins at the patient's present state and encourages the patient to avoid self-defeating behavior. The goal is to create social awareness for clients to use in coping with oppressive environments.

deferent duct. See **vas deferens.**

deferoxamine mesylate /dē'fərok'səmēn/, a chelating agent.

- INDICATIONS: It is prescribed in the treatment of acute iron intoxication and chronic iron overload.
- CONTRAINDICATIONS: Renal disease or anuria prohibits its use.
- ADVERSE EFFECTS: Among the most serious adverse reactions are hypotension, tachycardia, dysuria, visual difficulties, and allergic-type reactions.

defervescence /di'fərves'əns/ [L, *defervescere*, to reduce heat], the diminishing or disappearance of a fever. —**defervescent,** *adj.*

defibrillate /difi'brilāt, difib'-/ [L, *de* + *fibrilla*, little thread], to stop fibrillation of the ventricles by delivering an electric shock through the chest wall. See also **defibrillation.**

defibrillation /difi'brilā'shən/, the termination of ventricular fibrillation, by delivering an electric shock to the patient's precordium. It is a common emergency measure generally performed by a physician or specially trained nurse or paramedic. The defibrillator paddles are covered with a conductive paste or applied over special defibrillator pads. One paddle is placed to the right of the upper sternum below the clavicle, and the other is applied to the midaxillary line of the left lower rib cage. The defibrillator, usually a condenser-discharge system, is set to deliver between 200 and 400 joules. If shocks fail to restore a perfusion rhythm, cardiopulmonary resuscitation (CPR) is begun. Repeat shocks also are attempted periodically until defibrillation is successful. Successful defibrillation by electrical countershock can reverse life-threatening cardiac arrhythmias, especially ventricular fibrillation.

defibrillator /difi'brilā'tər, difib'-/, a device that delivers an electric shock at a preset voltage to the myocardium through the chest wall. It is used for restoring the normal cardiac rhythm and rate when the heart has stopped beating or is fibrillating.

deficiency disease /difish'ənsē/ [L, *de* + *facere*, to make; *dis*, opposite of; Fr, *aise*, ease], a condition resulting from the lack of one or more essential nutrients in the diet, from metabolic dysfunction, or from impaired digestion or absorption, excessive excretion, or increased biologic requirements. Compare **malnutrition.** See also **avitaminosis.**

deficiency of sweating [AS, *swaetan*], a failure of the sweat glands to secrete perspiration in normal amounts. The condition may be the result of a congenital defect, a blockage of the sweat ducts as a sequel to prickly heat, excessive heat, or conditions such as hemorrhage or diarrhea that cause a loss of body fluid. Also called **anhidrosis.**

deficit /def'isit/, any deficiency or difference from what is normal, such as an oxygen deficit, a cause of hypoxia.

definitive /difin'ətiv/ [L, *definitivus*, a limiting], **1.** final; clearly established without doubt or question. **2.** (in embryology) fully formed in the final differentiation of a tissue, structure, or organ. Compare **primitive. 3.** (in parasitology) of or pertaining to the host in which the parasite undergoes the sexual phase of its reproductive cycle.

definitive host, any animal in which the reproductive stages of a parasite develop. The female *Anopheles* mosquito is the definitive host for malaria. Humans are definitive hosts for pinworms, schistosomes, and tapeworms.

Also called **primary host.** Compare **dead-end host, intermediate host, reservoir host.** See also **host.**

definitive prosthesis, a permanent prosthetic device that replaces an immediate-fit appliance, such as a pylon. In some cases, a person may not be fitted with a definitive prosthesis until full weight-bearing on an artificial limb is feasible, which may require 6 to 10 weeks.

definitive treatment, any therapy generally accepted as a specific cure of a disease. Compare **expectant treatment, palliative treatment.**

defloration /def'lôrā'shən/ [L, *de* + *flos*, flower, *atio*, process], the rupture of the vaginal hymen. Defloration may occur during sexual intercourse, during a gynecologic examination, by the use of tampons, athletic sports activity, or by surgery if necessary to remove an obstruction to menstrual flow.

deformity /difôr'mitē/ [L, *deformis*, misshapen], a condition of being distorted, disfigured, flawed, malformed, or misshapen, which may affect the body in general or any part of it and may be the result of disease, injury, or birth defect, such as Arnold-Chiari deformity, in which a part of the brain protrudes through the base of the skull into the spinal canal, and seal-fin deformity, characterized by a deviation of the fingers as an effect of rheumatoid arthritis.

degeneration /dijen'ərā'shən/ [L, *degenerare*, to become unlike others], the gradual deterioration of normal cells and body functions.

degenerative /dijen'ərətiv/, [L, *degenerare*, to become unlike others], pertaining to or involving degeneration or changing to a lower form or dysfunctional form.

degenerative chorea. See **Huntington's chorea.**

degenerative disease any disease in which there is deterioration of structure or function of tissue. Some kinds of degenerative disease are **arteriosclerosis, cancer,** and **osteoarthritis.**

degenerative joint disease. See **osteoarthritis.**

degenerative lesion [L, *degenerare*, to deviate, *laesio*, hurting], an injury or disease state that results in loss of function.

degenerative neuralgia [L, *degenerare*, to deviate; Gk, *neuron*, nerve, *algos*, pain], a form of neuralgia caused by degenerative changes in nervous tissue, usually affecting older people.

degenerative neuritis [L, *degenerare*, to deviate; Gk, *neuron*, nerve, *itis*, inflammation], an inflammation caused by degenerative changes in nervous tissue.

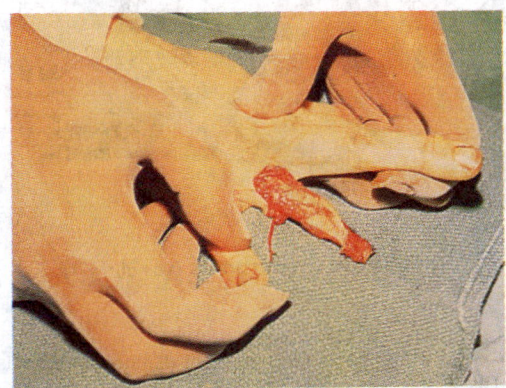

Degloving injury of finger (*Grossman, 1993*)

degloving /dēglov′ing/ [L, *de* + AS, *glof*], **1.** an injury to a finger in which the soft tissue down to the bone, including neurovascular bundles and sometimes tendons, is peeled off the finger. **2.** (in dentistry) the exposure of the bony mandibular anterior or posterior regions by oral surgery.

deglutition /di′glootish′ən/ [L, *deglutire,* to swallow], swallowing.

deglutition apnea, the normal absence of respiration during swallowing.

degradation /di′grədā′shən/ [L, *de* + *gradu,* step], the reduction of a chemical compound to a compound less complex, usually by splitting off one or more groups or subgroups of atoms, as deamination.

dehiscence /dihis′əns/ [L, *dehiscere,* to gape], the separation of a surgical incision or rupture of a wound closure.

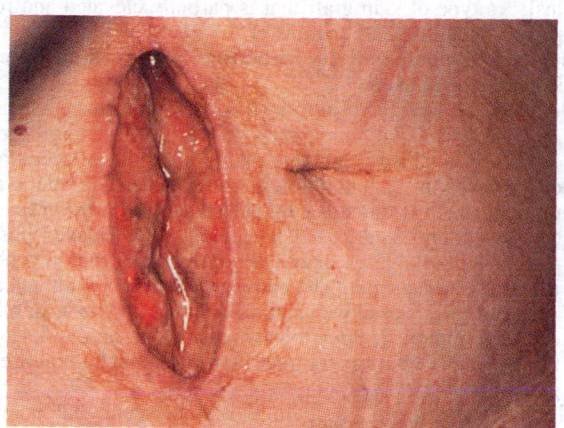

Wound dehiscence (Morison, 1992)

dehumanization /dihyo͞o′mənīzā′shən/ [L, *de,* from *humanitas,* human nature], the process of losing altruistic qualities, as may occur in some psychotic states.

dehydrate /dihī′drāt/ [L, *de* + Gk, *hydor,* water], **1.** to remove or lose water from a substance. **2.** to lose excessive water from the body. **-dehydration,** *n.*

dehydrated alcohol, a clear, colorless, highly hygroscopic liquid with a burning taste, containing at least 99.5% ethyl alcohol by volume. Also called **absolute alcohol.**

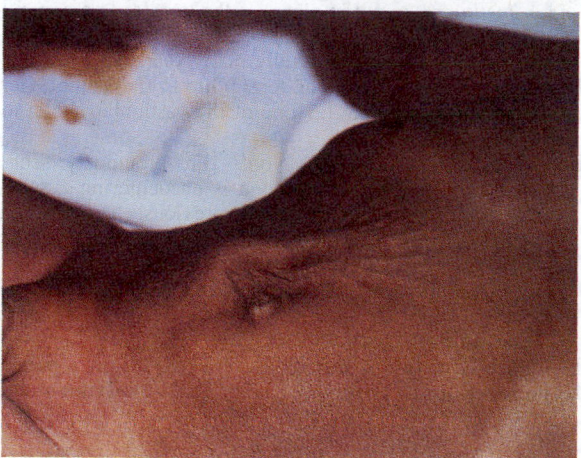

Poor skin turgor resulting from dehydration
(Zitelli, 1992)

dehydration /di′hīdrā′shən/, **1.** excessive loss of water from the body tissues. Dehydration is accompanied by a disturbance in the balance of essential electrolytes, particularly sodium, potassium, and chloride. Dehydration may follow prolonged fever, diarrhea, vomiting, acidosis, and any condition in which there is rapid depletion of body fluids. It is of particular concern among infants and young children, because their electrolyte balance is normally precarious. Signs of dehydration include poor skin turgor, flushed dry skin, coated tongue, oliguria, irritability, and confusion. Normal fluid volume and balanced electrolyte values are the primary goals of therapy. **2.** rendering a substance free from water.

Clinical manifestations of dehydration

	Isotonic (loss of water and salt)	Hypotonic (loss of salt in excess of water)	Hypertonic (loss of water in excess of salt)
Skin			
Color	Gray	Gray	Gray
Temperature	Cold	Cold	Cold or hot
Turgor	Poor	Very poor	Fair
Feel	Dry	Clammy	Thickened, doughy
Mucous membranes	Dry	Slightly moist	Parched
Tearing and salivation	Absent	Absent	Absent
Eyeball	Sunken	Sunken	Sunken
Fontanel	Sunken	Sunken	Sunken
Body temperature	Subnormal or elevated	Subnormal or elevated	Subnormal or elevated
Pulse	Rapid	Very rapid	Moderately rapid
Respirations	Rapid	Rapid	Rapid
Behavior	Irritable to lethargic	Lethargic to comatose; convulsions	Marked lethargy with extreme hyperirritability on stimulation

From Wong DL: *Whaley and Wong's essentials of pediatric nursing,* ed 4, St Louis, 1993, Mosby.

dehydration fever, a fever that frequently occurs in newborns, thought to be caused by dehydration. Also called **inanition fever.** Compare **inanition, starvation.**

dehydration of gingivae, the drying of gingival tissue, often the result of mouth breathing, which lowers the resistance of the gingival tissue to infection.

deinstitutionalization /dē·in′stityōō′shənal′īzā′shən/ [L, *de + instituere,* to put in place], the transfer to a community setting of a client who has been hospitalized for an extended period of time, generally many years.

Deiters' nucleus /dī′tərz, dē′terz/ [Otto F. C. Deiters, German anatomist, b. 1834], one of the vestibular nuclei located in the brainstem.

déjà vu /dāzhävY′, -vē′, -vōō′/ [Fr, previously seen], the sensation or illusion that one is encountering a set of circumstances or a place that was previously experienced. The phenomenon, which is normal in everyone but occurs more frequently or continuously in certain emotional and organic disorders, results from some unconscious emotional connection with the present experience. Compare **jamais vu, paramnesia.**

Déjérine-Klumpke's paralysis. See **Klumpke's palsy.**

Déjérine-Roussy syndrome. See **thalamic syndrome.**

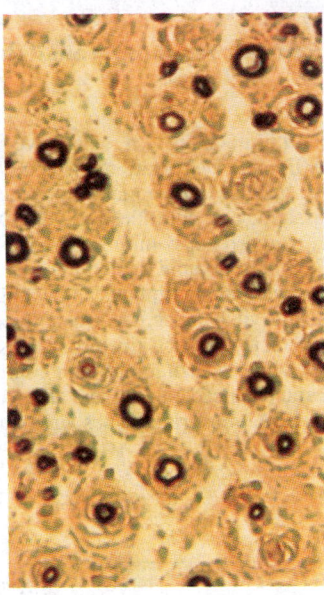

Déjérine-Sottas disease (Perkin, 1986)

Déjérine-Sottas disease /dezh′ərinsot′əz, -sotäz′/ [Joseph J. Dejerine, French neurologist, b. 1849; Jules Sottas, French neurologist, b. 1866], a rare, congenital spinocerebellar disorder characterized by the development of palpable thicken ings along peripheral nerves, degeneration of the peripheral nervous system, pain, paresthesia, ataxia, diminished sensation, and deep tendon reflexes. Diagnosis is made by a histologic examination of a peripheral nerve. There is no specific treatment. Also called **progressive interstitial hypertrophic neuropathy.**

deka-, a combining form indicating the multiple 10.

del, (in cytogenetics) abbreviation for **deletion.**

Delano, Jane A. (1862–1919), an American nurse who organized the American Red Cross Nursing Service, an organization formed to supply nurses to the military forces. In 1891 she became the director of the Nurses' Training School of the University of Pennsylvania and was later appointed the director of the Bellevue Hospital Training School for Nurses in New York, where she had been trained. On a trip to survey nursing conditions in Europe, she died after surgery for a mastoid infection at Base Hospital, Savenay, France, in March 1919.

delayed dentition. See **retarded dentition.**

delayed echolalia [Fr, *delai,* time extension; Gk, *echo,* sound, *lalein* to babble], a phenomenon, commonly seen in schizophrenia, involving the meaningless, automatic repetition of overheard words and phrases. It occurs hours, days, or even weeks after the original stimulus.

delayed graft [ME, *delaein,* to leave; Gk, *graphein,* stylus], a type of skin graft that is partially elevated and replaced for use in a later transfer.

delayed hypersensitivity reaction. See **cell-mediated immune response.**

delayed postpartum hemorrhage, hemorrhage occurring later than 24 hours after delivery. It is most often caused by retained fragments of the placenta, a laceration of the cervix or vagina that was not discovered or that was not completely sutured, or by subinvolution of the placental site within the uterus. Characteristics of delayed postpartum hemorrhage are heavy bleeding and signs of impending shock and anemia. The cause is diagnosed and treated. A laceration is closed with suture, retained fragments of placenta are removed, infection is treated with antibiotics, or the uterus is caused to contract by the administration of ergotrate or oxytocin.

delayed sensation, a feeling or impression that is not experienced immediately after a stimulus. See also **sensation.**

delayed symptom [Fr, *délai;* Gk, *symptoma,* that which happens], a symptom, such as shock, that may not appear until after the precipitating cause.

delayed treatment seeker, (in psychology) a person who delays seeking treatment for a problematic life event, such as a sexual assault, until months or years after the event, usually following a precipitating event such as an anniversary reaction.

Delecato-Doman theory, a therapeutic concept that full neurologic organization of a disabled or mentally retarded child requires that the child pass through developmental patterns covering progressively higher anatomic levels of the nervous system. The first five levels take the child from infantile reflexes through walking and the sixth covers cortical hemispheric dominance.

deleterious /del′itir′ē·əs/ [Gk, *deleterios,* destroyer], pertaining to something that is harmful or dangerous.

deletion (del) /dilē′shən/ [L, *deletionum,* destruction], (in cytogenetics) the loss of a piece of a chromosome because it has broken away from the genetic material.

deletion syndrome, any of a group of congenital autosomal anomalies that result from the loss of chromosomal genetic material, because of breakage of a chromatid during cell division, as the cat-cry syndrome, which results from the absence of the short arm of chromosome 5.

Delhi boil. See **oriental sore.**

deliberate biologic programing /dilib′ərit/ [L, *deliberare,* to weigh carefully], the Hayflick theory of aging based on studies showing that human cells contain biologic clocks that predetermine death after undergoing mitosis a finite number of times.

deliberate hypotension, an anesthetic process in which a short-acting hypotensive agent such as sodium nitroprusside or trimethaphan camsylate is given to reduce blood pressure and thus bleeding during surgery. The procedure facilitates surgery by making vessels and tissues more visible and reducing blood loss.

delinquency /diling′kwənsē/ [L, *delinquere,* to fail], **1.** negligence or failure to fulfill a duty or obligation. **2.** an offense, fault, misdemeanor, or misdeed; a tendency to commit such acts. See also **juvenile delinquency.**

delinquent /diling′kwənt/, **1.** characterized by neglect of duty or violation of law. **2.** one whose behavior is characterized by persistent antisocial, illegal, violent, or criminal acts; a juvenile delinquent.

délire de toucher /dālir′dətōōshā′/ [Fr], an abnormal desire or irresistible urge to touch objects.

-delirious. See **delirium.**

delirious mania /dilir′ē·əs/, an extreme form of the manic state in which activity is so frenzied, confused, and incoherent that it is difficult to discern any link between affect and behavior.

delirium /dilir′ē·əm/ [L, *delirare,* to rave], **1.** a state of frenzied excitement or wild enthusiasm. **2.** an acute organic mental disorder characterized by confusion, disorientation, restlessness, clouding of the consciousness, incoherence, fear, anxiety, excitement, and often illusions, hallucinations, usually of visual origin, and at times delusions. The condition is caused by disturbances in cerebral functions that may result from a wide range of metabolic disorders, including nutritional deficiencies and endocrine imbalances; postpartum or postoperative stress; the ingestion of toxic substances, as various gases, metals, or drugs, including alcohol; and other causes of physical and mental shock or exhaustion. The symptoms are usually of short duration and reversible with treatment of the underlying cause, although in extreme cases, where the toxic condition is exceedingly severe or prolonged, permanent brain damage may occur. Bed rest in a quiet environment is essential. The delirious patient must be protected from accidents and self-injury. In prolonged cases, dehydration and vitamin deficiency may occur. Sedatives or tranquilizing drugs are often used to relieve excitability. Kinds of delirium include **acute delirium, delirium tremens, exhaustion delirium, senile delirium,** and **traumatic delirium.** Compare **dementia. –delirious,** *adj.*

delirium of persecution [L, *delirare,* to rave, *persecutor,* to pursue], a state of clouded consciousness in which the patient believes others are threatening or conspiring against the person.

delirium tremens (DTs), an acute and sometimes fatal psychotic reaction caused by cessation of excessive intake of alcoholic beverages over a long period of time. Initial symptoms include loss of appetite, insomnia, and general restlessness, followed by agitation, excitement, disorientation, mental confusion, vivid and often frightening hallucinations, acute fear and anxiety, illusions and delusions, coarse tremors of the hands, feet, legs, and tongue, fever, increased heart rate, extreme perspiration, GI distress, and precordial pain. The episode, which usually constitutes a medical emergency, typically lasts from 3 to 6 days and is generally followed by a deep sleep. Treatment includes a quiet, nonstimulating environment in which the person is watched closely and protected from self-injury, not only

during the period of delirium but, more importantly, during convalescence, when depression and remorse often lead to attempted suicide. Extreme fatigue, pneumonia, respiratory infections, and heart failure are common complications, as are severe dehydration and nutritional deficiencies. Dietary supplements are often given; tube feeding and intravenous fluids may be needed. Sedatives and tranquilizing agents are useful for quieting the person. Compare **alcoholic hallucinosis, Stearns' alcoholic amentia.** See also **Korsakoff's psychosis.**

delivery /diliv′ərē/ [L, *de* + *liberare,* to free], (in obstetrics) the birth of a child; parturition.

delivery room, a unit of a hospital utilized for obstetric delivery and infant resuscitation.

DeLorme technique, a method of physical exercise with weights in which sets of repetitions are repeated with rests between sessions. The technique involves the use of heavier weights and fewer repetitions in successive sets.

delousing /dēlou′sing/ [L, *de,* from; AS, *lus*], to rid a person or object of an infestation of lice.

delta /del′tə/, Δ, δ, fourth letter of the Greek alphabet.

delta agent hepatitis /del′tə/ [L, *agere,* to do; Gk, *hepar,* liver, *itis,* inflammation], an infection caused by an RNA virus (δ Ag) associated with the hepatitis B surface antigen (HBsAg) in cases of chronic hepatitis and progressive liver damage. The delta agent apparently is able to induce the infection when it is present along with the B surface antigen.

delta hepatitis. See **viral hepatitis.**

delta-1-testolactone. See **testolactone.**

delta-9-tetrahydrocannabinol (THC), a pharmacologically active ingredient of cannabis that has been used in treating some cases of nausea and vomiting associated with cancer chemotherapy. See **cannabis.**

delta optical density analysis [Gk, *delta,* fourth letter of Greek alphabet; *optikos,* of sight; L, *densus,* thick; Gk, a loosening], a technique used to diagnose anemia in a fetus by measuring the proportion of bilirubin decomposition products in the amniotic fluid. The method involves spectrographic examination of a fluid sample. It measures the bilirubin and bilirubin-products concentration according to the wavelengths of light absorbed by the hemolytic products, as the bilirubin products alter the normal color of the amniotic fluid. The data are sometimes expressed in terms of $[Grk d]OD_{450}$, the number representing the wavelength in nm at which maximum absorption of light by bilirubin occurs. If the delta optical density analysis indicates the fetus is moderately to severely anemic, immediate delivery is usually recommended when the gestational age permits. Otherwise, intrauterine fetal blood transfusions may be recommended.

delta wave, 1. also called **delta rhythm.** the slowest of the four types of brain waves, characterized by a frequency of 4 Hz and a relatively high voltage. Delta waves are 'deepsleep waves' associated with a dreamless state from which an individual is not easily aroused. Compare **alpha wave, beta wave, theta wave. 2.** (in cardiology) a slurring of the QRS portion of an ECG tracing caused by preexcitation.

deltoid /del′toid/ [Gk, *delta,* triangular, *eidos,* form], **1.** triangular. **2.** of or pertaining to the deltoid muscle that covers the shoulder.

deltoideus. See **deltoid muscle.**

deltoid ligament [L, *ligamentum*], the medial ligament of the ankle joint.

deltoid muscle, a large, thick triangular muscle that covers the shoulder joint and abducts, flexes, extends, and rotates the arm. It arises from various surfaces on the clavicle, acromion, and scapula and inserts, with a thick tendon, into the humerus. Also called **deltoideus.**

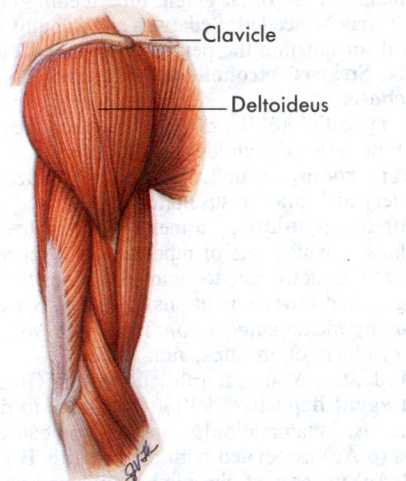

— Clavicle

— Deltoideus

Deltoid muscle (Thibodeau, 1993/John V Hagen)

delusion /diloo′zhən/ [L, *deludere*, to deceive], a persistent, aberrant belief or perception held inviolable by a person despite evidence to the contrary. Kinds of delusion include **delusion of being controlled, delusion of grandeur, delusion of persecution, nihilistic delusion,** and **somatic delusion.** Compare **illusion.**

delusion of being controlled, the false belief that one's feelings, beliefs, thoughts, and acts are governed by some external force, as seen in various forms of schizophrenia. See also **delusion.**

delusion of grandeur /grän′dyŏŏr/, the gross exaggeration of one's importance, wealth, power, or talents, as seen in such disorders as megalomania, general paresis, and paranoid schizophrenia. See also **delusion.**

delusion of persecution, a morbid belief that one is being mistreated, harassed, or conspired against, as seen in paranoia and paranoid schizophrenia. The patient may single out a person or group as the source of persecution. See also **delusion.**

delusion of poverty, (in psychology) a false belief by a person that he or she is impoverished.

delusion of reference. See **idea of reference.**

delusion stupor, the state of lethargy and unresponsiveness observed in catatonic schizophrenia.

demand pacemaker [L, *demandere*, to give in charge, *passus*, step; ME, *maken*], a device used to stimulate the heart electrically when the heart's own impulses are not sufficient. Pacemakers can be set to produce a heart beat when the heart's own impulses are not fast enough.

demarcation /dē′märkā′shən/ [L, *de*, from, *marcare*, to mark], the process of setting limits or boundaries.

demarcation current [L, *de* + *maracare*, to mark], an electric current that flows from an uninjured to an injured end of a muscle. Also called **current of injury.**

Demazin, a trademark for a respiratory, fixed-combination drug containing an adrenergic (phenylephrine hydrochloride) and an antihistaminic (chlorpheniramine maleate).

deme /dēm/ [Gk, *demos*, common population], a small, closely related, interbreeding population of organisms or individuals, usually occupying a circumscribed area. Also called **genetic population.**

demecarium bromide /dē′məker′ē·əm/, an ophthalmic anticholinesterase agent.

■ INDICATION: It is prescribed in the treatment of open-angle glaucoma.

■ CONTRAINDICATIONS: Active uveal inflammation and/or glaucoma, associated with iridocyclitis, bronchial asthma, peptic ulcer, epilepsy, recent myocardial infarction, pregnancy, or known hypersensitivity to this drug prohibits its use.

■ ADVERSE EFFECTS: Among the most serious adverse reactions are symptoms associated with systemic absorption of anticholinesterase agents (including certain insecticides), such as bradycardia and diarrhea. Eye irritation, hypotension, headache, formation of cysts, and lens opacities also may occur.

demeclocycline hydrochloride /dēmek′lōsī′klēn/, a tetracycline antibiotic.

■ INDICATIONS: It is prescribed in the treatment of a variety of infections, including infections in which use of penicillin is contraindicated.

■ CONTRAINDICATIONS: Renal or liver dysfunction, pregnancy, early childhood, or known hypersensitivity to this drug or to other tetracycline medication prohibits its use.

■ ADVERSE EFFECTS: Among the more serious adverse effects are blood disorders, GI disturbances, phototoxicity, potentially serious suprainfections, and hypersensitivity reactions. Discoloration of teeth may occur in children exposed to the drug in utero or before 8 years of age.

dementia /dimen′shə/ [L, *de* + *mens*, mind], a progressive, organic mental disorder characterized by chronic personality disintegration, confusion, disorientation, stupor, deterioration of intellectual capacity and function, and impairment of control of memory, judgment, and impulses. Dementia caused by drug intoxication, hyperthyroidism, pernicious anemia, paresis, subdural hematoma, benign brain tumor, hydrocephalus, insulin shock, and tumor of islet cells of the pancreas can be reversed by treating the condition; Alzheimer's disease, Pick's disease, Huntington's disease, and traumatic injuries to the brain are not amenable to treatment. Kinds of dementia include **Alzheimer's disease, dementia paralytica, Pick's disease, secondary dementia, senile dementia,** and **toxic dementia.**

dementia paralytica. See **general paresis.**

dementia praecox /prē′koks/, an obsolete term for schizophrenia, especially schizophrenia developing in adolescence or early adulthood. See also **schizophrenia.**

Demerol, a trademark for a narcotic analgesic (meperidine).

Demerol Hydrochloride, a trademark for a narcotic analgesic (meperidine hydrochloride).

-demic, a suffix meaning 'relating to people or a district': *interedemic, philodemic, prosodemic.*

demigauntlet bandage /dem′igônt′lit/ [L, *demidus*, half; Fr, *gant*, glove], a glovelike bandage covering only the hand and leaving the fingers free. See also **gauntlet bandage.**

demineralization /dēmin′əral′īzā′shən/ [L, *de* + *minera*, mine], a decrease in the amount of minerals or inorganic salts in tissues, as occurs in certain diseases.

demise /dimīz′/ [OFr, *démettre*], to put away], death, destruction, or ceasing to exist.

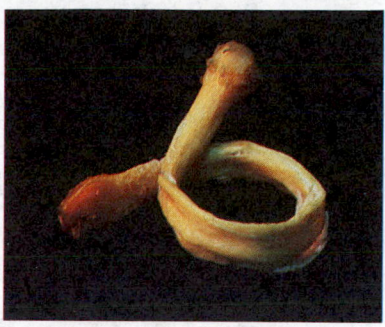

Demineralized bone (Seeley, 1992/Trent Stephens)

democratic style /dem′okrat′ik/, a people-centered leadership style in which the group participates openly in decision-making for group goals.

demography /dəmog′rəfē/ [Gk, *demos*, people, *graphein*, to record], the study of human populations, particularly the size, distribution, and characteristics of members of population groups. Demography is applied in studies of health problems involving ethnic groups, populations of a specific geographic region, religious groups with special dietary restrictions, such as Mormons (Church of Jesus Christ of Latter-Day Saints) or Seventh-Day Adventists, and members of population groups that may represent a typical cross-section of the entire nation, as in the continuing study of residents of Framingham, Massachusetts, by the National Institutes of Health. Compare **epidemiology.**

demonstrative /dimon′strətiv/, pertaining to an action, such as indicating the size of an object with the hands, that accompanies and illustrates speech. See also **circum-speech.**

De Morgan's spots. See **cherry angioma.**

Demser, a trademark for an antihypertensive (metyrosine).

demulcent /dimul′sənt/ [L, *demulcere*, to stroke down], **1.** any of several oily substances used for soothing and reducing irritation of surfaces that have been abraded or irritated. **2.** soothing, as a counterirritant or balm.

Demulen, a trademark for an oral contraceptive containing an estrogen (ethinyl estradiol) and a progestin (ethynodiol diacetate).

demyelination /dimī′əlinā′shən/ [L, *de* + Gk, *myelos*, marrow], the process of destruction or removal of the myelin sheath from a nerve or nerve fiber.

denaturation /dēnā′chərā′shən/ [L, *de* + *natura*, natural], **1.** the alteration of the basic nature or structure of a substance. **2.** the process of making a potential food or beverage substance unfit for human consumption although it may still be used for other purposes, such as a solvent.

denatured alcohol /dēnā′chərd/, ethyl alcohol made unfit for ingestion by the addition of acetone or methanol, used as a solvent and in chemical processes.

denatured protein [L, *de*, from, *natura, proteios*, first rank], a protein that has undergone change so that its original properties are lost. A protein can be denatured by radiation, heat, strong acids, or alcohol.

dendr-, a combining form meaning 'pertaining to a tree or branches': *dendriceptor, dendroid, dendrophobia.*

-dendria, a suffix meaning the 'twiglike branching of nerve fibers': *oligodendria, telodendria, zoodendria.*

dendrite /den′drīt/ [Gk, *dendron*, tree], a branching process that extends from the cell body of a neuron. Each neu-

ron usually possesses several dendrites, which receive impulses that are conducted to the cell body. The number of dendrites varies with the functions of a neuron. Compare **axon.**

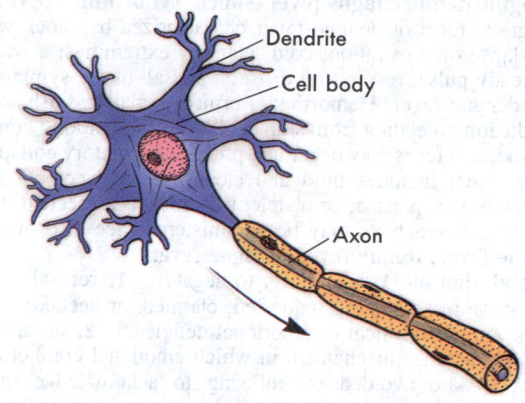

Dendrite (Thibodeau, 1993/Scott Bodell)

dendritic /dendrit′ik/, **1.** treelike, with branches that spread toward or into neighboring tissues, as dendritic keratitis. **2.** of or pertaining to a dendrite.

dendritic calculus [Gk, *dendron*, tree, *calculus*, pebble], a large calculus lodged in the pelvis of the kidney and shaped to fit the branches of the calyx. Also called **coral calculus**.

dendritic keratitis, a serious herpes virus infection of the eye, characterized by an ulceration of the surface of the cornea resembling a tree with knobs at the ends of the branches. Photophobia, the sensation of a foreign body in the eye, pain, and conjunctivitis are usual. Treatment includes application of idoxuridine (IDU), chemical debridement with an iodine tincture, or surgical removal of the involved layer of corneal tissue cells. Untreated dendritic keratitis may result in permanent scarring of the cornea with impaired vision or blindness. Also called **hepatic keratitis.**

dendrodendritic synapse /den′drōdendrit′ik/ [Gk, *dendron, dendron* + *synaptein*, to join], a type of synapse in which a dendrite of one neuron comes in contact with a dendrite of another neuron. Compare **axodendritic synapse.**

-dendron, a suffix meaning a 'the branching portion of a nerve cell receiving an impulse': *neurodendron, telodendron, toxicodendron.*

denervated /dēnur′vātid/ [L, *de, nervus*, nerve], a condition of having a nerve impulse route interrupted, as by excision or administration of a drug that blocks the pathway. This results in decreased or no transmission of impulses through this pathway.

dengue fever /deng′gē, den′gā/ [Sp, influenza; L, *febris*, fever], an acute arbovirus infection transmitted to humans by the *Aedes* mosquito and occurring in tropic and subtropic regions. The disease usually produces a triad of symptoms: fever, rash, and severe head, back, and muscle pain. Manifestations of dengue usually occur in two phases, separated by a day of remission. In the first attack, the patient experiences fever, extreme weakness, headache, sore throat, muscle pains, and edema of the hands and feet. The second attack is marked by a return of fever and by a bright-red scarlatiniform rash. Dengue is a self-limited illness, though it may take patients several weeks to recover. Treatment is symptomatic; analgesics may be given to relieve headache and other pains. Also called **Aden fever, bouquet fever, breakbone fever, dandy fever, solar fever.** See also *Aedes,* **arbovirus.**

dengue hemorrhagic fever shock syndrome (DHFS), a grave form of dengue fever characterized by shock with collapse or prostration; cold, clammy extremities; a weak, thready pulse; respiratory distress; and all of the symptoms of dengue fever. Hemorrhage, bruises, small reddish spots indicating bleeding from skin capillaries, and bloody vomit, urine, and feces may occur and precede circulatory collapse. Treatment includes fluid and electrolyte replacement and fresh blood, plasma, or platelet transfusions as needed. Oxygen and sedatives may be administered. See also **breakbone fever, dandy fever, dengue fever.**

denial /dinī′əl/ [L, *denegare,* to negate], **1.** refusal or restriction of something requested, claimed, or needed, often resulting in physical or emotional deficiency. **2.** an unconscious defense mechanism in which emotional conflict and anxiety are avoided by refusing to acknowledge those thoughts, feelings, desires, impulses, or external facts that are consciously intolerable.

denial, ineffective, a nursing diagnosis accepted by the Eighth National Conference on the Classification of Nursing Diagnoses. Ineffective denial is a conscious or unconscious attempt to disavow the knowledge or meaning of an event to reduce anxiety or fear to the detriment of health. The individual delays seeking or refuses medical attention and does not perceive personal relevance of symptoms or danger. Minor characteristics include the use of home remedies (self-treatment) to relieve symptoms, minimizing of symptoms, displacement of the source of symptoms to other organs, and displacement of fear of impact of the condition. The individual does not admit fear of death or invalidism, is unable to admit the impact of disease on his or her life pattern, makes dismissive gestures or comments when speaking of distressing events, and displays inappropriate affect. See also **nursing diagnosis.**

Denis Browne splint [Sir Denis J. W. Browne, English surgeon, b. 1892], a splint for the correction of talipes equinovarus (clubfoot), composed of a curved bar attached to the soles of a pair of high-top shoes. The splint is equipped with wing nuts, allowing abduction of each foot to be individualized. The splint is commonly applied nightly in late infancy after casting and manipulation have effectively reduced the deformity.

denitrogenation /dēnī′trōjənā′shən/, the elimination of nitrogen from the lungs and body tissues during a period of breathing pure oxygen.

Denman's spontaneous evolution [Thomas Denman, English physician, b. 1733; L, *sponte,* voluntarily; *evolvere,* to roll forth], a natural, unassisted turning of the fetus from the transverse presentation. The head rotates back and, as the breech descends, the shoulder ascends in the pelvis. The back of the fetus is generally posterior. Also called **Denman's method, Denman's spontaneous version.**

dens, *pl.* **dentes** /den′tēz/ [L, tooth], **1.** a tooth or toothlike structure or process. The term is sometimes modified to identify a particular tooth, as dens caninus or dens molaris. **2.** the cone-shaped odontoid process of the axis, or second cervical vertebra. It receives the atlantal ring to act as a pivot for the atlas, or first cervical vertebra. See also **dentition, tooth.**

dens deciduus. See **deciduous tooth.**

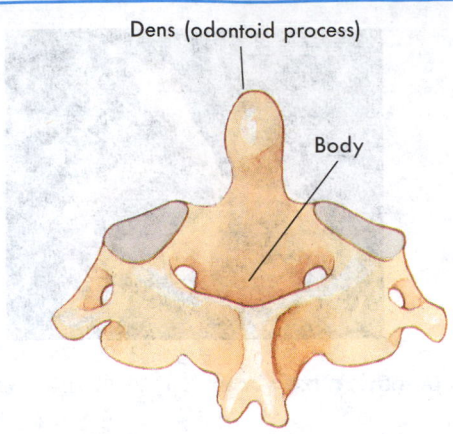

Dens of the axis *(Thibodeau, 1993/Yvonne Wylie Walston)*

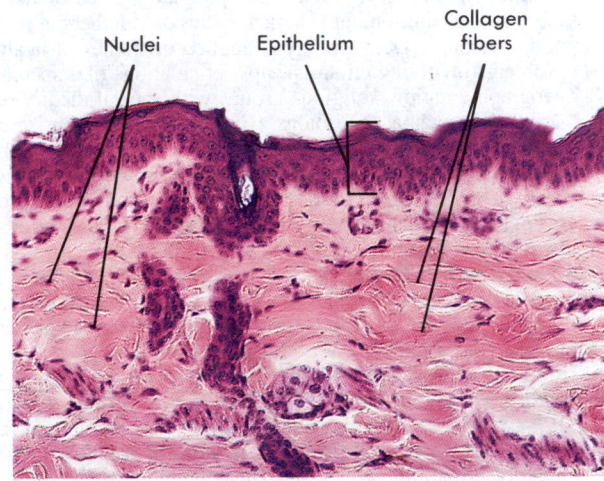

Dense irregular fibrous tissue *(Seeley, 1992/Ed Reschke)*

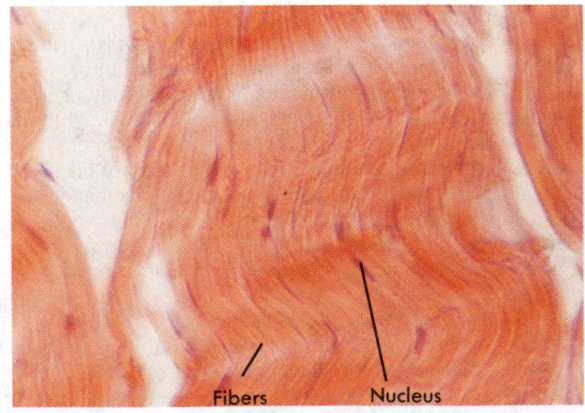

Dense regular fibrous tissue
(Seeley, 1992/Trent Stephens)

dense fibrous tissue [L, *densus*, thick], a fibrous connective tissue consisting of compact, strong, inelastic bundles of parallel collagenous fibers that have a glistening white color. Organized dense fibrous tissue comprises the tendons, the aponeuroses, and the ligaments; unorganized dense fibrous tissue comprises the fascial membranes, the dermis of the skin, the periosteum, and the capsules of organs. Compare **loose fibrous tissue.**

dens in dente /den′tə/, an anomaly of the teeth, found chiefly in the maxillary lateral incisors and characterized by invagination of the enamel. This condition results in a radiographic image suggestive of a tooth within a tooth. Also called **dens invaginatus, gestant odontoma.**

densitometer /den′sitom′ətər/ [L, *densus* + Gk, *metron*, measure], a device that uses a photoelectric cell to detect differences in the density of light transmitted through a liquid, as in spectrophotometric analysis of biologic substances.

density /den′sitē/ [L, *densus,* thick], **1.** the amount of mass of a substance in a given volume. The greater the mass in a given volume, the greater the density. See also **mass, volume. 2.** (in radiology) the degree of x-ray film blackening.

density gradient, a variation in the density of a solution due to a variationf the concentration of a solute in a confined solution.

dens serotinus. See **wisdom tooth.**

dent-, denta-. See **dento-.**

dental [L *dens* tooth], of or pertaining to a tooth or teeth.

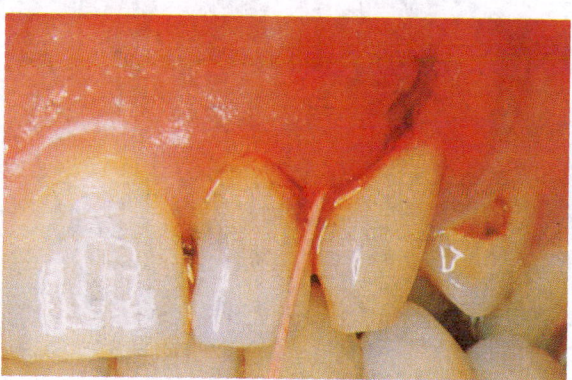

Dental abscess (*Grundy, 1992*)

dental abscess, an abscess that forms in bone or soft tisues of the jaw as a result of an infection that may follow dental caries or injury to a tooth. Symptoms include pain that may be continuous and exacerbated by hot or cold foods or the pressure of closing the jaws firmly. Untreated, the infection may spread to other structures of the mouth and jaw. Treatment may require analgesics, antibiotics, root canal therapy, or extraction of the tooth.

dental alveolus /alvē′ələs/, a tooth socket in the mandible or maxilla.

dental amalgam, an alloy of silver, tin, and mercury with small amounts of zinc and sometimes copper, used for filling tooth cavities.

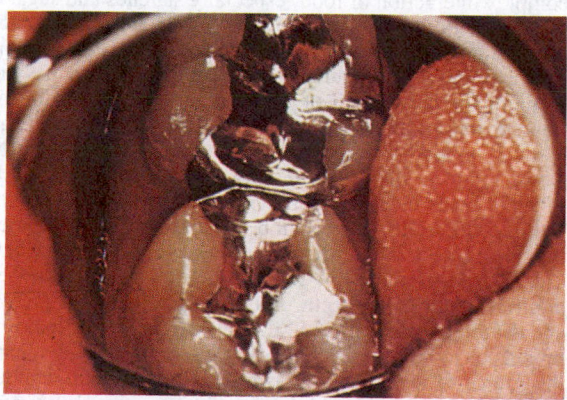

Dental amalgam (*Grundy, 1992*)

dental anesthesia, any of several anesthetic procedures used in dental surgery. Injectable local anesthetics have largely replaced the use of inhalational general anesthetics, especially of nitrous oxide.

dental anomaly, an aberration in which one or more teeth deviate from the normal in form, function, or position.

dental appliance, any device used by a dentist for a specific purpose, such as an orthodontic appliance used to correct malocclusion.

dental arch, the curving shape formed by the arrangement of a normal set of teeth in their proxinal position to each other in each jaw.

dental assistant, a person who assists a dentist in the performance of generalized tasks, including chairside assistance, clerical work, reception, and some radiography and dental laboratory work.

dental biomechanics, the field of biomechanics that deals with the biologic effects of dental restoration on oral structures.

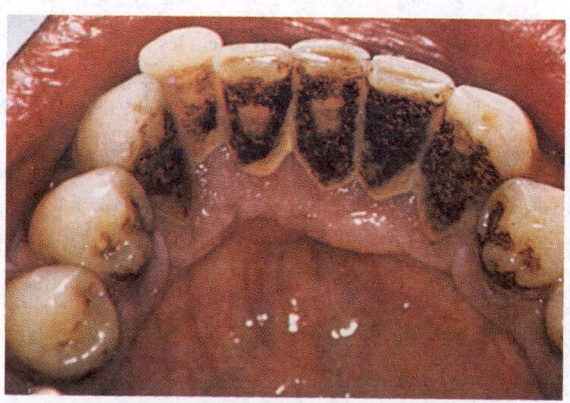

Dental calculus (*Grundy, 1992*)

dental calculus, a salivary deposit of calcium phosphate and calcium carbonate with organic matter on the teeth or a dental prosthesis. See also **calculus, subgingival calculus, supragingival calculus.**

dental caries, a plaque disease which is caused by the complex interaction of food, especially starches and sugars, with bacteria that form dental plaque. The term is also applied to any lesion caused by demineralization of a tooth. Plaque adheres to the surfaces of the teeth and provides the medium for the growth of bacteria and the production of organic acids that cause breaks in the enamel sheath of the tooth. Enzymes produced by the bacteria then attack the protein component of the tooth. This process, if untreated, ultimately leads to the formation of deep cavities and bacterial infection of the pulp chamber and nerves. Dental caries may be prevented by avoidance of sugar in the diet, regular brushing and removal of food particles from the surfaces and interstices of the teeth, fluoridation of drinking water, and the topical application of fluorides to the teeth. Removal of plaque by a dental hygienist is performed to eliminate the source of decay as well as to prevent infection and destruction of the peridontal tissues. Treatment of dental caries includes removal of the decayed material and the refilling of the cavity with an amalgam of silver or another restorative material. If the lesion has reached the nerve tissues of the tooth, it may be necessary to remove the nerve tissue to alleviate pain, to prevent the spread of infection to the rest of the body, and to allow the continued use of the natural tooth. Alternatively, the entire tooth may be extracted. The development of dental caries in a debilitated patient is a concern because of the danger that infections of the teeth or gingival tissues might spread to the rest of the body. In addition, missing, decayed, or painful teeth inhibit mastication and can lead to dietary changes, which may in turn cause nutritional and digestive disorders. Kinds of dental caries include **active caries, arrested caries, primary caries,** and **secondary caries.**

dental crypt, the space occupied by a developing tooth.

dental engine, an apparatus consisting of a hand instrument to which various rotating tools or drills can be fitted. It is driven by an electric motor via a continuous cordlike belt.

dental erosion, the chemical or mechanicochemical destruction of a tooth substance that causes variously shaped concavities at the cementoenamel junctions of teeth. The

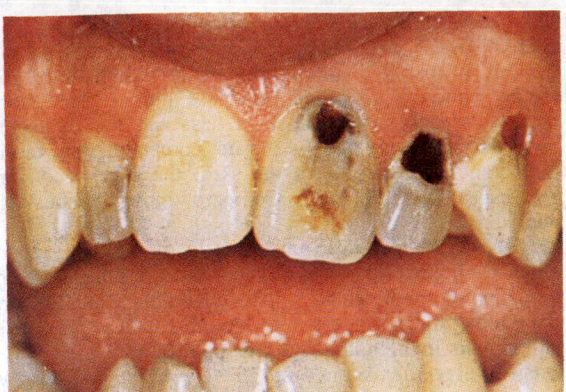

Recurrent dental caries (Grundy, 1992)

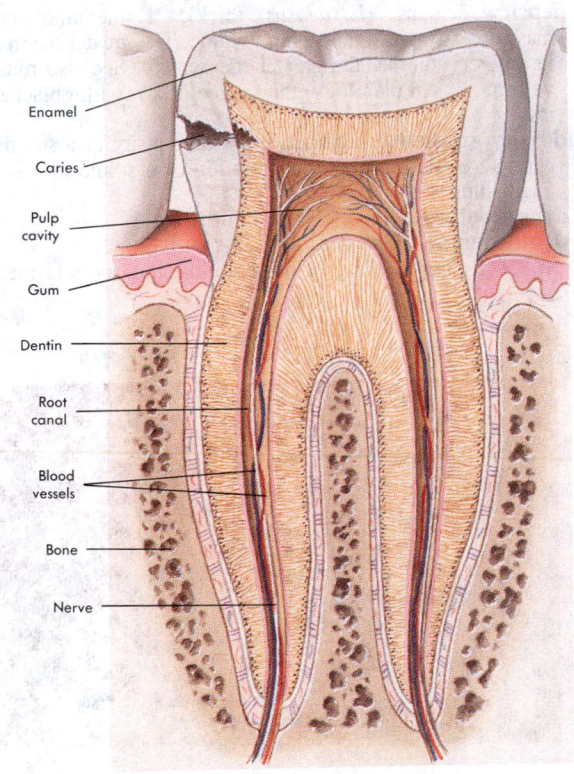

Dental decay (Wardlaw, 1993)

Black's system of classification of caries

Class I	Located in pits and fissures of the occlusal two thirds of posterior teeth or on the lingual surface of anterior teeth
Class II	Located on the proximal surfaces of premolars and molars
Class III	Located on the proximal surfaces of central and lateral incisors and cuspids
Class IV	Located at the gingival third of the facial or lingual surfaces of anterior or posterior teeth
Class V	Located at the gingival third of the facial or lingual surfaces of anterior or posterior teeth
Class VI	Located on cusp tips

Adapted from Woodall IR, Dafoe BR, Young NS, et al: *Comprehensive dental hygiene care,* ed 3, St Louis, 1989, Mosby.

surfaces of these depressions, unlike those of carious cavities, are hard and smooth.

dental ethics [L, *dens,* tooth; Gk, *ethos,* ethics], a sense of moral obligation and a system of moral principles governing the professional conduct of dental and dental hygiene practices.

dental extracting forceps, a type of forceps used for grasping teeth in extractions. Most forceps are designed for the extraction of a particular tooth in the maxilla or mandible.

dental film, a type of x-ray film made for either intraoral or extraoral exposure. Intraoral films are small, double-emulsion films without screens but with a lead foil backing to reduce patient dose. Extraoral films are large single-emulsion screen films.

dental fistula, an abnormal passage from the apical periodontal area of a tooth to the surface of oral mucous membrane, permitting the discharge of inflammatory or suppurative material. Also called **alveolar fistula.**

dental floss, a waxed or unwaxed thread used to clean interproximal tooth surfaces or spaces between the teeth.

dentalgia /dental'jē·ə/ [L, *dens,* tooth; Gk, *algos,* pain], toothache.

dental granuloma, a pathpological condition characterized by a mass of granulation tissue which is surrounded by a fibrous capsule attached to the apex of a pulp-involved tooth. On x-ray film it appears as a well-defined radiolucency.

dental hygienist, a person with special training to provide dental services under the supervision of a dentist. Services supplied by a dental hygienist include dental prophylaxis, radiography, application of medications, and provision of dental education at chairside and in the community.

dental identification [L, *dens,* tooth, *idem,* the same, *facere,* to make], the process of establishing the unique characteristics of the teeth and dental work of an individual, thereby leading to the identification of an individual by comparison with the person's dental charts and records.

dental implant, a plastic or metal device that is implanted in the jaw bones to provide permanent support for fixed bridges or dentures when there is insufficient bony ridge to support a denture.

dental jurisprudence [L, *dens,* tooth, *juris prudentia,* knowledge of the law], the application of the principles of law as they relate to the practice of dentistry, and the relations of dentists to patients, to society, and to each other.

dental laboratory technician, a person who makes dental prostheses and orthdodontic appliances as prescribed by a dentist. The dental laboratory technician may have a private laboratory or work in the premises of a dentist. Also called **dental technician.**

dental operculum [L, *dens,* tooth, *operculum,* a covering structure], a hood or flap of gingival tissue overlying the crown of an erupting tooth. This tissue disappears as the tooth erupts by being chewed away.

dental papilla [L, *dens,* tooth, *papilla,* a nippleshaped projection], a small mass of mesenchymal tissue in the enamel organ, which differentiates into dentin and dental pulp. The innermost layer consists of a cell-free zone of reticular fibers that form the basement membrane.

dental pathology [L, *dens,* tooth; Gk, *pathos,* disease, *logos,* science]. See **oral pathology, pathodontia.**

dental plaque. See **bacterial plaque.**

dental plate [L, *dens,* tooth; OFr, *plate,* a flat structure], a dental prosthesis made to the shape of the maxillary or mandibular jaw to support artificial teeth.

dental probe. See **periodontal probe.**

dental prosthesis [L, *dens,* tooth; Gk, *prosthesis,* an addition], a fixed or removable appliance to replace one or more lost natural teeth.

dental pulp, a small mass of connective tissue, blood vessels, and nerves located in a chamber within the dentin layer of a tooth. See also **pulp canal, pulp cavity.**

dental radiograph [L, *dens,* tooth; L, *radire,* to shine; Gk, *graphein,* to record], an intraoral and extraoral x-ray film

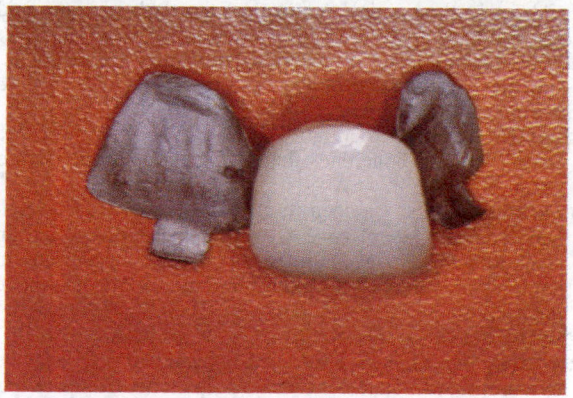

Dental prosthesis *(Jordan, 1993)*

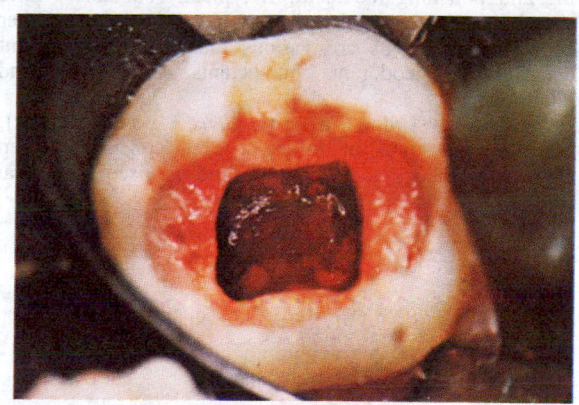

Dental pulp *(Grundy, 1992)*

of teeth and the bone surrounding them. See also **bite wing radiograph, periapical radiograph.**

dental restoration. See **restoration.**

dental root cyst. See **periodontal cyst.**

dental sealants /sē'lənts/, plastic film coatings that are applied and adhere to the chewing surfaces of teeth to seal pits and grooves where food and bacteria usually become trapped. The procedure involves isolation of the teeth to be treated to ensure that saliva contamination will not interfere with the process. The tooth surfaces are cleaned with a brush and pumice cleansing agent, then dried and etched with a phosphoric-acid solution. After the acid has been washed away, a resin sealant is applied. Dental sealants are reported to reduce the incidence of cavities in children's teeth by 50%. Also called **pit and fissure sealants.**

dental stone. See **artificial stone.**

dental surgeon [L, *dens,* tooth; Gk, *cheirourgos,* surgeon], a dentist who specializes in the teeth and surrounding oral tissues. An **operative dental surgeon** is concerned with the with the restoration of teeth that have been damaged. An **oral and maxillofacial surgeon** specializes in surgically reconstructing facial malformations caused by diseases of the head and neck or traumatic accidents. An **oral surgeon** specializes in the surgical removal of the teeth and surrounding oral tissues.

dental technician.   See **dental laboratory techician.**

-dentate, a suffix meaning 'possessing teeth': *edentate, multidentate, tridentate.*

dentate fracture /den'tāt/ [L, *dens*], any fracture that causes serrated bone ends that fit together like the teeth of gears.

dentate nucleus, a deep cerebellar nucleus. It receives fibers from the lateral zone of the cerebellar cortex and appears to act as a trigger for the motor cortex, governing intentional movements as well as properties of ongoing movements.

denti-, dentia-.   See **dento-.**

denticle /den'tikəl/, a calcified body in the pulp chamber of a tooth. Also called **endolith, pulp stone.** Compare **true denticle.**

dentifrice /den'tifris/ [L, *dens* + *fricare*, to rub], a pharmaceutic compound used with a toothbrush for cleaning and polishing the teeth. It typically contains a mild abrasive, a detergent, flavoring agent, and a binder. Other common ingredients are various medications to prevent dental caries, deodorants, humectants, desensitizers, and flavorings.

dentigerous cyst /dentij'ərəs/ [L, *dens* + *gerere*, to bear], one of three kinds of follicular cyst, consisting of an epithelium-lined sac, filled with fluid or viscous material that surrounds the crown of an unerupted tooth or odontoma. Compare **primordial cyst, multilocular cyst.**

dentin /den'tin/ [L, *dens*], the chief material of teeth, surrounding the pulp and situated inside of the enamel and cementum. Harder and denser than bone, it consists of solid organic substratum infiltrated with lime salts. Also spelled **dentine.**

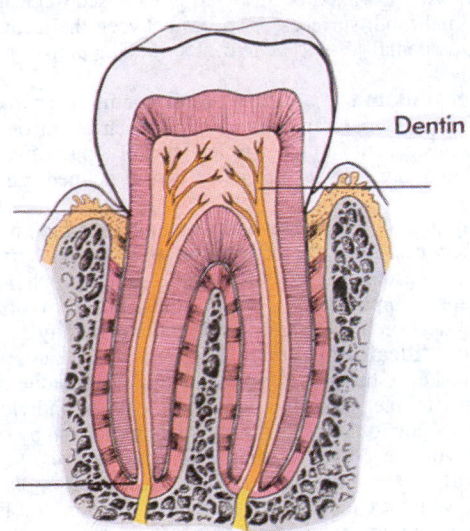

Position of dentin in a normal tooth *(Potter, 1993)*

dentin eburnation /ē'burnā'shən/, a change in carious teeth in which softened and decalcified dentin develops a hard, brown, polished appearance.

dentin globule, a small spheric body in peripheral dentin, created by early calcification.

dentinoenamel /den'tinō·inam'əl/ [L, *dens* + OFr, *enesmail*, enamel], pertaining to both the dentin and the enamel of the teeth.

dentinoenamel junction, the interface of the enamel and the dentin of a tooth crown, generally conforming to the shape of the crown. Also called **dentoenamel junction.**

dentinogenesis /den'tinōjen'əsis/ [L, *dens* + Gk, *genein*, to produce], the formation of the dentin of the teeth. **—dentinogenic,** *adj.*

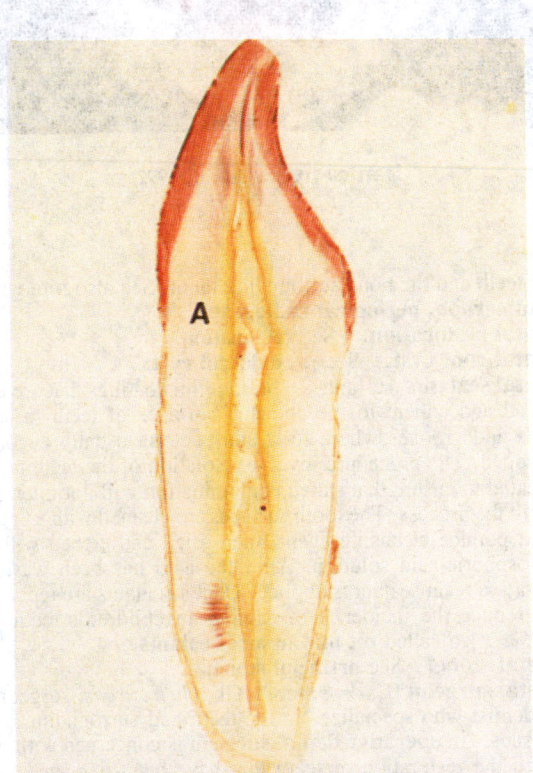

Distribution of dentin
(Berkovitz, 1992)

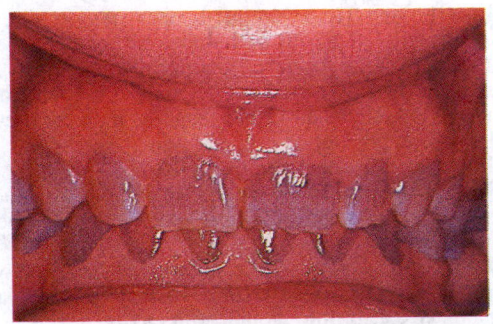

Dentinogenesis imperfecta *(Zitelli, 1992)*

dentinogenesis imperfecta, hereditary dysplasia of dentin of deciduous and permanent teeth in which brown, opalescent dentin overgrows and obliterates the pulp cavity. The teeth have short roots and wear rapidly. Early restorative dentistry is indicated. The condition is often associated with osteogenesis imperfecta and other congenital mesodermal dysplasias.

-dentinogenic. See **dentinogenesis.**

dentist [L, *dens*], a person who is qualified by training and licensed by the state to practice dentistry. Training requires a minimum of 2 years, preferably 4, in an undergraduate college and a satisfactory score on a Dental Aptitude Test (DAT), followed by 4 years at an ADA-accredited dental college. After completing dental college, a dentist is awarded a degree of either Doctor of Dental Surgery (D.D.S.) or Doctor of Dental Medicine (D.M.D.), which are equivalent degrees. Dental internships and residencies are not required for general practice, although written and practical examinations must be passed to obtain a state license. In various states, licensing requirements can be met by providing a certificate from the National Board of Dental Examiners in place of a written test and by taking the practical examination before a Regional Dental Examining Board rather than appearing before a state board. See also **dentistry.**

dentistry /den′tistrē/ [L, *dens*], the art and science of practicing the prevention and treatment of diseases and disorders of the teeth and surrounding structures of the oral cavity. Responsibilities include the repair and restoration of teeth and replacement of missing teeth, as well as the detection of signs of diseases, such as blood dyscrasias and tumors, that would require treatment by a physician. In addition to the general practice of dentistry, there are eight recognized specialties, each requiring additional training after graduation from a dental college: **endodontics, oral pathology, maxofacial surgery, orthodontics, pediatric dentistry, periodontics, prosthodontics,** and **public health dentistry.**

dentition /dentish′ən/ [L, *dentire*, to cut teeth], **1.** the development and eruption of the teeth. See also **teething. 2.** the arrangement, number, and kind of teeth as they appear in the dental arch of the mouth. **3.** the teeth of an individual or species as determined by their form and arrangement. Kinds of dentition include **artificial dentition, deciduous dentition, mixed dentition, natural dentition, permanent dentition, precocious dentition, predeciduous dentition,** and **retarded dentition.**

dento-, dent-, denta-, denti-, dentia-, a combining form meaning 'pertaining to a tooth or the teeth': *dentography, dentoidin, dentonomy.*

dentoalveolar abscess /den′tō·alvē′ələr/ [L, *dens + alveolus*, little hollow; *abscedere*, to go away], the formation and accumulation of pus in a tooth socket or the jawbone around the base of a tooth. The pus results from a bacterial infection that is usually secondary to an infection or injury to the tooth or alveolar tissues. Also called **periapical abscess.**

dentoalveolar cyst. See **periodontal cyst.**

dentoenamal junction. See **dentinoenamal junction.**

dentofacial /-fā′shəl/, of or pertaining to an oral or gnathic structure.

dentofacial anomaly, an abnormality in which an oral or gnathic structure deviates from the normal in form, function, or position.

PRIMARY TEETH	Eruption (mo)	Shedding (yr)
Central incisor	9.6	7.5
Lateral incisor	12.4	8
Cuspid (canine)	18.3	11.5
Bicuspid	15.7	10.5
Molar	26.2	10.5
Molar	26.0	11
Bicuspid	15.1	10
Cuspid (canine)	18.2	9.5
Lateral incisor	11.5	7
Central incisor	7.8	6

SECONDARY TEETH	Eruption (yr)
Central incisor	7.35
Lateral incisor	8.45
Cuspid (canine)	11.35
First bicuspid	10.2
Second bicuspid	11.05
First molar	6.3
Second molar	12.25
Third molar	(17-21) Variable
Third molar	11.9
Second molar	6.05
First molar	11.2
Second bicuspid	10.5
First biscuspid	10.35
Cuspid (canine)	7.5
Lateral incisor	6.4
Central incisor	(17-21) Variable

Dentition

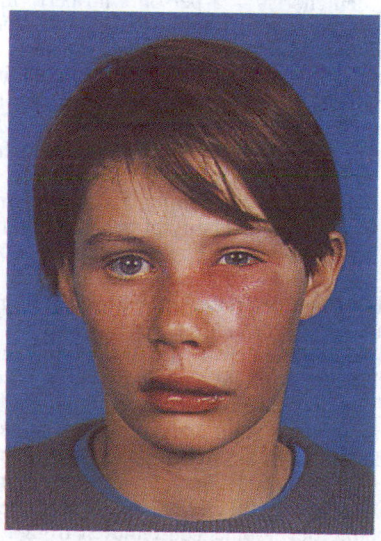

Facial swelling caused by dentoalveolar abscess
(Lamey, 1988)

dentogenesis imperfecta /-jen′əsis/, **1.** a genetic disturbance of the dentin, characterized by early calcification of the pulp chambers, marked attrition, and an opalescent hue to the teeth. **2.** a localized form of mesodermal dysplasia affecting the dentin of the teeth. It may be hereditary and associated with osteogenesis imperfecta. **3.** also called **hereditary opalescent dentin.** a genetic condition that produces defective dentin but normal tooth enamel.

dentogingival fiber /-jinjī′vəl/ [L, *dens + gingiva*, gum], any one of the many fibers that spread like a fan, emerge from the supraalveolar portion of the cementum, and terminate in the free gingiva.

dentogingival junction, the junction between the gingival attachment, a nonkeratinized epithelium, and the surface of the teeth.

dentoperiosteal fiber /den'tōper'ē·os'tē·əl/ [L *dens* + Gk *peri* around, *osteon* bone], any one of the many fibers that emerge from the supraalveolar part of the cementum of a tooth and extend apically beyond the alveolar crest into the mucoperiosteum of the attached gingiva.

dentulous /den'tyələs/ [L, *dens*, tooth, *-ulosus*, characterized by], possessing one or more natural teeth.

dentulous dental arch, a dental arch that contains natural teeth.

denture /den'chər/ [L, *dens*, tooth], an artificial tooth or a set of artificial teeth not permanently fixed or implanted. Compare **fixed bridgework.**

denture base, 1. the portion of a denture that fits the oral mucosa of the basal seat and supports artificial teeth. 2. the part of a denture that covers the soft tissue of the mouth, commonly made of resin or a combination of resins and metal.

denture-bearing area. See **basal seat area.**

denture flask, a sectional metal case in which plaster of paris or artificial stone is molded, and in which dentures or other resin restorations are processed.

denture packing, the laboratory procedure of filling and compressing a denture-base material into a mold in a flask.

denturist /den'chərist/, a person who performs the same type of work as a dental laboratory technician but without a dentist's prescription, providing dental prostheses directly to clients. In the United States, the practice is limited by laws to certain states. See also **dental laboratory technician.**

denucleated /dēnyo͞o'klē·ā'tid/ [L, *de*, from, *nucleus*, nut], pertaining to a condition in which the nucleus has been removed.

Denver Articulation Screening Examination (DASE), a test for evaluating the clarity of pronunciation in children between 2½ and 6 years of age. Each child's performance may be compared with a standardized norm for the age.

Denver classification, the system of identifying and classifying human chromosomes according to the criteria established at the Denver (1960), London (1963), and Chicago (1966) conferences of cytogeneticists. It is based on chromosome size and position of the centromere as determined during mitotic metaphase and is divided into seven major groups, designated A through G, which are arranged according to decreasing length. See **chromosome, karyotype.**

Denver Developmental Screening Test (DDST), a test for evaluating development in children from 1 month to 6 years of age. The developmental level of motor, social, and language skills may be discovered by comparing the child's performance with the average performance of other children. The score, or the developmental age, is expressed as a ratio in which the child's age is the denominator and the age at which the norm possesses skills equal to those of the child being tested is the numerator.

deodorant /dē·ō'dərənt/ [L, *de* + *odor*, smell], 1. destroying or masking odors. 2. a substance that destroys or masks odors. Underarm deodorants are available as sprays, creams, solid gels, and liquids containing an antiperspirant, as aluminum chloride, aluminum hydroxyl, aluminum sulfate, or aluminum zirconyl hydroxychloride. These aluminum salts form an obstructive hydroxide gel in sweat ducts. Aluminum salts may produce an allergic reaction in some

individuals, and hydrolyzed aluminum chloride can cause local tissue necrosis. Some underarm deodorants contain antibacterial agents or fragrances. Vaginal deodorant sprays contain a fatty ester emollient, a masking fragrance, and an antimicrobial agent, such as benzethonium chloride, chlorhexidine hydrochloride, or triacetin, and are often associated with allergic reactions. Room and breath deodorants contain masking agents, such as mint, pine, eucalyptus, lemon, lavender, rosemary, sassafras, or thyme. Ozone masks odors by decreasing olfactory sensitivity. Chlorophyll has a deodorizing action that is enhanced by croconic acid. Also called **antibromic.**

deodorized alcohol /dē·ō'dərīzd'/, a liquid, free of organic impurities, containing 92.5% absolute alcohol.

deontologism /dē'ontol'əgiz'əm/ [Gk, *deon*, obligation, *logos*, science], a doctrine of ethics that states that moral duty or obligation is binding; also, that which makes acts right are nonconsequential characteristics such as fidelity, veracity, justice, and honesty. Compare **natural law, utilitarianism.**

deossification /dē·os'ifikā'shən/, the loss of mineral matter from bones.

deoxy-, desoxy-, a prefix meaning 'containing a decreased amount of oxygen': *deoxygenation, desoxymorphine, desoxyribose.*

deoxygenation /dē·ōk'sijənā'shən/ [L, *de*, from; Gk, *oxys*, sharp, *genein*, to produce], the removal of oxygen from a chemical compound.

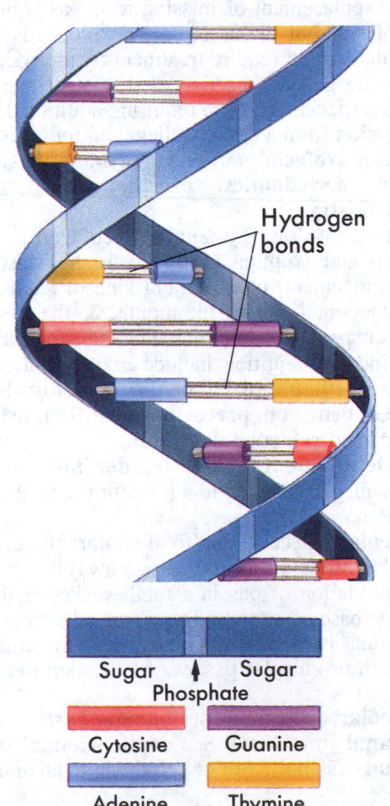

Hydrogen bonds

Sugar   Sugar
Phosphate

Cytosine   Guanine

Adenine   Thymine

Watson-Crick model of DNA
(Thibodeau, 1993/Joan M Beck)

deoxyribonucleic acid (DNA) /dē·ok′sirī′bōnooklē′ik/, a large nucleic acid molecule, found principally in the chromosomes of the nucleus of a cell, that is the carrier of genetic information. The genetic information is coded in the sequence of the nitrogenous, molecular subunits that are constituents of the deoxyribonucleic acid molecule. Also called **desoxyribonucleic acid.** See also **nucleic acid, ribonucleic acid.**

Depakene, a trademark for an anticonvulsant (valproic acid).

Department of Health and Human Services (DHHS), a cabinet-level department of the U.S. government with the responsibility for functions of various federal social welfare and health delivery agencies, such as the Food and Drug Administration (FDA). It also directs the U.S. Office of Consumer Affairs, Office of Civil Rights, Administration on Aging, Public Health Service, Indian Health Service, Social Security Administration, and National Institutes of Health.

Department of Transportation (DOT), a cabinet-level department of the U.S. government responsible for national transportation policies, including maritime, aviation, railroad, and highway safety and regulation of the transport of hazardous materials, such as medical gases.

-depend. See **dependent.**

dependence /dipen′dəns/ [L, de + pendere, to hang upon], **1.** the state of being dependent. **2.** the total psychophysical state of one addicted to drugs or alcohol who must receive an increasing amount of the substance to prevent the onset of abstinence symptoms.

dependency needs /dipen′dənsē/, the sum of the physical and emotional requirements of an infant for survival, including parenting, love, affection, shelter, protection, food, andwarmth. Reliance on others to satisfy these needs decreases with age and maturity; continuance in later years, in overt or latent form, is indicative of a pathologic emotional disorder. These needs may increase under stress, as during physical illness, in which case they do not reflect a psychopathologic condition. Compare **emotional need.**

dependent, of or pertaining to a condition of being reliant on someone or something else for help, support, favor, and other need, as a child is dependent on a parent, a narcotics addict is dependent on a drug, or one variable is dependent on another variable. **–depend,** v.

dependent differentiation. See **correlative differentiation.**

dependent edema [L, de, from, pendere, to hand; Gk, oidema, swelling], a fluid accumulation in the tissues influenced by gravity. It is usually greater in the lower part of the body than in tissues above the level of the heart.

dependent intervention, a therapeutic action based on the written or verbal orders of another health professional.

dependent personality, behavior characterized by excessive or compulsive needs for attention, acceptance, and approval from other people to maintain security and self-esteem.

dependent personality disorder, a mental state characterized by a lack of self-confidence and an inability to function independently.

dependent variable, (in research) a factor that is measured to learn the effect of one or more independent variables; for example, in a study of the effect of preoperative nursing intervention on postoperative vomiting, vomiting is the dependent variable measured to determine the effect of the nursing intervention. Compare **independent variable.**

depersonalization /dēpur′sənəlīzā′shən/ [L de + persona mask], a feeling of strangeness or unreality concerning oneself or the environment, often resulting from anxiety, stress, or fatigue. See also **alienation, depersonalization disorder.**

depersonalization disorder, an emotional disturbance characterized by depersonalization feelings in which a dreamlike atmosphere pervades the consciousness. The body may not feel like one's own, and dramatic and important events may be watched with equanimity. The reaction is commonly seen in various forms of schizophrenia and in severe depression.

depilation /dep′ilā′shən/ [L, de + pilum, hair], the removal or extraction of hair from the body, either temporarily by mechanical or chemical means or permanently, by electrolysis, which destroys the hair follicle. Also called **epilation. –depilate,** v.

depilatory /dipil′ətôrē/, **1.** of or pertaining to a substance or procedure that removes hair. **2.** a depilatory agent.

depilatory techniques [L, depilare, to deprive of hair; Gk, technikos, skillful], methods of removing unwanted body hair, such as by plucking, external application of chemicals, electrolyis, or the application of melted wax.

depolarization /dēpō′lərīzā′shən/, the reduction of a membrane potential to a less negative value. The positive current responsible for the buildup of positive ions on the inside of the cell is called a depolarizing current. In neurons and muscle fibers, volt-gated channels in the membranes of cells change shape in response to stimuli and allow the influx of sodium. In muscle cells, both sodium and calcium enter the cell during depolarization. Calcium is the cation responsible for muscle contractions.

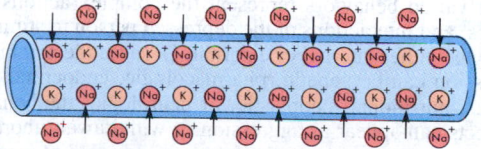

Depolarization and repolarization
(Thibodeau, 1993/Rolin Graphics)

deposition /dep′əzish′ən/ [L, deponere, to lay down], (in law) a sworn pretrial testimony given by a witness in response to oral or written questions and cross-examination. The deposition is transcribed and may be used for further pretrial investigation. It may also be presented at the trial if the witness cannot be present. Compare **discovery, interrogatories.**

depot /dē′pō, dep′ō/ [Fr, depository], **1.** any area of the body in which drugs or other substances, as fat, are stored and from which they can be distributed. **2.** (of a drug) injected or implanted to be slowly absorbed into the circulation.

depot injection, an intramuscular injection of a drug in an oil suspension that results in a gradual release of the medication over a period of several days.

depressant /dipres′ənt/ [L, deprimere, to press down], **1.** (of a drug) tending to decrease the function or activity of a system of the body. **2.** such a drug; for example, a cardiac depressant, central nervous system depressant, or a respiratory depressant.

depressed [L, deprimere, to press down], **1.** pertaining to a body structure that has been forced below the surface of surrounding parts, as in a fracture. **2.** pertaining to a condition in which general bodily activity is diminished, often accompanied by emotional dejection, loss of initiative, listlessness, loss of appetite, and concentration difficulty.

depressed fracture, any fracture of the skull in which fragments are depressed below the normal surface of the skull.

depression /dipresh′ən/ [L, *deprimere,* to press down], **1.** a depressed area, hollow, or fossa; downward or inward displacement. **2.** a decrease of vital functional activity. **3.** a mood disturbance characterized by feelings of sadness, despair, and discouragement resulting from and normally proportionate to some personal loss or tragedy. **4.** an abnormal emotional state characterized by exaggerated feelings of sadness, melancholy, dejection, worthlessness, emptiness, and hopelessness that are inappropriate and out of proportion to reality. The overt manifestations, which are extremely variable, range from a slight lack of motivation and inability to concentrate to severe physiologic alterations of body functions and may represent symptoms of a variety of mental and physical conditions, a syndrome of related symptoms associated with a particular disease, or a specific mental illness. The condition is neurotic when the precipitating cause is an intrapsychic conflict or a traumatic situation or event that is identifiable, even though the person is unable to explain the overreaction to it. The condition is psychotic when there is severe physical and mental functional impairment because of some unidentifiable intrapsychic conflict; it is often accompanied by hallucinations, delusions, and confusion concerning time, place, and identity. Depression may be expressed in a wide spectrum of affective, physiologic, cognitive, and behavioral manifestations. The varied behaviors represent the complex actions, reactions, and interactions of the depressed person to stimuli that may be either internal or external. Because the origin of depression can be genetic, pharmacologic, endocrinal, infectious, nutritional, neoplastic, or neurologic, the behavioral effects can appear as aggression or withdrawal, anorexia or overeating, anger or apathy or any of a myriad of responses. Kinds of depression include **agitated depression, anaclitic depression, endogenous depression, involutional melancholia, reactive depression,** and **retarded depression.** See also **bipolar disorder. -depressive,** *adj.*

depression with psychotic features [L, *deprimere,* to press down; Gk, *psyche,* mind, *osis,* condition], a psychosis in which a major diagnostic sign is depression.

-depressive. See **depression.**

depressor /dipres′ər/ [L, *deprimere,* to press down], any agent that reduces activity when applied to nerves and muscles. See also **depressant.**

depressor reflex [L, *deprimere,* to press down, *reflectere,* to bend back], a reflexive vasodilatation, or fall in arterial blood pressure, as may result from stimulation of the carotid sinus.

depressor septi /sep′tī/, one of the three muscles of the nose. Arising from the maxilla and inserting into the septum and the posterior aspect of the ala, it lies between the mucous membrane and the muscular structure of the lip and is a direct antagonist of the other muscles of the nose. It is innervated by buccal branches of the facial nerve and serves to draw the ala down, constricting the nostril. Compare **nasalis, procerus.**

deprivation /dep′rivā′shən/ [L, *deprivare,* to deprive], the loss of something considered valuable or necessary by taking it away or denying access to it. In experimental psychology, animal or human subjects may be deprived of something desired or expected for study of their reactions.

deprivation of sleep effects [L, *de, privare;* to deprive; ME, *slep;* L, *efficere,* to accomplish], the deliberate prevention of sleep resulting in progressive mental aberrations after 30 to 60 continuous hours. After this point, boring tasks become intolerable, speech begins to become slurred, and performance becomes increasingly poor. After a week of sleep deprivation, symptoms of psychosis may appear.

depth dose [AS, *diop;* Gk, *dosis,* giving], (in radiotherapy) the relationship between dose at any depth from a beam of radiation compared with the dose at the entrance from that beam.

depth electroencephalography. See **electroencephalography.**

depth perception, the ability to judge depth or the relative distance of objects in space and to orient one's position in relation to them. Binocular vision is essential to this ability.

depth psychology, any approach to psychology that emphasizes the study of personality and behavior in relation to unconscious motivation. See also **psychoanalysis.**

de Quervain's fracture /də kərvänz′/ [Fritz de Quervain, Swiss surgeon, b. 1868], fracture of the navicular bone of the hand, with dislocation of the lunate bone.

de Quervain's thyroiditis [Fritz de Quervain; Gk, *thyreos,* shield, *itis,* inflammation], an inflammatory condition of the thyroid, characterized by swelling and tenderness of the gland, fever, dysphagia, fatigue, and severe pain in the neck, ears, and jaw. The disorder often occurs after a viral infection of the upper respiratory tract and tends to remit spontaneously and to recur several times. The diagnosis may be made by a radiologic scan showing depressed uptake of radioactive iodine in involved areas. Occasionally, a needle biopsy of the thyroid is performed. Treatment may include antiinflammatory medication, such as aspirin or thyroid hormone, if the condition continues for more than a few days. Corticosteroids are prescribed for prolonged or severe cases. Also called **giant cell thyroiditis, granulomatous thyroiditis, subacute thyroiditis.**

der, (in cytogenetics) abbreviation for *derivative chromosome.*

der-, a prefix meaning 'pertaining to the neck': *deradelphus, deradenitis, deranencephalia.*

derailment /dirāl′mənt/, a pattern of speech in which incomprehensible, disconnected, and unrelated ideas replace logical and orderly thought.

derby hat fracture. See **dishpan fracture.**

dereflection /dē′rəflek′shən/ [L, *de* + *reflectere,* to bend backward], a technique of logotherapeutic psychology that is directed toward taking a person's mind off a certain goal through a positive redirection to another goal, with emphasis on assets and abilities rather than the problems at hand. Dereflection often results in accomplishment of the original goal.

dereistic thought /dē′rē·is′tik/ [L, *de* + *res,* thing], a type of mental activity in which fantasy is not modified by logic, experience, or reality.

derivative /dəriv′ətiv/ [L, *derivare,* to turn away], anything that is derived or obtained from another substance or object; for example, organs and tissues are derivatives of the primordial germ cells. Chemical derivatives may be produced to confirm identification of a compound.

derived protein /dirīvd′/,   a small protein obtained by enzymatic or chemical hydrolysis of a larger protein source, such as a proteose, peptone, or peptide.

derived quantity,   any secondary quantity derived from a combination of base quantities, such as mass, length, and time.

-derm,   a suffix meaning 'skin': *angioderm, mucoderm, paraderm.*

-derma, -dermia, -dermic,   1. a suffix meaning 'pertaining to the skin': *chrysderma, micoderma, sarcoderma.* **2.** a suffix meaning a '(specified) skin ailment or skin condition': *rhinoderma, syphiloderma, vaselinoderma.* **3.** a suffix meaning 'related to the variety of skin': *pachydermic.*

derma-.   See **dermato-.**

dermabrasion /dur′məbrā′zhən/ [Gk, *derma,* skin; L, *abradere,* to scrape],   a treatment for the removal of superficial scars on the skin by the use of revolving wire brushes or sandpaper. An aerosol spray is used to freeze the skin for this procedure. Dermabrasion is used to reduce facial scars of severe acne and to remove pigment from undesired tattoos.

Dermacentor /dur′məsen′tər/,   a genus of ticks. It includes species that transmit Rocky Mountain spotted fever, tularemia, brucellosis, and other infectious diseases. See also **Lyme disease.**

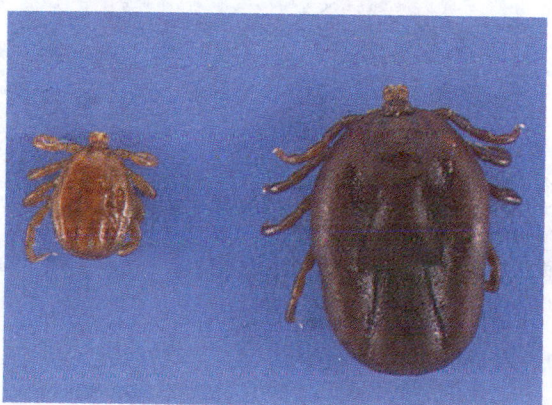

Dermacentor *(Muller, 1990)*

dermal /dur′məl/ [Gk, *derma,* skin],   pertaining to the skin.

dermal graft [Gk, *derma,* skin, *graphion,* stylus],   the transplantation of any living skin tissue that contains dermis and thus is capable of regenerating and secreting sweat and sebum, and generating new hair growth.

dermal papilla [Gk, *derma,* skin; L, *papilla,* nipple],   any small elevation in the skin, as the elongated alpine papilla seen in psoriasis.

dermat-.   See **dermato-.**

dermatitis /dur′mətī′tis/ [Gk, *derma* + *itis,* inflammation],   an inflammatory condition of the skin, characterized by erythema and pain or pruritus. Various cutaneous eruptions occur and may be unique to a particular allergen, disease, or infection. The condition may be chronic or acute; treatment is specific to the cause. Some kinds of dermatitis are **actinic dermatitis, contact dermatitis, rhus dermatitis,** and **seborrheic dermatitis.**

dermatitis exfoliativa neonatorum.   See **Ritter's disease.**

dermatitis herpetiformis,   a chronic, severely pruritic skin disease with symmetrically located groups of red, papulovesicular, vesicular, bullous, or urticarial lesions that leave hyperpigmented spots. It is occasionally associated with a malignancy of an internal organ or with celiac disease, patch, or IgA immunotherapy. Treatment may include a diet free of gluten and the administration of sulfone, dapsone, sulfapyridine, or antipruritic drugs.

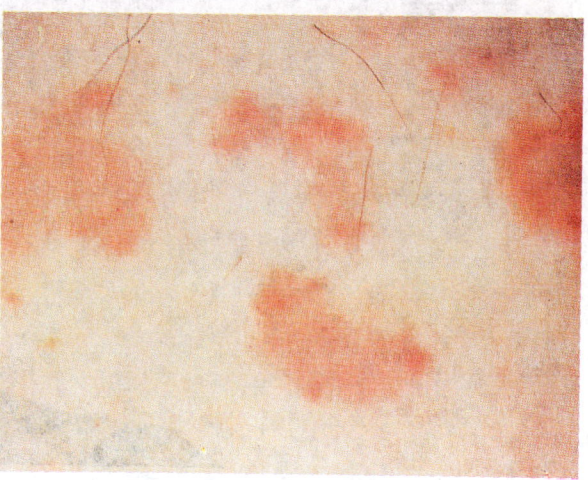

Dermatitis herpetiformis *(Epstein, 1992)*

dermatitis medicamentosa.   See **drug rash.**

dermatitis papillaris capillitii.   See **keloid acne.**

dermatitis venenata.   See **contact dermatitis.**

dermato-, derma-, dermat-, dermo-,   a combining form meaning 'pertaining to the skin': *dermatobiasis, dermatocele, dermatocyst.*

dermatocele /dur′mətōsēl′/ [Gk, *derma,* skin, *kele,* hernia],   an overgrowth of skin and subcutaneous tissue that hangs in pendulous folds.

dermatocyst /dur′mətōsist′/,   a cystic tumor of cutaneous tissues.

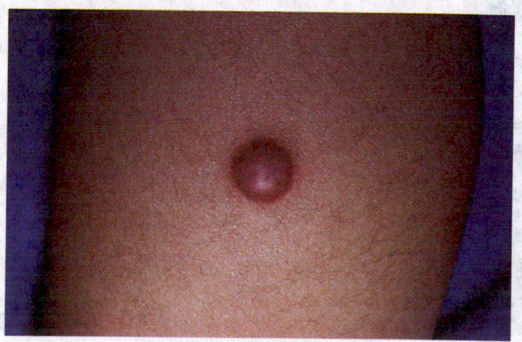

Dermatofibroma *(Weston, 1991)*

dermatofibroma /dur′mətōfībrō′mə/, *pl.* **dermatofibromas, dermatofibromata** [Gk, *derma* + L, *fibra*, fiber, *oma*, tumor], a cutaneous nodule that is painless, round, firm, gray or red, elevated and commonly found on the extremities. No treatment is required. Also called **fibrous histiocytoma.**

dermatofibrosarcoma /-fī′brōsärkō′mə/ [Gk, *derma*, skin; L, *fibra*, fiber; Gk, *sarx*, flesh, *oma*, tumor], a fibrosarcoma or fibrous tumor of the skin.

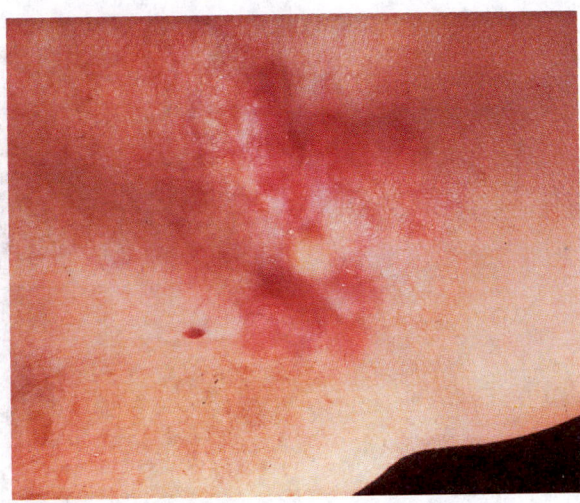

Dermatofibrosarcoma protuberans
(du Vivier, 1992/Courtesy Dr. Neil Smith)

dermatoglyphics /dur′mətōglif′iks/ [Gk, *derma* + *glyphe*, a carving], the study of the skin ridge patterns on fingers, toes, palms of hands, and soles of feet. The patterns are used as a basis of identification and also have diagnostic value because of associations between certain patterns and chromosomal anomalies.

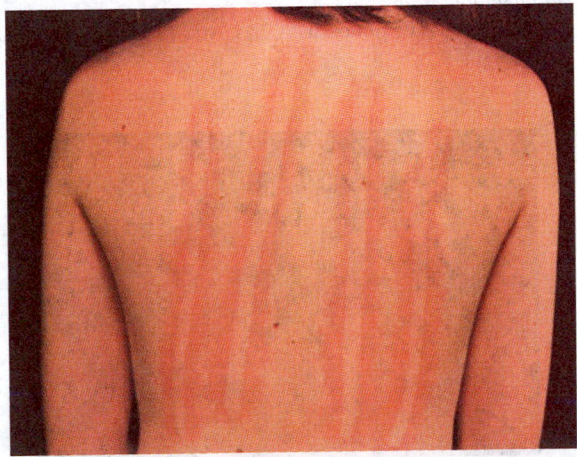

Dermatographia *(Cerio, 1992)*

dermatographia /dur′mətōgraf′ē·ə/ [Gk, *derma* + *graphein*, to record], a skin condition characterized by wheals that develop from tracing on the skin with the fingernail or a blunted instrument. This condition makes the skin especially susceptible to irritation and may be associated with urticaria. Also called **autographism, dermatographism, Ebbecke's reaction.**

dermatologist /dur′mətol′əjist/, a physician specializing in disorders of the skin.

dermatology /-ol′əjē/ [Gk, *derma* + *logos*, science], the study of the skin, including the anatomy, physiology, and pathology of the skin and the diagnosis and treatment of skin disorders.

dermatome /dur′mətōm/ [Gk, *derma* + *temnein*, to cut], **1.** (in embryology) the mesodermal layer in the early developing embryo that gives rise to the dermal layers of the skin. **2.** (in surgery) an instrument used to cut thin slices of skin for grafting. **3.** an area on the surface of a body innervated by afferent fibers from one spinal root.

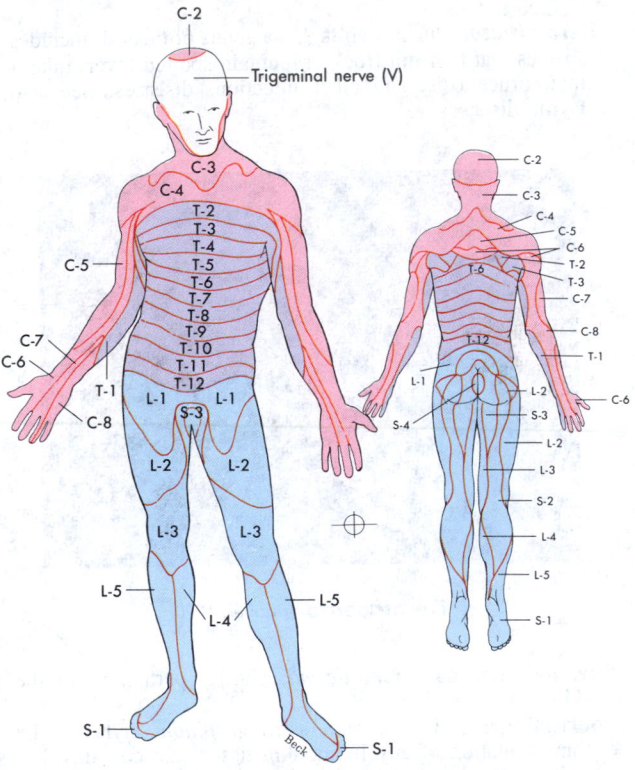

Dermatome distribution of spinal nerves
(Thibodeau, 1993/Ernest Beck)

dermatomycosis /dur′mətō′mīkō′sis/ [Gk, *derma* + *mykes*, fungus, *osis*, condition], a superficial fungal infection of the skin, characteristically found on parts that are moist and protected by clothing, such as the groin or feet. It is caused by a dermatophyte. See also **dermatophytosis.** —**dermatomycotic,** *adj.*

dermatomyositis /dur′mətōmī′ōsī′tis/ [Gk, *derma* + *mys*, muscle, *itis*, inflammation], a disease of the connective tissues, characterized by pruritic or eczematous inflammation of the skin and tenderness and weakness of the muscles. Muscle tissue is destroyed, and loss is often so severe that the person may become unable to walk or to perform simple tasks. Swelling of the eyelids and face and loss of weight are common manifestations. The cause is unknown, but in 15% of cases the condition develops with an internal malignancy. Viral infection and antibacterial medication are also associated with an increased incidence of dermatomyositis.

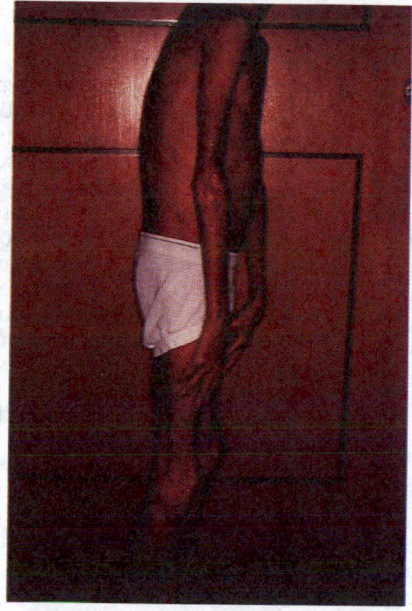

Dermatomyositis (Zitelli, 1992)

Dermatophagoides farinae /-fagoi′dēz/ [Gk, *derma* + *phagein*, to eat, *eidos*, form],   a ubiquitous species of household dust mite responsible for allergic reactions in sensitive individuals. Protection against the microscopically small mite includes use of insecticides, vacuum cleaning, and control of the temperature and humidity. The mites thrive on skin scales, hair, pet foods, carpets, and bedding, in addition to ordinary house dust.

dermatophyte /dur′mətōfīt′, dərmat′əfīt/,   any of several fungi that cause parasitic skin disease in humans. See also **dermatophytid**, and see specific fungal infections.

dermatophytid /dur′mətof′itid, dur′mətōfī′tid/ [Gk, *derma* + *phyton*, plant],   an allergic skin reaction characterized by small vesicles and associated with dermatomycosis. The lesions result from sensitization to the infection elsewhere on the skin and do not contain fungi. See also **dermatomycosis, dermatophyte.**

dermatophytosis /dur′mətō′fītō′sis/ [Gk, *derma* + *phyton*, plant, *osis*, condition],   a superficial fungus infection of the skin, caused by *Microsporum, Epidermophyton,* or *Trichophyton* species of dermatophyte. On the trunk and upper extremities it is commonly called 'ringworm' infection and is characterized by round or oval, scaly patches with slightly raised borders and clearing centers. On the feet small vesicles, cracking, itching, scaling, and often secondary bacte-

rial infections occur and are commonly called "athlete's foot." Treatment includes topical antifungal agents, as tolnaftate, clotrimazole, and undecylenic acid, and oral griseofulvin. Fingernails and toenails respond poorly to topical treatment. See also **tinea.**

dermatoplasty /dur′mətōplas′tē/,   a surgical procedure in which skin tissue is transplanted to a body surface damaged by disease or injury.

dermatosclerosis /-sklərō′sis/ [Gk, *derma* + *sklerosis,* hardening],   a skin disease characterized by fibrous infiltration of the fatty subcutaneous tissue, leading to patches of thick, leatherlike skin. See also **scleroderma.**

dermatosis /dur′mətō′sis/ [Gk, *derma* + *osis,* condition],   any disorder of the skin, especially those not associated with inflammation. Compare **dermatitis.**

dermatosis papulosa nigra,   a common skin condition in blacks consisting of multiple, tiny, benign, skin-colored or hyperpigmented papules on the cheeks. The lesions are permanent and increase in number with age.

dermis.   the layer of the skin, just below the epidermis, consisting of papillary and reticular layers and containing blood and lymphatic vessels, nerves and nerve endings, glands, and hair follicles. Formerly called **corium.**

-dermis,   a suffix meaning 'tissue or skin': *hypodermis, endepidermis, osteodermis.*

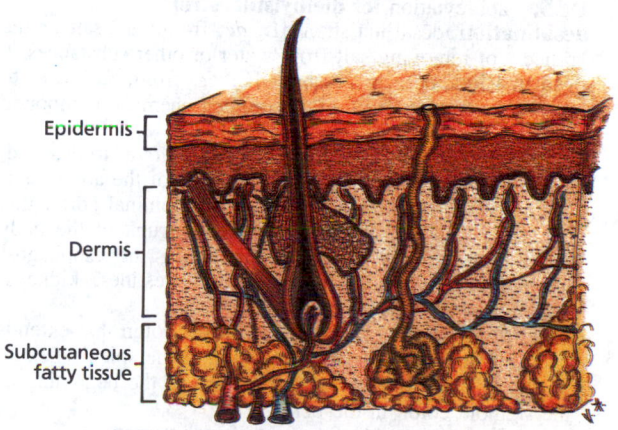

Dermis (Potter, 1993)

dermo-.   See **dermato-.**

dermographism.   See **dermatographia.**

dermoid /dur′moid/ [Gk, *derma* + *eidos,* form],   **1.** of or pertaining to the skin. **2.** *informal.* a dermoid cyst.

dermoid cyst,   a tumor, derived from embryonal tissues, consisting of a fibrous wall lined with epithelium and a cavity containing fatty material, hair, teeth, bits of bone, and cartilage. Kinds of dermoid cysts are **implantation dermoid cyst, inclusion dermoid cyst, thyroid dermoid cyst,** and **tubal dermoid cyst.** Also called **organoid tumor, teratoid tumor.** (See Fig. p. 464.)

-dermoma,   a suffix meaning a 'tumor of the skin layers': *epidermoma, monodermoma, tridermoma.*

derotation brace /dē′rōtā′shən/,   a customized orthosis that provides stability at the knee joint. It consists of a single-joint hinged bar on one side and a rotating dial pad on the opposite side. The rotating pad can be placed on ei-

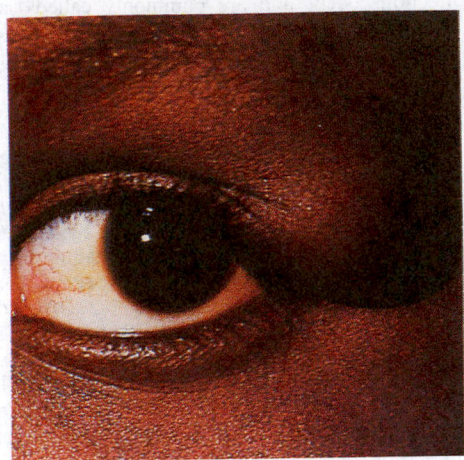

Dermoid cyst (*Zitelli, 1992*)

ther the medial or the lateral side, depending on the side with the primary instability. Each brace is designed individually, based on a negative plaster cast of the knee.

DES, abbreviation for **diethylstilbestrol.**

desalination /dēsal′inā′shən/ [L, *de*, from, *sal*, salt], the process of removing salt from water or other substances.

desaturation /dēsach′ərā′shən/ [L, *de*, from, *saturare*, to fill], the formation of an unsaturated chemical compound from a saturated one.

descending aorta /disen′ding/ [L, *descendere*, to descend; Gk, *aerein*, to raise], the main portion of the aorta, consisting of the thoracic aorta and the abdominal aorta, that continues from the aortic arch into the trunk of the body and supplies many structures, including the esophagus, lymph glands, ribs, stomach, liver, intestines, kidneys, spleen, and reproductive organs.

descending colon, the segment of the colon that extends from the end of the transverse colon at the splenic flexure on the left side of the abdomen down to the beginning of the sigmoid colon in the pelvis.

descending current. See **centrifugal current.**

descending myelitis [L, *descendere*, to descend; Gk, *myelos*, marrow, *itis*, inflammation], a form of myelitis in which the pathologic changes spread downward along the spinal cord.

descending neuritis [L, *descendere*, to descend; Gk, *neuron*, nerve, *itis*, inflammation], a form of neuritis that spreads downward from the upper part of the nervous system.

descending neuropathy [L, *descendere*, to descend; Gk, *neuron*, nerve, *pathos*, disease], a disease of the peripheral nervous system that spreads downward from the upper part of the body.

descending oblique muscle. See **obliquus externus abdominis.**

descending tract [L, *descendere*, to descend + *tractus*], a nerve tract found in the spinal cord that carries impulses away from the brain axis of the body or body part.

descending urography. See **intravenous pyelography.**

descensus /disen′səs/, the process of falling or descending; prolapse.

descent of testis /disent′/ [L, *descendere*, to descend + *testis*, testicle], the normal prenatal movement of the testis from the abdomen to the adult position in the scrotum. Incomplete descent is typically the result of hormonal or mechanical defects that may be surgically corrected in early childhood.

descriptive anatomy /diskrip′tiv/ [L, *describere*, to write], the study of the morphology and structure of the body by systems, such as the vascular system and the nervous system. Each system is composed of similar tissues that are essential to a particular function.

descriptive embryology, the study of the changes that occur in cells, tissues, and organs during the progressive stages of prenatal development.

descriptive epidemiology, the first stage of epidemiological investigation. It focuses on describing disease distribution by characteristics relating to time, place, and person.

descriptive psychiatry, the study of external, readily observable behavior. Compare **dynamic psychiatry.**

DES daughters, a group of women with increased susceptibility to cancer of the vagina and other reproductive organs because their mothers were given an estrogen medication, diethylstilbestrol (DES), from the 1940s through the 1960s to prevent miscarriage. Several other abnormalities have been reported among the DES daughters, including tissue that covers the cervix or a uterus that is too small to carry a pregnancy. Sons of women who took DES have an increased risk of undescended testes or other genital disorders.

Desenex, a trademark for a fixed-combination topical drug containing two antifungals (undecylenic acid and zinc undecylenate).

desensitization. See **systemic desensitization.**

desensitize /dēsen′sitīz/ [L, *de* + *sentire*, to feel], **1.** (in immunology) to render an individual insensitive to any of the various antigens. **2.** (in psychiatry) to relieve an emotionally disturbed person of the stress of phobias and neuroses by encouraging discussion of the anxieties and the stressful experiences that cause the emotional problems involved. **3.** (in dentistry) to remove or reduce the painful response of vital, exposed dentin to irritating substances and temperature changes.

deserpidine /disur′pədēn/, a rauwolfia alkaloid used as an antihypertensive.

■ INDICATIONS: It is prescribed for mild hypertension and for mild anxiety.

■ CONTRAINDICATIONS: Mental depression, peptic ulcer, ulcerative colitis, or known hypersensitivity to this drug prohibits its use. It interacts with monoamine oxidase inhibitors, which can increase hypertension and excitability.

■ ADVERSE EFFECTS: Among the more serious adverse reactions are orthostatic hypotension, potentially severe mental depression, and lethargy.

desert fever. See **coccidioidomycosis.**

desert rheumatism. See **coccidioidomycosis.**

Desferal Mesylate, a trademark for a chelating agent (deferoxamine mesylate).

desiccant /des′ikənt/ [L, *desiccare*, to dry thoroughly], any agent or procedure that promotes drying or causes a substance to dry up. Also called **exsiccant.**

desiccate /des′ikāt/, **1.** to dry thoroughly. **2.** to preserve by drying, especially food. Also **exsiccate.**

designer drugs [L, *de* + *signare*, to mark], synthetic organic compounds that are designed as analogs of illicit drugs, with the same narcotic or other dangerous effects. Because designer drugs are generally not listed as controlled substances by the United States Drug Enforcement Agency, prosecution of manufacturers, distributors, or users is frequently difficult.

desipramine hydrochloride /desip′rəmēn/, a tricyclic antidepressant.

■ INDICATION: It is prescribed in the treatment of mental depression.

■ CONTRAINDICATIONS: Concomitant administration of monoamine oxidase inhibitors, heart block, recent myocardial infarction, or known hypersensitivity to this drug or to tricyclic medication prohibits its use. It is used with caution in patients who have seizure disorders or cardiovascular disease.

■ ADVERSE EFFECTS: Among the more serious adverse reactions are sedation as well as GI, cardiovascular, and neurologic reactions. This drug interacts with many other drugs.

deslanoside /dislan′əsīd/, a cardiac glycoside.

■ INDICATIONS: It is prescribed for congestive heart failure and certain arrhythmias.

■ CONTRAINDICATIONS: Ventricular fibrillation, tachycardia, or known hypersensitivity to this drug prohibits its use.

■ ADVERSE EFFECTS: The most serious reactions are various cardiac arrhythmias.

-desma, a suffix meaning 'something bridging or connecting': *cytodesma, mesodesma, plasmodesma.*

desmo-, a combining form meaning 'pertaining to a ligament': *desmoma, desmorrhexis, desmotomy.*

desmocyte. See **fibroblast.**

desmoid tumor /dez′moid/ [Gk, *desmos*, band, *eidos*, form], a neoplasm in skeletal muscle and fascia that may occur in the head, neck, upper arm, abdomen, or lower extremities. The tumor is usually a firm, circumscribed, rubbery mass. Injury may be a factor in the development of this lesion, regarded as overproliferation of scar tissue.

desmopressin acetate /dez′mōpres′in/, an antidiuretic analog of vasopressin.

■ INDICATION: It is prescribed in the treatment of diabetes insipidus and nocturnal enuresis.

■ CONTRAINDICATION: Known hypersensitivity to this drug prohibits its use.

■ ADVERSE EFFECTS: Among the most serious adverse reactions are hyponatremia and water intoxication. Mild effects, such as headache, cramps, and nasal congestion, also may occur.

desmosis /dezmō′sis/, any disease of the connective tissue.

desmosome /dez′məsōm/ [Gk, *desmos*, band, *soma*, body], a small, circular, dense area within the intercellular bridge that forms the site of adhesion between certain epithelial cells, especially the stratified epithelium of the epidermis. Also called **macula adherens.**

desonide /des′ənīd/, a topical corticosteroid.

■ INDICATION: It is prescribed topically as an antiinflammatory agent.

■ CONTRAINDICATIONS: Viral and fungal diseases of the skin, impaired circulation, or known hypersensitivity to this drug or to steroid medication prohibits its use.

■ ADVERSE EFFECTS: Among the more serious adverse reactions, usually occurring after prolonged or excessive application, are striae, hypopigmentation or local irritation of the skin, and various systemic effects.

desoximetasone /desok′simet′əsōn/, a topical corticosteroid.

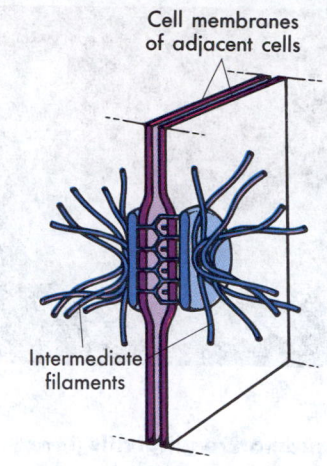

Desmosome (*Thibodeau, 1993/Michael P Schenk*)

■ INDICATION: It is prescribed topically as an antiinflammatory agent.

■ CONTRAINDICATIONS: Viral and fungal diseases of the skin, impaired circulation, or known hypersensitivity to this drug or to other steroid medication prohibits its use. Caution should be used in applying occlusive dressings over topical steroid medications.

■ ADVERSE EFFECTS: Among the more serious adverse reactions, usually occurring after prolonged or excessive application, are striae, hypopigmentation, or local irritation of the skin and various systemic effects.

desoxy-. See **deoxy-.**

desoxycorticosterone acetate /desok′sikôr′təkōstē′rōn/, a mineralocorticoid hormone.

■ INDICATIONS: It is prescribed in replacement therapy, in congenital adrenal hyperplasia, and in chronic primary adrenocortical insufficiency to prevent the excess loss of salt from the body.

■ CONTRAINDICATIONS: Hypertension, congestive heart failure, or known hypersensitivity to this drug prohibits its use.

■ ADVERSE EFFECTS: Among the more serious adverse reactions are excessive sodium and water retention and potassium loss, hypertension, edema, and heart failure.

Desoxyn, a trademark for a central nervous system stimulant (methamphetamine hydrochloride).

desoxyribonucleic acid. See **deoxyribonucleic acid.**

desquamation /des′kwəmā′shən/ [L, *desquamare*, to take off scales], a normal process in which the cornified layer of the epidermis is sloughed in fine scales. Certain conditions, injuries, and medications accelerate desquamation and may cause peeling and the loss of deeper layers of the skin. Also called **exfoliation.** **-desquamate,** *v.,* **desquamative** /deskwam′ətiv/, *adj.*

desquamative gingivitis, a gingival inflammation, characterized by peeling of the surface epithelium. It is a clinical rather than a pathologic condition and is most frequently associated with menopause. It may also be associated with any biologic stress. Compare **eruptive gingivitis.** (See Fig. p. 466.)

desquamative interstitial pneumonia, a respiratory disease characterized by an accumulation of cellular matter in

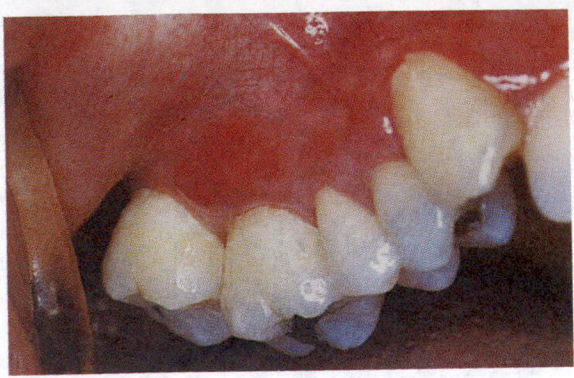

Desquamative gingivitis (Lamey, 1988)

the alveoli and bronchial tubes. It leads to a fibrotic condition with symptoms of coughing, chest pain, weight loss, and dyspnea. Treatment is with corticosteroids, oxygen, and supportive medical therapy.

destructive aggression /distruk′tiv/ [L, *destruere,* to destroy; *aggressio,* an attack], an act of hostility unnecessary for self-protection or preservation that is directed toward an external object or person. See also **aggression.**

destructive interference, (in ultrasonography) a phenomenon that results when propagated waves are out of phase so that maximum molecular compression for one wave occurs at the same point as the maximum rarefaction for the second wave and they cancel each other out.

destructive lesion [L, *destruere,* to destroy, *laesio,* a hurting], a disorder that leads to the damage or necrosis of an organ or tissue.

Desyrel, a trademark for an antidepressant (trazodone).

detached retina. See **retinal detachment.**

detection bias /ditek′shən/, a potential artifact in epidemiologic data due to the use of a particular diagnostic technique or equipment used. As an example, cancer rates may vary in different regions or time periods, not because of an actual difference in the incidence of the disease but because of different diagnostic technologies.

detergent /ditur′jənt/ [L, *detergere,* to cleanse], **1.** a cleansing agent. **2.** cleansing. **3.** (in respiratory therapy) a wetting agent that is administered to mediate the removal of respiratory tract secretions from airway walls. Examples include tyloxapol and acetylcysteine. See also **surfactant.**

deterioration /ditir′ē·ərā′shən/ [L, *deterior,* worse], a condition that is gradually worsening.

determinant evolution /ditur′minənt/ [L, *determinare,* to limit], the theory that evolution progresses according to a predetermined course. See also **orthogenesis.**

determinants of occlusion, (in dentistry) the classifiable factors that influence proper closure of the teeth. The common fixed factors are the intercondylar distance, anatomy, mandibular centricity, and relationship of the jaws. The common changeable factors are tooth shapes, tooth positions, and vertical dimensions of occlusion, cusp height, and fossa depth.

determinate cleavage /ditur′minit/, mitotic division of the fertilized ovum into blastomeres that are each destined to form a specific part of the embryo. If such cells are isolated, they are incapable of giving rise to an individual, complete embryo. Damage to or destruction of any of these cells results in a malformed organism. Also called **mosaic cleavage.** Compare **indeterminate cleavage.** See also **mosaic development.**

detoxification /dētok′sifikā′shən/ [L, *de* + Gk, *toxikon,* poison; L, *facere,* to make], the removal of a poison or its effects from a patient.

detoxification service, a hospital service providing treatment to diminish or remove from a patient's body the toxic effects of chemical substances, such as alcohol or drugs, usually as an initial step in the treatment of a chemical-dependent person. The service may also be used to remove poisonous substances to which a person may have been exposed. See also **alcoholism, drug addiction.**

detoxify /dētok′sifī/ [L, *de,* from; Gk, *toxikon,* poison], to make a poisonous substance harmless or to overcome the effects of a poison.

detrusor urinae muscle /ditr$\overline{oo}$′zər/ [L, *detruder,* to thrust; Gk, *ouron,* urine; L, *musculus*], a complex of longitudinal fibers that form the external layer of the muscular coat of the bladder. These fibers arise from the posterior surface of the pubis, traverse the inferior surface of the bladder, descend along the fundus, and attach to the prostate in men and to the front of the vagina in women. Along the sides of the bladder the fibers pass obliquely and intersect. The detrusor muscle is supplied by branches from the internal iliac artery and is innervated by medullated fibers from the third and fourth sacral nerves and by nonmedullated fibers from the hypogastric plexus.

deuterium (²H) /dy$\overline{oo}$tir′ē·əm/ [Gk, *deuteros,* second], a stable isotope of the hydrogen atom, used as a tracer. Also called **heavy hydrogen.** See also **tritium.**

deutero-, deuto-, a combining form meaning 'second': *deuteroalbumose, deuteroconidium, deuteroelastose.*

deuteroplasm. See **deutoplasm.**

deuto-. See **deutero-.**

deutoplasm /d$\overline{oo}$′təplaz′əm/ [Gk, *deuteros* + *plasma,* something formed], the inactive elements of the protoplasm, primarily the stored nutritive material contained in the yolk. Also called **deuteroplasm.**

DEV, abbreviation for **duck embryo vaccine.** See also **rabies vaccine.**

devascularization /dēvas′kyələr′izā′shən/ [L, *de,* from, *vasculum,* small vessel], the drawing away of blood from a body part or stopping the flow of blood to the part.

development [Fr, *développer,* to unfold], **1.** the gradual process of change and differentiation from a simple to a more advanced level of complexity. In humans the physical, mental, and emotional capacities that allow complex adaptation to the environment and function within society are acquired through growth, maturation, and learning. Kinds of development include **arrested development, mosaic development, psychomotor development, psychosexual development, psychosocial development,** and **regulative development. 2.** (in biology) the series of events that occur within an organism from the time of fertilization of the ovum to the adult stage. See also **film development. —developmental,** *adj.*

developmental age (DA) /divel′əpmen′təl/, an expression of a child's developmental progress stated in age and determined by standardized measurements, as of body size and dimensions, by social and psychologic functioning, by observations of motor skills, and by the giving of mental and aptitude tests. Compare **achievement age, developmental quotient, mental age.**

developmental agraphia, a deficiency in a child's ability to learn to form letters and to write. Other learning is normal, and the child usually has no musculoskeletal or neurologic problems.

developmental anatomy, the study of the differentiation and the growth of an organism from one cell to birth. Also called **embryology.**

developmental anomaly, any congenital defect that results from the interference with the normal growth and differentiation of the fetus. Such defects can arise at any stage of embryonic development, vary greatly in type and severity, and are caused by a wide variety of determining factors, including genetic mutations, chromosomal aberrations, teratogenic agents, and environmental factors. Developmental anomalies are classified either according to the organ system affected, such as congenital heart defects, or according to the way in which the defect occurred, such as developmental failure or arrest, failure to atrophy or subdivide, fusion, splitting, incorrect migration, and misplacement. Most developmental defects are apparent at birth, especially any structural malformation, but some, especially those involving the organ systems, do not become evident until days, weeks, or even years later.

developmental apraxia [L, *développer*, development; Gk, *a*, not, *prassein*, to do], a condition of ineffective motor planning and execution in children because of immaturity of the child's central nervous system.

developmental arrest. See **arrested development.**

developmental crisis, severe, usually transient, stress that occurs when a person is unable to complete the tasks of a psychosocial stage of development and is therefore unable to move on to the next stage. See also **psychosocial development.**

developmental disability (DD), a pathologic condition that starts developing before 18 years of age. Most developmental disabilities persist throughout the life of the individual, although many can be effectively treated. See also **congenital anomaly.**

developmental disorder, a form of mental retardation that develops in some children after they have progressed normally for the first 3 or 4 years of life. Onset of the mental deterioration usually begins with a vague viral infection or other similar disease symptoms.

developmental dyspraxia, a disorder of sensory integration characterized by an impaired ability to plan skilled nonhabitual movements.

developmental fog, (in radiology) an x-ray film that is dull, washed out, and lacking in contrast. Causes include temperature, timing, and developer concentration.

developmental groove, a fine recessed line in the enamel of a tooth that marks the union of the lobes of the crown in its development.

developmental guidance, (in dentistry) the comprehensive dentofacial orthopedic control over the growth of the jaws and the eruption of the teeth. It may require precisely timed active appliance therapy and supervisory examinations, including radiography and other diagnostic records, at various developmental stages. The control may be needed throughout the entire growth and maturation of the face, beginning at the earliest detection of a developing malformation.

developmental horizon, any one of 25 stages in the development of the human embryo from the one-cell stage at conception to the morphologically and physiologically complex organism at the end of the seventh week of gestation.

developmental model, 1. a conceptual framework devised to be used as a guide in making a diagnosis, in understanding a developmental process, and in forming a prognosis for continued development. It has five components. The 'identifiable state' describes the stage, level, phase, or period of the condition or process; the 'shift in state' identifies qualities of change as progressive, sudden, abrupt, or recurrent; and the 'form of progression' describes patterns of development as linear, spiral, or oscillating. The 'force' that triggers the change or the step in development may be self-actualization or any form of stress. Development is ultimately constrained by the fifth component, 'potentiality,' the genetic and environmental potential for growth. 2. (in nursing) a conceptual framework describing four stages, or processes, of development in the patient during therapy. In the first stage, called orientation, the patient begins a relationship with the nurse or other therapist and begins to clarify the problem with the help of the therapist. In the second stage, called identification, the patient develops a sense of closeness and attachment to the therapist. During this period the patient and the therapist work comfortably together. In the third stage, called exploitation, the patient makes full use of the nursing services offered, begins to assume some control of the interactions, and becomes more independent. During the last stage, called resolution, the therapeutic relationship is terminated; the patient is independent and no longer needs the nurse or therapist. With this model the nurse therapist may plan nursing interventions appropriate to the developmental level of the patient. The developmental model is one of the earliest nursing models to be developed. It views the person as a psychobiologic being whose needs are expressed in behavior and as one who is unique and capable of learning and changing. Health is viewed as a forward movement of personality development and other ongoing processes, reflected by the person's creative, constructive, and productive community living. Thus, the focus of nursing is to promote this forward movement by assisting the patient in self-repair and self-renewal.

developmental physiology, the study of the physiologic processes as they relate to embryonic development.

developmental quotient (DQ), the numeric expression of a child's developmental level as measured by dividing the developmental age by the chronologic age and multiplying by 100. Compare **intelligence quotient.** See also **developmental age.**

developmental sequence [Fr, *développer*; L, *sequi*, to follow], the order in which structure and function change during the process of growth and development of an organism. See also **ontogeny, phylogeny.**

developmental task, a physical or cognitive skill that a person must accomplish during a particular age period to continue developing, such as walking, which precedes the development of a sense of autonomy in the toddler period. The nurse may also outline developmental tasks for families.

developmental theory of aging, a concept based on the premise that traits and characteristics developed early in life tend to continue into the later years.

deviance /dē′vē·əns/ [L, *deviare*, to turn aside], behavior that is contrary to the accepted standards of a community or culture.

deviant /dē'vē·ənt/ [L, *deviare*, to turn aside],   pertaining to a person or object that departs from what is considered normal or standard.

deviant behavior,   actions that exceed the usual limits of accepted behavior and involve failure to comply with the social norm of the group.

deviate /dē'vē·it/ [L, *deviare*, to turn aside],   **1.** a person or an act that varies from that which is considered standard, such as a social or sexual deviate, or that which is within a statistic norm. **2.** to vary from that which is considered standard or within a statistic norm. –**deviant,** *adj.,* **deviation,** *n.*

deviated septum,   a shifted medial partition of the nasal cavity, a condition affecting many adults. The nasal septum more commonly shifts to the left during normal growth, but this deflection may be aggravated by a blow to the nose or by other trauma. A severe deflection of the septum may significantly obstruct the nasal passages and result in infection, sinusitis, shortness of breath, headache, or recurring nosebleeds. Severe septal deviation may be corrected by various surgical procedures, such as rhinoplasty or septoplasty. Postoperative care in such cases usually includes various measures, such as the maintenance of nasal packing, the administration of sedatives, and the placement of ice packs around the affected area to reduce swelling.

deviation, axis /dē'vē·ā'shən/ [L, *deviare*, to turn aside, *axle*],   in electrocardiography, deviation of the mean electric axis of the heart.

deviation from normal,   a quality, characteristic, symptom, or clinical finding that is different from what is commonly regarded as normal, such as an elevated temperature, multiple gestation, or an extra digit.

deviation of tongue [L, *deviare*, to turn aside; AS, *tunge*],   a tendency of the tongue to turn away from the midline when extended or protruded. The condition is associated with a hypoglossal nerve defect.

device /divīs'/ [OFr, *deviser*, to divide],   an item other than a drug that has application in the healing arts. The term is sometimes restricted to items used directly by, on, or in the patient and not surgical instruments or other equipment used for diagnosis and treatment. Devices include orthopedic appliances, crutches, artificial heart valves, pacemakers, prostheses, wheelchairs, cervical collars, hearing aids, and eye glasses.

devil's grip.   See **epidemic pleurodynia.**

devitalized /dēvī'təlīzd/,   pertaining to tissues with a reduced oxygen supply and blood flow.

devital tooth.   See **pulpless tooth.**

dewar /dyo͞o'ər/,   (in nuclear magnetic resonance imaging) a double chamber used to maintain the temperature of superconducting magnet coils at near absolute zero. The outer chamber is filled with liquid nitrogen at a temperature of near −196° C (−321° F) and the inner chamber is filled with a liquid helium at a temperature of −270° C (−454° F).

dew point /dyo͞o/,   the temperature at which air becomes saturated with water vapor and the water vapor condenses to liquid. In aerosol therapy, water may condense on containers, tubing, and other surfaces when the dew point is reached.

dexamethasone /dek'səmeth'əsōn/,   a glucocorticoid.

■ INDICATIONS: It is prescribed in the treatment of a variety of inflammatory conditions.

■ CONTRAINDICATIONS: Systemic fungal infections or known hypersensitivity to this drug prohibits its use.

■ ADVERSE EFFECTS: Among the more serious adverse reactions are GI, endocrine, neurologic, fluid, and electrolyte disturbances.

dexchlorpheniramine maleate /deks'klôrfənir'əmēn mal'ē·it/,   an antihistamine.

■ INDICATIONS: It is prescribed in the treatment of a variety of hypersensitivity reactions, including rhinitis, skin rash, and pruritus.

■ CONTRAINDICATIONS: Asthma or known hypersensitivity to this drug prohibits its use. It should not be given to newborn infants or lactating mothers.

■ ADVERSE EFFECTS: Drowsiness, skin rash, hypersensitivity reactions, dry mouth, and tachycardia may occur.

Dexedrine,   a trademark for a central nervous system stimulant (dextroamphetamine sulfate).

dexter /deks'tər/ [L, *dexter*, right],   pertaining to the right side, right.

dexterity /dekster'itē/ [L, *dexteritas*],   skillfulnes in the use of one's hands or body.

dextrad writing /deks'trad/ [L, *dexter*, right; ME, *writen*],   writing that moves from left to right.

dextrality.   See **right-handedness.**

dextran fermentation /dek'strən/ [L, *dexter*, right; *fermentare*, to cause to rise],   the conversion of dextrose to dextran by the action of *Leuconostoc mesenteroides* dextran (LMD) bacteria.

dextran preparation,   any of a group of solutions containing polysaccharides, water, and, in some preparations, electrolytes. These solutions are used as plasmavolume extenders in cases of hypovolemia from hemorrhage, dehydration, or another cause and are available for intravenous administration in several concentrations.

dextro-, dextr-,   a combining form meaning 'right': *dextrocardia, dextrocerebral, dextrogastria.*

dextroamphetamine sulfate /deks'trō·amfet'əmēn/,   a central nervous system stimulant.

■ INDICATIONS: It is prescribed in the treatment of narcolepsy and in the treatment of hyperkinetic disorders in children. It has also been prescribed as an anorexiant in treating exogenous obesity.

■ CONTRAINDICATIONS: Cardiovascular disease, glaucoma, hypertension, hyperthyroidism, agitation, history of drug abuse, concomitant administration of a monoamine oxidase inhibitor within 14 days, or known hypersensitivity to this drug prohibits its use.

■ ADVERSE EFFECTS: Among the more serious adverse reactions are various manifestations of central nervous system excitation, increased blood pressure, arrhythmias and other cardiovascular effects, nausea, anorexia, and drug dependence.

dextrocardia /-kär'dē·ə/,   the location of the heart in the right hemithorax, either as a result of displacement by disease or as a congenital defect.

dextrocardiogram /-kär'də·ōgram'/ [L, *dexter*, right; Gk, *kardia*, heart, *gramma*, record],   an electrocardiogram made from a unipolar electrode facing the right ventricle, producing a complex of a small R wave and a large S wave.

dextromethorphan hydrobromide /-methôr'fən/,   an antitussive derived from morphine, but lacking narcotic effects.

■ INDICATION: It is prescribed for the suppression of nonproductive cough.

- CONTRAINDICATIONS: Use of a monoamine oxidase inhibitor within the past 14 days or known hypersensitivity to this drug prohibits its use.
- ADVERSE EFFECTS: The most serious adverse reaction is respiratory depression resulting from large doses.

dextrose /dek′strōs/ [L, *dexter,* right side], a glucose available in various solutions for intravenous administration.

- INDICATIONS: It is prescribed to provide calories and fluid and to correct hypoglycemia.
- CONTRAINDICATIONS: Diabetic coma, intracranial or intraspinal hemorrhage, or delirium tremens prohibits its use.
- ADVERSE EFFECTS: Among the more serious adverse reactions are hyperglycemia, glycosuria, and phlebitis.

dextrose and sodium chloride injection, a fluid, nutrient, and electrolyte replenisher. It is available for parenteral use in a variety of concentrations.

dextrothyroxine sodium, an antihyperlipidemic.

- INDICATION: It is prescribed in the treatment of hyperlipidemia.
- CONTRAINDICATIONS: Known organic heart disease, hypertension, advanced liver or kidney disease, pregnancy, and a history of iodism prohibits its use. It is also prohibited for lactating mothers.
- ADVERSE EFFECTS: Among the most serious adverse reactions are angina pectoris, supraventricular tachycardia, cardiomegaly, myocardial infarction, insomnia, alopecia, hyperthermia, diuresis, dizziness, paresthesia, gallstones, and psychic changes.

D.H.E.-45, a trademark for an alpha-adrenergic blocking agent (dihydroergotamine mesylate).

DHFS, abbreviation for **dengue hemorrhagic fever shock syndrome.**

dhobie itch /dō′bē/ [Hindi, *dhobie,* laundryman; AS, *giccan*], a form of contact dermatitis associated with the use of laundry marking fluids.

di-, 1. a prefix meaning 'two, twice': *diacid, diamide, dimorphic.* **2.** also **dia-.** a prefix meaning 'apart, through': *diuresia, diactinism.* **3.** a prefix meaning 'apart, away from': *diffraction, discission, divergent.* See also, **di-, dis-.**

di-, dis-, 1. a prefix meaning 'reversal, apart, or to separate': *disacidify, dischronation, disinfect.* **2.** a prefix meaning 'two or duplication': *diplegia, dioxide, dissogeny.* **3.** a prefix meaning 'opposite': *disease.*

DiaBeta, a trademark for an oral antidiabetic drug (glyburide).

diabetes /dī′əbē′tēz/ [Gk, *diabainein,* to pass through], a clinical condition characterized by the excessive excretion of urine. The excess may be caused by a deficiency of antidiuretic hormone (ADH), as in diabetes insipidus, or it may be the polyuria resulting from the hyperglycemia occurring in diabetes mellitus.

diabetes insipidus /insip′idəs/, a metabolic disorder, characterized by extreme polyuria and polydipsia, caused by deficient production or secretion of the antidiuretic hormone (ADH) or an inability of the kidney tubules to respond to ADH. Rarely, the symptoms are self-induced by an excessive water intake. The condition may be acquired, familial, idiopathic, neurogenic, or nephrogenic.

- OBSERVATIONS: The onset may be dramatic and sudden, and urinary output may exceed 10 L in 24 hours. The patient is usually well and comfortable except for the annoyance of frequent urination and a constant need to drink. Diagnosis is established by a water deprivation test in which urine volume increases and urine osmolality decreases. A person

with diabetes insipidus who is unconscious because of trauma or surgery continues to produce massive quantities of urine. If fluids are not administered in adequate amounts, the patient becomes severely dehydrated and hypernatremic.

- INTERVENTIONS: In mild cases, no treatment is necessary. Vasopressin in an intramuscular injection or nasal spray is effective. Oral hypoglycemic agents improve the response of the kidneys to the decreased amount of available ADH in some cases, and thiazide diuretics, by inducing a state of salt depletion, sometimes decrease the diuresis of water by as much as 50%.
- NURSING CONSIDERATIONS: Infants and small children are particularly vulnerable to serious circulatory disturbances when dehydrated; therefore, exceedingly careful monitoring is essential in cases where the condition is suspected, especially after head surgery or trauma.

diabetes mellitus (DM) /məlī′təs/, a complex disorder of carbohydrate, fat, and protein metabolism that is primarily a result of a relative or complete lack of insulin secretion by the beta cells of the pancreas or of defects of the insulin receptors. The disease is often familial but may be acquired, such as in Cushing's syndrome, as a result of the administration of excessive glucocorticoid. The various forms of diabetes have been organized into a series of categories developed by the National Diabetes Data Group of the National Institutes of Health. Type I diabetes in this classification scheme includes patients dependent upon insulin to prevent ketosis. The category is also known as the insulin-dependent diabetes mellitus (IDDM) subclass. This group was previously called juvenile-onset diabetes, brittle diabetes, or ketosis-prone diabetes. Patients with Type II, or non-insulin-dependent diabetes mellitus (NIDDM), are those previously designated as having maturity-onset diabetes, adult-onset diabetes, ketosis-resistant diabetes, or stable diabetes. Those with gestational diabetes (GDM), are women who develop glucose intolerance when pregnant. Secondary diabetes, is diabetes associated with a pancreatic disease, hormonal changes, adverse effects of drugs, or genetic or other anomalies. A fifth subclass, the impaired glucose tolerance (IGT) group, includes persons whose plasma glucose levels are abnormal although not sufficiently beyond the normal range to be diagnosed as diabetic. Kinds of diabetes mellitus are **gestational diabetes, insulin-dependent diabetes,** and **non-insulin-dependent diabetes.** See also **impaired glucose tolerance, potential abnormality of glucose tolerance, previous abnormality of glucose tolerance.**

- OBSERVATIONS: The onset of diabetes mellitus (IDDM)is sudden in children and usually insidious in non-insulin-dependent diabetes mellitus (type II). Characteristically, the course is progressive and includes polyuria, polydipsia, weight loss, polyphagia, hyperglycemia, and glycosuria. The eyes, kidneys, nervous system, skin, and circulatory system may be affected, infections are common, and atherosclerosis often develops. In childhood and in the Type I, advanced stage of the disease, when no endogenous insulin is being secreted, ketoacidosis is a constant danger. The diagnosis is confirmed by glucose-tolerance tests, history, and urinalysis.
- INTERVENTIONS: The goal of treatment is to maintain insulin-glucose homeostasis. Mild early or late onset of the disease may be controlled by diet, with or without oral hypoglycemic agents, and exercise. In more severe diabetes, insulin is administered to keep blood-glucose levels below the point

Classification and characteristics of diabetes mellitus

Name	Previous synonyms	Characteristics
Type I Insulin-dependent diabetes mellitus (IDDM)	Juvenile diabetes Juvenile-onset diabetes Ketosis-prone diabetes Brittle diabetes Idiopathic diabetes	Abrupt onset of symptoms Individual prone to ketoacidosis Insulin dependent Viral etiology, autoimmune basis, genetic importance being investigated Often affects young Decrease in size and number of islet cells
Type II Non-insulin-dependent diabetes mellitus (NIDDM)	Adult-onset diabetes Maturity-onset diabetes Stable diabetes Ketosis-resistant diabetes	Usually not insulin dependent Individual not ketosis prone (but individual may form ketones under stress) Several syndromes, both nonobese and obese Generally occurs in those over the age of 40 Strong familial pattern being investigated
Secondary diabetes	Same	Cause established or strongly suspected May be associated with pancreatic disease, hormonal diseases, drugs and chemical agents, genetic syndromes, or malnutrition
Impaired glucose tolerance (IGT)	Asymptomatic diabetes Chemical diabetes Borderline diabetes Subclinical diabetes Latent diabetes	Show abnormal response to oral glucose tolerance test May revert to normal, remain impaired, or progress to diabetes Many with IGT are obese
Gestational diabetes mellitus (GDM)	Same	Glucose intolerance first recognized during pregnancy Following pregnancy, glucose may normalize, remain impaired, or progress to diabetes mellitus.
Statistical risk class: • Previously abnormal glucose level • Potential abnormal glucose tolerance	Latent diabetes Prediabetes Potential diabetes	Previous abnormality of oral glucose tolerance test or increased risk of developing diabetes because of genetic relationship with a diabetic

From McCance KL, Huether SE: *Pathophysiology: the biological basis for disease in adults and children,* St Louis, 1990, Mosby.

where ketoacidosis is likely. The Diabetes Control and Complications Trial, completed in mid-1993, demonstrated that tight control of blood glucose levels (i.e. frequent monitoring and maintenance at as close as possible to the level of nondiabetics) significantly reduces complications such as eye disease, kidney disease, and nerve damage. The kind and amount of insulin given varies with the person's condition. Stress of any kind may require an adjustment in the dosage. See also **diabetic foot and leg care.**

Nutritional principles in type I diabetes

1. Develop a basic daily meal plan that is relatively consistent in terms of:
   - Total energy (calorie) intake
   - Balance of energy-yielding nutrients (carbohydrates, fats, and proteins)
2. Provide for compensatory changes for nonbasal circumstances:
   - Extra food for extra activity
   - Extra insulin or activity for extra food
3. Avoid hyperglycemia by:
   - Omitting rapidly absorbed simple sugars from regular meal planning
4. Avoid hypoglycemia by:
   - Reasonably consistent meal timing
   - Provision of snacks

From Skyler, J.S.: Dietary planning in insulin-dependent diabetes mellitus, *Pediatr Ann* 12:652-657, 1983.

■ NURSING CONSIDERATIONS: Diabetic patients need extensive teaching and emotional support. The nurse may help the person to accept the diagnosis, to understand the disease, and to learn self-monitoring of glucose levels and self-administration of the medication. The person is also taught the need for continued medical supervision and for dietary carbohydrate, protein, fat, and calorie intake managements, and how to recognize the signs of impending coma: restlessness, thirst, hot dry skin, rapid pulse, fruity odor to the breath, and nausea. The patient also learns to recognize the signs of hypoglycemia and impending insulin shock: headache, nervousness, diaphoresis, thready pulse, and slurred speech. Certain safety precautions are emphasized; the patient should avoid infection, carry a supply of glucose at all times, wear a medical alert tag, and use sterile technique with insulin injection.

diabetic /dī'əbet'ik/, **1.** of or pertaining to diabetes. **2.** affected with diabetes. **3.** a person who has diabetes mellitus.

diabetic acidosis [Gk, *diabainein,* to pass through; L, *acidus,* acid; Gk, *osis,* condition], a type of acidosis that may occur in diabetes mellitus as a result of excessive production of ketone bodies during oxidation of fatty acids. See also **diabetic ketoacidosis (DKA).**

diabetic amaurosis [Gk, *diabainein,* to pass through; *amauroein,* to darken], blindness associated with diabetes, caused by a proliferative, hemorrhagic form of retinopathy that is characterized by capillary microaneurysms and hard or waxy exudates. Cataracts are also common in non-insulin-dependent diabetes, and, in insulin-dependent diabetes, snowflake cataract may progress until the entire lens is milky white.

diabetic coma, a life-threatening condition occurring in diabetics, caused by inadequate treatment, by failure to take prescribed insulin, excessive food intakes, or, most frequently, by infection, surgery, trauma, or other stressrs that increase the body's need for insulin. Without insulin to metabolize glucose, fats are utilized for energy, resulting in ketone waste accumulation and acidosis. The body's effort to counteract acidosis depletes the alkali reserve, causes a loss of sodium, chloride, potassium, and water, increases respiratory exhalation of carbon dioxide (Kussmaul breathing) and urinary excretion, and leads to dehydration and generalized hypoxia. Warning signs of diabetic coma include a dull headache, fatigue, inordinate thirst, epigastric pain, nausea, vomiting, parched lips, a flushed face, and sunken eyes. The temperature usually rises and then falls; the systolic blood pressure drops, and circulatory collapse may occur. Immediate treatment consists of administering rapid-acting insulin and replacing electrolytes and fluids to correct the acidosis and dehydration. Nonketotic coma may occur in patients with poorly controlled diabetes and high levels of blood glucose but no acetone in the urine. The plasma hyperosmolarity causes water to leave cells, and the dehydration of cerebral cells results in coma. See also **diabetic ketoacidosis, insulin shock.**

diabetic diet, a diet prescribed in the treatment of diabetes mellitus, usually containing limited amounts of simple sugars or readily digestible carbohydrates and increased amounts of proteins, complex carbohydrates, and unsaturated fats. Dietary regulation depends on the severity of the disease and on the type and extent of insulin therapy. The diet should be designed to prevent wide fluctuation in the amount of glucose in the blood, to preserve pancreatic function, and to prevent chronic diabetic complications. See also **diabetes mellitus, insulin.**

diabetic foot and leg care, the special attention given to prevent the circulatory disorders and infections that frequently occur in the lower extremities of diabetic patients.

■ METHOD: The patient's legs and feet are examined daily for signs of dry, scaly, red, itching, or cracked skin, blisters, corns, calluses, abrasions, infection, blueness and swelling around varicosities, and thickened, discolored nails. The feet are bathed daily in tepid water with mild or superfatted soap and are dried gently but thoroughly with a soft towel. A lanolin-based lotion is then applied, starting with the distal end of the toes; excess lotion is removed with a dry towel; vigorous rubbing and the use of alcohol preparations are avoided. The toenails are cut straight across above the level of soft tissue after the feet are soaked for 3 to 5 minutes in tepid water. The feet are also soaked in tepid water for several minutes before hardened areas are treated by applying soft soap and rubbing the area with a washcloth; calluses and corns are removed, and thickened, deformed nails are cut by a podiatrist.

■ NURSING INTERVENTION: The nurse provides foot and leg care while the diabetic patient is hospitalized. Before discharge, the patient is instructed to examine and bathe the feet daily according to the recommended method, to report abnormalities, to keep the feet dry at all times, to wear cotton socks or stockings with cotton feet, and to place clean lamb's wool or cotton between the toes if they perspire. The patient is

cautioned to avoid foot or leg trauma, walking barefoot, scratching insect bites, using a hot-water bottle or heating pad on the lower extremities, getting sunburned, wearing constricting garments, remaining in the same position for long periods, sitting at more than a right-angle bend, and crossing the knees. The diabetic individual is advised to alternate the wearing of two pairs of rubber-soled, well-fitted shoes wide enough to prevent pressure and rubbing, to air each pair of shoes between use, and to break in new shoes gradually. The patient is urged to walk to tolerance daily, to plan exercise periods after meals, to bend and straighten the knees and rotate the ankles occasionally when sitting, and, when standing, to shift weight from time to time and walk in place.

■ OUTCOME CRITERIA: Meticulous care of the feet and legs can prevent serious complications, including local infection, skin ulcers, cellulitis, and gangrene.

diabetic gangrene [Gk, *diabainein,* to pass through, *gaggraina*], gangrene, usually involving the lower extremities that develops secondary to peripheral vascular disease complications related to the diabetic disease process.

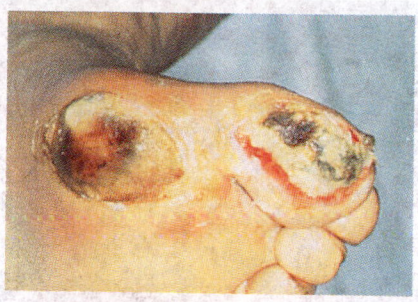

Diabetic gangrene (Morison, 1992)

diabetic glycosuria [Gk, *diabainein,* to pass through, *glykys,* sweet, *ouron,* urine], excessive excretion of sugar into the urine as an effect of diabetes mellitus.

diabetic ketoacidosis (DKA), diabetic coma, an acute, life-threatening complication of uncontrolled diabetes mellitus in which urinary loss of water, potassium, ammonium, and sodium results in hypovolemia, electrolyte imbalance, extremely high blood glucose levels, and the breakdown of free fatty acids causing acidosis, often with coma. Compare **insulin shock.**

■ OBSERVATIONS: The person appears flushed, has hot, dry skin, is restless, uncomfortable, agitated, diaphoretic, and has a fruity odor to the breath. Coma, confusion, and nausea are often noted. Diabetics who have no endogenous insulin are the most often affected, although the insulin concentration may be normal but inappropriately low for the degree of hyperglycemia. Untreated, the condition invariably proceeds to coma and death.

■ INTERVENTIONS: Intravenous insulin and hypotonic saline solution are administered immediately. Nasogastric intubation and bladder catheterization are usual. Blood glucose and ketone levels are determined hourly, and electrolyte and acid-base balance are monitored frequently. Bicarbonate or potassium may be given in dosages dependent on the degree of acidosis. Plasma or a plasma expander may be necessary to prevent or correct shock resulting from hypovolemia.

■ NURSING CONSIDERATIONS: The cause for the episode of ketoacidosis is sought. The most common precipitating factors are infection, GI upset, alcohol consumption, and the diabetic's failure to take insulin. In IIDM in childhood, diabetes characteristically begins suddenly and progresses rapidly; therefore, the diagnosis of insulin-dependent diabetes is usually made when the child is brought to the hospital in diabetic ketoacidosis. The care of a patient in the hospital after an episode of ketoacidosis is the same as for diabetes mellitus.

diabetic retinopathy, a disorder of retinal blood vessels characterized by capillary microaneurysms, hemorrhage, exudates, and the formation of new vessels and connective tissue. The disorder occurs most frequently in patients with long-standing, poorly controlled diabetes. Repeated hemorrhage may cause permanent opacity of the vitreous humor, and blindness may eventually result. Photocoagulation of damaged retinal blood vessels by a laser beam may be performed to prevent hemorrhage from the vessels. Rarely, cloudy vitreous humor is surgically removed by vitrectomy.

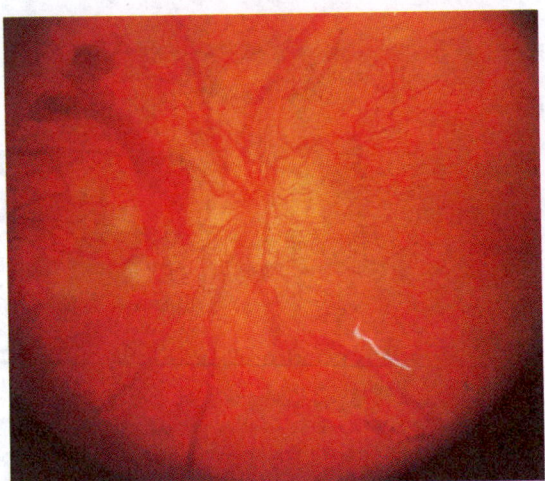

Diabetic retinopathy (Apple, 1991)

diabetic treatment, management of diabetes mellitus by means of a controlled carbohydrate diet, insulin injections, or oral hypoglycemic agents such as chlorpropamide, acetohexamide, tolbutamide, and tolazamide.

diabetic vulvovaginitis [Gk, *diabainein*, to pass through; L, *vulva*, wrapper + *vagina*, sheath; Gk, *itis*, inflammation], a form of mycotic inflammation of the vulva and vagina that is associated with diabetes.

diabetic xanthoma, an eruption of yellow papules or plaques on the skin in uncontrolled diabetes mellitus. The lesion disappears as the metabolic functions are stabilized and the disease is controlled.

diabetogenic state /dī′əbet′ōjen′ik/, a health condition manifested by signs and symptoms of diabetes.

Diabinese, a trademark for an oral antidiabetic (chlorpropamide).

diacet, abbreviation for a *carboxylate diacetate anion.*

diacetic acid. See **acetoacetic acid.**

diacondylar fracture /dī′əkon′dilər/ [Gk, *dia*, through,

kondylos, knuckle; L, *fractura,* break], any fracture that runs across the line of a condyle.

diadochokinesia /dī·ad′əkōkīnē′zhə/ [Gk, *diadochos*, successor, *kinesis*, motion], the normal ability of the muscles to move a limb alternately in opposite directions by flexion and extension.

Diagnex blue test, a trademark for a test for the presence of hydrochloric acid in gastric secretions. Diagnex blue tablets, which contain the dye azuresin, are taken by mouth. If the urine appears blue, it can be inferred that the stomach is secreting hydrochloric acid. See also **gastric analysis.**

diagnose /dī′agnōs/, to determine the type and cause of a health condition based on the signs and symptoms of the patient, data obtained from laboratory analysis of fluid, tissue specimens, and other tests, and family and occupational background information such as recent injuries or exposure to toxic substances.

diagnosis /dī′agnō′sis/, *pl.* **diagnoses** [Gk, *dia* + *gnosis*, knowledge], **1.** identification of a disease or condition by a scientific evaluation of physical signs, symptoms, history, laboratory tests, and procedures. Kinds of diagnoses are **clinical diagnosis, differential diagnosis, laboratory diagnosis, nursing diagnosis,** and **physical diagnosis. 2.** the art of naming a disease or condition. —**diagnostic,** *adj.,* **diagnose,** *v.*

diagnosis by exclusion [Gk, *dia*, through, *gnosis*, knowledge; L, *excludere*, to shut out], diagnosis made by eliminating other possible causes of disease symptoms.

diagnosis-related group (DRG), a group of patients classified for measuring a medical facility's delivery of care. The classifications, used to determine Medicare payments for inpatient care, are based on primary and secondary diagnosis, primary and secondary procedures, age, and length of hospitalization. See also **prospective payment system.**

diagnostic /dī′agnos′tik/, pertaining to a diagnosis.

Diagnostic and Statistical Manual of Mental Disorders (DSM), a manual, published by the American Psychiatric Association, listing the official diagnostic classifications of mental disorders. The *DSM* recommends the use of a multiaxial evaluation system as a holistic diagnostic approach. It consists of five axes, each of which refers to a different class of information, including mental and physical data. Axes I and II include all of the mental disorders, classified broadly as clinical syndromes and personality disorders; axis III contains physical disorders and conditions; and axes IV and V provide a coded outline of supplemental information on, for example, psychosocial stressors and adaptive functioning, which may be useful for planning individual treatment and predicting its outcome. Each of the classifications of the mental disorders contains a code that provides a reference to the WHO *International Classification of Diseases (ICD)* and offers such useful diagnostic criteria as essential and associated features of the disorder, age at onset, course, impairment, complications, predisposing factors, prevalence, sex ratio, familial patterns, and differential diagnoses. DSM-III-R is the revised version of the third edition of the manual, published in 1987.

diagnostic anesthesia, a procedure in which analgesia is induced to a depth adequate to comfortably permit performance of moderately painful diagnostic procedures of short duration. Awake anesthesia is often used for this purpose. See also **awake anesthesia.**

diagnostician /dī′agnostish′ən/, a person skilled and trained in making diagnoses.

Diagnostic Medical Sonographer, an allied health professional who provides patient services, using diagnostic ultrasound under the supervision of a doctor of medicine or osteopathy responsible for the use and interpretation of ultrasound procedures. The sonographer assists the physician in gathering sonographic data necessary to reach diagnostic decisions.

diagnostic position of gaze. See **cardinal position of gaze.**

diagnostic process, the act of determining a patient's health status and evaluating the factors influencing that status.

diagnostic radiology, medical imaging using external sources of radiation.

diagnostic radiopharmaceutical, a radioactive drug administered to a patient as a diagnostic tracer to differentiate normal from abnormal anatomic structures or biochemical or physiologic functions. Most diagnostic radioactive tracers indicate their position within the body by emitting gammarays. By monitoring the emissions with a collimated externalgamma-ray detector, the concentration of the tracer in different organs can be inferred and low-resolution images of the organs can be obtained. Tracers prepared with tritium, carbon 14, or phosphorus 32, which do not emit gamma rays, are used diagnostically by analyzing the concentration of the isotope in a metabolic end product in the patient's blood, urine, breath, or, in some cases, biopsy samples. When glucose containing 14C is administered, the subsequent monitoring of $14CO_2$ in the patient's breath can indicate the absorption of the compound, its metabolism, and elimination as a metabolic end product.

diagnostic related groups (DRG) See **diagnosis-related-group.**

diagnostic services, services related to the diagnosis made by a physician but which may be performed also by nurses or other health professionals.

diagonal conjugate /dī·ag′ənəl/, a radiographic measurement of the distance from the inferior border of the symphysis pubis to the sacral promontory. The measurement, which averages around 12.5 to 13.0 cm, may also be determined by vaginal examination. See also **conjugate, true conjugate.**

diakinesis /dī′əkinē′sis, dī′əkī-/ [Gk, *dia + kinesis,* motion], the final stage in the first meiotic prophase in gametogenesis in which the chromosomes achieve maximum contraction and are ready to separate. The chiasmata and nucleolus disappear, the nuclear membrane degenerates, and the spindle fibers form in preparation for the formation of dyads. See also **diplotene, leptotene, pachytene, zygotene.**

dialect /dī′əlekt/, a variation of a language different from other forms of the same language in pronunciation, syntax, and word meanings. A particular dialect is usually shared by members of an ethnic group or people living together in a geographic area.

dialogue /dī′əlog/ [L, *dialogus,* philosophic conversation], a complex form of computer-assisted instruction in which the student is actively engaged in "true conversation" with a computer.

Dialose, a trademark for a GI, fixed-combination drug containing a stool softener (docusate sodium sulfosuccinate) and a laxative (sodium carboxymethylcellulose).

dialy-, a prefix meaning 'pertaining to dialysis or dissolution': *dialytic, dialysate.*

dialysate /dī·al′isāt/, the solution subjected to dialysis.

dialysis /dī·al′isis/ [Gk *dia + lysis* a loosening], **1.** the process of separating colloids and crystalline substances in solution by the difference in their rate of diffusion through a semipermeable membrane. **2.** a medical procedure for the removal of certain elements from the blood or lymph by virtue of the difference in their rates of diffusion through an external semipermeable membrane or, in the case of peritoneal dialysis, through the peritoneum. Dialysis may be used to remove poisons and excessive amounts of drugs, to correct serious electrolyte and acid-base imbalances, and to remove urea, uric acid, and creatinine in patients with chronic end-stage renal disease. Dialysis involves diffusion of particles from an area of high to lower concentration, osmosis of fluid across the membrane from an area of lesser to greater concentration of particles, and the ultrafiltration or movement of the fluid across the membrane as a result of an artificially created pressure differential. See also **hemodialysis, peritoneal dialysis.**

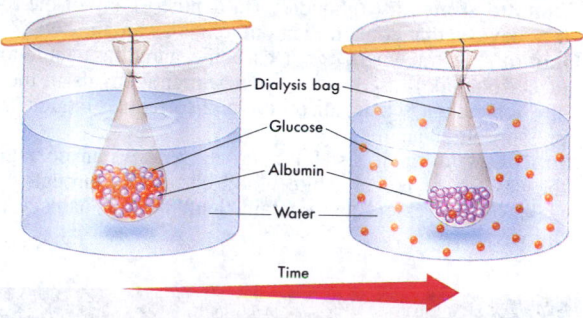

Dialysis *(Thibodeau, 1993/Rolin Graphics)*

dialysis dementia, a neurologic disorder that occurs in some patients undergoing dialysis. The precise cause is unknown, but the effect is believed to be related to chemicals in the dialyzing fluid, drugs administered to the dialysis patient, or both.

dialysis disequilibrium syndrome, a disorder caused by a rapid change in extracellular fluid composition during dialysis. The syndrome may be marked by cerebral or neurologic disturbances, cardiac arrhythmias, and pulmonary edema.

dialysis fluid, the solution that flows on the opposite side of a semipermeable membrane to blood.

dialysis shunt [Gk, *dia,* through + *lysis,* loosening; ME, *shunten*], an external artificial link between a peripheral artery and vein, either in an arm or leg, for use in hemodialysis.

dialysis technician [Gk, *dia,* through + *lysis,* loosening + *technikos,* skilful], an allied health professional who operates and maintains dialysis equipment for patients with kidney diseases.

dialyzer /dī′əlī′zər/ [Gk, *dia + lysis,* a loosening], **1.** a machine used in dialysis. **2.** a semipermeable membrane or porous diaphragm in a dialysis machine. See also **hemodialysis, peritoneal dialysis.**

diameter of fetal skull [Gk, *diametros*; L, *fetus*; AS, *skulle*, bowl],   the average distances between certain landmarks of the fetal skull as measured at term, such as biparietal, the fetal head between the two parietal eminences, 9.25 cm; occipitofrontal, from the external occipital protuberance to the most prominent point of the frontal midline, 11 cm; occipitomental, from the external occipital protuberance to the midpoint of the chin, 13 cm; and suboccipitobregmatic, from the lowest posterior point of the occipital bone to the center of the anterior fontanel, 9.5 cm.

Diameter-Index Safety System (DISS),   a system of standardized connections between cylinders of medical gases and flow meters or pressure regulators. Each gas has connections of a specific size to prevent accidental hookup of the wrong gas. Each type of gas and connector is assigned a DISS number, such as 1040 for nitrous oxide and 1240 for oxygen. See also **Pin-Index Safety System (PISS).**

Diamond-Blackfan syndrome,   a rare congenital disorder evident in the first 3 months of life, characterized by severe anemia, very low reticulocyte count, but normal numbers of platelets and white cells. It is caused by a deficiency of erythrocyte precursors. Also called **congenital hypoplastic anemia.** See also **anemia.**

diamond stone /dī'(ə)mənd/,   (in dentistry) any of the rotary devices that contain diamond chips as an abrasive.

Diamox,   a trademark for a carbonic anhydrase inhibitor (acetazolamide), used as an adjunct in anticonvulsant therapy for certain seizure disorders and to reduce intraocular pressure in glaucoma.

diapedesis /dī'əpidē'sis/ [Gk, *dia + pedesis*, an oozing],   the passage of red or white blood corpuscles through the walls of the vessels that contain them without damage to the vessels.

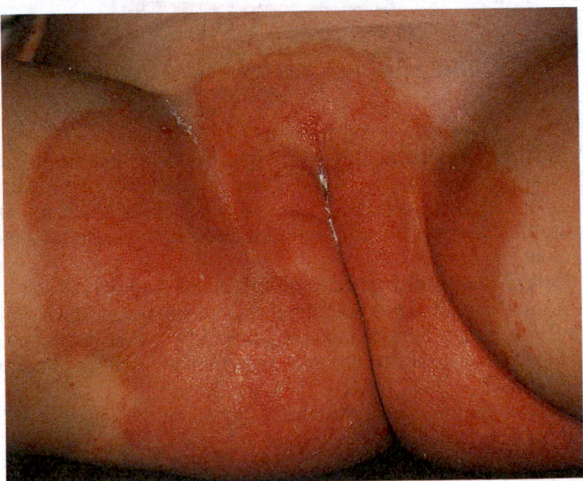

Diaper rash *(Habif, 1990)*

diaper rash [ME, *diapre*, patterned fabric],   a maculopapular and occasionally excoriated eruption in the diaper area of infants caused by irritation from feces, moisture, heat, or ammonia produced by the bacterial decomposition of urine. Secondary infection by *Candida albicans* is common. Principles of treatment include frequent diaper changes, dryness, cleanliness, coolness, and ventilation of the affected area. Specific topical antimicrobial medication may be prescribed for secondary infection. Also called **diaper dermatitis.**

diaper restraint,   a therapeutic device used especially in orthopedics for countertraction with lower extremity traction when other methods of countertraction are not effective. Diaper restraints are commonly used in treating children with orthopedic diseases and abnormalities and are designed to fit over the pelvic area like a diaper, with rings incorporated at each of four corners. A webbing strap is threaded through the rings and attached to the top side of the bedspring frame. Diaper restraints applied to incontinent patients are usually checked every half hour as a precaution against urinary tract infections that can develop from urinary wastes accumulating within such restraints. Diaper restraints are used with Russell traction and with split Russell traction if additional countertraction is required but are not usually used with other kinds of traction. Compare **jacket restraint, sling restraint.**

diaphanography /dī·af'ənog'rəfē/ [Gk, *diaphanes*, shining through, *graphein*, to record],   a type of transillumination used to examine the breast, using selected wavelengths of light and special imaging equipment. The images are still-frame recordings as in conventional radiography. See also **diaphanoscopy.**

diaphanoscopy /dī·af'ənos'kəpē/,   examination of an internal structure with a **diaphanoscope,** an instrument that transilluminates body tissues. It is sometimes used in the diagnosis of breast tumors.

diaphoresis /dī'əfərē'sis/ [Gk, *dia + pherein*, to carry],   the secretion of sweat, especially the profuse secretion associated with an elevated body temperature, physical exertion, exposure to heat, and mental or emotional stress. Sweating is centrally controlled by the sympathetic nervous system and is primarily a thermoregulatory mechanism, but the sweat glands on the palms and soles respond to emotional stimuli and do not participate in thermal sweating. The rate of sweating is generally not affected by water deficiency, but it may be reduced by severe dehydration and diminishes when salt intake exceeds salt loss. Also called **sweating.** See also **sudorific.**

diaphoretic.   See **sudorific.**

diaphragm /dī'əfram/ [Gk, *diaphragma*, a partition],   **1.** (in anatomy) a dome-shaped musculofibrous partition that separates the thoracic and the abdominal cavities. The convex cranial surface of the diaphragm forms the floor of the thoracic cavity, and the concave surface forms the roof of the abdominal cavity. This partition is pierced by various openings through which pass the aorta, esophagus, and vena cava. The diaphragm aids respiration by moving up and down. During inspiration it moves down and increases the volume of the thoracic cavity; during expiration it moves up, decreasing the volume. During deep inspiration and expiration the range of diaphragmatic movement in the adult is about 30 mm on the right side and about 28 mm on the left side. The height of this structure also varies with the degree of distension of the stomach and the intestines and with the size of the liver. It is innervated by the phrenic nerve from the cervical plexus. **2.** *informal*. a contraceptive diaphragm. **3.** (in optics) an opening that controls the amount of light passing through an optical network. **4.** a thin, membranous partition, as that employed in dialysis. **5.** (in radiography) a metal plate with a small opening that limits the diameter of the radiographic beam. **–diaphragmatic,** *adj.*

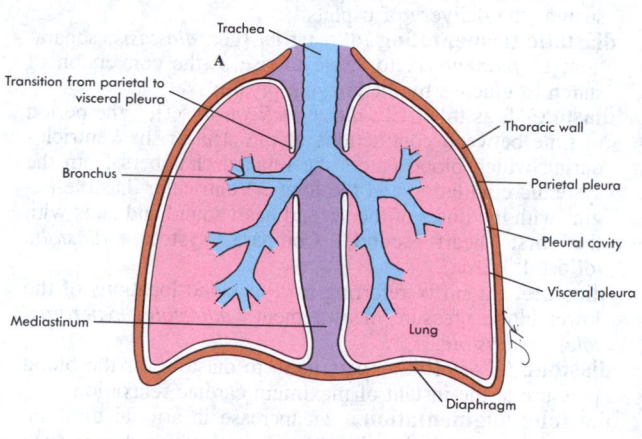

Diaphragm *(Seeley, 1992/Jody L Fulks)*

diaphragmatic breathing [Gk, *diaphragma*, partition], deliberate use of the diaphragm to control breathing. The technique is taught to patients with COPD to facilitate respiration. Also called **diaphragmatic respiration**.

diaphragmatic hernia [Gk, *diaphragma*, partition; L, rupture], the protrusion of part of the stomach through an opening in the diaphragm, most commonly an abnormally enlarged esophageal hiatus. In some cases the intestines may also herniate into the chest. The enlargement of the normal opening for the esophagus may be caused by trauma, congenital weakness, increased abdominal pressure, or relaxation of ligaments of skeletal muscles, and permits part of the stomach to slide into the thorax. A sliding hiatus hernia, one of the most common pathologic conditions of the upper GI tract, may occur at any age but is most frequent in elderly and middle-aged people. A kind of diaphragmatic hernia is **hiatus hernia**.

■ OBSERVATIONS: Symptoms of diaphragmatic hernia vary but usually include heartburn after meals, when the patient is in a supine position, and on exertion, especially when bending forward. There may be regurgitation of food, dysphagia, abdominal distention after eating, belching, rumbling in the intestines, rapid breathing, and a dull epigastric pain radiating to the shoulder. The similarity of some of the symptoms to those of myocardial infarction may make the patient fearful and anxious. The continued reflux of gastric juice into the esophagus may lead to ulceration with bleeding and the formation of fibrous tissue. Gastric contents regurgitated during sleep may be aspirated into the lungs. Rarely, a part of the stomach or other viscera becomes incarcerated in the chest.

■ INTERVENTIONS: The patient is placed in bed in a semi-Fowler's position and raised to a high Fowler's position during and after small, frequent meals of a bland diet. The individual is encouraged to chew slowly and thoroughly, to drink one or two glasses of water with a meal (unless contraindicated), and to avoid smoking. The blood pressure, pulse, respirations, and temperature are monitored. Medi-

cation for pain, an antacid, such as aluminum hydroxide gel, and diagnostic endoscopy and x-ray films may be ordered; to facilitate visualization of the hernia, the patient may be placed in a Trendelenburg position during studies of barium swallowing. If symptoms are severe and persistent and if they are unrelieved by conservative measures, the hernia may be repaired surgically.

■ NURSING CONSIDERATIONS: Diaphragmatic hernias are very common, especially among older people who are in the hospital for other indications. The recurrence of the symptoms of diaphragmatic hernia may often be prevented by instructing the patient, before discharge, to have frequent, small bland meals, not to recline after eating, to lose weight (if indicated), not to smoke, and to avoid constipation. Serious complications and severe discomfort may usually be avoided by the patient if the instructions are observed.

diaphragmatic node, a node in one of three groups of thoracic parietal lymph nodes, situated on the thoracic side of the diaphragm and consisting of the anterior set, the middle set, and the posterior set. The anterior set includes about three nodes dorsal to the base of the xiphoid process and one or two nodes on either side near the junction of the seventh rib. The nodes dorsal to the xiphoid process receive afferent lymphatic vessels from the convex surface of the liver. The afferents of the nodes near the seventh rib drain the ventral side of the diaphragm. The efferents of the anterior set pass to the sternal nodes. The middle set of about three nodes on each side is close to the diaphragmatic entry of the phrenic nerves. Some of the nodes of the middle set on the right side lie within the pericardium. The afferents of the middle set drain parts of the diaphragm and the liver. The efferents of the middle set pass to the posterior mediastinal nodes. The posterior set of diaphragmatic nodes consists of a few nodes on the crura of the diaphragm, connecting with the lumbar nodes and the posterior mediastinal nodes. Compare **intercostal node, sternal node.** See also **lymphatic system, lymph node.**

diaphragmatic respiration. See **diaphrogmatic breathing**

diaphragm pessary. See **pessary.**

diaphragm stethoscope, an instrument for auscultation of bodily sounds. Originally designed by René Laënnec, it consists of a vibrating disk, or diaphragm, which transmits sound waves through tubing to two earpieces. Also called **binaural stethoscope.** See also **stethoscope.**

diaphyseal aclasis /dī′əfiz′ē·əl ak′ləsis/ [Gk, *dia* + *phyein*, to grow; *a, klasis*, not breaking], a relatively rare abnormal condition that affects the skeletal system. Characterized by multiple exostoses or bony protrusions, it is hereditary, being transmitted as a dominant trait. Approximately half of the children of an individual with diaphyseal aclasis display varying degrees of its symptoms. The characteristic exostoses are radiographically and microscopically similar to osteochondromas. Evident involvement is diffuse, with the long bones usually affected more severely and more frequently than the short bones. Depending on the specific area involved, various angular or rotational deformities may result. Diaphyseal aclasis is usually bilateral and occurs more frequently in boys than in girls. Although this disease is hereditary, its signs and symptoms are not usually evident until the affected individual is 2 years of age or older. Children of a parent who has the disease are often routinely examined for symptoms. The major signs of the disease are the noticeable protrusions in the areas of the exostoses. Pain is not usually associated with the exostoses and, if present, is usually minimal. Deformities of the extremities may be evident, depending on the severity and the location of the exostoses. Radiographic examination reveals a broadened metaphyseal area, and the specific lesion is exhibited by abnormal continuity and decreased density. Asymptomatic lesions characteristic of diaphyseal aclasis usually require little or no treatment other than continued observation. The lesions located near the joints that interfere with joint motion or impair neurovascular function may be surgically excised. Angular and rotational deformities caused by the lesions may require surgical correction to facilitate improved function. Inequalities in the length of lower extremities resulting from unilateral involvement may require epiphysiodesis. A relatively small number of these lesions may become malignant. One form of the disorder, dyschondroplasia, results in dwarfism. Also called **hereditary deforming chondroplasia, multiple cartilaginous exostoses.**

diaphyseal dysplasia. See **Camurati-Engelmann disease.**

diaphysis /dī·af′isis/ [Gk, *dia* + *phyein*, to grow], the shaft of a long bone, consisting of a tube of compact bone enclosing the medullary cavity.

Diapid, a trademark for a pituitary antidiuretic hormone (lypressin).

diapositive. See **reversal film.**

diarrhea /dī′ərē′ə/ [Gk, *dia* + *rhein*, to flow], **1.** the frequent passage of loose, watery stools. The stool may also contain mucus, pus, blood, or excessive amounts of fat. Diarrhea is usually a symptom of some underlying disorder. Conditions in which diarrhea is an important symptom are dysenteric diseases, malabsorption syndrome, lactose intolerance, irritable bowel syndrome, GI tumors, and inflammatory bowel disease. In addition to stool frequency, patients may complain of abdominal cramps and generalized weakness. Untreated, severe diarrhea may lead to rapid dehydration and electrolyte imbalance and should be treated symptomatically until proper diagnosis can be made. Antidiarrheal preparations, such as diphenoxylate and paregoric, are helpful. If diarrhea is accompanied by vomiting, intravenous fluids may be necessary to prevent fluid depletion. **2.** a nursing diagnosis accepted by the Fourth National Conference on the Classification of Nursing Diagnoses. The cause of the condition, developed at the Fifth National Conference, includes stress and anxiety; dietary intake; the side effects of medications; inflammation, irritation, or malabsorption of the bowel; and the effects of toxins, contaminants, or radiation. The defining characteristics include abdominal pain, cramping, increased frequency of elimination, increased frequency of bowel sounds, loose or liquid stools, urgency of defecation, and a change in the color of the feces. See also **dehydration, nursing diagnosis. —diarrheal, diarrheic,** *adj.*

diarthrosis. See **synovial joint.**

diarticular /dī′ärtik′yələr/ [Gk, *di*, twice; L, *articulare*, to divide into joints], biarticular, or having two joints.

Diasone Sodium Enterab, a trademark for a leprostatic antibacterial (sulfoxone sodium).

diastasis /dī·as′təsis/ [Gk, separation], the forcible separation of two parts that normally are joined together, such as the separation of parts of a bone at an epiphysis or the separation of two bones that lack a synovial joint.

diastasis recti abdominis, the separation of the two rectus muscles along the median line of the abdominal wall. In a newborn infant, the condition is the result of incom-

plete development. In an adult woman, the abnormality is often caused by repeated pregnancies or a multiple birth, such as the delivery of triplets.

diastatic fermentation /dī′əstat′ik/ [Gk, *diastasis*, separation; L, *fermentare*, to cause to rise], the conversion of starch to glucose by the enzyme ptyalin.

diastole /dī·as′təlē/ [Gk, *dia* + *stellein*, to set], the period of time between contractions of the atria or the ventricles during which blood enters the relaxed chambers from the systemic circulation and the lungs. Ventricular diastole begins with the onset of the second heart sound and ends with the first heart sound. Compare **systole.** *diastolic* /dī′əstol′ik/, *adj.*

-diastole, a suffix referring to 'types and locations of the lower blood pressure measurement': *adiastole, hyperdiastole, prediastole.*

diastolic /dī′əstol′ik/, pertaining to diastole, or the blood pressure at the instant of maximum cardiac relaxation.

diastolic augmentation, an increase in arterial diastolic blood pressure produced by a counterpulsation device such as an intraaortic balloon pump. A balloon-tipped catheter positioned in the aorta inflates during ventricular diastole, forcing blood back toward the heart and augmenting diastolic pressure. Balloon deflation at the onset of ventricular systole creates a partial vaccum in the aorta, thereby assisting ventricular ejection and reducing systolice pressure.

diastolic blood pressure, the minimum level of blood pressure measured between contractions of the heart. Diastolic pressures for an individual may vary with age, sex, body weight, emotional state, and other factors.

diastolic filling pressure, the blood pressure in the ventricle during diastole.

diastolic murmur [Gk, *dia*, between, *stellein*, to set, L, *murmur*, humming], a murmur heard during ventricular diastole. It may indicate aortic or pulmonary valve incompetence or tricuspid or mitral valve stenosis.

diastrophic /dī′əstrof′ik/ [Gk, *diastrephein*, to distort], pertaining to a bent or curved condition of bones or distortion of other structures.

diastrophic dwarf, a person in whom short stature is caused by osteochondrodysplasia and is associated with various deformities of the bones and joints, including scoliosis, clubfoot, micromelia, hand defects, multiple joint contractures and subluxations, ear deformities, and cleft palate. The condition may be genetically related and transmitted as an autosomal recessive trait.

diathermy /dī′əthur′mē/ [Gk, *dia* + *therme*, heat], the production of heat in body tissues for therapeutic purposes by high-frequency currents that are insufficiently intense to destroy tissues or to impair their vitality. Diathermy is used in treating chronic arthritis, bursitis, fractures, gynecologic diseases, sinusitis, and other conditions.

diathesis /dī·əthē′sis/, *pl.* **diatheses** [Gk, arrangement], an inherited physical constitution predisposing to certain diseases or conditions, many of which are believed associated with the Y chromosome, because males appear to be more susceptible than females. A diasthesis may be bilious, indicating a familial tendency to develop GI distress, or gouty, indicating a predisposition to the accumulation of urates in the tissues, particularly in mature males.

diazepam /dī·az′əpam/, a benzodiazepam sedative and tranquilizer.

■ INDICATIONS: It is prescribed in the treatment of anxiety, nervous tension, and muscle spasm, and as an anticonvulsant.

■ CONTRAINDICATIONS: Acute narrow-angle glaucoma, psychosis, or known hypersensitivity to this drug or to any benzodiazepine medication prohibits its use.

■ ADVERSE EFFECTS: Among the more serious adverse reactions are withdrawal symptoms resulting from discontinuation of treatment. Hypotonia, respiratory depression, drowsiness, and fatigue commonly occur.

diazo-, a prefix indicating a chemical compound containing the group, -N=N-; *diazole, diazine.*

diazoxide /dī′əzok′sīd/, a vasodilator used as an antihypertensive.

■ INDICATIONS: It is prescribed for the emergency reduction of blood pressure in malignant hypertension when drastic reduction of the diastolic blood pressure is required and in some cases of hypoglycemia.

■ CONTRAINDICATIONS: Compensatory hypertension or known hypersensitivity to this drug or other thiazides prohibits its use. Caution is advised in heart disease, pregnancy, and impaired kidney function.

■ ADVERSE EFFECTS: Among the more serious adverse reactions are tachycardia, sodium and water retention, hyperglycemia, and severe hypotension.

■ NOTE: This drug is for intravenous use in hospitalized patients only. Severe hypotension may result.

Dibenzyline, a trademark for an alpha-adrenergic blocker (phenoxybenzamine hydrochloride).

dibucaine /dī′bəkān/, a topical anesthetic ointment.

dic, (in cytogenetics) abbreviation for *dicentric.*

DIC, abbreviation for **disseminated intravascular coagulation.**

dicalcium phosphate and calcium gluconate with vitamin D, /dīkal′sē·əm/ a source of calcium and phosphorus.

■ INDICATIONS: It is prescribed for hypocalcemia, especially in pregnancy and lactation.

■ CONTRAINDICATIONS: Hypoparathyroidism or known hypersensitivity to any of the ingredients of this drug prohibits its use.

■ ADVERSE EFFECTS: There are no known adverse reactions.

dicephaly /dīsef′əlē/ [Gk, *di,* twice, *kephale,* head], a developmental anomaly in which the fetus has two heads. –**dicephalous, dicephalic,** *adj.,* **dicephalus,** *n.*

dichlorodiphenyltrichloroethane. See **DDT.**

dichlorphenamide /dī′klôrfen′əmīd/, a carbonic anhydrase inhibitor.

■ INDICATION: It is prescribed in the treatment of chronic glaucoma.

■ CONTRAINDICATIONS: Liver and adrenocortical insufficiency, kidney failure, hyperchloremic acidosis, depressed sodium or potassium levels, pulmonary obstruction, Addison's disease, known or suspected pregnancy, or known hypersensitivity to this drug prohibits its use.

■ ADVERSE EFFECTS: Among the more serious adverse reactions are anorexia, GI disturbances, acidosis, ureteral calculus formation, and aplastic anemia.

dichorial twins, dichorionic twins. See **dizygotic twins.**

dichroic stain /dīkrō′ik/, a radiographic film artifact caused by a colored chemical stain. The color may range from yellow to purple and is usually the result of improper processing. See also **curtain effect.**

dichromatic vision /dī′krōmat′ik/ [Gk, *di,* two, *chroma,* color; L, *visio*], a form of color vision in which only two of the three primary colors are perceived. Also called **dichromasia; dichromatopsia.**

dichotomy /dīkot′əmē/ [Gk, *dicha,* in two, *temnein,* to cut], a division or separation into two equal parts.

Dick-Read method. See **Read method.**

Dick test [George F. Dick, b. 1881; Gladys R. H. Dick, b. 1881; American physicians], a skin test for determining sensitivity to an erythrotoxin produced by the group A streptococci that cause scarlet fever. A skin-test dose of the toxin is injected intradermally. An area of inflammation 1 cm in diameter indicates that the person is not immune, has no antitoxin, and therefore is susceptible to the toxin. Larger doses may then be given to induce immunity. Compare **Schultz-Charlton phenomenon.**

dicloxacillin sodium /dī′kloksəsil′in/, a penicillinase-resistant penicillin.

■ INDICATIONS: It is prescribed in the treatment of staphylococcal infections, especially those caused by penicillinase-producing strains of staphylococci.

■ CONTRAINDICATIONS: Known hypersensitivity to this drug or to any penicillin medication prohibits its use.

■ ADVERSE EFFECTS: The most serious adverse effect is hypersensitivity reaction. Other side effects include nausea, diarrhea, and epigastric distress.

Dicor, a trademark for a castable ceramic dental material.

dicrotic notch /dīkrot′ik/, a phenomenon observed on the downstroke of the arterial pressure waveform. It represents closure of the aortic valve at the onset of ventricular diastole. Also observed on the pulmonary artery pressure waveform, the interval represents closure of the pulmonic valve.

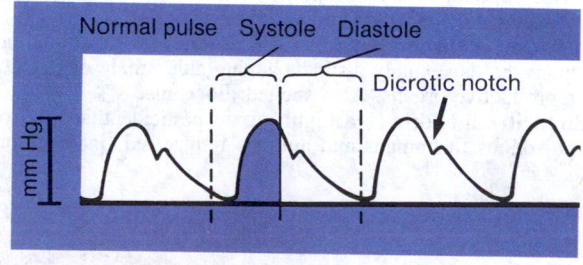

Dicrotic notch *(Canobbio, 1990)*

dicrotic pulse, a pulse with two separate peaks, the second usually weaker than the first. Compare **bisferien pulse.**

dicumarol /dīkyōō′mərol/, a synthetic anticoagulant.

■ INDICATIONS: It is prescribed for the prophylaxis and treatment of thrombosis and embolism.

■ CONTRAINDICATIONS: Risk of hemorrhage, peptic ulcer, ulcerative colitis, or known hypersensitivity to this drug prohibits its use.

■ ADVERSE EFFECTS: Among the more serious adverse reactions are GI disturbances, nausea, bleeding, and diarrhea.

dicyclomine hydrochloride /dīsī′kləmīn/, an anticholinergic.

■ INDICATION: It is prescribed as an adjunct to ulcer therapy.

■ CONTRAINDICATIONS: Narrow-angle glaucoma, asthma, obstruction of the genitourinary or GI tract, ulcerative colitis, or known hypersensitivity to this drug prohibits its use.

■ ADVERSE EFFECTS: Among the more serious adverse reac-

tions are blurred vision, central nervous system effects, tachycardia, dry mouth, decreased sweating, and hypersensitivity reactions.

didactic /dīdak′tik/ [Gr, *didaskein*, to teach], pertaining to teaching or instruction.

didanosine. See **dideoxyinosine (DDI).**

dideoxycytidine (ddC) /dī′dē·ok′sēsī′tidēn/, an antiretroviral drug that prevents the HIV virus from multiplying. It is chemically related to **dideoxyinosine (DDI).**

dideoxyinosine (DDI) /dī′dē·oksē·in′ōsēn/, an antiretroviral drug used in the treatment of HIV infections. DDI inhibits the enzyme reverse transcriptase, thereby restricting viral replication activity. Inside the body, DDI is converted to dideoxyadenosine, which becomes incorporated into the DNA chain, interrupting its normal sequence and making viral replication impossible. Also called **didanosine.**

Didrex, a trademark for an anorexiant (benzphetamine hydrochloride).

Didronel, a trademark for a calcium regulator (etidronate disodium).

didym-, **1.** a combining form meaning 'pertaining to a testis': *didymalgia, didymitis, didymodynia*. **2.** a combining form meaning 'paired or twin': *didymous*.

-didymis, -didymus-, **1.** a suffix meaning 'pertaining to the testicles': *epididymis*. **2.** a suffix meaning 'twins': *atlodidymus, pygodidymus*.

didymitis /did′əmī′tis/, an inflammation in a testicle.

didymus /did′iməs/, a testis.

-didymus, **1.** a suffix meaning a 'pair of twins joined at a (specified) part of the body': *gastrodidymus, thoracodidymus, vertebrodidymus*. **2.** a suffix meaning a 'fetal monster with supernumerary organ(s)': *atlodidymus, opodidymus, pygodidymus*.

diecious /dī·ē′shəs/ [Gk, *di + oikos*, house], an animal or plant that is sexually distinct, having either male or female reproductive organs. Also spelled **dioecious.**

dieldrin /dī·el′drin/, a highly toxic pesticide that is also poisonous to humans and animals if ingested, inhaled, or absorbed through the skin. It causes dysfunction of the central nervous system and is a possible carcinogen.

diencephalon /dī′ənsef′əlon/ [Gk, *di + enkephalon*, brain], the division of the brain between the cerebrum and the mesencephalon. It consists of the hypothalamus, thalamus, metathalamus, and the epithalamus and includes most of the third ventricle.

diener /dē′nər/ [Ger, man-servant], an individual who maintains the hospital laboratory or equipment and facilities. The morgue diener may also assist the pathologist in performing autopsies.

dienestrol /dī′ines′trôl/, an estrogen.

■ INDICATIONS: It is prescribed in the treatment of atrophic vaginitis and kraurosis vulvae.

■ CONTRAINDICATIONS: Pregnancy, known or suspected cancer of the breast, thrombophlebitis, unusual vaginal bleeding, or known hypersensitivity to this drug prohibits its use.

■ ADVERSE EFFECTS: Among the more serious adverse reactions are increased risk of cancer, thrombophlebitis, hepatic adenoma, embolism, and gallbladder disease.

diet /dī′it/ [Gk, *diaita*, a way of living], **1.** food and drink considered with regard to their nutritional qualities, composition, and effects on health. **2.** nutrients prescribed, regulated, orrestricted as to kind and amount for therapeutic or other purposes. **3.** the customary allowance of food and drink regularly provided or consumed. Compare **nutrition.** See also specific diets. **–dietetic,** *adj*.

dietary allowances /dī′əter′ē/, the recommended allowances of essential nutrients formulated by the Food and Nutrition Board of the National Research Council to serve as a guide for planning the diet to maintain good nutrition in healthy individuals. In general the recommended allowances exceed average nutritional requirements and are lower than the amounts needed in disease or deficiency states. See also **recommended dietary allowances (RDA).**

dietary amenorrhea [Gk, *diaita*, way of living, *a*, absence, *men*, month, *rhoia*, to flow], an interruption of menstru-

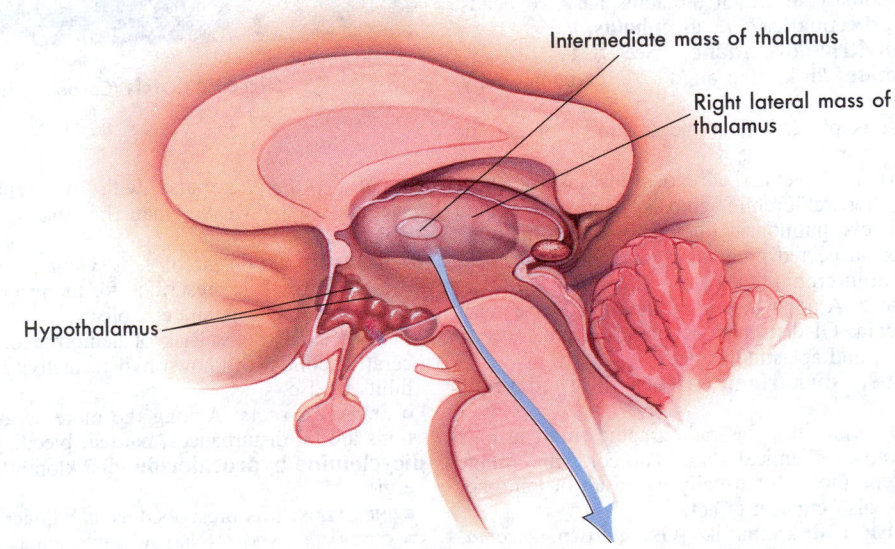

Diencephalon *(Thibodeau, 1993/Scott Bodell)*

Intermediate mass of thalamus

Right lateral mass of thalamus

Hypothalamus

ation because of malnutrition, starvation, or excessive voluntary dieting.

dietary fiber, a generic term for nondigestible chemical substances found in plant cell walls and surrounding cellular material, each with a different effect on the various GI functions, such as colon transit time, water absorption, and lipid metabolism. The main dietary fiber components are cellulose, lignin, hemicellulose, pectin, and gums. Foods high in dietary fiber are fruits; green leafy vegetables, such as lettuce, spinach, celery, and cabbage; root vegetables, such as carrots, turnips, and potatoes; legumes and whole-grain cereals and breads. Also called **bulk, roughage.**

-dietetic. See **diet.**

dietetic assistant /dī'ətet'ik/, a person who assists in providing food-service supervison and nutritional-care services under the guidance of a registered dietitian. A dietetic assistant is usually required to complete a training program approved by the American Dietetic Association in order to be qualified.

dietetic food, **1.** a specially prepared low-calorie food, often containing artificial sweeteners. **2.** a food prepared for any specific dietary need or restriction, such as salt-free or vegetarian foods. See also **dietetics.**

dietetic food diarrhea. See **osmotic diarrhea.**

dietetics /dī'itet'iks/, the science of applying nutritional principles to the planning and preparation of foods and regulation of the diet in relation to both health and disease.

dietetic technician, a person qualified by an associate degree program approved by the American Dietetic Association who may assist in providing food service management or nutritional-care services under the supervision of a registered dietitian.

diethylcarbamazine citrate /dī·eth'əlkärbam'əzēn/, an anthelmintic.

■ INDICATIONS: It is prescribed in the treatment of ascariasis, filariasis, onchocerciasis, loiasis, and tropic eosinophilia.

■ CONTRAINDICATIONS: Hypertension, severe heart, kidney, or liver impairment, or known hypersensitivity to this drug prohibits its use.

■ ADVERSE EFFECTS: The most serious adverse reactions are tachycardia, breathing difficulties, hypotension, and severe allergic reactions caused by the death of parasites.

diethyl ether. See **ether.**

diethylpropion hydrochloride /dī·eth'ilprō'pē·on/, an appetite suppressant.

■ INDICATION: It is prescribed in the treatment of exogenous obesity.

■ CONTRAINDICATIONS: Arteriosclerosis, hyperthyroidism, glaucoma, history of drug dependence, hypertension, concomitant administration of a monoamine oxidase inhibi tor within 14 days, or known hypersensitivity to this drug prohibits its use.

■ ADVERSE EFFECTS: Among the more serious adverse reactions are restlessness and insomnia, increased blood pressure, arrhythmias, cardiovascular effects, nausea, dry mouth, and drug dependence.

diethylstilbestrol (DES) /-stilbes'trol/, synthetic hormone with estrogenic properties. Also called **stilbestrol.**

diethylstilbestrol diphosphate, an antineoplastic agent.

■ INDICATION: It is prescribed for inoperable, progressing prostatic cancer.

■ CONTRAINDICATIONS: Present or previous conditions of markedly impaired liver, thrombophlebitis, thromboembolic disorders, or cerebral apoplexy prohibits its use.

■ ADVERSE EFFECTS: The most serious adverse reactions are thrombophlebitis, pulmonary embolism, cerebral thrombosis, cholestatic jaundice, mental depression, erythema nodosum and erythema multiforme, changes in libido, and dizziness.

dietitian /dī'ətish'ən/, a person who meets all the requirements for active membership in the American Dietetic Association after completing special educational training in the nutritional care of groups and individuals. A registered dietitian is one who has successfully completed an examination and maintains continuing education requirements of the Commission on Dietetic Registration.

Dietl's crisis /dē'təlz/ [Joseph Dietl, Polish physician, b. 1804; Gk *krisis* turning point], a sudden, excruciating pain in the kidney, caused by distention of the renal pelvis, by the rapid ingestion of very large amounts of liquid, or by a kinking of a ureter that produces temporary occlusion of the flow of urine from the kidney. The pain may be accompanied by nausea, vomiting, hematuria, and general collapse. See also **hydronephrosis.**

differential absorption /dif'əren'shəl/ [L, *differentia*, difference], (in radiology), the difference between those x-rays absorbed photoelectrically and those not absorbed at all, resulting in the x-ray image. In a radiograph of a body part, such as an arm, the image of the bone is produced because more x-rays are absorbed photoelectrically by bone than by the surrounding soft tissue. Differential absorption increases as the kVp is lowered, although lowering the kVp increases the patient dose. Also called **selective absorption.**

differential diagnosis, the distinguishing between two or more diseases with similar symptoms by systematically comparing their signs and symptoms. See also **diagnosis.**

differential growth, a comparison of the various increases in size or the different rates of growth of dissimilar organisms, tissues, or structures.

differential white blood cell count, an examination and enumeration of the distribution of leukocytes in a stained blood smear. The different kinds of white cells are counted and reported as percentages of the total examined. Compare **complete blood count.** See also **hematocrit, hemoglobin, leukocyte, red cell indexes.**

differentiation /dif'əren'shē·ā'shən/ [L, *differentia*, difference], **1.** (in embryology) a process in development in which unspecialized cells or tissues are systemically modified and altered to achieve specific and characteristic physical forms, physiologic functions, and chemical properties. Kinds of differentiation are **correlative differentiation, functional differentiation, invisible differentiation,** and **self-differentiation.** **2.** progressive diversification leading to complexity. **3.** the acquisition of functions and forms different from those of the original. **4.** the distinguishing of one thing or disease from another, as in differential diagnosis. **5.** (in psychology) a mental autonomy or separation of intellect and emotions so that one is not dominated by reactive anxiety of a family or group emotional system. **6.** the first subphase of the separation-individuation phase in Mahler's system of preoedipal development. It generally occurs between the ages of 5 months and 9 months, coinciding with the maturation of partial locomotor functioning and when the child begins to view the mother as a separate being. **–differentiate,** *v.*

diffraction /difrak'shən/ [L, *dis*, opposite of, *frangere*, to break], the bending and scattering of wavelengths of light or other radiation, such as the radiation that passes around obstacles in its path. X-ray diffraction is used in the study of the internal structure of cells. The x-rays are diffracted by cell parts into patterns that are indicative of chemical and physical structure. See also **refraction.**

diffuse /difyo͞oz/ [L, *diffundere,* to spread out], becoming widely spread, such as through a membrane or fluid.

diffuse fibrosing alveolitis. See **interstitial pneumonia.**

diffuse goiter, an enlargement of all parts of the thyroid gland.

diffuse hypersensitivity pneumonia, an immunologically mediated inflammatory reaction in the lungs induced by exposure to an allergen derived from a fungus, bird excreta, piscine, porcine, or bovine proteins, wood dust, or fur, or by an adverse reaction to a drug, such as chlorpropamide, hydrochlorothiazide, mecamylamine, mephenesin, methotrexate, nitrofurantoin, para-aminosalicylic acid, or penicillin. The disorder is characterized by cough, fever, dyspnea, malaise, pulmonary edema, and infiltration of the alveoli with eosinophils and large mononuclear cells. Also called **allergic alveolitis, allergic interstitial pneumonitis, extrinsic allergic pneumonia.** See also **bagassosis, P.I.E.**

diffuse idiopathic skeletal hyperostosis, a form of degenerative joint disease in which the ligaments along the spinal column become calcified and lose their flexibility.

diffuse lipoma, diffuse lipomatosis. See **multiple lipomatosis.**

diffuse myocardial fibrosis, a type of heart disease characterized by a generalized distribution of fibrous tissue that replaces normal heart muscle cells.

diffuse peritonitis [L, *diffundere,* to pour out; Gk, *peri,* near, *teinein,* to stretch, *itis,* inflammation], widespread peritonitis, affecting most of the peritoneum, usually caused by a ruptured stomach or appendix. Also called **generalized peritonitis.**

diffuse sclerosis [L, *diffundere,* to pour out; Gk, *sklerosis,* hardening], a form of sclerosis that extends through much of the central nervous system.

diffusing capacity /difyo͞o'sing/, the rate of gas transfer through a unit area of a permeable membrane per unit of gas pressure difference across it. It is affected by specific chemical reactions that may occur in the blood. Also called **diffusion factor, transfer factor of lungs.**

diffusing capacity of lungs (D_L), the number of milliliters of a gas that diffuse from the lung across the alveolar-capillary (A-C) membrane into the bloodstream each minute, for each 1 mm Hg difference in the pressure gradient across the membrane. The average normal D_L value for oxygen is 20 ml/min/mm Hg.

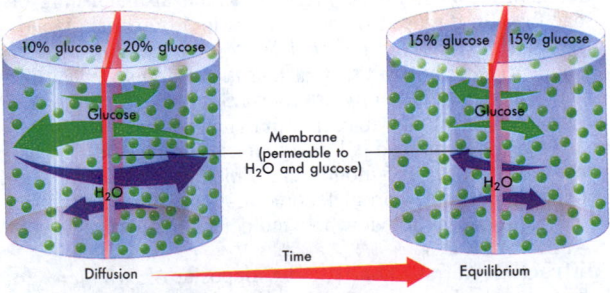

Diffusion *(Thibodeau, 1993/Rolin Graphics)*

diffusion /dify o͞o'zhən/ [L, *diffundere,* to spread out], the process in which solid, particulate matter in a fluid moves from an area of higher concentration to an area of lower concentration, resulting in an even distribution of the particles in the fluid. No energy is required.

diffusion coefficient. See **coefficient.**

diffusion constant, a mathematical constant relating to the ability of a substance to spread widely.

diffusion defect, any impairment of alveolar-capillary diffusion caused by pathologic changes in any of the structures of the alveolar-capillary membrane and resulting in fewer molecules of oxygen crossing the membrane. Specific causes may include fibrosis, granuloma, interstitial edema, and proliferation of connective tissue.

diffusion deposition, the impaction of an aerosol particle on the surface of an alveolar membrane or other airway structure, causing it to settle out of a vapor or gas.

diffusion factor. See **diffusing capacity.**

diffusion of gases, a natural process, essential in respiration, in which molecules of a gas pass from an area of high concentration to one of lower concentration.

diflorasone diacetate /dīflôr'əsōn dī·os'ətāt/, a topical corticosteroid.

■ INDICATION: It is prescribed topically as an antiinflammatory agent.

■ CONTRAINDICATIONS: Viral and fungal diseases of the skin, impaired circulation, or known hypersensitivity to this drug or to other steroidal medication prohibits its use.

■ ADVERSE EFFECTS: Among the more serious adverse reactions, usually occurring after prolonged or excessive application, are striae, hypopigmentation, local irritation of the skin, and various systemic effects.

Diflucan, trademark for a brand of fluconazole, a broad-spectrum bis-triazole antifungal agent used in the treatment of cryptococcal meningitis, oropharyngeal and esophageal candidiasis, and similar fungal infections.

diflunisal /dīflo͞o'nisal/, a nonsteroidal antiinflammatory agent.

■ INDICATIONS: It is prescribed for mild to moderate pain and inflammation in osteoarthritis and other musculoskeletal disorders.

■ CONTRAINDICATIONS: Hypersensitivity to aspirin and other nonsteroidal antiinflammatory drugs or known sensitivity to this drug prohibits its use.

■ ADVERSE EFFECTS: The most serious adverse reactions are GI pain, diarrhea, peptic ulcer, anorexia, and edema.

digastricus /dīgas'trikəs/ [Gk, *di,* twice, *gaster,* stomach], one of four suprahyoid muscles having two parts, an anterior belly and a posterior belly. The anterior belly originates in the lower border of the mandible and inserts in the body and great cornu of the hyoid bone. It is innervated by fibers of the mandibular branch of the trigeminal nerve. It acts to open the jaw and to draw the hyoid bone forward. The posterior belly originates in the mastoid notch of the temporal bone and inserts in the body and great cornu of the hyoid bone. It is innervated by fibers of the mandibular branch of the facial nerve and acts to draw back and to raise the hyoid bone. Also called **digastric muscle.** Compare **geniohyoideus, mylohyoideus, stylohyoideus.**

DiGeorge's syndrome /dijôrj'əz/ [Angelo M. DiGeorge, American physician, b. 1821], a congenital disorder characterized by severe immunodeficiency and structural abnormalities, including hypertelorism, notched, low-set ears, small mouth, downward slanting eyes, cardiovascular de-

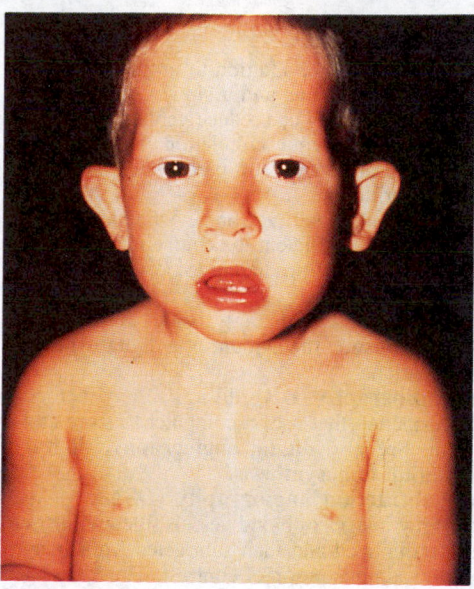

DiGeorge's syndrome *(Zitelli, 1992)*

fects, and the absence of the thymus and parathyroid glands. Death, often from infection, usually occurs before 2 years of age. Rarely, transplantation of a human fetal thymus is performed. Also called **thymic parathyroid aplasia.**

digest [L, *digere,* to digest], **1.** /dijest'/ to soften by heat and moisture. **2.** /dijest'/ to break into smaller parts and simpler compounds by mastication, hydrolysis, and the action of intestinal secretions and enzymes, especially in the way the body digests food for the absorption of nutrients required in metabolism. The small intestine digests food by enzymatic actions that produce absorbable amino acids, emulsified fat particles, and monosaccharides. **3.** /dī'jəst/ any material that results from digestion or hydrolysis.

digestant /dijes'tənt/, a substance, such as pepsin, that is added to the diet as an aid to the digestion of food.

digestion /dijes'chən/ [L, *digere,* to separate], the conversion of food into absorbable substances in the GI tract. Digestion is accomplished through the mechanical and chemical breakdown of food into smaller and smaller molecules, with the help of glands located both inside and outside the gut. **–digestive,** *adj.*

digestive enzyme /dijes'tiv/ [L, *digere,* to separate; Gk, *en, zyme,* ferment], any digestive system enzyme that hydrolyzes fats, proteins, and carbohydrates for absorption.

digestive fever, a slight rise in body temperature that normally accompanies the digestive process.

digestive gland, any one of the many structures that secretes reactive agents involved in the breaking down of food into the constituent absorbable substances needed for metabolism. Some kinds of digestive glands are the salivary glands, gastric glands, intestinal glands, liver, and pancreas. Some important secretions produced by different digestive glands are hydrochloric acid, bile, mucus, and various enzymes.

digestive system, the organs, structures, and accessory glands of the digestive tube of the body through which food passes from the mouth to the esophagus, stomach, and in-

testines. The accessory glands secrete the digestive enzymes, used by the digestive system to break down food substances in preparation for absorption into the bloodstream before carrying the waste to the intestines for excretion. See also the Color Atlas of Human Anatomy.

digestive tract, a musculomembranous tube, about 9 m long, extending from the mouth to the anus and lined with mucous membrane. Its various portions are the mouth, pharynx, esophagus, stomach, small intestine, and large intestine. The tube, which is part of the digestive system of the body, includes numerous accessory organs. Also called **alimentary canal, alimentary tract, digestive tube, GI tract, intestinal tract, intestinal tube.** See also **digestive system.**

Digibind, a trademark for the antibody used in the treatment of digoxin toxicity (digoxin immune fab, ovine).

digit-, a combining form meaning 'pertaining to a finger or toe': *digitate, digitigrade, digitoplantar.*

digital /dij'itəl/ [L, *digitus,* finger], **1.** of or pertaining to a digit, that is, a finger or toe. **2.** resembling a finger or toe. See also **digitate. 3.** the characterization or measurement of a signal in terms of a series of numbers rather than in terms of some continuously varying value.

digital angiography, a technique of producing enhanced x-ray images of the heart with computerized fluoroscopy equipment. After injection of contrast material through a large vein, a base mask image is digitized and stored in the digital memory. Successive digitized images are electronically subtracted from the mask image and amplified by a factor of 8 to 16 and displayed on a television monitor. The image is also recorded on videotape and can also be stored on a digital disk.

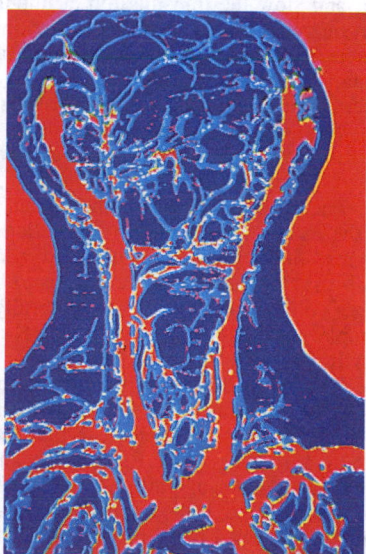

Digital subtraction angiography
(Seeley, 1992/Howard Sochurek)

digital compression [L, *digitus,* finger, *comprimere,* to press together], the act of pressing with the fingers, as when arresting the blood flow from a wound.

digital computer, a computer that processes information in numeric form. Compare **analog computer, hybrid computer.**

digital fluoroscopy, a method of conducting fluoroscopic examinations with an image intensifier–television system combined with a high-speed digital video image processor. The image intensifier has an input surface coated with a special x-ray–sensitive phosphor that is twice as efficient in detecting x-rays as conventional x-ray film. The visible light from the energized phosphor is electronically amplified and directed into a television camera. The television image is divided into pixels, which are in turn converted or digitized into binary numbers for storage or reproduction through an image processor.

digitalis /dij′ital′is/ [L, *digitus*, finger], a general term for cardiac glycoside.

■ INDICATIONS: It is prescribed in the treatment of congestive heart failure and certain cardiac arrhythmias.

■ CONTRAINDICATIONS: Ventricular fibrillation, ventricular tachycardia, or known hypersensitivity to this drug prohibits its use.

■ ADVERSE EFFECTS: The most serious reactions are various cardiac arrhythmias that are more common with concomitant diuretics.

digitalis glycoside. See **glycoside.**

digitalis poisoning [L, *digitalis*, of the fingers, *potio*, drink], the toxic effects of digitalis medications prescribed for heart disorders such as heart failure and atrial fibrillation. Toxicity may develop as a result of a cumulative effect of the drug. Symptoms include vomiting, headache, heart beat abnormalities, and visual color distortions.

digitalis therapy, the administration of a digitalis preparation to a person with a heart disorder to increase the force of myocardial contractions, produce a slower, more regular apical rate, and slow the transmission of impulses through the conduction system. It may be used in treating many cardiac disorders, including atrial fibrillation, atrial septal defect, coarctation of the aorta, congenital heart block, congestive heart failure, endocardial fibroelastosis, great vessel transposition, malformation of the tricuspid valve, myocarditis, paroxysmal atrial tachycardia, and patent ductus arteriosus.

■ METHOD: The completeness of the orders is ensured regarding the name of the digitalis preparation, the dosage in milligrams, the route and intervals of administration, and the pulse rate under which the drug is to be withheld. The dosage volume of the drug is carefully calculated by two people: two registered nurses, an RN and pharmacist, or an RN and physician. If the drug is to be given orally, the best method of ensuring that a child receives the full dose is determined: whether by spoon, nipple, or dropper. It is administered before feeding and is never mixed with the formula or food. Before each administration, the person's resting apical pulse is checked for rate and rhythm for a full minute; if the rate is slower than desired, if it is irregular or shows a rapid rise or fall, if there are any signs of toxicity, as anorexia, nausea, vomiting, or if there are visual disturbances, the drug is withheld and the problem is reported.

■ NURSING INTERVENTION: The nurse participates in calculating the dosage volume ordered, administers the drug, and observes for and reports any undesirable effects. Once the dosage is stabilized and before discharge, the nurse ensures that the patient understands the proper method, time, and purpose of administering the drug, as well as the need and the time to give the complete dose, when to withhold med-

ication, and how to recognize and report signs of toxicity to the drug.

■ OUTCOME CRITERIA: In addition to promoting more forceful myocardial contractions and a slower, more regular apical beat, digitalis therapy can reduce venous pressure, improve pulmonary and systemic circulation, increase urinary output, reduce edema, and stop paroxysmal atrial tachycardia and atrial fibrillation.

digitalization /dij′ətal′īzā′shən/, the administration of digitalis in doses sufficient to achieve maximum pharmacologic effects without producing toxic symptoms.

digitalized /dij′ətəlīzd′/, having a therapeutic total body level of digitalis, a cardiac glycoside.

digitalizing dose, the amount of a digitalis needed to digitalize a patient.

digital radiography (DR) /dij′itəl/, any method of x-ray image formation that uses a computer to store and manipulate data. See also **digital angiography, digital fluoroscopy, digital tomosynthesis.**

digital subtraction angiography (DSA), a method by which x-ray images of blood vessels filled with contrast material are digitized and then subtracted from images stored before the administration of contrast. Thus, the background is eliminated and only the vessels appear.

digital thermometer. See **thermometer.**

digital-to-analog converter, a device for converting digital information into analog form for representation as a continuous method of interpreting data, as from an ohmmeter or thermometer. Also called **D/A converter.**

digital tomosynthesis, a system of tomography using a computer and digital fluoroscopy unit, making it possible to synthesize any tomographic plane from a single tomographic pass. As only one tomographic slice is required, patient radiation exposure is reduced. Patient time in examination is also reduced as the recorded images can be synthesized and manipulated at a later time. See also **digital fluoroscopy.**

digitate /dij′itāt/ [L, *digitatus*, having fingers], having fingers or fingerlike projections. See also **digital.**

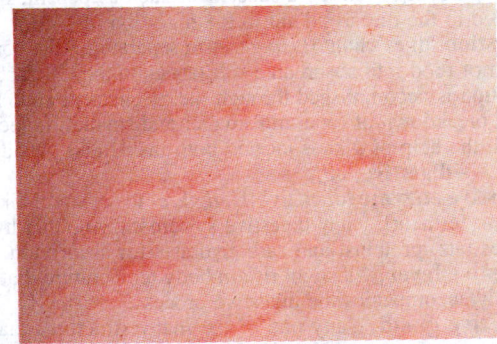

Digitate dermatosis (du Vivier, 1993)

digitate wart, a fingerlike, horny projection that arises from a pea-shaped base and occurs on the scalp or near the hairline. It is a benign viral infection of the skin and the adjacent mucous membrane. It may disappear spontaneously as the host develops an immune response, or it may require treatment, such as by electrodesiccation and curettage. Also called **filiform warts.**

digitoxin /dig'itok'sin/, a cardiac glycoside obtained from leaves of *Digitalis purpurea*.
- INDICATIONS: It is prescribed in the treatment of congestive heart failure and certain cardiac arrhythmias.
- CONTRAINDICATIONS: Ventricular fibrillation, ventricular tachycardia, or known hypersensitivity to this drug prohibits its use.
- ADVERSE EFFECTS: The most serious adverse reactions are cardiac arrhythmias and heart block.

diglyceride /dīglis'ərīd/, a chemical compound, an ester of glycerol in which the hydrogen in two of the hydroxyl groups is replaced by an acyl radical.

digoxin /digok'sin/, a cardiac glycoside obtained from leaves of *Digitalis lanata*.
- INDICATIONS: It is prescribed in the treatment of congestive heart failure and certain cardiac arrhythmias.
- CONTRAINDICATIONS: Ventricular fibrillation, ventricular tachycardia, or known hypersensitivity to this drug prohibits its use.
- ADVERSE EFFECTS: The most serious adverse reactions are cardiac arrhythmia and heart block.

digoxin immune Fab, ovine, a parenteral antidote for digoxin toxicity.
- INDICATIONS: It is prescribed for life-threatening digoxin or digitoxin toxicity.
- CONTRAINDICATIONS: Use of this product should be restricted to patients in shock or cardiac arrest or who show signs of severe ventricular dysrhythmias, progressive bradycardia, or potassium concentrations exceeding 5 mEq/L.
- ADVERSE EFFECTS: Among reported adverse reactions are possible low cardiac output, congestive heart failure exacerbated by withdrawal of digoxin's inotropic effect, possible rapid ventricular response due to withdrawal of the digitalis effect, and possible hypokalemia.

diGuglielmo's disease, diGuglielmo's syndrome. See **erythroleukemia.**

dihybrid /dī'hī'brid/ [Gk, *di,* twice; L, *hybrida,* mongrel offspring], (in genetics) pertaining to or describing a person, organism, or strain that is heterozygous for two specific traits, that is the offspring of parents differing in two specific gene pairs, or that is heterozygous for two particular traits or gene loci under consideration.

dihybrid cross, (in genetics) the mating of two individuals, organisms, or strains that have different gene pairs that determine two specific traits or in which two particular characteristics or gene loci are being followed.

dihydric alcohol /dīhī'drik/, an alcohol containing two hydroxyl groups.

dihydroergotamine mesylate /dīhī'drō·ərgot'əmēn me'silāt/, an alpha-adrenergic blocking agent.
- INDICATIONS: It is prescribed for migraine and for vascular headache.
- CONTRAINDICATIONS: Cardiovascular disease, hypertension, liver or kidney dysfunction, sepsis, pregnancy, or known hypersensitivity to this drug prohibits its use.
- ADVERSE EFFECTS: Among the more serious adverse reactions are gangrene and the toxicity of the ergot alkaloids.

dihydrotachysterol /dīhī'drōtəkis'tərol/, a rapid-acting form of vitamin D.
- INDICATIONS: It is prescribed in the treatment of hypocalcemia resulting from hypoparathyroidism and pseudohypoparathyroidism.
- CONTRAINDICATIONS: Hypercalcemia, hypocalcemia with kidney insufficiency, hyperphosphatemia, or known hyper-

sensitivity to this drug or to vitamin D prohibits its use. Caution is advised for lactating mothers.
- ADVERSE EFFECTS: The most serious adverse reaction is hypercalcemia. With overdosage, calcification of soft tissues, including those of the heart, or cardiovascular or kidney failure may occur.

diiodohydroxyquin. See **iodoquinol.**

dil-, -dil, a combining form for the name of a vasodilator.

Dilantin, a trademark for an anticonvulsant (phenytoin).

dilatation /dil'ətā'shən/ [L, *dilatare,* to widen], artificial increase in the diameter of such an opening either by medication, as in the use of cycloplegic eyedrops to open the pupil wide for examination of the retina, or by instrumentation as in the use of a dilator to open the uterine cervix to facilitate curettage. Also called **dilation** /dīlā'shən/. −**dilatate, dilate** /dī'lāt/, *v.,* **dilatator, dilator,** *n.*

dilatation and curettage (D & C), dilatation of the uterine cervix and scraping of the endometrium of the uterus, performed to diagnose disease of the uterus, to correct heavy or prolonged vaginal bleeding, or to empty uterine contents of the products of conception. It is also done to remove tumors, to rule out carcinoma of the uterus, to remove retained placental fragments postpartum or after an incomplete abortion, and to find the cause of infertility. The cervix is dilated with a series of dilators of increasing size to allow the insertion of a curet into the uterus. Vaginal packing may sometimes be inserted to slow bleeding but is not usually recommended. It may be left in place for 24 hours. A sterile perineal pad is applied. Postoperative care requires emotional support appropriate to the clinical situation and close observation for hemorrhage, infection, or dysuria. See also **abortion.**

dilatation of the heart [L, *dilatare,* to widen; AS, *heorte*], an enlargement of the heart caused by stretching the muscle tissue in the walls, as a result of a weakening of the myocardium. The condition is associated with acute pulmonary embolism and heart failure.

dilatator naris /dil'ətā'tər/, the alar portion of the nasalis muscle that dilates the nostril. Compare **compressor naris.**

dilatator pupillae, a muscle that contracts the iris of the eye and dilates the pupil. It is composed of radiating fibers, like spokes of a wheel, that converge from the circumference of the iris toward the center and blend with fibers of the sphincter pupillae near the margin of the pupil. The dilatator pupillae is innervated by nerve fibers from the sympathetic system. Compare **sphincter pupillae.**

dilate, to cause a normal physiologic increase in the diameter of a body opening, blood vessel, or tube, such as the widening of the pupil of the eye in response to decreased light or the widening of the opening of the uterine cervix during labor. Compare **dilatation.**

dilation. See **dilatation.**

dilation and evacuation (D&E) /dīlā'shən/ [L, *dilatare,* to widen, *evacuare,* to empty], the removal of the products of conception, using suction curretage and forceps, during the second trimester of pregnancy.

dilator /dī'lātər/ [L, *dilatare,* to widen], a device for expanding a body opening or cavity. Examples include a tent dilator, consisting of a sponge or bundle of seaweed that expands the cervical os, and a Barnes' dilator, a rubber bag that can be inserted into a body cavity and filled with water to produce pressure on the cavity walls. (See Fig. p. 484.)

Dilaudid Hydrochloride, a trademark for a narcotic analgesic (hydromorphone hydrochloride).

Dilor, a trademark for a bronchodilator (dyphylline).

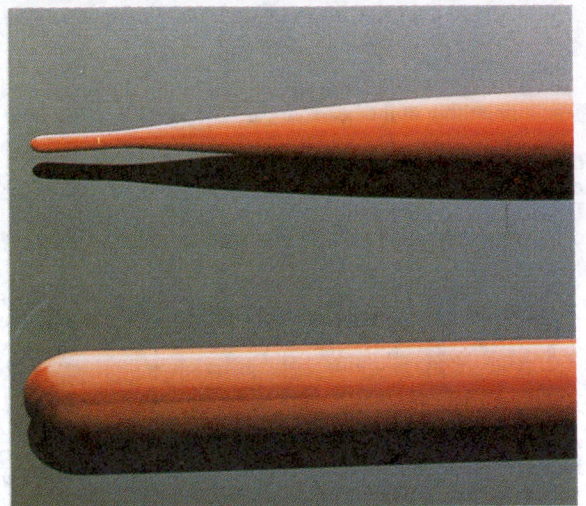

Mercury-filled dilators
(Winawer, 1992/Courtesy Pilling, Fort Washington PA)

diltiazem /diltī′əzam/, a slow calcium channel blocker or calcium antagonist.
- INDICATIONS: It is prescribed for the treatment of vasospastic and effort-associated angina.
- CONTRAINDICATIONS: Sick sinus syndrome, second- or third-degree atrioventricular block, or hypotension prohibits its use.
- ADVERSE EFFECTS: Among the more serious adverse reactions are edema, arrhythmia, bradycardia, hypotension, syncope, rash, headache, and dizziness.

diluent /dil′ōo·ənt, dil′yōo·ənt/ [L, *diluere*, to wash], a substance, generally a fluid, that makes a solution or mixture thinner, less viscous, or more liquid.

dilute /dilōot′, dī′lōot/ [L, *diluere*, to wash], pertaining to a solution in which there is a relatively small amount of solute in proportion to solvent.

diluting agent /dilōo′ting/, (in respiratory therapy) a substance that can modify the viscosity of secretions so that they can be removed easily. Examples include water and hypotonic saline, which can be aerosolized or nebulized.

dimenhydrinate /dim′ənhī′drināt/, an antihistamine.
- INDICATIONS: It is prescribed in the treatment of nausea and motion sickness.
- CONTRAINDICATIONS: Asthma or known hypersensitivity to this drug prohibits its use. It is not given to newborn infants or lactating mothers.
- ADVERSE EFFECTS: Among the more serious adverse reactions are skin rash, hypersensitivity reactions, and tachycardia. Drowsiness and dry mouth are common.

dimensional stability /dimen′shənəl/, (in radiology) the rigidity of the polyester base used for radiographic film and its resistance to image distortion from warping or changing size or shape during processing.

dimer /dī′mər/ [Gk, *di*, twice, *meros*, parts], a compound formed by the union of two radicals or two molecules of a simpler compound, as a polymer formed from two or more molecules of a monomer.

dimercaprol /dī′mərkap′rol/, a heavy-metal antagonist. Previously called **British antilewisite (BAL)**.

- INDICATIONS: It is prescribed in the treatment of Wilson's disease and in the treatment of acute arsenic, mercury, or gold poisoning, as from an overdosage with mercurial diuretics, arsenics, or gold salts or from an accidental ingestion of mercury, gold, or arsenic.
- CONTRAINDICATIONS: Hepatic or renal insufficiency, poisoning with cadmium, iron, or selenium, or known hypersensitivity to the drug prohibits its use.
- ADVERSE EFFECTS: Among the most serious adverse reactions are nephrotoxicity, acidosis, convulsions, and abnormal cardiovascular functions. Mild reactions include pain at the injection site, nausea, excessive salivation, and parasthesia.

Dimetane, a trademark for an antihistamine (brompheniramine maleate).

Dimetapp, a trademark for a fixed-combination drug containing two decongestants (phenylephrine hydrochloride and phenylpropanolamine hydrochloride) and an antihistamine (brompheniramine maleate).

dimethindene maleate /dīmeth′indēn/, an antihistamine.
- INDICATIONS: It is prescribed in the treatment of a variety of hypersensitivity reactions, including rhinitis, skin reactions, and itching.
- CONTRAINDICATIONS: The drug is not given to newborn infants or to lactating mothers. Asthma or known hypersensitivity to this drug prohibits its use.
- ADVERSE EFFECTS: Drowsiness, skin rash, hypersensitivity reactions, dry mouth, and tachycardia commonly occur.

dimethoxymethylamphetamine (DOM), /dī′məthok′-sēmeth′iləmfet′əmen/ a psychoactive or hallucinogenic agent.

dimethyl carbinol. See **isopropyl alcohol.**

dimethyl sulfoxide (DMSO) /dīmeth′il/, an antiinflammatory agent and organic solvent.
- INDICATIONS: It is prescribed in the treatment of interstitial cystitis and is being investigated as a topical antiinflammatory agent in orthopedic sports injuries.
- CONTRAINDICATION: Known hypersensitivity to this drug prohibits its use.
- ADVERSE EFFECTS: Among the most serious adverse reactions are GI disturbances, photophobia, disturbance of color vision, and headache. A garliclike body odor and taste in the mouth may occur. When applied to the skin, it can cause local irritations and carry toxins into the systemic circulation.

dimethyl tubocurarine iodide. See **metocurine iodide.**

Dimitri's disease. See **Sturge-Weber syndrome.**

dimorphous /dīmôr′fəs/ [Gk, *di*, two, *morphe*, form], (in biology, chemistry, genetics) pertaining to an organism or substance that exists in two distinct forms.

dimoxyline phosphate. See **dioxyline phosphate.**

dimpling [ME, *dympull*], small, abnormal indentations or depressions on the surface of a body or organ.

dinitrochlorobenzene (DNCB) /dīnī′trōklôr′ōben′zēn/, a substance applied topically as a test for delayed hypersensitivity reactions. The compound has also been used as an immunotherapeutic agent to treat skin tumors.

dioctyl calcium sulfosuccinate, dioctyl sodium sulfosuccinate. See **docusate.**

diode /dī′od/, (in radiology) an x-ray tube with two electrodes.

dioecious. See **diecious.**

diolamine /dī·ol′əmen/, abbreviated form for *diethanolamine.*

Dionysian /dē·onis′ē·ən/ [Gk, *Dionysos,* Greek god of wine], the personal attitude of one who is uninhibited, mystic, sensual, emotional, and irrational and who may seek to escape from the boundaries imposed by the limits of one's senses.

diopter /dī·op′tər/ [Gk *dioptra* optical measuring instrument], a metric measure of the refractive power of a lens. It is equal to the reciprocal of the focal length of the lens in meters. For example, a lens with a focal length of 0.5 m has a diopter measure of 2.0 (1/0.5) and when prescribed as a corrective lens for the eye should make printed matter most clearly focused when held 0.5 m from the eyes.

dioptric power /dī·op′trik/, the refractive power of an optic lens as measured in diopters.

Diothane, a trademark for a local anesthetic (diperodon monohydrate).

diovular. See **binovular.**

diovulatory /dī·ov′yələtôr′ē/ [Gk, *di,* twice; L, *ovum,* egg], routinely releasing two ova during each ovarian cycle. Compare **monovulatory.**

dioxide /dī·ok′sīd/[Gk, *di,* two, *oxys,* sharp, *genein,* to produce], an oxide that contains two oxygen atoms.

dioxin /dī·ok′sin/, a contaminant of the herbicide 2,4,5-trichlorophenoxyacetic acid (2,4,5-T), widely used throughout the world in forestry, on grassland, against woody shrubs and trees on industrial sites, and for rice and sugar-cane weed control. Because of its toxicity, it is no longer manufactured in the United States. Exposure to dioxin is associated with chloracne and porphyria cutanea tarda (PCT). Dioxin was a contaminant of the jungle defoliant Agent Orange sprayed by the United States military aircraft over areas of southeast Asia from 1965 to 1970. Also called **TCDD (2,3,7,8-tetrachlorodibenzopara-dioxin).**

dioxyline phosphate /dī·ok′silēn/, a synthetic antispasmodic and vasodilator. Also called **dimoxyline phosphate.**
- INDICATIONS: It is prescribed for the relief of angina pectoris and for spasm of blood vessels in arms, legs, or lungs.
- CONTRAINDICATION: Known hypersensitivity to this drug prohibits its use.
- ADVERSE EFFECTS: Among the most serious adverse reactions are nausea, dizziness, and flushing, which occur rarely.

DIP, abbreviation for **desquamative interstitial pneumonia.**

diphasic /dīfā′zik/ [Gk, *di,* two, *phasis,* appearance], pertaining to something that occurs in two stages or phases.

diphemanil methylsulfate /dīfē′mənil/, an anticholinergic.
- INDICATION: It is prescribed as an adjunct to ulcer therapy.
- CONTRAINDICATIONS: Narrow-angle glaucoma, asthma, obstruction of the genitourinary or GI tract, ulcerative colitis, or known hypersensitivity to this drug prohibits its use.
- ADVERSE EFFECTS: Among the more serious adverse reactions are blurred vision, central nervous system effects, tachycardia, dry mouth, decreased sweating, and hypersensitivity reactions.

diphenadione /dī′fənad′ē·ōn/, an anticoagulant.
- INDICATIONS: It is prescribed in the treatment of thrombosis and embolism.
- CONTRAINDICATIONS: Hemorrhage or known hypersensitivity to this drug prohibits its use.
- ADVERSE EFFECTS: The most serious adverse reaction is hemorrhage. This drug interacts with many other drugs.

diphenhydramine hydrochloride /dī′fənhī′drəmēn/, an antihistamine.
- INDICATIONS: It is prescribed in the treatment of a variety of hypersensitivity reactions, including rhinitis, skin rash, and pruritus, and in the treatment of motion sickness.
- CONTRAINDICATIONS: Asthma or known hypersensitivity to this drug prohibits its use. It is not given to newborn infants or lactating mothers.
- ADVERSE EFFECTS: Among the more serious adverse reactions are skin rash, hypersensitivity reactions, and tachycardia. Drowsiness and dry mouth commonly occur.

diphenidol /dīfē′nidol/, an antiemetic, antivertigo agent.
- INDICATIONS: It is prescribed in the treatment of vertigo and to control nausea and vomiting.
- CONTRAINDICATIONS: Anuria or known sensitivity to this drug prohibits its use.
- ADVERSE EFFECTS: Among the most serious adverse reactions are transient hypotension, hallucinations, disorientation, and mental confusion.

diphenoxylate hydrochloride /dī′fənok′silāt/, an antidiarrheal.
- INDICATIONS: It is prescribed in the treatment of noninfectious diarrhea and intestinal cramping.
- CONTRAINDICATIONS: Liver disease, antibiotic-associated diarrhea, or known hypersensitivity to this drug prohibits its use. It is not given to children under 2 years of age.
- ADVERSE EFFECTS: Among the more serious adverse reactions are abdominal discomfort, intestinal obstruction, skin rash, and nausea.

diphenylhydantoin. See **phenytoin.**

diphenylpyraline hydrochloride /dī′fenəlpī′rəlēn/, an antihistamine.
- INDICATIONS: It is prescribed in the treatment of a variety of hypersensitivity reactions, including rhinitis, skin rash, and pruritus.
- CONTRAINDICATIONS: Asthma or known hypersensitivity to this drug prohibits its use. It is not given to newborn infants or lactating mothers.
- ADVERSE EFFECTS: Among the more serious adverse reactions are skin rash, hypersensitivity reactions, and tachycardia. Drowsiness and dry mouth commonly occur.

2,3-diphosphoglyceric acid (DPG) /dīfos′fōgliser′ik/, a substance in the erythrocyte that affects the affinity of hemoglobin for oxygen. It is a chief end product of glucose metabolism and a link in the biochemical feedback control system that regulates the release of oxygen to the tissues.

diphtheria /difthir′ē·ə, dipthir′ē·ə/ [Gk, *diphthera,* leather membrane], an acute, contagious disease caused by the bacterium *Corynebacterium diphtheriae,* characterized by the production of a systemic toxin and a false membrane lining of the mucous membrane of the throat. The toxin is particularly damaging to the tissues of the heart and central nervous system, and the dense pseudomembrane in the throat may interfere with eating, drinking, and breathing. The membrane may occur in other body tissues. Lymph glands in the neck swell, and the neck becomes edematous. Untreated, the disease is often fatal, causing heart and kidney failure. Patients are usually hospitalized in isolation rooms. Treatment of the isolated patient may include administration of diphtheria antitoxin, antibiotics, bed rest, fluids, and an adequate diet. Tracheostomy is sometimes necessary. Recovery is slow, but it is usually complete. Immunization against diphtheria is available to all children in the United States and is usually given in conjunction with pertussis and tetanus immunization early in infancy. See also **Schick test.**

diphtheria and tetanus toxoids (DT),   an active immunizing agent.

■ INDICATIONS: It is prescribed for immunization against diphtheria and tetanus.

■ CONTRAINDICATIONS: Immunosuppression, acute infection, or concomitant use of corticosteroids prohibits its use.

■ ADVERSE EFFECTS: The most serious adverse reaction is anaphylaxis.

diphtheria and tetanus toxoids and pertussis vaccine (DTP),   an active immunizing agent.

■ INDICATIONS: It is prescribed for the routine immunization of children under 6 years of age against diphtheria, tetanus, and pertussis.

■ CONTRAINDICATIONS: Immunosuppressive therapy, active infection, or neurologic disorders prohibit its use.

■ ADVERSE EFFECT: The most serious adverse reaction is anaphylaxis.

diphtheria antitoxin [Gk, *diphtheria, anti,* anti, *toxikon,* poison],   an antitoxin prepared by immunizing horses with diphtheria toxoid and extracting. The serum is standardized for strength and quality.

diphtheria toxin [Gk, *diphtheria,* membrane + *toxikon,* poison]   the filtrate of a broth culture used to prepare an intradermal injectable form of toxin for Schick tests. A positive test is characterized by an inflammatory reaction, at the point of injection, whereas circulating antibodies in the blood result in a negative test result, indicating the person is immune.

diphtheritic croup /dif′thirit′ik/ [Gk, *diphtheria;* Scot, *croak,* to speak hoarsely],   a diphtheritic inflammation of the larynx. Also called **laryngeal diphtheria.** See **diphtheritic laryngitis.**

diphtheritic laryngitis [Gk, *diphtheria, larynx, itis,* inflammation],   an inflammation of the larynx caused by the Klebs-Loeffler bacillus (*Corynebacterium diphtheriae*). A serious complication is formation of a false membrane.

diphtheritic pharyngitis [Gk, *diphtheria, pharynx,* throat, *itis,* inflammation],   an inflammation of the pharynx caused by an infection of the Klebs-Loeffler bacillus (*Corynebacterium diphtheriae*) and associated with the formation of a false membrane.

diphtheroid /dif′thəroid′/ [Gk, *diphthera,* leather membrane, *eidos* form],   **1.** of or pertaining to diphtheria. **2.** resembling the bacillus *Corynebacterium diphtheriae.*

diphyllobothriasis.   See **fish tapeworm infection.**

Diphyllobothrium /dəfil′ōboth′rē·əm/ [Gk, *di,* twice, *phyllon,* leaf, *bothrion,* pit],   a genus of large, parasitic, intestinal flatworms having a scolex with two slitlike grooves. The species that most often infects humans is *Diphyllobothrium latum,* a giant freshwater fish tapeworm of North America and Europe. See also **fish tapeworm infection.**

Diphyllobothrium latum.   See **tapeworm.**

-dipine,   a suffix for the name of a phenylpyridine vasodilator.

dipivefrin /dī′pivef′rin/,   an ophthalmic adrenergic.

■ INDICATION: It is prescribed in the treatment of open-angle glaucoma.

■ CONTRAINDICATIONS: Narrow-angle glaucoma or known hypersensitivity to this drug prohibits its use.

■ ADVERSE EFFECTS: Among the most serious adverse effects are reactive hyperemia, conjunctivitis, allergic reactions, and macular edema. Systemic reactions, such as tachycardia, are possible.

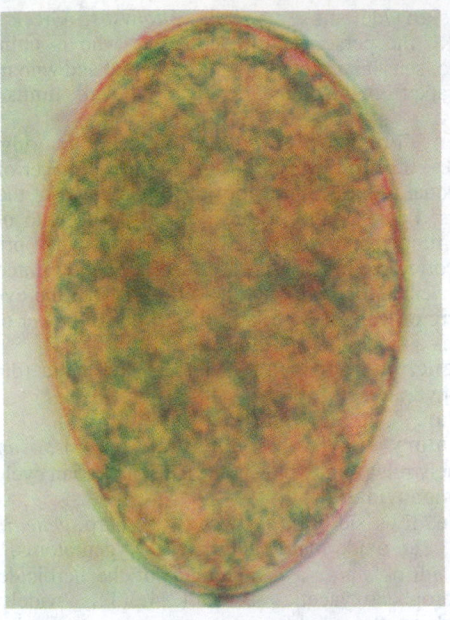

***Diphyllobothrium latum* egg**
(Murray, 1990/From Lennete EH, Ballows A, Hausler WJ, and Shadomy HJ: Manual of Clinical Microbiology, ed 4, Washington, DC 1985, American Society for Microbiology)

diplegia /dīplē′jē·ə/ [Gk, *di,* twice, *plege,* stroke],   bilateral paralysis of both sides of any part of the body or of like parts on the opposite sides of the body. A kind of diplegia is **facial diplegia.** Compare **hemiplegia.**   **−diplegic,** *adj.*

diplo-,   a combining form meaning 'double': *diplobacilli, diplococcus, diplokaryon.*

diplococcus /dip′lōkok′əs/, *pl.* **diplococci** /-kok′sī/ [Gk *diploos* double, *kokkos* berry],   a coccus of the *Coccaceae*

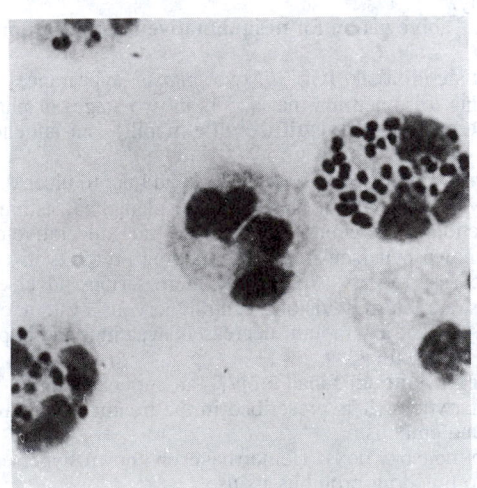

Diplococci (Baron, 1990)

family that occurs in pairs because of incomplete cell division. Diplococci are often found as parasites or saprophytes.

diploë /dip'lō·ē/, the loose tissue filled with red bone marrow between the two tables of the cranial bones.

diploid /dip'loid/ [Gk, *diploos* + *eidos*, form], of or pertaining to an individual, organism, strain, or cell that has two complete sets of homologous chromosomes, such as is normally found in the somatic cells and the primordial germ cells before maturation. In humans the normal diploid number is 46. Compare **haploid, tetraploid, triploid.** –**diploidic,** *adj.*

diploidy /dip'loidē/, the state or condition of having two complete sets of homologous chromosomes.

diplokaryon /dip'lōker'ē·on/ [Gk, *diploos* + *karyon,* nut], a nucleus that contains twice the diploid number of chromosomes.

diploma program in nursing, an educational program that is part of a hospital and designed to prepare nursing students for entry into practice, usually in 2 or 3 years. The recipient of a diploma is eligible to take the national certifying examination to become a registered nurse. In Canada, diploma programs are conducted in junior or community colleges, as well as in some hospital schools of nursing in the Atlantic provinces, Alberta and Manitoba.

diplomate /dip'ləmāt/, an individual who has earned a diploma or certificate, especially a physician who has been certified by a specialty board. See also **board certified.**

diplonema /dip'lənē'mə/ [Gk, *diploos,* + *nema,* thread], the looplike formation of the chromosomes in the diplotene stage of the first meiotic prophase of gametogenesis.

diplopagus /diplop'əgəs/ [Gk, *diploos* + *pagos,* something fixed], conjoined twins that are more or less equally developed, although one or several internal organs may be shared.

diplopia /diplō'pē·ə/ [Gk, *diploos* + *opsis,* vision], double vision caused by defective function of the extraocular muscles or a disorder of the nerves that innervate the muscles. Also called **ambiopia.** Compare **binocular vision.**

-diplopia, a suffix meaning '(condition of) double vision': *amphodiplopia, amphoterodiplopia, monodiplopia.*

diplornavirus /dī'plôrnəvī'rəs/, a double-stranded RNA virus that is the cause of Colorado tick fever. It is related to the reoviruses that are associated with various respiratory infections.

diplosomatia /dip'lōsōmā'shə/ [Gk, *diploos* + *soma,* body], a congenital anomaly in which fully formed twins are joined at one or more areas of their bodies. Also called **diplosomia.**

diplotene /dip'lətēn/ [Gk, *diploos* + *tainia,* ribbon], the fourth stage in the first meiotic prophase in gametogenesis in which the tetrads exhibit chiasmata between the chromatids of the paired homologous chromosomes and genetic crossing-over occurs. The chromosomes then begin to repel each other and separate longitudinally, forming loops. See also **diakinesis, leptotene, pachytene, zygotene.**

dipodia /dīpō'dē·ə/ [Gk, *di,* twice, *pous,* foot], a developmental anomaly characterized by the duplication of one or both feet.

dipolar ion. See **zwitterion.**

dipole /dī'pol/, a molecule with areas of opposing electric charges, as hydrogen chloride with a predominance of electrons about the chloride portion and a positive charge on the hydrogen side.

diprop, abbreviation for a *carboxylate dipropionate anion.*

diprosopus /dīpros'əpəs, dī'prəsō'pəs/ [Gk, *di,* twice, *prosopon,* face], a malformed fetus that has a double face showing varying degrees of development.

-dipsia, -dipsy, a combining form meaning '(condition of) thirst': *hydroadipsia, oligodipsia, polydipsia.*

dipsomania /dip'sōmā'nē·ə/ [Gk *dipsa* thirst, *mania* madness], an uncontrollable, often periodic craving for and indulgence in alcoholic beverages; alcoholism.

dipstick, a chemically treated strip of paper used in the analysis of urine or other fluids.

-dipsy. See **-dipsia.**

dipus /dī'pəs/, conjoined twins that have only two feet.

dipygus /dīpī'gəs, dip'əgəs/ [Gk, *di,* twice, *pyge,* rump], a malformed fetus that has a double pelvis, one of which is usually not fully developed.

dipyridamole /dī'pirid'əmōl/, a coronary vasodilator.

■ INDICATION: It is prescribed for the long-term treatment of angina.

■ CONTRAINDICATIONS: The drug should be used with caution in hypotension and anticoagulant therapy.

■ ADVERSE EFFECTS: The adverse reactions are mild and transient, such as headache, dizziness, rash, nausea, and flushing.

direct-access memory, access to computerized data independently of previously obtained data. The data transfer is directly between the computer memory and peripheral devices. See also **random-access memory (RAM).**

direct antagonist [L, *diregere,* to direct; Gk, *antagonisma,* struggle], one of a pair or a group of muscles that pull in opposite directions and whose combined action keeps the part from moving.

direct calorimetry, the measurement of the amount of heat directly generated by any oxidation reaction, especially one involving a living organism. Compare **indirect calorimetry.**

direct causal association, a cause-and-effect relationship between a causative factor and a disease with no other factors intervening in the process.

direct contact, mutual touching of two individuals or organisms. Many communicable diseases may be spread by the direct contact between an infected and a healthy person. Some kinds of diseases that may be spread by direct contact are gonorrhea, impetigo, staphylococcal skin infections, and syphilis. Other infections are transmitted by insect or animal vectors, airborne droplets, or contaminated food.

direct current (DC), an electric current that flows in one direction only and is substantially constant in value. Compare **alternating current.**

direct endometriosis [L, *diregire,* to direct; Gk, *endon,* within, *metra,* womb, *osis,* condition], an invasion of the myometrium of the uterus by the mucous membrane lining.

direct-exposure film, a type of x-ray film sometimes used to produce images of thin body parts, such as the hands and feet, that have a high subject contrast. The film is exposed directly by x-rays, rather than by indirect exposure.

direct fracture, any fracture occurring at a specific point of injury that is a direct result of that injury.

direct generation. See **asexual generation.**

direct gold, any form of pure gold that may be compacted or condensed directly into a prepared tooth cavity to form a restoration.

direct illumination. See **illumination.**

directive therapy [L, *diregere,* to direct; *therapeia,* treatment], a psychotherapeutic approach in which the psychotherapist directs the course of therapy by intervening to ask questions and offer interpretations. Compare **nondirective therapy.** See also **psychoanalysis.**

direct laryngoscopy [L, *diregire*, to direct; Gk, *larynx, skopein*, to watch], an examination of the larynx by means of a lighted tube inserted through the mouth.

direct lead /lēd/, **1.** an electrocardiographic conductor in which the exploring electrode is placed directly on the surface of the exposed heart. **2.** *informal.* a tracing produced by such a lead on an electrocardiograph.

direct light reflex, the constriction of a pupil receiving increased illumination, as by a flashlight during an ophthalmologic examination. Compare **consensual reaction to light.**

direct measurement of blood pressure [L, *diregire*, to direct, *mensura*, to measure; ME, *blod*; L, *premere*, to press], measurement of blood pressure in an artery by inserting a catheter into the blood vessel and recording the pressure directly, as opposed to the indirect method of using a pressure cuff, stethoscope, and sphygmomanometer.

direct nursing care functions, liaison nursing activities that are focused on a particular patient, patient's family, or a group for whom the nurse is directly responsible and accountable.

directory /direk'tərē/, a listing of the files in a computer storage device, such as a floppy disk.

direct patient care, (in nursing) care of a patient provided in person by a member of the staff. Direct patient care may involve any aspects of the health care of a patient, including treatments, counseling, self-care, patient education, and administration of medication.

direct percussion. See **percussion.**

direct provider reimbursement, a method of direct payment for health care services, as fee-for-service.

direct-question interview, an inquiry that usually requires simple one- or two-word responses.

direct relationship. See **positive relationship.**

direct retainer, a clasp, attachment, or assembly fastened to an abutment tooth for the purpose of maintaining a removable restoration in its planned position in relation to oral structures.

direct self-destructive behavior (DSDB), any form of suicidal activity, such as suicide threats, attempts, or gestures and the act of suicide itself. The intent of the behavior is death, and the person is aware of this as the desired outcome.

direct transfusion [L, *dirigere*, to direct + *transfundere*, to pour through], the transfer of whole blood directly from a vein of the donor to a vein of the recipient.

dirofilariasis /dī'rōfil'ərī'əsis/, a human infestation of the dog heartworm, *Dirofilaria immitis*, which may be transmitted through the bite of any of several species of mosquitoes. The filaria migrate through the bloodstream to the lung, producing pulmonary nodules and causing chest pain, coughing, and hemoptysis. The disease is rare among humans.

dis-, See **di-, dis-.**

disability /dis'əbil'itē/ [L, *dis*, opposite of, *habilis*, fit], the loss, absence, or impairment of physical or mental fitness. Compare **handicapped.**

disaccharidase deficiency. See **lactase deficiency.**

disaccharide /dīsak'ərīd/ [Gk, *di*, double, *sakcharon*,

sugar], a general term for simple carbohydrates formed by the union of two monosaccharide molecules.

disadvantaged /dis'ədvan'tijd/ [L, *dis* + *abante*, superior position], **1.** any group of people who lack money, education, literacy, or another status advantage. **2.** a euphemism for 'poor.'

disarticulation /dis'ärtik'yəlā'shən/ [L, *dis*, *articulare*, to divide into joints], the separation of a joint without cutting through a bone.

disaster-preparedness plan [L, *dis* + *astrum*, favorable stars; *praeparare*, to prepare], a formal plan of action, usually prepared in written form, for coordinating the response of a hospital staff in the event of a disaster within the hospital or the surrounding community.

disc. See **disk.**

discharge [OFr, *deschargier*, to expel], **1.** also **evacuate, excrete, secrete.** to release a substance or object. **2.** to release a patient from a hospital. **3.** to release an electric charge, which may be manifested by a spark or surge of electricity, from a storage battery, condenser, or other source. **4.** to release a burst of energy from or through a neuron. **5.** a release of emotions, often accompanied by a wide range of voluntary and involuntary reflexes, weeping, rage, or other emotional displays, called **affective discharge** in psychology. **6.** also called **evacuate, excretion, secretion.** a substance or object discharged.

discharge abstract /dis'chärj/, items of information compiled from medical records of patients discharged from a hospital, organized and recorded in a uniform format to provide data for statistical studies, reports, or research.

discharge coordinator, an individual who arranges with community agencies and institutions for the continuing care of patients after their discharge from a hospital.

discharge planning, the activities that facilitate a client's movement from one health care setting to another. It is a multidisciplinary process involving physicians, nurses, social workers, and possibly other health professionals and its goal is to enhance continuity of care.

discharge summary, a clinical report prepared by a physician or other health professional at the conclusion of a hospital stay or series of treatments, outlining the patient's chief complaint, the diagnostic findings, the therapy administered and the patient's response to it, and recommendations on discharge.

discharging lesion [OFr, *deschargier*; L, *laesio*, hurting], an injury or infection of the central nervous system that causes sudden abnormal episodes of discharging nerve impulses.

disciform keratitis /dis'ifôrm/ [Gk, *diskos*, flat plate; L, *forma*, form; Gk, *keras*, horn, *itis*, inflammation], an inflammatory condition of the eye that often follows an attack of dendritic keratitis and is believed to be an immunologic response to an ocular herpes simplex infection. The condition is characterized by disclike opacities in the cornea, usually with inflammation of the iris. See also **herpesvirus simplex.**

disclosing solution [L, *dis* + *claudere*, to close; *solutus*, dissolved], a topically applied dye, used in aqueous solution to stain and reveal plaque and other deposits on teeth.

disco-, a combining form meaning 'pertaining to a disk, disk-shaped': *discophorous, discopathy, discoplacenta.*

discoblastula /dis'kōblas'tyələ/ [Gk, *diskos*, flat plate, *blastos*, germ], a blastula formed from the partial cleavage that occurs in a fertilized ovum containing a large amount of yolk. It develops from the blastodisc and consists of a cellular cap, or blastoderm, separated from the uncleaved yolk mass by a small cavity, the blastocele.

discocyte /dis′kəsīt/ [Gk, *diskos + kytos,* cell], a mature, normal, erythrocyte, exhibiting one of many steady-state configurations, such as a biconcave disk without a nucleus.

discoid lupus erythematosus (DLE) /dis′koid/ [Gk, *diskos + eidos,* form; L, *lupus,* wolf; Gk, *erythema,* redness, *osis,* condition], a chronic, recurrent disease, primarily of the skin, characterized by red macules that are covered with scales and extend into follicles. The lesions are typically distributed in a butterfly pattern covering the cheeks and bridge of the nose but may also occur on other parts of the body. On healing, the lesions atrophy and leave hyperpigmented or hypopigmented scars, and, if hairy areas are involved, alopecia may result. The cause of the disease is not established, but there is evidence that it may be an autoimmune disorder, and some cases seem to be induced by certain drugs. It is at least five times more common in women than in men and occurs most frequently in the third and fourth decades of life. Treatment includes the use of a sunscreen lotion or ointment when exposure to sunlight cannot be avoided, the application of steroids to the lesions, and systemic antimalarial drugs, such as hydroxychloroquine; systemic corticosteroid agents may be used in severe cases. Also called **cutaneous lupus erythematosus.** See also **systemic lupus erythematosus.**

knee joint or that the knee joint gives way. These characteristics are often associated with an injury to the knee but occur also without any history of trauma. Examination demonstrates the 'clicking,' usually when the knee is moved from flexion to extension, during the last 15 to 20 degrees. Surgical excision of the meniscus is seldom warranted in treating this benign condition.

discoid placenta [Gk, *diskos,* quoit, *eidos,* form; L, *placenta,* flat cake], a round placenta.

disconfirmation /diskon′fərmā′shən/, a dysfunctional communication that negates, discounts, or ignores information received from another person.

discordance /diskôr′dəns/ [L, *discordare,* to disagree], (in genetics) the expression of one or more specific traits in only one member of a pair of twins. Compare **concordance.** –**discordant,** *adj.*

discordant twins, twins showing a marked difference in size (greater than 10% in weight) at birth usually caused by overperfusion of one twin and underperfusion of the other. It is fairly common in identical twins, but may also occur in dizygotic twins.

discovery /diskov′ərē/ [L, *dis + coopiere,* to cover], (in law) a pretrial procedure allowing one party to examine vital witnesses and documents held exclusively by the adverse party. Discovery is limited to materials, facts, and other resources that could not otherwise be reasonably expected to be discovered and that are necessary to the preparation of the case for trial. Also called **pretrial discovery.** Compare **deposition, interrogatories.**

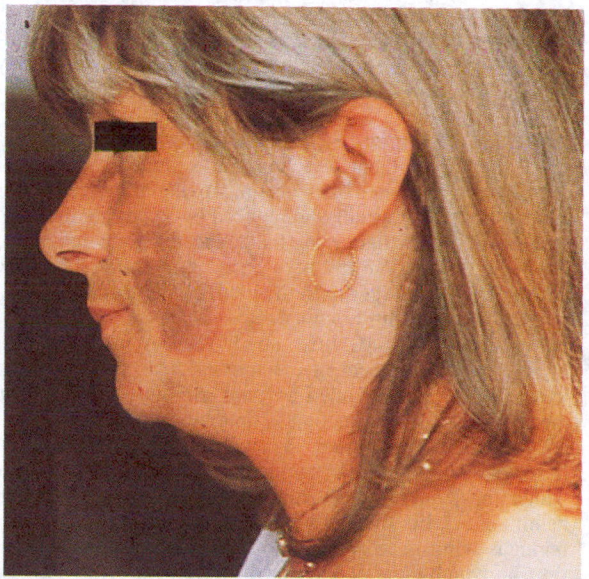

Discoid lupus erythematosus *(Shipley, 1993)*

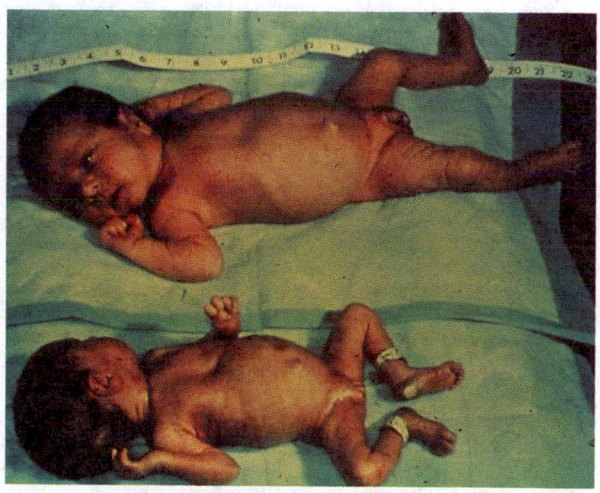

Discordant twins *(Zitelli, 1992)*

discoid meniscus, an abnormal condition characterized by a discoid rather than semilunar shape of the cartilaginous meniscus of the knee. The lateral meniscus is most often affected, although the medial meniscus may also become involved. The condition is a developmental anomaly, asymptomatic in the infant or in the young child, and occurs most frequently in children between 6 and 8 years of age. Common complaints are that a 'clicking' occurs in the

discrete x-rays. See **x-ray.**

discrimination /diskrim′inā′shən/ [L, *discrimen,* division], the act of distinguishing or differentiating. The ability to distinguish between touch or pressure at two nearby points on the body is known as two-point discrimination.

discriminator /diskrim′inā′tər/, (in nuclear medicine) an electronic device capable of accepting or rejecting a pulse of energy according to the pulse height of voltage. It is used to separate low-energy from high-energy radionuclides.

discus. See **disk.**

discus articularis /dis'kəs/,   a small oval plate between the condyle of the mandible and the mandibular fossa. Displacement of or injury to the plate may be a cause of temporomandibular joint (TMJ) pain.

discus interpubicus.   See **interpubic disk.**

discus nervi optici.   See **optic disc.**

disdiadochokinesia /dis'dī·ad'əkōkīnē'zhə/ [L, *dis*, apart, *diadochos*, successor, *kinesis*, movement],   an inability to quickly make fine coordinated motor movements. See also **diadochokinesia**.

disease [L, *dis* + Fr, *aise*, ease],   **1.** a condition of abnormal vital function involving any structure, part, or system of an organism. **2.** a specific illness or disorder characterized by a recognizable set of signs and symptoms, attributable to heredity, infection, diet, or environment. Compare **condition, diathesis.**

disease prevention,   activities designed to protect patients or other members of the public from actual or potential health threats and their harmful consequences.

disengagement /dis'engāj'mənt/ [Fr, *disengager*, to release from engagement],   **1.** an obstetrical manipulation in which the presenting part of the baby is dislodged from the maternal pelvis as part of an operative delivery. See also **Kielland rotation, version and extraction. 2.** the release or detachment of oneself from other persons or responsibilities. **3.** (in transactional family therapy) a role assumed by a nurse or other therapist in observing and restructuring intervention without becoming actively and directly involved in the problem.

disengagement theory,   the psychosocial concept that aging individuals and society normally withdraw from active engagement with each other. The theory also assumes that older adults are a homogenous group whose members prefer the company of others of their own age. See also **activity theory.**

disequilibrium /dīsē'kwilib'rē·əm/ [L, *dis*, apart, *aequilibrium*],   the loss of balance or adjustment, particularly mental or psychological balance.

dishpan fracture [AS, *disc*, plate; L, *patina*, dish; *fractura*, break],   a fracture that depresses the skull. Also called **derby hat fracture.**

disinfect /dis'infekt'/ [L, *dis*, apart, *inficere*, to infect],   to remove pathogens.

disinfectant /dis'infek'tənt/,   a chemical that can be applied to objects to destroy microorganisms.

disinfection /dis'infek'shən/,   the process of killing pathogenic organisms or of rendering them inert.

disinfection of thermometer [L, *dis*, *inficere*, to infect; Gk, *therme*, heat + *metron*, measure],   the destruction of infectious organisms that may be present on a clinical glass thermometer. The process usually involves the use of chemical germicides after thorough washing, following the Centers for Disease Guidelines for cleaning, disinfection, and sterilization of hospital equipment.

disinfestation /dis'infestā'shən/ [L, *dis*, apart, *infestare*, to infest],   elimination of a threat of infestation by vermin, rodents, lice, or other noxious organisms.

disinhibition /dis'inhibish'ən/ [L, *dis*, apart, *inhibere*, to restrain],   the removal of inhibition. See **inhibition**.

disintegrative psychosis /disin'təgrā'tiv/,   a mental disorder of childhood that usually has an onset after the age of 3 years and following normal development of speech, social behavior, and oth er traits. After a vague illness, the child becomes irritable and undergoes mental deterioration, even-

tually reaching a stage of severe mental retardation. The cause may be a viral infection. There is no specific treatment.

disjunction /disjungk'shən/ [L, *disjungere*, to disjoint], (in genetics) the separation of the paired homologous chromosomes during the anaphase stage of the first meiotic division or of the chromatids of a chromosome during anaphase of mitosis and the second meiotic division. Compare **nondisjunction.**

disk [Gk *diskos* flat plate],   **1.** also spelled (chiefly in ophthalmology) **disc.** a flat, circular platelike structure, as an articular disk or an optic disc. **2.** *informal.* an intervertebral disk. Also called *(Latin)* **discus.**

disk drive,   a computer device containing a disk that spins at high speeds, equipped with a head that allows electric impulses to be written onto and read from the electromagnetic surface.

diskette,   a semiflexible plastic, oxide-coated disk, contained in a special flat plastic box or jacket, for use in a computer disk drive. Diskettes for personal computers are either 5¼" or 3½" in diameter.

diskography /diskog'rəfē/,   the radiologic examination of individual intervertebral disks. It involves the injection of a small amount of water-soluble iodinated medium into the center of the disk by a double-needle entry. A local anesthetic is used.

dislocation /dis'lōkā'shən/ [L, *dis* + *locare*, to place],   the displacement of any part of the body from its normal position, particularly a bone from its normal articulation with a joint. See also **subluxation.** –**dislocate,** *v.*

dislocation of clavicle [L, *dis*, apart, *locare*, to place, *clavicula*, little key],   displacement of the collarbone. It may occur at the sternal end or the acromial or scapular extremity.

dislocation of finger [L, *dis*, apart, *locare*, to place; AS, *finger*],   displacement of a finger at a joint, as a result of trauma. In the absence of an accompanying fracture, the dislocated finger can usually be reduced by steadying the hand at the wrist and maneuvering the dislocated bone into place. After the dislocation has been reduced, a splint should be applied from the fingertip to the palm of the hand and a postreduction x-ray film obtained.

dislocation of hip [L, *dis*, apart, *locare*, to place; AS, *hype*],   a displacement of the femoral head out of the hip joint, usually accompanied by pain, rigidity, shortening of the leg, and loss of function. The dislocation can occur as an **obturator dislocation,** in which the head of the femur lies in the obturator foramen; a **perineal dislocation,** in which the head of the femur is displaced into the perineum; a **sciatic dislocation,** in which the head of the femur is lying in the sciatic notch; or a **subpubic dislocation,** in which there is anterior displacement of the femoral head.

dislocation of jaw [L, *dis*, apart, *locare*, to place; ME, *jowe*],   a displacement of the jaw, which may be unilateral or bilateral, as a result of a blow, a fall, or yawning. The mandible will appear fixed in an open position with only the back teeth in contact. If the mandible appears deviated to one side, the dislocation involves only one side. The dislocation is reduced manually, with or without injection of a local anesthetic.

dislocation of knee [L, *dis,* apart, *locare*, to place; AS, *cneow*],   a displacement of one of the bones of the knee joint. First aid treatment for the dislocation is the same as for a fracture: the joint is immobilized with splints, and the patient is moved quickly to a medical facility.

dislocation of shoulder [L, *dis, locare*; AS, *sculder*], any of several kinds of displacement of the shoulder joint, including acromial joint disruption and separation and dislocation of the glenohumeral joint with the humeral head displaced anteriorly and inferiorly.

dismiss [L *dis + mittere* to send], (in law) to discharge or dispose of an action, suit, or motion trial. **–dismissal,** *n.*

disobliterative endarterectomy. See **endarterectomy.**

disodium edetate. See **edetate disodium.**

Disophrol, a trademark for a respiratory, fixed-combination drug containing an antihistamine (dexbrompheniramine maleate) and an adrenergic bronchodilator (pseudoephedrine sulfate).

disopyramide phosphate /dī′sōpir′əmīd/, a cardiac antiarrhythmic depressant.

■ INDICATIONS: It is prescribed in the treatment of premature ventricular contractions and ventricular tachycardia.

■ CONTRAINDICATIONS: Heart failure, preexisting second- or third-degree heart block in the absence of a pacemaker, sick sinus syndrome, or known hypersensitivity to this drug prohibits its use.

■ ADVERSE EFFECTS: Among the more serious adverse reactions are severe hypotension, precipitation of heart failure, and aggravation of heart block. Urinary retention, dry mouth, and constipation commonly occur.

disorder [L, *dis,* apart, *ordo,* rank], a disruption of or interference with normal functions or established systems, as a mental disorder or nutritional disorder.

disorders of movement [L, *dis,* apart, *ordo,* rank, *movere,* to move], any perverse or abnormal functions of muscular action that may result from infection, injury, or congenital disability, such as ataxia, involuntary grimacing, or chorea.

disorders of sleep [L, *dis, ordo*; AS, *slaep*], any condition that interferes with normal sleep patterns, such as sleep apnea, phase shift, use of alcohol and certain drugs, excessive sleepiness, sleep walking, nightmares, Ekbom's syndrome, sleep paralysis, and narcolepsy. Treatment may include medications and therapy offered at sleep disorder clinics.

disorganized schizophrenia /disôr′gənīzd/ [L, *dis* + Gk, *organon,* organ], a subtype of schizophrenia characterized by an earlier age of onset, usually at puberty, and a more severe disintegration of the personality than occurs in other forms of the disease. The essential features include incoherence, loose associations, gross disorganization of behavior, and flat or inappropriate affect. Also called **hebephrenia, hebephrenic schizophrenia.** See also **schizophrenia.**

disorient /disôr′ē·ənt/, to cause to lose awareness or perception of space, time, or personal identity and relationships.

disorientation /-ā′shən/ [L, *dis* + *orienter,* to proceed from], a state of mental confusion characterized by inadequate or incorrect perceptions of place, time, or identity. Disorientation may occur in organic mental disorders, in drug and alcohol intoxication, and, less commonly, after severe stress.

disparate twins /dis′pərāt, disper′it/, twins who are distinctly different from each other in weight and other features.

dispense /dispens′/ [L, *dis,* apart, *pensare,* to weigh], to prepare and issue drugs or drug mixtures from a pharmaceutical outlet or department.

dispersing agent /dispur′sing/ [L, *dis + spargere,* to scatter; *agere* to do], a chemical additive used in pharmaceutics to cause the even distribution of the ingredients throughout the product, such as in dermatologic emulsions containing both oil and water. Dispersing agents commonly used in skin creams, lotions, and ointments include glyceryl monostearate, sodium lauryl sulfate, and polyethylene glycol derivatives, such as polysorbate 80 and polyoxyl 40 stearate. A dispersing agent may cause an allergic reaction or adverse effect in a hypersensitive person.

dispersion /dispur′shən/, the scattering or dissipation of finely divided material, as when particles of a substance are scattered throughout the volume of a fluid. Examples include colloids and gels, such as egg white, soap, and gelatin, which consist of large molecules or clumps of molecules that are able to attract and hold large numbers of water molecules.

dispersion forces. See **van der Waals forces.**

dispersion medium. See **continuous phase.** See also **medium.**

displaced fracture /displāst/ [Fr, *deplacement,* to remove], a traumatic bone break in which two ends of a fractured bone are separated from each other. The ends of broken bones in displaced fractures often pierce surrounding skin, as in an open fracture, or may be contained within the skin, as in a closed fracture.

displaced testis [Fr, *déplacement*; L, *testis,* testicle], a testis that is located in the pelvis, inguinal canal, or elsewhere after it normally would have descended into the scrotum.

displacement /displās′mənt/ [Fr, *deplacement,* to remove], **1.** the state of being displaced or the act of displacing. **2.** (in chemistry) a reaction in which an atom, molecule, or radical is removed from combination and replaced by another. **3.** (in physics) the displacing in space of one mass by another, such as the weight or volume of a fluid being displaced by a floating or submerged body. **4.** (in psychiatry) an unconscious defense mechanism for avoiding emotional conflict and anxiety by transferring emotions, ideas, or wishes from one object to a substitute that is less anxiety-producing. Compare **sublimation.** See also **percolation.**

displacement chromatography. See **chromatography.**

DISS, abbreviation for **Diameter-Index Safety System.**

dissect /disekt′/ [L, *dissecare,* to cut apart], to cut apart tissues for visual or microscopic study using a scalpel, a probe, or scissors. Compare **bisect. –dissection,** *n.*

dissecting aneurysm [L, *dissecare,* to cut apart; Gk, *aneurysma,* a widening], a localized dilatation of an artery, most commonly the aorta, characterized by a longitudinal dissection between the outer and middle layers of the vascular wall. Aortic dissecting aneurysms occur most frequently in men between the ages of 40 and 60 and are, in more than 90% of cases, preceded by hypertension. Blood entering a tear in the intimal lining of the vessel causes a separation of weakened elastic and fibromuscular elements in the medial layer and leads to the formation of cystic spaces filled with ground substance. Dissecting aneurysms in the thoracic aorta may extend into blood vessels of the neck. Rupture of a dissecting aneurysm may be fatal in less than 1 hour. Treatment consists

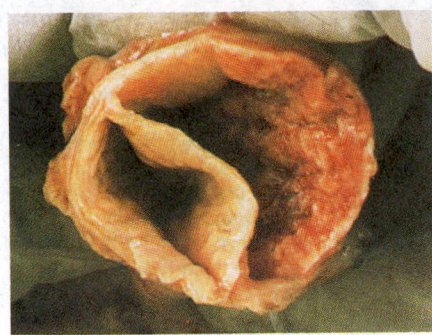

Dissecting aortic aneurysm (Fletcher, 1987)

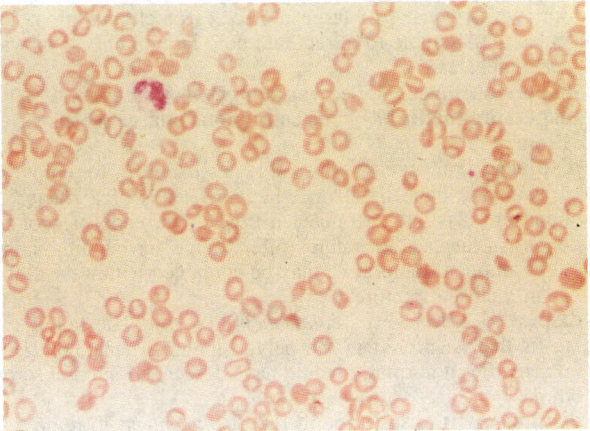

Disseminated intravascular coagulation (Zitelli, 1992)

of resection and replacement of the excised section of aorta with a synthetic prosthesis. See also **aortic aneurysm.**

-dissection. See **dissect.**

disseminated intravascular coagulation (DIC) /disem'i-nā'tid/ [L, *dis* + *seminare,* to sow; *intra,* within, *vasculum,* little vessel; *coagulare,* to curdle], a grave coagulopathy resulting from the overstimulation of clotting and anticlotting processes in response to disease or injury, such as septicemia, acute hypotension, poisonous snake bites, neoplasms, obstetric emergencies, severe trauma, extensive surgery, and hemorrhage. The primary disorder initiates generalized intravascular clotting, which in turn overstimulates fibrinolytic mechanisms; as a result the initial hypercoagulability is succeeded by a deficiency in clotting factors with hypocoagulability and hemorrhaging. Diagnosis is based on the presence of degredation products. Also called **consumption coagulopathy.**

■ OBSERVATIONS: Purpura on the chest and abdomen, reflecting fibrin deposits in capillaries, is a common first sign of DIC. Hemorrhagic bullae, acral cyanosis, and focal gangrene in the skin and mucous membranes may follow. Hemorrhages from incisions, catheter or injection sites, GI bleeding, hematuria, pulmonary edema, pulmonary embolism, progressive hypotension, tachycardia, absence of peripheral pulses, restlessness, convulsions, or coma may be present. Laboratory studies show generally a marked deficiency of blood platelets, low levels of fibrinogen and other clotting factors, prolonged prothrombin and partial thromboplastin times, and abnormal erythrocyte morphology.

■ INTERVENTIONS: Treatment of the primary disorder is essential in the management of DIC. Heparin may be infused intravenously to prevent clot formation, but, may increase bleeding. Heparin is not always used for surgical patients with DIC. Transfusions of whole blood, plasma, platelets, and other blood products are administered to replace depleted factors. Patients are maintained in a quiet, nonstressful environment and are protected from trauma and bleeding. The side rails of the bed are padded, foam or cotton swabs are used for mouth care.

■ NURSING CONSIDERATIONS: The care of a patient with life-threatening DIC requires monitoring of vital signs, observation for evidence of bleeding, extremely gentle handling, maintaining a safe environment, and giving emotional support.

disseminated lupus erythematosus. See **systemic lupus erythematosus.**

disseminated multiple sclerosis. See **multiple sclerosis.**

dissent /disent'/ [L, *dis* + *sentire,* to feel], (in law) a statement written by a judge who disagrees with the decision of the majority of the court. The dissent explicitly states the reasons for the dissenting judge's contrary opinion. **–dissenting,** *adj.*

dissimilar twins. See **dizygotic twins.**

dissociation /disō'shē·ā'shən/ [L, *dis* + *sociare,* to unite], **1.** the act of separating into parts or sections. **2.** an unconscious defense mechanism by which an idea, thought, emotion, or other mental process is separated from the consciousness and thereby loses emotional significance. See **dissociative disorder,** **–dissociative** /disō'shē·ətiv/, *adj.*

dissociative anesthesia /disō'shē·ətiv/, an anesthetic procedure characterized by analgesia and amnesia without loss of respiratory function. The patient does not appear to be anesthetized but is "dissociated" from the environment, The patient's eyes may remain open even while in a deep level of anesthesia. This form of anesthesia may be used to provide analgesia during brief, superficial operative procedures or diagnostic processes. It is especially useful for people who are sensitive to general or local anesthetics or for those who, for other reasons, may not be safely anesthetized with inhalant gases. Ketamine hydrochloride is a phencyclidine derivative used to produce the state of dissociative anesthesia. Emergence may be accompanied by delirium, excitement, disorientation, and confusion.

dissociative disorder, a disorder neurosis in which emotional conflicts are so repressed that a separation or split in the personality occurs, resulting in an altered state of consciousness or a confusion in identity. Symptoms include amnesia, somnambulism, fugue, dream state, or multiple personality. The disorder is caused by an inability to cope with severe stress or conflict and usually occurs suddenly, after a situation catastrophic to the person. Treatment may include hypnosis, especially when amnesia is the primary symptom, psychotherapy, and antianxiety medication. Also called **dissociative reaction.** Compare **conversion disorder.** See also **dissociation.**

dissolution /dis'əloo'shən/ [L, *dis*+*solvere,* to loosen], **1.** the separation of a complex chemical compound into simpler molecules. **2.** the liquifaction of organic substances. **3.** the loss of mental powers.

dissolved gas /disolvd'/ [L, *dis* + *solvere,* to loosen], gas in a simple physical solution, as distinguished from gas that has reacted chemically with a solvent or other solutes and is chemically combined.

distal /dis'təl/ [L, *distare,* to be distant], **1.** away from or being the farthest from a point of origin. **2.** away from or being the farthest from the midline or a central point, as a distal phalanx. Compare **proximal.**

distal latency, (in electroneuromyography) the time interval between the stimulation of a compound muscle and the observed response. Normal nerve conduction velocity is above 40 m/sec in the lower extremities and above 50 m/sec in the upper extremities, but age, muscle disease, temperature, and other factors can influence the velocity.

distal muscular dystrophy, a rare form of muscular dystrophy, usually affecting adults, characterized by moderate weakness and by wasting that begins in the arms and legs and then extends gradually to the proximal and facial muscles. Also called **Gowers' muscular dystrophy.**

distal phalanx, any one of the small distal bones in the third row of phalanges of the hand or the foot. Each one at the end of the finger has a convex dorsal surface and a flat palmar surface, with a rough elevation at the end of the palmar surface that supports a fingernail and its sensitive pulp. The distal phalanx of each of the toes is smaller and more flattened than that of a finger; it also has a rough elevation to support the toenail and its pulp. Also called **ungual phalanx.**

distal radioulnar articulation, the pivotlike articulation of the head of the ulna and the ulnar notch on the lower end of the radius, involving two ligaments. The joint allows rotation of the distal end of the radius around an axis that passes through the center of the head of the ulna. Also called **inferior radioulnar joint.** Compare **proximal radioulnar articulation.**

distal renal tubular acidosis (distal RTA), an abnormal condition characterized by excessive acid accumulation and bicarbonate excretion. It is caused by the inability of the distal tubules of the kidney to secrete hydrogen ions, thus decreasing the excretion of titratable acids and ammonium and increasing the urinary loss of potassium and bicarbonate. This condition may result in hypercalciuria and the formation of kidney stones. Treatment is as for renal tubular acidosis. **Primary distal RTA** occurs mostly in females, adolescents, older children, and young adults. It may occur sporadically or as the result of hereditary defects. **Secondary distal RTA** is associated with numerous disorders, such as cirrhosis of the liver, malnutrition, starvation, and various genetic problems. Compare **proximal renal tubular acidosis.**

distal sparing, a condition in which the spinal cord remains intact below a lesion. The reflex arc remains but is not modified by supraspinal influences. As a result there may be spastic movements distal to the level of the lesion.

distance regulation [L, *distantia; regula,* rule], behavior that is related to the control of personal space. Most humans establish a quantum of space between themselves and others that offers security from either psychologic or physical threat while not creating a feeling of isolation. The amount of social distance thus maintained varies with different individuals and in different cultures. A wild animal generally maintains a flight distance, the minimum it will allow between itself and a potential enemy before fleeing. Animals of the same species also maintain a personal distance from each other.

distance vision, the ability to see objects clearly from a distance, usually from more than 20 feet or 6 m away.

distemper /distem'pər/ [L, *dis,* apart, *temperare,* to regulate], **1.** any disorder or indisposition, mentally or physically. **2.** a potentially fatal viral disease of animals, characterized by rhinitis, fever, and a loss of appetite.

distend /distend'/ [L, *distendere,* to stretch], to make something enlarged or dilated.

distensibility /disten'sibil'itē/ [L, *distendere,* to stretch], pertaining to the ability of something to become stretched, dilated, or enlarged.

distension, /disten'shən/, the state of being distended or swollen.

distillate /distil'it/ [L, *distillare,* to drop down], the product of distillation. Also spelled *distention.*

distillation /dis'tilā'shən/ [L, *distillare,* to drop down], the process of vaporization followed by condensation in another part of the system.

distilled water /distild'/ [L, *distillare,* to drop down; AS, *waeter*], water that has been purified by being heated to a vapor form and then condensed into another container as liquid water free of nonvolatile solutes.

distortion /distôr'shən/ [L, *dis* + *torquere,* to twist], **1.** (in psychology) the process of shifting experience in one's perceptions. Distortions represent personal constructs of truth, validity, and right and wrong. The distortions of patients tend to influence their views of the world and themselves, as by altering a negative perception to one more favorable. **2.** (in radiology) x-ray image artifacts that may be caused by variations in the size and shape or the position of the object. Thick or curved objects result in greater distortion than thin, flat objects due to unequal magnification.

distractibility /distrak'tibil'itē/ [L, *dis, trahere,* to draw apart], a mental state in which attention does not remain fixed on any one subject but wavers or wanders.

distraction /distrak'shən/ [L, *distrahere,* to pull apart], **1.** procedures that prevent or lessen the perception of pain by focusing attention on sensations unrelated to pain. **2.** a method of straightening a spinal column by the forces of axial tension pulling on the joint surfaces, such as applied by a Milwaukee brace.

distraught /distrôt'/ [OFr, *destrait,* inattentive], a mental state of confusion, distraction, or absentmindedness.

distress /distres'/ [ME, *distressen,* to cause sorrow], an emotional or physical state of pain, sorrow, misery, suffering, or discomfort.

distress of the human spirit. See **spiritual distress.**

distributed processing /distrib'yətid/ [L, *distribuere,* to distribute], a combination of local and remote computers in a network connected to a central computer to distribute the processing and thereby reduce the load on the central computer.

distributive analysis and synthesis /distrib'yətiv/, the system of psychotherapy used by the psychobiologic school of psychiatry. It involves an extensive and systematic investigation and analysis of a person's total past experiences to discover the emotional factors underlying personality problems and how they can be synthesized into constructive behavioral patterns.

distributive care, a pattern of health care that is concerned with environment, heredity, living conditions, lifestyle, and early detection of pathologic effects. The system is usually directed toward continuous care of persons not confined to hospitals or other health care facilities.

district [L, *distringere*, to draw apart], **1.** (in hospital nursing) a group of patients in an area of the unit for whom a head nurse or primary nurse is responsible, usually a subdivision of a ward unit. Patients are customarily assigned to a district on the basis of certain shared needs for nursing care. **2.** the area of a city or town assigned to a public health nurse.

district nurse. See **public health nursing.**

disulfiram /dīsul′firam/, an alcohol-use deterrent.
- INDICATIONS: It is prescribed as a deterrent to drinking alcohol in the treatment of chronic alcoholism. It causes severe intestinal cramping, diaphoresis, and nausea if alcohol is ingested.
- CONTRAINDICATIONS: Alcoholic intoxication, recent or concomitant administration of metronidazole, paraldehyde, or alcohol, severe myocardial disease, coronary occlusion, psychosis, or known hypersensitivity to this drug prohibits its use.
- ADVERSE EFFECTS: The most serious adverse reactions occur after alcohol is ingested, including optic neuritis, psychotic reaction, and polyneuritis. Drowsiness, headache, and skin rash may occur. This drug interacts with several other drugs.

disuse phenomena /disyo̅o̅s′/ [L, *dis* + *usus*, to make use of; Gk, *phainein*, to show], the physical and the psychologic changes, usually degenerative, that result from the lack of use of a part of the body or a body system. Disuse phenomena are associated with confinement and immobility, especially in orthopedics. Individuals under treatment for fractures and other orthopedic disorders must often be confined to beds and immobilized in traction for long periods. Such patients are often deprived of interaction with the world around them and lose motivations, expectations, and even acquired abilities because of lack of practice. Such disorientation is compounded by pain and therapeutic narcotic drugs commonly associated with the treatment of many illnesses and abnormal conditions. The physical changes often induced by continued bed rest constitute problems affecting many key areas and systems of the body, such as the skin, the musculoskeletal system, the GI tract, the cardiovascular system, and the respiratory system. The skin of the patient on prolonged bed rest is commonly subjected to abnormal conditions, such as pressure exerted by the bed, moisture, friction, and inadequate nutrition. Pressure exerted on the skin by the bed is slightly higher than capillary hydrostatic pressure, often causing problems in blood circulation and inadequate airing of the skin surface. Any pressure that causes collapse of the superficial capillaries will lead to ischemia and eventual tissue necrosis. Of particular interest to the orthopedic nurse is the phenomenon, accompanying disuse, that may prevent the neurologically impaired patient from feeling pain. This phenomenon may be the first sign of ischemia followed by a rapid breakdown of the skin. Some indications of skin ischemia are redness, pain, edema, and skin breakdown. Elderly patients are often more susceptible to skin breakdown because of possible poor nutrition, more restricted mobility and generally poor skin condition. Unused muscles lose size and strength, often wasting away until they are unable to perform their vital functions of support and contraction. Contractures are usually caused by flexion, because patients flex knees and hips whenever possible to relax muscles, especially when cold or in pain. The immobilized patient may experience bone demineralization because of a restricted diet and de-

creased motility. Calcium and phosphorus are dependent on vitamin D for absorption from the gut and movement into the bones, and some nutritional experts describe calcium loss as a natural disuse phenomenon of bed rest. Muscle action is required to maintain the blood flow to the bones, and the immobilized patient may not be capable of sufficient muscular activity to assure such blood flow, with its attendant delivery of critical nutrients. The pooling of respiratory secretions is another disuse phenomenon caused by the immobility and the horizontal position of the bedrest patient. Some common therapeutic measures to deal with disuse phenomena are the improvement of diet and nutrition, proper positioning and regular movement of the bedrest patient, meticulous hygiene, scrupulous skin care, and positive social interaction with the patient. See also **hypostatic pneumonia.**

disuse syndrome, high risk for, a nursing diagnosis accepted by the Eighth National Conference on the Classification of Nursing Diagnoses. Potential for disuse syndrome is a state in which an individual is at risk for deterioration of body systems as the result of prescribed or unavoidable inactivity. The defining characteristics are the presence of risk factors such as paralysis, mechanical immobilization, prescribed immobilization, severe pain, and altered level of consciousness. See also **nursing diagnosis.**

Ditropan, a trademark for an antispasmodic (oxybutynin chloride).

Diucardin, a trademark for an antihypertensive and diuretic (hydroflumethiazide).

Diupres, a trademark for a fixed-combination drug containing a diuretic (chlorothiazide) and an antihypertensive (reserpine).

diuresis /dī′yo̅o̅rē′sis/ [Gk, *dia*, through, *ouron*, urine], increased formation and secretion of urine. Diuresis occurs in conditions such as diabetes mellitus and diabetes insipidus. It is normal in the first 48 hours postpartum. Coffee, tea, certain foods, diuretic drugs, anxiety, fear, and some steroids cause diuresis.

diuretic /dī′yo̅o̅ret′ik/, **1.** (of a drug or other substance) tending to promote the formation and excretion of urine. **2.** a drug that promotes the formation and excretion of urine. The more than 50 diuretic drugs available in the United States and Canada are classified by chemical structure and pharmacologic activity into these groups: aldosterone antagonists, carbonic anhydrase inhibitors, loop diuretics, mercurials, osmotics, potassium-sparing diuretics, and thiazides. A diuretic medication may contain drugs from one or more of these groups. Diuretics are prescribed to reduce the volume of extracellular fluid in the treatment of many disorders, including hypertension, congestive heart failure, and edema. The particular drug to be prescribed is selected according to the action desired and the physical status of the patient. Hypersensitivity to sulfonamides prohibits use of this class of drug, and diabetes mellitus may be aggravated by thiazide medications; thus, the presence of a particular condition may prohibit the use of a particular agent. Several adverse reactions are common to all diuretics, including hypovolemia and electrolyte imbalance. Mercurial diuretics are rarely used because of the nephrotoxicity, and carbonic anhydrase inhibitors have only a weak diuretic activity. Mannitol and urea osmotics are used primarily in emergency situations, as in the treatment of cerebral edema, rather than as hypertensive or cardiovascular medications.

Diuril, a trademark for a diuretic (chlorothiazide).

diurnal /dīyo͞or′nəl/ [L, *diurnalis,* of a day], happening daily, as sleeping and eating.

diurnal enuresis [L, *diurnalis,* daily; Gk, *enourein,* to urinate], involuntary voiding of urine during daylight hours.

diurnal mood variation, a change in mood that is related to the time of day. Examples are commonly found in differences between "night people" and "morning people."

diurnal rhythm [L, *diurnalis,* of a day; Gk, *rhythmos],* patterns of activity or behavior that follow day-night cycles, such as breakfast-lunch-dinner schedules.

diurnal variation, the range of the output or excretion rate of a substance in a specimen being collected for laboratory analysis over a 24-hour period.

divalent. See **bivalent.**

divergence /divur′jəns/ [L, *dis + vergere,* to incline], a separation or movement of objects away from each other, as in the simultaneous turning of the eyes outward due to an extraocular muscle defect.

divergent squint /divur′jənt/ [L, *di, vergere,* to incline; ME, *squint],* a visual disorder in which a deviating eye looks outward. The outward looking eye often is blind or has defective vision. Also called **divergent strabismus, exotropia, wall-eye.**

diversional activity deficit, a nursing diagnosis accepted by the Fourth National Conference on the Classification of Nursing Diagnoses. It is a state in which an individual experiences a decreased stimulation from or interest or engagement in recreational or leisure activities. The defining characteristics are boredom, a desire for something to do, and an inability to undertake usual hobbies. Related factors include an environmental lack of diversional activity, long-term hospitalization, and frequent, lengthy treatments. See also **nursing diagnosis.**

diverticula. See **diverticulum.**

diverticular. See **diverticulum.**

diverticular disease. See **diverticulitis, diverticulosis.**

diverticulitis /dī′vurtik′yo͞olī′tis/ [L, *diverticulare,* to turn aside; Gk, *itis,* inflammation], inflammation of one or more diverticula. The penetration of fecal matter through the thin-walled diverticula causes inflammation and abscess formation in the tissues surrounding the colon. With repeated inflammation, the lumen of the colon narrows and may become obstructed. During periods of inflammation, the patient will experience crampy pain, particularly over the sigmoid colon, fever, and leukocytosis. Barium enemas and proctoscopy are performed to rule out carcinoma of the colon, which exhibits some of the same symptoms. Conservative treatment includes bed rest, intravenous fluids, antibiotics, and nothing taken by mouth. In acute cases, bowel resection of the affected part greatly reduces mortality and morbidity. Compare **diverticulosis.**

diverticulosis /dī′vurtik′yo͞olō′sis/ [L, *diverticulare,* to turn aside; Gk, *osis,* condition], the presence of pouchlike herniations through the muscular layer of the colon, particularly the sigmoid colon. Diverticulosis affects increasing numbers of people over 50 years of age and may be the result of the modern, highly refined, low-residue diet. Most patients with this condition have few symptoms except for occasional bleeding from the rectum. Other reasons for bleeding, such as carcinoma and inflammatory bowel disease, must be ruled out. Barium enemas and proctoscopic examination are used in establishing diagnosis. An increase in the dietary fiber can aid in propelling the feces through the colon. Hemorrhage from bleeding diverticula can become quite severe, and the patient may require surgery. Diverticulosis may lead to diverticulitis. See also **diverticulitis.**

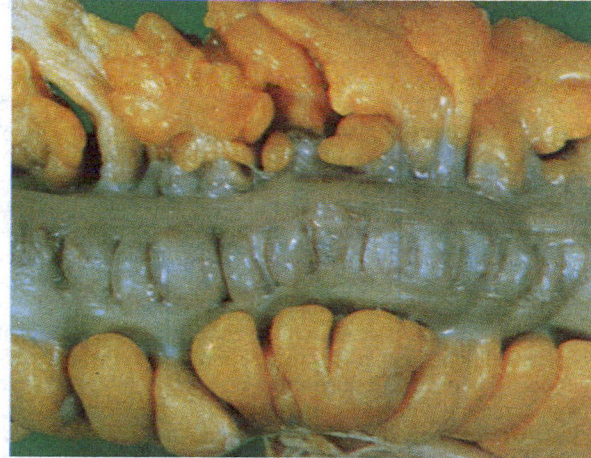

Diverticulosis (McLaren, 1992/Courtesy Dr. HM Gilmour)

diverticulum /dī′vurtik′yo͞oləm/, *pl.* **diverticula** [L, *diverticulare,* to turn aside], a pouchlike herniation through the muscular wall of a tubular organ. A diverticulum may be present in the stomach, in the small intestine, or, most commonly, the colon. See also **diverticulitis, diverticulosis, Meckel's diverticulum.** –**diverticular,** *adj.*

diving, the act of work or recreation in an underwater environment. The main health effects are related to the increased pressure to which the person is subjected as the ambient pressure generally increases by 1 atm (14.7 pounds per square inch) for each 33 feet of descent below the wa-

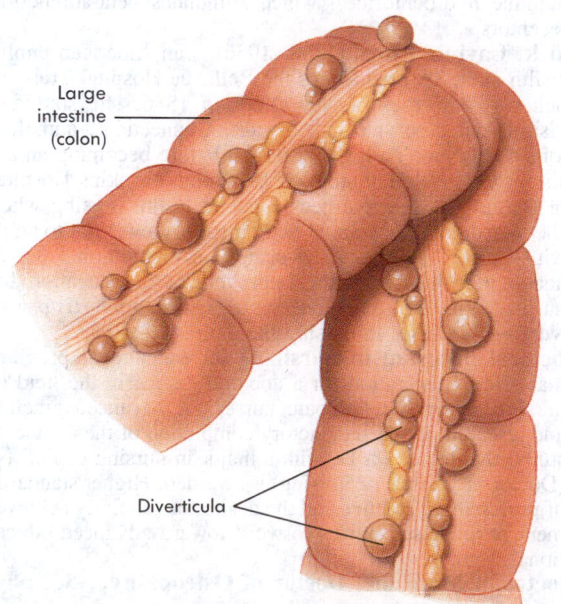

Large intestine (colon)

Diverticula

Diverticulitis (Wardlaw, 1993)

ter surface. Conditions that warrant caution against diving include obesity, diabetes, alcoholism, epilepsy, drug abuse, and respiratory disorders, including allergic rhinitis. See also **decompression sickness, diving reflex.**

diving goiter [AS, *dyypan,* to dip; L, *guttur,* throat], a large movable thyroid gland located at times above the sternal notch and at other times below the notch. Also called **plunging goiter, wandering goiter.**

diving reflex, an automatic change in the cardiovascular system that occurs when the face and nose are immersed in water. The heart rate decreases and the blood pressure remains stable or increases slightly, while blood flow to all parts of the body except the brain is reduced, thereby helping the body to conserve oxygen. The reflex occurs in both humans and other mammals.

division [L, *dividere,* to divide], **1.** an administrative subunit in a hospital, such as a division of medical nursing or a division of surgical nursing. **2.** (in public health nursing) an area that encompasses several geographic districts. **3.** the separation of something into two or more parts or sections, such as **cell division.**

divorce therapy, a type of counseling that attempts to help couples disengage from their former relationship and malicious behavior toward each other or their children.

Dix, Dorothea Lynde (1802–87), an American humanitarian who achieved fame as a social reformer, primarily for her work in improving prison conditions and care of the mentally ill. During her lifetime, she helped to establish mental institutions in 30 states and in Canada. During the Civil War, she was appointed superintendent of army nurses for government hospitals.

dizygotic /dī′zīgot′ik/ [Gk, *di,* twice, *zygotos,* yolked together], of or pertaining to twins from two fertilized ova. Compare **monozygotic.** See also **twinning.**

dizygotic twins, two offspring born of the same pregnancy and developed from two ova that were released from the ovary simultaneously and fertilized at the same time. They may be of the same or opposite sex, differ both physically and in genetic constitution, and have two separate and distinct placentas and membranes, both amnion and chorion. The frequency of dizygotic twinning varies according to ethnic origin, the highest incidence being in the black race, the lowest in Orientals, with the white races being intermediate; maternal age, the highest rate occurring when the mother is 35 to 39 years of age; and heredity, showing an increase in the female genetic line rather than the male, although fathers may transmit the disposition toward double ovulation to their daughters. In general, the overall ratio is two-thirds dizygotic twinning to one-third monozygotic. Also called **binovular twins, dissimilar twins, false twins, fraternal twins, heterologous twins.** Compare **monozygotic twins.**

dizziness [AS, *dysig,* stupid], a sensation of faintness or an inability to maintain normal balance in a standing or seated position, sometimes associated with giddiness, mental confusion, nausea, and weakness. A patient who experiences dizziness should be carefully lowered to a safe position on a bed, chair, or floor because of the danger of injury from falling. Compare **syncope.**

DKA, abbreviation for **diabetic ketoacidosis.**

DLE, abbreviation for **discoid lupus erythematosus.**

DM, abbreviation for **diabetes mellitus.**

D.M.D., abbreviation for *Doctor of Dental Medicine.*It is equivalent to a **D.D.S.** degree.

DMSO, abbreviation for **dimethyl sulfoxide.**

DNA, abbreviation for **deoxyribonucleic acid.**

DNA chimera /kīmē′rə/, (in molecular genetics) a recombinant molecule of DNA composed of segments from more than one source.

DNA ligase, an enzyme that can repair breaks in a strand of DNA by synthesizing a bond between adjoining nucleotides. Under some circumstances the enzyme can join together loose ends of DNA strands, and in some cases it can repair breaks in RNA.

DNA polymerase, (in molecular genetics) an enzyme that catalyzes the assembly of deoxyribonucleoside triphosphates into DNA, with single-stranded DNA serving as the template. The enzyme is often found in tumor cells. Also called **DNA nucleotidyltransferase.**

DNAR, abbreviation for **do not attempt resuscitation.**

DNCB, abbreviation for *dinitrochlorobenzene.*

DNR, abbreviation for *do not resuscitate.* See **no-code.**

D.O., abbreviation for *Doctor of Osteopathy.* See **physician.**

DOA, abbreviation for *dead on arrival.*

Dobie's globule /dō′bēz/ [William M. Dobie, English physician, b. 1828], a very small stainable body in the transparent disk of a striated muscle fiber. Also called **Krause's line, Z disk.**

dobutamine hydrochloride /dōbyōō′təmēn/, a beta-adrenergic stimulating agent.

■ INDICATIONS: It is prescribed to increase cardiac output in severe chronic congestive heart failure and as an adjunct in cardiac surgery.

■ CONTRAINDICATIONS: Idiopathic hypertrophic subaortic stenosis or known hypersensitivity to this drug prohibits its use. It is not recommended for use in pregnancy.

■ ADVERSE EFFECTS: Among the most serious adverse reactions are cardiovascular effects, including tachycardia, hypertension, arrythmias, and precipitation of angina. Nausea, vomiting, and headache may also occur.

Dobutrex, a trademark for a synthetic catecholamine (dobutamine hydrochloride), which stimulates beta-adrenergic receptors.

Dock, Lavinia Lloyd (1858–1956), an American public health nurse. A graduate of the Bellevue Hospital Training School for Nurses in New York in 1886, she started a visiting-nurse service in Norwalk, Connecticut, and then joined the New York City Mission before becoming an assistant to Isabel Hampton Robb at Johns Hopkins Hospital in Baltimore. She returned to public health nursing when she joined the Henry Street Settlement in New York to work with Lillian Wald. She advocated an international public health movement and the improvement of education for nurses. With M. Adelaide Nutting, she wrote *History of Nursing,* a classic in nursing literature.

doctoral program in nursing, an educational program that offers preparation for a doctoral degree in the field of nursing designed to prepare nurses for advanced practice and research. Upon satisfactory completion of the course of study, the degree Ph.D. with a major in nursing or D.S.N. (Doctor of Science in Nursing) is awarded. Higher standards of professional practice and the desire for scholarly achievement have caused nurses to work toward advanced educational degrees.

Doctor of Medicine, Doctor of Osteopathy. See **physician.**

documentation /dok′yəmentā′shən/ [L, *documentum,*

proof], written material associated with a computer or a program. Kinds of documentation include **user documentation,** an instruction manual that provides enough information for the individual to use the system; **system documentation,** a complete description of the hardware and the software that make up a system; and **program documentation,** a general and specific description of what a program does and how it does it.

docusate /dok'yo͞osāt/, a stool softener. Also called **dioctyl calcium sulfosuccinate, dioctyl sodium sulfosuccinate.**

■ INDICATION: It is prescribed in the treatment of constipation.

■ CONTRAINDICATIONS: Signs or symptoms of appendicitis, concomitant administration of mineral oil, or known hypersensitivity to the drug prohibits its use.

■ ADVERSE EFFECTS: No serious adverse reactions are known.

δOD, abbreviation for **delta optic density.**

Doederlein's bacillus /dā'dərlīnz, dō'dərlēnz/ [Albert S. Doederlein, German physician, b. 1860], a gram-positive bacterium present in normal vaginal secretions.

Doehle bodies /dā'lə, dōl/ [Karl G. P. Doehle, German pathologist, b. 1855], blue inclusions in the cytoplasm of some leukocytes in May-Hegglin anomaly and in blood smears from patients with acute viral infections.

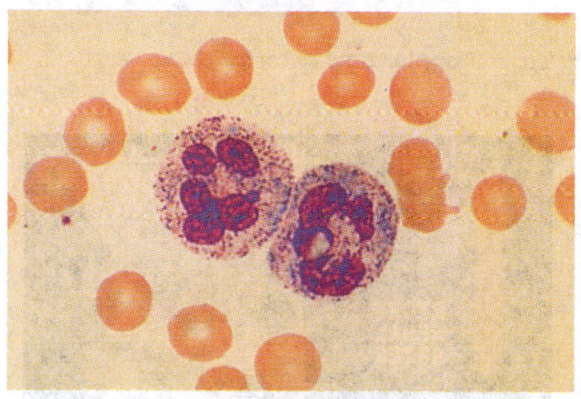

Doehle bodies (Hayhoe, 1992)

Döhle-Heller disease. See **syphilitic aortitis.**

Dolene, a trademark for an analgesic (propoxyphene hydrochloride).

dolicho-, a combining form meaning 'long': *dolichocephaly, dolichocolon, dolichomorphic*.

dolichocephaly. See **scaphocephaly.**

doll's-eye reflex, a normal response in newborns to keep the eyes stationary as the head is moved to the right or left. The reflex disappears as ocular fixation develops.

Dolobid, a trademark for an antiinflammatory agent (diflunisal).

Dolophine Hydrochloride, a trademark for a narcotic analgesic (methadone hydrochloride).

dolor /dō'lôr/ [L, pain], any condition of physical pain, mental anguish, or suffering from heat. It is one of the four signs of inflammation. The others are calor (heat), rubor (redness), and tumor (swelling).

DOM, abbreviation for **dimethoxymethylamphetamine.**

dome fracture [L, *domus*, house; *fractura*, break], any fracture of the acetabulum, specifically involving a weight-bearing surface.

dominance /dom'inəns/ [L, *dominari*, to rule], (in genetics) a basic principle stating that not all genes determining a given trait operate with equal vigor. If two genes at a given locus produce a different effect, such as eye color, they compete for expression. The gene that is manifest is dominant; it masks the effect of the other gene, which is recessive. See also **autosomal-dominant inheritance, independent assortment, recessive, segregation.** –**dominant,** *adj.*

dominant gene /dom'inənt/ [L, *dominari*, to rule; Gk, *genein* to produce], one that produces a phenotypic effect regardless of whether its allele is the same or different. Compare **recessive gene.**

dominant group, a social group that controls the value system and rewards in a particular society.

dominant trait, an inherited characteristic, such as eye color, that is likely to appear in an offspring although it may occur in only one parent. Thus, brown eye color is a dominant trait and is likely to appear in a child even if only one parent has brown eyes.

Donath-Landsteiner syndrome /dō'notland'stīnər/ [Julius Donath, Austrian physician, b. 1870; Karl Landsteiner, Austrian-American pathologist, b. 1868], a rare blood disorder marked by hemolysis minutes or hours after exposure to cold. Systemic symptoms include the passage of dark urine, severe pain in the back and legs, headache, vomiting, diarrhea, and moderate reticulocytosis. There may be temporary hepatosplenomegaly and mild hyperbilirubinemia following the onset of an attack. The condition may occur with congenital or acquired syphilis, in which case antisyphilitic treatment may be curative. Also called **paroxysmal cold hemoglobinuria.**

Don Juan, a seductive and sexually promiscuous man.

Donnatal, a trademark for a GI fixed-combination drug containing a sedative (phenobarbital) and three anticholinergics (hyoscyamine sulfate, atropine sulfate, and hyoscine hydrobromide), used to decrease the motility of the GI tract.

donor /dō'nər/ [L, *donare*, to give], **1.** a human or other organism that gives living tissue to be used in another body, for example, blood for transfusion or a kidney for transplantation. **2.** a substance or compound that gives part of itself to another substance. Compare **acceptor.** See also **universal donor.**

donor card [L, *donare*, to give, *charta*], a document in which a person offers to make an anatomic gift of body parts, at the time of death, for transplantation to recipients needing replacement of vital organs or tissues. The card is often incorporated into a state driver's license so the authorization will be immediately available if the donor dies in a traffic accident.

do not attempt resuscitation (DNAR), an advisory that resuscitation of a patient should not even be attempted. The order is more strictly defined than the **DNR** (do not resuscitate), which may be interpreted as authorizing an attempt at resuscitation.

Donovan bodies /don'əvan/ [Charles Donovan, Irish physician, b. 1863], encapsulated gram-negative rods of the species *Calymmatobacterium granulomatis,* present in the cytoplasm of mononuclear phagocytes obtained from the lesions of granuloma inguinale. They may be seen under the microscope in a Wright-stained smear of infected tissue. See also **granuloma inguinale.**

donut pad /dō′nut/, a pad designed to protect an injured joint. It is cut to fit over the site of the injury and cause force on the body part to be transferred to surrounding areas. It is most effective for protecting small areas, such as heels or elbows.

dopa /dō′pə/, an amino acid derived from tyrosine that occurs naturally in plants and animals. It is a precursor of dopamine, epinephrine, and norepinephrine. See also **dopamine hydrochloride, levodopa.**

dopamine hydrochloride /dō′pəmin/, a sympathomimetic catecholamine.
- INDICATIONS: It is prescribed in the treatment of shock, hypotension, and low cardiac output.
- CONTRAINDICATIONS: Pheochromocytoma, tachyarrhythmias, ventricular fibrillation, or known hypersensitivity to this drug prohibits its use.
- ADVERSE EFFECTS: Among the more serious adverse reactions are arrhythmias, hypotension, hypertension, and tachycardia.

dopaminergic /dō′pəminur′jik/, having the effect of dopamine.

dope [AS, *dyppan*, to dip], *slang,* morphine, heroin, or another narcotic, or marijuana or another substance illicitly bought, or sold, and often self-administered for sedative, hypnotic, euphoric, or other mood-altering purpose.

Doppler effect /dop′lər/ [Christian J. Doppler, Austrian scientist, b. 1803; L, *effectus*], the apparent change in frequency of sound or light waves emitted by a source as it moves away from or toward an observer. The frequency increases as the source moves toward the observer and decreases as it moves away, as the rising pitch of the whistle of an approaching train and the falling pitch of a departing train. The Doppler effect is also observed in electromagnetic radiation, such as light and radio waves. See also **electromagnetic radiation, ultrasonography, wavelength.**

Doppler scanning [Christian J. Doppler; L, *scandere,* to climb], a technique used in ultrasound imaging to monitor the behavior of a moving structure, such as flowing blood or a beating heart. The frequency of ultrasonic waves reflected from a moving surface is slightly different from that of the incident waves. The detected frequency shift yields information about the moving structure. Fetal heart detectors work on this principle.

Dorantamin, a trademark for an antihistamine (pyrilamine maleate).

Doriden, a trademark for a sedative (glutethimide).

dornase /dôr′nās/, a natural proteolytic substance that depolymerizes DNA molecules. Because as much as 70% of the solid matter of purulent material consists of DNA, dornase is used in respiratory therapy to help break off sputum accumulation in the airways. A principal source of dornase is beef pancreas.

dorsal /dôr′səl/ [L, *dorsum,* the back], pertaining to the back or posterior. Compare **ventral.** See also **dorsiflect. –dorsum,** *n.*

-dorsal, a suffix meaning 'the back of something' or 'the back': *predorsal, thoracodorsal, ventrodorsal.*

dorsal carpal ligament. See **retinaculum extensorum manus.**

dorsal cutaneous nerve, a nerve that is close to the surface of the foot and ankle, where it may be both visible and

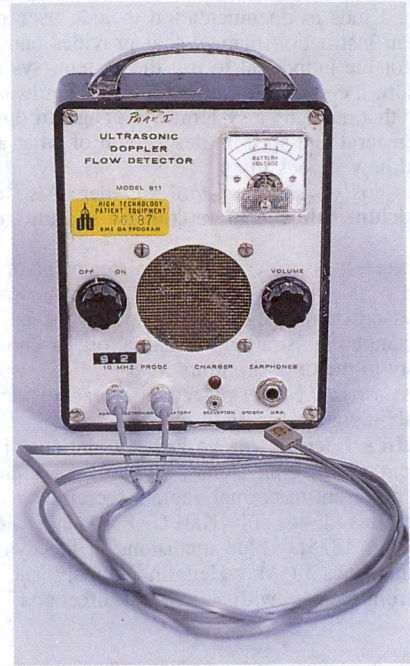

Doppler flow detector *(Seidel, 1991)*

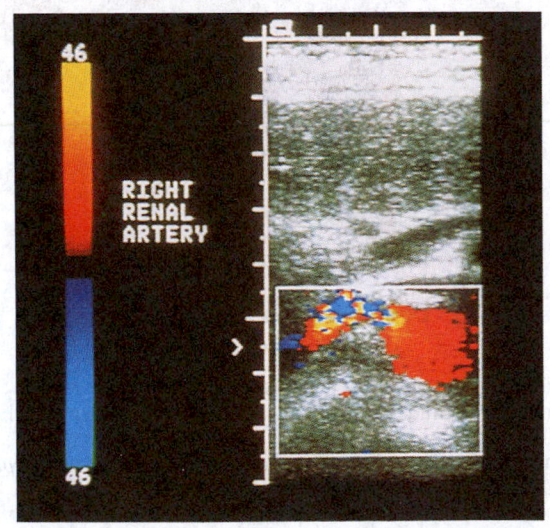

Image produced by doppler scanning *(Swales, 1991)*

palpable. Because of its location, it is vulnerable to injury and is the usual cause of pain in a sprained ankle.

dorsal decubitus position. See **supine.**

dorsal digital vein, one of the communicating veins along the sides of the fingers. The veins from the adjacent sides of the fingers unite to form three dorsal metacarpal veins, which end in a dorsal venous network on the back of the hand. Compare **basilic vein, cephalic vein, median antebrachial vein.**

dorsal flexure [L, *dorsalis*, back, *flectere*, to bend], the dorsal convexity of the thoracic region of the spine.

dorsal horn [L, *dorsalis*, back; AS, horn], a crescent-shaped projection of gray matter within the spinal cord, appearing as a horn in transverse sections. Also called **cornu posterius.**

dorsal inertia posture, a tendency of a debilitated or weak person to slip downward in bed when the head of the bed is raised. Because of loss of muscular strength or mental apathy, the person seems unable to adjust to a new position in bed.

dorsal interventricular artery, the arterial branch of the right coronary artery, branching to supply both ventricles. It runs down the dorsal sulcus two thirds of the way to the apex of the heart. Also called **right interventricular artery.**

dorsalis pedis artery, the continuation of the anterior tibial artery, starting at the ankle joint, dividing into five branches, and supplying various muscles of the foot and toes. Its branches are the lateral tarsal, medial tarsal, arcuate, first dorsal metatarsal, and deep plantar.

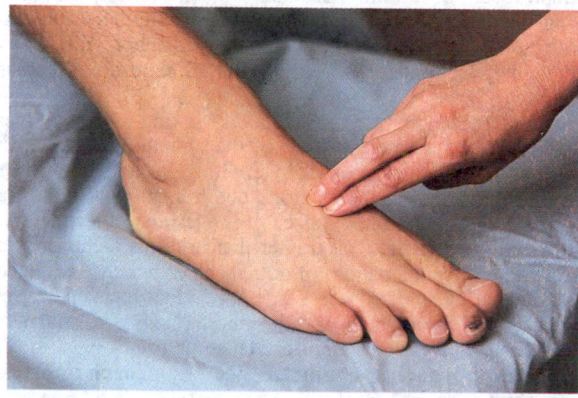

Palpation of the dorsalis pedis pulse (Seidel, 1991)

dorsalis pedis pulse, the pulse of the dorsalis pedis artery, palpable between the first and second metatarsal bones on the top of the foot. It can be felt in approximately 90% of people.

dorsal lip, the marginal fold of the blastopore during gastrulation in the early stages of embryonic development of many animals. It marks the dorsal limit of the developing embryo, constitutes the primary organizer, gives rise to neural tissue, and corresponds to the primitive node in humans and higher animals.

dorsal recumbent [L, *dorsalis*, back; *recumbere*, to lie down], lying on the back, as in a supine position.

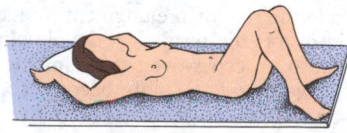

Dorsal recumbent position (Potter, 1993)

dorsal recumbent position [L, *dorsalis*, back, *positio*], the supine position with the person lying on the back, head, and shoulders.

dorsal reflex. See **erector spinae reflex.**

dorsal rigid posture, a position in which a patient lying in bed holds one or both legs drawn up to the chest. It often involves only the right leg and is intended to relieve the pain of appendicitis, peritonitis, kidney stones, or pelvic inflammation.

dorsal root [L, *dorsalis*, back; AS, *rot*], the sensory component or root of a spinal nerve.

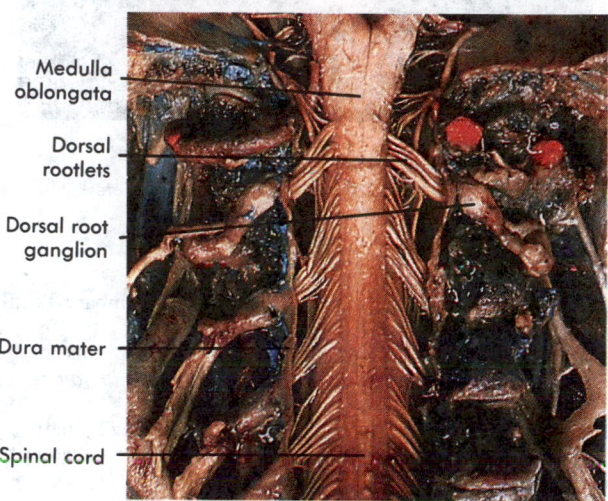

Medulla oblongata

Dorsal rootlets

Dorsal root ganglion

Dura mater

Spinal cord

Section of the spinal cord showing dorsal root and dorsal root ganglion
(Seeley, 1992/RT Hutchings)

dorsal root ganglion [L, *dorsalis*; AS, *rot*; Gk, *gagglion*, knot], a swelling consisting of sensory neuron cell bodies located on the dorsal root of a spinal nerve.

dorsal scapular nerve, one of a pair of supraclavicular branches from the roots of the brachial plexus. It arises from the fifth cervical nerve near the intervertebral foramen, pierces the scalenus medius, and runs dorsally and caudally to the vertebral border of the scapula. It supplies the rhomboideus major and the rhomboideus minor and sends a branch to the levator.

dorsi-. See **dorso-.**

dorsiflect /dôr′siflekt/ [L, *dorsum* + *flectere*, to bend], to bend or flex backward as in the upward bending of the fingers, wrist, foot, or toes.

dorsiflexion /dôr′siflek′shən/, flexion toward the back, as accomplished by a muscle. See also **dorsiflexor.** (See Fig. p. 500.)

dorsiflexor /dôr′siflek′sər/, a muscle causing backward flexion of a part of the body, as the hand or foot.

dorsiflexor gait, an abnormal gait caused by the weakness of the dorsiflexors of the ankle. It is characterized by foot-drop during the entire gait cycle and excessive knee and hip flexion to allow clearance of the involved extremity during the swing phase. The sole of the affected foot also slaps forcibly against the ground at the moment of heelstrike because of the inability of the dorsiflexor to decelerate the

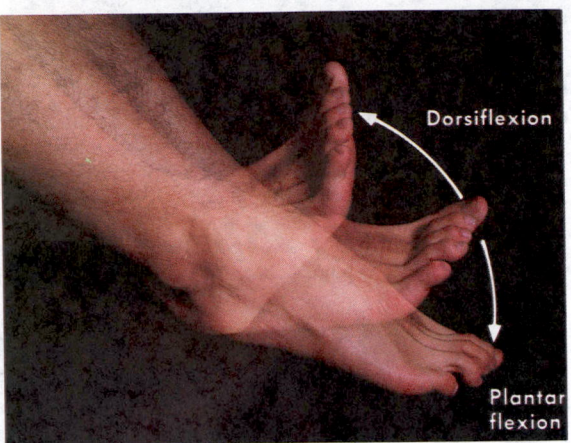

Dorsiflexion of the foot
(Thibodeau, 1993/Terry Cockerham & Associates)

body weight as the heel strikes the ground. Compare **Trendelenburg gait.**

dorso-, dorsi-, a combining form meaning 'pertaining to a dorsum or to the back': *dorsocephalad, dorsomesial, dorsoscapular.*

dorsodynia /dôr′sōdin′ē·ə/, a pain in the back, particularly in the muscles of the upper back area. Also called **dorsalgia.**

dorsosacral position. See **lithotomy position.**

dorsum /dôr′səm/ [L, *dorsum,* back], the back of the body, the posterior or upper surface of a body part.

dorsum sellae /sel′ē/, the posterior boundary of the sella turcica of the sphenoid bone. It bears the posterior clinoid process and is an anatomic marker for the location of the pituitary gland at the base of the skull.

DOS /dos/, abbreviation for *disk operating system.*

dosage [Gk, *didonai,* to give], the regimen governing the size, frequency, and number of doses of a therapeutic agent to be administered to a patient.

dosage compensation /dō′sij/, (in genetics) the mechanism that counterbalances the number of X-linked gene doses in the sex chromosomes so that they are equal in both the male, which has one X chromosome, and the female, which has two. In mammals this is accomplished by genetic activation of only one of the X chromosomes in the somatic cells of females. See also **Lyon hypothesis.**

dose /dōs/ [GK, *didonai,* to give], the amount of a drug or other substance to be administered at one time. See also **absorbed dose.**

dose equivalent (DE), a quantity used in radiation-safety work that equates on a unified scale the amount of radiation dose and the physical damages that it might produce. It is the product of the dose (in rad or gray) and modifying factors that are specific to the type and energy of the radiation delivering that dose. The unit of dose equivalent is the sievert (Sv) or the rem.

dose fractionation. See **fractionation,** def. 5.

dose-limiting recommendations, maximum permissible dose (MPD) of radiation exposure, which may vary for different body or organ exposures. For example, the MPD for the skin or forearms of a radiation worker is much higher than the whole-body exposure MPD.

dose rate, (in radiotherapy) the amount of delivered radiation absorbed per unit of time.

dose ratemeter /rāt′mētər/, (in radiotherapy) an instrument for measuring the dose rate of radiation.

dose response, a range of drug effects between the minimum dose needed to reach the threshold level, at which an effect is first observed, and a toxic dose level, where adverse effects result.

dose-response relationship, (in radiology) a mathematical relationship between the dose of radiation and the body's reaction to it. In a linear dose-response relationship, the response is proportional to the dose. Thus if the dose is doubled, the response is also doubled. In a linear nonthreshold relationship any dose, regardless of size, can theoretically cause a response.

dose threshold, (in radiotherapy) the minimum amount of absorbed radiation that produces a detectable degree of a given effect.

dose to skin, (in radiotherapy) the amount of absorbed radiation at the center of the irradiation field on the skin. It is the sum of the dose in the air and the scatter from body parts.

dosimeter /dōsim′ətr7 [L, *dosis* + Gk, *metron,* measure], an instrument to detect and measure accumulated radiation exposure. A pencil-sized ionization chamber with a self-reading electrometer is used to monitor exposure to personnel.

dosimetry /dōsim′ətrē/ [Gk, *dosis,* giving, *metron,* measure], **1.** the determination of the amount, rate, and distribution of radiation or radioactivity from a source of ionizing radiation. **2.** the accurate determination of medicinal doses, based upon body size, sex, age, and other factors.

dot-matrix printer, a printer that imprints a character by creating it from a pattern of dots, each of which is produced by actuating selected wires in a set so that their ends strike the paper through an inked ribbon. Compare **character printer, daisy-wheel printer, laser printer.**

double-approach conflict. See **approach-approach conflict.**

double-avoidant conflict. See **avoidance-avoidance conflict.**

double bind /bīnd/ [L, *duplus,* double; AS, *bindan,* to bind], a "no win" situation resulting from two conflicting messages from a person who is crucial to one's survival, such as a verbal message that differs from a nonverbal message. An example is the insistence of a mother that she is not angry about a child's behavior although she is perceived as being obviously angry and hostile.

double-blind study, an experiment designed to test the effect of a treatment or substance using groups of experimental and control subjects in which neither the subjects nor the investigators know which treatment or substance is being administered to which group. In a double-blind test of a new drug, the substance may be identified to the investigators by only a code. The purpose of a double-blind study is to eliminate the risk of prejudgment by the participants, which could distort the results. A double-blind study may be augmented by a **cross-over experiment,** in which experimental subjects unknowingly become control subjects, and vice versa, at some point in the study. See also **placebo.**

double-blind test [L, *duplus,* double; AS, *blind; testum,* crucible], an experimental design for drug testing in which neither the clients receiving the drugs nor the persons conducting the test know which subjects are receiving a new drug and which are getting a placebo, or sugar pill.

double-channel catheter [L, *duplus,* double; ME, *chanel*; Gk, *katheter,* a thing lowered into], a double-lumen catheter used to irrigate an internal cavity, with fluid entering one lumen and draining through the other. Also called **two-way catheter.**

double-contrast arthrography, a method of making anx-ray image of a joint by injecting two contrast agents intothe capsular space. A gaseous medium and a water-solubleiodinated agent are usually combined. The technique ismost commonly used in radiography of the knee joint.

double-contrast barium enema [L, *duplus,* double, *contra,* against, *stare,* to stand; Gk, *barys,* heavy, *enienai,* to inject], an enema of radiopaque barium followed by evacuation and injection of air. The purpose is to detail radiographically the mucosal lining of the large intestine.

double-contrast enema. See **double-contrast barium enema.**

double-emulsion film, x-ray film that is coated with gelatin emulsion on both sides.

double-flap amputation [L, *duplus,* double; ME, *flappe,* flap; L, *amputare*], an amputation in which two flaps are made from the soft tissues to cover an area that has lost its integument in surgery or accident.

double fracture, a fracture consisting of breaks or cracks in two places in a bone, resulting in more than two bone segments.

double gel diffusion. See **immunodiffusion.**

double innervation, innervation of effector organs by fibers of the sympathetic and parasympathetic divisions of the autonomic nervous system. The pelvic viscera, bronchioles, heart, eyes, and digestive system are all doubly innervated. The fibers of the two divisions operate at cross-purposes to achieve a state of balance and to maintain the homeostatic condition of the body. The mode of action of each division varies: in some structures one division is stimulating and the other inhibiting; in others, separate fibers from each division act to stimulate and inhibit complementary function.

double monster, a fetus that has developed from a single ovum but has two heads, trunks, and multiple limbs. Also called **twin monster.**

double-needle entry, a technique for injecting a contrast medium or other agent with two needles, one with a larger bore. In diskography, a 20-gauge needle is used to perform a spinal puncture and reach the annulus fibrosus of the disk, after which a longer, 26-gauge needle is passed through the guide needle to the injection target area.

double personality [L, *duplus,* double, *personalis,* of a person], a state of dissociation in which the individual presents personas to associates at different times as two different persons, each with different names and personality traits. The two personalities are generally independent, contrasting, and unaware of the existence of the other. Also called **dual personality.** See also **multiple personality disorder.**

double quartan fever, a form of malaria in which paroxysms of fever occur in a repeating pattern of 2 consecutive days followed by 1 day of remission. The pattern is usually the result of concurrent infections by two species of the genus *Plasmodium,* one causing paroxysms every 72 hours and the other every 48 hours. Compare **biduotertian fever.**

double setup, a nursing procedure in which an obstetric operating room is prepared for both vaginal delivery and cesarean section. The circulating and scrub nurses lay out the equipment required for both procedures, possibly including a vacuum aspirator, forceps, and cesarean-section packs. The scrub nurse remains scrubbed until the infant is delivered but does not participate unless a cesarean section is performed.

double vision. See **diplopia.**

double-void, a urinalysis procedure in which the first specimen is discarded and a second, obtained 30 to 45 minutes later, is tested. This method gives a more accurate measure of the amount of glucose in the urine at that particular time.

douche /dōōsh/ [Fr, shower-bath], **1.** a procedure in which a liter or more of a solution of a medication or cleansing agent in warm water is introduced into the vagina under low pressure. The woman often performs the procedure herself. Sitting on a toilet seat or semisitting in a bathtub, she introduces the douche tip into the vagina and releases a clamp on the tubing connected to the douche bag, which is suspended 2 feet above the introitus. She allows the solution to flow in, while holding the lips of the vagina closed to retain the fluid. As the accumulation of fluid distends the vagina, she clamps the tubing and, after a few minutes, allows the fluid to flow out. The process is repeated until the entire quantity of solution in the douche bag has been used. Douching may be recommended in the treatment of various pelvic and vaginal infections. **2.** to perform a douche.

doughnut pessary. See **pessary.**

Douglas' cul-de-sac [James Douglas, Scottish anatomist, b. 1675; Fr, bottom of the bag], a rectouterine pouch or recess formed by a fold of peritoneum that extends between the rectum and the uterus. Also called **excavatio rectouterina.**

down [AS, *adune,* off hill], (of a computer) not operating as a result of malfunction or maintenance or for other reasons.

download to transfer data or programs from a central computer to a peripheral unit.

Downey cells [Hal Downey, American physician, b. 1877], lymphocytes identified in one system of classification of the blood cells of patients with infectious mononucleosis. The cells are designated as Downey I, II, or III lymphocytes.

Down syndrome [John L. Down, English physician, b. 1828], a congenital condition characterized by varying degrees of mental retardation and multiple defects. It is the most common chromosomal abnormality of a generalized syndrome and is caused by the presence of an extra chromosome 21 in the G group or, in a small percentage of cases, by the translocation of chromosomes 14 or 15 in the D group and chromosomes 21 or 22. Also called **mongolism, mongoloid idiocy, trisomy G syndrome, trisomy 21.** Down's syndrome occurs in approximately 1 in 600 to 650 live births and is associated with advanced maternal age, particularly over 35 years of age. The incidence is as high as 1 in 80 for offspring of women older than 40 years. In those cases caused by translocation, which is a genetic aberration that is hereditary rather than a chromosomal aberration caused by nondisjunction during cell division, the incidence is not associated with maternal age, and the risk is low, about 1 in 5 if the mother is the carrier and 1 in 20 if the father is the carrier. The condition, which can be diagnosed prenatally by amniocentesis, also occurs as a mosaic variant, in which there is a mixture of trisomy 21 and normal cells. Such patients have fewer physical defects and less-severe retardation depending on the degree of mosaicism. Infants with the syndrome are small and hypotonic, with characteristic microcephaly, brachycephaly, a flattened occiput, and typical facies with a mongoloid slant to the eyes, depressed nasal bridge, low-set ears, and a large, protruding tongue that is furrowed and lacks the central fissure. The hands are short and broad with a transverse palmar or simian crease; the fingers are stubby and show clinodactyly, primarily of the fifth finger. The feet are broad and stubby with a wide space between the first and second toes and a prominent plantar crease. Other anomalies associated with the disorder are bowel defects, congenital heart disease (primarily septal defects), chronic respiratory infections, visual problems, abnormalities in tooth development, and susceptibility to acute leukemia. The most significant feature of the syndrome is mental retardation, which varies considerably, although the average IQ is in the range of 50 to 60, so that the child is generally trainable and in most instances can be reared at home. Those more severely affected are often institutionalized. The mortality rate is high within the first few years, especially in children with cardiac anomalies. Those who survive tend to be shorter than average and stocky in build, they show delayed or incomplete sexual development, and they can live to middle or old age, although adults with Down's syndrome are prone to respiratory infections, pneumonia, and lung disease.

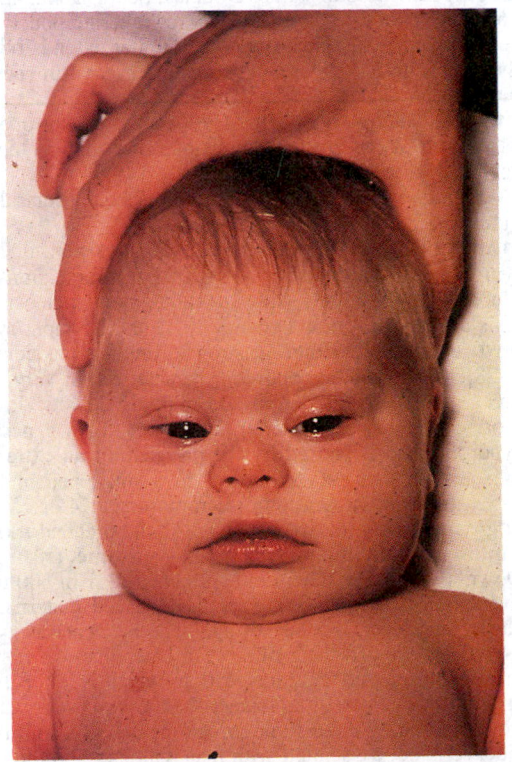

Typical face seen in Down syndrome (Zitelli, 1992)

down-time, a period during which a computer system is inoperable, for maintenance, as a result of malfunction, or for other reasons.

doxapram hydrochloride /dok'səpram/, a respiratory stimulant.
■ INDICATIONS: It is prescribed to improve respiratory function after anesthesia, in drug-induced central nervous system depression, and for chronic pulmonary disease associated with acute hypercapnia.
■ CONTRAINDICATIONS: Seizure disorder, pulmonary disease, coronary artery disease, hypertension, or known hypersensitivity to this drug prohibits its use.
■ ADVERSE EFFECTS: Among the more serious adverse reactions are convulsions, bronchospasm, cardiovascular symptoms, and phlebitis.

doxepin hydrochloride /dok'səpin/, a tricyclic antidepressant.
■ INDICATION: It is prescribed in the treatment of depression.
■ CONTRAINDICATIONS: Concomitant administration of monoamine oxidase inhibitors, recent myocardial infarction, seizure disorders, or known hypersensitivity to tricyclic medication prohibits its use.
■ ADVERSE EFFECTS: Among the more serious adverse reactions are GI, cardiovascular, and neurologic disturbances. Sedation, dry mouth, and many drug interactions may occur.

doxorubicin hydrochloride /dok'səroo'bisin/, an anthracycline antibiotic.
■ INDICATIONS: It is prescribed in the treatment of a variety of malignant neoplastic diseases.
■ CONTRAINDICATIONS: Myelosuppression, heart disease, concurrent administration of daunorubicin, or known hypersensitivity to this drug prohibits its use.
■ ADVERSE EFFECTS: Among the more serious adverse reactions are myelosuppression and cardiomyopathy. Stomatitis, GI disturbances, and alopecia commonly occur.

doxycycline /dok'sisī'klēn/, a tetracycline antibacterial.
■ INDICATIONS: It is prescribed in the treatment of a variety of infections.
■ CONTRAINDICATIONS: Renal or liver dysfunction or known hypersensitivity to this drug or to other tetracycline medication prohibits its use. It is not given during pregnancy or to children under 8 years of age.
■ ADVERSE EFFECTS: Among the more serious adverse reactions are GI disturbances, phototoxicity, potentially serious suprainfections, and hypersensitivity reactions. Discoloration of teeth may occur in children exposed to the drug in utero or under 8 years of age.

doxylamine succinate /dok'silam'ēn/, an antihistamine.
■ INDICATIONS: It is prescribed for the treatment of acute allergic symptoms produced by the release of histamine.
■ CONTRAINDICATIONS: Known hypersensitivity to this drug prohibits its use. It is not recommended for use during pregnancy or lactation and is not given to children under 6 years of age.
■ ADVERSE EFFECTS: Among the more serious reactions are sedation, ataxia, tachycardia, hemolytic anemia, and thrombocytopenia.

dp/dt, (in cardiology) the rate of pressure change per unit of time.

DPG, abbreviation for **2,3-diphosphoglyceric acid.**

D.P.H., abbreviation for *Diploma in Public Health.*

DPT vaccine, abbreviation for **diphtheria, tetanus toxoids, and pertussis vaccine.**

DQ, abbreviation for **developmental quotient.**

dr., **1.** abbreviation for **drachm.** **2.** abbreviation for **dram.**

drachm (dr.) [Gk, *drachme*, a weight of equal value]. See **dram.**

dracunculiasis /drakun'kyōōlī'əsis/ [Gk, *drakontion*, little dragon, *osis*, condition], a parasitic infection caused by infestation by the nematode *Dracunculus medinensis*. It is characterized by ulcerative skin lesions on the legs and feet that are produced by gravid female worms. People are infected by drinking contaminated water or eating contaminated shellfish. It is common in densely populated tropic and subtropic areas of the world. Also called **dracontiasis, guinea worm infection.**

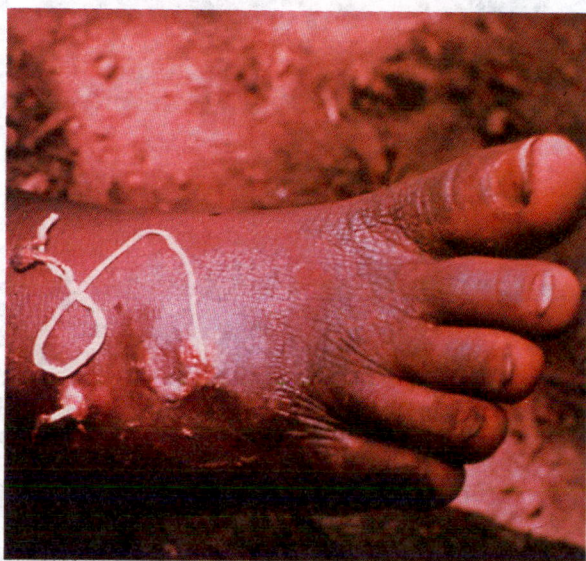

Dracunculiasis
(du Vivier, 1992/Courtesy Dr. R Muller)

Dracunculus medinensis /drakun'kyōōləs/, a parasitic nematode of the Mediterranean area that causes dracunculiasis. An American species is *Dracunculus insignis*. Also called **fiery serpent.**

drag-to gait [ME, *dragen, gate*, path], a method of walking with crutches in which the feet are dragged rather than lifted with each step.

drain, a tube or other opening used to remove air or a fluid from a body cavity or wound. The drain may be a closed system, designed to provide complete protection against contamination, or an open system.

drainage /drā'nij/ [AS, *drachen*, teardrop], the removal of fluids from a body cavity, wound, or other source of discharge by one or more methods. **Closed drainage** is a system of tubing and other apparatus attached to the body to remove fluid in an airtight circuit that prevents environmental contaminants from entering the wound or cavity. **Open drainage** is drainage in which discharge passes through an open-ended tube into a receptacle. **Suction drainage** utilizes a pump or other mechanic device to assist in extracting a fluid. **Tidal drainage** is drainage in which a body area is washed out by alternately flooding and then emptying it with the aid of gravity, a technique that may be used in treating a urinary bladder disorder. See also **postural drainage.**

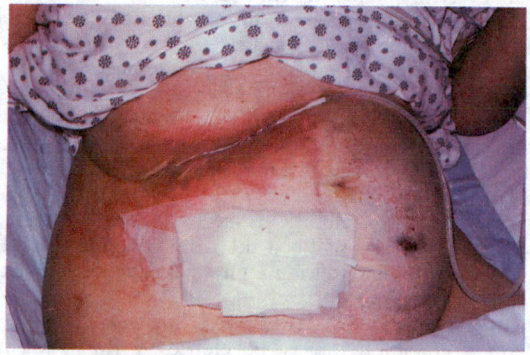

Closed wound drainage system
(Bryant, 1992/Courtesy Abbott Northwestern Hospital, Minneapolis)

drainage tube, a heavy-gauge catheter used for the evacuation of air or a fluid from a cavity or wound in the body. The tube may be attached to a suction device or simply allow flow by gravity into a receptacle.

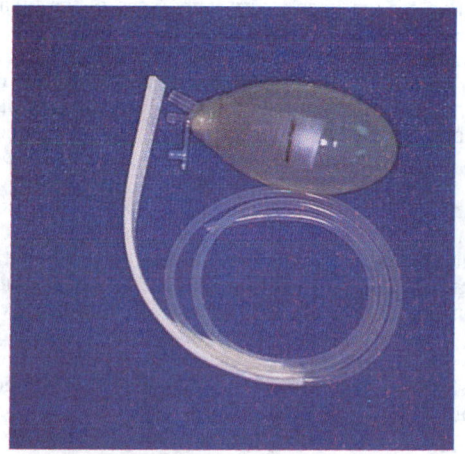

Jackson-Pratt silicon suction drain *(Grossman, 1993)*

draining sinus [AS, *drachen*, teardrop; L, *sinus*, hollow], an abnormal channel or fistula permitting the escape of exudate to the outside of the body.

Draize test /drāz/, a controversial method of testing the toxicity of pharmaceutic and other products to be used by humans by placing a small amount of the substance in the eyes of rabbits. The eye-irritancy potential of a substance is considered a measure of the possible effect the product could have on similar human tissues. The Draize in vivo test is recognized by the U.S. Food and Drug Administration as a reliable method of predicting the risk of new products to human eyesight, although alternative testing methods are being sought.

-dralazine, a suffix for the name of an antihypertensive.

dram (dr.) [Gk, *drachme*, weight of the same value], a unit of mass equivalent to an apothecaries' measure of 60 grains or ⅛ ounce and to 1/16 ounce or 27.34 grains avoirdupois. Also spelled **drachm (dr.).**

Dramamine, a trademark for an antihistamine (dimenhydrinate), used as an antiemetic.

dramatic play /dramat′ik/ [Gk, *drama*, deed; AS, *plegan*, game], an imitative activity in which a child fantasizes and acts out various domestic and social roles and situations, as rocking a doll, pretending to be a doctor or nurse, or teaching school. It is the predominant form of play among preschool children.

drape [ME, *drap*, cloth], a sheet of fabric or paper, usually the size of a small bed sheet, for covering all or a part of a person's body during a physical examination or treatment. **–drape,** *v.*

Draw-a-Person Test (DAP) [AS, *dragan*; L, *personalis*, *testum*, crucible], a test developed by Karen Machover [American psychologist, b. 1902] based on the interpretation of drawings of human figures of both sexes. Interpretation depends upon the subject's verbalizations, self-image, anxiety, and sexual conflicts and other factors. Also called **Machover Draw-a-Person Test.**

drawer sign [AS, *dragan*, to drag], a diagnostic sign of a ruptured or torn knee ligament. It is tested by having the patient flex the knee at a right angle while the examiner grasps the lower leg just below the knee and moves the leg first toward, then away from himself or herself. The test is positive for the knee injury if the head of the tibia can be moved more than a half inch from the joint.

drawing, *informal.* a vague sensation of muscle tension.

drawsheet, a sheet that is smaller than a bottom or top sheet of a bed and is usually placed over the middle of the bottom sheet to keep the mattress and bottom linens dry. The drawsheet can also be used to turn or move a patient in bed.

dream [ME, *dreem*, joyful noise], **1.** a sequence of ideas, thoughts, emotions, or images that pass through the mind during the rapid-eye-movement stage of sleep. **2.** the sleeping state in which this process occurs. **3.** a visionary creation of the imagination experienced during wakefulness. **4.** (in psychoanalysis) the expression of thoughts, emotions, memories, or impulses repressed from the consciousness. **5.** (in analytic psychology) the wishes, emotions, and impulses that reflect the personal unconscious and the archetypes that originate in the collective unconscious. See also **dream analysis, dream state.**

dream analysis, a process of gaining access to the unconscious mind by means of examining the content of dreams, usually through the method of free association.

dream association, a relationship of thoughts or emotions discovered or experienced when a dream is remembered or analyzed. See also **dream analysis.**

dream state, a condition of altered consciousness in which a person does not recognize the environment and reacts in a manner opposed to his or her usual behavior, as by flight or an act of violence. The state is seen in epilepsy and certain neuroses. See also **automatism, fugue.**

drepanocytic anemia /drep′ənōsit′ik/ [Gk, *drepane*, sickle, *kytos*, cell], sickle cell anemia.

dress code [OFr, *dresser*, to arrange; L, *codex*, book], the standards set by an institution for the dress of the members of the institution.

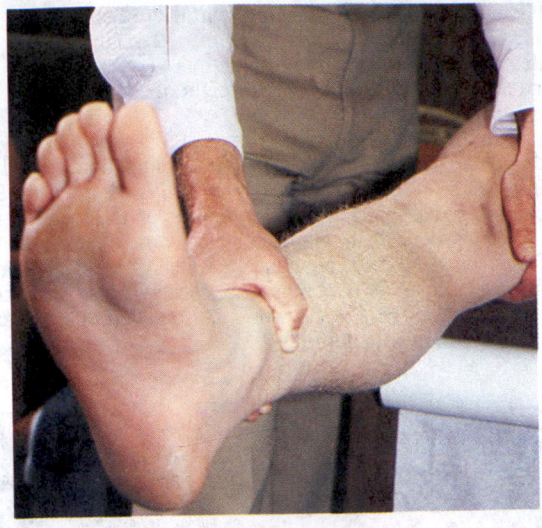

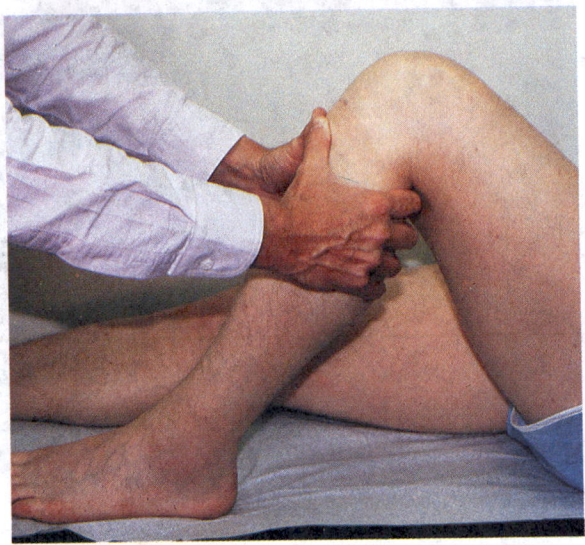

Drawer sign *(Seidel, 1991)*

dressing [OFr, *dresser*, to arrange], a clean or sterile covering applied directly to wounded or diseased tissue for absorption of secretions, for protection from trauma, for administration of medications, to keep the wound clean, or to stop bleeding. Kinds of dressings include **absorbent dressing, antiseptic dressing, occlusive dressing, pressure dressing,** and **wet dressing.**

dressing forceps, a kind of forceps that has narrow blades and blunt or notched teeth, designed for dressing wounds, removing drainage tubes, or extracting fragments of necrotic tissue.

Dressler's syndrome /dres′lərz/, an autoimmune disorder that may occur several days after acute coronary infarction, characterized by fever, pericarditis, pleurisy, pleural effusions, and joint pain. It results from the body's immunologic response to a damaged myocardium and pericardium.

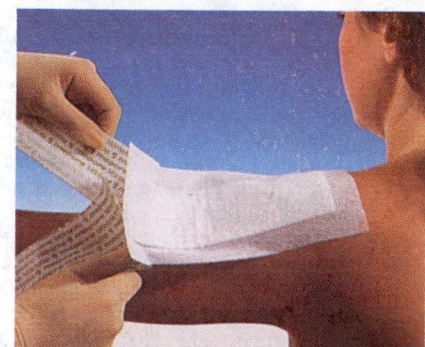

Mepore

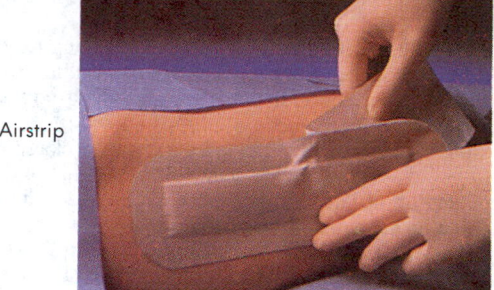

Airstrip

Simple dressings *(Morison, 1992)*

Treatment usually includes intensive aspirin therapy and, in severe cases, corticosteroids. A similar syndrome may occur after cardiac surgery.

DRG, abbreviation for **diagnosis related groups.**

drift [AS, *drifan,* to move forward], **1. antigenic drift,** a change that occurs in a strain of virus so that variations appear periodically with alterations in antigenic qualities. **2. genetic drift,** random variations in gene frequency of a population from one generation to the next.

drifting tooth, any one of the teeth that migrate from normal position in the associated dental arch. This anomaly may result from the loss of proximal support, loss of functional antagonists, occlusal traumatic tooth relationships, inflammatory and retrograde changes in the attachment apparatus, or oral habits, such as thumb-sucking and bruxism.

Drinker respirator [Philip Drinker, American engineer, b. 1893], an airtight respirator consisting of a metal tank that encloses the entire body, except for the head. Used for long-term therapy, it alternates positive and negative air pressure within the tank, providing artificial respiration by contracting and expanding the walls of the chest. Also called **artificial lung, iron lung.**

drip [AS, *dryppan,* to fall in drops], **1.** the process of a liquid or moisture forming and falling in drops. Kinds of drip are **nasal drip** and **postnasal drip. 2.** the slow but continuous infusion of a liquid into the body, as into the stomach or a vein. **3.** to infuse a liquid continuously into the body.

drip gavage, a method of feeding a liquid formula diet through a tube inserted through the nostrils to the stomach. The formula may be heated to about 100° F or administered at room temperature and is contained in a bag suspended from a stand. It may also be administered with the use of a feeding pump.

drip system, (in intravenous therapy) an apparatus for delivering specific volumes of intravenous solutions within predetermined periods of time and at a specific flow rate. See also **macrodrip, microdrip.**

drive [AS, *drifan,* to move forward], **1.** a basic, compelling urge. **Primary drive** refers to one that is innate and in close contact with physiologic processes. A **secondary drive** is one that evolves during the process of growth and that incites and directs behavior. **2.** an electromechanic device that holds a secondary-storage medium and allows for the transfer of data to and from the computer, such as a disk drive or tape drive.

Drixoral, a trademark for a fixed-combination drug containing an antihistamine (dexbrompheniramine maleate) and a vasoconstrictor and bronchodilator (pseudoephedrine sulfate), used for the relief of congestion of the upper respiratory tract.

-drome, a suffix meaning 'that which runs or moves together' in a specified way: *dermadrome, heterodrome, syndrome.*

dromo-, a combining form meaning 'pertaining to running or conduction': *dromomania, dromophobic, dromotropic.*

dromostanolone propionate /drō'mostan'əlōn/, a synthetic androgen.
■ INDICATION: It is prescribed for female breast cancer.
■ CONTRAINDICATIONS: It is not used for male breast cancer or in premenopausal women.
■ ADVERSE EFFECTS: Among the more serious adverse reactions are masculinization, edema, and hypercalcemia.

dronabinol /drōnab'inol/, an oral antiemetic.
■ INDICATIONS: It is prescribed for refractory nausea and vomiting caused by cancer chemotherapy.
■ CONTRAINDICATIONS: Dronabinol should not be given to persons who are hypersensitive to the product or to THC, the active ingredient of the drug.
■ ADVERSE EFFECTS: Dronabinol is a Schedule II controlled substance with a high potential for abuse. It can produce both physical and psychologic dependence. It is not recommended for patients taking a central nervous system depressant or other psychoactive drugs. Among adverse effects reported are drowsiness, dizziness, impaired coordination, and hallucinations.

drop [AS *dropa*], a small spherical mass of liquid. A drop may vary in size with differences in temperature, viscosity, and other factors. For therapeutic purposes, a drop is regarded as having a volume of .06 to 0.1 ml, or 1 to 1.5 minims.

drop arm test, a diagnostic test for a tear in the supraspinatus tendon. It is positive if the patient is unable to slowly and smoothly lower the affected arm from a position of 90 degrees of abduction.

drop attack, a form of transient ischemic attack (TIA) in which a brief interruption of cerebral blood flow results in a person falling to the floor without losing consciousness. The episode may affect the person's sense of balance or leg muscle tone, causing the collapse. A contributing factor may also be a weakness of the leg muscles or a hip or knee joint dysfunction.

droperidol /drəper'ədol/, an antipsychotic, sedative drug of the butyrophenone group, used most commonly with a narcotic analgesic (fentanyl) in neuroleptanesthesia.

drop foot. See **footdrop.**

droplet infection [AS, *dropa;* L, *inficere,* to infect], an infection acquired by the inhalation of pathogenic microorganisms suspended in particles of liquid exhaled, sneezed, or coughed by another infected person or animal. Some diseases spread by droplets are chickenpox, common cold, influenza, measles, and mumps.

dropped-beat pulse. See **intermittent pulse.**

dropped wrist. See **radial paralysis.**

dropper, a glass or plastic tube narrowed at one end so it will dispense a liquid medication one drop at a time.

dropsy. See **hydrops.**

Drosophila /drōsof'ilə/ [Gk, *drosos,* dew, *philein,* to love], a genus of fly, including *Drosophila melanogaster,* the Mediterranean fruit fly, useful in genetic experiments because of the large chromosomes found in its salivary glands and its sensitivity to environmental effects, as exposure to radiation.

drowning [ME, *drounen*], asphyxiation because of submersion in a liquid. See also **near drowning.**

drox, abbreviation for a *noncarboxylate hydroxide anion.*

drug [Fr, *drogue*], **1.** also called **medicine.** any substance taken by mouth, injected into a muscle, the skin, a blood vessel, or a cavity of the body, or applied topically to treat or prevent a disease or condition. **2.** *informal.* a narcotic substance.

drug absorption, the process whereby a drug moves from the muscle, digestive tract, or other site of entry into the body toward the circulatory system and the target organ or tissue.

drug abuse, the use of a drug for a nontherapeutic effect, especially one for which it was not prescribed or intended. Some of the most commonly abused drugs are alcohol, amphetamines, barbiturates, cocaine, methaqualone, and opium alkaloids. Drug abuse may lead to organ damage, addiction, and disturbed patterns of behavior. Some illicit drugs, such as heroin, lysergic acid diethylamide (LSD), and phencylidine hydrochloride (PCP), have no recognized therapeutic effect in humans. Use of these drugs often incurs criminal penalty in addition to the potential for physical, social, and psychologic harm. See also **drug addiction.**

drug action, the means by which a drug exerts a desired effect. Drugs are usually classified by their actions; for example, a vasodilator, prescribed to decrease the blood pressure, acts by dilating the blood vessels.

drug addiction, a condition characterized by an overwhelming desire to continue taking a drug to which one has become habituated through repeated consumption because it produces a particular effect, usually an alteration of mental activity, attitude, or outlook. Addiction is usually accompanied by a compulsion to obtain the drug, a tendency to increase the dose, a psychologic or physical dependence, and detrimental consequences for the individual and society. Common addictive drugs are barbiturates, alcohol, and morphine and other narcotics, especially heroin, which has slightly greater euphorigenic properties than other opium derivatives. See also **alcoholism, drug abuse.**

drug administration, the giving by a nurse or other authorized person of a single dose of a drug to a patient.

drug agonist, one of two similar drugs that may affect the same target organ or tissue, producing the same or a similar effect. If the drugs compete for the same receptor sites,

the two products may act as competitive antagonists, requiring larger than usual doses to achieve a desired effect.

drug allergy, hypersensitivity to a pharmacologic agent, manifested by reactions ranging from a mild rash to anaphylactic shock, depending on the individual, the allergen, and the dose. Allergic responses are frequently produced by contrast media containing iodine, aspirin, phenylbutazone, novobiocin, penicillin, and other antibiotics, but they may be caused by any drug.

drug clearance, the elimination of a drug from the body. It is commonly excreted by the kidneys, liver, lungs, and other routes. The rate of clearance helps determine the size and frequency of a dosage of a particular medication.

drug compliance, the reliability of the patient to use a prescribed medication exactly as ordered by the physician. Noncompliance occurs when a patient forgets or neglects to take the prescribed dosages at the recommended times or decides to discontinue the drug without consulting the physician.

drug dependence, a psychologic craving for or a physiologic reliance on a chemical agent, resulting from habituation, abuse, or addiction. See also **drug abuse, drug addiction.**

drug dispensing, the preparation, packaging, labeling, record keeping, and transfer of a prescription drug to a patient or an intermediary, such as a nurse, who is responsible for administration of the drug.

drug distribution, the pattern of absorption of drug molecules by various tissues after the chemical enters the circulatory system. Because of differences in pH, cell membrane functions, and other individual tissue factors, most drugs are not distributed equally in all parts of the body. For example, the acidity of aspirin influences a distribution pattern that is different from an alkaline product such as amphetamine.

drug-drug interaction, a modification of the effect of a drug when administered with another drug. The effect may be an increase or a decrease in the action of either substance, or it may be an adverse effect that is not normally associated with either drug. The particular interaction may be the result of a chemical-physical incompatibility of the two drugs or a change in the rate of absorption or the quantity absorbed in the body, the binding ability of either drug, or an alteration in the ability of receptor sites and cell membranes to bind either drug.

Drug Enforcement Agency (DEA), an agency of the Drug Enforcement Administration of the federal government, empowered to enforce regulations regarding the import or export of narcotic drugs and certain other substances or the traffic of these substances across state lines.

drug eruption. See **drug rash.**

drug fever, a fever caused by the pharmacologic action of a medication, its thermoregulatory action, a local complication of parenteral administration, or, most commonly, an immunologic reaction mediated by drug-induced antibodies. The onset of fever occurs usually between 7 and 10 days after the medication is begun; a return to normal is seen within 2 days of the discontinuance of the drug. The correct diagnosis of drug fever and the discontinuance of the medication are important to prevent further adverse reactions and to avoid possibly dangerous and expensive diagnostic and therapeutic interventions. See also **Jarisch-Herxheimer reaction.**

drug-food interaction, the effect produced when some

drugs and certain foods or beverages are taken at the same time, as in the example of monoamine oxidase inhibitors that can react dangerously with foods containing the amino acid tyramine.

drug-induced parkinsonism, a reversible syndrome with the clinical features of Parkinson's disease, but caused by the dopamine-blocking actions of antipsychotic drugs. See also **parkinsonism.**

drug metabolism, the transformation of a drug by the body tissues into a metabolite. Examples include aspirin, which is metabolized to salicylic acid, an analgesic, and codeine, which is converted to morphine.

drug monograph, a statement that specifies the kinds and amounts of ingredients a drug or class of drugs may contain, the directions for the drug's use, the conditions in which it may be used, and contraindications for its use.

drug overdose (O.D.) [Fr, *drogue,* drug; AS, *ofer;* Gk, *dosis,* giving], an accidental or purposeful dose of a drug large enough to cause severe adverse reactions. See also **dose-response relationship.**

drug potency, a measure of the effect of one drug as compared with a similar medication of the same dosage. The drug that produces the maximum effect with the smallest dose has the greater potency.

drug psychosis [Fr, *drogue,* drug; Gk, *psyche,* mind, *osis,* condition], a psychotic state induced by excessive dosage of certain therapeutic drugs as well as drugs of abuse. Therapeutic drugs often associated with drug-induced psychosis include belladonna, chloral hydrate, paraldehyde, steroids, and isoniazid.

drug rash, a skin eruption, usually an allergic reaction, that is caused by a particular drug. Nearly any drug can produce a skin reaction as a result of a gradual accumulation of the drug or because of the development of antibodies that reject a component of the medication. When a drug rash occurs as a sensitivity reaction, the skin rash does not occur the first time the drug is taken, but the effect is observed with subsequent uses of the same drug. Also called **dermatitis medicamentosa.** See also **fixed drug eruption.**

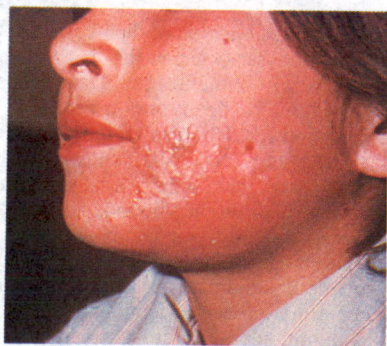

Drug rash (Thompson, 1989)

drug reaction [Fr, *drogue,* drug; L, *re, agere,* to act], any adverse effect of the body to therapeutic drugs, drugs of abuse, or by the interaction of two or more pharmacologically active agents within a short time span. Drugs most likely to cause adverse reactions include hypnotics, central

nervous system stimulants, antidepressants, tranquilizers, and muscle relaxants.

drug receptor, any part of a cell, usually a large protein molecule, with which a drug molecule interacts to trigger its desired response or effect on the cell surface or in the cytoplasm.

drug rehabilitation center, an agency that provides long-term care for a gradual return to the community of a person with a chemical or drug dependency.

drug-seeking behavior (DSB), a pattern of seeking narcotic pain medication or tranquilizers with forged prescriptions, false identification, repeatedly asking for replacement of "lost" drugs or prescriptions, complaining of severe pain without an organic basis, and being abusive or threatening when denied drugs.

drug sequestration, the process by which certain drugs are stored in the body tissues. Examples include tetracycline, which may be stored in bone tissue, and chloroquine, which is stored in the liver. Certain vitamins and other substances are stored in fat deposits.

drug tolerance, a condition of cellular adaptation to a pharmacologically active substance so that increasingly larger doses are required to produce the same physiologic or psychologic effect as obtained earlier with smaller doses.

drug trial, the process of determining an adequate and effective therapeutic dose of a specific drug for a particular patient. The trial culminates with (1) an acceptable clinical result, (2) intolerable adverse effects, (3) a poor response after an appropriate blood level is reached, or (4) administration of the drug for a specific time. The usual time required for trial of an antidepressant is 3 weeks; for an antipsychotic, 3 to 6 weeks.

drusen /drōō′zən/ [Ger, *Druse,* stony granule], small, white hyaline deposits that develop beneath the retinal pigment epithelium, sometimes appearing as nodules within the optic nerve head. They tend to occur most frequently in persons over the age of 60.

dry catarrh [AS, *dryge;* Gk, *kata,* down, *rhoia,* flow], a dry cough, accompanied by almost no expectoration that occurs in severe coughing spells. It is associated with asthma and emphysema in older people.

dry dressing, a plain dressing containing no medication, applied directly to an incision or a wound to prevent contamination or trauma or to absorb secretions. (See Fig. p. 508.)

dry eye syndrome, a dryness of the cornea and conjunctiva caused by a deficiency in tear production. The condition affects mainly women during menopausal years and later. The condition results in a sensation of a foreign body in the eye, burning eyes, keratitis, and erosion of the epithelial layers of the cornea and conjunctiva. See also **Sjögren's syndrome.** (See Fig. p. 508.)

dry gangrene. See **gangrene.**

dry gas (D), (in respiratory therapy) a gas that contains no water vapor.

dry heat sterilization [AS, *dryge + haetu;* L, *sterilis*], a method of sterilization using heated dry air at a temperature of 160° to 180° degrees C for 90 minutes to 3 hours.

dry ice, solid carbon dioxide, with a temperature of about -140° F. It is used in cryotherapy of various skin disorders, such as the removal of warts.

dry labor, *informal.* labor in which amniotic fluid has already escaped. As amniotic fluid is continually produced, no labor is really dry.

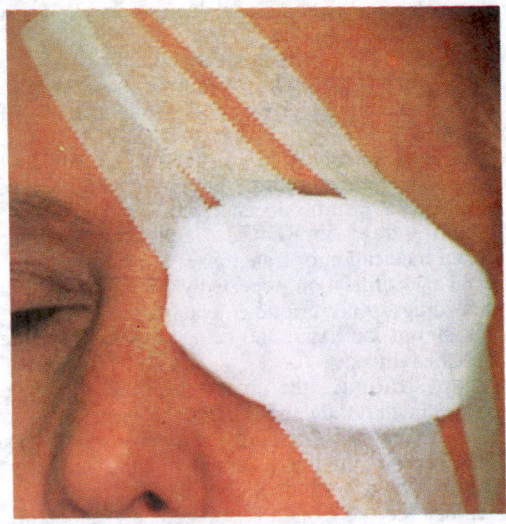

Dry dressing over the eye (Grossman, 1993)

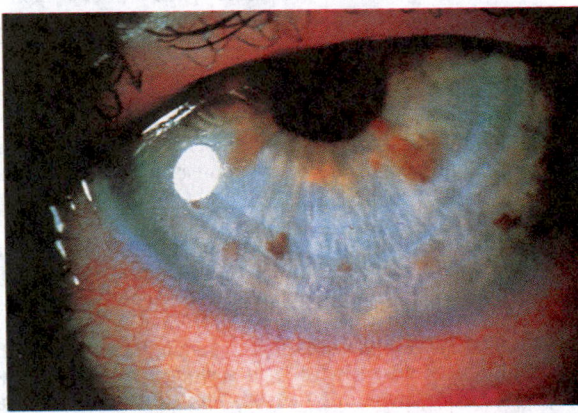

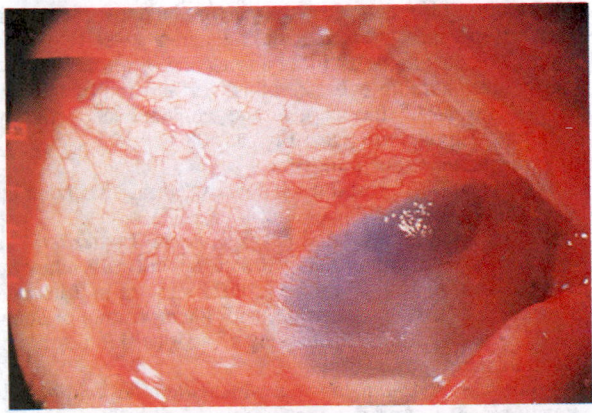

Dry eye syndrome (Schumacher, 1988)

dry pleurisy [AS, *dryge,* dry; Gk, *pleuritis*], an inflammation of the pleura without significant effusion. The cause may be a localized injury. It may also be an early sign of tuberculosis.

dry rale, (obsolete) an abnormal chest sound produced by air passing through a constricted bronchial tube. Compare **amphoric breath sound, atelectatic rale, bubbling rale.**

Drysdale's corpuscle /drīz′dālz/ [Thomas M. Drysdale, American gyndecologist, b. 1831], one of a number of transparent cells in the fluid of some ovarian cysts. Also called **Bennet's small corpuscle.**

dry skin, epidermis lacking moisture or sebum, often characterized by a pattern of fine lines, scaling, and itching. Causes include too frequent bathing, low humidity, decreased production of sebum in aging skin, and ichthyosis. Treatment includes decreased frequency of bathing, increased humidity, bath oils, emollients such as lanolin and glycerine, and hydrophilic ointments. Also called **xerosis** /zērō′sis/.

dry tooth socket, an inflamed condition of a tooth socket (alveolus) after extraction. Actually, the tooth socket is not dry but is filled with degenerating blood serum and infectious material. Normally, a blood clot forms over the alveolar bone at the base of the tooth socket after an extraction. If the clot fails to form properly or becomes dislodged, the bone tissue is exposed to the environment and can become infected, a usually painful condition requiring analgesics, sedatives, and drainage, in addition to treatment to cure the infection.

dry vomiting [AS, *dryge,* L, *vomere,* to vomit], nausea with retching that does not result in vomitus.

DSB, abbreviation for **drug-seeking behavior.**

DSDB, abbreviation for **direct self-destructive behavior.**

DSM, abbreviation for *Diagnostic and Statistical Manual of Mental Disorders.*

D.S.N., abbreviation for *Doctor of Science in Nursing.*

DSR, abbreviation for **dynamic spatial reconstructor.**

DT, abbreviation for **diphtheria and tetanus toxoids.**

dTc, abbreviation for *d-tubocurarine.*

DTIC-Dome, a trademark for an antineoplastic (dacarbazine).

DTP vaccine, a combination of diphtheria and tetanus toxoids and killed pertussis vaccine that is administered intramuscularly for active immunization against those diseases.

DTR, abbreviation for **deep tendon reflex.**

DTs, abbreviation for **delirium tremens.**

dual-energy imaging /dyo͞o′əl/, an x-ray imaging technique in which two radiographs are taken of the same target area using two different kilovoltages. Because the radiographic image of soft tissue and bone varies with the kilovoltage, one image isolating bone contrast and the other isolating soft tissue contrast, the combined x-ray films can help to make a more precise identification of an abnormality, such as a lung nodule calcification.

dual-focus tube, an x-ray tube used for diagnostic imaging. It has one large and one small focal spot. The large focal spot is used when techniques that produce high heat are required, and the small focal spot is used to produce fine, detailed images.

duality of central nervous system control /dyo͞o·al′itē/, a theory that the normal central nervous system is regulated by a check-and-balance feedback program. The theory is based on studies of posture-movement, mobility-stability, flexion-extension synergies, and similar action-reaction examples related to laws of basic physics. Duality theorists suggest that Central nervous system disorders result from imbalances in the feedback system.

dual personality. See **double personality.**

DUB,   **1.** abbreviation for **dysfunctional uterine bleeding. 2.** a genetically determined human blood factor that is associated with immunity to certain diseases.

Dubin-Johnson syndrome /dōō'binjon'sən/ [Isadore N. Dubin, American pathologist, b. 1913; Frank B. Johnson, American pathologist, b. 1919], a rare, chronic, hereditary hyperbilirubinemia, characterized by nonhemolytic jaundice, abnormal liver pigmentation, and abnormal function of the gallbladder. It is caused by an inability of the liver to excrete several organic anions. See also **hyperbilirubinemia of the newborn, Rotor syndrome.**

DuBois formula /dōōboiz'/, a logarithmic method of calculating the number of square meters of body surface area (BSA) of an individual from the height in centimeters, the weight in kilograms, and a constant, 0.007184.

Dubowitz assessment, a system of estimating the gestational age of a newborn child according to such factors as posture, ankle dorsiflexion, and arm and leg recoil.

Duchenne-Erb paralysis. See **Erb's palsy.**

Duchenne's disease /dōōshenz'/ [Guillaume B. A. Duchenne, French neurologist, b. 1806], a series of three different neurologic conditions: **spinal muscular atrophy, bulbar paralysis,** and **tabes dorsalis.** See also **muscular dystrophy.**

Duchenne-Aran disease /dōōshen'äräN'/, muscular atrophy caused by degeneration of the anterior horn cells of the spinal cord and affecting primarily the upper extremities. There is chronic muscle wasting and weakness that first appears in the hands and advances progressively to the arms and shoulders, eventually affecting the legs and other body areas. Several conditions may lead to this disease, such as the injection of toxins.

Duchenne's muscular dystrophy [Guillaume B. A. Duchenne], an abnormal congenital condition characterized by progressive symmetric wasting of the leg and pelvic muscles. This disease affects predominantly males and accounts for 50% of all muscular dystrophy diseases. It is an X-linked recessive disease that appears insidiously between 3 and 5 years of age and spreads from the leg and pelvic muscles to the involuntary muscles. Associated muscle weakness produces a waddling gait and pronounced lordosis. Muscles rapidly deteriorate, and calf muscles become firm and enlarged from fatty deposits. Affected children develop contractures, have difficulty climbing stairs, often stumble and fall, and display wing scapulae when they raise their arms. Such persons are usually confined to wheelchairs by 12 years of age, and progressive weakening of cardiac muscle causes tachycardia and pulmonary problems. The patients affected may also have cardiac murmurs, faint heart sounds, and chest pain and may suffer arrhythmias or infections that produce overt heart failure. Such complications, especially in the later stages of this disease, can cause sudden death. Duchenne's muscular dystrophy usually results in death within 10 to 15 years of the onset of symptoms. There is no successful treatment of the disease. Orthopedic appliances, exercise, physical therapy, and surgery to correct contractures can help preserve mobility. It cannot be detected by amniocentesis, but this procedure can determine the sex of the fetus and is often recommended for carriers who are pregnant. Nursing care involves the psychologic support of the patient and the family and the encouragement of the patient to avoid long periods of bed rest and inactivity to assure maximum physical activity. Splints, braces, grab bars, and overhead slings help the patient exercise. A wheelchair helps preserve mobility. Other devices that can increase comfort and help prevent footdrop include footboards, high-topped sneakers, and foot cradles. Also called **pseudohypertrophic muscular dystrophy.** (See Fig. below and on p. 510.)

Duchenne's paralysis [Guillaume B. A. Duchenne, French neurologist, b. 1806; Gk, *paralyein,* to be palsied], a form of motor neuron disease characterized by wasting and weakness in the laryngeal, pharyngeal, tongue, and facial muscles, leading to dysarthria and dysphagia. There may also be pyramidal tract involvement. Also called **Duchenne's syndrome, progressive bulbar paralysis.**

duck embryo vaccine. See **rabies vaccine.**

duck walk. See **metatarsus valgus.**

duct [L, *ducere,* to lead], a narrow tubular structure, especially one through which material is secreted or excreted.

duct carcinoma, a neoplasm developed of the epithelium of ducts, especially in the breast or pancreas.

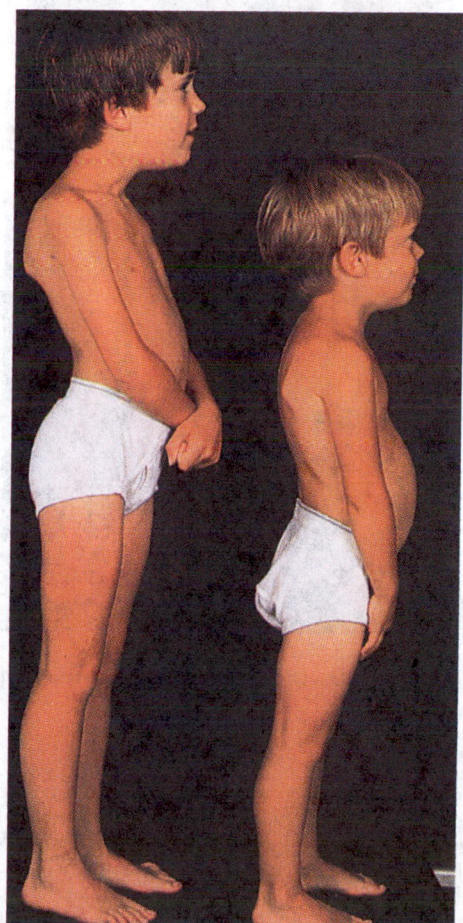

Duchenne muscular dystrophy—postural adjustments
(Zitelli, 1992)

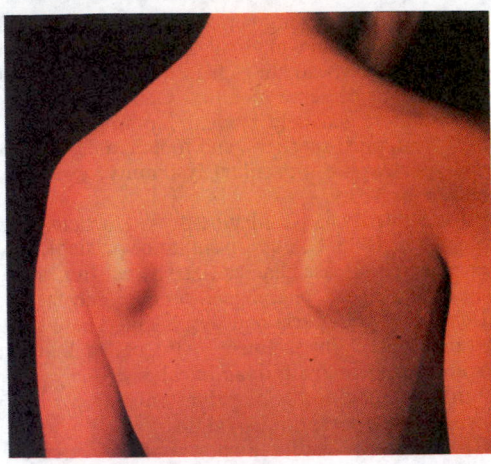

Duchenne muscular dystrophy—winged scapulae
(Zitelli, 1992)

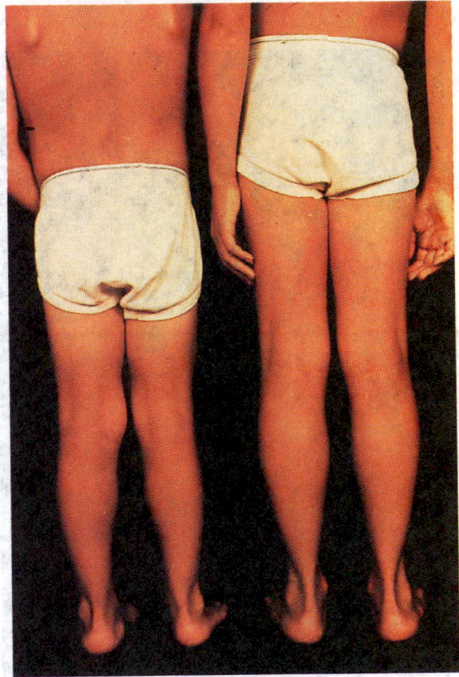

Duchenne muscular dystrophy—enlargement of calves
(Zitelli, 1992)

duct ectasia, an abnormal dilation of a duct by lipids and cellular debris. In a mammary duct the condition, which tends to affect mainly postmenopausal women, may be accompanied by inflammation and infiltration by plasma cells.

ductility /duktil′itē/, the property of a material that has a large elastic range and tends to deform before failing from stress.

duction /duk′shən/, the movement of an individual eyeball from the primary to secondary or tertiary positions of gaze.

ductless gland /dukt′les/, a gland lacking an excretory duct, such as an endocrine gland, which secretes hormones directly into blood or lymph.

duct of Rivinus /rivē′nəs/ [L, *ducere,* to lead; Augustus Q. Rivinus. German anatomist, b. 1652], one of the minor sublingual ducts. Compare **Bartholin's duct.**

duct of Wirsung. See **pancreatic duct.**

ductus /duk′təs/, *pl.* **ductus** /duk′tōōs/, the Latin term for duct.

ductus arteriosus, a vascular channel in the fetus that joins the pulmonary artery directly to the descending aorta.

ductus deferens. See **vas deferens.**

ductus epididymidis, a tube into which the efferent ductules of the testes empty.

ductus venosus, the vascular channel in the fetus passing through the liver and joining the umbilical vein with the inferior vena cava. Before birth, it carries highly oxygenated blood from the placenta to the fetal circulation. It closes shortly after birth as pulmonary circulation is established and as the vessels in the umbilical cord collapse and become occluded. See also **ductus arteriosus, foramen ovale.**

Duke diet. See **rice diet.**

Duke longitudinal study, a long-range in-depth research into the normal aging process of middle-aged and older men and women conducted at Duke University Medical Center. The Duke studies led to development of the "longevity quotient" (LQ) used to evaluate an individual's rate of aging. It is calculated by the number of years a person survives beyond a given point in time divided by the expected number of years derived from actuarial tables.

Dukes' classification, a system of identifying stages of colorectal tumors, from A to D, according to the degree of tissue invasion and metastasis. A Dukes' A tumor is one that is confined to the mucosa and submucosa. A B tumor is one that has invaded the musculature but has not involved the lymphatic system. C tumors have invaded the musculature with metastatic involvement of the regional lymph nodes. D tumors are those that have metastasized to distant organ tissues.

Dulcolax, a trademark for a laxative (bisacodyl).

dull pain [ME, *dul,* not sharp; L, *poena,* penalty], a mildly throbbing acute or chronic pain.

dumb terminal [AS, *tumb,* mute; L, *terminalis,* end], a computer terminal that serves as an input or output device only and is incapable of performing any data-processing functions by itself. Compare **intelligent terminal.**

dumdum fever. See **kala-azar.**

dump [ME, *dumpen,* to throw down], **1.** to preserve the contents of one computer memory by transferring it into another memory. **2.** to print out the contents of a computer memory or other computer-storage medium. **3.** the printout resulting from such an operation.

dumping syndrome [ME, *dumpen,* to throw down], the combination of profuse sweating, nausea, dizziness, and weakness experienced by patients who have had a subtotal gastrectomy. Symptoms are felt soon after eating, when the contents of the stomach empty too rapidly into the duodenum. A high-protein, high-calorie diet, with small meals taken frequently, should prevent discomfort and ensure adequate nutrition. See also **gastrectomy.**

Duncan's mechanism [James M. Duncan, English obstetrician, b. 1826; Gk, *mechane,* machine], a technique for delivery of the placenta with the maternal rather than the fetal surface presenting.

Dunlop skeletal traction, an orthopedic mechanism that helps immobilize the upper limb in the treatment of the contracture or the supracondylar fracture of the elbow. The mechanism employs a system of traction weights, pulleys, and ropes. The system is attached to the bone involved with a pin or wire; it may be further secured by adhesive or nonadhesive skin-traction components. Dunlop skeletal traction is usually applied unilaterally but may also be applied bilaterally. Compare **Dunlop skin traction.**

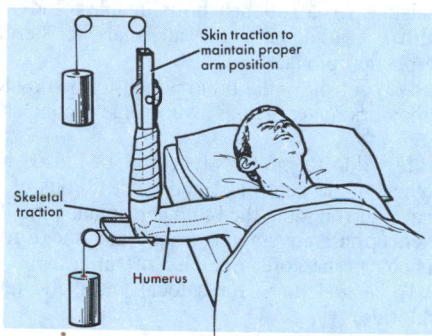

Dunlop skeletal traction

Dunlop skin traction, an orthopedic mechanism that helps immobilize the upper limb in the treatment of contracture and supracondylar fracture of the elbow. The mechanism employs a system of traction weights, pulleys, and ropes, usually applied unilaterally but sometimes bilaterally. Dunlop skin traction may be applied as adhesive skin traction or nonadhesive skin traction. Compare **Dunlop skeletal traction.**

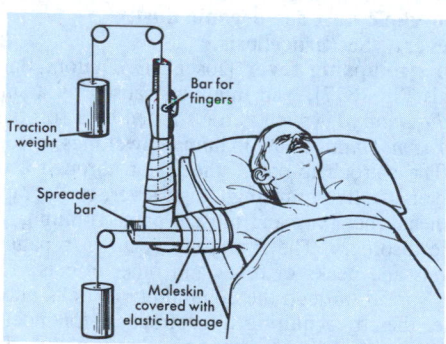

Dunlop skin traction

duodena. See **duodenum.**

duodenal /dōō′ədē′nəl/ [L, *duodeni*, 12 fingers long], of or pertaining to the duodenum.

duodenal bulb, the first part of the superior portion of the duodenum, which has a bulblike appearance on x-ray views of the small intestine.

duodenal digestion [L, *duodeni*, 12 fingers long, *digere*, to separate], digestion that occurs in the first intestinal segment beyond the pylorus, where secretions of the liver and pancreas are received and mixed with the partially digested food from the stomach. Chyle is formed, fats are emulsified, starch is hydrolyzed, and proteolytic enzymes begin to break down proteins.

duodenal mesentery. See **mesoduodenum.**

duodenal ulcer, an ulcer in the duodenum, the most common type of peptic ulcer. See also **peptic ulcer.**

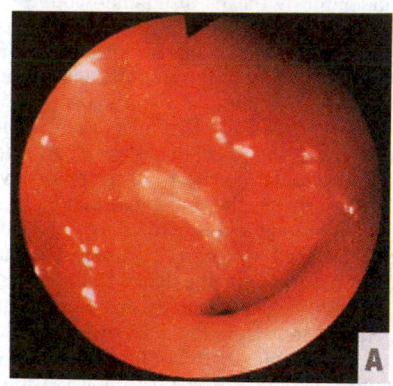

Duodenal ulcer—endoscopic appearance
(Winawer, 1992)

duodenectomy /dōō′ədēnek′təmē/ [L, *duodeni*, 12 fingers long, Gk, *ektome*, cutting out], the total or partial excision of the duodenum.

duodenitis /dōō′ədēnī′tis/ [L, *duodeni*, 12 fingers long, Gk, *itis*, inflammation], a condition of inflammation of the duodenum.

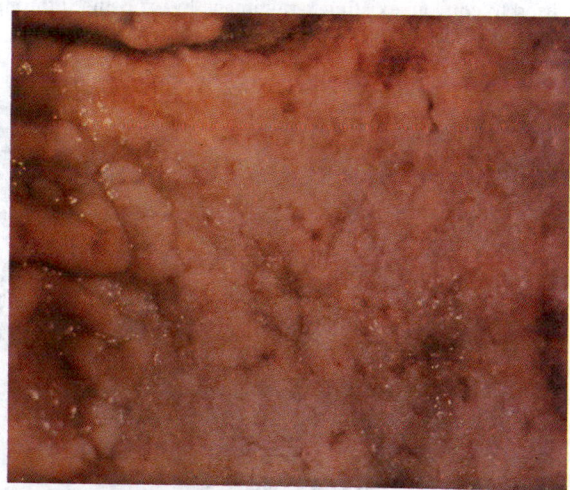

Duodenitis (Mitros, 1988)

duodeno-, a combining form meaning 'pertaining to the duodenum': *duodenocolic, duodenohepatic, duodenostomy.*

duodenography /dōō′ədənog′rəfē/ [L, *duodeni*, 12 fingers long, Gk, *graphein*, to record], the process of making an x-ray image of the duodenum and pancreas. It usually requires drug-induced paralysis of the duodenum to prevent peristaltic activity, use of a double-contrast medium, and maximum distention with the contrast medium so that the organ presses against and outlines the head of the pancreas.

duodenojejunal flexure. See **angle of Treitz.**

duodenoscope /dōō′ədē′nəskōp′/, an endoscopic instrument, usually fiberoptic, for the visual examination of the duodenum.

duodenoscopy /dōō′ədənos′kəpē/, the visual examination of the duodenum by means of an endoscope.

duodenostomy /dōō′ədenos′təmē/ [L, *duodeni*, 12 fingers each; Gk, *stoma*, mouth], the surgical creation of a direct opening to the duodenum through the abdominal wall.

duodenum /dōō′ədē′nəm, dōō·od′inəm/, *pl.* **duodena, duodenums** [L, *duodeni*, 12 fingers each], the shortest, widest, and most fixed portion of the small intestine, taking an almost circular course from the pyloric valve of the stomach so that its termination is close to its starting point. It is about 25 cm long and is divided into superior, descending, horizontal, and ascending portions. The superior portion is about 6 cm long and extends from the pylorus to the neck of the gallbladder. The descending portion is about 8 cm long and extends from the neck of the gallbladder at the level of the first lumbar vertebra to the cranial border of the fourth lumbar vertebra. The horizontal portion is about 7 cm long and passes from right to left, from the level of the fourth lumbar vertebra to the diaphragm. The ascending portion is about 4 cm long and rises on the left side of the aorta to the level of the second lumbar vertebra, turning ventrally to become the jejunum at the duodenojejunal flexure. Compare **jejunum, ileum.**

dup, (in cytogenetics) abbreviation for *duplication.*

duplex inheritance. See **amphigenous inheritance.**

duplex transmission [L, *duplex*, twofold], the passage of a neural impuse in both directions along a nerve fiber.

duplicating film /dōō′plikā′ting/, a single-emulsion film used to copy an existing x-ray image by exposing it through ultraviolet light.

duplicatus anterior. See **anadidymus.**

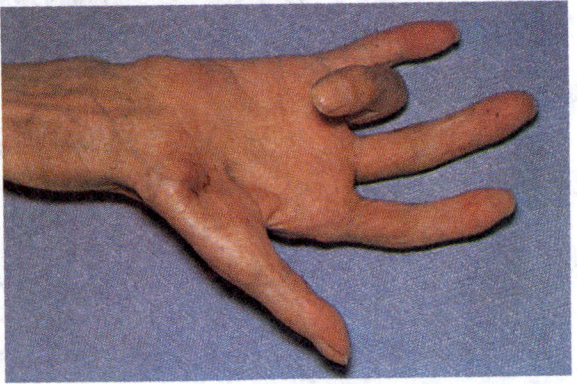

Dupuytren's contracture *(Kamal, 1991)*

Dupuytren's contracture /dYpY·itraNs′, dēpē·itranz′/ [Baron Guillaume Dupuytren, French surgeon, b. 1777; L *contractura* drawing together], a progressive, painless thickening and tightening of subcutaneous tissue of the palm, causing the fourth and fifth fingers to bend into the palm and resist extension. Tendons and nerves are not in-

volved. Although the condition begins in one hand, both will become symmetrically affected. Of unknown cause, it is most frequent in middle-aged males. Early surgical removal of the excess fibrous tissue under general anesthesia will restore full use of the hand. An incision is made into the palm, and the thickened tissue is excised carefully to avoid injury to adjacent ligaments.

Dupuytren's fracture. See **Galeazzi's fracture.**

dura /dōō′rə, dyōō′rə/ [L, *duras*, hard], a thick, tough membrane that surrounds the brain and spinal cord.

durable power of attorney for health /dyōōr′əbəl/, a document that designates an agent or proxy to make health-care decisions for a patient who is unable to do so.

Durabolin, a trademark for an anabolic steroid (nandrolone phenpropionate).

dural sac /dyōō′rəl/, the blind pouch formed by the lower end of the dura mater, at the level of the second sacral segment.

dura mater /dōō′rə mā′tər, dyōō′rə/ [L, *durus*, hard; *mater*, mother], the outermost and most fibrous of the three membranes surrounding the brain and spinal cord. The **dura mater encephali** covers the brain, and the **dura mater spinalis** covers the cord. See also **meninges.**

Duranest, a trademark for a local anesthetic (etidocaine hydrochloride).

duration tetany. See **tetany.**

duress /dyōōres′/ [L, *durus*, hard], (in law) an action compelling another person to do what otherwise would not be done voluntarily. A consent form signed under duress is not valid.

Duroziez's murmur /dY′rōzyās, dir′-, dōō′r-/, [Paul Louis Duroziez, French physician, b. 1826; L, *murmur*], a systolic murmur heard over the femoral or another large artery when the artery is compressed. The phenomenon is associated with high arterial pulse pressure or aortic insufficiency. A diastolic murmur may also be heard by increasing pressure on the artery distal to the stethoscope.

dust [AS], any fine, particulate, dry matter. Kinds of dust are **inorganic dust** and **organic dust.**

dust fever. See **brucellosis.**

Dutton's relapsing fever [Joseph E. Dutton, English pathologist, b. 1877], an infection caused by a spirochete, *Borrelia duttonii,* which is transmitted by a soft tick, *Ornithodoros moubata,* found in human dwellings in tropical Africa. The spirochete enters the lesion through a tick bite, characteristically producing a high fever, chills, rapid heartbeat, headache, joint and muscle pain, vomiting, and neurologic disorders. The symptoms recur in a pattern of remissions and peaks of fever and other effects. The infection is spread through the community as ticks bite infected people, thereby acquiring the spirochete for inoculation in others. Treatment with tetracycline is usually effective in curing the infection. Also called **African relapsing fever, Dutton's disease.** See also **relapsing fever.**

duty [ME, *duete*, conduct], (in law) an obligation owed by one party to another. Duty may be established by statute or other legal process, as by contract or oath supported by statute, or it may be voluntarily undertaken. Every person has a duty of care to all other people to avoid causing harm or injury by negligence.

Duverney's fracture /dōō′vərnāz′/ [Joseph G. Duverney, French anatomist, b. 1648], fracture of the ilium just below the anterior superior spine.

Duvoid, a trademark for **bethanechol chloride,** a cholinergic agonist.

dv/dt, (in cardiology) the rate of change of voltage with respect to time.

D.V.M., abbreviation for *Doctor of Veterinary Medicine*.

dwarf /dwôrf/ [AS, *dweorge*], **1.** also called **nanus.** an abnormally short, undersized person, especially one whose bodily parts are not proportional. Kinds of dwarfs include **achondroplastic dwarf, asexual dwarf, ateliotic dwarf, bird-headed dwarf, Brissaud's dwarf, cretin dwarf, diastrophic dwarf, phocomelic dwarf, pituitary dwarf, primordial dwarf, rachitic dwarf, renal dwarf, Russell dwarf, sexual dwarf, Silver dwarf,** and **thanatophoric dwarf. 2.** to prevent or retard, for example, normal growth.

dwarfism /dwôrf′izəm/, the abnormal underdevelopment of the body, characterized predominantly by extreme shortness of stature, although the condition is associated with numerous other defects and may involve varying degrees of mental retardation. Dwarfism has multiple causes, including genetic defects, endocrine dysfunction involving either the pituitary or thyroid glands, chronic diseases, such as rickets, renal failure, and intestinal malabsorption defects, and psychosocial stress, as in the maternal deprivation syndrome. See also **dwarf.**

dwarf tapeworm infection, a type of intestinal parasitic disease caused by an infestation of *Hymenolepsia nana*. It occurs mainly in the southern United States and usually affects children who ingest eggs by placing contaminated materials in the mouth. The disease may be asymptomatic or it may result in abdominal complaints and diarrhea. An infection may be treated with niclosamide or paromomycin.

Dwayne-Hunt law /dwān′hunt′/, (in radiology) the principle that x-ray energy is inversely proportional to the photon wavelength. As the photon wavelength increases, photon energy decreases, and vice versa. The minimum x-ray wavelength is associated with the maximum x-ray energy.

dwindles, *informal.* a condition of physical deterioration involving several systems of the body, usually in an elderly person.

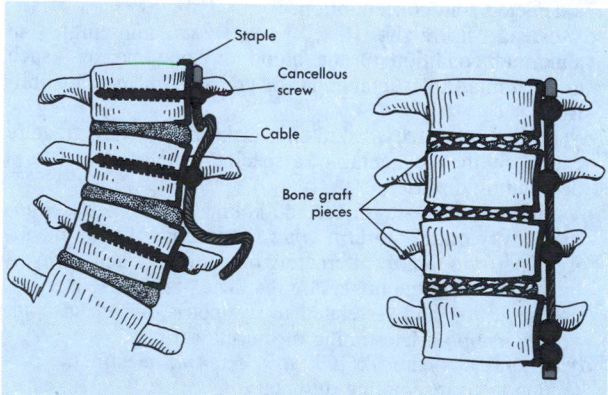

Dwyer instrumentation *(Phipps, 1991)*

Dwyer instrumentation /dwī′ər/, one method for correcting the spinal curvature associated with scoliosis. The Dwyer cable method uses a mechanical device that assists in obtaining the curvature correction. The device is inserted to assist in maintaining the corrected curvature while the fusion heals; it is not usually removed unless there is postoperative indication of displacement or a pattern of associated symptoms. Dwyer cable instrumentation involves surgical intervention through the pulmonary cavity and the rib cage and is accompanied by a relatively greater surgical risk than a posterior approach. It is often inadequate to correct the spinal curvature involved and must frequently be followed several weeks later by a posterior spinal fusion.

Dy, symbol for the element **dysprosium.**

dyad /dī′ad/ [Gk, *dyas*, two], (in genetics) one of the paired homologous chromosomes, consisting of two chromatids, which result from the division of a tetrad in the first meiotic division of gametogenesis. –**dyadic,** *adj.*

dyadic interpersonal communication /dī·ad′ik/, a process in which two people interact face to face as senders and receivers, as in a conversation.

Dyazide, a trademark for a fixed-combination drug containing two diuretic agents (triamterene and hydrochlorothiazide).

Dyclone, a trademark for a local anesthetic (dyclonine hydrochloride).

dyclonine hydrochloride /dī′klənīn/, a local anesthetic, with bactericidal and fungicidal properties, for oral pain, pruritis, insect bites, and minor skin burns and injuries.

dydrogesterone /dī′drəjes′tərōn/, a synthetic oral progestin.

■ INDICATIONS: It may be prescribed in the treatment of abnormal uterine bleeding, menopausal vasomotor symptoms, pickwickian syndrome, and endometrial cancer, and for contraception.

■ CONTRAINDICATIONS: Thrombophlebitis, breast cancer, missed abortion, known or suspected pregnancy, or known hypersensitivity to this drug prohibits its use.

■ ADVERSE EFFECTS: Among the more serious adverse reactions are thrombophlebitis, uterine fibroma, and embolism. Breakthrough bleeding may occur.

dye /dī/ [AS, *deag*], **1.** to apply coloring matter to a substance. **2.** a chemical compound capable of imparting color to a substance to which it is applied. Various dyes are used in medicine as stains for tissues, as test reagents, as therapeutic agents, and to color pharmaceutic preparations.

Dymelor, a trademark for an antidiabetic (acetohexamide).

-dynamia, -dynamy, a suffix meaning '(condition of) strength': *ataxiadynamia, hyperdynamia, plastodynamia.*

dynamic /dīnam′ik/ [Gk, *dynamis*, force], **1.** tending to change or to encourage change, such as a dynamic nurse-patient relationship. **2.** (in respiratory therapy) a condition of changing volume. Compare **static.**

dynamic cardiac work, the energy transfer that occurs during the process of ventricular ejection of blood.

dynamic compliance, the distensibility of the lung, as measured by plethysmography during the breathing cycle. See also **lung compliance.**

dynamic equilibrium, the ability of a patient to adjust to displacements of the body's center of gravity by changing the body's base of support.

dynamic ileus, an intestinal obstruction with associated recurrent and continuous muscle spasma. Also called **spastic ileus.**

dynamic imaging, (in ultrasonography) the imaging of an object in motion at a frame rate that does not cause significant blurring of any one image and at a repetition rate sufficient to adequately represent the movement pattern. Also called **real-time imaging.**

dynamic nurse-patient relationship, a conceptual framework in which the interpersonal aspects of the nurse-patient relationship are analyzed. The relationship is affected by many factors. Elements in the process include the behavior of the patient, the reaction of the nurse, and the actions of the nurse that are intended to aid the patient. Also examined are the means for validating nurses' perceptions and interpretations and for evaluating the effects of the nursing actions taken.

dynamic psychiatry, the study of motivational, emotional, and biologic factors as determinants of human behavior.

dynamic range, 1. (in radiology) the range of voltage or input signals that result in a digital output. 2. (in audiology) the range of decibels from the faintest sound a person can hear to the level of sound that causes pain.

dynamic response, the accuracy with which a physiologic monitoring system, such as an electrocardiograph, will simulate the actual event being recorded.

dynamic spatial reconstructor (DSR), a kind of radiographic machine used in research permitting moving three-dimensional images of human organs to be examined visually and from any direction.

dynamic splint [Gk, *dynamis*, force; D, *splinte*], any splint that incorporates springs, elastic bands, or other materials that produce a constant active force to counteract deforming forces of a splint.

dynamo-, a combining form meaning 'pertaining to power or strength': *dynamogenesis, dynamometer, dynamophore.*

dynamometer /dī'nəmom'ətər/ [Gk, *dynamis*, force, *metron*, measure], a device for measuring the degree of force expended in the contraction of a group of muscles, such as a squeeze dynamometer, which measures the gross grip strength of the hand muscles. Also called **ergometer.**

-dynamy. See **-dynamia.**

Dynapen, a trademark for an antibacterial (dicloxacillin sodium).

dyne /dīn/, a unit of force, specifically the force required to accelerate a free mass of 1 g at 1 cm per second. One dyne equals 10-5 newton.

-dynia, a suffix meaning 'pain': *cephalodynia, gastrodynia.*

dynode /dī'nōd/, one of a series of platelike elements that amplify electron pulses in a photomultiplier tube. For each electron that strikes each dynode, several secondary electrons are emitted. The dynode gain is the ratio of secondary electrons to incident electrons.

dyphylline /dī'fil'in/, a bronchodilator.

■ INDICATIONS: It is prescribed in the treatment of bronchospasm in acute bronchial asthma, bronchitis, and emphysema.

■ CONTRAINDICATIONS: It is used with caution in patients with peptic ulcer or cardiovascular disease. Known hypersensitivity to this or to other xanthines prohibits its use.

■ ADVERSE EFFECTS: Among the more serious adverse reactions are GI distress, dizziness, tachycardia, headache, and palpitations.

Dyrenium, a trademark for a diuretic (triamterene).

dys-, a prefix meaning 'bad, painful, disordered': *dysadrenia, dysbolism, dysmnesia.*

dysacousia. See **dysacusis.**

dysacousma. See **dysacusis.**

dysacusis /dis'əkōō'sis/ [Gk, *dys*, difficult, *akouein*, to hear], a condition in which loud sounds or noises can cause pain or discomfort. It is usually the result of damage to the cochlea. Also called **dysacousia, dysacousma.**

dysadrenia /dis'adrē'nē·ə/ [Gk, *dys*, bad; L, *ad*, to, *ren*, kidney], abnormal adrenal function characterized by decreased production of hormones, as in hypoadrenalism or hypoadrenocorticism, or by increased secretion of the products of the gland, as in hyperadrenalism or hyperadrenocorticism. Also called **dysadrenalism.**

dysarthria /disär'thrē·ə/ [Gk, *dys* + *arthroun*, to articulate], difficult, poorly articulated speech, resulting from interference in the control over the muscles of speech, usually because of damage to a central or peripheral motor nerve.

dysarthrosis /dis'ärthrō'sis/ [Gk, *dys*, difficult, *arthron*, joint], any disorder of a joint, including disease, dislocation, or deformity, that makes movement of the joint difficult.

dysautonomia /disô'tənō'mē·ə/ [Gk, *dys* + *autonomia*, self-government], a dysfunction of the autonomic nervous system that can be a clinical feature of diabetes, parkinsonism, Adie's syndrome, Shy-Drager syndrome, or Riley-Day syndrome. A fairly common effect is orthostatic hypotension with syncope and drop attacks. The condition may also be characterized by poor muscular coordination, impotence, incontinence, drooling, perspiration and tearing abnormalities, and emotional lability.

dysbarism /dis'bäriz'əm/, a reaction to a sudden change in ambient pressure, such as rapid exposure to the lower atmospheric pressures of high altitudes. It is marked by symptoms similar to those of decompression sickness.

dysbetalipoproteinemia /disbet'əlip'əprō'tinē'mē·ə/ an accumulation of abnormal beta-lipoprotein in the blood. See **broad beta disease.**

dyscholia /diskō'lē·ə/ [Gk, *dys* + *chole*, bile], any abnormal condition of the bile, either regarding the quantity secreted or the condition of the constituents.

dyschondroplasia. See **enchondromatosis.**

dyschroic film fault /diskrō'ik/, a defect in a radiograph that appears as a pinkish coloration when the film is viewed by transmitted light and as a green coloration when the film is viewed by reflected light. It is usually caused by incomplete fixation of the film or an overused fixing solution with a depleted acid concentration.

dyscrasia /diskrā'zhə/ [Gk, *dys* + *krasis*, mingling], an abnormal condition of the blood or bone marrow, such as leukemia, aplastic anemia, or prenatal Rh incompatibility.

dyscrasic fracture /diskrā'sik, diskraz'ik/, any fracture caused by the weakening of a specific bone as a result of a debilitating disease.

dysdiadochokinesia /dis'dī·ədō'kōkinē'zhə/ [Gk, *dys* + *diadochos*, working in turn, *kinesis*, movement], an inability to perform rapidly alternating movements, such as rhythmically tapping the fingers on the knee. The cause is a cerebellar lesion and is related to dysmetria, which also involves inappropriate timing of muscle activity.

dysenteric /dis'enter'ik/ [Gk, *dys*, *enteron*, intestine], pertaining to or resembling dysentery.

dysentery /dis'inter'ē/ [Gk, *dys* + *entron*, intestine], an inflammation of the intestine, especially of the colon, that may be caused by chemical irritants, bacteria, protozoa, or parasites. It is characterized by frequent and bloody stools, abdominal pain, and tenesmus. Dysentery is common in underdeveloped areas of the world and in times of disaster and social disorganization when sanitary living conditions, clean food, and safe water are not available. See also **amebic dysentery, shigellosis.**

dysergia /disur′jē·ə/ [Gk, *dys, ergon*, work], a condition in which the muscles, because of an efferent nerve irregularity, fail to function normally in certain voluntary movements.

dysesthesia /dis′esthē′zhə/, a common effect of spinal cord injury characterized by sensations of numbness, tingling, burning, or pain felt below the level of the lesion.

dysfunctional /disfungk′shənəl/ [Gk, *dys* + L, *functio*, performance], (of a body organ or system) unable to function normally. −**dysfunction,** *n.*

dysfunctional communication, a communication that results from inaccurate perceptions, faulty internal filters (personal interpretations of information), and social isolation. Communication behaviors of emotionally ill persons may have characteristics that prohibit their establishing and maintaining relationships with others.

dysfunctional stereotype, a stereotype in which the dysfunctional aspects of a culture are emphasized.

dysfunctional uterine bleeding (DUB), abnormal uterine bleeding that is not caused by a tumor, inflammation, or pregnancy. It may be characterized by painless, irregular, heavy bleeding or intermenstrual spotting or periods of amenorrhea. The condition is associated with anovulation and unopposed estrogen stimulation. The plan of treatment depends on the age of the patient and may include dilatation and curettage and the use of hormones and other medications.

dysgammaglobulinemia /disgam′əglob′yəlinē′mē·ə/, an inherited immune deficiency disease characterized by blood disorders and a tendency to experience repeated infections. The cause is a deficiency of immunoglobulins needed to produce antibodies.

dysgenesis /disjen′əsis/ [Gk, *dys* + *genein,* to produce], **1.** also called **dysgenesia.** defective or abnormal formation of an organ or part, primarily during embryonic development. **2.** impairment or loss of the ability to procreate. A kind of dysgenesis is **gonadal dysgenesis.** Compare **agenesis.** −**dysgenic,** *adj.*

dysgenics /disjen′iks/, the study of those factors or situations that are genetically detrimental to the future of a race or species. Compare **eugenics.**

dysgenitalism /disjen′itəliz′əm/ [Gk, *dys* + L, *genitalis,* belonging to birth], any condition involving the abnormal development of the genital organs.

dysgerminoma /dis′jərminō′mə/, *pl.* **dysgerminomas, dysgerminomata** [Gk, *dys* + L, *germen,* germ; Gk, *oma,* tumor], a rare malignant tumor of the ovary, found in young women, believed to arise from the undifferentiated germ cells of the embryonic gonad. The tumor is histologically identical to seminoma. Dysgerminomas are extremely sensitive to radiation and chemotherapy, and most patients retain their fertility. Also called **embryoma of the ovary, ovarian seminoma.**

dysgeusia /disgoo′zhə/ [Gk, *dys, geusis,* taste], an abnormal or impaired sense of taste.

dysgnathic anomaly /disnath′ik/ [Gk, dys + *gnathos,* jaw], (in dentistry) an abnormality that extends beyond the teeth, affecting the maxilla, the mandible, or both.

dysgraphia /disgraf′ē·ə/ [Gk, *dys* + *graphein,* to write], an impairment of the ability to write, caused by a pathologic disorder. Compare **agraphia.**

dyshidrosis /dis′hidrō′sis, dis′hī-/ [Gk, *dys* + *hidrosis,* sweating], a condition in which abnormal sweating occurs. Kinds of dyshidrosis are **hyperhidrosis** and **miliaria.**

Also called **pompholyx.** Compare **anhidrosis.** −**dyshidrotic,** *adj.*

dyskeratosis /dis′kerətō′sis/ [Gk, *dys* + *keras,* horn, *osis,* condition], an abnormal or premature keratinization of epithelial cells.

dyskinesia /dis′kinē′zhə/ [Gk, *dys* + *kinesis,* movement], an impairment of the ability to execute voluntary movements. Tardive dyskinesia is one type caused by an adverse effect of prolonged use of phenothiazine medications in elderly patients or those with brain injuries. See also **tardive dyskinesia.** −**dyskinetic** /-et′ik/, *adj.*

dyskinetic syndrome /dis′kinet′ik/, a form of cerebral palsy involving a basal ganglia disorder. Clinical features include athetoid movements of the extremities and sometimes the trunk. There may also be choreiform movements. The movements tend to increase with emotional tension and diminish during sleep.

dyslexia /dislek′sē·ə/ [Gk, *dys* + *lexis,* word], an impairment of the ability to read, as a result of a variety of pathologic conditions, some of which are associated with the central nervous system. Dyslexic persons often reverse letters and words, cannot adequately distinguish the letter sequences in written words, and have difficulty determining left from right. Compare **alexia.** −**dyslexic,** *adj.*

dysmaturity /dis′machoor′itē/ [Gk, *dys* + L, *maturare,* to make ripe], **1.** the failure of an organism to develop, ripen, or otherwise achieve maturity in structure or function. **2.** the condition of a fetus or newborn being abnormally small or large for its age of gestation. Kinds of dysmaturity are **small for gestational age** and **large for gestational age.** Compare **postmature, premature.** −**dysmature,** *adj.*

dysmegalopsia /dis′megalop′sē·ə/ [Gk, *dys, megas,* large, *opsis,* appearance], an inability to judge accurately the size or measure of an object. Also called **dysmetropsia.**

dysmelia /dismē′lyə/ [Gk, *dys* + *melos,* limb], an abnormal congenital condition characterized by missing or shortened extremities of the body and associated with abnormalities of the spine in some individuals. It is caused by abnormal metabolism during the development of the embryonic limbs. See also **phocomelia.**

dysmenorrhea /dis′menərē′ə/ [Gk, *dys* + *men,* month, *rhein,* to flow], pain associated with menstruation. Primary dysmenorrhea is menstrual pain that results from factors intrinsic to the uterus and the process of menstruation. It is extremely common, occurring at least occasionally in almost all women. If the painful episode is mild and brief, it is considered functional and normal and requires no treatment. In approximately 10% of women, dysmenorrhea is sufficiently severe to cause episodes of partial or total disability. The cause in most cases is poorly understood; various anatomic, neurohormonal, and psychosomatic abnormalities have been suggested. Pain occurs typically in the lower abdomen or back and is crampy, coming in successive waves—apparently in conjunction with intense uterine contractions and slight cervical dilatation. Pain usually begins just before, or at the onset of, menstrual flow and lasts from a few hours to 1 day or more; but it may persist through the entire period in a few women. Pain is frequently associated with nausea, vomiting, and frequent bowel movements with intestinal cramping. Dizziness, fainting, pallor, and obvious distress may also be observed. Treatment with an antiprostaglandin provides relief for many women if begun 1 to 3 days premenstrually and continued through the first day of the menses. Oral contraceptive steroids are also effective for many women and are taken through the full monthly cycle. Potent analgesics or narcotics may be required by a few women. Secondary dysmenorrhea is menstrual pain that occurs secondary to specific pelvic abnormalities, such as endometriosis, adenomyosis, chronic pelvic infection, chronic pelvic congestion, or degenerating fibroid tumors. Typically, the pain begins earlier in the cycle and lasts longer than the pain of primary dysmenorrhea. Painful bowel or bladder function may accompany the condition, depending on the location of the specific lesions. Diagnosis of the chief cause is made by pelvic examination, ultrasonography, laparoscopy, or laparotomy. Treatment, most often surgical, is directed at the specific organic disease involved.

dysmetria /dismē′trē·ə/ [Gk, *dys* + *metron*, measure], an abnormal condition that prevents the affected individual from properly measuring distances associated with muscular acts and from controlling muscular action. It is associated with cerebellar lesions and typically characterized by over- or underestimating the range of motion needed to place the limbs correctly during voluntary movement. A normal person with eyes closed can move the arms from a position of 90 degrees of flexion to a position over the head and then return the arms to the 90-degree position; a person with dysmetria is unable to perform this test accurately. See also **hypermetria, hypometria.**

dysmetropsia. See **dysmegalopsia.**

dysmnesic syndrome /disnē′sik/, a memory disorder characterized by an inability to learn simple new skills although the person can still perform highly complex skills learned before the onset of the condition. The cause is a disease or injury that affects only certain brain tissues associated with memory. The victim often confabulates about events of the recent past for which there is no clear memory. Also called **dysmnesia.**

dysmorphogenesis /dis′môrfōjen′əsis/, the development of ill-shaped or otherwise malformed body structures.

dysmorphophobia /-fō′bē·ə / [Gk, *dys* + *morphe*, form, *phobos*, fear], **1.** a fundamental delusion of body image. **2.** the morbid fear of deformity.

dysostosis /dis′ostō′sis/ [Gk, *dys* + *osteon*, bone, *osis*], an abnormal condition characterized by defective ossification, especially by defects in the normal ossification of fetal cartilages. Kinds of dysostoses include **cleidocranial dysostosis, craniofacial dysostosis, mandibulofacial dysostosis, metaphyseal dysostosis,** and **Nager's acrofacial dysostosis.**

dyspareunia /dis′pəroo͞o′nē·ə/ [Gk, *dys* + *pareunos*, mating], an abnormal pain during sexual intercourse. It may result from abnormal conditions of the genitalia, dysfunctional psychophysiologic reaction to sexual union, forcible coition, or incomplete sexual arousal. Dyspareunia is also associated with hormonal changes of the menopause and lactation that result in drying of the vaginal tissues as well as endometriosis. Painful adhesions around the vagina and ligaments may result, decreasing their flexibility during intercourse. Dryness is commonly relieved by the local application of water-soluble lubricants. See also **vaginismus.**

dyspepsia /dispep′sē·ə/ [Gk, *dys* + *peptein*, to digest], a vague feeling of epigastric discomfort, felt after eating. There is an uncomfortable feeling of fullness, heartburn, bloating, and nausea. Dyspepsia is not a distinct condition, but it may be a sign of underlying intestinal disorder, such

as peptic ulcer, gallbladder disease, or chronic appendicitis. Symptoms usually increase in times of stress. **–dyspeptic,** *adj.*

dysphagia /disfā′jē·ə/ [Gk, *dys* + *phagein*, to swallow], difficulty in swallowing, commonly associated with obstructive or motor disorders of the esophagus. Patients with obstructive disorders like esophageal tumor or lower esophageal ring are unable to swallow solids but can tolerate liquids. Persons with motor disorders, such as achalasia, are unable to swallow solids or liquids. Diagnosis of the underlying condition is made through barium studies, the observed clinical signs, and evaluation of the patient's symptoms. See also **achalasia, aphagia, corkscrew esophagus.**

dysphagia lusoria, an abnormal condition, characterized by difficulty in swallowing, caused by the compression of the esophagus from an anomalous right subclavian artery that arises from the descending aorta and courses behind or in front of the esophagus. Compare **contractile ring dysphagia, vallecular dysphagia.**

dysphasia /disfā′zhə/ [Gk, *dys* + *phasis*, speaking], an impairment of speech, not as severe as aphasia, usually the result of an injury to the speech area in the cerebral cortex of the brain. It may follow a stroke or brain tumor and may be accompanied by other language disorders, such as dysgraphia. Compare **dysarthria.**

dysphonia /disfō′nē·ə/ [Gk, *dys* + *phone*, voice], any abnormality in the speaking voice, such as hoarseness. Dysphonia puberum identifies the voice changes that occur in adolescent boys.

dysphoria /disfôr′ə·ə/, a disorder of affect characterized by depression and anguish.

dysplasia /displā′zhə/ [Gk, *dys* + *plassein*, to form], any abnormal development of tissues or organs.

-dysplasia, a combining form meaning '(condition of) abnormal development': *chondrodysplasia, epidermodysplasia, osteomyelodysplasia.*

dyspnea /dispnē′ə/ [Gk, *dys* + *pnoia*, breathing], a shortness of breath or a difficulty in breathing that may be caused by certain heart conditions, strenuous exercise, or anxiety. Compare **hyperpnea. –dyspneal, dyspneic,** *adj.*

dyspraxia /disprak′sē·ə/ [Gk, *dys* + *prassein*, to do], a partial loss of the ability to perform skilled, coordinated movements in the absence of any associated defect in motor or sensory functions. See also **apraxia.**

dysprosium (Dy) /disprō′sē·əm/ [Gk, *dys* + *prositos*, to approach], a rare-earth metallic element. Its atomic number is 66; its atomic weight is 162.50. Radioactive isotopes of dysprosium are used in radioisotope scanning, particularly in studies of the bones and joints.

dysproteinemia /disprō′tēnē′mē·ə/ [Gk, *dys* + *protos*, first, *haima* blood], an abnormally of the protein content of the blood, usually involving the immunoglobulins.

dysraphia /disrā′fē·ə/ [Gk, *dys* + *raphe*, seam], failure of a raphe to fuse completely, as in incomplete closure of the neural tube. Also called **status dysraphicus.**

dysraphic syndrome /disraf′ik/, a developmental disorder, usually involving the spinal cord, such as encephalocele or myelomenigocele. See also **Arnold-Chiari malformation.**

dysreflexia /dis′riflek′sē·ə/ [Gk, *dys* + L, *reflectere*, to bend backward], a nursing diagnosis accepted by the Eighth National Conference on the Classification of Nursing Diagnoses. The condition is a state in which an individual with a spinal cord injury at T7 or above experiences or is at risk to experience a life-threatening uninhibited sympathetic response of the nervous system to a noxious stimulus. The major defining characteristics of the diagnosis of an individual with spinal cord injury (T7 or above) are paroxysmal hypertension (sudden periodic elevated blood pressure in which systolic pressure is over 140 mmHg and diastolic is above 90 mmHg), bradycardia or tachycardia (pulse rate of less than 60 or over 100 beats per minute), diaphoresis above the injury, red splotches on the skin above the injury, and pallor below the injury. There is also a headache that is a diffuse pain in different portions of the head and not confined to any nerve distribution area. Minor characteristics include chilling (shivering accompanied by the sensation of coldness or pallor of the skin), conjunctival congestion (excessive amount of blood and tissue fluid in the conjunctiva), blurred vision, chest pain, a metallic taste in the mouth, nasal congestion, and pilomotor reflex (gooseflesh formation when skin is cooled). There can also be paresthesia (abnormal sensation such as numbness, prickling or tingling and increased sensitivity). Horner's syndrome caused by paralysis of the cervical sympathetic nerve trunk can also be a characteristic with contraction of the pupil, partial ptosis of the eyelid, enophthalmos and sometimes sweating over the affected side of the face. See also **nursing diagnosis. –dysreflexic,** *adj.*

dysrhythmia /disrith′mē·ə/, any disturbance or abnormality in a normal rhythmic pattern, specifically, irregularity in the brain waves or cadence of speech. Compare **arrhythmia.**

dyssebacea /disibā′shē·ə/ [Gk, *dys* + L, *sebum*, suet], a skin condition characterized by red, scaly, greasy patches on the nose, eyelids, scrotum, and labia. It results from a deficiency of vitamin B$_2$ and is most commonly associated with chronic alcoholism, liver disease, chronic diarrhea, and protein malnutrition. Also called (*informal*) **shark skin.**

dyssynergia /dis′inur′jē·ə/ [Gk, *dys* + *syn*, together, *ergein*, work], any disturbance in muscular coordination, such as in cases of ataxia.

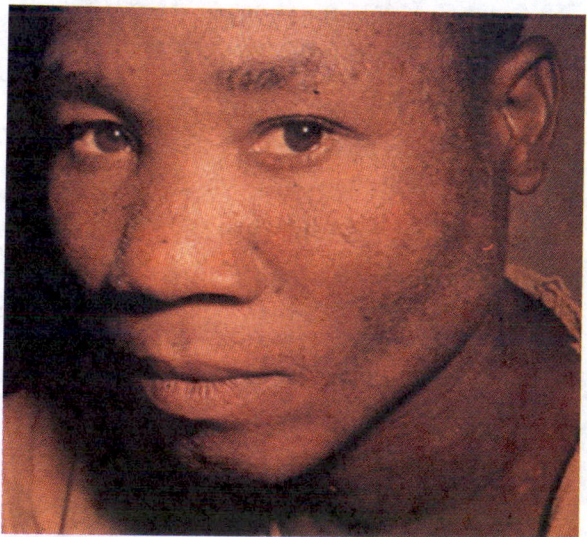

Dyssebacea *(McLaren, 1992)*

dystaxia /distak′sē·ə/ [Gk, *dys, taxis*, order], partial ataxia, such as dystaxia agitans in which there is a tremor caused by a spinal cord irritation but there is no paralysis.

dysthymia /disthim′ē·ə/ [Gk, *dys* + *thymos*, mind], a form of chronic unipolar depression that tends to occur in elderly persons with debilitating physical disorders, multiple interpersonal losses, and chronic marital difficulties. Several depressive episodes may merge into a low-grade chronic depressive state. The condition is sometimes treated with noradrenergic tricyclic compounds.

dysthymic disorder /disthim′ē·ə/ [Gk, *dys* + *thymos*, mind], a disorder of mood whereby the essential feature is a chronic disturbance of mood of at least two years duration, involving either depressed mood or loss of interest or pleasure in all or almost all usual activities and pastimes, and associated symptoms, but not of sufficient severity and duration to meet the criteria for a major depressive episode. Also called **neurotic depression.**

dystocia /distō′shə/ [Gk, *dys* + *tokos*, birth], pathologic or difficult labor, which may be caused by an obstruction or constriction of the birth passage or an abnormal size, shape, position, or condition of the fetus. See also **clinical pelvimetry, fetal presentation, x-ray pelvimetry.**

dystonia /distō′nē·ə/ [Gk, *dys* + *tonos*, tone], any impairment of muscle tone. The condition commonly involves the head, neck, and tongue, and often occurs as an adverse effect of a medication.

dystonia musculorum deformans, a rare abnormal condition characterized by intense, irregular torsion muscle spasms that contort the body. The muscles of the trunk, shoulder, and pelvis are commonly involved. This disease appears in several forms, generally classified as autosomal recessive or autosomal dominant. The cause of this disorder is not known; a biochemical dysfunction is suspected. The autosomal recessive form appears most often in Ashkenazic Jews and starts between 5 and 15 years of age, causing abnormalities of movement and speech. Muscle power and tone appear normal, but convulsive spasms make the involved muscles relatively useless. The autosomal recessive form of the disease commonly begins with intermittent spasmodic inversion of the foot, so that the affected individual has difficulty in placing the heel on the ground when walking and develops an odd, bowing gait. Lordosis and torsion of pelvis appear as the proximal muscles become more involved. Torticollis is often an early sign if the muscles of the neck and shoulder girdle are involved. The autosomal dominant form of the disease appears in early adult life, generally affects the axial musculature, and progresses more slowly than the autosomal recessive form. Some muscle-relaxing drugs, such as the benzodiazepines, have been helpful in treating both forms of the condition. Mild cases have been successfully controlled for long periods with treatments that combine the use of muscle-relaxing drugs and psychotherapy.

dystonic /diston′ik/, referring to an excessive increase in muscle tone, often resulting in postural abnormalities.

dystrophia. See **dystrophy.**

dystrophic /distrof′ik/ [Gk, *dys, trophe*, nourishment], pertaining to a usually congenital disorder of structure or function of an organ or tissue that is aggravated by torturous nutrition, such as accumulation of calcium salts in the cornea.

dystrophic calcification [Gk, *dys* + *trophe*, nourishment;

L, *calx*, lime, *facere*, to make], the pathologic accumulation of calcium salts in necrotic or degenerated tissues. Compare **metastatic calcification.**

dystrophy /dis′trəfē/ [Gk, *dys* + *trophe*, nourishment], any abnormal condition caused by defective nutrition, often applied to a developmental change in muscles that does not involve the nervous system, such as fatty degeneration associated with increased size but decreased strength. Also called **dystrophia.** −**dystrophic** /distrof′ik/, *adj.*

dysuria /disyo͞or′ē·ə/ [Gk, *dys* + *ouron*, urine], painful urination, usually the result of a bacterial infection or obstructive condition in the urinary tract. The patient complains of a burning sensation when passing urine, and laboratory examination may reveal the presence of blood, bacteria, or white blood cells. Dysuria is a symptom of such conditions as cystitis, urethritis, prostatitis, urinary tract tumors, some gynecologic disorders, and certain medications, such as opiates. Compare **hematuria, pyuria.**

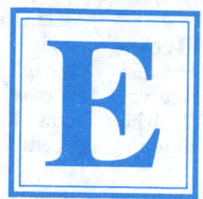

E, symbol for **expired gas.**

E1, symbol for **monomolecular elimination reaction.**

E2, symbol for **bimolecular elimination reaction.**

e-, a prefix meaning 'out from': *ebonation, egesta, emollient.*

E and GW, abbreviation for **Economic and General Welfare.**

ear [AS *eare*], the organ of hearing and balance, consisting of the internal, middle, and external ear. The external ear includes the skin-covered cartilaginous auricle visible on either side of the head and the portion of the external auditory canal that is outside the skull. Together they form a funnel that directs sound waves toward the eardrum, or tympanic membrane, which marks the boundary between the external ear and the air-filled middle ear. The middle ear contains three very small bones, the malleus, incus, and stapes, which transmit vibrations caused by sound waves reaching the tympanic membrane to the oval window of the inner ear. The leverage of the ossicles, or middle-ear bones, increases the intensity of sound vibrations by more than 25 dB. Because the inner ear is filled with fluid, the increased intensity helps compensate for the loss of signal normally caused by sound-wave reflection of the fluid. The inner ear contains two separate organs: the vestibular apparatus, which provides the sense of balance, and the organ of Corti, which receives vibrations from the middle ear and translates them into nerve impulses, which are again interpreted by brain cells as specific sounds.

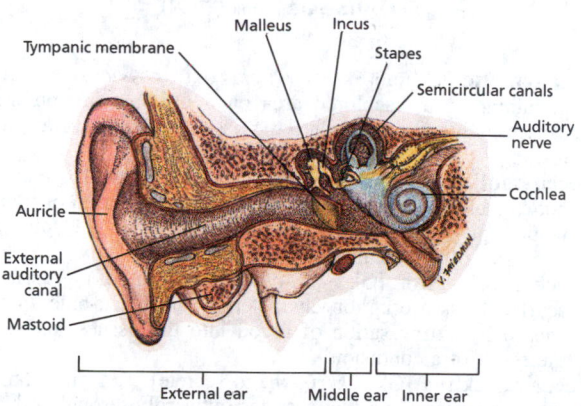

Structures of the ear (Potter, 1993)

earache /ir'āk/ [AS, *eare* + *acan*, to hurt], a pain in the ear, sensed as sharp, dull, burning, intermittent, or constant. The cause is not necessarily a disease of the ear, because infections and other disorders of the nose, oral cavity, larynx, and temporomandibular joint can produce referred pain in the ear. Also called **otalgia, otodynia.**

eardrop instillation, the instillation of a medicated solution into the external auditory canal of the ear. The patient is asked to turn the head to the side so that the ear being treated faces upward. The orifice is exposed, and the drops of medicine are directed toward the internal wall of the canal. The pinna is pulled up and back in a person over 3 years of age and down and back in a younger child. The tragus is then pushed against the ear canal to ensure that the drops stay in the canal.

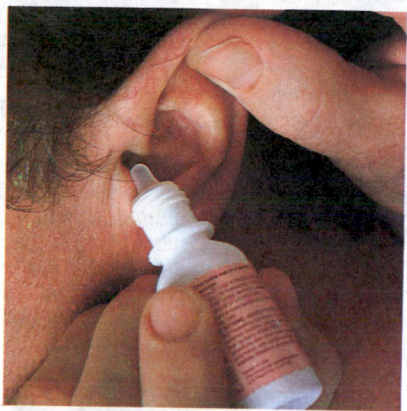

Instilling drops into the ear canal

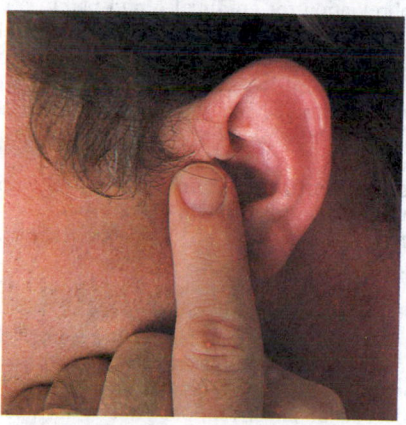

Pushing the tragus against the ear canal
Eardrop instillation (Potter, 1993)

eardrops [AS, *eare* + *dropa*], a topical, liquid form of medication for the local treatment of various conditions of the ear, such as inflammation or infection of the lining of the external auditory canal or impacted cerumen.

eardrum. See **tympanic membrane.**

Early and Periodic Screening Diagnosis and Treatment (EPSDT), a section of the Medicaid program that requires all states to maintain a program to determine the physical and mental defects of persons under age 21 who are covered by the program and to provide short- and long-range treatment. See also **Medicaid.**

ear oximeter [AS, *eare*; Gk, *oxys*, sharp, *genein*, to produce, *metron*, measure], a device placed over the ear lobe that transmits a beam of light through the ear lobe tissue to a receiver. It is a noninvasive method of measuring the level of saturated hemoglobin in the blood. As the amount of saturated hemoglobin in the blood alters the wavelengths of light transmitted through the ear lobe, analysis of the light received is translated into percentage of oxygen saturation (SO_2) of the blood.

ear speculum [AS, *eare*; L, *speculum*, mirror], a short, funnel-shaped tube attached to an otoscope for examining the ear canal.

ear thermometry, the measurement of the temperature of the tympanic membrane by detection of infrared radiation from the ear drum. See also **tympanic membrane thermometer.**

earwax. See **cerumen.**

East African Sleeping Sickness. See **Rhodesian trypanosomiasis.**

eastern equine encephalitis. See **equine encephalitis.**

eating disorders, a group of dysfunctional behaviors of nutrition, including anorexia, bulimia, or cravings for such nonfood items as ice, clay, or starch.

Eaton agent, an alternative name for *Mycoplasma pneumoniae*, a common cause of atypical pneumonia in humans. It is distinguished from other *Mycoplasma* organisms by its lack of a 'fried egg' appearance when cultured on agar. See also *Mycoplasma.*

Eaton agent pneumonia. See **mycoplasma pneumonia.**

Eaton-Lambert syndrome, a form of myasthenia that tends to be associated with lung cancer.

Ebbecke's reaction. See **dermatographia.**

EBP, abbreviation for **epidural blood patch.**

Ebstein's anomaly [Wilhelm Ebstein, German physician, b. 1836; Gk, *anomalia*, irregularity], a congenital heart defect in which the tricuspid valve is displaced downward into the right ventricle. The abnormality is often associated with right-to-left atrial shunting and Wolff-Parkinson-White syndrome.

eburnation of dentin. See **arrested dental caries.**

EBV, abbreviation for **Epstein-Barr virus.**

ec-, a prefix meaning 'out of': *ecbolic, eccephalosis, ecchondroma.*

ECC, **1.** abbreviation for **emergency cardiac care. 2.** abbreviation for *external cardiac compression.*

eccentric /eksen'trik/ [Gk, *ek*, out, *centre*, center], **1.** pertaining to an object or activity that departs from the usual course or practice. **2.** pertaining to behavior that may appear to be odd or unconventional but is not necessarily a disorder.

eccentric contraction, a type of muscle contraction that involves lengthening of the muscle fibers, such as when a weight is lowered through a range of motion. The muscle yields to the resistance, allowing itself to be stretched.

eccentric implantation [Gk, *ek*, out, *centre*, center], (in embryology) the embedding of the blastocyst within a fold or recess of the uterine wall, which then closes off from the main cavity.

eccentricity /ek'sentris'itē/, behavior that is regarded as odd or peculiar for a particular culture or community although not unusual enough to be considered pathologic.

eccentric jaw relation, (in dentistry) any jaw relation other than centric relation.

eccentric occlusion [Gk, *ek, centre*; L, *occludere*, to close up], an occlusion of the teeth in which the habitual voluntary closure pattern of the mandible does not coincide with centric relation, resulting in premature tooth contacts. Also called **acentric occlusion.**

ecchondroma /ek'əndrō'mə/ [Gk, *ek* + *chondros*, cartilage, *oma*, tumor], a benign tumor that develops on the surface of a cartilage or under the periosteum of bone.

ecchondrosis. See **ecchondroma.**

ecchymosis /ek'imō'sis/, *pl.* **ecchymoses** [Gk, *ek* + *chymos*, juice], discoloration of an area of the skin or mucous membrane caused by the extravasation of blood into the subcutaneous tissues as a result of trauma to the underlying blood vessels or by fragility of the vessel walls. Also called **bruise.** Compare **contusion, petechiae.**

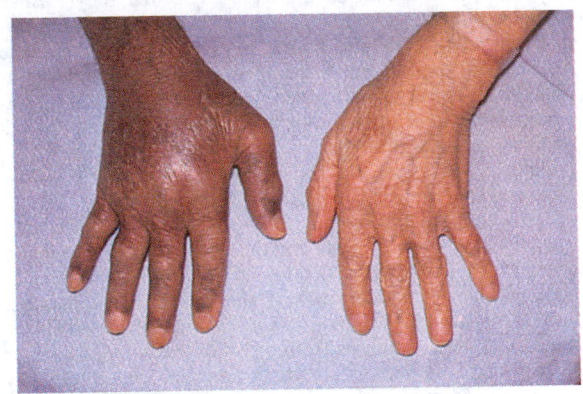

Ecchymosis (Kamal, 1991)

ecchymotic /ek'imot'ik/ [Gk, *ek*, out, *chymous*, juice], pertaining to a discolored area on the skin or membrane caused by blood seeping into the tissue as a result of a contusion.

ecchymotic mask [Gk, *ek, chymous*; Fr, *masque*], a cyanotic or bluish discoloration of the face of a victim of traumatic asphyxia, as in strangulation or choking. The color is the result of petechial hemorrhages.

ecchymotic rash [Gk, *ek, chymos*, juice; OFr, *rasche*, scurf], a skin eruption characterized by black-blue spots caused by extravasation of blood into the tissues, usually the result of a contusion.

eccrine /ek'rin/ [Gk, *ekkrinein*, to secrete], of or pertaining to a sweat gland that secretes outwardly through a duct to the surface of the skin. See also **exocrine.**

eccrine gland, one of two kinds of sweat glands in the corium of the skin. Such glands are unbranched, coiled, and tubular, and they are distributed throughout the dermal covering of the body. They promote cooling by evaporation of their secretion, which is clear, has a faint odor, and contains water, sodium chloride, and traces of albumin, urea, and other compounds. Compare **apocrine gland.**

eccyesis. See **ectopic pregnancy.**

ECF, 1. abbreviation for **extended care facility. 2.** abbreviation for **extracellular fluid.**

ECG, 1. abbreviation for **electrocardiogram. 2.** abbreviation for **electrocardiograph.**

ecgonine /ek'gōnēn/, the principal part of the cocaine molecule. It is obtained by hydrolysis of cocaine and is used as a topical anesthetic.

-echia, a suffix meaning a 'condition of holding': *asynechia, blepharosynechia, synechia.*

echino-, a combining form meaning 'pertaining to spines, or spiny': *echinochroma, echinosis, echinostomiasis.*

echinococcosis /ekī'nōkokō'sis/ [Gk, *echinos,* prickly husk, *kokkos,* berry, *osis,* condition], an infestation, usually of the liver, caused by the larval stage of a tapeworm of the genus *Echinococcus.* Dogs are the principal hosts of the adult worm; sheep, cattle, rodents, and deer are the natural intermediate hosts for the larvae. Humans, especially children, can become infested with larvae by ingesting eggs shed in the stool of infected dogs. The disease is most common in countries where domestic animals are raised with the help of dogs. Clinical manifestations and prognosis vary, depending upon the tissue invaded and the extent of infestation. Diagnosis is made by skin tests for sensitivity, serologic tests, radiologic evidence of cyst formation, and identification of larval cysts in infected tissue. Surgical excision of the cysts is the only treatment available. The disease can be prevented by avoiding contact with infected dogs, deworming pet animals, and preventing dogs from eating carcasses of infected intermediate hosts. Also called **hydatid disease, hydatidosis.** See also **cysticercosis, tapeworm infection.**

Echinococcus /ekī'nōkok'əs/ [Gk, *echinos,* prickly husk, *kokkos,* berry], a genus of small tapeworms that infects primarily canines. See also **echinococcosis, hydatid cyst.**

echinocyte. See **burr cell.**

echo /ek'ō/, *informal.* echoradiography.

echo beat [Gk, sound; AS, *beatan,* to throb], a reciprocal heart beat, or one that results from the return of an impulse to a chamber of origin.

echocardiogram /ek'ōkär'dē·əgram'/ [Gk, *echo,* sound, *kardia,* heart, *gramma,* record], a graphic outline of movements of the heart structures compiled from ultrasound vibrations that are echoed from these structures.

echocardiography /ek'ōkär'dē·og'rəfē/ [Gk, *echo* + *kardia,* heart, *graphein,* to record], a diagnostic procedure for studying the structure and motion of the heart. Ultrasonic waves directed through the heart are reflected backward, or echoed, when they pass from one type of tissue to another, such as from cardiac muscle to blood. The sound waves are transmitted from and received by a transducer and are recorded on a strip chart. Major diagnostic uses include the detection of atrial tumors and pericardial effusion, the measurement of the ventricular septa and the ventricular chambers, and the determination of mitral valve motion abnormalities and congenital lesions. Also called **ultrasonic cardiography.** See also **phonocardiograph, ultrasonography.**

echoencephalogram /ek'ō·ensef'ələgram'/ [Gk, *echo* + *enkephalos,* brain, *gramma,* record], a recording produced by an echoencephalograph.

echoencephalography /ek'ō·ensef'əlog'rəfē/, the use of ultrasound to study the intracranial structures of the brain. The technique is useful for showing ventricular dilatation and a major shift of midline structures as a result of an ex-

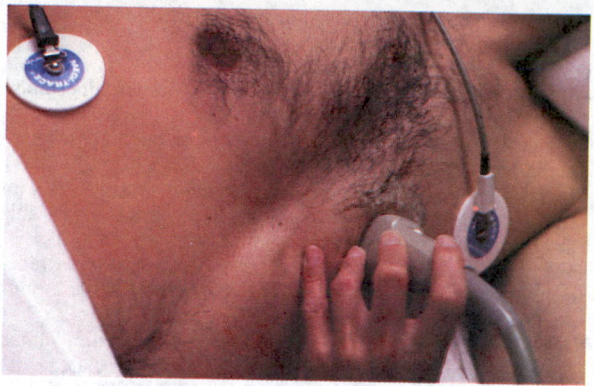

Echocardiography—placement of chest leads and transducer
(Canobbio, 1990)

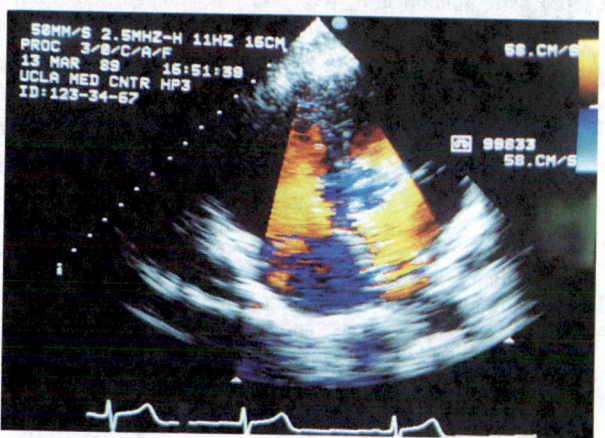

Color flow Doppler echocardiography
(Canobbio, 1990)

panding lesion. See also **ultrasonography.** —echoencephalographic, *adj.*

echogram /ek'ōgram/ [Gk, *echo,* sound, *gramma,* record], a recording of ultrasound echo patterns of body structures, such as a gravid uterus.

echography. See **ultrasonography.**

echolalia /ek'ōlā'lyə/ [Gk, *echo* + *lalein,* to babble], **1.** (in psychiatry) the automatic and meaningless repetition of another's words or phrases, especially as seen in schizophrenia. A kind of echolalia is **delayed echolalia. 2.** (in pediatrics) a baby's imitation or repetition of sounds or words produced by others. It occurs normally in early childhood development. Also called **echophrasia, echo speech.** —echolalic, *adj.*

echopraxia /ek'ōprak'sē·ə/ [Gk, *echo* + *prassein,* to practice], imitation or repetition of the body movements of another person, a behavior exhibited by some schizophrenic patients.

echoradiography /ek'ōrā'dē·og'rəfē/ [Gk, *echo* + L, *radius* ray; Gk, *graphein,* to record], a diagnostic procedure using ultrasonography and various devices for the visualization of internal structures of the body.

echo speech. See **echolalia.**

echothiophate iodide /-thī′ōfāt/, an anticholinesterase used for ophthalmic purposes.

■ INDICATIONS: It is prescribed for chronic open-angle glaucoma and accommodative esotropia.

■ CONTRAINDICATIONS: Uveal inflammation, most types of angle-closure glaucoma, or known hypersensitivity to this drug prohibits its use.

■ ADVERSE EFFECTS: Among the more serious adverse reactions are retinal detachment, nonreversible cataract, lens opacity, activation of iritis or uveitis, and iris cysts.

ECHO virus /ek′ōvī′rəs/ [enteric *c*ytopathicgenic *h*uman *o*rphan + L *virus* poison], a picornavirus associated with many clinical syndromes but not identified as the causative organism of any specific disease. There are many ECHO viruses. More than 30 serotypes have been identified. Many are harmless. Bacterial or viral disease may be complicated by ECHO virus infection, such as seen in aseptic meningitis accompanying some severe bacterial and viral infections.

eclampsia /iklamp′sē·ə/ [Gk, *ek*, out, *lampein*, to flash], the gravest form of pregnancy-induced hypertension, characterized by grand mal convulsion, coma, hypertension, proteinuria, and edema. The symptoms of impending convulsion often include body temperature of up to 104° F, anxiety, epigastric pain, severe headache, and blurred vision. The nurse is alert to persistently and extremely high blood pressure and to increasingly hyperactive deep-tendon reflexes, or clonus. Convulsions may be prevented by bed rest in a quiet, dimly lit room and parenteral administration of magnesium sulfate and antihypertensive medications. The nurse attentively monitors the mother's general condition, including respiration, deep tendon reflexes, blood pressure, magnesium sulfate levels, and urine and protein excretion, and the baby's heart rate. Treatment of a convulsion must include maintenance of the mother's airway, protection against self-injury, and administration of medication to check the convulsion and decrease the blood pressure. Once this is accomplished, delivery is indicated. Convulsions rarely occur in the puerperium. Complications of eclampsia include cerebral hemorrhage, pulmonary edema, renal failure, necrosis of the liver, abruptio placentae, hypofibrinogenemia, hemolysis, and retinal hemorrhages, sometimes with temporary blindness. Maternal mortality in eclampsia is 10%; fetal mortality is 25%. Eclampsia occurs in 0.2% of pregnancies. The cause is not known.

eclamptogenic toxemia /iklamp′tōjen′ik/ [Gk, *ek*, *lampein*, to flash + *genein*, to produce + *toxikon*, poison + *haima*, blood], a form of blood poisoning accompanied by convulsions that may occur during pregnancy. See **eclampsia.**

eclectic /iklek′tik/ [Gk, *eklektikos*, selecting], pertaining to a therapy that selects, combines, and incorporates diverse techniques from several systems or theories into an integrated approach.

eclipse scotoma /iklips′/ [Gk, *ekleipsis*, abandoning + *skotos*, darkness + *oma*, tumor], a small central area of depressed or lost vision resulting from looking directly at the sun without adequate protection.

ECM, abbreviation for **erythema chromicum migrans.**

-ecoia, a suffix meaning '(condition of the) sense of hearing': *bradyecoia, dysecoia, oxyecoia.*

ECMO, abbreviation for **extracorporeal membrane oxygenator.**

E. coli, abbreviation for *Escherichia coli.*

ecologic chemistry /ikəloj′ik/, the study of chemical compounds synthesized by plants that influence ecology because of their toxic effects.

ecologic fallacy, a false assumption that the presence of a pathogenic factor and a disease in a population can be accepted as proof of cause for the disease in a particular individual.

ecology /ikol′əjē/ [Gk, *oekos*, house, *logos*, science], the study of the interaction between living organisms and their environment.

econazole /ikon′əzōl/, an antifungal agent.

■ INDICATIONS: It is prescribed in the treatment of tinea and candidiasis.

■ CONTRAINDICATION: Known sensitivity to this drug prohibits its use.

■ ADVERSE EFFECTS: Among the most serious adverse reactions are local irritation and hypersensitivity of the skin.

Economic and General Welfare (E and GW), a unit of the American Nurses Association whose major goal is to upgrade the salaries, benefits, and working conditions of nurses.

ecosystem /ek′ōsis′təm/, the sum total of all living and nonliving things that support chain of life events within a particular area.

ecstasy /ek′stəsē/ [Gk, *ekstasis*, derangement], an emotional state characterized by exultation, rapturous delight, or frenzy. Compare **euphoria, mania.** **–ecstatic,** *adj.*

ECT, abbreviation for **electroconvulsive therapy.**

-ectas a combining form meaning 'dilatation, extension, or distension of an organ': *esophagectasia, lymphectasia, pharyngectasia.*

ecthyma /ek′thimə/ [Gk, *ek*, out, *thyein*, to rush], a superficial pyodermia evolving into firm crusts and shallow ulceration a deep, burrowing form of impetigo characterized by large pustules, crusts, and ulcerations surrounded by erythema. Staphylococci and streptococci are the offending bacteria, and the skin of the legs is most frequently affected. Treatment includes vigorous cleansing, application of compresses of cool Burow's solution to soften and remove crusts, and systematic administration of penicillin or

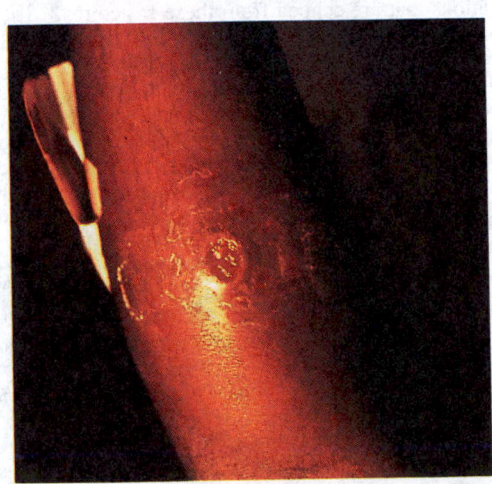

Ecthyma
(Zitelli, 1992/Courtesy Dr. Ellen Wald, Children's Hospital of Pittsburgh)

erythromycin given systemically. Compare **folliculitis, impetigo.**

ecto-, a prefix meaning 'outside': *ectoblast, ectocolon, ectodermal.*

ectoderm /ek′tədurm/ [Gk, *ektos,* outside, *derma,* skin], the outermost of the three primary cell layers of an embryo. The ectoderm gives rise to the nervous system; the organs of special sense, such as the eyes and ears; the epidermis and epidermal tissue, such as fingernails, hair, and skin glands; and the mucous membranes of the mouth and anus. See also **embryo, endoderm, mesoderm.** – **ectodermal, ectodermic,** *adj.*

ectodermal cloaca ek′tədur′məl/, a part of the cloaca in the developing embryo that lies external to the cloacal membrane and eventually gives rise to the anus and anal canal. Compare **endodermal cloaca.**

-ectodermic. See **ectoderm.**

ectomorph /ek′təmôrf′/ [Gk, *ektos* + *morphe,* form], a person whose physique is characterized by slenderness, fragility, and a predominance of structures derived from the ectoderm. Compare **endomorph, mesomorph.** See also **asthenic habitus.**

-ectomy, a suffix meaning the 'surgical removal' of something specified: *lobectomy, thrombectomy, thyroidectomy.*

ectoparasite /ek′tōper′əsīt/ [Gk, *ektos* + *parasitos,* guest], (in medical parasitology) an organism that lives on the outside of the body of the host, such as a louse.

-ectopia, a combining form meaning a 'condition in which a (specified) organ or part is out of its normal place': *corectopia, osteectopia, tarsectopia.*

ectopic /ektop′ik/ [Gk, *ektos* + *topos,* place], **1.** (of an object or organ) situated in an unusual place, away from its normal location; for example, an ectopic pregnancy is a pregnancy that occurs outside the uterus. **2.** (of an event) occurring at the wrong time, as a premature heart beat or premature ventricular contraction.

ectopic beat, [Gk, *ek,* out, *topos,* place; AS, *beatan*], a heartbeat which had its origin at some place other than the sino-atrial node.

ectopic focus, an abnormal cardiac impulse that produces abnormal, or ectopic, beats. Ectopic foci may occur in both healthy and diseased hearts and are usually associated with irritation of a small area of myocardial tissue. Ectopic foci are produced in association with myocardial ischemias, drug effects, emotional stress, and stimulation by foreign objects, including pacemaker catheters.

ectopic myelopoiesis. See **extramedullary myelopoiesis.**

ectopic pacemaker /pās′mā′kər/, [Gk, *ek,* out, *topos,* place; L, *passus,* step; ME, *maken*], abnormally located group of cardiac nerve cells that initiate a cardiac impulse and override the sinoatrial node. The ectopic sites may be in an atrium, ventricle, or atrioventricular node.

ectopic pregnancy, an abnormal pregnancy in which the conceptus implants outside the uterine cavity. Kinds of ectopic pregnancy are **abdominal pregnancy, ovarian pregnancy,** and **tubal pregnancy.** Also called **eccyesis** /ek′sī·ē′sis/.

ectopic rhythm [Gk, *ek, topos,* place + *rhythmos,* beat], an abnormal heart rhythm caused by formation of the impulse in a focus outside the usual pacemaker. An ectopic focus usually develops when the natural sinus node pacemaker is depressed.

ectopic tachycardia [Gk, *ek, topos,* place + *tachys,* swift + *kardia,* heart], an abnormally rapid heartbeat resulting from a stimulus from an ectopic focus, or one outside the sinoatrial node.

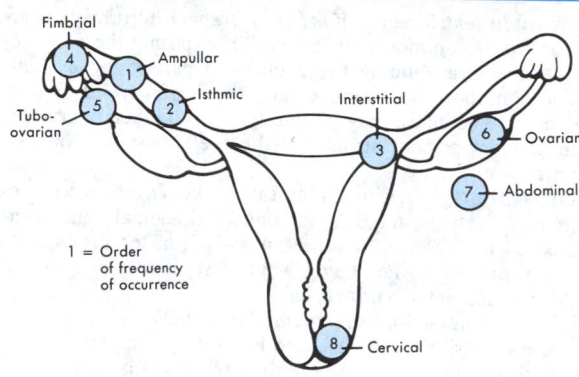

Ectopic pregnancy implantation sites *(Bobak, 1993)*

ectopic teratism, a congenital anomaly in which one or more parts are misplaced, such as dextrocardia, palatine teeth, and transposition of the great vessels.

ectopy /ek′təpē/ [Gk, *ek,* out, *topos,* place], a condition in which an organ or substance is not in its natural or proper place, such as an ectopic pregnancy that develops outside the uterus or ectopic heartbeats.

ectotoxin. See **exotoxin.**

ectro-, a prefix meaning 'pertaining to loss or absence of, miscarriage, abortion,' used primarily to indicate a loss of limbs or body parts: *ectrodactyly, ectromelia.*

ectrodactyly /ek′trōdak′təlē/ [Gk, *ektrosis,* miscarriage, *daktylos,* finger], a congenital anomaly characterized by the absence of part or all of one or more of the fingers or toes. Also called *ectrodactylia,* **ectrodactylism.**

-ectrogenic. See **ectrogeny.**

ectrogenic teratism /-jen′ik/ [Gk, *ektrosis* + *genein,* to produce; *teras,* monster], a congenital anomaly caused by developmental failure in which one or more parts or organs are missing.

ectrogeny /ektroj′ənē/ [Gk, *ektrosis* + *genein,* to produce], the congenital absence or defect of any organ or part of the body. – **ectrogenic,** *adj.*

ectromelia /ek′trōmē′lyə/ [Gk, *ektrosis* + *melos,* limb], the congenital absence or incomplete development of the long bones of one or more of the limbs. Kinds of ectromelia are **amelia, hemimelia,** and **phocomelia.** – **ectromelic,** *adj.,* **ectromelus,** *n.*

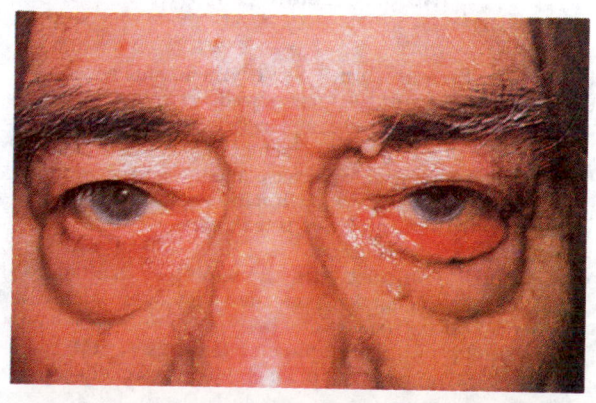

Ectropion *(Kamal, 1991)*

ectropion /ektrō′pē·on/ [Gk, *ek* + *trepein*, to turn], eversion, most commonly of the eyelid, exposing the conjunctival membrane lining the eyelid and part of the eyeball. The condition may involve only the lower eyelid or both eyelids. The cause may be paralysis of the facial nerve or, in an older person, atrophy of the eyelid tissues. Compare **entropion.**

ectrosyndactyly /ek′trōsindak′təlē/ [Gk, *ektrosis* + *syn*, together, *daktylos*, finger], a congenital anomaly characterized by the absence of some but not all of the digits, with those that are formed being webbed so as to appear fused. Also called **ectrosyndactylia.**

ECU, abbreviation for *extended care facility.*

eczema /ek′simə/ [Gk *ekzein* to boil over], superficial dermatitis of unknown cause. In the early stage it may be pruritic, erythematous, papulovesicular, edematous, and weeping. Later it becomes crusted, scaly, thickened, and lichenified. Eczema is not a distinct disease entity. See also **atopic dermatitis, nummular dermatitis.** —**eczematous,** *adj.*

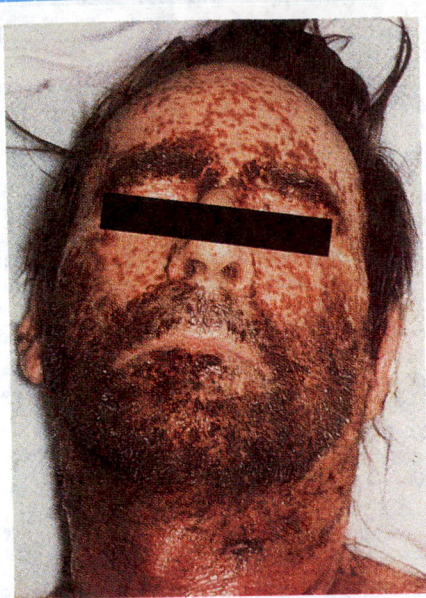

Eczema herpeticum *(Courtesy Professor Ross Barnetson)*

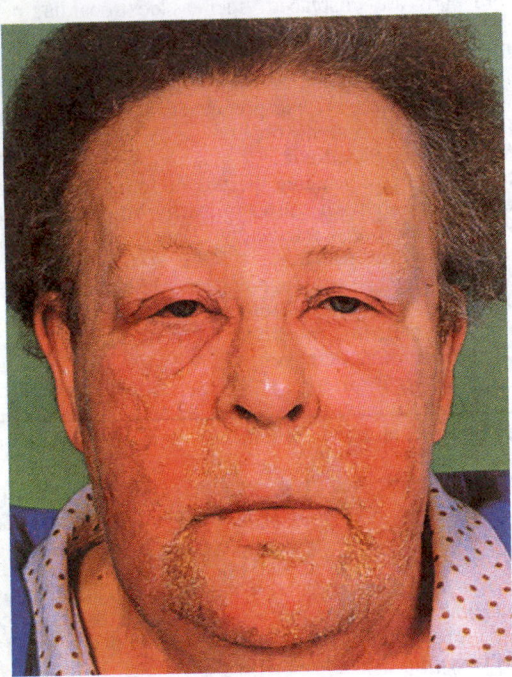

Atopic eczema *(Cerio, 1992)*

eczema erythematosum. See **erythematous eczema.**

eczema herpeticum, a generalized vesiculopustular skin disease caused by herpes simplex virus or vaccinia virus infection of a preexisting rash such as atopic dermatitis. Hospitalization is advisable because fatalities have occurred. Also called **Kaposi's varicelliform eruption.**

eczema marginatum. See **tinea cruris.**

-eczematous. See **eczema.**

eczematous conjunctivitis /eksem′ətəs/, conjunctival and corneal inflammation associated with multiple, tiny, ulcerated vesicles. The cause is believed to be a delayed hypersensitivity to bacterial protein. If untreated, the condition may lead to ingrowth of small blood vessels in the cornea, eventually obscuring vision. Treatment usually includes topical instillation of corticosteroids.

ED, abbreviation for **effective dose.**

E.D., abbreviation for **Emergency Department.**

ED50, symbol for **median effective dose.**

edaphon /ed′əfon/, the composite of organisms that live in the soil. —**edaphic,** *adj.*

EDB, abbreviation for **ethylene dibromide.**

EDC, abbreviation for **expected date of confinement.**

Edecrin, a trademark for a diuretic (ethacrynic acid).

Edecrin Sodium, a trademark for a loop diuretic (ethacrynate sodium).

edema /idē′mə/ [Gk, *oidema*, swelling], the abnormal accumulation of fluid in interstitial spaces of tissues, such as in the pericardial sac, intrapleural space, peritoneal cavity, or joint capsules. Edema may be caused by increased capillary fluid pressure, venous obstruction, such as occurs in varicosities, thrombophlebitis, or pressure from casts, tight bandages, or garters, congestive heart failure, overloading with parenteral fluids, renal failure, hepatic cirrhosis, hyperaldosteronism, such as in Cushing's syndrome, corticosteroid therapy, and inflammatory reactions. Edema may also occur because of loss of serum protein in burns, draining wounds, fistulas, hemorrhage, nephrotic syndrome, or

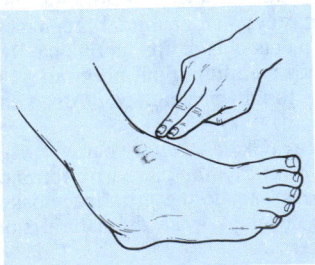

Pitting edema

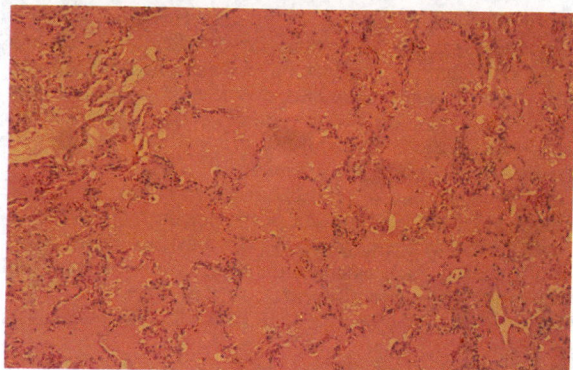

Edema—accumulation of fluid in interstitial spaces
(Christiansen, 1993)

chronic diarrhea; in malnutrition, especially kwashiorkor; in allergic reactions; and in blockage of lymphatic vessels caused by malignant diseases, filariasis, or other disorders. Treatment of edema is directed to correction of the basic cause. Potassium-sparing diuretics may be administered to promote excretion of sodium and water, and care should be exercised in protecting edematous parts of the body from prolonged pressure, injury, and temperature extremes. In the evaluation of tissue turgor, the nurse evaluates edema according to position change, specific location, and response to pressure, as in pitting edema in which pressing the fingers into the edematous area causes a temporary indentation. When a limb is edematous because of venous stasis, elevating the extremity and applying an elastic stocking or sleeve facilitates venous return. See also **anasarca, lymphedema.** —**edematous, edematose,** *adj.*

-edema, -edem, a combining form meaning 'swelling resulting from an excessive accumulation of serous fluid in the tissues of the body in (specified) locations': *cephaledema, dactyledema, papilledema.*

edema of glottis [Gk, *oidema,* swelling, *glossa,* tongue], a swelling caused by fluid accumulation in the soft tissues of the larynx. The condition, usually inflammatory, may result from an infection, injury, or inhalation of toxic gases. Also called **laryngeal edema.**

-edematous. See **edema.**

edematous /ēdem'ətəs/ [Gk, *oidema,* swelling], pertaining to or resembling edema, or excessive fluid accumulation in the tissues, causing swelling.

edentulous /ēden'chələs/, toothless.

edetate (EDTA) /ed'ətāt/, one of several salts of edetic acid, including calcium disodium edetate and edetate disodium, used as a chelating agent in treating poisoning with heavy metals.

edetate disodium, a parenteral chelating agent.
■ INDICATIONS: It is prescribed for hypercalcemic crisis, for ventricular arrhythmia and heart block resulting from digitalis toxicity, and for lead poisoning.
■ CONTRAINDICATIONS: Hypocalcemia, kidney disease, or known hypersensitivity to this drug prohibits its use.
■ ADVERSE EFFECTS: Among the more serious adverse reactions are hypocalcemia, thrombophlebitis, kidney damage, and hemorrhage associated with hypocoagulability.

edetic acid (EDTA) /idet'ik/, a chelating agent.
EDG, abbreviation for **electrodynograph.**
edge response function (ERF), the ability of a computed tomography system to reproduce accurately a high-contrast edge, such as the edge of the heart, with a sharp interface to show neighboring tissues.
edgewise fixed orthodontic appliance, an orthodontic appliance characterized by tooth attachment brackets with a rectangular slot that engages a round or rectangular arch wire. It is used to correct or improve malocclusion.

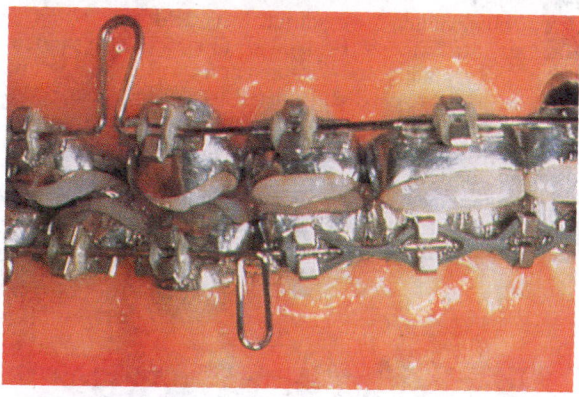

Edgewise fixed orthodontic appliance (Bennett, 1993)

edrophonium chloride /ed'rōfō'nē·əm/, a cholinesterase inhibitor that acts as an antidote to curare and is an aid in the diagnosis of myasthenia gravis.
■ INDICATIONS: It is prescribed in the treatment of curare toxicity, in the diagnosis of suspected myasthenia gravis, and to terminate paroxysmal supraventricular tachycardia.
■ CONTRAINDICATIONS: Obstruction of the GI or urinary tract, hypotension, bradycardia, or known hypersensitivity to this drug prohibits its use.
■ ADVERSE EFFECTS: Among the most serious adverse reactions are respiratory paralysis, hypotension, bradycardia, and bronchospasm.
edrophonium test, a test for myasthenia gravis by the injection of an IV solution of edrophonium chloride into a patient. A total of 10 mg of the cholinergic drug is prepared and a 2 mg dose is injected. If there is no reaction in 30 seconds, the remaining 8 mg is administered. A brief improvement in muscle activity is regarded as a positive result. Edrophonium chloride is also used to distinguish between myasthenia and a cholinergic crisis. Because edrophonium chloride can precipitate respiratory depression, the test should not be performed unless an anticholinergic antidote, such as atropine, and respiratory resuscitation equipment are available.
Edsall's disease [David L. Edsall, American physician, b. 1869], a cramping condition that is the result of excessive exposure to heat. Also called **heat cramp.**
EDTA, 1. abbreviation for **edetate.** 2. abbreviation for **edetic acid.**
educational psychology /ej'əkā'shənəl/ [L, *educatus,* to rear; Gk, *psyche,* mind, *logos,* science], the application of psychologic principles, techniques, and tests to educational problems, such as the determination of more effec-

tive instructional methods, the assessment of student advancement, and the selection of students for specialized programs.

Edwards' syndrome. See **trisomy 18.**

EEE, abbreviation for **eastern equine encephalitis.** See **equine encephalitis.**

EEG, 1. abbreviation for **electroencephalogram.** 2. abbreviation for **electroencephalography.**

EENT, abbreviation for *eyes, ears, nose, and throat.*

EEOC, abbreviation for **Equal Employment Opportunity Commission.**

ef-. See **ex-.**

EFA, abbreviation for **essential fatty acid.**

effacement /ifãs'mənt/ [Fr, *effacer*, to erase], the shortening of the vaginal portion of the cervix and thinning of its walls as it is stretched and dilated by the fetus during labor. When the cervix is fully effaced, the constrictive neck of the uterus is obliterated, the cervix being then continuous with the lower uterine segment. The extent of effacement, determined by vaginal examination, is expressed as a percentage of full effacement. See also **birth, cervix, dilatation, station.** (Figure, p. 406)

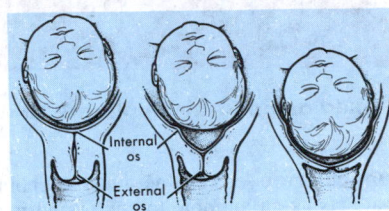

Cervical effacement *(Bobak, 1993)*
before labor, early effacement, complete effacement, complete dilatation

effective compliance /ifek'tiv/ [L, *effectus*, performance], the ratio of tidal volume to peak airway pressure.

effective dose (ED), the dosage of a drug that may be expected to cause a specific intensity of effect in the people to whom it is given.

effective half-life (ehl), (in radiotherapy) the time required for a radioactive element in an animal body to be diminished 50% as a result of the combined action of radioactive decay and biologic elimination. The effective half-life is equal to the product of the biologic half-life *(bhl)* and the radioactive half-life *(rhl)* divided by the product of the biologic half-life plus the radioactive half-life $ehl = (bhl [ti] rhl)/(bhl + rhl)$. See also **biologic half-life.**

effective refractory period, the period after the firing of an impulse during which a cell may respond to a stimulus but the response will not be propagated.

effector /ifek'tər/ [L, *efficere*, to accomplish], 1. an organ that produces an effect, such as glandular secretion, as a result of nerve stimulation. 2. a molecule, such as an enzyme, that can start or stop a chemical reaction.

effects of sleep deprivation [L, *effectus*; AS, *slaep*; L, *deprivare*, to deprive], interference with a basic physiologic urge to sleep, which appears to be governed by sleep centers in the hypothalamus and reticular activating system. The loss of sleep for 24 hours usually has no significant effect on physical or mental functioning. However, subjects kept awake for 30 or more hours have difficulty in handling boring tasks and performance on tests becomes increasingly poor. After several continuous sleepless days, subjects begin to show symptoms of psychoses, such as paranoid reactions and detachment from reality.

effeminate /ifem'init/ [L, *effeminare*, to make womanish], womanly or female in physical and mental characteristics, regardless of the biologic sex of the person.

efferent /ef'ərənt/ [L, *effere*, to carry out], directed away from a center, such as certain arteries, veins, nerves, and lymphatics. Compare **afferent.**

efferent duct, any duct through which a gland releases its secretions.

efferent nerve, a nerve that transmits impulses away or outward from a nerve center, such as the brain or spinal cord, usually resulting in a muscle contraction, release of a glandular secretion, or other activity.

efferent pathway [L, *effere*, to bear out; ME, *paeth, weg*], 1. the route of nerve fibers carrying impulses away from a nerve center. 2. the system of blood vessels that convey blood away from a body part. Compare **afferent.**

effervescence /ef'ərves'əns/ [L, *effervescere*, to foam up], the production of small bubbles or foam associated with the escape of gas from a fluid.

effervescent /ef'ərves'ənt/, producing and releasing gas bubbles.

efficacy /ef'əkəsē/ [L, *effectus*, performance], (of a drug or treatment) the maximum ability of a drug or treatment to produce a result, regardless of dosage. Narcotics have a nearly identical efficacy but require various dosages to obtain the effect.

effleurage /ef'ləräzh'/ [Fr, skimming the surface], a technique in massage in which long, light, or firm strokes are used, usually over the spine and back. Fingertip effleurage is a light technique performed with the tips of the fingers in a circular pattern over one part of the body or in long strokes over the back or an extremity. Fingertip effleurage of the abdomen is a technique commonly used in the Lamaze method of natural childbirth. Compare **pétrissage, rolling effleurage.**

effluent /ef'lōō·ənt/, a liquid, solid, or gaseous emission, such as the discharge or outflow from a machine or industrial process.

effluvium /iflōō'vē·əm/ [L, *effluvium*, a flowing out], an outflow of gas or vapor, usually malodorous or toxic.

effort syndrome [Fr, exertion; Gk, *syn*, together, *dromos*, course], an abnormal condition characterized by chest pain, dizziness, fatigue, and palpitations. This condition is often associated with soldiers in combat but occurs also in other individuals. The symptoms of effort syndrome often mimic angina pectoris but are more closely connected to anxiety states. Some indications that pain and other symptoms are related to effort syndrome rather than angina pectoris include cold, moist hands, sighing respiration, and chest pain after, rather than during, exercise. In some patients effort syndrome may be directly and obviously related to psychologic problems, but angina may also be associated with anxiety, and positive diagnosis may require an exercise electrocardiogram. Other chest pains that mimic effort syndrome and angina may be caused by musculoskeletal problems, as inflammation of the costochondral junctions, fractured ribs, and cervical spondylosis. Also called **neurocirculatory asthenia.**

effraction /ifrak'shən/, a breaking open or weakening.

effusion /ifyoo'zhən/ [L, *effundere*, to pour out], **1.** the escape of fluid from blood vessels because of rupture or seepage, usually into a body cavity. The condition is usually associated with a circulatory or renal disorder and is often an early sign of congestive heart disease. The term may be associated with an affected body area, as pleural or pericardial effusion. See also **edema, transudate. 2.** the outward spread of a bacterial growth.

eflornithine hydrochloride /eflôr'nithēn/, a drug used to treat *Pneumocystis carinii* pneumonia (PCP). It blocks the activity of ornithine decarboxylase, an enzyme required for polyamine synthesis in normal cell division and differentiation.

EFM, abbreviation for **electronic fetal monitor.**

Efudex, a trademark for an antineoplastic (fluorouracil).

egest /ijest'/ [L, *egerere*, to expel], to discharge or evacuate a substance from the body, especially to evacuate unabsorbed residue of foods from the intestines. **–egesta,** *n. pl.,* **egestive,** *adj.*

ego /ē'gō, eg'ō/ [Gk, I or self], **1.** the conscious sense of the self; those elements of a person, such as thinking, feeling, willing, and emotions, that distinguish the person as an individual. **2.** (in psychoanalysis) the part of the psyche that experiences and maintains conscious contact with reality and which tempers the primitive drives of the id and the demands of the superego with the social and physical needs of society. It represents the rational element of the personality, is the seat of such mental processes as perception and memory, and develops defense mechanisms against anxiety. See also **id, superego.**

ego-alien. See **ego-dystonic.**

ego analysis, (in psychoanalysis) the intensive study of the ego, especially the defense mechanisms.

ego boundary, (in psychiatry) a sense or awareness that there is a distinction between the self and others. In some psychoses the person does not have an ego boundary and cannot differentiate personal perceptions and feelings from other people's perceptions and feelings.

egocentric /ē'gōsen'trik/ [Gk, *ego* + *kentron*, center], **1.** regarding the self as the center, object, and norm of all experience and having little regard for the needs, interests, ideas, and attitudes of others. **2.** a person possessing these characteristics.

ego-defense mechanism. See **defense mechanism.**

ego-dystonic /ē'gōdiston'ik/, describing elements of a person's behavior, thoughts, impulses, drives, and attitudes that are unacceptable to the person and cause anxiety. Also called **ego-alien, self-alien.** Compare **ego-syntonic.**

ego-dystonic homosexuality, a psychosexual disorder in which there is a persistent desire to change sexual orientation from homosexuality to heterosexuality. See also **homosexual.**

ego ideal, the image of the self to which a person aspires both consciously and unconsciously and against which he measures himself and his performance. It is usually based on a positive identification with the significant and influential figures of the early childhood years. See also **identification.**

egoism /ē'gō·iz'əm, eg'-/, **1.** selfishness, an overvaluation of the importance of the self, expressed as a willingness to gain an advantage at the expense of others. See also **egotism. 2.** the belief that individual self-interest is, or ought to be, the basic motive for all conscious behavior.

egoist /ē'gō·ist, eg'-/, **1.** a selfish person, one who seeks to satisfy his or her own interests at the expense of others. See also **egotist. 2.** a person who believes in or follows the concept that all conscious action is justifiably motivated by self-interest. **–egoistic, egoistical,** *adj.*

ego libido, (in psychoanalysis) concentration of the libido on the self; self-love, narcissism.

egomania /ē'gōmā'nē·ə/ [Gk, *ego* I, madness], a pathologic preoccupation with the self and an exaggerated sense of one's own importance.

egophony /ēgof'ənē/, (in respiratory therapy) a change in the voice sound as heard on auscultation of a patient with pleural effusion. When the patient is asked to make 'ē-ē-ē' sounds, the sound is heard over the peripheral chest wall as 'ä-ä-ä,' particularly over an area of consolidated or compressed lung above a pleural effusion. Also called **tragophony.**

ego strength, (in psychotherapy) the ability to maintain the ego by a cluster of traits that together contribute to good mental health. The traits usually considered important include tolerance of the pain of loss, disappointment, shame, or guilt; forgiveness of those who have caused an injury, with feelings of compassion rather than anger and retaliation; acceptance of substitutes and the ability to defer gratification; persistence and perseverance in the pursuit of goals; openness, flexibility, and creativity in learning to adapt; and vitality and power in the activities of life. The psychiatric prognosis for a client correlates positively with ego strength.

ego-syntonic /ē'gōsinton'ik/, describing those elements of a person's behavior, thoughts, impulses, drives, and attitudes that are acceptable to the person and are consistent with the total personality. Compare **ego-dystonic.**

egotism /ē'gətiz'əm, eg'-/, vanity, conceit, or the overvaluation of the importance of the self and undervaluation or contempt of others. See also **egoism. –egotistic, egotistical,** *adj.*

egotist /ē'gətist, eg'-/, one who is vain or conceited or who places too much importance on the self and is boastful, egocentric, and arrogant. See also **egoist.**

-egotistic. See **egotism.**

-egotistical. See **egotism.**

egress /ē'gres/, the act of emerging or moving forward.

Egyptian ophthalmia. See **trachoma.**

EHD, abbreviation for **electrohemodynamics.**

ehl, abbreviation for **effective half-life.**

Ehlers-Danlos syndrome /ā'lərzdan'ləs/ [Edward Ehlers, Danish physician, b. 1863; Henri A. Danlos, French physician, b. 1844], a hereditary disorder of connective tissue, marked by hyperplasticity of skin, tissue fragility, and hypermotility of joints. Minor trauma may cause a gaping wound with little bleeding. Sprains, joint dislocations, and synovial effusions are common; life expectancy is usually normal. Nursing management includes emotional support of the patient and the family, with emphasis on avoiding trauma in childhood.

eicosanoic acid /ī'kōsənō'ik/ [Gk, *eikosa*, twenty], a fatty acid containing 20 carbon atoms in a straight chain, such as arachidic acid found in peanut oil, butter, and other fats.

eidetic /īdet'ik/ [Gk, *eidos*, a form or shape seen], **1.** pertaining to or characterized by the ability to visualize and reproduce accurately the image of objects or events previously seen or imagined. **2.** a person possessing such ability.

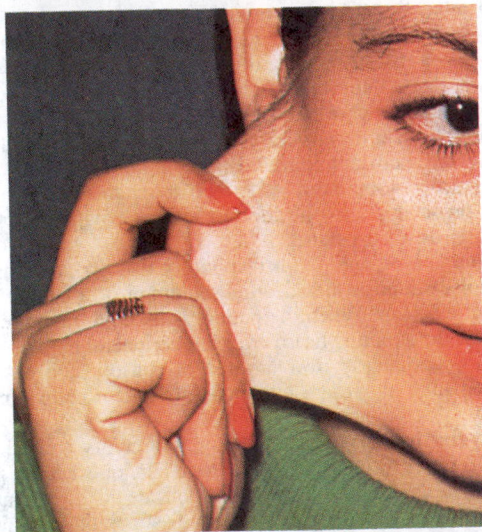

Ehler's Danlos syndrome (McKee, 1993)

eidetic image, an unusually vivid, elaborate, and apparently exact mental image resulting from a visual experience and occurring as a fantasy, dream, or memory. See also **image.**

eighth cranial nerve. See **acoustic nerve.**

einsteinium (Es) /īnstī′nē·əm/ [Albert Einstein, German-born scientist, b. 1879], a synthetic transuranic metallic element. Its atomic number is 99; its atomic weight is 254. Einsteinium was first found in the debris from a hydrogen bomb explosion. It decays rapidly into berkelium.

Einthoven's formula /īnt′hōvənz/ [Willem Einthoven, Dutch physician, b. 1860; L, *forma*, pattern], the theory that the heart lies in the center of an equilateral triangle **(Einthoven's triangle)** in the frontal plane of the body, defined by the right shoulder, left shoulder, and symphysis pubis (left leg). The potential difference in bipolar electrocardiograph lead II (right arm-left leg) is subtracted from the sum of the potential differences of the other bipolar leads.

Eisenmenger's complex /ī′sənmeng′ərz/ [Victor Eisenmenger, German physician, b. 1864; L, *complexus*, encirclement], a congenital heart disease in which there is a defect of the ventricular septum, a malpositioned aortic root which overrides the interventricular septum, and a dilated pulmonary artery. Also called **Eisenmenger's syndrome.**

ejaculate /ijak′yəlit/, the semen discharged in a single emission. See also **ejaculation. –ejaculate** /ijak′yəlāt/, *v.*

ejaculation /-ā′shən/ [L, *ejaculari*, to hurl out], the sudden emission of semen from the male urethra, usually occurring during copulation, masturbation, and nocturnal emission. It is a reflex action in two phases: First, sperm, seminal fluid, and prostatic and bulbourethral gland secretions are moved into the urethra; second, strong spasmodic peristaltic contractions force ejaculation. The sensation of ejaculation is commonly also called orgasm. The fluid volume of the ejaculate is usually between 2 and 5 ml; each milliliter usually contains 50 million to 150 million spermatozoa. **–ejaculatory** /ijak′yələtôr′ē/, *adj.*

ejaculatory duct /ijak′yələtôr′ē/, the passage through which semen enters the urethra.

ejaculator urinae. See **bulbocauernosus.**

ejection /ijek′shən/ [L, *ejicere*, to cast out], the forceful expulsion of something, such as blood from a ventricle of the heart.

ejection clicks, sharp clicking sounds from the heart, which may be caused by the sudden swelling of a pulmonary artery, the abrupt dilatation of the aorta, or the forceful opening of the aortic cusps. Ejection clicks, often heard during examinations of individuals with septal defects and in cases of patent ductus arteriosis, are associated with high pulmonary resistance and hypertension, but are common and of no clinical significance in pregnant women and in many other healthy people. See also **ejection sounds.**

ejection fraction (EF), the proportion of blood that is ejected during each ventricular contraction compared with the total ventricular filling volume. The EF is an index of left ventricular function, and the normal fraction is 65%.

ejection murmur. See **systolic murmur.**

ejection sounds, sharp clicking sounds heard early in systole, coinciding with the onset of either right or left ventricular systolic ejection and reflecting either dilatation of the pulmonary artery or aorta or the presence of valvular abnormalities. The term 'systolic click' is reserved for the nonejection sounds heard in mid or late systole. Aortic ejection sounds are commonly heard in the presence of aortic valvular stenosis, aortic insufficiency, coarctation of the aorta, and hypertension with aortic dilatation. Pulmonary ejection sounds are heard in mild to moderate pulmonary stenosis, in pulmonary hypertension, and in cases of dilatation of the pulmonary artery. See also **ejection clicks.**

Ekbom syndrome. See **restless legs syndrome.**

EKC, abbreviation for **epidemic keratoconjunctivitis.**

EKG, abbreviation for **electrocardiogram.**

elaborate /ilab′ərāt/[L, *elaborare*, to work out], (in endocrinology) a process by which a gland synthesizes a complex substance from simpler substances and secretes it, usually under the stimulation of a tropic hormone from the pituitary gland. This process, regulated by a negative feedback system, including the hypothalamus, pituitary, and target gland, serves to maintain homeostasis in body function. **–elaboration,** *n.*

Elase, a trademark for a topical, fixed-combination drug containing enzymes (fibrinolysin and desoxyribonuclease).

Elase with Chloromycetin, a trademark for a topical, fixed-combination drug containing two lytic enzymes and an antibacterial (chloramphenicol).

elastance /ilas′təns/ [Gk, *elaunein*, to drive], **1.** the quality of recoiling or returning to an original form after the removal of pressure. **2.** the degree to which an air-filled or fluid-filled organ, such as a lung, bladder, or blood vessel, can return to its original dimensions when a distending or compressing force is removed. **3.** the measurement of the unit volume of change in such an organ per unit of decreased pressure change. **4.** the reciprocal of compliance.

elastic bandage /ilas′tik/ [Gk, *elaunein*, to drive; Fr, *bande*, strip], a bandage of elasticized fabric that provides support and allows movement.

elastic-band fixation, a method of treatment of fractures of the jaw using rubber bands to connect metal splints or wires that are attached to the maxilla and mandible. The rubber bands produce traction and bring the teeth into occlusion and proper alignment while the fracture is healing. Rubber bands are safer than rigid wires in the event of vomiting. See also **maxillomandibular fixation, nasomandibular fixation.**

elastic bougie, a flexible bougie that can be passed through angular or winding channels.

elastic cartilage. See **yellow cartilage.**

elasticity /i'lastis'itē/, the ability of tissue to regain its original shape and size after being stretched, squeezed, or otherwise deformed. Muscle tissue is generally regarded as elastic because it is able to change size and shape and return to its original condition.

elastic membrane. See **cricothyroid membrane.**

elastic recoil /rē'koil/, the difference between intrapleural pressure and alveolar pressure at a given lung volume under static conditions.

elastic tissue [Gk, *elaunein,* to drive; OFr, *tissu*], a type of connective tissue containing elastic fibers. It is found in ligaments of the spinal column and in the walls of some large blood vessels.

elastic traction [Gk, *elaunein;* L, *trahere,* to draw], any therapeutic apparatus that uses an elastic device to pull on a limb.

elastin /ilas'tin/ [Gk, *elaunein,* to drive], a protein that forms the principal substance of yellow elastic tissue fibers.

elation /ilā'shən/ [L, *elatus,* a lifting up], an emotional reaction characterized by euphoria, excitement, extreme joyfulness, optimism, and self-satisfaction. It is considered to be of pathologic origin when such a response does not realistically reflect a person's actual circumstances. Thus an elated mood may be characteristic of a manic state.

Elavil, a trademark for an antidepressant (amitriptyline hydrochloride).

elbow [AS, *elboga*], the bend of the arm at the joint that connects the arm and forearm. It is a common site of inflammation and injuries, such as those incurred during participation in various sports. See also **elbow joint.**

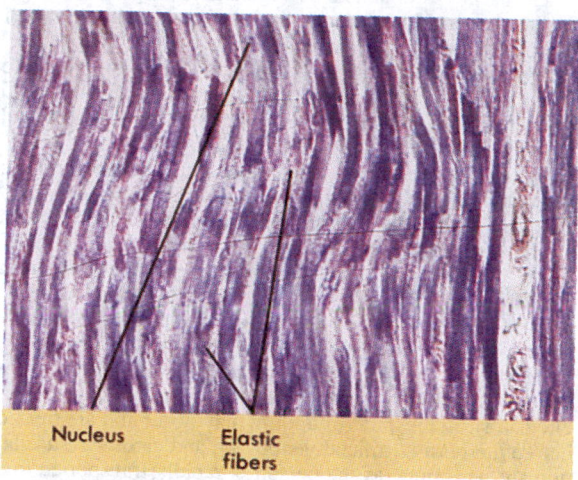

Dense regular elastic tissue *(Seeley, 1992/Trent Stephens)*

Nucleus   Elastic fibers

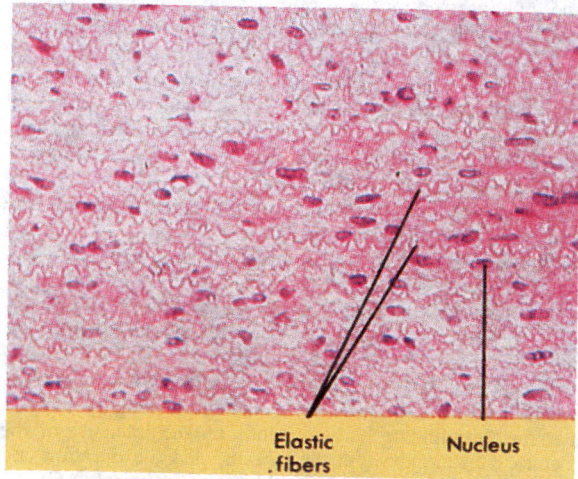

Elastic fibers   Nucleus

Dense irregular elastic tissue
(Seeley, 1992/Trent Stephens)

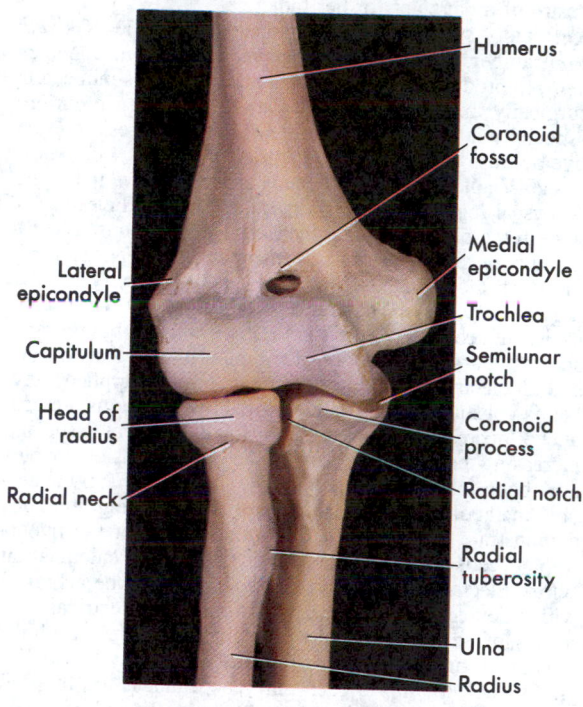

Humerus

Coronoid fossa

Medial epicondyle

Lateral epicondyle

Capitulum

Head of radius

Radial neck

Trochlea

Semilunar notch

Coronoid process

Radial notch

Radial tuberosity

Ulna

Radius

Elbow joint *(Vidic, 1984)*

elbow bone. See **ulna.**

elbow jerk [AS, *elboga,* elbow], a triceps reflex induced by tapping the triceps tendon near the insertion into the olecranon when the elbow is semiflexed. The reflex results in extension at the elbow joint. Also called **elbow reflex, triceps reflex.**

elbow joint, the hinged articulation of the humerus, the ulna, and the radius. It is covered by a protective capsule associated with three ligaments and an extensive synovial membrane. The elbow joint allows flexion and extension of the forearm and accommodates the radioulnar articulation. Also called **articulatio cubiti.**

elbow reflex. See **triceps reflex.**

elderly primagravida, a woman who becomes pregnant for the first time after the age of 34. Although an elderly primagravida was once at greater risk of adverse complications of a pregnancy, newer techniques and drugs have eliminated most of the risk and made it possible for even women of menopausal age to bear children.

Eldopaque, a trademark for a dermatologic bleaching agent (hydroquinone).

elective /ilek′tiv/ [L, *eligere*, to choose], of or pertaining to a procedure that is performed by choice but which is not essential, such as elective surgery.

elective abortion, induced termination of a pregnancy **(TOP),** usually before the fetus has developed enough to live if born, deemed necessary by the woman carrying it and performed at her request. Commonly (but incorrectly) called **therapeutic abortion.** See also **induced abortion, therapeutic abortion.**

elective induction of labor. See **induction of labor.**

Electra complex /ilek′trə/ (in psychiatry) the libidinous desire of a daughter for her father.

electrically stimulated osteogenesis /ilek′triklē/ [Gk, *elktron*, amber; L, *stimulare*, to incite; Gk, *osteon*, bone, *genein*, to produce], a bone regeneration process induced by surgically implanted electrodes conveying electric current, especially at nonunion fracture sites. The process is effective because of the different electrical potentials within bone tissue. Viable nonstressed bone is electronegative in the metaphyseal regions and over a fracture callus and electropositive in the diaphyses and other less active regions. Electric stimulation of fractures can accelerate osteogenesis, forming bone more quickly in the area of a surgically inserted negative electrode. The precise mechanisms by which electricity induces osteogenesis are not understood, but research shows that when cathodes are implanted at a fracture site and an electric potential of less than 1 volt is applied, oxygen is consumed at the cathode, and hydroxyl ions are produced, decreasing the oxygen tension of the local tissue and increasing the alkalinity. Low tissue-oxygen tension encourages bone formation, which follows a predominantly anaerobic metabolic pathway. Studies of bone-forming junctions demonstrate that an alkaline pH exists in the zone of hypertrophic cells of the bone growth plate when calcification starts. Electrically stimulated osteogenesis can be achieved with a device that stimulates the fracture site electrically by means of several surgically implanted cathodes. Cathode pins are connected to an external power supply that delivers 20 [Grk m]amp to each pin. The cathodes are inserted and positioned in the fracture space with the aid of image intensification or other radiographic techniques. Other methods for applying electric current to fractured bone involve open surgical procedures and the implantation of electrodes. The percutaneous technique involving the insertion of cathode pins is performed with a local anesthetic and usually involves less postoperative pain than open surgery methods. The number and the position of the cathodes in the percutaneous technique vary, depending on the bone involved. Generally two cathodes are used for nonunion fractures of small bones, such as the medial malleolus or the carpal navicular. Three or more cathodes are used in the clavicle and the bones of the forearm. Four cathodes are used in the treatment of large bones, such as the tibia, the femur, and the humerus. Cathodes are generally inserted from opposite directions into the nonunion site. If four cathodes are used, two are placed above and two below the fracture site, the exposed tips of the cathodes resting directly in the nonunion

space. Patients who receive such treatment are routinely released from the hospital the day after the procedure, and the stimulation of their fractures continues during the healing period from a portable power supply strapped to the skin over the fracture site. The osteogenesis is radiographically monitored, and after about 12 weeks the cathode pins are removed and the affected portion of the limb involved is placed in a weight-bearing cast. Use of the cathode-pin method of electrically stimulated osteogenesis is contraindicated in the treatment of pathologic fractures associated with benign or malignant tumors and in the treatment of congenital conditions, such as congenital pseudarthrosis and osteogenesis imperfecta. The cathode-pin method is also contraindicated in the presence of active systemic infections, clinically active osteomyelitis, proven patient sensitivity to the nickel or chromium from which the pins are made, or synovial pseudarthrosis, unless the fluid-filled cavity at the nonunion site is excised before the cathode pins are inserted. The success rate of treatment with the percutaneous method of electrically stimulated osteogenesis is significantly reduced in nonunions in which the gap is wider than one half the diameter of the bone involved.

electric blood warmer, a device for heating blood before infusions, especially massive transfusions in which cold blood might put the patient into shock. The electric blood warmer includes a receptacle containing an electric heater and space for the insertion of a disposable blood-warming bag composed of parallel plastic tubes. The warmer is also equipped with a temperature indicator, which shows when the heating bag reaches the proper temperature of 99° F (37.6° C). An intravenous Y-set is commonly employed in transfusions involving the electric blood warmer.

electric burns, the tissue damage resulting from heat of up to 5000° C generated by an electric current. The point of contact on the skin is burned, and the muscle and subcutaneous tissues may be damaged. If the burn is severe, circulatory and respiratory failure may occur and are treated before the burn. Artificial ventilation and cardiac resuscitation are performed as the person is rapidly transported to a medical facility.

electric cautery. See **electrocautery.**

electricity /i′lektris′itē/ [Gk, *elektron*, amber], a form of energy expressed by the activity of electrons and other subatomic particles in motion, as in dynamic electricity, or at rest, as in static electricity. Electricity can be produced by heat, generated by a voltaic cell, produced by induction, by rubbing nonconductors with dry materials, or by chemical activity. Electricity may be negative, when there is a surplus of electrons, or positive, when there is a surplus of protons or a deficiency of electrons.

electric potential gradient, the net difference in electric charge across the membrane of a cell.

electric shock, a traumatic physical state caused by the passage of electric current through the body. It usually involves accidental contact with exposed parts of electric circuits in home appliances and domestic power supplies but may also result from lightning or contact with high-voltage wires. About 1000 persons in the United States die from electric shock each year. The damage electricity does in passing through the body depends on the intensity of the electric current, the type of current, and the duration and the frequency of current flow. Alternating current (AC), direct current (DC), and mixed current cause different kinds and degrees of damage in passing through body tissues. High-frequency current produces more heat than low-frequency current and can cause burns, coagulation, and necrosis of affected body parts. Low-frequency current can burn tissues if the area of contact is small and concentrated. Severe electric shock commonly causes unconsciousness, respiratory paralysis, muscle contractions, bone fractures, and cardiac disorders. Even small electric currents passing through the heart can cause fibrillation. Treatment of electric shock commonly involves such measures as cardiopulmonary resuscitation, defibrillation, and the intravenous administration of electrolytes to help stabilize vital functions. See also **cardiogenic shock, hypovolemic shock.**

electric shock therapy. See **electroconvulsive therapy (ECT).**

electric spinal orthosis, an electric device that helps control curvature of the spine by stimulating back muscles. The portable, battery-powered machine does not correct scoliosis but prevents worsening of the condition.

electro-, a prefix meaning 'pertaining to electricity': *electrobiology, electrocatalysis, electrolepsy.*

electroanalgesia /ilek′trō·an′əljē′sē·ə/, the use of an electric current, applied to the spinal cord or a peripheral nerve, to relieve pain. Also called **transcutaneous electrical nerve stimulation (TENS).**

electroanalytic chemistry /-an′əlit′ik/ [Gk, *elektron* + *analysis*, a loosening; *chemeia*, alchemy], the branch of chemistry concerned with the analysis of compounds using electric current to produce characteristic, observable change in the substance being studied. See also **chemistry.**

electroanesthesia /-an′esthē′zhə/, the use of an electric current to produce local or general anesthesia.

electrocardiogram (ECG, EKG) /-kär′dē·əgram′/ [Gk, *elektron* + *kardia*, heart, *gramma*, record], a graphic record produced by an electrocardiograph.

electrocardiograph (ECG) /-kär′dē·əgraf′/, a device used for recording the electric activity of the myocardium to detect transmission of the cardiac impulse through the conductive tissues of the muscle. Electrocardiography allows diagnosis of specific cardiac abnormalities. Leads are affixed to certain anatomic points on the patient's chest, usually with an adhesive gel that promotes transmission of the electric impulse to the recording device. —**electrocardiographic,** *adj.*

electrocardiographic-auscultatory syndrome. See **Barlow's syndrome.**

electrocardiographic technician /-kär′dē·ōgraf′ik/, an allied health professional with special training and experience in operating and maintaining electrocardiographic equipment and providing recorded data for diagnostic review by a physician.

electrocardiograph lead /lēd/, 1. an electrode placed on part of the body and connected to an electrocardiograph. 2. a record, made by the electrocardiograph, that varies depending on the site of the electrode. Electrocardiography is generally performed with the use of three peripheral leads and six leads placed on the precordium. The peripheral or extremity leads are designated I, II, and III, and the chest leads are designated V_1, V_2, V_3, V_4, V_5, and V_6 to indicate the points on the precordium on which the electrodes are placed.

electrocardiography /-kär′dē·og′rəfē/ [Gk, *elektron, kardia,* heart, *graphein,* to record], a method of recording electrical activity generated by the heart muscle.

electrocautery /ilek′trōkô′tərē/ [Gk, *elektron* + *kauterion,* branding iron], the application of a needle or snare heated by electric current for the destruction of tissue, such as for the removal of warts or polyps and to cauterize small blood vessels to decrease blood loss during surgery. Also called **electric cautery, galvanic cautery, galvanocautery.** See also **diathermy.**

Correctly recorded ECG

Landmarks for ECG 6-lead placement

Suprasternal notch
Angle of Louis or sternal angle
Midclavicular line
Second rib
Second interspace

V_1
V_2
V_3
V_4
V_5
V_6

Landmarks for ECG 6-lead placement

Electrocardiogram (ECG)
Correctly recorded ECG,
Normal waveform (Berne, 1988),
Landmarks for ECG 6-lead placement

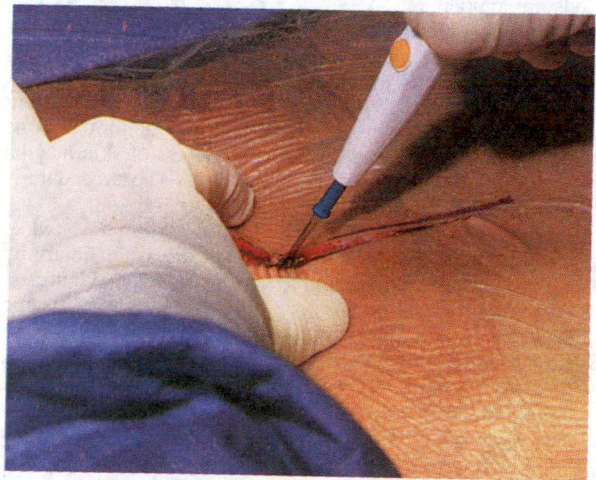

Electrocautery (Bray, 1993/Steve Young)

electrocoagulation /-kō·ag′yəlā′shən/ [Gk, *elektron* + L, *coagulare,* to curdle], a therapeutic, destructive form of electrosurgery in which tissue is hardened by the passage of high-frequency current from an electric cautery device. Also called **surgical diathermy.** Compare **electrodesiccation.**

electroconvulsive therapy (ECT) /-kənvul′siv/, the induction of a brief convulsion by passing an electric current through the brain for the treatment of affective disorders, especially in patients resistant to psychoactive-drug therapy. The patient is placed in a comfortable supine position with the limbs lightly restrained and with a padded tongue depressor between the back teeth, after premedication with succinylcholine to prevent fractures. Conductive paste is applied to the skin on both sides of the forehead where the electrodes are placed, and a 70 to 130 volt current is delivered for 0.1 to 0.5 seconds. The patient loses consciousness and undergoes tonic contractions for approximately 10 seconds, followed by a somewhat longer period of clonic convulsions accompanied by apnea; on awakening the individual has no memory of the shock. ECT is usually administered three times a week for 2 months and is used primarily for the treatment of acute depression. Also called **electric shock therapy (EST), electroshock therapy (EST), electrotherapy.**

electrocution /-kyo͞o′shən/, death caused by the passage of electric current through the body. See also **electric shock.**

electrode /ilek′trōd/ [Gk, *elektron* + *hodos*, way], **1.** a contact for the induction or detection of electric activity. **2.** a medium for conducting an electric current from the body to physiologic monitoring equipment.

electrodermal audiometry /-dur′məl/ [Gk, *elektron* + *derma*, skin; L, *audire*, to hear; Gk, *metron*, measure], a method of testing hearing in which a harmless electric shock is used to condition the subject to a pure tone; thereafter the tone, coupled with the anticipation of a shock, elicits a brief electrodermal response, which is recorded, and the lowest intensity of the sound producing the skin response is considered the subject's hearing threshold. It may be used for subjects who do not cooperate when conventional methods are applied.

electrodesiccation /-des′ikā′shən/ [Gk, *elektron* + *desiccare*, to dry up], a technique in electrosurgery in which tissue is destroyed by burning with an electric spark. It is used primarily for eliminating small superficial growths but may be used with curettage for eradicating abnormal tissue deeper in the skin. In the latter case, layers of skin may be burned, then successively scraped away. The procedure is performed under local anesthesia.

electrodiagnosis /-dī′agnō′sis/ [Gk, *elektron, dia,* twice, *gnosis,* knowledge], the diagnosis of disease or injury by applying electric stimulation to various nerves and muscles.

electrodynamics /-dīnam′iks/, the study of electrostatic charges in motion, such as the flow of electrons in an electric current. Compare **electrohemodynamics.**

electrodynograph (EDG) /-din′əgraf′/ [Gk, *elektron* + *dynamis,* force, *graphein,* to record], an electronic device used to measure pressures exerted in biologic activity, such as the pressures exerted by the human foot in walking, running, jogging, or climbing stairs.

electroencephalogram (EEG) /ilek′trō·ensef′ələgram′/ [Gk, *elektron* + *enkephalos,* brain, *gramma,* record], a graphic chart on which is traced the electric potential produced by the brain cells, as detected by electrodes placed on the scalp. The resulting brain waves are called alpha, beta, delta, and theta rhythms, according to the frequencies

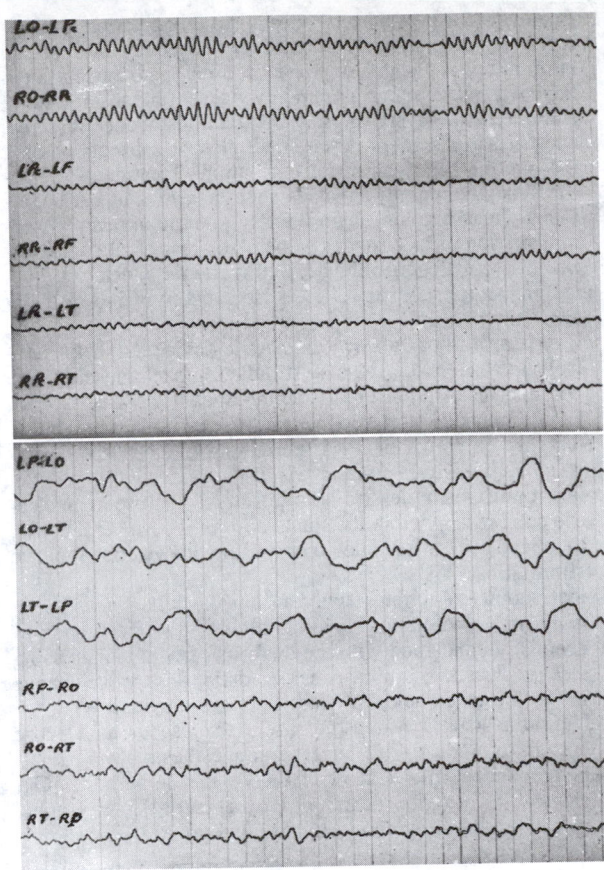

Electroencephalogram
top: normal; bottom: intracranial tumor

they produce, which range from 2 to 12 cps with an amplitude of up to 100 μV. Variations in brain-wave activity correlate with neurologic conditions, psychologic states, and level of consciousness. See also **encephalography.**

electroencephalograph /ilek′trō·ensef′ələgraf′/, an instrument for receiving and recording the electric potential produced by the brain cells. It consists of a vacuum-tube amplifier that magnifies the electric currents received through electrodes placed on the scalp and electromagnetically records the patterns on a graphic chart. See also **electroencephalography.**

electroencephalographic technologist /ilek′trō·ensef′-ələgraf′ik/, a person trained in the management of an electroencephalographic laboratory. The technologist may supervise electroencephalographic technicians, who are generally responsible for the operation and maintenance of the equipment.

electroencephalography (EEG) /ilek′trō·ensef′əlog′rəfē/, the process of recording brain-wave activity. Electrodes are attached to various areas of the patient's head with collodion. During the procedure the patient remains quiet, with eyes closed, and refrains from talking or moving, although, in certain cases, prescribed activities may be requested, especially hyperventilation. The test is used to diagnose seizure disorders, brainstem disorders, focal lesions, and impaired consciousness. During neurosurgery, the electrodes can be applied directly to the surface of the brain (intracranial electroencephalography) or placed within the brain tissue (depth electroencephalography) to detect lesions or tumors. See also **electroencephalogram.** −**electroencephalographic,** *adj.*

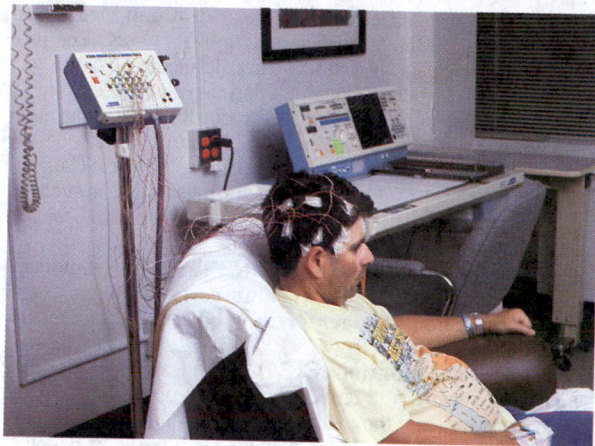

Electroencephalography (*Chipps, 1992*)

electrogram /ilek′trōgram′/ [Gk, *elektron* + *gramma,* record], a unipolar or bipolar record of electric activity of the heart as recorded from electrodes within the cardiac chambers or on the epicardium. Examples are atrial electrogram (AEG), ventricular electrogram (VEG), and His bundle electrogram (HBE).

electrohemodynamics (EHD) /ilek′trōhē′mōdīnam′iks/ [Gk, *elektron* + *haima,* blood, *dynamis,* force], a technique for noninvasively measuring the mechanical properties and hemodynamic characteristics of the vascular system, including arterial blood pressure, electric impedance, blood flow, and resistance to blood flow.

electroimmunodiffusion. See **immunodiffusion.**

electrolysis /il′ektrol′isis/ [Gk, *elektron* + *lysis,* loosening], a process in which electric energy causes a chemical change in a conducting medium, usually a solution or a molten substance. Electrodes, usually pieces of metal, induce the flow of electric energy through the medium. Electrons enter the solution through the cathode and leave the solution through the anode. Negatively charged ions, or anions, are attracted to the anode; positively charged ions, or cations, are attracted to the cathode. Various conducting mediums are used, such as solutions of copper, zinc, nickel, lead, and silver. Electric energy passing through such solutions causes deposition of pure metal at the cathode. Passing electric energy through solutions of alkali and alkaline-earth salts liberates hydrogen at the cathode. A metal anode causes metal ions to flow from the anode into the solution as the electric current passes through the medium. An inert electrode, as one of platinum, may liberate oxygen at the anode in an aqueous medium. A halogen salt solution liberates free bromine, chlorine, or iodine. Fluorine, which has a high oxidation potential, is not liberated by electrolysis. −**electrolytic,** *adj.*

electrolyte /ilek′trōlīt/ [Gk, *elektron* + *lytos,* soluble], an

Normal electrolyte content of body fluids*

Electrolytes (anions and cations)	Extracellular		Intracellular (mEq/L)
	Intravascular (mEq/L)	Interstitial (mEq/L)	
Sodium (Na^+)	142	146	15
Potassium (K^+)	5	5	150
Calcium (Ca^{++})	5	3	2
Magnesium (Mg^{++})	2	1	27
Chloride (Cl^-)	102	114	1
Bicarbonate (HCO_3^-)	27	30	10
Protein ($Prot^-$)	16	1	63
Phosphate ($HPO_4^=$)	2	2	100
Sulfate ($SO_4^=$)	1	1	20
Organic acids	5	8	0

*Note that the electrolyte level of the intravascular and interstitial fluids (extracellular) is approximately the same and that sodium and chloride contents are markedly higher in these fluids, whereas potassium, phosphate, and protein contents are markedly higher in intracellular fluid.
From Phipps WJ, Long BL, Woods NF, Cassmeyer VL: *Medical-surgical nursing: concepts and clinical practice, ed 4,* St Louis, 1991, Mosby.

element or compound that, when melted or dissolved in water or other solvent, dissociates into ions and is able to conduct an electric current. Electrolytes differ in their concentrations in blood plasma, interstitial fluid, and cell fluid and affect the movement of substances between those compartments. Proper quantities of principal electrolytes and balance among them are critical to normal metabolism and function. For example, calcium ($Ca++$) is necessary for the contraction of skeletal muscle and relaxation of cardiac muscle. Sodium ($Na+$) is essential in maintaining fluid balance. Certain diseases, conditions, and medications may lead to a deficiency of one or more electrolytes and to an imbalance among them; for example, certain diuretics and a low-sodium diet prescribed in hypertension may cause hypokalemic shock resulting from a loss of potassium. Diarrhea may cause a loss of many electrolytes, leading to hypovolemia and shock, especially in infants. Careful and regular monitoring of electrolytes and intravenous replacement of fluid and electrolytes are part of the acute care in many illnesses. −**electrolytic,** *adj.*

electrolyte balance, the equilibrium between electrolytes in the body.

electrolyte solution, any solution containing electrolytes prepared for oral, parenteral, or rectal administration for the replacement or supplementation of ions necessary for homeostasis. The loss of potassium ion ($K+$) by vomiting, by diarrhea, or by the action of certain medications, including diuretics and corticosteroids, may be corrected by administering a solution high in potassium. Other electrolyte solutions containing combinations of calcium, sodium, phosphate, chloride, or magnesium may be given to treat acid-base disturbance, as seen in chronic renal dysfunction or diabetic ketoacidosis. The solutions are available in a wide range of balanced formulas for replacement or maintenance, and most include various trace minerals.

-electrolytic. See **electrolysis.**

electromagnetic /-magnet′ik/ [Gk, *elektron, Magnesia,* ancient source of lodestone], pertaining to magnetism that is induced by an electric current.

electromagnetic induction [Gk, *elektron* + *magnes,* lodestone; L, *inducere,* to bring in], the production of electric current in a circuit when the circuit is passed through a changing magnetic field.

electromagnetic radiation, every kind of electric and magnetic radiation, regarded as a continuous spectrum of energy that includes energy with the shortest wavelength (gamma rays, with a wavelength of 0.0011 Å) to that with the longest wavelength (long radio waves, with a wavelength of more than 1 million kilometers). The visible part of the electromagnetic spectrum is between 3800 and 7600 Å. Ultraviolet radiation occurs beyond the short-wave (violet) end of the visible spectrum, having a wavelength of less than 4000 Å; x-rays have a much shorter wavelength (from 0.05 to a few hundred Å). Infrared radiation occurs just beyond the longer wave end of the visible spectrum, having a wavelength of 7000 Å or more.

electromagnetic tape. See **mag tape.**

electromallet condenser /-mal′ət/ [Gk, *elektron* + OFr, *mail* maul; L, *condensare*, to make dense], an electromechanic device for compacting direct-filling gold in prepared tooth cavities. The frequency of the blows delivered by this instrument may be varied from 200 to 3600 strokes per minute. The intensity of the blows is electrically controlled. Also called **McShirley's electromallet.**

electromotive force (EMF) /-mō′tiv/, the electric potential, or ability of electric energy to perform work. EMF is usually measured in joules per coulomb, or volts (V). The higher the voltage, the greater the potential of electric energy. Any device, such as a storage battery, that converts some form of energy into electricity is a source of EMF.

electromyogram (EMG) /ilek′trōmī′əgram′/, a record of the intrinsic electric activity in a skeletal muscle. Such data help in diagnosing neuromuscular problems and are obtained by applying surface electrodes or by inserting a needle electrode into the muscle and observing electric activity with an oscilloscope and a loudspeaker. Some electromyograms show abnormalities, such as spontaneous electric potentials within the muscle under study, and help pinpoint lesions of motor nerves. Electromyograms also measure electric poten tials induced by voluntary muscular contraction. See also **electroneuromyography.**

electron /ilek′tron/ [Gk, *elektron*, amber], **1.** a negatively charged elementary particle that has a specific charge, mass, and spin. The number of electrons associated with the nucleus of an atom is equal to the atomic number of the substance. **2.** a negative beta particle emitted from a radioactive substance. See also **atom, element, ion, neutron, proton.**

electronarcosis /ilek′trōnärkō′sis/ [Gk, *elektron* + *narkosis*, numbness], general anesthesia without the use of anesthetic gases or drugs. Narcosis is produced by passing an electric current through the brain, but adequate control and prevention of undesirable side effects, especially convulsions, remain a problem. The procedure is experimental. Compare **electrosleep therapy.**

electron capture, a radioactive decay process in which a nucleus with an excess of protons brings an electron into the nucleus, creating a neutron out of a proton, thus decreasing the atomic number of the atom by 1. The resulting atom is often unstable and gives off a gamma ray to achieve stability.

electroneurodiagnostic technologist, an allied health professional who specializes in recording and studying the electric activity of the brain. Working in collaboration with an electroencephalographer, the electroneurodiagnostic technologist takes and abstracts medical histories, applies adequate recording electrodes using EEG and EP techniques and understands the interface between EEG and EP equipment and other electrophysiologic devices. The responsibilities may also include laboratory management and supervision of EEG technicians.

electroneuromyography /ilek′trōnōōr′ōmī·og′rəfē/ [Gk, *elektron* + *neuron*, nerve, *mys*, muscle, *graphein*, to record], a procedure for testing and recording neuromuscular activity by the electric stimulation of nerves. The procedure involves the insertion of needle electrodes into any skeletal muscle being studied, applying electric current to the electrodes, and observing and recording neuromuscular functions by means of instruments, such as a cathode-ray oscilloscope and an appropriate recording device. The procedure is helpful in the study of neuromuscular conduction, the extent of nerve lesions, and reflex responses. See also **electromyogram.**

electronic bulletin board /ilektron′ik/ a computerized communications system that allows users to compose and store information to be retrieved by other users of the system.

electronic fetal monitor (EFM) [Gk, *elektron* + L, *fetus; monere*, to warn], a device that allows observation of the fetal heart rate and the maternal uterine contractions. It may be applied externally, in which case the fetal heart is detected by an ultrasound transducer positioned on the abdomen and the uterine contractions by a pressure sensor applied to the abdomen. Internal monitoring of the fetal heart rate is accomplished via an electrode clipped to the fetal scalp; the amplitude, frequency, and duration of the uterine contractions are detected by the use of an intrauterine catheter.

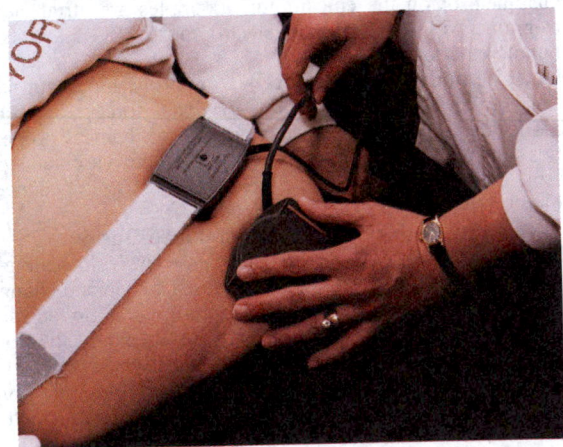

External fetal monitor

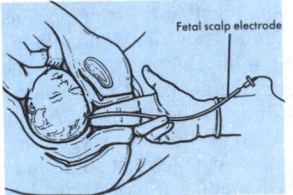

Internal fetal monitor

Electronic fetal monitoring (Dickason, 1994)

electronic mail (E-mail), messages sent by one user of an computerized communications system and retrieved instantaneously by another user. The messages may be transmitted via modem through telephone lines or, in some instances, by shortwave radio. See also **electronic bulletin board.**

electronic thermometer, a thermometer that registers temperature rapidly by electronic means.

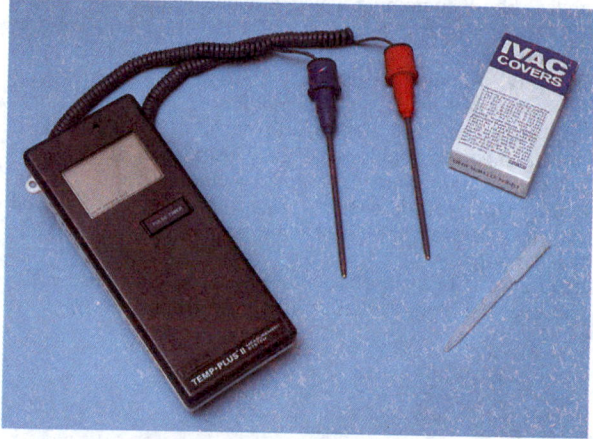

Electronic thermometer (Potter, 1993)

electron microscope, an instrument, similar to an optic microscope, that scans cell surfaces with a beam of electrons, instead of visible light, creating an image that can be photographed or viewed on a fluorescent screen. Compare **scanning electron microscope.** See also **electron microscopy.**

electron microscopy, a technique, using an electron microscope, in which a beam of electrons is focused by an electromagnetic lens and directed onto an extremely thin specimen. The electrons emerging are focused and directed by a second lens onto a fluorescent screen. The magnified image produced is 1000 times greater than with an optic microscope, and well resolved, but it is two-dimensional because of the thinness of the specimen. Also called **transmission electron microscopy.** Compare **scanning electron microscopy, transmission scanning electron microscopy.**

electron scanning microscope. See **scanning electron microscope.**

electron volt (eV), a unit of energy equal to the energy acquired by an electron in falling through a potential difference of one volt. One eV equals 1.6 [ti] 10[mi]12 erg or 1.6 [ti] 10[mi]19 J.

electronystagmography /ilek′trōnis′tagmog′rəfē/ [Gk, *elektron + nystagmos,* nodding, *graphein,* to record], a method of assessing and recording eye movements by measuring the electric activity of the extraocular muscles. See also **electroencephalogram, nystagmus.**

electrophoresis /ilek′trōfərē′sis/ [Gk, *elektron + pherein,* to bear], the movement of charged suspended particles through a liquid medium in response to changes in an electric field. Charged particles of a given substance migrate in a predictable direction and at a characteristic speed. The pattern of migration can be recorded in bands on an **electrophoretogram** /ilek′trōfəret′ōgram/. The technique is widely used to separate and identify serum proteins and other substances. *electrophoretic, adj.*

electrophysiology /-fis′ē·ol′əjē/ [Gk, *elektron, physis,* nature, *logos,* science], a branch of medical science concerned with the relationship between electric phenomena and human health.

electroporation /-pôrā′shən/, a type of osmotic transfection in which an electric current is used to produce holes in cell membranes so the alien DNA molecules can enter the cells. See also **transfection.**

electroresection /-risek′shən/ [Gk, *elektron* + L, *re,* again, *secare* to cut], a technique for the removal of bladder tumors by the insertion of an electric wire through the urethra. The electric wire is guided to the site with the aid of an optic probe. The electric lead is not energized until it is properly located in the tumor to be destroyed. The procedure is performed after administration of an anesthetic.

electroshock [Gk, *elektron;* Fr, *choc*], a condition of shock caused by accidental contact with an electric current. The symptoms are similar to those of shock by thermal burns, trauma, or coronary thrombosis.

electroshock therapy. See **electroconvulsive therapy (ECT).**

electrosleep therapy [Gk, *elektron* + AS, *slaep;* Gk, *therapeia,* treatment], a technique designed to induce sleep, especially in psychiatric patients, by administering a low-amplitude pulsating current to the brain. The cathode is placed supraorbitally, and the anode is placed over the mastoid process. The current, which is discharged for 15 to 20 minutes, produces a tingling sensation, but does not always induce sleep. The procedure is repeated from 5 to 30 times. Electrosleep therapy is said to be beneficial for patients with anxiety, depression, gastric distress, insomnia, personality disorders, and schizophrenia, but double-blind studies have yielded conflicting results. Compare **electronarcosis.**

electrostatic imaging /-stat′ik/ [Gk, *elektron* + *stasis,* standing still; L, *imago,* image], techniques for producing radiographic images in which the ionic charge liberated during the irradiation process is converted to a visible image using electronic read-out devices or by the use of liquid or powder 'toner' to convert a latent charge image into a visible one.

electrosurgery /-sur′jərē/ [Gk, *elektron* + *cheiourgos,* surgeon], surgery performed with various electric instruments that operate on high-frequency electric current. Kinds of electrosurgery include **electrocoagulation, electrodesiccation.**

electrotherapy. See **electroconvulsive therapy (ECT).**

electrotonic current [Gk, *elektron* + *tonos,* tension], a current induced in a nerve sheath by an action potential within the nerve or an adjacent nerve.

eleidin /əlē′ədin/ [Gk, *elaia,* olive tree], a transparent protein substance, resembling keratin, found in the stratum lucidum of the epidermis.

element [L, *elementum,* first principle], one of more than 100 primary, simple substances that cannot be broken down by chemical means into any other substance. Each atom of any element contains a specific number of electrons orbiting the nucleus. The nucleus contains a variable number of neutrons. A **stable element** contains an equal number of neutrons and electrons and does not easily give up neutrons. A **radioactive element** does not contain a balanced number of electrons and neutrons, and gives off neutrons readily. See also **atom, compound, molecule.**

element 104,　a synthetic, radioactive element, the twelfth transuranic element, and the first transactinide element. Also called **rutherfordium (Rf)** and **kurchatovium (Ku).**

element 105,　a synthetic element, and the thirteenth transuranic element. Also called **hahnium (Ha).**

element 106,　a synthetic radioactive element, with a half-life of 0.9 seconds. It was first synthesized in 1974 by scientists working independently in the United States and the Russia.

element 107,　an element reportedly synthesized in 1976 by Russian scientists who bombarded isotopes of bismuth with heavy nuclei of chromium 54. The finding was not confirmed by scientists of other nations.

eleo-,　a combining form meaning 'pertaining to oil': *eleoma, eleomyenchysis, eleopten.*

elephantiasis /el'əfəntī'əsis/ [Gk, *elephas*, elephant, *osis*, condition],　the end-stage lesion of filariasis, characterized by tremendous swelling, usually of the external genitalia and the legs. The overlying skin becomes dark, thick, and coarse. Elephantiasis results from filariasis that has lasted for many years. See also **filariasis.**

elephantoid fever.　See **elephantiasis, filariasis.**

eleventh nerve.　See **accessory nerve.**

elimination diet /ilim'inā'shən/ [L, *elininare*, to expel; Gk, *diata*, way of living],　a procedure for identifying a food or foods to which a person is allergic by successively omitting from the diet certain foods in order to detect those responsible for the symptoms.

ELISA /əlī'zə/,　abbreviation for **enzyme-linked immunosorbent assay.**

elixir /ilik'sər/ [Ar *il-iksir* seen as the 'philosopher's stone'],　a clear liquid containing water, alcohol, sweeteners, or flavors, used primarily as a vehicle for the oral administration of a drug.

Elixophyllin,　a trademark for a smooth muscle relaxant (theophylline), used as a bronchodilator.

Elliot forceps.　See **obstetric forceps.**

Elliot's position [John W. Elliott, American surgeon, b. 1852],　a supine posture assumed by the patient on the operating table, with a support placed under the lower costal margin to elevate the chest. The position is used in gallbladder surgery.

elliptocyte /ilip'təsīt/ [Gk, *elleipsis*, ellipse, *kytos*, cell],　an oval red blood cell. See also **elliptocytosis.**

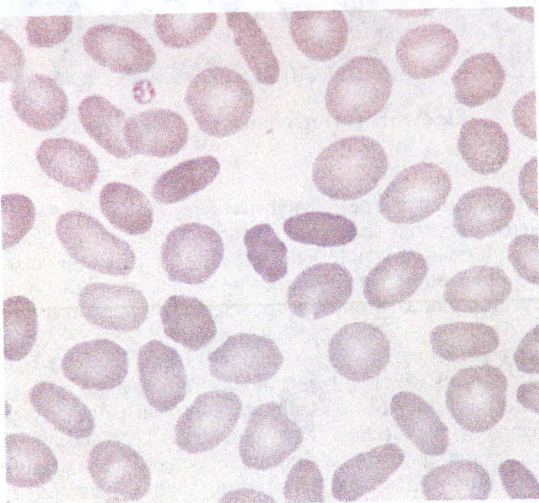

Elliptocytes (Bain, 1989)

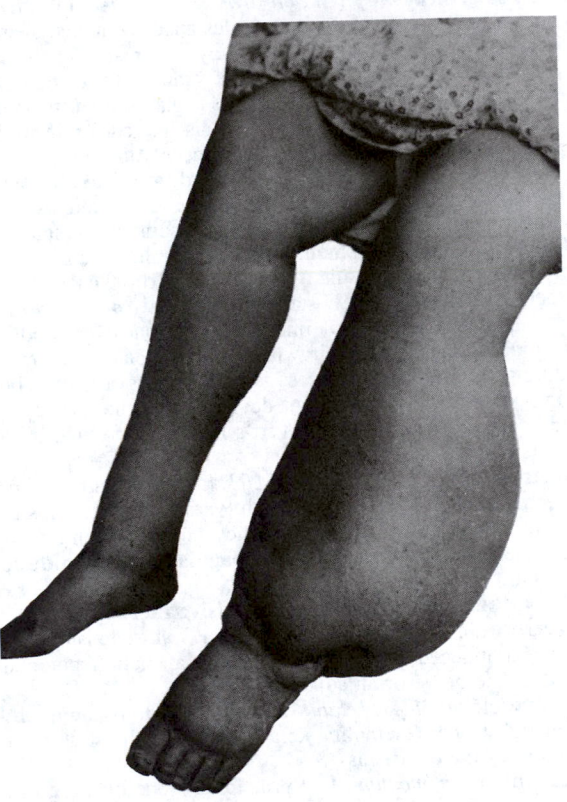

Elephantiasis

(Murray, 1990/from Binford CH and Conner DH: Pathology of tropical and extraordinary diseases. Washington, DC, 1976, Armed Forces Institute of Pathology)

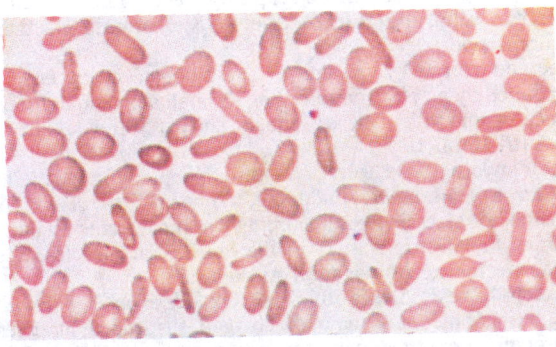

Elliptocytosis (Hayhoe, 1992)

elliptocytosis /ilip′tōsītō′sis/ [Gk, *elleipsis, kytos + osis,* condition], an abnormal condition of the blood characterized by increased numbers of elliptocytes or oval erythrocytes. Less than 15% of the red cells appear in this form in normal blood; modest increases occur in a variety of anemias, including a rare congenital disorder, hereditary elliptocytosis. Also called **ovalocytosis.** Compare **spherocytosis.** See **acanthocytosis, congenital nonspherocytic hemolytic anemia, sickle cell anemia, spherocytic anemia.**

Ellis-van Creveld syndrome. See **chondroectodermal dysplasia.**

elongation /i′longā′shən/ [L, *elongatio,* a prolonging], a state of being lengthened or extended.

elope /ilōp′/ [ME, *gantlopp,* to run away], *informal.* to leave a locked psychiatric institution without notice or permission.

Elspar, a trademark for an antineoplastic (asparaginase).

eluate /el′yo͞o·āt/ [L, *eluere,* to wash out], a solution or substance that results from an elution process. In column chromatography, the eluate is collected as it drips from the column.

eluent /el′yo͞o·ənt/, a solvent or solution used in an elution process, such as column chromatography.

elution /elo͞o′shən/, the removal of an absorbed substance from a porous bed or chromatographic column by means of a stream of liquid or gas or by the application of heat. The technique may consist of washing a material that dissolves out just one component of a mixture. The term is also applied to the removal of antibodies or radioactive tracers from erythrocytes. In heat elution of antibodies, red cells in a saline solution are heated to 56° C and then centrifuged. Liquid elution of antibodies usually employs ether as the solvent.

em, abbreviation for **extrinsic muscles.**

em-, a prefix meaning 'in, on': *embolism, empasma, emphysis.*

emaciation /imā′shi·ā′shən/ [L, *emaciare,* to make lean], excessive leanness caused by disease or lack of nutrition.

E-mail. See **electronic mail.**

emancipated minor /iman′sipā′tid/ [L, *emancipare,* to set free], a person who is not legally an adult but who, because he or she is married, in the military, or otherwise no longer dependent upon the parents, may not require parental permission for medical or surgical care. State and national laws vary in specific interpretations of the rule.

emasculation /imas′kyəlā′shən/, a loss of the testes or penis or both. See also **castration.**

embalming /embä′ming/, the practice of applying antiseptics and preservatives to a corpse to retard the natural decomposition of tissues.

Embden-Meyerhof defects /emb′denmī′ərhof/ [Gustav G. Embden, German biochemist, b. 1874; Otto F. Meyerhof, German biochemist, b. 1884], a group of hereditary hemolytic anemias caused by enzyme deficiencies. The most common form of the disorder is a pyruvate kinase deficiency. The condition is characterized by an absence of spherocytes and the presence of small numbers of crenated erythrocytes. The trait is transmitted as an autosomal recessive gene, and the hemolytic anemia occurs only in homozygotes.

Embden-Meyerhof pathway, a sequence of enzymatic reactions in the anaerobic conversion of glucose to lactic

acid, producing energy which is stored in the form of adenosine triphosphate.

embedded tooth, an unerupted tooth, usually completely covered with bone. Also called **imbedded tooth.** Compare **impacted tooth.**

embolectomy /em′bəlek′təmē/ [Gk, *embolos,* plug, *ektome,* excision], a surgical incision into an artery for the removal of an embolus or clot, performed as emergency treatment for arterial embolism. The operation is done within 4 to 6 hours of the onset of pain, if possible. Thrombi tend to lodge at the juncture of major arteries when the thrombi have broken away from a thrombophlebitis; more than half lodge in the aorta, in arteries of the lower extremities, in the common carotid arteries, or in the pulmonary arteries. Preoperatively, anticoagulants are administered, and an arteriogram is done to identify the affected artery. A longitudinal incision is made in the artery, and the embolus is removed. Postoperatively, the blood pressure is maintained close to the level of the preoperative baseline, as a decrease might predispose to new clot formation. A frequent complication of the procedure is hemorrhage from small arteries that may have been clogged with the embolus but overlooked while tying larger bleeding vessels.

embolic /embol′ik/ [Gk, *embolus,* plug], pertaining to or resembling an embolus or embolism.

embolic gangrene [Gk, *embolus, gaggraina*], the death and putrifaction of body tissues caused by an embolus blocking the blood supply to that part.

embolic thrombosis [Gk, *embolos,* plug + *thrombos,* lump, + *osis,* condition], a thrombosis that develops at the site of an impacted embolus in a blood vessel.

embolism /em′bəliz′əm/, an abnormal circulatory condition in which an embolus travels through the bloodstream and becomes lodged in a blood vessel. The symptoms vary with the degree of occlusion that results, the character of the embolus, and the size, nature, and location of the occluded vessel. Kinds of embolism include **air embolism** and **fat embolism.**

embolization agent, a substance used to occlude or drastically reduce blood flow within a vessel. Examples include vasoconstrictors, microfibrillar collagen, Gelfoam, polyvinyl alcohol, and silicone beads.

-emboloid. See **embolus.**

embolized atheroma, an embolized fat particle lodged in a blood vessel.

embolotherapy /em′bəlōther′əpē/, a technique of blocking a blood vessel with a balloon catheter. It is used for treating bleeding ulcers and blood vessel defects and, during surgery, to stop blood flow to a tumor.

embolus /em′bələs/, *pl.* **emboli** [Gk, *embolos,* plug], a foreign object, a quantity of air or gas, a bit of tissue or tumor, or a piece of a thrombus that circulates in the bloodstream until it becomes lodged in a vessel. Kinds of emboli include **air embolus** and **fat embolus.** –**embolic, emboloid,** *adj.*

embol- 1. a prefix meaning 'to throw in': *embolia, embole.* 2. a prefix meaning 'pertaining to an embolus or plug': *embolectomy.*

embrasure /embrā′zhər/, a normally occurring space formed between adjacent teeth because of variations in positions and contours.

embryatrics. See **fetology.**

embryectomy /em′brē·ek′təmē/ [Gk, *en,* in, *bryein,* to grow, *ektome*, excision], the surgical removal of an embryo, most commonly in an ectopic pregnancy.

embryo /em'brē·ō/ [Gk, *en*, in, *bryein*, to grow], **1.** any organism in the earliest stages of development. **2.** in humans, the stage of prenatal development between the time of implantation of the fertilized ovum about 2 weeks after conception until the end of the seventh or eighth week. The period is characterized by rapid growth, differentiation of the major organ systems, and development of the main external features. Compare **fetus, zygote.** —**embryonal, embryonoid, embryonic,** *adj*.

embryo-, a combining form meaning a 'fetus': *embryoctony, embryology*.

embryoctony /em'brē·ok'tənē/ [Gk, *en*, *bryein* + *kteinein*, to kill], the intentional destruction of the living embryo or fetus in utero. Also called **feticide.** See also **abortion.**

embryogenesis /em'brē·ōjen'əsis/ [Gk, *en*, *bryein* + *genein*, to produce], the process in sexual reproduction by which an embryo forms from the fertilization of an ovum. Also called **embryogeny** /em'brē·oj'ənē/. See also **heterogenesis, homogenesis.** —**embryogenetic, embryogenic.** *adj*.

-embryologic. See **embryology.**

-embryological. See **embryology.**

embryologic development /-loj'ik/, the various intrauterine stages and processes involved in the growth and differentiation of the conceptus from the time of fertilization of the ovum until the eighth week of gestation. The stages are related to the biologic status of the unborn child and are divided into two distinct periods. The first is embryogenesis, or the formation of the embryo, which occurs during the 10 days to 2 weeks after fertilization until implantation. The second period, organogenesis, involves the differentiation of the various cells, tissues, and organ systems and the development of the main external features of the embryo; it occurs from approximately the end of the second week to the eighth week of intrauterine life. The fetal stage follows these stages, beginning at about the ninth week of gestation. The entire process of the growth and development of the embryo and fetus is loosely called prenatal development. Embryogenesis is initiated shortly after fertilization by the formation of the zygote from the fusion of the pronuclei of the spermatozoon and the ovum. The zygote then divides by cleavage to form blastomeres, which eventually cluster into a solid mass of cells, called the morula, that are uniform in size, shape, and physiologic capabilities. With continued division the cells become unequal in size and shape, and fluid accumulates between them to produce the blastocyst. This hollow ball of cells consists of an outer layer, the trophoblast, and a localized inner cluster, the inner cell mass, which protrudes into the cavity. The inner cell mass contains two formative layers that differentiate into the primary germ layers and develop into the embryo. The trophoblastic cells contain the enzymes and other substances necessary for the implantation of the blastocyst onto the uterine wall and the formation of the extraembryonic structures, as the chorion and the placenta. By the time of implantation and the beginning of organogenesis, the endoderm, ectoderm, and mesoderm germ layers have differentiated into the embryonic disk and have formed the amniotic cavity and yolk sac cavity. During this stage, the embryo develops rapidly, changing from a flat, disklike shape into an elongated, cylindric, curved mass that contains the primitive structures, which will subsequently differentiate into all the organs and cavities of the body. By the fourth week of development, the primitive body includes the neural tube, which will develop into the brain, spinal cord, and other neural tissue of the central nervous system; the notochord, which will be replaced by the vertebral column; the somites, which will segment into skeletal and muscle tissue; the nephrotomes, which will form the urogenital system; the gut, which will differentiate into the digestive and respiratory systems; the coelom, which will subdivide into separate cavities for the heart, lungs, and abdominal viscera; and the primitive heart and tiny spaces within the mesoderm that will become the vessels of the circulatory and lymphatic systems. At 8 weeks of development, major differentiation of all the organs has occurred, and the main external features, such as the eyes, ears, nose, mouth, and digits, are recognizable. The embryo is now remarkably humanlike in appearance and at this stage is called a fetus. For the remaining 7 months of intrauterine life, the primary changes in the fetus are growth, further tissue differentiation, elaboration of structural detail, and specialization of organs and systems. See also **prenatal development.**

embryologist /em'brē·ol'əjist/, one who specializes in the study of embryology.

embryology /em'brē·ol'əjē/ [Gk, *en*, *bryein* + *logos*, science], the study of the origin, growth, development, and function of an organism from fertilization to birth. Kinds of embryology include **comparative embryology, descriptive embryology,** and **experimental embryology.** —**embryologic, embryological,** *adj*.

embryoma /em'brē·ō'mə/, *pl*. **embryomas, embryomata** [Gk, *en*, *bryein* + *oma*, tumor], a tumor arising from embryonic cells or tissues.

embryoma of the ovary. See **dysgerminoma**

-embryomas. See **embryoma.**

embryomata. See **embryo.**

embryomorph /embrē'əmôrf'/ [Gk, *en*, *bryein* + *morphe*, form], any structure that resembles an embryo, especially a mass of tissue that may represent an aborted conceptus. —**embryomorphous,** *adj*.

-embryonal. See **embryo.**

embryonal adenomyosarcoma, embryonal adenosarcoma. See **Wilms' tumor.**

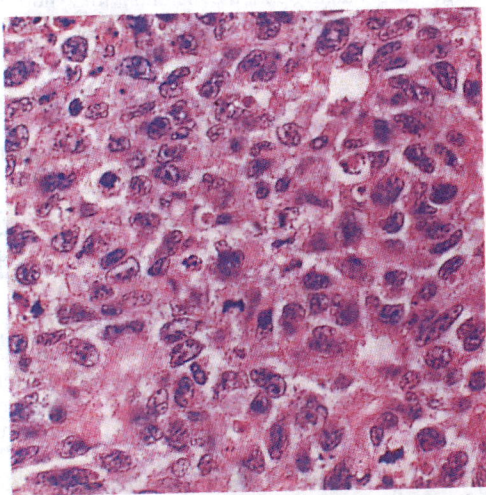

Embryonal carcinoma (Weiss, 1988)

embryonal carcinoma /em'brē·ənəl/, a malignant neoplasm derived from germinal cells, that usually develops in gonads, especially the testes. The tumor, a firm, nodular mass with hemorrhagic areas, is characterized histologically by large, undifferentiated cells with indistinct borders, eosinophilic cytoplasm, and prominent nucleoli in pleomorphic nuclei. Bodies resembling a 1- or 2-week-old embryo are occasionally seen in these tumors. The neoplasm is relatively resistant to radiation therapy. The tumor metastasizes by way of lymph channels. Surgery and chemotherapy are usually used in the treatment. See also **choriocarcinoma.**

embryonal leukemia. See **stem cell leukemia.**

embryonate /em'brē·ənāt'/ [Gk, *en, bryein* + L, *atus,* shaped like], **1.** impregnated; containing an embryo. **2.** of, pertaining to, or resembling an embryo.

embryonic /em'brē·on'ik/ [Gk, *en, bryein,* to grow], pertaining to or resembling an embryo.

embryonic abortion, 1. termination of pregnancy before the twentieth week of gestation. **2.** expelled products of conception before the twentieth week. Compare **fetal abortion.**

embryonic anideus [Gk, *en, bryein* + *an,* not, *eidos,* form], a blastoderm in which the axial elongation of the primitive streak and primitive groove fail to develop.

embryonic blastoderm, the area of the blastoderm that gives rise to the primitive streak from which the embryonic body develops. Compare **extraembryonic blastoderm.**

embryonic competence, the ability of an embryonic cell to react normally to the stimulation of an inductor, allowing continued, normal growth or differentiation of the embryo.

embryonic disk, the thickened plate from which the embryo develops in the second week of pregnancy. Scattered cells from the border of the disk migrate to the space between the trophoblast and yolk sac and become the embryonic mesoderm. The disk develops from the ectoderm and endoderm. Also called **gastrodisk, germ disk.**

embryonic layer, one of the three layers of cells in the embryo, the endoderm, the mesoderm, and the ectoderm. From these layers of cells arise all of the structures and organs and parts of the body. The endoderm is the first to develop, followed by the ectoderm. During the third week of gestation, the mesoderm arises between the ectoderm and the endoderm.

embryonic rest, a portion of embryonic tissue that remains in the adult organism. Such tissue may act as organ-specific indicators in certain types of cancer, can assist in the prediction of metastases, and can provide an objective therapeutic monitor. Also called **epithelial rest, fetal rest.**

embryonic stage, (in embryology) the interval of time from the end of the germinal stage, at 10 days of gestation, to the eighth week.

embryonic tissue [Gk, *en, bryein,* to grow; OFr, *tissu*], a loose, gelatinous mass of connective tissue cells. The gelatinous matrix is caused by the presence of mucopolysaccharides. Also called **mucous tissue; mucoid tissue.**

embryoniform /em'brē·on'ifôrm'/ [Gk, *en, bryein* + L, *forma,* form], resembling an embryo.

-embryonoid. See **embryo.**

embryopathy /em'brē·op'əthē/ [Gk, *en, bryein* + *pathos,* disease], any anomaly occurring in the embryo or fetus as a result of interference with normal intrauterine development. A kind of embryopathy is **rubella embryopathy.**

embryoplastic /em'brē·ōplas'tik/ [Gk, *en, bryein* + *plassein,* to mold], of or pertaining to the formation of an embryo, usually with reference to cells.

embryoscopy /em'brē·os'kəpē/, the examination of an embryo directly by insertion of a lighted instrument through the mother's abdominal wall and uterus. The technique may be used to obtain tissue specimens for analysis or to perform needed surgery.

embryotome /em'brē·ətōm'/ [Gk, *en, bryein* + *temnein,* to cut], an instrument used in embryotomy.

embryotomy /em'brē·ot'əmē/ [Gk, *en, bryein* + *temnein,* to cut], **1.** the dismemberment or mutilation of a fetus for removal from the uterus when normal delivery is not possible. **2.** the dissection of an embryo for examination and analysis.

embryotroph /em'brē·ətrof'/ [Gk, *en, bryein* + *trophe,* nourishment], the liquefied uterine nutritive material, composed of glandular secretions and degenerative tissue, that nourishes the mammalian embryo until placental circulation is established. Also called **embryotrophe** /-trōf'/, **histotroph, histotrophic nutrition.** Compare **hemotroph.**

embryotrophy /em'brē·ot'trəfē/, the nourishment of the embryo. See also **embryotroph, hemotroph. —embryotrophic,** *adj.*

embryulcia /em'brē·ul'sē·ə/ [Gk, *en, bryein* + *elkein,* to draw], the surgical extraction of the embryo or fetus from the uterus.

Emcyt, a trademark for an antineoplastic agent (estramustine phosphate sodium).

eme-, a combining form meaning 'to vomit': *emetocathartic, emetine.*

emergence /imur'jəns/ [L, *emergere,* to come forth], a stage in the process of recovery from general anesthesia that includes a return to spontaneous respiration, voluntary swallowing, and consciousness. See also **postoperative care.**

emergency /imur'jənsē/ [L, *emergere,* to come forth], a serious situation that arises suddenly and threatens the life or welfare of a person or a group of people, as a natural disaster or a medical crisis.

emergency cardiac care (ECC) [L, *emergens,* generally unexpected; Gk, *kardia;* ME, *caru,* sorrow], the concentration of personnel and facilities organized to sustain the cardiovascular and pulmonary systems when a heart attack occurs. The interventions assure prompt availability of basic life support (BLS), monitoring and treatment facilities, prevention of complications, and psychologic reassurance. If a heart attack occurs outside a hospital, efforts are devoted to stabilizing the patient's cardiovascular and pulmonary systems before removing the individual to a hospital.

emergency childbirth, a birth that occurs accidentally or precipitously in or out of the hospital, without standard obstetric preparations and procedures. Signs and symptoms of impending delivery include increased bloody show, frequent strong contractions, a desire on the part of the mother to bear down forcibly or her report that she feels as though she is going to defecate, visible bulging of the bag of waters, or crowning of the baby's head at the vaginal introitus.

■ METHOD: If time permits, equipment is readied, but the delivery is not delayed for such preparations. Useful equipment includes sterile gloves, towels, bulb syringe, receiving blankets, scissors, two Kelly clamps, cord clamp or tie, and a basin for the placenta. The mother's vital signs are taken, and her baby's heart tones are listened to if time permits and if equipment is available. The mother is reassured that emergency deliveries are usually simple and that all procedures and events will be explained. Despite her compelling urge to push and to deliver quickly, the mother is encouraged to ease the baby out slowly by not pushing and by blowing air forcibly out through pursed lips as she feels the strength of the urge building. As the head emerges, it is supported but allowed to rotate naturally. A check is made immediately to determine whether or not the umbilical cord is wound around the neck. If it is, a gentle attempt is made to slip it over the baby's head; if it is too tight, it is immediately clamped with two Kelly clamps placed 2 or 3 inches apart, cut between the clamps, and unwound from the neck. If the baby does not deliver immediately, mucus and fluid in the nose and the mouth are sucked out with a bulb syringe. The shoulders are delivered one at a time by guiding the head downward to deliver the anterior (upper) shoulder under the symphysis pubis, and then upward to deliver the posterior (lower) shoulder over the perineum. The rest of the baby is quickly born. If the membranes of the amniotic sac are intact, the sac is snipped or torn behind the baby's neck and peeled away from the face so that the baby can breathe. If necessary, the nares, nasopharynx, and mouth may be suctioned with the bulb syringe, taking care not to slow the heart rate by stimulating the vagus nerve with the tip of the syringe on the back of the throat. The baby is kept warm and held with the head lower than the chest; it may be laid skin-to-skin on the mother's abdomen. The baby may thus be positioned, observed, and warmed in one place as the nurse or other helper covers mother and baby with a dry blanket or towel and continues to provide emergency care as necessary through the third stage of labor. There is no urgent need to cut the cord or to deliver the placenta. When it is desired, the cord may be cut by clamping it in two places several inches from the baby and cutting it between the clamps with sterile scissors. The cord clamp may be put on later. If possible, an Apgar score is assigned first at 5 minutes of age, then at 10. The placenta is ready to be delivered when the cord is seen to advance a few inches, the uterus becomes firmer and rises in the abdomen, and a small gush of bright red blood is seen coming from the vagina. The mother may help expel it by bearing down. The placenta is lifted out of the vagina slowly, with care, so that all of the membranes are brought out with it. The placenta and membranes are kept for further evaluation. The uterus is massaged to ensure that it is well contracted, and the baby is put to breast if the mother wishes. The uterus is frequently palpated, and it is massaged when necessary. The baby is kept with the mother and observed for warmth, color, activity, and respiration. After delivery of the placenta, the perianal area is rinsed with warm sterile water and dried with a clean towel or cloth, and an ice pack and a sanitary pad or small towel are applied in such a way that the mother can hold them in place by bringing her legs together.

■ OUTCOME CRITERIA: Almost all births are normal and do not constitute true medical emergencies. If a mother is healthy and is not bleeding, if her vital signs are normal, and if the baby's heart tones are normal, there is no immediate cause for alarm, even if the birth is imminent. Emergency care is directed toward ensuring that the baby breathes well and is kept warm, that the mother is protected from hemorrhage, and that her privacy is maintained. The nurse is likely to be the person who must initially evaluate the situation and decide whether to attempt to transfer or transport the mother or to prepare for emergency delivery. If a mother says the baby is coming, the attendant is advised to believe her and to act accordingly. Throughout the delivery and the third stage of labor, the nurse works to help the mother to feel calm, confident, and well cared for.

emergency department (E.D.), (in a health care facility) a section of an institution that is staffed and equipped to provide rapid and varied emergency care, especially for those stricken with sudden and acute illness or those who are the victims of severe trauma. The emergency department may use a triage system of screening and classifying clients in order to determine priority needs for the most efficient use of available personnel and equipment.

emergency doctrine, (in law) a doctrine that assumes a person's consent to medical treatment when the person is in imminent danger and unable to give informed consent to treatment. Emergency doctrine assumes that the person would consent if able to do so.

emergency handling of radiation accidents, first aid treatment of a person who has received external body radiation through exposure to radioactive material or internal radiation contamination by inhaling or ingesting radioactive material. External radiation exposure is treated initially by cleansing and surgical isolation to protect others. One who has inhaled or ingested radioactive material should be given emergency treatment similiar to a person who has been exposed to chemical poisons. But body wastes should be collected and checked for radiation levels. If the victim has also suffered a wound, care must be taken to avoid cross-contamination of exposed surfaces. In general, except for taking special precautions to control the spread of radiation effects, the patient should be given any life-saving emergency treatment needed, and personnel handling the patient should wear surgical gowns, caps, and gloves.

Emergency Medical Service (EMS), a national network of services coordinated to provide aid and medical assistance from primary response to definitive care, involving personnel trained in the rescue, stabilization, transportation, and advanced treatment of traumatic or medical emergencies. Linked by a communications system that operates on both a local and regional level, EMS is a tiered system of care, which is usually initiated by citizen action in the form of a telephone call to an emergency number. Subsequent stages include the first medical responder, ambulance personnel, medium and heavy rescue equipment, and paramedic units, if necessary, continuing in the hospital with emergency room nurses, emergency room physicians, specialists, and critical care nurses and physicians. See also **emergency medical technician, emergency medical technician-advanced life support, emergency medical technician-intermediate, emergency medical technician-intravenous, emergency medical technician-paramedic.**

emergency medical technician (EMT), a person trained in and responsible for the administration of specialized emergency care and the transportation to a medical facility of victims of acute illness or injury. In addition to basic life-support skills, the EMT is trained in extrication and disentanglement, operation of emergency vehicles, basic anatomy, basic assessment of injury or illness, triage, care for specific injuries and illnesses, environmental emergencies, childbirth, and transport of the patient. EMT's undergo ongoing training in new procedures and must qualify for national recertification every 2 years. See also **emergency medical service.**

Emergency Medical Technician-Advanced Life Support (EMT-ALS), a third-level EMT. The EMT-ALS is locally certified in all the skills of the basic-level EMT and EMT-IV. Additionally, the EMT-ALS may administer certain medications following the orders of the hospital physician, with whom radio contact is maintained. An EMT-ALS is also trained in the use of advanced life-support systems, including electric defibrillation equipment. See also **emergency medical service.**

emergency medical technician-intermediate (EMT-I), a second-level emergency medical technician nationally certified as both an EMT-ALS and an EMT-IV. See also **emergency medical service**

emergency medical technician-intravenous (EMT-IV), a second-level emergency medical technician. The EMT-IV is trained and locally certified in intravenous therapy, endotracheal intubation, and the use of other antishock techniques. See also **emergency medical service.**

emergency medical technician-paramedic (EMT-P), an advanced-level emergency medical technician. The EMT-P is nationally certified in all the skills of EMTs of other levels, and has additional training in pharmacology and the administration of emergency drugs. See also **emergency medical service.**

emergency medicine, a branch of medicine concerned with the diagnosis and treatment of conditions resulting from trauma or sudden illness. The patient's condition is stabilized, and care of the patient is transferred to the primary physician or to a specialist. Emergency medicine requires a broad interdisciplinary training in the physiology and pathology of all of the systems of the body.

Emergency Nurses' Association (ENA), a national professional organization of emergency department nurses that defines and promotes emergency nursing practice. The Association, which was founded in 1970 and has more than 11,000 members, has written and implemented the Standards of Emergency Nursing Practice. The Association offers a certification examination and awards the designation Certified Emergency Nurse (CEN) to nurses who successfully complete it. ENA publishes the *Journal of Emergency Nursing (JEN)* and *Continuing Education Core Curriculum of Emergency Nursing Practice.* The Association, which has headquarters in Chicago, works closely with its members and with related associations to define practice and to prepare professionals to deliver emergency care.

emergency nursing, nursing care provided to prevent imminent severe damage or death or to avert serious injury. Activities that exemplify emergency nursing are basic life support, cardiopulmonary resuscitation, and control of hemorrhage.

emergency preparation of safe drinking water, methods of purifying unclean water for drinking purposes in emergencies. The three basic techniques include boiling the water and straining it through a cloth, adding three drops of tincture (alcoholic solution) of iodine per each quart of the water, and adding 10 drops of 1% chlorine bleach per each quart of water. When purifying chemicals are added, they should be thoroughly mixed with the water and the mixture allowed to stand for 30 minutes.

emergency room (ER, E.R.), a hospital area specially designed to receive and initially treat patients suffering from sudden trauma or medical problems, such as accidental hemorrhage, poisoning, fracture, heart attack, and respiratory failure. Also called **emergency department.**

emergent /imur′jənt/ [L, *emergens,* emerging], arising, often unexpectedly, or improving or modifying an existing thing.

emergent evolution, the theory that evolution occurs in a series of major changes at certain critical stages and results from the total rearrangement of existing elements so that completely new and unpredictable characteristics appear within the species. See also **saltatory evolution.**

Emery-Dreifuss syndrome /em′ərēdrī′fəs/, an X-linked recessive form of scapuloperoneal dystrophy that begins in early childhood and is characterized by joint contractures and cardiac conduction disorders. Patients who reach adulthood are often unable to work and require cardiac pacemakers to control arryhthmias.

emesis. See **vomit,** def. 2.

-emesis, a combining form meaning 'to vomit': *hyperemesis.*

emesis basin /em′əsis, əmē′sis/ [Gk, *emesis,* vomiting; Fr, *bassin,* hollow vessel], a kidney-shaped bowl or pan that fits against the neck to collect vomitus.

Emete-con, a trademark for an antiemetic (benzquinamide hydrochloride), used after anesthesia.

emetic /imet′ik/, **1.** of or pertaining to a substance that causes vomiting. **2.** an emetic agent. Apomorphine hydrochloride, acting through the central nervous system, induces vomiting 10 to 15 minutes after parenteral administration. Syrup of ipecac is used in the emergency treatment of drug overdosage and in certain cases of poisoning, but it can be cardiotoxic if it is absorbed and not vomited.

-emetic, -emetical, a combining form meaning 'pertaining to vomiting': *antiemetic, hematemetic, hyperemetic.*

Emetrol, a trademark for a fixed-combination drug containing fructose, glucose, and orthophosphoric acid, used to treat nausea and vomiting.

EMG, 1. abbreviation for **electromyogram. 2.** abbreviation for **exophthalmos, macroglossia, and gigantism.**

EMG syndrome, a hereditary disorder transmitted as an autosomal recessive trait. Clinical manifestations include exophthalmos, macroglossia, and gigantism, often accompanied by visceromegaly, dysplasia of the renal medulla, and enlargement of the cells of the adrenal cortex. Also called **Beckwith-Wiedemann syndrome, exophthalmos-macroglossia-gigantism syndrome.**

-emia, -aemia, -hemia, -haemia, a suffix meaning 'pertaining to a blood condition': *anemia, polycythemia, hyperemia.*

emissary veins /em′əser′ē/ [L, *emittere,* to send forth], the small vessels in the skull that connect the sinuses of the dura with the veins on the exterior of the skull through a series of anastomoses. The major emissary veins are the mastoid emissary vein, the parietal emissary vein, the internal carotid plexus, the rete canalis hypoglossi, the condyloid emissary vein, the rete foraminis ovalis, and the small veins passing through the foramen lacerum to connect the cavernous sinus with the pterygoid plexus. Also included in the emissary group is a vein passing through the foramen cecum, connecting the superior sagittal sinus with the veins of the nasal cavity.

emission /imish′ən/ [L, *emittere,* to send out], a discharge or release of something, as a fluid from the body, electronic signals from a radio transmitter, or an alpha or beta particle from an atomic nucleus during radioactive decay.

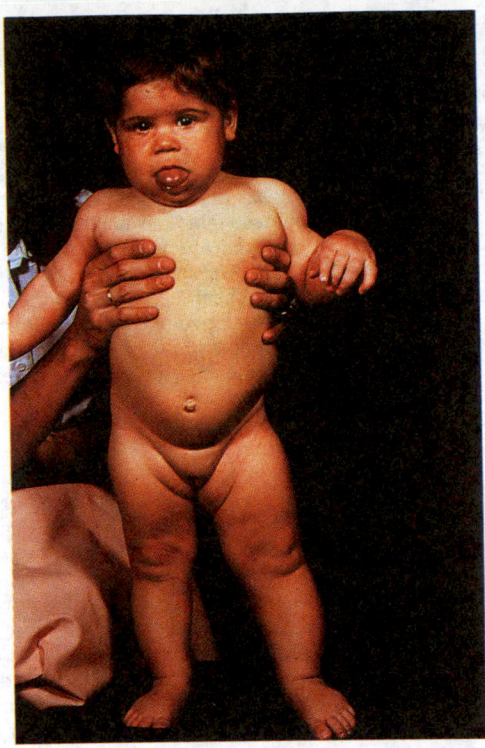

EMG syndrome (Zitelli, 1992/Courtesy Dr D Becker)

emission computed tomography (ECT) [L, *emittere*, to send forth; *computare*, to count; Gk, *tome*, section, *graphein*, to record], a form of tomography in which the emitted decay products, as positrons or gamma rays, of an ingested radioactive pharmaceutic are recorded in detectors outside the body. Computer reconstruction of the data yields a cross-sectional image of the body.

Emivan, a trademark for an analeptic agent (ethamivan).

emmetropia /em′ətrō′pē·ə/ [Gk, *emmetros*, proportioned, *opsis*, vision], a state of normal vision characterized by the proper relationship between the refractive system of the eyeball and its axial length. This correlation ensures that light rays entering the eye parallel to the optic axis are focused exactly on the retina. Compare **amblyopia, hyperopia, myopia.** **–emmetropic,** *adj.*

emmetr-, a combining form meaning 'the correct measure': *emmetropia, emmetrope.*

Emmet's operation, a surgical procedure for repair of a lacerated perineum or ruptured uterine cervix.

emollient /imol′yənt/ [L, *emolliere*, to soften], a substance that softens tissue, particularly the skin and mucous membranes.

emollient bath, a bath taken in water containing an emollient, such as bran, to relieve irritation and inflammation. See also **colloid bath.**

emotion /imō′shən/ [L, *emovere*, to disturb], the affective aspect of consciousness as compared with volition and cognition. Physiologic alterations often occur with a marked change of emotion regardless of whether the feelings are conscious or unconscious, expressed or unexpressed. See also **emotional need, emotional response.**

emotional abuse /imō′shənəl/, the debasement of a per-

son's feelings so that he perceives himself as inept, uncared for, and worthless.

emotional age [L, *emovere*, to disturb; L, *aetas*, age], the age of an individual as determined by the stage of emotional development reached.

emotional amalgam, an unconscious effort to deny or counteract anxiety.

emotional care of the dying patient, the compassionate, consistent support offered to help the terminally ill patient and the family cope with impending death. See also **stages of dying.**

■ METHOD: The professional person providing emotional support for the terminally ill encourages the expression of personal feelings, anxieties, and experiences regarding death, and empathizes with the patient and the family. The patient needs gentle, realistic care, but not all questions require answers, and the decision to tell the prognosis rests with the physician and family. To avoid conflicting statements, it is essential to know what the physician, other professionals, and family members tell the patient about the outcome. Effective support in terminal illness involves a nonjudgmental approach to the patient's relatives, an understanding of their problems, and efforts to assist them in the grieving process. The patient needs relief from pain, tender care, and continued attention through all the stages of dying: characteristically, a period of denial, followed by anger, bargaining, depression, and, finally, acceptance. When the patient denies the prognosis and refuses to follow directions, the nursing staff does not interfere with or support the denial mechanism but spends time with the sick person and encourages self-care. During the stage of anger, often manifested by refusal of care and food and by abusive language and negative criticism of the staff, the patient is not allowed to indulge in physically harmful behavior but is encouraged to verbalize the anger. In the period in which the patient tries to make bargains, such as "If I could live until. . . ," it is recognized that time is needed to accept death and that the person may appreciate discussing the importance of various events and people in earlier life. When depression, marked by apathy, insomnia, inability to concentrate, poor appetite, and weariness, sets in, efforts to cheer the patient or interrupt crying are inappropriate; the patient may want only the most beloved person to be present. In the final stage of acceptance, the patient usually experiences less pain and discomfort, seems peaceful and lacking in emotional affect, and appreciates care from people who are close and familiar.

■ NURSING INTERVENTION: The nurse has the major role in providing emotional care for the hospitalized, terminally ill patient and may help the family arrange for home care when it is possible and desirable for the person to die at home. The nurse may teach methods of care required at home, may assist the family in realizing the patient's need to live as normally and as long as possible, and may refer the family to the social service department and to community resources for assistance.

■ OUTCOME CRITERIA: Sensitive emotional support appropriate to the stage of dying may help the person to move more rapidly through the usual stages of acceptance of dying. The family usually goes through similar stages; therefore, support and counseling by an experienced person may greatly enhance the quality of life of the patient and the patient's family.

emotional deprivation [L, *emovere*, to disturb, *deprivare*, to deprive], a lack of adequate warmth, affection, and interest, especially on the part of a parent or significant other. It is a relatively common problem among institutionalized persons or children from broken homes.

emotional illness.   See **mental disorder.**

emotional need,   a psychologic or mental requirement of intrapsychic origin, usually centering on such basic feelings as love, fear, anger, sorrow, anxiety, frustration, and depression and involving the understanding, empathy, and support of one person for another. Such needs normally occur in everyone but usually are increased during periods of excessive stress or physical and mental illness and during various stages of life, as infancy, early childhood, and old age. If these needs are not routinely met by appropriate, socially accepted means, they can precipitate psychopathologic conditions. Appropriate measures common in nursing for anticipating and satisfying the emotional needs of patients in stress include physical closeness, especially remaining with the person during periods when the feeling is acute; empathic listening as the patient discusses the feeling; encouragement to talk; and planning activities that provide a constructive outlet for the feeling or the situation causing it. Compare **dependency needs.** See also **emotion.**

emotional response,   a reaction to a particular intrapsychic feeling or feelings, accompanied by physiologic changes that may or may not be outwardly manifest but that motivate or precipitate some action or behavioral response. See also **emotion.**

emotional support,   the sensitive, understanding approach that helps patients accept and deal with their illnesses, communicate their anxieties and fears, derive comfort from a gentle, sympathetic, caring person, and increase their ability to care for themselves.

■ METHOD: Essential in providing emotional support is recognizing and respecting the individuality, personal preferences, and human needs of each patient. Understanding the sick and appreciating the psychologic effects on the patient of the transition from health to illness are also important. The patient is encouraged to verbalize feelings and concerns, and the attentive listener avoids interjecting clichés, such as "Don't worry," "Take it easy," or "Everything will be all right." The nurse and other workers realize that the patient may express some fears but may act out others through anger, hostility, silence, or assumed joviality. Efforts to change the patient, negative criticism, a judgmental attitude, and facial expressions that may indicate rejection are carefully avoided. Opportunities to listen to the troubled patient and provide compassionate and realistic counseling and care are sought.

■ NURSING INTERVENTION: The nurse establishes means of communication, provides an atmosphere that invites the patient to discuss worrisome feelings, and presents a caring attitude. This is especially important when the illness damages the person's body image or self-concept. Care is administered by the nurse in a quiet, unhurried manner with the realization that a gentle touch is important and that the patient has a right to be informed of all procedures and their rationale.

■ OUTCOME CRITERIA: Emotional support frequently improves the patient's psychologic and physical state, often enabling the patient to accept the illness, to adjust with less anxiety, and to cope with the changes required.

empathic /empath'ik/ [Gk, en, into, pathos, feeling],   pertaining to or involving the entering of one person into the emotional state of another while remaining objective and distinctly separate.

empathy /em'pəthē/ [Gk, en, in, pathos, feeling],   the ability to recognize and to some extent share the emotions and states of mind of another and to understand the meaning and significance of that person's behavior. It is an essential quality for effective psychotherapy. Compare **sympathy.** —**empathic,** adj., **empathize,** v.

emphysema /em'fəsē'mə/ [Gk, en + physema, a blowing], an abnormal condition of the pulmonary system, characterized by overinflation and destructive changes of alveolar walls, resulting in a loss of lung elasticity and decreased gases. When emphysema occurs early in life, it is usually related to a rare genetic deficiency of serum alpha-1-antitrypsin, which inactivates the enzymes leukocyte collagenase and elastase. Acute emphysema may be caused by the rupture of alveoli by severe respiratory efforts, as in acute bronchopneumonia, suffocation, and whooping cough, and occasionally during labor. Chronic emphysema usually accompanies chronic bronchitis, a major cause of which is cigarette smoking. Emphysema is also seen after asthma or tuberculosis, conditions in which the lungs are overstretched until the elastic fibers of the alveolar walls are destroyed. In old age, the alveolar membranes atrophy and may collapse, resulting in large air-filled spaces with decreased total surface area of the pulmonary membranes.

■ OBSERVATIONS: The person may have shortness of breath, dyspnea, cough, cyanosis, orthopnea, unequal chest expansion, tachypnea, tachycardia, and an elevated temperature. Anxiety, carbon dioxide narcosis with a decreased pH, increased Pco_2, restlessness, confusion, weakness, anorexia, congestive heart failure, pulmonary edema, and respiratory failure are common in advanced cases.

■ NURSING INTERVENTION: The airway is kept open, and a low concentration of oxygen with humidification may be given for a prescribed number of minutes every hour. Bronchodilators, antibiotics, expectorants, and corticosteroids may be prescribed. Sedation is to be avoided, because most sedatives depress respiratory function. Postural drainage, cupping and vibration, and IPPB may improve pulmonary function.

■ NURSING CONSIDERATIONS: The patient is taught breathing exercises and encouraged to drink between 2000 and 3000 ml of fluids daily. Activity is encouraged to the limit of the patient's tolerance. Fatigue, constipation, and upper respiratory tract infection and irritation are to be avoided. A respirator and oxygen equipment may be prescribed for the patient's use at home. The patient is taught the adverse role that smoking plays in the disease and is encouraged to stop smoking.

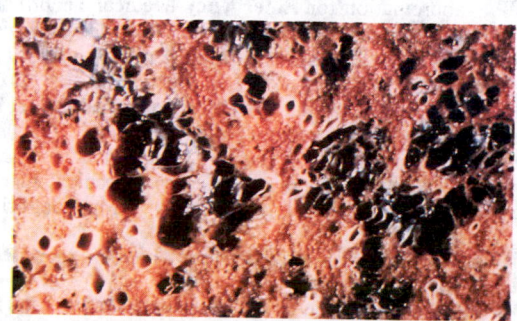

Alveoli ruptured as a result of emphysema
(Gottfried, 1993/M Moore, Visuals Unlimited)

emphysematous /em'fisem'ətəs/ [Gk, *en*, into, *physema*, a blowing], pertaining to or affected with emphysema.

emphysematous chest [Gk, *en*, *physema*; AS, *cest*, box], an atrophic type of emphysema accompanied by breathlessness but without a change in chest contour.

empiric /empir'ik/ [Gk, *empeirikos*, experimental], of or pertaining to a method of treating disease based on observations and experience without an understanding of the cause or mechanism of the disorder or the way the employed therapeutic agent or procedure effects improvement or cure. The empiric treatment of a new disease may be based on observations and experience gained in the management of analogous disorders. **–empirical,** *adj.*

empiricism /empir'isiz'əm/, a form of therapy based on personal experience and the experience of other practitioners. **–empiricist,** *n.*

empiric treatment. See **treatment.**

Empirin, a trademark for a fixed-combination drug containing two analgesic-antipyretics (aspirin and phenacetin) and a central nervous system stimulant (caffeine).

emprosthotonos /em'prosthot'ənəs/ [Gk, *emprosthen*, forward, *tenein*, to cut], a position of the body characterized by a forward, rigid flexure of the body at the waist. The position is the result of a prolonged, involuntary, muscle spasm that is most commonly associated with tetanus infection or strychnine poisoning.

empty end-feel. See **end-feel.**

empty sella syndrome [AS, *oemettig*, unoccupied; L, *sella*, saddle], an abnormal enlargement of the sella turcica in which no pituitary tumor is present; the gland may be smaller than normal, or it may be absent. Signs and symptoms of hormonal imbalance may be present, but some patients show no evidence of hypopituitarism or of any other endocrine abnormality. The condition is especially frequent in overweight, middle-aged, multiparous women. The diagnosis may be made by computerized axial tomography scan, skull x-ray study, or pneumoencephalography.

empyema /em'pī·ē'mə, em'pē·ē'mə/ [Gk, *en* + *ipyon*, pus], an accumulation of pus in a body cavity, especially the pleural space, as a result of bacterial infection, such as pleurisy or tuberculosis. It is usually removed by surgical incision, aspiration, and drainage. Antibiotics are administered to correct the cause of the underlying infection.

-empyema, a combining form meaning an 'accumulation of pus, especially thoracic': *arthroempyema, pneumoempyema, typhloempyema.*

EMS, 1. abbreviation for **Emergency Medical Service. 2.** abbreviation for **eosinophilia-myalgia syndrome.**

EMT, abbreviation for **Emergency Medical Technician.**

EMT-A, abbreviation for *emergency medical technician-ambulance,* a basic member of an emergency medical services crew.

EMT-ALS, abbreviation for **emergency medical technician-advanced life support.**

EMT-D, abbreviation for *emergency medical technician-defibrillator,* a member of an emergency medical services crew with special training in the use of cardiac defibrillating equipment.

EMT-I, abbreviation for **emergency medical technician-intermediate.**

EMT-IV, abbreviation for **emergency medical technician-intravenous.**

EMT-P, abbreviation for **emergency medical technician-paramedic.**

-emulsification. See **emulsify.**

emulsifier /imul'sifī'ər/ [L, *emulgere*, to milk out, *facere*, to make], a substance such as egg yolk or gum arabic that can cause oil to be suspended in water.

emulsify [L, *emulgere*, to milk out, *facere*, to make], to disperse a liquid into another liquid, making a colloidal suspension. Soaps and detergents emulsify by surrounding small globules of fat, preventing them from settling out. Bile acts as an emulsifying agent in the digestive tract by dispersing ingested fats into small globules. **–emulsification,** *n.*

emulsion /imul'shən/[L, *emulgere*, to drain], **1.** a system consisting of two immiscible liquids, one of which is dispersed in the other in the form of small droplets. **2.** (in photography) a composition sensitive to actinic rays of light, consisting of one or more silver halides suspended in gelatin applied in a thin layer to film.

E-Mycin, a trademark for an antibiotic (erythromycin).

en-, em- a prefix meaning 'in, on': *enanthema, encelialgia, enostosis.*

ENA. abbreviation for **Emergency Nurses' Association.**

enabler /enā'blər/, a significant other of a substance abuser who provides covert support of substance-abusing behavior.

enalapril maleate /enal'əpril/, an angiotensin-converting enzyme (ACE) inhibitor used as an oral antihypertensive drug.

■ INDICATIONS: It is prescribed in the treatment of hypertension.

■ CONTRAINDICATIONS: Enalapril maleate should not be started in a patient who is already taking a diuretic, although a diuretic may be added later in some cases. It should be used with caution in patients suffering severe salt or fluid depletion.

■ ADVERSE EFFECTS: Among adverse reactions reported are

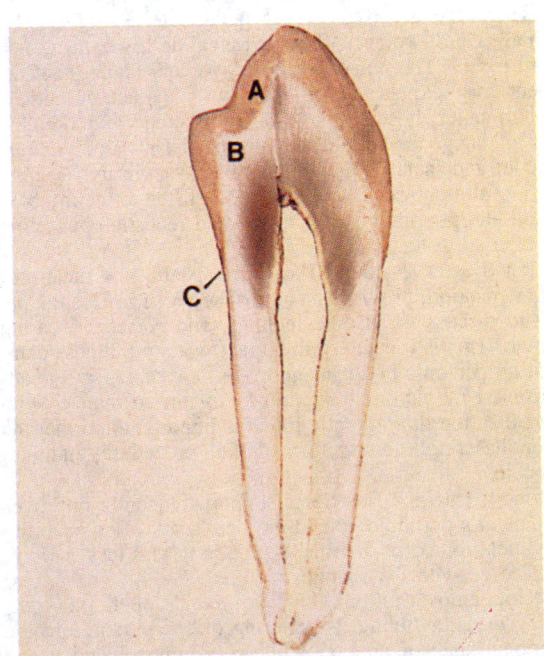

Distribution of enamel (*Berkovitz, 1992*)

mild, temporary headaches, dizziness, fatigue, diarrhea, rash, nausea, cough, and orthostatic hypotension.

enamel /inam'əl/ [OFr, *esmail*], a hard white substance that covers the dentin of the crown of a tooth. It is the outermost covering of the clinical and anatomic crown of a tooth, formed by ameloblasts during histologic development.

enamel hypocalcification, a hereditary dental defect in which the enamel of the teeth is soft and undercalcified in context yet normal in quantity, caused by defective maturation of the ameloblasts. The teeth are chalky in consistency, the surfaces wear down rapidly, and a yellow-to-brown stain appears as the underlying dentin is exposed. The condition affects both deciduous and permanent teeth. Compare **enamel hypoplasia.** See also **amelogenesis imperfecta.**

enamel hypoplasia, a developmental dental defect in which the enamel of the teeth is hard in context but thin and deficient in amount, caused by defective enamel matrix formation with a deficiency in the cementing substance. There is lack of contact between teeth, rapid breakdown of occlusive surfaces, and a yellowish brown stain that appears where the dentin is exposed. The condition, which affects both the deciduous and permanent teeth, is transmitted genetically or caused by environmental factors, such as vitamin deficiency, fluorosis, exanthematous diseases, congenital syphilis, or injury or trauma to the mouth. Administration of tetracyclines during the second half of pregnancy or during tooth development in the child can also cause the condition. Compare **enamel hypocalcification.** See also **amelogenesis imperfecta.**

enanthema /en'anthē'mə/ [Gk, *en* + *anthema*, blossoming], an eruptive lesion from the surface of a mucous membrane. Also called **enanthem** /ənan'thəm/.

enarthrosis. See **ball-and-socket joint.**

en bloc /enblok', äNblôk'/ [Fr, in a block], all together, or as a whole.

encainide /en'kānīd/, a sodium channel antagonist used as an antiarrhythmic agent.

■ INDICATIONS: It is prescribed in the treatment of life-threatening ventricular arrhythmias and other symptomatic ventricular arrhythmias.

■ CONTRAINDICATIONS: The product should not be given to patients with a known hypersensitivity to encainide or to similar sodium channel antagonists.

■ ADVERSE EFFECTS: Among the most commonly reported side effects are dizziness and blurred vision. Encainide potentiates other antiarrhythmics, and the dose of each may need to be adjusted to reduce adverse effects.

encapsulated /enkaps'yəlā'tid/ [Gk, *en* + L, *capsula*, little box], (of arteries, muscles, nerves, and other body parts) enclosed in fibrous or membranous sheaths. See also **fascia bulbi, synovial sheath.**

-ence. See **-ency.**

encephal-, a combining form meaning 'the brain': *encephalopathy, encephalitis.*

-encephalia, -encephaly, a suffix meaning '(condition of the) brain': *amyelencephalia, rhinencephalia, synencephalia.*

encephalitis /ensef'əlī'tis/, *pl.* **encephalitides** /-tidēz/ [Gk, *enkephalos*, brain, *itis*, inflammation], an inflammatory condition of the brain. The cause is usually an arbovirus infection transmitted by the bite of an infected mosquito, but it may be the result of lead or other poisoning or of hemorrhage. **Postinfectious encephalitis** occurs as a complica-

tion of another infection, such as chickenpox, influenza, or measles, or after smallpox vaccination. The condition is characterized by headache, neck pain, fever, nausea, and vomiting. Neurologic disturbances may occur, including seizures, personality change, irritability, lethargy, paralysis, weakness, and coma. The outcome depends on the cause, the age and condition of the person, and the extent of inflammation. Severe inflammation with destruction of nerve tissue may result in a seizure disorder, loss of a special sense or other permanent neurologic problem, or death. Usually, the inflammation involves the spinal cord and brain; hence, in most cases, a more accurate term is *encephalomyelitis*.

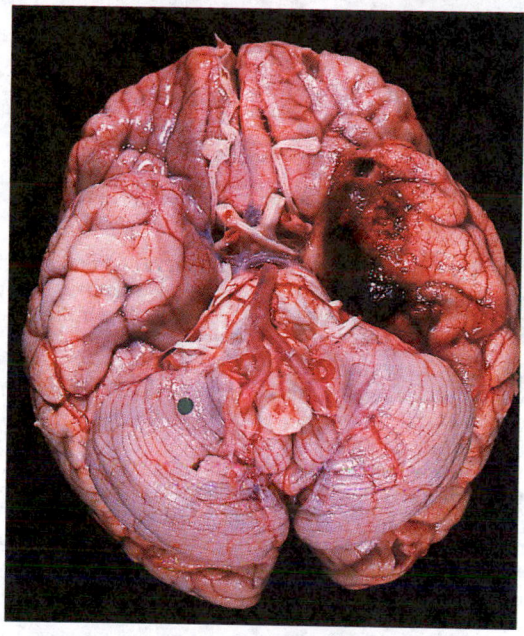

Encephalitis
(Okazaki, 1988/by permission of Mayo Foundation)

Compare **meningitis.** See also **encephalomyelitis, equine encephalitis.**

encephalitis lethargica. See **epidemic encephalitis.**

encephalitis neonatorum. See **neonatorum encephalitis.**

encephalitis periaxialis diffusa. See **Schilder's disease.**

encephalocele /ensef'ələsēl'/ [Gk, *enkephalos* + *koilia*, cavity], protrusion of the brain through a congenital defect in the skull; hernia of the brain. See also **neural tube defect.**

encephalodysplasia, any congenital anomaly of the brain.

encephalogram /ensef'ələgram'/ [Gk, *enkephalos* + *gramma*, record], a radiograph of the brain made during encephalography.

encephalography /ensef'əlog'rəfē/, radiographic delineation of the structures of the brain containing fluid after the cerebrospinal fluid is withdrawn and replaced by a gas, such as air, helium, or oxygen. The procedure is used mainly for indicating the site of cerebrospinal fluid obstruction in hydrocephalus or the structural abnormalities of the posterior fossa. Because of the risks involved, it is used only when computed tomography is not definitive. Kinds of en-

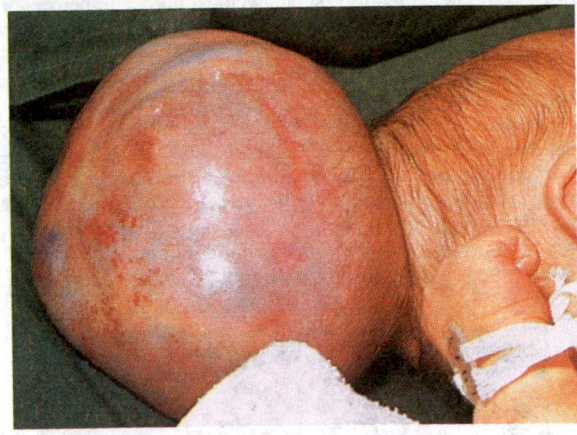

Encephalocele
(Zitelli, 1992/Courtesy Dr. Christine L. Williams, Scarsdale, New York)

cephalography are **pneumoencephalography** and **ventriculography**. Also called **air encephalography**. Compare **echoencephalography**, **electroencephalography**. —**encephalographic**, *adj*.

encephaloid carcinoma. See **medullary carcinoma**.

encephalomeningitis /-men'injī'tis/ [Gk, *enkephalos*, brain, *menigx*, membrane, *itis*, inflammation], an inflammation of the brain and meninges.

encephalomeningocele. See **meningoencephalocele**.

encephalomyelitis /ensef'əlōmī'əlī'tis/ [Gk, *enkephalos* + *myelos*, marrow, *itis*], an inflammatory condition of the brain and spinal cord characterized by fever, headache, stiff neck, back pain, and vomiting. Depending on the cause, the age and condition of the person, and the extent of the inflammation and irritation to the central nervous system, seizures, paralysis, personality changes, a decreased level of consciousness, coma, or death may occur. Sequelae, such as seizure disorders or decreased mental ability, may occur after severe inflammation that causes extensive damage to the cells and tissues of the nervous system. See also **encephalitis, equine encephalitis**.

encephalomyocarditis /ensef'əlōmī'ōkärdī'tis/ [Gk, *enkephalos* + *mys*, muscle, *kardia*, heart, *itis*, inflammation], an infectious disease of the central nervous system and heart tissue caused by a group of small RNA picornaviruses. Rodents are a major reservoir of the infection. Human illness ranges from asymptomatic infection to severe encephalomyelitis. Symptoms are generally similar to those of poliomyelitis. Myocarditis is not a feature of infection in humans, and most victims recover promptly without sequelae. Treatment is supportive. See also **picornavirus**.

encephalon [Gk, *enkephalos*, brain], **1.** the cerebrum and its related structures of cerebellum, pons, and medulla oblongata. **2.** the contents of the cranium.

encephalopathy /ensef'əlop'əthē/ [Gk, *enkephalos* + *pathos*, disease], any abnormal condition of the structure or function of tissues of the brain, especially chronic, destructive, or degenerative conditions, as Wernicke's encephalopathy or Schilder's disease.

encephalotrigeminal angiomatosis. See **Sturge-Weber syndrome**.

-encephaly. See **-encephalia**.

enchondroma /en'kəndrō'mə/, *pl.* **enchondromas, enchondromata** [Gk, *en* + *chondros*, cartilage, *oma*, tumor], a benign, slowly growing tumor of cartilage cells that arises in the extremity of the shaft of tubular bones in the hands or feet. The growth of the neoplasm may distend the bone. Also called **enchondrosis, true chondroma**.

enchondromatosis /en'kəndrō'mətō'sis/ [Gk, *en, chondros* + *oma*, tumor, *osis*, condition], a congenital disorder characterized by the proliferation of cartilage within the extremity of the shafts of bones, causing thinning of the cortex and distortion in length. Also called **dyschondroplasia, multiple enchondromatosis, Ollier's disease, skeletal enchondromatosis**. See also **Maffucci's syndrome**.

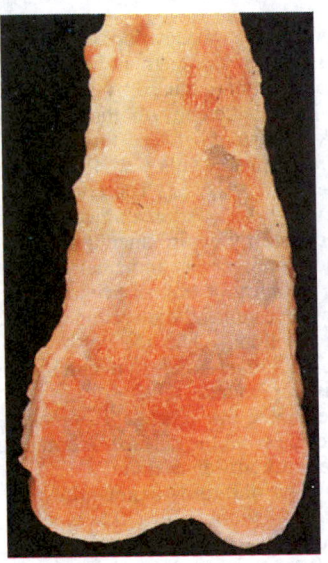

Enchondromatosis (Fletcher, 1987)

enchondromatous myxoma /en'kondrō'mətəs/, a tumor of the connective tissue, characterized by the presence of cartilage between the cells of connective tissue. See also **myxoma**.

enchondrosarcoma. See **central chondrosarcoma**.

enchondrosis. See **enchondroma**.

enchylema. See **hyaloplasm**.

-enchyma, a combining form meaning the 'liquid that nourishes tissue, or tissue itself': *karyenchyma, mesenchyma, sclerenchyma*.

encode /enkōd'/ [Gk, *en* + L, *caudex*, book], **1.** to translate a message, signal, or stimulus into a code. **2.** to rewrite, manually or automatically, such as by a computer program, information into a form that can be interpreted by a computer.

encoded message, (in communication theory) a message as transmitted by a sender to a receiver.

encopresis /en'kōprē'sis/, fecal incontinence. —**encopretic**, *adj*.

encounter [Gk, *en* + L, *contra*, against], (in psychotherapy) the interaction between a patient and a psychotherapist, such as occurs in existential therapy, or among several members of a small group, such as encounter or sensitivity training groups, in which emotional change and personal growth are brought about by the expression of strong feelings by the participants.

encounter group, (in psychology) a small group of people who meet to increase self-awareness, promote personal growth, and improve interpersonal communication. Members focus on becoming aware of their feelings and on developing the ability to express those feelings openly, honestly, and clearly. See also **group therapy, psychotherapy, sensitivity training group.**

enculturation /enkul′chərə′shən/ [Gk, *en* + L, *cultura*, cultivation], the process of learning the concepts, values, and behavioral standards of a particular culture.

-ency, -ance, -ancy, -ence, 1. a suffix meaning a 'quality or state': *deficiency, dependency.* 2. a suffix meaning a 'person or thing in a state': *latency.* 3. a suffix meaning an 'instance of a quality or state': *emergency.*

encyst /ensist′/, to form a cyst or capsule. See also **cyst.** —**encysted,** *adj.*

end /ē′en′dē′, end/, (in cytogenetics) abbreviation for *endoreduplication.*

end-. See **endo-.**

Endameba. See *Entamoeba.*

endamebiasis. See **amebiasis.**

Endamoeba. See *Entamoeba.*

endamoebiasis. See **amebiasis.**

endarterectomy /en′därtərek′təmē/ [Gk, *endon*, within, *arteria*, air pipe, *ektome*, excision], the surgical removal of the intimal lining of an artery. The procedure is done to clear a major artery that may be blocked by an accumulation of plaque. One technique, **disobliterative endarterectomy,** involves coring of the affected segment of the artery, removing the lining along with the obstructive material but leaving the remaining artery walls as a new passageway for blood flow. Another method is **gas endarterectomy,** in which carbon dioxide gas is injected between the intimal and medial layers of the artery wall, causing them to separate so the inner lining can be detached.

endarteritis /en′därtərī′tis/ [Gk, *endon*, *arteria* + *itis*, inflammation], an inflammatory disorder of the inner layer of one or more arteries, which may become partially or completely occluded.

endarteritis deformans. See **chronic endarteritis.**

endarteritis obliterans, an inflammatory condition of the lining of the arterial walls in which the intima proliferates, narrowing the lumen of the vessels and occluding the smaller vessels.

end bud [AS, *ende*; Gk, *bolbos*, onion], a mass of undifferentiated cells produced from the remnants of the primitive node and the primitive streak at the caudal end of the developing embryo after the formation of the somites is completed. In lower animals it gives rise to the tail or any other caudal appendage and part of the trunk; in humans it forms the caudal portion of the trunk. Also called **tail bud.**

end bulbs of Krause. See **Krause's corpuscles.**

end-diastolic pressure /-dī·əstol′ik/ [AS, *ende*; Gk, *dia, stellein*, to set; L, *premere*, to press], the pressure of the blood in the ventricles at the end of diastole and just before the next ventricular systole.

endemic /endem′ik/ [Gk, *endemos*, native], (of a disease or microorganism) indigenous to a geographic area or population. See also **epidemic, pandemic.**

endemic goiter, an enlargement of the thyroid gland caused by the intake of inadequate amounts of dietary iodine. Iodine deprivation leads to diminished production and secretion of thyroid hormone by the gland. The pituitary gland, operating on a negative feedback system, senses the deficiency and secretes increased amounts of thyroid-stimulating hormone, causing hyperplasia and hypertrophy of the thyroid gland. The goiter may grow during the winter months and shrink during the summer months when more iodine-bearing fresh vegetables are eaten. Initially, the goiter is diffuse; later, it becomes multinodular. Endemic goiter occurs occasionally in adolescents at puberty and widely in population groups in geographic areas in which limited amounts of iodine are present in the soil, water, and food. The use of iodized salt is a prophylactic treatment. Dessicated thyroid given orally may prevent further growth of adult goiters and may reduce the size of diffuse goiters. A large goiter may cause dysphagia, dyspnea, tracheal deviation, and cosmetic problems. See **goitrogens.**

endemic typhus. See **murine typhus.**

end-feel, the sensation imparted to the examiner's hands at the end point of the available range of motion. It varies according to the limiting structure or tissue. Types of end-feel include capsular, bone-on-bone, spasm, and springy block. **Empty end-feel** is the absence of an end-feel during a range of motion examination when the patient stops further movement of a joint before the examiner senses any organic resistance to the movement.

endo-, end-, ent-, ento-, a prefix meaning 'inward, within': *endobiotic, endocranial, endognathion.*

endocardia. See **endocardium.**

endobronchial anesthesia /en′dobrong′kē·əl/ [Gk, *endon* + *bronchos*, windpipe], a procedure, rarely performed, in which anesthetic gas is administered into the bronchi.

endocardial cushion defect /en′dōkär′dē·əl/, any cardiac defect resulting from the failure of the endocardial cushions in the embryonic heart to fuse and form the atrial septum. See also **atrial septal defect, congenital cardiac anomaly.**

endocardial cushions, a pair of thickened tissue sections in the embryonic atrial canal. During embryonic development, they meet and fuse to form a septum dividing the canal into two channels that eventually become the atrioventricular orifices.

endocardial fibroelastosis /fī′brō·ē′lastō′sis/ [Gk, *endon* + *kardia*, heart; L, *fibra*, fiber; Gk, *elaunein*, to drive, *osis*, condition], an abnormal condition characterized by the development of a thick, fibroelastic endocardium that can result in pump failure.

endocardial pacing See **pacing.**

endocarditis /en′dōkärdī′tis/ [Gk, *endon kardia*, heart, *itis*, inflammation], an abnormal condition that affects the endocardium and the heart valves and is characterized by lesions caused by a variety of diseases. The kinds of endocarditis are bacterial endocarditis, nonbacterial thrombotic endocarditis, and Libman-Sacks endocarditis. Untreated, all types of endocarditis are rapidly lethal, but they are often successfully treated by various antibacterial and surgical measures. With adequate treatment a majority of the patients with endocarditis survive. See also **bacterial endocarditis, subacute bacterial endocarditis.**

endocardium /en′dōkär′dē·əm/, *pl.* **endocardia,** the lining of the heart chambers, containing small blood vessels and a few bundles of smooth muscle. It is continuous with the endothelium of the great blood vessels. Compare **epicardium, myocardium.**

endocervical /-sur′fikəl/ [Gk, *endon* + L, *cervix*, neck], pertaining to the interior of the cervix and uterus.

endocervicitis /en'dōsur'visī'tis/, an abnormal condition characterized by inflammation of the epithelium and glands of the canal of the uterine cervix. See also **cervicitis.**

endocervix /en'dōsur'viks/, **1.** the membrane lining the canal of the uterine cervix. **2.** the opening of the cervix into the uterine cavity.

endochondral /-kon'drəl/ [Gk, *endon,* within, *chondros,* cartilage], pertaining to something within the cartilage.

endocrine /en'dəkrēn, -krīn/ [Gk, *endon + krinein,* to secrete], pertaining to a process in which a group of cells secrete into the blood or lymph circulation a substance that has a specific effect on tissues in another part of the body.

endocrine diabetes mellitus [Gk, *endon,* within, *krinein,* to secrete, *diabainein,* to pass through, *mellitus,* honeyed], a form of diabetes associated with diseases of other glands, such as the adrenals, pituitary, or thyroid.

endocrine fracture /en'dōkrīn, -krēn/, any fracture that results from weakness of a specific bone because of an endocrine disorder, such as hyperparathyroidism.

endocrine system [Gk, *endon + krinein,* to secrete; *systema*], the network of ductless glands and other structures that elaborate and secrete hormones directly into the bloodstream, affecting the function of specific target organs. Glands of the endocrine system include the thyroid and the parathyroid, the anterior pituitary, the posterior pituitary, the pancreas, the suprarenal glands, and the gonads. The pineal gland is also considered an endocrine gland because it is ductless, although its precise endocrine function is not established. The thymus gland, once considered an endocrine gland, is now classified in the lymphatic system. Various other organs have some endocrinologic function. Secretions from the endocrine glands affect various processes throughout the body, such as metabolism, growth, and secretions from other organs. Compare **exocrine.** See also the Color Atlas of Human Anatomy.

endocrine therapy. See **hormone therapy.**

endocrino- [Gk, *endon,* within, *krinein,* to secrete], a combining form 'pertaining to the endocrine system, endocrine structures or function': *endocrinology, endocrinal, endocrinopathy.*

endocrinologist /en'dōkrinol'əjist/, a physician who specializes in endocrinology.

endocrinology /-krinol'əjē/ [Gk, *endon + krinein,* to secrete, *logos* science], the study of the anatomy, physiology, and pathology of the endocrine system and of the treatment of endocrine problems.

endocrinopathy /-krinop'əthē/ [Gk, *endon,* within, *krinein,* to secrete, *pathos,* disease], a disease involving an endocrine gland or the quality or quantity of its secretion.

endoderm /en'dədurm/ [Gk, *endon + derma,* skin], (in embryology) the innermost of the cell layers that develop from the embryonic disk of the inner cell mass of the blastocyst. From the endoderm arises the epithelium of the trachea, bronchi, lungs, GI tract, liver, pancreas, urinary bladder and canal, pharynx, thyroid, tympanic cavity, tonsils, and parathyroid glands. The endoderm thus comprises the lining of the cavities and passages of the body and the covering for most of the internal organs. Compare **ectoderm, mesoderm.**

endodermal /-dur'məl/ [Gk, *endon,* within, *derma,* skin], pertaining to the inner of the three layers of the embryo, the epithelial lining of the respiratory system, the digestive tract, and other tissues. Also spelled **entodermal.**

endodermal cloaca, a part of the cloaca in the developing embryo that lies internal to the cloacal membrane and gives rise to the bladder and urogenital ducts. Compare **ectodermal cloaca.** See also **urogenital sinus.**

endodontia /-don'tē·ə/ [Gk, *endon,* within, *odous,* tooth], the diagnosis, treatment, and prevention of disorders of dental pulp, tooth root, and periapic tissues, and the associated practice of root canal therapy. Also called **endodontics, endodontology.**

endodontics, a branch of dentistry that specializes in the diagnosis and treatment of diseases in the dental pulp and its surrounding tissues, including root canal therapy.

endodontology. See **endodontia.**

endodontist /-don'tist/ [Gk, *endon,* within, *odous,* tooth], a dentist who specializes in the etiology, diagnosis, and treatment of diseases of the dental pulp, tooth root, and periapical tissues and performs root canal therapy.

endogenous /endoj'ənəs/ [Gk, *endon + genein,* to produce], **1.** growing within the body. **2.** originating from within the body or produced from internal causes, such as a disease caused by the structural or functional failure of an organ or system. Compare **exogenous.** –**endogenic,** *adj.*

endogenous carbon dioxide, carbon dioxide produced within the body by metabolic processes.

endogenous depression, a major disorder of mood characterized by a persistent dysphoric mood, anxiety, irritability, fear, brooding, appetite and sleep disturbances, weight loss, psychomotor agitation or retardation, decreased energy, feelings of worthlessness or guilt, difficulty in concentrating or thinking, occasional delusions and hallucinations, and thoughts of death or suicide. The disorder, which occurs in children, adolescents, and adults, may develop over a period of days, weeks, or months; episodes may occur in clusters or singly, separated by several years of normality. The causes of the disorder are multiple and complex and may involve biologic, psychologic, interpersonal, and sociocultural factors that lead to some unidentifiable intrapsychic conflict. Treatment includes the use of antidepressants, electroconvulsive therapy (ECT), followed by long-term psychotherapy. In severe cases, proper nursing care is needed for adequate nutrition, appropriate balance of fluid intake and output, good personal hygiene, and protection of the patient from self-injury. Also called **major depressive episode, unipolar disorder.** See also **bipolar mood disorder, depression, dysthymic disorder.**

endogenous infection, an infection caused by the reactivation of previously dormant organisms, as in coccidioidomycosis, histoplasmosis, and tuberculosis. Compare **germinal infection, mixed infection, retrograde infection, secondary infection.**

endogenous iritis. See **primary iritis.**

endogenous obesity, obesity resulting from dysfunction of the endocrine or metabolic systems. Compare **exogenous obesity.** See also **obesity.**

endogenous uric acid [Gk, *endon,* within + *genein,* to produce + *ouron,* urine; L, *acidus*], uric acid produced by the metabolism of purines in the body's own nucleoproteins, as distinguished from metabolism of purine products in foods.

endolith. See **denticle.**

endolymph /en'dəlimf/ [Gk, *endon + lympha,* water], the fluid in the membranous labyrinth (cochlear duct) of the internal ear. Compare **perilymph.**

endolymphatic duct /-limfat'ik/, a labyrinthine passage joining an endolymphatic sac with a utricle and saccule.

endolymphatic hydrops, an obsolete term for **Mé-nie[gv]re's disease.**

endometrial /en'dōmē'trē·əl/ [Gk, *endon* + *metra*, womb], **1.** of or pertaining to endometrium. **2.** of or pertaining to the uterine cavity.

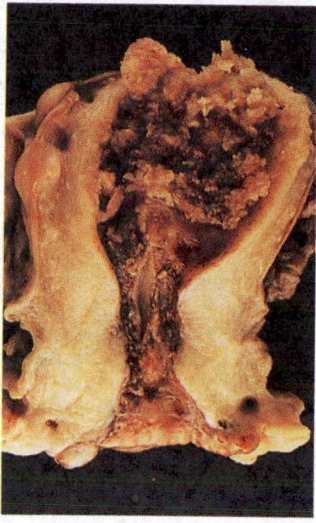

Endometrial adenocarcinoma
(Fletcher, 1987/Courtesy Prof PG Bullough, Cornell University Medical College, New York)

endometrial cancer, a malignant neoplastic disease of the endometrium of the uterus most often occurring in the fifth or sixth decade of life. Some of the factors associated with an increased incidence of the disease are a medical history of infertility, anovulation, administration of exogenous estrogen, uterine polyps, and a combination of diabetes, hypertension, and obesity. Abnormal vaginal bleeding, especially in a postmenopausal woman, is the cardinal symptom. There also may be lower abdominal and low back pain; a large, boggy uterus is often a sign of advanced disease. Less than half the patients with endometrial cancer have a positive Papanicolaou (Pap) test of the cervix and vagina, because the tumor cells rarely exfoliate in early stages of the lesion. A Pap test of cells removed from the endometrium obtained from jet washings of the uterine cavity provides more accurate data. Vacuum curettage is also used to extract endometrial cells for study, but the diagnostic technique most frequently recommended is a dilatation and curettage in which each section of the uterus is examined and curetted for biopsy specimens. Adenocarcinomas constitute roughly 90% of all endometrial tumors; mixed carcinomas, sarcomas, and benign adenoacanthomas comprise the rest. Endometrial lesions may spread to the cervix but rarely invade the vagina. They metastasize to the broad ligaments, fallopian tubes, and ovaries so frequently that bilateral salpingo-oophorectomy with abdominal hysterectomy is the usual treatment. Radiotherapy is usually administered preoperatively and postoperatively. High doses of a progestogen may be administered for palliation in advanced or inoperable cases.

endometrial cyst [Gk, *endon*, within, *metra*, womb, *kystis*, bag], **1.** an endometrial tumor. **2.** an ovarian cyst that develops as a distention of an endometrial gland.

endometrial hyperplasia, an abnormal condition characterized by overgrowth of the endometrium resulting from sustained stimulation by estrogen (of endogenous or exogenous origin) that is not opposed by progesterone. Estrogens act as growth hormone for the endometrium. Through a complex intercellular mechanism, endometrial cells bind estrogens preferentially and undergo changes characteristic of the proliferative phase of the menstrual cycle. If estrogen stimulation continues for 3 to 6 months without periodic cessation or counteractive progesterone stimulation, as occurs in anovulatory or perimenopausal women or in women receiving replacement estrogen without added progestogen, the endometrium becomes abnormally thickened and glandularized. Unremitting estrogen stimulation eventually causes cystic or adenomatous endometrial hyperplasia. The latter a premalignant lesion that undergoes malignant degeneration in approximately 25% of women having it. The causative relationship between estrogen and endometrial hyperplasia is well established; there is implication but not proof that estrogen also provokes the change from hyperplasia to neoplasia and malignancy. Endometrial hyperplasia often results in abnormal uterine bleeding; such bleeding, particularly in older women, constitutes an indication for biopsy or curettage of the endometrium to establish histopathologic diagnosis and to rule out malignancy. A functioning estrogen-secreting tumor is suspected if the woman is not taking estrogen medication. Progestogen therapy is effective in reversing the abnormal histopathologic changes of endometrial hyperplasia; if hyperplasia is adenomatous, hysterectomy is commonly performed.

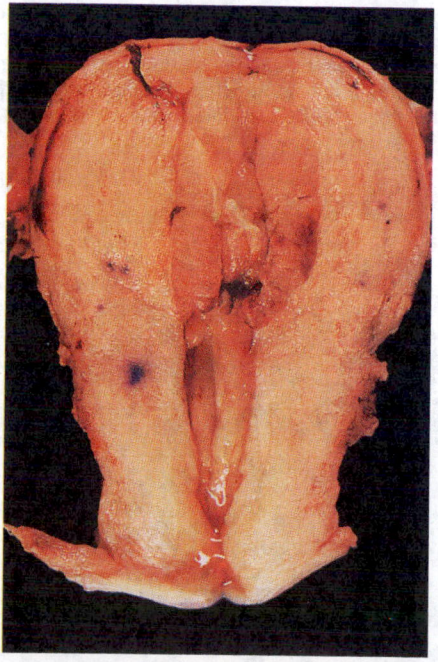

Endometrial hyperplasia *(Fletcher, 1987)*

endometrial polyp, a pedunculated overgrowth of endometrium, usually benign. Polyps are a common cause of vaginal bleeding in perimenopausal women and are often associated with other uterine abnormalities, such as endometrial hyperplasia or fibroids. They may occur singly or in clusters and are usually 1 cm or less in diameter, but they may become much larger and prolapse through the cervix. Treatment for the condition includes surgical dilatation and curettage.

endometrioma /-mē′trē·ō′mə/ [Gk, *endon,* within, *metra,* womb, *oma,* tumor], a tumor or mass of ectopic endometrial tissue that has no function in the uterus.

endometriosis /en′dōmē′trē·ō′sis/ [Gk, *endon + metra,* womb, *osis,* condition], an abnormal gynecologic condition characterized by ectopic growth and function of endometrial tissue. Precise incidence of the disease is unknown, but evidence of it is found in approximately 15% of women who undergo pelvic laparotomy for other indications. The average age of women found to have endometriosis is 37 years. Pregnancy may have an influence in preventing or ameliorating the disease. The causes of endometriosis are unknown; evidence suggests that the ectopic endometrium of endometriosis develops from vestigial tissue of the wolffian or müllerian ducts; other evidence strongly suggests that fragments of endometrium from the lining of the uterus are regurgitated during menstruation backward through the fallopian tubes into the peritoneal cavity, where they attach, grow, and function. Fragments of this tissue, which is microscopically similar to or identical with endometrium, having glands or glandlike structures, stroma, and areas of hemorrhage, may be found in the wall of the uterus or on its surface, in or on the tubes, ovaries, rectosigmoid, or pelvic peritoneum, or, occasionally, in remote extrapelvic areas. Foci of endometriosis have been found in surgical scars, the umbilicus, the bowel, the lung, the eye, and the brain. When endometriosis occurs in a critical location, it may result in grave dysfunction of the organ involved or, rarely, in death; intestinal obstruction is a common complication. The lesions of pelvic endometriosis are typically small cystic structures a few millimeters in diameter that appear individually or in clusters as black nodules on the visceral and parietal peritoneum.

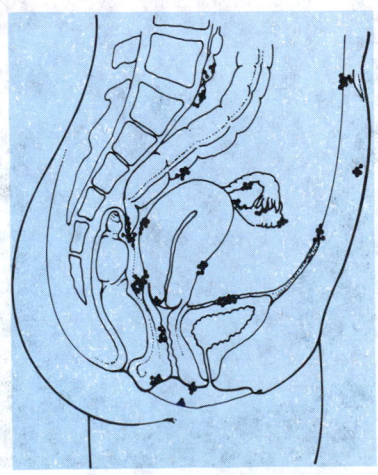

Common sites of endometriosis

endometriosis interna. See **primary endometriosis.**

endometritis /en′dōmitrī′tis/ [Gk, *endon + metra,* womb, *itis,* inflammation], an inflammatory condition of the endometrium, usually caused by bacterial infection, commonly gonococci or hemolytic streptococci. It is characterized by fever, abdominal pain, malodorous discharge, and enlargement of the uterus. It occurs most frequently after childbirth or abortion and in women fitted with an intrauterine contraceptive device. The diagnosis may be made by physical examination, history, laboratory analysis revealing an elevated white blood cell count, ultrasound, and bacteriologic identification of the pathogen. Treatment includes antibiotics, rest, analgesia, an adequate intake of fluids, and, if necessary, surgical drainage of a suppurating abscess, hysterectomy, or salpingo-oophorectomy. Endometritis may be mild and self-limited, chronic or acute, and unilateral or bilateral. It may result in sterility because of scar formation occluding the passage of the fallopian tubes. Septic abortion and puerperal fever are forms of endometritis that caused many deaths before antibiotics and asepsis became commonly available. A kind of endometritis is **decidua endometritis.** See also **pelvic inflammatory disease.**

endometritis dessicans, *obsolete.* endometritis characterized by ulceration and shedding of the endometrium of the uterus.

endometrium /en′dōmē′trē·əm/ [Gk, *endon + metra,* womb], the mucous membrane lining of the uterus, consisting of the stratum compactum, the stratum spongiosum, and the stratum basale. The endometrium changes in thickness and structure with the menstrual cycle. The stratum compactum and the stratum spongiosum comprise the pars functionalis and are shed with each menstrual flow. The pars functionalis is known as the decidua during pregnancy, when it underlies the placenta. Compare **parametrium.**

endomorph /en′dəmôrf′/ [Gk, *endon + morphe,* form], a person whose body build is characterized by a soft, round physique with a large trunk and thighs, tapering extremities, an accumulation of fat throughout the body, and a predominance of structures derived from the endoderm. Compare **ectomorph, mesomorph.** See also **pyknic.**

endomyocarditis /-mī′ōkärdī′tis/ [Gk, *endon,* within, *mys,* muscle, *kardia,* heart, *itis,* inflammation], an inflammation of the lining of the heart.

endoneurial nerve sheath. See **nerve sheath.**

endoparasite /en′dōper′əsīt/ [Gk, *endon + parasitos,* guest], (in medical parasitology) an organism that lives within the body of the host, such as a tapeworm.

endophthalmitis /endof′thalmī′tis/ [Gk, *endon + ophthalmos,* eye, *itis*], an inflammatory condition of the internal eye in which the eye becomes red, swollen, painful, and, sometimes, filled with pus. This condition may blur the vision and cause vomiting, fever, and headache. Endophthalmitis may result from bacterial or fungal infection, trauma, allergy, drug or chemical toxicity, or vascular disease. Depending on the cause, therapy requires surgical intervention or the administration of an antibiotic, atropine, or a corticosteroid. Also called **endophthalmia.**

endophthalmitis phacoanaphylactica /fak′ō·an′-əfilak′təkə/, an abnormal condition characterized by an acute autoimmune reaction of the eye. It is caused by hypersensitivity of the eye to the protein of the crystalline lens and commonly occurs after trauma to the crystalline lens or after a cataract operation. Associated symptoms include swelling and inflammation of the eye, severe pain, and

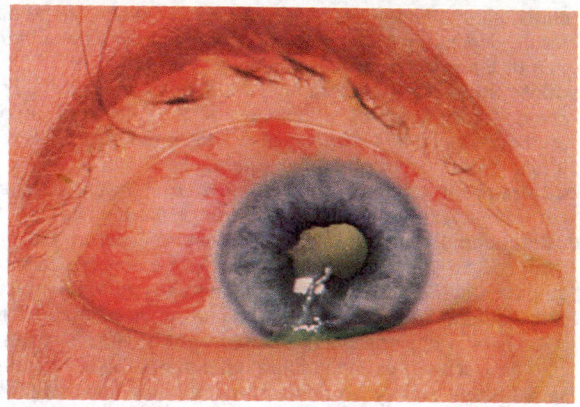

Endophthalmitis *(Bedford, 1986)*

blurred vision. The substance of the lens is invaded by poly-morphonuclear cells and mononuclear phagocytes. Sensitization of one eye often follows the extracapsular removal of the lens of the eye on the opposite side. Accurate diagnosis must differentiate between this condition and infectious endophthalmitis. Therapy is supportive and commonly includes the administration of corticosteroids and atropine. Refractory cases may require surgical removal of the lens. Compare **uveitis.**

endophytic /en'dōfit'ik/ [Gk, *endon* + *phyton*, plant], of or pertaining to the tendency to grow inward, such as an endophytic tumor that grows on the inside of an organ or structure.

endoplasm /en'doplaz'əm/ [Gk, *endon*, within, *plasma*, plasm], the inner portion of cytoplasm.

endoplasmic reticulum /-plaz'mik/ [Gk, *endon* + *plassein*, to mold], an extensive network of membrane-enclosed tubules in the cytoplasm of cells. The ultramicroscopic organelle, which can be seen only with an electron microscope, is classified as granular or rough-surfaced when ribosomes are attached to the surface of the membrane and agranular or smooth-surfaced when ribosomes are absent. The structure functions in the synthesis of proteins and lipids and in the transport of these metabolites within the cell.

endoprosthesis /-prosthē'sis, -pros'thəsis/ [Gk, *endon* + *prosthesis*, addition], a prosthetic device installed within the body, such as dentures or an internal cardiac pacemaker.

end-organ [AS, *ende*; Gk, *organon,* instrument], a nerve ending in which the terminal nerve filaments are encapsulated.

endorphin /endôr'fin/ [Gk, *endon* + Gk *morphe*, shape], any one of the neuropeptides composed of many amino acids, elaborated by the pituitary gland and acting on the central and the peripheral nervous systems to reduce pain. Endorphins isolated by researchers are alpha-endorphin, beta-endorphin, and gamma-endorphin, all chemicals producing pharmacologic effects similar to morphine. Beta-endorphin has been isolated in the brain and in the GI tract and seems to be the most potent of the endorphins. Beta-endorphin is composed of 31 amino acids that are identical to part of the sequence of 91 amino acids of the hormone beta-lipoprotein, also produced by the pituitary gland. Behavioral tests indicate that beta-endorphin is a powerful analgesic in humans and animals. Brain-stimulated analgesia in humans releases beta-endorphin into the cerebrospinal fluid. Compare **enkephalin.**

endorsement /endôrs'mənt/ [Gk, *en* + L, *dorsum,* the back], a statement of recognition of the license of a health practitioner in one state by another state. An endorsement relieves the health practitioner of the necessity of going through the full licensing procedure of the state in which practice is to be undertaken.

endoscope /en'dəskōp'/ [Gk, *endon* + *skopein*, to look], an illuminated optic instrument for the visualization of the interior of a body cavity or organ. Instruments are available in varying lengths, and the fiber-opticendoscope has great flexibility, reaching previously inaccessible areas. Although the endoscope is generally introduced through a natural opening in the body, it may also be inserted through an incision. Other instruments for viewing specific areas of the body include the bronchoscope, cystoscope, gastroscope, laparoscope, otoscope, and vaginoscope. See also **fiberoptics.** –**endoscopic,** *adj.*

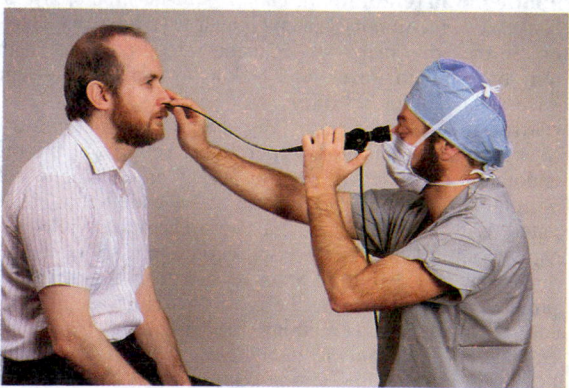

Endoscope *(Bingham, 1992)*

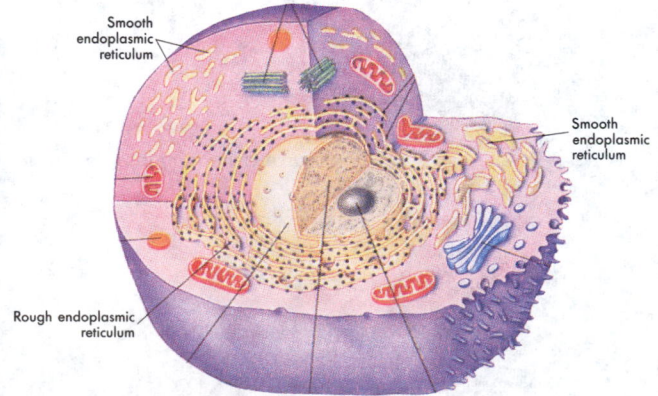

Endoplasmic reticulum *(Thibodeau, 1993/William Ober)*

Smooth endoplasmic reticulum

Smooth endoplasmic reticulum

Rough endoplasmic reticulum

endoscopic retrograde cholangiography /en'dəskop'ik/, (in radiology) a diagnostic procedure for outlining the common bile duct. A flexible fiberoptic duodenoscope is placed in the common bile duct. A radiopaque substance is instilled directly into the duct, and serial x-ray films are taken. See also **cholangiography.**

endoscopy /endos'kəpē/, the visualization of the interior of organs and cavities of the body with an endoscope. The procedure is indicated for the diagnosis of gastric ulcers with atypical radiologic features, to locate the source of upper GI bleeding, to establish the presence and extent of varices in the lower esophagus and stomach in patients with liver disease, and to detect abnormalities of the lower colon. For examination of the upper GI tract, the stomach of the patient is lavaged with ice water through a large-bore gastric tube, with the patient placed on the side to reduce the chance of aspiration. For examination of the lower colon, fecal material is removed by enema, laxative, or suppository. The patient is placed in the knee-chest position for the procedure and afterward is observed by the nurse for abdominal pain or rectal bleeding. Aseptic rather than sterile techniques are routinely followed. Endoscopy can also be used to obtain samples for cytologic and histologic examination and to follow the course of a disease, as the assessment of the healing of gastric and duodenal ulcers. See also **bronchoscopy, cystoscopy, gastroscopy, laparoscopy.**

endoskeletal prosthesis /-skel'ətəl/ [Gk, *endon* + *skeletos*, dried up; *prosthesis*, addition], a prosthetic device in which an internal pylon provides the actual support of the body. The pylon is usually covered with a lightweight plastic material, such as plastic foam. See also **pylon.**

endoskeleton, the internal network of bones, to which muscles are attached. Compare **exoskeleton.**

endosteal hyperostosis /endos'tē·əl/, an inherited bone disorder characterized by an overgrowth of the mandible and brow areas. The excessive bone growth can lead to entrapment of cranial nerves, resulting in facial palsy and loss of hearing. Also called **Van Buchem's syndrome.**

endostomy therapist. See **enterostomal therapist.**

endothelial /en'dōthē'lē·əl/ [Gk, *endon*, within, *thele*, nipple], pertaining to or resembling endothelium.

endothelial cell [Gk, *endon*, within, *thele*, nipple; L, *cella*, storeroom], a lining cell of a body cavity or of the cardiovascular system. It is usually seen as a flat nucleated cell.

endothelial myeloma [Gk, *endon* + *thele*, nipple; *myelos*, marrow, *oma*, tumor], a malignant myeloma that develops in the bone marrow, occurring most frequently in the long bones. Pain, fever, and leukocytosis may be present. Also called **Ewing's tumor.**

endothelin (ET) /-thē'lin/, any of a group of vasoconstrictive peptides produced by endothelial cells from pre-proendothelin by a cleavage performed by an endothelin converting enzyme (ACE). Three known endothelins designated as ET-1, ET-2, and ET-3 are chemically related to asp venom. ET-1 is the most potent vasopressor compound yet discovered, being 10 times greater than angiotensin-II, previously believed to be the most powerful vasopressor.

-endothelioma, a combining form meaning 'a tumor of endothelial tissue': *hemendothelioma, lymphendothelioma.*

endothelium /en'dōthē'lē·əm/ [Gk, *endon* + *thele*, nipple], the layer of simple squamous epithelial cells that lines the heart, the blood and the lymph vessels, and the serous cavities of the body. It is highly vascular, heals quickly, and is derived from the mesoderm.

endotoxin /en'dōtok'sin/ [Gk, *endon* + *toxikon*, poison], a toxin contained in the cell walls of some microorganisms, especially gram-negative bacteria, that is released when the bacterium dies and is broken down in the body. Fever,

chills, shock, leukopenia, and a variety of other symptoms result, depending on the particular organism and the condition of the infected person. Compare **exotoxin.**

endotoxin shock [Gk, *endon,* within, *toxikon,* poison; Fr, *choc*], a septic shock in response to the release of endotoxins produced by Gram-negative bacteria. The toxin is released on the death of the bacterial cell.

endotracheal /en'dōtrā'kē·əl/ [Gk, *endon* + *tracheia, arteria,* rough air pipe], within or through the trachea.

endotracheal anesthesia, inhalation anesthesia that is achieved by the passage of an anesthetic gas or mixture of gases through an endotracheal tube into the respiratory tract.

endotracheal intubation, the management of the patient with an airway catheter inserted through the mouth or nose into the trachea. An endotracheal tube may be used to maintain a patent airway, to prevent aspiration of material from the digestive tract in the unconscious or paralyzed patient, to permit suctioning of tracheobronchial secretions, or to administer positive-pressure ventilation that cannot be given effectively by a mask. Endotracheal tubes may be made of rubber or plastic and usually have an inflatable cuff to maintain a closed system with the ventilator.

■ METHOD: With the aid of paralytic agents to ease the passage, the endotracheal tube is inserted via the mouth or nose through the larynx into the trachea; if the oral route is used, a bite block may be required to keep the patient from biting and obstructing the tube. Breath sounds are auscultated immediately after insertion and every 1 or 2 hours thereafter to make certain the tube is properly positioned and is not obstructing one of the mainstem bronchi. Once the tube is correctly positioned, it is taped securely in place and checked for patency and slippage every 15 to 60 minutes.

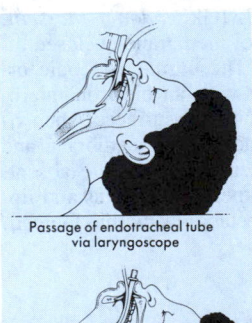

Passage of endotracheal tube via laryngoscope

Passage of endotracheal tube via laryngoscope

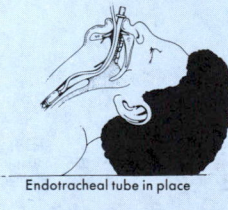

Endotracheal tube in place

Endotracheal tube in place

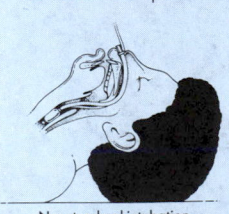

Nasotracheal intubation

Nasotracheal intubation

Endotracheal intubation

The trachea is suctioned every hour and irrigated with normal saline solution, if so ordered. The patient is usually on intermittent positive-pressure breathing (IPPB) or a volume respirator with the cuff of the endotracheal tube inflated; if the patient can breathe independently, the trachea and mouth are suctioned, the cuff is deflated, and the respiratory rate and quality are checked hourly. The patient is turned every 1 to 2 hours, with the blood pressure and pulse checked every 2 to 4 hours. Parenteral fluids are administered as ordered; nothing is given orally; the intake and output of fluids are measured and recorded. The patient's level of consciousness is determined hourly, and if he is sufficiently conscious, a method of communication is established.

■ NURSING ORDERS: The nurse monitors the position and patency of the endotracheal tube, performs the necessary suctioning, inflates and deflates the cuff at appropriate times, and administers IPPB or support with the volume respirator. The nurse checks the vital signs at the ordered intervals and provides emotional support as well as physical care for the patient, who is usually acutely ill, unable to communicate, and suffering from the discomfort of an endotracheal tube.

■ OUTCOME CRITERIA: Meticulous care of the patient with an endotracheal tube can result in the survival of a critically ill person.

endotracheal tube, a large-bore catheter inserted through the mouth or nose and into the trachea to a point above the bifurcation of the trachea proximal to the bronchi. It is used for delivering oxygen under pressure when ventilation must be totally controlled and in general anesthetic procedures. See also **endotracheal intubation.**

endoxin /endok′sin/, an endogenous analog of digoxin, occurring naturally in humans. It is a hormone that may regulate the excretion of salt.

end plate [AS, *ende*; ME, *plat*], in the nervous system, the motor end plate, located at the terminal membrane of an axon and the postjunctional membrane of the adjoining muscle tissue. Also called **myoneural junction.**

end-stage disease [AS, *ende*; OFr, *estage*; L, *dis*; Fr, *aise,* ease], a disease condition that is essentially terminal because of irreversible damage to vital tissues or organs. Kidney or renal end-stage disease is defined as a point at which the kidney is so badly damaged or scarred that hemodialysis or transplantation is required for patient survival.

end-tidal capnography /end′tīdəl/, (in respiratory therapy) the process of continuously recording the concentration or percentage of carbon dioxide in expired air. The percentage of carbon dioxide at the end of the breath can be estimated and gives a close approximation of the alveolar carbon dioxide concentration. The process requires the use of infrared spectroscopy. It is used in continuous monitoring of critically ill patients and also in pulmonary function testing. The data are typically automatically recorded on a strip of graph paper.

end-tidal CO_2. See **capnometry.**

end-tidal CO_2 determination, the concentration of carbon dioxide in a patient's end-tidal breath, assumed to reflect arterial carbon dioxide tension. A significant difference may indicate a change in ventilation/perfusion matching.

end-to-end anastomosis. See **anastomosis.**

endurance /endyŏŏr′əns/, the ability to continue an activity despite increasing physical or psychologic stress, as in the effort to perform additional numbers of muscle contractions before the onset of fatigue. Although endurance and strength are different qualities, weaker muscles tend to have less endurance than strong muscles.

Enduron, a trademark for a thiazide diuretic and antihypertensive (methyclothiazide).

Enduronyl, a trademark for a cardiovascular, fixed-combination drug containing a diuretic (methyclothiazide) and an antihypertensive (deserpidine).

-ene, a suffix used for naming hydrocarbons: *ethidene, somnifene, xanthene.*

enema /en′əmə/ [Gk, *enienai*, injection], a procedure in which a solution is introduced into the rectum for cleansing or therapeutic purposes. Enemas may be commercially packed disposable units or reusable equipment prepared just before use.

■ METHOD: The equipment is assembled; if disposable equipment is to be used, an 18-to-20 French gauge catheter, a 2- to 3-foot length of tubing, an enema can, the solution, a clamp, and a thermometer are collected and brought to the bedside. If a disposable set is to be used, no other equipment is necessary. The patient is positioned in the left lateral knee-chest or dorsal position. After air is expelled from the tubing, the tip of the catheter is lubricated. (Disposable units usually have prelubricated tips.) The patient is asked to bear down, as if to defecate, and the tip of the catheter is gently inserted 7.5 to 10 cm into the rectum, depending on the size of the patient and the purpose of the enema. The solution is allowed to flow from a height of 45 cm above the level of the hips, or, with some disposable enemas, the container is squeezed slowly to force the fluid into the rectum. The tip of the catheter or squeeze-bottle is withdrawn when all the solution has been administered, and light pressure is applied over the anus with a gauze pad. The fluid is held in by the patient for the prescribed length of time. It is then expelled as the patient sits on the toilet.

■ NURSING INTERVENTION: The reasons for performing the procedure and the steps to be taken are explained to the patient. The solution is warmed to 99° F (37.8° C) to 105° F (40.6° C) to reduce the stimulation of intestinal peristalsis

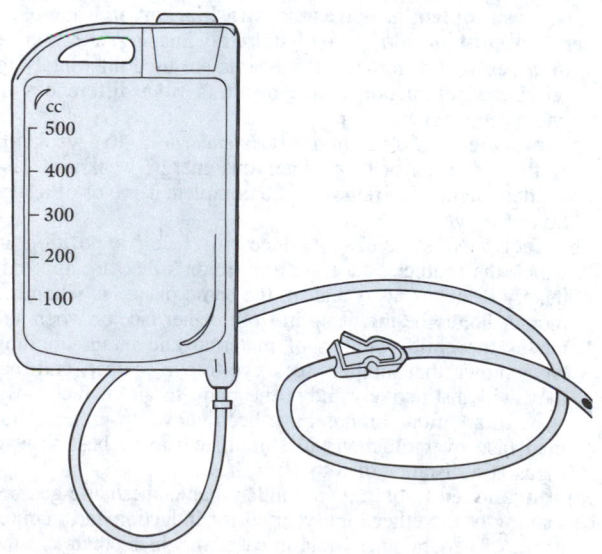

Enema kit (Sorrentino, 1992)

by a sudden change of temperature in the colon. The patient is warned that some discomfort may occur because the colon tends to contract when distended by the fluid. The enema is given slowly to avoid sudden distention that would cause peristalsis, or spasm, and increased discomfort. A call bell is kept within reach of the patient during expulsion of the enema because the discomfort of the procedure and the effort required to expel the enema may cause faintness. The color, consistency, and amount of material evacuated are evaluated. If nondisposable equipment is used, it is rinsed in cold water before being washed with warm soapy water and sterilized.

■ OUTCOME CRITERIA: Careful observation of the patient during the procedure, slow and gentle administration of the enema, evaluation of the results of the procedure, and a thorough explanation to the patient of all aspects of the procedure are important to achieve the desired effect of the enema.

energy /en′ərjē/ [Gk, *energia*], the capacity to do work or to perform vigorous activity. Energy may occur in the form of heat, light, movement, sound, or radiation. Human energy is usually expressed as muscle contractions and heat production, made possible by the metabolism of food that originally acquired the energy from sunlight. Chemical energy refers to the energy released as a result of a chemical reaction, as in the metabolism of food. Compare **anergy**. –**energetic**, *adj*.

energy conservation, a principle that energy cannot be created or destroyed although it can be changed from one form into another, as when heat energy is converted to light energy.

energy cost of activities, the metabolic cost in calories or kilojoules of various forms of physical activity. For example, the average metabolic equivalent of walking at a rate of 3 km/h is 2 METS per minute while the energy cost of walking at a speed of 6 km/h is 5 METs per minute. See also **MET**.

energy-protein malnutrition, a wasting condition resulting from a diet deficient in both calories and proteins. Also called **protein-calorie malnutrition**. See also **anorexia nervosa, bulemia, marasmic kwashiorkor, marasmus**.

energy subtraction, (in digital x-ray imaging) a technique in which two different x-ray beams are used alternately to provide a subtraction image resulting from differences in photoelectric interaction.

enervation /en′ərvā′shən/ [L, *enervare*, to weaken], **1.** the reduction or lack of nervous energy; weakness; lassitude; languor. **2.** removal of a complete nerve or of a section of nerve.

en face /äNfäs′, enfäs′/, 'face -to- face'; a position in which the mother's face and the infant's face are approximately 8 inches apart and on the same plane, as when the mother holds the infant up in front of her face or when she nurses the child. Studies of maternal and infant bonding have shown that mothers seek eye-to-eye contact, and that they will instinctively move the baby to an en face position. In addition, infants have been shown to prefer a human face over other visual stimuli and to be best able to focus at a distance of 8 to 10 inches.

enflurane /en′floorān′/, a nonflammable anesthetic gas belonging to the ether family, used for induction and maintenance of general anesthesia in cases in which ethers are the drugs of choice. A halogenated volatile liquid, enflurane is administered through vaporizers specially calibrated for de-livery via oxygen or an oxygen-nitrous oxide mixture, permitting close control of dosage. Because excitement may occur on induction, a hypnotic dose of short-acting barbiturate is sometimes used for premedication. Adverse reactions may include seizure activity, muscle fasciculation, hypotension, cardiac arrhythmia, shivering, and elevated white blood cell count. Nausea and vomiting on emergence from anesthesia sometimes occur.

engagement /engāj′mənt/ [Fr, a bonding], **1.** fixation of the presenting part of the fetus in the maternal true pelvis. The largest diameter of the presenting part is at or below the level of the ischial spines. **2.** fixation of the fetal head in the maternal midpelvis with the biparietal diameter of the head level with the ischial spines.

English position. See **lateral recumbent position.**

engorgement /engôrj′mənt/ [Fr, *engorger*, to fill up], distention or vascular congestion of body tissues, such as the swelling of breast tissue caused by an increased flow of blood and lymph preceding true lactation.

engram /en′gram/, **1.** a hypothetical neurophysiologic storage unit in the cerebrum that is the source of a particular memory. **2.** an interneuronal circuit involving specific neurons and muscle fibers that can be coordinated to perform specific motor activity patterns. Thousands of repetitions may be needed to establish an engram.

engrossment. See **bonding.**

enhancement /enhans′mənt/ [ME, *enhauncen,* to raise], to improve, heighten, or augment.

Enkaid, a trademark fo a sodium channel antagonist antiarrhythmic drug (encainide).

enkephalin /enkef′əlin/ [Gk, *enkepalos*, brain, *in*, within], one of two pain-relieving pentapeptides produced in the body. Researchers have isolated enkephalins in the pituitary gland, brain, and GI tract. The enkephalins are methionine-enkephalin and isoleucine-enkephalin, each composed of five amino acids, four of which are identical in both compounds. It is believed that these two neuropeptides can depress neurons throughout the central nervous system. Axon terminals that release enkephalins are concentrated in the posterior horn of the gray matter of the spinal cord, in the central part of the thalamus, and in the amygdala of the limbic system of the cerebrum. Enkephalins inhibit neurotransmitters in the pathway for pain perception, thereby reducing the emotional as well as the physical impact of pain. Although it is not known exactly how these two neuropeptides function, many experts believe that the enkephalins are natural pain killers and that they may be involved, with other neuropeptides, in the development of psychopathologic behavior in some cases. Compare **endorphin.**

enol /ē′nol/, an organic compound with an alcohol or hydroxyl group adjacent to a double bond. By transfer of the hydrogen atom, the enol form becomes the keto form. Such compounds usually exist as enol-keto tautomers.

enophthalmos /en′əfthal′məs/ [Gk, *en*, in, *ophthalmos*, eye], backward displacement of the eye in the bony socket, caused by traumatic injury or developmental defect. Ptosis may cause a false impression of enophthalmos. –**enophthalmic,** *adj*.

Enovid, a trademark for an oral contraceptive containing an estrogen (mestranol) and a progestin (norethynodrel).

ensiform process. See **xiphoid process.**

Ensure, a trademark for a lactose-free nutritional supplement containing protein, carbohydrate, fat, vitamins, and minerals.

ENT, abbreviation for *ear, nose, and throat.*

Entameba. See *Entamoeba.*

entamebiasis. See **amebiasis.**

Entamoeba /en'təmē'bə/ [Gk, *entos,* within, *amoibe,* change], a genus of intestinal amebic parasites of which several species are pathogenic to humans. Also spelled *Entameba.* See also *Entamoeba histolytica.*

Entamoeba histolytica /his'təlit'ikə/, a pathogenic species of ameba that causes amebic dysentery and hepatic amebiasis in humans. See also **amebiasis, amebic dysentery, hepatic amebiasis.**

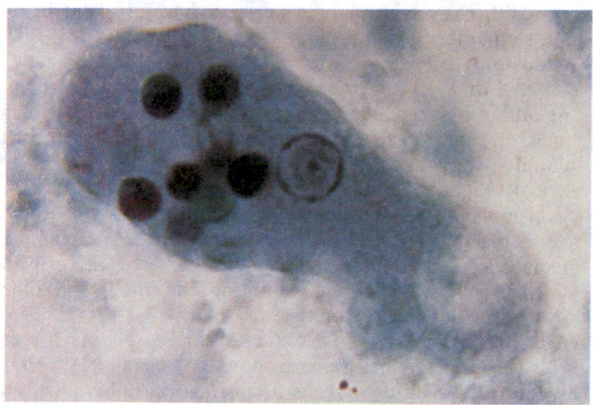

Entamoeba histolytica trophozoite
(Murray, 1990/From Lennette EH et al: Manual of clinical microbiology, ed. 4. Washington, DC, 1985, American Society for Microbiology)

entamoebiasis. See **amebiasis.**

enter-. See **entero-.**

enteral /enter'əl/ [Gk, *enteron,* bowel], within the small intestine, or via the small intestinal.

enteral nutrition, the provision of nutrients through the gastro-intestinal tract when the client cannot injest, chew, or swallow food, but can digest and absorb nutrients.

enteral tube feeding [Gk, *enteron,* bowel; L, *tubus;* AS, *faedan*], the introduction of food or nutritive material directly into the digestive tract by nasogastric or gastric tube.

enterectomy /en'tərek'təmē/ [Gk, *enteron,* intestine, *ektome,* excision], the surgical removal of a portion of intestine.

enteric /enter'ik/ [Gk, *enteron,* bowel], pertaining to the intestine.

enteric coating, a coating added to oral medications that are designed to be absorbed from the intestinal tract. The coating resists the effects of stomach juices, which can interact with or destroy certain drugs.

enteric cytopathogenic human orphan virus. See **ECHO virus.**

enteric fever. See **typhoid fever.**

enteric infection, a disease of the intestine caused by any infection. Symptoms similar to those caused by pathogens may be produced by chemical toxins in ingested foods and by allergic reactions to certain food substances. Among bacteria commonly involved in enteric infections are *Es-*

cherichia coli, Vibrio cholerae, and several species of *Salmonella, Shigella,* and anaerobic streptococci. Enteric infections are characterized by diarrhea, abdominal discomfort, nausea and vomiting, and anorexia. There may be a significant loss of fluid and electrolytes as a result of severe vomiting and diarrhea. Nothing is offered by mouth until vomiting has ceased. At that time, a clear fluid diet may be given. In severe cases, an IV solution containing glucose, saline, and electrolytes may be administered. Medication for sedation and relief of abdominal cramps may be prescribed. Antibiotics may be recommended, depending upon the specific microorganism causing the infection.

entericoid fever /enter'ikoid/ [Gk, *enteron + eidos,* form], a typhoidlike febrile disease characterized by intestinal inflammation and dysfunction. See also **enteric infection, typhoid fever.**

enteric orphan virus [Gk, *enteron,* bowel + *orphanos,* bereft; L, *virus,* poison], a GI disease virus that has been identified and isolated but was not originally associated with the disease. See also **ECHO virus.**

enteritis /en'tərī'tis/, inflammation of the mucosal lining of the small intestine, resulting from a variety of causes—bacterial, viral, functional, and inflammatory. Involvement of small and large intestine is called **enterocolitis.** Compare **gastroenteritis.**

entero-, enter-, a combining form meaning 'pertaining to the intestines': *enteric, enterobiliary, enteroptosis.*

Enterobacter cloacae /en'tirōbak'tər klō·ā'kē, klō·ā'sē/ [Gk, *enteron + bakterion,* small staff; L, *cloaca,* sewer], a common species of bacteria found in human and animal feces, dairy products, sewage, soil, and water. It is rarely the cause of disease. Also called *Aerobacter aerogenes* /ero-j'inēz/, *Enterobacter aerogenes.*

Enterobacteriaceae /en'tirōbaktir'ē·ā'si·ē/ [Gk, *enteron + bakterion,* small staff], a family of aerobic and anaerobic bacteria that includes both normal and pathogenic enteric microorganisms. Among the significant genera of the family are *Escherichia, Klebsiella, Proteus,* and *Salmonella.*

enterobacterial /-baktir'ē·əl/ [Gk, *enteron + bakterion,* small staff], of or pertaining to a species of bacteria found in the digestive tract.

enterobiasis /en'tirōbī'əsis/ [Gk, *enteron + bios,* life, *osis,* condition], a parasitic infestation with *Enterobius vermicularis,* the common pinworm. The worms infect the large intestine, and the females deposit eggs in the perianal area, causing pruritus and insomnia. Reinfection commonly occurs by transfer of eggs to the mouth by contaminated fingers. Airborne transmission is possible because eggs remain viable for two or three days in contaminated bedclothes. To make the diagnosis, the sticky side of an adhesive cellophane tape swab is pressed against the perianal skin and examined for eggs under a microscope. Therapy for the whole family may be necessary. Effective anthelmintics include piperazine, pyrantel pamoate, pyrvinium pamoate, and thiabendazole. Personal hygiene, including handwashing, is the best preventive measure. There appears to be little benefit from disinfection procedures for the home. Also called **oxyuriasis.**

Enterobius vermicularis /en'tərō'bē·əs/ [Gk, *enteron + bios,* life; L, *vermiculus,* small worm], a common parasitic nematode that resembles a white thread between 0.5 and 1 cm long. Also called **pinworm, seatworm, threadworm.**

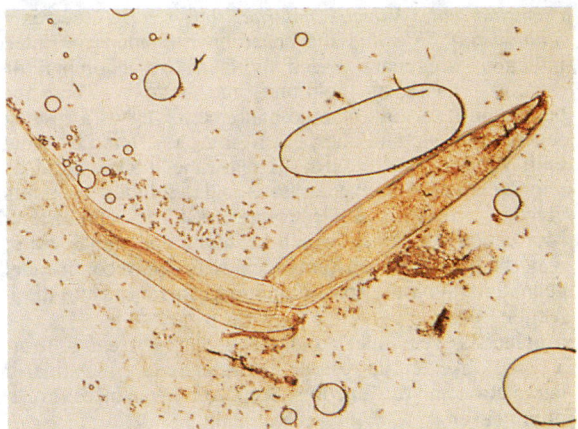

***Enterobius vermicularis*—mature worm surrounded by eggs**
(Zitelli, 1992)

enterochromaffin cell. See **argentaffin cell.**

enteroclysis /en'tərok'lisis/, a radiographic procedure in which a contrast medium is injected into the duodenum to examine the small intestine. In some patients, air is injected into the small intestine after the contrast medium has reached the cecum.

enterococcus /-kokəs/, *pl.* **enterococci** /-kok'sī, -kôk'ē/ [Gk, *enteron* + *kokkos*, berry], any *Streptococcus* that inhabits the intestinal tract.

enterocolitis /-kōlī'tis/ [Gk, *enteron* + *kolon*, bowel, *itis*], an inflammation involving both the large and small intestines. Also called **coloenteritis.**

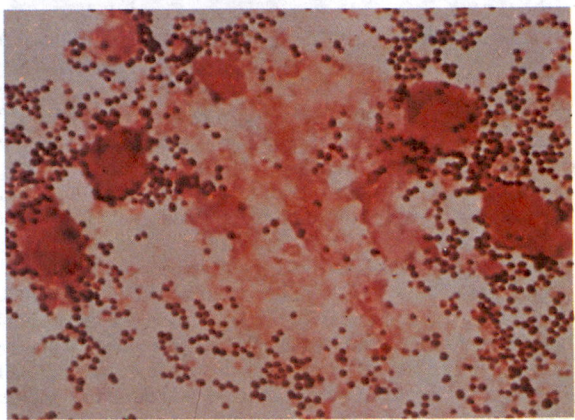

Enterocolitis *(Baron, 1990)*

enteroenterostomy /en'tərō·en'təros'təmē/, the surgical creation of an artificial connection between two segments of the intestine.

enterohepatic circulation /en'tərōhəpat'ik/, a route by which part of the bile produced by the liver enters the in-

testine to be reabsorbed by the liver and recycled back into the intestine. The remainder of the bile is excreted in feces.

enterokinase /en'tirōkī'nās/ [Gk, *enteron* + *kinesis*, movement, *ase*, enzyme], an intestinal juice enzyme that activates the proteolytic enzyme in pancreatic juice as they enter the duodenum.

enterolith /en'tərōlith'/ [Gk, *enteron* + *lithos*, stone], a stone consisting of ingested material found within the intestine. See also **calculus.**

enterolithiasis /en'tərōlithī'əsis/, the presence of enteroliths in the intestine.

enteropathy /en'tərop'əthē/, a disease or other disorder of the intestines.

enterostomal therapist /-stō'məl/, a registered nurse who is qualified by education in an accredited program in enterostomal therapy to provide care for patients. Also called **endostomy therapist.**

enterostomy /en'təros'təmē/ [Gk, *enteron* + *stoma*, mouth], a surgical procedure that produces an artificial anus or fistula in the intestine by incision through the abdominal wall. Compare **colostomy.**

enterotoxigenic /en'tirōtok'sijen'ik/, pertaining to an organism or other agent that produces a toxin causing an adverse reaction by cells of the intestinal mucosa. Examples include bacteria that produce enterotoxins, resulting in intestinal reactions such as vomiting, diarrhea, and other symptoms of food poisoning.

enterotoxin /-tok'sin/, a toxic substance specific for the cells of the intestinal mucosa, produced usually by certain species of bacteria, such as *Staphylococcus*. See also **enterotoxigenic.**

enterovirus /-vī'rəs/ [Gk, *enteron* + L, *virus*, poison], a virus that multiplies primarily in the intestinal tract. Kinds of enteroviruses are **coxsackievirus, ECHO virus,** and **poliovirus.** –**enteroviral,** *adj.*

enthesitis /en'thəsī'tis/, an inflammation of the insertion of a muscle with a strong tendency toward fibrosis and calcification. It is usually only painful when the involved muscle is activated.

ento-. See **endo-.**

entoderm. See **endoderm.**

entodermal. See **endodermal.**

Entozyme, a trademark for a GI fixed-combination drug containing bile salts and the digestive enzymes (pancreatin and pepsin).

entrainment /entrān'mənt/ [Fr, *entrainer*, to drag along], a phenomenon observed in the microanalysis of sound films in which the speaker moves several parts of the body and the listener responds to the sounds by moving in ways that are coordinated with the rhythm of the sounds. Infants have been observed to move in time to the rhythms of adult speech but not to random noises or disconnected words or vowels. Entrainment is thought to be an essential factor in the process of maternal-infant bonding.

entrance block /entrans'/ [Fr, *entrer*, to enter; AS, *blok*], (in cardiology) a theoretic zone surrounding a pacemaker focus, protecting it from discharge by an extraneous impulse that might trigger ectopic ventricular contractions.

entrance exposure, (in radiology) the skin dose of radiation. It may be expressed in milliroentgens.

entrapment neuropathy /entrap'mənt/ [OFr, *entraper*, to catch in a trap; Gk, *neuron*, nerve, *pathos*, disease], injury or inflammation of single nerves caused by pressure from surrounding tissues, such as ligaments and fascia.

entropion /entrō′pē·on/ [Gk, *en* + *tropos*, a turning],   turning inward or turning toward, usually a condition in which the eyelid turns inward toward the eye. **Cicatricial entropion** can occur in either the upper or lower eyelid as a result of scar tissue formation. **Spastic entropion** results from an inflammation or other factor that affects tissue tone. An inflammation of the eyelid may be the result of an infectious disease or irritation from an inverted eyelash. Compare **ectropion**. See also **blepharitis**.

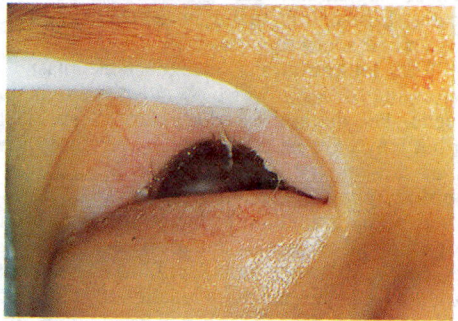

Entropion *(Zitelli, 1992)*

entropy /en′trəpē/ [Gk, *en* + *tropos*, a turning],   the tendency of a system to go from a state of order to a state of disorder, expressed in physics as a measure of the part of the energy in a thermodynamic system that is not available to perform work. Living organisms tend to go from a state of disorder to a state of order in their development and thus appear to reverse entropy. However, maintaining a living system requires the expenditure of energy, leaving less energy available for work, with the result that the entropy of the system and its surroundings increases.

ENT specialist,   a physician who specializes in the treatment of the ear, nose, and throat. See also **otolaryngologist.**

enucleation /inōo′klē·ā′shən/ [L, *e*, out of, *nucleus*, nut], **1.**   removal of an organ or tumor in one piece. **2.**   removal of the eyeball, performed for malignancy, severe infection, or extensive trauma or to control pain in glaucoma. Local or general anesthesia is used. The optic nerve and muscle attachments are cut; if possible, the surrounding layer of fascia is left with the muscles. A ball-shaped implant of silicone, plastic, or tantalum is inserted, and the muscles are sutured around it, providing a permanent stump to give support and motion to an artificial eye. Postoperatively, pressure dressings are kept in place for 1 or 2 days to prevent hemorrhage. Other possible complications include thrombosis of nearby blood vessels, which may lead to infection, including meningitis.

enucleator /inōo′klē·ā′tər/ [L, *e*, without, *nucleus*, nut],   a procedure or device for removing a nucleus from a cell.

enuresis /en′yŏorē′sis/ [Gk, *enourein*, to urinate],   incontinence of urine, especially in bed at night.

environment [Gk, *en*, in; L, *viron*, circle],   all of the many factors, as physical and psychologic, that influence or affect the life and survival of a person. See also **biome, climate.**

environmental carcinogen /envī′rənmen′təl/,   any of the natural or synthetic substances that can cause cancer. Such agents, or oncogens, may be divided into chemical agents, physical agents, hormones and viruses. Some environmental carcinogens are arsenic, asbestos, uranium, vinyl chloride, ionizing radiation, ultraviolet rays, x-rays, and coal tar derivatives. Carcinogenic effects of chemicals may be delayed as long as 30 years. Other carcinogens produce more immediate effects. Some studies indicate that the carcinogens in cigarette smoke are involved in 80% of all lung cancer. Most carcinogens are unreactive or secondary carcinogens but are converted to primary carcinogens in the body. Research indicates that numerous factors, such as heredity, affect the susceptibilities of different individuals to cancer-causing agents.

environmental control units,   control units that regulate various devices for handicapped persons from remote positions such as a bed or wheel chair. Examples include units (often with switches that can be manipulated by the lips, chin, or other functional body parts) that control lamps, television, radio, telephone, and alarm systems.

environmental health,   the total of various aspects of substances, forces, and conditions in and about a community that affect the health and well-being of the population.

environmental services,   a functional unit of a hospital or other health care facility. It has the responsibility for laundry, liquid and solid waste control, safe disposal of materials contaminated by radiation or pathogenic organisms, and general maintenance of safety and sanitation.

Enzactin,   a trademark for a topical antifungal (triacetin).

enzygotic twins.   See **monozygotic twins.**

enzymatic detergent asthma /en′zīmat′ik/,   a type of allergic reaction experienced by persons who have become sensitized to alcalase, an enzyme contained in some laundry detergents. Alcalase is produced by a bacterium, *Bacillus subtilis;* persons who are sensitive to the enzyme are also usually allergic to the bacterium. Asthmatic symptoms may progress in some severe cases to an allergic alveolitis. The most serious cases were originally among workers in plants manufacturing laundry detergents.

enzyme /en′zīm/ [Gk, *en*, in, *zyme*, ferment],   a protein produced by living cells that catalyzes chemical reactions in organic matter. Most enzymes are produced in minute quantities and catalyze reactions that take place within the cells. Digestive enzymes, however, are produced in relatively large quantities and act outside the cells in the lumen of the digestive tube.

enzyme induction [Gk, *en*, *zyme*, ferment; L, *inducere*, to lead in],   the increase in the rate of a specific enzyme synthesis from basal to maximum level caused by the presence of a substrate or substrate analog that acts as an inducer. The inducer may be a substance that inactivates a repressor chemical in the cell.

enzyme-linked immunosorbent assay (ELISA),   a laboratory technique for detecting specific antigens or antibodies, using enzyme-labeled immunoreactants and a solid-phase binding support, such as a test tube. A number of different enzymes can be used, including carbonic anhydrase, glucose oxidase, and alkaline phosphatase. Labeling is done by covalently binding the enzyme to the test substance through an enzyme-protein coupling agent, such as glutaraldehyde. Products of the reaction may be detected by fluorimetry or photometry. ELISA is nearly as sensitive as radioimmunoassay and more sensitive than complement-fixation, agglutination, and other techniques. It is commonly employed in the diagnosis of HIV infections.

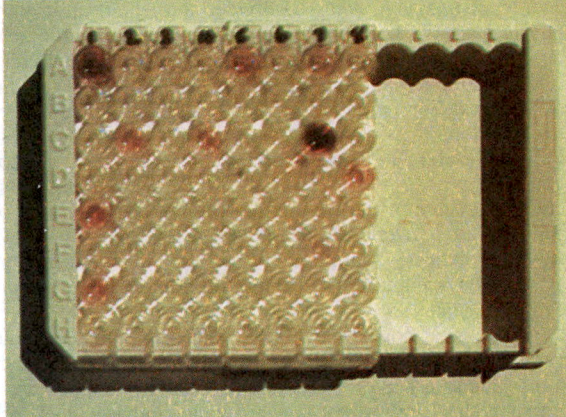

ELISA (Hart, 1992)

eosin /ē′əsin/, a group of red, acidic xanthine dyes often used in combination with a blue-purple, basic dye, such as hematoxylin, to stain tissue slides in the laboratory.

eosinophil /ē′əsin′əfil/ [Gk, *eos*, dawn, *philein*, to love], a granulocytic, bilobed leukocyte somewhat larger than a neutrophil characterized by large numbers of coarse, refractile, cytoplasmic granules that stain with the acid dye, eosin. Eosinophils constitute 1% to 3% of the white blood cells of the body. They increase in number with allergy and some parasitic infections and decrease with steroid administration. Compare **basophil, neutrophil.** –**eosinophilic,** *adj.*

eosinophilia /ē′əsin′ōfil′yə/, an increase in the number of eosinophils in the blood, accompanying inflammatory conditions. Substantial increases are considered a reflection of an allergic response.

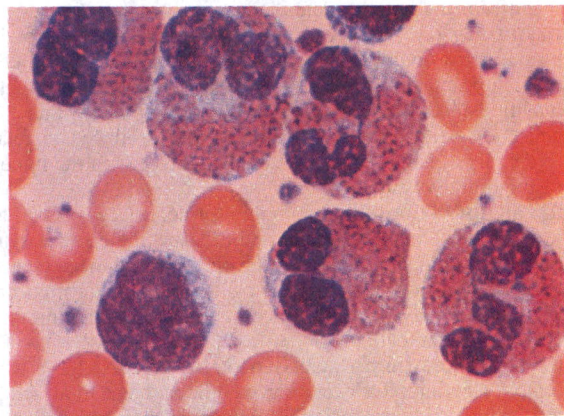

Eosinophilia (Hayhoe, 1992)

eosinophilia-myalgia syndrome, tryptophan-induced, a potentially fatal disorder characterized by a symptom complex of severe muscle pain, tenosynovitis, muscle edema, and skin rash lasting several weeks. The cause has been associated with a contaminant in L-tryptophan taken for sedation or psychotropic support.

eosinophilic /ē′əsin′əfil′ik/, **1.** the tendency of a cell, tissue, or organism to be readily stained by the dye eosin. **2.** of or pertaining to an eosinophilic leukocyte.

eosinophilic adenoma. See **acidophilic adenoma.**

eosinophilic enteropathy, a rare form of food allergy that is characterized by nausea, crampy abdominal pain, diarrhea, urticaria, an elevated eosinophil count in the blood, and eosinophilic infiltrates in the intestine. Diagnosis is made by an elimination diet; symptoms usually disappear when the offending food is removed from the diet.

eosinophilic granuloma, a simple or multiple growth in the bone or lung characterized by numerous eosinophils and histiocytes. Eosinophilic granulomas occur most frequently in children and adolescents.

eosinophilic leukemia, a malignant neoplasm of the blood-forming tissues in which eosinophils are the predominant cells. The disease resembles chronic myelocytic leukemia but may have an acute course even though no blast forms are present in the peripheral blood.

eosinophilic pneumonia, inflammation of the lungs, characterized by infiltration of the alveoli with eosinophils and large mononuclear cells, pulmonary edema, fever, night sweats, cough, dyspnea, and weight loss. The disease may be caused by a hypersensitivity reaction to spores of fungi, plant fibers, wood dust, bird droppings, porcine or bovine or piscine proteins, *Bacillus subtilis* enzyme in detergents, or certain drugs. Treatment consists of removal of the offending allergen and symptomatic and supportive therapy. Compare **bronchopneumonia.** See also **asthmatic eosinophilia.**

eosin-, a combining form meaning 'a rose, red, or dawn color': *eosinophil, eosinopenia, eosinophilic.*

-eous, a suffix meaning 'like' or 'composed of' or 'relating to' something specified: *anedeous, cutaneous, osseous.*

EP, abbreviation for **evoked potential.**

ep-. See **epi-.**

ependyma /ipen′dimə/ [Gk, an upper garment], a layer of ciliated epithelium that lines the central canal of the spinal cord and the ventricles of the brain. –**ependymal** /ipen′diməl/, *adj.*

ependymal glioma, a large, vascular, fairly solid glioma in the fourth ventricle.

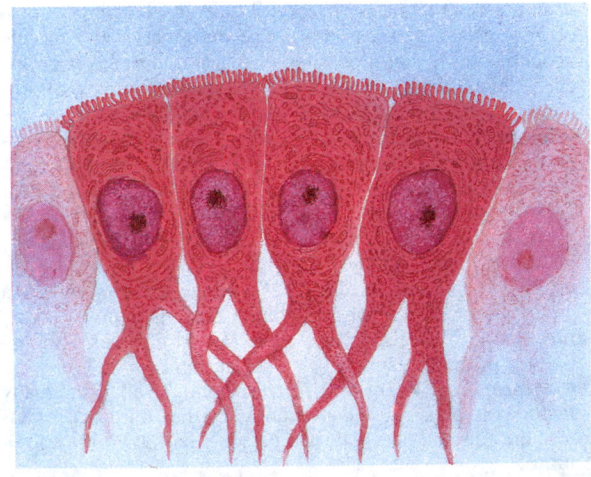

Ependyma cells (Chipps, 1992)

ependymoblastoma /ipen′dimōblastō′mə/, a malignant neoplasm composed of primitive cells of the ependyma. Also called **malignant ependymoma.**

ependymoma /ipen′dimō′mə/ [Gk, *ependyma*, an upper garment, *oma*, tumor], a neoplasm composed of differentiated cells of the ependyma. The tumor, which is usually a benign, pale, firm, encapsulated, somewhat nodular mass, commonly arises from the roof of the fourth ventricle and may extend to the spinal cord. Primary lesions may also develop in the spinal cord. Also called **ependymocytoma.**

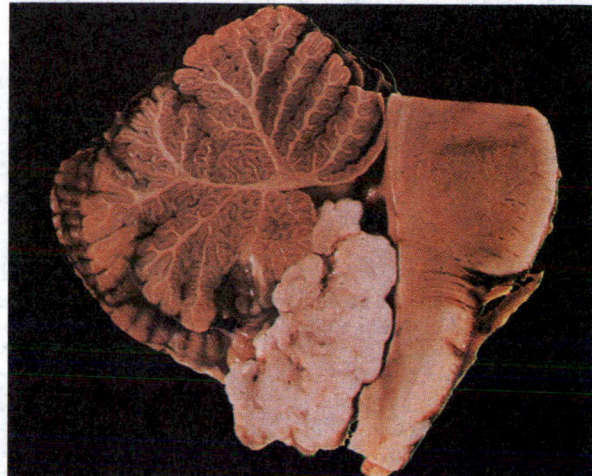

Ependymoma
(Fletcher, 1987/Prof PL Lantos, Dept of Neuropathology, Institute of Psychiatry, London)

ephapse /ef′aps/ [Gk, *ephasis*, a touching], a point of lateral contact between nerve fibers across which impulses may be transmitted directly through the membranes of the cells rather than across a synapse. Compare **synapse.** — **ephaptic,** *adj.*

ephaptic transmission /ifap′tik/, the passage of a neural impulse from one nerve fiber, axon, or dendrite to another through the membranes. The mechanism may be a factor in epileptic seizures. Compare **synaptic transmission.**

ephebiatrics /ēfeb′ē·at′riks/ [Gk, *ephebos*, puberty, *iatros*, physician], a branch of medicine that specializes in the health of adolescents.

ephedrine /ef′ədrēn/, an adrenergic bronchodilator.

■ INDICATIONS: It is prescribed in the treatment of asthma and bronchitis and is used topically as a nasal decongestant.

■ CONTRAINDICATIONS: Concomitant administration of monoamine oxidase inhibitors, hypertension, cardiac artery disease, cardiac arrhythmia, or known hypersensitivity to this drug prohibits its use.

■ ADVERSE EFFECTS: Among the more serious adverse reactions are nervousness, insomnia, anorexia, and increased blood pressure.

ephemeral /ifem′ərəl/ [Gk, *epi*, above, *hemera*, day], pertaining to a short-lived condition, such as a fever.

ephemeral fever, any febrile condition lasting only 24 to 48 hours that is uncomplicated and of unknown origin.

epi-, ep-, a prefix meaning 'on, upon': *epicanthus, epicostal, epidural.*

epiblast /ep′iblast′/ [Gk, *epi*, upon, *blastos*, germ], the primordial outer layer of the blastocyst or blastula, before differentiation of the germ layers, that gives rise to the ectoderm and contains cells capable of forming the endoderm and mesoderm. See also **ectoderm.** — **epiblastic,** *adj.*

epicanthus /ep′ikan′thəs/ [Gk, *epi* + *kanthos*, lip of a vessel], a vertical fold of skin over the angle of the inner canthus of the eye. It may be slight or marked, covering the canthus and the caruncle. It is normal in Oriental people and is of no clinical significance. Some infants with Down's syndrome have marked epicanthal folds. Also called **epicanthal fold, epicanthic fold.** — **epicanthal, epicanthic,** *adj.*

epicardia /-kär′dē·ə/ [Gk, *epi*, above, *kardia*, heart], the part of the esophagus that lies between the cardiac orifice of the stomach and the esophageal opening of the diaphragm.

-epicardial. See **epicardium.**

epicardial pacing. See **pacing.**

epicardium /ep′ikär′dē·əm/ [Gk, *epi* + *kardia*, heart], one of the three layers of tissue that form the wall of the heart. It is composed of a single sheet of squamous epithelial cells overlying delicate connective tissue. The epicardium is the visceral portion of the serous pericardium and folds back upon itself to form the parietal portion of the serous pericardium. Compare **myocardium.** — **epicardial,** *adj.*

-epicondylar. See **epicondyle.**

epicondylar fracture /-kon′dilər/, any fracture that involves the medial or the lateral epicondyle of a specific bone, such as the humerus.

epicondyle /ep′ikon′dəl/ [Gk, *epi* + *kondylos*, knuckle], a projection on the surface of a bone above its condyle. — **epicondylar,** *adj.*

epicondylitis /ep′ikon′dilī′tis/, a painful and sometimes disabling inflammation of the muscle and surrounding tissues of the elbow, caused by repeated strain on the forearm near the lateral epicondyle of the humerus, such as from violent extension or supination of the wrist against a resisting force. The strain may result from activities, such as tennis or golf, twisting a screwdriver, or carrying a heavy load with the arm extended. Treatment usually includes rest, injection of procaine with or without hydrocortisone, and, in some cases, surgery to release part of the muscle from the epicondyle. See also **lateral humeral epicondylitis.**

-epicranial. See **epicranium.**

epicranial aponeurosis /-krā′nē·əl/ [Gk, *epi* + *kranion*, skull; *apo*, away, *neuron*, tendon], a fibrous membrane that covers the cranium between the occipital and frontal muscles of the scalp. Also called **galea aponeurotica.**

epicranium /-krā′nē·əm/ [Gk, *epi* + *kranion*, skull], the complete scalp, including the integument, the muscular sheets, and the aponeuroses. Compare **epicranius.** — **epicranial,** *adj.*

epicranius [Gk, *epi* + *kranion*, skull], the broad, muscular, and tendinous layer of tissue covering the top and the sides of the skull from the occipital bone to the eyebrows. It consists of broad, thin muscular bellies, connected by an extensive aponeurosis. Innervation of the epicranius by branches of the facial nerves can draw back the scalp, raise the eyebrows, and move the ears. Compare **epicranium.** See also **epicranial aponeurosis, occipitofrontalis, temporoparietalis.**

epicritic /-krit'ik/, pertaining to the somatic sensations of fine discriminative touch, vibration, two-point discrimination, stereognosis, and conscious and unconscious proprioception.

epidemic /-dem'ik/ [Gk, *epi* + *demos*, people], **1.** affecting a significantly large number of people at the same time. **2.** a disease that spreads rapidly through a demographic segment of the human population, such as everyone in a given geographic area, a military base, or similar population unit, or everyone of a certain age or sex, such as the children or women of a region. **3.** a widespread disease that tends to occur periodically. Compare **endemic, epizootic, pandemic.**

epidemic diarrhea in newborn [Gk, *epi*, above, *demos*, the people, *dia*, through, *rhein*, flow; ME, *newe, beren*], any severe gastroenteritis epidemic among a community of newborns, as may occur in a hospial nursery.

epidemic encephalitis, any diffuse inflammation of the brain occurring in epidemic form. Two kinds of epidemic encephalitis are **Japanese encephalitis** and **St. Louis encephalitis.** See also **encephalitis.**

epidemic hemoglobinuria. See **hemoglobinuria.**

epidemic hemorrhagic conjunctivitis [Gk, *epi*, above, *demos*, the people, *haima*, blood, *rhegnynei*, to gush; L, *conjunctivus,* connecting; Gk, *itis*, inflammation], a highly contagious infection, commonly involving an enterovirus, that begins with eye pain, accompanied by swollen eyelids, hyperemia of the conjunctiva. It is a self-limiting disorder and there is no specific remedy.

epidemic hemorrhagic fever, a severe viral infection marked by fever and bleeding. The disorder develops rapidly, characterized initially by fever and muscle ache, possibly followed by hemorrhage, peripheral vascular collapse, hypovolemic shock, and acute kidney failure. The arbovirus or other pathogen is believed transmitted by mosquitoes, ticks, or mites. The pathophysiology of the hemorrhagic effect is uncertain, although it is assumed the disease organism causes the development of lesions in the lining of the capillaries. Among the various forms of epidemic hemorrhagic fevers are **Argentine hemorrhagic fever, Bolivian hemorrhagic fever, dengue hemorrhagic fever, Lassa fever,** and **yellow fever.** See also specific viral infections.

epidemic hysteria. See **major hysteria.**

epidemic keratoconjunctivitis (EKC) [Gk, *epi*, above, *demos*, the people, *keras*, horn; L, *conjunctivus*; Gk, *itis*, inflammation], an acute complex of keratitis and conjunctivitis transmitted by an adenovirus. A highly contagious form of keratoconjunctivitis, it often includes lymph node involvement. It is commonly spread by handling contaminated materials in eye clinics, particularly offices that handle emergency care of eye injuries. Also called **shipyard eye.**

epidemic myalgia, a disease caused by coxsackie B virus, characterized by sudden, acute chest or epigastric pain and fever lasting a few days, followed by complete, spontaneous recovery. Also called **devil's grip, epidemic myositis, epidemic pleurodynia.**

epidemic myositis. See **epidemic myalgia, epidemic pleurodynia.**

epidemic parotitis. See **mumps.**

epidemic pleurodynia, an infection caused by a coxsackievirus, affecting mainly children. It is characterized by severe intermittent pain in the abdomen or lower chest, fever, headache, sore throat, malaise, and extreme myalgia. The symptoms may continue for weeks or subside after a few days and recur for a period of weeks. Treatment is symptomatic; complete recovery is usual. Also called **Bornholm disease, devil's grip, epidemic myositis.**

epidemic typhus, an acute, severe rickettsial infection characterized by prolonged high fever, headache, and a dark maculopapular rash that covers most of the body. The causative organism, *Rickettsia prowazekii,* is transmitted indirectly as a result of the bite of the human body louse; the pathogen is contained in feces of the louse and enters the body tissues as the bite is scratched. An intense headache and a fever reaching 40° C (104° F) begin after an incubation period of 10 days to 2 weeks. The rash follows. Complications may include vascular collapse, renal failure, pneumonia, or gangrene. Mortality is high among older patients. Treatment may include chloramphenicol or tetracycline, aspirin, and supportive, symptomatic care. Also called **classic typhus, European typhus, jail fever, louse-borne typhus.** Compare **murine typhus.** See also **Brill-Zinsser disease, rickettsia, typhus.**

-epidemiologic. See **epidemiology.**

epidemiologist /-dē'mē·ol'əjist/, a physician or medical scientist who studies the incidence, prevalence, spread, prevention, and control of disease in a community or a specific group of individuals. In a hospital, a physician may be assigned as a staff epidemiologist with responsibility for directing infection control programs within the facility.

epidemiology /-dē'mē·ol'əjē/ [Gk, *epi* + *demos*, people, *logos* science], the study of the occurrence, distribution, and causes of disease in humankind. **–epidemiologic,** *adj.*

epiderm-, epidermo-, a combining form meaning 'of or pertaining to the epidermis': *epidermoid, epidermolysis, epidermolytic.*

-epidermal. See **epidermal nevus.**

epidermal nevus /-dur'məl/ [Gk, *epi, derma,* the skin; L, *naevus,* birthmark], a discrete discolored lesion caused by an overgrowth of epidermis. It may be seen in newborns. Also called **epithelial nevus, hard nevus.**

epidermis /ep'idur'mis/ [Gk, *epi* + *derma,* skin], the superficial, avascular layers of the skin, made up of an outer, dead, cornified portion and a deeper, living, cellular portion. Epidermal cells gradually move outward to the skin surface, undergoing change as they migrate, until they are desquamated as cornified flakes. Cells in various transitional stages make up the basal cell layer, the prickle cell layer, the granular layer, the clear cell layer, and the cornified layer. Altogether, these layers are between 0.5 and 1.1 mm in thickness. Also called **cuticle.** See **skin. –epidermal, epidermoid,** *adj.*

epidermoid carcinoma /-dur'moid/ [Gk, *epi, derma* + *eidos,* form], a malignant neoplasm in which the tumor cells tend to differentiate in the manner of epidermal cells, then form horny cells called prickle cells.

epidermoid cyst, a common, benign, variable, subcutaneous swelling lined by keratinizing epithelium and filled with a cheesy material composed of sebum and epithelial debris. The cyst is movable but attached to the skin by the remains of the duct of a sebaceous gland. Eepidermoid cysts frequently become infected. Treatment is surgical excision. Also called **sebaceous cyst, wen.** Compare **pilar cyst.**

epidermolysis bullosa /ep'idərmol'isis/ [Gk, *epi, derma* +

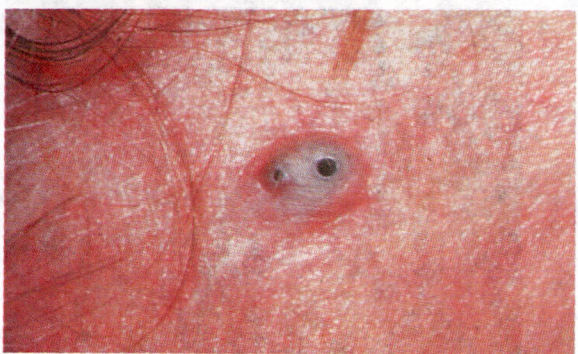

Epidermoid cyst
(McKee, 1993/Courtesy Dr. D McGibbon, St. Thomas' Hospital, London)

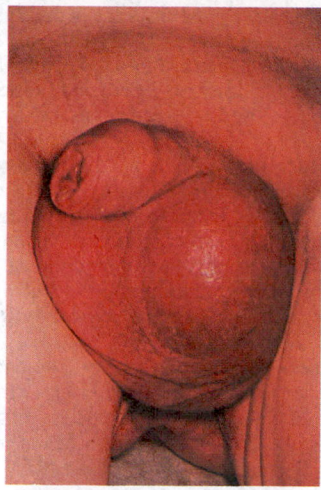

Epididymitis *(Lloyd-Davies, 1983)*

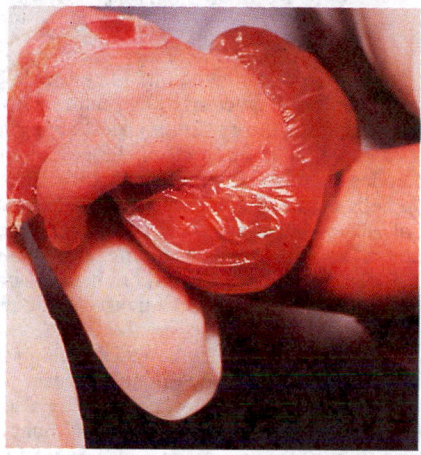

Junctional epidermolysis bullosa *(Zitelli, 1992)*

epididymoorchitis /ep'idid'imō'ôrkī'tis/ [Gk, *epi, didymos + orchis,* testis, *itis*], inflammation of the epididymis and of the testis. See also **epididymitis, orchitis.**

epididymovesiculography /ep'idid'imōves'ikyəlog'rəfē/, a radiologic examination of the seminal ducts usually performed in cases of sterility, cysts, tumors, abscesses, or inflammation. The contrast medium may be injected by catheter or by a surgical incision in the upper part of the scrotum to expose the ducts, which are directly injected with contrast medium.

epidural /ep'idŏōr'əl/ [Gk, *epi + dura,* hard], outside or above the dura mater.

epidural anesthesia, the process of achieving regional anesthesia of the pelvic, abdominal, genital, or other area by the injection of a local anesthetic into the epidural space of the spinal column.

lysis, loosening], a group of rare, hereditary or acquired skin diseases in which vesicles and bullae develop, usually at sites of trauma. Severe forms may also involve mucous membranes and may leave scars and contractures on healing. Basal cell and squamous cell carcinomas sometimes develop in the scar tissue.

epidermophytosis /ep'idur'mōfītō'sis/, a superficial fungus infection of the skin.

epididym-, a combining form meaning 'pertaining to the epididymis': *epididymectomy, epididymitis.*

epididymis /ep'idid'imis/, *pl.* **epidiymides** [Gk, *epi + didymos,* pair], one of a pair of long, tightly coiled ducts that carries sperm from the seminiferous tubules of the testes to the vas deferens.

epididymitis /ep'idid'imī'tis/ [Gk, *epi, didymos + itis,* inflammation], acute or chronic inflammation of the epididymis. It may result from venereal disease, urinary tract infection, prostatitis, or prostatectomy. Symptoms include fever and chills, pain in the groin, and tender, swollen epididymis. Treatment includes bed rest, scrotal support, and antibiotics, as appropriate.

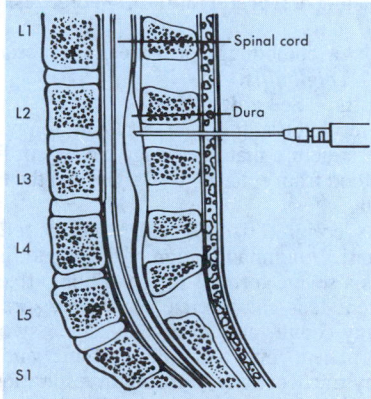

Epidural anesthesia

epidural blood patch, a patch repairing a tear or a hole in the dura mater around the spinal cord. The tear is usually the result of needle puncture during spinal anesthesia or lumbar puncture. Spinal fluid leaks through the hole, resulting in a spinal headache. To form a seal, 10 to 15 ml of the patient's blood is injected into the epidural space. A clot forms, covering the hole and preventing further loss of fluid. The technique is used to treat persistent or severe spinal headache.

epidural hemorrhage, a hemorrhage that results in a collection of blood outside the dura mater of the brain or spinal cord. Also called **extradural hemorrhage.**

epidural space, the space immediately above and surrounding the dura mater of the brain or spinal cord, beneath the periosteum of the cranium and the spinal column.

epigastric /-gas'trik/ [Gk, *epi*, above, *gaster*, stomach], pertaining to the epigastrium.

epigastric node [Gk, *epi* + *gaster*, stomach; L, *nodus*, knot], a node in one of the seven groups of parietal lymph nodes serving the abdomen and the pelvis, comprising about four nodes along the caudal portion of the inferior epigastric vessels. See also **lymph, lymphatic system, lymph node.**

epigastric pain [Gk, *epi*, above, *gaster*, stomach; L, *poena*, penalty], pain in the epigastric region of the abdomen.

epigastric reflex [Gk, *epi*, above, *gaster*, stomach; L, *reflectere*, to bend back], a contraction of the rectus abdominis muscle that occurs when the skin surface in the upper and middle abdominal region is stimulated. The reflex also may be induced when the axillary region of the 5th and 6th dorsal nerves is stimulated.

epigastric region, the part of the abdomen in the upper zone between the right and left hypochondriac regions. Also called **antecardium, epigastrium.** See also **abdominal regions.**

epigastric sensation, a weak, sinking feeling of undefined nature that is usually localized in the pit of the stomach but may occur throughout the abdominal region. See also **sensation,** def.1.

epigastrium. See **epigastric region.**

epigenesis /ep'ijen'əsis/ [Gk, *epi* + *genein*, to produce], (in embryology) a theory of development in which the organism grows from a simple to more complex form through the progressive differentiation of an undifferentiated cellular unit. Compare **preformation. −epigenesist,** *n.* *epigenetic, adj.*

epiglott-, a combining form meaning 'pertaining to the epiglottis': *epiglottitis.*

epiglottiditis. See **epiglottitis.**

epiglottis /ep'iglot'is/ [Gk, *epi* + *glossa*, tongue], the cartilaginous structure that overhangs the larynx like a lid and prevents food from entering the larynx and the trachea while swallowing.

epiglottitis /ep'igloti'tis/ [Gk, *epi* + *glossa*, tongue, *itis*, inflammation], an inflammation of the epiglottis. Acute epiglottitis is a severe form of the condition, affecting primarily children. It is characterized by fever, sore throat, stridor, croupy cough, and an erythematous, swollen epiglottis. The patient may become cyanotic and require an emergency tracheostomy to maintain respiration. The causative organism is usually *Haemophilus influenzae,* type B. Antibiotics, rest, oxygen, and supportive care are usually included in treatment. Also called **epiglottiditis.** See also **acute epiglottitis.**

epilating forceps /ep'ilā'ting/ [L, *e, pilus*, without hair], a kind of small spring forceps, used for removing unwanted hair.

epilation. See **depilation.**

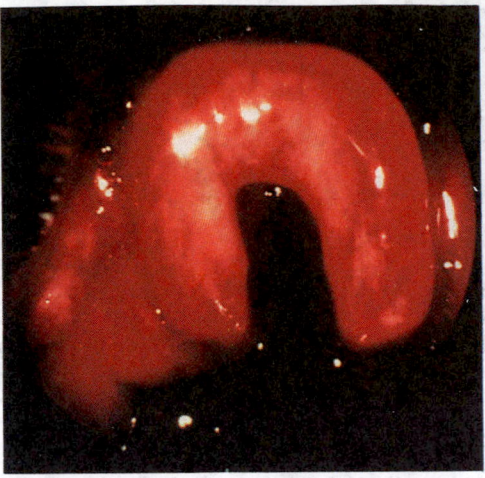

Acute epiglottitis (Zitelli, 1992)

epilepsy /ep'ilep'sē/ [Gk, *epilepsia*, seizure], a group of neurologic disorders characterized by recurrent episodes of convulsive seizures, sensory disturbances, abnormal behavior, loss of consciousness, or all of these. Common to all types of epilepsy is an uncontrolled electric discharge from the nerve cells of the cerebral cortex. Although most epilepsy is of unknown cause, it may sometimes be associated with cerebral trauma, intracranial infection, brain tumor, vascular disturbances, intoxication, or chemical imbalance. See also **absence seizure, focal seizure, tonic-clonic seizure, psychomotor seizure.**

■ OBSERVATIONS: The frequency of attacks may range from many times a day to intervals of several years. In predisposed individuals, seizures may occur during sleep or after physical stimulation, such as by a flickering light or sudden loud sound. Emotional disturbances also may be significant trigger factors. Some seizures are preceded by an aura, but others have no warning symptoms. Most epileptic attacks are brief. They may be localized or general, with or without clonic movements, and are often followed by drowsiness or confusion. Diagnosis is made by observation of the pattern of seizures and abnormalities on an electroencephalogram. Diagnosis is also aided by a system of classification of the criteria that characterize the different types of epileptic seizures. One major category in the classification scheme encompasses the partial seizures, which often begin focally, then spread to other brain areas. A second major category includes the generalized seizures, which usually begin deep in the brain and impair consciousness.

■ INTERVENTION: The kind of epilepsy determines the selection of preventive medication. Correctable lesions and metabolic causes are eliminated when possible. During an attack the patient should be protected from injury without being severely restrained.

■ NURSING CONSIDERATIONS: A nurse observing an epileptic attack, in addition to protecting the patient from injury, should carefully note and accurately describe the sequence of seizure activity. The patient and family must be fully informed and counseled about the disorder, the importance of regularly taking prescribed medication and never discontinuing treatment without professional advice, toxic effects of medication, wearing a medical identification tag, and continuing to live as normal a life as possible. Nurses also have a responsibility to help improve the public's attitude toward epilepsy and to correct misunderstanding that limits educational and occupational opportunities for patients with this diagnosis. See also **anticonvulsant, aura, central nervous system stimulant, clonus, ictus, tonic. —epileptic,** *adj.,* *n.*

epileptic dementia /epˈileptik/ [Gk, *epilepsia*, seizure; L, *de, mens*, mind], a loss of cognitive and intellectual functions that develop in some cases of incompletely controlled epilepsy. Symptoms include slowness and circumstantiality of speech and narrowed attention span.

epileptic mania, *obsolete*. a mood disorder characterized by attacks of violence that occur immediately before, after, or in place of an epileptic seizure. See also **epilepsy, mania.**

epileptic stupor, the state of unawareness and unresponsiveness after an epileptic seizure.

epileptic vertigo [Gk, *epilepsia*, seizure; L, *vertigo*, dizziness], an aura of dizziness that may precede, accompany, or follow an epileptic seizure.

epiloia. See **tuberous sclerosis.**

epimysium /epˈimizˈēˌəm/ [Gk, *epi* + *mys*, muscle], a fibrous sheath that enfolds a muscle and extends between the bundles of muscle fibers, such as the perimysium. It is sturdy in some areas but more delicate in others, such as those areas where the muscle moves freely under a strong sheet of fascia. The epimysium may also fuse with fascia that attaches a muscle to a bone.

epinephrine /epˈənefˈrin/ [Gk, *epi* + *nephros*, kidney], an endogenous adrenal hormone and synthetic adrenergic vasoconstrictor.

■ INDICATIONS: It is prescribed in the treatment of anaphylaxis, acute bronchial spasm, and nasal congestion and to increase the effectiveness of a local anesthetic.

■ CONTRAINDICATION: Known hypersensitivity to this drug prohibits its use.

■ ADVERSE EFFECTS: Among the most serious adverse reactions are arrhythmias, increases in blood pressure, and rebound congestion (when used as a decongestant).

International classification of epileptic seizures

Traditional terminology	New nomenclature
	Partial seizures (seizures beginning locally)
Focal motor; jacksonian seizures (occasionally become secondarily generalized)	Simple (without impairment of consciousness)
	With motor symptoms
	With special sensory or somatosensory symptoms
	With autonomic symptoms
	With psychic symptoms
Temporal lobe or psychomotor seizures	Complex (with impairment of consciousness)
	Simple partial onset followed by impairment of consciousness—with or without automatisms
	Impaired consciousness at onset—with or without automatisms
	Secondarily generalized (partial onset evolving to generalized tonic-clinic seizures)
	Generalized seizures (bilaterally symmetrical and without local onset)
Petit mal	Absences
Minor motor	Myoclonic
Limited grand mal	Clonic
	Tonic
Grand mal	Tonic-clonic
Drop attacks	Atonic
	Infantile spasms
	Unclassified seizures (because of incomplete data)
	Status epilepticus (prolonged partial or generalized seizures without recovery between attacks)

From Rothner AD, ed: *Recend developments in the treatment of epilepsy*, Philadelphia, 1983, Borland-Coogan Associates, Inc. (© Abbott Laboratories, Chicago).

epinephryl borate /-nefˈril/, an adrenergic.

■ INDICATIONS: It is prescribed in the treatment of primary open-angle glaucoma.

■ CONTRAINDICATIONS: Narrow-angle glaucoma, aphakia, or known hypersensitivity to this drug prohibits its use. It should not be given before peripheral iridectomy and should not be administered to eyes that are capable of angle closure.

■ ADVERSE EFFECTS: Among the more serious adverse reactions are tachycardia, hypertension, headache, blurred vision, and allergic reaction.

epiphora. See **tearing.**

epiphyseal /epˈfizˈēˌəl, ipifˈəsēˈəl/ [Gk, *epi*, above, *phyein*, to grow], pertaining to or resembling the epiphysis. Also spelled **epiphysial.**

epiphyseal fracture [Gk, *epi* + *phyein,* to grow; *fractura,* break], a fracture involving the epiphyseal growth plate of a long bone, resulting in separation or in fragmentation of the plate. Also called **Salter fracture.**

epiphyseal plate [Gk, *epi*, above, *phyein*, to grow, *platys,* flat], a thin layer of cartilage between the epiphysis, a sec-

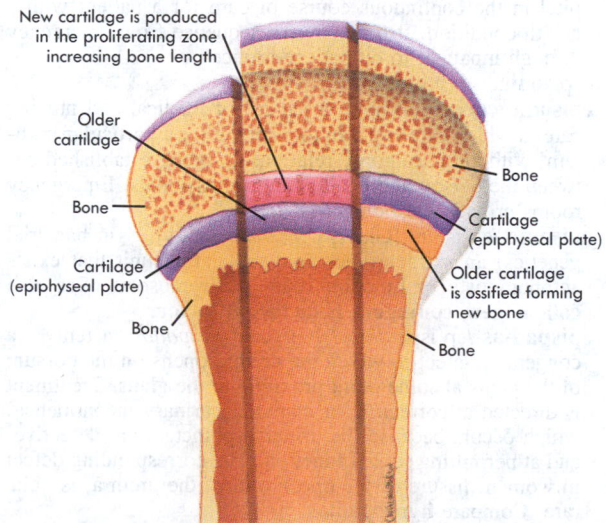

New cartilage is produced in the proliferating zone increasing bone length

Older cartilage

Bone

Cartilage (epiphyseal plate)

Bone

Bone

Cartilage (epiphyseal plate)

Older cartilage is ossified forming new bone

Bone

Epiphyseal plate (Seeley, 1992/Christine Oleksyk)

E-F

ondary bone-forming center, and the bone shaft. The new bone forms along the plate.

epiphysial. See **epiphyseal.**

epiphysis /epif'isis/, *pl.* **epiphyses** [Gk, *epi* + *phyein*, to grow], the head of a long bone that is separated from the shaft of the bone by the epiphyseal plate until the bone stops growing, the plate is obliterated, and the shaft and the head become united. Compare **diaphysis.** –**epiphyseal** /ipif'əsē'əl/, *adj.*

epiphysis cerebri. See **pineal body.**

epiphysitis /ipif'isī'tis/, an inflammation of the epiphysis, usually of a long bone, such as the femur or humerus. The disorder affects mainly children.

epiploic foramen /-plō'ik/ [Gk, *epiploon*, caul; L, *foramen*, a hole], a passage between the peritoneal cavity and the omental bursa. It is lined with peritoneum and is approximately 3 cm in diameter.

epipygus. See **pygomelus.**

episcleritis /ep'isklərī'tis/, inflammation of the outermost layers of the sclera and of the tissues overlying the posterior portions of this tough, white outer coat of the eyeball.

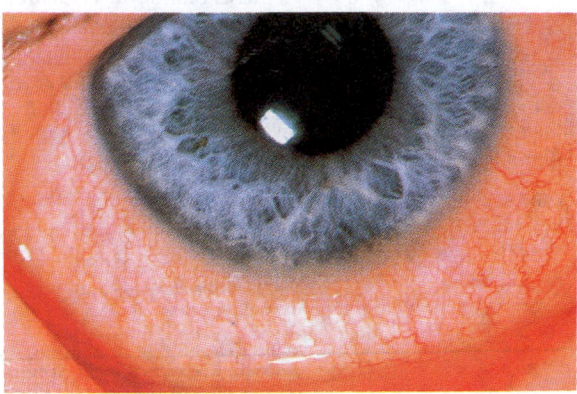

Episcleritis *(Schumacher, 1988)*

episi-, a combining form meaning 'pertaining to the vulva': *episioplast, episiotomy.*

episiotomy /epē'zē·ot'əmē/ [Gk, *episeion*, pubic region, *temnein*, to cut], a surgical procedure, usually required for forceps delivery, in which an incision is made in a woman's perineum to enlarge her vaginal opening for delivery, performed most often electively to prevent tearing of the perineum, to hasten or facilitate delivery of the baby, or to prevent stretching of perineal muscles and connective tissue thought to predispose to subsequent abnormalities of pelvic outlet relaxation, as cystocele, rectocele, and uterine prolapse; its prophylactic efficacy is debated. The incision into the vaginal and perineal tissue is closed with absorbable sutures that need not be removed. Deep incisions require closure in two or more layers. Immediate complications include hemorrhage and extension of the incision along the vaginal sulcus or into the anal sphincter or rectum. Delayed complications include hematoma and abscess. Application of cold packs to the perineum for several hours immediately postpartum minimizes swelling. Alternating applications later of heat and cold and warm sitz baths reduce discomfort, but sitz baths longer than 10 minutes soften tissue and prolong healing. A mediolateral episiotomy is an

episiotomy cut at an angle of approximately 45 degrees with the midline. Although it affords wide exposure for delivery, it is painful postpartum and is prone to hematoma and infection. A median or midline episiotomy is an incision in the perineum in the midline; although less painful postpartum, it affords less exposure for delivery and may extend into or through the anal sphincter and into the rectum.

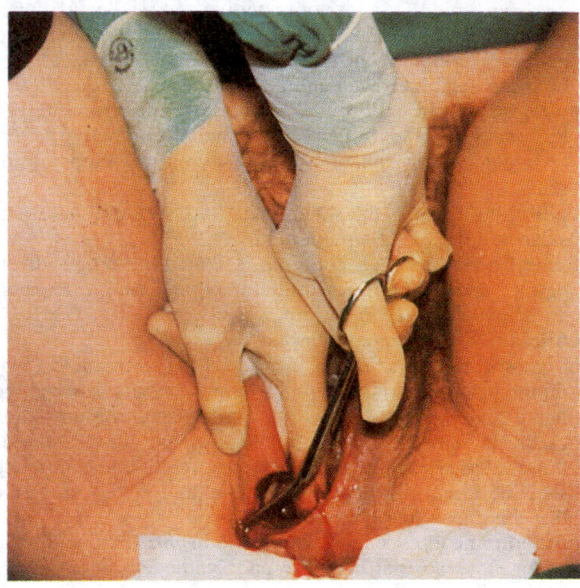

Episiotomy *(Al-Azzawi, 1991)*

episode /ep'isōd/ [Gk, *episodion*, coming in besides], an incident or event that stands out from the continuity of everyday life, such as an episode of illness or a traumatic episode in the course of a child's development. –**episodic,** *adj.*

episode of hospital care, the services provided by a hospital in the continuous course of care for a patient with a health condition. It may cover a sequence from emergency through inpatient to outpatient services.

-episodic. See **episode.**

episodic care /-sod'ik/, a pattern of medical and nursing care in which care is given to a person for a particular problem, without an ongoing relationship being established between the person and health care professionals. Emergency rooms provide episodic care.

episome /ep'isōm/ [Gk, *epi* + *soma*, body], (in bacterial genetics) an extrachromosomal replicating unit that exists autonomously or functions with a chromosome. See also **colicinogen, conjugon, F factor, R factor.**

epispadias /ep'ispā'dē·əs/ [Gk, *epi* + *spadon*, a rent], a congenital defect in which the urethra opens on the dorsum of the penis at some point proximal to the glans. Treatment is directed at correcting or managing urinary incontinence, which occurs because the urinary sphincters are defective, and at permitting sexual function. The corresponding defect in women, fissure of the upper wall of the urethra, is quite rare. Compare **hypospadias.**

epistasis /epis'təsis/ [Gk, a standing], (in genetics) a type of interaction between genes at different loci on a chromosome in which one is able to mask or suppress the expression of the other. The epistatic effect, which is nonallelic and therefore the opposite of the dominance relationship, may be caused by the presence of homozygous recessives at one gene pair, as occurs in the Bombay phenotype, or by the presence of a dominant allele that counteracts the expression of another dominant gene. Compare **dominance.** **–epistatic,** *adj.*

epistaxis /ep′istak′sis/ [Gk, a dropping], bleeding from the nose caused by local irritation of mucous membranes, violent sneezing, fragility of the mucous membrane or of the arterial walls, chronic infection, trauma, hypertension, leukemia, vitamin K deficiency, or, most often, picking of the nose. Also called **nosebleed.**

■ OBSERVATIONS: Epistaxis may result from rupture of tiny vessels in the anterior nasal septum; this occurs most frequently in early childhood and adolescence. In adults, it occurs more commonly in men than in women, may be severe in elderly persons, may be accompanied by respiratory distress, apprehension, restlessness, vertigo, and nausea, and may lead to syncope.

■ INTERVENTIONS: The patient suffering epistaxis is instructed to breathe through the mouth, to sit quietly with the head tilted slightly forward to prevent blood from entering the pharynx, and to avoid swallowing blood. The bleeding may be controlled by pinching the nose firmly with the fingers, by inserting a cotton ball soaked in a topical vasoconstrictor and applying pressure to the skin on both sides of the nose, occluding the blood supply to the nostrils, or by placing an ice compress over the nose. If bleeding continues, the clots may be removed by suction. The nasal mucosa may be anesthetized with topical lidocaine, cauterized with a silver nitrate stick or an electric cautery, and then sprayed with epinephrine. Severe bleeding, especially from the posterior nasal septum, may be treated by inserting packing, which generally is left in place for 1 to 3 days. During that period the patient is kept in high Fowler's position, the placement of the packing is checked frequently, and a sedative, antibiotics, vitamins C and K, and a cool, nonirritating liquid diet may be ordered. Persistent or recurrent profuse epistaxis may be treated by ligating an artery supplying the nose, such as the external carotid, ethmoid, or internal maxillary.

■ NURSING CONSIDERATIONS: The nurse administers first aid and ordered medication; assists in cauterization and nasal packing; checks the patient's blood pressure, pulse, and respiration every half hour until bleeding subsides; and then continues to check them every 4 hours. The nurse limits the patient's activity, avoids serving milk and hot liquids, encourages expectoration rather than swallowing of blood, and reports symptoms of respiratory distress, vertigo, and any bleeding. Before the patient is discharged, the nurse provides instruction on the prevention of epistaxis by using a vaporizer and applying petroleum jelly with a cotton swab gently to the mucous membrane lining the nostrils.

epistropheus. See **axis.**

epithalamus /ep′ithal′əməs/ [Gk, *epi* + *thalamos*, chamber], one of the portions of the diencephalon. It includes the trigonum habenulae, the pineal body, and the posterior commissure. Compare **hypothalamus, metathalamus, subthalamus, thalamus. –epithalamic,** *adj.*

epithelial /-thē′lē·əl/ [Gk, *epi*, above, *thele*, nipple], pertaining to or involving the outer layer of the skin.

epithelial cancer [Gk, *epi*, above, *thele*, nipple; L, *cancer*,

crab], a carcinoma that develops from squamous or transitional epithelium, or related tissues in the skin, esophagus, and other organs. Also called **epithelioma.**

epithelial cuff. See **junctional epithelium.**

epithelial debridement [Gk, *epi*, above, *thele*, nipple; Fr, *débridement*, an incision], the removal of the entire inner lining and the attachment from the gingival or periodontal pocket in gingival curettage. Also called **canal debridement, deepithelialization.**

epithelialization /-thē′lē·al′izā′shən/ [Gk, *epi*, above, *thele*, nipple; L, *ization*, process], the regrowth of skin over a wound.

epithelial nevus. See **epidermal nevus.**

epithelial peg [Gk, *epi* + *thele*, nipple]], any of the papillary projections of the epithelius that penetrate the underlying stroma of connecting tissue and normally develop in mucous membranes and dermal tissues. Also called **rete peg** /rē′tē/.

epithelial rest. See **embryonic rest.**

epithelial tissue [Gk, *epi*, above, *thele*, nipple; OFr, *tissu*], a closely packed single or stratified layer of cells covering the body and lining its cavities, with the exception of the blood and lymph vessels.

epitheliofibril. See **tonofibril.**

epithelioid leiomyoma /ep′ithē′lē·oid/ [Gk, *epi*, *thele* + *eidos*, form], an uncommon neoplasm of smooth muscle in which the cells are polygonal in shape. It usually develops in the stomach. Also called **bizarre leiomyoma, leiomyoblastoma.**

epithelioma /-thē′lē·ō′mə/ [Gk, *epi*, *thele* + *oma*, tumor], **1.** a neoplasm derived from the epithelium. **2.** *obsolete.* any carcinoma.

-epithelioma, a combining form meaning a 'tumor of epithelial tissue': *inoepithelioma, periepithelioma, trichoepithelioma.*

epithelioma adamantinum. See **ameloblastoma.**

epithelioma adenoides cysticum. See **trichoepithelioma.**

epithelium /-thē′lē·əm/ [Gk, *epi* + *thele*, nipple], the covering of the internal and the external organs of the body, also the lining of vessels, body cavities, glands, and organs. It consists of cells bound together by connective material and varies in the number of layers and the kinds of cells. Epithelium in different parts of the body is made of simple

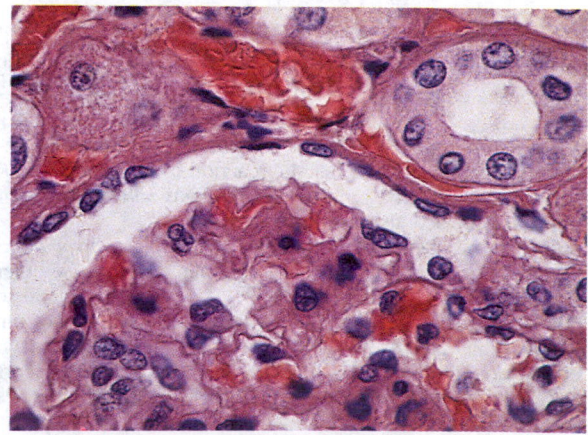

Photomicrograph of epithelium (Erlandsen, 1992)

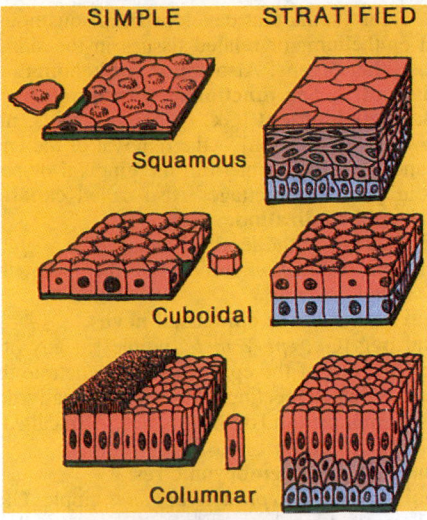

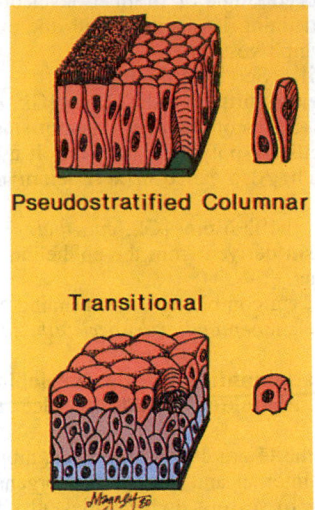

Classification of epithelium (Erlandsen, 1992)

squamous cells, simple cuboidal cells, and stratified columnar cells. The stratified squamous epithelium of the epidermis comprises five different cellular layers.—**epithelial,** *adj.*

epitope /ep′itōp/ [Gk *epi* + *topos* place], an antigenic determinant that causes a specific reaction by an immunoglobulin. It consists of a group of amino acids on the surface of the antigen. See also **antibody.**

epitympanic recess /-timpan′ik/ [Gk, *epi* + *tympanon*, drum], one of two areas of the tympanic cavity, the other being the tympanic cavity proper. The recess is cranial to the tympanic membrane and contains the upper half of the malleus and greater part of the incus. Also called **the attic.**

epizootic /ep′izō·ot′ik/, a disease or condition that occurs at about the same time in many of the animals of a species in a geographic area.

EPO, abbreviation for **erythropoietin.**

eponychium. See **cuticle,** def. 3.

eponym /ep′ənim/ [Gk, *epi*, above, *onyma*, name], a name for a disease, organ, procedure, or body function that is derived from the name of a person, usually a physician or scientist who first identified the condition or devised the object bearing the name. Examples include fallopian tube, Parkinson's disease, and Billing's method.

epoophorectomy /ep′ō·of′ərek′təmē/ [Gk, *epi* + *oophoron*, ovary, *temnein*, to cut], surgical removal of the epoophoron.

epoophoron /ep′ō·of′əron/ [Gk, *epi* + *oophoron*, ovary], a structure that is situated in the mesosalpinx between the ovary and the uterine tube. It is composed of a few short tubules. The ends of the tubules converge in one direction toward the ovary and, in the opposite direction, open into a rudimentary duct. The epoophoron is a persistent portion of the embryonic mesonephric duct. Also called **parovarium.**

epoxy, an organic chemical formula formed by the union of an oxygen atom and two other atoms, usually carbon. Epoxy resins are used as bonding agents. Also called **epoxide.**

EPSDT, abbreviation for **Early and Periodic Screening Diagnosis and Treatment.**

epsilon /ep′silon/, E, ∈, the fifth letter of the greek alphabet.

Epsom salt. See **magnesium sulfate.**

EPSP, abbreviation for *excitatory postsynaptic potential.*

Epstein-Barr virus (EBV) /ep′stīnbär′/ [Michael A. Epstein, English pathologist, b. 1921; Yvonne M. Barr, 20th-century English virologist; L, *virus*, poison], the herpesvirus that causes infectious mononucleosis, Burkitt's lymphoma, and other lymphoproliferative disorders, especially in tranplant patients. It is also thought to cause oral hairy leukoplakia. The virus resides in the salivary glands of the patient, is transmitted with saliva, and asymptomatically reactivates from time to time. EBV is ubiquitous and by age 40, 99% of the U.S. population has serological evidence of EBV infection.

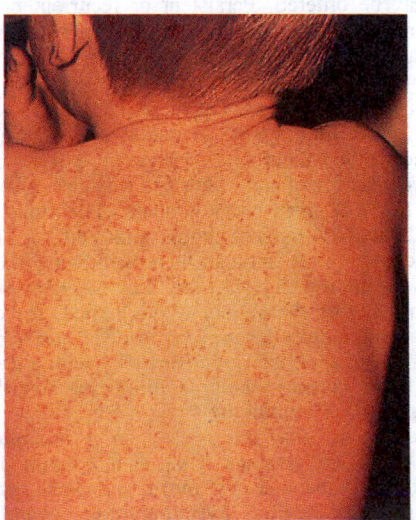

Maculopapular rash commonly seen in Epstein-Barr virus
(Zitelli, 1992/Courtesy Dr. M Sherlock)

Epstein's pearls [Alois Epstein, Czechoslovakian physician, b. 1849; L, *perla*, a mussel], small, white, pearl-like epithelial cysts that occur on both sides of the midline of the hard palate of the newborn baby. They are normal and usually disappear within a few weeks. Compare **Bednar's aphthae, thrush.**

e.p.t., a trademark for a human pregnancy test kit using monoclonal antibody technology to detect the presence of human chorionic gonadotropin (HCG) in urine.

epulis /epyoo'lis/, *pl.* **epulides** [Gk, *epi* + *oulon*, gum], any tumor or growth on the gingiva.

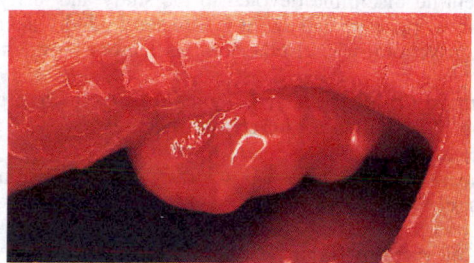

Epulis *(Zitelli, 1992)*

Equagesic, a trademark for a central nervous system, fixed-combination drug containing an analgesic (aspirin) and a sedative (meprobamate).

equal cleavage /ē'kwəl/ [L, *aequare*, to make alike; AS, *cleofan*], mitotic division of the fertilized ovum into blastomeres of identical size, as occurs in humans and most mammals. Compare **unequal cleavage.**

Equal Employment Opportunity Commission (EEOC), a commission appointed by the President of the United States to administer the Civil Rights Act of 1964, particularly to investigate complaints of discrimination in employment in businesses engaged in interstate commerce. Discrimination based on race, color, creed, or national origin is forbidden, but certain kinds of employers and certain conditions of employment allow exceptions to the act. Women and men must both be considered for a position that both can perform, and men and women must be paid equal wages for equal work.

Equanil, a trademark for a sedative (meprobamate).

equatorial plate /ēk'wətôr'ē·əl/ [L, *aequare*, to make alike; Fr, *flat, vessel*] the platelike configuration formed by the chromosomes at the center of the spindle during the metaphase stage of mitosis and meiosis.

equi-, a prefix meaning 'equality': *equilibrate, equilibrium.*

equianalgesic dose /ē'kwē·an'əljē'sik/, a dose of one analgesic that is equivalent in pain-relieving effects to another analgesic. This equivalence permits substitution of medications to avoid possible adverse effects of one of the drugs. The term is also applied to equivalent alternative dose sizes and routes of administration.

equilibration /ē'kwilibrā'shən/ [L, *aequus*, equal, *libra*, balance], the balancing and integrating of new experiences with those of the past in the psychologic development of an individual.

equilibrium /ē'kwilib're·əm/ [L, *aequilibrium*], **1.** a state of balance or rest resulting from the equal action of oppos-

ing forces, such as calcium and phosphorus in the body. **2.** (in psychiatry) a state of mental or emotional balance. **3.** (in radiotherapy) a point at which the rate of production of a daughter element is equal to the rate of decay of the parent element and the activities of parent and daughter are identical.

equilibrium reaction, any of several reflexes that enable the body to recover balance. Equilibrium reactions begin to develop around the age of 6 months.

equine encephalitis /ē'kwīn, ek'win/ [L, *equinus*, horse; Gk, *enkephalon*, brain, *itis*, inflammation], an arbovirus infection, characterized by inflammation of the nerve tissues of the brain and spinal cord, with high fever, headache, nausea, vomiting, myalgia and neurologic symptoms, such as visual disturbances, tremor, lethargy, and disorientation. The virus is transmitted by the bite of an infected mosquito. Horses are the primary host of the particular viruses that cause the infection; humans are secondary hosts. **Eastern equine encephalitis (EEE)** is a severe form of the infection. It occurs primarily along the eastern seaboard of the United States and lasts longer and causes more deaths and residual morbidity than **western equine encephalitis (WEE),** which occurs throughout the United States and results in a mild, brief illness, as does **Venezuelan equine encephalitis (VEE),** which is common in Central and South America, Florida, and Texas. See also **encephalitis, encephalomyelitis.**

equine gait [L, *equus*, horse; ONorse, *gata*, a way], a manner of walking characterized by drop foot. The condition is the result of damage to the peroneal nerve, causing the foot to hang in a toes-downward position.

equinus /ēkwī'nəs/ [L, horse], a condition characterized by tiptoe walking on one or both feet. It is usually associated with clubfoot.

equivalent weight [L, *a, equs, valere*, equal value; AS, *gewiht*], **1.** the weight of an element in any given unit (such as grams) that will displace a unit weight of hydrogen from a compound or combine with or replace a unit weight of hydrogen. **2.** the weight of an acid or base that will produce or react with 1.008 grams of hydrogen ion. **3.** the weight of an oxidizing or reducing agent that will produce or accept one electron in a chemical reaction.

equivocal symptom [L, *aequs*, equal + *vocare*, to call; Gk, *symptoma*, that which happens], a symptom that may be attributed to more than one cause or that may occur in several diseases.

Er, symbol for the element **erbium.**

ER,E.R., abbreviation for **emergency room.**

Erb-Duchenne paralysis. See **Erb's palsy.**

erbium (Er) /ur'bē·əm/ [Ytterby, Sweden], a rare-earth, metallic element. Its atomic number is 68; its atomic weight is 167.26.

Erb's muscular dystrophy [Wilhelm H. Erb, German neurologist, b. 1840], a form of muscular dystrophy that first affects the shoulder girdle and later often involves the pelvic girdle. It is a progressively crippling disease with onset in childhood or adolescence and is usually inherited as an autosomal recessive trait. It affects both sexes. In males, differential diagnosis between Erb's muscular dystrophy and Duchenne's muscular dystrophy may be difficult. Also called **scapulohumeral muscular dystrophy.**

Erb's palsy [Wilhelm H. Erb], a kind of paralysis caused by traumatic injury to the upper brachial plexus. It occurs most commonly in childbirth from forcible traction during delivery, with injury to one or more cervical nerve roots. The signs of Erb's palsy include loss of sensation in the arm and paralysis and atrophy of the deltoid, the biceps, and the brachialis muscles. The arm on the affected side hangs loosely with the elbow extended and the forearm pronated. Treatment initially requires that the arm and shoulder be immobilized to allow the swelling and inflammation of the associated neuritis to resolve. Physical therapy and splinting may be necessary to improve function of the muscles and to prevent flexion contracture of the elbow. Also called **Erb-Duchenne paralysis.**

Erb's point, a landmark of the brachial plexus on the upper trunk, located about 1 inch (2.5 cm) above the clavicle at about the level of the sixth cervical vertebra. The point locates an angle between the posterolateral border of the sternocleidomastoid muscle and the clavicle. Electrical stimulation at Erb's point causes contractions of the biceps, deltoid, and other arm muscles.

erectile /irek′til, -tīl/ [L, *erigere*, to erect], capable of being erected or raised to an erect position. The term is usually used to describe spongy tissue of the penis or clitoris that becomes turgid and erectile when filled with blood. It also may be used when referring to the epidermal tissue involved in the appearance of 'goose bumps' (piloerection) in response to fear, anger, cold, or other stimuli.

erectile myxoma, an angioma that contains areas of myxomatous tissue.

erection /irek′shən/ [L, *erigere*, to erect], the condition of hardness, swelling, and elevation observed in the penis and to a lesser degree in the clitoris, usually caused by sexual arousal but also occurring during sleep or as a result of physical stimulation. It occurs as additional blood enters the organ and blood pressure increases and is influenced by psychic and nerve stimulation. It is needed to enable the penis to enter the vagina and to emit semen. See also **ejaculation, nocturnal emission, priapism.**

erector spinae. See **sacrospinalis.**

erector spinae reflex [L, *erigere*, to erect, *spina*, spine, *reflectere*, to bend back], a reflex characterized by contraction of the sacrospinalis and other back muscles when the overlying skin is stimulated. Also called **dorsal reflex.**

erethistic idiocy /er′ithis′tik/, *obsolete*. severe mental retardation associated with continuous, purposeless activity and restlessness.

erg /urg, erg/, a unit of energy in the CGS (centimeter-gram-second) system equal to the work done by a force of 1 dyne through a distance of 1 cm. See also **joule.**

-erg-, a combining form denoting an ergot alkaloid derivative.

ergastoplasm /ərgas′təplaz′əm/ [Gk, *ergaster*, worker, *plassein*, to mold], a network of cytoplasmic structures that show basophilic staining properties; granular endoplasmic reticulum. See **endoplasmic reticulum.**

-ergic, -ergetic, a combining form meaning an 'effect of activity': *allergic, pathergic, telergic.*

ergo-, a combining form meaning 'pertaining to work': *ergodermatosis, ergomaniac, ergotropy.*

ergocalciferol. See **calciferol.**

ergoloid mesylates /ur′gōloid/, an adrenergic with psychotropic actions.

■ INDICATIONS: It is prescribed in the treatment of symptomatic decline in mental capacity for an unknown cause, as in senile dementia.

■ CONTRAINDICATIONS: Psychosis or known sensitivity to this drug prohibits its use.

■ ADVERSE EFFECTS: Among the most serious adverse reactions are sublingual irritation, transient nausea, and gastric disturbance.

ergometer. See **dynamometer.**

ergometrine maleate. See **ergonovine maleate.**

Ergomar, a trademark for an ergot alkaloid (ergotamine tartrate) used to treat migraine.

ergometry /ərgom′ətrē/, the study of physical work activity, including work performed by specific muscles or muscle groups. The studies may involve testing with equipment such as stationary bicycles, treadmills, or rowing machines.

ergonomics /ur′gonom′iks/ [Gk, *ergon*, work, *nomos*, law], a scientific discipline devoted to the study and analysis of human work, especially as it is affected by individual anatomy, psychology, and other human factors. –**ergonomic,** *adj.*

ergonovine maleate /ur′gōnō′vēn/, an oxytocic ergot alkaloid. Also called **ergometrine maleate.**

■ INDICATIONS: It is prescribed to contract the uterus in the treatment or prevention of postpartum or postabortion hemorrhage.

■ CONTRAINDICATIONS: Pregnancy, peripheral vascular disease, elevated blood pressure, or known hypersensitivity to this drug prohibits its use.

■ ADVERSE EFFECTS: Among the more serious adverse effects are hypertension, nausea, headache, blurred vision, and hypersensitivity reactions. Fetal death may occur if the drug is given in pregnancy.

ergosome. See **polysome.**

ergosterol /ərgos′tərôl/, an unsaturated hydrocarbon of the vitamin D group isolated from yeast, mushrooms, ergot, and other fungi. When treated with ultraviolet irradiation it is converted into vitamin D2[0E]. See also **calciferol, viosterol, vitamin D.**

ergot /ur′gət/ [L, *ergota*, a plant disease], (in pharmacology) the food storage body of a fungus, *Claviceps purpurea,* which commonly infects rye and other cereal grasses. It contains ergot alkaloids.

ergot alkaloid, one of a large group of alkaloids derived from a common fungus, *Claviceps purpurea,* that grows on rye and other grains throughout the temperate areas of the world. The alkaloids are divided into three groups; the amino acid alkaloids, typified by ergotamine; the dihydrogenated amino acid alkaloids, such as dihydroergotamine; and the amine alkaloids, such as ergonovine. Ergotamine and dihydroergotamine are not as effective oxytocics as ergonovine; therefore, ergonovine, given orally or intravenously, is currently used in obstetrics to treat or prevent postpartum uterine atony and to complete an incomplete or missed abortion. Ergotamine is prescribed to relieve migraine headache. It acts by reducing the amplitude of arterial pulsations in the external carotid branches of the cranial arteries. Dihydroergotamine was formerly used to enhance cerebral blood flow in elderly patients to improve mental function but is no longer thought to be a useful or effective drug for that purpose. Contraindications to the use of any of the ergot alkaloids include peripheral vascular disease, coronary artery disease, hypertension, renal or hepatic dysfunction, and sepsis. Pregnancy prohibits use of the drugs because contractions of the uterus and decreased blood flow to the fetus may result, causing fetal death. Ergot poisoning may occur with prolonged or excessive use of the drug or by accidental ingestion of contaminated grain. Signs of toxicity are thirst, diarrhea, dizziness, chest pain, abnormal and variable rate of cardiac contraction, nausea and vomiting, digital paresthesia, severe cramping, and seizures. Tissue anoxia and gangrene of the extremities may occur, as a result of prolonged vasoconstriction, if poisoning is severe.

ergotamine tartrate /ərgot′əmēn/, a vasoconstrictor and oxytocic.
- INDICATIONS: It is prescribed in the treatment of migraine and postpartum uterine atony.
- CONTRAINDICATIONS: Pregnancy, peripheral vascular disease, infectious disease, or known hypersensitivity to this drug prohibits its use.
- ADVERSE EFFECTS: Among the more serious adverse reactions are vomiting, diarrhea, thirst, tingling of fingers and toes, and increased blood pressure. Fetal death may occur if the drug is administered to a woman during pregnancy.

ergotherapy /ur′gōther′əpē/ [Gk, *ergon*, work, *therapeia*, treatment], the use of physical activity and exercise in the treatment of disease. By extension, the therapy includes any procedure that increases the blood supply to a diseased or injured part, such as massage or various types of hot baths. –**ergotherapeutic**, *adj.*

ergotism /ur′gətiz′əm/ [Fr, *argot*, a grain fungus], **1.** an acute or chronic disease caused by excessive dosages of medications containing ergot. Symptoms may include cerebrospinal symptoms such as spasms, cramps, and dry gangrene. **2.** a chronic disease caused by eating cereal products made with rye flour contaminated by ergot fungus.

ergot poisoning [Fr, *argot*, a grain fungus; L, *potio*, drink], the toxic effects of ingesting food or medications containing ergot alkaloids, particularly ergotamine. See **ergotism**.

ergotropic /ur′gōtrop′ik/, **1.** pertaining to an activity or work state involving somatic muscle, sympathetic nervous system, and cortical alpha rhythm activity. **2.** pertaining to the administration of medications or other therapies to energize the power of the body's blood and other tissues to resist infections.

-eridine, a combining form denoting an analgesic of the meperidine group.

-ergy, 1. a suffix meaning an 'action': *abioenergy, leukergy, synergy.* **2.** a combining form meaning an 'effect or result': *allergy, anabolergy, pathergy.*

erogenous /iroj′ənəs/ [Gk, *eros*, love, *genein*, to produce], pertaining to the production of erotic sensations or sexual excitement. Also called **erotogenic** /irot′ōjen′ik/.

erogenous zones, areas of the body in which sexual tension tends to become concentrated and can be relieved by manipulation of the region. The areas include the mouth, anus, and genitals.

Eros /ir′os, er′os/ [Gk, mythic love-inciting son of Aphrodite], a Freudian term for the drive or instinct for survival, including self-preservation and survival of the species through reproduction.

erosion /irō′zhən/ [L, *erodere*, to consume], the wearing away or gradual destruction of a surface, such as a mucosal or epidermal surface as a result of inflammation, injury, or other effects, usually marked by the appearance of an ulcer. See also **necrosis**.

erosive gastritis /irō′siv/, an inflammatory condition characterized by multiple erosions of the mucous membrane lining the stomach. Nausea, anorexia, pain, and gastric hemorrhage may occur. Treatment includes removal of the irritating substance, and supportive care includes intravenous fluids, electrolytes, and, if necessary, blood transfusion. See also **chemical gastritis, corrosive gastritis**.

erosive osteoarthritis. See **Kellgren's syndrome.**

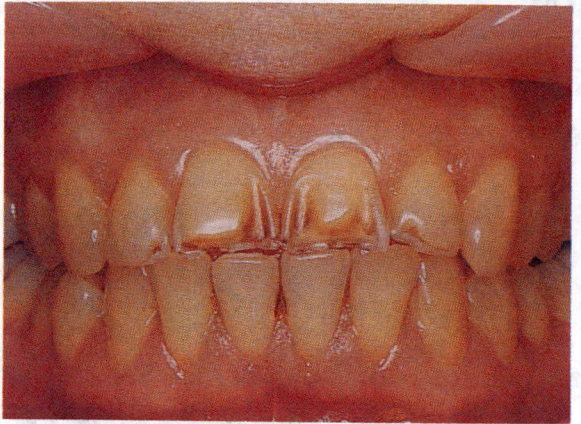

Erosion of tooth enamel (Lamey, 1988)

-erotic, a combining form meaning 'pertaining to sexual love or desire': *anterotic, homoerotic, hysteroerotic*.

eroticism /irot′isiz′əm/ [Gk, *erotikos*, sexual love], **1.** sexual impulse or desire. **2.** the arousal or attempt to arouse the sexual instinct through suggestive or symbolic means. **3.** the expression of sexual instinct or desire. **4.** an abnormally persistent sexual drive. Also called **erotism**. See also **anal eroticism, oral eroticism.**

eroto- /irot′ə-/, a combining form meaning 'pertaining to love or sexual desire': *erotogenic, erotopath, erotophobia*.

erotogenic. See **erogenous**.

erotomania /-mā′nē·ə/, *obsolete*. a psychopathologic state characterized by preoccupation with sexuality and sexual behavior.

erotomaniac /-mā′nē·ak/, *obsolete*. a person displaying characteristics of erotomania.

erratic /irat′ik/ [L, *erraticus*, wandering], deviating from the normal but with no apparent fixed course or purpose.

error [L, *errare*, to wander], (in research) a defect in the design of a study, in the development of measurements or instruments, or in the interpretation of the findings.

error message, a brief statement delivered by a computer via a peripheral device, such as a CRT or printer, that something has been done incorrectly.

ERT, abbreviation for **external radiation therapy.**

erucic acid /eroo′sik/, a fatty acid that has been associated with heart disease. It is present in rapeseed oil and is used in some countries as a vegetable oil for salad dressings, margarines, and mayonnaise.

eructation /ē′ruktā′shən/ [L, *eructare*, to belch], the act of bringing up air from the stomach with a characteristic sound through the mouth. Also called **belching**.

eruption /irup′shən/ [L, *eruptio*, bursting forth], the rapid development of a skin lesion, especially of a viral exanthem, or of the rash commonly accompanying a drug reaction.

eruptive fever /irup′tiv/ [L, *eruptio*, bursting forth; *febris*], any disease characterized by fever and a rash.

eruptive gingivitis, a gingival inflammation that may occur concurrently with the eruption of the permanent teeth. Compare **desquamative gingivitis.**

eruptive xanthoma, a skin disorder associated with elevated triglyceride levels in the blood. Erythematous or pale raised papules suddenly appear in large numbers on the trunk, legs, arms, and buttocks.

ERV, abbreviation for **expiratory reserve volume.**

erysipelas /er′isip′ələs/ [Gk, *erythros,* red, *pella,* skin], an infectious skin disease characterized by redness, swelling, vesicles, bullae, fever, pain, and lymphadenopathy. It is caused by a species of group A, beta-hemolytic streptococci. Treatment includes antibiotics, analgesics, and packs or dressings applied locally to the lesions.

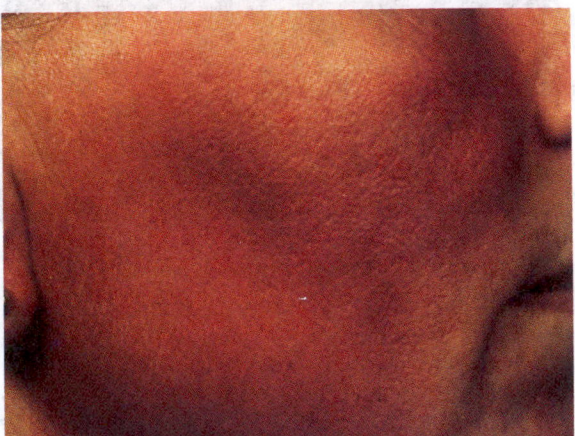

Erysipelas *(du Vivier, 1993/Courtesy King's College Hospital)*

erysipeloid /er′isip′əloid/ [Gk, *erhthros, pella + eidos,* form], an infection of the hands characterized by blue-red nodules or patches and, occasionally, by erythema. It is acquired by handling meat or fish infected with *Erysipelothrix rhusiopathiae.* The disease is self-limited, lasting about 3 weeks, but responds to penicillin. Also called **fish-handler's disease.** Compare **erysipelas.**

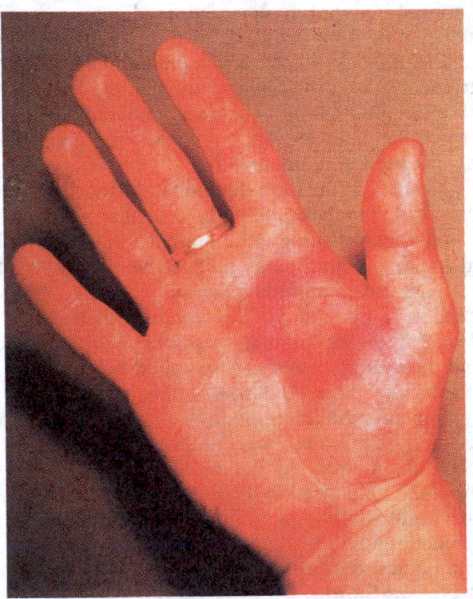

Erysipeloid *(London, 1990)*

erythema /er′ithē′mə/ [Gk, *erythros,* red], redness or inflammation of the skin or mucous membranes that is the result of dilatation and congestion of superficial capillaries. Examples of erythema are nervous blushes and mild sunburn. See also **erythroderma, rubor. –erythematous,** *adj.*

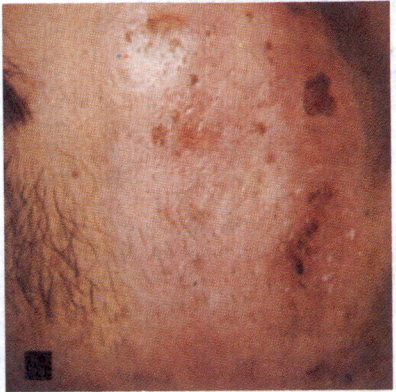

Erythema *(Zacarian, 1985)*

erythema chronicum migrans (ECM), a skin lesion that begins as a small papule and spreads peripherally, extending by a raised, red margin and clearing in the center. It marks the site of a deer tick bite and is a diagnostic sign of **Lyme disease.**

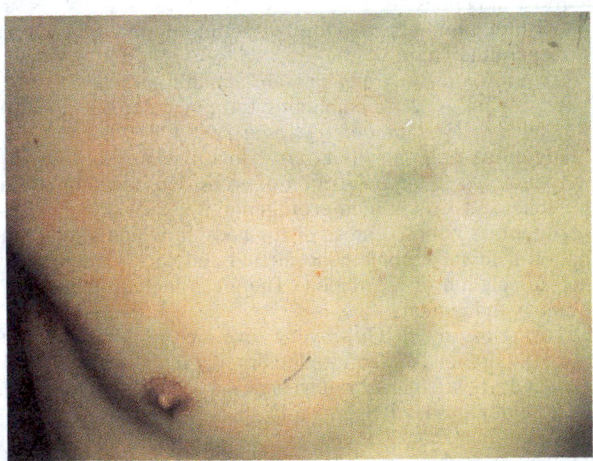

Erythema chronica migrans *(Shipley, 1993)*

erythema infectiosum, an acute, benign infectious disease, mainly of children, characterized by fever and an erythematous rash beginning on the cheeks and appearing later on the arms, thighs, buttocks, and trunk. As the rash progresses, earlier lesions fade. Sunlight aggravates the eruption, which usually lasts about 10 days. For a period of time the rash may reappear whenever the skin is irritated. It is caused by parvovirus B_{19}. No treatment is necessary, and prognosis is excellent. The isolation of patients is not required. Also called **fifth disease.**

with many infections, collagen diseases, drug sensitivities, allergies, and pregnancy. Definitive and preventive treatment depends on finding the specific cause, but topical or systemic corticosteroids are helpful in most cases. A severe form of this condition is **Stevens-Johnson syndrome.**

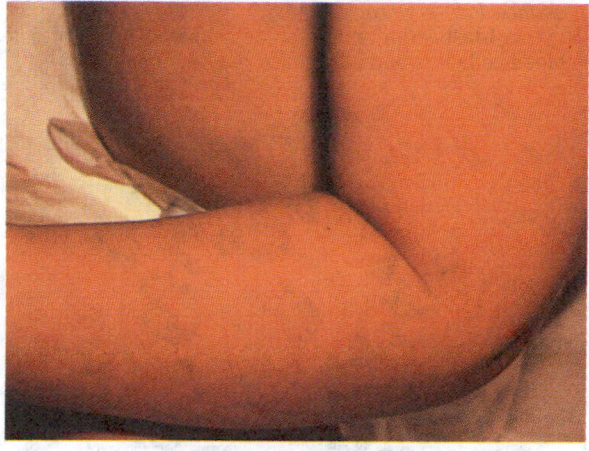

Erythema infectiosum
(Zitelli, 1992/Courtesy Dr. Michael Sherlock)

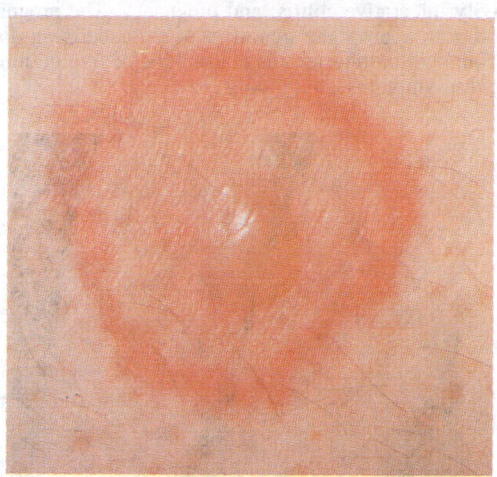

Erythema multiforme (McKee, 1993)

erythema marginatum, a variant of **erythema multiforme** seen in acute rheumatic fever characterized by temporary disk-shaped, nonpruritic, reddened macules that fade in the center, leaving raised margins.

erythema neonatorum, a common skin condition of neonates characterized by a pink papular rash frequently superimposed with vesicles or pustules. The rash appears within 24 to 48 hours after birth, is confined to the trunk, and disappears spontaneously after several days. A smear of the papules shows eosinophils rather than neutrophils which differentiates the condition from neonatal pustular melanosis.

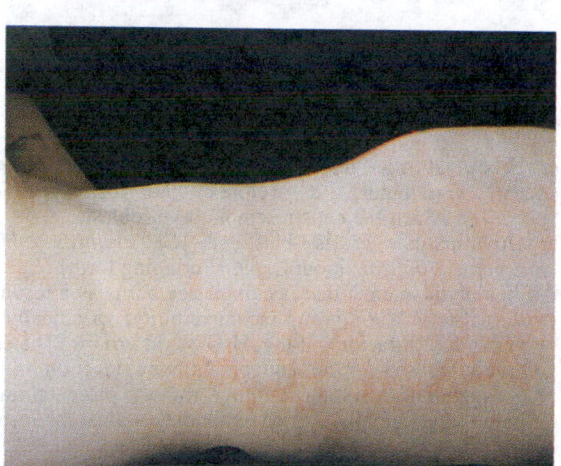

Erythema marginatum (Ansell, 1992)

erythema multiforme /mul´tifôr´mē, mo͞ol´tēfôr´mā/, a hypersensitivity syndrome characterized by polymorphous eruption of skin and mucous membranes. Macules, papules, nodules, vesicles or bullae, and target (bull's-eye-shaped) lesions are seen. Erythema multiforme has been associated

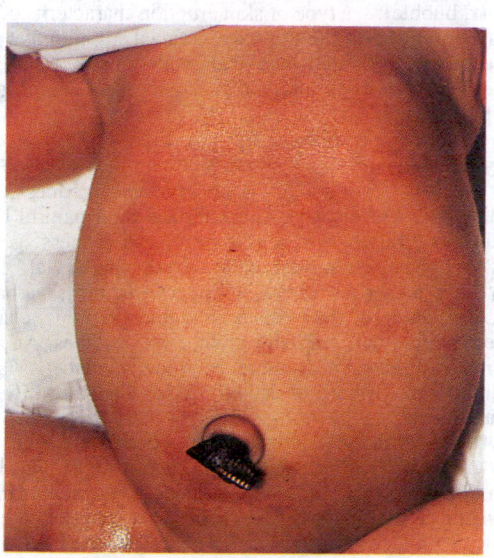

Erythema neonatorum (Zitelli, 1992)

erythema nodosum, a hypersensitivity vasculitis characterized by bilateral, reddened, tender, subcutaneous nodules on the shins and, occasionally, on other parts of the body. The nodules last for several days or weeks, never ulcerate, and are often associated with mild fever, malaise, and pains in muscles and joints. This condition may be seen with streptococcal infections, tuberculosis, sarcoidosis, drug sensitivity, ulcerative colitis, and pregnancy. The prognosis is good with appropriate treatment of the underlying disease. A course of corticosteroids is usually effective in diminishing the symptoms.

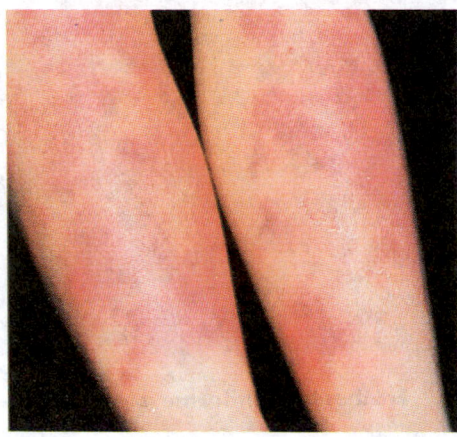

Erythema neonatorum (Zitelli, 1992)

erythema perstans, a persistent local redness of the skin, often caused by a fixed-combination drug eruption.

-erythematous. See **erythema.**

erythematous eczema /er′ithem′ətəs/ [Gk, *erythema*, redness, *ekzein*, to boil over], a scaly red skin eruption frequently accompanied by edema. Also called **eczema erythematosum.**

erythematous pemphigus [Gk, *erythema*, redness, *pemphix*, bubble], a type of skin eruption characterized by bullous eruptions on the trunk and a facial eruption that resembles lupus erythematosus. The condition may be accompanied by sebhorrheic dermatitis. Also called **pemphigus erythematosus.**

erythmo-, a combining form meaning 'red': *erythmatous, erythemogenic.*

erythralgia /er′ithral′jə/ [Gk, *erythema*, redness, *algos*, pain], a skin disorder characterized by a painful burning sensation, raised skin temperature, and redness, generally of the lower limbs. Also called **erythromelalgia.**

erythrasma /er′ithraz′mə/ [Gk, *erythros*, red], a bacterial skin infection of the axillary or inguinal regions, characterized by irregular, reddish-brown, raised patches. An asymptomatic disease, it is more common in diabetics and responds quickly to oral erythromycin. Compare **intertrigo, tinea cruris.**

erythroderma polyneuropathy. See **acrodynia.**

erythremia /er′ithrē′mē·ə/ [Gk, *erythros* + *haima*, blood], an abnormal increase in the number of red blood cells.

erythrityl tetranitrate /erith′ritil/, a coronary vasodilator.

■ INDICATIONS: It is prescribed in the treatment of angina pectoris.

■ CONTRAINDICATIONS: It is used with caution when glaucoma is present. Known hypersensitivity to this drug prohibits its use.

■ ADVERSE EFFECTS: Among the most serious adverse reactions are hypotension, allergic reactions, headache, and flushing.

erythro-, a combining form meaning 'red': *erythroblast, erythroclast, erythrocyte.*

erythroblast /erith′rəblast′/, an immature form of a red blood cell. It is normally found only in bone marrow.

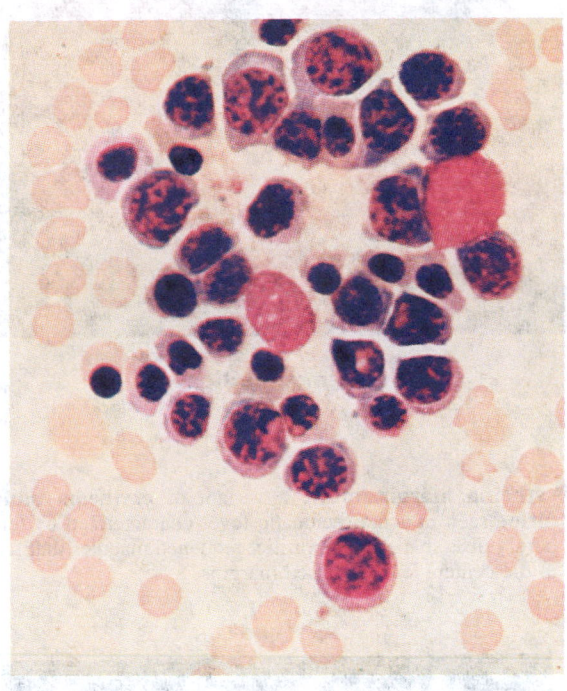

Erythroblasts (Hayhoe, 1992)

erythroblastoma /-blastō′mə/ [Gk, *erythros*, red, *blastos*, germ, *oma*, tumor], a myeloma tumor (osteolytic neoplasm) in which the cells resemble erythroblasts.

erythroblastosis fetalis /-blastō′sis/ [Gk, *erythros* + *blastos*, germ, *osis*, condition; L, *fetus*, bringing forth], a type of hemolytic anemia that occurs in newborns as a result of maternal-fetal blood group incompatibility, specifically involving the Rh factor and the ABO blood groups. The condition is caused by an antigen-antibody reaction in the bloodstream of the infant resulting from the placental transmission of maternally formed antibodies against the incompatible antigens of the fetal blood. In Rh factor incompatibility, the hemolytic reaction occurs only when the mother is Rh negative and the infant is Rh positive. The isoimmunization process rarely occurs with the first pregnancy, but there is increased risk with each succeeding pregnancy. However, maternal sensitization to the Rh factor can be prevented by injection of a high-titer anti-Rh gamma globulin preparation after delivery or abortion of an Rh positive fetus. No sensitization may occur in situations in which a strong placental barrier prevents transfer of fetal blood into the maternal circulation. In about 10% to 15% of sensitized mothers, there is no hemolytic reaction in the newborn. Clinical manifestations of the condition include severe anemia, jaundice, and enlargement of the liver and spleen, which, without intervention, can lead to hypoxia, cardiac failure, generalized edema, respiratory distress, and death. Prenatal diagnosis of the disease is confirmed through amniocentesis and analysis of bilirubin levels in amniotic fluid. Higher than normal levels result from the breakdown of hemoglobin from the lysed erythrocytes. Treatment consists of intrauterine transfusion when placental bilirubin levels progressively increase or immediate exchange transfusions after birth. Hemolytic reactions involving the ABO blood groups have similar manifestations but are generally less severe. See also **hydrops fetalis, hyperbilirubinemia of the newborn, Rh factor.**

Erythrocin, a trademark for an antibacterial (erythromycin).

erythrocyte /erith′rəsīt′/ [Gk, *erythros* + *kytos*, cell], a biconcave disk about 7 micrometers in diameter that contains hemoglobin confined within a lipoid membrane. The major cellular element of the circulating blood, its principal function is to transport oxygen. The number of cells per cubic millimeter of blood is usually maintained between 4.5 and 5.5 million in men and between 4.2 and 4.8 million in women. It varies with age, activity, and environmental conditions. For example, an increase to a level of 8 million/cu mm can normally occur at over 10,000 feet above sea level. An erythrocyte normally lives for 110 to 120 days, at which time it is removed from the bloodstream and broken down by the reticuloendothelial system. New erythrocytes are produced at a rate of slightly more than 1% a day; thus, a constant level is usually maintained. With acute blood loss, hemolytic anemia, or chronic oxygen deprivation, erythrocyte production may increase greatly. Erythrocytes originate in the marrow of the long bones. Maturation proceeds from a stem cell (promegaloblast) through the pronormoblast stage to the normoblast, the last stage before the mature adult cell develops. Kinds of erythrocyte include **burr cell, discocyte, macrocyte, meniscocyte,** and **spherocyte.** Also called **red blood cell, red cell, red corpuscle.** Compare **normoblast, reticulocyte.** See also **erythropoiesis, hemoglobin, red cell indices.**

erythrocyte sedimentation rate (ESR), the rate at which red blood cells settle out in a tube of unclotted blood, expressed in millimeters per hour. Blood is collected in an anticoagulant and allowed to form a sediment in a calibrated glass column. At the end of 1 hour, the laboratory technician measures the distance the erythrocytes have fallen in the tube. Elevated sedimentation rates are not specific for any disorder but indicate the presence of inflammation. Inflammation causes an alteration of the blood proteins, which makes the red blood cells aggregate, becoming heavier than normal. The speed with which they fall to the bottom of the tube corresponds to the degree of inflammation. Serial evaluations of erythrocyte sedimentation rate are useful in monitoring the course of inflammatory activity in rheumatic diseases and, when performed with a white blood cell count, can indicate infection. Certain noninflammatory conditions, such as pregnancy, are also characterized by high sedimentation rates. Two methods are used. The Wintrobe ESR is performed in a 10 cm Wintrobe tube, and the Westergren ESR is performed in a 200 mm Westergren tube. Values are higher for women in both methods and vary according to the method used. Normal findings by the Westergren method are up to 20 mm/hr for females and up to 15 mm/hr for males. Also called *(informal)* **sed. rate.** See also **inflammation.**

erythrocythemia /erith′rōsīthē′mē·ə/ [Gk, *erythros, kytos* + *haima*, blood]], an increase in the number of erythrocytes circulating in the blood.

erythrocytopenia /-sī′təpē′nē·ə/ [Gk, *erythros*, red, *kytos*, cell, *penes*, poor], a condition characterized by a deficiency of erythrocytes.

erythrocytosis /erith′rōsītō′sis/ [Gk, *erythros, kytos* + *osis*, condition], an abnormal increase in the number of circulating red cells. See also **polycythemia.**

erythroderma /erith′rōdur′mə/ [Gk, *erythros* + *derma*, skin], any dermatosis associated with abnormal redness of the skin. Compare **erythema, rubor.**

erythroleukemia /-lo͞okē′mē·ə/ [Gk, *erythros* + *leukos*, white, *haima*, blood], a malignant blood disorder characterized by a proliferation of erythropoietic elements in bone

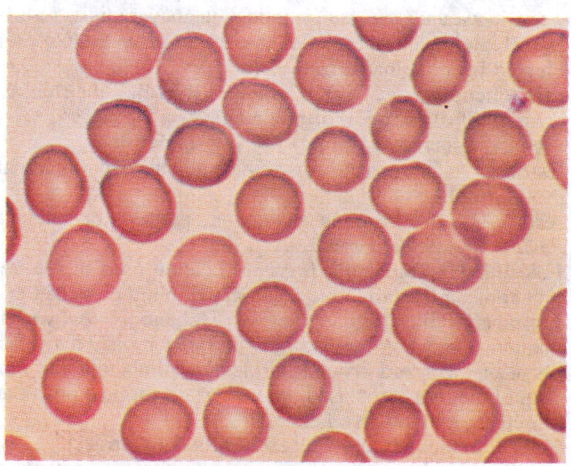

Erythrocytes *(Hayhoe, 1992)*

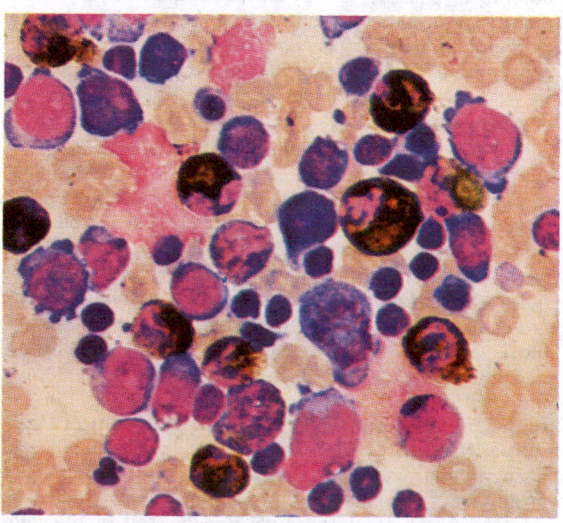

Erythroleukemia *(Hayhoe, 1992)*

marrow, erythroblasts with bizarre lobulated nuclei, and abnormal myeloblasts in peripheral blood. The disease may have an acute or chronic course. Also called **diGuglielmo's disease** /di'gōōlyel'mōs/, **diGuglielmo's syndrome, erythromyeloblastic leukemia.**

erythromelalgia /erith'rōmilal'jə/ [Gk, *erythros* + *melos*, limb, *algos*, pain], a rare disorder characterized by a paroxysmal dilatation of the peripheral blood vessels. It occurs bilaterally, usually in the extremities, and is associated with burning, redness of the skin, and pain. **—erythromelalgic,** *adj.*

erythromycin /erith'rōmī'sin/, an antibacterial antibiotic.

■ INDICATIONS: It is prescribed in the treatment of many bacterial and mycoplasmic infections, particularly infections that cannot be treated by penicillins.

■ CONTRAINDICATIONS: Liver disease or known hypersensitivity to this drug prohibits its use.

■ ADVERSE EFFECTS: Among the more serious adverse effects are cholestatic hepatitis and hypersensitivity reactions.

erythromyeloblastic leukemia. See **erythroleukemia.**

erythrophobia /-fō'bē·ə/ [Gk, *erythros* + *phobos*, fear], **1.** an anxiety disorder characterized by an irrational fear of blushing or of displaying embarrassment. **2.** a neurotic symptom manifested by blushing at the slightest provocation. **3.** a morbid fear of or aversion to the color red. **—erythrophobic,** *adj.*

erythroplasia of Queyrat /erith'rōplā'zhə/ [Gk, *erythros* + *plasis*, forming; Auguste Queyrat, French dematologist, b.1872], a premalignant lesion on the glans or corona of the penis. It is a well-circumscribed reddish patch on the skin. It is usually excised surgically. See also **Bowen's disease.**

erythropoiesis /erith'rōpō·ē'sis/ [Gk, *erythros* + *poiein*, to make], the process of erythrocyte production involving the maturation of a nucleated precursor into a hemoglobin-filled, nucleus-free erythrocyte that is regulated by erythropoietin, a hormone produced by the kidney. See also **erthrocyte, erythropoietin, hemoglobin, leukopoiesis. —erythropoietic,** *adj.*

erythropoietic porphyria. See **porphyria.**

erythropoietin (EPO) /erith'rōpō·ē'tin/ [Gk, *erythros* + *poiein*, to make], a glycoprotein hormone synthesized mainly in the kidneys and released into the bloodstream in response to anoxia. The hormone acts to stimulate and to regulate the production of erythrocytes and is thus able to increase the oxygen-carrying capacity of the blood. See also **erythropoiesis.**

Es, symbol for the element **einsteinium.**

escape beat [ME, *escapen*, to flee; *beten*, to beat], an automatic beat of the heart that occurs after an interval longer than the duration of the dominant cycle. Escape beats function as safety mechanisms, and anything that produces a pause in the prevailing heart cycle may allow an escape to occur. Some kinds of pauses in which escape beats occur are caused by sinoatrial (SA) block, atrioventricular (AV) block, and the completion of a paroxysm of tachycardia. Escape beats may arise from the atria, the AV junction, or the ventricles.

escape phenomenon. See **Marcus Gunn pupil sign.**

escape rhythm [OFr, *escaper*; Gk, *rhythmos*, beat], a heart rhythm that occurs when the atrioventricular junction or any ventricular muscle fiber assumes control because the rate set by the sinoatrial node is depressed or blocked, or when the ventricle assumes control because the rate set by the sinus or atrioventricular nodes are depressed or blocked.

escarronodulaire. See **Marseilles fever.**

-escent, 1. a suffix meaning 'beginning to be': *alkalescent, convalescent, turgescent.* **2.** a combining form meaning 'emitting or reflecting light': *incandescent, iridescent, opalescent.*

eschar /es'kär/ [Gk, *eschara*, scab], a scab or dry crust resulting from a thermal or chemical burn, infection, or excoriating skin disease. **—escharotic,** *adj.*

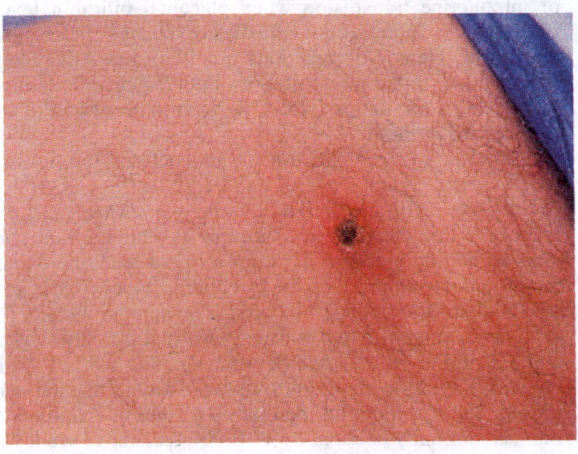

Eschar (Hart, 1992)

escharonodulaire. See **Marseilles fever.**

-escharotic. See **eschar.**

escharotomy /es'kärot'əmē/, a surgical incision into necrotic tissue resulting from a severe burn. It is sometimes necessary to prevent edema from building up sufficient interstitial pressure to impair capillary filling and cause ischemia.

Escherichia coli (E. coli) /eshirī'kē·ə kō'lī/ [Theodor Escherich, German physician, b. 1857; Gk, *kolon*, colon], a species of coliform bacteria of the family Enterobacteriaceae, normally present in the intestines and common in water, milk, and soil. *E. coli* is the most frequent cause of urinary tract infection and is a serious gram-negative pathogen in wounds. *E. coli* septicemia may rapidly result in shock and death because of the action of an endotoxin released from the bacteria.

escutcheon /eskuch'ən/ [L, *scutum*, shield], the shieldlike pattern of distribution of pubic hair.

eserine, eserine sulfate. See **physostigmine.**

Esidrix, a trademark for a thiazide diuretic (hydrochlorothiazide).

-esis, a suffix meaning an 'action, process, or result of': *enuresis, oxydesis, synthesis.*

Eskalith, a trademark for a medication used in the treatment of biploar affective disorders (lithium carbonate).

Esmarch's bandage /es'märks/ [Johann F. A. von Esmarch, German surgeon, b. 1823], a broad, flat, elastic bandage wrapped around an elevated limb to force blood out of the limb. It is used before certain surgical procedures to create a blood-free field.

ESO, abbreviation for **electric spinal orthosis.**

eso-, a combining form meaning 'within': *esocataphoria, esogastritis, esotropia.*

-esophageal. See **esophagus.**

esophageal atresia /əsof′əjē′əl, es′ofā′jē·əl/ [Gk, *oisophagos*, gullet], an abnormal esophagus that ends in a blind pouch or narrows to a thin cord and thus fails to provide a continuous passage to the stomach. It usually occurs as a congenital anomaly.

esophageal cancer, a malignant neoplastic disease of the esophagus that occurs three times more frequently in men than in women and more often in Asia and Africa than in North America. Risk factors associated with the disease are heavy consumption of alcohol, smoking, betel-nut chewing, Plummer-Vinson syndrome, hiatus hernia, and achalasia. Aflatoxin in moldy grain and peanuts or a dietary deficiency, especially of molybdenum, may be involved. Esophageal cancer does not often cause any symptoms in the early stages but in later stages causes painful dysphagia, anorexia, weight loss, regurgitation, cervical adenopathy, and, in some cases, a persistent cough. Left vocal cord paralysis and hemoptysis indicate an advanced state of the disease. The tumor may spread locally to invade the trachea, bronchi, pericardium, great blood vessels, and thoracic vertebrae or may metastasize to lymph nodes, the lungs, and the liver. Diagnostic measures include fluoroscopic observation of the esophagus as the patient swallows barium, fiberoptic esophagoscopy, and biopsy and cytologic examination of the primary lesion and regional nodes. Most esophageal tumors are poorly differentiated squamous cell carcinomas; adenocarcinomas occur less frequently and are usually found in the lower third of the esophagus as extensions of gastric cancer. Surgical treatment may require total or partial esophagectomy with the resected segment replaced by a Dacron graft or a section of the colon. If only the lower third of the esophagus is removed, the proximal end may be anastomosed to the stomach. A catheter inserted into the stomach through an incision or a nasogastric tube may be used to feed patients who have inoperable esophageal cancer. Radiotherapy may eradicate early local tumors and may effectively palliate the symptoms of advanced lesion. Methotrexate given before irradiation may increase the chances of survival. See also **esophagectomy.**

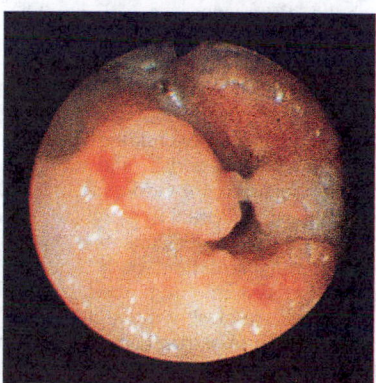

Esophageal cancer—endoscopic view (Geenen, 1992)

esophageal dysfunction, any disturbance, impairment, or abnormality that interferes with the normal functioning of the esophagus, such as dysphagia, esophagitis, or sphincter incompetence. The condition is one of the primary symptoms of scleroderma.

esophageal lead /lēd/, **1.** an electrocardiographic conductor in which the exploring electrode is placed within the lumen of the esophagus. It is used to detect sizable atrial deflections as an aid in identifying cardiac arrhythmias. **2.** *informal.* a tracing produced by such a lead on an electrocardiograph.

esophageal obturator airway, an emergency airway device that consists of a large tube that is inserted into the mouth through an airtight face mask. Holes in the tube open into the oropharynx when properly placed. The esophagus is blocked by inflating a balloon at the end of the tube. Because of the design, air passes only into the trachea.

esophageal speech [Gk, *oisophagos*, gullet; AS, *spaec*], alaryngeal sounds made by forcing air in and out of the esophagus, causing it to vibrate. It may be produced by a number of methods.

esophageal varices, a complex of longitudinal, tortuous veins at the lower end of the esophagus, enlarged and swollen as the result of portal hypertension. These vessels are especially susceptible to hemorrhage.

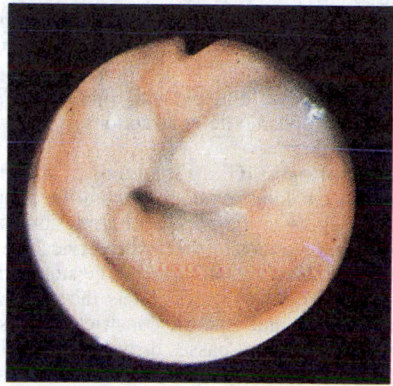

Esophageal varices—endoscopic view (Geenen, 1992)

esophageal web, a thin membrane that may develop across the lumen of the esophagus, usually near the level of the cricoid cartilage. The abnormal condition is generally associated with iron-deficiency anemia and usually disappears when the underlying problem is resolved. See also **Plummer-Vinson syndrome.**

esophagectomy /esof′əjek′təmē/ [Gk, *oisophagos* + *ektome*, excision], a surgical procedure in which all or part of the esophagus is removed, as may be required to treat severe, recurrent, bleeding, esophageal varices, or cancer of the esophagus.

esophagitis /esof′əjī′tis/ [Gk, *oisophagos* + *itis*], inflammation of the mucosal lining of the esophagus, caused by infection, irritation from a nasogastric tube, or, most commonly, backflow of gastric juice from the stomach. See also **gastroesophageal reflux.**

esophagogastronomy /esof′əgō′gastron′əmē/ [Gk, *oisophagos*, gullet, *gaster*, stomach, *stoma*, mouth], the surgical creation of a passage between the esophagus and the stomach.

esophagogastroscopy /-gastros′kəpē/ [Gk, *oisophagos*, gullet, *gaster*, stomach, *skopein*, to watch] the examination of the esophagus and stomach using an endoscope.

esophagojejunostomy /-jij′o·moos′təmē/ [Gk, *oisophagos*, gullet; L, *jejunum*, empty, *stoma*, mouth], the surgical

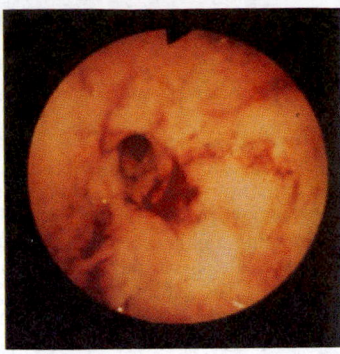

Esophagitis—endoscopic view (Mitros, 1988)

creation of a direct passage from the esophagus to the jejunum, bypassing the stomach. The procedure is used after total gastrectomy.

esophagoscopy /esof'əgos'kəpē/ [Gk, *oisophagos* + *skopein*, to look], examination of the esophagus with an endoscope.

esophagospasm /esof'əgōspaz'əm/ [Gk, *oisophagos*, gullet, *spasmos*], spasmodic contractions of the walls of the esophagus.

esophagus /esof'əgəs/ [Gk, *oisophagos*], the muscular canal, about 24 cm long, extending from the pharynx to the stomach. It begins in the neck at the inferior border of the cricoid cartilage, opposite the sixth cervical vertebra, and descends to the cardiac sphincter of the stomach in a vertical path with two slight curves. It is the narrowest part of the digestive tube and is most constricted at its beginning and at the point where it passes through the diaphragm. The esophagus is composed of a fibrous coat, a muscular coat, and a submucous coat and is lined with mucous membrane. Also called **gullet.** **–esophageal,** *adj.*

esophoria /es'əfôr'ē·ə/ [Gk, *eso*, inward, *pherein*, to bear], deviation of the visual axis of one eye toward that of the other eye in the absence of visual stimuli for fusion. Also called **cross-eye.** Compare **esotropia. –esophoric,** *adj.*

esotropia /es'ətrō'pē·ə/ [Gk, *eso* + *tropos*, turning], a kind of strabismus characterized by an inward deviation of one eye relative to the other eye. Also called **convergent strabismus, internal strabismus.** Compare **esophoria, exotropia.** See also **strabismus.** **–esotropic,** *adj.*

ESP, abbreviation for **extrasensory perception.**

espundia /espun'dē·ə/ [Sp, cancerous ulcer], a cutaneous form of American leishmaniasis most common in Brazil, caused by *Leishmania brasiliensis*. The primary lesion often disappears spontaneously followed by mucocutaneous lesions that destroy the mucosal surface of the nose, pharynx, and larynx. If the condition is left untreated, secondary bacterial infections that are potentially fatal may occur.

ESR, abbreviation for **erythrocyte sedimentation rate.**

essential amino acid /esen'shəl/ [L, *essentia*, quality], an organic compound not synthesized in the body that is essential for nitrogen equilibrium in adults and optimal growth in infants and children. Adults require isoleucine, leucine, lysine, methionine, phenylalanine, threonine, tryptophan, and valine. Infants need these eight amino acids plus arginine and histidine. Cysteine and tyrosine, limited substitutes respectively for methionine and phenylalanine, are considered quasi-essential. See also **amino acid.**

essential fatty acid (EFA), a polyunsaturated acid, such as linoleic, alpha-linolenic, and arachidonic, essential in the diet for the proper growth, maintenance, and functioning of the body. It is a precursor of the prostaglandins and has an important role in fat transport and metabolism and in maintaining the function and integrity of cellular membranes. It is also necessary for the normal functioning of the reproductive and endocrine systems and for the breaking up of cholesterol deposits on arterial walls. The best dietary sources are natural vegetable oils, such as safflower, soy, and corn oils; margarines blended with vegetable oils; wheat germ; edible seeds, such as pumpkin, sesame, and sunflower; poultry fat; and fish oils, especially cod-liver oil. A deficiency of essential fatty acids causes changes in cell structure and enzyme function resulting in decreased growth and other disorders. Symptoms include brittle and lusterless hair, nail problems, dandruff, allergic conditions, and dermatoses, especially eczema in infants. Excessive amounts may reduce the level of vitamin E in the tissues and cause other metabolic disturbances as well as abnormal weight gain.

essential fever, any fever of unknown origin.

essential hypertension, an elevated systemic arterial pressure for which no cause can be found and which is often the only significant clinical finding. Elevated blood pressure is always considered a risk, and individuals with elevated pressures are at risk for cardiovascular disease. In examining patients with essential hypertension, clinicians consider the normal complex mechanisms that control pressure, such as the arterial baroreflex, body fluid regulators, the renin-angiotensin system, and vascular autoregulation. These mechanisms are closely integrated, and it is not precisely clear how their impairment affects normotension and hypertension. Also called **primary hypertension.** See also **benign hypertension, malignant hypertension.**

essential nutrient, the carbohydrates, proteins, fats, minerals, vitamins, and water necessary for growth, normal function, and body maintenance. These substances are supplied by food, because some are not synthesized by the body in the quantities required for normal health.

essential pruritis [L, *essentia,* quality, *prurire,* to itch], localized or general pruritus that begins without any previous skin disorder.

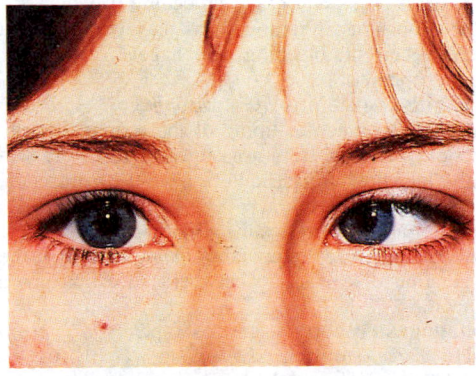

Esotropia (Zitelli, 1992)

essential tachycardia [L, *essentia*, quality; Gk, *tachys,* fast + *kardia,* heart], a heart rhythm with a consistently excessive rate despite the absence of an organic cause for the abnormality.

essential thrombocythemia. See **thrombocytosis.**

essential tremor, an involuntary fine shaking of the hand, the head, and the face, especially during routine movements of the body. It is a familial disorder inherited as an autosomal dominant trait and appears during adolescence or in middle age, slowly progressing as a more pronounced disorder. The precise cause of this condition is not known. Essential tremor is aggravated by activity and emotion and can be reduced in some patients by the administration of alcohol and mild sedatives, such as propranolol and diazepam. Also called **benign essential tremor, familial tremor.** Compare **parkinsonism.**

essential vertigo [L, *essentia*, quality + *vertigo,* dizziness], a form of vertigo for which no organic cause has been found.

EST. See **electroconvulsive therapy (ECT).**

established name, the name assigned to a drug by the U.S. Adopted Names Council. The established name, generally shorter than the chemical name, is the name by which the drug is known to health practitioners. Also called **generic name.** See also **chemical name, trademark.**

Estar, a trademark for a coal tar preparation used to treat eczema and psoriasis.

ester /es′tər/ [Ger Essigäther acetic ether], a class of chemical compounds formed by the bonding of an alcohol and one or more organic acids. Fats are esters, formed by the bonding of fatty acids with the alcohol glycerol.

esterase /es′tərās/, any enzyme that splits esters.

ester-compound local anesthetic, any one of four potent local anesthetics slightly different in chemical structure from the amide group of local anesthetics. Tetracaine is the most commonly used. Kinds of ester-compound local anesthetics are **chloroprocaine, cocaine hydrochloride,** and **procaine hydrochloride.**

esterified estrogen /ester′ifīd/, an ester of natural estrogen.
- INDICATIONS: It is prescribed in the treatment of menstrual irregularities, contraception, and menopausal symptoms.
- CONTRAINDICATIONS: Pregnancy, known or suspected breast cancer, thrombophlebitis, vaginal bleeding of unknown origin, or known hypersensitivity to this drug prohibit its use.
- ADVERSE EFFECTS: Among the more serious adverse reactions are gallbladder disease, thromboembolic disease, and a possible increase in risk of cancer.

esthesio-, a combining form meaning 'pertaining to feeling or to the perceptive faculties': *esthesiogenic, esthesioneure, esthesioscopy.*

-esthetic, -esthetical, -esthes, -aesthetic, -aesthetical, a combining form meaning 'pertaining to a person's consciousness of a sensation or something': *anesthesia, cenesthetic, photoesthetic, somatesthetic.*

esthetics /esthet′iks/ [Gk, *aisthetikos,* sensitivity], the branch of philosophy dealing with the forms and psychologic effects of beauty. In medicine, aesthetics may be applied to dental resconstruction and plastic surgery.

Estinyl, a trademark for an estrogen (ethinyl estradiol).

estr-, a combining form for the name of an estrogen.

Estrace, a trademark for an estrogen (estradiol).

estradiol /es′trədī′ôl/, the most potent naturally occurring human estrogen, also found in hog ovaries and in the urine of pregnant mares. Various esters of estradiol administered intramuscularly or orally are used as estrogens. See also **estrogen.**

Estradurin, a trademark for an antineoplastic estrogen (polyestradiol phosphate).

estramustine phosphate sodium /es′trəmus′tēn/, an antineoplastic agent.
- INDICATIONS: It is prescribed for metastatic or progressive carcinoma of the prostate.
- CONTRAINDICATIONS: Thromboembolytic disorders or known hypersensitivity to this drug prohibits its use.
- ADVERSE EFFECTS: The most serious adverse reactions are cerebrovascular accident, myocardial infarction, thrombophlebitis, pulmonary emboli, and congestive heart failure.

estrangement /estrānj′mənt/ [L, *extraneus,* not belonging], a psychologic effect caused by the required separation of a mother from her newborn child when the infant is ill, premature, or has a congenital defect, thereby diverting the mother from establishment of a normal relationship with her child.

Estratab, a trademark for esterified estrogens.

Estraval, a trademark for an estrogen (estradiol valerate).

estriol /es′trē·ôl/, a relatively weak, naturally occurring human estrogen found in high concentrations in urine. See also **estrogen.**

estrogen /es′trojən/ [Gk, *oistros,* gadfly, *genein,* to produce], one of a group of hormonal steroid compounds that promote the development of female secondary sex characteristics. Human estrogen is elaborated in the ovaries, adrenal cortices, testes, and fetoplacental unit. During the menstrual cycle estrogen renders the female genital tract suitable for fertilization, implantation, and nutrition of the early embryo. Pharmaceutic preparations of estrogen are used in oral contraceptives, to palliate postmenopausal breast cancer and prostatic cancer, to inhibit lactation, and to treat threatened abortion, osteoporosis, and ovarian disease. Estrogen is also prescribed to relieve discomforts of menopause, but its long-term, continued use increases the risk of endometrial carcinoma. Kinds of estrogen are **conjugated estrogen, esterified estrogen, estradiol, estriol,** and **estrone.** −**estrogenic,** *adj.*

estrone /es′trōn/, a relatively potent estrogen.
- INDICATIONS: It is prescribed in the treatment of menstrual cycle irregularities, prostatic cancer, and menopausal vasomotor symptoms, and to prevent pregnancy.
- CONTRAINDICATIONS: Thrombophlebitis, abnormal genital bleeding, known or suspected pregnancy, or known hypersensitivity to this drug prohibits its use.
- ADVERSE EFFECTS: Among the more serious adverse reactions are thrombophlebitis, embolism, and hypercalcemia.

estropipate /es′trəpip′āt/, an estrogen.
- INDICATIONS: It is prescribed in the treatment of vasomotor symptoms of menopause, atrophic vaginitis, kraurosis vulvae, female hypogonadism, female castration, and primary ovarian failure.
- CONTRAINDICATIONS: Known or suspected cancer of the breast or estrogen-dependent neoplasia, pregnancy, thrombophlebitis or thromboembolic disorders, undiagnosed abnormal genital bleeding, or complications from previous administration of estrogen prohibits its use.
- ADVERSE EFFECTS: Among the most serious adverse reactions are a possible increased risk of cancer, gallbladder disease, and thromboembolic disorders.

estrus /es′trəs/, the cyclic period of sexual activity in mammals other than primates.

estrus cycle [Gk, *oistros*, gadfly, *kyklos*, circle], the periodic changes in the female body that occur under the influence of sex hormones.

ESWL, abbreviation for **extracorporeal shock-wave lithotripsy**.

eta /ē′tə, ā′tə/, H, η, the seventh letter of the Greek alphabet.

-etanide, a combining form denoting an analgesic of the meperidine group.

état criblé /ātä′krēblā′/ [Fr, sievelike state], a condition or state of multiple sievelike perforations in swollen Peyer's patches of the intestine. It is a frequently fatal complication of untreated typhoid fever.

ethacrynate sodium. See **ethacrynic acid**.

ethacrynic acid /eth′əkrin′ik/, a potent loop diuretic.
- INDICATIONS: It is prescribed to relieve the effects of severe edema and hypertension.
- CONTRAINDICATIONS: Pregnancy, anuria, or known hypersensitivity to this drug prohibits its use. It is not given to infants.
- ADVERSE EFFECTS: Among the more serious adverse reactions are tetany, muscle weakness, cramps, and excessive diuresis. Hearing loss or deafness may occur.

ethambutol hydrochloride /eth′əmbyōō′təl/, a tuberculostatic antibiotic.
- INDICATION: It is prescribed in the treatment of pulmonary tuberculosis.
- CONTRAINDICATIONS: Optic neuritis or known hypersensitivity to this drug prohibits its use. It is not recommended for small children.
- ADVERSE EFFECTS: Among the most serious adverse reactions are diminished visual acuity and allergic reactions, such as rashes.

ethanoic acid. See **acetic acid**.

ethanol /eth′ənol/, ethyl alcohol. See also **alcohol**.

ethaverine hydrochloride /eth′əver′ēn/, a smooth muscle relaxant.
- INDICATIONS: It is prescribed to relieve spasm of the GI or genitourinary tract, arterial vasospasm, and cerebral insufficiency.
- CONTRAINDICATIONS: Liver disease, atrioventricular dissociation, or known hypersensitivity to this drug prohibits its use. It is used with caution in patients who have glaucoma.
- ADVERSE EFFECTS: Among the more serious adverse reactions are hypotension, abdominal distress, cardiac arrhythmia, and headache.

ethchlorvynol /ethklôr′vənôl/, a sedative and hypnotic.
- INDICATIONS: It is prescribed in the treatment of insomnia.
- CONTRAINDICATIONS: Porphyria or known hypersensitivity to this drug prohibits its use.
- ADVERSE EFFECTS: Among the most serious adverse effects are allergic reactions, nausea, dizziness, aftertaste, and drug hangover.

ethene. See **ethylene**.

ether /ē′thər/ [Gk, *aither*, air], a nonhalogenated, volatile liquid used as a general anesthetic. It provides such excellent analgesia and at high concentrations profound muscle relaxation that adjuncts to anesthesia, such as narcotic and neuromuscular blocking agents, are often unnecessary. Ether has a mild depressant effect on the respiratory and cardiovascular systems and may cause hyperglycemia, decreased excretion of urine, decreased intestinal tone and motility, and transient abnormalities in the function of the liver.

It has an irritating, pungent odor, is highly flammable and explosive, and frequently causes postoperative nausea and vomiting.

ethereal /ithir′ē·əl/ [Gk, *aither*, air], pertaining to or resembling ether.

ethics /eth′iks/ [Gk, *ethikos*, moral duty], the science or study of moral values or principles, including ideals of autonomy, beneficence, and justice.

ethinamate /ethin′əmāt/, a sedative.
- INDICATION: It is prescribed in the treatment of insomnia.
- CONTRAINDICATIONS: Known hypersensitivity to this drug prohibits its use. It is not recommended for pregnant women, for people under 15 years of age, or for persons with a history of drug abuse.
- ADVERSE EFFECTS: Among the more serious adverse reactions are thrombocytopenic purpura, physical and psychologic dependence, and skin rash.

ethinyl estradiol /eth′inil/, an estrogen.
- INDICATIONS: It is prescribed in the treatment of postmenopausal breast cancer, menstrual cycle irregularities and prostatic cancer, and hypogonadism, for contraception, and to relieve menopausal vasomotor symptoms.
- CONTRAINDICATIONS: Thrombophlebitis, abnormal genital bleeding, known or suspected pregnancy, or known hypersensitivity to this drug prohibits its use.
- ADVERSE EFFECTS: Among the more serious adverse reactions are thrombophlebitis, embolism, and hypercalcemia.

ethionamide /eth′ē·ənam′īd/, a tuberculostatic antibacterial.
- INDICATION: It is prescribed for tuberculosis.
- CONTRAINDICATIONS: Existing liver damage or known hypersensitivity to this drug prohibits its use.
- ADVERSE EFFECTS: Among the more serious adverse reactions are skin rash, jaundice, and mental depression. GI side effects are common.

ethmoid /eth′moid/ [Gk, *ethmos*, sieve, *eidos*, form], 1. pertaining to the ethmoid bone. 2. having a large number of sievelike openings.

ethmoidal air cell /ethmoi′dəl/ [Gk, *ethmos*, sieve, *eidos*, form], one of the numerous, small thin-walled cavities in the ethmoid bone of the skull, rimmed by the frontal maxilla, lacrimal, sphenoidal, and palatine bones. The cavities are lined with mucous membrane continuous with that of the nasal cavity and lie between the upper part of the nasal cavities and the orbits. They are divided bilaterally into anterior, middle, and posterior cavities. The anterior and the middle cavities open into the middle meatus of the nose; the posterior cavities open into the superior meatus. The ethmoidal air cells start to develop at birth. Compare **frontal sinus, maxillary sinus, sphenoidal sinus**.

ethmoid bone, the very light and spongy bone at the base of the cranium, forming most of the walls of the superior part of the nasal cavity and consisting of four parts: a horizontal plate, a perpendicular plate, and two lateral labyrinths.

ethnic group /eth′nik/, a population of individuals organized around an assumption of common cultural origin.

ethnocentrism /eth′nōsen′trizm/ [Gk, *ethnos*, nation, *kentron*, center], 1. a belief in the inherent superiority of the "race" or group to which one belongs. 2. a proclivity to consider other ethnic groups in terms of one's own racial origins.

ethoheptazine citrate /eth′ōhep′təzēn/, a nonnarcotic analgesic.

■ INDICATION: It is prescribed to relieve mild to moderate pain.

■ CONTRAINDICATION: Known hypersensitivity to this drug prohibits its use.

■ ADVERSE EFFECTS: Among the most common adverse reactions are GI distress and dizziness.

ethology /ethol′əjē/ [Gk, *ethos*, character, *logos*, science], **1.** (in zoology) the scientific study of the behavioral patterns of animals, specifically in their native habitat. **2.** (in psychology) the empiric study of human behavior, primarily social customs, manners, and mores. **–ethologic, ethological,** *adj.,* **ethologist,** *n.*

ethopropazine hydrochloride /eth′ōprō′pəzēn/, a phenothiazine anticholinergic agent.

■ INDICATIONS: It is prescribed in the treatment of extrapyramidal parkinsonism and other nervous system disorders.

■ CONTRAINDICATIONS: Narrow-angle glaucoma, asthma, obstruction of the genitourinary or GI tract, severe ulcerative colitis, or known hypersensitivity to this drug or to phenothiazine medication prohibits its use.

■ ADVERSE EFFECTS: Among the more serious adverse effects are blurred vision, central nervous system effects, tachycardia, dry mouth, decreased sweating, and hypersensitivity reactions.

ethosuximide /eth′ōsuk′simīd/, an anticonvulsant.

■ INDICATION: It is prescribed in the treatment of petit mal epilepsy.

■ CONTRAINDICATIONS: Known hypersensitivity to this drug or to any succinimide medication prohibits its use.

■ ADVERSE EFFECTS: Among the more serious adverse reactions are blood dyscrasias, GI disturbance, and hematopoietic complications.

ethotoin /eth′ōtō′in/, an anticonvulsant.

■ INDICATIONS: It is prescribed in the treatment of generalized tonic-clonic and complex-partial seizures.

■ CONTRAINDICATIONS: Liver disease, hematologic disorders, or known hypersensitivity to this drug or to any hydantoin prohibits its use. It is not recommended for use during pregnancy or lactation.

■ ADVERSE EFFECTS: Among the more serious adverse reactions are blood disorders, nausea, fatigue, skin rash, and chest pain.

Ethrane, a trademark for an inhalational general anesthetic (enflurane).

Ethril, a trademark for an antibacterial (erythromycin stearate).

ethyl alcohol. See **alcohol.**

ethyl aminobenzoate. See **benzocaine.**

ethyl chloride /eth′il/, a topical anesthetic for short operations.

■ INDICATIONS: It is prescribed in the treatment of skin irritations and in minor skin surgery.

■ CONTRAINDICATIONS: Known hypersensitivity to this drug prohibits its use. It is not used on broken skin or on mucous membrane.

■ ADVERSE EFFECTS: Among the more serious adverse reactions are pain, muscle spasm, and, from excessive use, frostbite.

■ NOTE: It is highly flammable.

ethylene /eth′əlēn/ [Gk, *aither*, air, *hyle*, stuff], a colorless, flammable gas that is lighter than air and has a slightly sweet odor and taste. It was previously used as a general anesthetic, being slightly more potent than nitrous oxide. Also called **ethene, olefiant gas.**

ethylenediamine /eth′ələndi·am′ēn/, a clear, thick liquid having the odor of ammonia. It is used as a solvent, an emulsifier, and a stabilizer with aminophylline injections.

ethylene dibromide (EDB), a volatile liquid used as an insecticide and gasoline additive. Because it has been found to be a cause of cancer in animals, the Environmental Protection Agency has restricted the use of EDB to control insect pests in grains and fruits intended for human use.

ethylene dichloride poisoning, the toxic effects of exposure to ethylene dichloride, a hydrocarbon solvent, diluent, and fumigant, and one of the most abundant of all chlorinated organic chemicals. It is an eye, ear, nose, throat, and skin irritant, and has produced cancers in laboratory animals. Inhalation or ingestion can lead to serious illness or death. The compound is metabolized into 2-chloroethanol and monochloroacetic acid, both more toxic than the original chemical.

ethylene glycol poisoning, the toxic reaction to ingestion of ethylene glycol or diethylene glycol, chemicals used in automobile antifreeze preparations. Symptoms in mild cases may resemble those of alcohol intoxication but without the breath odor of alcoholic beverages. There may also be vomiting, carpopedal spasm, lumbar pain, renal failure, respiratory distress, convulsions, and coma. Treatment may include emesis, gastric lavage, establishing electrolyte balance, and hemodialysis. In some cases, ethanol may be given because it impedes the metabolism of ethylene glycol.

ethylene oxide, a gas used to sterilize surgical instruments and other supplies.

ethylestrenol, an anabolic steroid.

ethylnorepinephrine hydrochloride /eth′ilnôrep′inef′rin/, a bronchodilator.

■ INDICATION: It is prescribed in the treatment of bronchial asthma.

■ CONTRAINDICATIONS: Known hypersensitivity to this drug or to other sympathomimetic medication prohibits its use.

■ ADVERSE EFFECTS: Among the more serious adverse reactions are increased or decreased blood pressure, palpitations, and an increase in heart rate.

ethyl oxide, an alternative name for diethyl ether.

ethynodiol diacetate /eth′inōdī′ôl/, a synthetic progestin derivative.

ethynodiol diacetate and ethinyl estradiol, an oral contraceptive.

■ INDICATION: It is prescribed for contraception.

■ CONTRAINDICATIONS: Thrombophlebitis, cardiovascular disease, breast or reproductive organ cancer, or known hypersensitivity to either ingredient prohibits its use.

■ ADVERSE EFFECTS: Among the more serious adverse reactions are thrombophlebitis, uterine fibroma, gallbladder disease, embolism, and hepatic lesions.

ethynodiol diacetate and mestranol, an oral contraceptive.

■ INDICATION: It is prescribed for contraception.

■ CONTRAINDICATIONS: Thrombophlebitis, cardiovascular disease, breast or reproductive organ cancer, or known hypersensitivity to either ingredient prohibits its use.

■ ADVERSE EFFECTS: Among the more serious adverse reactions are thrombophlebitis, uterine fibroma, gallbladder disease, embolism, and hepatic lesions.

-etic, a suffix used as the equivalent of *-ic* in forming adjectives: *enuretic, genetic, kinetic.*

etidronate disodium /etid′rənāt/, a regulator of calcium metabolism. Also called **sodium etidronate.**

■ INDICATIONS: It is prescribed in the treatment of Paget's disease, for heterotopic ossification caused by injury to the spinal cord, and after total hip replacement.

■ CONTRAINDICATIONS: There are no known contraindications.

■ ADVERSE EFFECTS: Among the more serious adverse reactions are bone pain at both Pagetic sites and previously asymptomatic sites, GI disturbances, and elevated serum phosphate concentrations.

etiodocaine. See **amide-compound local anesthesia.**

etiology /ē′tē·ol′əjē/ [Gk, *aitia*, cause, *logos*, science], **1.** the study of all factors that may be involved in the development of a disease, including susceptibility of the patient, the nature of the disease agent, and the way in which the patient's body is invaded by the agent. **2.** the cause of a disease. Compare **pathogenesis.** –**etiologic**, *adj.*

etomidate /etom′idāt/, a hypnotic and short-acting, nonbarbiturate intravenous induction agent for general anesthesia. It is reported to have minimal adverse cardiovascular and respiratory effects, thus providing a greater margin of safety in patients at risk because of heart disease. The damage may cause suppression of adrenal function.

Etrafon, a trademark for a central nervous system fixed-combination drug containing a tranquilizer (perphenazine) and an antidepressant (amitriptyline hydrochloride).

etretinate /etret′ināt/, a synthetic derivative of vitamin A used as an oral drug to treat psoriasis.

■ INDICATIONS: Etretinate is prescribed for severe recalcitrant psoriasis, including generalized pustular and erythrodermic psoriasis.

■ CONTRAINDICATIONS: It is contraindicated for women who are of childbearing age unless a pregnancy test within 2 weeks of the start of therapy has negative results. Because of the risk of hyperostosis, the drug should not be given to children unless all alternative therapies have been exhausted.

■ ADVERSE EFFECTS: Adverse reactions may include benign intracranial hypertension, hepatitis, visual abnormalities including corneal damage, skeletal hyperostosis, peeling skin and alopecia, muscle cramps, and headache.

etymology [Gk, *etymos*, base; L, *logos*, words], the study of the origin and development of words. An **etymon** (*pl.* **etyma**) is an earlier form of a word.

Eu, symbol for the element **europium.**

eu-, a prefix meaning 'well, easily, good, true': *euangiotic*, *eucrasia*, *euthyroid*.

eubiotics /yōo′bī·ot′iks/ [Gk, *eu*, well, *bios*, life], the science of healthy living.

eucalyptol /yōo′kəlip′tol/, a substance with an aromatic odor obtained from the volatile oil of *Eucalyptus* and used in nasal emollients. Also called **cajeputol.**

eucaryocyte. See **eukaryocyte.**

eucaryote. See **eukaryote.**

-eucaryotic. See **eukaryote.**

eucaryon. See **eukaryon.**

eucaryosis. See **eukaryosis.**

eucatropine hydrochloride /yōokat′rəpin/, an ophthalmic anticholinergic.

■ INDICATION: It is prescribed for dilating the pupil in an ophthalmoscopic examination of the eye.

■ CONTRAINDICATIONS: Known hypersensitivity to this drug or to other anticholinergics prohibits its use.

■ ADVERSE EFFECTS: Among the most serious adverse reactions are tachycardia and severe constipation. Dry mouth, heat intolerance, and other effects associated with systemic absorption of an anticholinergic agent may also occur.

eucholia /yōokō′lyə/ [Gk, *eu*, well, *chole*, bile], the nor-

mal state of the bile as to the quantity secreted and the condition of the constituents.

euchromatin /yōokrō′mətin/ [Gk, *eu* + *chroma*, color], that portion of chromosome material that is active in gene expression during cell division. It stains most deeply during mitosis when it is in a coiled, condensed state, and during each division of the cell it passes through a continuous cycle of condensation and dispersion. Compare **heterochromatin.** See also **chromatin.** –**euchromatic**, *adj.*

euchromosome. See **autosome.**

eugamy /yōo′gəmē/ [Gk, *eu* + *gamos*, marriage], the union of those gametes that contain the same haploid number of chromosomes. –**eugamic**, *adj.*

eugenics /yōojen′iks/ [Gk, *eu* + *genein*, to produce], the study of methods for controlling the characteristics of future human populations through selective breeding.

euglobulin /yōoglob′yəlin/ [Gk, *eu* + L, *globulus*, small sphere], a "true" globulin (a protein insoluble in distilled water). This is one of a number of different properties used to classify proteins. Compare **albumin, cryoglobulin.** See also **plasma protein, electrophoresis.**

eugnathic anomaly /yōonath′ik/ [Gk, *eu* + *gnathos*, jaw; *anomalia* irregularity], (in dentistry) an abnormality of the teeth and their alveolar supports. Compare **dysgnathic anomaly.**

eukaryocyte /yōoker′ē·ōsīt′/ [Gk, *eu* + *karyon*, nut, *kytos*, cell], a cell with a true nucleus, found in all higher organisms and in some microorganisms, as amebae, plasmodia, and trypanosomes. Also spelled **eucaryocyte.** Compare **prokaryocyte.** –**eukaryotic**, *adj.*

eukaryon /yōoker′ē·on/ [Gk, *eu*, good, *karyon*, nut], **1.** a nucleus that is highly complex, organized, and surrounded by a nuclear membrane, usually characteristic of higher organisms. **2.** an organism containing such a nucleus. Also spelled **eucaryon.** Compare **prokaryon.**

eukaryosis /yōoker′i·ō′sis/ [Gk, *eu* + *karyon*, nut, *osis*, condition], the state of having a highly complex, organized nucleus containing organelles surrounded by a nuclear membrane, such as is characteristic of all organisms except bacteria, viruses, and blue-green algae. Also spelled **eucaryosis.** Compare **prokaryosis.**

eukaryote /yōoker′ē·ot/ [Gk, *eu* + *karyon*, nut], an organism having cells that contain a true nucleus. Also spelled **eucaryote.** –**eukaryotic, eucaryotic**, *adj.*

-eukaryotic. See **eukaryocyte.**

eunuch /yōo′nək/ [Gk, *eune*, couch, *echein*, to guard], a male whose testicles have been destroyed or removed. If this occurs before puberty, secondary sex characteristics fail to develop and symptoms such as a feminine voice and absence of facial hair can stem from the absence of male hormones. See also **secondary sex characteristic.**

eunuchoidism /yōo′nəkoidiz′əm/, deficiency of the function of male hormone or of its formation by the testes. The deficiency leads to sterility and to abnormal tallness, small testes, and deficient development of secondary sexual characteristics, libido, and potency.

euphoretic /yōo′fəret′ik/ [Gk, *eu* + *pherein*, to bear], **1.** (of a substance or event) tending to produce a condition of euphoria. **2.** a substance tending to produce euphoria, as LSD, mescaline, marijuana, and other hallucinogenic drugs.

euphoria /yōofôr′ē·ə/ [Gk, *eu* + *pherein*, to bear], **1.** a feeling or state of well-being or elation. **2.** an exaggerated or abnormal sense of physical and emotional well-being not based on reality or truth, disproportionate to its cause, and inappropriate to the situation, as commonly seen in the

manic stage of bipolar disorder, in some forms of schizophrenia, in organic mental disorders, and in toxic and drug-
induced states. Compare **ecstasy.**

euploid /yōo´ploid/ [Gk, *eu* + *ploos*, multiple],   **1.** of or
pertaining to an individual, organism, strain, or cell with a
chromosome number that is an exact multiple of the normal, basic haploid number characteristic of the species, as
diploid, triploid, tetraploid, or polyploid. Variation occurs
through entire sets rather than individual chromosomes, so
that there is a balanced number of chromosomes. **2.** such
an individual, organism, strain, or cell. Compare **aneuploid.**

euploidy /yōo´ploidē/,   the state or condition of having a
variation in chromosome number that is an exact multiple
of the characteristic haploid number. Compare **aneuploidy.**

eupnea /yōop·nē´ə/ [Gk, *eu*, well, *pnein*, to breathe],   normal breathing.

Eurax,   a trademark for a scabicide (crotamiton).

European blastomycosis.   See **cryptococcosis.**

European typhus.   See **epidemic typhus.**

europium (Eu) /yōorō´pē·əm/ [Europe],   a rare-earth, metallic element. Its atomic number is 63; its atomic weight is
151.96.

eury-,   a combining form meaning 'wide, broad': *euryce-
phalic, eurygnathic, euryopia.*

eustachian tube /yōostā´shən/ [Bartolomeo Eustachio, Italian anatomist, b. 1520; L, *tubus*],   a tube, lined with mucous membrane, that joins the nasopharynx and the middle
ear cavity, allowing equalization of the air pressure in the
middle ear with atmospheric pressure. Also called **auditory
tube.**

eustress /yōo´stres/,   **1.** a positive form of stress. **2.** a balance between selfishness and altruism through which an individual develops the drive and energy to care for others.

euthanasia /yōo´thənā´zhə/ [Gk, *eu* + *thanatos*, death],
deliberately bringing about the death of a person who is suffering from an incurable disease or condition, actively, such
as by administering a lethal drug, or passively, by allowing the person to die by withholding treatment. Legal authorities, church leaders, philosophers, and commentators
on ethics and morality usually treat passive euthanasia
differently from active euthanasia. Also called **mercy
killing.**

euthenics /yōothen´iks/ [Gk, *eu* + *tithenai*, to place],   the
science that deals with improvement of the human species
through the control of environmental factors, as pollution,
malnutrition, disease, and drug abuse. Compare **eugenics.**

Euthroid,   a trademark for a thyroid hormone preparation
(liotrix; a combination of levothyroxine sodium and liothry-
onine sodium).

euthymism /yōothī´mizəm/ [Gk, *eu* + *thymos*, thyme flow-
ers],   the characteristic of normal mood responses.

euthyroid /yōothī´roid/ [Gk, *eu*, well, *thyreos*, oblong
shield],   pertaining to a normal thyroid gland.

Eutonyl,   a trademark for a monoamine oxidase inhibitor
(pargyline hydrochloride).

Eutron,   a trademark for a fixed-combination drug containing a diuretic (methyclothiazide) and a monoamine oxidase
inhibitor (pargyline hydrochloride), used as an antihypertensive.

evacuant /ivak´yōo·ənt/ [L, *evacuare*, to empty],   any
medicine or other agent that causes an organ to discharge
its contents, as an emetic or laxative.

evacuate /ivak´yōo·āt/ [L, *evacuare*, to empty],   **1.** to discharge or to remove a substance from a cavity, space, organ, or tract of the body. **2.** a substance discharged or removed from the body.   —**evacuation,** *n.*

evagination /ēvaj´inā´shən/,   the turning inside-out or protrusion of a body part or organ.

evaluating /ival´yōo·ā´shən/ [L, *ex*, away, *valare*, to be
strong],   (in five-step nursing process) a category of nursing behavior in which a determination is made and recorded
regarding the extent to which the established goals of care
have been met. To make this judgment, the nurse estimates
the degree of success in meeting the goals, evaluates the
implementation of nursing measures, investigates the client's compliance with therapy, and records the client's response to therapy. The nurse evaluates effects of the measures used, the need for change in goals of care, the accuracy of the implementation of nursing measures, and the
need for change in the client's environment or in the equipment or procedures used. The impact of the care or treatment on the client, the client's family, and the staff is evaluated, the accuracy of tests and measurements is checked,
and the client's and the family's understanding of the information given them is evaluated. The client's expressed and
observed response to care is recorded. Although evaluating
is considered the final step of the five-step nursing process,
after implementing, evaluating is, in practice, integral to effective nursing practice at all steps of the process. See also
**analyzing, assessing, implementing, nursing process,
planning.**

-evaporate.   See **evaporation.**

evaporated milk /ivap´ərā´tid/,   homogenized whole milk
from which 50% to 60% of the water content has been evaporated. It is fortified with vitamin D, canned, and sterilized.
When it is diluted with an equal amount of water, its nutritional value is comparable to that of fresh whole milk.

evaporation /ivap´ərā´shən/ [L, *ex* + *vapor*, steam],   the
change of a substance from a solid or liquid state to a gaseous state. The process of evaporation is hastened by an increase in temperature and a decrease in atmospheric pressure. See also **boiling point.**   —**evaporate,** *v.*

eventration /ē´vəntrā´shən/,   the protrusion of the intestines from the abdomen.

event-related potential (ERP) [L, *evenire*, to happen; *relatus*, carry back; *potentia*, power],   a type of brain wave
that is associated with a response to a specific stimulus, such
as a particular wave pattern observed when a patient hears
a clicking sound. See also **evoked potential.**

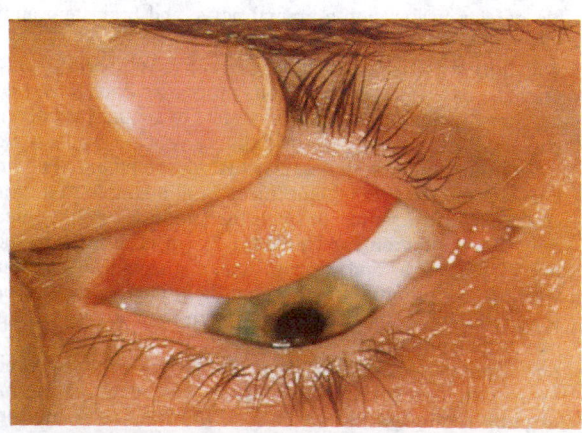

Eversion of the eyelid *(Eagling, 1986)*

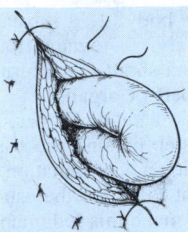

Wound evisceration

eversion /ivur′zhən/, a turning outward or inside-out, such as a turning of the foot outward at the ankle.

everywhere lines. See **Kerley lines.**

evisceration /ivis′ərā′shən/ [L, *ex* + *viscera*, entrails], **1.** the removal of the viscera from the abdominal cavity; disembowelment. **2.** the removal of the contents from an organ or an organ from its cavity. **3.** the protrusion of an internal organ through a wound or surgical incision, especially in the abdominal wall. **–eviscerate,** *v.*

evocation /ev′ōkā′shən/ [L, *evocare,* to call forth], (in embryology) a specific morphogenetic change within a developing embryo that occurs as a result of the action of a single evocator. See also **induction.**

evocator /ev′ōkā′tər/ [L, *evocare,* to call forth], a specific chemical substance or hormone that is emitted from the organizer part of the embryonic tissue and acts as a morphogenetic stimulus in the developing embryo.

evoked potential (EP) /ivōkt′/ [L, *evocare,* to call forth; *potentia,* power], an electrical response in the brainstem or cerebral cortex which is elicited by a specific stimulus. The stimulus may affect the visual, auditory, or somatosensory pathways, producing a characteristic brain wave pattern. The activity and function of the system may be monitored during surgery, while the patient is unconscious. The surgeon is thus able to avoid damage to the nerves during operative procedures. Evoked potentials are also used to diagnose multiple sclerosis and various disorders of hearing and of sight. Kinds of evoked potentials include **brainstem auditory evoked potential, somatosensory evoked potential,** and **visual evoked potential.** See also **brain electric activity map.**

evoked response audiometry, a method of testing hearing ability at the level of the brainstem and auditory cortex. Evoked response audiometry is useful in diagnosing possible defects in the eighth cranial nerve and brainstem auditory pathways.

evolution /ev′əloo′shən/ [L, *evolvere,* to roll forth], **1.** a gradual, orderly, and continuous process of change and development from one condition or state to another. It encompasses all aspects of life, including physical, psychologic, sociologic, cultural, and intellectual development, and involves a progressive advancement from a simple to a more complex form or state through the processes of modification, differentiation, and growth. **2.** (in genetics) the theory of the origin and propagation of all plant and animal species, including humans, and their development from lower to more complex forms through the natural selection of variants produced through genetic mutations, hybridization, and inbreeding. Kinds of evolution are **convergent evolution, determinant evolution, emergent evolution, organic evolution, orthogenic evolution,** and **saltatory evolution.** **–evolutionist,** *n.*

evolution of infarction the normal healing process after a myocardial infarction, as shown on successive electrocardiograms.

evulsed tooth. See **avulsed teeth.**

Ewing's sarcoma /yoo′ingz/ [James Ewing, American pathologist, b. 1866], a malignant tumor developing from bone marrow, usually in long bones or the pelvis. It occurs most frequently in adolescent boys and is characterized by pain, swelling, fever, and leukocytosis. The tumor, a soft, crumbly grayish mass that may invade surrounding soft tissues, is difficult to distinguish histologically from a neuroblastoma or a reticulum cell sarcoma. Radiotherapy often produces a dramatic initial response, but relapses are common. Surgical excision, often requiring amputation, may be recommended. Also called **Ewing's tumor.** See also **endothelial myeloma, neuroblastoma, reticulum cell sarcoma.**

ex-, a prefix meaning 'away from, outside, without': *exacrinous, excoriation, exfoliato.*

exa-, a prefix indicating the SI unit 10^{18}.

exacerbation /igzas′ərbā′shən/ [L, *exacerbare,* to provoke], an increase in the seriousness of a disease or disorder as marked by greater intensity in the signs or symptoms of the patient being treated.

exanthema /ig′zanthē′mə/ [Gk, eruption], a skin eruption or rash that may have specific diagnostic features of an infectious disease. Chickenpox, measles, roseola infantum, and rubella are usually characterized by a particular type of exanthema. Also called **exanthem.** Compare **enanthema.** **–exanthematous,** *adj.*

exanthematous /ig′zanthem′ətəs/ [Gk, *ex,* out, *anthema,* blossoming], pertaining to the skin rash accompanying an infectious disease.

exanthem subitum. See **roseola infantum.**

excavatio rectouterina. See **Douglas' cul-de-sac.**

excessive sweat /ikses′iv/ [L, *excedere,* to go out; AS, *swaeaten],* perspiration greater than normal for the ambient environment. It is usually a sign of septic fever, pulmonary tuberculosis, hyperthyroidism, chronic renal disease, or malaria. Abnormal sweating of the hands and feet is often a sign of nervous irritability or other emotional stress.

excess mortality /ikses′/ [L, *excedere,* to go out; *mortalis,* mortal], a premature death or one that occurs before the average life expectancy for a person of a particular demographic category.

exchange transfusion in the newborn /iks·chāng′/ [L, *ex* + *cambire,* to change], the introduction of whole blood in exchange for 75% to 85% of an infant's circulating blood that is repeatedly withdrawn in small amounts and replaced with equal amounts of donor blood. The procedure is performed to improve the oxygen-carrying capacity of the blood in the treatment of erythroblastosis neonatorum by removing Rh and ABO antibodies, sensitized erythrocytes producing hemolysis, and accumulated bilirubin.

■ METHOD: A radiant heat warmer, pacifier, and cardiac and respiratory monitors are prepared, and resuscitative equipment and drugs, including oxygen, a mask, a bag, suction apparatus, glucose, calcium, and sodium bicarbonate, are made readily available. The results of laboratory studies of the infant's bilirubin, hemoglobin, and calcium levels, hematocrit, blood culture, and random blood glucose test and the donor blood culture are checked. The donor blood is checked to make certain that it is not more than 48 hours old; if fresh whole blood is not used, stored blood is mixed in amounts as ordered with frozen plasma or plasmanate. Before exchange transfusion, nothing is administered by

mouth for 3 to 4 hours, or the contents of the infant's stomach are aspirated. The baby's extremities are restrained; the blood is warmed as ordered, and the physician is assisted with the insertion of an umbilical venous line, if one is not in place. The physician may administer albumin with the donor blood. The procedure may be carried out under phototherapy lights, and, unless contraindicated, the infant's parents may be in attendance. During the procedure the young patient is observed for bradycardia with less than 100 beats a minute, cyanosis, hypothermia, vomiting, aspiration, apnea, an air embolus, abdominal distention, or cardiac arrest. The respiratory and cardiac rates are checked every 5 minutes, the axillary temperature every 15 to 30 minutes. The integrity of all blood tubing connections is inspected periodically. The amount of blood withdrawn and infused is recorded, and the physician is notified when each 100 ml of blood has been exchanged. A repetition of laboratory studies is requested as ordered for the last amount of blood removed from the infant. After the procedure, the infant is observed for signs of tachycardia or bradycardia, tachypnea or bradypnea, hypothermia, lethargy, jitteriness, increasing jaundice, cyanosis, edema, dark urine, bleeding from the cord, convulsions, or complications, such as hemorrhage, hypocalcemia, heart failure, hypoglycemia, sepsis, acidosis, hyperkalemia, thrombus formation, or shock. The infant is maintained in a neutral thermal environment and is handled gently and minimally for the next 2 to 4 hours. The cardiac and respiratory rates are monitored every 15 minutes for 4 hours, then every 30 to 60 minutes for 24 to 48 hours or as ordered. The axillary temperature is checked every 1 to 3 hours for 48 hours, and the cord is observed for bleeding every 5 to 15 minutes for 1 to 2 hours after the procedure. Feeding, by gavage or a bottle having a soft nipple with a large enough hole to ensure adequate intake, is initiated 4 to 6 hours after the transfusion, as ordered; the infant is fed slowly and repositioned after each feeding. Intake and output of fluids are measured, and ongoing care is provided as for all high-risk infants.
■ NURSING INTERVENTION: The nurse prepares the equipment and infant for the exchange transfusion, assists the physician in the insertion of the umbilical venous line, and monitors the baby during and after the procedure.
■ OUTCOME CRITERIA: An exchange transfusion is usually administered only to a high-risk infant, but the procedure often effectively counteracts the hemolytic anemia and hyperbilirubinemia associated with erythroblastosis neonatorum.

excise /iksīz′/ [L, *ex* + *caedere*, to cut], to remove completely, as in the surgical excision of the palatine tonsils. Compare **resect.**

excision /iksish′ən/ [L, *ex* + *caedere*, to cut], **1.** the process of excising or amputating. **2.** (in molecular genetics) the process by which a genetic element is removed from a strand of DNA.

excitability /iksī′təbil′itē/ [L, *excitare*, to arouse], the property of a cell that enables it to react to irritation or stimulation, such as the reaction of a nerve or myocardial cell to an adequate stimulus.

excitant /eksī′tənt/, a drug or other agent that arouses the central nervous system or other body system in a particular manner. Excitants may be drugs or other substances, such as caffeine, or visual or auditory stimuli.

excitation /ek′sitā′shən/ [L, *excitare*, to rouse], a state of mental or physical excitement; nerve or muscle acting on impulse.

excitatory amino acids /eksī′tətôr′ē/, amino acids that af-

fect the central nervous system and may in some cases act as neurotoxins. Examples include glutamate and aspartate, which have depolarizing properties and may function as neurotransmitters but may also cause the death of neurons. Amino acids produced by plants and fungi also are capable of functioning both as neurotransmitters and as neurotoxins and may be responsible for hypoxic or hypoglycemic brain damage.

excited state /eksī′tid/ [L, *excitare*, to rouse + *status*], in nuclear physics, an energy level of a system that is higher than the ground state. The system decays to the ground state and emits the energy difference, usually in the form of photons.

excitement /eksīt′mənt/, (in psychiatry) a pathologic state marked by emotional intensity, impulsive behavior, anticipation, and arousal. Excitement in schizophrenic patients tends to result from blocked communications and hostile feelings between the patients and the hospital staff.

exciting eye, (in sympathetic ophthalmia) the eye that is primarily affected by an injury or infection in a bilateral disorder. Also called **inciting eye.**

excoriation /ekskôr′ē·ā′shən/ [L, *excoriare*, to flay], an injury to the surface of the skin or other part of the body caused by trauma, such as scratching, abrasion, chemical or thermal burns.

excreta /ekskrē′tə/ [L, *excernere*, to separate], any waste matter discharged from the body.

excrete /ekskrēt′/ [L, *excernere*, to separate], to evacuate a waste substance from the body, often via a normal secretion; for example, a drug may be excreted in breast milk.

excretion /ekskrē′shən/, the process of eliminating, shedding, or getting rid of substances by body organs or tissues, as part of a natural metabolic activity. Excretion usually begins at the cellular level where water, carbon dioxide, and other waste products of cellular life are emptied into the capillaries. The epidermis excretes dead skin cells by shedding them daily.

excretion urography [L, *excernere*, to separate; Gk, *ouron*, urine + *graphein*, to record], a radiographic examination in which an opaque medium is introduced and its pathways recorded as it is passes through the urinary tract. Also called **intravenous pyelography (IVP).**

excretory /eks′krətôr′ē/ [L, *excernere*, to separate], relating to the process of excretion, often used in combination with a term to identify an object or procedure associated with excretion, such as **excretory urography.**

excretory duct, a duct that is conductive but not secretory.

excretory urography. See **intravenous pyelography.**

excursion /ikskur′zhən/ [L, *ex*, out, *currere*, to run], a departure or deviation from a direct or normal course.

execute /ek′səkyoot/, (of a computer) to follow a set of instructions to complete a program or specified function.

executive physical /iksek′yətiv/, a physical examination including extensive laboratory, x-ray, and other tests that is provided periodically to management level personnel at employer expense. Such examinations may be detailed, expensive, and overly complete.

exercise /ek′sərsiz/ [L, *exercere*, to exercise], **1.** the performance of any physical activity for the purpose of conditioning the body, improving health, or maintaining fitness or as a means of therapy for correcting a deformity or restoring the organs and bodily functions to a state of health. **2.** any action, skill, or maneuver that exerts the muscles and is performed repeatedly in order to develop or strengthen the body or any of its parts. **3.** to use a muscle or part of the body in a repetitive way to maintain or develop its strength. The nurse constantly assesses the patient's needs and provides the proper type and amount of exercise, taking into account the patient's physical or mental limitations. Exercise has a beneficial effect on each of the body systems, although in excess it can lead to the breakdown of tissue and cause injury. Kinds of exercise are **active assisted exercise, active exercise, active resistance exercise, aerobic exercise, anaerobic exercise, corrective exercise, isometric exercise, isotonic exercise, muscle-setting exercise, passive exercise, progressive resistance exercise, range of motion exercise,** and **underwater exercise.**

exercise electrocardiogram (exercise ECG), a stress test that is important in the diagnosis of coronary artery disease. An exercise electrocardiogram is recorded as a person walks on a treadmill or pedals a stationary bicycle for a given length of time at a specific rate of speed. Abnormal changes in cardiac function that were absent during rest may appear with exercise.

exercise-induced asthma /-indyo͞ost′/, a form of asthma that produces symptoms after strenuous exercise. The condition usually occurs in persons who already have asthma, hay fever, or related hypersensitivity reactions. The effect may be acute but is reversible.

exercise prescription [L, *exercere, prae, scribere,* to write], an individualized schedule for physical fitness exercises.

exercise tolerance, the level of physical exertion an individual may be able to perform before reaching a state of exhaustion. Exercise-tolerance tests are commonly performed on a treadmill under the supervision of a health professional who can stop the test when signs of distress are observed.

exertional headache /igzur′shənəl/ [L, *exserere,* to stretch out; AS, *heafod, acan,* headache], an acute headache that occurs during strenuous exercise. It usually recedes when the level of effort is reduced or by taking an analgesic medication, or both.

exfoliation /eksfō′lē·ā′shən/ [L, *ex + folium,* leaf], peeling and sloughing off of tissue cells. This is a normal process that may be exaggerated in certain skin diseases or after a severe sunburn. See also **desquamation, exfoliative dermatitis. –exfoliative,** *adj.*

exfoliative cytology /eksfō′lē·ətiv/, the microscopic examination of desquamated cells for diagnostic purposes. The cells are obtained from lesions, sputum, secretions, urine, and other material by aspiration, scraping, a smear, or washings of the tissue. Compare **aspiration biopsy cytology.**

exfoliative dermatitis, any inflammatory skin disorder characterized by excessive peeling or shedding of skin. The cause is unknown in about half of the cases. Known causes include drug reactions, scarlet fever, leukemia, lymphoma, and generalized dermatitis. Treatment is individualized, but care is essential to prevent secondary infection, avoid further irritation, maintain fluid balance, and stabilize body temperature.

exhalation. See **expiration.**

exhale /eks·hāl′/ [L, *exhalare,* to breathe out], to breathe out or to let out with the breath. **–exhalation,** *n.*

exhaustion /igzôs′chən/ [L, *exhaurire,* to drain away], a state of extreme loss of physical or mental abilities caused by fatigue or illness.

exhaustion delirium, a delirium that may result from pro-

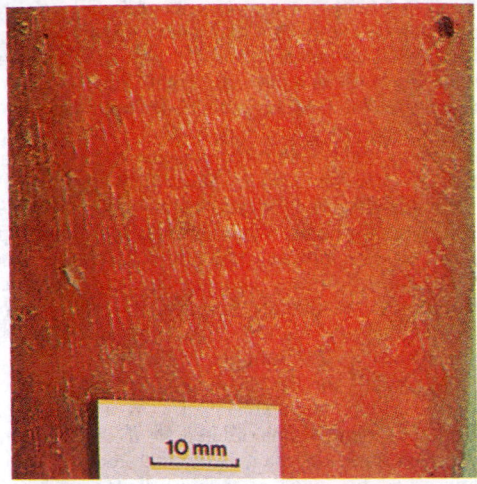

Exfoliative dermatitis *(Cerio, 1992)*

longed physical or emotional stress, fatigue, or shock associated with severe metabolic or nutritional problems. See also **delirium.**

exhaustion psychosis [L, *exhaurire,* to drain out; Gk, *psyche,* mind, *osis,* condition], an abnormal mental condition attributed to physical exhaustion. The main symptom, a delirious state, may develop in some explorers, mountain climbers, persons lost in the wilderness, and some terminally ill patients. See also **exhaustion delirium.**

exhibitionism /ek′sibish′əniz′əm/ [L, *exhibere,* to exhibit], **1.** the flaunting of oneself or one's abilities in order to attract attention. **2.** (in psychiatry) a psychosexual disorder occurring in men in which the repetitive act of exposing the genitals to unsuspecting women or girls in socially unacceptable situations is the preferred means of achieving sexual excitement and gratification. See also **paraphilia, scopophilia. –exhibitionist,** *n.*

eximer laser /ek′simir/, a small laser designed to break up organic molecules, such as cholesterol deposits, without producing intense heat.

existential humanistic psychotherapy. See **humanistic existential therapy.**

existential psychiatry /eg′zisten′shəl/ [L, *exsistere,* to spring forth; Gk, *psyche,* mind, *iatreia,* medical care], a school of psychiatry based on the philosophy of existentialism that emphasizes an analytic, holistic approach in which mental disorders are viewed as deviations within the total structure of an individual's existence rather than as caused by any biologically or culturally related factors.

existential therapy, a kind of psychotherapy that emphasizes the development of a sense of self-direction through choice, awareness, and acceptance of individual responsibility.

exit block [L, *exire,* to depart; Fr, *bloc*], (in cardiology) the failure of an expected impulse to emerge from its focus of origin and cause depolarization.

exit dose, (in radiotherapy) the amount of radiation at the side of the body opposite the surface to which the beam is directed.

Exna, a trademark for a diuretic and antihypertensive (benzthiazide).

exo-, a prefix meaning 'outside, outward': *exocataphoria, exohysteropexy, exotoxin.*

exocoelom. See **extraembryonic coelom.**

exocrine /ek'səkrin/ [Gk, *exo*, outside, *krinein*, to secrete], of or pertaining to the process of secreting outwardly through a duct to the surface of an organ or tissue or into a vessel, such as a gland that secretes through a duct. Compare **endocrine system.** See also **eccrine.**

exocrine gland, any of the multicellular glands that open onto the skin surface through ducts in the epithelium, as the sweat glands and the sebaceous glands. Exocrine glands also include other simple glands having only one duct and compound glands having more than one duct. See also **apocrine gland.**

exogenous /igzoj'ənəs/ [Gk, *exo* + *genein*, to produce], **1.** growing outside the body, **2.** originating outside the body or an organ of the body or produced from external causes, such as a disease caused by a bacterial or viral agent foreign to the body. Compare **endogenous.** —**exogenic,** *adj.*

exogenous depression. See **reactive depression.**

exogenous hemochromatosis [Gk, *exo,* outside + *genein,* to produce + *haima,* blood + *chroma,* color + *osis,* condition], a condition of bronzed pigmentation of the skin caused by accumulation of an iron pigment from excessive intake of iron-rich foods or blood transfusions. Also called **bronze diabetes.**

exogenous hypertriglyceridemia. See **hyperlipidemia type I.**

exogenous infection [Gk, *exo,* outside, *genein,* to produce; L, *inficere,* to infect], an infection that develops from bacteria normally outside the body that have gained access to the body.

exogenous obesity, obesity caused by a caloric intake greater than needed to meet the metabolic needs of the body. Compare **endogenous obesity.** See also **obesity.**

exogenous uric acid [Gk, *exo,* outside + *genein,* to produce + *ouron,* urine; L, *acidus*], the accumulation of uric acid in the body produced by the metabolism of purine-rich foods.

exon /ek'son/ [Gk, *exo* + *genein,* to produce], (in molecular genetics) the part of a DNA molecule that produces the code for the final messenger RNA.

exonuclease /ek'sōnōō'klē·ās/ [Gk, *exo* + L, *nucleus,* nut; *ase,* enzyme], (in molecular genetics) a nuclease that digests DNA or RNA from the ends of the strands.

exophoria /ek'səfôr'ē·ə/ [Gk, *exo* + *pherein,* to bear], deviation of the visual axis of one eye outward and away from that of the other eye, occurring in the absence of visual stimuli for fusion. Compare **exotropia.** —**exophoric,** *adj.*

exophthalmia /ek'softhal'mē·ə/ [Gk, *exo* + *ophthalmos,* eye], an abnormal condition characterized by a marked protrusion of the eyeballs (**exophthalmos, exophthalmus**), usually resulting from the increased volume of the orbital contents caused by a tumor; swelling associated with cerebral, intraocular, or intraorbital edema or hemorrhage; paralysis of or trauma to the extraocular muscles; or cavernous sinus thrombosis. It may also be caused by endocrine disorders, such as hyperthyroidism and Graves' disease, by varicose veins within the orbit, or by injury to orbital bones. Visual acuity may be impaired in exophthalmia; keratitis, ulceration, infection, and blindness may also occur. Treatment depends on the underlying cause. The outcome depends on the cause and the stage at which the condition is detected and treatment is begun. Acute advanced exophthalmia is often irreversible. Also called **proptosis, protrusio bulbi.** —**exophthalmic,** *adj.*

exophthalmic goiter /ek'softhal'mik/, exophthalmos occurring in association with goiter, as in Graves' disease.

exophthalmometer /ek'səfthalmom'ətər/ [Gk, *exo* + *ophthalmos,* eye, *metron,* measure], an instrument used for measuring the degree of forward displacement of the eye in exophthalmos. The device allows measurement of the distance from the center of the cornea to the lateral orbital rim. This distance is rarely more than 18 mm.

exophthalmos. See **exophthalmia.**

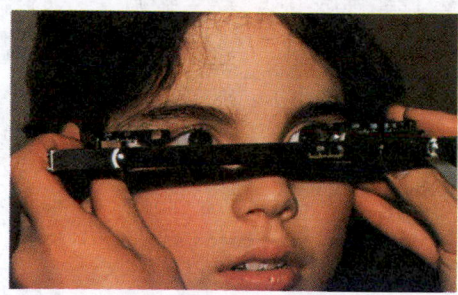

Exophthalmometer *(Zitelli, 1992)*

exophthalmos-macroglossia-gigantism syndrome. See **EMG syndrome.**

exophthalmus. See **exophthalmia.**

exophytic /ek'səfit'ik/ [Gk, *exo* + *phyton,* plant], of or pertaining to the tendency to grow outward, such as an exophytic tumor that grows on the surface or exterior portion of an organ or structure.

exophytic carcinoma, a malignant, epithelial neoplasm that resembles a papilloma or wart.

exoskeletal prosthesis /ek'səskel'ətəl/ [Gk, *exo* + *skeletos,* dried up; *prosthesis,* addition], a prosthetic device in which support is provided by an outside structure.

exoskeleton /ek'səskel'ətən/ [Gk, *exo,* outside, *skeletos,* dried up], the hard outer covering of many invertebrates, such as crustaceans, which lack the bony internal structures of vertebrates. Compare **endoskeleton.**

exostosis /ek'sostō'sis/ [Gk, *exo* + *osteon,* bone], an abnormal, benign growth on the surface of a bone. Also called **hyperostosis.** —**exostosed, exostotic,** *adj.*

exostosis cartilagines [Gk, *ex,* out, *osteon,* bone; L, *cartilago,* cartilage], an outgrowth of cartilage at the ends of long bones. Also called **cartilage capped exostosis.**

-exostotic. See **exostosis.**

exoteric /ek'səter'ik/ [Gk, *exoterikos,* external], pertaining to something outside the organism.

exotoxin /ek'sətok'sin/ [Gk, *exo* + *toxikon,* poison], a toxin that is secreted or excreted by a living microorganism. Compare **endotoxin.**

exotropia. See **divergent squint.**

expanded role [L, *expandere,* to spread out; OFr, *rolle,* an assumed character], the role of a nurse beyond the traditional limits of nursing practice legislation. Common roles are primary nurse and nurse practitioner, necessitating le-

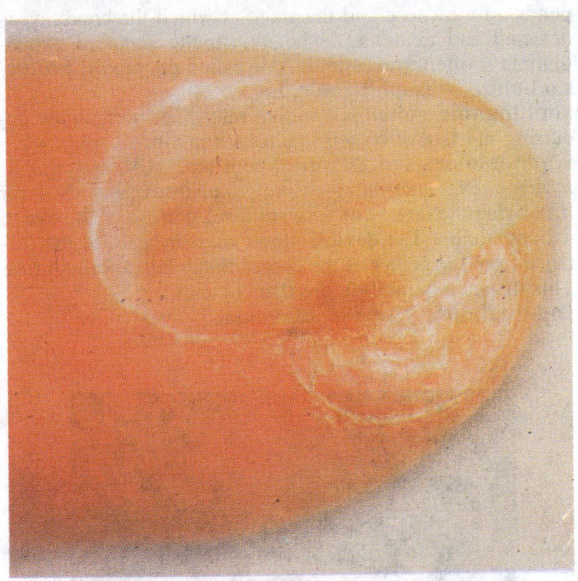

Subungual exostosis (Baran, 1991)

gal coverage through the establishment of standardized procedures or amendments or changes in nursing practice acts.

expectant treatment /ekspek'tənt/ [L, *exspectare*, to wait for; Fr, *traitment*], applying therapeutic measures to relieve symptoms as they arise in the course of a disease rather than treating the cause of the illness itself. Some kinds of expectant treatment are amputations for gangrene in a patient with diabetes, coronary bypass procedures in a patient with generalized atherosclerosis, and transplantation of tendons in a patient with severe rheumatoid arthritis. Compare **definitive treatment, palliative treatment, treatment.**

expectation /eks'pektā'shən/ [L, *exspectare*, to wait for], (in nursing) **1.** anticipation by the staff of a patient's behavior based on a knowledge and understanding of the person's abilities and problems. **2.** anticipation of the performance of the nursing staff in defined roles, as role expectation.

expectation of life, See **life expectancy.**

expected date of delivery (EDD), the predicted date of a pregnant woman's delivery. Pregnancy lasts approximately 266 days or 38 weeks from the day of fertilization but is considered clinically to last 280 days, or 40 weeks, or 10 lunar months, or 9⅓ calendar months from the first day of the last menstrual period (LMP). The EDD is usually calculated on the basis of 9⅓ calendar months, but if a woman is certain that coitus occurred only once during the month and if she knows the date on which it occurred, the EDD may be calculated as 38 weeks from that date. In the absence of a special calendar or device for calculating the EDD, it is arrived at by counting back 3 months from the first day of the LMP and then adding 7 days and 1 year; thus, if the first day of a woman's LMP was July 18, 1993, one counts back 3 months to April 18, 1993, then adds 7 days and 1 year to arrive at an EDD of April 25, 1994. Because calendar months differ in length, this calculation may give a date that is a few days more or less than 280 days

from the first day of the LMP, but it provides a very close approximation, and a trivial error will not be of clinical significance because of the variability of the actual durations of normal pregnancies. The expectant mother is advised that the EDD is only an estimate and that the chances are that she will give birth within 2 weeks before or, more commonly, after the calculated date. Formerly called **expected date of confinement, (EDC).**

expectorant /ikspek'tərənt/ [Gk, *ex*, out, *pectus*, breast], **1.** of or pertaining to a substance that promotes the ejection of mucus or other exudates from the lung, bronchi, and trachea. **2.** an agent that promotes expectoration by reducing the viscosity of pulmonary secretions or by decreasing the tenacity with which exudates adhere to the lower respiratory tract. Expectorant drugs include acetylcysteine, guaifenesin, terpin hydrate, and tyloxapol. Also called **mucolytic. –expectorate,** *v.*

expectoration /ekspek'tərā'shən/, the ejection of mucus, sputum, or fluids from the trachea and lungs by coughing or spitting.

experience rating /ikspir'ē·əns/ [L, *experientia*, testing; *rata*], a rating system used by an insurance company to set the premium to be paid by the insured, based on the risk to the insurance company of providing the insurance. Experience rating may lead to very high malpractice premiums in some medical specialties, for the insurance company calculates the premium on the basis of settlements made in related malpractice cases during a specified period. Experience rating is also used to set annual membership health maintenance fees in organizations in which the cost of providing the services in a previous accounting period is used to determine the premiums for the next fiscal year.

experimental design /eksper'imen'təl/ [L, *experimentum; designare*, to mark out], (in research) a study design used to test cause-and-effect relationships between variables. The classic experimental design specifies an experimental group and a control group. The independent variable is administered to the experimental group and not to the control group, and both groups are measured on the same dependent variable. Subsequent experimental designs have used more groups and more measurements over longer periods of time.

experimental embryology, the study and analysis through experimental techniques of the factors, mechanisms, and relationships that determine and influence prenatal development.

experimental epidemiology, a stage of epidemiologic investigation that uses an experimental model for studies to confirm a causal relationship suggested by observational studies.

experimental group. See **group.**

experimental medicine, a branch of the practice of medicine in which new drugs or treatments are evaluated for safety and efficacy in a clinical laboratory setting by using animals or, in certain cases, human subjects.

experimental physiology, a branch of the study of physiology in which the functions of various body systems are evaluated in a clinical laboratory setting by using animals or, in some cases, human subjects.

experimental psychology, the study of mental processes and phenomena by observation in a controlled environment using various tests, manipulations, and experiments. Compare **analytic psychology.**

experimental variable. See **independent variable.**

expertise /eks'pərtēz'/ [L, *experiri*, to try], pertaining to special skills or knowledge acquired by a person through education, training, or experience.

expert witness /ikspurt´, ek´spərt/ [L, *experiri,* to try; AS, *witnes,* knowledge], a person who has special knowledge of a subject about which a court requests testimony. Special knowledge may be acquired by experience, education, observation, or study but is not possessed by the average person. An expert witness gives expert testimony or expert evidence. This evidence often serves to educate the court and the jury in the subject under consideration.

expiration /ik´spirā´shən/ [L, *expirare,* to breathe out], **1.** also called **exhalation.** breathing out, normally a passive process, depending on the elastic qualities of lung tissue and the thorax. Compare **inspiration. 2.** termination or death. **–expire,** *v.*

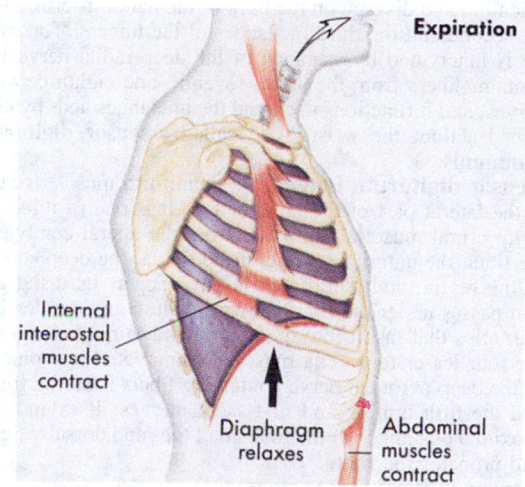

Expiration (Thibodeau, 1993/Christy Krames)

expiratory /ikspī´rətôr´ē/ [L, *expirare,* to exhale out], pertaining to the expiration of air from the lungs.

expiratory center [L, *expirare,* to breath out; Gk, *kentron,* center], one of several regions of the medulla responsible for the control of respiration. It is a subregion specifically involved in carrying out the activity of expiration.

expiratory dyspnea, a feeling of discomfort or distress in breathing because of bronchospasms of the bronchioles.

expiratory phase, the portion of the respiratory cycle that involves exhalation, or moving air out of the lungs. In a ventilated patient, the expiratory phase may be passive, depending on the recoil of elastic tissues in the lung to move air out, or active, applying positive pressure to the abdominal area or negative pressure to the upper airway.

expiratory reserve volume (ERV), the maximum volume of gas that can be expired from the resting expiratory level. See also **vital capacity.**

expiratory retard, (in respiratory care) a mode of mechanical ventilation that mimics the prolonged expiratory phase and pursed-lip breathing of emphysema. The method adds some resistance to expiration. Low levels of positive end-expiratory pressure may produce a similar effect. Also called **expiratory resistance.**

expire /ikspī´ər/ [L, *expirare,* exhale], **1.** to breathe out. **2.** to die.

expired gas (E), any gas exhaled from the lungs.

exploratory /iksplôr´ətôr´ē/ [L, *explorare,* to search out], pertaining to exploration, as in exploratory surgery.

exploratory operation [L, *explorare,* to search out; *operari,* to work], surgical intervention to find the cause of a disorder by opening a body cavity or organ and examining the interior.

explosive personality /iksplō´siv/ [L, *ex,* out, *plaudere,* to clap], behavior characterized by episodes of uncontrolled rage and physical abusiveness in reaction to relatively minor stressors.

explosive speech, abnormal speech characterized by slow, jerky articulation interspersed with the sudden loud enunciation of words, often seen in brain disorders.

exponent /ikspō´nənt/, a superscript on a number that indicates how many times a number is to be multiplied by itself (for example, $3^4 = 3 \times 3 \times 3 \times 3 = 81$). In medical or scientific reports, the number 10 is commonly used to indicate very large or very small numbers, such as in the examples 10^6 representing 1,000,000 or 10^{-6} representing 1/1,000,000. Exponents also are indicated by prefixes, such as mega- for 10^6 and micro- for 10^{-6}.

exposed pulp [L, *exponere,* to lay out; *pulpa,* flesh], dental pulp that becomes exposed to the external environment and potential bacterial infection. Causes include fracture of the crown through trauma or loss of a tooth crown or penetration of the dentin during restorative preparation.

exposure /ikspō´zhər/ [L, *exponere,* to lay out], (in radiotherapy) a measure of the ionization of air produced by a beam of radiation. Exposure is defined in coulomb per kilogram of air, but there is no special unit in the SI system for this concept. An older unit, the roentgen (R), was defined as 2.58 [ti] 10[mi]4 C/kg.

exposure angle, the angle of the arc described by the movement of the x-ray tube and film during tomography.

exposure switch, a control switch that is designed to interrupt the power automatically when pressure by the operator's hand or foot is released. The purpose is to prevent accidental continuing exposure of the patient to radiation. A typical exposure switch is a foot pedal.

exposure unit, any of the conventional or SI units used to measure radiation exposure. They include roentgen (R), rad, rem, curie (Ci), gray (Gy), sievert (Sv), and becquerel (Bq).

expression /ikspresh´ən/ [L, *exprimere,* to express], **1.** the indication of a physical or emotional state through facial appearance or vocal intonation. **2.** the act of pressing or squeezing to expel something, such as milk from the breast after pregnancy or the fetus from the uterus by exerting pressure on the abdominal wall. **3.** (in genetics) the detectable effect or appearance in the phenotype of a particular trait or condition. See also **expressivity. –express,** *v.*

expressive aphasia. See **motor aphasia.**

expressivity /eks´presiv´itē/ [L, *exprimere,* to make clear], (in genetics) the variability with which basic patterns of inheritance are modified, both in degree and in variety, by the effect of a given gene in people of the same genotype. Polydactyly may be expressed as extra toes in one generation and extra fingers in another.

expulsive stage of labor /ikspul´siv/ [L, *expellere,* to drive out; *stare* stand; *labor* work], the second stage of labor, during which the mother's uterine contractions are accompanied by a bearing-down reflex. It begins after full dilatation of the cervix and continues to the complete delivery of the infant.

exsanguinate /eksang′gwināt/ [L, *ex, sanguis,* blood], to drain away or deprive an organ or blood.

exsanguination /eksang′gwinā′shən/, a loss of blood.

exsiccant. See **desiccant.**

exsiccate. See **desiccate.**

extended arm. See **reacher.**

extended care facility [L, *extendere,* to stretch], an institution devoted to providing medical, nursing, or custodial care for an individual over a prolonged period of time, such as during the course of a chronic disease or during the rehabilitation phase after an acute illness. Kinds of extended care facilities are **intermediate care facility** and **skilled nursing facility.** Also called **convalescent home, nursing home.**

extended family, a family group consisting of the biologic or adoptive parents, their children, the grandparents, and other family members. The extended family is the basic family group in many societies. Among its characteristics are increased exchange of information from experienced older members to less experienced younger ones, care of the older family members in the home by the younger ones, and care by the older people for the children of the younger members. Compare **nuclear family.**

extended insulin-zinc suspension, a long-acting insulin that is slowly absorbed and slow to act.

Extendryl, a trademark for a fixed-combination nasal decongestant drug containing an adrenergic (phenylephrine hydrochloride), an antihistaminic (chlorpheniramine maleate), and an anticholinergic (methscopolamine nitrate).

extension /iksten′shən/ [L, *extendere,* to stretch], a movement allowed by certain joints of the skeleton that increases the angle between two adjoining bones, such as extending the leg, which increases the angle between the femur and the tibia. Compare **flexion.**

extension partial denture. See **partial denture.**

extensor /iksten′sər/ [L, *extendere,* to stretch out], any muscle that extends a body part, as the **extensor indicis** which extends the index finger.

extensor carpi radialis brevis [L, *extendere* + Gk, *karpos,* wrist; L, *radius,* ray, *brevis,* short], one of the muscles of the posterior forearm. Lying beneath the extensor carpi radialis longus, it arises from the lateral epicondyle of the humerus, from the radial collateral ligament of the elbow joint, and from various intermuscular septa. It inserts into the dorsal surface of the third metacarpal bone. The muscle is innervated by a branch of the radial nerve that contains fibers from the sixth and the seventh cervical nerves, and it functions to extend the hand.

extensor carpi radialis longus, one of the seven superficial muscles of the posterior forearm. Lying above the extensor carpi radialis brevis, it arises from the lateral supracondylar ridge of the humerus, from the lateral intermuscular septum, and from the common tendon of the extensor muscles of the forearm. It inserts into the dorsal surface of the second metacarpal bone. The muscle is innervated by a branch of the radial nerve that contains fibers from the sixth and seventh cervical nerves, and it serves to extend and flex the hand radially.

extensor carpi ulnaris, one of the muscles of the lateral forearm. It arises from the lateral epicondyle of the humerus and inserts by a tendon into the ulnar side of the fifth meta-

carpal bone. It is innervated by a branch of the deep radial nerve, containing fibers of the sixth, seventh, and eighth cervical nerves, and functions to extend and adduct the hand.

extensor digiti minimi, an extensor muscle of the posterior forearm. Located on the medial side of the extensor digitorum, it is a slender muscle that arises from the common extensor tendon and joins the expansion of the extensor digitorum tendon on the back of the first phalanx of the little finger. It is innervated by a branch of the deep radial nerve that contains fibers from the sixth, seventh, and eighth cervical nerves, and it functions to extend the little finger.

extensor digitorum, the principal muscle of the medial digits of the posterior forearm. Arising from the lateral epicondyle of the humerus, the intermuscular septa between it and adjacent muscles, and the antebrachial fascia, it divides distally into four tendons that pass through the extensor retinaculum and diverge on the back of the hand, inserting into the second and the third phalanges of the fingers. The muscle is innervated by a branch of the deep radial nerve that contains fibers from the sixth, seventh, and eighth cervical nerves, and it functions to extend the phalanges and, by continued action, the wrist. Also called **extensor digitorum communis.**

extensor digitorum longus, a penniform muscle located at the lateral part of the anterior leg. It is one of three anterior crural muscles and arises from the lateral condyle of the tibia, the anterior surface of the fibula, the deep surface of the fascia, and from intermuscular septa. Its distal tendon passes under the extensor retinaculum and divides into four slips that insert into the second and third phalanges of the four lesser toes. The muscle is innervated by branches of the deep peroneal nerve containing fibers from the fourth and the fifth lumbar and first sacral nerves. It extends the proximal phalanges of the four small toes and dorsally flexes and pronates the foot.

extensor indicis. See **extensor.**

extensor retinaculum of ankle, either of two thick layers of fascia holding tendons in the ankle. The inferior extensor retinaculum of the ankle is a Y-shaped band of fascia passing medially from the lateral side of the upper surface of the calcaneum and dividing into two bands, one going to the medial malleolus and the other to the plantar aponeurosis. The superior extensor retinaculum consists of thick fascia attached to the lower ends of the tibia and fibula and extending over the tendons of the extenor muscles.

extensor retinaculum of hand. See **retinaculum extensorum manus.**

extensor retinaculum of wrist, a broad thickening of deep fascia over the back of the wrist, over the extensor tendons.

extensor thrust, a spinal-level reflex present in a human in the first 2 months of life. It is an exaggeration of the positive support reflex and consists of an uncontrolled extension of a flexed leg when the sole of the foot is stimulated.

extern /eks′turn/ [L, *externus,* outward], a medical or dental student who lives outside the institution but provides medical or dental care to patients as an extracurricular activity under the professional supervision of hospital staff members. Compare **intern.**

external /ikstur′nəl/ [L, *externus,* outward], **1.** being on the outside or exterior of the body or an organ. **2.** acting from the outside, such as an external influence or exogenous factor. **3.** pertaining to the outward or visible appearance. Compare **internal.**

external abdominal region. See **lateral region.**

external absorption, the taking up of substances through the mucous membranes or the skin.

external acoustic meatus, the canal of the external ear, comprised of bone and cartilage, extending from the auricle to the tympanic membrane. Also called **external auditory canal.**

external aperture of aqueduct of vestibule, an external opening for the small canal extending from the vestibule of the inner ear, located on the internal surface of the petrous part of the temporal bone lateral to the opening for the internal acoustic passage.

external aperture of canaliculus of cochlea, an external opening of the cochlear channel on the margin of the jugular opening in the temporal bone.

external aperture of tympanic canaliculus, the lower opening of the tympanic channel on the inferior surface of the petrous part of the temporal bone.

external auditory canal, external auditory meatus. See **external acoustic meatus.**

external carotid artery, one of a pair of arteries with eight major temporal or maxillary branches, rising from the common carotid arteries and supplying various parts and tissues of the head and neck.

external carotid plexus, a network of nerves around the external carotid artery, formed by the external carotid nerves from the superior cervical ganglion and supplying sympathetic fibers associated with branches of the external carotid artery. Compare **common carotid plexus, internal carotid plexus.**

external cervical os, an external opening of the uterus that leads into the cavity of the cervix. This opening, bounded by the ventral lip and the dorsal lip, is in the center of the rounded extremity of the cervix that projects into the cavity of the vagina. Compare **internal cervical os.**

external conjugate, the distance measured with obstetric calipers from the depression below the lowest lumbar vertebra posteriorly to the upper border of the symphysis anteriorly (usually about 21 cm). Also called **Baudelocque's diameter.**

external counterpulsation, (in cardiology) a noninvasive technique for providing counterpulsation. In one technique, the limbs are placed in inflatable trousers. Inflation and deflation are synchronized with the cardiac cycle, resulting in augmented blood flow during diastole and assisted ejection during systole.

external cuneiform bone. See **lateral cuneiform bone.**

external ear, the outer structure of the ear, consisting of the auricle and the external acoustic meatus. Sound waves are funneled through the external ear to the middle ear. Compare **internal ear, middle ear.**

external fertilization, the union of male and female gametes outside of the bodies from which they originated, such as occurs in fish and frogs.

external fistula, an abnormal passage between an internal organ or structure and the cutaneous surface of the body.

external fixation, a method of holding together the fragments of a fractured bone by employing transfixing metal pins through the fragments and a compression device attached to the pins outside the skin surface. Nursing care includes regular cleansing of the skin around the pins and, often, the application of antibiotic solutions or ointments. The pins are removed at a later procedure when the fracture is healed. Compare **internal fixation.**

external iliac artery, a division of the common iliac ar-

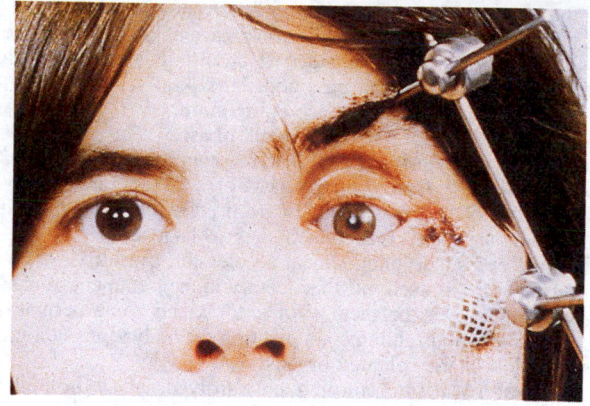

External fixation (Eagling, 1986)

tery descending into the thigh and becoming the femoral artery. The external iliac supplies the lower limb and is larger than the internal iliac, except in the fetus, where it is smaller. Compare **internal iliac artery.**

external iliac node, a node in one of the seven groups of parietal nodes serving the lymphatic system in the abdomen and the pelvis. About 10 external iliac nodes, arranged in three groups, lie along the external iliac vessels. Their afferent vessels drain lymph from numerous abdominal and pelvic structures, as the deep abdominal wall, the adductor region of the thigh, the prostate, and the vagina. Compare **common iliac node, iliac circumflex node, internal iliac node.** See also **lymph, lymphatic system, lymph node.**

external iliac vein, one of a pair of veins in the lower body that join the internal iliac vein to form the two common iliac veins. Each external iliac vein begins under the inguinal ligament, ascends along the brim of the lesser pelvis, and ends opposite the sacroiliac articulation by joining the internal iliac vein. In many individuals it contains at least one valve and sometimes two. It receives the inferior epigastric vein, the deep iliac circumflex vein, and the pubic veins. Compare **internal iliac vein.**

external jugular vein, one of a pair of large vessels in the neck that receive most of the blood from the exterior of the cranium and the deep tissues of the face. Each external jugular vein is formed by the junction of the retromandibular vein with the posterior auricular vein and arises in the parotid gland on a level with the angle of the mandible. It runs perpendicularly down the neck and joins the subclavian vein lateral or ventral to the scalenus anterior. It contains two pairs of valves, the inferior pair at the junction with the subclavian vein and the superior pair, usually about 4 cm above the clavicle. A sinus lies between the two sets of valves. Compare **internal jugular vein.**

external locus of control. See **locus of control.**

external malleolus [L, *externus,* outward, *malleolus,* little hammer], a rounded bony prominence on either side of the ankle joint. Also called **malleolus fibulae.**

external oblique muscle. See **obliquus externus abdominis.**

external pacemaker [L, *externus,* outward, *passus,* step; ME, *maken,* to make], **1.** a device used to stimulate the heart beat electrically by the discharge of impulses through the chest wall, as employed in emergency care of significant bradyarrythmias. **2.** a cardiac pacemaker in which the impulse generator is outside the chest but connected with the heart by wires that pass under the skin.

external perimysium. See **epimysium.**

external phase. See **continuous phase.**

external pterygoid muscle. See **pterygoideus lateralis.**

external radiation therapy (ERT), the therapeutic application of ionizing radiation from an external beam of a kilovoltage x-ray machine, a megavoltage cobalt 60 machine, or a supervoltage linear accelerator, cyclotron, or betatron. ERT is used most frequently in the treatment of cancer but also in the therapy of keloids and some dermatologic conditions and in counteracting the body's physiologic rejection of transplanted organs.

external rotation, turning outwardly or away from the midline of the body, such as when a leg is externally rotated with the toes turned outward or away from the body's midline.

external secretion. See **exocrine glands.**

external shunt, a device for the passage of a body fluid from one compartment of the body to another, consisting of a tube or catheter or a series of such containers that passes over the surface of the body from one compartment or cavity to another. See also **hemodialysis, hydrocephalus.**

external version, an obstetric procedure in which a fetus is turned, usually from a breech to a vertex presentation, by external manipulation of the fetus through the wall of the abdomen. Compare **version and extraction.**

exteroceptive /ek′stərōsep′tiv/ [L, *externus*, outside, *recipere*, to receive], pertaining to stimuli that originate from outside of the body or to the sensory receptors that they activate. Compare **interoceptive, proprioception.**

exteroceptor /ek′stərōsep′tər/ [L, *externus*, outside, *recipere*, to receive], any sensory nerve ending, as those located in the skin, mucous membranes, or sense organs, that responds to stimuli originating from outside of the body, such as touch, pressure, or sound. Compare **interoceptor, proprioceptor.** See also **chemoreceptor.**

extirpation /ek′stərpā′shən/ [L, *extirpare*, to root out], the total removal of a diseased organ or body part.

extra-, extro- ek′strə-/, a combining form meaning 'outside of, beyond, in addition to': *extrabronchial, extradural, extramarginal, extroversion.*

extraarticular /ek′strə·ärtik′yələr/ [L, *extra*, outside of, *articulare*, to divide into joints], pertaining to the area outside a joint or within the joint but not involving the joint structures.

extra beat [L, *extra*, outside; AS, *beatan*], an extra systole; an extra heart contraction.

extracapsular /-kaps′yələr/ [L, *extra*, outside, *capsula*, little box], pertaining to something outside a capsule, such as the articulare capsule of the knee joint.

extracapsular ankylosis. See **false ankylosis.**

extracapsular dendrite [L, *extra, capsula*; Gk, *dendron*, tree], pertaining to dendrites of some autonomic nerves that penetrate the boundary of the capsule and extend some distance from the cell body.

extracapsular fracture [L, *extra* + *capsula*, little box], any fracture that occurs near a joint but does not directly involve the joint capsule. This type of fracture is extremely common in the hip.

extracellular /-sel′yələr/ [L, *extra* + *cella*, storeroom], occurring outside a cell or cell tissue or in cavities or spaces between cell layers or groups of cells. See also **cell, edema, interstitial.**

extracellular fluid (ECF), the portion of the body fluid comprising the interstitial fluid and blood plasma. The adult body contains about 11.2 L of interstitial fluid, constituting about 16% of body weight, and about 2.8 L of plasma, constituting about 4% of body weight. Plasma and interstitial fluid are very similar chemically and, in conjunction with intracellular fluid, help control the movement of water and electrolytes throughout the body. Some of the important ionized components of extracellular fluid are protein, magnesium, potassium, chlorine, calcium, and certain sulfates.

extracoronal retainer /-kôr′ənəl/ [L, *extra* + *corona*, crown; *retinere*, to hold], **1.** a kind of dental retainer that incorporates a cast restoration lying largely external to the coronal portion of a tooth and complements the contour of the tooth crown. The retention or resistance to displacement is developed between the inner surfaces of the casting and the external walls of the prepared tooth. The restoration incorporating the extracoronal retainer may be a complete or partial crown. **2.** a direct clasp-type retainer that engages an abutment tooth on its external surface, used for the retention and stabilization of a removable partial denture. **3.** a manufactured direct retainer, the protruding portion of which is attached to the external surface of a cast crown on an abutment tooth.

extracorporeal /-kôrpôr′ē·əl/ [L, *extra* + *corpus*, body], something that is outside the body, such as extracorporeal circulation in which venous blood is diverted outside the body to a heart-lung machine and returned to the body through a femoral or other artery.

extracorporeal membrane oxygenator (ECMO), a device that oxygenates the blood of a patient outside the body and returns the blood to the patient's circulatory system. The technique may be used to support an impaired respiratory system.

extracorporeal oxygenation, the use of an artificial membrane outside the body by which to provide for oxygenation in a patient with severe lung disease.

extracorporeal shock-wave lithotripsy (ESWL) [L, *extra*, outside, *corpus*, body; Fr, *choc*; AS, *wafian*; Gk, *lithos*, stone, *tribein*, to wear away], Use of vibrations of powerful sound waves to break up calculi in the urinary tract.

extracorporeal technician. See **perfusion technologist.**

extracranial /-krā′nē·əl/ [L, *extra*, outside; Gk, *kranion*, cranium], pertaining to something outside the skull.

extract [L, *ex*, out, *trahere*, to draw], **1.** /ek′strakt/ a substance, usually a biologically active ingredient of a plant or animal tissue, prepared by the use of solvents or evaporation to separate the substance from the original material. Beef extract, belladonna, and cascara are examples of extracts. **2.** /ikstrakt′/ to remove a tooth from the oral cavity by means of elevators or forceps or both. /ikstrakt′/ —**extraction,** *n.*

extractor /ikstrak′tər/, a medical instrument, such as a forceps, used to remove a foreign body, tissue sample, or medical device that had been placed in a body cavity.

extradural /ek′trədŏŏr′əl/ [L, *extra* + *dura*, hard], outside the dura mater.

extradural anesthesia, anesthetic nerve block achieved by the injection of a local anesthetic solution into the space in the spinal canal outside the dura mater of the spinal cord, as in epidural, caudal, or paravertebral anesthesia.

extradural hemorrhage, See **epidural hemorrhage.**

extraembryonic blastoderm /-em'brē·on'ik/ [L, *extra* + Gk, *en*, in, *bryein*, to grow], the area of the blastoderm outside the embryo that gives rise to the membranes that surround the embryo during gestation. Compare **embryonic blastoderm.** See also **allantois, amnion, chorion, yolk sac.**

extraembryonic coelom, a cavity external to the developing embryo that forms between the mesoderm of the chorion and that covering the amniotic cavity and yolk sac. During early prenatal development, there is direct contact with the embryonic coelom at the umbilicus, but this junction is obliterated by the growth of the amnion and the closing of the body wall. Also called **exocoelom.**

extraembryonic mesoderm [L, *extra*, outside; Gk, *en*, *bryein*, to grow, *mesos*, middle, *derma*, skin], any mesoderm in the uterus that is not involved with the embryo itself. Included are mesoderms in the amnion, chorion, and yolk sac.

extramammary Paget's disease /-mam'ərē/ [L, *extra*, outside, *mamma*, breast; James Paget; L, *dis*; Fr, *aise*, ease], a gradually spreading red, scaly and crusted lesion resembling that of Paget's disease, but not occurring on the breast. A common area is the vulva. The lesions give rise to carcinoma.

extramedullary /-med'yələr'ē/ [L, *extra, medulla,* marrow], pertaining to something outside the medulla, particularly the medulla oblongata.

extramedullary myeloma [L, *extra,* + *medulla,* marrow], a plasma cell tumor that occurs outside of the bone marrow, usually affecting the visceral organs or the nasopharyngeal and oral mucosa. Also called **extramedullary plasmacytoma, peripheral plasma cell myeloma, plasma cell tumor.**

extramedullary myelopoiesis, the formation and development of myeloid tissue outside of the bone marrow. Also called **ectopic myelopoiesis.**

extramedullary plasmacytoma. See **extramedullary myeloma.**

extraocular /-ok'yōōlər/ [L, *extra* + *oculus,* eye], outside the eye.

extraocular muscle palsy, an abnormal condition characterized by paralysis of the extrinsic muscles of the eye, such as the superior, inferior, medial, and lateral rectus muscles, and the superior and the inferior oblique muscles. See also **strabismus.**

extraoral anchorage /-ôr'əl/ [L, *extra* + *oralis,* mouth; *ancora,* hook], an orthodontic anchorage outside the mouth, typically linking dental attachments to a wire bow or to hooks extending between the lips and attached by elastic to a cap, a neck strap, or another extraoral device.

extraoral orthodontic appliance, a device secured to a portion of the face, the neck, or the back of the head to deliver traction force to the teeth or jaws for changing the relative positions of dentitions.

extraperitoneal /-per'itənē'əl/ [L, *extra* + Gk, *peri,* near, around, *teinein* to stretch], occurring or located outside the peritoneal cavity.

extraperitoneal cesarean section, a method for surgically delivering a baby through an incision in the lower uterine segment without entering the peritoneal cavity. The uterus is approached through the paravesicle space. This procedure is performed most often to avoid spread of infection from the uterus into the peritoneal cavity. It is somewhat slower to perform than the low cervical or classical cesarean operations. Compare **classic cesarean section, low cervical cesarean section.** See also **cesarean section.**

extrapsychic conflict /-sī'kik/ [L, *extra* + Gk, *psyche,* mind; L *confligere* to strike together], an emotional conflict usually occurring when one's inner needs and desires do not coincide with the restrictions of the environment or society. Compare **intrapsychic conflict.** See also **conflict.**

extrapyramidal /ek'strəpiram'ədəl/ [L, *extra* + Gk, *pyramis,* pyramid], **1.** of or pertaining to the tissues and structures outside the cerebrospinal pyramidal tracts of the brain that are associated with movement of the body, excluding motor neurons, the motor cortex, and the corticospinal and corticobulbar tracts. **2.** of or pertaining to the function of these tissues and structures.

extrapyramidal disease, any of a large group of conditions affecting the extrapyramidal tracts and characterized by involuntary movement, changes in muscle tone, and abnormal posture, such as in tardive dyskinesia, chorea, athetosis, and Parkinson's disease.

extrapyramidal side effects, side effects caused by drugs that block dopamine receptor sites in the extrapyramidal system tract.

extrapyramidal system, the part of the nervous system that includes the basal ganglia, substantia nigra, subthalamic nucleus, part of the midbrain, and the motor neurons of the spine. See also **extrapyramidal tracts.**

extrapyramidal tracts, the tracts of motor nerves from the brain to the anterior horns of the spinal cord, except for the fibers of the pyramidal tracts. Within the brain, extrapyramidal tracts comprise various relays of motoneurons between motor areas of the cerebral cortex, the basal ganglia, the thalamus, the cerebellum, and the brainstem. The extrapyramidal tracts are functional rather than anatomic units, comprising the nuclei and the fibers and excluding the pyramidal tracts. They especially control and coordinate the postural, static, supporting, and locomotor mechanisms and cause contractions of muscle groups in sequence or simultaneously. The extrapyramidal tracts include the corpus striatum, the subthalamic nucleus, the substantia nigra, and the red nucleus, together with their interconnections with the reticular formation, the cerebellum, and the cerebrum. Compare **pyramidal tract.**

extrarenal uremia /-rē'nəl/ [L, *extra* + *ren,* kidney; Gk, *ouron,* urine + *haima,* blood], uremia that may be involved with kidney failure although the cause is outside the kidney, as in alkalosis from excessive alkali ingestion or severe vomiting.

extrasensory /-sen'sərē/ [L, *extra, sentire,* to feel], pertaining to alleged awareness of events that cannot be observed by any of the five basic senses. They include telepathy, clairvoyance, and psychokinesis.

extrasensory perception (ESP) [L, *extra* + *sentire,* to feel; *percipere,* to perceive], alleged awareness or knowledge acquired without using the physical senses. See also **clairvoyance, parapsychology, telepathy.**

extrasystole /-sis'təlē/ [L, *extra* + Gk, *systole,* contraction], an abnormal cardiac contraction that results from depolarization by an ectopic inpulse. Also called **ectopic beat.**

extrauterine /-yōō'tərin/ [L, *extra* + *uterus,* womb], occurring or located outside the uterus, as an ectopic pregnancy.

extravasation /ikstrav'əsā'shən/ [L, *extra* + *vas,* vessel], a passage or escape into the tissues, usually of blood, serum, or lymph. Compare **bleeding.** See also **exudate, transudate.** —**extravasate,** *v.*

extravascular fluid /-vas′kyələr/ [L, *extra,* outside, *vasculum,* small vessel, *fluere,* to flow], fluids in the body that are outside the blood vessels. Examples include lymph and cerebrospinal fluid.

extraventricular hydrocephalus. See **hydrocephalus.**

extravert. See **extrovert.**

extraverted personality. See **extroverted personality.**

extraversion. See **extroversion.**

extremity /ikstrem′itē/ [L, *extremitas*], an arm or a leg. The arm may be identified as an upper extremity and the leg as a lower extremity.

extrinsic /ikstrin′sik/ [L, *extrinsecus,* on the outside], pertaining to anything external or originating outside a structure or organism, including parts of an organ that are not wholly contained within it, as an extrinsic muscle.

extrinsic allergic alveolitis. See **hypersensitivity pneumonitis.**

extrinsic allergic pneumonia. See **diffuse hypersensitivity pneumonia.**

extrinsic asthma. See **allergic asthma.**

extrinsic factor. See **cyanocobalamin.**

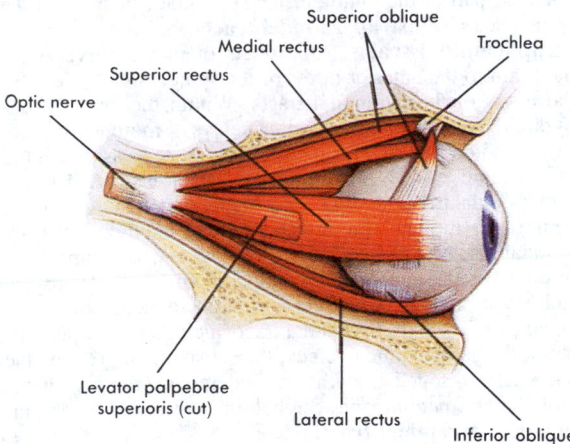

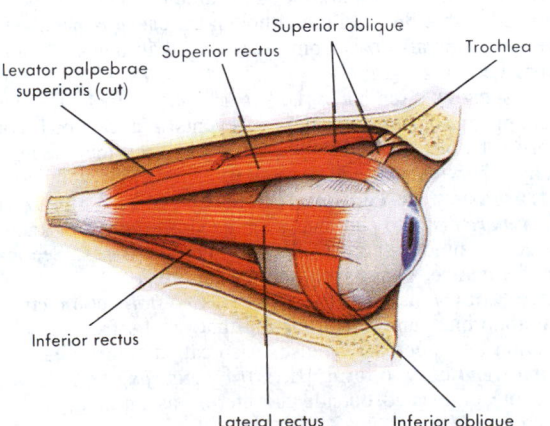

Extrinsic muscles of the eye *(Seeley, 1992/John V Hagen)*

extrinsic muscles (em) [L, *extrinsecus,* on the outside], **1.** muscles that are outside the organ they control, as the extraocular muscles that control eye movements. **2.** muscles that link a limb to the trunk of the body.

extro-. See **extra-.**

extroversion /-vur′zhən/ [L, *extra* + *vertere,* to turn], **1.** the tendency to direct one's interests and energies toward external values or things outside the self. **2.** the state of being totally or primarily concerned with what is outside the self. Also spelled **extraversion.** Compare **introversion.**

extrovert /ik′strəvurt′/, **1.** a person whose interests are directed away from the self and concerned primarily with external reality and the physical environment rather than with inner feelings and thoughts. This person is usually highly sociable, outgoing, impulsive, and emotionally expressive. **2.** a person characterized by extroversion. Also spelled **extravert.** Compare **introvert.**

extroverted personality /-vur′tid/ [L, *extra,* outside, *vertere,* to turn, *personalis,* of a person], a persona that is directed to a greater degree toward the outer world of people and events rather than the subjective inner world experience. Also called **extraverted personality.**

extrusion reflex /ekstrōō′zhən/ [L, *extrudere,* to push out; *reflectere* to bend backward], a normal response in infants to force the tongue outward when touched or depressed. The reflex begins to disappear by about 3 or 4 months of age. Before it fades, food must be placed well back in the mouth to be retained and swallowed. Constant protrusion of a large tongue may be a sign of Down's syndrome.

extubation /iks′t(y)ōōbā′shən/ [L, *ex,* out, *tuba,* tube], the process of withdrawing a tube from an orifice or cavity of the body. —**extubate,** *v.*

exuberant callus. See **heterotopic ossification.**

exudate /eks′yōōdāt/ [L, *exsudare,* to sweat out], fluid, cells, or other substances that have been slowly exuded, or discharged, from cells or blood vessels through small pores or breaks in cell membranes. Perspiration, pus, and serum are sometimes identified as exudates.

exudation /eks′yədā′shən/ [L, *exudare,* the discharge of fluid, pus, or serum. The exudate may or may not contain fibrous or coagulated material.

exudative /igzōō′dətiv/, relating to the exudation or oozing of fluid and other materials from cells and tissues, usually as a result of inflammation or injury.

exudative angina. See **croup.**

exudative enteropathy, diarrhea seen in diseases characterized by inflammation or destruction of intestinal mucosa. Crohn's disease, ulcerative colitis, tuberculosis, and some lymphomas cause an increase of plasma, blood, mucus, and protein to accumulate in the intestine, adding to fecal bulk and frequency. See also **diarrhea.**

exudative inflammation [L, *exudare,* to sweat out, *inflammare,* to set afire], an inflammation of a serous or raw cavity in which fluid is being released from the inflamed surface.

eye [AS *eage*], one of a pair of organs of sight, contained in a bony orbit at the front of the skull, embedded in orbital fat and innervated by one of a pair of optic nerves from the forebrain. Associated with the eye are certain accessory structures, such as the muscles, the fasciae, the eyebrow, the eyelids, the conjunctiva, and the lacrimal gland. The bulb of the eye is composed of segments of two spheres with nearly parallel axes that constitute the outside tunic and one of three fibrous layers enclosing two internal cavities separated by the crystalline lens. The smaller cavity anterior to the lens is divided by the iris into two chambers, both filled with aqueous humor. The posterior cavity is larger than the anterior cavity and contains the jellylike vitreous body that is divided by the hyaloid canal. The outside tunic of the bulb consists of the transparent cornea anteriorly, constituting one fifth of the tunic, and the opaque sclera posteriorly, constituting five sixths of the tunic. The intermediate vascular, pigmented tunic consists of the choroid, the ciliary body, and the iris. The internal tunic of nervous tissue is the retina. Light waves passing through the lens strike a layer of rods and cones in the retina creating impulses that are transmitted by the optic nerve to the brain. The transverse and the anteroposterior diameters of the eye bulb are slightly greaterthan the vertical diameter; the bulb in women is usually smaller than the bulb in men. Also called **bulbus oculi, eyeball.**

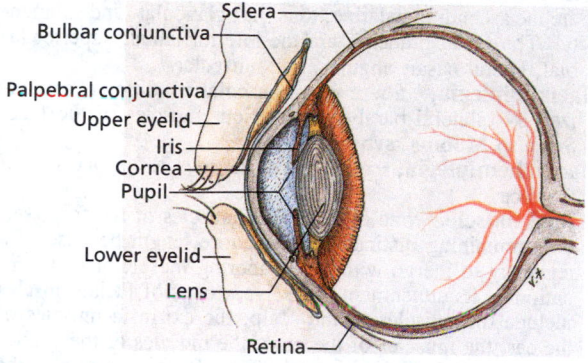

Cross-section of the eye (Potter, 1993)

eye bank [AS, *éage,* It, *banca,* bench],   a facility for collecting and storing corneas of eyes for transplantation to recipients.

eyebrow [AS, *eage* + *bru*],   **1.** the supraorbital arch of the frontal bone that separates the orbit of the eye from the forehead. **2.** the arch of hairs growing along the ridge formed by the supraorbital arch of the frontal bone.

eyecup,   a small vessel, or cup, that is shaped to fit over the eyeball and used to bathe the exposed surface of the organ.

eye deviation [AS, *éage;* L, *deviare,* to turn aside],   the movement of the two eyes in which their visual axes are not parallel. **Manifest deviation** is the amount in degrees that the visual axis of one eye deviates from that of the other in cases of squint, when both eyes are open.

eye dominance,   an unconscious preference to use one eye rather than the other for certain purposes, such as sighting a rifle or looking through a telescope.

eyedrops,   a liquid medicine that is administered by allowing it to fall in drops onto the conjunctival surface.

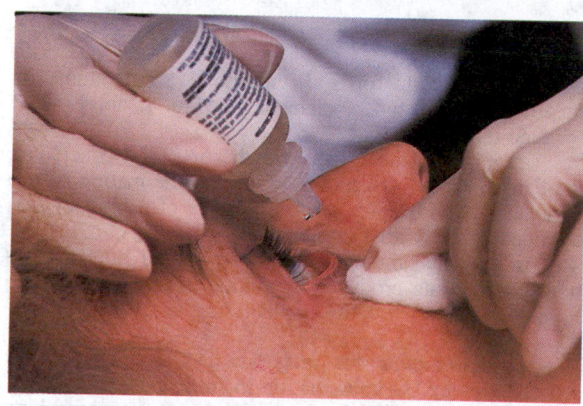

Eyedrop administration (Potter, 1993)

eye glasses,   transparent devices held in metal or plastic frames in front of the eyes to correct refractive errors or to protect the eyes from harmful electromagnetic waves or flying objects.

eyeground,   the fundus of the eye. See also **funduscopy.**

eyelash [AS, *eage* + ME, *lasche*],   one of many cilia growing in double or triple rows along the border of the eyelids in front of a row of ciliary glands that are in front of a row of meibomian glands.

eyelid [AS, *eage* + *hlid*],   a movable fold of thin skin over the eye, with eyelashes and ciliary and meibomian glands along its margin. It consists of loose connective tissue containing a thin plate of fibrous tissue lined with mucous membrane. The orbicularis oculi muscle and the oculomotor nerve control the opening and closing of the eyelid. The upper and lower eyelids are separated by the palpebral fissure. Also called **palpebra** /pal′pəbrə/.

eye memory.   See **visual memory.**

eye worm.   See *Loa loa.*

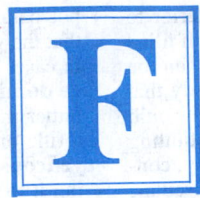

f, **1.** symbol for *breaths per unit time*. **2.** symbol for *respiratory frequency*.

F, **1.** abbreviation for **Fahrenheit**. **2.** abbreviation for **farad**. **3.** symbol for the element **fluorine**. **4.** abbreviation for **frequency**.

F₁, (in genetics) the symbol for the first filial generation; the heterozygous offspring produced by the mating of two unrelated individuals or by the crossing of a homozygous dominant strain with a homozygous recessive.

F₂, (in genetics) the symbol for the second filial generation the offspring produced by mating two members of the F_1 generation or, broadly, by crossing any two heterozygous strains.

FA, **1.** abbreviation for **fatty acid**. **2.** abbreviation for **femoral artery**. **3.** abbreviation for **folic acid**.

F.A.A.N., abbreviation for **Fellow of the American Academy of Nursing**.

Fabere's test /fā′bārāz/, a test for pain or dysfunction in the hip and sacroiliac joints in which overpressure is applied at the knee during flexion, abduction, and external rotation of the hip. While applying pressure on the knee, the examiner also applies counterpressure at the opposite anterior superior iliac spine. Also called **figure 4 test**.

fabrication /fab′rikā′shən/, a psychologic reaction in which false statements are contrived to mask memory defects. It is a clinical feature of Korsakoff's syndrome and other disorders. See also **confabulation**.

Fabry's disease, Fabry's syndrome. See **angiokeratoma corporis diffusum**.

FAC, an anticancer drug combination of fluorouracil, doxorubicin, and cyclophosphamide.

F.A.C.C.P., abbreviation for *Fellow of the American College of Chest Physicians*.

F.A.C.D., abbreviation for *Fellow of the American College of Dentists*.

face [L, *facies*], **1.** the front of the head from the chin to the brow, including the skin and muscles and structures of the forehead, eyes, nose, mouth, cheeks, and jaw. **2.** the visage. **3.** to direct the face toward something. See also **en face**. **–facial**, *adj*.

face-bow [L, *facies* + AS, *boga*], a device resembling a caliper, used for measuring the relationship of the maxillae to the temporomandibular joints, which is required for the fabrication of denture casts.

face lift, a plastic surgery procedure in which wrinkles and other signs of aging skin are eliminated. Also called **rhytidoplasty**.

face presentation [L, *facies*, face, *praesentare*, to show], an obstetrical presentation in which the chin of the fetus is the point of direction.

facet /fas′it/ [Fr, *facette*, little face], **1.** (in dentistry) a flattened, highly polished wear pattern on a tooth. **2.** a small, smooth-surfaced process for articulation.

-facial. See **face**.

facial angle /fāshəl/ [L, *facies; angulus*, a corner], an anthropomorphic expression of the degree of protrusion of the lower face, assessed by measuring the inclination of the facial plane relative to the horizontal reference plane.

facial artery, one of a pair of tortuous arteries that arise from the external carotid arteries, divide into four cervical and five facial branches, and supply various organs and tissues in the head. The cervical branches of the facial artery are the ascending palatine, tonsillar, glandular, and submental. The facial branches are the inferior labial, superior labial, lateral nasal, angular, and muscular.

facial diplegia, a rare neuromuscular condition characterized by bilateral paralysis of various muscles of the face. See also **Möbius' syndrome**.

facial hemiplegia, paralysis of the muscles of one side of the face.

facial muscle, one of numerous muscles of the face, seldom remaining distinct over its entire length because of a tendency to merge with a neighboring muscle at its termination or its attachment. The five groups of facial muscles include the muscles of the scalp, the extrinsic muscles of the ear, the muscles of the nose, the muscles of the eyelid, and the muscles of the mouth. The platysma is one of the facial group but is described with the muscles of the neck. Also called **muscle of expression**.

facial nerve, either of a pair of mixed sensory and motor cranial nerves that arise from the brainstem at the base of the pons and divide just in front of the ear into six branches, innervating the scalp, forehead, eyelids, muscles of facial expression, cheeks, and jaw. Also called **seventh cranial nerve**.

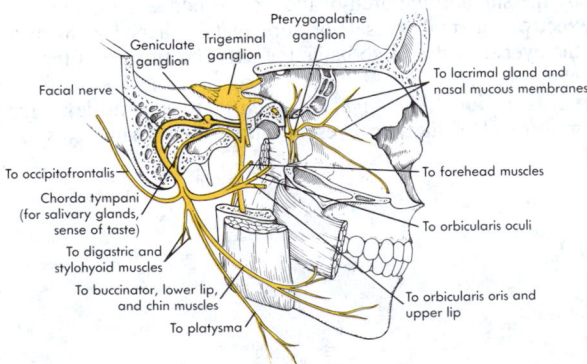

Facial nerve (Seeley, 1992/David J. Mascaro & Associates)

facial palsy [L, *facies*, face; Gk, *paralyein*, to be palsied], a loss of motor nerve function in the facial muscles. See **Bell's palsy**.

facial paralysis, an abnormal condition characterized by the partial or the total loss of the functions of the facial muscles or the loss of sensation in the face. It may be caused by disease or by trauma. The degree of paralysis depends on the nerves affected. Brain injury above the facial nerve nucleus usually does not block the innervation of the brow and the forehead muscles. Injury to the nucleus of the facial nerve or injury to its peripheral neurons paralyzes all the ipsilateral facial muscles. See also **Bell's palsy.**

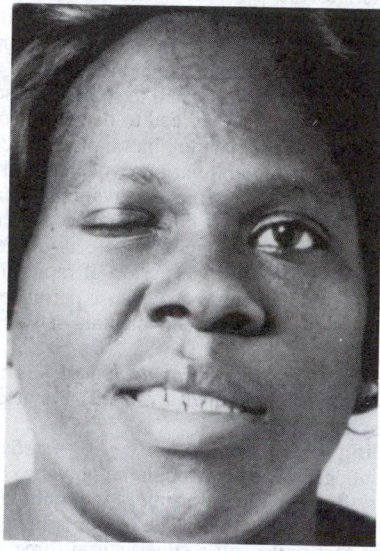

Facial paralysis (Dyken, 1980)

facial perception, the ability to judge the distance and direction of objects through the sensation felt in the skin of the face. The phenomenon is commonly experienced by those who are blind and is rarely experienced in the dark by those with sight. Also called **facial vision.**

facial tic [L, *facies,* face; Fr. *tic,* twitching], any repetitive spasmodic and involuntary contraction of groups of facial muscles. See **tic douloureux.**

facial vein, one of a pair of superficial veins that drain deoxygenated blood from the superficial structures of the face. Each facial vein starts as the angular vein at the union of the frontal and the supraorbital veins and accompanies the facial artery, passing deep to the zygomaticus major and the zygomaticus minor, following the border of the masseter, curving around the mandible into the neck, and communicating with the anterior jugular vein and the external jugular vein to empty into the internal jugular vein. The facial vein anastomoses with the cavernous sinus through various veins, such as the angular, the supraorbital, and the superior ophthalmic. Because the vein has no valves that prevent the backflow of blood, infections of the skin near the nose and mouth may progress into deeper tissues and lead to meningitis. Blood-borne organisms can reach the cavernous sinus through the anastomoses.

facial vision. See **facial perception.**

facies /fā'shē·ēs/, *pl.* **facies** /fā'shē·ēs/ [L, face], **1.** the face. **2.** the surface of any body structure, part, or organ. **3.** facial expression or appearance.

facilitation /fəsil'itā'shən/ [L, *facilitas,* easiness], **1.** the enhancement or reinforcement of any action or function so that it is carried out with increased ease. Compare **inhibition.** See also **summation. 2.** (in neurology) the phenomenon whereby two or more afferent impulses that individually are not strong enough to elicit a response in a neuron can collectively produce a reflex discharge greater than the sum of the separate responses.

facio-, a combining form meaning 'pertaining to the face': *faciocervical, faciolingual, facioplegia.*

F.A.C.O.G., abbreviation for *Fellow of the American College of Obstetricians and Gynecologists.*

F.A.C.P., abbreviation for *Fellow of the American College of Physicians.*

F.A.C.S. abbreviation for *Fellow of the American College of Surgeons.*

facsimile (fax) a method of transmitting images or printed matter by electronic means. Images are scanned, converted into electronic signals, and sent to a fax receiver which reconverts the electronic data into a duplicate of the original image.

F.A.C.S.M., abbreviation for *Fellow of the American College of Sports Medicine.*

-faction, a suffix meaning a 'process of making': *bilifaction, chylifaction, liquefaction.*

factitial /fakti'shəl/ [L, *facticius,* artificial], artificial or self-induced, such as a factitial dermatitis.

factitial dermatitis, a skin rash caused by the patient, usually for secondary gain or as a manifestation of a psychiatric illness.

factitious disorders /faktish'əs/, conditions marked by disease symptoms caused by deliberate efforts of a person to gain attention. Such attempts to gain attention may be repeated, even when the individual is aware of the hazards involved.

-factive, -fying, a suffix meaning 'making': *liquefactive, stupefactive, vasofactive.*

factor I. See **fibrinogen.**

factor II. See **prothrombin.**

factor III. See **thromboplastin.**

factor IV, a designation for calcium in the process of the coagulation of blood.

factor V, an unstable procoagulant needed to convert prothrombin rapidly to thrombin. Research indicates that during coagulation, factor V changes from an inactive agent to an active prothrombin accelerator. Also called **proaccelerin.**

factor VI, a hypothetic chemical agent that some suggest is derived from proaccelerin, or factor V, in the process of blood coagulation.

factor VII, a blood procoagulant present in the blood plasma and synthesized in the liver in the presence of vitamin K. Also called **proconvertin.**

factor VIII, a coagulation factor present in normal plasma but deficient in the blood of persons with hemophilia A. It is a macromolecular complex composed of two separate entities, one of which, when deficient, results in hemophilia A, and the other, when deficient, results in Von Willebrand's disease. See also **antihemophilic factor.**

factor IX, a coagulation factor present in normal plasma but deficient in the blood of persons with hemophilia B. Also called **Christmas factor.**

factor IX complex, a hemostatic containing factors II, VII, IX, and X.

■ INDICATION: It is prescribed in the treatment of hemophilia

B. It is a vitamin K-dependent protein synthesized in the liver.

■ CONTRAINDICATION: Liver disease with intravascular coagulation and fibrinolysis is the only contraindication.

■ ADVERSE EFFECTS: Among the more serious adverse reactions are hepatitis, intravascular coagulation, circulatory collapse, and hypersensitivity reaction.

factor X, a coagulation factor that occurs in normal plasma but is deficient in some inherited defects in coagulation. Factor X and prothrombin are closely related; both are synthesized in the liver in the presence of vitamin K. Also called **Stuart-Power factor.**

factor XI, a coagulation factor present in normal plasma. Deficiency results in hemophilia C.

factor XII, a coagulation factor present in normal plasma that triggers the formation of bradykinin and associated enzymatic reactions. Factor XII is required for rapid coagulation in vitro but is apparently not needed for hemostasis in vivo. It can be activated in the laboratory by contact with negatively charged surfaces, which can develop on glass and kaolin or on biologic material, such as collagen. Also called **activation factor, contact factor, glass factor, Hageman factor.**

factor XIII, a coagulation factor present in normal plasma that acts with calcium to produce an insoluble fibrin clot. Also called **fibrinase, fibrin stabilizing factor.**

factor-searching study, (in nursing research) a study design that produces a qualitative, narrative description including categories or classifications of phenomena. It may be used to describe various aspects of nursing practice, characteristics of a population, or both. Factor searching is often a preliminary step in a study at a higher level of inquiry.

facultative /fak′əltā′tiv/ [L, facultus, capability], not obligatory; having the ability to adapt to more than one condition, such as a facultative anaerobe.

facultative aerobe, an organism able to grow under anaerobic conditions but that develops most rapidly in an aerobic environment. Compare **obligate aerobe.** See **aerobe.**

facultative anaerobe, an organism able to grow under aerobic conditions but that develops most rapidly in an anaerobic environment. Compare **obligate anaerobe.** See also **anaerobe, anaerobic infection.**

facultative parasite. See **parasite.**

faculty /fak′əltē/ [L, facultus, capability], **1.** any normal physiologic function or natural ability of a living organism, such as the digestive faculty or the ability to perceive and distinguish sensory stimuli. **2.** an ability to do something specific, such as learn languages or remember names. **3.** any mental ability or power, such as memory or thought. **4.** a department in an institution of learning or the people who teach in a department of such an institution.

FAD. See **nonstress test.**

Faget's sign /fazhāz′/ [Jean C. Faget, American physician, b. 1818], a falling pulse rate associated with a constant temperature, or a constant pulse associated with a rising temperature. It is an unusual sign found in yellow fever. Also called **Faget's law.**

fagicladosporic acid /faj′iklad′ōspôr′ik/, a toxin produced by Cladosporium epiphyllum, a member of a genus of fungi that cause "black spot" in stored meat, tinea negra, and black degeneration of the brain.

Fahrenheit (F) /fer′ənhīt/ [Daniel G. Fahrenheit, German physicist, b. 1686], a scale for the measurement of temperature in which the boiling point of water is 212° and the freezing point of water is 32° at sea level. Compare **Celsius.**

failed forceps, an attempted mid-forceps operation that is abandoned because there is a greater degree of resistance to rotation or traction than anticipated, as a result of cephalopelvic disproportion. Cesarean section is performed to deliver the infant. Compare **trial forceps.** See also **cephalopelvic disproportion.**

failure to thrive (FTT) /fāl′yər/ [L, fallere, to deceive; ME, thriven, to grasp], the abnormal retardation of the growth and development of an infant resulting from conditions that interfere with normal metabolism, appetite, and activity. Causative factors include chromosomal abnormalities, as in Turner's syndrome and the various trisomies; major organ system defects that lead to deficiency or malfunction; systemic disease or acute illness; physical deprivation, primarily malnutrition; and various psychosocial factors, as seen in severe cases of maternal deprivation syndrome. Metabolic disturbances of short duration, as occur during acute illness, have usually no long-term effects on development and are usually followed by a period of rapid growth. Prolonged nutritional deficiency may cause permanent and irreversible retardation of physical, mental, or social development.

faint [OFr, faindre, to feign] nontechnical **1.** to lose consciousness, as in a syncopal attack. **2.** a syncopal attack. See also **syncope.**

faith healing [L, fidere, to trust; AS, hoelen, to make whole], alleged healing through the power to cause a cure or recovery from an illness or injury without the aid of conventional medical treatment. The healer is believed to have been given that power by a supernatural force.

falciform body. See **sporozoite.**

falciform ligament /fal′sifôrm/, a triangular or sickle-shaped ligament of the body, such as the ligamentum falciform hepatis. See **broad ligament of liver.**

falciform ligament of the liver. See **broad ligament of liver.**

falciparum malaria /falsip′ərəm/ [L, falx, sickle, forma, form; It, bad air], the most severe form of malaria, caused by the protozoan Plasmodium falciparum, which affects red blood cells and is characterized by extremely grave systemic symptoms, mental confusion, enlarged spleen, edema, GI symptoms, and anemia. Falciparum malaria does not last as long as other forms of malaria; if treatment is begun promptly, the disease may be mild and the recovery uneventful. Relapses are uncommon, but death may result from dehydration and anemia. The usual treatment is chloroquine, but patients known to have contracted malaria in an area that harbors drug-resistant P. falciparum are often treated with a combination of quinine, pyrimethamine, and mefloquine. Compare **quartan malaria, tertian malaria.** See also **algid malaria, blackwater fever, malaria.**

fallectomy /fəlek′təmē/, the surgical removal of one or both of the fallopian tubes. See **salpingectomy.**

fallopian canal [Gabriele Fallopius, Italian anatomist, b. 1523; L, canalis], a passageway for the facial nerve through the petrous bone. Also called **Fallopius' canal.**

fallopian tube /fəlō′pē·ən/ [Gabriele Fallopio, Italian anatomist, b. 1523], one of a pair of ducts opening at one end into the uterus and at the other end into the peritoneal cavity, over the ovary. Each tube serves as the passage through which an ovum is carried to the uterus and through which spermatozoa move out toward the ovary. The tube lies in the upper border of the broad ligament (the mesosalpinx).

Each tube has four parts: the fimbriae, the infundibulum, the ampulla, and the isthmus. The fimbriae drape in finger-like projections from the infundibulum over the ovary. Just proximal to the infundibulum is the ampulla, the widest portion of the tube. The ampulla is connected to the fundus of the uterus by the isthmus. Also called **oviduct, uterine tube.** See **tubal ligation.**

Fallopius' canal. See **fallopian canal.**

Fallot's syndrome. See **tetralogy of Fallot.**

fallout [AS, *feallan,* to fall, *ut*], the deposition of radioactive debris after a nuclear explosion. The debris from an atmospheric explosion of an atomic bomb may travel thousands of miles in the atmosphere and be deposited over a large geographic area.

false ankylosis [L, *fallere,* to deceive; Gk, *agkylosis,* joint stiffness], a type of joint immobility resulting from abnormal inflexibility of body parts outside the joint. Also called **extracapsular ankylosis.**

false anorexia. See **pseudoanorexia.**

false diverticulum [L, *fallere,* to deceive, *diverticulare,* to turn aside], a protrusion of mucous membrane through a muscular coat defect of a hollow organ.

false imprisonment [L, *falsus,* deceptive; ME, *imprisonen*], (in law) the intentional, unjustified, nonconsensual detention or confinement of a person for any length of time.

false joint [L, *fallere,* to deceive, *jungere,* to join], a joint that develops at the site of a former fracture. Also called **pseudarthrosis.**

false labor. See **Braxton Hicks contractions.**

false negative, an incorrect result of a diagnostic test or procedure that falsely indicates the absence of a finding, condition, or disease. The rate of occurrence of false negative results varies with the diagnostic accuracy and the specificity of the test or procedure. As the accuracy and specificity of a test increase, the rate of false negatives decreases. Certain tests are known to yield false negative results at a certain rate; in all tests, a small number will occur by chance alone. False negative results are more common than false positive results, because the person conducting the test is more likely to fail to observe a finding than to imagine seeing something that does not exist. Compare **false positive.**

false-negative rate [L, *fallere,* to deceive, *negare,* to deny, *ratum,* calculate], the rate of occurrence of negative test results in subjects known to have the disease or behavior for which the individual is being tested.

false neuroma, **1.** a neoplasm that does not contain nerve elements. **2.** a cystic neuroma.

false nucleolus. See **karyosome.**

false pelvis, the part of the pelvis superior to a plane passing through the linea terminalis.

false personification, (in psychiatry) the labeling and prejudgment of others without validating impressions.

false positive, a test result that wrongly indicates the presence of a disease or other condition the test is designed to reveal. Compare **false negative.**

false-positive rate [L, *fallere,* to deceive, *positivus, ratum,* calculate], the rate of occurrence of positive test results in tests of individuals known to be free of a disease or disorder for which the individual is being tested.

false pregnancy. See **pseudocyesis.**

false rib. See **rib.**

false suture, an immovable fibrous joint in which rough articulating surfaces form the connection between certain bones of the skull. Two kinds of false sutures are **sutura plana** and **sutura squamosa.** Compare **true suture.**

false transactions, in transactional analysis, transactions in which communication is stopped or distorted by one individual relating from a different ego state than was expected.

false twins. See **dizygotic twins.**

false vertebrae, the vertebral segments that form the sacrum and the coccyx. Also called **fixed vertebrae.**

false vocal cord, either of two thick folds of mucous membrane in the larynx separating the ventricle from the vestibule. Each fold encloses a narrow band of fibrous tissue (the ventricular ligament). Compare **vocal cord.**

falx /falks, fôlks,/ *pl.* **falces** /fal′sēz, fôl′sēz/ [L, sickle], **1.** a sickle-shaped structure. **2.** sickle-shaped.

falx cerebelli /ser′əbel′ī/, a small sickle-shaped process of the dura mater attached to the occipital bone above and projecting into the posterior cerebellar notch between the two cerebellar hemispheres.

falx cerebri /ser′əbrī/, a sickle-shaped fold of dura mater membrane extending into and following along the longitudinal fissure of the two hemispheres of the cerebrum.

falx inguinalis, transverse and internal oblique muscles.

falx ligamentosa, the broad ligament of the liver.

FAM, an anticancer drug combination of fluorouracil, doxorubicin, and mitomycin.

familial /fəmi′yəl/ [L, *familial′, household*], pertaining to a characteristic, condition, or disease that is present in some families and not others or that occurs in more family members than would be expected by chance. It is usually but not always hereditary. Compare **acquired, congenital, hereditary.**

familial adenomatous polyposis. See **adenomatous polyposis coli.**

familial cretinism, a rare genetic disorder caused by an inborn error of metabolism resulting from an enzyme deficiency that interferes with thyroid hormone biosynthesis. Clinical manifestations include lethargy, stunted growth, and mental retardation. The condition is transmitted as an autosomal recessive trait and is treated by early administration of thyroid hormone, if possible in utero, to reduce the abnormalities of mental development. See also **cretinism.**

familial histiocytic reticulosis [L, *familia,* household; Gk, *histion,* web, *kytos,* cell; L, *reticulum,* little net; Gk, *osis,* condition], a hereditary disease, transmitted as an autosomal recessive trait, characterized by anemia, granulocytopenia, and thrombocytopenia. Phagocytosis of blood cells and infiltration of bone marrow by histocytes commonly results in death in childhood. Also called **familial hemophagocytic reticulosis.**

familial hypercholesterolemia, an inherited disorder transmitted as a dominant trait and characterized by a high level of serum cholesterol, tendinous xanthomas, and early evidence of atherosclerosis, especially of the coronary arteries. Affected individuals at 50 years of age have three to ten times greater risk of ischemic heart disease than the general population. Cholesterol levels are elevated at birth, increase with age, and average 250 to 500 mg/dl in heterozygous adults and 500 to 1000 mg/dl in adults who are homozygous for the gene. Xanthomas begin to appear at 20 years of age and occur most frequently on the Achilles tendon, extensor tendons of the hands, elbows, and tibial tuberosities. In Type IIA familial hypercholesterolemia, only low-density lipoprotein (LDL) is elevated, while in Type

IIB, LDL and very low-density lipoprotein (VLDL) are increased. The disorder occurs in whites, blacks, and Orientals, and the prevalence of the gene in the United States is 1:1000. Treatment includes a low-cholesterol and low-saturated-fat diet. Cholestyramine may be given to patients with Type IIA familial hypercholesterolemia but not to those with Type IIB. Also called **hypercholesterolemic xanthomatosis, hyperlipidemia type IIA.**

familial hyperglyceridemia. See **hyperlipidemia type I.**

familial iminoglycinuria. See **iminoglycinuria.**

familial juvenile nephronophthisis. See **medullary cystic disease.**

familial lipoprotein lipase deficiency. See **hyperchylomicronemia.**

familial osteochondrodystrophy. See **Morquio's disease.**

familial periodic paralyis [L, *familia,* household; Gk, *peri,* near, *hodos,* way, *paralysein,* to be palsied], a rare inherited disorder in which clients suffer attacks of general flaccid paralysis following attacks of hypokalemia or potassium depletion. The attacks may follow administration of glucose and are relieved by the administration of potassium salts.

familial polyposis, an abnormal condition characterized by multiple polyps in the colon and rectum. The disease has a high malignancy potential and is inherited as a heterozygous, autosomal dominant trait. Total proctocolectomy eliminates the risk of cancer, which, if untreated, occurs before 40 years of age. Genetic counseling is advised. A kind of familial polyposis is **Gardner's syndrome.** See also **polyposis.**

familial spinal muscular atrophy. See **Werdnig-Hoffmann disease.**

familial tremor. See **essential tremor.**

family [L, *familia,* household], 1. a group of people related by heredity, such as parents, children, and siblings. The term sometimes is broadened to include persons related by marriage or those living in the same household, who are emotionally attached, interact regularly, and share concerns for the growth and development of the family and its individual members. 2. a group of persons having a common surname, such as the Anderson family. 3. a category of animals or plants situated on a taxonomic scale between order and genus. Humans are members of the genus *Homo sapiens,* which is a part of the hominid family which, in turn, is a division of the primate order of mammals. See also **genetics, heredity.** –**familial,** *adj.*

family Apgar, a family therapy rating system in which the name 'Apgar' gives the first letters of five words— adaptability, partnership, growth, affection, and resolve— representing the questionnaire categories. Each family member indicates a degree of satisfaction in each of the five categories on a scale of 0 to 2. The system is used most frequently in studies of families with a geriatric member. See also **Apgar score.**

family care leave, absence from a job that is permitted for an employee to care for a family member who is ill, disabled, or pregnant. The U.S. Family and Medical Leave Act of 1993 provides 12 weeks of unpaid leave per year from a job for the birth or adoption of a child; for the care of a seriously ill child, spouse, or parent; or for a serious illness afflicting the employee. The law applies only to companies with 50 or more employees. Employers must guaranteee that a worker can return to the same or a comparable job.

family-centered care, primary health care that includes an assessment of the health of an entire family, identification of actual or potential factors that might influence the health of its members, and implementation of actions needed to maintain or improve the health of the unit and its members.

family-centered maternity care, a system for the delivery of safe, high-quality health care adapted to the physical and psychosocial needs of the patient, the patient's entire family, and the newly born offspring.

family-centered nursing care, nursing care directed toward improving the potential health of a family or any of its members by assessing individual and family health needs and strengths, by identifying problems influencing the health care of the family as a whole and those influencing the individual members, by using family resources, by teaching and counseling, and by evaluating progress toward stated goals.

family counseling, a program of providing information and professional guidance to members of a family concerning specific health matters, such as care of a severely retarded child or the risk of transmitting a known genetic defect.

family disorganization, a breakdown of a family system. It may be associated with parental overburdening or loss of significant others who served as role models for children or support systems for family members. Family disorganization can contribute to the loss of social controls that families usually impose on their members.

family dynamics, the forces at work within the family that result in particular behaviors or symptoms.

family functions, processes by which the family operates as a whole, including communication and manipulation of the environment for problem solving.

family health, (in a health history) an account of the health of the members of the immediate family. Hereditary and familial diseases are especially noted. The age and health of each person, the ages at death, and the causes of death are charted. The family health history is obtained from the patient or family in the initial interview and becomes a part of the permanent record.

family history, an essential portion of a patient's medical history in which the patient is asked about the health of the other members of the family in a series of specific questions, such as "Has anyone in your family had tuberculosis? diabetes mellitus? breast cancer?," to discover any diseases to which the patient may be particularly vulnerable. Other questions, such as those concerning the age, sex, relationships of others in the household, and the marital history of the patient, may also be asked if the information has not already been secured.

family medicine, the branch of medicine that is concerned with the diagnosis and treatment of health problems in people of either sex and any age. Practitioners of family medicine are often called family practice physicians, family physicians, or, formerly, general practitioners. They often act as the primary health care providers, referring complicated problems to a specialist.

family myths, myths that are constructed to deny the reality of family situations.

family nurse practitioner (FNP), a nurse practitioner possessing skills necessary for the detection and management of acute self-limiting conditions and management of chronic stable conditions. An FNP provides primary, ambulatory care for families in collaboration with primary care physicians. The FNP provides direct health care and guides or counsels families as required. Consultation, copractice, and referral to associated physicians are aspects of the FNP's practice.

family of origin, the family into which a person is born.

family of procreation, the family a person forms through marriage and/or having children.

family physician, 1. a medical practitioner of the specialty of family medicine. **2.** a general practitioner. **3.** a family practice physician. See also **family medicine.**

family planning. See **contraception.**

family practice [L, *familia*, household; Gk, *praktikos*, ready for action], a medical specialty that encompasses several branches of medicine, including internal medicine, pediatrics, surgery, psychiatry, and obstetrics and gynecology; includes client management, counseling, and problem solving; and coordinates total health care delivery to all members of a family, regardless of sex or age of the patient.

family practice physician, a practitioner of family medicine, usually one who has completed a residency program in the specialty. See also **family medicine.**

family processes, altered, a nursing diagnosis accepted by the Fifth National Conference on the Classification of Nursing Diagnoses. The origin of the problem is a situational or developmental change or crisis within the family network. The defining characteristics include the inability of the family system to meet the physical, emotional, spiritual, or security needs of its members; the inability of family members to communicate adequately, to express or accept a wide range of feelings, or to relate to each other for mutual growth and maturation; the parents' disrespect for each other's views on child-rearing practices; family rigidity in function and roles and its uninvolvement in community activities; the inability of the family to accept or receive appropriate help, to adapt to change, or to deal with traumatic experience constructively; disrespect for individuality and autonomy; failure to accomplish current or past developmental tasks; ineffective decision-making processes; inappropriate or poorly communicated family rules, rituals, or symbols; and unexamined family myths. See also **nursing diagnosis.**

family structure, the composition and membership of the family and the organization and patterning of relationships among individual family members. In planning health care for a family member, or the entire family, an awareness of that family's structure may be important.

family therapy, (in psychiatry) a therapy modality that focuses treatment on the process between family members that supports and perpetuates symptoms; a way of conceptualizing human relationship problems that focuses on the context in which an emotional problem is generated.

famine fever. See **relapsing fever.**

famotidine /famot′idēn/, an oral and parenteral antiulcer drug.

■ INDICATIONS: It is prescribed for the short-term treatment of active duodenal ulcer, maintenance therapy for duodenal ulcer after healing, and for pathologic hypersecretory conditions such as Zollinger-Ellison syndrome.

■ CONTRAINDICATIONS: Famotidine should be used with caution in patients with impaired kidney function.

■ ADVERSE EFFECTS: Among adverse reactions reported are headache, dizziness, constipation, diarrhea, and temporary irritation of the injection site.

fan beam, a geometric pattern that results from collimating a spatially extended x-ray beam with a long, narrow slit.

FANCAP, *U.S.* a mnemonic device for helping student nurses learn to assess, provide, and evaluate direct patient care. It stands for fluids, aeration, nutrition, communication, activity, and pain. Occasionally a variant, FANCAS, is substituted for FANCAP, in which case the 'S' stands for stimulation.

Fanconi's anemia /fankō′nēs/ [Guido Fanconi, Swiss pediatrician, b. 1892], a rare, usually congenital disorder transmitted as an autosomal recessive trait, characterized by aplastic anemia in childhood or early adult life, bone abnormalities, chromatin breaks, and developmental anomalies. Children begin to show symptoms between the ages of 4 and 12 years. Also called **congenital pancytopenia, pancytopenia-dysmelia.**

Fanconi's syndrome, a group of disorders including renal tubular function, glycosuria, phosphaturia, and bicarbonate wasting. The condition is often marked by osteomalacia, acidosis, and hypokalemia. Two main types of the syndrome have been differentiated. Idiopathic Fanconi's syndrome is inherited and usually appears in early middle age. Acquired Fanconi's syndrome is usually the result of toxicity from various sources, including the ingestion of outdated tetracycline. Because of numerous variations of the syndrome, it is believed that different alleles are responsible for the different recessively inherited factors expressed as signs and symptoms of the group of disorders.

fango /fän′gō/ [It, mud], mud taken from thermal springs at Battaglia, Italy, and used to treat gout and other rheumatic diseases.

fan lateral projection, a technique for making an x-ray image of the hand without superimposition of the phalanges. The patient places the fingers about a sponge wedge designed so that each finger appears separately, in a fanlike pattern, on the x-ray film.

Fansidar, a trademark for a fixed-combination antimalarial agent (pyrimethamine and sulfadoxine).

fantasy /fan′təsē/ [Gk, *phantasia*, imagination], **1.** the unrestrained free play of the imagination; fancy. **2.** a mental image, usually distorted or grotesque in nature, often the result of the action of drugs or a disease of the central nervous system. **3.** the mental process of transforming undesirable experiences into imagined events or into a sequence of ideas in order to fulfill an unconscious wish, need, or desire or to give expression to unconscious conflicts, such as a daydream.

F.A.O.T.A., abbreviation for *Fellow of the American Occupational Therapy Association.*

F.A.P.T.A., abbreviation for *Fellow of the American Physical Therapy Association.*

farad (F) /fer′əd/ [Michael Faraday, English scientist, b. 1791], a unit of capacitance that increases the potential difference between the plates of a capacitor by 1 volt with a charge of 1 coulomb.

Faraday cage /fer′ədā/, (in nuclear magnetic resonance imaging) a wire-mesh cage that surrounds the MR scanner to shield it from stray radio frequency waves. The radio waves, which are generally present in the environment from commercial and other broadcasting sources, are not an immediate threat to the patient but can distort the results of MR imaging.

Farber test, a microscopic examination of newborn meconium for lanugo and squamous cells. The fetus normally swallows amniotic fluid containing these large proteins, which then pass through the digestive system to be excreted, usually after birth, in the first stools. The absence of hair or skin cells is suggestive of intestinal obstruction or atresia and requires further evaluation.

Far Eastern hemorrhagic fever, a form of epidemic hemorrhagic fever, indigenous to Asia, that is transmitted by a virus carried by an Asian rodent. The infection is characterized by chills, fever, headache, abdominal pain, nausea, vomiting, anorexia, and extreme thirst. Hypotensive shock may occur as the fever subsides. Thirst continues into the second week, oliguria develops, and the blood pressure returns to normal. Blood urea nitrogen levels increase hyperphosphatemia and hypercalcemia, and other complications occur. Diuresis follows the oliguric phase, resulting in an output of as much as 8 L a day of urine and in electrolyte imbalance. Mortality may be as high as 33%. There is no specific treatment.

far field. See **Fraunhofer zone.**

farmer's lung [L, *firmare,* to make firm], a respiratory disorder caused by the inhalation of actinomycetes or other organic dusts from moldy hay. It is a form of hypersensitivity pneumonitis, affecting individuals who have developed antibodies to the mold spores. It is characterized by coughing, dyspnea, cyanosis, tachycardia, nausea, chills, and fever. Treatment may include cromolyn sodium and a corticosteroid.

far point [ME, *farr;* L, *punctus,* pricked], **1.** the farthest distance from the eye that an object can be seen clearly when eye is at rest and accommodation is fully relaxed. **2.** the point at which the visual axes of the two eyes meet when at rest.

farsightedness. See **hyperopia.**

FAS, abbreviation for **fetal alcohol syndrome.**

fasci-, a combining form meaning 'pertaining to a band or bundle of fibrous tissue': *fasciagram, fascicular, fasciitis.*

fascia /fash′ē·ə/, *pl.* **fasciae** [L, band], the fibrous connective tissue of the body that may be separated from other specifically organized structures, such as the tendons, the aponeuroses, and the ligaments. It varies in thickness and density and in the amounts of fat, collagenous fiber, elastic fiber, and tissue fluid it contains. Kinds of fasciae are **deep fascia, subcutaneous fascia,** and **subserous fascia. –fascial,** *adj.*

fascia bulbi, a thin membranous socket that envelops the eyeball from the optic nerve to the ciliary region and allows the eyeball to move freely. The fascia bulbi has a smooth inner surface, pierced by vessels and nerves, and fuses with the sheath of the optic nerve and with the sclera. The lower part of the membrane thickens into the suspensory ligament, which attaches to the zygomatic arch and the lacrimal bones. Also called **Tenon's capsule.**

fasciae. See **fascia.**

fascial. See **fascia.**

fascial cleft /fash′ē·əl/ [L, *fascia* + ME, *clift*], a place of cleavage between two contiguous fascial surfaces, such as the deep fasciae and the subcutaneous fasciae. A fascial cleft is rich in fluid but poor in traversing fibers; thus, two fascial surfaces may move or be separated from each other easily. Compare **fascial compartment, fascial membrane lamination.**

fascial compartment, a part of the body that is walled off by fascial membranes, usually containing a muscle or group of muscles or an organ, just as the heart is contained by the mediastinum. Compare **fascial cleft, fascial membrane lamination.**

fascial membrane lamination, a pad of connective tissue that contains fat and an occasional blood vessel or a lymph node. It is found where a fascial membrane splits into two sheets, such as at the division of the outer cervical fascia above the sternum. Compare **fascial cleft, fascial compartment.**

fascia thoracolumbalis, the extensive subdivision of the vertebral fascia that sheaths the sacrospinalis muscle. It spreads caudally to become the glistening, white lumbar aponeurosis and the origin of the latissimus dorsi. Medially it attaches to the sacrum, laterally to the ribs and the intercostal fascia, and cranially to the ligamentum nuchae. Also called **lumbodorsal fascia.**

fascicle. See **fasciculus.**

fascicular /fəsik′yələr/ [L, *fasciculus,* a little bundle], pertaining to something arranged in bundles, such as groups of nerve or muscle fibers in a tract.

fascicular neuroma, a neoplasm composed of myelinated nerve fibers. Also called **medullated neuroma.**

fascicular twitching. See **twitching.**

fasciculation /fasik′yo͞olā′shən/ [L, *fasciculus,* little bundle, *atio* process], a localized, uncoordinated, uncontrollable twitching of a single muscle group innervated by a single motor nerve fiber or filament that may be palpated and seen under the skin. It results from a variety of drugs as a side effect with normal dosage or from an overdose, or it may be symptomatic of a number of disorders, including dietary deficiency, cerebral palsy, fever, neuralgia, polio, rheumatic heart disease, sodium deficiency, tic, or uremia. Fasciculation of the heart muscle is known as fibrillation. **–fascicular,** *adj.,* **fasciculate,** *v.*

fasciculus /fəsik′yələs/, *pl.* **fasciculi** [L, little bundle], a small bundle of muscle, tendon, or nerve fibers. The arrangement of fasciculi in a muscle is correlated with the power of the muscle and its range of motion. The patterns of muscular fasciculi are penniform, bipenniform, multipenniform, and radiated. **–fascicular,** *adj.*

fasciitis /fas′ē·ī′tis/, **1.** an inflamation of the connective tissue, which may be caused by streptococcal or other types of infection, an injury, or an autoimmune reaction. **2.** an abnormal, benign growth (*Pseudosarcomatous fasciitis*) resembling a tumor that develops in the subcutaneous oral tissues, usually in the cheek. Commonly growing rapidly and then regressing, it consists of young fibroblasts and many capillaries and may be mistaken for fibrosarcoma. Also called **fascitis** /fasī′tis/

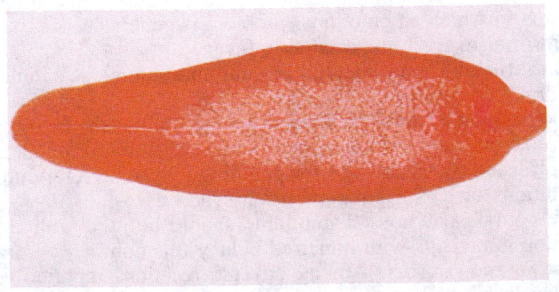

Fasciola hepatica (Muller, 1990)

fascioliasis /fas′ē·ōlī′əsis/ [L, *fasciola*, little band; Gk, *osis* condition], infection with the liver fluke *Fasciola hepatica*, characterized by epigastric pain, fever, jaundice, eosinophilia, urticaria, and diarrhea, with fibrosis of the liver a consequence of prolonged infection. It is acquired by ingestion of encysted forms of the fluke found on aquatic plants, such as raw watercress. The disease is prevalent in many parts of the world, including the southern and western United States. Bithionol, given orally, is the usual treatment.

fasciolopsiasis /fas′ē·ōlopsī′əsis/ [L, *fasciola*, little band; Gk, *opsis*, appearance, *osis*, condition], an intestinal infection, prevalent in the Far East, characterized by abdominal pain, diarrhea, constipation, eosinophilia, ascites, and, sometimes, edema; caused by the fluke *Fasciolopsis buski*. The disease is usually acquired by eating contaminated water plants, such as raw water chestnuts. It is easily treated with anthelmintics, such as piperazine.

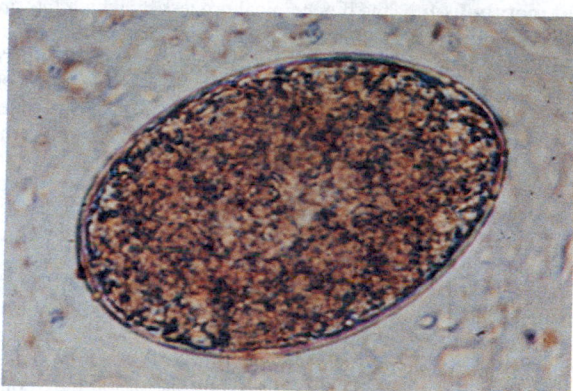

Fasciolopsis buski egg
(Murray, 1990; from Koneman EW, Allen SD, Dowell VR and Sommers HM: Color atlas and textbook of diagnostic mictobiology, ed. 2. Philadelphia, 1979, JB Lippincott Co.)

Fasciolopsis buski /fas′ē·əlop′sis bus′kē/, a species of flukes that is an important intestinal parasite endemic in the Orient and tropics. In the United States and other countries it is occasionally found in imported food products. See also **fasciolopsiasis**.

fascioscapulohumeral muscular dystrophy /fas′ē·ō·skap′yəlōhyōō′mərəl/ [L, *fasciculus*, little bundle, *scapula* shoulderblade, *humerus* shoulder], an abnormal congenital condition and one of the main types of muscular dystrophy. It is characterized by progressive symmetric wasting of the skeletal muscles, especially the muscles of the face, the shoulders, and the upper arms, without any associated neural or sensory disorders. This disease is not usually fatal but spreads to all the voluntary muscles and commonly produces a pendulous lower lip and the absence of the nasolabial fold. It is an autosomal dominant disease that may be transmitted to males and females. Also called **Landouzy-Déjérine muscular dystrophy.** Compare **Duchenne's muscular dystrophy.**

■ OBSERVATIONS: Fascioscapulohumeral dystrophy usually occurs before 10 years of age but may also develop during adolescence. Early symptoms include the inability to pucker the lips, abnormal facial movements when laughing or cry-

ing, facial flattening, winging of the scapulae, inability to raise the arms over the head, and, in infants, the inability to suckle. Diagnosis of this disease is based on the typical family and medical history and associated characteristic signs of abnormality. Confirming diagnosis is based on muscle biopsy showing abnormal deposits of fat and connective tissue. Electromyography may show attenuated electric activity, an inconclusive sign when considered alone but helpful in ruling out neurogenic muscle atrophy.

fasciotomy /fas′ē·ot′əmē/, a surgical incision into an area of fascia.

fascitis. See **fasciitis.**

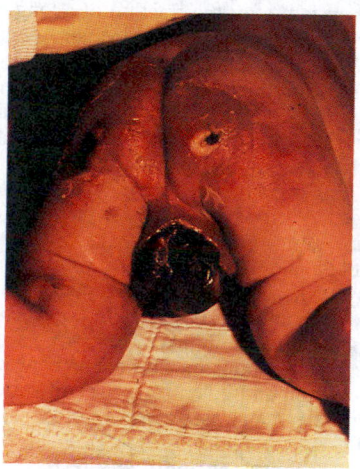

Necrotizing fasciitis
(Zitelli, 1992; Courtesy Dr. Michael Sherlock)

F.A.S.R.T., abbreviation for *Fellow of the American Society of Radiologic Technologists.*

fast [AS, *faest*, firm], **1.** resistant to change, especially to the action of a specific drug or chemical, as a staining agent. **2.** to abstain from all or certain foods. See also **fasting.**

fast-acting insulin, one of a group of insulin preparations in which the onset of action is rapid, approximately 1 hour, and the duration of the action is relatively brief, approximately 6 to 14 hours. Kinds of fast-acting insulins include **insulin regular** and **prompt insulin zinc suspension.**

fastigium /fastij′ē·əm/ [L, ridge], **1.** the highest point in the course of a fever, or the most symptomatic point in the course of an illness. **2.** the angle at the top of the roof of the fourth ventricle in the brain.

Fastin, a trademark for an anorexiant (phentermine hydrochloride).

fasting [AS, *foestan*, to observe], the act of abstaining from food for a specific period of time, usually for therapeutic or religious purposes.

fast-twitch (FT) fiber, a muscle fiber that can develop high tension rapidly. It is usually innervated by a single alpha neuron, and has low fatigue resistance, low capillary density, low levels of aerobic enzymes, and low oxygen availability. FT fibers are used in such activities as sprinting, jumping, and weight lifting. Also called **fast-twitch muscle fiber.** See also **slow-twitch (ST) fiber.**

fat [AS, *faett*], **1.** a substance composed of lipids or fatty acids and occurring in various forms or consistencies ranging from oil to tallow. **2.** a type of body tissue composed of cells containing stored fat (depot fat). Stored fat is usually identified as white fat, which is found in large cellular vesicles, or brown fat, which consists of lipid droplets. Stored fat contains more than twice as many calories per gram as sugars and serves as a source of quickly mobilized body energy. In addition, stored fat helps cushion and insulate vital organs. See also **adipose, obesity.**

fatal /fā′təl/ [L, *fatum,* what has been spoken], leading inevitably to death.

fat cell lipoma. See **hibernoma.**

fat embolism, a circulatory condition characterized by the blocking of an artery by an embolus of fat that entered the circulatory system after the fracture of a long bone or, less commonly, after traumatic injury to adipose tissue or to a fatty liver. A systemic condition may occur after extensive trauma, since lipid metabolism is altered by the injury and causes release of free fatty acids resulting in vasculitis with obstruction of many small pulmonary and cerebral arteries. Fat embolism usually occurs suddenly 12 to 36 hours after the injury and is characterized by symptoms related to the site occluded, such as severe chest pain, pallor, dyspnea, tachycardia, delirium, prostration, and, in some cases, coma. Anemia and thrombocytopenia are common. Classic signs of systemic fat embolism are petechial hemorrhages on the neck, shoulders, axillae, and conjunctivae, appearing 2 or 3 days after the injury. There is no specific therapy for systemic fat embolism; the patient is placed in a high Fowler's position and given oxygen, corticosteroids, blood transfusion, respiratory assistance, or other supportive care, as needed.

FA test. See **fluorescent antibody test.**

father complex [L, *pater; complecti,* to embrace], *nontechnical.* a repressed desire for an incestuous relationship with one's father.

father fixation, an arrest in psychosexual development characterized by an abnormally persistent, close, and often paralyzing emotional attachment to one's father. Compare **mother fixation.** See also **Freudian fixation.**

fatigability /fat′igəbil′itē/, a tendency to become tired or exhausted quickly or easily. Fatigability may occur in certain types of cells that undergo periods of excessive activity.

fatigue /fətēg′/ [L, *fatigare,* to tire], **1.** a state of exhaustion or a loss of strength or endurance, such as may follow strenuous physical activity. **2.** loss of ability of tissues to respond to stimuli that normally evoke muscular contraction or other activity. Muscle cells generally require a refractory or recovery period after activity, during which time cells restore their energy supplies and excrete metabolic waste products. **3.** an emotional state associated with extreme or extended exposure to psychic pressure, as in battle or combat fatigue. **4.** a nursing diagnosis accepted by the Eighth National Conference on the Classification of Nursing Diagnoses. Fatigue is defined as an overwhelming sense of exhaustion and decreased capacity for physical and mental work regardless of adequate sleep. The major defining characteristics are verbalization of fatigue or lack of energy and inability to maintain usual routines. Minor characteristics include a perceived need for additional energy to accomplish routine tasks, an increase in physical complaints, impaired ability to concentrate, decreased performance, and decreased libido. The individual with fatigue can also be emotionally labile or irritable, lethargic or list-

less, have disinterest in surroundings or introspection, and be accident prone. Related factors include overwhelming psychological or emotional demands; increased energy requirements to perform acitivity of daily living; excessive social or role demands; states of discomfort; decreased metabolic energy production; and altered body chemistry such as from medications or drug withdrawal. See also **nursing diagnosis.**

fatigue fever, a benign episode of fever and muscle pain after overexertion. The symptoms are caused by an accumulation of the metabolic waste products of muscle contractions and may persist for several days.

fatigue fracture, any fracture that results from excessive physical activity and not from any specific injury, as commonly occurs in the metatarsal bones of runners.

fatigue state [L, *fatigare,* to tire, *status,* condition], the state of lowest energy of a system. Also called **ground state.** See also **neuresthenia.**

fat-induced hyperlipidemia. See **hyperlipidemia type I.**

fat metabolism, the biochemical process by which fats are broken down and elaborated by the cells of the body. Fats provide more food energy than carbohydrates; the catabolism of 1 g of fat provides 9 kcal of heat as compared with 4.1 kcal yielded in the catabolism of 1 g of carbohydrate. Fat catabolism involves a series of chemical reactions, the last stages of which are similar to the final reactions of carbohydrate catabolism. Before the final reactions in fat catabolism can occur, fats must be hydrolyzed into fatty acids and glycerol. Conversion of glycerol provides a compound that can enter the citric acid cycle. Catabolism of fatty acids continues by beta-oxidation to produce acetyl-CoA, which also enters the citric acid cycle. The body synthesizes fats from fatty acids and glycerol or from compounds derived from excess glucose or from amino acids. Fat anabolism also includes the synthesis of complex compounds, such as phospholipid, an important component of cell membranes. The body can synthesize only saturated fatty acids. Essential unsaturated fatty acids can be supplied only by the diet. Certain hormones, such as insulin, growth hormone, adrenocorticotropic hormone, and the glucocorticoids, control fat metabolism. Fat catabolism is inversely related to the rate of carbohydrate catabolism, and in some conditions, such as diabetes mellitus, the secretion of these hormones increases to counter a decrease in carbohydrate catabolism.

fat necrosis [AS, *faett;* Gk, *nekros,* dead, *osis,* condition], a condition caused by trauma or infection in which neutral tissue fats are broken down into fatty acids and glycerol. Fat necrosis occurs most commonly in the breasts and subcutaneous areas. It also may develop in the abdominal cavity following an attack of pancreatitis causing a release of enzymes from the pancreas.

fat pad, a mass of closely packed fat cells surrounded by fibrous tissue septa. Fat pads may be generously supplied with capillaries and nerve endings. Intraarticular fat pads are also covered by a layer of synovial cells.

fatty acid [AS, *faett* + L, *acidus,* sour], any of several organic acids produced by the hydrolysis of neutral fats. In a living cell a fatty acid usually occurs in combination with another molecule rather than in a free state. Essential fatty acids are unsaturated molecules that cannot be produced by the body and must therefore be included in the diet. Some kinds of are **arachidonic** and **linoleic.** See also **saturated fatty acid, unsaturated fatty acid.**

fatty alcohol, a hydroxy derivative of a hydrocarbon from the paraffin series.

fatty ascites. See **chylous ascites.**

fatty cirrhosis [AS, *faett*, Gk, *kirrhos*, yellow, *osis*, condition], a form of cirrhosis that develops over a long period of poor nutrition resulting in fatty infiltration of the liver. See also **cirrhosis.**

fatty degeneration [AS, *faett*, L, *degenerare*, to deviate], the abnormal deposition of fat within cells or the fatty tissue invasion of organs. Also called **adipose degeneration.**

fatty infiltration, a normal phase of breast development, characterized by accumulation of increased amounts of fat around the parenchymal breast tissue. It is normally followed later in life by involution.

fatty infiltration of heart [AS, *faett*; L, *in, filtrare*; AS, *heorte*], an accumulation of large amounts of fat within the cells of the heart. The heart muscle may be marked by irregular streaks of pale areas of fatty infiltration. It is sometimes associated with severe and prolonged anemia.

fatty liver, an accumulation of triglycerides in the liver. The causes include obesity, diabetes, excessive consumption of alcohol, IV administration of drugs such as tetracycline and corticosteroids, and exposure to toxic substances, such as carbon tetrachloride and yellow phosphorus. Fatty liver is also seen in kwashiorkor and is a rare complication of unknown origin in late pregnancy. The symptoms are anorexia, hepatomegaly, and abdominal discomfort; fat cells can be seen under the microscope after liver biopsy. The condition is usually reversible after the underlying condition is corrected or the offending drug is withdrawn. See also **cirrhosis.**

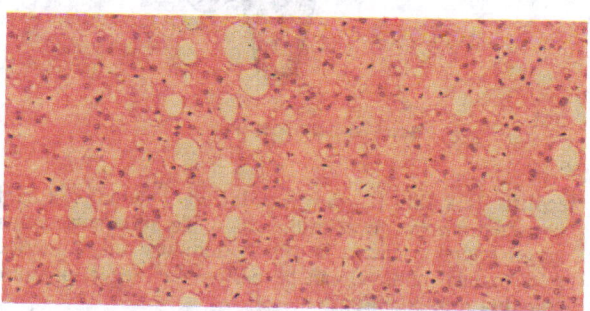

Fatty liver in kwashiorkor
(McLaren, 1992/Courtesy Prof JDL Hansen)

such as overhanging or incomplete tooth fillings, incorrect anatomy of occlusal and marginal ridge areas, and faulty clasps. Such faults may mar individual tooth restorations and fixed or removable prosthetics, which may cause inflammatory and dystrophic diseases of the teeth and periodontium. See also **restoration.**

favism /fā'vizəm/ [It, *fava*, bean], an acute hemolytic anemia caused by ingestion of the beans or inhalation of the pollen from the *Vicia faba* (fava) plant. Sensitive individuals show a deficiency of glucose-6-phosphate dehydrogenase, usually the result of a hereditary biochemical abnormality of the erythrocytes. Symptoms include dizziness, headache, vomiting, fever, jaundice, eosinophilia, and often diarrhea. The condition is found primarily in persons of southern Italian extraction and is treated by blood transfusion and avoidance of fava beans and pollen. See also **glucose-6-phosphate dehydrogenase deficiency.**

favus /fā'vəs/ [L, honeycomb], a fungal infection of the scalp, skin, or nails, more common in children than adults. It is caused by *Trichophyton* fungi. Favus is characterized by thick, yellow crusts with suppuration, a distinct 'mousy' odor, permanent scars, and alopecia. It is rarely seen in North America, common in the Middle East and Africa.

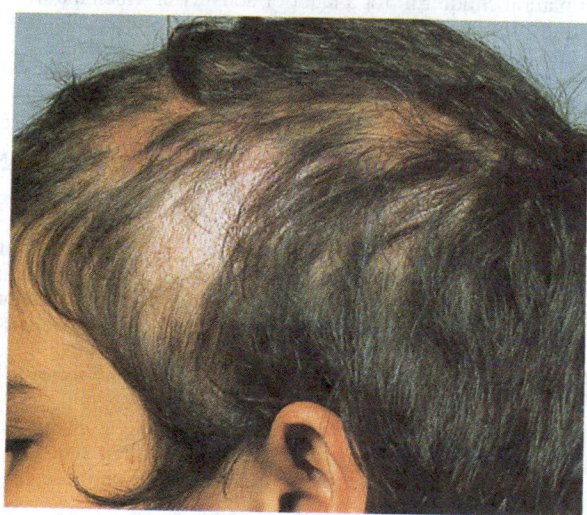

Favus (Baran, 1991)

fatty stool [AS, *faett, stol*, seat], a stool containing an abnormally large amount of fat, as indicated by a stool that floats on water.

fatty tissue [AS, *faett*; OFr, *tissu*], loose connective tissue with many cells containing fat droplets. Also called **adipose tissue.**

fauces /fô'sēz/ [L, *faux*, throat], the opening of the mouth into the pharynx. The anterior pillars of the fauces form the glossopalatine arch, and the posterior pillars form the pharyngopalatine arch.

faucial isthmus /fô'shəl/, an aperture between the pharynx and the mouth.

faulty restoration /fôl'tē/ [L, *fallere*, to deceive; *restaurare*, to renew], any dental restoration that contains flaws,

fax, abbreviation for **facsimile.**

F.C.A.P., abbreviation for *Fellow of the College of American Pathologists*.

Fc fragment, a part of a molecule of an antibody after it has been split by a proteolytic enzyme. It represents the relatively constant region, as distinguished from the Fab portion that contains the binding sites. The Fc portion is sometimes identified as the crystallizable fragment.

FDA, abbreviation for **Food and Drug Administration.**

Fe, symbol for the element **iron.**

fear [ME *fer* danger], a nursing diagnosis accepted by the Fourth National Conference on the Classification of Nursing Diagnoses. As a symptom, fear is a feeling of dread related to an identifiable source that the client is able to validate. The etiology of the problem, developed at the Fifth

National Conference, results from natural or innate origins, such as a sudden noise, loss of physical support, pain, heights, or other environmental stimuli; a learned or conditioned response; separation from a support system in a potentially threatening situation, such as hospitalization; knowledge defect or unfamiliarity; language barrier; sensory impairment; phobia or phobic stimulus. The defining characteristics may be subjective or objective. Subjective characteristics include increased tension, apprehension, impulsiveness, terror, panic, and decreased self-assurance. Objective characteristics are increased alertness and concentration on the source of fear; a wide-eyed, aggressive attack mode of behavior or withdrawal from the source of fear; and cardiovascular excitation, superficial vasoconstriction, and pupil dilatation. See also **nursing diagnosis.**

fear-tension-pain syndrome, a concept formulated by Grantly Dick-Read, M.D., to explain the pain commonly expected and reported in childbirth. The concept proposes that mistaken cultural attitudes induce anxiety before labor and cause fear in labor. This fear causes muscular and psychologic tension that interferes with the natural processes of dilatation and delivery, resulting in pain. He advocated education, exercise, and warm emotional and physical support in labor to counteract the syndrome, coining the term 'natural childbirth' for a labor or delivery in which the well-trained woman joyfully, comfortably, and with a calm, cooperative attitude, participates in the natural experience. Elements of his method of psychophysical preparation for childbirth are incorporated into most other methods of natural childbirth. See also **Bradley method, Lamaze method.**

febri-, a combining form meaning 'pertaining to a fever': *febricant, febrifugal, febriphobia.*

febrifuge. See **antipyretic.**

febrile /fē′bril, feb′ril/ [L, *febris,* fever], pertaining to or characterized by an elevated body temperature, such as a febrile reaction to an infectious agent. A body temperature of over 100° F is commonly regarded as febrile. **−febrility,** *n.*

-febrile, a combining form meaning 'pertaining to fever': *afebrile, nonfebrile, subfebrile.*

febrile delirium [L, *febris,* fever, *delirare,* to rave], a symptom of disordered central nervous system functions, with excitement, restlessness, and disorientation, accompanying some acute fevers.

febrile seizure, a seizure associated with a febrile illness. Treatment depends on the age of the patient and the number of seizures. Generalized recurrent febrile seizures in children may be treated as grand mal epilepsy.

febrile state [L, *febris,* fever, *status,* condition], a significant increase in body temperature accompanied by increased pulse and respiration rates, anorexia, constipation, insomnia, headache, pains, and irritability.

-febrility. See **febrile.**

fecal /fē′kəl/ [L, *faex,* waste matter], pertaining to the nature of feces or excrement.

fecal fistula [L, *faex,* dregs; *fistula,* pipe], an abnormal passage from the colon to the external surface of the body, discharging feces. Fistulas of this kind are usually created surgically in operations involving the removal of malignant or severely ulcerated bowel segments. See also **colostomy.**

fecal impaction, an accumulation of hardened or inspissated feces in the rectum or sigmoid colon that the individual is unable to move. Diarrhea may be a sign of fecal impaction since only liquid material is able to pass the obstruc-

tion. Occasionally, fecal impaction may cause urinary incontinence because of pressure on the bladder. Treatment includes oil and cleansing enemas and manual breaking up and removal of the stool by a gloved finger. Persons who are dehydrated, nutritionally depleted, on long periods of bedrest, receiving constipating medications such as iron or opiates, or undergoing barium x-ray studies are at risk of developing fecal impaction. Prevention includes adequate bulk food, fluids, exercise, regular bowel habits, privacy for defecation, and occasional stool softeners or laxatives. See also **constipation, obstipation.**

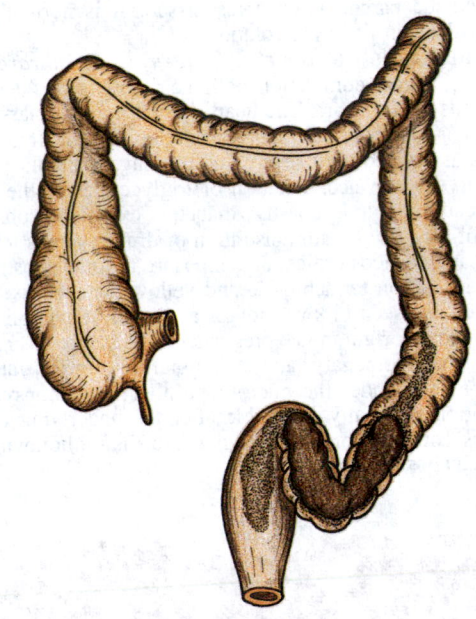

Fecal impaction (Potter, 1991)

fecalith /fē′kəlith/ [L, *faex* + Gk, *lithos,* stone], a hard, impacted mass of feces in the colon. To allow evacuation, an oil retention enema is usually administered; if ineffective, manual removal can be performed. See also **atonia constipation, constipation.**

fecal softener, a drug that lowers the surface tension of the fecal mass, allowing the intestinal fluids to penetrate and soften the stool. Also called **stool softener.**

feces /fē′sēz/ [L, *faex,* dregs], waste or excrement from the digestive tract that is formed in the intestine and expelled through the rectum. Feces consist of water, food residue, bacteria, and secretions of the intestines and liver. Gross examination of feces for color, odor, quantity, and consistency and microscopic examination for the presence of blood, fat, mucus, or parasites are common diagnostic procedures. Also called **stool.** See also **defecation. −fecal,** *adj.*

-fecund. See **fecundity.**

fecundation /fē′kəndā′shən, fek′-/ [L, *fecundare,* to make fruitful], impregnation or fertilization; the act of fertilizing. See also **artificial insemination. −fecundate,** *v.*

fecundity /fikun′ditē/, the ability to produce offspring, especially in large numbers and rapidly; fertility. **−fecund** /fek′ənd, fē′kənd/, *adj.*

Federal Register, a document published by the U.S. government each working day to inform the public of executive regulations, presidential orders, hearings and meetings schedules of various federal agencies, and related matters. The *Federal Register* contains announcements of the Food and Drug Administration, the Environmental Protection Agency, and other government bureaus that regulate matters of health and safety.

Federal Tort Claims Act, a statute passed in 1946 that allows the federal government to be sued for the wrongful action or negligence of its employees. The act, for most purposes, eliminates the doctrine of governmental immunity, which formerly prohibited the bringing of a suit against the federal government.

Federal Trade Commission (FTC), an agency in the executive branch of the federal government created to promote trade and to prevent practices that restrain free enterprise and competition. In the area of health care, the commission successfully challenged the American Medical Association's ban on physician advertising. The FTC held that competition among physicians and the free choice of the consumer were impaired by the antiadvertising policy.

Federation Licensing Examination (FLEX), the standardized licensing examination for state licensure of physicians. Developed by the Federation of State Medical Boards of the United States, the examination is based on National Board of Medical Examiners test materials.

Fede's disease. See **Riga-Fede disease.**

feeblemindedness. See **mental retardation.**

feedback [AS, *faedan, baec*], (in communication theory) information produced by a receiver and perceived by a sender that informs the sender about the receiver's reaction to the message. Feedback is a cyclic part of the process of communication that regulates and modifies the content of messages.

feeding [AS, *faedan*], the act or process of taking or giving food or nourishment. Kinds of feeding include **breast-feeding** and **forced feeding.** See also **alimentation, parenteral nutrition.**

fee-for-service [AS, *feoh*, property; L, *servitum*, slavery], **1.** a charge made for a professional activity, such as a physical examination, the fitting of a contraceptive diaphragm, or the monitoring of a person's blood pressure. **2.** a system for the payment of professional services in which the practitioner is paid for the particular service rendered, rather than receiving a salary for providing professional services as needed during scheduled hours of work or time on call.

Feer's disease. See **acrodynia.**

fee screen system, a method of establishing payment for physician services based on the usual, customary, or reasonable charge according to a regional evaluation. It allows physicians to establish their own reimbursement level for units of service.

feet. See **foot.**

Fehling's solution /fā'lingz/ [Hermann C. von Fehling, German chemist, b. 1812], a solution containing cupric sulfate with sodium hydroxide and potassium sodium tartrate, used for testing for the presence of glucose and other reducing substances in the urine. Also called **Fehling's reagent.**

Feingold diet /fīn'gōld/, a diet developed by American pediatrician Benjamin Feingold for treating hyperactive children. The diet excludes foods manufactured with synthetic colorings, flavorings, and preservatives and limits the intake of fruits and vegetables, that contain salicylates, such

as oranges, apricots, peaches, cucumbers, and tomatoes.

Feldene, a trademark for an antiinflammatory agent (piroxicam).

Feldenkrais therapy /fel'dənkrīs/, (in psychiatry) an alternative therapy based on establishment of a good self-image through awareness and correction of body movements.

feldspar /feld'spär/ [Ger, *feld*, field, *spath*, spar], a crystalline mineral of aluminum silicate with potassium, sodium, barium, and calcium. It melts over a range of 1100° F to 2000° F (593.5° C to 1093° C) and is an important component of dental porcelain.

F element. See **F factor.**

fellatio /fəlā'shō/, oral stimulation of the male genitalia.

fellow [ME, *felaghe*, friendly association], **1.** a member of a learned society. **2.** a graduate student who holds a position in a university or college. **3.** a peer, associate, or person of the same class or rank.

Fellow of the American Academy of Nursing (F.A.A.N.), a member of the American Academy of Nursing. The Academy was established in 1966 by the House of Delegates of the ANA to recognize significant contributions of individuals to the nursing profession.

fellowship /fel'ōship/ [As, *feolaga*, partnership], a grant given to a person for study or training or to allow payment for work on a special project, but not for study toward a degree. It provides a stipend and, in some cases, the miscellaneous expenses involved in the study, training, or project.

felon /fel'ən/ [L, *fel*, venom], a suppurative abscess on the distal phalanx of a finger.

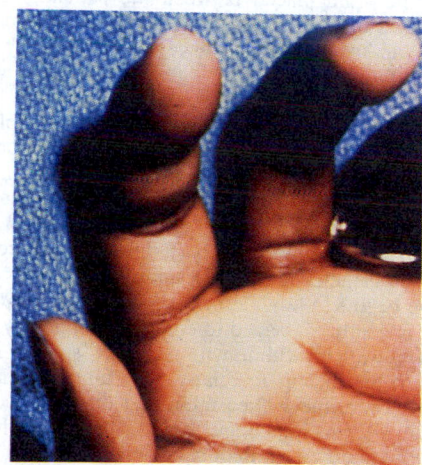

Felon (Lewis, 1989)

felonious assault. See **assault, felony.**

felony /fel'ənē/, (in criminal law) a crime declared by statute to be more serious than a misdemeanor and deserving of a more severe penalty. Conviction usually requires imprisonment in a penitentiary for longer than 1 year. Crimes of murder, rape, burglary, and arson are tried as felonies in most cases. Compare **misdemeanor.**

Felty's syndrome /fel'tēz/ [Augustus R. Felty, American physician, b. 1895], hypersplenism occurring with adult rheumatoid arthritis, characterized by splenomegaly, leukopenia, and frequent infections. The cause of the syndrome is unknown. Surgical resection of the spleen offers temporary improvement in about one half of the cases. See also **hypersplenism.**

female [L, *femella*, young woman], **1.** of or pertaining to the sex that has the ability to become pregnant and bear children; feminine. **2.** a female person.

female catheterization, a procedure for removing urine by means of a urinary catheter introduced through the urinary meatus and urethra into the bladder. The procedure is performed to relieve distention if voluntary micturition is not possible (such as after trauma or surgery), as a preparation for and during anesthesia, if a specimen of urine from the bladder is required, or if medication is to be instilled into the bladder. A straight catheter or a retention catheter with a balloon may be used. A French size 12 to 16 is usually selected for straight drainage. See also **catheterization, male catheterization.**

■ METHOD: The necessary sterile equipment is usually available in a sterile catheterization kit and includes cotton swabs, a bowl for collecting the urine, a disposable catheter, a sponge stick for holding the swabs, a disinfectant for washing the urinary meatus and the perineal area adjacent to it, gloves, a lubricant for the catheter tip, and a drape. Often, a preassembled kit of disposable sterile equipment is available, leaving only the separately packaged catheter to be selected. The patient is positioned on her back, with the knees flexed and the legs abducted, and is then draped. A bright light is directed at the perineum. The nurse then scrubs the hands, dries them well, and opens the catheterization kit or tray carefully, not touching the inside of the wrapper or the contents. Sterile gloves are put on, and the tray is lifted and placed between the patient's legs. The small sterile drape in the kit is placed over the patient so that the window in it allows access to the urinary meatus. With the thumb and the forefinger, the labia are separated and the tissues are retracted, exposing the meatus. The area is cleansed from the front to the back using one pledget or swab for each stroke. Each pledget is discarded before beginning another stroke; three or more strokes are used, and the location of the meatus is verified while the area is cleaned. The catheter is picked up approximately 4 cm from its tip, the tip is lubricated, and the end is placed in the basin. The catheter is inserted approximately 7.5 cm until the urine begins to flow. When the urine stops flowing, the bladder is gently massaged to empty it completely, and the catheter is slowly withdrawn. A sterile sponge is gently pressed to the meatus to remove any lubricant and to dry the area. The urine is measured, and the odor, color, and any abnormal precipitate are noted. A specimen for bacteriologic culture and antibiotic sensitivity is often secured, labeled, and sent to the laboratory.

■ NURSING INTERVENTION: Catheterization is ordered by a physician for an individual patient, or the conditions under which a catheterization is to be performed are stated in written standing orders. Catheterization is needlessly dreaded by many patients; careful explanation may allay the fears. Having the woman take a deep breath may cause the meatus to open slightly, revealing its presence, and asking her to bear down slightly may minimize the momentary discomfort that commonly accompanies the insertion of the catheter into the bladder. Voluntary micturition is almost always preferable, and the nurse encourages the woman to try to void spontaneously. Signs of

infection are carefully observed. If a woman is to be catheterized more than twice, an indwelling catheter is usually preferred to a third catheterization.

■ OUTCOME CRITERIA: Catheterization predisposes the urinary tract to infection, and traumatic catheterization further increases the risk. Care, gentleness, and asepsis are essential. If the bladder is distended with urine, the first 1000 ml may be withdrawn, the catheter clamped, as withdrawing more than that amount at once may cause damage to the bladder, chills, and shock. Certain conditions, including radical vulvectomy, postoperative swelling, or structural anomalies, may obscure the urinary meatus. The indication for catheterization, the age of the patient, and the condition and size of the urethra affect the choice of catheter style and size.

female reproductive system assessment, an evaluation of a patient's genital tract and breasts with an investigation of past and present disorders that may be factors in the individual's current gynecologic condition. See also **pelvic examination.**

■ METHOD: The patient is interviewed to determine if she has lower abdominal pain, cramps, vaginal bleeding, itching, swelling, redness, or a vaginal discharge that is mucoid, watery, frothy, or thick in consistency and white, yellow, greenish, bloody, or brown in color. She is asked if she experiences pain on intercourse and pain or burning on urination. Observations are recorded of her general appearance, vital signs, weight, breast symmetry, texture, and lumps or bumps, nipple color, and the presence of a serous, bloody, or purulent nipple discharge. The abdomen is examined for contour, symmetry, stretch marks, scars, lesions, and visible pulsations and peristaltic waves, and is auscultated for bowel sounds in each quadrant. Carefully noted are edema or redness of the external genitalia, cervix, and perineum, lumps or lesions on the labia majora, the size of the urethral orifice, the presence or absence of the hymenal ring, hymenal tags, perineal scars or excoriation, and a bloody, purulent, or odoriferous discharge. The normal mucoid secretion is distinguished from the thick, white, cheesy discharge typical of candidosis, the frothy, yellow-green, watery liquid characteristic of trichomoniasis, and the thick, yellow-green or brown, and bloody drainage typical of upper genital tract infection. The patient's age at onset of menses, the duration, spacing, and regularity of cycles, the amount and character of the flow, the date of the last menstrual period, and associated symptoms, such as pain and menorrhagia, are investigated. The complications and outcome of each of the patient's pregnancies, the kind of delivery, the incidence and outcome of any abortion, and the date of menopause and associated symptoms, such as hot flushes and dry vaginal mucosa, are explored. It is determined if the patient suffers from a venereal disease, constipation, hemorrhoids, hypothyroidism or hyperthyroidism, polycystic ovary syndrome, hypertension, or blood dyscrasias or has a history of gynecologic or other major abdominal surgery or a serious illness, especially one related to the endocrine system. The patient's smoking habits, sexual activity, use of oral contraceptives or an intrauterine device, her experience with estrogen therapy, and family history of gynecologic diseases and deaths are reported in the assessment. Diagnostic procedures indicated by the history may include a manual examination, Pap test, basal body temperature determination, culture of vaginal discharge, punch biopsy, endometrial biopsy, dilatation and curettage, cold-knife conizations, laparoscopy, ultrasound study, and tubal insufflation. Laboratory studies that may be performed include determinations of levels of human chorionic gonadotropin, serum luteinizing and follicle-stimulating hormones, 17-ketosteroids, and corticosteroids, tests for venereal diseases, and thyroid function tests, such as the basal metabolic rate and protein-bound iodine level.

■ NURSING INTERVENTION: The nurse conducts the interview, records observations of the patient, and collects the pertinent background information and the results of the diagnostic procedures and laboratory studies.

■ OUTCOME CRITERIA: A careful assessment of the patient's reproductive system is essential in establishing the diagnosis.

female sexual dysfunction, impaired or inadequate ability of a woman to engage in or enjoy satisfactory sexual intercourse and orgasm. Symptoms, usually psychologic in origin, include dyspareunia, vaginismus, persistent inability to reach orgasm, and inhibition in sexual arousal, so that congestion and vaginal lubrication are minimal or absent. Causes include anxiety, fear, negative emotions associated with sexual arousal and intercourse, and interpersonal problems. Treatment is focused on eliminating physical problems and sexual anxieties and on enhancing erotic sensitivities. Compare **male sexual dysfunction.** See also **sexual dysfunction.**

female sterility [L, *femella,* little woman, *sterilis,* barren], a condition of being an infertile woman because of congenital defects in the reproductive system, such as failure of the uterus to develop normally, or disease, injury, or corrective surgery affecting functioning of the ovaries, fallopian tubes, uterus, cervix, or vagina.

feminist therapy, an alternative therapy that is both a philosophical approach to the conduct of therapy and a specific type of therapy. The focus of both types is a consciousness raising that focuses on the presence of sexism and sex role stereotyping in society.

feminization /fem'inīzā'shən/ [L, *femina,* woman], **1.** the normal development or induction of female sex characteristics. **2.** the induction of female sex characteristics in a genotypic male. Testicular feminization may be caused by the inability of target tissues to respond to endogenous or administered androgen; some cases seem related to an absent or inadequate conversion of testosterone to dihydrotestosterone, which presumably is the active form of the androgen. Testicular feminization in males with an X and Y chromosome and a female phenotype may be caused by fetal hypogonadism and is often familial. Individuals with this defect usually have undescended or labial testes, a short, blind vaginal pouch, no uterus, well-developed breasts, sparse or absent axillary and pubic hair, normal plasma levels of testosterone and follicle-stimulating hormone, and increased concentrations of estradiol and luteinizing hormone. Treatment consists of orchiectomy because of the risk of cancer in gonads of these patients. Feminization may also be caused by adrenocortical estrogen-secreting tumor, by failure of the liver to inactivate endogenous estrogens, such as in advanced alcoholism, or by the administration of estrogen therapy for androgen-dependent neoplasms. Some testicular tumors may produce feminizing symptoms, and gynecomastia may be caused by Klinefelter's syndrome and by certain drugs, such as reserpine, digitalis, meprobamate, and cimetidine. Compare **virilization.** See also **pseudohermaphroditism.**

feminizing adrenal tumor /fem'inī'zing/, a rare neoplasm of the adrenal cortex, characterized in males by gy-

necomastia, hypertension, diffuse pigmentation, a high level of estrogen in urine, and loss of potency. Testicular atrophy frequently occurs, but the prostate and penis are usually normal in size. The tumor may be large enough to palpate or to be diagnosed by intravenous urography or arteriography. In most cases it is a carcinoma. Treatment includes surgical resection and chemotherapy with mitotane. In women, these tumors, which are extremely rare, are associated with precocious puberty.

femora. See **femur.**

femoral /fem'ərəl/ [L, *femur,* thigh], of or pertaining to the femur or the thigh.

femoral artery, an extension of the external iliac artery into the lower limb, starting just distal to the inguinal ligament and ending at the junction of the middle and lower thirds of the thigh. It divides into seven branches and supplies various parts of the lower limb and trunk, such as the groin and its organs. Its branches are the superficial epigastric, superficial iliac circumflex, superficial external pudendal, deep external pudendal, muscular, profundis femoris, and descending genicular.

femoral condyle, one of a pair of large flared prominences on the distal end of the femur. Identified as lateral and medial femoral condyles, they are covered with a thick layer of hyaline cartilage and articulate with the patella and the tibia at the knee joint.

femoral epiphysis, a secondary bone-forming center of the femur, separated from the main part of the bone by cartilage during the period of bone immaturity. In overweight adolescents there may be bone slippage along the femoral capital epiphysis, marked by pain and loss of range of motion.

femoral hernia, a hernia in which a loop of intestine descends through the femoral canal into the groin. Surgical repair, herniorrhaphy, is the usual treatment. See **hernia.**

femoral nerve, the largest of the seven nerves stemming from the lumbar plexus and the main nerve of the anterior part of the thigh. It arises from the dorsal parts of the ventral primary divisions of the second, third, and fourth lumbar nerves, passes through the lateral, distal fibers of the psoas major, and descends between the psoas major and the iliacus under the cover of the transversalis fascia. Lateral to the femoral artery, it passes under the inguinal ligament, enters the thigh, and breaks into the muscular branches, the anterior cutaneous branches, the intermediate cutaneous nerve, the medial cutaneous nerve, the nerve to the pectineus, the nerve to the sartorius, the saphenous nerve, the branches to the quadriceps femoris, the articular branch to the hip joint, and the articular branches to the knee joint. Also called **anterior crural nerve.**

femoral pulse, the pulse of the femoral artery, palpated in the groin.

femoral reflex [L, *femur,* thigh, *reflectere,* to bend back], an extension of the knee and a plantar flexion of the foot which occurs when the skin is stimulated on the upper anterior third of the thigh.

femoral torsion, an extreme lateral or a medial twisting rotation of the femur on its longitudinal axis, which may be caused by the action of the gluteal muscles. Compare **tibial torsion.**

femoral vein, a large vein in the thigh originating in the popliteal vein and accompanying the femoral artery in the proximal two thirds of the thigh. Its distal portion lies lateral to the artery; its proximal portion deeper to the artery.

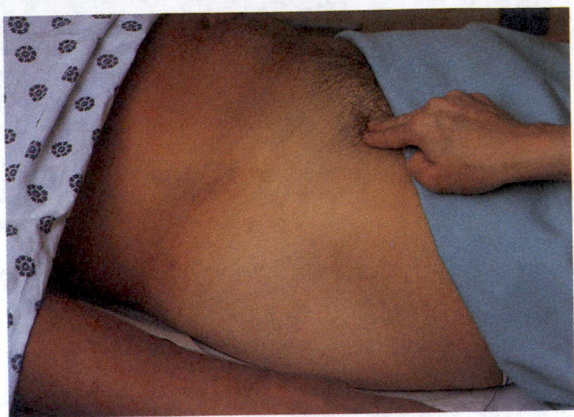

Palpation of femoral pulse (Potter, 1993)

About 4 cm below the inguinal ligament it is joined by the deep femoral vein. Near its termination it is joined by the great saphenous vein. It receives tributaries from the branches of the deep femoral artery and receives the medial and the lateral femoral circumflex veins. At the inguinal ligament it becomes the external iliac vein. The femoral vein has four valves.

Femstat, a trademark for an antifungal drug (butoconazole nitrate).

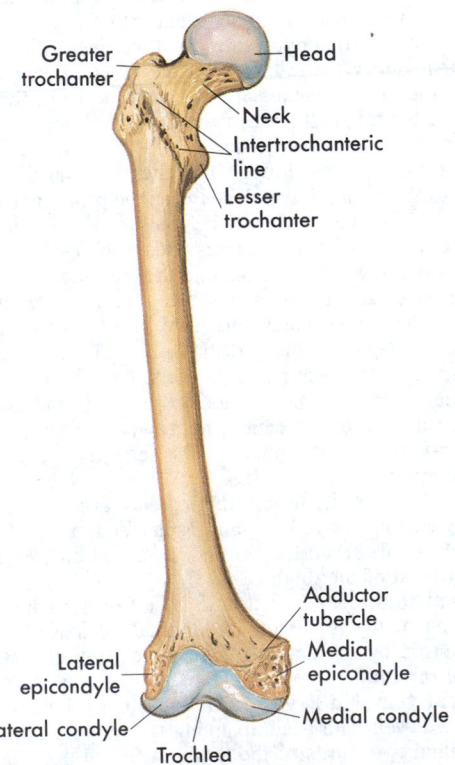

Femur (Thibodeau, 1993)

femur /fē'mər/, *pl.* **femora, femurs** [L, thigh], the thigh bone, which extends from the pelvis to the knee. It is largely cylindric and is the longest and strongest bone in the body. It has a large, round head that fits the acetabulum of the hip, and it displays a large neck and several prominences and ridges for muscle attachments. In an erect posture it inclines medially, bringing the knee joint near the line of gravity of the body. The degree of this inclination is usually greater in a woman than in a man. Also called **thigh bone.**

fenestra /fines'trə/, *pl.* **fenestrae** [L, window], an aperture, especially in a bandage or cast, that is often cut out to relieve pressure or to administer regular skin care.

fenestra cochlea, fenestra rotunda. See **round window.**

fenestrae. See **fenestra.**

-fenestrate. See **fenestration.**

fenestrated /fen'əstrā'tid/ [L, *fenestra,* window], pertaining to a membrane or other object that has numerous small holes or openings.

fenestrated drape, a drape with a round or slitlike opening in the center.

fenestration /fen'əstrā'shən/ [L, *fenestra,* window], **1.** a surgical procedure in which an opening is created in order to gain access to the cavity within an organ or a bone. **2.** an opening created surgically in a bone or organ of the body. Also called **window.** —**fenestrate,** *v.*

fenfluramine hydrochloride /fenfloor'əmēn/, a sympathomimetic anorectic agent.

■ INDICATION: It is prescribed to decrease the appetite in exogenous obesity.

■ CONTRAINDICATIONS: Glaucoma, alcoholism, severe hypertension, use of a monoamine oxidase inhibitor within 14 days, or known hypersensitivity to this drug or to other sympathomimetic medication prohibits its use.

■ ADVERSE EFFECTS: Among the more serious adverse reactions are drug dependence, diarrhea, mental confusion, and depression.

fenoprofen calcium /fē'nəprō'fen/, a nonsteroidal antiinflammatory agent and analgesic.

■ INDICATIONS: It is prescribed in the treatment of arthritis and other painful inflammatory conditions.

■ CONTRAINDICATIONS: Renal dysfunction, upper GI disease, or known hypersensitivity to this drug, to aspirin, or to nonsteroidal antiinflammatory medication prohibits its use.

■ ADVERSE EFFECTS: Among the more serious adverse reactions are GI disturbances, gastric or duodenal ulceration, dizziness, skin rash, and tinnitus. The drug interacts with many other drugs.

fenoterol /fen'ōter'ol/, a beta-adrenergic drug used in respiratory therapy. It reportedly induces a dose-related decrease in lung recoil pressure that can reduce the effort in breathing for some patients.

fentanyl, a potent, narcotic analgesic, used most commonly with the sedative and antipsychotic drug droperidol as an adjunct in anesthesia.

fentanyl citrate /fen'tənil/, a narcotic analgesic.

■ INDICATIONS: It is prescribed as an adjunct to general anesthesia, as a preoperative and postoperative analgesic, and as a component in neuroleptanesthesia and analgesia.

■ CONTRAINDICATIONS: Myasthenia gravis, use of a monoamine oxidase inhibitor within 14 days, or known hypersensitivity to this drug prohibits its use.

■ ADVERSE EFFECTS: Among the more serious adverse reactions are drug dependence, hypotension, pruritus, respiratory depression, and laryngospasm.

Feosol, a trademark for a hematinic (ferrous sulfate).

-fer, a combining form meaning 'something that carries something': *parasitifer, sonifer, vaccinifer.*

Fergon, a trademark for a hematinic (ferrous gluconate).

Ferguson's reflex, a contraction of the uterus after the cervix is stimulated. The reflex is an important function of labor.

fermentation /fur'məntā'shən/ [L, *fermentare,* to cause to rise], a chemical change that is brought about in a substance by the action of an enzyme or microorganism, especially the anaerobic conversion of foodstuffs to certain products. Kinds of fermentation are **acetic fermentation, alcoholic fermentation, ammoniacal fermentation, amylic fermentation, butyric fermentation, caseous fermentation, dextran fermentation, diastatic fermentation, lactic acid fermentation, propionic fermentation, storing fermentation,** and **viscous fermentation.**

fermentative dyspepsia /fərmen'tətiv/, an abnormal condition characterized by impaired digestion associated with the fermentation of digested food. See also **dyspepsia.**

fermium (Fm) /fur'mē·əm/ [Enrico Fermi, Italian physicist, b. 1901], a synthetic transuranic metallic element. Its atomic number is 100; its atomic weight is 257. Fermium was first detected in the debris from a hydrogen bomb explosion and later produced in a reactor. Ten isotopes of fermium have been identified.

ferning test /fur'ning/ [AS, *faern,* fern; L, *testum,* crucible], a technique used to determine the presence of estrogen in the uterine cervical mucus. It is often used as a test for ovulation; high levels of estrogen cause the cervical mucus to dry on a slide in a fernlike pattern. Also called **arborization test.**

-ferous, a suffix meaning 'producing or carrying' something specified: *lactiferous, sebiferous, tubiferous.*

ferr-, ferri-. See **ferro-.**

ferric /fer'ik/, pertaining to a compound of iron in which the metal is trivalent, such as ferric chloride and ferric hydroxide.

ferritin /fur'itin/ [L, *ferrum,* iron], an iron compound formed in the intestine and stored in the liver, spleen, and bone marrow for eventual incorporation into hemoglobin molecules. Serum ferritin levels are used as an indicator of the body's iron stores. Normal findings are 12-300 ng/ml for males and 10-150 ng/ml for females.

ferro-, ferr-, ferri-, a combining form meaning 'pertaining to iron': *ferrocyanide, ferropectic, ferrosilicon.*

ferromagnetic /fer'ōmagnat'ik/, pertaining to substances, such as iron, nickel, and cobalt, that are strongly affected by magnetism and may become magnetized by exposure to a magnetic field.

ferrous sulfate /fer'əs/, a hematinic agent.

■ INDICATION: It is prescribed in the treatment of iron deficiency anemia.

■ CONTRAINDICATIONS: There are no known contraindications.

■ ADVERSE EFFECTS: Among the most serious adverse reactions are gastrointesinal irritation, diarrhea, and constipation.

fertile /fur'təl/ [L, *fertilis,* fruitful], **1.** capable of reproducing or bearing offspring. **2.** (of a gamete) capable of inducing fertilization or being fertilized. **3.** prolific; fruitful; not sterile. **−fertility,** *n.,* **fertilize,** *v.*

fertile eunuch syndrome, a hypogonadotropic hormonal disorder occurring only in males in which the quantity of testosterone and follicle stimulating hormone is inadequate for the inducement of spermatogenesis and the development

of secondary sexual characteristics. If supplemental hormones are not prescribed, the affected person acquires the appearance of a eunuch.

fertile period, the time in the menstrual cycle during which fertilization may occur. Spermatozoa can survive for 48 to 72 hours; the ovum lives for 24 hours. Thus, the fertile period begins 2 to 3 days before ovulation and lasts for 2 to 3 days afterward. The fertile period may be identified by observation of the changes in the quantity and character of the cervical mucus or of changes in the basal body temperature, or it may be deleted. from a calendar record of six or more menstrual cycles, applying the fact that ovulation usually occurs 14 days before menstruation.

fertility /fərtil'itē/, the ability to reproduce.

fertility factor. See **F factor.**

fertility rate, the number of live births divided by the number of females aged 15 through 44. It is usually expressed as the number per 1000 women.

fertilization /fur'tilīzā'shən/ [L, *fertilis,* fruitful], the union of male and female gametes to form a zygote from which the embryo develops. The process usually takes place in the outer one-third of the fallopian tube of the female when a spermatozoon, carried in the seminal fluid discharged during coitus, comes in contact with and penetrates the ovum. Rapid chemical changes in the membrane of the ovum prevent the entrance of additional spermatozoa. Penetration by the spermatozoon stimulates the completion of the second meiotic division and formation of the pronucleus in the ovum. Fusion and synapsis of the male and female pronuclei restore the diploid number of chromosomes to the germ cell, resulting in the determination of the sex of the zygote and of the characteristics inherited from each parent, and stimulate the initiation of development through cleavage. Kinds of fertilization include **cross-fertilization, external fertilization,** and **internal fertilization.** See also **in-vitro fertilization, oogenesis, spermatogenesis.**

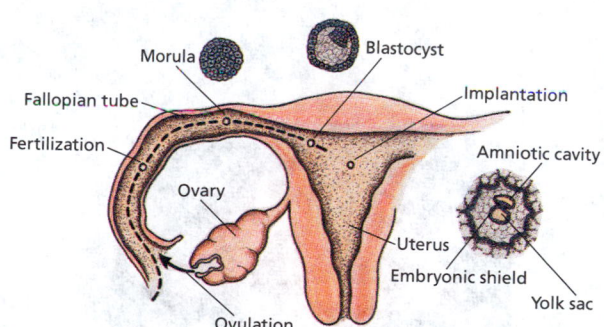

Fertilization cycle (Potter, 1991)

fertilization age. See **fetal age.**

fertilization membrane, a viscous membrane surrounding the fertilized ovum that prevents penetration of additional spermatozoa. It is formed by granules from the cytoplasm of the fertilized ovum adhering to the vitelline membrane.

fertilize. See **fertile.**

fertilizin /fərtil'izin/, a glycoprotein found on the plasma membrane of the ovum in various species. It was once thought that the specific agglutinizing receptor groups of the substance were complementary to antifertilizin, a substance extracted from the sperm, and were responsible for binding the spermatozoon to the ovum during the early stage of fertilization, but the theory has since been discarded. See also **acrosomal reaction.**

Festal, a trademark for a GI fixed-combination drug containing a group of digestive enzymes and bile constituents.

festinating gait [L, *festinare,* to hasten], a manner of walking in which the speed of the person increases in an unconscious effort to 'catch up' with a displaced center of gravity. It is a common characteristic of Parkinson's disease.

festoon [Fr *feston* scallop], a carving in the base material of a denture that simulates the contours of the natural gingival tissues. See also **gingival festoon, McCall's festoon.**

fetal /fē′təl/ [L, *fetus*], pertaining to the final stage of development of an embryonic mammal. In humans, the fetal period extends from the end of the eighth week of intrauterine life until birth.

fetal abortion [L, *fetus*], termination of pregnancy after the twentieth week of gestation but before the fetus has developed enough to live outside of the uterus. Compare **embryonic abortion.**

fetal activity determination. See **nonstress test.**

fetal advocate, a person who regards the health and well-being of the fetus as a matter of top priority.

fetal age, the age of the conceptus computed from the time elapsed since fertilization. Also called **fertilization age.** Compare **gestational age.**

fetal alcohol syndrome (FAS) [L, *fetus*; Ar, *alkohl,* essence; Gk, *syn,* together, *dromos,* course], a set of congenital psychological, behavioral, cognitive, and physical abnormalities that tend to appear in infants whose mothers consumed alcoholic beverages during pregnancy. It is characterized by typical craniofacial and limb defects, cardiovascular defects, intrauterine growth retardation, and re-

tarded development. The most serious cases have involved infants born to mothers who were chronic alcoholics and drank heavily during pregnancy. Women who drank less reportedly gave birth to infants with less serious malformations, or **fetal alcohol effects (FAE),** but it is not known if there is a lower limit to alcohol consumption during pregnancy or if there is a particular period in embryonic life when the offspring is most vulnerable to effects of alcohol.

fetal alveoli, the terminal pulmonary sacs of a fetus, which are filled with fluid before birth. The fluid is a transudate of fetal plasma.

fetal asphyxia, a condition of hypoxemia, hypercapnia, and respiratory and metabolic acidosis that may occur in the uterus. Among possible causes are uteroplacental insufficiency, abruptio placentae, placenta previa, uterine tetany, maternal hypotension, and compression of the umbilical cord.

fetal attitude, the relationship of the fetal parts to each other, such as the 'military' attitude, in which the fetal head is not flexed and the chin on chest is as usual but is held straight up. Compare **fetal position, fetal presentation.**

fetal bradycardia, an abnormally slow fetal heart rate, usually below 100 beats per minute.

fetal circulation, the pathway of blood circulation in the fetus. Oxygenated blood from the placenta travels through the umbilical vein to the liver and the ductus venosus, which carries it to the inferior vena cava and right atrium. The blood enters the right atrium at a pressure sufficient to di-

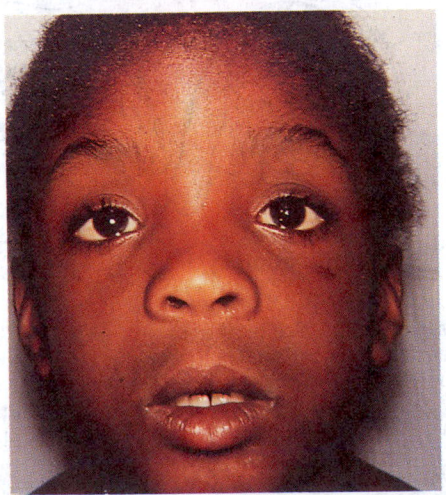

Fetal alcohol syndrome *(Zitelli, 1992)*

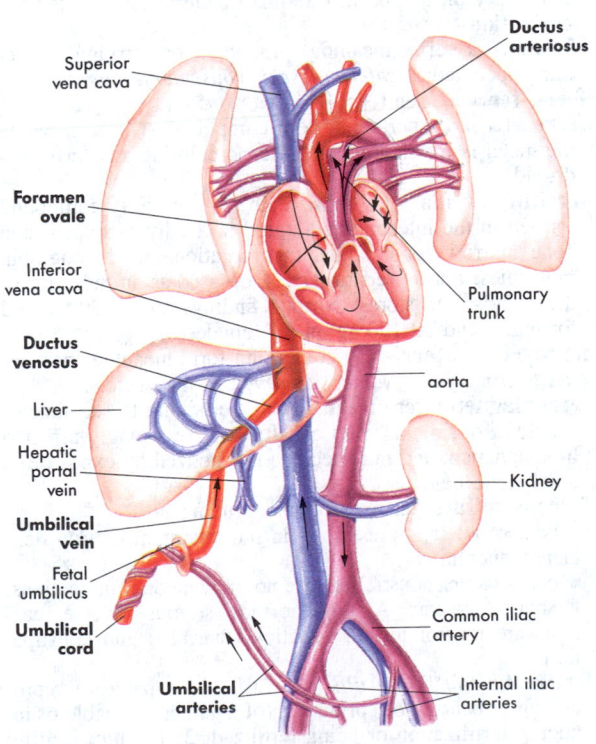

Fetal circulation
(Thibodeau, 1993/Molly Babich/John Dougherty)

rect the flow across the atrium and through the foramen ovale into the left atrium; thus, oxygenated blood is available for circulation through the left ventricle to the head and upper extremities. The blood returning from the head and arms enters the right atrium via the superior vena cava. It flows through the atrium at a relatively low pressure; passing the tricuspid valve, the blood falls into the right ventricle, from which it is pumped through the pulmonary artery and the ductus arteriosus into the descending aorta for circulation to the lower parts of the body. A small amount of blood in the pulmonary artery is not shunted through the ductus and is carried to the lungs. The blood is returned to the placenta through the umbilical arteries.

fetal death, the intrauterine death of a fetus, or the death of a fetus weighing at least 500 g or after 20 or more weeks of gestation.

fetal distress, a compromised condition of the fetus, usually discovered during labor, characterized by a markedly abnormal rate or rhythm of myocardial contraction. Some patterns, such as late decelerations of the fetal heart rate seen on records of electronic fetal monitoring, are indicative of fetal distress. If possible, the cause of the situation is identified and corrected and the acid-base balance of the fetal blood is tested. Labor is allowed to continue if the pH is within normal range and if the abnormal pattern does not recur or persist. Cesarean section may be necessary if the fetus is markedly alkalotic or acidotic or if the cause of the problem cannot be corrected. If possible, the baby is stabilized before being delivered by giving the mother oxygen, increased fluids, or a narcotic antagonist, a vasopressor, or an agent to relax the uterus. A pediatrician is required to attend the birth of a distressed baby to manage resuscitation and care immediately after delivery.

fetal dose, the estimated amount of radiation received by a fetus during an x-ray examination of a pregnant woman. It is calculated in millirads per 1000 milliroentgens of skin exposure and varies from less than 1 mrad when an extremity is being examined to nearly 300 mrad when the beam is directed toward the pelvis.

fetal heart rate (FHR), the number of heartbeats in the fetus occurring in a given unit of time. The FHR varies in cycles of fetal rest and activity and is affected by many factors, including maternal fever, uterine contractions, maternal-fetal hypotension, and many drugs. The normal FHR is more than 100 beats per minute and less than 160 beats per minute. In labor the FHR is monitored with a fetoscope or an electronic fetal monitor to detect abnormal alterations in the rate, especially recurrent decelerations that continue past the end of uterine contractions.

fetal heart sound [L, *fētus*; AS, *heorte*; L, *sonus*, sound], the beats of the fetal heart as detected by auscultation or by electronic fetal monitoring. The embryonic heart begins beating at about 14 days of intrauterine life.

fetal heart tones (fht), the pulsations of the fetal heart heard through the maternal abdomen in pregnancy. The rate, usually between 120 and 160 beats per minute, tends to increase briefly with or just after fetal movement.

fetal hemoglobin, hemoglobin F, the major hemoglobin present in the blood of a fetus and neonate. Hemoglobin F is present in only trace amounts in the blood of normal adults.

fetal hydantoin syndrome (FHS), a complex of birth defects associated with prenatal maternal ingestion of hydan-

toin derivatives. Symptoms of FHS include microcephaly, hypoplasia or absence of nails on the fingers or toes, abnormal facies, mental and physical retardation, and cardiac defects. The syndrome occurs to some degree in 10% to 40% of infants born of mothers for whom this anticonvulsant has been prescribed. Hydantoin sometimes appears to be associated with hemorrhage and, more rarely, with neural crest tumors in the newborn.

fetal hydrops. See **hydrops fetalis.**

fetal lie, the relationship of the long axis of the fetus to the long axis of the mother. See also **fetal presentation.**

fetal lipoma. See **hibernoma.**

fetal membranes, the structures that protect, support, and nourish the embryo and fetus, including the yolk sac, allantois, amnion, chorion, placenta, and umbilical cord.

fetal monitor. See **electronic fetal monitor.**

fetal mortality, the number of fetal deaths per 1000 births, or per live births.

fetal movements [L, *fētus, movere,* to move], muscular movements produced by the fetus *in utero* beginning around the fifth month of life. The early fetal movements can be felt by the mother.

fetal placenta [L, *fētus, placenta,* flat cake], the portion of the placenta that is formed from the shaggy chorion frondosum, the villi of which invade the decidua basalis. Also called **pars fetalis.**

fetal position, the relationship of the part of the fetus that presents in the pelvis to four quadrants of the maternal pelvis identified by initial L (left), R (right), A (anterior), and P (posterior). The presenting part is also identified by initial O (occiput), M (mentum), and S (sacrum). If a fetus presents with the occiput directed to the posterior aspect of the mother's right side, the fetal position is right occiput posterior (ROP). Compare **fetal attitude, fetal presentation.**

fetal presentation, the part of the fetus that first appears in the pelvis. Cephalic presentations include vertex, brow, and chin; breech presentations include frank breech, complete breech, and single or double footling breech. Shoulder presentations are rare and require cesarean section or turning before vaginal delivery. Compound presentation involves the entry of more than one part in the true pelvis; most commonly a hand next to the head. See also **fetal attitude, fetal lie, fetal position.**

fetal rest. See **embryonic rest.**

fetal rickets. See **achondroplasia.**

fetal rotation [L, *fētus, rotare,* to rotate], the turning of the head of the fetus as it begins the descent through the birth canal. The fetal head may be rotated by hand or with forceps if needed to guide the body in a proper position for delivery.

fetal stage, (in embryology) the interval of time from the end of the embryonic stage, at the end of the seventh week of gestation, to birth, 38 to 42 weeks after the first day of the last menstrual period.

fetal tachycardia, a fetal heart rate that continues at 160 or more beats per minute for more than 10 minutes.

feti-, feto-, foeti-, foeto-, a combining form meaning 'fetus or fetal': *feticide, fetochorionic, fetoscope.*

feticide. See **embryoctony.**

fetid /fet'id, fē'tid/ [L, *fetere,* to stink], pertaining to something that has a foul or putrid odor.

fetish [Fr, *fetiche,* artificial], **1.** any object or idea given unreasonable or excessive attention or reverence. **2.** (in psychology) any inanimate object or any part of the body not of a sexual nature that arouses erotic feelings or fixation. The erotic symbology is unique to the fetishist and results from unconscious associations. **—fetishism,** *n.*

fetishist /fet′ishist/, a person who believes in or receives erotic gratification from fetishes.

feto-. See **feti-.**

fetochorionic /fē′tōkôr′ē·on′ik/ [L, *fetus* + Gk, *chorion,* a skin], of or pertaining to the fetus and the chorion.

fetofetal transfusion. See **parabiotic syndrome.**

fetography /fētog′rəfē/ [L, *fetus* + Gk, *graphein,* to record], roentgenography of the fetus in utero. See also **fetometry.**

fetology /fētol′əjē/ [L, *fetus* + Gk, *logos,* science], the branch of medicine that is concerned with the fetus in utero, including the diagnosis of abnormalities, congenital anomalies, the prevention of teratogenic influences, and the treatment of certain disorders. Also called **embryatrics.**

fetometry /fētom′ətrē/ [L, *fetus* + Gk, *metron,* measure], the measurement of the size of the fetus, especially the diameter of the head and circumference of the trunk. A kind of fetometry is **roentgen fetometry.**

fetoplacental /-pləsen′təl/ [L, *fetus* + *placenta,* flat cake], of or pertaining to the fetus and the placenta.

fetoprotein /-prō′tēn/ [L, *fetus* + Gk, *proteios,* first rank], an antigen that occurs naturally in fetuses and occasionally in adults as the result of certain diseases. Leukemia, hepatoma, sarcoma, and other neoplasms are associated with **beta fetoprotein** in the blood of adults. An increased amount of **alpha fetoprotein** in the fetus is diagnostic for neural tube defects.

fetor hepaticus [L, stench; *hepar* liver], foul-smelling breath associated with severe liver disease. Also called **liver breath.**

fetoscope /fē′təskōp′/ [L, *fetus* + Gk, *skopein,* to look], a stethoscope for auscultating the fetal heartbeat through the mother's abdomen.

fetoscopy /fētos′kəpē/, a procedure in which a fetus may be directly observed in utero, using a fetoscope introduced through a small incision in the abdomen under local anesthesia. Photographs of the fetus may be taken, and amniotic fluid, fetal cells, or blood may be sampled for prenatal diagnosis of many congenital anomalies or genetic defects.

fetotoxic /-tok′sik/ [L, *fetus* + Gk, *toxikon,* poison], pertaining to anything that is poisonous to a fetus.

fetus /fē′təs/ [L, fruitful], the unborn offspring of any viviparous animal after it has attained the particular form of the species, more specifically, the human being in utero after the embryonic period and the beginning of the development of the major structural features, usually from the eighth week after fertilization until birth. Kinds of fetuses include **anideus, lithopedion, mummified fetus, parasitic fetus,** and **sirenomelia.** Also spelled **foetus.** Compare **embryo.** See also **prenatal development. —fetal, foetal,** *adj.*

fetus acardiacus, fetus acardius. See **acardia.**

fetus amorphus, a shapeless conceptus in which there are no formed or recognizable parts.

fetus anideus. See **anideus.**

fetus in fetu /infē′too/, a fetal anomaly in which a small, imperfectly formed twin, incapable of independent existence, is contained within the body of the normal twin, the autosite.

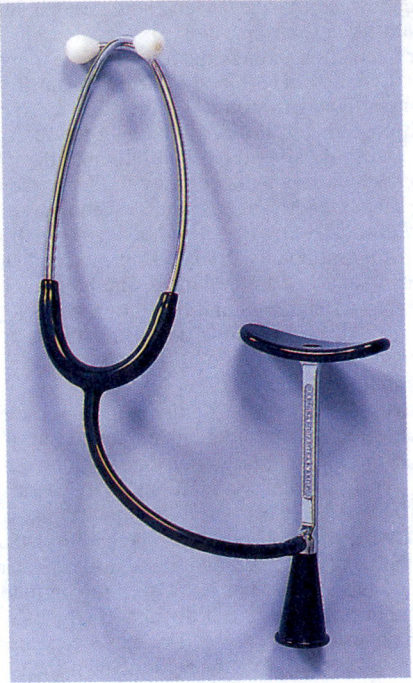

Fetoscope *(Seidel, 1991)*

fetus papyraceus, a twin fetus that has died in utero early in development and has been pressed flat against the uterine wall by the living fetus. Also called **paper-doll fetus, papyraceous fetus.**

fetus sanguinolentis /sang′gwinəlen′tis/, a darkly colored, partly macerated fetus that has died in utero.

FEV, abbreviation for **forced expiratory volume.**

fever [L, *febris*], an abnormal elevation of the temperature of the body above 37° C (98.6° F) because of disease. Fever results from an imbalance between the elimination and the production of heat. Exercise, anxiety, and dehydration may increase the temperature of healthy people. Infection, neurologic disease, malignancy, pernicious anemia, thromboembolic disease, paroxysmal tachycardia, congestive heart failure, crushing injury, severe trauma, and many drugs may cause the development of fever. No single theory explains the mechanism whereby the temperature is increased. Fever has no recognized function in conditions other than infection. It increases metabolic activity by 7% per degree Celsius, requiring a greater intake of food. Convulsions may occur in children whose fevers tend to rise abruptly, and delirium is seen with high fevers in adults and in children. Very high temperatures, as in heatstroke, may be fatal. The course of a fever varies with the cause and the condition of the patient and with the treatment given. The onset may be abrupt or gradual, and the period of maximum elevation, called the stadium or fastigium, may last for a few days or up to 3 weeks. The fever may resolve suddenly, by crisis, or gradually, by lysis. Certain diseases and conditions are associated with fevers that begin, rise, and fall in such characteristic curves that diagnosis may be made by studying a graphic record of the course of the fever. Kinds of hyperthermia include **habitual fever, inter-**

mittent fever, and relapsing fever. See also fever treatment, hyperpyrexia.

fever blister, a cold sore caused by herpesvirus I or II. Also called herpes simplex.

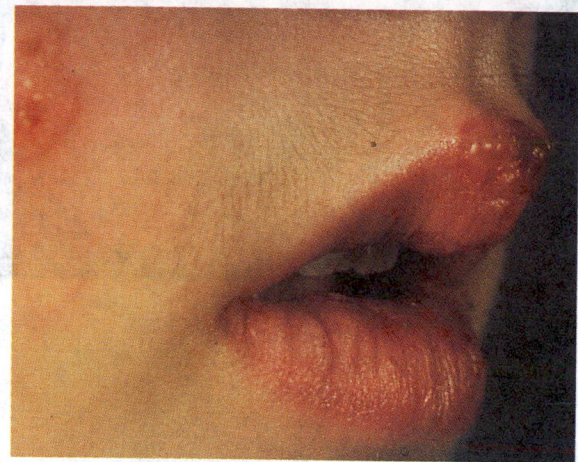

Fever blister (Epstein, 1992)

fever of unknown origin (FUO), a fever of at least 101° F (38.3 C) that persists for at least 3 weeks without discovery of the cause despite at least 1 week of intensive study.

fever therapy. See artificial fever.

fever treatment, the care and management of a person with an elevated temperature.

■ METHOD: The patient is observed for symptoms of fever, such as tachycardia; a full, bounding pulse or a weak, thready pulse; rapid breathing; hot, dry, hyperemic skin; chills; headache; diaphoresis; restlessness; delirium; dehydration; tremors; convulsions; and coma. Treatment may include the administration of antibiotic, antipyretic, and sedative drugs. If the temperature is extremely high, an alcohol sponge bath, cooling tub bath, cold wet sheet, ice packs, or hypothermia may be ordered. The patient's temperature is checked every 2 to 4 hours. Antipyretic and sedative therapy is continued as ordered and, if necessary, cooling measures are reinstituted; the room temperature is reduced, and air currents are increased by a fan. Increased amounts of fluids are given orally or parenterally, physical activity is reduced, and the skin is exposed to air.

■ INTERVENTIONS: The nurse observes and records the symptoms accompanying fever, administers the ordered medication and cooling measures, reassures the patient, and explains the importance of therapy and of drinking adequate fluids.

■ OUTCOME CRITERIA: Antipyretic drugs and cooling measures usually reduce the temperature, but the patient may require additional fluids and treatment for the underlying cause of the fever.

F factor, (in bacterial genetics) an episome present in conjugating male bacteria but absent in females. Also called F element, fertility factor, sex factor.

FFA, abbreviation for free fatty acid.

18F-FDG, symbol for [18F]-2-fluoro-2-deoxy-D-glucose, a sugar analog used in positron emission tomography to determine the local cerebral metabolic rate of glucose as a measure of neural activity in the brain.

FHR, abbreviation for fetal heart rate.

FHS, abbreviation for fetal hydantoin syndrome.

rhitidoplasty. See face lift.

fht, abbreviation for fetal heart tones.

fiber diet /fī'bər/ [L, fibra; Gk, diata, way of living], a diet that contains an abundance of fibrous material, such as cellulose, hemicellulose, pectin, and lignin, that resists digestion. Fibrous foods are found mainly in vegetables, fruits, and cereals. They add bulk to the diet, reduce the incidence of constipation, and reportedly reduce the risk of bowel cancer.

fiberoptic bronchoscopy /-op'tik/ [L, fibra + Gk, optikos, sight], the visual examination of the tracheobronchial tree through a fiberoptic bronchoscope. Also called bronchofibroscopy. See also bronchoscopy, fiberoptics.

fiberoptic duodenoscope, an instrument for visualizing the interior of the duodenum, consisting of an eyepiece, a flexible tube incorporating bundles of coated glass or plastic fibers with special optic properties, and a terminal light. When the duodenoscope is introduced into the patient's mouth and threaded through the upper digestive tract to the duodenum, the light illuminates the internal structures and any lesions present, and the fiberoptic bundles transmit the image to the observer's eyepiece.

fiberoptics /-op'tiks/, the technical process by which an internal organ or cavity can be viewed, using glass or plastic fibers to transmit light through a specially designed tube and reflect a magnified image. —fiberoptic, adj.

fiberscope /fī'bərskōp/ [L, fibra + Gk, skopein, to look], a flexible fiberoptic instrument having an inner shaft coated with light-conveying glass or plastic fibers for visualization of internal structures. Fiberscopes are specially designed for the examination of particular organs and cavities of the body and are used in bronchoscopy, endoscopy, and gastroscopy.

-fibrate, a combining form for clofibrate-type compounds.

fibril /fī'bril/ [L, fibrilla, small fiber], a small filamentous structure that often is a component of a cell, as in a mitotic spindle.

fibrillation /fī'brilā'shən/ [L, fibrilla, small fiber, atio, process], involuntary recurrent contraction of a single muscle fiber or of an isolated bundle of nerve fibers. Fibrillation of a chamber of the heart results in inefficient random contraction of that chamber and disruption of the normal sinus rhythm of the heart. Fibrillation is usually described by the part that is contracting abnormally, such as atrial fibrillation or ventricular fibrillation.

fibrillin /fibri'lin/ [L, fibrilla, small fiber], a major component of elastin-associated microfibrils linked to Marfan syndrome by immunohistochemical studies. Fibrillin is also associated with a disease similar to Marfan syndrome, arachnodactyly.

fibrin /fī'brin/ [L, fibra, fiber], a stringy, insoluble protein produced by the action of thrombin on fibrinogen in the clotting process. Fibrin is responsible for the semisolid character of a blood clot. Compare fibrinogen. See also blood clotting, coagulation, fibrinolysis, thrombin.

fibrinase. See factor XIII.

fibrinogen /fībrin'əjən/ [L, fibra, fiber; Gk, genein, to produce], a plasma protein that is converted into fibrin by thrombin in the presence of calcium ions. Compare fibrin. See also afibrinogenemia, blood clotting, fibrinolysis, thrombin.

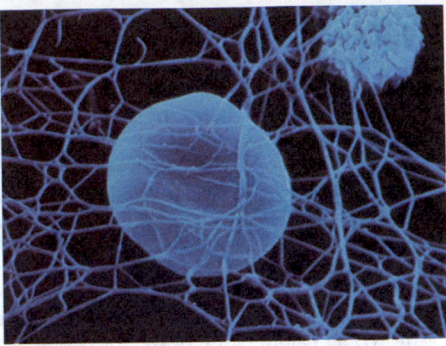

Fibrin (Gottfried, 1993/Manfred Kage/Peter Arnold, Inc)

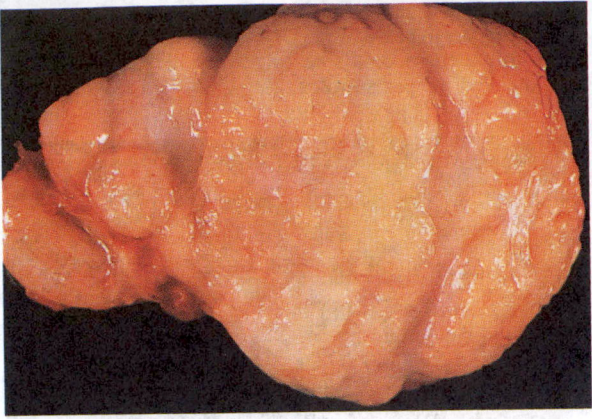

Fibroadenoma (Fletcher, 1987)

fibrinogenic [L, *fibra,* fiber; Gk, *genein,* to produce], See **fibrogenous; fibrinogenous**.

fibrinogenopenia /fī′brōjen′ōpē′nē·ə/ [L, *fibra* + Gk, *genein,* to produce, *penes,* poor], a condition in which a deficiency of fibrinogen in the blood exists.

fibrinogenous /fī′brinōj′ənəs/ [L, *fibra,* fiber; Gk, *genein,* to produce], pertaining to the characteristics or properties of fibrinogen, or the production of fibrin.

fibrinokinase /fī′brinōkī′nās/ [L, *fibra* + Gk, *kinesis,* motion], a non-water-soluble enzyme in animal tissue that activates plasminogen. Also called **tissue activator, tissue kinase.**

fibrinolysin /fī′brinol′isin/ [L, *fibra* + Gk, *lysein,* to loosen], a proteolytic enzyme that dissolves fibrin. It is formed from plasminogen in the blood plasma. Also called **plasmin.** See also **fibrinolysis.**

fibrinolysis /fī′brinol′isis/, the continual process of fibrin decomposition by fibrinolysin that is the normal mechanism for the removal of small fibrin clots. It is stimulated by anoxia, inflammatory reactions, and other kinds of stress. **–fibrinolytic,** *adj.*

fibrinopeptide /fī′brinōpep′tīd/ [L, *fibra* + Gk, *peptein,* to digest], a product of the action of thrombin on fibrinogen. The enzymatic cleavage responsible for the release of this protein fragment produces fibrin as well as the fibrinopeptides A and B. The latter consist of short peptides derived from the N-terminal ends of the alpha and beta chains of the fibrinogen molecule. See also **fibrinogen, thrombin.**

fibrinous pericarditis [L, *fibra,* fiber; Gk, *peri,* near, *kardia,* heart, *itis,* inflammation], a condition in which a lymph exudate accumulates on the pericardium and coagulates. The coagulated exudate may acquire a thick buttery appearance.

fibrin-stabilizing factor. See **factor XIII.**

fibro- /fī′brō-/, a combining form meaning 'pertaining to fiber': *fibroadipose, fibroblast, fibroelastosis.*

fibroadenoma /fī′brō·ad′inō′mə/, *pl.* **fibroadenomas, fibroadenomata** [L, *fibra* + Gk, *aden,* gland, *oma*], a benign tumor composed of dense epithelial and fibroblastic tissue. A fibroadenoma of the breast is nontender, encapsulated, round, movable, and firm. It occurs most frequently in women under 25 years of age and is caused by greater than usual amounts of estrogen. Surgical excision under local anesthesia and cytologic examination of the mass are usually performed to be sure it is not cancerous.

fibroangioma. See **angiofibroma.**

fibroareolar tissue. See **areolar tissue.**

fibroblast /fī′brəblast/ [L, *fibra* + Gk, *blastos,* germ], a flat, elongated undifferentiated cell in the connective tissue that gives rise to various precursor cells, such as the chondroblast, collagenoblast, and osteoblast, that form the fibrous, binding, and supporting tissue of the body. Also called **desmocyte, fibrocyte. –fibroblastic,** *adj.*

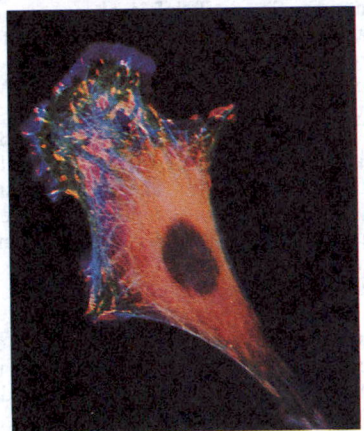

Fibroblast (Gottfried, 1993/JV Small & F Rinnerthaler)

fibroblastoma /-blastōma/, *pl.* **fibroblastomas, fibroblastomata** [L, *fibra* + Gk, *blastos,* germ, *oma*], a tumor derived from a fibroblast, now differentiated as a fibroma or a fibrosarcoma.

fibrocarcinoma. See **scirrhous carcinoma.**

fibrocartilage /-kär′tilij/ [L, *fibra* + *cartilago*]], cartilage that consists of a dense matrix of white collagenous fibers. Of the three kinds of cartilage in the body, fibrocartilage has the greatest tensile strength. Fibrocartilaginous disks between the vertebrae help to cushion the jolts to which the vertebral column is continually subjected. See also **hyaline cartilage. –fibrocartilaginous,** *adj.*

fibrocartilaginous joint. See **symphysis.**

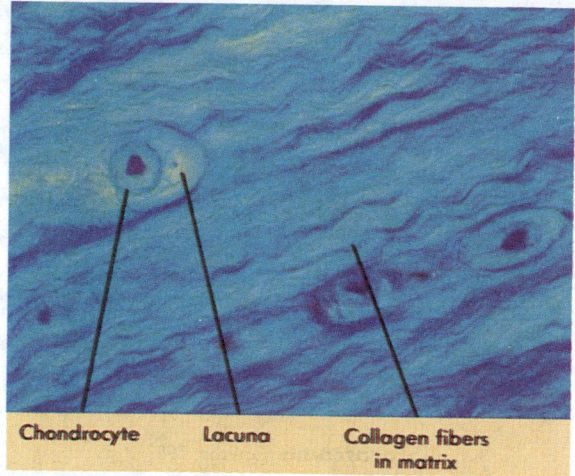

Fibrocartilage (Seeley, 1992/Ed Reschke)

Chondrocyte   Lacuna   Collagen fibers in matrix

fibrocystic disease /-sis'tik/ [L, *fibra* + Gk, *kystis* bag], **1.** (of the breast) the presence of single or multiple cysts that are palpable in the breasts. The cysts are benign and fairly common, yet must be considered potentially malignant and observed carefully for growth or change. Women with fibrocystic disease of the breast are at greater than usual risk of developing breast cancer later in life. The cysts can be aspirated and a biopsy performed. In most cases no treatment is required. The nurse must vigorously counsel women who have fibrocystic disease to examine their own breasts frequently. A woman is shown any cysts present, palpation is taught, and the importance of any change is emphasized. Reassurance should also be given that the condition is very common and generally not associated with cancer. Also called **chronic cystic mastitis. 2.** See **cystic fibrosis.**

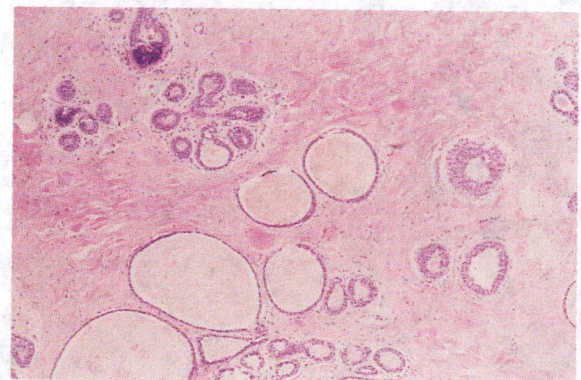

Fibrocystic disease of the breast (Skarin, 1991)

fibrocystic disease of the pancreas. See **cystic fibrosis.**
fibrocyte. See **fibroblast.**
fibroelastic tissue. See **fibrous tissue.**
fibroepithelial papilloma /-ep'ithē'lē·əl/ [L, *fibra* + Gk, *epi*, above, *thele*, nipple; L, *papilla*, nipple; Gk, *oma*, tumor], a benign epithelial tumor containing extensive fibrous tissue. Also called **fibropapilloma.**

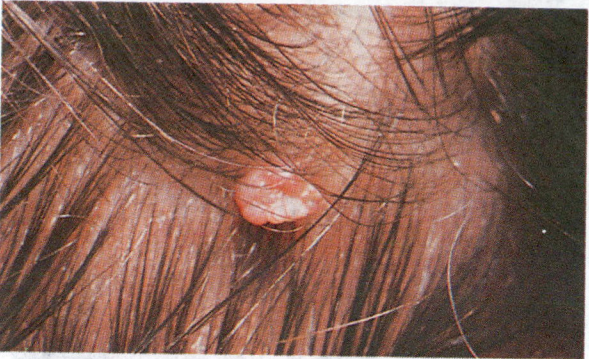

Fibroepithelial papilloma (Baran, 1991)

fibroepithelioma /fī'brō·ep'ithē'lē·ō'mə/, *pl.* **fibroepitheliomas, fibroepitheliomata** [L, *fibra*, + Gk, *epi*, above, *thele*, nipple, *oma*, tumor], a neoplasm consisting of fibrous and epithelial components. A kind of fibroepithelioma is **premalignant fibroepithelioma.**
fibroid /fī'broid/ [L, *fibra*, + Gk, *eidos*, form], **1.** having fibers. **2.** *informal.* a fibroma or myoma, particularly of the uterus.

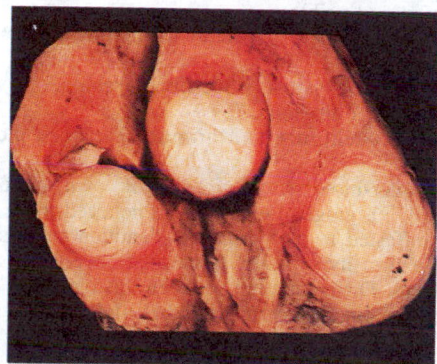

Fibroids (Fletcher, 1987)

fibroidectomy /fī'broidek'təmē/ [L, *fibra*, fiber; Gk, *eidos*, form, *ektome*, cutting out], the surgical removal of a fibrous tumor, such as a uterine fibromyoma.
fibroid tumor. See **fibroma.**
fibrolipoma /fī'brōlipō'mə/, a fibrous tumor that also contains fatty material.
fibroma /fībrō'mə/, *pl.* **fibromas, fibromata** [L, *fibra* + Gk, *oma*, tumor]], a benign neoplasm consisting largely of fibrous or fully developed connective tissue. See also specific fibromas.
-fibroma, a combining form meaning a 'benign tumor made up of fibrous tissue': *neurofibroma, hemangiofibroma, lymphangiofibroma.*
fibroma cavernosum, a tumor containing large vascular spaces, an excessive amount of fibrous tissue, and blood or lymph vessels.
fibroma cutis, a fibrous tumor of the skin.

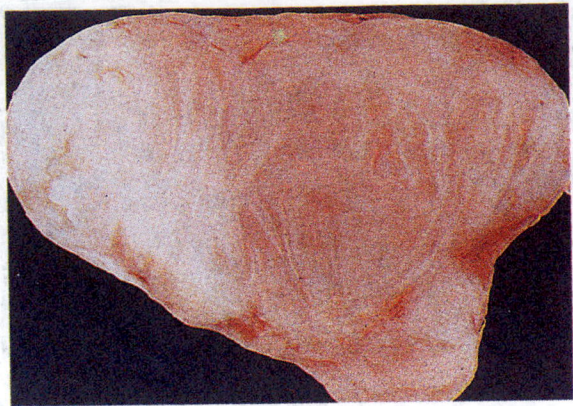

Ovarian fibroma (Fletcher, 1987)

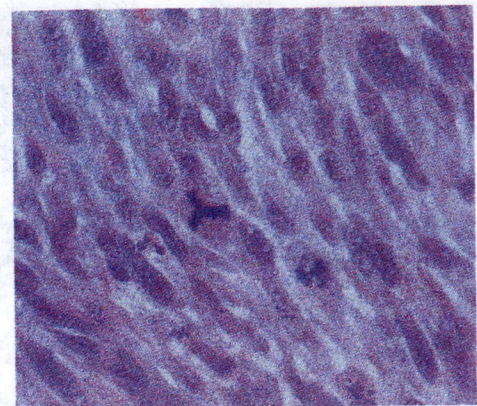

Fibrosarcoma (Cawson, 1987)

fibroma durum.   See **hard fibroma.**

fibroma molle.   See **soft fibroma.**

fibroma mucinosum,   a fibrous tumor in which mucoid material with degeneration is present.

fibroma myxomatodes.   See **myxofibroma.**

fibroma of breast [L, *fibra,* fiber; Gk, *oma,* tumor; AS, *braest*],   a connective tissue tumor of the breast. It is usually benign and painless.

fibroma pendulum,   a pendulous fibrous tumor of the skin.

fibroma sarcomatosum.   See **fibrosarcoma.**

fibromata.   See **fibroma.**

fibroma thecocellulare xanthomatodes.   See **theca cell tumor.**

fibromatosis /-mətō'sis/ [L, *fibra* + Gk, *oma,* tumor, *osis,* condition],   a gingival enlargement believed to be hereditary, manifested in the permanent dentition and characterized by a firm hyperplastic tissue that covers the surfaces of the teeth. Differentiation between this condition and diphenylhydantoin hyperplasia is based on a history of drug ingestion.

fibromyoma uteri.   See **leiomyoma uteri.**

fibromyomectomy /fī'brōmī'ōmek'təmē/,   a surgical procedure for removal of a uterine fibroma or other type of fibromyoma.

fibromyositis /fī'brōmī'əsī'tis/ [L, *fibra* + Gk, *mys,* muscle, *itis,* inflammation],   any one of a large number of disorders in which the common element is stiffness and joint or muscle pain, accompanied by localized inflammation of the muscle tissues and of the fibrous connective tissues. The condition may develop after climatic change, infection, or physical or emotional trauma. Fibromyositis may recur and become chronic. Treatment includes rest, heat, massage, salicylates, and, in severe cases, intraarticular injections of a corticosteroid and procaine. Kinds of fibromyositis include **lumbago, pleurodynia,** and **torticollis.** See **rheumatism.**

fibropapilloma.   See **fibroepithelial papilloma.**

fibrosarcoma /-särkō'mə/, *pl.* **fibrosarcomas, fibrosarcomata** [L, *fibra* + Gk, *sarx,* flesh, *oma,* tumor],   a sarcoma that contains connective tissue. The sarcoma develops suddenly from small nodules on the skin and metastases often occur before the nodules change.

fibrosing alveolitis /fī'brōsing/ [L, *fibra* + *alviolus,* small hollow; Gk, *itis,* inflammation],   a severe form of alveolitis characterized by dyspnea and hypoxia, occurring in advanced rheumatoid arthritis and other autoimmune diseases. X-ray films show thickening of the alveolar septa and diffuse pulmonary infiltrates. See also **alveolitis.**

fibrosis /fībrō'sis/ [L, *fibra* + Gk, *osis,* condition],   **1.** a proliferation of fibrous connective tissue. The process occurs normally in the formation of scar tissue to replace normal tissue lost through injury or infection. **2.** an abnormal condition in which fibrous connective tissue spreads over or replaces normal smooth muscle or other normal organ tissue. Fibrosis is most common in the heart, lung, peritoneum, and kidney. See also **cystic fibrosis, fibrositis.**

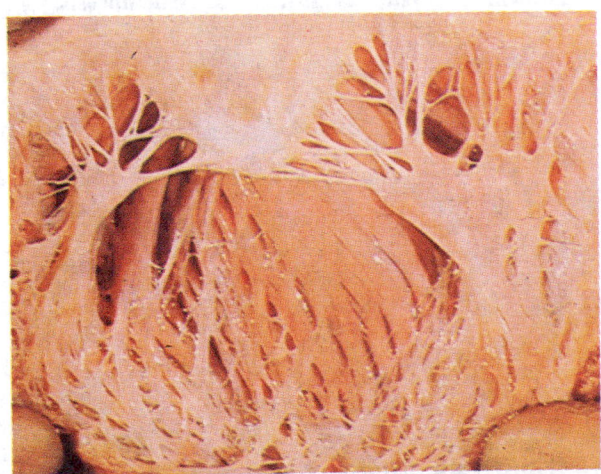

Cardiac fibrosis (Shipley, 1993)

fibrosis of the lungs [L, *fibra;* Gk, *osis,* condition; AS, *lungen,*   the formation of scar tissue in the connective tissue of the lungs as a sequel to any inflammation or irritation caused by tuberculosis, bronchopneumonia, or a pneumoconiosis. Localized fibrosis may be complicated by infarction, abscess, or bronchiectasis. Also called **pulmonary fibrosis**.

fibrositis /fī′brəsī′tis/, an inflammation of fibrous connective tissue, usually characterized by a poorly defined set of symptoms, including pain and stiffness of the neck, shoulder, and trunk. Fibrositis usually develops in middle age. There are no objectively measurable signs on radiologic examination. The person is often tense, and the origin of the condition may be psychogenic. Salicylates, sedatives, tranquilizers, muscle relaxants, and intraarticular injection of a local anesthetic may be prescribed in treatment. Compare **fibromyositis, myositis.**

fibrous /fī′brəs/ [L, *fibra,* fiber], consisting mainly of fibers or fiber-containing materials, such as fibrous connective tissue. See also **fibrosis.**

-fibrous, a combining form meaning 'composed of fibrous tissue': *cellulofibrous, fibrofibrous, interfibrous.*

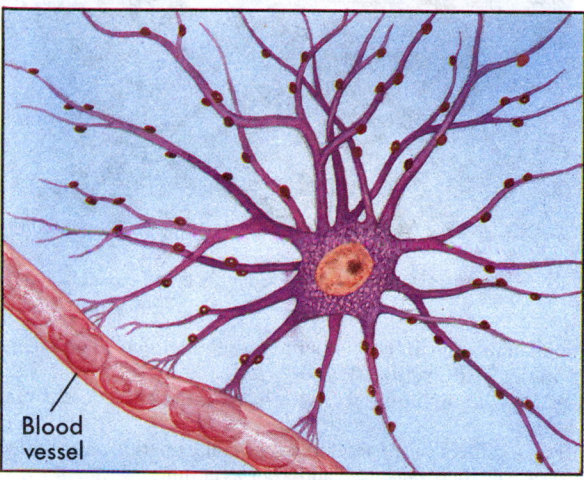

Fibrous astrocyte (*Chipps, 1992*)

fibrous capsule, 1. the external layer of an articular capsule. It surrounds the articulation of two adjoining bones. 2. the external, tough membranous envelope surrounding some visceral organs, such as the liver. Compare **synovial membrane.**

fibrous connective tissue. See **connective tissue.**

fibrous dysplasia, an abnormal condition characterized by the fibrous displacement of the osseous tissue within the bones affected. The specific cause of fibrous dysplasia is unknown, but indications are that the disease is of developmental or congenital origin. The distinct kinds of fibrous dysplasia are monostotic fibrous dysplasia, polyostotic fibrous dysplasia, and polyostotic fibrous dysplasia with associated endocrine disorders. Any bone may be affected with monostotic fibrous dysplasia. The polyostotic type usually displays a segmental distribution of the involved bones, all of which show varying degrees of the characteristic fibrous replacement of the osseous tissue. The onset of fibrous dysplasia is usually during childhood, progressing beyond puberty and through adulthood. The onset of symptoms is usually during childhood although diagnosis may be delayed until adolescence or even early adulthood if symptoms are minimal. The initial signs may be a limp, a pain, or a fracture on the affected side. Girls affected may have an early onset of menses and breast development and early epiphyseal closure. Albright's syndrome is usually diagnosed on the basis of a triad of symptoms, including the polyostotic type of fibrous dysplasia, café-au-lait patches on the skin, and precocious puberty. Pathologic fractures are frequently associated with this process, and angulation deformities may follow. The involved extremity may be shortened, and the classic 'shepherd's crook' deformity is common. Radiographic examination usually reveals a well-circumscribed lesion occupying all or a portion of the shaft of the long bone involved. Pathologic fractures in patients with fibrous dysplasia usually heal with conservative treatment, but residual deformities often remain. When symptoms are mild and limited, this disease usually progresses slowly. Radiation therapy is not employed because it may provoke malignant degeneration. Biopsies are commonly performed if pain increases or if alterations are seen on radiographic examination.

fibrous goiter, an enlargement of the thyroid gland, characterized by hyperplasia of the capsule and connective tissue.

fibrous gold. See **gold foil.**

fibrous histiocytoma. See **dermatofibroma.**

fibrous joint, any one of many immovable joints, such as those of the skull segments, in which a fibrous tissue or a hyaline cartilage connects the bones. The three kinds of articulation associated with fibrous joints are syndesmosis, sutura, and gomphosis. Also called **junctura fibrosa, synarthrosis.** Compare **cartilaginous joint, synovial joint.**

fibrous thyroiditis, a disorder characterized by slowly progressive fibrosis of an enlarged thyroid with replacement of normal thyroid tissue by dense fibrous tissue. The gland eventually becomes fixed to the adjacent muscles, nerves, blood vessels, and trachea by means of this fibrous tissue. The disease occurs more frequently in women than in men and usually arises after the age of 40. Symptoms include a choking sensation, dyspnea, dysphagia, and hypothyroidism, but in some patients the gland functions normally. Treatment includes surgical excision and thyroid hormone administered postoperatively, as required. Also called **ligneous thyroiditis, Riedel's struma, Riedel's thyroiditis.**

fibrous tissue, the fibrous connective tissue of the body, consisting of closely woven elastic fibers and fluid-filled areolae. Also called **fibroelastic tissue.** Compare **areolar tissue.**

fibula /fib′yələ/ [L, buckle], one of the two bones of the lower leg, lateral to and smaller than the tibia. In proportion to its length, it is the most slender of the long bones and presents three borders and three surfaces for attaching various muscles, including the peronei longus and brevis and the soleus longus. Also called **calf bone.**

fibular /fib′yələr/ [L, *fibula,* clasp], pertaining to the fibula.

Fick principle [Adolf E. Fick, German physiologist, b. 1829], a method for making indirect measurements, based on the law of conservation of mass. It is used specifically to determine cardiac output, in which the amount of oxygen uptake of each unit of blood as it passes through the lungs is equal to the oxygen concentration difference between arterial and mixed venous blood. Cardiac output is calculated by measuring the uptake of oxygen for a given period of time, noted as milliliters per minute, then dividing that ratio by the difference in oxygen saturation of arterial and mixed venous blood samples in milliliters per 100 ml of blood, and multiplying the total by 100.

Fick's law [Adolf E. Fick],   **1.** (in chemistry and physics) an observed law stating that the rate at which one substance diffuses through another is directly proportional to the concentration gradient of the diffusing substance. **2.** (in medicine) an observed law stating that the rate of diffusion across a membrane is directly proportional to the concentration gradient of the substance on the two sides of the membrane and inversely related to the thickness of the membrane.

fictive kin /fik'tiv/,   people who are regarded as being part of a family even though they are not related by either affinal or sanguinal bonds. Fictive kinship may bind people together in ties of affection, concern, obligation, and responsibility.

FID,   abbreviation for **free induction decay.**

field [AS, *feld*],   **1.** a defined space, area, or distance. The field of vision represents the total area that can be seen with one fixed eye. The binocular field is the area that can be seen with both eyes. **2.** an area within a computer record where a specified type of data is stored.

field fever,   a form of leptospirosis caused by *Leptospira grippotyphosa*, affecting primarily agricultural workers. It is characterized by fever, abdominal pain, diarrhea, vomiting, stupor, and conjunctivitis. Also called **canefield fever, harvest fever.** See also **leptospirosis.**

field of vision [AS, *feld*; L, *visio*, seeing],   the area of space in which objects are visible at the same time when the eye is fixed and the face is turned so as to exclude the limiting effects of the orbital margins and nose.

fiery serpent /fī'ərē/ [AS, *fyre*; L, *serpere*, to creep],   an informal term for *Dracunculus medinesis*. See also **dracunculiasis.**

fièvre boutonneuse.   See **African tick typhus.**

fifth disease.   See **erythema infectiosum.**

fifth cranial nerve.   See **trigeminal nerve.**

fight-or-flight.   See **flight-or-fight reaction.**

FIGLU,   abbreviation for **formiminoglutamic acid.**

figure 4 test.   See **Fabere's test.**

figure ground.   See **ground.**

figure-ground relationship /fig'(y)ər/ [L, *figura*, form; AS, *grund*; L, *relatus*, carry back],   a perceptual field that is divided into a figure, which is the object of focus, and a diffuse background.

figure-of-eight bandage,   a bandage with successive laps crossing over and around each other like the figure eight. See also **bandage.**

figure-of-eight suture [L, *sutura*],   a suture that begins at the deepest layer on each side of a wound, then crosses over to pass through the superficial layers on the opposite side before being tied.

fila-,   a combining form meaning 'pertaining to a thread, or threadlike': *filaceous, filamentous, filaria.*

filament /fil'əmənt/ [L, *filare*, to spin],   a fine threadlike fiber. Filaments are found in most tissues and cells of the body and serve various morphologic or physiologic functions.

filamentous /fil'əmen'təs/, [L, *filamentum*, thread],   pertaining to something that is threadlike or capable of being drawn out into a threadlike structure.

filariasis /fil'ərī'əsis/ [L, *filum*, thread; Gk, *osis*, condition],   a disease caused by the presence of filariae or microfilariae in the tissues of the body. Filarial worms are round, long, and threadlike and are common in most tropic and subtropic regions of the world. They tend to infest the lymph glands and channels after entering the body as microscopic larvae through the bite of a mosquito or other insect. The infection is characterized by occlusion of the lymphatic vessels, with swelling and pain of the limb distal to the blockage. After many years, the limb may become greatly swollen and the skin coarse and tough. Treatment is by oral administration of diethylcarbamazine. The most effective means of preventing infestation is mosquito control. See also **elephantiasis.**

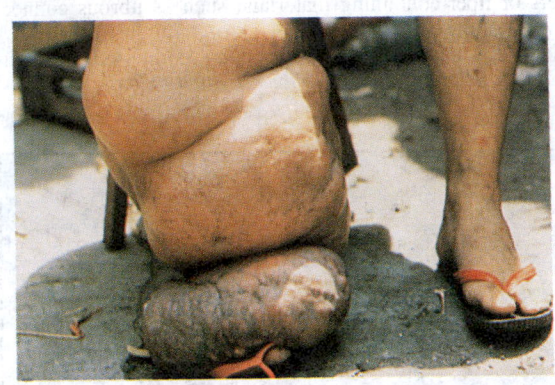

Filariasis *(Muller, 1990; Courtesy Dr AE Bianco)*

filariform /filer'ifôrm/,   pertaining to a structure or organism that is threadlike.

-filcon,   a combining form for hydrophilic contact lens material.

file,   a collection of related data or information, assembled for a specified purpose, and kept as a unit.

filial generation /fil'ē·əl/ [L, *filius*, son; *generare*, to beget],   the offspring produced from a given mating or cross in a genetic sequence. See also F_1, F_2.

filiform bougie /fil'ifôrm/ [L, *filum*, thread, *forma*, form; Fr, *bougie*, candle],   an extremely thin bougie for passage through a narrow stricture, such as a sinus tract.

filiform catheter,   a catheter with a slender, threadlike tip that allows the wider portion of the instrument to be passed through canals that are constricted or irregular because of an obstruction or an angulation in the canal. It may bypass obstructions or dilate strictures.

filiform papilla.   See **papilla.**

filiform warts.   See **digitate wart.**

filling factor [AS, *fyllan*, filling; L, *factor*, a maker],   a measure of the geometric relationship of a radiofrequency coil used in MR imaging and the body. This relationship affects the efficiency of irradiating the body and detecting MR signals, and thereby affects the signal-to-noise ratio and, ultimately, image quality. Achieving a high filling factor requires fitting the coil closely to the body, thus potentially decreasing patient comfort.

filling pressure,   the pressure in the left ventricle at the end of diastole.

film [AS, *filmen*, membrane],   **1.** a thin sheet or layer of any material, such as a coating of oil on a metal part. **2.** (in photography and radiography) a thin, flexible, transparent sheet of cellulose acetate or polyester plastic material coated with a light-sensitive emulsion, used to record images, such as organs, structures, and tissues that may be involved in disease and diagnoses.

film badge, a photographic film packet, sensitive to ionizing radiation, used for estimating the exposure of personnel working with x-rays and other radioactive sources.

film development, the processing of photographic or x-ray films to manifest the latent image resulting from exposure of the chemically treated gelatin emulsion to a pattern of electromagnetic radiation. Development involves wetting the film to loosen the emulsion, followed by a series of chemical baths, including reducing agents, activators, restrainers, preservatives, and hardeners. The reducing agents for radiographic films generally contain hydroquinone to produce black tones slowly and phenidone to produce shades of gray rapidly.

film fault, a defect in a photograph or radiograph, usually caused by a chemical, physical, or electric error in its production.

film on teeth, a collection of mucinous deposits adhering to the teeth, which contains microorganisms, desquamated tissue elements, blood cellular elements, and other debris. See also **plaque.**

film screen mammography, a breast x-ray technique in which a special single-emulsion film and high-detail intensifying screens are used. The technique provides a fine image at radiation exposure levels of less than 1 rad, compared with older methods that resulted in radiation levels of as much as 16 rad.

filter [Fr, *filtrer*, to strain], **1.** a device or material through which a gas or liquid is passed to separate out unwanted matter. **2.** (in radiology) a device added to x-ray equipment to selectively remove low-energy x-rays that have no chance of getting to the film. Examples include bow-tie, compensating, and conic filters.

filtered back projection, a mathematical technique used in NMR imaging and computed tomography to create images from a set of multiple projection profiles.

filtration /filtrā′shən/ [Fr, *filtrer*, to strain], the addition of sheets of metal into a beam of x-rays, altering the energy spectrum and thus the imaging characteristics and penetrating ability of the radiation. Filtration is generally provided by aluminum or copper at low to medium energies, and by tin, copper, and aluminum for higher energy beams.

filum /fī′ləm/, a threadlike structure, as the filum terminale that marks the lower end of the spinal cord.

fimbria /fim′brē·ə/ [L, fringe], any structure that forms a border or edge or that resembles a fringe. Kinds of fimbria are **fimbria hippocampi, fimbria ovarica,** and **fimbriae tubae.** See also **pilus,** def. 2.

fimbriae tubae /fim′bri·ī/, the branched, fingerlike projections at the distal end of each of the fallopian tubes. The projections are connected to the ovary and have epithelial cells with cilia that serve to move the ovum toward the uterus.

fimbria hippocampi, a band of efferent fibers formed by the alveus hippocampi that is continuous with the posterior pillar of the fornix.

fimbrial tubal pregnancy /fim′brē·əl/, a kind of tubal pregnancy in which implantation occurs in the fimbriated distal end of one of the fallopian tubes. See also **tubal pregnancy.**

fimbria ovarica, the longest of the fimbriae tubae. It extends from the infundibulum to the ovary. Also called **fimbriated extremity.**

fimbriated /fim′brē·ā′tid/ [L, *fimbria,* a fringe], pertaining to or resembling the fimbria or fringelike structure of the ovaries or the nerve fibers along the border of the hippocampus.

finastride /fin′əstrīd, finas′trīd/, a drug used to treat prostatic hypertrophy by reversing the progressive enlargement of the gland.

fine motor skills [Fr, *fin,* thin; L, *movere;* ONorse, *skilja,* to cut apart], the use of precise coordinated movements in such activities as writing, buttoning, cutting, tracing, or visual tracking.

fineness /fīn′nes/ [Fr, *fin,* thin], (in dentistry) a means of grading alloys relative to gold content. The fineness of an alloy is designated in parts per thousand of pure gold, which is 1000 fine. Gold alloys and pure gold may be used in dental restorations, such as tooth crowns and prepared tooth cavity fillings.

fine tremor [Fr, *fin,* thin; L, *tremor,* to tremble], a tremor that occurs after a voluntary movement or one that develops as a result of fatigue in the corresponding muscle group.

finger [AS, *fingar*], any of the digits of the hand. The fingers of the hand are composed of a metacarpal bone and three bony phalanges. Some anatomists regard the thumb as a finger, since its metacarpal bone ossifies in the same way as a phalanx. Other anatomists regard the thumb as being composed of a metacarpal bone and two phalanges. The digits of the hand are anatomically numbered 1 to 5, starting with the thumb.

finger agnosia, a neurologic disorder in which a patient is unable to distinguish between stimuli applied to two different fingers without visual clues. It is a feature of some types of dementia.

finger goniometer [AS, *finger;* Gk, *gonia,* angle, *metron,* meter], an instrument for measuring the angle of a finger joint, or of an arm or leg.

finger-nose test [AS, *finger, nosu;* L, *testum,* crucible], a test of the coordination of the arms. The patient is asked to bring the tip of the index finger quickly to the nose, first with the eyes open, then with the eyes closed. An inability to accurately perform the test may be an indication of cerebellar disease.

finger percussion. See **percussion.**

finger stick, the act of puncturing the tip of the finger to obtain a small sample of capillary blood. In some procedures, the hand may be first immersed in warm water for 10 minutes to 'arterialize' the capillary blood, or give it characteristics similar to arterial blood.

Finnish bath. See **Russian bath.**

FiO₂, 1. abbreviation for **fraction of inspired oxygen. 2.** the percentage of inspired oxygen a patient is receiving, usually expressed as a fraction.

Fiorinal, a trademark for a group of fixed-combination drugs containing a sedative-hypnotic (butalbital), an analgesic, antipyretic, and antiinflammatory (aspirin), an analgesic (phenacetin), and a central nervous system stimulant (caffeine).

fire damp. See **damp.**

fireman's cramp. See **heat cramp.**

first aid [AS, *fyrst;* Fr, *aider,* to help], the immediate care that is given to an injured or ill person before treatment by medically trained personnel. Attention is directed first to the most critical problems: evaluation of the patency of the airway, the presence of bleeding, and the adequacy of cardiac function. The patient is kept warm and as comfortable as possible. The conscious patient is reassured and is queried for significant details of his medical history, such as diabetes, a known heart condition, or allergic reactions to drugs; if the patient is unconscious, a medical identification card, bracelet, or necklace is sought. The patient is moved as little as possible, particularly if there is a possibility of fracture. If there is vomiting, the patient's head is moved to a position for the vomitus to exit easily to avoid aspiration. See also **cardiopulmonary resuscitation, control of hemorrhage, emergency medicine, emergency nursing.**

first cuneiform.   See **medial cuneiform bone.**

first dentition.   See **deciduous dentition.**

first-dollar coverage,   an insurance plan under which the third-party payer assumes liability for covered services as soon as the first dollar of expense for such services is incurred, without requiring the insured to pay a deductible.

first filial generation.   See **F$_1$.**

first-generation scanner,   an early type of computed tomography device that used a finely collimated x-ray beam and a single detector moving in a translate-rotate mode. It required 180 translations, each separated by a 1-degree rotation, and up to 5 minutes for one scan.

first intention.   See **intention.**

first metacarpal bone,   the metacarpal bone of the thumb.

first nerve.   See **olfactory nerve.**

first-order change,   a change within a system that itself remains unchanged.

first-order kinetics,   a chemical reaction in which the rate of decrease in the number of molecules of a substrate is proportional to the concentration of substrate molecules remaining. The rate of metabolism of most drugs follows the rule of first-order kinetics and is independent of the dose. Also called **first-order reaction.** See also **kinetics.**

first rib,   the highest rib of the thoracic cage. It moves about the axis of its neck, raising and lowering the sternum. First rib movement during quiet breathing is negligible, but under conditions of stress it can increase the anteroposterior diameter of the chest.

first stage of labor [ME, *fyrst*; OFr, *estage*; L, *labor*, work],   a period of 8 to 12 hours marked by the onset of regular contractions of the uterus with full dilation of the cervix and the appearance of a bit of blood-tinged mucus. Danger signs of the first stage include abnormal bleeding, abnormal fetal heart rate, and abnormal presentation and position of the fetus.

first-state cementoma.   See **periapical fibroma.**

Fishberg concentration test,   a test of the ability of the kidneys to concentrate urine, developed by American physician Arthur M. Fishberg. The test involves measuring the specific gravity of morning urine samples following overnight deprivation of fluid intake.

fishhandler's disease.   See **erysipeloid.**

fish poisoning,   toxic effects caused by ingestion of fish containing substances that may produce symptoms ranging from nausea and vomiting to respiratory paralysis. Scrombroid poisoning usually results from a histamine-like toxin produced by bacterial activity in mackerel, tuna, or bonito. An almost immediate reaction is characterized by facial flushing, nausea and vomiting, abdominal pain, and urticaria. Tetraodon poisoning, caused by a toxin in puffer fish, may result in myalgia, paresthesia, and other neuromuscular disorders. See also **ciguatera poisoning.**

fish skin disease.   See **ichthyosis.**

fish tapeworm infection [AS, *fisc*, fish],   an infection caused by the tapeworm *Diphyllobothrium latum* that is transmitted to humans when they eat contaminated raw or undercooked freshwater fish. Fish tapeworm infection is common in temperate zones throughout the world and is found in the Great Lakes region of the United States. Also called **diphyllobothriasis** /dəfil′ōbōthrī′əsis/. See also *Diphyllobothrium,* **tapeworm infection.**

fiss-,   a combining form meaning 'pertaining to a split or cleft': *fissile, fissiparous, fissula.*

fission /fish′ən/ [L, *fissio,* splitting],   **1.** the act or process of splitting or breaking up into parts. **2.** a type of asexual reproduction common in bacteria, protozoa, and other lower forms of life in which the cell divides into two or more equal components, each of which eventually develops into a complete organism. Kinds of fission are **binary fission** and **multiple fission. 3.** also called **nuclear fission.** (in physics) the splitting of the nucleus of an atom and subsequent release of energy.

fissiparous /fisip′ərəs/,   reproduced by fission.

fissura.   See **fissure.**

fissural angioma /fish′ərəl/ [L, *fissura,* cleft,   a tumor composed of a cluster of dilated blood vessels found on the lip, face, or neck in an embryonal fissure.

fissure /fish′ər/ [L, *fissura,* cleft],   **1.** a cleft or a groove on the surface of an organ, often marking division of the organ into parts, such as the lobes of the lung. **2.** a crack-like lesion of the skin, such as an anal fissure. **3.** a lineal fault on a bony surface occurring during the development of a part, such as a fissure in the enamel of a tooth. A fissure is usually deeper than a sulcus but, in the terminology of anatomy, *fissure* and *sulcus* are often used interchangeably. Also **fissura.** Compare **sulcus.**   **–fissured,** *adj.*

fissured tongue /fish′ərd/ [L, *fissura,* cleft; AS, *tunge*],   a tongue with deep surface furrows that may radiate outward. The condition may be inherited as an autosomal dominant trait.

fissure fracture,   any fracture in which a crack extends into the cortex of the bone but not through the entire bone.

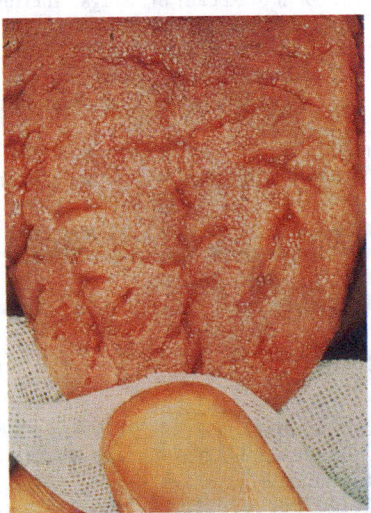

Fissured tongue (Lamey, 1988)

fissure-in-ano /-inā′nō/,   a painful linear ulcer at the margin of the anus.

fissure of Bichat.   See **transverse fissure.**

fissure of Rolando.   See **central sulcus.**

fissure of Sylvius.   See **lateral cerebral sulcus.**

fistula /fisʹchŏŏlə, -chələ/, *pl.* **fistulas, fistulae** [L, pipe], an abnormal passage from an internal organ to the body surface or between two internal organs, such as a hepatopleural or pulmonoperitoneal fistula, caused by a congenital defect, injury, infection, the spreading of a malignant lesion, radiotherapy of a cancerous growth, or trauma during childbirth. Fistulas may occur in many sites from the gingiva to the anus and may be created for therapeutic purposes or to obtain body secretions for physiologic studies. An arteriovenous fistula is commonly created to gain access to the patient's bloodstream for hemodialysis. Anal fistulas resulting from rupture or drainage of abscesses may be treated by fistulectomy or fistulotomy, and fistulas between the vagina and bladder, urethra, ureter, or rectum may be repaired surgically, but the results are not always successful. **–fistulous, fistular, fistulate,** *adj.*

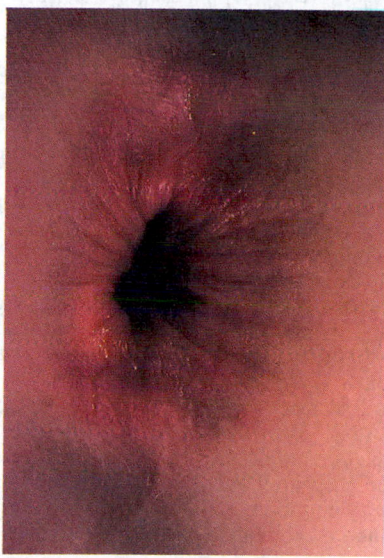

Anal fissure in child (400 Self-assessment picture tests, 1984)

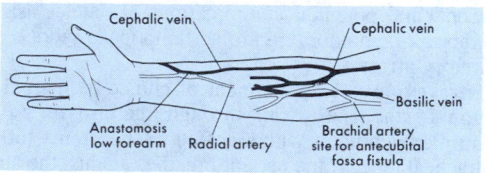

Arteriovenous fistula

fistula in ano.   See **anal fistula.**

-fistular.   See **fistula.**

fistulectomy /fisʹchələkʹtəmē/ [L, *fistula*, pipe; Gk, *ektome*, cutting out],   the surgical removal of a fistula.

-fistulate.   See **fistula.**

-fistulous.   See **fistula.**

fit,   1. *nontechnical.* a paroxysm or seizure. **2.** the sudden onset of an episode of symptoms, such as a fit of coughing. **3.** the manner in which one surface is aligned to another, such as the fit of a denture to the gingiva and jaw.

Fitzgerald factor,   a high molecular weight kinogen that may be required for the interaction of factors XII and XI in the coagulation process.

Fitzgerald treatment.   See **zone therapy.**

five-day fever,   *informal.* trench fever.

five-in-one repair.   See **Nicholas procedure.**

five-step nursing process,   a nursing process comprising five broad categories of nursing behaviors: assessing, analyzing, planning, implementing, and evaluating. The nurse gathers information about the client, identifies the specific needs of the client, develops a plan of care with the client to answer these needs, implements the plan of care, and evaluates the effects of the implementation. The nurse involves the client, the client's family, and significant others in each step of the process to the greatest extent possible and compensates for and acknowledges the factors that might influence the provision of care by the nurse and staff. Implicit in the nursing process is a therapeutic and personal relationship between the nurse, the client, the client's family, and significant others. See also **nursing process.**

-fixate.   See **fixation.**

fixated.   See **fixation.**

fixating eye /fikʹsāting/ [L, *figere*, to fasten; AS, *eage*],   (in strabismus) the normal eye that can be focused. Compare **squinting eye.**

fixation /fiksāʹshən/ [L, *figere*, to fasten, *atio*, process],   (in psychoanalysis) an arrest at a particular stage of psychosexual development, such as anal fixation.   **–fixate,** *v.,* **fixated,** *adj.*

fixation muscle,   a muscle that acts to hold a part of the body in appropriate position. Compare **antagonist, prime mover, synergist.**

fixative /fikʹsətiv/ [L, *figere*, to fasten],   **1.** any substance used to bind, glue, or stabilize. **2.** any substance used to preserve gross or histologic specimens of tissue for later examination.

fixed anions /fikst/,   anions that are not part of the body's buffer anions.

fixed bridgework,   a dental device incorporating artificial teeth permanently attached to natural teeth or implants in the upper or the lower jaw.

fixed cantilever.   See **partial denture.**

fixed cations,   cations that are not part of the body's metabolic buffering system.

fixed-combination drug [L, *figere*, to fasten; *combinare*, to combine; Fr, *drogue*],   any of a group of multiple-ingredient preparations that provides concomitant administration of specific amounts of two or more drugs.

fixed coupling,   a precise distance between a normal and ectopic beat that is duplicated each time the ectopic beat occurs.

fixed delusion [L, *figere*, to fasten, *deludere*, to deceive],   a delusion that is consistent and unaltered.

fixed dressing,   a dressing usually made of gauze impregnated with a hardening agent, such as plaster of paris, sodium silicate, starch, or dextrin, applied to support or immobilize a part of the body. The dressing is soaked in water, applied to the part to be immobilized, and allowed to harden. See also **cast.**

fixed-drug eruption,   well-defined red to purple lesions

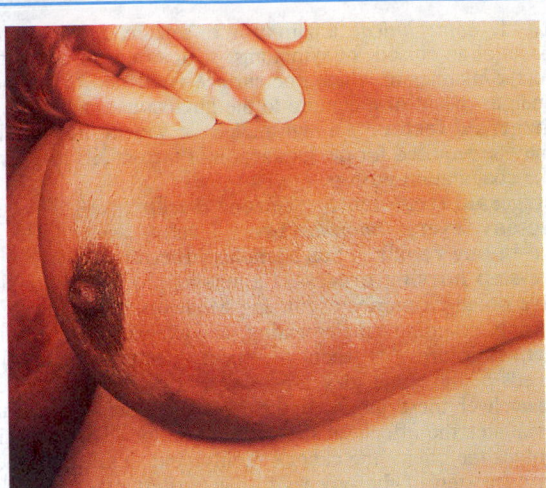

Fixed-drug eruption (Epstein, 1992)

that appear at the same sites on the skin and mucous membranes each time a particular drug is used. The reaction occurs most commonly in patients using tetracycline or phenolphthalein.

fixed fulcrum, a tomographic fulcrum that remains at a fixed height.

fixed idea, **1.** a persistent, obsessional thought or notion. **2.** in certain mental disorders, especially obsessive-compulsive neurosis, a delusional idea that dominates mental activity and persists despite contrary evidence or rational refutation. Also called **idée fixe** /idā′fiks′/.

fixed interval (FI) reinforcement, (in psychiatry) reinforcement given after a specific amount of time has elapsed.

fixed macrophage [L, *figere,* to fasten; Gk, *makros,* large, *pagein,* to eat], nonmotile mononuclear phagocyte in the liver sinuses, spleen, lymph glands, and other tissues.

fixed orthodontic appliance, a prosthetic device cemented to the teeth or attached by adhesive material, for changing the relative positions of dentitions.

fixed partial denture. See **partial denture.**

fixed-performance oxygen delivery system. See **high-flow oxygen delivery system.**

fixed phagocyte. See **phagocyte.**

fixed pupil [L, *figere,* to fasten, *pupilla,* little girl], an abnormal condition in which the pupils fail to dilate or contract when stimulated. The cause is commonly adhesions that bind the iris to the lens capsule, or because of interference with the nerve supply of the iris in acute glaucoma.

fixed rate pacemaker [L, *figere,* to fasten, *ratum,* calculate, *passus,* step; ME, *maken*], an artificial cardiac pacemaker that delivers impulses to the cardiac muscle at a preset rate regardless of the heart's independent activity.

fixed ratio (FR) reinforcement, (in psychiatry) reinforcement given after a specific number of responses have occurred.

fixed torticollis [L, *figere,* to fasten, *tortus,* twisted, *collum,* neck], a condition in which neck muscles on one side are so short that the head is held continuously in the same position. See also **torticollis.**

fixed vertebrae. See **false vertebrae.**

fixer, a chemical product used in processing photographic or x-ray film. Applied after the developing phase, it neutralizes any developer remaining on the film, removes un-developed silver halides, and hardens the emulsion.

flaccid /flak′sid/ [L, *flaccus,* flabby], weak, soft, and flabby; lacking normal muscle tone, such as flaccid muscles. **−flaccidity, flaccidness,** *n.*

flaccid bladder, a form of neurogenic bladder caused by interruption of the reflex pathways associated with the voiding reflex in the spinal cord. It is marked by continual filling and occasional overfilling of the bladder, absence of bladder sensation, and inability to urinate voluntarily. It is most often produced by trauma. The bladder can be emptied by pressure to the area. Also called **atonic bladder, autonomous bladder, nonreflex bladder.** Compare **spastic bladder.**

-flaccidity. See **flaccid.**

-flaccidness. See **flaccid.**

flaccid paralysis, an abnormal condition characterized by the weakening or the loss of muscle tone. It may be caused by disease or by trauma affecting the nerves associated with the involved muscles. Compare **spastic paralysis.**

flagell-, a combining form meaning 'pertaining to a whip-like process, tapping': *flagellation, flagelliform, flagellospore.*

flagella /flajel′ə/ [L, *flagellum,* whip], hairlike projections that extend from some unicellular organisms and aid in their movement.

flagellant /flaj′ələnt/, a person who receives sexual gratification from the practice of flagellation.

flagellate /flaj′əlāt′, -lit/ [L, *flagellum,* whip], a microorganism that propels itself by waving whiplike filaments or cilia behind its body, such as *Trypanosoma, Leishmania, Trichomonas,* and *Giardia.* See also **protozoa.**

flagellation /flaj′əlā′shən/, **1.** the act of whipping, beating, or flogging. **2.** a type of massage administered by tapping the body with the fingers. See **massage. 3.** a type of sexual deviation in which a person is erotically gratified by being whipped or by whipping another. See **masochism, sadism. 4.** the arrangement of flagella on an organism; ex-flagellation.

Flagyl, a trademark for an antiprotozoal (metronidazole).

flail chest /flāl/ [ME, *fleyl,* whip; AS, *cest,* box], a thorax in which multiple rib fractures cause instability in part of the chest wall and paradoxical breathing, with the lung underlying the injured area contracting on inspiration and bulging on expiration. If uncorrected, hypoxia will result.

■ OBSERVATIONS: Flail chest is characterized by sharp pain, uneven chest expansion, shallow, rapid respirations, and decreased breath sounds. Tachycardia and cyanosis may be present, and potential complications are atelectasis, pneumothorax, hemothorax, cardiac tamponade, shock, and respiratory arrest.

■ INTERVENTIONS: The treatment of choice is internal stabilization of the chest wall through the use of a volume-controlled ventilator with a cuffed tracheostomy tube or endotracheal tube. If the patient breathes against the automatic ventilator, a sedative and muscle relaxant may be ordered to achieve ventilatory control. Chest tubes may be required to remove air or fluid preventing expansion of the affected lung, and a nasogastric tube may be ordered to provide food and fluids. The patient's blood pressure, pulse, respirations, and breath sounds are checked every 1 to 2 hours, the rectal temperature every 2 to 4 hours, and arterial blood gases are determined as ordered. Traction is less frequently used in treating flail chest but may be applied by attaching a steel wire to the ribs or sternum under local anesthesia and connecting the wire to a rope, pulley, and weight.

■ NURSING CONSIDERATIONS: The patient with flail chest usually requires a long period of care involving frequent repositioning, scrupulous attention to the patency and cleanliness of the tracheostomy or endotracheal tube, skin care, oral hygiene, and emotional support. The nurse performs passive range-of-motion exercises to the extremities, explains the various procedures, and provides a pad and pencil or a magic slate so that the patient is able to communicate.

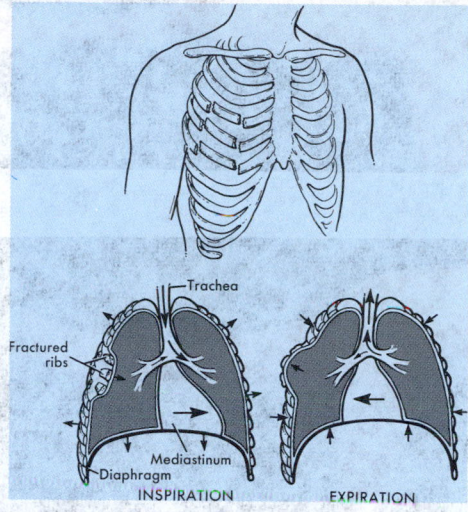

Flail chest

flame photometry [L, *flagrare*, to burn; Gk, *phos*, light, *metron*, measure], measurement of the wavelength of light rays emitted by excited metallic electrons exposed to the heat energy of a flame, used to identify characteristics in clinical specimens of body fluids. The intensity of the emitted light is proportional to the concentration of atoms in the fluid, and a quantitative analysis can be made on that basis. In the clinical laboratory, flame photometry is used to measure sodium, potassium, and lithium levels.

flange /flanj/, **1.** the part of a denture base that extends from the cervical ends of the teeth to the border of the denture. **2.** a prosthesis with a lateral vertical extension designed to direct a resected mandible into centric occlusion.

flank, the posterior portion of the body between the ribs and the ilium. Flank pain is sometimes associated with the kidney.

flapping tremor. See **asterixis.**

flare /fler/, **1.** a red blush on the skin at the periphery of an urticarial lesion seen in immediate hypersensitivity reactions. **2.** an expanding skin flush, spreading from an infective lesion or extending from the principal site of a reaction to an irritant. **3.** the sudden intensification of a disease.

flaring of nostrils, nasal flaring; a widening of the nostrils during inspiration, a sign of air hunger or respiratory distress.

flashback, a phenomenon experienced by persons who have taken hallucinogenic drugs and unexpectedly reexperience the drug effects.

flask closure [L, *vasculum*, small vessel; *claudere*, to close], (in dentistry) the joining of two halves of a flask that encloses and forms a mold for a denture base. Compare **closure, velopharyngeal closure.**

flat affect, the absence of emotional response to a situation that normally elicits emotion.

Flatau-Schilder disease. See **Schilder's disease.**

flat bone [AS, *flet*, floor], any of the bones that provide structural contours of the skeleton. Examples include ribs and bones of the skull.

flat electroencephalogram, a graphic chart on which no tracings were recorded during electroencephalography, indicating a lack of brain-wave activity. Flat readings are indicative of death except in cases of profound hypothermia and central nervous system depression. Also called **isoelectric electroencephalogram.**

flatfoot. See **pes planus.**

flat spring contraceptive diaphragm, a kind of contraceptive diaphragm in which the flexible metal spring that forms the rim is a thin, light, flat band made of stainless steel. The rubber dome is approximately 1.5 inches deep, and the diameter of the rubber-covered rim is between 5.5 and 10 cm. Ten sizes, in increments of 5 mm, allow the clinician to fit the diaphragm to each individual woman. This kind of diaphragm is prescribed for a woman whose vaginal musculature provides good support, whose uterus is in the normal position and not acutely retroflexed or anteflexed, and whose vagina, neither very long nor very short, has a shallow arch behind the symphysis pubis.

flatulence /flach′ələns/ [L, *flatus*, a blowing], the presence of an excessive amount of air or gas in the stomach and intestinal tract, causing distension of the organs and in some cases mild to moderate pain.

flatulent /flach′ələnt/ [L, *flatus*, a blowing], pertaining to gas or air in the digestive tract.

flatus /flā′təs/ [L, a blowing], air or gas in the intestine that is passed through the rectum. See also **aerophagy.**

flat wart. See **verruca plana.**

flav-, a prefix meaning 'yellow': *flavescens, flavin, flavism.*

flavone /flā′vōn/ [L, *flavus*, yellow], a colorless, crystalline, flavonoid derivative and component of bioflavonoid that increases capillary resistance.

flavoxate hydrochloride /flavok′sāt/, a smooth muscle relaxant.

■ INDICATION: It is prescribed for spastic conditions of the urinary tract.

■ CONTRAINDICATIONS: GI hemorrhage or obstruction, urinary tract obstruction, or known hypersensitivity to this drug prohibits its use.

■ ADVERSE EFFECTS: Among the more serious adverse reactions are nervousness, nausea, abdominal pain, fever, and tachycardia.

fl.dr., abbreviation for **fluid dram.**

flea [AS], a wingless, bloodsucking insect of the order Siphonaptera, some species of which transmit arboviruses to humans by acting as host or vector to the organism.

flea bite, a small puncture wound produced by a bloodsucking flea. Certain species of fleas transmit plague, murine typhus, and probably tularemia.

flea bites, *informal.* erythema toxicum neonatorum.

flea-borne typhus. See **murine typhus.**

flecainide acetate /flekā′nīd/, an oral antiarrhythmic drug.

■ INDICATIONS: It is prescribed for the treatment of ventricular dysrhythmias.

■ CONTRAINDICATIONS: This product is contraindicated for patients with preexisting second-or third-degree atrioventricular block, right bundle-branch block associated with a left

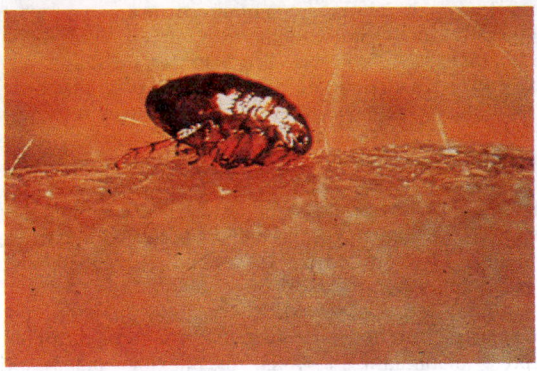

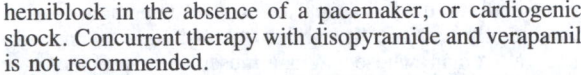

Rat flea *Xenopsylla* *(Muller, 1990)*

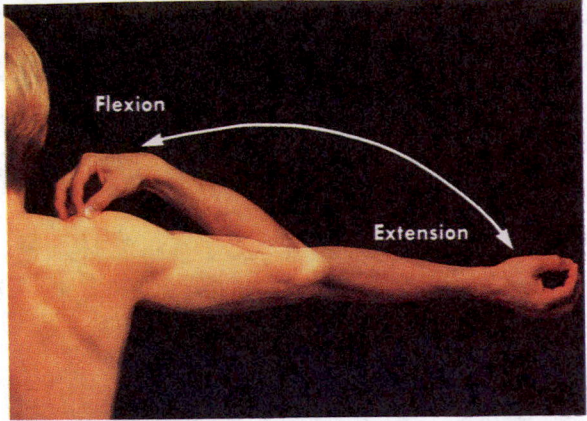

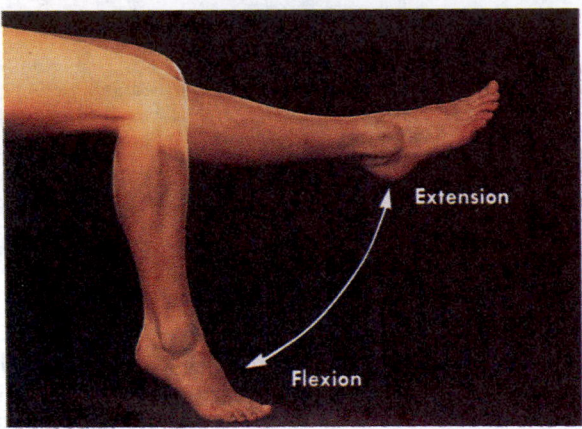

Flexion and extension of the knee
(Seeley, 1992/Terry Cockerham, Synapse Media Productions)

hemiblock in the absence of a pacemaker, or cardiogenic shock. Concurrent therapy with disopyramide and verapamil is not recommended.

■ ADVERSE EFFECTS: Among adverse reactions reported are new or increased dysrhythmias or congestive heart failure, dizziness, visual disturbances, dyspnea, headache, nausea, fatigue, tremor, constipation, and edema.

-flect, -flex, a combining form meaning 'to bend': *anteflect, circumflect.*

Fleet Enema, trademark for a manufactured enema formula containing 16 gm sodium biphosphate and 6 gm sodium phosphate per 100 ml solution made available in disposable plastic pouches fitted with prelubricated rectal tubes.

Fleischner method /flīsh′nər/, a technique for producing lordotic x-ray projections of the lungs. The patient is placed in P-A projection position while leaning backward from the waist to a nearly 45-degree posterior inclination.

Fletcher factor, a prekallikrein blood coagulation substance that interacts with both factor XII and Fitzgerald factor, activating both and accelerating thrombin formation.

FLEX, abbreviation for **Federation Licensing Examination.**

Flexeril, a trademark for a muscle relaxant (cyclobenzaprine hydrochloride).

Flex-Foot, a trademark for a stored-energy foot prosthesis. It contains a J-shaped plastic beam that acts like a spring when the wearer walks or runs. See also **stored-energy foot.**

flexibilitas cerea. See **cerea flexibilitas.**

flexitime. See **flextime.**

flexion /flek′shən/ [L, *flectere*, to bend], **1.** a movement allowed by certain joints of the skeleton that decreases the angle between two adjoining bones, such as bending the elbow, which decreases the angle between the humerus and the ulna. Compare **extension. 2.** (in obstetrics) a resistance to the descent of the fetus through the birth canal that causes the neck to flex so the chin approaches the chest. Thus the smallest diameter (suboccipitobregmatic) of the vertex presents.

flexion jacket, a corset designed to provide spinal immobility. A typical flexion jacket is fashioned out of a rigid material and provides three-point fixation in opposite directions, similar to a Jewett brace.

flexor /flek′sər/ [L, bender], a muscle that flexes a joint.

flexor carpi radialis [L, *flexor,* bender], a slender, superficial muscle of the forearm that lies on the ulnar side of the pronator teres. It arises from the medial epicondyle, the fascia of the forearm, and several intermuscular septa, and it inserts by a long tendon into the base of the second metacarpal bone. Fibers of the muscle extend to the base of the third metacarpal bone. The flexor carpi radialis is innervated by a branch of the median nerve that contains fibers from the sixth and the seventh cervical nerves, and it functions to flex and to help abduct the hand. Compare **flexor carpi ulnaris, palmaris longus.**

flexor carpi ulnaris, a superficial muscle lying along the ulnar side of the forearm that arises in a humeral and an ulnar head and inserts in a long tendon into the pisiform bone, extending by ligaments to the hamate and the fifth metacarpal bones. It is innervated by a branch of the ulnar nerve, which contains fibers from the eighth cervical and the first thoracic nerves. The flexor carpi ulnaris functions to flex and adduct the hand. Compare **flexor carpi radialis, palmaris longus.**

flexor digitorum superficialis, the largest superficial muscle of the forearm, lying on the ulnar side under the palmaris longus, arising by a humeral, an ulnar, and a radial head. The humeral head originates in the medial epicondyle of the humerus, in the ulnar collateral ligament of the elbow joint, and in various intermuscular septa; the ulnar head originates in the medial side of the coronoid process; the radial head originates in the oblique line of the radius. The muscle separates into a superficial layer and a deep layer and inserts by four tendons into the second phalanx of the fingers. The flexor digitorum superficialis is innervated by branches of the median nerve that contains fibers from the seventh and the eighth cervical and the first thoracic nerves. The muscle flexes the second phalanx of each finger and, by continued action, the hand. Also called **flexor digitorum sublimis.** Compare **flexor carpi radialis, flexor carpi ulnaris, palmaris longus, pronator teres.**

flexor retinaculum of ankle [L, *flexor,* bender, *retinaculum,* halter; AS, *ancleow*], an overgrowth of fascia from the medial malleolus to the calcaneum, passing over the long flexor tendons and blood vessels and nerves of the posterior tibia.

flexor retinaculum of the hand. See **retinaculum flexorum manus.**

flexor retinaculum of wrist [L, *flexor,* bender, *retinaculum,* halter; AS, *wrist*], a strong ligament across the front of the hollow of the carpus and over the flexor tendons of the fingers and median nerve.

flexor withdrawal reflex, a common cutaneous reflex consisting of a widespread contraction of physiologic flexor muscles and relaxation of physiologic extensor muscles. It is characterized by abrupt withdrawal of a body part in response to painful or injurious stimuli. A relatively innocuous stimulation of the skin may result in a weak contraction of one or more flexor muscles and a minimal withdrawal reflex.

flextime /fleks'tīm/ [L, *flectere,* to bend; AS, *tima*], a system of staffing that allows the individualization of work schedules. A person working days might choose to work from 7 to 3, 9 to 5, or other hours. Full staffing must be maintained, but within the group flextime can be arranged. Use of the system tends to improve morale and decrease turnover. Also called **flexitime.**

flexure /flek'shər/, a normal bend or curve in a body part, such as the colic flexure of the colon or the dorsal flexure of the spine.

flight into health [AS, *fleogan,* to fly], an abnormal but common reaction to an unpleasant physical sensation or symptom in which the person denies the reality of the feeling or observation, insisting that there is nothing wrong. See also **illness experience.**

flight of ideas, (in psychiatry) a continuous stream of talk in which the patient switches rapidly from one topic to another, each subject being incoherent and not related to the preceding one or stimulated by some environmental circumstance. The condition is frequently a symptom of acute manic states and schizophrenia. Compare **circumstantiality.**

flight-or-fight reaction [AS, *fleogan,* to fly; *feohtan,* to fight; L, *reagere,* to act again], **1.** (in physiology) the reaction of the body to stress, in which the sympathetic nervous system and the adrenal medulla act to increase the cardiac output, dilate the pupils of the eyes, increase the rate of the heartbeat, constrict the blood vessels of the skin, increase the glucose and fatty acids in the circulation, and induce an alert, aroused mental state. **2.** (in psychiatry) a person's reaction to stress by either fleeing from a situation or

remaining and attempting to deal with it.

flight to illness, the effort of the patient to convince the therapist that he or she is too ill to terminate therapy and that continued support is needed.

flip angle, in NMR imaging, the amount of rotation of the macroscopic magnetization vector produced by a radiofrequency pulse with respect to the direction of the static magnetic field.

floater [AS, *flotian,* to float], one or more spots that appear to drift in front of the eye, caused by a shadow cast on the retina by vitreous debris. Most floaters are benign and represent remnants of a network of blood vessels that existed prenatally in the vitreous cavity. The sudden onset of several floaters may indicate serious disease. Hemorrhage into the vitreous humor may cause a large number of big and little shadows and a red discoloration of vision. The cause is often traumatic injury, but spontaneous intraocular hemorrhage is seen in severe diabetes mellitus, hypertension, or increased intracranial pressure. Cancer, detachment of the retina, occlusion of a retinal vein, and other purely ocular diseases may also cause hemorrhage into the vitreous cavity. Inflammation of the retina resulting from chorioretinitis may cause entry of inflammatory cells into the vitreous humor. Inflammatory debris may adhere to the vitreous framework in netlike masses that are very disruptive of normal vision. Retinal detachment also causes a sudden appearance of lightninglike floaters and a diminished field of vision as a shower of red cells and pigment is released into the vitreous humor. Careful ophthalmologic examination through a well-dilated pupil is recommended for all people who experience a sudden occurrence of floaters, because each of the pathologic causes can be treated in the early stages and loss of vision can usually be avoided. Also called **muscae volitantes.**

floating head [AS, *flotian,* to float; *heafod*], unengaged fetal head. See also **ballottement, engagement.**

floating kidney, a kidney that is not securely fixed in the usual anatomic location because of congenital malplacement or traumatic injury. Compare **ptotic kidney.**

floating rib. See **rib.**

floating patella [AS, *flotian;* L, *patella,* small pan], a patella that has been forced away from the femoral condyle by an effusion into the knee joint.

float nurse, a nurse who is available for assignment to duty on an ad hoc basis, usually to assist in times of unusually heavy work loads or to assume the duties of absent nursing personnel. A float nurse is recruited from a group of nurses called a float pool. Also called **contingent nurse.**

flocculant /flok'yo̅o̅lənt/, an agent or substance that causes flocculation.

-flocculate. See **flocculent.**

flocculation. See **flocculent.**

flocculation test /flok'yo̅o̅lā'shən/ [L, *floccus,* flock of wool, a serologic test in which a positive result depends on the degree of flocculent precipitation produced in the material being tested. Many tests for syphilis, including the VDRL slide test, are flocculation tests.

flocculent /flok'yo̅o̅lənt/ [L, *floccus,* flock of wool], clumped or tufted, such as a cloud, or covered with a woolly, fuzzy surface. **—flocculate,** *v.,* **flocculation, floccule,** *n.*

flood fever. See **typhus.**

flooding [AS, *flod*], a technique used in behavior therapy for the reduction of anxiety associated with various phobias.

Exposure to a stimulus that usually provokes anxiety desensitizes a person to that stimulus, thereby reducing fear and anxiety. Also called **implosive therapy.** Compare **systemic desensitization.**

floppy, floppy disk. See **diskette.**

floppy infant syndrome [ME, *flappe*, slap; L, *infans*, speechless], a general term for juvenile spinal muscular atrophies, including Werdnig-Hoffmann disease and Wohlfart-Kugelberg-Welander disease.

flora /flôr'ə/, microorganisms that live on or within a body to compete with disease-producing microorganisms and provide a natural immunity against certain infections.

florid /flôr'id/ [L, *floridus*, flower], in human skin complexion or wound appearance, a bright red color.

Florone, a trademark for an antiinflammatory agent (diflorasone diacetate).

Floropryl, a trademark for an inhibitor of cholinesterase (isoflurophate), used ophthalmically.

flossing, the mechanical cleansing of interproximal tooth surfaces with stringlike, waxed or unwaxed dental floss.

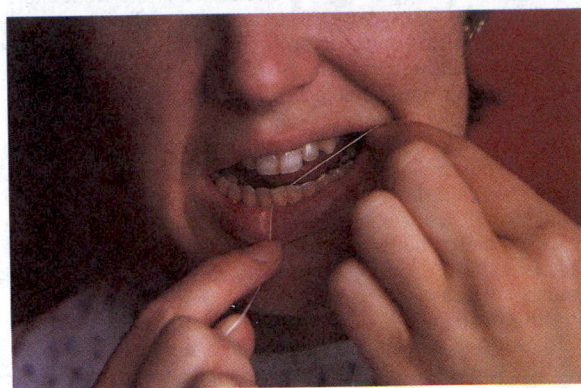

Flossing (Potter, 1993)

flotation device /flōtā'shən/ [Fr, *flotter*, to float], a foam mattress with a gel-like pad located in its center, designed to protect bony prominences and distribute pressure more evenly against the skin's surface.

flotation therapy, a state of semiweightlessness produced by various types of hospital equipment and used in the treatment and prevention of decubitus ulcers.

Flo-Trol clamp, a trademark of a triggerlike off-on control for intravenous and other infusion lines.

flow chart [AS, *flowan*; L, *charta*, paper], a graphic representation of a computer program sequence, an intermediate step between algorithm development and the writing of a computer program.

flowmeter. See **rotameter.**

flow sheet, (in a patient record) a graphic summary of several changing factors, especially the patient's vital signs or weight and the treatments and medications given. In labor, the flow sheet displays the progress of labor, including the centimeters of cervical dilatation, cervical effacement, the position of the baby's head, the baby's heart rate, the frequency of contractions, the mother's temperature and blood pressure, and any medications given or procedures performed.

flow transducer, a spirometer that calculates volume by dividing flow by time.

flow-volume curve, a graphic representation of the instantaneous volumetric flow rates achieved during a forced expiratory vital capacity maneuver. It is plotted as a function of the lung volume. It may be a maximum expiratory flow-volume curve (MEFV) or a partial expiratory flow-volume (PEFV) curve.

flow-volume loop, a pulmonary function test system in which the patient breathes into an electronic spirometer and performs a forced inspiratory and expiratory vital capacity maneuver while flow and volume are displayed on an oscilloscope screen. The data are displayed graphically as a loop whose shape indicates lung volume and other data through the complete respiratory cycle.

floxuridine /floksyŏŏr'ədēn/, an antineoplastic agent.

■ INDICATIONS: It is prescribed in the treatment of malignant neoplastic disease of the brain, breast, liver, and gallbladder.

■ CONTRAINDICATIONS: Bone marrow depression, infection, poor nutritional state, or known hypersensitivity to this drug prohibits its use.

■ ADVERSE EFFECTS: Among the more serious adverse reactions are severe depression of the bone marrow and acute GI disturbances, including nausea, vomiting, diarrhea, and stomatitis. Alopecia and dermatitis commonly occur.

fl.oz., abbreviation for **fluid ounce.**

flu /flōō/, *informal.* **1.** influenza. **2.** any viral infection, especially of the respiratory or intestinal system.

fluctuant /fluk'chōō·ənt/, pertaining to a wavelike motion that is detected when a structure containing a liquid is palpated.

fluctuation /fluk·chōō·ā'shən/ [L, *fluctuare*, to wave], **1.** a wavelike motion of fluid in a body cavity after succussion. **2.** a variation in a fixed value or mass.

flucytosine /flōōsī'təsēn/, an antifungal.

■ INDICATION: It is prescribed in the treatment of certain serious fungal infections.

■ CONTRAINDICATIONS: Known hypersensitivity to this drug prohibits its use. Close monitoring is required when administering this drug to patients with renal disorders or bone marrow depression.

■ ADVERSE EFFECTS: Among the more serious adverse reactions are GI disturbances, including enterocolitis, abnormal liver function, hepatomegaly, and bone marrow depression.

-fluent, a suffix meaning 'flowing': *diffluent, ossifluent.*

fluent aphasia /flōō'ənt/ [L, *fluere*, to flow; Gk, *a*, not, *phasis*, speech], forms of aphasia in which the patient says words easily although the words may be unintelligible or not be related to a particular stimulus. Types of fluent aphasia include **Wernicke's aphasia** and **conduction aphasia.**

fluid /flōō'id/ [L, *fluere*, to flow], **1.** a substance, such as a liquid or gas, that is able to flow and to adjust its shape to that of a container because it is composed of molecules that are able to change positions with respect to each other without separating from the total mass. **2.** a body fluid, either intracellular or extracellular, that is involved in the transport of electrolytes and other vital chemicals to, through, and from tissue cells. See also **blood, lymph, cerebrospinal fluid.**

fluid balance, a state of equilibrium in which the amount of fluid consumed equals the amount lost in urine, feces, perspiration, and exhaled water vapor.

fluid dram (fl.dr.), a unit of liquid measure equal to

3.696 milliliters (ml), 60 minims, or 1/8th of a fluid ounce.

fluidic ventilator /floo·id'ik/, a ventilator that applies the Coanda effect to the movement of the flow of air or gases. As the air stream passes a wall, a pocket of turbulence forms a low-pressure bubble next to the wall, causing the air stream to adhere to the wall. As a gas travels faster over the pocket of turbulence, the surrounding gas molecules not in the stream acquire a higher pressure, holding the stream against the wall. The gas flow tends to remain in that pattern until it is diverted by a different input pressure. See also **Coanda effect.**

fluid ounce (fl.oz.), a measure of liquid volume in the apothecaries' system, which is equal to 8 fluid drams or 29 ml, 480 minims, 1/20th of an Imperial pint, or the volume occupied by 437.5 grains of distilled water at a temmperature of 16.7°C. See also **apothecaries' measure, metric system.**

fluid retention, a failure to excrete excess fluid from the body. Causes may include renal, cardiovascular, or metabolic disorders. In uncomplicated cases, the condition can sometimes be corrected with diuretics and a low-salt diet.

fluid therapy, the regulation of water balance in patients with impaired renal, cardiovascular, or metabolic function by carefully measuring fluid intake against daily losses.

fluid volume deficit, 1. a nursing diagnosis accepted by the Fourth National Conference on the Classification of Nursing Diagnoses. The cause of the condition is a failure of the body's homeostatic mechanisms that regulate the retention and excretion of body fluids. The defining characteristics of the problem are dilute urine, increased output of urine, and a sudden loss of body weight. Several other characteristics may be observed, including hypotension, increased pulse rate, decreased turgor, increased body temperature, hemoconcentration, weakness, and thirst. **2.** a nursing diagnosis accepted by the Fourth National Conference on the Classification of Nursing Diagnoses. The cause of the condition is the active loss of excessive amounts of body fluid. The defining characteristics of the condition are decreased output of urine, high specific gravity of the urine, output of urine that is greater than the intake of fluid into the body, a sudden loss of weight, hemoconcentration, and increased serum levels of sodium. Other characteristics that may be observed are increased thirst, alteration in the mental state, dryness of skin and mucous membranes, elevated temperature, and an increased pulse rate. See also **nursing diagnosis.**

fluid volume deficit, high risk for, a nursing diagnosis accepted by the Fifth National Conference on the Classification of Nursing Diagnoses. Risk factors are advanced age; excessive weight; extreme loss of fluid through normal routes, such as diarrhea, or abnormal routes, such as indwelling tubes; the lack of intake of fluids, as happens during physical immobility; increased fluid needs, as created by hypermetabolic states; and the use of diuretics or other medications affecting the retention and excretion of body fluids. The defining characteristics of the condition include increased fluid output, urinary frequency, thirst, and any alteration in fluid intake. See also **nursing diagnosis.**

fluid volume excess, a nursing diagnosis accepted by the Fifth National Conference of the Classification of Nursing Diagnoses. Fluid volume excess is defined as a state in which an individual experiences increased fluid retention and edema. The defining characteristics of the condition include edema, effusion, weight gain, shortness of breath,

third heart sound, pulmonary congestion changes in respiratory pattern and abnormal breath sounds, decreased hemoglobin and hematocrit, blood pressure changes, an alteration in electrolyte balance, and restlessness, anxiety, and other changes in mental status. See also **nursing diagnosis.**

fluke /flook/, a parasitic flatworm of the class Trematoda, including the genus *Schistosoma*. See also **schistosomiasis.**

fluocinolone acetonide /floo'ōsin'əlōn/, a topical glucocorticoid.
- INDICATION: It is prescribed as an antiinflammatory agent.
- CONTRAINDICATIONS: Impaired circulation, viral and fungal diseases of the skin, or known hypersensitivity to this drug or to other steroid medication prohibits its use.
- ADVERSE EFFECTS: Among the more serious adverse reactions are systemic side effects resulting from prolonged use or excessive application. Various hypersensitivity reactions may occur.

fluocinonide /floo'ōsin'ənīd/, a synthetic corticosteroid.
- INDICATION: It is prescribed to reduce inflammation.
- CONTRAINDICATIONS: Viral and fungal diseases of the skin, tuberculosis of the skin, or known hypersensitivity to this drug prohibits its use.
- ADVERSE EFFECTS: Among the more serious adverse reactions are secondary infections, striae, miliaria, and contact dermatitis.

Fluonid, a trademark for a glucocorticoid (fluocinolone acetonide).

fluorescence /floores'əns/ [L, *flux*, a discharge], the emission of light of one wavelength (usually ultraviolet) when exposed to light of a different, usually shorter, wavelength, a property possessed by certain substances. Fluorescent substances that simultaneously absorb and emit light appear luminous. **–fluoresce,** *v.,* **fluorescent,** *adj.*

fluorescent antibody test (FA test) /floores'ənt/, a test in which a fluorescent dye is used to stain an antibody for

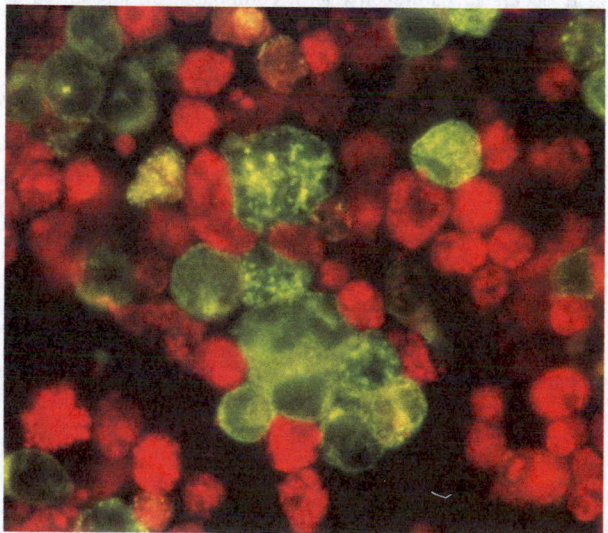

Fluorescent antibody test
(Baron, 1990; Courtesy Dr. Ellena Peterson, University of California, Irvine)

identification of clinical specimens. Fluorescent dyes conjugate with immunoglobulins without altering the antibody-antigen reaction, making the dyed organisms glow visibly when examined under a fluorescent microscope. The fluorescent antibody technique can be used to identify *Mycobacterium tuberculosis* and is used in the most common serologic screening test for syphilis. Kinds of fluorescent antibody tests include the **FTA-ABS test.** Also called **immunofluorescence test.**

fluorescent microscopy, examination with a fluorescent microscope equipped with a source of ultraviolet light rays, used to study specimens, such as tissues or microorganisms, that have been stained with fluorescent dye. Also called **ultraviolet microscopy.** See also **fluorescent antibody test.**

Fluorescent Treponemal Antibody Absorption Test (FTA-ABS test), a serologic test for syphilis. See also **fluorescent antibody test.**

fluoridation /floor'idā'shən/ [L, *fluere*, to flow], the process of adding fluoride, especially to a public water supply, to reduce tooth decay. See also **fluoride.**

fluoride /floor'īd/, a salt of hydrofluoric acid introduced into drinking water and applied directly to the teeth to prevent tooth decay.

fluoride dental treatment [L, *fluere*, to flow, *dens*, tooth; Fr, *traitment*], the direct oral application of fluoride compounds to reduce dental caries.

fluoride poisoning [L, *fluere*, to flow, *potio*, drink], the toxic effects of contact with compounds of fluorine, an intensely poisonous pale yellow gas. Sodium fluoroacetate is a powerful rodent poison while methyl fluoroacetate is regarded as too toxic to use as a pesticide. The fluoroacetate compounds inhibit enzymes of the citric-acid cycle. Inhalation of hydrogen fluoride can lead to bronchospasm, laryngospasm, and pulmonary edema.

fluorine (F) /floor'ēn/ /floo'ərēn/ [L, *fluere*, to flow], an element of the halogen family and the most reactive of the nonmetals. Its atomic number is 9; its atomic weight is 19. It occurs in nature only as a component of substances as fluorspar, cryolite, and phosphate rocks. It can be prepared by the electrolytic decomposition of hydrogen fluoride and in its pure form is a pale-yellow, flammable, toxic gas 1.6 times heavier than air. It is also a component of very stable fluorocarbons used in the manufacture of resins and plastics. As a component of fluorides it is widely distributed throughout the soils of the earth, enters plants, is ingested by humans, and is absorbed from the GI tract. Fluorides in the atmosphere and industrial dust are absorbed by the lungs and the skin. Relatively soluble compounds, such as sodium fluoride, are almost completely absorbed by humans. The relatively insoluble compounds, such as cryolite, are poorly absorbed. Small amounts of sodium fluoride are added to the water supply of many communities to harden tooth enamel and decrease dental caries. Excessive amounts of fluoride can mottle tooth enamel and cause osteosclerosis. Acute fluoride poisoning and death can result from the accidental ingestion of insecticides and rodenticides containing fluoride salts.

fluorination /floor'inā'shən/, the addition of a fluorine group to a compound, such as those commonly found in topical corticosteroids.

fluoroacetic acid /floor'ō·asē'tik, -aset'ik/, a colorless, water-soluble, highly toxic compound that blocks the Krebs' cycle, causing convulsions and ventricular fibrillation. It is

derived from a South African tree and is used in some potent pesticides.

fluorocarbons /floor'ōkär'bəns/ [L, *fluere*, to flow, *carbo*, coal], hydrocarbons that contain fluorine. Fluorocarbons are generally colorless, nonflammable gases, but some are liquids at room temperature. The compounds can produce mild upper respiratory tract irritation and excessive exposure has been cited as a cause of central nervous system depression.

fluorometry /floorom'ətrē/ [L, *fluere* + Gk, *metron*, measure], measurement of fluorescence emitted by compounds when exposed to ultraviolet or other intense radiant energy. The atoms of certain substances produce fluorescence of a characteristic color and wavelength, enabling identification and quantification of several clinically significant compounds in biologic specimens. Fluorometry is used to measure urinary estrogens, triglycerides, catecholamines, and other substances. Although it is a highly sensitive method of analysis, test interference by other compounds, especially drugs, may limit its usefulness in some situations. —**fluorometric,** *adj.*

Fluoroplex, a trademark for a topical preparation of antineoplastic (fluorouracil).

fluoroscope /floor'əskōp'/ [L, *fluere* + Gk, *skopein*, to look], a device used for the immediate projection of an x-ray image on a fluorescent screen for visual examination. —**fluoroscopic,** *adj.*

fluoroscopic compression device /floor'əskop'ik/, any of several objects that can be placed on a specific area of the patient's abdomen to compress the exterior surface during fluoroscopy of the digestive tract.

fluoroscopy /flooros'kəpē/, a technique in radiology for visually examining a part of the body or the function of an organ using a fluoroscope. The technique offers immediate, serial images that are invaluable in many clinical procedures, such as intrauterine fetal transfusion and cardiac catheterization.

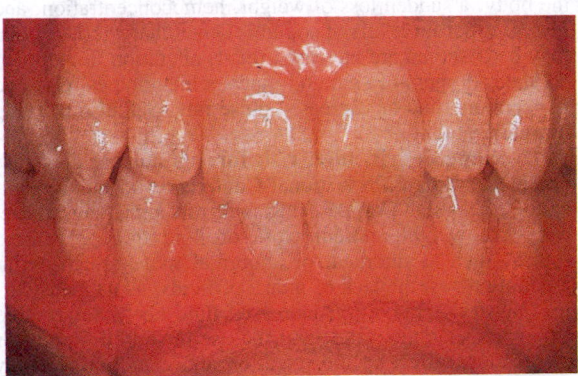

Fluorosis *(Jordon, 1993)*

fluorosis /floorō'sis/ [L, *fluere* + Gk, *osis*, condition], the condition that results from excessive, prolonged ingestion of fluorine. Unusually high concentration of fluorine in the drinking water typically causes mottled discoloration and pitting of the enamel of the permanent and deciduous teeth in children whose teeth developed while maternal intake of fluorinated water was high. Severe chronic fluorine poisoning will lead to osteosclerosis and other pathologic bone and joint changes in adults. See also **fluoridation, fluoride.**

fluorouracil /floor′oyōor′əsil/ /floo′ərōyōor′əsil/, an antineoplastic.
■ INDICATIONS: It is prescribed in the treatment of malignant neoplastic disease of the skin and internal organs.
■ CONTRAINDICATIONS: Bone marrow depression, infection, poor nutritional status, or known hypersensitivity to this drug prohibits its use.
■ ADVERSE EFFECTS: Among the more serious adverse reactions are severe depression of the bone marrow and acute GI disturbances, including nausea, vomiting, diarrhea, and stomatitis. Alopecia and dermatitis commonly occur.

Fluothane, a trademark for an inhalational general anesthetic (halothane).

fluoxymesterone /floo·ok′simes′tərōn/, an androgenic and anabolic steroid.
■ INDICATIONS: It is prescribed in the treatment of testosterone deficiency, breast cancer in females, and delayed puberty in males.
■ CONTRAINDICATIONS: Male breast or prostate cancer, liver disease, known or suspected pregnancy, or known hypersensitivity to this drug prohibits its use.
■ ADVERSE EFFECTS: Among the more serious adverse reactions are anaphylaxis, hypercalcemia, and jaundice.

fluphenazine hydrochloride /floofen′əzēn/, a phenothiazine tranquilizer.
■ INDICATION: It is prescribed in the treatment of psychotic disorders.
■ CONTRAINDICATIONS: Parkinson's disease, concurrent administration of central nervous system depressants, liver or renal dysfunction, severe hypotension, or known hypersensitivity to this drug or to other phenothiazine medication prohibits its use.
■ ADVERSE EFFECTS: Among the more serious adverse effects are hypotension, liver toxicity, a variety of extrapyramidal reactions, blood dyscrasias, and hypersensitivity reactions.

flurandrenolide /floo′randren′əlīd/, a topical glucocorticoid.
■ INDICATION: It is prescribed as an antiinflammatory agent.
■ CONTRAINDICATIONS: Impaired circulation, viral and fungal diseases of the skin, or known hypersensitivity to this drug or to steroid medication prohibits its use.
■ ADVERSE EFFECTS: Among the more serious adverse reactions are systemic side effects resulting from prolonged use or excessive application. Various hypersensitivity reactions may occur.

flurandrenolone. See **flurandrenolide.**

flurazepam hydrochloride /floo′raz′əpam/, a benzodiazepine minor tranquilizer.
■ INDICATION: It is prescribed in the treatment of insomnia.
■ CONTRAINDICATION: Known hypersensitivity to this drug prohibits its use.
■ ADVERSE EFFECTS: Among the most serious adverse reactions are possible physical and psychologic dependence. Dizziness and drug hangover may also occur.

flush [ME, *fluschen*], **1.** a blush or sudden reddening of the face and neck. **2.** a sudden, subjective feeling of heat. **3.** a prolonged reddening of the face such as may be seen with fever, certain drugs, or hyperthyroidism. **4.** a sudden, rapid flow of water or other liquid.

flush device, a device for the accurate transmission of a pressure wave from a catheter to a transducer in an IV line.

flutter, a rapid vibration or pulsation that may interfere with normal function.

flutter-fibrillation [AS, *fleotan,* to move quickly; L, *fibrilla,* small fiber], a type of atrial fibrillation in which the irregular fibrillatory line resembles atrial flutter.

flux gain /fluks/, (in radiology) the ratio between the number of light photons at the output phosphor of an image-intensifier tube to the number at the input phosphor.

fly [AS, *flyge*], a two-winged insect of the order Diptera, some species of which transmit arboviruses to humans.

fly bites, bites that may be caused by species of deer, horse, or sand flies. Such bites produce a small painful wound with swelling because of substances in the insect's saliva that are injected beneath the surface of the skin. Emergency treatment for fly bites includes cleaning the site and placing ice on it. The bite should be monitored for possible infections, as biting flies often transmit diseases.

Fm, symbol for the element **fermium.**

FMET, abbreviation for **formylmethionine.**

FMG, abbreviation for **foreign medical graduate.**

FML, a trademark for an ophthalmic glucocorticoid agent (fluorometholone).

FMR-1, the symbol for a gene associated with a mental retardation disorder of the **fragile X syndrome** disease. The normal function of the gene has not been determined.

FNP, abbreviation for **family nurse practitioner.**

foam bath [AS, *fam, baeth*], a bath taken in water containing a saporin substance that covers the surface of the liquid and through which air or oxygen is blown to form the foam.

focal /fō′kəl/ [L, *focus,* hearth], pertaining to a focus.

focal illumination. See **illumination.**

focal lesion [L, *focus, laesio,* hurting], an infection, tumor, or injury that develops at a restricted or circumscribed area of tissue.

focal plane, the plane of tissue that is in focus on a tomogram.

focal point [L, *focus,* hearth, *punctus,* pricked], a point at which rays of light meet when deflected, either by reflection or refraction.

focal seizure [L, *focus,* fireplace; OFr, *seisir*], a transitory disturbance in motor, sensory, or autonomic function resulting from abnormal neuronal discharges in a localized part of the brain, most frequently motor or sensory areas adjacent to the central sulcus. Focal motor seizures commonly begin as spasmodic movements in the hand, face, or foot and may spread progressively to other muscles to end in a generalized convulsion. Abnormal neuronal discharges arising in the motor area controlling mastication and salivation may be manifested by chewing, lip-smacking, swallowing movements, and by profuse salivation. Seizures originating in the eye-turning area of the brain may begin with a forced turning of the head and eyes away from the side of the focus or lesion. Abnormal electric activity in the sensory strip of the cortex may be evident initially as a numb, prickling, tingling, or crawling feeling, and the neuronal discharge may spread to motor areas. Focal seizures may be caused by localized anoxia or a small lesion in the brain. Also called **jacksonian seizure.** See also **epilepsy, motor seizure.**

focal spot, the area on the cathode of an x-ray tube or the target of an accelerator that is struck by electrons and from which the resulting x-rays are emitted. The shape and size of a focal spot influence the resolution of a diagnostic image. An increase in focal spot size, which may accompany deterioration of the x-ray tube, results in loss of ability to define small structures.

focal symptom [L, *focus,* hearth; Gk, *symptoma,* that which happens], a bodily function disturbance focused on a specific body system or part.

focal zone, (in ultrasonography) the distance along the beam axis of a focused transducer assembly, from the point where the beam area first becomes equal to 4 times the focal area to the point beyond the focal surface where the beam area again becomes equal to 4 times the focal area.

-focon, a combining form for hydrophobic contact lens material.

focus /fō'kəs/ [L, fireplace], a specific location, as the site of an infection or the point at which an electrochemical impulse originates.

focused activity /fō'kəst/, a therapeutic technique of actively leading the patient toward adaptive coping skills and away from maladaptive ones.

focused grid, (in radiography) an x-ray grid that has lead foils placed at an angle so that they all point toward a focus at a specific distance.

-foetal. See **fetus.**

foeti-, foeto-. See **feti-.**

foetus. See **fetus.**

fogged film fault /fogd/ [Dan *spray;* AS, *filmen,* membrane; L, *fallere,* to deceive], a defect in a photograph or radiograph, which appears as a foggy image or image area. It is usually caused by stray light or radiation, use of expired film, or an unsafe darkroom light.

fogging [ME, *fogge*], a method of determining refractive error, particularly in cases of astigmatism, by placing excessively convex or concave lenses in front of the eyes. The patient is made artificially myopic by means of plus spheres in order to relax all accommodation.

fog nebulizer /neb'yəlī'zer/, (in respiratory care) a device that humidifies by producing large volumes of particles.

foil assistant. See **foil holder.**

foil carrier. See **foil passer.**

foil holder [L, *folium,* leaf; AS, *haldan*], an instrument used for holding a foil pellet in place while it is being condensed or for retaining a bulk of gold while additions are being made to it for various dental restorations. Also called **foil assistant.** Compare **foil passer.**

foil passer, a pointed or forked instrument for carrying pellets of gold foil through an annealing flame or from the annealing tray to a prepared tooth cavity. Also called **foil carrier.** Compare **foil holder.**

foil pellet, a loosely rolled piece of gold foil, used for making various dental restorations, as a permanent tooth cavity filling or tooth crown. Pellets are prepared, as needed, from a piece of gold cut from foil that usually comes in 4 inch (10 cm) square sections. See also **fibrous gold, gold foil.**

folacin. See **folic acid, folate.**

folate /fō'lāt/, **1.** a salt of folic acid. **2.** any of a group of substances found in some foods and in mammalian cells that act as coenzymes and promote the chemical transfer of single carbon units from one molecule to another. Folates are often used as a dietarysupplement with iron during pregnancy.

folate deficiency. See **folic acid.**

Foley catheter /fō'lē/ [Frederick E. B. Foley, American

physician, b. 1891], a rubber catheter with a balloon tip to be filled with air or a sterile liquid after it has been placed in the bladder. This kind of catheter is used when continuous drainage of the bladder is desired, such as in surgery, or when repeated urinary catheterization would be necessary if an indwelling catheter were not used. Sterile technique is used in placing the catheter. See also **catheterization.**

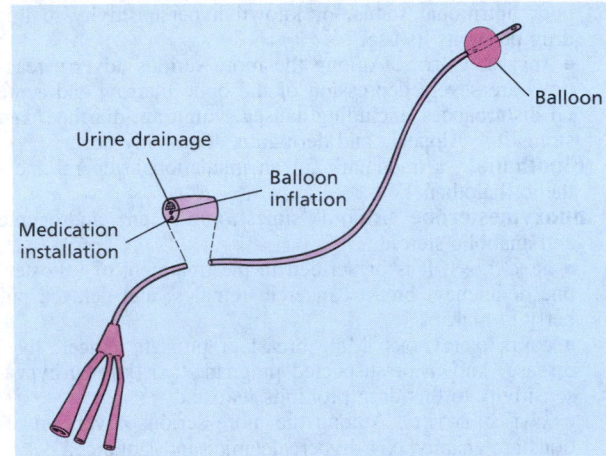

Foley catheter *(Potter, 1993)*

folic acid /fō'lik, fol'ik/, a yellow, crystalline, water-soluble vitamin of the B complex group essential for cell growth and reproduction. It functions as a coenzyme with vitamins B_{12} and C in the breakdown and utilization of proteins and in the formation of nucleic acids and heme in hemoglobin. It also increases the appetite and stimulates the production of hydrochloric acid in the digestive tract. The vitamin is stored in the liver and may be synthesized by the bacterial flora of the GI tract. Deficiency of the vitamin results in poor growth, graying hair, glossitis, stomatitis, GI lesions, and diarrhea, and it may lead to megaloblastic anemia. Deficiency is caused by inadequate dietary intake of the vitamin, malabsorption, or metabolic abnormalities.

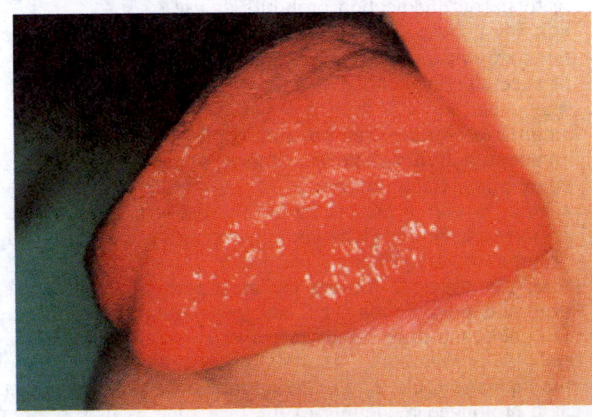

Glossitis in folic acid deficiency
(McLaren, 1992/Dr. WR Tyldesley)

Need for folic acid is increased in pregnancy, in infancy, and by stress. Rich dietary sources include spinach and other green leafy vegetables, liver, kidney, asparagus, lima beans, nuts, and whole-grain cereals. It is both heat and light labile, and considerable loss of the vitamin occurs when it has been stored for a long period. The vitamin, which is nontoxic, is effective in treating the specific deficiency states and may be beneficial in alleviating menstrual problems and leg ulcers. The adult RDA's for folate are 180-200 μg. Also called **folacin, pteroylglutamic acid, vitamin B$_9$**.

folic acid deficiency anemia, a form of megaloblastic (macrocytic) anemia caused by a lack of folic acid in the diet.

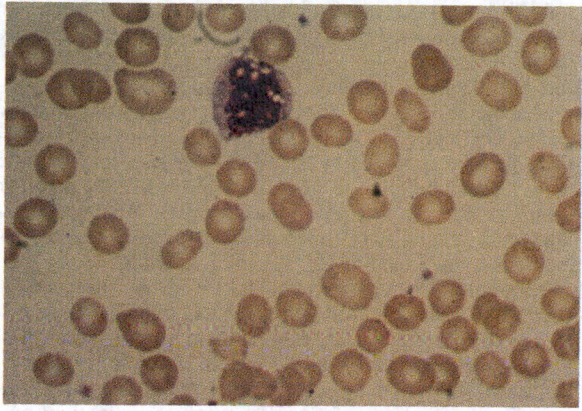

Folic acid deficiency anemia
(McLaren, 1992/Dr. AC Parker)

folie /fōlē'/ [Fr, madness], a mental disorder. Kinds of folie include **folie à deux, folie circulaire, folie du doute, folie du pourquoi, folie gemellaire, folie musculaire,** and **folie raisonnante.**

folie à deux. See **shared paranoid disorder.**

folie circulaire. See **bipolar disorder.**

folie du doute /dYdo͞ot'/ [Fr, madness of doubts], an extreme obsessive-compulsive reaction characterized by persistent doubting, vacillation, repetition of a particular act or behavior, and pathologic indecisiveness to the point of being unable to make even the most trifling decision.

folie du pourquoi /dYpo͞orkwô·ä'/ [Fr, madness of why], a psychopathologic condition characterized by the persistent tendency to ask questions, usually concerning unrelated topics.

folie gemellaire /zhemeler'/ [Fr, madness in twins], a psychotic condition occurring simultaneously in twins, sometimes in those not living together or closely associated at the time.

folie musculaire /mYskYler'/, severe chorea.

folie raisonnante /rezônäNt'/ [Fr, deliberating reason], a delusional form of any psychosis marked by an apparent logical thought process but lacking common sense.

folinic acid /fōlin'ik/, an active form of folic acid. Folinic acid is used in the treatment of megaloblastic anemias not caused by vitamin B$_{12}$ deficiency and to counteract the toxic effects of antineoplastic folic acid antagonists, such as methotrexate. Also called **citrovorum factor, leucovorin.**

folk illnesses /fōk/, health disorders that are attributed to nonscientific causes. The major categories are naturalistic illnesses, caused by impersonal factors such as yin-yang forces, and personalistic illnesses, caused by evil eye or other 'magic'.

follicle /fol'ikəl/ [L, *folliculus,* small bag], a pouchlike depression, such as the dental follicles that enclose the teeth before eruption or the hair follicles within the epidermis. **–follicular,** *adj.*

follicles of Lieberkuhn. See **Lieberkuhn's glands.**

follicle stimulating hormone (FSH), a gonadotropin, secreted by the anterior pituitary gland, that stimulates the growth and maturation of graafian follicles in the ovary and promotes spermatogenesis in the male. FSH-releasing factor produced in the median eminence of the hypothalamus controls the release of FSH by the pituitary. Increasing amounts of FSH are secreted in the postmenstrual or resting phase of the menstrual cycle, causing a primordial follicle to develop into a mature graafian follicle containing a mature ovum. The graafian follicle produces estrogen, which reaches a high level before ovulation and suppresses release of FSH. In males, FSH maintains the integrity of the seminiferous tubules and influences all the stages of spermatogenesis. FSH may be given in treating some conditions. One form is derived from the urine of postmenopausal women. Also called **menotropins.**

follicle-stimulating hormone releasing factor (FSH-RF) [L, *folliculus,* small bag, *stimulare,* to incite; Gk, *horaein,* to set in motion; ME, *relesen;* L, *facere,* to do], the gonadotropin releasing hormone.

follicular adenocarcinoma /fōlik'yələr/, a neoplasm characterized by a follicular arrangement of cells that are usually derived from the thyroid gland. The neoplasm has a tendency to metastasize distantly to the lungs and bones. Surgery is the preferred treatment; if complete excision of the primary tumor is not feasible, radioiodine therapy is indicated. See also **medullary carcinoma, papillary adenocarcinoma.**

follicular cyst, an odontogenic cyst that arises from the epithelium of a tooth bud and dental lamina. The kinds of follicular cysts are dentigerous, primordial, and multilocular.

follicular goiter, an enlargement of the thyroid gland characterized by proliferation of the follicles and epithelial tissue.

follicular phase, the first part of the menstrual cycle, when ovarian follicles grow to prepare for ovulation.

follicular tonsillitis [L, *folliculus,* a small bag, *tonsilla;* Gk, *itis,* inflammation], an inflammation of the tonsils accompanied by a purulent infection of the tonsillar crypts.

follicular vulvitis [L, *folliculus,* a small bag, *vulva,* a wapper; Gk, *itis,* inflammation], an inflammation of the skin follicles of the vulva.

folliculitis /fōlik'yo͞olī'tis/, inflammation of hair follicles, such as in sycosis barbae.

folliculoma. See **granulosa cell tumor.**

folliculosis /fōlik'yo͞olōsis/, a condition characterized by the development of a large number of lymph follicles, which may or may not be associated with an infection. In conjunctival folliculosis the large number of lymph follicles may give the conjunctival sac a granular appearance.

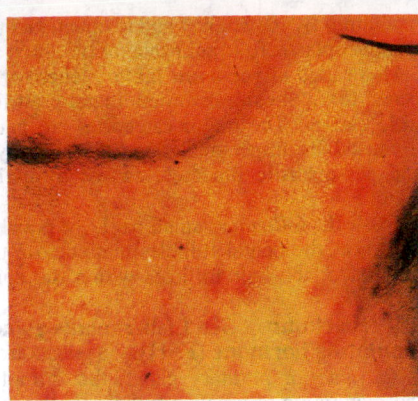

Folliculitis (Parkin, 1991)

Follutein, a trademark for a placental hormone (human chorionic gonadotropin).

fomentation /fō'mentā'shən/ [L, *fomentare,* to apply a poultice], **1.** a topical treatment for pain or inflammation with a warm, moist application. **2.** a substance or poultice that is used as a warm, moist application.

fomite /fō'mīt/ [L, *fomes,* tinder], nonliving material, such as bed linens, which may convey pathogenic organisms.

Fones' method /fōnz/, [Alfred C. Fones, American dentist, b. 1869], a toothbrushing technique that employs large, sweeping, scrubbing circles over occluded teeth, with the toothbrush held at right angles to the tooth surfaces. With the jaws parted, the palatal and lingual surfaces of the teeth are scrubbed in smaller circles. Occlusal surfaces of the teeth are scrubbed in an anteroposterior direction.

font, a set of type of one size and face.

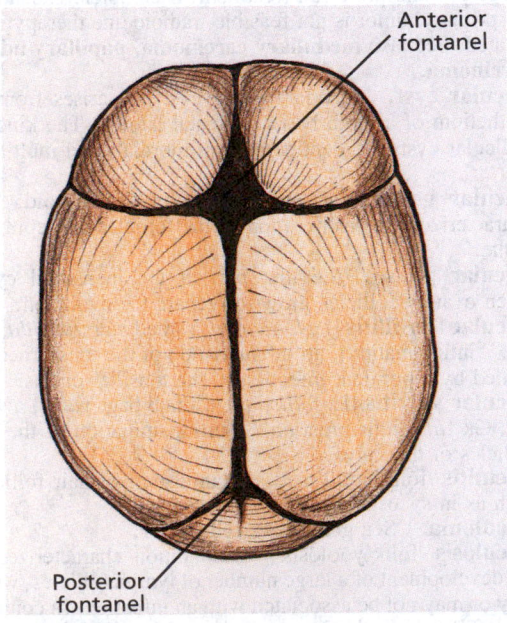

Fontanels (Potter, 1991)

fontanel /fon'tənel'/ [Fr, *fontaine,* fountain], a space covered by tough membranes between the bones of an infant's cranium. The anterior fontanel, roughly diamond-shaped, remains palpable until 18 to 24 months of age. The posterior fontanel, triangular in shape, closes about 2 months after birth. Increased intracranial pressure may cause a fontanel to become tense or bulge. A fontanel may be soft and depressed in the presence of dehydration. Also spelled **fontanelle.**

fonticulus /fontik'yələs/[L, little fountain], fontanel or fontanelle.

food [AS, *foda*], **1.** any substance, usually of plant or animal origin, consisting of carbohydrates, proteins, fats, and such supplementary elements as minerals and vitamins, that is ingested or otherwise taken into the body and assimilated to provide energy and to promote the growth, repair, and maintenance essential for sustaining life. **2.** nourishment in solid form as contrasted with liquid form. **3.** a particular kind of solid nourishment, such as breakfast food or snack food.

food additives, substances that are added to foods to prevent spoilage, improve appearance, enhance the flavor, or texture, or increase the nutritional value. Most food additives must be approved by the FDA after tests to determine if they could be a cause of cancer, birth defects, or other health problems. Examples include BHA (butylated hydroxyanisole) and BHT (butylated hydroxytoluene), antioxidants that are added to fats to retard rancidity.

food allergy, a hypersensitive state resulting from the ingestion of a specific food antigen. Symptoms of sensitivity to specific foods can include allergic rhinitis, bronchial asthma, urticaria, angioneurotic edema, dermatitis, pruritus, headache, labyrinthitis and conjunctivitis, nausea, vomiting, diarrhea, pylorospasm, colic, spastic constipation, mucous colitis, and perianal eczema. Food allergens are predominantly protein in nature. The most common foods causing allergic reactions are wheat, milk, eggs, fish and other sea foods, chocolate, corn, nuts, strawberries, chicken, pork, legumes, tomatoes, cucumbers, garlic, and citrus fruits. Foods that are rarely allergenic are rice, lamb, gelatin, peaches, pears, carrots, lettuce, artichokes, sesame oil, and apples. Diagnosis of a specific food allergy is obtained by a detailed food history, food diary, elimination diet, and cutaneous tests.

Food and Drug Administration (FDA), a federal agency responsible for the enforcement of federal regulations regarding the manufacture and distribution of food, drugs, and cosmetics as protection against the sale of impure or dangerous substances.

food and drug interactions, adverse health effects of certain combinations of foods and medications. A thiazide diuretic may cause depletion of potassium from body tissues, a vitamin C deficiency may reduce activity of drug-metabolizing enzymes, and isoniazid may interfere with the function of pyridoxine. Monoamine oxidase inhibitors may react with tyramine in certain cheeses, wines, and pickled seafood to produce a life-threatening hypertensive crisis.

food chain [ME, *fode, chaine*], an ecological sequence in which the various organisms within a community subsist upon a species lower in the sequence, as man eats the bird that eats the fish that eats the worm, and so on. Each level within the chain has a purpose and destruction of any one member in the chain affects the rest of the chain negatively.

food contaminants /kəntam'inənts/, substances that make

food unfit for human consumption. Examples include bacteria, toxic chemicals, carcinogens, teratogens, and radioactive materials. Also regarded as contaminants are basically harmless substances, such as water, that may be added to food to increase its weight.

food exchange list, a grouping of foods in which the carbohydrate, fat, and protein values are equal for the items listed. The list is used in meal planning for various diseases and deficiency states and was compiled by a joint committee of The American Dietetic Association, The American Diabetes Association, and the National Institutes of Health. The six groups of foods included on the list are milk, vegetables, fruits, grains, meats, and fats. Starchy vegetables and cereals are listed as bread exchanges; fish and cheese are meat exchanges.

food hypersensitivity reaction. See **food allergy.**

food poisoning, any of a large group of toxic processes resulting from the ingestion of a food contaminated by toxic substances or by bacteria containing toxins. Kinds of food poisoning include **bacterial food poisoning, ciguatera poisoning, Minamata disease, mushroom poisoning,** and **shellfish poisoning.** See also **botulism, ergot alkaloid, phalloidine poisoning, toadstool poisoning.**

food pyramid, a diagrammatic representation of human nutritional needs devised by the U.S. Department of Agriculture in 1992. It replaced the "four food groups" pie chart used since the 1950s. The USDA "Food Guide Pyramid" features a relatively wide base of 6 to 11 servings daily of grains and cereals beneath a layer representing 5 to 9 servings daily of fruits and vegetables. A third tapering level represents 4 to 6 daily servings of meats and dairy products. At the peak of the pyramid are fats and sweets, to be eaten sparingly.

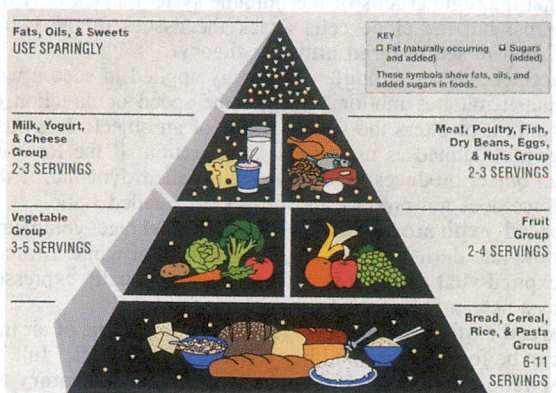

Food guide pyramid
(US Department of Agriculture: USDA Human Nutrition
Information Pub No. 249, Washington D.C., 1992,
US Government Printing Office)

food service administrator, a member of a hospital staff who is responsible for the planning and management of the food service system of the facility.

food service department, the department of a hospital or similar health facility that is responsible for food preparation and services to patients and personnel. It also provides nutritional care to patients.

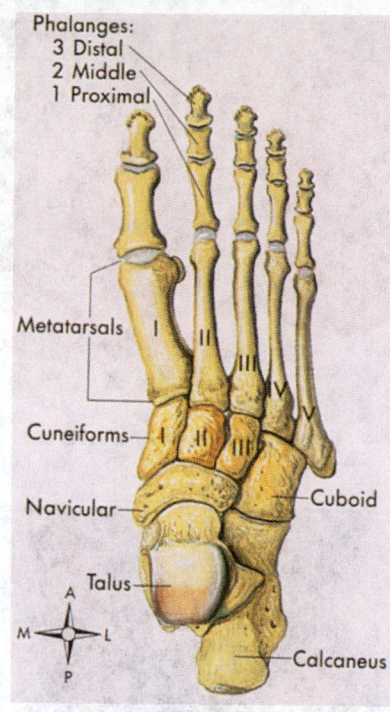

Foot
(Thibodeau, 1993/Ernest W. Beck)

foot [AS, *fot*], the distal extremity of the leg, consisting of the tarsus, the metatarsus, and the phalanges.

foot-and-mouth disease, an acute, extremely contagious, rhinovirus infection of cloven-hoofed animals. It is characterized by the development of ulcers on the skin around the mouth, on the mucous membrane in the mouth, and on the udders. Horses are immune. Uncommonly, the virus is transmitted to humans by direct contact with infected animals or their secretions or with contaminated milk. Symptoms and signs in humans include headache, fever, malaise, and vesicles on tongue, oral mucous membranes, hands, and feet. Generalized pruritus and painful ulcerations may occur; however, the temperature soon falls, the lesions subside in about a week, and total healing without scars is complete by 2 or 3 weeks. Treatment is symptomatic. Also called **aphthous fever** /af′thəs/. See also **picornavirus.**

footboard, a board or open box placed at the foot of a patient's bed and at a level above the top of the mattress to prevent the weight of the top sheet and blankets from resting on the feet. It is situated so that the feet rest firmly against the board, the legs at right angles to it, to maintain proper positioning of the feet while the patient is confined to bed. Its purpose is to help the bedfast patient retain normal posture and prevent footdrop. (See Fig. p. 634.)

footdrop /foot′drop/ [AS, *fot, dropa*], an abnormal neuromuscular condition of the lower leg and foot, characterized by an inability to dorsiflex, or evert, the foot because of damage to the common peroneal nerve. (See Fig. p. 634.)

-footed, a combining form meaning 'having feet' of a specified sort or number: *clubfooted, flatfooted, four-footed.*

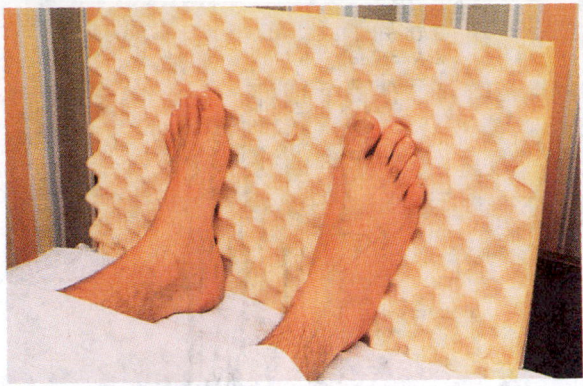

Footboard (Sorrentino, 1992)

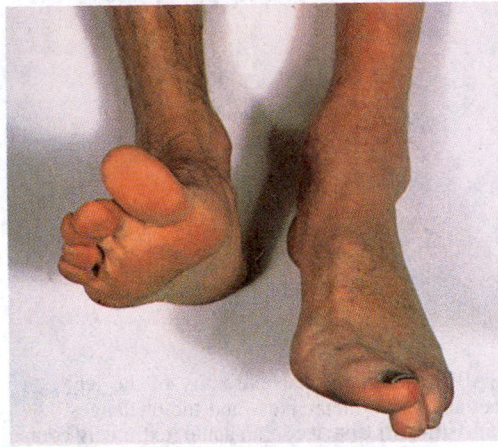

Footdrop (Perkin, 1986)

footling breech [AS, *fot;* ME, *brech*], an intrauterine position of the fetus in which one or both feet are folded under the buttocks at the inlet of the maternal pelvis, one foot presenting in a single footling breech, both feet in a double footling breech. Compare **frank breech.** See also **breech birth.**

foot-pound, a unit for the measurement of work or energy. One foot-pound is the amount of work required to move 1 pound a distance of 1 foot in the same direction as that of the applied force.

for-, a prefix meaning 'pertaining to an opening': *foramen, foramina, foration.*

foramen /fôrā′mən/, *pl.* **foramina** [L, hole], an opening or aperture in a membranous structure or bone, such as the apical dental foramen and the carotid foramen.

foramen magnum, a passage in the occipital bone through which the spinal cord enters the spinal column.

foramen of Monro /monrō′/, a passage between the lateral and third ventricles of the brain.

foramen ovale /ōvā′lē, ōvä′lā/, **1.** an opening in the septum between the right and the left atria in the fetal heart. This opening provides a bypass for blood that would otherwise flow to the fetal lungs. Most of the blood from the inferior vena cava in the fetus flows through the foramen

ovale into the left atrium. After birth, the foramen ovale functionally closes when the newborn takes the first breath and full circulation through the lungs begins. Complete closure of this opening takes about 9 months, and the foramen ovale eventually becomes the fossa ovale in the wall of the right atrial septum. See also **ductus arteriosus. 2.** an oval foramen situated laterally to the foramen rotundum of the sphenoid bone.

foramen rotundum, one of a pair of rounded apertures in the greater wings of the sphenoid bone.

foramen spinosum, a small opening near the posterior angle of the greater wing of the sphenoid bone. It is the smallest of three pairs of sphenoidal foramina that transmit nerves and blood vessels.

foramina. See **foramen.**

Forbes-Albright syndrome /fôrbsôl′brīt/ [A. P. Forbes; Fuller Albright, American physician, b. 1900], an endocrine disease characterized by amenorrhea, prolactinemia, and galactorrhea, caused by an adenoma of the anterior pituitary. Diagnosis is made by x-ray film of the anterior pituitary and a blood test for prolactin. Surgical resection of the adenoma is usually indicated. See also **galactorrhea, pituitary gland.**

Forbes' disease. See **Cori's disease.**

forbidden clone theory [AS, *forbeodan;* Gk, *klon,* a cutting; *theoria* speculation], a theory, associated with autoimmunity, based on the clonal evolution theory that at birth all the cells of the body that might react against the body have been eliminated, leaving only the cells that will react against foreign substances. The forbidden clone theory postulates that certain clone cells that can react against the body persist after birth and can be activated by a viral infection or by some metabolic change, especially if the viral organism is structurally similar to a body cell. The theory holds that the regular cells of the immune system attack only the virus, but the clone cells attack the tissues of the body. Compare **sequestered antigens theory.**

force [L, *fortis,* strong], **1.** energy applied in such a way that it initiates motion, changes the speed or direction of motion, or alters the size or shape of an object. **2.** a push or pull defined as mass times acceleration. If the force on an object produces movement, it is called dynamic; if the force does not produce movement, it is called static.

forced expiratory flow (FEF), the average volumetric flow rate during any stated volume interval while a forced expired vital capacity is performed. It is usually expressed as a percentage of vital capacity.

forced expiratory volume (FEV), the volume of air that can be forcibly expelled in a fixed time period after full inspiration. Compare **vital capacity.** See also **expiratory reserve volume.**

forced expired vital capacity (FEVC), a pulmonary function test of the maximal volume of gas that can be forcefully and rapidly exhaled starting from the position of full inspiration. Also called **forced vital capacity, time vital capacity.**

forced feeding, the administration of food by force, such as nasal feeding, to persons who cannot or will not eat.

forced-inhalation abdominal breathing, a respiratory therapy technique in which the patient is trained to inhale through the nose with an effort that is forceful enough to lift small sandbag weights placed on the abdomen. The technique is said to closely resemble the abdominal effort involved in normal breathing.

forced vital capacity. See **forced expired vital capacity.**

forceps, *pl.* forceps [L, pair of tongs], a pair of any of a large variety and number of surgical instruments, all of which have two handles or sides, each attached to a blade. The handles may be joined at one end, such as a pair of tweezers, or the two sides may be separate to be conjoined in use, such as obstetric forceps. Forceps are used to grasp, handle, compress, pull, or join tissue, equipment, or supplies. See specific forceps.

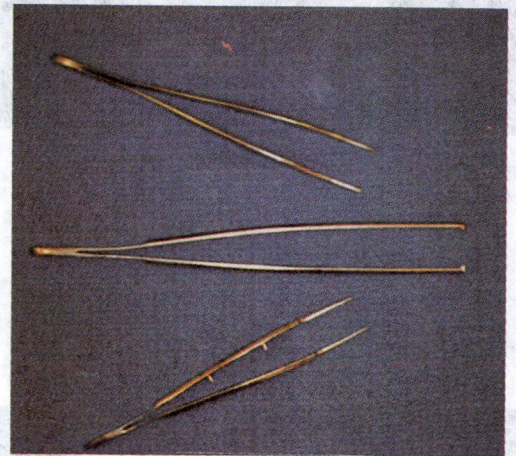

Forceps (Grossman, 1993)

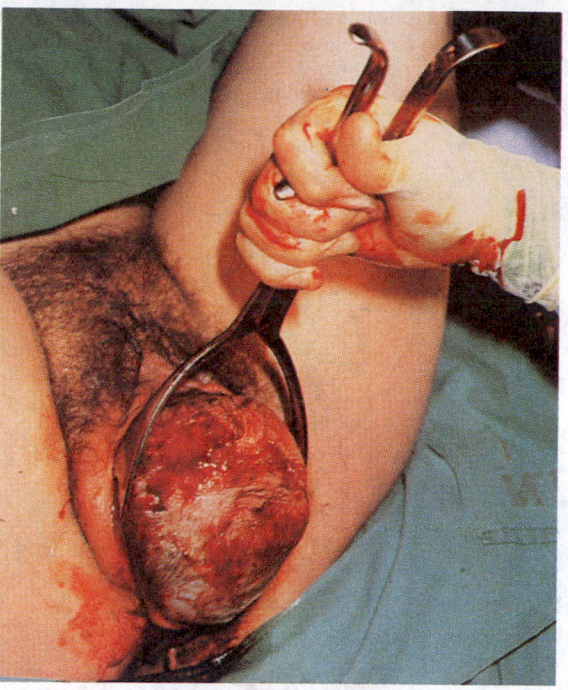

Forceps delivery (Al-Azzawi, 1991)

forceps delivery, an obstetric operation in which instruments are used to deliver a baby. It is performed to overcome dystocia, to quickly deliver a baby experiencing fetal distress, or, most often, to shorten normal labor. Local or regional anesthesia is usual, as is episiotomy. Prerequisites to forceps delivery include full dilatation of the cervix, engagement of the fetal head, and certain knowledge of the position of the head. The blades of the forceps are introduced into the vagina one at a time and applied symmetrically to opposite sides of the baby's head; the handles of the forceps are brought together so that the head is held firmly between the blades; the head is rotated, if necessary, to the occiput anterior or occiput posterior position; and traction is applied so as to draw the head from the birth passage. When the head has been delivered, the forceps are removed and the delivery is completed manually. Forceps produce marks on a baby's head and face; unless application has been imperfect, the marks are usually superficial and disappear in a few days. Because cesarean section is performed more often now than formerly, traumatic forceps deliveries are uncommon. Kinds of forceps delivery are **high forceps, low forceps,** and **mid forceps.** Compare **failed forceps, forceps rotation, trial forceps.** See also **obstetric forceps.**

forceps rotation, an obstetric operation in which forceps are used to turn a baby's head that is arrested in transverse or posterior position in the birth canal. It may be performed to facilitate spontaneous birth or as the first step in a forceps delivery. Kinds of forceps rotation are **Kielland rotation** and **Scanzoni rotation.** Compare **forceps delivery, manual rotation.** See also **obstetric forceps.**

forceps tenaculum. See **tenaculum.**

forcible inspiration [L, *fortis,* strong, *inspirare*],

breathing that is assisted by a mechanical ventilator that forces air into the lungs during inspiration but allows a return to ambient pressure as the patient exhales passively.

Fordyce-Fox disease /fôr′disfoks′/, an apocrine gland disorder producing symptoms similar to those of miliaria. It is characterized by intensely itchy follicular papules in the axillae, umbilicus, areolae of the breast, and pubic area.

Fordyce's disease, the presence of enlarged oil glands in the mucosal membranes of the lips, cheeks, gums, and genitalia. It is a common condition and may be symptomless. The ectopic sebaceous glands of the buccal mucosa appear as tiny, whitish yellow raised lesions (Fordyce spots).

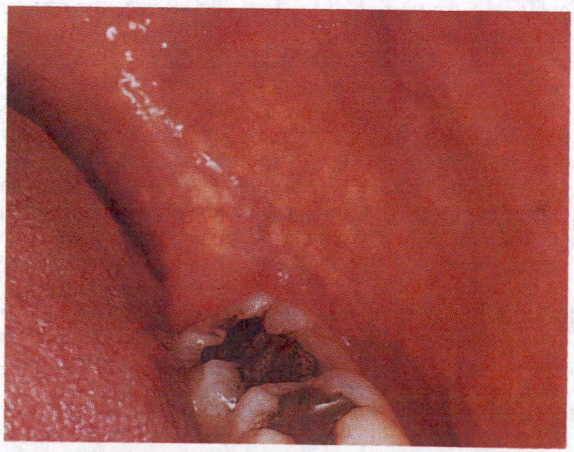

Fordyce's disease (Lamey, 1988)

fore-, a prefix meaning 'front or before': *forearm, foregut, forewaters.*

forearm, the portion of the upper extremity between the elbow and the wrist. It contains two long bones, the radius and ulna.

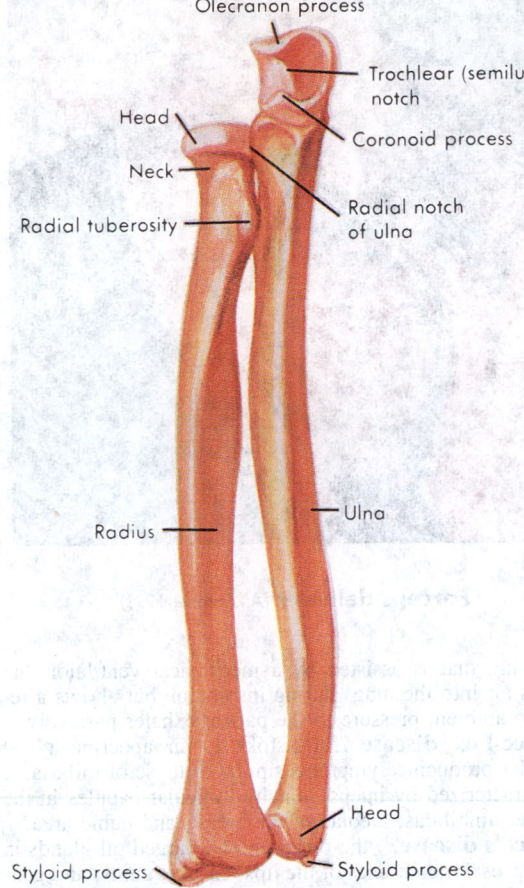

Forearm (Seeley, 1992/David J Mascaro & Associates)

forebrain. See **prosencephalon.**

forefinger, the first, or index, finger.

forefoot, the portion of the foot that includes the metatarsus and toes.

foregut /fôr′gut/ [AS, *fore*, in front, *guttas*], the cephalic portion of the embryonic alimentary canal. It consists of endodermal tissue and gives rise to the pharynx, esophagus, stomach, liver, pancreas, most of the small intestine, and the respiratory ducts. Compare **hindgut, midgut.**

foreign body /fôr′in/ [Fr, *forain*, alien; AS, *bodig*], any object or substance found in the body in an organ or tissue in which it does not belong under normal circumstances, such as a bolus of food in the trachea or a particle of dust in the eye.

foreign body granuloma [OFr, *forain*; AS, *bodig*; L, *granulum*, little grain; Gk, *oma*, tumor], a chronic inflammatory mass of tissue that accumulates around foreign bodies such as gravel, splinters, or bits of sutures.

foreign body in ear [OFr, *forain*; AS, *bodig, eare*], anything found in the ear that is not normally there, such as a bean or pebble.

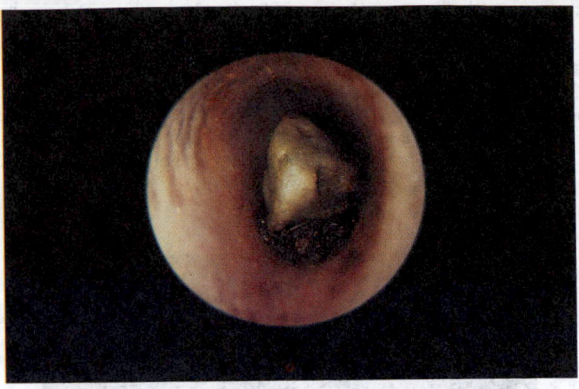

Foreign body in the ear
(Bingham, 1992/Courtesy Dr. Lalitha Shakar, St. Joseph's Health Centre, Toronto)

foreign body in esophagus [OFr, *forain*; AS, *bodig*; Gk, *oisophagos*, gullet], anything found in the esophagus that is not normally a part of the tissue.

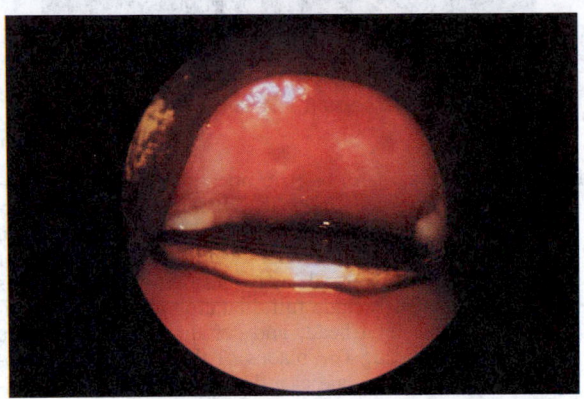

Foreign body in the esophagus
(Bingham, 1992/Courtesy Dr. Bruce Benjamin)

foreign body in eye [OFr, *forain*; AS, *bodig, éage*], anything found in the eye that is not a normal part of the tissue.

foreign body in larynx [OFr, *forain*; AS, *bodig*; Gk, *larynx*], anything found in the larynx tissues that is not normally present.

foreign body in throat [OFr, *forain*; AS, *bodig, throte*], anything found in throat tissue that is not normally present. A common foreign body in the throat is a posteriorly displaced tongue.

foreign body obstruction, a disturbance in normal function or a pathologic condition caused by an object lodged in a body orifice, passage, or organ. Most cases occur in children who suddenly inhale or swallow a foreign object or insert it in a body opening. In adults, large boluses of hastily eaten food frequently lodge in the esophagus, causing coughing, choking, and, if the airway is obstructed, asphyxia. Forceful blows to the victim's back between the

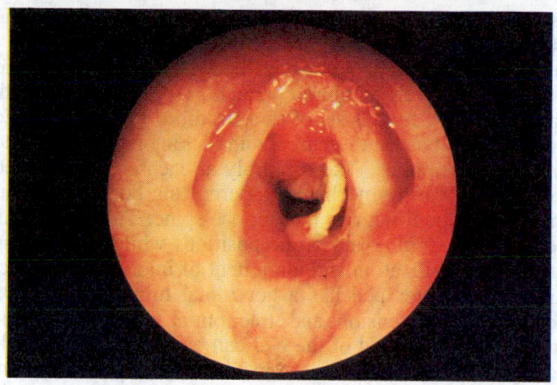

Foreign body in the larynx
(Bingham, 1992/Courtesy Dr. Bruce Benjamin)

shoulder blades or the Heimlich maneuver may dislodge the bolus. Esophageal foreign bodies usually produce an immediate reaction, but occasionally children have a long asymptomatic period before signs of obstruction or infection are evident. Laryngeal foreign bodies usually cause hoarseness, wheezing, and dyspnea; a sharp object, such as a chicken bone, may perforate the larynx and produce swelling and infection. Objects may be removed from the larynx, using a grasping forceps through a direct laryngoscope, with the patient under local or general anesthesia in the Trendelenburg position. A foreign body in the trachea may cause wheezing, an audible slap, coughing, and dyspnea; a small object may become lodged in a bronchus, producing coughing, which is often followed by an asymptomatic period before signs of obstruction and inflammation appear; vegetable foreign bodies produce earlier, more severe inflammatory symptoms than other objects. A bronchoscope with suitable forceps and general anesthesia are usually employed in removing bronchial foreign bodies, but thoracotomy may be required if the object is in the periphery of a lung. Objects that children sometimes insert in their nostrils may cause local obstruction, mild discomfort, or infection and may be removed by forceps or nasal suction. Needles and hairpins ingested by children often pass through the esophagus and stomach without incident but may become lodged at the turn of the duodenum and require removal by a magnetized nasogastric tube or by laparotomy; laxatives are contraindicated, and if tenderness, rigidity, pain, nausea, or vomiting ensues, immediate surgery is necessary. Coins, marbles, and closed safety pins usually pass through the digestive tract without creating problems; but hairballs, vegetable fibers, or shellac concretions, sometimes found in the stomach of emotionally disturbed or retarded patients, may cause anorexia, nausea, and vomiting. Hairballs may be fragmented with endoscope and removed by lavage; surgery may be required. Urethral inflammation and hematuria, sometimes caused by the introduction of a foreign body into the urethra during self-exploration, may be treated symptomatically.

foreign medical graduate (FMG), a physician trained in and graduated from a medical school outside the United States and Canada. United States citizens graduated from medical schools outside the United States and Canada are also classified as FMGs.

forensic /fôren′sik/ [L, *forum*, public place], pertaining to courts of law.

forensic dentistry, the branch of dentistry that deals with the legal aspects of professional dental practices and treatment, with particular emphasis on the use of dental records to identify victims of crimes or accidents.

forensic medicine [L *forum*, public place, *medicinus* physician], a branch of medicine that deals with the legal aspects of health care.

forensic psychiatry [L, *forum*, public place; Gk, *psyche*, mind + *iatreia*, treament], a branch of psychiatry concerned with the application of psychiatry to law, including criminal responsibility, guardianship, and competence to stand trial.

foreplay /fôr′plā/, sexual activities, such as kissing and fondling, that precede coitus.

foreshortened image /fôrshôr′tənd/, a distortion in x-ray imaging caused by inclination of an object or improper alignment of the x-ray tube, resulting in an image that is smaller than the object itself.

foreskin /for′skin/ [AS, *fore* + *skinn*], a loose fold of skin that covers the end of the penis or clitoris. Its removal constitutes circumcision. The nurse observes for any interference with urination in infants. Also called **prepuce.**

forest yaws /for′ist/ [L, *foris*, outside; Afr, *yaw*, strawberry], a cutaneous form of American leishmaniasis, common in South and Central America, caused by *Leishmania guyanensis*. The disease is chronic, with multiple deep skin ulcers that occasionally spread to the nasal mucosa. Also called **pian bois.**

forewaters /fôr′wôtərs/ [AS, *fore* + *waeter*], the amniotic fluid between the presenting part and the intact membranes.

forked tongue /fôrkt/ [L, *furca*; AS, *tunge*], a tongue divided by a longitudinal fissure. Also called **bifid tongue, slit tongue.**

-form, -forme, a suffix meaning 'having a (specified) shape or form': *linguiform, toruliform.*

formaldehyde /fôrmal′dəhīd/, a toxic, colorless, foul-smelling gas that is soluble in water and used in that form as a disinfectant, fixative, or preservative.

formalin /fôr′məlin/, a clear solution of formaldehyde in water. A 37% solution is used for fixing and preserving biologic specimens for pathologic and histologic examination.

format /fôr′mət/, a computer arrangement of data for storage or display. It may involve dividing the space on a disk into marked sectors for storage.

formation /fôrmā′shən/, a cluster of people that occupy and therefore define a quantum of space.

formative evaluation /fôr′mətiv/, judgments made about effectiveness of nursing interventions as they are implemented.

forme fruste /fôrm′ frYst′, fôrm′ frŌŌst′/, *pl.* **formes frustes,** [Fr, rough form] **1.** an incomplete or atypical form of a disease or a disease that is spontaneously arrested before it has run its usual course. **2.** (in genetics) an inherited disorder in which there is minimal expression of an abnormal trait.

formic acid /fôr′mik/, a colorless, pungent liquid found in nature in nettles, in ants, and in other insects. It is prepared commercially from oxalic acid and glycerin and from the oxidation of formaldehyde. Formerly used as a vesicant, it currently has no therapeutic applications.

formiminoglutamic acid (FIGLU) /fôrmim′inōglo͞ota-m′ik/, a compound formed in the metabolism of histidine, occurring in urine in elevated levels in folic acid deficiency. Increased excretion of FIGLU may indicate folic acid deficiency.

-formin, a combining form for phenformin-type oral hypoglycemics.

formol. See **formaldehyde.**

formula /fôr′m(y)ələ/ [L, *forma,* pattern], a simplified statement, generally using numerals and other symbols, expressing the constituents of a chemical compound, a method for preparing a substance, or a procedure for achieving a desired value or result. **–formulaic,** *adj.*

formulary /fôr′myəle′rē/ [L, *forma,* pattern], a listing of drugs intended to include a large enough range of drugs and sufficient information about them to enable health practitioners to prescribe treatment that is medically appropriate. Hospitals maintain formularies that list all drugs commonly stocked in the hospital pharmacy. Third-party organizations, such as insurance companies, usually maintain formularies listing drugs for which the company will pay in settlement of claims. See also **compendium,** *United States Pharmacopeia.*

formulation /fôr′myəlā′shən/ [L, *forma,* pattern], **1.** a pharmacologic substance prepared according to a formula. **2.** a systematic and precise statement of a problem, a theory, or a method of analysis in research.

formylmethionine (FMET) /fôr′milməthī′ənēn/, (in molecular genetics) the first amino acid in a protein sequence.

fornication /fôr′nikā′shən/ [L, *fornix,* arch], (in law) sexual intercourse between two people who are not married to each other. The specific legal definition varies from jurisdiction to jurisdiction. In some, both persons are unmarried; in some, one is unmarried; in some, the charge is adultery rather than fornication if the woman is married, regardless of the man's marital status.

fornix /fôr′niks/, *pl.* **fornices** /fôr′nisēz/ [L, arch], an archlike structure or space, such as the fornix cerebri, the superior or inferior conjunctival fornices, or the vaginal fornices.

fornix cerebri /ser′əbrī/, an archlike body of nerve fibers that lies beneath the corpus callosum of the cranium and serves as the efferent pathway from the hipppocampus.

fornix vaginae. See **vaginal fornix.**

forskolin (FSK), an activator of adenylate cyclase. FSK interacts directly with ion channels, increasing glutamate responses and amplitude and decay time of spontaneous excitatory postsynaptic currents.

Fortaz, a trademark for a cephalosporin antibiotic (ceftazidime).

Fort Bragg fever. See **pretibial fever.**

fortified milk [L, *fortis,* strong; AS *milc*], pasturized milk enriched with one or more nutrients, usually vitamins A and D, which has been standardized at 400 International Units per quart (**fortified vitamin D milk).**

forward-leaning posture, a respiratory therapy technique that is intended to reduce or eliminate accessory muscle activity in ambulatory patients with breathing difficulty. It involves walking in a slightly stooped, foward-leaning posture. For patients unable to tolerate functional walking, a special high walker with wheels is available.

Foscavir, trademark for an antiviral drug used in the treatment of cytomegalovirus retinitis.

fossa /fos′ə/, *pl.* **fossae** [L, ditch], a hollow or depression, especially on the surface of the end of a bone, such as the olecranon fossa or the coronoid fossa.

Foster bed /fos′tər/, a special bed used in the care and treatment of severely injured patients, especially those with spinal injuries. It consists of two Bradford frames mounted on a castered base and secured with locking bars to the head and foot assemblies. The assembly at each end is attached to a rotary bearing mechanism, permitting horizontal turning of the patient without moving the spine. The patient can be rotated to supine and prone positions while maintaining proper immobilization and alignment of injured body structures. The Foster bed has a horizontal turning frame that permits hyperextension and traction at each end of the frame, and either end of the bed can be elevated to provide countertraction. It can be used in posttraumatic management of patients with spinal instability, with or without cord damage, and in the management of the postoperative patient with multilevel spinal fusion when weight-bearing or ambulation is contraindicated. The Foster bed is also used in many scoliosis centers for halo-femoral traction, preparatory to spinal procedures with Harrington rods and Dwyer instrumentation. This preoperative technique permits stretching of the paravertebral soft tissues on the concavity of the spinal curve before operative correction and fusion. The bed also allows techniques for maintaining continuous cervical traction in flexion for selected patients with unstable cervical neck problems. The prone position with the use of a reading board permits self-feeding by the patient and participation in personal hygiene. Massage of the patient's forehead and chin areas toughens the skin and increases the patient's tolerance of the prone position. Foster bed patients sometimes display claustrophobia on being "sandwiched" between Foster frames, and skillful techniques to minimize the 'sandwiching' time are needed to ensure the greatest possible tranquillity of the patient. Frequent sensory stimulation with patient-staff interaction, discussions and games, and prism glasses that allow the patient to read and watch TV increase the person's comfort and tolerance of prolonged immobility. Compare **CircOlectric bed, hyperextension bed, Stryker wedge frame.**

foulage. See **pétrissage.**

foundation [L *fundamentum*], **1.** a charitable organization usually established to allocate private funds to worthy projects or to provide other services. **2.** (in dentistry) any device or material added to a remaining tooth structure to enhance the stability and retention of an overlying cast restoration, such as a pin retainer, amalgam, or a casting.

fourchette /fo͞orshet′/ [Fr, fork], a tense band of mucous membranes at the posterior angle of the vagina connecting the posterior ends of the labia minora.

four-handed dentistry, a technique of chairside operating in which four hands simultaneously perform tasks directly associated with dental work being accomplished in the oral cavity of a patient. The second pair of hands are those of a dental assistant or hygienist.

Fourier transform (FT) /fo͞oryā′/ [Jean B. J. Fourier, French mathematician, b. 1768; L, *transformare,* to change form], (in medical physics) a mathematic procedure that separates out the frequency components of a signal from its amplitudes as a function of time, or vice versa.

Fourier transform imaging, (in medical physics) NMR imaging techniques in which at least one dimension is phase encoded by applying variable gradient pulses along that dimension before 'reading out' the NMR signal with a gradient magnetic field perpendicular to the variable gradient. The Fourier transform is then used to reconstruct an image from the set of encoded NMR signals.

four-poster cast, a cast to immobilize the cervical vertebrae. It contains four verticle posts or poles on the anterior and posterior lateral sides of the head and is placed over the shoulders. The head is supported under the chin and occiput, and the posts prevent movement.

four-tailed bandage, a narrow piece of cloth with two ties on each end for wrapping a joint, such as an elbow or knee, or a prominence, such as the nose or chin.

fourth-generation scanner, a computed tomography machine in which the x-ray source rotates but the detector assembly does not. Radiation detection is accomplished through a fixed circular array of detectors that contains as many as 1000 individual elements. They may have scanning times as short as 1 second.

fourth nerve. See **trochlear nerve.**

fourth stage of labor [ME, *feower*, four; OFr, *estage*; L, *labor*, work], a postpartum period of about four hours following the third stage, or delivery of the placenta. Some complications, especially hemorrhage, occur at this time, requiring careful observation of the mother.

fourth ventricle [ME, *feower*, four; L, *ventriculum*, belly], a cavity with a diamond-shaped floor in the hindbrain, communicating below with the central canal of the spinal cord and above with the cerebral aqueduct of the midbrain. At the bottom of the ventricle are surfaces of the pons and medulla.

fovea capitis /fō′vē·ə/ [L, *fovea*, pit], 1. a depression on the proximal surface of the head of the radius where it meets the capitulum of the humerus. 2. a fovea on the head of the femur, where the ligamentum teres is attached.

fovea centralis an area at the center of the retina where cone cells are concentrated and there are no rod cells.

foxglove /foks′glov/, a common name for a plant that is a source of digitalis, *Digitalis purpura.*

Fowler's position /fou′lərz/ [George R. Fowler, American surgeon, b. 1848], the posture assumed by the patient when the head of the bed is raised 18 or 20 inches and the individual's knees are elevated.

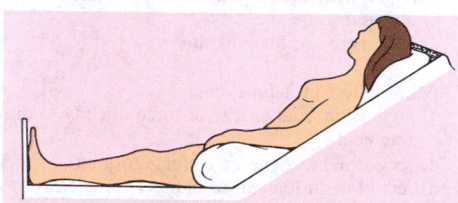

Fowler's position *(Potter, 1993)*

Fox's knife. See **Goldman-Fox knife.**

Fr, symbol for the element **francium.**

fract-, a combining form meaning 'pertaining to a breaking': *fractional, fractography, fracture.*

fractional anesthesia. See **continuous anesthesia.**

fractional dilatation and curettage /frak′shənəl/, a diagnostic technique in which each section of the uterus is examined and curetted to obtain specimens of the endometrium from all parts of the uterus. It is often performed under regional anesthesia in the diagnosis of endometrial cancer.

fractionation /frak′shənā′shən/ [L, *frangere*, to break], 1. (in neurology) a mechanism within the neural arch of the vertebrae whereby only a portion of the efferent nerves innervating a muscle reacts to a stimulus, even when the reflex requirement is maximal, so that there is a reserve of neurons to respond to additional stimuli. Through this phenomenon muscle tension is maintained. 2. (in chemistry) the separation of a substance into its basic constituents, by using such procedures as fractional distillation or crystallization. 3. (in bacteriology) the process of isolating a pure culture by successive culturing of a small portion of a colony of bacteria. 4. (in histology) the process of isolating the different components of living cells by centrifugation. 5. also called **dose fractionation, fractionation radiation.** (in radiology) the process of administering a dose of radiation in smaller units over a period of time to minimize tissue damage rather than in a single large dose.

fractionation radiation. See **fractionation.**

fraction of inspired oxygen (FiO₂) [L, *frangere*, to break, *inspirare*, to breathe in; Gk, *oxys*, sharp, *genein*, to produce], the proportion of oxygen in the air that is inspired.

fracture /frak′chər/ [L, *fractura*, break], a traumatic injury to a bone in which the continuity of the tissue of the bone is broken. A fracture is classified by the bone involved, the part of that bone, and the nature of the break, such as a comminuted fracture of the head of the tibia. See also specific types of fractures.

fracture-dislocation, a fracture involving the bony structures of any joint, with associated dislocation of the same joint.

fracture of clavicle [L, *fractura, clavicula*, little key], a break in the long bone of the shoulder girdle. It is usually accompanied by pain, swelling, and a protuberance and depression over the site of the injury. The patient usually supports the injured arm at the elbow. Treatment usually involves application of a clavicle strap or a figure-of-eight wrap.

fracture of olecranon [L, *fractura*; Gk, *olekranon*, point of the elbow], a fracture of the bony prominence of the ulna at the elbow joint. Different types of olecranon fractures may occur, depending upon the articular surfaces involved and possible displacement of the radius. The triceps, which normally extends the elbow, may become spastic as a result of the injury.

fracture of patella [L, *fractura, patella*, small pan], a break in the sesamoid knee cap. The fracture often occurs in automobile accidents in which the knee strikes the dashboard. The damage is complicated by the reflex bracing of the quadriceps femoris muscle that pulls the fragments apart. Treatment includes suturing the bone fragments and confining the patient in a lower body cast.

fracture of radius [L, *fractura, ray*] a fracture and dislocation of the lower end of the radius, usually with backward and radial displacement of the wrist and hand. The fracture commonly occurs when a falling person extends the arm and hand in an effort to cushion the impact. Also called **Colles' fracture.**

fracture of skull [L, *fractura*; AS, *skulle*, bowl], a break in the structure of one or more of the cranial bones. A fracture of bones in the vault of the skull is usually a compound fracture and complicated by possible damage to brain tissue, particularly if shards of cranial bones are driven into the brain by the force of the trauma.

fragile X syndrome /fraj′əl/, a reproductive disorder

Types and causes of fractures

Type	Description	Cause
Avulsed	Fracture that pulls bone and other tissues from usual attachments	Direct energy or force, with resisted extension of bone and joint
Bucket-handle	Double vertical fractures of pelvis on same side, resulting in pelvic dislocation	Direct blow or anterior compression force, with or without sacral torsion
Butterfly	Butterfly-shaped piece of fractured bone, usually accompanying comminuted fracture	Direct, indirect, or rotational force to bone
Comminuted	Fracture with more than two pieces; may have significant associated soft tissue trauma	Direct crushing injury or force to tissues and bone
Compound (open)	Skin broken over fracture; possible soft tissue trauma	Moderate to severe energy that is continuous and exceeds tissue tolerances
Compression	Fraction is squeezed or wedged together at one side	Compressive, axial energy or force applied directly from above fracture site
Displaced	Fracture with one, both or all fragments out of normal alignment	Direct energy or force to site
Greenstick	Break in only one cortex of bone	Minor direct or indirect energy
Impacted	Fracture with one end wedged into opposite end or inside fractured fragment	Compressive axial energy or force directly to distal fragment
Intraarticular	Fracture involving bones inside a joint	Direct or indirect energy or force to joint
Lead pipe (torus)	Fracture of one cortex of shafts of radius and ulna (one cortex of each bone), shown as wrinkle or buckle	Direct blow to forearm or indirect compressive force, as from fall
Linear	As a line, so can be transverse or oblique	Minor or moderate energy of force directly to bone
Neoplastic (pathologic)	Transverse, oblique, or spiral fracture of bone weakened by tumor pressure or presence	Minor energy or force, which may be direct or indirect
Oblique	Fracture at oblique angle across both cortices	Direct or indirect energy, with angulation and some compression
Occult	Fracture that is hidden or not readily discernible	Minor force or energy
Segmental	Fracture with two or more pieces or segments	Direct or indirect moderate to severe force
Spiral	Fracture that curves around cortices and may become displaced by twist	Direct or indirect twisting energy or force with distal part held or unable to move
Stellate	Central fracture point from which fissures radiate	Direct blow or force of moderate energy
Stress	Crack in one cortex of bone	Repetitive direct energy or force, as from jogging, running, or striking a lever, or from osteoporosis
Transverse	Horizontal break through bone	Direct or indirect energy toward bone

characterized by a nearly broken X chromosome, which has a tip hanging by a flimsy thread. It is the most common inherited cause of mental retardation. Tests for the broken chromosome are effective only about 75 percent of the time. Some healthy individuals may possess fragile x chromosomes without exhibiting symptoms and may transmit the condition to children or grandchildren.

fragilitas ossium.   See **osteogenesis imperfecta.**

fragmented fracture /frag'mentid/ [L, *frangere*, to break; *fractura* break],   a fracture that results in multiple bone fragments.

frail elderly,   an older person (usually over the age of 75) who is afflicted with physical or mental disabilities that may interfere the ability to independently perform activities of daily living.

frambesia.   See **yaws.**

frame of reference [AS, *framian*, to help; L, *referre*, to carry back],   the personal guidelines of an individual, taken as a whole. An individual frame of reference reflects the person's social status, cultural norms, and concepts.

Franceschetti's syndrome /fran'chesket'ēz/ [Adolphe Franceschetti, Swiss ophthalmologist, b. 1896],   a complete form of mandibulofacial dysostosis. See also **Treacher-Collins' syndrome.**

franchise dentistry /fran'chīz/ [Fr, exemption; L *dens,* tooth],   the practice of dentistry under a trade name, which has been purchased from another dentist or dental practice. Under a franchise license agreement the franchiser may use the trade name, the associated marketing products, and treatment techniques for a sum of money, in accordance with the franchise rules and regulations.

francium (Fr) /fran'sē·əm/ [France],   a metallic element of the alkali metal group. Its atomic number is 87; its atomic weight is 223. Formed from the decay of actinium, all of its 20 isotopes are radioactive and short-lived.

frank [L, *francus*, forthright],   obvious or clinically evident, such as the unequivocal presence of a condition or a disease.

Frank biopsy guide,   a device consisting of a long needle containing a hooked wire used to obtain biopsy samples of breast tissue. The needle is inserted into the breast until its tip nearly touches the lesion observed by mammography. The needle is withdrawn but the hooked wire remains to locate the tissue site. The surgeon cuts along the wire or otherwise approaches the hooked end of the wire and removes the tissue. See also **Kopans needle.**

frank breech [L, *francus* + ME, *brec*],   an intrauterine position of the fetus in which the buttocks present at the maternal pelvic inlet, the legs are straight up in front of the body, and the feet are at the shoulders. Babies born in this position tend to hold their feet near their heads for some days after birth. Compare **complete breech, footling breech.** See also **breech birth.**

Frankfort horizontal plane [Frankfurt-am-Main (anthropological) Agreement, 1882],   (in dentistry) a craniometric plane determined by the inferior borders of the bony orbits and the upper margin of the auditory meatus, passing through the two orbitales and the two tragions. It is commonly used as a reference plane in orthodontic diagnosis and treatment planning.

Frankfort-mandibular incisor angle (FMTA),   (in dentistry) the precumbency of the mandibular incisor tooth to the Frankfort horizontal plane.

Frank-Starling relationship [Otto Frank, German physiologist, b. 1865; Ernest H. Starling, English physiologist,

b. 1866],   an index for determining cardiac output, based on the length of the myocardial fibers at the onset of contraction. The force exerted per beat of the heart is directly proportional to the length or degree of stretch of the myocardial fiber so that improved performance is the result of a longer initial fiber length or a larger diastolic ventricular volume. Because there are no adequate in vivo methods of measuring fiber length or diastolic volume, pulmonary capillary wedge pressure (PCWP) or pulmonary artery end-diastolic pressure (PAEDP) are used as an indices of volume or stretch. Also called **Frank-Starling mechanism.**

fraternal twins.   See **dizygotic twins.**

fraud /frôd/ [L, *fraudare,* to cheat],   (in law) the act of intentionally misleading or deceiving another person by any means so as to cause him legal injury, usually the loss of something valuable or the surrender of a legal right.

Fraunhofer zone /froun'hōfər/,   (in ultrasonography) the zone farthest from the transducer face. It is characterized by a divergence of the ultrasound beam and a more uniform ultrasound intensity. Also called **far field.** See also **Fresnel zone.**

FRC,   abbreviation for **functional residual capacity.**

freckle [ME, *freken*],   a brown or tan macule on the skin that usually results from exposure to sunlight. There is an

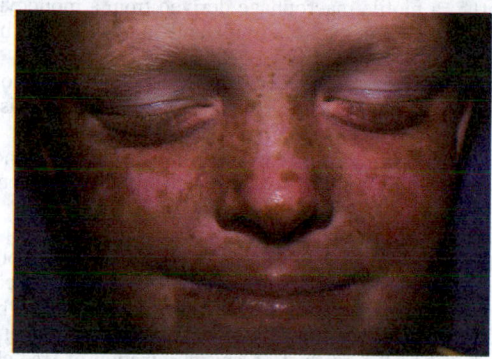

Freckles (Weston, 1991)

inherited tendency to freckling, and it is most frequently seen in persons with red hair. Freckles are harmless but people who freckle easily should avoid excessive sun exposure or use protective sunscreen lotions because they have a tendency to develop more serious actinic skin changes. Compare **lentigo.**

Fredet-Ramstedt's operation.   See **pyloromyotomy.**

free-air chamber [AS, *freo,* free; Gk, *aer,* air; L, *camera,* vault],   a device used as a primary standard for calibrating x-ray exposure. It is used in national calibration laboratories throughout the world.

free association, 1. the spontaneous, consciously unrestricted association of ideas, feelings, or mental images. 2. spontaneous verbalization of thoughts and emotions entering the consciousness during psychoanalysis.

freebase.   See **crack.**

freebasing,   a chemical process used to increase the stimulating effect of cocaine. The resulting product is smoked.

free clinic,   a clinic or health program, usually located in a neighborhood setting, that provides health care for ambulatory patients at nominal or no cost.

free fatty acid (FFA) [AS, *freo, faett*; L, *acidus,* sour], nonesterified fatty acids, released by the hydrolysis of triglycerides within adipose tissue. Free fatty acids can be used as an immediate source of energy by many organs and can be converted by the liver into ketone bodies.

free-floating anxiety, a generalized, persistent, pervasive fear that is not attributable to any specific object, event, or source. See also **anxiety, anxiety neurosis.**

free-form foot orthosis, an orthosis that is molded directly to a patient's foot. It requires less material and time but does not provide a positive model for a more exact fabrication of a balanced orthosis.

free gingiva, the unattached coronal portion of the gingiva that encircles a tooth and forms a gingival sulcus.

free gingival groove, a shallow line or depression on the gingival surface at the junction of the free and attached gingivae.

free graft [AS, *freo*; Gk, *graphein*, stylus], a graft completely removed from its original site and replaced at a new site in a single one-stage operation.

free-induction decay (FID), (in nuclear magnetic resonance imaging), a signal emitted by a tissue after a radio frequency (RF) pulse has excited the nuclear spins of the tissue at resonance. The decaying oscillation back to the normal state is the signal from which an NMR image is made.

free macrophage [AS, *freo*; Gk, *makros*, large, *phagein*, to eat], a motile macrophage derived from a monocyte. It responds to chemotactic stimuli and migrates from blood vessels to tissue spaces.

free nerve ending, a receptor nerve ending that is not enclosed in a capsule. A typical free nerve ending consists of a bare axon that may be myelinated or unmyelinated. It is often found in fibrous capsules, ligaments, or synovial spaces and may be sensitive to mechanical or biochemical stimuli.

free phagocyte. See **phagocyte.**

free radical, a compound with an unpaired electron or proton. It is unstable and reacts readily with other molecules.

free-radical theory of aging, a concept of aging based on the premise that the main causative factor is an imbalance between the production and elimination of free chemical radicals in the body tissues.

free thyroxine, the amount of the unbound, active thyroid hormone, thyroxine (T_4), circulating in the blood, measured by special laboratory procedures. See also **free thyroxine index.**

free thyroxine index, the amount of unbound, physiologically active thyroxine (T_4) in serum, determined by direct assay or, more frequently, calculated on the basis of an in vitro uptake test. In this test the uptake (by resin or charcoal) of labeled triiodothyronine (T_3) is measured; because T_3 is less strongly bound by serum, it is used rather than T_4. The free T_4 index is then obtained by multiplying the T_3 uptake by the total concentration of T_4 in serum.

freeway space [AS, *freo*, *wegan*; L, *spatiaum*], the interocclusal distance or separation between the occlusal surfaces of the teeth when the mandible is in its rest position.

freezing point [ME, *fresen*, to be cold; L, *punctus*, pricked], the temperature at which a substance changes from a liquid to a solid state. The freezing point for water is 32° on the **Fahrenheit** scale and 0° on the **Celsius** scale.

Freiberg's infarction [Albert H. Freiberg, American surgeon, b. 1868; L, *infarcire*, to stuff], an abnormal orthopedic condition characterized by osteochondritis or aseptic necrosis of bone tissue, most commonly affecting the head of the second metatarsal.

Frei test /frī/ [William S. Frei, German dermatologist, b. 1885], a test performed to confirm a diagnosis of lymphogranuloma venereum. Killed antigen, originally derived from infected patients, is injected intradermally in one forearm, and a control material is injected into the other arm. If a red, thickened papule develops at the site of injection of antigen, the test is positive. See also *Chlamydia.*

Frejka splint /frā'kə/, a corrective device consisting of a pillow that is belted between the legs of a baby born with dislocated hips to maintain abduction and articulation of the head of the femur with the acetabulum. See also **congenital dislocation of the hip.**

fremitus /frem'itəs/ [L, a growling], a tremulous vibration of the chest wall that can be auscultated or palpated during physical examination. Kinds of fremitus include **bronchial fremitus, coarse fremitus, tactile fremitus,** and **vocal fremitus.**

frena. See **frenum.**

frenectomy /frənek'təmē/ [L, *fraenum*, bridle; Gk, *ektome*, excision], a surgical procedure for excising a frenum or frenulum, such as the excision of the lingual frenum from its attachment into the mucoperiosteal covering of the alveolar process to correct ankyloglossia. Compare **frenotomy.**

Frenkel exercises, a system of slow repetitious exercises of increasing difficulty developed by a Swiss neurologist to treat ataxia in multiple sclerosis and similar disorders.

frenotomy /frənot'əmē/ [L, *fraenum* + Gk, *temnein*, to cut], a surgical procedure for repairing a defective frenum, such as the cutting or lengthening of the lingual frenum to correct ankyloglossia. Compare **frenectomy.**

frenulum. See **frenum.**

frenulum linguae. See **lingual frenum.**

frenulum of tongue /fren'yələm/ [L, *fraenum*, bridle; AS, *tunge*], a longitudinal fold of mucous membrane connecting the floor of the mouth to the underside of the tongue in midline. A congenital defect causes an abnormal shortness of the frenulum, resulting in tongue-tie, which can be surgically corrected.

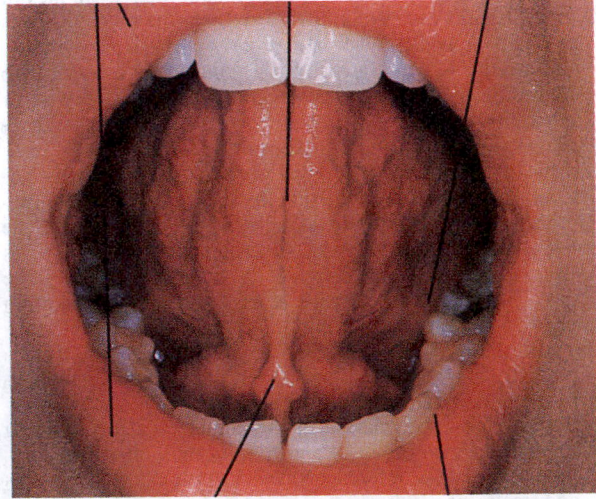

Frenulum

Frenulum of tongue (Seeley, 1992/Trent Stephens)

frenum /frē'nəm/, *pl.* **frenums, frena** [L, *fraenum*, bridle], a restraining portion or structure. Also called **frenulum.**

frequency (F) /frē′kwənsē/ [L, *frequens,* frequent], **1.** the number of repetitions of any phenomenon within a fixed period of time, such as the number of heart beats per minute. **2.** (in biometry) the proportion of the number of persons having a discrete characteristic to the total number of persons being studied. **3.** (in electronics) the number of cycles of a periodic quantity, such as alternating current, that occur in a period of 1 second. Electromagnetic frequencies, formerly expressed in cycles per second (cps), are now expressed in hertz (Hz).

fresh frozen plasma [ME, *fresen,* to be cold; Gk, *plassein,* to mold], an unconcentrated form of blood plasma containing all of the clotting factors except platelets. It can be used to supplement RBCs when whole blood is not available for exchange transfusion or to correct a bleeding problem of unknown etiology. See also **plasma.**

Fresnel zone /freznel′/, (in ultrasonography) the region nearest the transducer face. It is characterized by a highly collimated beam with great variation in ultrasound intensity and is generally the area of best image resolution. Also called **near field.**

Freud, Sigmund /froid/ [Austrian neurologist, 1856-1939], founder of a complex integrated theory of psychological causes of mental disorders, some, such as hysteria, with physical symptoms. Among tenets of Freudian theory: human beings are motivated by a pleasure principle; receive internal stimulation from a sex instinct and a death instinct; have personality structures that can be divided into ego, superego, and id; and have unconscious, preconscious, and conscious levels of mental activity. See also **freudian; freudian fixation; freudianism.**

freudian /froi′dē·ən/, **1.** of or pertaining to Sigmund Freud (1856–1939), his theories and doctrines, which stress the formative years of childhood as the basis for later psychoneurotic disorders, primarily through the unconscious repression of instinctual drives and sexual desires, and his system of psychoanalysis for treating such disturbances. **2.** anything that is easily interpreted according to the theories of Freud or in psychoanalytic terms. **3.** of or pertaining to the school of psychiatry based on Freud's teachings. **4.** one who adheres to Freud's school of psychiatry. See also **psychoanalysis.**

freudian fixation, an arrest in psychosexual development characterized by a firm emotional attachment to another person or object. Some kinds of freudian fixation are **father fixation** and **mother fixation.**

freudianism /froi′dē·əniz′əm/, the school of psychiatry based on the psychoanalytic theories and psychotherapeutic methods of treating psychoneurotic disorders developed by Sigmund Freud and his followers. Also called **freudism.** See also **psychoanalysis.**

friable /frī′əbəl/ [L, *friare,* to crumble], easily shattered, crumbled, or pulverized.

Fricke dosimeter, a chemical radiation dosimeter that uses the change of concentration of ferric ions in a solution subject to irradiation to quantify the amount of dose delivered to the sample.

friction /frik′shən/ [L, *fricare,* to rub], **1.** the act of rubbing one object against another. See also **attrition. 2.** a type of massage in which deeper tissues are stroked or rubbed, usually through strong circular movements of the hand. See also **massage.**

frictional force /frik′shənəl/, the force component parallel to the surfaces at the point of contact between two objects. The frictional component, in contact between curved objects, may be tangential to the surfaces. Frictional force may be increased or decreased by such factors as moisture on a surface.

friction burn, tissue injury caused by abrasion of the skin. See also **abrasion.**

friction rub, a dry, grating sound heard with a stethoscope during auscultation. It is a normal finding when heard over the liver and splenic areas. A friction rub auscultated over the pericardial area is suggestive of pericarditis; a rub over the pleural area may be present in lung disease.

Friedländer's bacillus /frēd′lendərz/ [Carl Friedländer, German pathologist, b. 1847], a bacterium of the species *Klebsiella pneumoniae,* which is associated with infection of the respiratory tract, especially lobar pneumonia.

Friedländer's disease, a severe arterial inflammation. There may be swelling and overgrowth of tissue cells lining the blood vessel, leading to complete obstruction of the artery. Also called **arteritis obliterans.**

Friedländer's pneumonia [Carl Friedländer. German pathologist, b.1847; Gk, *pneumon,* lung], a form of bronchopneumonia with a high mortality rate, particularly among older patients. The pneumonic patches tend to become confluent and those who survive may experience pulmonary abscesses and necrosis.

Friedman curve /frēd′mən/ [Emanuel A. Friedman, American obstetrician, b. 1926], a graph depicting the progress of labor, prepared by labor attendants to facilitate detection of dysfunctional labor. Observations of cervical dilatation and fetal descent are plotted on the vertical axis against time on the horizontal axis. The labor curve is divided into latent and active phases, with the latter subdivided into latent, acceleration, maximum slope, and deceleration phases.

Friedman's test [Maurice H. Friedman, American physiologist, b. 1903], a modification of the Aschheim-Zondek pregnancy test. A sample of urine from a woman is injected into a mature, unmated female rabbit. If, days later, the rabbit ovaries contain fresh corpora lutea or hemorrhaging corpora, the test is positive as a sign that the woman is pregnant.

Friedreich's ataxia /frēd′rīshs/ [Nickolaus Friedreich, German physician, b. 1825], an abnormal condition characterized by muscular weakness, loss of muscular control, weakness of the lower extremities, and an abnormal gait. Friedreich's ataxia, which may be hereditary, exhibits both dominant and recessive inheritance patterns. The primary

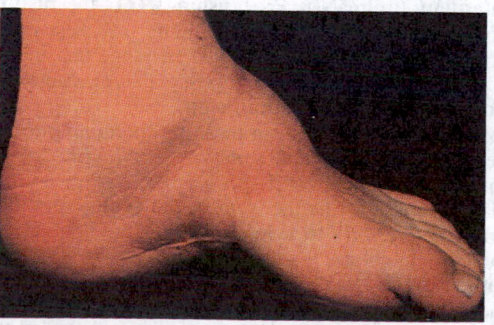

Pes cavus, common in Friedreich's ataxia
(Forbes, 1993)

pathologic feature of the disease is pronounced sclerosis of the posterior columns of the spinal cord with possible involvement of the spinocerebellar tracts and the corticospinal tracts. Friedreich's ataxia usually affects individuals between 5 and 20 years of age. The highest incidence of onset is at puberty. The characteristically ataxic gait may progress to severe disability. Over a period of years a child affected by Friedrich's ataxia may also develop ataxia of the upper extremities and have difficulty performing simple maneuvers, such as writing or handling silverware while eating. The characteristic gait of this disease is caused by a cavus deformity, or clawfoot. The gait and the stance of the affected individual are unsteady. A positive Romberg's sign may be evident, and Babinski's sign is present with absent or decreased deep reflexes. The condition may also cause slurred speech, head tremors, tachycardia, and cardiac failure. Thoracic scoliosis is present in approximately 80% to 90% of the patients afflicted. All the signs and symptoms are progressive. There is no curative treatment for Friedreich's ataxia. Orthoses may be useful to varying degrees in the prevention of associated deformities and the maintenance of an ambulatory status. Correction of the foot deformity allows the patient to remain ambulatory as long as possible and is preferred when the lack of progression of the disease process is demonstrated, thereby reducing the potential for recurrence. Spinal fusion may correct the associated scoliosis. Death in the progression of this disease is usually the result of myocardial failure.

Friedreich's sign [Nikolaus Friedreich, German physician, b. 1825; L, *signum*, sign], the diastolic collapse of the jugular veins in adherent pericardium.

Fried's rule, a method of estimating the dose of medicine for a child by multiplying the adult dose by the child's age in months and dividing the product by 150. See also **Clark's rule, Cowling's rule.**

frigid /frij′id/ [L, *frigidus*, cold], **1.** lacking warmth of feeling; unemotional; unimaginative; without passion or ardor and stiff or formal in manner. **2.** (of a woman) unresponsive to sexual advances or stimuli, abnormally indifferent or averse to sexual intercourse, or unable to have an orgasm during sexual intercourse. Compare **impotence.** See also **orgasm.** **–frigidity,** *n*.

fringe field /frinj/, (in magnetic resonance imaging) the part of a magnetic field that extends away from the confines of the magnet and cannot be used for imaging. However, it may affect nearby equipment and personnel.

frit /frit, frē/ [Fr, fried], a partially or wholly fused porcelain from which dental porcelain powders are made.

Fröhlich's syndrome. See **adiposogenital dystrophy.**

frôlement /frôlmäN′/ [Fr, brushing], **1.** the rustling type of sound often heard on auscultating the chest in diseases of the pericardium. **2.** a kind of massage that uses a light brushing stroke with the hand. See also **massage.**

Froment sign. See **thumb sign.**

front-, a combining form meaning 'pertaining to the forehead, or front': *frontad, frontalis, frontonasal.*

frontal bone /fron′təl/ [L, *frons*, forehead], a single cranial bone that forms the front of the skull, from above the orbits, posteriorly to a junction with the parietal bones at the coronal suture.

frontal lobe, the largest of five lobes constituting each of the two cerebral hemispheres. It lies beneath the frontal bone, occupies part of the lateral, the medial, and the inferior surfaces of each hemisphere, and extends posteriorly to the central sulcus and inferiorly to the lateral fissure. The frontal lobe significantly influences personality and is associated with the higher mental activities, such as planning, judgment, and conceptualizing. Research indicates that the right frontal and the right temporal lobes are associated with the nonverbal, specialized activities of the right cerebral hemisphere and that the left frontal and the left temporal lobes are associated with the verbal activities of the left cerebral hemisphere. The lateral surface of each frontal lobe contains the precentral, the superior, and the inferior sulci, which divide the lobe into the precentral, the superior, the middle, and the inferior frontal gyri. The left inferior frontal gyrus constitutes Broca's speech area and, in most individuals, is more convoluted than the right inferior frontal gyrus. An H-shaped orbital sulcus on the inferior surface of the frontal lobe divides its inferior surface into the medial, the anterior, the lateral, and the posterior orbital gyri. The olfactory sulcus on the inferior surface contains the olfactory tract and separates the gyrus rectus from the medial orbital gyrus. The medial surface of the frontal lobe is limited posteriorly by an imaginary line that extends downward and anteriorly to the corpus callosum from the intersection of the central sulcus with the superior margin of the lobe. The medial surface of the frontal lobe includes the superior frontal gyrus and part of the cingulate gyrus. The superior frontal gyrus extends posteriorly as the paracentral lobule into the parietal lobe of the hemisphere. Compare **central lobe, occipital lobe, parietal lobe, temporal lobe.**

frontal lobe syndrome, behavioral and personality changes usually observed after a neoplastic or traumatic frontal lobe lesion. The patient may become sociopathic, boastful, hypomanic, uninhibited, exhibitionistic, and subject to outbursts of irritability or violence; but in other cases the person may become depressed, apathetic, lacking in initiative, negligent about personal appearance, and inclined to perseverate. Partial frontal lobectomy was formerly performed by some psychosurgeons to reduce drive in extremely disturbed psychotic patients, but the results were highly questionable.

frontal plane, any one of the vertical planes passing through the body from the head to the feet, perpendicular to the sagittal planes, dividing the body into front and back portions. Also called **coronal plane.** Compare **median plane, sagittal plane, transverse plane.**

frontal pole [L, *frons*, forehead, *polus*], the anterior extremity of the frontal lobe of the cerebrum.

frontal section [L, *frons*, forehead, *sectio*, a cutting], a section of the head or other body part cut into anterior and posterior portions. Also called **coronal section.**

frontal sinus, one of a pair of small cavities in the frontal bone of the skull that communicates with the nasal cavity. The frontal sinuses, which are rarely symmetric, are situated behind the superciliary arches. Each sinus measures approximately 3 cm in height, 2.5 cm in width, and 2.5 cm in depth and is lined with a mucous membrane that is continuous with that of the nasal cavity. A large frontal sinus may project over most of the orbit. Each sinus opens into the anterior part of the middle meatus through the frontonasal duct. The frontal sinuses are absent at birth, well developed between the seventh and eighth years, and reach their full size after puberty. Compare **ethmoidal air cell, maxillary sinus, sphenoidal sinus.**

frontal vein, one of a pair of superficial veins of the face, arising in the plexus of the forehead. Each frontal vein communicates with the frontal tributaries of the superficial temporal vein and lies near the vein of the opposite side as it courses toward the root of the nose. The two frontal veins communicate by a transverse vessel before joining the supraorbital veins. Compare **angular vein, facial vein.**

frontocortical aphasia. See **motor aphasia.**

frostbite [AS, *frost, bitan*], traumatic effect of extreme cold on skin and subcutaneous tissues that is first recognized by distinct pallor of exposed skin surfaces, particularly the nose, ears, fingers, and toes. Vasoconstriction and damage to blood vessels impair local circulation and result in anoxia, edema, vesiculation, and necrosis. Gentle warming is appropriate first aid treatment; rubbing of the affected part is avoided. Later, therapy is similar to treatment of thermal burns. Iatrogenic frostbite is the result of excessive use of ethyl chloride sprays for local anesthesia for the relief of muscle and tendon strains. Compare **chilblain, immersion foot.**

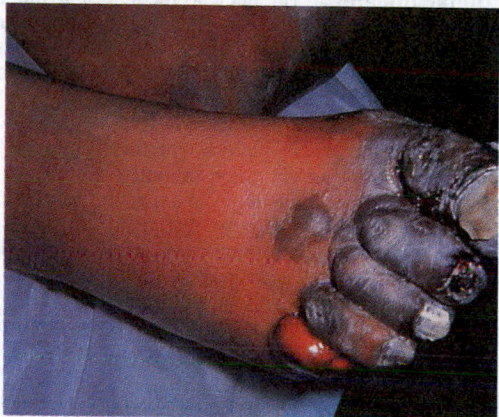

Frostbite (Grossman, 1993)

frostnip. See **frostbite.**

frottage /frôtäzh′/ [Fr, rubbing], sexual gratification obtained by rubbing (especially one's genital area) against the clothing of another person, as can occur in a crowd.

frotteur /frôtœr′/ [Fr], a person who obtains sexual gratification by the practice of frottage.

frozen blood. See **bank blood.**

frozen section [ME, *fresen*; L, *sectio*], a histological section of tissue that has been frozen by exposure to dry ice.

frozen section method [AS, *freosan*, to freeze; L, *sectio*, a cutting; Gk *meta* order, *hodos* path], (in surgical pathology) a method used in preparing a selected portion of tissue for pathologic examination. The tissue is moistened and, fixed or unfixed, is rapidly frozen and cut by a microtome in a cryostat. This method is very rapid, allowing the pathologist to examine the specimen during a surgical procedure.

F.R.S.C., abbreviation for *Fellow of the Royal Society of Canada.*

fructokinase /fruk′tōkī′nās/, an enzyme that catalyzes the transfer of a phosphate group from adenosine triphosphate to D-fructose.

fructose /fruk′tōs, frŏŏk′-/, a yellowish-to-white, crystalline, water-soluble levorotatory ketose monosaccharide that is sweeter than sucrose and found in honey, several fruits, and combined in many disaccharides and polysaccharides. It is used as a preservative. In the absence of insulin it is metabolized or converted in the body to glycogen. Also called **fruit sugar, levulose.**

fructose intolerance [L, *fructus*, fruit, *in, tolerare*, to bear], an inherited disorder marked by an absence of enzymes needed to metabolize fructose. Symptoms include sweating, tremors, confusion, and digestive distress, with vomiting, and failure of infants to grow. The condition is transmitted as an autosomal dominant trait.

fructosemia /frŏŏk′tōsē′mē·ə/ [L, *fructus*, fruit; Gk, *haima*, blood], the presence of fructose in the blood.

fructosuria /frŏŏk′tōsŏŏr′ē·ə/, presence of the sugar, fructose, in the urine. This usually harmless and asymptomatic condition is caused by the hereditary absence of the enzyme fructokinase, which normally helps metabolize fructose. Essential fructosuria is associated with symptoms of diabetes. Also called **levulosuria.**

fruit sugar. See **fructose.**

frustration /frustrā′shən/, a feeling that results from an interference with one's ability to attain a desired goal or satisfaction.

FSH, abbreviation for **follicle stimulating hormone.**

FSH-RF, abbreviation for **follicle-stimulating hormone releasing factor.**

FSK, abbreviation for **forskolin.**

FT, abbreviation for *fast-twitch.* See **fast-twitch fiber.**

FTA-ABS test. See **Fluorescent Treponemal Antibody Absorption Test.**

FTC, abbreviation for **Federal Trade Commission.**

FTT, abbreviation for **failure to thrive.**

fuchsin bodies. See **Russell's bodies.**

FUDR, a trademark for an antiviral and antineoplastic (floxuridine).

fugue /fyo͞og/ [L, *fuga*, running away], a state of dissociative reaction characterized by amnesia and physical flight from an intolerable situation. During the episode, the person appears normal and acts as though consciously aware of what may be very complex activities and behavior, but after the episode, the person has no recollection of the actions or behavior. The condition may last for only a few days or weeks, or it may continue for several years, during which the person wanders away from the customary environment, enters a new occupation, and undertakes an entirely different way of life. The syndrome appears to be caused by an inability to cope with a severe conflict or with a chronically stressful life situation. A form of fugue also occurs briefly after an epileptic seizure. See also **ambulatory automatism, automatism.**

fulcrum /fŏŏl′krəm, ful′-/ [L, *fulcire*, to support], **1.** the stable point or the position on which a lever, such as the ulna or the femur, turns. Numerous common movements of the body, such as raising the arm and walking, are combinations of lever actions involving fulcrums. The muscles of the body provide the forces that move the numerous bones acting as levers. **2.** (in radiology) an imaginary pivot point about which the x-ray tube and film move. During computed tomography, the fulcrum lies in the focal, or object plane, and only anatomic areas lying in this plane will be focused and imaged.

fulfillment [AS, *fullfyllan*, to make full], a perception of harmony in life that results when an individual has found meaning and leads a purposeful life.

fulgurate /ful′gyərāt/ [L, *fulgur*, lightning], **1.** pertaining to sudden, intense, sharp pain. **2.** the use of a movable electrode to destroy superficial tissue.

fulguration. See **electrodesiccation.**

full-arch wire, a wire that is attached to the teeth and extends from the molar region of one side of a dental arch to the other. It is used to cause or guide orthodontic tooth movement. A sectional arch wire or shorter version of the full arch wire may also be used.

full bath [AS, *fol; baeth*], a bath in which the patient's body is immersed in water up to the neck.

full denture [ME, *full*; L, *dens*, tooth], a removable dental prosthetic that replaces all of the natural teeth in the maxillary and/or mandibular arch. The denture is usually made of acrylic resin and completely supported by the mouth tissues.

full diet. See **regular diet.**

full-liquid diet, a diet consisting of only liquids and foods that liquefy at body temperature. It includes milk, milk drinks, carbonated beverages, coffee, tea, strained fruit juices, broth, strained cream soup, raw eggs, cream, melted butter or margarine, strained precooked infant cereals in milk, thin custards, gelatin desserts, ice cream, sherbet, strained vegetables in soup, honey, syrups, sugar, and dry skim milk dissolved in liquids. The diet is prescribed after surgery, in some acute infections of short duration, in the treatment of acute GI disorders, and for patients too ill to chew. See also **liquid diet.**

full-lung tomography, a technique of producing general tomographic surveys of both lungs to detect possible occult nodules of metastases. Such lesions usually cannot be visualized with conventional radiologic methods.

full pulse [ME, *full*; L, *pulsare*, to beat], a large volume pulse with a low pulse pressure. Also called **pulsus magnus**.

full term [ME, *full*; Gk, *terma*, limit], pertaining to the normal period of human gestation, between 38 and 41 weeks.

full weight-bearing (FWB) [ME, *full*; AS, *gewiht*; ME, *beren*], in radiology, a view that shows the response to stresses of a natural posture. Full weight-bearing views of the foot are useful in studying flatfoot or cave foot.

fulminant hepatitis, a rare and frequently fatal form of acute hepatitis β in which there is rapid deterioration in the condition of the patient, with hepatic encephalopathy, necrosis of the hepatic parenchyma, blood coagulation disorders, renal failure, and coma. The prognosis for adults is generally unfavorable.

fulminating /ful′minā′ting/ [L, *fulminare*, lightening flash], (of a disease or condition) rapid, sudden, severe, such as an infection, fever, or hemorrhage. Also **fulminant.** —**fulminate,** *v*.

Fulvicin, a trademark for an antifungal (griseofulvin).

fumagillin, fumigacin. See **helvolic acid.**

function /fungk′shən/ [L, *functio*, performance], **1.** an act, process, or series of processes that serve a purpose. **2.** to perform an activity or to work properly and normally.

functional /fungk′shənəl/ [L, *functio*, performance], **1.** pertaining to a function. **2.** affecting the functions but not the structure of an organism or organ system.

functional analysis, (in psychiatry) a type of therapy that traces the sequence of events involved in producing and maintaining undesirable behavior.

functional antagonism, (in pharmacology) a situation in which two agonists interact with different receptors and produce opposing effects.

functional assessment. See **health history.**

functional bowel syndrome. See **irritable bowel syndrome.**

functional contracture. See **hypertonic contracture.**

functional differentiation, (in embryology) the specialization or diversification as a result of the particular function of a cell or tissue.

functional disease, **1.** a disease that affects function or performance. **2.** a condition marked by signs or symptoms of an organic disease or disorder although careful examination fails to reveal any evidence of structural or physiologic abnormalities. The symptoms of a functional disorder are as real as those of an organic disease. Headache, impotence, certain heart murmurs, and constipation may be symptoms of organic disease or of functional disease.

functional dyspepsia, a condition characterized by impaired digestion caused by an atonic or a neurologic problem. See also **dyspepsia.**

functional health history. See **complete health history.**

functional imaging, (in nuclear medicine) a diagnostic procedure in which a sequence of radiographic or scintillation camera images of the distribution of an administered radioactive tracer delineates one or more physiologic processes in the body.

functional impotence. See **impotence.**

functional murmur [L, *functio*, performance], a heart murmur caused by an alteration of function without structural heart disease or damage, as in a murmur related to anemia rather than an organic heart disorder.

functional nursing, an organizational mode for assigning nursing personnel that is task and activity oriented, using auxiliary health workers trained in a variety of skills. Each person is assigned specific functions that are carried out for all patients in a given unit, and all are responsible to the head nurse.

functional occlusal harmony, an occlusal relationship of opposing teeth in all functional ranges and movements that provides the maximum masticatory efficiency without pathogenic force on the supporting oral structures.

functional overlay, an emotional aspect of an organic disease. It may occur as an overreaction to an illness and is characterized by symptoms that continue long after clinical signs of the disease have ended.

functional pathology [L, *functio*, performance; Gk, *pathos*, disease, *logos*, science], a study of the functional changes resulting from structural alterations in tissues.

functional position of the hand, a position for splinting the hand, including the wrist and fingers. It consists of dorsiflexing both the wrist between 20 and 35 degrees and the proximal interphalangeal joints between 45 and 60 degrees. The thumb is abducted and in opposition and alignment with the pads of the fingers.

functional progression, a rehabilitative sequence for a musculoskeletal or similar injury. With variations for individual cases, the program usually progresses from immobilization for primary healing through protection of range of motion to endurance and strengthening activities related to the patient's work and play requirements.

functional psychosis, a severe emotional disorder characterized by personality derangement and the loss of ability to function in reality, but without evidence that the disorder is related to the physical processes of the brain.

functional residual capacity, the volume of gas in the lungs at the end of a normal expiration. The functional residual capacity is equal to the residual volume plus the expiratory reserve volume.

functional splint [L, *functio,* performance; ME, *splent*], a splint that allows or assists a patient's movements. Also called **ambulatory splint, dynamic splint**.

fundal height /fun'dəl/ [L, *fundus,* bottom; AS, *heightho*], the height of the fundus, measured in centimeters from the top of the symphysis pubis to the highest point in the midline at the top of the uterus. Fundal height is measured at each prenatal visit with large, blunt calipers or with a tape measure. From the twentieth to the thirty-second weeks of pregnancy, the height in centimeters is equal to the gestation in weeks. Two measurements 2 weeks apart showing a deviation of more than 2 cm may indicate that the fetus is large or small for dates, that the estimated gestation is in error, or that the woman is carrying a multiple pregnancy.

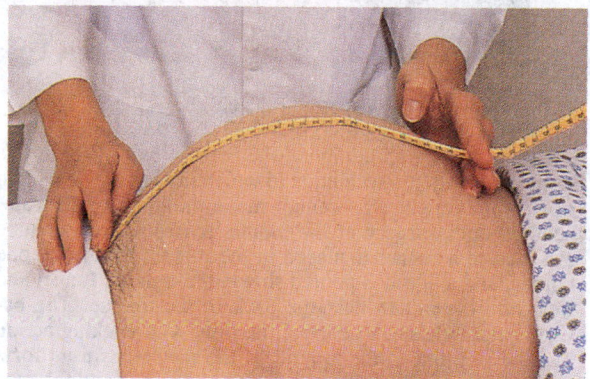

Measurement of fundal height (Seidel, 1991)

fundal placenta [L, *fundus,* bottom, *placenta,* flat cake], a placenta that is attached to the fundus of the uterus.

fundamentals of nursing /fun'dəmen'təls/, the basic principles and practices of nursing as taught in educational programs for nurses. In a course called 'the fundamentals of nursing,' traditionally required in the first semester of the program, the student attends classes and gives care to selected patients. It emphasizes the importance of knowledge and understanding of the fundamental needs of humans as well as competence in the basic skills as prerequisites to providing comprehensive nursing care.

fundi. See **fundus**.

fundoplication /fun'dəplikā'shən/ [L, *fundus,* bottom, *plicare,* to fold], a surgical procedure involving making tucks (plication) in the fundus of the stomach around the lower end of the esophagus. The operation is used in the treatment of gastric acid reflux into the esophagus. See also **plication**.

funduscopic. See **funduscopy**.

fundoscopy /fundos'kəpē/ [L, *fundus,* bottom; Gk, *skopein,* to view], an examination of the ocular fundus with an ophthalmoscope.

fundus /fun'dəs/, *pl.* **fundi** [L, bottom], the base or the deepest part of an organ; the portion farthest from the mouth of an organ, such as the fundus of the uterus or the fundus of an eye.

funduscope. See **ophthalmoscope**.

funduscopy /fundus'kəpē/ [L, *fundus* + Gk, *skopein,* to

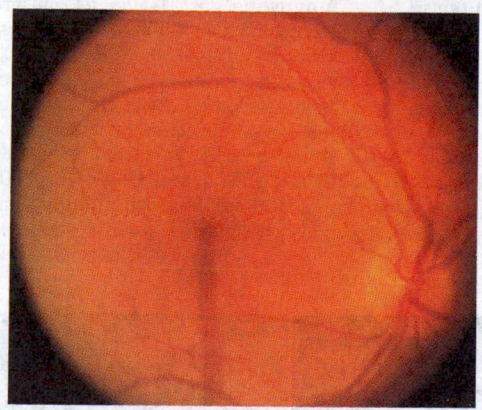

Normal fundus of the eye (Zitelli, 1992)

look], the examination and study of the fundus of the eye by means of an ophthalmoscope. **–fundoscopic, funduscopic,** *adj.*

fundus microscopy, examination of the base of the interior of the eye using an instrument that combines an ophthalmoscope and a lens with high magnifying power for observing minute structures in the cornea and iris.

fungal [L, *fungus*], pertaining to or resembling a fungus or fungi.

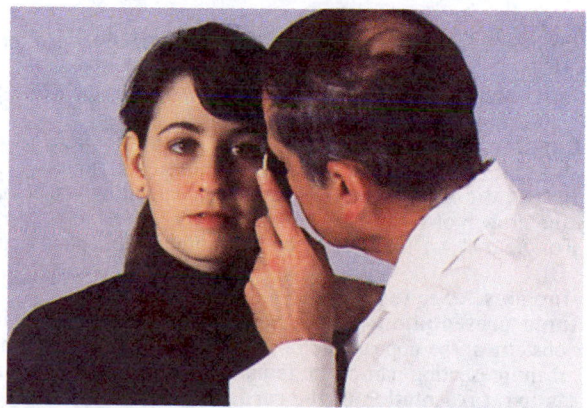

Direct funduscopy (Seidel, 1991)

fungal infection [L, *fungus,* mushroom, *inficere,* to stain], any inflammatory condition caused by a fungus. Most fungal infections are superficial and mild, though persistent and difficult to eradicate. Some, particularly in older, debilitated, or immunosuppressed people, may become systemic and life-threatening. Some kinds of fungal infections are **aspergillosis, blastomycosis, candidiasis, coccidioidomycosis,** and **histoplasmosis**.

fungal septicemia [L, *fungus;* Gk, *septikos,* putrid, *haima,* blood], a form of blood poisoning in which the causative agent is a fungus.

fungemia /funjē'mē·ə/ [L, *fungus* + Gk, *haima,* blood], the presence of fungi in the blood. Compare **bacteremia, parasitemia, viremia**.

fungi/fun′jī/, *sing.* **fungus**/fun′gəs/ [L, *fungus*, mushroom], a general term for a eukaryotic, thallus-forming organism that requires an external carbon source. Fungi lack both chlorophyll and chemolithotrophic systems. They may be saprophytes or parasites. A simple fungus reproduces by budding; multicellular fungi reproduce by spore formation. They may invade living organisms, including humans, as well as nonliving organic substances. Of the 100,000 identified species of fungi, 100 are common in humans and 10 are pathogenic. See also **fungal infection.** **–fungal, fungous,** *adj.*

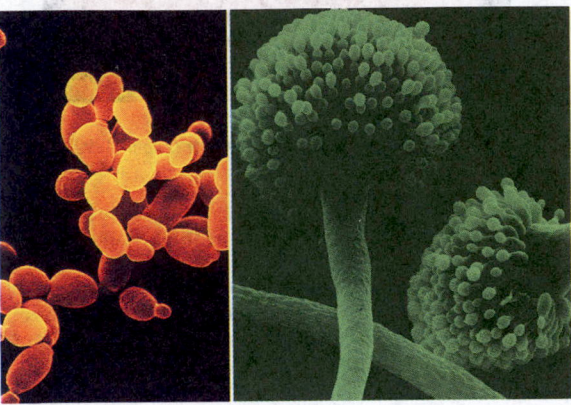

Fungi *(Thibodeau, 1993/David M Phillips/Visuals Unlimited)*

fungicide /fun′jisīd/, a drug that kills fungi. See also **antifungal,** def. 2. **–fungicidal,** *adj.*

fungiform /fun′ji/fôrm/ [L, *funis, forma*], shaped like a mushroom.

fungiform papilla. See **papilla.**

-fungin, a combining form for antifungal antibiotics.

fungistatic /fun′jēstat′ik/, having an inhibiting effect on the growth of fungi.

Fungizone, a trademark for an antifungal (amphotericin B).

-fungous. See **fungi.**

funic presentation [L, *funis, praesentare*, to show], in obstetrics, the appearance of the umbilical cord before the main presenting part of the fetus. Also called **cord presentation, presentation of the cord.**

funic souffle /fyōō′nik sōō′fəl/ [L, *funis*, cord; Fr, *souffle* breath], a soft, muffled blowing sound produced by blood rushing through the umbilical vessels and synchronous with the fetal heart sound.

funiculitis /fənik′yəlī′tis/, any abnormal inflammatory condition of a cordlike structure of the body, such as the spinal cord or spermatic cord.

funiculus /fənik′yələs/ [L, little cord], a division of the white matter of the spinal cord, consisting of fasciculi or fiber tracts.

funiculus umbilicalis. See **umbilical cord.**

funis /fyōō′nis, fōō′nis/, a cordlike structure, such as the umbilical cord.

funis presentation, See **funic presentation.**

funnel chest [L, *fundere*, to pour], a skeletal abnormality of the chest characterized by a depressed sternum. The deformity may not interfere with breathing, but surgical correction is often recommended for cosmetic reasons. Also called **pectus excavatum.**

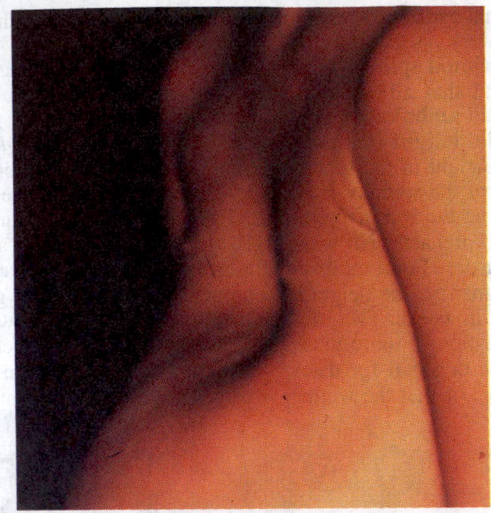

Funnel chest *(Zitelli, 1992)*

funnel feeding, a technique in which liquids may be given orally to a patient who cannot move the lips or masticate, such as after surgery at the mouth or lips. A rubber tube attached to a funnel is placed in the mouth, usually at one corner, and a liquid is poured slowly through the funnel and tube into the mouth near the back of the tongue. The patient quickly learns to control the flow with sucking action and the position of the tongue. If the method is used for a weak or young infant, a rubber bulb or a large syringe may be used instead of a funnel. The bulb or syringe is compressed gently, slowly, and continuously to control the rate of flow and prevent choking.

funny bone, a popular name for a point at the lower end of the humerus where the ulnar nerve is near the surface and subject to external pressure, resulting in a tingling sensation.

FUO, abbreviation for **fever of unknown origin.**

Furacin, a trademark for a topical antiinfective (nitrofurazone).

Furadantin, a trademark for an antibacterial (nitrofurantoin).

furazolidone /fōō′rəzol′idōn/, an antiinfective and antiprotozoal.

■ INDICATIONS: It is prescribed for certain bacterial or protozoal infections of the GI tract.

■ CONTRAINDICATIONS: Known hypersensitivity to this drug prohibits its use. It is not given to children under 1 month of age, and it is not used with drugs that are contraindicated with monoamine oxidase inhibitors.

■ ADVERSE EFFECTS: Among the more serious adverse reactions are hemolytic anemia and fever; skin rash and abdominal pain sometimes occur.

furcation /fərkā′shən/ [L, *furca*, fork], the region of division of the root portion of a tooth. It may exist as a bifurcation in a tooth with two roots or as a trifurcation in a tooth with three roots.

furfuraceous desquamation /fur′fərā′sē·əs/ [L, *furfur*, bran, *desquamare*, to scale off], the shedding of epidermis in large scales.

furosemide /fōōrō′səmīd fyərō′səmid/, a diuretic.

■ INDICATIONS: It is prescribed in the treatment of hypertension, renal failure, and edema.

■ CONTRAINDICATIONS: Anuria, pregnancy, lactation, electrolyte depletion, or known hypersensitivity to this drug prohibits its use.

■ ADVERSE EFFECTS: Among the more serious adverse reactions are fluid and electrolyte imbalance.

Furoxone, a trademark for an antiinfective antiprotozoal (furazolidone).

furred tongue [ME, *furre,* sheath; AS, *tunge*], a tongue, the surface of which is coated by a white to brown accumulation of desquamated epithelial cells, bacteria, mycelia, and other debris. It is a common occurrence in some fevers. Also called **coated tongue**.

furrow /fur′ō/ [AS, *furh*], a groove, such as the atrioventricular furrow that separates the atria from the ventricles of the heart.

furuncle /fyo͞or′ungkəl/ [L, *furunculus,* petty thief], a localized, suppurative staphylococcal skin infection originating in a gland or hair follicle that is characterized by pain, redness, and swelling. Necrosis deep in the center of the inflamed area forms a core of dead tissue that is spontaneously extruded, eventually resorbed, or surgically removed. It is important to avoid irritating or squeezing the lesion to prevent spread of the infection. Treatment may include antibiotics, local moist heat, and, when there is definite fluctuation and the hard white core is evident, incision and drainage. Also called **boil**. **—furunculous,** *adj.*

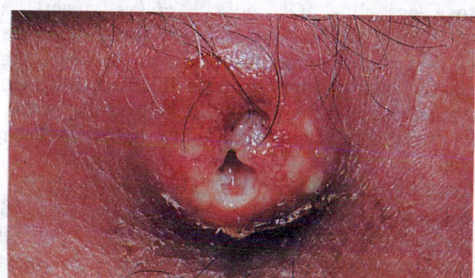

Furuncle
(Thompson, 1989; Courtesy Jaime A Tschen, MD, Baylor College of Medicine, Department of Dermatology, Houson)

furunculosis /fyo͞orung′kyo͞olō′sis/, an acute skin disease characterized by boils or successive crops of boils that are caused by staphylococci or streptococci.

-furunculosis. See **furuncle**.

-fuse, a suffix meaning 'to pour or flow': *diffuse, effuse, perfuse.*

fusiform /fyo͞o′sifôrm/ [L, *fusus,* spindle, *forma,* form], a structure that is tapered at both ends.

fusiform aneurysm, a localized dilatation of an artery in which the entire circumference of the vessel is distended. The result is an elongated tubular or spindlelike swelling. Also called **Richet's aneurysm**. Compare **saccular aneurysm**.

fusiform gyrus [L, *fusus,* spindle, *forma,* form; Gk, *gyros,* turn], a convolution of the cerebral hemispheres that lies below the collateral fissures and joins the occipital and temporal lobes.

fusimotor /fyo͞o′zimō′tər/ [L, *fusus* + *motare,* to move about], pertaining to the motor nerve fibers, or gamma efferent fibers, that innervate the intrafusal fibers of the muscle spindle.

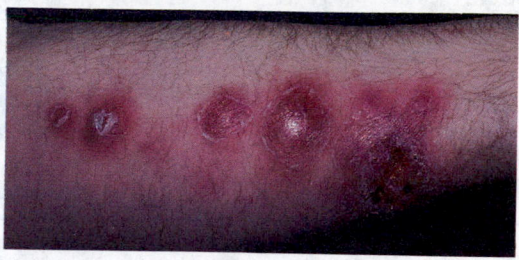

Furunculosis (Weston, 1991)

fusion /fyo͞o′zhən/ [L, *fusio,* outpouring], **1.** the bringing together into a single entity, as in optic fusion. **2.** also called **ankylosis**. the act of uniting two or more bones of a joint. **3.** the surgical joining together of two or more vertebrae, performed to stabilize a segment of the spinal column after severe trauma, a herniated disk, or degenerative disease. Under general anesthesia, the cartilage pads are removed from between the posterior portions of the involved vertebrae. Bone chips are cut from one of the patient's iliac crests and inserted in place of the cartilage, fusing the articulating surfaces into one segment of bone. Postoperative nursing care focuses on strict limitations of motion for the graft site until bony healing occurs. The patient's bed is completely flat; a Stryker frame may be used. In a standard bed the patient is log-rolled from side to side to avoid twisting the trunk. The nurse observes the dressing for any drainage of spinal fluid. Ambulation takes place before sitting. **4.** (in psychiatry) the tendency of two people experiencing an intense emotion to unite.

fusional amplitude. See **amplitude of convergence**.

fusion beat, (in electrocardiography) a P wave or QRS complex resulting from the concurrent activation of the atria or the ventricles by two stimuli in the same chamber. An atrial fusion beat results when the sinus beat coincides with an atrial ectopic beat, when two atrial ectopic beats coincide, or when an atrial or sinus beat coincides with retrograde conduction from a junctional focus. A ventricular fusion beat results when a ventricular beat coincides with a sinus beat, a ventricular ectopic beat, or a junctional beat.

fusospirochetal disease /fyo͞o′zōspī′rōke̅′təl/ [L, *fusus,* spindle; Gk, *speira,* coil, *chaite,* hair], any infection characterized by ulcerative lesions in which both a fusiform bacillus and a spirochete are found, such as trench mouth or Vincent's angina.

FVIII, (recombinant blood factor VIII), a large glycoprotein containing more than 2,300 amino acids, 24 cysteine residues, and 25 potential glycosylation sites. The factor is used to treat blood-clotting disorders, such as **hemophilia A,** in which the factor is deficient or missing.

f waves, (in cardiology) waves that represent fibrillation.

F wave, a wave form recorded in electroneuromyographic and nerve conduction tests. It appears on supramaximal stimulation of a motor nerve and is caused by antidromic transmission of a stimulus. The F wave is used in studies of motor nerve function in the arms and legs.

FWB, abbreviation for **full-weight bearing**.

-fy, a suffix meaning 'to make into' something specified: *acidify, decalcify, salify.*

-fying. See **-factive**.

-fylline, a combining form for theophylline derivatives.

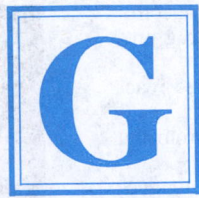

g, abbreviation for **gram.**

Ga, symbol for the element **gallium.**

GA, abbreviation for **general anesthesia.**

GABA, abbreviation for **gamma-aminobutyric acid.**

GABHS. See **group A beta-hemolytic streptococcal skin disease.**

gadolinium (Gd) /gad′əlin′ē·əm/ [Johan Gadolin, Finnish chemist, b. 1760], **1.** a rare earth metallic element. Its atomic number is 64; its atomic weight is 157.25. **2.** (in radiology)a phosphor used to intensify screens.

gag [ME, *gaggen*], **1.** a dental device for holding the jaws open during oral surgery or dental restoration. Also called **mouth prop. 2.** to retch or attempt to vomit.

gag reflex [ME, *gaggen*, to strangle; L, *reflectere*, to bend backward], a normal neural reflex elicited by touching the soft palate or posterior pharynx, the response being symmetrical elevation of the palate, retraction of the tongue, and contraction of the pharyngeal muscles. The reflex is used as a test of the integrity of the vagus and glossopharyngeal nerves. Also called **pharyngeal reflex.**

gait [ONor, *geta*, a way], the manner or style of walking, including rhythm, cadence, and speed.

gait determinant, one of a number of the kinetic anatomic factors that govern the locomotion of an individual in the process of walking. Some authorities have defined pelvic rotation, pelvic tilt, knee and hip flexion, knee and ankle interaction, and lateral pelvic displacement as the main determinants of gait. Such descriptions are often important in analyzing and correcting pathologic gaits of individuals afflicted by orthopedic diseases, deformities, or abnormal bone conditions.

gait disorder, an abnormality in the manner or style of walking, usually as a result of neuromuscular, arthritic, or other body changes. The body's center of gravity may change over the years, resulting in a difference in the degree of knee flexion needed to maintain one's balance when walking. Some individuals with neuromuscular disorders may walk with a shuffling gait or move with lurching actions. In some cases a gait disorder may be the result of a medication that causes confusion or loss of coordination or an eye or ear disturbance that affects the sense of balance.

galact-, galacta-. See galacto-.

-galactia, a combining form meaning a 'condition involving secretion of milk': *cacogalactia, dysgalactia, oligogalactia.*

galacto-, galact-, galacta-, a combining form meaning 'pertaining to milk': *galactochloral, galactogen, galactorrhea.*

galactocele /gəlak′təsēl′/, a cyst or hydrocele caused by blockage of a mammary gland milk duct.

galactokinase /gəlak′tōkī′nās/ [Gk, *gala*, milk, *kinesis*, movement; Fr, *diastase*, enzyme], an enzyme that functions in the metabolism of glycogen. Galactokinase catalyzes a metabolic step involving the transfer of a high-energy phosphate group from a donor molecule to a molecule of galactose, producing a molecule of D-galactose-1-phosphate.

galactokinase deficiency, an inherited disorder of carbohydrate metabolism in which the enzyme galactokinase is deficient or absent. As a result, dietary galactose is not metabolized, galactose accumulates in the blood, and cataracts may develop rapidly. Food containing galactose, such as milk and certain milk products, must be eliminated from the diet. Compare **lactase deficiency.**

galactophorous duct /-môr′fəs/ [Gk, *gala* + *pherein*, to bear; L, *ducere*, to lead], a passage for milk in the lobes of the breast.

galactorrhea /gəlak′tərē′ə/ [Gk, *gala* + *rhoia*, flowing], lactation not associated with childbirth or nursing. The condition is sometimes a symptom of a pituitary gland tumor. See also **Forbes-Albright syndrome.**

galactose /gəlak′tōs/ [Gk, *gala* + *glykys*, sweet], a simple sugar found in the dextrorotatory form in lactose (milk sugar), nerve cell membranes, sugar beets, gums, seaweed, and, in the levorotatory form, in flaxseed mucilage. Prepared galactose, a white crystalline substance, is less sweet and less soluble in water than glucose but is similar in other properties.

galactosemia /gəlak′tōsē′mē·ə/ [Gk, *gala* + *glykys*, sweet, *haima* blood], an inherited, autosomal recessive disorder of galactose metabolism, characterized by a deficiency of the enzyme galactose-1-phosphate uridyl transferase. Shortly after birth, an intolerance to milk occurs, evidenced by anorexia, nausea, vomiting, and diarrhea. Hepatosplenomegaly, cataracts, and mental retardation develop. Greater than normal amounts of galactose are present in the blood, the galactose tolerance test indicates an abnormality, and the red cells show deficient galactose-1-phosphate uridyl transferase activity. Because the elimination of galactose from the diet results in the rapid amelioration of all symptoms except mental retardation, early diagnosis and prompt therapy are essential. Pregnant women known to be carriers should exclude lactose and galactose from their diets. Compare **diabetes mellitus, glycogen storage disease.** See also **galactose, inborn error of metabolism.**

galactosuria /-sŏŏr′ē·ə/, the presence of galactose in the urine.

galactosyl ceramide lipidosis /gəlak′təsil/ [Gk, *gala* + *glykys*, sweet; L, *cera*, wax, *lipos*, fat, *osis*, condition], a rare, fatal, inherited disorder of lipid metabolism, present at birth. Infants become paralyzed, blind, deaf, and increasingly retarded, and eventually die of bulbar paralysis. There is no known treatment for the disorder, but it can be detected in pregnancy by amniocentesis. Also called **globoid leukodystrophy, Krabbe's disease.** Compare **Tay-Sachs disease.**

galacturia /gal′əktŏŏr′ē·ə/ [Gk, *gala*, milk, *ouron*, urine], a condition in which the urine has a milky color because of the abnormal presence of galactose, a monosaccharide, in the urine.

Galant reflex /gəlant'/, a normal response in the neonate to move the hips toward the stimulated side when the back is stroked along the spinal cord. The reflex disappears by about 4 weeks of age. Absence of the reflex may indicate spinal cord lesion. Also called **trunk incurvation reflex.**

galea aponeurotica. See **epicranial aponeurosis.**

Galeazzi's fracture /gal'ē·at'sēz/ [Riccardo Galeazzi, Italian surgeon, b. 1866], a fracture of the distal radius accompanied by dislocation of the radioulnar joint. Also called **Dupuytren's fracture.**

Galen's bandage /gā'lənz/ [Claudius Galen, Greek physician, b. 130 AD], a bandage for the head, consisting of a strip of cloth with each end divided into three pieces. The center of the cloth is placed on top of the head; the two strips in front are joined at the back of the neck; the two strips at the back are pulled up and fastened on the forehead; the remaining middle strips are fastened under the chin.

gall. See **bile.**

gallbladder /gôl'blad'ər/ [ME, gal; AS, blaedre], a pear-shaped excretory sac lodged in a fossa on the visceral surface of the right lobe of the liver. It serves as a reservoir for bile, which it receives from the liver via the hepatic duct. About 8 cm long and 2.5 cm wide at its thickest part, it holds about 32 ml of bile. During digestion of fats, the gallbladder contracts, ejecting bile through the common bile duct into the duodenum. The gallbladder is divided into a fundus, body, and neck and is covered by the peritoneum. Obstruction of the biliary system by gallstones may lead to jaundice and pain; it is a common condition in overweight, middle-aged women and may require surgical or other intervention.

gallbladder carcinoma, a malignant neoplasm of the bile reservoir, characterized by anorexia, nausea, vomiting, weight loss, progressively severe right upper quadrant pain, and, eventually, jaundice. Tumors of the gallbladder are predominantly adenocarcinomas; often associated with biliary calculi, they are three to four times more common in women than in men and rarely occur before 40 years of age. Physical examination reveals an enlarged gallbladder in about one half of the cases. X-ray film may aid in making a diagnosis, but obstruction of the biliary duct by the can-

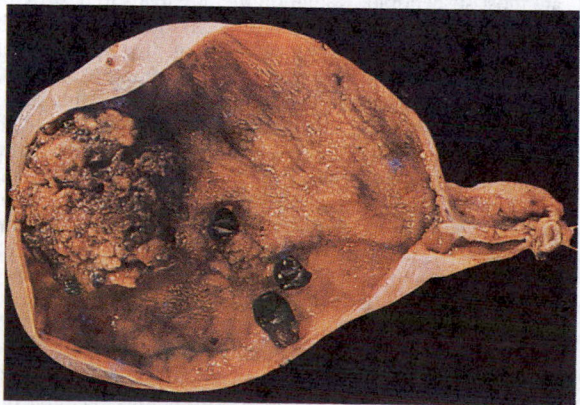

Gallbladder carcinoma (Fletcher, 1987)

cer or the inability of the gallbladder to concentrate the radiopaque dye often prevents visualization of the lesion, and the diagnosis is usually made during a laparotomy. Complete removal of the gallbladder may be curative, but partial hepatectomy may be required because the liver is often a site of early metastases. Surgery is contraindicated if there are distant metastases, as frequently occur in the lungs, bone, and adrenal glands. Radiotherapy may be palliative; chemotherapy is usually ineffective.

gallium (Ga) /gal'ē·əm/ [L, Gallia, Gaul], a metallic element. Its atomic number is 31; its atomic weight is 69.72. The melting point of gallium is 29.8° C (88.6° F); it will melt if held in the hand. Because of its high boiling point (1983° C; 3602° F), it is used in high-temperature thermometers. Radioisotopes of gallium are used in total body scanning procedures. Many of its compounds are poisonous.

gallop /gal'əp/ [Fr, galop], a third or fourth heart sound, which at certain heart rates sometimes sounds like the gait of a horse. The third heart sound (S3) may normally be heard in healthy children, but is pathologic in adults and may be the first sign of cardiac decompensation. An S3 gallop occurs early in diastole and is caused by the sudden deceleration of the diastolic filling wave as a result of a non-compliant ventricular wall. An S4 gallop follows atrial contraction and precedes the first heart sound. It is seldom normal and is related to either left or right atrial contraction and the resultant distension of a noncompliant ventricle just before systole.

gallop rhythm [Fr, galop; Gk, rhythmos], a cadence resembling that of a galloping horse produced by an abnormal third or fourth heart sound.

gallstone. See **biliary calculus.**

galvanic /galvan'ik/ [Luigi Galvani, Italian physician, b. 1737], pertaining to or involving electricity.

galvanic cautery, galvanocautery. See **electrocautery.**

galvanic electric stimulation [Luigi Galvani, Italian physiologist, b. 1737], the use of a high-voltage electric stimulator to treat muscle spasms, edema of acute injury, myofascial pain, and certain other disorders. See also **transcutaneous electric nerve stimulation.**

galvanic skin response (GSR) [Luigi Galvani, AS, scinn; L, respondere, to reply], a reaction to certain stimuli as indicated by a change in the electric resistance of the skin. The effect is related to unconscious activity of the sweat glands and may result from pleasant as well as unpleasant stimuli. The GSR is used in some polygraph examinations.

galvanoionization. See **iontophoresis.**

galvanometer /gal'vənom'ətər/ [Luigi Galvani], a device that indicates or measures electrical current by its effects on a needle or coil in a magnetic field. Galvanometers are employed in certain diagnostic instruments, such as electrocardiographs.

gam-. See **gamo-.**

Gambian trypanosomiasis /gam'bē·ən/, a usually chronic form of African trypanosomiasis, caused by the parasite Trypanosoma brucei gambiense. An infected individual may have relatively mild symptoms for months or years before developing the neurologic symptoms of the terminal stage. Also called **West African sleeping sickness.** Compare **Rhodesian trypanosomiasis.** See also **African trypanosomiasis.** (See Fig. p. 652.)

game knee [ME, gamen; AS, cneow], a common term for any injury or condition that interferes with normal function of the knee joint.

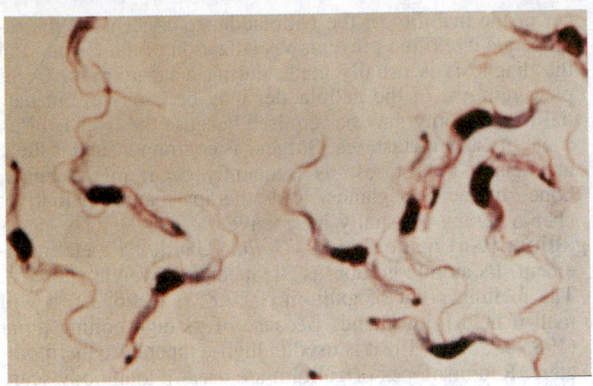

Trypanosoma gambiense in a blood smear
(Murray, 1990/Reproduced by permission from LR Ash and TC
Orihel, Atlas of human parasitology, ed. 2, copyright 1984 by the
American Society of Clinical Pathologists Press, Chicago)

gamet-. See **gameto-.**

gamete /gam′ēt/ [Gk, marriage partner], **1.** a mature male or female germ cell that is capable of functioning in fertilization or conjugation and contains the haploid number of chromosomes of the somatic cell. **2.** the ovum or spermatozoon. See also **meiosis.** –**gametic,** *adj.*

gamete intrafallopian transfer (GIFT), a human fertilization technique in which male and female gametes are injected through a laparoscope into the fimbriated ends of the fallopian tubes.

gametic /gəmat′ik/ [Gk,*gametes*/husband,*gamete*/wife], pertaining to a reproductive cell such as a spermatozoon or ovum.

gametic chromosome, any of the chromosomes contained in the haploid cell, specifically the spermatozoon or ovum, as contrasted with those in the diploid, or somatic cell.

gameto-, gamet-, a combining form meaning "reproductive cell": *gametocyte, gametophore, gametogenesis.*

gametocide /gəmē′tōsīd/ [Gk, *gamete* + L, *caedere,* to kill], any agent that is destructive to gametes or gametocytes, specifically to the malarial gametocytes. –**gametocidal,** *adj.*

gametocyte /gəmē′tōsīt/ [Gk, *gamete* + *kytos,* cell], (in genetics) any cell capable of dividing into or in the process of developing into a gamete, specifically an oocyte or spermatocyte.

gametogenesis /gam′itōjen′əsis/ [Gk, *gamete* + *genein,* to produce], the origin and maturation of gametes, which occurs through the process of meiosis. See also **oogenesis, spermatogenesis.** –**gametogenic, gametogenous,** *adj.*

gametophyte /gəmē′tōfīt/ [Gk, *gamete, phyton,* plant], a cell in the reproductive stage when the nuclei are in a haploid condition.

gamma /gam′ə/, Γ, γ, the third letter of the Greek alphabet. It is a symbol for photon, heavy-chain immunoglobulins, third in a series of certain chemical groups.

gamma-aminobutyric acid (GABA), an amino acid with neurotransmitter activity found in the brain and also in the heart, lungs, kidneys, and certain plants.

gamma-benzene hexachloride. See **lindane.**

gamma camera [Gk, *gamma,* third letter of Greek alphabet; L *camera* vault], a device that uses the emission of light from a crystal struck by gamma rays to produce an image of the distribution of radioactive material in a body organ. The light is detected by an array of light-sensitive electronic tubes and is converted to electric signals for further processing. The gamma camera is a workhorse of nuclear medicine departments, where it is used to produce scans of patients who have been injected with small amounts of radioactive materials.

gamma efferent fiber [Gk, *gamma* + L, *efferre,* to carry out; *fibra,* fiber], any of the motor nerve fibers that transmit impulses from the central nervous system to the intrafusal fibers of the muscle spindle. The gamma efferent fibers are responsible for deep tendon reflexes, spasticity, and rigidity but not for the degree of contractile response. They function in regulating the sensitivity of the spindle and the total tension of the muscle.

gamma globulin. See **immune gamma globulin.**

gamma-glutamyl transpeptidase (GGT), an enzyme that appears in the serum of patients with several types of liver or gallbladder disorders, including drug hepatotoxicity and biliary tract obstruction. Normal adult (after age 45) findings of GGT blood levels are 8-38 U/L.

gamma radiation [Gk, *gamma* + L, *radiare,* to emit rays], a very high frequency electromagnetic emission of photons from certain radioactive elements in the course of nuclear transition or from nuclear reactions. Gamma radiation is more penetrating than alpha radiation and beta radiation but has less ionizing power and is not deflected in electric and magnetic fields. The wavelengths of gamma rays emitted by radioactive substances are characteristic of the radioisotopes involved and range from about 4 [ti] 10[mi]10 to 5 [ti] 10[mi]13 m. High-voltage generators can produce x-rays of a wavelength much shorter than that of most gamma rays. The depth to which gamma rays penetrate depends on their wavelengths and energy. Gamma radiation and other forms of radiation can injure, distort, or destroy body cells and tissue, especially cell nuclei, but controlled radiation is used in the diagnosis and treatment of various diseases. Gamma radiation can penetrate thousands of meters of air and several centimeters of soft tissue and bone. Sixty percent of a dose of gamma radiation that enters the body tissue normally exits the same tissue. Radiation is an important form of therapy in the treatment of skin cancer and malignancies deep within the body. The ionizing effect of radiation affects all the cells of the body, but young, growing, and dividing cells are most susceptible. Radiation therapy tends to destroy the nuclei of rapidly dividing cancer cells by bombarding the nuclei with selective doses of radiation that spare normal slower dividing tissue. Any cell is vulnerable to injury if radiated while dividing, and the injury to the cells and tissue from radiation is basically the same, regardless of the type of radiant energy. There is no practical application of radiation in routine sterilization, but both heat and gamma radiation are employed to sterilize spacecraft. Body cells especially sensitive to radiation include lymphoid cells, bone marrow cells, cells that line the alimentary tract, and cells of the testes and the ovaries. Exposure of the entire body to sizable doses of radiation can cause acute radiation sickness. See also **ultraviolet radiation.**

gamma ray, an electromagnetic radiation of short wavelength emitted by the nucleus of an atom during a nuclear reaction. Composed of high-energy photons, gamma rays lack mass and an electric charge and travel at the speed of light. They are usually associated with alpha particles and beta rays (electrons ejected at high velocities from radioactive substances).

gammopathy /gamop'əthē/, an abnormal condition characterized by the presence of markedly increased levels of gamma globulin in the blood. Two different types of hypergammaglobulinemia can be distinguished. **Monoclonal gammopathy** is commonly associated with an electrophoretic pattern showing one sharp, homogenous electrophoretic band in the gamma globulin region. This reflects the presence of excessive amounts of one type of immunoglobulin secreted by a single clone of B cells. **Polyclonal gammopathy** reflects the presence of a diffuse hypergammaglobulinemia in which all immunoglobulin classes are proportionally increased. See also **Bence-Jones protein, multiple myeloma.**

gamo-, gam-, a combining form meaning 'pertaining to marriage or sexual union': *gamobium, gamont, gamophagia.*

gamogenesis /gam'ōjen'əsis/ [Gk, *gamos,* marriage, *genein,* to produce], sexual reproduction through the fusion of gametes. –**gamogenetic,** *adj.*

gamone /gam'ōn/ [Gk, *gamos,* marriage], a chemical substance secreted by the ova and spermatozoa that supposedly attracts the gametes of the opposite sex to facilitate union. Kinds of gamones are **androgamone** and **gynogamone.**

gampsodactyly. See **pes cavus.**

Gamulin Rh, a trademark for a passive immunizing agent, $Rh_o(D)$, immune human globulin.

-gamy, 1. a suffix meaning a '(specified) type of marriage': *endogamy, monogamy, pedogamy.* **2.** a suffix meaning 'possession of organs for reproduction': *cleistogamy, dichogamy, homogamy.* **3.** a suffix meaning a 'union for propagation': *hologamy, macrogamy, syngamy.*

gancyclovir /gansik'lōvir/ an acrylic nucleoside structurally related to acyclovir. It is used to prevent cytomegalovirus disease after allogenic bone marrow transplantation and in persons with AIDS.

gangli-. See **ganglio-.**

ganglia. See **ganglion.**

ganglio-, gangli-, a combining form meaning 'pertaining to a ganglion': *gangliocytoma, ganglioneuroma, ganglioplexus.*

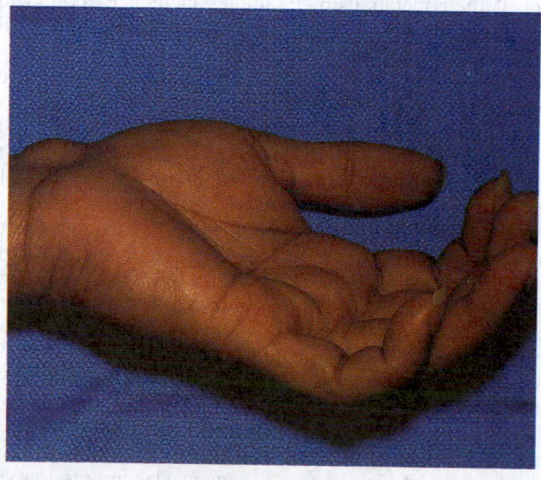

Ganglion *(Lewis, 1989)*

ganglion /gang'glē·on/, *pl.* **ganglia** [Gk, knot], **1.** a knot, or knotlike mass. **2.** one of the nerve cells, chiefly collected in groups outside the central nervous system. Individual cells and very small groups abound in association with alimentary organs. The two types of ganglia in the body are the sensory ganglia on the dorsal roots of spinal nerves and on the sensory roots of the trigeminal, facial, glossopharyngeal, and vagus nerves and the autonomic ganglia of the sympathetic and parasympathetic systems.

ganglionar neuroma /gang·glē'ənər/ [Gk, *ganglion* + *neuron,* nerve, *oma,* tumor], a tumor composed of a solid mass of ganglia and nerve fibers. Usually found in abdominal tissues, the tumor occurs most commonly in children. Chemotherapy or surgery is the recommended treatment. Also called **ganglionated neuroma, ganglionic neuroma.**

ganglionic blockade /gang'glē·on'ik/, the blocking of nerve impulses at synapses of autonomic ganglia, usually by the administration of ganglionic blocking agents.

ganglionic blocking agent, any one of a group of drugs prescribed to produce controlled hypotension, as required in certain surgical procedures or in emergency management of hypertensive crisis. The drugs act by occupying receptor sites on sympathetic and parasympathetic nerve endings of autonomic ganglia, preventing response of these nerves to the action of acetylcholine liberated by the presynaptic nerve endings. Trimethaphan and mecamylamine are the most commonly prescribed ganglionic blocking agents. They are used with great caution in treating patients who are affected with coronary, cerebrovascular, or renal insufficiency or who have a history of severe allergy. Adverse reactions to the drugs include sudden marked hypotension, paralytic ileus, urinary retention, constipation, visual disturbances, heartburn, and nausea.

ganglionic crest. See **neural crest.**

ganglionic glioma [Gk, *ganglion* + *glia,* glue, *oma,* tumor], a tumor composed of glial cells and ganglion cells that are nearly mature. See also **neuroblastoma.**

ganglionic neuroma. See **ganglionar neuroma.**

ganglionic ridge. See **neural crest.**

ganglionitis /gang'glē·ənī'tis/, an inflammation of a nerve or lymph ganglion.

ganglioside /gang'glē·əsīd'/, a glycolipid found in the brain and other nervous system tissues. Gangliosides are members of a group of galactose-containing cerebrosides with a basic composition of ceramide-glucose-galactose-N-acetyl neuraminic acid. Accumulation of gangliosides because of an inborn error of metabolism results in gangliosidosis or Tay-Sachs disease.

gangliosidosis type I. See **Tay-Sachs disease.**

gangliosidosis type II. See **Sandhoff's disease.**

gangrene /gang'grēn/ [Gk, *gangraina,* a gnawing sore], necrosis or death of tissue, usually the result of ischemia (loss of blood supply), bacterial invasion, and subsequent putrefaction. The extremities are most often affected, but it can occur in the intestines and gallbladder. Internally, gangrene may be a complication of strangulated hernia, appendicitis, cholecystitis, or thrombosis of the mesenteric arteries to the gut. **Dry gangrene** is a late complication of diabetes mellitus that is already complicated by arteriosclerosis in which the affected extremity becomes cold, dry, and shriveled and eventually turns black. **Moist gangrene** may follow a crushing injury or an obstruction of blood flow by an embolism, tight bandages, or tourniquet. This form of gangrene has an offensive odor, spreads rapidly, and may result in death in a few days. In all types of gangrene, surgical debridement is necessary to remove the necrotic tissue before healing can progress. Cleanliness and the maintenance of good circulation are nursing considerations essential in preventing this condition. See also **gas gangrene, open amputation.** – **gangrenous,** *adj.*

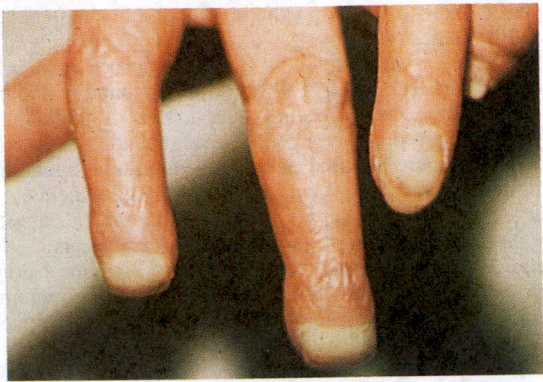

Gangrene *(Shipley, 1993)*

gangrenous appendicitis /gang′grənəs/ [Gk, *gaggraina*, a gnawing sore; L, *appendere*, to hang upon, Gk, *itis*, inflammation], a condition in which the appendix becomes gangrenous because obstruction of its lumen blocks the flow of blood to that body part.

gangrenous necrosis.   See **necrosis.**

gangrenous stomatitis.   See **noma.**

gangrenous vulvitis [Gk, *gaggraina;* L, *vulva,* wrapper; Gk, *itis,* inflammation], the death of tissues in the area of the vulva caused by a severe infection resulting in the sloughing of cells.

ganja.   See **cannabis.**

Gantanol, a trademark for an antibacterial (sulfamethoxazole).

Gantrisin, a trademark for an antibacterial (sulfisoxazole).

gantry assembly /gan′trē/, (in computed tomography) a subsystem consisting of the x-ray tube, the detector array, the high-voltage generator, the patient support and positioning couch, and the mechanical support for each.

gap [OE, *gapa,* a hole], (in molecular genetics) a short, missing segment in one strand of double-stranded DNA.

gap phenomenon, (in cardiology) a condition in which a premature stimulus encounters a block where an earlier or later stimulus could be conducted.

Garamycin, a trademark for an antibacterial (gentamicin sulfate).

Gardner, Mary Sewell (1871–1961), an American public health nurse who wrote the classic *Public Health Nurse.* She directed the Providence, Rhode Island, District Nursing Association and was instrumental in the development of the National Organization for Public Health Nursing and of public health nursing in the American Red Cross.

Gardner-Diamond syndrome, a condition resulting from autoerythrocyte sensitization, marked by large, painful, transient ecchymoses that appear without apparent cause but often accompany emotional upsets, various collagen disorders, and abnormalities of protein metabolism. Treatment includes topical and systemic corticosteroids. Also called **autoerythrocyte sensitization syndrome.**

Gardnerella vaginalis /gärd′nərel′ə/ [Herman L. Gardner, 20th century American bacteriologist; L, *vagina,* sheath], a genus of rodshaped Gram-negative bacteria normally found in the female genital tract. The bacteria, formerly identified as *haemophilus vaginalis,* may also be a cause of bacterial vaginitis.

Gardnerella vaginalis vaginitis [Herman Gardner, L, *vagina,* sheath; Gk, *itis,* inflammation], an infection of the female genital tract by bacteria of the Gardnerella vaginalis strain, often in combination with various anaerobic bacteria. It is assumed that the infection is sexually transmitted. The bacteria are also found in normal women without symptoms. The infection often produces a gray or yellow discharge with a 'fishy' odor that increases after washing the genitalia with alkaline soaps.

Gardner's syndrome [Eldon J. Gardner, American geneticist, b. 1909], familial polyposis of the large bowel, with fibrous dysplasia of the skull, extra teeth, osteomas, fibromas, and epidermal cysts. The condition is inherited as a dominant trait, and malignancies occur more often than usual in families having this syndrome.

Gardner-Wells tongs, braces that are attached to the skull of patients immobilized with cervical injuries. The tongs are used to apply traction to reduce a fracture or dislocation while the patient is in a special bed, such as a Stryker frame.

gargle /gär′gəl/ [Fr, *gargouille,* drainpipe], **1.** to hold and agitate a liquid at the back of the throat by tilting the head backward and forcing air through the solution. The procedure is used for cleansing or medicating the mouth and oropharynx. **2.** a solution used to rinse the mouth and oropharynx.

gargoylism.   See **Hurler's syndrome.**

Gartner's duct [Hermann T. Gartner, Danish anatomist, b. 1785], one of two vestigial, closed ducts, each one parallel to a uterine tube.

gas [Gk, *chaos*], an aeriform fluid possessing complete molecular mobility and the property of indefinite expansion. A gas has no definite shape, and its volume is determined by temperature and pressure. Compare **liquid, solid.**

gas bacillus [Gk, *chaos,* L, *bacillum,* small rod], any of several species of bacillus that produce a gas as a byproduct of their metabolism. Examples include E. coli, which ferments lactose and glucose, and the Clostridial species that produce gas gangrene.

gas chromatography, the separation and analysis of different substances according to their different affinities for a standard absorbent. In the process, a gaseous mixture of the substances is passed through a glass cylinder containing the absorbent, which may be dampened with a nonvolatile liquid solvent for one or more of the gaseous components. As the mixture passes through the absorbent, each substance is absorbed to a different extent and leaves a characteristic pigment. The bands of different colors left when all the gaseous mixture has moved through the absorbent constitute a chromatograph for analysis. Compare **column chromatography, ion-exchange chromatography.**

gas distention.   See **flatulence.**

gas embolism, an occlusion of one or more small blood vessels, especially in the muscles, tendons, and joints, caused by expanding bubbles of gases. Gas emboli can rupture tissue and blood vessels, causing decompression sickness and death. This phenomenon commonly affects deep-sea divers who rise too quickly to the surface without adequate decompression. Gas emboli are most dangerous in the central nervous system because of associated neurologic changes, such as syncope, paralysis, and aphasia. Such emboli are extremely painful. The prevention and treatment of gas emboli involve gradual decompression of atmospheric gases, especially nitrogen, that are dissolved in the blood. See also **air embolism, decompression sickness, embolism.**

gaseous /gas′ē·əs, gash′əs/ [Gk, *chaos,* pertaining to or resembling gas.

gas exchange, impaired, a nursing diagnosis accepted by the Fourth National Conference on the Classification of Nursing Diagnoses. Impaired gas exchange is the state in which the individual experiences a decreased passage of oxygen and/or carbon dioxide between the alveoli of the lungs and the vascular system. The cause of the condition is an imbalance in ventilatory perfusion. The defining characteristics are confusion, restlessness, irritability, somnolence, hypercapnea, and hypoxia. Additional related factors are altered oxygen supply, alveolar-capillary membrane changes, altered blood flow, and altered oxygen-carrying capacity of blood. See also **nursing diagnosis.**

gas gangrene, necrosis accompanied by gas bubbles in soft tissue after surgery or trauma. It is caused by anaerobic organisms, such as various species of *Clostridium,* particularly *C. perfringens.* Symptoms include pain, swelling, and tenderness of the wound area, moderate fever, tachycardia, and hypotension. The skin around the wound becomes necrotic and ruptures, revealing necrotic muscle. A characteristic finding is toxic delirium. If untreated, gas gangrene is rapidly fatal. Prompt treatment, including excision of gangrenous tissue and administration of penicillin G intravenously, saves 80% of patients. The disease is prevented by proper wound care. Also called **anaerobic myositis.**

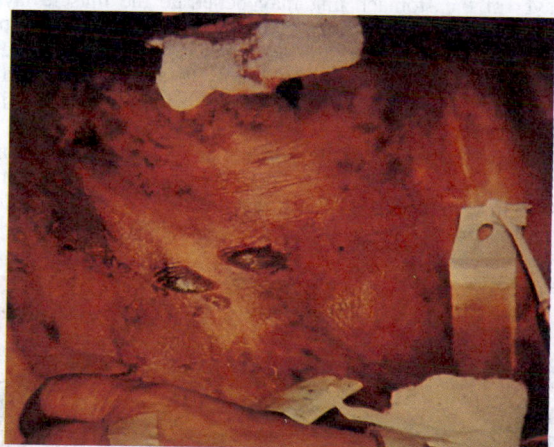

Gas gangrene *(Baron, 1990)*

gasoline poisoning. See **petroleum distillate poisoning.**
gas pains. See **flatulence.**
gas-scavenging system, the equipment and procedures used to eliminate anesthetic gases that escape into the atmosphere of the operating room. See also **trace gas.**
Gastaut's disease. See **Lennox-Gastaut syndrome.**

gas sterilization [Gk, *chaos,* gas; L, *sterilis,* barren] the use of a gas such as ethylene oxide, C_2H_4O, used to sterilize medical equipment.
gaster-, gastr-. See **gastro-.**
gas therapy, the use of medical gases in respiratory therapy. Kinds of gas therapy include **carbon dioxide therapy, controlled oxygen therapy, helium therapy,** and **hyperbaric oxygenation.**
gastralgia. See **stomach ache.**
gastrectasia /gas′trektā′zhə/ [Gk, *gaster,* stomach, *ektasis,* stretching], an abnormal dilatation of the stomach. It may be accompanied by pain, vomiting, rapid pulse, and falling body temperature. Causes can include overeating, obstruction of the pyloric valve, or a hernia.
gastrectomy /gastrek′əmē/, surgical excision of all or, more commonly, part of the stomach, performed to remove a chronic peptic ulcer, to stop hemorrhage in a perforating ulcer, or to remove a malignancy. Preoperatively, a GI series is done and a nasogastric tube is introduced. Under general anesthesia, one half to two thirds of the stomach is removed, including the ulcer and a large area of acid-secreting mucosa. A gastroenterostomy is then done, joining the remainder of the stomach to the jejunum or duodenum. Postoperatively, the nurse observes the drainage from the nasogastric suction tube for bright red blood, indicative of hemorrhage. The nurse encourages the patient to breathe deeply and to cough. With the return of peristalsis, water is given orally, and, if tolerated without pain or nausea, the tube is removed. A temperature elevation or dyspnea may indicate a leakage of the oral liquids from the incision into the abdomen. Complications of gastrectomy include fullness and discomfort after meals. A marginal ulcer may form where gastric acids come into contact with the mucous membrane of the anastomosis of the jejunum, causing painful contractions. The diet gradually progresses to six small, bland meals a day, with 120 ml of fluid hourly between meals. See also **dumping syndrome, gastroenterostomy, nasogastric tube, peptic ulcer.**
-gastria, a combining form meaning '(condition of) possessing a stomach or stomachs': *atretogastria, macrogastria, megalogastria.*
gastric /gas′trik/ [Gk, *gaster,* stomach], of or pertaining to the stomach.
-gastric, a combining form meaning a 'type of stomach or number of stomachs': *endogastric, paragastric, trigastric.*
gastric analysis, examination of the contents of the stomach, primarily to determine the quantity of acid present and incidentally to ascertain the presence of blood, bile, bacteria, and abnormal cells. A sample of gastric secretion is obtained via a nasogastric tube. The technique used varies according to the information desired. The total absence of hydrochloric acid is diagnostic of pernicious anemia. Patients with gastric ulcer and gastric cancer may secrete less acid than normal, whereas patients with duodenal ulcers secrete more. The composition and volume of the secretions may also provide diagnostic information. See also **Diagnex Blue test.**
gastric antacid. See **antacid.**
gastric atrophy. See **atrophic gastritis.**
gastric cancer, a malignancy of the stomach that is declining in incidence in North America and western Europe. Dietary factors, such as nitrates, smoked and salted fish and meats, and moldy foods containing aflatoxin are thought to cause gastric cancer, but the etiology remains unknown. The

incidence is higher in men than in women and peaks in the 50- to 59-year-old age group. The risk is increased in workers exposed to asbestos and in patients with pernicious anemia. Gastric ulcers may become malignant, and those that do may have originated as ulcerating cancerous lesions. Symptoms of gastric cancer are vague epigastric discomfort, anorexia, weight loss, and unexplained iron deficiency anemia; however, many cases are asymptomatic in the early stages, and metastatic enlargement of the left supraclavicular lymph node may be the first manifestation of a stomach lesion. Diagnostic measures include a test for occult blood in the stool, gastric analysis, x-ray films of the upper digestive tract after barium ingestion, examination of gastric mucosa with a flexible endoscope, biopsy, and cytologic studies of exfoliated tumor cells. Approximately 97% of stomach tumors are adenocarcinomas that may be ulcerating, polypoid, diffuse, and fibrous, or superficial spreading lesions; lymphomas and leiomyosarcomas account for less than 3%. Radical subtotal gastrectomy with excision of contiguous involved tissues and reconstruction by anastomosing the remainder of the stomach to the duodenum or jejunum is usually recommended. Total gastrectomy is associated with high morbidity and mortality, and usually leads to pernicious anemia. Radiotherapy and chemotherapy are usually not effective, but postoperative irradiation is recommended to control microscopic residual tumor; combinations of antineoplastic antimetabolites are used in treating advanced, metastatic gastric cancer.

gastric digestion [Gk, *gaster*, stomach; L, *digere*, to separate], digestion by gastric juice in the stomach.

gawtric dyspepsia, pain or discomfort localized in the stomach. See also **dyspepsia.**

gastric emesis [Gk, *gaster*, stomach; *emesis*, vomiting], vomiting associated with a stomach disorder, such as stomach cancer, stomach ulcer, or severe gastritis.

gastric fistula, an abnormal passage into the stomach, communicating most frequently with an opening on the external surface of the abdomen. A gastric fistula may be created surgically to provide tube feeding for patients with severe esophageal disorders.

gastric glands, glands in the stomach mucosa that secrete hydrochloric acid, mucin, and pepsinogen.

gastric inhibitory polypeptide (GIP), a gastrointestinal hormone found in the mucosa of the small intestine. Release of the hormone, mediated by the presence of glucose or fatty acids in the duodenum, results in the release of insulin by the pancreas and inhibition of gastric acid secretion.

gastric intubation, a procedure in which a Levine tube or other small-caliber catheter is passed into the esophagus and stomach for the introduction into the stomach of liquid formulas to provide nutrition for unconscious patients or for premature or sick newborn infants. Medication or a contrast medium may be instilled for treatment or for radiologic examination. Gastric intubation is most often performed to remove the contents of the stomach to prevent postoperative gastric distention, to prevent aspiration of gastric contents during general anesthesia, or to remove a poisonous substance and wash the stomach. See also **gastric lavage, Levine tube.**

gastric juice, digestive secretions of the gastric glands in the stomach, consisting chiefly of pepsin, hydrochloric acid, rennin, and mucin. The pH is strongly acid (0.9 to 1.5).

Achlorhydria (a deficiency of hydrochloric acid in gastric juice) is present in pernicious anemia and stomach cancer. Excessive secretion of gastric juice may lead to mucosal irritation and to peptic ulcer. See also **achlorhydria, gastric analysis, gastric ulcer.**

gastric lavage, the washing out of the stomach with sterile water or a saline solution. The procedure is performed before and after surgery to remove irritants or toxic substances and before such examinations as endoscopy or gastroscopy. See also **irrigation.**

gastric motility, the spontaneous peristaltic movements of the stomach that aid in digestion, moving food through the stomach and out through the pyloric sphincter into the duodenum. Excess gastric motility causes pain that is usually treated with antispasmodic medication. Less than normal motility is common in labor, after general anesthesia, and as a side effect of some sedative hypnotics.

gastric mucin [Gk, *gaster*, stomach; L, *mucus*], a viscous secretion of glycoproteins produced from the mucous membrane lining of swine stomachs and formerly used in the treatment of peptic ulcers.

gastric node, a node in one of three groups of lymph glands associated with the abdominal and pelvic viscera supplied by branches of the celiac artery. The gastric nodes accompany the left gastric artery and are divided into the superior and inferior gastric nodes. Compare **hepatic node, pancreaticolienal node.**

gastric partitioning, a surgical procedure in which a portion of the stomach is closed, reducing its capacity. It is used in the treatment of certain cases of obesity.

gastric resection [Gk, *gaster*, stomach; L, *re, secare*, to cut], the surgical removal of part or all of the stomach, usually performed in the treatment of stomach cancer or peptic ulcer.

gastric tetany. See **tetany.**

gastric ulcer, a circumscribed erosion of the mucosal layer of the stomach that may penetrate the muscle layer and perforate the stomach wall. It is characterized by episodes of burning epigastric pain, belching, and nausea, especially when the stomach is empty or after eating certain foods. Characteristically, antacid medication or milk quickly relieves the pain. Treatment includes medication to decrease the acidity of the stomach and to relieve symptomatic stress. If perforation and hemorrhage occur, surgical resection of part of the stomach may be necessary. Also called **peptic ulcer.**

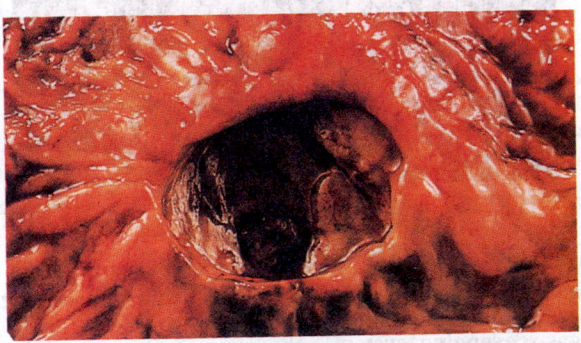

Chronic gastric ulcer (Fletcher, 1987)

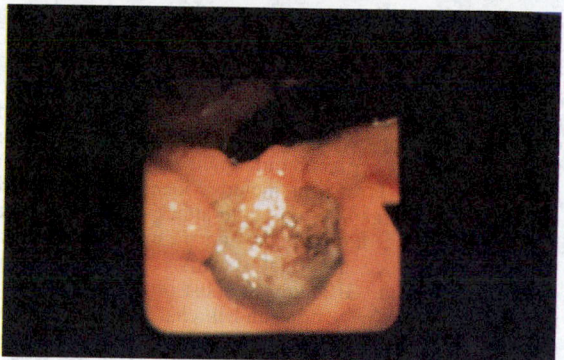

Malignant gastric ulcer—endoscopic view
(Kamal, 1991)

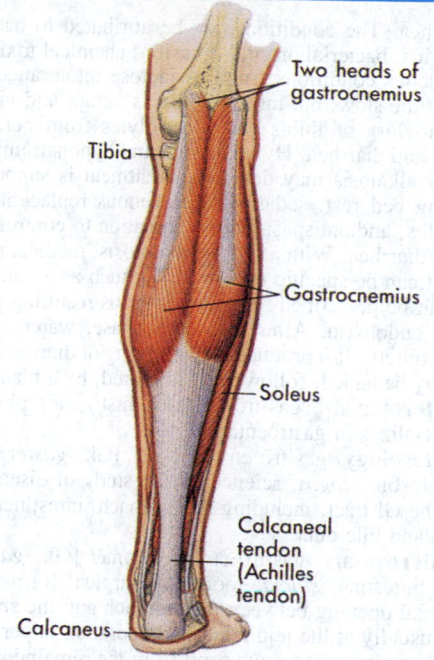

Gastrocnemius *(Thibodeau, 1993)*

gastrin /gas'trin/ [Gk, *gaster*, stomach], a polypeptide hormone, secreted by the pylorus, that stimulates the flow of gastric juice and contributes to the stimulus causing bile and pancreatic enzymes secretion. Normal findings of blood levels of gastrin are less than 200 pg/ml.

gastrinoma /gas'trinō'mə/, a tumor found in the pancreas and in the duodenum. It is associated with the presence of peptic ulcers.

gastritis /gastrī'tis/, an inflammation of the lining of the stomach that occurs in two forms. **Acute gastritis** may be caused by severe burns, major surgery, aspirin or other antiinflammatory agents, corticosteroids, drugs, food allergens, or viral, bacterial, or chemical toxins. The symptoms—anorexia, nausea, vomiting, and discomfort after eating—usually abate after the causative agent has been removed. **Chronic gastritis** is usually a sign of underlying disease, such as peptic ulcer, stomach cancer, Zollinger-Ellison syndrome, or pernicious anemia. Differential diagnosis is by endoscopy with biopsy. Kinds of gastritis include **atrophic gastritis, hemorrhagic gastritis,** and **hypertrophic gastritis.** Compare **peptic ulcer.**

gastro-, gaster-, gastr-, a combining form meaning 'pertaining to the stomach or abdomen': *gastroadynamia, gastrocolitis, gastrophrenic.*

gastrocamera /gas'trōkam'ərə/, a small camera that can be lowered into the stomach through the esophagus and retrieved after recording images of the stomach lining.

gastrocnemius /-knē'mē'əs/ [Gk, *gastroknemia*, calf of the leg], the most superficial muscle in the posterior part of the leg. It arises by a lateral head and a medial head and forms the greater part of the calf. The lateral head arises from the lateral condyle of the femur and the capsule of the knee. The medial head arises from the medial condyle of the femur and from the capsule of the knee. The fibers of both heads insert into a broad aponeurosis that narrows distally to join the tendon of the soleus as part of the tendo calcaneus. Compare **soleus, plantaris.**

gastrocnemius gait, an abnormal gait associated with a weakness of the gastrocnemius. It is characterized by the dropping of the pelvis on the affected side at the last moment of the stance phase in the walking cycle, accompanied by the lagging or the slowness of forward pelvic movement.

gastrocnemius test, a test of the function of the gastrocnemius muscle by ankle plantar flexion while the patient is in a prone position. The examiner places fingers for palpation on the posterior of the calf while the patient pulls the heel upward, thus plantar flexing the ankle. Flexion of the toes and forefoot before movement of the heel is evidence of muscle substitution.

gastrocoele. See **archenteron.**

gastrocolic omentum. See **greater omentum.**

gastrocolic reflex /-kol'ik/ [Gk, *gaster* + *kolon*, colon; L, *reflectere*, to bend backward], a mass peristaltic movement of the colon that often occurs 15 to 20 minutes after food enters the stomach. When an infant is fed, this reflex may result in a bowel movement.

gastrodidymus /-did'iməs/ [Gk, *gaster* + *didymos*, twin], conjoined, equally developed twins united at the abdominal region. Also called **omphalodidymus.**

gastrodisciasis /gas'trōdiskī'əsis/ [Gk, *gaster* + *diskos*, disk, *eidos* form, *osis* condition], an infection of trematodes of the genus *Gastrodiscoides*, which are digestive tract parasites. The species *G. hominis*, a reddish-orange fluke averaging 1 cm in length, is endemic in the hog populations of Southeast Asia and is transmitted to humans.

gastrodisk. See **embryonic disk.**

gastroduodenal /doo'ədē'nəl/ [Gk, *gaster*; L, *duodeni*, 12 fingers wide], pertaining to the stomach and duodenum.

gastroduodenitis /-doo'ədenī'tis/ [Gk, *gaster*, stomach; L, *duodeni*, 12 fingers; Gk, *itis*, inflammation], inflammation of the stomach and duodenum.

gastrodynia. See **stomach ache.**

gastroenteritis /gas'trō·en'tərī'tis/ [Gk, *gaster* + *enteron*, intestine, *itis* inflammation], inflammation of the stomach and intestines accompanying numerous GI disorders. Symptoms are anorexia, nausea, vomiting, abdominal discomfort, and diarrhea. The condition may be attributed to bacterial enterotoxins, bacterial or viral invasion, chemical toxins, or miscellaneous conditions, such as lactose intolerance. The onset may be slow, but more often it is abrupt and violent, with rapid loss of fluids and electrolytes from persistent vomiting and diarrhea. Hypokalemia and hyponatremia, acidosis, or alkalosis may develop. Treatment is supportive, employing bed rest, sedation, intravenous replacement of electrolytes, and antispasmodic medication to control vomiting and diarrhea. With a precise diagnosis, medication and treatment can be specific and curative, such as an antitoxin that might be prescribed for gastroenteritis resulting from a bacterial endotoxin. After the acute phase, water may be given by mouth. If it produces no vomiting or diarrhea, clear fluids may be added, followed, if tolerated, by a bland diet.

gastroenterologist /gas'trō·en'tərol'əjist/, a physician who specializes in gastroenterology.

gastroenterology /gas'trō·en'tərol'əjē/ [Gk, *gaster + enteron,* intestine, *logos,* science], the study of diseases affecting the GI tract, including the stomach, intestines, gallbladder, and bile duct.

gastroenterostomy /gas'trō·en'təros'təmē/ [Gk, *gaster + enteron,* intestine, *stoma,* mouth], surgical formation of an artificial opening between the stomach and the small intestine, usually at the jejunum. The operation is performed with a gastrectomy, to route food from the remainder of the stomach into the small intestine, or by itself, for perforating ulcer of the duodenum. A GI series is done preoperatively, and a nasogastric tube is inserted. The jejunum is pulled up and anastomosed with the stomach. A new opening is then made for food to pass from the stomach directly into the jejunum. Pancreatic juices and bile are still secreted into the duodenum and pass through its distal end to the jejunum. Postoperatively, drainage from the nasogastric suction tube is observed for bright red bleeding, indicative of hemorrhage. Deep breathing and coughing are encouraged. The nasogastric tube is removed when peristalsis returns and when water given orally does not cause pain or nausea. Temperature elevation or dyspnea may indicate a leakage of the fluids from the incision around the anastomosis. The diet is gradually increased to six small, bland meals a day, with 120 ml of fluids hourly between meals. Compare **gastrectomy.**

gastroesophageal /gas'trō·isof'əjē'əl/ [Gk, *gaster + oisophagos,* gullet], of or pertaining to the stomach and the esophagus.

gastroesophageal hemorrhage. See **Mallory-Weiss syndrome.**

gastroesophageal reflux, a backflow of contents of the stomach into the esophagus that is often the result of incompetence of the lower esophageal sphincter. Gastric juices are acid and therefore produce burning pain in the esophagus. Repeated episodes of reflux may cause esophagitis, peptic esophageal stricture, or esophageal ulcer. In uncomplicated cases, treatment consists of elevation of the head of the bed, avoidance of acid-stimulating foods, and regular administration of antacids. In complicated cases, surgical repair may provide relief. See also **chalasia, esophagitis, heartburn, hiatus hernia.**

gastrogavage. See **gastrostomy feeding.**

gastrohepatic omentum. See **lesser omentum.**

gastrointestinal (GI) /gas'trō·intes'tinəl/ [Gk, *gaster* + L, *intestinum,* intestine], of or pertaining to the organs of the GI tract, from mouth to anus.

gastrointestinal allergy, an immediate reaction of hypersensitivity after the ingestion of certain foods or drugs. GI allergy differs from food allergy, which can affect organ systems other than the digestive system. Characteristic symptoms include itching and swelling of the mouth and oral passages, nausea, vomiting, diarrhea (sometimes containing blood), severe abdominal pain, and, if severe, anaphylactic shock. Treatment includes identification and removal of the allergen. In an acute attack epinephrine may be administered as a stimulant, and muscle relaxants may be given to reduce intestinal spasms causing abdominal pain. In childhood, GI allergy is most often caused by hypersensitivity to cow's milk and is characterized by diarrhea and colicky pain, sometimes with vomiting, eczema, respiratory distress, and thrombocytopenia. See also **lactose intolerance.**

gastrointestinal bleeding, any bleeding from the GI tract. The most common underlying conditions are peptic ulcer, Mallory-Weiss syndrome, esophageal varices, diverticulosis, ulcerative colitis, and carcinoma of the stomach and colon. Vomiting of bright red blood or the passage of coffee ground vomitus indicates upper GI bleeding, usually from the esophagus, stomach, or upper duodenum. Aspiration of the gastric contents, lavage, and endoscopy are performed to determine the site and rate of bleeding. Tarry, black stools indicate a bleeding source in the upper GI tract; bright red blood from the rectum usually indicates bleeding in the distal colon. GI bleeding is treated as a potential emergency. Patients may require transfusions or fluid replacement and are watched carefully for signs of shock and hypovolemia. In all patients, blood loss is evaluated and ability to coagulate is tested. See also **coffee ground vomitus, hematochezia, melena.**

gastrointestinal gas. See **flatulence.**

gastrointestinal infection, any infection of the digestive tract caused by bacteria, viruses, or parasites. All may have common clinical features of nausea, vomiting, diarrhea, and anorexia. Treatment in most cases includes bed rest, easy access to a bathroom, and food and beverages to replenish loss of fluid and electrolytes.

gastrointestinal obstruction, any obstruction of the passage of intestinal contents, caused by mechanical blockage or failure of motility. Mechanical blockage may be caused by adhesions resulting from surgery or inflammatory bowel disease, an incarcerated hernia, fecal impaction, tumor, intussusception, or volvulus. Failure of motility may follow anesthesia, abdominal surgery, or occlusion of any of the mesenteric arteries to the gut. Symptoms vary with the cause of obstruction but generally include vomiting, abdominal pain, and increasing abdominal distention. Dehydration and prostration may follow. Characteristically, borborygmus is diminished or absent and abdominal guarding is prominent. A barium enema may be performed, but barium is never given by mouth in such cases because it would increase the volume of the obstruction. The objective of therapy is to remove the obstruction as quickly and safely as possible. A tube is inserted into the stomach or small intestine to aspirate contents and relieve distention. During these procedures, the patient is monitored for proper fluid and electrolyte balance. Surgical intervention may be necessary. The nurse helps the patient to understand that medication for pain can aggravate the condition by further decreasing motility of the GI tract and that it may not be prescribed in the acute period, before the location and extent of the obstruction is discovered.

gastrointestinal system assessment, an evaluation of the patient's digestive system and symptoms.

■ METHOD: Discussion of symptoms is encouraged, and the patient is asked whether there is or has been pain or tenderness in the oral cavity, gums, tongue, lips, or abdomen and whether there have been instances of dysphagia, belching, heartburn, anorexia, nausea, vomiting, constipation, diarrhea, or painful defecation. Information is elicited concerning any changes in eating, bowel habits, the color, character, and frequency of stools and urine, the use of laxatives or enemas, and the occurrence of fatigue, hemorrhoids, and edema of the extremities. The patient's general appearance, weight, and temperature are noted; the blood pressure, pulse, and respirations are checked in the supine, sitting, and standing positions; and the urinary output and color are determined. The presence of allergies, stomatitis, and halitosis; and the condition of the tongue, gums, oral mucosa, and teeth are recorded. The abdomen is examined for distention, rigidity, ascites, symmetry, hepatomegaly, keloid tissue, visible peristalsis, bowel sounds, masses, and the presence of an ostomy. The perianal area is inspected for its general condition, color, odor, and hemorrhoids; the sclera for signs of jaundice; and the skin for pruritus, spider angioma, purpura, palmar erythema, peripheral edema, jaundice, and distended, tortuous blood vessels. Relevant to the assessment are the patient's concurrent endocrine, cardiovascular, and neurologic disorders; severe burns, psychologic problems, carcinoma, alcohol or drug abuse, and previous GI surgery and illnesses, such as hepatitis, liver cirrhosis, or pancreatitis. The patient's personality type, attitude toward work, use of tobacco, antacids, laxatives, anticholinergics, steroids, antidiarrheals, antiemetics, sedatives, tranquilizers, barbiturates, antihypertensives, antibiotics, and aspirin are investigated. The family history, especially of GI disease, carcinoma, and diabetes, is an important aspect of the evaluation. Diagnostic aids include a complete blood count, stool examination, prothrombin time, and determinations of levels of alkaline phosphatase, serum and urine bilirubin, serum glutamic oxaloacetic transaminase (SGOT), serum glutamic pyruvic transaminase (SGPT), lactic acid dehydrogenase (LDH), blood urea nitrogen, serum lipase, cholinesterase, calcium, albumin, and glucose. Additional laboratory studies for the evaluation are the total protein level, a serum electrolyte profile; serum carotene, delta-xylose tolerance, galactose tolerance, hippuric acid, and bromosulphalein tests; the albumin-globulin ratio, serum flocculation, and thymol turbidity tests; urobilinogen level; the polyvinylpyrrolidone (PVP) test for protein loss, Sulkowitch's test for calcium in urine; and Schilling's test for GI absorption of vitamin B_{12}. Procedures that may be required for the diagnosis include upper GI, small bowel, and gallbladder series; esophageal and gastric endoscopy and biopsy; scans of the liver and pancreas; biopsies of the liver, colon, or rectum; gastric analysis, sigmoidoscopy, abdominal x-ray films, fluoroscopy, percutaneous transhepatic cholangiography, splenoportography, and digital rectal examinations.

■ INTERVENTIONS: The nurse conducts the interview, records observations of the patient, and assembles the results of the diagnostic laboratory studies and procedures.

■ OUTCOME CRITERIA: A well-conducted assessment of the patient's GI system is a valuable contribution to the diagnosis and plan of treatment.

gastrointestinal tract. See **digestive tract.**

gastromalacia /-məlā′shə/ [Gk, *gaster*, stomach, *malakia*, softness], an abnormal softening of the walls of the stomach.

gastromegaly /-meg′əlē/ [Gk, *gaster*, stomach, *megas*, large], an abnormal enlargement of the stomach or abdomen.

gastroplasty /gas′troplas′tē/ [Gk, *gaster*, stomach, *plassein*, to mold], any surgery performed to reshape or repair any stomach defect or deformity.

gastropore. See **blastopore.**

gastroschisis /gastros′kəsis/ [Gk, *gaster* + *schisis*, division], a congenital defect characterized by incomplete closure of the abdominal wall with protrusion of the viscera. Compare **omphalocele.**

gastroscope /gas′trōskōp′/ [Gk, *gaster* + *skopein*, to look], a fiberoptic instrument for examining the interior of the stomach. See also **fiberoptics.** –**gastroscopy,** *n.,* **gastroscopic,** *adj.*

gastroscopy /gastros′kəpē/, the visual inspection of the interior of the stomach by means of a gastroscope inserted through the esophagus. The flexible fiberoptic gastroscope has increased the visualization of the prepyloric antrum, but the fundus is still not visible. See also **endoscopy, fiberoptics.** –**gastroscopic,** *adj.*

gastrostomy /gastros′təmē/ [Gk, *gaster* + *stoma*, mouth], surgical creation of an artificial opening into the stomach through the abdominal wall, performed to feed a patient who has cancer of the esophagus or tracheoesophageal fistula or one who is expected to be unconscious for a prolonged period. The anterior wall of the stomach is drawn forward and sutured to the abdominal wall. A Foley catheter or other tube or a special prosthesis is then inserted into an incision in the stomach, and the opening is tightly sutured to prevent leakage of the contents of the stomach. The device is clamped, and opened when food is instilled. Postoperatively, glucose in water may be given, followed by a slow continuous feeding of a warm, blended formula to increase absorption. The skin is kept clean and dry around the site. Skin irritation indicates a leakage of gastric secretions and digestive enzymes. After 2 weeks the tube may be withdrawn after feeding and reinserted before the next meal.

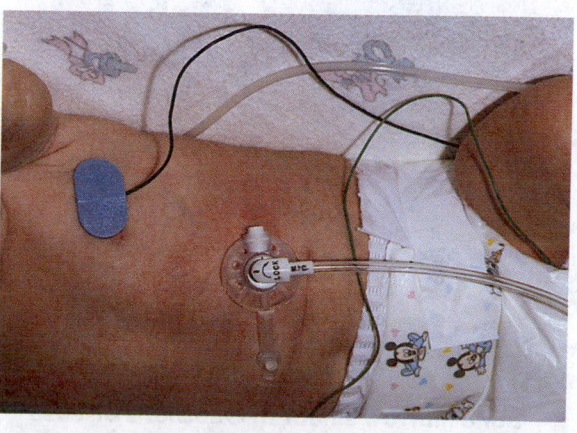

Gastrostomy device *(Wong, 1993)*

gastrostomy feeding, the introduction of a nutrient solution through a tube that has been surgically inserted into the stomach through the abdominal wall. Also called **gastrogavage.**

gastrostomy tube. See **stomach tube.**

gastrothoracopagus /gas′trōthôr′əkop′əgəs/ [Gk, *gaster* + *thorax*, chest, *pagos*, fixture], conjoined twins that are united at the thorax and abdomen.

gastrula /gas′trŏŏlə/ [Gk, *gaster*, stomach], the early embryonic stage formed by the invagination of the blastula. The cup-shaped gastrula consists of an outer layer of ectoderm and an inner layer of mesentoderm that subsequently differentiates into the mesoderm and endoderm. See also **blastula, embryonic layer.**

-gastrula, a combining form meaning an 'embryonic stage after the blastula': *amphigastrula, discogastrula, paragastrula.*

gastrulation /gas′trəlā′shən/ [Gk, *gaster*, stomach], the development of the gastrula in lower animals and the formation of the three germ layers in the embryo of humans and higher animals. It is characterized by an extensive series of coordinated morphogenetic movements within the blastula or blastocyst by which the primitive body plan of the organism is established and by which the areas that later differentiate into various structures and organs are in their proper position for development.

gatch bed /gach/ [William D. Gatch, American surgeon, b. 1879; AS, *bedd*], a bed that has an adjustable joint, allowing the knees to be flexed and the legs supported.

gate theory of pain. See **pain mechanism.**

gating, (in magnetic resonance imaging) organizing the data so that information used to construct an image comes from the same point in the cycle of a repeating motion, such as a heartbeat. The moving object is thus frozen at that phase of its motion, and image blurring is minimized.

gating mechanism, (in cardiology) the increasing duration of an action potential from the AV node to a point in the distal Purkinje system, beyond which it decreases.

Gaucher's disease /gōshāz′/ [Phillipe C. E. Gaucher,

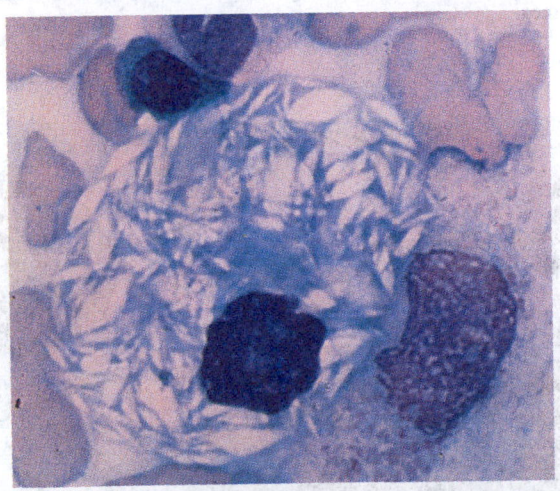

Bone marrow smear in Gaucher's disease
(Hayhoe, 1992)

French physician, b. 1854], a rare, familial disorder of fat metabolism, caused by an enzyme deficiency, characterized by widespread reticulum cell hyperplasia in the liver, spleen, lymph nodes, and bone marrow. Beginning in infancy or early childhood, splenomegaly, hepatomegaly, and abnormal bone growth develop. Diagnosis is made through biopsy of the liver, spleen, or bone marrow. Mortality is high, but children who survive adolescence may live for many years. Also called **glucosyl cerebroside lipidosis.**

gauntlet bandage /gônt′lit/ [Fr, *gantlet*, small glove; *bande*, strip], a glovelike bandage covering the hand and the fingers. See also **demigauntlet bandage.**

gauss /gôs, gous/ [J. K. F. Gauss, German physicist, b. 1777], a unit of magnetic field strength. It is equal to 1/10,000 of a tesla.

gauze /gôz/ [Fr, *gaze*], a transparent fabric of open weave and differing degrees of fineness, most often cotton muslin, used in surgical procedures and for bandages and dressings. It may be sterilized and permeated by an antiseptic or lotion. Kinds of gauze include **absorbable gauze, absorbent gauze,** and **petrolatum gauze.** See also **bandage.**

gauze sponge [Fr, *gaze;* Gk, *spoggia*], a piece of folded gauze used during surgery to wipe up bleeding surfaces and thereby help locate any sources of blood loss.

gavage /gäväzh′/ [Fr, *gaver*, to gorge], the process of feeding a patient through a nasogastric tube. See also **gastrostomy feeding.**

gavage feeding. See **tube feeding.**

gavage feeding of the newborn, a procedure in which a tube passed through the nose or mouth into the stomach is used to feed a newborn infant with weak sucking, uncoordinated sucking and swallowing, respiratory distress, tachypnea, or repeated apneic spells.

■ METHOD: After the gastric tube is inserted, its placement is checked by instilling air and auscultating the stomach for air sounds or by immersing the proximal end of the tube in water. If the amount of residual formula left in the infant's stomach at the time of the next feeding exceeds the quantity specified, the next feeding may be delayed or omitted. During feeding, the infant is held in a low Fowler's position, preferably by the mother, and is restrained only if necessary. The feeding syringe is held 6 to 8 inches above the infant's head, and the flow is initiated by pressure on the plunger. As the formula is slowly instilled, the baby is stroked and is offered a pacifier to promote gravity flow, exert a calming effect, and reinforce the relationship between sucking and feeding. If the infant gags, spits, chokes, regurgitates, vomits, or becomes cyanotic, the rate of flow of formula is reduced and the feeding may be stopped. To prevent air from entering the stomach when the feeding is completed, the tube is pinched closed as it is withdrawn. The infant is burped gently by patting or rubbing the back and then positioned on the right side in the crib; postural drainage and percussion are avoided for at least 1 hour after feeding. The time, amount, and kind of feeding and the size of tube used are entered in the nursing care plan.

■ INTERVENTIONS: The nurse administers intermittent gavage feeding to the infant, offers an explanation to the parents of the need for the procedure, and points out that nipple feedings may be instituted when the infant sucks on the gavage tube or pacifier, actively seeks nourishment, shows good suck and swallow coordination, gains weight, and has a respiratory rate of less than 60 breaths per minute.

■ OUTCOME CRITERIA: Intermittent gavage feedings can enable the high-risk infant to survive.

gay [Fr, *gai*, merry], **1.** any person who is homosexual. **2.** of or pertaining to homosexuality.

Gay-Lussac's law /gā'ləsaks'/ [Joseph L. Gay-Lussac, French scientist, b. 1778; L, *legu*, a rule], (in physics) a law stating that the volume of a specific mass of a gas will increase as the temperature is increased if the pressure remains constant. Also called **Charles' law.**

Gay Nurses' Alliance (GNA), a national organization of homosexual and lesbian nurses.

gaze /gāz/ [ME, *gazen*, to stare], a state of looking in one direction. A person with normal vision has six basic positions of gaze, each determined by control of different combinations of contractions of extraocular muscles.

gaze palsy, a partial or complete inability to move the eyes to all directions of gaze. A gaze palsy is often named for the absent direction of gaze, such as a right lateral gaze palsy.

GBIA. See **Guthrie test.**

g.c., *informal.* abbreviation for **gonococcus.**

Gd, symbol for the element **gadolinium.**

GDM, abbreviation for **gestational diabetes mellitus.**

Ge, symbol for the element **germanium.**

gegenhalten /gā'gənhäl'tən/ [Ger, counterpressure], the involuntary resistance to passive movement of the extremities. It may occur as a symptom of catatonia in which there is passive resistance to stretching movements, even when the patient attempts to cooperate. The effect may be psychogenic in origin or a sign of dementia or cerebral deterioration. Also called **paratonia.**

Geiger-Müller (GM) counter /gī'gərmil'ər/ [Hans Geiger, German physicist, b. 1882; Walther Müller, German physicist; Fr, *conter*, to tell], an electronic device that indicates the level of radioactivity of any substance by counting the number of subatomic particles, as electrons, emitted by the substance. It cannot identify the type or energy of a particle. The counter detects ionizing particles with a Geiger-Müller tube. As ionizing particles cross the tube, they ionize the gas within the tube and cause an electric discharge. Also called **Geiger counter.**

gel /jel/ [L, *gelare*, to congeal], a colloid that is firm even though it contains a large amount of liquid, used in many medicines as a demulcent, a vehicle for other drugs, an antacid, or an astringent, depending on the drug from which it is derived.

-gel [L, *gelare*, to congeal], a suffix for terms relating to jellylike substances formed by cooling a colloid into a semisolid state.

gelat-, a combining form meaning 'to freeze, congeal': *gelatigenous, gelatinoid, gelatum.*

gelatin buildup /jel'ətən/, an x-ray film artifact that may appear as a sharp area of either increased or reduced density.

gelatin film, absorbable, a hemostatic.

■ INDICATIONS: It is used to attain hemostasis during surgery, particularly neurologic, thoracic, and ophthalmic procedures.

■ CONTRAINDICATIONS: Infection or gross contamination of the surgical wound prohibits its use.

■ ADVERSE EFFECTS: There are no known adverse reactions.

gelatiniform carcinoma. See **mucinous carcinoma.**

gelatinous /jəlat'ənəs/ [L, *gelare*, to congeal], pertaining to or resembling a viscous, jellylike substance.

gelatinous carcinoma, a former term for **mucinous carcinoma.**

gelatin sponge, an absorbable local hemostatic.

■ INDICATIONS: It is prescribed to control bleeding in various surgical procedures and in the treatment of decubitus ulcers to promote healing and hemostasis.

■ CONTRAINDICATIONS: Frank infection, extensive and abnormal bleeding, postpartum bleeding, or menorrhagia prohibits its use.

■ ADVERSE EFFECTS: There are no known adverse reactions.

gel diffusion. See **immunodiffusion.**

Gelfoam, a trademark for an absorbable hemostatic gelatin sponge.

Gellhorn pessary. See **pessary.**

gemellary /jem'əler'ē/ [L, *gemellus*, twin], of or pertaining to twins.

gemellipara /jem'əlip'ərə/ [L, *gemellus* + *parare*, to give birth], a woman who has given birth to twins.

gemellology /jem'əlol'əjē/ [L, *gemellus* + Gk, *logos*, science], the study of twins and the phenomenon of twinning.

gemellus /jəmel'əs/, either of a pair of small muscles arising from the ischium. The gemellus superior inserts into the upper part of the tendon of the obturator internus, through which it is attached to the great trochanter of the femur. The gemellus inferior lies below and also inserts into the obturator internus. They rotate the thigh laterally.

gemellus test, a test of the function of the gemellus superior and gemellus inferior in hip external rotation while the patient is seated with the knees flexed. The examiner places one hand on the lateral aspect of the knee to prevent flexion or abduction of the hip while the patient rotates the thigh outward by moving the foot medially.

gemfibrozil /jemfī'brəzil/ an antihyperlipidemic agent.

■ INDICATION: It is prescribed for hyperlipidemia.

■ CONTRAINDICATIONS: Renal or hepatic dysfunction, gallbladder disease, or known hypersensitivity to this drug prohibits its use.

■ ADVERSE EFFECTS: Among the adverse reactions are abdominal or epigastric pain, urticaria, dizziness, and anemia.

gemin-, a combining form meaning 'pertaining to a twin, or double': *geminate, gemini, geminous.*

gemistocyte /gemis'təsīt/, an astrocyte with an eccentric nucleus and swollen cytoplasm, as seen in areas of nervous tissue affected by edema or infarction.

gemma /jem'ə/, *pl.* **gemmae** [L, bud], **1.** a budlike projection produced by lower forms of life during the budding process of asexual reproduction. **2.** any budlike or bulblike structure, such as a taste bud or end bulb. **−gemmaceous,** *adj.*

gemmate /jem'āt/ [L, *gemma* + *atus*, function], **1.** having buds or gemmae. **2.** to reproduce by budding.

gemmation /jemā'shən/ [L, *gemmare*, to produce buds], the process of cell reproduction by budding. Also called **gemmulation.**

gemmiferous /jemif'ərəs/ [L, *gemma* + *fer*, bearing], having buds or gemmae; gemmiparous.

gemmiform /jem'ifôrm'/, resembling a bud or gemma.

gemmipara /jemip'ərə/ [L, *gemma* + *parare*, to give birth], an animal that produces gemmae or reproduces by budding, such as the hydra. **−gemmiparous,** *adj.*

gemmulation. See **gemmation.**

gemmule /jem'yool/ [L, *gemmula*, small bud], **1.** the small, asexual reproductive structure produced by the parent during budding that eventually develops into an independent organism. **2.** [n](according to the early theory of pangenesis) any of the submicroscopic particles containing hereditary elements that are produced by each somatic cell of the parent, are transmitted through the bloodstream to the gametes, and, after fertilization, give rise to cells and tissues that have the exact same characteristics as those from which they originated. Compare **biophore.**

Gemonil, a trademark for an anticonvulsant (metharbital).

gen-, geno-, a combining form meaning 'to become or produce': *generic, genesiology, genophobia, genus.*

-gen, -gene, 1. a suffix meaning 'that which generates': *aerogen, proteinogen, venogen.* **2.** a combining form meaning 'that which is generated': *immunogen, ionogen, nitrogen.*

Genapax Tampon, a trademark for an antiinfective tampon (gentian violet).

gender /jen'dər/ [L, *genus*, kind], **1.** the classification of the sex of a person into male, female, or intersexual. **2.** the particular sex of a person. See also **sex.**

gender identity, the sense or awareness of knowing to which sex one belongs. The process begins in infancy, continues throughout childhood, and is reinforced during adolescence. Also called **core gender identity.**

gender identity disorder, a condition characterized by a persistent feeling of discomfort or inappropriateness concerning one's anatomic sex. The disorder typically begins in childhood with gender identity problems and is manifested in adolescence or adulthood as crossdressing.

gender role, the expression of a person's gender identity; the image that a person presents to both himself or herself and others demonstrating maleness or femaleness.

gender testing [L, *genus*, class, *testum*, crucible], a procedure for validating the sex of an individual by examining a tissue sample, usually obtained from oral mucous membrane cells, for the presence of a Y chromosome.

gene /jēn/ [Gk, *genein*, to produce], the biologic unit of genetic material and inheritance. The concept of the gene has undergone modification since the introduction of mendelian genetics. Changes continue as techniques for studying the molecular components of the cell are refined. The gene is now considered to be a particular nucleic acid sequence within a DNA molecule that occupies a precise locus on a chromosome and is capable of self-replication by coding for a specific polypeptide chain. In diploid organisms, which include humans and other mammals, genes occur as paired alleles and function in many capacities, primarily as structural and regulative components in controlling the differentiation of the cells and tissues of the body. Kinds of genes include **complementary genes, dominant gene, lethal gene, mutant gene, operator gene, pleiotropic gene, recessive gene, regulator gene, structural gene, sublethal gene, supplementary genes,** and **wild-type gene.** See also **chromosome, cistron, DNA, operon.**

-gene. See **-gen.**

gene amplification [Gk, *genein*, to produce; L, *amplus*, large], a gene duplicating process in which RNA molecules are transcribed many times in certain cells in response to defined signals or environmental stresses.

gene library, (in molecular genetics) a collection of all of the genetic information of a specific species, obtained from cloned fragments.

gene marker. See **genetic marker.**

gene pool [Gk, *genein*, to produce; AS, *pol*] the total number of genetic traits within a person or species population. In a population that reproduces by random sexual selection, the distribution of genetic traits follows a normal bell curve.

gene probe, a molecular biology device for locating a particular gene on a chromosome. It involves pairing a short known segment of DNA or RNA with a matching sequence of bases on a chromosome.

genera. See **genus.**

general adaptation syndrome (GAS) [L, *genus*, kind; L, *adaptare*, to fit; Gk, *syn*, together, *dromos*, course], the defense response of the body or the psyche to injury or prolonged stress, as described by Hans Selye (1907–1982). It consists of an initial stage of shock or alarm reaction, followed by a phase of increasing resistance or adaptation, using the various defense mechanisms of the body or mind, and culminating in either a state of adjustment and healing or of exhaustion and disintegration. Also called **adaptation syndrome.** See also **posttraumatic stress disorder, stress.**

general anesthesia, the absence of sensation and consciousness as induced by various anesthetic agents, given primarily by inhalation or intravenous injection. Four components of general anesthesia are analgesia, amnesia, muscle relaxation, and unconsciousness. The kind of anesthesia selected and the dose and route by which it is given depend on the indication for anesthesia. The depth of anesthesia is planned to allow the surgical procedure to be performed without the patient's experiencing pain or having any recall of the procedure. Endotracheal intubation and respiratory support are often necessary. General anesthesia may be administered only by a physician or a Certified Registered Nurse Anesthetist. See also **anesthesia, Guedel's signs, local anesthesia, regional anesthesia.**

generalization /jen'(ə)rəlīzā'shən/ [L, *genus*, kind; Gk, *izein*, to cause], the process of reducing or bringing under a general rule or statement, such as classifying items under general categories.

generalized actinomycosis. See **actinomycosis.**

generalized anaphylaxis /jen'(ə)rəlīzd'/, a severe reagin-mediated reaction to an allergen characterized by itching, edema, wheezing respirations, apprehension, cyanosis, dyspnea, pupillary dilation, a rapid, weak pulse, and falling blood pressure that may rapidly result in shock and death. Systemic anaphylaxis, the most extreme form of hypersensitivity, may be caused by insect stings, proteins in animal sera, food, or certain drugs; parenterally administered penicillin and contrast media containing iodide are frequent causes of anaphylactic shock, especially in individuals with a history of allergies. An anaphylactic reaction is mediated by reaginic antibodies (IgE) that form in response to an initial sensitizing dose of an allergen and render the individual hypersensitive to the allergen by binding it to mast cells and basophils. A subsequent challenging dose of the allergen, causing the cells to degranulate and release histamine, bradykinin, and other vasoactive amines, produces anaphylaxis; the severity of the reaction depends on several factors, including the amount and route of entrance of the sensitizing and challenging doses of the allergen. Treatment of generalized anaphylaxis consists of an immediate subcutaneous or intramuscular injection of 1:1000 epinephrine hydrochloride, the administration of an antihistamine, such as tripelennamine or diphenhydramine, and isoproterenol or aminophylline to relieve bronchial spasm. A vasopressor may be given to increase blood pressure, and a corticosteroid to suppress the immune response. The patient's legs are elevated to counteract shock; oxygen may be administered by a positive pressure mask, and, if tracheal edema is present, an endotracheal tube may be inserted or a tracheostomy performed. See also **reagin-mediated disorder.**

generalized peritonitis [L, *genus,* class; Gk, *peri,* near, *tenein,* to stretch, *itis,* inflammation], a bacterial infection of the peritoneum secondary to an infection in another organ, as when an appendix ruptures or an ulcer perforates the gastric wall. The symptoms are usually acute and severe.

generally recognized as effective (GRAE), one of the statutory criteria that must be met by a drug before it can be approved as a 'new drug.' Meeting these criteria relieves the manufacturer of the necessity of obtaining premarket approval as required by the Federal Food, Drug, and Cosmetic Act. To be recognized as effective, the drug must be, according to the Act, considered safe and effective by 'experts qualified by scientific training and experience.'

general paresis [L, *genus,* kind; Gk, paralysis], an organic mental disorder resulting from chronic syphilitic infection, characterized by degeneration of the cortical neurons; progressive dementia, tremor, and speech disturbances; muscular weakness; and, ultimately, generalized paralysis. It is often accompanied by periods of exultation and delusions of grandeur. Treatment usually consists of large doses of penicillin without which the outcome is almost invariably progressive deterioration and death. Also called **dementia paralytica,** *(obsolete)* **general paralysis of the insane, paretic dementia, syphilitic meningoencephalitis.**

general practitioner (GP) [L, *genus,* class; Gk, *praktikos,* qualified for action], a family practice physician. See also **family medicine.**

general relaxation [L, *genus,* class, *relaxare,* to ease], a slackening of strain or tension of the entire body, but particularly of the muscles.

general symptom [L, *genus;* Gk, *symptoma,* that which happens], a symptom that affects the entire body rather than a specific organ or location. Also called **constitutional symptom.**

generation /jen′ərā′shən/ [L, *generare,* to beget], **1.** the act or process of reproduction; procreation. **2.** a group of contemporary individuals, animals, or plants that are the same number of life cycles from a common ancestor. **3.** the period of time between the birth of one individual or organism and the birth of its offspring. Kinds of generation include **alternate generation, asexual generation, filial generation, parental generation, sexual generation,** and **spontaneous generation.**

generative /jen′ərā′tiv/ [L, *generare,* to beget], pertaining to activity that generates new physical or mental growth, such as creative problem solving.

generic /jənər′ik/ [L, *genus,* kind], **1.** of or pertaining to a genus. **2.** of or pertaining to a substance, product, or drug that is not protected by trademark. **3.** of or pertaining to the name of a kind of drug that is also the description of the drug, such as penicillin or tetracycline.

generic equivalent, a drug product sold under its generic name, identical in chemical composition to one or more others sold under a trademark but not necessarily equivalent in therapeutic effect.

generic name, the official, established nonproprietary name assigned to a drug. A given drug is licensed under its generic name, and all manufacturers of the drug list it by its generic name. However, a drug is usually marketed under a trademark chosen by the manufacturer. See also **chemical name, established name, trademark.**

generic nursing program, a program to prepare people with no previous professional nursing experience for entry into the field of nursing.

-genesia, 1. a suffix meaning a '(specified) condition concerning information': *agenesia, morphogenesia, paragenesia.* **2.** also **-genesis.** a combining form meaning 'the production or procreation of something (specified)': *algogenesia, palingenesia, syngenesia.*

genesis /jen′əsis/ [Gk, origin], **1.** the origin, generation, or developmental evolution of anything. **2.** the act of producing or procreating.

-genesis. See **-genesia.**

gene splicing /jēn/, (in molecular genetics) the process by which a segment of DNA is attached to or inserted in a strand of DNA from another source. In recombinant DNA technology genetic material from humans and other mammals is spliced into bacterial plasmids.

gene therapy a procedure that involves injection of "healthy genes" into the bloodstream of a patient to cure or treat a hereditary disease or similar illness. Blood is withdrawn from the patient and the white cells are separated and cultured in a laboratory, then inserted into modified viruses. Normal genes from a volunteer are inserted into the viruses, which, in turn, transfer the normal gene into the chromosomes of the patient's white cells. The white cells containing the normal genes are finally injected into the patient's bloodstream. Also called **somatic-cell gene therapy.**

genetic /jənet′ik/ [Gk, *genesis,* origin], **1.** pertaining to reproduction, birth, or origin. **2.** pertaining to genetics or heredity. **3.** pertaining to or produced by a gene; inherited.

-genetic, 1. a suffix meaning 'pertaining to generation by (specified) agents': *gamogenetic, mitogenetic, spermatogenetic.* **2.** a suffix meaning 'generating': *glycogenetic, ovigenetic, ureagenetic.* **3.** a suffix meaning 'pertaining to something generated by a (specified) agent': *biogenetic, ideogenetic, phylogenetic.*

genetic affinity, relationship by direct descent.

genetically significant dose (GSD) /jənet′iklē/, an arbitrary measure of the estimated annual gonadal radiation received by the population gene pool. In the United States the estimated GSD is 20 mrad. The figure is not intended to suggest possible genetic effects from exposure to that level of radiation.

genetic code, the information carried by the DNA molecules that determines the specific amino acids and their arrangement in the polypeptide chain of each protein synthesized by the cell. The code represents the sequence of nucleotides along the DNA molecule of each chromosome, and, during transcription, this arrangement is synthesized in messenger RNA and carried from the nucleus to the cytoplasm of the cell, where it is translated into protein at the site of the ribosomes. A unit of three consecutive nucleotides, or a codon, codes for each amino acid of the protein molecule. Any change in the code results in the incorrect arrangement of the amino acids in the protein, causing a mutation. See also **anticodon, transcription, translation.**

genetic colonization, the process by which a parasite introduces into its host genetic information that induces the host to synthesize products solely for the use of the parasite.

genetic counseling, the process of determining the occurrence or risk of occurrence of a genetic disorder within a family and of providing appropriate information and advice about the courses of action that are available, whether care of a child already affected, prenatal diagnosis, termination of a pregnancy, sterilization, or artificial insemination is involved. Effective genetic counseling requires an accurate diagnosis of the condition, sometimes necessitating special biochemical or cytogenetic tests, because many of the more than 3000 known inherited disorders have similar clinical manifestations but totally different modes of inheritance; a careful, detailed family history, recorded in the form of a pedigree chart; and an understanding of genetic principles, especially a knowledge of the risks related to multifactorial inheritance. The most efficient counseling services consist of a group of specialists, including physicians, geneticists, psychologists, biochemists, cytologists, nurses, and social workers. Nurses must be especially alert to those situations in which persons may need genetic counseling, must become familiar with facilities in the area that provide genetic counseling services, and must help couples arrive at tentative decisions regarding family planning or the care of a child with a genetic disorder. See also **genetic screening, prenatal diagnosis.**

genetic death, 1. the failure of an organism to survive as a result of its genetic makeup. 2. the removal of a gene or genotype from the gene pool of a population or a given familial descent because of sterility, failure of the individual or organism to reproduce, or death before sexual maturity.

genetic disorder. See **inherited disorder.**

genetic drift, the chance fluctuations in gene frequencies within a population. The smaller the population, the greater the tendency for variation within each generation, so that eventually small, isolated inbreeding groups become genetically quite different from the ancestors from which they derived. Also called **drift, random genetic drift.**

genetic engineering, the process of producing recombinant DNA so that the genotype and phenotype of organisms can be altered and controlled. Enzymes are used to break the DNA molecule into fragments so that genes from another organism can be inserted and the nucleotides rearranged in any desired sequence. Through genetic engineering using the recombinant DNA technique, such human proteins as the growth hormone, insulin, and interferon have been produced in bacteria. At present, genetic engineering represents a powerful tool for medical research and is possible only in microorganisms, but in the future, the technique may be applicable to higher organisms, with the possibility of controlling and eliminating genetic disorders and malformations in humans.

genetic equilibrium, the state within a population at which the frequency of genes and genotypes does not change from generation to generation. The condition routinely occurs in a large interbreeding population in which mating is random and there are no or relatively few mutations. See also **Hardy-Weinberg equilibrium principle.**

genetic homeostasis, the maintenance of genetic variability within a population through adaptation to varied or changing environments and conditions of life as a result of shifts or resistance to shifts in gene frequencies.

genetic immunity. See **natural immunity.**

genetic isolate, a group of plants, animals, or individuals that are genetically separated by geographic, racial, social, cultural, or any other barriers that prevent them from interbreeding with those outside of the group. Depending on the size of the group and the amount of inbreeding that occurs, genetic isolates generally show an increased incidence of otherwise rare, inherited defects. See also **deme.**

geneticist /jənet′isist/, one who specializes in the study or application of genetics.

genetic load, the average number of accumulated detrimental genes per individual within a population, including those caused by mutation and selection within a recent generation and those inherited from ancestors. Genetic load is measured according to lethal equivalents.

genetic map, the graphic representation of the linear arrangement of genes on a chromosome and the relative distance between them, as expressed in map or morgan units. Also called **linkage map.**

genetic marker, any specific gene that produces a readily recognizable genetic trait that can be used in family and population studies or in linkage analysis. Also called **gene marker, marker gene.**

genetic polymorphism, the recurrence within a population of two or more discontinuous genetic variants of a specific trait in such proportions that they cannot be maintained simply by mutation, such as the sickle cell trait, the Rh factor, and the blood groups. Compare **balanced polymorphism.**

genetic population. See **deme.**

genetics /jənet′iks/, 1. the science that studies the principles and mechanics of heredity, specifically the means by which traits are passed from parents to offspring and the causes of the similarities and differences between related organisms. 2. the total genetic makeup of a particular individual, family, group, or condition. Kinds of genetics are **clinical genetics, molecular genetics,** and **population genetics.** See also **cytogenetics, Mendel's laws.**

genetic screening, the process of investigating a specific population of persons for the purpose of detecting the presence of disease, either incipient or overt, such as the generalized screening of all newborn infants for phenylketonuria, of identifying those who possess defective genes, of gaining information concerning the incidence of a disorder in the population, and of providing reproductive information, specifically to those at risk, such as the close relatives of persons affected with inborn errors of metabolism or those in certain ethnic groups who have a high incidence of a particular disease, specifically sickle cell anemia in blacks and Tay-Sachs disease in Ashkenazic Jews. When accompanied by education and counseling, mass screening programs can be effective in the management of genetic disorders. See also **genetic counseling.**

gene transfer [Gk, *genein*, to produce; L, *transferre*, to bring across], a type of gene therapy in which a gene is transplanted from a donor organism into a recipient organism.

Genga's bandage. See **Theden's bandage.**

-genia, a suffix meaning '(condition or development of the) jaw': *microgenia, opisthogenia, progenia.*

-genic, 1. a suffix meaning 'causing, forming, producing': *collagenic, hemorrhagenic, phosphagenic.* 2. a suffix meaning 'produced by or formed from': *bacillogenic, coc-*

Selected genetic disorders

Disorder	Symptom	Defect	Dominant/ recessive	Frequency among human births
Cystic fibrosis	Mucus clogging lungs, liver, and pancreas	Failure of chloride ion transport mechanism	Recessive	$1/1800$ (whites)
Sickle cell anemia	Poor blood circulation	Abnormal hemoglobin molecules	Recessive	$1/1600$ (African-Americans)
Tay-Sachs disease	Deterioration of central nervous system in infancy	Defective form of enzyme hexosaminidase A	Recessive	$1/1600$ (Ashkenazic Jews)
Phenylketonuria	Failure of brain to develop in infancy	Defective form of enzyme phenylalanine hydroxylase	Recessive	$1/18,000$
Hemophilia (Royal)	Failure of blood to clot	Defective form of blood clotting factor IX	Sex-linked recessive	$1/7000$
Huntington's disease	Gradual deterioration of brain tissue in middle age	Production of an inhibitor of brain cell metabolism	Dominant	$1/10,000$
Muscular dystrophy (Duchenne)	Wasting away of muscles	Degradation of myelin coating of nerves stimulating muscles	Sex-linked recessive	$1/10,000$
Hypercholesterolemia	Excessive cholesterol levels in blood, leading to heart disease	Abnormal form of cholesterol cell-surface receptor	Dominant	$1/500$

From Raven PH, Johnson GB: *Biology*, ed 3, St. Louis, 1992, Mosby–Year Book.

cigenic, pituitarigenic. **3.** a suffix meaning 'related to a gene': *intragenic, polygenic, trigenic*.

geniculate neuralgia /jənik′yəlāt/ [L, *geniculum* little knee, Gk, *neuron*, nerve, *algos*, pain], a severe, debilitating, inflammatory condition of the geniculate ganglion of the facial nerve, characterized by pain, loss of the sense of taste, facial paralysis, and a decrease in salivation and lacrimation. It sometimes follows herpes zoster infection. See also **Ramsay Hunt's syndrome.**

geniculate zoster. See **herpes zoster.**

genio-, a combining form meaning 'pertaining to the chin':*genion, genioplasty.*

geniohyoideus /jē′nē·ōhī·oi′dē·əs/ [Gk, *genion*, chin, *hyoides*, Y-shaped], one of the four suprahyoid muscles, arising from the symphysis menti of the lower jaw and inserting into the body of the hyoid bone. A narrow muscle, it is innervated by a branch of the first cervical nerve, and it acts to draw the hyoid bone and the tongue forward. Also called **geniohyoid muscle.** Compare **digastricus, mylohyoideus, stylohyoideus.**

genit- [L, *genitalis*], a combining form pertaining to the generative organs or sexual reproduction: *genitourinary, genitalia.*

-genital. See **genitals.**

genital herpes. See **herpes genitalis, herpes simplex.**

genitalia. See **genitals.**

genital reflex. See **sexual reflex.**

genitals /jen′itəlz/ [L, *genitalis*], the sex, or reproductive, organs. In the female they include the vulva, mons veneris, labia majora, labia minora, clitoris, vagina, uterus, fallopian tubes, and ovaries. The male genitals include the penis, scrotum, testicles, epididymis, vas deferens, prostate gland, seminal vesicles, and Cowper's glands. Also called **genitalia. –genital,** adj.

genital self-examination. See **self-breast examination, testicular self-examination.**

genital stage /jen′itəl/ [L, *genitalis* + Fr, *stage*, trial period], (in psychoanalysis) the final period in psychosex-

ual development, beginning with adolescence and continuing through the adult years when the genitals are the predominant source of pleasurable stimulation. The most significant feature of this stage is direction of sexual interest not just toward self-satisfaction but toward the establishment of a stable and meaningful heterosexual relationship. See also **psychosexual development.**

genital wart [L, *genitalis*; AS, *wearte*], a small, soft, moist, pink or red swelling that becomes pedunculated. The growth may be solitary or there may be a cauliflower-like group in the same area of the prepuce or vulva. It is caused by a human papilloma virus (HPV) and is contagious. Atypical genital warts should be biopsied as possible carcinomas as they are associated with cervical cancer. No therapy has been shown to eradicate HPV. Also called **condyloma acuminatum, venereal wart, verruca acuminata.**

genit-, **1.** a combining form meaning 'pertaining to birth or reproduction': *genitalia*. **2.** a combining form meaning 'pertaining to organs of reproduction': *genitoplasty, genital.*

genitourinary (GU) /jen′itō·yŏŏr′iner′ē/ [L, *genitalis* + Gk, *ouron*, urine], referring to the genital and urinary systems of the body, the organ structures, functions, or both. Also called **urogenital.**

genitourinary system. See **urogenital system.**

genogram /jē′nōgram/, a diagram that depicts family relationships over at least three generations. It is useful as a tool for studying the process of a family system over time.

genome /jē′nōm/ [Gk, *genein*, to produce], the complete set of genes in the chromosomes of each cell of a particular organism.

genontopia. See **senopia.**

genotype /jē′nōtīp′/ [Gk, *genos*, birth, *typos*, mark], **1.** the complete genetic constitution of an organism or group, as determined by the particular combination and location of the genes on the chromosomes. **2.** the alleles situated at one or more sites on homologous chromosomes. The genetic information carried by a pair of alleles determines a specific characteristic or trait, usually designated by a letter or symbol, such as AA when the alleles are identical and Aa when they are different. **3.** a group or class of organisms having the same genetic makeup; the type species of a genus. Compare **phenotype.** **–genotypic,** *adj.*

-genous, a suffix meaning 'to originate from or to contain': *homogenous, hydrogenous.*

gentamicin sulfate /jen'təmī'sin/, an aminoglycoside antibiotic.

■ INDICATION: It is prescribed to relieve the effects of severe infections caused by organisms sensitive to gentamicin.

■ CONTRAINDICATIONS: Concomitant administration of other potentially ototoxic or nephrotoxic drugs or known hypersensitivity to this drug or to other aminoglycoside medications prohibits its use. It is used with caution in patients having impaired renal function.

■ ADVERSE EFFECTS: Among the more serious adverse reactions are nephrotoxicity, auditory or vestibular ototoxicity, impairment of neuromuscular transmission, and hypersensitivity reactions.

gentian violet /jen'shən/, an antibacterial antiinfective, antifungal, and anthelmintic.

■ INDICATIONS: It is prescribed in the treatment of pinworms, superficial infections of the skin, and vaginal infections.

■ CONTRAINDICATIONS: Known hypersensitivity to this drug prohibits its use. It is not applied to ulcerative lesions of the face.

■ ADVERSE EFFECTS: Among the most serious adverse reactions is permanent discoloration of the skin after topical exposure to the drug. GI distress and purple vomitus may occur after oral administration.

gentiotannic acid /jen'shē·ətan'ik/, a form of tannic acid once used as an astringent and in the treatment of burns but no longer recommended because the compound is hepatotoxic.

Gentran 40, a trademark for a plasma volume extender (dextran 40).

Gentran 75, a trademark for a plasma volume extender (dextran 75).

genu /jē'nōō/ [L, knee], the knee or any angular structure resembling the flexed knee.

genupectoral position /je'nōōpek'tərəl/ [L, *genu* + *pectus,* breast; *positio*], knee-chest position. To assume the genupectoral position, the person kneels so that the weight of the body is supported by the knees and chest, with the abdomen raised. The head is turned to one side and the arms are flexed so that the upper part of the body can be supported in part by the elbows.

genu recurvatum [L, *genu,* knee, *recurvare,* to bend back], a backward deformity, hyperextension, at the knee joint. Also called **back knee.**

genus /jē'nəs/, *pl.* **genera** /jen'ərə/ [L, kind], a subdivision of a family of animals or plants. A genus usually is composed of several closely related species, but the genus *Homo sapiens* has only one species, humans. See **family.**

genu valgum [L, knee; *valgus,* bowlegged], a deformity in which the legs are curved inward so that the knees are close together, knocking as the person walks, with the ankles widely separated. Also called **knock-knee.**

genu varum [L, knee; *varus,* bent outwards], a deformity in which one or both legs are bent outward at the knee. Also called **bowleg.** Compare **genu valgum.**

-geny, a combining form meaning 'production, generation, origin': *homogeny, hylogeny, morphogeny.*

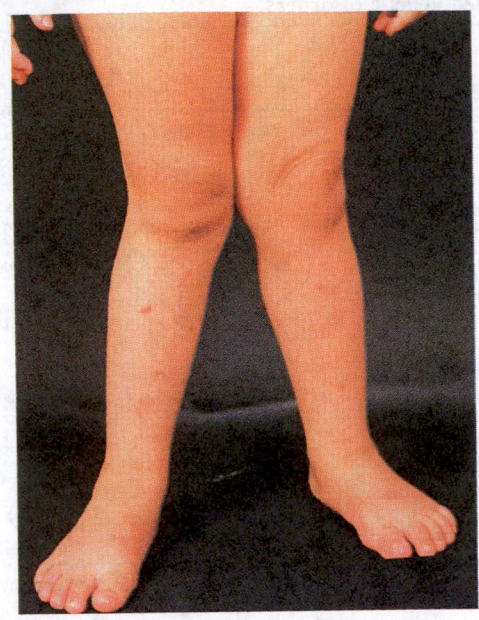

Genu valgum (Zitelli, 1992)

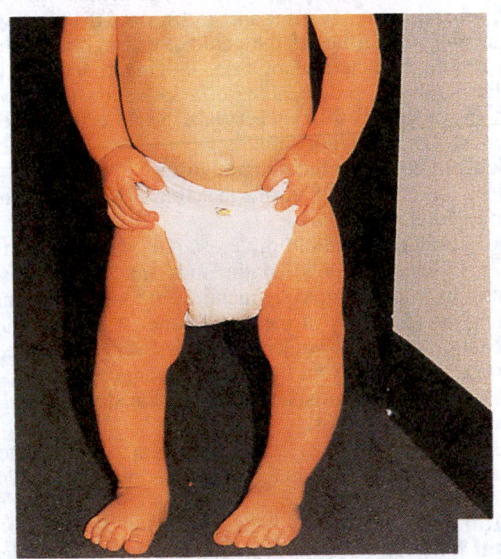

Genu varum (Zitelli, 1992)

geo-, a prefix meaning 'pertaining to the earth or soil': *geobiology, geophagia, geotropism.*

Geocillin, a trademark for an antibacterial (carbenicillin indanyl sodium).

geographic tongue /jē'əgraf'ik/ [Gk, *ge,* earth, *graphein,* to record; AS, *tunge*], an inflammatory disorder on the dorsal surface of the tongue characterized by numerous and continually changing areas of loss and regrowth of the filiform papillae. The wandering shape and outline of the denuded red patches surrounded by thickened white borders presents a geographic or maplike appearance. Also called **benign migratory glossitis.**

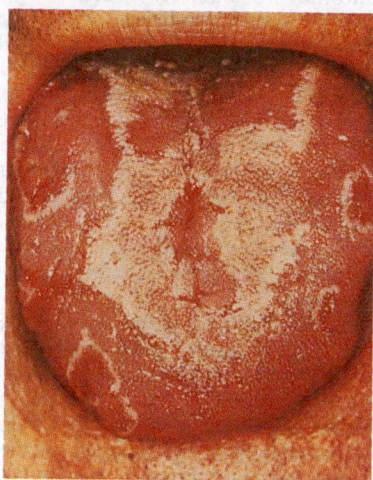

Geographic tongue (Lamey, 1988)

geometric mean. See **mean**

Geopen, a trademark for an antibacterial (carbenicillin disodium).

geotrichosis /jē'ōtrikō'sis/ [Gk, *ge*, earth, *thrix*, hair, *osis*, condition], a condition associated with the fungus *Geotrichum candidum* that may cause oral, bronchial, pharyngeal, and intestinal disorders. *Geotrichum candidum* is normally found in healthy individuals, the soil, and dairy products and is not necessarily pathogenic. Geotrichosis most commonly occurs in immunosuppressed individuals and in diabetics. Bronchopulmonary complications associated with this disorder may produce a cough with thick, bloody sputum. Geotrichosis has been associated with allergic asthmatic reactions similar to allergic aspergillosis and a type of intestinal disorder characterized by abdominal pain, diarrhea, and rectal bleeding. Oral lesions that may occur with this disorder are commonly treated with a solution of gentian violet; associated abdominal lesions are treated with the oral administration of gentian violet capsules; associated pulmonary lesions are treated with the oral administration of potassium iodide.

geriatric day care /jer'ē·at'rik/ [Gk, *geras*, old age; AS, *daeg*; L, *garrire*, chatter], an ambulatory health care facility for elderly people. It usually offers a broad range of professional and community services to maximize functional independence for the patients.

geriatrician /jer'ē·ətrish'ən/, a medical specialist in the field of geriatrics.

geriatric nurse practitioner, a registered nurse with additional education obtained through a master's degree program in nursing or a nondegree certificate program that prepares the nurse to deliver primary health care to elderly adults.

geriatrics /jer'ē·at'riks/, the branch of medicine dealing with the physiology of aging and the diagnosis and treatment of diseases affecting the aged.

germ /jurm/ [L, *germen*, sprout], **1.** any microorganism, especially one that is pathogenic. **2.** a unit of living matter able to develop into a self-sufficient organism, such as a seed, spore, or egg. **3.** (in embryology) the first stage in development, such as a spermatozoon or other germ cell.

germanium (Ge) /jərmā'nē·əm/ [Germany], a metallic element with some nonmetallic properties. Its atomic number is 32; its atomic weight is 72.59.

German measles. See **rubella.**

germ cell, 1. a sexual reproductive cell in any stage of development, from the primordial embryonic form to the mature gamete. **2.** an ovum or spermatozoon or any of their preceding forms. **3.** any cell undergoing gametogenesis. Also called **gonoblast, gonocyte.** Compare **somatic cell.**

germ disk. See **embryonic disk.**

germicide /jur'misīd/ [L, *germen*, sprout, *caedere*, to kill], a drug that kills pathogenic microorganisms. See also **antibacterial, antifungal, antiviral.** −**germicidal,** *adj.*

germinal /jur'minəl/ [L, *germen*, sprout], pertaining to or characteristic of a germ cell or to the early stages of development.

germinal center [L, *germen*, sprout; Gk, *kentron*, center], an antigen-localizing primary follicle with lymphoid tissue. It reacts to antigens, enlarging and becoming filled with lymphoblasts and macrophages at the center of a ring of small lymphocytes.

germinal disk. See **embryonic disk.**

germinal epithelium, 1. the epithelial layer covering the genital ridge from which the gonads are derived in early embryonic development. **2.** the epithelial covering of the ovary, formerly thought to be the site of the formation of the oogonia. See also **oogenesis.**

germinal infection, an infection transmitted to a child by the ovum or sperm of a parent. Compare **endogenous infection, mixed infection, retrograde infection, secondary infection.**

germinal membrane. See **blastoderm.**

germinal nucleus. See **pronucleus.**

germinal pole. See **animal pole.**

germinal spot, the nucleolus of a mature oocyte, before fertilization. See also **oogenesis, ovum.**

germinal stage, (in embryology) the interval of time from fertilization to implantation during which the ovum undergoes cell division several times, travels to the uterus, and, in the form of a blastocyst, begins to implant itself in the endometrium. The germinal stage is over at about 10 days of gestation.

germinal vesicle, the nucleus of a mature oocyte before fertilization. Much larger than the nucleus of other cells, it initiates the completion of meiotic division after fertilization. See also **oogenesis, ovum.**

germination /jur'minā'shən/ [L, *germinare*, to germinate], **1.** the initial growth and development of an organism from the time of fertilization to the formation of the embryo. **2.** the sprouting of a spore or the seed of a plant. −**germinate,** *v.*

germ layer, one of the three primordial cell layers formed during gastrulation in the early stages of embryonic development from which the entire range of body tissue is derived. Each layer has the potential for forming different cellular types that differentiate into the various structures and organs of the body. See also **ectoderm, endoderm, mesoderm.**

germ nucleus. See **pronucleus.**

germ plasm, 1. the protoplasm of the germ cells containing the basic reproductive and hereditary material; the sum total of the DNA in a particular cell or organism. The substance was first named by August Weismann (1834–1914) to indicate the material that originates in the germ cell, produces new organisms, transmits hereditary characteristics, and passes in direct continuity to germ cells of succeeding generations. 2. *nontechnical.* germ cells in any stage of development together with the tissues from which they originated. Compare **somatoplasm.** See also **weismannism.**

germ-plasm theory. See **weismannism.**

germ theory [L, *germen*, sprout; Gk, *theoria*, speculation], the concept that all infectious and contagious diseases are caused by living microorganisms.

gero-, geronto-, a combining form meaning 'pertaining to old age or the aged': *gerocomia, gerodontology, geromarasmus.*

-gerontic, -gerontal, a combining form meaning 'pertaining to old age': *paragerontic, phylogerontic, ungerontic.*

geronto-. See **gero-.**

Gerontologic Society of America (GSA), an organization of scientific and academic professionals interested in studies in the nature of the aging process and in the clinical manifestations of disease in the aging organism. GSA members participate with the International Association of Gerontology in periodic seminars at which worldwide research papers on longevity are presented.

gerontology /jer'əntol'əjē/ [Gk, *geras*, old age, *logos*, science], the study of all aspects of the aging process, including the clinical, psychologic, economic, and sociologic problems encountered by the elderly and their consequences for both the individual and society.

gerontoxon. See **arcus senilis.**

geropsychiatry /jer'ōsīkī'ətrē/ [Gk, *geras*, old age, *psyche*, mind], the study and treatment of mental illness in elderly people.

-gerous, a suffix meaning 'bearing, producing, or containing' something specified: *calcigerous, ovigerous, setigerous.*

Gerstmann-Straussler syndrome. See **human prion disease.**

Gesell Developmental Assessment, an evaluation program that provides information on gross motor, fine motor, language, personal-social, and cognitive development.

Gestalt /gəshtält'/, *pl.* **Gestalts, Gestalten** /gəshtäl'tən/ [Ger, form], a single physical, psychologic, or symbolic configuration, pattern, or experience consisting of a number of elements that has an effect as a whole different from that of the sum of its parts.

Gestalt psychology, a school of psychology, originating in Germany, that maintains that a psychologic phenomenon is perceived as a total configuration or pattern, rising from the relationships among its constituent elements, rather than as discrete elements possessing attributes of their own, and that the pattern, or Gestalt, cannot be derived from the summation of its constituents. Thus learning is regarded as resulting from insight, defined as a process or reorganization, rather than from association or trial and error, and behavior is seen as an integrated response to a unitary situation rather than as a series of reflexes and sensations. Also called **configurationism, Gestaltism.** See also **Gestalt.**

Gestalt therapy, a form of psychotherapy that stresses the unity of self-awareness, behavior, and experience. It incorporates elements of psychoanalytic, behavioristic, and humanistic existential therapy. See **Gestalt psychology.**

gestant anomaly. See **odontoma.**

gestant odontoma. See **dens in dente.**

gestate /jes'tāt/ [L, *gestare*, to bear], 1. to carry a developing fetus in the womb. 2. to grow and develop slowly toward maturity, such as a fetus in the womb.

gestation /jestā'shən/ [L, *gestare*, to bear], in viviparous animals, the period of time from the fertilization of the ovum until birth. Gestation varies with the species; in humans the average duration is 266 days or approximately 280 days from the onset of the last menstrual period. A gestation time of less than 37 weeks is regarded as premature and one that continues beyond 42 weeks is considered postmature, regardless of the size of the fetus or other factors. See also **pregnancy.**

gestational age /jestā'shənəl/ [L, *gestare* + *aetas*, time of life], the age of a fetus or a newborn, usually expressed in weeks dating from the first day of the mother's last menstrual period.

gestational assessment [L, *gestare*, to bear, *assidere*, to sit beside], calculation of the fetal age of the offspring, based on such factors as the menstrual history of the mother, the date that fetal heart sounds are first detected, and evaluation of ultrasound data. The information is important in planning emergency care in the event of premature birth signs.

gestational diabetes mellitus (GDM), a disorder characterized by an impaired ability to metabolize carbohydrate, usually caused by a deficiency of insulin, occurring in pregnancy and disappearing after delivery but, in some cases, returning years later. There is evidence that placental lactogen and considerable destruction of insulin by the placenta play a role in precipitating gestational diabetes. Treatment consists of insulin injections, a high-protein diet, and an adequate intake of calcium and iron, but no attempt is made to keep the patient's urine free of sugar. See also **diabetes mellitus.**

gestational psychosis [L, *gestare*, to bear; Gk, *psyche*, mind, *osis*, condition], any mental disorder that can be attributed to a pregnancy.

gestation period [L, *gestare*, to bear; Gk, *peri*, near, *hodos*, way], the time span between conception and labor in humans. The period is approximately 40 weeks.

Getman visuomotor theory, a concept that visual perception is based on developmental sequences of physiologic actions in children. The sequence of eight stages begins with innate response systems and advances to cognitive integration of perceptions, abstractions, and higher symbolic activity.

-geusia, -geustia, a suffix meaning, '(condition of the) sense of taste': *glycogeusia, hemiageusia, parageusia.*

GFR, abbreviation for **glomerular filtration rate.**

GH, abbreviation for **growth hormone.**

ghost cells [AS, *gast*; L, *cella*, storeroom], red blood cells that have lost their hemoglobin so that only the cell membranes are observed in microscopic examinations of urine samples. The hemoglobin is destroyed by the presence of urine. Also called **shadow cells.**

ghost teeth. See **adontodysplasia.**

GHRF, abbreviation for **growth hormone releasing factor.**

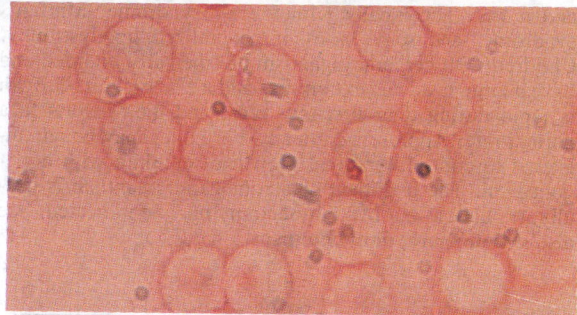

Ghost cells (Bain, 1989)

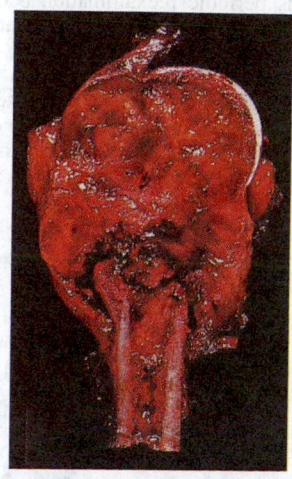

Specimen showing giant cell myeloma (Skarin, 1991)

GHRH, abbreviation for **growth hormone releasing hormone**.

GHRIH, abbreviation for *growth hormone release inhibiting hormone*. See **somatostatin.**

GI, abbreviation for **gastrointestinal.**

giant cell /jī'ənt/ [L, *gigant,* huge; *cella,* storeroom], an abnormally large tissue cell. It often contains more than one nucleus and may appear as a merger of several normal cells.

giant cell arteritis. See **temporal arteritis.**

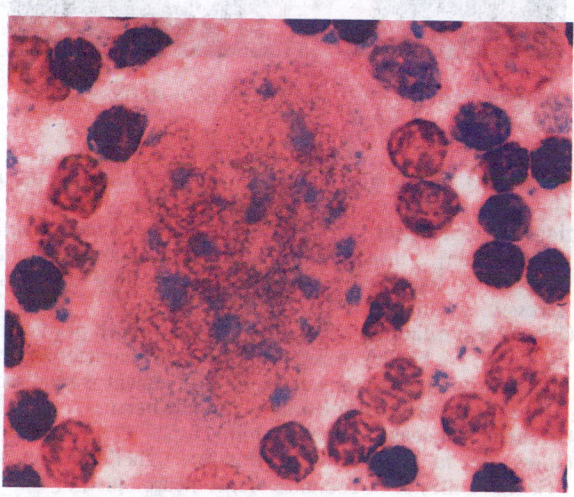

Giant cell (Hayhoe, 1992)

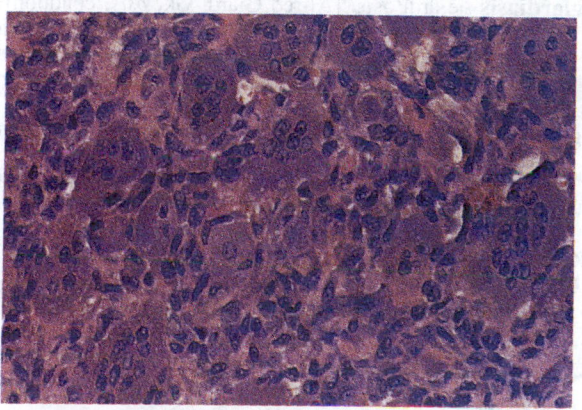

Photomicrograph of giant cell myelome
(Bullough, 1988)

giant cell carcinoma, a malignant epithelial neoplasm characteristically containing many large anaplastic cells. A small percentage of adenocarcinomas of the lung and liver also contain such cells. Also called **carcinoma gigantocellulare.**

giant cell interstitial pneumonia. See **interstitial pneumonia.**

giant cell myeloma, a bone tumor of multinucleated giant cells that resembles osteoclasts scattered in a matrix of spindle cells. Myelomas of this kind may be benign or malignant and may cause pain, functional disability, and pathologic fractures. Also called **giant cell tumor of bone.**

giant cell sarcoma. See **giant cell myeloma, osteoblastic sarcoma.**

giant cell thyroiditis. See **de Quervain's thyroiditis.**

giant cell tumor of bone. See **giant cell myeloma.**

giant chromosome, any of the excessively large chromosomes found in insects and the lower animals, specifically the lampbrush chromosome and polytene chromosome.

giant follicular lymphoma, a nodular, well-differentiated, lymphocytic, malignant lymphoma in which nodules distort the normal structure of a lymph node. Also called **Brill-Symmers disease, giant follicular lymphadenopathy, Symmers' disease.**

giant hypertrophic gastritis, a rare disease characterized by large folds of nodular gastric rugae that may cover the wall of the stomach, causing anorexia, nausea, vomiting, and abdominal distress. X-ray or endoscopic examination or surgery may be necessary for diagnosis. The nurse usually recommends periodic reexamination because the disease is associated with an incidence of stomach cancer that is greater than normal.

Giardia /jē·är′dē·ə/ [Alfred Giard, French biologist, b. 1846], a common genus of the flagellate protozoans. Many species of *Giardia* normally inhabit the digestive tract and cause inflammation in association with other factors that produce rapid proliferation of the organism. See also **giardiasis.**

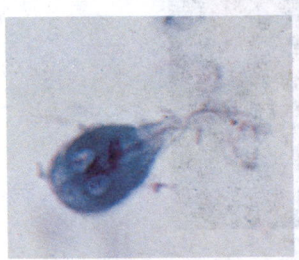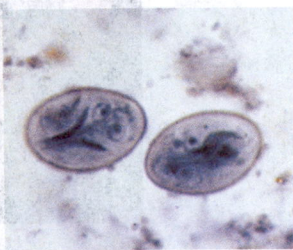

***Giardia lamblia* trophozoite and cyst** (Baron, 1990)

giardiasis /jē·ärdī′əsis/ [Alfred Giard; Gk, *osis*, condtion], an inflammatory, intestinal condition caused by overgrowth of the protozoan *Giardia lamblia*. The source of infection is usually untreated water contaminated with *G. lamblia* cysts. Also called **traveler's diarrhea.**

gibbus /gib′əs, jib′əs/ [L, hump], **1.** a hump, swelling, or enlargement on a body surface, usually confined to one side. **2.** a convex spinal curvature that may occur after the collapse of a vertebral body as may result from a fracture or tuberculosis of the spine.

Gibraltar fever. See **brucellosis.**

Gibson's murmur, a heart murmur that is heard continuously throughout the cardiac cycle. It waxes at the end of systole and wanes near the end of diastole and is often described as a "machinery-like" murmur. It is often accompanied by a thrill and occurs in patients with patent ductus arteriosus.

Gibson walking splint, a kind of Thomas splint that enables a patient to be ambulatory.

Giemsa's stain /gē·em′zəz/ [Gustav Giemsa, German chemist, b. 1867; Fr, *teindre*, to dye], an azure dye used as a stain in the microscopic examination of the blood for certain protozoan parasites, viral inclusion bodies, and rickettsia, and, more routinely, in the preparation of a smear for a differential white cell count.

GIFT, abbreviation for **gamete intrafallopian transfer.**

giga- a prefix meaning 'one billion (10^9)':*gigabit, gigabyte, gigahertz.*

gigantic acid /jīgan′tik/, an antibiotic substance derived from *Aspergillus giganteus*, a species of mold.

gigantism /jigan′tizəm/, [L, *gigas*, giant] an abnormal condition characterized by excessive size and stature, caused most frequently by hypersecretion of growth hormone (GH) and occurring to a lesser degree in hypogonadism and in certain genetic disorders. Gigantism with normal body proportions and normal sexual development usually results from hypersecretion of GH in early childhood. Hypogonadism, by delaying puberty and closure of the epiphyses, may lead to gigantism. Excessive linear growth often occurs in males with more than one Y chromosome,

and it may accompany Klinefelter's syndrome, Marfan's syndrome, and some cases of generalized lipodystrophy. Children with cerebral gigantism are mentally retarded and have a large head and extremities and a clumsy gait. Growth is rapid during their first few years and then reverts to a normal rate. Appropriate gonadal hormones may be administered to control abnormal growth of children with hypogonadism. The treatment of acromegalic gigantism is usually irradiation, but hypophysectomy may be indicated. See also **acromegaly, eunuchoidism.**

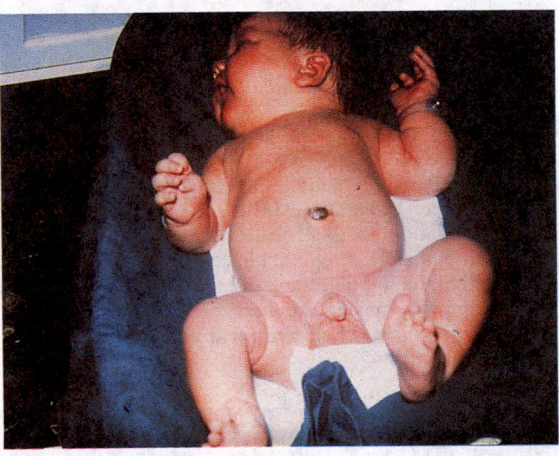

Gigantism (Bodansky, 1989/Courtesy Dr MI Drury, Dublin)

giganto-, a combining form meaning 'huge': *gigantoblast, gigantochromoblast, gigantocyte.*

giggle incontinence [Du, *giggelen*; L, *incontinentia*, inability to retain], urinary incontinence when intraabdominal pressure is increased by giggling or laughing. See also **stress incontinence.**

Gilbert's syndrome [Nicolas A. Gilbert, French physician, b. 1858], a benign, hereditary condition characterized by hyperbilirubinemia and jaundice. No treatment is required. See also **hyperbilirubinemia of the newborn.**

Gilchrist's disease. See **blastomycosis.**

Gilles de la Tourette's syndrome /zhēl′dəlätŏŏrets′/ [George Gilles de la Tourette, French neurologist, b. 1857], an abnormal condition characterized by facial grimaces, tics, and involuntary arm and shoulder movements. In adolescence, the condition worsens; the child may grunt, snort, and shout involuntarily. Coprolalia often develops, affecting judgment of the condition by the family and society. In adulthood the condition usually does not worsen; it comes and goes. Recently, treatment with dopamine antagonists has been found to be very effective, demonstrating an organic cause for this syndrome. Also called **Tourette's syndrome.**

Gillies' operation /gil′ēz/ [Harold D. Gillies, English surgeon, b. 1882], a surgical procedure for reducing fractures of the zygoma and zygomatic arch by making an incision in the temporal hairline.

gingiva /jinjī′və/, *pl.* **gingivae** [L, gum], the gingival tissues of the mouth, a mucous membrane with supporting fibrous tissue that overlies the crowns of unerupted teeth and

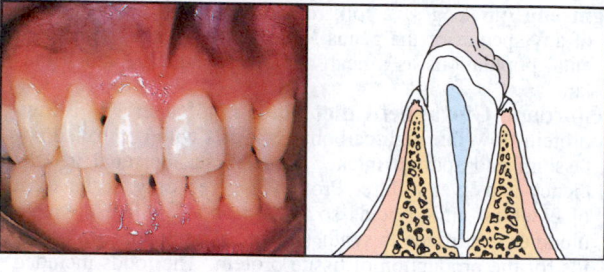

Normal gingiva (Murry, 1990)

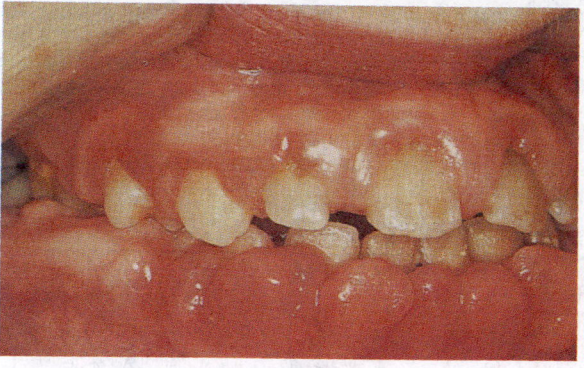

Gingival hyperplasia (Lamey, 1988)

encircles the necks of those that have erupted. **–gingival,** *adj.*

gingival blanching /jinjī′vəl/ [L, *gingiva;* Fr, *blanchir,* to whiten], the lightening of gingival color, usually temporary, caused by the stretching of gingival tissue with decreased blood supply.

gingival blood supply, the vascular supply to the gingivae, arising from blood vessels that pass on the gingival side of the outer periosteum of bone and anastomose with blood vessels of the periodontal membrane and intraalveolar blood vessels.

gingival cavity, a cavity that occurs in the gingival third of the clinical crown of the tooth.

gingival color, the color of healthy or diseased gingival tissues. It varies with the thickness and degree of keratinization of the epithelium, blood supply, pigmentation, and alterations produced by gingival diseases.

gingival consistency, the combination of visual and tactile characteristics of healthy gingival tissue. The visual characteristic varies from the look of smooth velvet to that of a finely or coarsely grained orange peel. The tactile consistency of healthy gingival tissue is firm and resilient. Compare **gingival color.**

gingival corium, the most stable connective tissue of the gingiva, lying between the periosteum and the lamina propria mucosae.

gingival crater, a depression in the gingival tissue, especially in the area of the former apex of interdental papilla. It is commonly caused by necrotizing ulcerative gingivitis and food impaction against the tissue subjacent to the contact areas of adjacent teeth.

gingival crevice, a normal space between the free gingiva and the tooth enamel. Also called **gingival sulcus.**

gingival cuff. See **junctional epithelium.**

gingival discoloration, a change in the normal coloration of the gingivae, associated with inflammation, reduced blood supply, abnormal pigmentation, and other problems.

gingival festoon, the distinct rounding and enlargement of the margins of the gingival tissue found in early gingival involvement. Compare **festoon, McCall's festoon.**

gingival hormonal enlargement, the enlargement of the gingivae associated with hormonal imbalance during pregnancy, puberty, and hormonal therapy. Also called **pregnancy epulis.**

gingival hyperplasia, overgrowth of the gingival tissue, often seen in patients treated with phenytoin for epileptic seizures.

gingival line [L, *gingiva,* gum, *linea*], the scalloped line formed by the free gingival margin at the neck of the teeth. Also called **gum line.**

gingival massage, the massage of gingival tissues for cleansing purposes, improving tissue tone and blood circulation, and for keratinization of the surface epithelium

gingival mat, the gingival connective tissue composed of coarse, broad collagen fibers that attach the gingivae to the teeth and hold the free gingivae in close approximation to the teeth.

gingival papilla. See **interdental gingiva.**

gingival physiology, the function of the gingivae as supportive and protective investments of the teeth and subjacent tissues. The gingival fiber apparatus serves as a barrier to apical migration of the epithelial attachment and binds the gingival tissues to the teeth. Normal gingival topograpy permits the free flow of food away from the occlusal surfaces and from the cervical and interproximal areas of the teeth.

gingival pocket. See **periodontal pocket.**

gingival position, the level of the gingival margin in relation to the teeth.

gingival shrinkage, the reduction in the size of gingival tissue, especially as the result of therapeutic elimination of subgingival deposits and curettement of the soft tissue wall of the gingival pocket.

gingival stippling, a series of small depressions in the surface of healthy gingivae, producing an appearance that varies from that of smooth, undulated velvet to that of an orange peel. See also **epithelial peg, gingival consistency, rete peg.**

gingival sulcus, any of the normal spaces between the free gingivae and the teeth.

gingivectomy /jin′jīvek′təmē/ [L, *gingiva* + Gk, *ektome,* excision], surgical removal of infected and diseased gingival tissue, performed to arrest the development of periodontal disease. With the patient under local anesthesia and sedation, all pockets around the teeth are scraped, and hypertrophied tissue is removed. The exposed surface of the gingival tissue is covered with packing to prevent trauma while eating and to allow new epithelial tissue to cover and fill in the areas. Moderate bleeding, discomfort. and pain are associated with the procedure. Postoperatively, the patient is closely observed for signs that may indicate hemorrhage, frequent swallowing, or a rise in pulse rate. The packing is removed 1 week later. Compare **gingivoplasty.**

gingivitis /jin′jivī′tis/ [L, *gingiva* + Gk, *itis,* inflammation], a condition in which the gums are red, swollen, and bleed ing. Most gingivitis is the result of poor oral hygiene and of the accumulation of bacterial plaque on the teeth, but gingivitis may be a sign of another condition, such as diabetes mellitus, leukemia, or vitamin deficiency. It is common in pregnancy, is usually painless, and may be acute or chronic. Frequent removal of plaque and regular visits to the dentist may be preventive. Compare **acute necrotizing ulcerative gingivitis.**

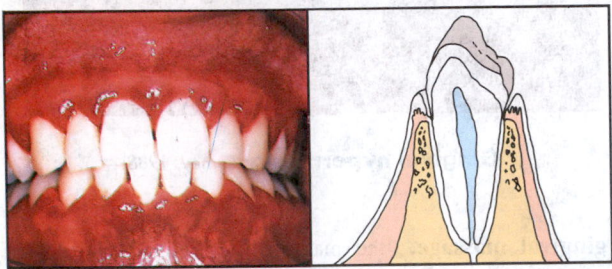

Gingivitis *(Murray, 1990)*

gingivo-, a combining form meaning 'pertaining to the gingiva': *gingivoglossitis, gingivolabial, gingivosis.*

gingivoplasty /jin′jivōplas′tē/ [L, *gingiva* + Gk, *plassein,* to shape], the surgical contouring of the gingival tissues to maintain healthy gingival tissue. Compare **gingivectomy.**

gingivostomatitis /jin′jivōstō′mətī′tis/ [L, *gingiva* + Gk, *stoma,* mouth, *itis,* inflammation], multiple, painful ulcers on the gums and mucous membranes of the mouth, the result of a herpesvirus infection. Seen most frequently in infants and young children, the condition usually subsides after 1 week, but in rare cases it may progress to a systemic viral infection. See also **herpes simplex.**

ginglymus joint. See **hinge joint.**

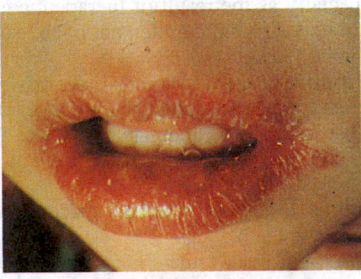

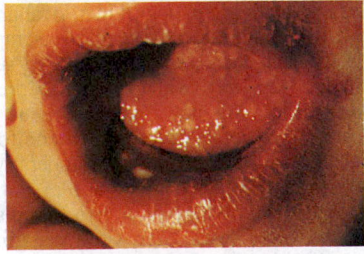

Gingivostomatitis *(Doughty, 1993)*

ginseng /jin′seng/, a folk remedy prepared from the root of any species of the genus *Panax.* It is used by some Oriental populations as a heart tonic, aphrodisiac, and stimulant.

Giordano-Giovannetti diet /jôrdä′nōjō′vənet′ē/, a low-protein, low-fat, high-carbohydrate diet with controlled potassium and sodium intake, used in chronic renal insufficiency and liver failure. Protein is given only in the form of essential amino acids so that the body will use excess blood urea nitrogen to synthesize the nonessential amino acids for the production of tissue protein. The foods included are eggs, small amounts of milk, low-protein bread, and some fruits and vegetables low in potassium, such as green beans, summer squash, cabbage, pears, grapefruit, and fresh or frozen blackberries, blueberries, and boysenberries. There are many modified forms of this diet depending on patient requirements and tolerance, usually varying in the amount and origin of the protein. Also called **Giovannetti diet.** See also **renal diet.**

gipoma /gipō′mə/, a pancreatic tumor that causes changes in secretion of gastric inhibitory polypeptide (GIP).

girdle /gur′dəl/, any curved or circular structure, such as the hipline formed by the bones and related tissues of the pelvis.

girdle pad, a pad that fits over the iliac crests and sacrum to protect the hip area in contact sports.

girdle sensation. See **zonesthesia.**

GI tract. See **digestive tract.**

glabella /gləbəl′ə/ [L, *glabrum,* bald], a flat triangular area of bone between the two superciliary ridges of the forehead. It is sometimes used as a baseline for cephalometric measurements.

glabrous skin /glā′brəs/ [L, *glaber,* smooth; AS, *scinn*], smooth, hairless skin.

glacial acetic acid /glā′shəl/, a clear, colorless liquid or crystalline substance (CH₃COOH) with a pungent odor. It is obtained by the destructive distillation of wood or from acetylene and water or by the oxidation of ethyl alcohol by aerobic bacteria, as in the production of vinegar. Glacial acetic acid is strongly corrosive and is potentially flammable with a low flash point. It is miscible in alcohol, ether, glycerol, and water, and is used as a solvent for organic compounds. Also called **vinegar acid.**

gland [L, *glans,* acorn], any one of many organs in the body, comprising specialized cells that secrete or excrete materials not related to their ordinary metabolism. Some glands lubricate; others, such as the pituitary gland, produce hormones; hematopoietic glands, such as the spleen and certain lymph nodes, take part in the production of blood components.

glanders [OFr, *glandres,* neck gland swelling], an infection caused by the bacillus *Pseudomonas mallei,* transmitted to humans from horses and other domestic animals. It is characterized by purulent inflammation of the mucous membranes and the development of skin nodules that ulcerate. If untreated with antibiotics, the infection may spread to the bones, liver, central nervous system, and other tissues and cause death. It is endemic in Africa, Asia, and South America but has been eradicated in Europe and North America.

glandes See **glans.**

gland of Montgomery. See **areolar gland.**

glands of Zeiss. See **ciliary gland.**

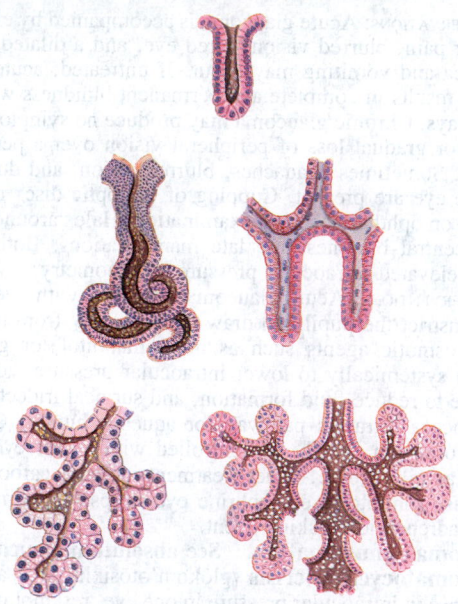

Glands *(Thibodeau, 1993/Ernest W Beck)*
**Simple tubular, simple coiled tubular,
compound tubular, compound alveolar,
compound tubuloalveolar**

glandular /glan'dyələr/ [L, *glandula*, small gland], pertaining to or resembling a gland.

glandular carcinoma. See **adenocarcinoma.**

glandular epithelium [L, *glandula*, small gland; Gk, *epi*, above, *thele*, nipple], epithelium that contains glandular cells.

glandular fever. See **infectious mononucleosis.**

glandular tissue [L, *glandula*, small gland; OFr, *tissu*], a group of epithelial secreting cells composing a definitive glandular organ, such as the thyroid.

glandula vestibularis major. See **Bartholin's gland.**

glans /glanz/, *pl.* **glandes** /glan'dēz/ [L, acorn], **1.** a general term for a small, rounded mass, or glandlike body. **2.** erectile tissue, as on the ends of the clitoris and the penis.

glans of clitoris [L, *glans;* Gk, *kleitoris*], the erectile tissue at the end of the clitoris, continuous with the intermediate part of the vaginal vestibular bulbs. It comprises two corpora cavernosa enclosed in a dense, fibrous membrane and connected to the pubis and ischium. Also called **glans clitoridis.**

glans penis [L], the conical tip of the penis that covers the end of the corpora cavernosa penis and the corpus spongiosom like a cap. The urethral orifice is normally located at the center of the distal tip of the glans penis; the corona glandis, the widest part of the glans penis, is around the base of the proximal portion. A fold of dark, thin, hairless skin forms the foreskin covering the glans penis.

Glanzmann's disease. See **thrombasthenia.**

Glasgow Coma Scale, a quick, practical, and standardized system for assessing the degree of conscious impairment in the critically ill and for predicting the duration and ultimate outcome of coma, primarily in patients with head injuries. The system involves three determinants: eye opening, verbal response, and motor response, all of which are evaluated independently according to a rank order that indicates the level of consciousness and degree of dysfunction. There are four grades of eye opening: spontaneous, which indicates that the arousal mechanisms in the brainstem are unimpaired, receives the highest score; opening in response to a verbal statement; opening in response to pain, which should be tested on the limbs, because facial pressure may cause eye closure; and no response. Verbal response has five grades: Orientation is indicated by the patient's awareness of self, location, and orientation, as well as the month and year; confused conversation is identified by the patient's verbal responses to questions accompanied by varying degrees of confusion and disorientation; inappropriate speech is indicated by the inability to sustain conversation, the shouting of intelligible words, and swearing; incomprehensible speech is identified by verbalization using unrecognizable 'words'; speechlessness is the fifth grade, in which the patient does not make any sound, even in response to a noxious stimulus. Motor responses also have five grades of dysfunction: The patient obeys commands, with care being taken not to confuse the grasp reflex or postural adjustment for a response; a localizing response is the result of a painful stimulus to more than one site causing a limb to move; flexor responses may be slow or rapid; extension responses are usually associated with adduction, internal rotation of the shoulder, and pronation of the forearm; no response indicates hypotonia, and spinal transection must be ruled out. The degree of consciousness may vary from determinant to determinant and is assessed numerically by the best response. The results are plotted on a graph to provide a visual representation of the improvement, stability, or deterioration of a patient's level of consciousness, which is crucial to predicting the eventual outcome of coma. The sum of the numeric values for each parameter can also be used as an overall objective measurement, with 14 being indicative of no impairment, 3 being compatible with brain death, and 7 usually accepted as a state of coma. The test score can also function as an indicator for certain diagnostic tests or treatments, such as the

Glasgow coma scale scoring

Eyes open
4 Spontaneously
3 On request
2 To pain stimuli (supraorbital or digital)
1 No opening

Best verbal response
5 Oriented to time, place, person
4 Engages in conversation, confused in content
3 Words spoken but conversation not sustained
2 Groans evoked by pain
1 No response

Best motor response
5 Obeys a command ("Hold out three fingers.")
4 Localizes a painful stimulus
3 Flexes either arm
2 Extends arm to painful stimulus
1 No response

From Phipps WJ, Long BC, Woods NF, Cassmeyer VL: *Medical surgical nursing concepts & clinical practice, ed 4,* St Louis, 1991, Mosby, p. 1758.

need for a CT scan, intracranial pressure monitoring, and intubation. The scale has a high degree of consistency even when used by staff of varied experience. (see Table, p. 673)

glass factor.   See **factor XII.**

glauco-,   a combining form meaning 'gray or silver': *glaucoma, glaucomatous.*

glaucoma /glôkō′mə, glou-/ [Gk, cataract], an abnormal condition of elevated pressure within an eye because of obstruction of the outflow of aqueous humor. **Acute (angle-closure, closed-angle,** or **narrow-angle) glaucoma** occurs if the pupil in an eye with a narrow angle between the iris and cornea dilates markedly, causing the folded iris to block the exit of aqueous humor from the anterior chamber. **Chronic (open-angle** or **wide-angle) glaucoma** is much more common, often bilateral; it develops slowly and is genetically determined. The obstruction is believed to be within the canal of Schlemm. –**glaucomatous,** *adj.*

■ OBSERVATIONS: Acute glaucoma is accompanied by extreme ocular pain, blurred vision, a red eye, and a dilated pupil. Nausea and vomiting may occur. If untreated, acute glaucoma results in complete and permanent blindness within 2 to 5 days. Chronic glaucoma may produce no symptoms except for gradual loss of peripheral vision over a period of years. Sometimes headaches, blurred vision, and dull pain in the eye are present. Cupping of the optic discs may be noted on ophthalmoscopic examination. Halos around lights and central blindness are late manifestations. Both types have elevated intraocular pressure by tonometry.

■ INTERVENTIONS: Acute glaucoma is treated with eye drops to constrict the pupil and draw the iris away from the cornea, osmotic agents such as urea, mannitol, or glycerol given systemically to lower intraocular pressure, acetazolamide to reduce fluid formation, and surgical iridectomy to produce a filtration pathway for aqueous humor. Chronic glaucoma can usually be controlled with miotic eye drops such as pilocarpine. Other treatment includes carbonic anhydrase inhibitors, epinephrine eye drops, and timolol, a beta-adrenergic blocking agent.

glaucoma connsumatum.   See **absolutum glaucoma.**

glaucomatocyclitic crisis /glôkom′ətōsiklit′ik/, a recurrent rise in intraocular pressure in one eye, resembling acute angle-closure glaucoma, and accompanied by signs of uveitis. Also called **Posner-Schlossman syndrome.**

-glaucomatous.   See **glaucoma.**

-glea, -gloea,   a suffix meaning a 'binding gelatinous medium': *ooglea, mesoglia, zooglea.*

glenohumeral /glē′nōhyōō′mərəl/, [Gk, *glene,* joint socket; L, *humerus,* shoulder], pertaining to the glenoid cavity and the humerus at the shoulder joint.

glenohumeral joint,   the shoulder joint, formed by the glenoid cavity of the scapula and the head of the humerus.

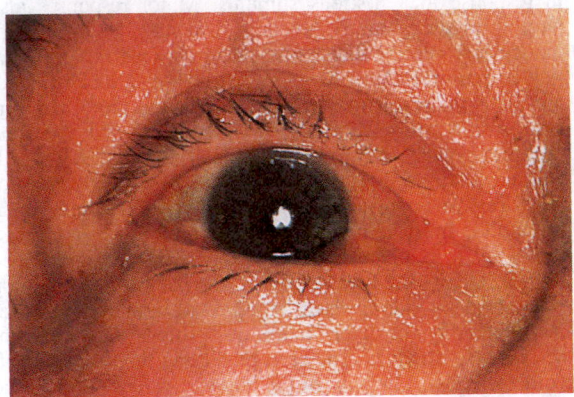

Appearance of the eye in acute glaucoma
(Kamal, 1991)

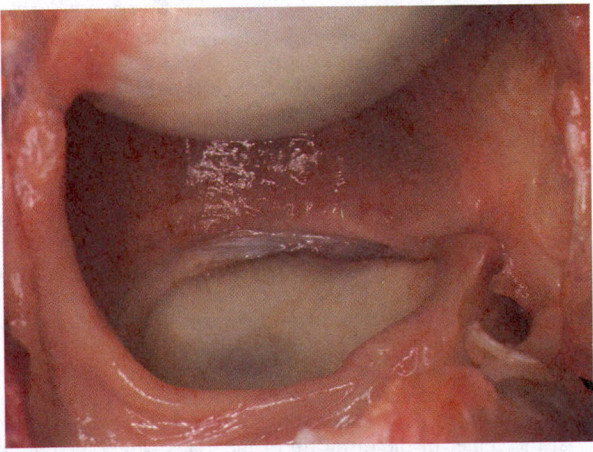

Glenohumeral joint *(Johnson, 1993)*

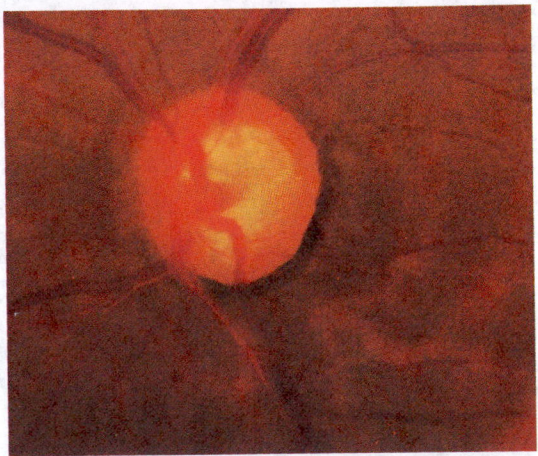

Appearance of the fundus in chronic open–angle glaucoma
(Apple, 1991)

glenohumeral ligaments [Gk, *glene,* joint socket, *humerus,* shoulder], three thickened bands of connective tissue attached proximally to the anterior margin of the glenoid cavity and labrum and distally to the lesser tuberosity and neck of the humerus.

glenoid cavity /glē′noid/ [Gk, *glene*, joint socket, *eidos*, form; L, *cavum*], a shallow depression with which the head of the humerus articulates. Also called **glenoid fossa**.

glia. See **neuroglia**.

glia cells /glī′ə, glē′ə/ [Gk, *glia*, glue; L, *cella*, storeroom], neural cells that have a connective tissue supporting function in the central nervous system. Examples include astrocytes and oligodendroglial cells of ectodermal origin and microglial cells of mesodermal origin.

gliadin /glī′ədin/ [Gk, *glia*, glue], a protein substance that is obtained from wheat and rye. Its solubility in diluted alcohol distinguishes gliadin from another grain protein, glutenin.

gliding [AS, *glidan*, to glide], **1.** a smooth, continuous movement. **2.** the simplest of the four basic movements allowed by various joints of the skeleton. It is common to all movable joints and allows one surface to move smoothly over an adjacent surface, regardless of shape. Gliding is the only motion allowed by most of the wrist and the ankle joints. Compare **angular movement, circumduction, rotation**.

gliding joint, a synovial joint in which articulation of contiguous bones allows only gliding movements, as in the wrist and the ankle. The ligaments or the osseous processes around each gliding joint limit movements of apposed plane surfaces or concavoconvex articulations. Also called **arthrodia, articulatio plana**. Compare **hinge joint, pivot joint**.

gliding zone, an articular cartilage surface area immediately adjacent to a joint space. It consists of a thin layer of densely packed collagen fibers lying parallel to the surface and covered by a fine, acellular, afibrillar membrane. At the periphery the fibrous components merge with the fibrous periosteum of the adjacent bone.

glio-, a combining form meaning 'pertaining to the neuroglia, or a gluey substance': *gliococcus, gliosarcoma, gliosome*.

glioblastoma. See **spongioblastoma**.

glioblastoma multiforme /glī′ōblastō′mə mul′tifôr′mē/

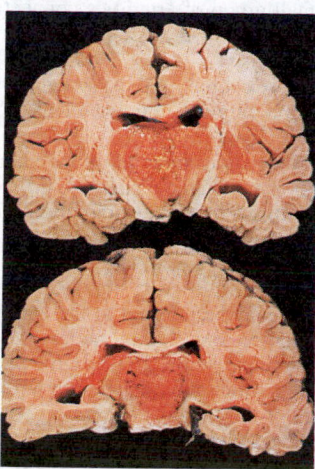

Glioblastoma multiforme *(Fletcher, 1987)*

[Gk, *glia*, glue, *blastos*, germ, *oma*, tumor; L, *multus*, many, *forma*, form], a malignant, rapidly growing, pulpy or cystic tumor of the cerebrum or the spinal cord. The lesion spreads with pseudopod-like projections. It is composed of a mixture of monocytes, pyriform cells, immature and mature astrocytes, and neural ectodermal cells with fibrous or protoplasmic processes. Also called **anaplastic astrocytoma, glioma multiforme**.

glioma /glī·ō′mə/, *pl.* **gliomas, gliomata** [Gk, *glia* + *oma*, tumor], any of the largest group of primary tumors of the brain, composed of malignant glial cells. Kinds of gliomas are **astrocytoma, ependymoma, glioblastoma multiforme, medulloblastoma,** and **oligodendroglioma**.

-glioma, a combining form meaning a 'tumor arising from the neuroglia': *angioglioma, fibroglioma, ganglioma*.

glioma multiforme. See **glioblastoma multiforme**.

glioma retinae. See **retinoblastoma**.

glioma sarcomatosum. See **gliosarcoma**.

gliomata. See **glioma**.

glioneuroma /glī′ōnŏŏrō′mə/, *pl.* **glioneuromas, glioneuromata** [Gk, *glia* + *neuron*, nerve, *oma* tumor], a neoplasm composed of nerve cells and elements of their supporting connective tissue.

gliosarcoma /glī′ōsärkō′mə/, *pl.* **gliosarcomas, gliosarcomata** [Gk, *glia* + *sarx,* flesh, *oma,* tumor], a tumor composed of spindle-shaped cells in the delicate supporting connective tissue of nerve cells. Also called **glioma, glioblastoma, spongioblastoma, spongiocytoma**.

gliosarcoma retinae. See **retinoblastoma**.

glipizide /glip′izīd/, an oral antidiabetic drug.

■ INDICATIONS: It is prescribed as an adjunct to diet and exercise in lowering blood glucose levels of patients with non-insulin-dependent diabetes.

■ CONTRAINDICATIONS: The dosage may have to be adjusted for patients taking drugs, such as diuretics, that increase blood glucose levels; elderly, debilitated, or malnourished patients are at risk of developing hypoglycemia.

■ ADVERSE EFFECTS: Among the most serious adverse reactions are nausea, heartburn, and skin allergies.

Glisson's capsule /glis′ənz/ [Francis Glisson, English physician, b. 1597; L, *capsula,* little box], the fibrous tissue sheath around lobules of the liver that carry branches of the hepatic artery, portal vein, and bile duct. Also called **hepatobiliary capsule**.

Glisson's sling [Francis Glisson, English physician, b. 1597], *obsolete.* an apparatus with a collar for the neck and chin, which is attached to weights and a pulley and used for traction of the cervical spine.

glitter cells [ME, *gliteren,* to shine], white blood cells in which movement of granules is observed in their cytoplasm. They are seen in microscopic examination of urine samples in cases of pyelonephritis or disorders marked by low osmolality.

Gln, abbreviation for **glutamine**.

global aphasia /glō′bəl/ [L, *globus,* ball; Gk, *a, phasis,* speech], a loss of ability to use any form of written or spoken language. The condition involves both sensory and motor nerve tracts. Communication is attempted through primitive gestures or the use of automatic words and phrases.

globin /glō′bin/ [L, *globus,* ball], a group of 4 globulin protein molecules that become bound by the iron in heme molecules to form hemoglobin or myoglobin.

-globin   a suffix meaning 'containing protein': *hemoglobin, myoglobin.*

-globinuria,   a combining form meaning '(condition involving) the presence of complex proteins in the urine': *hemoglobinuria, methemoglobinuria, myoglobinuria.*

globoid leukodystrophy.   See **galactosyl ceramide lipidosis.**

globule /glob′yool/ [L, *globulus,* small sphere],   a small spheric mass. Kinds of globules are **dentin globule, Dobie's globule, Marchi's globule, Margagni's globule, milk globule,** and **myelin globule.**

globulin /glob′yoolin/,   one of a broad category of simple proteins classified by solubility, electrophoretic mobility, and size. Compare **albumin.** See also **euglobulin, plasma protein.**

globulinuria /-oor′ē·ə/ [L, *globulus,* small globe; Gk, *ouron,* urine],   the presence of globulin class proteins in the urine.

globus hystericus /glō′bus/ [L, small sphere; Gk, *hystera,* womb],   a transitory sensation of a lump in the throat that cannot be swallowed or coughed up, often accompanying emotional conflict or acute anxiety. The condition is thought to be caused by a functional disturbance of the ninth cranial nerve and spasm of the inferior constrictor muscle that encircles the lower part of the throat. The physical examination tends to be normal, as does the barium esophagram.

globus pallidus /pal′idəs/ [L, small sphere; pale],   the smaller and more medial part of the lentiform nucleus of the brain, separated from the putamen by the lateral medullary lamina and divided into external and internal portions closely connected to the stratum, thalamus, and mesencephalon.

-gloea.   See **-glea.**

glomangioma /glōman′jē·ō′mə/, *pl.* **glomangiomas, glomangiomata** [L, *glomus,* ball of thread; Gk, *aggeion,* vessel, *oma*],   a benign tumor that develops from a cluster of blood cells in the skin. Also called **angiomyoneuroma, angioneuroma.**

glomera.   See **glomus.**

glomerular /glōmer′yoolər/ [L, *glomerulus,* small ball],   of or pertaining to a glomerulus, especially a renal glomerulus.

glomerular capsule.   See **Bowman's capsule.**

glomerular disease,   any of a group of diseases in which the glomerulus of the kidney is affected. Depending on the particular disease, there may be hyperplasia, atrophy, necrosis, scarring, or deposits in the glomeruli. The symptoms may be abrupt in onset or slowly progressive. See also **glomerulonephritis.**

glomerular filtration,   the renal process whereby fluid in the blood is filtered across the capillaries of the glomerulus and into the urinary space of Bowman's capsule.

glomerular filtration rate (GFR), [L, *glomerulus,* small ball; Fr, *filtre*; L, *ratus*],   a kidney function test in which results can be determined from the amount of ultrafiltrate formed by plasma flowing through the glomeruli of the kidney. It may be calculated from insulin and creatinine clearance, serum creatinine, and blood urea nitrogen (BUN). Normal values average around 170 L/day for men and 150 L/day for women, with variations caused by differences in age, muscle mass, and other factors.

glomeruli.   See **glomerulus.**

glomerulo-,   a combining form meaning 'pertaining to the kidney': *glomerulonephritis.*

glomerulonephritis /glōmer′yoolōnəfrī′tis/ [L, *glomerulus,* small ball; Gk, *nephros,* kidney, *itis*],   an inflammation of the glomerulus of the kidney, characterized by proteinuria, hematuria, decreased urine production, and edema. Kinds of glomerulonephritis are **acute glomerulonephritis, chronic glomerulonephritis,** and **subacute glomerulonephritis.**

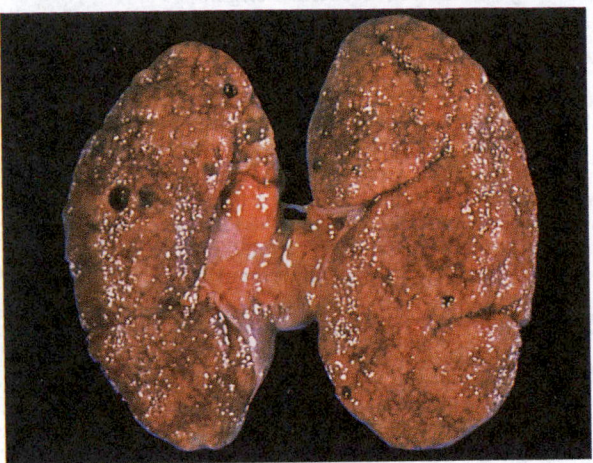

Chronic glomerulonephritis *(Fletcher, 1987)*

glomerulosclerosis /-sklərō′sis/ [L, *glomerulus,* small ball; Gk, *sklerosis,* a hardening, *osis,* condition],   a severe kidney disease in which glomerular function of blood filtration is lost as fibrous scar tissue replaces the glomeruli. The disease commonly follows an infection or arteriosclerosis.

glomerulus /glōmer′yooləs/, *pl.* **glomeruli** [L, small ball],   **1.** a tuft or cluster. **2.** a structure composed of blood vessels or nerve fibers, such as a renal glomerulus.

glomus /glō′məs/, *pl.* **glomera** /glom′ərə/ [L, ball of thread],   a small group of arterioles connecting directly to veins and having a rich nerve supply.

gloss-.   See **glosso-.**

glossectomy /glosek′təmē/ [Gk, *glossa,* tongue, *ektome,* cutting out],   the surgical removal of all or a part of the tongue.

-glossia,   **1.** a suffix meaning the 'possession of a specified type or condition of tongue': *cacoglossia, megaloglossia, schistoglossia.* **2.** a suffix meaning the 'possession of a specified number of tongues': *aglossia, diglossia.*

glossitis /glosī′tis/ [Gk, *glossa,* tongue, *itis*],   inflammation of the tongue. Acute glossitis, characterized by swelling, intense pain that may be referred to the ears, salivation, fever, and enlarged regional lymph nodes, may develop during an infectious disease or after a burn, bite, or other injury. Glossitis in which there is smooth atrophy of the surface and edges of the tongue is seen in pernicious anemia. Chronic superficial glossitis (Moeller's glossitis), in which irregular, bright red patches appear on the tip or sides of the tongue, occurs in middle-aged people, chiefly women. The condition causes pain or a burning sensation and sensitivity to hot or spicy foods; it often resists treatment. In congenital glossitis, there is a flat or slightly elevated patch or plaque anterior to the circumvallate papillae in the midline of the dorsal surface of the tongue.

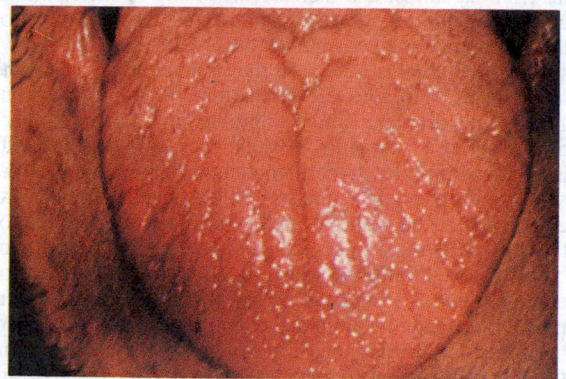

Glossitis *(McLaren, 1992/Courtesy Dr HH Sandstead)*

glossitis parasitica. See **parasitic glossitis.**

glossitis rhomboidea mediana. See **median rhomboid glossitis.**

glosso-, gloss-, a combining form meaning 'pertaining to the tongue': *glossocele, glossodynia, glossoplegia.*

glossodynia /glos'ōdin'ē·ə/ [Gk, *glossa* + *odyne*, pain], pain in the tongue, caused by acute or chronic inflammation, an abscess, or an ulcer.

glossodynia exfoliativa [Gk, *glossa, odyne* + L, *ex*, without, *folium*, leaf], a form of chronic glossitis, characterized by pain and sensitivity to spicy foods without any evidence of a pathologic condition. It occurs primarily in middle-aged women. Also called **Moeller's glossitis.**

glossoepiglottic /glos'ō·ep'iglot'ik/, pertaining to the epiglottis and the tongue.

glossohyal /glos'ōhī'əl/ [Gk, *glossa* + *hyoeides*, Y-shaped], of or pertaining to the tongue and the horseshoe-shaped hyoid bone at the base of the tongue immediately above the thyroid cartilage. Also called **hyoglossal.**

glossolalia /glos'ōlā'lyə/ [Gk, *glossa* + *lalein*, to babble], speech in an unknown 'language,' as 'speaking in tongues' during a state of religious ecstasy when the message being transmitted through the speaker is believed to be a message from a celestial spirit or from God.

glossoncus /glosong'kəs/ [Gk, *glossa* + *onkos*, swelling], a local swelling or general enlargement of the tongue.

glossopathy /glosop'əthē/ [Gk, *glossa* + *pathos*, disease], a pathologic condition of the tongue, such as acute inflammation caused by a burn, bite, injury, or infectious disease, enlargement resulting from congenital lymphangioma, or a disorder produced by mycotic infection, a malignant lesion, or a congenital anomaly.

glossopexy /glos'əpek'sē/ [Gk, *glossa* + *pexis*, fixation], an adhesion of the tongue to the lip.

glossopharyngeal /glos'ōfərin'jē·əl/ [Gk, *glossa* + *pharynx*, throat], of or pertaining to the tongue and pharynx. See also **glossopharyngeal nerve.**

glossopharyngeal nerve, either of a pair of cranial nerves

essential to the sense of taste, for sensation in some viscera, and for secretion from certain glands. The nerve has both sensory and motor fibers that pass from the tongue, parotid gland, and pharynx, communicate with the vagus nerve, and connect with two areas in the brain. Also called **nervus glossopharyngeus, ninth cranial nerve.**

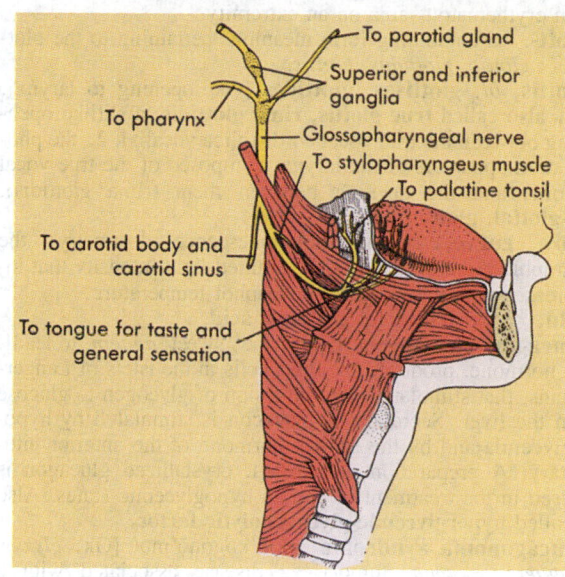

Glossopharyngeal nerve
(Seeley, 1992/David J Mascaro & Associates)

glossopharyngeal neuralgia, a disorder of unknown origin characterized by recurrent attacks of severe pain in the back of the pharynx, the tonsils, the base of the tongue, and the middle ear. It tends to affect men more than women, with an onset after the age of 40. Attacks lasting from a few seconds to minutes may be triggered by swallowing. The symptoms may be similar to those of trigeminal neuralgia. Treatment is usually pharmaceutical, but surgery may be recommended to sever involved nerve tracts.

glossophytia /glos'əfit'ē·ə/ [Gk, *glossa* + *phyton*, plant], a condition of the tongue characterized by a blackish patch on the dorsum on which filiform papillae are greatly elongated and thickened like bristly hairs. The usually painless condition may be caused by heavy smoking or the extensive use of broad-spectrum antibiotics. See also **parasitic glossitis.**

glossoplasty /glos'ōplas'tē/ [Gk, *glossa* + *plassein*, to mold], a surgical procedure or plastic operation on the tongue performed to correct a congenital anomaly, repair an injury, or restore a measure of function after excision of a malignant lesion.

glossoptosis /glos'optō'sis/ [Gk, *glossa* + *ptosis*, falling], the retraction or downward displacement of the tongue.

glossopyrosis /glos'ōpīrō'sis/ [Gk, *glossa* + *pyr*, fire, *osis*, condition], a burning sensation in the tongue caused by chronic inflammation, by exposure to extremely hot or spicy food, or by psychogenic glossitis.

glossorrhaphy /glosôr'əfē/ [Gk, *glossa* + *rhaphe*, seam], the surgical suturing of a wound in the tongue.

glossotrichia /glos'ətrik'ē·ə/ [Gk, *glossa* + *thrix*, hair], a condition of the tongue characterized by a hairlike appearance of the papillae. Also called **hairy tongue.**

glossy skin [[ONorse, *glosa*, smooth and shiny; AS, *scinn*], a shiny skin that is usually secondary to neuritis and may be associated with other integumentary disorders, including alopecia, skin fissuring, and ulceration. It usually begins as an erythematous area on an extremity.

glott-, a combining form meaning 'pertaining to the glottis': *glottic, glottidas, glottis.*

glottis, *pl.* **glottises, glottides** [Gk, opening to larynx], **1.** also called **true glottis, rima glottidis.** a slitlike opening between the true vocal cords (plica vocalis). **2.** the phonation apparatus of the larynx, composed of the true vocal cords and the opening between them (rima glottidis). –**glottal, glottic,** *adj.*

glow curve, (in thermoluminescence dosimetry) the graphic representation of the emitted light intensity that increases with the increasing phosphor temperature.

Glu, abbreviation for **glutamic acid.**

glucagon /glōō'kəgon/ [Gk, *glykys,* sweet, *agaein,* to lead], a hormone, produced by alpha cells in the islets of Langerhans, that stimulates the conversion of glycogen to glucose in the liver. Secretion of glucagon is stimulated by hypoglycemia and by the growth hormone of the anterior pituitary. A preparation of purified, crystallized glucagon is used in the treatment of certain hypoglycemic states. Also called **hyperglycemic-glycogenolytic factor.**

glucagonoma syndrome /glōō'kəgonō'mə/ [Gk, *glykys, agaein* + *oma,* tumor], a disease associated with a glucagon-secreting tumor of the islet cells of the pancreas, characterized by hyperglycemia, stomatitis, anemia, weight loss, and a characteristic rash.

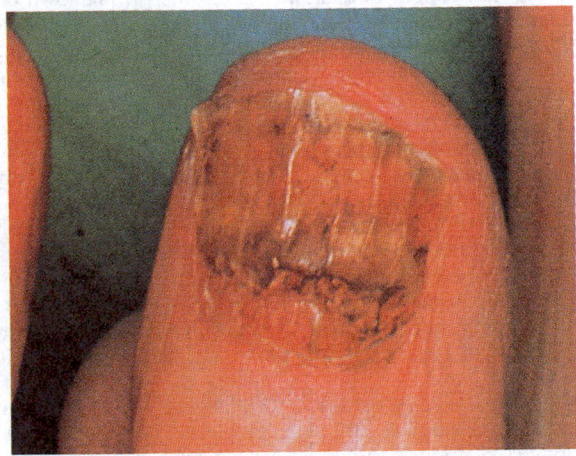

Fragmentation of the fingernails seen in glucagonoma syndrome
(Baran, 1991/Courtesy Prof J Hewitt)

gluco-, glyco-, a combining form meaning 'pertaining to sweetness or to glucose': *glucofuranose, glucokinetic, glucosuria.*

glucocorticoid /glōō'kōkôr'təkoid/ [Gk, *glykys* + L, *cortex,* bark; Gk, *eidos,* form], an adrenocortical steroid hormone that increases glyconeogenesis, exerts an antiinflam-

matory effect, and influences many body functions. The most important of the three glucocorticoids is cortisol (hydrocortisone); corticosterone is less active, and cortisone is inactive until converted to cortisol. Glucocorticoids promote the release of amino acids from muscle, mobilize fatty acids from fat stores, and increase the ability of skeletal muscles to maintain contractions and avoid fatigue. In vitro, these hormones are known to stabilize mitochondrial and lysosomal membranes, increase the production of adenosine triphosphate, promote the formation of certain liver enzymes, and decrease antibody production and the number of circulating eosinophils. A deficiency of glucocorticoids is characterized by hyperpigmentation (bronzing) of the skin, fasting hypoglycemia, weight loss, and apathy. An excess is associated with elevated serum glucose, thinning of the skin, ecchymosis, osteoporosis, poor wound healing, increased susceptibility to infection, and obesity. Glucocorticoid secretion is stimulated by the adrenocorticotropic hormone of the anterior pituitary, which in turn is regulated by the corticotropin-releasing factor of the hypothalamus. Synthetic or semisynthetic glucocorticoids, derived chiefly from cortisol, include prednisone, prednisolone, dexamethasone, methylprednisolone, triamcinolone, and betamethasone. Compare **mineralocorticoid.**

gluconeogenesis /glōō'kō·nē'ō·jen'əsis/, the formation of glycogen from fatty acids and proteins rather than carbohydrates.

glucosan /glōō'kəsan/ [Gk, *glykys,* sweet], any of a large group of anhydrous polysaccharides that on hydrolysis yield a hexose, primarily anhydrides of glucose. The glucosans include cellulose, glycogen, starch, and the dextrins.

glucose /glōō'kōs/ [Gk, *glykys,* sweet], a simple sugar found in certain foods, especially fruits, and a major source of energy occurring in human and animal body fluids. Glucose, when ingested or produced by the digestive hydrolysis of double sugars and starches, is absorbed into the blood from the intestines. Excess glucose in circulation is normally polymerized and stored in the liver and muscles as glycogen, which is depolymerized to glucose and liberated as needed. The determination of blood glucose levels is an important diagnostic test in diabetes and other disorders. Prepared glucose is a syrupy sweetening agent. Pharmaceutic preparations of glucose are widely used in the treatment of many disorders. Normal adult blood glucose levels range from less than 40 to more than 400 mg/dl, with generally higher levels after age 50. See also **dextrose, glycogen.**

glucose 1-phosphate, an intermediate compound in carbohydrate metabolism.

glucose 6-phosphate, an intermediate compound in carbohydrate metabolism.

glucose-6-phosphate dehydrogenase (G-6-PD) deficiency, an inherited disorder characterized by red cells partially or completely deficient in glucose-6-phosphate dehydrogenase, a critical enzyme in aerobic glycolysis. A sex-linked disorder, the defect is fully expressed in affected males despite a heterozygous pattern of inheritance. The disorder is associated with episodes of acute hemolysis under conditions of stress or in response to certain chemicals or drugs. The anemia that results is a kind of nonspherocytic hemolytic anemia. See also **congenital nonspherocytic hemolytic anemia, favism.**

glucose tolerance test, a test of the body's ability to metabolize carbohydrates by administering a standard dose of glucose and measuring the blood and urine for glucose at

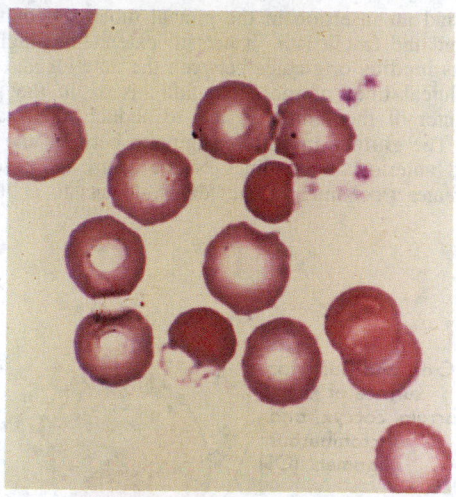

Glucose-6-phosphate dehydrogenase (G6PD) disease
(Zitelli, 1992)

regular intervals thereafter. The patient usually eats a high-carbohydrate diet for the 3 days preceding the test and fasts the night before. A fasting blood glucose is obtained the next morning, and then the patient drinks a 100 g dose of glucose. Blood and urine are collected periodically for up to 6 hours. The glucose tolerance test is most often used to assist in the diagnosis of diabetes or other disorders that affect carbohydrate metabolism.

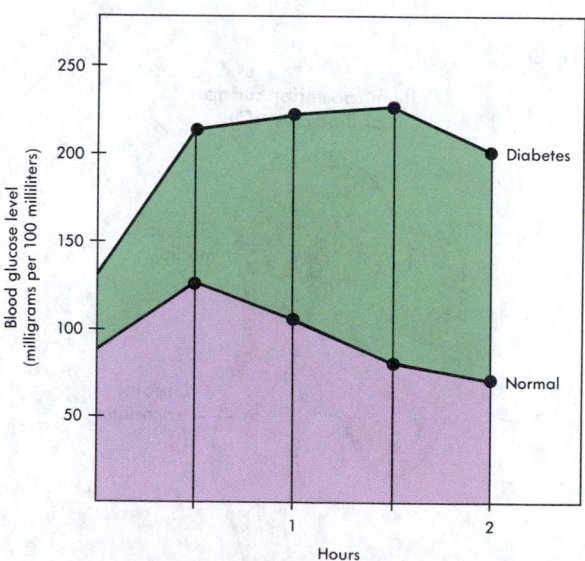

Typical responses seen after eating 50 grams (about 3 tablespoons) of glucose in normal and uncontrolled diabetic states.

Glucose tolerance test (Wardlaw, 1993)

glucosuria /glōō'kōsōōr'ē·ə/ [Gk, glykys + ouron, urine], abnormal presence of glucose in the urine resulting from the ingestion of large amounts of carbohydrate or from a kidney disease, such as nephrosis, or a metabolic disease, such as diabetes mellitus. See also **glycosuria.** –**glucosuric,** adj.

glucosyl cerebroside lipidosis. See **Gaucher's disease.**

Glucotrol, a trademark for an oral antidiabetic drug (glipizide).

glue sniffing [Gk, gloios; ME, sniffen], the practice of inhaling the vapors of toluene, a volatile organic compound used as a solvent in certain glues. The glue is squeezed into a plastic bag, which is then placed over the nose and mouth. Intoxication and dizziness result. Prolonged accidental or occupational exposure or repeated recreational use may damage a variety of organ systems. Death has been reported from asphyxiation by the plastic bag.

glutamate /glōō'təmāt/, a salt of glutamic acid.

glutamic acid (Glu) /glōōtam'ik/ [L, gluten, glue, amine, ammonia; acidus, sour], a nonessential amino acid occurring widely in a number of proteins. Preparations of glutamic acid are used as aids for digestion. See also **amino acid, protein.**

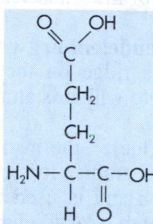

Chemical structure of glutamic acid

glutamicacidemia /glōōtam'ikas'idē'mē·ə/, an inherited disorder of amino acid metabolism resulting in an excessive level of glutamic acid. The precise enzyme defect is unknown, but the condition is characterized by mental and physical retardation, seizures, and fragile hair growth.

glutamic acid hydrochloride, a gastric acidifier.

■ INDICATION: It is prescribed for hypoacidity.

■ CONTRAINDICATIONS: Hyperacidity, peptic ulcer, or known hypersensitivity to this drug prohibits its use.

■ ADVERSE EFFECTS: The most serious adverse reaction is systemic acidosis resulting from overdose.

glutamic-oxaloacetic transaminase. See **aspartate aminotransferase.**

glutamic-pyruvic transaminase. See **alanine aminotransferase.**

glutamine (Gln) /glōō'təmēn/ [L, gluten + amine, ammonia], a nonessential amino acid found in many proteins in the body. It functions as an amino donor for many reactions and it is also a nontoxic transport for ammonia, being easily hydrolyzed to glutamic acid and free ammonia, the

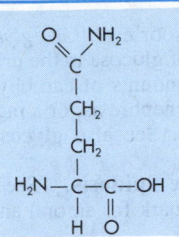

Chemical structure of glutamine

latter being excreted in the urine. See also **amino acid, protein.**

glutargin /glōōtär′gin/, arginine glutamate. See also **arginine.**

glutathione /glōō′təthī′ōn/ [L, *gluten* + Gk, *theione*, sulfur], an enzyme whose deficiency is commonly associated with hemolytic anemia.

gluteal /glōō′tē·əl/ [Gk, *gloutos*, buttocks], pertaining to the buttocks or to the muscles that form the buttocks.

gluteal gait. See **Trendelenburg gait.**

gluteal tuberosity, a ridge on the lateral posterior surface of the thigh bone to which is attached the gluteus maximus.

gluten /glōō′tən/ [L, glue], the insoluble protein constituent of wheat and other grains. It is obtained from flour by washing out the starch and is used as an adhesive agent, giving to dough its tough, elastic character. See also **celiac disease, food allergy.**

gluten-induced enteropathy. See **celiac disease.**

glutethimide /glōōteth′əmīd/, a sedative.

■ INDICATION: It is prescribed in the treatment of anxiety and insomnia.

■ CONTRAINDICATION: Known hypersensitivity to this drug prohibits its use.

■ ADVERSE EFFECTS: Among the most serious adverse reactions are physical and psychologic dependence. Rashes also may occur.

gluteus /glōōtē′əs/, any of the three muscles that form the buttocks. The **gluteus maximus** is a large muscle with an origin in the iliac, the sacrum, and the sacroturberus liga-

ment and an insertion in the gluteal tuberosity of the femur and the fascia lata. It acts to extend the thigh. The **gluteus medius** originates between the anterior and posterior gluteal lines of the ilium and inserts in the greater trochanter of the femur. It acts to abduct and rotate the thigh. The **gluteus minimus** originates between the inferior and anterior gluteal lines of the ilium and inserts in the greater trochanter of the femur. It acts to abduct the thigh.

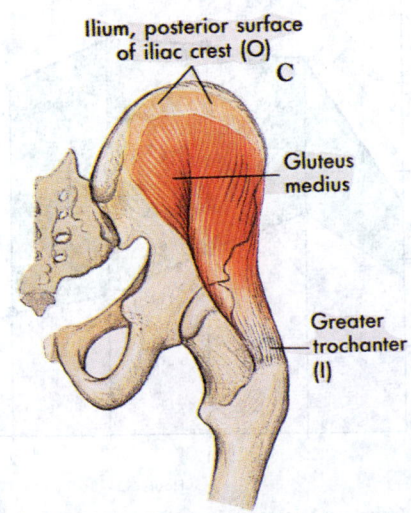

Gluteus maximus muscle
(Thibodeau, 1993/Ernest W Beck)

Gluteus medius muscle
(Thibodeau, 1993/Ernest W Beck)

Characteristics of a gluten-free diet for adult celiac disease

- All forms of wheat, rye, oat, buckwheat, and barley are omitted, except gluten-free wheat starch.
- All other foods are permitted freely, unless specified otherwise by the physician.
- The diet should be high in protein, calories, vitamins, and minerals.

From Williams SR: *Basic nutrition and diet therapy,* ed 9, St Louis, 1992, Mosby.

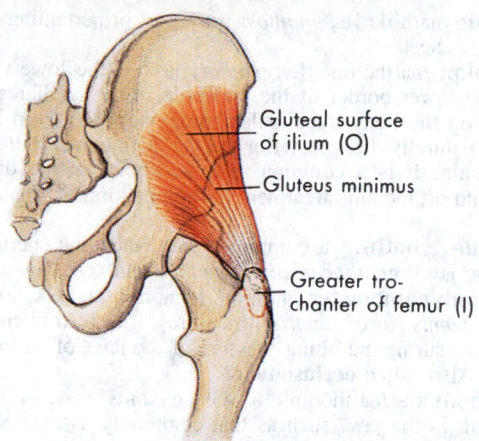

Gluteus minimus muscle
(Thibodeau, 1993/Ernest W Beck)

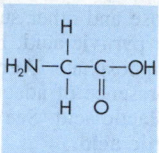

Chemical structure of glycine

Gly, abbreviation for **glycine.**

glyburide /glī′bərīd/, an oral antidiabetic drug.
- INDICATIONS: It is prescribed as an adjunct to diet and exercise in lowering blood glucose levels of patients with non-insulin-dependent diabetes.
- CONTRAINDICATIONS: Because of its long duration of action, glyburide may produce prolonged hypoglycemia; there is also a risk of severe hypoglycemia in elderly, debilitated, or malnourished patients. The dosage may need to be adjusted for patients taking other drugs that increase blood glucose levels.
- ADVERSE EFFECTS: Among the more serious adverse reactions are nausea, hypoglycemia, and skin allergies.

-glycemia, -glycaemia, a combining form meaning a 'condition of sugar in the blood': *dysglycemia, hepatoglycemia, hyperglycemia.*

glycerin /glis′ərin/ [Gk, *glykeros*, sweet], a sweet, colorless, oily fluid that is a pharmaceutic grade of glycerol. Glycerin is used as a moistening agent for chapped skin, as an ingredient of suppositories for constipation, and as a sweetening agent and vehicle for drug preparations. Also spelled **glycerine.**

glycerol /glis′ərôl/ [Gk, *glykeros*, sweet], an alcohol that is a component of fats. Glycerol is soluble in ethyl alcohol and water. See also **glycerin.**

glycerol kinase, an enzyme in the liver and kidneys that catalyzes the transfer of a phosphate group from adenosine triphosphate to form adenosine diphosphate and L-glycerol-3-phosphate.

glyceryl alcohol. See **glycerin.**

glyceryl guaiacolate. See **guaifenesin.**

glyceryl triacetate. See **triacetin.**

glycine (Gly) /glī′sin/ [Gk, *glykeros* + L, *amine*, ammonia], a nonessential amino acid occurring widely as a component of animal and plant proteins. Synthetically produced glycine is used in solutions for irrigation, in the treatment of various muscle diseases, and as an antacid and dietary supplement. See also **amino acid, protein.**

glyco-. See **gluco-.**

glycobiarsol /glī′kōbī′ərsol/, an antiamebic containing arsenic and bismuth, formerly used to treat intestinal amebiasis.

glycogen /glī′kəjən/ [Gk, *glykys*, sweet, *genein*, to produce], a polysaccharide that is the major carbohydrate stored in animal cells. It is formed from glucose and stored chiefly in the liver and, to a lesser extent, in muscle cells. Glycogen is depolymerized to glucose and released into circulation as needed by the body. Also called **animal starch, hepatin, tissue dextrin.** See also **glucose.**

glycogenesis /glī′kōjen′əsis/, the synthesis of glycogen from glucose.

glycogenolysis /glī′kōjenol′isis/ [Gk, *glykys, genein* + *lysis,* loosening], the breakdown of glycogen to glucose.

glycogenosis. See **glycogen storage disease.**

glycogen storage disease [Gk, *glykys, genein* + L, *instaurare,* to renew; *dis,* opposite of; Fr, *aise,* ease], any of a group of inherited disorders of glycogen metabolism. An enzyme deficiency causes glycogen to accumulate in abnormally large amounts in various parts of the body. Biopsy and chemical analysis reveal the missing enzyme. Also called **glycogenosis.**

glycogen storage disease, type I. See **von Gierke's disease.**

glycogen storage disease, type Ib, a form of glycogen storage disease in which excessive amounts of glycogen are deposited in the liver and leukocytes. Some symptoms are similar to, but less severe than, those of glycogen storage disease, **type Ia** (von Gierke's disease). Additional symptoms include neutropenia and recurrent GI infections. Biopsy of the affected organs reveals the absence of glucose-6-phosphatase translocase, an enzyme necessary for glycogen metabolism. See also **von Gierke's disease.**

glycogen storage disease, type II. See **Pompe's disease.**

glycogen storage disease, type III. See **Cori's disease.**

glycogen storage disease, type IV. See **Andersen's disease.**

glycogen storage disease, type V. See **McArdle's disease.**

glycogen storage disease, type VI. See **Hers' disease.**

glycogen storage disease, type VII. See **Tarui's disease.**

glycolic acid /glīkol′ik/ [Gk, *glykys* + L, *acidus,* sour], a substance in bile, formed by glycine and cholic acid, that aids in digestion and absorption of fats. Glycolic acid is used as a food additive and an emulsifying agent.

glycolipid /glī′kōlip′id/ [Gk, *glykys* + *lipos,* fat], a compound that consists of a lipid and a carbohydrate, usually galactose, found primarily in the tissue of the nervous system, especially the myelin sheath and the ganglion cells.

glycolysis /glīkol′isis/ [Gk, *glykys* + *lysis,* loosening], a series of enzymatically catalyzed reactions, occurring within cells, by which glucose and other sugars are broken down to yield lactic acid or pyruvic acid, releasing energy in the form of adenosine triphosphate. **Aerobic glycolysis** yields pyruvic acid in the presence of adequate oxygen. **Anaerobic glycolysis** yields lactic acid. See also **aldolase, Krebs' citric acid cycle, lactic acid.**

glycoprotein /glī'kōprō'tēn/ [Gk, *glykys* + *proteios*, first rank], any of the large group of conjugated proteins in which the nonprotein substance is a carbohydrate. These include the mucins, the mucoids, and the chondroproteins.

glycopyrrolate /glī'kōpir'əlāt/, an anticholinergic.
- INDICATION: It is prescribed as an adjunct to ulcer therapy.
- CONTRAINDICATIONS: Narrow-angle glaucoma, asthma, obstruction of the genitourinary or GI tract, ulcerative colitis, or known hypersensitivity to this drug prohibits its use.
- ADVERSE EFFECTS: Among the more serious adverse reactions are blurred vision, central nervous system effects, tachycardia, dry mouth, decreased sweating, and hypersensitivity reactions.

glycoside /glī'kəsīd/ [Gk, *glykys*, sweet], any of several carbohydrates that yield a sugar and a nonsugar on hydrolysis. The plant *Digitalis purpurea* yields a glycoside used in the treatment of heart disease.

glycosphingolipids /glī'kōsfing'gōlip'ids/, compounds formed from carbohydrates and ceramide, a fatty substance, found in tissues of the central nervous system and also in erythrocytes. Deficiency of an enzyme needed to metabolize glycosphingolipids leads to a potentially fatal disorder of the nervous system.

glycosuria /glī'kōsoōr'ē·ə/ [Gk, *glykys* + *ouron*, urine], abnormal presence of a sugar, especially glucose, in the urine. Glycosuria can result from the ingestion of large amounts of carbohydrate, or it may be the result of endocrine or renal disorders. It is a finding most routinely associated with diabetes mellitus. –**glycosuric,** *adj.*

glycosuric acid /-soōr'ik/ [Gk, *glykys* + *ouron*, urine; L, *acidus*, sour], a compound that is an intermediate product of the metabolism of tyrosine. It forms a melanin-like staining substance in the urine of people who have alkaptonuria.

glycosylated hemoglobin (GHb/Hb A$_{1c}$) /glīkō'silā'tid/, a hemoglobin A molecule with a glucose group on the N-terminal valine amino acid unit of the beta chain. The glycosylated hemoglobin concentration represents the average blood glucose level over the previous several weeks. In controlled diabetes mellitus the concentration of glycosylated hemoglobin is within the normal range, but in uncontrolled cases the level may be three to four times the normal concentration. Assays of Hb A$_{1c}$, which normally has a 4-month life span, reveal whether glucose levels have been properly controlled during a period of several weeks preceding the test. The normal range is 1.8% to 4.0% for children; 2.2% to 4.8% for adults.

glycyl alcohol. See **glycerin.**

gm, abbreviation for **gram.** Preferred is the abbreviation **g.**

GMENAC, abbreviation for **Graduate Medical Education National Advisory Committee.**

GMP, abbreviation for **guanosine monophosphate.**

GN. See **graduate nurse.**

GNA, abbreviation for **Gay Nurses' Alliance.**

gnath-. See **gnatho-.**

-gnathia, a combining form meaning a 'condition of the jaw': *brachygnathia, campylognathia, retrognathia.*

gnathic /nath'ik/ [L, *gnathos*, jaw], of or pertaining to the jaw or cheek.

gnathion /nā'thē·on/ [L, *gnathos*, jaw], the lowest point in the lower border of the mandible in the median plane. It is on the bony mandibular border palpated from below and naturally lies posterior to the tegumental border of the chin. It is a common reference point in the diagnosis and orthodontic treatment of various kinds of malocclusion.

gnatho-, gnath-, a combining form meaning 'pertaining to the jaw': *gnathocephalus, gnathodynia, gnathoplasty.*

gnathodynamometer /nā'thōdī'nəmom'ətər/ [Gk, *gnathos* + *dynamis*, force, *metron*, measure], an instrument used for measuring the biting pressure of the jaws of an individual. Also called **occlusometer.**

gnathodynia /nā'thōdin'ē·ə/ [Gk, *gnathos* + *odyne*, pain], a pain in the jaw, such as that commonly associated with an impacted wisdom tooth.

gnathology /nāthol'əjē/ [Gk, *gnathos* + *logos*, science], a field of dental or medical study that deals with the entire masticatory apparatus, including its anatomy, histology, morphology, physiology, pathology, and therapeutics.

gnathoschisis. See **cleft palate.**

gnathostatic cast /nā'thōstat'ik/ [Gk, *gnathos* + *statike*, weighing; ME, *casten*], a cast of the teeth trimmed so that its occlusal plane is in its normal oral attitude when the cast is set on a plane surface. It is used in orthodontic diagnosis based on the gnathostatic technique. See also **gnathostatics.**

gnathostatics /nā'thōstat'iks/ [Gk, *gnathos* + *statike*, weighing], a technique of orthodontic diagnosis based on an analysis of the relationships between the teeth and certain reference points on the skull. See also **gnathostatic cast.**

gno-, a combining form meaning 'to know or discern': *gnosia, gnosis.*

-gnomonic, -gnomonical, a combining form meaning 'signs or experience in knowing or judging (a condition)': *pathognomonic, physiognomonic, thanatognomonic.*

-gnomy, a combining form meaning the 'science or means of judging' something specified: *craniognomy, pathognomy, physiognomy.*

-gnosia, a combining form meaning a '(condition of) perceiving or recognizing': *acognosia, hypergnosia, topognosia.*

-gnosis, a combining form meaning 'knowledge': *acrognosis, diagnosis, topognosis.*

GnRH, abbreviation for **gonadotropin-releasing hormone.**

goal /gōl/ [ME, *gol*, limit], the purpose toward which an endeavor is directed, such as the outcome of diagnostic, therapeutic, and educational management of a patient's health problem.

goblet cell [ME, *gobelet*, small bowl], one of the many specialized cells that secrete mucus and form glands of the epithelium of the stomach, the intestine, and parts of the respiratory tract. Also called **beaker cell, chalice cell.** See also **gland.**

goiter [L, *guttur*, throat], a hypertrophic thyroid gland, usually evident as a pronounced swelling in the neck. The enlargement may be associated with hyperthyroidism, hypothyroidism, or normal levels of thyroid function. The goi-

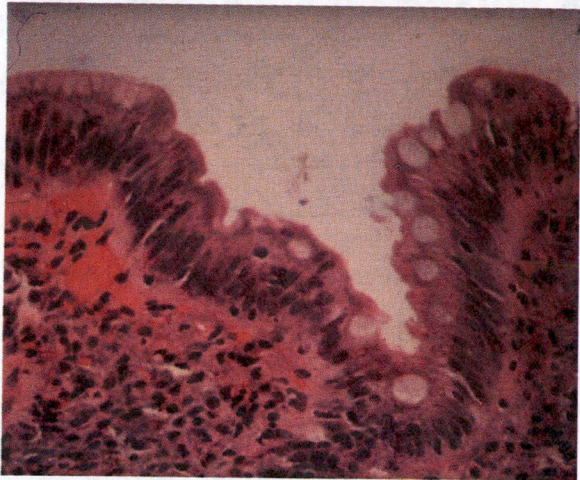

Goblet cells (Mitros, 1988)

ter may be cystic or fibrous, containing nodules or an increased number of follicles; it may surround a large blood vessel, or a part of the enlarged gland may be situated beneath the sternum or in the thoracic cavity. Treatment may include total or subtotal surgical removal, the administration of antithyroid drugs or radioiodine, or the use of thyroid hormone to block the hypothalamic mechanism that releases thyroid-stimulating hormone. After thyroidectomy, maintenance therapy with thyroid hormone may be required. See specific goiters. **–goitrous,** *adj.*

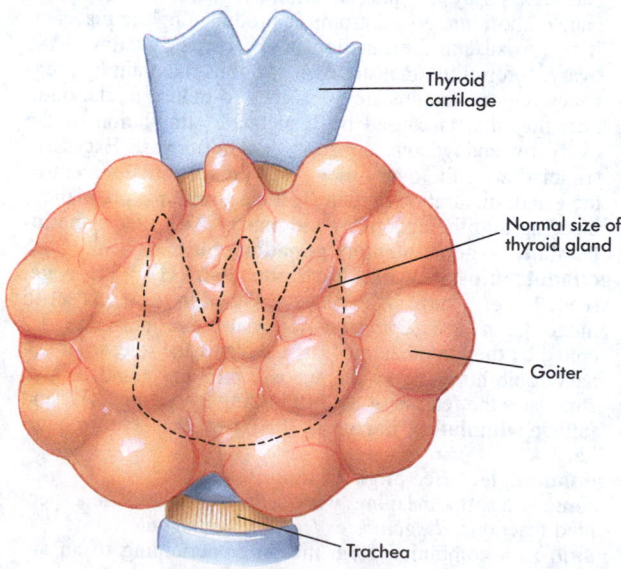

Thyroid cartilage

Normal size of thyroid gland

Goiter

Trachea

Goiter (Wardlaw, 1993)

Enlargement of the thyroid gland in goiter
(Gottfried, 1993/NMSB/Custom Medical Stock Photo, Inc.)

gold (Au) [AS, *geolu,* yellow], a yellowish, soft metallic element that occurs naturally as a free metal and as the telluride $AuAgTe_4$. Its atomic number is 79; its atomic weight is 197. Gold has been highly valued since antiquity and has been and is used for currency, for ornamentation, and as a dental restorative material. It is usually hardened by alloying it with small amounts of nickel or copper. Gold is highly resistive to oxidation but can be dissolved in aqua regia and aqueous potassium cyanide. Gold salts, in which gold is attached to sulfur, are often used in the treatment, or chrysotherapy, of patients with rheumatoid arthritis but cause serious toxicity in about 10% of patients and some toxicity in 25% to 50%. See also **chrysotherapy.**

gold 198, a radioactive gold antineoplastic.
■ INDICATIONS: It is prescribed for cancer of the prostate, cervix, and bladder and for the reduction of fluid accumulation secondary to a cancer.
■ CONTRAINDICATIONS: Ulcerative tumors, pregnancy, lactation, or unhealed surgical wounds prohibit its use. It is not prescribed for patients under 18 years of age.
■ ADVERSE EFFECTS: The most serious adverse reaction is radiation sickness.

Goldblatt kidney, an abnormal kidney in which constriction of a renal artery leads to ischemia and the release of renin, a pressor substance associated with hypertension.

gold compound, a drug containing gold salts, usually administered with other drugs in the treatment of rheumatoid arthritis. Gold is potentially toxic and is administered only under the supervision of a specialist in chrysotherapy. Toxic reactions range from mild dermatoses to lethal poisoning. Various radioisotopes of gold have been used in diagnostic radiology and in the radiologic treatment of certain malignant neoplastic diseases.

gold file, (in dentistry) an instrument designed for removing surplus gold from gold restorations in the mouth. It may be designed and used as either a pull-cut or push-cut file.

gold foil, (in dentistry) pure gold that has been rolled and beaten into a very thin sheet. The thickness of different gold foils varies from ¼₀,₀₀₀ inch for No. 2 foil to ½₀,₀₀₀ inch for No. 4 foil. The main types of gold foil are cohesive, semicohesive, and noncohesive. It is commonly compacted into a retentive tooth cavity form, using gold's property of cold welding. Also called **fibrous gold.**

gold inlay, an intracoronal cast restoration of gold alloy.

gold knife, an instrument that may be contraangled, with a blade or cutting edge, used for trimming excess metal and for developing contour in foil restorations.

Goldman-Fox knife, a dental surgical instrument with a sharp cutting edge, designed for the incision and contouring of gingival tissue.

gold sodium thiomalate, an antirheumatic.
- INDICATION: It is prescribed for rheumatoid arthritis.
- CONTRAINDICATIONS: Severe debilitation, systemic lupus erythematosus, renal or liver disease, blood dyscrasias, Sjögren's syndrome (in rheumatoid arthritis), or known hypersensitivity to this drug or to other gold or heavy metal salts prohibits its use.
- ADVERSE EFFECTS: Among the most serious adverse reactions are various blood dyscrasias, renal damage, and allergic reactions. Dermatitis, stomatitis, and lesions of the mucous membranes also may occur.

gold therapy. See **chrysotherapy.**

golfer's elbow, a popular term for medial epicondylitis associated with repeated use of the wrist flexors.

Golgi apparatus /gôl'jē/ [Camillo Golgi, Italian anatomist, b. 1844; L, *ad,* towards, *prepare,* to prepare], one of many small membranous structures found in most cells, composed of various elements associated with the formation of carbohydrate side chains of glycoproteins, mucopolysaccharides, and other substances. Saccules within each structure migrate through the cell membrane and release substances associated with external and internal secretion. Also called **Golgi body, Golgi complex.**

Golgi-Mazzoni corpuscles /gôl'jēmatsō'nē/ [Camillo Golgi; Vittori Mazzoni, Italian physician, b. 1823], a number of thin capsules enveloping terminal nerve fibrils in the subcutaneous tissue of the fingers. They have thicker cores than Pacini's corpuscles but are similar special sensory end organs. Also called **Krause's terminal bulbs.** Compare **Pacini's corpuscles, Ruffini's corpuscles.**

Golgi's cells [Camillo Golgi, Italian anatomist, b. 1844; L, *cella,* storeroom], **1. Golgi type I neurons,** nerve cells having long axons that leave the local neuropil area of the parent cell body, traverse the white matter, and project to the rest of the nervous system. **2. Golgi type II neurons,** nerve cells with short trajectory axons, like stellate cells of the cerebral and cerebellar cortex. They generally do not enter white matter but remain within the local neuropil in the cerebral and cerebellar cortices and the retina.

Golgi tendon organ, a sensory nerve ending that is sensitive to both tension and excessive passive stretch of a skeletal muscle.

Golgi type I neurons. See **Golgi's cells.**

Golgi type II neurons. See **Golgi's cells.**

gomphosis /gomfō'sis/, *pl.* **gomphoses** [Gk, *gomphos,* bolt], an articulation by the insertion of a conic process into a socket, such as the insertion of a root of a tooth into an alveolus of the mandible or the maxilla. Gomphosis is

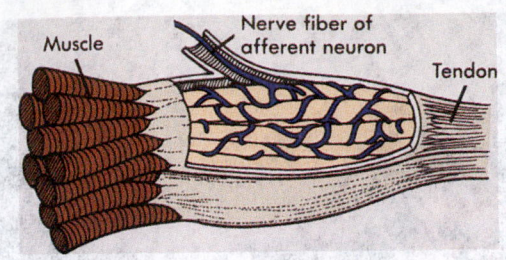

Golgi tendon organ *(Seeley, 1992/Michael Schenk)*

not a connection between true bones but is considered a type of fibrous joint. Compare **sutura, syndesmosis.**

gon-. See **gono-, gony-.**

gonad /gō'nad/ [Gk, *gone,* seed], a gamete-producing gland, such as an ovary or a testis. –**gonadal,** *adj.*

gonadal dysgenesis /gō'nədəl/, a general designation for a variety of conditions involving anomalies in the development of the gonads, such as Turner's syndrome, hermaphroditism, and gonadal aplasia.

gonadal dose, a measure of the dose of radiation received by the gonads as a result of an x-ray examination. It may vary from less than 1 mrad for a dental or chest radiograph to 225 mrad for a lumbar spine radiograph and 800 mrad for a fetus during pelvimetry.

gonadal shield, a specially designed contact or shadow shield used to protect the gonadal area of a patient from the primary radiation beam during x-ray procedures. It is generally used for all patients who are potentially reproductive, including all patients under the age of 40 and also older males.

gonadotropin /gō'nədōtrop'in/ [Gk, *gone* + *trophe,* nourishment], a hormonal substance that stimulates the function of the testes and the ovaries. The gonadotropic follicle stimulating hormone and luteinizing hormone are produced and secreted by the anterior pituitary gland. In early pregnancy, chorionic gonadotropin is produced by the placenta. It acts to sustain the function of the corpus luteum of the ovary, forestalling menstruation and thus maintaining pregnancy. Gonadotropins are prescribed to induce ovulation in infertility that is caused by inadequate stimulation of the ovary by endogenous gonadotropic hormones. Excessive stimulation of the ovary may result in vast enlargement of the gland, maturation of many follicles, multiple pregnancy, bleeding into the abdomen, and pain. Also called **gonadotrophin.** –**gonadotropic, gonadotrophic,** *adj.*

gonadotropin-releasing hormone (GnRH) [Gk, *gone,* seed, *trope,* a turn; ME, *relesen*; Gk, *hormaein,* to set in motion], a decapeptide hypophysiotropic hormone secreted by the hypothalamus. It stimulates the release of gonadotropin hormone by the anterior pituitary gland. It also stimulates the release of the **luteinizing hormone (LH)** and **follicle-stimulating hormone (FSH)** by the anterior pituitary.

gonial angle. See **angle of mandible.**

-gonic, a suffix meaning 'work required to facilitate a specified reaction': *dysgonic, endergonic, exergonic.*

gonio-, a combining form meaning 'pertaining to an angle': *goniocraniometry, goniometer, gonion.*

goniometer /gon'ē·om'ətər/, an instrument used to measure angles, particularly range-of-motion angles of a joint.

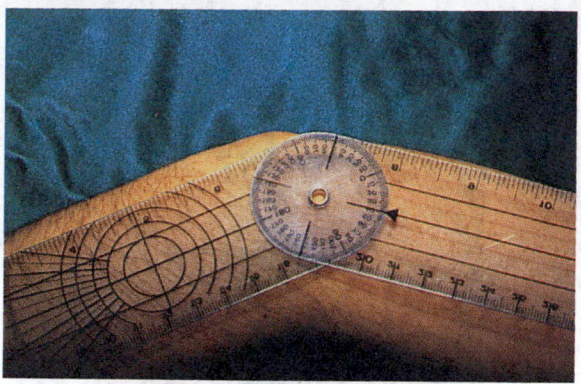

Goniometer (Schumacher, 1988)

goniometry /gon'ē·om'ətrē/ [Gk, *gonia*, angle, *metron*, measure], a system of testing for various labyrinthine diseases that affect the sense of balance. One test uses a plank, one end of which may be raised to any desired height. The patient stands on the plank as one end is gradually raised, and the point where the patient can no longer maintain balance is noted. **–goniometric,** *adj.*

gonioscope /gō'nē·əskōp'/ [Gk, *gonia* + *skopein,* to look], an ophthalmoscope used to examine the angle of the anterior chamber of the eye and for demonstrating ocular motility and rotation.

goniotomy /gōn'ē·ot'əmē/, an eye operation performed to remove any obstruction to the flow of aqueous humor in the front chamber of the eye. The procedure is commonly done in cases of glaucoma.

gono-, gon-, a prefix meaning 'pertaining to semen or seed': *gonococcin, gonophore, gonotome.*

gonoblast. See **germ cell.**

gonococcal /gon'əkok'əl/ [Gk, *gone,* seed, *kokkos,* berry], pertaining to or resembling gonococcus.

gonococcal pyomyositis [Gk, *gone,* seed, *kokkos,* berry; *pyon,* pus, *mys,* muscle, *itis,* inflammation], an acute inflammatory condition of a muscle caused by infection with a *Neisseria gonorrhoeae,* characterized by abscess formation and pain. It is an unusual form of gonorrhea and must be differentiated from sarcoma. The diagnosis is made by the discovery of the gonococcal diplococci within the abscess when a bacterial culture of a specimen is prepared after exploratory surgery. The patient is then usually found to be asymptomatically infected in the urogenital organs. Antibiotic treatment, most often with ceftriaxone, is rapidly effective in curing the infection.

gonococcal salpingitis [Gk, *gone,* seed, *kokkos,* berry, *salpigx,* tube, *itis,* inflammation], an inflammation of the fallopian tubes caused by a gonoccal infection. Also called **gonorrheal salpingitis.**

gonococcal urethritis [Gk, *gone,* seed, *kokkos,* berry, *ourethra,* urethra, *itis,* inflammation], an inflammation of the urethra caused by a gonococcal infection. Also called **gonorrheal urethritis.**

gonococcus /gon'əkok'əs/, *pl.* **gonococci** /gon'əkok'sī/ [Gk, *gone* + *kokkos,* berry], a gram-negative, intracellular diplococcus of the species *Neisseria gonorrhoeae,* the cause of gonorrhea. A nonmotile, aerobic microorganism of

the species *Neisseria gonorrhoeae.* It is a parasite of the mucous membrane and the cause of **gonorrhea.**

gonocyte. See **germ cell.**

gonorrhea /gon'ərē'ə/ [Gk, *gone* + *rhoia,* flow], a common sexually transmitted disease most often affecting the genitourinary tract and, occasionally, the pharynx, conjunctiva, or rectum. Infection results from contact with an infected person or by contact with secretions containing the causative organism *Neisseria gonorrhoeae.* Gonorrheal infections must be reported to local health departments in the United States **–gonorrheal, gonorrheic,** *adj.*

■ OBSERVATIONS: Urethritis, dysuria, purulent, greenish-yellow urethral or vaginal discharge, red or edematous urethral meatus, and itching, burning, or pain around the vaginal or urethral orifice are characteristic. The vagina may be massively swollen and red, and the lower abdomen may be tense and very tender. As the infection spreads, which is more common in women than in men, nausea, vomiting, fever, and tachycardia may occur as salpingitis, oophoritis, or peritonitis develops. Inflammation of the tissues surrounding the liver also may occur, causing pain in the upper right quadrant of the abdomen. Severe disseminated infection is also more common in women than in men and is characterized by signs of septicemia with polyarthritis, tender papillary lesions on the skin of the hands and feet, and inflammation of the tendons of the wrists, knees, and ankles. Gonoccocal ophthalmia involves infection of the conjunctiva and may lead to scarring and blindness. Gonorrhea is diagnosed by bacteriologic culture of the organism from a smear obtained from a specimen of exudate. In men a microscopic study of a gram-stained specimen of exudate that reveals gram-negative intracellular diplococci is diagnostic of gonorrheal infection, but this finding is not diagnostic in women.

■ INTERVENTIONS: The recommended regimen for uncomplicated gonorrhea is ceftriaxone 250 mg IM once plus Doxycycline 100 mg orally twice daily for 7 days. Generally, patients with gonorrhea infections should be treated simultaneously for presumptive chlamydial infections. Treatment

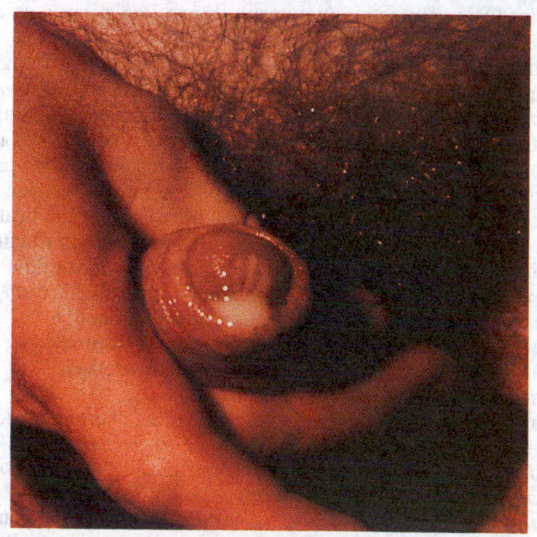

Gonorrhea in the male (Morse, 1990)

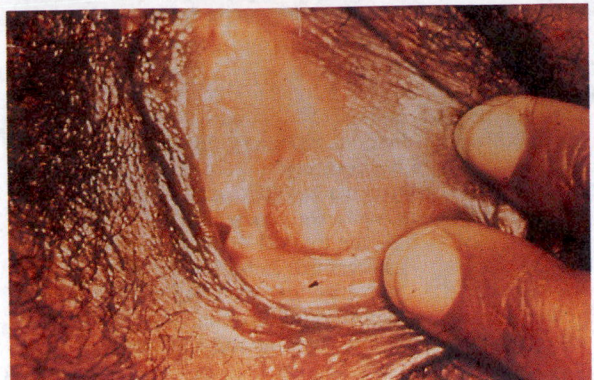

Gonorrhea in the female *(Morse, 1990)*

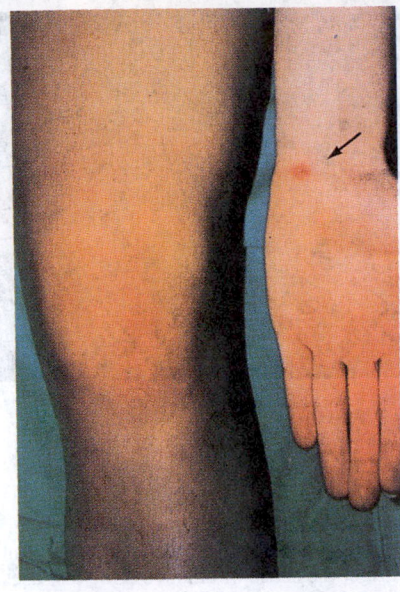

Gonorrheal arthritis of the knee
(Shipley, 1993/Courtesy Dr Rob Miller)

failure of this regimen is rare, therefore a follow-up culture for test-of-cure is not essential. The routine instillation of 1% silver nitrate in the eyes of the newborn provides effective prophylaxis against infection in the newborn period that might otherwise result from contact with the infected secretions of an asymptomatic infected mother during vaginal delivery.

■ NURSING CONSIDERATIONS: It is important that the patient's sexual contacts be treated. Before giving any antibiotic, it is ascertained that the patient does not have any known sensitivity to the drug being given and that equipment and drugs are available to treat any hypersensitivity reaction that may occur. The patient is alerted that precaution against spread of the disease is recommended in the future through condom use or monogamous sexual relations.

gonorrheal /gon′ərē′əl/ [Gk, *gone*, seed, *kokkos*], pertaining to or resembling gonorrhea.

gonorrheal arthritis [Gk, *gone*, seed, *kokkos*, berry, *arthron*, joint, *itis*, inflammation], a blood-borne gonococcal infection of the joints. It may affect one or several joints, may occur as a chronic or acute form, and often leads to joint fusion. Infection may result in pus formation in an affected joint.

gonorrheal conjunctivitis, a severe, destructive form of purulent conjunctivitis caused by the gonococcus *Neisseria gonorrhoeae*. Prompt treatment by the intravenous administration of antibiotics is required to prevent scarring of the cornea and blindness. Newborn infants receive routine prophylaxis of a topical instillation of 1% solution of silver nitrate or an antibiotic ointment, which has largely eradicated the infection in infants. See also **ophthalmia neonatorum.**

gonorrheal proctitis [Gk, *gone*, seed + *rhoia*, flow + *proktos*, anus + *itis*, inflammation], an inflammation of the rectum caused by an infection of gonorrhea.

gonorrheal salpingitis. See **gonococcal salpingitis.**

gonorrheal urethritis. See **gonococcal urethritis.**

gonnorheic. See **gonorrhea.**

gony-, gon-, a combining form meaning 'pertaining to a knee': *gonycampsis, gonyectyposis, gonyoncus.*

-gony, a suffix meaning 'birth, origin, or procreation': *amphigony, merogony, zoogony.*

Gonyaulax catanella /gon′ē-ô′laks/, a species of planktonic protozoa that produces a toxin ingested by shellfish along the coasts of North America, resulting in seafood poisoning. Also called **red tide** because it colors the sea red in an infected area.

Goodell's sign /gōōdelz′/ [William Goodell, American gynecologist, b. 1829], softening of the uterine cervix, a probable sign of pregnancy.

Goodpasture's syndrome /gŏŏd′pas·chər/ [Ernest W. Goodpasture, American pathologist, b. 1886], a chronic, relapsing pulmonary hemosiderosis, usually associated with glomerulonephritis and characterized by a cough with hemoptysis, dyspnea, anemia, and progressive renal failure. Mild forms of the syndrome may respond to corticosteroids or immunosuppressive drugs. Severe recurrent cases have a poor prognosis; hemodialysis and kidney transplantation are the only treatments.

Goodrich, Annie Warburton (1866–1954), an American nursing educator, instrumental in bringing nursing from an apprenticeship to a profession. She was superintendent of nurses at several New York hospitals before going to Teachers College, Columbia University, in 1914. In addition to teaching, she was associated with the Henry Street Settlement and the Nursing Department of the U.S. Army. In 1923 she became dean of the newly formed School of Nursing at Yale University, which awarded a degree similar to that awarded in other professions.

Good Samaritan legislation /səmar′itən/ [good Samaritan, from New Testament parable; L, *lex*, law, *lator*, proposer], laws enacted in some states to protect physicians, dentists, nuses, and some other health professionals from liability in rendering emergency medical or dental aid, unless there is proven willful wrong or gross negligence.

gooseflesh. See **pilomotor reflex.**

Gordon's elementary body [Mervyn H. Gordon, English physician, b. 1872], a particle found in tissues containing eosinophils once thought to be the viral cause of Hodgkin's disease. Also called **Gordon's encephalopathic agent.**

Gordon's reflex [Alfred Gordon, American neurologist, b.

1874], **1.** an abnormal variation of Babinski's reflex, elicited by compressing the calf muscles, characterized by extension of the great toe and fanning of the other toes. It is evidence of disease of the pyramidal tract. **2.** an abnormal reflex, elicited by compressing the forearm muscles, characterized by flexion of the fingers or of the thumb and index finger. It is seen in diseases of the pyramidal tract. Compare **Chaddock reflex, Oppenheim's reflex.** See also **Babinski's reflex.**

Gosselin's fracture /gôslaNz'/ [Leon A. Gosselin, French surgeon, b. 1815], a V-shaped fracture of the distal tibia, extending to the ankle.

GOT, abbreviation for **glutamic-oxaloacetic transaminase.**

goundou /gōōn'dōō/ [West African], a condition characterized by bony exostoses of the nasal and maxillary bones, usually occurring as a late sequela of yaws in people in Africa and Latin America.

gout [L, *gutta*, drop], a disease associated with an inborn error of uric acid metabolism that increases production or interferes with excretion of uric acid. Excess uric acid is converted to sodium urate crystals that precipitate from the blood and become deposited in joints and other tissues. Men are more often affected than women. The great toe is a common site for the accumulation of urate crystals. The condition can result in exceedingly painful swelling of a joint, accompanied by chills and fever. The symptoms are recurrent; episodes become longer each year. The disorder is disabling and, if untreated, can progress to the development of tophi and destructive joint changes. Treatment usually includes administration of colchicine, phenylbutazone, indomethacin, or glucocorticoid drugs, a diet that excludes purine-rich foods, such as organ meats, and may include surgical removal of tophi. Acquired gout is a condition having the signs and symptoms of gout but occurring as a result of another disorder or treatment for a different condition. Diuretic drugs can alter the concentration of uric acid so that uric acid salts precipitate from the blood and are carried to the joints. See also **chondrocalcinosis, Lesch-Nyhan syndrome, tophus.**

gouty /gou'tē/ [L, *gutta*, drop], pertaining to or resembling the condition of gout.

gouty arthritis. See **gout.**

Gowers' muscular dystrophy. See **distal muscular dystrophy.**

GP, abbreviation for **general practitioner.**

GPI, *obsolete.* abbreviation for *general paralysis of the insane.* See **general paresis.**

gp160, code for a glycoprotein that provides an outer coat for the HIV (human immunodeficiency virus). The outer coat, in turn, is composed of **gp120,** which protrudes from the virus surface, and **gp41,** which is embedded in the envelope coat.

GPT, abbreviation for **glutamic-pyruvic transaminase.** See **alanine aminotransferase.**

gr, abbreviation for **grain.**

graafian follicle /grä'fē·ən, -grä'-/ [Reijnier de Graaf, Dutch physician, b. 1641; L, *folliculus,* small bag] /gräf'/, a mature ovarian vesicle, measuring about 10 to 12 mm in diameter, that ruptures during ovulation to release the ovum. Many primary ovarian follicles, each containing an immature ovum about 35 [mu] in diameter, are imbedded near the surface of the ovary, just below the tunica albuginea. Under the influence of the follicle stimulating hormone from the adenohypophysis, one ovarian follicle ripens into a graafian follicle during the proliferative phase of each menstrual cycle. The cells that form the graafian follicle are arranged in a layer three to four cells thick around a relatively large volume of follicular fluid. Within the follicle the ovum grows to about 100 [mu] in diameter and, when the follicle ruptures, is swept into the fimbriated opening of the uterine tube. The cavity of the follicle collapses when the ovum is released, and the remaining follicular cells greatly enlarge to become the corpus luteum. If the ovum is fertilized, the corpus luteum grows and becomes the corpus luteum of pregnancy that, at the end of 9 months, has a diameter of about 30 mm. As the ovarian follicle ripens into the graafian follicle, it produces estrogen, which stimulates the proliferation of the endometrium and the enlargement of the uterine glands. The growing corpus luteum produces progesterone, which triggers endometrial gland secretion and prepares the uterus to receive the fertilized ovum. If the ovum is not fertilized, the graafian follicle forms the corpus luteum of menstruation, which degenerates, leaving the small scarred corpus albicans.

gracile /gras'il/, long, slender, and graceful.

gracilis /gras'ilis/, the most superficial of the five medial femoral muscles. A thin, flattened muscle that is broad proximally and narrow distally, it originates in a thin aponeurosis secured on the inferior aspect of the symphysis pubis and the superior half of the pubic arch. The muscle curves around the medial condyle of the tibia and inserts into the body of the tibia, distal to the condyle. It is innervated by a branch of the obturator nerve, which contains fibers from the third and fourth lumbar nerves, and it functions to adduct the thigh and flex the leg and to assist in the medial rotation of the leg after it is flexed. Compare **adductor brevis, adductor longus, adductor magnus, pectineus.**

gradation of activity /gradā'shən/, therapeutic activities that are appropriately paced and modified to demand maximal capacities at any point in progression or regression of the patient's condition.

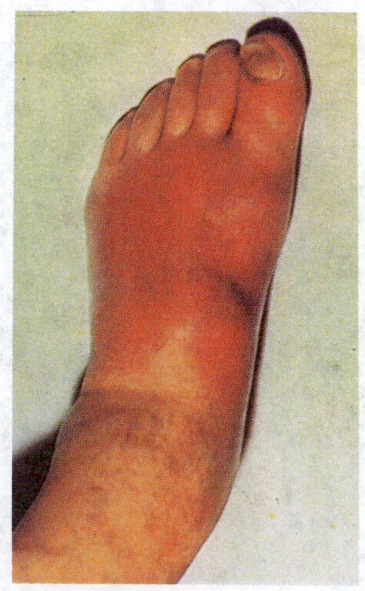

Gout *(Shipley, 1993)*

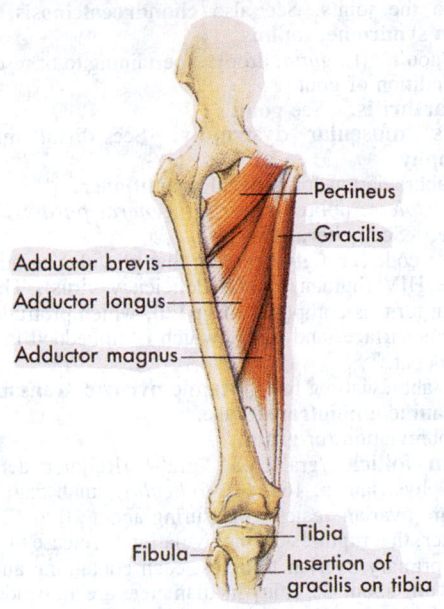

Gracilis muscle *(Thibodeau, 1993)*

Labels: Pectineus, Gracilis, Adductor brevis, Adductor longus, Adductor magnus, Tibia, Fibula, Insertion of gracilis on tibia

graded exercise test (GXT), a test given a cardiac patient during rehabilitation to assess prognosis and quantify maximal functional capacity. The test is given before discharge to determine guidelines for activity programs at home and work during convalescence. See also **exercise electrocardiogram.**

gradient /grā′dē·ənt/ [L, *gradus,* step], **1.** the rate of increase or decrease of a measurable phenomenon, such as temperature or pressure. **2.** a visual representation of the rate of change of a measurable phenomenon; a curve.

gradient magnetic field, a magnetic field that changes in strength in a certain given direction. Such fields are used in NMR imaging to select a region for imaging and also to encode the location of NMR signals received from the object being imaged.

graduated bath /graj′o͞o·a′tid/ [L, *gradus,* step; AS, *baeth*], a bath in which the temperature of the water is slowly reduced.

graduated resistance exercise. See **progressive resistance exercise.**

graduate medical education /graj′o͞o·it/, formal medical education pursued after receipt of M.D. or other professional degree in the medical sciences. Graduate medical education is usually obtained as an intern, resident, or fellow, or in continuing medical education programs.

Graduate Medical Education National Advisory Committee (GMENAC), a committee established by order of the Secretary of the Department of Health, Education and Welfare (now the Department of Health and Human Services) to study the personnel issues in medicine. The Committee issued its final report in September 1980. Among its conclusions was that the supply of nurses in expanded roles, including nurse practitioners and nurse midwives, should be increased.

graduate nurse (GN) [L, *gradus,* step, *nutrix,* nurse], a nurse who is a graduate of an accredited school of nursing.

Graduate Record Examination (GRE), an examination administered to graduates of institutions of higher learning. The scores are used as criteria for admission to masters and doctoral programs in many institutions and areas of specialization, including nursing. The examination tests verbal and mathematic aptitudes and abilities.

GRAE, abbreviation for **generally recognized as effective.**

graft [Gk, *graphion,* stylus], a tissue or an organ taken from a site or a person and inserted into a new site or person, performed to repair a defect in structure. The graft may be temporary, such as an emergency skin transplant for extensive burns, or permanent with the grafted tissue growing to become a part of the body. Skin, bone, cartilage, blood vessel, nerve, muscle, cornea, and whole organs, such as the kidney or the heart, may be grafted. Preoperative care focuses on a high protein diet and vitamins to ensure optimum physical condition and on freedom from infection. Under general or local anesthesia the tissue is transferred and sutured into place. Rejection is the major complication: fever, pain in the graft area, and evidence of loss of function 4 to 15 days after the procedure are indicative of rejection. Immunosuppressive drugs are given in large doses to suppress antibody production and rejection. Even if an early reaction is blocked, late rejection may occur 1 year or more after the graft is done. Also called **transplant.** See also **allograft, autograft, isograft, skin graft, xenograft.**

graft-versus-host reaction, a rejection response of certain grafts, especially bone marrow. It involves an incompatibility resulting from a deficiency in the immune response of some patients and is commonly associated with inadequate immunosuppressive therapy. Characteristic signs may include skin lesions with edema, erythema, ulceration, scal-

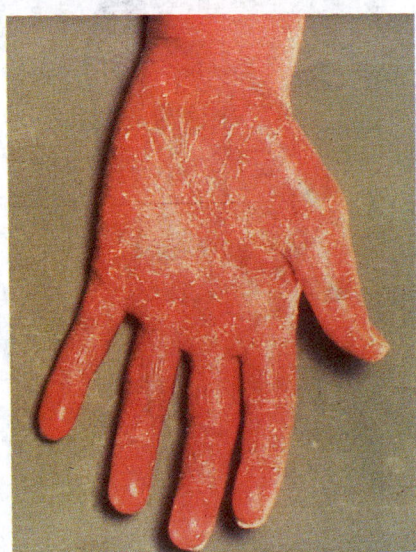

Graft versus host reaction *(Hewitt, 1985)*

ing, and loss of hair. Such reactions also may cause lesions of the joints and the heart and hemolytic anemia with a positive Coombs' reaction. The graft-versus-host reaction is similar to the type IV reaction in hypersensitive individuals who receive tuberculin injections. Some experts believe that it involves certain immunologically active cells that originate as the result of defective tolerance mechanisms or as the result of somatic mutation of certain host cells. Also called **homologous disease.**

Graham's law /grā′əmz/, the law stating that the rate of diffusion of a gas through a liquid (or the alveolar-capillary membrane) is directly proportional to its solubility coefficient and inversely proportional to the square root of its density.

grain (gr) [L, *granum*, seed], the smallest unit of mass in avoirdupois, troy, and apothecaries' weights, being the same in all and equal to 4.79891 mg. The troy and apothecaries' ounces contain 480 grains; the avoirdupois ounce contains 437.5 grains.

gram (g, gm) [L, *gramma*, small weight], a unit of mass in the metric system equal to 1/1000 of a kilogram, 15.432 grains, and 0.0353 ounce avoirdupois. The preferred abbreviation is *g*.

-gram, -gramme, **1.** a combining form meaning a 'drawing' or a written record: *cephalogram, mammogram, electroencephalogram.* **2.** a combining form meaning '1/1000 kilogram': *centigram, decagram, microgram.*

gram calorie. See **calorie.**

gram-equivalent weight (gEq), an equivalent weight of a substance calculated as the gram mass that contains, replaces, or reacts with (directly or indirectly) the Avogadro number of hydrogen atoms. As 1 atom of sulfur (atomic weight 32) combines with 2 atoms of hydrogen (atomic weight 1), the gram equivalent weight of sulfur is 32/2 = 16.

gram-molecular weight (gmW), a mass in grams numerically equal to the molecular weight of a substance, or the sum of all the atomic weights in its molecular formula. In the example of carbon dioxide (CO_2), its gram molecular weight is 12 (atomic weight of carbon) + 2 × 16 (atomic weight of oxygen), or 44 g. See also **mole, molecular weight.**

gram-negative [Hans C. J. Gram, Danish physician, b. 1853; L, *negare,* to say no], having the pink color of the

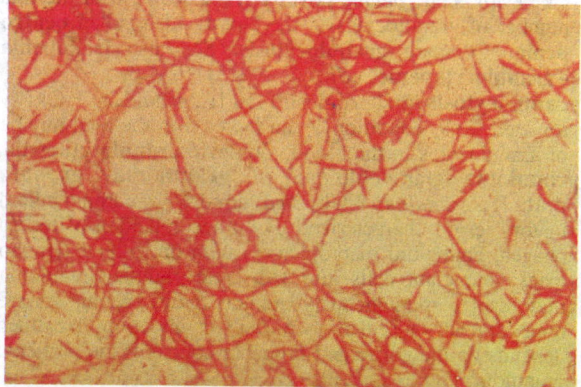

Gram-negative stain of *Fusobacterium nucleatum*
(Baron, 1990)

counterstain used in Gram's method of staining microorganisms. This property is a primary method of characterizing organisms in microbiology. Some of the most common gram-negative pathogenic bacteria are *Bacteroides fragilis, Brucella abortus, Escherichia coli, Haemophilus influenzae, Klebsiella pneumoniae, Neisseria gonorrhoeae, Proteus vulgaris, Pseudomonas aeruginosa, Salmonella typhi, Shigella dysenteriae,* and *Yersinia pestis.*

gram-positive [Hans C. J. Gram; L, *positivus*], retaining the violet color of the stain used in Gram's method of staining microorganisms. This property is a primary method of characterizing organisms in microbiology. Some of the most common kinds of gram-positive pathogenic bacteria are *Bacillus anthracis, Clostridium, Mycobacterium leprae, Mycobacterium tuberculosis, Staphylococcus aureus, Streptococcus pneumoniae,* and *Streptococcus pyogenes.*

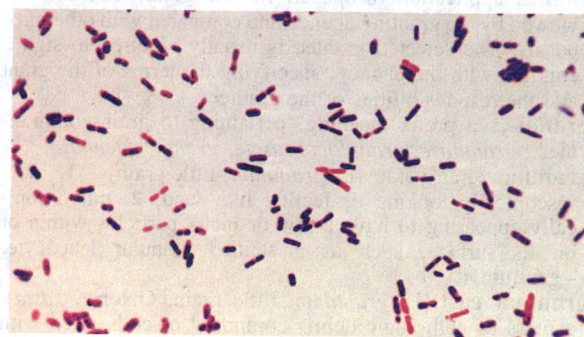

Gram-positive stain of *Clostridium perfringens*
(Baron 1990/from Sutter, VL, Citron, DM Edelstein, MAC, and Finegold SM, 1985. Wadsworth Anaerobic Bacteriology Manual, ed 4, Star Publishing Co., Belmont, CA)

Gram's stain [Hans C. J. Gram], the method of staining microorganisms using a violet stain, followed by an iodine solution, decolorizing with an alcohol or acetone solution, and counterstaining with safranin. The retention of either the violet color of the stain or the pink color of the counterstain serves as a primary means of identifying and classifying bacteria. Also called **Gram's method.** See also **gram-negative, gram-positive.**

grandiose /gran′dē·ōs′/ [L, *grandis,* great], pertaining to something or somebody imposing, impressive, magnificent, or also pompous and showy.

grand mal seizure /gräN·mäl′/ [Fr, great; illness; *saisir,* to seize], an epileptic seizure characterized by a generalized involuntary muscular contraction and cessation of respiration followed by tonic and clonic spasms of the muscles. Breathing resumes with noisy respirations. The teeth may be clenched, the tongue bitten, and control of the bladder or bowel lost. As this phase of the seizure passes, the person may fall asleep or experience confusion. Usually, the person has no recall of the seizure on awakening. A sensory warning, or aura, can precede each tonic-clonic seizure. These seizures may occur singly, at intervals, or in close succession. Anticonvulsant medications are usually prescribed as prophylaxis against tonic-clonic seizures. Also called **tonic-clonic seizure.** Compare **absence seizure, focal seizure, psychomotor seizure.**

grand multipara /grand/ [L, *grandis*, great, *multus*, many, *parere*, to give birth], a woman who has carried six or more pregnancies to a viable stage.

grand rounds [L, *grandis, rotundus*, wheel], a formal conference in which one usually expert person presents a lecture concerning a clinical issue intended to be educational for the listeners. Charts, tables, films, slides, tapes, and demonstrations are often used in presentation at grand rounds. Historically the patient was present. In some settings grand rounds may be formal teaching rounds conducted by an expert at the bedsides of selected patients.

grant [ME, *granten*, to believe a request], an award given to an institution, a project, or an individual usually consisting of a sum of money. A grant is given by a granting agency, the federal government, a foundation, private enterprise, or institution to provide financial support for research, service, or training. The applicant usually writes a formal application (proposal) for the grant, which is reviewed by the granting agency and compared with other proposals. The selected grantee is usually required to sign a contract with the agency, specifying the terms of the grant and the responsibilities of the grantee.

granul-, a prefix meaning 'pertaining to grains or granules': *granulase, granulocorpuscle, granulocytemia.*

granular /gran'yələr/ [L, *granulum*, little grain], **1.** macroscopically looking or feeling like sand. **2.** microscopically appearing to have a few or many particles within or on its surface, such as a stained granular leucocyte. **–granularity,** *n.*

granular cast [L, *granulum*, little grain, ONorse, *kasta*], a mass of pathologic debris composed of cells filled with protein and fatty granules.

granular conjunctivitis. See **trachoma.**

granular endoplasmic reticulum. See **endoplasmic reticulum.**

granularity. See **granular.**

granulation tissue /gran'yələ'shən/ [L, *granulum*, little grain], any soft, pink, fleshy projections that form during the healing process in a wound not healing by first intention. It consists of many capillaries surrounded by fibrous collagen. Overgrowth of granulation tissue results in proud flesh growing above the skin. See also **pyogenic granuloma.**

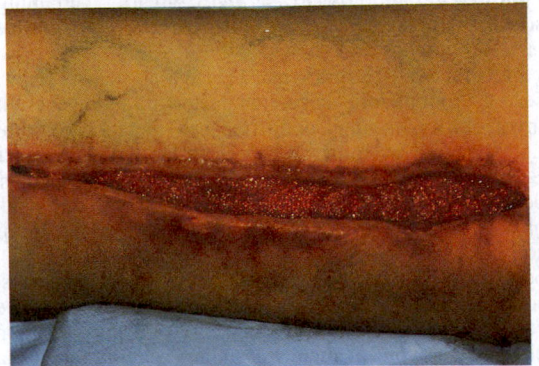

Granulation tissue
(Bryant, 1992/Courtesy Abbott Northwestern Hospital, Minneapolis)

granule /gran'yo͞ol/ [L, *granulum*, little grain], a particle, grain, or other small dry mass capable of free movement. Unlike powders, granules are usually free flowing because of small surface forces involved.

granulitis /gran'yəlī'tis/ [L, *granulum*, little grain; Gk, *itis*, inflammation], acute miliary tuberculosis.

granulocyte /gran'yo͞oləsīt'/ [L, *granulum* + Gk, *kytos*, cell], a type of leukocyte characterized by the presence of cytoplasmic granules. Kinds of granulocytes are **basophil, eosinophil,** and **neutrophil.** Compare **agranulocyte.**

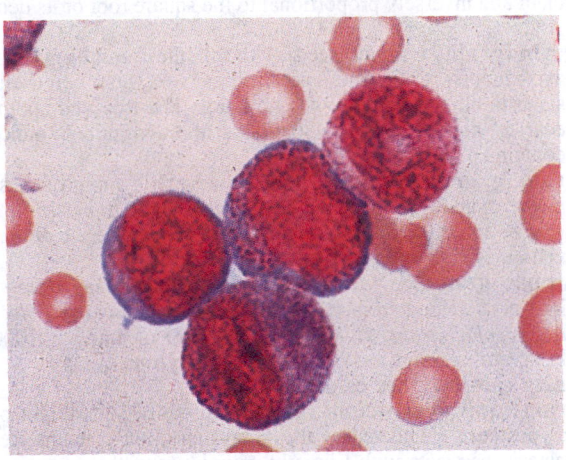

Granulocytes *(Hayhoe, 1992)*

granulocyte transfusion, the use of specially prepared leukocytes for the treatment of severe granulocytopenia and prophylactically for the prevention of serious infection in patients with leukemia or those receiving cancer chemotherapy. The procedure has the same risks as a blood transfusion. Also called **buffy coat transfusion.**

granulocytic leukemia. See **acute myelocytic leukemia, chronic myelocytic leukemia.**

granulocytic sarcoma. See **chloroma.**

granulocytopenia /gran'yo͞olōsī'tōpē'nē·ə/ [L, *granulum* + Gk, *kytos*, cell, *penia*, poverty], A decrease in the total number of granulocytes in the blood. Also called **neutropenia.** Compare **granulocytosis.** See also **leukopenia.** **–granulocytopenic,** *adj.*

granulocytosis /gran'yo͞olōsītō'sis/ [L, *granulum* + Gk, *kytos*, cell, *osis*, condition], an increase in the total number of granulocytes in the blood. Compare **granulocytopenia.**

granuloma /gran'yo͞olō'mə/, *pl.* **granulomas, granulomata** [L, *granulum* + Gk, *oma*, tumor], a chronic inflammatory lesion characterized by an accumulation of macrophages, epitheloid macrophages, with or without lymphocytes, and giant cells into a discrete granule. Granulomas may resolve spontaneously, remain static, become gangrenous, spread, or remain as a focus of infection. Treatment depends on the cause and probable course of the particular granuloma.

-granuloma, a combining form meaning a 'tumorlike mass or nodule of granulation tissue': *paragranuloma, ulcerogranuloma, xanthogranuloma.*

granuloma annulare, a self-limited, chronic skin disease of unknown cause that consists of reddish papules and nodules arranged in a ring. It is most commonly seen on the distal portions of the extremities in children. No treatment is necessary.

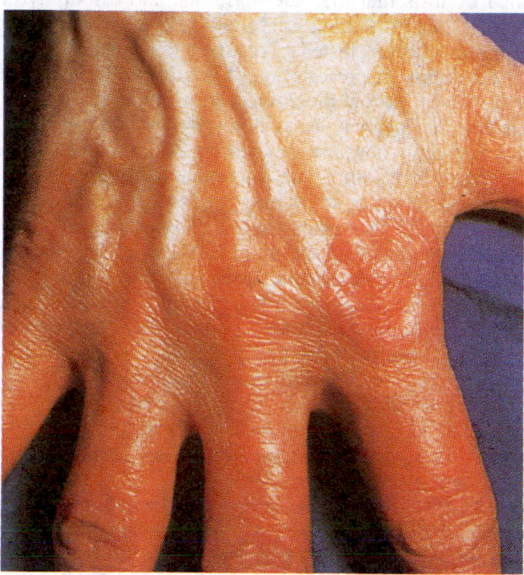

Granuloma annulare *(McKee, 1993)*

granuloma gluteale infantum, a skin condition of the neonate characterized by large, elevated bluish or brownish-red nodules on the buttocks, often occurring as a secondary reaction to the application of strong steroid salves over a period of time. The lesions routinely disappear within a couple of months after the use of the preparations is discontinued.

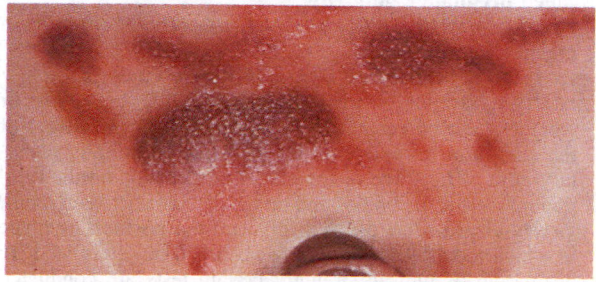

Granuloma gluteale infantum
(du Vivier, 1993/Courtesy David Atherton)

granuloma inguinale, a sexually transmitted disease characterized by ulcers of the skin and subcutaneous tissues of the groin and genitalia. It is caused by infection with *Calymmatobacterium granulomatis,* a small, gram-negative, rod-shaped bacillus. The diagnosis is made by the microscopic examination and identification of characteristic "safety-pin"-shaped bodies in the cytoplasm of phagocytes

taken from a lesion and dyed with Wright's stain. Untreated, the lesions spread, deepen, multiply, and become secondarily infected. Streptomycin is usually effective in treating the infection. All patients who have or are suspected of having granuloma inguinale are also tested for syphilis, because concurrent infection is common.

granulomatosis /gran′yŏŏlōmətō′sis/ [L, *granulum* + Gk, *oma*, tumor, *osis*, condition], a condition or disease characterized by the development of granulomas, such as **berylliosis, pulmonary Wegener's granulomatosis,** or **Wegener's granulomatosis.**

granulomatous /gran′yəlom′ətəs/ [L, *granulum*, little grain], pertaining to or resembling granulomas.

granulomatous lipophagia [L, *granulum*, little grain; Gk, *lipos*, fat, *phagein*, to eat], a disease in which enlarged intestinal and mesenteric lymph spaces become filled with fats and fatty acids.

granulomatous thyroiditis. See **de Quervain's thyroiditis.**

granulosa cell carcinoma. See **granulosa cell tumor.**

granulosa cell tumor /gran′yŏŏlō′sə/ [L, *granulum*, little grain], a fleshy ovarian tumor with yellow streaks that originates in cells of the primordial membrana granulosa and may grow to a large size. Excessive production of estrogen, resulting in endometrial hyperplasia and menorrhagia, may be associated with the tumor.

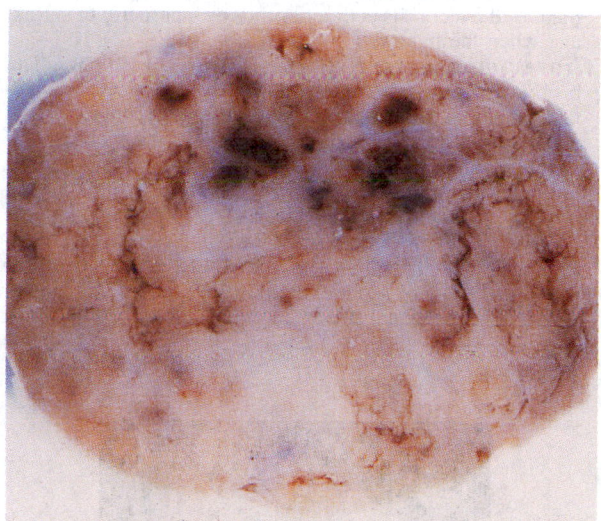

Granulosa cell tumor *(Turk, 1986)*

granulosa-theca cell tumor, an ovarian tumor composed of granulosa (follicular) cells or theca cells or both. The tumor is associated with excessive production of estrogen and hyperplasia of the breast and endometrium. See also **luteoma.**

granulosis /gran′yŏŏlō′sis/, any disorder characterized by an accumulation of granules in an area of body tissue, such as a skin eruption marked by tiny granules beneath the surface.

-graph, 1. a suffix meaning the 'product of drawing or writing': *hemophotograph, micrograph, retinograph.* **2.** a

-grapher, combining form meaning a 'machine for making something drawn': *clonograph, pneumograph, scopograph.*

-grapher, a suffix meaning 'one who writes about' something specified: *nosographer, syphilographer.*

-graphia, a suffix meaning an 'abnormality revealed through handwriting': *dysantigraphia, palingraphia.*

graphing /graf'ing/, the organization of data consisting of two or more variables along horizontal and vertical axes of a graph to show relationships between specific quantities or other specific factors.

grapho-, a combining form meaning 'pertaining to writing': *graphocatharsis, graphomania, graphophobia.*

graphospasm. See **writer's cramp.**

-graphy, a suffix meaning a 'kind of printing or process of recording': *arteriography, cardiography, dermagraphy.*

GRAS, abbreviation for *generally recognized as safe.*

grasp reflex [ME, *graspen,* grab; L, *reflectere,* to bend backward], a pathologic reflex induced by stroking the palm or sole with the result that the fingers or toes flex in a grasping motion. The reflex occurs in diseases of the premotor cortex. In young infants the tonic grasp reflex is normal: When an examiner strokes the infant's palms, the examiner's fingers are grasped so firmly that the child can be lifted into the air. Also called **darwinian reflex.**

grass. See **cannabis.**

grass-line ligature [AS, *graes;* L, *linea,* thread; *ligare,* to bind], a fine cord composed of the fibers of a grass-cloth plant, used in orthodontics for minor adjustments or movement of the teeth. Its action depends on a property of shrinkage when the ligature is wetted by saliva.

Graves' disease /grāvz/ [Robert J. Graves, Irish physician, b. 1796], a disorder characterized by pronounced hyperthyroidism usually associated with an enlarged thyroid gland and exophthalmos (abnormal protrusion of the eyeball). The origin is unknown, but the disease is familial and may be autoimmune; antibodies to thyroglobulin or to thyroid microsomes are found in more than 60% of patients with the disorder. Graves' disease, which is five times more common in women than in men, occurs most frequently between 20 and 40 years of age and often arises after an infection or physical or emotional stress. Typical signs are nervousness, a fine tremor of the hands, weight loss, fatigue, breathlessness, palpitations, increased heat intolerance, increased metabolic rate, and gastrointestinal motility. There may be an enlarged thymus, generalized hyperplasia of the lymph nodes, blurred or double vision, localized edema, atrial dysrhythmias, and osteoporosis. The diagnosis may be established by tests that measure thyroxine and triiodothyronine levels in serum. If necessary, radioactive iodine uptake in the gland may be tested. Treatment may include subtotal thyroidectomy or prescription of antithyroid drugs, such as methimazole, propylthiouracil, and iodine preparations. Radioactive iodine may be administered, but hospitalization for a few days is recommended for patients treated with a large dose. In patients with inadequately controlled Graves' disease, infection or stress may precipitate a life-threatening thyroid storm. The exophthalmia may or may not resolve with the treatment of the disease. Also called **exophthalmic goiter, thyrotoxicosis, toxic goiter.**

gravid /grav'id/ [L, *gravidus,* pregnant], pregnant; carrying fertilized eggs or a fetus. **–gravidity, gravidness,** *n.*

gravid-, a prefix meaning 'pertaining to pregnancy, or pregnant': *gravida, graviditas, gravidocardiac.*

gravida /grav'idə/ [L, *gravidus,* pregnant], a woman who is pregnant. The patient may be identified more specifically as **gravida I,** if pregnant for the first time, or **gravida II,** if pregnant a second time.

-gravida, a suffix meaning 'pregnant woman with (specified) quantity of pregnancies': *nonigravida, plurigravida, unigravida.*

gravida I or 1. See **primigravida.**

gravida II or 2. See **secundigravida.**

gravidarum chloasma /grav'ider'əm, grä'vidär'ōm/ [L, *gravidus,* pregnant; Gk, *chloazein,* to be green], a pigmentary change in the skin that occurs in some women during pregnancy. It usually occurs as patches of yellow, brown, or black discoloration.

gravidity, gravidness. See **gravid.**

gravidum gingivitis /grav'idəm/ [[L, *gravidus,* pregnant, *gingiva,* gums, *itis,* inflammation], a type of gum inflammation that is associated with plaque formation during pregnancy. It may be associated with hormonal changes. Also called **pregnancy gingivitis.**

gravid uterus [L, *gravidus,* pregnant, *uterus,* womb], a pregnant uterus.

gravimetric analysis. See **quantitative analysis.**

gravity /grav'itē/ [L, *gravis,* heavy], the heaviness or weight of an object resulting from the universal effect of the attraction between any body of matter and any planetary body. The force of the attraction depends on the relative masses of the bodies and on the distance between them.

gravity-eliminated plane, a supported position or plane in which the effect of gravity is absorbed or neutralized. In evaluation of muscle strength, certain tests are conducted in the gravity-eliminated plane. Other tests may involve movements against the force of gravity.

gray (Gy), the absorption of one joule per kilogram by material exposed to ionizing radiation. One gray equals 100 rad.

gray baby syndrome. See **gray syndrome.**

gray column. See **posterior column.**

gray hepatization. See **hepatization.**

gray matter. See **gray substance.**

gray scale, (in ultrasonograpy) a property of the display in which intensity information is recorded as changes in the brightness of the display.

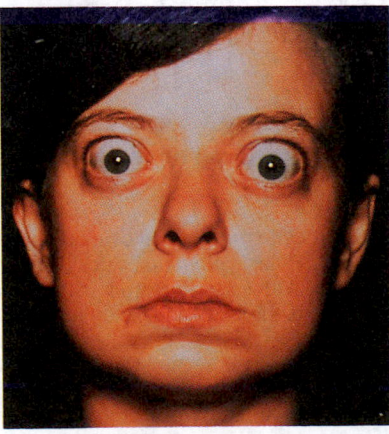

Graves' disease
(Seidel, 1991/Courtesy Paul W Ladenson, MD, The Johns Hopkins University and Hospital, Baltimore)

gray scale display, (in ultrasonography) a signal-processing method of selectively amplifying and displaying the level echoes from soft tissues at the expense of the larger echoes. Also called **compression amplification.**

gray substance [AS, *graeg;* L, *substantia*], the gray tissue that makes up the inner core of the spinal column, arranged in two large lateral masses connected across the midline by a narrow commissure. Each lateral portion of the gray substance splays outward, forming the posterior and anterior horns of the spinal cord. The horns consist primarily of cell bodies of interneurons and cell bodies of motor-neurons. The quantity of gray substance varies greatly at different levels of the cord, and its shape is characteristic at each level. In the thoracic region, the gray substance is small in comparison with surrounding white substance; in the cervical and the lumbar regions it is larger; and in the conus medullaris its proportion to the white substance is the greatest. Nuclei in the gray matter of the spinal cord function as centers for all spinal reflexes. Also called **gray matter.** Compare **white substance.** See also **spinal cord, spinal nerves.**

gray syndrome, a toxic condition in neonates, especially premature infants, caused by a reaction to chloramphenicol. Because the body's mechanisms for detoxification and excretion of drugs are immature, the infant has limited ability to conjugate and thus eliminate the chloramphenicol. The name of the condition comes from a characteristic ashen-gray cyanosis, which is accompanied by abdominal distention, hypothermia, vomiting, respiratory distress, and vascular collapse. The condition, which is fatal if the drug is continued, can be prevented by conservative dosages of the drug and by restricting its use in women during late pregnancy or labor (because chloramphenicol readily crosses the placental barrier) and in lactating mothers. Also called **gray baby syndrome.**

GRE, abbreviation for **Graduate Record Examination.**

great auricular nerve [AS, large; L, *auricula,* little ear, *nervus,* nerve], one of a pair of cutaneous branches of the cervical plexus, arising from the second and the third cranial nerves. It winds around the border of the sternocleido-mastoideus, perforates the deep fascia, and ascends on the surface of the muscle before dividing into the anterior branch and the posterior branch. The anterior branch is distributed to the skin of the face over the parotid gland, communicating within the gland with the facial nerve. The posterior branch supplies the skin of the mastoid process and the back of the auricula. It also communicates with the smaller occipital nerve, the auricular branch of the vagus nerve, and the posterior auricular branch of the facial nerve.

great calorie. See **calorie.**

great cardiac vein, one of the five tributaries of the coronary sinus, beginning at the apex of the heart and ascending along the anterior interventricular sulcus to the base of the ventricles. It then curves left in the coronary sulcus, reaches the back of the heart, and opens into the left part of the coronary sinus. It receives various tributaries from the left atrium, such as the large left marginal vein, which ascends along the left margin of the heart. The great cardiac vein drains the blood through its tributaries from the capillaries of the myocardium. Also called **vena cordis magna.** Compare **middle cardiac vein, small cardiac vein.**

greater multangular. See **trapezium.**

greater omentum [AS, *great,* large; L, *omentum,* entrails], a filmy, transparent extension of the peritoneum, draping the transverse colon and coils of the small intestine. It is attached along the greater curvature of the stomach and the first part of the duodenum, and between its two layers contains blood vessels and fat pads. Between the stomach and the colon the greater omentum forms the gastrocolic ligament, which contains the right and the left gastroepiploic blood vessels near the greater curvature of the stomach. The greater omentum is a very movable structure that spreads easily into areas of trauma, often sealing hernias and walling off infections that would otherwise cause general peritonitis, as can occur from a ruptured vermiform appendix. Also called **gastrocolic omentum.** Compare **lesser omentum.**

greater sciatic foramen [Gk, *ischiadikos,* hip joint; L, *foraminis,* a hole], an opening between the hip bone, sacrum, and sacrotuberous ligament.

greater sciatic notch [ME, *grete,* large; Gk, *ischiadikos,* hip joint; OFr, *enochier,* notch], a notch on the posterior border of the hip bone between the posterior inferior iliac spine and the spine of the ischium.

greater trochanter, a large projection of the femur, to which are attached various muscles, including the gluteus medius, gluteus maximus, and obturator internus. The greater trochanter projects from the angle formed by the neck and the body of the femur.

greater vestibular gland. See **Bartholin's gland.**

great saphenous vein, one of a pair of the longest veins in the body, containing 10 to 20 valves along its course through the leg and the thigh before ending in the femoral vein. It begins in the medial marginal vein of the dorsum of the foot and ascends anterior to the tibial malleolus and up the medial side of the leg in relation to the saphenous nerve. It runs posterior to the medial condyles of the tibia and the femur and passes through the hiatus saphenus just before joining the femoral vein. It contains more valves in the leg than in the thigh and receives many cutaneous veins and numerous tributaries, such as those from the sole of the foot. Near the saphenous hiatus it is joined by the superficial epigastric vein, the superficial epigastric circumflex, and the superficial external pudendal veins. Compare **common iliac vein, femoral vein.**

great vessels, the large arteries and veins entering and leaving the heart. They include the aorta, the pulmonary arteries and veins, and the superior and inferior venae cavae.

green cancer. See **chloroma.**

Greenfield's disease, a disorder of the white matter of the brain tissue, characterized by an accumulation of sphingolipid in both parenchymal and supportive tissues and a diffuse loss of myelination. An infantile form usually begins by the third year of life with symptoms that include loss of vision, rigidity, motor disorders, and mental deterioration. A juvenile form usually begins before the age of 10, and an adult form after the age of 16 marked by psychiatric symptoms that progress to dementia.

Greenough microscope. See **stereoscopic microscope.**

green soap [AS, *grene;,* L, *sapo*], a soft soap made from vegetable oils with sodium or potassium hydroxide with concentrations adjusted to retain the glycerol. The soap actually may be any color, depending on the ingredient oils added.

green soap tincture [AS, *grene,* L, *sapo,* soap, *tinctura,* dyeing], an alcoholic solution of green soap with lavendar oil added.

greenstick fracture [AS, *grene, stician*], an incomplete fracture in which the bone is bent but fractured only on the outer arc of the bend. Children are particularly likely to have greenstick fractures. Immobilization is usually effective, and healing is rapid. See also **fracture.**

-grel, a combining form for a platelet antiaggregate.

Grenz rays [Ger, *Grenze,* boundary; L, *radius,* emit rays], low-energy x-rays used for treatment of skin conditions. They have very little penetrating ability and are frequently applied by dermatologists rather than by radiotherapists.

Greulich-Pyle method /groi′lish-pīl′, grōo′lik-/, a technique for evaluating the bone age of children, using a single frontal radiograph of the left hand and wrist.

Grey Turner's sign, bruising of the skin of the loin in acute hemorrhagic pancreatitis. Also called **Turner's sign.**

grid [ME, *gredire,* a grate], (in radiology) a device used to absorb scattered radiation produced during an x-ray examination in the body of the patient. Such scatter does not contribute to the useful information and thus constitutes a source of unwanted noise. A grid selectively absorbs radiation that is not heading along straight lines from the x-ray source to the film. A **linear grid** is a simple x-ray grid consisting of parallel lead strips. Linear grids may result in variations in image density because of primary-photon attenuation. Density is at a maximum in the center of the film and decreases toward the edges.

grid cutoff, (in radiology) an undesirable absorption of primary-beam x-rays by the grid so that useful x-rays are literally cut off from the film. It is an effect of improper grid positioning but occurs most commonly with linear grids.

grief [L, *gravis,* heavy], a nearly universal pattern of physical and emotional responses to bereavement, separation, or loss. The physical components are similar to those of fear, hunger, rage, and pain. Stimulation of the sympathetic portion of the autonomic nervous system causes increased heart and respiratory rates, dilation of the pupils, sweating, bristling of the hair, increased flow of blood to the muscles, and increased reserves of energy. Digestion is slowed. The emotional components proceed in stages from alarm to disbelief and denial, to anger and guilt, to finding a source of comfort, and, finally, to adjustment to the loss. The way in which a grieving person behaves is greatly affected by the culture in which the person has been raised. See also **bereavement.**

grief reaction, a complex of somatic and psychologic symptoms associated with some extreme sorrow or loss, specifically the death of a loved one. Somatic symptoms include feelings of tightness in the throat and chest with choking and shortness of breath, abdominal distress, lack of muscular power, and extreme tiredness and lethargy. Psychologic reactions involve a generalized awareness of mental anguish and discomfort accompanied by feelings of guilt, anger, hostility, extreme restlessness, inability to concentrate, and the lack of capacity to initiate and maintain organized patterns of activities. Such symptoms may appear immediately after a crisis, or they may be delayed, exaggerated, or apparently absent, depending on the degree of involvement of the relationship and the physical and mental status of the person. Although both the somatic and psychologic reactions have the potential for developing into pathologic conditions, appropriate adaptive behavior and normal responses, such as sobbing or talking about the dead person or tragedy, are methods of working through the acute grief and lead to successful resolution of the crisis. Most acute grief reactions are resolved within 4 to 6 weeks, although the period varies and may be much longer, especially in cases of unexpected and sudden death. Interven-

tion by health care professionals, especially nurses, is necessary when individuals exhibit maladaptive behavioral patterns that avoid the resolution of grief and can lead to morbid reactions, including such accepted psychosomatic illnesses as asthma and ulcers. Also called **grief process.** See also **death, parental grief.**

grieving, anticipatory /an tis′əpətôr′ē/, a nursing diagnosis accepted by the Fourth National Conference on the Classification of Nursing Diagnoses. As a symptom, anticipatory grieving is grieving before an actual loss, as contrasted with grief in response to an actual loss. The cause of the condition, developed at the Fifth National Conference, is the perceived potential loss of a significant person in one's life, of one's physiopsychosocial well-being, or of one's personal possessions. The defining characteristics of the problem include the potential loss of something or someone important; expressions of distress; denial of potential loss; anger, guilt, or sorrow; and changes in eating habits, sleep patterns, activity level, libido, and patterns of communication. See also **nursing diagnosis.**

grieving, dysfunctional, a nursing diagnosis accepted by the Fourth National Conference on the Classification of Nursing Diagnoses. The cause of the problem is an actual or perceived loss of someone or something of great importance to the patient, thwarted grieving response to a loss, absence of anticipatory grieving, chronic fatal illness, or lack of resolution of a previous grieving response. The defining characteristics of the problem include expressions of distress or a denial of the loss; grief, anger, sadness, and weeping; changes in patterns and habits of sleeping, eating, and dreaming; and alterations in libido and activity levels. The lost person or object is idealized, past experience is relived, and concentration and purposeful work are diminished. The patient has a labile affect and seems to regress developmentally. See also **nursing diagnosis.**

griffe des orteils. See **pes cavus.**

Grifulvin, a trademark for an antifungal (griseofulvin).

grinder's asthma /grīn′dərz/ [ME, *grinden,* to crush; Gk, panting], a condition characterized by asthmatic symptoms caused by inhalation of fine particles produced by industrial grinding processes. See also **pneumoconiosis.**

grinder's disease. See **silicosis.**

grinding-in, a clinical corrective grinding of one or more natural or artificial teeth to improve centric and eccentric occlusions. Compare **selective grinding.**

grip and pinch strength, the measurable ability to exert pressure with the hand and fingers. It is measured by having a patient forcefully squeeze grip or pinch dynamometers, which may express results in either pounds or kilograms of pressure.

gripes /grīps/ [AS, *gripan,* to grasp], severe and usually spasmodic pain in the abdominal region caused by an intestinal disorder. Also called **gripping.**

grippe. See **influenza.**

gripping. See **gripes.**

Grisactin, a trademark for an antifungal (griseofulvin).

griseofulvin /gris′ē·ōful′vin/, an antifungal.

■ INDICATIONS: It is prescribed in the treatment of certain infections of the skin, hair, and nails.

■ CONTRAINDICATIONS: Liver dysfunction, porphyria, or known hypersensitivity to this drug prohibits its use.

■ ADVERSE EFFECTS: The most serious adverse reactions are blood dyscrasias. Headache, GI symptoms, and rashes also may occur.

Griswald brace, an orthosis for the control of vertebral body compression fractures. It is designed with two anterior forces with each equal to one half the posterior force to extend the spine. Also called **Jewett brace.**

Grocco's sign. See **Korányi's sign.**

Grocco triangle. See **Korányi's sign.**

grocer's itch [AS, *gican*, itch], a parasitic dermatitis caused by contact with mites found in grain, cheese, or dried foods. *Glyciphagus domesticus.*

groin [ME, *grynde*], each of two areas where the abdomen joins the thighs.

Grönblad-Strandberg syndrome /grōn′bladstrand′bərg/ [Ester E. Grönblad, Swedish ophthalmologist, b. 1898; James V. Strandberg, twentieth century Swedish dermatologist], an autosomal recessive disorder of connective tissue characterized by premature aging and breakdown of the skin, gray or brown streaks on the retina, and hemorrhagic arterial degeneration, including retinal bleeding that causes loss of vision. Angina pectoris and hypertension are common; weak pulse, episodic claudication, and fatigue with exertion may affect the extremities. The prognosis depends on vessel involvement, but life expectancy is shortened by the condition. Treatment is symptomatic. Also called **pseudoxanthoma elasticum.**

groove [AS, *grafan*, to dig], a shallow, linear depression in various structures throughout the body, as those that form channels for nerves along the bones, those in bones for the insertion of muscles, and those between certain areas of the brain.

gross [OFr, *gros*, large], **1.** macroscopic, as *gross pathology*, from the study of tissue changes without magnification by a microscope. **2.** large or obese. Compare **microscopic.**

gross anatomy, the study of the organs or parts of the body large enough to be seen with the naked eye. Also called **macroscopic anatomy.**

Grossman principle, (in tomography) the principle that when the fulcrum or axis of rotation remains at a fixed height, the focal place level is changed by raising or lowering the table top through this fixed point to the desired height.

gross motor skills [Fr, *gros*, big; L, *movere*, ONorse, *skilja*, to cut apart], the use of large muscle groups that coordinate body movements required for normal living, such as walking, running, jumping, throwing, and balance.

gross sensory testing, an evaluation procedure that usually precedes motor evaluation of a patient and includes assessment of passive motion sense in the shoulder, elbow, wrist, and fingers and ability to localize touch stimuli to specific fingers.

gross visual skills, the general ability of a person to track a large, bright object side-to-side or up-to-down without jerkiness, nystagmus, or convergence and to discriminate among various basic shapes and colors.

ground [AS, *grund*], **1.** (in electricity) a connection between the electric circuit and the ground, which becomes a part of the circuit. **2.** (in psychology) the background of a visual field that can enhance or inhibit the ability of a patient to focus on an object. See also **figure-ground.**

ground itch, pruritic papules, urticarial, vesiculo-pustular lesions secondary to penetration of the skin by hookworm larvae. The condition is prevalent in tropic and subtropic climates and may be prevented by wearing shoes and by establishing sanitary disposal of feces. See also **hookworm.**

ground stake. See **fatigue state.**

ground substance. See **matrix.**

group [Fr, *groupe*, cluster], (in research) any set of items or groups of people under study. An **experimental group** is studied to determine the effect of an event, a substance, or a technique. A **control group** serves as a standard or reference for comparison with an experimental group. A control group is similar to the experimental group in number and is identical in specified characteristics, such as sex, age, annual income, parity, or other factors. Subjects meeting the study criteria are selected from a larger group at random or by a protocol that ensures nonbiased selection.

group A beta-hemolytic streptococcal (GABHS) skin disease, a bacterial skin infection that affects mainly meat packers; symptoms range from mildly annoying to serious. The source of the bacteria is believed to be freshly butchered meat.

group dynamics [Fr, *groupe*; Gk, *dynamis*, force], the interactions and relationships that take place within groups as well as between the groups and the rest of society. It includes interdependence of group members, collective problem-solving and decision-making, and group conformity.

group function, (in dentistry) the simultaneous contacting of opposing teeth in a segment or a group.

group specificity. See **specificity.**

group therapy, the application of psychotherapeutic techniques within a small group of people who experience similar difficulties. Generally, a group leader directs the discussion of problems in an attempt to promote individual psychologic growth and favorable personality change. The procedure provides opportunities for treating a greater number of people in a shorter period of time than would be possible with individual therapy, and it is used in clinics, in institutions, and in private practice. Group therapy has been found to be particularly effective in the treatment of various addictions. A kind of group therapy is **psychodrama.** See also **Gestalt therapy, psychotherapy, self-help group, transactional analysis.**

growing fracture [AS, *growan*; L, *fractura*, to break], a fracture, usually linear, in which consecutive x-ray images show a gradual separation of the fracture edges with the passage of time. The cause often is pressure of soft tissues forcing the edges apart, as when arachnoid tissues expand through edges of a skull fracture.

growing pains, **1.** rheumatism-like pains that occur in the muscles and joints of children or adolescents as a result of fatigue, emotional problems, postural defects, and other causes that are not related to growth and that may be symptoms of various disorders. **2.** emotional and psychologic problems experienced during adolescence.

growth [AS, *growan*, to grow], **1.** an increase in the size of an organism or any of its parts, as measured in increments of weight, volume, or linear dimensions, that occurs as a result of hyperplasia or hypertrophy. **2.** the normal progressive anatomic, physiologic development from infancy to adulthood as a result of the gradual and normal processes of accretion and assimilation. The total of the numerous changes that occur during the lifetime of an individual constitute a dynamic and complex process that involves many interrelated components, notably heredity, environment, nutrition, hygiene, and disease, all of which are subject to a variety of influences. In childhood, growth is categorized according to the approximate age at which distinctive physical changes usually appear and at which specific developmental tasks are achieved. Such stages include the prenatal period, infancy, early childhood (including the toddler and the preschool child), middle childhood, and adolescence. There are two periods of accelerated growth: the first 12 months, in which the infant triples in weight, grows approximately 50% of the height at birth, and undergoes rapid motor, cognitive, and social development; the second, in the months around puberty, when the child approaches adult height and secondary sexual characteristics emerge. Physical growth may be abnormally accelerated or slowed by a defect in the hypophyseal or pituitary gland. **3.** any abnormal localized increase of the size or number of cells, as in a tumor or neoplasm. **4.** a proliferation of cells, specifically a bacterial culture or mold. Compare **development, differentiation, maturation.**

growth and development, altered, a nursing diagnosis accepted by the Seventh National Conference on the Classification of Nursing Diagnoses. Altered growth and development is defined as the state in which an individual demonstrates deviations in norms from his or her age group. The critical defining characteristics are delay or difficulty in performing skills (motor, social, or expressive) typical of the age group; altered physical growth; and inability to perform self-care or self-control activities appropriate for the age. Minor characteristics are flat affect, listlessness, and decreased responses. Related factors include inadequate caretaking; indifference, inconsistent responsiveness, multiple caretakers; separation from significant others; environmental and stimulation deficiencies; effects of physical disability; and prescribed dependence. See **nursing diagnosis.**

growth failure, a lack of normal physical and psychologic development as a result of genetic, nutritional, pathologic, or psychosocial factors. See also **failure to thrive, maternal deprivation syndrome.**

growth hormone (GH), a single-chain peptide secreted by the anterior pituitary gland in response to growth hormone releasing factor (GHRF) from the hypothalamus. Growth hormone promotes protein synthesis in all cells, increases fat mobilization and use of fatty acids for energy, and decreases use of carbohydrate. Growth effects depend on the presence of thyroid hormone, insulin, and carbohydrate. Somatomedins, proteins produced chiefly in the liver, play a vital role in GH-induced skeletal growth, but the hormone cannot cause elongation of long bones after the epiphyses close, so that stature does not increase after puberty. Growth hormone accelerates the transport of specific amino acids into cells, stimulates the synthesis of messenger RNA and ribosomal RNA, influences the activity of several enzymes, increases the storage of phosphorus and potassium, and promotes a moderate retention of sodium. The secretion of GH, controlled almost exclusively by the central nervous system, occurs in bursts with more than one half of the total daily amount released during early sleep. Somatostatin, an anterior pituitary regulating hormone produced in the hypothalamus, inhibits GH secretion as well as the secretion of insulin and gastrin. A deficiency of GH causes dwarfism; an excess results in gigantism or acromegaly. Also called **somatotropic hormone, somatotropin.** See also **acromegaly, dwarfism, gigantism, somatostatin.**

growth hormone release inhibiting hormone. See **somatostatin.**

growth hormone releasing factor (GHRF), somatotropin releasing factor released by the hypothalamus. Also called **somatoliberin.**

Grünfelder's reflex /grYn′feldərz, grēn′-/, an involuntary dorsal flexion of the great toe with a fanlike spreading

of the other toes, caused by continued pressure on the posterior lateral fontanel. The reflex occurs in children who have middle-ear disease.

grunting [ME, *grunten*], abnormal, short audible gruntlike breaks in exhalation that often accompany severe chest pain. The grunt occurs because the glottis briefly stops the flow of air, halting the movement of the lungs and their surrounding or supporting structures. Grunting is most often heard in a person who has pneumonia, pulmonary edema, or fractured or bruised ribs. Atelectasis in the newborn also causes grunting as a result of the effort required for the baby to fill the lungs.

GSA, abbreviation for **Gerontologic Society of America.**

G-6-PD deficiency, abbreviation for **glucose-6-phosphate dehydrogenase deficiency.**

GSR, abbreviation for **galvanic skin response.**

gt., abbreviation for the Latin word, *gutta*, a drop.

GTP, abbreviation for **guanosine triphosphate.**

gtt., abbreviation for the Latin word, *guttae*, drops.

G tube. See **stomach tube.**

GU, abbreviation for **genitourinary.**

guaiac /gwī′ak/, a wood resin, commonly used as a reagent in laboratory tests for the presence of occult blood.

guaiacol poisoning. See **phenol poisoning.**

guaiac test, a test, using guaiac as a reagent, performed on feces and urine for detecting occult blood in the intestinal and urinary tracts.

guaifenesin /gwī′əfen′əsin/, glyceryl guaiacolate, a white to slightly gray powder with a bitter taste and faint odor, widely used as an expectorant. Guaifenesin increases the flow of fluid in the respiratory tract, reducing the viscosity of bronchial and tracheal secretions and facilitating their removal by the cough reflex and ciliary action.

guanabenz acetate /gwan′abenz/, an antihypertensive agent.

■ INDICATION: It is prescribed for hypertension.

■ CONTRAINDICATION: Known hypersensitivity to this drug prohibits its use.

■ ADVERSE EFFECTS: Among adverse reactions are dizziness, sedation, and dry mouth.

guanadrel sulfate /gwan′ədril/, an antihypertensive agent.

■ INDICATION: It is prescribed in the treatment of hypertension in patients not responding to first-step agents.

■ CONTRAINDICATIONS: Pheochromocytoma, administration of monoamine oxidase antagonist inhibitors, frank congestive heart failure, or known sensitivity to this drug prohibits its use.

■ ADVERSE EFFECTS: Among the most serious adverse reactions are orthostatic hypotension and syncope.

guanase. See **guanine deaminase.**

guanethidine sulfate /gwaneth′idēn/, an antihypertensive.

■ INDICATION: It is prescribed in the treatment of moderate and severe hypertension.

■ CONTRAINDICATIONS: Heart failure, concomitant administration of monoamine oxidase inhibitors, pheochromocytoma, or known hypersensitivity to this drug prohibits its use.

■ ADVERSE EFFECTS: Among the more serious adverse reactions are orthostatic hypotension, salt and water retention, bradycardia, diarrhea, and an inability to ejaculate.

guanine /gwan′ēn/, a major purine base found in nucleotides and a fundamental constituent of DNA and RNA. In free or uncombined form it occurs in trace amounts in most cells, usually as a product of the enzymatic hydrolysis of nucleic acids and nucleotides. On enzymatic hydrolysis, it is first converted into xanthine and finally into uric acid, its end product. See also **adenine.**

guanine deaminase, an enzyme that catalyzes the hydrolysis of guanine to xanthine and ammonia. Also called **guanase** /gwan′ās/.

guanine deaminase assay, the measurement of an enzyme in the blood that commonly increases in patients with hepatitis and other types of liver disease and mononucleosis. The normal value in serum is less than 3 nm/ml/min.

guanosine /gwan′ōsēn/, a compound derived from a nucleic acid, composed of guanine and a sugar, D-ribose. It is a major molecular component of the nucleotides guanosine monophosphate and triphosphate and of DNA and RNA.

guanosine deaminase. See **deaminase.**

guanosine monophosphate (GMP), a nucleotide that plays an important role in various metabolic reactions and in the formation of RNA from DNA templates.

guanosine triphosphate (GTP), a high-energy nucleotide, similar to adenosine triphosphate, that functions in various metabolic reactions, such as the activation of fatty acids and the formation of the peptide bond in protein synthesis.

guaranine /gwərä′nin/, caffeine.

guardian ad litem /ad lī′təm/, (in law) a person who is appointed by a court to prosecute or defend a suit for an infant or an incapacitated person. A guardian ad litem is sometimes appointed when a person's life is in imminent danger and that person refuses treatment.

guardianship, a legal status that places the care and property of an individual in the hands of another person. Implementation of the law varies in different cases and jurisdictions. Some courts have held as legally incompetent mental patients who have jobs and live independently.

Gubbay test of motor proficiency, a screening test for the identification of developmental dyspraxia. It consists of eight activities, such as whistling, throwing a tennis ball, and fitting shapes into appropriate slots, the results of which discriminate between impaired motor function and normal development in children.

Guedel's signs /gōō′dəlz/ [Arthur E. Guedel, American anesthesiologist, b. 1883], a system for describing the stages and planes of anesthesia during an operative procedure. These stages are best seen with inhalation by ether and are difficult to delineate when combination anesthetics are given, such as intravenous barbiturate for induction of anesthesia followed by an inhalation anesthetic.

■ STAGE I: (amnesia and analgesia) begins with the administration of an anesthetic and continues to the loss of consciousness. respiration is quiet, though sometimes irregular, and reflexes are still present.

■ STAGE II: (delirium or excitement) begins with the loss of consciousness and includes the onset of total anesthesia. during this stage the patient may move the limbs, chatter incoherently, hold the breath, or become violent. vomiting, with the attendant danger of aspiration, may occur. no avoidable stimulation is allowed at this stage; the patient is brought to stage iii as quickly and smoothly as possible.

■ STAGE III: (surgical anesthesia) begins with establishment of a regular pattern of breathing and total loss of consciousness and includes the period during which signs of respiratory or cardiovascular failure first appear. this stage is divided into four planes: At *plane 1* all movements cease and respiration is regular and 'automatic.' Eyelid reflexes are lost, but eyeball movements are marked. Pharyngeal reflexes disappear, but laryngeal and peritoneal reflexes are still present. Tonicity of the abdominal muscles can be judged by the tonicity of the extraocular muscles. At *plane 2* the eyeballs become fixed centrally, conjunctivae lose their luster, and intercostal muscle activity diminishes. Respiration remains regular, with reduced tidal volume, and does not change in quality or rate in response to incision. Intubation no longer causes laryngospasm. At *plane 3* intercostal paralysis occurs, and respiration becomes solely diaphragmatic. The pupils no longer react to light, and total muscle relaxation is achieved. At *plane 4* deep anesthesia is achieved, with the cessation of spontaneous respiration and the absence of sensation.

■ STAGE IV: (premortem) signals danger. This stage is characterized by pupils that are maximally dilated and skin that is cold and ashen. blood pressure is extremely low, often unmeasurable, and the brachial pulse is feeble or entirely absent. cardiac arrest is imminent. anesthetic is reduced, the lungs are manually ventilated with 100% oxygen, and the reservoir bag is continually emptied. See also **anesthesia.**

Guérin's fracture /gāraNz′/ [Alphonse F.M. Guérin, French surgeon, b. 1816], a fracture of the maxilla. Also called **Le Fort I fracture** /ləfôr′/.

guide dog [ME, *guiden,* to guard; OE, *docga*], a dog trained to aid in the mobility of a blind person. Guide dogs are usually recruited from certain compatible breeds and tested at the age of 13 weeks. If qualified, the dog is then specially trained in private hands for 1 year and retested. Most dogs selected for training pass the final test. Guide dogs also may be trained to serve as "ears" for deaf persons. Also called **companion animals, Seeing Eye dog.**

guided imagery /gī′did/, a therapeutic technique in which a patient is encouraged to concentrate on an image that helps relieve pain or discomfort.

guide plane [ME, *guiden,* to guard; L, *planum,* level ground], **1.** a part of an orthodontic appliance that has an established inclined plane for changing the occlusal relation of the maxillary and mandibular teeth and for permitting their movement to normal positions. **2.** a plane that is developed on the occlusal sufaces of occlusion rims for positioning the mandible in centric relation. **3.** two or more vertically parallel surfaces of abutment teeth shaped to direct the path of placement and removal of a partial denture.

guide-shoe marks, an x-ray image artifact caused by pressure of the guide shoes, curved metal lips that guide x-ray film in automatic developing systems. The guide shoes sensitize the film and leave ridge lines in the image.

guidewire /gīd′wī·ər/ [ME, *guiden,* to guard; AS, *wir*], a device used to position an intravenous catheter.

Guillain-Barré syndrome /gēyaN′bärä′/ [Georges Guillain, French neurologist, b. 1876; Jean A. Barré, French neurologist, b. 1880], an idiopathic, peripheral polyneuritis occurring between 1 and 3 weeks after a mild episode of fever associated with a viral infection or with immunization. Symmetric pain and weakness affect the extremities, and paralysis may develop. The neuritis may spread, ascending to the trunk and involving the face, arms, and thoracic muscles. The course of the disease is variable; some people may have minimal symptoms, whereas others may have symptoms severe enough to require critical nursing care, including respiratory assistance and a CircOlectric

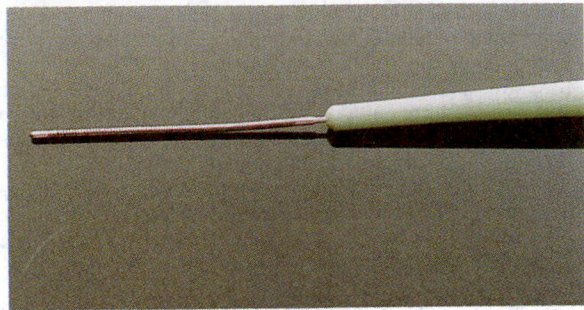

Guidewire
(Winawer, 1992/Courtesy Wilson-Cook, Inc, Winston-Salem, NC)

bed. The disease resolves itself completely in a few weeks or a few months. There is no treatment other than supportive care. Also called **acute febrile polyneuritis, acute idiopathic polyneuritis, infectious polyneuritis.**

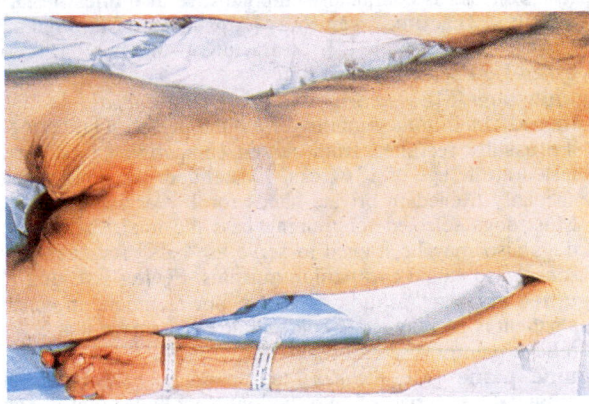

Limb-wasting in Guillain-Barré syndrome
(Perkin, 1986/Courtesy Dr PO Behan, Reader in Neurology, Institute of Neurological Sciences, Glaswow, UK)

guilt [AS *gylt* delinquency], a feeling caused by tension between the ego and superego when one falls below the standards set for oneself, or a remorseful awareness of having done something wrong.

guilty, (in criminal law) a verdict by the court, finding that to a moral certainty it is beyond reasonable doubt that the defendant committed the crime and is responsible for the offense as charged.

Guinea worm infection. See **dracunculiasis.**

gullet. See **esophagus.**

gum, 1. a sticky excretion from certain plants. 2. a firm layer of flesh covering the inside of the jaws and the base of the teeth. See **gingiva.**

gumboil [AS, *goma, byl*], an abscess of the gingiva and periosteum resulting from injury, infection, or dental decay. The gum is characteristically red, swollen, and tender. The abscess may rupture spontaneously, or it may require incision. Treatment may include antibiotics and hot mouthwashes. Also called **parulis.**

gum camphor. See **camphor.**

gum line [L, *gummi, linea*], the line formed by the gingival margin at the neck of the tooth. Also called **gingival line.**

gumma /gum′ə/, *pl.* **gummas, gummata** [L, *gummi,* gum], 1. a granuloma, characteristic of tertiary syphilis, varying from 1 mm to 1 cm in diameter. It is usually encapsulated and contains a central necrotic mass surrounded by inflammatory and fibrotic zones of tissue. Infectious organisms of the genus *treponema* may be found in a gumma. The lesion may be localized or diffuse, occurring on the trunk, legs, and face and on various internal organs, especially the liver. A ruptured gumma results in a shallow ulcer that heals slowly. 2. a soft granulomatous lesion sometimes occurring with tuberculosis.

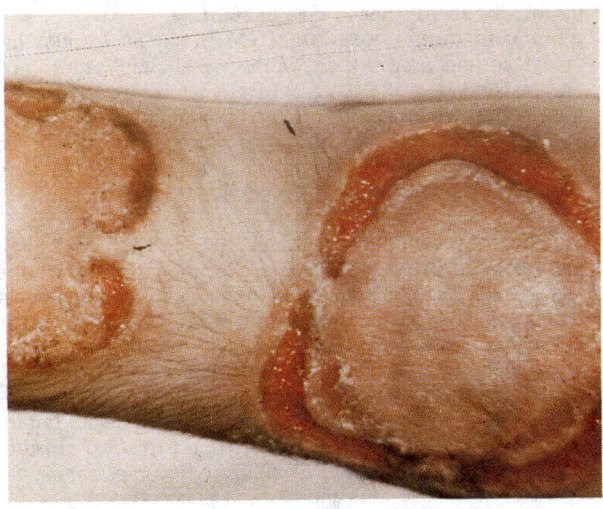

Gumma
(Morse, 1990/Centers for Disease Control, Atlanta, Georgia)

Gunning's splint [Thomas B. Gunning, American dentist, b. 1813; D, *splinte,* split], a maxillomandibular splint used for supporting the maxilla and the mandible in surgery of the jaws.

gunshot fracture [ME, *gunne;* AS, *sceotan* to shoot; L, *fractura,* break], a fracture caused by a bullet or similar missile.

Gunson method, (in radiology) a method of x-ray examination of the pharynx and upper esophagus during swallowing. A dark-colored shoestring is tied around the patient's throat just above the thyroid cartilage. The anterior and superior movement of the larynx is then shown by the elevation of the shoestring as the thyroid cartilage moves anteriorly, followed immediately by displacement of the shoestring as the cartilage passes superiorly.

Gunther's disease /gun′thərz/ [Hans Gunther, German physician, b. 1884], a rare congenital disorder of porphyrin metabolism that is associated with sunlight-induced skin lesions. See also **porphyria.**

gurgling rale [Fr, *gargouiller,* to gurgle; *rale,* rattle], an abnormal coarse sound heard during auscultation, especially over large cavities or over a trachea nearly filled with secretions.

gurry /gur′ē/, *slang.* the detritus incident to physical trauma or surgery, including body fluids, secretions, and tissue.

Gurvich radiation. See **mitogenetic radiation.**

gustation /gustā'shən/ [L, *gustare*, to taste], the sense and act of tasting foods, beverages, or other substances.

gustatory /gus'tətôr'ē/ [L, *gustare*, to taste], pertaining to the act or sense of taste or the organs of taste.

gustatory hallucination [L, *gustare*, to taste, *alucinari*, wandering mind], a false taste sensation either of food or beverage on the mucous membrane lining the empty mouth.

gustatory organ. See **taste bud.**

gustatory papilla [L, *gustare*, to taste, *papilla*, nipple], any of the small tissue elevations in the mouth that contain sense organs of taste such as the circumvallate papilla of the tongue.

gut [AS, *guttas*], **1.** intestine. **2.** *informal.* digestive tract. **3.** suture material manufactured from the intestines of sheep.

Guthrie test /guth'rē/, a screening for phenylketonuria used to detect the abnormal presence of phenylalanine metabolites in the blood. A small amount of blood is obtained and placed in a medium with a strain of *Bacillus subtilis*, a bacterium that cannot grow without phenylalanine. If phenylalanine metabolites are present, the bacteria reproduce and the test is positive, indicating that the patient has phenylketonuria. In most states, this test is done twice on all infants, once before discharge from the hospital and again at 2 weeks of age. See also **phenylketonuria.**

gutta (gt) /gut'ə, gōōt'ä/ [L, *drop*], one drop, or about one minim, of a medication, as eye drops or ear drops.

guttae (gtt) [L, *drops*], the plural of **gutta,** more than one drop, as in **guttae pro auribus,** or ear drops, or **guttae ophthalmicae,** or eye drops.

gutta-percha /gut'əpur'chə/ [Malay, *getah-percha*, latex sap], the coagulated, rubbery sap of various tropical trees, used for temporarily sealing the dressings of prepared tooth cavities. Small cones of gutta-percha may be used to fill dental root canals. When combined with fillers and coloring materials, it may be rolled into sheets and used to make temporary bases for dentures.

gutta-percha point, any of the fine, tapered cylinders of gutta-percha that may be used to fill a root canal. The radiopacity of gutta-percha points is an asset in their use as probes for determining the depth and topography of periodontal pockets by means of radiography.

guttate psoriasis /gut'āt/ [L, *gutta*, drop; Gk, itch], an acute form of psoriasis consisting of teardrop-shaped, red, scaly patches measuring 3 to 10 mm all over the body. A beta-hemolytic streptococcal pharyngitis or other upper respiratory infection may precipitate this reaction in susceptible individuals. Treatment is essential to prevent a more severe form of psoriasis. Compare **pustular psoriasis.** See also **psoriasis.**

guttural /gut'ərəl/ [L, *guttur*, throat], pertaining to or belonging to the throat, including low-pitched, raspy voice quality.

Guyon tunnel, a fibroosseous tunnel formed in part by the pisohamate ligament of the hand. It contains the ulnar artery and nerve, and may be the site of a compression injury.

gymno-, a combining form meaning 'pertaining to nakedness': *gymnocarpus, gymnocyte, gymnospore.*

gyn, *informal.* **1.** abbreviation for **gynecologist. 2.** abbreviation for **gynecology.**

gyn-. See **gyneco-.**

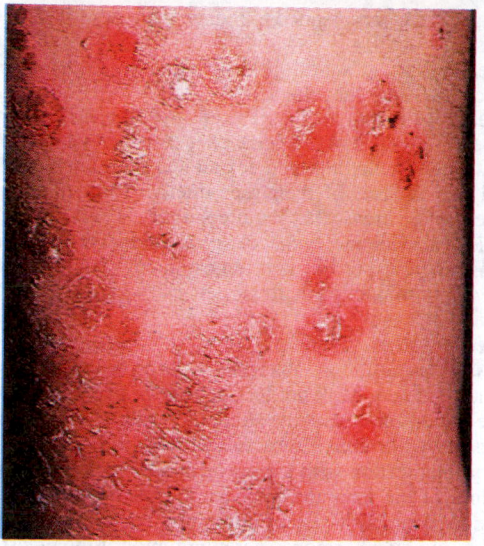

Guttate psoriasis (*Zitelli, 1992*)

gynandrous /gīnan'drəs, jī-/ [Gk, *gyne*, woman, *aner*, man], describing a man or a woman who has some of the physical characteristics usually attributed to the other sex, as a female pseudohermaphrodite. Compare **androgynous.** −**gynandry,** *n.*

gyne-. See **gyneco-.**

-gyne, -gyn, a suffix meaning '(specified) female characteristics': *androgyne, epigyne, trichogyne.*

gyneco-, gyn-, gyne-, gyno-, a combining form meaning 'pertaining to a woman or the female sex': *gynecoid, gynecomastia, gynotermon.*

gynecography /gī'nə-, jin'əkog'rəfē/, the radiologic examination of the female pelvic organs by means of intraperitoneal gas insufflation.

gynecoid pelvis /gī'nəkoid, jin'əkoid/ [Gk, *gyne* + *eidos*, form; L, *pelvis*, basin], a type of pelvis characteristic of the normal female and associated with the smallest incidence of fetopelvic disproportion. The inlet is nearly round, the sacrum is parallel to the posterior aspect of the symphysis pubis, the sidewalls are straight, and the ischial spines are blunt and do not encroach on the space in the true pelvis. It is the ideal pelvic type for childbirth.

gynecologic [Gk, *gynaikos*, of a woman], pertaining to gynecology or the study of diseases of the female reproductive organs and the breasts. Also **gynecological.**

gynecologic examination /gī'nə-, jin'əkəloj'ik/, pelvic examination.

gynecologic operative procedures [Gk, *gynaikos*, of a woman; L, *operari*, to work, *procedere*, to proceed], surgical intervention upon the female reproductive system. Gynecologic and obstetric problems account for one fifth of all female visits to physicians; many require surgical correction. Essential postoperative care demands that the patient be kept warm and quiet. Because of the risk of shock or hemorrhage, the patient should be closely monitored at frequent intervals during the first few hours. Fluids can be given when tolerated. Urine should be collected and measured periodically. Use of elastic stockings and suitable exercises are recommended to reduce the risk of thrombophlebitis.

gynecologist /gī′nəkol′əjist, jī′-, jin′-/, a physician who specializes in gynecology.

gynecology /gī′nəkol′əjē, jī′-, jin′-/ [Gk, *gyne* + *logos*, science], a branch of medicine concerned with the health care of women, including their sexual and reproductive function and the diseases of their reproductive organs, except diseases of the breast that require surgery. Unlike most specialities in medicine, gynecology encompasses surgical and nonsurgical expertise. It is almost always studied and practiced in conjunction with obstetrics. −**gynecologic, gynecological,** *adj.*

gynecomastia /gī′nəkōmas′tē·ə, jī′-, jin′-/ [Gk, *gyne* + *mastos*, breast], an abnormal enlargement of one or both breasts in men. Milk production may or may not be present. The condition is usually temporary and benign. It may be caused by hormonal imbalance, tumor of the testis or pituitary, medication with estrogens or steroidal compounds, or failure of the liver to inactivate circulating estrogen, as in alcoholic cirrhosis. Less commonly, the gynecomastia may be caused by a hormone-secreting tumor of the breast, lung, or other organ. It tends to remit spontaneously, but, if marked, may be corrected surgically for cosmetic or psychologic reasons. Biopsy may be performed to rule out the presence of cancer. Malignant neoplastic gynecomastia is usually inoperable and only briefly responsive to chemotherapy. Also called **gynecomasty.**

Gyne-Lotrimin, a trademark for an antifungal used for vaginal yeast infections (clotrimazole).

gynephobia /gī′nəfō′bē·ə, jī′-, jin′-/ [Gk, *gyne* + *phobos*, fear], an anxiety disorder characterized by a morbid fear of women or by a morbid aversion to the society of women. It is an obsessive, phobic phenomenon occurring almost entirely in men and may usually be traced to some frightening experience involving women that occurred in childhood. Treatment consists of psychotherapy to uncover the causative emotional conflict, followed by behavior therapy, specifically systemic desensitization and flooding to reduce anxiety.

-gynic, -gynous, a suffix meaning 'relating to the human female or to female characteristics': *androgynous, hologynic, monogynic, polygynic.*

gyno-. See **gyneco-.**

gynogamone /gī′nōgam′ōn/ [Gk, *gyne* + *gamos*, marriage], a gamone secreted by the female gamete.

-gynous, See **-gynic.**

gypsum /jip′səm/, a mineral composed mainly of crushed

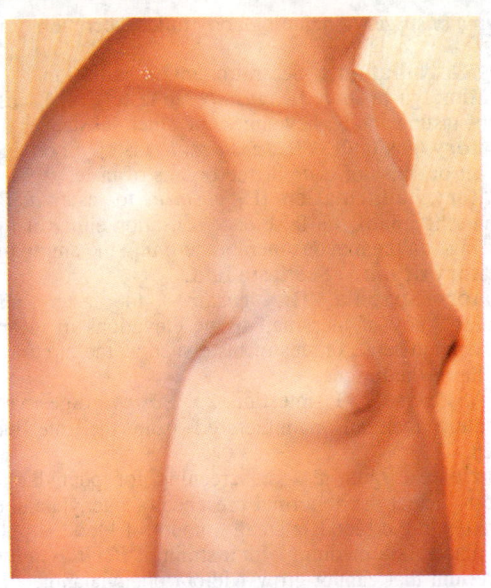

Prepubertal gynecomastia
(Seidel, 1991/Courtesy Wellington Hung, MD, Children's National Medical Center, Washington, DC)

calcium sulfate hemihydrate. It is used in making plaster of paris surgical casts and impressions for dentures. Gypsum dust has an irritant action on the mucous membranes of the respiratory tract and the conjunctiva.

gyrase /jī′rās/, an enzyme that enables certain DNA molecules to twist themselves into coils to replicate.

-gyria, a suffix meaning '(condition of the) development of the convolutions of the cerebral cortex': *oculogyria, polymicrogyria, ulegyria.*

gyri. See **gyrus.**

-gyria, a suffix meaning 'pertaining to a spiral or convolution': *oculogyria, polymicrogyria, ulegyria.*

gyri cerebri /jī′rī/ [Gk, *gyro*, circle; L, *cerebrum*, brain], the convolutions of the outer surface of the cerebral hemisphere, separated from each other by sulci, most of which appear during the sixth or seventh months of fetal life.

-gyro, a combining form meaning 'circle or spiral': *gyrus.*

gyrus /jī′rəs/, *pl.* **gyri** /jī′rī/ [Gk, *gyro*, circle], one of the tortuous convolutions of the surface of the brain caused by infolding of the cortex.

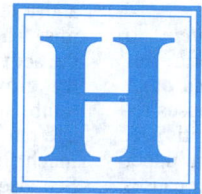

h, 1. abbreviation for **haustus. 2.** symbol for **hecto-. 3.** abbreviation for **height. 4.** symbol for *hora*, the Latin word for hour **5.** abbreviation for *horizontal*. **6.** abbreviation for **hyperopia.**

H, 1. symbol for the element **hydrogen. 2.** symbol for **henry.**

$_2$H, symbol for **deuterium.**

$_3$H, symbol for **tritium.**

[H$^+$], symbol for hydrogen ion concentration.

H$_2$, an abbreviation for a subtype of histamine receptor released in the stomach.

Ha, symbol for the element *hahnium*.

HaAg, abbreviation for *hepatitis A antigen*.

Haas method, a technique for producing x-ray images of the interior of the skull by having the patient rest the head with the forehead and nose on the table so that the beam enters the skull near the base of the occipital bone and emerges 1 inch above the nasion.

habeas corpus /hā'bē·əs kôr'pəs/, a right retained by all psychiatric patients that provides for the release of an individual who claims he or she is being deprived of his or her liberty and detained illegally. A hearing for this determination takes place in a court of law, and the patient's sanity is at issue.

habilitation /həbil'itā'shən/, the process of supplying a person with the means to develop maximum independence in activities of daily living through training or treatment.

habit [L, *habitus*, condition], **1.** a customary or particular practice, manner, or mode of behavior. **2.** an involuntary pattern of behavior or thought. **3.** also called **habitus.** *archaic*. appearance or physique, as pyknic habit. **4.** the habitual use of drugs or narcotics. See also **habit spasm, habit training.**

habitat /hab'itat/ [L, *habitare*, to dwell], a natural environment where a species of a plant or animal, including humans, may live and grow normally.

habit spasm, an involuntary twitching or tic usually involving a small muscle group of the face, neck, or shoulders and resulting in movements such as spasmodic blinking or rapid jerking of the head to the side. The movements are often generated by emotional conflicts rather than caused by any organic disorder. They may serve as a release for tension or anxiety.

habit tic [L, *habitus*, state; Fr, *tic*], a brief recurrent movement of a muscle group, such as a blink, grimace, or sudden head turning, that is of a psychogenic rather than organic cause.

habit training, the process of teaching a child how to adjust to the demands of the external world by forming certain habits, primarily those related to eating, sleeping, elimination, and dress.

habitual abortion /həbich'oo·əl/ [L, *habituare*, to become used to], spontaneous termination of three successive pregnancies before the twentieth week of gestation. Habitual abortion can result from chronic infection, abnormalities of the conceptus, maternal hormonal dysfunction, or uterine abnormalities such as cervical incompetence. See also **cerclage, incompetent cervix.**

habitual dislocation [L, *habitus*, state, *dis, locare,* to place], a dislocation that recurs repeatedly after reduction.

habitual fever. See **fever.**

habitual hyperthermia, a condition of unknown cause occurring in young females, characterized by body temperatures of 99° to 100.5° F regularly or intermittently for years, associated with fatigue, malaise, vague aches and pains, insomnia, bowel disturbances, and headaches. No organic cause can be found; the diagnosis is usually made only after a prolonged period of study and observation. No specific treatment is recommended. Reassurance and psychotherapy offer the best relief. Also called **habitual fever.**

habituation /həbich'oo·ā'shən/ [L, *habituare*, to become used to], **1.** an acquired tolerance from repeated exposure to a particular stimulus. **2.** also called **negative adaptation.** a decline and eventual elimination of a conditioned response by repetition of the conditioned stimulus. **3.** psychologic and emotional dependence on a drug, tobacco, or alcohol resulting from the repeated use of the substance but without the addictive, physiologic need to increase dosage. Compare **addiction.**

habitus /hab'itəs/, describing a person's appearance or physique, as an athletic habitus. See also **habit.**

hacking cough [AS, *haeccan, cohettan*], a short, weak repeating cough, often caused by irritation of the larynx by a postnasal drip.

Haeckel's law. See **recapitulation theory.**

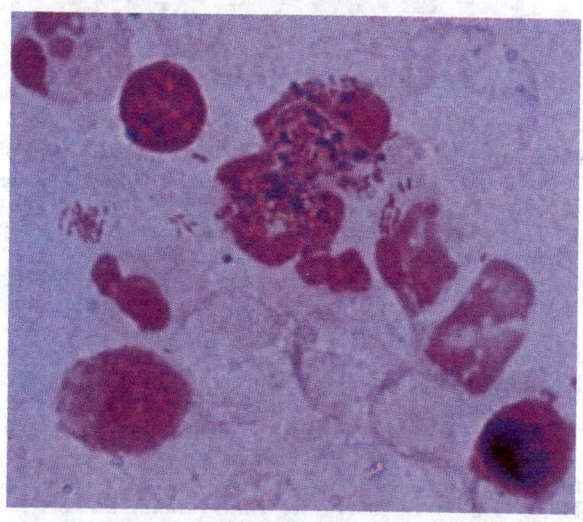

Haemophilus ducreyi (Baron, 1990)

-haemia. See **-emia.**

Haemophilus /hēmof'iləs/ [Gk, *haima*, blood, *philein*, to love], a genus of gram-negative pathogenic bacteria, frequently found in the respiratory tract of humans and other animals, such as *Haemophilus influenzae*, which causes respiratory tract infections and one form of meningitis, *H. haemolyticus*, a hemolytic species pathogenic in the upper respiratory tract of humans, and *H. ducreyi*, which causes chancroid. *Haemophilus* species are generally sensitive to cephalosporins, tetracyclines, and sulfonamides.

Haemophilus influenzae, a small, gram-negative, nonmotile, parasitic bacterium that occurs in two forms, encapsulated and nonencapsulated, and in six types, a, b, c, d, e, and f. Almost all infections are caused by encapsulated type b organisms. *Haemophilus influenzae* is found in the throats of 30% of healthy, normal people. In children and in debilitated older people, severe destructive inflammation of the larynx, trachea, and bronchi may result from infection. Subacute bacterial endocarditis and purulent meningitis also may be caused by it. Secondary infection by *H. influenzae* occurs in influenza and in many other respiratory diseases. Immunization is available for pediatric patients.

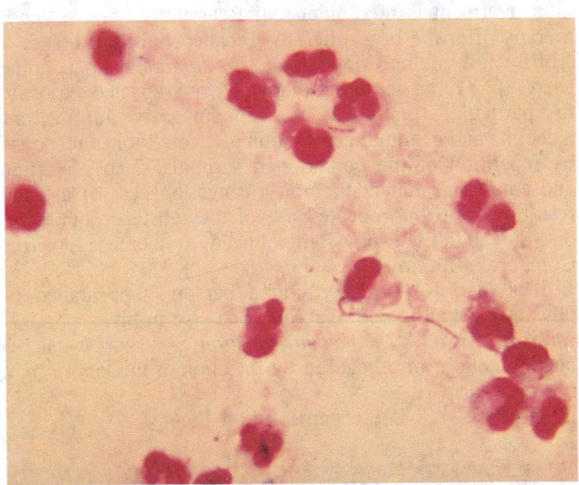

Haemophilus influenzae *(Baron, 1990)*

hafnium (Hf) /haf'nē·əm/ [Hafnia, Medieval Latin name of Copenhagen, Denmark], a hard, brittle, silver-gray metallic element of the first transition group. Its atomic number is 72; its atomic weight is 178.49. Elements in this group show some nonmetallic chemical characteristics.

Hagedorn needle /hä'gedôrn/ [Hans C. Hagedorn, Danish physician, b. 1888], a flat surgical needle with a cutting edge near its point and a very large eye at the other end.

Hageman factor. See **factor XII.**

Haglund's deformity, a foot disorder characterized by an enlarged posterior-superior lateral aspect of the calcaneus, often associated with an inverted subtalar joint. It is a common cause of posterior Achilles bursitis.

hahnium (Ha). See **element 105.**

Hailey-Halley disease. See *Hailey-Hailey disease.* See benign familial chronic pemphigus.

hair [AS *haer*], a filament of keratin consisting of a root

and a shaft formed in a specialized follicle in the epidermis. There are three stages of hair development: **anagen,** the active growing stage; **catagen,** a short interlude between the growth and resting phases; and **telogen,** the resting (club) stage before shedding. Scalp hair grows at an average rate of 1 mm every 3 days, body and eyebrow hair at a much slower rate. Hair plucking does not stop hair growth. See also **hirsutism, lanugo.**

hair analysis [AS, *haer*; Gk, a loosening], chemical analysis of a hair sample to find possible evidence of exposure to a toxic substance. Molecules of lead compounds and other chemicals are absorbed and stored in hair shafts. Hair analysis is also used to determine possible causes of malnutrition. Samples for analysis are taken from areas close to the scalp to eliminate chances that toxic chemicals found in the hair may have been absorbed from air pollutants.

hair follicle [AS, *haer*; L, *folliculus*, a small bag], a tiny tube of epidermal cells originating in the corium layer of the skin and containing the root of a hair shaft.

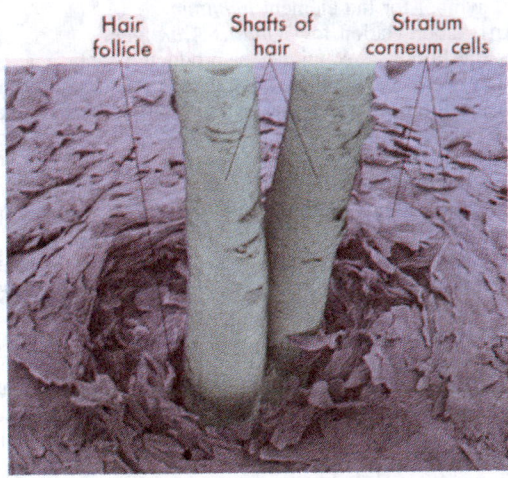

Hair follicle *(Thibodeau, 1993)*

hairline fracture [AS, *haer*; L, *linea, fractura*], a minor fracture that appears on x-ray film as a thin line between two segments of a bone. The segments remain in alignment and the fracture may not extend completely through the bone. A fatigue hairline fracture may develop without causing injury or in the absence of trauma.

hair matrix carcinoma. See **basal cell carcinoma.**

hair pulling. See **trichotillomania.**

hairy-cell leukemia [AS, *haer*; L, *cella*, storeroom; Gk, *leukos*, white, *haima*, blood], an uncommon neoplasm of blood-forming tissues, characterized by pancytopenia, an enlarged spleen, and the presence of reticulum cells with many fine projections on their surface in the blood and bone marrow. The disease occurs six times more frequently in men than in women and usually appears in the fifth decade with an insidious onset and a variable course marked by anemia, thrombocytopenia, and spontaneous bruising. Some cases may have long-term remission with alpha-interferon or chemotherapy using vincristine and prednisone. Also called **leukemic reticuloendotheliosis.**

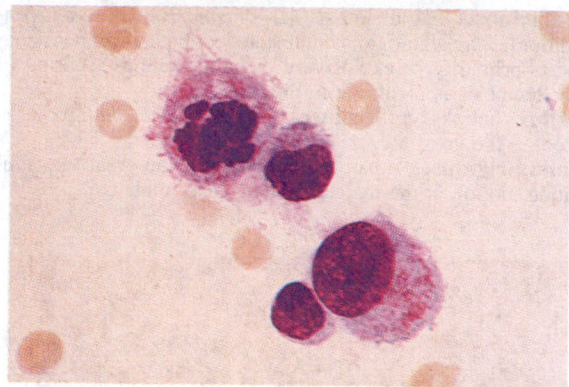

Hairy-cell leukemia *(Hayhoe, 1992)*

hairy leukoplakia, a form of leukoplakia characterized by a white plaque that is markedly folded in appearance or smooth and is often found on one or both lateral borders of the tongue. It is associated with severe immunodeficiency, occurs in HIV-infected patients, and is believed to result from the Epstein-Barr virus.

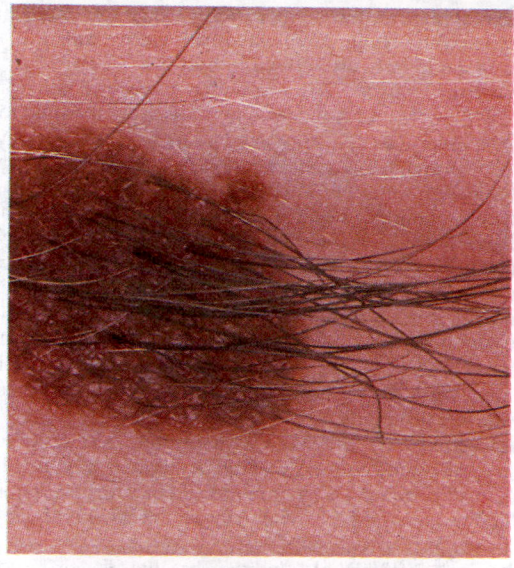

Hairy nevus *(du Vivier, 1992)*

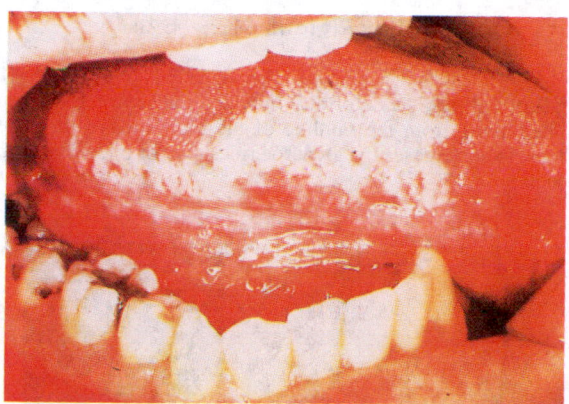

Hairy leukoplakia caused by EBV *(Murray, 1990)*

hairy nevus [AS, *haer*; L, *naevus*, birthmark], a mole, usually pigmented, with hairs growing from it.

hairy tongue, a dark, pigmented overgrowth of the filiform papillae of the tongue that is a benign and frequent side effect of some antibiotics. The condition gradually subsides, and no treatment is indicated. See also **glossitis.**

halcinonide /həlsin′ənīd/, a topical glucocorticoid.

■ INDICATION: It is prescribed topically as an antiinflammatory agent.

■ CONTRAINDICATIONS: Viral and fungal diseases of the skin, impaired circulation, or known hypersensitivity to this drug or to steroid medication prohibits its use.

■ ADVERSE EFFECTS: Among the more serious adverse effects are skin reactions and systemic side effects occurring from prolonged or excessive application.

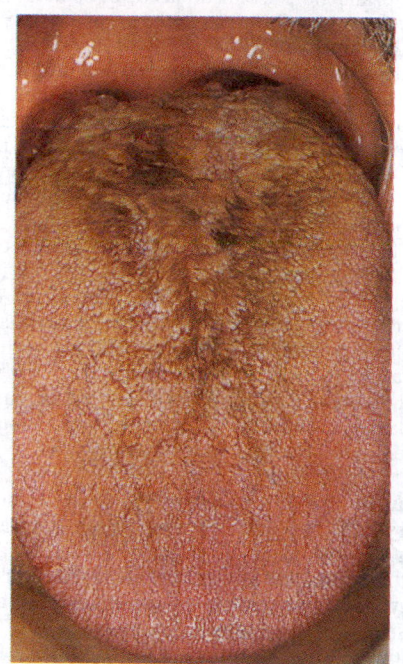

Hairy tongue *(Lamey, 1988)*

Halcion, a trademark for a hypnotic agent (triazolam).

Haldol, a trademark for a tranquilizer (haloperidol).

half-life (t½) [AS, *haelf, lif*], **1.** the time required for a radioactive substance to lose 50% of its activity through decay. Each radionuclide has a unique half-life. **2.** the amount of time required to reduce a drug level to one half of its initial value. Usually the term refers to time necessary to reduce the plasma value to one half of its initial value and is also applied to the disappearance of the total amount of drug from the body. Also called **radioactive half-life.** See also **biologic half-life, effective half-life.**

half-normal saline, (in respiratory therapy) a solution of 0.45% NaCl used for mucosal hydration. As the fluid tends to evaporate, the saline concentration increases, achieving nearly normal saline concentration in the respiratory tract.

half-sibling, one of two or more children who have one parent in common; a half brother or half sister. Also called **half-sib.**

half-value layer, the amount of material required to attenuate a beam of radiation to one half of its original level. Units are given in lengths, as centimeters.

halfway house, a specialized treatment facility, usually for psychiatric patients who no longer require complete hospitalization but who need some care and time to adjust to living independently.

halisteresis /həlis'tərē'sis/ [Gk, *hals*, salt, *steresis*, absence of], a theoretic process of bone resorption in which bone salts may be removed by humoral mechanisms and returned to body tissue fluids, leaving behind a decalcified bone matrix. See also **osteolysis.**

halitosis /hal'itō'sis/ [L, *halitus*, breath; Gk, *osis*, condition], offensive breath resulting from poor oral hygiene, dental or oral infections, the ingestion of certain foods, such as garlic or alcohol, use of tobacco, or some systemic diseases, such as the odor of acetone in diabetes and ammonia in liver disease.

Hallervorden-Spatz syndrome /hol'ərfôr'dən shpots/ [Julius Hallervorden, German neurologist, b. 1882; H. Spatz, German neurologist, b. 1888], a progressive neurologic disease of children, with symptoms of parkinsonism. It is characterized by rigidity, athetosis, and dementia. The cause is an accumulation of iron pigments in the globus pallidus and substantia nigra. Treatment is similar to that of Parkinson's disease and Huntington's chorea.

hallex. See **hallux.**

Hallpike caloric test /hôl'pīk/, a method for evaluating the function of the vestibule of the ear in patients with vertigo or hearing loss. Irrigation of the ears with cool and warm water or air mimics the stimulus of turning in the vestibular apparatus, causing nystagmus. Nystagmus can then be evaluated, and specific disorders of the vestibule may be diagnosed. See also **caloric test, nystagmus.**

halluces. See **hallux.**

hallucination /həloo'sinā'shən/ [L, *alucinari*, to ramble], a sensory perception that does not result from an external stimulus and that occurs in the waking state. It can occur in any of the senses and is classified accordingly as auditory, gustatory, olfactory, tactile, or visual. **–hallucinate,** /həloo'sənāt/ *v.*

hallucinogen /həloo'sənəjen', hal'əsin'əjən, hal'yəsin'əjən/ [L, *alucinari* + Gk, *genein*, to produce], a substance that causes excitation of the central nervous system, characterized by hallucination, mood change, anxiety, sensory distortion, delusion, depersonalization; increased pulse, temperature, and blood pressure, and dilatation of the pupils. Psychic dependence may occur, and depressive or suicidal psychotic states may result from the ingestion of hallucinogenic substances. Some kinds of hallucinogens are **lysergine, mescaline, peyote, phencyclidine hydrochloride,** and **psilocybin.**

hallucinogenesis /-jen'əsis/ [L, *alucinari*, a wandering mind; Gk, *genein*, to produce], a cause or source of hallucinations.

hallucinosis /haloo'sinō'sis/ [L, *alucinari* + Gk, *osis*, condition], a pathologic mental state in which awareness consists primarily or exclusively of hallucinations. A kind of hallucinosis is **alcoholic hallucinosis.**

hallux /hal'əks/, *pl.* **halluces** /hal'yoosēz/ [L, *hallex*, large toe], the great toe. Also spelled **hallex.**

hallux rigidus, a painful deformity of the great toe, limiting motion at the metatarsophalangeal joint.

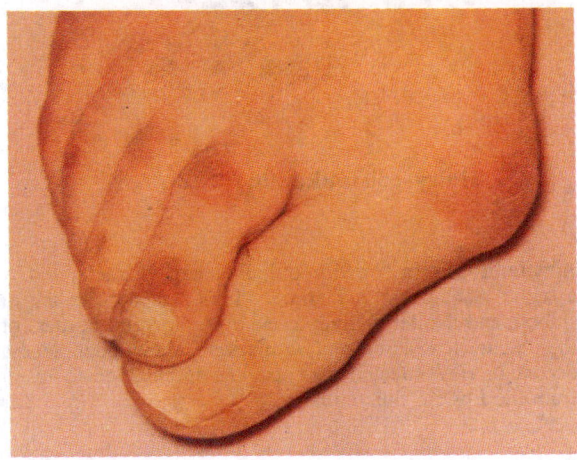

Hallux Rigidus *(Shipley, 1993)*

hallux valgus, a deformity in which the great toe is angulated away from the midline of the body toward the other toes; in some cases the great toe rides over or under the other toes.

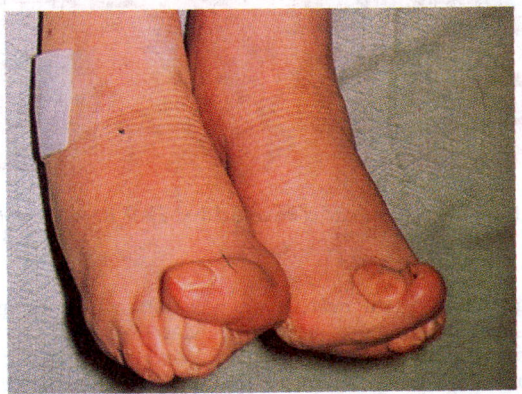

Hallux valgus *(Kamal, 1991)*

halo- /hal'ō-/, a combining form meaning 'salt': *halogen.*

halo cast /hā'lō/ [Gk, *halos*, circular floor; AS, *kasta*], an orthopedic device used to help immobilize the neck and head. It incorporates the trunk, usually with shoulder straps, and an apparatus by means of an outrigger within the cast to secure pins to a band around the skull. The halo cast is used to help the healing of cervical injuries and cervical dis-

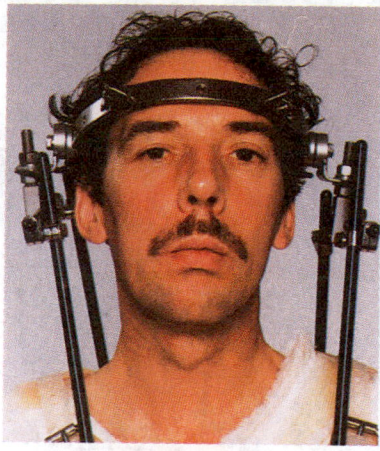

Halo cast (Houghton, 1989)

locations and for positioning and immobilization after cervical surgery.

halo effect, the beneficial effect of an interview or other encounter, as may occur in the course of a research project or a health care visit. The halo effect cannot be attributed to the content of the interview or to any specific act or treatment; it is the result of indefinable interpersonal factors present in the interaction.

Halog, a trademark for a topical glucocorticoid (halcinonide).

halogen /hal′ōjən/ [Gk, *hals,* salt, *genein,* to produce], any member of the group VII elements in the periodic table: fluorine, chlorine, bromine, iodine, and astatine. They are found in sea water as the corresponding halide ion.

halogenated hydrocarbon /həloj′ənā′tid/ [Gk, *hals*, salt, *genein*, to produce; *hydor*, water; L, *carbo*, coal], a volatile liquid used for general anesthesia, administered in combination with oxygen, or with oxygen in combination with nitrous oxide. Kinds of halogenated hydrocarbons are **enflurane, halothane, isoflurane, methoxyflurane,** and **trichloroethylene.**

haloperidol /hal′ōper′ədôl/, a butyrophenone tranquilizer.
- INDICATIONS: It is prescribed in the treatment of psychotic disorders and in the control of Gilles de la Tourette's syndrome.
- CONTRAINDICATIONS: Parkinson's disease, concurrent administration of central nervous system depressants, liver or renal dysfunction, severe hypotension, or known hypersensitivity to this drug prohibits its use.
- ADVERSE EFFECTS: Among the more serious adverse effects are hypotension and a variety of extrapyramidal and hypersensitivity reactions.

haloprogin /hā′lōprō′jin/, an antibacterial and antifungal.
- INDICATION: It is prescribed in the treatment of susceptible fungal infections, including athlete's foot.
- CONTRAINDICATION: Known hypersensitivity to this drug prohibits its use.
- ADVERSE EFFECTS: Among the most serious adverse reactions are exacerbation of existing lesions, formation of vesicles, and pruritus.

Halotestin, a trademark for an androgen (fluoxymesterone).

Halotex, a trademark for an antibacterial (haloprogin).

halothane /hal′əthān/, an inhalation anesthetic.
- INDICATION: It is prescribed for induction and maintenance of general anesthesia.
- CONTRAINDICATION: It is not recommended for obstetric anesthesia unless uterine relaxation is required.
- ADVERSE EFFECTS: Among the more serious but rare adverse reactions associated with halothane are hepatic necrosis, cardiac arrest or dysrhythmia, hypotension, malignant hyperpyrexia, nausea, and emesis.

halothane-related hepatitis, an adverse reaction of some patients to inhalation of halothane, a general anesthetic. The reaction is characterized by hepatitis and a severe fever that develops several days after exposure to the anesthetic. The risk is higher for obese patients, possibly because body fat tends to store the chemical.

Halsted's forceps /hal′stedz/ [William S. Halsted, American surgeon, b. 1852], **1.** also called **mosquito forceps.** a small, pointed hemostatic forceps. **2.** a forceps with slender jaws for grasping arteries and other blood vessels.

hamamelis water. See **witch hazel,** def 2.

hamate bone /ham′āt/ [L, *hamatus,* hooked], a carpal (wrist) bone that rests on the fourth and fifth metacarpal bones and projects a hooklike process, the hamulus, from its palmar surface. Its dorsal surface is rough for ligamentous attachment. The hamate bone articulates with the lunate proximally, the fourth and fifth metacarpal distally, the triangular medially, and the capitate laterally. Also called **os hamatum, unciform bone.**

Hamman's disease [Louis Virgil Hamman, American physician, b. 1877; L, *dis,* apart; Fr, *aise,* ease], progressive interstitial fibrosis of both lungs, causing right ventricular failure and ventilatory failure. Also called **Hamman-Rich syndrome.**

Hamman-Rich syndrome. See **interstitial pneumonia.**

hammer finger [AS, *hamer, finger*], a permanently flexed terminal phalanx resulting from an injury to the extensor tendon. Also called **mallet finger.**

hammertoe /ham′ər tō/ [AS, *hamer, ta*], a foot digit permanently flexed at the midphalangeal joint, resulting in a clawlike appearance. The anomaly may be present in more than one digit but is most common in the second toe.

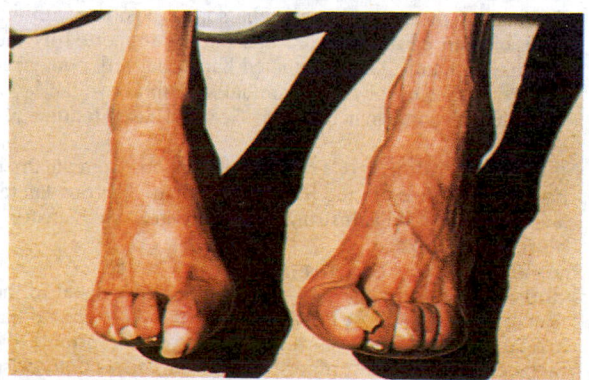

Hammertoe (Kamal, 1991)

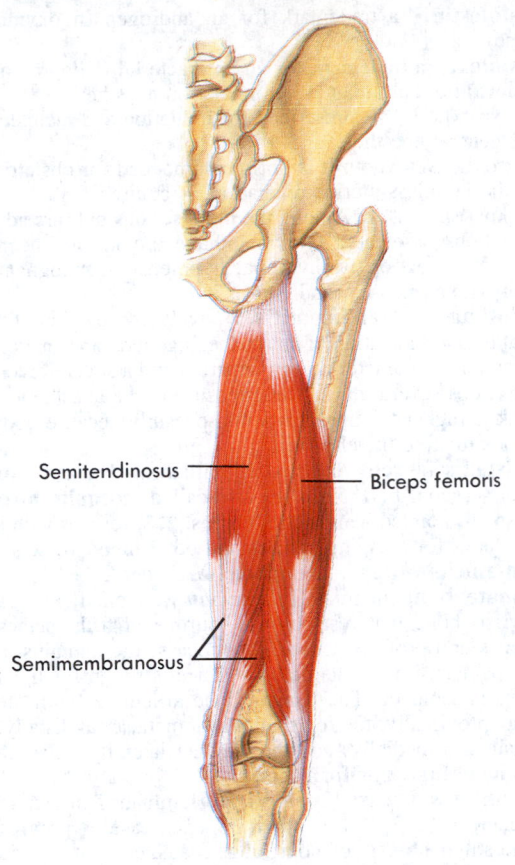

Hamstring muscle: semitendinosis, semimembranosus, and biceps femoris
(Seeley, 1992/John V Hagen)

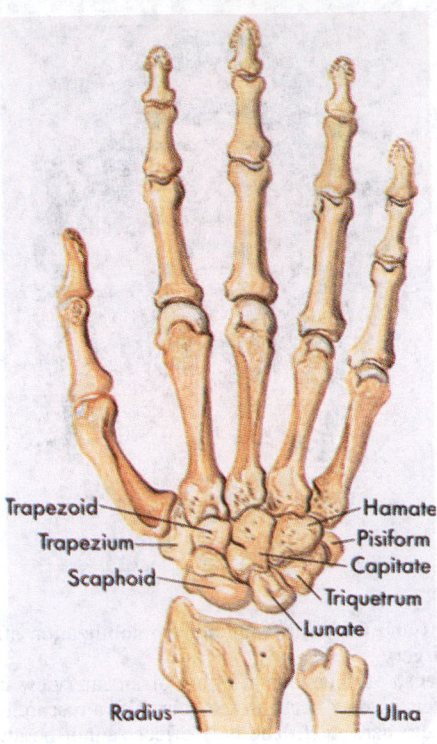

Hand *(Thibodeau, 1993/Ernest W Beck)*

hamstring muscle [AS, *hamm, streng;*], any one of three muscles at the back of the thigh; medially, the semimembranosus and the semitendinosus and laterally, the biceps femoris.

hamstring reflex, a normal deep tendon reflex elicited by tapping one of the hamstring tendons behind the knee, resulting in contraction of the tendon and flexion of the knee. The patient should be lying in the supine position with the knee and hip partially flexed and the leg supported by the examiner's hand. An accentuated hamstring reflex may result from a lesion of the pyramidal system above the level of the fourth lumbar nerve root. See also **deep tendon reflex.**

hamstring tendon, one of the three tendons from the three hamstring muscles in the back of the thigh. The one lateral and the two medial hamstring tendons connect the hamstring muscles to the knee.

hamular notch. See **pterygomaxillary notch.**

hand [AS, *hand*], the part of the upper limb distal to the forearm. It is the most flexible part of the skeleton and has a total of 27 bones, 8 forming the carpus, 5 forming the metacarpus, and 14 forming the phalangeal section. Also called **manus.**

handblock [AS, *hand* + Fr, *bloc*], a device made of a wood block several inches high with a firm handle that can be gripped by a disabled patient to provide a certain amount of body support in minor ambulatory activities, such as getting into or out of a bed.

hand condenser, (in dentistry) an instrument for compacting amalgams or gold foil using force applied by the operator, with or without supplementary force from a mallet of an assistant.

handedness /han'didnes/ [AS, *hand* + *ness*, condition], voluntary or involuntary preference for use of either the left or right hand. The preference is related to cerebral dominance, with left-handedness corresponding to dominance of the right side of the brain and vice versa. Also called **chirality, laterality.**

hand-foot-and-mouth disease, a Coxsackie viral infection characterized by the appearance of painful ulcers and vesicles on the mucous membranes of the mouth and on the hands and feet. The disease is highly contagious and affects mainly children, including infants. There is no specific cure.

hand-foot syndrome. See **sickle cell crisis.**

handicapped /han'dikapt/ [E, *hand in cap*, a game with forfeits], referring to a person who has a congenital or acquired mental or physical defect that interferes with normal functioning of the body system or the ability to be self-sufficient in modern society. Compare **disability.**

handpiece /hand'pēs/, a device for holding rotary instruments in a dental engine or condensing points in mechanical condensing units. It is connected by an arm, cable, belt, or tube to a power source, as a motor, or an air-pressure or water-pressure hose.

Hand-Schüller-Christian syndrome /hand'shoo'lər-kris'chən/, *obsolete*. a triad of symptoms, exophthalmos, diabetes insipidus, and bone destruction, which may occur in any of several disorders. See also **eosinophilic granu-loma, Letterer-Siwe disease.**

hanging drop preparation [ME, *hangen*, to hang; AS, *dropa*, to fall; L, *praeparer*, to make ready], a technique used for the examination and identification of certain microorganisms, such as spirochetes or trichomonads. The technique requires a cover slip, a microscope, and a special slide that has a central concavity. A specimen suspected of containing the microorganism is diluted with a sterile isotonic solution. A drop of this fluid mixture is placed on a glass cover slip, which is then inverted carefully and placed over the slide so that the drop is hanging from the slip into the concavity in the slide. The delicate structures and the method of movement characteristic of the species may then be viewed through the microscope.

hangman's fracture, a fracture of the posterior elements of the cervical vertebrae with dislocation of C2 or C3.

hangnail [AS, *angnaegl*, troublesome nail], a piece of partially disconnected epidermis of the cuticle or nail fold. Tearing the skin fragment causes a red, painful, easily infected sore. Early treatment is to trim the hangnail close with nail clippers. For inflamed cases an antibiotic ointment and protective bandage are used.

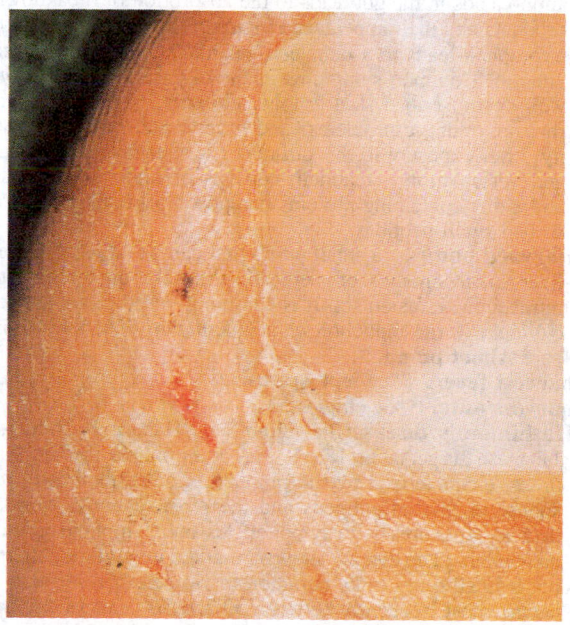

Hangnail *(Baran, 1991)*

hangover, a popular term for a group of symptoms, including nausea, thirst, fatigue, headache, and irritability, resulting from the use of alcohol and certain drugs.

Hanot's disease /hanōz'/ [Victor C. Hanot, French physician, b. 1844], primary biliary cirrhosis. See also **biliary cirrhosis.**

Hansen's bacillus [Gerard Henrik Armauer Hansen, Norwegian physician, b. 1841; L, *bacillum*, a small rod], the acid-fast *Mycobacterium leprae* that is the cause of leprosy.

Hansen's disease. See **leprosy.**

HA-1A, a genetically engineered antibody used in the treatment of certain blood infections. The HA-1A antibody attacks the bacterial toxin rather than the bacterium directly. It is relatively free of side effects.

Hantavirus, a newly added fifth genus within the *Bunyaviridae* family. The Hantavirus is the cause of several different forms of Hemorrhagic Fever with Renal Syndrome (HFRS). The severity of the illness is determined by the strain isolated through the use of IFA or ELISA. The Hantaan, Seoul, Puumala, Prospect Hill, and Porogia strains are five viruses within the Hantavirus genus. See also **Hemorrhagic fever.**

-haphia. See **-aphia.**

haploid /hap'loid/ [Gk, *haploos*, single, *eidos*, form], having only one complete set of nonhomologous chromosomes. Also called **monoploid.** –**haploidy,** *n.*

haploid nucleus [Gk, *haploos*, single, *eidos*, form; L, *nucleus*, nut], a nucleus possessing only half the normal somatic number of chromosomes. It may occur in a germ cell after reduction division and before fertilization.

-haploidy. See **haploid.**

hapten /hap'tən/ [Gk, *haptein*, to grasp], a nonproteinaceous substance that acts as an antigen by combining with particular bonding sites on an antibody. Unlike a true antigen, it does not induce the formation of antibodies. A hapten bonded to a carrier protein may induce an immune response. Also called **haptene** /hap'tēn/.

haptics /hap'tiks/ [Gk, *haptein*, to grasp], the science concerned with studying the sense of touch. –**haptic,** *adj.*

haptoglobin /hap'tōglō'bin/ [Gk, *haptein*, to grasp; L, *globus*, ball], a plasma protein whose only known function is to bind free hemoglobin. The quantity of haptoglobin is increased in certain chronic diseases and inflammatory disorders and is decreased or absent in hemolytic anemia. Normal adult findings range from 100 to 150 mg/dl. Compare **transferrin.** See also **hemoglobinemia, hemoglobinuria.**

hard chancre [AS, *heard*; Fr, *canker*], a syphilitic chancre or primary lesion that develops at the site of a syphilis infection. The lesion begins as a small red papule that gradually hardens and erodes into an extremely contagious ulcer. A secretion exuded by the sore contains *Treponema pallidum*, the organism that is the etiologic agent of syphilis in humans.

hard contact lens [AS, *heard*; L, *contingere*, to touch, *lentil*], a polymethylmethacryate, or rigid gas-permeable, contact lens that retains its form without support, in contrast with a soft contact lens that easily yields to pressure.

hard data, information about a patient that is obtained by observation and measurement, including laboratory data, as opposed to information collected by interviewing the patient or others.

hard disk, a computer data storage medium that consists of a rigid disk with an electromagnetic coating allowing information to be transcribed on it and from it. Usually permanently mounted in a dust-proof container, a hard disk has a storage capacity approximately 10 to 100 times that of a diskette. Compare **diskette.**

hardening of the arteries, arteriosclerosis.

hard fibroma, a neoplasm composed of fibrous tissue in which few cells are present. Also called **fibroma durum.**

hardness of x-rays, the relative penetrating power of x-rays. In general, the shorter the wavelength, the harder the radiation. Also called **hard radiation.** Compare **soft radiation.**

hard nevus. See **epidermal nevus.**

hard palate [AS, *heard*, hard; L, *palatum*], the bony portion of the roof of the mouth, continuous posteriorly with the soft palate and bounded anteriorly and laterally by the alveolar arches and the gums. The palatine process of the maxilla and the horizontal portion of the palatine bone form the bony support for the hard palate that is covered by periosteum and by the mucous membrane of the mouth. A linear raphe along its middle line ends anteriorly in a small papilla, which corresponds with the incisive canal. On each side and anterior to the raphe, the mucous membrane is thick, pale in color, and corrugated. Posteriorly the mucous membrane is thin, smooth, and darker. The hard palate is covered with squamous epithelium and furnished with numerous palatal glands lying between the mucous membrane and the surface of the bone. Compare **soft palate.**

hard radiation. See **hardness of x-rays.**

hardware, the tangible parts of a computer, such as chips, boards, wires, transformers, and peripheral devices. See also **software, wetware.**

hardware bug. See **bug.**

hard water [AS, *heard, waeter*], water that contains certain cations, particularly calcium and magnesium, that precipitate with soap solutions. The term is generally applied to tap water, and the degree of hardness varies with the source and previous treatment.

Hardy-Weinberg equilibrium principle /här′dē wīn′bərg/ [G. H. Hardy, English mathematician, b. 1877 Wilhelm Weinberg, German physician, b. 1862; L *aequilibris* equal weight; *principium* a beginning], the mathematic relationship between the frequency of genes and the resulting genotypes in populations. In a large interbreeding population characterized by random mating, mendelian inheritance, and the absence of migration, mutation, and selection, the ratio of individuals homozygous for a dominant gene to those heterozygous to those homozygous for a recessive gene is 1:2:1, at which point equilibrium is established; and the frequency of genes and genotypes remains relatively unchanged from generation to generation. See also **genetic equilibrium.**

harelip. See **cleft lip.**

hare's eye. See **lagophthalmos.**

harlequin color /här′lək(w)in/ [It, *arlecchino*, goblin; L, *color*, hue], a temporary flushing of the skin on the lower side of the body with pallor of the upward side. Commonly seen in normal young infants, it disappears as the child matures.

harlequin fetus, an infant whose skin at birth is completely covered with thick, horny scales that resemble armor and are divided by deep red fissures. The condition is the most severe form of lamellar exfoliation of the newborn, and the infant is stillborn or dies within a few days of birth. Also called **ichthyosis fetus.**

Harris tube [Franklin Harris, American surgeon, b. 1895], a tube used for gastric and intestinal decompression. It is a mercury-weighted, single-lumen tube that is passed through the nose and carried through the alimentary tract by gravity. The amount of mercury in the soft bag surrounding the tube varies from 2 to 5 ml according to the age, size, and condition of the patient. The location of the tube and its final placement are checked by fluoroscopy. The tube is lubricated before the procedure is begun, and the patient is positioned in such a way that gravity can aid advancement of the tube through the alimentary tract.

Hartmann's curet [Arthur Hartmann, German physician, b. 1849], a curet used for the removal of adenoids. See also **curet.**

Hartnup disease [Hartnup, family name of first patients di-

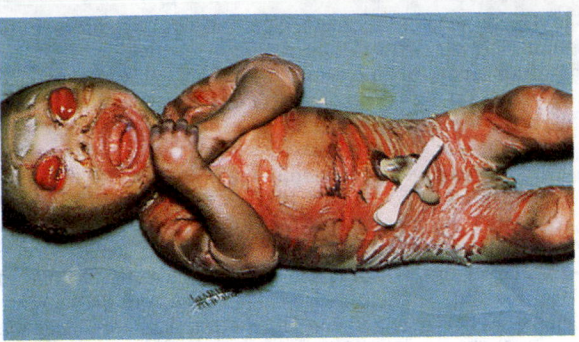

Harlequin fetus
(McKee, 1992/Courtesy Dr RA Marsden, St George's Hospital, London)

agnosed in England, 1956], a recessive genetic metabolic disorder characterized by pellagra-like skin lesions, transient cerebellar ataxia, and hyperaminoaciduria, caused by defects in intestinal absorption and renal reabsorption of neutral amino acids. Bacterial degradation of unabsorbed amino acids in the gut leads to the absorption of breakdown products and their appearance in urine; the unavailability of tryptophan leads to a deficiency of niacin, the antipellagra vitamin. Common symptoms of the disease are dry, scaly, well-circumscribed skin lesions, glossitis, stomatitis, diarrhea, psychiatric problems, and pronounced photosensitivity; brief exposure to the sun may cause erythema, edema, and vesiculation. Treatment consists of oral nicotinamide and a diet containing proteins composed of more easily absorbed small peptides.

Harvard pump, a small pump that can be adjusted to deliver small amounts of medication in solution through an intravenous infusion set. It is commonly used to administer oxytocin in the induction or augmentation of labor. Compare **Abbot pump.**

harvest fever. See **leptospirosis.**

harvest mite. See **chigger.**

Hashimoto's disease /hä′shimō′tōz/ [Hakaru Hashimoto, Japanese surgeon, b. 1881], an autoimmune thyroid disorder, characterized by the production of antibodies in response to thyroid antigens and the replacement of normal thyroid structures with lymphocytes and lymphoid germinal centers. The disease shows a marked hereditary pattern, but it is 20 times more common in women than in men. It occurs most frequently between 30 and 50 years of age but may arise in young children. The thyroid, typically enlarged, pale yellow, and lumpy on the surface, shows dense lymphocytic infiltration, and the remaining thyroid tissue frequently contains small empty follicles. The goiter is usually asymptomatic, but occasionally patients complain of dysphagia and a feeling of local pressure. The thymus is usually enlarged, and regional lymph nodes often show hyperplasia. A definitive diagnosis can be made if a fluorescent scan shows a decrease or absence of thyroid-stable iodine and if a hemagglutination test for thyroid antigens is positive. Replacement therapy with thyroid hormone is indicated for patients with thyroid deficiency and can prevent further enlargement of the goiter. Also called **Hashimoto's struma, Hashimoto's thyroiditis, lymphocytic thyroiditis, struma lymphomatosa.**

hashish. See **cannabis.**

Hasner's fold. See **lacrimal fold.**

haustus (h) /hôs′təs/, a draught of medicine.

HAV, abbreviation for *hepatitis A virus.* See **hepatitis A.**

Haverhill fever /hā′vəril/ [Haverhill, Massachusetts, disorder first diagnosed, 1925], a febrile disease, caused by infection with *Streptobacillus moniliformis,* transmitted by the bite of a rat. The spirochete-like bacterium is normally present in rat saliva. Characteristically the wound from the bite heals, but within 10 days fever, chills, vomiting, headache, muscle and joint pain, and a rash appear. Treatment with antibiotics is effective. *S. moniliformis* is identified by laboratory analysis using fluorescent antibody screening. Also called **streptobacillary ratbite fever.**

Haver's glands. See **haversian glands.**

haversian canal /havur′shən/ [Clopton Havers, English physician, b. 1650], one of the many tiny longitudinal canals in bone tissue, averaging about 0.05 mm in diameter. Each contains blood vessels, connective tissue, nerve filaments, and, occasionally, lymphatic vessels. The canals are interconnected and part of an intricate network. See also **haversian canaliculus, haversian system, Volkmann's canal.**

haversian canaliculus /kan′əlik′yələs/, any one of the many tiny passages radiating from the lacunae of bone tissue to larger haversian canals. See also **haversian canal, haversian system.**

haversian glands [Clopton Havers, English physician, b. 1650; L, *glans,* acorn], extrasynovial fat pads that may project into the joint space. Also called **Havers' glands.**

haversian lamella [Clopton Havers; L, *lamella,* a small plate], one of a series of lamellae (circular layers) arranged around the central haversian canal of an osteon, or cylindrical unit of bone structure. Also called **Havers' lamella.**

haversian system, a circular district of bone tissue, consisting of concentric lamellae in the bone around a central blood vessel canal. See also **haversian canal, haversian canaliculus, Volkmann's canal.**

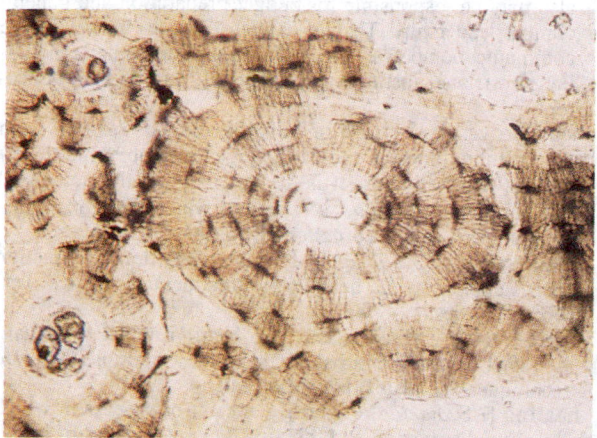

Haversian systems *(Seeley, 1992/Trent Steph*

Haver's lamella. See **haversian lamella.**

Hawthorne effect /hô′thôrn/, a general, unintentional, but usually beneficial effect on a person, a group of people, or the function of the system being studied. The Hawthorne effect is the effect of an encounter, as with an investigator or health care provider, or of a change in a program or facility, as by painting an office or changing the lighting system. The Hawthorne effect is likely to confound the results of a study or investigation, because it is usually present and difficult to identify. It was named for a study in industrial management at the Hawthorne (Illinois) facility of the Western Electric Company.

hay fever [AS, *heawan,* to hew; L, *febris,* fever], *informal.* an acute seasonal allergic rhinitis stimulated by tree, grass, or weed pollens. Also called **pollinosis.** See also **allergic rhinitis, organic dust.**

Hayflick limits [Leonard Hayflick, American scientist, b. 1928; L, *limes,* border], the concept that the lifespan of living organisms is limited by the number of times that somatic cells will subdivide. On the basis of human cells in cultures, where divisions occur about 50 times, it is estimated the average human life span is limited to around 115 years.

hazard /haz′ərd/ [Fr, *hasard,* chance], a condition or phenomenon that increases the probability of a loss that may result in injury or illness. **—hazardous,** *adj.*

Hb, abbreviation for **hemoglobin.**

HB, abbreviation for **hepatitis B.**

Hb A, abbreviation for **hemoglobin A.**

Hb A$_2$, abbreviation for **hemoglobin A$_2$.**

HB Ag, an abbreviation for *hepatitis B antigen.* See also **hepatitis B.**

Hb C, abbreviation for **hemoglobin C.**

HBE, abbreviation for **His bundle electrogram.**

Hb F, abbreviation for **hemoglobin F.**

HBIG, abbreviation for **hepatitis B immune globulin.**

Hb S, abbreviation for **hemoglobin S.**

HBsAG, abbreviation for **hepatitis B surface antigen.** See also **Australia antigen.**

Hb S-C, abbreviation for **hemoglobin S-C.**

HBV, abbreviation for *hepatitis B virus.* See **hepatitis B.**

HCG, abbreviation for **human chorionic gonadotropin.** See also **chorionic gonadotropin.**

HCG radioreceptor assay, a urine test to detect pregnancy or missed abortion, performed by measuring human chorionic gonadotropin, a chemical found only in the urine of pregnant women or in tumors that produce HCG. The normal values are negative (within 2 hours) if the patient is not pregnant and positive (within 1 hour) if the patient is pregnant. Also called **pregnancy test.**

HCl, abbreviation for **hydrochloric acid** or **hydrochloride.**

HCV, abbreviation for *hepatitis C virus.* See **hepatitis C.**

HDCV, abbreviation for **human diploid cell rabies vaccine.**

HDV, abbreviation for *hepatitis D virus.* See **hepatitis D.**

H deflection, (in cardiology) a deflection observed on the His electrogram that represents activation of the bundle of His.

HDL, abbreviation for **high-density lipoprotein.**

He, symbol for the element **helium.**

head [AS, *heafd*], the anteriormost part of the body, containing the brain, special sense organs, mouth, nose, and related structures. Most of the tissues are enclosed within the skull, composed of 22 bones. At birth the head is about half the size of an adult head; most of the changes after infancy involve growth of the facial area.

headache /hed′āk/ [AS, *heafd* + *acan,* to hurt], a pain in the head from any cause. Kinds of headaches include **func-**

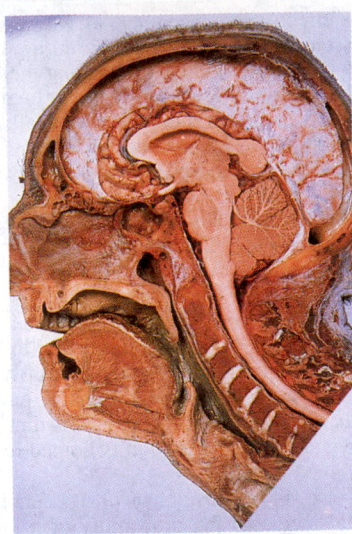

Midsagittal section of the head
(Seeley, 1992/RT Hutchings)

tional headache, histamine headache, migraine headache, organic headache, sinus headache, and **tension headache.** Also called **cephalalgia, cephalgia.**

head and neck cancer, any malignant neoplasms of the upper aerodigestive tract, facial features, and structures in the neck, presenting as masses, ulcerations, or flat lesions that usually produce early symptoms. Tumors of the oral cavity, lips, and tongue characteristically begin as a swelling or nonhealing ulcer and are most commonly epidermoid carcinomas that occur in men over 60 years of age; predisposing factors are chronic alcoholism, heavy use of tobacco, poor oral hygiene, syphilis, and Plummer-Vinson syndrome. Nasal and paranasal sinus malignancies, most often epidermoid cancers, cause a bloody discharge, obstruction in breathing, and facial and dental pain. Nasopharyngeal tumors, predominantly squamous cell and undifferentiated carcinomas occurring most frequently in Orientals, are associated with nasal obstruction, serous otitis media, hearing loss, lymphadenopathy, and cranial nerve involvement. Oropharyngeal and tonsillar neoplasms, usually squamous cell carcinomas and less frequently lymphomas, produce dysphagia, pain, dyspnea, and trismus. Most hypopharyngeal and laryngeal tumors are carcinomas that cause hoarseness, dysphagia, dyspnea, cough, and cervical adenopathy. Salivary gland carcinomas occur most frequently in the parotid gland and may cause facial palsy. Cancer of the mandible, including extremely painful osteosarcoma and, often, painless giant cell tumor, Ewing's sarcoma, and ameloblastoma, may erode through the gingiva, producing an intraoral ulcer, and may cause pathologic fractures. Ear neoplasms involve the auricle in most cases, usually occur in persons over 50 years of age, and are most commonly squamous cell carcinomas that cause pain, deafness, and facial nerve paralysis. Cancers of the lacrimal glands, lacrimal sacs, and parathyroid glands are rare, but hypercalcemia, hypercalcinuria, kidney stones, and renal and bone diseases are associated with parathyroid carcinoma. Tumors of the eye, as malignant melanoma in patients over 50 years of age and retinoblastoma in

children, are also rare. Head and neck tumors are diagnosed by clinical examination, x-ray examinations, tomograms, biopsies, arteriograms, supravital staining of lesions, and cytologic studies. Surgery and radiotherapy are the primary treatments, but their use may cause problems with swallowing and speaking; the effectiveness of chemotherapy is limited by the poor nutritional status of many patients with head or neck lesions. Plastic surgery and various prostheses are often essential in correcting deformities and restoring functions in patients who have undergone the excision or radiotherapy of a head or neck tumor. See also specific cancer.

head bobbing, a sign of respiratory distress in an infant. Head bobbing occurs as a result of attempting to use scaleni and sternocleidomastoid muscles to assist ventilation. Because neck extensor muscles are not strong enough to stabilize the head, accessory muscle use produces head bobbing.

head box, a clear plastic chamber that fits over a patient's head with an adjustable seal around the neck for mechanical ventilation. Humidified gas enters the chamber and excess gas is released through an outlet valve. The device may help prevent the need for intubation.

head, eye, ear, nose, and throat (HEENT), a specialty in medicine concerned with the anatomy, physiology, and pathology of the head, eyes, ears, nose, and throat and with the diagnosis and treatment of disorders of those structures.

head injury, any traumatic damage to the head resulting from blunt or penetrating trauma of the skull. Blood vessels, nerves, and meninges can be torn; bleeding, edema, and ischemia may result. See also **concussion.**

head kidney. See **pronephros.**

head louse. See **lice, pediculus humanus capitus.**

head nurse, the clinical and administrative leader of the nurses working in a given geographic division of an institution, usually a floor, ward, or unit. The responsibilities of a head nurse may include directing nursing care activities, scheduling of staff, evaluation of nursing personnel, and hiring, firing, or promoting staff nurses. The head nurse also may be responsible for budget preparation and general clinical leadership. The head nurse acts as liaison in the communication between the nursing staff and others, including physicians, institutional personnel, and nursing educators.

head process, a strand of cells that extends forward from the primitive node in the early stages of embryonic development in vertebrates. It is the precursor of the notochord and forms the primitive axis around which the embryo develops. Also called **notochordal plate.**

head traction [AS, *heafod*; L, *trahere*, to draw], traction that is applied to the head in the treatment of cervical vertebrae injuries.

Heaf test /hēf/ [Frederick R. G. Heaf, English physician, b. 1894], a tuberculin skin test using a multiple puncture technique. See also **tuberculin test.**

healing [AS, *haelan*, to cure], the act or process in which the normal structural and functional characteristics of health are restored to diseased, dysfunctional, or damaged tissues, organs, or systems of the body. See also **intention, wound repair.**

health [AS *haelth*], a condition of physical, mental, and social well-being and the absence of disease or other abnormal condition. It is not a static condition; constant change and adaptation to stress result in homeostasis. René Dubos, often quoted in nursing education, says, "The states of health or disease are the expressions of the success or failure experienced by the organism in its efforts to respond adaptively to environmental challenges." See also **high-level wellness, homeostasis.**

health assessment, an evaluation of the health status of an individual by performing a physical examination after obtaining a health history. Various laboratory tests also may be ordered to confirm a clinical impression or to screen for dysfunction. The depth of investigation and the frequency of the assessment vary with the condition and age of the client and the facility in which the assessment is performed. A significant part of the health assessment is counseling and education that may explain aspects of anatomy, physiology, and pathophysiology and that introduces or affirms the general tenets of a healthful way of life. The person's response to any dysfunction present is observed and noted. The techniques of the health assessment include: palpation, percussion, auscultation, and inspection, including sight, sound, and smell.

health behavior, an action taken by a person to maintain, attain, or regain good health and to prevent illness. Health behavior reflects a person's health beliefs. Some common health behaviors are exercising regularly, eating a balanced diet, and obtaining necessary inoculations.

health belief model, a conceptual framework that describes a person's health behavior as an expression of health beliefs. The model was designed to predict a person's health behavior, including the use of health services, and to justify intervention to alter maladaptive health behavior. Components of the model include the person's own perception of susceptibility to a disease or condition, the likelihood of contracting that disease or condition, the person's perception of the severity of the consequences of contracting the condition or the disease, the perceived benefits of care and barriers to preventive behavior, and the internal or external stimuli that result in appropriate health behavior by the person.

health care consumer, any actual or potential recipient of health care, such as a patient in a hospital, a client in a community mental health center, or a member of a prepaid health maintenance organization.

health care industry, the complex of preventive, remedial, and therapeutic services provided by hospitals and other institutions, nurses, doctors, dentists, government agencies, voluntary agencies, noninstitutional care facilities, pharmaceutic and medical equipment manufacturers, and health insurance companies.

health care provider, any individual who provides health services to health care consumers.

health care proxy [AS, *haelth*; ME, *caru*, sorrow; L, *procuratio*, a deputy], a person designated to make health care decisions for a patient who has become incapacitated.

health care system, the complete network of agencies, facilities, and all providers of health care in a specified geographic area. Nursing services are integral to all levels and patterns of care, and nurses form the largest number of providers in a health care system.

health certificate, a statement signed by a health care provider that attests to the state of health of a person.

health consumer. See **health care consumer.**

health councils. organizations initiated by the Canadian Minister of Health to plan and allocate health care failcities. Local participants are represented in the District Health Councils, funded by the Ministry of Health.

health culture, a system that attempts to explain and treat sickness and to maintain health. Health cultures are part of the larger culture or tradition of a people. It may be a popular or folk system, or it may be a technical or scientific one.

health economics, a social system that studies the supply and demand of health care resources and the effect of health services on a population.

health education, an educational program directed to the general public that attempts to improve, maintain, and safeguard the health of the community.

health hazard [AS, *haelth*; OFr, *hasard*], a danger to health resulting from exposure to environmental pollutants, such as asbestos or ionizing radiation, or to a lifestyle influence, such as cigarette smoking or chemical abuse.

health history, (in nursing and medicine) a collection of information obtained from the patient and from other sources concerning the patient's physical status and psychologic, social, and sexual functions. The history provides a data base on which a plan for management of the diagnosis, treatment, care, and follow-up of the patient may be made. The first part of the history describes the present illness (PI), including its signs and symptoms, onset and character, and any factors or behaviors that aggravate or ameliorate the symptoms. The patient's own words often serve as the best description and may be quoted. The second part of the history comprises an account of previous illnesses, conditions, allergies, transfusions, immunizations, screening tests, and hospitalizations. An occupational history, describing the patient's work and exposure to stress, toxins, radiation, or other occupational hazards, may be included. The effect of the current illness on the patient's work is also noted. A social history is taken in which the patient's social, cultural, and familial milieu are outlined, focusing on aspects that might have an effect on the current illness. In some instances a sexual history may be relevant. A review of systems may follow or be incorporated into the health history. Kinds of history include **complete health history, episodic health history,** and **interval health history.** Also called **functional assessment.** See also **occupational history, review of systems, sexual history.**

health maintenance, a program or procedure planned to prevent illness, to maintain maximal function, and to promote health. It is central to health care, especially to nursing care at all levels (primary, secondary, and tertiary) and in all patterns (preventive, episodic, acute, chronic, and catastrophic).

health maintenance, altered, a nursing diagnosis accepted by the Fifth National Conference on the Classification of Nursing Diagnoses. This diagnosis describes the condition in which the patient is unable to identify, manage, or seek help to maintain health. The causes of the problem include the lack of or significant alteration in written, verbal, or other communication skills; perceptual or cognitive impairment or the inability to make deliberate and thoughtful judgments; impairment or lack of motor skills; lack of material resources; or the inability to cope. The defining characteristics include a demonstrated lack of knowledge regarding basic health practices or the inability to take responsibility for meeting those needs, the inability to adapt to internal or external environmental change, a lack of financial or other resources or support systems, a history of a lack of health-seeking behavior, or an increased interest in improving health behavior. See also **nursing diagnosis.**

health maintenance organization (HMO), a type of group health care practice that provides basic and supplemental health maintenance and treatment services to voluntary enrollees who prepay a fixed periodic fee that is set without regard to the amount or kind of services received. Some of the first HMOs, Kaiser-Permanente among them, have demonstrated that high quality medical care often can be provided at less expense by such a system than by other health care systems. In addition to diagnostic and treatment services, including hospitalization and surgery, an HMO often offers supplemental services, such as dental, mental, and eye care, and prescription drugs. Federal financial support for the establishment of HMOs was provided under Title XIII of the 1973 U.S. Public Health Service Act.

health physicist, a health scientist who directs research, training, and management of programs in which patients and health professionals are exposed to potential hazards associated with the use of diagnostic and therapeutic equipment, such as radioactive materials.

health physics, the study of the effects of ionizing radiation on the body and the methods for protecting people from the undesirable effects of the radiation. Health physics is concerned with the development and evaluation of methods, techniques, materials, and procedures to be used to protect people from these untoward effects. Also called **medical physics.**

health policy, **1.** a statement of a decision regarding a goal in health care and a plan for achieving that goal; for example, to prevent an epidemic, a program for innoculating a population is developed and implemented. **2.** a field of study and practice in which the priorities and values underlying health resource allocation are determined.

health professional, any person who has completed a course of study in a field of health, such as a registered nurse, physical therapist, or physician. The person is usually licensed by a government agency or certified by a professional organization.

health-related services, services of a health facility other than medical care that may contribute directly or indirectly to the physical or mental health and well-being of patients, such as personal or social services.

health resources, all materials, personnel, facilities, funds, and anything else that can be used for providing health care and services.

health risk, a disease precursor associated with a higher than average morbidity or mortality. The disease precursors may include demographic variables, certain individual behaviors, familial and individual histories, and certain physiologic changes.

health risk appraisal, a process of gathering, analyzing, and comparing an individual's prognostic characteristics of health with a standard age group, thereby predicting the likelihood that a person may develop prematurely a health problem associated with a high morbidity and mortality rate.

health screening, a program designed to evaluate the health status and potential of an individual. In the process it may be found that a person has a particular disease or condition or is at greater-than-normal risk of developing it. Health screening may include taking a personal and family health history and performing a physical examination or tests, laboratory tests, or radiologic examination, and may be followed by counseling, education, referral, or further testing.

health seeking behaviors, a nursing diagnosis accepted by the Eighth National Conference on the Classification of Nursing Diagnoses. This diagnosis describes a state in which a client in stable health is actively seeking ways to alter personal health habits and the environment to move toward optimal health. The major defining characteristic is an expressed or observed desire to seek a higher level of wellness. Minor characteristics include (stated, demonstrated, or observed) unfamiliarity with wellness community resources, lack of knowledge in health promotion behaviors, desire for increased control of health practice, and concern about environmental conditions or health status. See also **nursing diagnosis.**

health service area, a geographic region designated under the National Health Planning and Resources Development Act of 1974, covering such factors as geography, political boundaries, population, and health resources, for the effective planning and development of health services.

health supervision, health teaching, counseling, or monitoring the status of the patient's health other than for physical care. Such supervision occurs in health care agencies, clinics, physicians' offices, or the patient's home. Compare **care of the sick.**

health systems agency (HSA), an agency established under the terms of the National Health Planning and Resources Development Act of 1974. Health planning agencies are intended to provide networks of health planning and resource development services in each of several health service areas established by the Act. Health systems agencies are nonprofit and include private organizations, public regional planning bodies, or local government agencies and consumers. See also **health systems plan.**

health systems plan, a plan in which the long-range health goals of a health services area are specified. Health systems plans are prepared by health systems agencies. See also **health policy.**

hearing [AS, *hieran*], the special sense that enables sound to be perceived. It is the major function of the ear. Any reduction in the ability to perceive sounds results in hearing loss, which can range from mild impairment to complete deafness. See also **deafness.**

hearing aid, an electronic device that amplifies sound for people with impaired hearing. The device consists of a microphone, a battery power supply, an amplifier, and a receiver. The microphone receives sound waves directed toward the person with hearing loss, the sound waves are converted to electric impulses that are amplified with the aid of the power supply, and the receiver converts the electric impulses back into sound vibrations.

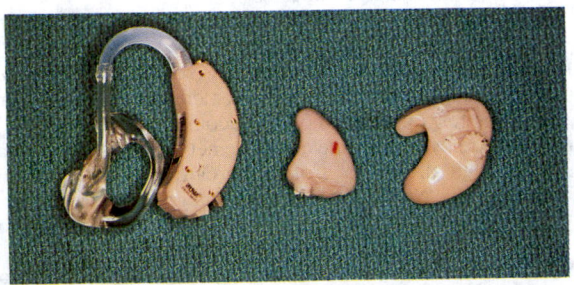

Hearing aids *(Bingham, 1992/Courtesy Dr Julian Nedzelski)*

hearing impairment loss of hearing that adversely affects an individual's ability to communicate.

hearing loss, an inability to perceive the normal range of sounds audible to an individual with normal hearing. Hearing loss may be greater at some frequencies than others, or all frequencies may be equally affected. **Conductive hearing loss** is a result of damage to the outer or middle ear, while **sensorineural hearing loss** results from damage to the inner ear or auditory nerve. The loss is measured in decibels and may be described as mild, moderate, severe, or profound.

heart [AS, *heorte*], the muscular, cone-shaped organ, about the size of a clenched fist, that pumps blood throughout the body and beats normally about 70 times per minute by coordinated nerve impulses and muscular contractions. Enclosed in pericardium, the heart rests on the diaphragm between the lower borders of the lungs, occupying the middle of the mediastinum. It is covered ventrally by the sternum and the adjoining parts of the third to the sixth costal cartilages. The organ is about 12 cm long, 8 cm wide at its broadest part, and 6 cm thick. The weight of the heart in men averages between 280 and 340 g and in women, between 230 and 280 g. The layers of the heart, starting from the outside, are the epicardium, the myocardium, and the endocardium. The epicardium includes the visceral pericardium and a layer of fibroelastic connective tissue interspersed with fat. The myocardium is composed of layers and bundles of cardiac muscle laced by blood vessels. The endocardium is continuous with the endothelial lining of the blood vessels and is composed of squamous endothelium. The chambers of the heart include two ventricles with thick muscular walls, making up the bulk of the organ, and two atria with thin muscular walls. A septum separates the ventricles and extends between the atria (interatrial septum), dividing the heart into the right and the left sides. The left side of the heart pumps oxygenated blood into the aorta and on to all parts of the body. The right side of the heart receives deoxygenated blood from the vena cavae and pumps it into the pulmonary arteries. The sinoatrial node in the right atrium of the heart initiates the cardiac impulse, causing the atria to contract. The atrioventricular node in the septal wall of the right atrium spreads the impulse over the bundle of His, causing the ventricles to contract. Both atria contract simultaneously, followed quickly by the simultaneous

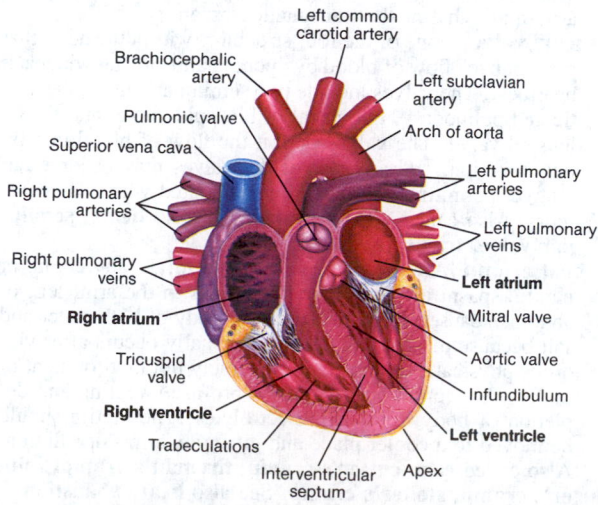

Right pulmonary arteries

Right pulmonary veins

Right atrium

Tricuspid valve

Right ventricle

Trabeculations

Interventricular septum

Apex

Brachiocephalic artery

Pulmonic valve

Superior vena cava

Left common carotid artery

Left subclavian artery

Arch of aorta

Left pulmonary arteries

Left pulmonary veins

Left atrium

Mitral valve

Aortic valve

Infundibulum

Left ventricle

Frontal section of the heart (Canobbio, 1990)

contraction of the ventricles. The valves of the heart include the tricuspid valve between the right atrium and the right ventricle, the bicuspid (mitral) valve between the left atrium and the left ventricle, the semilunar aortic valve at the exit of the left ventricle, and the semilunar pulmonary valve at the exit of the right ventricle. The sinoatrial node of the heartbeat sets the rate. Other factors affecting the heartbeat are emotion, exercise, hormones, temperature, pain, and stress.

heart block, an interference with the normal conduction of electric impulses that control activity of the heart muscle. Heart block usually is further defined as to the location of the block and the type, such as a first-degree AV block in which all atrial impulses that should be conducted to the ventricles reach the ventricles but are delayed by a fraction of a second. The delay or block can occur in the sinoatrial node, atria, atrioventricular node, the bundle of His, the fascicles, or a combination of these. See also **atrioventricular block, bundle branch block, cardiac conduction defect, infranodal block, intraatrial block, intraventricular block, sinoatrial block.**

heartburn, a painful burning sensation in the esophagus just below the sternum. Heartburn is usually caused by the reflux of gastric contents into the esophagus but may be caused by gastric hyperacidity or peptic ulcer. Antacids relieve the symptoms but do not cure the heartburn. Also called **pyrosis.** See also **gastroesophageal reflux, hiatus hernia.**

heart disease risk factors [AS, *heorte,* heart; L, *dis*; Fr, *aise,* ease, *risquer,* chance of injury; L, *facere,* to make], hereditary lifestyle and environmental influences that increase one's chances of developing heart disease. Examples include cigarette smoking, high blood pressure, obesity, foods that contribute exogenous fats, and hereditary factors.

heart failure, a condition in which the heart cannot pump enough blood to meet the metabolic requirements of body tissues. Many of the symptoms associated with heart failure are caused by the dysfunction of organs other than the heart, especially the lungs, kidneys, and liver. Ventricular dysfunction is usually the basic disorder in congestive heart failure and often triggers compensatory mechanisms that preserve cardiac output but produce symptoms and signs, such as dyspnea, orthopnea, rales, and edema. Heart failure is closely associated with many forms of heart disease. Most kinds of heart disease initially affect the left side of the heart, and clinicians commonly divide associated heart failure into left-sided heart failure and right-sided heart failure. Peripheral edema occurs in connection with right-sided heart failure and dyspnea in connection with left-sided heart failure. Current studies indicate that heart failure in infants and children is usually the result of congenital heart disease, but it also may be caused by myocarditis and ectopic tachycardia. Rheumatic mitral disease and aortic valve disease frequently cause congestive heart failure in young adults. Mitral valve disease, especially mitral stenosis, is the most common cause of heart failure and affects more young women than men. The common causes of heart failure after 40 years of age are coronary atherosclerosis with myocardial infarction, diastolic hypertension, valvular heart disease, pulmonary disease, and diffuse myocardial disease. Some individuals may suffer heart failure caused by a combination of congenital heart disease and acquired disease. After 50 years of age, a common cause of heart failure, especially in men, is calcific aortic stenosis. Some of the extracardiac signs of heart failure are ascites, bronchial wheezing, hydrothorax, edema, enlargement of the liver, moist rales, and splenomegaly. Some of the cardiac signs associated with heart failure are abnormalities in the jugular venous pulsation and the carotid pulse, and abnormal cardiographic tracings of the apex wave. The treatment for heart failure commonly involves the reduction of the workload of the heart, the administration of certain drugs, such as digitalis, to increase myocardial contractility and cardiac output, salt-restricted diets, diuretics, and surgical intervention. See also **compensated heart failure, congestive heart failure.**

heart-lung machine, an apparatus consisting of a pump and an oxygenator that takes over the functions of the heart and lungs, especially during cardiac surgery. The blood is shunted from the venous system through an oxygenator and returned to the arterial circulation.

heart massage. See **cardiac massage.**

heart murmur. See **cardiac murmur.**

heart rate, the pulse, calculated by counting the number of QRS complexes or contractions of the ventricles per minute. Tachycardia is a heart rate of more than 100 beats per minute; bradycardia is a heart rate of fewer than 60 beats per minute. See also **pulse.**

heart scan, a radiographic scan of the heart, performed after injecting a radioactive material into a vein, used for determining the size, shape, and location of the heart, for diagnosing pericarditis, and for viewing the chambers of the heart. See also **cardiography, echocardiography.**

heart sound, a normal noise produced within the heart during the cardiac cycle that can be heard over the precordium and may reveal abnormalities in cardiac structure or function. Cardiac auscultation is performed systematically from apex to base of the heart or from base to apex, using a stethoscope to listen initially with the diaphragm and then with the bell of the instrument. The first heart sound (S_1), a dull, prolonged 'lub,' occurs with the closure of the mitral and tricuspid valves and marks the onset of ventricular systole; the mitral valve sound is loudest at the apex of the heart and that of the tricuspid valve at the left sternal border in the fourth intercostal space. The second heart sound (S_2), a short, sharp 'dup,' occurs with the closing of the aortic and pulmonic valves at the beginning of ventricular diastole; the aortic valve closure is heard loudest on the right sternal border, and that of the pulmonic valve is most distinct on the left sternal border over the second intercostal space. A weak, low-pitched, dull third heart sound (S_3) is sometimes heard and is thought to be caused by vibrations of the walls of the ventricles when they are suddenly distended by blood from the atria. S_3, which is heard most clearly at the apex of the heart with the bell of a stethoscope, is called a ventricular or diastolic gallop; it may be normal in children, adolescents, or very thin adults, or it may be a sign of congestive heart failure or hypertension causing left ventricular failure. A left-sided fourth heart sound (S_4), which may be heard with the stethoscope's bell at the apex of the heart during expiration, is caused by vibrations of the atria after contraction. Called an atrial or presystolic gallop, S_4 is usually a sign of pathology, such as myocardial infarction or impending heart failure from another cause. Additional heart sounds include clicks, murmurs, rubs, and snaps.

heart surgery, any surgical procedure involving the heart, performed to correct acquired or congenital defects, to replace diseased valves, to open or bypass blocked vessels, or to graft a prosthesis or a transplant in place. Two major types of heart surgery are performed, closed and open. The closed technique is done through a small incision, without using the heart-lung machine. In the open technique the heart chambers are open and fully visible, and blood is detoured around the surgical field by the heart-lung machine. Preoperative care focuses on the correction of metabolic imbalances and cardiac and pulmonary ailments and on diagnostic and laboratory tests. General anesthesia is used, the chest cavity is opened, and the heart-lung machine is connected. Hypothermia also may be used to reduce the metabolic rate and the need of the tissues for oxygen. The heart is opened, and the defect is corrected. Postoperatively, constant observation is required in an intensive care unit for signs of hemorrhage, shock, fibrillation, dysrhythmia, sudden chest pain, and pulmonary edema. The blood pressure, all pulses, respirations, and venous and pulmonary artery pressures are monitored. If the blood pressure is high enough to assure cerebral profusion, the head of the patient's bed is lifted to a semi-Fowler's position to encourage chest drainage and lung expansion. Oxygen is given via the endotracheal tube for 18 to 24 hours. Chest tube drainage, urinary output, and temperature are noted hourly; and intravenous infusions and blood transfusions are often given. The patient may be kept heavily sedated for the first 12 hours. Narcotics help to control pain and allow coughing and deep breathing. Antibiotics are given to prevent infection. The mortality rate is highest during the first 48 hours after surgery. Kinds of heart surgery include **Blalock-Taussig procedure, coronary bypass,** and **endarterectomy.** See also **dysrhythmia, fibrillation, heart-lung machine, hypothermia, pulmonary edema.**

heart transplantation [AS, *hoerte*; L, *transplantare*], the surgical removal of a donor heart and transfer of the organ to a recipient. The procedure usually involves removal of a heart from a healthy individual who may have died in an accident or from another cause unrelated to heart disease and using it to replace a severely diseased heart of another person. Most recipients survive for more than 1 year with a transplanted heart, and nearly three-fourths of the recipients are able to return to work. Total ischemic time for a heart transplant is less than 6 hours between donor and recipient. The heart is transplanted with anastomoses of the aorta, pulmonary artery, and pulmonary vein while venous return is provided by an anastomosis between the recipient's right atrium and that of the transplanted organ.

heart valve, one of the four structures within the heart that prevent back flow of blood by opening and closing with each heartbeat. The valves include two semilunar valves, the aortic and pulmonary, the mitral or bicuspid valve, and the tricuspid valve. The valves permit the flow of blood in only one direction, and any one of the valves may become defective, permitting the backflow associated with heart murmurs. Also called **cardiac valve.** See also **heart, semilunar valve, tricuspid valve.**

heat cramp [AS, *haetu; crammian,* to fill], any cramp or painful spasm of the voluntary muscles in the arm, leg, or abdomen caused by depletion in the body of both water and salt because of heat exhaustion. It usually occurs after vigorous physical exertion in an extremely hot environment or under other conditions that cause profuse sweating and depletion of body fluids and electrolytes. The victim should be moved to a cooler place and given a warm salt solution. Also called **cane-cutter's cramp, fireman's cramp, miner's cramp, stoker's cramp.** See also **heat exhaustion.**

heated nebulization, a method of inhalation therapy using a heating device with a nebulizer that produces a spray with a higher water content than that of a cold atomizer. The mist may be administered through a mask or in a tent. Croup in infancy is often treated with a heated nebulizer.

heat exhaustion, an abnormal condition characterized by weakness, vertigo, nausea, muscle cramps, and loss of consciousness, caused by depletion of body fluid and electrolytes resulting from exposure to intense heat or the inability to acclimatize to heat. Body temperature is near normal blood pressure may drop but usually returns to normal as the person is placed in a recumbent position; the skin is cool, damp, and pale. The person usually recovers with rest and replacement of water and electrolytes. Also called **heat prostration.** Compare **heat hyperpyrexia.** See also **heat cramp.**

heat hyperpyrexia, a severe and sometimes fatal condition resulting from the failure of the temperature regulating capacity of the body, caused by prolonged exposure to the sun or to high temperatures. Reduction or cessation of sweating is an early symptom. Body temperature of 105° F or higher, tachycardia, hot and dry skin, headache, confusion, unconsciousness, and convulsions may occur. Treatment includes cooling, sedation, and fluid replacement. Also called **heatstroke, siriasis, sunstroke.** See also **hyperpyrexia.** Compare **heat exhaustion.**

heat labile. See **thermolabile.**

heat prostration. See **heat exhaustion.**

heat rash, a finely papular or vesicular inflammation of the skin resulting from prolonged exposure to heat and high humidity. Tingling and prickling sensations are common. Prevention and treatment include cool, dry temperatures, ventilation, and absorbent powders. See also **miliaria.**

heatstroke. See **heat hyperpyrexia.**

heaves /hēvz/ [AS, *hebban*, to lift], **1.** a chronic pulmonary disease of horses, similar to human pulmonary emphysema, characterized by wheezing, coughing, and dyspnea on exertion. The causes of the condition are unknown. **2.** *informal.* vomiting and retching.

heavy chain disease [AS, *heafig;* L, *catena,* chain; *dis,* opposite of; Fr, *aise,* ease], a plasma cell disorder characterized by a proliferation of immunoglobulin heavy chains. Excessive levels of alpha, gamma, delta, and mu chains are produced, and effects tend to vary according to the predominant type of heavy chain. Alpha heavy chain disease affects mainly children living in the Middle East, causing diffuse abdominal lymphoma and malabsorption disorders. Most gamma heavy chain disease patients are elderly men who have symptoms resembling those of malignant lymphoma: enlarged liver and spleen, fever, anemia, and increased susceptibility to infections. Delta heavy chain disease is rare and marked by symptoms similar to multiple myeloma. Mu heavy chain disease presents symptoms of chronic lymphocytic leukemia and is treated for those symptoms.

heavy function, (in dentistry) an increase in the functional activities of the teeth.

heavy hydrogen. See **deuterium.**

heavy metal, a metallic element with a specific gravity five or more times that of water. The heavy metals are antimony, arsenic, bismuth, cadmium, cerium, chromium, cobalt, copper, gallium, gold, iron, lead, manganese, mercury, nickel, platinum, silver, tellurium, thallium, tin, uranium, vanadium, and zinc. Small amounts of many of these elements are common and necessary in the diet. Large amounts of any of them may cause poisoning.

heavy metal poisoning, poisoning caused by the inges-

tion, inhalation, or absorption of various toxic heavy metals. Kinds of heavy metal poisoning include **antimony poisoning, arsenic poisoning, cadmium poisoning, lead poisoning,** and **mercury poisoning.** See also **heavy metal.**

heavy vaginal bleeding. See **vaginal bleeding.**

hebephrenia, hebephrenic schizophrenia. See **disorganized schizophrenia.**

Heberden's node /hē′bərdənz/ [William Heberden, English physician, b. 1710; L, *nodus,* knot], an abnormal cartilaginous or bony enlargement of a distal interphalangeal joint of a finger, usually occurring in degenerative diseases of the joints. Compare **Bouchard's node.**

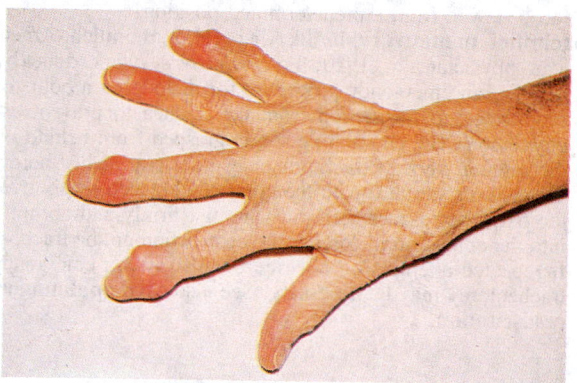

Heberden's nodes *(Kamal, 1991)*

hebetude /heb′itood′/ [L, *hebeo,* to be blunt], a state of dullness or lethargy, characteristic of some forms of schizophrenia.

heboid paranoia. See **paranoid schizophrenia.**

hecto. See **h.**

-hedonia, a combining form meaning '(condition of) pleasure, cheerfulness': *anhedonia, hyphedonia, parhedonia.*

-hedron, a suffix meaning a 'geometric figure with (specified) sides': *decahedron, octahedron, polyhedron.*

heel [AS, *hela*], the posterior part of the foot, formed by the largest tarsal bone, the calcaneus.

heel cup, a plastic device designed to help relieve pain of a heel spur or contusion by pushing the fat pad of the heel under the calcaneus to increase the cushioning effect.

heel-knee test [AS, *hela* + *cneow,* knee; L, *testum,* crucible], a method of assessing coordination of movements of the extremities. In the test the patient, lying supine, is asked to touch the knee of one leg with the heel of the other.

heel lift, a form of foot orthosis, usually made of sheets of cork, to correct a dysfunction that may be the result of anatomic limb length differences or decreased flexibility. The cause of dysfunction may be a compensatory pronation on the longer side in an attempt to equalize leg lengths or a flexibility deficiency caused by a tight gastrocnemius muscle

heel puncture [AS, *hela;* L, *punctura*], a method of obtaining a blood sample from a newborn or premature infant by a puncture in the lateral or medial areas of the plantar surface of the heel. Care must be exercised to avoid puncturing the posterior curvature of the heel and to make the puncture as shallow as feasible.

heel-shin test [AS, *hela* + *scinu,* shin; L, *testum,* crucible], a method of assessing coordination of movements of the extremities. In the test the patient, lying supine, is asked to pass the heel of one leg slowly down the shin of the other leg from the knee to the ankle.

HEENT,   abbreviation for **head, eye, ear, nose, and throat.**

Hegar's sign /hā'gärz/ [Alfred Hegar, German gynecologist, b. 1830; L, *signum*, sign],   a softening of the isthmus of the uterine cervix early in gestation. It is a probable sign of pregnancy.

height (ht) /hīt/ [AS, *hiehtho*],   the vertical measurement of a structure, organ, or other object from bottom to top, when it is placed or projected in an upright position.

height of contour,   the greatest convexity of a tooth surface, viewed from a predetermined position.

Heimlich maneuver /hīm'lik, -lish/ [H. J. Heimlich, American physician, b. 1920; Fr, *manœuvre*, work done by hand],   an emergency procedure for dislodging a bolus of food or other obstruction from the trachea to prevent asphyxiation. The choking person is grasped from behind by the rescuer whose fist, thumb side in, is placed just below the victim's sternum with the other hand placed firmly over the fist. The rescuer then pulls the fist firmly and abruptly into the epigastrium, forcing the obstruction up the trachea. If repeated attempts do not free the airway, an emergency tracheotomy may be necessary. See also **cardiopulmonary resuscitation.**

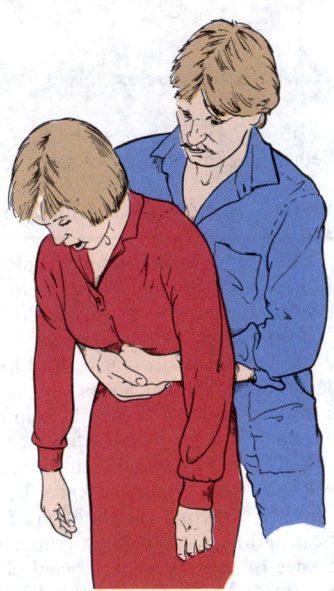

Heimlich maneuver (Thibodeau, 1993/Joan M Beck)

Heimlich sign [H.J. Heimlich, American physician, b. 1920; L, *signum*],   a universal distress signal that a person is choking and unable to speak, made by grasping the throat with a thumb and index finger, thereby attracting the attention of others nearby. Also called **universal choking signal.**

Heinz bodies /hīnts/ [Robert Heinz, German pathologist, b. 1865],   irregularly shaped bits of altered hemoglobin found in the red blood cells of people who are hypersensitive to certain chemicals, such as aniline, phenylhydrazine, and primaquine.

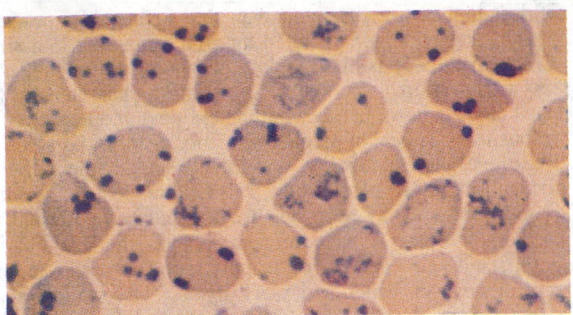

Heinz bodies (Hayhoe, 1992)

Helen, Sister (Helen Bowden),   a nurse who received her education in England and became the first director of the newly formed Bellevue Hospital Training School for Nurses in New York in 1873. Although she had not trained under Florence Nightingale, she set up the Bellevue school along Nightingale's principles. She was a member of the All Saints Sisterhood. After several years at Bellevue, having established one of the leading nursing schools in the United States, she went to South Africa.

Heliodorus' bandage.   See **T bandage.**

heliotherapy.   See **solar therapy.**

helium (He) /hē'lē·əm/ [Gk, *helios*, sun],   a colorless, odorless, gaseous element; the second lightest element after hydrogen. Its atomic number is 2; its atomic weight is 4. Helium is one of the rare or inert gases and does not usually combine with other elements. Most of the commercial helium in the world comes from natural gas reservoirs in Texas and Louisiana, where it is recovered after natural gas has been liquefied. It is produced in nature by the decay of radioactive elements and is produced in the sun from hydrogen. It occurs in the atmosphere in the ratio of five parts per million. Helium is used industrially in arc welding, refining, and other processes. Because of its lightness and lack of flammability it is also used to lift airships and balloons. The main physiologic and medical uses of helium are in respiratory therapy and testing and the prevention of nitrogen narcosis and decompression sickness in hyperbaric environments. A mixture of 80% helium and 20% oxygen is commonly breathed by deep-sea divers to prevent gas emboli and by patients undergoing treatment to clear obstructed respiratory tracts. Problems associated with such uses involve the high velocity of acoustic transmission in helium and the high thermal conductivity of the gas. These characteristics produce voice distortions and hypothermia in persons who inhale it. Helium is one third as soluble in lipids as nitrogen, which accounts for its preferred use in hyperbaric atmospheres, such as those associated with deep-sea diving. The low density of helium reduces the effort of breathing any gas mixture of which it is a component. Helium is used in pulmonary function testing to calculate the diffusing and residual capacities of the lungs.

helium therapy,   the use of helium-oxygen gas mixtures to treat patients with airway obstruction. Because of its low density, helium can negotiate an obstruction more easily. Less driving pressure is required to move helium, a lighter gas, than nitrogen.

helix /hē'liks/ [Gk, coil],   a coiled, spiral-like formation characteristic of many organic molecules, such as deoxyribonucleic acid (DNA).

Heller's test, a laboratory test for proteinuria in which urine is layered upon nitric acid. Appearance of a ring of precipitated protein at the junction of the fluids is a positive sign.

Hellin's law, a generalized formula for calculating the ratio of multiple births in any population, stating that if twin births occur at the rate of 1:N, then the rate of triplet births is approximately $1:N^2$, quadruplets $1:N^3$, quintuplets $1:N^4$, and so on, with the exponent of N being one less than the number in the multiple set. The constant N varies greatly with population, although it was originally set at 89 when the law was formulated. In general, twin births occur approximately once in every 80 pregnancies. Also called **Hellin-Zeleny law.**

helmet cells, fragmented red blood cells that have been 'scooped out' so they resemble helmets. They are found in patients with carcinomatosis, hemolytic anemia, and thrombotic thrombocytopenic purpura. Helmet cells can be seen in blood samples of people with prosthetic heart valves.

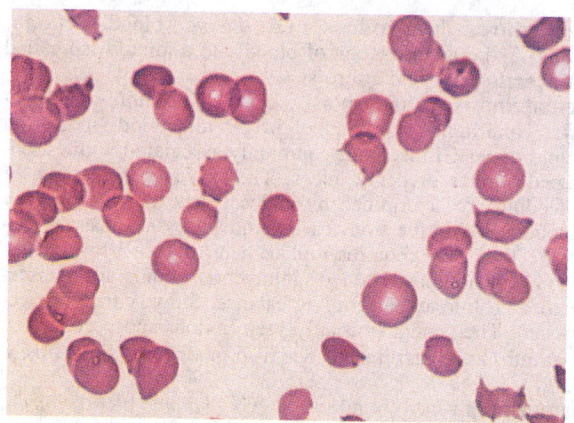

Helmet cells (Hayhoe, 1992)

helminth /hel′minth/ [Gk, *helmins*, worm], a worm, especially one of the pathogenic parasites of the division Metazoa fluke, including flukes, tapeworms, and roundworms.

-helminth, a suffix meaning 'worm': *nemathelminth, platyhelminth.*

helminthemesis /hel′minthem′əsis/ [Gk, *helmins,* worms, *emesis,* vomiting], the vomiting of intestinal worms.

helminthiasis /hel′minthī′əsis/ [Gk, *helmins,* worms, *osis* condition], a parasitic infestation of the body by helminths that may be cutaneous, visceral, or intestinal. Ascariasis, bilharziasis, filariasis, hookworm, and trichinosis are common forms of the disease.

helminthic /helmin′thik/ [Gk, *helmins,* worms], pertaining to worms.

helper T cell. See **T cell.**

helper virus, a virus that is necessary in a phenotypically mixed infection to mediate the replication of a defective virus. Viruses that mature by budding through the cell membrane, such as mammalian sarcoma viruses, require the coding of a helper virus.

helplessness /help′ləsnəs/, a feeling of a loss of control, usually after repeated failures, of being immobilized or fro-

zen by circumstances beyond one's control, with the result that one is unable to make autonomous choices.

Helsinki accords /helsing′kē/, a declaration signed by the representatives of 35 member nations of the Conference on Security and Cooperation in Europe in Helsinki, Finland, on August 1, 1975. The declared goals of the nonbinding document comprised four principal aspects of European security: economic cooperation, humanitarian issues, contact between the East and West, and provision for a later follow-up conference (held in Belgrade in 1978). Follow-up conferences were planned in part to allow the member nations to monitor each other's performance on humanitarian issues, such as the right to self-determination of all people and respect for the fundamental freedoms, including thought, conscience, and religion or belief, without regard to race, language, sex, or religion. The Helsinki accords grew from the precedent set by the judgments at the trials of the Nuremberg tribunals—that crimes against humanity are offenses subject to criminal prosecution. The principal and the practice of informed consent in health care grew from this precedent. Also called **Helsinki Declaration.** See also **Nuremberg tribunals.**

helvolic acid /helvol′ik/, an antibiotic, derived from the mold *Aspergillus fumigatus,* formerly used as an amebicide. Also called **fumagillin, fumigacin.**

hema- /hē′mə-, hem′ə-/, a prefix for terms relating to blood or blood vessels.

hema-, hemat-, a combining form meaning 'blood': *hematoma, hematophyte.*

hemacytometer /-sītom′ətər/ [Gk, *haima,* blood, *kytos,* cell, *metron,* measure], an apparatus for counting the number of cells in a known volume of blood or other fluid. See **Abbé-Zeiss apparatus.**

hemadsorption /hē′madsôrp′shən, hem′-/ [Gk, *haima,* blood; L, *ad* to, *sorbere,* to swallow], a process in which a substance or an agent, such as certain viruses and bacilli, adheres to the surface of an erythrocyte. The process occurs naturally, or it may be induced for laboratory identification of bacteriologic specimens.

hemagglutination /hē′məgloo′tinā′shən, hem′-/ [Gk, *haima,* + L, *agglutinare,* to glue], the coagulation of erythrocytes. See also **blood clotting.**

hemagglutinin [Gk, *haima* + L, *agglutinare*], a type of antibody that agglutinates red blood cells. It is classified according to the source of cells agglutinated as **autologous** (from the same organism), **homologous** (from an organism of the same species), and **heterologous** (from an organism of a different species). Some hemagglutinins clump red cells together as they are suspended in 0.85% sodium chloride solution; others will not agglutinate red cells unless hydrophilic colloids are added or unless the red cells have been treated with a proteolytic enzyme.

hemangi-, a combining form meaning 'pertaining to a condition of the blood vessel structure or a collection of blood vessels': *hemangioma, hemangiectesis.*

hemangioblastoma /hēman′jē·ōblastō′mə/, *pl.* **hemangioblastomas, hemangioblastomata** [Gk, *haima* + *aggeion,* small vessel, *blastos,* germ, *oma,* tumor], a brain tumor composed of a proliferation of capillaries and of disorganized clusters of capillary cells or angioblasts, usually occuring in the cerebellum.

hemangioendothelioma /hēman′jē·ō·en′dōthē′lē·ō′mə/, *pl.* **hemangioendotheliomas, hemangioendotheliomata** [Gk, *haima* + *endon,* inside, *thele,* nipple, *oma,* tumor], **1.** also called **angioendothelioma.** a tumor, consisting of

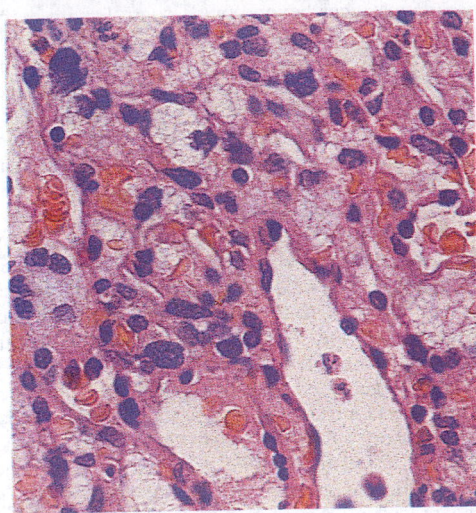

Hemangioblastoma
(Okazaki, 1988/by permission of Mayo Foundation)

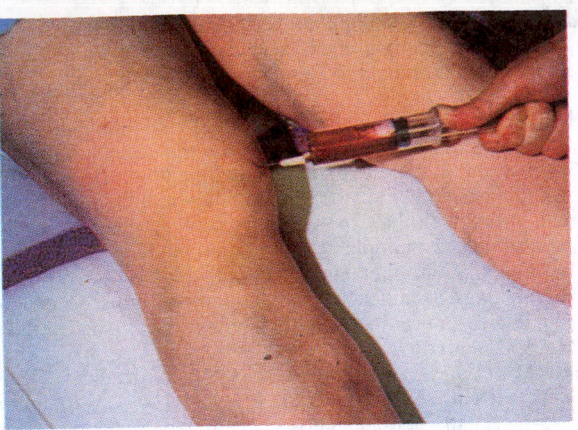

Hemarthros *(Shipley, 1993)*

endothelial cells, that grows around an artery or a vein. The benign form is seen in children and is usually cured by local excision. The tumor rarely becomes malignant. **2.** malignant hemangioendothelioma. See also **angiosarcoma.**

hemangiofibroma /-fībrō′mə/ [Gk, *haima,* blood; L, *fibra,* fiber; Gk, *oma,* tumor], a tumor that has the characteristics of both a hemangioma and a fibroma.

hemangioma /hēman′jē·ō′mə/, *pl.* **hemangiomas, hemangiomata** [Gk, *haima + aggeion,* small vessel, *oma*], a benign tumor consisting of a mass of blood vessels. Types of hemangiomas include **capillary hemangioma, cavernous hemangioma,** and **nevus flammeus.**

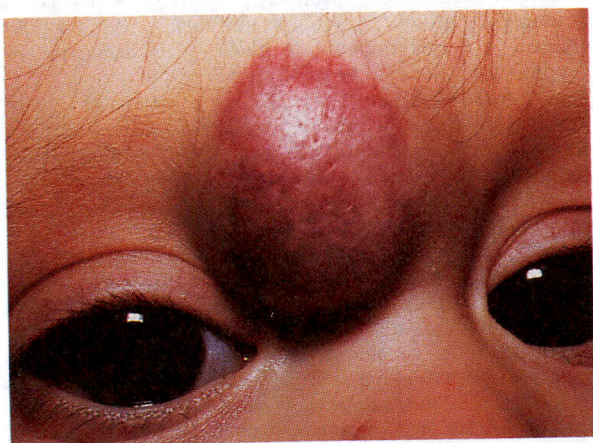

Mixed hemangioma *(Zitelli, 1992)*

hemangioma simplex. See **capillary hemangioma.**
hemangiosarcoma. See **angiosarcoma.**
hemapoiesis /hem′əpō·ē′sis/ [Gk, *haima,* blood, *poiein,* to make], the formation of blood cells.

hemarthros /hem′är′thrəs/ [Gk, *haima,* blood, *arthron,* joint], the extravasation of blood into a joint. Also called **hemarthrosis** /hem′ärthrō′sis/.

hematemesis /hē′mətem′əsis, hem′-/ [Gk, *haima + emesis,* vomiting], vomiting of bright red blood, indicating rapid upper GI bleeding, commonly associated with esophageal varices or peptic ulcer. The rate and the source of bleeding are determined by endoscopic examination. Any blood found in the stomach is removed by nasogastric suction. Treatment requires replacement of blood by transfusion and administration of intravenous fluids for maintenance of fluid and electrolyte balance. Surgery may be necessary. The patient is usually very anxious and needs quiet, warmth, and reassurance. See also **gastrointestinal bleeding.**

hematinuria /hem′ətinoor′ē·ə/ [Gk, *haima,* blood, *ouron,* urine], a dark colored urine resulting from the presence of hematin or hemoglobin. See also **hemoglobinuria.**

hemato- /hē′mətō-, hem′ətō-/ [Gk, *haima,* blood], a prefix for terms relating to blood or blood vessels.

hematocele /hem′ətōsēl′/, a cystlike accumulation of blood within the tunica vaginalis of the scrotum. It is usually caused by injury and may require surgery if the blood is not easily reabsorbed.

hematochezia /hem′ətōkē′zhə/ [Gk, *haima + chezo,* feces], the passage of red blood through the rectum. The cause is usually bleeding in the colon or rectum, but may result from the loss of blood higher in the digestive tract. Blood passed from the stomach or small intestine generally loses its red coloration through enzymatic activity on the erythrocytes. Cancer, colitis, and ulcers are among causes of hematochezia. Compare **melena.**

hematocrit /hemat′ōkrit/ [Gk, *haima + krinein,* to separate], a measure of the packed cell volume of red cells, expressed as a percentage of the total blood volume. The normal range is between 43% and 49% in men, and between 37% and 43% in women. See also **complete blood count, differential white blood cell count.**

hematocrit reading. See **packed cell volume.**

hematocyte /hem′ətōsīt/ [Gk, *haima,* blood, *kytos,* cell], a blood cell, particularly a red blood cell. Also called **hemocyte.**

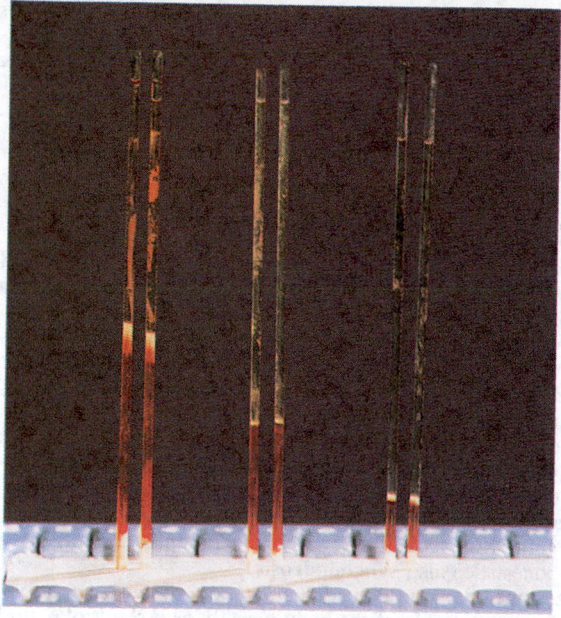

Hematocrit *(Bain, 1989)*

hematocytoblast /hem′ətōsī′təblast′/ [Gk, *haima*, blood, *kytos*, cell, *blastos*, germ], a large nucleated reticuloendothelial cell found in bone marrow. It is believed to be a common precursor of various blood elements. Also called **hemocytoblast.**

hematogenesis /-jen′əsis/ [Gk, *haima*, blood, *genein*, to produce], pertaining to the formation of blood cells or an increase in the production of blood elements. Also called **hemapoiesis.**

hematogenic shock /-jen′ik/ [Gk, *haima* + *genein*, to produce; Fe, *choc*], a condition of shock caused by the loss of blood or plasma.

hematogenous /hēmətoj′ənəs/ [Gk, *haima* + *genein*, to produce], originated or transported in the blood.

hematogenous pigment /hem′ətoj′ənəs/ [Gk, *haima*, blood, *genein*, to produce; L, *pingere*, to paint], the red color of erythrocytes caused by the presence of hemoglobin.

hematogenous tuberculosis [Gk, *haima*, blood, *genein*, to produce; L, *tuberculum*, a small swelling; Gk, *osis*, condition], a form of tuberculosis that is blood-borne.

-hematologic. See **hematology.**

-hematological. See **hematology.**

hematologic death syndrome /hem′ətōloj′ik/, a group of clinical signs and symptoms of radiation damage to the blood cells. The condition is characterized by nausea, vomiting, fever, diarrhea, infections, anemia, leukopenia, and hemorrhage. It can result from exposure to a dose of 200 to 1000 rad. The mean survival time for a person with hematologic death syndrome is estimated at between 10 and 60 days.

hematologic effect, (in radiology) the response of blood cells to radiation exposure. In general, all types of blood cells are destroyed by radiation, and the degree of cell depletion increases with increasing dose. However, lymphocytes are affected first and reduced in number within min-

utes or hours after exposure. Erythrocytes are less sensitive than other types of blood cells and may not show radiation effects for several weeks.

hematologist /hē′mətol′əjist, hem′-/, a medical specialist in the field of hematology.

hematology /hē′mətol′əjē, hem′-/ [Gk, *haima* + *logos*, science], the scientific study of blood and blood-forming tissues. **−hematologic, hematological,** *adj.*

hematolysis /hē′mətol′isis/ [Gk, *haima*, blood, *lysein*, to loosen], the release of hemoglobin from red blood cells by the breakdown of erythrocytes or by osmosis. Also called **hemolysis.**

hematoma /hē′mətō′mə, hem′-/, *pl.* **hematomas, hematomata** [Gk, *haima* + *oma*, tumor], a collection of extravasated blood trapped in the tissues of the skin or in an organ, resulting from trauma or incomplete hemostasis after surgery. Initially, there is frank bleeding into the space; if the space is limited, pressure slows and eventually stops the flow of blood. The blood clots, serum collects, the clot hardens, and the mass becomes palpable to the examiner and is often painful to the patient. A hematoma may be drained early in the process and bleeding arrested with pressure or, if necessary, with surgical ligation of the bleeding vessel. Considerable blood may be lost, and infection is a serious complication. Also called **blood blister.**

-hematoma, a combining form meaning a 'swelling containing blood': *cephalhematoma, episiohematoma, othematoma.*

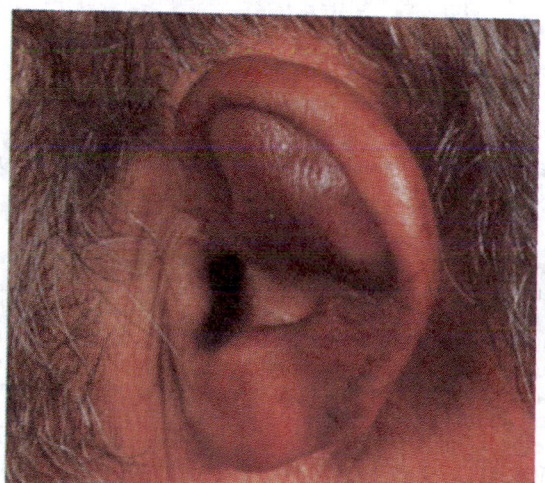

Hematoma *(Bingham, 1992)*

hematomyelia /hē′mətōmē′lē·ə/ [Gk, *haima* + *meylos*, marrow], the appearance of frank blood in the fluid of the spinal cord.

hematopericardium /per′ēkär′dē·əm/ [Gk, *haima*, blood, *peri*, near, *kardia*, heart], a seepage of blood into the pericardium. Also called **hemopericardium.**

hematoperitoneum /-per′itənē′əm/ [Gk, *haima*, blood, *peri*, near, *tenein*, to stretch], the effusion of blood into the peritoneal cavity.

hematopoiesis /hē′mətōpō·ē′sis, hem′-/ [Gk, *haima* + *poiein*, to make], the normal formation and development of blood cells in the bone marrow. In severe anemia and other hematologic disorders, cells may be produced in organs outside the marrow (extramedullary hematopoiesis). See also **erythropoiesis.** **–hematopoietic,** *adj.*

hematopoietic syndrome /-pō·et′ik/, a group of clinical features associated with effects of radiation on the blood and lymph tissues. It is characterized by nausea and vomiting, anorexia, lethargy, hemolysis and destruction of the bone marrow, and atrophy of the spleen and lymph nodes.

hematopoietic system [Gk, *haima*, blood, *poiein*, to make; L, *systema*], the system of body organs and tissues involved in the formation and functioning of blood elements. It includes the bone marrow and spleen.

hematospermia /-spur′mē·ə/, the presence of blood in the semen. Causes may include vascular congestion, an infection involving seminal vesicles, coitus interruptus, sexual abstinence, or frequent coitus. The condition is rarely serious and may respond to antibiotic therapy.

hematothorax. See **hemothorax.**

hematoxylin-eosin /hē′mətok′silin/ [*Haematoxylon campechianum*, logwood; Gk, *eos*, dawn], a stain commonly used to treat tissue sections on microscope slides.

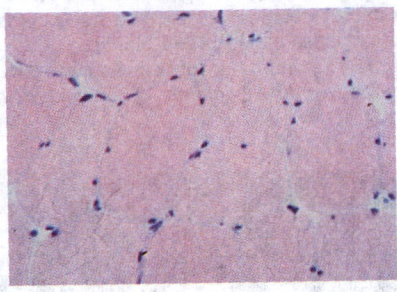

Hematoxylin-eosin stain of normal muscle tissue
(Shipley, 1993)

hematuria /hē′mətoor′ē·ə, hem′-/ [Gk, *haima* + *ouron*, urine], abnormal presence of blood in the urine. Hematuria is symptomatic of many renal diseases and disorders of the genitourinary system. Microscopic examination of the urine, culture and sensitivity of the urine, and physical examination of the patient are usually performed. **–hematuric,** *adj.*

heme /hēm/ [Gk, *haima*, blood], the pigmented, iron containing, nonprotein portion of the hemoglobin molecule. There are four heme groups in a hemoglobin molecule, each consisting of a cyclic structure of four pyrrole residues, called protoporphyrin, and an atom of iron in the center. Heme binds and carries oxygen in the red blood cells, releasing it to tissues that give off excess amounts of CO_2. See also **hemoglobin, porphobilinogen, protoporphyrin.**

hemeralopia /hem′ərəlō′pē·ə/ [Gk, *hemera*, day, *alaos*, blind, *ops*, eye], an abnormal visual condition in which bright light causes blurring of vision. Hemeralopia is an unpleasant side effect of certain anticonvulsant medications, including trimethadione, prescribed in treating children with petit mal epilepsy. Also called **day blindness, night sight.** **–hemeralopic,** *adj.*

hemi-, a prefix meaning 'half': *hemiplegia, hemiataxia, hemiopia.*

-hemia. See **-emia.**

hemiacephalus /hem′ē·āsef′ələs/ [Gk, *hemi*, half, *a*,

kephale, not head], a fetus in which the brain and most of the cranium are lacking. See also **anencephaly.**

hemiachromatosia /hem′ē·ak′rōmətō′zhə/, a state of being color blind in only one half of the visual field.

hemiamblyopia /hem′ē·am′blē·ō′pē·ə/ [Gk, *hemi*, half, *amblys*, dull, *ops*, eye], blindness in half of the normal visual field. Also called **hemianopia.**

hemianalgesia /hem′ē·an′əljē′sē·ə/ [Gk, *hemi*, half, *a*, not, *algos*, pain], a loss of feeling or sensitivity to pain affecting half of the body or one side of the body.

hemianesthesia /hem′ē·an′esthē′zhə/ /hem′ē·nō′pē·ə/ [Gk, *hemi* + *anaisthesia*, absence of feeling], a loss of feeling on one side of the body.

hemianopia [Gk, *hemi* + *a*, *opsis*, not vision], defective vision or blindness in one half of the visual field. Also called **hemiamblyopia.**

hemiarthroplasty /hem′ē·är′thrəplas′tē/, a surgical procedure for repair of an injured or diseased hip joint. It involves replacement of the head of the femur with a prosthesis without reconstruction of the acetabulum.

hemiarthrosis /hem′ē·ärthrō′sis/ [Gk, *hemi*, half, *arthron*, joint, *osis*, condition], a false articulation between two bones. See also **synchondrosis.**

hemiataxia /hem′ē·ətak′sē·ə/, a loss of muscle control affecting one side of the body, usually as a result of a stroke or cerebellar injury. The condition may be ipsilateral or contralateral.

hemiazygous vein /hem′ē·əzī′gəs/ [Gk, *hemi* + *a*, *zygon*, not yoke], one of the tributaries of the azygous vein of the thorax. It starts in the left ascending lumbar vein, enters the thorax through the left crus of the diaphragm, ascends on the left side of the vertebral column as high as the ninth thoracic vertebra, and passes dorsal to the aorta to enter the azygous. The hemiazygous vein receives about four of the caudal intercostal veins, the left subcostal vein, and some of the esophageal and the mediastinal veins.

hemiballismus. See **ballismus.**

hemicellulose /hem′ēsel′yōōlōs/ [Gk, *hemi* + L, *cellula*, little cell], any of a group of polysaccharides that constitute the chief part of the skeletal substances of the cell walls of plants and resemble cellulose but are more soluble and more easily extracted and decomposed. See also **dietary fiber.**

hemicephalia /-sefā′lyə/ [Gk, *hemi* + *kephale*, head], a congenital anomaly characterized by the absence of one side of the cerebrum, caused by severe arrest of brain development in the fetus. The cerebellum and basal ganglia may be present in rudimentary form.

hemicephalus /-sef′ələs/ [Gk, *hemi* + *kephale*, head], a fetus with congenital absence of one half of the cerebrum.

hemicrania /-krā′nē·ə/ [Gk, *hemi* + *kranion*, skull], **1.** a headache, usually migraine, that affects only one side of the head. **2.** a congenital anomaly characterized by the absence of one half of the skull in the fetus; incomplete anencephaly.

hemicraniectomy /-kran′ē·ek′təmē/ [Gk, *hemi*, half, *kranion*, skull, *ektome*, cutting out], a surgical procedure in which part or all of one half of the skull is excised and reflected as a preliminary step to certain types of brain operations.

hemidiaphragm /-dī′əfram/, either the left or right functional half of the diaphragm. Although the structure is a single anatomic unit, it is divided by the union of its central tendon and the pericardium into separate leaves, each with its own nerve supply, and each hemidiaphragm can function independently of the other.

hemiectromelia /hem′ē·ek′trōmē′lyə/ [Gk, *hemi* + *ektosis*, miscarriage, *melos*, limb], a congenital anomaly characterized by the incomplete development of the limbs on one side of the body. **–hemiectromelus,** *n.*

hemifacial spasm. See **convulsive tic.**

hemignathia /hem′ēnā′thē·ə/ [Gk, *hemi* + *gnathos*, jaw], **1.** a congenital anomaly characterized by incomplete development of the lower jaw on one side of the face. **2.** a condition of having only one jaw. **–hemignathus,** *n.*

hemihyperplasia /-hī′pərplā′zhə/ [Gk, *hemi* + *hyper*, excessive, *plassein* to form], overdevelopment or excessive growth of one half of a specific organ or part or all of the organs and parts on one side of the body.

hemihypertonia /-hī′pərtō′nē·ə/ [Gk, *hemi* + *hyper* + *tonikos*, stretching], exaggerated tension in the muscles on one side of the body, causing tonic contraction. In one form of the disorder, tonic spasms may occur occasionally in different muscle groups on one side of the body.

hemihypertrophy /-hī′pur′trəfē/ [Gk, *hemi* + *hyper* + *trophe*, nourishment], an abnormal enlargement or overgrowth of half of the body or half of a body part.

hemihypoplasia /-hī′pōplā′zhə/ [Gk, *hemi* + *hypo*, under, *plassein* to form], partial or incomplete development of one half of a specific organ or part or all of the organs and parts on one side of the body.

hemikaryon /hem′ēker′ē·on/ [Gk, *hemi* + *karyon*, nut], a cell nucleus that contains the haploid number of chromosomes, or one half of the diploid number, as that of the gametes. Compare **amphikaryon.** **–hemikaryotic,** *adj.*

hemimelia /-mē′lyə/ [Gk, *hemi* + *melos*], a developmental anomaly characterized by the absence or gross shortening of the lower portion of one or more of the limbs. The condition may involve either or both of the bones of the distal arm or leg and is designated according to which is absent or defective, as fibular, radial, tibial, or ulnar hemimelia. See also **ectromelia, phocomelia.**

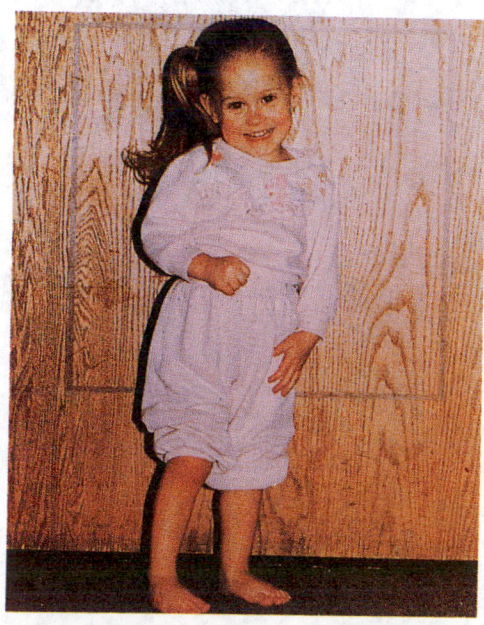

Hemiparesis (Zitelli, 1992)

hemiopia /hem′ē·ō′pē·ə/ [Gk, *hemi*, half, *ops*, eye], a condition involving only one eye or half the visual field.

hemipagus /hemip′əgəs/ [Gk, *hemi* + *pagos*, fixture], conjoined symmetric twins who are united at the thorax.

hemiparesis /-pərē′sis/ [Gk, *hemi* + *paralyein*, to be paralyzed], muscular weakness of one half of the body.

hemiparesthesia /-per′esthē′zhə/ [Gk, *hemi*, half, *para*, beside, *aisthesis*, sensation], a numbness or other abnormal or impaired sensation that is experienced on only one side of the body.

hemiplegia /hem′iplē′jə/ [Gk, *hemi* + *plege*, stroke], paralysis of one side of the body. Kinds of hemiplegia include **cerebral hemiplegia, facial hemiplegia,** and **spastic hemiplegia.** Compare **diplegia, paraplegia, quadriplegia.** **–hemiplegic,** *adj.*

hemiplegic gait /-plē′jik/ [Gk, *hemi*, half, *plege*, stroke; ONorse, *gata*, a way], a manner of walking in which an affected limb moves in a semicircle with each step.

hemisection /-sek′shən/ [Gk, *hemi*, half; L, *sectare*, to cut], half of a body or other object when divided along a longitudinal plane, producing two lateral halves.

hemisomus /hem′isō′məs/ [Gk, *hemi* + *soma*, body], a fetus or individual in which one side of the body is malformed, defective, or absent.

hemisphere /hem′isfir/ [Gk, *hemi* + *sphaira*, sphere], **1.** one half of a sphere or globe. **2.** the lateral half of the cerebrum or of the cerebellum. **–hemispherical,** *adj.*

hemiteras /hem′ēter′əs/, *pl.* **hemiterata** [Gk, *hemi* + *teras*, monster], any individual with a congenital malformation that is not so severe or disabling as to be classified as a monstrous or teratic condition. **–hemiteratic,** *adj.*

hemivertebra /-vur′təbrə/, an abnormal condition characterized by the congenital failure of a vertebra to develop completely, possibly caused by the complete failure of the growth center of one vertebral body. Usually one half of the vertebra involved is completely or partially developed and the other half is absent. One or more vertebrae may be involved, the different conditions producing varying degrees of balanced or unbalanced scoliosis. As a result of the developmental abnormality of the spine, a wedge-shaped vertebra develops, and adjacent vertebral bodies expand to fit the deformity or tilt to accommodate wedge-shaped articulation. Hemivertebra may be classified according to the degree of developmental failure of involved vertebral growth centers. There may be involvement of two vertebral bodies in which growth centers on the same side fail to develop, resulting in moderate to severe unbalanced congenital scoliosis, or there may be involvement of two vertebral bodies in which growth centers fail to develop on opposite sides, creating balanced congenital scoliosis. Singular hemivertebra may pose few if any signs and symptoms. Depending on the degree of congenital scoliosis involved, any associated deformity may become more apparent with growth. Other types of hemivertebra, especially those involving unbalanced congenital scoliosis, usually progress markedly with growth and have a relatively poor prognosis unless early spinal fusion prevents further spinal curvature. No treatment may be required for the form of the condition associated with balanced congenital scoliosis.

hemizygote /-zī′gōt/ [Gk, *hemi* + *zygon*, yoke], an individual, organism, or cell that has only one of a pair of genes for a specific characteristic. Such traits are expressed regardless of whether the genes transmitting them are dominant or recessive, such as with the X-linked genes on the single X chromosome in males, which have no alleles on the Y chromosome. **–hemizygosity,** *n.,* **hemizygous, hemizygotic,** *adj.*

hemo- /hē'mō-, hem'ō-/   a prefix relating to blood or blood vessels.

hemoagglutination /-əglōō'tinā'shən/ [Gk, *haima,* blood; L, *agglutinare,* to glue],   the coagulation of red blood cells.

hemoagglutinin /-əglōō'tinin/ [Gk, *haima,* blood; L, *agglutinare,* to glue],   an agglutinin that coagulates red blood cells.

hemoblastic leukemia.   See **stem cell leukemia.**

hemochromatosis /hē'mōkrō'mətō'sis, hem'-/ [Gk, *haima,* blood, *chroma,* color, *osis,* condition],   a rare disease of iron metabolism, characterized by excess iron deposits throughout the body. Hepatomegaly, skin pigmentation, diabetes mellitus, and cardiac failure may occur. The disease most often develops as a complication of some hemolytic anemia, such as sickle cell anemia. Multiple blood transfusions are required for treatment. Compare **hemosiderosis.** See also **iron metabolism, siderosis, thalassemia.**

hemoclip,   a malleable metal clip used to ligate small blood vessels during surgery. Hemoclips also may be used to mark the location of body structures in radiographic procedures.

hemoconcentration /-kon'səntrā'shən/ [Gk, *haima* + L, *cum,* together with, *centrum,* center],   an increase in the number of red blood cells resulting either from a decrease in plasma volume or increased production of erythrocytes.

hemocyanin /hē'mōsī'ənin/,   an oxygen-carrying protein molecule present in certain lower animals, particularly arthropods and mollusks. The molecule is similar to the hemoglobin molecule of human blood but utilizes copper atoms, rather than iron, and is less efficient than hemoglobin in requiring many more atoms to bind a single molecule of oxygen.

hemocyte.   See **hematocyte, hematocytoblast.**

hemocytoblast.   See **hematocytoblast.**

hemocytoblastic leukemia.   See **stem cell leukemia.**

hemocytology /-sītol'əjē/ [Gk, *haima,* blood, *kytos,* cell, *logos,* science],   the study of the components of blood.

hemodiafiltration /-dī'əfiltrā'shən/,   a technique similar to hemofiltration, used to treat uremia by convective transport of the solute rather than diffusion.

hemodialysis /hē'mōdī·al'isis, hem'-/ [Gk, *haima* + *dia,* apart, *lysis,* loosening],   a procedure in which impurities or wastes are removed from the blood, used in treating renal failure and various toxic conditions. The patient's blood is shunted from the body through a machine for diffusion and ultrafiltration and then returned to the patient's circulation. Hemodialysis requires access to the patient's bloodstream, a mechanism for the transport of the blood to and

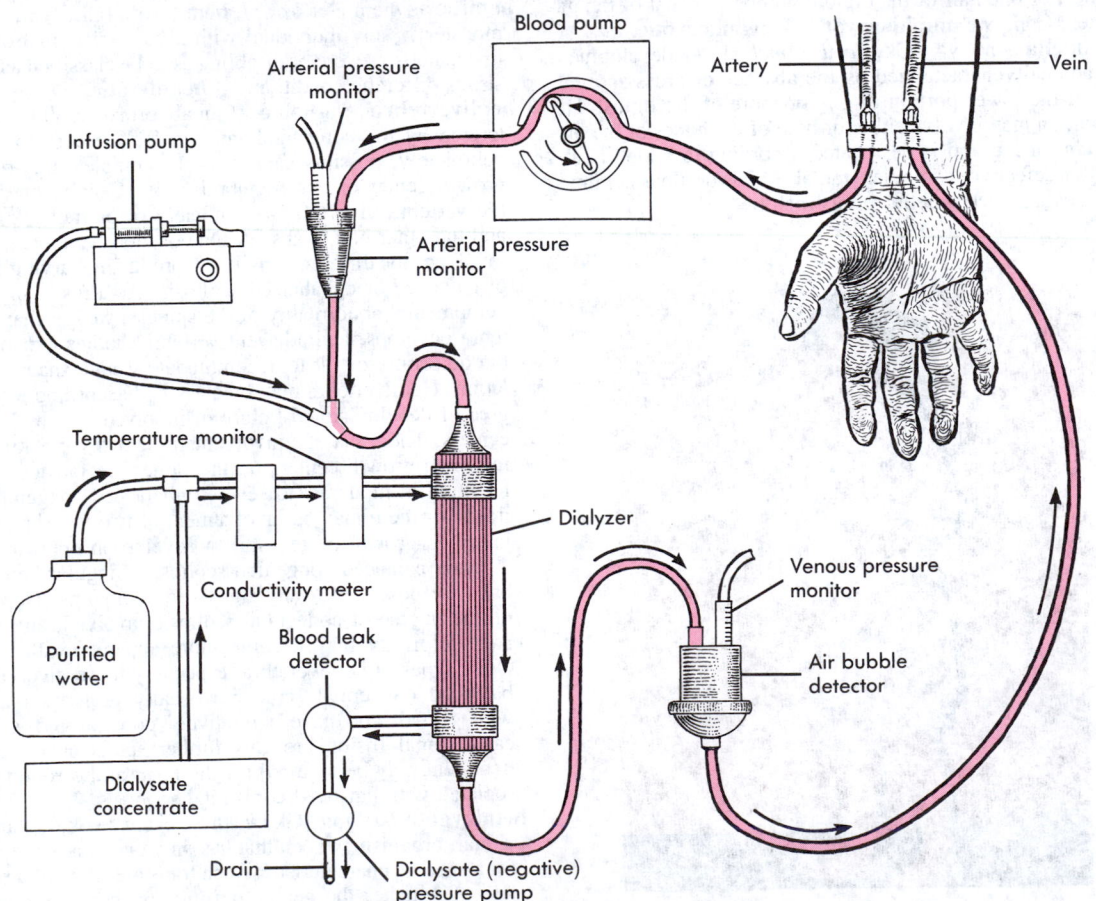

Components of a hemodialysis system *(Thelan, 1989)*

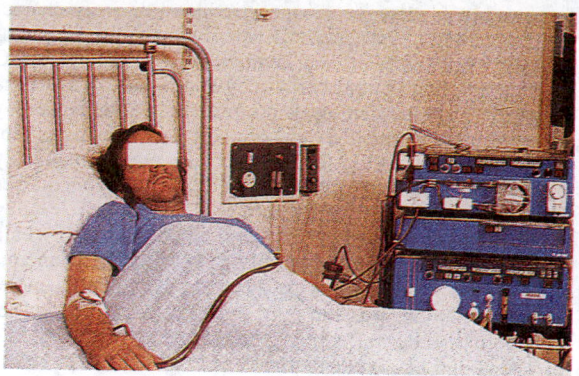

Patient undergoing hemodialysis
(Bodansky, 1989/Courtesy Dr EJ Will, Leeds)

from the dialyzer, and a dialyzer. See **arteriovenous fistula, external shunt.**

■ METHOD: Access may be achieved by an external shunt or an arteriovenous fistula. The external shunt is constructed by inserting two cannulas through the skin into a large vein and a large artery. When dialysis is not being performed, the cannulas are joined, allowing the blood to flow from artery to vein. When dialysis is being performed, the cannulas are separated, allowing the arterial blood to flow to the dialyzer and the dialyzed blood to return from the dialyzer to the circulation through the cannula in the vein. An arteriovenous fistula is created by the anastomosis of a large vein to an artery. Large-bore needles are threaded into superficial vessels enlarged by the increased flow caused by the fistula. Various dialyzers may be used. The procedure takes from 3 to 8 hours and may be necessary daily in acute situations or 2 or 3 times a week in chronic renal failure.

■ NURSING INTERVENTION: A decrease in the flow of blood through the shunt may result in clotting; therefore any factor that may result in a slowing of the flow is to be avoided. Some of these factors are systemic hypotension, infection of the shunt or fistula, compression of the shunt or fistula, thrombophlebitis, and prolonged inflation of a blood pressure cuff. Infection is avoided in the area around an external shunt by placing a sterile dressing over the shunt and changing the dressing daily. Before the procedure is begun, the patient is told how long the procedure will take, what pain or discomfort may be expected, what will be felt afterward, what food or activity will be allowed during the procedure, and whether family or friends may be present during treatment. Headache and nausea are common, especially during the procedure and for a few hours afterward. The patient usually feels the best on the day after hemodialysis. Rest, an antiemetic, and a mild analgesic may make the procedure more comfortable. Most patients need emotional support and some physical assistance during hemodialysis. The physical status of the patient is monitored frequently throughout; blood pressure, pulse, and blood tests for electrolyte and acid-base balance are performed. Normal saline may be administered to counteract hypotension that occurs as a result of a rapid removal of fluid from the intravascular compartment. The patient is weighed before and after the treatment to determine the amount of fluid lost during the procedure. An anticoagulant is usually given to prevent coagulation of the blood in the dialyzer, cannulas, or catheters; to prevent hemorrhage, protamine sulfate may be given after the procedure to reverse the effect of the anticoagulant. Any treatment that causes tissue trauma, such as dental extraction, venipuncture, or intramuscular injection, is not recommended during or immediately after dialysis.

■ OUTCOME CRITERIA: Infection and clotting of the shunt or erosion of the skin around the shunt are frequent complications of the external shunt; therefore the method using an arteriovenous fistula is more common. The discomfort before, during, and just after dialysis, the prolonged time of relative immobility during the procedure, and the dietary restrictions necessary in renal insufficiency all place considerable stress on the patient. Adjustments in the patterns of daily life are necessary and require the assistance of professionals with experience and training in the field.

hemodialysis technician, a registered health professional who has received special training in the operation of hemodialysis equipment and treatment of patients with kidney disorders.

hemodialyzer. See **dialyzer.**

hemodilution /-dilo͞o'shən/ [Gk, *haima,* blood; L, *diluare,* to wash away], a condition in which the concentration of erythrocytes or other blood elements is lowered.

hemodynamics /-dīnam'iks/ [Gk, *haima + dynamis,* force], the study of the physical aspects of blood circulation, including cardiac function and peripheral vascular physiology.

Hemofil, a trademark for human antihemophilic factor.

hemofiltration /-filtrā'shən/, a type of hemodialysis in which there is convective transport of the solute through ultrafiltration across the membrane. It is reported to be more effective than diffusion in removing larger molecular weight solutes from the blood, particularly in the treatment of uremia.

hemoglobin (Hb) /hē'məglō'bən/ [Gk, *haima* + L, *globus,* ball], a complex protein-iron compound in the blood that carries oxygen to the cells from the lungs and carbon dioxide away from the cells to the lungs. Each erythrocyte contains 200 to 300 molecules of hemoglobin, each molecule of hemoglobin contains several molecules of heme, and each molecule of heme can carry one molecule of oxygen. A hemoglobin molecule contains four globin polypeptide chains, designated in adults as the alpha (α), beta (β), gamma (γ), and delta (δ) chains. Each polypeptide chain is composed of several hundred amino acids, and the absence, replacement, or addition of only one amino acid modifies the properties of the hemoglobin. Different kinds of hemoglobin are identified by their specific combination of polypeptide chains, the number of chains of the different types in the molecule indicated by subscript numerals and superscript capital letters. More than 100 hemoglobins with different electrophoretic mobilities and characteristics have been identified and classified, such as S, C, D, E, G, H, I, J, K, L, M, N, and O. Improved research methods may reveal many more. The normal concentrations of hemoglobin in the blood are 12 to 16 g/dl in women and 13.5 to 18 g/dl in men. In an atmosphere of high oxygen concentration, such as in the lungs, hemoglobin binds with oxygen to form oxyhemoglobin. In an atmosphere of low oxygen concentration, such as in the peripheral tissues of the body, oxygen is replaced by carbon dioxide to form carboxyhemoglobin. Hemoglobin releases the carboxyhemoglobin in the lungs for excretion and picks up more oxygen for transport to the

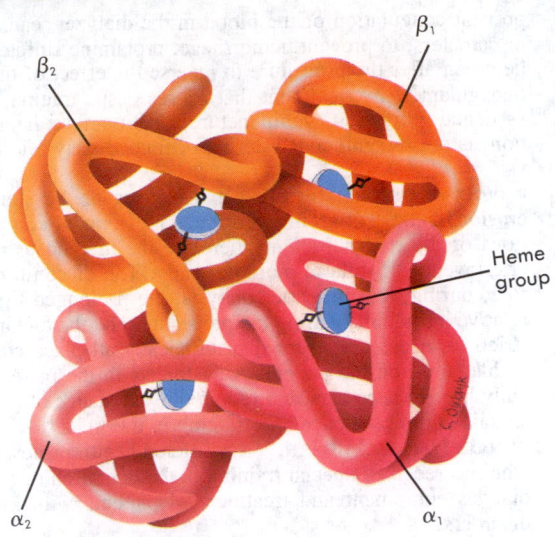

Hemoglobin (Thibodeau, 1993/Christine Oleksyk)

cells. See also **carboxyhemoglobin, complete blood count, differential white blood cell count, erythrocyte, erythropoiesis, heme, hemoglobinopathy, hemolysin, oxyhemoglobin,** and see specific hemoglobins.

hemoglobin_{Seattle}**,** an abnormal hemoglobin in which glutamic acid replaces alanine at position 76 of the β chain, decreasing the hemoglobin molecule's affinity for oxygen.

hemoglobin A (Hb A), a normal hemoglobin. Also called **adult hemoglobin.** Compare **hemoglobin F.** See also **hemoglobinopathy.**

hemoglobin A$_2$ (Hb A$_2$), a normal hemoglobin that occurs in small amounts in adults, characterized by the substitution of δ chains for β chains. Its concentration in the blood increases in various hematologic diseases. It normally constitutes 1.5% to 3.5% of the total hemoglobin.

hemoglobin C (Hb C), an abnormal type of hemoglobin characterized by the substitution of lysine for glutamic acid at position 6 of the [Grk b] chain of the hemoglobin molecule. Hemoglobin C moves slowly and reduces the plasticity of the erythrocytes.

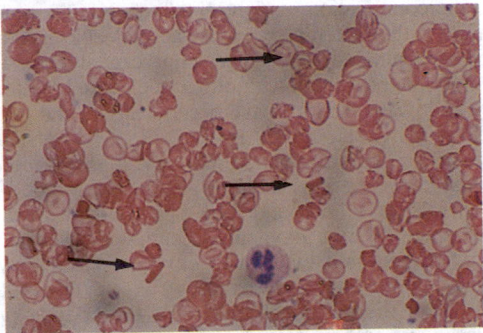

Hemoglobin C disease (Powers, 1989)

hemoglobin C disease, a genetic blood disorder characterized by a moderate, chronic hemolytic anemia and associated with the presence of hemoglobin C. Hemoglobin C is inherited as an autosomal codominant gene. No anemia or increased blood hemolysis are present. Target cells may be seen in microscopic examination of a blood smear. Abnormal hemoglobin C is accompanied by an approximately equal amount of its normal counterpart, hemoglobin A. See also **hemoglobin C, hemoglobin S-C disease.**

hemoglobin E disease [Gk, *haima,* blood; L, *globus,* ball; *E*; Gk, *dis,* not; Fr, *aise,* ease], a mild form of anemia caused by a genetic abnormality of the hemoglobin molecule. Worldwide, it is the third most common form of hemoglobin disorder, affecting primarily persons from Southeast Asia and black populations.

hemoglobin electrophoresis, a test to identify various abnormal hemoglobins in the blood, including certain genetic disorders, such as sickle cell anemia.

hemoglobinemia /hē′mōglō′binē′mē·ə, hem′-/, presence of free hemoglobin in the blood plasma.

hemoglobin F (Hb F), the normal hemoglobin of the fetus. Most Hb F is replaced by hemoglobin A in the first days after birth. Hb F has an increased capacity to carry oxygen and is present in increased amounts in some pathologic conditions, including sickle cell anemia, aplastic anemia, and leukemia. Small amounts are produced throughout life.

hemoglobin M disease [Gk, *haima,* blood; L, *globus,* ball; *M*; Gk, *dis,* not; Fr, *aise*, ease], a type of anemia in which part of the hemoglobin contains iron in the Fe^{+++} state and is unable to combine with oxygen. The patient may experience cyanosis but is able to function because part of the hemoglobin is normal. See **methemoglobin.**

hemoglobinometer /-om′ətər/ [Gk, *haima,* blood; L, *globus,* ball; Gk, *metron,* measure], any of several types of instruments designed to measure the percentage of hemoglobin in a blood sample. Some use colorimetric techniques of comparing the color of the blood sample with a standard red color.

hemoglobinopathy /hē′mōglō′binop′əthē, hem′-/ [Gk, *haima* + L, *globus,* ball; Gk, *pathos,* disease], a group of inherited disorders characterized by structural variations of the hemoglobin molecule. An abnormality may occur in the heterozygous or the homozygous form. The alteration appears as the substitution of one or more amino acids in the globin portion of the molecule at selected positions in the two alpha or two beta polypeptide chains. Although more than 100 variants have been described, only hemoglobins S, C, and D are commonly seen. In the heterozygous form, the normal adult pigment, hemoglobin A, and the variant both appear in the red cell; little or no clinical manifestation of disease may be present. In the homozygous form, only the variant hemoglobin is present, and the characteristic symptoms of that hemoglobinopathy appear. Mixed heterozygous forms are also known to occur. The normal hemoglobin A may be absent, and two or three hemoglobin variants may be present. Kinds of hemoglobinopathies include **hemoglobin C disease, hemoglobin S-C disease,** and **sickle cell anemia.** Compare **thalassemia.** See also **hemoglobin, hemoglobin A, sickle cell thalassemia, sickle cell trait.**

hemoglobin oxygen saturation, a quantitative measure of volume of oxygen per volume of blood, depending on the grams of hemoglobin per deciliter of blood. For example, two samples of blood, one with hemoglobin at 15 g/dl and the other at 7.5 g/dl, may both be 96% saturated with oxygen, but the hemoglobin oxygen saturation would be greater in the 15 g/dl sample.

hemoglobin S (Hb S), an abnormal type of hemoglobin, characterized by the substitution of the amino acid valine for glutamic acid in the β chain of the hemoglobin molecule. They move more slowly and are much less soluble than hemoglobin A. As the abnormal molecules become deoxygenated, because of decreased oxygen tension in the peripheral circulation, they become sickle-shaped, move slowly, clump together, and hemolyze. If the proportion of Hb S to Hb A is large, as in sickle cell anemia, local thrombosis and infarction may occur. See also **sickle cell anemia, sickle cell crisis, sickle cell trait.**

hemoglobin saturation, the amount of oxygen combined with hemoglobin in proportion to the amount of oxygen the hemoglobin is capable of carrying. It is expressed as a percentage of the ratio, content/capacity.

hemoglobin S-C (Hb S-C) disease, a genetic blood disorder in which two different abnormal alleles, one for hemoglobin S and one for hemoglobin C, are inherited. The disorder is characterized by a clinical course considerably less severe than sickle cell anemia despite the absence of normal hemoglobin. See also **hemoglobin C disease, sickle cell thalassemia.**

emphasizes the size, shape, special characteristics, and numbers of the solid components of the blood. See also **complete blood count.**

hemolysin /himol'əsin/ [Gk, *haima* + *lysis*, loosening], any one of the numerous substances that lyse or dissolve red blood cells. Hemolysins are produced by bacterial strains, including staphylococci and streptococci and are contained in venoms and vegetables. Bacterial hemolysins are divided into those that are filterable and those that cluster around the bacterial colony on a culture medium containing red blood cells. Hemolysins appear to aid the invasive power of bacteria. See also **hemoglobin, hemolysis.**

hemolysis /himol'isis/ [Gk, *haima* + *lysis*, loosening], the breakdown of red blood cells and the release of hemoglobin that occurs normally at the end of the life span of a red cell. Hemolysis may occur in antigen-antibody reactions, metabolic abnormalities of the red cell that significantly shorten red cell life span, and mechanical trauma, such as cardiac prosthesis. Dilution of the blood by intravenous administration of excessive amounts of hypotonic solutions, which cause progressive swelling and eventual rupture of the erythrocyte, also results in hemolysis. See also **hemolysin, hemolytic anemia, transfusion reaction.** —**hemolytic,** *adj.* Also called **hematolysis.**

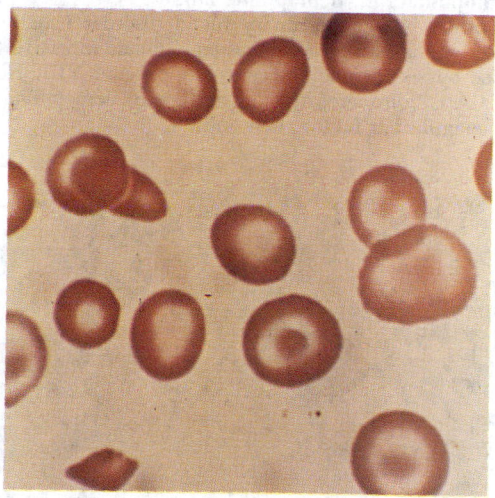

Hemoglobin S-C disease (Zitelli, 1992)

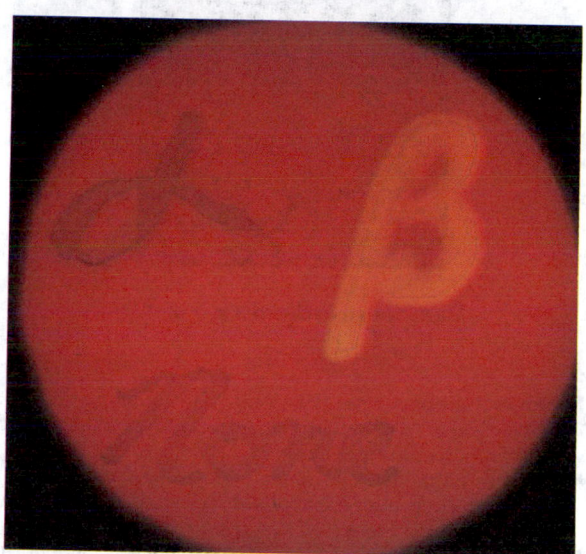

Hemolysis (Baron, 1990)

hemoglobinuria /-ōōr'ē·ə/ [Gk, *haima* + L, *globus*, ball; Gk, *ouron*, urine], an abnormal presence in the urine of hemoglobin that is unattached to red blood cells. Hemoglobinuria can result from various autoimmune diseases or episodic hemolytic disorders. It can be diagnosed using a dipstick reagent that is sensitive to free hemoglobin. Kinds of hemoglobinuria include **cold hemoglobinuria, march hemoglobinuria,** and **nocturnal hemoglobinuria.**

hemoglobinuric /-ōōr'ik/ [Gk, *haima*, blood; L, *globus*, ball; Gk, *ouron*, urine], pertaining to the presence of hemoglobin in the urine.

hemogram /hē'məgram/ [Gk, *haima* + *gramma*, record], a written or graphic record of a differential blood count that

hemolytic anemia /-lit'ik/ [Gk, *haima, lysis* + *a, haima,* not blood], a disorder characterized by chronic premature destruction of red blood cells. Anemia may be minimal or absent, reflecting the ability of the bone marrow to increase production of red blood cells. The condition may occur in association with some infectious diseases, with certain inherited red-cell disorders, or in response to drugs or other toxic agents. Compare **aplastic anemia, congenital nonspherocytic hemolytic anemia, iron deficiency anemia, myelophthisic anemia.** See also **anemia, hemolysis, spherocytosis.**

hemolytic jaundice, a yellowish discoloration of the skin caused by a breakdown of red blood cells, resulting in excessive bilirubin.

hemolytic jaundice of the newborn.   See **icterus gravis neonatorum.**

hemolytic uremia syndrome,   a rare kidney disorder marked by renal failure, microangiopathic hemolytic anemia, and platelet deficiency. The syndrome, the cause of which is unknown, usually occurs in infancy.

hemoperfusion /-pərfyōoˊzhən/,   the perfusion of blood through a sorbent device, such as activated charcoal or resin beads, rather than through dialysis equipment. Hemoperfusion may be used in treating uremia, liver failure, and certain forms of drug toxicity.

hemopericardium /-perˊikärˊdē·əm/ [Gk, *haima* + *peri*, around, *kardia*, heart],   an accumulation of blood within the pericardial sac surrounding the heart. Also called **hematopericardium.** /hēˊmətōperˊikärˊdē·əm/.

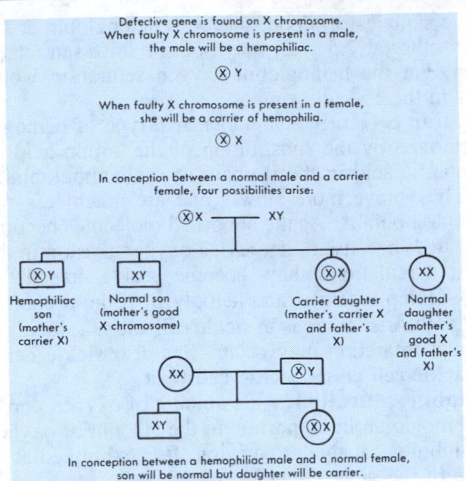

Defective gene is found on X chromosome.
When faulty X chromosome is present in a male, the male will be a hemophiliac.

⊗ Y

When faulty X chromosome is present in a female, she will be a carrier of hemophilia.

⊗ X

In conception between a normal male and a carrier female, four possibilities arise:

⊗ X ———— X Y

⊗ Y — Hemophiliac son (mother's carrier X)
X Y — Normal son (mother's good X chromosome)
⊗ X — Carrier daughter (mother's carrier X and father's X)
X X — Normal daughter (mother's good X and father's X)

X X ———— ⊗ Y

X Y   ⊗ X

In conception between a hemophiliac male and a normal female, son will be normal but daughter will be carrier.

Hemophilia inheritance pattern

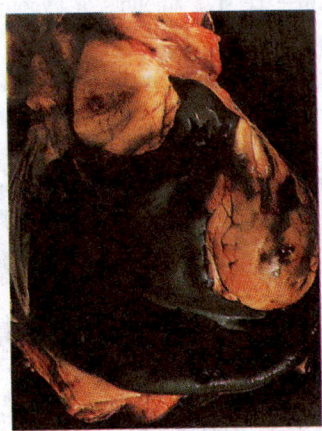

Hemopericardium *(Fletcher, 1987)*

injury. The nurse also provides assistance in coping with the disorder, refers parents for genetic counseling and to parent discussion groups, and implements home care. See **von Willebrand's disease,** and see specific blood factors. **—hemophiliac,** *n.,* **hemophilic,** *adj.*

hemophilia A,   a hereditary blood disorder usually expressed in males, transmitted as an X-linked recessive trait, caused by a deficiency of coagulation factor VIII. Hemophilia A is considered the classic type of hemophilia. See also **coagulation factor, hemophilia.**

hemoperitoneum /-perˊitōnēˊəm/ [Gk, *haima* + *peri*, around, *tenein*, to stretch],   the presence of extravasated blood in the peritoneal cavity.

hemophil /hēˊmōfil/ [Gk, *haima*, blood, *philein*, to love],   bacteria of the genus *Haemophilus*, which thrive in culture media containing blood.

hemophilia /hēˊmōfēˊlyə, hemˊ-/ [Gk, *haima* + *philein*, to love],   a group of hereditary bleeding disorders in which there is a deficiency of one of the factors necessary for coagulation of the blood. The two most common forms of the disorder are hemophilia A and hemophilia B. Hemophilia A (classic hemophilia) is the result of a deficiency or absence of antihemophilic factor VIII. Hemophilia B (Christmas disease) represents a deficiency of plasma thromboplastin component. The clinical severity of the disorder varies with the extent of the deficiency. Greater than usual loss of blood during dental procedures, epistaxis, hematoma, and hemarthrosis are common problems in patients with hemophilia. Severe nonsurgical internal hemorrhage and hematuria are less common. The primary objective of nursing care is to prevent bleeding and to make the environment as safe as possible. The nurse teaches measures for controlling bleeding and for limiting local joint damage and ways that the patient can be physically active without danger of

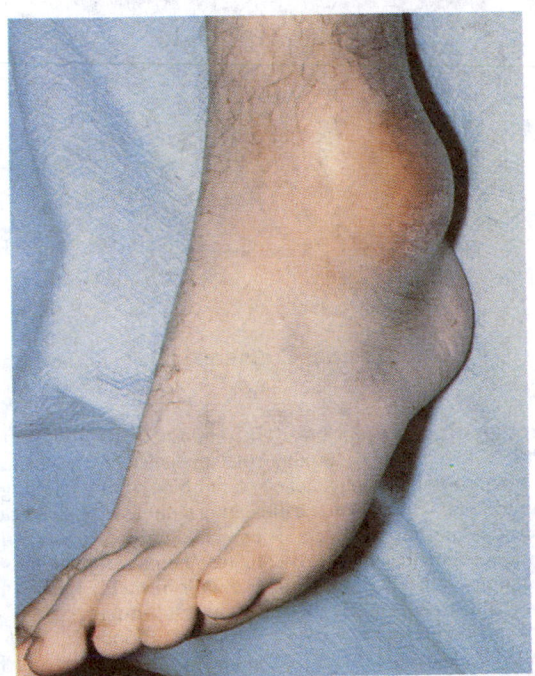

Bleeding over the external malleolus in a boy with hemophilia
(Ansell, 1992)

hemophilia B, a hereditary blood disorder, transmitted as an X-linked recessive trait, caused by a deficiency of factor IX, the plasma thromboplastin component. The condition is clinically similar to but less severe than hemophilia A. Also called **Christmas disease.** See **coagulation factor, hemophilia.**

hemophilia C, a hereditary blood disorder, transmitted as an X-linked recessive trait, caused by a deficiency of factor XI, the plasma thromboplastin antecedent. The condition is clinically similar to but may be less severe than hemophilia A. Also called **Rosenthal's syndrome.** See also **coagulation factor, hemophilia.**

hemophiliac /-fē'lē·ak/ [Gk, *haima*, blood, *philein*, to love], a person who has inherited the bleeding disease, **hemophilia.**

hemophilic. See **hemophilia.**

hemopneumopericardium /hē'mōnoo'mōper'ikär'dē·əm/ [Gk, *haima*, blood, *pneuma*, air, *kardia*, heart], an accumulation of both blood and air in the pericardium. Also called **pneumohemopericardium.**

hemopneumothorax /hē'mōnoo'mōthôr'aks/ [Gk, *haima*, blood, *pneuma*, air, *thorax*, chest], an accumulation of both air and blood in the pleural cavity.

hemopoietic /hē'mōpō·et'ik, hem'-/ [Gk, *haima* + *poiein*, to make], related to the process of formation and development of the various types of blood cells.

hemoptysis /himop'tisis/ [Gk, *haima* + *ptyein*, to spit], coughing up of blood from the respiratory tract. Blood-streaked sputum often occurs in minor upper respiratory infections or in bronchitis. More profuse bleeding may indicate *Aspergillus* infection, lung abscess, tuberculosis, or bronchogenic carcinoma. X-ray examination, endoscopy, and bronchoscopy are often used to diagnose hemoptysis. Treatment of significant hemoptysis includes monitoring the patient for signs of shock, preventing asphyxiation, and localizing and stopping the bleeding. Antibiotics and antitussives may be given. The frightened patient may be calmed by quiet and warmth; sedatives and tranquilizers are not given because of their tendency to depress respiration. Compare **hematemesis.**

hemorheology /-rē·ol'əjē/ [Gk, *haima*, blood; *rhoia*, flow; *logos*, science], the study of the effects of blood flow on the cellular components of blood and walls of blood vessels. Also spelled **hemorrheology.**

hemorrhage /hem'ərij/ [Gk, *haima* + *rhegnynei*, to break forth], a loss of a large amount of blood in a short period of time, either externally or internally. Hemorrhage may be arterial, venous, or capillary.

■ OBSERVATIONS: Symptoms of massive hemorrhage are related to hypovolemic shock: rapid, thready pulse; thirst; cold, clammy skin; sighing respirations; dizziness; syncope; pallor; apprehension; restlessness; and hypotension. If bleeding is contained within a cavity or joint, pain will develop as the capsule or cavity is stretched by the rapidly expanding volume of blood.

■ INTERVENTIONS: Effort is directed toward stopping the hemorrhage. If hemorrhage is external, pressure is applied directly to the wound or to the appropriate pressure points. The part of the body that is wounded may be elevated. Ice, applied directly to the wound, may slow bleeding by causing vasoconstriction. Body temperature may be maintained by keeping the person covered and flat. If an extremity is wounded, and if the bleeding is severe, a tourniquet may be applied proximal to the wound. **–hemorrhagic,** *adj.*

hemorrhagic diathesis /-raj'ik/, an inherited predisposition to any one of a number of abnormalities characterized by excessive bleeding. See also **Fanconi's syndrome, hemophilia, von Willebrand's disease.**

hemorrhagic disease of newborn, a bleeding disorder of neonates that is usually caused by a deficiency of vitamin K.

hemorrhagic familial angiomatosis. See **Osler-Weber-Rendu disease.**

hemorrhagic fever, group of viral aerosol infections, characterized by fever, chills, headache, malaise, and respiratory or GI symptoms, followed by capillary hemorrhages, and, in severe infection, oliguria, kidney failure, hypotension, and, possibly, death. Many forms of the disease occur in specific geographic areas.

hemorrhagic gastritis, a form of acute gastritis usually caused by a toxic agent, such as alcohol, aspirin or other drugs, or bacterial toxins that irritate the lining of the stomach. Nausea, vomiting, and epigastric distress may persist after the irritant is removed. Treatment is symptomatic; the nurse usually includes identification of the irritant and dietary counseling for a patient with hemorrhagic gastritis.

hemorrhagic infarct [Gk, *haima*, blood, *rhegnynei*, to gush; L, *infarcire*, to stuff], an infarct that has accumulated so much blood that it has a red color.

hemorrhagic jaundice [Gk, *haima*, blood, *rhegnynei*, to gush; Fr, *jaune*, yellow], a form of jaundice that occurs in **Weil's syndrome,** or other forms of **leptospirosis** in which there is capillary injury and anemia.

hemorrhagic lung. See **congestive atelectasis.**

hemorrhagic measles [Gk, *haima*, blood, *rhegnynei*, to gush; ME, *masalas*], a severe form of measles characterized by bleeding into the skin and mucous membranes. See also **black measles.**

hemorrhagic pericarditis [Gk, *haima*, blood, *rhegnynei*, to gush, *peri*, near, *kardia*, heart, *itis*, inflammation], an inflammation of the pericardium with a bloody effusion. The condition is frequently caused by tuberculosis or a tumor.

hemorrhagic plague [Gk, *haima*, blood, *rhegnynei*, to gush; L, *plaga*, stroke], a severe form of bubonic plague in which there is bleeding under the skin. Also called **black plague, bubonic plague.**

hemorrhagic pleurisy [Gk, *haima*, blood, *rhegnynei*, to gush, *pleuritis*], an inflammation of the pleura in which there in an effusion of blood into the tissues.

hemorrhagic purpura [Gk, *haima*, blood, *rhegnynei*, to gush; L, *purpura*, purple], a form of purpura associated with thrombocytopenia and prolonged bleeding time. Also called **thrombopenic purpura, thrombocytopenic purpura.**

hemorrhagic scurvy. See **infantile scurvy.**

hemorrhagic shock, a state of physical collapse and prostration associated with the sudden and rapid loss of significant amounts of blood. Severe traumatic injuries often cause such blood losses, which, in turn, produce low blood pressure in affected individuals. Death occurs within a relatively short time unless transfusion quickly restores normal blood volume. Hemorrhagic shock often accompanies secondary shock. Compare **primary shock.**

hemorrhagic urticaria [Gk, *haima*, blood, *rhegnynei*, to gush; L, *urtica*, nettle], a skin eruption in which there is bleeding in the wheals, usually as a complication of another disease, such as nephritis. In some cases, the bleeding occurs first and the wheals become superimposed. Also called **urticaria hemorrhagica.**

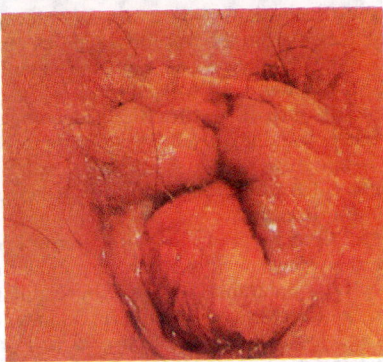

Primary internal hemorrhoids
(Seidel, 1991/Courtesy Gershon Efron, MD, Sinai Hospital
of Baltimore)

hemorrheology. See **hemorheology.**

hemorrhoid /hem′əroid/ [Gk, *haima* + *rhoia*, flow], a varicosity in the lower rectum or anus caused by congestion in the veins of the hemorrhoidal plexus.

■ OBSERVATIONS: Internal hemorrhoids originate above the internal sphincter of the anus. If they become large enough to protrude from the anus, they become constricted and painful. Small internal hemorrhoids may bleed with defecation. External hemorrhoids appear outside the anal sphincter. They are usually not painful, and bleeding does not occur unless a hemorrhoidal vein ruptures or thromboses.

■ INTERVENTIONS: Treatment includes local application of a topical medication to lubricate, anesthetize, and shrink the hemorrhoid; sitz baths and cold or hot compresses are also soothing. The hemorrhoids may require sclerosing by injection, ligation, or excision by a surgical procedure. Ligation is increasingly the preferred treatment: It is simple and effective, and does not require anesthesia. The hemorrhoid is grasped with a forceps, and a rubber band is slipped over the varicosity, causing tissue necrosis and sloughing of the hemorrhoid, usually within 1 week.

■ NURSING CONSIDERATIONS: Straining to defecate, constipation, and prolonged sitting contribute to the development of hemorrhoids. The client is counseled in ways to avoid these predisposing factors. Because pregnancy is associated with an increased incidence of hemorrhoids, the pregnant woman, in particular, is advised to avoid constipation.

hemorrhoidal /hem′əroi′dəl/ [Gk, *haimorrhois*, a vein that discharges blood], pertaining to or resembling hemorrhoids.

hemorrhoidectomy /hem′əroidek′təmē/ [Gk, *haimorrhois*, a vein that discharges blood, *ektome*, cutting out], a surgical procedure for excision of a hemorrhoid.

hemosalpinx /hē′mōsal′pinks/ [Gk, *haima*, blood, *salpinx*, tube], a collection of blood in a fallopian tube.

hemosiderin /hē′mōsid′ərin/ [Gk, *haima* + *sideros*, iron], an iron-rich pigment that is a product of red cell hemolysis. Iron is often stored in this form.

hemosiderosis /hē′mōsid′ərō′sis, hem′-/ [Gk, *haima* + *sideros*, iron, *osis*, condition], an increased deposition of iron in a variety of tissues, usually in the form of hemosiderin, and usually without tissue damage. Often associated with diseases involving chronic, extensive destruction of red blood cells, such as thalassemia major. Compare **hemochromatosis, sideroblastic anemia.** See also **ferritin, iron** transport, siderosis, thalassemia, transferrin.

hemostasis /himos′təsis, hē′məstā′sis/ [Gk, *haima* + *stasis*, halting], the termination of bleeding by mechanical or chemical means or by the complex coagulation process of the body, consisting of vasoconstriction, platelet aggregation, and thrombin and fibrin synthesis. Compare **blood clotting.** See also **platelet, thrombus, vasoconstriction.**

hemostat. See **Halsted's forceps.**

hemostatic /-stat′ik/ [Gk, *haima* + *stasis*, halting], of or pertaining to a procedure, device, or substance that arrests the flow of blood. Direct pressure, tourniquets, and surgical clamps are mechanical hemostatic measures. Cold applications are hemostatic and include the use of an ice bag on the abdomen to halt uterine bleeding and irrigation of the stomach with an iced solution to check gastric bleeding. Gelatin sponges, solutions of thrombin, and microfibrillar collagen, which causes the aggregation of platelets and the formation of clots, are used to arrest bleeding in surgical procedures. Aminocaproic acid is administered orally or intravenously in the treatment of excessive bleeding caused by systemic hyperfibrinolysis. Phytonadione (vitamin K_1) is used for the prevention and treatment of hemorrhagic disease in newborn infants and for the treatment of prothrombin deficiency induced by anticoagulants or other drugs.

hemostatic forceps. See **artery forceps.**

hemothorax /hē′mōthôr′aks, hem′-/ [Gk, *haima* + *thorax*, chest], an accumulation of blood and fluid in the pleural cavity, between the parietal and visceral pleura, usually the result of trauma. Hemothorax also may be caused by the rupture of small blood vessels as a result of inflammation from pneumonia, tuberculosis, or tumors. Shock from hemorrhage, pain, and respiratory failure follows if emergency care is not available. Also called **hematothorax** /hē′mətōthôr′aks/.

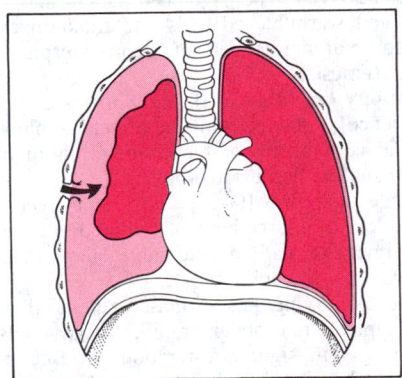

Traumatic hemothorax (Wilson, 1990)

hemotroph /hē′mətrof/, the total nutritive substances supplied to the embryo from the maternal circulation after the development of the placenta. Also spelled **hemotrophe.** Also called **hemotrophic nutrition.** Compare **embryotroph.** —**hemotrophic,** *adj.*

Henderson-Hasselbalch equation [Lawrence J. Henderson, American biochemist, b. 1878; Karl A. Hasselbach, Danish biochemist, b. 1874], the relationship between pH, the pK_a of a buffer system, and the ratio of the conjugate base and a weak acid.

Henderson, Virginia, a nursing theorist who introduced a holistic approach to nursing in 1966. It is based on the concepts that the body and mind are inseparable, no two individuals are alike, and the role of nursing is independent of the functions of the physician. The Henderson theory proposes that there are 14 components of basic nursing care that contribute to the health of a patient. The components relate to: (1) breathing, (2) eating and drinking, (3) elimination, (4) movement and posture, (5) sleep and rest, (6) clothing, (7) maintenance of body temperature, (8) cleaning and grooming the body, (9) avoiding environmental dangers and injury, (10) communication, (11) worship, (12) work, (13) play and recreation, and (14) learning and discovery.

Henle's fissure /hen'lēz/ [Friedrich G. J. Henle, German anatomist, b. 1809], one of many patches of connective tissue between the muscle fibers of the heart.

Henle's loop, a U-shaped portion of the renal tubule.

Henoch-Schönlein purpura /hen'ôkhshœn'līn/ [Eduard H. Henoch, German physician, b. 1820; Johannes L. Schönlein, German physician, b. 1793], a self-limited hypersensitivity vasculitis, chiefly of children, characterized by purpuric skin lesions that appear predominantly on the lower abdomen, buttocks, and legs, and usually associated with pain in the knees and ankles. Other joint involvement, GI bleeding, and hematuria are also common findings. The disease lasts up to 6 weeks and has no sequelae if renal involvement is not severe. Immunosuppressive drugs, such as corticosteroids, may help the nephropathy. Also called **anaphylactoid purpura, Schönlein-Henoch purpura.**

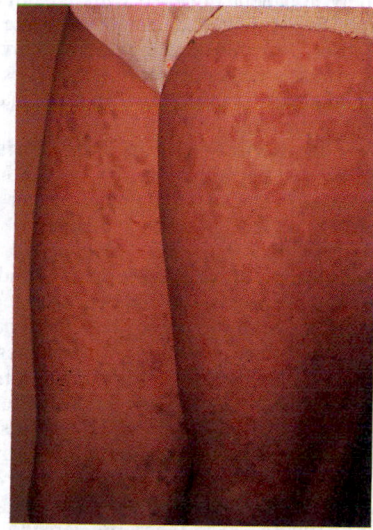

Henoch-Schönlein purpura (Zitelli, 1992)

Henry's law [William Henry, English chemist, b. 1774], (in physics) a law stating that the solubility of a gas in a liquid is proportional to the pressure of the gas if the temperature is constant and if the gas does not chemically react with the liquid.

Henschen method, (in radiology) a technique for positioning a patient's head in a true lateral position to produce an x-ray image of the mastoid and petrous portions of the head.

Hensen's knot, Hensen's node. See **primitive node.**

hen worker's lung. See **pigeon breeder's lung.**

heparin /hep'ərin/ [Gk, *hepar,* liver], a naturally occurring mucopolysaccharide that acts in the body as an antithrombin factor to prevent intravascular clotting. The substance is produced by basophils and mast cells, which are found in large numbers in the connective tissue surrounding capillaries, particularly in the lungs and liver. In the form of sodium salt, heparin is used therapeutically as an anticoagulant. See also **heparin sodium.**

heparin lock flush solution (USP) [Gk, *hepar,* liver; OE, *loc*; ME, *fluschen*; L, *solutus,* dissolved], a special sterile solution of heparin sodium, saline solution, and benzyl alcohol that is intended for use in maintaining patency in intravenous equipment. Not for use in anticoagulant therapy.

heparin rebound, the phenomenon of reactivation of heparin effect occurring from 5 minutes to 5 hours after neutralization with protamine sulfate.

heparin sodium, an anticoagulant.

■ INDICATIONS: It is prescribed in the treatment and prophylaxis of a variety of thromboembolic disorders.

■ CONTRAINDICATIONS: Known hypersensitivity to this drug prohibits its use. It is given only when frequent monitoring of the coagulation status of the patient's blood is possible.

■ ADVERSE EFFECTS: The most serious adverse reaction is hemorrhage. Vasospastic disorders may occur.

hepat-. See **hepato-.**

hepatectomy /hep'ətek'təmē/ [Gk, *hepar,* liver, *ektome,* cutting out], a surgical procedure to remove a portion of the liver.

-hepatia, a combining form meaning '(condition of the) liver or its functioning': *anhepatia, dyshepatia, hypohepatia.*

hepatic /hepat'ik/ [Gk, *hepar,* liver], of or pertaining to the liver.

hepatic adenoma, a rapidly growing tumor of the liver that may become very large and rupture, causing a lethal internal hemorrhage. The incidence is frequently associated with the use of oral contraceptives.

hepatic amebiasis, a disorder characterized by enlargement and tenderness of the liver that often occurs in association with amebic dysentery. The inflammation results from direct infection with *Entamoeba histolytica.* See also **amebiasis, amebic dysentery, Entamoeba histolytica.**

hepatic cells. See **hepatic cord.**

hepatic coma, a neuropsychiatric manifestation of extensive liver damage caused by chronic or acute liver disease. Either endogenous or exogenous waste toxic to the brain is not neutralized in the liver before being shunted back into the peripheral circulation of the blood, or substances required for cerebral function are not synthesized in the liver and therefore are not available to the brain. The condition is characterized by variable consciousness, lethargy, stupor, and coma; a tremor of the hands, personality change, memory loss, hyperreflexia, and hyperventilation. Respiratory alkalosis, mania convulsions, and death may occur. The outcome varies according to the pathogenesis of the condition and the treatment. Treatment in most cases includes cleansing enemas, low-protein diet, parenteral hydration with a balanced electrolyte solution, and specific treatment for the underlying cause. Also called **portal-systemic encephalopathy.** See also **cirrhosis, hepatitis.**

hepatic cord, a mass of cells, arranged in irregular radiating columns and plates, spreading outward from the central vein of the hepatic lobule. The cells are many-sided and contain one or, sometimes, two distinct nuclei. Many such cords join to form the parenchyma of the liver lobule. Each cell usually contains granules, some of which are protoplasmic whereas others consist of glycogen, fat, or an iron compound. Also called **hepatic cells.**

hepatic encephalopathy. See **hepatic coma.**

hepatic fistula, an abnormal passage from the liver to another organ or body structure.

hepatic keratitis. See **dendritic keratitis.**

hepatic lobes [Gk, *hepar,* liver, *lobos,* lobes], the large divisions of the liver, including caudate, quadrate, left, and right divisions.

hepatic node, a node in one of three groups of lymph glands associated with the abdominal and the pelvic viscera supplied by branches of the celiac artery. The hepatic nodes are divided into the hepatic and subpyloric groups. The hepatic group, on the stem of the hepatic artery, extends along the common bile duct, between the two layers of the lesser omentum, as far as the porta hepatis. The subpyloric group comprises about five nodes closely relating to the division of the gastroduodenal artery. Both groups receive materials from the stomach, the duodenum, the liver, the gallbladder, and the pancreas. Their efferent vessels join the celiac set of preaortic nodes. Compare **gastric node, pancreaticolienal node.**

hepatico-. See **hepato-.**

hepatic porphyria. See **porphyria.**

hepatic siderosis [Gk, *hepar,* liver, *sideros,* iron, *osis,* condition], a chronic disease in which hemosiderin, an iron-containing pigment, accumulates in the liver and causes a bronze skin pigmentation. Also called **hemochromatosis, bronzed diabetes.**

hepatic vein catheterization, the introduction of a long, fine catheter into a hepatic venule for the purpose of recording intrahepatic venous pressure. The catheter is inserted through a vein in the arm and is passed through the right atrium, inferior vena cava, and hepatic vein into the small hepatic vessel.

hepatic veins [Gk, *hepar,* liver; L, *vena*], the three main veins, the right, middle, and left, that drain the blood of the liver into the inferior vena cava.

hepatin. See **glycogen.**

hepatitis /hep'ətī'tis/ [Gk, *hepar* + *itis,* inflammation], an inflammatory condition of the liver, characterized by jaundice, hepatomegaly, anorexia, abdominal and gastric discomfort, abnormal liver function, clay-colored stools, and tea-colored urine. The condition may be caused by bacterial or viral infection, parasitic infestation, alcohol, drugs, toxins, or transfusion of incompatible blood. It may be mild and brief or severe, fulminant, and life-threatening. The liver usually is able to regenerate its tissue, but severe hepatitis may lead to cirrhosis and chronic liver dysfunction. Compare **anicteric hepatitis.** See also **viral hepatitis.**

hepatitis A, a form of infectious viral hepatitis caused by the hepatitis A virus (**HAV**), characterized by slow onset of signs and symptoms. The virus may be spread by direct contact through fecal-contaminated food or water. The infection most often occurs in young adults and is usually followed by complete recovery. Prophylaxis with immune globulin is effective in household and sexual contacts. Also called **acute infective hepatitis.** See **viral hepatitis.**

hepatitis B, a form of viral hepatitis caused by the hepatitis B virus (**HBV**). The virus is transmitted in contaminated serum in blood transfusion, by sexual contact with an infected person, or by the use of contaminated needles and

instruments. The infection may be severe and result in prolonged illness, destruction of liver cells, cirrhosis, or death. Also called **serum hepatitis.** See **viral hepatitis.**

hepatitis B immune globulin (HBIG), a passive immunizing agent.

■ INDICATION: It is prescribed for postexposure prophylaxis against infection by the hepatitis B virus.

■ CONTRAINDICATIONS: Known hypersensitivity to the drug or to gamma globulin prohibits its use.

■ ADVERSE EFFECTS: Among the most serious adverse reactions are severe hypersensitivity reactions. Pain and inflammation at the site of injection also may occur.

hepatitis B surface antigen. See **Australia antigen.**

hepatitis B vaccine, a vaccine prepared from the blood plasma of asymptomatic human carriers of hepatitis B virus or in yeast cells by recombinant DNA technology. A series of three doses is recommended to achieve immunity. The vaccine is particularly advised for people who are likely to have contact with blood or fluids of affected people, such as nurses, physicians, dentists, dental hygienists, and laboratory personnel.

hepatitis B vaccine (recombinant), a genetically engineered vaccine produced in yeast cells by recombinant DNA technology.

hepatitis C (non-A, non-B hepatitis HCV), a type of hepatitis transmitted largely by blood transfusion or percutaneous innoculation, such as with intravenous drug users sharing needles. The disease progresses to chronic hepatitis in up to 50% of the patients acutely infected. Diagnosis is made through identification of antibodies of HCV.

hepatitis D (delta hepatitis, HDV), a form of hepatitis that occurs only in patients infected with hepatitis B. HDV relies on HBV replication and cannot replicate independently. The disease usually develops into a chronic state. Diagnosis is made by detecting serum antibodies to HDV. It is transmitted sexually and through needle sharing. The only treatment is prevention of HBV.

hepatitis E (epidemic non-A, non-B hepatitis, HEV), a self-limited type of hepatitis that may occur after natural disasters because of fecal-contaminated water or food. There is currently no serologic test available.

hepatization /hep'ətīzā'shən/ [Gk, *hepatizein,* like the liver], transformation of lung tissue into a solid mass resembling the liver, as in early pneumococcal pneumonia in which consolidation and effusion of red blood cells in the alveoli produce **red hepatization.** In later stages of pneumococcal pneumonia, when white blood cells fill the alveoli, the consolidation becomes **gray hepatization,** or **yellow hepatization** when infiltrated by fat deposits.

hepato-, hepat-, hepatico-, a combining form meaning 'pertaining to the liver': *hepatobiliary, hepatocarcinogenic, hepatocellular.*

hepatobiliary capsule. See **Glisson's capsule.**

hepatoblastoma /hep'ətō'blastō'mə/, a cancer of the liver that tends to occur in children. It is usually detected during examination for causes of failing health and for the presence of a mass in the upper abdomen. Hepatoblastoma also may be associated with precocious puberty.

hepatocarcinoma, hepatocellular carcinoma. See **malignant hepatoma.**

hepatocele [Gk, *hepar,* liver, *kele,* hernia], a hernia of a portion of the liver through the diaphragm or the abdominal wall.

hepatocholangitis /hep'ətōkō'lanjī'tis/, an inflammation of both the liver and the bile ducts.

hepatocyte /hep'ətōsīt/ [Gk, *hepar* + *kytos*, cell], a parenchymal liver cell that performs all the functions ascribed to the liver.

hepatoduodenal ligament /hep'ətōdo͞o'ədē'nəl, -do͞o·-od'inəl/ [Gk *hepar* + L *duodeni* twelve fingers], the portion of the lesser omentum between the liver and the duodenum, containing the hepatic artery, the common bile duct, the portal vein, lymphatics, and the hepatic plexus of nerves. These structures are enclosed within a fibrous capsule between the two layers of the ligament. Compare **hepatogastric ligament.**

hepatogastric ligament /hep'ətōgas'trik/ [Gk, *hepar* + *gaster*, stomach], the portion of the lesser omentum between the liver and the stomach. Compare **hepatoduodenal ligament.**

hepatogenous jaundice /hep'ətoj'ənəs/ [Gk, *hepar*, liver; *genein*, to produce; Fr, *jaune*, yellow], a type of jaundice caused by a condition of the liver.

hepatojugular /hep'ətōjug'yo͞olər/ [Gk, *hepar*, liver; L, *jugulum*, neck], pertaining to the liver and the jugular vein.

hepatojugular reflux [Gk, *hepar* + L, *jugulum*, neck], an increase in jugular venous pressure when pressure is applied for 30 to 60 seconds over the abdomen, suggestive of right-sided heart failure.

hepatolienal fibrosis. See **congestive splenomegalia.**

hepatolenticular degeneration /həpat'ōlentik'yo͞olər/ [Gk, *hepar* + L, *lens*, lentil], an abnormal condition associated with defective copper metabolism in the body, characterized by decreased serum ceruloplasmin and copper levels and increased secretion of urinary copper. Individuals with this condition develop tissue deposits of copper associated with hepatic cirrhosis, deep marginal pigmentation of the cornea, and extensive degeneration of the central nervous system, especially the basal ganglions. Also called **Wilson's disease.**

hepatoma /hep'ətō'mə/, *pl.* **hepatomas, hepatomata** [Gk, *hepar* + *oma*, tumor], a primary malignant tumor of the liver characterized by hepatomegaly, pain, hypoglycemia, weight loss, anorexia, ascites, and the presence of alpha fetoprotein in the plasma. The tumor occurs most frequently in association with hepatitis or cirrhosis of the liver and, geographically, in those parts of the world where the mycotoxin, aflatoxin, is found. It is treated with resection when isolated to one lobe of the liver. Cyclophosphamide and liver transplants are used in experimental treatments.

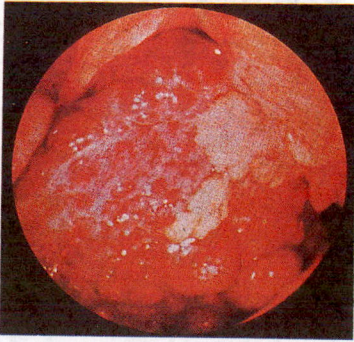

Hepatoma *(Misiewicz, 1985)*

hepatomegaly /hep'ətōmeg'əlē/ [Gk, *hepar* + *megas*, large], abnormal enlargement of the liver that is usually a sign of liver disease. It is often discovered by percussion and palpation as part of a physical examination: The liver is easily palpable below the ribs and may be tender to the touch. Hepatomegaly may be caused by hepatitis or other infection, fatty infiltration, as in alcoholism, biliary obstruction, or malignancy.

hepatopancreatic ampulla /-pan'krē·at'ik/ [Gk, *hepar* + *pan*, all, *kreas*, flesh], the dilatation formed by the junction of the pancreatic and bile ducts as they open into the lumen of the duodenum. Also called **ampulla of the bile duct, ampulla of Vater.**

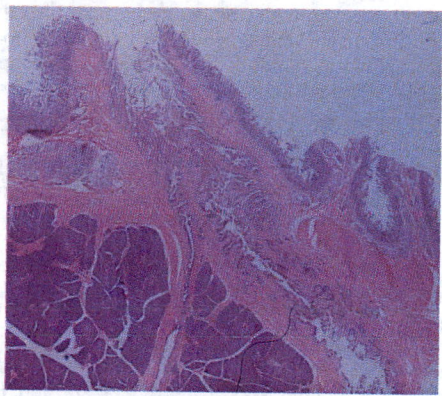

Hepatopancreatic ampulla *(Mitros, 1988)*

hepatorenal /hep'ətōrē'nəl/, [Gk, *hepar*, liver; L, *ren*, kidney], pertaining to the liver and the kidneys.

hepatorenal syndrome a type of kidney failure in which there is a gradual loss of function but no sign of tissue damage. It is associated with hepatitis or cirrhosis of the liver, but the exact cause is unknown.

hepatosplenomegaly /-splē'nōmeg'əlē/ [Gk, *hepar*, liver, *splen, megas,* large], enlargement of the spleen and liver.

hepatotoxic /-tok'sik/, potentially destructive of liver cells.

hepatotoxicity /hep'ətōtoksis'itē/ [Gk, *hepar* + *toxikon*, poison, the tendency of an agent, usually a drug or alcohol, to have a destructive effect on the liver.

hepta-, hept-, a combining form meaning 'seven': *heptachromic, heptadactylia, heptavalent.*

heptachlor poisoning /hep'təklôr'/ [Gk, *hepar*, seven; *chloros*, green; L, *potio*, drink], a form of chlorinated organic insecticide poisoning.

heptaploid. See **polyploid.**

herald patch. See **pityriasis rosea.**

herb bath /(h)urb/ [L, *herba*, grass; AS, *baeth*], a medicinal bath taken in water containing a decoction of aromatic herbs.

herbicide poisoning /hur'bisīd/ [L, *herba*, grass, *caedere*, to kill], a poisoning caused by the ingestion, inhalation, or absorption of a substance intended for use as a weed killer or defoliant. Many of the commonly used agricultural herbicides can produce symptoms ranging from skin irritation to hypotension, liver and kidney damage, and coma or convulsions. Estimated fatal doses may be as small as 1 to 10

g. If ingested, an emetic or gastric lavage is administered. Some herbicides contain extremely toxic substances; poisoning is characterized by dysphagia, burning stomach pain, throat constriction, diarrhea, or other severe symptoms. The substance is identified, the victim is rapidly taken to a medical facility, and therapy specific to the poison is promptly instituted.

herbivorous /hərbiv′ərəs/ [L, *herba*, grass, *vorare*, to devour], pertaining to feeding on plants or to animals that subsist mostly or entirely on plants. Also called **herbivore** /hur′bivôr/.

herd immunity [ME, *heord*, group; L, *immunis*, free from], the level of disease resistance of a community or population.

herd instinct [ME, *heord*; L, *instinctus*, impulse], the basic need of social animals, including humans, for the companionship of peers and a tendency to find compatibility with the behavioral standards of others in the group.

hereditability /həred′itəbil′itē/ [L, *hereditas*, inheritance], the degree to which a given trait is controlled by inheritance.

hereditary /həred′iter′ē/ [L, *hereditas*, inheritance], pertaining to a characteristic, condition, or disease transmitted from parent to offspring; inborn; inherited. Compare **acquired, congenital, familial.**

hereditary ataxia, one of a group of inherited degenerative diseases of the spinal cord, cerebellum, and, often, other parts of the nervous system, characterized by tremor, spasm, wasting of muscle, skeletal change, and sensory disturbances resulting in impaired motor activity. Kinds of hereditary ataxia include **ataxia telangiectasia** and **Friedreich's ataxia.**

hereditary brown enamel. See **amelogenesis imperfecta.**

hereditary deforming chondroplasia. See **diaphyseal aclasis.**

hereditary disorder. See **inherited disorder.**

hereditary elliptocytosis. See **elliptocytosis.**

hereditary enamel hypoplasia. See **amelogenesis imperfecta.**

hereditary essential tremor. See **essential tremor.**

hereditary hemorrhagic telangiectasia. See **Osler-Weber-Rendu disease.**

hereditary hyperuricemia. See **Lesch-Nyhan syndrome.**

hereditary multiple exostoses, a rare, familial, dyschondroplastic disease in which bony protruberances form on the shafts of the long bones and eventually develop into caps of cartilage covering the ends of the bones. The affected joints lose their mobility, and the bones stop growing. The disease begins in childhood and has no cure. Very rarely, a chondrosarcoma may develop from the cap of an exostosis. See also **Ollier's dyschondroplasia.**

hereditary opalescent dentin. See **dentinogenesis imperfecta.**

hereditary oral disease, any abnormal condition characterized by genetic defects of oral and paraoral structures, such as deformed dentition, ankyloglossia, hereditary gingivofibromatosis, or cleft palate. Many hereditary oral diseases are associated with generalized defects, such as Crouzon's disease, sickle cell anemia, gargoylism, familial amyloidosis, and achondroplasia.

hereditary protoporphyria. See **porphyria.**

hereditary spherocytosis. See **spherocytic anemia.**

hereditary tyrosinemia. See **tyrosinemia.**

heredity /həred′itē/ [L, *hereditas*, inheritance], **1.** the process by which particular traits or conditions are genetically transmitted from parents to offspring, resulting in resemblance of individuals related by descent. It involves the separation and recombination of genes during meiosis and fertilization and the further interaction of developmental influences and genetic material during embryogenesis. **2.** the total genetic constitution of an individual; the sum of the qualities inherited from ancestors and the potentialities of transmitting these qualities to offspring.

heredo-, a combining form meaning 'hereditary': *heredobiologic, heredosyphilitic, heredotrophedema.*

Hering-Breuer reflexes /her′ingbroi′ər/ [Karl E. K. Hering, Austrian physiologist, b. 1834; Joseph Breuer, Austrian psychiatrist, b. 1842], inhibitory and excitatory impulses that maintain the rhythm of respiration and prevent the overdistension of alveoli. The impulses originate in stretch receptors of the bronchi and bronchioles, travel via afferent fibers of the vagus nerves to the medullary respiratory centers, and back travel by motor neurons to the respiratory muscles of the chest. Hering-Breuer reflexes are well developed at birth. They are stimulated by distension of the airway, increased intratracheal pressures, or pulmonary inflation. The inflation reflex stops inspiration and stimulates expiration; the deflation reflex inhibits expiration and brings on inspiration. These reflexes are hyperactive in conditions of restrictive ventilatory insufficiency.

hermaphroditism /hərmaf′rəditiz′əm/ [Gk, *Hermaphrodites*, son of Hermes and Aphrodite], a rare condition in which both testicular and ovarian tissue exist in the same person, the testicular tissue containing seminiferous tubules or spermatozoa and the ovarian tissue containing follicles or corpora albicantia. The condition results from a chromosomal abnormality. Also called **hermaphrodism.** Compare **pseudohermaphroditism.**

hermetic /hərmet′ik/ [Gk, *Hermes*], from use in alchemy, pertaining to sealing a container so as to make it airtight.

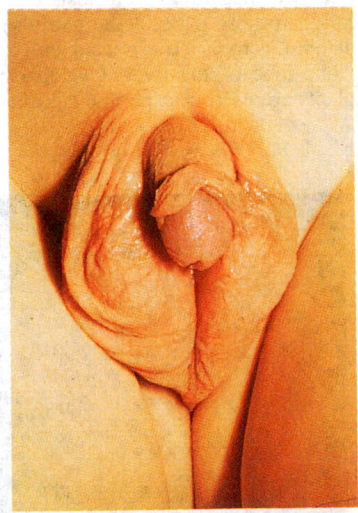

Hermaphroditism (Zitelli, 1992)

hernia /hur′nē·ə/ [L, rupture], protrusion of an organ through an abnormal opening in the muscle wall of the cavity that surrounds it. A hernia may be congenital, may result from the failure of certain structures to close after birth, or may be acquired later in life because of obesity, muscular weakness, surgery, or illness. Kinds of hernia include **abdominal hernia, diaphragmatic hernia, femoral hernia, hiatus hernia, inguinal hernia,** and **umbilical hernia.** See also **herniorrhaphy.**

hernial /hur′nē·əl/, pertaining to or resembling a hernia.

hernial sac [L, *hernia*; Gk, *sakkos,* sack], a pouch of peritoneum into which organs or other tissues pass to form a hernia.

herniated /hur′nē·ā′tid/, pertaining to a tear or abnormal bulge of an organ or organ part through a retaining tissue.

herniated disk, a rupture of the fibrocartilage surrounding an intervertebral disk, releasing the nucleus pulposus that cushions the vertebrae above and below. The resultant pressure on spinal nerve roots may cause considerable pain and damage the nerves. The condition most frequently occurs in the lumbar region. Also called **herniated nucleus pulposus, ruptured intervertebral disk, slipped disk.**

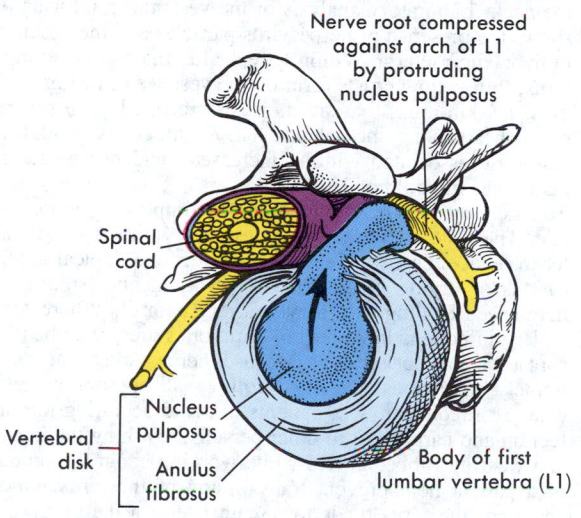

Herniated disk (Seeley, 1992/Karen Waldo)

herniated intervertebral disk. See **herniated disk.**

herniated nucleus. See **herniated disk.**

herniation /hur′nē·ā′shən/, a protrusion of a body organ or portion of an organ through an abnormal opening in a membrane, muscle, or other tissue. See also **hernia, hiatus.**

herniorrhaphy /hur′nē·ôr′əfē/, the surgical repair of a hernia.

herniotomy /hur′nē·ot′əmē/ [L, *hernia*; Gk, *tenein,* to cut], a surgical procedure to reduce a hernia.

heroin /her′ō·in/ [Ger, heroine, originally a trademark for diacetylmorphine], a morphinelike drug with no currently acceptable medical use in the United States. Heroin is included in Schedule I of the Comprehensive Drug Abuse Prevention and Control Act of 1970. As covered in this legislation, it may not be obtained by prescription but only for research and instructional use or for chemical analysis by application to the Drug Enforcement Administration of the Department of Justice. Heroin, like other opium alkaloids, can produce analgesia, respiratory depression, GI spasm, and physical dependence. It produces its major effects on the central nervous system and the bowel and alters the endocrine and the autonomic nervous systems. Illicitly obtained heroin is commonly used by individuals who become addicted and have a higher death rate than nonaddicts of similar age. Heroin, which loses much of its analgesic power when taken orally, is more powerful than morphine and acts more rapidly. Repeated use of this drug produces tolerance to most of the acute narcotic effects; physical dependence develops concurrently with tolerance. Withdrawal from heroin after relatively few exposures commonly produces acute abstinence syndrome. Withdrawal signs are usually observed shortly before the next planned dose and commonly include anxiety, restlessness, irritability, and craving for another dose. Other withdrawal signs that may appear 8 to 15 hours after the last dose include lacrimation, perspiration, yawning, and restless sleep. On awakening from such sleep the severely addicted heroin user may experience withdrawal signs, such as vomiting, pain in the bones, diarrhea, convulsions, and cardiovascular collapse. Withdrawal signs usually peak at between 36 and 48 hours and gradually subside during the following 10 days. Associated anxiety and depression may persist for months in many heroin addicts under treatment. Methadone is commonly used as a substitute drug in the treatment of heroin addiction. Also called **diacetylmorphine.**

herpangina /hur′panjī′nə/ [Gk, *herpein,* to creep; L, *angina,* quinsy], a viral infection, usually of young children, characterized by sore throat, headache, anorexia, and pain in the abdomen, neck, and extremities. Febrile convulsions and vomiting may occur in infants. Papules or vesicles may form in the pharynx and on the tongue, the palate, or the tonsils. The lesions evolve into shallow ulcers that heal spontaneously. The disease usually runs its course in less than 1 week. Treatment is symptomatic. The cause is often infection by a strain of coxsackievirus.

herpes genitalis /hur′pēz jen′ital′is/ [Gk, *herpein,* to creep; L, *genitalis,* genitalia], a chronic infection caused by type 2 herpes simplex virus (HSV2), usually transmitted by sexual contact, that causes painful vesicular eruptions on the

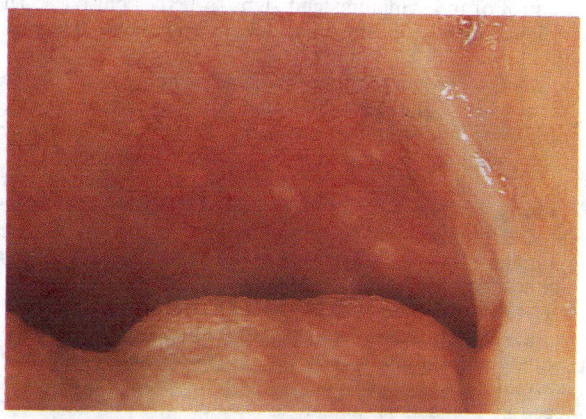

Herpangina (Lamey, 1988)

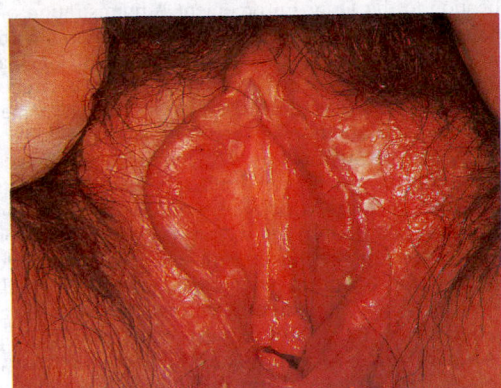

Herpes genitalis *(Habif, 1990)*

skin and mucous membranes of the genitalia of males and females. When acquired during pregnancy, HSV2 may be transmitted through the placenta to the fetus and to the newborn by direct contact with infected tissue during birth. HSV2 is a precursor of cervical cancer.

■ OBSERVATIONS: In the male, herpes genitalis infections may resemble penile ulcers. A small group of vesicular lesions surrounded by erythematous tissue may occur on the glans or prepuce. The lesions erupt into superficial ulcers that often heal in 5 to 7 days, although they also may become the sites of secondary infections. The lesions are painful and are often associated with a burning sensation, urinary dysfunction, fever, malaise, and swelling of the lymph nodes in the inguinal area. The female patient may exhibit the same or similar systemic effects, and members of both sexes may complain of painful sexual intercourse. In the female, herpes genitalis lesions are likely to appear as multiple superficial eruptions on the surfaces of the cervix, vagina, or perineum. There may be a discharge from the cervix. Vaginal lesions may appear as mucous patches with grayish ulcerations. Laboratory tests from smears of fluid taken from the base of lesions show a positive Tzanck reaction with multiple nucleated giant cells, which distinguishes HSV2 infections from other venereal diseases. HSV2 tends to recur.

■ INTERVENTIONS: Acyclovir taken orally results in partial control of the symptoms and signs of herpes episodes. The drug accelerates healing but does not eradicate the infection.

■ NURSING CONSIDERATIONS: Patients with genital herpes should be taught about the potential for recurrent episodes of lesions, and should be advised to abstain from sexual activity while the lesions are present. Sexual transmission has been documented during phases when no lesions were present. Women of childbearing age with genital herpes should inform their health care provider if they become pregnant. The nurse exercises extreme caution in contacts with infected patients.

herpes gestationis [Gk, *herpein;* L, *gestare*, to bear], a generalized, pruritic, vesicular or bullous rash appearing in the second or third trimester of pregnancy and disappearing several weeks postpartum. The lesions often recur with succeeding pregnancies and are associated with premature birth and increased fetal mortality. The disease closely resembles dermatitis herpetiformis.

herpes labialis. See **herpes simplex.**

herpes menstrualis [Gk, *herpein*, to creep; L, *menstruare*], a form of herpes simplex that tends to erupt during menstrual periods.

herpes simplex [Gk, *herpein;* L, *simplex*, uncomplicated], an infection caused by a herpes simplex virus (HSV), which has an affinity for the skin and nervous system and usually produces small, transient, irritating, and sometimes painful fluid-filled blisters on the skin and mucous membranes. HSV1 (oral herpes, herpes labialis) infections tend to occur in the facial area, particularly around the mouth and nose; HSV2 (herpes genitalis) infections are usually limited to the genital region.

■ OBSERVATIONS: The initial symptoms of a herpes simplex infection usually include burning, tingling, or itching sensations about the edges of the lips or nose within 1 or 2 weeks after contact with an infected person. Several hours later, small red papules develop in the irritated area, followed by the eruption of small vesicles, or fever blisters, filled with fluid. Several small vesicles may merge to form a larger blister. The vesicles generally are associated with itching, pain, or similar discomfort. Other effects often include a mild fever and enlargement of the lymph nodes in the neck. Laboratory analysis of the vesicular fluid usually shows the presence of herpesvirus particles and the absence of pyogenic bacteria. Within 1 week after the onset of symptoms, thin yellow crusts form on the vesicles as healing begins. In skin areas that are moist or protected or in severe cases, healing may be delayed. HSV2 infections in adolescence are associated with an increased incidence of cervical cancer in adulthood.

■ INTERVENTIONS: Treatment of herpes simplex is symptomatic. The lesions may be washed gently with soap and water to reduce the risk of secondary infection. Topical applications of drying medications, such as alcohol solutions, may speed healing, but they are very painful. Where secondary infections have begun, antibiotics are prescribed.

■ NURSING CONSIDERATIONS: Because herpesviruses are extremely contagious, the nurse follows all appropriate procedures in contacts with patients to avoid acquiring the infection and carrying it to other persons. Washing the hands and wearing rubber gloves while working about the mouth of a patient help prevent transmission of the virus. Once acquired, the virus tends to remain latent in the tissues of

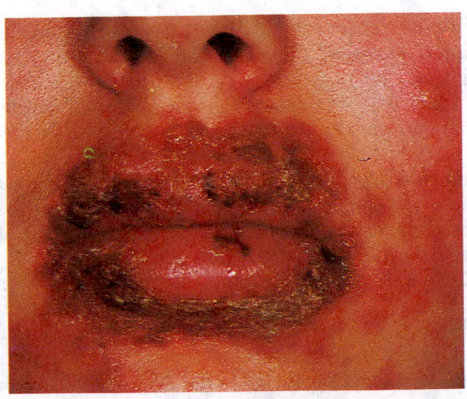

Herpes simplex *(Habif, 1990)*

the nervous system and may be reactivated by a variety of stimuli, including a febrile illness, physical or emotional stress, exposure to sunlight, or ingestion of certain foods or drugs. Topical sunscreen preparations offer some protection against exposure to the sun, and patients are advised to avoid repeated exposure to stimuli to which they are sensitive. The complications of herpetic infections may include encephalitis, herpes simplex keratitis, and gingivostomatitis. In cases involving systemic complications, intravenous acyclovir, blood transfusions, IV solutions, and other therapy may be required. In uncomplicated cases, the herpes attack is usually self-limiting and runs its course in 3 weeks or less.

herpes simplex keratitis. See **ocular herpes.**

herpesvirus /hur′pēzvī′rəs/ [Gk, *herpein* + L, *virus*, poison], any of seven related viruses including herpes simplex viruses 1 and 2, varicella zoster virus, Epstein-Barr virus, cytomegalovirus, HHV6, and HHV7.

herpesvirus hominis. See **herpes simplex.**

herpes virus simplex. See **disciform keratitis.**

herpes zoster /zos′tər/ [Gk, *herpein; zoster*, girdle], an acute infection caused by reactivation of the latent varicella zoster virus (VZV), affecting mainly adults and characterized by the development of painful vesicular skin eruptions that follow the underlying route of cranial or spinal nerves inflamed by the virus. Also called **shingles.** See also **herpes simplex, varicella zoster virus.**

■ OBSERVATIONS: Distribution of the pain and vesicular eruptions is usually unilateral, although both sides of the body may be involved. Any sensory nerve may be affected, but the virus in most cases tends to invade the posterior root ganglia associated with thoracic and trigeminal nerves. The pain, which may be constant or intermittent, superficial or deep, usually precedes other effects and may mimic other disorders, such as appendicitis or pleurisy. Early symptoms may include GI disturbances, malaise, fever, and headache. The vesicles usually evolve from small red macules along the path of a nerve, and the skin of the area is hypersensitive. All of the lesions may appear within a period of hours, but they most often develop gradually over a period of several days. The macules vesiculate and, after about 3 days, become turbid with cellular debris. Usually, at the end of the first week, the vesicles develop crusts. The symptoms

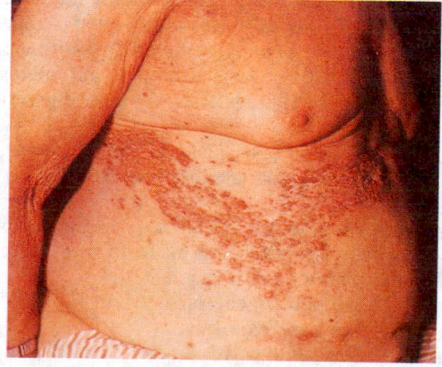

Herpes zoster
(Bryant, 1992/Courtesy Mary Brahman, Abbott Northwestern Hospital, Minneapolis)

may persist for 3 to 5 weeks, but in most cases they diminish after 2 weeks.

■ INTERVENTIONS: Treatment is primarily symptomatic and includes application of calamine lotion or similar medications to relieve itching and administration of analgesics for pain symptoms. Cool compresses may be applied to the affected skin areas. Topical corticosteroids may be prescribed for severe cases and for elderly patients who are potential candidates for a common sequela of postherpetic neuralgia. Surgical intervention to excise an affected nerve may be advised in cases of severe pain that fail to respond to more conservative treatment.

■ NURSING CONSIDERATIONS: The nurse encourages bed rest during the early stages of zoster infection, when fever and other systemic effects occur. Irritation of the vesicles may be exacerbated by contact with clothing or bed linen. The use of nonadherent dressings and of cradles to prevent direct contact of affected skin areas with irritating fabrics relieves discomfort. Older patients are most susceptible to complications, such as exhaustion and postherpetic neuralgia, which may persist for several months after the skin lesions have cleared. Other complications are geniculate zoster, with involvement of the ear, face, and soft palate, and ophthalmic herpes zoster, which can result in corneal damage. An attack of herpes zoster does not confer immunity, but most patients recover without permanent effects except for occasional scarring at sites of severe vesicular lesions. Evidence indicates VZV remains latent in the body of a person once infected, and a person lacking varicella immunity can acquire chickenpox from a herpes zoster patient.

herpes zoster ophthalmicus, a form of herpes zoster in which the virus invades the gasserian ganglion, causing pain and skin eruptions along the ophthalmic branch of the fifth cranial nerve. There also may be involvement of the third cranial nerve. The infection frequently leads to corneal ulceration or other ocular complications. Also called **ophthalmic herpes zoster.**

herpes zoster oticus, a herpes zoster infection of the eighth cervical nerve ganglia and geniculate ganglion, causing severe pain in the external ear structures and pain or paralysis along the facial nerve. The disease also may result in hearing loss and vertigo. The vertigo is usually transient, but the hearing loss and facial paralysis may be permanent. There may be vesicular eruptions along the external ear canal and ear pinna. Treatment is generally symptomatic, with diazepam administered for vertigo, analgesics for pain, and corticosteroids for other symptoms.

herpes zoster virus. See **chickenpox.**

herpetic keratitis [Gk, *herpein*, to creep, *keras*, horn, *itis*, inflammation], an inflammation of the cornea caused by a herpes virus. Also called **dendritic keratitis.**

herpetic neuralgia /hərpet′ik/ [Gk, *herpein*, to creep, *neuron*, nerve, *algos*, pain], a form of neuralgia with intractable pain that develops at the site of a previous eruption of herpes zoster.

herpetic stomatitis [Gk, *herpein*, to creep, *stoma*, mouth, *itis*, inflammation], a form of inflammation of the mouth caused by a herpes virus infection.

herpetiform /hərpet′ifôrm′/ [Gk, *herpein* + L, *forma*, form], having clusters of vesicles; resembling the skin lesions of some herpesvirus infections.

Herplex, a trademark for an antiviral (idoxuridine).

Hers' disease /herz, hurz/ [H. G. Hers, twentieth century French pathologist; L, *dis*, opposite of; Fr, *aise*, ease], an uncommon metabolic disorder of glycogen storage, characterized by hepatomegaly and an accumulation of abnormally large amounts of glycogen in the liver as a result of its inability to break down glycogen. The condition is inherited as an autosomal recessive trait. There is no known treatment. Also called **glycogen storage disease, type VI.** See also **glycogen storage disease.**

hertz (Hz) /hurts, herts/ [Heinrich R. Hertz, German physicist, b. 1857], a unit of measurement of wave frequency equal to one cycle per second (cps).

Herxheimer's reaction /herks'hī'mərz/, an increase in symptoms after administration of a drug. The reaction was originally discovered in penicillin treatment of syphilis, but has been found to occur with other diseases as well.

Herzog taping protocol, a procedure for immobilizing and balancing a foot with tape after a musculoskeletal injury. The protocol consists of step-by-step instructions for applying tape, beginning with the lateral aspect of the head of the fifth metatarsal and continuing through the lateral plantar aspect of the foot.

Heschl's gyrus /hesh'əl/ [Richard Ladislaus Heschl, Austrian pathologist, b. 1824; Gk, gyros, turn], any of several small gyri running transversely on the upper surface of the temporal operculum of the insula of the cortex.

hesperidin /hesper'idin/, a crystalline flavone glycoside found in bioflavonoid and occurring in most citrus fruits, especially in the spongy casing of oranges and lemons.

hetastarch /het'əstärch/, a plasma volume extender.
■ INDICATIONS: It is prescribed as an adjunct in shock and leukophoresis.
■ CONTRAINDICATIONS: Severe bleeding, severe heart or kidney dysfunction with oliguria or anuria, or known hypersensitivity to this drug prohibits its use.
■ ADVERSE EFFECTS: Among the more serious adverse reactions are influenza-like symptoms, muscle pain, edema, and anaphylaxis.

heter-. See **hetero-.**

heterauxesis. See **allometric growth.**

hetero-, heter-, a combining form meaning 'pertaining to another or different': *heteroalbumose, heterochronia, heterogamy.*

heteroallele /het'ərō·əlēl'/ [Gk, heteros, different, alleolon, of one another], one of a set of genes located at a specific locus on homologous chromosomes that differs from the other of the pair, resulting in a mutation. **–heteroallelic,** *adj.*

heteroblastic /het'ərōblas'tik/ [Gk, heteros + blastos, germ], developing from different germ layers or kinds of tissue rather than from a single type. Compare **homoblastic.**

heterocephalus /-sef'ələs/ [Gk, heteros + kephale, head], a malformed fetus that has two heads of unequal size. **–heterocephalous, heterocephalic,** *adj.*

heterochromatin /-krō'mətin/ [Gk, heteros + chroma, color], that portion of chromosome material that is inactive in gene expression but may function in controlling metabolic activities, transcription, and cell division. It stains most intensely during the interphase stage and usually remains in a condensed state throughout the cell cycle. It consists of two types, constitutive heterochromatin, which occurs in the centromeric region of the chromosome and is characteristic of the Y chromosome, and facultative heterochromatin, which is present in the inactivated X chromosome of the mammalian female. Compare **euchromatin.**

See also **chromatin. –heterchromatic,** *adj.*

heterochromatinization /-krō'mətīzā'shən/, the transformation of genetically active euchromatin into genetically inactive heterochromatin; the inactivation of one of the X chromosomes in the mammalian female during the early stages of embryogenesis. See also **Lyon hypothesis.**

heterochromosome /-krō'məsōm/, a sex chromosome. See also **heterotypic chromosomes. –heterochromosomal,** *adj.*

heterodidymus /het'ərōdid'iməs/ [Gk, heteros + didymos, twin], a conjoined twin fetus in which the parasitic elements consist of a head, neck, and thorax attached to the thoracic wall of the autosite. Also called **heterodymus.**

heteroduplex /-doo'pleks/ [Gk, heteros + L, duoplicare, to double], (in molecular genetics) a DNA molecule in which the two strands are derived from different individuals, with the result that some pairs or blocks of base pairs may not match.

heterodymus. See **heterodidymus.**

heteroeroticism /het'ərō·irot'isiz'əm/ [Gk, heteros + eros, love], sexual feeling or activity directed toward another individual. Also called **alloeroticism, heteroerotism.** Compare **autoeroticism.**

heterogamete /-gam'ēt/ [Gk, heteros + gamete, spouse], a gamete that differs considerably in size and structure from the one with which it unites, specifically denoting those of higher organisms as opposed to those of lower plants and animals. Compare **anisogamete, isogamete.**

heterogamy /het'ərog'əmē/ [Gk, heteros + gamos, marriage], 1. sexual reproduction in which there is fusion of dissimilar gametes, usually differing in size and structure. The word is used primarily to denote the reproductive processes of higher organisms as opposed to certain lower plants and animals. Compare **anisogamy, isogamy.** 2. reproduction by the alternation of sexual and asexual generations; heterogenesis. **–heterogamous,** *adj.*

heterogeneous /het'əroj'ənəs/ [Gk, heteros + genos, kind], 1. consisting of dissimilar elements or parts; unlike; incongruous. 2. not having a uniform quality throughout. Compare **homogeneous. –heterogeneity,** *adj.*

heterogenesis /-jen'əsis/ [Gk, heteros + genein, to produce], 1. also called **heterogeny, heterogony.** reproduction that differs in successive generations, such as the alternation of sexual with asexual reproduction, so that offspring have characteristics different from those of the parents. In the asexual stage, it often involves one or more parthenogenic or hermaphroditic generations, often with various hosts, as in the case of many trematode parasites. 2. asexual generation. 3. abiogenesis. Compare **autogenesis, homogenesis.** See also **metagenesis. –heterogenetic, heterogenic,** *adj.*

heterogenous /het'əroj'ənəs/ [Gk, heteros + genos, kind], derived or developed from another source or from two different sources.

heterogenous vaccine [Gk, heteros + genein, to produce; L, vaccinus, cow], a vaccine made from a source other than the patient's own tissues.

heterogeny. See **heterogenesis.**

heterogony. See **heterogenesis.**

heterograft. See **xenograft.**

heteroinfection /-infek'shən/ [Gk, heteros, different; L, inficere, to stain], an infection from a microorganism originating outside the body.

heterologous. See **xenogeneic.**

heterologous anaphylaxis /het′ərol′əgəs/ [Gk, *heteros*, different, *logos*, relation, *ana*, again, *phylaxis*, protection], a form of passive anaphylaxis involving the transfer of serum between two animals of the same species.

heterologous insemination. See **artificial insemination-donor.**

heterologous tumor [Gk, *heteros* + *logos*, relation], a neoplasm consisting of tissue different from that of its site.

heterologous twins. See **dizygotic twins.**

heterometropia /-mətrō′pē·ə/ [Gk, *heteros* + *metron*, measure, *ops*, eye], a generally mild visual disorder in which one eye refracts differently from the other, resulting in slightly different images being perceived by the right and left eyes.

heteronymous /het′əron′iməs/ [Gk, *heteros*, different, *onyma*, name], **1.** having different names; the opposite of synonymous. **2.** an optical phenomenon in which two images are produced by one object.

heterophil /het′ərofil′/ [Gk, *heteros*, different, *philein*, to love], having affinity for something unusual or abnormal, as an antibody that reacts to an antigen other than the one it is expected to challenge. Also **heterophile** /-fīl′/.

heterophil antibody test [Gk, *heteros* + *philein*, to love], a test for the presence of heterophil antibodies in the serum of patients suspected of having infectious mononucleosis, based on an agglutination reaction between heterophil antibodies in a person's serum and heterophil antigen, a normal component of sheep erythrocytes. This antibody eventually appears in the serum of more than 80% of the patients with mononucleosis, hence is highly diagnostic of the disease. See also **Epstein-Barr virus.**

heterophile. See **heterophil.**

heterophilic leukocyte /-fil′ik/ [Gk, *heteros*, different, *philein*, to love, *leukos*, white, *kytos*, cell], a neutrophil of certain animal species that takes an acid stain.

heteroplastic transplantation /-plas′tik/ [Gk, *heteros*, different, *plassein*, to mold; L, *transplantare*], the transfer of tissue from one animal to another of a different species. Compare **homoplastic transplantation.**

heteroploid /het′ərəploid′/ [Gk, *heteros* + *ploos*, times, *eidos*, form], **1.** of or pertaining to an individual, organism, strain, or cell that has a variation in the number of whole chromosomes characteristic for the somatic cell of the species. The change may involve entire sets of chromosomes or the addition or loss of single whole chromosomes. **2.** such an individual, organism, strain, or cell. See also **aneuploid, euploid.**

heteroploidy /het′ərəploi′dē/, the state or condition of having an abnormal number of chromosomes, either more or less than that characteristic of the somatic cell of the species.

heteropolymer /-pol′imir/ [Gk, *heteros* + *polys*, many, *meros* part], a compound formed from subunits that are not all the same, such as a protein composed of various amino acid subunits.

heterosexual /-sek′shəl/ [Gk, *heteros* + L, *sexus*, male or female], **1.** a person whose sexual desire or preference is for people of the opposite sex. **2.** of or pertaining to sexual desire or preference for people of the opposite sex. **—heterosexuality,** *n*.

heterosexual panic, an acute attack of anxiety resulting in the frantic pursuit of heterosexual activity in response to unconscious or latent homosexual impulses. Compare **homosexual panic.**

heterosis /het′ərō′sis/ [Gk, *heteros* + *osis*, condition], the superiority of first-generation hybrid plants and animals in respect to one or more traits when compared with either of the parent strains or with corresponding inbred strains. Also called **hybrid vigor.**

heterotopic ossification /-top′ik/ [Gk, *heteros* + *topos*, place], a nonmalignant overgrowth of bone, frequently occurring after a fracture, that is sometimes confused with certain bone tumors when visualized on x-ray film. Also called **exuberant callus, myositis ossificans.**

heterotopic transplantation [Gk, *heteros*, different, *topos*, place; L, *transplantare*], the transfer of tissue from one part of a body of a donor to another area of the body of a recipient.

heterotransplant /-trans′plant/ [Gk, *hetero*, different; L, *transplantare*], the transfer of tissue from one animal to another of a different species.

heterotypic /het′ərōtip′ik/ [Gk, *heteros* + *typos*, pattern], pertaining to or characteristic of a type differing from the usual or the normal, specifically regarding the first meiotic division of germ cells in gametogenesis as distinguished from the second or mitotic division. Also **heterotypical.** Compare **homeotypic.**

heterotypic chromosomes, any unmatched pair of chromosomes, specifically the sex chromosomes.

heterotypic mitosis, the division of bivalent chromosomes, as occurs in the first meiotic division of germ cells in gametogenesis; a reduction division. Compare **homeotypic mitosis.**

heterozygosis /het′ərōzīgō′sis/ [Gk, *heteros* + *zygotos*, yoked], **1.** the formation of a zygote by the union of two gametes that have dissimilar pairs of genes. **2.** the production of hybrids through crossbreeding. **—heterozygotic,** *adj*.

heterozygote /-zī′gōt/ [Gk, *heteros*, different, *zygotos*, yoked], an organism whose somatic cells have two different allelomorphic genes on the same locus of each pair of chromosomes. It can produce two different types of gametes.

heterozygote detection, the use of amniocentesis and other techniques to identify potential inherited X-linked recessive disorders, such as Hunter's syndrome or Duchenne's muscular dystrophy.

-heterozygotic. See heterozygosis.

heterozygous /het′ərəzī′gəs/ [Gk, *heteros* + *zygotos*, yoked], having two different genes at corresponding loci on homologous chromosomes. An individual who is heterozygous for a particular characteristic has inherited a gene for that characteristic from one parent and the alternative gene from the other parent. A person heterozygous for a genetic disease caused by a dominant gene, such as Huntington's chorea, manifests the disorder. An individual heterozygous for a hereditary disorder produced by a recessive gene, such as sickle cell anemia, is asymptomatic or exhibits reduced symptoms of the disease. The offspring of a heterozygous carrier of a genetic disorder have a 50% chance of inheriting the gene associated with the trait. Compare **homozygous.**

heuristic /hyŏŏris′tik/ [Gk, *heuriskein*, to discover], **1.** serving to stimulate interest for further investigation. **2.** a teaching method in which the student is encouraged to learn through independent research and investigation.

HEV, abbreviation for *hepatitis E virus*. See **hepatitis E.**

hex-, hexa-, a combining form meaning 'six': *hexabasic, hexavaccine, hexhydric.*

hexachlorophene /hek′səklôr′əfēn/, a topical antiinfective and detergent.
- INDICATIONS: It is used as an antiseptic scrub and as a disinfectant for inanimate objects.
- CONTRAINDICATIONS: Known hypersensitivity to this drug prohibits its use. Systemic absorption can occur when used on burns, broken skin, mucous membranes, and infant skin, with hemotoxic effects.
- ADVERSE EFFECTS: Among the more serious adverse reactions are skin rash and neurologic abnormalities.
- NOTE: The skin should be rinsed thoroughly to prevent systemic absorption.

hexacosanol. See **ceryl alcohol.**

hexadecanoic acid. See **palmitic acid.**

hexadecanol. See **cetyl alcohol.**

Hexadrol, a trademark for a glucocorticoid (dexamethasone).

hexafluorenium bromide /-floore′nē·əm/, an inhibitor of acetylcholinesterase.
- INDICATIONS: It is used as an adjunct to anesthesia to prolong the skeletal muscle relaxation caused by succinylcholine.
- CONTRAINDICATIONS: Known hypersensitivity to this drug or to bromides prohibits its use.
- ADVERSE EFFECTS: Among the more serious adverse reactions are excessive prolongation of muscle relaxation and resultant apnea, allergic reactions, and hypotension.

hexamethonium /-methō′nē·əm/, a cholinergic blocking agent used to control bleeding and in the treatment of peptic ulcers and hypertension. It produces ganglion blocking by occupying receptor sites.

hexamethylenamine. See **methenamine.**

hexamethylmelamine /-meth′ilmel′əmēn/, an experimental antineoplastic that has been used to treat bronchogenic, cervical, and ovarian carcinomas.

hexanoic acid. See **caproic acid.**

hexaploid. See **polyploid.**

hexenmilch. See **witch's milk.**

hexocyclium methylsulfate /-sī′klē·əm/, an anticholinergic.
- INDICATION: It is prescribed as an adjunct to ulcer therapy.
- CONTRAINDICATIONS: Narrow-angle glaucoma, asthma, obstruction of the genitourinary or GI tract, ulcerative colitis, or known hypersensitivity to this drug prohibits its use.
- ADVERSE EFFECTS: Among the more serious adverse reactions are blurred vision, central nervous system effects, tachycardia, dry mouth, decreased sweating, and hypersensitivity reactions.

hexokinase /hek′səkī′nās/ [Gk, hex, six, glykys, sweet, kinein, to move, ase, enzyme], an enzyme that catalyzes the transfer of a phosphate group from adenosine triphosphate to D-glucose.

hexose /hek′sōs/ [Gk, hex, six, glykys, sweet], a monosaccharide that contains six carbon atoms in the molecule. Glucose, maltose, and fructose are the principal hexoses found in nature, as well as being the principal absorbable endproducts of carbohydrate digestion.

hexylcaine hydrochloride /hek′silkān/, a local anesthetic for use on intact mucous membranes of the respiratory, upper GI, and urinary tracts.

hexylresorcinol /hek′ilrəsôr′sənol/, a topical skin anesthetic that is also administered for the treatment of certain types of worm infestations.

Hf, symbol for the element **hafnium.**

HFV, abbreviation for **high-frequency ventilation.**

HFJV, abbreviation for *high-frequency jet ventilation.* See **high-frequency ventilation.**

HFO, abbreviation for *high-frequency oscillation.* See **high-frequency oscillation.**

Hg, symbol for the element **mercury.**

HGF, **1.** an abbreviation for *human growth factor* **2.** abbreviation for *hyperglycemic-glycogenolytic factor.* See also **glucagon.**

HHS, abbreviation for **Department of Health and Human Services.**

hiatus /hī·ā′təs/ [L, gap], a usually normal opening in a membrane or other body tissue. **–hiatal,** *adj.*

hiatus aorticus [L, *hiare*, to yawn; Gk, *aerein*, to raise], an opening in the diaphragm for the aorta and thoracic duct.

hiatus esophagus [L, *hiare*, to yawn; Gk, *oisophagos*, gullet], the opening in the diaphragm for the esophagus.

hiatus hernia, protrusion of a portion of the stomach upward through the diaphragm. The condition occurs in about 40% of the population, and most people display few, if any, symptoms. The major difficulty in symptomatic patients is gastroesophageal reflux, the backflow of the acid contents of the stomach into the esophagus. Diagnosis is made easily on x-ray films. Surgical treatment is usually unnecessary, and efforts should be directed toward alleviating the discomfort associated with reflux. See also **diaphragmatic hernia, gastroesophageal reflux, heartburn.**

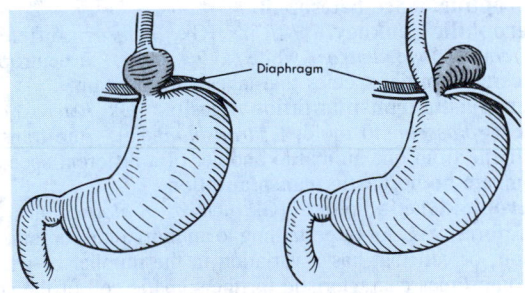

Hiatus hernia

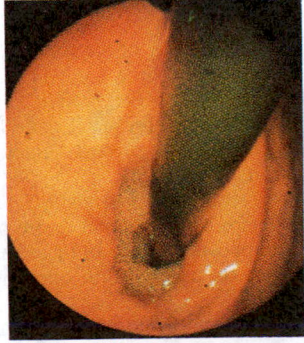

Hiatus hernia—endoscopic view *(Winawer, 1992)*

Hib disease, an infection caused by *Haemophilus influenzae* type b (Hib), which affects mainly children in the first 5 years of life. It is a leading cause of bacterial meningitis as well as pneumonia, joint or bone infections, and throat inflammations. More than two thirds of the U.S. cases of Hib disease have been attributed to exposure in day care centers. It is fatal in about 5% of infections. The infection can generally be prevented with a vaccine, b-Capsa-I, at 24 months.

hibakusha /hē′bäkoo′shä/ [Japanese], people who have been exposed to atomic bomb explosions. In 1985, some 370,000 hibakusha still lived in Hiroshima and Nagasaki, more than 40 years after the World War II. Their average age was over 60.

hibernoma /hī′bərnō′mə/, *pl.* **hibernomas, hibernomata** [L, *hibernus,* winter; Gk, *oma,* tumor], a benign tumor, usually on the hips or the back, composed of fat cells that are partly or entirely of fetal origin. Also called **fat cell lipoma, fetal lipoma.**

hiccup /hik′əp/, a characteristic sound that is produced by the involuntary contraction of the diaphragm, followed by rapid closure of the glottis. Hiccups have a variety of causes, including indigestion, rapid eating, certain types of surgery, and epidemic encephalitis. Most episodes of hiccups do not persist longer than a few minutes, but recurrent and prolonged attacks sometimes occur. The condition is most often seen in men. Sedatives are used in extreme cases. Also spelled **hiccough.** Also called **singultus.**

hickory stick fracture. See **greenstick fracture.**

hidradenitis. See **hydradenitis.**

hidro-, a combining form meaning 'pertaining to sweat or a sweat gland': *hidrocystoma, hidrosadenitis.*

hidrosis /hidrō′sis, hī-/ [Gk, *hidros,* sweat], sweat production and secretion. Also spelled **hydrosis.** Compare **anhidrosis, dyshidrosis, hyperhidrosis.** **–hidrotic,** *adj.*

hiero-, hier-, a combining form meaning 'pertaining to the sacrum, or to something sacred': *hierolisthesis, hieromania, hierotherapy.*

high-altitude edema [ME, *heigh;* L, *altitudo;* Gk, *oidema,* swelling], a form of pulmonary edema that occurs in people who move rapidly to higher altitudes. Fluid accumulates in the lungs as atmospheric pressure decreases.

high blood pressure. See **hypertension.**

high-calorie diet, a diet that provides 1000 or more calories a day beyond what is ordinarily recommended. It may be prescribed for nursing mothers, patients with severe weight loss caused by illness, or people with abnormally high metabolic rates or energy requirements, such as certain athletes or outdoor workers.

high-density lipoprotein (HDL) [AS, *heah,* top; L, *densus,* thick; Gk, *lipos,* fat, *proteios,* first rank], a plasma protein made in the liver and containing about 50% protein (apoprotein) with cholesterol and triglycerides. It may serve to stabilize very low-density lipoprotein and is involved in transporting cholesterol and other lipids from the body. See also **low-density lipoprotein, very low-density lipoprotein.**

high enema [ME, *heigh;* Gk, *einienai,* to send in], an enema that is inserted into the colon through a long catheter.

high-energy phosphate compound, a chemical compound containing a high-energy bond between phosphoric acid residues and certain organic substances. When the bond is hydrolyzed, a large amount of energy is released. Aden-osine triphosphate is the most powerful and ubiquitous of the high-energy phosphate compounds found in the body. All of these compounds liberate energy to fuel muscle contraction, active transport across cell membranes, and the synthesis of many substances in the body.

highest intercostal vein [AS, *heah,* top; L, *inter,* between, *costa* rib, *vena* vein], one of a pair of veins that drain the blood from the upper two or three intercostal spaces. The right vein descends and opens into the azygous vein. The left vein crosses the arch of the aorta and opens into the left brachiocephalic vein, usually receiving the left bronchial vein.

high-flow oxygen delivery system, respiratory care equipment that supplies inspired gases at a consistent preset oxygen concentration. It is generally not affected by changes in the ventilatory pattern. Also called **fixed-performance oxygen delivery system.**

high forceps, an obstetric operation in which forceps are used to deliver a baby whose head is not engaged in the birth canal. The procedure is considered hazardous and is generally condemned. Compare **low forceps, mid forceps.** See also **forceps delivery, obstetric forceps.**

high-Fowler's position [AS, *heah,* top; George R. Fowler, American surgeon, b. 1848], placement of the patient in a semisitting position by raising the head of the bed more than 20 inches.

high-frequency hearing loss [ME, *heigh;* L, *frequens;* AS, *déaf*], a loss of ability to hear high-frequency sounds. It is most commonly associated with aging or noise exposure. Hearing loss may begin in early adulthood with a loss of hearing to frequencies in the range of 18 to 20 kHz. Around the age of 60, loss of hearing may begin to affect lower frequencies, in the range of 4 to 8 kHz. Hearing loss caused by noise exposure is greatest at 4kHz.

high-frequency ventilation (HFV), a technique for providing ventilatory support to patients by operating at a breathing rate of 60 breaths per minute or more with small tidal volumes. It may be used during intraoperative procedures such as laryngoscopy or bronchoscopy, as well as for ventilation in patients with a bronchopleural fistula. **High-frequency jet ventilation (HFJV)** is a type using a high-pressure gas source that can be regulated to produce short, rapid jets of gas through a small-bore cannula into the airway above the carina. It has a respiratory rate of 100 to 400 cycles per minute. **High-frequency oscillation (HFO)** is a form of high-frequency ventilation that forces small impulses of gas in and out of the airway at frequencies of 400 to 4000 per minute.

high labial arch, a labial arch wire adapted to lie gingival to the anterior tooth crowns, having auxiliary springs that extend downward in contact with the teeth to be moved.

high-level wellness, a concept of optimal health that emphasizes the integration of body, mind, and environment to maximize the function of an individual.

high-potassium diet, a diet that contains foods rich in potassium, including all leafy green vegetables, brussels sprouts, citrus fruits, bananas, dates, raisins, legumes, meats, and whole grains. It is indicated for any condition resulting in the loss of extracellular fluid, such as acute diarrhea, congenital renal alkalosis, aldosteronism, hypokalemia, hypertension, and diabetic coma. It is also indicated for patients receiving thiazide or corticosteroid therapy.

high-protein diet, a diet that contains large amounts of protein, consisting largely of meats, fish, milk, legumes, and nuts. It may be indicated in protein depletion from any cause, as a preoperative preparation, in nephrotic syndromes, or in hepatic disorders. It may be contraindicated in liver failure or when function of the kidneys is so impaired that added protein could result in azotemia and acidosis.

high-residue diet /-rez′idyo͞o/ [ME, *heigh*; L, *residuum,* remaining; Gk, *diaita,* lifestyle], a diet that contains a greater than usual proportion of substances the digestive tract will not metabolize and absorb, such as fiber and other cellulose products.

high-resolution, the quality and accuracy of detail presented by a graphics system display, such as on CRT screen or a computer printout. Generally, resolution quality increases as the number of pixels, or image-forming units in the display, increases.

high-risk infant, any neonate, regardless of birth weight, size, or gestational age, who, because of preconceptual, prenatal, natal, or postnatal conditions or circumstances that interfere with the normal birth process or impede adjustment to extrauterine growth and development, has a greater than average chance of morbidity or mortality, especially within the first 28 days of life. See also **neonatal period, premature infant.**

high-speed handpiece, a rotary cutting instrument that operates at high speeds of up to 450,000 rpm. Modern high speed hand pieces are powered by miniature turbines driven by compressed air.

high-vitamin diet, a dietary regimen that includes a variety of foods that contain therapeutic amounts of all of the vitamins necessary for the metabolic processes of the body. It is often ordered in combination with other therapeutic diets containing larger than usual amounts of protein or calories, especially when treating severe or chronic infection, malnutrition, or vitamin deficiency.

hila. See **hilum.**

hilar /hī′lär/ [L, *hilum,* a little thing], pertaining to a hilum.

Hill-Burton Act, a 1946 amendment to the U.S. Public Health Service Act authorizing grants to states for surveying their hospital and public health center needs and for the planning and construction of additional facilities. Subsequent amendments authorized federal funding for as much as two thirds of the cost of construction projects and broadened the scope of the legislation to include diagnostic and treatment centers, long-term treatment centers, and nursing homes and to aid in modernization of existing hospitals. Also called **Hospital Survey and Construction Act.**

Hill-Burton programs, a cluster of programs created by legislation included in the National Health Planning and Resources Development Act of 1974. The programs allow federal monetary assistance for modernization of health facilities, construction of outpatient health centers, construction of inpatient facilities in underserved areas, and the conversion of existing health care facilities for the provision of new health services.

hilum /hī′ləm/ /hī′ləs/, *pl.* **hila** [L *hila* a trifle], a depression or pit at that part of an organ where vessels and nerves enter. Also called *(obsolete)* **hilus.**

hindbrain /hīnd′ brān/ [ME, *hind*; AS, *bragen*], the division in the brain of an embryo that eventually becomes the pons, the medulla oblongata, and the cerebellum.

hindgut /hīnd′ gut/ [ME, *hind;* AS, *guttas*], the caudal portion of the embryonic alimentary canal. Consisting of endodermal tissue, it is formed by the development of the tail fold and eventually gives rise to part of the small and large intestines, rectum, bladder, and urogenital ducts. Compare **foregut, midgut.** See also **cloaca.**

hind kidney. See **metanephros.**

hinge axis, the joint where the mandible meets the skull and the point of rotation of the mandible.

hinge axis-orbital plane, a craniofacial plane that is usually determined by marking three points on the face of the patient. Two of the points, one on each side of the face, are located on the hinge axis. The third point is located on the face at the level of the orbital rim just beneath the eye. The hinge axis-orbital plane is a reference plane for the diagnosis of various types of malocclusions and the development of associated prostheses.

hinged knee, an appliance designed to protect and support the knee during activity. It consists of an elastic sleeve with medial and lateral steel or aluminum bars hinged at the axis of the knee joint. The hinged bars are stabilized with leather or Velcro straps.

hinge joint [AS, *hangian,* to hang; ME, *jointe,* a connection], a synovial joint providing a connection in which articular surfaces are closely molded together in a manner that permits extensive motion in one plane. The distal bone of a hinge joint seldom moves in the same plane as that of the axis of the proximal bone. The interphalangeal joints are hinge joints. Also called **ginglymus joint.** Compare **gliding joint, pivot joint.**

hip. See **coxa.**

hip bath. See **sitz bath.**

hipbone. See **innominate bone.**

hip joint. See **coxal articulation.**

hip-joint disease [AS, *hype*; L, *jungere,* to join; Gk, *dis,* not; Fr, *aise,* ease], any abnormal condition of the hip joint, such as **Perthes' disease** or congenital dislocation of the hip.

Hippel's disease, von Hippel-Lindau disease [Eugen von Hippel, German ophthalmologist, b. 1867; Arvid Lindau, Swedish pathologist, b. 1892; Gk, *dis,* not; Fr, *aise,* ease], a familial disease involving the retina, first described by Hippel. It is characterized by hemangioblastomas of the cerebellar hemispheres, angiomatosis of the retina, and cysts of the kidneys and pancreas.

hippocampal /hip′ōkam′pəl/ [Gk, *hippokampos,* seahorse], pertaining to the hippocampus.

hippocampal commissure [Gk, *hippokampos,* seahorse; L, *commissura,* a joint], a thin, triangular layer of transverse fibers that connects the medial edges of the posterior pillars of the fornix in the brain.

hippocampal fissure, a fissure reaching from the posterior aspect of the corpus callosum to the tip of the temporal lobe.

hippocampal formation [Gk, *hippokampos,* seahorse; L, *formatio*], a part of the rhinencephalon, including the dentate gyrus, longitudinal striae, and hippocampus.

hippocampal gyrus [Gk, *hippokampos,* seahorse, *gyros,* turn], a convolution on the medial side of the temporal lobe of the cerebral cortex.

hippocampus /hip′ōkam′pəs/, *pl.* **hippocampi** [Gk, *hippokampos,* seahorse], a curved convoluted elevation of the floor of the inferior horn of the lateral ventricle of the brain. It is composed of gray substance covered by a layer of white fibers, the alveus, and functions as an important component of the limbic system. Its efferent projections form the fornix of the cerebrum. Also called **Ammon's horn, hippocampus major.**

hippocampus minor.   See **calcar avis.**

Hippocrates /hipok'rətēz/,   a Greek physician born about 460 BC on the island of Cos, a center for the worship of Æsculapius. Called the "Father of Medicine," Hippocrates introduced a scientific approach to healing by seeking physical causes for disease rather than magic or mythic relationships employed by members of the Æsculapian cults of the time. He also compiled case records of illnesses, including results of treatments administered, and developed the art of ethical bedside care. See **Æsculapius, Hippocratic oath.**

Hippocrates' bandage.   See **capeline bandage.**

Hippocratic oath /hip'əkrat'ik/,   an oath, attributed to Hippocrates, that serves as an ethical guide for the medical profession. It is traditionally incorporated into the graduation ceremonies of medical colleges and reads as follows:

I swear by Apollo the physician, by Æ sculapius, Hygeia, and Panacea, and I take to witness all the gods, and all the goddesses, to keep according to my ability and my judgment the following Oath:

To consider dear to me as my parents him who taught me this art; to live in common with him and if necessary to share my goods with him; to look upon his children as my own brothers, to teach them this art if they so desire without fee or written promise; to impart to my sons and the sons of the master who taught me and the disciples who have enrolled themselves and have agreed to the rules of the profession, but to these alone, the precepts and the instruction. I will prescribe regimen for the good of my patients according to my ability and my judgment and never do harm to anyone. To please no one will I prescribe a deadly drug, nor give advice which may cause his death. Nor will I give a woman a pessary to procure abortion. But I will preserve the purity of my life and my art. I will not cut for stone, even for patients in whom the disease is manifest; I will leave this operation to be performed by practitioners (specialists in this art). In every house where I come I will enter only for the good of my patients, keeping myself far from all intentional ill-doing and all seduction, and especially from the pleasures of love with women or with men, be they free or slaves. All that may come to my knowledge in the exercise of my profession or outside of my profession or in daily commerce with men, which ought not to be spread abroad, I will keep secret and will never reveal. If I keep this oath faithfully, may I enjoy my life and practice my art, respected by all men and in all times; but if I swerve from it or violate it, may the reverse be my lot. See also **Æsculapius, Hippocrates.**

hippuric acid [Gk, *hippos*, horse, *ouron*, urine; L, *acidus*, sour],   a detoxication product in the urine of some animals. It has been used as a medication in the treatment of arthritic diseases.

hip replacement [AS, *hype*],   replacement of the hip joint with an artificial ball and socket joint. Hip replacement is performed to relieve a chronically painful and stiff hip in advanced osteoarthritis, an improperly healed fracture, or degeneration of the joint. Antibiotic therapy is begun preoperatively, and the patient is taught to walk with crutches. During surgery, the femoral head, neck, and part of the shaft are removed, and the contours of the socket are smoothed. A prosthesis of a durable, hard metal alloy or stainless steel is shaped to resemble a head of a femur and is attached to

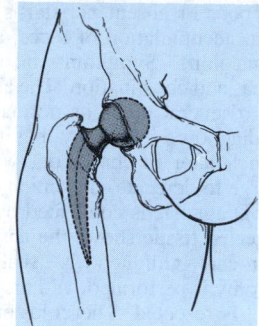

Hip replacement

the femur. A metal or a plastic acetabulum is implanted. Postoperatively, the patient may be placed in traction. The affected leg is kept abducted and in straight alignment with pillows; external rotation of the leg must be prevented. The nurse observes nerve function and circulation in the leg frequently during the first postoperative day. Support hose may be ordered and anticoagulant therapy begun. The most frequent complications are infection requiring removal of the new joint, or its dislocation. Ambulation begins gradually, with frequent short walks. Sitting for more than 1 hour is to be avoided, and hip flexion beyond 90 degrees may cause dislocation of the prosthesis. The patient continues an exercise program after discharge to maintain functional motion of the hip joint and to strengthen the abductor muscles.

Hiprex,   a trademark for a urinary antibacterial (methenamine hippurate).

Hirschberg's reflex /hursh'bərgz/,   a diagnostic test for pyramidal tract disease. The test result is regarded as positive if inversion of the foot occurs when the sole is stroked at the base of the great toe.

Hirschfeld-Dunlop file,   a kind of periodontal file, used with a pull stroke to remove tooth calculus. Various models with different angulations are available for different tooth surfaces.

Hirschfeld's method [Isador Hirschfeld, American dentist, b. 1881],   a tooth brushing technique in which the bristles are placed against the axial surfaces of the teeth at a slight incisal or occlusal angle and in contact with the teeth and gingivae, then vigorously rotated in very small circles.

Hirschsprung's disease /hirsh'spro͞ongz/ [Harald Hirschsprung, Danish physician, b. 1831],   the congenital absence of autonomic ganglia in the smooth muscle wall of the co-

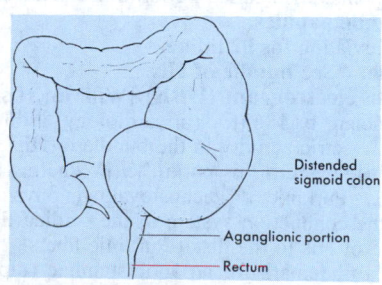

Hirschsprungs disease

lon, resulting in poor or absent peristalsis in the involved segment of colon, accumulation of feces, and dilatation of the bowel (megacolon). Symptoms include intermittent vomiting, diarrhea, and constipation. The abdomen may become distended to several times its normal size. The condition is usually diagnosed in infancy, but it may not be recognized until much later in childhood, when there is anorexia, lack of urge to defecate, distention of the abdomen, and poor health. Diagnosis is confirmed by barium enema; biopsy of the affected tissue shows the absence of ganglia. Surgical repair in early childhood is usually successful. A temporary colostomy is performed, and the aganglionic portion of the bowel is resected. The colostomy is almost always reversed a few months later. Also called **aganglionic megacolon, congenital megacolon.**

hirsutism /hur'sōotiz'əm/ [L, *hirsutus*, hairy], excessive body hair in a masculine distribution pattern as a result of heredity, hormonal dysfunction, porphyria, or medication. Treatment of the specific cause usually stops growth of more hair. Excess hair may be removed by electrolysis, chemical depilation, shaving, plucking, or rubbing with pumice. Fine facial hair may be most effectively minimized by bleaching. Also called **hypertrichosis.**   **–hirsute,** *adj.,* **hirsuteness,** *n.*

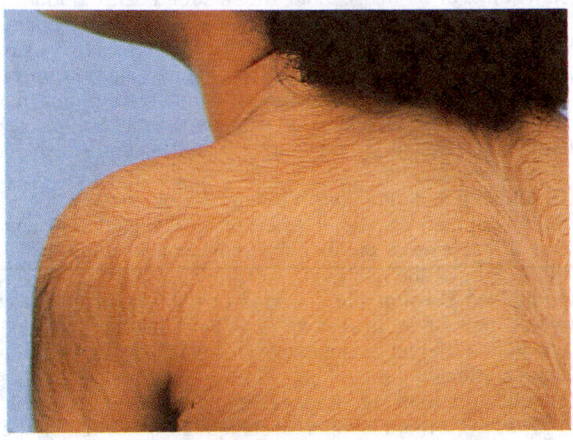

Hirsutism *(Baran, 1991)*

hirsutoid papilloma of the penis /hur'sōotoid/ [L, *hirsutus*, shaggy; Gk, *eidos*, form], a condition characterized by clusters of small, white papules on the coronal edge of the glans penis. Also called **papillomatosis coronae penis, pearly penile papules.**

His, abbreviation for **histidine.**

His bundle. See **bundle of His.**

His bundle electrogram (HBE) [Wilhelm His, Jr., German physician, b. 1863], (in cardiology) a direct recording of the electric activity in the bundle of His.

His-Purkinje system /his'pərkin'jē/ [Wilhelm His, Jr.; Johannes E. Purkinje, Czechoslovakian physiologist, b. 1787], the conduction system in the cardiac tissues from the bundle of His to the distal Purkinje fibers.

Hispril, a trademark for an antihistaminic (diphenylpyraline hydrochloride).

hist-. See **histo-.**

histamine /his'təmēn, -min/ [Gk, *histos*, tissue; L, *amine*, ammonia], a compound, found in all cells, produced by the breakdown of histidine. It is released in allergic, inflammatory reactions and causes dilatation of capillaries, decreased blood pressure, increased secretion of gastric juice, and constriction of smooth muscles of the bronchi and uterus.

histamine headache, a headache associated with the release of histamine from the body tissues and marked by symptoms of dilated carotid arteries, fluid accumulation under the eyes, tearing or lacrimation, and rhinorrhea (runny nose). Symptoms include sudden sharp pain on one side of the head, involving the facial area from the neck to the temple. Treatment includes the use of preparations of antihistamines and ergot that help constrict the arteries. Also called **cluster headache, Horton's histamine cephalalgia.** See also **cephalalgia.**

histamine-proved achlorhydria [Gk, *histos,* tissue, *amine, a,* not, *chlorhydria,* hydrochloric acid], the absence of normal hydrochloric acid production by cells in the lining of the stomach as demonstrated by the **histamine test.**

histamine test [Gk, *histos,* tissue, *amine*; L, *testum*, crucible], a test for achylia gastrica, or the lack of hydrochloric acid in the stomach. The stomach is emptied and washed out before subcutaneous injection of 0.1% histamine to stimulate gastric acid secretion. The stomach is aspirated continuously. If no acid is produced, it is considered evidence that the stomach is not producing hydrochloric acid.

-histechia, a combining form meaning a 'tissue retaining a (specified) substance': *cholesterohistechia, glycohistechia, uratohistechia.*

histidine (His) /his'tidēn/ [Gk, *histos,* tissue], a basic amino acid found in many proteins and a precursor of histamine. It is an essential amino acid in infants. See also **amino acid, protein.**

$$
\begin{array}{c}
HC = N \\
\| \qquad \diagdown \\
C - N \quad CH \\
\| \qquad \diagup \\
CH_2 \quad H \\
| \qquad | \\
H_2N - C - C - OH \\
| \qquad \| \\
H \quad O
\end{array}
$$

Chemical structure of histidine *(Seeley, 1992)*

histidinemia /his'tidinē'mē·ə/, an inherited metabolic disorder caused by an enzyme defect involving L-histidine ammonia lyase and affecting the amino acid histidine. The condition leads to retardation and nervous system disorders. It is controlled by diet that limits the intake of histidine.

histiocyte. See **macrophage.**

histiocytic leukemia. See **monocytic leukemia.**

histiocytic malignant lymphoma /his'tē·ōsit'ik/ [Gk, *histos* + *kytos,* cell], a lymphoid neoplasm containing undifferentiated primitive cells or differentiated reticulum cells. Also called **reticulum cell sarcoma.**

histiocytosis X /his'tē·ōsītō'sis/, *obsolete.* a cluster of conditions encompassing benign eosinophilic granuloma and several malignant lymphomatous diseases.

histiotypic growth /his′tē·ōtip′ik/ [Gk, *histos* + *typos*, mark], the uncontrolled proliferation of cells, as occurs in bacterial cultures and molds. Compare **organotypic growth.**

histo-, hist-, a combining form meaning 'pertaining to tissue': *histoclastic, histohematin, histonectomy.*

histocompatibility /his′tōkəmpat′ibil′itē/ [Gk, *histos,* tissue; L, *compatibilis,* agreeing], the compatibility of the antigens of donor and recipient of transplanted tissue.

histocompatibility antigens [Gk, *histos* + L, *compatibilis,* agreeable], a group of genetically determined antigens on the surface of many cells. Histocompatibility antigens are the cause of most graft rejections that occur in organ transplantation. See **isoantigen, histocompatibility locus.**

histocompatibility gene [Gk, *histos,* tissue; L, *compatibilis, genein,* to produce], the gene that determines histocompatibility between the donor and recipient of transplanted tissue.

histocompatibility locus, a set of positions on a chromosome occupied by a complex of genes that govern several tissue antigens. Together, the loci and the genes comprise the human leukocyte antigen complex.

histocyte /his′təsīt/ [Gk, *histion,* web, *kytos,* cell], a macrophage of connective tissue that plays a role in the body's immune system.

histogram /his′təgram′/ [Gk, *histos* + *gramma,* record], (in research) a graph showing the values of one or more variables plotted against time or against frequency of occurrence. A graph of a patient's temperature, pulse, and respiration is an example of a histogram.

histography /histog′rəfē/ [Gk, *histos, graphein,* to record], the process of describing or creating visualizations of tissues and cells. **–histographer,** *n.,* **histographic,** *adj.,* **histographically,** *adv.*

histoid neoplasm /his′toid/ [Gk, *histos* + *eidos,* form; *neos,* new, *plassein,* to mold], a growth that resembles the tissues in which it originates. Compare **organoid neoplasm.**

histoincompatible /his′tō·in′kəmpat′əbəl/, pertaining to host and donor tissues that have different genotypes and are therefore likely to induce an immune response, leading to rejection of a tissue graft or organ transplant.

histologic [Gk, *histos,* tissue, *logos,* science], pertaining to the study of the anatomy and physiology of tissue cells. **-histological.** See **histology.**

histologically. See **histology.**

histologic technician/technologist, an allied health professional who works in a clinical laboratory preparing sections of body tissue for examination by a pathologist. This includes preparation of tissue specimens of human and animal origin for diagnostic, research, or teaching purposes. The tissue sections enable the pathologist to diagnose body dysfunction and malignancy. Histotechnicians process sections of body tissue by fixation, dehydration, embedding, sectioning, decalcification, microincineration, mounting, and routine and special staining.

histologist /histol′əjist/, a medical scientist who specializes in the study of histology. See also **histology.**

histology /histol′əjē/ [Gk, *histos* + *logos,* science], **1.** the science dealing with the microscopic identification of cells and tissue. **2.** the structure of organ tissues, including the composition of cells and their organization into various body tissues. **–histologic, histological,** *adj.*

histolytic /his′tōlit′ik/ [Gk, *histos,* tissue, *lysis,* a loosening], breakdown or dissolution of living organic tissue.

histone /his′tōn/ [Gk, *histos,* tissue], any of a group of strongly basic, low molecular weight proteins that are soluble in water and insoluble in dilute ammonia, and combine with nucleic acid to form nucleoproteins. They are found in the cell nucleus, especially of glandular tissue, where they form a complex with deoxyribonucleic acid in the chromatin and function in regulating gene activity. Histones also interfere with coagulation of the blood and have been isolated from the urine of patients with leukemia and febrile conditions.

histopathology /his′tōpəthol′əjē/ [Gk, *histos,* tissue, *pathos,* disease, *logos,* science], the study of diseases involving the tissue cells.

histoplasma agglutinin /-plaz′mə/ [Gk, *histos* + *plasma,* a formation], an agglutinin associated with fungal lung infections.

Histoplasma capsulatum [Gk, *histos, plasma* + L, *capsula,* little box], a dimorphic fungal organism that is a single budding yeast at body temperature and a mold at room temperature. It is the causative organism in histoplasmosis, common in the Mississippi River Valley. The fungus, spread by airborne spores from soil contaminated with excreta from infected birds, acts as a parasite on the cells of the reticuloendothelial system.

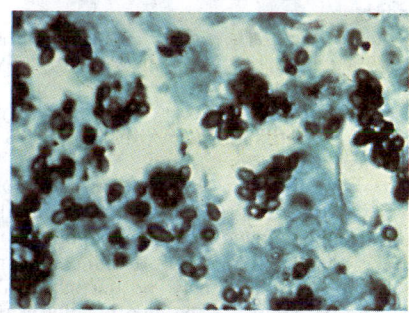

Histoplasma capsulatum in lung (Baron, 1990)

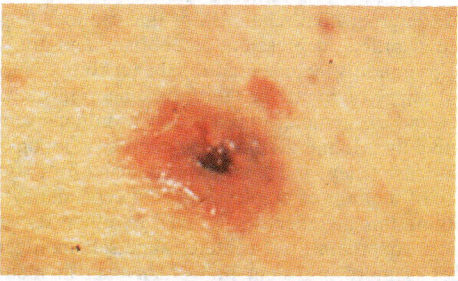

Pulmonary histoplasmosis (Parkin, 1991)

histoplasmosis /his′tōplazmō′sis/ [Gk, *histos, plasma* + *osis,* condition], an infection caused by inhalation of spores of the fungus *Histoplasma capsulatum.* **Primary histoplasmosis** is characterized by fever, malaise, cough, and lymphadenopathy. Spontaneous recovery is usual; small calcifications remain in the lungs and affected lymph glands.

Progressive histoplasmosis, the sometimes fatal, disseminated form of the infection, is characterized by ulcerating sores in the mouth and nose, enlargement of the spleen, liver, and lymph nodes, and severe and extensive infiltration of the lungs. The severe form is treated with amphotericin B, and less severe cases may be treated with ketoconazole. Infection confers immunity; a histoplasmin skin test may be performed to identify people who may safely work with contaminated soil. The disease is most common in the Mississippi and Ohio River Valleys.

history /his'tərē/ [L, *historia,* inquiry], **1.** a record of past events. **2.** a systematic account of the medical and psychosocial occurrences in a patient's life and of factors in family, ancestors, and environment that may have a bearing on the patient's condition.

history of present illness, an account obtained during the interview with the patient of the onset, duration, and character of the present illness, as well as of any acts or factors that aggravate or ameliorate the symptoms. The patient is asked what is believed to be the cause of the symptoms and whether a similar condition has occurred in the past.

histotoxin /-tok'sin/ [Gk, *histos* + *toxikon,* poison], any substance that is poisonous to the body tissues. It is usually generated from within the body rather than being introduced externally. **–histotoxic,** *adj.*

histotroph, histotrophe, histotrophic nutrition. See **embryotroph.**

histrionic /his'trē·on'ik/ [L, *histrio,* actor], pertaining to exaggerated facial expressions, speech, or body movements, such as used on the stage.

histrionic paralysis [L, *histrio,* actor; Gk, *paralyein*], a condition, such as **Bell's palsy,** in which paralysis of facial muscles results in a histrionic effect.

histrionic personality [L, *histrio,* actor; *persona,* role played], a personality characterized by behavioral patterns and attitudes that are overreactive, emotionally unstable, overly dramatic, and self-centered, exhibited as a means of attracting attention, consciously or unconsciously. Also called **hysteric personality.** See also **histrionic personality disorder.**

histrionic personality disorder, a disorder characterized by dramatic, reactive, and intensely exaggerated behavior, which is typically self-centered and results in severe disturbance in interpersonal relationships that can lead to psychosomatic disorders, depression, alcoholism, and drug dependency. Symptoms include emotional excitability, such as irrational angry outbursts or tantrums; abnormal craving for activity and excitement; overreaction to minor events; manipulative threats and gestures; egocentricity; inconsiderateness; inconsistency; and continuous demand for reassurance because of feelings of helplessness and dependency. A person having this disorder is perceived by others as vain, demanding, superficial, self-centered, and self-indulgent. The disorder is more prevalent in women than in men and is treated by various psychotherapies, depending on the individual and the severity of the condition. See also **narcissistic personality disorder.**

His-Werner disease [Wilhelm His, Jr., German physician, b. 1863; Heinrich Werner, German physician, b. 1874; Gk, *dis,* not; Fr, *aise,* ease], trench fever, an acute louse-borne infection that affected soldiers, mainly in World War I.

HIV, abbreviation for **human immunodeficiency virus.**

hives. See **urticaria.**

HLA, abbreviation for **human leukocyte antigen.**

HLA-A, abbreviation for *human leukocyte antigen A.* See **human leukocyte antigen.**

HLA-B, abbreviation for *human leukocyte antigen B.* See **human leukocyte antigen.**

HLA complex, human leukocyte group A, the major human histocompatibility complex that enables the immune system to differentiate tissues or proteins between 'self' and 'nonself.' It consists of groups of loci on the short arm of chromosome 6. They are identified by numbers and letters, such as HLA-B27. HLA-A, -B, and -C are cell surface antigens that occur on the surface of all nucleated cells and platelets and are important in tissue transplants. If donor and recipient HLA antigens do not match, the nonself antigens are recognized and destroyed by killer T cells.

HLA-D, abbreviation for *human leukocyte antigen D.* See **human leukocyte antigen.**

HLH, abbreviation for *human luteinizing hormone.*

HMD, abbreviation for *hyaline membrane disease.* See **respiratory distress syndrome of the newborn.**

HMG-CoA reductase, a rate-controlling enzyme of cholesterol synthesis. Activity of the enzyme may be as much as 60 times higher than normal in patients with familial hypercholesterolemia.

HMO, abbreviation for **health maintenance organization.**

HMS Liquifilm, a trademark for an ophthalmic preparation containing a glucocorticoid (medrysone).

Ho, symbol for the element **holmium.**

H₂O, symbol for **water.**

Hô, symbol for **null hypothesis.**

hod-, a prefix meaning 'pertaining to pathways': *hodology, hodoneuromere.*

Hodgkin's disease /hoj'kinz/ [Thomas Hodgkin, English physician, b. 1798], a malignant disorder characterized by painless, progressive enlargement of lymphoid tissue, usu-

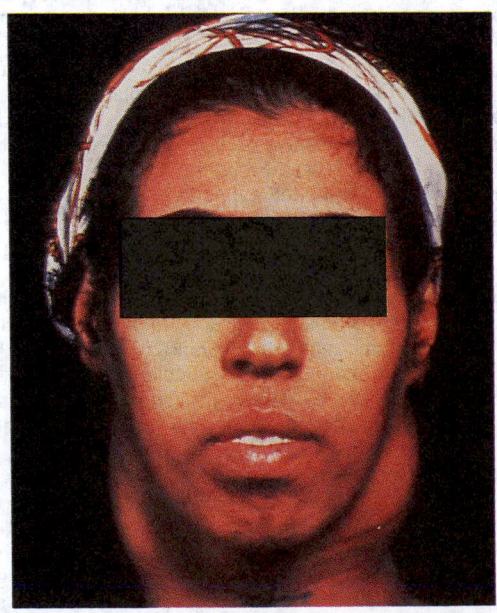

Hodgkin's disease—enlargment of lymph nodes
(Skarin, 1991)

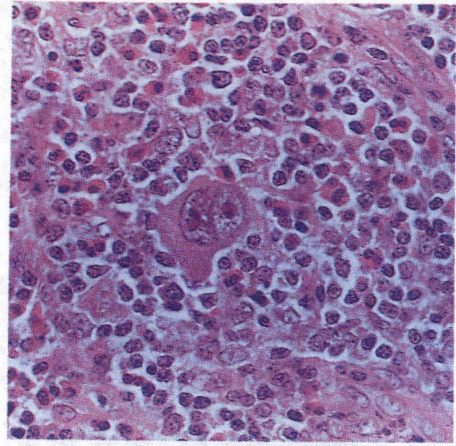

Hodgkin's disease—lymph node histology
(James, 1992)

ally first evident in cervical lymph nodes; splenomegaly; and the presence of Reed-Sternberg cells, large, atypical macrophages with multiple or hyperlobulated nuclei and prominent nucleoli. Symptoms include anorexia, weight loss, generalized pruritus, low-grade fever, night sweats, anemia, and leukocytosis. The disease is diagnosed in about 7100 Americans annually, causes approximately 1700 deaths a year, affects twice as many males as females, and usually develops between 15 and 35 years of age. The diagnosis is established by blood studies, x-ray films, lymphangiograms, lymph node biopsies, and ultrasonic and computerized tomographic scans. Total lymphoid radiotherapy, with a covering mantle to protect other organs, is the treatment of choice for early stages of the disease; combination chemotherapy is the treatment for advanced disease. Long-term remissions are achieved in more than one half of the patients treated, and 60% to 90% of those with localized disease may be cured. It is widely held that Hodgkin's disease may start as an inflammatory or infectious process and then become a neoplasm; according to another theory it may be an immune disorder. Clusters of cases have been reported, but there is no conclusive evidence of a causative infectious agent, and the cause of the disease remains an enigma.

Hodgson's disease /hoj'sənz/ [Joseph Hodgson, English physician, b. 1788; Gk, *dis,* not; Fr, *aise,* ease], an aneurysmal dilatation of the aorta.

Hoffmann's atrophy. See **Werdnig-Hoffmann disease.**

Hoffmann's reflex [Johann Hoffmann, German neurologist, b. 1857], an abnormal reflex elicited by sudden, forceful flicking of the nail of the index, middle, or ring finger, resulting in flexion of the thumb and of the middle and distal phalanges of one of the other fingers. It is indicative of pyramidal tract disease above the level of the seventh or eighth cervical and first thoracic vertebrae. Also called **Hoffmann's sign.**

hol-. See **holo-.**

holandric /holan'drik/ [Gk, *holos,* whole, *aner,* man], **1.** designating genes located on the nonhomologous portion of the Y chromosome. **2.** of or pertaining to traits or conditions transmitted only through the paternal line. Compare **hologynic.**

holandric inheritance, the acquisition or expression of traits or conditions only through the paternal line, transmitted by genes carried on the nonhomologous portion of the Y chromosome. Compare **hologynic inheritance.**

hold-relax, a technique of proprioceptive neuromuscular facilitation used in treating hypertonicity or motor dysfunction. It is often applied when there is muscle tightness on one side of a joint and when immobility is the result of pain.

holism /hō'lizəm/ [Gk, *holos,* whole], a philosophic concept in which an entity is seen as more than the sum of its parts. Holism is prominent in current approaches to psychology, biology, nursing, medicine, and other scientific, sociologic, and educational fields of study and practice. Also spelled **wholism.**

holistic /hōlis'tik/ [Gk, *holos*], of or pertaining to the whole; considering all factors, as holistic medicine. Also **wholistic.**

holistic counseling, an alternative form of psychotherapy that focuses on the whole person (mind, body, and spirit) and health; the goal is growth of the whole person.

holistic health care, a system of comprehensive or total patient care that considers the physical, emotional, social, economic, and spiritual needs of the person, the response to the illness, and the effect of the illness on the person's ability to meet self-care needs. Holistic nursing is the modern nursing practice that expresses this philosophy of care. Also called **comprehensive care.**

Hollenback condenser. See **pneumatic condenser.**

Holliday-Segar formula, a method of estimating the daily caloric needs of the average hospital patient under conditions of bed rest, based on the body weight in kilograms of the patient. Beginning at 100 kcal/kg for an infant, the formula plots a curve to 1,500 kcal plus 20 kcal/kg for each kilogram over 20 kg.

hollow cathode lamp [ME, *holg;* Gk, *kata,* down, *hodos,* way; *lampas*], a lamp consisting of a metal cathode and an inert gas. When an electric current is passed through the cathode, metal is dislodged. After colliding with the gas in the lamp, it emits a line spectrum of specific wavelengths related to the metal of the cathode.

holmium (Ho) /hōl'mē·əm/ [L, *Holmia,* Stockholm, Sweden], a rare earth metallic element. Its atomic number is 67; its atomic weight is 164.93.

holo-, hol-, a prefix meaning 'entire, or pertaining to the whole': *holodiastolic, holomastigote, holotonia.*

holoacardius /hol'ō·äkär'dē·əs/ [Gk, *holos* + *kardia,* heart], a separate, grossly defective monozygotic twin fetus, usually represented by a shapeless, nonformed mass in which the heart is absent and the circulation in utero is accomplished totally by the heart of the viable twin through a vascular shunt.

holoacardius acephalus, a grossly defective separate twin fetus that lacks a heart, a head, and most of the upper portion of the body.

holoacardius acormus, a grossly defective, separate twin fetus in which the trunk is malformed and little more than the head is recognizable.

holoacardius amorphus, a malformed separate twin fetus in which there are no recognizable or formed parts.

holoarthritis /-ärthrī'tis/, a form of arthritis that involves all or most of the joints.

holoblastic /hol'əblas'tik/ [Gk, *holos* + *blastos,* germ], of or pertaining to an ovum that contains little or no yolk and undergoes total cleavage. Compare **meroblastic.**

holocephalic /hō′lōsifal′ik/ [Gk, *holos* + *kephale*, head], a malformed fetus in which several parts are deficient although the head is complete.

holocrine /hol′əkrēn/ [Gk, *holos,* whole, *krienein,* to secrete], pertaining to a gland whose only function is to secrete or whose secretion consists of disintegrated cells of the gland itself.

holocrine secretion [Gk, *holos,* whole, *krienein,* to secrete], a secretion that consists of disintegrated or altered cells of the gland itself, as in the example of sebaceous glands.

holodiastolic. See **pandiastolic.**

holoenzyme /hol′ō·en′zīm/ [Gk, *holos* + *en,* in, *zymos,* ferment], a complete enzyme-cofactor complex that gives full catalytic activity.

holographic reconstruction /-graf′ik/, a method of producing three-dimensional images with diagnostic ultrasound equipment.

hologynic /hol′ōjin′ik/ [Gk, *holos* + *gyne,* female], **1.** designating genes located on attached X chromosomes. **2.** of or pertaining to traits or conditions transmitted only through the maternal line. Compare **holandric.**

hologynic inheritance, the acquisition or expression of traits or conditions only through the maternal line, transmitted by genes located on attached X chromosomes. The phenomenon is not known to occur in humans. Compare **holandric inheritance.**

holoprosencephaly /hol′ōpros′ensef′əlē/ [Gk, *holos* + *pro,* before, *enkephalos,* brain], a congenital defect caused by the failure of the prosencephalon to divide into hemispheres during embryonic development. It is characterized by multiple midline facial defects, including cyclopia in severe cases. It can also be caused by an extra chromosome in the 13-15 or D group, manifesting as one of many developmental defects. See also **trisomy 13.** –**holoprosencephalic, holoprosencephalous,** *adj.*

holorachischisis. See **complete rachischisis.**

holosystolic. See **pansystolic.**

Holter monitor [L, *monere,* to remind], a device for making prolonged electrocardiograph recordings on a portable tape recorder while the patient conducts normal daily activities. The patient also may keep an activity diary for the purpose of comparing daily events with ECG tracings. Also called **ambulatory electrocardiograph.**

Holthouse's hernia. See **inguinocrural hernia.**

Holtzman inkblot technique, a modification of the Rorschach test in which many more pictures of inkblots are used, the subject is permitted only one response to each design, and the scoring is predominantly objective rather than subjective.

Homans' sign [John Homans, American surgeon, b. 1877; L *signum* mark], pain in the calf with dorsiflexion of the foot, indicating thrombophlebitis or thrombosis.

home assessment [ME, *h]m*; L, *assidere,* to sit beside], an examination of the living area of a physically challenged person for the purposes of making recommendations about elimination of safety hazards and suggesting architectural or other modifications that would allow for independent functioning.

home care [AS, *ham,* village; L, *garrire,* to chatter], a health service provided in the patient's place of residence for the purpose of promoting, maintaining, or restoring health or minimizing the effects of illness and disability. Service may include such elements as medical, dental, and

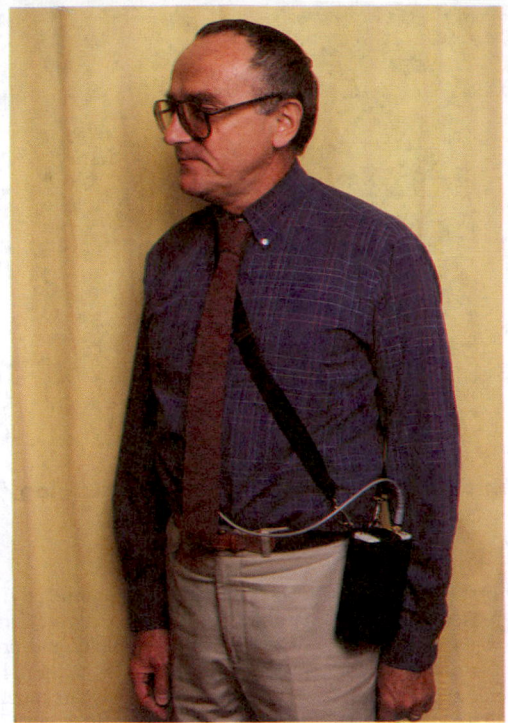

Holter monitor *(Canobbio, 1990)*

nursing care, speech and physical therapy, the homemaking services of a home health aide, or the provision of transportation. The level of care needed is determined by an assessment of the nature and extent of care needed and by the ability of the patient's family and friends to assume responsibility for the care needed. Nursing may be provided by a registered nurse, licensed practical nurse, or a home health aide. Some hospitals have home care services that include regular visits by a nurse and a physician to patients in their homes.

home health agency, an organization that provides health care in the home. Medicare certification for a home health agency depends on the providing of skilled nursing services and of at least one additional therapeutic service.

home maintenance management, impaired, a nursing diagnosis accepted by the Fourth National Conference on the Classification of Nursing Diagnoses. This diagnosis describes the situation in which a person is unable to maintain a safe, healthy home environment without help. The causes may include any of the following: disease or injury of a member of the family or household, disorganization of the family, inadequate finances, lack of knowledge of community or neighborhood resources, impaired or disordered emotional or cognitive function, inadequate support from others, lack of knowledge, or lack of role models competent in home maintenance. Among the defining characteristics reported by the patient and other members of the household are difficulty in maintaining the home in a comfortable condition, a need for help from the outside in maintaining the home, and the existence of debt or a financial crisis. Among the defining characteristics that may be observed in the home are disorder, an offensive odor, an inappropriate temperature, lack of necessary equipment or supplies, and the presence of rodents or vermin. The critical defining characteristics, at least one of which must be present for the diagnosis to be made, are unwashed or unavailable cooking utensils, clothes, or linens; the presence of accumulations of dirt, food, waste, and refuse; exhausted or distressed family or household members; and repeated infections and infestations resulting from a lack of hygiene. See also **nursing diagnosis.**

homeo-, homoeo-, homoio-, a combining form meaning 'sameness, similarity': *homeochrome, homeomorphus, homeothermal.*

homeodynamics /hō′mē·ədīnam′iks/ [Gk, *homoios,* similar, *dynamis,* force], the constantly changing interrelatedness of body components while maintaining an overall equilibrium.

homeopathic See **homeopathy.**

Homeopathic Pharmacopoeia of the United States, one of the three official drug compendia specified in the Federal Food, Drug, and Cosmetic Act. See also **compendium, National Formulary, United States Pharmacopoeia.**

homeopathist /hō′mē·op′əthist/, a physician who practices homeopathy.

homeopathy /hō′mē·op′əthē/ [Gk, *homoios + pathos,* disease], a system of therapeutics based on the theory that 'like cures like.' The theory was advanced in the late eighteenth century by Dr. Samuel Hahnemann, who believed that a large amount of a particular drug may cause symptoms of a disease and moderate dosage may reduce those symptoms; thus some disease symptoms could be treated by very small doses of medicine. In practice, homeopathists dilute drugs with milk sugar in ratios of 1 to 10 to achieve the smallest dose of a drug that seems necessary to control the symptoms in a patient and prescribe only one medication at a time. Compare **allopathy. –homeopathic,** *adj.*

homeostasis /hō′mē·əstā′sis/ [Gk, *homoios + stasis,* standing still], a relative constancy in the internal environment of the body, naturally maintained by adaptive responses that promote healthy survival. Various sensing, feedback, and control mechanisms function to effect this steady state. Some of the key control mechanisms are the reticular formation in the brainstem and the endocrine glands. Some of the functions controlled by homeostatic mechanisms are the heartbeat, hematopoiesis, blood pressure, body temperature, electrolytic balance, respiration, and glandular secretion. **–homeostatic,** *adj.*

homeotypic /hō′mē·ōtip′ik/ [Gk, *homoios + typos,* mark], pertaining to or characteristic of the regular or usual type, specifically applied to the second meiotic division of germ cells in gametogenesis as distinguished from the first meiotic division. Also **homeotypical.** Compare **heterotypic.**

homeotypic mitosis, the equational division of chromosomes, as occurs in the second meiotic division of germ cells in gametogenesis. Compare **heterotypic mitosis.**

Home's silver precipitation method, (in dentistry) a technique for depositing silver in enamel and dentin by the application of ammoniac silver nitrate solution and its reduction with formalin or eugenol.

homicide /hom′isīd/ [L, *homo,* man, *caedere,* to kill], the death of one human being caused by another human. Homicide is usually intentional and often violent.

hominal physiology /hom′inəl/ [L, *hominis,* human; Gk, *physis,* nature, *logos,* science], the study of the specific physical and chemical processes involved in the normal functioning of humans; human physiology.

hominid /hom′inid/ [L, *homo,* man; Gk, *eidos,* form], pertaining to the primate family, *Hominidae,* which includes humans.

homiothermal. See **warm-blooded.**

homiothermic /hom′ē·əthur′mik/ [Gk, *homos,* same, *therme,* heat], pertaining to the ability of warm-blooded animals to maintain a relatively stable internal temperature regardless of the temperature of the environment. This ability is not fully developed in newborn humans.

homo-, 1. a prefix meaning 'the same': *homocentric, homodont, homolysis.* **2.** a prefix meaning 'the addition of one CH_2 group to the main compound': *homochelidonine, homocystine, homoquinine.*

homoblastic /hō′mōblas′tik/ [Gk, *homos + blastos,* germ], developing from the same germ layer or a single type of tissue. Compare **heteroblastic.**

homochronous inheritance /hōmok′rənəs/ [Gk, *homos + chronos,* time], the appearance of traits or conditions in the offspring at the same age as they appeared in the parents.

homocystinuria /hō′mōsis′tinŏōr′ē·ə/ [Gk, *homos +* (cystine); Gk, *ouron,* urine], a rare biochemical abnormality characterized by the abnormal presence of homocystine, an amino acid, in the blood and urine, caused by any of several enzyme deficiencies in the metabolic pathway of methionine to cystine. The disease is inherited as an autosomal recessive trait, the clinical signs of the disease are similar to Marfan's syndrome, including mental retardation, osteoporosis leading to skeletal abnormalities, dislocated lenses, and thromboembolism. Treatment may include a diet low in methionine and supplementation with large doses of vitamin B_6. Long-term results of treatment are not available. **–homocystinuric,** *adj.*

homoeo-. See **homeo-.**

homogenate /hōmoj′ənit/, a tissue that is or has been made homogenous, as by grinding cells into a creamy consistency for laboratory studies. A homogenate usually lacks cell structure. Also called **broken cell preparation.**

homogeneous /hōmoj′ənəs/ [Gk, *homos + genos,* kind], **1.** consisting of similar elements or parts. **2.** having a uniform quality throughout. Compare **heterogeneous. –homogeneity,** *adj.*

homogenesis /hō′mōjen′əsis/ [Gk, *homos + genesis,* origin], reproduction by the same process in succeeding generations so that offspring are similar to the parents. Compare **heterogenesis.**

homogenetic /-jenet′ik/, **1.** of or pertaining to homogenesis. **2.** homogenous, def. 2.

homogenized /hōmoj′ənīzd/ [Gk, *homos,* same, *genein,* to produce], the state of having undergone homogenization, made the same texture or consistency throughout.

homogenized milk [Gk, *homos + genos,* kind], pasteurized milk that has been mechanically treated to reduce and emulsify the fat globules so that the cream cannot separate and the protein is more digestible.

homogenous /hōmoj′ənəs/ [Gk, *homos + genos,* kind], **1.** homogeneous. **2.** having a likeness in form or structure because of a common ancestral origin. Compare **heterogenous. 3.** homoplasty.

homogenous graft. See **homologous graft.**

homogentisic acid. See **glycosuric acid.**

homogeny /hōmoj′ənē/ [Gk, *homos + genos,* kind],

1. homogenesis. **2.** a likeness in structure or form because of a common ancestral origin. Compare **homoplasty.**

homograft. See **allograft.**

homoio-. See **homeo-.**

homiothermal. See **warm-blooded.**

homolateral /hō′mōlat′ərəl/, pertaining to the same side of the body.

homolateral limb synkinesis, a condition of hemiplegia in which there appears to be a mutual dependency between the affected upper and lower limbs. Efforts at flexion of an upper extremity cause flexion of the lower extremity.

homolog /hom′əlog/ [Gk, *homos*, same], **1.** any organ corresponding in function, origin, and structure to another organ, as the flippers of a seal that correspond to human hands. **2.** (in chemistry) one of a series of compounds, each formed by an added common element; for example, CO, carbon monoxide, is followed by CO_2, carbon dioxide, with the addition of an oxygen atom. Also spelled **homologue.** Compare **analog.** **–homologous,** *adj.*

homologous. See **hemagglutinin.**

homologous anaphylaxis /hōmol′əgəs/ [Gk, *homos*, same, *logos*, relation, *ana*, back, *phylaxis*, protection], a form of passive anaphylaxis in which serum from an animal of the same species is transferred.

homologous chromosomes [Gk, *homos*, same; *chroma* color, *soma* body], any two chromosomes in the diploid complement of the somatic cell that are identical in size, shape, and gene loci. In humans there are 22 pairs of homologous chromosomes and one pair of sex chromosomes, with one member of each pair being derived from the mother and the other from the father. Any deviation in the size, number, or genetic makeup of the chromosomes results in defects or disorders of varying severity in the affected individual.

homologous disease. See **graft-versus-host reaction.**

homologous graft [Gk, *homos*, same, *logos*, relation, *graphein*, stylus], a tissue removed from a donor for transplanting to a recipient of the same species. Also called **homogenous graft.**

homologous insemination. See **artificial insemination-husband.**

homologous organs, [Gk, *homos*, same, *logos*, relation, *organon*, instrument], body parts of different species that are structural equivalents, such as the arms of humans and the forelegs of dogs and cats.

homologous transplantation. See **homoplastic transplantation.**

homologous tumor, a neoplasm made up of cells resembling those of the tissue in which it is growing.

homologue. See **homolog.**

homonymous /hōmon′iməs/ [Gk, *homos*, same, *onyma*, name], having the same name or sound.

homonymous diplopia [Gk, *homos*, same, *onyma*, name, *diploos*, double, *opsis*, vision], a type of diplopia in which the image seen by the right eye is to the right of the image seen by the left eye.

homonymous hemianopia [Gk, *homos* + *onyma*, name], blindness or defective vision in the right or left halves of the visual fields of both eyes.

homophobia /hō′mōfō′bē·ə/ [Gk, *homos*, same, *phobos*, fear], the fear of or prejudice against homosexuals.

-homoplastic. See **homoplastic.**

homoplastic transplantation [Gk, *homos*, same, *plassein*, to mold; L, *transplantare*, to transplant], the homologous transplantation of tissue from one human to another or from one animal to another of the same species. Also called **homologous transplantation.**

homoplasty /hō′məplas′tē/ [Gk, *homos* + *plassein*, to mold], having a likeness in form or structure acquired through similar environmental conditions or parallel evolution rather than because of common ancestral origin. Compare **homogeny.** **–homoplastic,** *adj.*

homopolymer /hō′mōpol′imir/ [Gk, *homos* + *poly*, many, *meros* part], a compound formed from subunits that are the same, such as a carbohydrate composed of a series of glucose units.

Homo sapiens /hō′mō sā′pē·əns, sä′pē·ens/ [L, *homo*, human, *sapere*, to know or taste], the scientific term for the genus and species identifying humans.

homosexual /-sek′shəl/ [Gk, *homos* + L, *sexus*, sex, gender], **1.** of, pertaining to, or denoting the same sex. **2.** a person who is sexually attracted to members of the same sex. Compare **heterosexual.** See also **lesbian.**

homosexual panic, an acute attack of anxiety based on unconscious conflicts concerning gender identity and a fear of being homosexual. Compare **heterosexual panic.**

homosexual sexual intercourse [Gk, *homos*, same; L, *sexus*, male or female, *intercursus*, interposition], sexual activity between members of the same sex ranging from feelings and fantasies to kissing and genital, oral, or anal contact.

homothermal. See **warm-blooded.**

homovanillic acid /hō′mōvənil′ik/, an acid that is produced by normal metabolism of dopamine and may be elevated in the urine in association with tumors of the adrenal gland. Its normal accumulation in a 24-hour collection urine sample is 15 mg.

homozygosis /hō′mōzīgō′sis/ [Gk, *homos* + *zygon*, yoke], **1.** the formation of a zygote by the union of two gametes that have one or more pairs of identical genes. **2.** the production of purebred organisms or strains through the process of inbreeding.

homozygote /hō′məzī′gōt/ [Gk, *homos*, same, *zygon*, yoke], an organism whose somatic cells have identical genes on the same locus on one of the chromosome pairs.

homozygous /hō′məzī′gəs/ [Gk, *homos* + *zygon*, yoke], having two identical genes at corresponding loci on homologous chromosomes. An individual who is homozygous for a particular characteristic has inherited from each parent one of two identical genes for that characteristic. A person homozygous for a genetic disease caused by a pair of recessive genes, such as sickle cell anemia, manifests the disorder, and his or her offspring have a 100% chance of inheriting the gene for the disease. Compare **heterozygous.**

homunculus /hōmung′kyələs/, *pl.* **homunculi** [L, little man], **1.** a dwarf in whom all the body parts are proportionally developed and in which there is no deformity or abnormality. **2.** (in early embryologic theories of development, primarily preformation) a minute and complete human being contained in each of the germ cells that after fertilization grows from the microscopic to normal size; by extension, the human fetus. **3.** a small anatomic model of the human form; a manikin, specifically, one believed to have been produced by an alchemist and placed in a flask. **4.** (in psychiatry) a little man created by the imagination who possesses magical powers.

hook grasp, a type of prehension in which an object is

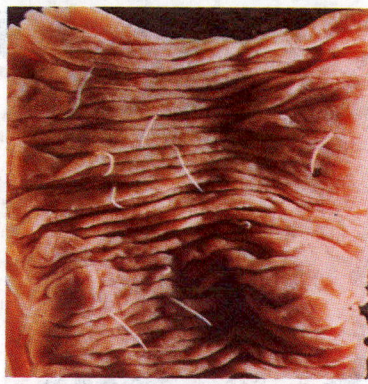

Hookworm infection (Peters, 1989)

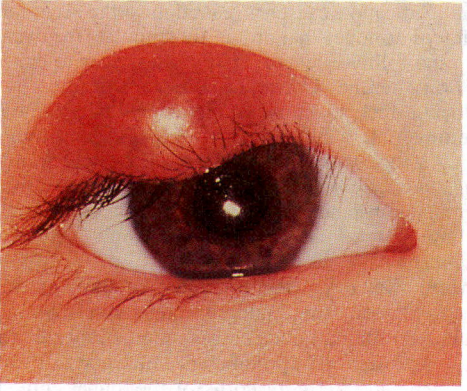

Hordeolum (Zitelli, 1992)

grasped with the fingers alone, excluding use of the thumb and palm.

hookworm [AS, *hok, wyrm*], *nontechnical*. a nematode of the genera *Ancylostoma, Necator,* or *Uncinaria.* Most hookworm infections in the Western Hemisphere are caused by the species *Necator americanus.*

hookworm disease [AS, *hok, wyrm*; Gk, *dis,* not; Fr, *aise,* ease], a roundworm infestation that may involve either of two serious intestinal parasites of humans, *Ancylostoma duodenale* or *Necator americanus.* Both forms of the disease are characterized by abdominal pain and iron-deficiency anemia. The worms enter the human body as larvae by penetrating the skin, traveling to the lungs via the circulatory system, and ascending the respiratory tract, where they are swallowed. In the intestinal tract, the hookworms attach their mouths to the mucosa and subsist on the blood of the host.

hopelessness [AS, *hopian,* to hope, *laes,* less, *ness,* condition], a nursing diagnosis accepted by the Seventh National Conference on the Classification of Nursing Diagnoses. Hopelessness describes a state in which an individual sees limited or no alternatives or personal choices available and is unable to mobilize energy on his or her own behalf. The defining characteristics include passivity, decreased verbalization, decreased affect, lack of initiative, decreased response to stimuli, turning away from the speaker, shrugging in response to the speaker, closing eyes, decreased appetite, increased or decreased sleep, and a lack of involvement in care. Related factors include prolonged activity restriction, failing or deteriorating physiological condition, long-term stress, abandonment, and a loss of belief in trascendent values. See also **nursing diagnosis.**

hordeolum /hôrdē′ələm/ [L, *hordeum,* barley], a furuncle of the margin of the eyelid originating in the sebaceous gland of an eyelash. Treatment includes hot compresses and antibiotic ophthalmic preparations; it occasionally requires incision and drainage. Also called **sty.** Compare **chalazion.**

horizon /hôri′zən/ [Gk, *horizein,* to encircle], a specific stage of human embryonic development based on the appearance and ultimate formation of certain anatomic characteristics. The classification comprises 23 stages, each lasting 2 to 3 days, beginning with the fertilization of the ovum and ending 7 to 9 weeks later with the initiation of the fetal period of intrauterine life.

horizontal angulation /hor′izon′təl/ [Gk, *horizein,* to en-

circle; L, *angularis,* angle], (in dentistry) the measured angle within the occlusal plane at which the primary x-ray beam is directed, relative to a reference in the vertical or sagittal plane. Compare **vertical angulation.**

horizontal fissure of the right lung, a cleft that marks the separation of the upper and middle lobes of the right lung.

horizontal plane [Gk, *horizein,* to encircle; L, *planum,* level ground], **1.** any plane of the erect body parallel to the horizon, dividing the body into upper and lower parts. **2.** a plane passing through a tooth at right angles to its long axis.

horizontal pursuit, a visual screening test in which the patient is asked to follow with both eyes a target moving in a horizontal plane while the examiner observes accuracy of alignment, supportive head movements, and other factors.

horizontal resorption, a pattern of bone reduction in marginal periodontitis whereby the marginal crest of the alveolar bone between adjacent teeth remains level and the bases of the periodontal pockets are supracrestal. Compare **vertical resorption.** See also **resorption.**

horizontal transmission, the spread of an infectious agent from one person or group to another, usually through contact with contaminated material, such as sputum or feces.

horm-, a prefix meaning 'an impulse, to urge or stimulate': *hormesis, hormonal, hormothyrin.*

hormic psychology /hôr′mic/ [Gk, *hormaien,* to begin action], (in psychology) the school that stresses the purposive, goal-oriented nature of human behavior. Also called **hormism.**

hormonal /hôr′mōnəl/ [Gk, *hormaein,* to set in motion], pertaining to or resembling hormones.

hormone /hôr′mōn/ [Gk, *hormaien,* to begin action], a complex chemical substance produced in one part or organ of the body that initiates or regulates the activity of an organ or a group of cells in another part of the body. Hormones secreted by the endocrine glands are carried through the bloodstream to the target organ. Secretion of these hormones is regulated by other hormones, by neurotransmitters, and by a negative-feedback system in which an excess of target organ activity signals a decreased need for the stimulating hormone. This principal is integral to oral contraceptive pills. A steady supply of estrogen and progesterone in the medication causes a reduction in the secretion of the pituitary hormones that ordinarily stimulate the ovary to develop the follicle, release the egg, and secrete the estrogen and progesterone. Other hormones are released by organs for local effect, most commonly in the digestive tract.

-hormone, **1.** a suffix meaning a 'chemical substance possessing a regulatory effect' classified by source: *necrohormone, phytohormone, zoohormone.* **2.** a suffix meaning a 'chemical substance possessing a regulatory effect' classified by activity affected: *cytohormone, neurohormone, parathormone.*

hormone therapy, the treatment of diseases with hormones obtained from endocrine glands or substances that simulate hormonal effects. Also called **endocrine therapy.**

horn, a projection or protuberance on a body structure. Examples include the gray horns of the spinal cord, horn of the hyoid bone, and iliac horn.

Horner's syndrome [Johann F. Horner, Swiss ophthalmologist, b. 1831], a neurologic condition characterized by miotic pupils, ptosis, and facial anhidrosis, resulting from a lesion in the spinal cord, with damage to a cervical nerve. In the case of traumatic injury, the person is carried prone or supine with as little movement as possible.

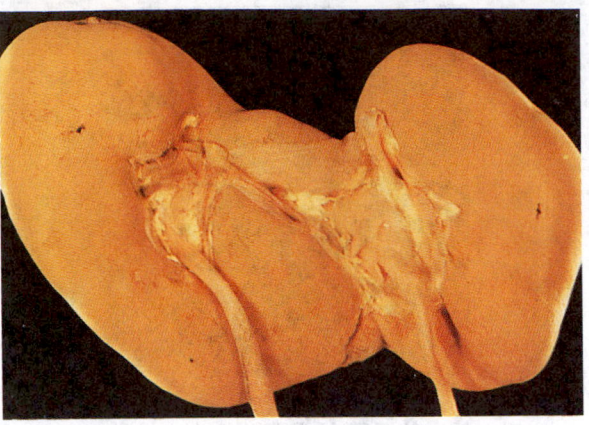

Horseshoe kidney (Fletcher, 1987)

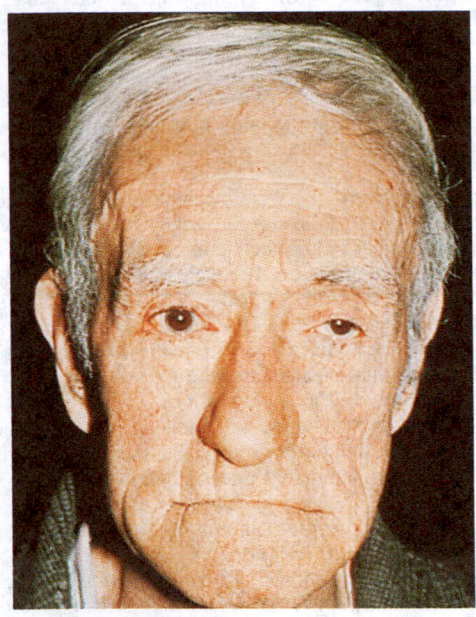

Horner's syndrome (Kamal, 1991)

horny layer. See **stratum corneum.**
horripilation. See **pilomotor reflex.**
horse serum [AS, *hors;* L, *serum,* whey], immune serum prepared from the blood of a horse, especially tetanus antitoxin. Because many people are sensitive to horse serum, a skin test for sensitivity is usually performed before immunization. Tetanus immune globulin prepared from human immune serum is preferred.
horseshoe fistula /hôrs′shoo/ [AS, *hors, scoh,* shoe], an abnormal, semicircular passage in the perianal area with both openings on the surface of the skin.

horseshoe kidney, a relatively common congenital anomaly characterized by an isthmus of parenchymal tissue connecting the two kidneys at the lower poles. The condition may result in obstruction of the ureters, hydronephrosis, and abdominal pain. The condition is corrected by surgery to separate and reposition the kidneys.
Hortega cells. See **microglia.**
Horton's arteritis. See **temporal arteritis.**
Horton's headache. See **migrainous cranial neuralgia.**
Horton's histamine cephalalgia. See **histamine headache.**
hospice /hos′pis/ [L, *hospes,* host], a system of family-centered care designed to assist the chronically ill person to be comfortable and to maintain a satisfactory lifestyle through the terminal phases of dying. Hospice care is multidisciplinary and includes home visits, professional health care available on call, teaching and emotional support of the family, and physical care of the client. Some hospice programs provide care in a center, as well as in the home. See also **emotional care of the dying patient, stages of dying.**
hospital /hos′pitəl/ [L, *hospitium,* guesthouse], a health-care facility that provides inpatient beds, continuous nursing services, and an organized medical staff. Diagnosis and treatment are provided to both surgical and medical patients for a variety of diseases and disorders.
hospital-acquired infection. See **nosocomial infection.**
hospitalism /hos′pitəliz′əm/, the physical or mental effects of hospitalization or institutionalization on patients, especially infants and children in whom the condition is characterized by social regression, personality disorders, and stunted growth. See also **anaclitic depression.**
Hospital Survey and Construction Act. See **Hill-Burton Act.**
host /hōst/ [L, *hospes*], **1.** an organism in which another, usually parasitic, organism is nourished and harbored. A **primary** or **definitive host** is one in which the adult parasite lives and reproduces. A **secondary,** or **intermediate host** is one in which the parasite exists in its nonsexual, larval stage. A **reservoir host** is a primary animal host for organisms that are sometimes parasitic in humans and from which humans may become infected. **2.** the recipient of a transplanted organ or tissue. Compare **donor.**

host defense mechanisms, a group of body protective systems, including physical barriers and the immune response, that normally guard against infective organisms.

hostility /hostil'itē/ [L, *hostilis*, hostile], the tendency of an organism to threaten harm to another or to itself. The hostility may be expressed passively and actively.

hot bath [AS, *hat, baeth*], a bath in which the temperature of the water is gradually raised to about 106° F.

hot compress [AS, *hat*; L, *comprimere*, to press together], a heated pad of damp, thickly folded cloth applied to an area to reduce pain or inflammation. See also **fomentation.**

hot flash, a transient sensation of warmth experienced by some women during or after menopause. Hot flashes result from autonomic vasomotor disturbances that accompany changes in the neurohormonal activity of the ovaries, hypothalamus, and pituitary. The exact causative mechanism is not known. Most menopausal women do not experience hot flashes; among those who do, the frequency, duration, and intensity of flashes vary widely. Although physically harmless, the symptom may be extremely disturbing or, rarely, disabling. Hot flashes may be alleviated by cyclic administration of exogenous estrogen. Also called **hot flush.** See **menopause.**

hot line, a means of contacting a trained counselor or specific agency for help with a particular problem, such as a rape hot line or a battered child hot line. The person needing help calls a telephone number and speaks to a counselor who remains anonymous and who offers emotional support, specific recommendations for action, and referral to other medical, social, or community services. Such services are usually maintained by volunteers who answer telephones 24 hours a day, 7 days a week.

hot spot, **1.** (in molecular genetics) a site in a gene sequence at which mutations occur with an unusually high frequency. **2.** (in nuclear medicine) an area on a nuclear medicine image that has an abnormally high amount of detected radiation as the result of increased absorption of radionuclide.

Hounsfield unit /hounz'fēld/, (in computed tomography) the numeric information contained in each pixel. It has a relationship to the composition and nature of the tissue imaged and is used to represent the density of tissue. Also called **CT number, Hounsfield number.**

hour glass uterus [Gk, *hora*; AS, *glaes*;], a uterus in which a segment of circular muscle fibers contracts during labor, causing constriction ring dystocia. The condition is marked by lack of progress despite adequate labor contractions and recession of the presenting part during a contraction rather than descent of the presenting part.

housekeeping department, a unit of a hospital staff responsible for cleaning the hospital premises and furnishings, including control of pathogenic organisms.

housemaid's knee [AS, *hus, maeden; cneow*, knee], a chronic inflammation of the bursa in front of the kneecap, characterized by redness and swelling. It is caused by prolonged and repetitive pressure of the knee on a hard surface.

house organ, a publication designed for distribution to the employees or members of an institution or business. A house organ may be prepared by a staff within the institution or business, or by an outside agency.

house physician [AS, *hus*; Gk, *physikos*, natural], a physician on call and immediately available in a hospital or other health care facility.

house staff, the interns and residents who are employed at a hospital while receiving additional training after graduation from medical college.

house surgeon, a surgeon on call and immediately available on the premises of a hospital.

housewives' eczema [AS, *hus, wif*; Gk, *ekzein*, to boil over], *nontechnical.* contact dermatitis of the hands caused and exacerbated by their frequent immersion in water and by the use of soaps and detergents.

Houston's valves. See **plicae transversales recti.**

Howell-Jolly bodies /hou'əljol'ē/, spheric and granular inclusions in the erythrocytes observed on microscopic examination of stained blood smears. They are most commonly seen in people who have hemolytic or pernicious anemia, leukemia, thalassemia, or congenital absence of the spleen and in those who have had a splenectomy.

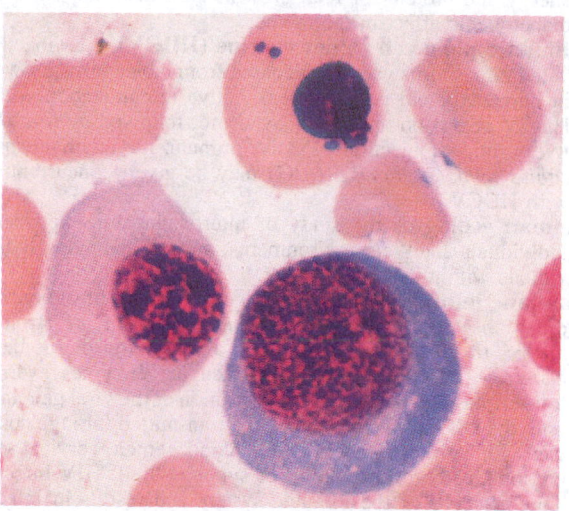

Howell-Jolly bodies *(Hayhoe, 1992)*

HPG, abbreviation for *human pituitary gonadotropin.*

HPL, abbreviation for **human placental lactogen.**

HPV, **1.** abbreviation for **human papilloma virus. 2.** abbreviation for **human parvovirus.**

hr, abbreviation for *hour.*

HRIG, abbreviation for *human rabies immune globulin* vaccine.

hs, h.s., abbreviation for the Latin *hora somni*, at bedtime.

HSA, abbreviation for **health systems agency.**

HSV, abbreviation for *herpes simplex virus*. See **herpes genitalis, herpes simplex.**

HSV1, abbreviation for *herpes simplex type 1*. See **herpes simplex.**

ht, abbreviation for **height.**

Hubbard tank [Carl P. Hubbard, American engineer, b. 1857; Port, *tanque,*], a tank containing warm water in which patients perform underwater exercise. The water provides buoyancy and heat for the benefit of weakened or painful muscles, or joints with limited active range of motion. See also **whirlpool bath.**

huffing, a type of forced expiration with an open glottis to replace coughing when pain limits normal coughing.

Huhner test /hōō′nər/, a test for male fertility in which a semen sample is examined for spermatozoa activity.

Huhn's gland, an anterior lingual gland imbedded in tissues on the inferior surface and near the apex and midline of the tongue.

human bite /h(y)ōō′mən/ [L, *humanus;* AS, *bitan*], a wound caused by the piercing of skin by human teeth. Bacteria are usually present, and serious infection often follows. The area is thoroughly washed, using an antiseptic, and rinsed well. The wound is examined frequently, and appropriate antibiotic therapy instituted, if necessary.

human chorionic gonadotropin. See **chorionic gonadotropin.**

human chorionic somatomammotropin (HCS), a hormone produced by the syncytiotrophoblast during pregnancy. It regulates carbohydrate and protein metabolism of the mother to ensure the delivery to the fetus of glucose for energy and protein for fetal growth. HCS also may have a diabetogenic effect in the mother.

human diploid cell rabies vaccine (HDCV), an inactivated rabies virus vaccine prepared from rabies virus grown in human diploid cell cultures. Active immunization with HDCV begins on the day of exposure, followed by four or five additional injections. Passive immunization with *human rabies immune globulin (RIG)* may be given concurrently with HDCV.

human ecology, the study of interrelationships between individuals and their environments, as well as among individuals within the environment.

human immunodeficiency virus (HIV) /im′yōōnō′difish′ənsē/ [L, *humanus, immunis,* free from, *de,* from, *facere,* to make, *virus,* poison], a type of retrovirus that causes AIDS. Retroviruses produce the enzyme reverse transcriptase, which allows transcription of the viral genome onto the DNA of the host cell. It is transmitted through contact with an infected individual's blood, semen, cervical secretions, cerebrospinal fluid, or synovial fluid. HIV infects T-helper cells of the immune system and results in infection with a long incubation perion, averaging 10 years. With the immune system destroyed, AIDS develops as opportunistic infections such as **Kaposi's sarcoma, pneumocystis carinii pneumonia, candidias,** and **tuberculosis,** that attack organ systems throughout the body. Aside from the initial antibody tests that establish the diagnosis for HIV infection, the most important laboratory test for monitoring the infection is the CD4 lymphocyte test. It determines the percentage of T lymphocytes that are CD4 positive; CD4

Signs and symptoms of HIV infection

Chills and fever	Malaise
Night sweats	Fatigue
Dry productive cough	Oral lesions
Dyspnea	Skin rashes
Lethargy	Abdominal discomfort
Confusion	Diarrhea
Stiff neck	Weight loss
Seizures	Lymphadenopathy
Headache	Progressive generalized edema

From Phipps WJ, Long BL, Woods NF, and Cassmeyer VL: *Medical-surgical nursing: concepts and clinical practice,* ed 4, St Louis, 1991, Mosby.

Spectrum of illness in HIV infection

Group	Category	Description
I	Acute infection	Mononucleosis-like "seroconversion" illness
		Meningitis symptoms
		HIV seropositivity signals infection has occurred
II	Asymptomatic infection	Apparently well
		Evidence of HIV infection is detectable in antibody tests
III	Persistent generalized lymphadenopathy (PGL)	≥1 cm at two or more extrainguinal sites
		Other symptoms may occur but lymphadenopathy predominates
		HIV infection detectable in antibody tests
IV	Other disease	HIV infection detectable
	Subgroup A	Constitutional disease or ARC: fever, weight loss, diarrhea
	Subgroup B	Neurologic disease, including AIDS dementia complex
	Subgroup C	Secondary infectious disease, including *Pneumocystis carinii* pneumonia (PCP)
	Subgroup D	Secondary cancers, including Kaposi's sarcoma (KS)
	Subgroup E	Other conditions

From Price SA, Wilson LM: *Pathophysiology: clinical concepts of disease processes,* ed 4, St Louis, 1992, Mosby.

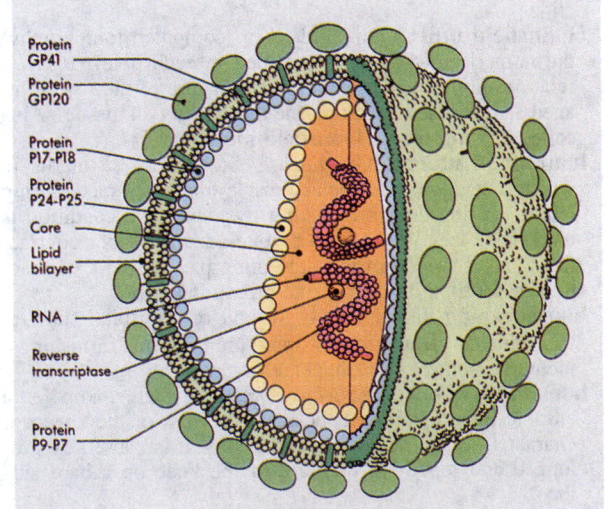

Cross-section of HIV
(Murray, 1990/Redrawn from Gallo RC and Montagnier L: Aci Am 259:41-51, 1988)

counts of greater than 500 per cubic mm are considered most likely to respond to treatment with alpha-interferon and/or zidovudine. A significant drop in the CD4 count is a signal for therapeutic intervention with antiretroviral therapy. Vaccines based on gp120 and gp160 HIV coat glycoproteins, to boost the immune system of people already infected with HIV, are being investigated. See also **acquired immuno-deficiency syndrome (AIDS).**

human insulin, a biosynthetic product manufactured from *Escherichia coli* using recombinant DNA technology. The advantages of human insulin are in eliminating allergic reactions that occur with the use of animal insulins, especially in patients who are noninsulin-dependent but who require insulin on a short-term basis. See also **insulin,** def.2.

human investigations committee, a committee established in a hospital, school, or university to review research proposals involving human subjects to protect the rights of the people to be studied. Also called **human subjects review committee.**

humanistic existential therapy /hyŏŏ'mənis'tik/, a kind of psychotherapy that promotes self-awareness and personal growth by stressing current reality and by analyzing and altering specific patterns of response to help realize the potential of a person. This process may be facilitated in a group setting, where additional aspects of problems are revealed through interaction with others. Kinds of humanistic existential psychotherapy are **client-oriented therapy, existential therapy, Gestalt therapy.** Also called **existential humanistic psychotherapy.**

humanistic nursing model, a conceptual framework in which the nurse-patient relationship is analyzed as a human-to-human event rather than a nurse-to-patient interaction. The nurse makes therapeutic use of herself or himself, understanding the effects of nursing actions. Four phases are recognized in the development of the therapeutic relationship. The encounter phase is followed by the phase in which the identities of the nurse and patient emerge. The nurse empathizes and then sympathizes with the patient. The meaning of the patient's experience is important; hope and suffering are seen as central to that experience. Self-knowledge and self-awareness on the part of the nurse are essential. Nursing intervention proceeds in five steps: observation of the need for intervention; validation of this observation; determination of the ability of the nurse to meet the necessity for referral; formulation of a plan for meeting the need; and evaluation of the degree to which the need was met.

humanistic psychology, a branch of psychology that emphasizes a person's struggle to develop and maintain an integrated, harmonious personality as the primary motivational force in human behavior. See also **self-actualization.**

human leukocyte antigen (HLA), any one of four significant genetic markers identified as specific loci on chromosome 6. They are HLA-A, HLA-B, HLA-C, and HLA-D. Each locus has several genetically determined alleles; each of these is associated with certain diseases or conditions; for example, HLA-B27 is usually present in people who have ankylosing spondylitis. The HLA system is used to assess tissue compatibility. White blood cells are used for testing. Perfect tissue compatibility exists only between identical twins.

human liver fluke   See **liver fluke.**

human natural killer cells, lymphocytes that are able to lyse tumor and virally infected cells as part of the body's

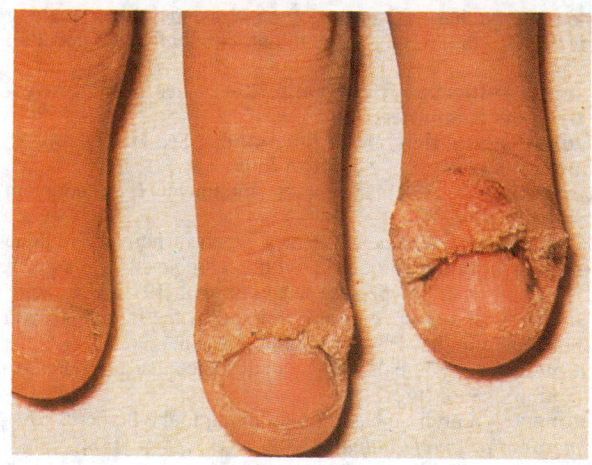

Warts caused by human papilloma virus
(Parkin, 1991)

natural defense against malignancy and invasion by pathogens.

human papilloma virus (HPV), a virus that is the cause of common warts of the hands and feet, as well as lesions of the mucous membranes of the oral, anal, and genital cavities. More than 50 types of HPV have been identified, some of which are associated with cancerous and precancerous conditions. The virus can be transmitted through sexual contact and is a precursor to cancer of the cervix. Transmission has occurred without the presence of warts, indicating that transmission may occur through body fluids, such as semen or cervical secretions. There is no specific cure for an HPV infection, but the virus often can be controlled by podophyllin or interferon and the warts can be removed by cryosurgery, laser treatment, or conventional surgery.

human parvovirus (HPV), a small, single-stranded DNA virion that has been associated with several diseases, including erythema infectiosum and aplastic crises of chronic hemolytic anemias. Parvoviruses of various types also infect wild and domestic animals and may replicate in susceptible cells without a helper virus. See also **helper virus, virion.**

human placental lactogen (HPL), a placental hormone that may be deficient in certain abnormalities of pregnancy. The normal concentrations of this hormone in serum after the fifth week of pregnancy are 0.5 mcg/ml and increase to approximately 8 mcg/ml at the time of delivery.

human prion diseases [L, *humanus, Proteinaceous Infection Particle,* Gk, *dis,* not; Fr, *aise,* ease], a group of neurodegenerative diseases that are unique in having both infectious and genetic causes. Examples include **Creutzfeldt-Jakob disease (CJD)** and **Gerstmann-Straussler syndrome.** A homozygous prion protein genotype predisposes in the diseases.

human protein C, an anticoagulant that inactivates coagulation cofactors 5 and 8c and mediates clot lysis by tissue plasminogen activator (t-PA).

human rhinovirus 14, the common cold virus. It has a complex protein coat containing "sticky sites" that help attach the virus to cell receptors in the upper respiratory system. More than 100 strains of the virus are known, making it difficult to devise a vaccine that would protect against all variations.

human subjects review committee. See **human investigations committee.**

human synthetic growth hormone. See **Humatrope.**

humanus capitus. See **head louse.**

Humatin, a trademark for an antiamebic (paromomycin sulfate).

Humatrope, a trademark for a brand of human synthetic growth hormone produced with recombinant DNA techniques. It is a polypeptide hormone with 191 amino acids in the same sequence as **somatotropin,** the human growth hormone produced by the pituitary gland.

humectant /hyoōmek'tənt/, a substance that promotes retention of moisture.

humer-, a prefix meaning 'pertaining to the humerus': *humeroradial, humeroulnar.*

humeral. See **humerus.**

humeral articulation. See **shoulder joint.**

humerus /hyoō'mərəs/, *pl.* **humeri** [L, shoulder], the bone of the upper arm, comprising a body, a head, and a condyle. The body is almost cylindric proximally and prismatic and flattened distally, and has two borders and three surfaces. The nearly hemispheric head articulates with the glenoid cavity of the scapula and has a constriction called the surgical neck, frequently the seat of a fracture. The condyle at the distal end has several depressions into which articulate the radius and ulna. Also called **arm bone.** −**humeral,** *adj.*

humidification /hyoōmid'ifikā'shən/ [L, *humiditas,* moist; *facere,* to make], the process of increasing the relative humidity of the atmosphere around a patient through the use of aerosol generators or steam inhalators that exert an antitussive effect. Humidification acts by decreasing the viscosity of bronchial secretions, whereas added medications or sodium chloride may stimulate coughing by an irritant effect.

humidifier /hyoōmid'ifi'ər/ [L, *humidus,* moist, *facere,* to make], a machine designed to adjust the amount of moisture in the atmosphere of a room or respiratory device.

humidity /hyoōmid'itē/ [L, *humidus,* moist], pertaining to the level of moisture in the atmosphere, the amount varying with the temperature. The percentage is usually represented in terms of **relative humidity,** with 100 percent being the point of air saturation or the level at which the air can absorb no additional water.

humor /hyoō'mər/ [L, *humidus,* moist], any body fluid such as blood or lymph. The term is often used in referring to the **aqueous humor** or the **vitreous humor** of the eye.

humoral immunity /hyoō'mərəl/ [L, *humor,* liquid; *immunis,* freedom], one of the two forms of immunity that respond to antigens such as bacteria and foreign tissue. Humoral immunity is the result of the development and the continuing presence of circulating antibodies carried in the immunoglobulins IgA, IgB, and IgM. Circulating antibodies are produced by the plasma cells of the reticuloendothelial system. Compare **cellular immunity.**

humoral response, one of a broad category of hypersensitivity reactions. Humoral responses are mediated by B cell lymphocytes and occur in type I, type II, and type III hypersensitivity reactions. Compare **cell-mediated immunity.**

Humorsol, a trademark for an ophthalmic anticholinesterase agent (demecarium bromide).

Humulin, a trademark for a brand of human insulin of recombinant DNA origin.

hung-up reflex, a deep tendon reflex in which, after a stimulus is given and the reflex action takes place, there is a slow return of the limb to its neutral position. This prolonged relaxation phase is characteristic of the reflexes in persons with hypothyroidism. See also **deep tendon reflex.**

Hunner's ulcer. See **interstitial cystitis.**

Hunter's canal. See **adductor canal.**

Hunter's syndrome [Charles Hunter, twentieth century Canadian physician; Gk, *syn,* together, *dromos,* course], a hereditary defect in mucopolysaccharide metabolism affecting only males, characterized by dwarfism, kyphosis, gargoylism, and mental retardation. It is transmitted as an X-linked recessive trait. Females who carry the gene can be identified by biochemical tests, and known carriers may choose to abort if amniocentesis reveals a male fetus, because males born of women who carry the trait have a 50% chance of having the syndrome. Also called **MPS II.** See also **mucopolysaccharidosis.**

Huntington's chorea [George S. Huntington, American physician, b. 1851; Gk, *choreia,* dance], a rare, abnormal hereditary condition characterized by chronic, progressive chorea and mental deterioration that terminates in dementia. An individual afflicted with the condition usually shows the first signs in the fourth decade of life and dies usually within 15 years. The condition is transmitted as an autosomal trait. There is no known effective treatment but symptoms can be relieved with medications.

Hunt's tremor. See **cerebellar tremor.**

Hurler's syndrome [Gertrude Hurler, German physician, b. 1920], a type of mucopolysaccharidosis, transmitted as an autosomal-recessive trait, that results in severe mental retardation. The onset of the symptoms of Hurler's syndrome occurs within the first few months of life. Characteristic signs of the disease are enlargement of the liver and

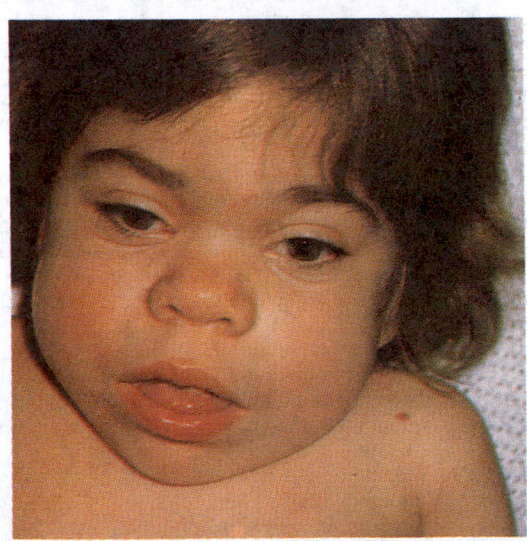

Hurler's syndrome *(Ansell, 1992)*

the spleen, often with cardiovascular involvement. Facial characteristics of individuals affected by Hurler's syndrome include a low forehead and enlargement of the head, sometimes resulting from hydrocephalus. Corneal clouding is common, and the neck is short. Marked kyphosis is apparent at the dorsolumbar level, and the hands and the fingers are short and broad. Flexion contractures are common with this disease. Hurler's syndrome usually results in death during childhood from cardiac complications or pulmonary disorders. Also called **gargoylism, MPS I.** See also **mucopolysaccharidosis.**

Hürthle cell adenoma /hirt′lə, hōorth′lē/ [Karl W. Hürthle, German histologist, b. 1860], a benign tumor of the thyroid gland composed of large cells with granular eosinophilic cytoplasm (Hürthle cells). Compare **Hürthle cell carcinoma.**

Hürthle cell carcinoma, a malignant neoplasm of the thyroid gland composed of Hürthle cells. These tumors, which occur more often in women than in men, are encapsulated, resemble adenomas, and are locally invasive. See also **Hürthle cell adenoma.**

Hürthle cell tumor, a neoplasm of the thyroid gland composed of large cells with granular eosinophilic cytoplasm (Hürthle cells); it may be benign (Hürthle cell adenoma) or malignant (Hürthle cell carcinoma).

husband-coached childbirth. See **Bradley method.**

Hutchinson's disease. See **angioma serpiginosum.**

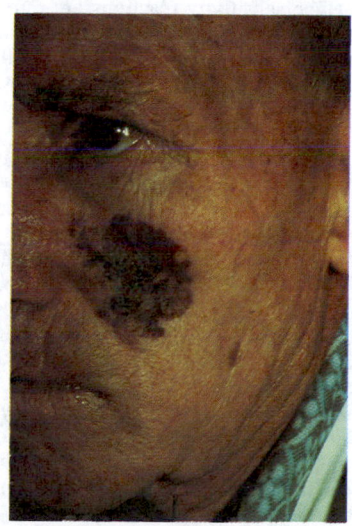

Hutchinson's freckle *(Belcher, 1992)*

Hutchinson's freckle [Sir Jonathan Hutchinson, English surgeon, b. 1828], a tan patch on the skin that grows slowly and becomes mottled, dark, thick, and nodular. The lesion is usually seen on one side of the face of an elderly person. Local excision is recommended because it often becomes malignant. Also called **lentigo maligna.** See also **melanoma.**

Hutchinson's teeth [Sir Jonathan Hutchinson, English physician, b. 1828], a characteristic of congenital syphilis in which the permanent lateral incisor teeth are peg-shaped,

widely spaced, and notched at the end with a centrally placed crescent-shaped deformity. See also **syphilis.**

Hutchinson's triad [Sir Jonathan Hutchinson], the interstitial keratitis, notched teeth, and deafness characteristic of congenital syphilis. See also **syphilis.**

Hutchison-type neuroblastoma [Sir Robert G. Hutchison, English physician, b. 1871; Gk *typos* mark], a neuroblastoma that has metastasized to the cranium.

HVA, abbreviation for **homovanillic acid.**

HV interval /in′tərvəl/, (in cardiology) the conduction time through the His-Purkinje system, measured from the onset of the His potential to the onset of ventricular activation as recorded on an electrogram.

hyal-. See **hyalo-.**

hyaline /hī′əlin/ [Gk, *hyalos,* glass], pertaining to substances that are clear or glasslike.

hyaline bodies [Gk, *hyalos;* AS, *bodig*], **1.** the residue of colloidal degeneration found in some cells. **2.** globules of neurosecretory material found in the posterior lobe of the pituitary. **3.** deposits of homogenous eosinophilic material found in renal tubular epithelium and representing excess protein molecules that cannot be metabolized or transported.

hyaline cartilage [Gk, *hyalos,* glass; L, *cartilago*], a type of elastic connective tissue composed of specialized cells in a translucent, pearly-blue matrix. Hyaline cartilage thinly covers the articulating ends of bones, connects the ribs to the sternum, and supports the nose, the trachea, and part of the larynx. It is covered by a membranous perichondrium, except where it coats the ends of bones, and tends to calcify in advanced age. Compare **yellow cartilage, white fibrocartilage.**

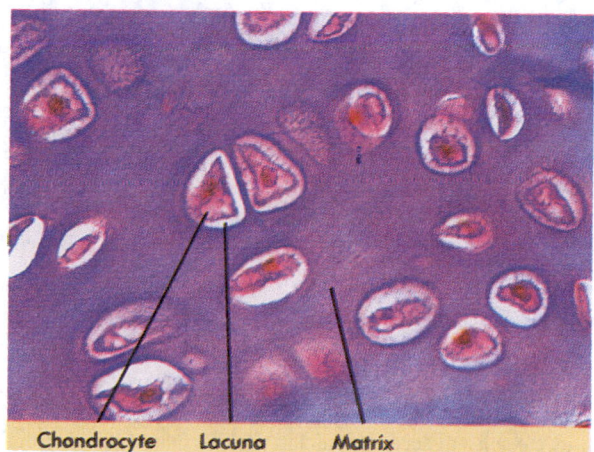

Chondrocyte   Lacuna   Matrix

Hyaline cartilage *(Seeley, 1992/Ed Reschke)*

hyaline cast, a transparent cast composed of mucoprotein.

hyaline membrane [Gk, *hyalos,* glass; L, *membrana*], a fibrous covering of acinar epithelium in premature infants caused by a lack of pulmonary surfactant associated with prematurity and low-birth-weight delivery. Hyaline membrane disease **(HMD)** or ideopathic respiratory distress syndrome **(IRDS)** is associated with cesarean section delivery, maternal diabetes, maternal hemorrhage, and asphyxia at birth.

hyaline membrane disease. See **respiratory distress syndrome of the newborn.**

hyaline thrombus, a translucent, colorless mass consisting of hemolyzed erythrocytes.

hyalinization /hī´əlin´īzā´shən/ [Gk, *hyalos*, glass], the development of glassy homogenous material within a cell.

hyalinuria /-ŏŏr´ē-ə/ [Gk, *hyalos*, glass, *ouron*, urine], the presence of hyaline casts of protein in the acid pH of urine.

hyalo-, hyal-, a prefix meaning 'resembling glass': *hyaloenchondroma, hyaloplasm, hyaloid.*

hyaloid /hī´əloid/ [Gk, *hyalos*, glass, *eidos*, form], pertaining to or resembling hyaline.

hyaloid artery [Gk, *hyalos* + *eidos*, form], an embryonic blood vessel that branches to supply the vitreous body of the eye and develops part of the blood supply to the capsula vasculosa lentis. The hyaloid artery disappears from the fetus in the ninth month of pregnancy, leaving a vestigial remnant, the hyaloid canal, which persists in the adult as a narrow passage through the vitreous body from the optic disc to the posterior surface of the crystalline lens.

hyaloid membrane [Gk, *hyalos*, glass; L, *membrana*], a surface layer of the vitreous body of the eye, at the interface between the primary and secondary vitreous and at the boundaries of the hyaloid canal.

hyaloplasm /hī´əlōplaz´əm/ [Gk, *hyalos* + *plasma*, formation], the portion of the cytoplasm that is clear and more fluid, as opposed to the granular and reticular part. Also called **cytohyaloplasm, cytolymph, enchylema, hyalotome, interfilar mass, interfibrillar mass of Flemming, paramitome, paraplasm.**

hyaluronic acid /hī´əlyŏŏron´ik/, a mucopolysaccharide formed by the polymerization of acetylglucosamine and glucuronic acid, occurring in vitreous humor, synovial fluids, and various tissues. Known as the cement substance of tissues, it forms a gel in intercellular spaces.

hyaluronidase /hī´əlyŏŏron´ədās/, an enzyme that hydrolyzes hyaluronic acid.
■ INDICATIONS: It is prescribed to increase the absorption and dispersion of other parenteral drugs, for hypodermoclysis, and for improving resorption of radiopaque agents.
■ CONTRAINDICATIONS: Acute inflammation, infection, or known hypersensitivity to this drug prohibits its use.
■ ADVERSE EFFECTS: The most serious adverse reaction is hypersensitivity.

hybrid /hī´brid/ [L, *hybrida*, offspring], **1.** an offspring produced from mating plants or animals from different species, varieties, or genotypes. **2.** of or pertaining to such a plant or animal.

hybrid computer, a computer that combines the characteristics of a digital computer and an analog computer by its capacity to accept input and provide output in either digital or analog form and to process information digitally. Compare **analog computer, digital computer.**

hybridization /hī´bridīzā´shən/, **1.** the process of producing hybrids by crossbreeding. **2.** (in molecular genetics) the process of combining single-stranded nucleic acids whose base composition is identical but whose base sequence is different to form stable double-stranded duplex molecules. The technique involves the fragmentation and separation of the double-stranded molecules by heating, then recombination through cooling. The resulting hybrids can be of a DNA-DNA, DNA-RNA, or RNA-RNA nature.

hybridoma /hī´bridō´mə/, a hybrid cell formed by the fusion of a myeloma cell and an antibody-producing cell. Hy-

bridomas are used in the production of monoclonal antibodies.

hybrid subtraction, a two-step subtraction method for producing digitalized x-ray images that uses at least four images. Both energy and temporal subtraction steps are used to mitigate patient motion artifacts.

hybrid vigor. See **heterosis.**

Hycodan, a trademark for a fixed-combination drug containing an anticholinergic (homatropine methylbromide) and an antitussive (hydrocodone bitartrate), used for cough relief.

Hycomine, a trademark for a fixed-combination drug containing an adrenergic (phenylpropanolamine hydrochloride) and an antitussive (hydrocodone bitartrate), used to treat coughs.

hydantoin /hīdan´tō·in/, any one of a group of anticonvulsant medications, chemically and pharmacologically similar to the barbiturates, that act to limit seizure activity and reduce the spread of the abnormal electric excitation from the focus of the seizure. A primary drug in the management of almost all forms of epilepsy, the most common hydantoin in current use is phenytoin, formerly known as diphenylhydantoin. Toxic effects of the drug include cardiovascular collapse and central nervous system depression when it is given in excessive dosage intravenously, as may occur in the emergency treatment of status epilepticus. Chronic toxicity, which is related to the dosage and the route of administration, may result in behavioral change, GI disturbance, osteomalacia, gingival hyperplasia, or megaloblastic anemia. Hypersensitivity reactions are rare but serious. Frequent observation for the blood concentrations of hydantoin are necessary. Seizures are usually controlled at a level of 10 [mu]g/ml; higher levels are associated with toxic effects. Phenytoin interacts with many drugs, including chloramphenicol, dicumarol, disulfiram, isoniazid, salicylates, phenylbutazone, antihistamines, and some sulfonamides. The interaction usually has the adverse effect of increasing the concentration of phenytoin in the blood, resulting in toxicity. Phenytoin is sometimes also prescribed in the treatment of trigeminal neuralgia and cardiac dysrhythmias.

hydatid /hī´dətid/ [Gk, *hydatis*, water drop], a cyst or cystlike structure that usually is filled with fluid, especially the cyst formed around the developing scolex of the dog tapeworm *Echinococcus granulosus.* Humans and sheep can become hosts to the larval stage by ingesting the eggs. Hydatid cysts may be identified by palpation; they occur most commonly in the liver. An acute anaphylactoid allergic reaction may occur if the cyst ruptures. See also **hydatid cyst, hydatid mole, hydatidosis.** **–hydatidiform,** *adj.*

hydatid cyst, a cyst in the liver that contains larvae of the tapeworm *Echinococcus granulosus,* whose eggs are carried from the intestinal tract to the liver via the portal circulation. Patients are generally asymptomatic, except for hepatomegaly and a dull ache over the right upper quadrant of the abdomen. Radiologic tests are employed in diagnosis, and because no medical treatment is available, surgical removal of the cyst is indicated. Compare **hydatid mole.**

hydatid disease. See **echinococcosis.**

-hydatidiform. See **hydatid.**

hydatid mole, an intrauterine neoplastic mass of grapelike enlarged chorionic villi occurring in approximately one in 1500 pregnancies in the United States and eight times more frequently in some oriental countries. Molar pregnancies are more common in older and younger women than in those

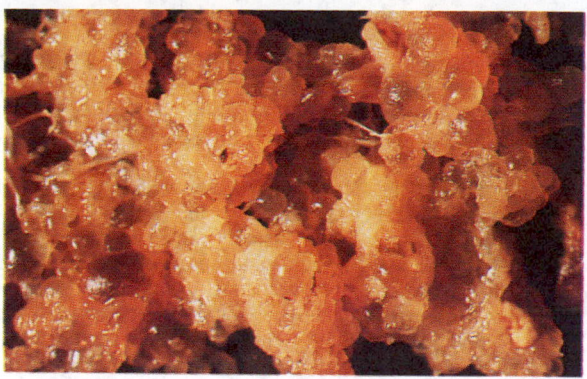

Hydatid mole *(Fletcher, 1987)*

between 20 and 40 years of age. The cause of the degenerative disorder is not known; it may be the result of a primary ovular defect, an intrauterine abnormality, or nutritional deficiency. Characteristic signs of the condition are extreme nausea, uterine bleeding, anemia, hyperthyroidism, an unusually large uterus for the duration of pregnancy, absence of fetal heart sounds, edema, and high blood pressure. Diagnostic measures include ultrasonography, amniography, and serial bioassay of chorionic gonadotropin in the blood. In most cases the mole is discovered when abortion is threatened or in progress. Oxytocin may be used to stimulate the evacuation of a mole that is not spontaneously aborted, and curettage is usually performed several days later to be certain that no molar tissue remains in the uterus. It is important that pregnancy be avoided for at least 1 year and that assays for chorionic gonadotropin be performed to minimize the risk of developing trophoblastic choriocarcinoma. Also called **hydatidiform mole.** See also **trophoblastic disease.**

hydatidosis /hī′dətidō′sis/ [Gk, *hydatis + osis*, condition], infestation with the tapeworm *Echinococcus granulosus.* See also **hydatid cyst.**

hydatiform /hīdat′ifôrm/ [Gk, *hydatis,* drop of water; L, *forma*], having the appearance or form of a **hydatid.** Also spelled **hydatidiform,** /hī′dətid′ifôrm/.

Hydeltrasol, a trademark for a glucocorticoid (prednisolone sodium phosphate).

Hydeltra TBA, a trademark for a glucocorticoid (prednisolone tebutate).

Hydergine, a trademark for a fixed-combination drug containing various ergoloid mesylates.

hydr-. See **hydro-.**

hydradenitis /hī′dradənī′tis/ [Gk, *hydos,* water, *aden,* gland, *itis* inflammation], an infection or inflammation of the sweat glands. Also spelled **hidradenitis.**

hydralazine /hīdral′əzēn/, an antihypertensive.
- INDICATION: It is prescribed in the treatment of hypertension.
- CONTRAINDICATIONS: Coronary artery disease, mitral valvular rheumatic heart disease, or known sensitivity to this drug prohibits its use.
- ADVERSE EFFECTS: Among the most serious adverse reactions are angina pectoris, palpitations, tachycardia, anorexia, tremors, blood dyscrasias, depression, nausea, and peripheral neuritis.

hydralazine hydrochloride, a vasodilator.
- INDICATION: It is prescribed in the treatment of high blood pressure.
- CONTRAINDICATIONS: Coronary artery disease, mitral valvular rheumatic heart disease, or known hypersensitivity to this drug prohibits its use.
- ADVERSE EFFECTS: Among the more serious adverse reactions are headache, anorexia, tachycardia, GI disturbances, and a syndrome resembling lupus erythematosus.

hydramnios /hīdram′nē·əs/ [Gk, *hydos + amnos,* lamb's caul], an abnormal condition of pregnancy characterized by an excess of amniotic fluid. It occurs in less than 1% of pregnancies and is diagnosed by palpation, ultrasound, or x-ray examination. It is associated with maternal disorders, including toxemia of pregnancy and diabetes mellitus. Some fetal disorders, including anomalies of the GI tract, respiratory tract, and cardiovascular system, may interfere with normal exchange of amniotic fluid, resulting in hydramnios. Fetal hydrops and multiple gestation are also associated with the condition. The incidence of premature rupture of the membranes, premature labor, and perinatal mortality are increased. Periodic amniocentesis may be necessary. Also called **hydramnion, polyhydramnios.** Compare **oligohydramnios.**

hydranencephaly /hī′dran′ənsef′əlē/, a neurologic disorder in which the cerebral hemispheres are lacking although the cerebellum, brainstem, and other central nervous system tissues may be normal. The newborn with hydranencephaly may show normal neurologic functions but fails to develop, and CT scans show absence of cerebral tissue.

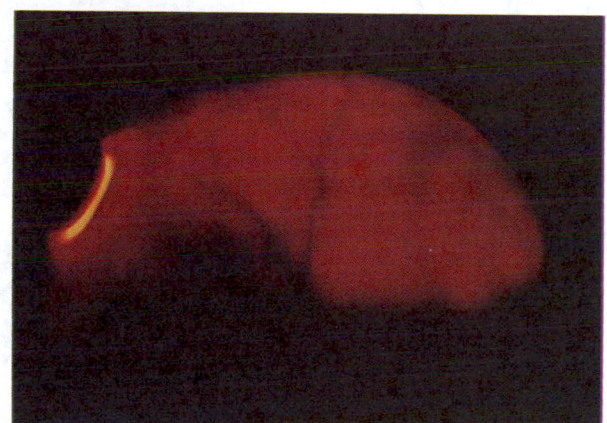

Hydranencephaly *(Zitelli, 1992)*

hydrargyrism. See **mercury poisoning.**

hydrate /hī′drāt/ [Gk, *hydor,* water], **1.** a combination of a substance with one or more water molecules. **2.** a molecular association of a substance with water.

hydration /hīdrā′shən/ [Gk, *hydor,* water], a chemical process in which water is taken up without disrupting the rest of the molecule.

Hydrea, a trademark for an antineoplastic (hydroxyurea).

hydremic ascites /hīdrem′ik/ [Gk, *hydor + haima,* blood; *askos,* bag], an abnormal accumulation of fluid within the peritoneal cavity accompanied by hemodilution, as in protein calorie malnutrition. See also **ascites.**

-hydria, a combining form meaning 'level of fluid in the body': *histohydria, isohydria, oligohydria.*

hydro-, hydr-, a prefix meaning 'pertaining to water or hydrogen': *hydroadipsia, hydrocele, hydropexis.*

hydroa /hīdrō′ə/ [Gk, *hydor + oon*, egg], an unusual vesicular and bullous skin condition of childhood that recurs each summer after exposure to sunlight, sometimes accompanied by itching and lichenification. Hydroa usually disappears soon after puberty. Treatment includes use of sunscreen preparations and the avoidance of exposure to sunlight.

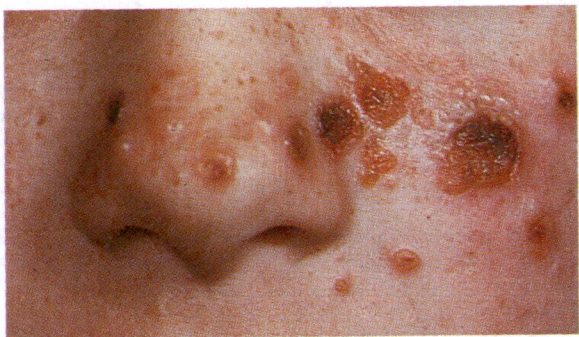

Hydroa vacciniforme *(du Vivier, 1993)*

hydrobilirubin /hī′drōbil′irōō′bin/ [Gk, *hydor,* water; L, *bilis,* bile, *ruber,* red], a reddish-brown bile pigment produced by the reduction of bilirubin.

hydrocarbon /-kär′bən/ [Gk, *hydor* + L, *carbo,* charcoal], any one of a large group of organic compounds, the molecules of which are composed of hydrogen and carbon, many of which are derived from petroleum.

hydrocele /hī′drōsēl′/ [Gk, *hydor + kele,* hernia], an accumulation of fluid in any saclike cavity or duct, specifically in the tunica vaginalis testis or along the spermatic cord. The condition is caused by inflammation of the epididymis or testis or by lymphatic or venous obstruction in the cord. Congenital hydrocele is caused by failure of the canal between the peritoneal cavity and the scrotum to close completely during prenatal development. In some newborn infants the defect may resolve spontaneously after neonatal obliteration of the communication. Treatment for persistent hydrocele is surgery. Aspiration is only a temporary measure and may induce secondary infection. See also **inguinal hernia.**

hydrocephalus /-sef′ələs/ [Gk, *hydor + kephale,* head], a pathologic condition characterized by an abnormal accumulation of cerebrospinal fluid, usually under increased pressure, within the cranial vault and subsequent dilatation of the ventricles. Interference with the normal flow of cerebrospinal fluid may be caused by increased secretion of the fluid, obstruction within the ventricular system (noncommunicating or intraventricular hydrocephalus), or defective reabsorption from the cerebral subarachnoid space (communicating or extraventricular hydrocephalus), resulting from developmental anomalies, infection, trauma, or brain tumors. Also called **hydrocephaly. —hydrocephalic,** /-səfal′ik/ *adj., n.*

■ OBSERVATIONS: The condition may be congenital with rapid onset of symptoms or it may progress slowly so that neurologic manifestations do not appear until early to late childhood or even until early adulthood. In infants, the head grows at an abnormal rate with separation of the sutures, bulging fontanelles, and dilated scalp veins; the face becomes disproportionately small, and the eyes appear depressed within the sockets. Typical behavior includes irritability with lethargy and vomiting, opisthotonos, lower extremity spasticity, and failure to perform normal reflex actions. If the condition progresses, lower brainstem function is disrupted, the skull becomes enormous, the cortex is destroyed, and the infant displays somnolence, seizures, and cardiopulmonary obstruction, usually not surviving the neonatal period. At later onset, after the cranial sutures have fused and the skull has formed, symptoms are primarily neurologic and include headache, edema of the optic disc, strabismus, and loss of muscular coordination. Hydrocephalus in infants is suspected when head growth is observed to be in excess of the normal rate. In all age groups diagnosis is confirmed by such procedures as cerebrospinal fluid examination, computed tomography, air encephalography, arteriography, and echoencephalography.

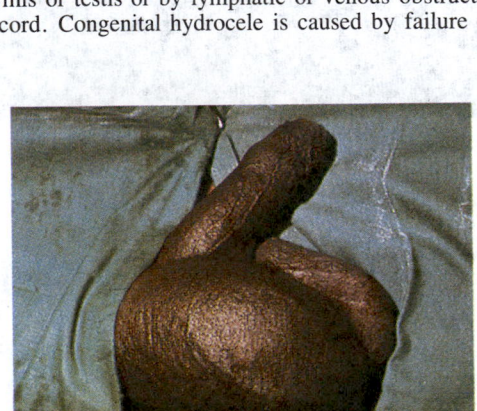

Hydrocele *(Lloyd-Davies, 1984)*

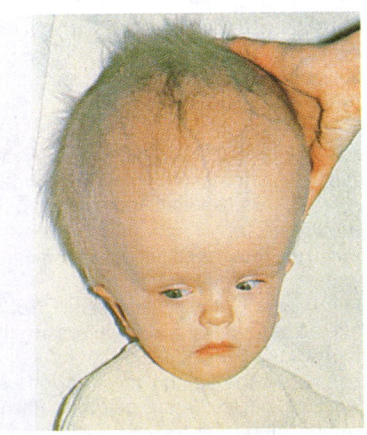

Hydrocephalus *(Hart, 1992)*

■ INTERVENTIONS: Treatment consists almost exclusively of surgical intervention to correct the ventricular obstruction, reduce the production of cerebrospinal fluid, or shunt the excess fluid by ventricular bypass to the right atrium of the heart or to the peritoneal cavity. Surgically treated hydrocephalus with continued neurosurgical and medical management has a survival rate of approximately 80%, although prognosis depends largely on the cause of the condition. Hydrocephalus is frequently associated with myelomeningocele, in which case there is a less favorable prognosis.

■ NURSING CONSIDERATIONS: Primary care of the child with hydrocephalus consists of maintaining adequate nutrition, proper positioning and support to prevent extra strain on the neck, and assistance with diagnostic evaluation and procedures. Postoperatively, in addition to routine care and observation to prevent complications, especially infection, the nurse gives support to the parents and teaches them how to care for a child with a functioning shunt, specifically how to recognize signs that indicate shunt malfunction or infection and how to pump the shunt.

hydrochloric acid /-klôr′ik/ [Gk, hydor + chloros, green], a compound consisting of hydrogen and chlorine. Hydrochloric acid is secreted in the stomach and is a major component of gastric juice.

hydrochloride. See **cyclobenzaprine.**

hydrochlorothiazide /-klôr′ōthī′əzīd/, a diuretic and antihypertensive.

■ INDICATIONS: It is prescribed in the treatment of hypertension and edema.

■ CONTRAINDICATIONS: Anuria or known hypersensitivity to this drug, to other thiazide medication, or to sulfonamide derivatives prohibits its use.

■ ADVERSE EFFECTS: Among the more serious adverse effects are hypoglycemia, hyperglycemia, hyperuricemia, and hypersensitivity reactions.

hydrocholeretics /-kō′lərct′iks/ [Gk, hydor + chloe, bile, eresis, removal], drugs that stimulate the production of bile with a low specific gravity, or with a minimal proportion of solid constituents.

Hydrocil, a trademark for a laxative (psyllium hydrophilic muciloid).

hydrocodone bitartrate /-kō′dōn/, a narcotic antitussive.

■ INDICATION: It is prescribed in the treatment of cough.

■ CONTRAINDICATIONS: Drug dependence or known hypersensitivity to this drug prohibits its use.

■ ADVERSE EFFECTS: Among the more serious adverse reactions are drug dependence and respiratory and circulatory depression.

hydrocortisone, hydrocortisone acetate, hydrocortisone cyclopentylpropionate, hydrocortisone sodium succinate. See **cortisol.**

hydrocortisone valerate /-kôr′tisōn/, a topical corticosteroid.

■ INDICATION: Used topically as an antiinflammatory agent.

■ CONTRAINDICATIONS: Viral and fungal diseases of the skin that occur where circulation is impaired or known hypersensitivity to steroids prohibits its use.

■ ADVERSE REACTIONS: Among the more serious adverse reactions are various systemic side effects that may occur from prolonged or excessive use. Local irritation of the skin may occur.

Hydrocortone, a trademark for a glucocorticoid (hydrocortisone acetate).

Hydro Diuril, a trademark for a diuretic (hydrochlorothiazide).

hydroflumethiazide /-floo′methī′əzīd/, a diuretic and antihypertensive.

■ INDICATIONS: It is prescribed in the treatment of hypertension and edema.

■ CONTRAINDICATIONS: Anuria or known hypersensitivity to this drug, to other thiazide medication, or to sulfonamide derivatives prohibits its use.

■ ADVERSE EFFECTS: Among the more serious adverse effects are blood disorders, hypotension, hypokalemia, hyperglycemia, hyperuricemia, and hypersensitivity reactions.

hydrogen (H) /hī′drəjən/ [Gk, hydor + genein, to produce], a gaseous, univalent element. Its atomic number is 1; its atomic weight is 1.008. It is the simplest and the lightest of the elements and is normally a colorless, odorless, highly inflammable diatomic gas. It occurs in pure form only sparsely in the earth and the atmosphere but is plentiful in the sun and in many other stars. Hydrogen is a component of numerous compounds, many of them produced by the body. As a component of water, hydrogen is crucial in the metabolic interaction of acids, bases, and salts within the body and in the fluid balance necessary for the body to survive.

hydrogenase /hī′drōjənās′/ [Gk, hydor, water, genein, to produce, ase, suffix indicating an enzyme], an enzyme that catalyzes reduction of molecules by combining them with molecular hydrogen.

hydrogenation. See **reduction.**

hydrogen bonding, the attractive force of compounds in which a hydrogen atom covalently linked to an electronegative element, such as oxygen, nitrogen, or sulfur, has a large degree of positive character relative to the electronegative atom, thereby causing the compound to possess a large dipole.

hydrogen ion [H⁺], a positively charged hydrogen atom nucleus.

hydrogen ion concentration of blood, a measure of blood pH and its effect on the ability of the hemoglobin molecule to hold oxygen. See also **Bohr effect.**

hydrogen peroxide, a topical antiinfective.

■ INDICATIONS: It is prescribed to cleanse open wounds, as a mouthwash, and to aid in the removal of cerumen in the external ear.

■ CONTRAINDICATIONS: Irritations to skin or mucous membranes or known hypersensitivity to this agent prohibits its use.

■ ADVERSE EFFECTS: There are no known adverse effects.

hydrokinetics /-kinet′iks/ [Gk, hydor, water, kinesis, motion], the study of movement of fluids.

hydrolase /hī′drōlās/, an enzyme that cleaves ester bonds by the addition of water.

hydrolysis /hīdrol′isis/ [Gk, hydor + lysis, loosening], the chemical alteration or decomposition of a compound with water.

hydrolytic /-lit′ik/ [Gk, hydor, water, lysis, loosening], pertaining to or having the ability to produce hydrolysis.

hydrolyze /hī′drōlīz/ [Gk, hydor, water, lysis, loosening], **1.** to cause or bring about hydrolysis. **2.** to cause a substance to split into component parts by the addition of water.

hydrometer /hīdrom′ətər/ [Gk, hydor + metron, measure], a device that determines the specific gravity or density of a liquid by a comparison of its weight with that of an equal volume of water. A calibrated, hollow glass device is placed in the liquid being examined, and the depth to which the device settles in the liquid is noted.

hydromorphone hydrochloride /-môr′fōn/, a narcotic analgesic.

- INDICATION: It is used to treat moderate to severe pain.
- CONTRAINDICATIONS: It is used with caution in many conditions, including head injuries, asthma, impaired renal or hepatic function, or unstable cardiovascular status. Known hypersensitivity to this drug prohibits its use.
- ADVERSE EFFECTS: Among the most serious adverse reactions are drowsiness, dizziness, nausea, constipation, respiratory and circulatory depression, and drug addiction.

hydronephrosis /hī′drōnefrō′sis/ [Gk, *hydor* + *nephros*, kidney, *osis*, condition], distention of the pelvis and calyces of the kidney by urine that cannot flow past an obstruction in a ureter. Ureteral obstruction may be caused by a tumor, a calculus lodged in the ureter, inflammation of the prostate gland, or edema caused by a urinary tract infection. The person may experience pain in the flank and, in some cases, hematuria, pyuria, and hyperpyrexia. Intravenous pyelography, cytoscopy, or retrograde pyelography may be used in diagnosis. Surgical repair or removal of the obstruction may be necessary. Prolonged hydronephrosis will result in atrophy and eventual loss of kidney function. See also **urinary calculus.** –**hydronephrotic**, *adj.*

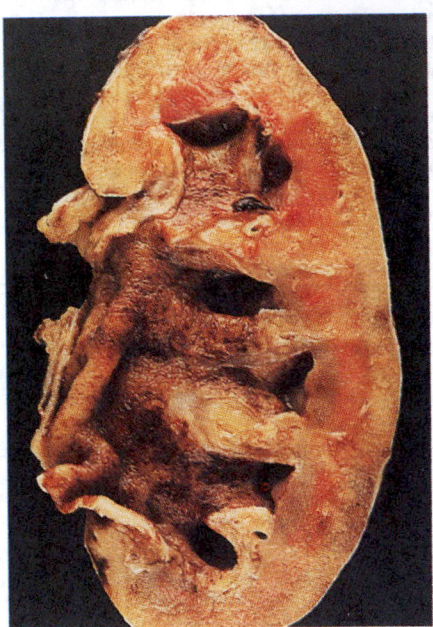

Hydronephrosis *(Fletcher, 1987)*

hydropenia /-pē′nē·ə/, lack of water in the body tissues.
hydrophilic /-fil′ik/ [Gk, *hydor* + *philein*, to love], pertaining to the property of attracting water molecules, possessed by polar radicals or ions. Compare **hydrophobic.**
hydrophobia /-fō′bē·ə/ [Gk, *hydor* + *phobos*, fear], **1.** *nontechnical.* rabies. **2.** a morbid, extreme fear of water.
hydrophobic [Gk, *hydor* + *phobos*, fear], pertaining to the property of repelling water molecules, a quality possessed by nonpolar radicals or molecules that are more sol-

uble in organic solvents than in water. Compare **hydrophilic.**
hydrophthalmos. See **congenital glaucoma.**
hydropic /hīdrop′ik/ [Gk, *hydrops*], pertaining to the condition of dropsy.
Hydropres, a trademark for a fixed-combination drug containing a diuretic (hydrochlorothiazide) and an antihypertensive (reserpine).
hydrops /hī′drops/ [Gk, dropsy], an abnormal accumulation of clear, watery fluid in a body tissue or cavity, such as a joint, a graafian follicle, a fallopian tube, the abdomen, the middle ear, or the gallbladder. Hydrops in the entire body may occur in infants born with thalassemia or severe Rh sensitization. Formerly called **dropsy.**
hydrops endolymphatic. See **endolymphatic hydrops.**
hydrops fetalis, massive edema in the fetus or newborn, usually in association with severe erythroblastosis fetalis. Severe anemia and effusions of the pericardial, pleural, and peritoneal spaces also occur. The condition usually leads to death, even with immediate exchange transfusions after delivery. Also called **fetal hydrops.**
hydrops gravidarum [Gk, *hydor*, water; L, *gravidus*, pregnant], edema due to pregnancy.
hydrops tubae profluens. See **intermittent hydrosalpinx.**
hydroquinone /hī′drōkwin′ōn/, a dermatologic bleaching agent.

- INDICATIONS: It is prescribed to reduce pigmentation of the skin in certain skin conditions in which an excess of melanin causes hyperpigmentation.
- CONTRAINDICATIONS: Sunburn, prickly heat, other irritation of the skin, or known hypersensitivity to this drug prohibits its use.
- ADVERSE EFFECTS: Among the more serious adverse reactions are tingling, erythema, burning, and severe inflammation of the skin.

hydrosalpinx /hī′drōsal′pingks/ [Gk, *hydor* + *salpinx*, tube], an abnormal condition of the fallopian tube in which the tube is cystically enlarged and filled with clear fluid, the end result of an infection that has previously occluded the tube at both ends. The purulent material produced

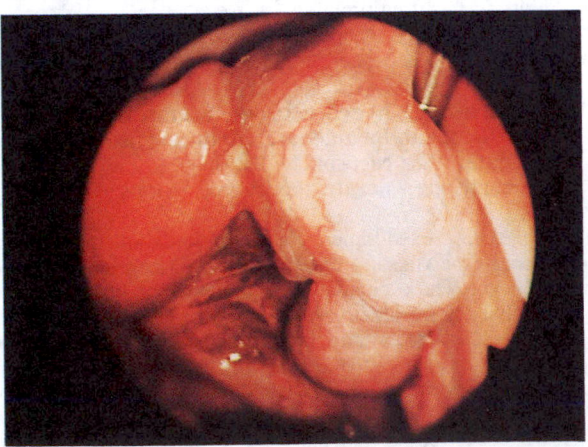

Hydrosalpinx *(Hunt, 1992/Courtesy Robert B Hunt, Boston)*

by the infection undergoes liquefaction during resolution of the acute phase of the inflammatory process.

Hydro-Sphere Nebulizer, a trademark for a type of nebulizer in which a source gas enters a hollow sphere coated with a film of water. The gas exits through slits at the top of the sphere as an aerosol jet, carrying particles of fluid from the sphere's surface.

hydrosis [Gk, *hydor,* water, *osis,* condition], pertaining to the production of sweat. Also spelled **hidrosis.**

hydrostatic /-stat′ik/ [Gk, *hydor,* water, *statos,* standing], pertaining to fluids at rest or in equilibrium and the pressure they exert.

hydrostatic pressure, the pressure exerted by a liquid.

hydrostatic dosimetry, the weighing of a person under water to determine the ratio of lean to fat body weight.

hydrotherapy /-ther′əpē/ [Gk, *hydor* + *therapeia,* treatment], the use of water in the treatment of various mental and physical disorders. Hydrotherapy may include continuous tub baths, wet sheet packs, or shower sprays.

hydrothorax /-thôr′aks/ [Gk, *hydor* + *thorax,* chest], a noninflammatory accumulation of serous fluid in one or both plural cavities.

hydrotropism /-trō′pizəm/ [Gk, *hydor* + *trope,* turning], the tendency of a cell or organism to turn or move in a certain direction under the influence of a water stimulus.

hydrous /hī′drəs/ [Gk, *hydor,* water], pertaining to a substance or object that contains water or is moist.

hydrous wool fat. See **lanolin.**

hydroxide /hīdrok′sīd/, an ionic compound that contains the OH[mi] ion, usually consisting of metals or the metal equivalent of the ammonium cation (NH$_4$−) that inactivates an acid.

hydroxyamphetamine hydrobromide /hīdrok′sē·əmfet′-əmēn/, an adrenergic and mydriatic.

■ INDICATIONS: It is prescribed for dilatation of the pupil for ophthalmoscopy and as a diagnostic aid in Horner's syndrome.

■ CONTRAINDICATIONS: Narrow-angle glaucoma or known hypersensitivity to this drug prohibits its use.

■ ADVERSE EFFECTS: Among the more serious adverse reactions are increased intraocular pressure and photophobia.

hydroxyandrosterone /hīdrok′sē·andros′tərōn/ [Gk *hydor* + *andros* male, *stereos* solid], a sex hormone that is secreted by the testes and adrenal glands. Its normal accumu-

lation in the urine of men after 24-hour collection is 0.1 to 8 mg; in women, 0 to 0.5 mg.

hydroxyapatite /hīdrok′sē·ap′ətīt/, an inorganic compound composed of calcium, phosphate, and hydroxide. It is found in the bones and teeth in a crystallized latticelike form that gives these structures rigidity.

hydroxybenzene. See carbolic acid.

hydroxychloroquine sulfate /-klôr′əkwīn/, an antiprotozoal, antirheumatic drug that is also a suppressant of lupus erythematosus and of polymorphous light eruption.

■ INDICATIONS: It is prescribed in the treatment of malaria and for the suppression of acute paroxysmal attacks of the disease, in the treatment of extraintestinal, usually hepatic, amebiasis, and in the reduction of symptoms of lupus erythematosus and rheumatoid arthritis.

■ CONTRAINDICATIONS: Concurrent use of other 4-aminoquinolones or of gold salts or a known hypersensitivity to this drug or to other 4-aminoquinolones prohibits its use. It is used with caution in people with alcoholism, blood dyscrasia, severe neurologic disorder, retinal or visual field damage, psoriasis, or porphyria. The drug is not usually recommended in pregnancy because it has been associated with damage to the central nervous system of the fetus.

■ ADVERSE EFFECTS: Among the many severe adverse reactions are retinopathy, corneal opacity, polyneuritis, seizure, agranulocytosis, and hepatitis. The incidence and severity of these and many other adverse effects increase with the dosage and prolonged duration of treatment.

17-hydroxycorticosteroid /-kôr′tikos′təroid/, any of the hormones, such as cortisol, secreted by adrenal glands and measured in the urine in a test for determining adrenal function and diagnosing hypoadrenalism or hyperadrenalism. The normal accumulation of this hormone in the urine of men after 24-hour collection is 5.5 to 14.5 μg; in women, 4.9 to 12.9 μg; and in children, slightly less. The levels are two to four times higher in all cases after injection of 25 USP units of adrenocorticotropic hormone.

11-hydroxyetiocholanolone /hīdrok′sē·ē′tē·ōkolan′əlōn/, a sex hormone secreted by the testes and adrenal glands. The normal accumulation in the urine of men after 24-hour collection is 0.2 to 0.6 mg; in women, 0.1 to 1 mg.

5-hydroxyindoleacetic acid /hīdrok′sē·in′dōle·əset′ik/, an acid produced by serotonin metabolism, measured in the blood and urine to aid in the diagnosis of certain kinds of tumors. It commonly rises above normal levels in whole blood in association with asthma, diarrhea, rapid heartbeat, and other symptoms and is elevated in the urine of patients with carcinoid syndrome. Its normal concentrations in whole blood are 0.05 to 0.20 [mu]g/ml; in urine after 24-hour collection, 1 to 5 mg.

hydroxyl (OH) /hīdrok′sil/, a radical compound containing an oxygen atom and a hydrogen atom.

hydroxyprogesterone caproate /-prōjes′tərōn/, a progestational steroid.

■ INDICATIONS: It is prescribed in the treatment of advanced adenocarcinoma of the uterine corpus, amenorrhea, and abnormal uterine bleeding caused by hormonal imbalance in the absence of organic disease.

■ CONTRAINDICATIONS: Markedly impaired liver function, carcinoma of the breast, undiagnosed abnormal genital bleeding, near abortion, thromboembolitic disorders, or known sensitivity to this drug prohibits its use.

■ ADVERSE EFFECTS: Among the most serious adverse reac-

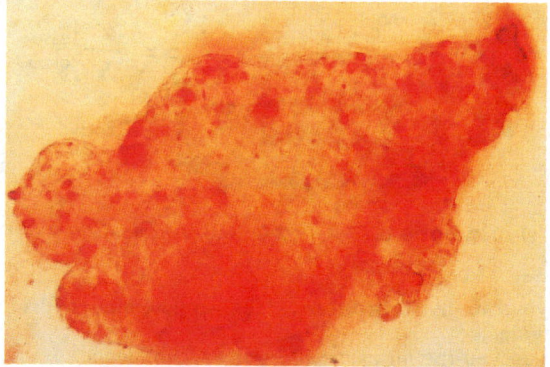

Hydroxyapatite *(Schumacher, 1988)*

tions are thrombophlebitis, pulmonary embolism, cerebrovascular accident, neuroocular lesions, anorexia, edema, hypertension, cholestatic jaundice, and depression.

hydroxyproline /-prō'lēn/, an amino acid that is elevated in the urine in diseases of the bone and certain genetic disorders, such as Marfan's syndrome. Its normal accumulations in urine after 24-hour collection are 10 to 75 mg.

5-hydroxytryptamine. See **serotonin.**

hydroxyurea /hīdrok'siyŏŏrē'ə/, an antineoplastic.
- INDICATION: It is prescribed in the treatment of a variety of neoplasms.
- CONTRAINDICATIONS: Bone marrow depression or known hypersensitivity to this drug prohibits its use. It is not to be given to women who are or might become pregnant.
- ADVERSE EFFECTS: The most serious adverse reaction is bone marrow depression. GI disturbances and dermatitis also may occur.

hydroxyzine hydrochloride /hīdrok'səzēn/, a minor tranquilizer.
- INDICATIONS: It is prescribed to relieve anxiety, nervous tension, hyperkinesis, and motion sickness.
- CONTRAINDICATION: Known hypersensitivity to this drug is the only contraindication.
- ADVERSE EFFECTS: No serious adverse reactions have been observed. Decreased mental alertness is sometimes seen.

hygiene /hī'jēn [Gk, *Hygieia,* the goddess of health], the principles and science of the preservation of health and prevention of disease.

hygienist /hī'jənist, hījē'nist/ [Gk, *Hygieia*], one who practices the principles and laws of **hygiene.**

hygro- /hī'grō-/ [Gk, *hygros,* moist], prefix for terms relating to moistness or moisture.

hygrometer /hīgrom'ətər/ [Gk, *hygros,* moist, *metron,* measure], an instrument that directly measures relative humidity of the atmosphere or the proportion of water in a specific gas or gas mixture, without extracting the moisture.

hygroscopic humidifier /-skop'ik/, a humidifying device attached to the tubing circuit of a mechanical ventilator or anesthesia gas machine to maintain a constant rate of humidity in the patient's trachea.

Hygroton, a trademark for a diuretic (chlorthalidone).

Hylorel, a trademark for an antihypertensive (guanadrel sulfate).

hymen /hī'mən/ [Gk, membrane], a fold of mucous membrane, skin, and fibrous tissue at the introitus of the vagina. It may be absent, small, thin and pliant, or, rarely, tough and dense, completely occluding the introitus. When the hymen is ruptured, small rounded elevations remain. See also **carunculae hymenales.**

hymenal /hī'mənəl/ [Gk, *hymen,* membrane], pertaining or belonging to the hymen.

hymenal tag, normal, redundant hymenal tissue protruding from the floor of the vagina during the first weeks after birth. It eventually disappears without treatment.

hymenectomy /hī'mənek'təmē/ [Gk, *hymen,* membrane, *ektome,* cutting out], the surgical excision of a membrane, particularly the hymen.

Hymenolepis /hī'minol'əpis/ [Gk, *hymen* + *lepis,* rind], a genus of intestinal tapeworms infesting humans, such as *Hymenolepis nana,* the dwarf tapeworm, and *H. diminuta.* Heavy infestation by *H. nana* may cause abdominal pain, bloody stools, and disorders of the nervous system, especially in children. Contaminated food spreads the disease, which is endemic in the United States. Quinacrine hydro-

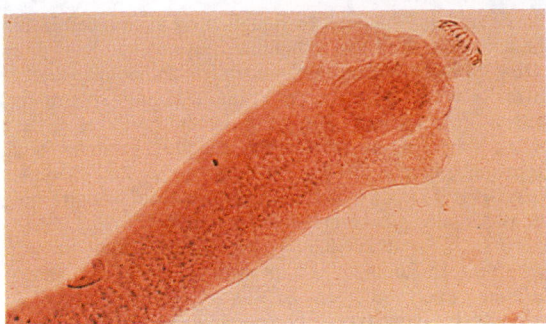

Hymenolepis nana *(Muller, 1990)*

chloride or hexylresorcinol is used to treat the infestation.

hymenotomy /hī'mənot'əmē/ [Gk, *hymen* + *temnein,* to cut], the surgical incision of the hymen.

hyo- /hī'ō-/ [Gk, *hyoeides,* shaped like the Greek letter Y], a prefix meaning 'shaped like the letter "u" or pertaining to the hyoid bone': *hyobasioglossus, hyoglossus.*

hyoglossal. See **glossohyal.**

hyoglossus /-glos'əs/ [Gk, *hyoeides, glossa,* tongue], a depressor muscle of the tongue arising from the hyoid bone.

hyoid /hī'oid/ [Gk, *hyoeides,* shaped like the Greek letter Y], **1.** the hyoid bone. **2.** pertaining to the hyoid bone.

hyoid arch [Gk, *hyoeides;* L, *arcus,* bow], the second pharyngeal or branchial arch. It is present in typical form in the embryo, but the skeletal elements develop into the stapes and styloid process of the temporal bone of the adult.

hyoid bone /hī'oid/ [Gk, *hyoeides,* upsilon, U-shaped; AS, *ban,* bone], a single U-shaped bone suspended from the styloid processes of the temporal bones. The body of the hyoid is square and flat, its ventral surface convex and angled cranially. Two greater wings of the bone attach to the lateral thyroid ligaments, and the body of the bone attaches to various muscles, such as the hypoglossus and the sternohyoideus. The hyoid is palpable in the neck. Also called **lingual bone, os hyoideum.**

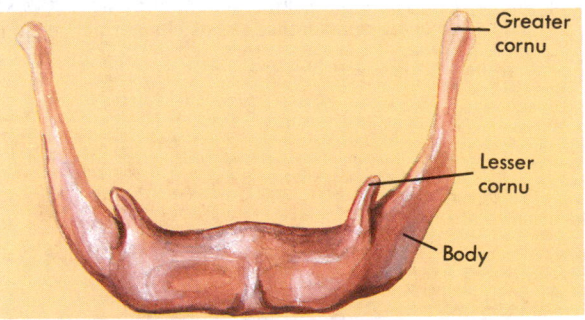

Hyoid bone *(Seeley, 1992/David J Mascaro & Associates)*

hyoscine hydrobromide. See **scopolamine hydrobromide.**

hyoscyamine /hī'əsī'əmēn/, an anticholinergic.
- INDICATIONS: It is prescribed in the treatment of hypermotility of the GI and the lower urinary tracts.

■ CONTRAINDICATIONS: Narrow-angle glaucoma, asthma, obstruction of the genitourinary or GI tracts, severe ulcerative colitis, or known hypersensitivity to this drug prohibits its use.

■ ADVERSE EFFECTS: Among the more serious adverse reactions are blurred vision, central nervous system effects, tachycardia, dry mouth, decreased sweating, and hypersensitivity reactions.

hyp-. See **hypo-.**

hypalgesia /hī'paljē'zē-ə/ [Gk, *hypo*, below, *algesis*, pain], the perception of a painful stimulus to a degree that varies significantly from a normal perception of the same stimulus.

hyper- /hī'pər-/, a prefix meaning 'excessive, above, or beyond': *hyperacidaminuria, hyperalkalinity, hyperechema.*

Hyperab, a trademark for a passive immunizing agent (rabies immune globulin).

hyperacidity /-əsid'itē/ [Gk, *hyper*, excess; L, *acidus*, sour], an excessive amount of acidity, as in the stomach. See also **hyperchlorhydria.**

hyperactive child syndrome /-ak'tiv/ [Gk, *hyper*, excess; L, *agere*, to do; AS, *cild*; Gk, *syn*, together, *dromos*, course], a childhood mental disorder with onset before age 7 and involving inattention, impulsivity, and hyperactivity. Also called **attention-deficit hyperactivity disorder.**

hyperactivity /-aktiv'itē/ [Gk, *hyper* + L, *activus*, active], any abnormally increased activity involving either the entire organism or a particular organ, as the heart or thyroid. Compare **hypoactivity.** See also **attention deficit disorder.**

hyperacuity /akyoo'itē/ [Gk, *hyper*, excessive, *akouien*, to hear], excessive sensitivity to sounds.

hyperadenosis /-ad'ənō'sis/ [Gk, *hyper*, excessive, *aden*, gland, *osis*, condition], a condition characterized by enlarged glands.

hyperadrenalism. See **Cushing's disease.**

hyperadrenocorticism. See **Cushing's syndrome.**

hyperaldosteronism. See **aldosteronism.**

hyperalimentation /-al'iməntā'shən/ [Gk, *hyper* + L, *alimentum*, nourishment], **1.** overfeeding or the ingestion or administration of an amount of nutrients in excess of the demands of the appetite. **2.** See **total parenteral nutrition.**

hyperammonemia /hī'pəram'ōnē'mē-ə/ [Gk, *hyper* + (ammonia), *haima*, blood], abnormally high levels of ammonia in the blood. Ammonia is produced primarily in the intestine, absorbed into the blood, and detoxified in the liver. If there is an increased production of ammonia or a decreased ability to detoxify it, levels of ammonia in the blood may increase. The disorder is controlled by low-protein diets, including essential amino-acid mixtures. Untreated, the condition leads to asterixis, vomiting, lethargy, coma, and death.

hyperbaric chamber /-ber'ik/ [Gk, *hyper*, excess, *baros*, weight, *kamara*, arched roof], an airtight chamber containing an oxygen atmosphere under high pressure. A patient may be placed in the chamber for the treatment of certain infections, tumors, and cardiovascular diseases in which atmospheric oxygen pressures up to three times normal may have therapeutic value.

hyperbaric oxygenation [Gk, *hyper* + *baros*, weight; *oxys*, sharp, *genein*, to produce], the administration of oxygen at greater than normal atmospheric pressure. The procedure is performed in specially designed chambers that permit the delivery of 100% oxygen at atmospheric pressure

that is three times normal. The technique is employed to overcome the natural limit of oxygen solubility in blood, which is about 0.3 ml of oxygen per 100 ml of blood. In hyperbaric oxygenation, dissolved oxygen can be increased to almost 6 ml per 100 ml and the Po_2 in blood may be nearly 2000 mm Hg at 3 atmospheres absolute. Hyperbaric oxygenation has been used to treat carbon monoxide poisoning, air embolism, smoke inhalation, acute cyanide poisoning, decompression sickness, Clostridial myonecrosis, and certain cases of blood loss or anemia in which increased oxygen transport may compensate in part for the hemoglobin deficiency. Factors limiting the usefulness of hyperbaric oxygenation include the hazards of fire and explosive decompression, pulmonary damage and neurologic toxicity at high atmospheric pressures, cardiovascular debility of the patient, and the need to interrupt treatments repeatedly because exposures at maximum atmospheric pressures must be limited to 90 minutes. Also called **hyperbaric oxygen therapy.**

hyperbaric oxygen therapy. See **hyperbaric oxygenation.**

hyperbaric solution [Gk, *hyper*, excess, *baros*, weight], a type of spinal anesthetic that has a specific gravity greater than the cerebrospinal fluid so it will settle into the lowest parts of the spinal canal.

hyperbarism /-ber'izəm/, any disorder resulting from exposure to increased ambient pressure, usually from sudden exposure to or a significant increase in pressure. See also **barotrauma, decompression sickness.**

hyperbasemia /-basē'mē-ə/, elevated arterial bicarbonate concentration that is caused by metabolic or nonrespiratory factors.

hyperbetalipoproteinemia /hī'pərbā'təlip'ōprō'tēnē'mē-ə/ [Gk, *hyper* + *beta*, second letter of Greek alphabet, *lipos*, fat, *proteios*, first rank, *haima*, blood], type II hyperlipoproteinemia, a genetic disorder of lipid metabolism, in which there are abnormally high levels of serum cholesterol, and xanthomas appear on the tendons of the heels, knees, and fingers. There is a marked tendency to develop atherosclerosis and early myocardial infarction, especially among males. Treatment attempts to reduce blood cholesterol levels in the hope of lowering the risk of early death from heart disease. The patient is usually counseled to avoid most meats, eggs, milk products, and all saturated fats and is encouraged to eat fish, grains, fruits, vegetables, lean poultry, and unsaturated fats. Exercise may be recommended, and drugs may be prescribed in some cases. See also **cholesterolemia.**

hyperbilirubinemia /hī'pərbil'iroo'binē'mē-ə/ [Gk, *hyper* + L, *bilis*, bile, *ruber*, red; Gk, *haima*, blood], greater than normal amounts of the bile pigment bilirubin in the blood, often characterized by jaundice, anorexia, and malaise. Hyperbilirubinemia is most often associated with liver disease or biliary obstruction, but it also occurs when there is excessive destruction of red blood cells, as in hemolytic anemia. Treatment is specific to the underlying condition. When bilirubin levels are high, treatment includes phototherapy and hydration. See also **jaundice.**

hyperbilirubinemia of the newborn, an excess of bilirubin in the blood of the neonate. It is usually caused by a deficiency of an enzyme, resulting from physiologic immaturity, or increased hemolysis, especially from blood group incompatibility, which, in severe cases, can lead to kernicterus. Also called **neonatal hyperbilirubinemia.** See also **breast milk jaundice, cholestasis, Crigler-Najjar syndrome, Dubin-Johnson syndrome, erythroblastosis fetalis (hydrops fetalis), Gilbert's syndrome, kernicterus, phototherapy in the newborn, Rotor syndrome.**

■ OBSERVATIONS: Serum bilirubin levels are elevated in the normal newborn because the concentration of circulating erythrocytes is greater and because infants have a decreased ability to conjugate and excrete bilirubin because of a lack of the enzyme glucuronyl transferase, a reduced albumin concentration, and a lack of intestinal bacteria. Jaundice appears when blood levels of bilirubin exceed 5 mg/100 ml, usually not before 24 hours in full-term neonates. Clinically observable jaundice or serum bilirubin levels exceeding 5 mg/100 ml within the first 24 hours of life are abnormal and indicate a pathologic cause of hyperbilirubinemia. In erythroblastosis fetalis, jaundice is evident shortly after birth and bilirubin levels rise rapidly. Severely affected infants also show hepatosplenomegaly and signs of anemia, which quickly worsen, causing decreased oxygen carrying capacity that may lead to cardiac failure and shock. Early symptoms of kernicterus are lethargy, poor feeding, and vomiting, followed by severe neurologic excitation or depression, including tremors, twitching, convulsion, opisthotonos, a high pitched cry, hypotonia, diminished deep tendon reflexes, and the absence of Moro and sucking reflexes. Brain damage generally does not occur at serum bilirubin levels below 20 mg/100 ml. Factors such as metabolic acidosis, lowered albumin levels, hypoxia, hypothermia, free fatty acids, and certain drugs, especially salicylates and sulfonamides, increase the risk at much lower levels. The mortality may reach 50%. Sequelae of kernicterus include mental retardation, minimal brain dysfunction, cerebral palsy, delayed or abnormal motor development, hearing loss, ataxia, athetosis, perceptual problems, and behavioral disorders.

■ INTERVENTIONS: Such preventive measures as frequent feedings during the first 6 to 12 hours of life to increase GI motility have little justification. Infants with mild jaundice require no treatment, only observation. Phototherapy is the usual treatment for severe or increasing hyperbilirubinemia. If hyperbilirubinemia is the result of increased hemolysis caused by blood group incompatibility, exchange transfusion may be done. It is usually indicated if laboratory analysis reveals a positive antiglobulin test, a hemoglobin concentration of the cord blood below 12 g/100 ml, or a bilirubin level of 20 mg/100 ml or more in a full-term infant or 15 mg/100 ml or more in a premature infant. Phototherapy may be used in conjunction with exchange transfusion, except in Rh incompatibility. If used immediately after the initial exchange transfusion, phototherapy may remove enough bilirubin from the tissues to make subsequent transfusions unnecessary. Pharmacologic management, such as the use of barbiturates to stimulate protein synthesis that, in turn, increases albumin for conjugating bilirubin and promotes hepatic glucuronyl transferase synthesis, is indicated in some instances, although this form of therapy is controversial because of the known side effects of the drugs.

■ NURSING CONSIDERATIONS: An initial concern is to identify high-risk infants who may develop hyperbilirubinemia and kernicterus. The nurse may monitor the serum bilirubin levels and observe for evidence of jaundice, anemia, central nervous system irritability, and such conditions as acidosis, hypoxia, and hypothermia. In erythroblastosis fetalis, exchange transfusion may be necessary. The amounts of blood infused and withdrawn, the vital signs, and any signs of exchange reactions are noted. Resuscitative equipment is kept available. Optimal body temperature is maintained: Hypothermia increases oxygen and glucose consumption, causing metabolic acidosis, and hyperthermia damages the donor's erythrocytes, causing an elevation in the amount of free potassium, which may lead to infant cardiac arrest. After the procedure, a sterile dressing is applied to the catheter site.

hypercalcemia /hī'pərkalsē'mē·ə/ [Gk, *hyper* + L, *calx*, lime; Gk, *haima*, blood], greater than normal amounts of calcium in the blood, most often resulting from excessive bone resorption and release of calcium, as occurs in hyperparathyroidism, metastatic tumors of bone, Paget's disease, and osteoporosis. Clinically, patients with hypercalcemia are confused and have anorexia, abdominal pain, muscle pain, and weakness. Extremely high levels of blood calcium may result in shock, kidney failure, and death. Hypercalciuria is also found in most patients with elevated blood calcium. Prednisone, diuretics, isotonic saline, and other drugs may be used in treatment. **–hypercalcemic,** *adj.*

hypercalcemic nephropathy /-kalsē'mik/ [Gk, *hyper,* excessive; L, *calx,* lime, *haima,* blood; Gk, *nephros,* kidney, *pathos,* disease], a progressive disorder of kidney function caused by excessive calcium in the blood. The calcium causes cumulative functional and histological abnormalities leading to a decreased glomerular filtration rate and kidney failure.

hypercalciuria /hī'pərkal'sēyŏŏr'ē·ə/ [Gk, *hyper* + L, *calx,* lime; Gk, *ouron,* urine], the presence of abnormally great amounts of calcium in the urine, resulting from conditions such as sarcoid, hyperparathyroidism, or certain types of arthritis, characterized by augmented bone resorption. Immobilized patients are often hypercalciuric. Some people absorb more calcium than is normal and therefore excrete greater than normal amounts into their urine. Concentrated amounts of calcium in the urinary tract may form kidney stones. Treatment is directed toward correcting any underlying disease condition and limiting dietary intake of calcium. Also called **hypercalcinuria.** Compare **hypercalcemia.** **–hypercalciuric,** *adj.*

hypercapnia /hī'pərkap'nē·ə/ [Gk, *hyper* + *kapnos,* vapor], greater than normal amounts of carbon dioxide in the blood. Also called **hypercarbia.**

hypercapnic acidosis /-kap'nik/ [Gk, *hyper,* excessive, *kapnos,* vapor; L, *acidus,* sour, *osis,* condition], an excessive acidity in body fluids caused by an increase in carbon dioxide tension in the blood. The condition may be secondary to pulmonary insufficiency; as carbon dioxide accumulates in the blood its acidity increases.

hypercarbia /-kär'bē·ə/ [Gk, *hyper,* excessive, *carbo,* coal], an abnormally high concentration of carbon dioxide in the blood.

hyperchloremia /-klôrē'mē·ə/ [Gk, *hyper* + *chloros,* green, *haima,* blood], an excessive level of chloride in the blood.

hyperchlorhydria /-klôrhid'rē·ə [Gk, *hyper, chloros* + *hydor,* water], the excessive secretion of hydrochloric acid by cells lining the stomach. See also **hyperacidity.**

hypercholesterolemia /-kōles'tərōlē'mē·ə/ [Gk, *hyper* + *chole,* bile, *stereos,* solid, *haima,* blood], a condition in which greater than normal amounts of cholesterol are present in the blood. High levels of cholesterol and other lipids may lead to the development of atherosclerosis. Hypercholesterolemia may be reduced or prevented by avoiding saturated fats, which are found in red meats, eggs, and dairy products.

hypercholesterolemic xanthomatosis. See **familial hypercholesterolemia.**

hyperchromia /-krō′mē·ə/ [Gk, *hyper,* excessive, *chroma,* color], an increase of hemoglobin in the erythrocytes.

hyperchromic /-krō′mik/ [Gk, *hyper + chroma,* color], having a greater density of color or pigment.

hyperchylomicronemia /-kī′lōmī′krōnē′mē·ə/ [Gk, *hyper + chylos,* juice, *mikros,* small, *haima,* blood], type I hyperlipoproteinemia, a rare congenital deficiency of an enzyme essential to fat metabolism. Fat accumulates in the blood as chylomicrons. The condition affects children and young adults, who develop xanthomas (fatty deposits) in the skin, hepatomegaly, and abdominal pain. Pancreatitis is the most significant complication. Strict limitation of dietary fat may allow the person to avoid discomfort and complications. Also called **familial lipoprotein lipase deficiency.** See also **chylomicron.**

hypercoagulability /-kō·ag′yələbil′itē/ [Gk, *hyper + L, coagulare,* to curdle, *habilis,* able], a tendency of the blood to coagulate more rapidly than is normal.

hyperdactyly. See **polydactyly.**

hyperdiploid. See **hyperploid.**

hyperdynamic syndrome /-dīnam′ik/ [Gk, *hyper + dynamis,* force], a cluster of symptoms that signal the onset of septic shock, often including a shaking chill, rapid rise in temperature, flushing of the skin, galloping pulse, and alternating rise and fall of the blood pressure. This is a medical emergency that requires expert medical support in a hospital. Emergency measures include keeping the patient warm and elevating the feet to assist venous return. Usually, it is ordered that nothing be given by mouth and that the patient's head be turned to avoid aspiration if there is vomiting. See also **septic shock.**

hyperemesis gravidarum /hī′pərem′isis/ [Gk, *hyper + emesis,* vomiting; L, *gravida,* pregnant], an abnormal condition of pregnancy characterized by protracted vomiting, weight loss, and fluid and electrolyte imbalance. If the condition is severe and intractable, brain damage, liver and kidney failure, and death may result. The cause of the condition is not known; an increase in chorionic gonadotropins or other hormones, an immunologic sensitivity to products of conception, or aggravation of preexisting emotional conflicts has been suggested, but a causal relationship has not been proven. It occurs in approximately three of every 1000 pregnancies, its incidence having diminished in recent years.

■ OBSERVATIONS: Women are frightened of and uncomfortable and embarrassed about their illness. Dry mucous membranes are a sign of dehydration. Other signs include decreased skin elasticity, a rapid pulse, and falling blood pressure. The specific gravity of the urine rises, and the volume of urine excreted falls. The hematocrit is elevated because of hemoconcentration. Loss of electrolytes in vomitus leads to metabolic acidosis with hypokalemia, hypochloremia, and hyponatremia. Severe potassium deficit alters myocardial function; the electrocardiogram may show prolonged P-R and Q-T intervals and inverted T waves. In addition to weight loss, undernourishment causes fever, ketosis, and acetonuria. Severe vitamin B deficiency may result in encephalopathy manifested by confusion and, eventually, coma. Laboratory analyses of blood indicate increased concentrations of metabolic products normally cleared from the blood by the liver and kidneys. Forceful vomiting may cause retinal hemorrhages that impair vision and gastroesophageal tears that bleed and result in hematemesis or melena.

■ INTERVENTIONS: Effective therapy arrests vomiting and achieves rehydration, adequate nutrition, and emotional stabilization. Women are placed at bed rest. Antiemetics safe for the fetus are administered. Fluids, electrolytes, nutrients, and vitamins are given parenterally if the woman is unable to retain fluids by mouth. The fetal heart rate is measured frequently. Psychiatric consultation and therapy are sometimes beneficial. Termination of pregnancy is curative but almost never required.

■ NURSING CONSIDERATIONS: Visitors are encouraged; formerly recommended isolation is not desirable. Sympathetic listening and supportive, nonjudgmental care are provided. The woman and her family are told often that the prognosis is excellent for both mother and baby. She is weighed regularly, and her weight is accurately recorded, for the best evidence of recovery is steady weight gain.

hyperemia /hī′pərē′mē·ə/ [Gk, *hyper + haima,* blood], increased blood in part of the body, caused by increased blood flow, as in the inflammatory response, local relaxation of arterioles, or obstruction of the outflow of blood from an area. Skin overlying a hyperemic area usually becomes reddened and warm. **–hyperemic,** *adj.*

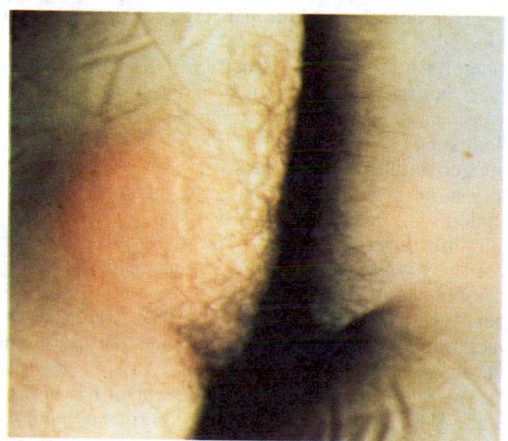

Hyperemia
(Potter, 1993/From Pires M, Muller M: Progressions 3(3):3, 1991

hyperesthesia /-esthē′zhə/, an extreme sensitivity of one of the body's sense organs, such as pain or touch receptors in the skin.

hyperextension /-ikten′shən/ [Gk, *hyper + L, extendere,* to stretch out], (of a joint) a position of maximum extension.

hyperextension bed, a bed used in pediatric orthopedics to maintain any correction achieved by suspension of a body part and to increase the range of motion of the hips after an operative muscle release procedure. The hyperextension bed may be purchased or it may be converted from a regular hospital bed. Removal of the mattress from a regular hospital bed and the addition of three half mattresses allow sufficient height to permit alternating prone and supine positions and the concomitant alternating flexion and extension of the hips. The bilateral extremities of the patient, in casts, are suspended over the lower half of the bed with rings and traction apparatus. The position of the patient's hips is alternated at 2-hour intervals; abduction and adduction can be controlled by the position of the pulleys. Restraints are required to maintain the child in position so that the horizontal, gluteal folds are even with the bottom edge of the stacked mattresses. Also called **Schwartz bed.** Compare **CircOlectric bed, Foster bed, Stryker wedge frame.**

hyperextension suspension, an orthopedic procedure used in the postoperative positioning of hip muscles. The procedure uses traction equipment, including metal frames, ropes, and pulleys to relieve the weight of the lower limbs and to position properly the muscles of the hip, without applying traction to the lower limbs involved. The ropes used to suspend the lower limbs in this procedure are attached by rings to long leg casts encasing the lower limbs of the patient. Compare **balanced suspension, lower extremity suspension, upper extremity suspension.**

hyperflexia /-flek'shə/ [Gk, *hyper* + L, *flectere*, to bend], the forcible overflexion or bending of a limb.

hyperfunction /-fungk'shən/ [Gk, *hyper* + L, *functio*, performance], increased function of any organ or system.

hypergenesis /-jen'əsis/ [Gk, *hyper* + *genesis*, origin], excessive growth or overdevelopment. The condition may involve the entire body, as in gigantism, or any particular part or it may result in the formation of extra parts, such as the development of additional fingers or toes. **–hypergenetic,** *adj.*

hypergenetic teratism /-jənet'ik/ [Gk, *hyper, genesis* + *teras*, monster], a congenital anomaly in which there is excessive growth of a part, organ, or the entire body, as in gigantism.

hypergenitalism /-jen'itəliz'əm/, the presence of abnormally large external genitalia. The condition is usually associated with precocious puberty.

hyperglobulinemia /-glob'yəline'mē·ə/ [Gk, *hyper,* excessive; L, *globulus,* small globe, *haima,* blood], an excess of globulin in the blood.

hyperglycemia /hī'pərglīsē'mē·ə/ [Gk, *hyper* + *glykys,* sweet, *haima,* blood], a greater than normal amount of glucose in the blood. Most frequently associated with diabetes mellitus, the condition may occur in newborns, after the administration of glucocorticoid hormones, and with an excess infusion of intravenous solutions containing glucose, especially in poorly monitored, long-term hyperalimentation. Compare **hypoglycemia.**

hyperglycemic-glycogenolytic factor. See **glucagon.**

hyperglycemic-hyperosmolar nonketotic coma /-glīsē'mik/ [Gk, *hyper, glykys* + *hyper, osmos,* impulse; L, *non,* not, (ketone); Gk, deep sleep], a diabetic coma in which the level of ketone bodies is normal; caused by hyperosmolarity of extracellular fluid and resulting in dehydration of intracellular fluid, often a consequence of overtreatment with hyperosmolar solutions.

hyperglyceridemia /-glī'səridē'mē·ə/ [Gk, *hyper,* excessive, *glykeros, haima,* blood], an excess of glycerides, particularly triglycerides, in the blood.

hypergonadism /-gō'nədiz'əm/ [Gk, *hyper,* excessive, *gone,* seed], excessive activity of the ovaries or testes.

HyperHep, a trademark for a hepatitis B immune globulin (human) that is administered intramuscularly to provide passive immunization for people who have been exposed to the hepatitis B virus.

hyperhidrosis /hī'pərhīdrō'sis, -hidrō'sis/ [Gk, *hyper* + *hidros,* perspiration], excessive perspiration often caused by heat, hyperthyroidism, strong emotion, menopause, or infection. Symptomatic therapy usually includes topical antiperspirants and may involve surgery to remove axillary sweat glands.

hyperimmune /-imyŌn'/ [Gk, *hyper* + L, *immunis,* freedom], a characteristic associated with an unusual abundance of antibodies, producing a greater than normal immunity.

hyperinsulinism /-in'səliniz'əm/ [Gk, *hyper* + L, *insula,* island], an excessive amount of insulin in the body, as may occur when a greater than required dose is administered or when an insulin-secreting tumor is present in the islets of Langerhans. Symptoms include hypoglycemia, hunger, shakiness, diaphoresis. See **insulin shock.**

hyperirritability /-irit'əbil'itē/ [Gk, *hyper,* excessive; L, *irritare,* to tease], excessive excitability or sensitivity, or exaggerated response to a stimulus.

hyperkalemia /hī'pərkəlē'mē·ə/ [Gk, *hyper* + L, *kalium,* potassium; Gk, *haima,* blood], greater than normal amounts of potassium in the blood. This condition is seen frequently in acute renal failure. Early signs are nausea, diarrhea, and muscle weakness. As potassium levels increase, marked cardiac changes are observed in the ECG. Treatment of severe hyperkalemia includes the intravenous administration of sodium bicarbonate, calcium salts, and dextrose. Hemodialysis is used if these measures fail.

hyperkalemic periodic paralysis. See **adynamia episodica heriditaria.**

hyperkeratinization /-ker'ətinīzā'shən/ [Gk, *hyper,* excessive, *keras,* horn], an abnormal horny thickening of the epithelium of the palms and soles.

hyperkeratosis /-ker'ətō'sis/ [Gk, *hyper* + *keras,* horn, *osis,* condition], overgrowth of the cornified epithelial layer of the skin. See also **callus, corn.**

hyperkinesis. See **attention deficit disorder.**

hyperlipemia /-lipē'mē·ə/, an excessive level of blood fats, usually caused by a lipoprotein lipase deficiency or a defect in the conversion of low-density lipoproteins (LDL) to high-density lipoproteins (HDL). The condition occurs in nephrotic syndrome and hypoalbuminemia.

hyperlipidemia /-lip'idē'mē·ə/ [Gk, *hyper* + *lipos,* fat, *haima,* blood], an excess of lipids in the plasma, including the glycolipids, lipoproteins, and phospholipids. See also **antilipidemic.**

hyperlipidemia type I, a condition of elevated lipid levels in the blood, characterized by an increase in both cholesterol and triglycerides, and caused by the presence of chylomicrons. It is inherited as an autosomal recessive trait with a low risk of atherosclerosis. It results in recurrent bouts of acute pancreatitis. The symptoms begin in childhood. The accumulation of triglycerides is generally proportional to the amount of dietary fat. Treatment is primarily dietary; both saturated and unsaturated fats are restricted to amounts that produce less than 500 mg/dl of blood, evaluated after an overnight fast. Also called **exogenous hypertriglyceridemia, familial hyperglyceridemia, fat-induced hyperlipidemia.**

hyperlipidemia type IIA, hyperlipidemia type IIB. See **familial hypercholesterolemia.**

hyperlipidemia type III. See **broad beta disease.**

hyperlipidemia type IV, a relatively common form of hyperlipoproteinemia characterized by a slight elevation in cholesterol levels, a moderate elevation of triglycerides, and an elevation of the normal triglyceride carrier protein VLDL. It is sometimes familial and is associated with an increased risk factor for coronary atherosclerosis. The condition is controlled with weight reduction, a low-carbohydrate diet, drugs, niacin, and avoidance of alcoholic beverages. Also called **endogenous hypertriglyceridemia.**

hyperlipidemia type V, a condition of elevated blood lipids, characterized by slightly increased cholesterol, greatly increased triglycerides, elevation of the triglyceride carrier protein VLDL, and chylomicrons. It is a genetically heterogenous disorder that apparently does not increase the risk of atherosclerosis. Treatment includes weight control, a low-fat diet, drugs, niacin, and abstinence from alcohol. Also called **mixed hypertriglyderidemia, mixed hyperlipemia.**

hyperlipoproteinemia /hī′pərlip′ōprō′tēnē′mē·ə/ [Gk, *hyper* + *lipos*, fat, *proteios*, first rank, *haima*, blood], any of a large group of inherited and acquired disorders of lipoprotein metabolism characterized by greater than normal amounts of certain protein-bound lipids and other fatty substances in the blood. The treatment includes diet to control obesity; diet may reduce lipoprotein levels in the blood. Medication and other treatment vary according to the specific metabolic defect, its cause, and its prognosis.

hypermagnesemia /hī′pərmag′nisē′mē·ə/ [Gk *hyper* + *magnesia* magnesium, *haima* blood], a greater than normal amount of magnesium in the plasma, found in people with kidney failure and in those who use large doses of drugs containing magnesium, such as antacids. Toxic levels of magnesium cause cardiac dysrhythmias and depression of deep tendon reflexes and respiration. Treatment often includes intravenous fluids, a diuretic, and hemodialysis.

hypermature cataract /-məcho͞or′/ [Gk, *hyper*, excessive; L, *maturare,* to make ripe; Gk, *katarrhaktes,* portcullis], an opaque lens that has lost water and has become reduced in size and soft.

hypermenorrhea. See **menorrhagia.**

hypermetria /hī′pərmē′trē·ə/ [Gk, *hyper* + *metron*, measure], an abnormal condition, a form of dysmetria, characterized by a dysfunction of the power to control the range of muscular action, resulting in movements that overreach the intended goal of the affected individual. Compare **hypometria.**

hypermetropia, hypermetropy, See **hyperopia.**

hypermobility /-mōbil′itē/ [Gk, *hyper*, excessive; L, *mobilis,* movable], a form of joint laxity characterized by an abnormally wide range of movement of the joints. The condition is seen in children and may be associated with **Marfan's syndrome** or degenerative joint diseases.

hypermorph /hī′pərmôrf′/ [Gk, *hyper* + *morphe*, form], **1.** a person whose arms and legs are disproportionately long in relation to the trunk, and whose sitting height is disproportionate to the standing height. **2.** (in genetics) a mutant gene that shows an increased activity in the expression of a trait. Compare **amorph, antimorph, hypomorph.**

hypermotility /-motil′itē/, an excessive movement of the involuntary muscles, particularly in the gastrointestinal tract.

hypernatremia /hī′pərnatrē′mē·ə/ [Gk, *hyper* + L, *natrium*, sodium], a greater than normal concentration of so-

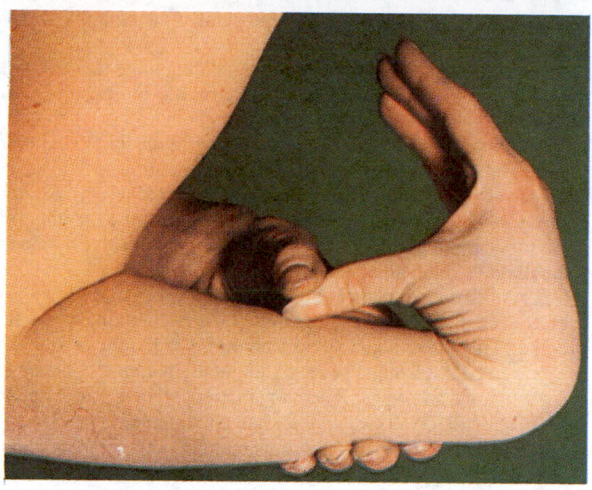

Hypermobility syndrome *(Shipley, 1993)*

dium in the blood, caused by excessive loss of water and electrolytes resulting from polyuria, diarrhea, excessive sweating, or inadequate water intake. When water loss is caused by kidney dysfunction, urine is profuse and dilute. If water loss is not through the kidneys, such as in diarrhea and excessive sweating, the urine is scanty and highly concentrated. People with hypernatremia may become mentally confused, have seizures, and lapse into coma. The treatment is restoration of fluid and electrolyte balance by mouth or by IV infusion. Care must be taken to restore water balance slowly, because further electrolyte imbalances may occur. See also **diabetes insipidus.**

hyperopia /-ō′pē·ə/ [Gk, *hyper* + *ops*, eye], farsightedness, a condition resulting from an error of refraction in which rays of light entering the eye are brought into focus behind the retina. Also called **farsightedness, hypermetropia, hypermetropy.** Compare **myopia.**

hyperosmia

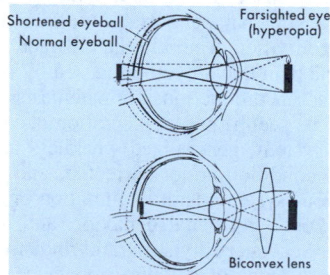

Hyperopia

hyperorchidism /-ôr′kidiz′əm/ [Gk, *hyper*, excessive, *orchis*, testis], excessive endocrine activity of the testes.

hyperornithinemia /-ôr′nithinē′mē·ə/, a metabolic disorder involving the amino acid ornithine, which tends to accumulate in the tissues, causing seizures and retardation. It is treated with a low-protein diet.

hyperosmia /-oz′mē·ə/,   an abnormally increased sensitivity to odors. Compare **anosmia.**

hyperosmolarity /-oz′məler′itē/ [Gk, *hyper* + *osmos*, impulse],   a state or condition of abnormally increased osmolarity.   –**hyperosmolar,** *adj.*

hyperosmotic /-osmot′ik/,   pertaining to an increased concentration of osmotically active components.

hyperostosis /-ostō′sis/ [Gk, *hyper,* excessive, *osteon,* bone, *osis,* condition],   an overgrowth of bone. It may occur as a bone swelling or an osteoma, or involve adjacent cartilage. Also called **exostosis.**

hyperoxaluria /-ok′səlŏŏr′ē·ə/,   an excessive level of oxalic acid or oxalates, primarily calcium oxalate, in the urine. The cause is usually an inherited deficiency of an enzyme needed to metabolize oxalic acid, which is present in many fruits and vegetables, or a disorder of fat absorption in the small intestine. An excess of oxalates may lead to the formation of renal calculi. Treatment may include pyridoxine, forced fluids, and a low-oxalate diet.

hyperoxemia /-oksē′mē·ə/ [Gk, *hyper,* excessive, *oxys,* sharp, *haima,* blood],   increased oxygen content of the blood.

hyperoxia /-ok′sē·ə/,   a condition of abnormally high oxygen tension in the blood.

hyperoxygenation /-ok′sijənā′shən/ [Gk, *hyper* + *oxys,* sharp, *genein,* to produce],   the use of high concentrations of inspired oxygen before and after endotracheal aspiration.

hyperparathyroidism /-per′əthī′roidiz′əm/ [Gk, *hyper* + *para,* beside, *thyreos,* shield, *eidos,* form],   an abnormal endocrine condition characterized by hyperactivity of any of the four parathyroid glands with excessive secretion of parathyroid hormone (PTH), increased resorption of calcium from the skeletal system and increased absorption of calcium by the kidneys and GI system. The condition may be primary, originating in one or more of the parathyroid glands, or secondary, resulting from an abnormal hypocalcemia-producing condition in another part of the body causing a compensatory hyperactivity of the parathyroid glands.

■ OBSERVATIONS: Hypercalcemia in primary hyperparathyroidism results in dysfunction of most of the systems of the body. In the kidneys, tissue calcifies, calculi form, and renal failure may ensue. In the bones and joints, osteoporosis develops, causing pain and fragility; fractures, synovitis, and pseudogout often occur. In the GI tract, chronic, piercing epigastric pain may develop, caused by pancreatitis and increased gastrin production. Hematemesis, anorexia, and nausea may be seen if peptic ulceration occurs. In the neuromuscular system, generalized weakness and atrophy develop if the condition is not corrected, and changes in the central nervous system result in alteration of consciousness, coma, psychosis, abnormal behavior, and disturbances of personality. Secondary hyperparathyroidism may result in many of these signs of calcium imbalance and in various abnormalities of the long bones, as in rickets. The diagnosis of primary hyperparathyroidism is made by laboratory findings of increased levels of PTH and calcium in the blood and by the characteristic appearance of the bones on x-ray films. Calcium in the blood and urine and chloride and alkaline phosphatase in the blood are present in excessive amounts; phosphorus is present in the serum in less than normal amounts.

■ INTERVENTIONS: Primary parathyroidism that is the result of an adenoma of one of the glands is treated by excision of

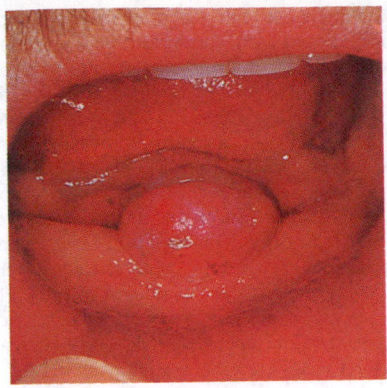

Hyperparathyroidism (Lamey, 1988)

the tumor; other causes of primary disease might require excision of up to one half of the glandular tissue. Dietary intake of calcium may be limited, and diuretics that promote urinary excretion of calcium and sodium may be administered. Calcitonin may be administered in severe hypercalcemia to lower the serum calcium level. Postoperatively, calcium levels in the blood may drop rapidly to dangerously low levels if frequent laboratory evaluations are not made and supplemental calcium is not given as required. Secondary hyperparathyroidism is treated by treating the underlying cause of hypertrophy of the gland. Vitamin D is frequently given, and peritoneal dialysis may be necessary to remove excess calcium from the circulation.

■ NURSING CONSIDERATIONS: Frequent laboratory evaluations of blood levels of calcium, phosphorus, potassium, and magnesium are necessary throughout the course of treatment. Because fractures occur easily and are common, great care is taken to avoid trauma for the patient. Intravenous hydration is usually performed to dilute the concentration of calcium, and the lungs are auscultated and percussed regularly to detect pulmonary edema in its earliest stages. Tetany is a warning sign of severe hypoglycemia; calcium gluconate is kept available for immediate use postoperatively. Walking and moving about cause pain to the patient but accelerate healing of the affected bones and are therefore encouraged.

hyperperistalis /-per′istal′is/ [Gk, *hyper,* excessive, *peristellein,* to clasp],   a state of excessive motility of the waves of alternate contractions and relaxations that propel contents forward through the digestive tract.

hyperphenylalaninemia /hī′pərfen′ilal′əninē′mē·ə/ [Gk, *hyper* + (phenylalanine), *haima,* blood],   an abnormally high concentration of phenylalanine in the blood. This symptom may be the result of one of several defects in the metabolic process of breaking down phenylalanine. See also **phenylketonuria.**

hyperphoria /hī′pərfôr′ē·ə/ [Gk, *hyper* + *pherein,* to bear],   the tendency of an eye to deviate upward.

hyperpigmentation /-pig′məntā′shən/ [Gk, *hyper* + L, *pigmentum,* paint],   unusual darkening of the skin. Causes include heredity, drugs, exposure to the sun, and adrenal insufficiency. Compare **hypopigmentation.** See also **chloasma, melanocyte stimulating hormone.**

hyperpituitarism /-pityŏŏ′itəriz′əm/ [Gk, *hyper,* excessive; L, *pituita,* phlegm],   overactivity of the anterior lobe

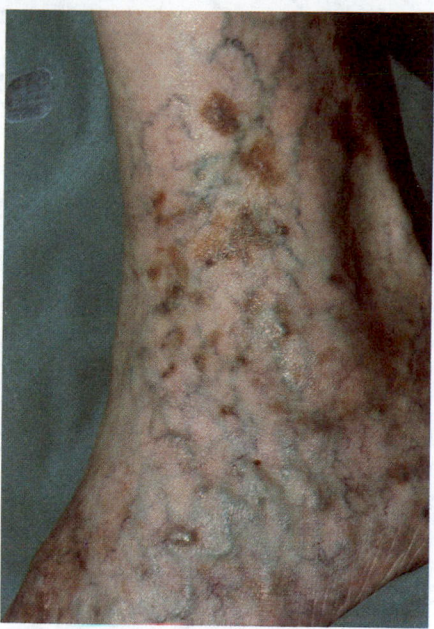

Hyperpigmentation *(Goldman, 1991)*

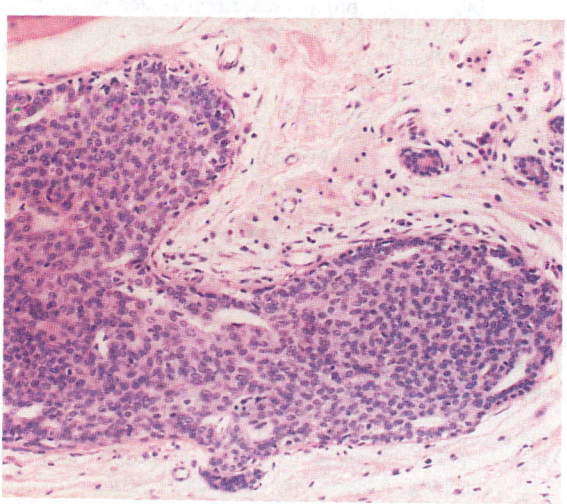

Epithelial hyperplasia *(Skarin, 1991)*

of the pituitary gland, leading to such conditions as **acromegaly** and **Cushing's disease.**

hyperplasia /hī′pərplā′zhə/ [Gk, *hyper* + *plassein,* to mold], an increase in the number of cells of a body part. Compare **hypertrophy, hypoplasia.**

hyperplastic endometritis /-plas′tik/, *obsolete.* endometritis with endometrial hyperplasia.

hyperplastic gingivitis [Gk, *hyper,* excessive, *plassein,* to mold; L, *gingiva,* gum; Gk, *itis,* inflammation], a condition of enlarged and inflamed gigival tissue, resulting from an increase in the number of cells, usually as a result of dental plaque accumulation.

hyperploid /hī′pərploid/ [Gk, *hyper* + *eidos,* form], **1.** of or pertaining to an individual, organism, strain, or cell that has one or more chromosomes in excess of the basic haploid number or of an exact multiple of the haploid number characteristic of the species. The result is unbalanced sets of chromosomes, which are referred to as hyperdiploid, hypertriploid, hypertetraploid, and so on, depending on the number of multiples of the haploid chromosomes they contain. **2.** such an individual, organism, strain, or cell. Compare **hypoploid.** See also **trisomy.**

hyperploidy /hī′pərploi′dē/, any increase in chromosome number that involves individual chromosomes rather than entire sets, resulting in more than the normal haploid number characteristic of the species, as in Downs syndrome. Compare **hypoploidy.**

hyperpnea /hī′pərpnē′ə/ [Gk, *hyper* + *pnoe,* blowing], a deep, rapid, or labored respiration. It occurs normally with exercise and abnormally with pain, fever, hysteria, or any condition in which the supply of oxygen is inadequate, such as cardiac disease and respiratory disease. Also spelled **hyperpnoea.** Compare **dyspnea, hypopnea, orthopnea.** See also **respiratory rate. —hyperpneic, hyperpnoic,** *adj.*

hyperprolactinemia /-prōlak′tinē′mē·ə/ [Gk, *hyper* + L, *pro,* before, *lac,* milk; Gk, *haima,* blood], an excessive amount of prolactin in the blood. The condition is caused by a hypothalamic-pituitary dysfunction. In women it is usually associated with gynecomastia, galactorrhea, and secondary amenorrhea; in men it may be a factor in decreased libido and impotence. It may be a result of endocrine side effects related to certain antipsychotic medications.

hyperproteinemia /-prō′tēnē′mē·ə/ [Gk, *hyper,* excessive, *proteios,* first rank, *haima,* blood], an abnormally high level of protein elements in the blood.

hyperptyalism. See **ptyalism.**

hyperpyrexia /hī′pərpīrek′sē·ə/ [Gk, *hyper* + *pyressein,* to be feverish], an extremely elevated temperature sometimes occurring in acute infectious diseases, especially in young children. Malignant hyperpyrexia, characterized by a rapid rise in temperature, tachycardia, tachypnea, sweating, rigidity, and blotchy cyanosis, occasionally occurs in patients undergoing general anesthesia. A high temperature may be reduced by sponging the body with tepid water and alcohol, by giving a tepid tub bath, by hypothermia treatment, or by administering antipyretic medication, such as aspirin or acetaminophen. See also **fever. —hyperpyretic,** *adj.*

hyperreactivity /-rē′aktiv′itē/ [Gk, *hyper* + L, *re,* again, *activus,* active], an abnormal condition in which responses to stimuli are exaggerated.

hyperreflection /-riflek′shən/, a compulsion to devote excessive attention to oneself.

hyperreflexia /-riflek′sē·ə/ [Gk, *hyper* + L, *reflectere,* to bend backward], increased reflex reactions.

hypersensitivity /-sen′sitiv′itē/ [Gk, *hyper* + L, *sentire,* to feel], an abnormal condition characterized by an excessive reaction to a particular stimulus. See also **allergy. —hypersensitive,** *adj.*

hypersensitivity pneumonitis. an inflammatory form of interstitial pneumonia that results from an immunologic reaction in a hypersensitive person. The reaction may be provoked by a variety of inhaled organic dusts, often those containing fungal spores. The disease can be prevented by avoiding contact with the causative agents. Hypersensitivity pneumonitis is a disease in which classification is based solely on the character of the immune response rather than on its clinical manifestations. A wide variety of symptoms may occur, including asthma, fever, chills, malaise, and muscle aches, which usually develop 4 to 6 hours after exposure. On laboratory examination of the blood, leukocytosis is commonly found. Recovery is usually spontaneous. In an acute attack, corticosteroids may be given to diminish the inflammatory response. Kinds of hypersensitivity pneumonitis include **bagassosis, cork worker's lung, farmer's lung, humidifier lung,** and **mushroom worker's lung.** Also called **extrinsic allergic alveolitis.** See also **Arthus reaction.**

hypersensitivity reaction,   an inappropriate and excessive response of the immune system to a sensitizing antigen. The antigenic stimulant is an allergen. There are several factors that determine the degree of an allergic response: the responsiveness of the host to the allergen, the amount of allergen, the kind of allergen, its route of entrance into the body, the timing of the exposures, and the site of the allergen-immune mediator reaction. Hypersensitivity reactions are classified by the components of the immune system involved in their mediation. Humoral reactions, mediated by the circulating B lymphocytes, are immediate and include three types: anaphylactic hypersensitivity, cytotoxic hypersensitivity, and immune system hypersensitivity. Cellular reactions, mediated by the T lymphocytes, are delayed, cell-mediated hypersensitivity reactions.

hypersensitization /-sen'sitīzā'shən/ [Gk, *hyper*, excessive; L, *sentire*, to feel],   a state of increased reactivity or sensitivity to a stimulus.

hypersomnia /hī'pərsom'nē·ə/ [Gk, *hyper* + L, *somnus*, sleep],   **1.** sleep of excessive depth or abnormal duration, usually caused by psychologic rather than physical factors and characterized by a state of confusion on awakening. **2.** extreme drowsiness, often associated with lethargy. **3.** a condition characterized by periods of deep, long sleep. Compare **narcolepsy.**

hyperspadias.   See **epispadias.**

hypersplenism /hī'pərsplē'nizəm/ [Gk, *hyper* + *splen*, spleen],   a syndrome consisting of splenomegaly and a deficiency of one or more types of blood cells. The numerous causes of this syndrome include portal hypertension, the lymphomas, the hemolytic anemias, malaria, tuberculosis, and various connective tissue and inflammatory diseases. Patients complain of abdominal pain on the left side and often experience fullness after eating very little, because the greatly enlarged spleen is pressing against the stomach. On physical examination the enlarged spleen is felt and abnormal bruits (vascular sounds) are heard with a stethoscope over the epigastric area. Treatment of the underlying disorder may cure the syndrome. Splenectomy is usually performed only in treating the hemolytic anemias or when splenic enlargement is severe and the danger of vascular accident is significant. See also **splenectomy.**

Hyperstat,   a trademark for a vasodilator (diazoxide).

hypersthenic /hī'pərsthen'ik/,   **1.** pertaining to a condition of excessive strength or tonicity of the body or a body part. **2.** pertaining to a body type characterized by massive proportions.

hypertelorism /hī'pərtel'əriz'əm/ [Gk, *hyper* + *tele*, far, *horizo* separate],   a developmental defect characterized by an abnormally wide space between two organs or parts. A kind of hypertelorism is **ocular hypertelorism.** Compare **hypotelorism.**

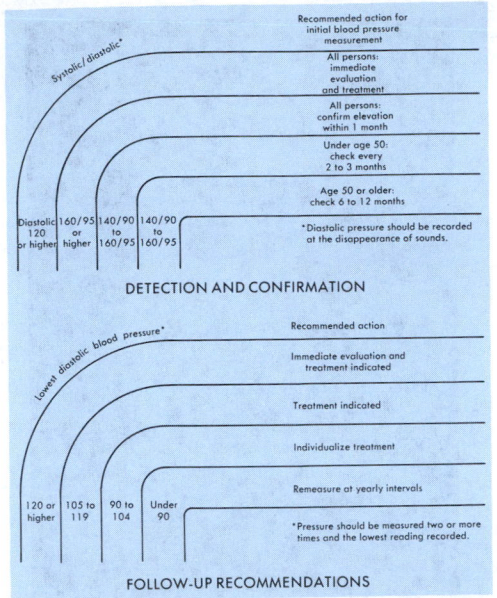

High blood pressure

hypertension /-ten'shən/ [Gk, *hyper* + L, *tendere*, to stretch],   a common, often asymptomatic disorder characterized by elevated blood pressure persistently exceeding 140/90 mm Hg. Essential hypertension, the most frequent kind, has no single identifiable cause, but the risk of the disorder is increased by obesity, a high serum sodium level, hypercholesterolemia, and a family history of high blood pressure. Known causes of hypertension include adrenal disorders, such as aldosteronism, Cushing's syndrome, and pheochromocytoma, thyrotoxicosis, toxemia of pregnancy, and chronic glomerulonephritis. The incidence of hypertension is higher in men than in women and is twice as great in blacks as in whites. People with mild or moderate hypertension may be asymptomatic or may experience suboccipital headaches, especially on rising, tinnitus, lightheadedness, easy fatigability, and palpitations. With sustained hypertension arterial walls become thickened, inelastic, and resistant to blood flow, and, as a result, the left ventricle becomes distended and hypertrophied in its efforts to maintain normal circulation. Inadequate blood supply to the coronary arteries may cause angina or myocardial infarction. Left ventricular hypertrophy may lead to congestive heart failure. Malignant hypertension, characterized by a diastolic pressure higher than 120 mm Hg, severe headaches, blurred vision, and confusion, may result in fatal uremia, myocardial infarction, congestive heart failure, or a cerebrovascular accident. Drugs used to treat hypertension include diuretics, such as furosemide and thiazide derivatives; vasodilators, such as hydralazine and prazosin; sympathetic nervous system (SNS) depressants, such as rauwolfia alkaloids; SNS inhibitors, such as guanethidine and methyldopa; angiotensin converting enzyme (ACE) inhibitors, calcium channel blockers, and ganglionic blocking agents, such as clonidine and propranolol. Patients with high blood pressure are advised to follow a low-sodium, low-saturated-fat diet, to reduce calories to control obesity, to exercise, to avoid stress, and to take adequate rest. See also **blood pressure.**

Classification of hypertension by age-group

Age-group	Significant hypertension (mM Hg)	Severe hypertension (mM Hg)
Newborns		
7 days	Systolic BP ≥ 96	Systolic BP ≥ 106
8-30 days	Systolic BP ≥ 104	Systolic BP ≥ 110
Infants (<2 yr)	Systolic BP ≥ 112	Systolic BP ≥ 118
	Diastolic BP ≥ 74	Diastolic BP ≥ 82
Children		
(3-5 yr)	Systolic BP ≥ 116	Systolic BP ≥ 124
	Diastolic BP ≥ 76	Diastolic BP ≥ 84
(6-9 yr)	Systolic BP ≥ 122	Systolic BP ≥ 130
	Diastolic BP ≥ 78	Diastolic BP ≥ 86
(10-12 yr)	Systolic BP ≥ 126	Systolic BP ≥ 134
	Diastolic BP ≥ 82	Diastolic BP ≥ 90
Adolescents		
(13-15 yr)	Systolic BP ≥ 136	Systolic BP ≥ 144
	Diastolic BP ≥ 86	Diastolic BP ≥ 92
(16-18 yr)	Systolic BP ≥ 142	Systolic BP ≥ 150
	Diastolic BP ≥ 92	Diastolic BP ≥ 98
Adults	Systolic BP ≥ 160	Systolic BP ≥ 240
	Diastolic BP ≥ 90	Diastolic BP ≥ 115

Calculation of systolic blood pressure expected for children over 1 year of age can be estimated with the following formula:

$$80 + (2 \times \text{child's age in years})$$

For example, the calculation of the expected systolic blood pressure of a 5-year-old would be as follows:

$$80 + (2 \times 5) = 90$$

Although this calculation gives a figure below the expected mean, it is still considered within normal limits for a 5-year-old child.

Modified from National Heart, Lung, and Blood Institute: Report of the second task force on blood pressure control in children—1987, *Pediatrics* 79:1, 1987. From Seidel HM, Ball JW, Dains JE, Benedict WG: *Mosby's guide to physical examination,* ed 2, St Louis, 1991, Mosby.

hypertensive /-ten′siv/ [Gk, *hyper,* excessive; L, *tendere,* to stretch], pertaining to high blood pressure, its cause, or its effects.

hypertensive crisis [Gk, *hyper* + L, *tendere,* to stretch; Gk, *krisi,* turning point], a sudden severe increase in blood pressure to a level exceeding 200/120 mm Hg, occurring most frequently in untreated hypertension and in patients who have stopped taking prescribed antihypertensive medication.

■ OBSERVATIONS: Characteristic signs include severe headache, vertigo, diplopia, tinnitus, nosebleed, twitching muscles, tachycardia or other cardiac dysrhythmia, distended neck veins, narrowed pulse pressure, nausea, and vomiting. The patient may be confused, irritable, or stuporous, and the condition may lead to convulsions, coma, myocardial infarction, renal failure, cardiac arrest, or stroke.

■ INTERVENTIONS: Treatment consists of antihypertensive drugs, administered intravenously or intramuscularly, and diuretics and may include the use of anticonvulsants, sedatives, and antiemetics, if indicated. The patient is usually placed on a cardiac monitor in a bed with the head elevated and is maintained in a quiet environment. The diet is low in calories, and sodium and fluids may be restricted. As the condition improves, the patient is permitted progressive ambulation but is carefully observed for symptoms of ortho-static hypotension, such as pallor, diaphoresis, or faintness.

■ NURSING CONSIDERATIONS: A major concern in caring for patients who have suffered a hypertensive crisis is observing and reporting of any sign of hypotension. In preparation for discharge the nurse advises the patient to recognize symptoms of any dramatic increase or decrease in blood pressure, to adhere to the prescribed diet and medication and to avoid fatigue, heavy lifting, smoking, and stressful situations.

hypertensive encephalopathy [Gk, *hyper* + L, *tendere,* to stretch; Gk, *enkephalos,* brain, *pathos,* disease], a set of symptoms, including headache, convulsions, and coma, associated with glomerulonephritis.

hypertensive retinopathy [Gk, *hyper;* L, *tendere,* to stretch, *rete net,* web; Gk, *pathos,* disease], a condition in which retinal changes occur in association with arterial hypertension. The changes may include blood vessel alterations, hemorrhages, exudates, and retinal edema.

hypertetraploid. See **hyperploid.**

hyperthermia /hī′pərthur′mē·ə/ [Gk, *hyper* + *therme,* heat], **1.** a much higher than normal body temperature induced therapeutically or iatrogenically. **2.** *nontechnical.* malignant hyperthermia. **3.** a nursing diagnosis accepted by the Seventh National Conference on the Classification of Nursing Diagnoses. The condition is defined as a state in which an individual's body temperature is elevated above his or her normal range. The increase in body temperature is the major defining characteristic. Minor characteristics include flushed skin, skin warm to the touch, increased respiratory rate, tachycardia, and seizures or convulsions. Related factors include exposure to a hot environment, vigorous activity, medications or anesthesia, inappropriate clothing, increased metabolic rate, illness or trauma, dehydration, and inability or decreased ability to perspire. See also **nursing diagnosis.**

hyperthyroidism /-thī′roidiz′əm/ [Gk, *hyper* + *thyreos,* shield, *eidos,* form], a condition characterized by hyperactivity of the thyroid gland. The gland is usually enlarged, secreting greater than normal amounts of thyroid hormones, and the metabolic processes of the body are accelerated. Nervousness, exophthalmos, tremor, constant hunger, weight loss, fatigue, heat intolerance, palpitations, and diarrhea may develop. Antithyroid drugs, as propylthiouracil or methimazole, are usually prescribed. Radioactive iodine may be prescribed in certain cases. Surgical ablation of the gland is sometimes necessary. Untreated hyperthyroidism may lead to death because of cardiac failure. See also **Graves' disease, thyroid storm, thyrotoxicosis.**

hypertonia /-tō′nē·ə/, **1.** abnormally increased muscle tone or strength. The condition is sometimes associated with genetic disorders, such as trisomy 18, and may be expressed in arm or leg deformities. **2.** a condition of excessive pressure, such as the intraocular pressure of glaucoma.

hypertonic /hī′pərton′ik/ [Gk, *hyper* + *tonos,* stretching], (of a solution) having a greater concentration of solute than another solution, hence exerting more osmotic pressure than that solution, such as a hypertonic saline solution that contains more salt than is found in intracellular and extracellular fluid. Cells shrink in a hypertonic solution. Compare **isotonic.**

hypertonic bladder [Gk, *hyper,* excessive, *tonos,* tone; AS, *blaedre*], a condition of hypertonicity in the detrusor muscle of the bladder, usually because of an irritant, such as a calculus.

hypertonic contracture, prolonged muscle contraction as a result of continuous nerve stimulation in spastic paralysis. Anesthesia or sleep eliminates this condition. Also called **functional contracture.**

hypertonicity /-tənis′itē/ [Gk, *hyper,* excessive, *tonos,* tone], **1.** (in ophthalmology) increased intraocular pressure. **2.** excessive tension of the arteries or muscles.

hypertonic saline, a saline solution that contains 1% to 15% sodium chloride (compared with normal saline at 0.9%). It is used as a bronchial lavage to stimulate sputum production by increasing movement of fluid into the mucosal blanket and also causing irritation that promotes coughing.

hypertonic solution, a solution that increases the degree of osmotic pressure on a semipermeable membrane.

hypertrichosis. See **hirsutism.**

hypertriglyceridemia. See **hyperchylomicronemia.**

hypertriploid. See **hyperploid.**

hypertrophic /-trof′ik/ [Gk, *hyper,* excessive, *trophe,* nourishment], pertaining to an increase in cell size.

hypertrophic angioma. See **hemangioendothelioma.**

hypertrophic cardiomyopathy, an abnormality in the structure and function of heart muscle characterized by gross hypertrophy of the interventricular septum and left ventricular free wall. Ventricular outflow obstruction results in impaired diastolic filling and reduced cardiac output. Signs and symptoms, such as fatigue and syncope, are often associated with exercise when the demand for increased cardiac output cannot be met. See also **idiopathic hypertrophic subaortic stenosis (IHSS).**

hypertrophic catarrh [Gk, *hyper* + *trophe,* nourishment; *kata,* down, *rhoia,* flow], a chronic condition characterized by inflammation and discharge from a mucous membrane, accompanied by the thickening of the mucosal and submucosal tissue. Compare **atrophic catarrh.** See also **catarrh.**

hypertrophic cicatrization. See **hypertrophic scarring.**

hypertrophic endometritis, *obsolete.* endometritis with endometrial hyperplasia.

hypertrophic gastritis, an inflammatory condition of the stomach characterized by epigastric pain, nausea, vomiting, and distention. It is differentiated from other forms of gastritis by the presence of prominent rugae (folds), enlarged glands, and nodules on the wall of the stomach. This condition often occurs with peptic ulcer, Zollinger-Ellison syndrome, or gastric hypersecretion.

hypertrophic gingivitis Gk, *hyper,* excessive; *trophe,* nourishment] a condition in which the gingiva become enlarged and inflamed, usually because of an underlying systemic disorder. The enlargement is the result of an increase in the size of cells rather than the number of cells. Compare **hyperplastic gingivitis, gingivitis.**

hypertrophic obstructive cardiomyopathy. See **hypertrophic cardiomyopathy; idiopathic hypertrophic subaortic stenosis.**

hypertrophic scarring, scarring caused by excessive formation of new tissue in the healing of a wound. It has the appearance of a hard, tumorlike keloid. Also called **hypertrophic cicatrization.**

hypertrophy /hīpur′trəfē/ [Gk, *hyper* + *trophe,* nourishment], an increase in the size of an organ caused by an increase in the size of the cells rather than the number of cells. Kinds of hypertrophy include **adaptive hypertrophy, compensatory hypertrophy, Marie's hypertrophy, physiologic hypertrophy,** and **unilateral hypertrophy.** Also

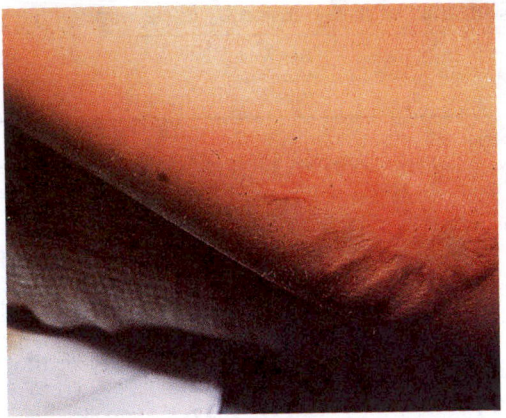

Hypertrophic scar *(Grossman, 1993)*

called **overgrowth.** Compare **atrophy, hyperplasia.** —**hypertrophic,** *adj.*

hypertrophy of heart [Gk, *hyper,* excessive, *trophe,* nourishment; AS, *heorte*], an increase in the size of the heart secondary to enlargement of the heart muscle, but without an increase in the size of the heart chambers.

hypertropia. See **anoopsia.**

hyperuricemia. See **gout.**

hyperventilation /-ven′tilā′shən/ [Gk, *hyper* + *ventilare,* to wave], a pulmonary ventilation rate that is greater than that metabolically necessary for the exchange of pulmonary gases. It is the result of an increased frequency of breathing, an increased tidal volume, or a combination of both, and causes excessive intake of oxygen and elimination of carbon dioxide. Hypocapnia and respiratory alkalosis then occur, leading to dizziness, faintness, numbness of the fingers and toes, possible syncope, and psychomotor impairment. Causes of hyperventilation include asthma or early emphysema; increased metabolism because of exercise, fever, hyperthyroidism, or infections; lesions of the central nervous system, as in cerebral thrombosis, encephalitis, head injuries, or meningitis; hypoxia or metabolic acidosis; hormones and drugs, such as epinephrine, progesterone, and salicylates; difficulties with mechanic respirators; and psychogenic factors, such as acute anxiety or pain. Compare **hypoventilation.** See also **respiratory center.**

hyperventilation tetany. See **tetany.**

hyperviscosity /-viskos′itē/ [Gk, *hyper,* excessive; L, *viscosus,* sticky], pertaining to an extremely viscous or thick fluid.

hypervitaminosis /-vī′təminō′sis/, an abnormal condition resulting from excessive intake of toxic amounts of one or more vitamins, especially over a long period of time. Serious effects may result from overdoses of fat-soluble vitamins A, D, E, or K, but adverse reactions are less likely with the water-soluble B and C vitamins, except when taken in megadoses. Compare **avitaminosis.** See also specific vitamins.

hypervolemia /-vōlē′mē·ə/ [Gk, *hyper* + L, *volumen,* paper roll; Gk, *haima,* blood], an increase in the amount of intravascular fluid, particularly in the volume of circulating blood or its components.

hypesthesia /hī′pəristhē′zhə/ [Gk, *hypo,* under, *aisthesis,* feeling], a decrease in sensation in response to stimulation of the sensory nerves or bodily organs or areas they innervate. Also called **hypoesthesia.–hypesthetic,** *adj.*

hypha /hī'fə/, *pl.* **hyphae** [Gk, *hyphe*, web], the threadlike structure of the mycelium in a fungus.

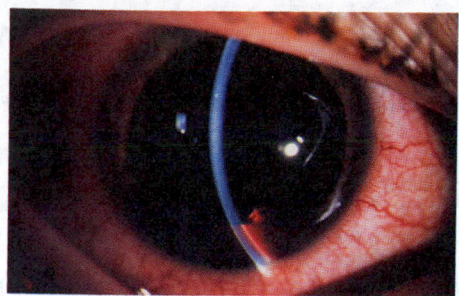

Hyphema *(Zitelli, 1992)*

hyphema /hīfē'mə/ [Gk, *hypo*, under *haima*, blood], a hemorrhage into the anterior chamber of the eye, usually caused by a blunt or percussive injury. Bedrest and a sedative are indicated. The patient is treated by an ophthalmologist, who evaluates the need for evacuation of the blood, and the use of mydriatic or miotic medications, or a carbonic anhydrase inhibitor. Glaucoma may result from recurrent bleeding. Also called **hyphemia** /hīfē'mē·ə/.

-hynagogic. See **hypnagogic.**

hypnagogic hallucination /hip'nəgoj'ik/ [Gk, *hypnos*, sleep, *agogos*, leading], a vivid image that occurs in the period between wakefulness and sleep. Compare **hallucination.**

hypnagogue /hip'nəgog/ [Gk, *hypnos* + *agogos*, leading], an agent or substance that tends to induce sleep or the feeling of dreamy sleepiness, as occurs before falling asleep. See also **hypnotic. –hypnagogic,** *adj.*

hypno-, a prefix meaning 'pertaining to sleep': *hypnagogic, hypnalgia.*

hypnoanalysis /hip'nə·anal'isis/ [Gk, *hypnos* + *analyein*, to loosen], the use of hypnosis as an adjunct to other techniques in psychoanalysis.

hypnosis /hipnō'sis/ [Gk, *hypnos*, sleep], a passive, trancelike state that resembles normal sleep during which perception and memory are altered, resulting in increased responsiveness to suggestion. The condition is usually induced by the monotonous repetition of words and gestures while the subject is completely relaxed.

hypnotherapy /hip'nəther'əpē/ [Gk, *hypnos* + *therapeia*, treatment], the use of hypnosis as an adjunct to other techniques in psychotherapy.

-hypnotic, a combining form meaning 'pertaining to sleep or hypnosis': *anhypnotic, autohypnotic, posthypnotic.*

hypnotics /hipnot'iks/ [Gk *hypnos* sleep], a class of drugs often used as sedatives.

hypnotic sleep /hipnot'ik/ [Gk, *hypnos*, sleep; ME, *slep*], sleep induced by hypnosis through the administration of hypnotic medicines.

hypnotic suggestion [Gk, *hypnos*, sleep; L, *suggerere*, to suggest], a suggestion implanted in the mind of a person under hypnosis.

hypnotic trance, an artificially induced sleeplike state, as in hypnosis.

hypnotism /hip'nətiz'əm/ [Gk, *hypnos*, sleep], the study or practice of inducing hypnosis.

hypnotist /hip'nətist/, one who practices hypnotism.

hypnotize /hip'nətīz/, **1.** to put into a state of hypnosis. **2.** to fascinate, entrance, or control through personal charm.

hypo-, hyp-, a prefix meaning 'under, below, beneath, deficient,' or, in chemistry, 'lacking oxygen': *hypochlorite, hypodermic, hypodontia.*

hypoacidity /hī'pō·əsid'itē/, a deficiency of acid.

hypoactivity /-aktiv'itē/ [Gk, *hypo*, under; L, *activus*, active], any abnormally diminished activity of the body or its organs, such as decreased cardiac output, thyroid secretion, or peristalsis. Compare **hyperactivity,** def. 1.

hypoacusis /-əkoo͞'sis/ [Gk, *hypo*, under, *akouein*, to hear], a reduced sensitivity to sounds; it could be conductive or sensorineural in nature.

hypoadrenalism. See **Addison's disease.**

hypoalbuminemia /-alboo͞'minē'mē·ə/, a condition of abnormally low levels of albumin in the blood. The condition may occur in celiac disease, tropical sprue, malnutrition, and some forms of liver or kidney impairment.

hypoalimentation /-al'iməntā'shən/ [Gk, *hypo* + L, *alimentum*, nourishment], a condition of insufficient or inadequate nourishment.

hypoallergenic /-al'ərjen'ik/ [Gk, *hypo*, under, *allos*, other, *ergein*, to work], pertaining to a lowered potential for producing an allergic reaction.

hypobarism /-ber'izəm/, air pressure that is significantly less than sea level normal of 760 mm Hg. See also **barotrauma, decompression sickness.**

hypobasemia /-basē'mē·ə/, reduced arterial bicarbonate concentration that is caused by metabolic or nonrespiratory factors.

hypobetalipoproteinemia /hī'pōbā'təlip'ōprō'tēnē'mē·ə/ [Gk, *hypo* + *beta*, second letter of Greek alphabet, *lipos*, fat, *proteios*, first rank, *haima*, blood], an inherited disorder in which there are less than normal amounts of beta-lipoprotein in the serum. Blood lipids and cholesterol are present at less than the expected levels regardless of dietary intake of fats. There are no clinical signs, and treatment is unnecessary. Compare **hyperbetalipoproteinemia.**

hypocalcemia /hī'pōkalsē'mē·ə/ [Gk, *hypo* + L, *calx*, lime; Gk, *haima*, blood], a deficiency of calcium in the serum that may be caused by hypoparathyroidism, vitamin D deficiency, kidney failure, acute pancreatitis, or inadequate plasma magnesium and protein. Mild hypocalcemia is asymptomatic. Severe hypocalcemia is characterized by cardiac dysrhythmias and tetany with hyperparesthesia of the hands, feet, lips, and tongue. The underlying disorder is diagnosed and treated, and calcium is given by mouth or by intravenous infusion. Hypocalcemia is also seen in dysmature newborns, in infants born of mothers with diabetes, or in normal babies delivered by normal mothers after a long or stressful labor and delivery. It is recognized by vomiting, twitching of extremities, poor muscle tone, high-pitched crying, and difficulty in breathing. See also **tetany. –hypocalcemic,** *adj.*

hypocalcemic tetany /-kalsē'mik/ [Gk, *hypo*, under, *calx*, calcium, *haima*, blood, *tetanos*, convulsive tension], a disease caused by an abnormally low level of calcium in the blood. It is characterized by hyperexcitability of the neuromuscular system. A common cause is a deficiency of parathyroid secretion.

hypocalciuria /-kal'siuŏŏr'ē·ə/ [Gk, *hypo,* under; L, *calx,* lime; Gk, *ouron,* urine], a diminished level of calcium in the urine.

hypocapnia /-kap'nē·ə/, an abnormally low arterial carbon dioxide level. Also called **hypocarbia.**

hypochloremia /-klôrē'mē·ə/ [Gk, *hypo* + *chloros,* green; *haima,* blood], a decrease in the chloride level in the blood serum, below 95 mEq/L. The condition may occur as a result of prolonged gastric suctioning.

hypochloremic alkalosis /-klôrē'mik/, a metabolic disorder resulting from increased blood bicarbonate secondary to loss of chloride from the body.

hypochlorhydria /-klôrhid'rē·ə/ [Gk, *hypo* + *chloros,* green, *hydor,* water], a deficiency of hydrochloric acid in the stomach's gastric juice.

hypochlorite poisoning /-klôr'īt/, toxic effects of ingestion of or skin contact with household or commercial bleaches or similar chlorinated products. Symptoms include pain and inflammation of the mouth and digestive tract, vomiting, and breathing difficulty. Skin contact may produce blisters. The recommended emergency treatment is dilution of ingested hypochlorite products with milk.

hypochlorous acid /-klôr'əs/ [Gk, *hypo* + *chloros,* green; L, *acidus,* sour], a greenish-yellow liquid derived from an aqueous solution of lime. An unstable compound that decomposes to hydrochloric acid and water, hypochlorous acid is used as a bleaching agent and disinfectant.

hypochondria, hypochondriac neurosis. See **hypochondriasis.**

hypochondriac /-kon'drē·ak/ [Gk, *hypo,* under, *chondros,* cartilage], **1.** pertaining to the region of the upper abdomen beneath the lower ribs. See **hypochondriac region. 2.** a person who is so preoccupied with health matters that this state of mind becomes a disability. **–hypochondriacal** /-kəndrī'əkəl/, *adj.*

hypochondriac region [Gk, *hypo* + *chondros,* cartilage; L, *regio,* direction], the part of the abdomen in the upper zone on both sides of the epigastric region and beneath the cartilages of the lower ribs. Also called **hypochondrium.** See also **abdominal regions.**

hypochondriasis /hī'pōkəndrī'əsis/ [Gk, *hypo* + *chondros,* cartilage, *osis,* condition], a chronic, abnormal concern about the health of the body, characterized by extreme anxiety, depression, and an unrealistic interpretation of real or imagined physical symptoms as indications of a serious illness or disease despite rational medical evidence that no disorder is present. The condition is caused by some unresolved intrapsychic conflict and may involve a specific organ, such as the heart, lungs, or eyes, or several body systems at various times or simultaneously. In severe cases, the distorted body-mind relationship is so strong that actual symptoms and disease may develop. Treatment usually consists of psychotherapy to uncover the underlying emotional conflict.

hypochondrium. See **hypochondriac region.**

hypochondroplasia /-kon'drōplā'zhə/, an inherited form of dwarfism that resembles a mild form of achondroplasia. It is relatively uncommon and is transmitted as an autosomal dominant trait.

hypochromic /hī'pōkrō'mik/ [Gk, *hypo* + *chroma,* color], pertaining to less than normal color. The term usually describes a red blood cell and characterizes anemias associated with decreased synthesis of hemoglobin. Compare **normochromic.** See also **hypochromic anemia, red cell indices.**

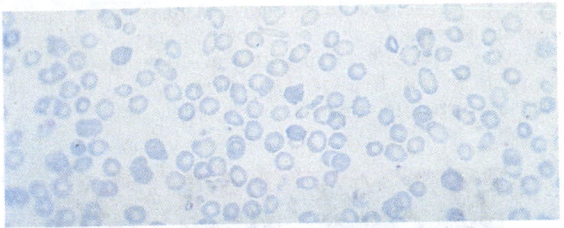

Hypochromic anemia *(Kamal, 1991/Courtesy Dr D Prangell)*

hypochromic anemia, a group of anemias characterized by a decreased concentration of hemoglobin in the red blood cells. See also **anemia, red cell indices.**

hypocycloidal motion /-sī'kloidəl/, (in computed tomography) a complex circular pattern of movement of the x-ray tube and film that results in excellent blurring of structures outside the focal plane and elimination of ghost images.

hypocytic leukemia. See **aleukemic leukemia.**

hypodermatoclysis. See **hypodermoclysis.**

hypodermic /-durmic/ [Gk, *hypo* + *derma,* skin], of or pertaining to the area below the skin, such as a hypodermic injection.

hypodermic implantation [Gk, *hypo,* under, *derma,* skin; L, *implantare,* to set into], the introduction of a solid medicine under the skin, usually on the chest or abdominal wall, to ensure local action or slow absorption.

hypodermic needle, a short, thin, hollow needle that attaches to a syringe for injecting a drug or medication under the skin or into vessels and for withdrawing a fluid, such as blood, for examination.

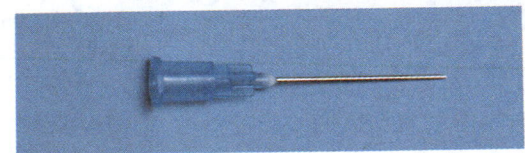

Hypodermic needle *(Potter, 1993)*

hypodermic syringe [Gk, *hypo,* under, *derma,* skin, *syrigx,* tube], an instrument designed to direct fluid under the skin into subcutaneous tissue through a fine hollow needle.

hypodermoclysis /hī'pōdərmok'lisis/ [Gk, *hypo* + *derma,* skin, *klysis,* flushing out], the injection of an isotonic or hypotonic solution into subcutaneous tissue to supply the patient with a continuous and large amount of fluid, electrolytes, and nutrients. The procedure is used to replace the loss or inadequate intake of water and salt during illness or surgery or after shock or hemorrhage and is performed only when the patient is unable to take fluids intravenously, orally, or rectally. The rate of absorption into the circulatory system is increased with the addition to the solution of the enzyme hyaluronidase. The most common sites of administration are the anterior thighs, the abdominal wall along the crest of the ilium, below the breasts in women, and directly over the scapula in children; sites should be changed when multiple infusions are given. The patient is placed in a comfortable position, because the procedure takes a long time. The nurse observes for signs of circulatory collapse, respiratory difficulty, and edema at the site of injection. Also called **hypodermatoclysis, interstitial infusion, subcutaneous infusion.**

hypodiploid. See **hypoploid.**

hypoesthesia. See **hypesthesia.**

hypofibrinogenemia /-fī′brinōjənē′mē·ə/ [Gk, *hypo* + L, *fibra*, fiber; Gk, *genein*, to produce, *haima*, blood], a deficiency of fibrinogen, a blood clotting factor, in the blood. The condition may occur as a complication of abruptio placentae.

hypofunction /-fungk′shən/ [Gk, *hypo*, under; L, *functio*, performance], a diminished or inadequate level of activity on the part of an organ system or its parts.

hypogammaglobulinemia /-gam′əglō′byəlinē′mē·ə/ [Gk, *hypo* + *gamma*, third letter in Greek alphabet; L, *globus*, small sphere; Gk, *haima*, blood], a less than normal concentration of gamma globulin in the blood, usually the result of increased protein catabolism or the loss of protein in the urine. The condition is associated with a decreased resistance to infection. Compare **agammaglobulinemia.**

hypogastric /-gas′trik/ [Gk, *hypo*, under, *gaster*, stomach], pertaining to the hypogastrium, or the lower abdominal region below the umbilical region and between the right and left iliac regions.

hypogastric artery. See **internal iliac artery.**

hypogastrium. See **pubic region.**

hypogenitalism /-jen′itəliz′əm/ [Gk, *hypo* + L, *genitalis*, fruitful], a condition of retarded sexual development caused by a defect in male or female hormonal production in the testis or ovary.

hypogeusia /-gōō′zē·ə/, reduced taste.

hypoglossal /-glos′əl/ [Gk, *hypo*, under, *glossa*, tongue], pertaining to nerves or other structures under the tongue.

hypoglossal nerve [Gk, *hypo* + *glossa*, tongue], either of a pair of cranial nerves essential for swallowing and for moving the tongue. Each nerve has four major branches, communicates with the vagus nerve, and connects to nucleus XII in the brain. Also called **nervus hypoglossus, twelfth cranial nerve.**

hypoglossus /-glos′əs/, **1.** a muscle that retracts and pulls down the side of the tongue. **2.** the hypoglossal nerve.

hypoglycemia /hī′pōglīsē′mē·ə/ [Gk, *hypo* + *glykys*, sweet, *haima*, blood], a less than normal amount of glucose in

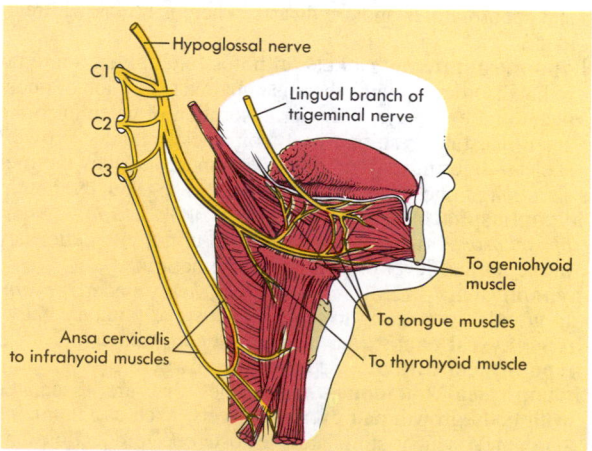

Hypoglossal nerve *(Seeley, 1992)*

Signs and symptoms of hypoglycemia

Sympathetic nervous system activity

Pallor	Palpitation	Weakness*
Perspiration*	Nervousness*	Trembling
Piloerection	Irritability	Hunger
Tachycardia		

Central nervous system activity

Headache	Fatigue
Blurred vision	Numbness of lips, tongue
Diplopia	Mental confusion*
Incoherent speech	Convulsions*
Emotional changes	Coma

*Signs most commonly reported by patients.
From Phipps WJ, Long BL, Woods NF, Cassmeyer VL: *Medical-surgical nursing: concepts and clinical practice,* ed 4. St Louis, 1991, Mosby.

the blood, usually caused by administration of too much insulin, excessive secretion of insulin by the islet cells of the pancreas, or dietary deficiency. The condition may result in weakness, headache, hunger, visual disturbances, ataxia, anxiety, personality changes, and, if untreated, delirium, coma, and death. The treatment is the administration of glucose in orange juice by mouth if the person is conscious or in an intravenous glucose solution if the person is unconscious. Compare **diabetic coma.**

hypoglycemic /-glīsē′mik/, [Gk, *hypo*, under, *glykys*, sweet, *haima*, blood], pertaining to or resembling a state of low blood sugar.

hypoglycemic agent any of a large heterogeneous group of drugs prescribed to decrease the amount of glucose circulating in the blood. Hypoglycemic agents include insulin, the sulfonylureas, and the biguanides. Insulin in its various forms is given parenterally and acts by increasing the use of carbohydrates and the metabolism of fats and protein. The sulfonylureas, including tolbutamide, tolazamide, chlorpropamide, and acetohexamide, act by stimulating the release of endogenous insulin from the pancreas.

hypoglycemic coma [Gk, *hypo*, under, *glykys*, sweet, *koma*, deep sleep], a loss of consciousness that results from abnormally low blood sugar levels.

hypogonadism /-gō′nədiz′əm/, a deficiency in the secretory activity of the ovary or testis. The condition may be primary, caused by a gonadal dysfunction involving the Leydig cells in the male, or secondary to a hypothalamic-pituitary disorder. Secondary hypogonadism is sometimes further differentiated into pituitary hypogonadism and hypothalamic hypogonadism.

hypoinsulinism /-in′səliniz′əm/ [Gk, *hypo*, under; L, *insula*, island (of Langerhans)], a deficiency of insulin secretion by cells of the pancreas and associated signs and symptoms of diabetes.

hypokalemia /hī′pōkəlē′mē·ə/ [Gk, *hypo* + L, *kalium*, potassium; Gk, *haima*, blood], a condition in which an inadequate amount of potassium, the major intracellular cation, is found in the circulating bloodstream. Hypokalemia is characterized by abnormal ECG, weakness, and flaccid paralysis and may be caused by starvation, treatment of diabetic acidosis, adrenal tumor, or diuretic therapy. Mild hypokalemia may resolve itself when the underlying disorder is corrected. Severe hypokalemia may be treated by the administration of potassium chloride, orally or parenterally, and by a diet high in potassium. Compare **hyperkalemia.** See also **electrolyte balance. hypokalemic,** *adj.*

hypokalemic alkalosis /-kalē'mik/, a pathologic condition resulting from the accumulation of base or the loss of acid from the body associated with a low level of serum potassium. The retention of alkali or the loss of acid occurs primarily in extracellular fluid, but the pH of intracellular fluid may also be subnormal. See also **hypokalemia.**

hypokalemic periodic paralysis [Gk, *hypo,* under; L, *kalium,* potassium; Gk, *peri,* near, *hodos,* way, *paralyein,* to be palsied], a state of recurring attacks of muscular weakness associated with low blood levels of potassium.

hypokinesia /-kīnē'zhə/, a condition of abnormally diminished motor activity.

hypokinetic /-kinet'ik/ [Gk, *hypo,* under, *kinesis,* movement], pertaining to diminished power of movement or motor function, which may or may not be accompanied by a mild form of paralysis.

hypolipoproteinemia /hī'pōlip'ōprō'tēnē'mē·ə/ [Gk, *hypo* + *lipos,* fat, *proteios,* first rank, *haima,* blood], a group of defects of lipoprotein metabolism that result in varying complexes of signs. Primary, or hereditary, hypolipoproteinemia factors include abnormal transport of triglycerides in the blood, low levels of high-density lipoproteins, high levels of low-density lipoproteins, and abnormal deposition of lipids in the body, especially in the kidneys and the liver. In some of the syndromes ocular, intestinal, and neurologic effects are also present. The condition also may be secondary to anemia, malabsorption syndromes, or malnutrition. Kinds of hypolipoproteinemias are **abetalipoproteinemia, hypobetalipoproteinemia, lecithin-cholesterol acyltransferase deficiency,** and **Tangier disease.**

hypomagnesemia /hī'pōmag'nisē'mē·ə/, an abnormally low concentration of magnesium in the blood plasma, resulting in nausea, vomiting, muscle weakness, tremors, tetany, and lethargy. Mild hypomagnesemia is usually the result of inadequate absorption of magnesium in the kidney or intestine, although it is also seen after prolonged parenteral feeding and during lactation. A more severe form is associated with malabsorption syndrome, protein malnutrition, and parathyroid disease. Magnesium salts to correct the deficiency may be given orally or intravenously.

hypomania /-mā'nē·ə/ [Gk, *hypo* + *mania,* madness], a mild degree of mania characterized by optimism, excitability, energetic, productive behavior, marked hyperactivity and talkativeness, heightened sexual interest, quick anger and irritability, and a decreased need for sleep. **—hypomaniac,** *n.,* **hypomanic,** *adj.*

hypometria /hī'pōmē'trē·ə/ [Gk, *hypo* + *metron,* measure], an abnormal condition, a form of dysmetria, characterized by a dysfunction of the power to control the range of muscular action, resulting in movements that fall short of the intended goals of the affected individual. Compare **hypermetria.**

hypomobility /-mōbil'itē/, a lack of normal movement of a joint or body part, as may result from an articular surface dysfunction or from disease or injury affecting a bone or muscle.

hypomorph /hī'pōmôrf/ [Gk, *hypo* + *morphe,* form], **1.** a person whose legs are disproportionately short in relation to the trunk and whose sitting height is greater in proportion than the person's standing height. **2.** (in genetics) a mutant allele that has a reduced effect on the expression of a trait but at a level too low to result in abnormal development. Also called **leaky gene.** Compare **amorph, antimorph, hypermorph.**

hypomotility /-mōtil'itē/ [Gk, *hypo,* under; L, *motare,* to move frequently], a state of diminished motility or loss of power to move about. Also called **hypokinesia.**

hyponatremia /hī'pōnatrē'mē·ə/ [Gk, *hypo* + L, *natrium,* sodium; Gk, *haima,* blood], a less than normal concentration of sodium in the blood, caused by inadequate excretion of water or by excessive water in the circulating bloodstream. In a severe case, the person may develop water intoxication, with confusion and lethargy, leading to muscle excitability, convulsions, and coma. Fluid and electrolyte balance may be restored by intravenous infusion of a balanced solution.

hypoosmolarity /hī'pō·os'mōler'itē/ [Gk, *hypo* + *osmos,* impulse], a state or condition of abnormally reduced osmolarity.

hypoparathyroidism /-per'əthī'roidiz'əm/ [Gk, *hypo* + *para,* beside, *thyreos,* shield, *eidos,* form], a condition of diminished parathyroid function, which can be caused by primary parathyroid dysfunction or by elevated serum calcium levels.

hypoperistalsis /-per'istal'sis/ [Gk, *hypo,* under, *peristellein,* to clasp], a state of abnormally slow motility of waves of alternate contraction and relaxation that impel contents forward through the digestive tract.

hypopharyngeal /-fərin'jē·əl/ [Gk, *hypo* + *pharynx,* throat], **1.** of, pertaining to, or involving the hypopharynx. **2.** situated below the pharynx.

hypopharynx /-fer'ingks/, the inferior portion of the pharynx, between the epiglottis and the larynx. It corresponds to the height of the epiglottis and is a critical dividing point in separating solids and fluids from air entering the region.

hypophonia /-fō'nē·ə/ [Gk, *hypo,* under, *phone,* voice], a weak or whispered voice.

hypophoria /-fôr'ē·ə/, a type of strabismus in which the patient may not show signs of ocular muscle imbalance until the affected eye is covered, resulting in a downward deviation. Otherwise, the central nervous system may attempt to compensate for the defect through a fusion of the images received from each of the eyes.

hypophosphatasia /hī'pōfos'fətā'zhə/ [Gk, *hypo* + *phosphoros,* lightbearing], congenital absence of alkaline phosphatase, an enzyme essential to the calcification of bone tissue. Affected newborns vomit, grow slowly, and often die in infancy. Children who survive have numerous skeletal abnormalities and are dwarfs. There is no known treatment.

hypophosphatemic rickets /hī'pōfos'fətē'mik/, a rare familial disorder in which there is impaired resorption of phosphate in the kidneys and poor absorption of calcium in the small intestine, resulting in osteomalacia, retarded growth, skeletal deformities, and pain. Treatment includes the prescription of phosphate and vitamin D, to be taken by mouth.

hypophosphaturia /-fos'fətoōr'ē·ə/ [Gk, *hypo,* under, *phosphoros,* bringer of light, *ouron,* urine], a deficiency in the normal level of phosphates in the urine.

hypophyseal /-fizē'əl, -fiz'ē·əl/ [Gk, *hypo,* under, *phyein,* to grow], pertaining to the hypophysis or pituitary body.

hypophyseal cachexia. See **panhypopituitarism.**

hypophyseal dwarf. See **pituitary dwarf.**

hypophyseal hormones, hormones that are associated with body growth and exercise effects, such as luteinizing hormone, which stimulates testosterone production and muscular hypertrophy, growth hormone, and antidiuretic hormone.

hypophysectomy /hīpof′əsek′təmē/ [Gk, *hypo* + *phyein*, to grow, *ektome*, excision], surgical removal of the pituitary gland. It may be performed to slow the growth and spread of endocrine-dependent malignant tumors or to excise a pituitary tumor. The gland is removed only if other treatment, such as x-ray therapy, radioactive implants, or cryosurgery, fails to destroy all pituitary tissue. General anesthesia is given and the gland is completely removed. Postoperative nursing care is as for a craniotomy. Hormone levels, including thyroid stimulating hormone, adrenocorticotropic hormone, and antidiuretic hormone, are monitored, and replacement therapy is begun as needed. Urinary output is measured every 2 hours for several days, and an amount in excess of 300 ml in any 2-hour period is reported. The patient is closely monitored for early signs of thyroid crisis, addisonian crisis, electrolyte imbalance, hemorrhage, and meningitis. —**hypophysectomize,** *v.*

hypophysis /hīpof′isis/ [Gk, *hypo*, under, *phyein*, to grow], the pituitary body (gland). The anterior lobe is sometimes identified as the **adenohypophysis** and the posterior lobe as the **neurohypophysis.**

hypophysis cerebri. See **pituitary gland.**

hypopigmentation /-pig′məntā′shən/ [Gk, *hypo* + L, *pigmentum*, paint], unusual lack of skin color, seen in albinism or vitiligo. Compare **hyperpigmentation.**

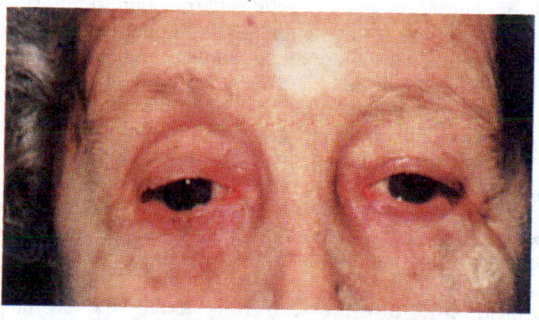

Hypopigmentation (Zacarian, 1985)

hypopituitarism /-pityoo′iteriz′əm/ [Gk, *hypo* + L, *pituita*, phlegm], an abnormal condition caused by diminished activity of the pituitary gland and marked by excessive deposits of fat and persistence or acquisition of adolescent characteristics. Serum levels of pituitary hormones are lower than normal.

hypoplasia /hī′pōplā′zhə/ [Gk, *hypo* + *plassein*, to mold], incomplete or underdeveloped organ or tissue, usually the result of a decrease in the number of cells. Kinds of hypoplasia are **cartilage-hair hypoplasia** and **enamel hypoplasia.** Also called **hypoplasty.** Compare **aplasia, hyperplasia.** See also **oligomeganephronia, osteogenesis imperfecta.** —**hypoplastic,** *adj.*

hypoplasia of the mesenchyme. See **osteogenesis imperfecta.**

-hypoplastic. See **hypoplasia.**

hypoplastic anemia /-plas′tik/, a broad category of anemias characterized by decreased production of red blood cells. Compare **aplastic anemia, polycythemia.** See also **anemia.**

hypoplastic dwarf. See **primordial dwarf.**

hypoplasty. See **hypoplasia.**

hypoploid /hī′pəploid/ [Gk, *hypo* + *eidos*, form], **1.** also **hypoploidic.** of or pertaining to an individual, organism, strain, or cell that has fewer than the normal haploid number or an exact multiple of the haploid number of chromosomes characteristic of the species. The result is unbalanced sets of chromosomes, which are referred to as hypodiploid, hypotriploid, hypotetraploid, and so on, depending on the number of multiples of the haploid chromosomes they contain. **2.** such an individual, organism, strain, or cell. Compare **hyperploid.** See also **monosomy.**

hypoploidy /hī′pōploi′dē/, any decrease in chromosome number that involves individual chromosomes rather than entire sets, resulting in fewer than the normal haploid number characteristic of the species, as in Turner's syndrome. Compare **hyperploidy.**

hypopnea /hīpop′nē·ə, hī′pōnē′ə/ [Gk, *hypo* + *pnoe*, breath], shallow or slow respiration. In well-conditioned athletes it may be normal and is accompanied by a slow pulse; otherwise, it is characteristic of damage to the brainstem, in which case it is accompanied by a rapid, weak pulse and is a grave sign. See also **respiratory rate.**

hypopotassemia /-pot′əsē′mē·ə/ [Gk, *hypo* + Dutch, *potasschen*, potash; Gk, *haima*, blood], a deficiency of potassium in the blood.

hypoproliferative anemias /-prolif′ərətiv′/, a group of anemias caused by inadequate production of erythrocytes. The condition is associated with protein deficiencies, renal diesease, and myxedema.

hypoproteinemia /hī′pōprō′tēnē′mē·ə/ [Gk, *hypo* + *proteios*, first rank, *haima*, blood], a disorder characterized by a decrease in the amount of protein in the blood to an abnormally low level, accompanied by edema, nausea, vomiting, diarrhea, and abdominal pain. It may be caused by an inadequate dietary supply of protein, by intestinal lymphangiectasia, or by renal failure. Also called **intestinal lymphangiectasia.**

hypoprothrombinemia /hī′pōprōthrom′binē′mē·ə/ [Gk, *hypo* + L, *pro*, before; Gk, *thrombos*, lump, *haima*, blood], an abnormal reduction in the amount of prothrombin (factor II) in the circulating blood, characterized by poor clot formation, longer bleeding time, and possible hemorrhage. The condition is usually the result of inadequate synthesis of prothrombin in the liver, most often the result of a deficiency of vitamin K caused by severe liver disease, or by anticoagulant therapy with the drug dicumarol, or in newborn infants. See also **blood clotting.**

hypoptyalism /hī′pōtī′əliz′əm/ [Gk, *hypo* + *ptyalon*, spittle], a condition in which there is a decrease in the amount of saliva secreted by the salivary glands. See also **hyposalivation, ptyalism.**

hypopyon /hīpō′pē·on/ [Gk, *hypo* + *pyon*, pus], an accumulation of pus in the anterior chamber of an eye, appearing as a gray fluid between the cornea and the iris. It may occur as a complication of conjunctivitis, herpetic keratitis, or corneal ulcer. (See Fig. p. 778.)

hyporeflexia /-riflek′sē·əl/ [Gk, *hypo* + L, *reflectere*, to bend backward], decreased reflex reactions.

hyposalivation /-sal′ivā′shən/ [Gk, *hypo* + L, *saliva*, spittle], a decreased flow of saliva that may be associated with dehydration, radiation therapy of the salivary gland regions, anxiety, the use of drugs, such as atropine and antihistamines, vitamin deficiency, various forms of parotitis, or various syndromes, such as Plummer-Vinson syndrome. Also called **xerostomia, asialorrhea.**

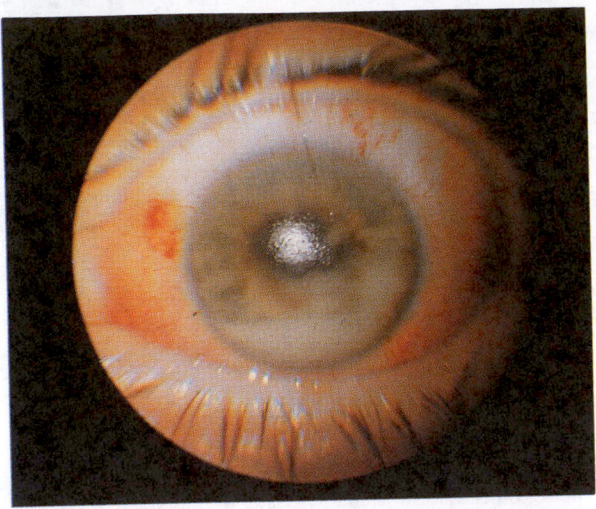

Hypopyon (Eagling, 1986)

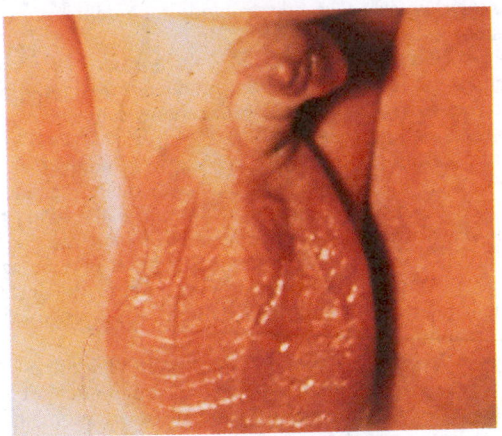

Hypospadias (Zitelli, 1992/Courtesy Dr Christine L Williams, New York Medical College)

hyposensitization. See **immunotherapy.**

hypospadias /hī′pəspā′dē·əs/ [Gk, *hypo* + *spadon*, a split], a congenital defect in which the urinary meatus is on the underside of the penis. Incontinence does not occur because the sphincters are not defective. The opening may be off center or anywhere along the underside of the penis or on the perineum. Surgical correction is performed as necessary for cosmetic, urologic, or reproductive indications. A corresponding defect in women is rare but recognized by the location of the urinary meatus in the vagina. Compare **epispadias.**

hypostatic /-stat′ik/ [Gk, *hypo* + *stasis*, standing still], pertaining to an accumulation of deposits of substances or congestion in a body area resulting from a lack of activity.

hypostatic lung collapse [Gk, *hypo*, under, *stasis*, standing still; AS, *lungen*; L, *collabi*, to fall together], a lung disorder in which the settling or pooling of fluids or suspended solids results in congestion caused by the effects of gravity in a dependent part.

hypostatic pneumonia, a type of pneumonia associated with elderly or debilitated people who remain in the same position for long periods. Gravity tends to accelerate fluid congestion in one area of the lungs, increasing the susceptibility to infection.

hyposthenic /hī′pōsthen′ik/, **1.** pertaining to a lack of strength or muscle tone. **2.** pertaining to a body type characterized by a slender build.

hypotelorism /hī′pōtel′əriz′əm/ [Gk, *hypo* + *tele*, far, *horizo*, separate], a developmental defect characterized by an abnormally decreased distance between two organs or parts. A kind of hypotelorism is **ocular hypotelorism.** Compare **hypertelorism.**

hypotension /-ten′shən/ [Gk, *hypo* + L, *tendere*, to stretch], an abnormal condition in which the blood pressure is not adequate for normal perfusion and oxygenation of the tissues. An expanded intravascular space, a decreased intravascular volume, or diminished cardiac output may be the cause.

hypotensive /-ten′siv/ [Gk, *hypo*, under; L, *tendere*, to stretch], pertaining to abnormally low blood pressure.

hypotensive anesthesia. See **deliberate hypotension.**

hypotetraploid. See **hypoploid.**

-hypothalamic. See **hypothalamus.**

hypothalamic amenorrhea /-thalam′ik/ [Gk, *hypo* + *thalamos*, chamber], cessation of menses caused by disorders that inhibit the hypothalamus from initiating the cycle of neurohormonal interactions of the brain, pituitary, and ovary necessary for ovulation and subsequent menstruation. Examples of causes are stress, anxiety, and acute weight loss. See **amenorrhea.**

hypothalamic hormones, a group of hormones secreted by the hypothalamus, including vasopressin, oxytocin, and the thyrotropin-releasing and gonadotropin-releasing hormones.

hypothalamic obesity [Gk, *hypo*, under, *thalamos*, chamber; L, *obesitas*, fatness], obesity that is caused by damage or a functional disturbance involving the hypothalamus.

hypothalamic-pituitary-adrenal axis, the combined system of neuroendocrine units that in a negative feedback network regulate the body's hormonal activities.

hypothalamus /hī′pōthal′əməs/ [Gk, *hypo* + *thalamos*, chamber], a portion of the diencephalon of the brain, forming the floor and part of the lateral wall of the third ventricle. It activates, controls, and integrates the peripheral autonomic nervous system, endocrine processes, and many somatic functions, such as body temperature, sleep, and appetite. Compare **epithalamus, metathalamus, subthalamus, thalamus. –hypothalamic,** *adj.*

hypothenar /hīpoth′ənär, hī′pōthē′när/ [Gk, *hypo* + *thenar*, palm], an eminence or fleshy elevation on the ulnar side of the palm of the hand.

hypothermal /-thur′mə/ [Gk, *hypo*, under, *therme*, heat], **1.** pertaining to a condition in which the body temperature is significantly below normal or has been reduced markedly for surgical or therapeutic purposes. **2.** pertaining to temperatures that are tepid to slightly warm.

hypothermia /hī′pōthur′mē·ə/ [Gk *hypo* + *therme* heat], **1.** an abnormal and dangerous condition in which the temperature of the body is below 95° F (35° C), usually caused by prolonged exposure to cold. Respiration is shallow and slow, and the heart rate is faint and slow. The person is very pale and may appear to be dead. People who are very old or very young, people who have cardiovascular problems, and people who are hungry, tired, or under the influence of alcohol are most susceptible to hypothermia. Treatment includes slowly warming the person. Hospitalization is necessary for evaluating and treating any metabolic abnormalities that may result from hypothermia. **2.** the deliberate and controlled reduction of body temperature with cooling mattresses or ice as preparation for some surgical procedures. **3.** a nursing diagnosis accepted by the Eighth National Conference on the Classification of Nursing Diagnoses. This diagnosis is defined as the state in which an individual's body temperature is reduced below his or her normal range but not below 96° F (rectal) or 97.5° F (rectal newborn). Major defining characteristics are mild shivering, cool skin, and moderate pallor. Minor characteristics include slow capillary refill, tachycardia, cyanotic nail beds, hypertension, and piloerection. Other related factors include exposure to a cool or cold environment, illness or trauma, inability or decreased ability to shiver, malnutrition, inadequate clothing, consumption of alcohol, medications causing vasodilation, evaporation from skin in cool environment, decreased metabolic rate, inactivity, and aging. See also **nursing diagnosis.**

hypothermia blanket, a covering used to conserve heat in the body of a patient suffering from hypothermia.

hypothermia therapy, the reduction of a patient's body temperature to counteract high prolonged fever caused by an infectious or neurologic disease, or, less frequently, as an adjunct to anesthesia in heart or brain surgery.
■ METHOD: Hypothermia may be produced by placing crushed ice around the patient, by immersing the body in ice water, by autotransfusing blood after it is circulated through coils submerged in a refrigerant, or, most commonly, by applying cooling blankets or vinyl pads containing coils through which cold water and alcohol are circulated by a pump. The cooling unit is placed in an open area; any kinks or twists in the tubing are removed, and the blanket is checked for leaks. The patient is wrapped in bath blankets and then covered with the cooling blanket; the patient's temperature, registered by means of a probe inserted in the rectum, is read and recorded before hypothermia is initiated, every 5 minutes until the desired reduction is achieved, and then every 15 minutes. The blood pressure, pulse, respirations, and neurologic status are checked every 5 to 10 minutes until the temperature is stabilized, then every 30 minutes for 2 hours, every 4 hours in the next 24 hours, and subsequently as required. Every 1 to 2 hours the patient is assisted in turning, coughing, and deep breathing. At similar intervals the chest is auscultated for breath sounds, and oral, nose, and skin care are administered; the skin is lubricated with oil or lotion before and during the procedure. An indwelling catheter is connected to a closed gravity drainage system, as ordered, and fluid intake and output are measured; if less than 30 ml of urine per hour is excreted, the physician is notified. If the patient's temperature is less than 90° F (32.2° C), the gag reflex is tested before any oral fluids or foods are administered. Naso-oral suction is performed as indicated; body alignment is maintained, and passive or active range-of-motion exercises are performed every 4 hours. Because shivering increases body heat, medication for its prevention, such as chlorpromazine hydrochloride, may be ordered. The patient is observed for medication reactions, decreased blood pressure, bradycardia, dysrhythmias, bradypnea, respiratory failure, unequal pupils, in-

creased intracranial pressure, changes in consciousness, intestinal ileus, and frostbite. Any changes in skin color or signs of edema and induration are reported to the physician immediately. At the termination of hypothermia, the cooling blanket is replaced by regular blankets and the patient usually warms at his or her own rate. As the patient's temperature approaches normal, the warming blankets are removed, but the temperature probe remains in place until the body temperature is stable.
■ NURSING INTERVENTION: The nurse administers hypothermia, carefully monitoring the patient's vital signs and any evidence of complications.
■ OUTCOME CRITERIA: Hypothermia used in the treatment of high fever associated with generalized severe infections reduces body heat by decreasing metabolism and also inhibits the multiplication of the causative pathogenic organisms. Patients with a high temperature caused by a neurologic disease may be maintained in a state of mild hypothermia (87° to 95° F or 30.6° to 35° C) for as long as 5 days. The procedure is successful if the fever is broken and complications do not occur.

hypothesis /hīpoth′isis/ [Gk, groundwork], (in research) a statement derived from a theory that predicts the relationship among variables representing concepts, constructs, or events. Kinds of hypotheses include **causal hypothesis, null hypothesis,** and **predictive hypothesis.**

hypothrombinemia /-throm′binē′mē·ə/, a deficiency of the clotting factor thrombin in the blood.

hypothyroid /-thī′roid/ [Gk, *hypo,* under, *thyreos,* shield, *eidos,* form], pertaining to or resembling thyroid deficiency.

hypothyroid dwarf. See **cretin dwarf.**

hypothyroidism /-thī′roidiz′əm/ [Gk, *hypo* + *thyreos,* shield, *eidos,* form], a condition characterized by decreased activity of the thyroid gland. It is caused by surgical removal of all or part of the gland, overdosage with antithyroid medication, decreased effect of thyroid releasing hormone secreted by the hypothalamus, decreased secretion of thyroid stimulating hormone by the pituitary gland, or by atrophy of the thyroid gland itself. Weight gain, mental and physical lethargy, dryness of the skin, constipation, arthritis, and slowing of the metabolic processes of the body may occur. Untreated, hypothyroidism leads to myxedema, coma, and death. Treatment is by administration of the deficient hormone. Dosage is adjusted to maintain normal serum levels of thyroid hormones. See **myxedema, Hashimoto's disease.**

hypotonia /-tō′nē·ə/ [Gk, *hypo,* under, *tonos,* stretching], a condition of diminished tone or tension that may involve any body structure.

hypotonic /hī′pōton′ik/ [Gk, *hypo* + *tonikos,* a stretching], (of a solution) having a smaller concentration of solute than another solution, hence exerting less osmotic pressure than that solution, such as a hypotonic saline solution that contains less salt than is found in intracellular or extracellular fluid. Cells expand in a hypotonic solution.

hypotonic saline [Gk, *hypo,* under, *tonos,* tone; L, *sal,* salt], a saline solution that is less than isotonic in strength.

hypotriploid. See **hypoploid.**

hypoventilation /-ven′tilā′shən/ [Gk, *hypo* + L, *ventilare,* to wave], an abnormal condition of the respiratory system, characterized by cyanosis, polycythemia, increased carbon dioxide arterial tension, and generalized decreased respiratory function. It occurs when the volume of air that enters

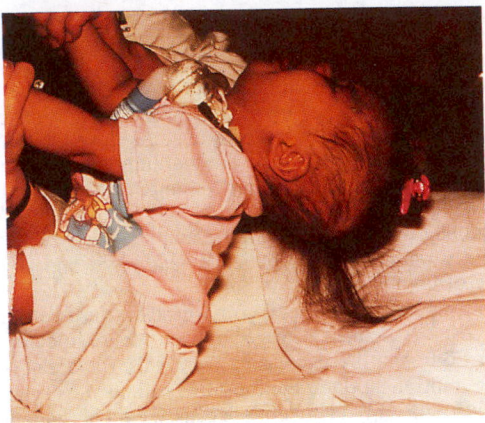

Hypotonic infant (Zitelli, 1992)

the alveoli and takes part in gas exchanges is not adequate for the metabolic needs of the body. Hypoventilation may be caused by uneven distribution of inspired air (such as in bronchitis), obesity, neuromuscular or skeletal disease affecting the thorax, decreased response of the respiratory center to carbon dioxide, and reduced functional lung tissue, such as in atelectasis, emphysema, and pleural effusion. The result of hypoventilation is hypoxia, hypercapnia, pulmonary hypertension with cor pulmonale, and respiratory acidosis. Treatment includes weight reduction in cases of obesity, artificial respiration, and possibly tracheostomy. Compare **hyperventilation.** See also **respiratory center.**

hypovitaminosis. See **avitaminosis.**

hypovolemia /-vōlē'mē·ə/ [Gk, *hypo* + L, *volumen*, whirl; Gk, *haima*, blood], an abnormally low circulating blood volume.

hypovolemic shock /-vōlē·mik/, a state of physical collapse and prostration caused by massive blood loss, circulatory dysfunction, and inadequate tissue perfusion. The loss of about one fifth of total blood volume in the affected individual can produce this condition. The common signs include low blood pressure, feeble pulse, clammy skin, tachycardia, rapid breathing, and reduced urinary output. The associated blood losses may stem from GI bleeding, internal hemorrhage, external hemorrhage, or excessive reduction of intravascular plasma volume and body fluids. Disorders that may cause hypovolemic shock are dehydration from excessive perspiration, severe diarrhea, protracted vomiting, intestinal obstruction, peritonitis, acute pancreatitis, and severe burns, which deplete body fluids. Associated effects may include metabolic acidosis with the accumulation of lactic acid, irreversible cerebral and renal damage, and disseminated intravascular coagulation. Treatment of hypovolemic shock focuses on prompt replacement of blood and fluid volumes, identification of bleeding sites, and the control of bleeding. Without fast aggressive treatment there is further collapse that can cause death. Compare **cardiogenic shock.** See also **electric shock, shock.**

hypoxemia /hī'poksē'mē·ə/ [Gk, *hypo* + *oxys*, sharp, *genein*, to produce, *haima*, blood], an abnormal deficiency of oxygen in the arterial blood. Symptoms of acute hypoxemia are cyanosis, restlessness, stupor, coma, Cheyne-Stokes breathing, apnea, increased blood pressure, tachycardia, and an initial increase in cardiac output that later falls, resulting in hypotension and ventricular fibrillation or

asystole. Chronic hypoxemia stimulates red blood cell production by the bone marrow, leading to secondary polycythemia. Hypoxemia caused by decreased alveolar oxygen tension or underventilation improves with oxygen therapy. Hypoxemia resulting from shunting of blood from the right side of the heart to the left side of the heart without exchange of gases in the lungs is treated with bronchial hygiene and positive end expiratory pressure therapy. Compare **hypoxia.** See also **anoxia, asphyxia.**

hypoxia /hīpok'sē·ə/ [Gk, *hypo* + *oxys*, sharp, *genein*, to produce], inadequate oxygen at the cellular level, characterized by cyanosis, tachycardia, hypertension, peripheral vasoconstriction, dizziness, and mental confusion. Mild hypoxia stimulates the peripheral chemoreceptors to increase heart and respiratory rates. However, the central mechanisms that regulate breathing fail in severe hypoxia, leading to irregular respiration, Cheyne-Stokes breathing, apnea, and respiratory and cardiac failure. Increased sensitivity to the depressant effect on the respiratory system by certain drugs is common in chronic hypoxia, resulting in severe depression or apnea from relatively small doses of opiates. If the amounts of oxygen are not adequate for aerobic cellular metabolism, energy is provided by less efficient anaerobic pathways that produce metabolites other than carbon dioxide and water. The tissues most sensitive to hypoxia are the brain, heart, pulmonary vessels, and liver. Treatment may include cardiotonic and respiratory stimulant drugs, oxygen therapy, mechanic ventilation, and frequent analysis of blood gases. Compare **hypoxemia.** See also **anoxia, chemoreceptor, hyperventilation, respiratory center.**

hypoxic drive /-hīpok'sik/, the low arterial oxygen pressure stimulus to respiration that is mediated through the carotid and aortic bodies.

hypsi-, a prefix meaning 'high': *hypsicephalia, hypsiconchous, hypsistaphylie.*

hypsibrachycephaly /hips'ibrakisef'əlē/ [Gk, *hypsi*, high, *brachys*, short, *kephale*, head], the condition of having a skull that is high with a broad forehead. See also **brachycephaly, oxycephaly.** —**hypsibrachycephalic,** *adj., n.*

hypsicephaly. See **oxycephaly.**

hypso-, a prefix meaning 'pertaining to height': *hypsonosus, hypsophobia, hypsotherapy.*

hyster-. See **hystero-.**

hysterectomy /his'tərek'təmē/ [Gk, *hystera*, womb, *ektome*, excision], surgical removal of the uterus, performed to remove fibroid tumors of the uterus or to treat chronic pelvic inflammatory disease, severe recurrent endometrial hyperplasia, uterine hemorrhage, and precancerous and cancerous conditions of the uterus. Types of hysterectomy include **total hysterectomy,** in which the uterus and cervix are removed, and **radical hysterectomy,** in which ovaries, oviducts, lymph nodes, and lymph channels are removed with the uterus and cervix. Menstruation ceases after either type is performed. A vaginal douche may be given preoperatively. During surgery, the uterus is excised and removed, either through the abdominal wall or through the vagina. One or both ovaries and oviducts may be removed at the same time. Postoperatively, the nurse will frequently observe the abdominal dressing, if present, for bleeding. Food and oral fluids are restricted to prevent abdominal distention. Toe to knee elastic stockings or bandages may be used to prevent circulatory stasis. The lower half of the bed is kept flat, and the patient is instructed to avoid sharply flexing the thighs or knees, because thrombophlebitis of the blood vessels of the pelvis and upper thigh is a frequent complication. Low back pain or scanty urine may indicate a ligated ureter. A kind of hysterectomy is **cesarean hysterectomy.** Compare **hysterosalpingo-oophorectomy.** **–hysterectomize,** *v.*

hysteresis /his′tərē′sis/ [Gk, *hysterein*, to be late], **1.** a lagging or retardation of one of two associated phenomena, or a failure to act in unison. **2.** the influence of the previous condition or treatment of the body on its subsequent response to a given force, as in the example of the elastic property of a lung. At any given lung volume, the elastic recoil pressure within the airways during expiration is less than that which exists at the same lung volume during inspiration.

hysteria /histir′ē·ə/ [Gk, *hystera*, womb], a general state of tension or excitement in a person or a group, characterized by unmanageable fear and temporary loss of control over the emotions.

hysteric /hister′ik/ [Gk, *hystera*, womb], pertaining to or resembling hysteria. Also **hysterical.**

hysterical aphonia [Gk, *hystera*, womb, *a*, not, *phone*, voice], an inability to produce vocal sounds, usually psychogenic in nature.

hysterical blindness. See **psychic blindness.**

hysterical deafness. See **psychic deafness.**

hysterical tremor [Gk, *hystera*, womb; L, *tremere*, to tremble], **1.** a fine tremor in one extremity or of a generalized nature that may be an expression of fear, anxiety, or hysteria. **2.** a coarse irregular tremor that increases with voluntary movements. **3.** a tremor that is transient and is caused by exposure to drugs or toxic substances rather than an organic disorder.

hysteric amaurosis [Gk, *hystera* + *amauroein*, to darken], monocular or, more rarely, binocular blindness occurring after an emotional shock. It may last for hours, days, or months.

hysteric ataxia [Gk, *hystera*, womb, *ataxia*, lack of order], a loss of control over voluntary movements in walking or standing although the involved muscles function normally when the person is lying or sitting down. See also **astasia-abasia.**

hysteric chorea [Gk, *hystera*, womb, *choreia*, dance], a condition in which an individual shows choreiform movements, usually associated with the person's occupation, although the actions are the result of hysteria rather than true chorea.

hysteric lethargy [Gk, *hystera* + *lethargia*, drowsiness], a sleep induced by hypnosis. See also **hypnosis, lethargy.**

hysteric paralysis [Gk, *hystera*, womb, *paralyein*, to be palsied], a loss of movement or muscular weakness that is due to hysteria rather than an identifiable organic defect.

hysteric personality. See **histrionic personality.**

hysteritis /his′tərī′tis/ [Gk, *hystera*, womb, *itis*, inflammation], an inflammation of the uterus.

hystero-, hyster-, a combining form meaning 'pertaining to the uterus': *hysterocarcinoma, hysterocleisis, hysterolith.*

hysterogram /his′tərōgram′/ [Gk, *hystera* + *gramma*, record], the radiographic record of a uterus made after the injection of a contrast medium into the uterine cavity. See also **hysterosalpingogram.**

hysterography /his′tərog′rəfē/ [Gk, *hystera*, womb, *graphein*, to record], the use of x-ray film and other instruments to make a medical assessment of the condition of the uterus.

hysterolaparotomy /his′tərōlap′ərot′əmē/ [Gk, *hystera* + *lapara*, loin, *temnein*, to cut], abdominal hysterectomy or hysterotomy.

hystero-oophorectomy /-ō′əfərek′təmē/ [Gk, *hystera*, womb, *oophoron*, ovary, *ektome*, cutting out], the surgical removal of both the uterus and the ovaries.

hysteropathy /his′tərop′əthē/ [Gk, *hystera*, womb, *pathos*, disease], any disease of the uterus.

hysterosalpingogram /his′tərō′salping′gōgram′/ [Gk, *hystera* + *salpinx*, tube, *gramma*, record], an x-ray film of the uterus and the fallopian tubes using gas or a radiopaque substance introduced through the cervix to allow visualization of the cavity of the uterus and the passageway of the tubes. A blockage of a structure is demonstrated on the film because the radiopaque substance cannot pass to the more distal structures and escape from the ends of the tubes into the peritoneal cavity. Serial hysterosalpingograms are useful in the diagnosis of the cause of infertility.

hysterosalpingography /his′tərōsal′ping·gog′rəfē/, a method of producing x-ray images of the uterus and fallopian tubes as part of the diagnosis of abnormalities in the reproductive tract of a nonpregnant woman. The technique outlines the size, shape, and position of the organs, including any tumors, fistulas, or polyps. It also reveals any obstructions in the fallopian tubes.

hysterosalpingo-oophorectomy /-salping′gō·ō′əfərek′-təmē/ [Gk, *hystera* + *salpinx*, tube; *oophoron*, ovary, *ektome*, excision], surgical removal of one or both ovaries and oviducts along with the uterus, performed commonly to treat malignant neoplastic disease of the reproductive tract and chronic endometriosis, and routinely done with a hysterectomy on menopausal or postmenopausal women. To avoid the severe symptoms of sudden menopause, a portion of one ovary is left, unless a malignancy is present. The uterus, one or both oviducts, and one or both ovaries are removed. If both ovaries are removed and no malignancy is present, estrogen replacement therapy is often begun immediately. Elastic stockings or bandages may be applied to the legs twice a day to prevent circulatory stasis because thrombophlebitis of the blood vessels of the pelvis or thigh is a frequent complication. The lower half of the bed is kept flat, and the patient is instructed to avoid flexing of the thighs or knees. Low back pain or scanty urine may indicate a ligated ureter. Compare **hysterectomy.**

hysteroscopy /his′təros′kəpē/ [Gk, *hystera* + *skopein*, to look], direct visual inspection of the cervical canal and uterine cavity through a hysteroscope. Hysteroscopy is performed to examine the endometrium, to secure a specimen for biopsy, to remove an intrauterine device, or to excise cervical polyps. The endoscope is passed through the vagina and into the uterus, and the surrounding tissues are examined. The procedure is contraindicated in pregnancy, acute pelvic inflammatory disease, chronic upper genital tract infection, recent uterine perforation, and known or suspected cervical malignancy. **–hysteroscope,** *n.,* **hysteroscopic,** *adj.*

hysterospasm /his′tərōspaz′əm/ [Gk, *hystera*, womb, *spasmos*], a spasmodic contraction of the uterus.

hysterotome /his′tərotom′/ [Gk, *hystera*, womb, *temnein*, to cut], a surgical knife used for certain procedures involving the uterus.

hysterotomy /his′tərot′əmē/ [Gk, *hystera* + *temnein*, to cut], surgical incision of the uterus, performed as a method of abortion in a pregnancy beyond the first trimester of gestation in which a saline-injection abortion was incomplete, or in which a tubal sterilization is to be done with the abortion. During surgery, the lower segment of the uterus is incised, and the products of conception are withdrawn. Postoperative care includes close observation for excessive vaginal bleeding.

hysterovaginoenterocele /-vaj'inō·en'tərōsēl'/ [Gk, *hystera*, womb; L, *vagina*, sheath; Gk, *enteron*, bowel, *kele*, hernia], a hernia involving the uterus, vagina, and intestines.

Hytone, a trademark for a glucocorticoid (hydrocortisone), used in a topical ointment for dermatitis.

Hz, abbreviation for **hertz.**

HZV, abbreviation for *herpes zoster virus*. See **chickenpox, herpes zoster.**

I, 1. symbol for *inspired gas.* **2.** symbol for the element iodine.

¹³¹I, symbol for *radioactive iodine, atomic weight 131.*

¹³²I, symbol for *radioactive iodine, atomic weight 132.*

-i, a plural-forming suffix used in native and later scientific Latin words: *bacilli, bronchi, plumbi,* and in scientific terms derived through Latin from Greek: *encephali, pylori, tympani.*

-ia, a suffix meaning a 'specified condition of a disease or process': *athrombia, phrenoblabia, pontobulbia.*

IABP, abbreviation for **intraaortic balloon pump.**

I.A.D.R., abbreviation for **International Association for Dental Research.**

I and O, abbreviation for *intake and output.*

-iasis, a suffix meaning 'the formation or presence of an abnormal condition or disease': *dicrocoeliasis, elephantiasis.*

-iatria. See **-iatry.**

-iatric, -iatrical, a combining form meaning 'relating to medicine, physicians, or to medical treatment': *neuropsychiatric, orthopsychiatric, pithiatric.*

-iatrist, -iatrician, a combining form meaning 'one who treats or a physician': *hydriatrist, pediatrist, podiatrist.*

iatro-, a combining form meaning 'pertaining to a physician or to treatment': *iatrogenic, iatrophysics, iatrotechnics.*

iatrogenic /ī′atrōjen′ik, yat-/ [Gk, *iatros,* physician, *genein,* to produce], caused by treatment or diagnostic procedures. An iatrogenic disorder is a condition caused by medical personnel or procedures or through exposure to the environment of a health-care facility, including fears instilled in patients by remarks or questions of examining physicians. See also **nosocomial. –iatrogenesis, iatrogeny** *n.*

iatrology, the science of medicine.

-iatry, -iatria, a combining form meaning a '(specified) type of medical treatment, the medical profession or physicians': *andriatry, pediatry, pithiatry.*

I band [ME, *band,* flat strip], an isotropic band of striated muscle fiber that appears dark in polarized light but light when stained.

IBC, abbreviation for *iron-binding capacity.*

-ible. See **-able.**

ibuprofen /ībyoo′prəfin/, a nonsteroidal antiinflammatory agent.

■ INDICATIONS: It is prescribed in the treatment of rheumatoid and osteoarthritis conditions, muscle aches, and menstrual cramps.

■ CONTRAINDICATIONS: Renal dysfunction, disorders of the GI tract, or known hypersensitivity to this drug, to other nonsteroidal antiinflammatory drugs, or to aspirin prohibits its use.

■ ADVERSE EFFECTS: Among the more serious adverse reactions are GI disturbances, gastric or duodenal ulceration,

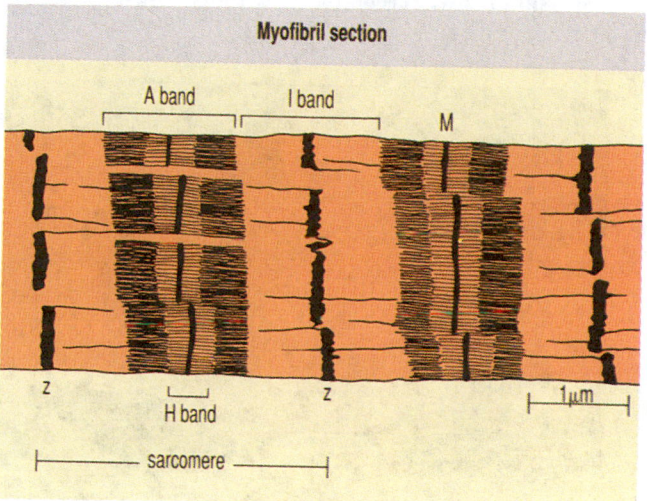

Myofibril section

I band (Epstein, 1992)

dizziness, skin rash, and tinnitus. Ibuprofen may interact with other drugs.

IBW, abbreviation for *ideal body weight.*

IC, abbreviation for **inspiratory capacity.**

-ic, -ac, a suffix meaning 'pertaining to, similar to': *allelic, cadaveric, hypochondriac.*

-icam, a suffix for antiinflammatory agents of the isoxicam group.

ICD, 1. abbreviation for **intraventricular conduction defect. 2.** abbreviation for *International Classification of Diseases.*

ICDA, abbreviation for *International Classification of Diseases Adapted for Use in the United States.*

Iceland disease /īs′land/, a group of symptoms associated with effects of a viral infection of the nervous system, including muscular pain and weakness, depression, and sensory changes. It affects mainly young adults. The exact cause is unknown. Also called **benign myalgic encephalomyelitis, chronic fatigue syndrome, royal free disease.**

ice pack [ME, *is + pakke*], a container of crushed ice used to reduce tissue temperatures, relieve pain, soothe inflamed tissues or control bleeding.

ICF, abbreviation for **intermediate care facility.**

ICF/MR, abbreviation for **intermediate care facility for the mentally retarded.**

ichthammol /ik′thəmôl/, a topical antiinfective used for treating certain skin diseases.

ichthyo-, a combining form meaning 'pertaining to fish': *ichthyocolla, ichthyophagy, ichthyotoxic.*

ichthyoid /ik′thē·oid/ [Gk, *ichthys,* fish, *eidos* form], pertaining to objects or structures that are fish-shaped or fish-like.

ichthyosis /ik′thē·ō′sis/ [Gk, *ichthys,* fish, *osis,* condition], any of several inherited dermatologic conditions in which the skin is dry, hyperkeratotic, and fissured, resembling fish scales. It usually appears at or shortly after birth and may be part of one of several rare syndromes. Some types respond temporarily to bath oils, topical retinoic acid, or propylene glycol. A rare acquired variety occurs in adults accompanying a lymphoma or multiple myeloma. Also called **fish skin disease, xeroderma.** **—ichthyotic,** *adj.*

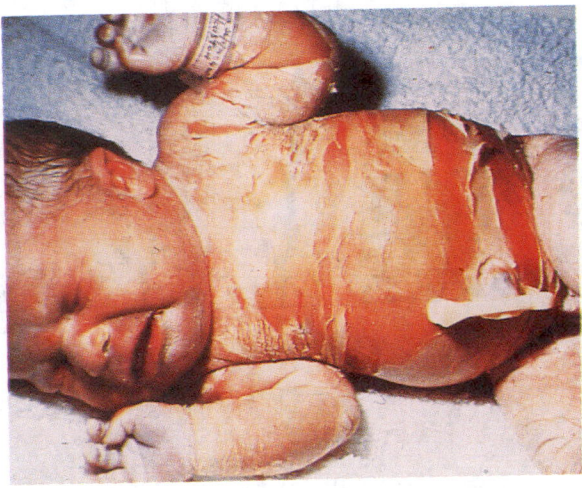

Ichthyosis
(McKee, 1993/Courtesy Dr M Beare, Royal Victoria Hospital, Belfast)

ichthyosis congenita, ichthyosis fetalis. See **lamellar exfoliation of the newborn.**

ichthyosis fetus. See **harlequin fetus.**

ichthyosis vulgaris [Gk, *ichthys, osis;* L, *vulgaris,* common], a hereditary skin disorder characterized by large,

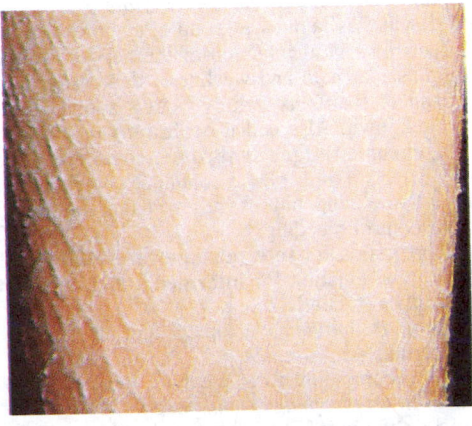

Ichthyosis vulgaris *(Zitelli, 1992)*

dry, dark scales that cover the face, neck, scalp, ears, back, and extensor surfaces but not the flexor surfaces of the body. The condition is transmitted as an autosomal dominant trait; not present at birth, it appears several months to 1 year after birth. Management consists of topical application of emollients and the use of keratolytic agents to facilitate removal of the scales. Also called **ichthyosis simplex.** See also **sex-linked ichthyosis.**

-ichthyotic. See **ichthyosis.**

-ician, a suffix meaning a 'specialist in a field': *clinician, pediatrician, technician.*

ICN, abbreviation for **International Council of Nurses.**

icon /ī′kən/, an image on the screen of a computer terminal representing a specific command. Also spelled **eikon.**

ICP, abbreviation for **intracranial pressure.**

-ics, a combining form meaning the 'systematic formulation of a body of knowledge': *bionomics, osmics, psychics.*

I.C.S., abbreviation for **International Congress of Surgeons.**

ICSH, abbreviation for **interstitial cell-stimulating hormone.** See **luteinizing hormone.**

ictal /ik′təl/ [Gk, *ikteros,* jaundice], pertaining to a sudden, acute onset, as convulsions of an epileptic seizure.

icteric /ikter′ik/ [Gk, *ikteros,* jaundice], pertaining to or resembling jaundice.

icterus. See **jaundice.**

icterus gravis neonatorum /ik′tərəs/ [Gk, *ikteros,* jaundice; L, *gravis,* weight, *neonatus,* newborn], a hemolytic jaundice of the newborn caused by incompatibility between the mother's serum and the red corpuscles of the infant.

icterus index [Gk, *ikteros;* L, *index,* pointer], a liver function test in which the blood serum is compared in intensity of color with that of potassium dichromate, normal being recorded in a numeric range of 3 to 5. When an excessive amount of bilirubin is present and jaundice becomes apparent, the index is usually 15 or higher; subnormal values are associated with various anemias.

icterus neonatorum, a jaundice condition in a newborn infant.

ictus /ik′təs/, *pl.* **ictuses, ictus** [L, stroke], **1.** a seizure. **2.** a cerebrovascular accident. **—ictal, ictic,** *adj.*

-ictal, a combining form meaning 'to be caused by a sudden attack, blow, or stroke': *postictal.*

icter-, a combining form meaning 'pertaining to jaundice': *icterohepatitis.*

ICU, abbreviation for **intensive care unit.**

id [L, it], **1.** (in psychoanalysis) the part of the psyche functioning in the unconscious that is the source of instinctive energy, impulses, and drives. It is based on the pleasure principle and has strong tendencies toward self-preservation. Compare **ego, superego. 2.** the true unconscious.

ID, abbreviation for *infectious disease.*

-id, **1.** a suffix meaning 'pertaining to a structure or body': *plasmid, protoconid, talonid, trigonid.* **2.** a suffix 'pertaining to a member of a group': *tuberculid.*

IDDM, abbreviation for **insulin-dependent diabetes mellitus.**

-ide, a suffix meaning 'a compoound of': *chloride, monoxide, sulfide.*

idea [Gk, form], any thought, concept, intention, or impression that exists in the mind as a result of awareness, understanding, or other mental activity.

ideal gas law /īdē′əl/ [Gk, *idea*, form, *chaos*, gas; AS, *lagu*, law], the rule that PV = nRT, with the product of pressure (P) and volume (V) equal to the product of the number of moles of gas (n), temperature (T), and a gas constant (R).

idealized image /īdē′əlizd/, a self-concept of a person with a compulsive craving for perfection and admiration. It results in high unrealistic and unattainable goals.

idea of influence, an idea held less firmly than a delusion, often seen in paranoid disorders, that external forces or persons are controlling one's thoughts, actions, and feelings.

idea of persecution, an idea held less firmly than a delusion, often seen in paranoid disorders, that one is being threatened, discriminated against, or mistreated by other persons or by external forces.

idea of reference, a delusion that the statements or actions of others refer to oneself, usually taken to be depreciatory, often seen in paranoid disorders. Also called **delusion of reference, referential idea.**

ideational apraxia /ī′dē·ā′shənəl/ [Gk, *idea*, form; *a*, *prassein*, not to do], a condition in which the conceptual process is lost, often because of a lesion in the submarginal gyrus of the parietal lobe. The individual is unable to formulate a plan of movement and does not know the proper use of an object because of a lack of perception of its purpose. There is no loss of motor movement, but the reason for the movement is confused. Also called **sensory apraxia.** See also **apraxia.**

idée fixe. See **fixed idea.**

identical twins. See **monozygotic twins.**

identification /īden′tifikā′shən/ [L, *idem*, the same, *facere*, to make], an unconscious defense mechanism by which a person patterns his or her personality on that of another person, assuming the person's qualities, characteristics, and actions. The process is a normal function of personality development and learning, and it contributes to the acquisition of interests and ideals.

identity /īden′titē/, a component of self-concept characterized by one's persisting consciousness of being oneself, separate and distinct from others. **Identity diffusion** is a lack of clarity and consistency in one's perception of the self, resulting in a high degreee of anxiety.

identity crisis [L, *idem*, the same; Gk, *krisis*, turning point], a period of disorientation concerning an individual's sense of self and role in society, occurring most frequently in the transition from one stage of life to the next.

identity diffusion. See **identity.**

ideo- [Gr, *idea*], a prefix meaning 'pertaining to ideas': *ideogram.*

ideokinetic apraxia. See **ideomotor apraxia.**

ideology /ī′de·ol′əjē/ [Gk, *idea*], a scheme of ideas or systematic organization of ideas associated with doctrine and philosophy.

ideomotor apraxia /īdē·əmō′tor/ [Gk, *idea* + L, *motare*, to move about; Gk *a*, *prassein*, not to do], the inability to translate an idea into motion, resulting from some interference with the transmission of the appropriate impulses from the brain to the motor centers. There is no loss of the ability to perform an action automatically, such as tying the shoelaces, but the action cannot be performed on request. The condition is often caused by diffuse cortical disease. Also called **ideokinetic apraxia, limb-kinetic apraxia, transcortical apraxia.** See also **apraxia.**

ideophobia /-fō′bē·ə/ [Gk, *idea* + *phobos*, fear], an anx-

iety disorder characterized by the irrational fear or distrust of ideas or reason. See also **phobia.**

idio-, a prefix meaning 'private, distinctive, peculiar,: *idiopathic.*

idiocrasy. See **idiosyncrasy.**

idiocy /id′ē·əsē/ [Gk, *idios*, ignoramus], an obsolete term for the lowest level of human intelligence or mental ability. Previously, the term was defined to include persons with an IQ of less than 20 and a maximum social and intellectual level of a 2-year-old.

idiogram /id′ē·əgram′/, a diagram or graphic representation of a karyotype, showing the number, relative sizes, and morphology of the chromosomes of a species, individual, or cell.

idiojunctional rhythm /-jungk′shənəl/ [Gk, *idios*, own; L, *jungere*, to join; Gk, *rhythmos*], a heart rhythm emanating from the AV junction but without retrograde conduction to the atria.

idiomere. See **chromomere.**

idiopathic /-path′ik/ [Gk, *idios* + *pathos*, disease], without a known cause.

idiopathic disease, a disease that develops without an apparent or known cause, although it may have a recognizable pattern of signs and symptoms and may be curable.

idiopathic gangrene [Gk, *idios*, own, *pathos*, disease, *gaggraina*], a gangrenous condition of unknown cause.

idiopathic hypertrophic subaortic stenosis (IHSS), a cardiomyopathic disorder, usually involving the left ventricle of the heart, that obstructs emptying. Also called **hypertrophic cardiomyopathy.**

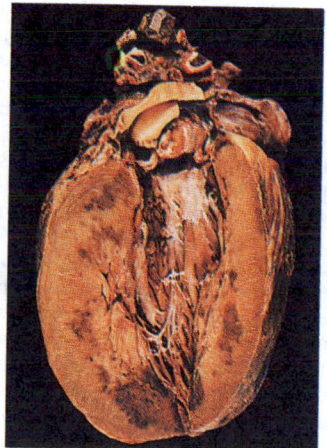

Idiopathic hypertrophic subaortic stenosis
(Fletcher, 1987)

idiopathic multiple pigmented hemorrhagic sarcoma. See **Kaposi's sarcoma.**

idiopathic nephrotic syndrome [Gk, *idios*, own, *pathos*, disease, *nephros*, kidney, *syn* together, *dromos*, course], a kidney disease of unknown origin, characterized by hematuria, albuminuria, edema, and blood pressure, and changes in the glomeruli capillaries.

idiopathic neuralgia [Gk, *idios*, own, *pathos*, disease, *neuron*, nerve, *algos*, pain], a form of neuralgia that occurs without any identifiable structural nerve lesion.

idiopathic pericarditis [Gk, *idios*, own, *pathos*, disease, *peri*, near, *kardia*, heart, *itis*, inflammation], an inflammation of the pericardium that occurs without a known cause.

idiopathic pulmonary fibrosis [Gk, *idios*, own, *pathos*, disease; L, *pulmoneus*, the lungs, *fibra*, fiber], fibrosis of the lungs that may follow an earlier inflammation or disease, such as tuberculosis or pneumoconiosis.

idiopathic respiratory distress syndrome. See **respiratory distress syndrome of the newborn.**

idiopathic scoliosis, an abnormal condition characterized by a lateral curvature of the spine. It is the most common type of scoliosis, evident in 70% of all patients with scoliosis and up to 80% of those with structural scoliosis. It may occur at any age, but three types are commonly associated with certain age groups. The infantile type affects 1- to 3-year-olds. The juvenile type affects 3- to 10-year-olds. The adolescent type affects preadolescents and adolescents. The main factors in diagnosing idiopathic scoliosis are the degree, balance, and rotational component of the curvature. The rotational component may contribute to rib cage deformities and impingement on the pulmonary and the cardiac systems. The most common type is the adolescent type. Early diagnosis is difficult because the associated curvature is often hidden by clothing. Scoliosis screening programs help in early detection of this condition. The signs commonly associated with scoliosis include unlevel shoulders, a prominent scapula, a prominent breast, a prominent flank area, an unlevel or a prominent hip, poor posture, and an obvious curvature. During diagnosis it is necessary to view the patient from the front and from the back and while the patient is bending. Other signs that may be associated with idiopathic scoliosis are occasional transient pain and fatigue and decreased pulmonary function. Radiographic films of the spine in the bending position are important in ascertaining the flexibility of the curvature and the potential of spontaneous correction. Neurologic deficits are commonly associated with severe curvature and vary according to the extent to which the curvature has impinged on the spinal cord. Some signs of such impingement are reflex, sensation, and motor alterations of the lower extremities. Nonsurgical intervention commonly employs observation, an exercise program, and a Milwaukee brace. Observation and an exercise program often suffice; the observation is implemented by frequent physical examinations and radiographic monitoring of the progress of the curvature. Exercise programs are designed to promote the maximum correction possible, as indicated by the degree of flexibility shown in the initial x-ray examination. Observation and the exercise program are employed with patients who have a curvature under 15 to 20 degrees. Greater degrees of curvature usually require the use of a Milwaukee brace in addition to observation and an exercise program. The Milwaukee brace, which is usually worn 23 hours a day, is used to control the progress of the curvature. The exercise program is implemented when the adolescent is out of the brace, and additional exercises are performed while in the brace. Surgical intervention may be required if the curvature has progressed to 40 degrees or more at the time of diagnosis or if a slightly lesser degree of curvature exists with a high degree of rotational component or imbalance. Approximately 5% to 10% of patients with idiopathic scoliosis require surgical intervention, which involves fusing of the involved vertebrae to prevent progress of the deformity. Preoperative traction, such as Cotrel traction and halo-femoral traction, may also be used to encourage gradual tissue alterations and to decrease postoperative complications. The patient involved may be placed in Cotrel traction for a period of 5 to 10 days preoperatively. If halo-femoral traction is used, the patient may be placed in traction 1 to 3 weeks preoperatively. Some physicians apply a preoperative cast to their patients with idiopathic scoliosis to achieve immobilization and adjustment, especially if surgery must be postponed for a considerable period after diagnosis. Common surgical intervention techniques for this condition are Harrington rod instrumentation technique and Dwyer cable instrumentation technique, the former being more common. Initial postoperative immobilization is achieved with a posterior plaster shell, a Milwaukee brace, or a windowed cast. A Stryker frame, Foster frame, or CircOlectric bed may also be used. Additional postoperative immobilization by means of cast therapy is often required

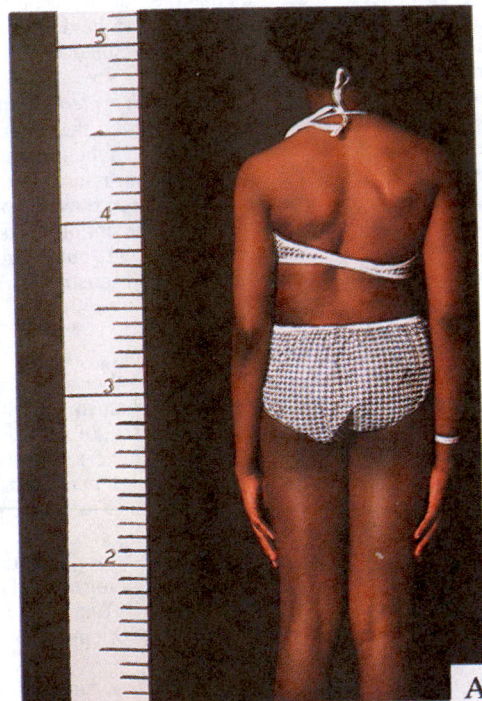
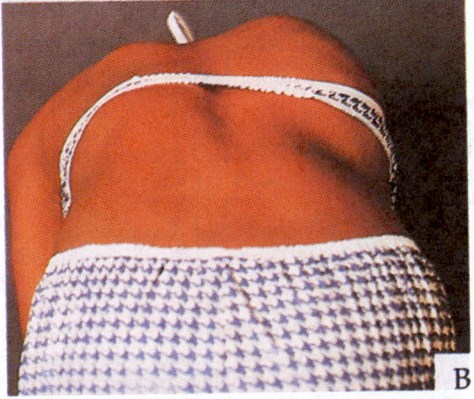

Idiopathic scoliosis: scapular asymmetry and rib hump deformity
(Zitelli, 1992)

for 8 to 12 months or until the bony union of the fused area is absolutely assured. The usual type of cast in this application is a Risser localizer cast, applied with a degree of traction. The Risser turnbuckle cast may also be used when instrumentation has not been employed. A Milwaukee brace or a plastic body jacket may be used when less immobilization is desired.

idiopathic steatorrhea [Gk, *idios*, own, *pathos*, disease, *stear*, fat, *rhoia*, flow],   excess fat in the stools, particularly as in celiac disease in adults.

idiopathic tetanus [Gk, *idios*, own, *pathos*, disease, *tetanos*, convulsive tension],   a tetanus infection of unknown cause.

idiopathic thrombocytopenic purpura (ITP),   a deficiency of platelets that results in bleeding into the skin and other organs. **Acute ITP** is a disease of children that may follow a viral infection, lasts a few weeks to a few months, and usually has no residual effects. **Chronic ITP** is more common in adolescents and adults, begins more insidiously, and lasts longer. Antibodies to platelets are found in patients with ITP; the condition may be transmitted to the fetus if the mother is affected. Treatment includes hemopheresis, corticosteroids, therapeutic plasma pheresis, and splenectomy. See also **thrombocytopenia, thrombocytopenic purpura.**

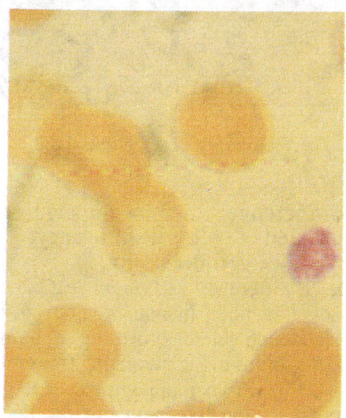

Bone marrow aspirate in ITP *(Zitelli, 1992)*

idiopathy /id′ē·op′əthē/,   any primary disease that arises without an apparent cause. **—idiopathic,** *adj.*

idiosyncrasy /-sin′krəsē/ [Gk, *idios* + *synkrasis*, mixing together],   **1.** a physical or behavioral characteristic or manner that is unique to an individual or to a group. **2.** an individual's unique hypersensitivity to a particular drug, food, or other substance. Also called **idiocrasy** /id′ē·ok′rəsē/. See also **allergy.** **—idiosyncratic,** *adj.*

idiosyncracy to a drug [Gk, *idios*, own, *sygkrasis*, mixing together; Fr, *drogue*],   an individual sensitivity to effects of a drug caused by inherited or other bodily constitution factors. In some cases, a drug may have indiosyncratic effects that are contrary to the expected results.

idiosyncratic /-sinkrat′ik/ [Gk, *idios*, own, *sygkrasis*, mixing together],   pertaining to personal peculiarities or mannerisms.

idiot savant /idē·ō′ savänt′/, *pl.* **idiot savants, idiots savants,**   an individual with mental retardation who is none-

theless capable of performing certain unusual mental feats, primarily those involving music, puzzle-solving, or the manipulation of numbers.

idiotype /id′ē·ətīp′/ [Gk, *idios* + *typos*, mark],   the portion of an immunoglobulin molecule conferring unique character; most often including its binding site.

idioventricular /-ventrik′yələr/ [Gk, *idios* + L, *ventriculum*, belly],   originating in a ventricle.

idioventricular rhythm [Gk, *idios*, own; L *ventriculum*, a chamber; Gk, *rhythmos*],   a slow heart rhythm caused by a repeated discharge of impulses from a focus within a ventricle. The condition occurs in heart block and sinus arrest.

-idium,   a noun-forming suffix: *coracidium, parorchidium, thrombidium.*

IDL (intermediate-density lipoprotein),   a lipid-protein complex with a density between VLDL (very-low-density lipoprotein) and LDL (low-density lipoprotein). The product has a relatively very short half-life and is normally in the blood in very low concentrations. In a type III hyperlipoproteinemic state, the IDL concentration in the blood is elevated.

IDM,   abbreviation for *infant of a diabetic mother.*

idoxuridine /ī′doksyŏŏr′əden/,   an ophthalmic antiviral.
- INDICATION: It is prescribed for herpes simplex keratitis.
- CONTRAINDICATIONS: Deep ulceration of the cornea or known hypersensitivity to this drug prohibits its use.
- ADVERSE EFFECTS: Among the more serious adverse reactions are visual disturbances and eye discomfort.

id reaction,   the autosensitization resulting from a fungal infection that causes pruritus and vesicular lesions. These secondary lesions are caused by circulating antigens and are usually distant from the primary fungal infection.

I:E ratio,   (in respiratory therapy) the duration of inspiration to expiration. A range of 1:1.5 to 1:2 for an adult is considered acceptable for mechanical ventilation. Ratio increases to 1:1 or 2:1 or higher may cause hemodynamic complications, whereas values of 1:2, 1:3, and lower indicate lower mean airway pressure and fewer associated hazards.

-ifene,   a combining form for antiestrogen products of the clomifene and tamoxifen group.

-iform,   a suffix meaning 'in the form of': *amebiform, bulbiform, nucleiform.*

Ig,   abbreviation for **immunoglobulin.**

IgA,   abbreviation for **immunoglobulin A.**

IgA deficiency,   a selective lack of immunoglobulin A, the most common type of immunoglobulin deficiency, appearing in about 1 in 400 individuals. Immunoglobulin A is a major protein antibody in the saliva and the mucous membranes of the intestines and the bronchi. It protects against bacterial and viral infections. A deficiency of immunoglobulin A is associated with autosomal dominant or autosomal recessive inheritance, and with autoimmune abnormalities. The IgA deficiency is common in patients with rheumatoid arthritis and in patients with systemic lupus erythematosus. Many individuals with this deficiency have normal numbers of peripheral blood lymphocytes with IgA receptors and normal amounts of other immunoglobulins. Normality accompanied by IgA deficiency suggests that the B lymphocytes of the involved patient may not secrete IgA. In some patients with this deficiency, T cells seem to depress the synthesis of IgA.
- OBSERVATIONS: Symptoms of IgA deficiency are often lacking in patients whose humoral immune systems may be compensating for low IgA with extra amounts of IgM to

assure adequate defenses. Common symptoms are respiratory allergies associated with chronic sinopulmonary infection, GI diseases, such as celiac disease and regional enteritis, autoimmune diseases, such as rheumatoid arthritis, systemic lupus erythematosus, and chronic hepatitis, malignant tumors, such as squamous cell carcinoma of the lungs, reticulum cell sarcoma, and thymoma. The age of onset varies. Some children with IgA deficiency may begin to synthesize the immunoglobulin spontaneously when their recurrent infections wane and their conditions improve. Diagnoses of IgA-deficient patients depend on the results of tests that commonly show normal IgE and IgM levels while IgA levels are below 5 mg/dl in serum. Cell-mediated response and circulating B cells commonly appear normal, although tests may indicate autoantibodies and antibodies against IgG, IgM, and cow's milk. T cell interferon production may be decreased in some patients with IgA deficiency, increasing the chances of infection.

■ INTERVENTIONS: There is no known cure for selective IgA deficiency; treatment usually involves the effort to control associated diseases, such as respiratory and GI infections.

■ NURSING CONSIDERATIONS: The patient with IgA deficiency should not receive gamma globulin because associated sensitization may cause anaphylaxis during administration of blood products. When the IgA deficient patient requires a blood transfusion, the risk of any harmful reaction can be reduced by using washed red blood cells. Using the cross-matched blood of an IgA-deficient donor in such a transfusion is considered a safer method and completely avoids the risk of an adverse reaction. The IgA deficiency is a lifelong condition, and patients with this disorder are commonly instructed to identify its symptoms and to seek treatment promptly.

IgD, abbreviation for **immunoglobulin D.**

IgE, abbreviation for **immunoglobulin E.**

IgG, abbreviation for **immunoglobulin G.**

IgM, abbreviation for **immunoglobulin M.**

IGT, abbreviation for **impaired glucose tolerance.**

I.H., an abbreviation for *infectious hepatitis.* See **hepatitis A.**

Ikwa fever. See **trench fever.**

ILD, abbreviation for **interstitial lung disease; interstitial lung disorders.**

Ile, abbreviation for **isoleucine.**

ilea. See **ileum.**

ileac, ileal. See **ileum.**

ileal bypass /il'ē·əl/ [L, *ilium,* intestine; AS, *bi,* near; Fr, *passer*], a surgical procedure for treating obesity by anastomosing the upper portion of the small intestine to a part closer to the end of the small intestine, thereby bypassing much of the length of the ileum that normally absorbs nutrients.

ileal conduit [Fr, *conduire,* to guide], a method of urinary diversion through intestinal tract tissue. Ureters are implanted in a section of dissected ileum. This section is sutured closed on one end and the other end is brought through the abdominal wall (RLQ) and a stoma is created. The patient wears a pouch to collect the urine.

ileitis /il'ē·ī'tis/ [L, *ileum,* intestine; Gk, *itis*], inflammation of the ileum. See also **Crohn's disease.**

ileo-, a combining form meaning 'pertaining to the ileum': *ileocecum, ileorectostomy, ileotomy.*

ileoanal anastomosis /il'ē·ō·ā'nəl/, a surgical procedure in which the colon and rectum are removed but the anus is left intact along with the anal sphincter. An anastomosis is formed between the lower end of the small intestine and the anus. The operation is an alternative to proctocolectomy for the treatment of ulcerative colitis.

ileocecal /il'ē·ōsē'kəl/ [L, *ilium,* intestine, *caecus,* blind], pertaining to both the ileum and the cecum and the region where they are joined.

ileocecal valve [L, *ileum,* intestine, *caecus,* blind; *valvarum,* folding door], the valve between the ileum of the small intestine and the cecum of the large intestine. The valve consists of two flaps that project into the lumen of the large intestine, just above the vermiform appendix, allowing the contents of the intestine to pass only in a forward direction.

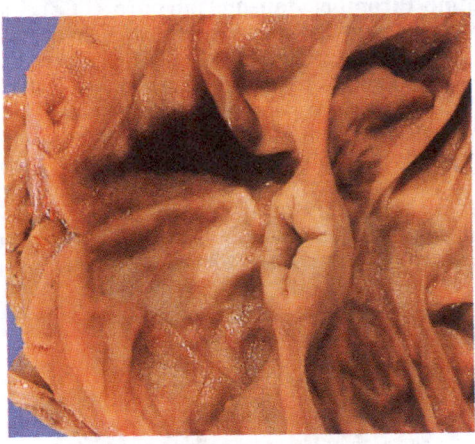

Ileocecal valve *(Mitros, 1988)*

ileocecal incompetence. See **incompetence.**

ileocecal insufficiency. See **insufficiency.**

ileocecostomy. See **cecoileostomy.**

ileocolic node /il'ē·ōkol'ik/ [L, *ileum* + Gk, *kolon,* colon; L, *nodus,* knot], a node in one of three groups of superior mesenteric lymph glands, forming a chain of approximately 15 nodes around the ileocolic (mesenteric) artery. They tend to form in two main groups, one near the duodenum, the other on the lower part of the ileocolic artery. The chain breaks into several groups where the artery divides into its terminal branches. The ileocolic nodes receive materials from the jejunum, ileum, cecum, vermiform appendix, ascending colon, and transverse colon. Their efferent vessels pass to the preaortic nodes. Compare **mesenteric node, mesocolic node.**

ileocystoplasty /-sis'təplas'tē/ [L, *ileum* + Gk, *kystis,* bag, *plassein,* to mold], a surgical procedure in which the bladder is reconstructed using a segment of the ileum for the bladder wall.

ileocystostomy /-sistos'təmē/ [L, *ilium* + intestines; Gk, *kystis,* bag, *stoma,* mouth], a surgical procedure to form a passage to direct urine through the abdominal wall using a segment of small intestine as a tube from the bladder.

ileostomate /il'ē·os'təmāt/, a person who has undergone an ileostomy.

ileostomy /il'ē·os'təmē/ [L, *ileum* + Gk, *stoma,* mouth, *temnein,* to cut], surgical formation of an opening of the ileum onto the surface of the abdomen, through which fecal matter is emptied. The operation is performed in advanced or recurrent ulcerative colitis, Crohn's disease, or cancer of the large bowel. A low-residue diet is given preoperatively and is reduced to fluids 24 hours before surgery to decrease intestinal residue. Intestinal antibiotics are given to decrease the bacterial count. A nasogastric or intestinal tube is passed. The diseased portion of the large bowel is removed in a permanent ileostomy; occasionally, the distal and proximal segments of bowel may be reconnected after ulcerated areas have healed. A loop of the proximal ileum is then brought out onto the abdomen and sutured in place, and a stoma is formed. A pouch may be made with part of the terminal ileum, in which the open end is woven through the rectus muscles to form a valve and then opens onto the abdomen. Postoperatively, the patient wears a temporary disposable bag to collect the semiliquid fecal matter, which begins to drain once peristalsis is restored and the tube is removed. Since the secretions contain digestive enzymes that can ulcerate the skin around the stoma, the nurse ensures that nothing leaks from the bag. The nurse instructs the patient how to apply and care for the stoma and the ileostomy bag. If a pouch is present, it is irrigated or drained three or four times a day through a small irrigating catheter through the valve. Compare **colostomy.** See also **enterostomy, ostomy irrigation, stoma.**

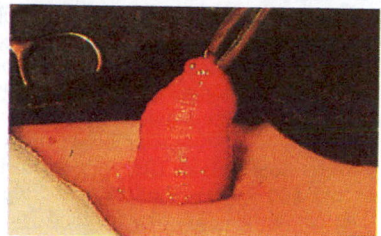

Ileostomy (Winawer, 1992)

ileum /il′ē·əm/, *pl.* **ilea** [L, intestine], the distal portion of the small intestine, extending from the jejunum to the cecum. It has a few small circular folds and numerous clusters of lymph nodes. It ends in the right iliac fossa, opening into the medial side of the large intestine. See **ileocecal valve.** −**ileac, ileal,** *adj.*

ileus /il′ē·əs/ [L; Gk, *eilein*, to twist], an obstruction of the intestines, such as an adynamic ileus caused by immobility of the bowel, or a mechanical ileus in which the intestine is blocked by mechanic means.

ilia. See **ilium.**

-iliac, a combining form meaning 'pertaining to the ilium': *occipitoiliac, subiliac, vertebroiliac.*

iliac circumflex node /il′ē·ak/ [L *ilium* + flank; *circum,* around, *flectere,* to bend; *nodus,* knot], a node in one of the seven clusters of parietal lymph nodes of the abdomen. This node is one of a group found along the course of the deep iliac circumflex vessels. Compare **common iliac node, external iliac node, internal iliac node.** See also **lymph, lymphatic system, lymph node.**

iliac crest [L, *ilia,* intestines; ME; *creste*], the upper elevated margins of the ilium.

iliac fascia, the portion of the endoabdominal fascia that is attached with the iliacus to the crest of the ilium and passes under the inguinal ligament into the thigh.

iliac region. See **inguinal region.**

iliacus /ilī′əkəs/ [L, *ilium,* flank], a flat, triangular muscle that covers the inner curved surface of the iliac fossa. It arises from the inner aspect of the superior iliac crest, from the anterior and the iliolumbar ligaments, and from the sa-

crum. It joins the psoas major to form the iliopsoas at the inguinal ligament. The iliacus is innervated by branches of the femoral nerve that contain fibers from the second and the third lumbar nerves. It acts to flex and laterally rotate the thigh. Compare **psoas major, psoas minor.**

ilio-, a combining form meaning 'of or pertaining to the ilium or flank': *iliocostal, iliolumbar, iliometer.*

iliofemoral /il′ē·ōfem′ərəl/, of or pertaining to the ilium and femur.

iliofemoral ligament [L, *ilium* + flank, *femur,* thigh, *ligamentum*], a triangular band of connective tissue attached by its apex to the anterior inferior spine of the ilium and acetabular margin and by its base to the interotrochanteric line of the femur.

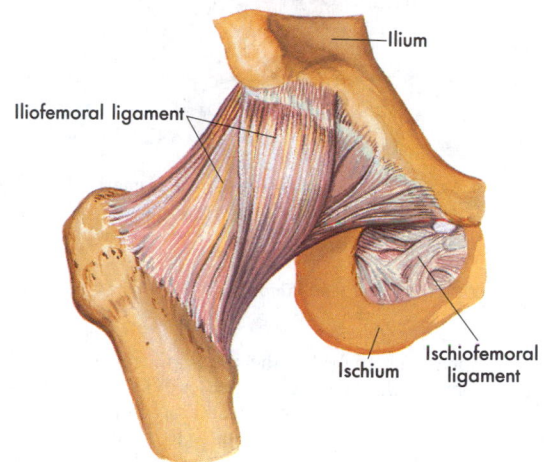

Iliofemoral ligament (Thibodeau, 1993/Ernest W Beck)

ilioinguinal /il′ē·ō·ing′gwinəl/ [L, *ilium* + *inguen,* groin], of or pertaining to the hip and inguinal regions.

iliolumbar ligament /-lum′bər/ [L, *ilium* + *lumbus,* loin; *ligare,* to bind], one of a pair of ligaments forming part of the connection between the vertebral column and the pelvis. Each iliolumbar ligament attaches to a transverse process of the fifth lumbar vertebra and passes to the base of the sacrum.

iliopectineal line /-pek′tənəl/ [L, *ilium* + *pectus,* breast; *linea*], a bony ridge on the inner surface of the ilium and pubic bones that divides the true and false pelvises. Also called **brim of true pelvic cavity, inlet.**

iliopsoas /il′ē·ōsō′əs/ [L, *ilium* + Gk, *psoa,* loin muscle], one of the pair of muscle complexes that flexes the thigh and the lumbar vertebral column. Each complex is composed of the psoas major, the psoas minor, and the iliacus, although the psoas minor is often absent. The psoas major is a long fusiform muscle, arising from certain lumbar vertebrae and inserting into the femur. The iliacus is a flat, triangular muscle arising from the iliac fossa and inserting into the femur and the tendon of the psoas major. The psoas minor is a long slender muscle ventral to the psoas major.

iliopsoas abscess [L, *ilium,* intestine], an abscess, possibly tuberculous in origin, that spreads from the thoracic or lumbar spine to the upper leg muscles.

iliotibial band /-tib′ē·əl/ [L, *ilium,* flank, *tibia,* shinbone], a layer of connective tissue that extends from the iliac crest to the knee and links the gluteus maximus to the tibia.

ilium /il′ē·əm/, *pl.* **ilia** [L, flank], the uppermost of the

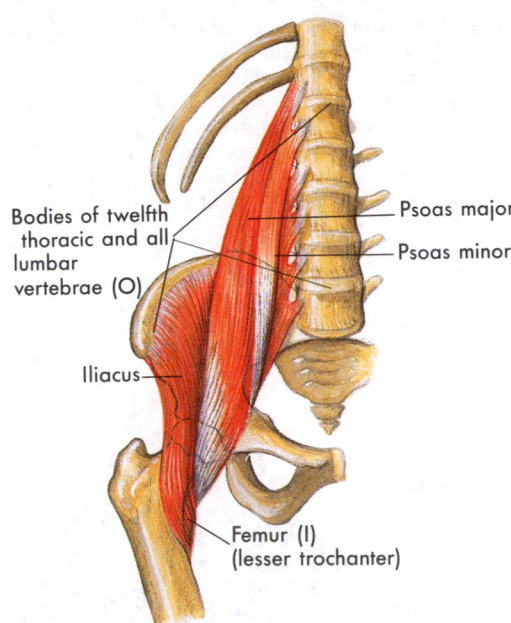

Bodies of twelfth
thoracic and all
lumbar
vertebrae (O)

Psoas major

Psoas minor

Iliacus

Femur (I)
(lesser trochanter)

Iliopsoas muscle *(Thibodeau, 1993/Ernest W Beck)*

three bones that make up the innominate bone. The ilium forms part of the acetabulum and provides attachment for several muscles, including the obturator internus, the gluteals, the iliacus, and the sartorius. The ilium is divided into the body, which forms less than two fifths of the acetabulum, and the ala ossis ilii, which is the large, winglike portion of the greater pelvis. The ala contains the iliac fossa and the greater sciatic notch and presents various prominences for muscle attachment, such as the iliac crest, the anterior superior and the posterior superior iliac spines, and the anterior inferior and the posterior inferior iliac spines. Compare **ischium, pubis.** **–iliac,** *adj.*

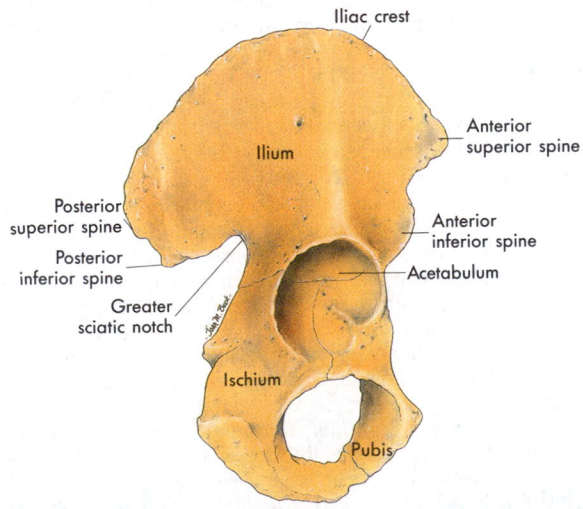

Iliac crest

Anterior
superior spine

Ilium

Posterior
superior spine

Anterior
inferior spine

Posterior
inferior spine

Acetabulum

Greater
sciatic notch

Ischium

Pubis

Ilium *(Thibodeau, 1993/Joan M Beck)*

illegitimate /il'ejit'imit/ [L, *in, legitimatus.* not lawful], **1.** not authorized by law. **2.** born out of wedlock. **3.** abnormal.

illicit /ilis'it/ [L, *illicitus,* unlawful], pertaining to an act that is unlawful or otherwise not permitted.

illness [ME, unhealthy condition], an abnormal process in which aspects of the social, physical, emotional, or intellectual condition and function of a person are diminished or impaired, compared with that person's previous condition.

illness behavior, the manner in which individuals monitor the structure and functions of their own bodies, interpret symptoms, take remedial action, and make use of health care facilities.

illness experience, the process of being ill, comprising five stages: phase I, experiencing a symptom; phase II, assuming a sick role; phase III, making contact for health care; phase IV, being dependent (a patient); and phase V, recovering or being rehabilitated. Each stage is characterized by certain decisions, behaviors, and end points. During phase I, in which a symptom is experienced, the person decides that something is wrong and tries to remedy the situation. Phase I ends with the person accepting the reality of the symptom, no longer delaying any action toward help or denying the symptom (flight into health). During phase II the person decides that the illness is real and that care is necessary. Advice, guidance, and validation are sought. This gives the person permission to act sick and to be excused temporarily from usual obligations. The outcome of this phase is acceptance of the role—or denial of its necessity. In phase III professional advice is sought; authoritative declarations identify and validate the illness and legitimize the sick role. The person usually asks for help and negotiates for treatment. Denial may still occur and the patient may 'shop' further for medical care or may accept the illness, the medical authority, and the plan for treatment. In phase IV professional treatment is performed and accepted by the person, who is now perceived as a patient. At any time during this phase the dependent patient may develop ambivalent feelings and may decide to reject the treatment, the care giver, and the illness. More often, care is accepted with ambivalence. The patient has a particular need to be informed and to be given emotional support during this phase. During phase V, the last stage of the illness experience, the patient relinquishes the sick role. The usual tasks and roles are resumed to the greatest degree possible. Some people do not willingly give up the sick role, becoming, in their own eyes, chronically ill, or, for secondary gain, they malinger, acting sick. Most people accept the recovery and work toward rehabilitation.

illness prevention, a system of health education programs and activities directed toward protecting patients from real or potential health threats, minimizing risk factors and promoting healthy behavior.

illumination /iloo'minā'shən/ [L, *illuminare,* to make light], the lighting up of a part of the body or of an object under a microscope for the purpose of examination. **–illuminate,** *v.*

illusion /iloo'zhən/ [L, *illudere,* to mock], a false interpretation of an external sensory stimulus, usually visual or auditory, such as a mirage in the desert or voices on the wind. Compare **delusion, hallucination.**

Ilopan, a trademark for a precursor of coenzyme A (dexpanthenol).

Ilosone, a trademark for an antibacterial (erythromycin estolate).

IL-6, abbreviation for *interleukin 6,* an antiviral compound also used in the treatment of some types of cancer. Also called **beta$_2$-interferon.**

im-, a prefix in chemistry indicating the bivalent group NH: *imadyl, imide, imperialine.*

I.M., abbreviation for *intramuscular.*

I.M.A., abbreviation for **Industrial Medical Association.**

image /im′ij/ [L, *imago,* likeness], **1.** a representation or visual reproduction of the likeness of someone or something, such as a painting, photograph, or sculpture. **2.** an optic representation of an object, such as that produced by refraction or reflection. **3.** a person or thing that closely resembles another; semblance. **4.** a mental picture, representation, idea, or concept of an objective reality. **5.** (in psychology) a mental representation of something previously perceived and subsequently modified by other experiences, resulting from intrapsychic or extrapsychic stimuli, or both.

image acquistion time, the time required to carry out an NMR imaging procedure comprising only the data acquisition time. The additional image reconstruction time will also be important to determine how quickly the image can be viewed. In comparing sequential plane imaging and volume imaging techniques, the equivalent image acquisition time per slice must be considered, as well as the actual image acquisition time.

image foreshortening, (in radiology) an x-ray image distortion caused by improper positioning of the object or the x-ray tube. It results in an image that is smaller than the object itself, and the reduction increases as the angle between the object and image planes increases.

image format, (in computed tomography) the manner in which an image is stored, such as on a floppy disk, magnetic tape, or film.

image intensifier, an electronic device used to produce a fluoroscopic image with a low-radiation exposure. A beam of x-rays passing through the patient is converted in a special vacuum tube into a pattern of electrons. The electrons are accelerated and concentrated onto a small fluorescent screen where they present a bright image. This is generally displayed on a TV monitor.

image matrix, (in radiology) an arrangement of columns or rows of imaginary cells, or pixels, forming a digital image. The size of the image matrix is determined by characteristics of the imaging equipment and by the capacity of the computer and may vary from 2562 to 10242. A 2562 image contains 65,536 pixels.

imagery /im′ijrē/ [L, *imago*], (in psychiatry) the formation of mental concepts, figures, ideas; any product of the imagination.

imagination /imaj′inā′shən/ [L, *imaginare,* picture to oneself, **1.** the ability to form, or the act or process of forming, mental images or conscious concepts of things that are not immediately available to the senses. **2.** (in psychology) the ability to reproduce images or ideas stored in the memory by the stimulation or suggestion of associated ideas or to regroup former ideas and concepts to form new images and ideas concerned with a particular goal or problem. See also **fantasy.**

imaging /im′ijing/ [L, *imago*], the formation of a mental picture or representation of someone or something using the imagination. See also **fantasy.**

imago /imā′gō/ [L, likeness], (in analytic psychology) an unconscious, usually idealized mental image of a significant individual, such as one's mother, in a person's early, formative years. See also **identification.**

imbalance /imbal′əns/ [L, *im,* not, *bilanx,* having two scales], **1.** lack of balance between opposing muscle groups, such as in the imbalance of extraocular muscles leading to strabismus. **2.** an abnormal balance of fluid and electrolytes in the body tissues. **3.** an unequal distribution of subjects in a population group, such as an only girl in a large family of boys. **4.** a person with mental abilities that are remarkable in one area but deficient in others, as an idiot savant.

imbedded tooth. See **embedded tooth.**

imbricate /im′brikāt/ [L, *imbrex,* roofing tile], to build a surface with overlapping layers of material. Surgeons may imbricate with layers of tissue when closing a wound or other opening in a body part. **−imbrication,** *n.*

Imferon, a trademark for an injectable hematinic (iron dextran).

imide-, imido-, a combining form indicating the presence in a chemical compound of the bivalent group > NH: *imidogen.*

imino-, a combining form indicating the presence of the bivalent group > NH attached to a nonacid radical: *iminourea.*

iminoglycinuria /im′inōglī′sinŏŏr′ē·ə/, a benign familial condition characterized by the abnormal urinary excretion of the amino acids glycine, proline, and hydroxyproline.

imipenem-cilastatin sodium /im′ipē′nəm sil′əstat′in/, a broad spectrum parenteral antibiotic.

■ INDICATIONS: It is prescribed for the treatment of infections caused by susceptible organisms in the lower respiratory or urinary tracts, skin, abdomen, reproductive organs, bones, or joints. It is also used in the treatment of endocarditis and septicemia.

■ CONTRAINDICATIONS: This product is not recommended for children. Caution should be used in administering the drug to patients with pseudomembranous colitis, hypersensitivity reactions, or a history of seizures.

■ ADVERSE EFFECTS: The most common adverse reactions include phlebitis, thrombophlebitis, nausea, vomiting, diarrhea, rash, fever, and central nervous system symptoms.

imipramine hydrochloride /imip′rəmēn/, a tricyclic antidepressant with a slow onset of action.

■ INDICATION: It is prescribed in the treatment of mental depression.

■ CONTRAINDICATIONS: Concomitant administration of monoamine oxidase inhibitors, recent myocardial infarction, cardiovascular disease or seizure disorder, or known hypersensitivity to this drug or to other tricyclic medication prohibits its use.

■ ADVERSE EFFECTS: Among the more serious adverse reactions are sedation, GI disturbances, and cardiovascular and neurologic reactions. It should not be withdrawn abruptly. This drug interacts with many other drugs.

immature baby /imə chŏŏr′/ [L, *in,* not, *maturare,* to make ripe], a term sometimes applied to an infant weighing less than 1134 g (2.5 lb) and who is considerably underdeveloped at birth.

immature cataract [L, *in, maturus,* ripe; Gk, *katarrhaktes*], a cataract at an early stage of development when the lens absorbs fluid and increases in swelling. Only part of the lens is opaque.

immature erythrocyte [L, *in, maturus,* ripe; Gk, *erythros,* red, *kytos,* cell], any of the intermediate blood cells between the hemocytoblasts and nonnucleated red blood cells. They may be found in the blood circulation after birth of the fetus.

immediate auscultation /imē′dē·it/ [L, *in* + *medius,* middle; *auscultare,* to listen], a method of examining a patient by placing an ear or stethoscope on the skin directly over the body part being studied.

immediate automatism, a state in which a person acts spontaneously and automatically without having any recollection of the behavior.

immediate denture [L, *in, medius, dens,* tooth], a removable artificial denture that is placed in the mouth immediately after removal of the natural teeth to maintain normal appearance and ability to masticate food. The immediate denture may be full or partial.

immediate hypersensitivity, an allergic reaction that occurs within minutes after exposure to an allergen.

immediate percussion. See **percussion.**

immediate postoperative fit prosthesis (IPOF), a temporary or preparatory prosthesis, such as a pylon.

immediate posttraumatic automatism, a posttraumatic state in which a person acts spontaneously and automatically without having any recollection of the behavior.

immersion /imur′zhən/ [L, *im* + *mergere,* to dip], the placing of a body or an object into water or other liquid so that it is completely covered by the liquid. —**immerse,** *v.*

immersion foot, an abnormal condition of the feet characterized by damage to the muscles, nerves, skin and blood vessels, caused by prolonged exposure to dampness or by prolonged immersion in cold water. See also **frostbite, trench foot.**

imminent abortion. See **inevitable abortion.**

immiscible /imis′əbəl/ [L, *im* + *miscere,* to mix], not capable of being mixed, such as oil and water. Compare **miscible.**

immotile cilia syndrome /imō′til/ [L, *in, motilis,* movable, *cilia,* eyelashes; Gk, *syn,* together, *dromos,* course], a condition in which the hairlike processes of epithelial cells and others fail to function normally. As a result, the patient has difficulty in moving dust and other airborne debris from the respiratory system.

immune /imyo͞on′/ [L, *immunis,* free from], being protected against infective or allergic diseases by a system of antibody molecules and related resistance factors.

immune body, See **antibody.**

immune complex hypersensitivity [L, *immunis,* free; *complexus,* embrace; Gk, *hyper,* excess; L, *sentire,* to feel], an IgG or IgM complement dependent, immediate acting humoral hypersensitivity to certain soluble antigens. An intradermal skin test results in erythema and edema within 3 to 8 hours and an acute inflammatory reaction with an increase in polymorphonuclear leukocytes. It is seen in serum sickness, Arthus reaction, and glomerulonephritis. Also called **type III hypersensitivity.** Compare **anaphylactic hypersensitivity, cell-mediated immune response, cytotoxic hypersensitivity.**

immune cytolysis, cell destruction mediated by a particular antibody in conjunction with complement.

immune gamma globulin, passive immunizing agents obtained from pooled human plasma. Also called **immune globulin.** See also **immunoglobulin G.**

■ INDICATIONS: It is prescribed for immunization against measles, poliomyelitis, chickenpox, serum hepatitis following transfusion, hepatitis A, agammaglobulinemia, and hypogammaglobulinemia.

■ CONTRAINDICATION: Known hypersensitivity to gamma globulins prohibits its use.

■ ADVERSE EFFECTS: Among the more serious adverse reactions are pain and inflammation at the site of injection and allergic reactions.

immune globulin. See **immune gamma globulin.**

immune human globulin, a sterile solution of globulins that is used as a passive immunizing agent and derived from adult human blood.

immune proteins [L, *immunis,* free from; Gk, *proteios,* first rank], proteins in the form of antibodies or antitoxins that contribute to the immunity of a host.

immune response, a defense function of the body that produces antibodies to destroy invading antigens and malignancies. Important components of the immune system and response are immunoglobulins, lymphocytes, phagocytes, complement, properdin, the migratory inhibitory factor, and interferon. Antigens, which are largely foreign protein macromolecules, trigger the immune response during interaction with countless cells of the reticuloendothelial system of the body. The kinds of immune response are humoral immune response, involving B lymphocytes or B cells, and cell-mediated immune response, involving T lymphocytes or T cells. The B cells and the T cells derive from the hemopoietic stem cells, which originate in the embryonic yolk sac. Every normal baby is born with many different clones of B cells in the bone marrow, the lymph nodes, and the spleen. All the cells of each clone synthesize a specific antibody with a different sequence of amino acids from that of any of the other numerous clones of B cells. The receptor sites on the surface membranes of the B cells are the combining sites of immunoglobulin molecules. The classes of immunoglobulins, identified by letter names, are M, G, A, E, and D. Immunoglobulin M, the antibody that immature B cells synthesize and incorporate in their cytoplasmic membranes, is the predominant antibody produced after initial contact with an antigen. The T cells develop in the thymus gland and proliferate with antigen receptors on their surface membranes. The T cells assist in the antigen-antibody reaction of the B cells and control the cell-mediated response associated with the reduction of tissue inflammation. The cell-mediated response is also effective against fungi, viruses, and tumors and is the major reaction in the rejection of organ transplants. In transplant surgery, certain methods, such as the administration of appropriate drugs and radiation, suppress transplant rejection. The T cells have little or no immunoglobulin on their surfaces and always maintain their leukocyte structure. They are divided into circulating T cells, noncirculating T cells, and memory T cells. Circulating T cells function within circulating fluids; noncirculating T cells include those that produce lymphokines and selectively migrate to inflamed tissue sites. Memory T cells recognize antigens as foreign and mobilize tissue macrophages in the presence of the migratory inhibitory factor. Humoral immune response protects the body against bacterial and viral infections through the stimulation of antibodies associated with the B cells. Plasma cells, which derive from B cells through the stimulation of antigens, secrete trillions of antibody molecules that aid the humoral immune response. Such molecules recognize microinvaders of the body as "foreigners" when the antigens bind to them. The antigen-antibody reaction may transform the toxic antigen into a harmless substance, or it may agglutinate antigens, allowing macrophages and other phagocytes to digest large numbers of antigens at one time. The antigen-antibody reactions of the humoral immune response also activate the complement in the blood serum, which triggers a nonspecific series of chemical reactions to amplify the humoral immune response. Activated discrete plasma proteins C1 to C3 in the complement system cause lysis of the antigenic cell and opsonize the antigen for phagocytosis. Humoral immune response may begin immediately with antigen contact or may be delayed for as long as 48 hours. The speed of humoral response is demonstrated in anaphylaxis. Other proteins associated with the immune response are properdin and interferon. Properdin provides an alternate process for activating complement. Interferon is synthesized by body cells after viral invasion acts to combat viruses and may retard the growth of cancer cells. Humoral immune response and cell-mediated immune response immunity are interdependent. The former can influence the function of T cells and the latter the function of B cells. Humoral and cell-mediated immunity can be natural or acquired. Natural immunity, or genetically inherited resistance to specific infectious organisms, can be affected by diet, mental health, environment, metabolism, and the virulence of invading pathogens. Also called **immune reaction.**

immune serum. See **antiserum.**

immune serum globulin. See **chickenpox, immune human globulin.**

immune system, a biochemical complex that protects the body against pathogenic organisms and other foreign bodies. The system incorporates the humoral immune response, which produces antibodies to react with specific antigens, and the cell-mediated response, which uses T cells to mobilize tissue macrophages in the presence of a foreign body. The immune system also protects the body from invasion by creating local barriers and inflammation. The local barriers provide chemical and mechanical defenses through the skin, the mucous membranes, and the conjunctiva. Inflammation draws polymorphonuclear leukocytes and neutrophils to the site of injury where these phagocytes engulf the invading organism. The humoral response and the cell-mediated response develop if these first-line defenses fail or are inadequate to protect the body. The humoral immune response is especially effective against bacterial and viral invasions and employs B cells that produce appropriate antibodies. The principal organs of the immune response system include the bone marrow, the thymus, and the lymphoid tissues. The system also employs peripheral organs, such as the lymph nodes, the spleen, and the lymphatic vessels. The antigen-antibody reactions of the immune system activate the complement system, which removes antigens from the body. The complement system contains several discrete proteins that function to produce lysis of the antigenic cells. The humoral response may begin immediately on invasion by the antigen or may start as long as 48 hours later.

immunity /imyŏŏ'nĭtē/ [L, *immunis,* free], **1.** (in civil law) exemption from a duty or an obligation generally required by law, as an exemption from taxation, exemption from penalty for wrongdoing, or protection against liability. **2.** the quality of being insusceptible to or unaffected by a particular disease or condition. Kinds of immunity are **active immunity** and **passive immunity.** –**immune,** *adj.*

immunization /im'yənīzā'shən/ [L, *immunis,* free], a process by which resistance to an infectious disease is induced or augmented.

immunoassay /im'yənō·as'ā/ [L, *immunis,* + Fr, *essayer,* to try], a competitive-binding assay in which the binding protein is an antibody.

immunocompetence /-kom'pətəns/, the ability of an immune system to mobilize and deploy its antibodies and other responses to stimulation by an antigen. Immunocompetence may be weakened in older individuals as a result of age-related attenuation in T cell function. It may also be diminished by viruses, radiation, and chemotherapeutic drugs.

immunocompromised /-kom'prəmīzd'/ [L, *immunis,* free from, *compromittere,* to promise mutually], pertaining to an immune response that has been weakened by a disease or immunosuppressive agent.

immunodeficiency disease /-difish'ənsē/ any of a group of health conditions caused by a defect in the immune system and generally characterized by susceptibility to infections and chronic diseases. The diseases are sometimes classified as B cell (antibody) deficiencies, T cell (cellular) deficiencies, combined T and B cell deficiencies, defects of cell movement, and defects of microbicidal activity.

immunodeficient /-difish'ənt/ [L, *immunis + de,* from, *facere,* to make], pertaining to an abnormal condition of the immune system in which cellular or humoral immunity is inadequate and resistance to infection is decreased. Kinds of immunodeficient conditions are **hypogammaglobulinemia** and **lymphoid aplasia.**

immunodiagnosis. See **serologic diagnosis.**

immunodiagnostic /-dī'əgnos'tik/ [L, *immunis* + Gk, *dia,* through, *gnosis* knowledge], pertaining to or characterizing a diagnosis based on an antigen-antibody reaction. In many cases a tumor releases a discrete antigenic substance into the blood; detection of a particular antigen can provide an immunodiagnostic sign of the presence of the tumor associated with that antigen.

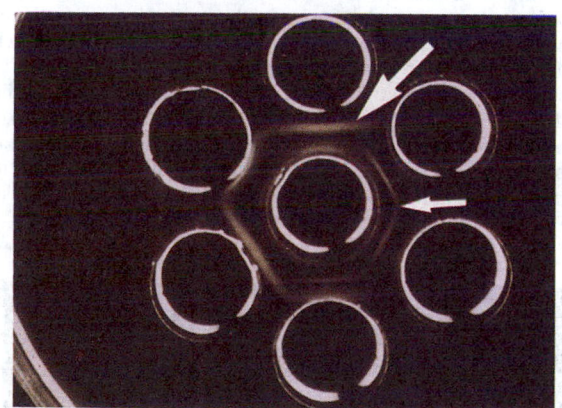

Immunodiffusion (Murray, 1990)

immunodiffusion /-dify ŏŏ'zhən/ [L, *immunis + diffundere,* to spread], a technique for the identification and quantification of any of the immunoglobulins. It is based on the presence of a visible precipitate that results from an antigen-antibody combination under certain circumstances. **Gel diffusion** is a technique that involves evaluation of the precipitin reaction in a clear gel, seen when an antigen placed in a hole in the agarose diffuses evenly into the medium. An obvious ring forms where the antigen meets the anti-

Properties of immunoglobulin classes

Property	Immunoglobulin class				
	IgG	IgM	IgA	IgE	IgD
Principal site found	Internal body fluids	Serum	Serum and exocrine secretions	Tissue bound	Bound to lymphocyte surface
Principal functions	Agglutination, detoxification, virus neutralization; enhances phagocytosis	Agglutination, cytolysis, enhances phagocytosis	Protection of mucosal surfaces	Mediates immediate type of hypersensitivity	Control of lymphocytic activation and suppression

Adapted from Phipps WJ, Long BC, Woods NF, Cassmeyer VL: *Medical-surgical nursing: concepts and clinical practice,* ed 4, St Louis, 1991, Mosby.

body. **Electroimmunodiffusion** is a gel diffusion to which an electric field is applied, accelerating the reaction. **Double gel diffusion** is a technique that permits identification of antibodies in mixed specimens. In an agar plate antigen is placed in one well, antibody in another. Antigen and antibody diffuse out of their wells. In mixed antigen specimens, each antigen-antibody combination forms a separate line; observation of the location, shape, and thickness of a line permits identification and quantification of the antibody. **immunoelectrodiffusion.** See **immunodiffusion.**

immunoelectrophoresis /-ilek′trōfôrē′sis/ [L, *immunis* + Gk, *elektron,* amber, *pherein,* to bear], a technique that combines electrophoresis and immunodiffusion to separate and allow identification of complex proteins. The proteins in the test serum are spread out in agar and separated by electrophoresis. Wells or troughs are then cut into the agar, and parts of antibody are placed in the troughs and allowed to diffuse toward the separated proteins. A visible precipitin will form in a series of arcs in the agar when an antigen-antibody reaction occurs. The shape and location of each arc are specific for known proteins. Unusual arcs are representative of abnormal or unknown protein. Although the density of the precipitation corresponds to the concentration of protein in each electrophoretic band, immunoelectrophoresis does not accurately quantify the amount of protein in the test serum. **–immunoelectrophoretic,** *adj.*

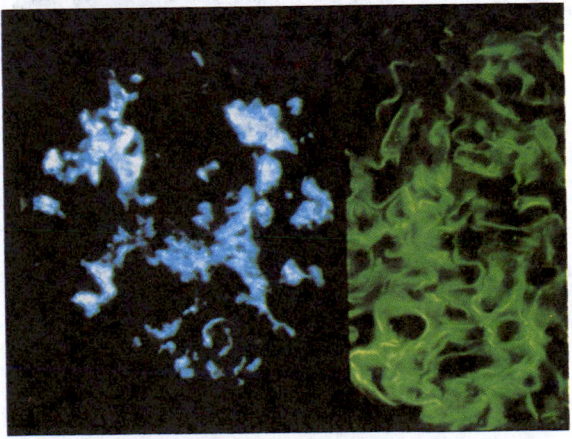

Immunofluorescence (Mudge, 1992)

immunofluorescence /-floores′əns/ [L, *immunis* + *fluere,* to flow], a technique used for the rapid identification of an antigen by exposing it to known antibodies tagged with the fluorescent dye fluorescein and observing the characteristic antigen-antibody reaction of precipitation. As the fluorescent antibody reacts with its specific antigen, the precipitate appears luminous in the ultraviolet light projected by a fluorescent microscope. Many of the most common infectious organisms can be identified using this technique. Among them are *Candida albicans, Haemophilus influenzae, Neisseria gonorrhoeae, Shigella, Staphylococcus aureus,* and several viruses, including rabies virus and many enteroviruses. See also **fluorescent microscopy. –immunofluorescent,** *adj.*

immunofluorescence test. See **fluorescent antibody test.**

-immunfluorescent. See **immunofluorescence.**

immunofluorescent microscopy. See **fluorescent microscopy, immunofluorescence.**

immunogen /imyoo′nəjən/ [L, *immunis* + Gk, *genein,* to produce], any agent or substance capable of provoking an immune response or producing immunity. **–immunogenic,** *adj.*

immunoglobulin /-glob′yəlin/ [L, *immunis* + *globus,* small sphere], any of five structurally and antigenically distinct antibodies present in the serum and external secretions of the body. In response to specific antigens, immunoglobulins are formed in the bone marrow, spleen, and all lymphoid tissue of the body except the thymus. Kinds of immunoglobulins are **IgA, IgD, IgE, IgG,** and **IgM.** Also called **immune serum globulin.** See also **antibody, antigen, immunity.**

immunoglobulin A (IgA), one of the five classes of humoral antibodies produced by the body and one of the most prevalent. It is found in all secretions of the body and is the major antibody in the mucous membrane lining the intestines and in the bronchi, saliva, and tears. IgA combines with a protein in the mucosa and defends body surfaces against invading microorganisms. Research indicates that it protects body tissues by seeking out foreign microorganisms and triggering an antigen-antibody reaction. The normal concentration of IgA in serum is 50 to 250 mg/dl. Compare **immunoglobulin D, immunoglobulin E, immunoglobulin G, immunoglobulin M.**

immunoglobulin D (IgD), one of the five classes of humoral antibodies produced by the body. It is a specialized protein found in small amounts in serum tissue. The precise function of IgD is not known, but it increases in quantity during allergic reactions to milk, insulin, penicillin, and various toxins. The normal concentration of IgD in serum is 0.5 to 3 mg/dl. Compare **immunoglobulin A, immunoglobulin E, immunoglobulin G, immunoglobulin M.**

immunoglobulin E (IgE), one of the five classes of humoral antibodies produced by the body. It is concentrated in the lung, the skin, and the cells of mucous membranes. It provides the primary defense against environmental antigens and is believed to be responsive to immunoglobulin A. IgE reacts with certain antigens to release certain chemical mediators that cause Type I hypersensitivity reactions characterized by wheal and flare. The normal concentration of IgE in serum is 0.01 to 0.04 mg/dl. Compare **immunoglobulin A, immunoglobulin D, immunoglobulin G, immunoglobulin M.**

immunoglobulin G (IgG), one of the five classes of humoral antibodies produced by the body. It is a specialized protein synthesized by the body in response to invasions by bacteria, fungi, and viruses. IgG crosses the placenta and protects against red cell antigens and white cell antigens. The normal concentration of IgG in serum is 800 to 1600 mg/dl. Compare **immunoglobulin A, immunoglobulin D, immunoglobulin E, immunoglobulin M.**

immunoglobulin M (IgM), one of the five classes of humoral antibodies produced by the body and the largest in molecular structure. It is the first immunoglobulin the body produces when challenged by antigens and is found in circulating fluids. IgM triggers the increased production of immunoglobulin G and the complement fixation required for effective antibody response. It is the dominant antibody in ABO incompatibilities. The normal concentration of IgM in serum is 40 to 120 mg/dl. Compare **immunoglobulin A, immunoglobulin D, immunoglobulin E, immunoglobulin G.**

immunohematology /-hem′ətol′əjē/ [L, *immunis* + Gk, *haima*, blood, *logos*, science], the study of antigen-antibody reactions and their effects on blood.

immunologic disease /-loj′ik/ [L, *immunis*, free from; Gk, *logos*, science; L, *dis*; Fr, *aise*, ease], the signs and symptoms of reactions of antibodies to antigens, as in anaphylaxis.

immunologic surveillance [L, *immunis*, free from; Gk, *logos*, science; Fr, *surveiller*, to watch over], the theory that the immune system destroys tumor cells, which are constantly arising during the life of the individual.

immunologic tests [L, *immunis* + *testum*, crucible], tests based on the principles of antigen-antibody reactions.

immunologic theory of aging, a concept based on the premise that normal cells are unrecognized as such, thereby triggering immune reactions within the individual's own body.

immunologist /im′yənol′əjist/, a specialist in immunology.

immunology /im′yənol′əjē/ [L, *immunis* + Gk, *logos*, science], the study of the reaction of tissues of the immune system of the body to antigenic stimulation.

immunomodulator /-mod′yəlā′tər/ [L, *immunis* + *modulus*, little measure], a substance that acts to alter the immune response by augmenting or reducing the ability of the immune system to produce specifically modified serum antibodies or sensitized cells that recognize and react with the antigen that initiated their production. Corticosteroids, cytotoxic agents, thymosin, and the immunoglobulins are among the immunomodulating substances. Some immuno-

modulating substances are naturally present in the body; some of these are available in various pharmacologic preparations. −**immunomodulation,** *n.*

immunopotency /-pō′tənsē/ [L, *immunis* + *potentia*, power], the ability of an antigen to elicit an immune response.

immunoselection /-silek′shən/ [L, *immunis* + *seligere*, to select], 1. the survival of certain cells because they lack surface antigens that would otherwise make them vulnerable to attack and destruction by antibodies of an immune system. 2. the chance of survival of a fetus because its genotype is compatible with that of the mother's immune system. See also **erythroblastosis fetalis, Rh factor.**

immunosuppression /-səpresh′ən/ [L, *immunis* + *supprimere*, to press down], 1. the administration of agents that significantly interfere with the ability of the immune system to respond to antigenic stimulation by inhibiting cellular and humoral immunity. Corticosteroid hormones given in large amounts, cytotoxic drugs, including antimetabolites and alkylating agents, antilymphocytic serum (ALS), and irradiation may result in immunosuppression. Immunosuppression may be deliberate, such as in preparation for bone marrow or other transplantation to prevent rejection by the host of the donor tissue, or incidental, such as often results from chemotherapy for the treatment of cancer. 2. an abnormal condition of the immune system characterized by markedly inhibited ability to respond to antigenic stimuli. −**immunosuppressed,** *adj.*

immunosuppressive /-səpres′iv/, 1. of or pertaining to a substance or procedure that lessens or prevents an immune response. 2. an immunosuppressive agent. The immunosuppressive drugs used most frequently to prevent homograft rejection are the cytotoxic purine antimetabolite azathioprine, the alkylating agent cyclophosphamide, and the adrenocorticosteroid prednisone. Methotrexate, cytarabine, dactinomycin, thioguanine, and antilymphocyte globulin are also potent immunosuppressives. The use of some of these agents is being explored for the treatment of autoimmune diseases, such as systemic lupus erythematosus, and for many other disorders.

immunosurveillance /-sərvā′ləns/ [L, *immunis* + Fr, *surveiller*, to watch over], the continuous detection and protection activity of the immune system in guarding against the presence of "non-self," or foreign proteins in the body tissues.

immunotherapy /-ther′əpē/ [L, *immunis* + Gk, *therapeia*, treatment], a special treatment of allergic responses that administers increasingly large doses of the offending allergens to gradually develop immunity. Immunotherapy is based on the premise that low doses of the offending allergen will bind with IgG to prevent an allergic reaction by damping the action of IgE by fostering the synthesis of the blocking IgG antibody. The individual who is exposed to the offending allergen develops an amount of blocking antibody in proportion to the extent of the exposure. The blocking antibody binds to the circulating antigen and seems to decrease the allergic response, or it eliminates the allergic response by producing an immunologic tolerance toward the antigen. In immunotherapy low doses of the offending allergen are gradually increased throughout the year or during a 3- to 6-month period before the allergy season starts; it usually continues until the patient shows no significant allergic response for 2 to 5 years. Also called **hyposensitization.** −**immunotherapeutic,** *adj.*

immunotoxin (IT) /-tok'sin/, a plant or animal toxin that is attached to a monoclonal antibody and used to destroy a specific target cell. An example is the bonding of the plant toxin ricin to an antibody that will guide ricin molecules to tumor cells. The toxic effect of the molecular A chain of ricin is its ability to inhibit cellular production of proteins.

Imodium, a trademark for an intestinal antiperistaltic (loperamide hydrochloride), used as an antidiarrheal agent.

Imovax, a trademark for a rabies virus vaccine (rabies human diploid cell vaccine).

impacted /impak'tid/ [L, *impingere*, to drive against], tightly or firmly wedged in a limited amount of space. –**impact,** *v.,* **impaction,** *n.*

impacted fracture, a bone break in which the adjacent fragmented ends of the fractured bone are wedged together.

impacted tooth, a tooth so positioned against another tooth, bone, or soft tissue that its complete and normal eruption is impossible or unlikely. An impacted third molar tooth may be further described according to its position, as buccoangular, distoangular, or vertical. Compare **embedded tooth.**

impaction /impak'shən/, **1.** an obstacle or malposition that prevents a tooth from erupting. **2.** the presence of a large or hard fecal mass in the rectum or colon.

impact printer /im'pakt/, a mechanical printer that imprints computer characters on paper by striking it as a typewriter does, usually through an inked ribbon. Compare **nonimpact printer.**

impaired glucose tolerance (IGT) /imperd'/ [L, *impejorare*, to make worse; Gk, *glykys*, sweet; L, *tolerare*, to endure], a condition in which fasting plasma glucose levels are higher than normal but lower than those diagnostic of diabetes mellitus. In some patients this represents a stage in the natural history of diabetes, but in a substantial number of persons IGT either does not progress or reverts to normal. See also **diabetes mellitus.**

impairment [L, *impejorare*, to make worse], any disorder in structure or function resulting from anatomic, physiologic, or psychologic abnormalities that interfere with normal activities.

impedance /impē'dəns/ [L, *impedire*, to entangle], a form of electric resistance observed in an alternating current that is analogous to the classic electric resistance that occurs in a direct current circuit. It is expressed as a ratio of voltage applied to a circuit to the current it produces, as an alternating current oscillates ahead of or behind the voltage.

impedance audiometry. See **audiometry.**

impedance plethysmography, a technique for detecting blood vessel occlusion that determines volumetric changes in the limb by measuring changes in its girth as indicated by changes in the electric impedance of mercury-containing Silastic tubes in a pressure cuff. The method is based on the principle that any circumferential rate of change in a limb segment is directly proportional to the volumetric rate of change, which in turn reflects occlusion of venous and arterial blood flow. However, the technique does not accurately indicate the presence or absence of partially obstructing thrombi in major vessels.

imperative conception /imper'ətiv/ [L, *imperare*, to command], a thought or impression that appears spontaneously in the mind and cannot be eliminated, such as an obsession.

imperative idea. See **compulsive idea.**

imperforate /impur'fərit/ [L, *im*, not, *perforare*, to pierce], lacking a normal opening in a body organ or passageway. An infant may be born with an imperforate anus. Compare **perforate.**

imperforate anus, any of several congenital, developmental malformations of the anorectal portion of the GI tract.

■ OBSERVATION: The most common form is anal agenesis, in which the rectal pouch ends blindly above the surface of the perineum. An anal fistula is present in 80% to 90% of cases. Other forms include anal stenosis, in which the anal aperture is small, and anal membrane atresia, in which the anal membrane covers the aperture, creating an obstruction.

■ INTERVENTIONS: The defect is usually discovered at birth; inspection reveals an absence of the anus or the presence of a thin translucent membrane covering it. Digital and endoscopic examination allows identification of the anatomic character of the malformation. X-ray examination is performed to outline the rectal pouch. A radiopaque marker is placed at the usual site of the anus, and the infant is held upside down. Air moving through the intestines into the distal portion of the bowel or the rectum is visible on the x-ray film. Anal stenosis is treated with daily digital dilatation begun in the hospital and continued at home by the parents. An imperforate anal membrane is excised, and digital dilatation is performed daily as the skin heals. Surgical reconstruction is performed to treat anal agenesis in infants in whom the pouch is below the puborectalis of the levator ani; an anus is created surgically by an anoplasty. Anal atresia in which the pouch at the end of the bowel is high above the perineum may require a colostomy.

■ NURSING CONSIDERATIONS: Often it is the nurse who identifies the anal malformation during the routine newborn assessment. A newborn who does not pass any stool in the first 24 hours requires further evaluation for the possibility of the defect. The passage of meconium from the vagina or urinary meatus clearly indicates the presence of anal fistula and usually occurs in association with an imperforate anus. Postoperative care in the newborn treated surgically for any of these conditions requires scrupulous perineal care.

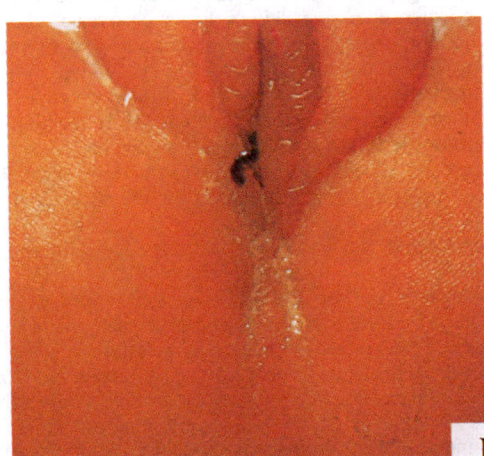

Imperforate anus
(Zetilli, 1992/Courtesy Dr Christine L Williams, New York Medical College)

imperforate hymen [L, *in*, *perforare*, to pierce through; Gk, *hymen*, membrane], a hymen that completely encloses the external orifice of the vagina.

impermeable /impur′mē·əbəl/ [L, *im*, not, *permeare*, to pass through], (of a tissue, membrane, or film) preventing the passage of a substance through it.

impetigo /im′pətī′gō/ [L, *impetus*, an attack], a streptococcal, staphylococcal, or combined infection of the skin beginning as focal erythema and progressing to pruritic vesicles, erosions, and honey-colored crusts. Lesions usually form on the face and spread locally. The disorder is highly contagious by contact with the discharge from the lesions. Acute glomerulonephritis is an occasional complication. Treatment includes thorough cleansing with antibacterial soap and water, compresses of Burow's solution, removal of crusts, and topical or oral antibiotics. treatment of the sores, use of individual wash cloths and linens, and scrupulous hand washing helps prevent spread of the infection. **–impetiginous** /im′petij′inəs/, *adj*.

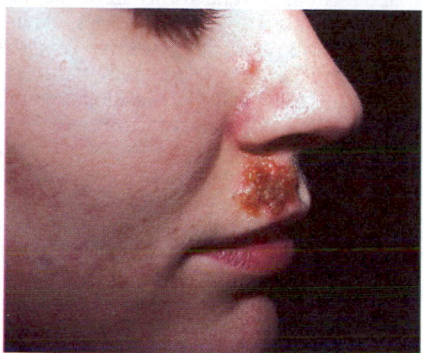

Impetigo *(Weston, 1991)*

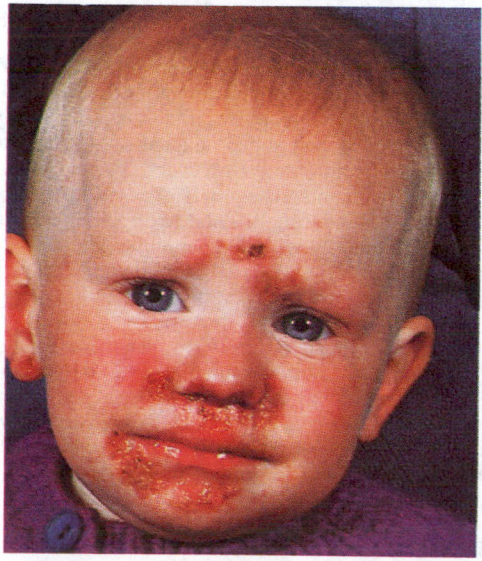

Impetigo contagiosa *(du Vivier, 1993)*

impetigo contagiosa [L, *impetus*, attack; *contingere*, to touch], an acute, contagious, superficial infection of the skin. It is characterized by vesicles that rupture, leaving a purulent exudate that dries into golden crusts.

impetigo herpetiformis [L, *impetus*, attack; Gk, *herpein*, to creep; L, *forma*], an acute form of impetigo that affects mainly pregnant women, beginning as an eruption in the genitofemoral area and spreading to other areas. The eruptions are usually irregular or circular groups of pustules that tend to coalesce.

implant /im′plant, implant′/ [L, *im*, within, *plantare*, to set], **1.** (in radiotherapy) an encapsulated radioactive substance embedded in tissue for therapy. Seeds containing iodine 125 may be implanted permanently in prostate and chest tumors and seeds of iridium 192 in ribbons or wire may be embedded temporarily in head and neck cancers. Sealed sources of cesium 137 or radium 226 may be implanted in the body cavity temporarily in the treatment of gynecologic malignancies; strontium 90 in sealed sources may be embedded for a brief period (usually less than 2 minutes) in the treatment of eye tumors; needles containing radium 226 may be used as temporary interstitial implants. Patients with radioactive implants are isolated from other patients whenever possible. **2.** (in surgery) material inserted or grafted into an organ or structure of the body. The implant may be of tissue, such as in a blood vessel graft, or of an artificial substance, such as in a hip prosthesis, a cardiac pacemaker, or a container of radioactive material.

implantation, (in embryology) the process involving the attachment, penetration, and embedding of the blastocyst in the lining of the uterine wall during the early stages of prenatal development. The degree of invasiveness required for an adequate maternal-fetal exchange varies greatly among species. In humans, the process occurs over a period of a few days, beginning about the seventh or eighth day after fertilization, and consists of the complete embedding of the conceptus within the uterine endometrium. Kinds of implantation include **eccentric implantation, interstitial implantation,** and **superficial implantation.** Also called **nidation.**

implantation dermoid cyst, a tumor derived from embryonal tissues, caused by an injury that forces part of the ectoderm into the body.

implantation endometriosis [L, *implantare*, to set into; Gk, *endon*, within, *metra*, womb, *osis*, condition], ectopic endometrial tissue found throughout the peritoneal cavity. Also called **peritoneal endometriosis**.

implant denture, an artificial or partial denture that consists of a subperiosteally or intraperiosteally implanted framework in contact with alveolar bone. A variety of designs exist, depending on manufacturers. One or more protrusions through the connective tissues and mucous membranes allow the prosthesis to be attached to the framework by posts over which the prosthesis fits. This type of solution to loss of natural teeth requires a strong commitment by the patient to practice effective oral hygiene measures.

implanted-fusion port, a self-sealing silicone septum encased in a metal or plastic case with an attached silicone catheter. It is used for long term venous access for infusion of medications, parenteral nutrition, or IV solutions. (See Fig. p. 798.)

implanted suture [L, *implantare*, to set into, *sutura*], a suture formed by inserting pins on opposite sides of a wound and bringing the edges of the wound together by winding thread tightly around the pins.

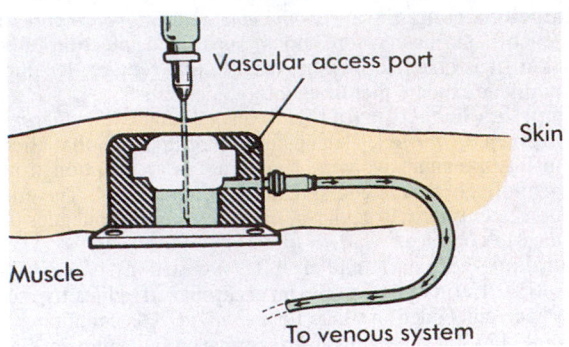

Implanted infusion port *(Potter, 1993)*

implant restoration, a single-tooth implant crown or multiple-tooth implant crown or bridge that replaces a missing tooth or teeth.

implementation /im′pləməntā′shən/ [L, *implere*, to fill], a deliberate action performed to achieve a goal, such as carrying out a plan in caring for a patient.

implementation mechanism, the means by which innovations are transferred from the planners to the units of service.

implementing /im′pləmen′ting/ [L, *implere*, to fill], (in five-step nursing process) a category of nursing behavior in which the actions necessary for accomplishing the health care plan are initiated and completed. Implementing includes the performance or assisting in the performance of the patient's activities of daily living; counseling and teaching the patient or the patient's family; giving care to achieve therapeutic goals and to optimize the achievement of health goals by the patient; supervising and evaluating the work of staff members; and recording and exchanging information relevant to the patient's continued health care. The patient may require assistance in performing certain activities of daily living. The nurse helps the patient to maintain optimal function, while instituting measures for the patient's comfort as necessary. The nurse helps the patient and the patient's family to recognize and manage the emotional and psychologic stress attendant on the patient's condition and facilitates the relationships of the patient, patient's family, staff, and other significant people. Correct principles, procedures, and techniques of health care are taught, and the patient is informed about the current status of health. If necessary, the patient or the patient's family is referred to a health or social resource in the community. Care is given to achieve therapeutic goals, including acting to compensate for adverse reactions; using preventive and precautionary measures and correct technique in administering care; preparing the patient for surgery, delivery, or other procedure; or initiating life-saving measures for emergency situations. Care is given to the patient in a manner and to a degree that best promotes attainment of the goals by the patient by providing an environment that is conducive to attaining the goals; by adjusting the care given according to the patient's needs; by stimulating and motivating the patient to achieve independence; by encouraging the patient to comply with and accept the regimen of care; and by compensating for the staff reactions to factors that influence the relationship with the patient and the therapy planned. Implementing follows planning and precedes evaluating in the five-step nursing process. See also **analyzing, assessing, evaluating, nursing process, planning.**

implied consent /implīd′/ [L, *implicare*, to involve, *consentire*, to feel], the granting of permission for health care without a formal agreement between the patient and health care provider. An example is an appointment made with a physician by a patient with a physical complaint; it is implied that by making the appointment the patient gives consent to the physician to make a diagnosis and offer treatment.

implosion /implō′zhən/ [L, *im*, within, *plaudere*, to strike], 1. a bursting inward. 2. a psychiatric treatment for people disabled by phobias and anxiety in which the person is desensitized to anxiety-producing stimuli by repeated intense exposure in imagination or reality, until the stimuli are no longer stressful. Also called **flooding.** –**implode,** *v.*

implosive therapy. See **flooding.**

impotence /im′pətəns/ [L, *im*, not, *potentia*, power], 1. weakness. 2. inability of the adult male to achieve penile erection or, less commonly, to ejaculate having achieved an erection. Several forms are recognized. **Functional impotence** has a psychologic basis. **Anatomic impotence** results from physically defective genitalia. **Atonic impotence** involves disturbed neuromuscular function. Poor health, age, drugs, and fatigue can inhibit normal sexual function. Also called **impotency.** –**impotent,** *adj.*

impregnate /impreg′nāt/ [L, *impregnare*, to make pregnant], 1. to inseminate and make pregnant; to fertilize. 2. to saturate or mix with another substance. –**impregnable,** *adj.*, **impregnation,** *n.*

impression /impresh′ən/ [L, *imprimere*, to press into], 1. (in dentistry and prosthetic medicine) a mold of a part of the mouth or other part of the body from which a replacement or prosthesis may be formed. 2. (in the medical record) the examiner's diagnosis or assessment of a problem, disease, or condition. 3. a strong sensation or effect on the mind, intellect, or feelings.

impression material [L, *imprimere*, to press into + *materia*, stuff], any material used for making impressions of teeth and oral structures for the purpose of producing dental restorations.

imprinting [Fr, *empreindre*, to impress], (in ethology) a special type of learning that occurs at critical points during the early stages of development in animals. It involves behavioral patterning and social attachment, is characterized by rapid acquisition and irreversibility, and is usually species-specific, although animals exposed to members of a different species during this short period may become attached to and identify with that particular species instead of their own. The degree to which imprinting occurs in human development has not been determined. See also **bonding.**

imprisonment /impriz′ənment/ [Fr, *emprisonner*, to confine], (in law) the act of confining, detaining, or arresting a person or in any way restraining personal liberty and preventing free exercise of movement. Imprisonment may be in a prison or other special facility, but every confinement is an imprisonment.

impulse /im′puls/ [L, *impellere*, to drive], 1. (in psychology) a sudden, irresistible, often irrational inclination, urge, desire, or action resulting from a particular feeling or mental state. 2. also called **nerve impulse, neural impulse.** (in physiology) the electrochemical process involved in neural transmission. –**impulsive,** *adj.*

impulse-conducting system [L, *impellere*, to drive before; *conducere*, to conduct; Gk, *systema*], the Purkinje fibers within the heart muscle that conduct impulses controlling the contractions of the atria and ventricles.

impulsion /impul′shən/ [L, *impellere*, to drive], an abnormal, irrational urge to commit an unlawful or socially unacceptable act.

-impulsive. See **impulse.**

Imuran, a trademark for an immunosuppressive (azathioprine).

IMV, abbreviation for **intermittent mandatory ventilation.**

In, symbol for the element **indium.**

in-, 1. a combining form meaning 'of or pertaining to fibers': *inaxon, inemia, initis.* 2. a prefix meaning 'in, on, within, into or toward': *inborn, inbreeding.* 3. a prefix meaning 'not, lack of, opposite of': *inarticulate.*

-in, 1. a suffix meaning 'pertaining to a neutral substance': *albumin, gelatin, bacitracin.*

-in, -ine, 1. a combining form meaning an 'antibiotic': *bacitracin, penicillin, streptomycin.* 2. a combining form meaning a 'pharmaceutic product': *aspirin, niacin.* 3. a combining form meaning a 'chemical compound': *albumin, gelatin, palmitin.* 4. a combining form meaning an 'enzyme': *emulsin, pepsin, myrosin.*

inactivated measles virus vaccine /inak′tivā′tid/ [L, *in*, *activus*; OE, *masala*, blister; L, *virus*, poison; *vaccinus*, of a cow], a measles vaccine virus that has been treated so that it is no longer capable of replication. It is an alternative to live attenuated measles vaccine, which is contraindicated for some individuals, such as those who are immunocompromised.

inactivation /inak′tivā′shən/ [L, *in*, not, *activus*, active], a reversible denaturation of a protein.

inactivation of complement [L, *in*, *activus*, *complere*, to complete], the loss of activity of the enzymatic proteins in blood, achieved by heating the serum to about 55° C. Inactivation of complement is a step in the process of **complement fixation.**

inactive colon /inak′tiv/ [L, *in*, not, *activus*, active; Gk, *kolon*, colon], hypotonicity of the bowel resulting in decreased contractions and propulsive movements and a delay in the normal 12-hour transit time of luminal contents from cecum to anus. Colonic inactivity may be caused by acquired or congenital megacolon, anticholinergic drugs, depression, faulty habits of elimination, inadequate fluid intake, lack of exercise, a low-residue or starvation diet, neuroendocrine response to surgical stress, prolonged bed rest, or a neurologic disease, such as diabetic visceral neuropathy, multiple sclerosis, parkinsonism, and spinal cord lesions. Normal motility of the colon is frequently compromised by the continued use of laxatives. Acquired megacolon, characterized by an abnormally large, inactive bowel and chronic constipation, is common in retarded children and adults with chronic mental illness. In congenital megacolon (Hirschsprung's disease) congenital absence of myenteric innervation in a distal segment of the colon results in loss of motility and causes massive dilatation of the proximal segment of the large bowel and extreme constipation. The disorder is more common in males than females and in severe cases retards growth. Treatment of colonic inactivity includes a stimulus-response training program to establish regular bowel habits, the use of stool softeners and hydrophilic colloids to increase fecal bulk, and a diet containing adequate roughage.

inadequate personality /inad′əkwit/ [L, *in*, not, *adaequare*, to equal; *personalis*, of a person], a personality characterized by a lack of physical stamina, emotional immaturity, social instability, poor judgment, reduced motivation, ineptness—especially in interpersonal relationships—and an inability to adapt or react effectively to new or stressful situations.

inanimate /inan′imit/ [L, *in*, not, *animus*, life spirit], not alive; lacking signs of life.

inanition /in′ənish′ən/ [L, *inanis*, empty], 1. an exhausted condition resulting from lack of food and water or a defect in assimilation; starvation. 2. a state of lethargy characterized by a loss of vitality or vigor in all aspects of social, moral, and intellectual life.

inanition fever, a temporary, mild, febrile condition of the newborn in the first few days after birth, usually caused by dehydration.

inborn /in′bôrn/ [L, *in*, within; AS, *beran*, to bear], innate; acquired or occurring during intrauterine life, with reference to both normally inherited traits and developmental or genetically transmitted anomalies. See also **congenital, hereditary, inborn error of metabolism.**

inborn error of metabolism, one of many abnormal metabolic conditions caused by an inherited defect of a single enzyme or other protein. Though people with such diseases are each defective in only protein, they generally display a large number of physical signs that are characteristic of the genetic trait. The diseases are rare. Kinds of inborn errors of metabolism include **phenylketonuria, Tay-Sachs disease, Lesch-Nyhan syndrome, galactosemia,** and **glucose-6-phosphate dehydrogenase deficiency.**

■ OBSERVATIONS: Inborn errors of metabolism may be detected in the fetus in utero by the examination of squamous and blood cells obtained by amniocentesis and fetoscopy. Laboratory tests after birth often show higher than normal levels of particular metabolites in the blood and urine, such as phenylpyruvic acid and phenylalanine in PKU and galactose in galactosemia. The values are higher in homozygous than in heterozygous carriers. Physical stigmata of the various defects are usually seen only in homozygous carriers.

■ INTERVENTIONS: Treatment for some pathologic inborn errors may be initiated by removing dietary precursors of the nondegradable metabolite to prevent its accumulation. Removal of dietary phenylalanine in PKU and galactose in galactosemia is effective in preventing the development of symptoms if treatment is begun early. In those cases of inborn errors of metabolism in which the nondegradable metabolite is endogenous, such as in the mucopolysaccaridoses, there is no treatment available.

inborn reflex. See **unconditioned response.**

inbreeding /in′brēding/ [L, *in*, within; AS, *bredan*, to reproduce], the production of offspring by the mating of closely related individuals, organisms, or plants; self-fertilization is the most extreme form, which normally occurs in certain plants and lower animals. The practice provides a greater chance for recessive genes for both desirable and undesirable traits to become homozygous and to be expressed phenotypically. In humans, the amount of inbreeding in a specific population is largely controlled by tradition and cultural practices. In plants and animals, inbreeding is a standard method for developing desirable genotypes and pure lines. Compare **outbreeding.**

incandescent [L, *incandescere*, to begin to glow], hot to the point of glowing or emitting intense light rays, as an incandescent light bulb.

incarcerate /inkar'sərāt/ [L, *in*, within, *carcerare*, to imprison], to trap, imprison, or confine, such as a loop of intestine in an inguinal hernia. See also **hernia.**

incarcerated hernia [L, *in, carcerare*, to imprison, *hernia*, rupture], a loop of bowel with ends occluded so that solids cannot pass and the hernia will not return to its normal position without manipulation or surgery. Also called **irreducible hernia.**

incentive spirometry /insen'tiv/, spirometric therapy in which the patient is given special encouragement to achieve a maximum inspiratory capacity. Using a specially designed spirometer, the patient inhales until a preset volume is reached, and then sustains the inspiratory volume by holding the breath for 3 to 5 seconds. Incentive spirometry reduces the risk of atelectasis and pulmonary consolidation.

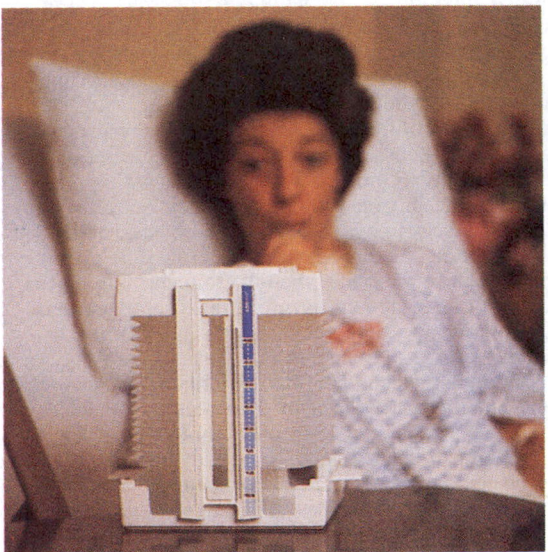

Incentive spirometry *(Potter, 1993)*

inception /insep'shən/ [L, *incipere*, to begin], the origin or beginning of anything.

incest /in'sest/ [L, *incestum*, defiled], sexual intercourse between members of the same family who are so closely related as to be legally prohibited from marrying one another by reason of their consanguinity. —**incestuous,** *adj.*

incidence /in'sidəus/ [L, *incidere*, to happen], **1.** the number of times an event occurs. **2.** (in epidemiology) the number of new cases in a particular period of time. Incidence is often expressed as a ratio, in which the number of cases is the numerator and the population at risk is the denominator. See also **rate.**

incidence rate, the rate of new cases of a disease in a specified population over a defined period of time.

incidental additives /in'siden'təl/ [L, *incidere*, to happen; *additio* something added], food additives caused by the use of pesticides, herbicides, or chemicals involved in food processing.

incident report, a document, usually confidential, describing any accident or deviation from policies or orders involving a patient, employee, visitor, or student on the premises of a health care facility.

incineration /insin'ərā'shən/ [L, *incinerare*, to burn to ashes], the removal or reduction of waste materials by burning.

incipient /insip'ē·ənt/ [L, *incipire*, to commence], coming into existence; at an initial stage; beginning to appear, such as a symptom or disease.

incipient dental caries, a dental condition in which a lesion of tooth decay is initially detectable.

incisal angle /insī'səl/ [L, *incidere*, to cut into; *angulus*, corner], the degree of slope between the axis-orbital plane and the discluding surface of the maxillary incisor teeth.

incisal guide, the part of a dental articulator that maintains the incisal guide angle. Also called **anterior guide.**

incisal guide pin, a metal rod, attached to the upper member of an articulator, that touches the incisal guide table to maintain the established vertical separation of the upper and lower members of the articulator.

incision /insizh'ən/ [L, *incidere*, to cut into], **1.** a cut produced surgically by a sharp instrument creating an opening into an organ or space in the body. **2.** the act of making an incision.

incisional hernia /insish'ənəl/ [L, *incidere*, to cut into, *hernia*, rupture], a herniation through a surgical scar.

incisor /insī'zər/, one of the eight front teeth, four in each dental arch, that first appear as primary teeth during infancy, are replaced by permanent incisors during childhood, and last until old age. The crown of the incisor is chisel shaped and has a sharp cutting edge. Its labial surface is convex, smooth, and highly polished; its lingual surface is concave and, in many individuals, is marked by an inverted V-shaped basal ridge near the gum of the upper arch. The neck of the incisor is constricted. The root is single, long, and conic. The upper incisors are larger and stronger than the lower and are directed obliquely downward and forward. Compare **canine tooth, molar, premolar.**

incisura /in'sisyoo'rə/ [L, *incidere*, to cut into], a notch or indentation on an organ or body part.

inciting eye. See **exciting eye.**

inclusion /inkloo'zhən/ [L, *in*, within, *claudere*, to shut], **1.** the act of enclosing or the condition of being enclosed. **2.** a structure within another, such as inclusions in the cytoplasm of the cells.

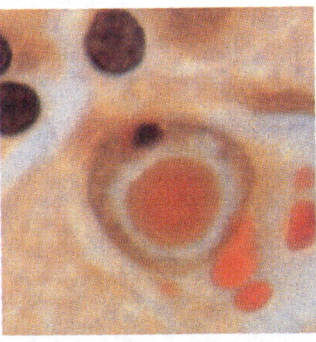

Inclusion body *(Perkin, 1986)*

inclusion bodies,   microscopic objects of various shapes and sizes observed in the nucleus or cytoplasm of blood cells or other tissue cells, depending on the type of disease.

inclusion conjunctivitis,   an acute, purulent, conjunctival infection caused by *Chlamydia* organisms. It occurs in two forms: the infection in infants is characterized by bilateral chemosis, redness, and purulent discharge; the adult variety is unilateral, less severe and less purulent, and is associated with preauricular lymphadenopathy. Local instillation of antibiotics is effective treatment.

inclusion dermoid cyst,   a tumor derived from embryonal tissues, caused by the inclusion of foreign tissue when a developmental cleft closes.

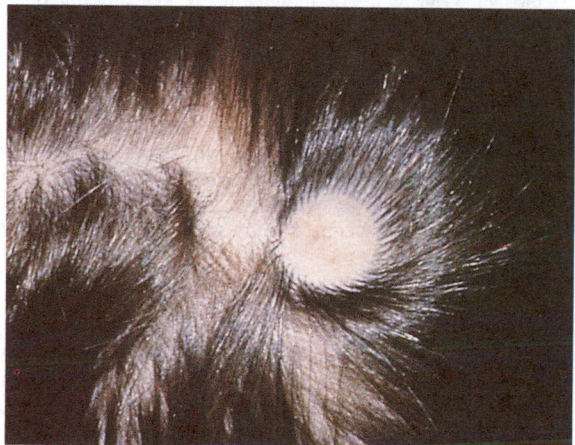

Inclusion dermoid cyst *(Baran, 1991)*

inclusiveness principle /inkloo′sivnəs/ [L, *in*, within, *claudere*, to shut; *principium*, a beginning],   a rule that response to various objects in the environment is proportional to the amount of stimulus provided by each object.

inclusive rate /inkloo′siv/,   a method of calculating inpatient hospital charges in which a fixed amount covers all services, regardless of the number or intensity of services provided.

incoherent /in′kōhir′ənt/ [L, *in*, not, *cohaere*, to hold together],   **1.** disordered; without logical connection; disjointed; lacking orderly continuity or relevance. **2.** unable to express one's thoughts or ideas in an orderly, intelligible manner, usually as a result of emotional stress.

incompatibility /in′kəmpat′ibil′itē/ [L, *in*, *compatibulus*, agreeing],   a state of not being able to exist in harmony, as when transfused blood produces adverse effects because the donor and recipient blood groups are in conflict with each other.

incompatible /in′kəmpat′əbəl/ [L, *in*, not, *compatibilis*, agreement],   unable to coexist. A tissue transplant may be rejected because recipient and donor antibody factors are incompatible.

incompetence /inkom′pətəns/ [L, *in*, not, *competentia*, capable],   lack of ability. Body organs that do not function adequately may be described as incompetent. Kinds of incompetence include **aortic incompetence, ileocecal incompetence,** and **valvular incompetence.** **–incompetent,** *adj.*

incompetency /inkomp′ətənsē/,   legal status of a person declared to be unable to provide for his or her own needs and protection. The status must be proved in a special court hearing, as a result of which the person can be deprived of certain civil rights. Incompetency can be reversed in another court hearing that may find the same person competent.

-incompetent.   See **incompetence.**

incompetent cervix [L, *in*, not, *competentia*, capable; *cervix*, neck],   (in obstetrics) a condition characterized by painless dilatation of the cervical os of the uterus before term without labor or contractions of the uterus. Miscarriage or premature delivery may result. Incompetent cervix is treated prophylactically by a Shirodkar or other procedure in which the cervix is held closed by a surgically implanted suture.

incomplete abortion /in′kəmplēt′/ [L, *in*, not, *complere*, to fill; *ab*, from, *oriri*, to be born],   termination of pregnancy in which the products of conception are not entirely expelled or removed, often causing hemorrhage that may require surgical evacuation by curettage, oxytocics, and blood replacement. Infection is also a frequent complication of incomplete abortion. Compare **complete abortion.**

incomplete dislocation [L, *in* , *complere*, to fill up, *dis*, *locare*, to place],   a partial abnormal separation of the articular surfaces of a joint. Also called **subluxation.**

incomplete fistula.   See **blind fistula.**

incomplete fracture,   a bone break in which the crack in the osseous tissue does not completely traverse the width of the affected bone but may angle off in one or more directions.

incomplete hernia [L, *in*, *complere*, to fill up, *hernia*, rupture],   a hernia that has not yet protruded through a weak spot or opening.

incongruent communication /inkong′groo·ənt/,   a communication pattern in which the sender gives conflicting messages on verbal and nonverbal levels and the listener does not know which message to accept. See **double bind.**

incontinence /inkon′tinəns/ [L, *incontinentia*, inability to retain],   the inability to control urination or defecation. Urinary incontinence may be caused by cerebral clouding in the aged, infection, lesions in the brain or spinal cord, damage to peripheral nerves of the bladder, or injury to the sphincter or perineal structures, sometimes occurring in childbirth. Treatment includes bladder retraining, the implantation of an artificial sphincter, and the use of internal or external drainage devices. Stress incontinence precipitated by coughing, straining, or heavy lifting occurs more often in women than in men, and mild cases may be treated by exercises involving tightening and relaxing perineal and gluteal muscles, or they may respond to sympathomimetic drug therapy. Severe cases may require surgery to correct the underlying anatomic defect. Fecal incontinence may result from relaxation of the anal sphincter or by central nervous system or spinal cord disorders and may be treated by a program of bowel training. A Bradford frame with an opening for a bedpan or urinal may be used for bedridden incontinent patients. See also **bowel training.** **–incontinent,** *adj.*

incontinence, bowel,   a nursing diagnosis accepted by the Fourth National Conference on the Classification of Nursing Diagnoses. The condition is defined as a state in which an individual experiences a change in normal bowel habits characterized by involuntary passage of stool. The cause of the condition, developed at the Fifth National Conference, is neuromuscular or musculoskeletal impairment; depression, severe anxiety, or perceptive or cognitive impairment; multiple life changes; inadequate relaxation; little or no exercise; poor nutrition; work-related tensions; no vacations; unmet expectations; unrealistic perceptions; and inadequate support systems or coping methods. See also **nursing diagnosis.**

incontinence, functional, a nursing diagnosis accepted by the Seventh National Conference on the Classification of Nursing Diagnoses. The condition is defined as the state in which an individual experiences an involuntary, unpredictable passage of urine. The critical defining characteristics are the urge to void or bladder contractions sufficiently strong to result in loss of urine before reaching an appropriate receptacle. Related factors include altered environment; and sensory, cognitive, or mobility deficits. See also **nursing diagnosis.**

incontinence, reflex, a nursing diagnosis accepted by the Seventh National Conference on the Classification of Nursing Diagnoses. The diagnosis describes the state in which an individual experiences an involuntary loss of urine occuring at somewhat predictable intervals when a specific bladder volume is reached. Defining characteristics include no awareness of bladder filling; no urge to void or feelings of bladder fullness; or uninhibited bladder contractions/spasms at regular intervals. Related factors include neurologic impairment, as a spinal cord lesion which interferes with conduction of cerebral messages above the level of the reflex arc. See also **nursing diagnosis.**

incontinence, stress, a nursing diagnosis accepted by the Seventh National Conference on the Classification of Nursing Diagnoses. The condition is defined as the state in which an individual experiences a loss of urine of less than 50 ml occurring with increased abdominal pressure. The major defining characteristic is reported or observed dribbling with increased abdominal pressure. Minor characteristics include urinary urgency or urinary frequency (more often than every 2 hours). Related factors are degenerative changes in pelvic muscles and structural supports associated with increased age high intraabdominal pressure, such as obesity, or gravid uterus; incompetent bladder outlet; overdistention between voidings; and weak pelvic muscles and structural supports. See also **nursing diagnosis.**

incontinence, total, a nursing diagnosis accepted by the Seventh National Conference on the Classification of Nursing Diagnoses. The condition is defined as the state in which an individual experiences a continuous and unpredictable loss of urine. Major defining characteristics include a constant flow of urine occurring at unpredictable times without distention or unihibited bladder contractions or spasms, unsuccessful incontinence refractory treatments, and nocturia. Minor characteristics are lack of perineal or bladder awareness and unawareness of incontinence. Related factors include neuropathy preventing transmission of a reflex indicating bladder fullness; neurologic dysfunction causing triggering of micturation at unpredictable times; independent contraction of detruser reflex due to surgery; trauma or disease affecting spinal cord nerves; and an anatomic factor, such as a fistula. See also **nursing diagnosis.**

incontinence, urge, a nursing diagnosis accepted by the Seventh National Conference on the Classification of Nursing Diagnoses. Urge incontinence is defined as the state in which an individual experiences involuntary passage of urine occurring soon after a strong sense of urgency to void.

Critical defining characteristics are urinary urgency, frequency (voiding more often than every 2 hours), and bladder contractions or spasms. Minor characteristics include nocturia (urination more than 2 times per night), voiding in small amounts (less than 100 ml) or in large amounts (500 ml), and an inability to reach a toilet on time. Related factors include decreased bladder capacity, as with a history of PID, abdominal surgery, or an indwelling urinary catheter; irritation of bladder stretch receptors causing spasm, as with a bladder infection; alcohol; caffeine; increased fluids; increased urine concentration; and overdistention of the bladder. See also **nursing diagnosis.**

-incontinent. See **incontinence.**

increment [L, *incresere,* to grow], **1.** an increase or gain. **2.** the act of growing or increasing. **3.** the amount of an increase or gain in intrauterine pressure as uterine contractions begin in labor. **–incremental,** *adj.*

incrustation, hardened exudate, scale, or scab.

incubation period /in'kyəbā'shən/ [L, *incubare,* to lie on; Gk, *peri,* around, *hodos,* way], **1.** the time between exposure to a pathogenic organism and the onset of symptoms of a disease. **2.** the time required to induce the development of an embryo in an egg or to induce the development and replication of tissue cells or microorganisms being grown in culture media or other special laboratory environment. **3.** the time allowed for a chemical reaction or process to proceed.

incubator /in'kyəbā'tər/, an apparatus used to provide a controlled environment, especially a particular temperature. Other environmental components, such as darkness, light, oxygen, moisture, or dryness, may also be provided, as in an incubator for the cultivation of eggs or microorganisms in a laboratory or an incubator for premature infants.

incud-, a combining form meaning 'of or pertaining to an anvil (the incus)': *incudectomy, incudiform, incudomalleal.*

incudectomy /in'kyo͞odek'təmē/ [L, *incus,* anvil, *ektome,* incision], surgical removal of the incus, performed to treat conductive hearing loss resulting from necrosis of the tip of the incus. Local or general anesthesia is used. The defective incus is excised and replaced with a bone chip graft so that sound vibrations are again transmitted. Postoperatively, the nurse instructs patient to change position slowly to avoid dizziness, avoid blowing the nose and sneezing, and report any fever, headache, dizziness, or pain in the ear.

incus /ing'kəs/, *pl.* **incudes** /inko͞o'dēz/ [L, anvil], one of the three ossicles in the middle ear, resembling an anvil. It communicates sound vibrations from the malleus to the stapes. Compare **malleus, stapes.** See also **middle ear.**

IND, abbreviation for **investigational new drug.**

indandione derivative /indan'dē·on'/, one of a small group of oral anticoagulants designed for long-term therapeutic use in patients who cannot tolerate other oral anticoagulants. The indandiones are difficult to control and may cause grave adverse effects, including severe renal and hepatic toxicity, agranulocytosis, and leukopenia. For this reason coumarin derivatives are preferred. Regular evaluations of prothrombin are necessary. Extreme fatigue, sore throat, chills, and fever are signs of impending toxicity and require discontinuation of the drug. Compare **coumarin.**

indentation /in'dəntā'shən/ [L, *in,* within, *dens,* tooth], a notch, pit, or depression in the surface of an object, such as toothmarks on the tongue or skin. **–indent,** *v.*

independence /in'dəpen'dəns/ [L, *in,* not, *de,* from, *pendere,* to hang], **1.** the state or quality of being independent; autonomy; free from the influence, guidance, or control of a person or a group. **2.** a lack of requirement or reliance on another for physical existence or emotional needs. **–independent,** *adj.*

independent assortment [L, *in*, not, *dependere*, to hang from; *ad*, towards, *sortiri*, to cast lots], (in genetics) a basic principle stating that the members of a pair of genes are randomly distributed in the gametes, independent of the distribution of other pairs of genes. See also **dominance, segregation.**

independent intervention. See **intervention.**

independent living centers, rehabilitation facilities in which disabled persons can receive special education and training in the performance of all or most activities of daily living with a particular handicap. A typical independent living center may contain a completely furnished multi-room apartment, including a kitchen with cabinets and cooking facilities that can be reached easily by a person in a wheelchair, designed for training patients in homemaking skills.

independent practice, (in nursing) the practice of certain aspects of professional nursing that are encompassed by applicable licensure and law and require no supervision or direction from others. Nurses in independent practice may have an office in which they see patients and charge fees for service. In all nursing settings, state practice acts define certain aspects of nursing practice that are independent and may define those that must be done only under supervision or direction of another individual, usually a physician.

independent practice association (IPA), a prepaid health service system in which office-based physicians contract for the care of patients on a prenegotiated fee-for-service basis. See also **health maintenance organization.**

independent variable, (in research) a variable that is manipulated by the researcher and evaluated by its measurable effect on the dependent variable or variables; for example, in a study of the effect of nursing intervention on postoperative vomiting, nursing intervention is the independent variable evaluated by its effect on the incidence of postoperative vomiting. Also called **experimental variable, predictor variable.** Compare **dependent variable.**

Inderal, a trademark for a beta-adrenergic blocking agent (propranolol).

indeterminate cleavage /in′ditur′minit/ [L, *in*, not, *determinare*, to fix limits; AS, *cleofan*, to split], mitotic division of the fertilized ovum into blastomeres that have similar developmental potential and, if isolated, can give rise to a complete individual embryo. Also called **regulative cleavage.** Compare **determinate cleavage.** See also **regulative development.**

index astigmatism [L, *indicare*, to indicate, *a*, *stigma*, point], an astigmatism caused by unequal refractive indices in different parts of the lens.

index case [L, pointer], (in epidemiology) the first case of a disease as contrasted with the appearance of subsequent cases. See also **propositus.**

Index Medicus, an index published monthly by the National Library of Medicine, which lists articles from the medical literature from throughout the world by subject and by author. An annual edition, the *Cumulative Index Medicus,* is published yearly; it contains the citations in all 12 issues of the *Index Medicus.*

index myopia, a kind of nearsightedness caused by a variation in the index of refraction of the media of the eye.

Indian Health Service, a bureau within the Department of Health and Human Services for providing public health and medical services to Native Americans in the United States. In Canada, the services are provided by the **Ministry of Indian Affairs.**

Indian tick fever. See **Marseilles fever.**

indican /in′dikən/ [Gk, *indikon*, indigo], a substance (potassium indoxyl sulfate) produced in the intestine by the decomposition of tryptophan, absorbed by the intestinal wall, and excreted in the urine. It may be elevated in the urine of patients on high-protein diets or those suffering from GI disease. The normal accumulation of indican in urine after 24-hour collection is 10 to 20 mg.

indication /in′dikā′shən/ [L, *indicare*, to make known], a reason to prescribe a medication or perform a treatment, as a bacterial infection may be an indication for the prescription of a specific antibiotic or as appendicitis is an indication for appendectomy. **–indicate,** *v.*

indicator /in′dikā′tər/, a tape, paper, tablet, or any other substance that is used to test for a particular reaction because it changes in a predictable visible way. Some kinds of indicators are **autoclave indicator, dipsticks,** and **litmus paper.** Also called **reagent.**

indigence /in′dijəns/ [L, *indigere*, to need], a condition of having insufficient income to pay for adequate medical care without depriving oneself or one's dependents of food, clothing, shelter, or other living essentials.

indigenous /indij′ənəs/ [L, *indigena*, a native], native to or occurring naturally in a specified area or environment, as certain species of bacteria in the human digestive tract.

indigestible /in′dijes′təbəl/ [L, *in*, not, *digerere*, to separate], pertaining to a food substance that cannot be broken down by the digestive tract and converted into an absorbable nutrient.

indigestion. See **dyspepsia.**

indirect anaphylaxis [L, *in*, not, *directus*, straight; Gk, *ana*, again, *phylaxis*, protection], an exaggerated reaction of hypersensitivity to a person's own antigen that occurs because the antigen has been altered in some way.

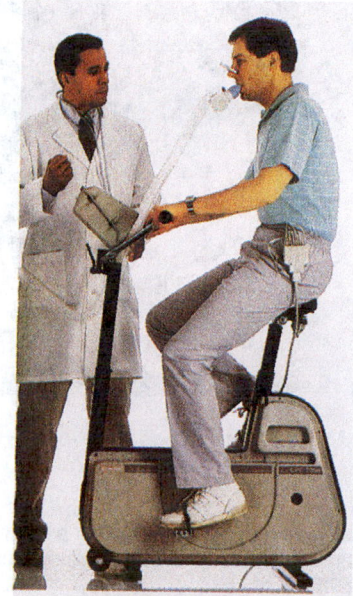

Indirect calorimetry
(Wardlaw, 1993/Medical Graphics Corporation, St. Paul, Minn.)

indirect calorimetry, the measurement of the amount of heat generated in an oxidation reaction by determining the intake or consumption of oxygen or by measuring the amount of carbon dioxide or the amount of nitrogen released and translating these quantities into a heat equivalent. Compare **direct calorimetry.**

indirect division. See **mitosis.**

indirect laryngoscopy [L, *in, directus,* straight; Gk, *larynx, skopein,* to view], a method of examining the larynx with a mirror.

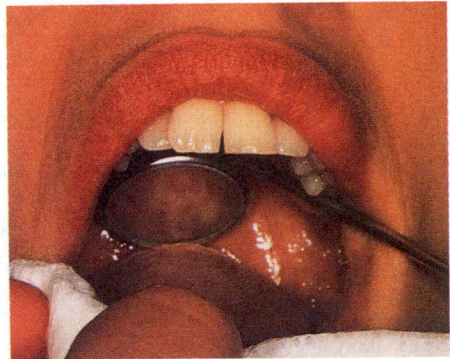

Indirect laryngoscopy *(Epstein, 1992)*

indirect nursing care functions, liaison nurse activities used to solve problems with a consultee who is responsible and accountable for implementing and evaluating any recommended changes.

indirect ophthalmoscope, an ophthalmoscope with a biconvex lens that produces a reversed direct image.

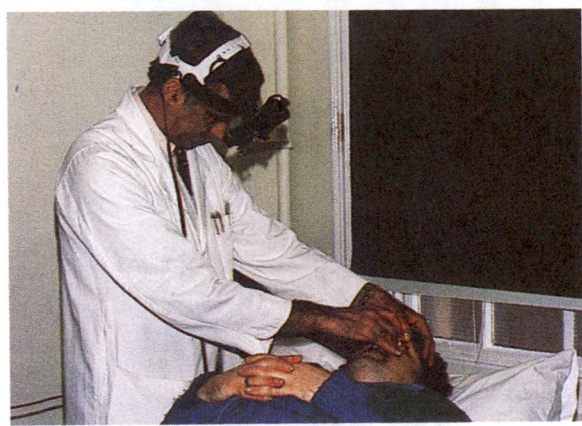

Indirect ophthalmoscope *(Eagling, 1986)*

indirect percussion. See **percussion.**

indirect provider reimbursement, a method of payment to an agency for health services delivered by providers, such as nurses.

indirect restorative method, the technique for fabricating a restoration on a cast of the original, such as the indi-

rect construction of an inlay. After a die is made from an impression of the prepared tooth, a wax pattern is formed and inverted. The cast inlay is then fitted and finished on the die and then cemented into the tooth.

indirect retainer, a portion of a removable partial denture that resists movement of a distal extension away from its tissue support by means of lever action opposite the fulcrum line of the direct retention.

indirect transfusion [L, *in, directus,* straight, *transfundere,* to pour through], the transfusion of blood to a recipient after the donor blood has been prepared with anticoagulants, defibrinating agents, or other substances, as opposed to transfusing blood directly from donor to recipient.

indirect vision [L, *in, directus,* straight, *visio,* seeing], a visual sensation caused by stimulation of the extramacular portion of the retina. Also called **peripheral vision**.

indium (In) [L, *indicum,* indigo], a silvery metallic element with some nonmetallic chemical properties. Its atomic number is 49; its atomic weight is 114.82. It is used in electronic semiconductors.

individual immunity /in'divij'oo·əl/ [L, *individuus,* indivisible; *immunis,* free], a form of natural immunity not shared by most other members of the race and species. It is rare and probably occurs as the result of the person having had an infection that went unrecognized. Compare **racial immunity, species immunity.**

individual psychology, a modified system of psychoanalysis, developed by Alfred Adler, that views maladaptive behavior and personality disorders as resulting from a conflict between the desire to dominate and feelings of inferiority. See also **inferiority complex.**

Indocin, a trademark for an antiinflammatory agent (indomethacin).

indoleacetic acid /in'dōləsē'tik, -əset'ik/, a major terminal metabolite of tryptophan that is present in very small amounts in normal urine and excreted in elevated quantities by patients with carcinoid tumors.

indolent /in'dələnt/ [L, *in, dolere,* to suffer pain], pertaining to an organic disorder that is accompanied by little or no pain.

indomethacin /in'dōmeth'əsin/, a nonsteroidal antiinflammatory agent.

■ INDICATIONS: It is prescribed in the treatment of arthritis and certain other inflammatory conditions.

■ CONTRAINDICATIONS: Upper GI disease or known hypersensitivity to this drug or to aspirin prohibits its use. It is not given to children under 15 years of age or to pregnant or lactating women.

■ ADVERSE EFFECTS: The most serious adverse reaction is peptic ulcers. GI upset, dizziness, tinnitus, and rashes also may occur.

induce /ind(y)oos'/ [L, *inducere,* to bring in], to cause or stimulate the start of an activity, as an enzyme induces a metabolic activity. See also **induced fever. —inducer, induction,** *n.*

induced abortion, an intentional termination of pregnancy before the fetus has developed enough to live if born. From 20% to 50% of pregnancies are terminated deliberately, at the request of the mother or for medical indications—during the first trimester by curettage, or during the second trimester by induction of labor or hysterotomy. Termination of pregnancy by a trained person under proper conditions is safe. Unskilled abortions can be extremely hazardous because of the susceptibility of the uterus to infection and laceration. Puerperal sepsis and hemorrhage after criminal abortion have been leading causes of maternal death. Compare **spontaneous abortion.** See also **criminal abortion, septic abortion, therapeutic abortion.**

induced fever, a deliberate elevation of body temperature by application of heat or by inoculation with a fever-producing organism in order to kill heat-sensitive pathogens.

induced hypotension. See **deliberate hypotension.**

induced lethargy, a trancelike state produced during hypnosis. See also **hypnosis, lethargy.**

induced mutation [L, *inducere,* to lead in, *mutare,* to change], a mutation that has been produced by treatment with a physical or chemical agent that affects the DNA molecules of a living organism.

induced phagocytosis [L, *inducere,* to lead in; Gk, *phagein,* to eat, *kytos,* cell], the ingestion of microorganisms and other foreign particles by cells of the reticuloendothelial system.

induced trance, a somnambulistic state resulting from hypnotism.

induced vomiting [L, *inducere,* to lead in; *vomere,* to vomit], vomiting produced by administration of ipecac syrup, soapy water, or handwashing liquid detergent, or by inserting a finger or blunt instrument into the throat. Vomiting may be medically indicated in cases of ingested noncaustic poisons but may also be self-induced by patients afflicted with **bulimia.**

inducer /indoo′sər/, (in molecular genetics) a substance, usually a molecular substrate of a specific enzyme, that combines with and deactivates the active repressor produced by the regulator gene. The result of this combination is the activation of the operator gene, which was previously inactivated by the active repressor, and initiation of the transcription of the amino acid sequence in the structural gene for the eventual synthesis of protein.

induction /induk′shən/ [L, *inducere,* to bring in], (in embryology) the process of stimulating and determining morphogenetic differentiation in a developing embryo through the action of chemical substances transmitted from one to another of the embryonic parts. See also **evocation.**

induction of anesthesia, all portions of the anesthetic process that occur before attaining the desired level of anesthesia, including the administration of a sedative, hypnotic, tranquilizer, or curariform adjunct to anesthesia; intubation; administration of oxygen; and administration of the anesthetic.

induction of labor, an obstetric procedure in which labor is initiated artificially by means of amniotomy or the administration of oxytocics. It is performed electively or for fetal or maternal indications. Elective induction is carried out for the convenience of the mother or the obstetrician, often to avert the possibility of delivery outside of the hospital when labor is judged to be imminent and the mother is expected to have an unusually rapid birth. Elective inductions are performed less often now than in the past. Prerequisites for elective induction are a term gestation, a fetal weight of at least 2500 g, a cervix judged ready to dilate, a vertex presentation, and engagement of the presenting part of the fetus in the pelvis. Errors in the estimation of gestational age and fetal weight may result in the delivery of an unexpectedly immature or low birth weight infant. Indicated induction is performed when the risk of induction is judged to be less than that of continuing the pregnancy in such con-

ditions as premature rupture of the membranes, severe maternal diabetes, and intractable preeclampsia. Surgical induction is effected by amniotomy, often with stripping of the membranes and digital stretching of the cervix; it is very often carried out in conjunction with medical induction. Medical induction is achieved through the administration of oxytocin, almost always by intravenous infusion, in a carefully controlled manner using microdrip equipment or an infusion pump. Beginning with very small amounts of oxytocin in an intravenous solution, the dosage is increased by gradual increments of the rate or concentration of infusion until effective labor is established. Oxytocin can be administered but prostaglandins are more commonly used to induce labor, particularly for therapeutic abortions in the second trimester. With intravenous oxytocin inductions, a secondary, piggyback infusion without medication is always attached to the tubing so that an unmedicated infusion can be maintained if oxytocin is stopped. Electronic fetal and uterine monitoring is usually instituted during induction of labor to avoid hyperstimulation of the uterus and fetal distress. Ideally, induced labor mimics natural labor, but in practice this is not usually achieved. Longer and harder contractions commonly occur. In addition to unexpected fetal immaturity, complications of induction of labor include umbilical cord prolapse after amniotomy, tumultuous labor, tetanic uterine contractions, rupture of the uterus, placental abruption, fetal maternal hypotension, water intoxication, postpartum uterine atony and hemorrhage, and fetal asphyxia, hypoxia, or death. If the induction fails to produce effective labor, cesarean section is often required to prevent the adverse sequelae of the procedures used in the induction. For this reason, it is usually recommended that induction of labor not be attempted unless delivery must be accomplished to avoid severe fetal or maternal morbidity.

induction phase, the period of time during which a normal cell becomes transformed into a cancerous cell.

inductive approach /induk′tiv/, the analysis of data and examination of practice problems within their own context rather than from a predetermined theoretical basis.

inductor /induk′tər/ [L, *inducere,* to bring in], (in embryology) a tissue or cell that emits a chemical substance that stimulates some morphogenetic effect in the developing embryo. See also **evocator, organizer.**

induration /in′dyərā′shən/ [L, *indurare,* to make hard], hardening of a tissue, particularly the skin, because of edema, inflammation, or infiltration by a neoplasm. **−indurated,** *adj.*

indurative myocarditis /in′dyərē′tiv/ [L, *indurare,* to make hard; Gk, *mys,* muscle, *kardia,* heart, *itis,* inflammation], a form of myocarditis in which the inflammation leads to a hardening of the muscles of the heart walls.

industrial health [Fr, *industriel;* ME, *helthe*], the health concerns associated with the workplace, such as exposure to asbestos, mining and milling dusts, metal and acid vapors, lighting and ergonomics.

Industrial Medical Association (I.M.A.), a professional organization whose members are concerned with the identification, prevention, diagnosis, and treatment of disorders associated with technology and industry.

industrial psychology [L, *industria,* diligence, the application of psychologic principles and techniques to the problems of business and industry, including the selection of personnel, the motivation of workers, and the development of training programs.

indwelling catheter /in′dweling/ [L, *in*, within; AS, *dwellan*, to remain], any catheter designed to be left in place for a prolonged period. See also **self-retaining catheter.**

-ine, a suffix meaning a 'chemical substance': *chlorine, pyrroline, strychnine.*

inebriant /inē′brē·ənt/ [L, *inebriare*, to make drunk], substance inducing inebriation or intoxication, as does ethanol.

inebriate /inē′brē·āt/, to make drunk.

inert /inurt′/ [L, *iners*, idle], 1. not moving or acting, such as inert matter. 2. (of a chemical substance) not taking part in a chemical reaction or acting as a catalyst, such as neon or an inert gas. 3. (of a medical ingredient) not active pharmacologically; serving only as a bulking, binding, or sweetening agent or other excipient in a medication.

inert gas, a chemically inactive gaseous element. The inert gases are argon, helium, krypton, neon, radon, and xenon. Also called **noble gas.**

inertia /inur′shə/ [L, idleness], 1. the tendency of a body at rest to remain at rest unless acted on by an outside force, and the tendency of a body in motion to remain at motion in the direction in which it is moving unless acted on by an outside force. 2. an abnormal condition characterized by a general inactivity or sluggishness, such as colonic inertia or uterine inertia.

inertial impaction /inur′shəl/, the deposition of large aerosol particles on the walls of an airway conduit. The impaction caused by inertia tends to occur where the airway direction changes. Small particles are more likely to be carried around corners and continue in the path of the airflow.

inevitable abortion /inev′itəbəl/ [L, *inevitablilis*, unavoidable], a condition of pregnancy in which spontaneous termination is imminent and cannot be prevented. It is characterized by bleeding, uterine cramping, dilatation of the cervix, and presentation of the conceptus in the cervical os. If heavy bleeding supervenes, immediate evacuation of the uterus may be required. The point at which an inevitable abortion becomes an incomplete abortion is of medicolegal interest because of the statutory difference between spontaneous and induced abortion. In clinical practice precise differentiation is seldom practicable. Compare **incomplete abortion, threatened abortion.**

in extremis ′ in the extremity, or at the point of death.

infant /in′fənt/ [L, *infans*, unable to speak], 1. a child who is in the earliest stage of extrauterine life, a time extending from the first month after birth to approximately 12 months of age, when the baby is able to assume an erect posture; some extend the period to 24 months of age. 2. (in law) a person not of full legal age; a minor. 3. of or pertaining to infancy; in an early stage of development. –**infantile,** *adj.*

infant botulism, an intoxication from neurotoxins produced by *Clostridium botulinum* that occurs in children less than 6 months of age. The condition is characterized by severe hypotonicity of all muscles, constipation, lethargy, and feeding difficulties, and it may lead to respiratory insufficiency. The botulism neurotoxin is usually found in the GI tract rather than in the blood, indicating that it is probably produced in the gut rather than ingested, although the epidemiology and pathophysiology of the syndrome are not clearly understood. Treatment is supportive, including optimal management of fluids, electrolytes, and nutrition. Ventilatory support may also be necessary. There is no evidence that antitoxin therapy is helpful, and it is usually not recommended.

infant death, the death of a live-born infant before 1 year of age.

infant feeder, a device for feeding small or weak infants who cannot suck hard enough to nurse from the breast or to get milk from a bottle. The feeder resembles a bulb syringe with a long soft nipple on the end. The bulb is squeezed slowly and gently, permitting the baby to suck and swallow without great effort and preventing the escape of fluid into the infant's trachea, where it might cause asphyxiation or aspiration pneumonia.

infant feeding. See **bottle feeding, breast feeding.**

infant feeding pattern, ineffective, a nursing diagnosis accepted by the Tenth National Conference on the Classification of Nursing Diagnoses. It is defined as a state in which an infant demonstrates an impaired ability to suck or coordinate the suck-swallow response. The defining characteristics are an inability to initiate or sustain an effective suck and inability to coordinate sucking, swallowing, and breathing. Related factors are prematurity, neurologic impairment or delay, oral hypersensitivity, prolonged NPO status, and anatomic abnormalities. See also **nursing diagnosis.**

infanticide /infan′tisīd/ [L, *infans*, unable to speak, *caedere*, to kill], 1. the killing of an infant or young child. The act is usually a psychotic reaction often associated with severe depression, such as occurs in bipolar disorder and, occasionally, in extreme postpartum disturbances. Infanticide may become a neurotic obsession among mothers who do not want the baby or who do not feel physically, mentally, or emotionally capable of caring for or coping with the infant. 2. one who takes the life of an infant or young child. –**infanticidal,** *adj.*

infantile /in′fəntīl/ [L, *infans*, unable to speak], 1. of, relating to, or characteristic of infants or infancy. 2. lacking maturity, sophistication, or reasonableness. 3. affected with infantilism. 4. being in a very early stage of development.

infantile amnesia, (in psychology) the inability to remember events from early childhood. It is explained by a theory that a memory for skills develops earlier than a fact-memory system, which may not develop until the third year. Thus a person may learn skills without remembering how the skills were acquired.

infantile arteritis, a disorder in infants and young children characterized by inflammation of many arteries in which atherosclerotic lesions are rarely present.

infantile autism, a disability characterized by abnormal emotional, social, and linguistic development in a child. It may result from organic brain dysfunction, in which case it occurs before 3 years of age.

infantile celiac disease. See **celiac disease.**

infantile cerebral ataxic paralysis [L, *infans*, unable to speak; *cerebrum*, the brain; Gk, *ataxia*, lack of order; *paralyein*, to be palsied], a form of congenital diplegia, characterized by cerebral maldevelopment, ataxia, spasticity of the legs, and possible mental deficiency.

infantile cerebral sphingolipidosis. See **Tay-Sachs disease.**

infantile colic [L, *infans*, unable to speak; Gk, *kolikos*, pain in the colon], a descriptive term for a suggested intestinal cause of discomfort in a newborn infant. However, specific causes and mechanisms have not been defined. The typical infantile colic patient eats and gains weight but may also appear excessively hungry. Aerophagia from crying may lead to flatulence and abdominal distention.

infantile cortical hyperostosis, a familial disorder characterized in infants by bony swellings and tenderness in the affected areas. The child also tends to be feverish and irritable. The mandible is most commonly involved. Radiographs indicate areas of new bone growth beneath the periosteum. Also called **Caffey's disease.**

infantile dwarf, a person whose mental and physical development is greatly retarded as a result of various causes, such as genetic or developmental defects.

infantile eczema. See **atopic dermatitis.**

infantile encephalitis [L, *infans,* unable to speak; Gk, *enkephalos,* brain, *itis,* inflammation], any of a group of brain inflammation conditions affecting infants. The cause may be a direct viral infection or a secondary encephalitis that is a complication of measles, chickenpox, rubella, or other diseases.

infantile hemiplegia, paralysis of one side of the body that may occur at birth from a cerebral hemorrhage, in utero from lack of oxygen, or during a febrile illness in infancy.

infantile hydrocele [L, *infans;* Gk, *hydor,* water, *kele,* hernia], an accumulation of fluid in the tunica vaginalis. It may be present at birth or acquired.

infantile paralysis. See **poliomyelitis.**

infantile pellagra. See **kwashiorkor.**

infantile poliomyelitis. See **acute atrophic paralysis.**

infantile scurvy, a nutritional disease caused by an inadequate dietary supply of vitamin C, most commonly occurring because cow's milk unfortified with vitamin C is the principal food in an infant's diet. Families are counseled to feed their children foods rich in vitamin C or to use a formula supplemented with this vitamin. Also called **Barlow's disease, hemorrhagic scurvy.** See also **ascorbic acid, citric acid, scurvy.**

infantile spinal muscular atrophy. See **Werdnig-Hoffmann disease.**

infantile spinal paralysis [L, *infans,* unable to speak; *spina;* Gk, *paralyein,* to be palsied], acute anterior poliomyelitis, a viral infection characterized by nonspecific illnesses, aseptic meningitis, and flaccid weakness of muscle groups.

infantile uterus, a uterus that has failed to attain adult characteristics.

infantilism /infan′tiliz′əm/ [L, *infans,* unable to speak], **1.** a condition in which various anatomic, physiologic, and psychologic characteristics of childhood persist in the adult. It is characterized by mental retardation, underdeveloped sexual organs, and, usually, small stature. Compare **progeria. 2.** a condition, usually of psychologic rather than organic origin, characterized by speech and voice patterns in an older child or adult that are typical of very young children.

infant mortality, the statistical rate of infant death during the first year after live birth, expressed as the number of such births per 1000 live births in a specific geographic area or institution in a given period of time. Neonatal mortality accounts for 70% of infant mortality.

infant of addicted mother, a newborn infant showing withdrawal symptoms, usually within the first 24 hours of life, most commonly caused by maternal antepartum dependence on heroin, methadone, diazepam, phenobarbital, or alcohol. See also **fetal alcohol syndrome.**

■ OBSERVATIONS: Characteristic symptoms include tremors, irritability, hyperactive reflexes, increased muscle tone, twitching, increased mucus production, nasal congestion, respiratory distress, excessive sweating, elevated tempera-

ture, vomiting, diarrhea, and dehydration. The infants cry shrilly, often sneeze, frantically suck their fists but feed poorly, and frequently yawn but have difficulty falling asleep. They are usually pale, are often born with nose and knee abrasions, and are subject to convulsions.

■ INTERVENTIONS: The infant is kept warm, snugly swaddled in a padded crib, and exposed to minimal visual, auditory, and tactile stimulation. The baby is handled only when necessary and is then held firmly, close to the body.

■ NURSING CONSIDERATIONS: These high-risk infants require special attention, and it is important for the mother to be encouraged to participate in her baby's care as soon as possible. The nurse may help to promote parent-child bonding.

infant stimulation [L, *infans,* unable to speak; *stimulare,* to incite], the testing of sensory inputs for newborns, usually through the performance of tasks involving coordination and manipulation.

infarct /infärkt′/ [L, *infarcire,* to stuff], a localized area of necrosis in a tissue, vessel, organ, or part resulting from tissue anoxia caused by an interruption in the blood supply to the area, or, less frequently, by circulatory stasis produced by the occlusion of a vein that ordinarily carries blood away from the area. An infarct may resemble a red swollen bruise, because of hemorrhage and an accumulation of blood in the area. Some infarcts are pale and white, caused by a lack of circulation to the area.

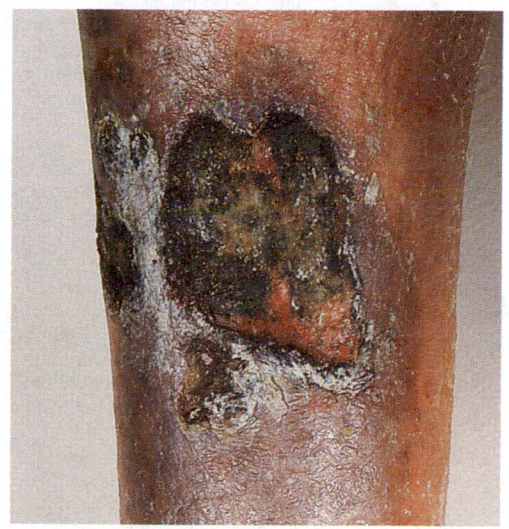

Infarct *(du Vivier, 1993)*

infarct extension, a myocardial infarction that has spread beyond the original area, usually as a result of the death of cells in the ischemic margin of the infarct zone.

infarction /infärk′shən/ [L, *infarcire,* to stuff], **1.** the development and formation of an infarct. **2.** an infarct. Kinds of infarction include **myocardial infarction** and **pulmonary infarction.**

infect [L, *inficere,* to taint], to transmit a pathogen that may induce development of an infectious disease in another person.

infected abortion, a spontaneous or induced termination

of an immature pregnancy in which the products of conception have become infected, causing fever and requiring antibiotic therapy and evacuation of the uterus. Compare **septic abortion.**

infection /infek'shən/[L, *inficere*, to taint], **1.** the invasion of the body by pathogenic microorganisms that reproduce and multiply, causing disease by local cellular injury, secretion of a toxin, or antigen-antibody reaction in the host. **2.** a disease caused by the invasion of the body by pathogenic microorganisms. Compare **infestation.** –**infectious,** *adj.*

infection control, the policies and procedures of a hospital or other health facility to minimize the risk of nosocomial or community-acquired infections spreading to patients or members of the staff.

infection control committee, a group of hospital health professionals composed of infection control personnel, with medical, nursing, administrative, and occasionally dietary and housekeeping department representatives, who plan and supervise infection control activities.

infection control nurse, a registered nurse who is assigned responsibility for surveillance and infection prevention and control activities.

infection, high risk for, a nursing diagnosis accepted by the Seventh National Conference on the Classification of Nursing Diagnoses. High risk for infection is defined as the state in which an individual is at increased risk for being invaded by pathogenic organisms. Risk factors include inadequate primary defenses, such as broken skin, traumatized tissue, decrease in ciliary action, stasis of body fluids, change in pH secretions, and altered peristalsis; inadequate secondary defenses, such as decreased hemoglobin, leukopenia, suppressed inflammatory response, and immunosuppression; inadequate acquired immunity; tissue destruction and increased environmental exposure; chronic disease; invasive procedures; malnutrition; pharmaceutical agents; trauma; rupture of amniotic membranes; and insufficient knowledge to avoid exposure to pathogens. See also **nursing diagnosis.**

infections following splenectomy [L, *inficere*, to stain; ME, *folwen*; Gk, *splen, ektome,* cutting out], infections that may follow removal of the spleen, an organ that plays a vital role in the body's immune system. The spleen is a major phagocytic organ of the reticuloendothelial network and also serves as an important site of antibody production. Splenectomized patients are particularly prone to certain bacterial infections.

infectious /infek'chəs/, **1.** capable of causing an infection. **2.** caused by an infection.

infectious bulbar paralysis [L, *inficere*, to stain; *bulbus,* swollen root; Gk, *paralyein,* to be palsied], a herpesvirus disease of animals that may cause a mild pruritis when transmitted to humans. Also called **pseudorabies.**

infectious disease [L, *inficere*, to stain; *dis*; Fr, *aise,* ease], any communicable disease, or one that can be transmitted from one human being to another, or from animal to human, by direct or indirect contact.

infectious-exhaustive syndrome. See **postinfectious psychosis.**

infectious granuloma [L, *inficere*, to stain; *granulum,* little grain; Gk, *oma,* tumor], a lumpy lesion of granuloma tissue that may develop in diseases such as tuberculosis, syphilis, and actinomycosis.

infectious hepatitis. See **hepatitis A.**

infectious isolation [L, *inficere*, to stain; It, *isolare,* to detach], a practice of confining a patient with a particularly virulent disease to an isolated room or other area so as to reduce the risk of contact and spread of the disease among hospital personnel.

infectious mononucleosis [L, *inficere*, to taint; Gk, *monos,* single; L, *nucleus,* nut; Gk, *osis,* condition], an acute herpesvirus infection caused by the Epstein-Barr virus (EBV). It is characterized by fever, sore throat, swollen lymph glands, atypical lymphocytes, splenomegaly, hepatomegaly, abnormal liver function, and bruising. The disease is usually transmitted by droplet infection but is not highly or predictably contagious. Young people are most often affected. In childhood, the disease is mild and usually unnoticed; the older the person, the more severe the symptoms are likely to be. Infection confers permanent immunity. Treatment is primarily symptomatic, with enforced bed rest to prevent serious complications of the liver or spleen, analgesics to control pain, and saline gargles for throat discomfort. Rupture of the spleen may occur, requiring imme-

Defenses against infection

Type of defense	Specific mechanism
Surface defenses	Physical barriers: skin, conjunctivae, mucous membranes
	Mechanical removal: desquamation of skin, tears, mucus, ciliary action, coughing, salivation, swallowing, urination, defecation
	Normal bacterial flora: antibacterial factors
	Chemical inhibitors: gastric acid, lactic acid, fatty acids, spermine, lactoperoxidase, bile salts
	Antimicrobial substances: lysozyme, secretory IgA
Nonspecific resistance factors	Fever, interferons, complement, lysozyme, C-reactive protein (reacts with bacterial surface polysaccharides and activates complement), lactoferrin (binds and removes iron as a bacterial nutrient), α-l-antitrypsin (inhibits bacterial enzymes)
Inflammation	Soluble factors:
	Clotting system: Hageman factor (factor XII)
	Complement system: chemotactic factors, anaphylatoxins
	Kinin system: bradykinin
	Phagocytes
	Circulating neutrophils, eosinophils, monocytes, macrophages
	Fixed cells (of mononuclear phagocyte system) in alveoli, spleen, liver, bone marrow
Immune response	Humoral immune response: B cells, plasma cells, immunoglobulins
	Cell-mediated immune response: T cells, lymphokines

From McCance KL, Huether SE: *Pathophysiology: the biological basis for disease in adults and children,* St Louis, *1990, Mosby.*

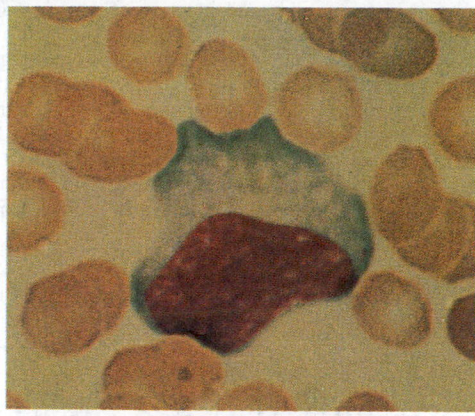

Infectious mononucleosis (Zitelli, 1992)

diate surgery and blood transfusion. See also **Epstein-Barr virus, viral infection.**

infectious myringitis, an inflammatory, contagious condition of the eardrum caused by viral or bacterial infection, characterized by the development of painful vesicles on the drum. Also called **bullous myringitis.**

infectious nucleic acid, DNA or, more commonly, viral RNA that is able to infect the nucleic acid of a cell and to induce the host to produce viruses.

infectious parotitis. See **mumps.**

infectious polyneuritis. See **Guillain-Barré syndrome.**

infective endocarditis /infek'tiv/ [L, *inficere*, to stain; Gk, *endon*, within; *kardia*, heart; *itis*, inflammation], a bacterial infection of the innermost lining of the heart, usually after rheumatic fever or another febrile disease. Subacute bacterial endocarditis may lead to vegetation on the heart valves or ulceration of the valve cusps. Also called **bacterial endocarditis.**

infective tubulointerstitial nephritis [L, *inficere*, to taint;

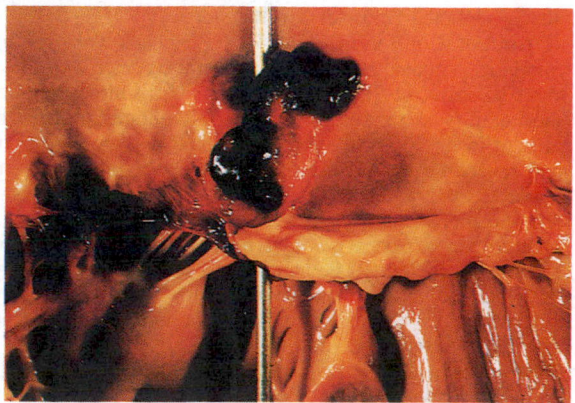

Infective endocarditis (Fletcher, 1987)

tubulus, tubule, *interstitium*, space between], an acute inflammation of the kidneys caused by an infection by *Escherichia coli* or other pyogenic pathogen. The condition is characterized by chills, fever, nausea and vomiting, flank pain, dysuria, proteinuria, and hematuria. The kidney may become enlarged, and portions of the renal cortex may be destroyed. Infection is usually the result of bacterial contamination of a urinary catheter, but it may occur in any condition characterized by urinary stasis.

infectivity /infektiv'itē/ [L, *inficere*, to taint], the ability of a pathogen to spread rapidly from one host to another.

inferior /infir'ē·ər/ [L, *inferus*, lower], **1.** situated below or lower than a given point of reference, as the feet are inferior to the legs. **2.** of poorer quality or value. Compare **superior.**

inferior alveolar artery, an artery that descends with the inferior alveolar nerve from the first or mandibular portion of the maxillary artery to the mandibular foramen on the medial surface of the ramus of the mandible. It enters the mandibular canal and runs through to the first premolar tooth where it divides into the mental and incisor branches. Also called **arteria alveolaris inferior.**

inferior aperture of minor pelvis, an irregular aperture bounded by the coccyx, the sacrotuberous ligaments, part of the ischium, the sides of the pubic arch, and the pubic symphysis.

inferior aperture of thorax, an irregular opening bounded by the twelfth thoracic vertebra, the eleventh and twelfth ribs, and the edge of the costal cartilages as they meet the sternum.

inferior carotid triangle [L, *inferior*, lower; Gk, *karos*, heavy sleep; L, *triangulus*, three-cornered], a triangular area bounded by the midline of the neck, the superior belly of the omohyoid muscle above and the sternocleidomastoid muscle behind. Also called **muscular triangle.**

inferior conjunctival fornix, the space in the fold of conjunctiva created by the reflection of the conjunctiva covering the eyeball and the lining of the lower eyelid. Compare **superior conjunctival fornix.**

inferior gastric node, a node in one of two groups of gastric lymph glands, lying between the two layers of the lesser omentum along the pyloric half of the greater curvature of the stomach. Compare **hepatic node, superior gastric node.**

inferiority complex /infir'ē·ôr'itē/, **1.** a feeling of fear and resentment resulting from a sense of being physically inadequate, characterized by a variety of abnormal behaviors. **2.** (in psychoanalysis) a complex characterized by striving for unrealistic goals because of an unresolved Oedipus complex. **3.** *informal.* a feeling of being inferior.

inferior maxillary bone. See **mandible.**

inferior mesenteric artery, a visceral branch of the abdominal aorta, arising just above the division into the common iliacs and supplying the left half of the transverse colon, all of the descending and iliac colons, and most of the rectum. It has left colic, sigmoid, and superior rectal branches.

inferior mesenteric node, a node in one of the three groups of visceral lymph glands serving the viscera of the abdomen and the pelvis. The inferior mesenteric nodes are associated with the branches of the inferior mesenteric artery and are divided into a group of small nodes along the branches of the left colic and sigmoid arteries, another group in the sigmoid mesocolon, and a pararectal group touching the muscular coat of the rectum. The inferior mesenteric nodes drain the descending colon, the iliac and sigmoid parts of the colon, and the upper part of the rectum. Their efferent vessels pass to the preaortic nodes. Compare **gastric node, superior mesenteric node.**

inferior mesenteric vein,   the vein in the lower body that returns the blood from the rectum, the sigmoid and descending colons, and part of the transverse colon. It begins in the rectum as the superior rectal vein, ascends through the lesser pelvis, and continues upward as the inferior mesenteric vein. It passes dorsal to the pancreas and opens into the lienal vein. It receives the sigmoid veins from the sigmoid colon and the iliac colon and the left colic vein from the descending colon and the left colic flexure. Compare **superior mesenteric vein.**

inferior olivary nucleus [L, *inferior*, lower; *oliva*, olive; *nucleus*, nut],   a small purse-shaped collection of nerve cells lying posterolateral to the pyramid, just below the level of the pons. It is a source of cerebellar climbing fibers.

inferior orbital fissure,   a groove in the inferolateral wall of the orbit that contains the infraorbital and zygomatic nerves and the infraorbital vessels.

inferior phrenic artery,   a small, visceral branch of the abdominal aorta, arising from the aorta itself, the renal artery, or the celiac artery. It divides into the medial and lateral branches and supplies the diaphragm. A few vessels of the inferior vena cava stem from the lateral branch of the right phrenic artery. Some branches of the left phrenic artery supply the esophagus.

inferior pole of kidney.   See **poles of kidney.**

inferior radioulnar joint.   See **distal radioulnar articulation.**

inferior sagittal sinus,   one of the six venous channels of the posterior dura mater, draining blood from the brain into the internal jugular vein. It is a cylindric sinus contained in the posterior portion of the free margin of the falx cerebri, increases in size as it courses posteriorly, and ends in the straight sinus. It receives deoxygenated blood from several veins from the falx cerebri and, in some individuals, a few veins from the cerebral hemispheres. Compare **straight sinus, superior sagittal sinus, transverse sinus.**

inferior subscapular nerve /subskap′yo̅o̅lər/,   one of two small nerves on opposite sides of the back that arise from the posterior cord of the brachial plexus. It supplies the distal part of the subscapularis and ends in the teres major. Compare **superior subscapular nerve.**

inferior thyroid vein,   one of the few veins that arises in the venous plexus on the thyroid gland and forms a plexus ventral to the trachea, under the sternothyroideus muscle. A left vein descends from this plexus to join the left brachiocephalic trunk; a right vein descends obliquely to open into the right brachiocephalic vein at its junction with the superior vena cava. The inferior thyroid veins contain valves at their terminations and receive the esophageal, the tracheal, and the inferior laryngeal veins.

inferior ulnar collateral artery,   one of a pair of branches of the deep brachial arteries, arising about 5 cm from the elbow, passing inward to form an arch with the deep brachial artery, and carrying blood to the muscles of the forearm. Compare **superior ulnar collateral artery.**

inferior vena cava,   the large vein that returns deoxygenated blood to the heart from parts of the body below the diaphragm. It is formed by the junction of the two common iliac veins at the right of the fifth lumbar vertebra and ascends along the vertebral column, pierces the diaphragm and opens into the right atrium of the heart. As it passes through the diaphragm, it receives a covering of serous pericardium. The inferior vena cava contains a semilunar valve that is rudimentary in the adult but very large and important in the fetus. The vessel receives blood from the two common iliacs, the lumbar veins, and the testicular veins. Compare **superior vena cava.**

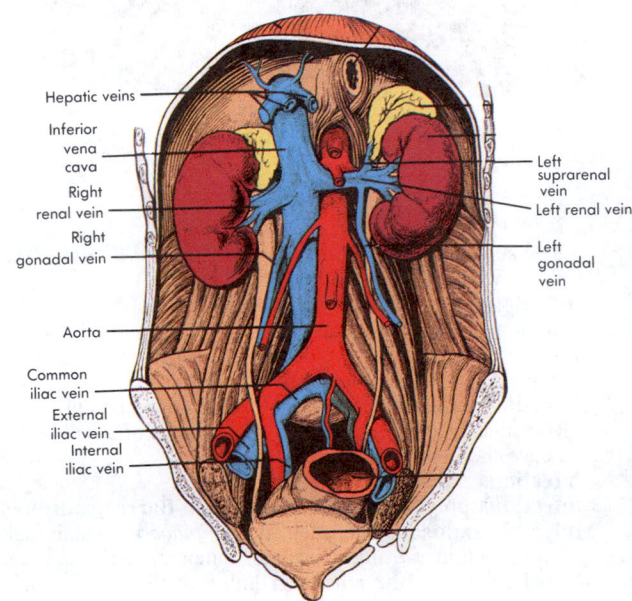

Hepatic veins

Inferior vena cava

Right renal vein

Right gonadal vein

Aorta

Common iliac vein

External iliac vein

Internal iliac vein

Left suprarenal vein

Left renal vein

Left gonadal vein

Inferior vena cava
(Seeley, 1992/David J Mascaro & Associates)

infero-,   a prefix meaning 'low': *inferolateral, inferomedial, inferoposterior.*

inferolateral /in′fərōlat′ərəl/ [L, *inferus*, lower, *latus*, side],   situated below and to the side.

inferomedial /in′fərōmē′dē·əl/ [L, *inferus*, lower, *medius*, middle],   situated below and toward the center.

infertile /infur′təl/ [L, *in*, not, *fertilis*, fruitful],   denoting the inability to produce offspring. This condition may be present in one or both sex partners and may be temporary and reversible. The cause may be physical, including immature sexual organs, abnormalities of the reproductive system, hormonal imbalance, and dysfunction or anomalies in other organ systems, or may result from psychologic or emotional problems. The condition is classified as primary, in which pregnancy has never occurred, and secondary, when there have been one or more pregnancies. Compare **sterile. –infertility.** *n.*

infest /infest′/,   to attack, invade, and subsist on the skin or in the internal organs of a host. Compare **infect.**

infestation in′festā′shən/ [L, *infestare*, to attack],   the presence of animal parasites in the environment, on the skin, or in the hair of a host.

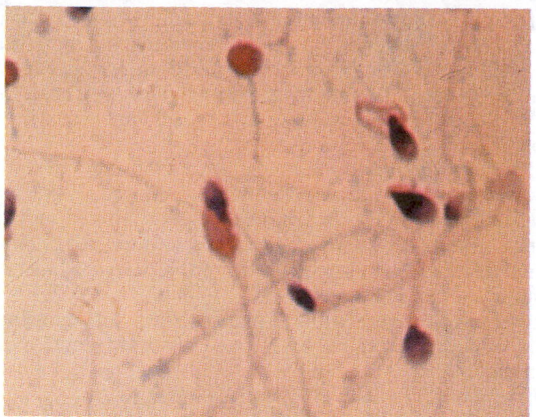

**Abnormal forms of spermotozoa from a patient
with a high degree of infertility**
(Besser, 1989)

infiltrate /in'filtrāt, infil'trāt/ [L, *in*, *filtrare*, to strainthrough], **1.** to perform the process of infiltration. **2.** a substance that seeps through a filter.

infiltration /in'filtrāshən/ [L, *in*, within, *filtare*, to strain through], the process whereby a fluid passes into the tissues, such as when a local anesthetic is administered or an IV infusion infiltrates.

infirmary /infur'mərē/ [L, *infirmus*, weak], a hospital, originally a part of a monastery, that provides care for sick or infirm persons, particularly indigent patients.

inflammation [L, *inflammare*, to set afire], the protective response of the tissues of the body to irritation or injury. Inflammation may be acute or chronic; its cardinal signs are redness (rubor), heat (calor), swelling (tumor), and pain (dolor), accompanied by loss of function. The process begins with a transitory vasoconstriction, then is followed by a brief increase in vascular permeability. The second stage is prolonged and consists of sustained increase in vascular permeability, exudation of fluids from the vessels, clustering of leukocytes along the vessel walls, phagocytosis of microorganisms, deposition of fibrin in the vessel, disposal of the accumulated debris by macrophages, and, finally, the migration of fibroblasts to the area and the development of new, normal cells. The severity, timing, and local character of any particular inflammatory response depend on the cause, the area affected, and the condition of the host. Histamine, kinins, and various other substances mediate the inflammatory process.

inflammation of the liver. See **hepatitis**.

inflammatory /inflam'ətôr'ē/ [L, *inflammare*, to set afire], pertaining to or resembling inflammation.

inflammatory bowel disease. See **ulcerative colitis**.

inflammatory dysmenorrhea [L, *inflammare*; Gk, *dys*, *men*, month, *rhein*, to flow], dysmenorrhea that accompanies pelvic infection, fibroids, or endometritis. Also called **secondary dysmenorrhea**.

inflammatory fracture [L, *inflammare*, to set afire; *fractura*, break], a fracture of bone tissue weakened by inflammation.

inflammatory response, a tissue reaction to injury or an antigen. The response may include pain, swelling, itching,

redness, heat, loss of function, or a combination of symptoms. There may be dilation of blood vessels, leakage of fluid from the vessels causing edema, leukocytic exudation, and the release of plasma proteases and vasoactive amines, such as histamine.

inflammatory scoliosis [L, *inflammare*; Gk, *skoliosis*, curvature], a form of scoliosis caused by muscle spasms associated with acute inflammation.

inflatable pessary. See **pessary**.

inflatable splint /inflā'təbəl/ [L, *in flare*, to blow; ME, *splente*], a tubular device that is placed around a patient's extremity and inflated with air to maintain rigidity. Also called **pneumatic splint**.

influenza /in'flōō·en'zə/ [It, influence], a highly contagious infection of the respiratory tract caused by a myxovirus and transmitted by airborne droplet infection. It occurs in isolated cases, epidemics, and pandemics. Symptoms include sore throat, cough, fever, muscular pains, and weakness. The incubation period is brief (from 1 to 3 days), and the onset is usually sudden, with chills, fever, and general malaise. Treatment is symptomatic and usually involves bed rest, aspirin, and drinking of fluids. Fever and constitutional symptoms distinguish influenza from the common cold. Complete recovery in from 3 to 10 days is the rule, but bacterial pneumonia may occur among high-risk patients, such as the elderly, the very young, and people who have chronic pulmonary disease. Three main strains of influenza virus have been recognized: type A, type B, and type C. New strains of the virus emerge at regular intervals and are named according to their geographic origin. **Asian flu** is a type A influenza. Yearly vaccination with the currently prevalent strain of influenza virus is recommended for elderly or debilitated persons and health care personnel. Treatment or prpophylaxis in high-risk patients may be achieved with amantadine. Also called **grippe, la grippe,** (informal) **flu**.

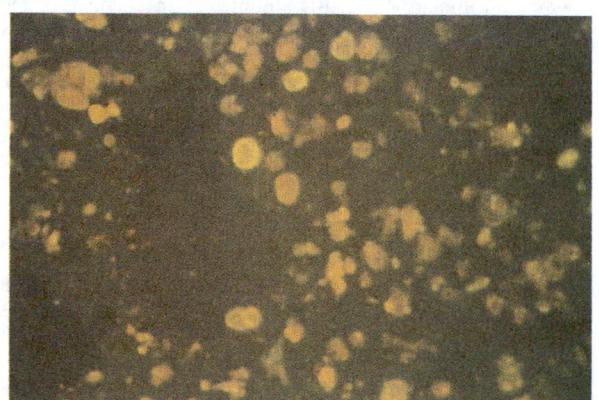

Respiratory secretion showing influenza A
(Murray, 1990/Courtesy Richard Thomson, Akron, Ohio)

influenza-virus vaccine, an active immunizing agent.
■ INDICATION: It is prescribed for immunization against influenza.
■ CONTRAINDICATIONS: Acute infection or allergy to eggs prohibits its use.

■ ADVERSE EFFECTS: Among the more serious adverse reactions are anaphylaxis and Guillain-Barré syndrome.

informal.   See **bipolar lead.**

informal admission,   a type of admission to a psychiatric hospital in which there is no formal or written application and the patient is free to leave at any time. See also **involuntary patient.**

information systems director [L, *informatio*, idea],   a person who directs and administers the data processing facilities of a hospital or other health facility.

informed consent [L, *informare*, to give form; *consentire*, to sense],   permission obtained from a patient to perform a specific test or procedure. Informed consent is required before performing most invasive procedures and before admitting a patient to a research study. The document used must be written in a language understood by the patient and be dated and signed by the patient and at least one witness. Included in the document are clear, rational statements that describe the procedure or test. Also required is a statement that care will not be withheld if the patient does not consent; informed consent is voluntary. By law, informed consent must be obtained more than a given number of days or hours before certain procedures, including therapeutic abortion and sterilization, and must always be obtained when the patient is fully competent.

infra-,   a prefix meaning 'situated, formed, or occurring beneath': *infraclavicular, infracortical, infratemporal.*

infrabony pocket.   See **periodontal pocket.**

infraclavicular fossa /in'frakləvik'yələr/,   a small pocket or indentation just below the clavicle on both sides of the body.

infraction fracture /infrak'shən/ [L, *infractio*, a breaking; *fractura* break],   a pathologic fracture characterized by a small radiolucent line and most commonly associated with a disorder of metabolism. See also **greenstick fracture.**

infranodal block /in'frənō'dəl/ [L, *infra*, below, *nodus*, knot; Fr, *bloc*],   a type of atrioventricular (AV) block in which an impairment of the stimulatory mechanism of the heart causes blockage of the impulse in the bundle of His or in both bundle branches after leaving the AV node. The condition is often the result of arteriosclerosis, degenerative diseases, a defect in the conduction system, or tumor; it is most often seen in older patients. Symptoms include frequent episodes of fainting and a pulse rate of between 20 and 50 beats per minute. Diagnosis is made by an electrocardiogram, which shows intraventricular conduction disturbances during sinus rhythm and distinguishes nodal from infranodal block. The usual therapy is the implantation of a pacemaker of the demand type. Compare **bundle branch block, intraventricular block.** See also **Adams-Stokes syndrome, atrioventricular block, cardiac conduction defect, heart block, intraatrial block, sinoatrial block.**

infraorbital /in'frə·ô'bitəl/ [L, *infra*, below; *orbita*, wheeltrack],   pertaining to the area beneath the floor of the bony cavity in which the eyeball is located.

infraorbital foramen [L, *infra*, below; *orbita*, wheeltrack; *foramen*, hole or aperture],   an opening on the anterior aspect of the maxilla. Through it pass the inferior orbital nerves and blood vessels.

infrapatellar fat pad /in'frəpatel'ər/,   an area of palpable soft tissue in front of the joint space on either side of the patellar tendon.

infraradian rhythm /in'frərā'dē·ən/ [L, *infra* + *radians*, diverging from center; Gk, *rhythmos*],   a biorhythm that repeats in patterns greater than 24-hour periods.

infrared radiation /in'frəred'/ [L, *infra* + AS, *read*, red; L, *radiare*, to emit rays],   electromagnetic radiation in which the wavelengths are between 10[mi]5 m and 10[mi]4 m, or longer than those of visible light waves but shorter than those of radio waves. Infrared radiation striking the body surface is perceived as heat.

infrared therapy,   treatment by exposure to various wavelengths of infrared radiation. Hot water bottles and heating pads of all kinds emit longwave infrared radiation; incandescent lights emit shortwave infrared radiation. Infrared treatment is performed to relieve pain and to stimulate circulation of blood.

infrared thermography,   measurement of temperature through the detection of infrared radiation emitted from heated tissue.

infraspinous fossa.   See **supraspinous fossa.**

infundibula.   See **infundibulum.**

infundibular stalk /in'fundib'yələr/ [L, *infundibulum*, funnel; ME, *stalke*],   an elongated funnel-shaped structure that connects the diencephalon with the pituitary gland.

infundibulum /in'fundib'yələm/ *pl.* **infundibula,** [L, funnel],   a funnel-shaped structure or passage, such as the cavity formed by the fimbriae tubae at the distal end of the fallopian tubes, the stalk that extends from the posterior lobe of the pituitary gland, or the passage connecting the middle meatus of the nose with the frontal sinus.

infusate /infyōō'sāt/,   a parenteral fluid infused into a patient over a specific time period.

infusion /infyōō'zhən/ [L, *in*, within, *fundere*, to pour],   **1.** the introduction of a substance, such as a fluid, electrolyte, nutrient, or drug, directly into a vein or interstitially by means of gravity flow. Sterile techniques are maintained, the equipment is periodically checked for mechanical difficulties, and the patient is observed for swelling at the site of injection and for cardiac or respiratory difficulties. Compare **injection, instillation, insufflation. 2.** the substance introduced into the body by infusion. **3.** the steeping of a substance, such as an herb, to extract its medicinal properties. **4.** the extract obtained by the steeping process. **—infuse,** *v.*

infusion pump,   an apparatus designed to deliver measured amounts of a drug or IV solution through injection over a period of time. Some kinds of infusion pumps can be implanted surgically.

ingestion /injes'chən/ [L, *in*, *gerere*, to carry],   the oral taking of substances into the body. The term is generally applied to both nutrients and medications.

ingrown hair [L, *in*, within; AS, *growen*, to grow; *haer*],   a hair that fails to follow the normal follicle channel to the surface, with the free end becoming embedded in the skin. The hair then acts like a foreign body, and inflammation and suppuration follow.

ingrown toenail,   a toenail whose free distal margin grows or is pressed into the skin of the toe, causing an inflammatory reaction. Granulation tissue may develop, and secondary infection is common. Treatment includes wider shoes, proper trimming of the nail, and various surgical procedures to narrow the nail or to reduce the size of the lateral nail fold.

inguinal /ing'gwinəl/ [L, *inguen*, groin],   of or pertaining to the groin.

inguinal canal,   the tubular passage through the lower muscular layers of the abdominal wall that contains the spermatic cord in the male and the round ligament in the female. It is a common site for hernias.

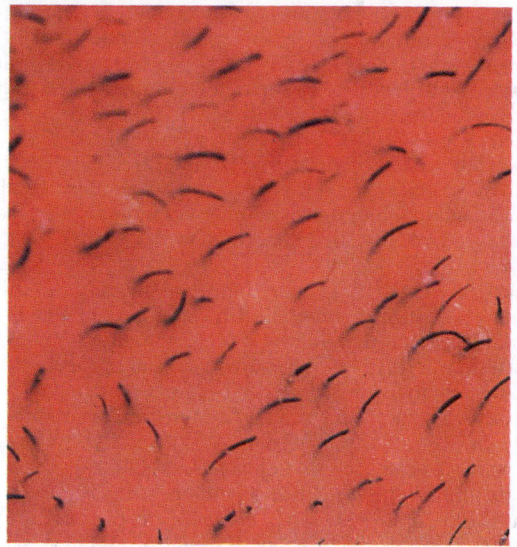

Ingrown hairs
(du Vivier, 1993/Courtesy Institute of Dermatology)

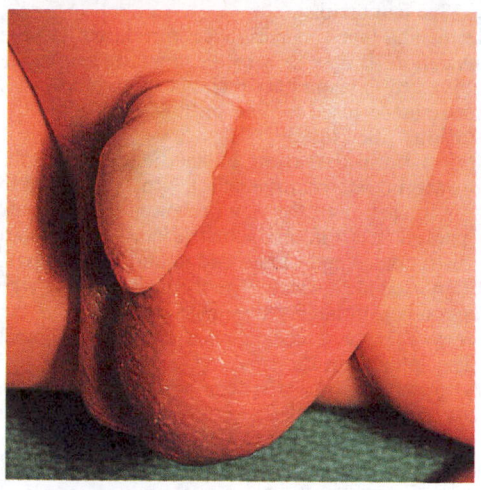

Inguinal hernia *(Zitelli, 1992)*

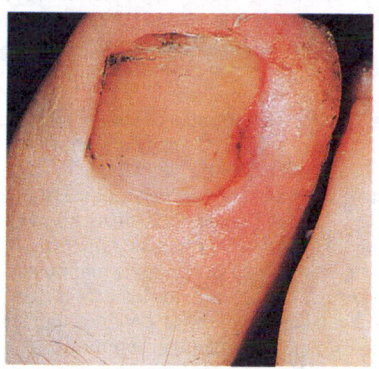

Ingrown toenail *(Habif, 1990)*

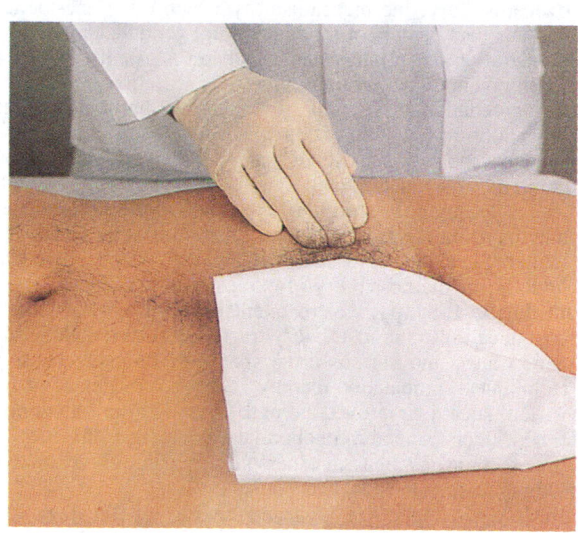

Palpation of inguinal nodes *(Seidel, 1991)*

inguinal falx, the inferior terminal portion of the common aponeurosis of the obliquus internus abdominis and the transverse abdominis. It is inserted into the crest of the pubis, just under the superficial inguinal ring, and strengthens that part of the anterior abdominal wall. The width and the strength of the inguinal falx vary. Also called **conjoined tendon.**

inguinal hernia, a hernia in which a loop of intestine enters the inguinal canal, sometimes filling, in a male, the entire scrotal sac. An inguinal hernia is usually repaired surgically to prevent the herniated segment from becoming strangulated, gangrenous, or obstructive, thereby blocking passage of waste through the bowel. Of all hernias, 75% to 80% are inguinal hernias. See also **hernia.**

inguinal node, one of approximately 18 nodes in the group of lymph glands in the upper femoral triangle of the thigh. These nodes are divided into the superficial inguinal nodes and the subinguinal nodes. Compare **anterior tibial node, popliteal node.**

inguinal region, the part of the abdomen surrounding the inguinal canal, in the lower zone on both sides of the pubic region. Also called **iliac region.** See also **abdominal regions.**

inguinal ring, either of the two apertures of the inguinal canal, the internal end opening into the abdominal wall and the external end opening into the aponeurosis of the obliquus externus abdominis above the pubis.

inguino-, a combining form meaning 'of or pertaining to the groin': *inguinocrural, inguinodynia, inguinoscrotal.*

inguinocrural hernia /ing′gwinəlkrōō′rəl/ [L, *inguen,* groin; *crus,* thigh; *hernia,* rupture], an inguinal hernia that has turned from the inguinal canal laterally over the groin. Also called **Holthouse's hernia.**

INH. See **isoniazid.**

inhalant /inhā′lənt/, a substance introduced into the body by inhalation. It may be a medication, such as an aerosol, adminis tered in respiratory therapy, or a volatile chemical, such as toluene, used in glue sniffing.

-inhalation. See **inhale.**

inhalation administration of medication /in′həlā′shən/ [L, *in*, within, *halare*, to breathe], the administration of a drug by inhalation of the vapor released from a fragile ampule packed in a fine mesh that is crushed for immediate administration. Amyl nitrate and ammonia act quickly and are often used in this way. The medication is absorbed into the circulation through the mucous membrane of the nasal passages. Vaporized medication is also given by inhalation. See also **inhalation therapy.**

inhalation analgesia, the occasional administration of anesthetic gas during the second stage of labor to reduce pain. Consciousness is retained to allow the woman to follow instructions and to avoid the adverse effects of general anesthesia.

inhalation anesthesia, surgical narcosis achieved by the administration of an anesthetic gas or a volatile anesthetic liquid via a carrier gas. Although general anesthesia by gas inhalation has been used to permit surgical operations for over a century, the mechanism by which these anesthetics dull the pain centers of the brain is not yet understood. Administration of an inhalation anesthetic is usually preceded by intravenous or intramuscular administration of a short-acting sedative or hypnotic drug, often a barbiturate. The procedure may require endotracheal intubation. Among the principal inhalation anesthetics are nitrous oxide, halothane, enflurane, and isoflurane. Some other inhalation anesthetics, including chloroform, ether, ethyl chloride, fluroxene, methoxyflurane, and trichloroethylene are not used in the United States today because of adverse effects, potential toxicity, or the possibility of explosion.

inhalation therapy, a treatment in which a substance is introduced into the respiratory tract with inspired air. Oxygen, water, and various drugs may be administered using techniques of inhalation therapy. The goals of treatment are varied, such as improved strength of respiratory function in a bedridden patient, bronchodilatation in an asthmatic, or liquefaction of mucus in a person with chronic obstructive lung disease.

inhale /inhāl′/ [L, *in*, within, *halare*, to breathe], to breathe in or to draw in with the breath. **–inhalation,** *n*.

inhaler [L, *in*, *halare*; to breathe], a device for administering medications to be inhaled, such as vapors, fine powders, or volatile substances. An inhaler also may be designed to administer anesthetic gases.

inherent /inhir′ənt/ [L, *inhaerere*, to cling to], inborn, innate; natural to an environment. Compare **indigenous.**

inherent rate, the frequency of impulse formation attributed to a given pacemaker location. The following are representative of the adult heart: SA node: 60-100/minute; AV junction: 40-60/minute; ventricle: 15-40/minute.

inheritance /inher′itəns/ [L, *in*, within, *hereditare*, to inherit], **1.** the acquisition or expression of traits or conditions by transmission of genetic material from parents to offspring. **2.** the sum total of the genetic qualities or traits transmitted from parents to offspring; the total genetic makeup of the fertilized ovum. Kinds of inheritance include **alternative inheritance, amphigenous inheritance, autosomal inheritance, blending inheritance, codominant inheritance, complemental inheritance, crisscross inheri-**

tance, cytoplasmic inheritance, holandric inheritance, hologynic inheritance, homochronous inheritance, maternal inheritance mendelism, monofactorial inheritance, multifactorial inheritance, supplemental inheritance, and x-linked inheritance. **–inherited,** *adj*. **inherit,** *v*.

inherited disorder /inher′itid/, any disease or condition that is genetically determined and involves either a single gene mutation, multifactorial inheritance, or a chromosomal aberration. Also called **genetic disorder, hereditary disorder.**

inherited trait [L, *in*, *hereditare*, to inherit; Fr, *trait*, a draft], a distinguishing quality or characteristic that is transmitted genetically from one generation to the next.

inhibin /inhib′in/, a reproductive system hormone that inhibits activity of the follicle stimulating hormone.

inhibiting gene /inhib′iting/ [L, *inhibere*, to restrain; Gk, *genein*, to produce], a gene that prevents the expression of another gene. See also **epistasis.**

inhibiting hormone. See **hormone.**

inhibition /in′hibish′ən/ [L, *inhibere*, to restrain], **1.** (in psychology) the unconscious restraint of a behavioral process, usually resulting from the social or cultural forces of the environment; the condition inducing such restraint. **2.** (in psychoanalysis) the process in which the superego prevents the conscious expression of an unconscious instinctual drive, thought, or urge. **3.** (in physiology) restraining, checking, or arresting the action of an organ or cell or the reducing of a physiologic activity by an antagonistic stimulation. **4.** (in chemistry) the stopping or slowing down of the rate of a chemical reaction.

inhibition assay, an immunoassay in which an excess of antigens prevents or inhibits the completion of either the initial or indicator phase of the reaction.

inhibition of reflexes [L, *inhibere*, to restrain; *reflectere*, to bend back], **1.** the prevention of a reflex action, requiring a series of biochemical mechanisms to restrict the flow of excitatory impulses at presynaptic and postsynaptic points in the system. **2.** a negative reflex effect that may become established during differential conditioning. The negative conditioned reflex represents an inhibition of a conditioned reflex.

inhibitor /inhib′itər/, a drug or other agent that prevents or restricts a certain action.

inhibitory /inhib′itôr′ē/ [L, *inhibere*, to restrain], tending to stop or slow a process, such as a neuron that suppresses the intensity of a nerve impulse. Compare **induce.**

inhibitory enzyme [L, *inhibere*, to restrain; Gk, *en*, within; *zyme*, ferment], an enzyme that blocks rather than catalyzes a chemical reaction.

inio-, a combining form meaning 'of or pertaining to the occiput': *iniodymus, iniopagus, iniops.*

inion /in′ē·on/ [Gk], the most prominent point of the back of the head, where the occipital bone protrudes the farthest.

initial contact stance stage /inish′əl/ [L, *initium*, beginning; *contigere*, to touch], one of the five stages in the stance phase of walking or gait, specifically associated with the moment when the foot touches the ground or floor, and the leg prepares to accept the weight of the body. The initial contact stance stage figures in the diagnoses of many abnormal orthopedic conditions and is often correlated with electromyographic studies of the muscles used in walking, such as the pretibial muscle and the gluteus maximus. Compare **loading response stance stage, midstance, preswing**

stance stage, terminal stance. See also **swing phase of gait.**

initial lesion. See **primary lesion.**

initiation codon /inish′ē·ā′shən kō′don/ [L, *initium*, beginning; *caudex*, book], (in molecular genetics) the triplet of nucleotides, usually adenine-uracil-guanine (AUG) or, in some cases, guanine-uracil-guanine (GUG), that code for formylmethionine, the first amino acid in protein sequences. Also called **start codon.**

initiator /inish′ē·ā′tər/, a cocarcinogenic factor that causes a usually irreversible genetic mutation in a normal cell and primes it for uncontrolled growth. Examples include radiation, aflatoxins, urethane, and nitrosamines.

inject. See **injection.**

injectable silicone /injek′təbəl/ [L, *in*, *jacere*, to throw; *silex*, silicon], polymeric organic compounds of silicone that are used in plastic surgery. The silicones are injected beneath the skin for cosmetic benefits.

injection /injek′shən/ [L, *in*, within, *jacere*, to throw], **1.** the act of forcing a liquid into the body by means of a needle and syringe. Injections are designated according to the anatomic site involved; the most common are intraarterial, intradermal, intramuscular, intravenous, and subcutaneous. Parenteral injections are usually given for therapeutic reasons, although they may be used diagnostically. Sterile technique is maintained. Compare **infusion, instillation, insufflate. 2.** the substance injected. **3.** redness and swelling observed in the physical examination of a part of the body, caused by dilatation of the blood vessels secondary to an inflammatory or infectious process. **−inject,** *v.*

injection cap, a rubber diaphragm covering a plastic cap. It permits needle insertion into a catheter or vial.

injection technique. See **intradermal injection, intramuscular injection, intrathecal injection, intravenous injection, subcutaneous injection,** and see other specific injection techniques.

injunction /injungk′shən/ [L, *injungere*, to enjoin], a court order that prevents a party from performing a particular act.

injury, high risk for /in′jərē/, a nursing diagnosis accepted by the Fourth National Conference on the Classification of Nursing Diagnoses. It is defined as a state in which an individual is at risk of injury as a result of environmental conditions interacting with the individual's adaptive and defensive resources. The cause of the condition may be somatic (internal) or environmental (external). The somatic factors may be biologic, chemical, physiologic, psychologic, or developmental; the environmental factors may be biologic, chemical, physiologic, psychologic, or interpersonal. The defining characteristics of a somatic risk for injury include abnormal sensory function, autoimmune condition, malnutrition, hemoglobinopathy or other abnormal hematologic condition, broken skin, developmental abnormality, or psychologic dysfunction. The defining characteristics of an environmental risk for injury include lack of immunization; presence of pathogenic microorganisms, chemical pollutants, poisons, alcohol, nicotine, or food additives; modes of transportation; physical aspects of the community, buildings, equipment, or facilities; nosocomial agents; nonavailability of assistance; and various psychologic factors. See also **nursing diagnosis.**

inlay splint [L, *in*, within; AS, *lecan*, lay], a casting for fixing or supporting one or more approximating teeth. It is composed of two or more inlays soldered together or a sin-gle casting for prepared cavities in approximating teeth.

inlet [L, *in*, within; ME, *leten*], a passage leading into a cavity, such as the pelvic inlet that marks the brim of the pelvic cavity.

inlet contraction. See **contraction.**

in loco parentis /in lō′kō pəren′tis/ [L, *in*, *locus*, place; *parentis*, parent], the assumption by a person or institution of the parental obligations of caring for a child without adoption.

innate /in′āt, ināt′/ [L, *innatus*, inborn], **1.** existing in or belonging to a person from birth; inborn; hereditary; congenital. **2.** a natural and essential characteristic of something or someone; inherent. **3.** originating in or produced by the intellect or the mind.

innate immunity. See **natural immunity.**

inner cell mass [AS, *innera*, within; L, *cella*, storeroom; *massa*, lump], a cluster of cells localized around the animal pole of the blastocyst of placental mammals from which the embryo develops. See also **trophoblast.**

inner ear. See **internal ear.**

innervate /in′ərvāt/ [L, *in*, *nervus*], to supply a body part or organ with nerves or nervous stimuli.

innervation /in′ərvā′shən/ [L, *in*, within, *nervus*, nerve], the distribution or supply of nerve fibers or nerve impulses to a part of the body.

innervation apraxia. See **motor apraxia.**

innidation. See **nidation.**

innocent /in′əsənt/ [L, *innocens*, harmless], benign, innocuous, or functional; not malignant, such as an innocent heart murmur.

innocuous /inok′yōō·əs/ [L, *innocuus*, harmless], pertaining to use of a substance or procedure that would cause no ill effects.

innominate /inom′ināt/ [L, *innominatum*, nameless], without a name; unnamed. The term is traditionally applied to certain anatomic structures, often identified by their descriptive name, such as the hipbone, brachiocephalic artery, and brachiocephalic vein.

innominate artery, one of the three arteries branching from the arch of the aorta, running about 5 cm from the level of the cranial border of the second right costal cartilage, ascending cranially, dorsally, and obliquely to the right, and dividing into the right common carotid and the right subclavian arteries. Also called **brachiocephalic artery, brachiocephalic trunk.**

innominate bone, the hipbone. It consists of the ilium, ischium, and pubis and unites with the sacrum and coccyx to form the pelvis. Also called **os coxae.**

innominate vein, a large vein on either side of the neck that is formed by the union of the internal jugular and subclavian veins. The two veins drain blood from the head, neck, and upper extremities and unite to form the superior vena cava. Also called **brachiocephalic vein.**

Inocor, a trademark for a cardiac inotropic drug (amrinone lactate).

inocula. See **inoculum.**

inoculant. See **inoculum.**

inoculate /inok′yəlāt/ [L, *inoculare*, to graft], to introduce a substance (inoculum) into the body to produce or to increase immunity to the disease or condition associated with the substance. It is introduced by making multiple scratches in the skin after placing a drop of the substance on the skin, by puncture of the skin with an implement bearing multiple short tines, or by intradermal, subcutaneous, or intramuscular injection.

inoculum /inok´yo͞oləm/, *pl.* **inocula** [L, *inocuus*, harm], a substance introduced into the body to cause or to increase immunity to a specific disease or condition. It may be a toxin; a live, attenuated, or killed virus or bacterium; or an immune serum. Also called **inoculant.** See also **immune system.**

inoperable /inop´ərəbəl/[L, *in, operari*, to work], pertaining to a medical condition that would not benefit from surgical intervention or for which the risk would outweigh the benefits.

inorganic /in´ôrgan´ik/ [L, *in*, not; Gk, *organikos*, natural], (in chemistry) a chemical compound that does not contain carbon.

inorganic acid, a compound containing no carbon that is composed of hydrogen and an electronegative element, such as chlorine. An example is hydrochloric acid. Some organic acids, such as carbonic acid, contain carbon dioxide.

inorganic chemistry, the study of the properties and reactions of all chemical elements and compounds other than hydrocarbons.

inorganic dust, dry, finely powdered particles of an inorganic substance, especially dust, which, when inhaled, can cause abnormal conditions of the lungs. See also **anthracosis, asbestosis, berylliosis, pneumoconiosis, silicosis.**

inorganic phosphorus, phosphorus that may be measured in the blood as phosphate ions. Its increased concentration may indicate bone, kidney, or glandular diseases; decreased concentration may be associated with alcoholism, vitamin deficiency, and other problems. Normal concentrations in the serum of adults are 1.8 to 2.6 mEq/L. See also **phosphorus.**

inosine /in´əsēn, -sīn/, a nucleoside, derived from animal tissue, especially intestines, originally used in food processing and flavoring. It has been used in the treatment of cardiac disorders and now is under investigation in studies of cancer and virology chemotherapy. See also **inosiplex.**

inosiplex /inō´sipleks/, a form of inosine that acts as a stimulator of the immune system. It is currently under investigation for use in cancer therapy and in the treatment of herpesvirus and rhinovirus infections. Also called **methisoprinol.**

inositol /inō´sətōl, inos´-/, an isomer of glucose that occurs widely in plant and animal cells. Although inositol has no current therapeutic use, it may be an essential cell constituent.

inotropic /in´ōtrop´ik/ [Gk, *inos*, fiber, *trope*, turning], pertaining to the force or energy of muscular contractions, particularly contractions of the heart muscle. An inotropic agent increases myocardial contractility.

inpatient /in´pāshənt/ [L, *in*, within, *patior*, to suffer], **1.** a patient who has been admitted to a hospital or other health care facility for at least an overnight stay. **2.** of or pertaining to the treatment or care of such a patient or to a health care facility to which a patient may be admitted for 24-hour care. Compare **outpatient.**

inpatient care unit, a unit of a hospital organized for medical and continuous nursing services for a group of inpatients who are usually grouped according to diagnosis or other common characteristics, such as maternity or surgical patients.

input, the information or material that enters a system.

input device [L, *in*, within; ME, *putten*, to place], a device that allows for the entry of commands or information for processing in a form acceptable to a computer, such as a typewriter, keyboard, tape drive, disk drive, microphone, or light pen.

inquest /in´kwest/ [L, *in, quaerere*, to seek], a legal inquiry into the cause, manner, and circumstances of a sudden, unexpected, or violent death.

insane /insān´/ [L, *in, sanus*, sound], a legal term for unsound, diseased, or deranged mental functioning, particularly said of a person who is unable to provide adequate self-care if there is a need to protect the patient and the public from each other. In the United States, the precise definition of this legal term varies from state to state.

insanity, /insan´itē/ [L, *in*, not, *sanus*, sound] *informal.* a severe mental disorder, such as a psychosis. The term is used more in legal and social than in medical terminology and refers to those mental illnesses that are of such a serious or debilitating nature as to interfere with one's capability of functioning within the legal limits of society and performing the normal activities of daily living.

insatiable /insā´sh(ē)əbəl/ [L, *insatiatus*], not satisfied], pertaining to an appetite for food or other needs that cannot be satisfied.

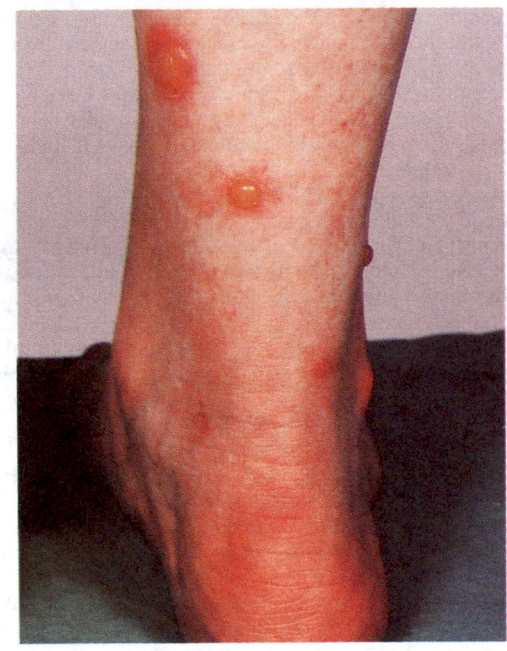

Insect bite *(du Vivier, 1993)*

insect bite [L, *in*, within, *secare*, to cut], the bite of any parasitic or venomous arthropod such as a louse, flea, mite, tick, or arachnid. Many arthropods inject venom that produces poisoning or severe local reaction, saliva that may contain viruses, or substances that produce mild irritation. The degree of irritation of an insect's bite is affected by the design and shape of its mouthparts: A horsefly, for example, makes a short lateral and coarse wound, whereas a tick takes hold with its backward curved teeth, making its removal difficult. Spiders inflict a sharp pinprick bite that may remain unnoticed until the injected venom has begun to produce a painful reaction. Treatment of a bite depends on the species of insect, the reaction to the bite, and the risk of sequelae from it. First aid treatment is generally symptomatic and includes ice or cold packs, careful cleaning of the wound, and antihistamines or specific antivenin as necessary.

insecticide /insek'tisīd/, a chemical agent that kills insects.

insecticide poisoning. See **chlorinated organic insecticide poisoning.**

insemination /insem'inā'shən/, the injection of semen into the uterine canal. It may involve an artificial process unrelated to sexual intercourse.

insenescence /in'sines'əns/ [L, insenescere, to begin to grow old], 1. the process of aging. 2. the state of being chronologically old but retaining the vitality of a person with a younger biologic age.

insensible /insen'sibəl/ [L, in, sentire, to feel], 1. pertaining to a person who is unconscious for any reason. 2. pertaining to a person who is apathetic or deprived of normal sense perceptions.

insensible perspiration [L, in, not, sentire, to feel; per, through, spirare, to breath], the loss of fluid from the body by evaporation, such as normally occurs during respiration. A small amount of perspiration is continually excreted by the sweat glands in the skin; the portion that evaporates before it may be observed also contributes to insensible perspiration. Also called **insensible water loss.**

insertion /insur'shən/ [L, inserere, to introduce], (in anatomy) the place of attachment, such as of a muscle to the bone it moves.

insertion forceps. See **point forceps.**

insertion site, the point in a vein where a needle or catheter is inserted.

in-service education [L, in, within, servus, a slave; educare, to rear], a program of instruction or training that is provided by an agency or institution for its employees. The program is held in the institution or at the agency and is intended to increase the skills and competence of the employees in a specific area. In-service education may be a part of any program of staff development. See also **staff development.**

insidious /insid'ē·əs/ [L, insidiosus, cunning], of, pertaining to, or describing a development that is gradual, subtle, or imperceptible. Certain chronic diseases, such as glaucoma, can develop insidiously with symptoms that are not detected by the patient until the disorder is established. Compare **acute.**

insight /in'sīt/ [L, in, within; AS, gesihth, sight], 1. the capacity of comprehending the true nature of a situation or of penetrating an underlying truth. 2. an instance of penetrating or comprehending an underlying truth, primarily through intuitive understanding. 3. (in psychology) a type of self-understanding encompassing both an intellectual and emotional awareness of the unconscious nature, origin, and mechanisms of one's attitudes, feelings, and behavior. It is one of the most important goals of psychotherapy and, with integration, leads to modification of maladaptive behavioral patterns. See also **integration.**

insipid /insip'id/ [L, in, sapidus, savory], dull, tasteless, or lifeless.

in situ /in sī'too, sit'oo/ [L, in, within; situs, position], 1. in the natural or usual place. 2. describing a cancer that has not metastasized or invaded neighboring tissues, such as carcinoma in situ.

insoluble /insol'yəbəl/ [L, in, not, solubilis, soluble], un-

able to be dissolved, usually in a specific solvent, such as a substance that is insoluble in water.

insomnia /insom'nē·ə/ [L, in, not, somnus, sleep], chronic inability to sleep or to remain asleep throughout the night; wakefulness; sleeplessness. Also called (formerly) **agrypnia.**

insomniac /insom'nē·ak/, 1. a person with insomnia. 2. pertaining to, causing, or associated with insomnia. 3. characteristic of or occurring during a period of sleeplessness.

inspiration /in'spirā'shən/ [L, in, within, spirare, to breathe], the act of drawing air into the lungs in order to exchange oxygen for carbon dioxide, the end product of tissue metabolism. The major muscle of inspiration is the diaphragm, the contraction of which creates a negative pressure in the chest, causing the normal lungs to expand and air to flow inward. Accessory inspiratory muscles include the external intercostals, scaleni, scapular elevators, and sternocleidomastoids. Since expiration is usually a passive process, these muscles of inspiration alone perform normal respiration. Lungs at maximal inspiration have an average total capacity of 5500 to 6000 ml of air. Compare **expiration.** See also **inspiratory reserve volume.**

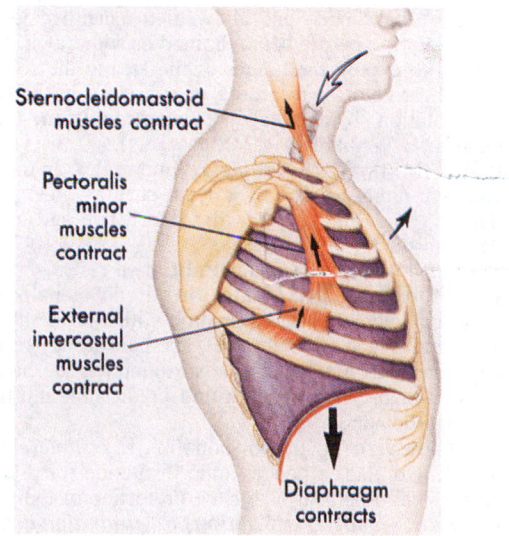

Inspiration (Thibodeau, 1993/Christy Krames)

inspiratory /inspī'rətôr'ē/ [L, in, within, spirare, to breathe], of or pertaining to inspiration.

inspiratory capacity (IC), the maximum volume of gas that can be inhaled from the resting expiratory level. Equal to the sum of the tidal volume and the inspiratory reserve volume, it is measured with a spirometer.

inspiratory dyspnea [L, inspirare, to breathe in; Gk, dys, without; pnoia, breath], a form of breathing difficulty caused by an obstruction in the larynx, trachea, or bronchi. The patient attempts to compensate for this deficiency with prolonged deep inspirations.

inspiratory hold, either of two kinds of modification in an intermittent positive pressure breathing (IPPB) pressure waveform. They are: (1) a pressure hold, in which a preset pressure is reached and held for a designated period, and (2) a volume hold, in which a predetermined volume is delivered and then held for a designated period.

inspiratory reserve volume, the maximum volume of gas that can be inspired from the end-tidal inspiratory level.

inspiratory resistance muscle training, exercises that require inhalation against some type of resisting force, such as abdominal breathing practice with the Pflex or threshold inspiratory muscle trainer. The amount of resistance is gradually increased over a period of several weeks during the abdominal muscle training. Resistance may also be used against expansion of the rib cage by the costal musculature during inspiration. The resistance may be provided by a therapist pushing against the ribs or by applying tightly a belt or swathe about the costal margin.

inspirometer /in'spirom'ətər/ [L, *inspirare*, to breathe in; Gk, *metron*, measure], an apparatus used to measure the volume, force, and frequency of a patient's inspirations.

inspissate /inspis'āt/ [L, *inspissare*, to thicken], (of a fluid) to thicken or harden through the absorption or evaporation of the liquid portion, such as milk in an inspissated milk duct. –**inspissation,** *n.*

instillation /in'stilā'shən/ [L, *instillare*, to drip], **1.** a procedure in which a fluid is slowly introduced into a cavity or passage of the body and allowed to remain for a specific length of time before being drained or withdrawn. It is performed to expose the tissues of the area to the solution, to warmth or cold, or to a drug or substance in the solution. **2.** a solution so introduced. Compare **infusion, injection, insufflate.** –**instill,** *v.*

instinct /in'stingkt/ [L, *instinctus*, impulse], an inborn psychologic representation of a need, such as life instincts of hunger, thirst, and sex, and the destructive and aggressive death instincts.

instinctive reflex. See **unconditioned reflex.**

institutionalism syndrome /in'stityōō'shənəliz'əm/, a condition characterized by apathy, withdrawal, submissiveness, and a lack of inititiative. The person may resist leaving a hospital, even when the surroundings are barely adequate, because it is familiar and predictable and there are minimal demands.

institutionalize /in'stityōō'shənəlīz'/ [L, *instituere*, to put in place], to place a person in an institution for psychologic or physical treatment or for the protection of the person or society. –**institutionalization,** *n., **institutionalized,** adj.*

institutional licensure /in'stityōō'shənəl/ [L, *instituere*, to put in place; *licere*, to be permitted], a proposed procedure in which licensure for almost all health professions would be abandoned and the responsibility for assessing professional competence would fall to the health care facility where the health professional is employed. Proponents of the procedure maintain that health needs would be better and more flexibly served. Opponents maintain that knowledge, judgment, and competency are the products of a good basic education in the profession and that educators cannot teach the profession without a set of standardized expectations, as are now provided by government-controlled licensing procedures and certifying examinations. In addition, health care facilities may not have the expertise or resources necessary to evaluate the various kinds of health care providers.

institutional review board (IRB), a federally approved committee that reviews all research proposals before submission of requests for funding by granting agencies.

instrument /in'strəmənt/ [L, *instrumentum* tool], a surgical tool or device designed to perform a specific function, such as cutting, dissecting, grasping, holding, retracting, or suturing. Surgical instruments are usually made of steel and are specially treated to be durable, heat-resistant, rust-resistant, and stain-proof. Proper care of surgical instruments is essential and includes correct use, careful handling, inspection for defects, adequate and appropriate sterilization, and proper labeling, dating, and storage. Some kinds of instruments are **clamp, needle holder, retractor,** and **speculum.**

instrumental conditioning. See **operant conditioning.**

instrumental labor /in'strəmen'təl/ [L, *instrumentum*, tool; *labor*, work], child delivery in which the use of instruments, such as forceps or perforators, is required.

instrumentation /in'strəməntā'shən/, the use of instruments for treatment and diagnosis.

insufficiency /in'səfish'ənsē/ [L, *in*, not, *sufficere*, to be adequate], inability to perform a necessary function adequately. Some kinds of insufficiency are **adrenal insufficiency, aortic insufficiency, ileocecal insufficiency, pulmonary insufficiency,** and **valvular insufficiency.**

insufflate /in'səflāt insuf'lāt/ [L, *insufflare*, to blow into], to blow a gas or powder into a tube, cavity, or organ to allow visual examination, to remove an obstruction, or to apply medication. See also **Rubin's test.** –**insufflation,** *n.*

insufflator /in'səflā'tər/ [L, *insufflare*, to blow into], an apparatus used to blow air or gas into a body cavity.

insul-, a combining form meaning 'of or pertaining to an island, or island-shaped': *insula, insulin, insuloma.*

insulation /in'sələ'shən/, a nonconducting substance that offers a barrier to the passage of heat or electricity.

insulin /in'səlin/ [L, *insula*, island], **1.** a naturally occurring hormone secreted by the beta cells of the islands of Langerhans in the pancreas in response to increased levels of glucose in the blood. The hormone acts to regulate the metabolism of glucose and the processes necessary for the intermediary metabolism of fats, carbohydrates, and proteins. Insulin lowers blood glucose levels and promotes transport and entry of glucose into the muscle cells and other tissues. Inadequate secretion of insulin results in hyperglycemia, hyperlipemia, ketonemia, and azoturia and in the characteristic signs of diabetes mellitus, including polyphagia, polydipsia, polyuria, and, eventually, lethargy and weight loss. Uncorrected severe deficiency of insulin is incompatible with life. Normal findings of insulin assay in adults show levels of 5 to 24 μU/ml. **2.** a pharmacologic preparation of the hormone administered in treating diabetes mellitus. The various preparations of insulin available for prescription vary in promptness, intensity, and duration of action. They are termed rapid-acting, intermediate-acting and long-acting. Most replacement insulin is given by subcutaneous injection in individualized dosage schedules. Insulin can be replaced intravenously. Adverse reactions include hypoglycemia and insulin shock from excess dosage and hyperglycemia and diabetic ketoacidosis from inadequate dosage. Many drugs interact with insulin, among them the monoamine oxidase inhibitors, corticosteroids, salicylates, thiazide diuretics, and phenytoin. Fever, stress, infection, pregnancy, surgery, and hyperthyroidism may significantly increase insulin requirements; liver disease, hy-

Insulins

Type	Description	Effect on blood glucose (hours after administration)		
		Onset	Peak	Termination
Short acting				
Regular (crystalline zinc)	Clear	Immediate	2 to 4	6 to 8
Semilente (SL)*	Cloudy: amorphous insulin zinc suspension, no protamine	1	4 to 6	12 to 16
Intermediate acting				
NPH†	Cloudy: crystalline zinc insulin suspension, 50% saturated with protamine	2 to 3	8 to 12	18 to 24
Lente	Cloudy: mixture 30% SL + 70% UL, no protamine	2 to 3	8 to 12	18 to 24
Long acting				
PZI†	Cloudy: excess protamine	6	14 to 20	24 to 36
Ultralente (UL)*	Cloudy: crystalline insulin suspension, high zinc content, no protamine	6	16 to 18	30 to 36

*Lente insulins (semi and ultra) do not contain protamine and are prepared in sodium acetate buffer. Their time of action depends on their variable zinc content and crystal size.
†Delayed action of NPH and PZI is controlled by their protamine content; they are prepared in sodium phosphate buffer.
From Price SA, Wilson LM: *Pathophysiology: clinical concepts of disease processes,* ed 4, St. Louis, 1992, Mosby, p. 887.

pothyroidism, vomiting, and renal disease may decrease the need for insulin. Urine or blood tests for glucose and ketones are performed to determine the need for adjustment of the dosage or of the schedule of administration. See also **human insulin.**

insulin-dependent diabetes mellitus (IDDM), an inability to metabolize carbohydrate caused by an overt insulin deficiency, occurring in children and adults and characterized by polydipsia, polyuria, polyphagia, loss of weight, diminished strength, and marked irritability. The onset is usually rapid, but approximately one third of the patients have a remission within 3 months; this stage may continue for days or years, but diabetes then progresses quickly to a state of total dependence on insulin. Occasionally, the disease is asymptomatic and is discovered only by postprandial hyperglycemia or abnormal glucose tolerance tests. Insulin-dependent diabetes mellitus tends to be unstable and brittle, with the patients quite sensitive to insulin and physical activity and diet and liable to develop ketoacidosis. Recent evidence suggests that insulin-dependent diabetes mellitus may be caused by environmental factors, such as a viral infection or autoimmune disease. Previously called brittle diabetes, juvenile diabetes, juvenile-onset diabetes, JOD, juvenile-onset-type diabetes, ketosis-prone diabetes. Compare **non-insulin-dependent diabetes mellitus.** See also **diabetes mellitus.**

insulinemia /in′səlinēmē·ə/ [L, *insula,* island (of Langerhans); Gk, *haima,* blood], an abnormally high level of insulin in the blood.

insulin injection sites, body tissue areas that offer optimum use of subcutaneous injections of insulin. The choice of sites can affect the rate of absorption and peak action times, but repeated use of the same injection sites can lead to localized tissue damage, resulting in malabsorption of insulin and misdiagnosis of insulin resistance. These problems

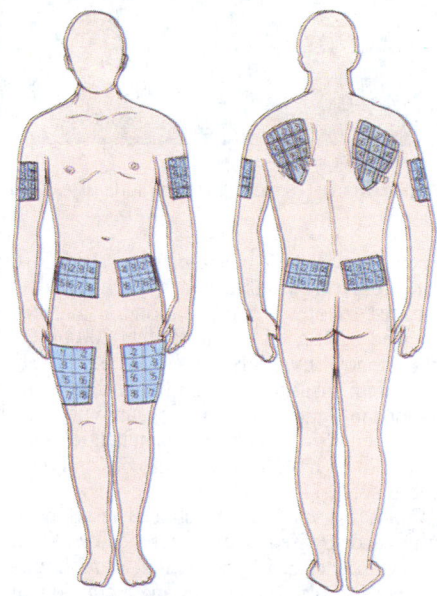

Insulin injection sites (Potter, 1993)

are minimized by systematic rotation of injection sites.

insulin kinase, an enzyme, assumed to be present in the liver, that activates insulin.

insulin lipodystrophy [L, *insula,* island; Gk, *lipos,* fat; *dys,* bad, *trophe,* nourishment], the loss of local fat deposits in diabetes patients as a complication of repeated insulin injections.

insulinogenic /in'səlin'ōjen'ik/ [L, *insula* + Gk, *genein*, to produce], promoting the production and release of insulin by the islands of Langerhans in the pancreas.

insulinoma /in'səlinō'mə/ *pl.* **insulinomas, insulinomata** [L, *insula* + Gk, *oma*, tumor], a benign tumor of the insulin-secreting cells of the islands of Langerhans. Surgical resection of the tumor may be possible, thus limiting the development of hypoglycemia. Also called **insuloma, islet cell adenoma.** Compare **islet cell tumor.**

insulin pump [L, *insula*, island; ME, *pumpe*], a portable battery-powered instrument that delivers a measured amount of insulin through the abdominal wall. It can be programmed to deliver varied doses of insulin according to the body's needs at the time.

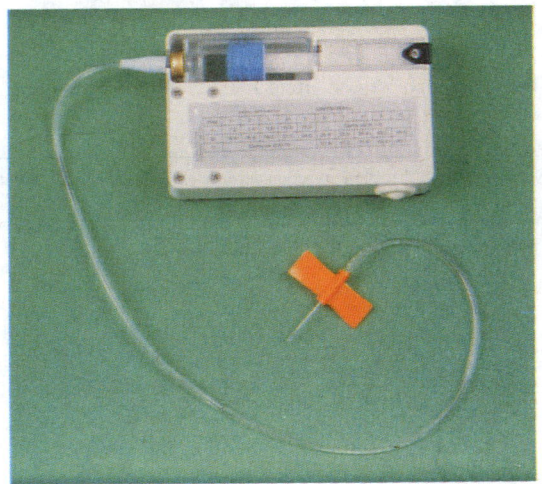

Insulin injection pump (Bodansky, 1989)

insulin reaction, the adverse effects caused by excessive levels of circulating insulin. See **hyperinsulinism.**

insulin resistance, a complication of diabetes mellitus characterized by a need for more than 200 units of insulin per day to control hyperglycemia and ketosis. The cause is associated with insulin binding by high levels of antibody. Insulin-resistant states also may occur with acanthosis nigrans, Werner's syndrome, ataxia telangiectasia, Älstrom syndrome, pineal hyperplasia syndrome, and various lipodystrophic disorders.

insulin shock, hypoglycemic shock caused by an overdose of insulin, a decreased intake of food, or excessive exercise. It is characterized by sweating, trembling, chilliness, nervousness, irritability, hunger, hallucination, numbness, and pallor. Uncorrected, it will progress to convulsions, coma, and death. Treatment requires an immediate dose of glucose orally or parenterally. Compare **diabetic coma, ketoacidosis.**

insulin tolerance test, a test of the body's ability to use insulin, in which insulin is given and blood glucose is measured at regular intervals. Thirty minutes after the insulin is given, blood glucose is usually lower but not less than half of the fasting glucose level. Glucose levels usually return to normal after about 90 minutes. In people with hypoglycemia, the glucose levels may drop lower and be slower to return to normal.

insulintropin /in'səlintrop'in/ [L, *insula*, island], a naturally occurring hormone produced in the intestines when food is ingested. It causes the release of insulin from the pancreas, which, in turn, regulates blood-sugar levels. It has been administered to Type II diabetes patients, but it would not be useful in its present form in the treatment of Type I diabetes patients because their pancreases do not secrete insulin.

insuloma. See **insulinoma.**

intake [L, *in*, within; AS, *tacan*, to take], **1.** the process in which a person is admitted to a clinic or hospital or is signed in for an office visit. The reason for the visit and various identifying data about the patient are noted. Certain preliminary, routine procedures may be performed, such as obtaining a blood pressure reading or a urine specimen. In some clinical settings, the intake may also include obtaining such additional information as the patient's basic health history and previous source of care. **2.** (in nursing) the amount of food or fluids ingested in a given period of time. Intake is measured and noted in milliliters or grams per 8- or 24-hour period.

Intal, a trademark for an antiasthmatic (cromolyn sodium).

integral dose /in'təgrəl/ [L, *integrare*, to make whole; Gk, *dosis*, giving], (in radiotherapy) the total amount of energy absorbed by a patient or object during exposure to radiation. Also called **volume dose.**

-integrate. See **integration.**

integrated system /in'təgrā'tid/, a group of interconnected units that form a functioning computer system.

integrating dose meter /in'təgrā'ting/, (in radiotherapy) an ionization chamber, usually designed to be placed on the patient's skin, with a measuring system for determining the total radiation administered during an exposure. A device may be included to terminate the exposure when the desired value is reached.

integration /in'təgrā'shən/ [L, *integrare*, to make whole], **1.** the act or process of unifying or bringing together. **2.** (in psychology) the organization of all elements of the personality into a coordinated, functional whole that is in harmony with the environment, one of the primary goals in psychotherapy. It involves the assimilation of insight and the coordination of new and old data, experiences, and emotional reactions so that an effective change can occur in behavior, thinking, or feeling. See also **insight.** – **integrate,** *v.*

integration of self, one of the components of high-level wellness. It is a prerequisite for the achievement of maturity and is characterized by the integration of mind, body, and spirit into one harmoniously functioning unit.

integument /integ'yo͞oment/ [L, *integumentum*, a covering], a covering or skin. – **integumentary,** *adj.*

integumentary system /integ'yəmen'tərē/, the skin and its appendages, hair, nails, and sweat and sebaceous glands. See also the Color Atlas of Human Anatomy.

integumentary system assessment, an evaluation of the general condition of a patient's integument and of factors or abnormalities that may contribute to the presence of a dermatologic disorder.

■ METHOD: The nurse askes if the patient suffers from itching, pain, rashes, blisters, or boils; if the skin usually is dry, oily, thin, rough, bumpy, or puffy; or if it feels hot or cold, peels, changes in color, or is marked with dark liver (aging) spots. Observations are made of the intactness, turgor, elasticity, temperature, cleanliness, odor, wetness or dryness, and color of the skin. Cyanosis of the lips, circumoral

area, or mucous membranes, earlobes, or nailbeds; jaundice of the sclera; pale conjunctivae; the distribution of pigment; and evidence of plethora are noted. Indications of rashes, edema, needle marks, insect bites, scabies, acne, sclerema, decubiti, uremic frost on the beard or eyebrows, or pressure areas over bony prominences are recorded. The nails are examined for brittleness, lines, a convex ram's horn or concave spoon shape, and the condition of surrounding tissue, including clubbing of the fingers and toes. The existence and characteristics of maculae, papules, vesicles, pustules, bullae, hives, warts, moles, ulcers, scars, keloids, petechiae, lipomas, crusts of dried exudate, flakes of dead epidermis, excoriations, blackheads, or a chancre are noted. The patient's exposure to parasites, to internal allergens in food and drugs, and to external allergens in cosmetics, soaps, topical medication, and plants, as well as a family history of allergies, is investigated. The patient's currently used medication, creams, lotions, ointments, hygienic measures, and sexual practices are ascertained. Diagnostic aids contributing to the evaluation are skin and lesion cultures, punch biopsies, skin tests for allergies, a lupus erythematosus preparation, and a blood culture.
■ NURSING ORDERS: the nurse conducts the interview to obtain subjective data on the patient's condition, makes the necessary observations, and assembles the background information and the results of the diagnostic tests.
■ OUTCOME CRITERIA: A well-conducted assessment of the patient's integument is a valuable aid in diagnosing a dermatologic disorder.

intellect /in'təlekt/ [L, *intellectus,* perception], **1.** the power and ability of the mind for knowing and understanding, as contrasted with feeling or with willing. **2.** a person possessing a great capacity for thought and knowledge. —**intellectual,** *adj., n.*

intellectualization /in'təlek'choo·əlīzā'shən/ [L, *intellectus* + Gk, *izein,* to cause], (in psychiatry) a defense mechanism in which reasoning is used as a means of blocking a confrontation with an unconscious conflict and the emotional stress associated with it.

intelligence /intel'ijəns/ [L, *intelligentia,* perception], **1.** the potential ability and capacity to acquire, retain, and apply experience, understanding, knowledge, reasoning, and judgment in coping with new experiences and in solving problems. **2.** the manifestation of such ability. See also **intelligence quotient.** —**intelligent,** *adj.*

intelligence quotient (IQ), a numeric expression of a person's intellectual level as measured against the statistical average of his or her age group. On several of the traditional scales it is determined by dividing the mental age, derived through psychologic testing, by the chronologic age and multiplying the result by 100. Average IQ is considered to be 100.

intelligence test, any of a variety of standarized tests designed to determine the mental age of an individual by measuring the relative capacity to absorb information and to solve problems.

-intelligent. See **intelligence.**

intelligent terminal, a computer terminal that can function as a processing device in addition to providing input/output facilities, whether operated independently or connected to a main computer.

intemperance /intem'pərəns/ [L, *in, temperare,* to moderate], excessive indulgence in eating, drinking, or other lifestyle functions.

intensifying screen /inten'sifī'ing/ [L, *intensus,* tighten,

facere, to make; ME, *screne*], a device consisting of fluorescent material, which is placed in contact with the film in a radiographic cassette. Radiation from a therapeutic process interacts with the fluorescent phosphor, releasing light photons. These expose the film with greater efficiency than would the radiation alone. Thus patient exposure can be reduced.

intensive care /inten'siv/ [L, *intensus,* tightened, *garrire,* to chatter], constant, complex, detailed health care as provided in various acute life-threatening conditions, such as multiple trauma, severe burns, myocardial infarction, or after certain kinds of surgery. Special training is necessary to provide intensive care. Care is most frequently given in an intensive care unit equipped with various advanced machines and devices for treating and monitoring the patient. Also called **critical care.**

intensive care unit (ICU), a hospital unit in which patients requiring close monitoring and intensive care are housed for as long as needed. An ICU contains highly technical and sophisticated monitoring devices and equipment, and the staff in the unit is educated to give critical care as needed by the patients. A large tertiary care facility usually has separate units specifically designed for the intensive care of adults, infants, children or newborns or for other groups of patients requiring a certain kind of treatment. See also **coronary care unit.**

intention /inten'shən/ [L, *intendere,* to aim], a kind of healing process. Healing by **first intention** is the primary union of the edges of a wound, progressing to complete healing without scar formation or granulation. Healing by **second intention** is wound closure in which the edges are separated, granulation tissue develops to fill the gap, and epithelium grows in over the granulations, producing a scar. Healing by **third intention** is wound closure in which granulation tissue fills the gap between the edges of the wound, with epithelium growing over the granulation at a slower rate and producing a larger scar than results from healing from second intention. Suppuration is also usually found.

intentional additives, substances that are deliberately added in the manufacture of food or pharmaceutical products to improve or maintain flavor, color, texture, or consistency, or to enhance or conserve nutritional value. Compare **incidental additives.**

intention tremor, fine, rhythmic, purposeless movements that tend to increase during voluntary movements. Compare **resting tremor.** See also **tremor.**

inter- /in'tər-/, a prefix meaning 'situated, formed, or occurring between': *interacinar, intercalary, intercartilaginous.*

interactional model /-ak'shənəl/ [L, *inter,* between, *agere,* to do], a family therapy model that views the family as a communication system comprising interlocking subsystems of family members. Family dysfunction occurs when the rules governing family interaction become vague and ambiguous. The therapeutic goal is to help the family clarify the rules governing family relationships.

interactionist theory /-ak'shənist/, an aging theory that views age-related changes as resulting from the interaction between the individual characteristics of the person, the circumstances in society, and the history of social interaction patterns of the person.

interaction processes, a component of the theory of effective practice. The processes consist of a series of interactions between a nurse and a patient. The series occurs in a sequence of actions and reactions until the patient and the nurse both understand what is wanted and the desired behavior or act is achieved.

interaction theme.   See **communication theme.**

interactive terminal /-ak′tiv/,   a data processing terminal that is integrated into a system to alow two-way communication between the user and the system. Also called **interactive system, user interaction.**

interalveolar /-alvē′ələr/ [L, *inter*, between; *alveolus*, little hollow],   pertaining to the area between alveoli.

interarticular /-ärtik′yələr/ [L, *inter*, between; *articulus*, joint],   pertaining to the areas between two joints or between facing surfaces of a joint.

interarticular fibrocartilage [L, *inter* + *articulus*, joint],   one of four kinds of fibrocartilage, consisting of flattened fibrocartilaginous plates between the articular cartilage of the most active joints, such as the sternoclavicular, wrist, and knee joints. The synovial surfaces extend over the fibrocartilaginous plates and attach to surrounding ligaments. The fibrocartilaginous plates absorb shocks and increase mobility. Compare **circumferential fibrocartilage, connecting fibrocartilage, stratiform fibrocartilage.**

intercalary /intur′kəler′ē, in′tərkal′ərē/ [L, *intercalare*, to insert],   occurring between two others, such as the absence of the middle part of a bone with the proximal and the distal parts present.

intercalate /intur′kəlāt/ [L, *intercalare*],   to insert between adjacent surfaces or structures. **–intercalation,** *n.*

intercapillary glomerulosclerosis /-kap′iler′ē/ [L, *inter* + *capillaris*, hairlike; *gomerulus*, small ball; Gk, *sklerosis*, a hardening],   an abnormal condition characterized by degeneration of the renal glomeruli. It is associated with diabetes and often produces albuminuria, nephrotic edema, hypertension, and renal insufficiency. Also called **Kimmelstiel-Wilson disease.**

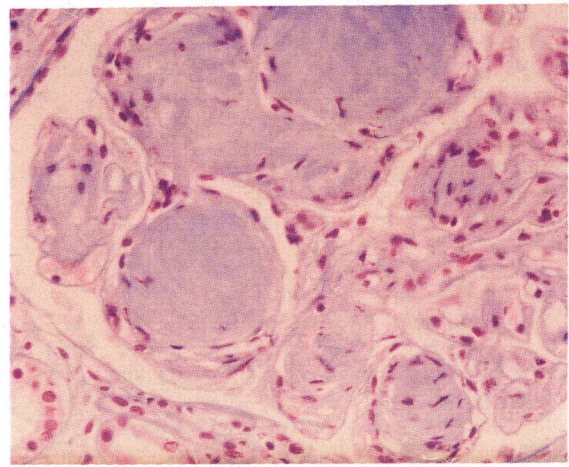

Intercapillary glomerulosclerosis
(Bodansky, 1990/Courtesy Dr JT Ireland, Glasgow)

intercavernous sinuses /-kav′ərnəs/ [L, *inter*, between; *caverna*, cavity; *sinus*, curve],   the cavities through which the cavernous sinuses of the dura mater communicate.

intercellular /-sel′yələr/ [L, *inter* + *cella*, storeroom],   between or among cells.

intercellular bridge,   a structure that connects adjacent cells, occurring primarily in the epithelium and other stratified squamous epithelia. It consists of slender strands of cytoplasm that project from the surfaces of adjacent cells and merge at the desmosome. Also called **cytoplasmic bridge.**

intercerebral /-ser′əbəl/ [L, *inter*, between; *cerebrum*, brain],   pertaining to the area between the left and right cerebral hemispheres.

interchange.   See **reciprocal translocation.**

interclavicular /-kləvik′yələr/ [L, *inter*, between; *clavicula*, little key],   pertaining to the area between the clavicles.

interconceptional gynecologic care /-kənsep′shənəl/ [L, *inter* + *concipere*, to take in],   health care of a woman during her reproductive years, between pregnancies, and after 6 weeks after delivery. Papanicolaou testing for cervical cancer, breast and pelvic examinations, evaluation of general health, and laboratory determination of glucosuria and proteinuria and of the hematocrit or hemoglobin are common and routine aspects of interconceptional care. Testing and treatment for pelvic, vaginal, or genital infections may be required. A contraceptive method may also be discussed, taught, prescribed, or provided. Ordinarily, the basic examination is performed annually. The method of contraception may be adjusted or changed at interim visits; infections or other complaints are investigated, diagnosed, and treated as symptoms appear. Interconceptional care is increasingly given by nurse practitioners or nurse midwives who follow protocols for treatment and referral formulated in consultation with a supervising gynecologist.

intercondylar fracture /in′tərkon′dilər/ [L, *inter* + Gk, *kondylos*, knuckle],   a fracture of the tissue between condyles.

intercostal /-kos′təl/ [L, *inter* + *costa*, rib],   of or pertaining to the space between two ribs.

intercostal bulging,   the visible bulging of the soft tissues of the intercostal spaces that occurs when increased expiratory effort is needed to exhale, as in asthma, cystic fibrosis, or obstruction of an airway by a foreign body. Compare **retraction of the chest.**

intercostal muscles,   the muscles between adjacent ribs. They are designated as external and internal, and function as secondary ventilatory muscles.

intercostal node,   a node in one of three groups of thoracic parietal lymph nodes situated near the dorsal parts of the intercostal spaces. The nodes are associated with lymphatic vessels that drain the posterolateral area of the chest. The efferent vessels from the nodes in the caudal four or five spaces form a descending trunk that opens into the dilated origin of the thoracic duct. The efferent vessels from the nodes in the upper intercostal spaces on the left side connect with the thoracic duct; those on the right side end in the right lymphatic duct. Compare **diaphragmatic node, sternal node.** See also **lymphatic system, lymph node.**

intercostal space [L, *inter*, between; *costa*, rib; *spatium*],   the region between the ribs.

intercourse /in′tərkôrs′/ [L, *intercursus*, running between],   *informal.* sexual intercourse. See **coitus.**

intercristal /-kris′təl/ [L, *inter* + *crista*, ridge],   of or pertaining to the space between two crests.

intercurrent disease /-kur′ənt/ [L, *intercurrere*, to run be-

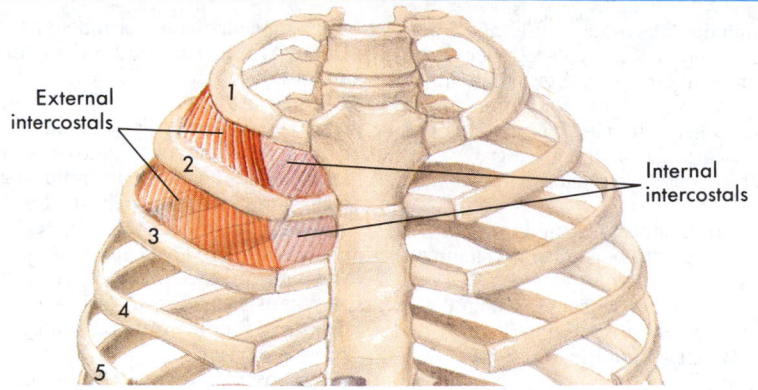

Intercostal muscles *(Thibodeau, 1993/John V Hagen)*

tween], a disease that develops in and may alter the course of another disease.

interdental canal /-den'tə/ [L, *inter* + *dens*, tooth], any one of the nutrient channels that pass upward to the teeth through the body of the mandible. Also called **nutrient canal.**

interdental gingiva, the soft supporting tissue, consisting of prominent horizontal collagen fibers, that normally fills the space between two approximating teeth.

interdental groove, a linear, vertical depression on the surface of the interdental papillae, which functions as a sluiceway for the egress of food from the interproximal areas.

interdental spillway, a sluiceway formed by the interproximal contours of adjoining teeth and their investing tissues.

interdependent intervention. See **intervention.**

interface /in'tərfās/ [L, *inter* + *facies*, face], the connection between different elements of a computer system or between different computers.

interference /-fir'əns/ [L, *inter* + *ferire*, to strike], the effect of a component on the accuracy of measurement of the desired analyte.

interferent /-fir'ənt/ [L, *inter* + *ferire*, to strike], any chemical or physical phenomena that can interfere or disrupt a reaction or process.

interferential current therapy /-fərən'shəl/, a form of electric stimulation therapy using two or three distinctively different currents that are passed through a tissue from surface electrodes. Portions of each current are canceled by the other, resulting in a different net current applied to the target tissue.

interferon /-fir'on/ [L, *inter* + *ferire*, to strike], a natural cellular protein formed when cells are exposed to a virus or other foreign particle of nucleic acid. It induces the production of translation inhibitory protein (TIP) in noninfected cells. TIP blocks translation of viral RNA, thus giving other cells protection against both the original and other viruses. Interferon is species specific.

interferon alpha-2a, recombinant, a parenteral antineoplastic drug.

■ INDICATIONS: It is administered in the treatment of hair cell leukemia.

■ CONTRAINDICATIONS: Caution is recommended in prescribing this product for patients with severe cardiovascular disease.

■ ADVERSE EFFECTS: Among reported adverse reactions are influenzalike symptoms, particularly at the beginning of therapy with the drug, confusion, dizziness, nervousness, depression, anorexia, nausea, vomiting, diarrhea, throat inflammation, dry and itching skin, alopecia, diaphoresis, blood pressure changes, and tachycardia.

interferon alpha-2b, recombinant, a parenteral antineoplastic drug with indications, contraindications, and adverse effects similar to those of **interferon alpha-2a, recombinant.**

interferon nomenclature, a system recommended by the International Interferon Nomenclature Committee for identifying interferon compounds. For a specific isolated product, "interferon" is the first word of the name. It is followed by a Greek letter, spelled out, an arabic number, and a lower case letter appended by a dash, as in the example: interferon alpha-2a.

interfibrillar mass of Flemming /-fī'brilər/, **interfilar mass.** See **hyaloplasm.**

interim rate /in'tərim/ [L, meanwhile; *ratum* calculate], a method of third-party payment for costs of hospital services in which an amount is paid periodically pending an accounting of actual costs at the end of a designated period.

interiorization /intir'ē·ərīzā'shən/ [L, *interior*, inner; Gk, *izein*, to cause], the merging of reflex and cognitive processes as a response to the environment.

interior mesenteric artery [L, inner; Gk, *mesos*, middle; *enteron*, intestine; *arteria*, air pipe], a visceral branch of the abdominal aorta, arising just above the division into the common iliacs and supplying the left half of the transverse colon, all of the descending and iliac colons, and most of the rectum. It has left colic, sigmoid, and superior rectal branches.

interkinesis /in'tərkinē'sis, -kīnē'sis/ [L, *inter* + Gk, *kinein*, to move], the interval between the first and second nuclear divisions in meiosis. See also **interphase.**

interlace mode /-lās'/, (in radiology) a process whereby a conventional TV camera tube reads off its target assembly so that two fields of 262.5 lines each are read in 17 ms to form a 525-line video frame in 33 ms. Each field represents repeated adjacent active traces and horizontal retraces of the electron beam across a TV screen.

interleukin-1 (IL-1) /-loo'kin/, a protein with numerous immune system functions, including activation of resting T cells, and endothelial and macrophage cells, mediation of inflammation, and stimulation of synthesis of lymphokines, collagen, and collagenases. It can also induce fever, sleep, ACTH release, and nonspecific resistance to infection.

interleukin-2 (IL-2), a protein with various immunologic functions, including the ability to initiate proliferation of activated T cells. IL-2 is used in the laboratory to grow T cell clones with specific helper, cytotoxic, and suppressor functions.

interleukin-3 (IL-3), an immune response protein that supports the growth of pluripotent bone marrow stem cells and is a growth factor for mast cells.

interleukin-4 (IL-4), an immune response protein that is a growth factor for activated B cells, resting T cells, and mast cells. Also called **B cell stimulating factor-1.**

interleukin-6. See **IL-6.**

interlobular duct /-lob′yələr/ [L, *inter* + *lobulus,* small lobe], any duct connecting or draining the lobules of a gland.

interlocked twins [L, *inter* + AS, *loc,* a fastening], monozygotic twins so positioned in the uterus that the neck of one becomes entwined with that of the other during presentation so that vaginal delivery is not possible. Such interlocking occurs when one fetus is a breech presentation and the other a vertex presentation. Also called **interlocking twins.**

intermediary /-mē′dē·er′ē/ [L, *inter* + *mediare,* to divide], a Blue Cross plan, private insurance company, or public or private agency selected by health care providers to pay claims under Medicare.

intermediary metabolism [L, *inter,* between; *mediary,* to divide; Gk, *metabole,* change], the metabolic processes involved in the synthesis of cellular components between digestion of food and excretion of waste products.

intermediate-acting insulin [L, *inter* + *mediare,* to divide; *activus,* active], a preparation of the antidiabetic principle of beef pancreas or pork pancreas modified by interaction with zinc under specific chemical conditions and having an intermediate range of action. The action of semilente insulin begins within 1 hour of injection, reaches a peak in 6 to 10 hours, and lasts for 12 to 16 hours. Three other intermediate-acting preparations begin to act 2 to 4 hours after injection; globin zinc insulin reaches a peak in 6 to 10 hours and lasts for 18 to 24 hours; neutral protamine Hagedorn insulin (NPH) has a peak action in 8 to 12 hours and a duration of action of 28 to 32 hours, whereas lente insulin has a similar peak interval and a slightly shorter duration of action. See also **insulin.** Compare **long-acting insulin, short-acting insulin.**

intermediate care /-mē′dē·it/, a level of medical care for certain chronically ill or disabled individuals in which room and board are provided but skilled nursing care is not. Title XI of U.S. Medicaid legislation mandates standards and federal subsidies for intermediate care of the recipients of public assistance.

intermediate care facility, a health facility that provides medical-related services to persons with a variety of physical or emotional conditions requiring institutional facilities but without the degree of care provided by a hospital or skilled nursing facility. An example is a health care facility for mentally retarded persons.

intermediate cell mass. See **nephrotome.**

intermediate cuneiform bone, the smallest of the three cuneiform bones of the foot, located between the medial and the lateral cuneiform bones. It has six surfaces, is attached to various ligaments, and articulates with the navicular, me-

dial, and lateral cuneiform bones and with the second metatarsal. Also called **middle cuneiform bone, second cuneiform bone.**

intermediate disk. See **Z disk.**

intermediate host, any animal in which the larval or intermediate stages of a parasite develop. Certain snails are intermediate hosts for liver flukes and schistosomes. Humans are intermediate hosts for malaria parasites. Also called **secondary host.** Compare **dead-end host, definitive host, reservoir host.** See also **host,** def. 1.

intermediate mesoderm. See **nephrotome.**

intermenstrual /-men′strōō·əl/ [L, *inter* + *menstruum,* menstrual fluid], of or pertaining to the time between menstrual periods.

intermenstrual fever, the normal, slight elevation of temperature that marks ovulation, usually occurring about 14 days before the onset of menses.

intermittent /-mit′ənt/ [L, *inter* + *mittere,* to send], occurring at intervals; alternating between periods of activity and inactivity, such as rheumatoid arthritis, which is marked by periods of signs and symptoms followed by periods of remission.

intermittent assisted ventilation (IAV), (in respiratory therapy) a system in which an assisted rate is combined with spontaneous breathing. Also called **intermittent demand ventilation (IDV).**

intermittent claudication. See **claudication.**

intermittent demand ventilation. See **intermittent assisted ventilation.**

intermittent fever, a fever that recurs in cycles of paroxysms and remissions, such as in malaria. Kinds of intermittent fever include **biduotertian malaria, double quartan malaria,** and **quartan malaria.**

intermittent hydrosalpinx /-hī′drōsal′pingks/ [L, *inter,* between; *mittere,* to send; Gk, *hydor,* water; *salpigx,* tube], a fluid accumulation in a fallopian tube. The fluid is released periodically through the uterine cavity. Also called **hydrops tubae profluens.**

intermittent incontinence [L, *inter,* between; *mittere,* to send; *incontinentia,* inability to retain], urinary incontinence that occurs only when there is pressure on the bladder or during muscular effort.

intermittent mandatory ventilation (IMV), a mode of mechanical ventilation in which the patient is allowed to breathe independently and then, at certain prescribed intervals, a ventilator delivers a breath either under positive pressure or in a measured volume. Compare **intermittent positive pressure breathing.** See also **respiratory therapy.**

intermittent positive pressure breathing. See **IPPB.**

intermittent positive pressure breathing unit. See **IPPB unit.**

intermittent positive pressure ventilation. See **IPPB.**

intermittent pulse [L, *inter,* between; *mittere,* to send; *pulsare,* to beat], a pulse in which an occasional beat is absent. It tends to occur with second degree heart block or extrasystole. Also called **dropped-beat pulse.**

intermittent torticollis [L, *inter,* between; *mittere,* to send; *tortus,* twisted; *collum,* neck], intermittent spasms of the neck muscles, drawing the head to one side. The powerful contractions usually occur in the sternocleidomastoid muscle.

intermittent tremor [L, *inter,* between; mittere, to send; *tremor,* trembling], a rhythmic involuntary shaking that occurs intermittently or tremor that occurs after a voluntary movement is attempted.

intern /in′turn/ [L, *internus*, inward], **1.** a physician in the first postgraduate year, learning medical practice under supervision before beginning a residency program. **2.** any immediate postgraduate trainee in a clinical program. **3.** to work as an intern. Also spelled **interne.**

internal /intur′nəl/ [L, *internus*, inward], within or inside. −**internally,** *adv.*

internal aperture of tympanic canaliculus, the upper opening of the tympanic channel in the temporal bone, leading to the tympanum.

internal bleeding [L, *internus*, inward; AS, *blod*], any hemorrhage from an internal organ or tissue, such as intraperitoneal bleeding into the peritoneal cavity or intestinal bleeding into the bowel.

internal carotid artery, each of two arteries starting at the bifurcation of the common carotid arteries, opposite the cranial border of the thyroid cartilage, through which blood circulates to many structures and organs in the head. Each artery includes cervical, petrous, cavernous, and cerebral portions and divides into 11 branches. There are no branches from the cervical portion. The four branches from the petrous portion are the caroticotympanic, the artery of the pterygoid canal, the cavernous, and the hypophyseal. The five branches from the cavernous portion are the ganglionic, anterior meningeal, ophthalmic, anterior cerebral, and middle cerebral. The two branches from the cerebral portion are the posterior communicating and the anterior choroidal.

internal carotid plexus, a network of nerves on the internal carotid artery, formed by the internal carotid nerve. The internal carotid plexus supplies sympathetic fibers to the branches of the internal carotid artery, the tympanic plexus, the nerves of the cavernous sinus, and the cranial parasympathetic ganglia through which the fibers pass. Compare **common carotid plexus, external carotid plexus.**

internal cervical os, an internal opening of the uterus that corresponds to the slight constriction or isthmus of that organ about midway in its length. The internal cervical os separates the body of the uterus from the cervix. Compare **external cervical os.**

internal cuneiform bone. See **medial cuneiform bone.**

internal ear, the complex inner structure of the ear, containing receptors for two different fubctions. The maculae and crystae cells help maintain equilibrium while the organ of Corti cells translate sound vibrations into impulses for the sense of hearing. Ther auditory receptor cells are innervated by the cochlear nerve. Also called **inner ear, labyrinth.** Compare **external ear, middle ear.**

internal fertilization, the union of gametes within the body of the female after insemination. See also **artificial insemination.**

internal fistula, an abnormal passage between two internal organs or structures.

internal fixation, any method of holding together the fragments of a fractured bone without the use of appliances external to the skin. After open reduction of the fracture, smooth or threaded pins, Kirschner wires, screws, plates attached by screws, or medullary nails may be used to stabilize the fragments. In some instances the device is removed at a later operation, but sometimes it may remain in the body permanently. Compare **external pin fixation.**

internal iliac artery, a division of the common iliac artery, supplying the walls of the pelvis, the pelvic viscera, the genital organs, and part of the medial thigh. The pattern of its branches is the most variable of any artery in the

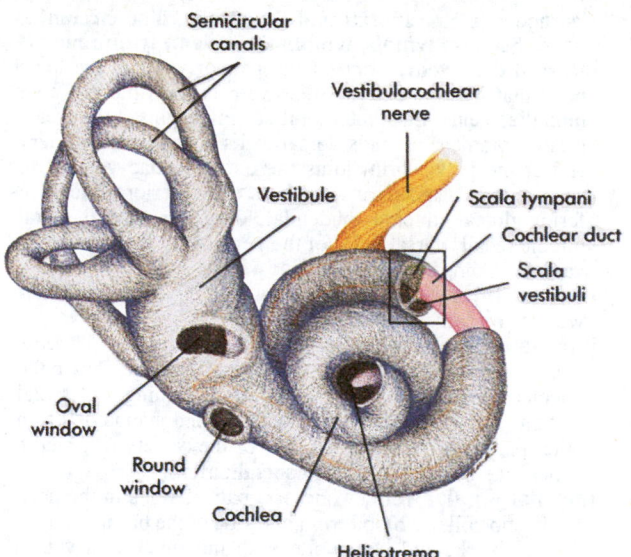

Internal ear (Seeley, 1992/Lisa Chuch/Michael Schenk)

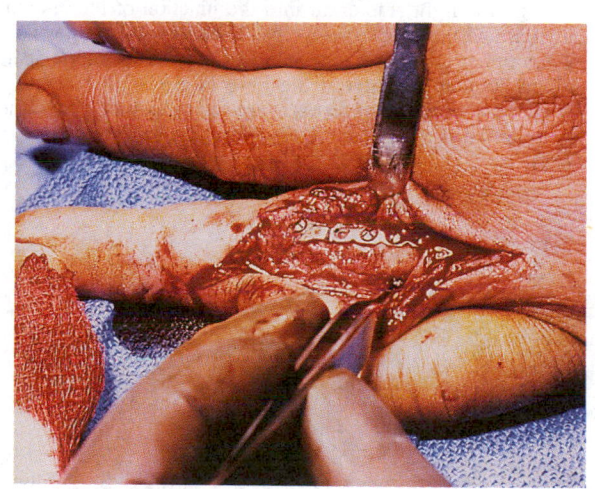

Internal fixation (Bray, 1993/Steve Young)

body. Its 10 most common branches are umbilical, inferior vesical, middle rectal, uterine, obturator, internal pudendal, iliolumbar, lateral sacral, superior gluteal, and inferior gluteal. In the fetus, the internal iliac artery is twice as large as the external iliac and is the direct continuation of the common iliac artery. After birth, the internal iliac becomes smaller than the external iliac. Also called **hypogastric artery.** Compare **external iliac artery.**

internal iliac node, a node in one of seven groups of parietal lymph nodes serving the abdomen and the pelvis. The internal iliac nodes surround the internal iliac vessels and receive lymphatic vessels corresponding to the branches of the internal iliac artery. Their afferent vessels drain lymph from the pelvic viscera, the buttocks, and dorsal portions of the thighs. Their efferent vessels end in the common iliac nodes. Compare **external iliac node, iliac circumflex node.** See also **lymph, lymphatic system, lymph node.**

internal iliac vein, one of the pair of veins in the lower body that join the external iliac vein to form the two common iliac veins. Each internal iliac vein begins at the greater sciatic foramen, ascends dorsal to its corresponding artery, and at the pelvic brim joins the external iliac vein. It receives various tributaries, such as the superior gluteal, inferior gluteal, internal pudendal, obturator, lateral sacral, middle rectal, dorsal veins of the penis, vesical, uterine, and vaginal. Compare **external iliac vein.**

internal injury [L, *internus*, inward; *injuria*], any hurt, wound, or damage to the viscera.

internalization /intur'nəlīzā'shən/ [L, *internus* + Gk, *izein*, to cause], the process of adopting within the self, either unconsciously or consciously through learning and socialization, the attitudes, beliefs, values, and standards of another person or, more generally, of the society or group to which one belongs. See also **socialization.**

internal jugular vein, one of a pair of veins in the neck. Each vein collects blood from one side of the brain, the face, and the neck, and both unite with the subclavian vein to form the brachiocephalic vein. The left internal jugular vein is usually smaller than the right, and each vein contains a pair of valves located about 2.5 cm above its termination. The thoracic duct on the left side and the right lymphatic duct on the right side drain into the junction of the internal jugular and the subclavian veins. Each internal jugular vein is continuous with the transverse sinus in the posterior part of the jugular foramen at the base of the skull where, in some people, the vein forms a jugular bulb. Just above the termination is the inferior bulb. Compare **external jugular vein.**

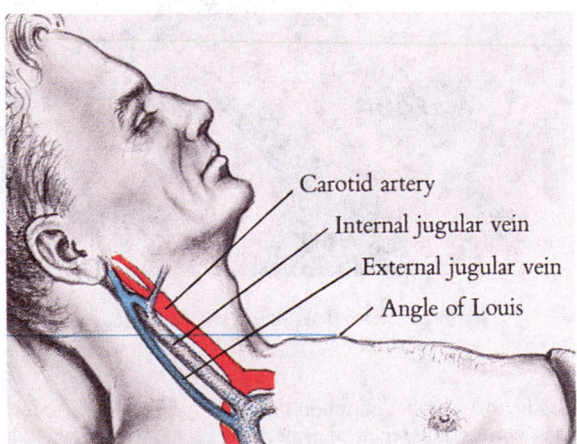

Carotid artery
Internal jugular vein
External jugular vein
Angle of Louis

Internal jugular vein *(Thompson, 1993)*

internal locus of control. See **locus of control.**

-internally. See **internal.**

internal malleolus [L, *internus*, inward; *malleolus*, little hammer], the rounded process of the tibia forming the internal surface of the ankle joint. Also called **medial malleolus.**

internal mammary artery bypass, a surgical procedure to correct a coronary artery obstruction. The internal mam-

mary artery in situ and still attached to the subclavian artery is anastomosed to the coronary artery beyond the obstruction.

internal medicine, the branch of medicine concerned with the study of the physiology and pathology of the internal organs and with the medical diagnosis and treatment of disorders of these organs.

internal oblique muscle. See **obliquus internus abdominis.**

internal os, the internal opening of the cervical canal.

internal podalic version and total breech extraction. See **version and extraction.**

internal pterygoid muscle. See **pterygoideus medialis.**

internal respiratory nerve of Bell. See **phrenic nerve.**

internal rotation, the turning of a limb toward the midline of the body.

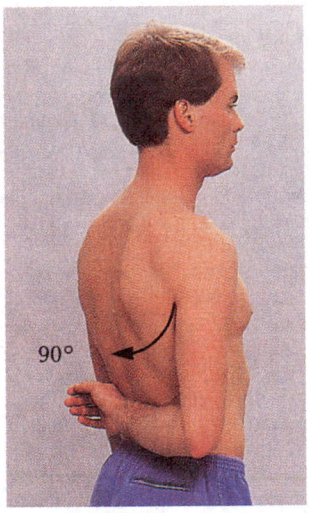

90°

Internal rotation *(Seidel, 1991)*

internal secretion [L, *internus*, inward; *secernere*, to separate], a type of secretion in which substances pass directly from a gland into the bloodstream.

internal standard, an element or compound added in a known amount to yield a signal against which an instrument or an analyte to be measured can be calibrated.

internal strabismus. See **esotropia.**

internal strangulation [L, *internus*, inward; *strangulare*, to choke], a state of extreme constriction of an organ, such as a loop of intestine trapped in an opening, resulting in an interruption in the blood supply and ischemia.

internal thoracic artery, one of a pair of arteries that arise from the first portions of the subclavian arteries, descend to the margin of the sternum, and divide into the musculophrenic and superior gastric arteries at the level of the sixth intercostal space. The artery supplies the pectoral muscles, the breasts, the pericardium, and the abdominal muscles. Each artery has eight branches: pericardiophrenic, mediastinal, thymic, sternal, anterior intercostal, perforating, musculophrenic, and superior epigastric.

internal thoracic vein, one of a pair of veins that accompanies the internal thoracic artery, receiving tributaries that correspond to those of the artery. It forms a single trunk that runs up on the medial side of the artery and ends in the corresponding brachiocephalic vein. The superior phrenic vein usually opens into the internal thoracic vein.

International Association for Dental Research (I.A.D.R.), an international organization concerned with research in dentistry and the exchange of information regarding such research.

International Classification of Disease Adapted for Use in the United States (ICDA), a classification system adapted by the U.S. Public Health Service from the parent system developed by the World Health Organization. The system is used in categorizing and indexing hospital records. Each disease is listed as belonging to a major section, such as infectious disease or neoplastic disease, and then further coded into major disease categories and subdivisions. The system is updated every 10 years.

International Classification of Diseases (ICD), an official list of categories of diseases, physical and mental, issued by the World Health Organization (WHO). It is used primarily for statistic purposes in the classification of morbidity and mortality data. Any nation belonging to WHO may adjust the classification to meet specific needs; for example, in the United States, the *ICD-9-CM,* a clinical modification of the 1975 revision, *ICD-9,* was adopted to provide additional data required by clinicians, research workers, epidemiologists, medical record librarians, and administrators of inpatient, outpatient, and community programs. See also *Diagnostic and Statistical Manual of Mental Disorders.*

International Commission on Radiation Protection (ICRP), a nongovernmental organization founded in England in 1928 to provide general guidance on the safe use of radiation sources, including appropriate protective measures and codes of practice for medical radiology. The ICRP was originally established as a source of information about the hazards of x-rays and radium in medicine but was reorganized in 1950 to include effects of nuclear energy.

International Congress of Surgeons (I.C.S.), an international professional organization of surgeons.

International Council of Nurses (ICN), the oldest international health organization. It is a federation of nurses' associations from 93 nations and was one of the first health organizations to develop strict policies of nondiscrimination based on nationality, race, creed, color, politics, sex, or social status. The objectives of the ICN include promotion of national associations of nurses, improvement of standards of nursing and competence of nurses, improvement of the status of nurses within their countries, and provision of an authoritative international voice for nurses. The following ICN definition of the nurse is accepted internationally and serves as a pattern in developing nursing practice and nursing education throughout the world: 'A nurse is a person who has completed a program of basic education and is qualified and authorized in her/his country to practice nursing. Basic nursing education is a formally recognized program of study that provides a broad and sound foundation for the practice of nursing, and for postbasic education, which develops specific competency. At the first level, the educational program prepares the nurse, through study of behavior, life, and nursing sciences and clinical experience, for effective practice and direction of nursing care and for the leadership role. The first level nurse is responsible for planning, providing, and evaluating nursing care in all set-

tings for the promotion of health, prevention of illness, care of the sick, and rehabilitation; and functions as a member of the health team. In countries with more than one level of nursing personnel, the second level program prepares the nurse, through study of nursing theory and clinical practice, to give nursing care in cooperation with and under the supervision of a first level nurse.' The ICN is active in the World Health Organization (WHO), the United Nations Educational, Scientific, and Cultural Organization (UNESCO), and other international organizations.

International Red Cross Society, an international philanthropic organization, based in Geneva, Switzerland, concerned primarily with the humane treatment and welfare of the victims of war and calamity and with the neutrality of hospitals and medical personnel in times of war. See also **American Red Cross.**

International System of Units (SI), an internationally accepted scientific system of expressing length, mass, and time in basic units (I.U.) of centimeters, grams, and seconds, replacing the old centimeter-gram-second system (**CGS**). The SI system also includes as standard measurements, **ampere, kelvin, candela,** and **mole.**

International Unit (IU, I.U.), a unit of measure in the International System of Units. See also **SI units.**

internist /intur′nist, in′turnist/ [L, *internus,* inward], a physician who specializes in internal medicine.

internship /in′turnship′/, a period of apprenticeship for a medical school graduate who serves in a hospital for a specified period before beginning a professional practice.

internuncial neuron /-nun′sē·əl/ [L, *inter* + *nuntius,* messenger], a connecting neuron in a neural pathway, usually serving as a link between two other neurons.

interocclusal record /-əklo͞o′səl/, a record of the positional relation of opposing teeth or jaws to each other, made on the occlusal surfaces of occlusal rims or teeth with a plastic material that hardens, such as plaster of paris, wax, zinc oxide-eugenol paste, or acrylic resin.

interoceptive /in′tərōsep′tiv/ [L, *internus,* inward, *capere,* to take], pertaining to stimuli originating from within the body regarding the functioning of the internal organs or to the receptors they activate. Compare **exteroceptive, proprioception.**

interoceptor /-sep′tər/ [L, *internus* + *capere,* to take], any sensory nerve ending located in cells in the viscera that responds to stimuli originating from within the body regarding the function of the internal organs, such as digestion, excretion, and blood pressure. Compare **exteroceptor, proprioceptor.**

interosseous /-os′ē·əs/ [L, *inter,* between; *os,* bone], pertaining to an area between bones or pertaining to a structure, such as a ligament, connecting two bones.

interparietal fissure. See **intraparietal sulcus.**

interparoxysmal /-per′əksis′məl/ [L, *inter,* between; *paroxysmos,* irritation], pertaining to something that happens between paroxysms.

interperiosteal fracture /in′tərper′ē·os′tē·əl/ [L, *inter* + Gk, *peri,* around, *osteon,* bone], an incomplete fracture in which the periosteum is not disrupted.

interpersonal /-pur′sənəl/ [L, *inter,* between; *personalis*], pertaining to the interactions between individuals.

interpersonal psychiatry [L, *inter* + *persona,* mask], a theory of psychiatry introduced by Sullivan that stresses the nature and quality of relationships with significant others as the most critical factor in personality development.

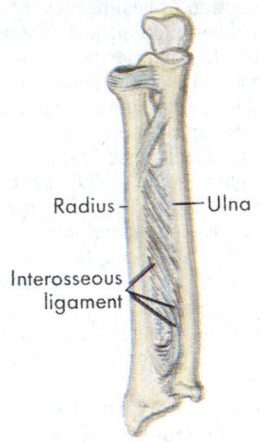

Interosseus ligament
(Thibodeau, 1993/David J Mascaro & Associates)

interpersonal therapy, a kind of psychotherapy that views faulty communications, interactions, and interrelationships as basic factors in maladaptive behavior. A kind of interpersonal therapy is **transactional analysis.**

interphase /in′tərfās′/ [L, *inter* + Gk, *phasis*, phase], the metabolic stage in the cell cycle during which the cell is not dividing, the chromosomes are not individually distinguishable, and such biochemical and physiologic activities as DNA synthesis occur. The stage follows telophase of one division and extends to the beginning of prophase of the next division. See also **anaphase, interkinesis, metaphase, mitosis, prophase, telophase.**

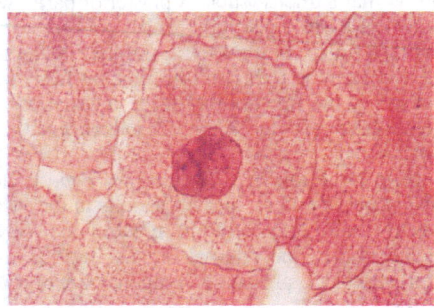

Interphase
(Seeley, 1992/Ed Reschke/Michael Abbey, Science Source)

interpleural space /-ploor′əl/ [L, *inter*, between; Gk, *pleura*, rib; L, *spatium*], the potential space of the mediastinum between the two pleural linings.

interpolated PVC /intur′pəlā′tid/ [L, *interpolare*, to refurbish], a ventricular extrasystole sandwiched between two consecutive sinus-conducted beats. Also called **interpolated VPB.**

interpolation /intur′pəlā′shən/, **1.** the transfer of tissues, as in plastic surgery or transplants. **2.** in statistics, the introduction of an estimated intermediate value of a variable between known values of the variable.

interpreter /intur′prətər/ [Fr, *interpréter*, to translate], a

computer program that remains in the memory and interprets or executes higher-level language.

interproximal film. See **bite-wing film.**

interpubic disk /-pyōō′bik/ [L, *inter* + *os pubis*, pubic bone; Gk, *diskos*, flat plate], the fibrocartilaginous plate connecting the opposed surfaces of the pubic bones at the pubic symphysis. Varying in thickness, it is strengthened by interlacing fibers and often contains a cavity that usually appears after the tenth year of life. Also called **discus interpubicus.**

interradicular space /-radik′yələr/ [L, *inter* + *radix*, root; *spatium*], the area between the roots of a multirooted tooth, normally occupied by a bony septum and the periodontal membrane.

interrogatories /in′tərog′ətôr′ēz/ [L, *inter* + *rogare*, to ask], (in law) a series of written questions submitted to a witness or other person having information of interest to the court. The answers are transcribed and are sworn to under oath. Interrogatories are used during pretrial preparation as a means of discovery. They differ from depositions in that there is no opportunity for cross-examination. Compare **discovery, deposition.**

interrupted suture /in′tərup′tid/ [L, *interrumpere*, to sever; *sutura*], a single suture tied separately, as distinguished from a continuous suture.

intersex /in′tərseks′/ [L, *inter* + *sexus*, sex, gender], any individual who has anatomic characteristics of both sexes or whose external genitalia are ambiguous or inappropriate for either the normal male or female. See also **intersexuality, pseudohermaphroditism.**

intersexuality /-sek′shōō·al′itē/ [L, *inter* + *sexus*, male or female], the condition in which an individual has both male and female anatomic characteristics to varying degrees or in which the appearance of the external genitalia is ambiguous or differs from the gonadal or genetic sex. See also **hermaphroditism, pseudohermaphroditism. —intersexual,** *adj.*

interspinal ligament /-spī′nəl/ [L, *inter* + *spina*, spine; *ligare*, to bind], one of many thin, narrow membranous ligaments that connect adjoining spinous processes and extend from the root of each process to the apex. The interspinal ligaments meet the ligamenta flava ventrally and the supraspinal ligament dorsally and are only slightly developed in the neck.

interspinous /-spī′nəs/ [L, *interstitium*, space between], of or pertaining to the space between any spinous processes.

interstitial /in′tərstish′əl/ [L, *inter* + *sistere*, to stand], of or pertaining to the space between tissues, as interstitial fluid.

interstitial cell-stimulating hormone (ICSH), the luteinizing hormone that also stimulates the production of testosterone by the Leydig, or interstitial, cells of the testis.

interstitial cystitis, an inflammation of the bladder, believed to be associated with an autoimmune or allergic response. The bladder wall becomes inflamed, ulcerated, and scarred, causing frequent, painful urination. Hematuria often occurs. Treatment may include distention of the bladder and cauterization of the ulcers or weekly lavage of the bladder until the inflammation clears. Both procedures are performed with the patient under anesthesia. Corticosteroids are often prescribed to control inflammation. Ulceration is rarely severe enough to require cystectomy with urinary diversion. The condition occurs most often in women of middle age and may resemble the early stages of cancer of the bladder. Cystoscopy and biopsy are required for a diagnosis. Also called **Hunner's ulcer.**

interstitial emphysema, a form of emphysema in which air or gas escapes into the interstitial tissues of the lung after a penetrating injury or as the result of a rupture in an alveolar wall. Since the alveoli must be decompressed, there is danger that the pleura will be torn, resulting in a pneumothorax. The condition is diagnosed by chest x-ray films. See also **pneumothorax.**

interstitial fibroid [L, *interstitium*, space between; *fibra*, fiber; Gk, *eidos*, form], a fibrous tumor that develops in the muscular wall of the uterus and tends to grow inward.

interstitial fluid, an extracellular fluid that fills the spaces between most of the cells of the body and provides a substantial portion of the liquid environment of the body. Formed by filtration through the blood capillaries, it is drained away as lymph. It closely resembles blood plasmain composition but contains less protein. Compare **intracellular fluid, lymph, plasma.**

interstitial growth, an increase in size by hyperplasia or hypertrophy within the interior of a part or structure that is already formed. Compare **appositional growth.**

interstitial hypertrophic neuropathy. See **Dejerine-Sottas disease.**

interstitial implantation, (in embryology) the complete embedding of the blastocyst within the endometrium of the uterine wall.

interstitial inflammation [L, *interstitium*, space between; *inflammare*, to set afire], an inflammation in an area of connective tissues.

interstitial infusion. See **hypodermoclysis.**

interstitial keratitis, an uncommon inflammation within the layers of the cornea. The first symptom is a diffuse haziness. Blood vessels may grow into the area and cause permanent opacities. The causes are syphilis, tuberculosis, leprosy, and vascular hypersensitivity. Treatment is specific to the infection or condition.

interstitial lung disease, a respiratory disorder characterized by a dry, unproductive cough and dyspnea on exertion. The patient may have swallowing disorders or joint and muscle pain and a history of industrial exposure to inorganic dusts, such as asbestos or silica. X-ray films usually show fibrotic infiltrates in the lung tissue, usually in the lower lobes. The fibrosing or scarring of lung tissue is often the result of an immune reaction to an inhaled substance. However, interstitial lung disease may result from viral, bacterial, or other types of infections, uremic pneumonitis,cancers, congenital or inherited disorders, or circulatoryimpairment. The condition may be self-limiting, progressto respiratory or cardiac failure, or undergo spontaneousrecovery.

interstitial mastitis [L, *interstitium*, space between; Gk, *mastos*, breast], an inflammation of the connective tissue between the ducts of the breast.

interstitial myositis. See **myositis.**

interstitial nephritis, inflammation of the interstitial tissue of the kidney, including the tubules. The condition may be acute or chronic. **Acute interstitial nephritis** is an immunologic, adverse reaction to certain drugs, often sulfonamide or methicillin. Acute renal failure, fever, rash, and proteinuria are characteristic of this condition. Most people regain normal function of the kidneys when the offending drug is removed. **Chronic interstitial nephritis** is a syndrome of interstitial inflammation and structural changes,

sometimes associated with such conditions as ureteral obstruction, pyelonephritis, exposure of the kidney to a toxin, rejection of a transplant, and certain systemic diseases. Gradually, renal failure, nausea, vomiting, weight loss, fatigue, and anemia develop. Acidosis and hyperkalemia may follow. The nurse watches carefully for signs of electrolyte imbalance, dehydration, and hypovolemia, especially if there is frequent vomiting. Fluids and electrolytes may be replaced intravenously. Treatment includes correction of the underlying cause. If the cause is an obstruction of the urinary tract, rapid recovery may follow removal of the obstruction; in other cases hemodialysis and kidney transplantation may be necessary.

interstitial plasma cell pneumonia. See **pneumocystosis.**

interstitial pneumonia, a diffuse, chronic inflammation of the lungs beyond the terminal bronchioles, characterized by fibrosis and collagen formation in the alveolar walls and by the presence of large mononuclear cells in the alveolar spaces. The symptoms of this condition are progressive dyspnea, clubbing of the fingers, cyanosis, and fever. The disease may result from a hypersensitive reaction to busulfan, chlorambucil, hexamethonium, or methotrexate. Interstitial pneumonia may also be an autoimmune reaction, since it often accompanies celiac disease, rheumatoid arthritis, Sjögren's syndrome, and systemic sclerosis. X-ray films of the lungs show patchy shadows and mottling, as in bronchopneumonia. Later stages of the disease reveal bronchiectasis, dilatation of the bronchi, and shrinkage of the lungs. Treatment includes bed rest, oxygen therapy, and corticosteroids. Most patients die within 6 months to a few years, usually from cardiac or respiratory failure. Also called **diffuse fibrosing alveolitis, giant cell interstitial pneumonia, Hamman-Rich syndrome.** Compare **bronchopneumonia.**

interstitial pregnancy. See **ectopic pregnancy.**

interstitial therapy, radiotherapy in which needles or wires that contain radioactive material are implanted directly into tumor areas.

interstitial tissues [L, *interstitium*, space between; OFr, *tissu*], the connective and supporting tissue within and surrounding major functional elements of an organ.

interstitial tubal pregnancy, a kind of tubal pregnancy in which implantation occurs in the proximal, interstitial portion of one of the fallopian tubes. See also **tubal pregnancy.**

intertransverse ligament /-transvurz'/ [L, *inter* + *transversus*, cross-direction], one of many fibrous bands connecting the transverse processes of vertebrae. In the cervical region, intertransverse ligaments consist of a few scattered fibers; in the thoracic region, they are rounded cords intimately connected with the deep muscles of the back; in the lumbar region, they are thin and membranous.

intertrigo /in'tərtrī'gō/ [L, *inter* + *terere*, to scour], an erythematous irritation of opposing skin surfaces caused by friction. Common sites are the axillae, the folds beneath large or pendulous breasts, and the inner aspects of the thighs. Maceration and monilial infection may be complications if the area is also warm and moist. Prevention is by weight reduction, powdering, cleansing, and antifungal topical medication when necessary. **–intertriginous,** *adj.*

intertrochanteric crest /in'tərtrō'kanter'ik/ [L, *inter* + *trochanter*, runner; *crista*, ridge], one of a pair of ridges along the thigh bones, curving obliquely from the greater

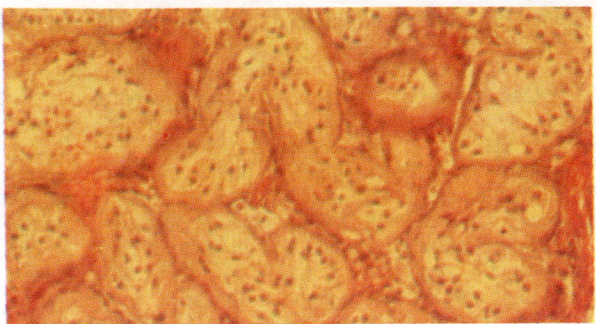

Interstitial tissue (Besser, 1987/Courtesy Dr AB Jenson)

intervertebral disk, one of the fibrous disks found between adjacent spinal vertebrae, except the axis and the atlas. The disks vary in size, shape, thickness, and number depending on the location in the back and on the particular vertebrae they separate.

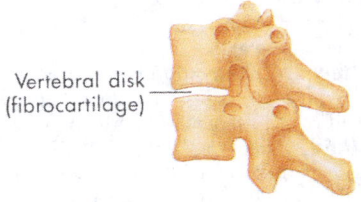

Vertebral disk
(fibrocartilage)

Intervertebral disk (Thibodeau, 1993)

to the lesser trochanter. Immediately distal to the crest a slight ridge, the linea quadrata, receives the insertion of the quadratus femoris and a few fibers of the adductor magnus.

intertrochanteric fracture, a fracture characterized by a crack in the tissue of the proximal femur between the greater and the lesser trochanters.

intertrochanteric line, a line that runs across the anterior surface of the thigh bone from the greater to the lesser trochanter, winding around the medial surface, and ending in the linea aspera. The proximal half of the intertrochanteric line is the attachment for the iliofemoral ligament; the distal half holds the vastus medialis muscle.

intertuberous diameter /-tōō'bərəs/ [L, *inter + tuber*, swelling; Gk, *dia*, across, *metron*, measure], the distance between the ischial tuberosities, a factor used in determining the dimensions, including the narrowest diameter, of the pelvic outlet.

interval /in'tərval/ [L, *intervallum*, space between ramparts], a space between things or events, or a break or interruption in an otherwise continuous flow.

interval health history [L, *intervallum*, space between], a kind of health history that notes the general condition of a client during the period between visits and is not limited to facts relevant to a particular condition. The interval health history provides an ongoing account of a person's health, serving to bring the data base up to date.

intervention /in'tərven'shən/ [L, *inter + venire*, to come], any act performed to prevent harm from occurring to a patient or to improve the mental, emotional, or physical function of a patient. A physiologic process may be monitored or enhanced, or a pathologic process may be arrested or controlled. **Independent intervention** is any health care activity pertaining to certain aspects of professional practice that are encompassed by applicable licensure and law and require no supervision or direction from others. **Interdependent intervention** refers to any health care activity carried out by one health care professional in collaboration with another. See also **nursing intervention**.

interventricular /-ventrik'yələr/ [L, *inter*, between; *ventriculum*, chamber], located between the ventricles, as the septum of the heart.

interventricular septum [L, *inter*, between; *ventriculum*, chamber; *saeptum*, fence], the wall between the ventricles of the heart. Also called **ventricular septum**.

intervertebral /in'tərvur'təbrəl/ [L, *inter + vertebra*, back joint], of or pertaining to the space between any two vertebrae, such as the fibrocartilaginous disks.

intervertebral fibrocartilage. See **intervertebral disk.**

intervertebral foramen, any of the passages between adjacent vertebrae through which the spinal nerves and vessels pass.

intervertebral ganglion [L, *inter*, between; *vertebra*, joint; Gk, *gagglion*, knot], the ganglionic enlargement of a spinal nerve root between adjacent vertebrae.

interview /in'tərvyōō/, a communication with a patient initiated for a specific purpose and focused on a specific content area. A **problem-seeking interview** is an inquiry that focuses on gathering data to identify problems the patient needs to resolve. A **problem-solving interview** focuses on problems that have been identified by the patient or health care professional.

intervillous space /in'tərvil'əs/ [L, *inter + villus*, hair; *spatium*], one of many spaces between the chorionic villi of the endometrium of the gravid uterus, beneath the placenta. The intervillous spaces act as small reservoirs for oxygenated maternal blood from which the fetal circulation may take up the nutrients and gases by osmosis, hydrostatic pressure, and diffusion. The spaces form early in gestation, when the trophoblastic layer of the embryo embeds itself in the wall of the uterus.

intestinal /intes'tinəl/ [L, *intestinum*], pertaining to the intestines.

intestinal absorption [L, *intestinum*, intestine; *absorbare* to swallow], the passage of the products of digestion from the lumen of the small intestine into the blood and lymphatic vessels in the wall of the gut. The surface area of the intestine is greatly increased by the presence of fingerlike projections, called villi, each of which contains capillaries and a lymphatic vessel, or lacteal. Most dissolved nutrients pass quickly into the capillary bed for transport through the portal circulation to the liver. Lipids enter the lymphatic channels, which eventually rejoin the venous circulation at the thoracic duct in the neck.

intestinal amebiasis. See **amebic dysentery.**

intestinal angina, chronic vascular insufficiency of the mesentery caused by atherosclerosis and resulting ischemia of the smooth muscle of the small bowel. Also called **chronic intestinal ischemia.**

intestinal apoplexy, the sudden occlusion of one of the three principal arteries to the intestine by an embolism or a thrombus. This condition leads rapidly to necrosis of intestinal tissue and is often fatal. Treatment is usually surgical:

The occlusion is removed, and often the affected portion of the bowel is resected. See also **atherosclerosis**.

intestinal atresia [L, *intestinum*; Gk, *a*, *tresis*, boring], a pathologic obstruction of the continuous lumen of the intestinal tract due to a defect in development in utero.

intestinal bypass surgery [L, *intestinum*; AS, *bi*; Fr, *passer*; Gk, *cheirourgos*], a surgical procedure to shorten the digestive tract so that less intestinal surface will be available to absorb nutrients from the digested food passing through, or to bypass a blocked or diseased portion of the intestine. The technique usually involves anastomosing the jejunum to the ileum.

intestinal colic [L, *intestinum*; Gk, *kolikos*, colonic pain], spasmodic pain in intestinal disorders.

intestinal dyspepsia, an abnormal condition characterized by impaired digestion associated with a problem that originates in the intestines. See also **dyspepsia**.

intestinal fistula, an abnormal passage from the intestine to an external abdominal opening or stoma, usually created surgically for the exit of feces after removal of a malignant or severely ulcerated segment of the bowel. See also **colostomy**.

intestinal flora [L, *intestinum*; *flos*, flowers], the natural bacterial content of the inside of the digestive tract.

intestinal flu, a viral gastroenteritis, usually caused by infection by an enterovirus. It is characterized by abdominal cramps, diarrhea, nausea, and vomiting. Outbreaks may be sporadic or epidemic, and the disease usually is mild and self-limited. Treatment is symptomatic. Control of diarrhea may be achieved with antidiarrheal medication and a diet limited to clear fluids. See also **enteric infection, gastroenteritis**.

intestinal fluke [L, *intestinum*; AS, *floc*], any internal parasite of the genera *Fasciolopsis*, *Heterophyes*, and *Metagonimus*, in North America and of other genera in the Orient and in tropical countries. They enter the body through the mouth as encysted larvae in aquatic vegetation or freshwater fish. Symptoms of intestinal fluke infestation usually include abdominal pain and obstruction and diarrhea.

intestinal gases [L, *intestinum*], gas in the digestive tract arising from three sources swallowed air, gas produced by digestive processes, and blood gases diffused into the intestinal lumen. Gases produced in the intestine and diffused from blood are mainly hydrogen, H_2, most of which is a bacterial fermentation product of ingested carbohydrates, carbon dioxide, CO_2, and methane, CH_4.

intestinal glands. See **Lieberkühn's glands**.

intestinal infarction. See **intestinal strangulation**.

intestinal juices, the secretions of glands lining the intestine.

intestinal lipodystrophy. See **lipodystrophy**.

intestinal lymphangiectasia. See **hypoproteinemia**.

intestinal obstruction, any obstruction that results in failure of the contents of the intestine to pass through the lumen of the bowel. The most common cause is a mechanical blockage resulting from adhesions, impacted feces, tumor of the bowel, hernia, intussusception, volvulus, or the strictures of inflammatory bowel disease. Obstruction may also be the result of paralytic ileus. Obstruction of the small bowel may cause severe pain, vomiting of fecal matter, dehydration, and eventually a drop in blood pressure. Obstruction of the colon causes less severe pain, marked abdominal distention, and constipation. X-ray examination reveals the level of obstruction and its cause. Treatment includes the evacuation of intestinal contents by means of an intestinal tube. Surgical repair is sometimes necessary. Fluid balance and electrolyte balance are restored by carefully monitored intravenous infusion. Nonnarcotic analgesics are usually prescribed to avoid the decrease in intestinal motility that often accompanies the administration of narcotic analgesics. Also called *(informal)* **ileus**. See also **hernia, intussusception, volvulus**.

intestinal perforation [L, *intestinum*; *perforare*, to pierce], the escape of digestive tract contents into the peritoneal cavity due to trauma or a disease condition, such as a ruptured appendix or perforated ulcer. The condition inevitably leads to peritonitis.

intestinal strangulation, the arrest of blood flow to the bowel, resulting in edema, cyanosis, and gangrene of the affected loop of bowel. This condition is usually caused by a hernia, intussusception, or volvulus. Early signs of intestinal strangulation resemble those of intestinal obstruction, but peritonitis, shock, and the presence of a tender mass in the abdomen are important in making a differential diagnosis. In addition to surgery, treatment includes the immediate correction of fluid and electrolyte imbalance. Also called **intestinal infarction**.

intestinal tonsil, one of a group of lymphatic nodules forming a single layer in the mucous membrane of the ileum opposite the mesenteric attachment. They are oval patches about 1 cm wide and extend for about 4 cm along the intestine. In most individuals they appear in the distal ileum but also appear in the jejunum of a few individuals. Also called **Peyer's patches**. Compare **lingual tonsil, palatine tonsil, pharyngeal tonsil**.

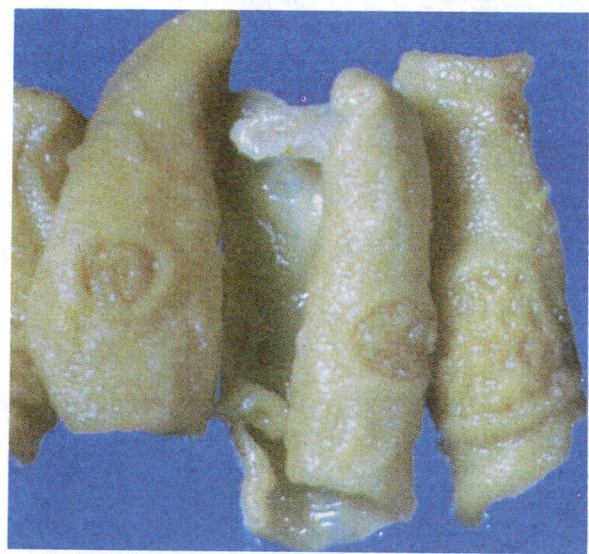

Intestinal tonsil (*Mitros, 1988*)

intestinal tract [L, *intestinum*; *tractus*], the segments of small and large intestines between the pyloric valve and the rectum. Also called **alimentary tract, digestive tract, GI tract**.

intestinal tubes [L, *intestinum*; *tubus*], the alimentary canal or digestive tract.

intestine /intes′tin/ [L, *intestinum*], the portion of the alimentary canal extending from the pyloric opening of the stomach to the anus. It includes the small and large intestines. **−intestinal**, *adj.*

intima /in′timə/, *pl.* **intimae** [L, *intimus*, innermost], the innermost layer of a structure, such as the lining membraneof an artery, vein, lymphatic, or organ. **−intimal**, *adj.*

intimal sclerosis [L, *intimus*, inmost; Gk, *sklerosis*, hardening], a hardening of the intimal layer of a blood vessel. See **atherosclerosis**.

intoe. See **metatarsus varus.**

intolerance /intol′ərəns/ [L, *in*, not, *tolerare*, to bear], a condition characterized by inability to absorb or metabolize a nutrient or medication. Exposure to the substance may cause an adverse reaction, as in lactose intolerance. Compare **allergy,atopic.**

intoxicant /intok′sikənt/ [L, *in*; Gk, *toxikon*, poison], any agent that can cause intoxication or poisoning.

intoxication /intok′sikā′shən/ [L, *in*, within; Gk, *toxikon*, poison], **1.** the state of being poisoned by a drug or other toxic substance. **2.** the state of being inebriated because of an excessive consumption of alcohol. **3.** a state of mental or emotional hyperexcitability, usually euphoric.

intra- /in′trə-/, a prefix meaning 'situated, formed, or occurring within': *intrabronchial, intracutaneous, intramatrical.*

intraabdominal pressure /in′trə·abdom′inəl/ [L, *intra*, within, *abdomen*, belly], the degree of pressure within the abdominal cavity.

intraalveolar pocket. See **periodontal pocket.**

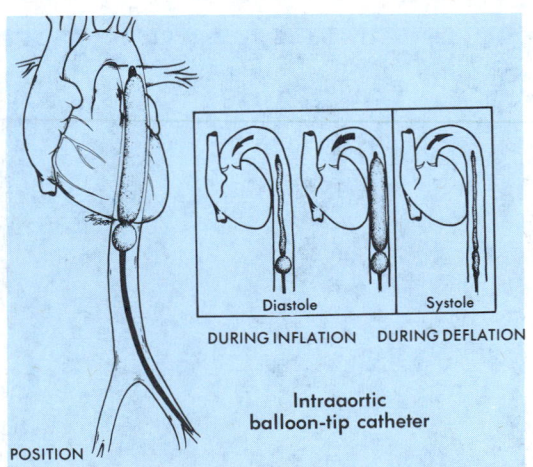

Diastole   Systole

DURING INFLATION   DURING DEFLATION

Intraaortic
balloon-tip catheter

POSITION

Intraaortic balloon-tip catheter

intraaortic balloon pump /in′trə·ā·ôr′tik/ [L, *intra* + *aeirein*, to rise], a counterpulsation device that provides temporary cardiac assist in the management of refractory left ventricular failure, as may follow myocardial infarction or occur in preinfarction angina. The balloon is attached to a catheter inserted in the aorta and is automatically inflated during diastole and deflated during systole. See also **counterpulsation.**

intraarterial /in′trə·ärtir′ē·əl/, pertaining to a structure or action inside an artery.

intraarticular /in′trə·ärtik′yələr/ [L, *intra* + *articulus*, joint], within a joint.

intraarticular fracture, a fracture involving the articular surfaces of a joint.

intraarticular injection, the injection of a medication into a joint space, usually to reduce inflammation, such as in bursitis or fibromyositis. With the same technique, abnormally excessive fluid may be withdrawn from the joint space. The fluid may be a result of trauma or inflammation.

intraarticular ligament, a ligament that forms part of the joints between 16 of the 24 ribs, dividing the joints into two cavities, each containing a synovial membrane. Each intraarticular ligament consists of a short, flattened band of fibers inside the joint, attached by one extremity to the rib and by the other to the intervertebral disk. Intraarticular ligaments are not present in the joints of the first, tenth, eleventh, and twelfth ribs, each of which has only one synovial cavity. Compare **radiate ligament.**

intraatrial /in′trə·ā′trē·əl/ [L, *intra* + *atrium*, entrance hall], within an atrium in the heart.

intraatrial block, delayed or abnormal conduction within the atria, identified on an electrocardiogram by a prolonged and often notched P wave. See also **atrioventricular block, heart block, intraventricular block, sinoatrial block.**

intrabony pocket. See **periodontal pocket.**

intracanalicular fibroma /-kan′əlik′yələr/ [L, *intra* + *canaliculus*, small channel], a tumor containing glandular epithelium and fibrous tissue, occurring in the breast.

intracanicular papilloma /-kənik′yələr/, a benign warty growth in certain glands, especially the breast.

intracapsular fracture /-kap′syələr/ [L, *intra* + *capsula*, little box], a fracture within the capsule of a joint.

intracardiac /-kar′dē·ak/ [L, *intra*, within; Gk, *kardia*, heart], pertaining to the interior of the heart chambers.

intracardiac catheter. See **cardiac catheter.**

intracardiac lead /lēd/ [L, *intra* + Gk, *kardia*, heart; AS, *laedan*, lead], **1.** an electrocardiographic conductor in which the exploring electrode is placed within one of the cardiac chambers, usually by means of cardiac catheterization. **2.** *informal.* a tracing produced by such a lead on an electrocardiograph.

intracartilaginous ossification. See **ossification.**

intracatheter /-kath′ətər/ [L, *intra* + Gk, *katheter*, something lowered], a thin, flexible plastic catheter introduced and threaded into a blood vessel to infuse blood, fluid, or medication. Also called *(informal)* **intracath.**

intracavitary /in′trəkav′itər′ē/ [L, *intra* + *cavum*, cave], pertaining to the space within a body cavity.

intracavitary therapy, a kind of radiotherapy in which one or more radioactive sources are placed, usually with the help of an applicator or holding device, within a body cavity to irradiate the walls of the cavity or adjacent tissues.

intracellular /-sel′yələr/ [L, *intra*, within; *cella*, storeroom], pertaining to the interior of a cell.

intracellular fluid [L, *intra* + *cella*, storeroom; *fluere*, to flow], a fluid within cell membranes throughout most of the body, containing dissolved solutes that are essential to electrolytic balance and to healthy metabolism. Also called **intracellular water (ICW).** Compare **extracellular fluid, interstitial fluid, lymph, plasma.**

intracerebral /-ser′əbrəl/ [L, *intra* + *cerebrum*, brain], within the tissue of the brain, inside the bony skull.

intracistronic /in′trəsistron′ik/ [L, *intra* + *cis*, this side, *trans*, across], within a cistron.

intracoronal retainer /-kôr′ənəl/ [L, *intra* + *corona*, crown], **1.** a retainer in which the prepared tooth cavity and its cast restoration lie largely within the body of the coronal portion of a tooth and within the contour of the tooth crown, such as an inlay. The retention or resistance to displacement is developed between the casting and the internal walls of the prepared tooth cavity. **2.** a direct retainer used in the construction of removable partial dentures. It consists of a female portion within the coronal segment of the crown of an abutment and a fitted male portion attached to the denture proper.

intracranial /-krā′nē·əl/ [L, *intra*, within; Gk, *kranion*, skull], within the cranium.

intracranial abscess. See **brain abscess.**

intracranial aneurysm, any aneurysm of any of the cerebral arteries. Rupture of an intracranial aneurysm results in mortality approaching 50%, and there is a high risk of recurrence in survivors of a rupture. Characteristics of the condition include sudden severe headache, stiff neck, nausea, vomiting, and, sometimes, loss of consciousness. Some forms of intracranial aneurysm may be treated surgically. Kinds of intracranial aneurysms include **berry aneurysm, fusiform aneurysm,** and **mycotic aneurysm.**

intracranial electroencephalography. See **electroencephalography.**

intracranial hemorrhage [L, *intra*, within; Gk, *kranion*, skull; *haima*, blood], a hemorrhage within the cranium.

intracranial pressure, pressure that occurs within the cranium.

intractable /intrak′təbəl/ [L, *intractabilis*, hard to manage], having no relief, such as a symptom or a disease that remains unrelieved by the therapeutic measures employed.

intractable pain [L, *intractabilis*, hard to manage; *poena*, penalty], pain that is unrelieved by ordinary medical and surgical measures. The pain is often chronic, persistent, and psychogenic in nature.

intracutaneous /-kyo̅o̅tā′nē·əs/ [L, *intra* + *cutis*, skin], within the layers of the skin.

intracystic papilloma /-sis′tik/ [L, *intra* + Gk, *kystis*, bag], a benign epithelial tumor formed with a cystic adenoma.

intradermal /-dur′məl/ [L, *intra*, within, Gk, *derma*, skin], within the tissue of the skin.

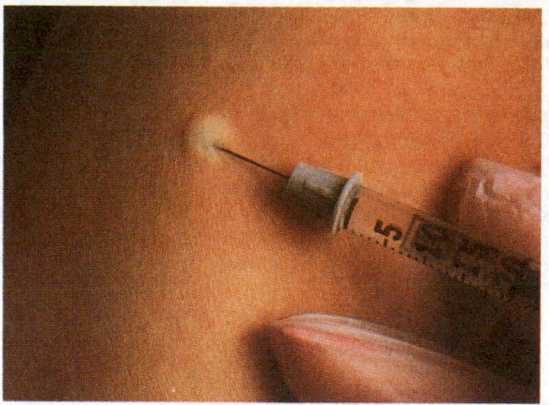

Formation of bleb following intradermal injection
(Potter, 1993)

intradermal injection, the introduction of a hypodermic needle into the dermis for the purpose of instilling a substance, such as a serum or vaccine.

intradermal test [L, *intra* + Gk, *derma*, skin], a procedure used to identify suspected allergens by subcutaneously injecting the patient with small amounts of extracts of the suspected allergens. The injections are made at spaced intervals, usually in the forearm or in the scapular region. The patient is concurrently injected with the diluent alone as a control procedure. The test is positive if, within 15 to 30 minutes, the injection of extract produces a wheal surrounded by erythema and the control injection produces no symptoms. The intradermal test is started with highly diluted solutions, and, if the initial test is negative, the procedure is repeated with stronger solutions. This gradual method is used to prevent a systemic reaction, which is more of a risk with intradermal testing than with other kinds of allergy testing, such as the scratch test. Intradermal testing tends to be more accurate than the scratch test and is often performed if scratch test results are negative or unclear. Intradermal testing also limits to between 20 and 30 the number of suspected allergens that can be examined simultaneously in the skin of one patient. Also called **subcutaneous test.** Compare **patch test, scratch test.** See also **conjunctival test, use test.**

intraductal carcinoma [L, *intra* + *ductus*, duct], a large neoplasm occurring most often in the breast. The lesion on cross section usually shows well-differentiated tumor cells in calcified and dilated ducts of the breast.

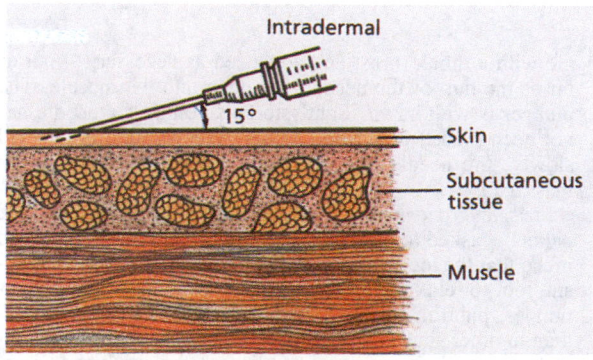

Intradermal injection showing angle of needle and placement in skin
(Potter, 1993)

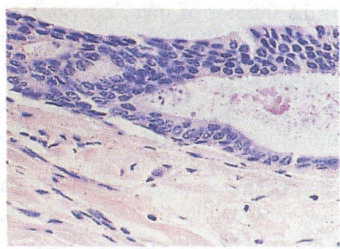

Intraductal carcinoma *(Skarin, 1991)*

intradural lipoma [L, *intra* + *dura*, hard], a fatty tumor in or beneath the dura mater of the spine or sacrum that tends to infiltrate the dorsal column and roots of spinal nerves, causing pain and dysfunction.

intraepidermal carcinoma /in'trə·ep'idur'məl/ [L, *intra* + Gk, *epi*, above, *derma*, skin], a neoplasm of squamous epidermal cells that does not proliferate into the basal area and often occurs in many sites simultaneously. The lesions, which enlarge slowly, are resistant to chemotherapy and to radiation. Also called **Bowen's disease, Bowen's precancerous dermatosis, precancerous dermatitis.**

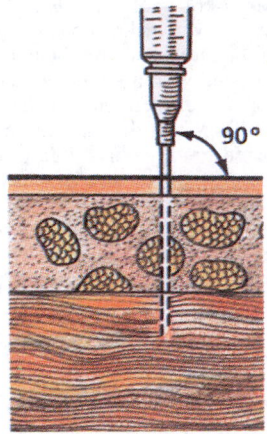

Intramuscular injection showing angle of needle and placement in skin
(Potter, 1993)

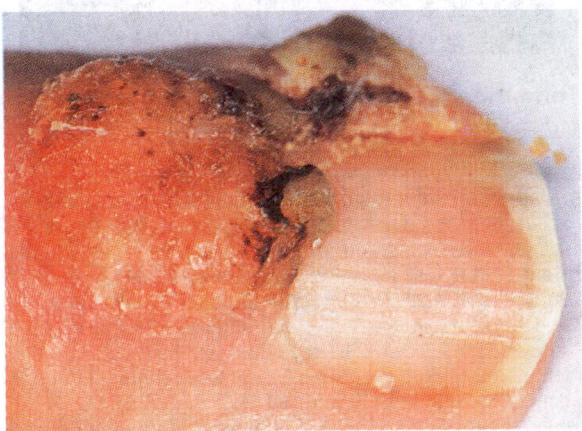

Intraepidermal carcinoma *(Baran, 1991)*

intraepidermal vesicle, a fluid-filled blisterlike cavity within the epidermis. It is usually less than 1 cm in diameter.

intraepithelial carcinoma. See **carcinoma in situ.**

intrafusal muscle fiber /-fyo͞o'zəl/, the striated muscle fiber within a muscle spindle.

intramembranous ossification. See **ossification.**

intramenstrual pain /-men'stro͞o·əl/ [L, *intra*, within; *menstrualis*, monthly; *poena*, penalty], pelvic or lower abdominal pain that occurs about midway between menses and may be associated with ovulation. See also **mittelschmerz**.

intramural /-myo͞o'rəl/ [L, *intra*, within; *murus*, wall], pertaining to events or structures within the walls of an organ or body part or cavity.

intramuscular /-mus'kyələr/ [L, *intra*, within; *musculus*], pertaining to the interior of muscle tissue.

intramuscular injection [L, *intra* + *musculus*, muscle], the introduction of a hypodermic needle into a muscle to administer a medication.

■ METHOD: The equipment is selected and the medication drawn up into the syringe. The site that has been selected is prepared by cleansing with alcohol. The sites most commonly used are the upper, outer quadrant of the gluteal area, the ventrogluteal area, the vastus lateralis of the thigh, or the deltoid muscle. The skin is stretched between the thumb and forefinger. The needle is introduced at a 90-degree an-

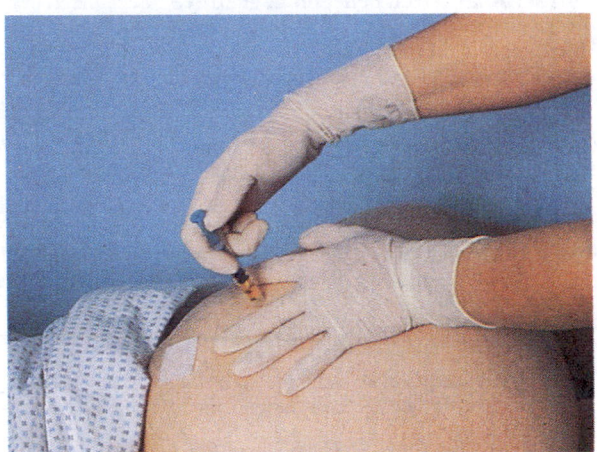

Hand position for administration of intramuscular injection
(Potter, 1993)

gle with a quick thrust and advanced as necessary—not as far as the hub of the needle, but deep into the muscle. The plunger is withdrawn slightly to be sure that the needle has not been placed in a blood vessel. The solution is injected slowly, the needle is withdrawn, and the injection site is massaged.

■ NURSING INTERVENTION: If the gluteal area is chosen, the patient is asked to lie prone with ankles bent and feet curved in, so that the toes of each foot are directed toward the opposite foot to relax the gluteal muscles, thus making the injection less painful. Injection in deltoid muscles is more painful than in other sites and is avoided if possible. The ventrogluteal area and the vastus lateralis are the preferred injection sites in infants. Care is taken not to hit the femur with the tip of the needle when injecting into the vastus lateralis. Needles and syringes are always disposed of in a safe way; they are usually destroyed.

■ OUTCOME CRITERIA: Infection may result from nonaseptic technique; care is taken not to contaminate the needle before injection or suffer a needlestick. Certain medications can cause tissue necrosis if injected into the subcutaneous tissues. Many medications may be given intravenously or intramuscularly, but the intravenous dose may be much smaller; inadvertent injection into a blood vessel could result in severe systemic reactions of an overdose. Often, biologicals may leave a knot in the muscle that is not painful and that subsides slowly over several weeks or months, though it may cause concern in the patient or in the parents of younger patients. The lump should not grow larger or become more painful; if it does, it may be assumed that an abscess has formed.

intraocular /-ok'yələr/ [L, *intra* + *oculus*, eye], pertaining to structures or substances within the eyeball.

intraocular pressure, the internal pressure of the eye, regulated by resistance to the flow of aqueous humor through the fine sieve of the trabecular meshwork. Contraction or relaxation of the longitudinal muscles of the ciliary body affects the size of the apertures in the meshwork. In older persons, the trabecular meshwork may become sclerotic and obstructed, preventing the normal flow of aqueous humor from passing out at the proper rate and causing an increase in the intraocular pressure. See also **glaucoma.**

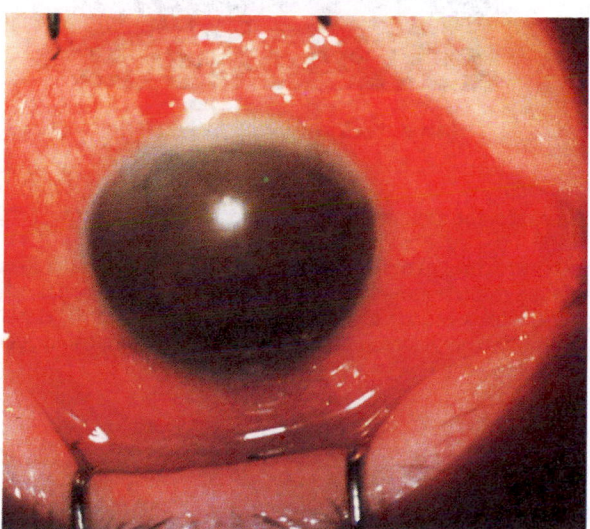

Increased intraocular pressure *(Eagling, 1986)*

intraoperative /-op'ərətiv'/ [L, *intra* + *operari*, to work], pertaining to the period of time during a surgical procedure.

intraoperative hyperthermia /-op'ərətiv/ [L, *intro* + *operari*, to work], hyperthermia delivered to internal sites that have been exposed by a surgical procedure. After heating the patient is "closed."

intraoperative ultrasound, a diagnostic technique that uses a portable ultrasound device to scan the spinal cord during spinal surgery. The method enables surgeons to locate and identify the size of tumors of the central nervous system that may not be detected by computed tomography or other techniques. Intraoperative ultrasound can distinguish between syrinxes, or fluid-filled cysts, and neoplastic growths in nervous system tissue.

intraoral examination. See **dental examination.**

intraoral orthodontic appliance /in'trə·ôr'əl/ [L, *intra* + *oralis*, mouth], an orthodontic device placed inside the mouth to correct or alleviate malocclusion.

intraosseous /in'trə·os'ē·əs/ [L, *intra*, within; *os*, bone], pertaining to the interior of bone.

intraosseous infusion, the injection of blood, medications, or fluids into bone marrow rather than into a vein. The technique may be performed in emergency treatment of a child when IV infusion is not feasible.

intraparietal sulcus /-perī'ətəl/ [L, *intra* + *paries*, wall; *sulcus*, groove], an irregular groove on the convex surface of the parietal lobe that marks the division of the inferior and superior parietal lobules. Also called **interparietal fissure.**

intrapartal care /-pär'təl/ [L, *intra* + *partus*, birth], care of a pregnant woman from the onset of labor to the completion of the 4th stage of labor with the expulsion of the placenta. See also **antepartal care, newborn intrapartal care, postpartal care.**

■ METHOD: The signs and symptoms of true labor are observed. Uterine contractions increase in frequency, duration, and strength. Pressure of the presenting part of the fetus causes dilatation and effacement of the cervix and contractions of the amniotic sac, producing a bloody discharge called 'bloody show.' A physical examination of the mother is performed, urine is measured regularly through labor and may be tested for ketones, protein, glucose, and specific gravity. A microhematocrit is often done. The position, attitude, and presentation of the fetus is ascertained by abdominal palpation. The cervical effacement and dilatation and the station of the presenting part of the fetus are determined periodically by vaginal examination, using careful aseptic technique. If the amniotic sac has broken, the color, character, and quantity of the amniotic fluid is noted. The fetal heart rate is counted, and variations are noted in relation to the timing and intensity of contractions. See also **emergency childbirth.**

■ NURSING INTERVENTION: Emotional support and measures to increase physical comfort are provided by the nurse throughout labor and delivery. Asepsis is maintained, the progress of labor is monitored, and the well-being of the fetus and the mother are continually observed. After delivery of the infant, the mother is observed; the uterine fundus may need to be massaged to cause it to contract. The placenta is weighed and examined for completeness. The episiotomy, if performed, or any laceration that occurred is usually repaired after delivery of the placenta. Depending on the mother's preference and condition and the policy of the maternity service, the infant may be placed in a warmer or on the mother's abdomen. The mother and infant are observed for a brief period in the delivery area before being transferred to the postpartum unit.

■ OUTCOME CRITERIA: During labor and delivery several danger signs alert the observer to problems. These danger signs include strong, continuous uterine contractions, marked variation of the fetal heart rate, sudden, excessive fetal movement, continuous abdominal pain with increased fundal height, vaginal bleeding, protrusion of the umbilical cord, a large amount of amniotic fluid, meconium-stained amniotic fluid, or an elevation or drop in the mother's temperature, pulse, or blood pressure. Observation for these danger signs is important in providing intrapartal care, but normal spontaneous vaginal delivery of a healthy baby from a healthy mother is the usual outcome of this period.

intrapartal period, the period spanning labor and birth.

intrapartum /-pär′təm/, pertaining to the period of labor and delivery.

intraperiosteal fracture /in′trəper′ē·os′tē·əl/ [L, *intra* + Gk, *peri*, around, *osteon*, bone], a fracture that does not rupture the periosteum.

intrapleural space /-plŏŏr′əl/ [L, *intra* , within; Gk, *pleura*, rib; L, *spatium*], pertaining to the cavity of the pleura.

intrapsychic conflict /-sī′kik/ [L, *intra* + Gk, *psyche*, mind], an emotional conflict within oneself. See also **conflict.**

intrapulmonary /-pul′məner′ē/ [L, *intra*, within; *pulma*, lung], pertaining to the interior of the lungs.

intrapulmonary shunt [L, *intra* + *pulmoneus*, relating to the lung], (in respiratory therapy) a condition of perfusion without ventilation, expressed as a ratio of QS/QT, with QS reflecting the difference between end capillary oxygen content and mixed venous oxygen content, and QT representing cardiac output. The condition may occur in atelectasis, pneumonia, pulmonary edema, and adult respiratory distress syndrome (ARDS).

intrarenal hemodynamics /-rē′nəl/ [L, *intra* + *ren*, kidney], the pattern of blood flow or distribution in the various parts of the kidney. Normally the renal cortex and outer medulla receive the major portion of renal blood flow.

intraspinal hypodermic /-spī′nəl/ [L, *intra*, within; *spina*, spine; *hypo*, under, *derma*, skin], pertaining to the injection of a substance into the spinal canal.

intrathecal /in′trəthē′kəl/ [L, *intra* + *theca*, sheath], of or pertaining to a structure, process, or substance within a sheath, such as within the spinal canal.

intrathecal injection, the introduction of a hypodermic needle into the subarachnoid space for the purpose of instilling a material for diffusion throughout the spinal fluid.

intrathoracic goiter /-thôras′ik/ [L, *intra* + Gk, *thorax*, chest; L, *guttur*, throat], an enlargement of the thyroid gland that protrudes into the thoracic cavity.

intrauterine /in′trəyŏŏ′tərin/ [L, *intra*, within; *uterus*, womb], pertaining to the inside of the uterus.

intrauterine catheter. See **catheter.**

intrauterine device (IUD) [L, *intra* + *uterus*, womb; Fr, *devise*], a contraceptive device consisting of a bent strip of radiopaque plastic with a fine monofilament tail that is inserted and left in the uterine cavity for the purpose of altering the physiology of the uterus and fallopian tubes to prevent pregnancy. The mechanism of action is not known. Insertion is performed during or just after menstruation when the cervix is slightly open and menstruation assures that a pregnancy does not exist. The tail string of the IUD is left projecting a few centimeters from the cervix. By feeling the string with her finger at least once each menstrual cycle the wearer can be sure the device is in place. The string also provides a hold for removing the IUD. The rate of failure for the IUD method of contraception is approxi-

mately two to four unplanned pregnancies in 100 women using the device for 1 year. IUDs can cause complications, the most serious being pelvic infection (PID). Such infections occurring in pregnancy may be overwhelming and lethal; therefore the IUD is removed if pregnancy is suspected. Some other complications are cervicitis, perforation of the uterus, salpingitis causing sterility, ectopic pregnancy, abortion, embedding of the device in the wall of the uterus, endometritis, bleeding, pain, cramping, undetected expulsion, and irritation of the penis. Also called **intrauterine contraceptive device (IUCD),** *(informal)* **coil,** *(informal)* **loop.**

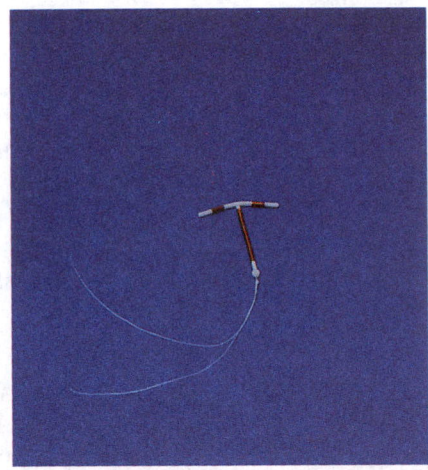

Intrauterine device *(Edge, 1994)*

intrauterine fracture, a fracture that occurs during fetal life.

intrauterine growth curve, a line on a standardized graph representing the mean weight for gestational age through pregnancy to term. It provides a method for classifying infants according to their state of maturity and fetal development.

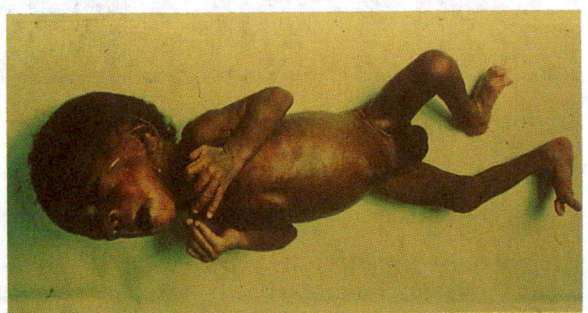

Intrauterine growth retardation
(Zitelli, 1992/Courtesy TALC, Institute of Child Health)

intrauterine growth retardation, an abnormal process in which the development and maturation of the fetus is impeded or delayed by genetic factors, maternal disease, or fetal malnutrition caused by placental insufficiency. See also **small for gestational age infant.**

intravascular /-vas′kyələr/ [L, *intra, vasculum,* little vessel], pertaining to the inside of a blood vessel.

intravascular coagulation test [L, *intra + vasculum,* little vessel], a test for detecting internal coagulation of blood.

intravenous (IV) /-vē′nəs/ [L, *intra + vena,* vein], of or pertaining to the inside of a vein, as of a thrombus or an injection, infusion, or catheter.

intravenous alimentation. See **total parenteral nutrition.**

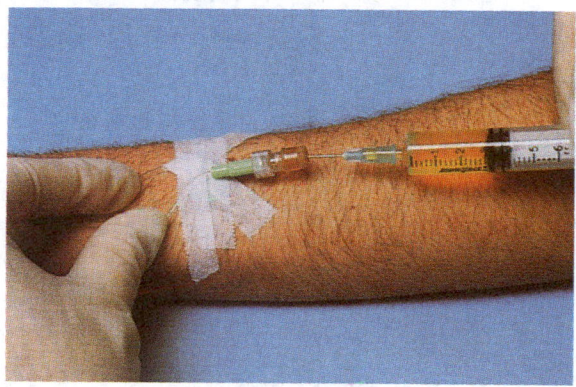

Administration of medication by intravenous bolus
(Potter, 1993)

intravenous bolus, a relatively large dose of medication administered IV in a short period of time, usually within 1 to 30 minutes. The IV bolus is commonly used when administration of a medication is needed quickly, such as in an emergency, when drugs are administered that cannot be diluted, such as many cancer chemotherapeutic drugs, and when the therapeutic purpose is to achieve a peak drug level in the bloodstream of the patient. The IV bolus is not used when the medication involved must be diluted in a large-volume parenteral fluid before entering the bloodstream or when the rapid administration of a medication, such as potassium chloride, could be life-threatening. The IV bolus is normally not used for patients with decreased cardiac outputs, decreased urinary outputs, pulmonary congestion, orsystemic edema. Such patients have decreased tolerances to medications, which therefore must be diluted more than usual and administered at slower rates. A wristwatch with a second hand is recommended for the timing of all IV bolus injections. The amount of medication to be delivered per minute is determined by dividing the total amount of medication to be injected by the prescribed time for delivery. The IV bolus site is prepared with an appropriate antiseptic, and the site is entered with a venipuncture needle, using sterile technique. A winged-tip needle is used for administering an IV bolus because it is small enough to lessen

the risk of collapsing the vein and causing trauma and is more stable than a syringe needle. If a primary IV line is already established, the IV bolus is administered by mixing the prescribed drug with the appropriate amount of diluent and then administering the drug into the primary line, after first determining whether the drug is compatible with the primary IV solution. Also called **intravenous push.**

intravenous catheter [L, *intra,* within; *vena,* vein; Gk, *katheter,* a thing lowered], a catheter that is inserted into a vein to supply medications or nutrients directly into the bloodstream, or for diagnostic purposes such as studying blood pressure.

intravenous cholangiography (IVC), (in diagnostic radiology) a procedure for outlining the major bile ducts. A radiopaque contrast material is injected intravenously, and serial x-ray films are taken. See also **cholangiography.**

intravenous controller, any one of several devices that automatically deliver IV fluid at selectable flow rates, usually between 1 and 69 drops per minute. The controller is commonly equipped with a rate selector, drop sensor, drop indicator, and drop alarm. When the infusion does not flow at the prescribed rate, the drop alarm emits a visual and an audible signal. The IV controller works by gravity so that the IV container must be placed at least 30 inches above the venipuncture site. The controller cannot exert the positive pressure of a true pump and is not recommended for the delivery of highly viscous fluid or for keeping an arterial line open. Compare **intravenous peristaltic pump, intravenous piston pump, intravenous syringe pump.**

intravenous DSA (IV-DSA), a form of digital subtraction angiography in which radiopaque dye is injected into a vein, rather than an artery, in order to visualize arteries in the body.

intravenous fat emulsion, a preparation of 10% fat administered intravenously to help maintain the weight of an adult patient or the weight and growth of a younger patient. Such fat emulsions are prepared from refined soybean oil and egg-yolk phospholipids and may contain such major fatty acids as linoleic, oleic, palmitic, and linolenic acids. The IV fat emulsion is isotonic and may be administered into a peripheral vein, but it is not mixed with other solutions employed in parenteral alimentation. IV fat emulsions are often administered when hyperalimentation is not sufficient to maintain adequate treatment of a patient or when the patient needs calories but cannot tolerate the high percentage of dextrose contained in hyperalimentation solutions. Such emulsions may also be administered to patients who need more essential fatty acids than are contained in hyperalimentation solutions or to patients who need general nutritional improvement, especially postoperative patients. IV emulsions are not administered to patients suffering from disturbances of normal fat metabolism (such as hyperlipemia), severe hepatic diseases, blood coagulation defectscaused by decreased blood-platelet counts, pulmonary diseases, lipoid nephrosis, hepatocellular damage, or bone marrow dyscrasia, or to patients being treated with anabolic inhibitory drugs. If possible, the IV fat emulsion is usually administered during the daytime hours so that the patient may follow a normal eating pattern with rest during the night and a lower nocturnal urinary flow. Once the primary IV line has been established, IV fat emulsions are usually administered with the aid of an electronic control device to maintain an even flow rate and avoid any fatty-acid overload. The patient's fluid intake and output are regularly measured during the delivery of such an emulsion, and daily blood studies are conducted to determine the level of free-floating triglycerides. Hepatic function tests are performed if the patient receives consecutive IV fat emulsion infusions over a long period of time. Immediate adverse reactions or those that may occur up to 2½ hours after the onset of the infusion may include temperature rise, flushing, sweating, pressure sensations over the eyes, nausea, vomiting, headache, chest and back pains, dyspnea, and cyanosis. Delayed adverse reactions or those that may occur within 10 days of the onset of such infusions may include hepatomegaly, splenomegaly, thrombocytopenia, focal seizures, hyperlipemia, hepatic damage, jaundice, hemorrhagic diathesis, and gastroduodenal ulcer.

intravenous feeding, the administration of nutrients through a vein or veins.

necting the bottle to a catheter or a needle in the patient's vein. **2.** the process of administering a solution intravenously. Swelling of the limb around and distal to the site of injection may indicate that the tip of the catheter or needle is in the subcutaneous tissue and not in the vein. The fluid may be infiltrating the tissue spaces. It should be withdrawn and the limb elevated. Redness, swelling, heat, and pain around the vein at the site of injection or proximal to it may indicate thrombophlebitis. The infusion should be discontinued and the inflammatory condition treated. The infusion is usually begun again at another site. See also **venipuncture.**

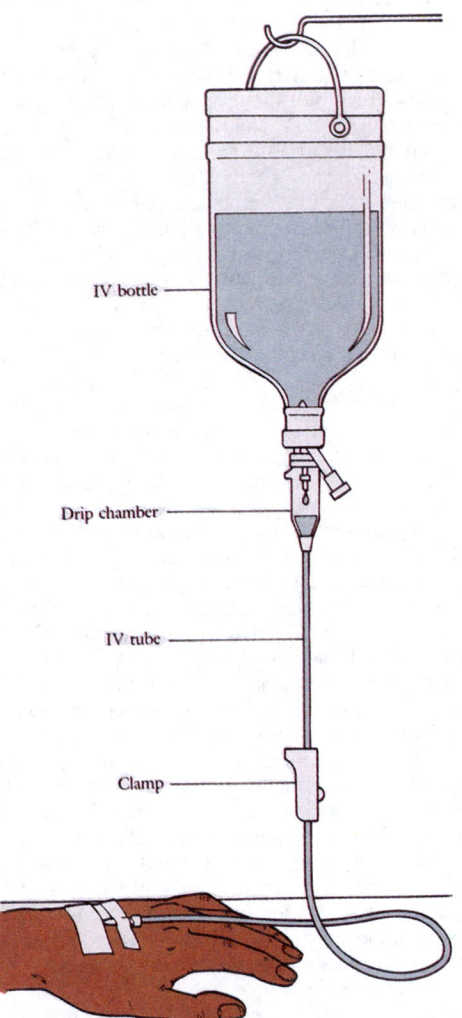

Intravenous equipment (Sorrentino, 1992)

intravenous infusion, **1.** a solution administered intravenously through an infusion set that includes a plastic or glass vacuum bottle or bag containing the solution and tubing con-

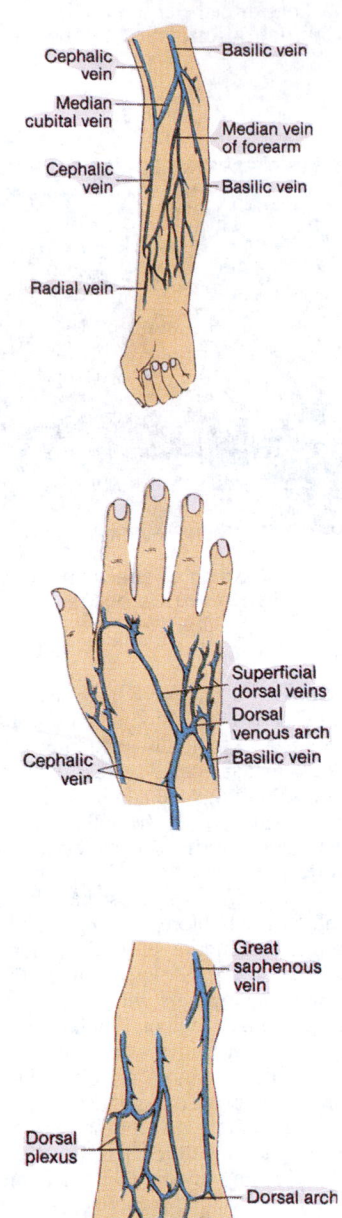

Common intravenous sites (Potter, 1993)

intravenous infusion filter, any one of the numerous devices used in helping to ensure the purity of an IV solution. IV filters strain the IV solution to remove such contaminants as dissolved impurities (detergents, proteins, and polysaccharides), extraneous salts, microorganisms, particles, precipitates, and undissolved drug powders. Any such contaminants may complicate the IV therapy and the recovery of the patient. Some filters are built into the primary IV tubing; others must be attached. Manufacturers' instructions come with most filters to assure proper use. One of the main criteria for selecting a filter is the assurance that the filter is not too fine for the IV solution to be strained. Filters that are too fine will clog. The size of filter membranes vary from 5 [Grk m] to 0.22 [Grk m]. Filters of 1 to 5 [Grk m] will remove most particulate debris but not most fungi or bacteria. Filters that are 0.45 [Grk m] or less will remove fungi and most bacteria; filters that are 0.22 [Grk m] will remove all fungi and bacteria but will also reduce the flow rate of the IV solution, which is crucial when rapid delivery is required. Aseptic techniques are essential in attaching all filters to the IV delivery system. Once attached, filters must be primed according to manufacturers' instructions. Most filters should be upright to function properly, but some filters must be inverted. See also **needle filter.**

intravenous infusion technique, the calculations for determining the delivery rate of IV fluid for the individual patient and the necessary spiking of the container and priming of the tubing before venipuncture and administration of the fluid.

■ METHOD: The rate at which solution is to be administered by IV infusion can be determined from the procedure formula. The hands are washed thoroughly before assembling the container of IV solution, the IV pole, and the proper tubing with the flow clamp placed in a position directly beneath the drip chamber and clamped. If a bottle with a rubber stopper is used, the protective metal cap is removed, and, with the bottle held securely on a stable surface, the spike of the tubing is pushed firmly into the stopper. To spike an IV bottle with an indwelling vent and latex diaphragm, the metal cap and diaphragm are removed and the spike is inserted into the nonvented hole; if a hiss, indicating a vacuum, is not heard, the bottle is contaminated and should be discarded. Nonvented tubing is used with this-kind of bottle. A plastic bag of IV fluid is hung on a hook-for spiking; the cap is removed by pulling it smoothly to the right, and a nonvented spike is inserted into the port using one quick, even motion to prevent the escape of fluid. An IV bag with a firm, easily grasped port with a lip to prevent touch contamination may be spiked before hanging by grasping the port firmly; squeezing the bag may expel air and is carefully avoided. After the hanging bag or bottle is spiked, the drip chamber is gently squeezed until it is half full before the tubing is primed. The end of the tubing is held over a sink or wastebasket as the protective cap is removed, and the cap is kept uncontaminated for reuse. The flow clamp is released, and the tubing is allowed to fill with fluid until all air bubbles are expelled; if a backcheck valve is on the tubing, the valve is inverted during priming. The flow clamp is then closed, the protective cap is replaced, and the tubing is looped over the IV pole so that it is out of the way during venipuncture. Once the needle or intracatheter is inserted and connected to the tubing, the fluid container is hung securely from the IV pole or a hook at a height 3 feet above the insertion site. The flow clamp is opened and adjusted to deliver the proper rate of delivery of fluid by counting the number of drops entering the drip chamber in a minute. Throughout the administration of IV fluid, the rate of flow is checked periodically and any necessary readjustments of the clamp are made.

■ NURSING INTERVENTION: The nurse assembles the apparatus for the IV infusion, spikes the fluid container, primes the tubing, calculates the proper rate for the patient, and ensures that the rate of delivery and asepsis are maintained. The nurse carefully observes the patient for signs of circulatory overload, such as a bounding pulse, engorged peripheral veins, dyspnea, cough, and pulmonary edema, indicating that the infusion rate is too rapid and requires adjustment.

■ OUTCOME CRITERIA: IV solutions administered to maintain normal body fluid levels and the electrolyte balance do not overload the circulation when delivered at the flow rate required by the individual patient.

Complications of intravenous fluid therapy

Complication	Observations	Nursing actions
Circulatory overload	Bounding pulse, venous distention, hoarseness, dyspnea, cough, pulmonary rales, restlessness	Notify physician Reduce flow to "keep open" rate Raise head of bed to facilitate breathing
Local infiltration	Decreased rate or cessation of fluid flow Tissue around needle or catheter site cold, pale, swollen, hard Complaint of local pain	Stop infusion Arrange to restart infusion at another site Apply moist heat Elevate lower arm
Thrombophlebitis	Pain, redness, warmth, edema along vein	Same as for local infiltration Cold compresses may be applied initially
Pyrogenic reaction	Fever, chills, general malaise, nausea, and vomiting 30 min after infusion started Hypotension (if severe)	Switch to another infusion solution and run at "keep open" rate Notify physician Monitor vital signs Save infusion fluid for culture
Anaphylactic reaction (with proteins)	Apprehension, dyspnea, wheezing, tightness of chest, itching, hypotension	Switch infusion to nonprotein solution and run at "keep open" rate Notify physician Monitor vital signs

From Phipps WJ, Long BC, Woods NF, Cassmeyer VL: *Medical-surgical nursing: concepts and clinical practice,* ed 4, St Louis, 1991, Mosby.

intravenous injection, a hypodermic injection into a vein for the purpose of instilling a single dose of medication, injecting a contrast medium, or beginning an IV infusion of blood, medication, or a fluid solution, such as saline or dextrose in water. See also **venipuncture.**

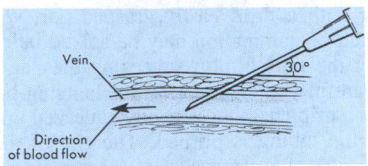

Intravenous injection (note bevel direction of needle)

intravenous medication [L, *intra*, within, *vena*, vein; *medicare*, medicine], the delivery of a medication directly into the bloodstream via a vein.

intravenous peristaltic pump, any one of several devices for administering IV fluids by exerting pressure on the IV tubing rather than on the fluid itself. Most peristaltic pumps operate with normal IV tubing and deliver fluid at a selectable drop-per-minute rate. This device typically can infuse between 1 and 99 drops of IV fluid per minute and is equipped with a drop sensor, rate selector, power switch indicator lamp, and drop indicator and alarm. The drop indicator flashes whenever a drop of IV fluid passes the drop sensor. The drop alarm sounds when the infusion does not flow at the prescribed rate. Compare **intravenous controller, intravenous piston pump, intravenous syringe pump.**

intravenous piston pump, any one of several devices that accurately control the infusion of IV fluids by piston action. Most IV piston pumps can be operated by battery, as well as by electric current, and require special tubing. Some models are portable. IV piston pumps are commonly equipped with controls that allow selectable flow rates and indicators that display flow rates, dose limits, and cumulative fluid volumes. Such pumps commonly monitor the patient's skin for infiltration by IV fluid and are equipped with infiltration and flow alarms. The IV piston pump monitors the actual volume of IV fluid administered instead of counting drops of fluid. Hence its accuracy is not affected by drop size, temperature, or fluid viscosity. The pump is designed to reduce the delivery rate to a keep-vein-open rate if the proper flow rate or the dose limit is exceeded. The pump also stops delivery of the IV fluid if the IV line is clogged or if infiltration is detected. Compare **intravenous controller, intravenous peristaltic pump, intravenous syringe pump.**

intravenous pump, a pump designed to regulate the rate of flow of a fluid given intravenously through an intracatheter or a scalp vein needle. See also **Abbot pump, Harvard pump.**

intravenous push. See **intravenous bolus.**

intravenous pyelography (IVP), a technique in radiology for examining the structures and evaluating the function of the urinary system. A contrast medium is injected intravenously, and serial x-ray films are taken as the medium is cleared from the blood by glomerular filtration. The renal calyces, renal pelvis, ureters, and urinary bladder are all visible on the x-ray films. Tumors, cysts, stones, and many structural and functional abnormalities may be diagnosed using this technique. A cathartic or an enema is usually given the day before the procedure, because the kidneys lie retroperitoneally and gas or fecal material in the bowel may prevent visualization of the urinary tract. The patient is given nothing by mouth from midnight before the test to induce a moderate state of dehydration, thereby allowing concentration of the contrast medium in the collecting structures. The patient may also be asked to void immediately before injection of the dye to avoid dilution of the medium in the bladder and immediately afterward to check residual urine in the bladder. Also called **descending urography, excretory urography.**

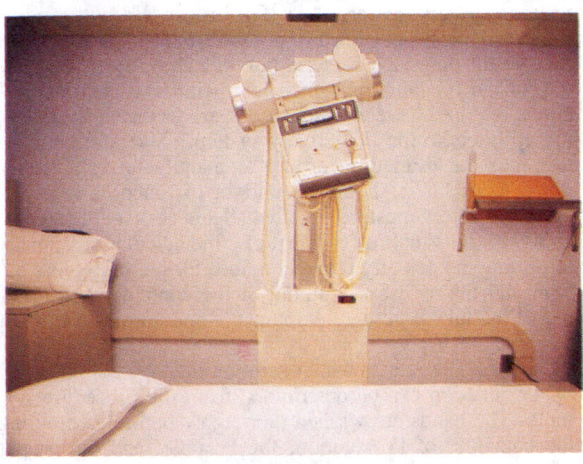

IVP equipment *(Gray, 1992)*

intravenous syringe pump, any one of several devices that automatically compress a syringe plunger at a controlled rate. Such devices are used with disposable syringes that can deliver blood, medications, or nutrients by IV, arterial, or subcutaneous routes. IV syringe pumps can deliver small volumes of fluid at rates as low as 0.01 ml/hour and are often used in the treatment of infants. They are ideal for keeping arterial lines open and are usually battery-operated and portable. They are especially useful in treating ambulatory patients. Compare **intravenous controller, intravenous peristaltic pump, intravenous piston pump.**

intravenous team, a group of registered nurses and licensed practical nurses with special training who administer IV therapy under the direction of a physician. State laws may restrict practice of IV therapy to specific categories of health professionals.

intravenous therapy, the administration of fluids or drugs, or both, into the general circulation through a venipuncture.

intravenous urography. See **intravenous pyelography.**

intraventricular /-ventrik'yələr/ [L, *intra* + *ventriculum*, belly], of or pertaining to the space within a ventricle.

intraventricular block, the altered conduction of the cardiac impulse, within the ventricles. The block can occur as a right bundle branch block, a left bundle branch block, or left anterior or posterior fascicular block. The block is identified on an electrocardiogram, when the QRS duration is wider than normal. The block can be caused by coronary artery disease, valvular heart disease, ventricular hypertrophy and fibrosis, cardiomyopathy, or degeneration of the conduction system. Prognosis is based on the underlying cardiac condition. Kinds of intraventricular block include **bundle branch block** and **fascicular block**. See also **heart block, intraatrial block, sinoatrial block.**

intraventricular conduction defect (ICD), a delay in conduction of a ventricular contraction impulse that may occur beyond the Purkinje myocardial gates. It is seen in patients with acute myocardial infarction and is caused by faulty cell-to-cell conduction of the impulse.

intraventricular hydrocephalus. See **hydrocephalus.**

intraventricular pressure [L, *intra*, within; *ventriculum*], the pressure of the blood within the heart's ventricles. It varies with the phase of the cardiac cycle.

intrinsic /intrin'sik/ [L, *intrinsecus*, inside], **1.** denoting a natural or inherent part or quality. **2.** originating from or situated within an organ or tissue.

intrinsic asthma, a nonseasonal, nonallergic form of asthma, usually first occurring later in life than allergic asthma, that tends to be chronic and persistent rather than episodic. The precipitating factors include inhalation of irritating pollutants in the atmosphere, such as dust particles, smoke, aerosols, strong cooking odors, paint fumes, and other volatile substances. Bronchospasm may also occur in cold, damp weather, after the sudden inhalation of cold, dry air, and after physical exercise or violent coughing or laughing. Respiratory infections, such as the common cold, and psychologic factors, such as anxiety, may also induce an attack. Compare **allergic asthma.** See also **asthma.**

intrinsic factor, a substance secreted by the gastric mucosa that is essential for the intestinal absorption of cyanocobalamin. Intrinsic factor forms a bond with molecules of cyanocobalamin and transports them across the membranes of the ileum. A deficiency of intrinsic factor, caused by gastrectomy, myxedema, or atrophy of the gastric mucosa, results in pernicious anemia. See also **pernicious anemia.**

intrinsic minus hand deformity, an abnormality that results from interruption of the ulnar and median nerves at the wrist. It causes metacarpophalangeal joint hyperextension and interphalangeal joint flexion.

intrinsic muscles, muscles that are entirely within the body part or segment moved by them, as the tongue muscles.

intro-, a prefix meaning 'into or within': *introgastric, introjection, introspection.*

introitus /intrō'itəs/ [L, *intro*, inside, *ire*, to go], an entrance or orifice to a cavity or a hollow tubular structure of the body, such as the vaginal introitus.

introjection /-jek'shən/ [L, *intro* + *jacere*, to throw], an ego defense mechanism whereby an individual unconsciously incorporates into his own ego structure the qualities of another person.

intromission /-mish'ən/, the insertion of one object into another, such as the introduction of the penis into the vagina.

intron /in'tron/ [L, *intra*, within, *regin*, region], (in molecular genetics) a sequence of base pairs in DNA that interrupts the continuity of genetic information. Some genes contain a number of long intervening sequences.

Intron A, a trademark for a parenteral antineoplastic (interferon alfa-2b, recombinant).

Intropin, a trademark for an adrenergic (dopamine hydrochloride).

introspection /-spek'shən/ [L, *introspicere*, to look into], **1.** the act of examining one's own thoughts and emotions by concentrating on the inner self. **2.** a tendency to look inward and view the inner self. —**introspective,** *adj.*

introsusception /-susep'shən/ [L, *intro*, inside; *suscipere*, to receive], the telescoping or invagination of one segment of the digestive tract into another segment, usually a lower segment. The result can be obstruction and strangulation of the bowel.

introversion /-vur'zhən/ [L, *intro* + *vertere*, to turn], **1.** the tendency to direct one's interests, thoughts, and energies inward or toward things concerned with the self. **2.** the state of being totally or primarily concerned with one's own intrapsychic experience. Also spelled **intraversion.** Compare **extroversion.**

introvert /in'trəvurt/ [L, *intro* + *vertere*, to turn], **1.** a person whose interests are directed inward and who is shy, withdrawn, emotionally reserved, and self-absorbed. **2.** to turn inward or to direct one's interests and thoughts toward oneself. Compare **ambivert, extrovert.** See also **egocentric.**

introverted personality /-vur'tid/ [L, *intro*, inside; *vertere*, to turn; *personalis*], a personality that is preoccupied with inner thoughts and fantasies rather than with the outer world of people and things.

intubate /in'tyōōbāt/ [L, *in*, *tubus*], to catheterize or insert a tube into an organ or body part.

intubation [L, *in*, within, *tubus*, tube, *atio*, process], passage of a tube into a body aperture, specifically the insertion of a breathing tube through the mouth or nose or into the trachea to ensure a patent airway for the delivery of anesthetic gases and oxygen. **Blind intubation** is the insertion of a breathing tube without the use of a laryngoscope. Kinds of intubation are **endotracheal intubation, nasogastric intubation.**

intussusception /in'təsəsep'shən/ [L, *intus*, within, *suscipere*, to receive], prolapse of one segment of bowel into the lumen of another segment. This kind of intestinal obstruction may involve segments of the small intestine, the colon, or the terminal ileum and cecum. Intussusception occurs most often in infants and small children and is characterized by abdominal pain, vomiting, and bloody mucus in the stool. Barium enema is used to confirm the diagnosis, and surgery is usually necessary to correct the obstruction. See also **intestinal obstruction.**

inulin /in'yōolin/, a fructose-derived substance used as a diagnostic aid in tests of kidney function, specifically glomerular filtration. It is not metabolized or absorbed by the body but is readily filtered through the kidney.

inulin clearance, a test of the rate of filtration of a starch, inulin, in the glomerulus of the kidney. Inulin is given by mouth, and the glomerular filtration rate can be estimated from the length of time needed for the inulin to appear in the urine. The normal clearance rate of inulin in urine is 100 to 150 ml/minute.

inunction /inungk'shən/ [L, *in*, within, *ungere*, to smear], **1.** the rubbing of a drug mixed with an oil or fatty substance into the skin, with absorption of the active ingredient. **2.** any compound so applied.

inundation fever. See **scrub typhus.**

in utero /inyōo'tərō/, inside the uterus.

invagination /invaj'ənā'shən/ [L, *in*, within, *vagina*, sheath], **1.** a condition in which one part of a structure telescopes into another part, as the intestine during peristalsis. If the invagination is extensive or involves a tumor or polyps, it may cause an intestinal obstruction, and surgery is indicated. **2.** surgery for repair of a hernia by replacing the contents of the hernial sac in the abdominal cavity. General or spinal anesthesia may be used. No upper respiratory infection, chronic cough, or allergy with sneezing can be present, because it will weaken the repair. Postoperatively, the nurse checks for retention of urine. See also **hernia, intestinal obstruction, peristalsis.** **−invaginate,** v.

invariable behavior /invər′ē·əbəl/ [L, in, not, variare, to vary], behavior that results from physiologic response to a stimulus and is not modified by individual experience, such as a reflex. Compare **variable behavior.**

invasion /invā′zhən/ [L, in, within, vadere, to go], the process by which malignant cells move through the basement membrane and gain access to blood vessels and lymphatic channels.

invasion of privacy, (in law) the violation of another person's right to be left alone and free from unwarranted publicity and intrusion.

invasive /invā′siv/ [L, in, within, vadere, to go], characterized by a tendency to spread, infiltrate, and intrude.

invasive carcinoma, a malignant neoplasm composed of epithelial cells that infiltrate and destroy surrounding tissues.

invasive mole. See **chorioadenoma destruens.**

invasive procedure [L, in, vadere, to go; procedere, to proceed], a diagnostic or therapeutic technique that requires entering a body cavity or an interruption of normal body functions. Examples include the Pap test and colonoscopy.

invasive thermometry, measurement of tissue temperature using probes placed directly in the tissue.

inverse anaphylaxis /invurs′, in′vurs/, an exaggerated reaction of hypersensitivity induced by an antibody rather than by an antigen. Also called **reverse anaphylaxis.**

inverse I:E ratio, an inspiratory/expiratory ratio in which the duration of inspiration is prolonged relative to time allowed for exhalation. This procedure is sometimes instituted to improve oxygenation, as in the care of infants with idiopathic respiratory distress syndrome, and adults in whom conventional ventilator techniques fail. I:E ratios in such cases may be on the order of 2:1 or 3:1. Also called **reversed I:E ratio.** See also **I:E ratio.**

inverse relationship. See **negative relationship.**

inverse square law, a law stating that the amount of radiation emitted is inversely proportional to the square of the distance between the source and the irradiated surface, such as a person 2 feet from a patient being treated with radium is exposed to four times more radiation than he or she would be exposed to at 4 feet.

Inversine, a trademark for a ganglionic blocking agent (mecamylamine hydrochloride).

inversion /invur′zhən/ [L, invertere, to turn over], **1.** an abnormal condition in which an organ is turned inside out, such as a uterine inversion. **2.** a chromosomal defect in which two or more segments of a chromosome break off and become separated. They rejoin the chromosome in the wrong order, causing the genes carried on one arm of the chromosome to be in a position and sequence different from those on the other arm.

invert /in′vurt/ [L, invertere, to turn over], to turn something upside down or inside out.

invert sugar [L, invertere, to turn upside down; Gk, sakcharon], a mixture of glucose and fructose produced by the hydrolysis of sucrose. The process results in an inversion of optical rotation from dextrorotation of sucrose to levorotation of the mixture.

investigational device exemption (I.D.E.) /inves′tigā′shənəl/ [L, investigare, to search for], an agreement through which the federal government permits the testing of new medical devices.

investigational new drug (IND), a drug not yet approved for marketing by the Food and Drug Administration and available only for use in experiments to determine its safety and effectiveness. The use of an investigational new drug in human subjects requires approval by the Food and Drug Administration of an application that includes reports of animal toxicity tests, descriptions of proposed clinical trials, and a list of the investigators and their qualifications.

invisible differentiation /inviz′ibəl/ [L, in, not, visibilis, visible; differentia, difference], (in embryology) a fixed determination for specialization and diversification that exists in embryonic cells but is not yet visibly apparent. See also **chemodifferentiation.**

in vitro /invē′trō/ [L, in, within; vitreus, glassware], (of a biologic reaction) occurring in laboratory apparatus. Compare **in vivo.**

in vitro fertilization (IVF), a method of fertilizing human ova outside the body by collecting the mature ova and placing them in a dish with a sample of spermatozoa. After the ova are allowed to incubate over a period of 48 to 72 hours, the fertilized ova are injected into the uterus through the cervix. The procedure takes from 2 to 3 days. See also **gamete intrafallopian transfer.**

in vivo /invē′vō/ [L, in, within, vivo, alive], (of a biologic reaction) occurring in a living organism. Compare **in vitro.**

in vivo tracer study, (in nuclear medicine) a diagnostic procedure in which a series of radiograms of an administered radioactive tracer as it passes through a compartment in the patient's body demonstrates normal or abnormal structures or processes. A strip chart recording of an in vivo tracer study, such as a radionuclide angiocardiogram, shows the passage of the tracer through the central circulation.

involucrum /in′vəlo͞o′krəm/, pl. **involucra** [L, involvere, to wrap up], a sheath or coating, such as that encasing a sequestrum of necrotic bone.

involuntary /invol′ənter′ē/ [L, in, not, voluntas, will], occurring without conscious control or direction. See also **autonomy.**

involuntary muscle. See **smooth muscle.**

involuntary nervous system. See **visceral nervous system.**

involuntary patient, a patient admitted to a psychiatric facility against his will. See also **informal admission.**

involution /in′vəlo͞o′shən/ [L, involvere, to wrap up], **1.** a normal process characterized by a decrease in the size of an organ caused by a decrease in the size of its cells, such as postpartum involution of the uterus. **2.** (in embryology) a developmental process in which a group of cells grows over the rim at the border of the organ or part and, rolling inward, rejoins the organ or part to form a tube, such as in the heart or bladder.

involutional melancholia [L, involvere + Gk, melas, black, chole, bile], a state of depression occurring during the climacteric. The disorder begins gradually and is characterized by pessimism, irritability, insomnia, loss of appetite, feelings of anxiety, and an increase in motor activity, ranging from mere restlessness to extreme agitation. In the rare instances where treatment is necessary, antidepressant drugs, electroconvulsive treatment, and various forms of psychotherapy may be used. Also called **climacteric melancholia, involutional depression, involutional psychosis.** See also **depression.**

involutional psychosis /in'vəloo'shənəl/ [L, *in, volere,* to roll up; Gk, *psyche,* mind, *osis,* condition], an obsolete term for a disorder that tends to develop late in life, characterized by severe depression and, occasionally, paranoia. Symptoms include agitation, apprehension, despair, loss of appetite, and chronic fatigue.

inward aggression /in'wərd/ [AS, *inweard*], destructive behavior that is directed against oneself. See also **aggression, masochism.**

-io, 1. a noun-forming combining form: *abrasio, evulsio, injectio.* 2. a combining form for iodine-containing contrast media.

iodide /ī'ədīd/ [Gk, *ioeides.* violetlike], any salt of hydroiodic acid. Sodium and potassium iodide are the salts most commonly used in medicine.

iodinated 125I serum albumin /ī'ədinā'tid/, a sterile, buffered isotonic solution containing radioiodinated normal human serum adjusted to provide not more than 1 mCi of radioactivity per milliliter in diagnostic tests of blood volume and cardiac output.

iodine (I) /ī'ədīn/ [Gk, *ioeides,* violet], a nonmetallic element of the halogen group. Its atomic number is 53; its atomic weight is 126.90. Iodine is a bluish-black solid that becomes a violet vapor on heating without going through a liquid phase. An essential micronutrient or trace element, almost 80% of the iodine present in the body is in the thyroid gland, mostly in the form of thyroglobulin. Iodine deficiency can result in goiter or cretinism. Iodine is found in seafoods, iodized salt, and some dairy products. Radioisotopes of iodine are used in radioisotope scanning procedures and in palliative treatment of cancer of the thyroid.

iodine poisoning [Gk, *ioeides,* violetlike; L, *potio,* drink], toxic effects of ingesting iodine, a potent antiseptic with a low tissue toxicity. Symptoms include burning pain in the mouth and esophagus, abdominal pain, vomiting, diarrhea, shock, nephritis, laryngeal edema, and circulatory collapse. The mucous membranes are stained brown by the iodine.

iodism /ī'ədiz'əm/ [Gk, *ioeides* + *ismos,* process], a condition produced by excessive amounts of iodine in the body. It is characterized by increased lacrimation and salivation, rhinitis, weakness, and a typical skin eruption.

iodize /ī'ədīz/ [Gk, *ioeides* + *izein,* to cause], to treat or impregnate with iodine or an iodide. Table salt is iodized to prevent the occurrence of goiter in areas with insufficient iodine in the drinking water or food. Iodized oil, a viscous liquid with the odor of garlic, has been used as a contrast medium in radiology.

iodized salt [Gk, *ioeides,* violetlike; AS, *sealt*], table salt to which potassium or sodium iodide has been added as a preventive measure to protect against goiter, particularly in regions where there is a low iodine content in the soil and drinking water. The iodides are added in a ratio of approximately 100 ppm.

iodo-, a combining form meaning 'of or pertaining to iodine': *iododerma, iodogenic, iodolography.*

iodochlorhydroxyquin /ī·ō'dōklôrhīdrok'səkwin/, an antiamebic and topical antiinfective.

■ INDICATIONS: It is prescribed in the treatment of eczema, athlete's foot, and other fungal infections.

■ CONTRAINDICATIONS: The presence of tuberculosis or viral skin conditions or known hypersensitivity to this drug or to iodine prohibits its use.

■ ADVERSE EFFECTS: The most serious adverse reaction is irritation to sensitive skin.

iododerma /ī·ō'dōdur'mə/ [Gk, *ioeides* + *derma,* skin], a skin rash caused by a hypersensitivity to ingested iodides. The lesions may be acneiform, bullous, or fungating. Treatment requires removal of iodides from the diet.

iodoform /ī·ō'dəfôrm/ [Gk, *ioeides* + (chloroform)], a topical antiinfective used as an antiseptic.

iodophor /ī·ōdəfôr/ [Gk, *ioeides* + *phoros,* bearer], an antiseptic or disinfectant that combines iodine with another agent, such as a detergent.

iodopsin /ī'ōdop'sin/ [Gk, *ioeides* + *optikos,* vision], a photosensitive chemical in the cones of the retina that reacts in association with other chemicals and plays a part in color vision. Iodopsin is more stable when exposed to bright light than rhodopsin, which is found in the rods of the retina. Color vision, a synthesis of red, green, and blue light, is induced by changes within the pigments of different types of cones during a photochemical process in which coded nerve impulses are sent to the brain. Research continues into color vision, and the exact role of iodopsin is still unknown.

iodoquinol /ī'ōdō·kwinol/, an amebicide.

■ INDICATION: It is prescribed in the treatment of intestinal amebiasis.

■ CONTRAINDICATIONS: Hepatic disease and known hypersensitivity to iodine or 8-hydroxyquinolines prohibit its use.

■ ADVERSE EFFECTS: Among the most serious adverse reactions are dizziness, thyroid enlargement, optic neuropathy, optic atrophy, and peripheral neuropathy.

ion /ī'ən, ī'on/ [Gk, *ienai,* to go], an atom or group of atoms that has acquired an electric charge through the gain or loss of an electron or electrons.

-ion, 1. a suffix meaning an 'electrically charged particle': *anion, cation, ion.* 2. a noun-forming combining form: *endognathion, osteopedion, parhelion.*

Ionamin, a trademark for an anoretic (phentermine).

ion exchange chromatography, the process of separating and analyzing different substances according to their affinities for chemically stable but very reactive synthetic exchangers, which are composed largely of polystyrene and cellulose. The process uses an absorbent containing ionizing groups and accommodates the exchange of ions between a solution of substances to be analyzed and the absorbent. Ion exchange chromatography is often used to separate components of nucleic acids and proteins elaborated by various structures throughout the body. Different ions deposited in the absorbent during the exchange produce bands of different colors, which constitute a chromatograph. Compare **column chromatography, gas chromatography.**

ionic bonding /ī·on'ik/ [Gk, *ienai* + ME, *band,* to bind], an electrostatic force between ions.Ionic compounds do not form true molecules and in aqueous solution break down into their constituent ions.

ionic dissociation, a phenomenon whereby ions in ionic compounds in an aqueous solution are freed from their mutual attractions and distribute themselves uniformly throughout the solvent.

ionic strength, the sum of the concentrations of all ions in a solution, weighted by the squares of their charges.

ionization /ī'ənīzā'shən/ [Gk, *ienai* + *izein*, to cause], the process in which a neutral atom or molecule gains or loses electrons and thus acquires a negative or positive electric charge. Ionization occurs when atoms or molecules dissociate in solution or when those of gases dissociate in an electric field. Ionizing radiation produces ionization in its passage through body tissue or other matter. Ionization can also cause cell death or mutation.

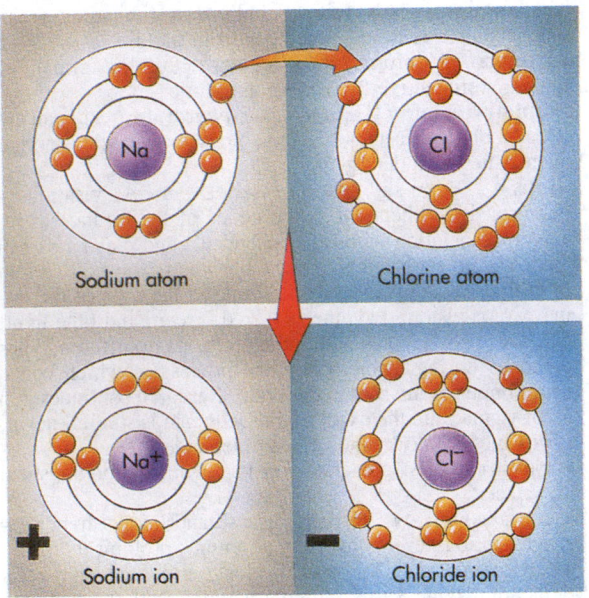

Ionization *(Raven, 1992/Nadine Sokol)*

ionization chamber, a small cavity filled with air that has the capability of collecting the ionic charge liberated during irradiation. A measure of this charge combined with knowledge of the mass of air in the chamber is a means of determining exposure and dose.

ionization constant (K), after establishment of ionic equilibrium, the product of the molar concentration of the ions divided by the molar concentration of the nonionized molecules.

ionize /ī'ənīz/ [Gk, *ienai* + *izein*, to cause], to separate or change into ions. See also **ion.**

ionized calcium, the ionized, unbound, noncomplexed fraction of serum calcium that is biologically active.

ionizing energy /ī·ənī'zing/, the average energy lost by ionizing radiation in producing an ion pair in a gas. In air, the value is approximately 33.73 electron-volts (eV).

ionizing radiation, high-energy electromagnetic waves (such as x-rays and gamma rays) and particulate rays (such as alpha particles, beta rays, electrons, neutrons, positrons, protons, and heavy nuclei) that dissociate substances in their paths into ions. The spatial distribution of the ionization depends on the kind of radiation, its penetrating power, the location of the source, and the nature of the irradiated material. High energy x-rays penetrate deeply, most beta particles penetrate only a few millimeters, and alpha particles penetrate only a fraction of a millimeter, but they all pro-

duce intense ionization along their tracks. Ionizing radiation directly affects living organisms by killing cells or retarding their development; its indirect effects include the production of gene mutations and chromosome breaks by striking a DNA molecule in the path of a particle ray. Animal tissues containing elements with relatively high atomic weights, such as calcium in bones and teeth, absorb much higher doses from a given radiation than are absorbed by soft tissue.

ionizing radiation injury [Gk, *ion*, going; L, *radiare*, to shine; *injuria*], damage or ill effects suffered by exposure to ionizing radiation, including cellular harm resulting from radiation for diagnostic or therapeutic application. The risk of cell death or injury from radiation depends upon the type of tissue cells, the stage of cell division at the time of exposure, the intensity and time span of exposure, and the type of radiation administered.

ionophoresis. See **iontophoresis.**

ion-selective electrode, a potentiometric electrode that develops a potential in the presence of one ion (or class of ions) but not in the presence of a similar concentration of other ions.

iontophoresis /ī·on'tōfôrē·sis/ [Gk, *ion*, going; *pherein*, to carry], the introduction of ions of soluble salts into the tissues by direct current. Also called **galvanoionization, medical ionization.** Also called **ionophoresis** /ī·ō'nō-/.

iontophoretic pilocarpine test [Gk, *ienai* + *pherein*, to carry], a sweat test used in the diagnosis of cystic fibrosis. Pilocarpine iontophoresis is employed to stimulate production of sweat, which is absorbed from the forearm in a previously weighed gauze pad. The sweat sample is then analyzed for concentrations of sodium and chloride electrolytes.

iota /ī·ō'təl/, I, ι, the ninth letter of the Greek alphabet.

Iowa trumpet /ī'əwə/, a kind of needle guide used in performing a pudendal block. It consists of a long thin cylinder through which a needle may be passed. A ring is attached to the proximal end of the guide, allowing the operator to hold it securely.

IPA, abbreviation for **independent practice association.**

ipecac /ip'əkak/, an emetic.

■ INDICATIONS: It is prescribed to cause emesis in certain types of poisoning and drug overdose.

■ CONTRAINDICATIONS: Known hypersensitivity to this drug prohibits its use. It is not used in unconscious patients or for poisoning by petroleum distillates, strong alkalis, acids, or strychnine.

■ ADVERSE EFFECT: The most serious adverse reaction is cardiotoxicity if vomiting does not occur and the substance is retained.

■ NOTE: If vomiting does not occur, the ipecac is recovered by gastric lavage.

IPOF, abbreviation for **immediate postoperative fit prosthesis.**

ipomea /ipəmē'ə/, a resin prepared from the dried root of *Ipomoea orizabensis,* formerly used as a cathartic.

IPPB (intermittent positive pressure breathing), a form of assisted or controlled respiration produced by a ventilatory apparatus in which compressed gas is delivered under positive pressure into the person's airways until a preset pressure is reached. Passive exhalation is allowed through a valve, and the cycle begins again as the flow of gas is triggered by inhalation. Also called **(IPPV) intermittent positive pressure ventilation.**

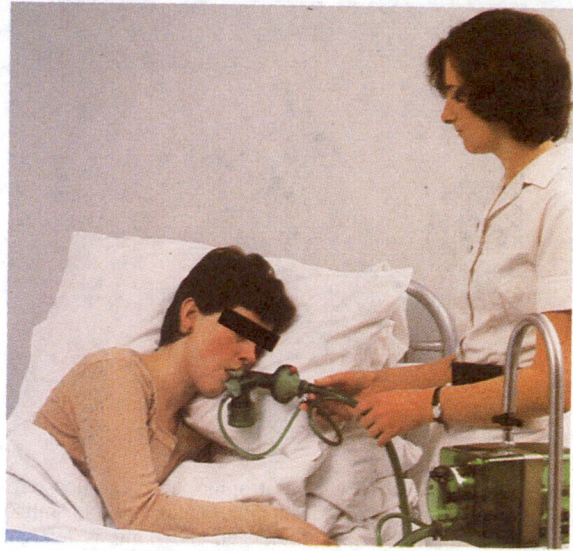

IPPB *(Turner-Warwick, 1989)*

■ METHOD: The use of the IPPB unit involves the combined efforts of the physician, the inhalation therapist or technician, and the nurse. The specific pressure and volume and the use of nebulizing or other attachments are ordered individually. The equipment is tested and is introduced to the patient by the inhalation therapist. The nurse observes that the patient closes the lips around the mouthpiece and does not allow air to escape from the nose or mouth during inspiration and that the therapy is effective.

■ NURSING ORDERS: The patient may require reassurance that the machine will automatically shut off the flow of air at the end of inspiration and encouragement to relax and allow the lungs to be completely filled by the machine. The patient is cautioned not to manipulate any of the controls.

■ OUTCOME CRITERIA: Ventilation may be greatly improved by the use of the IPPB unit. Secretions may be thinned and cleared, and the passages may be humidified, allowing greater comfort and a better exchange of gases.

IPPB unit, a pressure-cycled ventilator for providing a flow of air into the lungs at a predetermined pressure. As the pressure is attained, the flow is stopped, pressure is released, and the patient exhales. The device is used to prevent postoperative atelectasis, to promote full expansion of the lungs, to improve oxygenation, and to administer nebulized medications into the respiratory passages.

IPPV, abbreviation for **intermittent positive pressure ventilation.** See **IPPB.**

ipsi-, a prefix meaning 'the same, or self': *ipsilateral.*

ipsilateral [L, *ipse,* same, *latus,* side], pertaining to the same side of the body. Compare **contralateral.**

IPSP, abbreviation for *inhibitory postsynaptic potential.*

IQ, abbreviation for **intelligence quotient.**

Ir, symbol for the element **iridium.**

iralgia /iral′jə/ [Gk, *iris,* rainbow, *algos,* pain], *obsolete.* any pain or inflammation in the iris. Also called *(obsolete)* **iridalgia. –iralgic, iridalgic,** *adj.*

IRB, abbreviation for **institutional review board.**

Ir g, abbreviation for *immune response function gene.* See **immune response.**

iridalgia. See **iralgia.**

iridalgic. See **iralgia.**

iridectomy /ī′ridek′təmē/ [Gk, *iris* + *ektome,* excision], surgical removal of part of the iris of the eye, performed most often to restore drainage of the aqueous humor in glaucoma or to remove a foreign body or a malignant tumor. An incision is made through the cornea, and the iris is grasped with forceps or a hook and drawn out through the incision. The area involved is cut away, and the elastic iris is allowed to slip back into place. Atropine and an antibiotic are instilled, and a dressing and a shield are applied. Postoperatively, the patient is observed for signs of local hemorrhage or excessive pain.

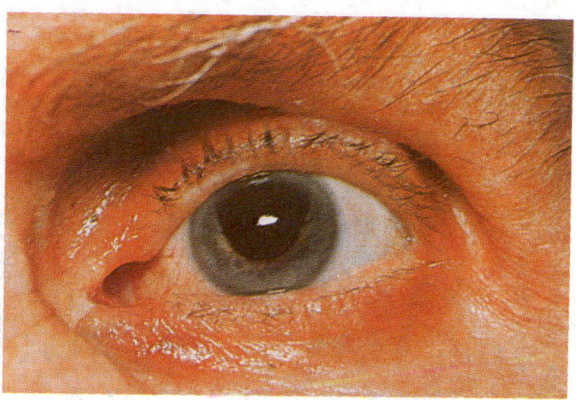

Pupil abnormality caused by iridectomy
(Kamal, 1991)

iridescence /ir′ides′əns/ [L, *iridescere,* to shine like a rainbow], the property of light interference or ability to break up light waves into colors of the spectrum.

-iridic. See **iris.**

iridium (Ir) /irid′ē·əm/ [Gk, *iris,* rainbow], a silvery-bluish metallic element. Its atomic number is 77; its atomic weight is 192.2.

irido-, iro-, a combining form meaning 'of or pertaining to the iris, or to a colored circle': *iridocele, iridokeratitis, iridoplegia.*

iridology /ī′ridol′əjē/ [Gk, *iris,* rainbow; *logos,* science], the science that specializes in relations between disease and the shape, color, and other individual characteristics of the iris.

iridoplegia /ī′ridōplē′jə/ [Gk, *iris,* rainbow; *plege,* stroke], a condition of paralysis of the sphincter muscle of the iris or the dilator muscle, or both.

iridotomy /ī′ridot′əmē/ [Gk, *iris* + *temnein,* to cut], a surgical incision into the iris of the eye, performed to relieve occlusion of the pupil, to enlarge the pupil in cataract extraction, or to treat postoperative glaucoma. Local or general anesthesia is used. An incision is made through the cornea, and a cut is made transversely across the sphincter fibers of the iris. Atropine and an antibiotic are instilled, and a dressing and shield are applied. Postoperatively, the dressing is observed for signs of drainage. Excessive pain is abnormal. See also **iridectomy, iris.**

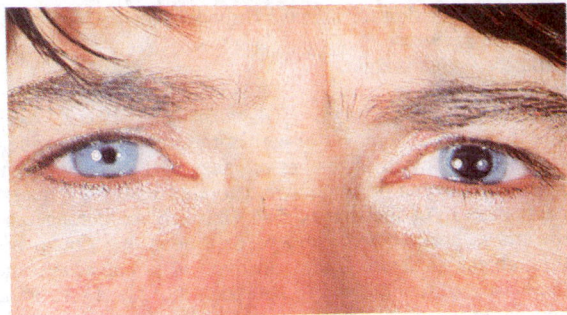

Iridoplegia *(Perkin, 1986)*

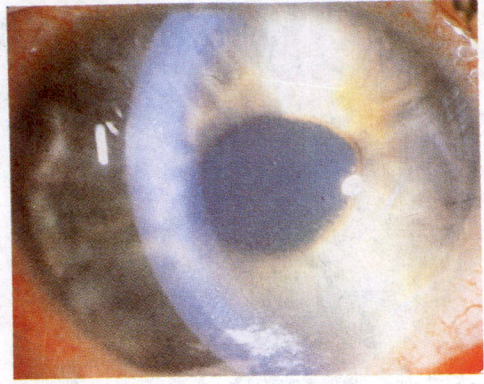

Iritis *(Zitelli, 1992)*

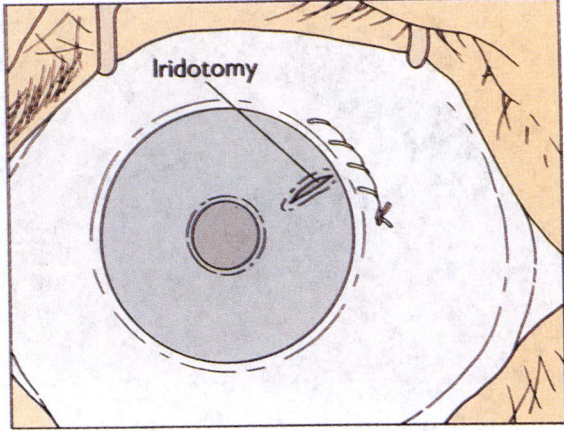

Iridotomy *(Jaffe, 1990)*

iris /ī′ris/ [Gk, rainbow], a circular, contractile disc suspended in aqueous humor between the cornea and the crystalline lens of the eye and perforated by a circular pupil. Muscle fibers of the iris contract and relax to allow more or less light to enter the eye through the pupil. The periphery of the iris is continuous with the ciliary body and is connected to the cornea by the pectinate ligament. The iris divides the space between the lens and the cornea into an anterior and a posterior chamber. In the adult, the two chambers communicate through the pupil, but they are separated in the fetus, up to the seventh month, by the membrana pupillaris. The involuntary muscle of the iris is composed of circular fibers and radiating fibers. Dark pigment cells under the translucent tissue of the iris are variously arranged in different people to produce different colored irises. The pigment is absent in albinos. In blue eyes the pigment cells are confined to the posterior surface of the iris, but in gray eyes, brown eyes, and black eyes the pigment cells appear in the anterior layer of epithelium and in the stroma. See also **dilatator pupillae, sphincter pupillae.** —**iridic,** *adj.*

iritis /īrī′tis/ [Gk, *iris + itis*], an inflammatory condition of the iris of the eye characterized by pain, lacrimation, photophobia, and, if severe, diminished visual acuity. On ophthalmic examination the eye looks cloudy, the iris bulges, and the pupil is contracted. The underlying cause is treated if known, but the condition is most often idiopathic. The pupil is dilated, usually with atropine, and a corticosteroid may be prescribed to reduce inflammation. If the inflammation is allowed to continue and the pupil is left constricted, permanent scarring may occur, causing an opacity over the lens and diminished vision.

iro-,   See **irido-.**

iron (Fe) /ī′ərn/ [AS, *iren*], a common metallic element essential for the synthesis of hemoglobin. Its atomic number is 26; its atomic weight is 55.85. It is used as a hematinic in the form of its salts and complexes, as ferrocholinate, ferrous fumarate, ferrous gluconate, ferrous sulfate, and iron-dextran. Normal blood levels of iron are 60 to 190 μg/dl.

iron deficiency anemia, a microcytic, hypochromic anemia caused by inadequate supplies of iron needed to synthesize hemoglobin, characterized by pallor, fatigue, and weakness. Laboratory diagnosis includes hemoglobin, hematocrit, transferrin, and serum iron evaluation. Iron deficiency may be the result of an inadequate dietary supply of iron, of poor absorption of iron in the digestive system, or of chronic bleeding. Replacement iron can be supplied by ferrous sulfate, the oral form being preferable. The anemia

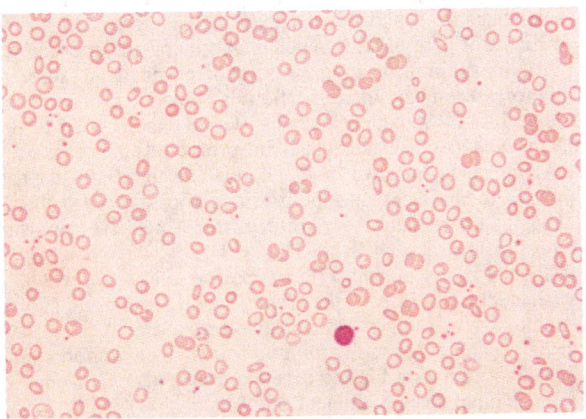

Iron deficiency anemia *(Zitelli, 1992)*

should be corrected in 2 months, but therapy is continued for another 4 months to replace tissue stores. Compare **hemolytic anemia, hypoplastic anemia.** See also **anemia, iron metabolism, nutritional anemia, red cell indices.**

iron dextran, an injectable hematinic.

■ INDICATION: It is prescribed in the treatment of iron deficiency anemia not responsive to oral iron therapy.

■ CONTRAINDICATIONS: Early pregnancy, anemias other than iron deficiency anemia, or known hypersensitivity to this drug prohibits its use.

■ ADVERSE EFFECTS: Among the more serious adverse effects are severe hypersensitivity reactions, including fatal anaphylaxis. Inflammation or phlebitis at the site of injection, arthralgia, headache, GI distress, fever, and lesser hypersensitivity reactions may occur.

iron lung. See **Drinker respirator.**

iron metabolism, a series of processes involved in the entry of iron into the body and its absorption, transport, storage, utilization in the formation of hemoglobin and other iron compounds, and eventual excretion. Iron normally enters the body through the epithelium of the intestinal mucosa, being oxidized from ferrous to ferric iron in the process. The rate at which iron enters is modulated by this absorption mechanism. When iron stores are high, iron no longer passes through but is trapped by the mucosal cells of the intestine to be eliminated. Once in the blood, iron cycles between the plasma and the reticuloendothelial or erythropoietic system. Plasma iron is delivered to the normoblast for hemoglobin synthesis where it remains up to 4 months, trapped in the hemoglobin molecules of a mature red cell. Senescent red cells then deteriorate and break down. The iron is released from the hemoglobin by the reticuloendothelial system to reenter the transport pool for recycling. The normal iron distribution in a 70 kg adult (male) totals approximately 3.7 g with more than 65% of this in circulating hemoglobin. Another 27% is found in the storage pool as hemosiderin or ferritin. The body normally conserves iron so well that loss, usually only through the feces, is normally limited to about 1 mg/day. This amount is easily provided by a dietary intake of only 10 mg/day. Iron deficiency may follow extended intervals of inadequate iron intake (especially in women) or after excessive blood loss. Iron overload sometimes occurs in disorders in which normal regulation of absorption of iron is impaired. It is most commonly produced iatrogenically through the parenteral administration of large amounts of iron or blood for therapeutic purposes. See also **anemia, hemochromatosis, iron deficiency anemia, iron transport.**

iron poisoning [AS, *iren*, L, *potio*, drink], toxic effects of ingesting iron salts, particularly ferrous sulfate and ferrous chloride. Ferrous sulfate tablets, sometimes mistaken for candy, can cause vomiting, collapse, and liver necrosis. Ferrous chloride, a corrosive substance, when taken internally, causes vomiting, diarrhea, and hemorrhages. Iron encephalopathy has occurred from excessive use of iron preparations.

iron-rich food, any nutrient containing a relatively large amount of iron. The best source of dietary iron is liver, with oysters, clams, heart, kidney, lean meat, seafood, and iron-fortified foods. Leafy green vegetables, whole grains, and legumes are the best plant sources. See also **iron, iron deficiency anemia.**

iron salts poisoning, poisoning caused by overdose of ferric or ferrous salts, characterized by vomiting, bloody diarrhea, cyanosis, and gastric and intestinal pain. Therapy includes gastric lavage, administration of an emetic, deferoxamine, and supportive therapy as indicated by the severity of the symptoms.

iron saturation, the capacity of iron to saturate transferrin, measured in the blood to detect iron excess or deficiency. The normal iron saturation capacity in serum is 20% to 55%. See also **total iron.**

iron transport, the process whereby iron is carried from the intestinal mucosa to sites of utilization and storage. Iron binds with transferrin and shuttles to storage and utilization sites. Transferrin becomes attached to exogenous iron entering through the intestinal villi or to iron reentering the plasma from the sinusoids of the spleen. The iron is then released to the normoblasts, and the transferrin is freed for additional transport functions that may involve iron stored as ferritin or hemosiderin. See also **hemosiderosis, iron metabolism, transferrin.**

irradiation /irā'dē·ā'shən/ [L, *irradiare*, to emit rays], exposure to any form of radiant energy like heat, light, or x-ray. Radioactive sources of radiant energy, such as x-rays or isotopes of iodine or cobalt, are used diagnostically to examine internal body structures, using knowledge of the ways in which various tissues absorb or reflect radioactive emissions. The same or similar sources of radioactivity in larger amounts are used to destroy microorganisms or tissue cells that have become cancerous. Infrared or ultraviolet light may be used to produce heat in body tissues to relieve pain and soreness or to treat acne, psoriasis, or other skin ailments. Ultraviolet light is also used to identify certain bacteria and toxic molds. See also **radiation sickness, radioactivity, ultraviolet.** −**irradiate,** *v.*

irrational /irash'ənəl/ [L, *irrationalis*, contrary to reason], pertaining to events, conditions, or behavior that may be considered unreasonable.

irreducible /ir'əd(y)ōō'sibəl/ [L, *in*, not, *reducere*, to bring back], unable to be returned to the normal position or condition, as an irreducible hernia. See also **incarcerate.**

irreducible hernia. See **incarcerated hernia.**

irregular pulse /ireg'yələr/ [L, *in*, *regula*, rule, *pulsare*, to beat], any pulse that is of irregular force or rhythm.

irreversible /ir'əvur'sibəl/ [L, *irrevertere*, to not turn back], pertaining to a situation or condition that cannot be reversed.

irreversible coma. See **brain death.**

irrigate /ir'igāt/ [L, *irrigare*, to supply water], to flush with a fluid, usually with a slow steady pressure on a syringe plunger. It may be done to cleanse a wound or to clear tubing.

irrigation /ir'igā'shən/, the process of washing out a body cavity or wounded area with a stream of water or other fluid. It is also used to cleanse a tube or drain inserted into the body, such as an indwelling catheter. The procedure is most commonly performed with water, saline, aminoacetic acid, or antiseptic solutions on the eye, ear, throat, vagina, and urinary tract. Gentle pressure is applied in the introduction of the fluid, except in the debridement of wounds, and the solution is removed from internal cavities through suction or by drainage. See also **lavage.** −**irrigate,** *v.*

irrigator /ir'igā'tər/, an apparatus with a flexible tube for flushing or washing out a body cavity.

irritability /ir'itəbil'itē/ [L, *irritare*, to tease], a condition of abnormal excitability or sensitivity.

irritable bladder /ir'itəbəl/ [L, *irritare*, to tease; AS, *blaedre*], a condition in which there is a nearly constant urge

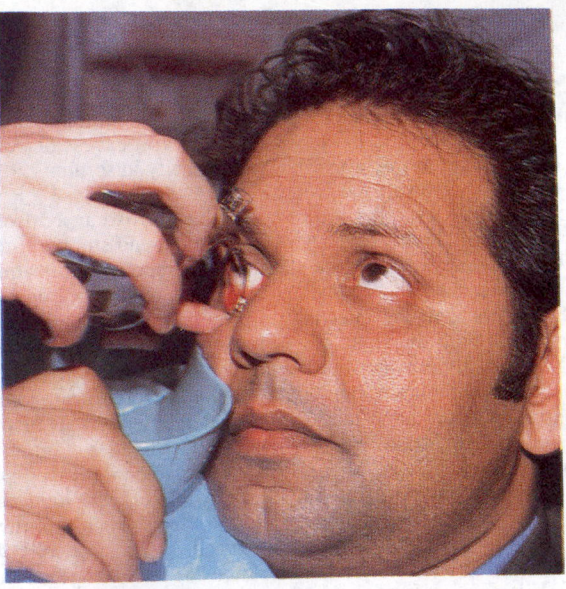

Eye irrigation (Eagling, 1986)

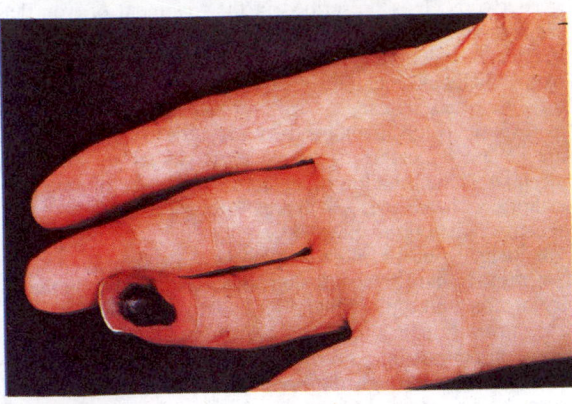

Ischemia of the fingertip (Schumacher, 1988)

to urinate despite the lack of evidence of a cause, such as inflammation or a kidney stone.

irritable bowel syndrome [L, *irritare*, to tease; OFr, *boel*; Gk, *syn*, together, *dromos*, course], abnormally increased motility of the small and large intestines, generally associated with emotional stress. Most of those affected are young adults, who complain of diarrhea and, occasionally, pain in the lower abdomen. The pain is usually relieved by moving the bowels. In diagnosing irritable bowel syndrome, other more serious conditions, such as dysentery, lactose intolerance, and the inflammatory bowel diseases, must be ruled out. Because there is no organic disease present in irritable bowel syndrome, no specific treatment is necessary. Many persons benefit from the use of bulk-producing agents in the diet, because bulk tends to stabilize the water content of the stool. Antidiarrheal drugs are helpful in decreasing the frequency of stool. Although this is a functional disorder, patients experience pain and discomfort and need emotional support. Mild tranquilizers or antidepressants are sometimes given to relieve anxiety or depression. Also called **functional bowel syndrome, mucous colitis, spastic colon.**

irritant /ir'itənt/ [L, *irritare*, to tease], an agent that produces inflammation or irritation.

irritant poisons [L, *irritare*, to tease; *potio*, drink], any of a large number of toxic substances in the environment that can cause pain in the digestive tract, diarrhea, vomiting, abdominal cramps, and urinary tract disorders. Some irritant chemicals are industrial gases, such as ammonia, chlorine, phosgene, sulfur dioxide, hydrogen sulfide, and nitrogen dioxide that may leak into the atmosphere.

irritation fibroma /ir'itā'shən/, a localized peripheral, tumorlike enlargement of connective tissue caused by prolonged irritation. It commonly develops on the gingivae or the buccal mucosa.

IRV, abbreviation for *inspiratory reserve volume*. See **pulmonary function test.**

ischemia /iskē'mē·ə/ [Gk, *ischein*, to hold back, *haima*, blood], a decreased supply of oxygenated blood to a body

organ or part, often marked by pain and organ dysfunction, as in ischemic heart disease. Some causes of ischemia are arterial embolism, atherosclerosis, thrombosis, and vasoconstriction. Compare **infarction.   – ischemic,** *adj.*

ischemic contracture.   See **Volkmann's contracture.**

ischemic heart disease /iskē'mik/, a pathologic condition of the myocardium caused by lack of oxygen reaching the tissue cells.

ischemic lumbago, a pain in the lower back and buttocks caused by vascular insufficiency, as in occlusion of the abdominal aorta.

ischemic pain, the unpleasant, often excruciating sensation associated with ischemia, resulting from peripheral vascular disease, from decreased blood flow caused by mechanical obstruction, constricting orthopedic casts, or from insufficient blood flow caused by surgical trauma or accidental injury. Ischemic pain caused by occlusive arterial disease is often severe and may not be relieved, even with narcotics. The individual with peripheral vascular disease may experience ischemic pain only while exercising because the metabolic demands for oxygen cannot be met due to occluded blood flow. The ischemic pain of partial arterial occlusion is not as severe as the abrupt, excruciating pain associated with a complete blocking of the artery, such as by an embolism. See also **pain intervention, pain mechanism.**

ischemic pericarditis [Gk, *ischein*, to hold back; *haima*, blood; *peri*, near, *kardia*, heart, *itis*, inflammation], an inflammation of the pericardium caused by interruption of its blood supply during myocardial infarction.

ischia.   See **ischium.**

ischial spines /is'kē·əl/ [Gk, *ischion*, hip joint; L, *spina*, thorn], two relatively sharp bony projections into the pelvic outlet from the ischial bones that form the lower border of the pelvis.

ischial tuberosity [Gk, *ischion*, hip joint; L, *tuber*, swelling], a rounded protuberance of the lower part of the ischium. It forms a bony area on which the human body rests when in a sitting position.

ischio-, a combining form meaning 'of or pertaining to the ischium, or to the hip': *ischioanal, ischiodidymus, ischiopagus.*

ischium /is'kē·əm/, pl. *ischia* [L; Gk, *ischion*, hip joint], one of the three parts of the hip bone, joining the ilium and the pubis to form the acetabulum. The ischium comprises the dorsal part of the hip bone and is divided into the body of the ischium, which forms two fifths of the acetabulum, and the ramus, which joins the inferior ramus of the pubis. The spine of the ischium provides attachment for various muscles, such as the gemellus superior, the coccygeus, and the levator ani. The greater sciatic notch above the spine transmits the superior and the inferior gluteal vessels and various nerves, such as gluteal nerves, the sciatic nerve, and the nerves to the obturator internus and the quadratus femoris. A notch below the spine of the ischium transmits various ligaments, vessels, and nerves for other parts. The large dorsal tuberosity of the ischium provides attachment for various muscles, such as the adductor longus, the semimembranosus, the biceps femoris, and the semitendinosus. Compare **ilium, pubis.**

ischo-, a prefix meaning 'restraint or suppression': *ischemia, ischesis.*

I.S.C.L.T., abbreviation for *International Society of Clinical Laboratory Technologists.*

ISG, abbreviation for **immune serum globulin.**

Ishihara color test /ish′ēhä′rə/ [Shinobu Ishihara, Japanese ophthalmologist, b. 1879], a test of color vision using a series of plates on which are printed round dots in a variety of colors and patterns. People with normal color vision are able to discern specific numbers or patterns on the plates;

the inability to pick out a given number or shape is symptomatic of a specific deficiency in color perception.

ISIS, abbreviation for *International Study of Infarct Survival.*

island fever. See **scrub typhus.**

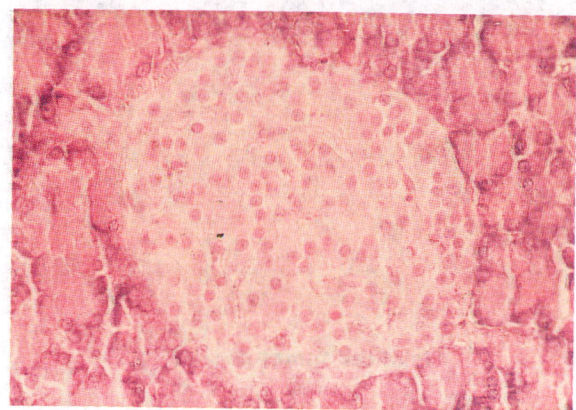

Island of Langerhans—normal islet
(Bodansky, 1989/Prof KD Buchanan, Belfast)

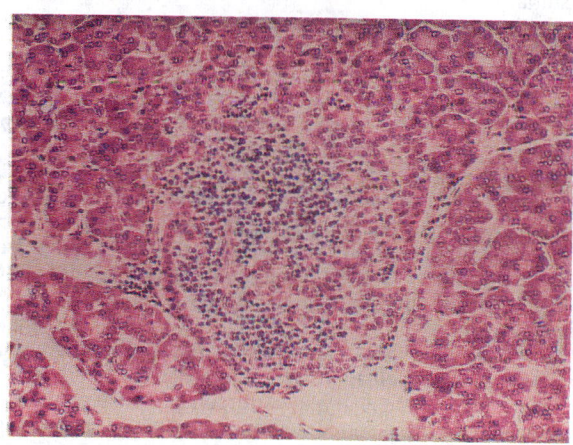

Island of Langerhans in IDDM
(Bodansky, 1989/Prof W Gepts, Brussels)

islands of Langerhans /lang′gərhanz/ [AS, *igland,* island; Paul Langerhans, German pathologist, b. 1847], clusters of cells within the pancreas that produce insulin, glucagon, and pancreatic polypeptide. They form the endocrine portion of the gland and their hormonal secretions released into the bloodstream are balanced, important regulators of carbohydrate metabolism. The islands of Langerhans are scattered throughout the pancreas; the beta cells, which secrete insulin, usually appear in the center of each of the lobules. Alpha cells secrete glucagon, and pancreatic peptide cells secrete pancreatic peptide. The cells comprising the islands are arranged in plates interspersed by capillaries. Also called **islets of Langerhans.**

islet cell adenoma. See **insulinoma.**

islet cell antibody /ī′lit/ [OFr, *islette,* little island], an im-

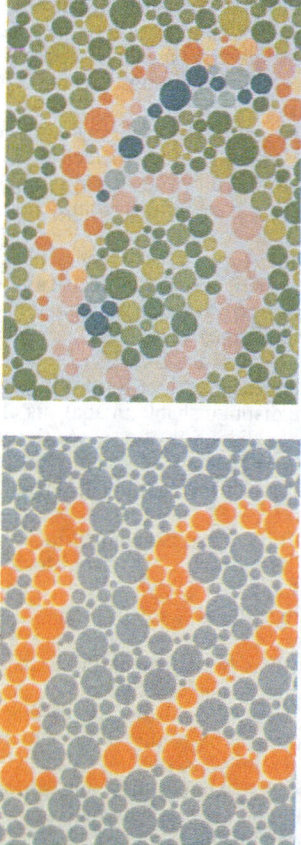

Ishihara color test (Epstein, 1992)

munoglobulin that reacts with the cytoplasm of all of the cells of the pancreatic islets. These antibodies occur in about 60% to 70% of newly diagnosed insulin-dependent diabetic patients, and the presence of the antibody is transient.

islet cell tumor, any tumor of the islands of Langerhans.

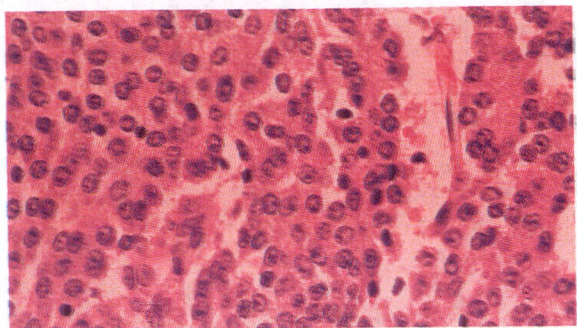

Islet cell tumor *(Skarin, 1991)*

islets of Langerhans. See **islands of Langerhans.**

-ism, -ismus, a suffix meaning 'condition of, practice of, theory of': *hyperthyroidism, hypopituitarism, strabismus.*

Ismelin, a trademark for an antihypertensive (guanethidine sulfate).

iso- /ī'sō-/, a prefix meaning 'equal': *isobar, isochromatic, isohydric.*

isoagglutination /ī'sō·əglōō'tinā'shən/ [Gk, *isos*, equal; L, *agglutinare*, to glue], the clumping of erythrocytes by agglutinins from the blood of another individual of the same species.

isoagglutinin /ī'sō·əglōō'tinin/ [Gk, *isos*, equal; L, *agglutinare*, to glue], an antibody that causes agglutination of erythrocytes in other members of the same species that carry an isoagglutinogen on their erythrocytes. Also called **isohemagglutinin.** Compare **isoagglutinogen.** See also **ABO blood groups, antibody.**

isoagglutinogen /ī'sō·əglōō'tin'əjən/ [Gk, *isos* + L, *agglutinare*, to glue; Gk, *genein*, to produce], an antigen that causes the agglutination of erythrocytes in others of the same species that carry a corresponding isoagglutinin in their serum. Also called **isohemagglutinin.** Compare **agglutinin.** See also **ABO blood groups.**

isoamyl alcohol. See **amyl alcohol.**

isoantibody /ī'sō·an'tibod'ē/ [Gk, *isos* + *anti*, against; AS, *bodig*, body], an antibody to isoantigens found in other members of the same species. See also **autoimmune disease, tissue typing.**

isoantigen /ī'sō·an'tijən/ [Gk, *isos* + *anti*, against; AS, *bodig*, body; Gk, *genein*, to produce], a substance that interacts with isoantibodies in other members of the same species. Compare **autoantigen, autoimmune disease.** See also **antigen, isoagglutinogen.**

isobar /ī'səbär/ [Gk, *isos* + *baros*, weight], **1.** a line connecting points of equal pressure on a graph, as lines connecting points of equal carbon dioxide tension on a pH-bicarbonate diagram. **2.** (in nuclear medicine) one of a group of nuclides having the same total number of neutrons and protons in the nucleus but so proportioned as to result in different values of the atomic number.

isobaric /-bär'ik/ [Gk, *isos*, equal, *baros*, weight], **1.** per-

taining to two substances or solutions of the same specific gravity. **2.** pertaining to two isotopes having the same mass number but different atomic numbers.

isobutyl alcohol /ī'sōbyōō'til/ [Gk, *isos* + *boutyron*, butter, *hyle*, matter; AR, *alkohl*, essence], a clear, colorless liquid that is miscible with ethyl alcohol or ether.

isocapnic /-kap'nik/, pertaining to a steady level of carbon dioxide in the tissues despite changing levels of ventilation.

isocarboxazid /-kärbok'səzid/, a monoamine oxidase inhibitor.

■ INDICATION: It is prescribed in the treatment of mental depression.

■ CONTRAINDICATIONS: Liver or kidney dysfunction, congestive heart failure, pheochromocytoma, concomitant use of a sympathomimetic drug or foods high in tryptophan or tyramine, or known hypersensitivity to drug prohibits its use.

■ ADVERSE EFFECTS: Among the more serious adverse reactions are hyperactivity, cardiac arrhythmia, hypotension, vertigo, dryness of mouth, constipation, and blurred vision. Monoamine oxidase inhibitors produce many adverse drug interactions.

isochromosome /-krō'məsōm/, a chromosome with identical arms on either side of the centromere.

isodose chart /ī'sədōs/ [Gk, *isos* + *dosis*, giving; *charta*, paper], (in radiotherapy) a graphic representation of the distribution of radiation in a medium; lines are drawn through points receiving equal doses. Isodose charts are determined for x-rays traversing the body, for radium applicators used in intracavitary or interstitial treatment, and for working areas where x-rays or radionuclides are employed.

isoelectric /ī'sō·ilek'trik/ [Gk, *isos* + *elektron*, amber], pertaining to the electric base line of an electrocardiogram.

isoelectric electroencephalogram. See **flat electroencephalogram.**

isoelectric focusing, the ordering and concentration of substances according to their isoelectric points.

isoelectric period, a period in physiologic activity, such as nerve conduction or muscle contraction, when there is no variation in electrical potential.

isoelectric point, the pH at which a molecule containing two or more ionizable groups is electrically neutral. The average number of positive charges equals the average number of negative charges.

isoenzyme /ī'sō·en'zīm/ [Gk, *isos* + *en*, in, *zyme*, ferment], a chemically distinct form of an enzyme. The various forms are distinguishable in analysis of blood samples, which aids in the diagnosis of diseases. Isoenzymes that catalyze the same physiologic reaction may also appear in different forms in different animal species. Also called **isozyme.**

isohemagglutinin. See **isoagglutinin.**

isoetharine, isoetharine hydrochloride. See **isoetharine mesylate.**

isoetharine mesylate /ī'sō·eth'ərēn/, a beta-adrenergic bronchodilator.

■ INDICATIONS: It is prescribed in the treatment of bronchial asthma, bronchitis, and emphysema.

■ CONTRAINDICATIONS: A history of cardiac arrhythmias or known hypersensitivity to this drug or to sympathomimetic medications prohibits its use.

■ ADVERSE EFFECTS: Among the more serious adverse reactions are palpitations, tachycardia, arrhythmias, vertigo, nervousness, and headache.

isoexposure lines /ī'sō·ikpō'zhər/, (in radiology) imaginary lines representing positions of equal exposure to radiation in the area around fluoroscopic equipment.

isoflows /ī′səflōz/, (in respiratory therapy) a measure of early small airways dysfunction in a patient made by comparing forced expiratory flow rates between air and helium at fixed points in time.

isoflurophate /-floo′rōfāt/, a cholinesterase inhibitor.
■ INDICATIONS: It is prescribed in the treatment of open-angle glaucoma and esotropia.
■ CONTRAINDICATIONS: Uveal inflammation or known hypersensitivity to this drug or to other organophosphates prohibits its use.
■ ADVERSE EFFECTS: Among the more serious adverse reactions are systemic cholinergic effects, visual disturbances, a paradoxical increase in intraocular pressure, and, with long-term administration, the development of cataracts.

isofosfamide. See isophosphamide.

isogamete /ī′sōgam′ēt/ [Gk, isos + gamete, wife], a reproductive cell of the same size and structure as the one with which it unites. Compare **anisogamete, heterogamete. –isogametic,** adj.

isogamy /īsog′əmē/ [Gk, isos + gamos, marriage], sexual reproduction in which there is fusion of gametes of the same size and structure, such as in certain algae, fungi, and protozoa. Compare **anisogamy, heterogamy. –isogamous,** adj.

isogeneic. See syngeneic.

isogenesis /-jen′əsis/ [Gk, isos + genein, to produce], development from a common origin and according to similar processes. Also called **isogeny** /īsoj′ənē/. **–isogenetic, isogenic,** adj.

isograft /ī′səgraft′/ [Gk, isos + graphion, stylus], surgical transplantation of histocompatible tissue obtained from genetically identical individuals, such as between a patient and identical twin or between animals of a highly inbred strain. Compare **allograft, autograft, xenograft.** See also **graft.**

isohemagglutinin. See isoagglutinin.

isohydric shift [Gk, isos + hydor, water: AS, sciftan, to divide], the series of reactions in red blood cells in which CO_2 is taken up and oxygen is released without the production of excess hydrogen ions.

isoimmunization /ī′so·im′yənīzā′shən/, the development of antibodies against antigens from the same species (isoantigens), such as the development of anti-Rh antibodies in an Rh-negative person. See also **erythroblastosis fetalis.**

isokinetic /-kinet′ik/, pertaining to a concentric or eccentric contraction that occurs at a set speed against a force of maximal resistance produced at all points in the range of motion.

isokinetic exercise [Gk, isos, equal; kinesis, motion; L, exercere, to keep at work], a form of exercise in which maximum force is exerted by a muscle at each point throughout the range of motion as the muscle contracts. The effort of the patient to resist the movement is measured.

isolate /ī′səlāt/ [It, isolare, to detach], **1.** to separate a pure chemical substance from contamination by foreign matter. **2.** to derive from any source a pure culture of a micro-organism. **3.** to prevent an individual from having contact with the rest of a population.

isolation /-lā′shən/ [L, insula, island], the separation of a seriously ill patient from others to prevent the spread of an infection or to protect the patient from irritating environmental factors. A patient undergoing radiation therapy may

also be isolated to reduce the exposure of hospital personnel to effects of radioactive materials.

isolation incubator, an incubator bed regularly maintained for premature or other infants who require isolation.

isolation ward [It, isolare, to detach; ME, warden], a room or section of a hospital in which certain categories of patients, particularly those infected with acute contagious diseases, can be treated with a minimum of contact with the rest of the patients and hospital personnel.

Isolette, a trademark for a self-contained incubator unit that provides a controlled heat, humidity, and oxygen microenvironment for the isolation and care of premature and low birth-weight neonates. The apparatus is made of a clear plastic material and has a large door and portholes for easy access to the infant with a minimum of heat and oxygen loss. A servocontrol mechanism constantly monitors the infant's temperature and controls the heat within the unit.

isoleucine (Ile) /ī′sōloo′sēn/ [Gk, isos + leukos, white], an amino acid, occurring in most dietary proteins, that is essential for proper growth in infants and for nitrogen balance in adults. See also **amino acid, maple syrup urine disease, protein.**

Chemical structure of isoleucine (Seeley, 1992)

isologous graft /īsol′əgəs/ [Gk, isos, equal; logos, relation; graphion, stylus], a tissue transplant between two individuals who are genetically identical, as identical twins.

isomeric /-mer′ik/ [Gk, isos, equal; meros, part], pertaining to a chemical phenomenon in which two compounds of the same proportion of elements and molecular weight may differ in chemical and physical properties. The difference is the result of the arrangement of atoms in the respective molecules, either the connections between the atoms or in the arrangements of the atoms in three-dimensional space.

isomers /ī′səmərz/, molecules that have the same molecular weight and formula but different structures, resulting in different properties.

isometheptene hydrochloride /-məthep′tēn/, an antispasmodic and vasoconstrictor drug that is a component in some fixed-combination drugs used to treat migraine.

isometric /ī′səmet′rik/ [Gk, isos + metron, measure], maintaining the same length or dimension.

isometric contraction [Gk, isos, equal; metron, measure; L, contractio, a drawing together], muscular contraction not accompanied by movement of the joint. The muscle is neither lengthened or shortened but tension changes alone can be measured.

isometric exercise, a form of active exercise that increases muscle tension by applying pressure against stable resistance. This may be accomplished by opposing different muscles in the same individual, such as by pressing the hands together or by making a limb push or pull against an immovable object. There is no joint movement and the length of the muscle remains unchanged, but muscle strength and tone are maintained or improved. Compare **isotonic exercise.** See also **exercise.**

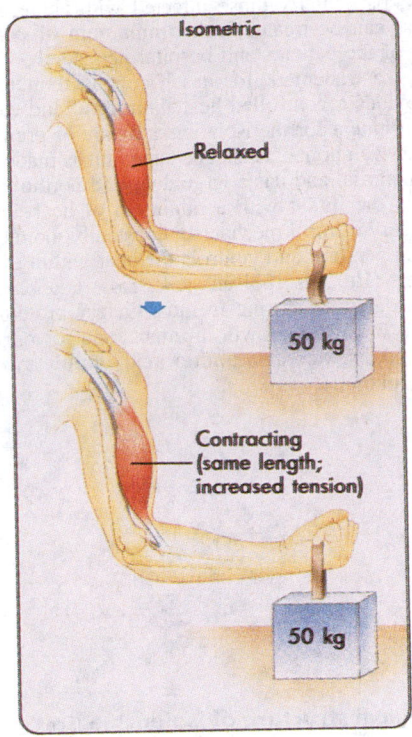

Isometric exercise (Thibodeau, 1993/Rolin Graphics)

isometric growth, an increase in size of different organs or parts of an organism at the same rate. Compare **allometric growth.**

isoniazid /ī′sənī′əzid/, a tuberculostatic antibacterial. Also called **INH (isonicotinic acid hydrazide).**
- INDICATION: It is prescribed in the treatment of tuberculosis caused by mycobacteria sensitive to the drug.
- CONTRAINDICATIONS: Liver disease, a previous history of a hepatotoxic reaction to isoniazid, or known hypersensitivity to this drug prohibits its use.
- ADVERSE EFFECTS: Among the more serious adverse reactions in long-term treatment are hepatoxicity and peripheral neuropathy. Rashes, fever, and central nervous system effects commonly occur.

isoosmotic solution /ī′sō·osmot′ik/ [Gk, *isos*, equal; L, *solutus*, dissolved], a solution with electrolytes that will exert the same osmotic pressure as another solution. Also called **isosmotic solution.**

isopentoic acid. See **isovaleric acid.**

isophane insulin suspension /ī′səfān/ [Gk, *isos* + *phanein*, to show; L, *insula*, island; *suspendere*, to hang up], a modified form of protamine zinc insulin suspension. It is an intermediate-acting insulin that is a stable, commonly prescribed preparation. Also called **NPH insulin.**

isophosphamide /-fos′fəmīd/, an antineoplastic that is a derivative of cyclophosphamide and used similarly to cyclophosphamide. Also called **isofosfamide.** See also **cyclophosphamide.**

isoprenaline. See **isoproterenol hydrochloride.**

isopropamide iodide /-prō′pəmīd/, an anticholinergic.
- INDICATION: It is prescribed as an adjunct to ulcer therapy.
- CONTRAINDICATIONS: Narrow-angle glaucoma, asthma, obstruction of the genitourinary or GI tract, ulcerative colitis, or known hypersensitivity to this drug prohibits its use.
- ADVERSE EFFECTS: Among the more serious adverse reactions are blurred vision, central nervous system effects, tachycardia, dry mouth, decreased sweating, and hypersensitivity reactions.

isopropanol. See **isopropyl alcohol.**

isopropylacetic acid. See **isovaleric acid.**

isopropyl alcohol /ī′sōprō′pil/, a clear, colorless, bitter aromatic liquid that is miscible with water, ether, chloroform, and ethyl alcohol. A solution of approximately 70% isopropyl alcohol in water is used as a rubbing compound. Also called **avantin, dimethyl carbinol, isopropanol.** See also **alcohol.**

isopropylaminoacetic acid. See **valine.**

isoproterenol hydrochloride /ī′sōprəter′ənol/, a beta-adrenergic stimulant.
- INDICATIONS: It is used as a bronchodilator and as a cardiac stimulant.
- CONTRAINDICATIONS: Cardiac arrhythmia or known hypersensitivity to this drug prohibits its use.
- ADVERSE EFFECTS: Among the more serious adverse reactions are arrhythmias, tachycardia, hypotension, and intensification of angina.

Isoptin, a trademark for a slow channel blocker or calcium ion antagonist (verapamil).

Isopto Atropine, a trademark for an anticholinergic (atropine sulfate).

Isopto Carbachol, a trademark for a cholinergic (carbachol).

Isopto Carpine, a trademark for a cholinergic (pilocarpine hydrochloride).

Isopto Cetamide, a trademark for an antibacterial (sulfacetamide sodium).

Isopto Homatropine, a trademark for an anticholinergic (homatropine hydrobromide).

Isopto Hyoscine, a trademark for an anticholinergic (scopolamine hydrobromide).

Isordil, a trademark for an antianginal agent (isosorbide dinitrate).

isosmotic. See **isotonic.**

isosmotic solution. See **isosmotic solution.**

isosorbide dinitrate /-sôr′bīd/, an antianginal agent.
- INDICATION: It is prescribed as a coronary vasodilator in the treatment of angina pectoris and congestive heart failure.
- CONTRAINDICATION: Known hypersensitivity to this drug prohibits its use.
- ADVERSE EFFECTS: The most serious reaction is occasional marked hypotension. Flushing, headache, and dizziness also may occur.

isotachophoresis /-tak′ōfôrē′sis/ [Gk, *isos* + *tachos*, speed, *pherein*, to bear], the ordering and concentration of substances of intermediate effective mobilities between an ion of high effective mobility and one of much lower effective mobility, followed by their migration at a uniform speed.

isothermal /-thur′məl/ [Gk, *isos*, equal; *therme*, heat], having the same temperature.

isotones /ī'sətōnz'/, atoms that have the same number of neutrons but different numbers of protons.

isotonic /ī'səton'ik/ [Gk, *isos* + *tonikos*, stretching], (of a solution) having the same concentration of solute as another solution, hence exerting the same amount of osmotic pressure as that solution, such as an isotonic saline solution that contains an amount of salt equal to that found in the intra- and extracellular fluid. Also **isosmotic.** Compare **hypertonic, hypotonic.**

isotonic exercise, a form of active exercise in which the muscle contracts and causes movement. Throughout the procedure there is no significant change in the resistance so that the force of the contraction remains constant. Such exercise greatly improves joint mobility and helps to improve muscle strength and tone. Compare **isometric exercise.** See also **exercise.**

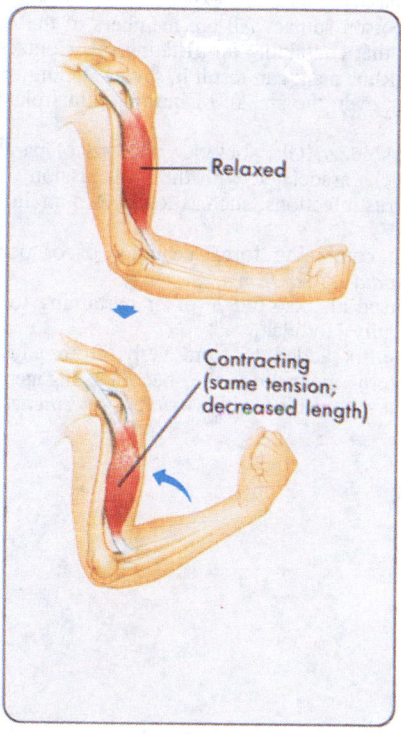

Isotonic exercises *(Thibodeau, 1993/Rolin Graphics)*

isotonic solutions [Gk, *isos*, equal; *tonos*, tone; *solutus*, dissolved], solutions exerting equal osmotic pressures.

isotope /ī'sətōp/ [Gk, *isos* + *topos*, place], one of two or more forms of a chemical element having almost identical properties: They have the same number of protons in the atomic nucleus and the same atomic number, but they differ in the number of their nuclear neutrons and atomic weights. Carbon (12C) has six nuclear neutrons, while its isotope 14C has eight. Many hundreds of radioactive isotopes are used in diagnostic and therapeutic procedures.

isotopic tracer /ī'sətop'ik/ [Gk, *isos* + *topos*, place; Fr, *tracer*, to track], an isotope or artificial mixture of isotopes of an element incorporated into a sample to permit observation of the course of the element, alone or in com-

bination, through a chemical, physical, or biologic process. The observations may be made by measuring the radioactivity or the abundance of the isotope.

isotretinoin /-trətin'ō·in/, an antiacne agent.
- INDICATION: It is prescribed for cystic acne.
- CONTRAINDICATIONS: Pregnancy or sensitivity to hydroxybenzoic acid esters prohibits its use.
- ADVERSE EFFECTS: The most serious adverse reactions are epistaxis, cheilitis, conjunctivitis, paresthesia, dizziness, serum lipid, and hematologic disturbances.

isovaleric acid /-vəler'ik/ [Gk, *isos* + L, *valeriana*, herb, *acidus*, sour], a fatty acid with a pungent taste and disagreeable odor that is found in valerian and other plant products, as well as in cheese. It also occurs as a metabolite of the amino acid leucine and is found in the sweat of feet and in urine of patients with smallpox, hepatitis, and typhus. It has been used commercially in a variety of drugs, perfumes, and flavorings. Isovaleric acidemia occurs in patients who have inherited a deficiency of the enzyme isovaleryl coA dehydrogenase, resulting in abnormally high levels of isovaleric acid in the blood and urine. The condition is treated with diets that contain low-leucine foods. Also called **isopentoic acid, isopropylacetic acid.**

isovolume pressure-flow curve /-vol'yəm/, a curve on a graph describing the relationship of driving pressure to the resulting volumetric flow rate in the airways at any given lung inflation.

isovolumic contraction /-vəloo'mik/ [Gk, *isos* + L, *volumen*, paper roll; *contractio*, drawing together], (in cardiology) an early phase of systole in which the left ventricle is generating enough tension to overcome the resistance of the aortic end-diastolic pressure. See also **afterload.**

isoxsuprine hydrochloride /īsok'səprēn/, a peripheral vasodilator.
- INDICATIONS: It is prescribed for the symptomatic relief of cerebrovascular insufficiency and to improve the circulation in arteriosclerosis, Raynaud's disease, and Buerger's disease.
- CONTRAINDICATION: Known hypersensitivity to this drug is the only contraindication.
- ADVERSE EFFECTS: Among the more serious adverse reactions are tachycardia, hypotension, and dermatitis.

-ist, a suffix meaning a 'practitioner of a science': *audiologist, pharmacist, psychosomaticist.*

isthmus /is'məs/, *pl.* **isthmuses, isthmi** [Gk, *isthmos*], a narrow connection between two larger bodies or parts, such as the isthmus of the auditory tube in the ear, which connects the bony and the cartilaginous parts of the tube.

isthmus of thyroid [Gk, *isthmos*, a short narrow body part or constriction; *thyreos*, *eidos*, form], a part of the thyroid gland, anterior to the trachea, which joins the two lateral lobes of the gland.

Isuprel, a trademark for a beta-adrenergic stimulant (isoproterenol).

IT, abbreviation for **immunotoxin.**

itch [AS, *giccan*], **1.** to feel a sensation, usually on the skin, that makes one want to scratch. **2.** a tingling, annoying sensation on an area of the skin that makes one want to scratch it, such as may be caused in some people by rhus dermatitis, a mosquito bite, or an allergic reaction. **3.** the pruritic condition of the skin caused by infestation with the parasitic mite *Sarcoptes scabiei.* —**itchy,** *adj.*

itch mite [AS, *giccan, mite*], a tiny eight-legged insect with piercing and sucking mouth parts. At least three genera of itch mites are recognized. They are *Chorioptes*, *Notoëdres*, and *Sarcoptes*.

-itchy. See **itch.**

-ite, **1.** a suffix meaning 'compounds': *nitrite, phosphite, sulfite.* **2.** a combining form meaning a 'body part': *chondriomite, osteite, zygoite.*

ithy-, a combining form meaning 'erect or straight': *ithylordosis, ithyokyphosis.*

ithycyphosis /ith'ēsifrō'sis/ [Gk, *ithys*, straight; *kyphosis*, humpback], a backward angular displacement of the spine without lateral displacement. Also called **ithyokyphosis** /ith'ē·ōkīfō'sis/.

-itic, a suffix meaning 'of or related to something specified': *encephalitic, nephritic, syphilitic.*

-itis, a suffix meaning an 'inflammation of a (specified) organ': *carditis, cecitis, sarcitis.*

ITP, abbreviation for **idiopathic thrombocytopenic purpura.**

IU, I.U., abbreviation for **International Unit.**

IUCD, abbreviation for *intrauterine contraceptive device.* See **intrauterine device.**

IUD, abbreviation for **intrauterine device.**

-ium, **1.** a suffix used to name metallic elements: *aluminum, radium, sodium.* **2.** a suffix for quaternary ammonium derivatives.

IV, **1.** abbreviation for **intravenous** or **intravenously.** **2.** *informal.* equipment consisting of a bottle of fluid, infusion set with tubing, and an intracatheter, used in intravenous therapy. **3.** intravenous administration of fluids or medication by injection into a vein.

IVAC pump, a trademark for a portable IV pump that electronically regulates and monitors the flow of fluid. It is usually attached to the IV stand. See also **intravenous pump.**

IVC, abbreviation for **intravenous cholangiography.**

IVF, abbreviation for **in vitro fertilization.**

ivory bones. See **osteopetrosis.**

IVP, abbreviation for *intravenous pyelography.*

IV push, a technique in which a bolus of medication or a large volume of IV fluid is given rapidly via IV injection or infusion. Methergine may be given in this way to cause immediate contraction of the uterus in postpartum hemorrhage. See also *intravenous injection.*

I.V.T., abbreviation for **intravenous transfusion.**

IV-type traction frame, a metal support that holds traction equipment consisting of two metal uprights, one at each end of the bed, which support an overhead metal bar. Each upright is clamped to a horizontal bar that fits into holders inserting at the corners of the bed. Compare **claw-type traction frame.** See also **traction frame.**

ivy poisoning [OE, *ifig*; L, *potio*, drink], a form of contact dermatitis caused by exposure to poison ivy, poison oak, or poison sumac. All are members of the *Rhus* genus of plants that containing an irritating oil. Contact with any part of a Rhus plant can result in severe itching, rashes, and blistering; even the smoke of burning Rhus plants may be toxic.

Ixodes /iksō'dēz/ [Gk, sticky], a genus of parasitic hard-shelled ticks associated with the transmission of a variety of arbovirus infections, such as Rocky Mountain spotted fever.

ixodi-, a combining form meaning 'of or pertaining to ticks': *ixodiasis, ixodism.*

ixodid /iksod'id, iksō'did/, of or pertaining to hard ticks of the family Ixodidae.

-ize, a suffix added to form verbs from adjectives and nouns. Verbs mean 'to make, become, engage in, or use, or to treat or combine with': *oxidize, anesthetize.*

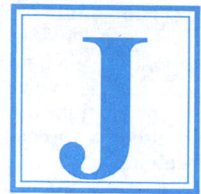

J, abbreviation for **joule.**

Jaccoud's dissociated fever /zhäko͞oz'/ [Sigismond Jaccoud, French physician, b. 1830], a form of meningitic fever accompanied by a paradoxical slow pulse rate.

jacket/ [Fr *jaquette*], a supportive or confining therapeutic casing or garment for the torso. Some kinds of jackets are **Minerva jacket** and **Sayre's jacket.**

jacket restraint, an orthopedic device used to help immobilize the trunk of a patient in traction and to discourage the patient from sitting up in bed. The jacket restraint is attached to both sides of the bedspring frame by means of buckled webbing straps that are sewn into the side seams of the restraint. The jacket restraint may be used with most kinds of traction but is not usually used with Dunlop skin traction or Dunlop skeletal traction, Bryant traction, halo-femoral traction, or halo-pelvic traction. Compare **diaper restraint, sling restraint.**

jackknife position /jak'nīf/, an anatomic position in which the patient is placed on the back in a semisitting position, with the shoulders elevated and the thighs flexed at right angles to the abdomen. Examination and instrumentation of the male urethra is facilitated by this position.

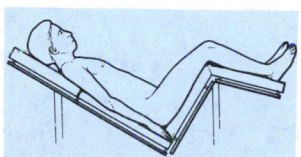

Jackknife position

Jackson crib, a removable orthodontic appliance retained in position by crib-shaped wires.

jacksonian seizure. See **focal seizure.**

Jackson tracheostomy tube, a silver tracheostomy tube with a rubber cuff built onto the tube. The design is intended to prevent accidental migration of the cuff off the end of the tube, resulting in interference with air flow to the patient.

Jacob's membrane [Arthur Jacob, Irish surgeon, b. 1790; L *membrana* thin skin], the outermost of the nine layers of the retina, composed of rods and cones interacting directly with the optic nerve.

Jacquemier's sign /zhäkmē·āz'/ [Jean M. Jacquemier, French obstetrician, b. 1806], a deepening of the color of the vaginal mucosa just below the urethral orifice. It may sometimes be noted after the fourth week of pregnancy, but it is not a reliable sign of pregnancy.

jactitation /jak'titā'shən/ [L, *jactare*, show off, display], twitchings or spasms of muscles or muscle groups, as observed in the restless body movements of a patient with a severe fever.

JADA, abbreviation for *Journal of the American Dental Association.*

jail fever. See **epidemic typhus.**

Jakob-Creutzfeldt disease. See **Creutzfeldt-Jakob disease.**

JAMA /jä'mä, jam'ə, jā'ā'em'ā'/, abbreviation for *Journal of the American Medical Association.*

jamais vu /zhämävY', -vē', -vo͞o'/ [Fr, never seen], the sensation of being a stranger when with a person one knows or when in a familiar place. The phenomenon occurs occasionally in normal people but more frequently in people who have temporal lobe epilepsy. Compare **déjà vu.**

Janeway lesion /jān'wā/ [Edward G. Janeway, American Physician, b. 1841; L, *laedere*, to injure], a small erythematous or hemorrhagic macule occurring on the palms or soles. It is diagnostic of subacute bacterial endocarditis.

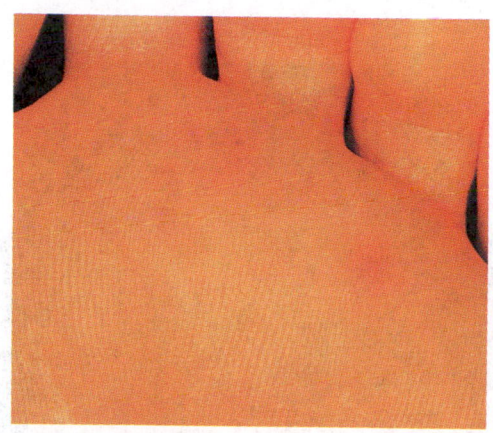

Janeway lesion *(Zitelli, 1992)*

janiceps /jan'əseps/ [L, *Janus*, two-faced Roman god, *caput*, head], a conjoined, twin fetus in which the heads are fused, with the faces looking in opposite directions. The faces and bodies of both twins may be fully formed or one member may be only partially formed and act as a parasite on the more fully developed fetus.

Jansen's disease. See **metaphyseal dysostosis.**

Japanese encephalitis, a severe epidemic infection of brain tissue seen in East Asia and the South Pacific, including Australia and New Zealand, characterized by shaking chills, paralysis, and weight loss, and caused by a group of B arboviruses transmitted by mosquitoes. Mortality may be as high as 33%. Various neurologic and psychiatric sequelae are common. There is no specific treatment. Also called **Japanese B encephalitis.**

Japanese flood fever, Japanese river fever.   See **scrub typhus**.

JAPHA /jaf'ə, jā'ā'pē'ăch'ā'/,   abbreviation for *Journal of the American Public Health Association*.

jargon (jar.) /jär'gən/ [Fr, **jargonner**, to speak indistinctly],   **1.** incoherent speech or gibberish. **2.** a language used by scientists, artists, or others of a professional subculture that is not understood by the general population.

jargon aphasia [Fr, *jargonner*; Gk, *a. phasis*, speech],   a form of speech in which several words are combined in a single word but in a jumbled manner with incorrect accents or words mixed with neologisms. Although outwardly incomprehensible, the speech may be meaningful when analyzed by a psychotherapist. Also called **word hash, word salad**.

Jarisch-Herxheimer reaction /jä'risherks'hīmər/ [Adolph Jarisch, Austrian dermatologist, b. 1850; Karl Herxheimer, German dermatologist, b. 1861],   a an acute febrile reaction that may occur after therapy for syphilis. It is often accompanied by headache and myalgia and is more common in patients with early syphilis. No proven methods for prevention exist. Pregnant women should be warned that early labor may occur.

Jarotzky's treatment /jərot'skēz/ [Alexander Jarotsky, Russian physician, b. 1866],   therapy of gastric ulcer using a bland diet consisting of egg whites, fresh butter, bread, milk, and noodles.

Jarvik-7 [Robert K. Jarvik, American physician, b. 1946],   an artificial heart designed by R.K. Jarvik for use in humans. The Jarvik-7 was an early model that depended on air pressure to drive the ventricles.

jaundice /jôn'dis, jän'dis/ [Fr, *jaune*, yellow],   a yellow discoloration of the skin, mucous membranes, and sclerae of the eyes, caused by greater than normal amounts of bilirubin in the blood. Persons with jaundice may also experience nausea, vomiting, and abdominal pain and may pass dark urine. Jaundice is a symptom of many disorders, including liver diseases, biliary obstruction, and the hemolytic anemias. Newborns commonly develop physiologic jaundice, which disappears after a few days. Rarer disorders causing jaundice are Crigler-Najjar syndrome and Gilbert's syndrome. Useful diagnostic procedures include a clinical evaluation of the signs and symptoms, tests of liver function, and techniques for direct or indirect visualization such as x-ray film, CT scan, ultrasound, endoscopy or exploratory surgery, and biopsy. Also called **icterus** /ik'tərəs/. See also **anicteric hepatitis, hyperbilirubinemia**. **–jaundiced**, *adj.*

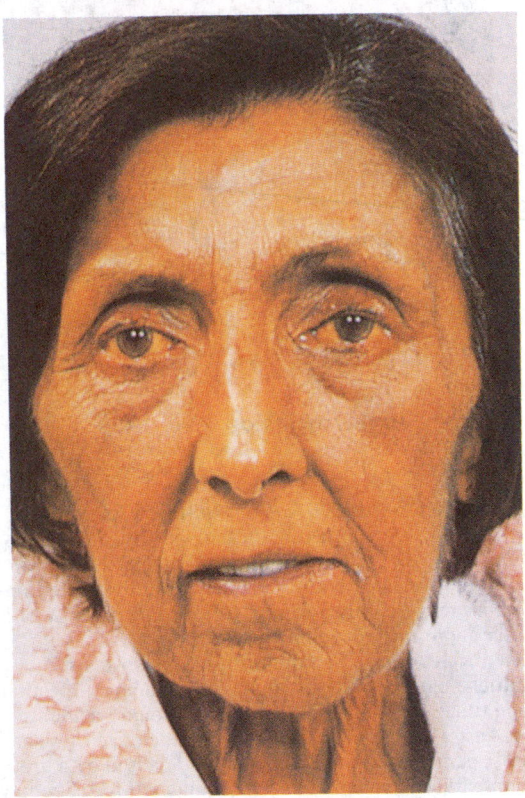

Severe jaundice *(Kamal, 1991)*

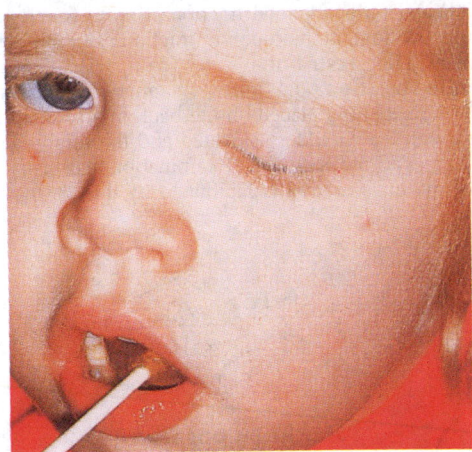

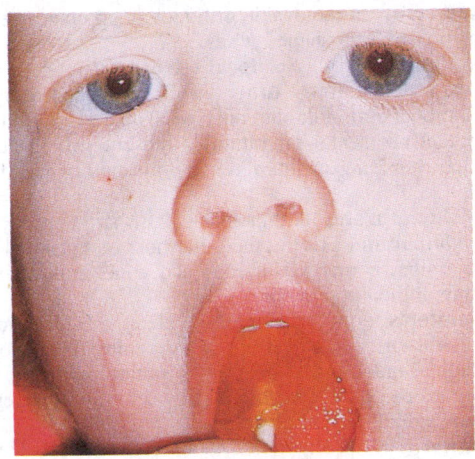

Jaw-winking *(Zitelli, 1992)*

jaw [AS, *ceowan*, to chew], a common term used to describe the maxillae and the mandible and the soft tissue that covers these structures. See also **jaw relation.**

jaw reflex, an abnormal reflex elicited by tapping the chin with a rubber hammer while the mouth is half open and the jaw muscles are relaxed. A quick snapping shut of the jaw implies damage to the area of cerebral cortex governing motor activity of the fifth cranial nerve. Also called **chin reflex, jaw jerk, mandibular reflex.**

jaw relation, any relation of the mandible to the maxillae.

jaw-winking, an involuntary facial movement phenomenon in which the eyelid droops, usually on one side of the face, when the jaw is closed but raises when the jaw is opened or when the jaw is moved from side to side. The raising of the eyelid often appears exaggerated. Also called **Marcus Gunn syndrome.** See also **Marin Amat syndrome.**

JCAHO, abbreviation for **Joint Commission on Accreditation of Health Care Organizations.**

J chain, the portion of the IgM molecule possibly holding the structure together, thus "joining chain."

J/deg, abbreviation for *joules per degree.*

Jefferson fracture, a fracture characterized by bursting of the ring of the atlas.

jejuna. See **jejunum.**

jejunal /jijo͞o′nəl/ [L, *jejunus,* empty], pertaining to the **jejunum,** the length of intestine between the duodenum and the ileum.

jejunal feeding tube, a hollow tube inserted into the jejunum through the abdominal wall for administration of liquified foods to patients who have a high risk of aspiration.

jejuno-, a combining form meaning 'of or pertaining to the jejunum': *jejunocecostomy, jejunocolostomy, jejunotomy.*

jejunoileitis. See **Crohn's disease.**

jejunostomy /jij′o͞onos′təmē/, a surgical procedure to create an artificial opening to the jejunum through the abdominal wall. It may be a permanent or a temporary opening.

jejunostomy feeding. See **tube feeding.**

jejunum /jijo͞o′nəm/, *pl.* **jejuna** [L, *jejunus,* empty], the intermediate or middle of the three portions of the small intestine, connecting proximally with the duodenum and distally with the ileum. The jejunum has a slightly larger diameter, a deeper color, and a thicker wall than the ileum and contains heavy, circular folds that are absent in the lower part of the ileum. The jejunum also has larger villi than the ileum. Compare **ileum.** –**jejunal,** *adj.*

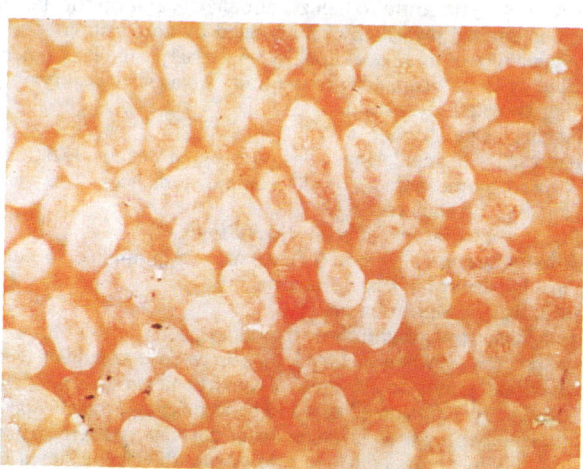

Jejunal mucosa *(Winawer, 1992)*

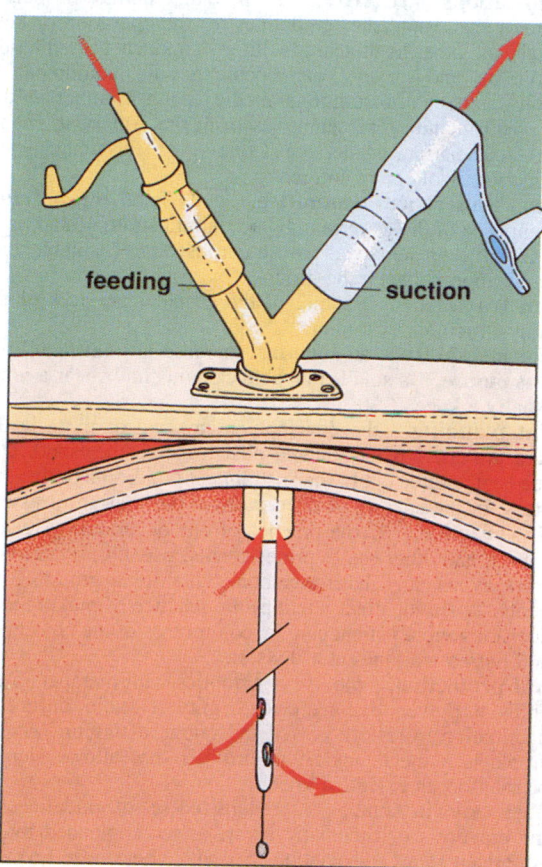

Placement of jejunal feeding tube *(Geenen, 1992)*

jellyfish sting [L, *gelare,* to congeal; AS, *fisc; stingan*], a wound caused by skin contact with a jellyfish, a sea animal with a bell-shaped gelatinous body and suspended numerous long tentacles containing stinging structures. In most cases a tender, red welt develops on the affected skin. In some cases, depending on the sensitivity of the person and the particular species of jellyfish, severe localized pain and nausea, weakness, excessive lacrimation, nasal discharge, muscle spasm, perspiration, and dyspnea may occur. Treatment includes carefully removing any tentacles and applying a compress of alcohol, aromatic spirits of ammonia, or Dakin's solution. Calcium gluconate may be administered to control muscle spasms.

Jendrassik's maneuver /yendrä′shiks/ [Ernst Jendrassik, Hungarian physician, b. 1858; Fr, *manoeuvre,* action], (in neurology) a diagnostic procedure in which the patient hooks the flexed fingers of the two hands together and forcibly tries to pull them apart. While this tension is being exerted, the lower extremity reflexes are tested, particularly the patellar reflex.

jet humidifier, a humidifier that increases the surface area for exposure of water to gas by breaking the water into small aerosol droplets. Air, or a gas, passes through a restriction after entering the humidifier, producing a foaming mixture of liquid and gas. Gas issuing from the unit has a maximum amount of water vapor and a minimum of liquid water particles.

jet lag [L, *jacere*, to throw; Norw, *lagga*, to fall behind], a condition characterized by fatigue, insomnia, and sluggish body functions caused by disruption of the normal circadian rhythm resulting from air travel across several time zones.

jet nebulizer [L, *nebula*, mist], a humidifier that uses the Bernoulli effect to convert a source of liquid into a fine mist of aerosol particles. The Bernoulli effect is produced by projecting a jet stream of gas at high velocity across the end of a capillary tube. The gas jet alters the pressure surrounding the tube, forcing the liquid to the top where it is continuously blown off as aerosol particles that enter the outflow passage to the person being treated.

Jeune's syndrome /zhœnz, zhoonz/, a form of lethal short-limbed dwarfism characterized by constriction of the upper thorax and, occasionally, polydactylism. It is inherited as an autosomal recessive trait. Also called **asphyxiating thoracic dysplasia.**

jigger. See **chigoe.**

jitters, 1. irregularities in ultrasound echo locations caused by mechanical or electronic disturbances. **2.** a very uneasy, nervous feeling.

jkg, abbreviation for *joules per kilogram.*

Jobst garment, a type of pressure wrap applied to control hypertrophic scar formation.

jock itch. See **tinea cruris.**

Jod-Basedow phenomenon /jod'bä'zədō'/, thyrotoxicosis occurring when dietary iodine is given to a patient with endemic goiter in an area of environmental iodine deficiency. It is presumed that iodine deficiency protects some patients with endemic goiter from developing thyrotoxicosis. The phenomenon may also occur when large doses of iodine are given to patients with nontoxic multinodular goiter in areas with sufficient environmental iodine.

jogger's heel [ME, *joggen*, to shake; AS, *hela*, heel], a painful condition, common among joggers and distance runners. It is characterized by bruising, bursitis, fasciitis, or calcaneal spurs, caused by repetitive and forceful strikes of the heel on the ground. Judicious selection of well-fitting running shoes and avoidance of running on hard surfaces are recommended to avoid occurrence or recurrence of the condition. Rest, heat, or corticosteroid medication or aspirin may be recommended.

Johnson's method, (in dentistry) a technique for filling root canals, in which gutta-percha cones are dissolved in a chloroform-rosin solution in the root canal to form a plastic mass. The plastic material is forced into the apex of the root canal with more added until the canal is sealed.

joint [L, *jungere*, to join], any one of the connections between bones. Each is classified according to structure and movability as fibrous, cartilaginous, or synovial. Fibrous joints are immovable, cartilaginous joints slightly movable, and synovial joints freely movable. Typical immovable joints are those connecting most of the bones of the skull with a sutural ligament. Typical slightly movable joints are those connecting the vertebrae and the pubic bones. Most of the joints in the body are freely movable and allow gliding, circumduction, rotation, and angular movement. Also called **articulation.** See also **cartilaginous joint, fibrous joint, synovial joint.**

joint and several liability, (in law) a condition in which several persons share the liability for a plaintiff's injury and may be found liable individually or as a group.

joint appointment, 1. a faculty appointment to two institutions within a university or system, as to the schools of nursing and medicine of the same university. **2.** (in academic nursing) the appointment of a member of the faculty of a university to a clinical service of an associated service institution. A psychiatric nurse might hold appointment in a university as an assistant professor and might also be a clinical nurse specialist in a service institution. The practice of joint appointments is said to have begun at Case Western Reserve University, University Hospital. See also **unification model.**

joint audit. See **nursing audit.**

joint capsule [L, *jungere*, to join; *capsula*, little box], a fibrous connective tissue envelope surrounding a joint.

joint chondroma, a cartilaginous mass that develops in the synovial membrane of a joint.

Joint Commission on Accreditation of Health Care Organizations (JCAHO), a private, nongovernmental agency that establishes guidelines for the operation of hospitals and other health care facilities, conducts accreditation programs and surveys, and encourages the attainment of high standards of institutional medical care. Members of the JCAHO include representatives from the American Medical Association, American College of Physicians, and American College of Surgeons.

joint conference committee, a hospital organization composed of the governing board, administration, and medical staff representatives whose purpose is to facilitate communication between the groups.

joint fracture, a fracture of the articular surfaces of the bony structures of a joint.

joint instability, an abnormal increase in joint mobility.

joint mouse, a small, movable calculus in or near a joint, usually a knee.

joint planning, the development by two or more health care providers of a strategic plan to serve the health care needs of an area while sharing clinical or administrative services, or the sharing of data, without the sharing of assets.

joint practice, 1. the practice of one or more physicians, nurses, and other health professionals, usually private, who work as a team, sharing responsibility for a group of patients. **2.** (in inpatient nursing) the practice of making joint decisions about patient care by committees of the physicians and nurses working on a division.

joint protection, the use of orthotics with therapeutic exercise to prevent damage or deformity of a joint during rehabilitation to restore power and range of motion. An example is a metal ankle-foot orthosis that allows weight-bearing on an extended knee.

Jones criteria /jōnz/, a standardized set of guidelines for the diagnosis of rheumatic fever, as recommended by the American Heart Association. See also **rheumatic fever.**

joule /jool/ [James P. Joule, English physicist, b. 1818], a unit of energy or work in the MKS (meter-kilogram-second) system. It is equivalent to 10^7 ergs or 1 watt second.

joystick, a vertical stick or lever that can be manipulated

Classification of joints

Type of joint	Example	Description
Fibroid (synarthrosis)		No movement is permitted
Suture	Cranial sutures	United by thin layer of fibrous tissue
Synchondrosis	Joint between the epiphysis and diaphysis of long bones	A temporary joint in which the cartilage is replaced by bone later in life
Cartilaginous (amphiarthrosis)		Slightly movable joint
Symphysis	Symphysis pubis	Bones are connected by a fibrocartilage disk
Syndesmosis	Radius-ulna articulation	Bones are connected by ligaments
Synovial (diarthrosis)		Freely movable; enclosed by joint capsule, lined with synovial membrane
Ball and socket	Hip	Widest range of motion, movement in all planes
Hinge	Elbow	Motion limited to flexion and extension in a single plane
Pivot	Atlantoaxis	Motion limited to rotation
Condyloid	Wrist between radius and carpals	Motion in two planes at right angles to each other, but no radial rotation
Saddle	Thumb at carpal-metacarpal joint	Motion in two planes at right angles to each other, but no axial rotation
Gliding	Intervertebral	Motion limited to gliding

Joint types (Thibodeau, 1993/Rolin Graphics)

Adapted from Seidel HM, Ball JW, Dains JE, Benedict GW: *Mosby's guide to physical examination,* ed 2, St Louis, 1991, Mosby.

in various directions to control cursor movement on a computer screen or the direction of an electric wheelchair. See also **mouse, trackball.**

J-pouch, a fecal reservoir formed surgically by folding over the lower end of the ileum in an ileoanal anastomosis.

JRA, abbreviation for **juvenile rheumatoid arthritis.**

Judd method, (in radiology) a technique for positioning

a patient for x-ray examination of the atlas and odontoid process.

judgment /juj′mənt/ [L, *judicare*, to judge], **1.** (in law) the final decision of the court regarding the case before it. **2.** the reason given by the court for its decision; an opinion. **3.** an award, penalty, or other sentence of law given by the court. **4.** (in psychiatry) the ability to recognize the relationships of ideas and to form correct conclusions from those data as well as from those acquired from experience.

judgment call,   *slang.* a decision based on experience, especially a judgment that resolves a serious problem in which the data are inconclusive or equivocal.

jug-,   **1.** a combining form meaning 'pertaining to a yoke type of connection': *jugal, jugum, conjugal.* **2.** a combining form meaning 'pertaining to the collarbone, throat, neck': *jugular, jugate.*

jugu-,   a combining form meaning 'to kill': *jugulate, jugulation.*

jugular /jug'yələr/ [L, *jugulum*, neck],   **1.** pertaining to or involving the neck. **2.** *informal* the jugular vein.

jugular foramen [L, *jugulum*, neck; *foramen*, hole],   one of a pair of openings between the lateral part of the occipital bone and the petrous part of the temporal bones in the skull. The foramen contains the inferior petrosal sinus, the transverse sinus, some meningeal branches of the occipital and ascending pharyngeal arteries, and the glossopharyngeal, vagus, and accessory nerves.

jugular foramen syndrome.   See **Vernet's syndrome.**

jugular fossa,   a deep depression adjacent to the interior surface of the petrosa of the temporal bone of the skull.

jugular process,   a portion of the occipital bone that projects laterally from the squamous part. On its anterior border a deep notch forms the posterior and medial boundary of the jugular foramen.

jugular pulse,   a pulsation in the jugular vein caused by comditions that inhibit diastolic filling of the right side of the heart.

jugular venous pressure (JVP),   blood pressure in the **jugular vein,** which reflects the volume and pressure of venous blood. JVP is estimated by positioning the head of a supine patient at a 45-degree angle and observing the neck

sues of animals or plants. In humans, it usually refers to the secretions of the digestive glands. Kinds of juices include **gastric juice, intestinal juice,** and **pancreatic juice.**

jumentous /jo͞omen'təs/ [L, *jumentum*, beast of burden], having a strong animal odor, especially that of a horse. The term is used to describe the odor of urine during certain disease conditions.

jumping gene,   (in molecular genetics) a unit of genetic information associated with a segment of DNA that can move from one position in the genome to another.

junction /jungk'shən/ [L, *jungere*, to join],   an interface or meeting place for tissues or structures.

junctional bigeminy /jungk'shənəl/ [L, *jungere*, to join; *bis*, twice, *geminus*, twin],   a condition in which events occur in pairs, as a bigeminal pulse or nodal extrasystoles, with origination from the junction.

junctional epithelium [L, *jungere*, to join; Gk, *epi, thele,* nipple],   an area of epithelial soft tissue surrounding the abutment post of a tooth. Also called **attached epithelial cuff, epithelial cuff, gingival cuff.**

junctional extrasystole [L, *jungere*, to join; *extra*, beyond; Gk, *systole*, contraction],   an extrasystole arising from the atrioventricular junction. See also **atrioventricular junction.**

junctional rhythm,   the cardiac rhythm originating in the atrioventricular junction.

junctional tachycardia,   an automatic heart rhythm of greater than 100 beats/minute, emanating from the AV junction. The mechanism is enhanced automatically, and may be caused by digitalis toxicity.

junction lines,   (in radiology) vertical lines that appear in the mediastinum on a P-A (posterior-anterior) projection x-ray image.

junction nevus [L, *jungere*, to join; *naevus*, birthmark],   a hairless, flat or slightly raised, brown skin blemish arising from pigment cells at the epidermal-dermal junction. A junction nevus may be found anywhere on the surface of the body. All nevi of the palms and soles and all pigmented nevi in early childhood are of this type. Malignant change may be signaled by increase in size, hardness or darkening, bleeding, or the appearance of satellite discoloration around the nevus. Junction nevi undergoing these changes and lesions found in areas subject to trauma should be removed.

Measurement of jugular venous pressure
(Seidel, 1991)

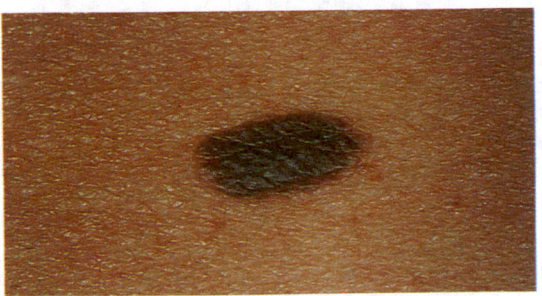

Junction nevus *(Habif, 1990)*

veins. If the neck veins are filled only to a point a few millimeters above the clavicle at the end of exhalation, JVP is usually normal. With elevated JVP the neck veins may be distended as high as the angle of the jaw.

juice /jo͞os/ [L, *jus*, broth],   any fluid secreted by the tis-

junctura cartilaginea.   See **cartilaginous joint.**
junctura fibrosa.   See **fibrous joint.**
junctura synovialis.   See **synovial joint.**
Jungian psychology.   See **analytic psychology.**

Junin fever. See **Argentine hemorrhagic fever.**

juniper tar /joo'nipər/ [L, *juniperus;* AS, *teoru*], a dark oily liquid obtained by the destructive distillation of the wood of *Juniperus oxycedrus* trees. It is used as an antiseptic stimulant in ointments for skin disorders such as psoriasis and eczema. Also called **Cade oil.**

junk, *slang.* **heroin.**

jurisprudence /joo'risproo'dəns/ [L, *jus*, law, *prudentia,* knowledge], the science and philosophy of law. **Medical jurisprudence** relates to the interfacing of medicine with criminal and civil law.

justo major /jus'tō mā'jər/ [L, *justus*, right; *major*, greater], *archaic.* atypically large, such as a woman's bony pelvis.

juvenile /joo'vənəl, -vənīl/ [L, *juvenus*, youthful], **1.** a young person; youth; child; youngster. **2.** of, pertaining to, characteristic of, or suitable for a young person; youthful. **3.** physiologically underdeveloped or immature. **4.** denoting psychologic or intellectual immaturity; childish.

juvenile alveolar rhabdomyosarcoma, a rapidly growing tumor of striated muscle occurring in children and adolescents, chiefly in the extremities. The prognosis is grave.

juvenile angiofibroma. See **nasopharyngeal angiofibroma.**

juvenile delinquency, persistent antisocial, illegal, or criminal behavior by children or adolescents to the degree that it cannot be controlled or corrected by the parents, it endangers others in the community, and it becomes the concern of a law enforcement agency.

juvenile delinquent, a person who performs illegal acts and who has not reached an age at which treatment as an adult can be accorded under the laws of the community having jurisdiction. Also called **juvenile offender, young offender.**

juvenile diabetes. See **insulin-dependent diabetes mellitus.**

juvenile glaucoma [L, *juvenis*, young man; Gk, *glaukcos*, bluish-gray], increased intraocular tension in a young adult because of developing structural defects that restrict the outflow of fluid.

juvenile kyphosis. See **Scheuermann's disease.**

juvenile lentigo. See **lentigo.**

juvenile myxedema. See **childhood myxedema.**

juvenile offender. See **juvenile delinquent.**

juvenile periodontitis, an abnormal condition that may affect the dental alveoli, especially in the anterior and first molar regions of children and adolescents. It is character-

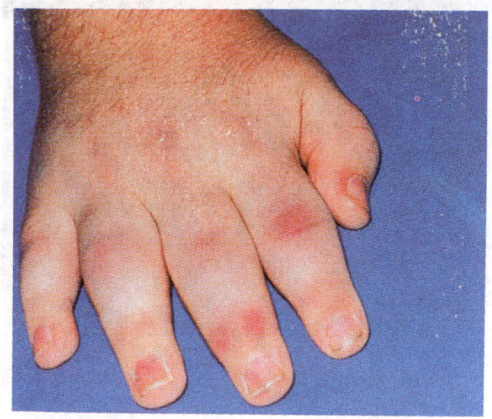

Juvenile rheumatoid arthritis *(Zitelli, 1992)*

ized by severe pocketing and bone loss. Formerly called **periodontosis.**

juvenile rheumatoid arthritis (JRA), a form of rheumatoid arthritis, usually affecting the larger joints of children under 16 years of age. As bone growth in children is dependent on the epiphyseal plates of the distal epiphyses, skeletal development may be impaired if these structures are damaged. Treatment includes analgesia, antiinflammatory medication, and rest. The recovery rate in this juvenile form is better than in the adult forms of rheumatoid arthritis. Also called **Still's disease.**

juvenile spinal muscular atrophy, a disorder beginning in childhood in which progressive degeneration of anterior horn and medullary nerve cells leads to skeletal muscle wasting. The condition usually begins in the legs and pelvis. Also called **Wohlfart-Kugelberg-Welander disease.**

juvenile xanthogranuloma, a skin disorder characterized by groups of yellow, red, or brown papules or nodules on the extensor surfaces of the arms and legs, and in some cases

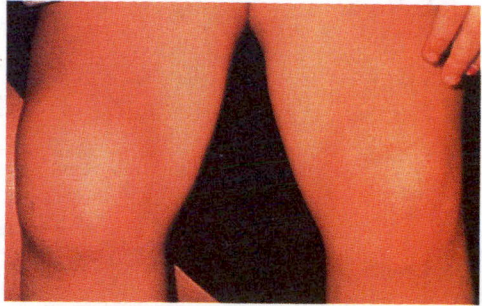

Juvenile rheumatoid arthritis *(Zitelli, 1992)*

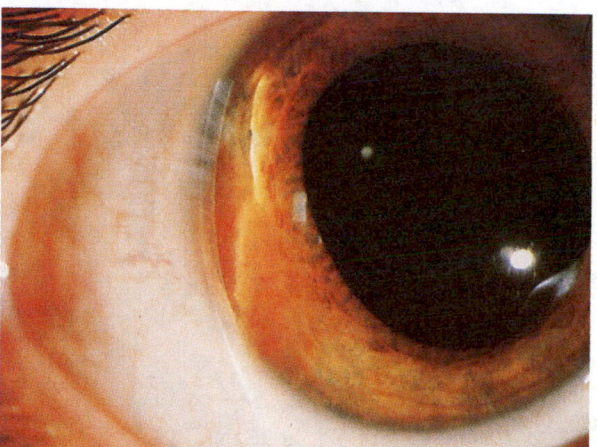

Juvenile xanthogranuloma
(Zitelli, 1992)

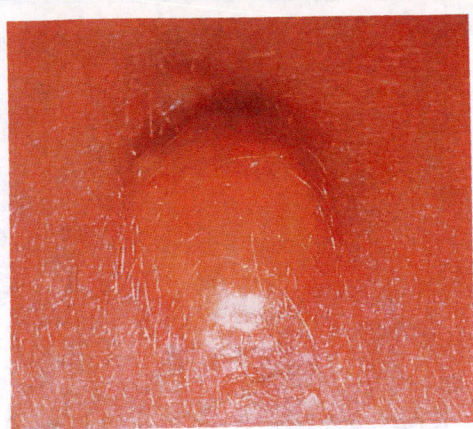

Juvenile xanthogranuloma (Zitelli, 1992)

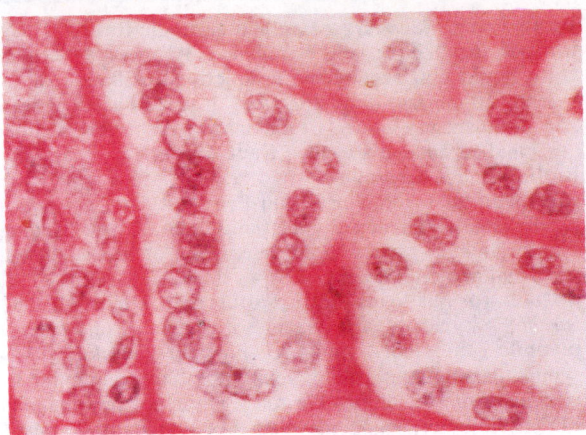

Juxtaglomerular cells (Swales, 1991)

on the eyeball, meninges, and testes. The lesions typically appear in infancy or early childhood and usually disappear in a few years.

juxta-, a prefix meaning 'near': *juxtaglomerular, juxtangina, juxtaposition.*

juxtaarticular /juk′stə·ärtik′yələr/ [L, *juxta,* adjacent; *articulus,* joint], pertaining to a location near a joint.

juxtaglomerular /-glōmer′ələr/ [L, *juxta,* adjacent; *glomerulus,* small ball], pertaining to an area between the afferent and efferent arterioles of the kidney glomerulus.

juxtaglomerular cells [L, *juxta,* near, *glomerulus,* small sphere; *cella,* storeroom], smooth muscle cells lining the glomerular end of the afferent arterioles in the kidney that are in opposition to the macula densa region of the early distal tubule. These cells synthesize and store renin and release it in response to decreased renal perfusion pressure, increased sympathetic nerve stimulation of the kidneys, or decreased sodium concentration in fluid in the distal tubule.

juxtaposition /-pəzish′ən/, the placement of objects side by side or end to end.

JVP, abbreviation for **jugular venous pressure.**

K, **1.** symbol for *ionization constant.* **2.** symbol for **Kelvin scale.** **3.** abbreviation for **kilo,** 1000, or 10^3. **4.** symbol for the element **potassium** (kalium). **5.** abbreviation for **kilobyte.** **6.** symbol in electronics for **1,024 (2^{10}).** **7.** abbreviation for **katal.**

K_m, symbol for *Michaelis-Menten constant.*

ka, abbreviation for *kiloampere.*

-kacin, suffix for antibiotics derived from *Streptomyces kanamyceticus.*

Kahn test [Reuben L. Kahn, American bacteriologist, b. 1887], **1.** one of the older serologic tests for syphilis. The appearance of a white precipitate in a serum sample allowed to stand overnight in a mixture with a sensitized antigen is regarded as a positive reaction. **2.** a test for the presence of cancer by measuring the proportion of albumin A in a blood sample.

kainate /kī'nāt/, a non-NMDA (N-methyl-D-aspartate) receptor agonist.

kak-, a combining form meaning 'bad': *kakidrosis, kakosmia.*

kakke disease. See **beriberi.**

kakosmia. See **cacosmia.**

kala-azar /kä'lə·äzär'/ [Hindi, *kala,* black; Assamese, *azar,* fever], a disease caused by the protozoan *Leishmania donovani,* transmitted to humans, particularly to children, by the bite of the sand fly. Kala-azar occurs primarily in Asia, parts of Africa, several South and Central American countries, and in the Mediterranean region. The liver and spleen are the main sites of infection; signs and symptoms include anemia, hepatomegaly, splenomegaly, irregular fever, and emaciation. Patients with kala-azar are also susceptible to secondary bacterial infections. Untreated, the disease has an extremely high mortality. Treatment includes sodium antimony gluconate, blood transfusions (for anemia), bed rest, and adequate nutrition. Also called **Assam fever, black fever, dumdum fever, ponos, visceral leishmaniasis.** See also **leishmaniasis.**

kalemia /kəlē'mē·ə/, the presence of potassium in the blood.

kali-, a combining form meaning 'of or pertaining to potassium': *kaligenous, kalinite, kalium.*

kaliuresis /kal'iyŏorē'sis/, the excretion of potassium in the urine.

kallikrein-kinin system /kalik'rē·in-/, a proposed hormonal system that functions within the kidney, with the enzyme kallikrein in the renal cortex mediating production of bradykinin, which acts as a vasodilator peptide.

Kallmann's syndrome [Franz J. Kallman, American psychiatrist, b. 1897], a condition characterized by the absence of the sense of smell because of agenesis of the olfactory bulbs and by secondary hypogonadism because of the lack of LHRH.

kanamycin /kan'əmī'sin/, an antibacterial substance derived from *Streptomyces kanamyceticus.*

kanamycin sulfate, an aminoglycoside antibiotic.

■ INDICATIONS: It is prescribed in the treatment of certain severe infections and those resistant to other antibiotics.

■ CONTRAINDICATIONS: Concomitant administration of ototoxic drugs or known hypersensitivity to this drug or to other aminoglycoside antibiotics prohibits its use. It is used with caution in patients having impaired renal function and in the elderly.

■ ADVERSE EFFECTS: Among the more serious adverse reactions are nephrotoxicity, vestibular and auditory ototoxicity, neuromuscular blockade, and hypersensitivity reactions.

Kanner's syndrome, a form of infantile psychosis with an onset in the first 30 months of life. It is characterized by infantile autism, with signs of lack of attachment, avoidance of eye contact, and general failure to develop social relationships; rituals and compulsive behavior manifested by a resistance to change and repetitive acts; general intellectual retardation; and language disorders, which may range from muteness to echolalia. Treatment may include psychotherapy and special education, depending on the intelligence level of the child.

Kantrex, a trademark for an antibacterial (kanamycin sulfate).

Kanulase, a trademark for a GI, fixed-combination drug containing various antiflatulent ingredients.

Kaochlor, a trademark for an electrolyte-replacement solution (potassium chloride).

kaodzera. See **Rhodesian trypanosomiasis.**

kaolin /kā'əlin/ [Chin, *kao-ling,* high ridge], an adsorbent used internally to treat diarrhea, often in combination with pectin. Kaolin in an ointment base is also used topically as an absorbent and a protective emollient.

Kaon, a trademark for the electrolyte-replacement solution (potassium chloride).

Kaopectate, a trademark for an antidiarrheal fixed-combination drug containing an adsorbent (kaolin) and an emollient (pectin).

Kaposi's disease /kap'əsēz/ [Moritz K. Kaposi, Austrian dermatologist, b. 1837; L, *dis*; Fr, *aise,* ease], a rare inherited skin disorder that begins in childhood and involves mainly exposed skin areas. Exposure to sunlight results in erythema and vesiculation, followed by increased pigmentation and telangiectasia, skin ulcers, warts, and, malignant epitheliomas. Also called **xeroderma pigmentosum.**

Kaposi's sarcoma (KS, ks) [Moritz J. Kaposi, Austrian dermatologist, b. 1837], a malignant, multifocal neoplasm of reticuloendothelial cells that begins as soft, brownish or purple papules on the feet and slowly spreads in the skin, metastasizing to the lymph nodes and viscera. It occurs most often in men and is occasionally associated with diabetes, malignant lymphoma, AIDS, or other disorders. Radiotherapy and chemotherapy are usually recommended. Also called **idiopathic multiple pigmented hemorrhagic sarcoma, multiple idiopathic hemorrhagic sarcoma.**

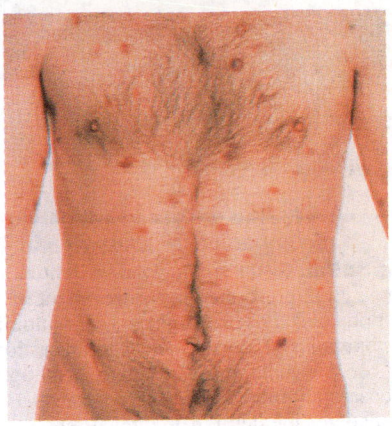

Kaposi's sarcoma (Wisdom, 1990)

Kaposi's varicelliform eruption. See **eczema herpeticum.**

kappa /kap'ə/, K, κ, tenth letter of the Greek alphabet.

kaps-. See **caps-.**

karaya powder /kär'äyä/ [Hindi, *karayal*, resin; L, *pulvis*, dust], a dried form of *Sterculia urens* or other species of *Sterculia*, used as a bulk cathartic. Like other bulk-forming agents, karaya powder reduces the intraluminal rectosigmoid pressure and helps relieve symptoms in patients with irritable bowel disease and diverticular disease of the colon. Relief of pain and other symptoms may occur progressively over several months. Because of its ability to absorb water and form an emollient intestinal mass, karaya powder also may be useful in relieving the symptoms of acute diarrhea, in modifying the effluent in the patient with an ileostomy or a colostomy, and in the care of skin surfaces around a stoma. The use of such a bulk-forming cathartic may also increase the loss of sodium, potassium, and water in such patients. With some individuals the use of karaya powder may cause allergic reactions, such as urticaria, rhinitis, dermatitis, and asthma. Methylcellulose has largely replaced this drug in modern use. Externally, it is used as a drying agent for stage I and stage II decubitus ulcers.

Kardex. a trademark for a card-filing system that allows quick reference to the particular needs of each patient for certain aspects of nursing care. Included on the card may be a schedule of medications, level of activity allowed, ability to perform basic self-care, diet, any special problems, a schedule of treatments and procedures, and a care plan. The Kardex is updated as necessary and is usually kept at the nurses' station.

Kartagener's syndrome /kärtag'ənərz/, an inherited disorder characterized by bronchiectasis, chronic paranasal sinusitis, and transposed viscera, usually dextrocardia.

karyenchyma. See **karyolymph.**

karyo- /ker'ē·ō-/, a combining form meaning 'of or pertaining to a nucleus': *karyochrome, karyokinesis, karyolymph.*

karyoclasis. See **karyoklasis.**

karyoclastic. See **karyoklasis.**

karyocyte /ker'ē·əsīt'/ [Gk, *karyon*, nut; *kytos*, cell], a normoblast, or developing red blood cell with a nucleus condensed into a homogenous staining body. It is normally found in the red bone marrow.

karyogamy /ker'ē·og'əmē/ [Gk, *karyon*, nut, *gamos*, marriage], the fusion of cell nuclei, as in conjugation and zygosis. **–karyogamic,** *adj.*

karyogenesis /ker'ē·ōjen'əsis/ [Gk, *karyon* + *genein*, to produce], the formation and development of the nucleus of a cell. **–karyogenetic,** *adj.*

karyokinesis /ker'ē·ōkinē'sis, -kīnē'sis/ [Gk, *karyon* + *kinesis*, motion], the division of the nucleus and equal distribution of nuclear material during mitosis and meiosis. The process involves the four stages of prophase, metaphase, anaphase, and telophase, and it precedes the division of the cytoplasm. Also called **karyomitosis.** See also **cytokinesis. –karyokinetic,** *adj.*

karyoklasis /ker'ē·ok'ləsis/ [Gk, *karyon* + *klasis*, breaking], **1.** the disintegration of the cell nucleus or nuclear membrane. **2.** the interruption of mitosis. Also spelled **karyoclasis. –karyoklastic, karyoclastic,** *adj.*

karyology /ker'ē·ol'əjē/ [Gk, *karyon* + *logos*, science], the branch of cytology that concentrates on the study of the cell nucleus, especially the structure and function of the chromosomes. **–karyologic, karyological,** *adj.,* **karyologist,** *n.*

karyolymph /ker'ē·əlimf'/ [Gk, *karyon* + *lympha*, water], the clear, usually nonstaining, fluid substance of the nucleus. It consists primarily of proteinaceous, colloidal material in which the nucleolus, chromatin, linin, and various submicroscopic particles are dispersed. Also called **karyenchyma, nuclear hyaloplasm, nuclear sap, nucleochyme. –karyolymphatic,** *adj.*

karyolysis /ker'ē·ol'isis/ [Gk, *karyon* + *lysis*, loosening], the dissolution of the cell nucleus. It occurs normally, both as a form of necrobiosis and during the generation of new cells through mitosis and meiosis.

karyolytic /ker'ē·əlit'ik/, **1.** of or pertaining to karyolysis. **2.** that which causes the destruction of the cell nucleus.

karyomere /ker'ē·əmir'/ [Gk, *karyon* + *meros*, part], **1.** a saclike structure containing an unequal portion of the nuclear material after atypical mitosis. **2.** a segment of the chromosome. See also **chromomere.**

karyometry /ker'ē·om'ətrē/, the measurement of the nucleus of a cell. **–karyometric,** *adj.*

karyomit /ker'ē·əmit'/ [Gk, *karyon* + *mitos*, thread], **1.** a single chromatin fibril of the network within the nucleus of a cell. **2.** a chromosome.

karyomitome /ker'ē·om'itōm/ [Gk, *karyon* + *mitos*, thread], the fibrillar chromatin network within the nucleus of a cell. Also called **karyoreticulum.**

karyomitosis. See **karyokinesis.**

karyomorphism /-môr'fizəm/ [Gk, *karyon* + *morphe*, form], the shape or form of a cell nucleus, especially that of the leukocyte. **–karyomorphic,** *adj.*

karyon /ker'ē·on/ [Gk, nucleus, nut], the nucleus of a cell. **–karyontic,** *adj.*

karyophage /ker'ē·ōfāj'/ [Gk, *karyon* + *phagein*, to eat], an intracellular protozoan parasite that destroys the nucleus of the cell it infects. **–karyophagic, karyophagous,** *adj.*

karyoplasm. See **nucleoplasm.**

karyoplasmic ratio. See **nucleocytoplasmic ratio.**

karyopyknosis /-piknō'sis/ [Gk, *karyon* + *pyknos*, thick], the state of a cell in which the nucleus has shrunk and the chromatin has condensed into solid masses, as in cornified cells of stratified squamous epithelium. **–karyopyknotic,** *adj.*

karyoreticulum. See **karyomitome.**

karyorrhexis /-rck′sis/ [Gk, *karyon* + *rhexis*, rupture], the fragmentation of chromatin and distribution of it throughout the cytoplasm as a result of nuclear disintegration. **–karyorrhectic,** *adj.*

karyosome /ker′ē·əsōm′/ [Gk, *karyon* + *soma*, body], a dense irregular mass of chromatin filaments in the cell nucleus. It is often seen during interphase and may be confused with the nucleolus because of similar staining properties. Also called **chromatin nucleolus, chromocenter, false nucleolus, prochromosome.**

karyospherical /-sfer′ikəl/ [Gk, *karyon* + *sphaira,* ball], **1.** of or pertaining to a nucleus that is spherical in shape. **2.** such a nucleus.

karyostasis /ker′ē·os′təsis/ [Gk, *karyon* + *stasis,* standing], the resting stage of the nucleus between cell division. See also **interphase. –karyostatic,** *adj.*

karyotheca /-thē′kə/ [Gk, *karyon* + *theke,* sheath], the membrane that encloses a cell nucleus. **–karyothecal,** *adj.*

karyotin. See **chromatin.**

karyotype /ker′ē·ətīp′/ [Gk, *karyon* + *typos,* mark], **1.** the total morphologic characteristics of the somatic chromosome complement of an individual or species, described in terms of number, form, size, and arrangement within the nucleus, as determined by a microphotograph taken during the metaphase stage of mitosis. **2.** a diagrammatic representation of the chromosome complement of an individual or species, arranged in pairs in descending order of size and according to the position of the centromere. See also **chromosome, Denver classification. –karyotypic,** *adj.*

osteoarthrosis afflicting mainly children living in China, Korea, and eastern Siberia. It is believed to be caused by eating foods made with wheat contaminated by a fungus, *Fusarium sporotrichiella.* Also spelled **Kaschin-Beck disease.** Also called **osteoarthritis deformans edemica.**

kat, abbreviation for **katal.**

kat-, kata-, cat-, cata-, a prefix meaning 'to go down, to go against, or to reverse': *katadidymus, katakinetomeric, katolysis.*

katadidymus /kat′ədid′əməs/ [Gk, *kata,* down, *didymos,* twin], conjoined twins that are united in the lower portion of the body and separated at the top.

katal (K, kat) /kat′al/ [Gk, *kata,* down], an enzyme unit in moles per second defined by the SI system: 1 K = 6.6 [ti] 109 U.

Kawasaki disease. See **mucocutaneous lymph node syndrome.**

Kay Ciel, a trademark for an electrolyte replacement solution (potassium chloride).

Kayser-Fleischer ring /kī′zərflī′shər/ [Bernhard Kayser, German ophthalmologist, b. 1869; Bruno Fleischer, German ophthalmologist, b. 1874], a gray-green to red-goldpigmented ring at the outer margin of the cornea, pathognomonic of hepatolenticular degeneration, a rare progressivedisease caused by a defect in copper metabolism and transmitted as an autosomal recessive trait. The disease is characterized by cerebral degenerative changes, liver cirrhosis, splenomegaly, involuntary movements, muscle rigidity, psychic disturbances, and dysphagia. See also **Wilson's disease.**

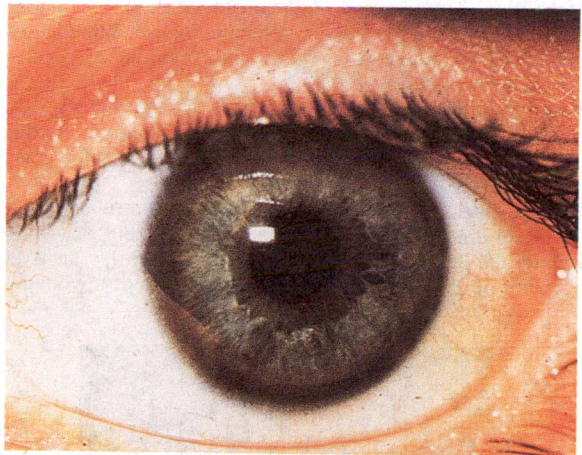

Kayser-Fleischer ring as seen in Wilson's disease
(Perkin, 1986)

Human karyotype
(Raven, 1992/Photo Researchers, Science Photo Library)

Kasabach method /kas′əbak/, (in radiology) a technique for positioning a patient for x-ray examination of the odontoid process.

Kasai operation. See **portoenterostomy.**

Kashin-Bek disease [Nikolai I. Kashin, Russian orthopedist, b. 1825; E.V. Bek; L, *dis,* Fr, *aise,* ease], a form of

Kazanjian's operation /kasan′jē·ənz/ [Varstad J. Kazanjian, American dentist and physician, b. 1879], a surgical procedure for extending the vestibular sulcus to improve prosthetic foundation of edentulous ridges.

kb, abbreviation for **kilobyte.**

kbe, abbreviation for *keyboard entry.*

kbs, abbreviation for *kilobits per second.*

kcal, abbreviation for **kilocalorie.**

K cell. See **null cell.**

kCi, abbreviation for *kiloCurie*.

ke, abbreviation for **kinetic energy.**

Kedani fever. See **scrub typhus.**

keel, (in prosthetics) a device in a stored-energy foot prosthesis that functions as a cantilever spring, bending the foot upward when weight is applied to the toe. See also **carina, Seattle Foot, stored-energy foot.**

kefir /kef'ər/ [Russ, fermented milk], a slightly effervescent, acidulous beverage prepared from the milk of cows, sheep, or goats through fermentation by kefir grains, which contain yeasts and lactobacilli. It is an important source of the bacteria necessary in the GI tract to synthesize vitamin K. Also spelled **kephir.**

Keflex, a trademark for an antibacterial (cephalexin).

Kefzol, a trademark for an antibacterial (cefazolin sodium).

Kegel exercises. See **pubococcygeus exercises.**

Keith-Flack node. See **sinoatrial node.**

Keith-Wegener-Barker classification system, a method of classifying the degree of hypertension in a patient on the basis of retinal changes. The stages are group 1, identified by constriction of the retinal arterioles; group 2, constriction and sclerosis of the retinal arterioles; group 3, characterized by hemorrhages and exudates in addition to group 2 conditions; and group 4, papilledema of the retinal arterioles.

kel-, a combining form meaning 'of or pertaining to a tumor or fibrous growth': *kelectome, keloid, keloplasty.*

Kellgren's syndrome /kel'grinz/ [Henry Kellgren, Swedish physician, b. 1827], a form of osteoarthritis affecting the proximal and distal interphalangeal joints, the first metatarsophalangeal and carpometacarpal joints, the knees, and the spine. The absence of rheumatoid factor and rheumatoid nodules and the lack of systemic involvement differentiate this syndrome from rheumatoid arthritis. Also called **erosive osteoarthritis.**

Kelly clamp [Howard A. Kelly, American gynecologist, b. 1858; AS *clam* to fasten], a curved hemostat without teeth, used primarily in gynecologic procedures for grasping vascular tissue.

Kelly's pad, a horseshoe-shaped, inflatable rubber drainage pad used in a bed or on the operating table.

keloid /kē'loid/ [Gk, *kelis*, spot, *eidos*, form], an overgrowth of collagenous scar tissue at the site of a wound of

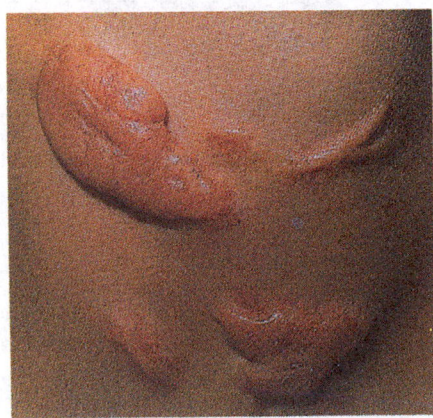

Keloids *(Zitelli, 1992)*

the skin. The new tissue is elevated, rounded, and firm, with irregular, clawlike margins. Young women and blacks are particularly susceptible to keloid formation. Most keloids flatten and become less noticeable over a period of years. Types of therapy include solid carbon dioxide, liquid nitrogen, intralesional corticosteroid injections, radiation, and surgery. Treatment may worsen the condition and should be performed only by skilled professionals. Also spelled **cheloid. –keloidal, cheloidal,** *adj.*

keloid acne [Gk, *kelis,* spot; *akme,* point], a chronic irritating skin eruption on the nape of the neck that begins as folliculitis and progresses through papulation to a condition of keloid plaques. Also called **dermatitis papillaris capillitii.**

-keloidal. See **keloid.**

keloidal scar. See **keloid scar.**

keloidosis /kē'loidō'sis/ [Gk, *kelis, eidos + osis,* condition], habitual or multiple formation of keloids. Also spelled **cheloidosis.**

keloid scar [Gk, *kelis,* spot; *eidos,* form; *eschara,* scab], an overgrowth of tissue in a scar at the site of skin injury, particularly a wound or a surgical incision. The amount of tissue growth is excessive for the need to repair the wound and is partially caused by an accumulation of collagen at the site. Also called **keloidal scar.**

kelp [ME, *culp*], **1.** any of the brown seaweeds species of *Laminaria* found on the Atlantic coast of Europe. **2.** the ashes of *Laminaria* seaweeds burned in a process of extracting iodine and potassium salts.

Kelvin scale (K) [Lord Kelvin (William Thomson), British physicist, b. 1824], an absolute temperature scale calculated in Celsius units from the point at which molecular activity apparently ceases, −273° C. To convert Celsius degrees to Kelvin, add 273.

Kemadrin, a trademark for an antiparkinsonian skeletal muscle relaxant (procyclidine hydrochloride).

Kempner rice-fruit diet. See **rice diet.**

Kenalog, a trademark for a glucocorticoid (triamcinolone acetonide).

Kennedy classification [Edward Kennedy, American dentist, b. 1883], a method of classifying edentulous conditions and partial dentures, based on the position of the spaces of the missing teeth in relation to the remaining teeth.

Kenny treatment. See **Sister Kenny's treatment.**

keno-, a combining form meaning 'empty': *kenophobia, kenotoxin, kenotron.*

kenogenesis. See **cenogenesis.**

kenophobia /kē'nōfō'bē·ə/ [Gk, *kenos,* empty, *phobos,* fear], the morbid fear of large and open spaces; agoraphobia. Also called **cenophobia** /sē'nō-/.

Kent bundle [Albert F. S. Kent, English physiologist, b. 1863; AS *byndel* to bind], an accessory pathway between atria and ventricles outside of the conduction system. This congenital anomaly causes Wolff-Parkinson-White syndrome. Compare **bundle of His.**

Kenya fever. See **Marseilles fever.**

kephal-. See **cephalo-.**

kephir. See **kefir.**

kera-, a combining form meaning 'horn': *keracele, keraphyllocele, keratosis, keratin.*

kerasin /ker'əsin/ [L, *cera,* wax], a cerebroside, found in brain tissue, that consists of a fatty acid, galactose, and sphingosine.

kerat-, kerato-,   **1.** a combining form meaning 'horny, cornified': *keratolysis, keratoma, keratonosis.* **2.** a combining form meaning 'cornea, corneal': *keratoiritis, keratoleukoma, keratome.*

keratectomy /ker'ətek'təmē/ [Gk, *keras* horn, *ektome* excision], surgical removal of a portion of the cornea, performed to excise a small, superficial lesion that does not warrant a corneal graft. Local anesthesia is used. The scar is excised, and an antibiotic is injected under the conjunctiva. A topical steroid is given, and a light pressure dressing is applied. Postoperatively, the dressings are changed daily. Corneal epithelium grows rapidly, filling a small surgical area in about 60 hours.

keratic /kərat'ik/ [Gk, *keras,* horn; L, *icus,* like], **1.** of or pertaining to keratin. **2.** of or pertaining to the cornea.

keratic precipitate, a group of inflammatory cells deposited on the endothelial surface of the cornea after trauma or inflammation, sometimes obscuring vision.

keratin /ker'ətin/ [Gk, *keras,* horn], a fibrous, sulfur-containing protein that is the primary component of the epidermis, hair, nails, enamel of the teeth, and horny tissue of animals. The protein is insoluble in most solvents and is not dissolved by the gastric juice. For this reason, it is often used as a coating for pills that must pass through the stomach unchanged in order to be dissolved in the intestines.

keratinization /-īzā'shən/ [Gk, *keras* + L, *izein,* to cause], a process by which epithelial cells exposed to the external environment lose their moisture and are replaced by horny tissue. **–keratinize** /ker'ətinīz/.

keratinocyte /kerat'inōsīt'/ [Gk, *keras* + *kytos,* cell], an epidermal cell that synthesizes keratin and other proteins and sterols. These cells constitute 95% of the epidermis, being formed as undifferentiated, or basal, cells at the dermal-epidermal junction. In its various successive stages keratin forms the prickle cell layer and the granular cell layer, in which the cells become flattened and slowly die to form the final layer, the stratum corneum, which gradually exfoliates.

keratitis /ker'ətī'tis/, any inflammation of the cornea. Kinds of keratitis include **dendritic keratitis, interstitial keratitis, keratoconjunctivitis sicca,** and **trachoma.** Compare **keratopathy. –keratic,** *adj.*

keratoacanthoma /ker'ətō·ak'antho[-]'mə/, *pl.* **keratoacanthomas, keratoacanthomata** [Gk, *keras* + *akantha,* thorn, *oma,* tumor], a benign, rapidly growing, flesh-colored papule of the skin with a central plug of keratin. The lesion is most common on the face or the back of the hands and arms. It disappears spontaneously in 4 to 6 months, leaving a slightly depressed scar. Biopsy is often necessary to differentiate it from a squamous carcinoma.

keratoconjunctivitis /ker'əto[-]kənjungk'tivī'tis/ [Gk, *keras* + L, *conjunctivus,* connecting; Gk, *itis*], inflammation of the cornea and the conjunctiva. Kinds of keratoconjunctivitis include **eczematous conjunctivitis, epidemic keratoconjunctivitis,** and **keratoconjunctivitis sicca.**

keratoconjunctivitis sicca, dryness of the cornea caused by a deficiency of tear secretion in which the corneal surface appears dull and rough, and the eye feels gritty and irritated. The condition may be associated with erythema multiforme, Sjögren's syndrome, trachoma, and vitamin A deficiency. Methylcellulose artificial tears may give some relief.

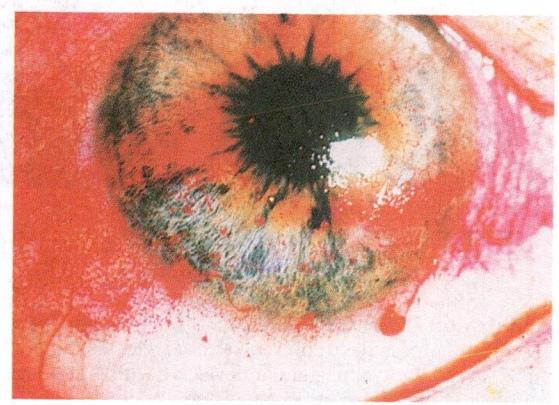

Keratoconjunctivitis sicca (Shipley, 1993)

keratoconus /ker'ətōkō'nəs/ [Gk, *keras* + *konos,* cone], a noninflammatory protrusion of the central part of the cornea. More common in females, it may cause marked astigmatism; contact lenses usually restore visual acuity. The cause of the condition is unknown.

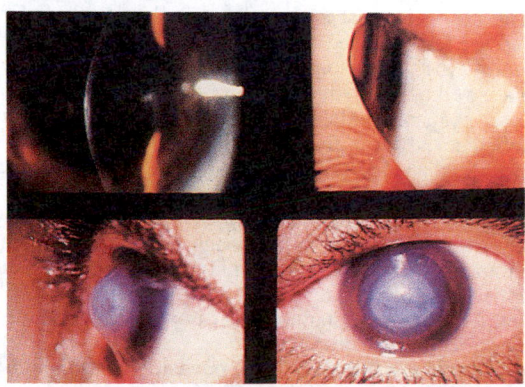

Keratoconus
(Apple, 1991)

Keratoacanthoma (Sharville, 1984)

keratoderma blennorrhagica /-dur′mə/,   the development of hyperkeratotic skin lesions of the palms, soles, and nails. The condition tends to occur in some patients with Reiter's syndrome.

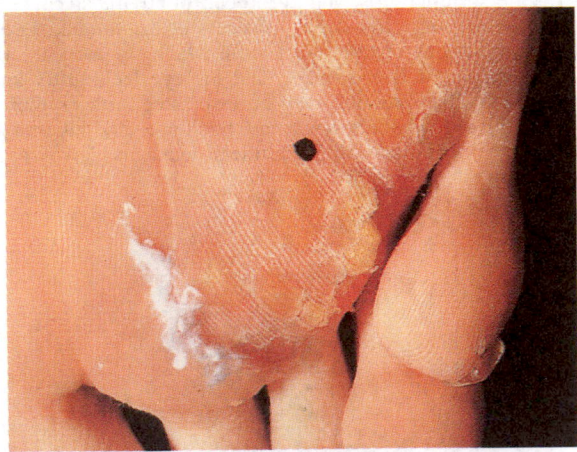

Keratoderma blennorrhagica (Schumacher, 1988)

keratohyalin /-hī′əlin/ [Gk, *keras* + *hyalos*, glass],   a substance in the granules found in keratinocytes of the epidermis. The keratohyalin granule develops within and around the fibrillar protein, contributing in an unknown manner to the functional maturity of keratin.

keratolysis /ker′ətol′sis/ [Gk, *keras* + *lysis*, loosening],   the loosening and shedding of the outer layer of the skin, which may occur normally by exfoliation or as a congenital condition in which the skin is shed at periodic intervals. **–keratolytic,** *adj.*

keratomalacia /-məlā′shə/ [Gk, *keras* + *malakia*, softness],   a condition, characterized by xerosis and ulceration of the cornea, resulting from severe vitamin A deficiency. It commonly occurs as a secondary result of diseases that affect vitamin A absorption or storage, such as ulcerative colitis, celiac syndrome, cystic fibrosis, or sprue. Also at risk are infants and children who are given dilute formula, who are malnourished, or who are allergic to whole milk and are fed skimmed milk, which is a poor source of vitamin A. Early symptoms include night blindness, photophobia, swelling and redness of the eyelids, and drying, roughness, pain, and wrinkling of the conjunctiva. In advanced deficiency, Bitot's spots appear, the cornea becomes dull, lusterless, and hazy, and, without adequate therapy, it eventually softens and perforates, resulting in blindness. Treatment consists of vitamin A supplements determined by the severity of the condition, although prolonged daily administration of large doses, especially to infants, may result in hypervitaminosis. An adequate diet containing whole milk and foods high in vitamin A or carotenes prevents the condition. See also **vitamin A.**

keratomycosis linguae.   See **parasitic glossitis.**

keratopathy /ker′ətop′əthē/ [Gk, *keras* + *pathos*, disease],   any noninflammatory disease of the cornea. Compare **keratitis.**

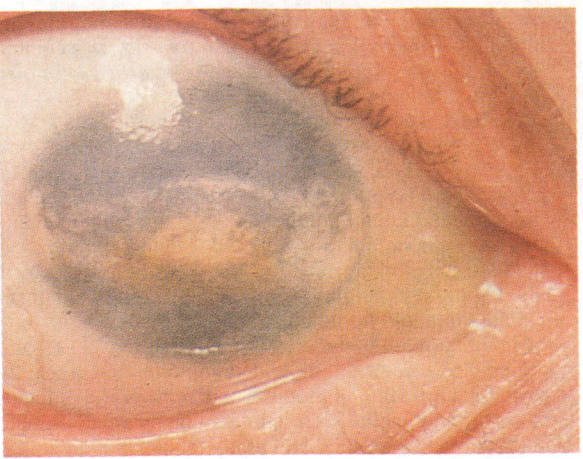

Band keratopathy (Shipley, 1993)

keratoplasty /ker′ətōplas′tē/ [Gk, *keras* + *plassein*, to mold],   a procedure in ophthalmologic surgery in which an opaque portion of the cornea is excised.

keratosis /ker′ətō′sis/ [Gk, *keras* + *osis*, condition],   any skin condition in which there is overgrowth and thickening of the cornified epithelium. Kinds of keratosis include **actinic keratosis, keratosis senilis,** and **seborrheic keratosis. –keratotic,** *adj.*

keratosis follicularis,   a name of several skin disorders characterized by keratotic papules that coalesce to form brown or black, crusted, wartlike patches. These vegetations may spread widely, ulcerate, and become covered with a purulent exudate. Treatment includes large doses of vitamin A orally, topical vitamin A acid cream, and oral or topical corticosteroids. Also called **Darier's disease.**

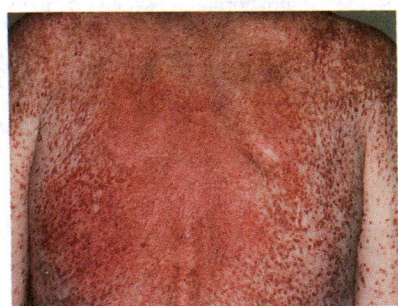

Keratosis follicularis
(Holgate, 1993/Courtesy Dr. Tony Ormerod)

keratosis seborrheica.   See **seborrheic keratosis.**

keratosis senilis.   See **keratosis.**

-keratotic.   See **keratosis.**

kerauno-,   a combining form meaning 'of or pertaining to lightning': *keraunoneurosis, keraunophobia.*

kerion /kir′ē·on/ [Gk, honeycomb],   an inflamed, boggy granuloma that develops as an immune reaction to a superficial fungus infection, generally in association with *Tinea capitis* of the scalp. The lesion heals within a short time without treatment.

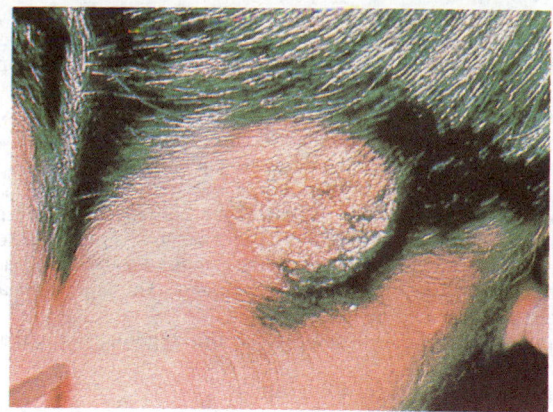

Kerion *(Hart, 1992)*

Kerley lines /kur′lē/, (in radiology) lines resembling interstitial infiltrate that appear on chest x-ray images and are associated with certain disease conditions. They are several centimeters in length and may be oriented in many directions. Kerley lines may occur with congestive heart failure and pleural lymphatic engorgement. Also called **everywhere lines.**

KERMA, abbreviation for *kinetic energy released in the medium,* a quantity that describes the transfer of energy from a photon to a medium as the ratio of energy transferred per unit mass at each point of interaction.

kernicterus /kərnik′tərəs/ [Ger, *Kern,* kernel; Gk, *ikteros,* jaundice], an abnormal toxic accumulation of bilirubin in central nervous system tissues caused by hyperbilirubinemia. See also **hyperbilirubinemia of the newborn.**

Kernig's sign /ker′niks/ [Vladimir M. Kernig, Russian physician, b. 1840], a diagnostic sign for meningitis marked by a loss of the ability of a seated or supine patient to completely extend the leg when the thigh is flexed on the abdomen. However, the patient usually can extend the leg completely when the thigh is not flexed on the abdomen.

kerosene poisoning /ker′əsēn/ [Gk, *keros,* wax; L, *potio,* drink], a toxic condition caused by the ingestion of kerosene or the inhalation of its fumes. Symptoms after ingestion include drowsiness, fever, a rapid heartbeat, tremors, and severe pneumonitis if the fluid is aspirated. Vomiting is not induced. Treatment for ingestion may include 1 or 2 ounces of vegetable oil to prevent absorption of the kerosene in the stomach and gastric lavage with copious amounts of water, a 3% sodium bicarbonate solution, or normal saline. Treatment for poisoning by inhalation includes fresh air, oxygen, and respiratory assistance if necessary. See also **petroleum distillate poisoning.**

Ketalar, a trademark for a general anesthetic (ketamine hydrochloride).

ketamine hydrochloride /kē′təmēn/, a nonbarbiturate general anesthetic administered parenterally to achieve dissociative anesthesia. Because ketamine hydrochloride does not cause muscle relaxation, intubation is usually not required. Ketamine hydrochloride is particularly useful for brief, minor surgical procedures and for the induction of inhalation anesthesia in pediatric, geriatric, and disturbed patients. Hallucinations, confusion, and disorientation may occur on emergence from anesthesia. Other potential disadvantages attending use of this drug include increased blood pressure, increased cerebrospinal fluid pressure, increased intracranial pressure, and a tendency toward potentiation of the effects of alcohol, barbiturates, and narcotics. See also **dissociative anesthesia.**

keto- /kē′tō-/, a combining form indicating possession of the carbonyl (:C:O) group: *ketoheptose, ketolysis, ketonuria.*

ketoacidosis /-as′idō′sis/ [Gk, *keton,* form of acetone; L, *acidus,* sour, *osis,* condition], acidosis accompanied by an accumulation of ketones in the body, resulting from faulty carbohydrate metabolism. It occurs primarily as a complication of diabetes mellitus and is characterized by a fruity odor of acetone on the breath, mental confusion, dyspnea, nausea, vomiting, dehydration, weight loss, and, if untreated, coma. Emergency treatment includes the administration of insulin and IV fluids and the evaluation and correction of electrolyte imbalance. Nasogastric intubation and bladder catheterization may be required if the patient is comatose. Before discharge of the patient from the hospital, the nurse carefully reviews the diet, activity, urine testing, and insulin schedule prescribed, emphasizing to the patient that ketoacidosis may be life threatening and is largely avoidable by strict adherence to the patient's prescribed diabetic regimen. See also **diabetes mellitus, ketosis. −ketoacidotic,** *adj.*

ketoaciduria /-as′idōōr′ē·ə/ [Gk, *keton* + L, *acidus,* sour; Gk, *ouron,* urine], presence in the urine of excessive amounts of ketone bodies, occurring as a result of uncontrolled diabetes mellitus, starvation, or any other metabolic condition in which fats are rapidly catabolized. The condition can be diagnosed with a dipstick reagent or acetone test tablet. Also called **ketonuria.** See also **Acetest, ketosis. −ketoaciduric,** *adj.*

11-ketoandrosterone /-andros′tərōn/, a sex hormone, secreted by the testes and adrenal glands, that may be measured in the urine to assess hormonal and adrenal functions. Normal amounts in the urine of men after 24-hour collection are 0.2 to 1 mg; in women, 0.2 to 0.8 mg.

ketoconazole /kō′nəzōl/, an antifungal agent.
■ INDICATIONS: It is prescribed for the treatment of candidosis, coccidioidomycosis, histoplasmosis, and other fungal diseases.
■ CONTRAINDICATIONS: Known hypersensitivity to this drug prohibits its use. It should not be used for fungal meningitis.
■ ADVERSE EFFECTS: The most serious adverse reactions are liver disorders.

11-ketoetiocholanolone /kē′tō·ē′tē·ōkəlan′əlōn/, a sex hormone, secreted by the testes and adrenal glands, that may be measured in the urine to assess hormonal and adrenal functions. Normal amounts in the urine of men after 24-hour collection are 0.2 to 1 mg; in women, 0.2 to 0.8 mg.

ketogenesis /-jen′əsis/ [Fr, *acétone;* Gk, *genein,* to produce], the formation or production of ketone bodies.

ketogenic diet /-jen′ik/, a diet that is high in fats and low in carbohydrates.

ketone /kē′tōn/ [Fr, *acétone*], an organic chemical compound characterized by having in its structure a carbonyl, or keto, group, $=CO$, attached to two alkyl groups. It is produced by oxidation of secondary alcohols.

ketone alcohol [Gk, *keton* + Ar, *alkohl,* essence], an alcohol containing the ketone group.

ketone bodies, the normal metabolic products, [Grk b]-hydroxybutyric acid and aminoacetic acid, from which acetone may arise spontaneously. The two acids are products of lipid pyruvate metabolism, via acetyl-CoA in the liver, and are oxidized by the muscles. Excessive production of these bodies leads to their excretion in urine, as in diabetes mellitus. Also called **acetone bodies.**

ketone group, the chemical carbonyl group with attached hydrocarbons.

ketonemia /kē′tōnē′mē·ə/, the presence of ketones, mainly acetone, in the blood. It is characterized by the fruity breath odor of ketoacidosis.

ketonuria. See **ketoaciduria.**

ketoprofen /-prō′fən/, a nonsteroidal antiinflammatory drug with analgesic and antipyretic actions.

■ INDICATIONS: It is prescribed for the treatment of rheumatoid and osteoarthritis and related conditions.

■ CONTRAINDICATIONS: Hypersensitivity to ketoprofen or to aspirin or other nonsteroidal antiinflammatory drugs prohibits its use.

■ ADVERSE EFFECTS: Among the more serious adverse reactions are GI disturbances, including peptic ulcer and GI bleeding, central nervous system effects of headache, dizziness, and drowsiness, and skin rash.

ketose /kē′tōs/ [Gk, *keton* + *glykys*, sweet], the chemical form of a monosaccharide in which the carbonyl group is a ketone.

ketosis /kitō′sis/ [Gk, *keton* + *glykys*, sweet, *osis*, condition], the abnormal accumulation of ketones in the body as a result of a deficiency or inadequate utilization of carbohydrates. Fatty acids are metabolized instead, and the end products, ketones, begin to accumulate. This condition is seen in starvation, occasionally in pregnancy, if the intake of protein and carbohydrates is inadequate, and, most frequently, in diabetes mellitus. It is characterized by ketonuria, loss of potassium in the urine, and a fruity odor of acetone on the breath. Untreated, ketosis may progress to ketoacidosis, coma, and death. See also **diabetes mellitus, ketoacidosis, starvation.** −**ketotic,** *adj.*

ketosis-prone diabetes. See **insulin-dependent diabetes mellitus.**

ketosis-resistant diabetes. See **non-insulin-dependent diabetes mellitus.**

17-ketosteroid /kētō′stəroid/, any of the adrenal cortical hormones, or ketosteroids, that has a ketone group attached to its seventeenth carbon atom, commonly measured in the blood and urine to aid the diagnoses of Addison's disease, Cushing's syndrome, stress, and endocrine problems associated with precocious puberty, feminization in men, and excessive hair growth. Measured in patients in the morning, the normal concentration in plasma is less than 30 [μg/dl; in the evening, less than 10 [μg/dl. The normal amounts in the urine of men after 24-hour collection are 8 to 15 mg; in women, 6 to 11.5 mg; in children 12 to 15 years of age, 5 to 12 mg; in children less than 12 years of age, less than 5 mg. Levels of 17-ketosteroids increase 50% to 100% after an injection of ACTH.

ketotic /kētot′ik/ [Fr, *acétone*], **1.** pertaining to the presence of ketone in the body. **2.** denoting the presence of a carbonyl group in a chemical compound.

keV, an abbreviation for *kiloelectron volts,* an energy unit equivalent to 1000 electron volts. Also **kev.**

Kew Gardens spotted fever. See **rickettsialpox.**

keyboard, a computer input device consisting of rows of switches with keytops marked as letters or numbers. Manual pressure on a series or combination of the keys generates an electronic code representing words, data, commands, or other input.

keypad, a numeric keyboard consisting of the numerals 1 to 9 arranged in three ranks of three keys each and an additional key for zero, as on some calculators.

key pinch. See **lateral pinch.**

key points of control, areas of the body that can be handled by a therapist in a specific manner to change an abnormal pattern, to reduce spasticity throughout the body, and to guide the patient's active movements. The key points are the shoulder and pelvic girdles.

key ridge, the lowest point of the zygomaticomaxillary ridge.

kg, abbreviation for **kilogram.**

kG, abbreviation for *kilogauss.*

kg cal, abbreviation for *kilogram calorie.* See **calorie.**

kHz, abbreviation for *kilohertz.*

kidney [ME, *kidnere*], one of a pair of bean-shaped urinary organs in the dorsal part of the abdomen, one on each side of the vertebral column. The cranial extremities of the kidneys are on a level with the cranial border of the twelfth thoracic vertebra, and the caudal extremities are on a level with the third lumbar vertebra. In most individuals, the right kidney is slightly more caudal (lower) than the left. Each kidney is about 11 cm long, 6 cm wide, and 2.5 cm thick. In men, each kidney weighs from 125 to 170 g; in women, each kidney weighs from 115 to 155 g. In the newborn, the kidneys are about three times as large in proportion to the body weight as in the adult. The kidneys produce and eliminate urine through a complex filtration network and reabsorption system comprising more than 2 million nephrons.

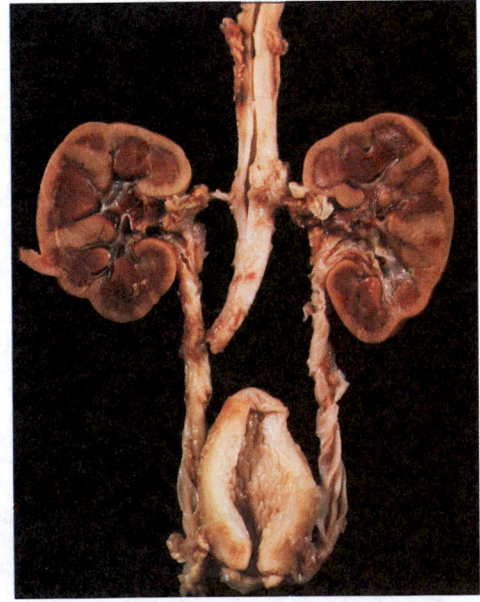

Normal kidney
(Brundage, 1992/Courtesy Department of Pathology, Duke University Medical Center, Durham, North Carolina)

The nephrons are composed of glomeruli and renal tubules that filter blood under high pressure, removing urea, salts, and other soluble wastes from blood plasma and returning the purified filtrate to the blood. More than 2500 pints of blood pass through the kidneys every day, entering the kidneys through the renal arteries and leaving through the renal veins. All the blood in the body passes through the kidneys about 20 times every hour but only about one fifth of the plasma is filtered by the nephrons during that period. The kidneys remove water as urine and return water that has been filtered to the blood plasma, thus helping to maintain the water balance of the body. Hormones, especially the antidiuretic hormone (ADH), produced by the pituitary gland, control the function of the kidneys in regulating the water content of the body. ADH reaches the renal tubules in the blood and stimulates the reabsorption of water from the filtrate into the blood. If water intake is inadequate to compensate for the water lost in perspiration and in respiration, the change in concentration in the blood is detected by the brain and the pituitary gland releases more ADH, thus reducing the loss of water in urine. If the blood is too dilute, the pituitary gland reduces the secretion of ADH, producing a large flow of dilute urine to restore the water balance.

kidney cancer, a malignant neoplasm of the renal parenchyma or renal pelvis. Factors associated with an increased incidence of disease are exposure to aromatic hydrocarbons or tobacco smoke and the use of drugs containing phenacetin. A long asymptomatic period may precede the onset of the characteristic symptoms, which include hematuria, flank pain, fever, and the detection of a palpable mass. Diagnostic measures include urinalysis, excretory urography, nephrotomography, ultrasonography, renal arteriography, and microscopic and cytologic studies of cells from the renal pelvis. Adenocarcinoma of the renal parenchyma accounts for 80% of kidney tumors, occurring twice as frequently in men as in women; transitional cell or squamous cell carcinomas in the renal pelvis account for approximately 15% and are equally frequent in men and women. Radical nephrectomy with lymph node dissection is usually recommended for tumors of the parenchyma; nephroureterectomy is usually recommended for operable tumors of the renal pelvis. Radiotherapy may be used preoperatively or postoperatively and as palliation for inoperable tumors. Chemotherapeutic agents that may induce temporary remission are cyclophosphamide, bleomycin, hydroxyurea, and vinblastine. See also **Wilms' tumor.**

kidney dialysis. See **hemodialysis.**

kidney disease, any one of a large group of conditions including infectious, inflammatory, obstructive, vascular, and neoplastic disorders of the kidney. Characteristics of kidney disease are hematuria, persistent proteinuria, pyuria, edema, dysuria, and pain in the flank. Specific symptoms vary with the type of disorder. For example: Hematuria with severe, colicky pain suggests obstruction by a kidney stone; hematuria without pain may indicate renal carcinoma; proteinuria is generally a sign of disease in the glomerulus, or filtration unit of the kidney; pyuria indicates infectious disease; and edema is characteristic of the nephrotic syndrome. Diagnosis of kidney disease is made after laboratory tests and other procedures have been performed. Among the special tests for kidney disorders are excretory urography, intravenous pyelography, tests of the glomerular filtration rate, biopsy, and ultrasound examination. Treatment de-

pends upon the type of kidney disease diagnosed. Some forms of advanced kidney disease may lead to renal failure, coma, and death unless hemodialysis is started. See also **glomerulonephritis, nephrotic syndrome, renal failure, urinary calculus.**

kidney failure, *informal.* **renal failure.**

kidney machine. See **artificial kidney, dialyzer,** def. 1.

kidney stone. See **renal calculus.**

Kielland forceps. See **obstetric forceps.**

Kielland rotation /kē′land/ [Christian Kielland, Norwegian obstetrician, b. 1871], an obstetric operation in which Kielland forceps are used in turning the head of the fetus from an occiput posterior or occiput transverse position to an occiput anterior position. It is performed most commonly to correct an arrest in the active stage of labor. The rotation is done at the midplane of the pelvis. As it is associated with increased harm to the mother and to the baby, cesarean section is often preferred. See also **forceps delivery, obstetric forceps.**

Kiesselbach's plexus /kē′səlbäkhs′, -bäks′/, a convergence of small, fragile arteries and veins located superficially on the anterosuperior portion of the nasal septum.

killed vaccine [ME, *killen*; L, *vaccinus*, of a cow], a vaccine prepared from dead microorganisms. Killed vaccines are generally used to provide immunization from organisms that are too virulent to be used in the living attenuated state. The immune system reacts to the presence of the pathogen in the same manner, whether the organism is live or dead. However, immunity produced by a live, attenuated vaccine, when possible, is usually more effective.

killer cell. See **null cell.**

kilo- /kil′ə-/, a prefix meaning 'one thousand': *kilocalorie, kilogram, kilometer.*

kilobyte (K, Kb) /-bīt/, one thousand (or, more precisely, 1024) bytes.

kilocalorie /-kal′ərē/ [Gk, *chilioi*, thousand; L, *calor*, heat], a unit of heat equal to 1,000 small calories (c) or 4,186 joules. Also called **large calorie (C).**

kilogram (kg) /-gram/ /kil′əgram/ [Gk, *chilioi*, thousand; Fr, *gramme*], a unit for the measurement of mass in the metric system. One kilogram is equal to 1000 grams or to 2.2046 pounds avoirdupois.

kilogram calorie. See **calorie.**

kilohertz (kHz) /-hurts/ [Gk, *chilioi*, thousand; *hertz*; Heinrich Rudolf Hertz, German physicist b. 1857], 1000 hertz cycles per second.

kiloliter (kL) /lē′tər/ [Gk, *chilioi*, thousand; Fr, *litre*], unit of volume equivalent to 1057 quarts, 1000 liters. Also spelled **kilolitre.**

kilometer (km) /-mē′tər/ [Gk, *chilioi*, thousand; *metron*], measure equivalent to 39.37 inches, 1000 meters (about 0.62 miles).

kilovolt (kv) /-volt/ [Gk, *chilioi*, thousand; Count Alessandro Volta, Italian scientist, b. 1745], measure of electrical potential, 1000 volts.

kilovolt peak (kVp), a measure of the maximum electrical potential in kilovolts across an x-ray tube. Most x-ray machines are operated at maximum voltages ranging from 40 to 150 kVp and at tube currents of 25 to 1200 milliamperes (mA). X-ray equipment is usually operated at the minimum kVp, mA, and exposure time necessary for an examination.

Kimmelstiel-Wilson disease. See **intercapillary glomerulosclerosis.**

kinase /kī′nās/ [Gk, *kinesis*, motion, (ase), enzyme],   **1.** an enzyme that catalyzes the transfer of a phosphate group or another high-energy molecular group to an acceptor molecule. Each of these kinases is named for its receptor, such as acetate kinase, fructokinase, or hexokinase. **2.** an enzyme that activates a preenzyme (zymogen). Each of these kinases is named for its source, such as bacterial kinase, enterokinase, fibrinokinase, insulin kinase, staphylokinase, streptokinase, streptokinase-streptodornase, or urokinase.

kind firmness,   (in psychology) a direct, clear, and confident approach to a patient in which rules and regulations are calmly cited in response to infractions and requests.

kine-.   See **kinesio-.**

kinematic face-bow /kin′əmat′ik/,   an adjustable caliper-like device, used for precisely locating the axis of rotation of a mandible through the sagittal plane.

kinematics /kin′əmat′iks, kī-′/ [Gk, *kinema*, motion],   (in physiology) the geometry of the motion of the body without regard to the forces acting to produce the motion. Kinematics deals with the description and the measurement of body motion and the means of recording it. Recordings of body motions are defined in one-plane relationships, although natural motions of the body often occur in more than one plane. Kinematics considers the motions of all body parts relative to the segments of the part involved in the motion and not necessarily in relation to the standard anatomic position; for example, the movements of the fingers are considered in relation to the midline of the hand, not the midline of the body. The most common types of motions studied in kinematics are flexion, extension, adduction, abduction, internal rotation, and external rotation. Kinematics is especially important in orthopedics and rehabilitation medicine. Also called **cinematics.** Compare **kinetics.**

kinesia /kīnē′zhə/ [Gk, *kinein*, to move],   any feeling of nausea caused by the sensation of motion, as in sea sickness or car sickness. Also called **cinesia** /sīnē′zhə/.

-kinesia,   a suffix meaning 'pertaining to movement': *hypekinesia.*

kinesic behavior /kīnē′sik/,   nonverbal cues of communication that function to achieve and maintain bonds of attachments between people.

kinesics /kīnē′siks/ [Gk, *kinesis*, motion],   the study of body position and movement in relation to communication. The observance of nonverbal interactional behavior is an integral part of nursing assessment and is used especially in mental health assessment as an objective and measurable tool for diagnosing disturbances of communication and behavioral disorders. See also **body language, communication.**

kinesio-, kine-,   a combining form meaning 'pertaining to movement': *kinesiology, kinesioneurosis, kinesiotherapy.*

kinesiologic electromyography /kinē′sē·oloj′ik/,   the study of muscle activity involved in body movements.

kinesiology /-ol′əjē/ [Gk, *kinesis* + *logos*, science],   the scientific study of muscular activity and of the anatomy, physiology, and mechanics of the movement of body parts.

-kinesis, -cinesia, -cinesis, -kinesia,   a suffix meaning an 'activation': *angiokinesis, lymphokinesis, thrombokinesis.*

kinesthesia /kin′esthē′zhə/ [Gk, *kinein*, to move, *aisthesis*, feeling],   the perception of one's own body parts, weight, and movement.

kinesthetic memory /kin′esthet′ik/,   the recollection of movement, weight, resistance, and position of the body or parts of the body.

kinesthetic sense [Gk, *kinesis*, movement; L, *sentire*, to feel],   an ability to be aware of muscular movement and position. By providing information through receptors about muscles, tendons, joints, and other body parts, the kinesthetic sense helps control and coordinate such activities as walking and talking.

-kinetic, -cinetic, -cinetical, -kinetical,   a suffix meaning 'pertaining to movement': *akinetic, parakinetic, synkinetic.*

kinetic analysis /kinet′ik/,   analysis in which the change of the monitored parameter with time is related to concentration, such as change of absorbance per minute.

kinetic energy (ke) [Gk, *kinesis*, movement; *energeia*],   the energy possessed by an object by virtue of its motion. It is expressed by the formula $E = 1/2mv^2$, where *m* represents the mass of the object and **v** is its velocity.

kinetic hallucination [Gk, *kinesis*, movement; L, *allucinari*, a wandering mind],   a false perception of body movement.

kinetic reflex [Gk, *kinesis*, movement; L, *reflectere*, to bend back],   a postural response resulting from stimulation of the vestibular apparatus. Also called **labyrinthine reflex.**

kinetics /kinet′iks/ [Gk, *kinesis* + L, *icus*, like],   (in physiology) the study of the forces that produce, arrest, or modify the motions of the body. Newton's first and third laws of inertia are especially applicable to kinetics. Newton's first law states that bodies at rest tend to stay at rest and bodies in motion tend to keep moving. Newton's third law states that action and reaction are equal in magnitude but opposite in direction. These two laws are applicable to the forces produced by muscles of the body that act on joints. The reaction forces of the muscles contribute to the equilibrium and the motion of the body. Compare **kinematics.**

kineto-,   a combining form meaning 'movable': *kinetochore, kinetogenic, kinetoplasm.*

kinetochore.   See **centromere.**

kinetotherapeutic bath /kinet′ōthur′əpyo̅o̅′tik/ [Gk, *kinesis* + *therapeutike*, medical practice; AS, *baeth*],   a bath in which underwater exercises are performed to strengthen weak or partially paralyzed muscles.

kin group,   family members who are related genetically or by marriage.

kinky hair disease [Du, *kink*, short twist, AS, *haer*, L, *dis*, Fr, *aise*, ease],   an inherited condition characterized by short, sparse, poorly pigmented hair with shafts that are twisted and broken. Other mental and physical disorders are usually associated with the disease.

kino-, kinesi/o-, [Gk, *kinein*, to move],   combining forms meaning 'related to movement': *kinematics, kinesiology, hyperkinesia.*

kinomere.   See **centromere.**

kinship model family group,   a family unit comprising the biologic parents and their offspring. It is like a nuclear family but is more closely tied to an extended family. Characteristics of this family group include dominance by the maternal grandmother, who raises the children and makes most of the decisions, clearly delineated sex roles, and resistance to change.

Kirkland knife [Olin Kirkland, American dentist, b. 1876; AS *cnif*],   a surgical knife with a heart-shaped blade, sharp on all edges, used for a primary gingivectomy incision.

Kirklin staging system,   a system for determining the prognosis of colon cancer, based on the extent to which the tumor has penetrated the bowel area. See also **cancer staging, Dukes' classification, TNM.**

Kirschner's wire /kursh'nərz/ [Martin Kirschner, German surgeon, b. 1879; AS, *wir*], a threaded or smooth metallic wire available in three diameters and 22.86 cm long. The wire is used in internal fixation of fractures or for skeletal traction.

Kite method, (in radiology) a technique for positioning the leg of a patient with congenital clubfoot for x-ray examination.

kiting /kī'ting/, *informal.* the improper and illegal practice of altering a drug prescription to indicate that more of a drug was prescribed than was actually ordered by the physician. Kiting may be done by a patient seeking greater quantities of drugs, especially narcotics, than the physician prescribed, or may be done by the pharmacist to increase reimbursement from a third party, such as an insurance company.

KJ, abbreviation for *knee jerk.*

kL, abbreviation for **kiloliter.**

klang association. See **clang association.**

Klebsiella /kleb'zē·el'ə/ [Theodore A. E. Klebs, German bacteriologist, b. 1834], a genus of diplococcal bacteria that appear as small, plump rods with rounded ends. Several respiratory diseases, including bronchitis, sinusitis, and some forms of pneumonia, are caused by infection by species of *Klebsiella*.

Klebsiella pneumonia [Theodore Albrecht Edwin Klebs, German bacteriologist, b. 1834; Gk, *pneumon*, lung], a species of bacteria, also called Friedländer's bacillus, found in soil, water, cereal grains, and the intestinal tract of humans and other animals. It is associated with several pathologic conditions, including pneumonia.

Klebs-Loeffler bacillus /klebz'lef'lər/ [Theodore A. E. Klebs; Friederich A. J. Loeffler, German bacteriologist, b. 1852; L, *bacillum*, small rod], *Corynebacterium diphtheriae.*

kleeblattschädel deformity syndrome. See **cloverleaf skull deformity.**

Kleine-Levin syndrome /klīn'lev'in/ [Willi Kleine, 20th century German psychiatrist; Max Levin, Russian-born American neurologist, b. 1901], a disorder of unknown cause often associated with psychotic conditions, characterized by episodic somnolence, abnormal hunger, and hyperactivity. The episodes of sleep may last for several hours or days and are followed by confusion on awakening. There is no specific treatment. Compare **narcolepsy.**

klepto-, a prefix meaning 'of or pertaining to theft or stealing': *kleptolagnia, kleptomania.*

kleptolagnia /klep'tōlag'nē·ə/ [Gk, *kleptein*, to steal, *lagneia*, lust], sexual excitement or gratification produced by stealing.

kleptomania /-mā'nē·ə/ [Gk, *kleptein*, to steal, *mania*, madness], a neurosis characterized by an abnormal, uncontrollable, and recurrent urge to steal. The objects, taken not for their monetary value, immediate need, or utility but because of a symbolic meaning usually associated with some unconscious emotional conflict, are usually given away, returned surreptitiously, or kept and hidden. People who have the condition experience an increased sense of tension before committing the theft and intense gratification during the act. Afterward, they display signs of depression, guilt, and anxiety over the possibility of being apprehended and losing status in society. In less severe cases, the impulse is expressed by the continuous borrowing of objects and not re-

turning them. Treatment consists of psychotherapy to uncover the underlying emotional problems. Also spelled **cleptomania. –kleptomaniac,** *n.*

Klinefelter's syndrome /klīn'feltərz/ [Harry F. Klinefelter, American physician, b. 1912], a syndrome of gonadal defects, appearing in males, with an extra X chromosome in at least one cell line. Characteristics are small, firm testes, long legs, gynecomastia, poor social adaptation, subnormal intelligence, chronic pulmonary disease, and varicose veins. The severity of the abnormalities increases with greater numbers of X chromosomes. The most common abnormality is a 47 XXY karyotype. Men with the karyotype XXXXY have marked congenital malformations and mental retardation.

Klippel-Feil syndrome /klipel'fel', klip'əlfīl'/ [Maurice Klippel, French neurologist, b. 1858; Andre Feil, French neurologist, b. 1884], a condition of short neck and limited neck movements because of congenital fusion of the cervical vertebrae. Also called **Klippel-Feil disease, Klippel-Feil malformation.** See **congenital short neck syndrome.**

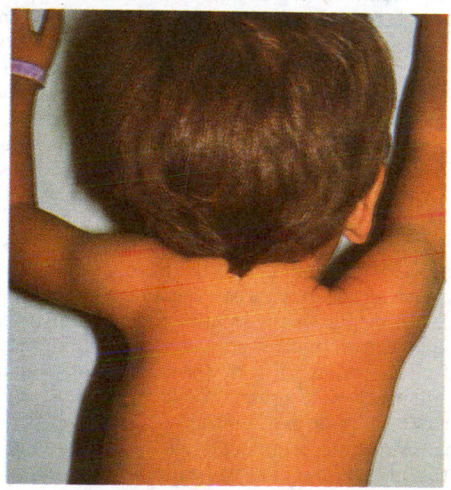

Klippel-Feil syndrome (Zitelli, 1992)

Kloehn cervical extraoral orthodontic appliance, a cervical extraoral traction appliance for correcting or improving malocclusion. It consists of a relatively light and flexible 0.045 inch (1.15 mm) inner arch rigidly attached to a long outer bow.

Klonopin, a trademark for an anticonvulsant (clonazepam).

Klor, a trademark for an electrolyte replacement solution (potassium chloride).

Klorvess, a trademark for an electrolyte replenisher (potassium chloride).

Klumpke's palsy /klŏŏmp'kēz/, atrophic paralysis of the forearm. It is present at birth and involves the seventh and eighth cervical nerves and the first thoracic nerve. The condition may be accompanied by Horner's syndrome, ptosis, and miosis because of involvement of sympathetic nerves. Also called **Dejerine-Klumpke's paralysis.**

K-Lyte/Cl, a trademark for an electrolyte replacement solution (potassium chloride).

km, abbreviation for **kilometer.**

kneading /nē'ding/ [AS, *cnedan*], a grasping, rolling, and pressing movement, as is used in massaging the muscles. See also **massage.**

knee /nē/ [AS, *cneow*], a joint complex that connects the thigh with the lower leg. It consists of three condyloid joints, 12 ligaments, 13 bursae, and the patella. Two of the condyloid joints constituting the knee are between the condyles of the femur and the corresponding menisci and condyles of the tibia. The third condyloid joint within the knee is a partially arthrodial joint between the patella and the femur. The motion of this joint is not a simple gliding motion, because the articular surfaces of the bones involved are not mutually adapted to each other. The ligaments of the knee include the articular capsule, the patellar ligament, the oblique popliteal ligament, the arcuate popliteal ligament, the tibial collateral ligament, the fibular collateral ligament, the anterior cruciate ligament, the posterior cruciate ligament, the medial and the lateral menisci, the transverse ligament, and the coronary ligament. Four of the bursae of the knee are located in front, four laterally, and five medially. The largest bursa is the prepatellar bursa between the patellar ligament and the skin. The painful condition 'housemaid's knee' is caused by inflammation of the prepatellar bursa. The knee is relatively unprotected by surrounding muscles and is often injured by blows, sudden stops, and turns, especially those associated with sports. Ligamental tears of the knee joint are extremely common in athletes and produce a variety of signs and symptoms, such as effusion surrounding the knee joint, varying degrees of edema, differences in the shape of the knee joint, tenderness on palpation, crepitation, instability of the knee joint, and possible ecchymosis. Radiographic examination may reveal varying degrees of displacement from ligamental tears, but the primary ligamentous injuries are not visible on x-ray films. Ligamental tears are a form of sprain and are treated according to the degree of trauma. Mild tears involving only a few fibers usually do not require any treatment and heal with time. Moderate ligamental tears require protective treatment, with rest essential to healing. Aspiration of ex-

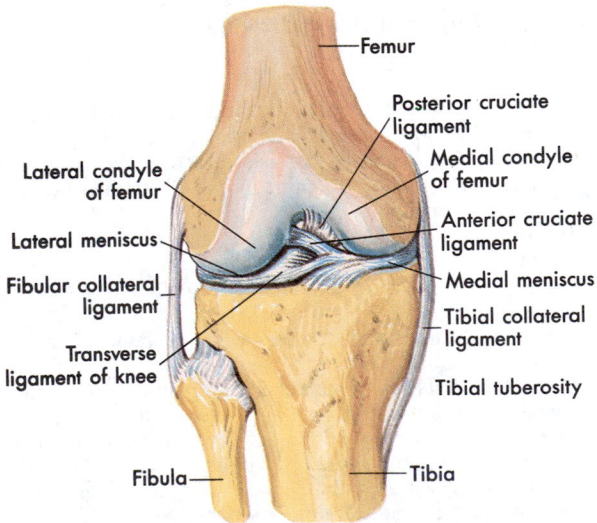

Knee joint (Thibodeau, 1993/Ernest W Beck)

cessive joint fluid and compression of the joint may be performed to control swelling. Sports injuries of this kind are commonly taped in a special way or treated with splints. Surgical intervention is often necessary to repair severe ligamentous tears, and postoperative exercises are prescribed to strengthen knee structures. Torn menisci are very common sports injuries and can cause severe pain, limping, edema, and greatly reduced motion. Surgical intervention, such as a meniscectomy, may be required. Various orthopedic conditions, such as arthritis, commonly affect the knee, especially in elderly individuals, and require continuing treatment and special maintenance.

knee-ankle interaction, one of the five major kinetic determinants of gait, which helps to minimize the displacement of the center of gravity of the body during the walking cycle. The knee and the foot work simultaneously to lower the center of gravity of the body. When the heel of the foot is in contact with the ground, the foot is dorsiflexed and the knee is fully extended so that the associated limb is at its maximum length with the center of gravity at its lower point. Plantar flexion of the foot with the initiation of knee flexion maintains the center of gravity in its forward progression at about the same level, also helping to minimize the vertical displacement of the center of gravity. Knee-ankle interaction is often a factor in the diagnosis and treatment of various orthopedic diseases, deformities, and abnormal conditions, and in the analysis and the correction of pathologic gaits. Compare **knee-hip flexion, lateral pelvic displacement, pelvic rotation, pelvic tilt.**

kneecap. See **patella.**

knee-chest position. See **genupectoral position.**

knee-elbow position [AS, *cneow, elboga*], a position in which a patient being examined rests on the knees and elbows with the head supported on the hands.

knee-hip flexion, one of the five major kinematic determinants of gait, which allows the passage of body weight over the supporting extremity during the walking cycle. Knee-hip flexion occurs during the stance and the swing phases of the cycle. The knee first locks into extension as the heel of the weight-bearing limb strikes the ground and is unlocked by final flexion and initiation of the swing phase in the walking cycle. Hip flexion is synchronized with these movements, which help to minimize the vertical displacement of the center of gravity of the body in the act of walking. Knee-hip flexion is often a factor in the diagnosis and treatment of various orthopedic diseases, deformities, and abnormal conditions and in the analysis and correction of pathologic gaits. Compare **knee-ankle interaction, lateral pelvic displacement, pelvic rotation, pelvic tilt.**

knee-jerk reflex. See **patellar reflex.**

knee joint, the complex, hinged joint at the knee, regarded as three articulations in one, comprising condyloid joints connecting the femur and the tibia and a partly arthrodial joint connecting the patella and the femur. The knee joint and its ligaments permit flexion, extension, and, in certain positions, medial and lateral rotation. It is a common site for sprain and dislocation. Also called **articulatio genus.**

knee replacement, the surgical insertion of a hinged prosthesis, performed to relieve pain and restore motion to a knee severely affected by osteoarthritis, rheumatoid arthritis, or trauma. Under inhalation anesthesia, the diseased surfaces are removed and a two-piece metallic hinge is cemented into the medullary cavities of the femur and tibia. Postoperatively, the knee is held in a position of maximum extension, usually with a plaster cast. Progressive exercise and whirlpool baths are prescribed through physical therapy. Possible complications include infection, fat embolism, peroneal nerve palsy, loosening of the prosthesis, and flexion contractures. To prevent contractures, the nurse cautions the patient to keep the leg extended in bed; a blanket roll along the femur prevents external rotation. The mobility and range of motion of the joint increase slowly. See also **arthroplasty, hip replacement, osteoarthritis, plastic surgery.**

knee sling, a leg support in sling form used under the knee for Russell's traction.

knife needle /nīf/ [AS, *cnif; naedl*], a slender surgical knife with a needle point, used in the discission of a cataract and in other ophthalmic procedures, such as goniotomy and goniopuncture.

knock-knee. See **genu valgum.**

Knoop hardness test /nŏop/ [Frederick Knoop, 20th century American metallurgist], a method of measuring surface hardness by resistance to the penetration of an indenting tool made of diamond. The test produces a diamond-shaped indentation in the material involved and is commonly used for testing the hardness of tooth structure.

knot /not/ [AS, *cnotta*], (in surgery) the interlacing of the ends of a ligature or suture so that they remain in place without slipping or becoming detached. The ends of the suture are passed twice around each other before being pulled taut to make a simple surgeon's knot. For additional stability, the ends may be recrossed and a second simple knot made over the first. There are many kinds of knots, some of which are interlocking.

knowledge deficit /nol'ij/, a nursing diagnosis accepted by the Fourth National Conference on the Classification of Nursing Diagnoses. It is defined as a state in which specific information is lacking. The defining characteristics include verbalization by the person that the deficit exists, or that there is a misconception concerning the information, an observed failure on the part of the client to follow through on instructions, the observation of an inadequate performance by the client on a test, a request by the person for information, or the observation of inappropriate or exaggerated behavior on the part of the client. Related factors include a lack of exposure to information, a lack of ability to recall the information, a misinterpretation of the information, a cognitive or perceptual limitation in the ability to learn or to understand the information, a lack of interest in acquiring the information, or an unfamiliarity with the resources necessary to gain the information. See also **nursing diagnosis.**

Kocher's forceps /kō'kərz/ [Emil T. Kocher, Swiss surgeon, b. 1841], a kind of surgical forceps that has notched jaws, interlocking teeth, and thick, curved or straight, powerful handles.

Koch's bacillus /kōks/ [Robert Koch, German bacteriologist, b. 1843; L, *bacillum*, small rod], the *Mycobacterium tuberculosis* microorganism.

Koch's phenomenon [Robert Koch; Gk, *phainomenon*, anything seen], a tuberculin reaction that occurs when a culture of tubercle bacilli is injected into subjects already infected with the disease. In humans, a positive tuberculin reaction indicates sensitization resulting from a tuberculosis infection. Also called **Koch's reaction.**

Koch's postulates [Robert Koch, German bacteriologist, b. 1843; L, *postulare*, to demand], the prerequisites for establishing that a specific microorganism causes a particular disease. The conditions are the following: (1) the microor-

ganism must be observed in all cases of the disease; (2) the microorganism must be isolated and grown in pure culture; (3) microorganisms from the pure culture, when inoculated into a susceptible animal, must reproduce the disease; (4) the microorganism must be observed in and recovered from the experimentally diseased animal.

Koch's reaction. See **Koch's phenomenon.**

Koebner phenomenon /kōb'nər/ [Heinrich Koebner, Polish dermatologist, b. 1838; Gk, *phainomenon*, something observed], the development of isomorphic lesions at the site of an injury occurring in psoriasis, lichen nitidus, lichen planus, and verruca plana.

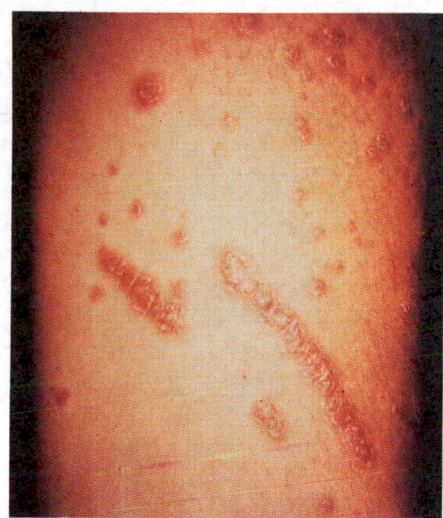

Koebner phenomenon *(Zitelli, 1992)*

KOH, chemical symbol for **potassium hydroxide.**

Kohnstamm's phenomenon. See **aftermovement.**

koilo-, a combining form meaning 'hollow or concave': *koilonychia, koilorrhachic, koilosternia.*

koilonychia /koi'lōnik'ē·ə/ [Gk, *koilos*, hollow, *onyx*, nail], spoon nails; a condition in which nails are thin and con-

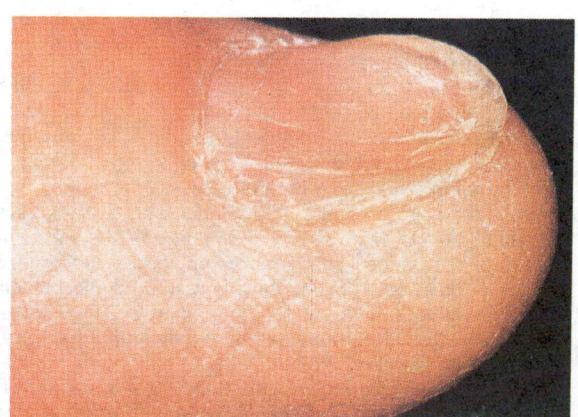

Koilonychia *(Baran, 1991)*

cave from side to side. It is usually familial but may occur with iron deficiency anemia and Raynaud's phenomenon.

koinoni-, a combining form meaning 'of or pertaining to a community': *koinonia, koinoniphobia.*

kolpo-. See **colpo-.**

koly-, a combining form meaning 'to hinder': *kolypeptic, kolyphrenia, kolyseptic.*

kon-, a combining form meaning 'of or pertaining to dust': *konometer, koniocortex.*

Konakion, a trademark for a vitamin K formulation (phytonadione).

Kopan's needle /kō'pənz/, a long biopsy needle used to locate the position of a breast tumor on x-ray film. The needle is inserted into the approximate location of the tumor and is left in place during radiography so that it can be repositioned if necessary. In some cases the site is further identified for the surgeon by injecting a colored dye, such as methylene blue.

Koplik's spots /kop'liks/ [Henry Koplik, American pediatrician, b. 1858], small red spots with bluish white centers on the lingual and buccal mucosa, characteristic of measles. The rash of measles usually erupts a day or two after the appearance of Koplik's spots.

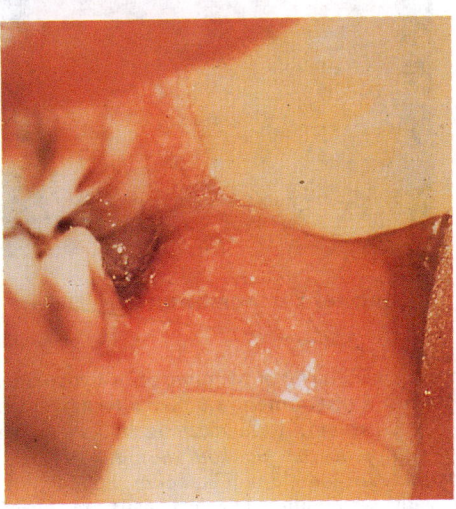

Koplick's spots (Zitelli, 1992)

kopr-, kopra-. See **copro-.**

Koranyi's sign /kôr'ənyēz/ [Friedrich von Korányi, Hungarian physician, b. 1828; L, *signum*], a paravertebral area of dullness found posteriorly on the side opposite a pleural effusion. Also called **Grocco's sign, Korányi-Grocco triangle, triangular dullness.**

Korotkoff sounds /kôrot'kôf/ [Nickolai Korotkoff, Russian physician, b. 1874], sounds heard during the taking of blood pressure using a sphygmomanometer and stethoscope. As air is released from the cuff, pressure on the brachial artery is reduced, and the blood is heard pulsing through the vessel. See also **blood pressure, diastole, sphygmomanometer, systole.**

Korsakoff's psychosis /kôr'səkôfs/ [Sergei S. Korsakoff, Russian psychiatrist, b. 1854], a form of amnesia often seen in chronic alcoholics, characterized by a loss of short-

term memory and an inability to learn new skills. The person is usually disoriented, may present with delirium and hallucinations, and confabulates to conceal the condition. The cause of the condition can often be traced to degenerative changes in the thalamus as a result of a deficiency of B complex vitamins, especially thiamine and B_{12}. Compare **Wernicke's encephalopathy.**

kosher [Heb, *kasher,* fit or proper], pertaining to the preparation and serving of foods according to Jewish dietary laws. Inherently kosher foods include common fruits, vegetables, and cereals, as well as tea and coffee. Foods that are not kosher include pork, birds of prey, and seafood that lacks fins and scales, such as lobster and eels. Some not inherently kosher foods can become kosher if properly processed; they include most domestic poultry and meat products, excluding pork.

Kr, symbol for the element **krypton.**

Krabbe's disease. See **galactosyl ceramide lipidosis.**

Kraske position /kras'kə/ [Paul Kraske, Swiss surgeon, b. 1851], an anatomic position in which the patient is prone, with hips flexed and elevated, head and feet down. The position is used for renal surgery, as it enlarges the costovertebral angle, allowing the surgeon to have optimal access to the kidneys.

kraurosis /krôrō'sis/ [Gk, *krauros,* dry, *osis,* condition], a thickening and shriveling of the skin. See also **kraurosis vulvae.**

kraurosis vulvae, a skin disease of aged women characterized by dryness, itching, and atrophy of the external genitalia. It is a condition that exhibits a predisposition to leukoplakia and carcinoma of the vulva. See also **lichen sclerosis et atrophicus.**

Krause's corpuscles/ [Wilhelm J. F. Krause, German anatomist, b. 1833; L, *corpusculum,* little body], a number of sensory end organs in the conjunctiva of the eye, mucous membranes of the lips and tongue, epineurium of nerve trunks, the penis, and the clitoris, and the synovial membranes of certain joints. Krause's corpuscles are tiny cylindric oval bodies with a capsule formed by the expansion of the connective tissue sheath of a medullated fiber. They contain a soft, semifluid core in which the axon terminates either in a bulbous extremity or in a coiled mass. Also called **end bulbs of Krause.** Compare **Golgi-Mazzoni corpuscles, Pacini's corpuscles.**

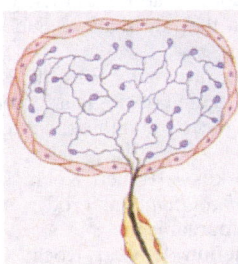

Krause's corpuscles (Thibodeau, 1993/Rolin Graphics)

Krause's membrane. See **z disk.**

Krebs' cycle /krebz/ [Hans A. Krebs, English biochemist, b. 1900; Gk, *kitron,* citron; L, *acidus,* sour; Gk, *kyklos,* circle], a sequence of enzymatic reactions involving the metabolism of carbon chains of sugars, fatty acids, and amino acids to yield carbon dioxide, water, and high-energy phosphate bonds. The cycle is initiated when pyruvate combines with coenzyme A (CoA) to form a two-carbon unit, acetyl-CoA, which enters the cycle by combining with four-carbon oxaloacetic acid to form six-carbon citric acid. In subsequent steps isocitric acid, produced from citric acid, is oxidized to oxalosuccinic acid, which loses carbon dioxide to form alpha-ketoglutaric acid. Succinic acid, resulting from the oxidative decarboxylation of alpha-ketoglutaric acid, is oxidized to fumaric acid, and its oxidation regenerates oxaloacetic acid, which condenses with acetyl-CoA, closing the cycle. The Krebs' cycle provides a major source of adenosine triphosphate energy and also produces intermediate molecules that are starting points for a number of vital metabolic pathways including amino acid synthesis. Also called **citric acid cycle, tricarboxylic acid cycle.** See also **acetylcoenzyme A.**

Krebs-Henseleit cycle. See **urea cycle.**

Krukenberg's tumor /kroo'kənbərgz/ [Georg P. H. Krukenberg, German gynecologist, b. 1856], a neoplasm of the ovary that is a metastasis of a GI malignancy, usually stomach cancer. Cytologic examination reveals mucoid degeneration and many large cells shaped like signet rings. Also called **carcinoma mucocellulare.**

krypto-. See **crypto-.**

krypton (Kr) /krip'ton/, a generally inert rare gaseous element present in air. Its atomic number is 36; its atomic weight is 83.80.

KS, ks abbreviation for Kaposi's sarcoma.

KUB, abbreviation for *kidney, ureter, and bladder,* a term used in a radiographic examination to determine the location and size of the kidneys.

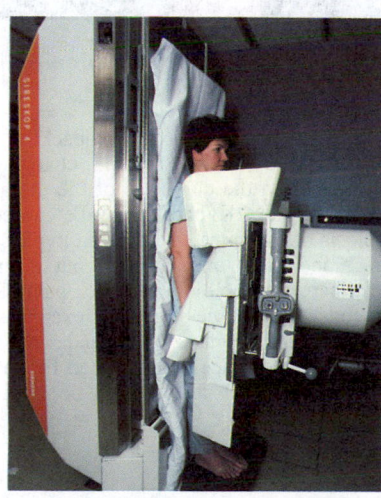

KUB equipment *(Brundage, 1992)*

Kuchendorf method /koo'kəndôrf/ (in radiology) a technique for positioning a patient for radiography of the patella.

Kufs' disease /koofs/ [H. Kufs, German psychiatrist, b. 1871; L, *dis,* Fr, *aise,* ease], an adult form of hereditary

cerebral sphingolipidosis (amaurotic familial idiocy), characterized by cerebromacular degeneration, hypertonicity, and progressive spastic paralysis. Also called **adult ceroid lipofuscinosis.**

Kulchitsky cell carcinoma. See **carcinoid.**

Kulchitsky's cell. See **argentaffin cell.**

Kümmell's disease /kim'əlz/ [Hermann Kümmell, German surgeon, b. 1852; L, *dis;* Fr, *aise,* ease], a set of symptoms that develop after a compression fracture of the vertebrae. They include spinal pain, intercostal neuralgia, kyphosis, and weakness in the legs. Also called **Kummell's spondylitis, posttraumatic spondylitis, traumatic spondylopathy.**

Küntscher nail /koon'chər, kin'chər/ [Gerhard Küntscher, German surgeon, b. 1902; AS, *naegel*], a stainless steel nail used in orthopedic surgery for the fixation of fractures of the long bones, especially the femur. Also called **Küntscher intramedullary nail.**

Kupffer's cells /koop'fərz/ [Karl W. von Kupffer, German anatomist, b. 1829], specialized cells of the reticuloendothelial system lining the sinusoids of the liver. The function of Kupffer's cells is to filter bacteria and other small, foreign proteins out of the blood.

Kurchatovium (Ku). See **element 104.**

kuru /koo'roo/ [New Guinea, trembling], a slow, progressive, fatal infection of the central nervous system seen only in natives of the New Guinea highlands. The incubation period may be 30 or more years, but death usually occurs within months of the onset of symptoms. Characteristic of kuru are ataxia and decreased coordination progressing to paralysis, dementia, slurring of speech, and visual disturbances. Transmission of the disease is probably the result of cannibalism, as brain tissue from infected people produces the disease when inoculated in primates in the laboratory and incidence of the disease has declined with the decline of cannibalism.

Kussmaul breathing /koos'moul/ [Adolf Kussmaul, French physician, b. 1822; AS, *braeth*], abnormally deep, very rapid sighing respirations characteristic of diabetic ketoacidosis (DKA).

Kussmaul's coma [Adolf Kussmaul, German physician, b. 1822; Gk, *koma,* deep sleep], a diabetic coma characterized by acidosis and deep breathing or extreme hypernea.

Kussmaul's sign [Adolf Kussmaul; L, *signum,* mark], **1.** a paradoxical rise in venous pressure with distention of the jugular veins during inspiration, as seen in constrictive pericarditis or mediastinal tumor. **2.** conditions of convulsions and coma associated with a GI disorder caused by absorption of a toxic substance.

kv, abbreviation for **kilovolt.**

Kveim reaction [Morton A. Kveim, Norwegian physician, b. 1892; L, *re,* again, *agere,* to act], a reaction used in a diagnostic test for sarcoidosis, based on an intradermal injection of antigen derived from a lymph node known to be sarcoid. If a noncaseating granuloma appears on the skin at the test site in 4 to 8 weeks, the reaction is said to be positive evidence that the patient has sarcoidosis.

kVp, abbreviation for **kilovolt peak.**

kVp test cassette, (in radiology) a cassette containing a copper filter, a series of stepwedges, and an optical attenuator, used to test the accuracy of kVp settings for peak electrical potential across an x-ray tube.

kwashiorkor /kwä'shē·ôr'kôr/ [Afr], a malnutrition disease, primarily of children, caused by severe protein defi-

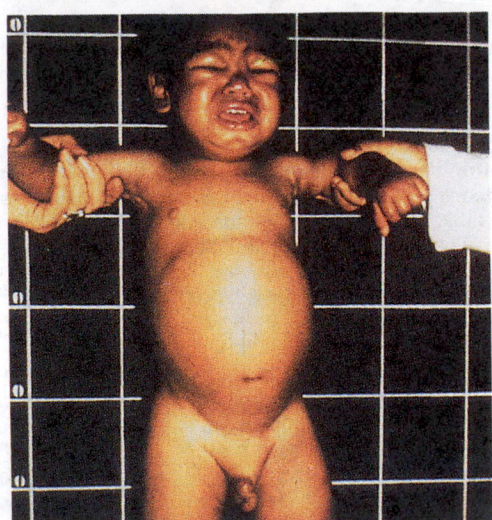

Kwashiorkor (Zitelli, 1992)

ciency, usually occurring when the child is weaned from the breast. Because calorie-rich starches like breadfruit are available, the child does not lose weight as dramatically and does not look as sick as a marasmic child, who lacks protein and calories. Eventually the following symptoms occur: retarded growth, changes in skin and hair pigmentation, diarrhea, loss of appetite, nervous irritability, edema, anemia, fatty degeneration of the liver, necrosis, dermatoses, and fibrosis, often accompanied by infection and multivitamin deficiencies. Because dietary fats are poorly tolerated in kwashiorkor, a skimmed milk formula is used in initial feedings, followed by additional foods until a full, well-balanced diet is achieved. Also called **infantile pellagra, malignant malnutrition.** See also **marasmic kwashiorkor, marasmus.**

Kwell, a trademark for a pediculicide and scabicide (gamma benzene hexachloride).

Kyasanur Forest disease, an arbovirus infection transmitted by the bite of a tick that is harbored by shrews and other forest animals in western tropical India. Characteristics of the infection include fever, headache, muscle ache, cough, abdominal and eye pain, and photophobia. Treatment is symptomatic.

kymo-, a combining form meaning 'of or pertaining to waves': *kymograph, kymoscope, kymotrichous.*

kymography /kēmog′rəfē/ [Gk, *kyma,* wave, *graphein,* to record], a technique for graphically recording motions of body organs, as of the heart and the great blood vessels.

kyno-, a combining form meaning 'of or pertaining to dogs': *kynocephalus, kynophobia.*

kypho-, a combining form meaning 'of or pertaining to a hump': *kyphoscoliosis, kyphosis, kyphotone.*

kyphos /kī′fəs/ [Gk, *kyphos,* hunchbacked], the hump in the thoracic vertebral column that is associated with kyphosis.

kyphoscoliosis /kī′fōskō′lē·ō′sis/ [Gk, *kyphos,* hunchbacked, *skolios* curved, *osis* condition], an abnormal condition characterized by an anteroposterior curvature and a lateral curvature of the spine. It occurs in children and adults, often associated with cor pulmonale. Compare **kyphosis, scoliosis.** —**kyphoscoliotic,** *adj.*

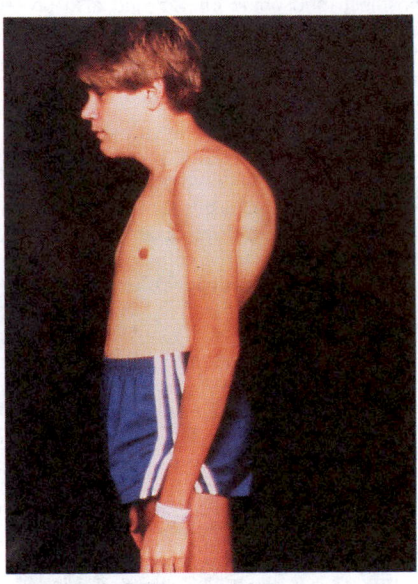

Severe kyphosis of thoracic spine (Zitelli, 1992)

kyphosis /kīfō′sis/ [Gk, *kyphos,* hunchbacked], an abnormal condition of the vertebral column, characterized by increased convexity in the curvature of the thoracic spine as viewed from the side. Kyphosis may be caused by rickets or tuberculosis of the spine. Adolescent kyphosis is usually self-limiting and often undiagnosed, but if the curvature progresses, there may be moderate back pain. Conservative treatment consists of spine-stretching exercises and sleeping without a pillow, with a board under the mattress. A modified Milwaukee brace may be used for severe kyphosis, and, rarely, spinal fusion may be required. —**kyphotic,** *adj.*

kysth-, kystho-. See **colpo-.**

kyto-. See **cyt-.**

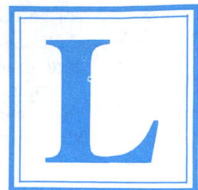

L, 1. symbol for *kinetic potential*. **2.** abbreviation for *Lactobacillus*. **3.** symbol for *lambert*. **4.** abbreviation for *Latin*. **5.** symbol for *liter*. **6.** abbreviation for **lung.**

La, symbol for the element **lanthanum.**

LA, abbreviation for *left atrium*.

L & A, abbreviation for *reaction of the pupil to light accommodation*.

lab, abbreviation for **laboratory.**

label [ME, band], **1.** a substance with a special affinity for an organ, tissue, cell, or microorganism in which it may become deposited and fixed. **2.** the process of depositing and fixing a substance in an organ, tissue, cell, or microorganism. **3.** an atom or molecule attached to either a ligand or binding protein and capable of generating a signal for monitoring in the binding reaction. **4.** the process of attaching a radio isotope to a compound for the purpose of tracing it during a physiological action in the body.

labeled compound, a chemical substance in which part of the molecules are labeled with a radionuclide so that observations of the radioactivity or isotopic composition make it possible to follow the compound or its fragments through physical, chemical, or biologic processes.

labeling, 1. the providing of information on a drug, food, device, or cosmetic to the purchaser or user. The information may be in any one of various forms, including printing on a carton, adhesive label, package insert, and monograph. Regulations for labeling are provided by the Food and Drug Administration. The label must contain directions for use, unless such directions are exempted by regulation, as well as warnings or contraindications. It must not contain false or misleading information. **2.** the assignment of a word or term to a form of behavior. **3.** the act of classifying a patient according to a diagnostic category. Labeling can be misleading because not all cases conform to defined characteristics of standard diagnostic categories.

la belle indifference /lä bel eNdifäräNs'/[Fr, nice indifference], an air of unconcern displayed by some patients toward their physical symptoms. It is believed the physical symptoms may relieve anxiety and result in secondary gains in the form of sympathy or attention.

labetalol hydrochloride /ləbet'əlol/, an antihypertensive drug.

■ INDICATIONS: It is prescribed for the treatment of hypertension.

■ CONTRAINDICATIONS: The presence of asthma or emphysema prohibits its use. It should be used with caution in patients with diabetes as it may mask symptoms of hypoglycemia, particularly tachycardia.

■ ADVERSE EFFECTS: Among the most serious adverse reactions are orthostatic hypotension, fatigue, headache, skin rashes, scalp paresthesia, nausea, vomiting, and constipation.

labia /lā'bē·ə/ *sing.* **labium** [L, lip], **1.** the lips; the fleshy, liplike edges of an organ or tissue. **2.** the folds of skin at the opening of the vagina.

-labial, a combining form meaning 'of or pertaining to lips': *alveololabial, glossolabial, maxillolabial*.

labial bar /lā'bē·əl/, a major connector that is installed labial or buccal to the dental arch and joins bilateral parts of a mandibular removable partial denture.

labial flange, the part of a denture flange that occupies the labial vestibule of the mouth.

labial glands [L, *labium*, lip; *glans*, acorn], small mucous or serous glands embedded in the lips.

labial notch, a depression in the denture border that accommodates the labial frenum.

labia majora /major'ə/, *sing.* **labium majus** /mā'jəs/, two long lips of skin, one on each side of the vaginal orifice outside the labia minora. They extend from the anterior labial commissure to the posterior labial commissure and form the lateral boundaries of the pudendal cleft. Each labium contains areolar tissue, fat, and a thin layer of nonstriated muscle. In some women the outer surface of each lip may be covered with coarse pubic hair. The embryologic derivations of the labia majora and the scrotum are homologous.

labia minora /minôr'ə/, *sing.* **labium minus** /mē'nəs/, two folds of skin between the labia majora, extending from the clitoris backward on both sides of the vaginal orifice, ending between it and the labia majora. Anteriorly, each labium divides into an upper and a lower division. The upper divisions pass above the clitoris and meet to form the preputium clitoridis; the lower divisions pass beneath the clitoris and unite to form the frenulum of the clitoris. Opposed surfaces of the labia minora contain sebaceous follicles.

labile /lā'bil/ [L, *loðilis*, slipping], **1.** unstable; characterized by a tendency to change or to be altered or modified. **2.** (in psychiatry) characterized by rapidly shifting or changing emotions, as in bipolar disorder and certain types of schizophrenia; emotionally unstable. **–lability,** *n.*

-labile, a combining form meaning 'unstable, subject to change': *frigolabile, siccolabile, thixolabile*.

-lability. See **labile.**

labio-, a combining form meaning 'of or pertaining to the lips, particularly the lips of the mouth': *labiocervical, labiodental, labiomental*.

labiodental /lā'bē·ōden'təl/ [L, *labium*, lip; *dens*, tooth], **1.** pertaining to the labial surfaces of the 12 anterior teeth. **2.** in speech therapy, sounds of speech that require a special coordination of teeth and lips.

labioglossolaryngeal paralysis. See **bulbar paralysis.**

labiolingual fixed orthodontic appliance /lā'bē·ō·ling'gwəl/ [L, *labium*, lip, *lingua*, tongue], an orthodontic appliance for correcting or improving malocclusion, characterized by anchorage to the maxillary and mandibular first permanent molars and by labial and lingual arches 0.09 to 0.10 cm in diameter. The labial arches fit into horizontal buccal tubes attached to anchor bands. The lingual arches are fastened to the lingual side of the anchor bands.

labium.   See **labia.**

labium majus.   See **labia majora.**

labium minus.   See **labia minora.**

labor [L, work],   the time and the processes that occur during parturition from the beginning of cervical dilatation to the delivery of the placenta. See also **birth, cardinal movements of labor, station.**

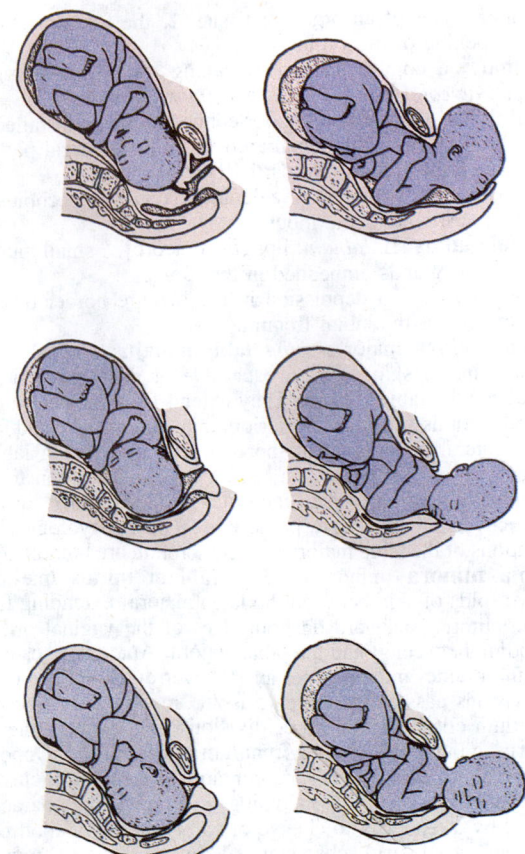

Mechanisms of labor, engagement and descent, flexion, internal rotation, extension, external rotation beginning, external rotation
(Bobak, 1993)

labor, abnormal.   See **dystocia.**

laboratory (lab) /lab′(ə)rətôr′e/ [L, *laborare,* to labor], **1.** a facility, room, building, or part of a building in which scientific research, experimentation, testing, or other investigative activities are carried out. **2.** of or pertaining to a laboratory.

laboratory core.   See **core.**

laboratory diagnosis,   a diagnosis arrived at after study of secretions, excretions, or tissue through chemical, microscopic, or bacteriologic means or by biopsy. See also **diagnosis.**

laboratory error,   any error made by the personnel in a clinical laboratory in the performance of a test, in the inter-

pretation of the data, or in reporting or recording the results. Laboratory error must always be considered a possible explanation for findings that are at variance with the composite clinical condition of the patient or that are widely divergent from previous laboratory tests.

laboratory medicine,   the branch of medicine in which specimens of tissue, fluid, or other body substance are examined outside of the person, usually in the laboratory. Some fields of laboratory medicine are **chemistry, cytology, hematology, histology,** and **pathology.**

laboratory test,   a procedure, usually conducted in a laboratory, that is intended to detect, identify, or quantify one or more significant substances, evaluate organ functions, or establish the nature of a condition or disease. Laboratory tests range from quite simple to extremely sophisticated. In modern medical practice, they are commonly used to help establish or confirm a diagnosis and often aid in the management of disease.

labor coach,   a person who assists a woman in labor and delivery by closely attending to her emotional needs and by encouraging her to use properly the breathing patterns, concentration techniques, body positions, and massage techniques that were taught in a program of psychophysical preparation for childbirth. The task of a labor coach is to minimize the need for pharmacologic pain relief used to decrease or eliminate the use of analgesia or anesthesia. Usually, the coach is the father of the baby or a close friend of the mother, but a professional labor coach, often a registered nurse specially trained in a method, may fill the role. See also **monitrice.**

labored breathing,   abnormal respiration characterized by evidence of increased effort, including use of the accessory muscles of respiration of the chest wall, stridor, grunting, or nasal flaring.

labor pains [L, *labor,* work + *poena,* penalty],   pain associated with contraction of the uterus in labor.

labyrinth-,   a combining form meaning 'pertaining to the labyrinth or inner ear': *labyrinthitis, labyrinthectomy.*

labyrinth.   See **internal ear.**

labyrinthine /lab′ərin′thin/ [Gk, *labyrinthos,* maze],   pertaining to or resembling a labyrinth or maze, such as the structure of the inner ear.

labyrinthine reflex.   See **kinetic reflex.**

labyrinthine righting,   one of the five basic neuromuscular reactions involved in a change of body positions. The change stimulates cells in the semicircular canals of the inner ear causing neck muscle to respond by automatically adjusting the head to the new position.

labyrinthitis /lab′ərinthī′tis/ [Gk, *labyrinthos,* maze, *itis*],   inflammation of the labyrinthine canals of the inner ear, resulting in vertigo.

labyrinthus osseus.   See **osseous labyrinth.**

laceration /las′ərā′shən/ [L, *lacerare,* to tear to pieces],   **1.** the act of tearing or lacerating. **2.** a torn, jagged wound. **–lacerate,** *v.,* **lacerated,** *adj.*

laceration of cervix [L, *lacerare,* to tear; *cervix,* neck],   a wound or irregular tear of the cervix uteri during childbirth.

laceration of the perineum [L, *lacerare,* to tear; Gk, *perineos*],   a wound or irregular tear of the perineal tissues during childbirth.

lachrymal.   See **lacrimal.**

lachrymation.   See **lacrimation.**

lacri-, lachry-,   a combining form meaning 'of or pertaining to tears': *lacrimalin, lacrimator, lacrimotomy.*

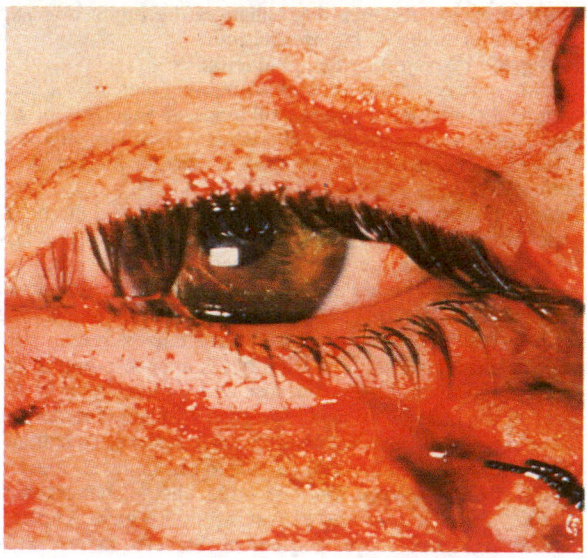

Laceration of the eye (Bedford, 1986)

lacrimal /lak'riməl/ [L, *lacrima*, tear], of or pertaining to tears. Also spelled **lachrymal.**

lacrimal apparatus, a network of structures of the eye that secrete tears and drain them from the surface of the eyeball. These parts include the lacrimal glands, the lacrimal ducts, the lacrimal sacs, and the nasolacrimal ducts.

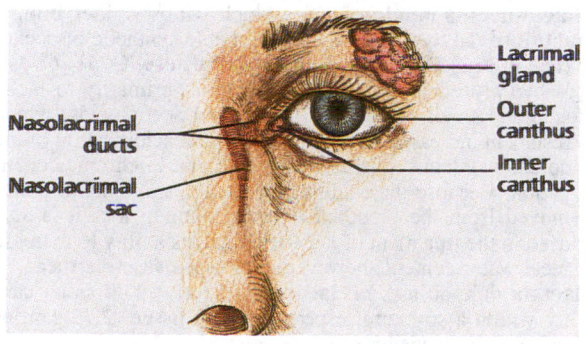

Lacrimal apparatus (Potter, 1993)

lacrimal bone, one of the smallest and most fragile bones of the face, located at the anterior part of the medial wall of the orbit. It unites with the maxilla to form the lacrimal fossa, which contains the lacrimal duct.

lacrimal canaliculus. See **lacrimal duct.**

lacrimal caruncle, the small, reddish, fleshy protuberance that fills the triangular space between the medial margins of the upper and the lower eyelids. It contains sebaceous and sudoriferous glands and secretes a whitish substance that collects in the corner of the eye.

lacrimal duct, either one of the two channels through which tears pass from the lacrimal lake to the lacrimal sac of each eye. Also called **lacrimal canaliculus.**

lacrimal fold [L, *lacrima*, tear; AS, *fealdan*], a valvelike fold of mucous membrane at the lower part of the nasolacrimal duct. Also called **Hasner's fold.**

lacrimal gland, one of a pair of glands situated superior and lateral to the eye bulb in the lacrimal fossa. It is an oval structure about the size of an almond and is divided into an orbital part and a palpebral part. The orbital part is connected to the periosteum of the orbit by a few fibrous bands and rests on the tendons of the recti superioris and the recti lateralis, which separate the gland from the eye bulb. The palpebral part is separated from the orbital part by a fibrous septum and projects into the back portion of the upper eyelid. The gland has about 10 ducts that run obliquely beneath the conjunctiva and open along the upper and lateral half of the superior conjunctival fornix. The watery secretion from the gland consists of the tears, slightly alkaline and saline, that moisten the conjunctiva.

lacrimal papilla, the small conic elevation on the medial margin of each eyelid, supporting an apex pierced by the punctum lacrimale through which tears emerge to moisten the conjunctiva.

lacrimal reflex [L, *lacrima*, tear; *reflectere*, to bend back], a release of tears in response to stimulation or irritation of the corneal conjunctiva.

lacrimal sac, the dilated end of each of the two nasolacrimal ducts. Each sac is lodged in a deep groove formed by the lacrimal bone and the frontal process of the maxilla. The sac is ovoid and about 13 mm long. Its upper end is closed and rounded, its lower end continuous with the nasolacrimal duct. The lacrimal sacs fill with tears secreted by the lacrimal glands and conveyed through the lacrimal ducts.

lacrimation /lak'rimā'shən/, **1.** the normal continuous secretion of tears by the lacrimal glands. **2.** an excessive amount of tear production, as in crying or weeping. Also spelled **lachrymation.**

lact-. See **lacto-.**

lactalbumin /lak'təlbyo̅o̅'min/ [L, *lac*, milk, *albus*, white], a simple, highly nutritious protein found in milk. It is similar to serum albumin. See also **albumin, serum albumin.**

lactam /lak'təm/, a cyclic amide created by the elimination of a molecule of water from aminocarboxylic acid. Also spelled **lactim.**

lactase /lak'tās/ [L, *lac* + Fr, *diastase*, enzyme], an enzyme that catalyzes the hydrolysis of lactose to glucose and galactose. Lactase is concentrated in the kidney, liver, and intestinal mucosa. Also called **beta-galactosidase.**

lactase deficiency, an inherited abnormality in which the amount of the digestive enzyme lactase is deficient, resulting in the inability to digest lactose, except for the bacterial breakdown of lactose in the large intestine. The deficiency occurs in infancy in severe form and persists throughout life. In adults, a relative deficiency may appear as a natural process of aging; it occurs more frequently in persons of Asiatic and African heritage. A lactase deficiency may result from subtotal gastrectomy, any disease of the small intestine in which structural changes occur, such as tropical sprue, ulcerative colitis, infectious hepatitis, and kwashiorkor, from malnutrition, or from some types of antibiotic therapy. Also called **alactasia** /al'əktā'zhə/. See also **lactose intolerance.**

lactate /lak'tāt/, a salt of lactic acid.

lactate dehydrogenase (LDH), an enzyme that is found in the cytoplasm of almost all body tissues, where its main function is to catalyze the oxidation of L-lactate to pyruvate. It is assayed as a measure of anaerobic carbohydrate metabolism and as one of several serum indicators of myocardial infarction and muscular dystrophies. Serum levels of LDH usually rise 12 to 18 hours after myocardial cell necrosis. See also **CPK isoenzyme fraction, Duchenne's muscular dystrophy, serum glutamic oxaloacetic transaminase (SGOT).**

lactation /laktā′shən/ [L, *lac*, milk, *atio*, process], the process of the synthesis and secretion of milk from the breasts in the nourishment of an infant or child. See also **breastfeeding.**

lactation mastitis. See **caked breast.**

lacteal /lak′tē·əl/, of or pertaining to milk.

lacteal fistula, an abnormal passage opening into a lacteal duct.

lacteal vessel, one of the many central lymphatic capillaries in the villi of the small intestine. They open into the lymphatic vessels in the submucosa. The capillary is filled with chyle that turns milky white during the absorption of fat.

lactic /lak′tik/ [L, *lac* + *icus*, like], referring to milk and milk products. See also **lactic acid, lactose.**

lactic acid, a three-carbon organic acid produced by anaerobic respiration. There are three forms: L-lactic acid in muscle and blood is a product of glucose and glycogen metabolism; D-lactic acid is produced by the fermentation of dextrose by a species of micrococcus; DL-lactic acid is a racemic mixture found in the stomach, in sour milk, and in certain other foods, such as sauerkraut, prepared by bacterial fermentation. Also called **alpha-hydroxypropionic acid.** See also **glycolysis.**

lactic acid fermentation, **1.** the production of lactic acid from sugars by various bacteria. **2.** the souring of milk.

lactic acidosis, a disorder characterized by an accumulation of lactic acid in the blood, resulting in a lowered pH in muscle and serum. The condition occurs most commonly in tissue hypoxia, but may also result from liver impairment, respiratory failure, neoplasms, and cardiovascular diseases.

lactiferous /laktif′ərəs/ [L, *lac* + *ferre*, to bear], of or pertaining to a structure that produces or conveys milk, such as the tubules of the breasts.

lactiferous duct, one of many channels carrying milk from the lobes of each breast to the nipple.

lactiferous glands [L, *lac*, milk; *ferre*, to carry; *glans*, acorn], glands that secrete or convey milk, such as mammary glands.

lactim. See **lactam.**

lactin. See **lactose.**

Lactinex, a trademark for a GI, fixed-combination drug containing antidiarrheals (*Lactobacillus acidophilus* and *Lactobacillus bulgaricus*).

lacto-, lact-, a combining form meaning 'of or pertaining to milk or lactic acid': *Lactobacillus, lactopeptin, lactotoxin.*

Lactobacillus /lak′tobəsil′us/ [L, *lac* + *bacillum*, small rod], any one of a group of nonpathogenic, gram-positive, rod-shaped bacteria that produce lactic acid from carbohydrates. Many species are normally found in the human intestinal tract and vagina.

Lactobacillus acidophilus [L, *lac*, milk; *bacillum*, small rod; *acidus*, sour; Gk, *philein*, to love], a bacterium found in milk and dairy products, feces of bottlefed babies and adults, saliva, and carious teeth. The strain is used to manufacture a fermented milk product.

lactogen /lak′təjən/ [L, *lac* + Gk, *genein*, to produce], a

drug or other substance that enhances the production and secretion of milk. —**lactogenic,** *adj.*

lactogenic hormone. See **prolactin.**

lacto-ovo-vegetarian /lak′tō·ōv′ōvej′əter′ē·ən/, one whose diet consists primarily of foods of vegetable origin and also includes some animal products, such as eggs *(ovo)*, milk, and cheese *(lacto),* but no meat, fish, or poultry. Also called **ovo-lacto-vegetarian.**

lactose /lak′tos/ [L, *lac* + Gk, *glykys*, sweet], a disaccharide found in the milk of all mammals. On hydrolysis lactose yields the monosaccharides glucose and galactose. Lactose is used as a laxative, as a diuretic, and as a component of formulas for infants. Also called **lactin, milk sugar.** See also **lactase deficiency, lactose intolerance, sugar.**

lactose intolerance, a sensitivity disorder resulting in the inability to digest lactose because of a deficiency of or defect in the enzyme lactase. Symptoms of the disorder are bloating, flatus, nausea, diarrhea, and abdominal cramps. The diet is adjusted according to the tolerance level, restricting such milk-derived foods as milk, cheese, butter, margarine, and any products containing milk, such as cakes, ice cream, cream soups, and sauces. See also **lactase deficiency.**

lactosuria /lak′təsŏŏr′ē·ə/ [L, *lac* + Gk, *glykys*, sweet, *ouron*, urine], the presence of lactose in the urine, a condition that may occur in late pregnancy or during lactation.

lactotherapy /-ther′əpē/ [L, *lac*, milk; Gk, *therapeia*, treatment], any treatment that depends upon a diet consisting exclusively or nearly so on milk.

lacto-vegetarian /-vej′əter′ē·ən/, one whose diet consists of milk and milk products *(lacto)* in addition to foods of vegetable origin but does not include eggs, meat, fish, or poultry.

Lacto-dectus mactans. See **black widow spider bite.**

lactulose /lak′tyəlōs/, a nonabsorbable synthetic disaccharide, 4-0-[β]-D-galactopyranosyl-D-fructose, $C_{12}H_{22}O_{11}$. It is hydrolyzed in the colon by bacteria, primarily to lactic acid and small amounts of formic and acetic acids, which results in increased osmotic pressure and acidification of the colonic contents. It is used as a cathartic in chronic constipation. Because the acidification causes ammonia to be removed from the blood to form ammonium ion, it is also used in the treatment of hepatic coma. Its ability to increase fecal water content, however, may also cause diarrhea.

lacuna /ləkyōō′nə/, *pl.* **lacunae** [L, pit], **1.** a small cavity within a structure, especially bony tissue. **2.** a gap, as in the field of vision.

lacunar /lakyōō′nər/ [L, *lacuna*, pit], pertaining to or characterized by the presence of pits, depressions, hollows, or spaces.

lacunar state, a pseudobulbar disorder characterized by the appearance of small, smooth-walled cavities in the brain tissue. The condition usually follows a series of small strokes, particularly in older adults with arterial hypertension and arteriosclerosis. Also called **status lacunaris.**

lacus lacrimalis /lā′kəs lak′rimā′ləs/ [L, *lacus*, lake; *lacrimalis*, tears], a triangular space separating the medial ends of the upper and the lower eyelids. It is an extension of the medial canthus and contains the lacrimal caruncle.

LAD, abbreviation for *left anterior descending.*

LADME /lad′mē/, an abbreviation for the time course of drug distribution, representing the terms *liberation, absorption, distribution, metabolism,* and *elimination.*

Laënnec's catarrh /lā′əneks′/ [Rene T. H. Laënnec,

French physician, b. 1781; Gk, *kata,* down, *rhoia,* flow], a form of bronchial asthma characterized by the discharge of small, round, viscous, beadlike bodies of sputum. These bodies, **Laënnec's pearls,** are formed in the bronchioles and appear in the asthmatic person's expectorated bronchial secretions.

Laënnec's cirrhosis [René T. H. Laennec, French physician, b. 1781; Gk, *kirrhos,* yellow; *osis,* condition], a fibrotic form of cirrhosis precipitated by alcohol abuse. Also called **alcoholic cirrhosis.** See **cirrhosis.**

Laënnic's pearls. See **Laënnec's catarrh.**

Laetrile /lā′ətril/, a substance composed primarily of amygdalin, a cyanogenic glycoside derived from apricot pits. Laetrile has been offered as a cancer medication despite clinical studies by the National Cancer Institute that failed to show benefits from its use. It is claimed that amygdalin is hydrolyzed by enzymes in cancer cells to produce benzaldehyde and hydrogen cyanide, which kill the cancer cells. Also called **vitamin B₁₇.**

laevo-. See **levo-.**

laf, abbreviation for **laminar air flow.**

lagen-, a combining form meaning 'flasklike': *lageniform.*

-lagnia, -lagny, a suffix meaning 'lust or a sexual predilection': *osmolagnia, pyrolagnia, scoptolagnia.*

lagophthalmos /lag′əfthal′məs/ [Gk, *lagos,* hare, *ophthalmos,* eye], an abnormal condition in which an eye may not be fully closed because of a neurologic or muscular disorder. Also called **hare's eye.**

lag phase [Dan, *lakke,* go slowly; Gk, *phasis,* appearance], a time span during which bacteria injected into a fresh medium have not begun to multiply although they may enlarge.

la grippe. See **influenza.**

laity /lā′itē/ [Gk, *laikos,* of the people], a nonprofessional segment of the population, as viewed from the perspective of a member of a particular profession. A clergyman may regard a physician as a member of the laity, and vice versa.

LAK, abbreviation for **lymphokine-activated killer cells.**

laked blood /lākt/ [Fr *laque* a deep red color], blood that is clear, red, and homogenous because of hemolysis of the red blood cells, as may occur in poisoning and severe, extensive burns.

lal-, lalio-, lalo-, a prefix meaning 'talk, babble': *laliatry, lalognosis, lalopathology.*

La Leche League International /lä lech′ā/ [Sp, *la leche,* the milk], an organization that promotes and provides education about breastfeeding.

-lalia, a suffix meaning a 'disorder of speech': *agitolalia, echolalia, oxylalia.*

lalio-. See **lal-.**

lallation /lalā′shən/ [L, *lallare,* to babble], **1.** babbling, repetitive, unintelligible utterances, like the babbling of an infant, and the mumbled speech of schizophrenics, alcoholics, and the severely mentally retarded. **2.** a speech disorder characterized by a defective pronunciation of words containing the sound /l/ or by the use of the sound /l/ in place of the sound /r/. Compare **lambdacism, rhotacism.**

lalo-. See **lal-.**

lalophobia /lal′ōfō′bē·ə/ [Gk, *lalia,* speech, *phobos,* fear], a morbid dread of talking caused by fear and anxiety that one will stammer or stutter.

lamarckism /ləmär′kizəm/ [Jean B. P. de Lamarck, French naturalist, b. 1744; Gk, *ismos,* practice], the theory postulated that organic evolution results from structural changes in plants and animals that are caused by adaptation to environmental conditions and that these acquired characteristics are transmitted to offspring. Also called **lamarckianism, Lamarck's theory.** Compare **darwinism.** **–lamarckian,** *adj., n.*

Lamaze method /ləmäz′/, a method of psychophysical preparation for childbirth developed in the 1950s by a French obstetrician, Fernand Lamaze. It requires classes, practice at home, and coaching during labor and delivery, often by a trained coach called a 'monitrice.' The classes, given during pregnancy, teach the physiology of pregnancy and childbirth, exercises to develop strength in the abdominal muscles and control of isolated muscles of the vagina and perineum, and techniques of breathing and relaxation to promote control and relaxation during labor. The woman is conditioned by repetition and practice to dissociate herself from the source of a stimulus by concentration on a focal point, by consciously relaxing all muscles, and by breathing in a special way at a particular rate—thereby training herself not to pay attention to the stimuli associated with labor. The kind and rate of breathing changes with the advancing stages of labor. During the early part of the first stage of labor, when the uterine cervix is dilated less than 5 cm and the contractions occur every 2 to 4 minutes, last 40 to 60 seconds, and are of mild to moderate strength, the mother does slow chest breathing during contractions. Her fingers may rest lightly on her lower ribs to feel them rise and fall. The abdominal wall does not move with respiration. She may perform an effleurage, or rhythmic fingertip massage, of her lower abdomen during the contractions. The rate of respiration is 10 or fewer breaths a minute, increasing to 12 per minute as labor intensifies. A deep 'cleansing breath' is taken before and after each contraction. During the active part of the first stage of labor up to the transition to the second stage, the cervix is from 5 cm to nearly fully dilated, the interval between contractions is from 1½ to 4 minutes, and the duration of contractions is from 45 to 90 seconds. (The interval decreases and the intensity and duration increase as labor progresses.) During contractions, the mother breathes quietly and shallowly in her chest. The rate of her breathing varies with the strength of the contractions, increasing during a contraction to as fast as once a second at the peak and slowing to every 6 seconds as the uterus relaxes. She is coached to concentrate on the focal point she has selected, to perform the effleurage of her abdomen, to relax her perineal and vaginal muscles, and to take a cleansing breath at the beginning and end of each contraction. At the end of the first stage of labor, when the cervix is almost completely dilated and the contractions are strong, occurring every 1½ to 2 minutes and lasting 60 to 90 seconds, the mother begins to feel the urge to bear down and push during contractions. She avoids pushing before full dilatation by combining several light, shallow breaths in the chest with short puffing exhalations as the urge increases during the contractions. During the second stage of labor, the cervix is fully dilated and contractions are strong, frequent, and expulsive. The mother's head and shoulders are supported on pillows. During contractions, she is helped to draw her legs back, flexing the thighs against the abdomen, holding them behind the lower thigh with her hands. Her chin is tucked on her chest, the air is blocked from escaping from her lungs, her perineum is relaxed, and she bears down forcibly. Depending on the length of the contraction, several pushes of 10 to 15 or more seconds may be possible during the contraction. As the ba-

K-L

by's head crowns, she is asked to pant lightly so that the head may be delivered slowly. The advantages of the method include the need for little or no analgesia for relief of pain and participation in the labor by the mother, giving her a great sense of self-satisfaction at delivery. The father of the baby also benefits by participating in the birth of his child. Compare **Bradley method, Read method.**

lambda /lam'də/, **1.** Λ, λ, the eleventh letter of the Greek alphabet. **2.** a posterior fontanel of the skull marking the point where the sagittal and lambdoidal sutures meet.

lambda chain, one of the immunoglobulin light chains.

lambdacism /lam'dəsiz'əm/ [Gk, *lambda* + *ismos*, practice], a speech disorder characterized by a defective pronunciation of words containing the sound /l/, or by the excessive use of the sound, or by the substitution of the sound /r/ for /l/. Compare **lallation, rhotacism.**

lambda wave, a low-voltage occipital wave recorded by electroencephalography during visual activity.

lambdoid /lam'doid/, having the shape of the Greek letter lambda. See also **lambdoidal suture.**

lambdoidal suture /lamdoi'dəl/, the serrated connection between the occipital bone and the parietal bones of the skull. It is continuous with the occipitomastoid suture between the occipital and the mastoid portions of the temporal bones.

lamella /ləmel'ə/, *pl.* lamellae [L, small plate], **1.** a thin leaf or plate, as of bone. **2.** a medicated disk, prepared from glycerin and an alkaloid, for insertion under the eyelid, where it dissolves and is absorbed.

lamellar /ləmel'ər/ [L, *lamella*, small plate], pertaining to or characterized by lamella.

lamellar exfoliation of the newborn [L, *lamella* + *ex*, without, *folium*, leaf; AS, *niwe*, new, *boren*, born], a congenital skin disorder transmitted as an autosomal recessive trait in which a parchmentlike, scaly membrane that covers the infant peels off within 24 hours of birth. Complete healing or a progressively less severe process of reforming and shedding of the scales then occurs. Also called **ichthyosis congenita, ichthyosis fetalis, lamellar desquamation of the newborn, lamellar ichthyosis of the newborn.** See also **collodion baby.**

lameness /lām'nəs/ [ME, *lama*, to break], a condition of being crippled or disabled, particularly because of a foot or leg injury. The term may also be applied to a stiff or painful back that makes walking difficult.

lamin-, a combining form meaning 'layer and pertaining to lamina': *laminagram, laminated, laminotomy.*

lamina /lam'inə/, *pl.* **laminae** [L, plate], any thin, flat layer of membrane or other tissue. It may be structureless or part of a structure, as the laminae of the vertebral arch.

lamina dura, a sheet of compact alveolar bone that lies adjacent to the periodontal membrane, the lining of the tooth socket.

lamina propria, a layer of connective tissue that lies just under the epithelium of the mucous membrane.

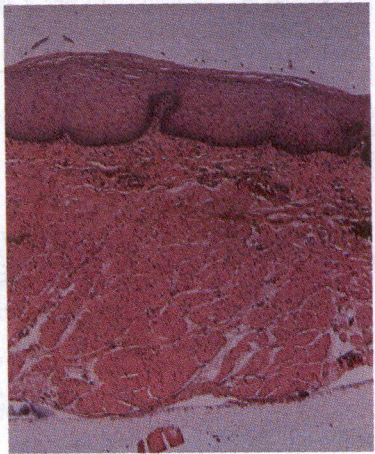

Lamina propria of a normal esophagus
(Mitros, 1988)

laminar air flow /lam'iner/ (laf) [L, *lamina*, thin plate; Gk, *aer*; AS, *flowan*], a system of circulating filtered air in parallel flow planes in hospitals or other health care facilities. The system reduces the risk of bacterial contamination or exposure to chemical pollutants in surgical theaters, food preparation areas, hospital pharmacies, and laboratories.

laminar flow. See **laminar air flow (laf).**

laminaria /lam'iner'ē·ə/ [L, *lamina*, plate], a type of seaweed that swells on absorption of water.

laminaria tent, a cone of dried seaweed that swells as it absorbs water and therefore is used to dilate the cervix nontraumatically in preparation for induced abortion or induced labor.

laminated thrombus /lam'inā'tid/, a thrombus composed of an aggregation of blood platelets, fibrin, clotting factors, and cellular elements, arranged in layers apparently formed at different times.

laminectomy /lam'inek'təmē/ [L, *lamina* + Gk, *ektome*, excision], surgical removal of the bony arches of one or more vertebrae, performed to relieve compression of the spinal cord, as caused by a bone displaced in an injury, as the result of degeneration of a disk, or to reach and remove a displaced intervertebral disk. With the patient prone and under general anesthesia, the laminae are removed and the underlying problem is corrected. Spinal fusion may be neces-

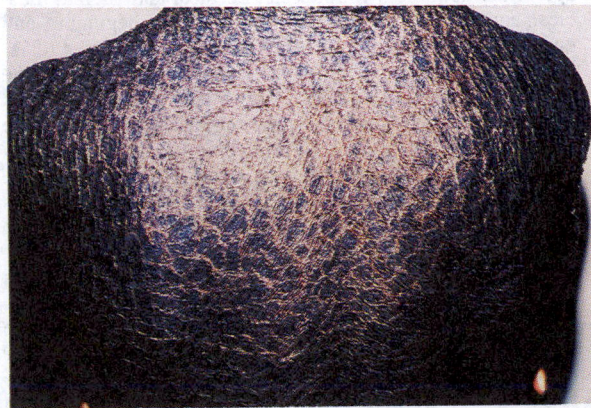

Lamellar exfoliation of the newborn *(Zitelli, 1992)*

sary for stability of the spine if several laminae are removed. After surgery, the bed is kept flat to hold the patient's spine in correct alignment. If the procedure was a cervical laminectomy, the patient is observed for signs of respiratory distress caused by cord edema. Motor function and sensation in the extremities are evaluated every 2 to 4 hours for 48 hours. The dressing is examined frequently for hemorrhage or leakage of cerebrospinal fluid. A sheet is used to logroll the patient without twisting the spine or hips. **–laminectomize,** v.

lampbrush chromosome [Gk, *lampas*, torch; AS, *bryst*, bristle], an excessively large type of chromosome found in the oocytes of many lower animals. It has long, threadlike projecting loops, giving it a hairy, brushlike appearance. See also **giant chromosome.**

lampro-, a combining form meaning 'clear': *lamprophonia, lamprophonic.*

LAN, an abbreviation for **local area network.**

lance [L *lancea* spear], to incise a furuncle or an abscess to release accumulated pus. A topical anesthetic is applied, the lesion is incised, and the pus is drained. A drain is inserted if the infection is deep. The bacteria involved are most often staphylococci. The nurse uses aseptic technique. An antibiotic is given systemically if the boil is facial to prevent infection from spreading into the cranial sinuses. Infected drainage is kept off surrounding skin to prevent a recurrence. The nurse teaches the patient and family stringent handwashing techniques.

Lancefield's classification [Rebecca C. Lancefield, American bacteriologist, b. 1895], a serologic classification of streptococci based on their antigenic characteristics. The bacteria are divided into 13 groups by the identification of their pathologic action. Group A contains most of the streptococci that cause infection in humans. Groups B to T are less pathogenic and are often present without causing disease. Most are hemolytic; of those, the beta subgroup is the most likely to be the cause of infection.

lancet /lan'sit/ [Fr, *lancette*], **1.** *obsolete.* a very small, pointed, surgical knife, sharp on both sides. **2.** a short pointed blade used to obtain a drop of blood for a capillary sample. It has a guard above the blade that prevents deep incision, and it is usually disposable.

lancinating /lan'sinā'ting/ [L, *lancinare*, to tear to pieces], sharply cutting or tearing, such as lancinating pain.

Landau reflex /lan'dou/, a normal response of infants when held in a horizontal prone position to maintain a convex arc with the head raised and the legs slightly flexed. The reflex is poor in those with floppy infant syndrome and exaggerated in hypertonic and opisthotonic infants.

landmark position [AS, *land, meark*, mark; L, *positio*], the correct placement of the hands on the chest in cardiopulmonary resuscitation. See also **cardiopulmonary resuscitation.**

Landouzy-Dejerine muscular dystrophy. See **facioscapulohumeral muscular dystrophy.**

Landsteiner's classification /land'stī'nərz/ [Karl Landsteiner, American pathologist, b. 1868], the classification of blood groups A, B, AB, and O on the basis of the presence or absence of the two agglutinogens A and B on the erythrocytes in human blood.

Langer's line. See **cleavage line.**

Langhans' layer. See **cytotrophoblast.**

language /lang'gwij/ [L, *lingua*, tongue], **1.** a defined set of characters that when used alone or in combinations form a meaningful set of words and symbols. **2.** a unified, related set of commands or instructions that a computer can accept.

lano-, a combining form meaning 'of or pertaining to wool': *lanolin, lanonol, lanosterol.*

lanolin /lan'əlin/ [L, *lana*, wool, *oleum*, oil], a fatlike substance from the wool of sheep. It contains about 25% water as a water-in-oil emulsion and is used as an ointment base and an emollient for the skin. Also called **hydrous wool fat.**

Lanoxin, a trademark for a cardiotonic (digoxin).

lanthanum (La) /lan'thənəm/ [Gk, *lanthanein*, to escape notice], a rare earth metallic element. Its atomic number is 57; its atomic weight is 138.91.

lanuginous /lənoo'jinəs/ [L, *lanugo*, down], pertaining to lanugo.

lanugo /lanyoo'gō/ [L, down], **1.** the soft, downy hair covering a normal fetus that begins in the fifth month of gestation and almost entirely shed by the ninth month. **2.** the fine, soft hair covering all parts of the body except palms, soles, and areas where other types of hair are normally found. Also called **vellus hair.**

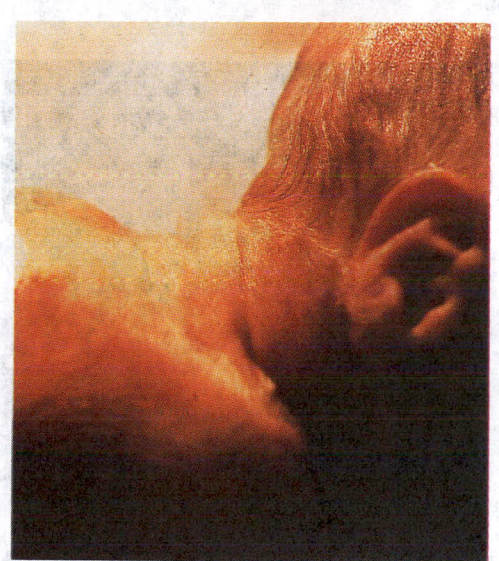

Lanugo *(Zitelli, 1992)*

lanulous /lan'yoolos/ [L, *lana*, wool, *osus*, filled with], downy or covered with short, fine wooly hair, such as the skin of a fetus. See also **lanugo.**

lap, 1. abbreviation for **laparotomy. 2.** abbreviation for *left atrial pressure.*

laparo- /lap'əro-/, a combining form meaning 'of or pertaining to the abdomen or abdominal wall': *laparectomy, laparotomy, laparorrhaphy.*

laparoenterostomy /-en'təros'təmē/ [Gk, *lapara*, loin; *enteron*, bowel; *stoma*, mouth], the surgical installation of a tube through an external opening in the abdomen in order to drain the bowel. A similar procedure may be used to supply nutrients to a patient with an upper digstive tract obstruction.

laparohysterectomy /-his'tərek'təmē/ [Gk, *lapara*, loin; *hystera*, womb; *ektome*, excision], a hysterectomy performed by making an excision through the abdominal wall.

laparoscope /lap'ərəskōp'/ [Gk, *lapara*, loin, *skopein*, to look], a type of endoscope, consisting of an illuminated tube with an optical system, that is inserted through the abdominal wall for examining the peritoneal cavity. Also called **celioscope, peritoneoscope.** –**laparoscopic,** *adj.,* **laparoscopy,** *n.*

laparoscopic sterilization /-skop'ik/ [Gk, *lapara*, loin + *skopein*, to view; L, *sterilis*, barren], the process of rendering a woman incapable of reproduction by inserting a specialized endoscope through a small incision in the abdominal wall. Sterilization may be performed through the incision with clips to occlude the fallopian tubes or by electrocoagulation and severance.

laparoscopy /lap'əros'kəpē/, the examination of the abdominal cavity with a laparoscope through a small incision in the abdominal wall. The procedure is also used for examining the ovaries and fallopian tubes and as a gynecologic sterilization technique for fulgurating the oviducts. Also called **abdominoscopy.** See also **endoscopy, laparoscope.**

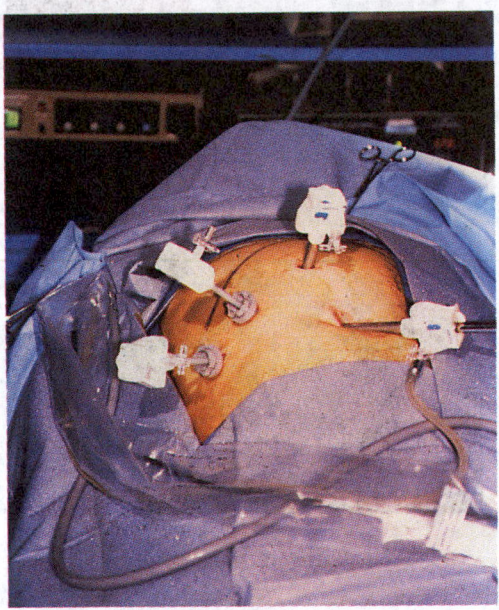

Laparoscopic cholecystectomy (Rosato, 1992)

laparotomy (lap) /lap'ərot'əmē/ [Gk, *lapara* + *temnein*, to cut], any surgical incision into the peritoneal cavity, usually performed under general or regional anesthesia, often on an exploratory basis. Before surgery, a complete blood count and a urinalysis are done; the skin is shaved and cleansed from the nipple line to the pubis. Food and oral fluids by mouth are withheld for several hours preoperatively. If the intestine is to be opened, a nasogastric tube is passed. Frequent observation of vital signs and drainage systems is essential. Intake and output of fluids are recorded. The patient is turned and helped to cough and breathe deeply every hour; medication is given as needed for relief of pain. Some kinds of laparotomy are **appendectomy, cholecystectomy,** and **colostomy.** –**laparotomize,** *v.*

lap-board [ME, *lappa*, *bord*, plank], a flat board placed over the lap to serve as a temporary desk or table.

Laplace's law /läpläs'/ [Pierre Simon Marquis de Laplace, French physicist, b. 1749], a principle of physics that the tension on the wall of a sphere is the product of the pressure times the radius of the chamber and the tension is inversely related to the thickness of the wall.

-lapse, a suffix meaning 'a slip or fall backward': *collapse, prolapse, relapse.*

large calorie. See **calorie.**

large for gestational age (LGA) infant, an infant whose fetal growth was accelerated and whose size and weight at birth fall above the ninetieth percentile of appropriate for gestational age infants, whether delivered prematurely, at term, or later than term. Factors other than genetic influences that cause accelerated intrauterine growth include maternal diabetes mellitus and Beckwith's syndrome. LGA infants born of diabetic mothers are generally obese and plethoric, with very pink skin and red, shiny cheeks. They are often listless and limp, feed poorly, and become hypoglycemic within the first few hours. A major problem is that preterm LGA infants, because of their size, are not recognized as high-risk neonates with immature organ system development. Often these infants develop respiratory distress syndrome because pulmonary maturation occurs later in gestation. In cases of Beckwith's syndrome, the infant is characterized by gigantism, macroglossia, omphalocele or umbilical hernia, and visceromegaly. Compare **small for gestational age infant.**

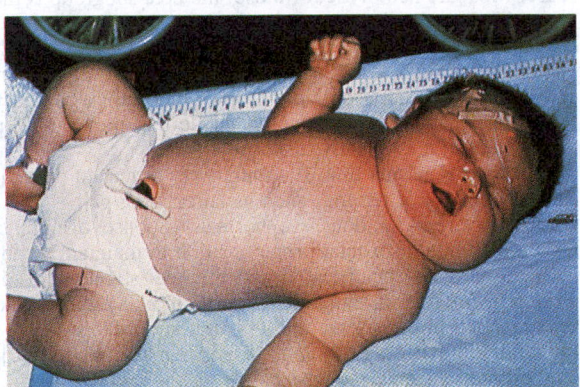

Large for gestational age infant (Zitelli, 1992)

large intestine [L, *largus*, abundant, *intestinum*], the portion of the digestive tract comprising the cecum, appendix, the ascending, transverse, and descending colons, and the rectum. The ileocecal valve separates the cecum from the ileum.

lariat structure /ler'ē·ət/, a ring of intron segments that have been spliced out of an mRNA molecule by enzymes. Some introns form a long tail attached to the ring, giving the structure the appearance of a microscopic cowboy lariat.

Larmor frequency [Sir Joseph Larmor, Irish physicist, b. 1857], the frequency of the precession of a charged particle when its motion comes under the influence of an applied magnetic field and a central force.

Larodopa, a trademark for an antiparkinsonian (levodopa).

larva /lär′və/ [L, specter], the early immature form of an animal, which undergoes metamorphosis to an adult form.

larva migrans. See **cutaneous larva migrans, visceral larva migrans.**

laryng-. See **laryngo-.**

laryngeal /lerin′jē·əl/ [Gk, *larynx*], pertaining to the larynx.

laryngeal cancer [Gk, *larynx* + L, *cancer*, crab], a malignant neoplastic disease characterized by a tumor arising from the epithelium of the structures of the larynx. Laryngeal tumors are almost 20 times more common in men than in women and occur most frequently between 50 and 70 years of age. Chronic alcoholism and heavy use of tobacco increase the risk of developing the cancer. Persistent hoarseness is usually the first sign; advanced lesions may cause a sore throat, dyspnea, dysphagia, and unilateral cervical adenopathy. Diagnostic measures include direct laryngoscopy, biopsy, and radiologic examination, including tomographic studies and chest films. Malignant tumors of the larynx are epidermoid carcinomas. Radiation is generally recommended for small lesions; total laryngectomy, often combined with radiotherapy, is indicated for extensive lesions. After the operation, many persons with laryngectomies learn esophageal speech; some use an electric larynx, and a few undergo surgical reconstruction. See also **laryngectomy.**

laryngeal catheterization, the insertion of a catheter into the larynx for the purpose of removing secretions or introducing gases.

laryngeal dyphtheria. See **diphtheritic croup.**

laryngeal edema. See **edema of glottis.**

laryngeal polyp [Gk, *larynx* + *poly,* many + *pous,* foot], a polyp on the vocal cords that causes hoarseness due to vocal abuse or smoking.

laryngeal prominence. See **Adam's apple.**

laryngeal reflex [Gk, *larynx*; L, *reflectere,* to bend back], a cough reflex caused by irritation of the fauces and larynx.

laryngeal vertigo [Gk, *larynx*; L, *vertere,* to turn], a short episode of dizziness or unconsciousness following a paroxysmal attack of coughing or laryngeal spasm. Also called **cough syncope.**

laryngectomy /ler′injek′təmē/ [Gk, *larynx* + *ektome,* excision], surgical removal of the larynx, performed to treat cancer of the larynx. Before surgery, the patient is referred to a speech pathologist to discuss esophageal speech and prostheses. Antibiotics are usually administered to reduce the risk of infection. Under regional or general anesthesia, the trachea is sutured to the skin, as in a tracheostomy, to ensure an adequate airway. In a partial laryngectomy only the vocal cords are removed, and the tracheostomy is closed within several days. If the malignancy is extensive, the entire larynx is removed, along with the thyroid cartilage and epiglottis; the tracheostomy is permanent, and a laryngectomy tube left in place. After surgery the patient is observed for excessive coughing or any vomiting of blood, and the laryngectomy tube is kept free of mucus. A humidifier or vaporizer is useful to decrease coughing and the production of mucus. IV fluids are given, and liquid feedings may be given via nasogastric tube. A Magic Slate is useful for communication between patient, staff, and family. The laryngectomy tube is removed 3 to 6 weeks after surgery. Compare **neck dissection, radical neck dissection. –laryngectomize,** *v.*

laryngismus /ler′injiz′məs/ [Gk, *laryngismos,* whooping], spasm of the larynx. **Laryngismus stridulus,** a condition characterized by sudden laryngeal spasm with a crowing sound on inspiration and the development of cyanosis, occurs in inflammation of the larynx. The relatively small larynx of the infant and young child is susceptible to spasm when infected or irritated and readily becomes partially or totally obstructed.

laryngitis /ler′injī′tis/ [Gk, *larynx* + *itis*], inflammation of the mucous membrane lining the larynx, accompanied by edema of the vocal cords with hoarseness or loss of voice, occurring as an acute disorder caused by a cold, by irritating fumes, by sudden temperature changes, or as a chronic condition resulting from excessive use of the voice, heavy smoking, or exposure to irritating fumes. In acute laryngitis, there may be a cough, and the throat usually feels scratchy and painful. The patient is advised to remain in an environment with an even temperature, to avoid talking and exposure to tobacco smoke, and to inhale steam containing aromatic vapors, such as tincture of benzoin, oil of pine, or menthol. Acute laryngitis may cause severe respiratory distress in children under 5 years of age because the relatively small larynx of the young child is subject to spasm when irritated or infected and readily becomes partially or totally obstructed. The youngster may develop a hoarse, barking cough and an inspiratory stridor and may become restless, gasping for air. Treatment consists of the administration of copious amounts of vaporized cool mist. Chronic laryngitis may be treated by removal of irritants, avoidance of smoking, voice rest, correction of faulty voice habits, cough medication, steam inhalations, and spraying the throat with an astringent antiseptic, such as hexylresorcinol.

laryngo- /lering′gō-/, **laryng-,** a combining form meaning 'of or pertaining to the larynx': *laryngocentesis, laryngograph.*

laryngocele /lering′gōsēl′/, an abnormal air-containing cavity connected to the laryngeal ventricle. It is caused by an evagination of the mucous membrane of the ventricle and may displace and enlarge the false vocal cord, resulting in hoarseness and airway obstruction. Because a laryngocele is also a potential reservoir of infection, it is usually excised.

laryngography. See **laryngopharyngography.**

laryngology (laryngol) /ler′ing·gol′əjē/, [Gk, *larynx; logos,* science], the branch of medicine that specializes in the causes and treatments of disorders of the larynx.

-laryngopharyngeal. See **laryngopharynx.**

laryngopharyngitis /lering′gōfer′injī′tis/ [Gk, *larynx* + *pharynx,* throat, *itis*], inflammation of the larynx and pharynx. See also **laryngitis, pharyngitis.**

laryngopharyngography /lering′gōfer′ingog′rəfē/ [Gk, *larynx, pharynx* + *graphein,* to record], the radiographic examination of the larynx and the pharynx. Also called **laryngography.**

laryngopharynx /lering′gōfer′ingks/ [Gk, *larynx* + *pharynx,* throat], one of the three regions of the throat, extending from the hyoid bone to the esophagus. Compare **nasopharynx, oropharynx. laryngopharyngeal** /lering′gōferin′jē·əl/, *adj.*

laryngoscope /ləring′gəskōp/, an endoscope for examining the larynx.

laryngoscopic /-skop′ik/ [Gk, *larynx; skopein,* to view], pertaining to the use of a laryngoscope.

laryngoscopy /ler′ing·gos′kəpē/ [Gk, *larynx; skopein,* to view], the use of a laryngoscope to view the larynx.

laryngospasm /ləring′gōspaz′əm/ [Gk, *larynx + spasmos,* spasm], a spasmodic closure of the larynx.

laryngostasis. See **croup.**

laryngotomy /ler′ing·got′əmē/ [Gk, *larynx; temnein,* to cut], a surgical incision into the larynx through the cricovocal membrane. It is usually an emergency procedure that is performed when a standard tracheotomy cannot be done.

laryngotracheobronchitis (LTB) /lering′gōtrā′kē·ō′brongkī′tis/ [Gk, *larynx* + L, *tractus,* trachea; Gk, *bronchos,* windpipe, *itis*], an inflammation of the major respiratory passages, usually causing hoarseness, nonproductive cough, and dyspnea. Among the causes are infections by coxsackieviruses, echoviruses, *Haemophilus influenzae,* and *Corynebacterium diphtheriae.* Treatment usually includes steam inhalations, cough suppressants, and, for bacterial infections, appropriate antibiotics. See also **croup.**

larynx /ler′ingks/ [Gk], the organ of voice that is part of the air passage connecting the pharynx with the trachea. It accounts for a large bump in the neck called the Adam's apple and is larger in men than in women although remaining the same size in men and women until puberty. The larynx forms the caudal portion of the anterior wall of the pharynx and is lined with mucous membrane that is continuous with that of the pharynx and the trachea. The larynx extends vertically to the fourth, fifth, and sixth cervical vertebrae and is somewhat higher in the female and during childhood. It is composed of three single cartilages and three paired cartilages, all connected together by ligaments and moved by various muscles. The single cartilages are the thyroid, cricoid, and epiglottis. The three paired cartilages are the arytenoid, corniculate, and cuneiform, which form the vocal folds. The larynx is broad above and narrow and cylindric at its caudal extremity. **—laryngeal,** *adj.*

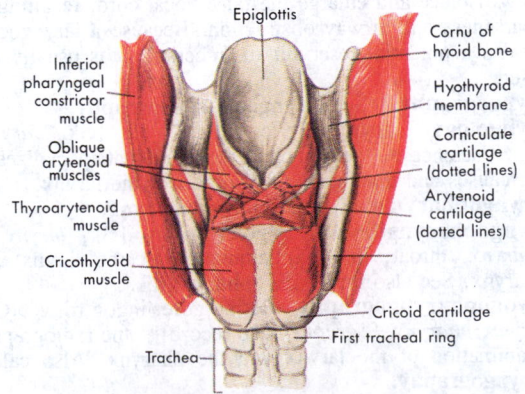

Posterior view of the larynx
(Thibodeau, 1993/Ernest W Beck)

LAS, abbreviation for **lymphadenopathy syndrome.**

Lasan, a trademark for an antipsoriatic (anthralin).

laser /lā′zər/, acronym for *light amplification by stimulated emission of radiation,* a source of intense radiation of the visible, ultraviolet, or infrared portions of the spectrum. Lasers are used in surgery to divide or to cause adhesions or to destroy or to fix tissue in place. Also called **optic laser.**

laser bronchoscopy, bronchoscopy that is performed with the aid of a carbon dioxide laser beam directed through fiberoptic equipment in the diagnosis and treatment of bronchial disorders. Neodymium-yttrium aluminum garnet (Nd-YAG) lasers have also been used in the treatment of tracheobronchial tumors and subglottic stenosis.

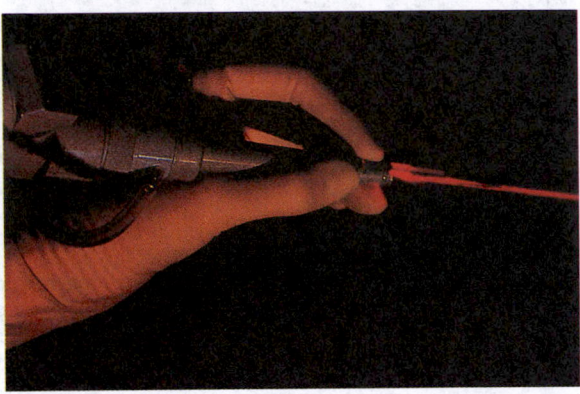

Carbon dioxide laser handpiece *(Ball, 1990)*

laser disk, a plastic-coated disk that stores computer data as tiny pits etched in the surface. A laser beam scanning the pits translates the data into a computer language.

laser printer, a high-speed output device for computers utilizing a technique in which laser beams focus images on photosensitive drums. The technology is similar to that of xerographic photocopiers. Compare **daisy wheel printer, dot matrix printer.**

Lasix, a trademark for a diuretic (furosemide).

Lassa fever /lä′sə/ [Lassa, Nigeria; L, *febris,* fever], a highly contagious disease caused by a virulent arenavirus. It is characterized by fever, pharyngitis, dysphagia, and ecchymoses. Pleural effusion, edema and renal involvement, mental disorientation, confusion, and death from cardiac failure often ensue. Stringent precautions are taken against the spread of infection. Supportive, symptomatic care is the only treatment available. See also **arenavirus, Argentine hemorrhagic fever, Bolivian hemorrhagic fever.**

last sacraments [ME, *laste*; L, *sacramentum,* solemn oath], a religious ceremony performed by a member of the clergy in behalf of a person about to die. Also called **last rites.**

latchkey children, minors who are often at home alone because their parents are at work. They carry a key to their home and are more likely to become involved in accidents or antisocial behavior than children who are supervised by adults when not in school.

late dyspituitary eunuchism. See **acromegalic eunuchoidism.**

latency period /lā′tənsē/ [L, *latere,* to keep out of sight; Gk, *peri, hodos,* way], **1.** the period between contact with a pathogen and development of symptoms. Also called **incubation period. 2.** the time between stimulus and response. Also called **latency of response. 3.** a period between early childhood and puberty when there is little overt interest in the opposite sex. Also called **latency stage.**

latency stage [L, *latere*, to be concealed; Fr, *estage*, stage], (in psychoanalysis) a period in psychosexual development occurring between early childhood and puberty when sexual motivation and expression are repressed or transferred, through sublimation, to the feelings and behavioral patterns expected as typical of the age.

latent /lā'tənt/ [L, *latere*, to be concealed], dormant; existing as a potential; for example, tuberculosis may be latent for extended periods of time and become active under certain conditions.

latent carcinoma.   See **occult carcinoma.**

latent diabetes.   See **impaired glucose tolerance, previous abnormality of glucose tolerance.**

latent energy [L, *latere*, to keep out of sight; Gk, *energeia*], the energy contained in an object due to its position in space, internal structure, and stresses imposed on it. Also called **potential energy.**

latent heat [L, *latere*, to keep out of sight; AS, *haetu*], the heat absorbed by a substance when it changes from a solid to a liquid, or from a liquid to a gas without an accompanying rise in temperature.

latent image, (in radiology), an invisible image produced in the x-ray film emulsion by x-rays or visible light that can be converted to a visible image by development.

latent learning [L, *latere*, to keep out of sight; ME, *lernen*], learning acquired unintentionally. It may remain in the subconscious, or latent, until a need for the knowledge arises.

latent malaria [L, *latere*, to keep out of sight; It, *mal + aria*, bad air], a continuing infection without clinical symptoms resulting from a balance established between the parasite and the body's immune system. See also **malaria.**

latent period, (in radiology) an interval of seeming inactivity between the time of exposure to an injurious dose of radiation and the response.

latent phase, the early stage of labor that is characterized by irregular, infrequent, and mild contractions and little or no dilatation of the cervix or descent of the fetus. Also called **prodromal labor.** See also **Friedman curve.**

latent syphilis [L, *latere*, to keep out of sight; Gk, *syn*, together + *philein*, to love], a stage of syphilis infection in which no clinical symptoms appear but serological tests indicate the presence of the syphilis spirochete.

latent tetany [L, *latere*, to keep out of sight; Gk, *tetanos*, convulsive tension], a form of tetany that is elicited only by mechanical or electrical stimuli.

lateral /lat'ərəl/ [L, *latus*, side], **1.** on the side. **2.** away from the midsagittal plane. **3.** farther from the midsagittal plane. **4.** to the right or left of the midsagittal plane.

lateral abdominal region.   See **lateral region.**

lateral aortic node, a lumbar lymph node in any of three clusters of nodes serving the pelvis and abdomen. The right lateral aortic nodes are situated partly ventral to the inferior vena cava, near the termination of the renal vein, and partly dorsal to the inferior vena cava on the right crus of the diaphragm. The left lateral aortic nodes form a chain on the left side of the abdominal aorta, ventral to the origin of the psoas major and ventral to the right crus of the diaphragm. The afferent vessels from both sides drain various structures, such as the testes, ovaries, kidneys, and lateral abdominal muscles. Most of the efferent vessels from the lateral aortic nodes converge to form the right and the left lumbar trunks, which join the cisterna chyli. Compare **preaortic node, retroaortic node.**

lateral aperture of the fourth ventricle, an opening between the end of each lateral recess of the fourth ventricle and the subarachnoid space.

lateral cerebral sulcus, a deep cleft marking the division of the temporal, frontal, and parietal lobes of brain. Also called **fissure of Sylvius.**

lateral condensation method, a technique for filling and sealing tooth root canals. A preselected gutta-percha cone is sealed into the apex of the root; other cones are forced laterally with a spreader until the canal is filled.

lateral cuneiform bone, one of the three cuneiform bones of the foot, located in the center of the front row of tarsal bones between the intermediate cuneiform bone medially, the cuboid bone laterally, the scaphoid bone posteriorly, and the third metatarsal anteriorly. It also articulates with the second and fourth metatarsals. Also called **external cuneiform bone, third cuneiform bone.**

lateral decentering, (in radiology) an error in positioning of a focused grid, resulting in partial grid cutoff over the entire film. The error may also be a result of improperly positioning the tube head rather than the grid.

lateral geniculate body, one of two elevations of the lateral posterior thalamus receiving visual impulses from the retina via the optic nerves and tracts and relaying the impulses to the calcarine cortex.

lateral humeral epicondylitis, inflammation of the tissue at the lower end of the humerus at the elbow joint, caused by the repetitive flexing of the wrist against resistance. It may result from athletic activity or manual manipulation of tools or other equipment. Pain radiates from the elbow joint. Treatment includes rest, correction of body mechanics, infiltration of a long-acting anesthetic, or serial injections of hydrocortisone, depending on the severity of the condition. Surgery is rarely indicated. Also called **tennis elbow.** See also **epicondylitis.**

lateral incisal guide angle, (in dentistry) the inclination of the incisal guide in the frontal plane.

laterality.   See **handedness.**

lateralization /lat'ərəl'īzā'shən/, the tendency for certain processes to be more highly developed on one side of the brain than the other, such as development of spatial and musical thoughts in the right hemisphere and verbal and logical processes in the left hemisphere in most persons.

lateral lobes of thyroid gland [L, *latus*, side; Gk, *lobos*; *thyreos*, shield; L, *glans*, acorn], the left and right lobes of a highly vascular thyroid gland situated in front of the neck. The two conical lobes lying on either side of and attached to the larynx are connected by a narrow isthmus.

lateral nystagmus [L, *latus*, side; Gk, *nystagmos*, nodding], an involuntary jerky movement in which the eyes move from side to side.

lateral pectoral nerve, one of a pair of branches from the brachial plexus that, with the medial pectoral nerve, supplies the pectoral muscles. It lies lateral to the axillary artery and arises from the lateral cord of the plexus or from the anterior divisions of the superior and the middle trunks just before they unite into the cord. It passes above to the first part of the axillary artery and the axillary vein, gives a filament to the inferior pectoral branch, pierces the clavipectoral fascia, and ends on the deep surface of the clavicular and the cranial sternocostal parts of the pectoralis major. Compare **medial pectoral nerve.**

lateral pelvic displacement, one of the five major kinetic determinants of gait. It helps to synchronize the rhythmic movements of walking and is produced by the horizontal shift of the pelvis or by relative hip abduction. It is often a factor in the diagnosis and treatment of various orthopedic diseases, deformities, and abnormal conditions, and in the analysis and the correction of dysfunctional gaits. Compare **knee-ankle interaction, knee-hip flexion, pelvic rotation, pelvic tilt.**

lateral pinch, a grasp in which the thumb is opposed to the middle phalanx of the index finger. Also called **key pinch.** See also **palmar pinch, pinch, tip pinch.**

lateral projection, (in radiology) a position of a patient between the x-ray tube and the film cassette so the beam will travel from the left to the right side of the body, or vice versa. The projection may be identified as right lateral if the right side of the body, or left lateral if the left side, is adjacent to the cassette.

lateral recumbent position, the posture assumed by the patient lying on the left side with the right thigh and knee drawn up. Also called **English position, obstetric position.**

lateral region, the part of the abdomen in the middle zone on both sides of the umbilical region. Also called **external abdominal region, lateral abdominal region, lumbar region.** See also **abdominal regions.**

lateral resolution, (in ultrasonography) the resolution of objects in a plane perpendicular to the axis of the beam. It is a measure of the ability of the system to detect closely separated objects such as adjacent blood vessels.

lateral rocking, a sideways rocking of the body used to move the body forward or backward when normal muscle action is not possible. The technique is used by some handicapped patients to move the body to or from the edge of a chair or to a different sitting position on a bed. The rocking is performed while leaning the trunk forward with the arms in front and the head in line above the knees and feet, which are pulled back.

lateral rotation, a turning away from the midline of the body. Compare **medial rotation.** See also **rotation.**

lateral sinus [L, *latus,* side + *sinus,* hollow], one of the transverse bilateral sinuses of the dura mater that lie along the attached margin of the tentorium cerebelli. They receive the superior sagittal and straight sinuses and drain into the internal jugular veins.

lateral spinal curvature [L, *latus,* side + *spina,* backbone + *curvatura,* bend], a bending or abnormal curve of the vertebral column to the right or left side.

lateral umbilical fold, a fold in the peritoneum produced by a slight protrusion of the inferior epigastric artery and the interfoveolar ligament. The lateral umbilical fold is about 3 cm lateral to the middle umbilical fold. Also called **plica umbilicalis lateralis.**

lateral ventricle [L, *latus,* side + *ventriculum*], a cavity in each cerebral hemisphere that communicates with the third ventricle through the interventricular foramen.

late rickets [Gk, *rhachis,* backbone], a form of rickets in which bone changes because of a kidney defect that result in a vitamin D or calcium deficiency. The disorder tends to affect older children.

latero-, a prefix meaning 'of or pertaining to the side': *laterodeviation, lateroduction, laterotorsion.*

latex /lā′teks/ [L, liquid], an emulsion or fluidlike sap produced in special cells or vessels of certain plants. Latex contains resins, proteins, and other substances and is a source of rubber.

latex fixation test [L, *latex,* fluid; *figere,* to fasten], a serologic test used in the diagnosis of rheumatoid arthritis in which antigen-coated latex particles agglutinate with rheumatoid factors in a slide specimen of serum or synovial fluid. If positive, the screening slide test is followed by titration. Also called **RA latex test, RF test.** See also **rheumatoid factor.**

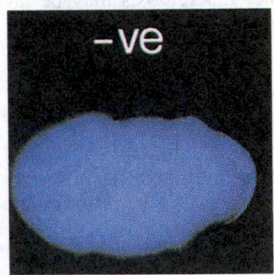 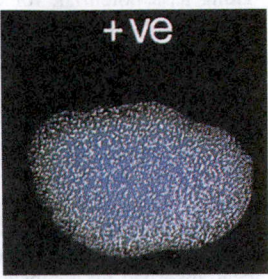

**Negative (left) and positive (right)
latex fixation tests**
(Shipley, 1984)

Lathrop, Rose Hawthorne (1851–1926), an American nurse, who was a daughter of Nathaniel Hawthorne. She established a home in New York for incurable cancer patients, mostly those who were poor and who were not accepted in hospitals because of the nature of their disease. Later, she became a member of the Third Order of St. Dominic and founded the order of sisters called Servants of Relief for Incurable Cancer. The order founded hospitals wherever there was sufficient need and offered quality care to their patients.

latissimus dorsi /latis′iməs dôr′sī/ [L, widest; *dorsum* the back], one of a pair of large triangular muscles on the thoracic and lumbar areas of the back. The base of the triangle inserts through lumbar aponeuroses to the spines of lumbar and sacral vertebrae and in the supraspinous ligaments, posterior iliac crest, and the lower four ribs. The fibers of the muscle twist as they pass the scapula and converge at the base of the intertubercular groove of the humerus. The latissimus dorsi extends, adducts, and rotates the arm medially, draws the shoulder back and down, and, with the pectoralis major, draws the body up when climbing. It is innervated by the thoracodorsal nerve. Compare **levator scapulae, rhomboideus major, rhomboideus minor, trapezius.**

latitude [L, *latitudio,* breadth], the ability of an x-ray imaging system to produce acceptable images over a range of exposures. If a system has wide latitude, it is possible to image parts of the body that vary in thickness or density with only one exposure. A system of lesser latitude would require a lower exposure over the thin section and a greater exposure where the absorption was greater.

LATS, abbreviation for **long-acting thyroid stimulator.**

LATS-P, abbreviation for *long-acting thyroid stimulator protector.*

lattice formation [OFr, *lattis,* geometric design], a three-

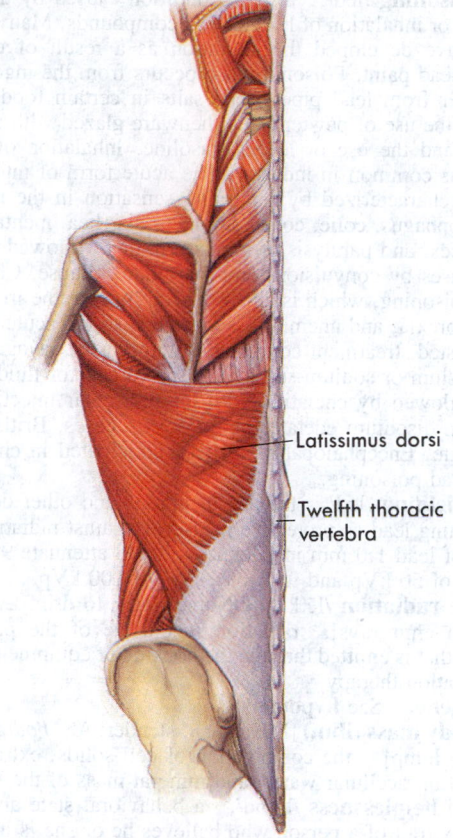

Latissimus dorsi

Twelfth thoracic vertebra

Latissimus dorsi (Thibodeau, 1993/John V Hagen)

dimensional cross-linked structure formed by the reaction of multivalent antigens with antibodies.

laudanum /lôd′(ə)nəm/ [Gk, landanon, a gum resin], a tincture of opium, made from a solution of macerated raw opium and 50% alcohol. It is believed to have originated as a secret remedy of Paracelsus, sixteenth century Swiss alchemist and physician.

Lauenstein method,   (in radiology) a technique for positioning a patient in order to x-ray the hip joint with emphasis on the relationship of the femur to the acetabulum. The knee of the affected leg is flexed and the thigh drawn up to a near right angle. Also called **frog leg position.**

laughing gas /laf′ing/,   informal. nitrous oxide, a side effect of which is laughter or giggling when administered in less than anesthetizing amounts.

Laurence-Moon-Bardet-Biedl syndrome /lôr′əns mōōn′ bärdā′ bē′dəl/ [John Z. Laurence, English ophthalmologist, b. 1830; Robert C. Moon, American ophthalmologist, b. 1844; Georges Bardet, French physician, b. 1885; Artur Biedl, Czechoslovakian physician, b. 1869],   an abnormal condition characterized by obesity, hypogenitalism, mental deficiency, polydactylism, and retinitis pigmentosa. It is an inherited disorder, transmitted as an autosomal recessive trait.

lavage /ləväzh′/ [Fr, washing], **1.** the process of washing out an organ, usually the bladder, bowel, paranasal sinuses, or stomach for therapeutic purposes. **2.** to perform a lavage. Kinds of lavage are **blood lavage, gastric lavage,** and **peritoneal dialysis.** See also **irrigation.**

law [AS, lagu], **1.** (in a field of study) a rule, standard, or principle that states a fact or a relationship between factors, such as Dalton's law regarding partial pressures of gas or Koch's law regarding the specificity of a pathogen. **2.** a rule, principle, or regulation established and promulgated by a government to protect or to restrict the people affected; the field of study concerned with such laws; or the collected body of the laws of a people, derived from custom and from legislation.

Law method,   (in radiology) any of several techniques for positioning a patient for x-ray examination of the facial bones, sinuses, and relationship of the teeth to the jaw bones.

law of definite composition,   (in chemistry) a law stating that a given compound is always made of the same elements present in the same proportion.

law of dominance,   formerly considered as a separate principle of Mendel's laws of inheritance, but in modern genetics it is incorporated as part of the first Mendelian law, the law of segregation. See also **Mendel's laws.**

law of independent assortment, law of segregation. See **Mendel's laws.**

law of universal gravitation,   (in physics) the law stating that the force with which bodies are attracted to each other is directly proportional to the masses of the objects and inversely proportional to the square of the distance by which they are separated. See also **gravity, mass.**

lawrencium (Lr) /lôren′sē·əm/ [Ernest O. Lawrence, American physicist, b. 1901],   a synthetic transuranic metallic element. Its atomic number is 103; its atomic weight is 257.

lax, 1. abbreviation for **laxative. 2.** a condition of relaxation or looseness.

laxative (lax) /lak′sətiv/ [L, laxare, to loosen], **1.** of or pertaining to a substance that causes evacuation of the bowel by a mild action. **2.** a laxative agent that promotes bowel evacuation by increasing the bulk of the feces, by softening the stool, or by lubricating the intestinal wall. Compare **cathartic.**

lay referral system,   an illness referral system through which a person passes from the first recognition of an abnormality to an announcement to the family, to members of the community, then to traditional or culturally recognized healers, and then to the regular medical system that includes nurses and physicians. Depending on the culture and the medical care available, some steps may be omitted.

lazy colon. See **atonia constipation.**

lazy leukocyte syndrome,   an immunodeficiency disease of children characterized by recurrent stomatitis, gingivitis, otitis media, and low-grade fever with severe neutropenia. The condition has been associated with abnormal chemotaxis. It is treated with normal human serum transfusions.

lb [L, libra],   abbreviation for **pound.**

lb ap,   abbreviation for apothecary pound.

lb avdp,   abbreviation for avoirdupois pound.

LBBB,   abbreviation for left bundle branch block.

LBW,   abbreviation for low birth weight. See **low birth weight infant.**

lb cal,   abbreviation for pound calorie.

lbd,   abbreviation for lower back disorder.

lbf,   abbreviation for pound-force.

lbf/ft²,   abbreviation for *pound-force per square foot.*

lbf/in²,   abbreviation for *pound-force per square inch.*

lbm,   abbreviation for **lean body mass.**

lbp,   **1.** abbreviation for **low back pain. 2.** abbreviation for *low blood pressure.*

L-carnitine /elkär'nitēn/,   an oral drug for carnitine deficiency.

■ INDICATIONS: The product is prescribed for the treatment of primary systemic carnitine deficiency.

■ CONTRAINDICATIONS: It should not be given to patients with a known hypersensitivity to carnitine.

■ ADVERSE EFFECTS: Nausea, vomiting, abdominal cramps, diarrhea, and body odor are included in adverse reactions.

LCAT,   abbreviation for *lecithin-cholesterol acetyltransferase.*

LCBF   abbreviation for **local cerebral blood flow.**

LCMRG   abbreviation for **local cerebral metabolic rate of glucose utilization.**

LD,   abbreviation for *lethal dose.*

LD50,   (in toxicology) the amount of a substance sufficient to kill one half of the population of test subjects.

LDH,   abbreviation for **lactate dehydrogenase.**

LDL,   abbreviation for **low-density lipoprotein.**

L-dopa.   See **levodopa.**

le,   abbreviation for *left eye.*

LE,   abbreviation for *lupus erythematosus.* See **systemic lupus erythematosus.**

lead (Pb) /led/ [ME, *leed*],   a common soft, blue-gray, metallic element. Its atomic number is 82; its atomic weight is 207.19. In its metallic form, lead is used as a protective shielding against x-rays. Lead is poisonous, a characteristic that has led to a reduction in the use of lead compounds as pigments for paints and inks. Normal concentrations in whole blood are 0 to 5 [Grk m]g/dl. The normal amount in urine after 24-hour collection is less the 100 [Grk m]g.

lead /lēd/ [As, *laedan*, to lead],   an electric connection attached to the body to record electric activity, especially of the heart or brain. See also **electrocardiograph, electroencephalograph.**

lead apron /led/ [AS, *led*; Fr, *napperon*],   a protective shield of lead and rubber that may be worn by a patient, radiologic technician, or radiologist, or both, during exposure to x-rays or other diagnostic or therapeutic radiation. It is intended to guard against excessive exposure of the genitalia and other vital body organs to ionizing radiation. Also called **protective apron.**

lead encephalopathy /led/ [AS, *led*; Gk, *enkephalos*, brain; *pathos,* disease],   a condition of brain structure and function as a result of lead poisoning, including exposure to tetraethyl lead. Children are commonly afflicted after eating chips of lead-based paints. The untreated disorder is characterized by delirium, convulsions, mania, cortical blindness, and coma.

lead equivalent /led/,   (in radiology) the thickness of lead required to achieve the same shielding effect against radiation, under specified conditions, as that provided by a given material.

leadership [AS, *leadan*, to lead, *scieppan*, to shape],   the ability to influence others to the attainment of goals. Kinds of leadership include authoritarian, democratic, participative, and permissive.

lead pipe fracture /led/,   a fracture that compresses the bony tissue at the point of impact and creates a linear fracture on the opposite side of the bone involved.

lead poisoning /led/,   a toxic condition caused by the ingestion or inhalation of lead or lead compounds. Many children have developed the condition as a result of eating flaked lead paint. Poisoning also occurs from the ingestion of water from lead pipes, lead salts in certain foods and wines, the use of pewter or earthenware glazed with a lead glaze, and the use of leaded gasoline. Inhalation of lead fumes is common in industry. The acute form of intoxication is characterized by a burning sensation in the mouth and esophagus, colic, constipation, or diarrhea, mental disturbances, and paralysis of the extremities, followed in severe cases by convulsions and muscular collapse. Chronic lead poisoning, which is characterized by extreme irritability, anorexia, and anemia, may progress to the acute form. If ingested, treatment commences with gastric lavage with magnesium or sodium sulfate. All cases call for fluid therapy followed by chelation with intramuscular injection of calcium disodium edetate, or for severe cases, British antilewisite. Encephalopathy must be anticipated in children with lead poisoning.

lead shielding /led/,   the use of aprons and other devices containing lead as protective measures against radiation. A layer of lead 1.0 mm in thickness should attenuate 99% of x-rays of 50 kVp and 94% of x-rays of 100 kVp.

leakage radiation /lē'kij/ [ONorse, *leka*, to drip; L, *radiare*, to emit rays],   radiation, exclusive of the primary beam, that is emitted through the housing of equipment used in radiation therapy.

leaky gene.   See **hypomorph.**

lean body mass (lbm) [ME, *lenen*, slender; AS, *bodig*; ME, *massa*, lump],   the combination of cell solids, extracellular and intracellular water, and mineral mass of the body.

learned helplessness /lurnd/,   a behavioral state and personality trait of a person who believes he or she is ineffectual, responses are futile, and control over reinforcers in the environment has been lost.

learning [AS, *leornian*, to learn],   **1.** the act or process of acquiring knowledge or some skill by means of study, practice, or experience. **2.** knowledge, wisdom, or a skill acquired through systematic study or instruction. **3.** (in psychology) the modification of behavior through practice, experience, or training. See also **conditioning.**

learning disability,   an abnormal condition often affecting children of normal or above-average intelligence, characterized by difficulty in learning such fundamental procedures as reading, writing, and numeric calculation. The condition may result from psychologic or organic causes and is usually related to slow development of perceptual motor skills. See also **attention deficit disorder, dysgraphia, dyslexia.**

learning theory [AS, *leornian,* to learn; Gl, *theoria,* speculation],   a group of concepts and principles that attempts to explain the learning process. One concept, Guthrie's contiguous conditioning premise, postulates that each response becomes permanently linked with stimuli present at the time so that contiguity rather than reinforcement is a part of the learning process.

leather-bottle stomach.   See **linitis plastica.**

Leber's congenital amaurosis /lā'bərz/ [Theodor von Leber, German ophthalmologist, b. 1840; L, *congenitus,* born with; Gk, *amauroein,* to darken],   a rare kind of blindness or severely impaired vision caused by a defect transmitted as an autosomal recessive trait and occurring at birth or shortly thereafter. The eyes appear normal externally, but pupillary constriction to light is sluggish or absent and retinal pigment is degenerated. Pendular nystagmus, photophobia, cataract, and keratoconus may be present, and the ophthalmic disorder may be associated with mental retardation and epilepsy. One kind of Leber's amaurosis results in complete blindness, but with a second kind the pathology does not progress and the patient has very slight vision. Also called **amaurosis congenita of Leber.**

Leboyer method of delivery /ləboiyā'/, an approach to the delivery of an infant formulated by the French obstetrician Charles Leboyer. It has four aspects: a gentle, controlled delivery in a quiet, dimly lit room, avoidance of pulling on the head, avoidance of overstimulation of the infant's sensorium, and encouragement of maternal-infant bonding. The goal of the method is to minimize the trauma of birth by gently and pleasantly introducing the newborn to life outside the womb. Unnecessary intervention in the process of birth is eschewed. After delivery, the baby is gently laid on the mother's abdomen, the back is massaged as the cord stops pulsating, and, when regular spontaneous respirations are established, the baby is gently supported in a warm tub of water by the father. Many birth centers and obstetric services in the United States have found that no adverse effects result from this method. Some studies in France have suggested superior psychologic, social, and intellectual development in young children delivered by this method. Compare **Bradley method, Lamaze method, Read method.**

L.E. cell (lupus erythematosus cell), a neutrophil that has phagocytosed the nucleus of another leukocyte that has already been altered by interacting with the L.E. factor in the bloodstream.

lecithin /les'ithin/ [Gk, *lekithos*, yolk], any of a group of phospholipids common in plants and animals. Lecithins are found in the liver, nerve tissue, semen, and in smaller amounts in bile and blood. They are essential for the metabolism of fats and are used in the processing of foods, pharmaceutical products, cosmetics, and inks. Rich dietary sources are soybeans, egg yolk, and corn. Deficiency leads to hepatic and renal disorders, high serum cholesterol levels, atherosclerosis, and arteriosclerosis. See also **choline, inositol.**

lecithin/sphingomyelin ratio, the ratio of two components of amniotic fluid, used for predicting fetal lung maturity. The normal ratio in amniotic fluid is 2:1 or greater when fetal lungs are mature.

lecitho-, a combining form meaning 'of or pertaining to the yolk of an egg, or to the ovum': *lecithoblast, lecithoprotein, lecithovitellin.*

lectin /lek'tin/, a protein substance occurring in seeds and other parts of certain plants that binds with glycoproteins and glycolipids on the surface of animal cells causing agglutination. Some lectins cause agglutination of erythrocytes in specific blood groups, and others stimulate the production of T lymphocytes.

Ledercillin VK, a trademark for an antibacterial (penicillin V potassium).

Lee-Davidsohn test, a heterophil antibody test for infectious mononucleosis using horse red blood cells. See also **heterophil antibody test.**

Leeuwenhoekia australiensis [Anton van Leeuwenhoek, Dutch microscopist, b. 1632; Australia], a mite indigenous to New South Wales that burrows into the skin, producing severe irritation. Also called **scrub itch.**

Lee-White method [Roger I. Lee, American physician, b.

1881; Paul D. White, American physician, b. 1886; Gk, *meta*, beyond, *hodos*, way], a method of determining the length of time required for a clot to form in a test tube of venous blood. It is not specific for any coagulation disorder but is often used to monitor coagulation during heparin therapy. Because normal values and precise methodology vary, instructions are provided by most laboratories. See also **clotting time.**

LeFort I fracture. See **Guérin's fracture.**

left atrioventricular valve. See **mitral valve.**

left brachiocephalic vein [ME, *left*, weak; Gk, *brachys*, short, *kephale*, head], a vessel, about 6 cm long, that starts in the root of the neck at the junction of the internal jugular and the subclavian veins on the left side and runs obliquely across the thorax to join the right brachiocephalic vein and form the superior vena cava. The left brachiocephalic vein, which is longer than the right, receives various tributaries, such as the vertebral vein, the internal thoracic vein, and the inferior thyroid vein. Also called **left innominate vein.** Compare **right brachiocephalic vein.**

left common carotid artery, the longer of the two common carotid arteries, springing from the aortic arch and having cervical and thoracic portions. The cervical portion passes obliquely from the level of the sternoclavicular articulation to the cranial border of the thyroid cartilage, dividing into the left internal and the left external carotid arteries. Compare **right common carotid artery.**

left coronary artery, one of a pair of branches from the ascending aorta, arising in the left posterior aortic sinus, dividing into the left interventricular artery and the circumflex branch, supplying both ventricles and the left atrium. Compare **right coronary artery.**

left-handedness /left'han'didnes/, a natural tendency by some persons to favor the use of the left hand in performing certain tasks. Also called **sinistrality.** See also **cerebral dominance, handedness.**

left-heart failure, an abnormal cardiac condition characterized by the impairment of the left side of the heart and by elevated pressure and congestion in the pulmonary veins and capillaries. Left-heart failure may be related to right-heart failure, because both sides of the heart are part of a circuit and the impairment of one side will eventually affect the other. However, research indicates that experimentally produced pure failure of one ventricle may produce significant hemodynamic and biochemical abnormalities of the opposite ventricle, even without the usual signs of failure. In 'pure' left-heart failure, the body retains significant amounts of sodium and water and consequently develops peripheral edema without clinical evidence of right-heart failure. Also called **left-sided failure.** Compare **right-heart failure.**

left hepatic duct, the duct that drains the bile from the left lobe of the liver into the common bile duct.

left innominate vein. See **left brachiocephalic vein.**

left lateral recumbent position [ME, *left*; L, *latus*, side + *recumbere*, to lie down + *positio*], a position in which the patient lies on the left side with the upper knee and thigh drawn upward.

left lymphatic duct. See **thoracic duct.**

left pulmonary artery, the shorter and smaller of two arteries conveying venous blood from the heart to the lungs, rising from the pulmonary trunk, connecting to the left lung, and tending to have more separate branches than the right pulmonary artery. In the fetus it is larger and more important than the right pulmonary artery because it provides the ductus arteriosus that degenerates to become a ligament after birth. Compare **right pulmonary artery.**

left-sided failure. See **left-heart failure.**

left subclavian artery, an artery, divided into three parts, that arises from the aortic arch dorsal to the left common carotid at the level of the fourth thoracic vertebra, ascends to the root of the neck, arches laterally to the scalenus anterior, and forms six main branches to supply the vertebral column, spinal cord, ear, and brain. The short second portion lies dorsal to the scalenus anterior and forms the arch described by the vessel. The third portion runs from the scalenus anterior to the first rib where it becomes the axillary artery. See also **subclavian artery.** Compare **right subclavian artery.**

left ventricle (LV), the thick-walled chamber of the heart that pumps blood through the aorta and the systemic arteries, the capillaries, and back through the veins to the right atrium. It has walls about three times thicker than those of the right ventricle and contains a mitral valve with two flaps that controls the flow of blood from the left atrium. The left ventricle occupies about half the diaphragmatic surface of the heart and is longer and more conical than the right ventricle, narrowing caudally to form the apex. The chordae tendineae of the left ventricle are thicker, stronger, and less numerous than those in the right ventricle. See also **chordae tendineae.**

left ventricular assist device (LVAD), a mechanical pump that temporarily and artificially aids the natural pumping action of the left ventricle.

left ventricular failure, heart failure in which the left ventricle fails to contract forcefully enough to maintain a normal cardiac output and peripheral perfusion. Pulmonary congestion and edema develop from back pressure of accumulated blood in the left ventricle. Signs include breathlessness, pallor, sweating, and peripheral vasoconstriction. The heart is usually enlarged. A prominent third heart sound (gallop), normal in children and young adults, is a sign of left ventricular failure in older adults with heart disease. Hypertension is common and may be a causative factor or a result of pulmonary edema. Treatment includes meperidine or morphine for sedation, diuretics, digitalis, and rest. See **congestive heart failure.**

legacy /leg'əsē/ [L, *legatum*, bequest], something that is handed down from the past or is intended to be bestowed on future generations.

legal [L, *lex*], actions or conditions that are permitted or authorized by law.

legal blindness [L, *lex*, law; ME, *blend*, sightless], a state of visual acuity in which no better than 20/200 is measured in the better eye with corrective lenses, or a visual field of not more than 20 degrees is obtained.

legal death. See **death.**

leg cylinder cast [ONorse, *leggr;* Gk, *kylindros;* ONorse, *kasta*], an orthopedic device of plaster of paris or fiberglass used to immobilize the leg in treating fractures in the legs from the ankle to the upper thigh. It is especially used for fractures and dislocations of the knee, for the soft tissue trauma around the knee, for postoperative positioning and immobilization of the knee, and for correction or maintenance of correction of deformities of the knee. The long-leg cast may be used for these same conditions rather than the leg cylinder cast because it encases the foot and ensures greater immobilization.

Legg-Calvé-Perthes disease. See **Perthes disease.**

Legionella pneumonia /lē'jənel'ə/ [American Legion; Gk, *pneumon*, lung], a form of pneumonia caused by a gram-negative bacillus identified as *Legionella pneumophila*. It was discovered after an outbreak of the disease among veterans attending a 1976 convention of the American Legion. See also *Legionella pneumophila*, **Legionnaire's disease.**

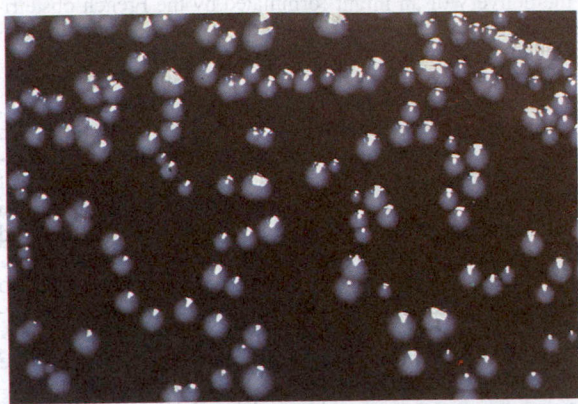

Legionella pneumophilia
(Baron, 1990/Courtesy Dr. Clifford Mintz)

Legionella pneumophila /nōōmof'ələ/, a small, gram-negative, rod-shaped bacterium that is the causative agent in **Legionnaires' disease.**

Legionnaires' disease /lē'jənerz'/ [L, *legionarius*, member of a legion], an acute bacterial pneumonia caused by infection with *Legionella pneumophila* and characterized by an influenza-like illness followed within a week by high fever, chills, muscle aches, and headache. The symptoms may progress to dry cough, pleurisy, and sometimes diarrhea. Usually the disease is self-limited, but mortality has been 15% to 20% in a few localized epidemics. Contaminated air conditioning cooling towers and stagnant water supplies, including water vaporizers and water sonicators may be a source of organisms. Person-to-person contagion has not occurred. Risk of infection is increased by the presence of other conditions, such as cardiopulmonary diseases. Treatment includes supportive care and erythromycin. Also called **legionellosis.**

legume /leg'yōōm/ [L, *legumen*, pulse], any of the members of the *Fabales* order of dicotyledenous plants, including dried peas, beans, and lentils.

leio-, lio-, a prefix meaning 'smooth': *leiodermia, leiodystonia, leiomyofibroma.*

leiomyoblastoma. See **epithelioid leiomyoma.**

leiomyofibroma /lī'ōmī'ōfībrō'mə/, *pl.* **leiomyofibromas, leiomyofibromata** [Gk, *leios*, smooth, *mys*, muscle; L, *fibra*, fiber; Gk, *oma*, tumor], a tumor consisting of smooth muscle cells and fibrous connective tissue, commonly occurring in the uterus in middle-aged women. See also **fibroid.**

leiomyoma /lī'ōmī·ō'mə/, *pl.* **leiomyomas, leiomyomata,** a benign smooth muscle tumor occurring most commonly in the stomach, esophagus, or small intestine. Surgical resection is necessary only when the tumor undergoes central necrosis, causing sudden and severe hemorrhage.

leiomyoma cutis, a neoplasm of the smooth muscles of the skin. The lesion is characterized by many small, tender, red nodules.

leiomyoma uteri, a benign neoplasm of the smooth muscle of the uterus. The tumor is characteristically firm, well circumscribed, round, and gray-white. Histologically, a pattern of whorls is present. Tumors of this kind develop in the myometrium and occur in women between 30 and 50 years of age. Also called **fibromyoma uteri, myoma previum, (informal) fibroids.**

leiomyosarcoma /-särkō′mə/ [Gk, *leios,* smooth; *mys,* muscle; *sarx,* flesh; *oma,* tumor], a sarcoma that contains large spindle cells of unstriated muscle.

leipo-. See **lip-.**

Leishman-Donovan body /lēsh′məndon′əvən/ [Sir William B. Leishman, English pathologist, b. 1865; Charles Donovan, Scottish physician, b. 1863], the resting stage of an intracellular, nonflagellated protozoan parasite *(Leishmania donovani)* that causes kala-azar, or visceral leishmaniasis as it appears in infected tissue specimens.

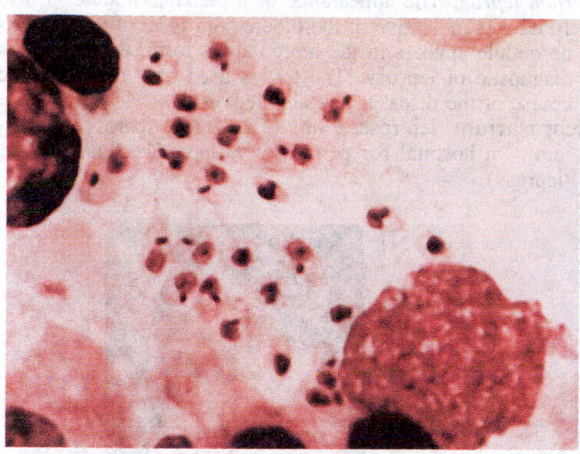

Leishman-Donovan bodies
(Murray, 1990/Reproduced by permission from LR Ash and TC Orihel, Atlas of Human Parasitology, ed 2, 1984, by the American Society of Clinical Pathologists Press, Chicago)

Leishmania /lēshmä′nē·ə/ [Sir William B. Leishman], a genus of protozoan parasites. These organisms are transmitted to humans by any of several species of sand flies.

leishmaniasis /lēsh′mənī′əsis/ [Sir William B. Leishman], infection with any species of protozoan of the genus *Leishmania.* The diseases caused by these organisms may be cutaneous or visceral. Diagnosis is made by microscopic identification of the intracellular, nonflagellated protozoan on a Giemsa-stained smear taken from a cutaneous lesion or visceral biopsy. Kinds of leishmaniasis are **American leishmaniasis, kala-azar,** and **oriental sore.** See also *Leishmania.* **–leishmanial,** *adj.*

-lemma, a combining form meaning a 'confining membrane': *axiolemma, epilemma, neurolemma.*

lemniscal system /lemnis′kəl/ [Gk, *lemniskos,* fillet; *systema*], a part of the somatosensory network of large diameter myelinated A fibers. It includes the dorsal columns

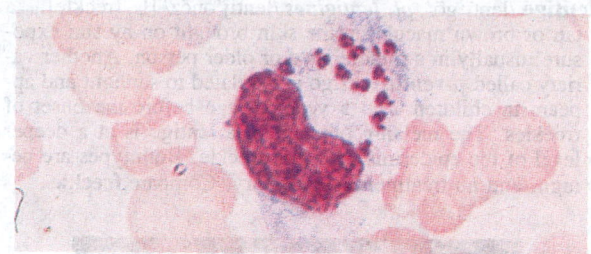

Leishmania donovani amastiagotes in a macrophage
(Hayhoe, 1992)

and the neospinothalamic tract extending from the spinal cord to the thalamus and cortex.

lemniscus /lemnis′kəs/ [Gk, *lemniskos,* fillet], a band or tract of central nervous system fibers, particularly the ascending axons of secondary sensory neurons leading to the thalamus.

length of stay (LOS), the period of time a patient remains in a hospital or other health care facility as an inpatient.

lens [L, lentil], **1.** a curved transparent piece of plastic or glass that is shaped, molded, or ground to refract light in a specific way, as in eyeglasses, microscopes, or cameras. **2.** *informal.* the crystalline lens of the eye. **–lenticular,** *adj.*

lens capsule, the clear thin elastic capsule that surrounds the lens of the eye. Also called **capsule of the lens.**

lens implant, an artifical lens that is usually implanted at the time of cataract extraction but may also be used for patients with extreme myopia, diplopia, ocular albinism, and certain other abnormalities. The operation may be performed with a local anesthetic. Eyedrops containing an antibiotic, such as neomycin, are applied preoperatively to prevent infection, and several times a day for a number of weeks postoperatively. After extraction of the cataract, the lens is inserted through a corneal incision; it may be held in place in the anterior chamber by extremely fine sutures to the iris, or, if the lens is implanted into the capsular sac, a miotic agent, such as pilocarpine, is used to prevent the iris from dilating too widely, which would allow the implant to slip. The implanted lens does not cause the problems with abnormal peripheral vision associated with cataract spectacles. The implanted lens produces only 2% larger images on the retina than the normal lens, compared with a 24% enlargement produced by cataract spectacles and an 8% enlargement produced by contact lenses. A low rate of complications is reported in implant surgery and in some cases of glaucoma.

Lente Insulin, a trademark for an intermediate-acting insulin.

lenticonus /len′tikō′nəs/, an abnormal spherical or conical protrusion on the lens of the eye. It is a congenital defect found in Alport's syndrome.

-lenticular. See **lens.**

lenticular nucleus /lentik′yələr/ [L, *lentil,* lens + *nucleus,* nut], biconvex basal ganglia of the cerebrum, composed of lateral putamen and medial globus pallidus tissue as part of the corpus striatum.

lentiform /len′tifôrm/ [L, *lens; forma*], pertaining to or resembling a lentil shape, such as the lens of the eye.

lentigo /lentī′gō/, *pl.* **lentigines** /lentij′ənēz/ [L, freckle], a tan or brown macule on the skin brought on by sun exposure, usually in a middle-aged or older person. Another variety called **juvenile lentigo** is unrelated to sunlight and appears in children 2 to 5 years of age before the onset of freckles. The melanin pigment in a lentigo is at a deeper level of the epidermis than in a freckle. Both types are benign, and no treatment is necessary. Compare **freckle.**

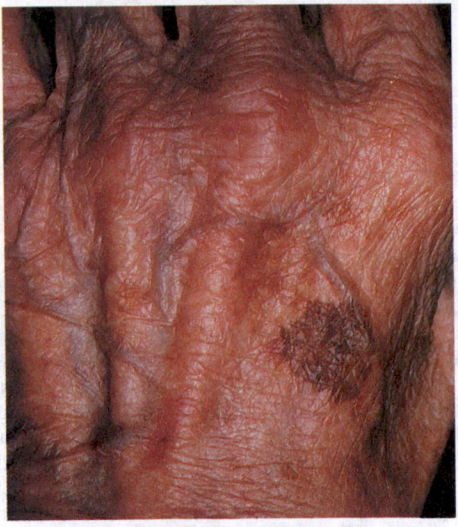

Lentigo *(Habif, 1990)*

lentigo maligna. See **Hutchinson's freckle.**
lentigo maligna melanoma, a neoplasm developing from Hutchinson's freckle on the face or other exposed surfaces of the skin in elderly patients. It is asymptomatic, flat, and tan or brown, with irregular darker spots and frequent hypopigmentation. It is one of the three major clinical types

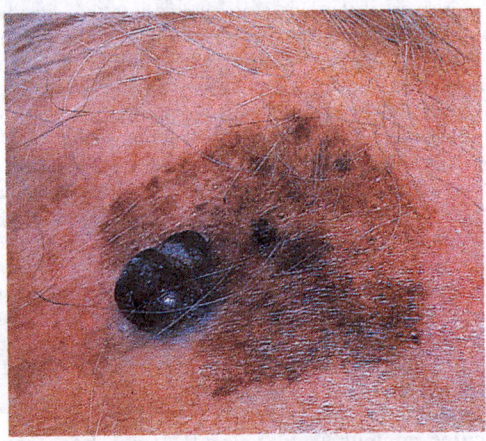

Lentigo maligna melanoma *(du Vivier, 1986)*

of melanoma and occurs in 10% to 15% of melanoma patients. See also **nodular melanoma, superficial spreading melanoma.**

lentivirus /len′tivī′rəs/, a member of a subfamily of retroviruses that includes the AIDS virus. Lentiviruses are usually slow viruses, with long incubation periods that may delay the onset of symptoms until several years after exposure.
Leopold's maneuver [Christian Gerhard Leopold, German physician, b. 1846], a series of four steps used in palpating the abdomen of a pregnant woman to determine the position and presentation of the fetus.
leper /lep′ər/ [Gk, *lepis*, scaly], an outdated term for a person afflicted with Hansen's disease (leprosy).
lepido-, a prefix meaning 'of or pertaining to a flake or scale': *lepidoma, lepidosis.*
LE prep, abbreviation for **lupus erythematosus preparation.**
lepro-, a prefix meaning 'of or pertaining to leprosy': *leprologist, lepromatous, leprosarium.*
-lepromatous. See **leprosy.**
lepromatous leprosy. See **leprosy.**
lepromin test /leprō′min/, a skin sensitivity test used to distinguish between the lepromatous and tuberculoid forms of leprosy. The test consists of intradermal injection of lepromin, which is prepared from heat-sterilized *Mycobacterium leprae.* The appearance of a palpable nodule in 8 to 10 days is indicative of the tuberculoid form of leprosy. As no nodule appears in the lepromatous form, the test is not diagnostic of leprosy. The test is used only to follow the course of the disease. See also **leprosy.**
leprosarium /lep′rōser′ē·əm/ [Gk, *lepra*, leprosy; sanitarium], a hospital for persons who have Hansen's disease (leprosy).

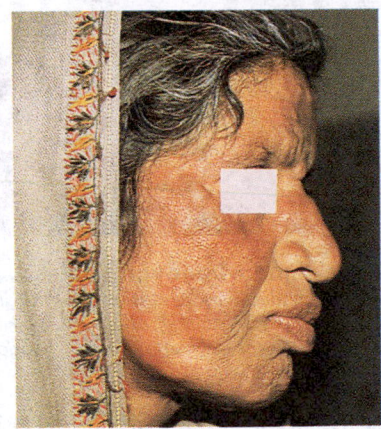

Lepromatous leprosy
(McKee, 1993/Courtesy Dr S Lucas, University College Hospital, London)

leprosy /lep′rəsē/ [Gk, *lepra*], a chronic, communicable disease, caused by *Mycobacterium leprae,* that may take either of two forms, depending on the degree of immunity of the host. **Tuberculoid leprosy,** seen in those with high resistance, presents as thickening of cutaneous nerves and anesthetic, saucer-shaped skin lesions. **Lepromatous leprosy,** seen in those with little resistance, involves many systems of the body, with widespread plaques and nodules in the skin, iritis, keratitis, destruction of nasal cartilage and bone, testicular atrophy, peripheral edema, and involvement of the reticuloendothelial system. Blindness may result. Death is rare unless amyloidosis or tuberculosis occurs concurrently.

Contrary to traditional belief, leprosy is not very contagious, and prolonged, intimate contact is required for it to be spread between individuals. Children are more susceptible than adults. Plastic surgery, physical therapy, and psychotherapy are often necessary. Treatment with sulfones, such as dapsone, continued for several years results usually in improvement of skin lesions, but recovery from nerve impairment is limited. The disease is found mostly in underdeveloped tropic and subtropic countries. In the United States, patients may be referred to the U.S. Public Health Service leprosarium in Carville, Louisiana. BCG vaccine may protect against leprosy. Also called **Hansen's disease.** See also *Mycobacterium*. **—lepromatous, leprotic, leprous,** *adj.*

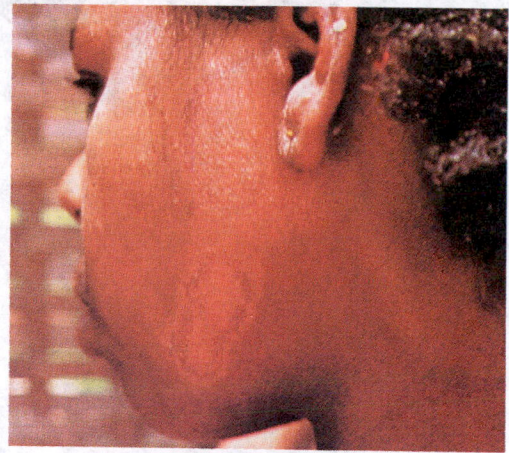

Tuberculoid leprosy
(Perkin, 1986/Courtesy Dr R St. C Barnetson, Consultant Dermatologist, Department of Dermatology, Edinburgh Royal Infirmary, Edinburgh, UK)

-lepsy, -lepsia, -lepsis, a suffix meaning a 'seizure': *deolepsy, electrolepsy, pyknolepsy.*

-leptic, a suffix meaning 'pertaining to a (specified) type of seizure': *cataleptic, epileptic, hypnoleptic.*

lepto- /lep′tō-/, a combining form meaning 'slender, small, thin, or delicate': *leptodermic, leptodactylosis.*

leptocyte. See **target cell.**

leptocytosis /lep′tōsītō′sis/ [Gk, *leptos*, thin, *kytos*, cell, *osis*, condition], a hematologic condition in which target cells are present in the blood. Thalassemia, some forms of liver disease, and absence of the spleen are associated with leptocytosis.

leptomeninges /lep′tōminin′jēz/ [Gk, *leptos* + *meninx*, membrane], the arachnoid membrane and the pia mater, two of the three layers covering the brain and spinal cord. Compare **meninges.**

leptonema /lep′tənē′mə/ [Gk, *leptos* + *nema*, thread], the threadlike chromosome formation in the leptotene stage in the first meiotic prophase of gametogenesis before the beginning of synapsis.

Leptospira /-spī′rə/ [Gk, *leptos* + *speira*, coil], a genus of the family Treponemataceae, order Spirochaetales, tightly coiled microorganisms having spirals with hooked ends. The spirochete thrives in the urine of infected animals, especially rodents, is pathogenic to humans and other mammals, and may cause hepatitis, jaundice, skin hemorrhages, fever, renal failure, mental status changes, and muscular illness. See also **leptospirosis.**

Leptospira agglutinin, an agglutinin found in the blood of patients with leptospirosis.

leptospirosis /lep′tōspīrō′sis/ [Gk, *leptos, speira* + *osis*, condition], an acute infectious disease caused by several serotypes of the spirochete *Leptospira interrogans*, transmitted in the urine of wild or domestic animals, especially rats and dogs. Human infections arise directly from contact with an infected animal's urine or tissues or indirectly from contact with contaminated water or soil. Clinical symptoms may include hepatitis, jaundice, hemorrhage into the skin, fever, chills, renal failure, meningitis with mental status changes, and muscular pain. The spirochete can be isolated from the urine or blood during the acute stage of the disease, and antibodies can be found in the patient's blood during convalescence. Treatment with antibiotics, usually penicillin or tetracycline, may be effective if they are administered during the first few days of the disease. Fluid and electrolyte replacement is essential if jaundice or other signs of severe illness are present. The disease is usually short-lived and mild, but severe infections can damage the kidneys and the liver. Blood pressure and vital signs should be monitored, and the patient's urine should be disposed of carefully to prevent spread of the organism. The most serious form of the disease is called **Weil's disease.** Also called **autumn fever.** See also **nanukayami.**

leptotene /lep′tətēn/ [Gk, *leptos* + *tainia*, ribbon], the initial stage in the first meiotic prophase in gametogenesis in which the chromosomes become visible as single thin filaments. See also **diakinesis, diplotene, pachytene, zygotene.**

Leriche's syndrome /lərēshs′/ [Rene Leriche, French surgeon, b. 1879], a vascular disorder marked by gradual occlusion of the terminal aorta, intermittent claudication in the buttocks, thighs, or calves, absence of pulsation in femoral arteries, pallor and coldness of the legs, gangrene of the toes, and, in men, impotence. Symptoms are the result of chronic tissue hypoxia caused by inadequate arterial perfusion of the affected areas. Treatment may include endarterectomy, embolectomy, or synthetic bypass graft at the bifurcation of the aorta.

lesbian /lez′bē·ən/ [Gk, island of Lesbos, home of Sappho], **1.** a female homosexual. **2.** of or pertaining to the sexual preference or desire of one woman for another. **—lesbianism,** *n.*

Lesch-Nyhan syndrome /lesh′nī′han/ [Michael Lesch, American pediatrician, b. 1939; William L. Nyhan, Jr., American pediatrician, b. 1926], a hereditary disorder of purine metabolism, characterized by mental retardation, self-mutilation of the fingers and lips by biting, impaired renal function, and abnormal physical development. It is transmitted as a recessive, sex-linked trait.

lesion /lē′zhen/ [L, *laesus*, an injury], **1.** a wound, injury, or pathologic change in body tissue. **2.** any visible, local abnormality of the tissues of the skin, such as a wound, sore, rash, or boil. A lesion may be described as benign, cancerous, gross, occult, or primary. (Table, pp. 686-687)

lesser circulation. See **pulmonary circulation.**

lesser multangular bone. See **trapezoid bone.**

lesser occipital nerve [AS, *losian*, to lose; L, *occiput*, back of the head, *nervus*, nerve], one of a pair of cutaneous branches of the cervical plexus, arising from the second cervical nerve, curving around the sternocleidomastoideus muscle, and ascending along the side of the head behind the ear to supply the skin. It communicates with the greater

Types of skin lesions

Observed skin changes	Differentiation	Term	Example
Change in color or texture			
Spot	Circumscribed, flat, color change	Macule	Freckle
Discoloration (reddish purple)	Bleeding beneath the surface, injury to tissue	Contusion	Bruise
Soft whitening	Caused by repeated wetting of skin	Maceration	Between toes after soaking
Flake	Dry cells of surface	Scale	Dandruff
Roughness from dried fluid	Dry exudate over lesions	Crust	Eczema, impetigo
Roughness from cells	Leathery thickening of outer skin layer	Lichenification	Callus on foot
Silvery scale	Buildup of scale	Plaque	Psoriasis
Change in shape			
Solid mass, cellular growth	Less than 5 mm	Papule	Small mole, raised rash
	5 mm to 2 cm	Nodule	Enlarged lymph node

Illustrations from Seidel HM, Ball JB, Davis JE, and Benedict GW, *Mosby's Guide to Physical Examination, Ed. 2.* St. Louis, 1991, Mosby–Year Book, Inc.

Types of skin lesions—cont'd

Observed skin changes	Differentiation	Term	Example
Change in shape— cont'd			
Solid mass, cellular growth —cont'd	Greater than 2 cm	Tumor	Benign or malignant tumor
	Excess connective tissue over scar	Keloid	Overgrown scar
Fluid-filled lesions	Less than 1 cm, clear fluid	Vesicle	Blister, chickenpox
	Greater than 1 cm, clear fluid	Bulla	Large blister, pemphigus
	Small, thick yellowish fluid (pus)	Pustule	Acne
	Semisolid	Cyst	Sebaceous cyst
Swelling of tissue	Generalized swelling; fluid between cells	Edema	Inflammation, swelling of feet

Continued.

Types of skin lesions—cont'd

Observed skin changes	Differentiation	Term	Example	
Change in shape—cont'd				
Swelling of tissue—cont'd	Circumscribed surface edema, transient, some itching	Wheal	Allergic reaction	
Breaks in skin surfaces				
Oozing, scraped surface	Loss of superficial surface of skin	Abrasion	"Floor burn," scrape	
Linear crack or cleft	Slit or splitting of skin layers	Fissure	Athlete's foot	
Scooped-out depression	Loss of deeper layers of skin	Ulcer	Decubitus, stasis ulcer	

Types of skin lesions—cont'd

Observed skin changes	Differentiation	Term	Example
Breaks in skin surfaces—cont'd			
Superficial linear skin breaks	Scratch marks, frequently by fingernails	Excoriations	Scratching

Observed skin changes	Differentiation	Term	Example
Jagged cut	Tearing of skin surface	Laceration	Accidental cut by blunt object
Linear cut, edges approximated	Cutting by sharp instrument	Incision	Knife cut
Vascular lesions			
Small, flat, round, purplish red spot	Intradermal or submucous hemorrhage	Petechia	Bleeding tendency, vitamin C deficiency

Observed skin changes	Differentiation	Term	Example
Spiderlike, red, small	Dilatation of capillaries, arterioles, or venules	Telangiectasis	Liver disease, vitamin B deficiency, sun-damaged skin

Observed skin changes	Differentiation	Term	Example
Discoloration, (reddish purple)	Escape of blood into tissue	Ecchymosis	Trauma to blood vessels

occipital and the great auricular nerves and with the posterior auricular branch of the facial nerve.

lesser omentum [AS, *losian*, to lose; L, *omentum*, entrails], a membranous extension of the peritoneum from the peritoneal layers covering the ventral and the dorsal surfaces of the stomach and the first part of the duodenum. The lesser omentum extends from the portal fissure of the liver to the diaphragm where the layers separate to enclose the end of the esophagus. It also forms two ligaments, one associated with the liver, the ligamentum hepatogastricum, and the other, the ligamentum hepatoduodenale, with the duodenum. Also called **gastrohepatic omentum, small omentum.**

lesser sciatic notch [ME, *les*; Gk, *ischiadikos*, hip joint; OFr, *enochier*], a notch on the posterior border of the hip bone. It is smooth, is coated with cartilage, and has several ridges corresponding to subdivisions of the obturator internus tendon.

lesser trochanter, one of a pair of conic projections at the base of the neck of the femur, providing insertion of the tendon of psoas major. Compare **greater trochanter.**

let-down, a sensation in the breasts of lactating women that often occurs as the milk flows into the ducts. It may occur when the infant begins to suck or when the mother hears the baby cry or even thinks of nursing the child.

let-down reflex. See **milk ejection reflex.**

lethal /lē'thəl/, deadly, capable of causing death.

lethal equivalent [L, *letum*, death; *aequus*, equal, *valere*, to be strong], any recessive gene carried in the heterozygous state that, if homozygous, would be lethal and result in the death of the individual or organism. It is estimated that any person carries from 3 to 8 lethal equivalents or any combination of genes, each with slightly deleterious effects, that are equivalent to 3 to 8 recessive genes.

lethal gene, any gene that produces a phenotypic effect that causes the death of the organism at some stage of development from fertilization of the egg to adulthood. The gene may be dominant, incompletely dominant, or recessive. In humans, examples of diseases caused by lethal genes are Huntington's chorea, which is transmitted as an autosomal dominant, and sickle cell anemia, which shows recessive lethality. Compare **sublethal gene.** See also **lethal equivalent.**

lethality /lēthal'itē/, the probability that a person threatening suicide will succeed, based on the method described, the specificity of the plan, and the availability of the means.

lethargic. See **lethary.**

lethargic encephalitis. See **epidemic encephalitis.**

lethargic stupor /lithär'gik/ [Gk, *lethargia*, drowsiness; L, *stupor,* numbness], *obsolete.* Any stupor accompanied by lethargy.

lethargy /leth'ərjē/ [Gk, *lethargos*, forgetful], **1.** the state or quality of being indifferent, apathetic, or sluggish. **2.** stupor or coma resulting from disease or hypnosis. —**lethargic,** *adj.*

Letterer-Siwe syndrome /let'ərərzē'və/ [Erich Letterer, German pathologist, b. 1895; Sture A. Siwe, Swedish physician, b. 1897], any of a group of malignant neoplastic diseases of unknown origin, characterized by histiocytic elements. The syndrome, which is fatal, occurs in infancy and is not familial. Anemia, hemorrhage, splenomegaly, lymphadenopathy, and localized tumefactions over bones are usually present.

letter quality printer, an electronic printer that produces

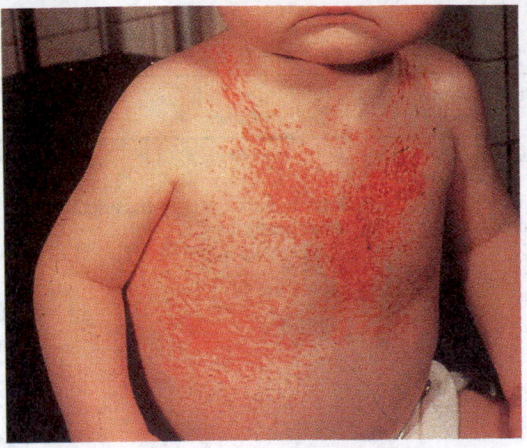

Letterer-Siwe syndrome
(McKee/Courtesy Prof D Burrows, Royal Victoria Hospital, Belfast)

characters resembling those of a typewriter in production quality. See **daisy wheel.**

leucine (Leu) /lōō'sēn/ [Gk, *leukos*, white], a white, crystalline amino acid essential for optimal growth in infants and nitrogen equilibrium in adults. It cannot be synthesized by the body and is obtained by the hydrolysis of food protein during pancreatic enzyme digestion. An inherited defect in one of the enzymes involved in the process results in a rare disorder called maple syrup urine disease. See also **amino acid, leucinosis, maple syrup urine disease.**

Chemical structure of leucine *(Seeley, 1992)*

leucinosis /lōō'sinō'sis/ [Gk, *leukos* + *osis*, condition], a condition in which the pathways for the degradation of leucine are blocked and large amounts of the amino acid accumulate in body tissue. See also **leucine.**

leuco-. See **leuko-.**

leucocyte. See **leukocyte.**

leucocytopenia. See **leukopenia.**

leucovorin. See **folinic acid.**

leucovorin calcium /lōō'kəvôr'in/, an antianemic.

■ INDICATIONS: It is prescribed in the treatment of an overdose of a folic acid antagonist and certain cases of megaloblastic anemia.

■ CONTRAINDICATIONS: Anemia caused by vitamin B12[0E] deficiency or known hypersensitivity to this drug prohibits its use.

■ ADVERSE EFFECTS: Hypersensitivity reactions may occur.

leukapheresis /lōō'kəfərē'sis/ [Gk, *leukos* + *aphairesis*, removal], a process by which blood is withdrawn from a vein, white blood cells are selectively removed, and the remaining blood is reinfused in the donor. The white blood cells may be used for treating patients with blood deficiencies or for research. Compare **plasmapheresis, plateletpheresis.** See also **apheresis.**

leukemia /lōōkē′mē·ə/ [Gk, *leukos* + *haima*, blood], a malignant neoplasm of blood-forming tissues characterized by diffuse replacement of bone marrow with proliferating leukocyte precursors, abnormal numbers and forms of immature white cells in circulation, and infiltration of lymph nodes, the spleen and liver. Approximately 20,500 new cases in adults and 2500 in children are diagnosed annually in the United States, and the disease causes about 15,900 deaths a year. Males are affected twice as frequently as females. The origin of leukemia is not clear, but it may result from exposure to ionizing radiation, benzene, or other chemicals that are toxic to bone marrow. The risk of the disease is increased in individuals with Down's syndrome, Fanconi's syndrome, ataxia-telangiectasia, Bloom's syndrome, or some other forms of congenital aneuploidy, and in an identical twin of a leukemia victim. Leukemia is classified according to the predominant proliferating cells, the clinical course, and the duration of the disease. Acute leukemia usually has a sudden onset and rapidly progresses from early signs, such as fatigue, pallor, weight loss, and easy bruising, to fever, hemorrhages, extreme weakness, bone or joint pain, and repeated infections. Chronic leukemia develops slowly, and signs similar to those of the acute forms of the disease may not appear for years. Diagnoses of acute and chronic forms are made by blood tests and bone marrow biopsies. Involved marrow may range in color from muddy red-brown to pale gray, and changes are usually first evident in the vertebrae, ribs, sternum, and pelvis. The most effective treatment includes intensive combination chemotherapy, the use of antibiotics to prevent infections, and blood transfusions to replace red cells and platelets. See also **acute childhood leukemia, acute lymphocytic leukemia, acute myelocytic anemia.** —**leukemic,** *adj.*

-leukemia, a combining form meaning an 'increased number of leukocytes in the tissues and/or in the blood': *chloroleukemia, erythroleukemia, hypoleukemia.*

leukemia cutis, a condition of the skin in which yellow-brown, red, or purple nodular lesions form localized or general diffuse infiltrations. Also called **lymphoderma perniciosa.**

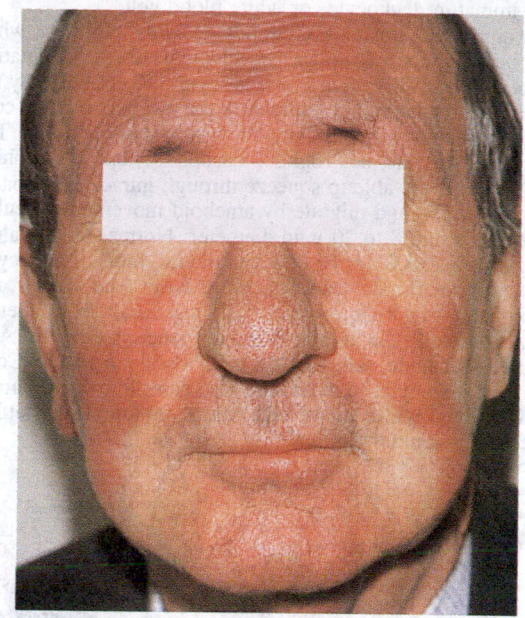

Leukemia cutis (McKee, 1993)

-leukemic. See **leukemia.**

leukemic reticuloendotheliosis. See **hairy-cell leukemia.**

leukemoid /lōōkē′moid/, resembling leukemia.

leukemoid reaction [Gk, *leukos* + *eidos*, form; L, *re,* again, *agere,* to act], a clinical syndrome resembling leukemia in which the white blood cell count is elevated in re-

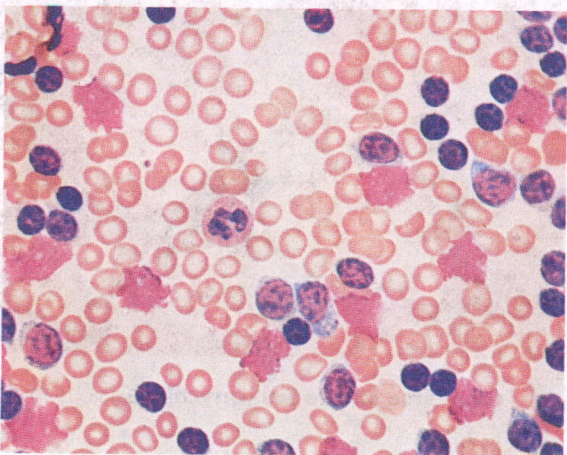

Peripheral blood smear showing chronic lymphocytic leukemia (Hayhoe, 1992)

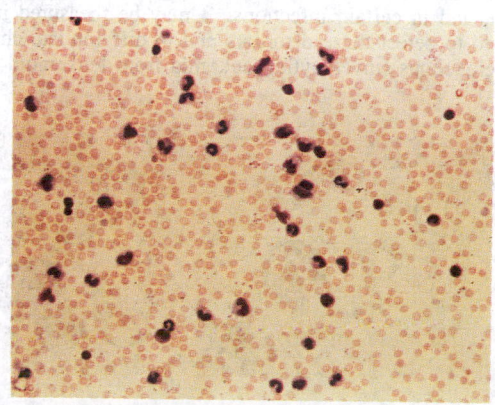

Leukemoid reaction (Zitelli, 1992)

sponse to an allergy, inflammatory disease, infection, poison, hemorrhage, burn, or severe physical stress. Compare **leukemia.**

Leukeran, a trademark for an antineoplastic (chlorambucil).

-leukin, a combining form for interleukin-2-type products.

leuko-, leuco-, a combining form meaning 'pertaining to a white corpuscle, or white': *leukocytopenia, leukocytosis.*

leukoblast /loo'kəblast/ [Gk, *leukos,* white; *blastos,* germ], an immature leukocyte, or white blood cell.

leukocyte /loo'kəsīt/ [Gk, *leukos + kytos,* cell], a white blood cell, one of the formed elements of the circulating blood system. Five types of leukocytes are classified by the presence or absence of granules in the cytoplasm of the cell. The agranulocytes are lymphocytes and monocytes. The granulocytes are neutrophils, basophils, and eosinophils. White cells are able to squeeze through intracellular spaces by diapedesis and migrate by ameboid movements. Leukocytes measure 8 to 20 μ in diameter. Normal blood values vary from 5000 to 10,000 leukocytes mm^3. Leukocytes function as phagocytes of bacteria, fungi, and viruses, detoxification of toxic proteins that may result from allergic reactions and cellular injury, and immune system cells. Also called **leucocyte, white blood cell, white corpuscle.** Compare **erythrocyte, platelet.** See also **complete blood count, differential white blood cell count, leukocytosis, leukopenia.** **−leukocytic,** *adj.*

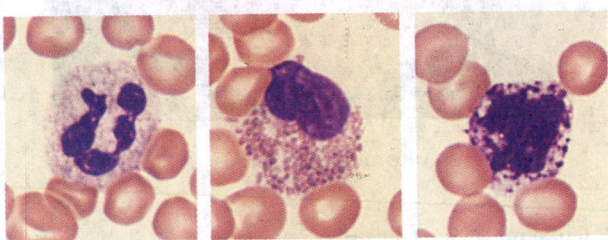

Examples of leukocytes: neutrophil, eosinophil, and basophil
(Erlandsen, 1992)

leukocyte alkaline phosphatase, an enzyme that is elevated in various diseases, such as cirrhosis and polycythemia, and in certain infections. It may be measured in the blood to detect these disorders and to differentiate chronic myelogenous (myelocytic) leukemia from leukemoid reac-

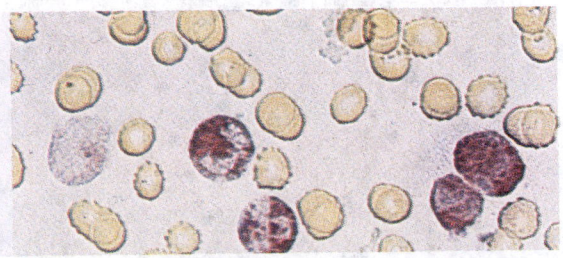

Increased leukocyte alkaline phosphatase reaction
(Hayhoe, 1992)

tions. Normal amounts of this enzyme in a smear of fresh venous blood are 50 to 150 units. Also called **neutrophil alkaline phosphatase.**

leukocythemia. See **leukemia.**

-leukocytic. See **leukocyte.**

leukocytic crystal. See **Charcot-Leyden crystal.**

leukocytopenia. See **leukopenia.**

leukocytosis /loo'kōsītō'sis/ [Gk, *leukos + kytos,* cell, *osis,* condition], an abnormal increase in the number of circulating white blood cells. An increase often accompanies bacterial, but not usually viral, infections. The normal range is 5000 to 10,000 white cells per cubic millimeter of blood. Leukemia may be associated with a white blood cell count as high as 500,000 to 1 million per cubic millimeter of blood, the increase being either equally or disproportionately distributed among all types. Kinds of leukocytosis include **basophilia, eosinophilia,** and **neutrophilia.** Compare **leukemia, leukemoid reaction, leukopenia.** See also **leukocyte.**

leukoderma /loo'kōdur'mə/ [Gk, *leukos + derma,* skin], localized loss of skin pigment caused by several specific causes. Compare **vitiligo.**

leukodystrophy /-dis'trəfē/ [Gk, *leukos,* white; *dys, trophe,* nourishment], a disease of the white matter of the brain, characterized by demyelination.

leukoerythroblastic anemia /loo'kō·erith'rōblas'tik/ [Gk, *leukos + erythros,* red, *blastos,* germ; *a, haima,* not blood], an abnormal condition in which large numbers of immature white and red blood cells are present. It is characteristic of some anemias that occur as a result of the replacement of normal bone marrow with malignant tumor. See also **myeloid metaplasia, myelophthisic anemia.**

leukonychia /loo'kōnik'ē·ə/ [Gk, *leukos + onyx,* nail], a benign, congenital condition in which white patches appear under the nails. Trauma, infection, and many systemic disorders can cause white spots or streaks on nails. A common cause is the presence of air bubbles under the nails.

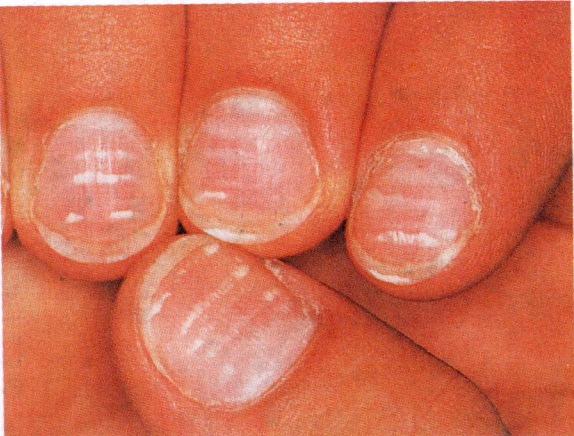

Transverse striate leukonychia *(Baran, 1991)*

leukopenia /loo'kōpē'nē·ə/ [Gk, *leukos + penes,* poor], an abnormal decrease in the number of white blood cells to fewer than 5000 cells per cubic millimeter. The condition may be caused by an adverse drug reaction, radiation poisoning, or pathologic conditions. One or all kinds of white blood cells may be affected. The two most common forms of leukopenia are neutrophilic leukopenia and lymphocytic leukopenia. Also called **leucocytopenia.** Compare **aleukia, leukocytosis.** See also **aplastic anemia, leukocyte.** —**leukopenic,** *adj.*

leukopenic leukemia. See **aleukemic leukemia.**

leukophlegmasia. See **phlegmasia alba dolens.**

leukophoresis /loo´kōfərē´sis/ [Gk, *leukos* + *phoresis*, being transmitted], a laboratory procedure in which white blood cells are separated by electrophoresis for identification and an evaluation of the types of cells and their proportions.

leukoplakia /loo´kōplā´kē·ə/ [Gk, *leukos* + *plax*, plate], a precancerous, slowly developing change in a mucous membrane characterized by thickened, white, firmly attached patches that are slightly raised and sharply circumscribed. They may occur on the penis or vulva; those appearing on the lips and buccal mucosa are associated with pipe smoking. Malignant potential is evaluated by microscopic study of biopsied tissue. Compare **lichen planus.** See also **lichen sclerosis et atrophicus.**

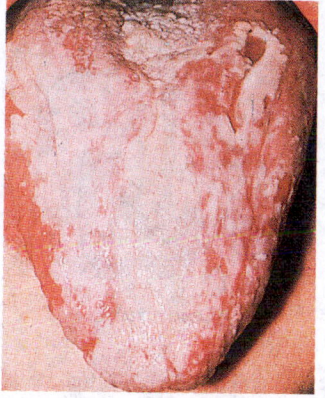

Oral leukoplakia
(Fletcher, 1987/Courtesy Prof FV O'Brien, School of Dentistry, Queen's University, Belfast)

leukoplakic vulvitis /-plā´kik/ [Gk, *leukos,* white + *plakos,* plate + *vulva* + *itis,* inflammation], a condition in which the skin of the vulva becomes thick and white, develops bleeding fissures, and later becomes atrophic. The condition may progress to cancer.

leukopoiesis /loo´kōpō·ē´sis/ [Gk, *leukos* + *poiein,* to make], the process by which white blood cells form and develop. Neutrophils, basophils, and eosinophils are produced in myeloid tissue in the bone marrow. Lymphocytes and monocytes are normally derived from hemocytoblasts in lymphoid tissue, but a few develop in the marrow. —**leukopoietic,** *adj.*

leukorrhea /loo´kərē´ə/ [Gk, *leukos* + *rhoia,* flow], a white discharge from the vagina. Normally, vaginal discharge occurs in regular variations of amount and consistency during the course of the menstrual cycle. A greater than usual amount is normal in pregnancy and a decrease is to be expected after delivery, during lactation, and after menopause. Leukorrhea is the most common reason for women to seek gynecologic care. See also **vaginal discharge.**

leukotomy. See **lobotomy.**

leukotoxin /loo´kətok´sin/ [Gk, *leukos* + *toxikon,* poison], a substance that can inactivate or destroy leukocytes. —**leukotoxic,** *adj.*

leukotrienes /-trī´ēnz/, a class of biologically active compounds that occur naturally in leukocytes and that produce allergic and inflammatory reactions. They are thought to play a role in the development of allergic and autoallergic disease, such as asthma and rheumatoid arthritis.

leukovirus /-vī´rus/ [Gk, *leukos,* white; L, *virus,* poison], any of a group of RNA virus that cause disease in animals. The diseases include Rous sarcoma and murine leukemia.

leuprolide acetate /loo´prōlīd/, a parenteral antineoplastic drug.

■ INDICATIONS: It is prescribed for the palliative treatment of advanced prostatic cancer.

■ CONTRAINDICATIONS: Caution should be exercised during the beginning of leuprolide acetate therapy when symptoms of bone pain, urinary obstruction, and neurologic problems may increase.

■ ADVERSE EFFECTS: Among adverse reactions reported are hot flashes, transient increases in testosterone levels, dizziness, pain, headache, decreased libido, impotence, and injection site irritation.

levamfetamine. See **levamphetamine.**

levamisole, a new drug used as an anthelmintic agent against a wide variety of nematodes. It has also been used in the treatment of bacterial and viral infections.

levamphetamine /lev´əmfet´əmēn/, an isomer of amphetamine, formerly used as an anorexiant. Also spelled **levamfetamine.**

levarterenol bitartrate. See **norepinephrine bitartrate.**

levator /livā´tər/, *pl.* **levatores** /lev´ətôr´ēz/ [L, *levare,* to lift up], **1.** a muscle that raises a structure of the body, as the levator ani raises parts of the pelvic diaphragm. **2.** a surgical instrument used to lift depressed bony fragments in fractures of the skull and other bones.

levator ani, one of a pair of muscles of the pelvic diaphragm that stretches across the bottom of the pelvic cavity like a hammock, supporting the pelvic organs. It is a broad, thin muscle that separates into the pubococcygeus and the iliococcygeus. It originates from the ramus of the pubic bone, the spine of the ischium, and a band of fascia between the pubis and the ischium; it inserts into the last two segments of the coccyx, the anococcygeal raphe, the sphincter ani externus, and the central tendinous point of the perineum. The left and right levator ani muscles are divided ventrally but converge as a single sheet across the midline dorsally, forming most of the pelvic diaphragm. The levator ani is innervated by branches of the pudendal plexus, which contains fibers from the fourth sacral nerve, and it functions to support and slightly raise the pelvic floor. The pubococcygeus draws the anus toward the pubis and constricts it. Compare **coccygeus.**

levatores. See **levatore.**

levator palpebrae superioris, one of the three muscles of the eyelid, also considered a muscle of the eye. It is thin and flat and rises from the small wing of the sphenoid. It splits into three lamellae: The superficial lamella extends to the upper eyelid; the middle lamella inserts into the superior tarsus; and the deep lamella is attached to the conjunctiva. It is innervated by the oculomotor nerve, raises the upper eyelid, and is the antagonist of the orbicularis oculi. Compare **corrugator supercilii, orbicularis oculi.**

levator scapulae, a muscle of the dorsal and lateral aspects of the neck. It arises from the axis and the atlas, and it inserts into the transverse processes of the four upper cervical vertebrae. It is innervated by the third and fourth cervical nerves and acts to raise the scapula and pull it toward the midline.

LeVeen shunt, a tube that is surgically implanted to connect the peritoneal cavity and the superior vena cava to drain an accumulation of fluid in the peritoneal cavity in cirrhosis of the liver, right-sided heart failure, or cancer of the abdomen. Before surgery, a sodium-restricted diet and diuretics are given to decrease sodium and water retention. Under general anesthesia, a silicone rubber tube is inserted under the subcutaneous tissue from the peritoneum to the superior vena cava. As the patient inhales, the fluid pressure in the peritoneal cavity rises and that in the blood vessel falls, allowing peritoneal fluid to enter the shunt valve. After surgery the patient is closely observed for signs of occlusion of the shunt, GI bleeding, or leakage of peritoneal fluid from the incision. Excessive dilution of the blood may lead to abnormalities of coagulation.

level of activities [OFr, *livel*; L, *activus*], pertaining to the hierarchy of nervous system activity which determines the level responsible for certain functions while also being controlled by another higher level above it, as in the sequence of events in a reflex action.

level of consciousness (L.O.C.) a degree of cognitive function involving arousal mechanisms of the reticular formation of the brain. Impaired L.O.C. may be expressed in obtundation or reduced alertness, stupor, syncope, or unresponsiveness. See also **Glasgow coma scale.**

level of inquiry [L, *libella*, carpenter's level; *inquirere*, to ask about], (in nursing research) one of the levels in a rank-ordered system of classification and organization of the questions to be answered in a research study. The level of inquiry is determined by an analysis of the theory to be developed or tested and the kinds of data to be collected. Studies that describe comprise the first level whereas those that explain comprise the second level. Those that prescribe or predict are the most difficult to answer or to support.

levels of care, a classification of health care service levels by the kind of care given, the number of people served, and the people providing the care. Kinds of health care service levels are **primary health care, secondary health care,** and **tertiary health care.**

levels of consciousness [OFr, *livel*; L, *conscire*, to be aware of], the stages of response of the mind to stimuli, varying from unconsciousness through vague awareness to full attention. The usual standard levels include coma, in which the patient does not appear to be aware of the environment; stupor, in which the patient is vaguely aware of the environment; drowsiness, in which the patient responds to stimuli but may be slow to react, and alert wakefulness. See also **preconscious; subconscious.**

lever /lē′vər, lev′ər/ [L, *levare*, to lift up], (in physiology) any one of the numerous bones and associated joints of the body that act together as a lever so that force applied to one end of the bone to lift a weight at another point tends to rotate the bone in the direction opposite from that of the applied force. The basic components of a lever are the fulcrum, the force arm, the weight arm, and the force moment. A first-class lever, such as the hip, has a fulcrum between the weight and the applied force. A third-class lever, such as that situated at all the joints of the upper and the lower extremities of the body, accommodates forces between the fulcrum and the weight. The body contains few second-class levers in which the force arm is longer than the weight arm. The muscles of the body produce the forces that move the levers. The body uses its third-class levers for speed and first-class levers to gain either force or speed, depending on the force applied to the weight arm. The moment of force produced by the weight of any body part involved in a lever action can be determined if the center of gravity of the part is known. Charts are available that list the center of gravity of various body parts.

Lévi-Lorain dwarf. See **pituitary dwarf.**

Levin tube /lev′in/ [Abraham L. Levin, American physician, b. 1880], a #16 French, plastic catheter, used in gastric intubation for gastric decompression or gavage feeding. It has a closed, weighted tip and an opening on the side. Compare **Miller-Abbott tube.** See also **gastric intubation.**

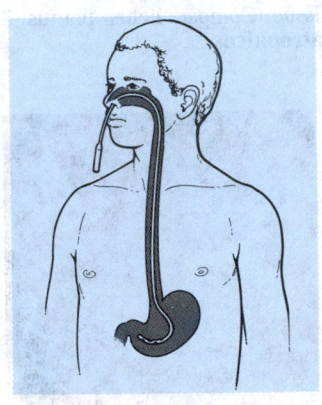

Levin tube

levitation /lev′itā′shən/ [L, *levitas*, lightness, *atus*, process], (in psychiatry) a hallucinatory sensation of floating or rising in the air. **–levitate,** *v.*

levo- /lē′vō-/, a prefix meaning 'left': *levocardia, levoclination, levotorsion.*

levobunolol hydrochloride /-bun′əlol/, a topical ophthalmic beta-adrenergic blocker drug for glaucoma.

■ INDICATIONS: It is prescribed for the treatment of chronic open-angle glaucoma and ocular hypertension.

■ CONTRAINDICATIONS: Levobunolol hydrochloride is contraindicated for patients with bronchial asthma, severe chronic obstructive pulmonary disease, sinus bradycardia, second- or third-degree atrioventricular block, overt cardiac failure, or cardiogenic shock.

■ ADVERSE EFFECTS: Adverse reactions may include transient ocular burning or stinging, bradycardia, pulmonary edema, and blepharoconjunctivitis.

levodopa /lē′vōdō′pə/, an antiparkinsonian.

■ INDICATIONS: It is prescribed in the treatment of Parkinson's disease, juvenile forms of Huntington's disease, and chronic manganese poisoning.

■ CONTRAINDICATIONS: Narrow-angle glaucoma, concomitant use of a monoamine oxidase inhibitor, suspected melanoma, or known hypersensitivity to this drug prohibits its use.

■ ADVERSE EFFECTS: Among the more serious adverse reactions are severe GI disturbances, hypotension, various movement disorders, emotional changes, cardiac arrhythmia, and anorexia.

Levo-Dromoran, a trademark for a narcotic analgesic (levorphanol tartrate).

Levophed Bitartrate, a trademark for an adrenergic (norepinephrine bitartrate).

levopropoxyphene napsylate /-prōpək′sifēn/, an antitussive.
- INDICATION: It is prescribed for cough.
- CONTRAINDICATIONS: Its use is prohibited during the first trimester of pregnancy, after surgery, or in cases of known hypersensitivity to this drug.
- ADVERSE EFFECTS: Among the more serious adverse reactions are skin rash, muscle tremor, and vomiting.

levorphanol tartrate /lē′vôrfā′nol/, a narcotic analgesic.
- INDICATIONS: It is prescribed for pain and preoperative analgesia.
- CONTRAINDICATIONS: Alcoholism, asthma, increased intracranial pressure, respiratory depression, anoxia, or known hypersensitivity to this drug prohibits its use.
- ADVERSE EFFECTS: Among the more serious adverse reactions are drug dependence, orthostatic hypotension, cardiac arrhythmia, and retention of urine.

levothyroxine sodium /-thī′rəksēn/, a thyroid hormone.
- INDICATION: It is prescribed in the treatment of hypothyroidism.
- CONTRAINDICATIONS: Recent myocardial infarction, normal thyroid function, or known hypersensitivity to this drug prohibits its use.
- ADVERSE EFFECTS: The most serious adverse reactions are angina, tachycardia, arrhythmias, and tremors.

Levsinex, a trademark for an anticholinergic (hyoscyamine sulfate).

levulose. See **fructose.**

levulosuria. See **fructosuria.**

lewisite /lōō′isīt/ [Winford L. Lewis, American chemist, b. 1878], 2-chlorovinyl arsine; a poisonous blister gas, used in World War I, that causes irritation of the lungs, dyspnea, damage to the tissues of the respiratory tract, tears, and pain.

-lexia, a suffix meaning 'reading': *alexia, bradylexia, dyslexia.*

Leyden-Moebius muscular dystrophy /lī′dən-m′bē·əs, -mē′bē·əs/, a form of limb-girdle muscular dystrophy that begins in the pelvic girdle. Also called **pelvifemoral muscular dystrophy.**

Leydig cells /lī′dig/ [Franz von Leydig, German anatomist, b. 1821], cells of the interstitial tissue of the testes that secrete testosterone.

Leydig cell tumor, a generally benign neoplasm of interstitial cells of a testis that may cause gynecomastia in adults and precocious sexual development if the lesion occurs before puberty. The tumor is usually a circumscribed, lobulated, palpable mass.

LF, abbreviation for *low frequency.*

L.F.A., abbreviation for *left frontoanterior fetal position.*

L.F.P., abbreviation for *left frontoposterior fetal position.*

LFT, abbreviation for **liver function test.**

LGA, abbreviation for *large for gestational age.* See **large gestational infant.**

LGV, abbreviation for **lymphogranuloma venereum.**

LH, abbreviation for **luteinizing hormone.**

Lhermitte's sign /ler′mits/ [Jacques J. Lhermitte, French neurologist, b. 1877], sudden, transient, electric-like

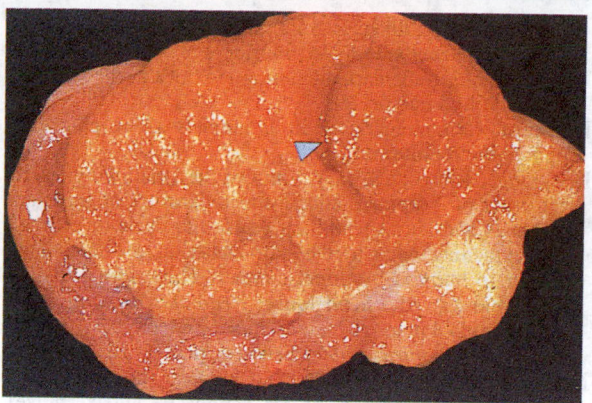

Leydig cell tumor (Weiss, 1988)

shocks spreading down the body when the head is flexed forward, occurring chiefly in multiple sclerosis but also in compression disorders of the cervical spinal cord.

LHRH, abbreviation for **luteinizing hormone-releasing hormone.**

Li, symbol for the element **lithium.**

liability /līəbil′itē/ [L, *ligare*, to bind], 1. something one is obligated to do or an obligation required to be fulfilled by law, usually financial in nature. 2. the amount of money required to fulfill a financial obligation.

liaison nursing /lē·ā′zən/, an arrangement with clinical specialists in psychiatric nursing whereby nurses and health professionals in other disciplines obtain consultation services in medical-surgical, parent-child, and geriatric settings.

libel /lī′bəl/ [L, *libellus*, little book], a false accusation written, printed, or typewritten, or presented in a picture or a sign that is made with malicious intent to defame the reputation of a person who is living or the memory of a person who is dead, resulting in public embarrassment, contempt, ridicule, or hatred.

liberation /lib′ərā′shən/ [L, *liber*, free], the process of drug release from the dosage form.

libidinal. See **libidinous.**

libidinal development. See **psychosexual development.**

libidinous /libid′inəs/ [L, *libidinosus*, lustful], 1. pertaining to or belonging to the libido. 2. having or characterized by sexual desire. Also **libidinal.** –**libidinize,** *v.*

libido /libē′dō, libī′dō/, 1. the psychic energy or instinctual drive associated with sexual desire, pleasure, or creativity. 2. (in psychoanalysis) the instinctual drives of the id. 3. lustful desire or striving.

Libman-Sacks endocarditis /lib′mənsaks′/ [Emanuel Libman, American physician, b. 1872; Benjamin Sacks, American physician, b. 1896], an abnormal condition and the most common manifestation of lupus erythematosus, characterized by verrucous lesions that develop near the heart valves but rarely affect valvular action. The lesions usually are dry and granular, with a pink or tawny color, contain basophilic cellular debris, and develop in the angle of the atrioventricular valves and at the base of the mitral valve. Also called **Libman-Sacks disease, Libman-Sacks syndrome.**

Librax, a trademark for a GI, fixed-combination drug containing an anticholinergic (clidinium bromide) and a sedative (chlordiazepoxide hydrochloride).

Libritabs, a trademark for an antianxiety agent (chlordiazepoxide hydrochloride).

Librium, a trademark for an antianxiety agent (chlordiazepoxide hydrochloride).

lice, *sing.,* **louse** [AS, *lus*], any of the small wingless insect order of *Anoplura*. Lice are ectoparasites of birds and mammals and may spend their entire life cycle on a single host, attaching eggs to the hair shafts or feathers. They transfer to humans by direct contact. Three forms that infect humans are the **head louse,** *Pediculus humanus capitis;* the **body louse,** *Pediculus humanus corporis,* and the **crab louse,** *Phthirus pubis.* See also **pediculosis.**

licensed practical nurse (LPN) /lī'sənst/ [L, *licere*, to be allowed; Gk, *praktikos*, fit for action; L, *nutrix*, nurse], *U.S.* a person trained in basic nursing techniques and direct patient care who practices under the supervision of a registered nurse. The course of training usually lasts 1 year. In Canada an LPN is called a certified nursing assistant. Also called *(U.S.)* **licensed vocational nurse.**

licensed psychologist, a person who has earned a PhD in psychology from an accredited graduate school and who has completed 2 to 3 years of postgraduate training with special emphasis on the diagnosis and treatment of psychologic disorders. Also called **clinical psychologist.** See also **psychotherapist.**

licensed vocational nurse. See **licensed practical nurse.**

licensure /lī'sənshŏŏr/ [L, *licere*, to be allowed], the granting of permission by a competent authority (usually a government agency) to an organization or individual to engage in a practice or activity that would otherwise be illegal. Kinds of licensure include the issuing of licenses for general hospitals or nursing homes, for health professionals, as physicians, and for the production or distribution of biologic products. Licensure is usually granted on the basis of education and examination rather than performance. It is usually permanent, but a periodic fee, demonstration of competence, or continuing education may be required. Licensure may be revoked by the granting agency for incompetence, criminal acts, or other reasons stipulated in the rules governing the specific area of licensure.

lichenification /līken'ifikā'shən/ [Gk, *leichen*, lichen; *facere*, to make], thickening and hardening of the skin, often resulting from the irritation caused by repeated scratching of a pruritic lesion. **–lichenified,** *adj.*

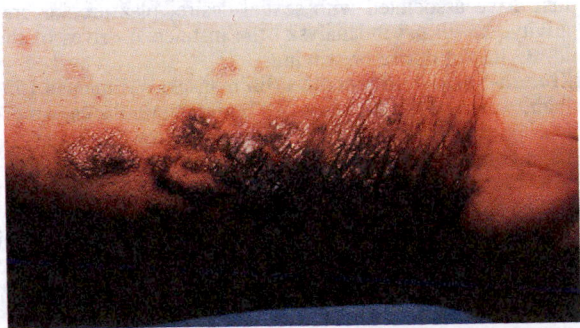

Lichenification *(Zitelli, 1992)*

lichen nitidus /lī'kən/ [Gk, *leichen* + L, *nitidus*, bright], a rare skin disorder characterized by numerous flat, glistening, pale, discrete papules measuring 2 to 3 mm in diameter. Also called **Pinkus' disease.**

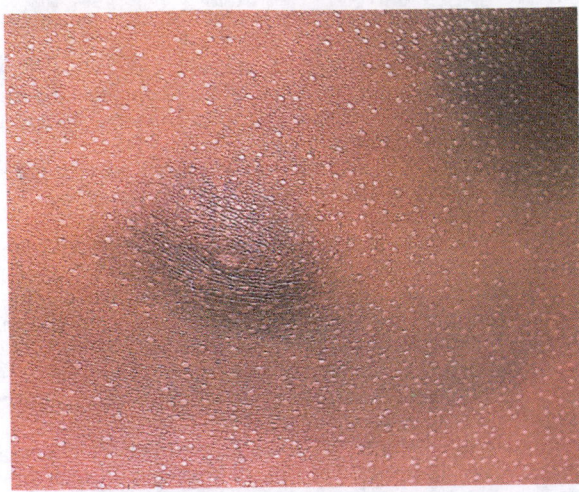

Lichen nitidus *(McKee, 1993)*

lichen planus, a nonmalignant, chronic, pruritic skin disease of unknown cause that is characterized by small, flat, purplish papules or plaques with fine, gray lines on the surface. Common sites are flexor surfaces of wrists, forearms, ankles, abdomen, and sacrum. On mucous membranes the lesions appear gray and lacy. Nails may have longitudinal ridges. Episodes of disease activity vary but may last for months and may recur. Compare **leukoplakia.**

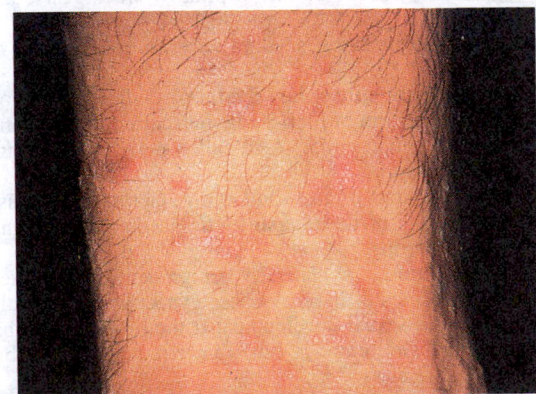

Lichen planus on the forearm *(Habif, 1990)*

lichen sclerosis et atrophicus, a chronic skin disease characterized by white, flat papules with an erythematous halo and black, hard follicular plugs. In advanced cases, the papules tend to coalesce into large, white patches of thin, pruritic skin. Lesions often occur on the torso and, almost inevitably, in the anogenital regions. In the latter case the

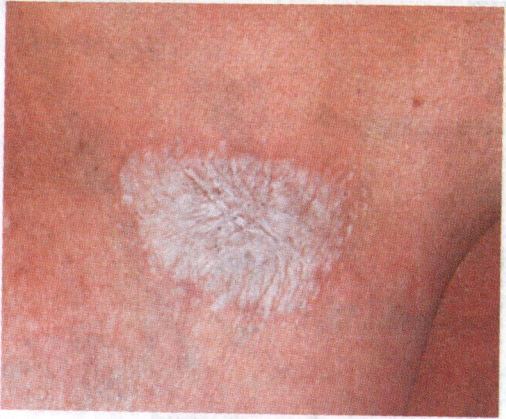

Lichen sclerosus et atrophicus on the torso
(McKee, 1993)

disease is called kraurosis vulvae. Corticosteroids are applied topically to reduce itching.

lichen simplex chronicus, a form of neurodermatitis characterized by a patch of pruritic, confluent papules. Psychogenic factors and mechanical trauma, such as scratching, contribute to its chronicity. Treatment may include topical or intralesional application of corticosteroids to relieve the pruritus.

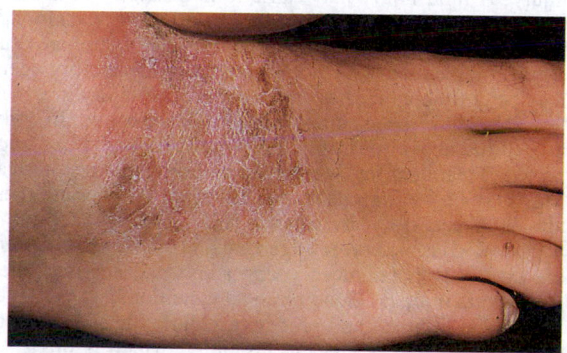

Lichen simplex chronicus on the foot (Habif, 1990)

licorice /lik'ərish, -ris/ [Gk, *glykys*, sweet, *rhiza*, root], a dried root of gummy texture from the leguminous plant *Glycyrrhiza glabra*. It has a sweet, astringent taste and is used as a flavoring agent in medicines, especially in cough syrups and laxatives, confectionery, and tobacco. It may cause an elevation of blood pressure. Also spelled **liquorice.**

lid. See **eyelid.**

Lidex, a trademark for a glucocorticoid (fluocinonide).

lidocaine hydrochloride /lī'dəkān/, a local anesthetic agent.

■ INDICATIONS: It is prescribed as a local anesthetic for topical administration to skin or to mucous membranes. It is used parenterally as an antiarrhythmic agent.

■ CONTRAINDICATIONS: Known hypersensitivity to this drug prohibits its topical use. Heart block or known hypersensitivity to this drug prohibits its systemic use.

■ ADVERSE EFFECTS: Among the more serious adverse reactions to the systemic administration of the drug are central nervous system disturbances, hypotension, bradycardia, and cardiac arrest. A variety of hypersensitivity reactions may occur from topical administration of this drug. Eating and drinking is avoided for 1 hour after topical application of this drug to the pharynx or the esophagus.

lid poppers, *slang.* amphetamines.

lie [AS, *licgan*, position], the relationship between the long axis of the fetus and the long axis of the mother. In a longitudinal lie the fetus is lying lengthwise, or vertically, in the uterus, whereas in a transverse lie the fetus is lying crosswise, or horizontally.

Lieberkühn's glands /lē'bərkēnz/ [Johann Nathanael Lieberkühn, German anatomist, b. 1711; L, *glans*, acorn], tubular glands between the bases of the villi of the small intestine and on the surface of the epithelium of the large intestine. Also called **intestinal glands; crypts of Lieberkühn; follicles of Lieberkühn.**

lie detector [AS, *leogan*, untruth; L, *detegere*, to uncover], an electronic device or instrument used to detect lying or anxiety in regard to specific questions. A commonly used lie detector is the polygraph recorder that senses and records pulse, respiratory rate, blood pressure, and perspiration. Some experts hold that certain patterns indicate the presence of anxiety, guilt, or fear, emotions that are likely to occur when the subject is lying.

lien. See **spleen.**

lienal vein /lī'ənəl, lē·ē'nəl/ [L, *lien*, spleen; *vena*], a large vein of the lower body that unites with the superior mesenteric vein to form the portal vein. It returns blood from the spleen and arises from about six large tributaries that unite to form the single vessel passing from left to right across the superior, dorsal part of the pancreas. It receives the short gastric veins, the left gastroepiploic vein, the pancreatic veins, and the inferior mesenteric veins. Also called **splenic vein.**

lieno-, a combining form meaning 'of or pertaining to the spleen': *lienomalacia, lienomedullary, lienopathy.*

lienography /lē'ənog'rəfē/, the radiographic examination of the spleen after it has been injected with a contrast medium.

life [AS, *lif*], the energy that enables organisms to grow, reproduce, absorb and use nutrients, evolve, and, in some organisms, achieve mobility, express consciousness, and demonstrate a voluntary use of the senses.

life costs [AS, *lif*; L, *constare*, constant], the mortality, morbidity, and suffering associated with a given disease or medical procedure.

life expectancy, the probable number of years a person will live after a given age, as determined by the mortality rate in a specific geographic area. It may be individually qualified by the person's condition or race, sex, age, or other demographic factors. Also called **expectation of life.**

life extension [AS, *lif*, life; L, *extenere*, to stretch out], the process of extending the life span of an individual or population by intervention that promotes better use of preventive medicine and use of established diagnostic and therapeutic facilities.

life island, a plastic bubble enclosing a bed, used to provide a germ-free environment for a patient.

life review,   **1.** (in psychiatry) a progressive return to consciousness of past experiences. **2.** reminiscences that occur in old age as a consequence of the realization of the inevitability of death. Also called **reminisence therapy.**

lifesaving measure,   any independent, interdependent, or dependent nursing intervention that is implemented when a patient's physical or psychologic status is threatened.

life science,   the study of the laws and properties of living matter. Some kinds of life science are **anatomy, bacteriology,** and **biology.** Compare **physical science.**

life space,   a term introduced by American psychologist Kurt Lewin to describe simultaneous influences that may affect individual behavior. The totality of the influences make up the life space.

life-style-induced health problems,   diseases with natural histories that include conscious exposure to certain health-compromising or risk factors. An example is heart disease associated with cigarette smoking, poor dietary habits, lack of exercise, and sustaining unbuffered stress.

life support [AS, *lif,* life; L, *supportare,* to bring up to], the use of any therapeutic technique or device to maintain life functions.

lifetime reserve [AS, *lif, tid,* time; L, *re,* again, *servare,* to keep],   a lifetime total of days of inpatient hospitalization benefits that may be drawn on by a patient who has exhausted the maximum benefits allowed under Medicare for a single spell of illness.

lift assessment [AS, *lyft,* loft; L, *assidere,* to sit beside], the selection of the most appropriate lift method to use when moving a patient, as from the bed to a chair. The assessment involves consideration of such factors as whether the patient is conscious or unconscious, if the patient has a visual or hearing impairment, the need for special care in handling patient attachments, as IV lines or monitors, and whether the patient has full range of motion or flaccid or spastic limbs.

ligament /lig′əmənt/ [L, *ligare,* to bind],   **1.** one of many predominantly white, shiny, flexible bands of fibrous tissue binding joints together and connecting various bones and cartilages. Such ligaments are slightly elastic and composed of parallel collagenous bundles. When part of the synovial membrane of a joint, they are covered with fibroelastic tissue that blends with surrounding connective tissue. Yellow elastic ligaments, such as the ligamenta flava, connect certain parts of adjoining vertebrae. Compare **tendon. 2.** a layer of serous membrane with little or no tensile strength, extending from one visceral organ to another, such as the ligaments of the peritoneum. See also **broad ligament.** Also called **ligamentum. –ligamentous,** *adj.*

ligamenta flava [L, *ligare* + *flavus,* yellow],   the bands of yellow elastic tissue connecting the laminae of adjacent vertebrae from the axis to the first segment of the sacrum. They are thin, broad, and long in the cervical region, thicker in the thoracic region, and thickest in the lumbar region. They help to hold the body erect.

ligamental tear /lig′əmen′təl/ [L, *ligare,* to bind; AS, *teran,* to destroy],   a complete or a partial tear of a ligamentous structure connecting and surrounding the bones of a joint, caused by an injury to the joint, as by a sudden twisting motion or by a forceful blow.

■ OBSERVATIONS: Ligamental tears may occur at any joint but are most common in the knees. The pathologic features of ligamental tears of the knee are dependent on the location and severity of the injury. The most common ligaments in-

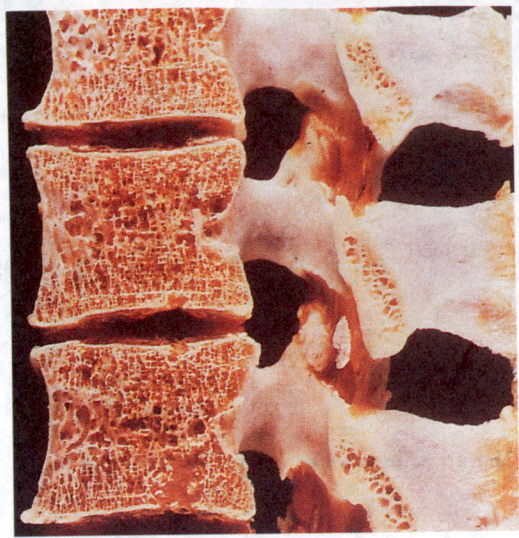

Ligamenta flava (Bullough, 1988)

volved in knee injuries are the medial, lateral, and posterior ligaments and the anterior and posterior cruciate ligaments. Usually, the injury involves more than one structure because of the way in which the structures connect with and support each other.

■ INTERVENTIONS: Treatment depends on the severity of the injury. A mild injury may cause little damage with tenderness, swelling, and pain with stress. Rest, compression, applications of heat and cold, elevation, and early use are usually recommended. Injection of an anti-inflammatory agent may be desirable. Treatment for a moderate injury in which few fibers have been completely torn is protective. In addition to the above measures, the joint is aspirated and supported. Treatment for a severe, complete tear is restorative. This may be by immobilization followed by physical therapy or, if necessary, by surgical repair.

■ NURSING CONSIDERATIONS: Ligamental tears of the knee joint are extremely common in young adults and are associated with sports injuries. Good physical condition may help prevent many injuries, and proper care during healing is necessary to prevent permanent disability, which is often accompanied by instability, stiffness, or pain in the joint.

ligament of the neck of the rib,   one of five ligaments of each costotransverse joint, consisting of short, strong fibers passing from the neck of the rib to the transverse process of the adjacent vertebra. Also called **middle costotransverse ligament.**

ligament of the tubercle of the rib,   one of the five ligaments of each costotransverse joint, comprising a short, thick fasciculus passing obliquely from the transverse process of a vertebra to the tubercle of the associated rib. Compare **ligament of the neck of the rib.**

ligamentous /lig′əmen′təs/ [L, *ligare,* to bind],   pertaining to or having the characteristics of a ligament.

ligamentum.   See **ligament.**

ligamentum falciforme hepatitis.   See **broad ligament of liver.**

ligamentum latum uteri.   See **broad ligament.**

ligamentum nuchae /lig′əmen′təm/,   the fibrous membrane that reaches from the external occipital protuberance and median nuchal line to the spinous process of the seventh vertebra. A fibrous lamina from the ligament attaches to the posterior tubercle of the atlas and to the spinous processes of the cervical vertebrae, forming a septum between muscles on either side of the neck.

ligand /lig'ənd, lī'gənd/ [L, *ligare*, to bind], **1.** a molecule, ion, or group bound to the central atom of a chemical compound, such as the oxygen molecule in hemoglobin, which is bound to the central iron atom. **2.** an organic molecule attached to a specific site on a surface or to a tracer element. The binding is reversible in a competitive binding assay. It may be the analyte or a cross-reactant. Examples include vitamin B$_{12}$, a ligand with intrinsic factor as the binding protein, and various antigens, which are ligands with antibody binding proteins.

ligases /lī'gāsəz/ [L, *ligare* + Fr, *diastase*, enzyme], a group of enzymes that catalyze the formation of a bond between substrate molecules coupled with the breakdown of a pyrophosphate bond in ATP or a similar donor molecule. Examples of ligases include the synthetase enzymes.

ligation /līgā'shən/ [L, *ligare*, to bind], the procedure of tying off a blood vessel or duct with a suture or wire ligature. It may be performed to stop or prevent bleeding during surgery, to stop spontaneous or traumatic hemorrhage, or to prevent passage of material through a duct, as in tubal ligation or to treat varicosities. In venous ligation, the saphenous vein is tied above the varicosed portion, and the distal portions are removed. After surgery, the nurse observes the patient's feet and legs for circulatory impairment; the foot of the bed is raised to encourage venous return. Ambulation is begun the day of surgery, with elastic bandages for firm support. Analgesics are given as necessary for pain and discomfort. See also **ligature, tubal ligation, varicose veins. –ligate,** *v.*

ligature /lig'əchər/ [L, *ligare*, to bind], **1.** a suture. **2.** a wire, as used in orthodontics.

ligature needle, a long, thin, curved needle used for passing a suture underneath an artery for ligation of the vessel.

ligature wire [L, *ligare*, to bind; AS, *wir*], a soft, thin wire used in dental procedures, particularly to connet brackets or attachments in orthodontic appliances.

light [AS, *leoht*], **1.** electromagnetic radiation of the wavelength and frequency that stimulate visual receptor cells in the retina to produce nerve impulses that are perceived as vision. **2.** electromagnetic radiation with wavelengths shorter than ultraviolet light and longer than infrared light, the range of visible light generally in the range of 400 to 800 nm.

light-adapted eye [AS, *leoht*; L, *adaptatio*; AS, *éage*], an eye that has been exposed to bright light long enough for chemical and physiologic changes to take place, such as bleaching of the rhodopsin or visual purple. The loss of cone sensitivity to light may require increased light intensity to obtain the same degree of visual acuity. Also called **photopic eye.**

light bath, the exposure of the patient's uncovered skin to the sun or to actinic light rays from an artificial source for therapeutic purposes.

light chain, a subunit of an immunoglobulin molecule composed of a polypeptide chain of about 22,000 daltons, or atomic mass units. An example of a light chain is a Bence Jones protein molecule associated with multiple myeloma.

light chain disease, a type of multiple myeloma in which plasma cell tumors produce only monoclonal light chain proteins. Persons with light chain disease may develop lytic bone lesions, hypercalcemia, impaired kidney function, and amyloidosis. See also **gammopathy, heavy chain disease, multiple myeloma.**

light diet, a diet suitable for convalescent or bedridden patients taking little or no exercise. It consists of simple, moderate quantities of soft-cooked and easily digested foods, including meats, potatoes, rice, eggs, pasta, some fruits, refined cereals, and breads. It avoids all highly seasoned and fried foods.

lightening /lī'təning/ [AS, *leoht*, light in weight], a subjective sensation reported by many women late in pregnancy as the fetus settles lower in the true pelvis, leaving more space in the upper abdomen. The diaphragm, no longer restricted by the fundus of the uterus beneath it, can move down more fully during inspiration, allowing deeper breaths to be taken. The stomach, too, is less compressed, so the woman can comfortably eat more food at each meal. Urinary frequency occurs as the fetus drops. The profile of the abdomen changes with lightening, because the round, full uterus is visibly lower. The baby is then said to have "dropped."

light film fault [AS, *leoht*, light; *filmen*, membrane; L, *fallere*, to deceive], a defect in a radiograph or developed photographic film that appears as a barely distinct and inadequate image. It is caused by underexposure, underdevelopment, development in too-cold solutions, or use of the wrong film speed.

light microscope [AS, *leoht*; Gk, *mikros*, small + *skopein*, to view], a microscope that uses visible light to view objects too small for the naked eye to see.

light pen, an electric device, resembling a pen, that may be used with a computer terminal to enter or modify information displayed on the screen.

light reflex, the mechanism by which the pupil of the eye constricts in response to direct or consensual stimulation with light. Also called **pupillary reflex.** Compare **consensual light reflex.** See also **consensual reaction to light, direct reaction to light.**

light therapy [AS, *leoht*; Gk, *therapeia*, treatment], exposure of the body to electromagnetic waves of the infrared, ultraviolet, or visible spectrum for therapeutic purposes. In the winter months, light therapy may be used to treat depressive disorders.

light-touch palpations [AS, *leoht*; Fr, *toucher*; L, *palpare*, to touch gently], a method of examination by gently depressing the abdomen 1-2 cm in order to outline the size and position of abdominal organs.

light vaginal bleeding. See **vaginal bleeding.**

ligneous /lig'nē·əs/ [L, *ligum*, wood], woody or resembling wood in texture or other characteristics.

ligneous thyroiditis. See **fibrous thyroiditis.**

lignin /lig'nin/ [L, *lignum*, wood], a polysaccharide that with cellulose and hemicellulose forms the chief part of the skeletal substances of the cell walls of plants. It provides bulk in the diet necessary for proper GI functioning. See also **dietary fiber.**

lignocaine. See **lidocaine hydrochloride.**

lilliputian hallucination /lil'ipyoo'shən/ [Lilliput, mythic island in Swift's *Gulliver's Travels*], a hallucination in which things seem smaller than they actually are. See also **hallucination.**

limb /lim/ [AS, *lim*], **1.** an appendage or extremity of the body, such as an arm or leg. **2.** a branch of an internal organ, such as a loop of a nephron.

limb-girdle muscular dystrophy [AS, *lim*, limb; *gyrdel*], a form of muscular dystrophy transmitted as an autosomal recessive trait. The characteristic weakness and degeneration of the muscles begins in the shoulder girdle or in the pelvic girdle. The condition is progressive, regardless of the area in which it is first manifest. Kinds of limb-girdle muscular dystrophy are **Erb's muscular dystrophy, Leyden-Moebius muscular dystrophy.**

limbic /lim'bik/ [L, *limbus*, edge or border], pertaining to something that is marginal or at a junction between structures.

limbic lobe [L, *limbus*, edge; Gk, *lobos*, lobe], the marginal section of the cerebral hemispheres on the medial aspects. It forms a ring of neural tissue around the hypothalamus and some nuclei.

limbic system [L, *limus*, border], a group of structures within the rhinencephalon of the brain that are associated with various emotions and feelings, such as anger, fear, sexual arousal, pleasure, and sadness. The structures of the limbic system include the cingulate gyrus, the isthmus, the hippocampal gyrus, the uncus, and the amygdala. The structures connect with various other parts of the brain, such as the septum and the hypothalamus. Unless the limbic system is modulated by other cortical areas, periodic attacks of uncontrollable rage may occur in some individuals. The function of the system is poorly understood.

limb kinetic apraxia. See **ideomotor apraxia.**

limb lead /lēd/ [AS, *lim*, limb; *laeden*, lead], in electrocardiography, an electrode that is attached to an arm or a leg.

lime [AS, *lim*], **1.** any of several oxides and hydroxides of calcium. The various kinds of lime have many uses, including the treatment of sewage, purification of water and refining of sugar, and the manufacture of materials such as plaster and fertilizers. **2.** a citrus fruit yielding a juice with a high ascorbic acid content. Lime juice was one of the first effective agents to be used in the treatment of scurvy. See also **ascorbic acid, scurvy.**

limen. See **threshold stimulus.**

liminal stimulus. See **threshold stimulus.**

limitation of motion /lim'itā'shən/ [L, *limes*, limit], the restriction or reduction to a normal range of motion of a body part caused by disease or injury.

limited fluctuation method of dosing [L, *limes*, limit; *fluctuare*, to wave], a method of drug administration in which the dose is not allowed to rise or fall beyond specified maximum and minimum limits.

limiting charge, the maximum amount that can be charged in the United States for the services of a physician who does not accept the restrictions on fees established by Medicare laws. Also called **billing limit.**

limiting resolution, (in computed tomography) the spatial frequency at a modulation transfer function (MTF) equal to 0.1. The absolute object size that can be resolved by a scanner is equal to the reciprocal of the spatial frequency.

limo-, a combining form meaning 'of or pertaining to hunger': *limophthisis, limosis, limotherapy.*

limp [ME, not firm], an abnormal pattern of ambulation in which the two phases of gait are markedly asymmetric. See also **stance phase of gait, swing phase of gait.**

LINAC, abbreviation for **linear accelerator.**

Lincocin, a trademark for an antibacterial (lincomycin hydrochloride).

lincomycin hydrochloride /lin'kəmī'sin/, an antibiotic.

■ INDICATIONS: It is prescribed in the treatment of certain infections.

■ CONTRAINDICATIONS: Known hypersensitivity to this drug or to clindamycin prohibits its use.

■ ADVERSE EFFECTS: Among the more serious adverse reactions are blood disorders, diarrhea, and the development of life-threatening pseudomembranous colitis caused by suprainfection.

lindane /lin'dān/, gamma-benzene hexachloride.

■ INDICATIONS: It is prescribed in the treatment of pediculosis and scabies.

■ CONTRAINDICATIONS: It is not usually given to infants or pregnant women and is not applied to the face. Known hypersensitivity to this drug prohibits its use.

■ ADVERSE EFFECTS: Among the most serious adverse reactions are neurologic damage and aplastic anemia. Given topically, irritation of eyes, skin, and mucosa may occur.

Lindau-von Hippel disease. See **cerebroretinal angiomatosis.**

Lindbergh pump [Charles A. Lindbergh, American technician, b. 1902; ME, *pumpe*], a pump used to preserve an organ of the body by perfusing its tissues with oxygen and other essential nutrients, usually during the transport of an organ from a donor to a recipient. Also called **Carrel-Lindbergh pump.**

line [L, *linea*], **1.** a connection between two points. **2.** a stripe, streak, or narrow ridge, often imaginary, that serves to connect reference points or to separate various parts of the body, as the hairline or nipple line. **3.** a black absorption line in a continuous spectrum passing through a medium. **4.** an accretion line in the enamel of a tooth marking successive layers of calcification. **5.** a catheter or wire that may be inserted in a vein, as an intravenous line. **6.** the base line of an electrocardiogram when neither positive nor negative potentials are recorded. **7.** line of sight. Also called **linea.** See also **Frankfort horizontal plane.**

linea [L, *(Latin)* line], a line defining anatomical features, such as the **linea alba** of the abdomen, the **linea albicantes** or **linea nigra** seen on the abdomen during pregnancy, or the **linea vitalis** curving across the palm at the base of the thumb.

linea alba /lin'ē·ə/ [L, *linea*, line; *albus*, white], the portion of the anterior abdominal aponeurosis in the middle line of the abdomen, representing the fusion of three aponeuroses into a single tendinous band extending from the xiphoid process to the symphysis pubis. It contains the umbilicus. Also called **Hunter's line, white line.** Compare **linea semilunaris.**

linea albicantes, lines, white to pink or gray in color, that occur on the abdomen, buttocks, breasts, and thighs and are caused by the stretching of the skin and weakening or rupturing of the underlying elastic tissue. The condition is usually associated with pregnancy, excessive obesity, rapid growth during adolescence, Cushing's syndrome, or prolonged adrenal cortical hormone therapy. Also called **stria atrophica.**

linea arcuata, the curved tendinous band in the sheath of the rectus abdominis below the umbilicus. It is usually derived from the aponeurosis of the transversus abdominis or the obliquus internus, sometimes from both those muscles. It inserts into the linea alba. Compare **linea semilunaris.**

linea aspera, the posterior crest of the thigh bone, extending proximally into three ridges to which are attached various muscles, including the gluteus maximus, pectineus, and iliacus.

linea nigra,   a dark line appearing longitudinally on the abdomen of a pregnant woman during the latter 24 weeks of term. It usually extends from the symphysis pubis midline to the umbilicus, and sometimes as far as the sternum.

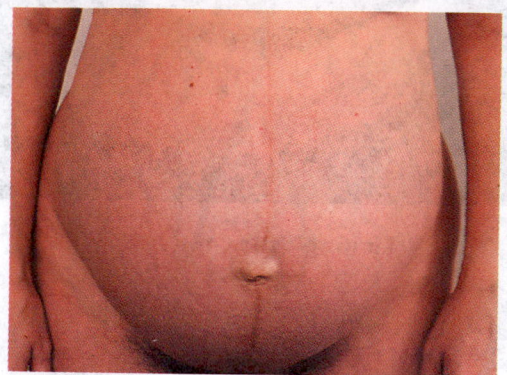

Linea nigra on the abdomen of a pregnant woman
(Seidel, 1991)

linear /lin'ē·ər/ [L, *linea*, line],   pertaining to a line or lines, particularly straight lines.

linear accelerator (LINAC) [L, *linea*, line; *accelerare*, to quicken],   an apparatus for accelerating charged subatomic particles used in radiotherapy, physics research, and the production of radionuclides. In a linear accelerator a pulsed electron beam generated by an electron gun passes through a straight long vacuum tube containing alternating hollow electrodes. The electrodes are so arranged that when their high-frequency potentials are properly varied, the particles passing through the vacuum tube waveguide receive successive increments of energy. The electrons are stopped abruptly by a heavy metal target at the end of the waveguide and are directed by a collimator to deliver supervoltage x-rays to the patient receiving radiotherapy.

linear array,   (in radiology) a contiguous sequence of identical discrete detectors, either gas-filled ionization chambers or solid-state semiconductors, used with a fan beam x-ray generator. The detectors read off once for each x-ray pulse. The resulting electronic signal is converted to a digital number and stored in a computer memory.

linear energy transfer (LET),   (in radiology) the rate at which energy is transfered from ionizing radiation to soft tissue. It is expressed in terms of kiloelectron volts (keV) per micrometer of track length in soft tissue. The LET of diagnostic x-rays is about 3 keV per micrometer, compared with 100 keV per micrometer for 5 MeV alpha particles.

linear flow velocity,   the velocity of a particle carried in a moving stream, usually measured in centimeters per second.

linear fracture,   a fracture that extends parallel to the long axis of a bone but does not displace the bone tissue.

linear grid.   See **grid.**

linearity /lin'ē·er'itē/,   (in radiology) the ability to obtain the same exposure for the same milliampere-seconds (mAs), regardless of mA and exposure time used.

linear regression,   a statistical procedure in which a straight line is established through a data set that best rep-

resents a relationship between two subsets or two methods. This mathematical technique minimizes the sum of the squares of the differences between the observed y values and the y values predicted by the regression line for a given x value.

linear scan,   (in ultrasonography) the motion of the transducer at a constant speed along a straight line at right angles to the beam.

linear tomography,   tomography that produces a blurring pattern with linear, or unidirectional, motion. The pattern is caused by elongation of structures outside the focal plane so that they become indistinguishable linear streaks or blurs over the focal plane image.

linea semilunaris,   the slightly curved line on the ventral abdominal wall, approximately parallel to the median line and lying about halfway between the median line and the side of the body. It marks the lateral border of the rectus abdominis and can be seen as a shallow groove when that muscle is tensed. Compare **linea alba.**

linea terminalis,   a hypothetical line dividing the upper, or false, pelvis, from the lower, or true, pelvis.

linea vitalis.   See **linea.**

line compensator,   an electrical device that monitors electric power for medical devices, such as x-ray equipment, and makes automatic adjustments for voltage fluctuations.

line of demarcation [L, *linea*; L, *de, marcare*, to mark],   a line that indicates a change in the condition of tissues, such as the boundary between gangrenous and healthy tissues.

line of gravity,   an imaginary line that extends from the center of gravity to the base of support.

line pair (lp),   (in computed tomography) a factor in determining spatial frequency. It consists of a bar, or line, and its adjacent equal width interspace, forming a pair. As line pairs per centimeter increase, the fidelity of the line pair image decreases.

Lineweaver-Burk transformation /lī'nwē'vərburk'/ [Hans Lineweaver, American chemist, b. 1907; Dean Burk, American scientist, b. 1904; L, *transformare*, to change shape],   a method of converting experimental data from studies of enzyme activity so that they can be displayed on a linear plot. The linear form is derived by using reciprocals of both sides of the equation.

lingu-, linguo-,   a combining form meaning 'of or pertaining to the tongue': *linguiform, lingulectomy, linguodental.*

lingua.   See **tongue.**

lingual /ling'gwəl/ [L, *lingua*, tongue],   pertaining to or resembling the tongue.

lingual artery [L, *lingua*, tongue],   one of a pair of arteries that arises from the external carotid arteries, divides into four branches, and supplies the tongue and surrounding muscles. The branches of the lingual artery are the suprahyoid, dorsal lingual, sublingual, and the deep lingual.

lingual bar,   a major connector that is installed lingual to the dental arch and joins bilateral parts of a mandibular removable partial denture.

lingual bone.   See **hyoid bone.**

lingual crib,   an orthodontic appliance consisting of a wire frame suspended lingually to the maxillary incisor teeth. It is used for obstructing undesirable thumb and tongue habits that can produce malocclusions, especially in youngsters.

lingual flange,   the part of a mandibular denture that occupies the space adjacent to the residual ridge and next to the mouth.

lingual frenum, a band of tissue that extends from the floor of the mouth to the inferior surface of the tongue. Also called **frenulum linguae.**

lingual gingiva [L, *lingua,* tongue; *gingiva,* gum], the gum covering the teeth on the surfaces facing the tongue.

lingual goiter, a tumor at the back of the tongue formed by an enlargement of the primordial thyrolingual duct.

lingualis leukoplakia [L, *lingua,* tongue; Gk, *leukos,* white; *plax,* plate], a chronic inflammatory lesion characterized by smooth, thick, white patches on the surface of the tongue, generally attributed to excessive use of alcohol and tobacco. The lesions may be a precursor of epithelioma.

lingual papilla. See **papilla.**

lingual rest, a metallic extension onto the lingual surface of an anterior tooth to provide support or indirect retention for a removable partial denture.

lingual tonsil, a mass of lymphoid follicles near the root of the tongue. Each follicle forms a rounded eminence containing a small opening leading into a funnel-shaped cavity surrounded by lymphoid tissue.

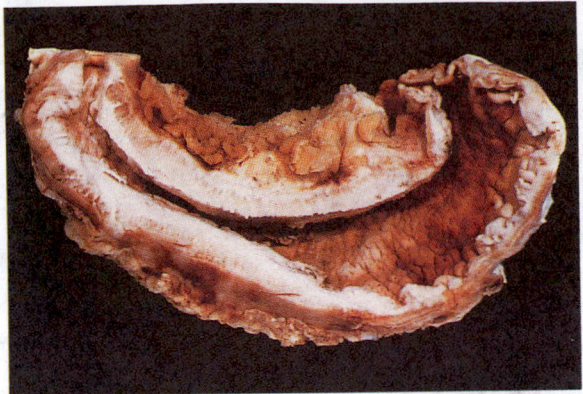

Linitis plastica *(Turk, 1986)*

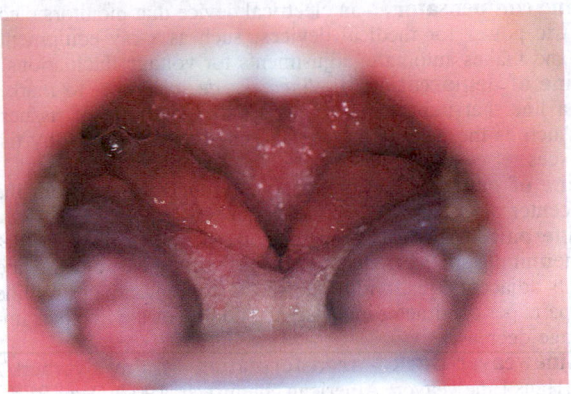

Lingual tonsil *(Bingham, 1992)*

lingua villosa nigra. See **parasitic glossitis.**

lingula /ling′gyələ/ [L, small tongue], any anatomical structure that resembles a tongue.

lingula of the lung [L, *lingula,* small tongue; AS, *lungen*], a tonguelike projection from the costal surface of the upper lobe of the left lung.

liniment /lin′imənt/ [L, *linere,* to smear], a preparation, usually containing an alcoholic, oily, or soapy vehicle, that is rubbed on the skin as a counterirritant.

linin /li′nin/ [Gk, *linon,* flax, thread], the faintly staining threads seen in the nuclei of cells, with granules of chromatin attached to the threads. See also **karyolymph.**

linitis /lini′tis/ [Gk, *linon,* flax, thread, *itis,* inflammation], inflammation of cellular tissue of the stomach as in linitis plastica, seen frequently in adenocarcinoma of the stomach.

linitis plastica, a diffuse fibrosis and thickening of the wall of the stomach, resulting in a rigid, inelastic organ. The layer of connective tissue of the stomach becomes fibrotic and thick, and the stomach wall becomes shrunken and rigid. Causes of this condition include infiltrating undifferentiated carcinoma, syphilis, and Crohn's disease involving the stomach. Also called **leather bottle stomach.**

linkage /ling′kij/ [Gk, *linke,* connection], **1.** (in genetics) the location of two or more genes on the same chromosome so that they do not segregate independently during meiosis but tend to be transmitted together as a unit. The closer the loci of the genes, the more likely they are to be inherited as a group and associated with a specific trait, whereas the farther apart they are, the greater the chance that they will be separated bycrossing over and carried on homologous chromosomes. The concept of linkage, which opposes the independent assortment theory of mendelian genetics, led to the foundation of the modern chromosome theory of genetics. See also **synteny. 2.** (in psychology) the association between a stimulus and the response it elicits. **3.** (in chemistry) the bond between two atoms or radicals in a chemical compound or the lines used to designate valency connections between the atoms in structural formulas.

linkage group, (in genetics) a group of genes located on the same chromosome that tends to be inherited as a unit. Theoretically, without crossing over, all of the genes on a given chromosome constitute a linkage group and are equal to the number of autosomes in the haploid cell.

linkage map. See **genetic map.**

linked genes [Me, *linke* + Gk, *genein,* to produce], genes that are located on the same chromosome and whose position is close enough so that they tend to be transmitted as a linkage group.

linker [ME, *linke,* connection], (in molecular genetics) a small segment of synthetic DNA having a place on its surface that can be ligated to DNA fragments in cloning. Some linkers are commercially available.

linoleic acid /lin′ələ′ik/ [L, *linum,* flax, *oleum,* oil], a colorless to straw-colored essential fatty acid with two unsaturated bonds, occurring in linseed and safflower oils. Commercially produced linoleic acid is used in margarine, animal feeds, emulsifying agents, soaps, and drugs.

linolenic acid /lin′ōlen′ik/ [L, *linum,* flax, *oleum,* oil], an unsaturated fatty acid essential for normal human nutrition. It occurs in glycerides of linseed and other vegetable oils.

lio-. See **leio-.**

Lioresal, a trademark for an antispastic agent (baclofen).

liothyronine sodium /li′ōthī′rənēn/, a synthetic thyroid hormone.

■ INDICATIONS: It is prescribed in the treatment of primary

hypothyroidism, myxedema, simple goiter, cretinism, and secondary hypothyroidism.

■ CONTRAINDICATIONS: Hyperthyroidism, thyrotoxicosis, acute myocardial infarction, or known hypersensitivity to this drug prohibits its use. It is used with caution in patients with diabetes mellitus or cardiovascular disease.

■ ADVERSE EFFECTS: Among the serious adverse reactions, usually caused by overdosage, are tachycardia, arrhythmias, thyrotoxicosis, nausea, vomiting, hypertension, nervousness, and loss of weight.

liotrix /lī'ətriks/, a uniform mixture of the thyroid hormones T_3 and T_4.

■ INDICATION: It is prescribed in the treatment of hypothyroid conditions.

■ CONTRAINDICATIONS: Most diseases and abnormal conditions of the myocardium or known hypersensitivity to this drug prohibits its use.

■ ADVERSE EFFECTS: Among the more serious adverse reactions are symptoms of thyrotoxicosis, including tachycardia, nervousness, insomnia, and fever.

lip [AS, *lippa*], **1.** either the upper or lower fleshy structure surrounding the opening of the oral cavity. **2.** any rimlike structure bordering a cavity or groove; labium.

lip-, See **lipo-.**

LIP, abbreviation for *lipoid interstitial pneumonia.*

lipase /lī'pās, lip'ās/ [Gk, *lipos* + Fr, *diastase*, enzyme], any of several enzymes, produced by the organs of the digestive system, that catalyze the breakdown of lipids through the hydrolysis of the linkages between fatty acids and glycerol in triglycerides and phospholipids. Normal blood levels of lipase range from 0 to 110 units/L. See also **fat, fatty acid, glycerol, phospholipid, triglyceride.**

lipectomy /lipek'təmē/ [Gk, *lipos* + *ektome*, excision], an excision of subcutaneous fat, as from the abdominal wall. Also called **adipectomy.**

lipedema /lip'ədē'mə/, a condition in which fat deposits accumulate in the lower extremities, from the hips to the ankles, accompanied by symptoms of tenderness in the affected areas. Treatment is dietary.

lipemia /lipē'mē·ə/ [Gk, *lipos* + *haima*, blood], a condition in which increased amounts of lipids are present in the blood, a normal occurrence after eating.

lipid /lip'id, lī'pid/ [Gk, *lipos* + *eidos*, form], any of the free fatty acid fractions in the blood. Lipids are insoluble in water but soluble in alcohol, chloroform, ether, and other solvents. They are stored in the body and serve as an energy reserve, but are elevated in various diseases, such as atherosclerosis. Kinds of lipids are **cholesterol, fatty acids, neutral fat, phospholipids, phospholipid as phosphorus,** and **triglycerides.** The normal concentrations of total lipids in serum are 400 to 800 mg/dl; cholesterol, 150 to 250 mg/dl; fatty acids, 9 to 15 mM/L; neutral fat, 0 to 200 mg/dl; phospholipids, 150 to 380 mg/dl; phospholipid as phosphorus, 9 to 16 mg/dl; triglycerides, 10 to 190 mg/dl.

lipidosis /lip'idō'sis/ [Gk, *lipos* + *osis*, condition], a general term including several rare familial disorders of fat metabolism. The chief characteristic of these disorders is the accumulation of abnormal levels of certain lipids in the body. Kinds of lipidoses are **Gaucher's disease, Krabbe's disease, Niemann-Pick disease,** and **Tay-Sachs disease.**

lipiduria /lip'idōōr'ē·ə/, the presence of lipids (fatty bodies) in the urine.

lipo-, lip- a prefix meaning 'fat': *lipase, lipodystrohy, lipoma.*

lipoatrophic diabetes /lip'ō·atrof'ik/, an inherited disease characterized by insulin-resistant diabetes mellitus, loss of body fat, acanthosis nigricans, and hypertrophied musculature. It is associated with a disorder of the hypothalamus resulting in excessive blood levels of growth hormone and ACTH releasing hormones.

lipoatrophy /lip'ō·at'rəfē/, a breakdown of subcutaneous fat at the site of an insulin injection. It usually occurs after several injections at the same site. Compare **lipohypertrophy.**

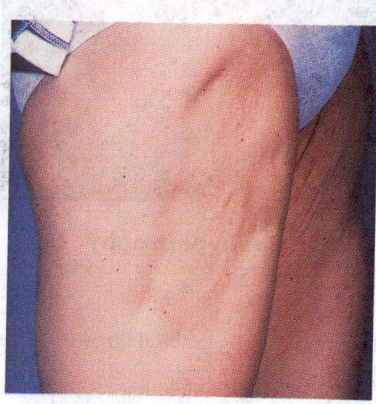

Lipoatrophy
(Bodansky, 1989/Courtesy Professor AG Cudworth, London)

lipocele. See **adipocele.**

lipochondrodystrophy. See **Hurler's syndrome.**

lipochrome /lip'əkrōm/ [Gk, *lipos* + *chroma*, color], any of the naturally occurring pigments that contain a lipid, and which give a yellow color to fats, such as carotene.

lipodystrophia progressiva /-distrō'fē·ə/ [Gk, *lipos* + *dys*, bad, *trophe*, nourishment; L, *progredior*, to go forth], an abnormal accumulation of fat around the buttocks and thighs and a progressive, symmetric disappearance of subcutaneous fat from areas above the pelvis and on the face. Also called **lipomatosis atrophicans.**

lipodystrophy /lip'ōdis'trəfē/ [Gk, *lipos* + *dys*, bad, *trophe*, nourishment], any abnormality in the metabolism or deposition of fats. Kinds of lipodystrophy are **bitrochanteric lipodystrophy, insulin lipodystrophy,** and **intestinal lipodystrophy.**

lip of hip fracture, a fracture of the posterior lip of the acetabulum, often associated with displacement of the hip.

lipofuscin /lip'əfus'in/, a class of fatty pigments consisting mostly of oxidized fats that are found in abundance in the cells of adults. Studies suggest that lipofuscins contribute to the aging process in a cell.

lipogenesis /-jen'əsis/ [Gk, *lipos*, fat; *genein*, to produce], the production and accumulation of fat.

lipogranuloma /lip'ōgran'yoōlō'mə/, *pl.* **lipogranulomas, lipogranulomata** [Gk, *lipos* + L, *granulum*, little grain; Gk, *oma*, tumor], a nodule of necrotic, fatty tissue associated with granulomatous inflammation or a foreign-body reaction around a deposit of injected material containing an oily substance.

lipohypertrophy /lip′ōhīpur′trəfē/, a buildup of subcutaneous fat tissue at the site of an insulin injection. Compare **lipoatrophy.**

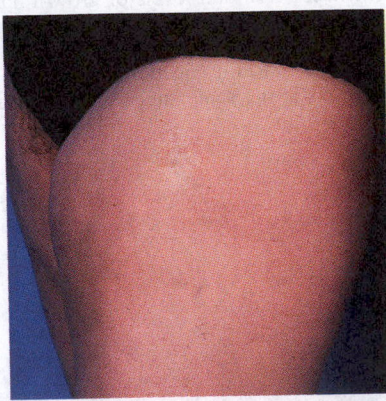

Lipohypertrophy
(Bodansky, 1989/Courtesy Professor AG Cudworth, London)

lipoic acid /lipō′ik/, a bacterial growth factor found in liver and yeast.

lipoid /lip′oid/, any substance that resembles a lipid.

lipolysis /lipol′isis/, the breakdown or destruction of lipids or fats.

lipolytic /-lit′ik/ [*lipos,* fat; *lysis,* loosening], the chemical breakdown of fat.

lipoma /lipō′mə/, *pl.* **lipomas, lipomata** [Gk, *lipos + oma,* tumor], a benign tumor consisting of mature fat cells. Also called **adipose tumor.** See also **multiple lipomatosis.** **–lipomatous,** *adj.*

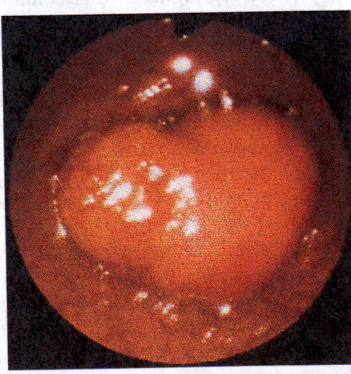

Endoscopic view of a lipoma (Mitros, 1988)

-lipoma, a combining form meaning a 'tumor made up of fatty tissue': *angiolipoma, fibrolipoma, osteolipoma.*

lipoma annulare colli, a diffuse, symmetric accumulation of fat around the neck, not a true lipoma. Also called **Madelung's neck.**

lipoma arborescens, a fatty tumor of a joint, characterized by a treelike distribution of fat cells.

lipoma capsulare, a benign neoplasm characterized by the abnormal presence of fat cells in the capsule of an organ.

lipoma cavernosum. See **angiolipoma.**

lipoma diffusum renis. See **lipomatous nephritis.**

lipoma dolorosa. See **lipomatosis dolorosa.**

lipoma fibrosum, a fatty tumor containing masses of fibrous tissue.

lipoma myxomatodes. See **lipomyxoma.**

lipoma sarcomatodes. See **liposarcoma.**

lipomata. See **lipoma.**

lipomatosis /lip′ōmətō′sis/ [Gk, *lipos + oma,* tumor, *osis,* condition], a disorder characterized by abnormal tumorlike accumulations of fat in body tissues.

lipomatosis atrophicans. See **lipodystrophia progressiva, lipomatosis.**

lipomatosis dolorosa, a disorder characterized by the abnormal accumulation of painful or tender fat deposits. Also called **lipoma dolorosa.**

lipomatosis gigantea, a condition characterized by massive deposits of fat.

lipomatosis renis. See **lipomatous nephritis.**

lipomatous /lipō′mətəs/ [Gk, *lipos,* fat; *oma,* tumor], pertaining to or resembling a benign tumor made up of mature fat cells.

lipomatous myxoma, a tumor containing fatty tissue that arises in connective tissue.

lipomatous nephritis, a rare condition in which the renal nephrons are replaced by fatty tissue. Kidney failure may result. Also called **lipoma diffusum renis, lipomatosis renis.**

lipometabolism /-metab′əliz′əm/ [Gk, *lipos,* fat; *metabole,* change], the chemical processes involved in building up or breaking down fat molecules.

lipomyoma /-mī·ō′mə/ [Gk, *lipos,* fat; *mys,* muscle; *oma,* tumor], a tumor that combines characteristics of a lipoma and myoma.

lipomyxoma /lip′ōmiksō′mə/, *pl.* **lipomyxomas, lipomyxomata** [Gk, *lipos + myxa,* mucus, *oma,* tumor], a myxoma that contains fat cells. Also called **lipoma myxomatodes.**

lipophilia /-fil′yə/ [Gk, *lipos,* fat; *philein,* to love], a tendency to attract or absorb fat.

lipoprotein /lip′ōprō′tēn/ [Gk, *lipos + proteios,* first rank], a conjugated protein in which lipids form an integral part of the molecule. They are synthesized primarily in the liver, contain varying amounts of triglycerides, cholesterol, phospholipids, and protein, and are classified according to their composition and density. Practically all of the plasma lipids are present as lipoprotein complexes. The elevation of low-density lipoproteins in plasma is asociated with an increased risk of atheroslcerosis. Normal adult levels of lipoproteins include: HDL, greater than 45 mg/dl; LDL, 60-180 mg/dl; VLDL, 25%-50%. Kinds of lipoproteins are **chylomicrons, high-density lipoproteins, low-density lipoproteins,** and **very low-density lipoproteins.** See also **proteolipid.**

liposarcoma /lip′ōsärkō′mə/, *pl.* **liposarcomas, liposarcomata** [Gk, *lipos + sarx,* flesh, *oma,* tumor], a malignant growth of primitive fat cells. Also called **lipoma sarcomatodes.**

liposis. See **lipomatosis.**

liposoluble /-sol′yəbəl/ [Gk, *lipos,* fat; L, *solubilis*], fat soluble.

liposome /lip′əsōm/ [Gk, *lipos,* fat; *soma,* body], a mul-

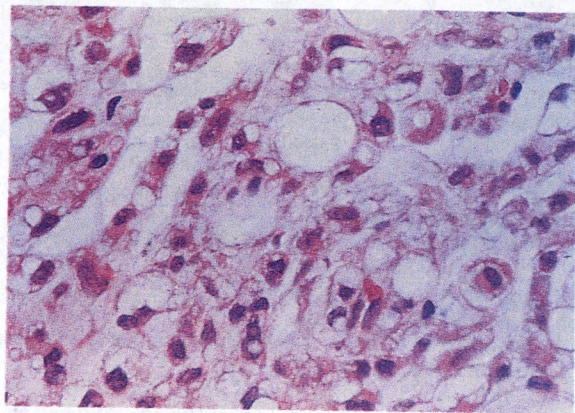

Liposarcoma (Cawson, 1987)

tilayered spherical particle of a lipid in an aqueous medium in a cell. It is formed when a phopholipid encounters water and develops sphere of bimolecular, hydrophilic and hydrophobic layers.

liposuction /-suk′shən/, a technique for removing adipose tissue from obese patients with a suction-pump device. It is used primarily to remove or reduce localized areas of fat around the abdomen, breasts, legs, face, and upper arms where the skin is contractile enough to redrape in a normal manner. Also called **suction lipectomy.**

lip reading, a former name for **speech reading.**

-lipsis, -lipse, a combining form meaning 'to leave out, fail, omit': *eclipsis, ellipsis, menolipsis.*

Liquaemin Sodium, a trademark for an anticoagulant (heparin sodium).

liquefaction /lik′wəfak′shən/ [L, *liquere*, to flow, *facere*, to make], the process in which a solid or a gas is made liquid.

liquid /lik′wid/ [L, *liquere*, to flow], a state of matter, intermediate between solid and gas, in which the substance flows freely with little application of force and assumes the shape of the vessel in which it is contained. Compare **fluid.** See also **gas, solid.**

liquid diet, a diet consisting of foods that can be served in liquid or strained form plus custard, ice cream, pudding, tapioca, and soft-cooked eggs. It is prescribed in acute infections, in acute inflammatory conditions of the GI tract, and for patients unable to consume soft or semifluid foods, usually after surgery. See also **full liquid diet.**

liquid glucose, a thick, syrupy, odorless, and colorless or yellowish liquid obtained by the incomplete hydrolysis of starch primarily consisting of dextrose with dextrins, maltose, and water. It is used as a flavoring agent and may be used as a calorie source, chiefly in treating dehydration.

liquid nitrogen. See **cryogen.**

liquor /lik′ər/, any fluid or liquid, such as liquor amnii, the amniotic fluid.

liquor amnii. See **amniotic fluid.**

liquorice. See **licorice.**

Lisfranc's fracture /lisfrangks′/ [Jacque Lisfranc, French surgeon, b. 1790], a fracture dislocation of the foot in which one or all of the proximal metatarsals are displaced.

lisping, the defective pronunciation of one or more of the sibilant consonant sounds, usually |s| and |z|.

Lister, Baron Joseph (born 1827), [Scottish surgeon], introduced the use of antiseptic surgery in London hospitals in 1867. Lister operations were performed under a spray of diluted carbolic acid, instruments were dipped in carbolic acid, and wounds were dressed with gauze similarly treated.

Listeria monocytogenes /lister′ē·ə/ /mon′ōsītoj′inēz/ [Baron Joseph Lister, Scottish surgeon, b. 1827; Gk, *mono*, single, *kytos*, cell, *genein*, to produce], a common species of gram-positive, motile bacillus that causes listeriosis.

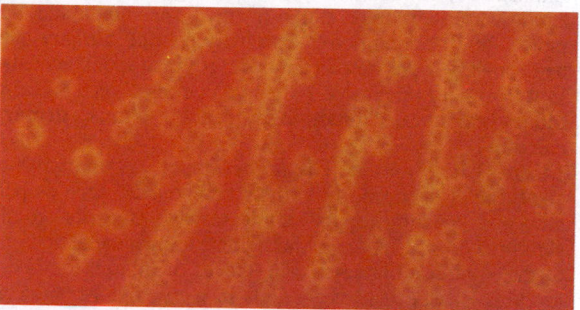

Colonies of *Listeria monocytogenes* (Baron, 1990)

listeriosis /listir′ē·ō′sis/ [Baron Joseph Lister; Gk, *osis*, condition], an infectious disease caused by a genus of gram-positive motile bacteria that are nonsporulating. *Listeria monocytogenes* infects shellfish, birds, spiders, and mammals in all areas of the world, but infection in humans is uncommon. Transmitted by direct contact from infected animals to humans, through ingesting contaminated meat and dairy products, by inhalation of dust, or by contact with mud, sewage, or soil contaminated with the organism, it is characterized by circulatory collapse, shock, endocarditis, hepatosplenomegaly, and a dark red rash over the trunk and the legs. Fever, bacteremia, malaise, and lethargy are commonly seen. Newborns and immunosuppressed, debilitated older people are more vulnerable to infection than are immunocompetent children and young or middle-aged adults. The signs of infection and the severity of the disease vary according to the site of infection and the age and condition of the person. Pregnant women characteristically experience a mild, brief episode of illness, but fetal infection acquired through the placental circulation in utero is usually fatal. Infection in the newborn apparently results from exposure to the organism in the birth canal of an infected mother. Meningitis and encephalitis occur in 75% of cases. Treatment may include ampicillin, penicillin, tetracycline, or erythromycin, given intramuscularly or intravenously. If infection is suspected in a pregnant woman, treatment is begun immediately, even before bacteriologic culture of the blood, spinal fluid, or vaginal secretions can confirm the diagnosis. All secretions from the patient may contain the organism. Also called **listerosis.**

Liston's forceps [Robert Liston, Scottish surgeon, b. 1794], a kind of bone cutting forceps.

liter (L) /lē′tər/ [Fr], a unit of volume equivalent to 1.057 quarts and defined as the volume occupied by a mass of one kilogram of water at standard temperature and pressure.

lith. See **litho-.**

-lith, a suffix meaning 'a calculus': *pneumolith, ptyalith, tonsillolith*.

Lithane, a trademark for an antimanic drug (lithium carbonate).

-lithiasis-, a suffix meaning 'pertaining to the presence, condition, or formation of stones': *cholelithiasis, uterolithiasis*.

lithiasis /lithī'əsis/ [Gk, *lithos*, stone, *osis*, condition], the formation of calculi in the hollow organs or ducts of the body. Calculi are formed of mineral salts and may irritate, inflame, or obstruct the organ in which they form or lodge. Lithiasis occurs most commonly in the gallbladder, kidney, and lower urinary tract. Lithiasis may be asymptomatic, but more often the condition is extremely painful. Surgery may be necessary if the stones cannot be excreted spontaneously. Lower urinary tract calculi often can be dissolved. See also **biliary calculus, cholelithiasis, renal calculus, urinary calculus.**

lithium (Li) /lith'ē·əm/ [Gk, *lithos*, stone], a silvery white alkali metal occurring in various compounds, such as petalite and spodumene. Its atomic number is 3; its atomic weight is 6.94. Lithium is the lightest known metal and one of the most reactive elements. Traces of lithium ion occur in animal tissue, and it abounds in many alkaline mineral spring waters. Its salts are used in the treatment of manias, but the mechanisms by which these compounds help to stabilize psychologic moods are not understood. Lithium carbonate is a salt commonly used for psychiatric purposes in the United States; it has been effective in the prevention of recurrent attacks of manic-depressive illnesses. It has helped to correct sleep disorders in manic patients, apparently by suppressing the rapid eye movement phases of sleep. Therapeutic concentrations of lithium have no observable psychotropic effects on normal individuals. In manic patients, lithium salts also produce high-voltage slow waves in the electroencephalograph, often with superimposed beta waves. An important feature of the lithium ion is its relatively small gradient of distribution across biologic membranes. Although it can replace sodium in supporting a nerve cell action potential, it cannot adequately prime the sodium pump and maintain membrane potentials. Lithium ions are quickly and almost completely absorbed from the GI tract, producing peak concentrations in plasma within 2 to 4 hours. The ion first spreads through the extracellular fluid and then gradually disperses in varying concentrations through different tissues. The ion passes slowly through the blood-brain barrier, and, when a steady state is achieved, the concentration of lithium in the cerebrospinal fluid is about 40% of the lithium concentration in the plasma. About 95% of a single dose of lithium salts is eliminated in the urine. The lithium ion has such a low therapeutic index that safe treatment requires daily determination of plasma concentrations. Intoxication may result if levels rise beyond peak concentrations, which can be 2 to 3 times higher than steady-state concentrations. Acute intoxication by lithium may cause seizure and death. Side effects may include polyuria, polydipsia, and benign enlargement of the thyroid. Mixed and inconclusive results have followed lithium treatment of disorders other than manias, such as premenstrual tension, alcoholism, episodic anger, and anorexia nervosa. Patients suffering severe manic attacks are hospitalized so that they can receive proper medical maintenance; treatments start with large doses of antipsychotic drugs, which are followed by the gradual and safe introduction of lithium therapy. Ideally, lithium treatment is prescribed only for patients with normal sodium intake and normal heart and kidney function.

lithium carbonate, an antimanic agent.
- INDICATION: It is prescribed in the treatment of manic episodes of manic-depressive disorder.
- CONTRAINDICATIONS: It is used with caution in the presence of renal or cardiovascular disease and is not recommended for children under 12 years of age. Known hypersensitivity to this drug prohibits its use.
- ADVERSE EFFECTS: Among the most serious adverse reactions are renal damage, polydipsia and polyuria, and impairment of mental and physical abilities. Retention of sodium and fluid may occur.

lithium fluoride (LiF), a compound commonly used for thermoluminescent dosimetry.

litho-, lith-, a combining form meaning 'of or pertaining to a stone, or to a calculus': *litholysis, lithomyl, lithophone*.

lithogenesis /lith'əjen'əsis/ [Gk, *lithokos*, stone; *genein*, to produce], the origin of the formation of a calculus.

lithopedion /lith'əpē'dē·ən/ [Gk, *lithos* + *paidion*, child], a fetus that has died in utero and has become calcified or ossified. Also called **lithopedium, calcified fetus, ostembryon, osteopedion.**

lithotomy /lithot'əmē/ [Gk, *lithos* + *temnein*, to cut], the surgical excision of a calculus, especially one from the urinary tract.

lithotomy forceps, a forceps for the extraction of a calculus, usually from the urinary tract.

lithotomy position, the posture assumed by the patient lying supine with the hips and the knees flexed and the thighs abducted and rotated externally. Also called **dorsosacral position.**

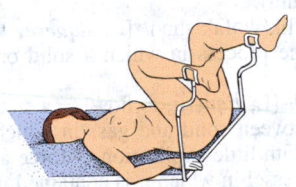

Lithotomy position *(Potter, 1993)*

lithotripsy /lith'ətrip'sē/ [Gk, *lithokos*, stone; *tribein*, to wear away], a procedure for eliminating a kidney stone by crushing or dissolving it in situ.

lithotrite /lith'ətrīt/ [Gk, *lithos* + L, *terere*, to rub], an instrument for crushing a stone in the urinary bladder. Also called **lithotriptor. –lithotrity,** *n*.

litigant /lit'əgənt/ [L, *litigare*, to go to law], (in law) a party to a lawsuit. See also **defendant, plaintiff.**

litigate /lit'əgāt/, (in law) to carry on a suit or to contest.

litigious paranoia [L, *litigare*, to go to law; Gk, *paranous*, madness], a form of paranoia in which the person seeks legal proof or justification for systematized delusions.

litmus paper /lit'məs/ [ONorse, *litmosi*, coloring herb; L, *papyrus*, paper], absorbent paper coated with litmus, a blue dye, that is used to determine pH. Acid substances or solutions turn blue litmus to red. Alkaline substances or solutions do not cause a color change in blue litmus. The pH range is 4.5 (red) to 8.5 (blue).

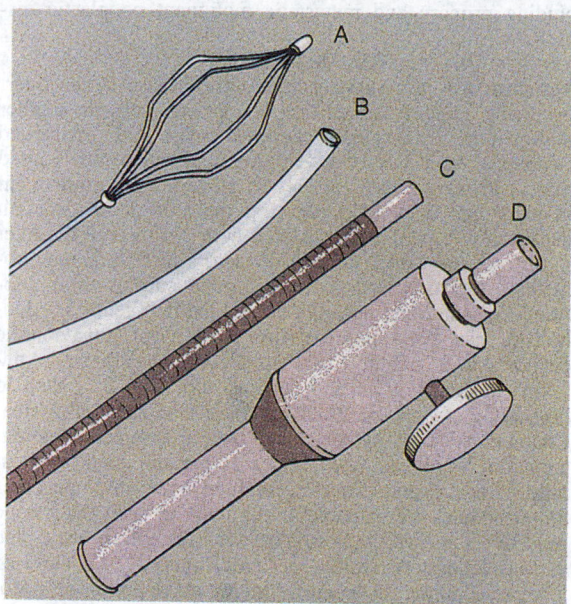

Mechanical lithotrite assembly: A. basket wire; B. polyethylene catheter; C. metal sheath or cable; D. crank device
(Geenen, 1992)

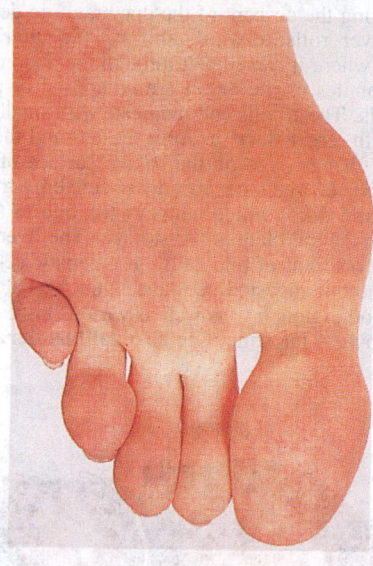

Livedo reticularis seen on the foot *(Schumacher, 1988)*

litter [Fr *lit* bed], a stretcher.

Little's disease. See **cerebral palsy.**

Litzmann's obliquity. See **asynclitism.**

live attenuated measles virus vaccine, a vaccine prepared from live strains of measles virus that have been cultured under conditions that cause them to lose their virulence without losing their ability to induce immunity. The vaccine is not recommended for pregnant women or others who may have certain medical conditions that tend to diminish immunity.

live birth [AS, *libben*, to be alive; ONorse, *byrth*], the birth of an infant, irrespective of the duration of gestation, that exhibits any sign of life, such as respiration, heartbeat, umbilical pulsation, or movement of voluntary muscles. A live birth is not always a viable birth.

livedo /livē′dō/ [L, *liveo*, bluish spot], a blue or reddish mottling of the skin that worsens in cold weather and is probably caused by arteriolar spasm. **Cutis marmorata** is a transient form of livedo. See also **livedo reticularis.**

livedo reticularis, a vasospastic disorder accentuated by exposure to cold and presenting with a characteristic reddish blue mottling with a typical 'fishnet' appearance. The condition involves the entire leg and, less often, the arms. See also **livedo.**

livedo vasculitis. See **segmented hyalinizing vasculitis.**

live measles and mumps virus vaccine, a vaccine prepared from live strains of measles and mumps viruses. The vaccine is commonly combined with live rubella viruses as **MMR vaccine** and administered to normal infants at the age of 15 months.

live oral poliovirus vaccine, a vaccine prepared from three strains (trivalent) of live polioviruses. Primary immunization with the vaccine usually begins at the age of two months.

liver [AS, *lifer*], the largest gland of the body and one of its most complex organs. More than 500 of its functions have been identified. It is divided into four lobes, contains as many as 100,000 lobules, and is served by two distinct blood supplies. The hepatic artery conveys oxygenated blood to the liver, and the hepatic portal vein conveys nutrient-filled blood from the stomach and the intestines. At any given moment the liver holds about one pint of blood or approximately 13% of the total blood supply of the body. Some of the major functions performed by the liver are the production of bile by hepatic cells, the secretion of glucose, proteins, vitamins, fats, and most of the other compounds used by the body, the processing of hemoglobin for vital use of its iron content, and the conversion of poisonous ammonia to urea. Bile from the liver is stored in the gallbladder, which is connected to the liver by connective tissue, in the hepatic duct, and in numerous blood vessels. The liver is located in the cranial, right portion of the abdominal cavity, occupying almost the entire right hypochondrium, the greater part of the epigastrium, and in many individuals extends into the left hypochondrium as far as the mammary line. The liver develops in the embryo as a hollow projection from the ventral surface of the primitive gut, which eventually becomes the descending portion of the duodenum. The adult liver in men weighs about 1.8 kg; in women, about 1.3 kg. It has a soft, solid consistency, is shaped like an irregular hemisphere, and is dark reddish brown in color. The right lobe of the liver is much larger than the left lobe or the caudate and the quadrate lobes. The ventral portion of the liver is separated by the diaphragm from the sixth to the tenth ribs on the right side and from the seventh and the eighth costal cartilages on the left side. It is completely covered by peritoneum except along the line of attachment of the falciform ligament. The dorsal part of the organ is wide and rounded on the right but narrow on the left, and the central section has a deep concavity that fits the vertebral column and the crura of the diaphragm. The liver attaches to the diaphragm by the coronary and the triangular ligaments. During the descent of the diaphragm in deep breathing, the liver rolls forward, shifting the inferior border downward where it can be felt through the abdominal wall. The tiny lobules of the organ are composed of polyhedral hepatic cells. These cells communicate with small ducts that connect with larger ducts to form the left and the right hepatic ducts that emerge on the caudal surface of the liver. The left and the right hepatic ducts converge to form the single hepatic duct, which conveys the bile to the duodenum and to the gallbladder for storage. The liver cells produce about one pint of bile daily. The hepatic cells also detoxify numerous ingested substances, such as alcohol, nicotine, and other poisons, as well as various toxic substances produced by the intestine. See also **gallbladder.**

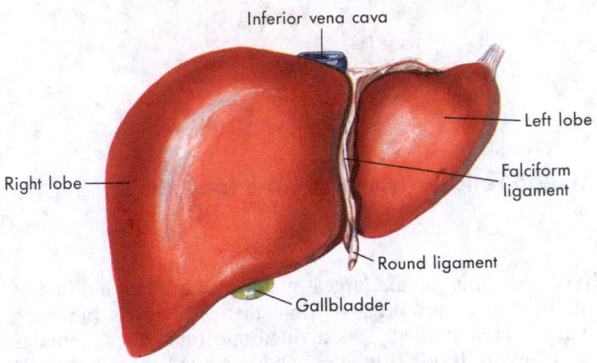

Inferior vena cava

Left lobe

Falciform ligament

Right lobe

Round ligament

Gallbladder

Anterior view of the liver
(Thibodeau, 1993/David J Mascaro & Associates)

liver biopsy, a diagnostic procedure in which a special needle is introduced into the liver under local anesthesia to obtain a specimen for pathologic examination.

■ METHOD: Before a liver biopsy is performed by the physician, the procedure is explained to the patient, whose baseline vital signs are recorded and who is taught how to inhale and hold the breath during insertion of the needle. After the patient's possible allergy to the local anesthetic is checked and results of bleeding, clotting, and prothrombin tests are obtained, an analgesic or sedative is administered as ordered. On completion of the biopsy, pressure is applied to the site for 15 minutes; the patient is positioned on the right side for the first 2 hours and remains in a supine position in bed for the next 22 hours. The blood pressure, pulse, and respirations are checked every 15 minutes for the first hour, then every 30 minutes for the next 2 hours, and subsequently every 4 hours or as ordered. The biopsy site is observed every 30 minutes for bleeding, swelling, or increased pain; epigastric or referred shoulder pain may occur. Analgesia and vitamin K may be given as ordered, and the recumbent patient is assisted with eating and other activities as needed.

■ INTERVENTIONS: The nurse reinforces explanations of the biopsy and its purpose, provides care before and after the procedure, and closely observes the patient for postbiopsy complications, such as intraperitoneal hemorrhage, shock, and pneumothorax.

■ OUTCOME CRITERIA: An uneventful liver biopsy is a valuable aid in establishing a diagnosis of hepatic disease, including primary and metastatic malignant neoplastic disease.

liver breath. See **fetor hepaticus.**

liver cancer, a malignant neoplastic disease of the liver, occurring most frequently as a metastasis from another malignancy. Primary liver cancer is common in Africa and Southeast Asia but relatively uncommon in the United States. Primary tumors are six to 10 times more prevalent in men than in women, develop most often in the sixth decade of life, and are associated with cirrhosis of the liver in 70% of the cases. Other risk factors include hemochromatosis, hepatitis, schistosomiasis, exposure to vinyl chloride or arsenic, and possibly nutritional deficiencies. Alcoholism may be a predisposing factor, but nonalcoholic cirrhosis is a greater risk than alcoholic cirrhosis. Aflatoxins in moldy grain and peanuts appear to be linked to high rates of hepatocellular carcinoma in parts of Africa. Characteristics of liver cancer are abdominal bloating, anorexia, weakness, dull upper abdominal pain, ascites, mild jaundice, and a tender enlarged liver; in some cases tumor nodules are palpable on the liver surface. Diagnostic procedures include radioisotope scan, needle biopsy, and various laboratory studies of liver function. An elevated level of alkaline phosphatase, increased retention of sulfobromophthalein, and the presence of alpha fetoprotein in the blood suggest liver cancer. All primary liver tumors are adenocarcinomas, classified as hepatomas when derived from hepatic cells, and cholangiomas if they originate in cells of the bile duct. They form large single nodules or satellite nodules surrounding a central lesion and are found more often in the right lobe than in the left. Primary lesions spread centrifugally in the liver, invade the portal vein and lymphatic vessels, and metastasize to lymph nodes, the lungs, brain, and other sites. Total hepatic lobectomy is the treatment of choice for primary tumors; because the liver is able to regenerate, 80% of it may be resected. Systemic chemotherapy such as methotrexate, cyclophosphamide, and 5-fluorouracil infused through a catheter in the hepatic artery may result in temporary tumor regression. Irradiation is very destructive to liver cells and not very toxic to tumor cells in the liver.

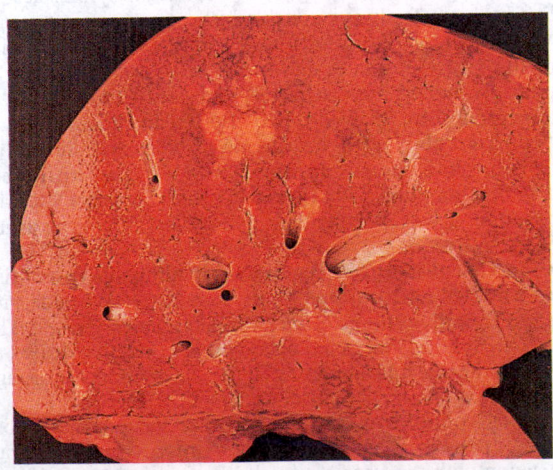

Primary liver cancer *(Fletcher, 1987)*

liver cell carcinoma. See **malignant hepatoma.**

liver disease, any one of a group of disorders of the liver. Characteristics of liver disease are jaundice, anorexia, hepatomegaly, ascites, and impaired consciousness. The exact diagnosis of liver disease is made through a combination of laboratory tests and clinical findings. See also **cholestasis, cirrhosis, hepatitis.**

liver failure [AS, *lifer*, L, *fallere,* to deceive], a condition in which the liver fails to fulfill its function or is unable to meet the demands made on it. Anorexia, fatigue, and weakness are common symptoms of liver cell failure while jaundice indicates a biliary obstruction and fever may accompany viral or alcoholic liver diseases.

liver flap. See **asterixis.**

liver fluke [AS, *lifer*; *floc*], a parasitic Trematode with six genera that may infest the liver. The most important species affecting humans in industrialized countries is *Clonorchis sinensis,* which is usually acquired by eating freshwater fish containing the encysted larvae. The larvae are released in the duodenum, enter the common bile duct, and migrate to other bile ducts, the gall bladder, and pancreatic ducts. The liver fluke may survive for many years in the human biliary tree, releasing eggs into the feces. Infestations are most likely to result from ingestion of raw, dried, salted, or pickled freshwater fish and can be prevented by thorough cooking of such fish.

liver function test (LFT), a test used to evaluate various functions of the liver—for example, metabolism, storage, filtration, and excretion. Kinds of liver function tests include **alkaline phosphatase, bromsulfalein test, prothrombin time, serum bilirubin,** and **serum glutamic pyruvic transaminase.**

liver scan, a noninvasive technique of visualizing the size, shape, and consistency of the liver by the intravenous injection of a radioactively labeled compound that is readily taken up and trapped in the Kupffer cells of the liver. The radiation emitted by the compound is recorded by a radiation detector and can be photographed with a scintillation camera or filmed with x-ray. Liver scans are most useful for diagnosing three-dimensional lesions such as abscesses or tumors.

liver spot, *nontechnical.* a senile lentigo or actinic keratosis.

liver transplantation, a treatment for end-stage hepatic dysfunction in which a donor liver from a previously healthy but brain-dead individual is matched in size and blood group to the recipient. The transplanted organ may be introduced as an auxiliary liver or as a total replacement. The procedure requires five anastomoses and many units of blood. Because of a shortage of child-size livers, pediatric transplants often are performed with a segment of an adult liver.

livid /liv'id/ [L, *lividus,* bluish], pertaining to an injury that is congested and discolored.

lividity /livid'itē/ [L, *lividus,* bluish], a tissue condition of being red or blue because of venous congestion, as in a contusion.

living-in unit [AS, *libben,* to be alive; L, *in,* within; *unus,* one], a room provided in some hospitals for mothers who want to assume immediate care of their newborn infants under the supervision of nursing personnel.

living will [AS, *libben* + *willa,* wish], a written agreement between a patient and physician to withhold heroic measures if the patient's condition is found to be irreversible.

livor mortis /lī'vər/, a purple discoloration of the skin in some dependent body areas following death as a result of blood cell destruction.

lizard /liz'ərd/ [L, *lacerta*], a scaly-skinned reptile with a long body and tail and two pairs of legs. The large Gila monster of Arizona, New Mexico, and Utah, and the beaded lizard of Mexico are the only lizards known to be venomous. The symptoms of their bites and the recommended treatment are similar to those of the bites from moderately poisonous snakes.

LLD factor. See **cyanocobalamin.**

LLE, abbreviation for *left lower extremity.*

LLQ, abbreviation for *left lower quadrant of abdomen.*

LMA, abbreviation for *left mentoanterior fetal position.*

LMD. See **dextran preparation.**

L.M.D., abbreviation for *local medical doctor,* used by house staff or others to distinguish a patient's primary physician from university faculty, attending specialist physicians, or house staff. Also called **P.M.D.**

LMP, 1. abbreviation for *last menstrual period.* 2. abbreviation for *left mentoposterior fetal position.*

LMT, abbreviation for *left mentotransverse fetal position.*

LOA, abbreviation for *left occipitoanterior fetal position.*

loading response stance stage [AS, *lad,* support; L, *responsum,* reply], one of the five stages of the stance phase of walking or gait, specifically associated with the moment when the leg reacts to and accepts the weight of the body. The loading response stance stage is one of the factors in the diagnoses of many abnormal orthopedic conditions and is often studied in conjunction with analyses of the electromyographic activity of the muscles used in walking. Compare **initial contact stance stage, midstance, preswing stance stage, terminal stance.**

loads [AS, *lad,* support], *slang.* a fixed combination of a sedative hypnotic, glutethimide, and a major narcotic analgesic, codeine. The medications are taken orally by drug abusers for a euphoric effect reported to be similar to that produced by heroin, but longer lasting. Toxicity may develop, characterized by nystagmus, slurred speech, seizures, coma, pulmonary edema, or sudden apnea and death. Detoxification of an addicted person is managed under close medical supervision with methadone and phenobarbital, as sudden withdrawal can cause death.

Loa loa /lō'älō'ä/, a parasitic worm of western and central Africa that causes loiasis. Also called **eye worm.**

-lobar. See **lobe.**

lobar bronchus /lō'bär [Gk, *lobos,* lobe; *bronchos,* windpipe], a bronchus extending from a primary bronchus to a segmental bronchus into one of the lobes of the right or left lung.

lobar pneumonia, a severe infection of one or more of the five major lobes of the lungs that, if untreated, eventually results in consolidation of lung tissue. The disease is characterized by fever, chills, cough, rusty sputum, rapid shallow breathing, cyanosis, nausea, vomiting, and pleurisy. *Streptococcus pneumoniae* is the usual cause but *Klebsiella pneumoniae, Haemophilus influenzae,* and other streptococci can produce the disease. If the diagnosis is made early, appropriate antibiotic therapy is highly successful. Complications include lung abscess, atelectasis, empyema, pericarditis, and pleural effusion. Precautions against spread of the contagious disease are important. Because the fatality rate in the elderly and those with underlying systemic illness is high, prophylactic polyvalent pneumococcal vaccine is recommended for them. Compare **bronchopneumonia.**

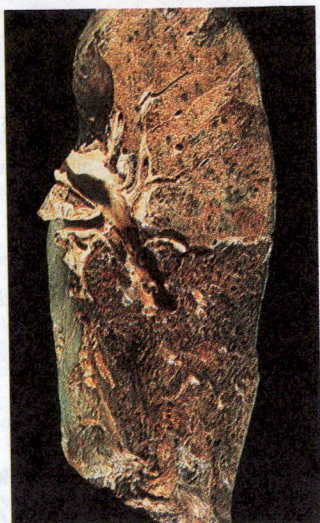

**Consolidation of lung tissue from
lobar pneumonia**
*(Fletcher, 1987/Courtesy Dr JM Sloan, Senior Lecturer/Consultant
Pathologist, Royal Victoria Hospital, Belfast)*

lobe /lōb/ [Gk, *lobos*], **1.** a roundish projection of any structure. **2.** a portion of any organ, demarcated by sulci, fissures, or connective tissue, as the lobes of the brain, liver, and lungs. **—lobar, lobular,** *adj.*

lobe-, -lobe, a combining form meaning a 'rounded prominence', a lobe: *lobotany gonilobe, multilobe.*

lobectomy /lōbek′təmē/ [Gk, *lobos + ektome,* excision], a type of chest surgery in which a lobe of a lung is excised, performed to remove a malignant tumor and to treat uncontrolled bronchiectasis, trauma with hemorrhage, or intractable tuberculosis. Any respiratory infection is cleared before surgery. Administration of antibiotics is begun. General anesthesia is administered via an endotracheal tube. The chest cavity is entered through a long back-to-front incision, and the diseased lobe is removed. A large-caliber tube remains in the wound and is connected to a water-sealed drainage system. Oxygen is given during the first 24 hours after surgery. The vital signs are closely monitored, coughing and deep breathing are encouraged hourly, blood transfusion may be given, and IV fluids are continued. Care is taken that the chest tube remain open and that the drainage system be sealed and functional. The chest tube is removed 2 to 3 days after surgery. Some compensatory emphysema is expected as the remaining lung tissue overexpands to fill the new space. **—lobectomize,** *v.*

lobe of ear [Gk, *lobos,* lobe; AS, *eare*], the lower portion of the auricle that contains no cartilage.

lobotomy /lōbot′əmē/ [Gk, *lobos + temnein,* to cut], a neurosurgical procedure in which the nerve fibers in the bundle of white matter in the frontal lobe of the brain are severed to interrupt the transmission of various affective responses. Severe intractable depression and pain are among the indications for the operation. It is seldom performed, because it has many unpredictable and undesirable effects, including personality change, aggression, socially unacceptable behavior, incontinence, apathy, and lack of consider-

ation for others. Because lobotomy is simple to perform, it was overused in the treatment of mental patients in the past. A cannula is passed through the bony orbit of the eye, and a wire loop is inserted through the cannula to the cingulum. The nerve fibers are severed with the wire loop. Also called **leukotomy.**

lobster claw deformity. See **bidactyly.**

-lobular. See **lobe.**

lobular carcinoma /lob′yələr/ [Gk, *lobos + karkinos,* crab, *oma,* tumor], a neoplasm that often forms a diffuse mass and accounts for a small percentage of breast tumors.

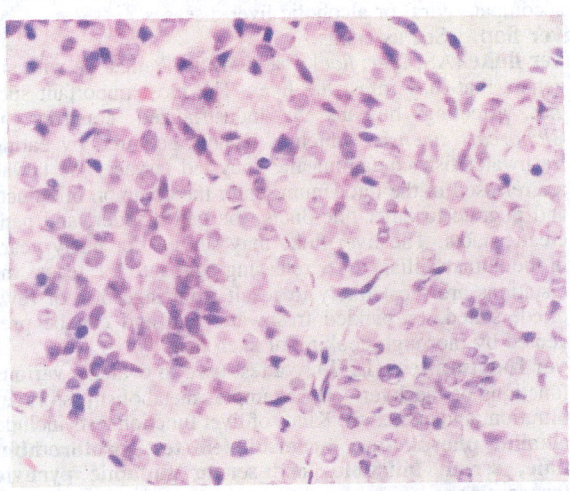

Lobular carcinoma *(Skarin, 1991)*

lobule /lob′yо̄оl/, a small lobe, such as the soft, lower, pendulous part of the external ear. **—lobular,** *adj.*

loc-, a prefix meaning 'from a place': *locomotor, locum, locus.*

L.O.C., abbreviation for **level of consciousness.**

local [L *locus* place], **1.** of or pertaining to a small circumscribed area of the body. **2.** of or pertaining to a treatment or drug applied locally. **3.** *informal.* a local anesthetic.

local adaptation syndrome (LAS), the localized response of a tissue, organ, or system that occurs as a reaction to stress. See also **general adaptation syndrome.**

local anaphylaxis [L, *locus,* place; Gk, *ana, phylaxis*], a condition in which injections of an antigen result in local swellings and localized necrosis of the skin and subcutaneous tissues.

local anesthesia, the direct administration of an anesthetic agent to tissues to induce the absence of sensation in a small area of the body. Brief surgical or dental procedures are the most common indications for local anesthesia. The anesthetic may be applied topically to the surface of the skin or membrane or injected subcutaneously through an intradermal weal. The principal drawbacks to the use of local anesthesia are the incidence of allergic reactions to certain agents, and the occasional difficulty encountered in achieving adequate anesthesia. The advantages include low cost, ease of administration, low toxicity, and safety. A conscious patient can cooperate and does not require respiratory support or intubation. To avoid general anesthesia, major surgical procedures are occasionally performed under local anesthesia. The tissues are anesthetized layer by layer, as the surgeon approaches the deeper structures of the body. Regional anesthesia has largely replaced this procedure. In all cases, the recommended dosage of any agent is the smallest possible to achieve the desired effect, because toxicity is directly related to the total amount of drug given rather than to the initial amount or the concentration of the agent used. Each anesthetic agent also carries a recommended maximum allowable dose that is not safely exceeded. Compare **general anesthesia, regional anesthesia, topical anesthesia.**

local anesthetic, a substance used to reduce or eliminate neural sensation, specifically pain, in a limited area of the body. Local anesthetics act by blocking transmission of nerve impulses. More than 100 drugs are available for local anesthesia; they are classified as members of the alcohol-ester or the aminoamide family. Principal representatives of the alcohol-ester group are phenols and benzyl, ethyl, and salicylic alcohol; these have generally been replaced by the less toxic esters (chloroprocaine, cocaine, procaine, tetracaine) and the amides (dibucaine, bupivacaine, lidocaine, mepivacaine, prilocaine, etidocaine). Specific preparations are available for use for topical administration, for infiltration, and for various kinds of regional administration, including field block, regional nerve block, epidural nerve block, and spinal nerve block. Any substance sufficiently potent to induce local anesthesia has potential for causing adverse side effects, ranging from easily reversible dermatitis to lethal anaphylaxis or simultaneous respiratory and cardiac arrest. Among the factors that are involved in an adverse reaction to a local anesthetic are hypersensitivity to the drug, the vascularity of the injection site, the speed with which the drug is given, the rapidity of action of the drug, and the presence of epinephrine in the solution. Serious adverse results have occurred related to the epinephrine used with a local anesthetic. Some people who are sensitive to local anesthetics of the amide group, which are metabolized in the liver, can tolerate local anesthetics of the ester group, which are metabolized in the plasma. Vasopressors should also be at hand in case of hypotension or other forms of circulatory depression. A patient who has a severe adverse reaction to a particular local anesthetic is advised to avoid this class of drug in the future.

local area network (LAN), a system of linking together computers and other electronic office equipment within an office or building.

local cerebral blood flow (LCBF), (in positron emission tomography) the parametric image of blood flow through the brain. It is expressed in units of milliliters of blood flow per minute.

local cerebral metabolic rate of glucose utilization (LCMRG), (in positron emission tomography) a parametric image of the brain expressed in units of milligrams of glucose utilization per minute per 100 g of brain tissue.

local control, the arrest of cancer growth at the site of origin.

local hypothermia, the heating of a local area of tissue to therapeutic temperatures.

local infection [L, *locus*, place + *inficere*, to stain], an infection involving bacteria that invade the body at a specific point and remain there, multiplying, until eliminated.

localization /lō′kəlīzā′shən/ [L, *locus*, place], **1.** the designation of a particular site for a lesion or organ function. **2.** the determination of the site of a biological function.

3. the assignment of a position to an object detected by radiography.

localization audiometry. See **audiometry.**

localization film [L, *locus*, place; Gk, *izein*, to cause; AS, *filmen*, membrane], (in radiotherapy) a diagnostic film taken to confirm a treatment effect or to view the position of an intracavitary or interstitial implant, especially for the purpose of computing the dose delivered.

localized scleroderma. See **morphea.**

localizer image, (in computed tomography) an image used to localize a specific body part.

localizing symptom, local symptom. See **symptom.**

local lesion [L, *locus*, place; *laesio*, hurting], a lesion of the central nervous system characterized by distinctive local symptoms.

local reaction [L, *locus*, place + *re, agere*, to act], a reaction to treatment that occurs at the site where it was administered.

location [L, *locus*, place, *atus*, process], a specific place in the memory of a computer where a unit of information is stored.

lochia /lō′kē·ə/ [Gk, *lochos*, childbirth], the discharge that flows from the vagina after childbirth. During the first 3 or 4 days post partum, the lochia is red (**lochia rubra**) and is made up of blood, endometrial decidua, and fetal lanugo, vernix, and sometimes meconium, small shreds of placental tissue and membranes. After the third day the amount of blood diminishes, the placental site exudes serous material and lymph, and the lochia becomes darker and thinner (**lochia fusca**), and then serous (**lochia serosa**) as evacuation of particulate material is completed. During the second week white blood cells and bacteria appear in large numbers along with fatty, mucinous decidual material, causing the lochia to appear yellow (**lochia flava** or **lochia purulenta**). During the third week and thereafter, as endometrial epithelialization progresses, the amount of lochia decreases markedly and takes on a seromucinous consistency and a gray-white color (**lochia alba**). Cessation of the flow of lochia at about 6 weeks is usual. –**lochial,** *adj.*

loci. See **locus.**

locked-in syndrome [ME, *loc*; Gk, *syn*, together, *dromos*, course], a paralytic condition in which a person may be conscious and alert but unable to communicate except by eye movements or blinking. Bilateral destruction of the medulla oblongata or pons has rendered the individual unable to speak or move any of the limbs.

locked knee [AS, *loc + cneow*], a condition in which the knee cannot be fully extended, often caused by longitudinal splitting of the medial meniscus. Also called **trick knee.**

locked twins. See **interlocked twins.**

lock forceps. See **point forceps.**

locking point [AS, *loc*, lock; L, *punctum*, puncture], a point on the body at which light pressure can be applied to help a weak or debilitated patient maintain a desired posture or position. A basic locking point is the body's center of gravity, at the level of the second sacral vertebra, where mild pressure can assist a patient in standing or walking erect.

lockjaw, *informal.* See **tetanus.**

locomotion [L, *locus*, place; *motio*, movement], movement or the ability to move from one place or position to another.

locomotor [L, *locus; motio*], pertaining to locomotion.

locomotor ataxia. See **tabes dorsalis.**

loculate /lok'yo͞olāt/ [L, *loculus*, little place], divided into small spaces or cavities.

loculus /lok'yo͞oləs/ [L, little place], a small chamber, pocket, or cavity, such as the interior of a polyp.

locum tenens /lō'kəm ten'ənz/ [L, *locus*, place; *tenere*, to hold], a temporary substitute for a physician who is away from the practice.

locus, *pl.* **loci** /lō'sī, lō'kē/ [L, place], a specific place or position, such as the locus of a particular gene on a chromosome.

locus ceruleus [L, *locus*, place; *ceruleus*, heaven], a deeply pigmented group of several thousand neurons in the floor of the fourth ventricle. It is part of a major norepinephrine route of the central nervous system.

locus of control [L, *locus*, place; Fr, *contrôle*], a center of responsibility for one's behavior. Individuals with an **internal locus of control** believe they can control events related to their life while those with an **external locus of control** tend to believe that real power resides in forces outside themselves and determines their life.

locus of infection, a site in the body where an infection originates.

Loestrin, a trademark for an oral contraceptive containing an estrogen (ethinyl estradiol) and a progestin (norethindrone acetate).

Lofenalac, a trademark for a commercial milk-substitute formula that is low in phenylalanine and used for infants with phenylketonuria. It is made from hydrolyzed casein and is supplemented with tyrosine and fortified with added fat, carbohydrate, minerals, and vitamins to balance the formula. A common problem with the formula is diarrhea, which may appear after the first few feedings but generally disappears in a few days.

Löffler's syndrome /lef'lərz/ [Wilhelm Löffler, Swiss physician, b. 1887], a benign, idiopathic disorder marked by episodes of pulmonary eosinophilia, transient opacities in the lungs, anorexia, breathlessness, fever, and weight loss. Recovery is spontaneous and prompt. See also **P.I.E.**

log-, logo-, -log, -logue, a combining form meaning 'word, speech, thought': *logagnosia, logorrhea, dialog, dialogue*.

logad-, a combining form meaning 'of or pertaining to the whites of the eyes': *logadectomy, logaditis, logadoblennorrhea*.

-logia. See **-logy.**

logo-. See **log-.**

logotherapy /log'ōther'əpē/ [Gk, *logos*, word, *therapeia*, treatment], a treatment modality based on the application of humanistic and existential psychology to assist a patient in finding meaning and purpose in life and unique life experiences.

log roll [ME, *logge*; L, *roto*, turn around], a maneuver used to turn a reclining patient from one side to the other or completely over without flexing the spinal column. The arms of the patient are folded across the chest and the legs extended. A draw sheet under the patient is manipulated by attending nursing personnel to facilitate the procedure.

-logue See **-log.**

-logy, -logia, a suffix meaning 'a science or study of': *mammalogy, metabology, neonatology*.

loiasis /lō·ī'əsis/, a form of filariasis caused by the worm *Loa loa*, which may migrate for 10 to 15 years in subcutaneous tissue, producing localized inflammation known as Calabar swellings. Occasionally, the migrating worms may be visible beneath the conjunctiva. The disease is acquired through the bite of an infected African deer fly. Treatment with diethylcarbamazine usually results in cure and may also be successful as prophylaxis. See also **filariasis, onchocerciasis.**

loin [ME, *loyn*, flank], a part of the body on each side of the spinal column between the false ribs and the hip bones.

Lomotil, a trademark for an antidiarrheal fixed-combination drug containing an antiperistaltic (diphenoxylate hydrochloride) and an anticholinergic (atropine sulfate).

lomustine /lōmus'tēn/, an antineoplastic alkylating agent.
- INDICATIONS: It is prescribed in the treatment of a variety of malignant neoplastic diseases.
- CONTRAINDICATION: Known hypersensitivity to this drug prohibits its use.
- ADVERSE EFFECTS: Among the more serious adverse reactions are bone marrow depression, nausea, and vomiting.

Lonalac, a trademark for a low-sodium, nutritional supplement.

long-acting drug [AS, *lang;* L, *agere*, to do; Fr, *drogue*, drug], a pharmacologic agent with a prolonged effect because of a formulation resulting in the slow release of the active principle or the continued absorption of small amounts of the dosage of the drug over an extended period.

long-acting insulin, a preparation of the antidiabetic principle of beef pancreas or pork pancreas modified by an interaction with zinc under specific chemical conditions and supplied as a suspension with a prolonged action. An injection of the preparation takes effect within 8 hours, reaches a peak of action in 16 to 24 hours, and has a duration of action of more than 36 hours. Also called **slow-acting insulin, ultralente insulin.** See also **insulin.** Compare **intermediate-acting insulin, short-acting insulin.**

long-acting thyroid stimulator (LATS), an immunoglobulin, probably an autoantibody, that exerts a prolonged stimulatory effect on the thyroid gland, causing rapid growth of the gland and excess activity of thyroid function resulting in hyperthyroidism. It is found circulating in the blood of 50% of people with Graves' disease.

long-arm cast [As, *lang + earm*, arm; ONorse, *kasta*], an orthopedic cast applied to immobilize upper extremities from the hand to the upper arm. It is used in the treatment of fractures of the forearm and the elbow, fractures of the humerus, for postoperative positioning of the distal arm, the elbow, or the upper arm, and for correction or for maintenance of correction of deformities of the distal arm, the wrist, or the elbow. Compare **short-arm cast.**

long bones, the bones that contribute to the height or length of an extremity, particularly the bones of the legs and arms.

longevity /lonjev'itē/ [L, *longus*, long; *aveum*, age], the number of years an average person of a particular age can expect to continue living. It is determined by statistical tables based on mortality rates of various population groups.

longitudinal /lon'jəto͞o'dənəl/ [L, *longitudo*, length], **1.** a measurement in the direction of the long axis of an object, body, or organ, such as the longitudinal arch of the foot. **2.** a scientific study that is conducted over a long period of time, such as the Framingham (Massachusetts) Study of heart disease.

longitudinal diffusion, the diffusion of solute molecules in the direction of flow of the mobile phase.

longitudinal dissociation, (in cardiology) the insulation of parallel pathways of impulses from each other, usually in the AV junction.

longitudinal fissure [L, *longitudo*, length; *fissura*, cleft], the largest and deepest groove between the medial surfaces of the cerebral hemispheres.

longitudinal presentation [L, *longitudo*, length + *praesentare*, to show], the normal presentation of a fetus, with the long axis of the infant body parallel to that of the mother.

longitudinal sound waves, pressure waves formed by the oscillation of particles or molecules parallel to the axis of wave propagation. The compression and expansion of such longitudinal waves at high frequencies is the principle on which ultrasonography is based.

long-leg cast, an orthopedic cast applied to immobilize the leg from the toes to the upper thigh. It is used in treating fractures and dislocations of the knee, for postoperative positioning and immobilization of the knee, distal leg, and ankle, and for correction or for maintenance of correction of the foot, distal leg, and knee. Compare **short-leg cast.**

long-leg cast with walker, an orthopedic cast applied to immobilize the lower extremities from the toes to the upper thigh in treating certain fractures of the leg. This type of cast is the same as the long-leg cast but incorporates a rubber walker, allowing the patient to walk while the leg is encased in the cast and when weight-bearing ambulation is allowed.

long-term care (LTC), the provision of medical, social, and personal care services on a recurring or continuing basis to persons with chronic physical or mental disorders. The care may be provided in environments ranging from institutions to private homes. Long-term care services usually include symptomatic treatment, maintenance, and rehabilitation for patients of all age groups.

long-term memory, the ability to recall sensations, events, ideas, and other information for long periods of time without apparent effort.

long thoracic nerve, one of a pair of supraclavicular branches from the roots of the brachial plexus. It arises by three roots, from the fifth, the sixth, and the seventh cervical nerves. Its fibers from the fifth and the sixth cervical nerves join just after they pierce the scalenus medius and are united with its fibers from the seventh cervical nerve at the level of the first rib. Compare **phrenic nerve.**

long tract signs, neurologic signs, such as clonus, muscle spasticity, or bladder involvement, that usually indicate a lesion in the middle or upper portions of the spinal cord or in the brain.

Loniten, a trademark for an antihypertensive (minoxidil).

loop [ME, *loupe*], **1.** a set of instructions in a computer program that causes certain commands to be executed repeatedly if specified criteria are met. **2.** *informal.* intrauterine device.

loop colostomy [ME, *loupe*; Gk, *kolon*, colon, *stoma*, mouth], a type of temporary colostomy performed as part of the surgical repair of some colon diseases. To perform the procedure, an intact segment of colon anterior to the repair is brought through an abdominal incision and sutured onto the abdomen. A loop is formed and held in position by placing a piece of glass rod between the segment and the abdomen. The two ends of the rod are connected with a piece of rubber tubing to prevent the rod from slipping. The stomal opening is made on the exterior surface of the segment. The colostomy is reversed after resolution of the orig-

inal pathology. See also **colostomy irrigation, Hirschsprung's disease.**

loop diuretic. See **diuretic.**

loop of Henle /hen′lē/ [ME, *loupe*; Friedrich G. J. Henle, German anatomist, b. 1809], the U-shaped portion of a renal tubule, consisting of a thin descending limb and a thick ascending limb.

loose association. See **loosening.**

loose fibrous tissue [ME, *lous*, not fastened], a constrictive, pliable fibrous connective tissue consisting of interwoven elastic and collagenous fibers, interspersed with fluid-filled areolae. It is found in adipose tissue, areolar tissue, reticular tissue, and fibroelastic tissue. Compare **dense fibrous tissue.**

loosening [ME, *lous*], (in psychiatry) a disturbance of thinking in which the association of ideas and thought patterns become so vague, diffuse, and unfocused as to lack any logical sequences or relationship to any preceding concepts or themes. When severe, speech may be incoherent. Also called **loose association.**

loose-pack joint position, a point in the range of motion at which articulating surfaces are the least congruent and the supporting structures are the most lax.

Lo/Ovral, a trademark for an oral contraceptive containing an estrogen (ethinyl estradiol) and a progestin (norgestrel).

LOP, abbreviation for *left occipitoposterior fetal position.*

loperamide hydrochloride /lōper′əmīd/, an antiperistaltic.

■ INDICATION: It is prescribed in the treatment of diarrhea.

■ CONTRAINDICATIONS: Known hypersensitivity to this drug prohibits its use. It is not given to patients in whom constipation must be avoided.

■ ADVERSE EFFECTS: Among the most serious reactions are abdominal pain, constipation, nausea, and vomiting.

loph-, a combining form meaning 'of or pertaining to a ridge': *lophius, lophodont, lophotrichous.*

Lopid, a trademark for a lipid regulating agent (gemfibrozil).

Lopressor, a trademark for a beta-adrenergic receptor blocking agent (metoprolol tartrate).

Loprox, a trademark for an antifungal (ciclopirox olamine).

lorazepam /lôrā′zəpam/, a benzodiazepine tranquilizer.

■ INDICATIONS: It is prescribed as a minor tranquilizer in the treatment of anxiety, nervous tension, and insomnia.

■ CONTRAINDICATIONS: Acute glaucoma, psychosis, or known hypersensitivity to this drug or to any benzodiazepine prohibits its use.

■ ADVERSE EFFECTS: Among the more serious adverse reactions are drowsiness and fatigue. Withdrawal symptoms may occur on discontinuation of the drug, especially after prolonged use or high dosage.

lordoscoliosis /lôr′dōskō′lē·ō′sis/ [Gk, *lordos*, bent; *skoliosis*, curvature], a combination of lordosis and scoliosis.

lordosis /lôrdō′sis/ [Gk, *lordos*, bent forward, *osis*, condition], **1.** the normal curvature of the lumbar and cervical spine, seen as an anterior concavity if the person is observed from the side. **2.** an abnormal, increased degree of curvature of any part of the back.

lordotic pelvis /lôrdot′ik/ [Gk, *lordos*, convex in front; L, *pelvis*, basin], a pelvis that is inadequate for childbirth because the spinal column bends forward in the lumbar region.

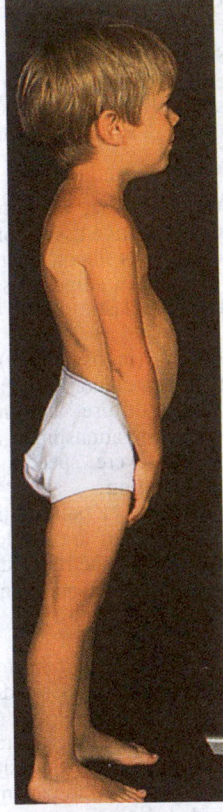

Lordosis *(Zitelli, 1992)*

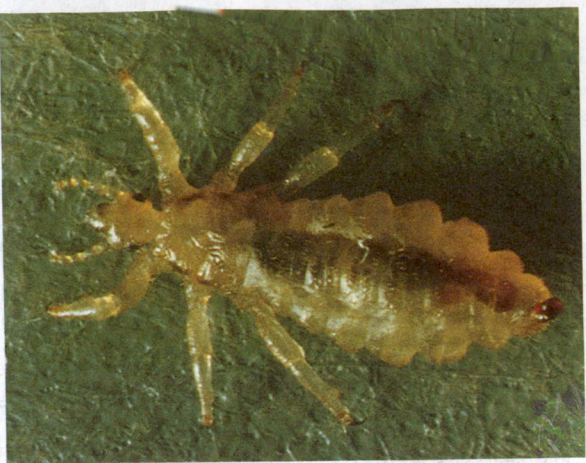

Human body louse
(Habif, 1990/Courtesy Ken Gray, Oregon State University Extension Services)

Lorelco, a trademark for an anticholesteremic (probucol).
LOS, abbreviation for *length of stay*.
loss of consortium [ME, *lossen*, to lose; L, *consortionis*, companionship], (in law) a claim for damages sought in recompense for the loss of conjugal relations, including society, affection, and assistance, and impairment or loss of sexual relations. Loss of consortium may be charged against a person whose negligence or malfeasance caused injury to the spouse or against a person who caused a marriage to break up.
LOT, abbreviation for *left occipitotransverse fetal position*.
lotion [L, *lotio*, a washing], a liquid preparation applied externally to protect the skin or to treat a dermatologic disorder.
Lotrimin, a trademark for an antifungal (clotrimazole).
Lotusate, a trademark for a barbiturate (talbutal).
Lou Gehrig's disease. See **amyotrophic lateral sclerosis.**
Louis-Bar syndrome. See **ataxia-telangiectasia.**
loupe /lo͞op/ [Fr, magnifying glass], a magnifying lens mounted in a frame worn on the head, as used to examine the eyes.
louse See **lice.**
louse bite, a minute puncture wound produced by a louse that may transmit typhus, trench fever, and relapsing fever. Secondary infection may result from scratching the affected area. Head and body lice are the most common and are fre-

quently found among schoolchildren. Washing and bathing, application of an approved insecticide, and the washing or cleaning of clothes and bed linens are recommended procedures for treatment and prophylaxis against spread of the infestation. See also **pediculosis.**
louse-borne typhus. See **epidemic typhus.**
low back pain (lbp) [ME, *low;* AS, *baec;* L, *poena,* penalty], local or referred pain at the base of the spine caused by a sprain, strain, osteoarthritis, ankylosing spondylitis, a neoplasm, or a prolapsed intervertebral disk. Low back pain is a common complaint and is often associated with poor posture, obesity, sagging abdominal muscles, or sitting for prolonged periods of time.
■ OBSERVATIONS: Pain may be localized and static; it may be accompanied by muscle weakness or spasms; or it may radiate down the back of one or both legs, as in sciatica. It may be initiated or increased by coughing, sneezing, rising from a seated position, lifting, stretching, bending, or turning. To guard against the pain, the person may decrease the range of motion of the spine. If an intervertebral disk is prolapsed, deep pressure over the interspace generally causes pain, and flexion of the hip elicits sciatic pain when the knee is extended but not when the knee is flexed (Lase[gv]gue's sign).
■ INTERVENTIONS: The patient is placed in a semi-Fowler's position on a firm mattress with the knees flexed and supported. Analgesics, muscle relaxants, and tranquilizers may be administered, and dry or moist heat is applied. Diagnostic x-ray examinations; pelvic traction and physiotherapy, consisting of hydrotherapy, diathermy, or the application of hot paraffin; and a myelogram may be performed if a herniated disk is suspected. When the acute pain subsides, the patient may increase activity as tolerated, fatigue is avoided, and a corset or back brace may be ordered. The patient is instructed to use a straight-backed chair, not to sit with legs crossed or extended on a footstool, and to sleep on the side or back with knees flexed and a small pillow under the head. Before discharge the patient is advised to maintain a normal weight, to follow the ordered exercise program, to wear flatheeled shoes, and to avoid constipation by using natural laxatives, if required.

■ NURSING CONSIDERATIONS: The nurse encourages the patient to follow the recommended regimen. Correct body mechanics, adequate and appropriate exercise, and the elimination of excess weight are emphasized.

low birth weight (LBW) infant, an infant whose weight at birth is less than 2500 g, regardless of gestational age. These babies are at risk for the development of hypoxia during labor, hypoglycemia, and respiratory distress syndrome (RDS) after birth, and growth retardation in childhood, especially if the condition is the result of prolonged placental insufficiency, maternal malnutrition, or drug addiction. Many low birth weight infants have no problems and develop normally, their smallness being genetic or idiopathic, or the problem that caused their slowed growth being mild or brief.

low blood, *informal.* anemia.

low-calcium diet, a diet that restricts the use of calcium and that eliminates most of the dairy foods, all breads made with milk or dry skimmed milk, and deep-green leafy vegetables. It is prescribed for patients who form renal calculi. Meats, including beef, lamb, pork, veal, and poultry, fish, vegetables, legumes, and fruits are recommended.

low-caloric diet, a diet that is prescribed to limit the intake of calories, usually to cause a reduction in body weight. Such diets may be designated as 800 calorie, 1000 calorie, or other specific numbers of calories. Exchange lists may be used to allow the patient to select preferred foods from groups of foods categorized as carbohydrate, protein, and fat.

low cervical cesarean section, a method for surgically delivering a baby through a transverse incision in the thin supracervical portion of the lower uterine segment, behind the bladder and the bladder flap. This incision bleeds less during surgery and heals with a stronger scar than the higher vertical scar of the classic cesarean section. Compare **extraperitoneal cesarean section.** See also **cesarean section.**

low-cholesterol diet, a diet that restricts foods containing animal fats and saturated fatty acids, such as egg yolk, cream, butter, milk, muscle and organ meats, and shellfish, and concentrates on poultry, fish, vegetables, fruits, cottage cheese, and polyunsaturated fats. The diet is indicated for persons with high serum cholesterol levels, cardiovascular disorders, obesity, hyperlipidemia, hypercholesterolemia, or hyperlipoproteinemia. Also called **low-saturated-fat diet.**

low-density lipoprotein (LDL), a plasma protein containing relatively more cholesterol and triglycerides than protein. It is derived in part, if not completely, from the intravascular breakdown of the very low-density lipoproteins and delivers lipids to the body tissues. The high cholesterol content may account for its greater atherogenic potential as compared with the very low-density lipoproteins and chylomicrons.

lower extremity suspension [ME, *low;* L, *extremitas; suspendere,* to hang], an orthopedic procedure used in the treatment of bone fractures and in the correction of orthopedic abnormalities of the lower limbs. The procedure uses traction equipment, including metal frames, ropes, and pulleys, to relieve the weight of the lower limb involved rather than to exert traction pull. Lower extremity suspension may be either unilateral or bilateral and is used in the postoperative, posttraumatic, or postreduction control of edema. Compare **balanced suspension, hyperextension suspension, upper extremity suspension.**

lower level discriminator (LLD), (in nuclear medicine) a radiation energy-sensitive device used to discriminate against all radionuclide pulses whose heights are below the accepted level.

lower motor neuron paralysis, an injury to or lesion that damages the cell bodies or axons, or both, of the lower motor neurons, which are located in the anterior horn cells of the spinal cord and the spinal and peripheral nerves. If complete transection of the spinal cord occurs, voluntary muscle control is totally lost. In partial transection, function is altered in varying degrees, depending on the areas innervated by the nerves involved. In lower motor neuron paralysis the reflex arcs are permanently damaged, causing decreased muscle tone and flaccidity, diminished or absent reflexes, absence of pathologic reflexes, local twitching of muscle groups, and progressive atrophy of the atonic muscles. Compare **upper motor neuron paralysis.**

lower respiratory infection. See **respiratory tract infection.**

lower respiratory tract, one of the two divisions of the respiratory system. The lower respiratory tract includes the left and the right bronchi and the alveoli where the exchange of oxygen and carbon dioxide occurs during the respiratory cycle. The bronchi divide into smaller bronchioles in the lungs, the bronchioles into alveolar ducts, the ducts into alveolar sacs, and the sacs into alveoli. The alveolar sacs and the alveoli present a total lung surface of about 850 square feet for the exchange of oxygen and carbon dioxide, which occurs between the most internal alveolar surface and the tiny capillaries surrounding the external alveolar wall. The lower respiratory tract is a continuation of the upper respiratory tract and is a common site of infections, obstructive conditions, and neoplastic disease. Compare **upper respiratory tract.** See also **lung.**

low-fat diet [ME, *low;* AS, *faett;* Gk, *diaita,* life-style], a diet containing limited amounts of fat and consisting chiefly of easily digestible foods of high carbohydrate content. It includes all vegetables, lean meats, fish, fowl, pasta, cereals, and whole wheat or enriched bread. Egg yolk and fatty meats are restricted. Cream, fried foods, foods prepared in oil, gravy, cheese, peanut butter, nuts, and olives are among the foods omitted. The diet may be indicated in gallbladder disease and malabsorption syndromes and hyperlipidemia.

low-fat milk, milk containing 1% to 2% fat, making it an intermediate in fat content between whole and skimmed milk.

low-fiber diet. See **low-residue diet.**

low-flow oxygen delivery system, respiratory care equipment that does not supply all the inspired gases. The patient inhales some room air along with the oxygen being delivered. As the patient's ventilatory pattern changes, different amounts of air are mixed with the constant flow of oxygen and thus the inspired oxygen concentration varies. Also called **variable-performance oxygen delivery system.**

low forceps [ME, *low;* L, *forceps,* pair of tongs], an obstetric operation in which forceps are used to deliver a baby whose head is on the pelvic floor. The procedure is performed most often as an elective procedure to shorten normal labor and to control delivery, usually in conjunction with anesthesia and episiotomy. It is commonly required for the delivery of mothers whose expulsive powers have been weakened by analgesia, anesthesia, or fatigue. Also called **outlet forceps, prophylactic forceps.** Compare **high for-**

ceps, mid forceps, natural childbirth, spontaneous delivery. See also **forceps delivery, obstetric forceps.**

low-grade fever, a temperature that is above 98.6° F but lower than 100.4° F for 24 hours.

low-grade infection [ME, *lah*; L, *gradus*, degree + *inficere*, to stain], a subacute or chronic infection with mild fever and no pus production.

low-level language, a computer language employing mathematic logic but requiring precise manipulation of binary numbers. Compare **high-level language.**

Lown-Ganong-Levine syndrome (LGL) /loun'-gənong'ləvēn'/ [Bernard Lown, American physician, b. 1921; William F. Ganong, American physiologist, b. 1924; S. A. Levine, American physician, b. 1891], a disorder of the atrioventricular (AV) conduction system, marked by ventricular preexcitation. Part or all of the AV nodal connection is bypassed by an abnormal AV connection from the atrial muscle to the bundle of His. The condition may be discovered by routine ECG or may be seen in association with paroxysmal atrial arrhythmias, supraventricular tachycardia, atrial flutter, and fibrillation. Treatments include the use of antiarrhythmic drugs, such as quinidine sulfate, procainamide, and propranolol, surgical interruption of the abnormal AV pathway, and implantation of a pacemaker. Compare **Wolff-Parkinson-White syndrome.**

low-power field, the low magnification field of vision under a light microscope.

low-protein diet [ME, *lah*, low; Gk, *proteios*, first rank; *diaita*, lifestyle], a diet proportionally low in protein, usually designed for persons who must restrict their intake of protein because of a metabolic abnormality associated with kidney failure or a liver disease.

low-residue diet, a diet that will leave a minimal residue in the lower intestinal tract after digestion and absorption. It consists of tender meats, poultry, fish, eggs, white bread, pasta, simple desserts, clear soups, tea, and coffee. Omitted are highly seasoned or fried foods, all fruits and fruit juices, raw vegetables, whole grain cereals and bread, nuts, jams, and, usually, milk. The diet is prescribed in cases of diverticulitis, GI irritability or inflammation, and before and after GI surgery. Because it is lacking in calcium, iron, and vitamins, it should be used only for a limited period of time or with nutrient supplementation. Also called **low-fiber diet.**

low-salt diet. See **low-sodium diet.**

low-saturated-fat diet. See **low-cholesterol diet.**

low-sodium diet, a diet that restricts the use of sodium chloride plus other compounds containing sodium, such as baking powder or soda, monosodium glutamate, sodium citrate, sodium propionate, and sodium sulfate. It is indicated in hypertension, edematous states (especially when associated with cardiovascular disease), renal or liver disease, and therapy with corticosteroids. The degree of sodium restriction depends on the severity of the condition. Foods included in the diet are eggs, skimmed milk, beef, poultry, lamb, pork, veal, fish, potatoes, green beans, broccoli, asparagus, peas, salad ingredients, and fresh fruits. Many flavoring extracts, spices, and herbs can be used to add taste to the diet. Foods to be avoided include fresh or canned shellfish, ham, bacon, frankfurters, luncheon meats, sausage, cheese, salted butter or margarine, any breads or cereals made with salt, beets, carrots, celery, sauerkraut, spinach, and most canned or frozen foods—unless prepared without sodium. Also to be avoided are many drugs, such as laxatives, sedatives, and alkalizers, which contain sodium, and drinking water from a source using a water softener, because this appliance adds sodium to the water. Also called **low-salt diet, salt-free diet, sodium-restricted diet.**

loxapine /lok'səpēn/, a tranquilizer.

■ INDICATION: It is prescribed in the treatment of schizophrenia.

■ CONTRAINDICATIONS: Parkinson's disease, concurrent administration of central nervous system depressants, liver or kidney dysfunction, severe hypotension, or known hypersensitivity to this drug prohibits its use.

■ ADVERSE EFFECTS: Among the more serious adverse effects are hypotension, liver toxicity, a variety of extrapyramidal reactions, and hypersensitivity reactions.

Loxitane, a trademark for a tranquilizer (loxapine succinate).

loxo-, a combining form meaning 'oblique, slanting': *loxophthalmus, loxotic, loxotomy.*

lozenge. See **troche.**

lpm, abbreviation for *liters per minute.*

LP, abbreviation for **lumbar puncture.**

LPN, abbreviation for **licensed practical nurse.**

LPO, abbreviation for *left posterior oblique position.*

LPS Act, a California law named for sponsors of the legislation (Lanterman, Petris, and Short) that provides for the protection and treatment of persons judged to be 'gravely disabled' and, thus, unable to provide food, clothing, or shelter for themselves. The legislation was designed to safeguard the constitutional rights of persons threatened with involuntary commitment on the basis of a psychiatric diagnosis.

Lr, symbol for the element **lawrencium.**

LSD, abbreviation for *lysergic acid diethylamide.* See **lysergide.**

L/S ratio, the lecithin/sphingomyelin ratio, used in a test for fetal lung maturity.

LTB, abbreviation for **laryngotracheobronchitis.** See **croup.**

LTC, abbreviation for **long-term care.**

LTH, abbreviation for *luteotropic hormone.*

L-Trp, abbreviation for *L-tryptophan.* See **tryptophan.**

Lu, symbol for the element **lutetium.**

lubb-dupp, in auscultation, an imitation of the two basic sounds heard in the cardiac cycle. Lubb represents the first sound, and is made by closure of the mitral and tricuspid valves. It is lower in pitch and lasts slightly longer than the second sound, dupp, which is made by closure of the aortic valve.

lubricant /loo'brikənt/ [L, *lubricans*, making slippery], a fluid, ointment, or other agent capable of diminishing friction and making a surface slippery.

lubricating enema /loo'brəkā'ting/ [L, *lubricans*, making slippery; Gk, *enienai*], an enema used to lubricate the anal canal after surgery for hemorrhoids or to prevent fecal impaction. The enema solution may be made with warm olive oil.

luc-, a combining form meaning 'of or pertaining to light': *lucifugal, lucipetal, lucotherapy.*

-lucent, a suffix meaning 'light-admitting': *radiolucent, translucent.*

lucid /loo'sid/ [L, *lucidus*, clear], clear, rational, and able to be understood. See also **lucid interval.**

lucid interval, a period of relative mental clarity between periods of irrationality, especially in organic mental disorders, such as delirium and dementia.

lucidity /lōosid′itē/ [L, *lucidus,* clear], pertaining to clarity of mind, perception, or intelligibility.

lucid lethargy, a mental state characterized by a loss of will; hence, an inability to act, even though the person is conscious and intellectual function is normal. See also **lethargy.**

Ludiomil, a trademark for an antidepressant (maprotiline hydrochloride).

Ludwig's angina /lōōd′vigz/ [Wilhelm F. von Ludwig, German surgeon, b. 1790; L, *angina,* quinsy], acute streptococcal cellulitis of the floor of the mouth. It is treated with penicillin.

lue-, a combining form meaning 'of or pertaining to syphilis': *luetic, luetin, luetism.*

LUE, abbreviation for *left upper extremity.*

Luer-Lok syringe /lōō′ərlōk′/, a glass or plastic syringe for injection having a simple screw lock mechanism that securely holds the needle in place. Also called **Luer's syringe.**

lues. See **syphilis.**

-luetic, -luic, a suffix meaning 'pertaining to syphilis': *antiluetic, heredoluetic, paraluetic.*

luetic aortitis. See **syphilitic aortitis.**

Lufyllin, a trademark for a smooth muscle relaxant (dyphylline).

Lugol's solution [Jean G. A. Lugol, French physician, b. 1786; L, *solutus,* unbound], an aqueous solution of iodine (5%) and potassium iodide (10%).

-luic. See **luetic.**

Lukes-Collins classification, a system of identifying non-Hodgkin's lymphomas according to B cell, T cell, true, and unclassifiable types. B cell types include lymphocytic, plasmacytic, follicular cell lymphomas, and B cell —derived immunoblastic sarcoma. T cell types include T cell —derived immunoblastic sarcoma and convoluted cell lymphoma. True types are of histiocytic origin.

lukewarm bath [ME, *luke;* AS, *wearm, baeth*], a bath in which the temperature of the water is between 90° and 96° F.

lumbago /lumbā′gō/ [L, *lumbus,* loin], pain in the lumbar region caused by a muscle strain, rheumatoid arthritis, osteoarthritis, or a herniated intravertebral disk. Ischemic lumbago, characterized by pain in the lower back and buttocks, is caused by vascular insufficiency, as in terminal aortic occlusion. See also **low back pain.**

lumbar /lum′bər, lum′bär/ [L, *lumbus,* loin], of or pertaining to the part of the body between the thorax and the pelvis.

lumbar nerves, the five pairs of spinal nerves rising in the lumbar region. They become increasingly large the more caudal their location and pass laterally and downward under the cover of the psoas major or between its fasciculi. The first three lumbar nerves and the larger part of the fourth are connected by communicating loops and, in many individuals, communicate with the twelfth thoracic nerve, forming the lumbar plexus. The ventral primary divisions of the lumbar nerves give rise to muscular branches that supply the psoas major and the quadratus lumborum before the nerves enter the lumbar plexus. The smaller section of the fourth lumbar nerve joins the fifth lumbar nerve to form the lumbosacral trunk that comprises part of the sacral plexus. Only the first two lumbar nerves extend white rami to the sympathetic trunk. All lumbar nerves receive gray rami. The lumbar ganglia follow no fixed pattern, and massive fusions of ganglia are common. When occurring independently, the lumbar ganglia lie on the body's corresponding vertebrae or intervertebral disks caudally. The ganglion on the second lumbar vertebra is the largest, the most constant, and the most easily palpated.

lumbar node, a node in one of the seven groups of parietal lymph nodes serving the abdomen and the pelvis. The lumbar nodes are very numerous and are divided into the lateral aortic nodes, the preaortic nodes, and the retroaortic nodes. They receive the afferent vessels from many different structures, such as the kidneys, the internal reproductive organs, the lateral abdominal muscles, and certain vertebrae, and pass efferents that form lymphatic trunks. Compare **sacral node.** See also **lymph, lymphatic system, lymph node.**

lumbar plexus, a network of nerves formed by the ventral anterior primary divisions of the first three and the greater part of the fourth lumbar nerves. It is located on the inside of the posterior abdominal wall, either dorsal to the psoas major or among its fibers and ventral to the transverse processes of the lumbar vertebrae. The plexus develops from the splitting of various lumbar nerves. The first lumbar nerve splits into the cranial and the caudal branches. The cranial branch forms the iliohypogastric and the ilioinguinal nerves. The caudal branch unites with a branch from the second lumbar nerve to form the genitofemoral nerve. The rest of the second nerve and the third and the fourth nerves each split into a small ventral and a large dorsal section. The ventral portions unite to form the obturator nerve. The dorsal portions of the second and the third nerves each divide into two smaller branches to form the lateral femoral cutaneous nerve and two larger branches that join the dorsal portion of the fourth lumbar nerve to form the femoral nerve. Part of the fourth lumbar nerve joins the fifth lumbar nerve in the lumbosacral trunk. The branches of the lumbar plexus are the iliohypogastric nerve, the ilioinguinal nerve, the genitofemoral nerve, the lateral femoral cutaneous nerve, the obturator nerve, the accessory obturator nerve, and the femoral nerve. The iliohypogastric, the ilioinguinal, and the genitofemoral nerves supply the caudal part of the abdominal wall. The lateral femoral cutaneous, the obturator, the accessory obturator, and the femoral nerves supply the anterior thigh and the middle of the leg. The accessory obturator nerve is present in only 20% of individuals and comes from the third and the fourth lumbar nerves. Compare **sacral plexus.**

lumbar puncture (LP), the introduction of a hollow needle and stylet into the subarachnoid space of the lumbar portion of the spinal canal. With the use of strict aseptic technique, it is performed in various therapeutic and diagnostic procedures. Diagnostic indications include measuring of cerebrospinal fluid (CSF) pressure, obtaining CSF for laboratory analysis, evaluating the canal for the pressure of a tumor, and injecting air, oxygen, or a radiopaque substance for radiographic visualization of the structures of the nervous system of spinal canal and meninges and brain. Therapeutic indications for lumbar puncture include removing blood or pus from the subarachnoid space, injecting sera or drugs, withdrawing CSF to reduce intracranial pressure, introducing a local anesthetic to induce spinal anesthesia, and placing a small amount of the patient's blood in the subarachnoid space to form a clot to patch a rent or hole in the dura to prevent leak of CSF into the epidural space.

■ METHOD: The skin over the interspace of the third and fourth lumbar vertebrae is cleansed. A fenestrated sterile drape is placed over the back, the window over the punc-

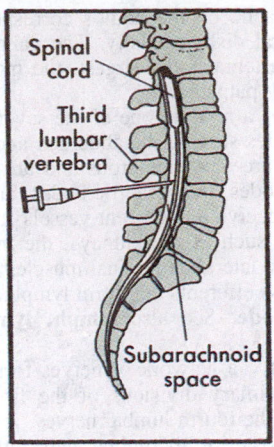

Position of needle for lumbar puncture (Beare, 1990)

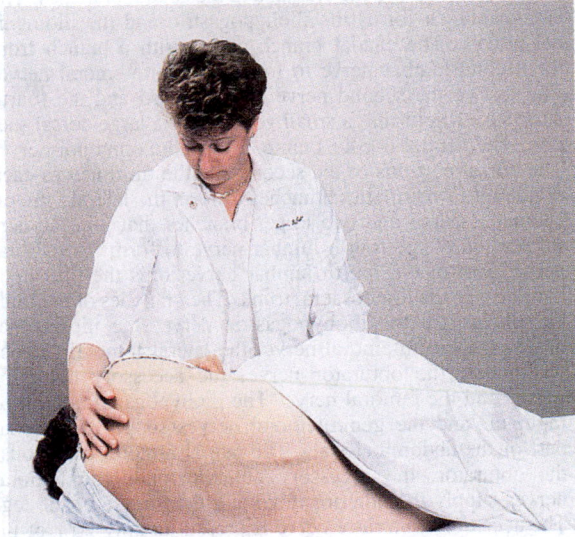

Position of patient for lumbar puncture
(Grimes, 1991)

ture site. The needle is inserted through the interspace to the subarachnoid space, and the stylet is withdrawn. If the needle is in the proper place, clear, straw-colored CSF will begin to drip out through the needle. Depending on the indication for the procedure, various techniques follow. The pressure of the CSF may be measured using a manometer attached to a catheter and stopcock, or fluid may be withdrawn, visually examined, and sent to the laboratory for chemical or bacteriologic analysis.
■ INTERVENTIONS: The nurse is often responsible for obtaining the patient's written permission for the physician to perform a lumbar puncture. The patient, if apprehensive, is given a sedative one half hour before the procedure. The techniques to be used and the treatments to be given or the information to be obtained are explained. The patient is placed in a lateral recumbent position, the back as near the edge of the bed as possible. The legs are flexed on the

thighs, the thighs are flexed on the abdomen, and the head and shoulders are bent down, curving the spine convexly to afford the greatest space between the vertebrae. If the patient is hirsute, a dry shave of the lumbar area is performed before draping the area. After the procedure, significant signs to be observed by the nurse include pain, change in mentation or alertness, leakage of CSF from the puncture site, fever, and urinary retention. The patient is usually kept flat in bed, often in a prone position, for 4 to 6 hours after the procedure.
■ OUTCOME CRITERIA: Lumbar puncture is contraindicated if the procedure will not contribute to the diagnosis or treatment of the illness, if intracranial tumor is suspected and there is evidence of greatly increased intracranial pressure, if there are signs of infection at the site of puncture, or, to avoid a second puncture, if encephalography or myelography is planned in the near future. Infection, leakage of CSF, headache, nausea, vomiting, dysuria, or signs of meningeal irritation occur in approximately 25% of patients.
lumbar region. See **lateral region.**
lumbar subarachnoid peritoneostomy, a surgical procedure for draining cerebrospinal fluid in hydrocephalus, usually in the newborn. It spares the kidney but is a somewhat less effective method than a lumbar subarachnoid ureterostomy. The procedure may be used when a temporary shunt is needed. First a lumbar laminectomy is performed, then a polyethylene tube is passed from the subarachnoid space around the flank and into the peritoneum. This procedure is performed to correct a communicating type of hydrocephalus.
lumbar subarachnoid ureterostomy, a surgical procedure for draining excess cerebrospinal fluid through the ureter to the bladder in hydrocephalus, usually in the newborn. The procedure first completes a lumbar laminectomy and a left nephrectomy, after which a polyethylene tube is passed from the lumbar subarachnoid space through the paraspinal muscles and into the free ureter. The procedure is performed to correct a communicating type of hydrocephalus.
lumbar veins, four pairs of veins that collect blood by dorsal tributaries from the loins and by abdominal tributaries from the walls of the abdomen. They receive veins from the vertebral plexus, pass ventrally around the vertebrae, dorsal to the psoas major, and end in the inferior vena cava. The left lumbar veins are longer than the right and pass dorsal to the aorta. The lumbar veins are connected by the ascending lumbar vein that runs ventral to the transverse processes of the lumbar vertebrae.
lumbar vertebra, one of the five largest segments of the movable part of the vertebral column, distinguished by the absence of a foramen in the transverse process and by vertebral bodies without facets. The body of each lumbar vertebra is flattened or slightly concave superiorly and inferiorly and is deeply constricted ventrally at the sides. The spinous process of each is thick, broad, and somewhat quadrilateral. The body of the fifth lumbar vertebra is much deeper ventrally than dorsally, and in some individuals is defective, tending to weaken the spinal column. Compare **cervical vertebra, coccygeal vertebra, sacral vertebra, thoracic vertebra.**
lumbo-, a combining form meaning 'of or pertaining to the loins': *lumbocolostomy, lumbocostal, lumbosacral.*
lumbodorsal fascia. See **fascia thoracolumbalis.**
lumbosacral /lum′bōsā′krəl/ [L, *lumbus,* loin; *sacrum,* sacred], pertaining to the lumbar vertebrae and the sacrum.
lumbosacral plexus [L, *lumbus,* loin, *sacrum,* sacred;

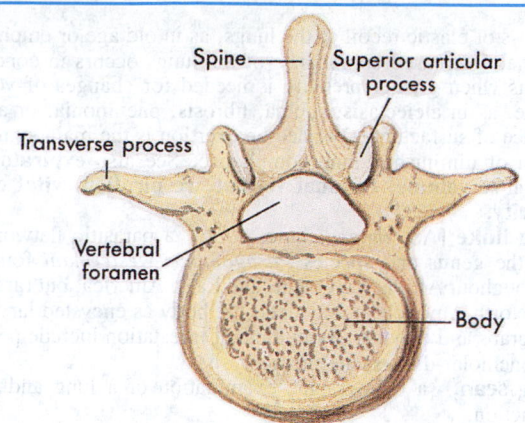

Superior view of a lumbar vertebra
(Thibodeau, 1993/Ernest W Beck)

Labels: Spine, Superior articular process, Transverse process, Vertebral foramen, Body

plexus, braided], the combination of all the ventral anterior primary divisions of the lumbar, the sacral, and the coccygeal nerves. The lumbar and the sacral plexuses supply the lower limb. The sacral nerves also supply the perineum through the pudendal plexus and the coccygeal area through the coccygeal plexus. See also **lumbar plexus, sacral plexus.**

lumbrical, See **vermiform.**

lumbrical plus deformity /lum′brikəl/, a complication of rheumatoid arthritis in which the lumbricals (muscles in the hands and feet) become contracted, with a resultant action of extension rather than flexion. A main effect of the dysfunction is metacarpophalangeal joint flexion and interphalangeal joint extension.

lumen /loo′mən/, *pl.* ***lumina, lumens*** [L, light], **1.** a cavity or the channel within any organ or structure of the body. **2.** a unit of luminous flux that equals the flux emitted in a unit solid angle by a point source of one candle intensity. **–lumenal, luminal,** *adj.*

lumin-, a combining form meaning 'of or pertaining to light': *luminescence, luminiferous, luminophore.*

luminescence /loo′mines′əns/ [L, *lumen,* light, *escens,* beginning], **1.** the emission of light by a material after excitation by some stimulus. **2.** (in radiology) the emission of light by intensifying screen phosphors after x-ray interaction. See also **thermoluminescent dosimetry.**

luminiferous /loo′minif′ərəs/ [L, *lumen,* light; *ferre,* to bear], pertaining to a medium that will transmit light.

lumpectomy /lumpek′təmē/ [ME, *lump,* mass; *ektome,* excision], surgical excision of a tumor without removal of large amounts of surrounding tissue or adjacent lymph nodes. See also **breast cancer.**

lumpy jaw [ME, *lump,* mass; *ceowan,* to chew], *nontechnical.* actinomycosis of cows, caused by infection with *Actinomyces bovis* and not communicable to humans.

lun-, a combining form meaning 'of or pertaining to the moon': *lunacy, lunate, lunatism.*

lunar month /loo′nər/ [L, *luna,* moon; AS, *monath,* month], a period of 4 weeks or 28 days, approximately the time required for the moon to revolve about the earth.

lunate bone /loo′nāt/ [L, *luna,* moon; AS, *ban*], the carpal bone in the center of the proximal row of carpal bones between the scaphoid and triangular bones. It articulates with five bones, the radius proximally, the capitate and the hamate distally, the scaphoid laterally, and the triangular medially. Also called **os lunatum, semilunar bone.**

Lundh test, a pancreatic function test in which the pancreas is stimulated by oral intake of a formula diet and lipase values are measured in aspirate from the duodenum.

lung (L) [AS, *lungen*], one of a pair of light, spongy organs in the thorax, constituting the main component of the respiratory system. The two highly elastic lungs are the main mechanisms in the body for inspiring air from which oxygen is extracted for the arterial blood system and for exhaling carbon dioxide dispersed from the venous system. The lungs are composed of lobes that are smooth and shiny on their surface. The right lung contains three lobes; the left lung two lobes. Each lung is composed of an external serous coat, a subserous layer of areolar tissue, and the parenchyma. The serous coat comprises the thin, visceral pleura. The subserous areolar tissue contains many elastic fibers and invests the entire surface of the organ. The parenchyma is composed of secondary lobules divided into primary lobules, each of which consists of blood vessels, lymphatics, nerves, and an alveolar duct connecting with air spaces. The color of the lungs at birth is pinkish white, and darkens in later life. The coloring is from carbon granules deposited in the areolar tissue near the surface of the lung. The carbon deposits increase with age and are more abundant in men than women. The lungs of men are usually heavier than the lungs of women and usually have a greater capacity. The quantity of air that can be exhaled from the lungs after the deepest inspiration, the vital capacity, averages 3700 cc. Each lung is conical and has an apex, a base, three borders, and two surfaces. The apex is rounded and extends into the root of the neck about 4 cm above the first rib. The base of the lung is broad and concave, rests on the convex surface of the diaphragm, and with the diaphragm moves up during expiration and down during inspiration. The surfaces of the lungs are partially concave, with a cardiac impression that cradles the heart. The bronchial arteries supply blood to nourish the lungs and are derived from the ventral side of the thoracic aorta or from the aortic intercostal arteries. The bronchial vein is formed at the root of the lung. Most of the blood supplied by the bronchial arteries are returned by the pulmonary veins to the left atrium of the heart.

lung abscess [AS, *lungen;* L, *abscedere,* to go away], a complication of an inflammation and infection of the lung, often caused by aspiration of infected material from the mouth.

lung cancer, a pulmonary malignancy attributable to cigarette smoking in 50% of cases. Other predisposing factors are exposure to acronitrile, arsenic, asbestos, beryllium, chloromethyl ether, chromium, coal products, ionizing radiation, iron oxide, mustard gas, nickel, petroleum, uranium, and vinyl chloride. Lung cancer develops most often in scarred or chronically diseased lungs, and is usually far advanced when detected, because metastases may precede the detection of the primary lesion in the lung. Symptoms of lung cancer include persistent cough, dyspnea, purulent or blood-streaked sputum, chest pain, and repeated attacks of bronchitis or pneumonia. Diagnostic measures include x-ray films, fluoroscopy, tomography, bronchography, angiography, cytologic studies of sputum, bronchial washings or brushings, and needle biopsy. Epidermoid cancers and adenocarcinomas each account for approximately 30% of lung tumors, about 25% are small or oat cell carcinomas, and 15% are large-cell anaplastic cancers. Epidermoid tumors tend to remain in the thorax, but other lung lesions metastasize widely; small cell carcinomas frequently invade bone marrow and the central nervous system, and large-cell cancers frequently metastasize to mediastinal nodes and gastrointestinal mucosa. Surgery is the most effective treatment, but only one half of the cases are operable at the time of diagnosis and of these 50% are not resectable. Thoracotomy is contraindicated if metastases are found in contralateral or scalene lymph nodes. Irradiation is used to treat localized lesions and unresectable intrathoracic tumors and as palliative therapy for metastatic lesions. Radiotherapy may also be administered postoperatively to destroy remaining tumor cells and may be combined with chemotherapy. Remissions are obtained in some cases treated with chemotherapeutic agents, such as cyclophosphamide, procarbazine, cisplatinum, VP-16, doxorubicin hydrochloride, and bleomycin. Chemotherapy is especially indicated for small cell carcinoma. Postoperatively, bacillus Calmette-Guérin vaccine, an antituberculosis drug that stimulates the immune system, is administered to some patients with early stage lung cancer.

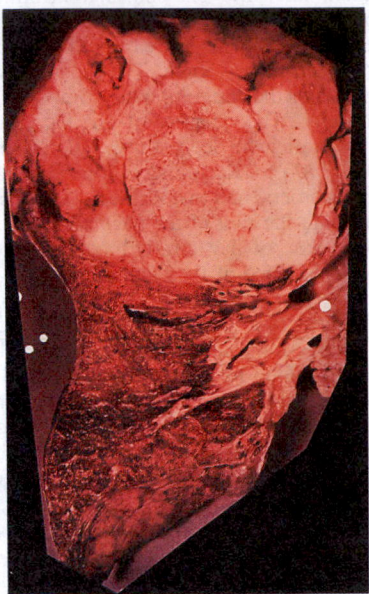

Lung cancer in top half of the lung
(Raven, 1992/Courtesy American Cancer Society)

lung capacities, lung volumes that consist of two or more of the four primary nonoverlapping volumes. Functional residual capacity is the sum of residual volume and expiratory reserve volume. Inspiratory capacity is the sum of the tidal volume and inspiratory reserve volume. Vital capacity is the sum of the expiratory reserve volume, the tidal volume, and the inspiratory reserve volume. Total lung capacity, at the end of maximal inspiration, is the sum of the functional residual capacity and the inspiratory capacity.

lung compliance, a measure of the ease of expansion by the lungs and thorax. It is determined by pulmonary volume and elasticity, a high degree of compliance indicating

a loss of elastic recoil of the lungs, as in old age or emphysema. Decreased compliance of the lungs occurs in conditions when greater pressure is needed for changes of volume, as in atelectasis, edema, fibrosis, pneumonia, or absence of surfactant. Dyspnea on exertion is the main symptom of diminished lung compliance. See also **expiratory reserve volume, residual volume, respiration, vital capacity.**

lung fluke [AS, *lungen*, lung, *floc*], a parasitic flatworm of the genus and species *Paragonimus westermani* found throughout Africa, the Orient, and Latin America, but rarely in North America. It may enter the body as encysted larvae in crabs and crayfish. Symptoms of infestation include peribronchiolar distress and hemoptysis.

lung scan, a radiographic examination of a lung and its function.

lunula /loon′yələ/, *pl.* **lunulae** [L, *luna*, moon], a semilunar structure, such as the crescent-shaped pale area at the base of the nail of a finger or toe.

lupoid. See **lupus.**

lupoid hepatitis. See **hepatitis.**

Lupron, a trademark for a parenteral antineoplastic drug (leuprolide acetate).

lupus /loo′pəs/ [L, wolf], **1.** *nontechnical*, lupus erythematosus. **2.** *obsolete.* any chronic skin condition in which ulcerative lesions spread over the body over a long period of time. **−lupoid,** *adj.*

lupus erythematosus. See **systemic lupus erythematosus.**

lupus erythematosus cell. See **LE cell.**

lupus erythematosus preparation (LE prep), a laboratory test for lupus erythematosus in which normal neutrophils are incubated with a specimen of the patient's serum resulting in the appearance of large, spherical, phagocytized inclusions within the neutrophils if the patient has lupus erythematosus.

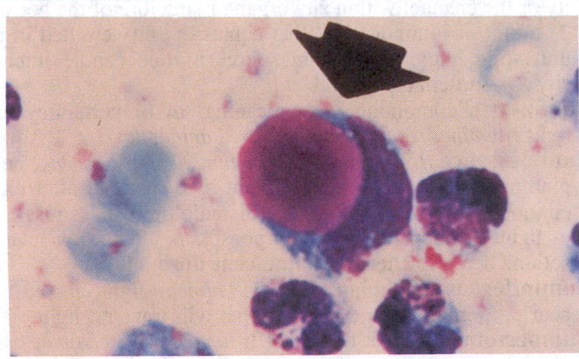

Lupus erythematosus preparation *(Tilton, 1992)*

lupus vulgaris, a rare cutaneous form of tuberculosis in which areas of the skin become ulcerated and heal slowly, leaving deeply scarred tissue. The disease is not related to lupus erythematosus.

LUQ, abbreviation for *left upper quadrant of abdomen.*

Luride, a trademark for a chemical prophylactic (sodium fluoride) that reduces dental caries.

lusus naturae /loo′səs/ [L, *lusus*, sport; *natura*, nature], a congenital anomaly; teratism.

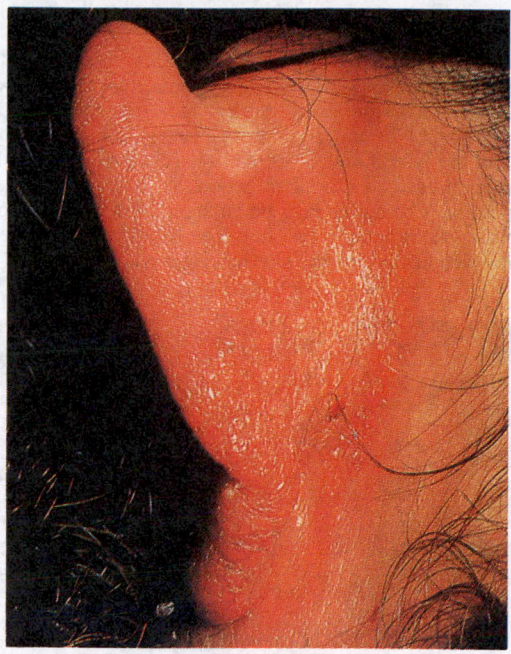

Lupus vulgaris (McKee, 1993)

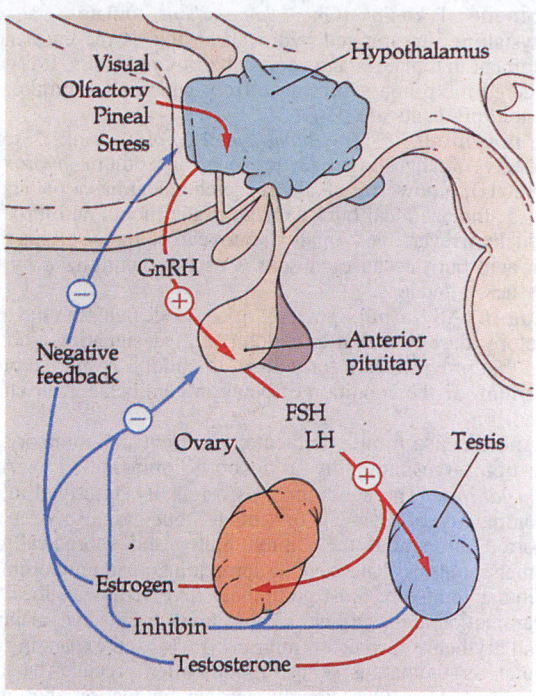

Feedback regulation of luteinizing hormone
(Zitelli, 1992)

luteal /lōō′tē·əl/, of or pertaining to the corpus luteum or its functions or effects.

luteal hormone [L, *luteus,* yellow; Gk, *hormaein,* to set in motion], a hormone produced by the **corpus luteum.** See also **progesterone.**

luteal phase. See **secretory phase.**

lutein /lōō′tē·in/ [L, *luteus,* yellow], a yellow-red, crystalline, carotenoid pigment found in plants with carotenes and chlorophylls and also in animal fats, egg yolk, the corpus luteum, or any lipochrome.

luteinization /lōō′tē·in′izā′shən/ [L, *luteus,* yellow], the formation of the corpus luteum from an ovarian follicle that had recently discharged an ovum. The process involves the hypertrophy of the follicular lutein cells and the development of blood vessels and conective tissue at the site.

luteinizing hormone (LH) /lōō′tē·ini′zing/ [L, *luteus,* yellow; Gk, *izein,* to cause; Gk, *hormein,* to begin activity], a glycoprotein hormone, produced by the anterior pituitary, that stimulates the secretion of sex hormones by the ovary and the testes and is involved in the maturation of spermatozoa and ova. In men, it induces the secretion of testosterone by the interstitial cells of the testes. Testosterone, together with follicle stimulating hormone (FSH), induces the maturation of seminiferous tubules and stimulates them to produce sperm. In females, LH, working together with FSH, stimulates the growing follicle in the ovary to secrete estrogen. High concentrations of estrogen stimulate the release of a surge of LH, which stimulates ovulation. LH then induces the development of the ruptured follicle into the corpus luteum, which continues to secrete estrogen and progesterone. The normal LH concentration in the plasma of men is less than 11 mIU/ml. In women, it is, premenopausal, less than 25 mIU/ml; at midcycle peak, greater than

three times the baseline concentration; postmenopausal, more than 25 mIU/ml. See also **interstitial cell-stimulating hormone, menstrual cycle.**

luteinizing hormone–releasing hormone (LHRH), a neurohormone of the hypothalamus that stimulates and regulates the pituitary gland's release of the luteinizing hormone (LH).

luteoma /lōō′tē·ō′mə/, *pl.* **luteomas, luteomata** [L, *luteus,* + Gk, *oma,* tumor], **1.** a granulosa or theca cell tumor whose cells resemble those of the corpus luteum. **2.** also called **pregnancy luteoma.** a unilateral or bilateral nodular hyperplasia of ovarian lutein cells, occasionally developing during the last trimester of pregnancy.

luteotropin. See **prolactin.**

lutetium (Lu) /lōōtē′shē·əm/ [L, *Lutetia,* Paris], a rare earth metallic element. Its atomic number is 71; and its atomic weight is 174.97.

luxated joint /luk′sātid/, a condition of complete dislocation, with no contact between articular surfaces of the joint.

LV, abbreviation for **left ventricle.**

LVAD, abbreviation for **left ventricular assist device.**

LVN, abbreviation for **licensed vocational nurse.** See **licensed practical nurse.**

lyases /lē′āsis [Gk, *lyein,* to loosen; Fr, *disastase,* enzyme], a group of enzymes that reversibly split carbon bonds with carbon, nitrogen, or oxygen without hydrolysis or oxygen reduction reactions. The activity results in two subunits in which one or both may contain a double-bonded carbon. An example of a lyase is deaminase.

lyco-, a combining form meaning 'of or pertaining to a wolf': *lycomania, lycorexia.*

lycopene /lī′kəpin/ [Gk, *lykopersikon*, tomato], a red, crystalline, unsaturated hydrocarbon that is the carotenoid pigment in tomatoes and various berries and fruits. It is considered the primary substance from which all natural carotenoid pigments are derived.

lye poisoning /lī/ [AS, *leah*, lye; L, *potio*, drink], toxic effects of ingesting caustic soda or sodium hydroxide (NaOH), a powerful alkali. If the chemical has a pH above 11.5, the chemical burn damage to the mouth and throat is usually irreversible. An alkali burn can be more serious than an acid burn because an acid is usually neutralized by the tissues it contacts.

lying-in [AS, *licgan*, lying; L, *in*], **1.** designating the time before, during, and after childbirth. **2.** designating a hospital that provides care for women in childbirth and the puerperium. **3.** the condition of being in confinement, or childbed.

Lyme disease /līm/, an acute, recurrent inflammatory infection, transmitted by a tickborne spirochete, *Borrelia burgdorferi*. The condition was originally described in the community of Lyme, Connecticut, but has also been reported throughout the United States and sporadically in other countries. Knees, other large joints, and temporomandibular joints are most commonly involved, with local inflammation and swelling. Chills, fever, headache, malaise, and erythema chronicum migrans (ECM), an expanding annular, erythematous skin eruption, often precede the joint manifestations. Occasionally cardiac conduction abnormalities, aseptic meningitis, and Bell's palsy are associated conditions. Symptoms appear in recurrent episodes, lasting usually about 1 week, at intervals of from 1 to several weeks, declining in severity over a 2- or 3-year period. Treatment includes tetracycline or amoxycillin/probenicid for early symptoms and intravenous ceftriaxone for later complications, such as meningitis or atrioventricular block, if necessary, and nonsteroidal antiinflammatory drugs for joint symptoms. Also called **Lyme arthritis.**

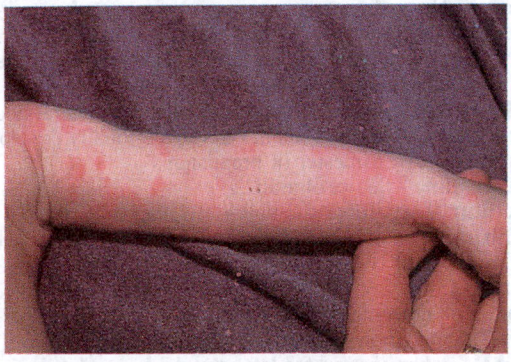

**Skin eruption (erythema chronicum migrans)
commonly seen in Lyme disease**
(Weston, 1991)

lymph /limf/ [L, *lympha*, water], a thin opalescent fluid originating in organs and tissues of the body that circulates through the lymphatic vessels and is filtered by the lymph nodes. Lymph enters the bloodstream at the junction of the internal jugular and subclavian veins. Lymph contains chyle, erythrocytes, and leukocytes, most of which are lymphocytes. See also **chyle.**

lymph-, lympho-, -lymph, a combining meaning a 'pertaining to the lymph': *lymphoduct, neurolymph, perilymph.*

lymphadenitis /limfad′inī′tis, lim′fəd-/ [L, *lympha* + Gk, *aden*, gland, *itis*, inflammation], an inflammatory condition of the lymph nodes, usually the result of systemic neoplastic disease, bacterial infection, or other inflammatory condition. The nodes may be enlarged, hard, smooth or irregular, red, and may feel hot. The location of the affected node is indicative of the site or origin of disease.

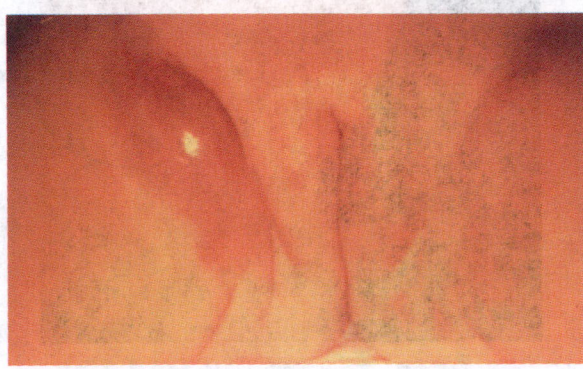

Acute suppurative lymphadenitis
(Zitelli, 1992/Courtesy Dr M Sherlock)

lymphadenoma, lymphadenoma venerum. See **lymphogranulomatosis.**

lymphadenopathy /limfad′inop′əthē/, any disorder of the lymph nodes or lymph vessels.

lymphadenopathy syndrome (LAS), a persistent, generalized swelling of the lymph nodes. It is often a part of the AIDS-related complex.

lymphangiectasia /limfan′jē·ektā′zhə/ [L, *lympha* + Gk, *aggeion*, vessel, *ektasis*, stretching], dilatation of the smaller lymphatic vessels, characterized by diarrhea, steatorrhea, and protein malabsorption. It usually results from obstruction in the larger vessels, such as in pelvic tuberculosis, mesenteric node metastases, and certain protozoan diseases.

lymphangiogram /limfan′jē·əgram′/ [L, *lympha*, water; Gk, *aggeion*, vessel; *gramma*, record], a radiographic visualization of a part of the lymphatic system.

lymphangiography /-jē·og′rəfē/ [L, *lympha* + Gk, *aggeion*, vessel, *graphein*, to record], the x-ray examination of lymph glands and lymphatic vessels after an injection of contrast medium. Also called **lymphography.**

lymphangioma /limfan′jē·ō′mə/, *pl.* **lymphangiomas, lymphangiomata** [L, *lympha* + Gk, *aggeion*, vessel, *oma*, tumor], a benign, yellowish tan tumor on the skin, composed of a mass of dilated lymph vessels. The tumor is removed by excision or electrocoagulation for cosmetic reasons. Also called **angioma lymphaticum.** Compare **hemangioma.**

lymphangioma cavernosum, a tumor formed by dilated lymphatic vessels and filled with lymph mixed with coagulated blood. The lesion, which is often congenital, may cause extensive enlargement of the affected tissue, especially of the tongue and lips. Also called **cavernous lymphangioma.**

lymphangioma circumscriptum, a benign skin lesion that develops from superficial hypertrophic lymph vessels. Most commonly seen in children, the lesion is characteristically pigmented and may grow to several centimeters in diameter.

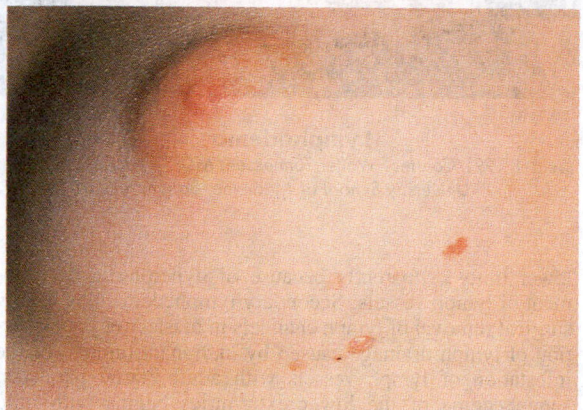

Lymphangioma circumscriptum (McKee, 1993)

lymphangioma cysticum. See **cystic lymphangioma.**
lymphangiomata. See **lymphangioma.**
lymphangioma simplex, a growth formed by moderately dilated lymph vessels in a circumscribed area, on the skin.
lymphangiosarcoma /limfan′jē·ō′särkō′mə/ [L, *lympha,* water; Gk, *aggeion,* vessel + *sarx,* flesh + *oma,* tumor], a tumor arising from the lymphatic vessels.

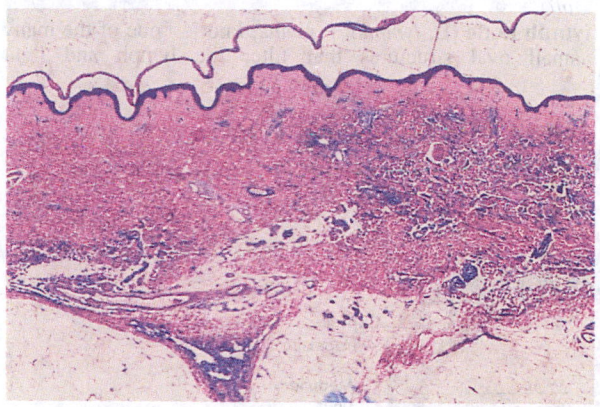

Lymphangiosarcoma—skin biopsy (Skarin, 1991)

lymphangitis /lim′fanjī′tis/ [L, *lympha* + Gk, *aggeion,* vessel, *itis*], an inflammation of one or more lymphatic vessels, usually resulting from an acute streptococcal infection of one of the extremities. It is characterized by fine red streaks extending from the infected area to the axilla or groin, and by fever, chills, headache, and myalgia. The infection may spread to the bloodstream. Penicillin and hot

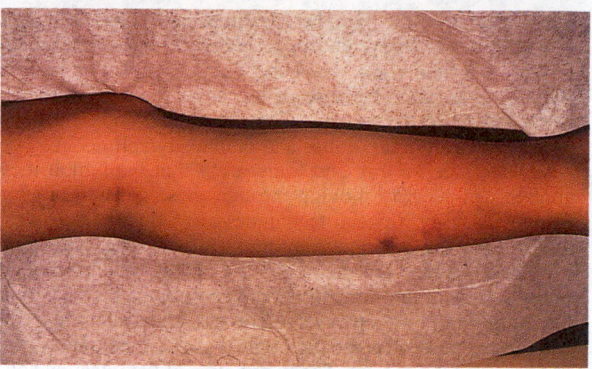

Lymphangitis (Zitelli, 1992)

soaks are usually prescribed; aseptic technique is important to avoid contagion.

lymphatic /limfat′ik/ [L, *lympha* + *icus,* form], **1.** of or pertaining to the lymphatic system of the body, consisting of a vast network of tubes transporting lymph. **2.** any one of the vessels associated with the lymphatic network.

lymphatic capillary plexus, one of the numerous networks of lymphatic capillaries that collect lymph from the intercellular fluid and constitute the beginning of the lymphatic system. The lymphatic vessels arise from the capillary plexuses, which vary in size and number in different regions and organs of the body. The capillary networks do not contain lymphatic valves as do the vessels. The plexuses are especially abundant in the dermis of the skin but also lace many other areas such as the mucous membranes of the respiratory and digestive systems, testes, ovaries, liver, kidneys, and heart. See also **lymphatic system.**

lymphatic leukemia. See **acute lymphocytic leukemia, chronic lymphocytic leukemia.**

lymphatic nodule. See **malpighian body.**

lymphatic organ [L, *lympha,* water; Gk, *organon,* instrument], any body structure composed of lymphatic tissue, such as the thymus, spleen, tonsils, and lymph nodes.

lymphatic system, a vast, complex network of capillaries, thin vessels, valves, ducts, nodes, and organs that helps to protect and maintain the internal fluid environment of the entire body by producing, filtering, and conveying lymph and by producing various blood cells. The lymphatic network also transports fats, proteins, and other substances to the blood system and restores 60% of the fluid that filters out of the blood capillaries into interstitial spaces during normal metabolism. The peripheral parts of the lymphatic complex do not directly communicate with the venous system into which the lymph flows, but the endothelium of the veins at the junction of the blood and the lymphatic networks is continuous with the endothelium of the lymphatic vessels. Small semilunar valves throughout the lymphatic network help to control the flow of lymph and, at the junction with the venous system, prevent venous blood from flowing into the lymphatic vessels. The lymph collected from throughout the body drains into the blood through two ducts situated in the neck. Various body dynamics, such as respiratory pressure changes, muscular contractions, and movements of organs surrounding lymphatic vessels combine to pump the lymph through the lymphatic system. The thoracic duct that rises into the left side of the neck is the major vessel of the lymphatic system and conveys lymph from the whole body, except for the right quadrant, which is served by the right lymphatic duct. Lymphatics have a beaded appearance because of sinuses associated with the many valves in the vessels. They resemble veins but have more valves, thinner walls, and contain lymph nodes. The lymphatics are so thin and transparent that the lymph they contain can be seen moving through these delicate tubules in a living body. Special techniques are required, however, to examine the lymphatic system closely. The lymphatic capillaries, which are the beginning of the system, abound in the dermis of the skin, forming a continuous network over the entire body, except for the cornea. The system also includes specialized lymphatic organs, such as the tonsils, the thymus, and the spleen. The lymphatics of the intestine contain a special substance, especially during the digestion of fatty foods. Lymph flows into the general circulation through the thoracic duct at a rate of about 125 ml per hour during routine exertion. The rate may jump to as high as 1800 ml per hour during vigorous exercise. See also **lymph, lymph node, spleen, thymus,** and see the Color Atlas of Human Anatomy.

lymphatic vessels [L, *lympha*, water + *vascellum*, little vase], fine transparent valved channels distributed through most tissues. They are often distinguished by their beaded appearance, which is caused by an irregular lumen. The collecting branches form two systems, one generally running with the superficial veins and the other below the deep fascia and including the intestinal lacteals. They drain through a thoracic duct and a right lymphatic duct into the venous system near the base of the neck.

lymph cell   See **lymphocyte.**

lymphedema /lim′fidē′mə/ [L, *lympha* + Gk, *oidema*, swelling], a primary or secondary disorder characterized by the accumulation of lymph in soft tissue and swelling, caused by inflammation, obstruction, or removal of lymph channels. Congenital lymphedema (Milroy's disease) is a hereditary disorder characterized by chronic lymphatic obstruction. Lymphedema praecox occurs in adolescence, chiefly in females, and causes puffiness and swelling of the

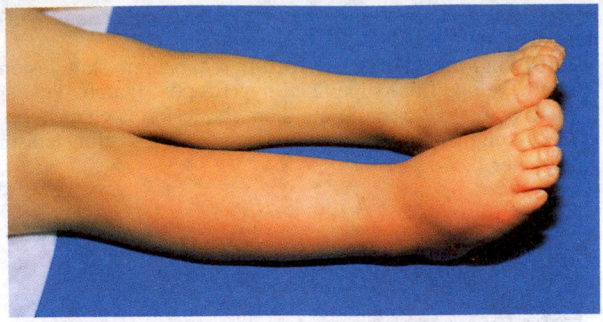

Lymphedema
(Seidel, 1991/Courtesy Walter Tunnessen, MD, The Johns Hopkins University School of Medicine, Baltimore)

lower limbs, apparently because of hyperplastic development of lymph vessels. Secondary lymphedema may follow surgical removal of lymph channels in mastectomy, obstruction of lymph drainage caused by malignant tumors, or the infestation of lymph vessels with adult filarial parasites. Lymphedema of the lower extremities begins with mild swelling of the foot, gradually extends to the entire limb, and is aggravated by prolonged standing, pregnancy, obesity, warm weather, and the menstrual period. There is no cure for the disorder, but lymph drainage from the extremity can be improved if the patient sleeps with the foot of the bed elevated 4 to 8 inches, wears elastic stockings, and takes moderate exercise regularly. Light massage in the direction of the lymph flow and thiazide diuretics may be prescribed; constricting clothing and salty or spicy foods that increase thirst are contraindicated. Surgery may be performed to remove hypertrophied lymph channels and disfiguring tissue. **–lymphedematous, lymphedematose,** *adj.*

lymph node [L, *lympha* + *nodus*, knot], one of the many small oval structures that filter the lymph and fight

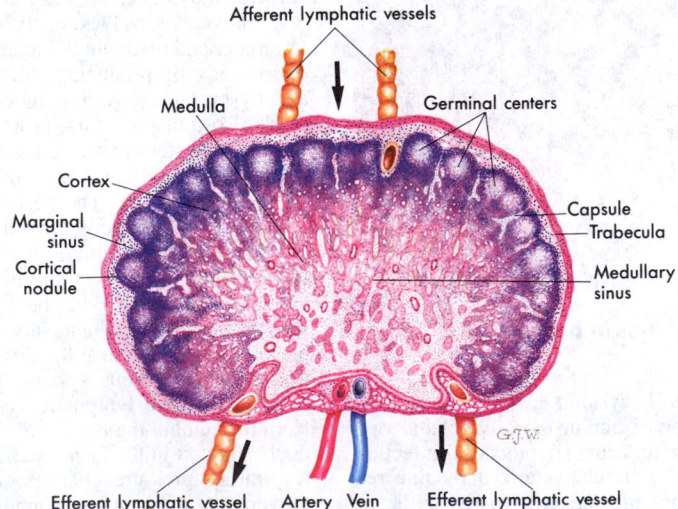

Afferent lymphatic vessels

Medulla   Germinal centers

Cortex

Marginal sinus

Cortical nodule

Capsule

Trabecula

Medullary sinus

Efferent lymphatic vessel   Artery   Vein   Efferent lymphatic vessel

Structures of a lymph node *(Belcher, 1992)*

infection, and in which there are formed lymphocytes, monocytes, and plasma cells. The lymph nodes are of different sizes, some as small as pinheads, others as large as lima beans. Each node is enclosed in a capsule, is composed of a lighter colored cortical portion and a darker medullary portion, and consists of closely packed lymphocytes, reticular connective tissue laced by trabeculae, and three kinds of sinuses, subcapsular, cortical, and medullary. Lymph flows into the node through afferent lymphatic vessels that open into the subcapsular sinuses. Efferent lymphatic vessels arise from the medullary sinuses of the node and emerge through a small peripheral hilum that also receives blood vessels. The sinuses and meshes of reticular fibers retard the flow of lymph to which lymphocytes are added from germinal centers within the node that multiply those cells by mitosis. Most lymph nodes are clustered in (specific) areas, such as the mouth, the neck, the lower arm, the axilla, and the groin. The lymphatic network and nodes of the breast are especially crucial in the diagnosis and treatment of breast cancer. Cancer cells from a 'primary' breast tumor often spread through the lymphatic system to other parts of the body. Also called **lymph gland.**

lymph nodule [L, *lympha,* water; *nodulus,* small knot], any of the small densely packed spherical nodes or aggregations of lymph cells embedded in the reticular meshwork of the lymphatic system, mainly in the tonsils, spleen, and thymus.

lympho- See **lymph-.**

lymphoblastic lymphoma, lymphoblastic lymphosarcoma, lymphoblastoma. See **poorly differentiated lymphocytic malignant lymphoma.**

lymphocyte /lim'fəsīt/ [L, *lympha* + Gk, *kytos,* cell], small, agranulocytic leukocytes, originating from fetal stem cells and developing in the bone marrow. Lymphocytes normally comprise 25% of the total white blood cell count but increase in number in response to infection. Two forms occur: B cells and T cells. B cells circulate in an immature form and synthesize antibodies for insertion into their own cytoplasmic membranes. Both reproduce mitotically, each of the clones displaying identical antibodies on their surface membranes. When an immature B cell is exposed to a specific antigen, the cell is activated, traveling to the spleen or to the lymph nodes, differentiating, and rapidly producing **plasma cells** and **memory cells.** Plasma cells synthesize and secrete antibody. Memory cells do not secrete antibody, but on reexposure to the specific antigen, develop into antibody-secreting plasma cells. T cells are lymphocytes that have circulated through the thymus gland and have differentiated to become thymocytes. When exposed to an antigen, they divide rapidly and produce large numbers of new T cells sensitized to that antigen. Some T cells are often called 'killer cells' because they secrete immunologically essential chemical compounds and assist B cells in destroying foreign protein. T cells also appear to play a significant role in the body's resistance to the proliferation of cancer cells. Also called **lymph cell.** See also **lymphokine.**

lymphocyte transformation, an in vitro immunity test process in which a patient's lymphocytes are placed in a culture with an antigen. The rate of transformation, in terms of proliferation and enlargement of T memory cells, is measured by the uptake of radioactive thymidine by the lymphocytes, indicating protein synthesis.

lymphocytic choriomeningitis /lim'fəsit'ik/ [L, *lympha* + Gk, *kytos,* cell; *chorion,* skin, *meninx,* membrane, *itis,* inflammation], an arenavirus infection of the meninges and the cerebrospinal fluid, caused by the lymphocytic choriomeningitis virus and characterized by fever, headache, and stiff neck. The infection occurs primarily in young adults, most often in the fall and winter months. Recovery usually takes place within 2 weeks.

lymphocytic leukemia. See **acute lymphocytic leukemia, chronic lymphocytic leukemia.**

lymphocytic lymphoma, lymphocytic lymphosarcoma. See **well-differentiated lymphocytic malignant lymphoma.**

lymphocytic thyroiditis. See **Hashimoto's disease.**

lymphocytoma. See **well-differentiated lymphocytic malignant lymphoma.**

lymphocytopenia /lim'fōsī'təpē'nē·ə/ [L, *lympha* + Gk, *kytos,* cell, *penes,* poor], a decreased number of lymphocytes in the peripheral circulation, occurring as a primary hematologic disorder or in association with nutritional deficiency, malignancy, or infectious mononucleosis. Compare **alymphocytosis.** See also **agranulocyte.**

lymphocytosis /lim'fōsītō'sis/, a proliferation of lymphocytes, as occurs in certain chronic diseases and during convalescence from acute infections.

lymphoderma perniciosa. See **leukemia cutis.**

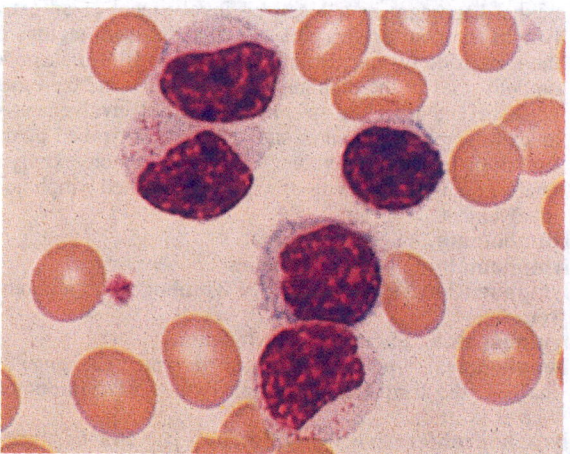

Normal lymphocytes *(Hayhoe, 1992)*

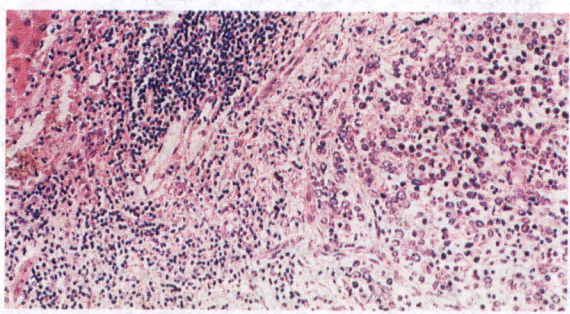

Lymphoepithelioma *(Skarin, 1991)*

lymphoepithelioma /lim′fō·ep′ithē′lē·ō′mə/ [L, *lympha* + Gk, *epi*, above, *thele*, nipple, *oma*, tumor], a poorly differentiated neoplasm developing from the epithelium overlying lymphoid tissue in the nasopharynx. It occurs most frequently in young Oriental people. Also called **lymphoepithelial carcinoma.**

lymphogenous leukemia. See **acute lymphocytic leukemia, chronic lymphocytic leukemia.**

lymphogranulomatosis /-gran′yəlō′mətō′sis/ [L, *lympha*, water; *granulum*, small grain; Gk, *oma*, tumor; *osis*, condition], an infectious granuloma of the lymphatic system. The term is used to identify several inflammatory granulomata or sarcomata disorders, such as **Hodgkin's disease, sarcoidosis, lymphadenoma,** and **lymphadenoma venereum.**

lymphogranuloma venereum (LGV) /-gran′yəlō′mə/ [L, *lympha* + *granulum*, small grain; Gk, *oma*, tumor; L, *Venus*, goddess of love], a sexually transmitted disease caused by a strain of the bacterium *Chlamydia trachomatis.* It is characterized by ulcerative genital lesions, marked swelling of the lymph nodes in the groin, headache, fever, and malaise. Ulcerations of the rectal wall occur less commonly. The disease is diagnosed by isolating the organism from an infected node, demonstrating LGV antibodies by serologic blood test. Doxycycline is usually prescribed for the patient and for any person with whom there has been sexual contact. When changing dressings, aseptic technique is used. Also called **lymphopathia venereum.** See also *Chlamydia.*

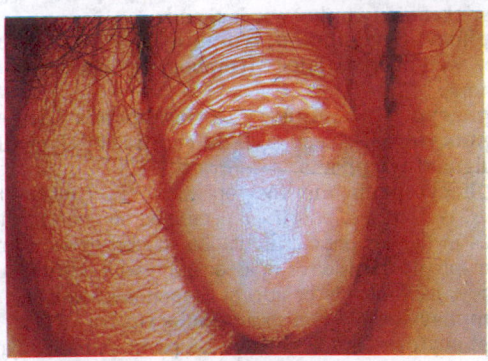

Lymphogranuloma venereum *(Meheus, 1982)*

lymphography. See **lymphangiography.**

lymphoid /lim′foid/ [L, *lympha*, water; Gk, *eidos*, form], pertaining to lymph or lymphatics.

lymphoid aplasia. See **immunodeficient.**

lymphoid interstitial pneumonia (LIP), a form of pneumonia that involves the lower lobes with extensive alveolar infiltration by mature lymphocytes, plasma cells, and histiocytes. It is associated with AIDS, dysproteinemia, and Sjögren's syndrome.

lymphoid leukemia. See **acute lymphocytic leukemia, chronic lymphocytic leukemia.**

lymphoidocytic leukemia. See **stem cell leukemia.**

lymphoid ring. See **Waldeyer's throat ring.**

lymphoid tissue [L, *lympha*, water; Gk, *eidos*, form; OFr, *tissu*], tissue that consists of lymphocytes on a framework of reticular cells and fibers, as the tonsils and adenoids.

lymphokine /lim′fōkīn/ [L, *lympha* + Gk, *kinesis*, motion], one of the chemical factors produced and released by T lymphocytes that attract macrophages to the site of infection or inflammation and prepare them for attack. Kinds of lymphokines include **chemotactic factor, lymphotoxin, migration inhibiting factor,** and **mitogenic factor.**

lymphokine-activated killer (LAK) cells, nonspecific cytotoxic cells that are generated in the presence of interleukin-2 and in the absence of antigen. They are distinct from human natural killer cells, peripheral T lymphocytes, or memory cytotoxic thymus-derived lymphocytes. A deficiency of LAK cells has been found in patients with hypogam maglobulinemia, who are also at a much greater than average risk of developing cancer.

lympholysis /limfol′əsis/ [L, *lympha* + Gk, *lysein*, to loosen], cellular destruction of lymphocytes, especially of certain lymphocytes in the process of an immune response. **–lympholytic,** *adj.*

lymphoma /limfō′mə/, *pl.* **lymphomas, lymphomata** [L, *lympha* + Gk, *oma*, tumor], a neoplasm of lymphoid tissue that is usually malignant but, in rare cases, may be benign. The various lymphomas differ in degree of cellular differentiation and content, but the manifestations are similar in all types. Characteristically, the appearance of a painless, enlarged lymph node or nodes is followed by weakness, fever, weight loss, and anemia. With widespread involvement of lymphoid tissue, the spleen and liver usually enlarge, and gastrointestinal disturbances, malabsorption, and bone lesions frequently develop. Men are more likely than women to develop lymphoid tumors. Treatment for lymphoma includes intensive radiotherapy and chemotherapy. Kinds of lymphoma include **Burkitt's lymphoma, giant follicular lymphoma, histiocytic malignant lymphoma, Hodgkin's disease, mixed cell malignant lymphoma. –lymphomatoid,** *adj.*

-lymphoma, a combining form meaning a 'tumor or neoplastic disorder of lymphoid tissue': *adenolymphoma, angiolymphoma, cystadenolymphoma.*

lymphoma staging, a system for classifying lymphomas according to the extent of the disease for the purpose of treatment and prognosis. Stage I is characterized by the involvement of a single lymph node region or one extralymphatic organ or site. Stage II is characterized by the involvement of two or more lymph node regions on the same side of the diaphragm or a localized involvement of an extralymphatic organ or site plus one or more node regions on the same side of the diaphragm. In stage III lymph nodes on both sides of the diaphragm are affected, and there may be involvement of the spleen or localized involvement of an extralymphatic organ or site. Stage IV is typified by diffuse or disseminated involvement of one or more extralymphatic organs or sites with or without associated lymph node involvement.

lymphomata. See **lymphoma.**

lymphomatoid. See **lymphoma.**

lymphopathia venereum. See **lymphogranuloma venereum.**

lymphopenia. See **lymphocytopenia.**

lymphopoiesis /-pō·ē′sis/ [L, *lympha*, water; Gk, *poien*, to make], the formation of lymphocytes. **–lymphopoietic** /-pō·et′ik/, *adj.*

lymphoproliferative /-prōlif′ərətiv/ [L, *lympha*, water; *prolles*, offspring; *ferre*, to bear], pertaining to the proliferation of lymphoid tissue.

lymphoreticulosis /-retik′yəlō′sis/ [L, *lympha* + *reticulum*, little net; Gk, *osis*, condition], subacute granulomatous inflammation of lymphoid tissue with proliferation of reticuloendothelial cells, occurring most commonly as the result of a cat scratch. No causative agent is known. The disorder is characterized by the formation of an ulcerated papule at the site of the scratch, fever, and tender lymphadenopathy, sometimes progressing to suppuration. Also called **cat scratch fever.**

lymphosarcoma. See **non-Hodgkin's lymphoma.**

lymphosarcoma cell leukemia /-särkō′mə/ [L, *lympha* + Gk, *sarx*, flesh, *oma*, tumor], a malignancy of blood-forming tissues characterized by many lymphosarcoma cells in the peripheral circulation that tend to infiltrate surrounding tissues. These cells are extremely immature, larger, and more reticulated than lymphocytes. The disease may accompany lymphoma or exist as a separate entity with bone marrow involvement. Also called **lymphoblastic lymphoma.**

lymphotoxin. See **lymphokine.**

lymph sinuses [L, *lympha*, water + *sinus*, hollow], continuous small endothelial-lined spaces just below the capsule of the lymph node. The sinuses slow the flow of lymph through the nodes.

lyo-, a combining form meaning 'to loosen or dissolve': *lyogel, lyophobe, lyotropic.*

Lyon hypothesis /lī′ən/ [Mary L. Lyon, English geneticist, b. 1925], (in genetics) a hypothesis stating that only one of the two X chromosomes in a female is functional, the other having become inactive early in development. A female is mosaic in regard to X chromosomes; some are from her father, some from her mother. Sex-linked genes may therefore appear on some of her cells and not on others.

lyonization /lī′ənīzā′shən/ [Mary L. Lyon; Gk, *izein*, to cause], the process of random inactivation of one of the X chromosomes in the female gamete to compensate for the presence of the double X gene complement. See also **Lyon hypothesis.**

Lyon's ring, a type of congenital uropathy in females in which submeatal or distal urethral stenosis causes enuresis, dysuria, and recurring infections. The disorder is treated surgically.

lyophilic /lī′ōfil′ik/ [Gk, *lyein*, to dissolve; *philein*, to love], pertaining to substances having an affinity for stability, in solution. Lyophilic substances are used to stabilize colloids.

lypressin /līpres′in/, an antidiuretic and vasoconstrictor.

■ INDICATION: It is prescribed in diabetes insipidus to decrease urinary water loss.

■ CONTRAINDICATIONS: Vascular disease or known hypersensitivity to this drug prohibits its use.

■ ADVERSE EFFECTS: Among the most serious adverse reactions are angina in people with cardiovascular disease, nausea, cramping, and marked facial pallor.

Lys, abbreviation for **lysine.**

-lyse. See **-lyze.**

lysergide /līsur′jīd/, a psychotomimetic, semisynthetic derivative of ergot that acts at multiple sites in the central nervous system from the cortex to the spinal cord. In susceptible individuals, as little as 20 to 25 μg of the potent drug may cause pupillary dilatation, increased blood pressure, hyperreflexia, tremor, muscle weakness, piloerection, and increased body temperature. Larger doses also produce dizziness, drowsiness, paresthesia, euphoria or dysphoria, and synesthesias; colors may be heard, sounds visualized, and time is felt to pass slowly. Psychologic dependence may de-

velop, and use of lysergide is associated with significant hazards, such as panic, serious depression, paranoid behavior, and prolonged psychotic episodes. called **LSD** (an abbreviation of the original German name, (*Lyserg-Säure-Diäthylamid*) **lysergic acid diethylamide,** *(slang)* **acid.** See also **hallucinogen.**

Lysholm method, (in radiology) any of several techniques for positioning a patient for x-ray examination of the cranial base, the mastoid and petrous regions of the temporal bone, and the optic foramen and orbital fissure.

-lysin, a suffix meaning a 'cell-dissolving antibody': *antilysin, betalysin, paralysin.*

lysine (Lys) /lī′sēn, lī′sin/, an essential amino acid needed for proper growth in infants and for maintenance of nitrogen balance in adults. See also **amino acid, protein.**

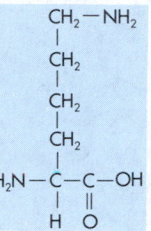

Chemical structure of lysine *(Seeley, 1992)*

lysine intolerance, a congenital disorder resulting in the inability to use the essential amino acid lysine because of an enzyme deficiency or defect. The disorder is characterized by weakness, vomiting, and coma and is treated by adjusting the protein content of the diet, restricting those foods especially high in lysine. See also **lysinemia.**

lysinemia /lī′sinē′mē·ə/, a condition caused by an inborn error of metabolism and resulting in the inability to use the essential amino acid lysine because of an enzyme defect or deficiency. It is characterized by muscle weakness and mental retardation. Treatment consists of a diet that controls the intake of lysine by reducing dietary proteins and including such foods as fruits, vegetables, and rice.

lysine monohydrochloride, a salt of the amino acid lysine, used as a dietary supplement to increase the use of vegetable proteins, such as corn, rice, and wheat.

lysis /lī′sis/ [Gk, *lysein*, to loosen], **1.** destruction or dissolution of a cell or molecule through the action of a specific agent. Cell lysis is frequently caused by a lysin. **2.** gradual diminution in the symptoms of a disease. Compare **crisis.**

-lysis, a suffix meaning a 'breaking down or detachment': *cytolysis, dialysis, osteolysis.*

lysis of adhesions, surgery performed to free adhesions of tissues.

lyso-, a combining form meaning 'of or pertaining to dissolution': *lysocephalin, lysotype, lysozyme.*

Lysodren, a trademark for an antineoplastic (mitotane).

lysogenesis /lī′səjen′əsis/ [Gk, *lysis*, loosening; *genein*, to produce], the formation of lysins, or antibodies that cause partial or complete dissolution of the target cell.

lysosome /lī′səsōm/ [Gk, *lysein* + *soma*, body], a cytoplasmic, membrane-bound particle that contains hydrolytic enzymes that function in intracellular digestive processes.

The organelles are found in most cells but are particularly prominent in leukocytes and in the cells of the liver and kidney. If the hydrolytic enzymes are released into the cytoplasm, they cause self-digestion of the cell so that lysosomes may play an important role in certain self-destructive diseases characterized by the wasting of tissue, such as muscular dystrophy.

lysozyme /lī′səzīm/ [Gk, *lysein* + *en*, within, *zyme*, ferment], an enzyme with antiseptic actions that destroys some foreign organisms. It is found in granulocytic and monocytic blood cells and is normally present in saliva, sweat, breast milk, and tears.

lysso-, a combining form meaning 'of or pertaining to rabies, or hydrophobia': *lyssodexis, lyssoid, lyssophobia.*

-lyte, 1. a suffix pertaining to 'electrolyte': *ampholyte.* 2. a suffix meaning a 'substance capable of or resulting from decomposition': *cytolyte, sarcolyte.*

lytes /līts/, an informal abbreviation of *electrolytes*, especially the levels of potassium, sodium, phosphorus, magnesium, and calcium in the blood, as determined by laboratory testing.

-lytic, a suffix meaning 'pertaining to or effecting decomposition': *fibrillolytic, leukolytic, myelolytic.*

lytic cocktail /lit′ik/, an informal name for a neuroleptic compound of chlorpromazine, meperidine, and promethazine that blocks the autonomic nervous system, depresses the circulatory system, and induces neuroplegia.

Lytren, a trademark for a nutritional supplement containing various electrolytes.

-lyze, -lyse, a suffix meaning 'to produce decomposition': *bacteriolyze, hemolyze, paralyze.*

M

m, 1. abbreviation for **meter.** 2. abbreviation for **milli-.**

M, 1. abbreviation for *mega.* 2. abbreviation for **molar,** def. 2. 3. abbreviation for *metastasis* in the TNM (tumor, node, metastasis) system for staging malignant neoplastic disease. See also **cancer staging.**

ma, MA, abbreviation for **milliampere.**

MA, abbreviation for **mental age.**

M.A., abbreviation for *Master of Arts* degree.

MAA, abbreviation for *methacrylic acid.*

Maass, Clara (1876–1901), an American nurse. After training and working at the Newark German Hospital, which has since been renamed for her, she volunteered for military service at the outbreak of the Spanish-American War. After working at Army camps where soldiers were dying of yellow fever, she volunteered to go to Havana to participate in the experiments being done to determine the cause of that disease. She was bitten by a mosquito and died 10 days later of yellow fever. She was one of the first nurses to be inducted into the Hall of Fame of the American Nurses' Association.

Mab, abbreviation for **monoclonal antibody.**

mabp, abbreviation for *mean arterial blood pressure.* See **mean arterial pressure.**

MAC, 1. abbreviation for **midupper arm circumference.** 2. abbreviation for **minimum alveolar concentration.**

MAC AWAKE, the concentration of an inhaled anesthetic that allows a patient to respond rationally to questions and verbal instructions.

macerate /mas′ərāt/ [L, *macerare,* to soften], to soften something solid by soaking. **–maceration,** *n.*

maceration /-ā′shən/, the softening and breaking down of skin from prolonged exposure to moisture. It may be caused by prolonged exposure to amniotic fluid in a postterm infant or dead fetus.

machinery murmur /məshēn′ərē/ [L, *machina; murmur,* humming], a continuous murmur heard throughout systole and diastole, with systolic accentuation. It is heard to the left of the sternum in patients with a ductus arteriosus condition.

machismo /mächis′mō/, (in psychology) a concept of the male that includes both culturally desirable traits of courage and fearlessness and the dysfunctional behaviors of heavy drinking, seduction of women, and domineering and abusive spouse behavior.

Machover Draw-A-Person Test. See **Draw-A-Person Test.**

Machupo. See **Bolivian hemorrhagic fever.**

macrencephaly /mak′rənsef′əlē/ [Gk, *makros,* large, *enkephalos,* brain], a congenital anomaly characterized by abnormal largeness of the brain. Also called **macroencephaly.** See also **macrocephaly.** **—macrencephalic, macroencephalic,** *adj.*

macro-, makro- /mak′rō-/, a prefix meaning 'large, or abnormal size': *macrobiosis, macrocardius, macrophage.*

macrobiosis /-bī·ō′sis/ [Gk, *makros,* long; *bios,* life], a long life.

macroblepharia /mak′rōblifer′ē·ə/ [Gk, *makros* + *blepharon,* eyelid], the condition of having abnormally large eyelids.

macrocephaly /mak′rōsef′əlē/ [Gk, *makros* + *kephale,* head], a congenital anomaly characterized by abnormal largeness of the head and brain in relation to the rest of the body, resulting in some degree of mental and growth retardation. The head is more than two standard deviations above the average circumference size for age, sex, race, and period of gestation, with excessively wide fontanelles; the facial features are usually normal. The condition may be caused by some defect in formation during embryonic development, or it may be the result of progressive degeneration processes, such as Schilder's disease, Greenfield's disease, or congenital lipoidosis. In macrocephaly there is symmetric overgrowth at the head without increased intracranial pressure, as differentiated from hydrocephalus, in which the lateral, asymmetric growth of the head is caused by excessive accumulation of cerebrospinal fluid, usually under increased pressure. Specific diagnostic tests may be necessary to differentiate the two conditions. Treatment is primarily symptomatic, with nursing care concentrated specifically on helping parents learn to care for a brain-damaged child. Also called **macrocephalia, megalocephaly.** Compare **microcephaly.** See also **hydrocephalus.** **—macrocephalic, macrocephalous,** *adj.,* **macrocephalus,** *n.*

macrocyte /mak′rəsīt/ [Gk, *makros* + *kytos,* cell], an abnormally large, mature erythrocyte usually exceeding 9 μm in diameter that is commonly seen in megaloblastic anemias. Compare **microcyte.** See also **macrocytic anemia.**

macrocytic /mak′rōsit′ik/ [Gk, *makros, kytos* + L, *icus,* form], (of a cell) larger than normal, such as the erythrocytes in macrocytic anemia.

macrocytic anemia, a disorder of the blood characterized by impaired erythropoiesis and the presence of large red blood cells in the circulation. Macrocytic anemia is most often the result of a deficiency of folic acid or vitamin B_{12}. Compare **microcytic anemia.**

macrocytosis /mak′rōsītō′sis/ [Gk, *makros, kytos* + *osis,* condition], an abnormal proliferation of macrocytes in the peripheral blood. Compare **poikilocytosis.** See also **anisocytosis.** (See Fig. p. 942.)

Macrodantin, a trademark for a urinary antibacterial (nitrofurantoin).

Macrodex, a trademark for a plasma expander (dextran).

macrodrip /mak′rōdrip/ [Gk, *makros* + AS, *drypan,* to fall in drops], (in intravenous therapy) an apparatus that is used to deliver measured amounts of IV solutions at specific flow rates based on the size of drops of the solution. The size of the drops is controlled by the fixed diameter of a plastic delivery tube. The drops delivered by a macrodrip are larger than those delivered by a microdrip. Different

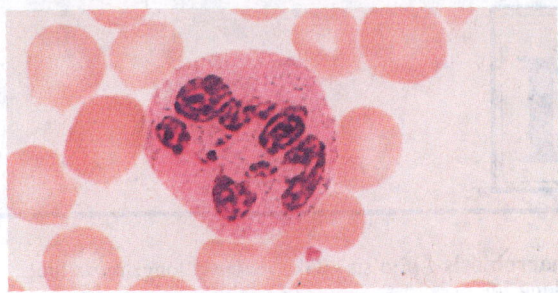

Macrocytosis *(Hayhoe, 1992)*

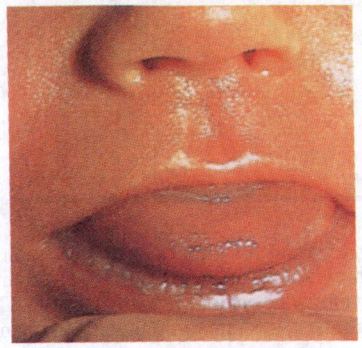

Macroglossia
(Zitelli, 1992/Courtesy Dr. Christine L Williams, New York Medical College)

macrodrips deliver 10, 15, or 20 drops per milliliter of solution. Macrodrips are not usually used to deliver a small amount of IV solution or to keep a vein open, because the time between drips is so long that a clot may form at the tip of the IV catheter. Compare **microdrip.**

macroelement. See **macronutrient.**

macroencephalic. See **macrencephaly.**

macroencephalic, macroencephaly. See **macrencephaly.**

macrogamete /-gam′ēt/ [Gk, *makros* + *gamete*, spouse], a large, nonmotile female gamete of certain thallophytes and sporozoa, specifically the malarial parasite *Plasmodium*. It corresponds to the ovum of the higher animals and is fertilized by the smaller, motile male gamete. See also **microgamete.**

macrogametocyte /-gamē′təsīt/ [Gk, *makros, gamete* + *kytos*, cell], an enlarged merozoite that undergoes meiosis to form the mature female gamete during the sexual phase of the life cycle of certain thallophytes and sporozoa, specifically the malarial parasite *Plasmodium*. Macrogametocytes are found in the red blood cells of a person infected with the malarial parasite, but they must be ingested by a female *Anopheles* mosquito to complete the maturation process and develop into a macrogamete.

macrogenitosomia /mak′rōjen′itōsō′mē·ə/ [Gk, *makros* + L, *genitalis*, genitalia; Gk, *soma*, body], a congenital condition in which the genitalia are abnormal because of an excess of androgen during fetal development. It is characterized in boys by enlarged external genitalia and in girls by pseudohermaphroditism.

macroglobulinemia /mak′rōglob′yōōline′mē·ə/ [Gk, *makros* + L, *globulus*, small ball; Gk, *haima*, blood], a form of monoclonal gammopathy in which immunoglobulin (IgM) is overproduced by the clones of a plasma B cell in response to an antigenic signal. Increased viscosity of the blood may result in circulatory impairment, weakness, neurologic disorders, and fatigue. Normal immunoglobulin synthesis is decreased, and the person is susceptible to infection, particularly bacterial pneumonia and septicemia. Treatment may include therapeutic plasma exchange to lower the viscosity. Also called **Waldenström's macroglobulinemia.** See also **multiple myeloma.**

macroglossia /mak′rōglos′ē·ə/ [Gk, *makros* + *glossa*, tongue], a congenital anomaly characterized by excessive size of the tongue, as seen in certain syndromes of congenital defects, including Down's syndrome.

macrognathia /mak′rōnā′thē·ə/ [Gk, *makros* + *gnathos*, jaw], an abnormally large growth of the jaw. Compare **micrognathia.** –**macrognathic,** *adj.*

macrolide /ma′krōlīd/, any of a group of antibiotics produced by actinomycetes. They include erythromycin and troleandomycin. Macrolides are generally used against gram-positive bacteria and in patients allergic to penicillins.

macromolecule /-mol′əkyōōl/ [Gk, *makros* + L, *moles*, mass], a molecule of colloidal size, such as proteins, nucleic acids, or polysaccharides.

macronucleus /-nōō′klē·əs/ [Gk, *makros* + L, *nucleus*, nut], **1.** a large nucleus. **2.** (in protozoa) the larger of two nuclei in each cell; it governs cell metabolism and growth as opposed to the micronucleus, which functions in sexual reproduction.

macronutrient /-nōō′triənt/ [Gk, *makros* + L, *nutriens*, nourishing], a chemical element required in relatively large quantities for the normal physiologic processes of the body. Macronutrients include carbon, hydrogen, oxygen, nitrogen, potassium, sodium, calcium, chloride, magnesium, phosphorus, and sulfur. Also called **macroelement, major element.** Compare **micronutrient.**

macrophage /mak′rəfāj/ [Gk, *makros* + *phagein*, to eat], any phagocytic cell of the reticuloendothelial system including specialized Kupffer's cells in the liver and spleen, and histocyte in loose connective tissue. See also **phagocyte, reticuloendothelial system.**

macrophage activating factor (MAF) [Gk. *makros*, long; *phagein*, to eat; L, *activus*, active; *facere*, to make], a

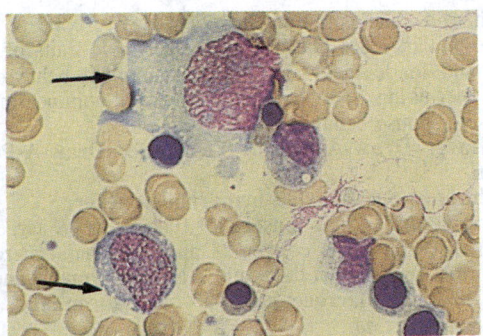

Macrophages in bone marrow *(Powers, 1989)*

lymphokine released from a sensitized leukocyte that induces changes in the appearance and function of macrophages as needed to make them active against certain antigens.

macrophage migration inhibiting factor [Gk, *makros,* large; *phagein,* to eat; L, *migrare,* to wander; *inhibere,* to restrain; *facere,* to make], a lymphokine produced by leukocytes that immobilizes marcophages after contact with an antigen. Also called **macrophage inhibition factor (MIF).**

macropsia /makrop′sē·ə/ [Gk, *makros,* large; *opsis,* vision], a visual abnormality in which objects appear larger than they actually are.

macroreentry /mak′rōrĕ·en′trē/ [Gk, *makros* + L, *re,* again; Fr, *entree,* entry], (in cardiology) a reentry circuit with anterograde conduction down one of the bundle branches and retrograde conduction up another. It causes ventricular tachycardia with a BBB pattern and a relatively narrow QRS.

macroscopic /-skop′ik/ [Gk, *makros,* large; *skopein,* to view], large enough to be examined with the naked eye.

macroscopic anatomy. See **gross anatomy.**

macrosis /makrō′sis/ [Gk, *makros,* large; *osis,* condition], an increase in the size or volume of an object.

macrosomia. See **gigantism.**

macula /mak′yələ/, *pl.* **maculae** [L, spot], **1.** a small pigmented area or a spot that appears separate or different from the surrounding tissue. **2.** See **macula lutea.**

macula adherens. See **desmosome.**

macula albidae [L, *macula,* spot; *albidare,* to make white], small white areas in the serous membranes of the pericardium or in the peritoneum or pleura. Also called **milk patch, tache laiteuse** /täsh′latœs′/.

macula cerulea. See **blue spot,** def. 1.

macula densa [L, *macula,* spot; *densus,* thick], a thickening in the wall of a distal tubule of the kidney nephron at a point where it is in contact with the afferent glomerulus. It may be part of a negative-feedback system for sodium.

macula lutea, an oval yellow spot at the center of the retina 2 mm from the optic nerve. It contains a pit, no blood vessels, and the fovea centralis. Central vision occurs when an image is focused directly on the fovea centralis of the macula lutea. Also called *(informal)* **macula.**

macular degeneration /mak′yələr/ [L, *macula,* spot; *degenerare,* to deviate], a progressive deterioration of the maculae of the retina and choroid of the eye. The condition is an effect of several diseases, such as **retinitis pigmentosa.**

macular rash [L, *macula,* spot; OFr, *rasche*], a skin eruption in which the lesions are flat and less than one centimeter in diameter.

macula solaris [L, *macula,* spot; *solaris,* sun], a freckle.

macule /mak′yōōl/ [L, *macula,* spot], **1.** a small, flat blemish or discoloration that is flush with the skin surface. Examples are freckles and the rashes of measles and roseola. Compare **papule. 2.** a gray scar on the cornea that is visible without magnification. **—macular,** *adj.*

maculopapular rash /mak′yəlōpap′yələr/ [L, *macula,* spot + *papula,* pimple; OFr, *rasche*], a skin eruption with distinctive macules or papules, or both.

maculopathy /mak′yəlop′əthē/ [L, *macula,* spot; Gk, *pathos,* disease], a form of macular degeneration involving primarily the macula lutea.

Madelung's neck. See **lipoma annulare colli.**

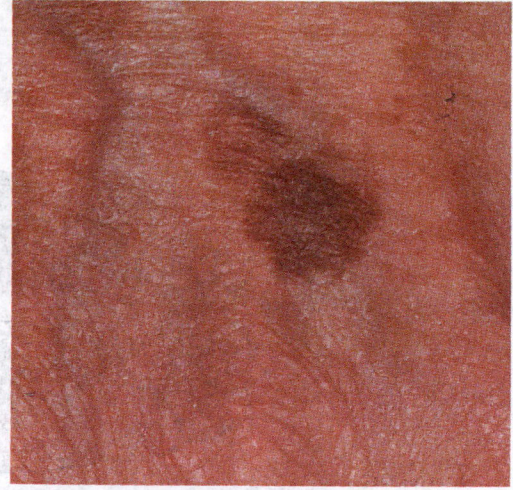

Macule *(du Vivier, 1993)*

mad hatter's disease. See **mercury poisoning.**

Madura foot /maj′ŏŏr′e/ [Madura, India; AS, *fot,* foot], a progressive, destructive, tropical fungal infection of the foot, named for a district in India. Also called **maduromycosis.** See also **mycetoma.** (See Fig. p. 944.)

MAF, abbreviation for **macrophage activating factor.**

mafenide acetate /maf′ənīd/, a topical antiinfective.

- INDICATION: It is prescribed in the treatment of burns.
- CONTRAINDICATIONS: Known hypersensitivity to this drug or to sulfonamide prohibits its use.
- ADVERSE EFFECTS: Among the more serious adverse effects are hypersensitivity reactions and suprainfections particularly by *Candida albicans.*

Maffuci's syndrome. See **enchondromatosis.**

magaldrate /mag′əldrāte/, an antacid containing a combination of magnesium and aluminum compounds.

- INDICATIONS: It is prescribed in the treatment of hypersensitivity and stomach upset associated with heartburn, sour stomach, or acid indigestion.
- CONTRAINDICATIONS: It may alter the absorption of several drugs, such as tetracyclines.
- ADVERSE EFFECTS: There may be a change in bowel function.

Magendie's law. See **Bell's law.**

magical thinking /maj′ikəl/, (in psychology) a belief that merely thinking about an event in the external world can cause it to occur. It is regarded as a form of regression to an early phase of development. It may be part of ideas of reference or may reach delusional proportions when the individual maintains a firm conviction about the belief, despite evidence to the contrary.

magic-bullet approach [Gk, *magikos,* sorcerer; Fr, *boulette,* small ball; L, *ad,* toward, *prope,* near], **1.** a therapeutic or diagnostic method that makes use of a specific relationship between a drug and a disease or organ. **2.** (in clinical medicine) the administration of a specific drug to cure or ameliorate a given disease or condition. **3.** (in traditional diagnostic radiology) the administration of a specific dye to facilitate the visualization by x-ray of a given organ, such as the intravenous injection of a specific dye

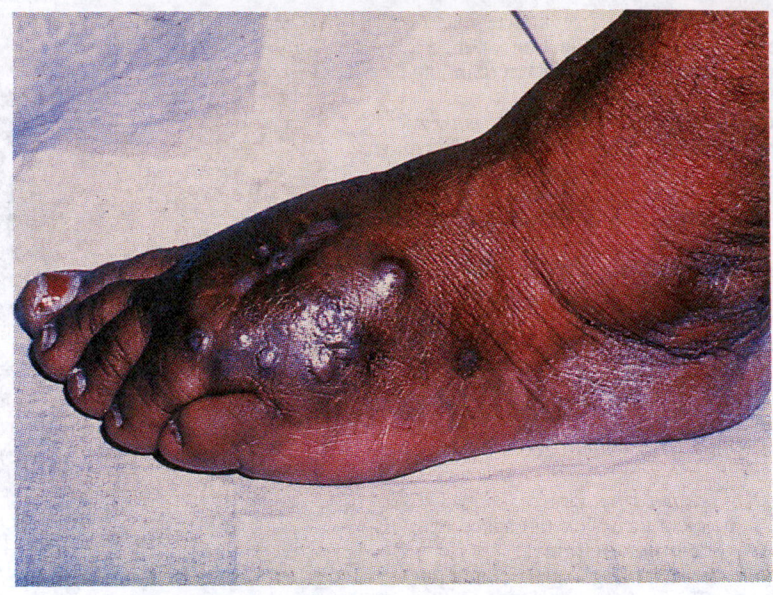

Madura foot (du Vivier, 1993/Courtesy Dr. Rod Hay)

for renal studies. **4.** (in nuclear medicine) the administration of a specific radionuclide tagged to an appropriate carrier to provide a scintillation camera image of a given organ or structure, such as the use of a substance containing phosphate and technetium for bone scanning.

magnesemia /mag′nəsē′mē·ə/, the presence of magnesium in the blood.

magnesia magma. See **milk of magnesia.**

magnesium (Mg) /magnē′sē·əm, magnē′zhəm/ [Magnesia, ancient Greek town], a silver-white mineral element. Its atomic number is 12; its atomic weight is 24.32. Magnesium occurs abundantly in nature, always in combination with other elements, in sea water, bones, seeds, in the chlorophyll in the green parts of plants, and in minerals, such as magnesite, dolomite, and carnalite. It is obtained chiefly by the electrolysis of fused salts containing magnesium chloride or by the thermal reduction of magnesia and is used in photography, metallurgy, and various medicines, such as magnesium sulfate. Magnesium is the second most abundant cation of the intracellular fluids in the body and is essential for many enzyme activities. It also is important to neurochemical transmissions and muscular excitability. The body of the average 145-pound adult contains about 2000 mEq of magnesium, about 50% of which is in the bones, 45% existing as intracellular cations, and about 5% in the extracellular fluid. Intracellular concentrations of magnesium range from 5 to 30 mEq per kilogram, depending on the type of tissue. The concentration of magnesium in plasma is 1.5 to 2.2 mEq per liter, with about two thirds as free cation and one third bound to plasma proteins. Very little is known about the exchange of magnesium between the plasma, the intracellular capsule, and the bone. About 30% of the magnesium in the skeleton represents an exchangeable pool. The average adult in the United States ingests between 20 and 40 mEq of magnesium daily, and about one third of the quantity ingested is absorbed from the GI tract. Absorption occurs in the upper small bowel by means of an active process closely related to the transport system for calcium. Magnesium is excreted mainly by the kidney, and 3% to 5% of the magnesium is excreted in the urine. Most of the reabsorption of magnesium takes place in the proximal tubules of the kidney. Renal excretion of magnesium increases during diuresis induced by ammonium chloride, glucose, and organic mercurials. Diuretic therapy can cause hypomagnesemia. Small amounts of magnesium are excreted in milk and in the saliva. The element influences many enzymes in the body and is a cofactor of all enzymes participating in phosphate transfer reactions involving adenosine triphosphate and other nucleotide triphosphates, such as substrates. It is also essential to the interaction of intracellular particles and the binding of macromolecules to subcellular organelles, such as the binding of messenger RNA to ribosomes. Magnesium affects the central nervous, neuromuscular, and cardiovascular systems. Hypomagnesemia increases central nervous system irritability and may cause disorientation, convulsions, and psychosis. Some researchers report abnormally high concentrations of magnesium in the plasma of manic-depressive and schizophrenic individuals and abnormally low magnesium concentrations in the plasma of patients with endogenous and neurotic depressions. Magnesium tends to depress the action of skeletal muscle, and excessive magnesium inhibits the release of acetylcholine by motor nerve impulses. Insufficient magnesium in extracellular fluid increases the release of acetylcholine, increases muscular excitability, and can cause tetany. Excess magnesium in the body can slow the heartbeat, and concentrations of magnesium greater than 15 mEq per liter can produce cardiac arrest in diastole. Excess magnesium also causes vasodilation by directly affecting the blood vessels and by ganglionic blockade. Hypomagnesemia can cause changes in cardiac muscles and skeletal muscle and can cause nephrocalcinosis. Some of the abnormal conditions that can produce hypomagnesemia are diarrhea, steatorrhea, chronic alcoholism, and diabetes mellitus. Hypomagnesemia also may be associated with new-borns and infants who are fed cow's milk or artificial for-mulas, apparently because of the high phosphate-magnesium ratio in such diets. Hypomagnesemia is often treated with parenteral fluids containing magnesium sulfate or magnesium chloride. Hypermagnesemia is usually caused by renal insufficiency and is manifested by hypotension, electrocardiogram changes, muscle weakness, sedation, and a confused mental state.

magnesium sulfate, a salt of magnesium. Also called **Epsom salts.**

■ INDICATIONS: It is prescribed parenterally to prevent sei-zures, especially in preeclampsia, and orally to treat consti-pation and heartburn and to correct deficiency of magne-sium in the body.

■ CONTRAINDICATIONS: It is used with caution in patients with renal impairment or hypersensitivity to the drug. Re-spiratory depression, severe cardiac myopathy, heart block, or symptoms of appendicitis or fecal impaction prohibit its use.

■ ADVERSE EFFECTS: The most serious adverse reaction is cir-culatory collapse from excessive serum concentrations of magnesium. Respiratory depression, confusion, and muscle weakness also may occur.

magnetic field /magnet'ik/ [Gk, *magnesia* (lodestone); AS, *feld*], the region around any magnet in which its effects can be detected.

magnetic lines of force [Gk, *magnesia* (lodestone); L, *linea*, line; *fortis*, strong], theoretical lines of magnetism that surround a magnet or fill a magnetic field. The pres-ence of the magnetic force along the imaginary lines can be demonstrated by inserting a sensitive material such as iron filings into the lines of magnetic effect.

magnetic moment [L, *lapis*, *Magnes*, lodestone; *momen-tum*, movement], a measure of the net magnetic field pro-duced by an elementary particle or an atomic nucleus spin-ning about its own axis. These fields are similar to those produced by a bar magnet. It is the basis for nuclear mag-netic resonance imaging.

magnetic resonance (MR), **1.** a phenomenon in which the atomic nuclei of certain materials placed in a strong, static magnetic field will absorb radio waves supplied by a transmitter at particular frequencies. The energy of the ra-dio frequency photons promotes the nucleus from a low-energy state, in which the nuclear spin is aligned parallel to the strong magnetic field, to a higher energy state in which the nuclear spin has a component transverse or opposed to the field. These nuclei will occasionally revert to the lower energy state by emitting photons at characteristic (reso-nance) frequencies, providing information about the local magnetic field at the nucleus. The rate at which the nuclei revert, or relax, to the lower energy state when the source of radio waves is turned off is another important factor. See also **relaxation time. 2.** spectra emitted by phosphorus in body tissues as measured and imaged on phosphorus nuclear magnetic resonance instruments.

magnetic resonance imaging (MRI) [L, *lapis*, *Magnes*, lodestone; *resonare*, to sound again; *imago*, image], med-ical imaging that uses radiofrequency radiation as its source of energy. See also **nuclear magnetic resonance.**

magnetic susceptibility, a measure of the ability of a sub-stance to become magnetized.

magnetization /mag'nətīzā'shən/ [L, *lapis*, *Magnes*, lode-stone; Gk, *izein*, to cause], the magnetic polarization of a

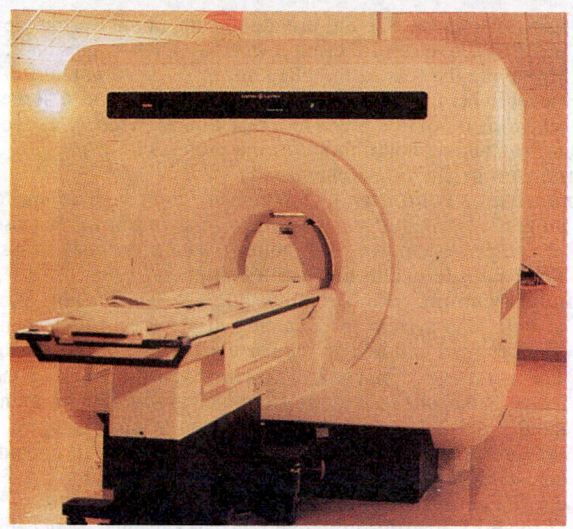

Clinical setting for magnetic resonance imaging
(Mourad, 1991)

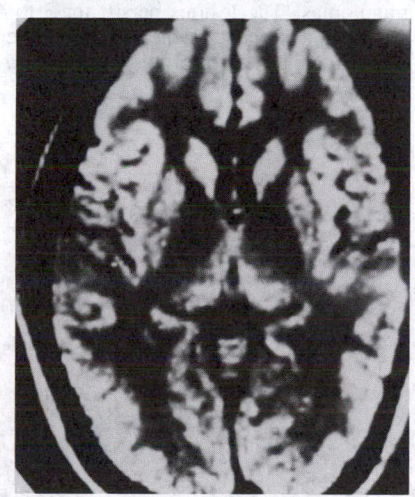

Magnetic resonance imaging

material produced by a magnetic field (magnetic moment per unit volume).

magnetron /mag'nətron/ [L, *lapis*, *Magnes*, lodestone, *trum*, device], a source of microwave energy used in med-ical linear accelerators to accelerate electrons to the thera-peutic energies.

magnification /mag'nifikā'shən/, (in psychology) cogni-tive distortion in which the effects of one's behavior are magnified. See also **minimization.**

magnification factor, (in radiology) the image size di-vided by the object size.

Mahaim fibers, conductive tracts in cardiac tissue running between the AV node or His bundle and the muscle of the ventricular septum. They conduct early excitation impulses.

Mahoney, Mary Eliza (1845–1926), the first black

American nurse. She did private nursing in the Boston area and was active in furthering intergroup relationships and in improving the role of the black nurse in the community. A medal in her name, established after her death, was first presented in 1936; it is given to a black nurse in recognition of an outstanding contribution to the profession.

main en griffe. See **clawhand.**

mainframe computer [AS, *maegen*, strength, *framian*, to progress; L, *computare*, to count], a large general-purpose computer system for high-volume data processing tasks. Compare **microcomputer, minicomputer.**

mainstreaming /mān′strēming/ [OE, *maegan*, might; ME, *strem*], the system of educating disabled or mildly mentally retarded children in regular classrooms, but with special assistance as needed. The term is also applied to the return of persons recovering from mental illness to the community.

maintenance dose /mān′tənəns/ [Fr, *maintenir*, to uphold; Gk, *dosis*, giving], the amount of drug required to keep a desired mean steady-state concentration in the tissues.

Majocchi's granuloma /mäjok′ēz/ [Domenico Majocchi, Italian dermatologist, b. 1849; L, *granulum*, small grain; Gk, *oma*, tumor], a rare type of tinea corporis that mainly affects the lower legs. It is caused by the fungus *Trichophyton*, which infects the hairs of the affected site and raises spongy granulomas. The lesions persist for 3 to 4 months and are gradually absorbed, or they necrose, often leaving deep scars. Also called **trichophytic granuloma.**

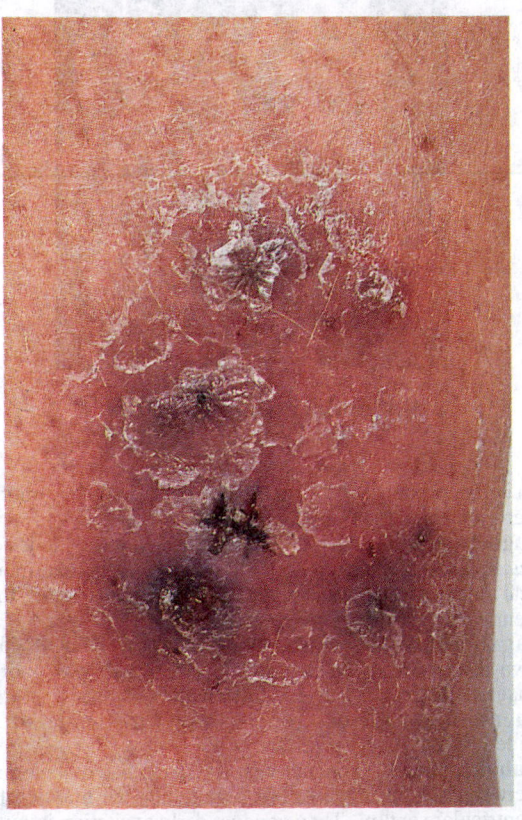

Majocci's granuloma *(du Vivier, 1993)*

major affective disorder [L, *magnus*, great; *affectus*, state of mind; *dis*, opposite of, *ordo*, rank], any of a group of psychotic disorders characterized by severe and inappropriate emotional responses, by prolonged and persistent disturbances of mood and related thought distortions, and by other symptoms associated with either depressed or manic states, such as occurs in bipolar disorder, depression, and involutional melancholia. The disorder is usually episodic but may be chronic or cyclic, as in the case of bipolar disorder.

major connector, a metal plate or bar, used for joining the components of one side of a removable partial denture to those on the opposite side of the dental arch.

major depressive episode. See **endogenous depression.**

major element. See **macronutrient.**

major histocompatibility complex (MHC) [L, *magnus*, great; Gk, *histos*, tissue; L, *compatibilis*, agreement; *complexus*, embrace], a group of proteins on the outer membrane of a cell that helps identify self and nonself (invading) molecules. MHC Class I molecules normally help the immune system discriminate between healthy body cells and those that may be precancerous or infected by viruses. MHC Class II molecules normally recognize foreign proteins. The MHC Class II molecules resemble the gp120 molecules on the outer membranes of HIV viruses, leading confused antibodies to attack the body's own T helper cells. Individuals with Type I diabetes have lower than normal levels of MHC Class I proteins, a susceptibility marker. Their immune systems fail to recognize their own beta cells.

major hysteria [ME, *maiour*, great; Gk, *hystera*, womb], an episode of psychogenic illness affecting a large group of individuals at the same time. Examples include the witchcraft trials of the seventeenth century and irrational mass reaction to the 1938 radio show based on H.G. Well's science-fiction novel, *War of the Worlds*. Also called **collective hysteria, epidemic hysteria, mass hysteria, mass panic, mass psychogenic illness.**

major medical insurance, insurance coverage designed to offset the costs of prolonged or catastrophic illness and injury. Most major medical insurance policies are written to pay a certain percentage of costs up to a predetermined figure, beyond which payment is in full up to a maximum amount, at which point payment ceases. Many require the insured to pay a specified initial, or deductible, amount.

major renal calyx. See **renal calyx.**

major surgery, any surgical procedure that requires general anesthesia or respiratory assistance. Compare **minor surgery.**

makro-. See **macro-.**

mal /mal, mäl/ [L, *malus*, bad], an illness or disease, such as grand mal or petit mal.

mal-, a prefix meaning 'bad, poor, or abnormal': *maladjustment, malalignment, malignant.*

malabsorption /mal′əbsôrp′shən/ [L, *malus* + *absorbere*, to swallow], impaired absorption of nutrients from the GI tract. It occurs in celiac disease, sprue, dysentery, diarrhea, and other disorders and may result from an inborn error of metabolism, malnutrition, or any chemical or anatomic condition of the digestive system that prevents normal absorption. See **inborn error of metabolism, malnutrition.**

malabsorption syndrome, a complex of symptoms resulting from disorders in the intestinal absorption of nutrients, characterized by anorexia, weight loss, bloating of the abdomen, muscle cramps, bone pain, and steatorrhea. Anemia, weakness, and fatigue occur because iron, folic acid, and vitamin B$_{12}$ are not absorbed in sufficient amounts. Among the many conditions causing this syndrome are gastric or small bowel resection, celiac disease, tropical sprue, Whipple's disease, intestinal lymphangiectasia, and cystic fibrosis. Treatment and prognosis are determined by the underlying condition. See also **celiac disease, cystic fibrosis, hypoproteinemia, tropical sprue.**

malacia /məlā′shə/ [Gk, *malakia*, softness], **1.** a morbid softening or a sponginess in any part or any tissue of the body. **2.** a craving for spicy foods, such as mustard, hot peppers, or pickles. **−malacic,** *adj.*

-malacia, a suffix meaning the 'softening of tissue': *cardiomalacia, esophagomalacia, tracheomalacia.*

malaco-, a combining form meaning 'a condition of abnormal softness': *malacoplakia, malacosarcosis.*

maladaptation /mal′adəptā′shən/ [L, *malus* + *adaptatio*], faulty intrapersonal adaptation to stress or change. It may involve a failure to make necessary changes in the desires, values, needs, and attitudes or an inability to make necessary adjustments in the external world. Illness often provokes maladaptive behavior that worsens the problems accompanying the illness.

maladjusted /mal′adjus′tid/ [L, *malus*, bad; *adjuxtare*, to bring together], appearing unable to maintain effective relationships needed to fit into the environment, and showing irritability, depression, and other psychogenic influences.

malady /mal′ədē/ [ME, *maladie*, sick], a disease or illness.

malaise /malāz′/ [Fr, discomfort], a vague feeling of bodily weakness or discomfort, often marking the onset of disease.

malalignment /mal′əlīn′mənt/ [L, *malus* + *ad*, to, *linea*, line], a failure of parts of the body to align normally, such as the teeth in the dental arch.

malar /mā′lər/ [L, *mala*, cheek], of or pertaining to the cheek or the cheek bone.

malaria /məler′ē·ə/ [L, *malus*, bad, *aer*, air], a serious infectious illness caused by one or more of at least four species of the protozoan genus *Plasmodium*, characterized by chills, fever, anemia, an enlarged spleen, and a tendency to recur. The disease is transmitted from human to human by a bite from an infected *Anopheles* mosquito. Malarial infection can also be spread by blood transfusion from an infected patient or by the use of an infected hypodermic needle. Although the endemic disease is limited largely to tropical areas of South and Central America, Africa, and Asia, a number of new cases are brought to the United States by refugees, military personnel, and travelers returning from malarial areas. *Plasmodium* parasites penetrate the erythrocytes of the human host, where they mature, reproduce, and burst out periodically. Malarial paroxysms occur at regular intervals, coinciding with the development of a new generation of parasites in the body. Because the life cycle of the infecting parasite varies according to species, the clinical patterns of chills and fever differ as do the course and severity of the disease. Bouts of malaria usually last from 1 to 4 weeks, with attacks occurring less frequently as the disease progresses. Relapse is common, and the disease can persist for years. Diagnosis is made by demonstrating the *Plasmodium* parasite in a blood smear. The organism is most likely to be seen in the blood during an acute attack. The exact species of *Plasmodium* must be identified, because the treatment and prognosis vary according to the strain found. Chloroquine, given orally or intramuscularly,

is the drug of choice for all but those strains of *Plasmodium* resistant to chloroquine, which are treated with a combination of quinine, pyrimethamine, and one of the sulfonamides or sulfones. Modern antimalarial drugs can suppress symptoms or cure malaria completely. Symptoms of headache, nausea, muscle ache, and high fever can be relieved with cold compresses, aspirin, and fluids. Through the use of insecticides and by destroying the swampy habitat of *Anopheles*, the disease has been eliminated from many parts of the world where it has been endemic. Worldwide eradication of the disease has not been possible, however, and insecticide-resistant mosquitoes and drug-resistant malarial protozoa have arisen. Prophylaxis with antimalarial drugs is still important for those visiting endemic areas. The use of netting and mosquito repellent is also encouraged. See also **antimalarial, biduotertian fever, blackwater fever, falciparum malaria,** *Plasmodium,* **quartan malaria, tertian malaria. −malarial,** *adj.*

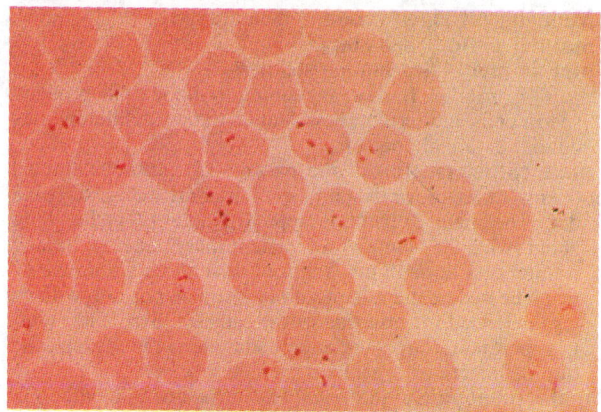

Malaria—presence of *plasmodium falciparum* in the blood
(Murray, 1990)

malarial hemoglobinuria. See **blackwater fever.**

malarial parasite /məler′ē·əl/ [It, *malaria*, bad air; Gk, *parasitos*, guest], one of four known species of *Plasmodium* that may be injected into the human bloodstream by an anopheline mosquito to begin the cycle of malarial disease.

Malassezia /mal′əsē′zē·ə/ [Louis C. Malassez, French physiologist, b. 1842], a genus of fungi. *M. furfur* causes tinea versicolor (previous name: *Pityrosporum oviculare*). *M. ovalis* is a nonpathogenic organism found in sebaceous areas (previous name: *Pityrosporum ovale*). (See Fig. p. 948.)

malathion poisoning /malā′thē·on, məl′əthī′on/, a toxic condition caused by the ingestion or absorption through the skin of malathion, an organophosphorus insecticide. Symptoms include vomiting, nausea, abdominal cramps, headache, dizziness, weakness, confusion, convulsions, and respiratory difficulties. Treatment includes immediate intravenous administration of atropine, followed by pralidoxime chloride, gastric lavage, a saline cathartic, respiratory assistance, and oxygen. Malathion is much less toxic than parathion and is the only organophosphorus insecticide approved for household use.

malaxation. See **pétrissage.**

M-N

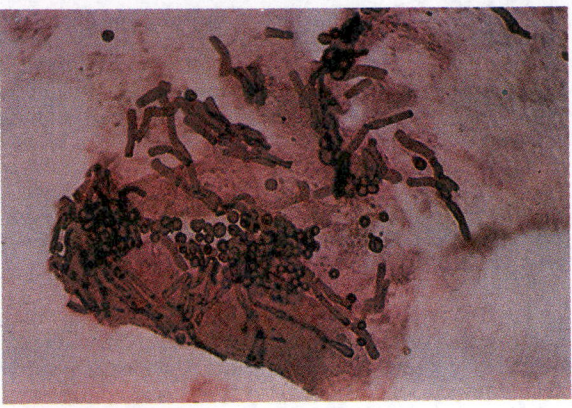

Malassezia furfur (Murray, 1990)

Malayan pit viper venom. See **ancrod.**

mal del pinto. See **pinta.**

mal de mer. See **motion sickness.**

male [L, *mas*], **1.** of or pertaining to the sex that produces sperm cells and fertilizes the female to beget children; masculine. **2.** a male person.

male catheterization, the passage of a catheter through the male urethra for the purpose of draining the urinary bladder. The male catheter is approximately 12 inches long, about twice the length of a female urinary catheter, because it must pass through the length of the urethra within the penis. The male patient is placed in a supine position with the legs extended for insertion of the catheter. Sterile technique is important throughout the procedure to avoid the introduction of infectious organisms into the bladder.

male menopause [L, *mas,* male; *mensis,* month; Gk, *pauein,* to cease], a late middle-age psychogenic condition affecting some men who experience anxiety over diminished potency, increased fatigue, thinning and graying hair, and other signs of aging. Also called **male climacterium.**

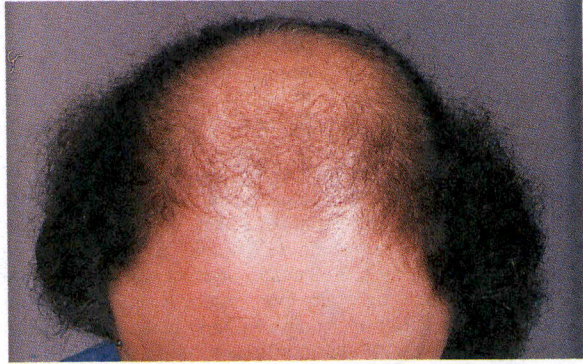

Male pattern alopecia (du Vivier, 1993)

male pattern alopecia [L, *mas,* male; ME, *patron*; Gk, *alopex,* fox mange], a common form of baldness in males, beginning at the front and spreading gradually until a fringe

remains around the back and temples. Individual differences are determined by heredity, androgenic stimulation, and aging. A similar hair loss pattern may develop in women after menopause. Also called **male pattern baldness.**

male reproductive system assessment, an evaluation of the condition of the patient's genitalia, reproductive history, and past and present genitourinary infections and disorders.
■ METHOD: In a relaxed, professional interview the procedures to be conducted are explained and the patient is reassured that his privacy will be scrupulously maintained. He is questioned about his offspring, sexual activity, the existence of nocturia, urgency, frequency, dysuria, urethral discharge, hernia, genital sores, discomfort or pain in the groin, lower back, or legs, and past treatment for epididymitis, gonorrhea, herpes genitalis, hydrocele, nonspecific urethritis, orchitis, prostatitis, syphilis, and varicocele. The examiner, while inspecting the genitalia, wears rubber gloves to prevent infection. The penis is examined for swelling, inflammation, and lesions, such as herpes vesicles or a syphilitic sore, chancre, or scar. Anomalies that may be noted include hypospadias or epispadias, resulting from failed closure of the urethra, elongation of the foreskin constricting the urinary meatus, or swelling of the glans caused by a retracted, tight foreskin. The urethral orifice is inspected for a purulent or bloody discharge, and the scrotum is observed for symmetry and shape; in elderly or debilitated men the scrotum may be elongated and flat. The normally smooth testes, epididymes, and spermatic cords are palpated for the presence of beading, varicosities, and the size, location, and consistency of any scrotal mass; fluid felt around the testes may be seen by darkening the room and illuminating the scrotum with a flashlight. The patient is asked to cough or bear down to reveal a hernia, and the abdomen is palpated above the symphysis pubis to determine if the bladder is distended. The inguinal lymph nodes are palpated, and the amount and distribution of pubic hair is observed. The prostate may be examined with the patient in the Sims' knee-chest position or lithotomy position, but, when possible, it is preferable for the patient to stand bent at a right angle over a table as the examiner's well-lubricated gloved forefinger sweeps the rectal circumference and palpates the lobes and medial sulcus of the gland. The size, consistency, and any localized nodule suggesting a neoplasm of the normally smooth, firm prostate are carefully noted, and the findings are recorded as on a clock dial with the symphysis pubis representing 12 o'clock. When additional studies are indicated, a smear is prepared from the first urine voided after massage of the prostate. Enzyme tests showing elevated phosphatase levels in serum suggest prostate cancer, but a diagnosis is usually established by a biopsy. Tissue may be obtained by a perineal, transurethral, or transrectal needle biopsy, but the most accurate method is an open perineal biopsy, which permits identification of the suspect lesion and the removal of multiple specimens. The assessment includes laboratory studies of discharge from the penis. A gram-stained smear usually confirms or rules out a diagnosis of gonorrhea, and a fluorescent-tagged antibody method may be required if the result is equivocal. Cultures may be needed to determine whether nonspecific urethritis (NSU) is caused by *Escherichia coli, Pseudomonas, Staphylococcus, Streptococcus,* or organisms of other pathogenic genera. Syphilis may be diagnosed by the Venereal Disease Research Laboratory serologic test, but the Fluorescent Treponemal Antibody-Absorption test is the

most sensitive and specific diagnostic measure. If infertility is a problem, examinations of multiple semen samples are conducted; each specimen collected after 3 days of abstinence is inspected in the laboratory to determine if the volume of the ejaculate approximates the normal 3.5 ml average and if the semen has a pH of 7.7 and a sperm count of 60 to 150 million per milliliter.

■ INTERVENTIONS: The nurse conducts the interview and examination, assembles the results of laboratory studies, and urges the patient to inform his sex partner, or partners, if an infectious disease is diagnosed. Throughout the assessment the nurse recognizes that the patient may be reluctant to discuss his symptoms and activities and may be sensitive about the necessary procedures.

■ OUTCOME CRITERIA: A careful, understanding evaluation of the male patient's reproductive system helps to establish the diagnosis and plan the treatment and aids in allaying the patient's anxiety. The assessment also serves as a public health measure by encouraging the reporting of a sexually transmitted disease to the patient's contacts and proper authorities.

male sexual dysfunction, impaired or inadequate ability of a man to carry on his sex life to his own satisfaction. Symptoms, often psychologic in origin, include difficulties in starting and maintaining an erection, premature ejaculation, inability to ejaculate, and even loss of desire. Men are often embarrassed by the problem and ask the physician to treat a 'prostate problem,' hoping that the covert message becomes clear. Compare **female sexual dysfunction.** See also **impotence, premature ejaculation, sexual dysfunction.**

male sterility [L, *mas* + *sterilis*, barren], the inability of a man to produce sperm. Causes may include environmental factors such as exposure to heat or radiation, undescended testes, varicocele, prolonged fever, endocrine disorders, and abuse of alcohol or marijuana. See also **infertility.**

malfeasance /malfē′zəns/ [Fr, *malfaire*, to do evil], performance of an unlawful, wrongful act. Compare **misfeasance, nonfeasance.**

malformation /mal′fôrmā′shən/ [L, *malus* + *forma*, shape], an anomalous structure in the body. See also **congenital anomaly.**

malfunction /mal′fungk′shən/ [L, *malus*, bad; *functio*, performance], **1.** the inability to function normally. **2.** not to function normally.

Malgaigne's fracture of pelvis /malgā′nyəz/ [Joseph F. Malgaigne, French surgeon, b. 1806], trauma involving multiple pelvic fractures, including fracture of the wing of the ilium or sacrum and fracture of the ipsilateral pubic rami, with associated upper displacement of the hemipelvis.

malicious prosecution /məlish′əs/ [L, *malitia*, wickedness; *prosequi*, to pursue], (in law) a suit begun in malice and pursued without sufficient cause. It is usually an action for damages. Malicious prosecution is a wrongful civil proceeding, and a person who takes an active part in initiating or continuing it is subject to liability.

malign /məlīn′/ [ME, *malignen*, deceptive], to show ill will or maliciousness, to act viciously, to harm.

malignant /məlig′nənt/ [L, *malignus*, ill-disposed], **1.** also **virulent.** tending to become worse and cause death. **2.** (describing a cancer) anaplastic, invasive, and metastatic. **–malignancy,** *n.*

malignant dysentery [L, *malignus*, bad disposition; Gk, *dys*, bad; *enteron*, bowel], a potentially fatal form of dysentery in which symptoms are severe.

malignant endocarditis [L, *malignus*, bad disposition; Gk, *endon*, within; *kardia*, heart; *itis*, inflammation], a bacterial infection of the innermost layer of the heart but affecting primarily the valves after they have already been damaged by rheumatic fever or another disease. The valve cusps may be perforated or ulcerated. The patient usually experiences fever and sweating, emboli, and possible septicemia. Also called **bacterial endocarditis.**

malignant ependymoma. See **ependymoblastoma.**

malignant granuloma [L, *malignus*, bad disposition; *granulum*, little grain; *oma*, tumor], a malignant lymphoma, such as Hodgkin's disease, or a lymphosarcoma.

malignant hemangioendothelioma. See **angiosarcoma.**

malignant hepatoma, a malignant tumor of the liver. Primary liver cancer is relatively rare in the United States, occurring one sixth to one fifth as often as in Africa and the Far East. The only effective treatment is surgical excision of the tumor. This is often not feasible, because the tumors grow rapidly and spread through both lobes of the liver. The prognosis is poor. Also called **hepatocarcinoma, hepatocellular carcinoma, liver cell carcinoma.**

malignant hypertension, the most lethal form of hypertension. It is a fulminating condition, characterized by severely elevated blood pressure that commonly damages the intima of small vessels, the brain, retina, heart, and kidneys. It affects more blacks than whites and may be caused by a variety of factors, such as stress, genetic predisposition, obesity, the use of tobacco, the use of oral contraceptives, high intake of sodium chloride, a sedentary lifestyle, and aging. Many patients with this condition exhibit signs of hypokalemia, alkalosis, and aldosterone secretion rates even higher than those associated with primary aldosteronism. See also **essential hypertension.**

malignant hyperthermia (MH), an autosomal dominant trait characterized by often fatal hyperthermia with rigidity of the muscles occurring in affected people exposed to certain anesthetic agents, particularly halothane and succinylcholine. Treatment includes the administration of dantrolene, 100% oxygen, cooling procedures, and the correction of acidosis and hyperkalemia. Patients who have malignant hyperthermia are informed of their condition so that close relatives who may be susceptible may be tested.

malignant malnutrition. See **kwashiorkor.**

malignant melanoma. See **melanoma.**

malignant mesenchymoma, a sarcoma that contains mesenchymal elements.

malignant mole. See **melanoma.**

malignant neoplasm, a tumor that tends to grow, invade, and metastasize. The tumor usually has an irregular shape and is composed of poorly differentiated cells. If untreated, it may result in the death of the organism.

malignant neuroma. See **neurosarcoma.**

malignant pustule. See **anthrax.**

malignant tumor, a neoplasm that characteristically invades surrounding tissue, metastasizes to distant sites, and contains anaplastic cells. A malignant tumor may result in the death of the host if treatment does not intervene.

malingering /məling′gəring/ [Fr, *malingre*, puny, weak], a willful and deliberate feigning of the symptoms of a disease or injury to gain some consciously desired end.

Compare **compensation neurosis.** −**malinger,** *v.,* **malingerer,** *n.*

malleable /mal'ē·əbəl/ [L, *malleare,* to beat], able to be pressed, hammered, or otherwise forced into a shape without breaking.

malleolus /məlē'ələs/, *pl.* **malleoli** [L, little hammer], a rounded bony process, such as the protuberance on each side of the ankle.

malleolus fibulae. See **external malleolus.**

mallet deformity [ME, *maillet,* maul], a flexion abnormality of the distal joint of a finger or toe. It may be caused by severe damage such as rupture of the terminal tendon and is characterized by a loss of normal extension ability. See also **hammertoe.**

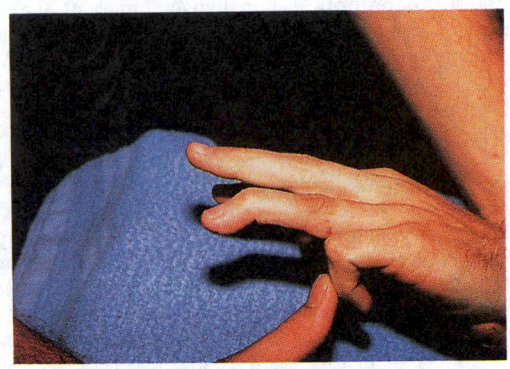

Mallet deformity *(Grossman, 1993)*

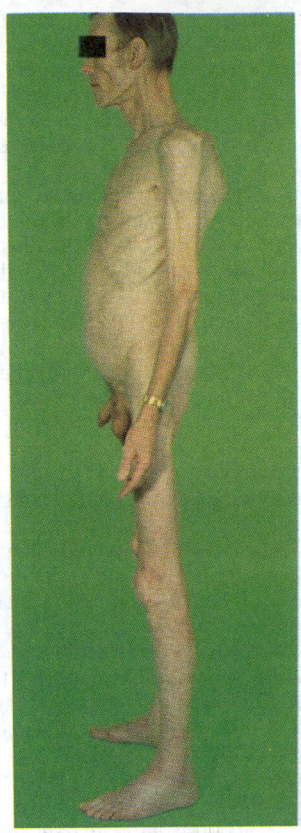

Malnutrition resulting in severe weight loss
(Forbes, 1993)

mallet finger. See **hammer finger.**

mallet fracture, avulsion fracture of the dorsal base of a distal phalanx of the hand or foot, involving the associated extensor apparatus and causing dropped flexion of the distal segment.

malleus /mal'ē·əs/, *pl.* **mallei** [L, hammer], one of the three ossicles in the middle ear, resembling a hammer with a head, neck, and three processes. It is connected to the tympanic membrane and transmits sound vibrations to the incus, which communicates with the stapes. Compare **incus, stapes.** See also **middle ear.**

Mallory bodies /mal'ərē/ [Frank B. Mallory, American pathologist, b. 1862; AS, *bodig,* body], an eosinophilic cytoplasmic inclusion, alcoholic hyalin, found in the liver cells. It is typically, but not always, associated with acute alcoholic liver injury. See also **cirrhosis.**

Mallory-Weiss syndrome [G. Kenneth Mallory, American pathologist, b. 1926; Soma Weiss, American physician, b. 1899], a condition characterized by massive bleeding after a tear in the mucous membrane at the junction of the esophagus and the stomach. The laceration is usually caused by protracted vomiting, most commonly in alcoholics or in people whose pylorus is obstructed. The esophageal tear is located by esophagoscopy or arteriography. Surgery is rarely necessary to stop the bleeding. After repair, the prognosis is excellent.

malnutrition /mal'nōōtrish'ən/ [L, *malus* + *nutrire,* to nourish], any disorder of nutrition. It may result from an unbalanced, insufficient, or excessive diet or from the impaired absorption, assimilation, or use of foods. Compare **deficiency disease.**

malocclusion /mal'əklōō'zhən/ [L, *malus* + *occludere,* to shut up], abnormal contact of the teeth of the upper jaw with the teeth of the lower jaw. See also **occlusion.**

malonic acid /məlō'nik/, a white, crystalline, highly toxic substance used as an intermediate compound in the production of barbiturates.

malpighian body /malpig'ē·ən/ [Marcello Malpighi, Italian physician, b. 1628; AS, *bodig,* body], **1.** the renal corpuscle, which includes a glomerulus with Bowman's capsule. **2.** also called **lymphatic nodule.** lymphoid tissue surrounding the arteries of the spleen.

malpighian corpuscle [Marcello Malpighi; L, *corpusculum,* little body], one of a number of small, round, deepred bodies in the cortex of the kidney, each communicating with a renal tubule. Malpighian corpuscles average about 0.2 mm in diameter, each capsule composed of two parts: a central glomerulus and a glomerular capsule. The corpuscles are thought to be part of a filtering system through which nonprotein components of blood plasma enter the tubules for urinary excretion. Also called **malpighian body, renal corpuscle.**

malpractice /malprak'tis/ [L, *malus* + Gk, *praktikos,* performance], (in law) professional negligence that is the proximate cause of injury or harm to a patient, resulting from a lack of professional knowledge, experience, or skill that can be expected in others in the profession or from a failure to exercise reasonable care or judgment in the application of professional knowledge, experience, or skill.

malpresentation /malpres'əntā'shən/ [L, *malus*, bad; *praesentare*, to show], an abnormal position of the fetus in the birth canal.

malrotation /mal'rōtā'shən/, **1.** any abnormal rotation of an organ or body part, such as the vertebral column or a tooth. **2.** a failure of the intestinal tract or other viscera to undergo normal rotation during embryonic development.

Malta fever. See **brucellosis.**

malunion /malyōō'nyən/ [L, *malus* + *unus*, one], an imperfect union of previously fragmented bone or other tissue.

mamm-, a combining form meaning 'of or pertaining to the mammary gland; the breast': *mammectomy, mammogram, mammotropic.*

mamma. See **mammary gland.**

mammary /mam'ərē/ [L, *mamma*, breast], pertaining to or resembling the mammary gland.

mammary duct. See **lactiferous duct.**

mammary gland [L, *mamma*, breast; *glans*, acorn], one of two discoid, hemispheric glands on the chest of mature females, present in rudimentary form in children and in males. Glandular tissue forms a radius of lobes containing alveoli, each lobe having a system of ducts for the passage of milk from the alveoli to the nipple. The central portion of the breast is filled with glandular tissue; the periphery is made up mostly of adipose tissue. The left breast is usually larger than the right. Also called **breast, mamma.** See also **lactation.**

mammary papilla. See **nipple.**

mammillary body /mam'iler'ē/ [L, *mammilla*, nipple; AS, *bodig*, body], either of the two small round masses of gray matter in the hypothalamus located close to one another in the interpeduncular space.

mammogram /mam'əgram/ [L, *mamma* + Gk, *gramma*, record], an x-ray film of the soft tissues of the breast.

mammography /mamog'rəfē/, radiography of the soft tissues of the breast to allow identification of various benign and malignant neoplastic processes.

mammoplasty /mam'əplas'tē/ [L, *mamma* + Gk, *plassein*, to mold], plastic reshaping of the breasts, performed to reduce or lift enlarged or sagging breasts, to enlarge small breasts, or to reconstruct a breast after removal of a tumor. To reduce the size of the breasts and raise them, excess tissue is removed from the underside of the breasts; the breast is then lifted and the nipple brought through an opening in an overhanging skin flap. To enlarge a breast, a plastic prosthesis is inserted in a pouch formed beneath the breast on the chest wall. The complications after surgery are infection and, with the use of implants, rejection reaction of tissues to the foreign body. The nurse observes the nipples for signs of vascular insufficiency or congestion, applies a firm supporting breast binder, and instructs the patient not to use her arms to lift herself.

mammothermography /mam'ōthərmog'rəfē/ [L, *mamma* + Gk, *therme*, heat, *graphein*, to record], a diagnostic procedure in which thermography is used for examining the breast to detect abnormal growths. Compare **mammography.** See also **thermography.**

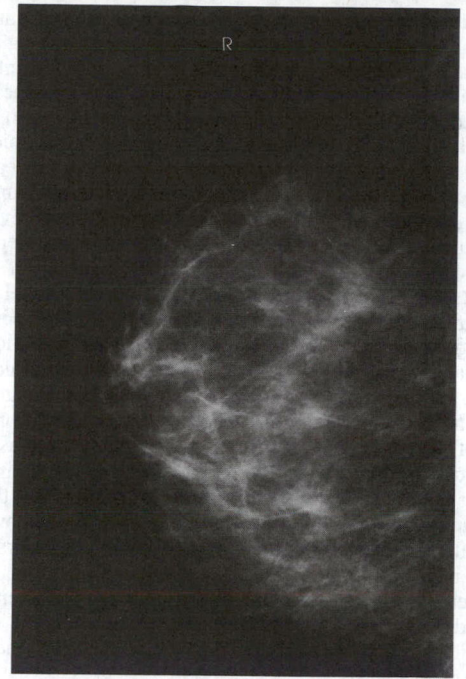

Mammogram

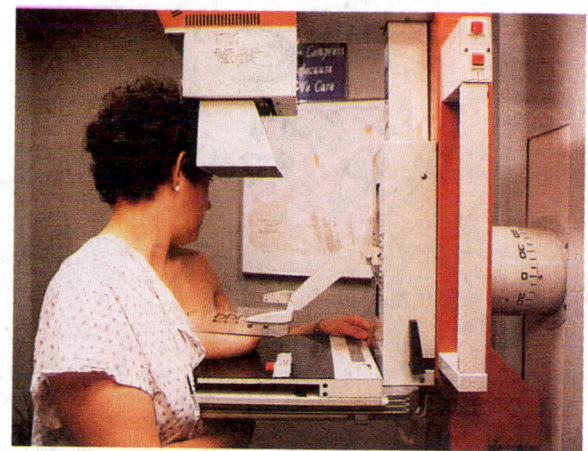

Clinical setting for mammography (Belcher, 1992)

man-, a combining form meaning 'of or referring to the hand': *manoptoscope, manual, manudynamometer.*

managed care, a health care system in which there is administrative control over primary health care services in a medical group practice. Redundant facilities and services are eliminated and costs are reduced. Health education and preventive medicine are emphasized. Patients may pay a flat fee for basic family care but may be charged additional fees for secondary care services of specialists. See also **health maintenance organizations.**

management of therapeutic regimen (individual), in-

effective, a nursing diagnosis accepted by the Tenth National Conference on the Classification of Nursing Diagnoses. It is defined as a pattern of regulating and integrating into daily living a program for treatment of illness and the sequelae of illness that is unsatisfactory for meeting specific health goals. Defining characteristics are choices of daily living ineffective for meeting the goals of a treatment or prevention program, acceleration of illness symptoms, verbalized desire to manage the treatment and prevention of sequelae, verbalized difficulty with regulation/integration of one or more prescribed regimens for treatment of illness and its effects or prevention of complications, verbalization that intimates that the patient would not attempt to include treatment regimens in daily routines, and verbalization that intimates that the patient would not attempt to reduce risk factors for progression of illness and sequelae. Related factors include complexity of the health care system, complexity of the therapeutic regimen, decisional conflicts, economic difficulties, excessive demands made on the individual or family, family conflict, family patterns of health care, inadequate number and types of cues to action, knowledge deficits, mistrust of regimen and/or health care personnel, perceived seriousness, perceived susceptibility, perceived barriers, perceived benefits, powerlessness, and social support deficits. See also **nursing diagnosis.**

Mandelamine, a trademark for an antibacterial (methenamine mandelate).

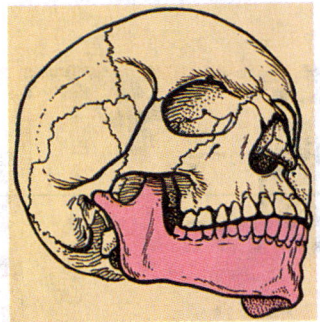

Mandible (Seeley, 1992)

mandible /man'dibəl/ [L, *mandere,* to chew], a large bone constituting the lower jaw. It contains the lower teeth and consists of a horizontal portion, a body, and two perpendicular rami that join the body at almost right angles. The body of the mandible is curved, somewhat resembling a horseshoe, and has two surfaces and two borders. The external surface is marked by the symphysis menti, indicating the junction of the two halves of the mandible in the fetus. Each ramus is topped by the anterior coronoid process and the posterior condyle, prominences separated by the mandibular notch. The superior border of the mandible contains sockets for the 16 lower teeth. The inferior border provides a groove for the facial artery. The mandible and its rami provide attachment for various muscles, such as the masseter, temporalis, pterygoideus lateralis, digastricus, mentalis, genioglossi, geniohyoidei, and mylohyoideus. Also called **inferior maxillary bone.** Compare **maxilla. –mandibular,** *adj.*

mandibular arch /mandib'yələr/ [L, *mandere,* to chew; *ar-*

cus, bow], the first visceral arch from which the lower jaw bone develops.

mandibular canal [L, *mandere + canalis,* channel], (in dentistry) a passage or channel that extends from the mandibular foramen on the medial surface of the ramus of the mandible to the mental foramen. It holds mandibular blood vessels and a portion of the mandibular branch of the trigeminal nerve.

mandibular notch, a depression in the inferior border of the mandible, anterior to the attachments of the masseter muscle, where the external facial muscles cross the lower border of the mandible. It is a landmark that may be accentuated by arrested condylar growth and developmental disturbances of the mandible.

mandibular process [L, *mandere,* to chew + *processus*], **1.** the upper alveolar part of the mandible. **2.** the projection of the upper posterior part of the ramus of the mandible bearing the condyle.

mandibular ramus [L, *mandere,* to chew + *ramus,* branch], a broad quadrilateral portion of the mandible projecting upward from the posterior end of the body behind the lower teeth. It has two surfaces, four borders, and two processes.

mandibular reflex [L, *mandere,* to chew; *reflectere,* to bend back], a reflex contraction of the masseter muscle after a downward tap on the point of the jaw while the mouth is open. Also called **chin reflex; chin-jerk reflex; jaw jerk.**

mandibular retrusion, mandibular retroposition. See **retrognathia.**

mandibular sling, the connection between the mandible and the maxilla, formed by the masseter and the pterygoideus at the angle of the mandible. When the mouth is opened and closed, the mandible moves around a center of rotation formed by the mandibular sling and the sphenomandibular ligament.

mandibulofacial dysostosis /mandib'yəlofā'shəl/ [L, *mandere + facies,* face; Gk, *dys,* bad, *osteon,* bone], an abnormal hereditary condition characterized by an antimongoloid slant of the palpebral fissures, colomboma of the lower lid, micrognathia and hypoplasia of the zygomatic arches, and microtia. Evidence indicates that this disorder is transmitted as an autosomal dominant trait. The condition occurs in the complete form as Franceschetti's syndrome and in the incomplete form as Treacher Collins' syndrome. See also **dysostosis.**

Mandol, a trademark for a cephalosporin antibiotic (cefamandole nafate).

mandrel /man'drəl/ [Fr, *mandrin,* boring tool], a shaft secured in a handpiece or lathe to support an object to be rotated, such as a dental polishing disk, cutting device, or sharpening stone.

maneuver /mənoo'vər/ [Fr, *manœuvre,* action], **1.** an adroit or skillful manipulation or procedure. **2.** (in obstetrics) a manipulation of the fetus performed to aid in delivery.

manganese (Mn) /mang'gənēs/ [L, *manganesium,* associated with magnesium], a common metallic element found in trace amounts in tissues of the body where it aids in the functions of various enzymes. Its atomic number is 25; its atomic weight is 54.938.

mani-, a prefix meaning 'mental aberration or madness': *mania, maniaphobia.*

mania /mā'nē·ə/ [Gk, madness], a state characterized by

an expansive emotional state, extreme excitement, excessive elation, hyperactivity, agitation, overtalkativeness, flight of ideas, increased psychomotor activity, fleeting attention, and sometimes violent, destructive, and self-destructive behavior.

-mania, -manic **1.** a suffix meaning a 'state of mental disorder'. **2.** a suffix meaning 'a state of psychosis': *hypermania, melanomanic.*

-maniac, **1.** a suffix meaning a 'person exhibiting a type of psychosis': *kleptomaniac, narcomaniac,* or *toxicomaniac.* **2.** a suffix meaning a 'person revealing an inordinate interest in something': *ergomaniac, nymphomaniac, opiomaniac.*

manic depressive /mä′nik dipres′iv, man′ik/ [Gk, *mania* madness; L, *deprimere,* to sink down], See **bipolar disorder.**

manifest deviation. See **eye deviation.**

manipulation /mənip′yəlā′shən/ [L *manipulare* to work with the hands], the skillful use of the hands in therapeutic or diagnostic procedures, such as palpation, reducing a dislocation, turning the position of the fetus, or various treatments in physical therapy and osteopathy. A kind of manipulation is **conjoined manipulation.** See also **massage.**

mannitol /man′itol/, a poorly metabolized sugar used as an osmotic diuretic and in kidney function tests.

■ INDICATIONS: It is prescribed to promote diuresis, to decrease intraocular and intracranial pressure, to promote the excretion of poisons and other toxic wastes, and to evaluate renal function.

■ CONTRAINDICATIONS: Pulmonary edema, dehydration, or known hypersensitivity to this drug prohibits its use.

■ ADVERSE EFFECTS: Among the more serious adverse reactions are pulmonary edema, heart failure, hyponatremia, headache, vomiting, and confusion.

-manometer, a combining form meaning 'an instrument to measure pressure': *sphygmomanometer.*

manometer /mənom′ətər/ [Gk, *manos,* thin, *metron,* measure], a device for measuring the pressure of a fluid, consisting of a tube marked with a scale and containing a relatively incompressible fluid, such as mercury. The level of the fluid in the tube varies with the pressure of the fluid being measured. Kinds of manometers are **aneroid manometer** and **sphygmomanometer.**

Mansonella ozzardi /man′sənel′ə/, a parasitic worm that is indigenous to much of Latin America and the Caribbean islands. It is a relatively benign nematode that infects humans, sometimes causing hydrocele or lymphadenopathy. The larvae live in the bloodstream, and adult worms are found in the visceral mesenteries. The intermediate hosts are biting flies of the genus *Culicoides.*

Mantadil, a trademark for a topical, fixed-combination drug containing a glucocorticoid (hydrocortisone acetate) and an antihistaminic (chlorcyclizine hydrochloride).

Mantoux test /mantoo′/ [Charles Mantoux, French physician, b. 1877], a tuberculin skin test that consists of intradermal injection of a purified protein derivative of the tubercle bacillus. A hardened, raised red area of 8 to 10 mm, appearing 24 to 72 hours after injection, is a positive reaction. This method is the most reliable means of testing tuberculin sensitivity. See also **tuberculin test.**

manual rotation /man′yoo·əl/ [L, *manualis,* hand; *rotare,* to turn], an obstetric maneuver in which a baby's head is turned by hand from a transverse to an anteroposterior po-

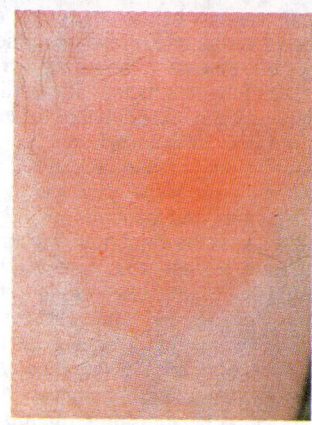

Positive Mantoux test *(Hart, 1992)*

sition in the birth canal to facilitate delivery. Compare **forceps rotation.**

manubriosternal articulation /mənoo′brē·ōstur′nəl/ [L, *manubrium,* handle; Gk, *sternum,* chest; L, *articularis,* pertaining to joints], the fibrocartilaginous connection between manubrium and the body of the sternum. This joint usually closes by the age of 25 years. Compare **xiphisternal articulation.**

manubrium /mənoo′brē·əm/ [L, handle], the most anterior of the three bones of the sternum, presenting a broad quadrangular shape that narrows caudally at its articulation with the superior end of the body of the sternum. The pectoralis major and the sternocleidomastoideus are attached to the manubrium. Compare **xiphoid process.** **–manubrial,** *adj.*

manudynamometer /man′oodīnə′mom′ətər/ [L, *manus,* hand; Gk, *dynamis,* force; *metron,* measure], a device for measuring the force or extent of thrust.

manus. See **hand.**

many-tailed bandage [AS, *manig,* many, *taegel,* tail; Fr, *bande,* strip], **1.** a broad, evenly shaped bandage with both ends split into strips of equal size and number. As the bandage is placed on the abdomen, chest, or limb, the ends may be overlapped and secured. **2.** an irregularly shaped bandage with torn or cut ends that are secured together. See also **Scultetus bandage.**

MAO, abbreviation for **monoamine oxidase.**

MAOI, abbreviation for **monoamine oxidase inhibitor.**

Maolate, a trademark for a skeletal muscle relaxant (chlorphenesin carbamate).

MAP, **1.** abbreviation for *medical aid post.* **2.** abbreviation for **mean arterial pressure.**

map distance. See **map unit.**

maple bark disease [AS, *mapul;* ONorse, *bark;* L, *dis,* opposite of; Fr, *aise,* ease], a hypersensitivity pneumonitis caused by exposure to the mold *Cryptostroma corticale,* found in the bark of maple trees. In the susceptible person, the condition may be acute, accompanied by fever, cough, dyspnea, and vomiting, or it may be chronic, characterized by fatigue, weight loss, dyspnea on exertion, and a productive cough. Although differential diagnosis may be difficult, a good occupational history may reveal the cause and the source of exposure. In an acute or severe case, a short course of prednisone may be used to control the symptoms; avoiding exposure to the bark prevents further reaction.

maple syrup urine disease [AS, *mapul;* Ar, *sharab;* Gk, *ouron,* urine], an inherited metabolic disorder in which an enzyme necessary for the breakdown of the amino acids valine, leucine, and isoleucine is lacking. The disease is usually diagnosed in infancy, being recognized by the characteristic maple syrup odor of the urine and by hyperreflexia. Stress, fever, infection, and the ingestion of lysine, leucine, or isoleucine aggravate the condition. Treatment includes a diet avoiding these amino acids and, rarely, dialysis or transfusion. Also called **branched chain ketoaciduria.**

mapping [L, *mappa,* napkin], (in genetics) the process of locating the relative position of genes on a chromosome through the analysis of genetic recombination. Distances between genes in a linkage group are expressed in map or morgan units. Also called **chromosome mapping.**

maprotiline hydrochloride /maprō′tilēn/, an antidepressant similar to the tricyclics.

- INDICATION: It is prescribed for the treatment of depression.
- CONTRAINDICATIONS: It is used with caution in conditions in which anticholinergics are contraindicated, in seizure disorders, and in patients with cardiovascular disorders. Concomitant administration of monoamine oxidase inhibitors, recent myocardial infarction, or known hypersensitivity to this drug prohibits its use.
- ADVERSE EFFECTS: Among the more serious adverse reactions are sedation and anticholinergic side effects. A variety of GI, cardiovascular, and neurologic reactions (including convulsions) may occur. The drug, like the tricyclics, is involved in many potential drug interactions.

map unit [L, *mappa,* napkin; *unus,* one], (in genetics) an arbitrary unit of measure used to designate the distance between genes on a chromosome. It is calculated from the percentage of recombinations that occur between specific genes so that 1% of crossing over represents one unit on a genetic map or approximately the number of new combinations that can be detected. The measurement is accurate only for small distances, because double crossovers do not appear as new recombinations. Also called **map distance.** See also **morgan.**

marasmic kwashiorkor /məraz′mik/ [Gk, *marasmos,* a wasting; Afr], a malnutrition disease, primarily of children, resulting from the deficiency of both calories and protein. The condition is characterized by severe tissue wasting, dehydration, loss of subcutaneous fat, lethargy, and growth retardation.See also **marasmus.**

marasmus /məraz′məs/ [Gk, *marasmos,* a wasting], a condition of extreme malnutrition and emaciation, occurring chiefly in young children, that is characterized by progressive wasting of subcutaneous tissue and muscle. It results from a lack of adequate calories and proteins and is seen in children with failure to thrive and in starvation. Less commonly, marasmus occurs as a result of an inability to assimilate or use protein because of a defect in metabolism. Care of the marasmic child involves the reestablishment of fluid and electrolyte balance, followed by the slow and gradual addition of foods as they are tolerated. Stimulation appropriate to the developmental age should be provided. As much of the care of the child as possible should be given consistently by one person, because it must be assumed that the physically starved child has also been emotionally deprived. See also **failure to thrive, kwashiorkor.**

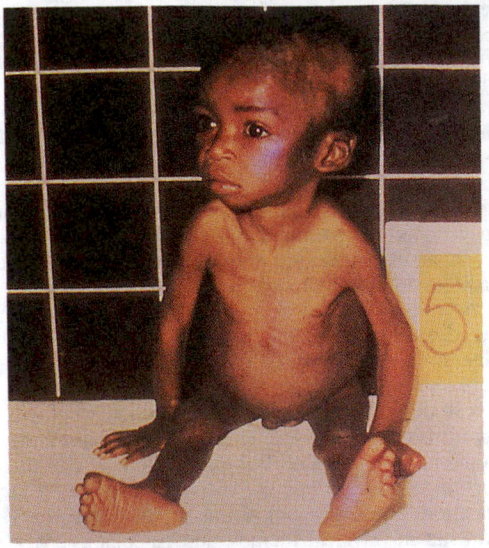

Marasmus (Zitelli, 1992)

marathon encounter group /mer′əthon/ [Marathon, Greece; L, *in,* in, *contra,* against; Fr, *groupe*], an intensive group experience that accelerates self-awareness and promotes personal growth and behavioral change through the continuous interaction of group members for a period ranging from 16 to more than 40 hours. See also **encounter group.**

Marax, a trademark for a respiratory, fixed-combination drug containing a smooth muscle relaxant (theophylline), an adrenergic (ephedrine sulfate), and a tranquilizer (hydroxyzine hydrochloride).

marble bones. See **osteopetrosis.**

Marburg-Ebola virus disease /mär′bərgeb′ələ/, a serious febrile disease characterized by rash and severe GI hemorrhages. An epidemic in Marburg, Germany, in 1967, was apparently contracted from imported African green monkeys. In 1976, in the Ebola River District of Zaire and Sudan, an explosive epidemic occurred with a mortality of 85%. This disease may be transmitted to hospital personnel by improper handling of contaminated needles or from hemorrhagic lesions of patients. The diagnosis is made through serologic abnormalities. There is no effective treatment. Also called **hemorrhagic fever.**

Marcaine Hydrochloride, a trademark for a local anesthetic (bupivacaine hydrochloride).

march foot [Fr, *marcher,* to walk; AS, *fot*], an abnormal condition of the foot caused by excessive use, such as in a long march. The forefoot is swollen and painful, and one or more of the metatarsal bones may be broken. See also **stress fracture.**

march fracture. See **metatarsal stress fracture.**

march hemoglobinuria, a rare, abnormal condition, characterized by the presence of hemoglobin in the urine, that occurs after strenuous physical exertion or prolonged exercise, such as marching or distance running. See also **hemolysis.**

Marchiafava-Micheli disease /mär′kyəfä′vəmikā′lē/ [Ettore Marchiafava, Italian physician, b. 1847; F. Micheli,

Italian physician, b. 1872], a rare disorder of unknown origin characterized by episodic hemoglobinuria, occurring usually, but not always, at night.

Marchi's method /mär'kēz/ [Vittoria Marchi, Italian physician, b. 1851], a laboratory staining procedure for demonstrating degenerated nerve fibers. The tissue specimen is first fixed in a solution of potassium bichromate (Mueller's fluid), which prevents normal nerve fibers from being stained with osmic acid; osmic acid is then applied as a definitive black stain for abnormal nerve fibers.

Marcus Gunn pupil sign [Robert Marcus Gunn, English ophthalmologist, b. 1850], paradoxical dilation of the pupils in an ophthalmologic examination in response to afferent visual stimuli. In a dark room a beam of light is moved from one eye to the other. Normal miosis is caused by the consensual pupil reaction when the normal eye is illuminated; but as the light is moved to the opposite, abnormal eye, the direct reaction to light is weaker than the consensual reaction; hence both pupils dilate.

Marcus Gunn-syndrome. See **jaw winking.**

Marezine, a trademark for an antiemetic (cyclizine hydrochloride).

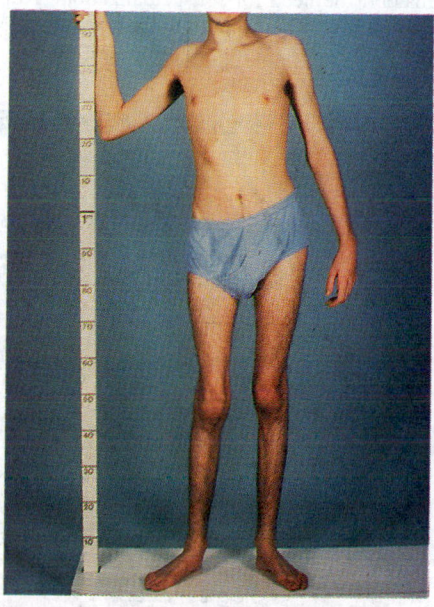

Marfan's syndrome
(Epstein, 1992/Courtesy Department of Clinical Genetics, Royal Free NHS Trust)

Marfan's syndrome /märfäNz'/ [Bernard-Jean A. Marfan, French pediatrician, b. 1858], an abnormal condition characterized by elongation of the bones, often with associated abnormalities of the eyes and the cardiovascular system. Marfan's syndrome is inherited as an autosomal-dominant trait. The disease causes major pathologic musculoskeletal disturbances, such as muscular underdevelopment, ligamentous laxity, joint hypermobility, and bone elongation. With Marfan's syndrome pathologic alterations of the cardiovascular system appear to produce fragmentation of the elastic fibers in the media of the aorta, which

may lead to aneurysm. Ocular changes associated with the disease include a variety of disorders, including dislocation of the lens. Cardiac and ocular involvement occurs in approximately one half of the patients affected. The disease affects men and women equally, elongating the limbs so that most adult patients with the disease are over 6 feet tall. The extremities of individuals with Marfan's syndrome are very long and spiderlike, with greatly extended metacarpals, metatarsals, and phalanges. The skulls of such patients are usually asymmetric. Pectus excavatum is common, and a lateral curvature of the spine may develop and increase during years of rapid vertebral growth, with kyphoscoliosis developing to varying degrees. The severe ligamental laxity and the joint hypermobility associated with Marfan's syndrome may be seen by radiographic examination and often results in pes valgus and genu recurvatum. No specific treatment is advocated for Marfan's syndrome, and symptomatic management of the associated problems is the usual alternative. Resulting deformities, such as kyphoscoliosis, may be treated with orthoses or other surgical procedures, as indicated.

marginal gingiva /mär'jənəl/ [L, *margo*, margin; *gingiva*, gum], the uppermost of the free gingiva that overlaps the neck and base of the crown of the tooth.

marginal gyrus [L, *margo*, margin; Gk, *gyros*, turn], the superior frontal convolution on the surface of the cerebral hemispheres.

marginal peptic ulcer [L, *margo*, border; Gk, *peptein*, to digest; L, *ulcus*, ulcer], an ulcer that develops postoperatively at the surgical anastomosis of the stomach and jejunum. See also **peptic ulcer.**

marginal placenta previa, placenta previa in which the placenta is implanted in the lower uterine segment, with its margin touching or spreading to some degree over the internal os of the uterine cervix. During labor, as the cervix dilates, bleeding may occur from the separation of the edge of the placenta from the uterus beneath it. Bleeding may be so scant as to pose no clinical problem. In some cases frank severe hemorrhage may occur, but the pressure of the presenting part of the baby is often sufficient to act as a tamponade, arresting the hemorrhage. Diagnosis of marginal placenta previa may be suggested by the apparent location of the placenta on ultrasonic visualization. Cesarean section is not usually necessary. See also **placenta previa.**

marginal rale. See **atelectatic rale.**

marginal ridge, an elevation of enamel that forms the proximal boundary of the occlusal surface of a tooth.

marginal sinus [L, *margo* + *sinus*, hollow], a sinus that may encircle the placenta. Also called **placental sinus.**

Marie's hypertrophy [Pierre Marie, French neurologist, b. 1853; Gk, *hyper*, excess, *trophe*, nourishment], chronic enlargement of the joints caused by periostitis. Also called **hypertrophic pulmonary osteopathy.**

Marie-Strümpell disease. See **ankylosing spondylitis.**

marijuana. See **cannabis.**

Marin Amat syndrome [Manuel Marin Amat, Spanish Opthalmologist, b. 1879] an involuntary facial movement phenomenon in which the eyes close when the mouth opens or when the jaws move in mastication. The effect results from a facial nerve paralysis. Also called **inverse Marcus Gunn syndrome.**

Marinol, a trademark for an oral antiemetic (dronabinol).

marital rape [L, *rapere*, to seize], forcible sexual intercourse by a man with his wife.

mark [AS, *mearc*], any nevus or birthmark.

marker gene. See **genetic marker.**

markers [AS, *mearc*], body language movements that serve as indicators and punctuation marks in interpersonal communication.

Marplan, a trademark for an antidepressant (isocarboxazid).

marrow. See **bone marrow.**

Marseilles fever /märsālz′, märsā/ [Marseilles, France; L, *febris*, fever], a disease endemic around the Mediterranean, in Africa, in the Crimea, and in India, caused by *Rickettsia conorii* transmitted by the brown dog tick (*Rhipicephalus sanguineus*). Characteristic symptoms are chills, fever, an ulcer covered with a black crust at the site of the tick bite, and a rash appearing on the second to fourth day. Also called **boutonneuse fever, Bruch's disease, Conor's disease, escharonodulaire, Indian tick fever, Kenya fever.**

Marshall-Marchetti operation [Victor F. Marshall, American urologist, b. 1913; Andrew A. Marchetti, American obstetrician, b. 1901], a surgical procedure performed to correct a condition of stress incontinence. The procedure, a vesicourethropexy, involves a retropubic incision and suturing of the urethra, vesicle neck, and bladder to the posterior surface of the pubic bone. Also called **Marshall-Marchetti-Krantz operation.**

marsupialize /märsōō′pē·əlīz/ [L, *marsupium*, pouch; Gk, *izein*, to cause], to form a pouch surgically to treat a cyst when simple removal would not be effective, such as in a pancreatic or a pilonidal cyst. With the patient under general or local anesthesia, the cyst sac is opened and emptied. Its edges are sutured to adjacent tissues, and a drain is left in place. Secretions decrease over a period of several months and may eventually cease.

Martorell's syndrome. See **Takayasu's arteritis.**

masculine /mas′kyəlin/ [L, *masculinus*, male], having the characteristics of a male.

masculinization /mas′kyəlin′īzā′shən/ [L, *masculinus* + Gk, *izein*, to cause], the normal development or induction of male sex characteristics. See also **virilization.** —**masculinize,** *v.*

MASER /mā′sər/, acronym for *microwave amplification by stimulated emission of radiation.*

MASH /mash/, acronym for *mobile army surgical hospital.*

mask [Fr, *masque*], **1.** to obscure, as in symptomatic treatment that may mask the development of a disease. **2.** to cover, as does a skin-toned cosmetic that may mask a pigmented nevus. **3.** a cover worn over the nose and mouth to prevent inhalation of toxic or irritating materials, to control delivery of oxygen or anesthetic gas, or (by medical personnel) to shield a patient during aseptic procedures from pathogenic organisms normally exhaled from the respiratory tract.

mask image, (in digital fluoroscopy) an x-ray image made immediately after contrast material has been injected but before it reaches the anatomic site being examined. The image thus produced is stored in the computer memory and displayed on a video monitor. The initial mask image is then subtracted electronically from a series of additional images. The technique has the effect of enhancing the image of the tissues being studied. See also **remasking.**

masking, **1.** the covering or concealing of a disorder by a second condition, such as when a person begins a weight-loss diet while an undiagnosed wasting disease such as cancer has developed. The loss of body weight is attributed to the diet, masking the disease and delaying diagnosis and treatment. **2.** the unconscious display of a personality trait that conceals a behavioral aberration.

masking agent, a cosmetic preparation for covering nevi, surgical scars, and other blemishes. Masking agents are generally composed of a flesh-colored pigment in a lotion or cream base.

masklike facies [Fr, *masque*; L, *facies*, face], an immobile expressionless face with staring eyes and slightly open mouth. It is sometimes associated with parkinsonism.

mask of pregnancy. See **chloasma.**

Maslow's hierarchy of needs /mas′lōz/ [Abraham H. Maslow, American psychiatrist, b. 1908; Gk, *hierarches*, position of authority; AS, *nied*, obligation], (in psychology) a hierarchic categorization of the basic needs of humans. The most basic needs on the scale are the physiologic or biologic, such as the need for air, food, or water. Of second priority are the safety needs, including protection and freedom from fear and anxiety. The subsequent order of needs in the hierarchic progression are the need to belong, to love, and to be loved; the need for self-esteem; and ultimately, the need for self-actualization. To progress from one need to another, the more basic need must first be satisfied.

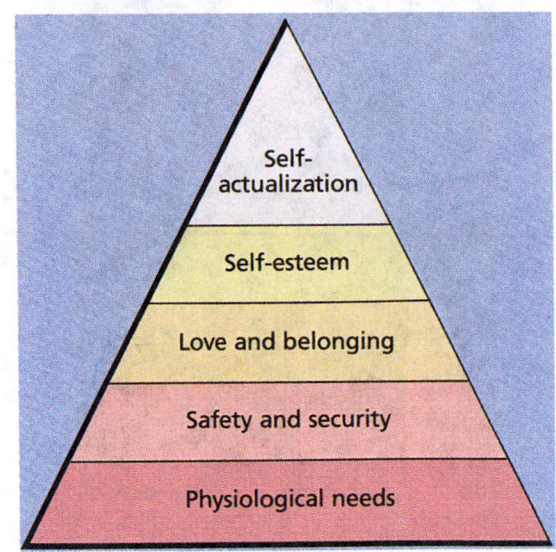

Maslow's hierarchy of needs (Potter, 1993)

masochism /mas′ōkiz′əm/ [Leopold von Sacher-Masoch, Austrian author, b. 1836], pleasure or gratification derived from receiving physical, mental, or emotional abuse. The maltreatment may be inflicted by another person or by oneself. It may involve a need to experience emotional or physical pain, in reality or fantasy, to become sexually aroused. Also called **passive algolagnia.** Compare **sadism.** See also **algolagnia, sadomasochism.** —**masochistic,** *adj.*

masochist /mas′ōkist/ [Leopold von Sacher-Masoch], a person deriving pleasure or gratification from masochistic acts or abuse. See also **masochism.**

mass [L, *massa*],   **1.** the physical property of matter that gives it weight and inertia. **2.** (in pharmacology) a mixture from which pills are formed. **3.** an aggregate of cells clumped together, such as a tumor. Compare **weight.** See also **inertia.**

massage /məsäzh, məsäj'/ [Fr, *masser*, to stroke],   the manipulation of the soft tissue of the body through stroking, rubbing, kneading, or tapping, to increase circulation, to improve muscle tone, and to relax the patient. The procedure is performed either with the bare hands or through some mechanical means, such as a vibrator. The most common sites for massage are the back, knees, elbows, and heels. Care is taken not to massage inflamed areas, particularly of the extremities, because of the danger of loosening blood clots; open wounds and areas of rash, tumor, or excessive sensitivity are avoided. The procedure is performed with the patient prone or on the side, comfortably positioned, with an emollient lotion or cream applied to the area to be massaged. The nurse's hands are warm, and excessive pressure is avoided so as not to cause pain or injury. Kinds of massage are **cardiac massage, effleurage, flagellation, friction, frôlement, pétrissage, tapotement,** and **vibration.**

-massage,   a combining form meaning a 'therapeutic kneading of the body': *electromassage, hydromassage, phonomassage.*

masseter /masē'tər/ [Gk, one who chews],   the thick, rectangular muscle in the cheek that functions to close the jaw. It is one of the four muscles of mastication and consists of a superficial portion and a deep portion, each arising from the zygomatic arch and inserting into the mandible. The deep portion is the smaller and more muscular of the two parts. The masseter is innervated by the masseteric nerve from the mandibular division of the trigeminal nerve.

mass fragment [L, *massa*, lump; *frangere*, to shatter],   a degraded portion of a molecule containing one or more charges.

mass hysteria.   See **major hysteria.**

mass number (A),   the sum of the number of protons and neutrons in the nucleus of an atom or isotope. See also **atomic number, atomic weight.**

mass panic, mass psychogenic illness.   See **major hysteria.**

mass reflex,   an abnormal condition, seen in patients with transection of the spinal cord, characterized by a widespread nerve discharge, resulting in flexor muscle spasms, incontinence of urine and feces, priapism, hypertension, and profuse sweating.

■ OBSERVATIONS: A mass reflex may be triggered by scratching or other painful stimulus to the skin, overdistention of the bladder or intestines, cold weather, prolonged sitting, or emotional stress. Muscle spasms may be so violent as to throw the patient off a bed or stretcher.

■ INTERVENTIONS: Medications to reduce mass reflexes include diazepam, dantraline, chlordiazepoxide, and meprobamate. Hubbard baths and exercises in warm water also help. Occasionally chordotomy, rhizotomy, peripheral nerve transection, or tenotomy may be necessary.

■ NURSING CONSIDERATIONS: Nurses should avoid stimulating areas that trigger mass reflexes and should be prepared to accept them when they occur and to explain the cause to the patient. It is important to prevent decubitus ulcers and bladder infections in paraplegic and quadriplegic patients

because they may also serve as triggers to initiate mass reflexes.

mass spectrometer,   an analytic instrument for identifying a substance by sorting a stream of charged particles (ions) according to their mass. The sorting is usually accomplished by deflecting a stream of charged particles into a semicircular path as it enters a magnetic field and ultimately strikes a photographic plate or a photomultiplier tube sensor.

mass spectrometry,   (in chemistry) a technique for the analysis of a substance in which the constituents are identified and quantified using a mass spectrometer. See also **spectrometry, spectrophotometry.**

mass transfer,   the movement of mass from one phase to another.

mast-.   See **masto.**

MAST.   See **military antishock trousers.**

mastalgia /mastal'jə/ [Gk, *mastos*, breast, *algos*, pain],   pain in the breast caused by congestion or 'caking' during lactation, an infection, fibrocystic disease, especially during or before menstruation, or advanced cancer. The early stages of breast cancer are rarely accompanied by pain. **–mastalgic,** *adj.*

mast cell [Ger, *Mast*, fattening; L, *cella*, storeroom],   a constituent of connective tissue containing large basophilic granules that contain heparin, serotonin, bradykinin, and histamine. These substances are released from the mast cell in response to injury and infection.

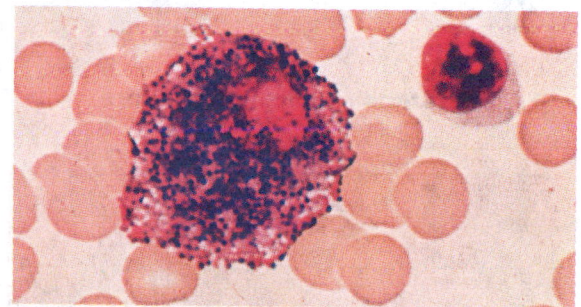

Mast cell in bone marrow (Hayhoe, 1992)

mast cell leukemia,   a malignant neoplasm of leukocytes characterized by connective tissue mast cells in circulating blood.

mast cell tumor [Ger, *Mastzelle*, food cell; L, *tumor*],   a connective tissue tumor composed of mast cells. Granules of the cells stain metachromatically with toluidine blue.

mastectomy /mastek'təmē/ [Gk, *mastos*, breast, *ektome*, excision],   the surgical removal of one or both breasts, most commonly performed to remove a malignant tumor. In a simple mastectomy, only breast tissue is removed. In a radical mastectomy, some of the muscles of the chest are removed with the breast with all lymph nodes in the axilla. In a modified radical mastectomy, the large muscles of the chest that move the arm are preserved. A biopsy of tissue taken from the tumor is performed before the mastectomy. If the specimen shows a malignancy, the tumor and adjacent tissues are removed in one piece. After surgery, a drainage catheter is placed in the wound. The nurse inspects the wound for swelling or excessive bleeding and encourages the patient to take deep breaths and to cough at frequent intervals. The affected arm is positioned with the hand pointed upward or on pillows so that the hand is higher than the lower arm, with the lower arm above heart level. Hand and wrist movements and flexion and extension of the elbow are begun within 24 hours and performed regularly. The patient may be fitted with a prosthesis when the wound is completely healed or at the time of the mastectomy. Emotional support and counseling are essential. See also **breast cancer, modified radical mastectomy, radical mastectomy, simple mastectomy.**   **-mastectomize,** *v.*

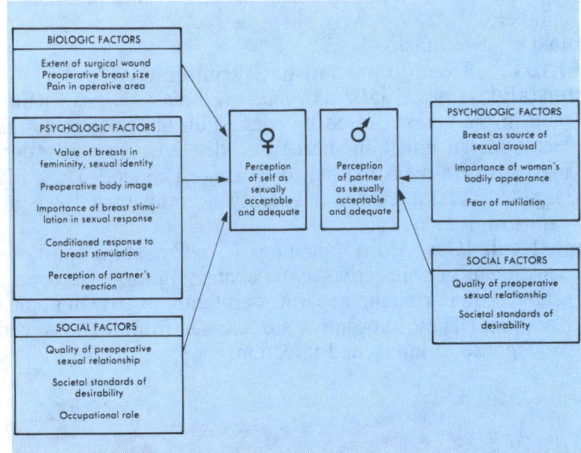

Mastectomy adaptation factors

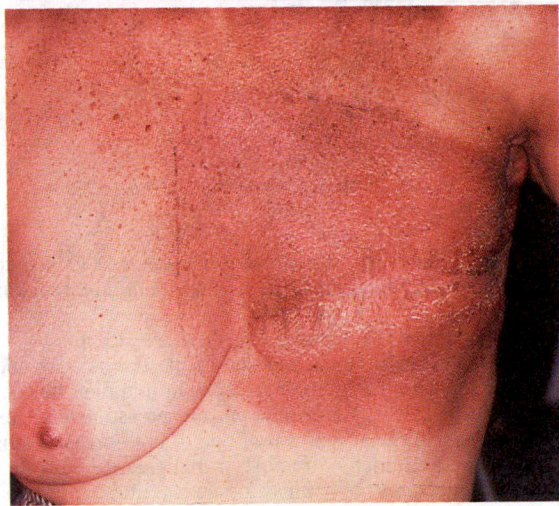

Modified radical mastectomy *(Skarin, 1991)*

master problem list, a list of a patient's problems that serves as an index to the patient's record. Each problem, the date the problem was first noted, the treatment, and the outcome are added to the master problem list as each be-

comes known. Thus the master problem list provides an ongoing guide for reviewing the health status of the patient and for planning care for the patient.

master's degree program in nursing, a postgraduate program in a school of nursing, based in a university setting, that grants the degree Master of Science in Nursing to successful candidates. Most programs include theory of nursing and techniques in nursing research as integral parts of the curriculum. The degree may be awarded for work in maternal-newborn nursing, medical-surgical nursing, pediatric nursing, psychiatric nursing, or other fields of nursing. Nurses with this degree function in leadership roles in clinical nursing, as consultants in various settings, in faculty positions in schools of nursing, and as nurse practitioners in the various specialties.

mastery /mas′tərē/ [L, *magister*, chief], being in command or control of a situation, as in learning accomplishment.

-mastia. See **-mazia.**

mastication /mas′tikā′shən/ [L, *masticare*, to chew], chewing, tearing, or grinding food with the teeth while it becomes mixed with saliva. See also **bolus, digestion, ptyalin.**

masticatory surface. See **occlusal surface.**

masticatory system /mas′tikətôr′ē/ [L, *masticare*, to chew; Gk, *systema*], the combination of organs, structures, and nerves involved in chewing. It includes but is not limited to the jaws, the teeth and their supporting structures, the mandibular musculature, the mandible, the maxillae, the temporomandibular joints, the tongue, the lips, the cheeks, the oral mucosa, and cranial nerves. Also called **masticatory apparatus.** Compare **stomatognathic system.**

mastigophora. See **protozoa.**

mastitis /mastī′tis/ [Gk, *mastos*, breast, *itis*, inflammation], an inflammatory condition of the breast, usually caused by streptococcal or staphylococcal infection. **Acute mastitis,** most common in the first 2 months of lactation, is characterized by pain, swelling, redness, axillary lymphadenopathy, fever, and malaise. If untreated or inadequately treated, abscesses may form. Antibiotics, rest, analgesia, and warm soaks are usually prescribed. Usually, breast feeding may continue. **Chronic tuberculous mastitis** is rare; when it occurs, it represents extension of tuberculosis from the lungs and ribs beneath the breast.

masto-, mast-, a prefix meaning 'of or pertaining to the breast': *mastochondroma, mastologist, mastoplasia.*

mastocytosis /mas′təsītō′sis/ [Ger, *Mast*, fattening; Gk, *kytos*, cell, *osis*, condition], local or systemic overproduction of mast cells, which, in rare instances, may infiltrate liver, spleen, bones, the GI system, and skin. Systemic mastocytosis may precede mast cell leukemia.

mastoid /mas′toid/ [Gk, *mastos*, breast, *eidos*, form], **1.** of or pertaining to the mastoid process of the temporal bone. **2.** breast-shaped.

mastoid-, a prefix meaning 'pertaining to the mastoid process': *mastoidectomy.*

mastoid cells [Gk, *mastos*, breast; *eidos*, form; L, *cella*, storeroom], air cells in the mastoid process of the temporal bone. Also called **mastoid air cells.**

mastoidectomy /mas′toidek′təmē/ [Gk, *mastos* + *eidos*, form, *ektome*, excision], surgical excision of a portion of the mastoid part of the temporal bone, performed to treat chronic suppurative otitis media or mastoiditis when systemic antibiotics are ineffective. Entry is made through the

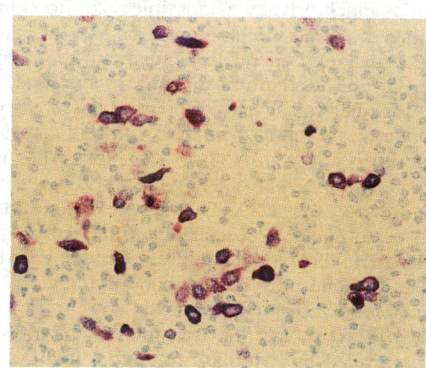

Mastocytosis infiltration into the spleen
(Holgate, 1993/Courtesy Dr. Tony Ormerod)

ear canal or from behind the ear. In a simple mastoidectomy, with the patient under general anesthesia, infected bone cells are removed and the eardrum is incised to drain the middle ear. Topical antibiotics are then instilled in the ear. In a radical procedure, the eardrum and most middle ear structures are removed; the stapes is left intact so that a hearing aid may be used. The opening to the eustachian tube is plugged. In a modified radical procedure, the eardrum and the middle ear structures are saved, and the patient will hear better than after a radical mastoidectomy. After surgery any bright red blood on the dressing may indicate hemorrhage. A stiff neck or disorientation may signal the onset of meningitis. Dizziness is usual and may be expected to last for several days.

mastoid fontanel, a posterolateral fontanel that is usually not palpable. See also **fontanel.**

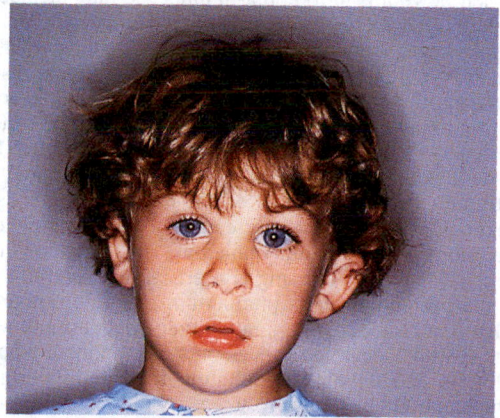

Mastoiditis (Zitelli, 1992)

mastoiditis /mas'toidī'tis/ [Gk, *mastos* + *eidos*, form, *itis*, inflammation], an infection of one of the mastoid bones, usually an extension of a middle ear infection, characterized by earache, fever, headache, and malaise. Swelling of the mastoid process often displaces the pinna anteriorly and inferiorly. The infection is difficult to treat, often requiring antibiotics administered intravenously for several days. Children are most often affected. Residual hearing loss may follow the infection.

mastoid process, the conic projection of the caudal, posterior portion of the temporal bone, serving as the attachment for various muscles, including the sternocleidomastoideus, splenius capitis, and longissimus capitis. A hollow section of the process contains air cells that are distinguished from a large, irregular tympanic antrum in the superior anterior portion of the process. See also **temporal bone.**

masturbation /mas'tərbā'shən/ [L, *masturbari*, to masturbate], sexual activity in which the penis or clitoris is stimulated, usually to orgasm, by means other than coitus. It is performed, at least occasionally, by most people and is considered to be normal and harmless. —**masturbate,** *v*, **masturbatic, masturbatory,** *adj*.

-masty. See **-mazia.**

mat., 1. abbreviation for **matunity.** 2. abbreviation for **maturity.**

matched group. See **group.**

materia /matir'ē·ə/, matter or material, such as materia medica.

material fact /mətir'ē·əl/ [L, *materia*, matter; *factum*], (in law) a fact that establishes or refutes an element essential to the complaint, charge, or defense. The presence of a material fact in a case being tried precludes granting of a summary judgment.

materia medica, 1. the study of drugs and other substances used in medicine, their origins, preparation, uses, and effects. 2. a substance or a drug used in medical treatment.

matern., 1. abbreviation for **maternal.** 2. abbreviation for **maternity.**

Materna, a trademark for an antenatal multivitamin supplement with calcium and iron.

maternal (matern) /mətur'nəl/ [L, *maternus,* motherhood], 1. inherited, derived, or received from a mother. 2. motherly in behavior. 3. related through the mother's side of the family, such as a maternal grandfather.

maternal and child health (MCH) services, various facilities and programs organized for the purpose of providing medical and social services for mothers and children. Medical services include prenatal, postnatal, family planning care, and pediatric care in infancy.

maternal-child attachment. See **maternal-infant bonding.**

maternal-child separation syndrome. See **separation anxiety.**

maternal death, the death of a woman during the childbearing cycle.

maternal deprivation syndrome [L, *mater,* mother; *deprivare,* to deprive; Gk, *syn,* together *dromos,* course], a condition characterized by developmental retardation that occurs as a result of physical or emotional deprivation. It is seen primarily in infants. Typical symptoms include lack of physical growth, with weight below the third percentile for age and size, malnutrition, pronounced withdrawal, silence, apathy, and irritability, and a characteristic posture and body language, featuring unnatural stiffness and rigidity with a slow response reaction to others. Causes of the syndrome are usually multiple and complex, involving such factors as parental indifference, emotional instability or insecurity of the mother, lack of or delayed development of the mother-child attachment process, unrealistic expectations or disappointment concerning the sex, appearance, or adaptability of the child, or unfavorable socioeconomic conditions within the family. Treatment often requires hospitalization, especially in cases of severe malnutrition. Care includes assessment of the family situation, and treatment often involves psychotherapy, counseling, or special nursing instruction to help the parents learn to deal with and provide for the child. The nature and extent of the effects of the condition on later physical, emotional, intellectual, and social development vary considerably and depend on the age at which deprivation occurs, the degree and duration of the situation, the constitutional makeup of the child, and the substituted care that is provided. Emotionally deprived children often remain below normal in intellectual development, fail to learn acceptable social behavior, and are unable to form trusting, meaningful relationships with others. In severe cases of early and prolonged deprivation, the damage to an infant may be irreversible. See also **failure to thrive.**

maternal effect.   See **maternal inheritance.**

maternal-infant bonding,   the complex process of attachment of a mother to her newborn baby. Disastrous effects of the disruption or absence of this attachment have long been known. The specific steps in its development and the factors that disturb or encourage it have been identified and described by anthropologists, pediatricians, psychologists, nurses, midwives, and sociologists. The process begins before birth as the parents plan for the pregnancy or discover that the mother is pregnant. The mother feels fetal movement, begins to accept the fetus as an individual, and makes plans for the baby after birth. In the first minutes and hours after birth, a sensitive period occurs during which the baby and the mother become intimately involved with each other through behaviors and stimuli that are complementary and that provoke further interactions. The mother touches the baby and holds it en face to achieve eye-to-eye contact. The infant looks back eye to eye. The mother speaks in a quiet, high-pitched voice. The mother and the baby move in turn to the voice and sounds of the other, a process known as entrainment; it can be likened to a dance. The infant's movements constitute a response to the mother's voice, and she is encouraged to continue the process. The secretion of oxytocin and prolactin by the maternal pituitary gland is stimulated by the baby's sucking or licking of the mother's breasts; T and B lymphocytes and macrophages are given to the baby in the mother's milk, promoting resistance to infection. The child is also colonized by the normal flora of the mother's skin and nasal passages, improving the baby's ability to fend off infection. Physically, the mother provides her body heat for the baby's warmth and comfort. Thus the extended contact in the newborn period satisfies physical and emotional needs of the mother and baby. Experts have made the following recommendations to increase the development of maternal-infant bonding: The special needs of the mother are assessed before delivery; the parents are given classes to prepare them for labor, delivery, and the puerperium; and discussions are held regarding the stresses of pregnancy and the postpartum period. In labor and delivery, a companion is encouraged to stay with the mother. After the baby is born, silver nitrate drops or other medications are not placed in the baby's eyes until the mother and the baby have had time to be together en face, with eye contact for an extended period of time, because the drops cause a film to form over the eyes, dimming vision. During the first hour after birth the parents and the infant are not separated and

are given as much privacy as possible. Skin-to-skin contact is encouraged; various methods may be used to maintain an ambient temperature adequate to maintain the baby's temperature. On the postpartum unit the mother and the baby are kept together for at least 5 hours a day, but optimally for 24 hours a day in a 24-hour rooming-in care unit. The entire family is allowed to visit. The mother has responsibility for the care of her baby, with consultation available from a midwife or a nurse. The staff does not criticize the mother's performance, because it is to the baby's inestimable benefit that the mother believes her baby is the best, most beautiful, and most perfect baby in the world and that she feels able to care for her baby.

maternal inheritance,   the transmission of traits or conditions controlled by cytoplasmic factors within the ovum that are not self-replicating and are determined by genes within the nucleus. An example of such a characteristic is the direction of coiling in the shells of snails. Also called **maternal effect.**

maternal mortality,   **1.** the death of a woman as a result of childbearing. **2.** the number of maternal deaths per 100,000 births.

maternal placenta [L, *mater*, mother + *placenta*, flat cake],   the portion of the placenta that develops from the decidua basalis of the uterus and is usually shed along with the fetal elements.

maternity (mat., matern.) /mətur′nitē/ [L, *maternus*, motherhood],   motherhood, the character and quality of a mother.

maternity cycle [L, *mater*, mother; Gk, *kyklos*, circle],   the antepartal, intrapartal, and postpartal periods of pregnancy and the puerperium, from conception to 6 weeks after birth.

maternity nursing,   nursing care of women and their families during pregnancy, during parturition, and through the first days of the puerperium. Increasingly, postpartum maternity nursing includes the supervision of the mothers' care of their newborns in rooming-in units and may include care of normal newborns in the nursery when they are not with their mothers. Maternity nursing requires extensive instruction of the mothers in the usual behavior and needs of a newborn, in expected patterns of growth and development of the infant during the first week, and in details of care needed by the mother during the first weeks after birth. Breast-feeding, bottle-feeding, baby baths, perineal care, nutrition, and danger signs of the puerperium are usually taught by the maternity nurse. Observation for abnormal conditions, such as thrombophlebitis, mastitis, and other infections, is a daily ongoing concern of the maternity nurse on the postpartum unit. Intrapartum maternity nursing involves the care of mothers in labor and delivery, as well as high-risk technical nursing, emotional support in labor and delivery, and ongoing observation for abnormal signs or symptoms. Often, pregnant women with medical problems associated with pregnancy are cared for on a special high-risk antepartum unit by specially educated maternity nurses.

mat gold [Fr, *mat*, dull; AS, *geolu*, yellow],   a noncohesive form of pure gold, which is prepared by electrodeposition and may be used in the base of some dental restorations, then veneered or overlaid with cohesive foil. Also called **crystal gold, sponge gold.**

mating /mā′ting/ [MDu, *mate*, companion],   the pairing of individuals of the opposite sex, primarily for purposes of reproduction.

mat. med.,　abbreviation for **materia medica.**

matrifocal family /mat′rifō′kəl/ [L, *mater*, mother, *focus*, hearth; *familia*, household],　a family unit composed of a mother and her children. Biologic fathers have a temporary place in the family during the first years of the children's lives, but they maintain a more permanent position in their own original families. Common characteristics of this kind of family include living at a subsistence level, because of irregular employment of the fathers and unreliable economic support from them, and child care by older female relatives so that the mother of the children is free to work.

matrix /mā′triks, mat′riks/ [L, womb],　**1.** an intercellular substance **2.** also called **ground substance.** a basic substance from which a specific organ or kind of tissue develops. **3.** a form used in shaping a tooth surface in dental procedures.

matrix retainer,　a mechanical device used to secure the ends of a matrix around a tooth to provide a substitute wall where a portion of the tooth is missing and help compact a restoration in a tooth cavity. Also called *matrix holder*. See also **retainer.**

matrix unguis.　See **nailbed.**

matter [L, *materia*],　**1.** anything that has mass and occupies space. **2.** any substance not otherwise identified as to its constituents, such as gray matter, pus, or serum exuding from a wound.

Matulane,　a trademark for an antineoplastic (procarbazine hydrochloride).

maturation /mach′ərā′shən/ [L, *maturare*, to ripen],　**1.** the process or condition of attaining complete development. In humans it is the unfolding of full physical, emotional, and intellectual capacities that enable a person to function at a higher level of competency and adaptability within the environment. **2.** the final stages in the meiotic formation of germ cells in which the number of chromosomes in each cell is reduced to the haploid number characteristic of the species. See also **meiosis, oogenesis, spermatogenesis. 3.** suppuration.　-**maturate**, *v.*

maturational crisis /mach′ərā′shənəl/,　a transitional or developmental period within a person's life, such as puberty, when psychologic equilibrium is upset.

mature /məchŏŏr′/ [L, *maturus*, ripe],　**1.** to become fully developed; to ripen. **2.** fully developed or ripened.

mature cell leukemia.　See **polymorphocytic leukemia.**

maturity (mat.) /məchŏŏ′ritē/ [L, *maturus*, ripe],　**1.** a state of complete growth or development, usually designated as the period of life between adolescence and old age. **2.** the stage at which an organism is capable of reproduction.

maturity-onset diabetes.　See **non-insulin-dependent diabetes mellitus**

max,　**1.** abbreviation for *maxima.* **2.** abbreviation for *maximum.*

maxilla /maksil′ə/, *pl.* **maxillae** [L *mala* jaw],　one of a pair of large bones that form the upper jaw, consisting of a pyramidal body and four processes: the zygomatic, frontal, alveolar, and palatine.

-maxilla,　a combining form meaning the 'upper jaw or the bones composing it': *intermaxilla, submaxilla, supermaxilla.*

maxillary /mak′sələr′ē/ [L, *maxilla*, jaw],　pertaining to the upper jawbone.

maxillary arch [L, *maxilla*, upper jaw; *arcus*, bow],　the curved bony ridge of the upper jaw bone, in the shape of a horseshoe, including the dentition and supporting structures.

maxillary artery [L, *mala*, upper jaw; Gk, *arteria*, air pipe],　either of two larger terminal branches of the external carotid arteries that rise from the neck of the mandible near the parotid gland and divide into three branches, supplying the deep structures of the face.

maxillary fossa.　See **canine fossa.**

maxillary process [L, *maxilla*, jaw + *processus*],　**1.** the alveolar process of the upper jaw that contains the tooth sockets. **2.** the frontal process that extends upward to articulate with the frontal and nasal bones. **3.** the palatine process that helps form the hard palate. **4.** the zygomatic process or anterior surface that articulates with the zygomatic bone.

maxillary sinus,　one of the pair of large air cells forming a pyramidal cavity in the body of the maxilla. The apex of each sinus extends into the zygomatic arch, and its floor, formed by the alveolar process, is usually 1 to 10 mm below the floor of the nose. In the adult the volume of the sinus averages 14.75 cc. The mucous membrane of the sinus is continuous with that of the nasal cavity; an opening in the medial wall of the sinus communicates with the middle meatus. In the fourth month of gestation the embryonic sinus appears as a shallow groove on the medial surface of the bone but does not reach full size until after the second teething. Also called **antrum of Highmore.** Compare **ethmoidal air cell, frontal sinus, sphenoidal sinus.**

maxillary vein,　one of a pair of deep veins of the face, accompanying the maxillary artery and passing between the condyle of the mandible and the sphenomandibular ligament. Each maxillary vein is formed by the confluence of veins in the pterygoid plexus and joins the superficial temporal vein to form the retromandibular vein. Each maxillary vein is a tributary of the internal jugular and the external jugular veins.

maxillofacial /mak′silōfā′shəl/ [L, *maxilla*, jaw; *facies*, face],　pertaining to the maxilla and face.

maxillofacial prosthesis [L *mala* upper jaw, *facies* face],　a prosthetic replacement for part, or all, of the upper jaw, nose, or cheek. It is applied when surgical repair alone is inadequate.

maxillofacial surgery.　See **oral surgery.**

maxillomandibular fixation /maksil′ōmandib′yŏŏlər/ [L, *mala*, upper jaw, *mandere*, to chew; *figere*, to fasten],　stabilization of fractures of the face or jaw by temporarily connecting the maxilla and mandible by wires, elastic bands, or metal splints. See also **elastic band fixation, nasomandibular fixation.**

maximal breathing capacity (MBC) /mak′siməl/ [L, *maximus*, greatest; AS, *braeth;* L, *capacitas*],　the amount of gas exchanged per minute with maximal rate and depth of respiration.

maximal diastolic membrane potential,　(in cardiology) the greatest degree of negative transmembrane potential achieved by a cell during repolarization.

maximal expiratory flow rate (MEFR),　the rate of the most rapid flow of gas from the lungs during a forced vital capacity maneuver.

maximal midexpiratory flow rate,　the average volumetric rate of gas flow during the middle half (in terms of volume) of a forced expiratory vital capacity maneuver. It is used in pulmonary function tests to detect and evaluate chronic diffuse obstructive bronchopulmonary diseases, such as bronchitis, emphysema, and asthma.

maximal voluntary ventilation, the maximal volume of gas that a person can ventilate by voluntary effort per unit of time breathing as quickly and deeply as possible. It is used in pulmonary function tests. The results are expressed in volume units per minute.

maximum diastolic potential. See **maximal diastolic membrane potential.**

maximum inspiratory pressure (MIP) /mak'səməm/ [L, *maximus,* greatest; *inspirare,* to breathe in; *premere,* to press], the maximum pressure within the alveoli of the lungs that occurs during a maximum inspiratory effort.

maximum oxygen uptake, the greatest amount of oxygen that can be transported from the lungs to the working muscle tissue. Also called **aerobic capacity.**

maximum permissible dose (MPD), the estimated maximum amount of radiation to which a person may be exposed with a minimum risk of experiencing leukemia, cancer, or genetic effects based on data obtained from dose-response models and actual experience accumulated in more than 50 years. The MPD for the general population is 500 mrem per year, a figure that is 10% of the whole-body MPD of 5000 mrem per year for radiation workers. Other MPDs range from 50 mrem for the gestation period of a pregnant woman to 75 rem in any 1 year, or 25 rem in a 3-month period, for the hands of an occupationally exposed person. Also called **allowable dose, tolerance dose.** See also **accumulated dose equivalent.**

maxofacial surgery. See **dentistry.**

Mayer's reflex /mā'ərz/ [Karl Mayer, Austrian neurologist, b. 1862], a normal reflex elicited by grasping the ring finger and flexing it at the metacarpophalangeal joint of a person whose hand is relaxed with thumb abducted. The normal response is adduction and apposition of the thumb. The reflex is absent in disease of the pyramidal system.

Mayo scissors. See **scissors.**

-mazia, -mastia, -masty, a combining form meaning '(condition of the) breasts': *macromazia, pleomazia, polymazia.*

mazindol /mā'zindōl/, an anorexiant.

  ■ INDICATION: It is prescribed to decrease the appetite in the treatment of exogenous obesity.

  ■ CONTRAINDICATIONS: Glaucoma, history of drug abuse, concomitant use of a monoamine oxidase inhibitor, or known hypersensitivity to this drug prohibits its use.

  ■ ADVERSE EFFECTS: Among the more serious adverse reactions are insomnia, palpitation, dizziness, dry mouth, tachycardia, and hypersensitivity reactions.

mazo-, a combining form meaning 'of or pertaining to the breast': *mazodynia, mazology, mazopexy.*

mb, mbar, abbreviation for *millibar.*

M.B., abbreviation for *Bachelor of Medicine.*

MBC, abbreviation for **maximal breathing capacity.**

MBD, M.B.D., abbreviation for *minimal brain dysfunction.* See **attention deficit disorder.**

mbp, abbreviation for *mean blood pressure.*

mbt, abbreviation for *mean body temperature.*

mc, 1. abbreviation for *millicycle;* **2.** abbreviation for **millicurie.**

mC, abbreviation for **millicoulomb.**

Mc, abbreviation for *megacycle.*

MC, 1. abbreviation for *medical certificate.* **2.** abbreviation for *Medical Corps.*

McArdle's disease /məkär'dəlz/ [Brian McArdle, twentieth century English neurologist], an inherited metabolic disease marked by an absence of myophosphorylase B and abnormally large amounts of glycogen in skeletal muscle. It is milder than other glycogen storage diseases, characterized only by muscle weakness and cramping after exercise. There is no known treatment. Also called **glycogen storage disease, type V.** See also **glycogen storage disease.**

MCAT, abbreviation for **Medical College Aptitude Test.**

McBurney's point /makbur'nēz/ [Charles McBurney, American surgeon, b. 1845; L, *pungere,* to puncture], a site of extreme sensitivity in acute appendicitis, situated in the normal area of the appendix about 2 inches from the right anterior superior spine of the ilium, on a line between that spine and the umbilicus. See also **appendicitis.**

McBurney's sign, a reaction of the patient indicating severe pain and extreme tenderness when McBurney's point is palpated. Such a reaction indicates appendicitis.

McCall's festoon /məkôlz'/, (in dentistry) any one of the enlargements of the gingival margins that may be associated with occlusal trauma.

mcg, abbreviation for **microgram.**

M.Ch., abbreviation for *Master of Surgery.*

MCH, 1. abbreviation for **maternal and child health.** **2.** abbreviation for **mean corpuscular hemoglobin.**

MCHC, abbreviation for **mean corpuscular hemoglobin concentration.**

mc hr, abbreviation for *millicurie hour.*

mCi, abbreviation for **millicurie.**

McManus, R. Louise (b. 1885), an American nurse who established the first national testing service for the nursing profession, currently the second largest educational testing program in the nation. She was also instrumental in developing a means of evaluating the nursing programs in community and junior colleges, and she established a center for education in nursing research at Teachers College, Columbia University.

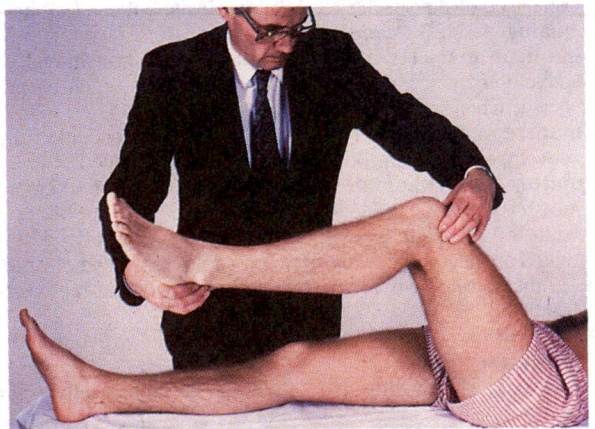

McMurray's sign *(Epstein, 1992)*

McMurray's sign /makmur'ēz/ [Thomas P. McMurray, English surgeon, b. 1887], an audible click heard when rotating the tibia on the femur, indicating injury to meniscal structures.

M.C.P., abbreviation for **metacarpophalangeal joint.**

McShirley's electromallet. See **electromallet condenser.**

MCTD, abbreviation for **mixed connective tissue disease.**

MCV, abbreviation for **mean corpuscular volume.**

Md, symbol for the element **mendelevium.**

MD, abbreviation for **muscular dystrophy.**

M.D., abbreviation for *Doctor of Medicine.* See **physician.**

MDA, abbreviation for *Muscular Dystrophy Association.*

MDR, abbreviation for **minimum daily requirement.**

M.D.V., abbreviation for **Doctor of Veterinary Medicine.**

Me, abbreviation for the methyl radical CH_3..

Meals on Wheels, a program designed to deliver hot meals to elderly, physically disabled, or other people who lack the resources to provide themselves with nutritionally adequate warm meals on a daily basis.

mean [ME, *mene,* in the middle], occupying a position midway between two extremes of a set of values or data. The **arithmetic mean** is a value that is derived by dividing the total of a set of values by the number of items in the set. The **geometric mean** is a value that is between the first and last of a set of values organized in a geometric progression.

mean arterial pressure (MAP), the arithmetic mean of the blood pressure in the arterial portion of the circulation.

mean corpuscular hemoglobin (MCH), an estimate of the amount of hemoglobin in an average erythrocyte, derived from the ratio between the amount of hemoglobin and the number of erythrocytes present. The normal value of MCH is between 28 and 32 picograms of hemoglobin per red blood cell. See also **hypochromic anemia, iron deficiency anemia.**

mean corpuscular hemoglobin concentration (MCHC), an estimation of the concentration of hemoglobin in grams per 100 ml of packed red blood cells, derived from the ratio of the hemoglobin to the hematocrit. The normal MCHC is between 32% and 36%.

mean corpuscular volume (MCV), an evaluation of the average volume of each red cell, derived from the ratio of the volume of packed red cells (the hematocrit) to the total number of red blood cells. The normal MCV is between 82 and 92 $\mu m3$.

mean marrow dose (MMD), an arbitrary measure of the estimated average annual somatic radiation received by the population of the United States. The figure is 77 mrad and represents a weighted average for both people exposed to radiation and people not exposed during the period. It is expressed in terms of bone marrow because irradiation of that tissue is assumed to be a cause of leukemia.

measles /mēʹzəlz/ [ME, *meseles,* skin spots], an acute, highly contagious, viral disease involving the respiratory tract and characterized by a spreading maculopapular cutaneous rash that occurs primarily in young children who have not been immunized. Measles is caused by a paramyxovirus and is transmitted by direct contact with droplets spread from the nose, throat, and mouth of infected people, usually in the prodromal stage of the disease. Indirect transmission by uninfected people or by contaminated articles is unusual. Diagnosis is confirmed by the identification of Koplik's spots on the buccal mucosa and by bacteriologic culture or serologic examination. Also called **morbilli, rubeola.** See also **roseola infantum, rubella.**

■ OBSERVATIONS: An incubation period of 7 to 14 days is followed by the prodromal stage, characterized by fever,

malaise, coryza, cough, conjunctivitis, photophobia, anorexia, and the pathognomonic Koplik's spots, which appear 1 to 2 days before onset of the rash. Pharyngitis and inflammation of the laryngeal and tracheobronchial mucosa develop, the temperature may rise to 103° or 104° F, and there is marked granulocytic leukopenia. The papules of the rash first appear as irregular brownish-pink spots around the hairline, the ears, and the neck, then spread rapidly, within 24 to 48 hours, to the trunk and extremities, becoming red, maculopapular, and dense, giving a blotchy appearance. Within 3 to 5 days, the fever subsides and the lesions flatten, turn a brownish color, and begin to fade, causing a fine desquamation, especially over heavily affected areas.

■ INTERVENTIONS: Routine treatment consists of bed rest, antipyretics, antibiotics to control secondary bacterial infection, and, when necessary, application of calamine lotion, corn starch solution, oatmeal, baking soda, or cool water to relieve itching. Preventive measures include active immunization with measles virus vaccine after the infant is 1 year old. Passive immunization with immune serum globulin is recommended for unvaccinated individuals exposed to the disease. One attack of the disease confers lifelong immunity.

■ NURSING CONSIDERATIONS: Bed rest, isolation, and quiet activity are recommended as long as fever and rash persist. Acetaminophen, fluids, cool sponge baths, nose drops, and cough medication may be necessary to counteract fever and respiratory symptoms. Bright sunlight may be irritating to the eyes. Special attention is given to the care and cleansing of the eyes and skin, especially in cases of severe papular eruption. An important nursing function is instruction of the parents in the proper home care of the child, because most cases are not serious enough to require hospitalization. The disease is usually benign, and mortality is rare. Complications sometimes occur, the most common of which are otitis media, pneumonia, bronchiolitis, obstructive laryngitis, laryngotracheitis, and, occasionally, encephalitis and appendicitis. Rarely, but most gravely, the virus causes subacute sclerosing panencephalitis several years after the acute attack of measles has occurred.

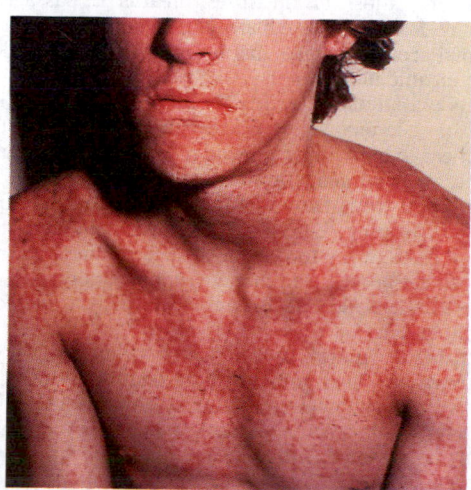

Measles *(Zitelli, 1992/Courtesy Dr. M. Sherlock)*

measles and rubella virus vaccine live, an active immunizing agent.

■ INDICATIONS: It is prescribed for immunization against measles and rubella.

■ CONTRAINDICATIONS: Immunosuppression, concomitant administration of corticosteroids, tuberculosis, known or suspected pregnancy, hypersensitivity to neomycin, neoplasms of the lymphatic system or bone marrow, or active infection prohibits its use. It should not be given for 3 months after the use of whole blood, plasma, or immune serum globulin, or for 1 month before or after immunization with other live virus vaccines, except mumps vaccine.

■ ADVERSE EFFECT: The most serious adverse reaction is anaphylaxis.

measles immune globulin. See **immune gamma globulin.**

measles, mumps, and rubella virus vaccine live (MMR), an active immunizing agent.

■ INDICATION: It is prescribed for simultaneous immunization against measles, mumps, and rubella.

■ CONTRAINDICATIONS: Immunosuppression, concomitant administration of corticosteroids, tuberculosis, hypersensitivity to neomycin, neoplasms of the lymphatic system or bone marrow, known or suspected pregnancy, or acute infection prohibits its use. It is not given for 3 months after the use of whole blood, plasma, or immune serum globulin, and it is not given for 1 month before or after immunization with other live virus vaccines.

■ ADVERSE EFFECTS: The most serious adverse reaction is anaphylaxis.

measurement /mezh′ərment/ [L, *mensura*], the determination, expressed numerically, of the extent or quantity of a substance, energy, or time. See also **international unit, metric system.**

meatal /mē·ā′təl/ [L, *meatus*, channel], pertaining to a meatus.

meatorrhaphy /mē′ətôr′əfē/ [L, *meatus*, channel; Gk, *rhaphe*, suture], the suturing of the cut end of the urethra to the glans penis after surgery to enlarge the urethral meatus.

meatoscopy /mē′ətos′kəpē/ [L, *meatus* + Gk, *skopein*, to look], the visual examination of any meatus, especially the urethra, usually performed with the aid of a speculum.

meatus /mē·ā′təs/, *pl.* **meatuses, meatus** [L, passage], an opening or tunnel through any part of the body, such as the external acoustic meatus that leads from the external ear to the tympanic membrane.

meatus acusticus externus [L, *meatus*, channel; Gk, *akoustikos*, hearing; L, *externus*], the passage from the external ear to the tympanic membrane. Also called **auditory canal, external acoustic meatus.**

meatus acusticus internus [L, *meatus*, channel; Gk, *akoustikos*, hearing; L, *internus*], the internal acoustic meatus, a passageway for the facial, intermediate, and vestibulocochlear nerves, and the labyrinthine artery.

Mebaral, a trademark for an anticonvulsant and sedative (mephobarbital).

mebendazole /məben′dəzōl/, an anthelmintic.

■ INDICATIONS: It is prescribed in treatment of pinworm, whipworm, roundworm, and hookworm infestations.

■ CONTRAINDICATIONS: Pregnancy or known hypersensitivity to this drug prohibits its use.

■ ADVERSE EFFECTS: Among the most serious adverse reactions are abdominal pain and diarrhea.

MEC, abbreviation for *minimum effective concentration,*

or the minimum inhibitory concentration for a drug to be active. The drug is effective at any level above this threshold value.

mecamylamine hydrochloride /mek′əmil′əmēn/, a ganglionic blocking agent.

■ INDICATION: It is prescribed in the management of hypertensive cardiac disease.

■ CONTRAINDICATIONS: Coronary or cerebrovascular insufficiency, recent myocardial infarction, uremia, pyelonephritis, glaucoma, or known hypersensitivity to this drug prohibits its use.

■ ADVERSE EFFECTS: Among the most serious adverse reactions are orthostatic hypotension, paralytic ileus, urinary retention, and cycloplegia. The incidence of side effects is very high because the drug reduces all autonomic activity.

mechanical advantage [Gk, *mechane*, machine; L, *abante*, superior position], (in physiology) the ratio of the output force developed by the muscles to the input force applied to the body structures that the muscles move, especially the ratio of these forces associated with the body structures that act as levers. Variations in the sizes of muscles and the lengths of bones in different individuals partially account for the different mechanical advantages from one body type to another and their different physical capabilities, such as speed and strength.

mechanical condenser, a device that delivers automatically controlled impacts for condensing restorative material in the filling of tooth cavities. It may be spring activated, pneumatic, or electrically controlled. Also called **automatic mallet condenser.**

mechanical dead air space [Gk, *mechane*; AS, *déad*; Gk, *aer*; L, *spatium*], the volume of air that fills the breathing circuits of a mechanical ventilator. The mechanical dead space may be increased if necessary to control hypocapnia and respiratory alkalosis.

mechanical heart-lung, a device connected to the circulatory system to maintain oxygenated blood flow during surgery that requires interruption of normal heart-lung functions. See also **blood pump.**

mechanical restraint [Gk, *mechane;* L, *restringere*, to confine], a straitjacket, chair, bed, or other device used to enforce confinement of a patient, as opposed to the use of chemical restraints, such as neuroleptic medications, for the same purpose.

mechanical vector. See **vector.**

mechanism /mek′əniz′əm/, **1.** an instrument or process by which something is done, results, or comes into being. **2.** a machine or machinelike system. **3.** a stimulus-response system. **4.** a habit or drive.

mechanism of labor. See **cardinal movements of labor.**

mechano-, a combining form meaning 'mechanical': *mechanocyte, mechanotherapy, mechanothermy.*

mechanoreceptor /mek′ənō′risep′tər/ [Gk, *mechane*, machine; L, *recipere*, to receive], any sensory nerve ending that responds to mechanical stimuli, such as touch, pressure, sound, and muscular contractions. See also **proprioceptor.**

mechlorethamine hydrochloride /mek′ôreth′əmēn/, an antineoplastic alkylating agent. Also called **nitrogen mustard.**

■ INDICATIONS: It is prescribed in the treatment of a variety of neoplasms.

■ CONTRAINDICATIONS: Bone marrow depression, pregnancy,

infection, or known hypersensitivity to this drug prohibits its use.

■ ADVERSE EFFECTS: Among the most serious adverse reactions are bone marrow depression and inflammation caused by extravasation at the site of injection. Nausea, vomiting, and alopecia also may occur.

Meckel's diverticulum [Johann F. Meckel, German anatomist, b. 1781], an anomalous sac protruding from the wall of the ileum between 30 and 90 cm from the ileocecal sphincter. It is congenital, resulting from the incomplete closure of the yolk stalk, and occurs in 1% to 2% of the population. The diverticulum is usually asymptomatic, but the condition is suggested by signs of appendicitis in infancy, by sudden and painless bleeding, usually in childhood, or by symptoms of intestinal obstruction. Symptomatic diverticula are most commonly resected. Surgical resection of asymptomatic diverticula is also recommended to avoid diverticulitis, obstruction, and blood loss, which may occur. Many Meckel's diverticula are discovered incidentally during surgery for other causes and on postmortem examination.

used with caution in patients having upper GI disease or impaired renal function.

■ ADVERSE EFFECTS: Among the more serious adverse reactions are GI distress, peptic ulcers, dizziness, rashes, and tinnitus. This drug interacts with many other drugs.

Meclomen, a trademark for an antiinflammatory agent (meclofenamate sodium).

mecocephaly. See **scaphocephaly.**

meconium /mikō′nē·əm/ [Gk, *mekon,* poppy], a material that collects in the intestines of a fetus and forms the first stools of a newborn. It is thick and sticky in consistency, usually greenish to black in color, and composed of secretions of the intestinal glands, some amniotic fluid, and intrauterine debris, such as bile pigments, fatty acids, epithelial cells, mucus, lanugo, and blood. With ingestion of breast milk or formula and the proper functioning of the GI tract, the color, consistency, and frequency of the stools change by the third or fourth day after the initiation of feedings. The presence of meconium in the amniotic fluid during labor may indicate fetal distress.

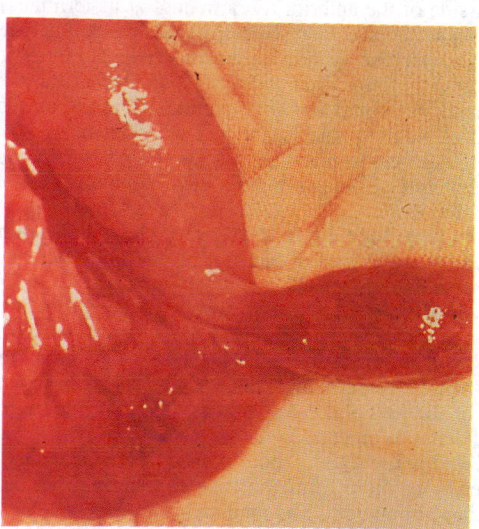

Meckel's diverticulum (Zitelli, 1992)

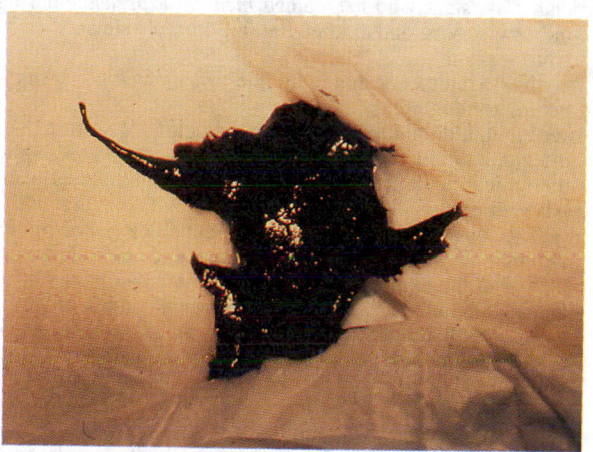

Meconium (Zitelli, 1992)

Meclan, a trademark for an antibacterial (meclocycline sulfosalicylate).

meclizine hydrochloride /mek′lizēn/, an antihistamine.

■ INDICATION: It is prescribed in the prevention and treatment of motion sickness.

■ CONTRAINDICATIONS: Newborn infants and lactating mothers are not given this drug. Asthma or known hypersensitivity to this drug prohibits its use.

■ ADVERSE EFFECTS: Among the more serious adverse effects are drowsiness, skin rash, hypersensitivity reactions, dry mouth, tachycardia, and nervousness.

meclofenamate sodium /mek′lōfen′əmāt/, a nonsteroidal antiinflammatory agent.

■ INDICATIONS: It is prescribed in the treatment of rheumatoid arthritis and osteoarthritis.

■ CONTRAINDICATIONS: Known hypersensitivity to aspirin or to nonsteroidal antiinflammatory drugs prohibits its use. It is

meconium aspiration, the inhalation of meconium by the fetus or newborn, which can block the air passages and result in failure of the lungs to expand or cause other pulmonary dysfunction, such as pneumonia or emphysema.

meconium ileus, obstruction of the small intestine in the newborn caused by impaction of thick, dry, tenacious meconium, usually at or near the ileocecal valve. Symptoms include abdominal distention, vomiting, failure to pass meconium within the first 24 to 48 hours after birth, and rapid dehydration with associated electrolyte imbalance. The condition results from a deficiency in pancreatic enzymes and is the earliest manifestation of cystic fibrosis. In uncomplicated cases in which perforation, volvulus, or atresia does not occur, the obstruction may be relieved by giving enemas with a contrast medium, such as a hypertonic solution of meglumine diatrizoate and sodium diatrizoate, under fluoroscopy. Fluid loss is replaced intravenously to prevent dehydration. If two or three enemas do not dislodge the obstruction, surgery is necessary. See also **meconium plug syndrome.**

meconium plug syndrome, obstruction of the large intestine in the newborn caused by thick, rubbery meconium that may fill the entire colon and part of the terminal ileum. Symptoms include failure to pass meconium within the first 24 to 48 hours after birth, abdominal distention, and vomiting if complete intestinal blockage occurs. A barium enema will indicate the presence of a plug and in most cases will dislodge it from the bowel wall. Subsequent gentle saline enemas may be needed to expel it. The condition may be an indication of Hirschsprung's disease or cystic fibrosis. See also **meconium ileus.**

med, 1. abbreviation for *medical.* 2. abbreviation for *medicine.* 3. abbreviation for *minimum effective dose.*

MED, 1. abbreviation for *minimal effective dose;* 2. abbreviation for *minimal erythema dose.* See **threshold dose.**

medcard /med′kärd/, (in nursing) a small card listing the name, dose, and schedule of administration of each patient's medications, used in dispensing medication to each patient.

medevac, abbreviation for *medical evacuation.*

MEDEX /med′eks/, 1. an educational program accredited by the AMA for training military personnel with *medical experience* to become physician's assistants. 2. a physician's assistant who has gained *medical experience* during military service and further training in a physician's assistant program.

medi-, a prefix meaning 'middle': *medialecithal, medicinerea, mediotarsal.*

medial /mē′dē·əl/ [L, *medianus,* middle], 1. situated or oriented toward the midline of the body. 2. pertaining to the tunica media, the middle layer of a blood vessel wall. Also **mesial.**

medial antebrachial cutaneous nerve, a nerve of the arm that arises from the medial cord of the brachial plexus, medial to the axillary artery. Near the axilla it passes a filament to supply the skin over the biceps almost as far as the elbow. It descends on the ulnar side of the arm medial to the brachial artery, pierces the deep fascia with the basilic vein about the middle of the arm, and divides into the anterior branch and the ulnar branch. The anterior branch is the larger of the two branches and continues on the anterior part of the ulnar side of the arm, distributes filaments to the skin as far as the wrist, and communicates with the palmar cutaneous branch of the ulnar nerve. The ulnar branch descends on the medial side of the basilic nerve as far as the wrist, innervates the skin, and communicates with branches of the ulnar nerve. Compare **medial brachial cutaneous nerve.**

medial arteriosclerosis. See **Mönckeberg's arteriosclerosis.**

medial brachial cutaneous nerve, a nerve of the arm arising from the medial cord of the brachial plexus and distributed to the medial side of the arm. It passes through the axilla, pierces the deep fascia in the middle of the arm, and supplies the skin of the arm as far as the olecranon. Compare **medial antebrachial cutaneous nerve.**

medial cuneiform bone, the largest of three cuneiform bones of the foot, situated on the medial side of the tarsus, between the scaphoid bone and the first metatarsal. It serves as the attachment for various ligaments, the tendons of the tibialis anterior, and the peroneus longus. It articulates with the scaphoid, the intermediate cuneiform, and the first and second metatarsals. Also called **internal cuneiform bone.**

medial geniculate body, either of the two areas on the posterior dorsal thalamus, relaying auditory impulses from the lateral lemniscus to the auditory cortex.

medialis /mē′dē·ā′lis/ [L, *medius,* middle], pertaining to the middle or to the median plane.

medial malleolus. See **internal malleolus.**

medial pectoral nerve, a branch of the brachial plexus that, with the lateral pectoral nerve, supplies the pectoral muscles. It arises from the medial cord of the plexus, medial to the axillary artery, passes between the axillary artery and the axillary vein, and joins the lateral pectoral nerve to form a loop around the artery before ending deep in the pectoralis minor. The loop branches to supply the pectoralis minor and the pectoralis major. Compare **lateral pectoral nerve.**

medial rotation, a turning toward the midline of the body. Compare **lateral rotation.** See also **rotation.**

median /mē′dē·ən/ [L, *medianus,* middle], (in statistics) the number representing the middle value of the scores in a sample. In an odd number of scores arrayed in ascending order, it is the middle score; in an even number of scores so arrayed, it is the average of the two central scores.

median antebrachial vein /an′tēbrā′kē·əl/, one of the superficial veins of the upper limb that drains the venous plexus on the palmar surface of the hand. It ascends on the ulnar side of the anterior forearm and, at its terminus, joins the median cubital vein. In many individuals it divides into two vessels, one joining the basilic vein, the other joining the cephalic vein distal to the elbow. One of the veins of the median cubital complex commonly anastomoses with the deep veins of the forearm. The anastomosis holds the superficial vein in place and makes it a practical choice for venipuncture. Compare **basilic vein, cephalic vein, dorsal digital vein.**

median aperture of fourth ventricle, an opening between the lower part of the roof of the fourth ventricle and the subarachnoid space.

median atlantoaxial joint, one of three points of articulation of the atlas and the axis. The median atlantoaxial joint is a pivot articulation between the dens, the axis, and the ring of the atlas and involves five ligaments. It allows rotation of the axis and the skull, the extent of rotation limited by the alar ligaments.

median basilic vein, one of the superficial veins of the upper limb, often formed as one of two branches from the median cubital vein. The median basilic vein courses across the palmar surface of the forearm near the elbow and is commonly used for venipuncture, phlebotomy, or intravenous infusion. Compare **basilic vein.**

median effective dose (ED$_{50}$), the dose of a drug that may be expected to cause a specific intensity of effect in one half of the patients to whom it is given.

median glossitis. See **median rhomboid glossitis.**

median jaw relation, (in dentistry) any jaw relation that exists when the mandible is in the median sagittal plane.

median lethal dose (MLD, LD$_{50}$), (in radiotherapy) the amount of radiation that kills 50% of the individuals in a large group of animals or organisms within a specified period of time.

median nerve, one of the terminal branches of the brachial plexus that extends along the radial portions of the forearm and the hand and supplies various muscles and the skin of these parts. It arises from the brachial plexus by two large roots, one from the lateral and one from the medial cord. The roots unite to form the trunk of the nerve that courses down the arm with the brachial artery. In the forearm it passes between the two heads of the pronator teres and passes through the flexor retinaculum into the palm of the hand, where it is covered only by the skin and the palmar aponeu rosis. Emerging from the retinaculum, it is enlarged and flattened and splits into digital and muscular branches. The median nerve usually has no branches above the elbow, but in some individuals the nerve to the pronator teres arises there. The median nerve gives off a few articular branches to the elbow joint and muscular branches to the forearm, the anterior interosseous nerve, the palmar branch, the muscular branch in the hand, the first, second, and third palmar digital nerves, and the proper digital nerves. Compare **musculocutaneous nerve, radial nerve, ulnar nerve.**

median palatine suture, the line of junction between the horizontal portions of the palatine bones that extends from both sides of the skull to form the posterior part of the hard palate.

median plane, a vertical plane that divides the body into right and left halves and passes approximately through the sagittal suture of the skull. Also called **cardinal sagittal plane, midsagittal plane.** Compare **frontal plane, sagittal plane, transverse plane.**

median rhomboid glossitis, a red, depressed, diamond-shaped area on the dorsum of the tongue, frequently irritated by alcohol, hot drinks, or spicy foods. The condition is most often seen in adult men and may be caused by candidiasis.

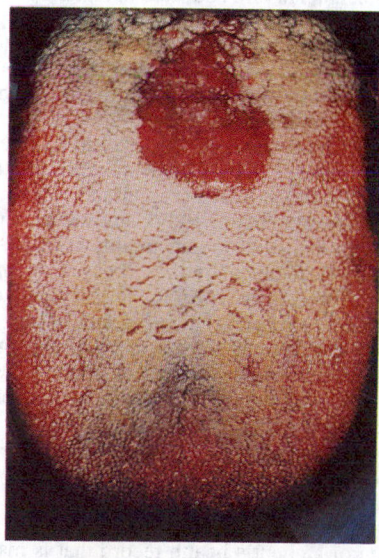

Median rhomboid glossitis (Lamey, 1988)

median sternotomy, a chest surgery technique in which an incision is made from the suprasternal notch to below the xiphoid process. The sternum is then opened with a saw. Closure requires reunion of the sternum with stainless steel sutures. The procedure is used for coronary artery bypass and valve replacement operations. Compare **anterolateral thoracotomy, posterolateral thoracotomy.**

median toxic dose (TD$_{50}$), the dosage that may be expected to cause a toxic effect in one half of the patients to whom it is given.

mediastinal /mē′dē·əstī′nəl/ [L, *mediastinus*, midway], pertaining to a median septum or space between two parts of the body, such as the interval between the pleural sacs.

mediastinitis, an inflammation of the mediastinum.

mediastinoscopy /mē′dē·as′tinos′kəpē/ [L, *mediastinus*, midway; Gk, *skopein*, to view], an examination of the mediastinum through an incision in the suprasternum, using an endoscope with light and lenses.

mediastinum /mē′dē·əstī′nəm/, pl. **mediastina** [L, *mediastinus*, midway], a portion of the thoracic cavity in the middle of the thorax, between the pleural sacs containing the two lungs. It extends from the sternum to the vertebral column and contains all the thoracic viscera except the lungs. It is enclosed in a thick extension of the thoracic subserous fascia and is divided into the cranial portion and the caudal portion by a plane extending from the sternal angle to the caudal border of the fourth thoracic vertebra. The caudal portion is divided into the anterior mediastinum, ventral to the pericardium, the middle mediastinum, containing the pericardium, and the posterior mediastinum, dorsal to the pericardium. —**mediastinal,** *adj.*

mediate /mē′dē·āt/ [L, *medio*, in the middle], **1.** to cause a change to occur, as in stimulation by a hormone. **2.** to settle a dispute, as in collective bargaining. **3.** situated between two places, things, parts, or terms. **4.** (in psychology) an event that follows one process or event and precedes another; for example, in the process of cognition, perception follows stimulation and precedes thinking. —**mediating,** *adj.,* **mediator,** *n.*

Mediatric, a trademark for a nutritional supplement containing multivitamins, minerals, hormones, and a central nervous system stimulant (methamphetamine hydrochloride).

medic, abbreviation for **paramedic.** See also **medical corpsman.**

Medicaid /med′ikād/, a federally funded, state operated program of medical assistance to people with low incomes, authorized by Title XIX of the Social Security Act. Under broad federal guidelines, the individual states determine benefits, eligibility, rates of payment, and methods of administration.

medical abortion. See **abortion.**

Medicaid mill, *informal.* a health program or facility that solely or primarily serves people eligible for Medicaid. Such facilities are found mainly in depressed areas where there are few other health services.

medical assistant /med′ikəl/ [L, *medicare*, to heal; *assistere*, to stand by], a person who, under the direction of a physician, performs various routine administrative and nontechnical clinical tasks in a hospital, clinic, or similar facility.

medical care, the provision by a physician of services related to the maintenance of health, prevention of illness, and treatment of illness or injury.

medical care plan [L, *medicare*; OE, *caru*, sorrow; *planus,* floor], a long-range program of professional medical guidance designed to meet specific health objectives.

medical center, **1.** a health care facility. **2.** a hospital, especially one staffed and equipped to care for many patients and for a large number of kinds of diseases and dysfunctions, using sophisticated technology.

Medical College Aptitude Test (MCAT), an examination taken by persons applying to medical school, the score on this examination being an important criterion for acceptance. Basic science, intellectual ability, and mathematic and verbal aptitude and knowledge are tested.

medical consultation, a procedure whereby, on request by one physician, another physician reviews a patient's medical history, examines the patient, and makes recommendations as to care and treatment. The medical consultant often is a specialist with expertise in a particular field of medicine.

medical corpsman /kōr'man/ [L, *medicare,* to heal; *corpus,* body], **1.** a member of a military medical unit. **2.** a paramedic. Also called **medic.**

medical decision level, the concentration of analyte, or body fluid sample being analyzed, at which some medical action is indicated for proper patient care. There may be several medical decision levels for a given analyte.

medical diagnosis [L, *medicare;* Gk, *dia,* through; *gnosis,* knowledge], the determination of the cause of a patient's illness or suffering by the combined use of physical examination, patient interview, laboratory tests, review of the patient's medical records, a knowledge of the cause of observed signs and symptoms, and differential elimination of similar possible causes.

medical diathermy [L, *medicare, dia,* through, *thereme,* heat], the application of high-frequency electrical currents to generate therapeutic heat in diseased tissues.

medical directive, a general term for documents that provide direction on the type of care a person desires. See **advance directive, living will.**

medical director, a physician who is usually employed by a hospital to serve in a medical and administrative capacity as head of the organized medical staff. The medical director also may serve as liaison for the medical staff with the hospital's administration and governing board.

medical engineering, a field of study that involves biomedical engineering and technologic concepts to develop equipment and instruments required in health care delivery.

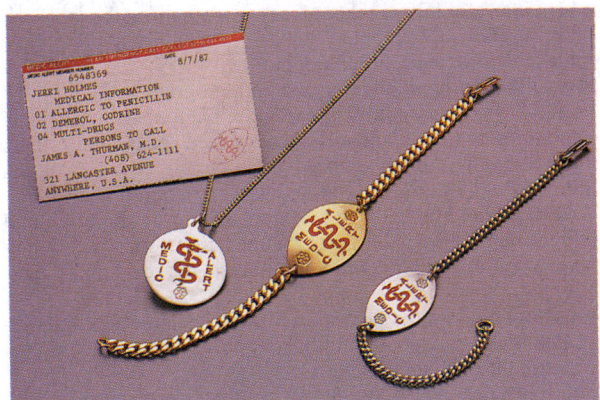

Medic Alert^R *(Judd, 1988)*

Medic Alert,® a nonprofit U.S. organization that maintains a huge database of information about individuals who are taking one or more medications for a chronic disorder. The database also includes emergency telephone numbers for physicians treating the patients and provides bracelets

or pendants to alert paramedics, interns, or other emergency medical personnel of the patient's medical condition and prescription drugs taken by the patient, who may be unconscious or confused after an accident or episode of illness. Medic Alert maintains access to the database for emergency medical personnel through a 24-hour telephone service.

medical ethics [L, *medicare;* Gk, *ethikos*], the moral conduct and principles that govern members of the medical profession.

medical examiner. See **coroner.**

medical genetics. See **clinical genetics.**

medical history. See **health history.**

medical illustrator, an artist qualified by special training in preparing illustrations of organs, tissues, and medical phenomena in normal and abnormal states.

medical indigency /in'dijen'sē/, the lack of financial reserves adequate to pay for medical care, especially a person or family able to manage other basic living expenses.

medical induction of labor. See **induction of labor.**

medical ionization. See **iontophoresis.**

medical jurisprudence [L, *medicare; jus,* law; *prudentia,* knowledge], the interaction of medicine with civil and criminal law.

medical laboratory technician, a person who, under the supervision of a medical technologist or physician, performs microscopic and bacteriologic tests of human blood, tissue, and fluids for diagnostic and research purposes. Medical laboratory technicians are educated in either a 12-month certificate program or a 2-year associate degree program, with associate degree graduates able to perform and interpret tests requiring discrimination between similar items.

medical model, the traditional approach to the diagnosis and treatment of illness as practiced by physicians in the Western world since the time of Koch and Pasteur. The physician focuses on the defect, or dysfunction, within the patient, using a problem-solving approach. The medical history, physical examination, and diagnostic tests provide the basis for the identification and treatment of a specific illness. The medical model is thus focused on the physical and biologic aspects of specific diseases and conditions. Nursing differs from the medical model in that the patient is perceived primarily as a social person relating to the environment; nursing care is formulated on the basis of a nursing assessment that assumes multiple causes for the problems experienced by the patient.

medical pathology [L, *medicare;* Gk, *pathos,* disease + *logos,* science], the study of diseases not easily treated by surgical procedures.

medical record [L, *medicare;* ME, *recorden,* to report], that portion of a client's health record that is made by physicians and is a written or transcribed history of various illnesses or injuries requiring medical care, inoculations, allergies, treatments, prognosis, and, frequently, health information about parents, siblings, occupation, and military service. The record may be reviewed by a physician in diagnosing the condition. See also **chart.**

medical record administrator, a person who maintains records of patients' medical histories, diagnoses, treatment, and outcome in a condition that meets medical, administrative, legal, ethical, regulatory, and institutional requirements.

medical record technician, a health professional responsible for maintaining components of health information systems consistent with the medical, administrative, ethical, legal, accreditation, and regulatory requirements of the health care delivery system.

medical secretary, a person who prepares and maintains medical records and performs related secretarial duties.

medical staff, physicians and dentists who are approved and given privileges to provide health care to patients in a hospital or other health care facility. Medical staff personnel may be full time or part time, and may be employed by the facility, or simply granted admitting priveleges to practice.

medical staff, courtesy, physicians and dentists who meet certain qualifications of the medical staff of a hospital but who admit patients only occasionally or act as consultants. They are ineligible to participate in medical staff activities.

medical staff, honorary, physicians and dentists, usually retired, who are recognized by the hospital medical staff for their noteworthy contributions but who may not admit patients to the hospital or participate in medical staff activities.

medical-surgical nursing, the nursing care of adult patients whose conditions or disorders are treated pharmacologically or surgically.

medical technologist, a person who, under the direction of a pathologist or other physician or medical scientist, performs specialized chemical, microscopic, and bacteriologic tests of blood, tissue, and fluids. A medical technologist who has successfully completed an examination by the Board of Registry of the American Society of Clinical Pathologists, or a similar professional body, may be designated a certified medical technologist.

medical transcriptionist, a health professional who prepares a written record of patient data that has been dictated by a physician. A **certified medical transcriptionist** is one who has met the qualifying standards of the American Association of Medical Transcription.

medical vagotomy [L, *medicare + vagus*; Gk, *temnein,* to cut]. See **pharmacologic vagotomy.**

medical waste, any discarded biologic product, such as blood or tissues, removed from operating rooms, morgues, laboratories, or other medical facilities. The term may also be applied to bedding, bandages, syringes, and similar materials that have been used in treating patients and animal carcasses or body parts used in research.

Medical Women's International Association (M.W.I.A.), an international professional organization of women physicians.

medicamentosus /med'ikəmen'tōsəs/ [L, *medicamentum,* drug], pertaining to a drug, particularly to an adverse reaction attributed to a medication.

Medicare /med'iker/, a federally funded national health insurance program in the United States for people over 65 years of age. The program is administered in two parts. Part A provides basic protection against costs of medical, surgical, and psychiatric hospital care. Part B is a voluntary medical insurance program financed in part from federal funds and in part from premiums contributed by people enrolled in the program. Medicare enrollment is offered to people 65 years of age or older who are entitled to receive Social Security or railroad retirement benefits. Other people over 65, such as federal employees and aliens, may not be eligible. Medicare was authorized by Title XVIII of the Social Security Act of 1965.

medicate /med'ikāt/ [L, *medicare,* to heal], to treat an illness by administering drugs.

medicated bougie /med'ikātid/ [L, *medicare,* to heal; Fr, candle], **1.** a bougie containing a medicated agent. **2.** *obsolete.* a suppository.

medicated enema, a medication administered via an enema. It is usually used preoperatively with patients scheduled for bowel surgery.

medicated tub bath, a therapeutic bath in which medication is dispersed in water, usually in the treatment of dermatologic disorders.

■ METHOD: The amount of medication and the amount and temperature of the water are specified in the order for the bath. The water is run, the medication is added, and the solution is stirred with a bath thermometer to disperse the medication in the water while testing the temperature. The temperature is usually between 35.6° C (96° F) and 37.8° C (100° F) but may be as high as 39.4° C (103° F), as in the treatment of psoriasis vulgaris. Most medicated baths are prescribed as half-hour treatments. A folded towel or waterproof pillow is placed behind the head, and a towel is draped over the shoulders to add to the patient's comfort. In certain conditions, the patient may be asked to scrub affected areas with a brush and washcloth; in others, the patient is instructed not to scrub at all. After the bath the skin is patted dry and any ointment, cream, or other topical prescription is applied.

■ NURSING INTERVENTION: The reason for the treatment is explained to the patient, and instructions are given not to get out of the tub without assistance and not to add water without calling the nurse. If the patient is to scrub the affected areas, the necessary equipment is brought to the bath. The tub is thoroughly scrubbed and rinsed before and after the treatment.

■ OUTCOME CRITERIA: The medicated bath is usually soothing, relaxing, and comforting for the patient. Close attention to instructing the patient fully and to ensuring comfort during the procedure improves the patient's compliance with the treatment.

medication /med'ikā'shən/ [L, *medicare,* to heal], **1.** a drug or other substance that is used as a medicine. **2.** the administration of a medicine.

medication error, any incorrect or wrongful administration of a medication, such as a mistake in dosage or route of administration, a failure to prescribe or administer the correct drug or formulation for a particular disease or condition, the use of outdated drugs, failure to observe the correct time for administration of the drug, or lack of awareness of adverse effects of certain drug combinations. Causes of medication error may include difficulty in reading handwritten orders, confusion about different drugs with similar names, and lack of information about a patient's drug allergies or sensitivities. When the nurse is in doubt, administration of a drug should be delayed until specifically authorized by a physician.

medication order, a written order by a physician, dentist, or other designated health professional for a medication to be dispensed by a hospital pharmacy for administration to an inpatient.

medicinal restraint /mədis'ənəl/ [L, *medicina + restringere,* to confine], the use of hypnotics or other sedatives to control a potentially violent patient. Also called **chemical restraint.**

medicinal treatment, therapy of disorders based chiefly on the use of appropriate pharmacologic agents.

medicine [L, *medicina*, art of healing], **1.** a drug or a remedy for illness. **2.** the art and science of the diagnosis, treatment, and prevention of disease and the maintenance of good health. **3.** the art or technique of treating disease without surgery. Two major divisions of medicine are academic medicine and clinical medicine. Some of the many branches of medicine include **environmental medicine, family medicine, forensic medicine, internal medicine,** and **physical medicine.** –**medical,** *adj.*

medicolegal /med′ikōlē′gəl/ [L, *medicina*, art of healing, *lex*, law], of or pertaining to both medicine and law. Medicolegal considerations are a significant part of the process of making many patient care decisions and in determining definitions and policies regarding the treatment of mentally incompetent people and minors, the performance of sterilization or therapeutic abortion, and the care of terminally ill patients. Medicolegal considerations, decisions, definitions, and policies provide the framework for informed consent, professional liability, and many other aspects of current practice in the health care field.

Medihaler-Epi, a trademark for an adrenergic (epinephrine bitartrate).

Medihaler-Ergotamine Aerosol, a trademark for an analgesic (ergotamine tartrate).

Medimmune, trademark for a recombinant form of **bacille Calmette-Guerin (BCG),** a live bovine bacterium used to immunize against tuberculosis. It is inexpensive to produce and can be given orally.

medio- [L, *medius*, middle], a prefix meaning 'pertaining to the middle': *mediopalatine, mediastinum*.

meditation /med′itā′shən/ [L, *meditari*, to consider], a state of consciousness in which the individual eliminates environmental stimuli from awareness so that the mind can focus on a single thing, producing a state of relaxation and relief from stress. A wide variety of techniques are used to clear the mind of stressful outside interferences.

meditation therapy, a method of achieving relaxation and consciouness expansion by focusing on a mantra or a key word, sound, or image while eliminating outside stimuli from one's awareness.

Mediterranean anemia. See **thalassemia.**

Mediterranean fever. See **brucellosis.**

medium, /mē′dē·əm/, *pl.* **media** [L, *medius*, middle], a substance through which something moves or through which it acts. A **contrast medium** is a substance that has a density different from that of body tissues, permitting visual comparison of structures when used with imaging techniques such as x-ray film. A **culture medium** is a substance that provides a nutritional environment for the growth of microorganisms or cells. A **dispersion medium** is the substance in which a colloid is dispersed. A **refractory medium** is the transparent tissues and fluid of the eye that refract light.

medium-chain triglyceride (MCT), a glycerine ester combined with an acid and distinguished from other triglycerides by having 8 to 10 carbon atoms and that can be absorbed directly into the portal system. MCTs in foods are usually high in calories and easily digested.

MEDLARS /med′lärs/, abbreviation for *Medical Literature Analysis and Retrieval System,* a computerized literature retrieval service of the National Library of Medicine in Bethesda, Maryland. MEDLARS contains more than 4,500,000 references to medical articles found in professional journals and books published since 1966. The references are made available on request to more than 1000 hospitals, universities, government agencies, and other interested parties throughout the world by means of a network of computer terminals. The references are filed in 15 data bases, including MEDLINE, TOXLINE, CHEMLINE, RTECS, CANCERLIT, and EPILEPSYLINE. See also **MEDLINE.**

MEDLINE /med′līn/, a National Library of Medicine computer data base that covers approximately 600,000 references to biomedical journal articles published currently and in the 2 preceding years. The files duplicate the contents of the monthly and annual volumes of the *Unabridged Index Medicus,* also published by the National Library of Medicine, which indexes medical reports from 3000 professional journals in more than 70 countries. See also **MEDLARS.**

MedRC, abbreviation for *medical reserve corps.*

Medrol, a trademark for a glucocorticoid (methylprednisolone disodium phosphate).

Medrol Acetate, a trademark for a glucocorticoid (methylprednisolone acetate).

medroxyprogesterone acetate /medrok′sēprōjes′tərōn/, a progestin.
■ INDICATION: It is prescribed in the treatment of menstrual disorders caused by hormone imbalance.
■ CONTRAINDICATIONS: Known or suspected pregnancy, thrombophlebitis, embolism, stroke, liver dysfunction, cancer of the breast or genitals, abnormal vaginal bleeding, missed abortion, or known hypersensitivity to this drug prohibits its use.
■ ADVERSE EFFECTS: Among the more serious adverse reactions are thrombophlebitis, pulmonary embolism, stroke, hepatitis, and cerebral thrombosis.

Med.Sc.D., abbreviation for *Doctor of Medical Science.*

Med Tech, abbreviation for *medical technician.*

medulla /mədul′ə/, *pl.* **medullas, medullae** [L, marrow], **1.** the most internal part of a structure or organ, such as the spinal medulla. **2.** *informal.* medulla oblongata.

medulla oblongata, the most vital part of the entire brain, continuing as the bulbous portion of the spinal cord just above the foramen magnum and separated from the pons by a horizontal groove. It is one of three parts of the brainstem and contains mostly white substance with some mixture of gray substance. The medulla contains the cardiac, the vasomotor, and the respiratory centers of the brain, and medullary injury or disease often proves fatal. Compare **mesencephalon, pons.**

medulla of the kidney [L, *medulla,* marrow; ME, *kidenei*], a part of the parenchyma of the kidney, beneath the cortex, including the renal pyramids and columns. It contains few, if any, glomeruli. An inner layer contains the papillae, and the outer portion, which extends as far as the arcuate vessels, contains the thick ascending limbs of the loop of Henle.

medullary /med′ələr′ē, mədul′erē, med′yəler′ē/ [L, *medulla,* marrow], **1.** of or pertaining to the medulla of the brain. **2.** of or pertaining to the bone marrow. **3.** of or pertaining to the spinal cord and central nervous system. Also **medullar.**

medullary carcinoma, a soft, malignant neoplasm of the epithelium containing little or no fibrous tissue. Also called **carcinoma medullare, carcinoma molle, encephaloid carcinoma.**

medullary chemoreceptor. See **central chemoreceptor.**

medullary cystic disease, a chronic familial disease of the kidney, characterized by the slow onset of uremia. The disease appears in young children or adolescents, who pass large volumes of dilute urine with greater than normal amounts of sodium. Hemodialysis is the usual treatment for the disease as the uremia progresses and becomes severe. See also **uremia.**

medullary fold. See **neural fold.**

medullary groove. See **neural groove.**

medullary nerve sheath. See **nerve sheath.**

medullary plate. See **neural plate.**

medullary sponge kidney, a congenital defect of the kidney, leading to cystic dilatation of the collecting tubules. People with this defect often develop a kidney stone or an infection of the kidney caused by urinary stasis. The condition is diagnosed using urographic techniques. Treatment includes drugs to acidify the urine and a diet low in calcium and high in fluids to discourage formation of stones.

medullary tube. See **neural tube.**

medulla spinalis. See **spinal cord.**

medullated /med'yəlā'tid/ [L, *medulla,* marrow], enclosed by a marrowlike substance, such as the myelin sheath of a nerve fiber.

medullated neuroma. See **fascicular neuroma.**

medulloblastoma /mədul'ōblastō'mə/ [L, *medulla* + Gk, *blastos,* germ, *oma,* tumor], a poorly differentiated malignant neoplasm composed of tightly packed cells of spongioblastic and neuroblastic lineage. The tumor usually arises in the cerebellum, occurs most frequently between 5 and 9 years of age, and affects more boys than girls. Medulloblastomas are extremely radiosensitive and grow rapidly, and prognosis is poor.

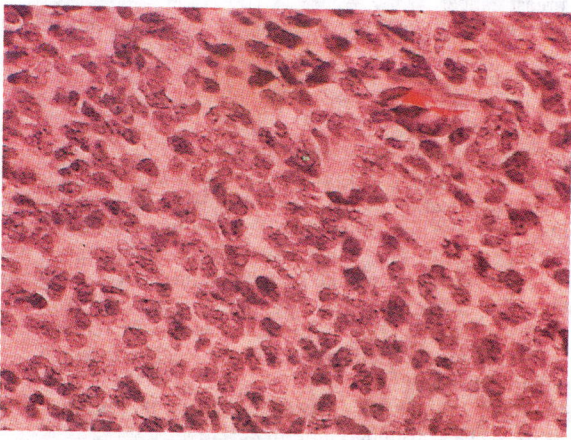

Medulloblastoma
(Okazaki, 1988/by permission of Mayo Foundation)

medulloepithelioma. See **neurocytoma.**

mefenamic acid /mef'ənam'ik/, a nonsteroidal antiinflammatory agent and analgesic.

■ INDICATION: It is prescribed in the treatment of mild to moderate pain.

■ CONTRAINDICATIONS: GI ulceration or inflammation, impaired renal function, or known hypersensitivity to this drug prohibits its use. It is used with caution in patients with asthma.

■ ADVERSE EFFECTS: Dyspepsia and diarrhea are the most common adverse effects. Other GI symptoms, dizziness, drowsiness, or skin rash occasionally occur. Rarely, serious blood dyscrasias occur.

mefloquine /mef'ləkēn/, an antimalarial that has been shown to be effective in the prophylaxis and treatment of chloroquine-resistant falciparum and vivax malaria.

Mefoxin, a trademark for a cephalosporin antibiotic (cefoxitin sodium).

MEFR, abbreviation for **maximal expiratory flow rate.**

mega-, megalo-, mego-, a prefix meaning 'great or huge': *megacardia, megacoccus, megadyne.*

megabladder. See **megalocystis.**

megacaryocyte /meg'əker'ē·əsīt'/ [Gk, *megas,* large, *karyon,* nut, *kytos,* cell], an extremely large bone marrow cell measuring between 35 and 160 [mu] in diameter and having a nucleus with many lobes. Megacaryocytes are essential for the production and proliferation of platelets in the marrow and are normally not present in the circulating blood. Also spelled **megakaryocyte.** See also **platelet.** **–megacaryocytic,** *adj.*

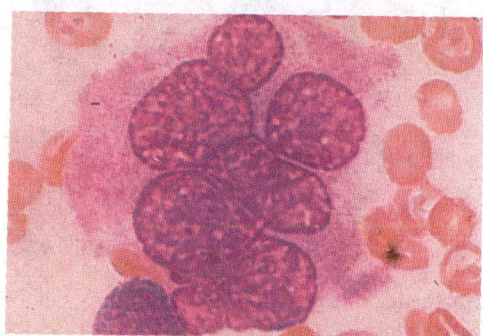

Megacaryocyte *(Powers, 1989)*

Megace, a trademark for an antineoplastic progestational agent (megestrol acetate).

megacolon /meg'əkōlən/ [Gk, *megas* + *kolon,* colon], massive, abnormal dilation of the colon that may be congenital, toxic, or acquired. **Congenital megacolon** (Hirschsprung's disease) is caused by the absence of autonomic ganglia in the smooth muscle wall of the colon. **Toxic megacolon** is a grave complication of ulcerative colitis and may result in perforation of the colon, septicemia, and death. Colonoscopy and surgery are the usual treatments for toxic and congenital megacolon. **Acquired megacolon** is the result of a chronic refusal to defecate, usually occurring in children who are psychotic or mentally retarded. The colon becomes dilated by an accumulation of impacted feces. Laxatives, enemas, and psychiatric treatment are often necessary. See also **Hirschsprung's disease.**

megacycle. See **megahertz.**

megadose /meg'ədōs/, a dose that is greatly in excess of the amount usually prescribed or recommended.

megaesophagus /meg'ə·isof'əgəs/ [Gk, *megas* + *oisophagos,* gullet], abnormal dilatation of the lower segments of the esophagus caused by distention resulting from the failure of the cardiac sphincter to relax and allow the passage of food into the stomach. See also **achalasia.**

megahertz (MHz) /meg'əhurts/ [Gk, *megas,* large, *hertz,* a number of cycles per second], a unit of frequency equal to a million cycles per second. Also called **megacycle.** See also **hertz (Hz).**

megakaryocytic leukemia /meg′əker′ē·ōsit′ik/ [Gk, *megas* + *karyon*, nut, *kytos*, cell], a rare malignancy of blood-forming tissue in which megakaryocytes proliferate in the bone marrow and circulate in the blood in large numbers.

megalencephaly /meg′ələnsef′əlē/ [Gk, *megas* + *enkephalos*, brain], a condition characterized by pathologic parenchymal overgrowth of the brain. In some cases generalized cerebral hyperplasia is associated with mental retardation or a brain disorder, such as epilepsy. Also called **macrencephaly, macroencephaly.** **–megalencephalic, megalencephalous,** *adj.*

-megalia. See **-megaly.**

megalo-. See **mega-.**

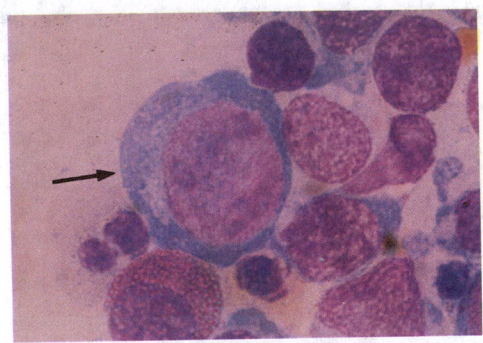

Megaloblast in pernicious anemia *(Powers 1989)*

megaloblast /meg′əlōblast′/ [Gk, *megas* + *blastos*, germ], an abnormally large nucleated immature erythrocyte that develops in large numbers in the bone marrow and is plentiful in the circulation in anemias associated with deficiency of vitamin B_{12}, folic acid, or intrinsic factor. Effective treatment is the intramuscular injection of vitamin B_{12}. **–megaloblastic,** *adj.*

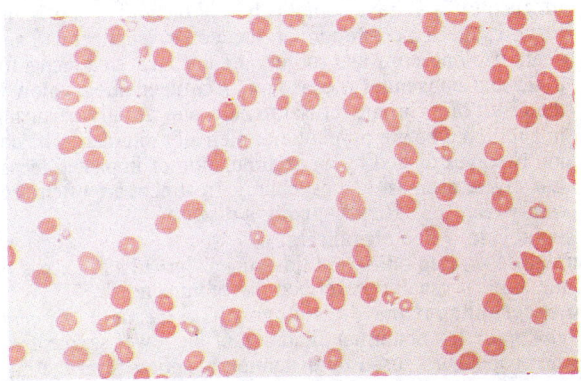

Megaloblastic anemia *(Kamal, 1991)*

megaloblastic anemia /-blas′tik/, a hematologic disorder characterized by the production and peripheral proliferation of immature, large, and dysfunctional erythrocytes. Megaloblasts are usually associated with severe pernicious anemia or folic acid deficiency anemia. See also **nutritional anemia.**

megalocephaly. See **macrocephaly.**

megalocystis /meg′əlōsis′tis/ [Gk, *megas* + *kystis*, bag], an abnormal condition occurring primarily in girls, characterized by an enlarged and thin-walled bladder. Reduction of the size of the bladder or diversion of the flow of urine through the ileum may be surgically performed to correct this condition. Also called **megabladder.**

megalomania /meg′əlōmā′nē·ə/ [Gk, *megas* + *mania*, madness], an abnormal mental state characterized by delusions of grandeur in which one believes oneself to be a person of great importance, power, fame, or wealth. See also **grandiosity, mania.**

megalaureter /meg′əlōyŏŏrē′tər/ [Gk, *megas* + *oureter*, ureter], an abnormal condition characterized by marked dilation of one or both ureters, resulting from dysfunctional peristaltic action of the smooth muscle in the ureters. Treatment may include surgical resection.

-megaly, -megalia, a suffix meaning an 'enlargement of a (specified) body part': *cardiomegaly, dactylomegaly, gastromegaly.*

megavitamin therapy /-vī′təmin/, a type of treatment that involves the administration of large doses of certain vitamins and minerals.

megestrol acetate /məjes′trōl/, an antineoplastic progestational agent.

■ INDICATIONS: It is prescribed to treat endometrial cancer and, more commonly, to palliate advanced endometrial and breast cancer.

■ CONTRAINDICATION: Hypersensitivity to the drug prohibits its use.

■ ADVERSE EFFECTS: There are no known serious adverse reactions.

mego-. See **mega-.**

meibomian cyst. See **chalazion.**

meibomian gland /mēbō′mē·ən/ [Heinrich Meibom, German physician, b. 1638], one of several sebaceous glands that secrete sebum from their ducts on the posterior margin of each eyelid. The glands are embedded in the tarsal plate of each eyelid. Also called **tarsal gland, palpebral gland.**

Meigs' syndrome /megz/ [Joseph V. Meigs, American gynecologist, b. 1892], ascites and hydrothorax associated with a fibroma of the ovaries or other pelvic tumor.

meio-. See **mio-.**

meiocyte /mī′əsīt/ [Gk, *meiosis*, becoming smaller, *kytos*, cell], any cell undergoing meiosis.

meiogenic /mī′əjen′ik/ [Gk, *meiosis* + *genein*, to produce], producing or causing meiosis.

meiosis /mī·ō′sis/ [Gk, becoming smaller], the division of a sex cell, as it matures, into two, then four gametes, the nucleus of each receiving one half of the number of chromosomes present in the somatic cells of the species. Also called **meiotic division.** Compare **mitosis.** See also **anaphase, metaphase, oogenesis, prophase, telophase.** **–meiotic** /mī·ot′ik/, *adj.*

Meissner's corpuscle. See **tactile corpuscle.**

Meissner's plexus /mīs′nərz/, [Georg Meissner, German anatomist, b. 1829; L, *plaited*], small aggregations of ganglion cells located in the submucosa of the intestine.

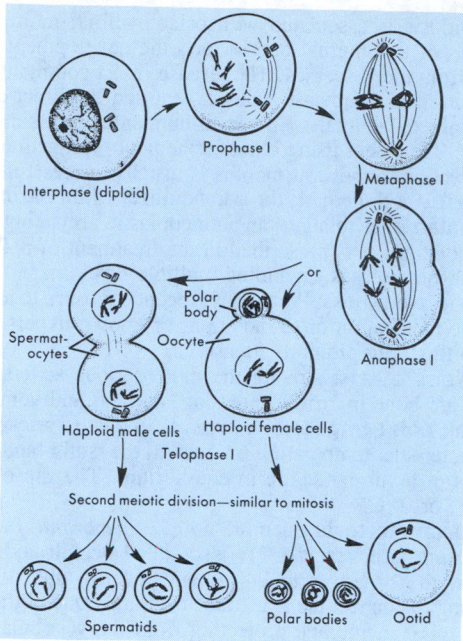

Meiosis

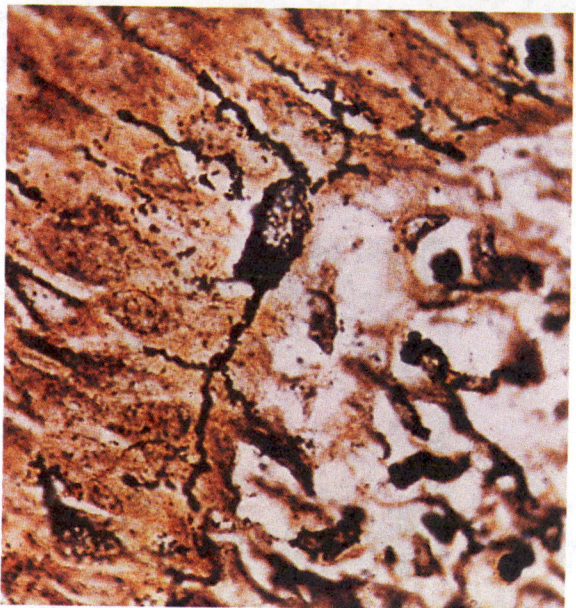

Melanocyte (du Vivier, 1993/Warthin-Starry)

mel-, melo- combining forms meaning 'pertaining to limb or limbs': *melalgia, phocomelia.*

mel [L], honey, a mixture of invert sugars and polysaccharides produced from the nectar of flowers by enzymes secreted by the honey bee, *Apis mellifica.*

melan-. See **melano-.**

melancholia /mel′angkō′lē·ə/ [Gk, *melas*, black, *chole*, bile], extreme sadness.

melaniferous /mel′ənif′ərəs/ [Gk, *melas*, black; L, *ferre*, to bear], pertaining to a black pigment.

melanin /mel′ənin/ [Gk, *melas*, black], a black or dark brown pigment that occurs naturally in the hair, skin, and the iris and choroid of the eye. See also **melanocyte.**

melano-, melan-, mel-, a combining form meaning 'black': *melanoderm, melanoleukoderma, melanophore.*

melanoblast /mel′ənōblast′/ [Gk, *melas*, black; *blastos*, germ], an epithelial tissue cell containing black granules. It develops into a melanocyte.

melanocyte /mel′ənōsīt′, mələn′ōsīt/ [Gk, *melas* + *kytos*, cell], a body cell capable of producing melanin. Melanocytes are distributed throughout the basal cell layer of the epidermis and form melanin pigment from tyrosine, an amino acid. Melanin granules are then transferred to adjacent basal cells and to hair. Melanocyte- stimulating hormone from the pituitary controls the amount of melanin produced.

melanocyte stimulating hormone (MSH), a polypeptide hormone, secreted by the anterior pituitary gland, that controls the intensity of pigmentation in pigmented cells. It is synthesized on the same large precursor polypeptide as adrenocorticotrophic hormone and the enkephalins.

melanoderma /mel′ənōdur′mə/ [Gk, *melas* + *derma*, skin], any abnormal darkening of the skin caused by increased deposits of melanin or the salts of iron or silver.

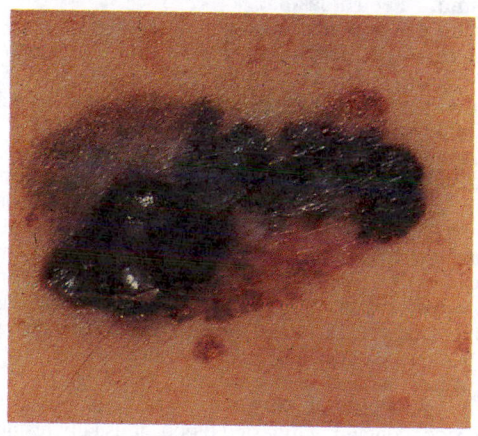

Melanoma (Zitelli, 1992)

melanoma /mel′ənō′mə/ [Gk, *melas* + *oma*, tumor], any of a group of malignant neoplasms, primarily of the skin, that are composed of melanocytes. Most melanomas develop from a pigmented nevus over a period of several months or years and occur most commonly in fair-skinned people having light-colored eyes. A previous sunburn also increases a person's risk. Any black or brown spot having an irregular border, pigment appearing to radiate beyond that border, a red, black, and blue coloration observable on close examination, or a nodular surface is suggestive of melanoma and is usually excised for biopsy. Prognosis depends on the kind of melanoma, its size, depth of invasion, and location, and the age and condition of the patient. Kinds of melanoma are **amelanotic melanoma, benign juvenile**

melanoma, lentigo maligna melanoma, nodular melanoma, primary cutaneous melanoma, and **superficial spreading melanoma.** Compare **blue nevus.** See also **Hutchinson's freckle.**

melanosis coli /mel′ənō′sis/, an abnormal condition in which the mucous membrane of the colon is pigmented with melanin.

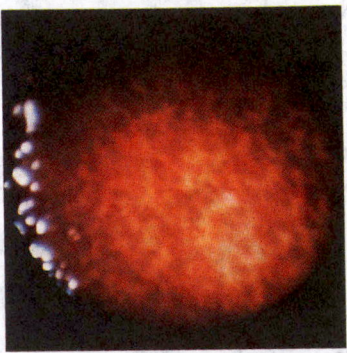

Melanosis coli—endoscopic view (Mitros, 1988)

melanotrichia linguae. See **parasitic glossitis.**

melasma. See **chloasma.**

melasma gravidarum /məlaz′mə/ [Gk, *melas*, black spot; L, *gravida*, pregnant], a dark pigment or discoloration that may appear on the skin of pregnant women.

melatonin /mel′ətō′nin/ [Gk, *melas* + *tonikos*, stretching], the only hormone secreted into the bloodstream by the pineal gland. It has marked diurnal rhythm; blood levels are up to 10 times greater at night than during the day. The hormone appears to inhibit numerous endocrine functions, including the gonadotropic hormones, and to decrease the pigmentation of the skin. When injected, exogenous melatonin causes drowsiness. Decreased secretion of melatonin occurs when calcification or tumor formation destroys or damages the pineal gland. A marked decrease results in precocious puberty, especially in boys, and in diabetes insipidus, hypogonadism, and optic atrophy.

melena /məlē′nə/ [Gk, *melaina*, black], abnormal, black, tarry stool containing digested blood. It usually results from bleeding in the upper GI tract and is often a sign of peptic ulcer or small bowel disease. See also **gastrointestinal bleeding.**

melena neonatorum [Gk, *melas*, black; *neos*, new; L, *natus*, born], the passage of dark tarry stools by a newborn. The cause is usually the altered blood pigments associated with hemorrhage. Normal meconium stools are greenish to black.

meli-, a prefix meaning 'sweet, or related to honey': *melicera, melitagra, melitoptyalism.*

-melia, a suffix meaning 'related to the limbs': *acromelia, dolichomelia, phocomelia.*

melioidosis /mel′ē·oidō′sis/ [Gk, *melis*, glanders, *eidos*, form, *osis*, condition], an infection that is uncommon in humans and is caused by the gram-negative bacillus *Malleomyces pseudomallei.* **Acute melioidasis** is fulminant and usually characterized by pneumonia, empyema, lung abscess, septicemia, and liver or spleen involvement. **Chronic**

melioidosis is associated with osteomyelitis, multiple abscesses of the internal organs, and the development of fistulas from the abscesses. The disease, most commonly seen in China and Southeast Asia, is acquired by direct contact with infected animals. Human-to-human transmission is unlikely. Treatment using chloramphenicol, sulfonamides, or tetracycline for several months is usually successful.

Mellaril, a trademark for a tranquilizer (thioridazine).

melphalan /mel′fələn/, an antineoplastic alkylating agent.
- INDICATIONS: It is prescribed in the treatment of malignant neoplastic diseases, including multiple myeloma.
- CONTRAINDICATIONS: Pregnancy, recent exposure to antineoplastic medication or to radiation, or known hypersensitivity to this drug prohibits its use.
- ADVERSE EFFECTS: Among the more serious adverse reactions are bone marrow depression, nausea, and vomiting.

melting point (mp) [AS, *meltan*; L, *punctus,* pricked], a characteristic temperature at which the solid and liquid forms of a substance are in equilibrium. The mp of ice is 32° F, or 0° C.

membrana tectoria /membrā′nə/ [L, *membrana,* thin skin; *tectorium,* a covering], **1.** also called **occipitoaxial ligament.** the broad, strong ligament covering the dens and helping to connect the axis to the occipital bone of the skull. **2.** a spiral membrane projecting from the vestibular lip of the cochlea over the organ of Corti.

membrana tympani. See **tympanic membrane.**

membrane /mem′brān/ [L, *membrana,* thin skin], a thin layer of tissue that covers a surface, lines a cavity, or divides a space, such as the abdominal membrane that lines the abdominal wall and Descemet's membrane between the substantia propria and the endothelium of the cornea. The principal kinds of membranes are **mucous membrane, serous membrane, synovial membrane,** and **cutaneous membrane.**

membrane conductance, (in cardiology) the degree of permeability of a cellular membrane to certain ions.

membrane diffusion coefficient, a component of total pulmonary diffusing capacity. It includes qualitative and quantitative characteristics of the functioning alveolarcapillary membrane.

membrane potential [L, *membrana* + *potentia*], the difference in electrical polarization or charge between two sides of a membrane or a cell wall.

membrane responsiveness, (in cardiology) the relationship between the membrane potential at the time of stimulation and the maximal rate of depolarization of the action potential.

membranous /mem′brənəs/ [L, *membrana*], resembling or consisting of a membrane.

membranous dysmenorrhea [L, *membrana*; Gk, *dys*, bad; *mens*, month; *men*, month, *rhein*, to flow], a form of spasmodic dysmenorrhea in which a cast of the uterine cavity is passed.

membranous labyrinth [L, *membrana* + *labyrinthos*, a maze], a network of three fluid-filled, membranous, semicircular ducts suspended within the bony semicircular canals of the inner ear, associated with the sense of balance. The ducts, which contain endolymph, follow the contours of the bony canals and are about one fourth of the diameter of the canals.

membranous pharyngitis [L, *membrana*; Gk, *pharynx*, throat], a diphtheric inflammation of the pharynx with the formation of a false membrane in the throat.

membranous stomatitis. See **pseudomembranous stomatitis.**

memory /mem′ərē/ [L *memoria*], **1.** the mental faculty or power that enables one to retain and to recall, through unconscious associative processes, previously experienced sensations, impressions, ideas, concepts, and all information that has been consciously learned. **2.** the reservoir of all past experiences and knowledge that may be recollected or recalled at will. **3.** the recollection of a past event, ideas, sensations, or previously learned knowledge. Kinds of memory include **affect memory, anterograde memory, kinesthetic memory, long-term memory, screen memory, short-term memory,** and **visual memory.** See also **amnesia, déjà vu.**

memory cell. See **lymphocyte.**

memory image, a sensation, impression, or sense perception as it is recalled in the memory.

menadiol sodium diphosphate /men′ədī′ol/, a water-soluble analog of vitamin K. See **menadione.**

menadione, menaphthone /men′ədī′ōn/, a synthetic form of vitamin K₃. A water-soluble injectable form of the product is menadiol sodium diphosphate.

menarche /menär′kē/ [Gk, *mēn*, month, *archaios* from the beginning], the first menstruation and the commencement of cyclic menstrual function. It usually occurs between 9 and 17 years of age. See also **pubarche.**

menarcheal age /menär′kē·əl/ [Gk, *mēn*, month, *archaios*, beginning; L, *aetas*, age], the age at which menstruation begins. The normal range is from 9 to 17 years. See also **puberty.**

mendelevium (Md) /men′dəlē′vē·əm/ [Dimitri I. Mendeleyev, Russian chemist, b. 1834], a synthetic element in the actinide group. Its atomic number is 101. The atomic weight of its most stable isotope is 256. It is the ninth transuranic element.

mendelian /mendē′lē·ən/ **genetics, Mendelian laws.** See **Mendel's laws.**

mendelism /men′dəliz′əm/ [Gregor J. Mendel, Austrian geneticist, b. 1822], the concept of inheritance derived from the application of Mendel's laws. Also called **mendelianism,** *adj.* **–mendelian,** *adj.*

Mendel's laws [Gregor J. Mendel], the basic principles of inheritance based on the breeding experiments of garden peas by the nineteenth century Austrian monk Gregor Mendel. These are usually stated as two laws, commonly called the law of segregation and the law of independent assortment. According to the first, each characteristic of a species is represented in the somatic cells by a pair of units, now known as genes, which separate during meiosis so that each gamete receives only one gene for each trait. In any monohybrid crossing, the possible ratio for the phenotypic expression of a particular dominant characteristic is 3:1, whereas the ratio of pure dominants to dominant hybrids to pure recessives is 1:2:1. According to the second law, the members of a gene pair on different chromosomes segregate independently from other pairs during meiosis, so that the gametes show all possible combinations of factors. Genes on the same chromosome are affected by linkage and segregate in blocks according to the amount of crossing over that occurs, a discovery made after Mendel. Also called **mendelian genetics, mendelian laws.** See also **chromosome, crossing over, dominant gene, linkage, meiosis, recessive gene.**

Mendelson's syndrome [Curtis L. Mendelson, American obstetrician, b. 1913], a respiratory condition caused by the chemical pneumonia resulting from the aspiration of acid gastric contents into the lungs. It usually occurs when a person vomits when inebriated, when stuporous from anesthesia, or when unconscious, such as during a seizure. Also called **pulmonary acid aspiration syndrome.**

Ménétrier's disease. See **giant hypertrophic gastritis.**

-menia, a suffix meaning '(condition of) menstrual activity': *catamenia, ischomenia, pausimenia.*

Méniére's disease /mānē·erz′/ [Prosper Méniére, French physician, b. 1799], a chronic disease of the inner ear characterized by recurrent episodes of vertigo, progressive sensorineural hearing loss, which may be bilateral, and tinnitus. Also called **Méniére's syndrome,** paroxysmal labyrinthine vertigo.

■ OBSERVATIONS: The cause is unknown, although occasionally the condition follows middle ear infection or trauma to the head. There also may be associated nausea, vomiting, and profuse sweating. Attacks last from a few minutes to several hours.

meningeal /mənin′jē·əl/ [Gk, *menigx*, membrane], pertaining to the meninges, the three layers of membranes covering the brain and spinal cord.

meningeal hydrops. See **pseudotumor cerebri.**

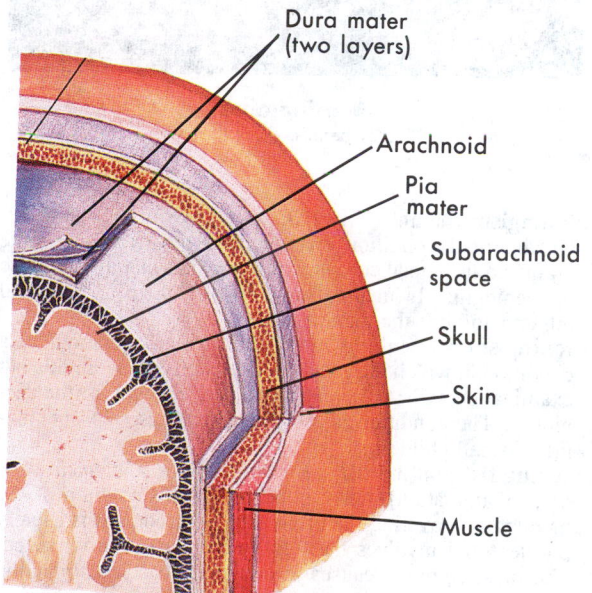

Dura mater (two layers)
Arachnoid
Pia mater
Subarachnoid space
Skull
Skin
Muscle

Meningeal layers of the brain (Chipps, 1992)

meninges /minin′jēz/, *sing.* **meninx** /mē′ningks, men′-/ [Gk *menix* membrane], the three membranes enclosing the brain and the spinal cord, comprising the dura mater, the pia mater, and the arachnoid. The pia mater and the arachnoid can become inflamed by bacterial meningitis, causing serious complications that may be life threatening. **–meningeal,** *adj.*

meningioma /minin′jē·ō′mə/, *pl.* **meningiomas, meningiomata** [Gk, *menigx* + *oma*, tumor], a mesenchymal fibroblastic tumor of the membranes enveloping the brain and spinal cord. Meningiomas grow slowly, are usually vascular, and occur most commonly near the superior longitudinal transverse and cavernous sinuses of the dura mater of the brain. The tumors may be nodular, plaquelike, or diffuse lesions that invade the skull, causing bone erosion and compression of brain tissue. Meningiomas usually occur in adults.

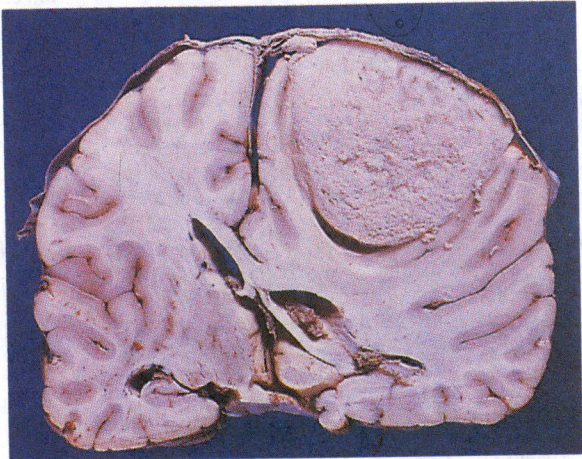

Meningioma
(Okazaki, 1988/by permission of Mayo Foundation)

meningism /minin'jizəm/ [Gk, *menigx* + *ismos*, process], an abnormal condition characterized by irritation of the brain and the spinal cord and by symptoms that mimic those of meningitis. In meningism, however, there is no actual inflammation of the meninges.

meningismus /men'injis'məs/ [Gk, *menigx*, membrane; a condition in which the patient shows signs of meningitis but examination fails to reveal pathologic changes in the meninges. The condition is associated with cases of pneumonia in small children.

meningitis /min'inji'tis/, *pl.* **meningitides** [Gk, *menigx* + *itis*, inflammation], any infection or inflammation of the membranes covering the brain and spinal cord. It is usually purulent and involves the fluid in the subarachnoid space. The most common causes in adults are bacterial infection with *Streptococcus pneumoniae*, *Neisseria meningitidis*, or *Haemophilus influenzae*. Aseptic meningitis may be caused by chemical irritation, by neoplasm, or by viruses. Many of these diseases are benign and self-limited, such as meningitis caused by strains of coxsackievirus or echovirus. Others are more severe, such as those involving arboviruses, herpesviruses, or poliomyelitis viruses. Yeasts such as *Candida* and *Cryptococcus* may cause a severe, often fatal, meningitis. A kind of meningitis is **tuberculous meningitis.** Compare **encephalitis.**

■ OBSERVATIONS: The onset of meningitis is usually sudden and characterized by severe headache, stiffness of the neck, irritability, malaise, and restlessness. Nausea, vomiting, delirium, and complete disorientation may develop quickly. Temperature, pulse rate, and respirations are increased. Re-

sidual damage may include deafness, blindness, paralysis, and mental retardation. Hydrocephalus also may develop.

■ INTERVENTIONS: Bacterial meningitis is treated promptly with antibiotics specific for the causative organism; they are administered intravenously or intrathecally. Antifungal medications, such as amphotericin B, given intravenously or intrathecally for several weeks, may prevent death from fungal meningitis, but serious neurologic sequelae may occur.

■ CONSIDERATIONS: Constant skilled nursing attention is necessary to ensure early recognition of rising intracranial pressure, to prevent aspiration in the event of convulsive seizures, and to avoid airway obstruction. Except for the first day or two of meningococcal disease, strict isolation procedures are unnecessary. Intravenous fluids and nasogastric tube feeding may be necessary for a prolonged period. Sedatives and narcotic analgesics may obscure important neurologic signs in addition to depressing vital functions.

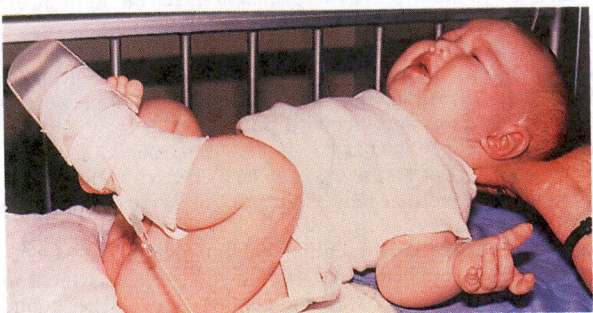

Stiffness commonly seen in meningitis *(Zitelli, 1992)*

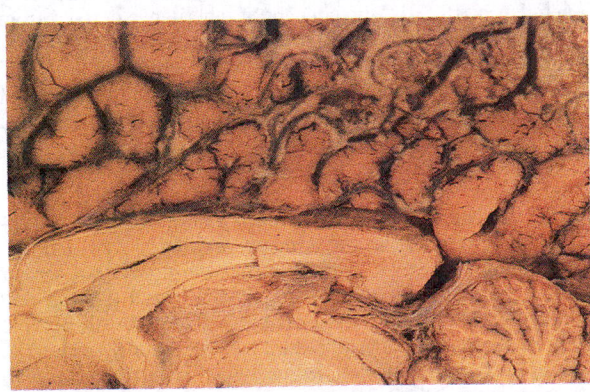

Tuberculous meningitis *(Fletcher, 1987)*

meningo-, a combining form meaning 'pertaining to membranes covering the brain or spinal cord or to other membranes': *meningocele, meningococcus, meningopathy.*

meningocele /mining'gōsēl'/ [Gk, *menigx* + *kele*, hernia], a saclike protrusion of either the cerebral or spinal meninges through a congenital defect in the skull or the vertebral column. It forms a hernial cyst that is filled with cerebrospinal fluid but does not contain neural tissue. The anomaly is designated a cranial meningocele or spinal meningocele, depending on the site of the defect; it can be easily repaired by surgery. See also **myelomeningocele, neural tube defect.**

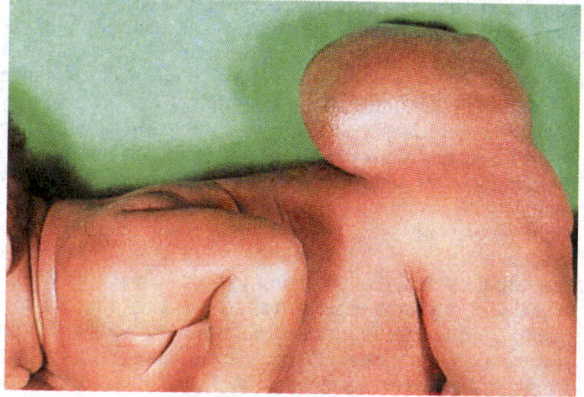

Meningocele *(Zitelli, 1987)*

meningococcal polysaccharide vaccine /-kok'əl/, either of two active immunizing agents against group A and group C meningococcal organisms.

■ INDICATION: It is prescribed for immunization against meningococcal meningitis.

■ CONTRAINDICATIONS: Immunosuppression or acute infection prohibits its use.

■ ADVERSE EFFECTS: The most serious adverse reaction is anaphylaxis.

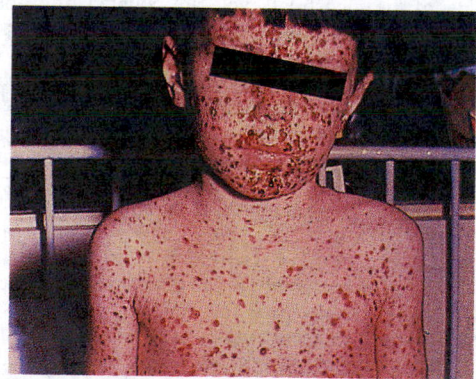

Meningococcemia *(Zitelli, 1992)*

meningococcemia /mining'gōkoksē'mē·ə/ [Gk, *menigx + kokkos*, berry, *haima*, blood], a disease caused by *Neisseria meningitidis* in the bloodstream. Onset is sudden, with chills, pain in the muscles and joints, headache, petechiae, sore throat, and severe prostration. Tachycardia is present, respirations and pulse rate are increased, and fever is intermittent. Treatment of choice is penicillin G; peripheral cir-

culatory collapse or Waterhouse-Friderichsen syndrome may occur, which is fatal if not aggressively treated.

meningococcus /mining'gōkok'əs/, *pl.* **meningococci** /-kok'sī/ [Gk, *menigx + kokkos*, berry], a bacterium of the genus *Neisseria meningitidis*, a nonmotile, gram-negative diplococcus, frequently found in the nasopharynx of asymptomatic carriers, that may cause septicemia or epidemic cerebrospinal meningitis. Meningococcal infections are not highly communicable; however, crowded conditions, such as may be found in army camps, concentrate the number of carriers and reduce individual resistance to the organism. Hemorrhagic skin lesions are significant clues to the diagnosis. Stained smears of these lesions or of cerebrospinal fluid must be examined quickly because meningococci are fragile and lyse easily. Early treatment with appropriate antibiotics, such as penicillin G, is essential for cure. Several meningococcal vaccines are available. See also **meningitis. –meningococcal,** *adj.*

meningoencephalitis /-ensef'əlī'tis/ [Gk, *menigx,* membrane; *enkephalos,* brain; *itis,* inflammation], an inflammation of both the brain and the meninges, usually caused by a bacterial infection.

meningoencephalocele /mining'gō·ensef'əlōsēl'/ [Gk, *menigx + enkephalos,* brain, *kele,* hernia], a saclike cyst containing brain tissue, cerebrospinal fluid, and meninges that protrudes through a congenital defect in the skull. It may or may not contain portions of the ventricular system and is commonly associated with defects in the brain. Also called **encephalomeningocele.** See **neural tube defect.**

meningomyelitis /-mī'əlī'tis/ [Gk, *menigx,* membrane; *myelos,* marrow; *itis,* inflammation], an inflammation of the spinal cord and its surrounding membranes.

meningomyelocele. See **myelomeningocele.**

meningovascular neurosyphilis /-vas'kyələr/ [Gk, *menigx,* membrane; L, *vasculum,* little vessel; Gk, *neuron,* nerve + *syn,* together + *philein,* to love], a neurosyphilis inflammation of the supporting and nutrient tissues of the central nervous system.

meniscectomy /men'isek'təmē/ [Gk, *meniskos,* crescent, *ektome,* excision], surgical excision of one of the crescent-shaped cartilages of the knee joint, performed when a torn cartilage results in chronic pain and in instability or locking of the joint. After surgery, the leg is kept elevated to reduce swelling and exercises are performed to maintain muscle strength. Crutch walking usually begins about the fourth day and full ambulation about the twelfth day. See also **arthroscopy.**

meniscocyte. See **erythrocyte.**

meniscocytosis. See **sickle cell anemia.**

meniscus /minis'kəs/, *pl.* **menisci** [Gk, *meniskos,* crescent], 1. the interface between a liquid and air. 2. a lens with both convex and concave aspects. 3. a curved, fibrous cartilage in the knees and other joints. See also **meniscectomy.**

Menkes' kinky hair syndrome /men'kēz/ [John H. Menkes, American neurologist, b. 1928; Dutch, *kinke,* tight twist; AS, *haer*], a familial disorder affecting the normal absorption of copper from the intestine, characterized by the growth of sparse, kinky hair. Infants with the syndrome suffer cerebral degeneration, retarded growth, and early death. Early diagnosis and intravenous administration of copper may prevent irreversible damage.

meno-, a combining form meaning 'of or related to the menses': *menolipsis, menopause, menorrhea.*

menometrorrhagia /men'ōmet'rōrā'jē·ə/ [L, *mensis,*

month; Gk, *metra*, womb, *rhegynein*, to burst forth], excessive menstrual and uterine bleeding other than that caused by menstruation. It is a combination of metrorrhagia and menorrhagia and may be a sign of a urogenital malignancy, especially cancer of the cervix.

menopause /men'əpôz/ [L, *mensis*, month; Gk, *pausis*, to cease], strictly, the cessation of menses, but commonly used to refer to the period of the female climacteric. Menses stop naturally with the decline of cyclic hormonal production and function between 35 and 60 years of age but may stop earlier in life as a result of illness or the surgical removal of the uterus or both ovaries. As the production of ovarian estrogen and pituitary gonadotropins decreases, ovulation and menstruation become less frequent and eventually stop. Fluctuations in the circulating levels of these hormones occur as the levels decline. Hot flashes are the only nearly universal symptom of the menopause. They often can be controlled with estrogen but are seldom so severe as to require therapy and will cease in time without hormonal treatment. Occasionally, heavy irregular bleeding occurs at this time, usually associated with myomata (fibroids) or other uterine pathologic condition. Estrogens given in large parenteral doses may be effective, but hysterectomy is sometimes required for control of the bleeding.

menorrhagia /men'ərā'jē·ə/ [L, *mensis* + *rhegynein*, to burst forth], abnormally heavy or long menstrual periods. Menorrhagia occurs occasionally during the reproductive years of most women's lives. If the condition becomes chronic, anemia from recurrent excessive blood loss may result. Abnormal bleeding after menopause always warrants investigation to rule out malignancy. Menorrhagia is a relatively common complication of benign uterine fibromyomata; it may be so severe, or intractable, as to require hysterectomy. Also called **hypermenorrhea.** Compare **metrorrhagia, oligomenorrhea. –menorrhagic,** *adj*.

menorrhea /men'ôrē'ə/ [L, *mensis* + Gk, *rhoia*, flow], the normal discharge of blood and tissue from the uterus. See also **menorrhagia, menstruation.**

menostasis /minos'təsis/ [L, *mensis* + Gk, *stasis*, stand still], an abnormal condition in which the products of menstruation cannot escape the uterus or vagina because of stenosis, an occlusion of the cervix, or the introitus of the vagina. An imperforate hymen is a rare cause of menostasis. **–menostatic,** *adj*.

menotropins /men'ōtrop'inz/ [L, *mensis* + Gk, *trepein*, to turn], a preparation of gonadotropic hormones from the urine of postmenopausal women.
■ INDICATION: It is prescribed with chorionic gonadotropin to induce ovulation.
■ CONTRAINDICATIONS: Elevated gonadotropin levels in the urine, thyroid or adrenal dysfunction, pituitary tumor, abnormal bleeding, ovarian cysts, pregnancy, or known hypersensitivity to this drug prohibits its use.
■ ADVERSE EFFECTS: Among the more serious adverse reactions are ovarian hyperstimulation syndrome, hemoperitoneum, arterial thromboembolism, multiple gestation, and possible birth defects.

menoxenia /men'oksē'nē·ə/ [L, *mensis* + Gk, *xenos*, strange], any abnormality relating to menstruation.

Menrium, a trademark for a fixed-combination drug for menopausal symptoms, containing esterified estrogens and a sedative (chlordiazepoxide).

menses /men'sēz/ [L, *mensis*, month], the normal flow of

blood and decidua that occurs during menstruation. The first day of the flow of the menses is the first day of the menstrual cycle. Also called **catamenia,** (nontechnical) **period.**

menstrual /men'stroo·əl/ [L, *menstrualis*, monthly], pertaining to menstruation.

menstrual age [L, *menstrualis*, monthly; *aetas*, lifetime], the age of an embryo or fetus as calculated from the first day of the last menstrual period.

menstrual colic [L, *menstrualis*, monthly; Gk, *kolikos*, colon pain], a form of dysmenorrhea characterized by abdominal pain during or just before menstruation.

menstrual cramps, low abdominal pain that may range from a colicky feeling to a constant dull ache. The pain may radiate to the lower back and legs. Menstrual cramps are often associated with the beginning of menses, reaching a peak in 24 hours and subsiding after 2 days. Treatment may include administration of ibuprofen or other drugs immediately before and after the start of menses. See also **dysmenorrhea.**

menstrual cycle, the recurring cycle of change in the endometrium during which the decidual layer of the endometrium is shed, then regrows, proliferates, is maintained for several days, and sheds again at menstruation. The average length of the cycle, from the first day of bleeding of one cycle to the first of another, is 28 days. The duration and character vary greatly among women. Menstrual cycles begin at menarche and end with menopause. The uterine phases of the cycle are the **proliferative-follicular phase, secretory-luteal phase,** and **follicular/ovulatory/luteal-ovarian phases.** See also **oogenesis.**

menstrual period [L, *menstrualis*, monthly; Gk, *peri, hodos,* way], the periodic discharge of blood and cellular debris from the uterus.

menstrual phase, the final of the three phases of the menstrual cycle, the one in which menstruation occurs. The necrotic mucosa of the endometrium is shed, leaving the stratum basale; bleeding, primarily from the spiral arteries, occurs. The average blood loss is 30 ml. For convenience, the days of the menstrual cycle are counted from the first day of the menstrual phase. Compare **proliferative phase, secretory phase.**

menstrual sponge, a small natural sponge or a piece of a sponge of synthetic material to which a loop of string is attached. It is inserted in the vagina to absorb the menstrual flow and is removed by pulling the string. It may be washed, squeezed dry, and reused as necessary through menstruation. Menstrual sponges are not commonly used.

menstruation /men'stroo·ā'shən/ [L, *menstruare*, to menstruate], the periodic discharge through the vagina of a bloody secretion containing tissue debris from the shedding of the endometrium from the nonpregnant uterus. The average duration of menstruation is 4 to 5 days, and it recurs at approximately 4-week intervals throughout the reproductive life of nonpregnant women. Kinds of menstruation are **anovular menstruation, retrograde menstruation,** and **vicarious menstruation.** See also **menstrual cycle. –menstruate,** *v*.

ment-, a prefix meaning 'mind': *mental, menticide, mentimeter*.

mental¹ /men'təl/ [L, *mens*, mind], **1.** of, relating to, or characteristic of the mind or psyche. **2.** existing in the mind; performed or accomplished by the mind. **3.** of, relating to, or characterized by a disorder of the mind.

mental² [L, *mentum*, chin], of or pertaining to the chin.

mental age (MA), the age level at which one functions intellectually, as determined by standardized psychologic and intelligence tests and expressed as the age at which that level is average. Compare **achievement age.** See also **developmental age.**

mental deficiency. See **mental retardation.**

mental disorder, any disturbance of emotional equilibrium, as manifested in maladaptive behavior and impaired functioning, caused by genetic, physical, chemical, biologic, psychologic, or social and cultural factors. Also called **emotional illness, mental illness, psychiatric disorder.**

mental handicap, any mental defect or characteristic resulting from a congenital abnormality, traumatic injury, or disease that impairs normal intellectual functioning and prevents a person from participating normally in activities appropriate for a particular age group. See also **mental retardation.**

mental health, a relative state of mind in which a person who is healthy is able to cope with and adjust to the recurrent stresses of everyday living in an acceptable way.

Mental Health Association (MHA), a voluntary, non-professional agency dedicated to the improvement of mental health facilities and services in community clinics and hospitals, the recruitment and training of volunteers, and the promotion of mental health legislation. Formerly called the **National Association for Mental Health.**

mental health consultation, any interaction between two or more health care professionals regarding an issue.

mental health nursing. See **psychiatric nursing.**

mental health service, any one of a group of government, professional, or lay organizations operating at a community, state, national, or international level to aid in the prevention and treatment of mental disorders. See also **community mental health center.**

mental hygiene, the study concerned with the development of healthy mental and emotional habits, attitudes, and behavior and with the prevention of mental illness. Also called **psychophylaxis.**

mental illness. See **mental disorder.**

mental image, any concept or sensation produced in the mind through memory or imagination.

mentality /mental'itē/ [L, *mens*, mind], **1.** the functional power and the capacity of the mind. **2.** intellectual character.

mental retardation, a disorder characterized by subaverage general intellectual function with deficits or impairments in the ability to learn and to adapt socially. The cause may be genetic, biologic, psychosocial, or sociocultural.

mental ridge [L, *mentum*, chin; AS, *hyrcg*], (in dentistry) a dense elevation that extends from the symphysis to the premolar area on the anterolateral aspect of the body of the mandible.

mental status, the degree of competence shown by a person in intellectual, emotional, psychologic, and personality functioning as measured by psychologic testing with reference to a statistical norm. See also **mental status examination.**

mental status examination, a diagnostic procedure for determining the mental status of a person. The trained interviewer poses certain questions in a carefully standardized manner and evaluates the verbal responses and behavioral reactions.

mentation /mentā'shən/ [L, *mens*, mind, *atus*, process],

any mental activity, including conscious and unconscious processes.

menthol /men'thol/ [L, *menta*, mint], a topical antipruritic with a cooling effect that relieves itching. It is an ingredient in many topical creams and ointments.

mentholated camphor /men'thəlā'tid/, a mixture of equal parts of camphor and menthol, used as a local counterirritant.

-mentia, a suffix meaning '(condition of the) mind': *dementia, moramentia, pseudodementia.*

menton /men'ton/ [L, *mentum*, chin], the most inferior point on the chin in the lateral view. It is a cephalometric landmark.

mentor /men'tər/ [Gk, *Mentor*, mythic educator], an older, trusted adviser or counselor who offers helpful guidance to younger colleagues.

mentum /men'təm/ [L, chin], **1.** the chin, especially of the fetus. **2.** a fetal reference point in designating the position of the fetus with respect to the maternal pelvis; for example, left mentum anterior (L,MA) indicates the fetal chin is presenting in the left anterior quadrant of the pelvis.

menu /men'yōō/ [Fr, small], a list of optional computer applications displayed for selection by the operator, who indicates the next action to be taken by signaling through the keyboard or another device a choice of the options.

mep, abbreviation for *mean effective pressure.*

mepenzolate bromide /mepen'zəlāt/, an anticholinergic agent.

■ INDICATIONS: It is prescribed in the treatment of GI hypermotility and as an adjunct in treating peptic ulcer.

■ CONTRAINDICATIONS: Narrow-angle glaucoma, asthma, obstruction of the genitourinary or GI tract, severe ulcerative colitis, or known hypersensitivity to this drug prohibits its use.

■ ADVERSE EFFECTS: Blurred vision, central nervous system effects, tachycardia, dry mouth, decreased sweating, or hypersensitivity reactions may occur.

Mepergan, a trademark for a central nervous system fixed-combination drug containing a narcotic analgesic (meperidine hydrochloride) and an antihistaminic (promethazine hydrochloride).

meperidine hydrochloride /meper'idēn/, a narcotic analgesic.

■ INDICATIONS: It is used to treat moderate to severe pain and as preoperative medication to relieve pain and allay anxiety.

■ CONTRAINDICATIONS: It is used with caution in many conditions, including head injuries, asthma, impaired renal or hepatic function, or unstable cardiovascular status. Concomitant use of a monoamine oxidase inhibitor or known hypersensitivity to this drug prohibits its use.

■ ADVERSE EFFECTS: Among the most serious adverse reactions are drowsiness, dizziness, nausea, constipation, sweating, respiratory and circulatory depression, and drug addiction.

mephenesin /mifen'isin/, a curare-like skeletal muscle relaxant sometimes prescribed in the relief of muscle spasm.

mephenytoin /mifen'ətō'in/, an anticonvulsant.

■ INDICATION: It is prescribed for the control of seizures in epilepsy when less toxic medications have not been effective.

■ CONTRAINDICATIONS: It is not usually recommended in pregnancy. Known hypersensitivity to this drug or to any hydantoin prohibits its use.

■ ADVERSE EFFECTS: Among the most serious adverse reactions are morbilliform rash, fever, hepatotoxicity, and various blood dyscrasias. The frequent occurrence of adverse reactions limits the use of this drug.

mephobarbital /mef'ōbär'bitol/, an anticonvulsant and sedative.

■ INDICATIONS: It is prescribed in the treatment of anxiety, nervous tension, insomnia, and epilepsy.

■ CONTRAINDICATIONS: Porphyria or known hypersensitivity to this drug or to barbiturates prohibits its use.

■ ADVERSE EFFECTS: Among the more serious adverse reactions are drug dependence, deficiency in vitamin D, paradoxical excitement, skin rash, and GI disturbance.

Mephyton, a trademark for a vitamin K product (phytonadione).

mepivacaine. See **amide-compound local anesthetic.**

meprednisone /mepred'nisōn/, an oral glucocorticoid prescribed in the treatment of a large number of inflammatory conditions.

meprobamate /miprō'bəmāt/, a sedative.

■ INDICATIONS: It is prescribed in the treatment of anxiety and tension and as a muscle relaxant.

■ CONTRAINDICATIONS: Intermittent porphyria or known hypersensitivity to this drug or to the chemically related drugs tybamate, mebutamate, and carisoprodol prohibits its use.

■ ADVERSE EFFECTS: Among the most serious adverse reactions are exacerbation of intermittent porphyria, augmentation of effects of other central nervous system depressants, and various allergic reactions. Drowsiness and ataxia commonly occur.

mEq, abbreviation for **milliequivalent.**

mEq/L,, abbreviation for **milliequivalent per liter.**

-mer, -mere, 1. a combining form meaning 'part, portion': *isomer, monomer.* 2. a combining form meaning 'polymer'.

meralgia /miral'jə/ [Gk, *meros,* thigh, *algos,* pain], the presence of pain in the thigh.

meralgia paresthetica /per'esthet'ikə/, a condition characterized by pain, paresthesia, and numbness on the lateral surface of the thigh in the region supplied by the lateral femoral cutaneous nerve. The cause of the condition is ischemia of the nerve caused by its entrapped position in the inguinal ligament.

mercaptopurine /mərkap'təpyōōr'ēn/, an antineoplastic and immunosuppressive.

■ INDICATIONS: It is prescribed in the treatment of a variety of malignant neoplastic diseases, including acute lymphocytic leukemia.

■ CONTRAINDICATIONS: Known hypersensitivity to this drug prohibits its use.

■ ADVERSE EFFECTS: Among the more severe adverse reactions are bone marrow depression and acute GI disturbances, including nausea, vomiting, diarrhea, and stomatitis.

mercurial /mərkyōōr'ē·əl/, 1. of or pertaining to mercury, particularly a medicine containing the element mercury. 2. an adverse effect associated with the administration of a mercurial medication, such as a mercurial tremor caused by mercury poisoning.

mercurial diuretic, any one of several diuretic agents that contain mercury in an organic chemical form. The principal use for the drugs is in treating edema of cardiac origin, ascites associated with cirrhosis, or oliguria in the nephrotic stage of glomerulonephritis. Immediate fatal reactions have occurred, usually because of ventricular failure after intravascular injection and transient high concentration of mercury in the blood. Flushing, urticaria, fever, and nausea and vomiting are common side effects. Thrombocytopenia, neutropenia, agranulocytosis, systemic mercury poisoning, and severe hypersensitivity reactions are among the more serious adverse effects of the mercurial diuretics: The drugs are contraindicated for use in the presence of renal insufficiency or acute nephritis. Because of the toxicity of these drugs, current practice usually recommends their replacement with more convenient and less toxic diuretics.

mercurialism. See **mercury poisoning.**

-mercuric, a combining form meaning 'molecules of bivalent mercury or its compounds': *phenylmercuric, potassiomercuric, trimercuric.*

mercury (Hg) /mur'kyərē/ [L, *Mercurius,* mythic messenger of the gods], a metallic element. Its atomic number is 80; its atomic weight is 200.6. It is the only common metal that is liquid at room temperature, and it occurs in nature almost entirely in the form of its sulfide, cinnabar. Mercury is produced commercially and is used in dental amalgams, thermometers, barometers, and other measuring instruments. It forms many poisonous compounds. The air, soil, and water in many areas of the world have become contaminated by mercury because of the burning of fossil fuels that contain the element and because of the greater use of mercury in industry and agriculture. The major toxic forms of this metal are mercury vapor, mercuric salts, and organic mercurials. Elemental mercury is only mildly toxic when ingested, because it is poorly absorbed. The vapor of elemental mercury, however, is readily absorbed through the lungs and enters the brain before it is oxidized. The kidneys retain mercury longer than any of the other body tissues.

mercury poisoning, a toxic condition caused by the ingestion or inhalation of mercury or a mercury compound. The chronic form, resulting from inhalation of the vapors or dust of mercurial compounds or from repeated ingestion of very small amounts, is characterized by irritability, excessive saliva, loosened teeth, gum disorders, slurred speech, tremors, and staggering. Symptoms of acute mercury poisoning appear in a few to 30 minutes and include a metallic taste in the mouth, thirst, nausea, vomiting, severe abdominal pain, bloody diarrhea, and renal failure that may result in death. The presence of mercury in the body is determined by a urine test. Treatment varies. Free mercury, such as in thermometers, is not absorbed in the GI tract, but because it is very volatile, hazardous vapors may penetrate ordinary toxic dust respirators, causing poisoning by inhalation. Mercury compounds are found in agricultural fungicides and in certain antiseptics and pigments; they are used extensively in industry. Industrial wastes containing mercury have been identified in some areas, and seafood from contaminated waters has caused serious public health problems. Also called **hydrargyrism, mercurialism.** See also **Minamata disease.**

mercury thermometer [L,, *Mercurius,* messenger of the gods; Gk,, *therme,* heat + *metron,* measure], a thermometer in which the expandable indicator is mercury.

mercy killing. See **euthanasia.**

merergasia /mer'ərgā'zhə/ [Gk, *meros,* part, *ergein,* to work], a mild mental incapacity characterized by some emotional instability and some anxiety. **–merergastic,** *adj.*

merethoxylline procaine /mer'əthok'silēn/, a diuretic.

-meria, a suffix meaning 'related to parts': *platymeria, polymeria*.

merisis /mer'isis/ [Gk, *merizein*, to divide into parts], an increase in size as a result of cell division and the addition of new material rather than of cell expansion. Also called **multiplicative growth**. Compare **auxesis**. See also **hyperplasia**.

mero-, a combining form meaning 'part': *meroacrania, merocyte, meropia*.

meroblastic /mer'əblas'tik/ [Gk, *meros* + *blastos*, germ], pertaining to or characterizing an ovum that contains a large amount of yolk and in which cleavage is restricted to a part of the cytoplasm. Compare **holoblastic**.

merocrine secretion /mer'əkrin/ [Gk, *meros*, part + *krinein*, to separate; L, *secernere*, to separate], a secretion in which the secreting cell remains intact while producing and releasing the secretory product. Compare **apocrine secretion**.

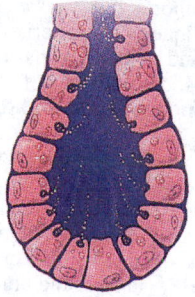

Merocrine gland *(Thibodeau, 1993/Joan M Beck)*

meromelia /mer'əmē'lyə/ [Gk, *meros* + *melos*, limb], a general designation for the congenital absence of any part of a limb. It is used in reference to such conditions as adactyly, hemimelia, or phocomelia. Compare **amelia**.

merozoite /mer'əzō'īt/ [Gk, *meros* + *zoon*, animal], an organism produced from segmentation of a schizont during the asexual reproductive phase of the life cycle of a sporozoan, specifically the malarial parasite *Plasmodium*. Merozoites can either continue the asexual phase of the life cycle by developing into trophozoites and repeating the process of schizogony, or differentiate into male and female gametes and enter the sexual stage. See also *Plasmodium*.

merozygote /mer'əzī'gōt/, an incomplete zygote that contains only part of the genetic material of one of the parents. It occurs in bacterial genetics, where part of the donor chromosome is excluded by the transfer mechanism.

Merrifield's knife, a surgical knife with a long, narrow, triangular blade set into a shank, used for gingivectomy incisions.

Meruvax, a trademark for an active immunizing agent (live rubella virus vaccine).

mes-, mesio-, meso-, a prefix meaning 'pertaining to the middle or median': *mesoderm, mesencephalon, mesiodens*.

mesangial IgA nephropathy. See **Berger's disease**.

mesangium /mesan'jē·əm/, a cellular network in the renal glomerulus that helps support the capillary loops. The mesangial cells are phagocytic and frequently contain macromolecules or inflammatory agents that may aid in diagnosis of a kidney disorder when examined in a laboratory.

Mesantoin, a trademark for an anticonvulsant (mephenytoin).

mescaline /mes'kəlēn, -lin/ [Mex, *mezcal*], a psychoactive, poisonous alkaloid derived from a colorless alkaline oil in the flowering heads of the cactus *L,ophophora williamsii*. Closely related chemically to epinephrine, mescaline causes heart palpitations, diaphoresis, pupillary dilation, and anxiety. The drug, taken in capsules or dissolved in a drink, produces visual hallucinations, such as color patterns and spatial distortions, but it does not ordinarily induce disorientation. Mescaline is used in some religious ceremonies to produce euphoria and a feeling of ecstasy. Also called **peyote**.

mescalism /mes'kəliz'əm/ [Mex, *mezcal*], a type of chemical dependence on the effects of mescal, an intoxicant spirit obtained from a species of cactus.

mesencephalon /mes'ensef'əlon/ [Gk, *mesos*, middle, *enkephalos*, brain], one of the three parts of the brainstem, lying just below the cerebrum and just above the pons. It consists primarily of white substance with some gray substance around the cerebral aqueduct. A red nucleus lies within the reticular formation of the mesencephalon and contains the terminations of fibers from the cerebellum and the frontal lobe of the cerebral cortex. The ventral part of the mesencephalon is formed by the cerebral peduncles; the dorsal part is formed by the corpora quadrigemina. The cerebral peduncles are two twisted masses of white substance that extend from the pons to the undersurface of the cerebral hemispheres. Deep within the mesencephalon are nuclei of the third and the fourth cranial nerves and the anterior part of the fifth cranial nerve. The mesencephalon also contains nuclei for certain auditory and certain visual reflexes. Also called **midbrain**. **–mesencephalic** /mes'ensifal'ik/, *adj*.

mesenchymal chondrosarcoma /meseng'kəməl/ [Gk, *mesos*, middle, *enchyma*, infusion; *chondros*, cartilage, *sarx*, flesh, *oma*, tumor], a malignant cartilaginous tumor that develops in many sites.

mesenchyme /mes'engkīm/ [Gk, *mesos* + *enchyma*, infusion], a diffuse network of tissue derived from the embryonic mesoderm. It consists of stellate cells embedded in gelatinous ground substance with reticular fibers.

mesenchymoma /mes'engkimō'mə/ [Gk, *mesos* + *enchyma*, infusion, *ioma*, tumor], a mixed mesenchymal neoplasm composed of two or more cellular elements not usually associated and fibrous tissue. See also **benign mesenchymoma, malignant mesenchymoma**.

mesenteric /mes'enter'ik/ [Gk, *mesos*, middle; *enteron*, intestine], pertaining to the mesentery, the double layer of peritoneum connecting the intestine to the posterior abdominal wall.

mesenteric adenitis. See **adenitis**.

mesenteric node [Gk, *mesos* + *enteron*, intestine; L, *nodus*, knot], a node in one of three groups of superior mesenteric lymph glands serving parts of the intestine. An average of 125 mesenteric nodes in three different groups lie between the layers of the mesentery. The first group lies close to the wall of the small intestine, among the terminal twigs of the superior mesenteric artery. The second group is located in relation to the loops and primary branches of the artery. The third group lies along the trunk of the artery. The mesenteric nodes receive afferent vessels from the jejunum, ileum, cecum, vermiform appendix, ascending colon, and transverse colon. Their efferent vessels pass to the preaortic nodes. Compare **ileocolic node, mesocolic node.**

mesentery proper /mez'ənter'ē/ [Gk, *mesos* + *enteron*, intestine; L, *propius*, more suitable], a broad, fan-shaped fold of peritoneum connecting the jejunum and the ileum with the dorsal wall of the abdomen. The root of the mesentery proper is about 15 cm long and is connected to certain structures ventral to the vertebral column. The intestinal border of the mesentery proper is about 6 m long and separates to enclose the intestine. The cranial part of the mesentery is narrow but widens to about 20 cm and suspends the small intestine and various nerves and arteries. Compare **sigmoid mesocolon, transverse mesocolon.**

MESH /mesh/, an acronym derived from *Medical Subject Headings,* the list of medical terms used by the U.S. National L,ibrary of Medicine (NL,M) for its computerized system of storage and retrieval of published medical reports. The system is also used for indexing medical references published in the monthly and annual volumes of *Index Medicus,* published by the NL,M. Also spelled **MeSH.** See also **MEDL,ARS.**

mesial. See **medial.**

mesiobucco-occlusal /mē'zē·ōbuk'ō·okloo'zəl/ [Gk, *mesos,* middle; L, *bucca,* cheek; L, *occludere,* to close up], pertaining to the angle formed by the mesial, buccal, and occlusal surfaces of a tooth. Also called **mesiolinguo-occlusal.**

mesiocclusion /mē'zē·okloo'zhən/ [Gk, *mesos* + L, *occludere,* to close up], an occlusal relationship in which the lower teeth are positioned mesially.

mesiodens /mē'zē·ədenz/ [Gk, *mesos* + L, *dens,* tooth], a supernumerary erupted or unerupted tooth that develops between two maxillary central incisors.

mesiolinguo-occlusal. See **mesiobucco-occlusal.**

mesioversion /mē'zē·ōvur'zhən/ [Gk, *mesos* + L, *vertere,* to turn], **1.** a condition in which one or more teeth are closer than normal to the midline. **2.** a condition in which the maxillae or mandible is positioned more anteriorly than normal.

mesmerism /mez'məriz'əm/ [Franz Anton Mesmer, Austrian physician, b. 1734], a practice of hypnotism introduced by Mesmer, who believed human health was affected by "celestial magnetic forces." Some patients were reported cured or experienced diminished symptoms by undergoing a "grand crisis," or seizure, while under hypnosis. Mesmer was regarded as a fraud by the medical profession, but his work led to serious studies of the health effects of the power of suggestion.

meso- /mez'ō-/, a prefix meaning 'middle': *mesocardium, mesocecum, mesoderm.*

mesocolic node /mes'ōkol'ik/ [Gk, *mesos* + *kolon,* colon; L, *nodus,* knot], a node in one of three groups of superior mesenteric lymph glands, proliferating between the layers of the transverse mesocolon, close to the transverse colon. They are best developed near the right and the left colic flexures and receive afferents from the jejunum, ileum, cecum, vermiform appendix, ascending colon, and transverse colon. Their efferents pass to the preaortic nodes. Compare **mesenteric node.**

mesocolopexy /mes'ōkō'ləpek'sē/ [Gk, *mesos* + *kolon,* co-

lon, *pexis,* fixation], suspension or fixation of the mesocolon.

mesoderm /mes'ōdurm/ [Gk, *mesos* + *derma,* skin], (in embryology) the middle of the three cell layers of the developing embryo. It lies between the ectoderm and the endoderm. Bone, connective tissue, muscle, blood, vascular and lymphatic tissue, and the pleurae of the pericardium and peritoneum are all derived from the mesoderm.

mesoduodenum /-doo'ədē'nəm/ [Gk, *mesos,* middle; L, *duodeni,* 12 fingers], a fold of tissue that joins the duodenum to the wall of the abdomen of the fetus. The membrane sometimes persists in later life as the **duodenal mesentery.**

mesogastric /-gas'trik/ [Gk, *mesos,* middle; *gaster,* belly], pertaining to the **mesogastrium,** a mesentery of the embryonic stomach.

mesoglia. See **microglia.**

mesomere /mez'əmir/ [Gk, *mesos,* middle; *meros,* part], a row of mesodermal cells between the mesothelium and epimere of the embryo. It develops into the renal tubules.

mesometritis. See **myometritis.**

mesomorph /mes'əmôrf'/ [Gk, *mesos* + *morphe,* form], a person whose physique is characterized by a predominance of muscle, bone, and connective tissue, structures that develop from the mesodermal layer of the embryo. Compare **ectomorph, endomorph.** See also **athletic habitus.**

mesonephric duct /-nef'rik/ [Gk, *mesos* + *nephros,* kidney; L, *ducere,* to lead], (in embryology) a duct that, in the male, gives rise to the ducts of the reproductive system (ductus epididymidis, ductus deferens, seminal vesicle, ejaculatory duct). In the female, it persists vestigially as **Gartner's duct.** Also called **wolffian duct.**

mesonephric tubule, any of the embryonic renal tubules comprising the mesonephros. They function as excretory structures during the early embryonic development of humans and other mammals but are later incorporated into the reproductive system. In males the tubules give rise to the efferent and aberrant ductules of the testes, the appendix epididymis, and paradidymis, and in females to the epoophoron, paroophoron, and vesicular appendices. All of the structures are vestigial except the efferent ductules of the testes.

mesonephros /-nef'rəs/, *pl.* **mesonephroi, mesonephra** [Gk, *mesos* + *nephros,* kidney], the second type of excretory organ to develop in the vertebrate embryo. It consists of a series of twisting tubules that arise from the nephrogenic cord caudal to the pronephros and that at one end form the glomerulus and at the other connect with the excretory mesonephric duct. The organ is the permanent kidney in lower animals, but in humans and various other mammals it is functional only during early embryonic development and is later replaced by the metanephros, although the duct system is retained and incorporated into the male reproductive system. Also called **mesonephron, middle kidney, wolffian body.** See also **metanephros, pronephros.** —**mesonephric, mesonephroid,** *adj.*

mesoridazine /mez'ərid'əzēn/, a phenothiazine tranquilizer.

■ INDICATIONS: It is prescribed in the treatment of psychotic disorders, behavioral problems in mental retardation, and alcoholism.

■ CONTRAINDICATIONS: Parkinson's disease, concurrent administration of central nervous system depressants, liver or renal dysfunction, severe hypotension, or known hypersensitivity to this drug or to other phenothiazine medications prohibits its use.

■ ADVERSE EFFECTS: Among the more serious adverse effects are hypotension, liver toxicity, a variety of extrapyramidal reactions, persistent tardive dyskinesia, blood dyscrasias, and hypersensitivity reactions.

mesosalpinx /mes′ōsal′pingks/ [Gk, *mesos* + *salpinx*, tube], the cephalic, free border of the broad ligament in which the uterine tubes lie.

mesothelioma /mes′ōthē′lē·ō′mə/, *pl.* **mesotheliomas, mesotheliomata** [Gk, *mesos* + *epi*, above, *thele*, nipple, *oma*, tumor], a rare, malignant tumor of the mesothelium of the pleura or peritoneum, associated with exposure to asbestos. The lesion, composed of spindle cells or fibrous tissue, may form thick sheets covering the viscera. The prognosis is poor. Also called **celothelioma**.

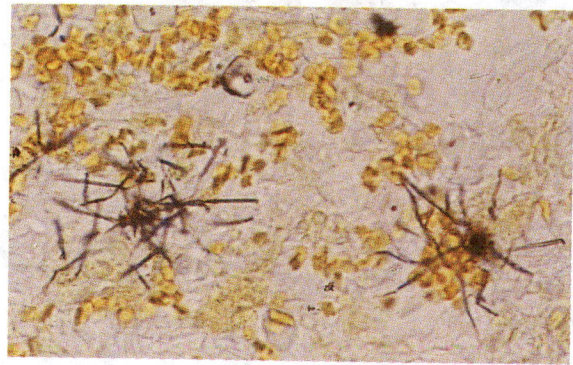

Mesothelioma
(Skarin, 1991/Courtesy Pathology Department, Brigham and Women's Hospital, Boston)

mesothelium /mes′ōthē′lē·əm/ [Gk, *mesos* + *epi*, above, *thele*, nipple], a layer of cells that lines the body cavities of the embryo and continues as a layer of squamous epithelial cells covering the serous membranes of the adult.

messenger RNA (mRNA) /mes′ənjər/ [ME, *messangere*, message bearer; *RNA*, ribonucleic acid], (in molecular genetics) an RNA fraction that transmits information from DNA to the protein-synthesizing ribosomes of cells. mRNA contains codons that are eventually encoded into amino acids via the translation process.

Mestinon, a trademark for a neuromuscular blocking agent (pyridostigmine), used as an adjunct to anesthesia and in the treatment of myasthenia gravis.

mestranol /mes′trənōl/, an estrogen prescribed in fixed-combination drugs with a progestin as an oral contraceptive.

Met, abbreviation for the amino acid **methionine**.

MET, abbreviation for **metabolic equivalent**.

meta- /met′ə-/, 1. a prefix meaning 'change or exchange': *metabasis, metallaxis, metamorphosis*. 2. a prefix meaning 'after or next': *metachemical, metapneumonic, metapsychics*. 3. a prefix meaning 'the 1, 3 position in derivative of benzine': *metacetone, metachloridine, metacresol*.

metabolic /met′əbol′ik/ [Gk, *metabole*, change], of or pertaining to **metabolism**.

metabolic acidosis, acidosis in which excess acid is added

to the body fluids or bicarbonate is lost from them. Acidosis is indicated by a pH of blood below 7.4. In starvation and in uncontrolled diabetes mellitus, glucose is not present or is not available for oxidation for cellular nutrition. The plasma bicarbonate of the body is used up in neutralizing the ketones that result from the breakdown of body fat for energy that occurs in compensation for the lack of glucose. Metabolic acidosis also occurs when oxidation takes place without adequate oxygen, as in heart failure or shock. Severe diarrhea, renal failure, and lactic acidosis also may result in metabolic acidosis. Hyperkalemia often accompanies the condition. See **diabetic ketoacidosis.**

metabolic alkalosis, an abnormal condition characterized by the significant loss of acid in the body or by increased levels of base bicarbonate. The reduction of acid may be caused by excessive vomiting, insufficient replacement of electrolytes, hyperadrenocorticism, and Cushing's disease. An increase in base bicarbonate may be caused by various problems, such as the ingestion of excessive bicarbonate of soda and other antacids during the treatment of peptic ulcers, and by the administration of excessive intravenous fluids containing high concentrations of bicarbonate. Severe, untreated metabolic alkalosis can lead to coma and death. Compare **respiratory alkalosis.** See also **metabolic acidosis, respiratory acidosis.**

■ OBSERVATIONS: Signs and symptoms of metabolic alkalosis may include apnea, headache, lethargy, irritability, nausea, vomiting, and atrial tachycardia. Confirmation of the diagnosis is commonly based on laboratory findings that show a blood pH level greater than 7.45, a carbonic acid concentration greater than 29 mEq/L, and alkaline urine. The electrocardiogram of a patient with this condition may show atrial tachycardia with a low T wave merging with a P wave.

■ INTERVENTIONS: Treatment seeks to eliminate the underlying cause of alkalosis and may include the intravenous administration of ammonium chloride to release hydrogen chloride and restore chloride levels. Potassium chloride and normal saline solutions usually replace fluid losses from gastric drainage but are contraindicated in patients with associated congestive heart failure.

■ NURSING CONSIDERATIONS: Nurses closely monitor the status of the patient and cautiously administer any prescribed intravenous solutions. The intravenous administration of ammonium chloride is usually contraindicated in patients with liver or kidney disease. Too rapid infusion of ammonium chloride may hemolyze the red blood cells, and excessive dosage may overcorrect alkalosis and cause acidosis. The fluid intake and output of the patient are carefully noted, and the respiration rate is regularly checked. Decreased respiratory rate indicates an effort to compensate for alkalosis and may cause respiratory acidosis.

metabolic balance [Gk, *metabole*, change; L, *bilanx*, having two scale trays], an equilibrium between the intake of nutrients and their eventual loss through absorption or excretion. If the intake of a nutrient exceeds its loss, it is called a positive balance, and a negative balance indicates that a nutrient is used or excreted faster than it is consumed in the diet.

metabolic component, the bicarbonate component of plasma.

metabolic disorder, any pathophysiologic dysfunction that results in a loss of metabolic control of homeostasis in the body.

metabolic equivalent (MET), a unit of measurement of

heat production by the body. One MET is equal to 50 kilogram calories (kcal) per hour per square meter of body surface of a resting individual.

metabolic rate, the amount of energy liberated or expended in a given unit of time. Energy is stored in the body in energy-rich phosphate compounds (adenosine triphosphate, adenosine monophosphate, and adenosine diphosphate) and in proteins, fats, and complex carbohydrates. See also **basal metabolic rate.**

metabolic respiratory quotient (R), the ratio of production of CO_2 to the corresponding consumption of O_2. The values of R change according to the fuel being burned; the R of fat is lower than that of glucose, whereas the R of protein is between that of glucose and fat.

metabolic waste products [Gk, *metabole*, change; L, *vastare*, to destroy + *producere*, to produce], the products of metabolic activity after oxygen and nutrients have been supplied to a cell. These include mainly water and carbon dioxide, along with sodium chloride and soluble nitrogenous salts, which are excreted in urine, feces, and exhaled air.

metabolism /mətab′əliz′əm/ [Gk, *metabole*, change, *ismos*, process], the aggregate of all chemical processes that take place in living organisms, resulting in growth, generation of energy, elimination of wastes, and other bodily functions as they relate to the distribution of nutrients in the blood after digestion. Metabolism takes place in two steps: anabolism, the constructive phase, in which smaller molecules (such as amino acids) are converted to larger molecules (such as proteins); and catabolism, the destructive phase, in which larger molecules (such as glycogen) are converted to smaller molecules (such as pyruvic acid). Exercise, elevated body temperature, hormonal activity, and digestion can increase the metabolic rate, which is the rate determined when a person is at complete rest, physically and mentally. The metabolic rate is customarily expressed (in calories) as the heat liberated in the course of metabolism. See also **acid-base metabolism, anabolism, basal metabolism, catabolism.**

metabolite /mitab′əlīt/ [Gk, *metabole*, change], a substance produced by metabolic action or necessary for a metabolic process. An essential metabolite is one required for a vital metabolic process.

metabolize /mətab′əlīz/ [Gk, *metabole*, change], to undergo metabolism, the breaking down of carbohydrates, proteins, and fats into smaller units, reorganizing those units as tissue building blocks or as energy sources and eliminating waste products of the processes.

metacarpal phalanx /-kär′pəl/ [Gk, *meta, karpos,* wrist + *phalagx,* line of soldiers], the hands and fingers, particularly phalanges that articulate with carpal bones.

metacarpophalangeal /-kar′pōfəlan′jē·əl/ [Gk, *meta,* beyond; *karpos,* wrist; *phalagx,* line of soldiers], pertaining to the metacarpal bones of the hand and the phalanges of fingers, as in metacarpophalangeal joints.

metacarpophalangeal joint (MCP) dislocation [Gk, *meta, karpos, phalagx;* L, *jungere,* to join; *dis, locare,* to place], the dislocation of a finger, usually with damage to tendons and other structures.

metacarpus /met′əkär′pəs/ [Gk, *meta,* beyond, *karpos,* wrist], the middle portion of the hand, consisting of five slender bones numbered from the thumb side, metacarpals I through V. Each metacarpal consists of a body and two extremities. —**metacarpal,** *adj., n.*

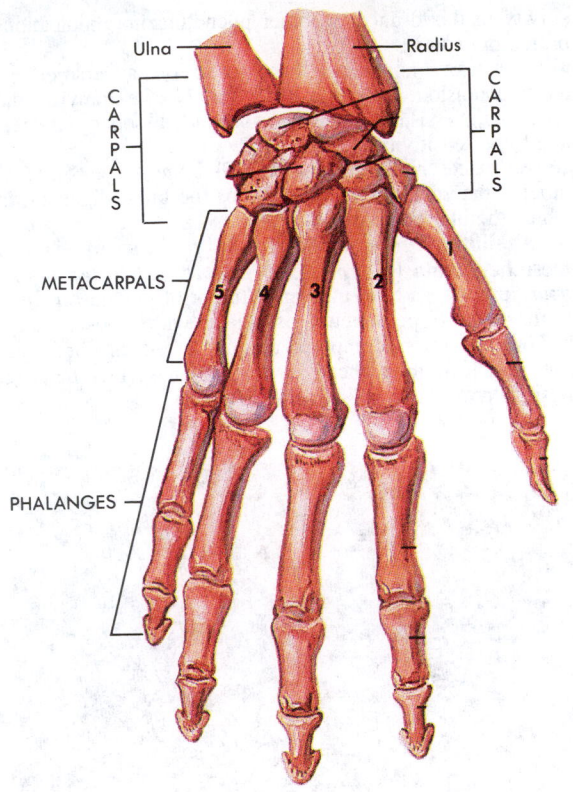

Metacarpal bones
(Seeley, 1992/David J Mascaro & Associates)

metacentric /met′əsen′trik/ [Gk, *meta + kentron,* center], pertaining to a chromosome in which the centromere is located near the center so that the arms of the chromatids are of approximately equal length. Compare **acrocentric, submetacentric, telocentric.**

metachromasia /-krōmā′zhē·ə/ [Gk, *meta,* beyond; *chroma,* color], a tissue staining phenomenon in which cells being examined acquire a color other than that of the dye used. Cartilage cells, for example, may appear red after being stained with a blue dye. The cause is an interaction between the dye molecules and the acidic radicals of the tissue cells. Also called **metachromism.**

metachromatic lipids /-krōmat′ik/ [Gk, *meta,* beyond; *chroma,* color; *lipos,* fat], lipid molecules that accumulate in the central nervous system, peripheral nerves, and internal organs of infants who inherit a lipidosis disorder. See also **cerebroside sulfatase.**

metachromatic stain [Gk, *meta + chroma,* color; OFr, *desteindre,* to dye], a basic dye, such as toluidine, that can stain substances a different color than that of the stain.

metachromism. See **metachromasia.**

-metacin, a combining form for indomethacin-type antiinflammatory substances.

metacommunication /-kəmyōō′nikā′shən/ [Gk, *meta* + L, *communicare,* to inform], communication that indicates how verbal communication should be interpreted. It may support or contradict verbal communication.

metagenesis /met′əjen′əsis/ [Gk, *meta* + *genein,* to produce], the regular alternation of sexual with asexual methods of reproduction within the same species. **−metagenetic, metagenic,** *adj.*

Metahydrin, a trademark for a diuretic and antihypertensive (trichlormethiazide).

metal [Gk, *metallon*, a mine], any element that conducts heat and electricity, is malleable and ductile, and forms positively charged ions (cations) in solution.

metal fume fever, an occupational disorder caused by the inhalation of fumes of metallic oxides and characterized by symptoms similar to those of influenza. The condition occurs among workers engaged in welding, metal fabrication, casting, and other occupations dealing with the manipulation of metals. Access to fresh air and treatment of the symptoms usually alleviate the condition. Also called **brass founder's ague, zinc chill.** Compare **siderosis.**

metallesthesia /met′əlesthē′zhə/ [Gk, *metallon*, mine; *aisthesia*, perception], an ability to identify a metal through the sense of touch.

metallurgy /met′əlur′jē/ [Gk, *metallon*, mine; *ergein*, to work], the theoretic and applied sciences of the nature and uses of metals.

metamorphopsia /met′əmôrfop′sē·ə/ [Gk, *meta* + *morphe*, form, *opsis*, sight], a defect in vision in which objects are seen as distorted in shape, resulting from disease of the retina or imperfection of the media.

metamorphosis /met′əmôr′fəsis/ [Gk, *meta* + *morphe*, form], a change in shape or structure, especially a change from one stage of development to another, such as the transition from the larval to the adult stage.

metamyelocyte /met′əmī′əlōsīt′/ [Gk, *meta* + *myelos*, marrow, *kytos*, cell], a stage in the development of the granulocyte series of leukocytes, between the myelocyte stage and the mature granulocyte. See also **leukocyte, myeloblast, myelocyte.**

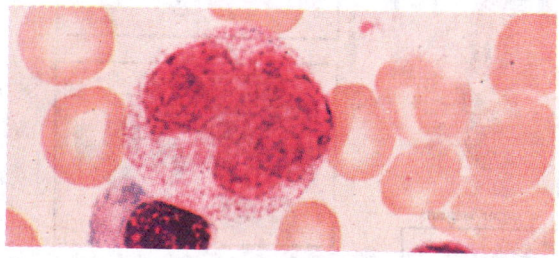

Metamyelocyte *(Hayhoe, 1992)*

Metandren, a trademark for an androgen (methyltestosterone).

metanephrine /met′ənef′rin/, one of the two principal urinary metabolites of epinephrine and norepinephrine in the urine, the other being vanillylmandelic acid. The 24-hour normal value for total metanephrine is 1.3 mg. Normally, less than 1.3 mg of metanephrine is excreted in 24 hours.

metanephrogenic /met′ənef′rəjen′ik/ [Gk, *meta* + *nephros*, kidney, *genein*, to produce], capable of forming the metanephros, or fetal kidney.

metanephros /-nef′rəs/, *pl.* **metanephroi, metanephra** [Gk, *meta* + *nephros*, kidney], the third, and permanent, excretory organ to develop in the vertebrate embryo. It con-

sists of a complex structure of secretory and collecting tubules that develop into the kidney and are formed later than the mesonephros from the caudal end of the nephrogenic cord and the mesonephric duct. In most mammals there is limited functional use of the metanephric kidney during fetal life, because waste materials are transferred across the placenta to the mother for elimination. Also called **metanephron, hind kidney.** See also **kidney, mesonephros, pronephros.**

metaphase /met′əfāz/ [Gk, *meta* + *phasis*, appearance], the second of the four stages of nuclear division in mitosis and in each of the two divisions of meiosis, during which the chromosomes become arranged in the equatorial plane of the spindle to form the equatorial plate, with the centromeres attached to the spindle fibers in preparation for separation. See also **anaphase, interphase, meiosis, mitosis, prophase, telophase.**

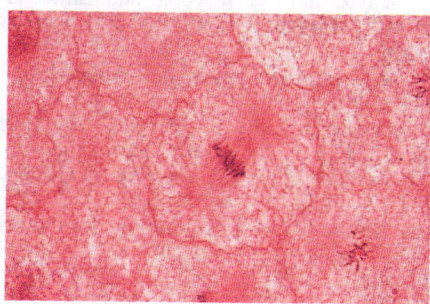

Metaphase
(Seeley, 1992/Ed Reschke/Michael Abbey, Science Source)

metaphyseal dysostosis /mətaf′izē′əl, met′əfiz′ē·əl/ [Gk, *meta* + *phyein*, to grow; *dys*, bad, *osteon*, bone], an abnormal condition that affects the skeletal system and is characterized by a disturbance of the mineralization of the metaphyseal area of the bones, resulting in dwarfism. Metaphyseal dysostosis is classified as the Gansen type, Schmidt type, Spahar-Hartmann type, or cartilage-hair hypoplasia. The Gansen type is characterized by metaphyseal alterations similar to those of achondroplasia but not involving the skull or the epiphyses of the long bones. The Schmidt type of metaphyseal dysostosis is characterized by developmental changes from the weight-bearing age to approximately 5 years of age. The metaphyseal alterations associated with the Schmidt type are similar to those of achondroplasia, resulting in moderate dwarfism. The Spahar-Hartmann type is characterized by skeletal changes and severe genu varum. Cartilage-hair hypoplasia is characterized by severe dwarfism and hair that is sparse, short, and brittle. Mental retardation is not usually associated with metaphyseal dysostosis. Radiographic examination of all types of the disease reveals characteristic widening of the metaphyses of the tubular bones, with normal diaphyseal and epiphyseal ossification centers. Treatment is supportive and symptomatic with no specific modality.

metaphyseal dysplasia, an abnormal condition characterized by disordered modeling of the cylindric bones. The involvement of this disease is limited to the long bones and displays a characteristic radiographic image of the "Erlenmeyer flask" deformity in which the metaphyseal circumference is enlarged and the medullary area of the affected bone is reduced. Metaphyseal dysplasia most often affects the distal femur or the proximal tibia.

metaphysis /mətaf′əsis/ [Gk, *meta* + *phyein*, to grow], a region of bone in which diaphysis and epiphysis converge.

metaplasia /met′əplā′zhə/, the conversion of normal tissue cells into an abnormal form in response to chronic stress or injury.

Metaprel, a trademark for a bronchodilator (metaproterenol sulfate).

metaproterenol sulfate /met′əprōter′inôl/, a beta-adrenergic bronchodilator.

■ INDICATION: It is prescribed in the treatment of bronchial asthma.

■ CONTRAINDICATIONS: Dysrhythmias associated with tachycardia or known hypersensitivity to this drug prohibits its use.

■ ADVERSE EFFECTS: Among the more serious adverse reactions are tachycardia, hypertension, and cardiac arrest.

metaraminol bitartrate /met′äram′inol/, an adrenergic vasopressor.

■ INDICATION: It is prescribed in the treatment of hypotension and shock.

■ CONTRAINDICATIONS: Known hypersensitivity to this drug prohibits its use. It is not used with cyclopropane or halothane anesthesia or as the sole drug for hypovolemic hypotension.

■ ADVERSE EFFECTS: Among the more serious adverse reac-

tions are cardiac dysrhythmia, tissue necrosis at the site of injection, hypertension, tremors, and nausea.

metarubricyte /-rōō′brisīt/ [Gk, *meta* + L, *ruber*, red, *kytos*, cell]], a red blood cell possessing a nucleus. Such cells, also known as normoblasts, are not normally found in circulating blood.

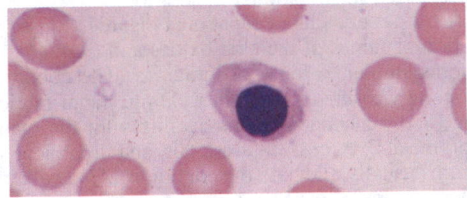

Metarubricyte (Powers, 1989)

metastable solution. See **supersaturate solution.**

metastasis /mətas′təsis/, *pl.* **metastases** [Gk, *meta* + *stasis*, standing], **1.** the process by which tumor cells spread to distant parts of the body. Because malignant tumors have no enclosing capsule, cells may escape, become emboli, and be transported by the lymphatic circulation or the bloodstream to implant lymph nodes and other organs far from the primary tumor. **2.** a tumor that develops away from the

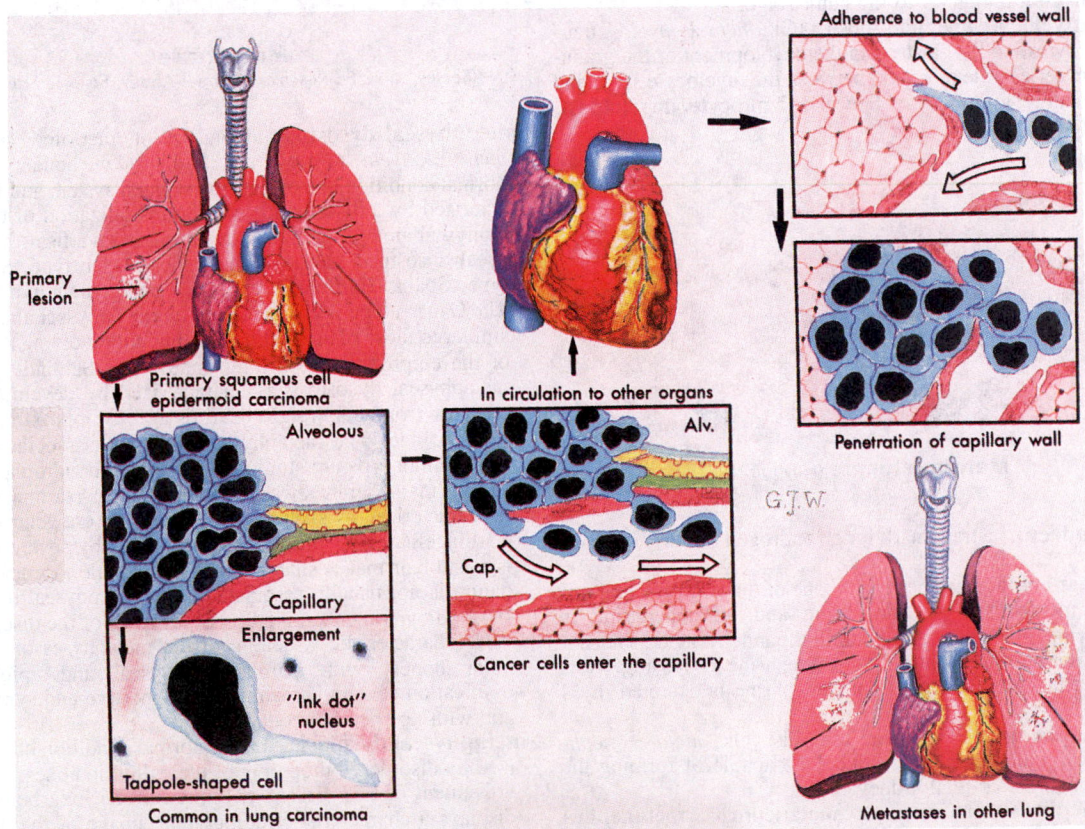

Metastasis of cancer (Belcher, 1992)

site of origin. Compare **anaplasia.** **–metastatic,** *adj.,*
metastasize (metas) /mətas'təsīz/, *v.*

metastasizing mole. See **chorioadenoma destruens.**

metastatic abscess /-stat'ik/ [Gk, *meta,* beyond; *stasis,*
standing; L, *abscedere,* to go away], any secondary abscess that develops at a point distant from an original infection, the infectious particles being transported to other locations in the bloodstream.

metastatic calcification [Gk, *meta* + *stasis,* standing; L,
calx, lime, *facere,* to make], the pathologic process-
whereby calcium salts accumulate in previously healthy tissues. It is caused by excessive levels of blood calcium, such
as in hyperparathyroidism.

metastatic endometriosis [Gk, *meta,* beyond; *stasis,* standing; *endon,* within; *metra,* womb; *osis,* condition], extraperitoneal lesions that resemble metastases from a carcinoma.

metastatic ophthalmia. See **sympathetic ophthalmia.**

metastatic survey [Gk, *meta,* beyond; *stasis,*standing; OFr,
surveoir, to examine], a method of monitoring the spread
of a cancer by taking a periodic series of x-ray films.

metatarsal /met'ətär'səl/ [Gk, *meta* + *tarsos,* plate],
1. of or pertaining to the metatarsus of the foot. **2.** any one
of the five bones making up the metatarsus.

metatarsalgia /met'ətärsal'jə/ [Gk, *meta, tarsos* + *algos,*
pain], a painful condition around the metatarsal bones
caused by an abnormality of the foot or recalcification of
degenerated heads of metatarsal bones. See also **Morton's
foot, Morton's neuroma, Morton's toe.**

metatarsal phalanx /-tär'səl/ [Gk, *meta* + *tarsos,* sole of
foot + *phalagx,* line of soldiers], the bones of the foot
and toes.

metatarsal stress fracture, a break or rupture of a meta-
tarsal bone, resulting from prolonged running or walking.
The condition is often difficult to diagnose with x-ray films.
Also called **fatigue fracture, march fracture.**

metatarsus /-tär'sis/ [Gk, *meta* + *tarsos,* plate], a part of
the foot, consisting of five bones numbered I to V, from
the medial side. Each bone has a long, slender body, a
wedge-shaped proximal end, a convex distal end, and flattened, grooved sides for the attachment of ligaments. The
metatarsal bones articulate with the tarsus proximally and
the first row of phalanges distally. Kinds of metatarsus include **metatarsus valgus** and **metatarsus varus.** **–metatarsal,** *adj.*

metatarsus adductus. See **metatarsus varus.**

metatarsus valgus, a congenital deformity of the foot in
which the forepart rotates outward away from the midline
of the body and the heel remains straight. Also called **duck
walk, toeing out.**

metatarsus varus, a congenital deformity of the foot in
which the forepart rotates inward toward the midline of the
body and the heel remains straight. Also called **intoe, metatarsus adductus, pigeon-toed, toeing in.**

Metatensin, a trademark for a cardiovascular, fixed-
combination drug containing a diuretic (trichlormethiazide)
and an antihypertensive (reserpine).

metathalamus /met'əthal'əməs/ [Gk, *meta* + *thalamos,*
chamber], one of five parts of the diencephalon. It is composed of a medial geniculate body and a lateral geniculate
body on each side. The medial geniculate body acts as a
relay station for nerve impulses between the inferior brachium and the auditory cortex. The lateral geniculate body
is an oval bulge at the posterior end of the thalamus, which

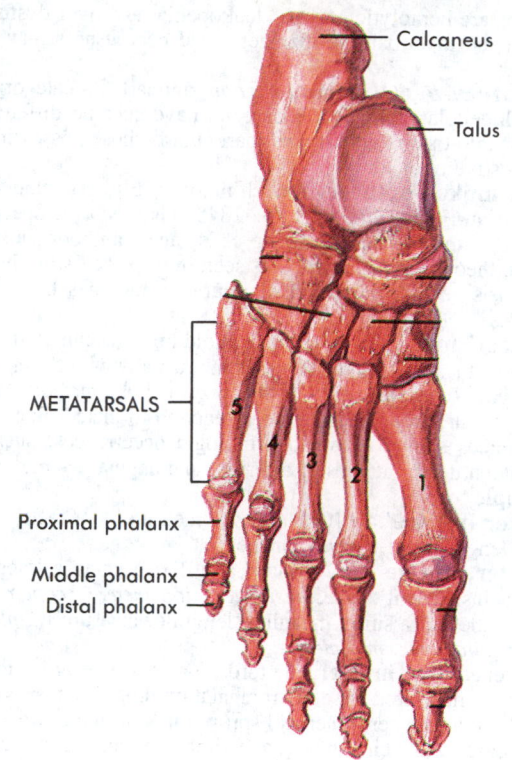

Metatarsal bones
(Seeley, 1992/David J Mascaro & Associates)

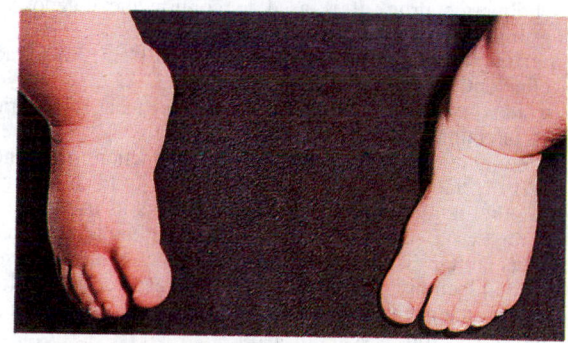

Metatarsus varus *(Zitelli, 1992)*

accommodates the terminal ends of the fibers of the optic
tract. Compare **epithalamus, hypothalamus, subthalamus.** **–metathalamic,** *adj.*

metaxalone /metak'səlōn/, a skeletal muscle relaxant.
■ INDICATION: It is prescribed as an adjunct in the treatment
of acute skeletal muscle spasm.
■ CONTRAINDICATIONS: Significantly impaired renal or hepatic
function, susceptibility to drug-induced hemolytic anemia,
or known hypersensitivity to this drug prohibits its use.
■ ADVERSE EFFECTS: Among the more serious adverse reac-

tions are hemolytic anemia, leukopenia, and liver dysfunction. GI disturbances, dizziness, and nervousness may occur.

metazoa /-zō′ə/ [Gk, *meta + zoon*, animal], a category of multicellular animals whose cells have become differentiated into tissues and organs, particularly those possessing a digestive tract.

Metchnikoff's theory /mech′nikofs/ [Elie Metchnikoff, Russian-French biologist, b. 1845; Gk, *theoria*, speculation], the theory that living cells ingest microorganisms. The theory proved correct, as seen in the process of phagocytosis and the ingestion of injurious microbes by leukocytes.

meteorism [Gk, *meteorizein*, to hold up], accumulation of gas in the abdomen or the intestine, usually with distention.

meteorotropism /mē′tē·ərətrō′pizəm/ [Gk, *meteors*, high in the air, *trope*, turning], a reaction to meteorologic influences shown by various biologic occurrences, such as sudden death, attacks of arthritis, and angina. **—meteorotropic,** *adj*.

meter (m) /mē′tər/ [Gk, *metron*, measure], a metric unit of length equal to 39.37 inches.

-meter, -metre **1.** /-m′ətər/ a suffix meaning a 'measuring instrument': *anesthesimeter, ionometer, scopometer*. **2.** /-mē′tər/ a suffix meaning 'length or measure': *centimeter, kilometer, millimeter*.

metered dose inhaler /mē′tərd/, a device designed to deliver a measured dose of an inhalation drug. It consists usually of a canister of aerosol spray, mist, or fine powder that releases a specific dose each time the canister is pushed against a dispensing valve. It is intended to reduce the risk of overmedication by the person.

methacholine challenge /meth′əkō′lēn/, a method of measuring airway activity by an inhalation challenge test. It consists of inhaling a saline aerosol as a control, followed by increasing concentrations of methacholine chloride, a cholinergic drug. It is used to confirm the diagnosis of asthma when symptoms are present.

methacycline hydrochloride /meth′əsī′klēn/, a tetracycline antibiotic.
- INDICATIONS: It is prescribed in the treatment of a variety of infections.
- CONTRAINDICATIONS: Renal or liver dysfunction, pregnancy, early childhood, or known hypersensitivity to this drug or to other tetracycline medications prohibits its use.
- ADVERSE EFFECTS: Among the more serious adverse reactions are GI disturbances, phototoxicity, potentially serious suprainfections, and hypersensitivity reactions. Discoloration of teeth may occur in children exposed to the drug in utero or before 8 years of age.

methadone /meth′ədōn/, a synthetic narcotic analgesic.
- INDICATIONS: It is prescribed for relief of severe pain, for treatment in detoxification, and in treatment programs for opiate-addicted patients.
- CONTRAINDICATIONS: It is used with caution in many conditions, including head injuries, asthma, impaired renal or hepatic function, or unstable cardiovascular status. Known hypersensitivity to this drug prohibits its use.
- ADVERSE EFFECTS: Among the more serious adverse reactions are drowsiness, dizziness, nausea, constipation, respiratory and circulatory depression, and drug addiction.

methadone hydrochloride, a narcotic analgesic used for anesthesia or as a substitute for heroin, permitting withdrawal without development of acute abstinence syndrome.

Methadone does not produce marked euphoria, sedation, or narcosis. It is not given to pregnant women or to patients with liver disease.

methamphetamine hydrochloride /meth′amfet′əmēn/, a central nervous system stimulant.
- INDICATIONS: It is prescribed in the treatment of narcolepsy and hyperkinesis and to reduce the appetite in exogenous obesity.
- CONTRAINDICATIONS: Glaucoma, arteriosclerosis, cardiovascular disease, hypertension, hyperthyroidism, history of drug abuse, concomitant use of a monoamine oxidase inhibitor, or known hypersensitivity to this drug or to other sympathomimetic drugs prohibits its use.
- ADVERSE EFFECTS: Among the more serious adverse reactions are various manifestations of central nervous system excitation, increase in blood pressure, dysrhythmia and other cardiovascular effects, nausea, and drug dependence.

methandriol /methan′drē·ol/, an anabolic hormone used as adjunctive therapy in senile and postmenopausal osteoporosis.

methanol /meth′ənol/, a clear, colorless, toxic, liquid distillate of wood miscible with water, alcohol, and ether. It is widely used as a solvent and in the production of formaldehyde. Ingestion of methanol paralyzes the optic nerve and may cause death. Also called **wood alcohol.**

methanol extractable residue, an immunotherapeutic substance, prepared from a methanol extracted fraction of the bacillus Calmette-Guérin (BCG).

methaqualone /methak′wəlōn/, a sedative-hypnotic.
- INDICATIONS: It is prescribed in the treatment of anxiety and insomnia.
- CONTRAINDICATIONS: It is not given to children or to pregnant women. Known hypersensitivity to this drug prohibits its use.
- ADVERSE EFFECTS: Among the more serious adverse reactions are GI distress, drug hangover, peripheral neuropathy, loss of inhibition, and drug dependence.

metharbital /methär′bitəl/, an anticonvulsant.
- INDICATION: It is prescribed in the treatment of epilepsy.
- CONTRAINDICATIONS: Porphyria or known hypersensitivity to barbiturates prohibits its use. It is prescribed with caution in pregnancy or hepatic impairment.
- ADVERSE EFFECTS: Among the more serious adverse reactions are ataxia, irritability in children, and confusion in elderly patients. Rashes and other allergic reactions also may occur.

methazolamide /meth′əzō′ləmīd/, a carbonic anhydrase inhibitor.
- INDICATION: It is prescribed in the treatment of glaucoma.
- CONTRAINDICATIONS: Hyponatremia, hypokalemia, Addison's disease, severe pulmonary obstruction, adrenocortical insufficiency, or known hypersensitivity to this drug prohibits its use.
- ADVERSE EFFECTS: Among the more serious adverse effects are aplastic anemia, drowsiness, paresthesia, hypersensitivity reactions, and acidosis.

methdilazine /methdil′əzēn/, a phenothiazine antihistamine.
- INDICATION: It is prescribed to relieve itching.
- CONTRAINDICATIONS: Asthma, glaucoma, or known hypersensitivity to this drug or to phenothiazine medications prohibits its use. It is not given to newborn infants or lactating mothers.
- ADVERSE EFFECTS: Among the more serious adverse reac-

tions are bone marrow depression and extrapyramidal reactions. Dry mouth and sedation commonly occur.

methemoglobin /met'hēməglō'bin, met·he'məglō'bin/, a form of hemoglobin in which the iron component has been oxidized from the ferrous to the ferric state. Methemoglobin cannot carry oxygen. Methemoglobin is a product of various oxidative reactions that constitute normal metabolic activity. Normally present in only trace amounts (about 1%) in the blood, maintainance of levels occurs by an active enzymatic reducing capability, the NADH-methemoglobin reductase system present in normal red cells. See also **hemoglobin.**

methemoglobinemia /-ē'mē·ə/, the presence of methemoglobin in the blood.

methemoglobinuria /-o͝or'ē·ə/ [Gk, *meta,* beyond, *haima,* blood; L, *globus,* ball; Gk, *ouron,* urine], the presence of methemoglobin in the urine.

methenamine /methē'nəmēn/, a urinary antibacterial.

■ INDICATION: It is prescribed in the treatment of urinary tract infections.

■ CONTRAINDICATIONS: Liver or kidney dysfunction or known hypersensitivity to this drug or to mandelic acid prohibits its use.

■ ADVERSE EFFECTS: Among the most serious adverse reactions are severe GI disturbances and rashes.

Methergine, a trademark for an oxytocic (methylergonovine maleate).

methionine (Met) /methī'ənēn/, an essential amino acid needed for proper growth in infants and for maintenance of nitrogen balance in adults. It is a source for methyl groups and sulfur in the body. It is also administered as adjunctive treatment in liver diseases. See also **amino acid, protein.**

Chemical structure of methionine (Seeley, 1992)

methocarbamol /meth'əkär'bəmol/, a skeletal muscle relaxant.

■ INDICATION: It is prescribed in the treatment of skeletal muscle spasm.

■ CONTRAINDICATIONS: Renal dysfunction, central nervous system depression, or known hypersensitivity to this drug prohibits its use.

■ ADVERSE EFFECTS: Among the more serious adverse reactions are hypotension and tachycardia. Drowsiness, dizziness, vertigo, and nausea may occur.

method /meth'əd/ [Gk, *meta,* beyond, *hodos,* way], a technique or procedure for producing a desired effect, such as a surgical procedure, a laboratory test, or a diagnostic technique.

methodology /meth'ədol'əjē/ [Gk, *meta, hodos* + *logos,* science], **1.** a system of principles or methods of procedure in any discipline, such as education, research, diagnosis, or treatment. **2.** the section of a research proposal in which the methods to be used are described. The research design, the population to be studied, and the research instruments, or tools, to be used are discussed in the methodology. **–methodologic,** *adj.*

methohexital sodium /meth'ōhek'sitôl/, an intravenous barbiturate.

■ INDICATION: It is prescribed for the induction of anesthesia in short surgical procedures as a supplement to other anesthetics.

■ CONTRAINDICATIONS: Porphyria, status asthmaticus, or known hypersensitivity to this drug or to any barbiturate prohibits its use.

■ ADVERSE EFFECTS: Among the more serious adverse reactions are respiratory depression, skin rash, and cardiovascular dysfunction.

methotrexate /meth'ōtrek'sāt/, an antineoplastic antimetabolite.

■ INDICATIONS: It is prescribed in the treatment of severe psoriasis and a variety of malignant neoplastic diseases.

■ CONTRAINDICATIONS: Blood dyscrasias, severe renal or hepatic impairment, or known hypersensitivity to this drug prohibits its use.

■ ADVERSE EFFECTS: Among the more serious adverse reactions are diarrhea, ulcerative stomatis, bone marrow depression, hepatotoxicity, and skin rash.

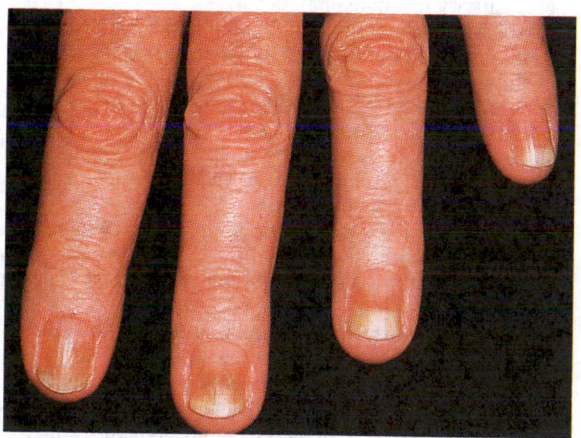

Methotrexate toxicity (du Vivier, 1993)

methoxamine hydrochloride /methok'səmēn/, an adrenergic that acts as a vasoconstrictor.

■ INDICATION: It is prescribed for use during anesthesia to maintain blood pressure and in the treatment of paroxysmal supraventricular tachycardia.

■ CONTRAINDICATIONS: It is not recommended for use as a vasoconstrictor with local anesthetics. Known hypersensitivity to this drug prohibits its use.

■ ADVERSE EFFECTS: Among the most serious adverse reactions are hypertension, bradycardia, cardiac depression, severe headache, and vomiting.

methoxsalen /methok'sələn/, a pigmentation agent.

- INDICATIONS: It is used topically to enhance pigmentation or for repigmentation in vitiligo.
- CONTRAINDICATIONS: Liver impairment, concomitant use of a drug that may cause photosensitization, or known hypersensitivity to this drug prohibits its use.
- ADVERSE EFFECTS: Among the most serious adverse reactions are central nervous system effects and burns. GI discomfort and allergic reactions also may occur.

3-methoxy-4-hydroxymandelic acid /methok'sē-hīdrok'sēməndel'ik/, a product of metabolism that may be measured in the urine to determine the levels of the catecholamines (adrenaline and noradrenaline). Increased concentrations of this acid may raise the blood pressure; indicate the presence of tumors of the adrenal glands or nervous system, muscular dystrophy, and myasthenia gravis; or be caused by stress, exercise, or certain drugs or foods. Normal amounts in the urine of adults after 24-hour collection are 1.5 to 7.5 mg; in the urine of infants, 83 [mu]g/kg of body weight.

methscopolamine bromide /meth'skōpō'ləmēn/, an anticholinergic.
- INDICATIONS: It is prescribed in the treatment of hypermotility of the GI tract and as an adjunct in treating peptic ulcer.
- CONTRAINDICATIONS: Narrow-angle glaucoma, asthma, obstruction of the genitourinary or GI tract, severe ulcerative colitis, or known hypersensitivity to this drug prohibits its use.
- ADVERSE EFFECTS: Blurred vision, central nervous system effects, tachycardia, dry mouth, decreased sweating, or hypersensitivity reactions may occur.

methsuximide /methsuk'simīd/, an anticonvulsant.
- INDICATION: It is prescribed in the treatment of refractory petit mal epilepsy.
- CONTRAINDICATIONS: Known hypersensitivity to this drug or to any succinimide prohibits its use.
- ADVERSE EFFECTS: Among the more serious adverse reactions are blood dyscrasias, liver and kidney damage, and systemic lupus erythematosus.

methyclothiazide /məthī'klōthī'əzīd/ /meth'əklōthī'əzīd/, a diuretic and antihypertensive.
- INDICATIONS: It is prescribed in the treatment of hypertension and edema.
- CONTRAINDICATIONS: Anemia, renal or urinary disorders, or known hypersensitivity to this drug, to other thiazide medications, or to sulfonamide derivatives prohibits its use.
- ADVERSE EFFECTS: Among the more serious adverse reactions are hypokalemia, hyperglycemia, hyperuricemia, hypotension, and hypersensitivity reactions.

methyl (Me) /meth'il/, the chemical radical CH_3.

methyl alcohol. See **methanol.**

methylate /meth'ilāt/ [Gk, *methy*, wine; *hyle*, matter], to add a methyl group, CH_3-, to a chemical compound.

methylation /-lā'shən/ [Gk, *methy*, wine; *hyle*, matter], **1.** the introduction of a methyl group, CH_3-, to a chemical compound. **2.** the addition of methyl alcohol and naphtha to ethanol to produce denatured alcohol.

methylbenzethonium chloride /ben'zəthō'nē·əm/, a topical antiinfective.
- INDICATIONS: It is prescribed for the prevention and treatment of diaper rash and other dermatoses.
- CONTRAINDICATION: Known hypersensitivity to this drug is the only contraindication.
- ADVERSE EFFECTS: There are no known adverse reactions. Local skin irritation may occur.

methyldopa /-dō'pə/, an antihypertensive.
- INDICATION: It is prescribed for the reduction of high blood pressure.
- CONTRAINDICATIONS: Use of monoamine oxidase inhibitors, liver dysfunction, or known hypersensitivity to this drug prohibits its use.
- ADVERSE EFFECTS: Among the more serious adverse reactions are liver toxicity and blood dyscrasias. Sedation, dry mouth, nasal stuffiness, and postural hypotension may occur.

methylene blue /meth'ələn/, a bluish-green crystalline substance used as a histologic stain and as a laboratory indicator. It is also used in the treatment of cyanide poisoning and methemoglobinemia.

methylergonovine maleate /-ərgon'əvēn/, a synthetic ergot alkaloid.
- INDICATIONS: It is prescribed as an oxytocic to prevent or to treat postpartum uterine atony, hemorrhage, or subinvolution.
- CONTRAINDICATIONS: It is not prescribed during pregnancy or given intravenously, except in life-threatening situations. Hypertension, toxemia, or known hypersensitivity to ergot alkaloids prohibits its use.
- ADVERSE EFFECTS: Among the most serious adverse reactions are convulsions and death. Hypertension, nausea, blurred vision, and headaches also may occur. Adverse effects are more common after IV administration.

methylphenidate hydrochloride /-fen'idāt/, a central nervous system stimulant.
- INDICATIONS: It is prescribed in the treatment of hyperkinesis in children and in the treatment of narcolepsy in adults.
- CONTRAINDICATIONS: Glaucoma, severe anxiety, tension, mental depression, or known hypersensitivity to this drug prohibits its use. It is not given to children under 6 years of age.
- ADVERSE EFFECTS: Among the more serious adverse reactions are nervousness, insomnia, and anorexia. Hypersensitivity reactions and tachycardia may occur.

methylprednisolone /-prednis'əlōn/, a glucocorticoid.
- INDICATIONS: It is prescribed in the treatment of inflammatory conditions, including rheumatic fever and rheumatoid arthritis.
- CONTRAINDICATIONS: Fungal infections or known hypersensitivity to this drug prohibits its systemic use. Viral or fungal infections of the skin, impaired circulation, or known hypersensitivity to this drug prohibits its topical use.
- ADVERSE EFFECTS: Among the more serious adverse reactions to the systemic administration of the drug are GI, endocrine, neurologic, fluid, and electrolyte disturbances. A variety of skin reactions may occur from topical administration of this drug.

methylrosaniline chloride. See **gentian violet.**

methyl salicylate Also called **Wintergreen oil.**

methyltestosterone /meth'iltəstos'tərōn/, an androgen.
- INDICATIONS: It is prescribed in the treatment of testosterone deficiency, osteoporosis, and female breast cancer, and to stimulate growth, weight gain, and red blood cell production.
- CONTRAINDICATIONS: Cancer of the male breast or prostate, cardiac, renal, or hepatic disease, hypercalcemia, known or suspected pregnancy, lactation, or known hypersensitivity to this drug prohibits its use.
- ADVERSE EFFECTS: Among the more serious adverse reactions are hypercalcemia, edema, irreversible masculinization of female patients, and jaundice.

methyprylon /meth′əprī′lon/, a sedative and hypnotic.
- INDICATION: It is prescribed in the treatment of insomnia.
- CONTRAINDICATIONS: It is not given to children under 3 months of age. Intermittent porphyria or known hypersensitivity to this drug prohibits its use.
- ADVERSE EFFECTS: Among the most serious adverse reactions are physical dependence and paradoxical excitement. Dizziness, headache, rash, and GI upset also may occur.

methysergide maleate /meth′isur′jīd/, a vasoconstrictor.
- INDICATION: It is prescribed for relief of migraine headache.
- CONTRAINDICATIONS: Pregnancy, severe infection, liver or kidney dysfunction, cardiovascular or lung disease, or known hypersensitivity to this drug prohibits its use. It is not recommended for use in children.
- ADVERSE EFFECTS: Among the more serious adverse reactions are retroperitoneal fibrosis, hallucinations, abnormally low white cell count, pulmonary and cardiac complications, hemolytic anemia, leg cramps, and pain in the chest, abdomen, back, hands, or feet.

Meticorten, a trademark for a glucocorticoid (prednisone).

metoclopramide hydrochloride /met′əklō′prəmīd/, a GI stimulant.
- INDICATIONS: It is prescribed to stimulate motility and to increase the tone of gastric contractions of the upper GI tract and as an antiemetic.
- CONTRAINDICATIONS: Epilepsy; concomitant use of drugs that cause extrapyramidal reactions, pheochromocytoma, GI hemorrhage, obstruction, or perforation, or known hypersensitivity to this drug prohibits its use.
- ADVERSE EFFECTS: Among the more serious adverse reactions are extrapyramidal reactions, usually in children, and GI disturbances. Drowsiness and allergic reactions with a rash also may occur.

metocurine iodide /met′əkyōō′rēn/, a potent neuromuscular blocking agent. Also called **dimethyl tubocurarine iodide.**
- INDICATIONS: It is given to produce flaccid paralysis as an adjunct to anesthesia, to reduce muscle spasm in tetanus, and to assist controlled ventilation.
- CONTRAINDICATIONS: Asthma or known hypersensitivity to this drug or to iodides prohibits its use. It is given only by medical personnel trained and equipped to maintain assisted mechanic ventilation.
- ADVERSE EFFECTS: Among the more serious adverse reactions are hypotension, respiratory or circulatory depression, and bronchospasm.

metolazone /mətō′ləzōn/, a diuretic and antihypertensive.
- INDICATIONS: It is prescribed for the treatment of edema and high blood pressure.
- CONTRAINDICATIONS: Anuria or known hypersensitivity to this drug, to thiazides, or to sulfonamide drugs prohibits its use.
- ADVERSE EFFECTS: Among the more serious adverse reactions are hypokalemia, hyperglycemia, hyperuricemia, and various allergic reactions.

"me-too" drug, *informal.* a drug product that is similar, identical, or closely related to a drug for which a manufacturer has obtained a new drug application. The drug is placed on the market by a company or companies other than the holder of the new drug application. On the assumption that the new drug has been recognized as safe and effective, clinical trials required of the original manufacturer are not required of the new supplier, but information regarding the manufacture, bioavailability, and labeling of the prod-

uct is required to complete the abbreviated procedure for approval by the Food and Drug Administration.

metopic /mətə′pik/, of or pertaining to the forehead.

metopo-, a combining form meaning 'of or related to the forehead': *metopodynia, metopopagus, metopoplasty.*

metoprolol tartrate /metop′rəlol/, an antiadrenergic (beta-receptor).
- INDICATION: It is prescribed in the treatment of hypertension.
- CONTRAINDICATIONS: Bradycardia, cardiogenic shock, overt cardiac failure, bronchospastic disease, or known hypersensitivity to this drug prohibits its use.
- ADVERSE EFFECTS: Among the more serious adverse reactions are fatigue, bradycardia, bronchospasms, and GI upset.

metr-, a combining form meaning 'measure': *metrechoscopy, metric, metrology.*

metra-. See **metro-.**

metralgia /mətral′jə/ [Gk, *metra,* womb, *algos,* pain], tenderness or pain in the uterus. Also called **metrodynia.**

-metria[1], a suffix meaning '(condition of the) ability to measure muscular acts': *dysmetria, hypermetria, hypometria.*

-metria[2], a suffix meaning '(condition of the) uterus': *ametria, atretometria, dimetria.*

metric /met′rik/, of or pertaining to a system of measurement that uses the meter as a basis. See also **metric system.**

metric equivalent [Gk, *metron,* measure; L, *aequus,* equal, *valare,* to be strong], any value in metric units of measurement that equals the same value in English units, for example, 2.54 cm equals 1 inch, or 1 L equals 1.0567 quarts.

metric system, a decimal system of measurement based on the meter (39.37 inches) as the unit of length, on the gram (15.432 grains) as the unit of weight or mass, and, as a derived unit, on the liter (0.908 U.S. dry quart or 1.0567 U.S. liquid quart) as the unit of volume.

metritis /mətrī′tis/ [Gk, *metra,* womb, *itis,* inflammation], inflammation of the walls of the uterus. Kinds of metritis are **endometritis** and **parametritis.** Also called **uteritis.** See also **puerperal fever.**

metro-, metra-, a prefix meaning 'of or related to the uterus': *metrocele, metrofibroma, metromalacoma.*

metrocarcinoma /met′rōkär′sinō′mə/ [Gk, *metra,* womb; *karkinos,* crab; *oma;* tumor], a cancer of the uterus.

metrodynia. See **metralgia.**

metronidazole /met′rəni′dəzōl/, an antimicrobial.
- INDICATIONS: It is prescribed in the treatment of amebiasis, trichomonas, and certain bacterial infections.
- CONTRAINDICATIONS: First trimester of pregnancy, blood dyscrasias, organic disease, central nervous system disorders, or known hypersensitivity to this drug prohibits its use.
- ADVERSE EFFECTS: Among the more serious adverse reactions are severe GI distress, dizziness, neutropenia, and neurologic disturbances. A metallic taste in the mouth is commonly noted.

metronoscope /mətron′əskōp/, **1.** a tachistoscope, or device that exposes a small amount of reading matter to the eyes for brief preset time periods. It is used in testing and to help increase reading speed. **2.** an apparatus that exercises the eyes rhythmically to improve binocular coordination.

-metropia, -metropy, a suffix meaning '(condition of the) refraction of the eye': *allometropia, antimetropia, isometropia.*

metrorrhagia /met′rōrä′jē·ə/ [Gk, *metra*, womb, *rhyegnynai*, to burst forth], uterine bleeding other than that caused by menstruation. It may be caused by uterine lesions and may be a sign of a urogenital malignancy, especially cervical cancer.

-metry, -metria, a suffix meaning the 'process of measuring something' specified: *oncometry, pelvimetry, symmetry*.

Metubine, a trademark for a neuromuscular blocking agent (metocurine iodide), used as an adjunct to anesthesia.

metyrapone /metir′əpōn/, a diagnostic test drug.
■ INDICATION: It is used to test hypothalamicpituitary function.
■ CONTRAINDICATIONS: Adrenal cortical insufficiency or hypersensitivity prohibits its use.
■ ADVERSE EFFECTS: Among the most serious adverse reactions are nausea, dizziness, and allergic rash.

metyrosine /mətir′əsēn/, an antihypertensive.
■ INDICATION: It is prescribed in the treatment of pheochromocytoma.
■ CONTRAINDICATION: Known hypersensitivity to this drug prohibits its use.
■ ADVERSE EFFECTS: Among the more serious adverse reactions are extrapyramidal reactions, including tremor, drooling, and crystalluria. Sedation is common, and diarrhea and anxiety may occur.

Metzenbaum scissors. See **scissors.**

Meuse fever. See **trench fever.**

mev, MeV, abbreviation for *million electron volts,* the equivalent of 3.82×10^{-14} small calories, or $1.6 \ 10^{-6}$ ergs.

mevalonate kinase /məval′ənāt/, an enzyme in the liver and in yeast that catalyzes the transfer of a phosphate group from adenosine triphosphate to produce adenosine diphosphate and 5-phosphomevalonate.

Mexate, a trademark for an antineoplastic (methotrexate).

Mexican typhus [Gk, *typhos,* fever], a form of epidemic typhus carried by lice in Mexico. Also called **tabardillo.**

mexiletine hydrochloride /mek′silē′tin/, an oral antidysrhythmic drug.
■ INDICATIONS: It is prescribed for the treatment of symptomatic ventricular dysrhythmias.
■ CONTRAINDICATIONS: It is contraindicated in patients with cardiogenic shock or preexisting second- or third-degree atrioventricular block in the absence of a pacemaker.
■ ADVERSE EFFECTS: Among adverse reactions reported are upper gastrointestinal distress, lightheadedness, tremor, loss of coordination, diarrhea, sleep disorders, headache, visual disturbances, and palpitations.

Mexitil, a trademark for an oral antidysrhythmic drug (mexiletine hydrochloride).

Meynet's node /mānāz′/, any one of the numerous nodules that may develop within the capsules surrounding joints and in tendons affected by rheumatic diseases, especially in children.

Mezlin, a trademark for a semisynthetic penicillin antibiotic (mezlocillin sodium).

mezlocillin sodium /mezlos′ilin/, a semisynthetic penicillin antibiotic.
■ INDICATIONS: It is prescribed for lower respiratory tract, intraabdominal, urinary tract, gynecologic, and skin infections and bacterial septicemia caused by susceptible strains of multiple microorganisms.
■ CONTRAINDICATION: Hypersensitivity to any of the penicillins prohibits its use.

■ ADVERSE EFFECTS: The most serious adverse reactions are anaphylactic reactions, convulsive seizures, epigastric pain, reduction in blood elements, and elevation in hepatic and renal parameters.

mF, abbreviation for *millifarad;* see **Farad.**

MFCC, abbreviation for *Marriage, Family, and Child Counselor*.

mfd, abbreviation for **microfarad.**

MFD, abbreviation for *minimum fatal dose. See* **minimum lethal dose.**

μg, abbreviation for **microgram.** unit of weight equal to one millionth of a gram.

mg, abbreviation for **milligram.**

Mg, symbol for the element **magnesium.**

MH, 1. abbreviation for **malignant hyperthermia. 2.** abbreviation for **mental health.**

MHA, abbreviation for **Mental Health Association.**

MHC, abbreviation for **major histocompatibility complex.**

MHz, abbreviation for **megahertz.**

MI, abbreviation for **myocardial infarction.**

miasma /mī·az′mə/ [Gk, *miainein*, defilement], an unwholesome, polluted atmosphere or environment, such as a marsh or swamp with rotting organic matter. Also called **miasm** /mī′əzəm/.

MIC, abbreviation for **minimal inhibitory concentration.**

micellar chromatography /mīsel′ər/, a method of monitoring minute quantities of drugs in whole body fluids by using micellar or colloidial compounds to keep proteins in solution. The technique eliminates the need to remove proteins that usually interfere with chromatographic analysis of blood serum, urine, or saliva. Micellar chromatography is used to monitor levels of prescribed drugs, as well as illicit drugs such as LSD and THC.

Michaelis-Menten kinetics [Leonor Michaelis, American biochemist, b. 1875; Maud R. Menten, American physician, b. 1879], a method of transforming drug plasma levels into a linear relationship using the parameters of drug concentration and a constant, K_m, which is a measure of enzyme-substrate affinity.

-micin, a combining form for antibiotics produced by Micromonospora strains.

miconazole nitrate /mīkon′əzōl/, an antifungal.
■ INDICATIONS: It is used topically in the treatment of certain fungal infections of the skin and vagina and parenterally to treat systemic fungal infections.
■ CONTRAINDICATION: Known hypersensitivity to this drug prohibits its use.
■ ADVERSE EFFECTS: Among the more serious adverse reactions to topical or vaginal application are irritation, burning, and maceration of the skin. When used systemically, nausea, pruritus, phlebitis, and anemia may occur.

micr-. See **micro-.**

micrencephalia. See **microcephaly.**

micrencephalon /mī′krənsef′əlon/, 1. an abnormally small brain. See also **microcephaly. 2.** *obsolete.* the cerebellum. **–micrencephalic,** *adj., n.*

micrencephaly. See **microcephaly.**

micro-, micr-, mikro-, a prefix meaning 'small': *microadenopathy, microanalysis, microglossia*.

microabscess /mīkrō·ab′ses/ [Gk, *mikros,* small; L, *abscedere*, to go away], a very small abscess.

microaerophile /mī′krō·er′ōfil/ [Gk, *mikros*, small, *aer,* air, *philein,* to love], a microorganism that requires free oxygen for growth but at a lower concentration than that contained in the atmosphere. Compare **aerobe, anaerobe.** **–microaerophilic,** *adj.*

microaerotonometer /mī′krō·er′ətonom′ətər/ [Gk, *mikros* + *aer*, air, *tonos*, tension, *metron*, measure], instrument for measuring the volume of gases in blood or other fluids.

microaggregate recipient set /mi′krō·ag′rəgāt/ [Gk, *mikros* + L, *ad*, to, *gregare*, to collect; *recipere*, to receive; AS, *settan*], a device composed of plastic components for the intravenous delivery of large volumes of stored whole blood or of packed blood cells. The components of the set include the plastic tubing, the roller clamp, and the special filter that prevents the microaggregates or deteriorated red blood cells of stored whole blood from entering and clogging the circulatory system of the patient. The plastic tubing of this device has a larger lumen than the tubing of most other intravenous sets, which allows the blood to be delivered more rapidly. Compare **component drip set, component syringe set, straight line blood set, Y set.**

microampere /mī′krō·am′pir/, one millionth of an ampere.

microaneurysm /mi′krō·an′yəriz′əm/ [Gk, *mikros* + *aneurysma*, widening], a microscopic aneurysm characteristic of thrombotic purpura.

microangiopathy /mī′krō·an′jē·op′əthē/ [Gk, *mikros* + *aggerion*, vessel, *pathos*, disease], a disease of the small blood vessels, such as diabetic microangiopathy, in which the basement membrane of capillaries thickens, or thrombotic microangiopathy, in which thrombi form in the arterioles and the capillaries.

microbe /mī′krōb/, a microorganism. **–microbial,** *adj.*

-microbe, a suffix meaning a 'small living organism': *aeromicrobe, inframicrobe, ultramicrobe.*

-microbic, a suffix meaning 'referring to or consisting of microbes': *amicrobic, monomicrobic, polymicrobic.*

microbicide /mīkrō′bisīd/ [Gk, *mikros*, small; *bios*, life; L, *cadere*, to kill], any drug, chemical, or other agent that can kill microorganisms.

microbiology /mī′krōbī·ol′əjē/ [Gk, *mikros* + *bios*, life, *logos*, science], the branch of biology concerned with the study of microorganisms, including algae, bacteria, viruses, protozoa, fungi, and rickettsiae.

microbiology technologist, a medical technologist who specializes in the identification of bacteria and other microorganisms found in patient tissues and other specimens.

microblast /mī′krōblast′/ [Gk, *mikros*, small; *blastos*, germ], a very small immature red blood cell.

microbrachia /mī′krōbrā′kē·ə/ [Gk, *mikros* + *brachion*, arm], a developmental defect characterized by abnormal smallness of the arms. **–microbrachius,** *n.*

microcentrum. See **centrosome.**

microcephaly /mī′krōsef′əlē/ [Gk, *mikros* + *kephale*, head], a congenital anomaly characterized by abnormal smallness of the head in relation to the rest of the body and by underdevelopment of the brain, resulting in some degree of mental retardation. The head is more than two standard deviations below the average circumference size for age, sex, race, and period of gestation, and it has a narrow, receding forehead, a flattened occiput, and a pointed vertex. The facial features are generally normal. The condition may be caused by an autosomal recessive disorder, a chromosomal abnormality, a toxic stimulus, such as irradiation, chemical agents, or maternal infection during prenatal development, or any trauma, especially during the third trimester of pregnancy or early infancy. There is no treatment, and nursing care is primarily supportive and educational,

helping parents learn to care for a brain-damaged child. Also called **microcephalia, microcephalism.** Compare **macrocephaly.** **–microcephalic, microcephalous,** *adj.,* **microcephalic, microcephalus,** *n.*

microcheiria /mī′krōkī′rē·ə/ [Gk, *mikros* + *cheir*, hand], a developmental defect characterized by abnormal smallness of the hands. The condition is usually associated with other congenital malformations or with bone and muscle disorders. Also spelled **microchiria.**

microcirculation /-sur′kyəlē′shən/, the flow of blood throughout the system of smaller vessels of the body, particularly the capillaries.

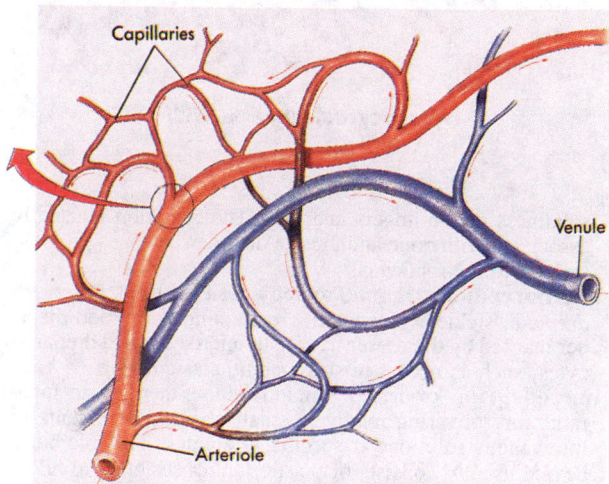

Microcirculation *(Thibodeau, 1993/Bill Ober)*

microcomputer /-kəmpyōō′tər/, a complete multiuse electronic digital computer system consisting of a central processing unit, storage facilities, I/O ports, and a chip with megabytes of high-speed internal storage. Compare **mainframe computer, minicomputer.**

microcurie (μCi, μc) /mī′krōkyōōr′ē/ [Gk, *mikros* + *curie*, Marie and Pierre Curie], a unit of radiation equal to one millionth (10^{-6}) of a curie.

microcyte /mī′krəsīt/ [Gk, *mikros* + *kytos*, cell], an abnormally small erythrocyte with a mean corpuscular volume of less than 80 μm^3, often occurring in iron deficiency anemias.

microcythemia /-thē′mē·ə/ [Gk, *mikros*, small; *kytos*, cell; *haima*, blood], an excessive amount of microcytes in the blood.

microcytic /mī′krōsit′ik/ [Gk, *mikros* + *kytos*, cell], (of a cell) pertaining to smaller than normal cells.

microcytic anemia, a hematologic disorder characterized by abnormally small erythrocytes, usually associated with chronic blood loss or a nutritional anemia, such as iron deficiency anemia. Compare **macrocytic anemia.**

microcytosis /mī′krōsītō′sis/ [Gk, *mikros, kytos* + *osis*, condition], a hematologic condition characterized by erythrocytes that are smaller than normal. Microcytosis is found in iron deficiency anemia. Compare **poikilocytosis.** See also **anisocytosis.** **–microcytic,** *adj.* (See Fig. p. 993.)

microdactyly /mī′krōdak′təlē/ [Gk, *mikros* + *dactylos*, finger], a developmental defect characterized by abnormal

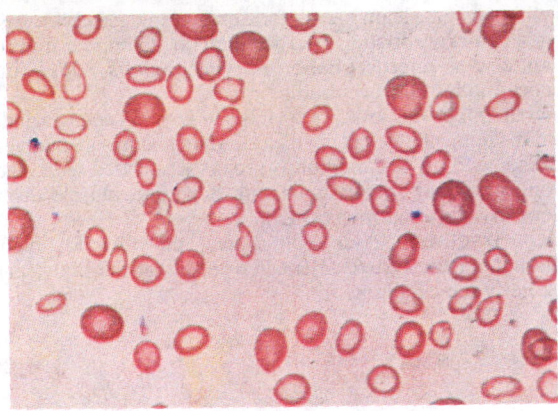

Microcytosis (Hayhoe, 1992)

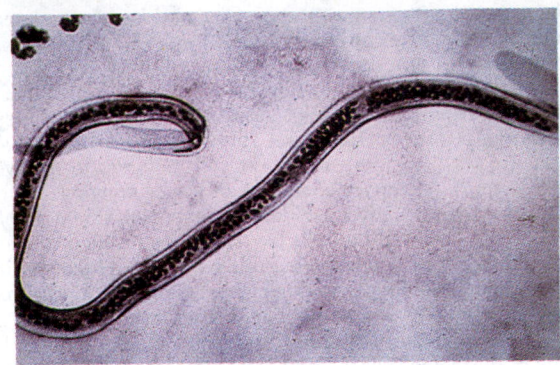

Microfilaria of *Wuchereria bancrofti* in stained blood smear
(Muller, 1990)

smallness of the fingers and toes. The condition is usually associated with bone and muscle disorders, such as progressive myositis ossificans.

microdrepanocytic /mī'krōdrep'ənōsit'ik/ [Gk, *mikros* + *drepane*, sickle, *kytos*, cell], pertaining to a blood disorder marked by the presence of both microcytes and drepanocytes, such as occurs in sickle cell-thalassemia.

microdrip /mī'krōdrip'/, (in intravenous therapy) an apparatus for delivering relatively small, measured amounts of intravenous solutions at specific flow rates. The microdrip device usually consists of plastic tubing designed to allow small drops of solution to pass into the primary intravenous tubing through a clear plastic housing. A microdrip is usually used to deliver small volumes of solution over a long time. With a microdrip, 60 drops deliver 1 ml of solution. Compare **macrodrip**.

microelement. See **micronutrient**.

microencapsulation /mī'krō·enkap'syəlā'shən/ [Gk, *mikros* + *en*, in; L, *capsula*, little box], a laboratory technique used in the bioassay of hormones in which certain antibodies are encapsulated with a perforated membrane. The antibodies cannot escape through the tiny perforations, but hormones that bind with the antibodies may enter the structure to bind with them. Technicians then can measure the amount of hormone present in the specimen. The technique is used for encapsulating unstable enzymes and in the preparation of some drugs in slow- or timed-release forms.

microencephaly /mī'krō·ensef'əlē/ [Gk, *mikros,* small; *egkephalos,* brain], an infant born with an abnormally small brain.

microfarad (mfd) /mī'krōfer'əd/ [Gk, *mikros* + *farad*, Michael Faraday], a unit of capacitance that equals one millionth of a farad.

microfiche /mī'krōfēsh'/ [Gk, *mikros* + Fr, *fiche*, peg], a sheet of microfilm that contains several separate photographic reproductions. The sheet is a convenient size for filing and enables large amounts of data to be stored in a relatively small space. See also **microfilm**.

microfilament /-fil'əmənt/, any of the submicroscopic cellular filaments, such as the tonofibrils, found in the cytoplasm of most cells, that function primarily as a supportive system. Compare **microtubule**.

microfilaria /mī'krōfiler'ē·ə/, *pl*. **microfilariae** [Gk, *mikros* + L, *filum*, thread], the prelarval form of any filarial

worm. Certain blood-sucking insects ingest these forms from an infected host, and the microfilariae then develop in the body of the insect and become infective larvae. See also **filariasis, loiasis, onchocerciasis, *Wuchereria***.

microfilm /mī'krəfilm/, a strip of 16 mm or 35 mm film that contains photographic reproductions of pages of books, documents, or other library or medical records in greatly reduced size. The film is viewed through special machines that enlarge the photographic images to normal reading size.

microfluorometry. See **cytophotometry**.

microgamete /-gam'ēt/, the small, motile male gamete of certain thallophytes and sporozoa, specifically the malarial parasite *Plasmodium*. It corresponds to the sperm of the higher animals and unites in conjugation with the larger, nonmotile female gamete. See also **macrogamete**.

microgametocyte /-gamē'təsīt/ [Gk, *mikros* + *gamete,* spouse, *kytos*, cell], an enlarged merozoite that undergoes meiosis to form the mature male gamete during the sexual phase of the life cycle of certain thallophytes and sporozoa, specifically the malarial parasite *Plasmodium*. Microgametocytes are found in the red blood cells of a person infected with the malarial parasite, but they must be ingested by a female *Anopheles* mosquito to complete the maturation process and develop into a microgamete.

microgenitalia /-jen'itā'lē·ə/, a condition characterized by abnormally small external genitalia.

microglia /mīkrog'lē·ə/ [Gk, *mikros* + *glia*, glue], small migratory interstitial cells that form part of the central nervous system. They have various forms and slender, branched processes. Microglia serve as phagocytes that collect waste products of the nerve tissue of the body. Also called **Hortega cells, mesoglia**.

micrognathia /mī'krōnā'thē·ə/ [Gk, *mikros* + *gnathos*, jaw], underdevelopment of the jaw, especially the mandible. Compare **macrognathia**. **–micrognathic,** *adj*.

microgram (μg), /mī'krəgram/, a unit of measurement of mass equal to one millionth (10^{-6}) of a gram. See also **gram**.

microgyria /mī'krōjī'rē·ə/ [Gk, *mikros* + *gyros*, turn], a developmental defect of the brain in which the convolutions are abnormally small, resulting in structural malformation of the cortex. The condition is usually associated with mental retardation and physical defects. Also called **polymicrogyria**.

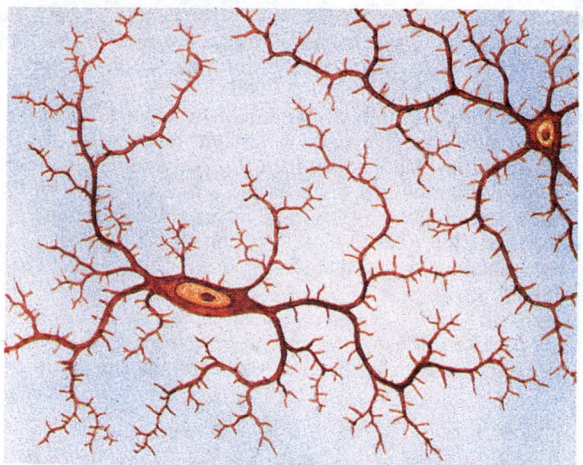

Microglia (Chipps, 1992)

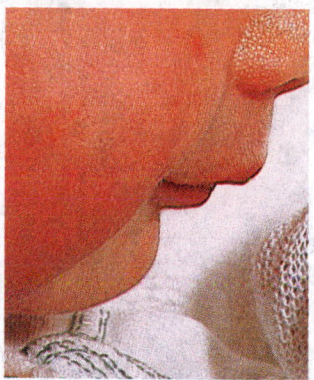

Micrognathia
(Zitelli, 1992/Courtesy Dr. Christine Williams, Scarsdale, NY)

microgyrus /mī′krōjī′rəs/, *pl.* **microgyri,** an underdeveloped, malformed convolution of the brain.

microhm /mī′krōm/ [Gk, *mikros* + *ohm,* George Ohm], a unit of electric resistance equal to one millionth of an ohm.

microinvasive carcinoma /mī′krō·invā′siv/ [Gk, *mikros* + L, *in,* within, *vadere,* to go], a squamous epithelial neoplasm that has penetrated the basement membrane, the first stage in invasive cancer. See also **carcinoma in situ.**

microlevel interventions /-lev′əl/, health-generating changes performed at the individual level, such as in conditioning or stimulus control therapies.

microliter (μL) /mī′krəlē′tər/, a unit of liquid volume equal to one millionth of a liter.

microlith /mī′krəlith/ [Gk, *mikros* + *lithos,* stone], a small rounded mass of mineral matter or calcified stone.

micromelic dwarf /-mē′lik/ [Gk, *mikros* + *melos,* limb], a dwarf whose limbs are abnormally short.

micrometer, 1. /mīkrom′ətər/, **1.** 1.an instrument used for measuring small angles or distances on objects being observed through a microscope or telescope.
2. /mī′krōmē′tər/, a unit of measurement, commonly referred to as a *micron,* that is, one thousandth (10^{-3}) of a millimeter.

micromicro- (μμ), a combining form meaning '10^{-12}': *micromicron.*

micromillimeter /-mil′imē′tər/ [Gk, *mikros,* small; L, mille, thousand; Gk, *metron*], a nanometer.

micromyeloblastic leukemia /mī′krōmī′əlōblas′tik/ [Gk, *mikros* + *myelos,* marrow, *blastos,* germ], a malignant neoplasm of blood-forming tissues, characterized by the proliferation of small myeloblasts distinguishable from lymphocytes only by special staining techniques and microscopic examination.

micron (μ, mu) /mī′kron/ [Gk, *mikros,* small], **1.** a metric unit of length equal to one millionth of a meter; micrometer (def. 2). **2.** (in physical chemistry), a colloidal particle with a diameter of between 0.2 and 10 microns.

Micronase, a trademark for an oral antidiabetic drug (glyburide).

Micronor, a trademark for an oral contraceptive containing a progestin (norethindrone).

micronucleus /-nōō′klē·əs/, **1.** a small or minute nucleus. **2.** (in protozoa) the smaller of two nuclei in each cell; it functions in sexual reproduction as opposed to the macronucleus, which governs cell metabolism and growth. **3.** See **nucleolus.**

micronutrient /-nōōtrē·ənt/, an organic compound, such as a vitamin, or a chemical element, such as zinc or iodine, essential only in minute amounts for the normal physiologic processes of the body. Also called **microelement, minor element, trace element.**

microorganism /-ôr′gəniz′əm/ [Gk, *mikros* + *organon,* instrument], any tiny, usually microscopic entity capable of carrying on living processes. It may be pathogenic. Kinds of microorganisms include **bacteria, fungi, protozoa,** and **viruses.**

micropenis. See **microphallus.**

microphage /mī′krəfāj/ [Gk, *mikros* + *phagein,* to eat], a neutrophil capable of ingesting small things, such as bacteria. Compare **macrophage.** –**microphagic,** *adj.*

microphallus /-fal′əs/ [Gk, *mikros* + *phallos,* penis], an abnormally small penis. When it is observed in the newborn, the nurse examines the child for other signs of ambiguous genitalia. Also called **micropenis.** See also **ambiguous genitalia.**

microphthalmos /mī′krəfthal′məs/ [Gk, *mikros* + *ophthalmos,* eye], a developmental anomaly characterized by abnormal smallness of one or both eyes. When the condition occurs in the absence of other ocular defects, it is called pure microphthalmos or nanophthalmos. Also spelled **microphthalmus.** Also called **microphthalmia.** –**microphthalmic,** *adj.*

microplasia. See **dwarfism.**

micropodia /-pō′dē·ə/ [Gk, *mikros* + *pous,* foot], a developmental anomaly characterized by abnormal smallness of the feet. The condition is often associated with other congenital malformations or with bone and skeletal disorders.

microprosopus /mī′krōprō′səpəs, -prəsō′pəs/ [Gk, *mikros* + *prosopon,* face], a fetus in which the face is abnormally small or underdeveloped.

micropsia /mīkrop′sē·ə/ [Gk, *mikros* + *opsis,* sight], a condition of vision by which a person perceives objects as smaller than they really are. **microptic,** *adj.*

microreentry /-rē·en′trē/ [Gk, *mikros* + L, *re,* again; Fr, *entree,* entry], (in cardiology) pertaining to abnormal transmission of electrical impulses, and involving a very small circuit, such as within Purkinje fibers.

microscope /mī′krəskōp′/ [Gk, *mikros*, small; *skopein*, to view], an instrument with lenses for viewing very small objects. An electron microscope uses a beam of electrons instead of visible light.

microscopic /mī′krəskop′ik/ [Gk, *mikros* + *skopein*, to look], **1.** of or pertaining to a microscope. **2.** very small; visible only when magnified and illuminated by a microscope. Compare **gross.**

microscopic anatomy, the study of the microscopic structure of the tissues and cells. Kinds of microscopic anatomy are **cytology** and **histology.**

microscopy /mīkros′kəpē/ [Gk, *mikros* + *skopein*, to look], a technique for observing minute materials using a microscope. Kinds of microscopy include **darkfield microscopy, electron microscopy,** and **immunofluorescent microscopy.**

microshock /mī′krəshok/, the passage of current directly into the cardiac tissue.

microsomal enzymes /-sō′məl/, a group of enzymes associated with a certain particulate fraction of liver homogenate that plays a role in the metabolism of many drugs.

microsomia /-sō′mē·ə/ [Gk, *mikros* + *soma*, body], the condition of having an abnormally small and underdeveloped yet otherwise perfectly formed body with normal proportionate relationships of the various parts. See also **primordial dwarf.**

Microsporum /-spôr′əm/ [Gk, *mikros* + *sporos*, seed], a genus of dermatophytes of the family Moniliaceae. The spores are multiseptate and variable in shape, and have thin or thick walls. One type species is *M. audouinii*, which causes epidemic tinea capitis in children; others are *m. canis* and *m. gypseum*. Formerly called *Microsporon.*

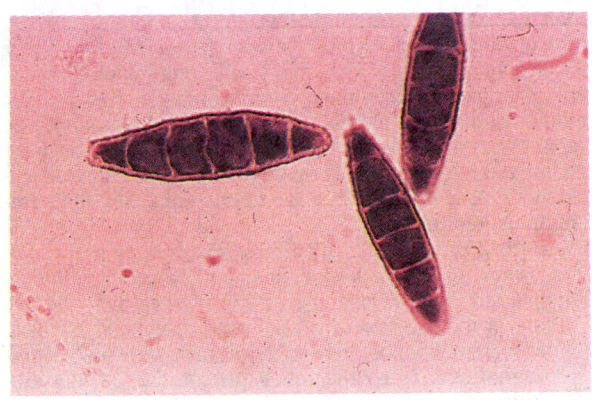

Microsporum gypseum (Murray, 1990)

microstomia /-stō′mē·ə/ [Gk, *mikros*, small; *stoma*, mouth], the condition of having an abnormally small mouth.

microsurgery /-sur′jərē/ [Gk, *mikros*, small; *cheirourgos*, surgery], surgery that involves microdissection and micromanipulation of tissues.

microthermy /-thur′mē/ [Gk, *mikros* + *therme*, heat], a form of therapy in which heat generated by radio wave conversion is used in physical therapy.

microtome /mī′krətōm/ [Gk, *mikros* + *temnein*, to cut], a device that cuts specimens of tissue prepared in paraffin blocks into extremely thin slices for microscopic study by a surgical pathologist.

microtubule. a hollow cylindrical structure (200 to 300 angstrom in diameter and of variable length) that occurs widely within plant and animal cells. Microtubules increase in number during cell division and are associated with the movement of DNA material. Compare **microfilament.**

microvascular /-vas′kyələr/, pertaining to the portion of the circulatory system that is composed of the capillary network.

microvilli /-vil′ī/ [Gk, *mikros*, small; L, *villus*, shaggy hair], tiny hairlike processes that extend from the surface of many cells. They are visible with an electron microscope.

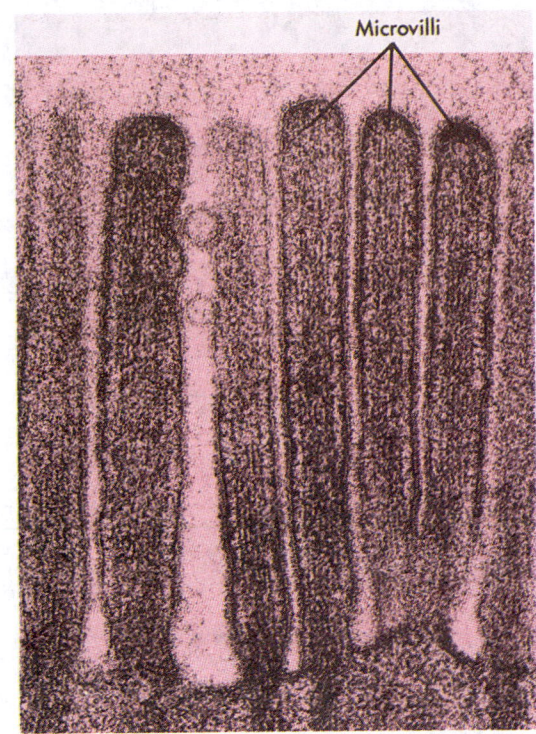

Microvilli
(Thibodeau, 1993/Courtesy Susumo Ito, Harvard Medical School)

microwave interstitial system /mī′krəwāv/ [Gk, *mikros* + AS, *wafian*, wave], a microwave-generated hyperthermia system that employs up to eight 50-watt applicators to create a heat field in certain accessible tumors no more than 2 inches beneath the skin. The microwaves produce a temperature of about 109° F to destroy the tumor cells. The treatment can be monitored on a video terminal that shows location of the tumor and heat applicators.

microwaves, electromagnetic radiation in the frequency range of 300 to 2450 MHz.

microwave thermography, measurement of temperature through the detection of microwave radiation emitted from heated tissue.

micturate, micturition. See **urination.**

micturition reflex /mik'chərish'ən/ [L, *micturire*, to urinate; *reflectere*, to bend backward], a normal reaction to a rise in pressure within the bladder, resulting in contraction of the bladder wall and relaxation of the urethral sphincter. Voluntary inhibition normally prevents incontinence, with urination occurring on withdrawal of this inhibition.

micturition syncope [L, *micturire*, to make water; Gk, *syn*, together; *koptein*, to cut], a temporary loss of consciousness that tends to affect some adult males after arising from a reclining posture to urinate in an upright posture. The effect is due to a brief interruption of blood flow to the brain and is often associated with the use of alcohol, which contributes to vasodilation. See also **hypotension; orthostatic hypotension.**

MICU, abbreviation for *medical intensive care unit.*

mid-, a prefix pertaining to 'the middle': *midsagittal.*

Midamor, a trademark for a diuretic (amiloride hydrochloride).

midarm muscle circumference, an indication of muscle wasting in the upper arm calculated by subtracting the triceps skin fold (TSF) from the midupper arm circumference (MAC) measurement.

midaxillary line /midak'siler'ē/, an imaginary vertical line that passes midway between the anterior and posterior axillary folds.

midazolam hydrochloride /midaz'əlam/, a parenteral central nervous system depressant.

■ INDICATIONS: It is prescribed for preoperative sedation and impairment of memory of preoperative events, and for conscious sedation before short diagnostic or endoscopic procedures.

■ CONTRAINDICATIONS: This product is contraindicated for patients with acute narrow-angle glaucoma. It should be used with caution in patients with open-angle glaucoma.

■ ADVERSE EFFECTS: Possible adverse reactions include decreased tidal volume, decreased respiratory rate, apnea, hypotension, hiccups, nausea, vomiting, oversedation, and tenderness at the site of injection.

midbody, 1. the middle of the body, or the midregion of the trunk. 2. a mass of granules that appears in the middle of the spindle during mitotic anaphase.

midbrain. See **mesencephalon.**

midclavicular line /mid'kləvik'yo͞olər/ [AS, *midd*; L, *clavicula*, little key; *linea*, line], (in anatomy) an imaginary line that extends downward over the trunk from the midpoint of the clavicle, dividing each side of the anterior chest into two parts. The left midclavicular line is an important marker in describing the location of various cardiac phenomena, including the point of maximum impulse.

middle adult [AS, *middel*; L, *adultus*, grown up], an individual in the transitional age span between young adult and elderly, whose psychologic task is generativity versus stagnation.

middle cardiac vein, one of the five tributaries of the coronary sinus that drains blood from the capillary bed of the myocardium. It starts at the apex of the heart, rises in the posterior interventricular sulcus, receives tributaries from both ventricles, and ends in the right extremity of the coronary sinus. Compare **great cardiac vein, small cardiac vein.**

middle costotransverse ligament. See **ligament of the neck of the rib.**

middle cuneiform bone. See **intermediate cuneiform bone.**

middle ear, the tympanic cavity and the auditory ossicles contained in an irregular space in the temporal bone. It is separated from the external ear by the tympanic membrane and from the inner ear by the oval window. The eustachian tube carries air from the posterior pharynx into the middle ear. Compare **external ear, internal ear.**

middle kidney. See **mesonephros.**

middle lobe syndrome, localized atelectasis of the middle lobe of the right lung, characterized by chronic infection, cough, dyspnea, wheezing, and obstructive pneumonitis. Asymptomatic obstruction of the bronchus may occur. The condition is caused by enlargement of the surrounding cuff of lymphatic glands, because of nonspecific or tuberculous inflammation during childhood. The middle lobe bronchus is thus compressed, with bronchiectasis developing in the obstructed part of the lung. Treatment includes antituberculosis chemotherapy, corticosteroids, or surgical excision. See also **atelectasis.**

middle mediastinum, the widest part of the mediastinum containing the heart, ascending aorta, lower half of the superior vena cava, pulmonary trunk, and phrenic nerves. It is one of three caudal portions of the mediastinum. Compare **anterior mediastinum, posterior mediastinum, superior mediastinum.**

middle plate. See **nephrotome.**

middle sacral artery, a small, visceral branch of the abdominal aorta, descending to the fourth and fifth lumbar vertebrae, the sacrum, and the coccyx. Minute branches are said to supply the posterior surface of the rectum.

middle suprarenal artery, one of a pair of small, visceral branches of the abdominal aorta, arising opposite the superior mesenteric artery, and supplying the suprarenal gland.

middle temporal artery, one of the branches of the superficial temporal artery on each side of the head. It arises just above the zygomatic arch, pierces the temporal fascia, branches to the temporalis, and anastomoses with the deep temporal branches of the maxillary artery. Compare **deep temporal artery, superficial temporal artery.**

middle temporal gyrus [AS, *middel*; L, *tempus*, time; Gk, *gyros*, turn], the middle of three gyri of the temporal area of the surface of the brain. It runs horizontal in direction and lies between the inferior and superior temporal sulci of the temporal lobe.

middle umbilical fold, the fold of peritoneum over the urachal remnant within the abdomen. Approximately 3 cm lateral to the middle umbilical fold is the lateral umbilical fold. Between the lateral and the middle folds is the medial umbilical fold. Also called **plica umbilicalis mediana.**

mid forceps [AS, *midd*; L, *forceps*, pair of tongs], an obstetric operation in which forceps are applied to the head of the baby when the head has reached the midplane of the mother's pelvis. An episiotomy is usually performed, and local, regional, or inhalation anesthesia is provided. In some cases, such as severe fetal distress, mid forceps may be the most rapid and the safest means of delivery, but astute selection of cases, skill, and experience are essential. Difficult mid forceps delivery is likely to be more traumatic to the baby and the mother than cesarean section. Compare **high forceps, low forceps.** See also **failed forceps, forceps delivery, obstetric forceps, trial forceps.**

midgut [AS, *midd, guttas*], the middle portion of the embryonic alimentary canal. It consists of endodermal tissue, is connected to the yolk sac during early prenatal development, and eventually gives rise to some of the small intestine and part of the large intestine. Compare **foregut, hindgut.**

midlife transition, a period between early adulthood and middle adulthood that occurs between 40 and 45 years of age.

midline /mid'līn/ [AS, *midd;* L, *linea,* line], an imaginary line that divides the body into right and left halves.

midline episiotomy. See **episiotomy.**

midpelvic contraction. See **contraction.**

midposition /mid'pəzish'ən/, the end-expiratory or end-tidal level or position of the lung-chest system under any given conditions, defining the patient's functional residual capacity.

Midrin, a trademark for a central nervous system, fixed-combination drug containing an adrenergic (isometheptene mucate), a hypnotic (dichloralphenazone), and an analgesic (acetaminophen), used in the treatment of migraine.

midsagittal plane. See **median plane.**

midstance /mid'stanz/ [AS, *midd;* L, *stare,* to stand], one of the five stages in the stance phase of walking, or gait, directly associated with the period of single-leg support of body weight or the period during which the body advances over the stationary foot. During midstance the tibialis posterior and the flexor hallucis longus display their greatest activity. The midstance phase is considered in the diagnosis of many abnormal orthopedic conditions and in the analysis of the associated weaknesses of certain muscles and muscle groups. Compare **initial contact stance stage, loading response stance stage, preswing stance stage, terminal stance.** See also **swing phase of gait.**

midsternum /midstur'nəm/ [AS, *midd;* Gk, *sternon,* chest], the body of the breast bone, or sternum.

midstream catch urine specimen [AS, *midd, stream;* L, *captere,* to capture], a urine specimen collected during the middle of a flow of urine, after the urinary opening has been carefully cleaned.

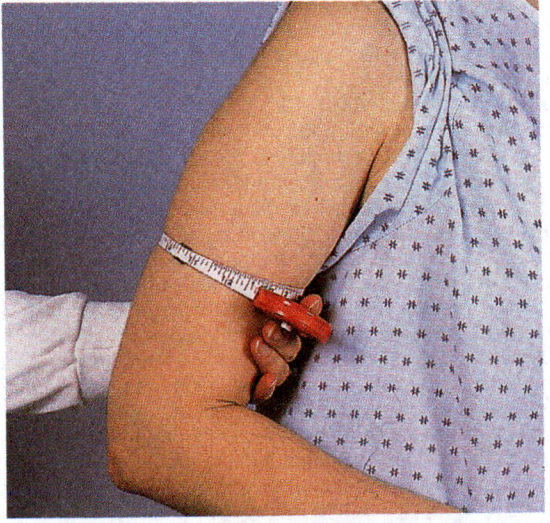

Measurement of midupper arm circumference
(Seidel, 1991)

midupper arm circumference (MAC), an indication of upper arm muscle wasting based on measurement of the circumference of the arm at a midpoint between the tip of the acromial process of the scapula and the olecranon process of the ulna.

midwife [AS, *midd, wif*], **1.** also called **obstetrix.** (in traditional use) a (female) person who assists women in childbirth. **2.** (according to the International Confederation of Midwives, World Health Organization, and Federation of International Gynecologists and Obstetricians) "a person who, having been regularly admitted to a midwifery educational program fully recognized in the country in which it is located, has successfully completed the prescribed course of studies in midwifery and has acquired the requisite qualifications to be registered and/or legally licensed to practice midwifery." Among the responsibilities of the midwife are supervision of the woman's pregnancy, labor, delivery, and puerperium. The midwife conducts the delivery independently, cares for the newborn, procures medical assistance when necessary, executes emergency measures as required, and may practice in a hospital, clinic, maternity home, or in a woman's home. The midwife, whose practice may include well-child care, family planning, and some aspects of gynecology, is often an important source of health counseling in the community. **3.** a lay midwife. **4.** a nurse midwife or Certified Nurse Midwife.

midwifery /mid'wīf(ə)rē/ [AS, *midd;* wif], the employment of a person who is qualified by special training and experience to assist a woman in childbirth. See **midwife.**

MIF, abbreviation for **macrophage inhibition factor.** See **macrophage migration inhibiting factor.**

migraine /mī'grān/ [Gk, *hemi,* half, *kranion,* skull], a recurring vascular headache characterized by a prodromal aura, unilateral onset, and severe pain, photophobia, and autonomic disturbances during the acute phase, which may last for hours or days. The disorder occurs more frequently in women than in men, and a predisposition to migraine may be inherited. The exact mechanism responsible for the disorder is not known, but the head pain is related to dilatation of extracranial blood vessels, which may be the result of chemical changes that cause spasms of intracranial vessels. A greatly increased amount of a vasodilating polypeptide related to bradykinin is found in tissue fluid of patients during migraine attacks. Allergic reactions, excess carbohydrates, iodine-rich foods, alcohol, bright lights, or loud noises may trigger attacks, which often occur during a period of relaxation after physical or psychic stress. An impending attack may be heralded by visual disturbances, such as flashing lights or wavy lines, or by a strange taste or odor, numbness, tingling, vertigo, tinnitus, or a feeling that part of the body is distorted in size or shape. The acute phase may be accompanied by nausea, vomiting, chills, polyuria, sweating, facial edema, irritability, and extreme fatigue. After an attack the individual often has dull head and neck pains and a great need for sleep. Aspirin seldom provides relief during an attack, but ergotamine tartrate preparations that constrict cranial arteries can usually prevent the headache from developing if administered early in the onset via injection, suppository, or tablet. Ergotamine tartrate is also available combined with other drugs, such as caffeine, phenobarbital, and belladonna; migraine patients unable to tolerate ergot preparations may use other analgesics, including acetaminophen, phenacetin, and propoxyphene.

migrainous cranial neuralgia /mī'grānəs, mīgrā'nəs/ [Gk, *hemi*, half, *kranion*, skull; L, *osus*, having], a variant of migraine, characterized by closely spaced episodes of excruciating, throbbing, unilateral headaches often accompanied by dilation of temporal blood vessels, flushing, sweating, lacrimation, nasal congestion or rhinorrhea, ptosis, and facial edema. Repeated episodes usually occur in clusters within a few days or weeks and may be followed by a relatively long remission period. A typical attack begins abruptly without prodromal signs, as a burning sensation in an orbit or temple, and the resulting radiating intense pain may last 1 or 2 hours. Histamine diphosphate injected subcutaneously in people subject to these headaches produces symptoms identical to those occurring in a spontaneous attack. The pain may be relieved by antihistamines, and ergotamine tartrate preparations may be helpful if administered at the onset of an attack. Also called **cluster headache, histamine headache, Horton's headache.** See also **migraine.**

migrating phlebitis /mī'grāting/ [L, *migrare,* to wander; Gk, *phleps,* vein + *itis,* inflammation], a form of phlebitis characterized by inflammation in one part of a vein and, after remission, in another part of the vein.

migration /mīgrā'shən/ [L, *migrare,* to wander], the passage of the ovum from the ovary into a fallopian tube and then into the uterus.

migratory gonorrheal polyarthritis. See **migratory polyarthritis.**

migratory ophthalmia. See **sympathetic ophthalmia.**

migratory polyarthritis /mī'grətôr'ē/, arthritis progressively affecting a number of joints and finally settling in one or more, occurring in patients with gonorrhea and developing a few days to a few weeks after the onset of gonorrheal urethritis. The patient usually has a moderate fever and 1 to 5 days of migratory polyarthralgia with variable signs of inflammation. In more prolonged episodes, initially arthritic sites may clear as new areas are affected, but persistently involved joints are usually severely inflamed and swollen. Large joints are most affected; after the swelling subsides, the overlying skin may peel. Treatment with penicillin or tetracycline generally produces some response in 24 to 72 hours. Also called **migratory gonorrheal polyarthritis.**

migratory thrombophlebitis, an abnormal condition in which multiple thromboses appear in both superficial and deep veins. It may be associated with malignancy, especially carcinoma of the pancreas, often preceding other evidence of cancer by several months. Pulmonary embolism is uncommon with this condition. Also called **thrombophlebitis migrans.** See also **thrombophlebitis.**

mikro-. See **micro-.**

Mikulicz's syndrome /mik'yo͞olich'ēz/ [Johann von Miculicz-Radecki, Polish surgeon, b. 1850], an abnormal bilateral enlargement of the salivary and lacrimal glands, found in a variety of diseases, including leukemia, tuberculosis, and sarcoidosis. Also called **Mikulicz's disease.** Compare **Sjögren's syndrome.**

mild [AS *milde* soft], gentle, subtle, or of low intensity, such as a mild infection.

milia. See **milium.**

milia neonatorum [L, *milium,* millet; Gk, *neo,* new; L, *natus,* born], a nonpathologic dermatologic condition characterized by minute epidermal cysts consisting of keratinous debris that occur on the face and, occasionally, the trunk of the newborn. They are eliminated by normal desquamation of the skin within a few weeks after birth and leave no scars.

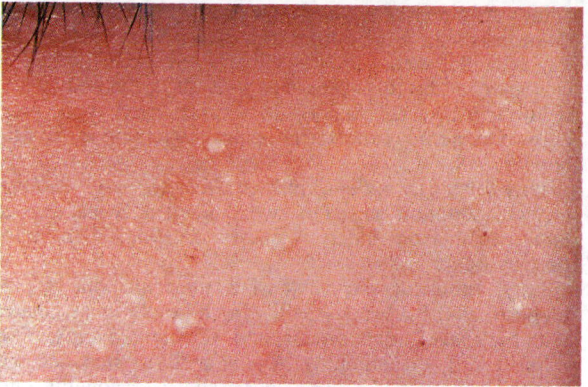

Milia *(du Vivier, 1993)*

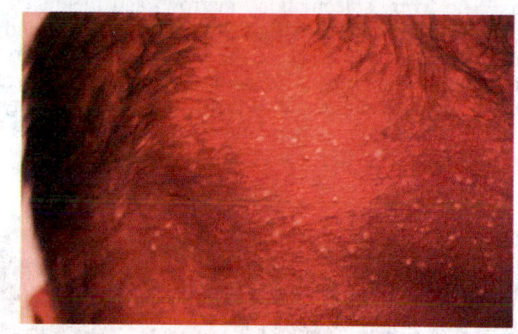

Milia neonatorum *(Weston, 1991)*

miliaria /mil'ē·er'ē·ə/ [L, *milium,* millet], minute vesicles and papules, often with surrounding erythema, caused by occlusion of sweat ducts during times of exposure to heat and high humidity. Backup pressure may cause sweat to escape into adjacent tissue producing itching and prickling. Prevention and treatment include cool environment, ventilation, colloidal baths, and dusting powders. Also called **prickly heat.**

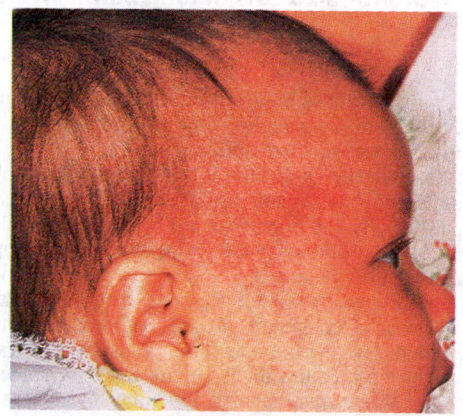

Miliaria in infant *(Habif, 1990)*

miliary /mil′ē·er′ē/ [L, *milium*, millet], describing a condition marked by the appearance of very small lesions the size of millet seeds, such as miliary tuberculosis, which is characterized by tiny tubercules throughout the body.

miliary carcinosis, a condition characterized by the presence of numerous cancerous nodules resembling miliary tubercles.

miliary fever [L, *milium*, millet; L, *febris*], an inflammatory skin eruption caused by sweat retention. Sweat trapped in the dermis or epidermis causes irritation. Also called **prickly heat.**

miliary tuberculosis, extensive dissemination by the bloodstream of tubercle bacilli. In children it is associated with high fever, night sweats, and, often, meningitis, pleural effusions, or peritonitis. A similar illness may occur in adults but with a less abrupt onset and, occasionally, with weeks or months of nonspecific symptoms, such as weight loss, weakness, and low-grade fever. Multiple small opacities resembling millet seeds may be evident on chest x-ray films. The liver, spleen, bone marrow, and meninges are often affected. The tuberculin test may be negative, and diagnosis is made by biopsy of the infected tissue or organ. Combined drug therapy with isoniazid rifampin and pyrazinamide is usually successful if the diagnosis is not delayed. Concurrent tuberculous meningitis makes the prognosis less favorable. See also *Mycobacterium*, **tuberculosis.**

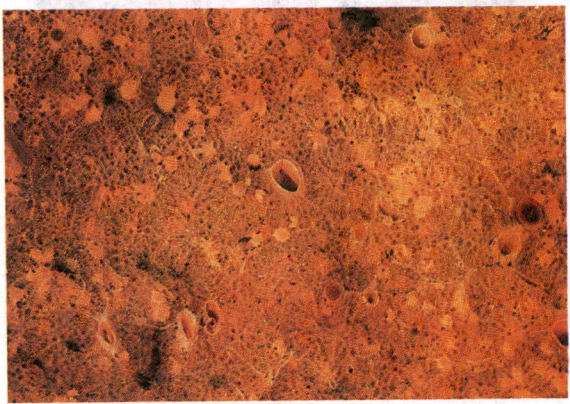

Miliary tuberculosis of lung parenchyma
(Fletcher, 1987)

milieu /milyœ, milyōō′/, *pl.* **milieus, milieux** [Fr, middle], the environment, surroundings, or setting. Kinds of milieus are **milieu extérieur** and **milieu intérieur.**

milieu extérieur /eksterē·œr′/, the external or physical surroundings of an organism, including the social environment, especially the home, school, and recreational facilities, that play a dominant role in personality development.

milieu intérieur /aNterē·œr′/, the basic concept in physiology, originated by Claude Bernard, that multicellular organisms exist in an aqueous internal environment composed of the blood, lymph, and interstitial fluid that bathes all cells and provides a medium for the elementary exchange of nutrients and waste material. All fundamental processes necessary for the maintenance and life of the tissue elements depend on the stability and balance of this environment.

milieu therapy, a type of psychotherapy in which the to-

tal environment is used in treating mental and behavioral disorders. It is primarily conducted in a hospital or other institutional setting where the entire facility acts as a therapeutic community. The emphasis is on providing pleasant physical surroundings, structured activities, and a stable social environment where behavioral modification and personal growth are promoted through patient-group interaction, staff support and understanding, and a total, humanistic approach. Individual daily routines and treatment modalities, such as drug therapy, occupational therapy, and sensitivity training, are determined by the patient's emotional and interpersonal needs. See also **situational therapy.**

military antishock trousers (MAST) /mil′iter′ē/ [L, *miliaris; ante,* opposed; Fr, *choc;* Gael, *triubhas,* trews], a garment designed to produce pressure on the lower part of the body, thereby preventing the pooling of blood in the legs and abdomen during aviation maneuvers or weightlessness experienced in space travel. The trousers have also been used in treating postural hypotension and to control internal bleeding. Also called **anti-G suit.**

milium /mil′ē·əm/, *pl.* **milia** [L, millet], a minute, white cyst of the epidermis caused by obstruction of hair follicles and eccrine sweat glands. One variety is seen in newborn infants and disappears within a few weeks. Another type is found primarily on the faces of middle-aged women. Milia may be treated with an abrasive cleanser or by incision and drainage. Also called **whitehead.** Compare **comedo, miliaria.**

milk [AS, *meoluc*], a liquid secreted by the mammary glands or udders of animals that suckle their young. After breast feeding, people consume the milk of the cow, as well as that of many other animals, including the goat, camel, mare, reindeer, llama, and yak. Milk is a basic food containing carbohydrate (in the form of lactose), protein (mainly casein, with small amounts of lactalbumin and lactoglobulin), suspended fat, the minerals calcium and phosphorus, the vitamins A, riboflavin, niacin, thiamine, and, when the milk is fortified, vitamin D. It is a valuable nutrient for adults and nearly a complete food for infants, especially breast milk. Milk does not contain a significant amount of iron; its ascorbic acid content depends on the amount ingested by the mother or by the animal producing the milk. Some individuals show a sensitivity reaction to milk caused by a deficiency of the enzyme lactase. See also **breast milk.**

milk-alkali syndrome, a condition of alkalosis caused by the excessive ingestion of milk, antacid medications containing calcium, or other sources of absorbable alkaline substances. The condition results in hypercalcemia, hypocalciuria, and calcium deposits in the kidneys and other tissues. The patient may experience symptoms of nausea, headache, weakness, and kidney damage. Milk-alkali syndrome tends to occur most frequently in older adults with peptic ulcers.

milk baby, an infant with iron deficiency anemia caused by ingestion of excessive amounts of milk and the delayed or inadequate addition of iron-rich foods to the diet. Milk babies are overweight, have pale skin and poor muscle development, and are highly susceptible to infection. See also **anemia.**

milk bath, a bath taken in milk for cosmetic or emollient reasons.

milk ejection reflex, a normal reflex in a lactating woman elicited by tactile stimulation of the nipple, resulting in release of milk from the glands of the breast. This reflex requires intact nerve connections from nipple to hypothalamus and the release of the hormone oxytocin from the posterior pituitary into the bloodstream. Also called **let-down reflex.** See also **oxytocin.**

milker's nodule, a smooth, brownish-red papilloma of the fingers or palm that begins as a macule and progresses through a vesicular stage to become a nodule. The disease is acquired from pustular lesions on the udder of a cow infected with poxvirus. No treatment is necessary because immunity is produced after primary infection.

milk fever, *nontechnical.* postpartum fever that begins with the onset of lactation and lasts only a few hours. It was formerly considered a normal reaction to lactation. Maternal oral temperature during the puerperium does not normally exceed 100.4] F; continued high readings may indicate infection.

milk globule, a spherical droplet of fat in milk that tends to separate out as cream.

milk patch. See **macula albidae.**

milking, a procedure used to express the contents of a duct or tube, to test for tenderness, or to obtain a specimen for study. The examiner compresses the structure with a finger and moves the finger firmly along the duct or tube to its opening. Also called **stripping.**

milk leg. See **phlegmasia alba dolens.**

Milkman's syndrome [Louis A. Milkman, American Radiologist, b. 1895], a form of osteomalacia characterized by multiple, bilateral, symmetric absorption stripes, indicating pseudofractures, in hypocalcified long bones and the pelvis and scapula. The abnormalities appear on x-ray films.

milk of magnesia, a laxative and antacid containing magnesium hydroxide.

■ INDICATIONS: It is prescribed to relieve constipation and acid indigestion.

■ CONTRAINDICATIONS: Renal impairment, symptoms of appendicitis, or known hypersensitivity to the drug prohibits its use.

■ ADVERSE EFFECTS: Among the most serious adverse reactions are diarrhea and hypermagnesemia, usually occuring in patients who have impaired renal function.

milk patch. See **macula albidae.**

milkpox. See **alastrim.**

milk sugar. See **lactose.**

milk therapy, a nutritional treatment used in the therapy of Curling's ulcer in patients who have been severely burned. Cool, homogenized milk is administered in doses of 1 to 2 ounces every hour through a nasogastric tube. After instillation the tube is clamped for 5 minutes and then unclamped. Milk remaining in the stomach is allowed to flow into a basin. As the milk is better absorbed and tolerated, feedings are increased to 150 ml of milk per kilogram of body weight daily. The interval between feedings is gradually lengthened to 4 hours. As the condition improves, the nasogastric tube is withdrawn, and milk may be continued by mouth.

milk tooth. See **deciduous tooth.**

milky ascites. See **chylous ascites.**

Miller-Abbott tube [Thomas G. Miller, American physician, b. 1886; William O. Abbott, American physician, b. 1902], a long, small-caliber, double-lumen catheter, used in intestinal intubation for decompression. It has several openings on the side of its tip and a balloon above the tip. Compare **Harris tube.** See also **gastric intubation.**

milli- /mil′ē-/, a prefix meaning '1/1000 part': *milliampere, millibar, milliliter.*

milliampere (ma) /-am′pir/ [L, *mille*, thousand; Andre Am-

pere], a unit of electric current that is one thousandth of an ampere.

milliampere seconds (mAs), the product obtained by multiplying the electric quantity in milliamperes by the time in seconds. It is used to describe the exposure setting of an x-ray machine. It determines the density of the radiographic image.

millicoulomb (mC) /-kōō′lōm/ [L, *mille*, thousand; Charles A. de Coulomb], a unit of electric charge that is one thousandth of a coulomb.

millicurie (mCi, mc) /-kōōr′ē/ [L, *mille*, thousand; Marie and Pierre Curie], a unit of radioactivity that is equal to one thousandth of a curie, or 3.70×10^{-7} disintegrations per second.

milliequivalent (mEq) /-ikwiv′ələnt/ [L, *mille* + *aequus*, equal, *valere*, to be strong], **1.** the number of grams of solute dissolved in 1 ml of a normal solution. **2.** one thousandth of a gram equivalent.

milliequivalent per liter (mEq/L), one thousandth of 1 gram of a specific substance dissolved in 1 L of plasma.

milligram (mg) /-gram/ [L, *mille* + Fr, *gramme*, small weight], a metric unit of weight equal to one thousandth (10^{-3}) of a gram.

milliliter (ml) /-lē′tər/ [L, *mille* + Fr, *litre*, a measure], a metric unit of volume that is one thousandth (10^{-3}) of a liter.

millimeter (mm) /-mē′tər/, a metric unit of length equal to one thousandth (10^{-3}) of a meter.

millimicro- (mμ), a combining form meaning 'billionth (10^{-9})': *millimicrogram, millimicroliter.* This combining form is now generally replaced by **nano-.**

millimole (mmol) /-mōl/ [L, *mille* + *moles*, mass], a unit of metric measurement of mass that is equal to one thousandth (10^{-3}) of a mole.

milliosmol /mil′ē·oz′mōl/, a unit of measure representing the concentration of an ion in a solution, expressed in milligrams per liter divided by atomic weight. See also **osmol, osmolality, osmolarity.** **–milliosmolar,** *adj.*

millipede /mil′ipēd/ [L, *mille* + *pes*, foot], a manylegged, wormlike arthropod. Certain species squirt irritating fluids that may cause dermatitis.

millirad /-rad/, one thousandth (10^{-3}) of a rad, a unit of measurement of absorbed dose of ionizing radiation.

milliroentgen (mR, mr) /mil′irent′gən, -jən/ [L, *mille*, thousand; William von Roentgen], a unit of radiation that is equal to one thousandth (10^{-3}) of a roentgen.

millisecond (msec) /-sek′ənd/ [L, *milli*, thousand; ME, *seconde*, small part], one one-thousandth of a second.

millivolt (mV, mv) /-vōlt/ [L, *mille*, thousand; Alessandro Volta, b. 1745], a unit of electromotive force equal to one thousandth of a volt.

Milontin, a trademark for an anticonvulsant (phensuximide).

Miltown, a trademark for a sedative (meprobamate).

Milwaukee brace /milwô′kē/ [Milwaukee, Wisconsin; OFr *bracier* to embrace], an orthotic device that helps immobilize the torso and the neck of a patient in the treatment or correction of scoliosis, lordosis, or kyphosis. It is usually constructed of strong but light metal and fiberglass supports lined with rubber to protect against abrasion. Milwaukee braces, which may be employed in the treatment of orthopedic bed patients or ambulatory patients, commonly connect cervical supports, rib supports, and hip supports with rigid bars of metal that hold the trunk and the neck erect while controlling cervical flexion and hip movements.

-mimesis, a suffix meaning 'simulation, imitation': *necromimesis, neuromimesis, pathomimesis*.

-mimetic, a suffix meaning 'pertaining to simulation of (specified) effects': *andromimetic, neuromimetic, vagomimetic*.

-mimia, a suffix meaning '(condition of) ability to express thought through gestures': *macromimia, paramimia, pathomimia*.

mimic spasm /mim'ik/ [Gk, *mimetikos*, imitative; *spasmos*, spasm], involuntary, stereotyped movements of a small group of muscles, such as of the face. The spasm is usually psychogenic and may be aggravated by stress or anxiety but is generally controllable momentarily. Multiple grimacing and blinking mimic spasms occur in Gilles de la Tourette's syndrome. Also called **tic.**

min, abbreviation for **minim.**

Minamata disease /min'əmä'tə/, a severe, degenerative, neurologic disorder caused by the ingestion of seed grain heated with alkyl compounds of mercury or of seafood taken from waters polluted with industrial wastes contaminated by soluble mercuric salts. The term is derived from a tragedy involving Japanese who ate seafood from Minamata Bay. Mercury passes the placental barrier, causing the congenital form of the disease. Symptoms may not appear for several weeks or months; they include paresthesia of the mouth and extremities; tunnel vision; difficulties with speech, hearing, muscular coordination, and concentration; weakness; emotional instability; and stupor. Continued ingestion causes serious damage to the renal tubules and corrosion of the GI tract. Acute cases may result in coma and death. See also **mercury poisoning.**

mind [AS, *gemynd*], **1.** the part of the brain that is the seat of mental activity and that enables one to know, reason, understand, remember, think, feel, react to, and adapt to surroundings and all external and internal stimuli. **2.** the totality of all conscious and unconscious processes of the individual that influence and direct mental and physical behavior. **3.** the faculty of the intellect or understanding in contrast to emotion and will. See also **brain, intellect, psyche.**

mine damp. See **damp.**

mineral /min'ərəl/ [L, *minera*, mine], **1.** an inorganic substance occurring naturally in the earth's crust, having a characteristic chemical composition and (usually) crystalline structure. **2.** (in nutrition) a mineral usually referred to by the name of a metal, nonmetal, radical, or phosphate rather than by the name of the compound of which it is a part, and that is ingested as a compound, such as sodium chloride (table salt), rather than as a free element. Minerals play a vital role in regulating many body functions.

mineral deficiency, the inability to use one or more of the mineral elements essential in human nutrition because of a genetic defect, malabsorption dysfunction, or lack of that mineral in the diet. The symptoms and manifestations vary, depending on the specific function or functions of the element in promoting growth and maintaining body health. Minerals are constituents of all the body tissues and fluids, and they are important factors in maintaining physiologic processes. They act as catalysts in nerve response, muscle contraction, and the metabolism of nutrients in foods, they regulate electrolyte balance and hormonal production, and they strengthen skeletal structures. All mineral deficiencies are treated by adding the specific element to the diet, either in supplementary form or in the appropriate foods. See also specific minerals.

mineralization /-īzā'shən/ [L, *minera* + Gk, *izein*, to cause], the addition of any mineral to the body.

mineralocorticoid /min'əral'ōkôr'tikoid/ [L, *minera* + *cortex*, bark; Gk, *eidos*, form], a hormone, secreted by the adrenal cortex, that maintains normal blood volume, promotes sodium and water retention, and increases urinary excretion of potassium and hydrogen ions. Aldosterone, the most potent mineralocorticoid in regard to electrolyte balance, and corticosterone, a glucocorticoid and a mineralocorticoid, act on the distal tubules of the kidneys to enhance the reabsorption of sodium into the plasma. Trauma and stress increase mineralocorticoid secretion. The synthetic mineralocorticoids desoxycorticosterone, which does not influence carbohydrate metabolism, and fluorocortisone, which also has glucocorticoid activity, are used in treating the salt-losing adrenogenital syndrome and the severe corticoid deficiency characteristic of Addison's disease. See also **glucocorticoid.**

mineral oil, a laxative, stool softener, emollient, and pharmaceutic aid used as a solvent.

■ INDICATIONS: It is prescribed to prevent constipation, to treat mild constipation, to prepare the bowel for surgery or examination, and as a solvent for various preparations.

■ CONTRAINDICATIONS: Symptoms of appendicitis, fecal impaction, obstruction or perforation of the intestinal tract, pregnancy, or known hypersensitivity to this drug prohibits its use.

■ ADVERSE EFFECTS: Among the more serious adverse reactions are laxative dependence, lipid pneumonitis, fat-soluble vitamin deficiency, and abdominal cramps.

mineral soap. See **bentonite.**

miner's cramp. See **heat cramp.**

miner's elbow [L, *minera* + AS, *elboga*], an inflammation of the olecranon bursa, caused by resting the weight of the body on the elbow, as in some coal mining activities. The condition is sometimes seen in school children who lean on their elbows. Compare **lateral humeral epicondylitis.** See also **bursitis.**

miner's pneumoconiosis. See **anthracosis.**

Minerva cast /minur'və/ [L, *Minerva*, Roman goddess of wisdom; ONorse, *kasta*], an orthopedic cast applied to the trunk and the head, with spaces cut out for the face area and the ears. The section encasing the trunk extends to the sternum and the distal rib border anteriorly and across the distal rib border posteriorly. The cast is used for immobilizing the head and part of the trunk in the treatment of torticollis, cervical and thoracic injuries, and cervical spinal infections. It is not used as frequently as it once was because of advancement in the field of orthotics. Also called **Minerva jacket.**

minicomputer /min'ikəmpyōō'tər/ [L, *minimum*, smallest, *computare*, to calculate], a medium-sized computer, intermediate in size and processing capacity between a microcomputer and a mainframe computer. Compare **mainframe computer, microcomputer.**

minim (min) /min'im/ [L, *minimum*, smallest], a measurement of volume in the apothecaries' system, originally one drop (of water). Sixty minims equal 1 fluid dram. One minim equals 0.06 ml.

minimal bactericidal concentration. See **minimal inhibitory concentration.**

minimal brain dysfunction. See **attention deficit disorder.**

minimal care unit /min'iməl/ [L, *minimum*, smallest], a unit for the treatment of inpatients who are ambulatory and able to meet many of their own daily living needs but require minimal nursing care.

minimal dose [L, *minimum,* smallest; Gk, *dosis,* giving], the smallest dose of a drug or other agent necessary to produce a desired effect. Because of individual variations in drug response, the minimal dose for one person may be either excessive or insufficient for another patient.

minimal erythema dose. See **threshold dose.**

minimal inhibitory concentration (MIC), the lowest concentration of an antibiotic medication in the blood that is effective against an infection, determined by injecting infected venous blood into a culture medium containing various concentrations of a proposed antibiotic. The lowest antibiotic concentration that stops microbial growth may be used in further treatment of the patient. Typical antibiotic test concentrations in the culture medium range from 0.195 to 100 µg/ml. Also called **minimal bactericidal concentration.**

minimal occlusive volume (MOV), the volume of endotracheal or tracheostomy tube cuff inflation that just obliterates an air leak during the inspiratory phase of ventilation. Also called **minimal occlusive pressure.**

Mini-Mental State Examination, a brief psychologic test designed to differentiate between dementia, psychosis, and affective disorders. It may include ability to count backward by 7s from 100, to identify common objects such as a pencil and a watch, to write a sentence, to spell simple words backward, and to demonstrate orientation by identifying the day, month, and year, as well as town and country.

minimization /min'imīzā'shən/ [L, *minimum,* smallest; Gk, *izein,* to cause], (in psychology) cognitive distortion in which the effects of one's behavior are minimized. See also **magnification.**

minimum alveolar concentration (MAC) /min'iməm/, the smallest amount of a gas detected and measured in the alveoli of the lungs.

minimum daily requirement (MDR) [L, *minimum;* OE, *daeglie;* L, *requirere,* to seek], the daily human requirements of nutrients, for health and as needed to prevent a deficiency disease. The figures, established by the U.S. Food and Drug Administration, are generally extrapolated from experimental animal studies, and include an added small margin for safety.

minimum lethal dose (MLD) [L, *minimum,* smallest; *lethum,* death; Gk, *dosis,* giving], the smallest dose of a drug, relative to body weight, that will kill an experimental animal. The MLD may vary with the species of animal tested. Also called **minimum fatal dose (MFD).** See also **median lethal dose (LD$_{50}$).**

Minipress, a trademark for an antihypertensive (prazosin hydrochloride).

Minnesota Multiphasic Personality Inventory (MMPI), a commonly used psychologic test that includes 550 statements for interpretation by the subject, used clinically for evaluating personality and for detecting various disorders.

Minocin, a trademark for an antibacterial (minocycline hydrochloride).

minocycline hydrochloride /min'əsī'klēn/, a tetracycline antibiotic active against bacteria, rickettsia, and other organisms.

■ INDICATIONS: It is prescribed in the treatment of a variety of infections.

■ CONTRAINDICATIONS: It must be used with caution with re-

nal or hepatic dysfunction. Known hypersensitivity to this or other tetracyclines prohibits its use.

■ ADVERSE EFFECTS: Among the more serious adverse reactions are GI disturbances, phototoxicity, vestibular toxicity, potentially serious suprainfections, and various allergic reactions. Use during pregnancy or in children under 8 years of age may result in discoloration of teeth.

minor /mī'nər/ [L, smaller], (in law) a person not of legal age; a person beneath the age of majority. Minors usually cannot consent to their own medical treatment unless theyare substantially independent from their parents, are married, support themselves, or satisfy other requirements as provided by statute. A kind of minor is **emancipated minor.**

minor connector, (in dentistry) a device that links the major connector or base of a removable partial denture to other denture units, such as rests and direct and indirect retainers.

minor element. See **micronutrient.**

minor epilepsy. See **petit mal epilepsy.**

minor hysteria [Gk, *hystera,* womb], a mild disorder that may be expressed in emotional outbursts, repressed anxieties, or conversion of unconscious conflicts into physical symptoms.

minor renal calyx. See **renal calyx.**

minor surgery, any surgical procedure that does not require general anesthesia or respiratory assistance.

minoxidil /mīnok'sidil/, a vasodilator.

■ INDICATION: It is prescribed in the treatment of severe refractory hypertension.

■ CONTRAINDICATIONS: Pheochromocytoma or known hypersensitivity to this drug prohibits its use.

■ ADVERSE EFFECTS: Among the most serious adverse reactions are tachycardia, pericardial effusion, cardiac tamponade, salt and water retention, and excessive hair growth. GI disturbances also may occur.

Mintezol, a trademark for an anthelmintic (thiabendazole).

minute ventilation /min'it/ [L, *minus,* very small], the total ventilation per minute, the product of tidal volume and respiratory rate as measured by expired gas collection for a period of 1 to 3 minutes. The normal rate is 5 to 10 liters per minute.

mio-, meio-, a combining form meaning 'less': *miolecithal, mioplasmia, miosphygmia.*

miosis /mī·ō'sis/ [Gk, *meiosis,* becoming less], **1.** contraction of the sphincter muscle of the iris, causing the pupil to become smaller. Certain drugs and stimulation of the pupillary light reflex by an increase in light result in miosis. **2.** an abnormal condition characterized by excessive constriction of the sphincter muscle of the iris, resulting in very small, pinpoint pupils. Compare **mydriasis.**

miotic /mē·ot'ik/, **1.** of or pertaining to miosis. **2.** causing constriction of the pupil of the eye. **3.** any substance or pharmaceutic, such as pilocarpine, that causes constriction of the pupil of the eye. Such agents are used in the treatment of glaucoma.

MIP, abbreviation for **maximum inspiratory pressure.**

miracidium /mir'əsid'ē·əm/, *pl.* **miracidia** [Gk, *meirakidion,* youthfulness], the ciliated larva of a parasitic trematode that hatches from an egg and can survive only by penetrating and further developing within a host snail, whereupon the larva further develops into a maternal sporocyte that produces more larvae.

mirage /miräzh'/ [L, *mirari,* to look at], an optical illusion caused by the refraction of light through air layers of different temperatures, such as the illusionary sheets of water that seem to shimmer over stretches of hot sand and pavement. This phenomenon is caused by horizontal light waves being bent upward from the layer of heated air directly over the hot surface. Wind rippling the air layers may produce surprising changes in the shapes and sizes of such mirages. Individuals under severe stress are especially susceptible to interpreting these optic phenomena in bizarre, unrealistic ways.

mirror image /mir′ər/ [L, *mirare*, to look at; *imago*], **1.** an image formed by a reflection in a plane mirror. **2.** a kind of reversed asymmetry of characteristics often found in sets of monzygotic twins. **3.** chemical molecules with the same composition but with asymmetrical arrangement of the atoms.

mirror speech [L, *mirari*, to look at; AS, *spaec*, speech], abnormal speech characterized by the reversal of the order of syllables in a word.

mis-, a prefix meaning ′wrongly or badly.′

miscarriage. See **spontaneous abortion.**

miscible /mis′ibəl/ [L, *miscere*, to mix], able to be mixed or mingled with another substance. Compare **immiscible.**

misdemeanor /mis′dəmē′nər/ [AS, *missan*, to miss; ME, *demenen*, conduct], (in criminal law) an offense that is considered less serious than a felony and carries with it a lesser penalty, usually a fine or imprisonment for less than 1 year. Conviction for a misdemeanor does not prohibit the person from holding public office or from practicing a licensed occupation.

misfeasance /misfē′zəns/ [AS, *missan*, to miss; L, *facere*, to do], an improper performance of a lawful act, especially in a way that might cause damage or injury. Compare **malfeasance, nonfeasance.**

miso-, a combining form meaning ′hatred of′: *misocainia, misogyny, misopedia.*

misogamy /misog′əmē/ [Gk, *misein*, to hate, *gamos*, marriage], an aversion to marriage. **–misogamic, misogamous,** *adj.,* **misogamist,** *n.*

misogyny /misoj′inē/ [Gk, *misein* + *gyne*, women], an aversion to women. **–misogynist,** *n.,* **misogynistic,** *adj.*

misopedia /mis′ōpē′dē·ə/ [Gk, *misein* + *pais*, children], an aversion to children. **–misopedic,** *adj.,* **misopedist,** *n.*

misophobia. See **mysophobia.**

missed abortion [AS, *missan*, to miss; L, *aboriri*, to miscarry], a condition in which a dead, immature embryo or fetus is not expelled from the uterus for 2 or more months. The uterus diminishes in size, and symptoms of pregnancy abate; infection and disorders of the clotting of the mother′s blood may follow. The fetus and placenta may become necrotic, or, less commonly, the fetus becomes calcified and the rest of the products of conception are resorbed.

missed period [ME, *missen*, to change; Gk, *peri, hodos,* way], an unexplained interruption in the menstrual cycle.

missile fracture [L, *mittere*, to throw], a penetration fracture caused by a projectile, such as a bullet or a piece of shrapnel.

mistura /mistyoo̅′rə/ [L, mixture], any of a number of mixtures of drugs, usually containing suspensions of insoluble substances intended for internal use. Examples include **mistura kaolini et morphinae,** a mixture of kaolin and morphine, and **mistura cretae pro infantibus,** a mixture of chalk, tragacanth, chloroform water, and other ingredients formulated for the treatment of GI disorders in infants.

mite /mīt/ [AS], a minute arachnid with a flat, almost transparent body and four pairs of legs. Many species of these relatives of ticks and spiders are parasitic, including the chigger and *Sarcoptes scabiei,* which cause localized pruritus and inflammation. Some female mites burrow into the skin and lay eggs that hatch into larvae; the movements of the larvae cause intense itching. See also **scabies.**

mite typhus. See **scrub typhus.**

Mithracin, a trademark for an antineoplastic (plicamycin).

mithramycin. See **plicamycin.**

mithridatism. See **tachyphylaxis.**

mitleiden /mit′līdən/ [Ger, *mit,* with, *leiden,* to suffer], psychosomatic symptoms sometimes experienced by expectant fathers.

mito-, a combining form meaning ′threadlike′: *mitochondria, mitokinetic, mitoplasm.*

mitochondrion /mī′tōkon′drē·on/, *pl.* **mitochondria** [Gk, *mitos,* thread, *chondros,* cartilage], a small rodlike, threadlike, or granular organelle within the cytoplasm that functions in cellular metabolism and respiration and occurs in varying numbers in all living cells except bacteria, viruses, blue-green algae, and mature erythrocytes. It consists of two sets of membranes, a smooth outer one and a convoluted inner one, arranged in folds to form projections, or cristae, that extend into the matrix. Mitochondria provide the principal source of cellular energy through oxidative phosphorylation and adenosine triphosphate synthesis. They also contain the enzymes involved with electron transport and the citric and fatty acid cycles. Mitochondria are self-replicating and contain an extranuclear source of DNA, RNA polymerase, transfer RNA, and ribosomes. Also called **chondriosome. –mitochondrial,** *adj.*

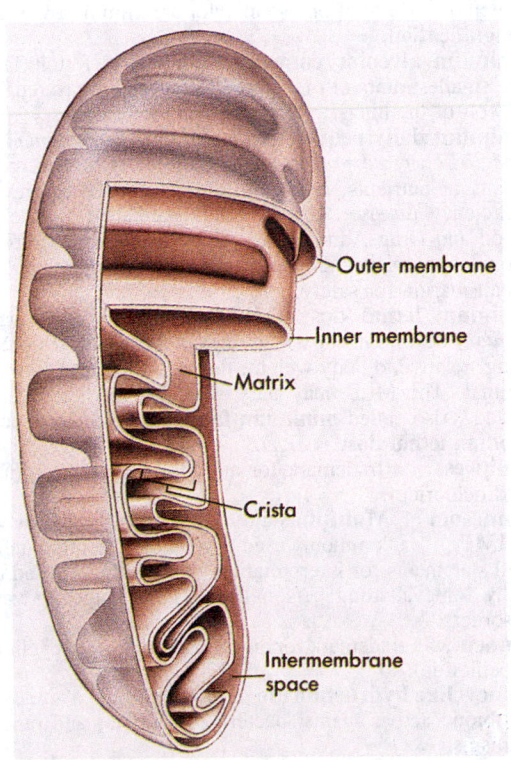

Mitochondrion (Thibodeau, 1993/William Ober)

mitogen /mī'təjən, mit'-/ [Gk, *mitos* + *genein*, to produce], an agent that triggers mitosis. **mitogenic,** *adj.*

mitogenesia /mī'tōjənē'zhə/ [Gk, *mitos* + *genein*, to produce], the production by or formation resulting from mitosis.

mitogenesis /mī'tōjen'əsis/, the induction of mitosis in a cell. **–mitogenetic,** *adj.*

mitogenetic radiation /-jənet'ik/, the force or specific energy that is supposedly given off by cells undergoing division. It may, in turn, stimulate the process of mitosis in other cells. Also called **mitogenic radiation, Gurvich radiation.**

mitogenic factor /-jen'ik/, a lymphokine that is released from activated T lymphocytes and stimulates the production of normal unsensitized lymphocytes.

mitogenic radiation. See **mitogenetic radiation.**

mitome /mī'tōm/, the reticular network sometimes observed within the cytoplasm and nucleoplasm of fixed cells. See also **cytomitome, karyomitome.**

mitomycin /mītəmī'sin/, an antineoplastic antibiotic.

■ INDICATIONS: It is prescribed in the treatment of a variety of malignant neoplastic diseases.

■ CONTRAINDICATIONS: Clotting deficiency, thrombocytopenia, or known hypersensitivity to this drug prohibits its use.

■ ADVERSE EFFECTS: The most serious adverse reaction is bone marrow depression. GI disturbances, alopecia, and skin reactions commonly occur.

mitosis /mītō'sis, mit-/ [Gk, *mitos,* thread], a type of cell division that occurs in somatic cells and results in the formation of two genetically identical daughter cells containing the diploid number of chromosomes characteristic of the species. It consists of the division of the nucleus through the four stages of prophase, metaphase, anaphase, and telophase, during which the two chromatids of the chromosomes separate and migrate to opposite ends of the cell, followed by the division of the cytoplasm. Mitosis is the process by which the body produces new cells for both growth and repair of injured tissue. Kinds of mitosis are **heterotypic mitosis, homeotypic mitosis, multipolar mitosis,** and **pathologic mitosis.** Also called **indirect division.**

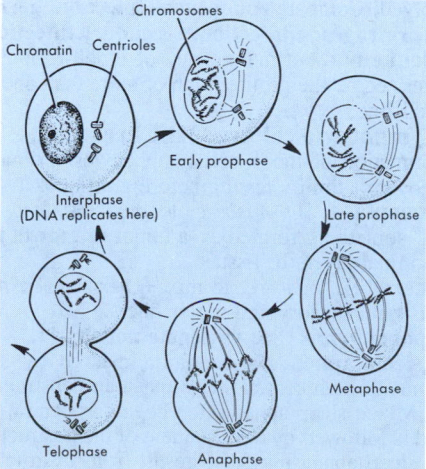

Mitosis

Compare **meiosis.** See also **anaphase, interphase, metaphase, prophase, telophase.** **–mitotic,** *adj.*

mitotane /mī'tətān/, an antineoplastic that destroys normal and neoplastic adrenal cortical cells.

■ INDICATION: It is prescribed in the treatment of carcinoma of the adrenal cortex.

■ CONTRAINDICATION: Known hypersensitivity to this drug is the only contraindication.

■ ADVERSE EFFECTS: Among the more serious adverse reactions are GI symptoms, lethargy, and adrenal insufficiency.

mitotic /mītot'ik/ [Gk, *mitos,* thread], pertaining to or characterized by mitosis, the process of cell division in the formation of identical daughter cells.

mitotic figure [Gk, *mitos* + L, *figura,* form], any chromosome or chromosome aggregation during any of the stages of mitosis.

mitotic index, the number of cells per unit (usually 1000) undergoing mitosis during a given time. The ratio is used primarily as an estimation of the rate of tissue growth.

mitral /mī'trəl/ [L, *mitra,* head dress], **1.** of or pertaining to the mitral valve of the heart. **2.** shaped like a miter.

mitral communissurotomy [L, *mitra,* turban; *commissura,* joining together; Gk, *temnein,* to cut], a closed-heart surgical procedure in which the mitral valve is divided at the junction of its cusps for the treatment of mitral stenosis.

mitral gradient, the difference in pressure in the left atrium and left ventricle during diastole.

mitral insufficiency. See **mitral regurgitation.**

mitral murmur [L, *mitra,* turban; *murmur,* humming], a heart murmur caused by a defective mitral valve.

mitral regurgitation, a backflow of blood from the left ventricle into the left atrium in systole across a diseased valve. The condition may result from congenital valve abnormalities, rheumatic fever, mitral valve prolapse, endocardial fibroelastosis, dilation of the left ventricle because of severe anemia, myocarditis, or myocardiopathy. Symptoms include dyspnea, fatigue, intolerance to exercise, and heart palpitations. Congestive heart failure may ultimately occur. Treatment depends on the severity of the condition. Surgery may be necessary in cases of refractory congestive heart failure, progressive cardiomegaly, and pulmonary hypertension. Also called **mitral insufficiency.** See also **valvular heart disease.**

mitral stenosis. See **mitral valve stenosis.**

mitral valve, a bicuspid valve situated between the left atrium and the left ventricle; the only valve with two, rather than three, cusps. The mitral valve allows blood to flow from the left atrium into the left ventricle but prevents blood from flowing back into the atrium. Ventricular contraction in systole forces the blood against the valve, closing the two cusps and assuring the flow of blood from the ventricle into the aorta. The ventral cusp of the mitral valve is longer than the dorsal cusp. Also called **bicuspid valve, left atrioventricular valve.** Compare **aortic valve, pulmonary valve, semilunar valve, tricuspid valve.**

mitral valve prolapse (MVP), protrusion of one or both cusps of the mitral valve back into the left atrium during ventricular systole, resulting in incomplete closure of the valve and mitral insufficiency. The condition is caused by pleating or scalloplike folds of extraneous mitral cusp tissue, frequently with myxomatous degeneration, that form along the surface of the valve. The lesions may be primary, occurring in patients with Marfan's syndrome or as an associated anomaly with atrial septal defect, or they may be secondary to previous rheumatic fever, ischemic heart disease, cardiomyopathy, or ruptured chordae tendinae. Most patients are asymptomatic, although some may experience chest pain, palpitations, fatigue, or dyspnea. The condition may lead to progressive mitral regurgitation, resulting in enlargement of the left atrium and ventricle. Also called **Barlow's syndrome.** See also **valvular heart disease.**

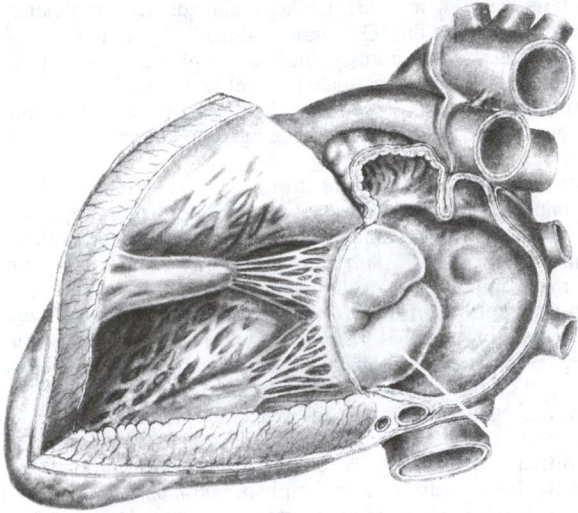

Mitral valve prolapse (Cannobio, 1990)

mitral valve stenosis, an obstructive lesion in the mitral valve caused by adhesions on the leaflets of the valve, usually the result of recurrent episodes of rheumatic endocarditis or age-related calcification of the valve leaflets.. Hypertrophy of the left atrium develops and may be followed by right-sided heart failure and pulmonary edema (cor pulmonale). Reduced cardiac output characteristically produces fatigue, dyspnea, orthopnea, and cyanosis. Surgical correction of the defective valve may be necessary. The valve may be freed of the adhesions in a commissurotomy, or it may be replaced by a prosthetic valve. See also **atrioventricular valve, valvular heart disease, valvular stenosis.**

mittelschmerz /mit′əlshmerts/ [Ger, *Mitte,* middle, *Schmerz,* pain], abdominal pain in the region of an ovary during ovulation, which usually occurs midway through the menstrual cycle. Present in many women, mittelschmerz is useful for identifying ovulation, thus pinpointing the fertile period of the cycle.

Mittendorf's dot, an eye anomaly characterized by the presence of a small dense floating opacity behind the posterior lens capsule. It is a remnant of the hyaloid artery that was present in the eye during embryonic development. The object usually does not affect vision.

mixed anesthesia. See **balanced anesthesia.**

mixed aneurysm. See **compound aneurysm.**

mixed cell malignant lymphoma [L, *miscere,* to mix], a lymphoid neoplasm containing lymphocytes and histiocytes (macrophages).

mixed cell sarcoma, a tumor consisting of two or more cellular elements, excluding fibrous tissue. Also called **malignant mesenchymoma.**

mixed connective tissue disease (MCTD), a systemic disease characterized by the combined symptoms of various collagen diseases, such as synovitis, polymyositis, scleroderma, and systemic lupus erythematosus. This condition involves a high concentration of antibodies of ribonucleoprotein and may produce arthralgia, inflammation of the muscles, nondeforming arthritis, swollen hands, esophageal hypomotility, and reduced diffusing capacity of the lungs. Treatment often includes the administration of corticosteroids. Recurrence is common when the steroid medication is discontinued.

mixed culture [L, *miscere,* to mix; *colere,* to cultivate], a laboratory culture that contains two or more different strains of organisms.

mixed dentition, a phase of dentition during which some of the teeth are permanent and some are deciduous.

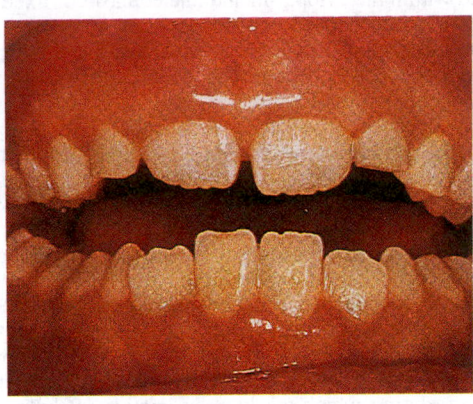

Mixed dentition (Zitelli, 1992)

mixed glioma, a tumor, composed of glial cells, that contains more than one kind of cell, the most common being nonneural cells of ectodermal origin.

mixed infection, an infection by several microorganisms, as in some abscesses, pneumonia, and infections of wounds. Numerous combinations of bacteria, viruses, and fungi may be involved. Compare **endogenous infection, germinal infection, retrograde infection, secondary infection.**

mixed leukemia, a malignancy of blood-forming tissues characterized by the proliferation of more than one predominant cell line.

mixed lymphocyte culture (MLC) reaction, an assay of the function of the T cell lymphocytes, primarily used for histocompatibility testing before grafting.

mixed neoplasm [L, *miscere,* to mix; Gk, *neos,* new + *plasma,* something formed], a tumor or growth involving two germinal layers of tissue.

mixed nerve [L, *miscere,* to mix + *nervus*], a nerve that contains both sensory and motor fibers.

mixed porphyria. See **variegate porphyria.**

mixed sleep apnea, a condition marked by signs and symptoms of both central sleep apnea and obstructive sleep apnea. Mixed sleep apnea often begins as central sleep apnea and is followed by development of the obstructive form. Mixed sleep apnea may also result from obstructive sleep apnea as hypoxia and hypercapnia induce signs and symptoms of the central form. See also **central sleep apnea, obstructive sleep apnea.**

mixed tumor, a growth composed of more than one kind of neoplastic tissue.

mixed venous blood, blood that is composed of the venous blood from the heart and all systemic tissues in proportion to their venous returns. In the absence of abnormalities, mixed venous blood is present in the main pulmonary artery.

-mixis, -mixia, -mixie, -mixy, a combining form meaning 'related to intercourse.': *amphimixis, automixis, endomixis.*

mixture /miks'chər/ [L, *miscere,* to mix], **1.** a substance composed of ingredients that are not chemically combined and do not necessarily occur in a fixed proportion. **2.** (in pharmacology) a liquid containing one or more medications in suspension. The proportions of the ingredients are specific to each mixture. Compare **compound, solution.** See also **mistura.**

-mixy. See **-mixis.**

ml, abbreviation for **milliliter.**

MLC, abbreviation for **mixed lymphocyte culture.** See **mixed lymphocyte culture reaction.**

MLD, abbreviation for **minimum lethal dose.**

mm, abbreviation for **millimeter.**

MMEF, abbreviation for *maximal midexpiratory flow.*

M-mode, abbreviation for *motion mode,* a variation of B-mode ultrasound scanning. It is used in echocardiography. See also **B-mode.**

mmol, abbreviation for **millimole.**

MMPI, abbreviation for **Minnesota Multiphasic Personality Inventory.**

MMR, abbreviation for **measles, mumps, and rubella virus vaccine live.**

MMWR, abbreviation for *Morbidity and Mortality Weekly Report.*

Mn, symbol for the element **manganese.**

mne-, a combining form meaning 'of or pertaining to memory': *mnemic, mnemism, mnemonic.*

mnemonics [Gk, *mnemonikos*], a system of memory training by linking a new concept or image with one already established in the memory, such as associating the numbers of a combination lock with a birthday or telephone number.

-mnesia, a suffix meaning '(condition or type of) memory': *acousmatamnesia, ecmnesia, logamnesia.*

-mnestic, -mnesic, a suffix meaning 'pertaining to memory': *amnestic, anamnestic, catamnestic.*

Mo, symbol for the element **molybdenum.**

Moban, a trademark for an antipsychotic agent (molindone hydrochloride).

mobile arm support /mō'bəl, mōbēl'/, a forearm support device that enables people with upper extremity disabilities to fulfill some activities of daily living, such as by helping to position the hand properly for self-feeding. The orthotic device may be mounted on a wheelchair.

mobility /mōbil'itē/ [L, *mobilis,* movable], the velocity a particle or ion attains for a given applied voltage and a relative measure of how quickly an ion may move in an electric field.

-mobility. See **-motility.**

mobility, impaired physical, a nursing diagnosis accepted by the Fourth National Conference on the Classification of Nursing Diagnoses. It is defined as a state in which an individual experiences a limitation of ability for independent physical movement. The defining characteristics of the condition include an inability to achieve a functional level of mobility in the environment, a reluctance to move, a limited range of motion of the limbs or extremities, a decrease in the strength or control of the musculoskeletal system, abnormal or impaired ability to coordinate movements, or any of a large number of imposed restrictions on movement, such as medically required bed rest or traction. It is suggested that the limitation of injury be ranked from 0, "completely independent," to 4, "dependent, does not participate in any activity." Related factors include a decrease in the person's strength or endurance, the presence of pain or discomfort, impaired cognition or perception, depression or severe anxiety, or impaired neuromuscular or musculoskeletal function. See also **nursing diagnosis.**

Mobitz I heart block /mō'bits/ [Woldemar Mobitz, German physician, b. 1889; AS, *hoerte,* heart; Fr, *bloc,* block], second-degree or partial atrioventricular (AV) block in which the PR interval increases progressively until the propagation of an atrial impulse does not occur and the corresponding ventricular beat drops out. Mobitz I heart block is caused by abnormal conduction of the cardiac impulse in the AV node and may be precipitated by increased vagal tone, by AV nodal ischemia, or by digitalis therapy. It may be a complication of inferior myocardial infarction. Also called **AV Wenckebach heart block,** or **type I AV block.**

Mobitz II heart block, second-degree or partial atrioventricular block, characterized by the sudden nonconduction of an atrial impulse and a periodic dropped beat without prior lengthening of the PR interval. This kind of block usually results from impaired conduction in the bundle branches and may be caused by anterior myocardial infarction, myocarditis, drug toxicity, electrolyte disturbances, rheumatoid nodules, and various degenerative diseases. Syncopal attacks, occurring without warning when the patient is upright or recumbent, are common in Mobitz II block, which may be transient or suddenly progress to complete block. Long-term therapy requires the implantation of a **pacemaker.** Also called **type II AV block.**

Möbius' syndrome /mē'bē·əs/ [Paul J. Möbius, German neurologist, b. 1853], a rare developmental disorder characterized by congenital bilateral facial palsy usually associated with oculomotor or other neurologic dysfunctions, speech disorders, and various anomalies of the extremities. The condition is caused by a developmental defect involving the motor nuclei of the cranial nerves. Also called **congenital facial diplegia, congenital oculofacial paralysis, nuclear agenesis.**

mode /mōd/ [L, *modus,* measure], a value or term in a set of data that occurs more frequently than other values or terms.

model /mod'əl/ [L, *modulus,* small measure], (in nursing research) a symbolic representation of the interrelations exhibited by a phenomenon within a system or a process. The model is presented as a conceptual framework or a theory that explains a phenomenon and allows predictions to be made about a patient or a process. A model is analogous to an equation in mathematics. Nursing models usually describe person, environment, health, and nursing.

modeling /mod'əling/, a technique used in behavior therapy in which a person learns a desired response by observing it performed.

modem, /mō'dəm/, abbreviation for *modulate/demodulate.* It is a device for transforming serial binary numbers into an audible tone, and vice versa, for transmission over a telephone line to another computer. Also spelled **MODEM.** Also called **data set.**

moderator band /mod'ərā'tər/ [L, *moderari,* to restrain; AS, *bindan,* to bind], a thick bundle of muscle in the central part of the right ventricle of the heart. Missing in some individuals and varying in size in different people, it usually contains part of the atrioventricular conduction bundle. Also called **trabecula septomarginalis.**

Modicon, a trademark for an oral contraceptive containing an estrogen (ethinyl estradiol) and a progestin (norethindrone).

modification allele. See **modifying gene.**

modified milk /mod'ifīd/ [L, *modus,* measure, *facere,* to make], cow's milk in which the protein content has been reduced and the fat content increased to correspond to the composition of breast milk. See also **formula, infant.**

modified radical mastectomy, a surgical procedure in which a breast is completely removed with the underlying pectoralis minor and some of the adjacent lymph nodes. The pectoralis major is not excised. The operation is performed in treating early and well-localized malignant neoplasms of the breast. It appears to be as curative as the more extensive radical mastectomy when the tumor meets these criteria. Care of the woman before and after a modified radical mastectomy is similar to that for a radical mastectomy. Compare **radical mastectomy, simple mastectomy.** See also **mastectomy.**

modifying gene /mod'ifī'ing/ b[L, *modus,* measure; Gk, *genein,* to produce], a gene that alters or influences the expression function of another gene, including the suppression or reduction of the usual function of the modified gene. Also called **modification allele.**

Modrastane, a trademark for an oral drug used to treat Cushing's syndrome (trilostane).

modulation transfer function (MTF) /mod'yəlā'shən/ [L, *modulus,* small measure; L, *transferre,* to carry; *functio,* performance], a quantitative measure of the ability of an imaging system to reproduce patterns that vary in spatial frequency. The MTF is useful in predicting image degradation in a series of radiographic components.

Moeller's glossitis /mel'ərz/ [Julius O. L. Moeller, German surgeon, b. 1819], a form of chronic glossitis, characterized by burning or pain in the tongue and an increased sensitivity to hot or spicy foods. Also called **glossodynia exfoliativa.** See also **glossitis.**

mogi-, a combining form meaning 'difficult, or with difficulty': *mogiarthria, mogigraphia, mogilalia.*

mohel /mō'əl, môhāl'/, an ordained Jewish circumciser.

moiety /moi'itē/ [L, *medietas,* middle], a part of a molecule that exhibits a particular set of chemical and pharmacologic characteristics.

moist gangrene. See **gangrene.**

moist heat [OFr, *moiste;* AS, *haetu*], the use of hot water, towels soaked in hot water, or hot water vapors to reduce inflammation and pain, stimulate circulation, and/or relieve symptoms as directed by a physician. Hot towels should be wrung out to remove surplus moisture and should not be too hot to be held in the hands of the person applying moist heat.

moist rale [OFr, *moiste,* fresh + *rale,* rattle], an abnormal breathing sound heard on auscultation when air bubbles through fluid or secretions in the bronchi or trachea.

mol. See **mole².**

molality /mōlal'itē/ [L, *moles,* mass], the numbers of moles of solute per kilogram of water or other solvent.

molal volume. See **mole volume.**

molar /mō'lər/ [L, *moles,* mass], **1.** any one of the 12 molar teeth, six in each dental arch, three located posterior to

the premolar teeth. The crown of each molar is nearly cubical, convex on its buccal surface and its lingual surface and flattened on its surfaces of contact. It is surmounted by four or five cusps separated by cruciate depressions and has a large rounded neck. Each of the upper molars has three roots, two of which are buccal and the other lingual. The roots of the third upper molar are more or less fused. The lower molars are larger than the upper, and each has two roots, an anterior, almost vertical root and a posterior root directed almost obliquely backward. The roots of the third lower molar tend to fuse. **2.** (M) of or pertaining to the gram molecular weight of a substance. See also **mole².**

molarity /mōler'itē/ [L, *moles,* mass], the number of moles of solute per liter of water or other solvent.

molar pregnancy, pregnancy in which a hydatid mole develops from the trophoblastic tissue of the early embryonic stage of development. The signs of pregnancy are all exaggerated: the uterus grows more rapidly than is normal, morning sickness is often severe and constant, blood pressure is likely to be elevated, and blood levels of chorionic gonadotropins are extremely high. The uterus must be evacuated, because the mole may develop into a malignant trophoblastic disease, choriocarcinoma. See also **hydatid mole.**

molar solution, a solution that contains one mole of solute per liter of solution.

molar volume. See **mole volume.**

mold¹, **1.** a fungus. **2.** a growth of fungi.

mold², a hollow form for casting or shaping an object, as a prosthesis.

molding /mōl'ding/ [ME, *moulde,* shaping], the natural process by which a baby's head is shaped during labor as it is squeezed into and through the birth passage by the forces of labor. The head often becomes quite elongated, and the bones of the skull may be caused to overlap slightly at the suture lines. The biparietal diameter of the head may be compressed as much as 0.5 cm without intracranial damage. Most of the changes caused by molding resolve themselves during the first few days of life. Compare **caput succedaneum.** See also **cephalhematoma.**

mole¹ [L, mass], *informal.* **1.** a pigmented nevus. **2.** (in obstetrics) a hydatidiform mole.

mole² [L, *molecula,* small mass], the standard unit used to measure the amount of a substance. A mole of a substance is the amount containing the same number of elementary particles (atoms, electrons, ions, molecules, or other particles) as there are atoms in 12 g of carbon 12. Also spelled **mol.** **–molar,** *adj.*

molecular biology /məlek'yələr/ [L, *moles,* mass; Gk, *bios,* life; *logos,* science], the study of biology from the viewpoint of the physical and chemical interactions of molecules involved in life functions.

molecular genetics [L, *molecula,* small mass; Gk, *genesis,* origin], the branch of genetics that focuses on the chemical structure and the functions, replication, and mutations of the molecules involved in the transmission of genetic information, such as DNA and RNA. Molecular genetics is concerned with the arrangement of genes on DNA, the double helix molecule's replication and transcription into RNA, and the way RNA directs the formation of proteins. See also **recombinant DNA.**

molecular lesion. See **point lesion.**

molecular pathology [L, *moles,* mass; Gk, *pathos,* disease

+ *logos,* science], the branch of the science of disease that is concerned with the health effects of specific molecules.

molecular weight (mol. wt.), the total of the atomic weights of the atoms in a molecule. See also **atom, atomic weight, molecule.**

molecule /mol′əkyo͞ol/ [L, *molecula,* small mass], the smallest unit that exhibits the properties of an element or compound. A molecule is composed of two or more atoms that are chemically combined. See also **atom, compound.**

mole percent, a percentage calculation expressed in terms of moles of a substance in a mixture or solution rather than in terms of molecular weight.

mole volume, the volume occupied by one mole of a substance, which may be a solid, liquid, or gas. It is numerically equal to the molecular weight divided by the density. Also called **molal volume, molar volume.**

molindone hydrochloride /mol′indōn/, an antipsychotic agent.

■ INDICATION: It is prescribed in the treatment of schizophrenia.

■ CONTRAINDICATIONS: Severe central nervous system depression or known hypersensitivity to this drug prohibits its use.

■ ADVERSE EFFECTS: Among the most serious adverse reactions are extrapyramidal reactions, hypotension, sedation, and other reactions characteristic of the phenothiazine antipsychotics.

molluscum /məlus′kəm/ [L, *molluscus,* soft], any skin disease having soft, rounded masses or nodules. See also **molluscum contagiosum.**

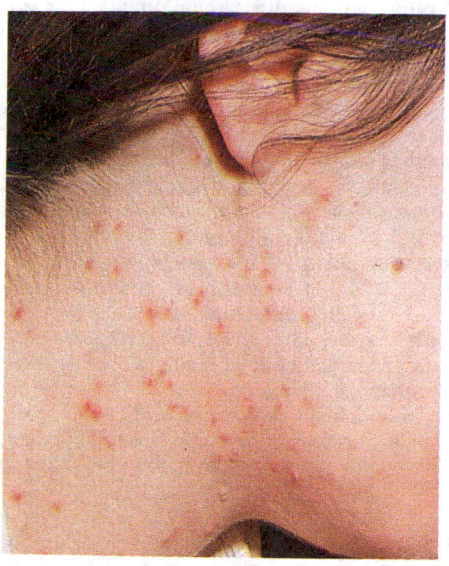

Molluscum contagiosum *(Cerio, 1992)*

only 6 to 8 weeks. Diagnosis is easily made by electron microscopy. Curettage or electric or chemical dessication helps to clear the lesions, but untreated lesions eventually resolve spontaneously without scarring.

mol.wt., abbreviation for **molecular weight.**

molybdenum (Mo) /məlib′dənəm/ [Gk, *molybdos,* lead], a grayish metallic element. Its atomic number is 42; its atomic weight is 95.94. Molybdenum is poisonous if ingested in large quantities.

molybdenum 99, the radionuclide that is the parent of technetium 99, and as such is present as a generator in all nuclear medicine departments.

-monab, a combining form for monoclonal antibodies.

Monactin, a trademark for a gallstone dissolving agent (monooctanoin).

-monam, a combining form for monobactam (monocyclic beta-lactam) antibiotics.

monarthritis /mon′ärthrī′tis/ [Gk, *monos,* single; *arthron,* joint; *itis,* inflammation], arthritis affecting only one joint.

monarticular /mon′ärtik′yələr/ [Gk, *monos,* single; L, *articulus,* joint], pertaining to only one joint.

monaural /monôr′əl/ [Gk, *monos,* single; L, *auris,* ear], pertaining to one ear.

Mönckeberg's arteriosclerosis /meng′kəbərgz/ [Johann G. Mönckeberg, German pathologist, b. 1877], a form of arteriosclerosis in which extensive calcium deposits are found in the media of the artery with little obstruction of the lumen. Also called **medial arteriosclerosis.**

Monday morning fever. See **byssinosis.**

Monge's disease. See **altitude sickness.**

Mongolian spot /mong·gōlē·ən/ [*Mongol,* Asian ethnic group; ME, *spotte,* stain], a benign, bluish-black macule, between 2 and 8 cm, occurring over the sacrum and on the buttocks of some newborns. It is especially common in blacks, Native Americans, southern Europeans, and Orientals and usually disappears during early childhood.

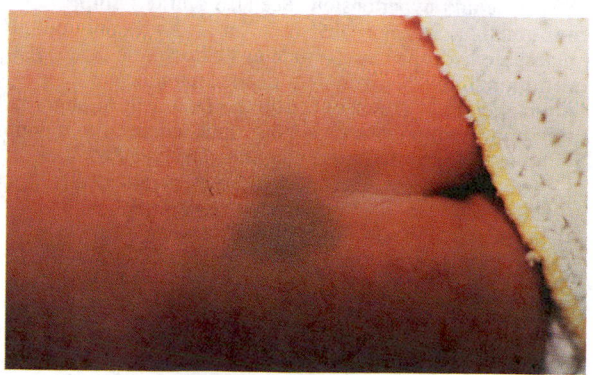

Mongolian spot *(Zitelli, 1992)*

molluscum contagiosum, a disease of the skin and mucous membranes, caused by a poxvirus and found all over the world. It is characterized by scattered flesh-toned white papules. Palms of the hands and soles of the feet are not affected. The disease most frequently occurs in children and in adults with an impaired immune response. It is transmitted from person to person by direct or indirect contact and lasts up to 3 years, although individual lesions persist for

mongolism, mongoloid idiocy. See **Down's syndrome.**

Monilia. See *Candida albicans.*

monilial vulvovaginitis, moniliasis. See **candidiasis.**

Monistat, a trademark for an antifungal (miconazole nitrate).

monitor /mon′ətər/ [L, *monere,* to warn], **1.** to observe and evaluate a function of the body closely and constantly. **2.** a mechanical device that provides a visual or audible signal or a graphic record of a particular function, such as a cardiac monitor or a fetal monitor.

monitrice /mon'itris'/ [Fr, female instructor], a labor coach, usually a registered nurse, who is specially trained in the Lamaze method of childbirth. The coach provides emotional support and leads the mother through labor and delivery, using the specific techniques for breathing, concentration, and massage taught by the Lamaze method in classes for the psychophysical preparation for childbirth.

mono, abbreviation for **mononucleosis.**

mono- /mon'ō-/, a prefix meaning 'one': *monobacillary, monodal, mononeuritis.*

monoamine /mon'ō·am'in/, an amine containing one amine group.

monoamine oxidase (MAO), an enzyme that catalyzes the oxidation of amines. See also **monoamine oxidase inhibitor.**

monoamine oxidase (MAO) inhibitor, any of a chemically heterogeneous group of drugs used primarily in the treatment of depression. These drugs also exert an antianxiety effect, especially anxiety associated with phobia. The effects of the drugs vary greatly from patient to patient, and their specific actions leading to clinical benefits are poorly understood. Among the most common adverse effects are drowsiness, dry mouth, orthostatic hypotension, and constipation. Overdosage may cause tremor, euphoria, or manic behavior. MAO inhibitors interact with many drugs and with foods containing large amounts of the amino acid tyramine. Ingestion of these foods by a person taking a MAO inhibitor is likely to cause a severe hypertensive episode associated with headache, palpitations, and nausea. Among these foods are cheeses, red wine, smoked or pickled herring, beer, and yogurt. Among the drugs that interact with MAO inhibitors are dopamine, meperidine, and the indirect acting sympathomimetics, one of which, ephedrine, is an ingredient in many common cold remedies. MAO inhibitors are also sometimes used in the treatment of migraine headache and hypertension. See also **amine pump.**

monobasic acid /mon'ōbā'sik/, an acid with only one replaceable hydrogen atom, such as hydrochloric acid (HCl).

monobenzone /-ben'zōn/, a depigmenting agent.
- ■ INDICATIONS: It is prescribed in the treatment of abnormal skin pigmentation, such as in disseminated vitiligo. It is not to be used for more trivial conditions, such as freckles.
- ■ CONTRAINDICATION: Known hypersensitivity to this drug prohibits its use.
- ■ ADVERSE EFFECTS: The most serious adverse reaction is excessive and irreversible hypopigmentation. Common reactions are irritation and allergic reactions of the skin.

monoblast /mon'əblast/ [Gk, *monos* single, *blastos* germ], an immature monocyte. Increased production of monoblasts in the marrow and the presence of these forms in the peripheral circulation are found in certain leukemias. Compare **megaloblast, myeloblast.** See also **bone marrow, leukocyte. –monoblastic,** *adj.*

monoblastic leukemia, /blas'tik/ a malignancy of blood-forming organs, characterized by the proliferation of monoblasts and monocytes. The disease occurs in children and adults and develops late in the course of a small but significant number of cases of plasma cell myeloma. Also called **monocytic leukemia, Schilling's leukemia.**

monocephalus. See **syncephalus.**

monochorial twins, monochorionic twins. See **monozygotic twins.**

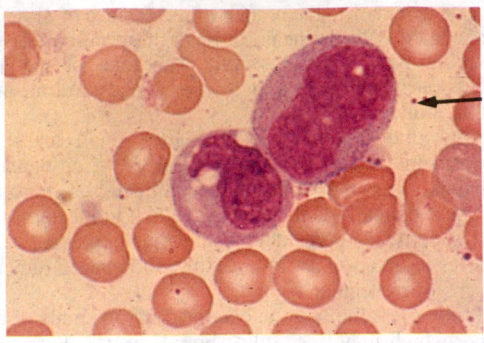

Monoblast (Powers, 1989)

monochrotic pulse /-krot'ik/ [Gk, *monos*, single + *krotein,* to strike; L, *pulsare,* to beat], a pulse characterized by a single wave.

Monocid, a trademark for a cephalosporin-type antibiotic (cefonicid sodium).

monoclonal /mon'əklō'nəl/ [Gk, *monos* + *klon,* graft], of, pertaining to, or designating a group of identical cells or organisms derived from a single cell.

monoclonal antibody (MOAB) [Gk, *monos,* single; *klon,* a twig; Gk, *anti,* AS, *bodig,* body], antibodies produced by a hybridoma or antibody-producing cell source for a specific antigen.

monoclonal gammopathy. See **gammopathy.**

monocomponent insulin /-kəmpō'nənt/ [Gk, *monos,* single; L, *componere,* to bring together + *insula,* island of Langerhans], See **single component insulin.**

monocular diplopia /monok'yələr/ [Gk, *monos,* one + *oculus,* eye; Gk, *diploos,* double + *opsis,* vision], a condition in which a double image is perceived with one eye. The cause is a disorder in the refracting medium of the eye, such as cataracts, or partial dislocation of the lens. In rare cases, more than two images may be seen with one eye. Also called **uniocular diplopia.**

monocular strabismus [Gk, *monos,* single; L, *oculus,* eye; Gk, *strabismos*], a squint that is confined to one particular eye. Also called **uniocular squint.**

monocular vision [Gk, *monos,* single; L, *oculus,* eye + *visio,* seeing], a condition of seeing with only one eye. Also called **uniocular vision.**

monocyte /mon'əsīt/ [Gk, *monos* + *kytos,* cell], a large mononuclear leukocyte, 13 to 25 [Grk m]m in diameter with an ovoid or kidney-shaped nucleus, containing chromatin

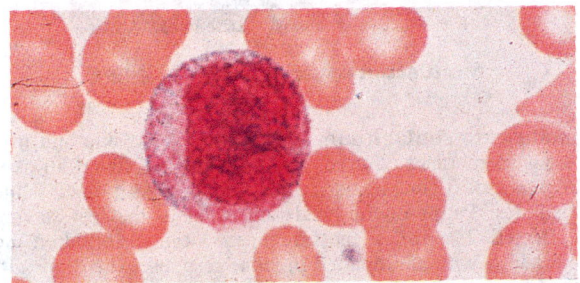

Monocyte (Hayhoe, 1992)

material with a lacy pattern and abundant gray-blue cytoplasm filled with fine, reddish, and azurophilic granules. See also **monocytosis.**

monocytic leukemia /mon′əsit′ik/, a malignancy of blood-forming tissues in which the predominant cells are monocytes. The disease has an erratic course characterized by malaise, fatigue, fever, anorexia, weight loss, splenomegaly, bleeding gums, dermal petechiae, anemia, and unresponsiveness to therapy. There are two forms: **Schilling's leukemia,** in which most of the cells are monocytes that probably arise from the reticuloendothelial system, and the more common **Naegeli's leukemia,** in which a large number of the cells resemble myeloblasts. Also called **histiocytic leukemia.**

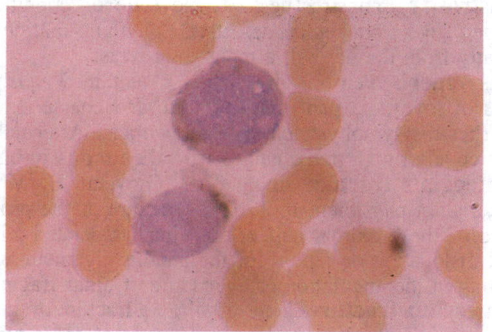

Monocytic leukemia (Powers, 1989)

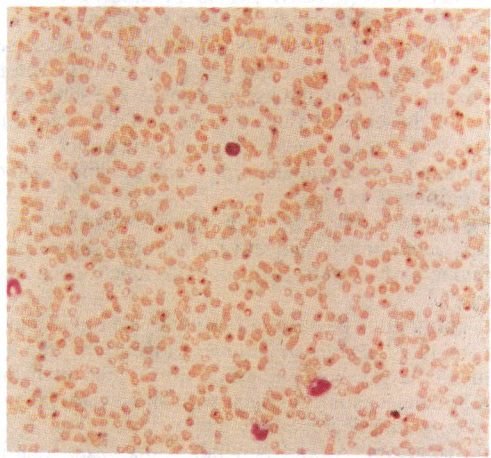

Monocytosis (Zitelli, 1992)

monocytosis /mon′ōsītō′sis/, an increased proportion of monocytes in the circulation.

monodactylism /-dak′tiliz′əm/ [Gk, monos, single; daktylos, finger or toe], a congenital defect in which the person is born with only one finger on the hand or one toe on the foot.

monoethanolamine /mon′ō·eth′ənol′əmēn/, an amino alcohol formed by the decarboxylation of serine. It is a component of certain cephalins and phospholipids and is used as a surfactant in pharmaceutical products.

monofactorial inheritance /-faktôr′ē·əl/ [Gk, monos + L, factare, to make], the acquisition or expression of a trait or condition that depends on the transmission of a single specific gene. Compare **multifactorial inheritance.**

monohybrid /-hī′brid/ [Gk, monos + L, hybrida, mixed offspring], pertaining to or describing an individual, organism, or strain that is heterozygous for only one specific trait or that is heterozygous for the single trait or gene locus under consideration.

monohybrid cross, the mating of two individuals, organisms, or strains that have different gene pairs for only one specific trait or in which only one particular characteristic or gene locus is being followed.

monohydric alcohol /-hī′drik/, an alcohol containing one hydroxyl group.

monomer /mon′əmər/ [Gk, monos + meros, part], a molecule that repeats itself to form a polymer, such as the molecules of fibrin monomer that polymerize to form fibrin in the blood-clotting process. —**monomeric,** adj.

monomolecular elimination reaction (E1) /-məlek′yələr/, a first-order chemical kinetic reaction in which only one molecule is involved in the slow step reaction. Also called **unimolecular reaction.**

monomphalus /mənom′fələs/ [Gk, monos + omphalos, navel], conjoined twins that are united at the umbilicus. Also called **omphalopagus.**

mononeuritis multiplex. See **multiple mononeuropathy.**

mononeuropathy /-nŏŏrop′əthē/ [Gk, monos + neuron, nerve, pathos, disease], any disease or disorder that affects a single nerve trunk. Some common causes of disorders involving single nerve trunks are electric shock, radiation, and fractured bones that may compress or lacerate nerve fibers. Casts and tourniquets that are too tight may also damage a nerve by compression or by ischemia. Accidental injection of penicillin and other medications into the sciatic nerve can seriously injure the nerve, especially if the injected medication is an oil-based drug. The peripheral nerve trunks are especially vulnerable to compression and entrapment.

mononuclear /-nyŏŏ′klē·ər/ [Gk, monos, single; L, nucleus, nut], pertaining to one nucleus, such as a monocyte.

mononuclear cell [Gk, monos + L, nucleus, nut kernel, cella, storeroom], Leukocytes, including lymphocytes and monocytes, with round or oval nuclei.

mononucleosis (mono) /mon′ōnŏŏ′klē·ō′sis/ [Gk, monos + L, nucleus; Gk, osis, condition], **1.** an abnormal increase in the number of mononuclear leukocytes in the blood. **2.** See **infectious mononucleosis.**

monooctanoin /mon′ō·ok′tənō′in/, a gallstone-dissolving agent.

■ INDICATIONS: It is used to dissolve cholesterol gallstones.

■ CONTRAINDICATIONS: The product is contraindicated in patients with jaundice, a severe biliary tract infection, or a history of recent duodenal ulcer or jejunitis.

■ ADVERSE EFFECTS: Adverse reactions may include nausea, vomiting, diarrhea, and gastrointestinal pain.

monoovular. See **uniovular.**

monophasic /-fā′sik/, having one phase, part, aspect, or stage.

monoploid /mon′əploid/, haploid. Also **monoploidic.**

monopodial symmelia. See **sympus monopus.**

monopus /mon'əpəs/ [Gk, *monos* + *pous*, foot], a fetus or individual with the congenital absence of a foot or leg.

monorchid /monôr'kid/, a male who has monorchism.

monorchism /mon'ôrkiz'əm/ [Gk, *monos* + *orchis*, testicle, *ismos*, state], a condition in which only one testicle has descended into the scrotum. Also called **monorchidism.** See also **cryptorchidism.** –**monorchidic,** *adj.*

monosaccharide /-sak'ərīd/ [Gk, *monos* + *sakcharon*, sugar], a simple carbohydrate consisting of a single basic unit with the general formula $C_n(H_2O)_n$, with n ranging from 3 to 8.

monosome /mon'əsōm/ [Gk, *monos* + *soma*, body], **1.** also called **accessory chromosome.** an unpaired X or Y sex chromosome. **2.** the single, unpaired chromosome in monosomy.

monosomy /mon'əsō'mē/ [Gk, *monos* + *soma*, body], a chromosomal aberration characterized by the absence of one chromosome from the normal diploid complement. In humans, the monosomic cell contains 45 chromosomes and is designated 2n[mi]1, such as occurs in the XO condition in Turner's syndrome. Compare **trisomy.** See also **aneuploidy.** –**monosomic,** *adj.*

monosomy X. See **Turner's syndrome.**

monospecific /-spəsif'ik/ [Gk, *monos* + L, *species*, form, *facere*, to make], an antibody that will react with only one type of antigen.

monosynaptic reflex /-sinap'tik/ [Gk, *monos*, single + *synaptein*, to join; L, *reflectere*, to bend back], a reflex requiring only one afferent and one efferent neuron.

monotropy /mənot'rəpē/ [Gk, *monos* + *trepein*, to turn], a concept named by J. Bowlby, describing the phenomenon in which a mother appears to be able to bond with only one infant at a time. The concept is used by Marshall Klaus and John Kennell in their studies of maternal-infant bonding in mothers of twins. When one twin is taken home from the hospital earlier than the other, the mother often reports that she does not feel that the baby discharged later is hers. The second baby to reach the home is much more likely to fail to thrive or to be neglected or abused. Nurses working in intensive care nurseries and adoption homes are also known to become attached to only one child at a time. Monotropy also may explain a mother's common tendency to dress twins alike, in effect making them one. –**monotropic,** *adj.*

monounsaturated fatty acid. See **unsaturated fatty acid.**

monovular. See **uniovular.**

monovulatory /mənō'vyələtôr'ē/ [Gk, *monos* + L, *ovulum*, small egg, *orius*, characterized by], routinely releasing one ovum during each ovarian cycle. Compare **diovulatory.**

monozygotic (MZ) /-zīgō'tik/ [Gk, *monos* + *zygon*, yoke], pertaining to or developed from a single fertilized ovum, or zygote, such as occurs in identical twins. Compare **dizygotic.** –**monozygosity,** *n.,* **monozygous,** *adj.*

monozygotic twins, two offspring born of the same pregnancy and developed from a single fertilized ovum that splits into equal halves during an early cleavage phase in embryonic development, giving rise to separate fetuses. Such twins are always of the same sex, have the same genetic constitution, possess identical blood groups, and closely resemble each other in physical, psychologic, and mental characteristics. Monozygotic twins may have single or separate placentas and membranes, depending on the time during development when division occurred. Monozygotic twinning occurs with relatively uniform frequency in all races, is unaffected by heredity, and represents approximately one third of all twin births. Also called **enzygotic twins, identical twins, true twins, uniovular twins.** Compare **dizygotic twins.** See also **Siamese twins.**

mons /mons/ [L, mountain], a mound or slight elevation.

Monson curve [George S. Monson, American dentist, b. 1869; L, *curvus*, a bend], the curve of occlusion in which each tooth cusp and incisal edge conform to a segment of the surface of a sphere 8 inches (20 cm) in diameter, with its center in the region of the glabella.

mons pubis. See **mons veneris.**

monster [L, *monstrum*], a fetus that is grossly malformed and usually nonviable. Kinds of monsters include **compound monster, double monster,** and **single monster.**

monstrosity /monstros'itē/, **1.** the state or condition of having severe congenital defects. **2.** anything that deviates greatly from the normal; a monster or teras.

mons veneris /ven'əris/ [L, *mons*, mountain; *Venus*, goddess of love], a pad of fatty tissue and coarse skin that overlies the symphysis pubis in the woman. After puberty, it is covered with pubic hair. Also called **mons pubis.**

Monteggia's fracture /montej'əz/ [Giovanni B. Monteggia, Italian physician, b. 1762], fracture of the proximal third of the proximal half of the ulna, associated with radial dislocation or rupture of the annular ligament and resulting in the angulation or overriding of ulnar fragments.

Montercaux fracture /mont'ərkō'/, a fracture of the neck of the fibula associated with the diastasis of ankle mortise.

Montgomery's gland. See **Montgomery's tubercle.**

Montgomery straps /mont·gom'ərē/, bands of adhesive tape that are used to secure dressings that must be changed frequently. Also called **Montgomery tapes.**

Montgomery's tubercle [William F. Montgomery, Irish gynecologist, b. 1797; L, *tuber*, swelling], one of several sebaceous glands on the areolae of the breasts. The tubercles normally enlarge during pregnancy. The sebaceous material that is secreted from the ducts of the glands to the skin of each areola serves to lubricate and protect the breast from infection and trauma during breast feeding. Also called **Montgomery's gland.**

Montgomery tapes. See **Montgomery straps.**

mood, a prolonged subjective emotional state that influences one's whole personality and life functioning. See also **affect.**

mood-congruent psychotic features /-kon'grōō·ənt/ [AS, *mod,* mind; L, *congruere,* to come together], the characteristics of a psychosis in which the content of hallucinations or delusions is consistent with an elevated, expansive mood or with a depression.

mood disorders [AS, *mod,* mind; L, *dis, ordo,* rank], an affective state characterized by any of a variety of periods of depression or depression elation. If mild and occasional, the feelings may be normal. If more severe, they may be a sign of a dysthymic reaction or symptomatic of an affective disorder.

mood theme. See **communication, impaired verbal.**

moon face [AS, *mona,* moon; L, *facies,* face], a condition characterized by a rounded, puffy face, occurring in people treated with large doses of corticosteroids, such as those with chronic asthma, rheumatoid arthritis or acute childhood leukemia. The features return to normal when the medication is stopped. Moon face is symptomatic in Cushing's disease and Cushing's syndrome.

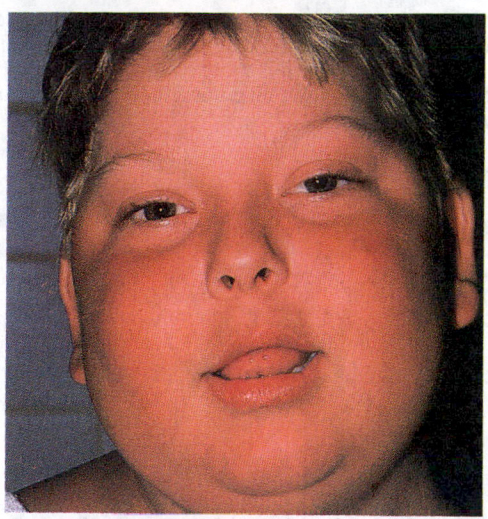

Moon face (Zitelli, 1992)

morbilliform /môrbil′ifôrm/ [L, *morbilli*, little disease, *forma*, form], describing a skin condition that resembles the erythematous, maculopapular rash of measles.

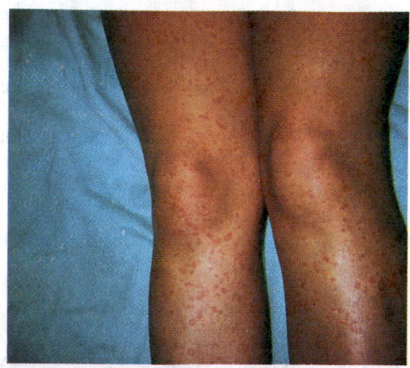

Morbilliform eruption on legs (Weston, 1991)

Moore's fracture [Edward M. Moore, American surgeon, b. 1814], a fracture of the distal radius with associated dislocation of the ulnar head, resulting in the securement of the styloid process under the annular ligaments of the wrist.

MOPP /mop/, an abbreviation for a combination drug regimen used in the treatment of cancer, containing three antineoplastics, Mustargen (mechlorethamine), Oncovin (vincristine sulfate), and Matulane (procarbazine hydrochloride), and prednisone (a glucocorticoid). MOPP is prescribed in the treatment of Hodgkin's disease.

morbid [L, *morbidus*, diseased], pertaining to a pathologic or diseased condition, either physical or mental.

morbid anatomy. See **pathologic anatomy.**

morbidity /môrbid′itē/ [L, *morbidus*, diseased], **1.** an illness or an abnormal condition or quality. **2.** (in statistics) the rate at which an illness or abnormality occurs, calculated by dividing the entire number of people in a group by the number in that group who are affected with the illness or abnormality. **3.** the rate at which an illness occurs in a particular area or population.

Morbidity and Mortaility Weekly Report (MMWR), a weekly epidemiologic report on the incidence of communicable diseases and deaths in 120 urban areas of the United States. It is published by the Centers for Disease Control and Prevention in Atlanta, Georgia. The publication also includes information on accident rates and important international health data.

morbidity rate [L, *morbidus*, diseased; *ratum*, calculation], the number of cases of a particular disease occurring in a single year per a specified population unit, as x cases per 1000. It also may be calculated on the basis of age groups, sex, occupation, or other population unit.

morbidity statistics [L, *morbidus*, diseased + *status*, condition], a branch of statistics that is concerned with the disease rate of a population or geographic region.

morbid obesity [L, *morbidus*, diseased + *obesitas*, fatness], an excess of body fat that threatens normal body functions such as respiration.

morbid physiology. See **pathologic physiology.**

morbilli. See **measles.**

Morgagni's globule /môrgan′yēz/ [Giovanni B. Morgagni, Italian anatomist, b. 1682], a minute opaque sphere that may form from fluid coagulation between the eye lens and its capsule, especially in cataract.

Morgagni's tubercle [Giovanni B. Morgagni], one of several small, soft nodules on the surface of each of the areola in women. The tubercles are produced by large sebaceous glands just under the surface of the areolae. They secrete a bacteriostatic, lubricating substance during pregnancy and lactation.

morgan /môr′gən/ [Thomas H. Morgan, American biologist, b. 1896], (in genetics) a unit of measure used in mapping the relative distances between genes on a chromosome. The measurement, named after the biologist Thomas Hunt Morgan, uses the total crossover value as the basic unit so that one morgan equals 100% crossing over or one centimorgan equals 1% recombination. One centimorgan is also equal to one map unit.

morgue /môrg/ [Fr, mortuary], a unit of a hospital with facilities for the storage and autopsy of the dead.

-moria, a combining form meaning '(condition of) dementia': *monomoria, phantasmatomoria.*

moribund /môr′ibund/ [L, *moribundus*, dying], near death or in the act of dying.

Morita therapy /môrē′tä/, an alternative therapy founded by Shoma Morita that has as its focus the symptoms of the patient. The goal of the therapy is character building, which enables the patient to live responsibly and constructively, even if the symptoms persist.

morning after pill [AS, *morgen; aefter; pilian*, to peel], *informal.* A large dose of an estrogen given orally, over a short period of time, to a woman within 24 to 72 hours after sexual intercourse to prevent conception, most commonly in an emergency situation such as rape or incest. The woman is warned that the medication may cause the formation of clots, severe nausea and vomiting, and teratogenic and carcinogenic effects on the fetus if pregnancy already exists or if contraception fails. See also **diethylstilbestrol.**

morning dip, a significant decline in respiratory function observed in some asthmatic people during the early morning hours. A similar fall in peak expiratory flow rate (PEFR) can occur in normal people after reaching a peak in the afternoon. The PEFR in an asthmatic person tends to follow a circadian rhythm with a morning dip and a high point in midafternoon.

morning sickness.   See **nausea and vomiting of pregnancy.**

morning stiffness [OE, *morgen*; *stif*],   a period of muscular stiffness after awakening in the morning, a common complaint of patients with arthritis or similar musculoskeletal disorders.

Moro reflex /môr′ō/ [Ernst Moro, German pediatrician, b. 1874],   a normal mass reflex in a young infant elicited by a sudden loud noise, such as by striking the table next to the child or raising the head slightly and allowing it to drop. A normal response consists of flexion of the legs, an embracing posture of the arms, and usually a brief cry. Also called **startle reflex.**

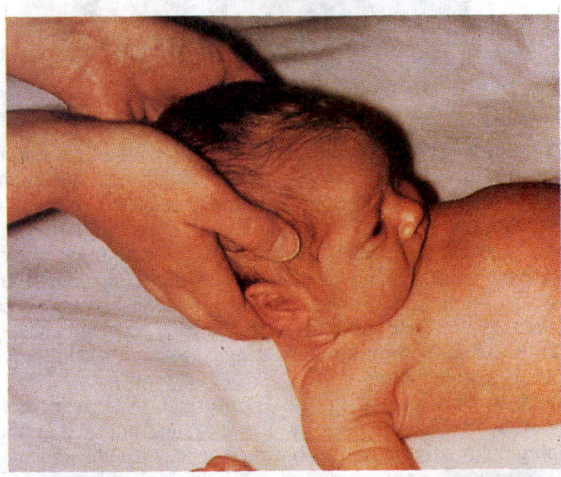

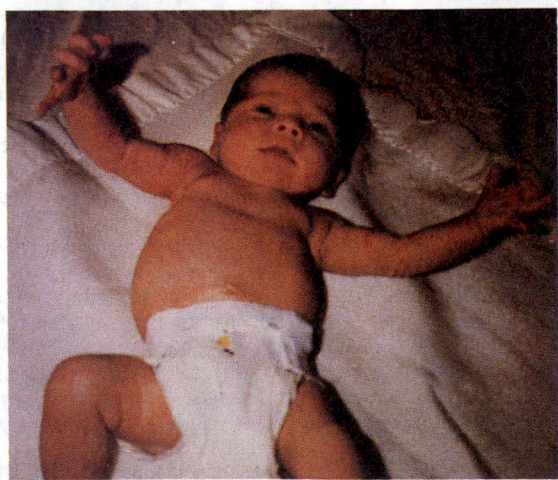

Moro reflex *(Zitelli, 1992)*

morph-, morpho-, -morph,   a combining form meaning 'form or shape': *morphallaxis, morphea, morphogenesis, endomorph.*

morphea /môr′fē·ə/ [Gk, *morphe*, form],   localized scleroderma consisting of patches of yellowish or ivory-colored, rigid, dry, smooth skin. It is more common in females. Also called **Addison's keloid, circumscribed scleroderma, localized scleroderma.**

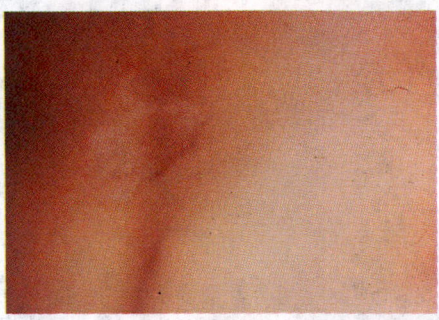

Morphea *(Zitelli, 1992)*

-morphia, -morphy,   a suffix meaning a 'condition of form': *pantamorphia, prosopodysmorphia, theromorphia.*

morphine sulfate /môr′fēn/,   a narcotic analgesic.
- INDICATION: It is prescribed to reduce pain.
- CONTRAINDICATIONS: Drug dependence or known hypersensitivity to this drug prohibits its use.
- ADVERSE EFFECTS: Among the more serious adverse reactions are increased intracranial pressure, cardiovascular disturbances, respiratory depression, and drug dependence.

-morphism,   a suffix meaning the 'condition of having a (specified) shape': *amorphism, isomorphism, pedomorphism.*

morpho-,   See **morph-.**

morphogenesis /môr′fəjen′əsis/ [Gk, *morphe* + *genein*, to produce],   the development and differentiation of the structures and the form of an organism, specifically the changes that occur in the cells and tissue during embryonic development. Also called **morphogeny** /môrfoj′ənē/.

morphogenetic /-jənet′ik/,   (in embryology) of or pertaining to a substance or hormone that acts as an evocator in differentiation. Also **morphogenic.**

morphogeny.   See **morphogenesis.**

morphology /môrfol′əjē/ [Gk, *morphe* + *logos*, science],   the study of the physical shape and size of a specimen, plant, or animal.   **—morphologic** /môr′fəloj′ik/, *adj.*

-morphosis,   a suffix meaning a 'development or change': *chemomorphosis, epimorphosis, heteromorphosis.*

Morquio's disease /môrkē′ōz/ [Luis Morquio, Uruguayan physician, b. 1867],   a familial form of mucopolysaccharidosis that results in abnormal musculoskeletal development in childhood. Dwarfism, hunchback, enlarged sternum, and knock-knees may occur. The disease may first be evident as the child, learning to walk, displays an abnormal, waddling gait. Also called **MPS IV.** See also **mucopolysaccharidosis.**

mortal [L, *mortalis*, to die],   **1.** liable to die. **2.** causing death.

mortality [L, *mortalis*, perishable],   **1.** the condition of being subject to death. **2.** the death rate, which reflects the number of deaths per unit of population in any specific region, age group, disease, or other classification, usually expressed as deaths per 1000, 10,000, or 100,000.

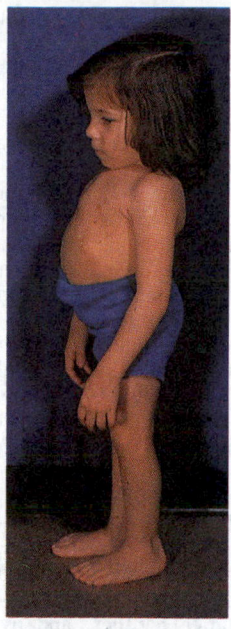

Morquio's syndrome (Lewis, 1989)

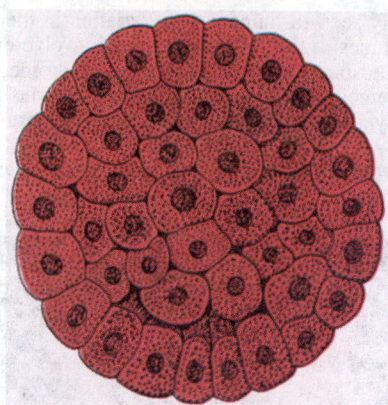

Morula (Thibodeau, 1993)

mortar /môr′tər/ [L, *mortarium*], a cup-shaped vessel in which materials are ground or crushed by a pestle in the preparation of drugs.

mortinatality /môr′tinātal′itē/ [L, *mors*, death; *natus*, birth], the stillbirth rate. It is calculated by multiplying the number of stillbirths by 1000 and dividing by the total number of births per year. Also called **natimortality**.

mortise joint /môr′tis/ [ME, *mortays*, fixed in; *jungere*, to join], the *articulatio talocruralis* joint of the ankle.

Morton's disease [Thomas George Morton, American surgeon, b. 1835; L, *dis*, Fr, *aise*, ease], a form of foot neuralgia caused by a falling metatarsal arch and pressure on the digital branches of the lateral plantar nerve. Also called **Morton's neuralgia; Morton's toe.** See also **metatarsalgia.**

Morton's foot. See **metatarsalgia.**

Morton's neuralgia. See **Morton's disease.**

Morton's neuroma. See **metatarsalgia.**

Morton's plantar neuralgia [Thomas G. Morton, American surgeon, b. 1835; L, *planta*, foot sole; Gk, *neuron*, nerve, *algos*, pain], a severe throbbing pain that affects the anastomotoc nerve branch between the medial and the lateral plantar nerves. Also called *(obsolete)* **Morton's plantar neuroma.**

Morton's syndrome [Dudley J. Morton, American orthopedist, b. 1884; Gk, *syn*, together; *dromos*, course], a congenital foreshortening of the first metatarsal segment, causing pain and deformity of the forefoot.

Morton's toe. See **metatarsalgia.**

morula /môr′ələ/, *pl.* **morulas, morulae** [L, *morulus*, blackberry], a solid, spherical mass of cells resulting from the cleavage of the fertilized ovum in the early stages of embryonic development. It represents an intermediate stage between the zygote and the blastocyst and consists of blastomeres that are uniform in size, shape, and physiologic capabilities. **morular,** *adj.*

-morula, a suffix meaning a 'clump of blastomeres formed by cleavage of a fertilized ovum': *amphimorula, archimorula, pseudomorula.*

Morvan's disease, a form of syringomyelia with tissue changes in the extremities, such as a paresthesia of the forearms and hands, and progressive painless ulceration of the fingertips.

mosaic /mōzā′ik/ [L, *Musa*, goddess of the arts], **1.** (in genetics) an individual or organism that developed from a single zygote but that has two or more kinds of genetically different cell populations. Such a condition results from a mutation, crossing-over, or, more commonly in humans, nondisjunction of the chromosomes during early embryogenesis, which causes a variation in the number of chromosomes in the cells. The type of chromosomal aberration and its ratio depend on whether nondisjunction occurred in the first or later mitotic divisions of the zygote. Because monosomic cells are nonviable, except in X monosomic conditions, most mosaic conditions in humans represent a mixture of normal and trisomic cells, regardless of whether an autosome or the sex chromosomes are involved. The degree of clinical involvement depends on the type of tissue containing the abnormality and may vary from near normal to full manifestation of a syndrome, such as Down's syndrome or Turner's syndrome. Compare **chimera.** See also **monosomy, sex chromosome mosaic, trisomy. 2.** (in embryology) a fertilized ovum that undergoes determinate cleavage. See also **mosaic development.**

mosaic bone, bone tissue appearing to be made up of many tiny pieces cemented together, as seen on microscopic examination of an x-ray film of the affected bone. It is characteristic of Paget's disease of the bone.

mosaic cleavage. See **determinate cleavage.**

mosaic development, a kind of embryonic development occurring in the blastocyst. The fertilized ovum undergoes determinate cleavage, developing according to a precise, unalterable plan in which each blastomere has a characteristic position and limited developmental potency, and is a precursor of a definite part of the embryo. Damage to or destruction of these cells results in a defective organism. Compare **regulative development.**

mosaicism /mōzā′isiz′əm/ [L, *Musa*, goddess of the arts], (in genetics) a condition in which an individual or an organism that develops from a single zygote has two or more cell populations that differ in genetic constitution. Most commonly seen in humans is a variation in the number of chromosomes in the cells, which may involve either a particular autosome, such as in Down's syndrome, or the sex chromosomes, such as in Turner's syndrome and Kleinfelter's syndrome. See also **mosaic, sex chromosome mosaic.**

mosaic wart, a group of contiguous plantar warts.

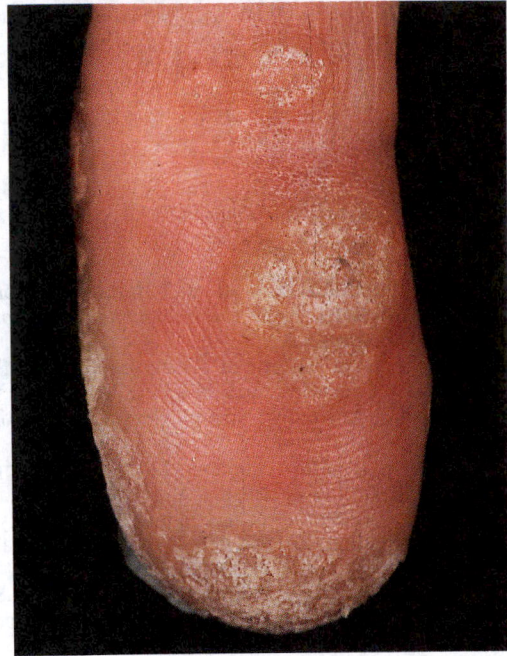

Mosaic wart (du Vivier, 1993)

mosquito bite /məskē′tō/ [L, *musca,* a fly; AS, *bitan,* to bite], a bite of a bloodsucking arthropod of the subfamily Culicidae that may result in a systemic allergic reaction in a hypersensitive person, an infection, or, most often, a pruritic wheal. Mosquitoes, which are attracted to hosts by moisture, carbon dioxide, estrogens, sweat, or warmth, are vectors of many infectious diseases.

mosquito forceps, a small hemostatic forceps. See also **Halsted's forceps,** def. 1.

Mössbauer spectrometer /mes′bou·ər, ms′bou·ər/ [Rudolf L. Mössbauer, German physicist, b. 1929], an instrument that can detect small changes between an atomic nucleus and its environment, such as caused by changes in temperature, pressure, or chemical state. The device is used in chemical and physical research with applications in medicine.

mot-, a prefix meaning 'of or related to movement': *motoneuron, motorgraphic, motoricity.*

mother fixation [AS, *modor,* mother; L, *figere,* to fasten], an arrest in psychosexual development characterized by an abnormally persistent, close, and often paralyzing emotional attachment to one's mother. Compare **father fixation.** See also **freudian fixation.**

mother yaw. See **yaw.**

motile /mō′til/ [L, *motare,* to move often], capable of

spontaneous but unconscious or involuntary movement. **–motility,** *n.*

-motility, -mobility, a suffix meaning the 'condition of being capable of movement': *cardiomotility, hypermotility, supermotility.*

-motine, a combining form for antiviral quinoline derivatives.

motion sickness /mō′shən/ [L, *motio,* movement; AS, *seoc,* sick, OE, *nes,* condition], a condition caused by erratic or rhythmic motions in any combination of directions, such as in a boat or a car. Severe cases are characterized by nausea, vomiting, vertigo, and headache, mild cases by headache and general discomfort. Various antihistamines are used prophylactically. Kinds of motion sickness are air sickness, car sickness, and seasickness (mal de mer).

motivation /mō′tivā′shən/ [L, *movere,* to move], conscious or unconscious needs, interests, rewards, or other incentives that arouse, channel, or maintain a particular behavior.

motivational conflict /mō′tivā′shənəl/ [L, *motus,* cause of motion, *alis,* relating to; *confluere,* to come together], a conflict resulting from the arousal of two or more motives that direct behavior toward incompatible goals. Kinds of motivational conflict include **approach-approach conflict, approach-avoidance conflict,** and **avoidance-avoidance conflict.**

motoneuron /mō′tōnŏŏr′on/ [L, *movere,* to move; Gk, *neuron,* nerve], a motor neuron, or a neuron whose axon ends in muscle fibers or other effector organs.

motor [L, *motare,* to move about], **1.** of or pertaining to motion, the body apparatus involved in movement, or the brain functions that direct purposeful activities. **2.** of or pertaining to a muscle, nerve, or brain center that produces or subserves motion.

-motor, a suffix meaning 'pertaining to the effects of activity in a body part': *nervimotor, psychomotor, viscerimotor.*

motor aphasia, the inability to utter remembered words, caused by a cerebral lesion in the inferior frontal gyrus (Broca's motor speech area) of the left hemisphere in right-handed individuals. The condition most commonly is the result of a stroke. The patient knows what to say but cannot articulate the words. Also called **ataxic aphasia, expressive aphasia, frontocortical aphasia, verbal aphasia.**

motor apraxia, the inability to carry out planned movements or to handle small objects, although the proper use of the object is recognized. The condition results from a lesion in the premotor frontal cortex on the opposite side of the affected limb. Also called **innervation apraxia.** See also **apraxia.**

motor area, a portion of the cerebral cortex that includes the precentral gyrus and the posterior part of the frontal gyri and that causes the contraction of the voluntary muscles on stimulation with electrodes. It corresponds to Brodmann's areas IV and VI and is characterized histologically by the absence of the granular layer in the cortex. It contains the giant pyramidal cells of Betz in layer V. Normal voluntary activity requires associations between the motor area and other parts of the cortex; removal of the motor area from one cerebral hemisphere causes paralysis of voluntary muscles, especially of the opposite side of the body. Various parts of the motor area are associated with different body structures, such as the lower limb, the face, the mouth, and the hand. The parts associated with more delicate, compli-

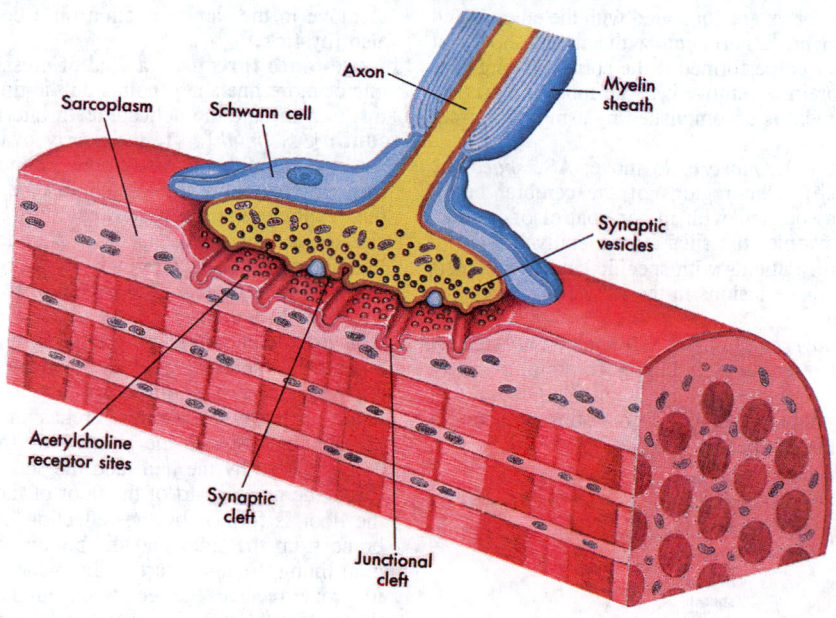

Motor end plate (Mourad, 1991)

cated movements, such as those of the hand, are larger than those associated with more general movements.

motor coordination, the coordination of body functions that involve movement, including gross motor movement, fine motor movement, and motor planning.

motor depressant [L, *motus*, mover; *deprimere*, to press down], a drug or agent that reduces the normal functioning level of motor neurons, mainly in voluntary muscles.

motor end plate, a broad band of terminal fibers of the motor nerves of the voluntary muscles. Motor nerves derived from the cranial and spinal nerves enter the sheaths of striated muscle fibers, lose their myelin sheaths, and ramify like the roots of a tree. In forming the motor end plate, the neurilemma of the nerve fiber merges with the sarcolemma of the muscle, and the axon synapses with the muscle fibers.

motor fiber, one of the fibers in the spinal nerves that transmit impulses to muscle fibers.

motor hallucination [L, *motus*, mover; *alucinari*, wandering mind], the subjective experience of movement when there is no movement.

motor image, a visual concept of one's bodily movements, real or imagined.

motor nerve. See **motor neuron.**

motor neuron, one of various efferent nerve cells that transmit nerve impulses from the brain or from the spinal cord to muscular or glandular tissue. According to location, some kinds of motor neurons are the peripheral motor neurons and the upper motor neurons. Also called **motoneuron.** Compare **sensory nerve.** See also **nervous system.**

motor neuron disease [L, *movere,* to move; *neuron,* nerve; L, *dis,* Fr, *aise,* ease], a progressive disease that tends to affect middle-age men with degeneration of anterior horn cells, motor cranial nerve nuclei, and pyramidal tracts. An example is **amyotrophic lateral sclerosis (ALS).**

motor neuron paralysis, an injury to the spinal cord that causes damage to the motor neurons and results in various degrees of functional impairment depending on the site of the lesion. See **lower motor neuron paralysis, upper motor neuron paralysis.**

motor nucleus [L, *movere,* to move + *nucleus,* nut], the nucleus of a motor nerve or a collection of motor neurons.

motor pathway [L, *movere,* to move; AS, *paeth*], the route of motor nerve impulses, from the central neuron to a muscle or gland.

motor planning, the ability to plan and execute skilled nonhabitual tasks. Also called **motor praxis.**

motor point, **1.** a point at which a motor nerve enters the muscle it innervates. **2.** a point at which electric stimulation will cause contraction of a muscle. Compare **motor end plate.** See also **motor neuron, nervous system.**

motor praxis. See **motor planning.**

motor root [L, *movere,* to move; AS, *rot*], the proximal end of a motor nerve at its attachment to the spinal cord.

motor seizure, a transitory disturbance in brain function caused by abnormal neuronal discharges that arise initially in a localized motor area of the cerebral cortex. The manifestations depend on the site of the abnormal electric activity, such as tonic contractures of the thumb, caused by excessive discharges in the motor area of the cortex controlling the first digit, or chewing movements resulting from discharges in the lower part of the motor strip controlling mastication. The disturbance may spread, or it may end in a shower of clonic movements or a generalized convulsion. See also **epilepsy, focal seizure.**

motor sense, the feeling or perception enabling a person to accomplish a purposeful movement, presumably achieved by evoking a sensory engram or memory of the pattern for that specific movement. Proprioceptive signals transmitted by feedback pathways through the cerebellum and sensory areas of the motor cortex are compared with the engram and modify the movement. Experiments with animals show that a movement cannot be performed if the corresponding sensory area of the brain is removed; if the motor area is removed, the movement is accomplished by using a different group of muscles.

motor speech area [L, *movere,* to move; AS, *spaec;* L, *area,* vacant place], the regions of the cerebral hemispheres that are associated with motor control of speech. For right-handed people, the sites are generally located in the left hemisphere. Patients with specific language defects often are found to have lesions in the left hemisphere. See also **Broca's area.**

motor tract [L, *movere,* to move + *tractus*], an efferent nerve pathway that conveys impulses controlling movement.

motor unit, a functional structure consisting of a motor neuron and the muscle fibers it innervates.

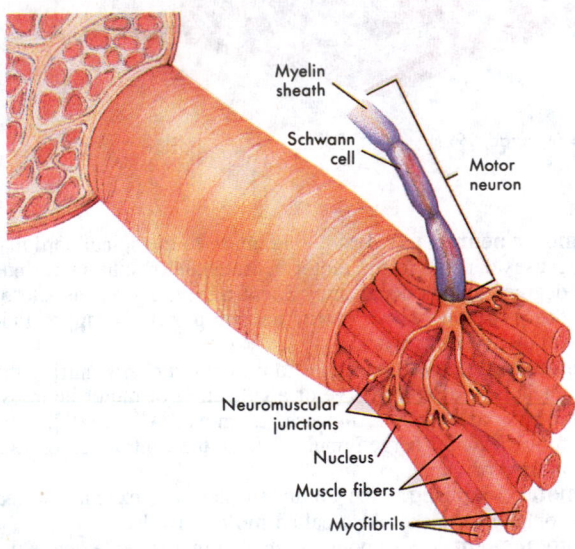

Motor unit (Thibodeau, 1993/Laurie O'Keefe/John Daugherty)

Motrin, a trademark for an antiinflammatory (ibuprofen).

mottle [ME, *motley,* mixed colors], an effect observed in radiologic imaging when the dose of radiation employed is reduced to a level where individual quantum effects can be seen. Instead of a uniform beam of radiation, the number of photons being produced is so low that the statistical variations in x-ray production can be visualized. Also called **noise, quantum mottle.**

mountain fever, mountain tick fever. See **Colorado tick fever, Rocky Mountain spotted fever.**

mountain sickness [L, *montana,* AS, *seoc*]. See **altitude sickness.**

mourning /mōr′ning/ [AS, *murnan,* to mourn], a psychologic process of reaction activated by an individual to assist in overcoming a great personal loss. The process is finally resolved when a new object relationship is established.

mouse [AS, *mus*], a hand-controlled cursor movement device. Rolling the device on a flat surface causes the cursor

to move in the same direction on a computer screen. See also **joystick.**

mouse-tooth forceps, a kind of dressing forceps that has one or more fine sharp points on the tip of each blade. The tips turn in, and the delicate teeth interlock.

mouth [AS, *muth*], **1.** the nearly oval oral cavity at the anterior end of the digestive tube, bounded anteriorly by the lips and containing the tongue and the teeth. It consists of the vestibule and the mouth cavity proper. The vestibule, situated in front of the teeth, is bounded externally by the lips and the cheeks, internally by the gums and the teeth. The vestibule receives the secretion from the parotid salivary glands and communicates, when the jaws are closed, with the mouth cavity proper by an aperture on each side behind the molar teeth and by narrow clefts between opposing teeth. The mouth cavity proper is bounded ventrally and laterally by the alveolar arches and the teeth, communicates dorsally with the pharynx by the ischium faucium, and is roofed by the hard and the soft palates. The tongue forms the greater part of the floor of the cavity. The rest of the floor is formed by the reflection of the mucous membrane from the sides and the bottom of the tongue to the gum lining the inner part of the mandible. The mouth cavity proper receives the secretion from the submandibular and the sublingual salivary glands. **2.** an orifice.

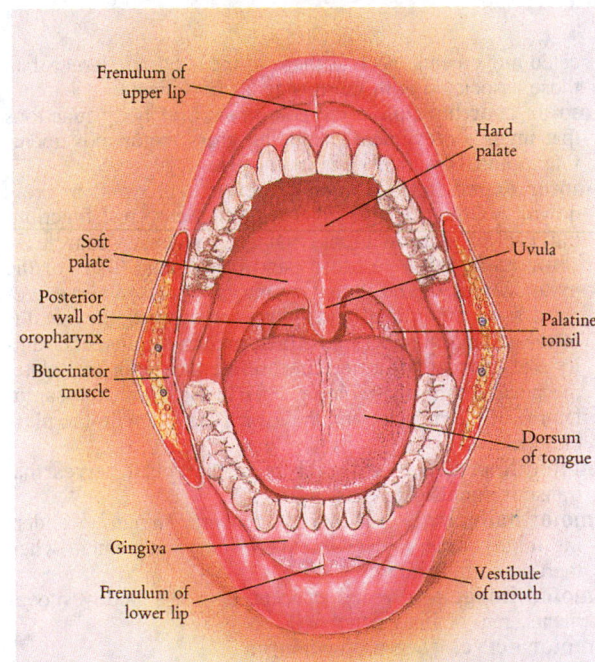

Mouth structures (Seidel, 1991)

mouth guard, a soft plastic intraoral appliance that covers all the occlusal surfaces and the palate. It is worn in contact sports to limit damage to tissues of the mouth, lips, and other oral surfaces.

mouthstick, a device that can be manipulated with the mouth and can be used to type, push buttons, turn pages, or operate power wheelchairs and other equipment for paralyzed patients.

mouth-to-mouth resuscitation, a procedure in artificial resuscitation, performed most often with cardiac massage. The victim's nose is sealed by pinching the nostrils closed, the head is extended, and air is breathed by the rescuer through the mouth into the lungs. See also **cardiopulmonary resuscitation.**

mouth-to-nose resuscitation, a procedure in artificial resuscitation in which the mouth of the victim is covered and held closed and air is breathed through the victim's nose. See also **mouth-to-mouth resuscitation.**

MOV, abbreviation for **minimal occlusive volume.**

movement decomposition [L *movere* to go; *de* away, *componere* to assemble], a distortion in voluntary movement in which the movement occurs in a distinct sequence of isolated steps, rather than in a normal, smooth, flowing pattern.

moving grid, (in radiography) an x-ray grid that is continuously moved or oscillated throughout the exposure of a radiographic film.

moxibustion /mok′səbus′chən/ [Jpn *moe kusa* burning herb; L *comburere* to burn up], a method of producing analgesia or altering the function of a system of the body achieved by igniting moxa, wormwood, or other combustible, slow-burning substance and holding it as near the point on the skin as possible without causing pain or burning. It is also sometimes used in conjunction with acupuncture.

MPD, M.P.D., abbreviation for **maximum permissible dose.**

M.P.H., abbreviation for *Master of Public Health.*

MPL + PRED, an anticancer drug combination of melphalan and prednisone.

MPS, abbreviation for **mucopolysaccharidosis.**

MPS I, abbreviation for *mucopolysaccharidosis I.* See **Hurler's syndrome.**

MPS II, abbreviation for *mucopolysaccharidosis II.* See **Hunter's syndrome.**

MPS IV, abbreviation for *mucopolysaccharidosis IV.* See **Morquio's disease.**

MQF, abbreviation for *mobile quarantine facility.*

mr, mR, abbreviation for **milliroentgen.**

mrad, abbreviation for **millirad.**

mrem, abbreviation for *millirem.*

MRI, abbreviation for **magnetic resonance imaging.**

mRNA, abbreviation for **messenger RNA.**

MS, abbreviation for **multiple sclerosis.**

M.S., **1.** abbreviation for *Master of Science.* **2.** abbreviation for *Master of Surgery.*

msec, abbreviation for **millisecond.**

MSH, abbreviation for **melanocyte stimulating hormone.**

M.S.N., abbreviation for *Master of Science in Nursing.* See **master's degree program in nursing.**

M.T., abbreviation for **medical technologist.**

MTX + MP + CTX, an anticancer drug combination of methotrexate, mercaptopurine, and cyclophosphamide.

mu, /myōō, mōō/, **1.** μ, the twelfth letter of the greek alphabet. **2.** symbol for **micron.**

muc-, muco-, a combining form meaning 'relating to mucus': *mucolytic, mucoid.*

Much's granules /mōōks, mōōkhs/ [Hans C. Much, German physician, b. 1880], granules and rods, found in tuberculosis sputum, that stain with gram stain but not by the usual methods for acid-fast bacilli.

mucin /myōō′sin/ [L, *mucus*, slime], a mucopolysaccharide, the chief ingredient in mucus. Mucin is present in most glands that secrete mucus and is the lubricant protecting body surfaces from friction or erosion.

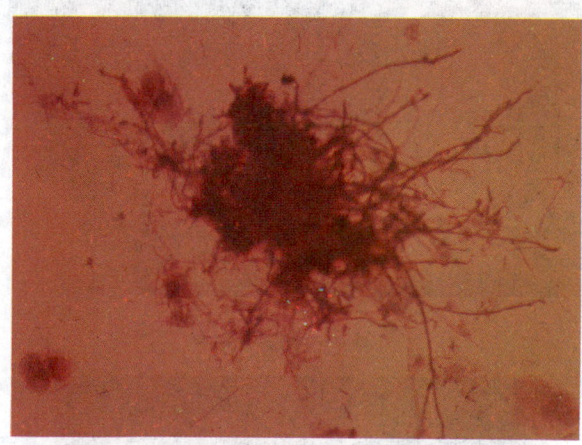

mucinous carcinoma *(Berkovitz, 1992)*

mucinoid /myōō′sinoid/ [L, *mucus* + Gk, *eidos*, form], resembling mucin. See also **mucoid,** def. 2.

mucinous adenocarcinoma /myōō′sinəs/. See **mucinous carcinoma.**

mucinous carcinoma, an epithelial neoplasm characterized by a sticky gelatinous consistency caused by copious mucin secretion. Also called **colloid carcinoma, gelatiniform carcinoma, gelatinous carcinoma.**

muco-. See **muc-.**

mucocutaneous /myōō′kōkyōōtā′nē·əs/ [L, *mucus* + *cutis*, skin, *osus,* having], of or pertaining to the mucous membrane and the skin.

mucocutaneous leishmaniasis. See **American leishmaniasis.**

mucocutaneous lymph node syndrome (MLNS), an acute, febrile illness, primarily of young children, characterized by inflamed mucous membranes of the mouth, 'strawberry tongue,' cervical lymphadenopathy, polymorphous rash on the trunk, and edema, erythema, and desquamation of the skin on the extremities. Other commonly associated findings include arthralgia, diarrhea, otitis, pneumonia, photophobia, meningitis, and electrocardiographic changes. The cause is unknown; no clear-cut environmental, seasonal, or geographic factors have been discovered, and person-to-person transmission is unproven. A genetic predisposition has been indicated. Treatment includes aspirin in large doses, which may be prescribed over a long period of time, and supportive care. Also called **Kawasaki disease.** (See Figs. p. 1020.)

mucoepidermoid carcinoma /myōō′kō·ep′idur′moid/ [L, *mucus* + Gk, *epi,* above, *derma,* skin, *eidos,* form], a malignant neoplasm of glandular tissues, especially the ducts of the salivary glands. The tumor contains mucinous and epidermoid squamous cells.

mucogingival junction /myōō′kōjinjī′vəl/ [L, *mucus* + *gingiva,* gum; *jungere,* to join], the scalloped linear area

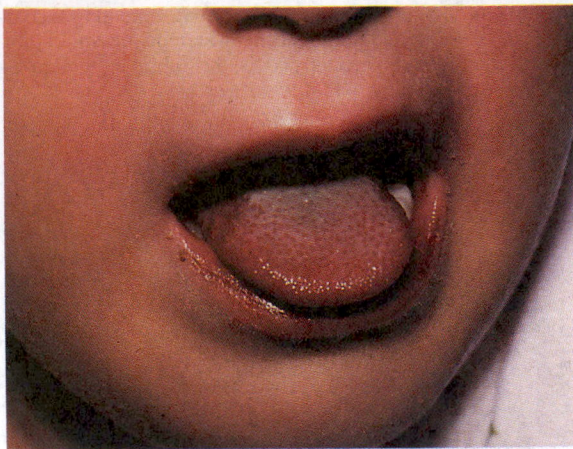

Strawberry tongue

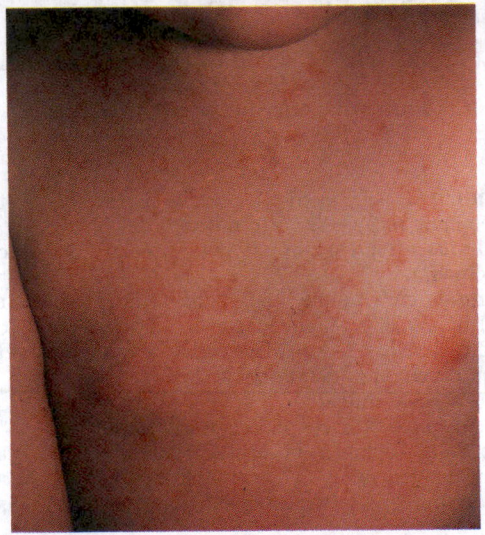

Morbilliform rash
**Mucocutaneous lymph node syndrome
(Kawasaki disease)**
(Zitelli, 1992)

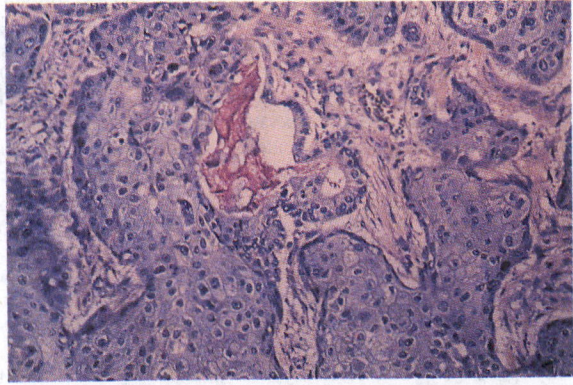

Mucoepidermoid carcinoma (Mitros, 1988)

of the gums that separates the gingivae from the alveolar mucosa.

mucoid /myoo̅'koid/ [L, *mucus* + Gk, *eidos,* form],   **1.** resembling mucus. **2.** also **mucinoid.** a group of glycoproteins, including colloid and ovomucoid, similar to the mucins, the primary difference being in solubility.

mucoid cyst [L, *mucus*; Gk, *eidos,* form; *kytis,* bag],   a cyst formed by an overgrowth of a mucus gland or by the spread of mucus into the interstitial tissues. Also called **mucous cyst.**

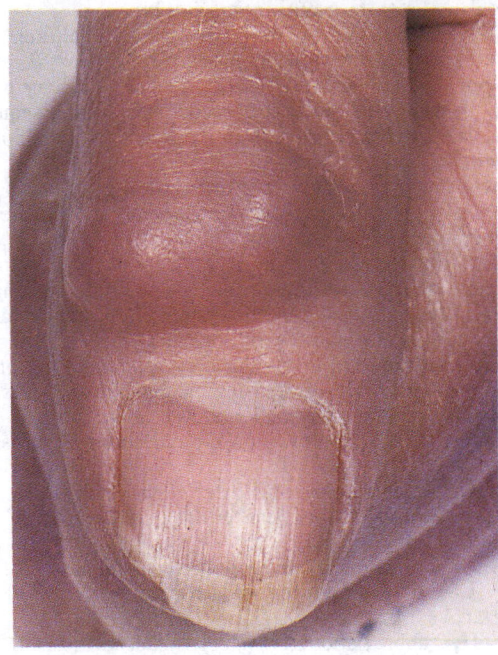

Mucoid cyst (du Vivier, 1993)

mucoid tissue.   See **embryonic tissue.**

mucolytic /myoo̅'kəlit'ik/ [L, *mucus* + Gk, *lysis,* loosening],   **1.** exerting a destructive effect on the mucus. **2.** any agent that dissolves or destroys the mucus.

mucomembranous /myoo̅'kəmem'brənəs/ [L, *mucus* + *membrana,* thin skin, *osus,* having],   of or pertaining to a mucous membrane, such as that of the small intestine or the bladder.

Mucomyst,   a trademark for a mucolytic (acetylcysteine), used as an adjunct to anesthesia and as adjuvant therapy for patients with abnormal, viscid, or inspissated mucous secretions. It is also used in the treatment of acetaminophen toxicity.

mucopolysaccharide /myoo̅'kōpol'ēsak'ərīd/ [L, *mucus*; Gk, *polys,* many; *sakcharon,* sugar],   a polysaccharide containing hexosamine and sometimes occurring with protein, such as mucins.

mucopolysaccharidosis   (MPS)   /myoo̅'kōpol'ēsak' ərīdō'sis/, *pl.* **mucopolysaccharidoses** [L, *mucus* + *polys,* many, *sakcharon,* sugar, *osis,* condition],   one of a group of genetic disorders characterized by greater than normal accumulations of mucopolysaccharides in the tissues, with other symptoms specific to each type. The disorders are numbered MPS I through MPS VII, and each type has a specific eponym. In all types there is pronounced skeletal deformity (especially of the face), mental and physical retardation, and decreased life expectancy. The disorders may be detected before birth by testing fetal cells present in amniotic fluid. After birth, diagnosis is established through urine testing, skeletal changes observed on x-ray films, and family history. There is no successful treatment. Kinds of mucopolysaccharidosis include **Hunter's syndrome (MPS II), Hurler's syndrome (MPS I),** and **Morquio's disease (MPS IV).**

mucoprotein /myōō′kōprō′tēn, -tē·in/ [L, *mucus* + Gk, *proteios,* first rank], a compound, present in all connective and supporting tissue, that contains polysaccharides combined with protein and is relatively resistant to denaturation.

mucopurulent /myōō′kōpyōōr′yələnt/ [L, *mucus* + *purulentus,* pus], characteristic of a combination of mucus and pus.

mucormycosis. See **zygomycosis.**

mucosa /myōōkō′sə/, *pl.* **mucosae,** mucous membrane. **–mucosal,** *adj.*

mucositis /myōō′kōsī′tis/, any inflammation of a mucous membrane, such as the lining of the mouth and throat.

mucous. See **mucus.**

-mucous, a suffix meaning 'containing or composed of mucus': *fibromucous, puromucous, seromucous.*

mucous colitis. See **irritable bowel syndrome.**

mucous cyst. See **mucoid cyst.**

mucous membrane /myōō′kəs/ [L, *mucus* + *membrana,* thin skin], any one of four major kinds of thin sheets of tissue that cover or line various parts of the body. Mucous membranes line cavities or canals of the body that open to the outside, such as the linings of the mouth, the digestive tube, the respiratory passages, and the genitourinary tract. It consists of a surface layer of epithelial tissue covering a deeper layer of connective tissue and protects the underlying structure, secretes mucus, and absorbs water, salts, and other solutes. Compare **serous membrane, skin, synovial membrane.**

mucous plug, (in obstetrics) a collection of thick mucus in the uterine cervix that is often expelled at the onset of dilation of the cervix, just before labor begins or in its early hours. The plug may be dry and firm, following the shape of the endocervical canal, but, more often, it is semifluid and mucoid, streaked with blood.

mucous shreds. See **shreds.**

mucous tissue. See **embryonic tissue.**

mucous tumor. See **myxoma.**

mucoviscidosis. See **cystic fibrosis.**

mucus /myōō′kəs/ [L, slime], the viscous, slippery secretions of mucous membranes and glands, containing mucin, white blood cells, water, inorganic salts, and exfoliated cells. **—mucoid,** *adj.,* **mucous** /myōō′kəs/, *adj.*

mucus cyst. See **mucoid cyst.**

mucus trap suction apparatus, a catheter containing a trap to prevent mucus being aspirated from the nasopharynx and trachea of a newborn infant from entering the mouth of the person operating the device.

mud bath, the application of warm mud to the body for therapeutic purposes.

Mudrane, a trademark for a respiratory, fixed-combination drug containing a smooth muscle relaxant (theophylline), an adrenergic (ephedrine hydrochloride), an expectorant (potassium iodide), and a sedative-hypnotic (phenobarbital).

mulibrey nanism /mul′ibrī/, a rare genetic disorder, transmitted as an autosomal recessive trait, characterized by dwarfism, constrictive pericarditis, muscular hypotonia, anomalies of the skull and face, and characteristic yellow dots in the ocular fundus. The name of the condition is an acronym composed of the first two letters of the anatomic sites of the principal defects: *mu*scle, *li*ver, *br*ain, and *eye*s.

müllerian duct /miler′ē·ən, mYl-/ [Johannes P. Müller, German physiologist, b. 1801], one of a pair of embryonic ducts that become the fallopian tubes, uterus, and vagina in females and that atrophy in males.

Müller's maneuver [Johannes P. Müller], an inspiratory effort against a closed airway or glottis. The effort decreases intrapulmonary and intrathoracic pressures and expands pulmonary gas.

multi- /mul′ti-/, a prefix meaning 'many': *multicapsular, multifamilial, multipara.*

multicentric mitosis. See **multipolar mitosis.**

multidisciplinary health care team /-dis′ipliner′ē/, a group of health care workers who are members of different disciplines, each one providing specific services to the patient.

multifactorial /-faktôr′ē·əl/ [L, *multus,* many, *facere,* to make], of, pertaining to, or characteristic of any condition or disease resulting from the interaction of many factors, specifically the interaction of several genes, usually polygenes, with or without the involvement of environmental factors. Many disorders, such as spina bifida, neural tube defects, and Hirschsprung's disease, are considered to be multifactorial.

multifactorial inheritance, the tendency to develop a physical appearance, disease, or condition that is a condition of many genetic and environmental factors, such as stature and blood pressure. See also **polygene.**

multifocal -fō′kəl/ [L, *multus* + *focus,* hearth], an action, such as the transmission of an impulse, that arises from more than two foci.

multiform /mul′tifôrm/ [L, *multus,* many, *forma*], an organ, tissue, or other object that may appear in more than one shape.

multigenerational model /-jen′ərā′shənəl/, a model of family therapy that focuses on reciprocal role relationships over a period of time and thus takes a longitudinal approach. The family is viewed as an emotional system where patterns of interacting and coping, as well as unresolved issues, can be passed down from one generation to the next and can cause stress to the family members on whom they are projected.

multigenerational transmission process, the repetition of relationship patterns, including divorce, suicide, or alcoholism, associated with emotional dysfunction that can be traced through several generations of the same family.

multigravida /mul′tigrav′idə/ [L, *multus* + *gravidare,* to impregnate], a woman who has been pregnant more than once. Compare **multipara, primigravida.**

multihospital system /-hos′pitəl/, a group of two or more hospitals owned, sponsored, or managed by a central organization.

multiinfarct dementia /-infärkt′/ [L, *multus* + *infarcire,* to stuff; *de,* away, *mens,* mind], a form of organic brain disease characterized by the rapid deterioration of intellectual functioning, caused by vascular disease. Symptoms include emotional lability; disturbances in memory, abstract thinking, judgment, and impulse control; and focal neurologic impairment, such as gait abnormalities, pseudobulbar palsy, and paresthesia.

multilocular cyst /-lok'yələr/ [L, *multus* + *locilus*, little place; Gk, *kystis*, bag], one of three kinds of follicular cyst, containing many spaces and not associated with a tooth. Compare **dentigerous cyst, primordial cyst.**

multipara /multip'ərə/, *pl.* **multiparae** [L *multus* + *parere* to bear], a woman who has delivered more than one viable infant. Also called **pluripara.** Compare **multigravida, nullipara, primipara.**

multiparity /-per'itē/ [L, *multus*, many; *parere*, to give birth], the status of a mother of more than one child.

multiparous /multip'ərous/ [L, *multus*, many; *parere*, to give birth], having given birth to more than one child.

multipenniform /-pen'ifôrm/ [L, *multus* + *penna*, feather, *forma*], (of a bodily structure) having a shape resembling a pattern of many feathers, especially the pattern formed by the muscular fasciculi that converge to several tendons. Compare **bipenniform, penniform.**

multiphasic screening /-fā'sik/ [L, *multus* + *phasis*, appearance; ME, *scren*], a technique of screening populations for diseases in which there is combined use of a battery of screening tests. The technique serves to identify any of several diseases being screened for in a population that is apparently healthy.

multiple benign cystic epithelioma. See **trichoepithelioma.**

multiple cartilaginous exostoses. See **diaphyseal aclasis.**

multiple enchondromatosis. See **enchondromatosis.**

multiple endocrine adenomatosis. See **adenomatosis.**

multiple factor. See **polygene.**

multiple family therapy /mul'tipəl/ [L, *multus* + *plica*, fold], psychotherapy in which four or five families meet weekly to confront and deal with problems or issues that they have in common.

multiple fission, cell division in which the nucleus first divides into several equal parts followed by the division of the cytoplasm into as many cells as there are nuclei. It is the common form of asexual reproduction in certain unicellular organisms. Compare **binary fission.**

multiple fracture, **1.** a fracture extending several fracture lines in one bone. **2.** the fracture of several bones at one time or from the same injury.

multiple gene. See **polygene.**

multiple idiopathic hemorrhagic sarcoma. See **Kaposi's sarcoma.**

multiple lipomatosis, a rare, inherited disorder characterized by discrete, localized, subcutaneous deposits of fat in the tissues of the body. This fat is not available for metabolic use, even in starvation.

multiple mononeuropathy, an abnormal condition characterized by dysfunction of several individual nerve trunks. It may be caused by various diseases, such as necrotizing angiopathy, uremia, diabetes mellitus, and some inflammatory immunologic disorders. Also called *(obsolete)* **mononeuritis multiplex.**

multiple myeloma, a malignant neoplasm of the bone marrow. The tumor, composed of plasma cells, destroys osseous tissue, especially in flat bones, causing pain, fractures, hypercalcemia, and skeletal deformities. Characteristically, abnormal proteins in the plasma and urine, anemia, weight loss, pulmonary complications secondary to rib fractures, and kidney failure are present. Also called **multiple plasmacytoma of bone, myelomatosis, plasma cell myeloma.**

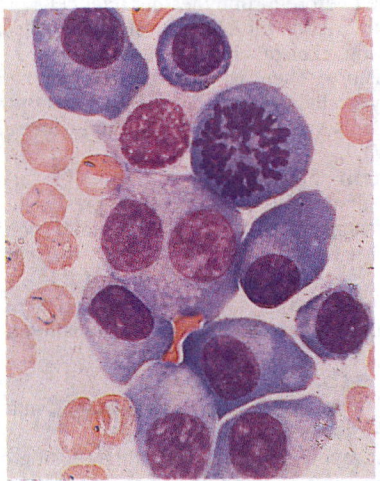

Multiple myeloma—bone marrow aspirate
(Hoffbrand, 1987)

multiple myositis. See **polymyositis.**

multiple neuroma. See **neuromatosis.**

multiple peripheral neuritis, acute or subacute disseminated inflammation or degeneration of symmetrically distributed peripheral nerves, characterized initially by numbness, tingling in the extremities, hot and cold sensations, and slight fever, progressing to pain, weakness, diminished reflexes, and in some cases flaccid paralysis. The disorder may be caused by toxic substances, such as antimony, arsenic, carbon monoxide, copper, lead, mercury, nitrobenzol, organophosphates, and thallium; or various drugs, including diphenylhydantoin, isoniazid, nitrofurantoin, thalidomide, and vincristine. Multiple peripheral neuritis may occur in alcoholism, arteriosclerosis, beriberi, chronic GI disease, diabetes, leprosy, pellagra, porphyria, rheumatoid arthritis, systemic lupus erythematosus, and many infectious diseases. Therapy consists of removal of the toxic agent or treatment of the causative disease, rest, and medication for pain. Guillain-Barré syndrome sometimes occurs after an influenza vaccination. See also **Guillain-Barré syndrome.**

multiple personality, an abnormal condition in which the organization of the personality is fragmented. It is characterized by the presence of two or more distinct subpersonalities. Also called **split personality.**

multiple personality disorder, a dissociative disorder characterized by the existence of two or more distinct, clearly differentiated personality structures within the same individual, any of which may dominate at a particular time. Each personality is a complex unit with separate, well-developed emotional and thought processes, behavior patterns, and social relationships. The various subpersonalities are usually dramatically different from one another and may or may not be aware of the existence of the others.

multiple plasmacytoma of bone. See **multiple myeloma.**

multiple pregnancy, a pregnancy in which there is more than one fetus in the uterus at the same time.

multiple sclerosis (MS) [L, *multus* + *plica*, fold; Gk, *sclerosis,* hardening], a progressive disease characterized by disseminated demyelination of nerve fibers of the brain and spinal cord. It begins slowly, usually in young adulthood, and continues throughout life with periods of exacerbation and remission. The first signs are paresthesias, or abnormal sensations in the extremities or on one side of the face. Other early signs are muscle weakness, vertigo, and visual disturbances, such as nystagmus, diplopia (double vision), and partial blindness. Later in the course of disease there may be extreme emotional lability, ataxia, abnormal reflexes, and difficulty in urinating. Because many other conditions affect the nervous system and produce similar symptoms, the diagnosis of MS is difficult to make. A history of exacerbation and remission of symptoms and the presence of greater than normal amounts of protein in cerebrospinal fluid are characteristic. As the disease progresses, the intervals between exacerbations grow shorter and disability becomes greater. There is no specific treatment for the disease; corticosteroids and other drugs are used to treat the symptoms accompanying acute episodes. Physical therapy may help to postpone or prevent specific disabilities. The patient is encouraged to live as normal and active a life as possible. Also called **disseminated multiple sclerosis.**

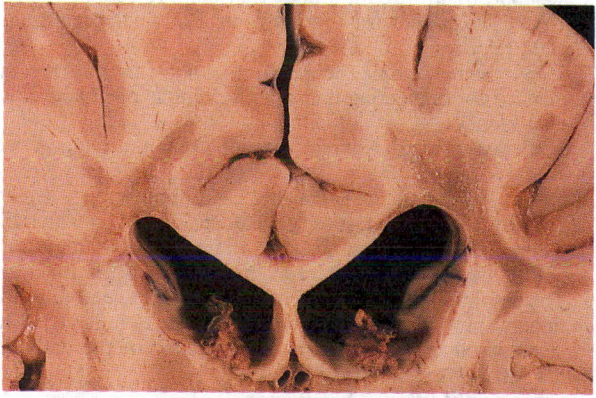

**Multiple sclerosis—demyelination in the
white matter**
(Okazaki, 1983)

multiple self-healing squamous epithelioma. See **keratoacanthoma.**

multiple transfusion syndrome [L, *multus,* many + *plica,* fold + *transfundere,* to pour through; Gk, *syn,* together + *dromos,* course], a hemorrhagic reaction to massive transfusions of platelet-poor stored blood. Other clotting factors seldom contribute to the condition. Platelet concentrates may be given to correct the deficiency.

multiplicative growth. See **merisis.**

multipolar mitosis /-pō′lər/ [L, *multus* + *polus,* pole], cell division in which the spindle has three or more poles and results in the formation of a corresponding number of daughter cells. Also called **multicentric mitosis, pluripolar mitosis.** See also **trisomy.**

multisource drug /mul′tisôrs/ [L, *multus* + OFr, *sourse,* origin], a drug that can be purchased under any of several trademarks from different manufacturers or distributors. See also **generic equivalent, generic name.**

multisynaptic /-sinap′tik/ [L, *multus* + Gk, *synaptein,* to join], pertaining to a nervous process or system of nerve cells requiring a series of synapses.

multivalent /mul′tivā′lənt/ [L, *multus* + *valere,* to be strong], **1.** (in chemistry) denoting the capacity of an element to combine with three or more univalent atoms. **2.** (in immunology) able to act against more than one strain of organism. Compare **valence.**

multivalent vaccine [L, *multus,* many + *valere,* value + *vaccinus,* cow], a vaccine prepared from several antigenic types within a species. Also called **polyvalent vaccine.**

mummification /mum′ifikā′shən/ [Per, *mum,* wax; L, *facere,* to make], a dried-up state, such as occurs in dry gangrene or a dead fetus in utero.

mummified fetus /mum′ifīd/, a fetus that has died in utero and has shriveled and dried up.

mumps [D, *mompen,* to sulk], an acute viral disease, characterized by a swelling of the parotid glands, caused by a paramyxovirus. It is most likely to affect children between 5 and 15 years of age, but it may occur at any age. In adulthood the infection may be severe. Passive immunity from maternal antibodies usually prevents this disease in children under 1 year of age. The incidence of mumps is highest during the late winter and early spring. The mumps paramyxovirus lives in the saliva of the affected individual and is transmitted in droplets or by direct contact. The virus is present in the saliva from 6 days before to 9 days after the onset of the swelling of the parotid gland. The time of maximum communicability is believed to be the 48-hour period immediately before the start of parotid swelling. The prognosis in mumps is good, but the disease sometimes involves complications, such as arthritis, pancreatitis, myocarditis, oophoritis, and nephritis. About one half of the men with mumps-induced orchitis suffer some atrophy of the testicles, but because the condition is usually unilateral, sterility rarely results. Also called **epidemic parotitis, infectious parotitis.**

■ OBSERVATIONS: The common symptoms of mumps usually last for about 24 hours and include anorexia, headache, malaise, and low-grade fever. These signs are commonly followed by earache, parotid gland swelling, and a temperature of 101° to 104° F (38.3° to 40° C). The patient also experiences pain when drinking acidic liquids or when chewing. The salivary glands also may become swollen. Complications, such as epididymoorchitis and mumps meningitis, may develop. About 25% of the postpubertal men who contract mumps develop epididymoorchitis with associated testicular swelling and tenderness that may persist for several weeks. Mumps meningitis develops in 10% of the patients with mumps and occurs in three to five times as many males as females. Diagnosis of mumps is usually based on typical symptoms, especially parotid gland swelling. If the parotid gland is not swollen, confirming diagnosis may be based on serologic antibody tests.

■ INTERVENTIONS: The treatment of mumps commonly includes the respiratory isolation of the patient and the administration of analgesics, antipyretics, and a fluid intake adequate to prevent dehydration associated with fever and anorexia. Intravenous fluids may be administered to the patient who cannot swallow as the result of severe parotitis.

■ NURSING CONSIDERATIONS: The patient is confined to bed and may be given antipyretics and tepid sponge baths to reduce fever. Patients with mumps are also encouraged to drink fluids and to avoid spicy foods and those that require considerable chewing. During the acute phase of the disease, the nurse is especially alert to any signs of central nervous system involvement, such as nuchal rigidity and altered consciousness. All cases of mumps are routinely reported to local health authorities. Nurses aid public health education by stressing the importance of immunization with live attenuated mumps virus for children at 15 months of age and for susceptible people, especially males who are approaching puberty or who are past puberty. Immunization within 24 hours of exposure may prevent the disease or may minimize its effects.

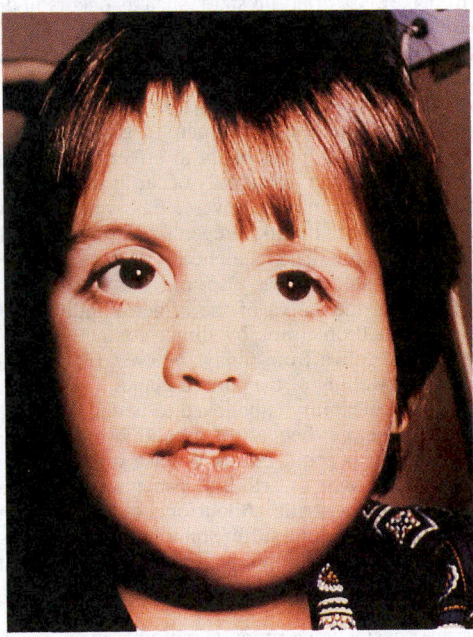

Mumps (Zitelli, 1992, Courtesy Dr. GDW McKendrik)

Mumpsvax,   a trademark for an active immunizing agent (live mumps virus vaccine).

mumps virus vaccine live,   an active immunizing agent.
- INDICATION: It is prescribed for immunization against mumps.
- CONTRAINDICATIONS: Immunosuppression, concomitant use of corticosteroids, acute infection, pregnancy, or known hypersensitivity to chicken proteins, neomycin, or this drug prohibits its use.
- ADVERSE EFFECTS: Among the most serious adverse effects are fevers, parotitis, and allergic reactions.

Munchausen's syndrome /mun′chousənz/ [Baron von Münchausen, b. 1720, German adventurer and confabulator],   an unusual condition characterized by habitual pleas for treatment and hospitalization for a symptomatic but imaginary acute illness. The affected person may logically and convincingly present the symptoms and history of a real disease. Symptoms resolve with treatment, but the person may seek further treatment for another imaginary disease. Also called **pathomimicry.**

mural /myoo′rəl/ [L, murus, wall],   something that is found on or against the wall of a cavity, such as a mural thrombus on an interior wall of the heart.

muriatic acid /moo′rē·at′ik/ [L, muria, brine; acidus, sour],   hydrochloric acid.

Murchison fever.   See **Pel-Ebstein fever.**

murine typhus /myoo′rēn/ [L, mus, mouse; Gk, typhos, stupor],   an acute arbovirus infection caused by Rickettsia typhi and transmitted by the bite of an infected flea. The disease is similar to epidemic typhus but less severe. It is characterized by headache, chills, fever, myalgia, and rash. After an 8- to 16-day incubation period, fever develops and lasts about 12 days. A dull-red, maculopapular rash, mainly on the trunk, appears about the fifth day and lasts for 4 to 8 days. Recovery is usually rapid and complete, but death has occurred in elderly or debilitated people. Weil-Felix and complement fixation tests aid in the diagnosis. Chloramphenicol or tetracycline is usually prescribed in treatment. Prevention involves the elimination of the rodents that are the natural host of the organism and the use of appropriate insecticides to control fleas. Also called **endemic typhus, flea-borne typhus, New World typhus, rat typhus, urban typhus.** Compare **epidemic typhus, Rocky Mountain spotted fever.** See also **Brill-Zinsser disease.**

murmur /mur′mər/ [L, a humming],   a low-pitched fluttering or humming sound, such as a heart murmur.

muromonab-CD3 /myoo′rəmon′ab/,   a parenteral immunosuppressant drug for kidney transplant rejection.
- INDICATIONS: It is used in the control of acute renal transplant rejection.
- CONTRAINDICATIONS: The product is not currently recommended for preventing transplant rejections of organs other than kidneys.
- ADVERSE EFFECTS: Adverse reactions reported include pulmonary edema, fever, chills, breathing difficulty, chest pain, vomiting, nausea, diarrhea, and tremors.

Murphy's sign,   a test for gallbladder disease in which the patient is asked to inspire while the examiner's fingers are held under the liver border at the bottom of the rib cage. The inspiration causes the gallbladder to descend onto the fingers, producing pain if the gallbladder is inflamed. The test is used in the diagnosis of carcinoma of the gallbladder, as well as cholecystitis.

muscae volitantes.   See **floater.**

muscarine /mus′kəren/ [L, musca, fly],   a choline-related alkaloid present in the poisonous mushroom Amanita muscaria. It is similar pharmacologically to acetylcholine, although it is not used in therapeutics.

muscarinic /mus′kərin′ik/ [L, musca, fly],   stimulating the postganglionic parasympathetic receptor.

muscle /mus′əl/ [L, musculus],   a kind of tissue composed of fibers that are able to contract, causing and allowing movement of the parts and organs of the body. Muscle fibers are richly vascular, irritable, conductive, and elastic. There are two basic kinds, striated muscle and smooth muscle. Striated muscle, which comprises all skeletal muscles except for the myocardium, is long and voluntary; it responds very quickly to stimulation and is paralyzed by interruption of its innervation. Smooth muscle, which comprises all visceral muscles, is short and involuntary; it reacts slowly to all stimuli and does not entirely lose its tone if innervation is interrupted. The myocardium is sometimes classified as a third (cardiac) kind of muscle, but it is basically a striated muscle that does not contract as quickly as the striated muscle of the rest of the body, and it is not completely paralyzed if it loses its neural stimuli. See also **cardiac muscle, smooth muscle, striated muscle.**

muscle albumin,   albumin present in muscle.

muscle biopsy [L, *musculus*; Gk, *bios,* life, *opsis,* view], an examination of surgically removed muscle tissue for diagnosis.

muscle bridge,   a band of myocardial tissue over one or more of the large epicardial coronary vessels. It may cause constriction of the artery during systole.

muscle of expression.   See **facial muscle.**

muscle reeducation,   the use of physical therapeutic exercises to restore muscle tone and strength after an injury or disease.

muscle relaxant,   a chemotherapeutic agent that reduces the contractility of muscle fibers. Curare derivatives and succinylcholine compete with acetylcholine and block neural transmission at the myoneural junction. These drugs are used during anesthesia, in the management of patients undergoing mechanical ventilation, and in shock therapy, to reduce muscle contractions in pharmacologically or electrically induced seizures. Quinine sulfate, prescribed for the prevention and treatment of nocturnal leg cramps, reduces muscle tension by increasing the refractory period of muscle fibers and by decreasing the excitability of the motor end plate. Several drugs that relieve muscle spasms act at various levels in the central nervous system: Baclofen inhibits monosynaptic and polysynaptic reflexes at the spinal level; cyclobenzaprine acts primarily in the brainstem; chlorzoxazone inhibits multisynaptic arcs in the spinal cord and subcortical areas of the brain; and the benzodiazepines reduce muscle tension, chiefly by acting on reticular neuronal mechanisms that control muscle tone. Dantrolene acts directly on muscles in reducing contraction and apparently achieves its effect by interfering with the release of calcium from the sarcoplasmic reticulum.

muscle-setting exercise,   a method of maintaining muscle strength and tonality by alternately contracting and relaxing a skeletal muscle or any group of muscles without moving the associated part of the body. Such activity is useful in preventing atrophy of the muscles, especially in patients with conditions involving the joints.

muscles of ventilation [L, *musculus* + *respirare,* to breathe],   muscles that provide inspiration, partly by increasing the volume of the chest cavity so that air is drawn into the lungs, including the diaphragm and external intercostals. They are aided during forced breathing by the scaleni, levatores costarum, sternocleidomastoideus, greater pectoral, platysma myoides, and superior posterior serratus. Muscles of forced expiration include the external and internal oblique, rectus abdominus and transverse abdominus.

muscle spindle [L, *musculus*; AS, *spinel*],   a specialized proprioceptive sensory organ composed of a bundle of fine striated intrafusal muscle fibers innervated by gamma nerve fibers. Their nuclei are gathered together near the center of each fiber to form a nuclear sac, which is surrounded in turn by sensory, annulospiral nerve endings, all enclosed in a fibrous sheath.

muscle testing,   a method of evaluating the contractile unit, including the muscle, tendons, and associated tissues, of a moving part of the body by neurologic or resistance testing. The tests may include shortened, middle, and lengthened range-of-motion ability; isokinetic measurement of muscle strength, power, and endurance; and functional tests, such as jogging or specific agility drills, as well as radiograpy, arthroscopy, electromyography, and other medical tests.

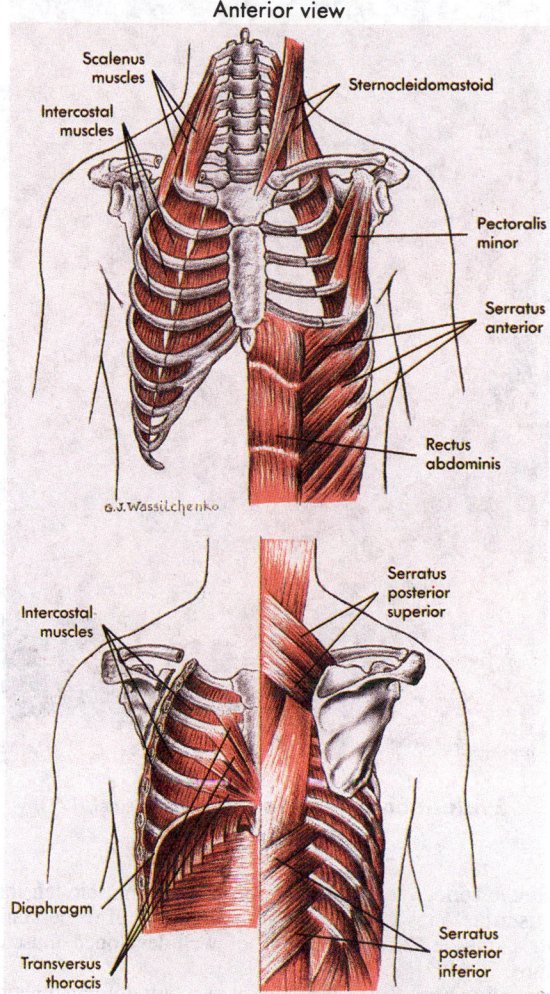

Anterior view

Scalenus muscles

Intercostal muscles

Sternocleidomastoid

Pectoralis minor

Serratus anterior

Rectus abdominis

G.J.Wassilchenko

Serratus posterior superior

Intercostal muscles

Diaphragm

Transversus thoracis

Serratus posterior inferior

Posterior view
Muscles of ventilation
(Wilson, 1990)

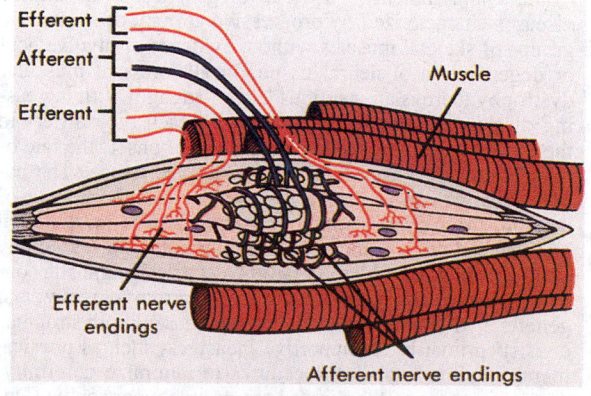

Efferent

Afferent

Efferent

Muscle

Efferent nerve endings

Afferent nerve endings

Muscle spindle *(Seeley, 1992/Michael Schenk)*

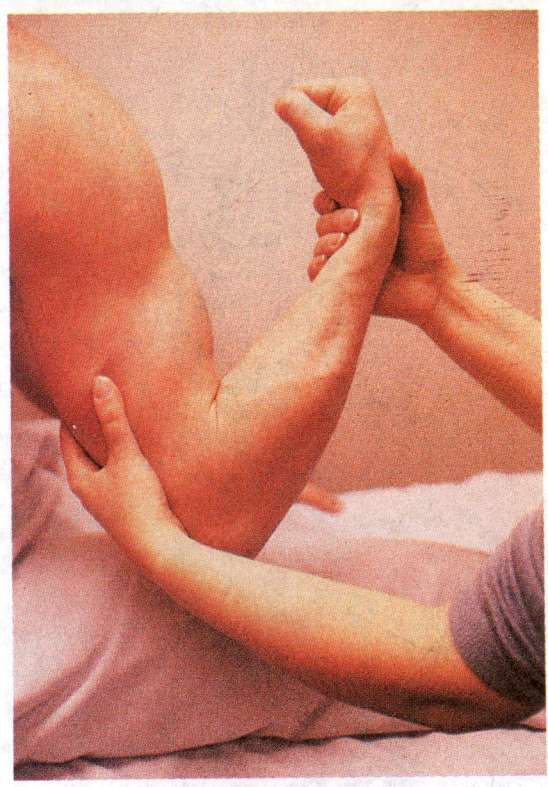

Evaluation of muscle strength *(Seidel, 1991)*

muscle tone,   a normal state of balanced muscle tension.

muscular /mus′kyələr/ [L, *musculus*],   **1.** of or pertaining to a muscle. **2.** characteristic of well-developed musculature.

muscular atrophy,   a condition of motor unit dysfunction, usually the result of a loss of efferent innervation.

muscular branch of the deep brachial artery,   one of several similar branches of the deep brachial artery, supplying certain arm muscles, such as the coracobrachialis, biceps brachii, and brachialis.

muscular dystrophy (MD) [L, *musculus* + Gk, *dys*, bad, *trophe*, nourishment],   a group of genetically transmitted diseases characterized by progressive atrophy of symmetric groups of skeletal muscles without evidence of involvement or degeneration of neural tissue. In all forms of muscular dystrophy there is an insidious loss of strength with increasing disability and deformity, although each type differs in the groups of muscles affected, the age of onset, the rate of progression, and the mode of genetic inheritance. The basic cause is unknown but appears to be an inborn error of metabolism. Serum creatine phosphokinase is increased in affected individuals and acts as a diagnostic aid, especially in asymptomatic children in families at risk. Diagnostic confirmation is made by muscle biopsy, electromyography, and genetic pedigree. Treatment of the muscular dystrophies consists primarily of supportive measures, such as physical therapy and orthopedic procedures to minimize deformity. The main types of the disease are pseudohypertrophic (Du-

chenne) muscular dystrophy, limb-girdle muscular dystrophy, and facioscapulohumeral (Landouzy-Déjérine) muscular dystrophy. Rarer forms include Becker's muscular dystrophy, distal muscular dystrophy, ocular myopathy, and myotonic muscular dystrophy. See also **myotonic myopathy.**

muscular incompetence [L, *musculus*; *incompetens*],   a failure of a cardiac valve to close properly because of incompetence of the papillary muscles of the heart.

muscular sarcoidosis,   sarcoidosis of the skeletal muscles in which there is interstitial inflammation, fibrosis, atrophy, and damage of the muscle fibers as sarcoid tubercles form within and replace normal muscle cells. See also **sarcoidosis.**

muscular system,   all of the muscles of the body, including the smooth, cardiac, and striated muscles, considered as an interrelated structural group. See also the Color Atlas of Human Anatomy.

muscular tension [L, *musculus* + *tendere*, to stretch],   strain that results from muscular contractions. Internal tension is caused by crossbridge activity between the actin and myosin filaments within the muscle fiber. The force generated by these contractile elements is transmitted to the bones via tendons and connective tissue. The bones move and produce external tension.

muscular tone [L, *musculus*; Gk, *tonos*, stretching],   a normal degree of tension in muscles at rest.

muscular tremor [L, *musculus* + *tremor*, shaking],   minute regular involuntary contraction of individual muscle fasciculi. If the tremors are mild and occasional, the cause may be physiologic. Profuse, persistent or recurrent widespread muscular twitching often indicates a motor neuron disorder.

muscular triangle.   See **inferior carotid triangle.**

muscular tumor.   See **myoma.**

musculature /mus′kyəlā′chər/,   the arrangement and condition of the muscles.

musculo- /mus′kyəlō-/,   a combining form meaning 'muscle'.

musculocutaneous nerve /mus′kyo͞olōyo͞otā′nē·əs/ [L, *musculus* + *cutis*, skin, *osus*, having],   one of the terminal branches of the brachial plexus. It is formed on each side by division of the lateral cord of the plexus into two branches. It pierces the coracobrachialis and crosses to the lateral side of the arm, where it pierces the deep fascia just above the elbow and continues into the forearm as the lateral antebrachial cutaneous nerve. Various branches and filaments supply different structures, such as the biceps, the brachialis, the humerus, and the skin of the forearm. The branches of the musculocutaneous nerve are the coracobrachialis branch, the muscular branches, an articular filament to the elbow joint, a filament to the humerus, the lateral antebrachial cutaneous nerve, the anterior branch, and the dorsal branch. Compare **median nerve, radial nerve, ulnar nerve.**

musculoskeletal /mus′kyo͞olōskel′ətəl/ [L, *musculus* + Gk, *skeletos*, dried up],   of or pertaining to the muscles and the skeleton.

musculoskeletal system,   all of the muscles, bones, joints, and related structures, such as the tendons and connective tissue, that function in the movement of the parts and organs of the body. See also the Color Atlas of Human Anatomy.

musculoskeletal system assessment, an evaluation of the condition and functioning of the patient's muscles, joints, and bones and of factors that may contribute to abnormalities in these body structures.

■ METHOD: The patient is questioned about any pain and edema in muscles, joints, and bones, weakness in extremities, limitations in movements and activities, unsteadiness on the feet, fatigability, insomnia, anorexia, weight loss, and feelings of frustration. The individual's general appearance, age, blood pressure, pulse, respirations, body alignment, ability or inability to move in bed, gait, need for assistance in walking, handgrip, range of motion, and internal and external rotation of extremities are observed. The presence of contractures, deformities, paralysis, contusions, lacerations, wounds, footdrop, wristdrop, paralysis, crutches, brace, cast, prosthesis, cane, walker, decubiti, allergies, skin rash, or tenseness is noted. It is ascertained whether the patient can perform activities of daily living and is able to sit up, turn, and use the trapeze in bed; whether constipation is a complaint; and whether the individual is independent or dependent. Concurrent diseases or conditions investigated include injury to the spinal cord, nerve impairment, cerebrovascular accident, rheumatoid arthritis, osteoarthritis, bursitis, polyneuritis, multiple sclerosis, muscular dystrophy, myasthenia gravis, fracture, ruptured disk, Méniére's disease, and labyrinthitis. It is determined whether the patient previously had orthopedic or spinal surgery, poliomyelitis, hemiplegia, cerebral palsy, parkinsonism, a cerebrovascular accident, ataxia, syphilis, hyperparathyroidism, osteoporosis, rickets, osteomalacia, tuberculosis, alcoholism, and impaired vision or hearing. A family history of carcinoma, diabetes, or tuberculosis, the patient's involvement in a hazardous job or recreation, history of previous accidents, and the use of tobacco or medications, such as steroids, sedatives, tranquilizers, analgesics, antimalarials, acetylsalicylic acid, or indomethacin, are determined. Laboratory studies important for the assessment are assays of serum and urine calcium and phosphorus and of alkaline

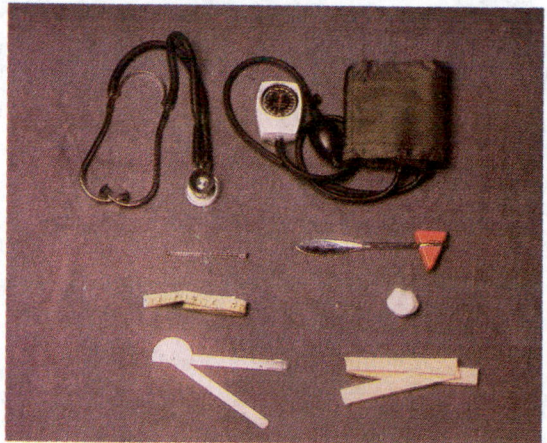

Equipment for musculoskeletal system assessment
(Mourad, 1991)

phosphatase serum level. Diagnostic procedures that may be required include x-ray films of bones, arthrograms, myelograms, arteriograms, arthroscopy, biopsies of bone or muscle, incision and drainage of joints, and electromyograms of muscles.

■ NURSING INTERVENTION: The nurse conducts the interview to obtain subjective data, makes the necessary observations of the patient, and assembles the information on concurrent and previous disorders, the family history, the patient's social and medication background, and the results of laboratory studies and diagnostic procedures.

■ OUTCOME CRITERIA: A meticulous assessment of the patient's musculoskeletal system is a valuable aid in diagnosis, in planning the course of therapy, and in predicting the prognosis.

musculospiral nerve. See **radial nerve.**

mush bite, a procedure used in making dental impressions for the construction of full or partial dentures. The patient brings his upper and lower jaws together into a block of softened wax, thus supplying a spatial relationship between the maxilla and mandible.

mushroom [ME, *mucheron*], the fruiting body of the fungus of the class Basidomycetes, especially edible members of the order Agaricales, commonly known as the field mushrooms or meadow mushrooms. Although mushrooms contain some protein and minerals, they are composed largely of water and are of limited nutritional value. Fungal poisoning is caused by ingestion of mushrooms of the genus *Amanita,* in particular *A. muscaria* and *A. phalloides.* Symptoms, caused by toxic peptides, may appear within a few minutes of ingestion and consist of severe abdominal pain, vomiting, extreme nausea, salivation, sweating, diarrhea, excessive thirst, coma, and, occasionally, convulsion. Extensive damage to the liver, kidneys, and central nervous system may occur. Some mushrooms, especially *Psilocybe mexicana,* contain substances that produce hallucinatory states.

mushroom poisoning, a toxic condition caused by the ingestion of certain mushrooms, particularly two species of the genus *Amanita.* Muscarine in *Amanita muscaria* produces intoxication in from a few minutes to 2 hours. Symptoms include lacrimation, salivation, sweating, vomiting, labored breathing, abdominal cramps, diarrhea, and, in severe cases, convulsions, coma, and circulatory failure. Atropine is usually administered in treatment. More deadly but slower-acting phalloidine in *A. phalloides* and *A. verna* causes similar symptoms, as well as liver damage, renal failure, and death in 30% to 50% of the cases. Treatment varies. Intensive care, as for kidney or liver failure, and hemodialysis may reduce mortality. In some people, the consumption of alcohol complicates mushroom poisoning, and the combination has the effect of disulfiram.

music therapy [Gk, *mousike,* music; *therapeia,* treatment], a form of adjunctive psychotherapy in which music is used as a means of recreation and communication, especially with autistic children, and as a means to elevate the mood of depressed and psychotic patients.

mustard gas /mus'tərd/, a poisonous gas used in chemical warfare during World War I. It causes corrosive destruction of the skin and mucous membranes, often resulting in permanent respiratory damage and death.

mustard plaster [L, *mustum;* Gk, *emplastron*], a mustard medication in a fabric base that can be placed close to the skin for a period of time as a counter-irritant in the form of a poultice.

Mustargen, a trademark for an antineoplastic (mechlorethamine hydrochloride).

-mustine, a combining form for antineoplastic agents, particularly [B-chlorethyl] amine derivatives.

mutacism /myōō'təsiz'əm/, mimmation, or the incorrect use of /m/ sounds.

mutagen /myōō'təjən/ [L, *mutare*, to change, *genein*, to produce], any chemical or physical environmental agent that induces a genetic mutation or increases the mutation rate. **—mutagenic,** *adj.,* **mutagenicity,** *n.*

mutagenesis /myōō'təjen'əsis/, the induction or occurrence of a genetic mutation. See also **teratogenesis.**

Mutamycin, a trademark for an antineoplastic (mitomycin).

mutant /myōō'tənt/ [L, *mutare*, to change], **1.** any individual or organism with genetic material that has undergone mutation. **2.** relating to or produced by mutation.

mutant gene, any gene that has undergone a change, such as the loss, gain, or exchange of genetic material, that affects the normal transmission and expression of a trait. Such genes can become inactive or show reduced, increased, or antagonistic activity. Kinds of mutant genes are **amorph, antimorph, hypermorph, hypomorph.**

mutase /myōō'tās/, any enzyme that catalyzes the shifting of a chemical group or radical from one position to another within the same molecule or, occasionally, from one molecule to another.

mutation /myōōtā'shən/ [L, *mutare*, to change], an unusual change in genetic material occurring spontaneously or by induction. The alteration changes the original expression of the gene. Genes are stable units, but when a mutation occurs, it often is transmitted to future generations. **—mutate,** *v.,* **mutational,** adj.

mutism /myōō'tizəm/ [L, *mutus*, mute], the inability to speak because of a physical defect or emotional problem.

muton /myōō'ton/, (in molecular genetics), the smallest DNA segment whose alteration can result in a mutation.

mutually exclusive categories /myōō'chōō·əlē/, categories on a research instrument that are sufficiently precise to allow each subject, factor, or variable to be classified in only one category.

mutual support group, a type of group in which members organize to solve their own problems. They are led by the group members themselves who share a common goal and use their own strengths to gain control over their lives.

mv, mV, abbreviation for **millivolt.**

mVo₂, symbol for *myocardial oxygen consumption*.

MVV, abbreviation for *maximal voluntary ventilation*. See **maximal breathing capacity.**

M.W.I.A., abbreviation for **Medical Women's International Association.**

MX gene, a human gene that helps the body resist viral infections. When exposed to interferon, the MX gene inhibits the production of viral protein and nucleic acid necessary for the proliferation of new viral particles. Presence of the gene helps explain why some individuals are better able to resist certain viral infections, such as influenza, than other people.

my-. See **myo-.**

myalgia /mī·al'jə/ [Gk, *mys*, muscle, *algos*, pain], diffuse muscle pain, usually accompanied by malaise.

myalgic asthenia /mī·al'jik/ [Gk, *mys* + *algos*, pain; *a,*

sthenos, not strength], a condition characterized by a general feeling of fatigue and muscular pain, often resulting from or associated with psychologic stress.

Myambutol, a trademark for an antibacterial (ethambutol hydrochloride).

myasthenia /mī'əsthē'nē·ə/ [Gk, *mys* + *a, sthenos,* not strength], a condition characterized by an abnormal weakness of a muscle or a group of muscles that may be the result of a systemic myoneural disturbance, such as in myasthenia gravis, or myasthenia laryngis involving the vocal cord tensor muscles. **—myasthenic,** *adj.*

myasthenia gravis, an abnormal condition characterized by the chronic fatigability and weakness of muscles, especially in the face and throat, as a result of a defect in the conduction of nerve impulses at the myoneural junction.

■ OBSERVATIONS: Muscular fatigability in myasthenia gravis is caused by the inability of receptors at the myoneural junction to depolarize because of a deficiency of acetylcholine; hence the diagnosis may be made by administering an anticholinesterase drug and observing improved muscle strength and stamina. The onset of symptoms is usually gradual, with ptosis of the upper eyelids, diplopia, and weakness of the facial muscles. The weakness may then extend to other muscles innervated by the cranial nerves, particularly the respiratory muscles. Muscular exertion aggravates the symptoms, which typically vary over the course of the day. The disease occurs in younger women more often than in older women and in men over 60 years of age more often than in younger men.

■ INTERVENTIONS: Anticholinesterase drugs are given. The edrophonium test is used to determine the optimal maintenance dose. Neostigmine or pyridostigmine is the drug most often used.

■ NURSING CONSIDERATIONS: Physical activity is restricted, and bed rest encouraged. Anticholinesterase drugs are usually administered before meals, and the patient is monitored for toxic side effects. Myasthenic crisis may require emergency

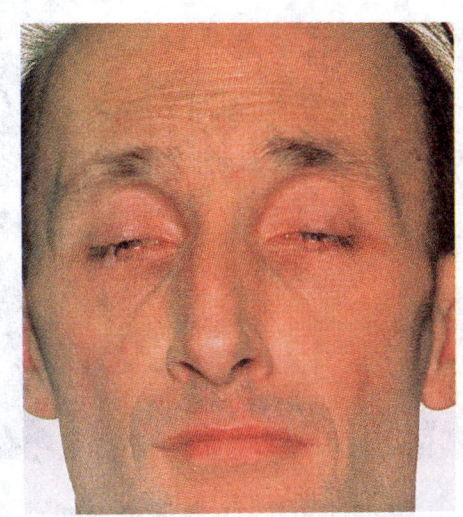

Myasthenia gravis (Perkin, 1986)

respiratory assistance. The patient's diet may have to be adjusted if the ability to chew and swallow is affected.

myasthenia gravis crisis, acute exacerbation of the muscular weakness characterizing the disease, triggered by infection, surgery, emotional stress, or an overdose or insufficiency of anticholinesterase medication.

■ OBSERVATIONS: Typical signs and symptoms include respiratory distress progressing to periods of apnea, extreme fatigue, increased muscular weakness, dysphagia, dysarthria, and fever. The patient may be anxious, restless, irritable, and unable to move the jaws or to raise one or both eyelids. If the condition is caused by anticholinesterase toxicity, there may be anorexia, nausea, vomiting, abdominal cramps, diarrhea, excessive salivation, sweating, lacrimation, blurred vision, vertigo, and muscle cramps and spasms, as well as general weakness, dysarthria, and respiratory distress.

■ INTERVENTIONS: Initial treatment is directed to maintaining patency of the airway. Oxygen with assisted or controlled ventilation is administered, procedures such as a tracheostomy may be performed, and bronchoscopy may be indicated. The patient is placed in a bed in which the head is elevated 30 degrees. The withdrawal or reduction of anticholinergic drugs may be ordered, or they may be given to differentiate the kind of crisis. Respiratory secretions and saliva are suctioned, and blood pressure, pulse, and respiration are carefully observed. The chest is auscultated, and the rectal temperature is taken every 2 to 4 hours; cooling measures may be necessary. Parenteral fluids, antibiotics, nasogastric feeding, and the insertion of an indwelling catheter with closed gravity drainage may be ordered. The patient is turned every 2 hours and given mouth and skin care every 2 to 4 hours; the lips are kept well lubricated and decubiti are avoided by using an air mattress and by keeping the skin dry at all times. If an eyelid is affected, the eye may be covered with a patch; crusts are removed whenever required, and soothing eyedrops may be administered. To enable the patient to communicate, the call bell and a pad and pencil or magic slate are placed within reach. When the acute crisis subsides, the patient may progress from clear liquids to a soft diet but may require help in eating. Nourishment is offered between meals, and a daily intake of up to 2000 ml of fluids is encouraged. Walking as tolerated and other activities are planned at the time of the maximum effect of medication. Active or passive range-of-motion exercises of all extremities are performed several times a day, but rest periods are maintained to avoid fatigue and relapse.

■ NURSING CONSIDERATIONS: Before discharge the patient is instructed on the importance of taking the prescribed medication with milk, crackers, or bread at the scheduled time and of reporting toxic side effects and symptoms of recurrent or progressive disease. The nurse points out the need to maintain a regular diet, to exercise to tolerance, to rest, and to avoid infections and exposure to hot or cold weather and the use of alcohol and tobacco. The nurse's help in planning a schedule that conserves energy for essential activities can enable the patient to be relatively independent and self-sufficient.

myasthenic crisis /mī'asthen'ik/, an acute episode of muscular weakness.

myc-. See **myco-.**

mycelium /mīsē'lē·əm/, *pl.* **mycelia** [Gk, *mykes*, fungus, *helos*, nail], a mass of interwoven, branched, threadlike filaments that make up most fungi. Also called **hypha.**

mycetismus /mī'sitiz'məs/, mushroom poisoning.

myceto-. See **myco-.**

mycetoma /mī'sətō'mə/ [Gk, *mykes* + *oma*, tumor], a serious fungal infection involving skin, subcutaneous tissue, fascia, and bone. One kind of mycetoma is **Madura foot.**

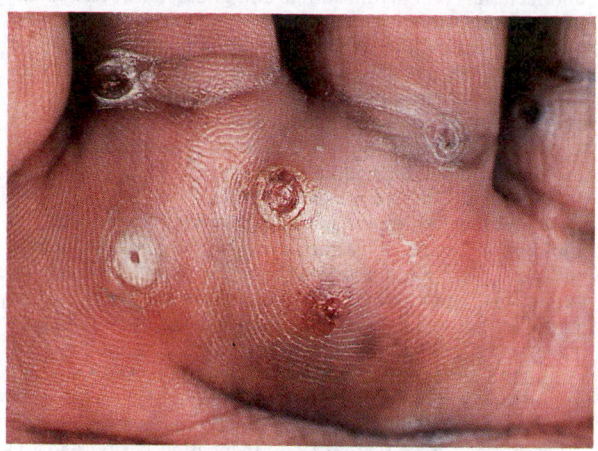

Mycetoma (du Vivier, 1993, Courtesy Dr. Rod Hay)

-mycin, a suffix for antibiotics produced by Streptomyces strains.

Mycitracin, a trademark for a topical, fixed-combination drug containing antibacterials (polymyxin B sulfate, bacitracin, and neomycin sulfate).

myco-, myc-, myceto-, myko-, a combining form meaning 'related to fungus': *mycobacteriosis, mycohemia, mycophage.*

mycobacteria /mī'kōbaktir'ē·ə/ [Gk, *mykes* + *bakterion*, little rod], acid-fast microorganisms belonging to the genus *Mycobacterium*. **—mycobacterial,** *adj.*

mycobacteriosis /mī'kōbak'tirē·ō'sis/ [Gk, *mykes, bakterion* + *osis*, condition], a tuberculosislike disease caused by mycobacteria other than *Mycobacterium tuberculosis*.

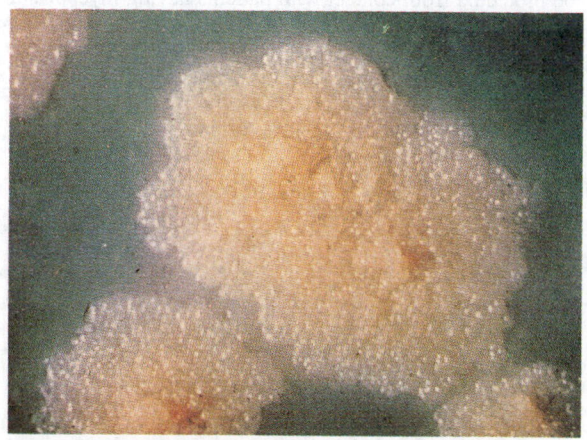

***Mycobacterium tuberculosis* colonies** (Baron, 1990)

Mycobacterium /mī′kōbaktir′ē·əm/ [Gk, *mykes* + *bakterion*, little rod], a genus of rod-shaped, acid-fast bacteria having two significant pathogenic species: *Mycobacterium leprae* causes leprosy; *M. tuberculosis* causes tuberculosis.

Mycolog, a trademark for a topical fixed-combination drug containing a glucocorticoid (triamcinolone acetonide), two antibacterials (neomycin sulfate and gramicidin), and an antifungal (nystatin).

mycology /mīkol′əjē/ [Gk, *mykes* + *logos*, science], the study of fungi and fungoid diseases. —**mycologic, mycological,** *adj.,* **mycologist,** *n.*

mycomyringitis. See **myringomycosis.**

mycophenolic acid /mī′kōfinō′lik/, a bacteriostatic and fungistatic crystalline antibiotic obtained from *Pencillium brevi compactum* and related species.

Mycoplasma /mī′kōplaz′mə/ [Gk, *mykes* + *plassein*, to mold], a genus of ultramicroscopic organisms lacking rigid cell walls and considered to be the smallest free-living organisms. Some are saprophytes, some are parasites, and many are pathogens. One species is a cause of mycoplasma pneumonia, tracheobronchitis, pharyngitis, and bullous myringitis. See also **pleuropneumonia-like organism.**

mycoplasma pneumonia, a contagious disease of children and young adults caused by *Mycoplasma pneumoniae,* characterized by a 9- to 12-day incubation period and followed by symptoms of an upper respiratory infection, dry cough, and fever. Also called **Eaton-agent pneumonia, primary atypical pneumonia, walking pneumonia.** See also **cold agglutinin.**

■ OBSERVATIONS: Harsh or diminished breath sounds and fine inspiratory rales are frequently heard. Pulmonary infiltrates visible on chest x-ray films may resemble bacterial or viral pneumonia and may persist for 3 weeks in untreated cases. Rarely, complications, such as sinusitis, pleurisy, polyneuritis, myocarditis, or Stevens-Johnson syndrome, may follow the pneumonia. In untreated adults prolonged cough, weakness, and malaise are common. Diagnosis is suggested by physical examination and by observation of the clinical course and elevated cold agglutinins and is confirmed by a complement fixation test. Prognosis is favorable.

■ INTERVENTIONS: Erythromycin or tetracycline, bed rest, a high-protein diet, and an adequate intake of fluids are recommended. It is important that infants and people for whom a respiratory illness would be a particular hazard avoid or be protected from contact with patients having mycoplasma pneumonia.

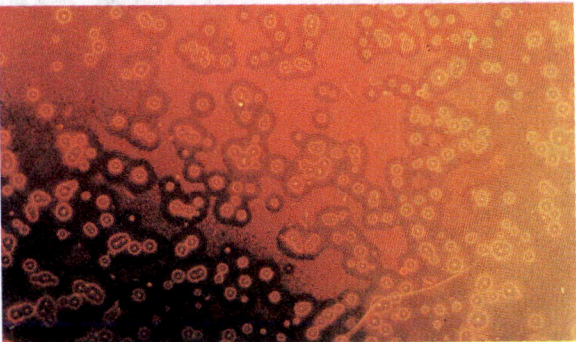

Mycoplasma pneumoniae (Baron, 1990)

mycosis /mīkō′sis/ [Gk, *mykes* + *osis*, condition], any disease caused by a fungus. Some kinds of mycoses are **athlete's foot, candidiasis,** and **coccidioidomycosis.** —**mycotic,** *adj.*

mycosis fungoides /fung·goi′dēz/, a rare, chronic, lymphomatous skin malignancy resembling eczema or a cutaneous tumor that is followed by microabscesses in the epidermis and lesions simulating those of Hodgkin's disease in lymph nodes and viscera. The condition is considered a distinctive entity by some specialists and a cutaneous manifestation of a malignant lymphoma by others.

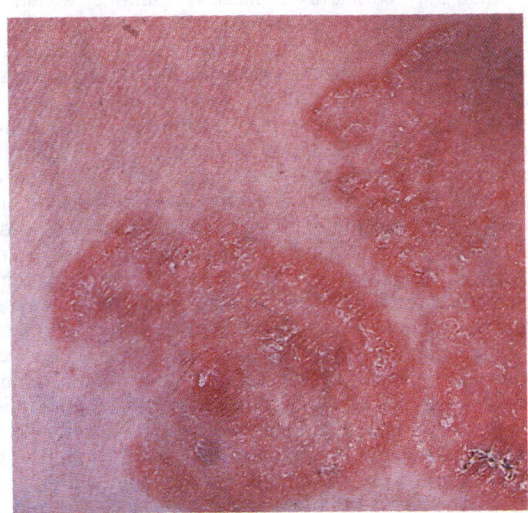

Mycosis fungoides (du Vivier, 1986)

Mycostatin, a trademark for an antifungal (nystatin).

mycotic /mīkot′ik/ [Gk, *mykes*, fungus], pertaining to a disease caused by a fungus.

mycotic aneurysm, a localized dilatation in the wall of a blood vessel caused by the growth of a fungus, usually occurring as a complication of bacterial endocarditis. See also **bacterial aneurysm.**

mycotoxicosis /mī′kōtok′sikō′sis/ [Gk, *mykes* + *toxikon,* poison, *osis,* condition], a systemic poisoning caused by toxins produced by fungal organisms.

mydriasis /midrī′əsis/ [Gk, *mydros,* hot mass], **1.** dilatation of the pupil of the eye caused by contraction of the dilator muscle of the iris, a muscular sheath that radiates outward like the spokes of a wheel from the center of the iris around the pupil. With a decrease in light or the pharmacologic action of certain drugs the dilator acts to pull the iris outward, enlarging the pupil. **2.** an abnormal condition characterized by contraction of the dilator muscle, resulting in widely dilated pupils. Compare **miosis.** —**mydriatic** /mid′rē·at′ik/, *adj.*

mydriatic and cycloplegic agent [Gk, *mydros* + *kyklos,* circle, *plege,* stroke], any one of several ophthalmic pharmaceutic preparations that dilate the pupil and paralyze the ocular muscles of accommodation. Mydriatics stimulate the sympathetic nerve fibers or block parasympathetic nerve fibers of the eye, temporarily paralyzing the iris sphincter muscle. Cycloplegics temporarily paralyze accommodation while relaxing the ciliary muscle. These drugs are used in diagnostic and refractive examination of the eye, before and after various procedures in eye surgery, in some tests for glaucoma, in the treatment of anterior uveitis, and in treating certain kinds of glaucoma. Blurred vision, thirst, flushing, fever, and rash may occur. In children and elderly people, ataxia, somnolence, delirium, and hallucination may occur but are rare. Among these drugs are atropine, cyclopentolate, homatropine, scopolamine, and tropicamide; they are prepared in solution for topical ophthalmic application.

myel-.   See **myelo-.**

myelacephalus /mī'ələsef'ələs/ [Gk, *myelos*, marrow, *a, kephale*, not head], a fetal monster, usually a separate monozygotic twin, whose form and parts are barely recognizable; a slightly differentiated amorphous mass. **—myelacephalous,** *adj.*

myelatelia /mī'əlatē'lē·ə/ [Gk, *myelos* + *atelia*, unfinished], any developmental defect involving the spinal cord.

myelauxe /mī'əlôk'sē/ [Gk, *myelos* + *auxe* increasing], a developmental anomaly characterized by hypertrophy of the spinal cord.

myelencephalon /mī'əlensef'əlon/, the lower part of the embryonic hindbrain from which the medulla oblongata develops.

-myelia, a suffix meaning '(condition of the) spinal cord': *atelomyelia, hydromyelia, syringomyelia.*

myelin /mī'əlin/ [Gk, *myelos*, marrow], a substance constituting the sheaths of various nerve fibers throughout the body. It is largely composed of fat, which gives the fibers a white, creamy color. **—myelinic,** *adj.*

myelinated /mī'əlinā'tid/, (of a nerve) having a myelin sheath.

myelination /mī'əlinā'shən/ [Gk, *myelos* + L, *atio*, process], the process of furnishing or taking on myelin.

myelin globule, a fatlike droplet found in some sputum.

myelinic /mī'əlin'ik/ [Gk, *myelos* + L, *icus*, form of], of or pertaining to myelin.

myelinic neuroma, a neuroma neoplasm composed of myelinated nerve fibers.

myelinization /mī'əlin'īzā'shən/ [Gk, *myelos* + *izein*, to cause], development of the myelin sheath around a nerve fiber. Also called **myelinogenesis.**

myelinolysis /mī'əlinol'isis/ [Gk, *myelos* + *lysein*, to loosen], a pathologic process that dissolves the myelin sheaths around certain nerve fibers, such as those of the pons in alcoholic and undernourished people who are afflicted with central pontine myelinolysis.

myelin sheath, a segmented, fatty lamination composed of myelin that wraps the axons of many nerves in the body. In myelinated peripheral nerves, the sheaths are composed of Schwann cells. The myelin sheaths around the central nerve fibers are composed of oligodendroglia. Their lipoid content gives these coverings a whitish appearance. In the peripheral nerves the sheaths are interrupted every 1 to 2 cm by the nodes of Ranvier, which occur only rarely in the fibers of the central nervous system. The usual thickness of the myelin sheath is between 2 and 10 μm. Various diseases, such as multiple sclerosis, can destroy these myelin wrappings.

myelitis /mī'əlī'tis/, an abnormal condition characterized by inflammation of the spinal cord with associated motor or sensory dysfunction. Some kinds of myelitis are **acute transverse myelitis, leukomyelitis,** and **poliomyelitis. —myelitic,** *adj.*

myelo- /mī'əlō-/, **myel-,** a prefix meaning 'related to the spinal cord or bone marrow': *myeloblast, myelocyte, myelomenia.*

myeloblast /mī'əlōblast'/ [Gk, *myelos* + *blastos*, germ], one of the earliest precursors of the granulocytic leukocytes. The cytoplasm appears light blue, scanty, and nongranular when seen in a stained blood smear through a microscope. The nucleus contains distinct chromatin material in strands, together with several nucleoli. In certain leukemias, a marked increase in myeloblasts is observed in the marrow and in the peripheral blood. Compare **megaloblast, myelocyte, normoblast.** See also **myelocytic leukemia. —myeloblastic,** *adj.*

myeloblastemia. See **myeloblastosis.**

myeloblastic leukemia /-blas'tik/, a malignant neoplasm

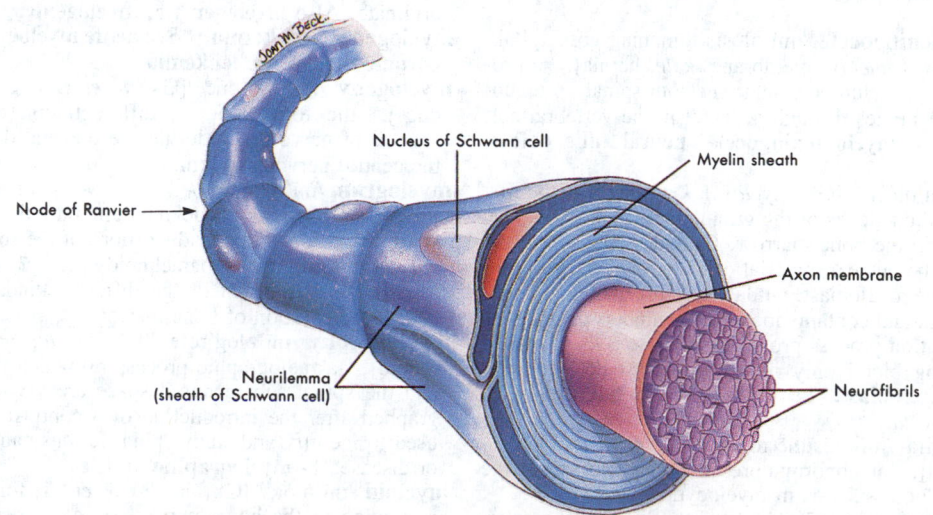

Myelin sheath *(Thibodeau, 1993/Joan M Beck)*

Node of Ranvier

Nucleus of Schwann cell

Myelin sheath

Axon membrane

Neurilemma (sheath of Schwann cell)

Neurofibrils

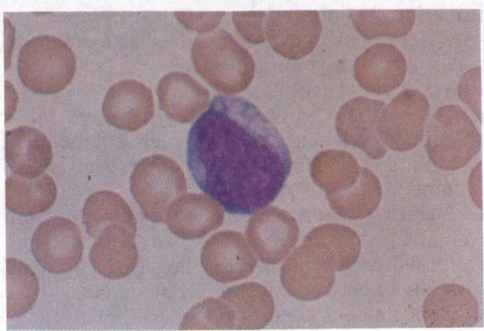

Myeloblast (Powers, 1989)

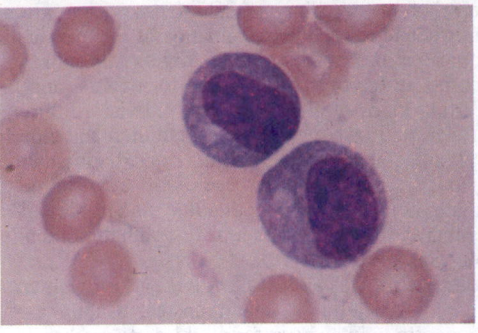

Myelocyte (Powers, 1989)

of blood-forming tissues, characterized by many myeloblasts in the circulating blood and tissues. The disease may be a terminal event in the course of chronic granulocytic leukemia.

myeloblastomatosis /mī'əlōblas'tōmətō'sis/ [Gk, *myelos, blastos* + *oma*, tumor, *osis*, condition],   abnormal, localized clusters of myeloblasts in the peripheral circulation.

myeloblastosis /mī'əloblastō'sis/ [Gk, *myelos, blastos* + *osis*, condition],   the abnormal presence of myeloblasts in the circulation.

myelocele /mī'əlōsēl'/ [Gk, *myelos* + *kele*, hernia],   a saclike protrusion of the spinal cord through a congenital defect in the vertebral column. See also **myelomeningocele, neural tube defect.**

myeloclast /mī'əlōclast'/ [Gk, *myelos* + *klastos*, broken],   a cell that breaks down the myelin sheaths of nerves.

myelocyst /mī'əlōsist'/ [Gk, *myelos* + *kystis*, cyst],   any benign cyst that is formed from the rudimentary medullary canals that give rise to the vertebral canal during embryonic development.

myelocystocele /mī'əlōsis'təsēl'/ [Gk, *myelos, kystis* + *kele*, hernia],   a protrusion of a cystic tumor containing spinal cord substance through a defect in the vertebral column. See also **myelomeningocele, neural tube defect, spina bifida.**

myelocystomeningocele /mī'əlōsis'tōməning'gōsēl/ [Gk, *myelos, kystis* + *menix*, membrane, *kele*, hernia],   a protrusion of a cystic tumor containing both spinal cord substance and meninges through a defect in the vertebral column. See also **myelomeningocele, neural tube defect, spina bifida.**

myelocyte /mī'əlōsīt'/ [Gk, *myelos* + *kytos*, cell],   the first of the maturation stages of the granulocytic leukocytes normally found in the bone marrow. Granules are seen in the cytoplasm. The nuclear material of the myelocyte is denser than that of the myeloblast, but lacks a definable membrane. The cell is flat and contains increasing numbers of granules as the maturation process progresses. These cells appear in the circulating blood only in certain forms of leukemia. Compare **myeloblast.** See also **myelocytic leukemia.** **–myelocytic,** *adj.*

myelocythemia /mī'əlōsīthē'mē·ə/ [Gk, *myelos, kytos* + *haima*, blood],   an abnormal presence of myelocytes in the circulating blood, such as in myelocytic leukemia.

myelocytic leukemia /mī'əlōsit'ik/,   a disorder characterized by the unregulated and excessive production of leukocytes. Also called **granulocytic leukemia, myelogenous**

leukemia. Compare **leukemoid reaction, acute lymphocytic leukemia, chronic lymphocytic leukemia.** See also **leukocytosis.**

myelocytoma /mī'əlō'sītō'mə/ [Gk, *myelos* + *kytos*, cell, *oma*, tumor],   a localized cluster of myelocytes in the peripheral vasculature that may occur in myelocytic leukemia.

myelocytosis.   See **myelocythemia.**

myelodiastasis /mī'əlōdī·as'təsis/ [Gk, *myelos* + *diastasis*, separation],   disintegration and necrosis of the spinal cord.

myelodysplasia /-displā'zhə/ [Gk, *myelos* + *dys*, bad, *plassis*, formation],   a general designation for the defective development of any part of the spinal cord. The term is used primarily to describe abnormalities without gross superficial defects, especially of the lower segment, specifically spina bifida occulta.

myelofibrosis.   See **myeloid metaplasia.**

myelogenesis /-jen'əsis/ [Gk, *myelos* + *genein*, to produce],   **1.** the formation and differentiation of the nervous system during prenatal development, in particular the brain and spinal cord. See also **neural tube formation. 2.** the development of the myelin sheath around the nerve fiber. See also **myelinization.**

myelogenous /mī'əloj'ənəs/,   pertaining to the cells produced in bone marrow or to the tissue from which such cells originate. Also **myelogenetic, myelogenic.**

myelogenous leukemia.   See **acute myelocytic leukemia, chronic myelocytic leukemia.**

myelogeny /mī'əloj'ənē/ [Gk, *myelos* + *genein*, to produce],   the formation and differentiation of the myelin sheaths of nerve fibers during the prenatal development of the central nervous system.

myelogram /mī'əlōgram'/,   **1.** an x-ray film taken after the injection of a radiopaque medium into the subarachnoid space to demonstrate any distortions of the spinal cord, spinal nerve roots, and subarachnoid space. **2.** a graphic representation of a count of the different kinds of cells in a stained preparation of bone marrow.

myelography /mī'əlog'rəfē/ [Gk, *myelos* + *graphein*, to record],   a radiographic process by which the spinal cord and the spinal subarachnoid space are viewed and photographed after the introduction of a contrast medium. It is used to identify and study spinal lesions caused by trauma or disease.   **–myelographic,** *adj.*

myeloid /mī'əloid/ [Gk, *myelos* + *eidos*, form],   **1.** of or pertaining to the bone marrow. **2.** of or pertaining to the spinal cord. **3.** of or pertaining to myelocytic forms that do not necessarily originate in the bone marrow.

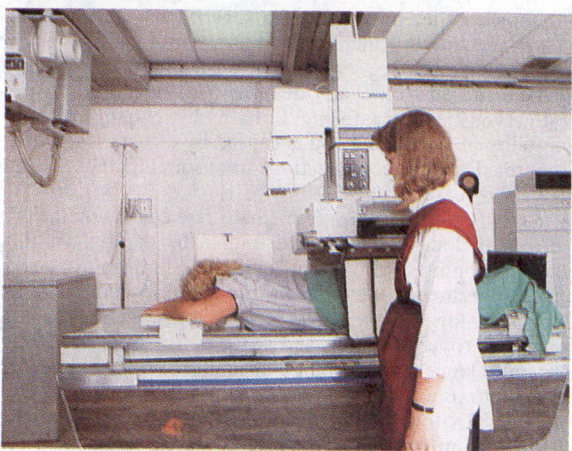

Positioning of patient for a myelogram
(Chipps, 1992, Courtesy Doctors Hospital, Columbus, Ohio)

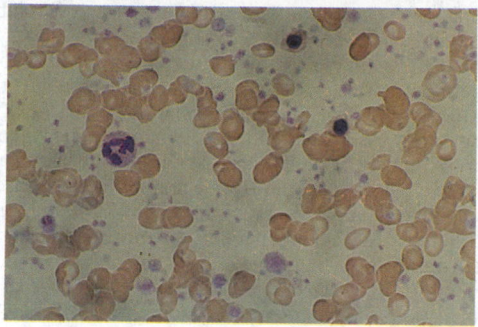

Immature red blood cells of myeloid metaplasia
(Powers, 1989)

myeloid leukemia. See **acute myelocytic leukemia, chronic myelocytic leukemia.**

myeloid metaplasia, a disorder in which bone marrow tissue develops in abnormal sites. Characteristics of the condition are anemia, splenomegaly, immature blood cells in the circulation, and hematopoiesis occurring in the liver and spleen. Myeloid metaplasia may be secondary to carcinoma, leukemia, polycythemia vera, or tuberculosis. The primary form is also called **agnogenic myeloid metaplasia, myelofibrosis.**

myeloidosis /mī′əloidō′sis/ [Gk, *myelos* + *eidos*, form, *osis*, condition], an abnormal condition characterized by general hyperplasia of the myeloid tissue. See also **Hodgkin's disease, multiple myeloma.**

myeloma /mī′əlō′mə/ [Gk, *myelos* + *oma*, tumor], an osteolytic neoplasm consisting of a profusion of cells typical of the bone marrow that may develop in many sites and cause extensive destruction of the bone. The tumor occurs most frequently in the ribs, vertebrae, pelvic bones, and flat bones of the skull. Intense pain and spontaneous fractures are common. The tumor is radiosensitive, and local lesions are curable. Kinds of myeloma are **endothelial myeloma, extramedullary myeloma, giant cell myeloma, multiple myeloma,** and **osteogenic myeloma.**

-myeloma, a suffix meaning a 'tumor composed of cells normally found in bone marrow': *globomyeloma, lymphomyeloma, orchiomyeloma.*

myelomalacia /mī′əlōmələā′shə/ [Gk, *myelos* + *malakia*, softening], abnormal softening of the spinal cord, caused primarily by inadequate blood supply.

myelomatosis. See **multiple myeloma.**

myelomeningocele /mī′əlō′məning′gōsēl/ [Gk, *myelos* + *menix*, membrane, *kele*, hernia], a developmental defect of the central nervous system in which a hernial sac containing a portion of the spinal cord, its meninges, and cerebrospinal fluid protrudes through a congenital cleft in the vertebral column. The condition is caused primarily by the failure of the neural tube to close during embryonic development, although in some instances it may result from the reopening of the tube from an abnormal increase in cerebrospinal fluid pressure. Also called **meningomyelocele.** Compare **meningocele.** See also **neural tube defect, spina bifida cystica.** (See Fig. p. 1034.)

■ OBSERVATIONS: The defect, which occurs in approximately 2 in every 1000 live births, is readily apparent and easily diagnosed at birth. Although the opening may be located at any point along the spinal column, the anomaly characteristically occurs in the lumbar, low thoracic, or sacral region and extends for three to six vertebral segments. The saclike structure may be covered with a thin layer of skin or with a fine membrane that can be easily ruptured, increasing the risk of meningeal infection. The severity of neurologic dysfunction is directly related to the amount of neural tissue involved, which can be roughly estimated by the degree of the transillumination of the mass. Usually the condition is accompanied by varying degrees of paralysis of the lower

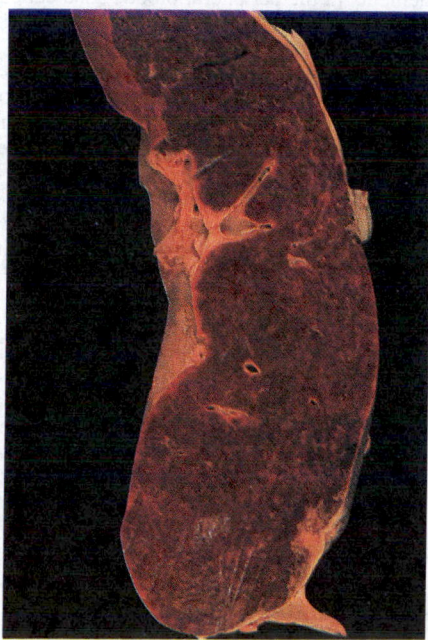

Myelometaplasia resulting in splenomegaly
(Fletcher, 1987)

extremities, by musculoskeletal defects, such as clubfoot, flexion and joint deformities, or hip dysplasia, and by anal and bladder sphincter dysfunction, which can lead to serious genitourinary disorders. Hydrocephalus, frequently related to the Arnold-Chiari malformation, is the most common anomaly associated with myelomeningocele and occurs in approximately 90% of the cases in which the spinal lesion is located in the lumbosacral region. In most cases hydrocephalus is apparent at birth, although it may appear shortly afterward. Supplementary diagnostic procedures include x-ray film of the spine, skull, and chest to determine the extent of the vertebral defect and the presence of other malformations in other organ systems, a computed tomographic (CT) scan of the brain to establish the ventricular size and the presence of any structural congenital anomalies, and laboratory examinations, especially urine analysis, culture, blood urea nitrogen evaluation, and creatinine clearance determination. Amniocentesis is recommended for all pregnant women who have had a child with a neural tube defect.

■ INTERVENTIONS: Immediate surgical repair is essential if the defect is leaking cerebrospinal fluid. However, surgical intervention may not be appropriate if neurologic involvement is extreme, if the lesion is infected, or if associated problems, such as hydrocephalus, are severe. When surgical repair of the spinal defect is recommended, associated problems are managed by appropriate measures, including shunt procedures for correction of hydrocephalus; antibiotic therapy to reduce the incidence of meningitis, urinary tract infections, and pneumonia, casting, bracing, traction, and surgical techniques for correction of hip, knee, and foot deformities, and prevention and treatment of renal complications.

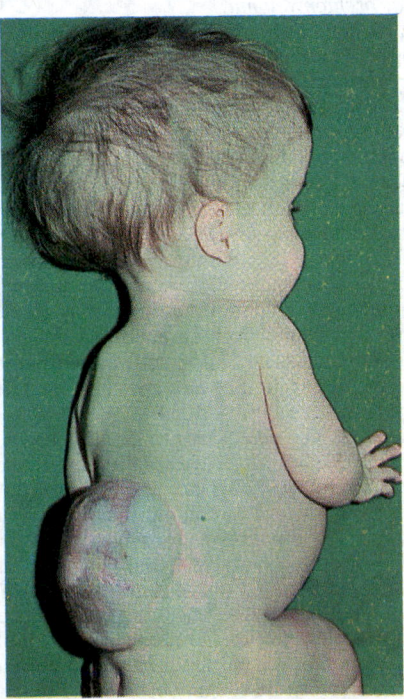

Myelomeningocele (Milner, 1991)

Prognosis is determined by the severity of neurologic involvement and the number of associated anomalies. With proper care and long-term maintenance, most children can survive and do well. Early death is usually caused by central nervous system infection or by hydrocephalus, whereas mortality in later childhood is caused by urinary tract infection, renal failure, complications from shunt therapy, or pulmonary disease.

■ NURSING CONSIDERATIONS: Immediate care centers on the prevention of local infection and trauma by careful handling and positioning of the infant, applying sterile moist dressings to the membranous sac, avoiding fecal contamination and breakdown of sensitive skin areas, and maintaining warmth, proper nutrition, and adequate hydration and electrolyte balance. Gentle range-of-motion exercises are carried out to prevent or minimize hip and lower extremity deformity. An important function of the nurse is to involve the parents in the care of the infant as soon as possible and to teach them the essential procedures for adequate home care, including how to observe for signs of complications. The nurse also helps the parents in long-term management by planning activities appropriate to the developmental age and physical limitations of the child, and by providing information for teaching all family members about the condition.

myelomere /mī′əlōmir′/ [Gk, *myelos* + *meros*, part], any of the embryonic segments of the brain or spinal cord during prenatal development.

myelomonocytic leukemia. See **monocytic leukemia.**

myelopathic anemia. See **myelophthisic anemia.**

myelopathy /mī′əlop′əthē/, **1.** any disease of the spinal cord. **2.** any disease of the myelopoietic tissues.

myelophthisic anemia /mī′əlofthiz′ik/ [Gk, myelos + *phthisis*, wasting], a disorder characterized by anemia and the appearance of immature granulocytes and nucleated erythroid elements in the peripheral blood. Also called **myelopathic anemia.** Compare **hemolytic anemia, leukoerythroblastic anemia.**

myelopoiesis /mī′əlō′pō·ē′sis/ [Gk, *myelos* + *poiein*, to form], the formation and development of the bone marrow or the cells that originate from it. A kind of myelopoiesis is **extramedullary myelopoiesis. −myelopoietic,** /-pō·et′ik/ *adj.*

myeloradiculodysplasia /mī′əlō′rədik′yəlōdis′plā′zhə/ [Gk, *myelos* + L, *radiculus*, small root; Gk, *dys*, bad, *plassein*, to form], any developmental abnormality of the spinal cord and spinal nerve roots. See also **myelomeningocele, neural tube defect.**

myeloschisis /mī′əlos′kəsis/ [Gk, *myelos* + *schisis*, cleft], a developmental defect characterized by a cleft spinal cord that results from the failure of the neural plate to fuse and form a complete neural tube. See also **neural tube defect, neural tube formation, myelomeningocele, rachischisis, spina bifida.**

myelosuppression /-səpresh′ən/, the inhibition of the process of production of blood cells and platelets in the bone marrow.

myenteric plexus /mī′enter′ik/ [Gk, *mys*, muscle + *enteron*, bowel; L, *plexus*, plaited], a group of autonomic nerve fibers and ganglion cells in the muscular coat of the intestine.

myesthesia /mī′esthē′zhə/, perception of any sensation in a muscle, such as touch, direction, proprioception, contraction, relaxation, or extension.

myiasis /mī′yəsis/ [Gk, *myia*, fly, *osis*, condition], infection or infestation of the body by the larvae of flies, usually through a wound or an ulcer, but, rarely, through the intact skin.

myitis. See **myositis.**

myko-. See **myco-.**

Myleran, a trademark for an antineoplastic (busulfan).

Mylicon, a trademark for an antiflatulent (simethicone).

mylohyoideus /mī′lōhī·oi′dē·əs/ [Gk, *myle*, mill, *hyoeides*, U-shaped], one of a pair of flat triangular muscles that form the floor of the cavity of the mouth. Immediately superior to the digastricus, it arises from the whole length of the mylohyoid line of the mandible and inserts into the hyoid bone. It is innervated by the mylohyoid nerve and acts to raise the hyoid bone and the tongue. Also called **mylohyoid muscle.** Compare **digastricus, geniohyoideus, stylohyoideus.**

myo- /mī′ō-/, **my-,** a prefix meaning 'relating to muscle': *myocardia, myocele, myolipoma.*

myocardial infarction (MI) /mī′ōkär′dē·əl/ [Gk, *mys*, muscle, *kardia*, heart; L, *infarcire*, to stuff], necrosis of a portion of cardiac muscle caused by obstruction in a coronary artery from either atherosclerosis or an embolis. Also called **heart attack.**

■ OBSERVATIONS: The onset of MI is characterized by a crushing, viselike chest pain that may radiate to the left arm, neck, or epigastrium and sometimes stimulates the sensation of acute indigestion or a gallbladder attack. The patient usually becomes ashen, clammy, short of breath, faint, and anxious and often feels that death is imminent. Typical

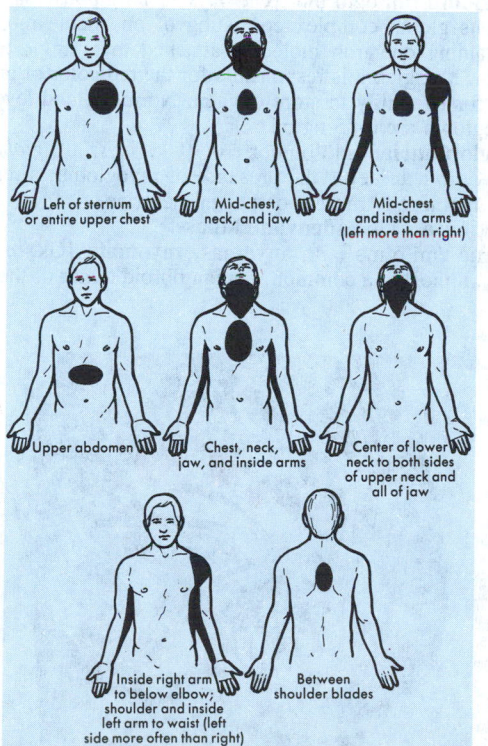

Locations of pain from myocardial infarction

Left of sternum or entire upper chest

Mid-chest, neck, and jaw

Mid-chest and inside arms (left more than right)

Upper abdomen

Chest, neck, jaw, and inside arms

Center of lower neck to both sides of upper neck and all of jaw

Inside right arm to below elbow; shoulder and inside left arm to waist (left side more often than right)

Between shoulder blades

signs are tachycardia, a barely perceptible pulse, low blood pressure, and elevated temperature, cardiac dysrhythmia, and electrocardiographic evidence of elevation of the ST segment and Q wave. Laboratory studies usually show an increased sedimentation rate, leukocytosis, and elevated serum levels of creatine phosphokinase, lactic dehydrogenase, and glutamic-oxaloacetic transaminase. Potential complications in MI are pulmonary or systemic embolism, pulmonary edema, shock, and cardiac arrest.

■ INTERVENTIONS: Emergency treatment of MI may require cardiopulmonary resuscitation before the patient is admitted to an intensive cardiac care unit and placed on a cardiac monitor. In the acute phase, oxygen, cardiotonic drugs, antidysrhythmic agents, and anticoagulants are usually administered and sedatives and analgesics may be indicated. Blood pressure, temperature, respiration, and apical pulse are checked frequently. Parenteral fluids may be administered; iced drinks and cold foods are avoided, and the patient is usually served a low-sodium, low-cholesterol diet. Stool softeners and laxatives may be indicated to prevent straining.

■ NURSING CONSIDERATIONS: The nurse's role in helping the patient and family understand the nature and treatment of the disease is extremely important. Before discharge, discussions regarding the need to adhere to the prescribed diet and medication, to limit activities, to rest at regular periods, and to avoid caffeine, nicotine, large meals, and emotional stress can facilitate the patient's convalescence.

myocardiopathy /mī′ōkär′dē·op′əthē/ [Gk, *mys*, muscle, *kardia*, heart, *pathos*, disease], any disease of the myocardium causing enlargement. Also called **cardiomyopathy.**

myocarditis /mī′ōkärdī′tis/ [Gk, *mys, kardia* + *itis*, inflammation], an inflammatory condition of the myocardium caused by viral, bacterial, or fungal infection, serum sickness, rheumatic fever, or chemical agent, or as a complication of a collagen disease. Myocarditis most frequently occurs in an acute viral form and is self-limited, but it may lead to acute heart failure. Management includes treatment of the cause, analgesia, oxygen, antiinflammatory agents, constant monitoring, and rest to prevent shock or heart failure.

myocardium /mī′ōkär′dē·əm/ [Gk, *mys*, muscle, *kardia*, heart], a thick, contractile, middle layer of uniquely constructed and arranged muscle cells that forms the bulk of the heart wall. The myocardium contains a minimum of other tissue, except for the blood vessels, and is covered interiorly by the endocardium. The contractile tissue of the myocardium is composed of fibers with the characteristic cross-striations of muscular tissue. The fibers, which are about one third as large in diameter as those of skeletal muscle and contain more sarcoplasm, branch frequently and are interconnected to form a network that is continuous except where the bundles and the laminae are attached at their origins and insertions into the fibrous trigone of the heart. The bundles of myocardial fibers are spiral-shaped; the individual muscle fibers contain fibrillae that are more concentrated at the periphery of each fiber. The central cores of the fibers contain the nuclei and may also contain concentrated sarcoplasm rich in sarcosomes. Myocardial muscle fibers also contain characteristic intercalated disks. Electron microscope studies reveal that these disks represent cell boundaries and may cross an entire fiber in a straight line or may be arranged in a steplike configuration. Myocardial muscle contains less connective tissue than does skeletal muscle. The fibers of the connective tissue are covered by a delicate fibrillar net with few elastic fibers. Collagenous fibers run between the muscular bundles and the associated blood vessels. Specially modified fibers of myocardial muscle constitute the conduction system of the heart, including the sinoatrial node, the atrioventricular node, the atrioventricular bundle, and the Purkinje fibers. Most of the myocardial fibers function to contract the heart. Contraction involves the action of calcium ions and sodium ions and a complex electrochemical process still not precisely understood. Defects in the kinetics of intracellular calcium may cause myocardial dysfunctions in patients with heart failure. The metabolic processes of the myocardium are almost exclusively aerobic and constantly supply the heart muscle with high-energy phosphate bonds for mechanical and chemical functions. The heart uses free fatty acids as its predominant fuel, as well as important quantities of glucose, lactate, pyruvate, and ketone bodies, and a very small amount of amino acids. Many key enzymatic reactions of the heart, such as the citric acid cycle and oxidative phosphorylation, take place in the highly concentrated myocardial sarcosomes. The major anaerobic processes of glycolysis occur in the sarcoplasm. The process of oxidative phosphorylation produces adenosine triphosphate, the immediate energy source for myocardial contraction. Oxygen, which significantly affects contractibility, is the most important metabolic nutrient for the myocardium, which consumes from 6.5 to 10 ml/100 g of tissue per minute. Without this oxygen supply, myocardial contractions decrease in a few minutes. Ventricular pressure and heart rate together determine myocardial oxygen consumption. The heart normally extracts about 70% of the oxygen reaching it by the coronary arteries. This leaves only about 30% in coronary sinus blood and limits the amount of additional oxygen the heart can extract from its blood supply. In heart failure caused by hypertension, valvular heart disease, or coronary atherosclerosis, the myocardial oxygen consumption per gram of tissue is usually normal, but the total oxygen consumption per minute often increases significantly because the weight of the heart often increases with such diseases. Myocardial oxygen consumption increases in hyperthyroidism and decreases in hypothy-

roidism. The myocardium maintains a relatively constant level of glycogen in the form of sarcoplasmic granules. Hypoxia rapidly depletes this supply and produces lactate and hexosemonophosphate. In anemia, the total consumption of myocardial oxygen may significantly increase because of increased hemodynamic demands resulting from the disorder. Myocardial hypertrophy may develop if the anemia is chronic. Compare **epicardium**.   –**myocardial**, *adj.*

Myochrysine,   a trademark for an antirheumatic (gold sodium thiomalate).

myoclonus /mī′ŏklō′nəs/ [Gk, *mys* + *klonos*, contraction], a spasm of a muscle or a group of muscles.   –**myoclonic**, *adj.*

myodiastasis /mī′ōdī·as′təsis/ [Gk, *mys* + *diastasis*, separation], an abnormal condition in which there is separation of muscle bundles.

myoedema /mī′ō·idē′mə/, *pl.* **myoedemas, myoedemata,** muscle edema. Compare **myxedema.**

myofibril /-fī′bril/ [Gk, *mys* + L, *fibrilla*, small fiber], a slender striated strand of muscle tissue. Myofibrils occur in groups of branching threads running parallel to the cellular long axis.

myogelosis /mī′ōjəlō′sis/ [Gk, *mys* + L, *gelare*, to freeze; Gk, *osis*], a condition in which there are hardened areas or nodules within muscles, especially the gluteal muscles. There are no serious consequences of this condition, and no treatment is necessary.

myogenic /mī′ōjen′ik/ [Gk, *mys* + *genesis*, origin], pertaining to muscles, particularly cardiac and smooth muscles that do not require nerves to initiate and maintain contractions.

myoglobin /mī′ŏglō′bin/ [Gk, *mys* + L, *globus*, ball], a ferrous globin complex consisting of one heme molecule containing one iron molecule attached to a single globin chain. Myoglobin is responsible for the red color of muscle and for its ability to store oxygen. Normal blood levels of myoglobin are 0-85 ng/ml.

myoglobinuria /-glō′binŏŏr′ē·ə/ [Gk, *mys*; L, *globus* + Gk, *ouron*, urine], the presence of myoglobin, a respiratory pigment of muscle tissue, in the urine.

myokinase.   See **adenylate kinase.**

myoma /mī·ō′mə/, *pl.* **myomas, myomata** [Gk, *mys* + *oma*, tumor], a common, benign fibroid tumor of the uter-

Pericardial space

Myocardium

Endocardium

Myocardium *(Cannobio, 1990)*

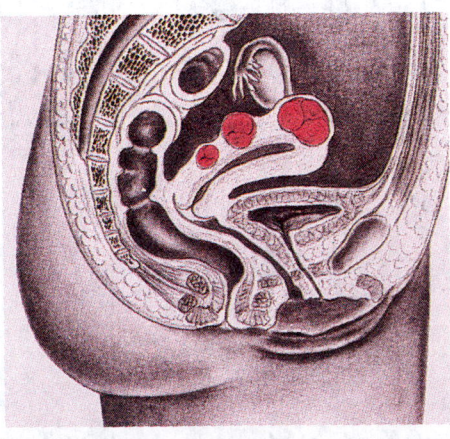

Myomas of the uterus *(Seidel, 1991)*

ine muscle. The tumor develops most frequently after 30 years of age in women, especially black women, who have never been pregnant. Menorrhagia, backache, constipation, dysmenorrhea, dyspareunia, and other symptoms develop in proportion to the size, location, and rate of growth of the tumor.

myoma previum.   See **leiomyoma uteri.**

myoma striocellulare.   See **rhabdomyoma.**

myomectomy /mī′ōmek′təmē/,   the surgical removal of muscle tissue.

myomere.   See **myotome.**

myometritis /mī′ōmətrī′tis/,   an inflammation or infection of the myometrium of the uterus.

myometrium /mī′ōmē′trē·əm/, *pl.* **myometria** [Gk, *mys + metra*, womb],   the muscular layer of the wall of the uterus. The fibers of the myometrium course around the uterus horizontally, vertically, and diagonally.

myonecrosis /mī′ōnekrō′sis/ [Gk, *mys + necrosis*, death],   the death of muscle fibers. **Progressive** or **clostridial myonecrosis** is caused by the anaerobic bacteria of the genus *Clostridium.* Seen in deep wound infections, progressive myonecrosis is accompanied by pain, tenderness, a brown serous exudate, and a rapid accumulation of gas within the tissue of the muscle. The affected muscle turns a blackish-green color. Treatment includes thorough wound debridement, IV administration of penicillin, and the use of hyperbaric oxygen therapy to destroy the anaerobe and to promote healing.

myoneural /mī′ōnŏŏr′əl/ [Gk, *mys + neuron*, nerve],   of or pertaining to a muscle and its associated nerve, especially to nerve endings in muscles.

myoneural junction   See **end plate.**

myopathy /mī·op′əthē/ [Gk, *mys + pathos*, disease],   an abnormal condition of skeletal muscle characterized by muscle weakness, wasting, and histologic changes within muscle tissue, such as seen in any of the muscular dystrophies. A myopathy is distinct from a muscle disorder caused by nerve dysfunction. The specific diagnosis of any myopathy is made using tests of serum enzymes, electromyography, and muscle biopsy. See also **muscular dystrophy.** —**myopathic,** *adj.*

myope /mī′ōp/,   an individual who is nearsighted or afflicted with myopia.

myophosphorylase deficiency glycogenosis.   See **McArdle's disease.**

myopia /mī·ō′pē·ə/ [Gk, *myops*, nearsighted],   a condition of nearsightedness caused by the elongation of the eyeball or by an error in refraction so that parallel rays are focused in front of the retina. Some kinds of myopia are **chronic**

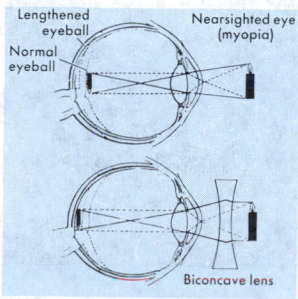

Myopia

myopia, curvature myopia, index myopia, and **pathologic myopia.** Also called **nearsightedness, shortsight.** —**myopic,** *adj.*

myorrhaphy /mī·ôr′əfē/ [Gk, *mys + rhaphe*, suture],   suturing of a wound in a muscle.

myorrhexis /mī′ərek′sis/ [Gk, *mys + rhexis*, rupture],   a tearing in any muscle. —**myorrhectic,** *adj.*

myosarcoma /mī′ōsärkō′mə/ [Gk, *mys + sarx*, flesh, *oma*, tumor],   a malignant tumor of muscular tissue.

myosin /mī′əsin/ [Gk, *mys + in*, within],   a cardiac and skeletal muscle protein that makes up close to one half of the proteins that occur in muscle tissue. The interaction of myosin and actin is essential for muscle contraction.

myositis /mī′əsī′tis/,   inflammation of muscle tissue, usually of the voluntary muscles. Causes of myositis include infection, trauma, and infestation by parasites. Kinds of myositis include **epidemic myositis, interstitial myositis, parenchymatous myositis, polymyositis,** and **traumatic myositis.** Also called **myitis** /mī·ī′tis/. Compare **fibrositis.**

myositis fibrosa,   an uncommon inflammation of the muscles, characterized by abnormal formation of connective tissue. Also called **interstitial myositis.** See also **myositis.**

myositis ossificans /əsif′əkanz/,   a rare, inherited disease in which muscle tissue is replaced by bone. It begins in childhood, with stiffness in the neck and back and progresses to rigidity of the spine, trunk, and limbs. The administration of diphosphonates may prevent the abnormal deposition of bone, but there is no cure after it has occurred. Metabolism of calcium and phosphate remains normal throughout the course of the disease. Compare **myositis.**

myositis purulenta,   any bacterial infection of muscle tissue. This condition may result in the formation of an abscess or multiple abscesses.

myositis trichinosa /trik′ənō′sə/,   inflammation of the muscles resulting from infection by the parasite *Trichinella spiralis.* See also **trichinosis.**

myostasis /mī′ōstā′sis/ [Gk, *mys + stasis*, standing],   an abnormal condition of weakened muscle in which there is a relatively fixed length of muscle fibers in the relaxed state. In normal muscle the force of contraction is greatest at the resting length of the muscle; in myostasis the resting length is shorter than normal, and there is a shorter acting length in which the contractile force can work. —**myostatic,** *adj.*

myostatic reflex.   See **deep tendon reflex.**

myostroma /mī′əstrō′mə/ [Gk, *mys + stroma*, covering],   the framework of muscle tissue.

myotenotomy /-tenot′əmē/ [Gk, *mys + tenon*, tendon, *temnein*, to cut],   surgical division of the whole or part of a muscle by cutting through its main tendon.

myotherapy /-ther′əpē/   a technique of corrective muscle exercises involving pressure on fingers and joints to relieve pain or spasms.

myotome /mī′ətōm/ [Gk, *mys + temnein*, to cut],   **1.** also called **myomere.** The muscle plate of an embryonic somite that develops into a voluntary muscle. **2.** a group of muscles innervated by a single spinal segment. **3.** an instrument for cutting or dissecting a muscle.

myotomic muscle /-tom′ik/,   any of the numerous muscles of the trunk of the body, derived from the myotomes and divided into the deep muscles of the back and the thoracoabdominal muscles.

myotomy /mī·ot′əmē/ [Gk, *mys + temnein*, to cut],   the cutting of a muscle, performed to gain access to underlying tissues or to relieve constriction in a sphincter, such as in severe esophagitis or pyloric stenosis. With the patient under general anesthesia, a longitudinal cut is made through the sphincter muscle but not through the mucosa lining the stomach. See also **abdominal surgery.**

Myotonachol, a trademark for a cholinergic (bethanechol chloride).

myotonia /mī′ətō′nē·ə/ [Gk, *mys* + *tonos*, tone], any condition in which a muscle or a group of muscles does not readily relax after contracting. **—myotonic,** *adj.*

myotonia atrophica. See **myotonic muscular dystrophy.**

myotonia congenita /konjen′itə/, a rare, mild, and nonprogressive form of myotonic myopathy evident early in life. The only effects of the disorder are hypertrophy and stiffness of the muscles. Also called **Thomsen's disease.**

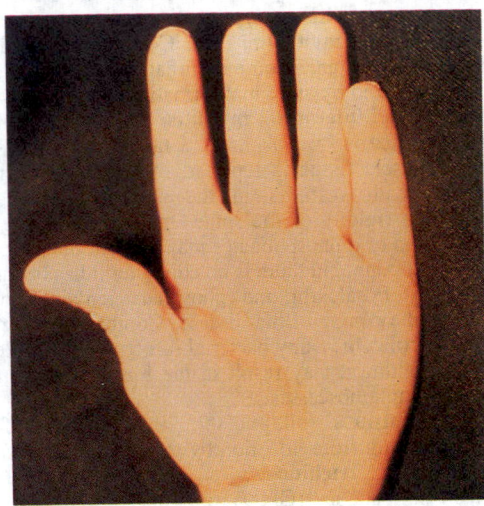

Mytonia congenita (Zitelli, 1992)

myotonic muscular dystrophy /-ton′ik/, a severe form of muscular dystrophy marked by ptosis, facial weakness, and dysarthria. Weakness of the hands and feet precedes that in the shoulders and hips. Myotonia of the hands is usually present. Electromyography is helpful in establishing the diagnosis. Although there is no specific treatment, active and passive exercises are used to alleviate symptoms. Also called **myotonia atrophica, Steinert's disease.**

myotonic myopathy, any of a group of disorders characterized by increased skeletal muscle tone and decreased relaxation of muscle after contraction. Kinds of myotonic myopathy include **myotonia congenita, myotonic muscular dystrophy.**

myria-, a combining form meaning 'a great number': *myriapod.*

myringa. See **tympanic membrane.**

myringectomy /mir′injek′təmē/ [L, *myringa*, eardrum; Gk, *ektome*, excision], excision of the tympanic membrane.

myringitis /mir′injī′tis/ [L, *myringa* + Gk, *itis*], inflammation or infection of the tympanic membrane.

myringo-, a combining form meaning 'related to the tym-

panic membrane': *myringodectomy, myringoplasty, myringoscope.*

myringomycosis /miring′gōmīkō′sis/ [L, *myringa* + Gk, *mykes*, fungus, *osis*, condition], a fungal infection of the tympanic membrane. Also called **mycomyringitis.**

myringoplasty /miring′gōplas′tē/ [L, *myringa* + Gk, *plassein*, to mold], surgical repair of perforations of the eardrum with a tissue graft, performed to correct hearing loss. With the patient under local or general anesthesia, the openings in the eardrum are enlarged, and the grafting material is sutured over them. Topical antibiotics are applied, and then a packing of absorbable gelatin sponge is applied to hold the graft in position. After surgery, an antihistamine with an ephedrine derivative is given. The nurse keeps the outer ear clean and dry. Debris is removed by gentle suctioning about 12 days after surgery. See also **myringotomy, tympanoplasty.**

myringotomy /mir′ing·got′əmē/ [L, *myringa* + Gk, *temnein*, to cut], surgical incision of the eardrum, performed to relieve pressure and release pus or fluid from the middle ear. Antibiotics are given before surgery and continued afterward. The drum is incised, and cultures may be taken; fluid is gently suctioned from the middle ear. Ear drops may be instilled to improve drainage. Tubes may be inserted to allow for drainage. The nurse cautions against putting cotton in the canal, because the ear must drain freely. The outer ear is kept clean and dry; careful handwashing is essential to prevent infection. If pain increases, the procedure may have to be repeated. Severe headache or disorientation must be reported. Also called **tympanotomy.** See also **myringoplasty.**

Mysoline, a trademark for an anticonvulsant (primidone).

mysophobia /mē′sə-/ [Gk, *mysos*, anything disgusting, *phobos*, fear], an anxiety disorder characterized by an overreaction to the slightest uncleanliness, or an irrational fear of dirt, contamination, or defilement. Also spelled **misophobia. —mysophobic, misophobic,** *adj.*

myx-, myxo-, a combining form meaning 'relating to mucus': *myxoblastoma, myxocyte, myxoma.*

myxedema /mik′sədē′mə/ [Gk, *myxa*, mucus, *oidema*, swelling], the most severe form of hypothyroidism. It is

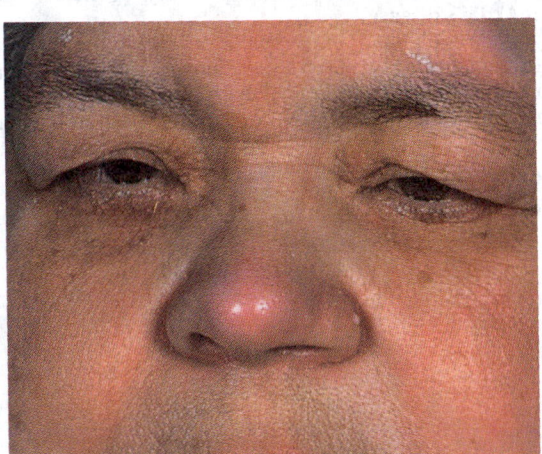

Myxedema (Epstein, 1992)

characterized by swelling of the hand, face, feet, and periorbital tissues. At this stage, the disease may lead to coma and death.

myxofibroma /mik'sōfībrō'mə/ [Gk, *myxa* + L, *fibra,* fiber; Gk, *oma,* tumor],   a fibrous tumor that contains myxomatous tissue. Also called **myxoma fibrosum.**

myxoid.   See **mucoid,** def. 1.

myxoma /miksō'mə/ [Gk, *myxa* + *oma,* tumor],   a neoplasm of the connective tissue, characteristically composed of stellate cells in a loose mucoid matrix crossed by delicate reticulum fibers. These tumors may grow to enormous size and may occur under the skin but are also found in bones, the genitourinary tract, and the retroperitoneal area. **–myxomatous,** *adj.*

-myxoma,   a suffix meaning a 'soft tumor made up of primitive connective tissues': *adenomyxoma, gliomyxoma, lipomyxoma.*

myxoma fibrosum.   See **myxofibroma.**

myxoma sarcomatosum.   See **myxosarcoma.**

myxomatous.   See **myxoma.**

myxopoiesis /mik'sōpō·ē'sis/ [Gk, *myxa* + *poiein,* to make],   the production of mucus.

myxosarcoma /mik'sōsärkō'mə/ [Gk, *myxa* + *sarx,* flesh, *oma* tumor],   a sarcoma that contains some myxomatous tissue. Also called **myxoma sarcomatosum.**

myxovirus /mik'sōvī'rəs/ [Gk, *myxa* + L, *virus,* poison], any of a group of medium-size RNA viruses that are further divided into orthomyxoviruses and paramyxoviruses. Infection with these viruses is usually caused by transmission of the respiratory secretions of an infected host. Some kinds of myxoviruses are the viruses that cause influenza, mumps, and parainfluenza.

MZ,   abbreviation for **monozygotic.**

N

n, 2n, 3n, 4n, symbols for the haploid, diploid, triploid, and tetraploid number of chromosomes in a cell, organism, strain, or individual.

N, 1. symbol for **the element nitrogen. 2.** abbreviation for **normal. 3.** abbreviation for *node* in the TNM system for staging malignant neoplastic disease. See also **cancer staging. 4.** symbol for **Avogadro's number. 5.** symbol for **magnetic flux**.

N/1, symbol for **normal solution**.

nA, abbreviation for *nanoampere*.

Na, chemical symbol for the element **sodium**.

NAACOG, abbreviation for **Nurses Association of the American College of Obstetrics and Gynecology.**

-nab, a combining form for cannabinol derivatives.

nabothian cyst /nəbō′thē·ən/ [Martin Naboth, German physician, b. 1675; Gk, *kystis*, bag], a cyst formed in a nabothian gland of the uterine cervix. It is a common finding on routine pelvic examination of women of reproductive age, especially in women who have borne children. The cyst, which is pearly white and firm, seldom results in adverse or pathologic effects. Also called **cervical cyst**.

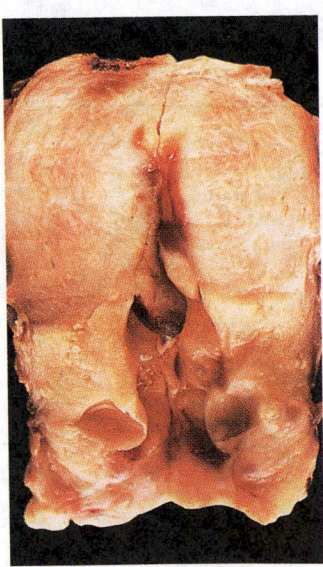

Nabothian cysts *(Fletcher, 1987)*

nabothian gland /nəbō′thē·ən/ [Martin Naboth; L, *glans*, acorn], one of many small, mucus-secreting glands of the uterine cervix.

N.A.D.. abbreviation for *no appreciable disease*.

NADH, abbreviation for *nicotine adenine dinucleotide, reduced*.

nadir /nā′dər/, the lowest point, such as the blood count after it has been depressed by chemotherapy.

nadolol /nad′ənol/, a beta-adrenergic blocking agent.
■ INDICATIONS: It is prescribed for long-term management of angina pectoris and for hypertension.
■ CONTRAINDICATIONS: Bronchial asthma, sinus bradycardia, greater than first-degree conduction block, cardiogenic shock, overt cardiac failure, or known hypersensitivity to this drug prohibits its use.
■ ADVERSE EFFECTS: Among the more serious adverse reactions are bronchospasm, bradycardia, precipitation of heart failure, cardiac dysrhythmia, masking of signs of hypoglycemia in diabetics, fatigue, and lethargy. GI disturbances, rashes, and other allergic reactions also may occur.

NADPH, abbreviation for *nicotine adenine disphosphonucleotide, reduced*.

Naegeli's leukemia. See **monocytic leukemia**.

nafcillin sodium /nafsil′in/, an antibacterial.
■ INDICATIONS: It is prescribed in the treatment of infections caused by penicillinase-producing staphylococci.
■ CONTRAINDICATIONS: Known hypersensitivity to this drug or to other penicillins prohibits its use.
■ ADVERSE EFFECTS: Among the more serious adverse reactions are hypersensitivity reactions, nausea, and vomiting.

Naffziger sign /naf′zigər/, a diagnostic sign for sciatica or a herniated nucleus pulposus. Nerve root irritation is produced by the examiner through external jugular venous compression.

Naffziger syndrome, a condition of scalene muscle spasms secondary to intervertebral disk disease, cervical rib, or other disorder. The spasms result in pressure on the major nerve plexus of the arm, and the patient experiences pain in the neck, shoulder, arm, and hand. Also called **scalenus anticus syndrome**.

Nägele's obliquity. See **asynclitism**.

Nägele's rule /nä′gələz/ [Franz K. Nägele, German obstetrician, b. 1778; L, *regula*, model], a method for calculating the estimated date of delivery based on a mean length of gestation. Three months are subtracted from the first day of the last normal menstrual period, and 1 year plus 7 days are added to that date.

Nager's acrofacial dysostosis /nä′gərz/ [F. R. Nager, twentieth century Swiss physician; Gk, *akron*, extremity; L, *facies*, face; Gk, *dys*, bad, *osteon*, bone, *osis*, condition], an abnormal congenital condition characterized by limb deformities, such as radioulnar synostosis, hypoplasia, and the absence of the radius or of the thumbs. Also called **dysostosis mandibularis**. Compare **cleidocranial dysostosis, craniofacial dysostosis, mandibulofacial dysostosis**.

Nahrungs-Einheit-Milch (nem) /nä′rŏŏngz in′hīt milsh, milkh/ [Ger, *Nahrung*, food; *Einheit*, unit; *Milch*, milk], a nutritional unit in Pirquet's system of feeding that is equivalent to 1 g of breast milk.

nail [AS, *naegel*], **1.** also called **unguis.** a flattened, elastic structure with a horny texture at the end of a finger or a toe. Each nail is comprised of a root, body, and free edge at the distal extremity. The root fastens the nail to the finger or the toe by fitting into a groove in the skin and is closely molded to the surface of the corium. The nail matrix beneath the body and the root projects longitudinal vascular ridges, which are easily visible through the translucent tissue of the body. The matrix firmly attaches the body of the nail to the underlying connective tissue. The whitish lunula near the root contains irregularly arranged papillae that are less firmly attached to the connective tissue than the rest of the matrix. The cuticle is attached to the surface of the nail just ahead of the root. The superficial horny part of the nail consists of the thick stratum lucidum, the thin stratum corneum, which forms the cuticle overlapping the lunula, and the stratum mucosum. The nails grow longer by proliferation of the cells in the stratum germinativum at the root. They grow thicker from proliferation of that part of the stratum germinativum underlying the lunula. **2.** any of various metallic nails used in orthopedics to fasten together bones or pieces of bone.

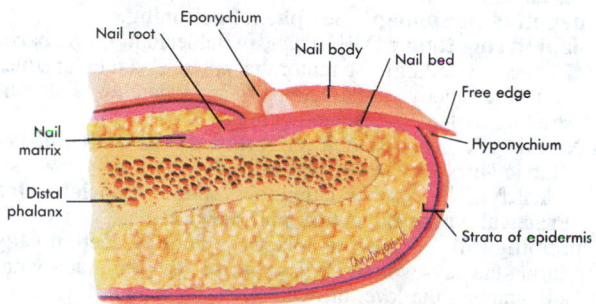

Nail *(Seeley, 1992/Marsha J Dohrmann)*

nailbed [AS, *naegle*, nail; *bedd*, bed], the corium beneath the nail. It appears through the clear nail as a series of longitudinal ridges. Also called **matrix unguis**.

nail fold, a fold of skin supporting the nail at its base.

nail groove [AS, *naegle*; Du, *groeve*, groove], a shallow depression between the nail bed and the nail wall.

nail matrix. See nail bed.

nail plate, the hard portion of the dorsum of the fingers and thumb, a rigid outer covering that extends about 8 mm under the nail fold and arises from the nail bed.

nail plate avulsion, a temporary partial or complete removal of the nail plate without disrupting the underlying matrix cells.

nal-, a prefix meaning 'narcotic agonists or antagonists related to normorphine.'

Naldecon, a trademark for a fixed-combination drug containing two adrenergics (phenylpropanolamine hydrochloride and phenylephrine hydrochloride) and two antihistamines (chlorpheniramine maleate and phenyltoloxamine citrate).

Nalebuff arthrodesis, an arthrodesis of the wrist in which fusion includes the use of a Steinmann pin.

Nalfon, a trademark for an antiinflammatory agent (fenoprofen calcium).

nalidixic acid /nal'idik'sik/, an antibacterial.

■ INDICATIONS: It is prescribed in the treatment of certain urinary tract infections.

■ CONTRAINDICATIONS: Renal or hepatic insufficiency, a history of convulsive disorders, or known hypersensitivity to this drug prohibits its use.

■ ADVERSE EFFECTS: Among the more serious adverse reactions are mild neurologic disturbances, GI disturbances, and hemolytic anemia in glucose-6-phosphate dehydrogenase deficiency. Convulsions and increased cranial pressure may occur. Among the more serious reactions are increased intracranial pressure, seizures, hemolytic anemia in people affected with glucose-6-phosphate dehydrogenase deficiency, and GI and neurologic disturbances.

naloxone hydrochloride /nal'əksōn/, a narcotic antagonist.

■ INDICATIONS: It is prescribed for reversal of narcotic depression, or for acute narcotic intoxication.

■ CONTRAINDICATION: Known hypersensitivity to this drug prohibits its use.

■ ADVERSE EFFECTS: Among the most serious adverse reactions when given to narcotic-dependent patients are side effects associated with narcotic withdrawal.

naltrexone hydrochloride /naltrek'sōn/, an oral opioid antagonist.

■ INDICATIONS: It is prescribed to block the effects of opioid analgesics, including heroin, morphine, and methadone in patients recovering from addiction.

■ CONTRAINDICATIONS: Acute hepatitis or liver failure prohibits the use of the drug. Periodic liver function tests are recommended for all patients. Patients must be completely free of opioids before taking naltrexone to prevent severe withdrawal symptoms. Respiratory depression may be deep and prolonged in a patient given a large emergency dose of an opioid analgesic after taking naltrexone.

■ ADVERSE EFFECTS: The most serious adverse reactions are abdominal pain, cramps, nausea, vomiting, headache, sleep disorders, and joint and muscle pain. Some adverse effects may actually be withdrawal symptoms rather than reactions to naltrexone.

Namaqualand hip dysplasia, an autosomal dominant genetic defect found in African children. It is characterized by a growth failure in the femoral epiphysis, resulting in pain and early degenerative arthritis of the hip.

NAMI, abbreviation for **National Alliance for the Mentally Ill.**

NANB, abbreviation for **non-A, non-B hepatitis.**

NANDA, abbreviation for **North American Nursing Diagnosis Association.**

nandrolone decanoate /nan'drəlōn/, an androgen.

■ INDICATIONS: It is prescribed in the treatment of testosterone deficiency, osteoporosis, and female breast cancer, and to stimulate growth, weight gain, and the production of red cells.

■ CONTRAINDICATIONS: Cancer of the male breast or prostate, liver disease, pregnancy, suspected pregnancy, or known hypersensitivity to this drug prohibits its use.

■ ADVERSE EFFECTS: Among the most serious adverse effects are various endocrine disturbances, depending on the age of the patient. Hirsutism, acne, liver toxicity, and electrolyte imbalances also occur.

nandrolone phenpropionate, an anabolic steroid with androgenic properties.

■ INDICATIONS: It is prescribed in the treatment of osteoporosis, in certain anemias, in metastatic breast cancers of women, and for protein-sparing effects in many situations.

■ CONTRAINDICATIONS: Carcinoma of the breast in males and some females, pregnancy, nephrosis, or known hypersensitivity to this drug prohibits its use.

■ ADVERSE EFFECTS: Among the more serious adverse reactions are hirsutism, acne, various endocrine effects depending on the age and sex of the patient, masculinization, liver dysfunction, hypercalcemia in women taking the drug for breast cancer, and fluid and salt retention.

nanism /nā′nizəm, nan′-/ [Gk, *nanos*, dwarf], an abnormal smallness or underdevelopment of the body; dwarfism. Kinds of nanism are **mulibrey nanism, Paltauf's nanism, pituitary nanism, renal nanism, senile nanism,** and **symptomatic nanism.** Also called **nanosomia.**

nano-, **1.** /nā′nō-/ a prefix meaning 'small, or related to smallness or dwarfism': *nanocephalia, nanomelia.* **2.** /nan′ə-/ a combining form used in measurement to mean 'billionth (10^{-9})': *nanocurie, nanogram, nanometer.*

nanocephalic dwarf. See **bird-headed dwarf.**

nanocephaly /nā′nōsef′əlē, nan′-/ [Gk, *nanos* + *kephale*, head], a developmental defect characterized by abnormal smallness of the head. Also called **nanocephalia, nanocephalism.** —**nanocephalous,** *adj.,* **nanocephalus,** *n.*

nanocormia /nā′nōkôr′mē·ə/ [Gk, *nanos* + *kormos*, trunk], abnormal disproportionate smallness of the trunk of the body in comparison with the head and limbs. —**nanocormus,** *n.*

nanocurie (nc, nC) /nan′əkyŏŏr′ē/ [Gk, *nanos*, dwarf; Marie and Pierre Curie], a unit of radiation equal to one billionth of a curie.

nanogram (ng) /nan′əgram/ [Gk, *nanos* + Fr, *gramme*, small weight], a unit of weight equal to one billionth of a gram.

nanomelia /nā′nōmē′lyə, nan′-/ [Gk, *nanos* + *melos*, limb], a developmental defect characterized by abnormally small limbs in comparison with the size of the head and trunk. —**nanomelous,** *adj.,* **nanomelus,** *n.*

nanometer (nm) /nan′əmē′tər/ [Gk, *nanos* + *metron*, measure], a unit of length equal to one billionth of a meter.

nanophthalmos /nā′nofthal′məs, nan′-/ [Gk, *nanos* + *ophthalmos*, eye], the condition in which one or both eyes are abnormally small, although other ocular defects are not present. Also called **nanophthalmia.** See also **microphthalmos.**

nanosecond (ns) /nan′əsek′ənd/ [Gk, *nanos*, dwarf; L, *secundus*, second], one billionth (10^{-9}) of a second.

nanosomia. See **nanism.**

nanosomus /nā′nōsō′məs/ [Gk, *nanos* + *soma*, body], a person of very short stature; a dwarf.

nanukayami /nä′nŏŏkäyä′mē/ [Jpn], an acute, infectious disease caused by one of the serotypes of the spirochete *Leptospira* that is indigenous to Japan. See also **leptospirosis.**

nanus /nā′nəs/, **1.** a dwarf. **2.** a pygmy. —**nanoid** /nā′noid/, *adj.*

napalm /nā′päm/, abbreviation for *napthenate palmitate,* a form of jellied gasoline used in warfare.

napalm burn [AS, *baernan,* burn], a thermal burn caused by contact with flaming **napalm.**

nape [ME], the back of the neck.

naphazoline hydrochloride /nəfaz′əlēn/, an adrenergic vasoconstrictor.

■ INDICATIONS: It is prescribed in the treatment of nasal congestion and as an ophthalmic vasoconstrictor.

■ CONTRAINDICATIONS: Glaucoma or known hypersensitivity to this drug or abnormal sensitivity to sympathomimetic drugs prohibits its use.

■ ADVERSE EFFECTS: Among the most serious adverse reactions are those associated with systemic absorption, including sedation and cardiovascular effects. Irritation to mucosa and rebound congestion also may occur.

naphthalene poisoning /naf′thəlēn/ [Gk, *naptha,* flammable liquid; L, *potio,* drink], a toxic condition, caused by the ingestion of naphthalene or paradichlorobenzene, that may cause nausea, vomiting, headache, abdominal pain, spasm, and convulsions. Treatment varies. Blood transfusion and fluid replacement may be necessary. Diazepam is indicated for the control of involuntary muscular contractions. Naphthalene and paradichlorobenzene are common ingredients in mothballs and moth crystals; paradichlorobenzene is also used as an insecticide in agriculture.

naphthol camphor /naf′thol/, a syrupy mixture of two parts of camphor and one part betanaphthol, used externally as an antiseptic.

naphthol poisoning. See **phenol poisoning.**

napkin ring tumor [ME, *nappekin,* tablecloth, *hring,* band; L, *tumor,* swelling], a tumor that encircles a tubular structure of the body, usually impairing its function and constricting its lumen to some degree.

NAP-NAP, abbreviation for **National Association of Pediatric Nurse Associates/Practitioners.**

N.A.P.N.E.S., abbreviation for **National Association for Practical Nurse Education and Services.**

napping [ME, *nappen,* to doze], periods of sleep, usually during the day, which may last from 15 to 60 minutes without attaining the level of deep sleep.

Naprosyn, a trademark for a nonsteroidal antiinflammatory, antipyretic, and analgesic (naproxen).

naproxen /naprok′sən/, a nonsteroidal antiinflammatory agent.

■ INDICATION: It is prescribed for the relief of inflammatory symptoms of arthritis.

■ CONTRAINDICATIONS: Impaired renal function, GI disease, or known hypersensitivity to this drug, to aspirin, or to nonsteroidal antiinflammatory drugs prohibits its use.

■ ADVERSE EFFECTS: Among the more serious adverse reactions are GI disorders and peptic ulcers. Dizziness, rashes, and tinnitus commonly occur. This drug interacts with many other drugs.

N.A.P.T., abbreviation for *National Association of Physical Therapists.* See also **A.P.T.A.**

Naqua, a trademark for a diuretic and antihypertensive (trichlormethiazide).

Naquival, a trademark for an antihypertensive, fixed-combination drug containing a diuretic (trichlormethiazide) and an antihypertensive (reserpine).

narc, abbreviation for **narcotic.**

Narcan, a trademark for a narcotic antagonist (naloxone hydrochloride).

narcissism /när′sisiz′əm/ [Gk, *Narcissus,* mythic youth in love with himself],   **1.** an abnormal interest in oneself, especially in one's own body and sexual characteristics; self-love. **2.** (in psychoanalysis) sexual self-interest that is a normal characteristic of the phallic stage of psychosexual development, occurring as the infantile ego acquires a libido. Narcissism in the adult is abnormal, representing fixation at this stage of development or regression to it. Compare **egotism.** See also **narcissistic personality, narcissistic personality disorder.**

narcissistic personality /när′sisis′tik/,   a personality characterized by behavior and attitudes that indicate an abnormal love of the self. Such a person is self-centered and self-absorbed, is extremely unrealistic concerning attributes and goals, vacillates between overidealizing and devaluing others, and, in general, assumes that he or she is entitled to more than is reasonable in relationships with others. Compare **narcissism.**

narcissistic personality disorder,   a condition characterized by an exaggerated sense of self-importance and uniqueness, an abnormal need for attention and admiration, preoccupation with grandiose fantasies concerning the self, and disturbances in interpersonal relationships, usually involving the exploitation of others and a lack of empathy for them.

narco- /när′kō/,   a prefix meaning 'related to stupor or a stuporous state': *narcolepsy, narcomania, narcotic.*

narcoanalysis /-ənal′isis/,   an interview conducted while the patient is deeply sedated with medication so that inhibitions are reduced and responses will be more truthful.

narcoanesthesia.   See **basal anesthesia.**

narcohypnosis /-hipnō′sis/ [Gk, *narke,* stupor; *hypnos,* sleep],   hypnosis induced with the aid of a narcotic drug, such as sodium amobarbital or sodium pentothal.

narcolepsy /när′kəlep′sē/ [Gk, *narke,* stupor, *lambanein,* to seize],   a syndrome characterized by sudden sleep attacks, cataplexy, sleep paralysis, and visual or auditory hallucinations at the onset of sleep. The syndrome begins in adolescence or young adulthood and persists throughout life. Its cause is unknown, and no pathologic lesions are found in the brain. Persons with narcolepsy experience an uncontrollable desire to sleep, sometimes many times in one day. Episodes may last from a few minutes to several hours. Momentary loss of muscle tone occurs during waking hours (cataplexy), or while the person is asleep. Narcolepsy may be difficult to diagnose because all people with the disorder do not experience all four symptoms. EEG or other brain studies may be used to distinguish narcolepsy from an intracranial mass or encephalitis. Amphetamines and other stimulant drugs are prescribed effectively to prevent the attacks.

narcoleptic /när′kəlep′tik/,   **1.** of or pertaining to a condition or substance that causes an uncontrollable desire for sleep. **2.** a narcoleptic drug. **3.** a person suffering from narcolepsy.

Narcon,   abbreviation for *Narcotics Anonymous.*

narcosis /närkō′sis/ [Gk *narkosis* numbness],   a state of insensibility or stupor caused by narcotic drugs. See also **narcotic.**

narcotic (narc) /närkot′ik [Gk, *narkotikos,* benumbing],   **1.** of or pertaining to a substance that produces insensibility or stupor. **2.** a narcotic drug. Narcotic analgesics, derived from opium or produced synthetically, alter perception of pain; induce euphoria, mood changes, mental cloud-

ing, and deep sleep; depress respiration and the cough reflex; constrict the pupils; and cause smooth muscle spasm, decreased peristalsis, emesis, and nausea. Repeated use of narcotics may result in physical and psychologic dependence. Among the narcotic drugs administered clinically for relief of pain are butorphanol tartrate, hydromorphone hydrochloride, morphine sulfate, pentazocine lactate, and meperidine hydrochloride. These drugs act by binding to opiate receptors in the central nervous system; narcotic antagonists, such as naloxone hydrochloride, which is used in treating narcotic overdosage, apparently displace opiates from receptor sites.

-narcotic, -narcotical,   a suffix meaning 'pertaining to analgesic or soporific drugs': *antinarcotic, prenarcotic, pseudonarcotic.*

narcotic analgesic.   See **analgesic.**

narcotic antagonist,   a drug that is used primarily in the treatment of narcotic-induced respiratory depression. The narcotic antagonists nalorphine, levallorphan, and naloxone are usually administered parenterally.

narcotic antitussive.   See **antitussive.**

narcotic poisoning [Gk, *narke,* stupor; L, *potio,* drink],   the toxic effects of a narcotic drug that depresses the brain centers, causing unconsciousness or coma. Narcotic drugs are generally derived from opium, but other drugs, including alcohol, can produce similar effects.

Nardil,   a trademark for an antidepressant (phenelzine sulfate).

nares /ner′ēz/, *sing.* **naris,**   the pairs of anterior openings and posterior openings in the nose that allow the passage of air from the nose to the pharynx and the lungs during respiration. See also **anterior nares, posterior nares.**

narrow-angle glaucoma.   See **glaucoma.**

nas-.   See **naso-.**

nasal (nas) /nā′zəl/ [L, *nasus,* nose],   of or pertaining to the nose and the nasal cavity. **nasally,** *adv.*

nasal airway,   a flexible, curved piece of rubber or plastic, with one wide, trumpetlike end and one narrow end that can be inserted through the nose into the pharynx.

nasal cannula,   a device for delivering oxygen by way of two small tubes that are inserted into the nares.

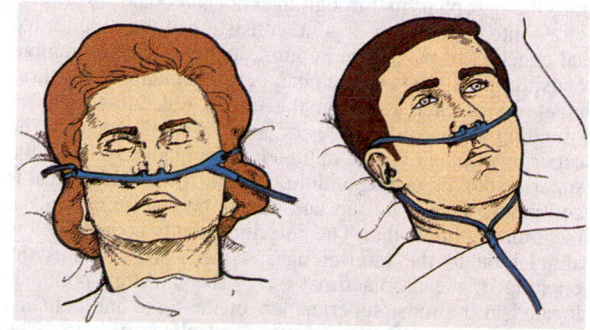

Nasal cannulas *(Wade, 1983)*

nasal cartilage [L, *nasus,* nose; *cartilago*],   a flat plate of cartilage in the lower anterior portion of the nasal septum. Also called **septal cartilage.**

nasal cavity,   one of a pair of cavities that open on the face

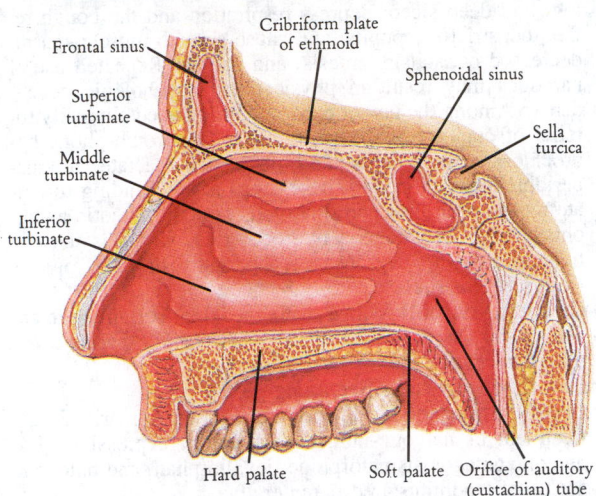

Frontal sinus
Superior turbinate
Middle turbinate
Inferior turbinate
Cribriform plate of ethmoid
Sphenoidal sinus
Sella turcica
Hard palate
Soft palate
Orifice of auditory (eustachian) tube

Nasal cavity *(Seidel, 1991)*

through the pear-shaped anterior nasal aperture and communicate with the pharynx. Each cavity is narrower at the top than at the bottom.

nasal decongestant, a drug that provides temporary relief of nasal symptoms in acute and chronic rhinitis and sinusitis. Most are over-the-counter products compounded with a small amount of vasoconstrictor, such as ephedrine or phenylephrine. An antihistamine may enhance the value of a nasal decongestant in allergic rhinitis, and a corticosteroid may reduce inflammation. Prolonged use or dosage greater than recommended on the package may cause rebound vasodilatation and severe congestion.

nasal drip, a method of slowly infusing liquid into a dehydrated infant by means of a catheter inserted through the nose down the esophagus.

nasal fossa, one of the pair of approximately equal chambers of the nasal cavity that are separated by the nasal septum and open externally through the nostrils and internally into the nasopharynx through the choanae. Each fossa is divided into an olfactory region, consisting of the superior nasal concha and part of the septum, and a respiratory region, constituting the rest of the chamber. Overhanging the three meatuses of each fossa on the lateral wall are the corresponding superior, middle, and inferior nasal conchae. The superior meatus extends obliquely about halfway along the superior border of the middle concha. The middle meatus continues into the atrium and bulges on the lateral wall at the bulla ethmoidalis. The inferior meatus courses below and lateral to the inferior nasal concha and contains the opening of the nasolacrimal duct. The olfactory region is located in the most superior part of the fossa and contains olfactory cells, olfactory nerves, and olfactory hairs. The respiratory region is lined with mucous membrane, numerous glands, nerves, a plexus of dilated veins, and blood spaces. The plexus is easily irritated, causing the membrane to swell, blocking the meatuses and the openings of sinuses.

nasal glioma, a neoplasm characterized by the ectopic growth of neural tissue in the nasal cavity.

nasal instillation of medication, the instillation of a medicated solution into the nostrils by drops from a drop-

per or by an atomized spray from a squeeze bottle. Drops are instilled in each nostril as the patient's neck is hyperextended and the head tilted back over the edge of the bed. The patient's mouth should remain open during the procedure, and the head should stay in the tilted back position for several minutes to allow spread of the medication through the nasal passages. Nasal spray is administered to the patient in a sitting position. The patient is asked to expectorate any solution that runs down the posterior nares into the throat.

nasalis /nāzal'is/ [L, *nasus*, nose], one of the three muscles of the nose, divided into a transverse part and an alar part. The transverse portion arises from the maxilla and covers the bridge of the nose; the alar part attaches at one end to the greater alar cartilage and at the other end to skin at the end of the nose. The transverse part serves to depress the cartilaginous portion of the nose and to draw the alar toward the septum. The alar part serves to dilate the nostril. The nasalis is innervated by buccal branches of the facial nerve. Compare **depressor septi, procerus.**

nasal obstruction [L, *nasus*, nose; *obstruere*], a narrowing of the nasal cavity, thereby reducing the breathing capacity, caused by an irregular septum, nasal polyps, foreign bodies, or enlarged turbinates. Sinusitis is a common complication of the condition.

nasal polyp, a rounded, elongated bit of boggy, dependent mucosa that projects into the nasal cavity.

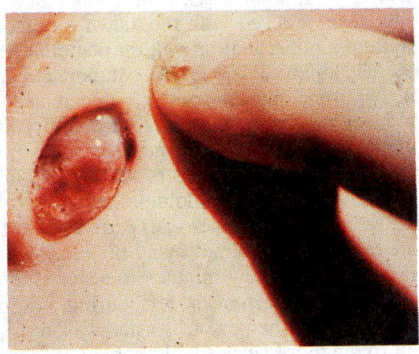

Nasal polyp
(Holgate, 1993/Courtesy D Gatland, St. Bartholomew's Hospital, London)

nasal septum, the partition dividing the nostrils. It is composed of bone and cartilage covered by mucous membrane.

nasal sinus, any one of the numerous cavities in various bones of the skull, lined with ciliated mucous membrane continuous with that of the nasal cavity. The membrane is very sensitive; easily irritated, it may cause swelling that blocks the sinuses. The nasal sinuses are divided into frontal sinuses, ethmoidal air cells, sphenoidal sinuses, and maxillary sinus.

nascent /nas'ənt, nā'sənt/ [L, *nasci*, to be born], **1.** just born; beginning to exist; incipient. **2.** (in chemistry) pertaining to any substance liberated during a chemical reac-

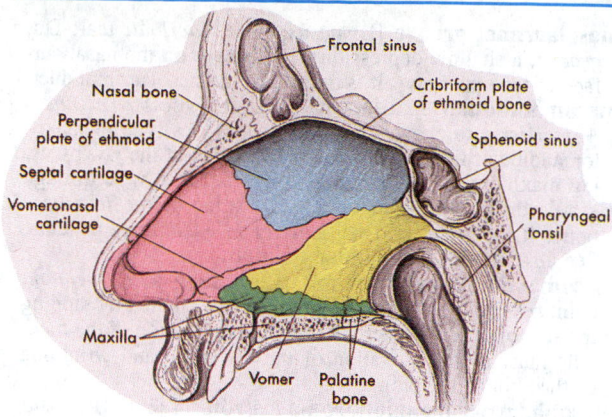

Nasal septum (*Thibodeau, 1993/Ernest W. Beck*)

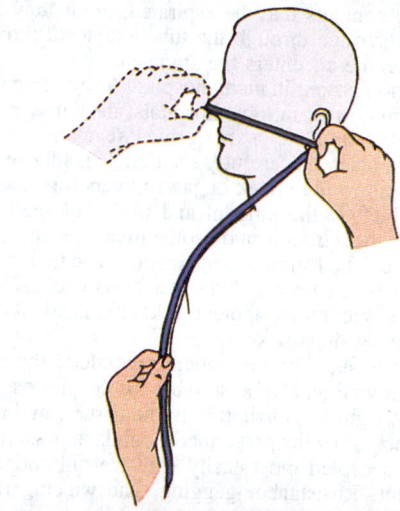

tion, which, because of its uncombined state, is more reactive.

nascent oxygen, oxygen that has just been liberated from a chemical compound.

nasion /nā′zē·on/ [L, *nasus*, nose], **1.** the anthropometric reference point at the front of the skull where the midsagittal plane intersects a horizontal line tangential to the highest points in the superior palpebral sulci. **2.** the depression at the root of the nose that indicates the junction of the intranasal and the frontonasal sutures.

naso- /nā′zō-/, **nas-,** a combining form meaning 'of or pertaining to the nose': *nasociliary, nasolabial, nasonnement.*

nasogastric feeding /nā′zōgas′trik/ [L, *nasus*, nose; Gk, *gaster*, stomach; AS, *faedan*, to feed], the process of introducing nutrients in a liquid form directly into the stomach via a nasogastric tube. Also called **gavage feeding.** See also **nasogastric intubation.**

nasogastric intubation, the placement of a nasogastric tube through the nose into the stomach to relieve gastric distention by removing gas, gastric secretions, or food; to instill medication, food, or fluids; or to obtain a specimen for laboratory analysis. After surgery and in any condition in which the person is able to digest food but not eat it, the tube may be introduced and left in place for tube feeding until the ability to eat normally is restored.

■ METHOD: A French size 12 to 18 plastic or rubber catheter is selected. The procedure is explained to the patient. If the catheter is rubber, it is soaked in ice water to stiffen and lubricate it. The patient is placed in an upright sitting position, and a towel or bib is placed over the chest. The necessary length of tube is marked off; it is the same as the distance from the tip of the nose to the earlobe. The tip of the tube may be lubricated with a water-soluble lubricating jelly, but, if a specimen is to be obtained for cytologic study, water or saline solution is preferred. The tube is grasped and held 7.5 cm from the tip and is placed in the nostril, where it is advanced forward and downward. When it has been passed 7.5 cm, it is in the pharynx. The patient is then asked to bend the neck forward, to take shallow, rapid breaths, and to help advance the tube by swallowing. The placement of the tube is checked after it has been inserted the predetermined distance to be sure that the tube is in the stomach and not in the lungs. This may be done in several ways: Fluoroscopy allows visualization of the place-

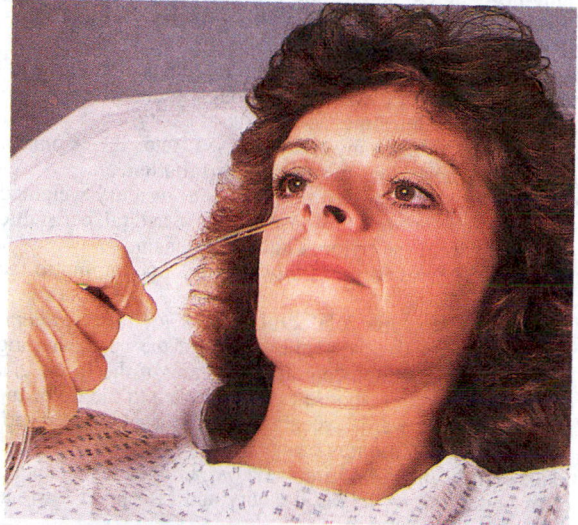

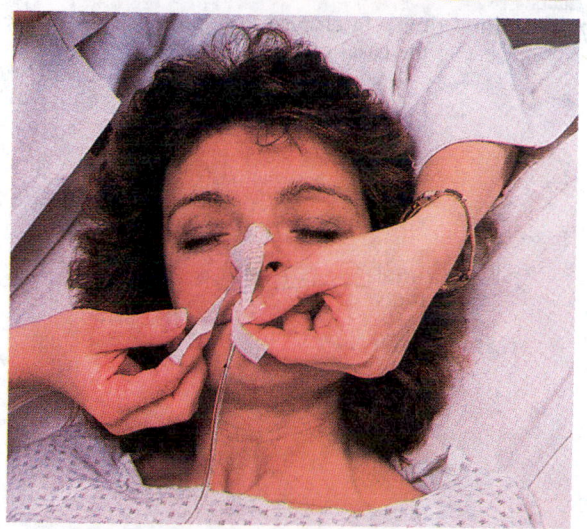

Nasogastric intubation (*Potter, 1993*)

ment; gastric contents may be aspirated; or air may be injected with a syringe through the tube and heard through a stethoscope as the air enters the stomach.

■ NURSING INTERVENTION: In many hospitals a physician inserts the tube the first time; in most hospitals, the nurse inserts it thereafter. Oral hygiene is performed regularly, and the tube, if left in place, is carefully secured with adhesive tape to the nose and to the cheek or jaw. Orders for tube feeding usually include the amount and timing of feeding, as well as the concentration and, sometimes, the ingredients of the formula. The formula is refrigerated and then warmed in a bowl of warm water. If the person is unconscious or unresponsive, suction equipment is kept at hand. An exact record of the feedings is kept.

■ OUTCOME CRITERIA: For the patient's comfort, the tube is selected to fit well and to be suitable for the purpose of the procedure: A tight fit is irritating to the tissues, and a small tube might not allow the prescribed formula to pass through. The tube is accepted most easily with the full cooperation of the patient. Resistance, gagging, and wincing may be minimized by explaining the procedure, by a slow steady progress, and by proper lubrication of the tube and positioning of the patient.

nasogastric suction, the removal by suction of solids, fluids, or gases from the GI tract through a tube inserted into the stomach or intestines via the nasal cavity.

nasogastric tube, any tube passed into the stomach through the nose. See **nasogastric intubation.**

nasojejunal tube /nā′zōjijo͞o′nəl/, a mercury-weighted tube inserted through the nose to allow natural peristaltic movement from the pylorus into the jejunum.

nasolabial [L, *nasus*, nose; *labium*, lip], pertaining to the nose and lip.

nasolabial reflex /nā′zōlā′bē·əl/ [L, *nasus*, nose, *labium*, lip], a sudden backward movement of the head, arching of the back, and extension and stretching of the limbs that occur in infants in response to a light touch to the tip of the nose with an upward sweeping motion. The reflex disappears by about 5 months of age.

nasolacrimal /nā′zōlak′riməl/ [L, *nasus* + *lacrima*, tears], of or pertaining to the nasal cavity and associated lacrimal ducts.

nasolacrimal duct, a channel that carries tears from the lacrimal sac to the nasal cavity.

nasolacrimal groove [L, *nasus*, nose; *lacrima*, tear; Du, *groeve*, a shallow depression], a groove on the nasal surface of the upper jaw. It is the site of the nasolacrimal duct.

nasomandibular fixation /nā′zōmandib′yo͞olər/ [L, *nasus* + *mandere*, to chew; *figere*, to fasten], a type of maxillomandibular fixation to stabilize fractures of the jaw by using maxillomandibular splints connected to a wire through a hole drilled in the anterior nasal spine of the maxillary bone. It has been used particularly in edentulous patients. See also **maxillomandibular fixation.**

nasomental reflex /-men′təl/ [L, *nasus*, nose; *mentum*, chin; *reflectere*, to bend back], a reflex elicited by tapping the side of the nose, thereby causing contraction of the mentalis muscle with elevation of the lower lip and wrinkling of the skin of the chin.

nasopharyngeal angiofibroma /nā′zōfərin′jē·əl/ [L, *nasus* + Gk, *pharynx*, throat], a benign tumor of the nasopharynx, consisting of fibrous connective tissue with many vascular spaces. The tumor usually arises in puberty and is more common in boys than in girls. Typical signs are nasal and eustachian tube obstruction, adenoidal speech, and dysphagia. Also called **juvenile angiofibroma, nasopharyngeal fibroangioma.**

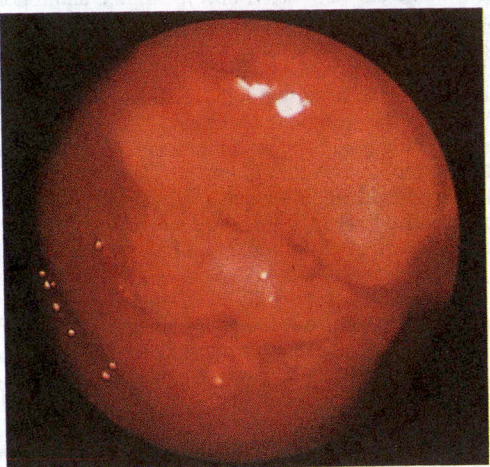

Squamous cell carcinoma of the nasopharynx
(Hawke, 1987)

nasopharyngeal cancer, a malignant neoplastic disease of the nasopharynx. Depending on the site of a nasopharyngeal tumor, there may be nasal obstruction, otitis media, hearing loss, sensory or motor nerve damage, bony destruction of the skull, or deep cervical lymphadenopathy. Diagnostic measures include nasopharyngoscopy, biopsy, and radiologic examination of the skull with tomographic studies. Squamous cell and undifferentiated carcinomas are the most common lesions. Nasopharyngeal cancer occurs rarely in the United States and very frequently in southern China. Exposure to dusts of nickel, chromium, wood, and leather and to isopropyl oil increases the risk of developing nasopharyngeal cancer. High titers of antibodies to the Epstein-Barr virus are found in Chinese patients with the cancer, and there is evidence of genetic susceptibility, because a certain histocompatibility antigen is associated with

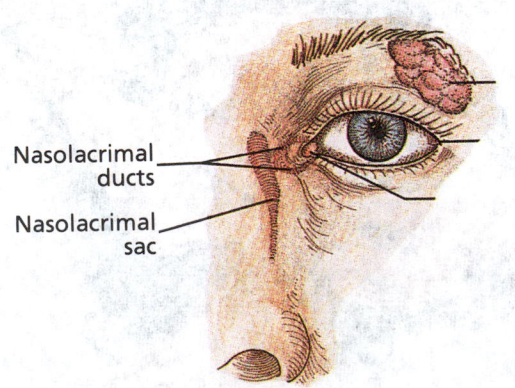

Nasolacrimal ducts

Nasolacrimal sac

Nasolacrimal ducts *(Potter, 1993)*

the disease and multiple cases occur in some families. Radiation is the most effective therapy, and 5-fluorouracil and adriamycin are also used.

nasopharyngeal fibroangioma. See **nasopharyngeal angiofibroma.**

nasopharyngography /-fer′ingog′rəfē/ [L, *nasus* + Gk, *pharynx*, throat, *graphein*, to record], radiographic imaging and examination of the nasopharynx.

nasopharyngoscopy /nā′zōfer′ing·gos′kəpē/ [L, *nasus* + Gk, *pharynx*, throat, *skopein*, to look], a technique in physical examination in which the nose and throat are visually examined using a laryngoscope, a fiberoptic device, a flashlight, and a dilator for the nares. **—nasopharyngoscopic,** *adj.*

nasopharynx /nā′zōfer′ingks/ [L, *nasus* + Gk, *pharynx*, throat], the uppermost of the three regions of the throat, or pharynx, situated behind the nose and extending from the posterior nares to the level of the soft palate. On the posterior wall of the nasopharynx, opposite the posterior nares, are the pharyngeal tonsils. Swollen or enlarged pharyngeal tonsils can fill the space behind the posterior nares and may completely block the passage of air from the nose into the throat. Compare **laryngopharynx, oropharynx.** See also **tonsil. —nasopharyngeal,** *adj.*

nasotracheal tube /-trā′kē·əl/ [L, *nasus* + Gk, *tracheia*, rough artery; L, *tubus*], a catheter inserted into the trachea through the nasal cavity and the pharynx. It is commonly used to administer oxygen and in other respiratory therapy.

nat-, a prefix meaning 'pertaining to birth': *natal, natality.*

natal /nā′təl/, **1.** [L, *natus*] of or pertaining to birth. **2.** [L *nates*] of or pertaining to the nates, or buttocks.

nates /nā′tēz/, *sing.* **natis** [L, buttocks], the large fleshy protuberances at the lower posterior portion of the torso comprising fat and the gluteal muscles. Also called **buttocks.**

natimortality. See **mortinatality.**

National Alliance for the Mentally Ill (NAMI), a national organization for family members of psychotic patients.

National Association for Mental Health. See **Mental Health Association.**

National Association for Practical Nurse Education and Services (N.A.P.N.E.S.), a national organization concerned with the education of practical nurses and with the services provided by licensed practical nurses.

National Association of Pediatric Nurse Associates/ Practitioners (NAP-NAP), a national organization of nurses who are prepared by training or experience to give primary care to pediatric patients. NAP-NAP works in conjunction with American Academy of Pediatrics.

National Bureau of Standards (NBS), a federal agency in the Department of Commerce that sets accurate measurement standards for commerce, industry, and science in the United States. The NBS compares and coordinates its standards with those of other countries and provides research and technical service to improve computer science, materials technology, building construction, and consumer product safety. The Bureau also provides measurement services and standards for other federal agencies and for state and local governments.

National Council Licensure Examination (NCLEX), a comprehensive integrated examination, developed and administered by the National Council of State Boards of Nurs-

ing, designed to test basic competency for nursing practice. The NCLEX-RN test plan has three components including nursing behaviors grouped under nursing process categories, the process of decision making that defines nursing's role, and levels of cognitive ability.

National Eye Institute (NEI), a division of the National Institutes of Health. NEI was established in 1968 to support research in the normal functioning of the human eye and visual system, the pathology of visual disorders, and the rehabilitation of the visually handicapped. See also **eye, vision.**

National Formulary (N.F.), a publication containing the official standards for the preparation of various pharmaceutics not listed in the *United States Pharmacopoeia.* It is revised every 5 years.

national health insurance, a health insurance program that is financed by taxes and administered by the government to provide comprehensive health care that is accessible to all citizens of that nation.

National Health Planning and Resources Development Act of 1974, U.S congressional legislation (PL 93-641) that established a nationwide network of health systems agencies. The act provides for the coordination and direction of national health policy through state and regional regulatory agencies.

National Health Service Corps (NHSC), a program of the United States Public Health Service (USPHS) in which health care personnel are placed in areas that are underserved. The Corps was established by the Emergency Health Personnel Act of 1970. The provisions of the Act are updated as needed. Nurses, physicians, and dentists serve in rural and urban areas, usually as employees of local health care agencies. The USPHS pays most of the salary of each corps member.

National Institute of Child Health and Human Development (N.I.C.H.H.D.), a branch of the National Institutes of Health that is concerned with all aspects of the growth, development, and health of the children of the United States.

National Institute of Mental Health (NIMH), a branch of the (U.S.) National Institutes of Health within the Alcohol, Drug Abuse, and Mental Health Administration. It is responsible for federal research and education programs dealing with mental health.

National Institutes of Health (N.I.H.), an agency within the United States Public Health Service made up of several institutions and constituent divisions, including the Bureau of Health Manpower Education, the National Library of Medicine, the National Cancer Institute, and several research institutes and divisions.

National League for Nursing (NLN), an organization concerned with the improvement of nursing education, nursing service, and the provision of health care in the United States. Among its many activities are accreditation of nursing programs, preadmission and achievement tests for nursing students, and compilation of statistic data on nursing personnel and on trends in health care delivery. It acts as the testing service for the State Board Test Pool Examinations for registered and practical nurse licensure. The Research Division and the Public Affairs Office are among the other sections of NLN. A monthly refereed journal, *Nursing and Health Care,* is the official publication of the organization.

National Male Nurses' Association (NMNA), a national organization that promotes the interests and practice of male nurses.

National Marrow Donor Program (NMDP), a coordinating center for bone marrow transplants, providing links with national and international registries of prospective volunteer donors of HLA-compatible bone tissue.

National Organization of Victims Assistance, a private, nonprofit organization of victims and witness assistance practitioners, criminal justice professionals, researchers, former victims, and others committed to the recognition of victims' rights.

National Society of Critical Care Nurses of Canada (NSCCN), an organization of Canadian critical care nurses, established originally in 1975 as the Toronto Chapter of the American Association of Critical-Care Nurses. The group became an independent Canadian organization in 1983. Publications include a bimonthly journal, *Critical Care Nurse,* and a newsletter, *CriticaList.*

National Student Nurses Association (NSNA), a national organization of students in the field of nursing. Among its purposes are the improvement of nursing education to improve health care, to aid in the development of the nursing student, and to encourage optimal achievement in the professional role of the nurse and the health care of people. It publishes a journal, *Imprint,* five times a year, participates in legislative activities at all levels, and gives scholarships, awards, and career workshops.

natriuresis /nā′trēyŏŏrē′sis/ [L, *natrium,* sodium; Gk, *ouresis,* urination], the excretion of greater than normal amounts of sodium in the urine, such as from the administration of natriuretic diuretic drugs or from various metabolic or endocrine disorders.

natriuretic /nā′trēyŏŏret′ik/, **1.** of or pertaining to the process of natriuresis. **2.** a substance that inhibits the resorption of sodium ions from the glomerular filtrate in the kidneys, thus allowing more sodium to be excreted with the urine.

natural antibody /nach′(ə)rəl/ [L, *natura,* nature; Gk, *anti*; AS, *bodig,* body], an antibody that is present in serum in the absence of an apparent specific antigen contact.

natural childbirth [L, *natura,* nature; AS, *cild,* child; ME, *bwith,* birth], labor and parturition accomplished by a mother with little or no medical intervention. It is generally considered the optimal way of giving birth and being born, safest for the baby and most satisfying for the mother. Prerequisites include normal gestation, an adequate birth canal, strong maternal motivation, physical and emotional preparation, and constant and intensive support of the mother during labor and birth. See also **Lamaze method.**

natural dentition, the entire array of natural teeth in the dental arch at any given time, consisting of deciduous or permanent teeth or a mixture of the two. See also **tooth.**

natural family planning method, any one of several methods of family planning that does not rely on a medication or a device for effectiveness in avoiding pregnancy. Some of the methods are also used to pinpoint the time of ovulation to increase the chance of fertilization when artificial insemination or extraction of an oocyte for in vitro fertilization is to be performed. Natural family planning methods require thorough instruction, the cooperation and self-motivation of the couple, and the diligent, accurate observation and recording of the data relevant to the method. Kinds of natural family-planning include **basal body tem-**

perature method of family planning, calendar method of family planning, ovulation method of family planning, and symptothermal method of family planning.

natural immunity, a usually innate and permanent form of immunity to a specific disease. Kinds of natural immunity include **individual immunity, racial immunity,** and **species immunity.** Also called **genetic immunity, innate immunity.** Compare **acquired immunity.**

naturalistic illness /nach′ərəlis′tik/, an illness thought to be caused by impersonal factors, such as a disturbance in the Oriental yin and yang equilibrium or the Hispanic model of hot and cold forces.

natural killer cells (NK) [L, *natura*; ME, *kullen,* to kill; *cella,* storeroom], effector cells that have the capacity for spontaneous cytotoxicity toward various target cells. These cells are lymphocytes that are capable of binding to and killing virus-infected and tumor cells by a mechanism not yet understood.

natural law, a doctrine that holds there is a natural moral order or natural moral law inherent in the structure of the universe.

naturally acquired immunity. See **acquired immunity.**

natural network, (in psychiatric nursing) a patient's natural contacts in the community, including church and social groups, friends, family, and occupation that support the person's function outside the hospital environment.

natural pacemaker, any cardiac pacing site in the heart tissues.

natural radiation, radioactivity that emanates from the soil and rocks or particles and rays that reach the earth from cosmic sources, such as actinic radiation from the sun and neutrinos from beyond the solar system.

natural selection, the natural evolutionary processes by which those organisms best suited for adaptation to the environment tend to survive and propagate the species, whereas those unfit are eliminated. Compare **artificial selection.**

Naturetin, a trademark for a diuretic and antihypertensive (bendroflumethiazide).

nature versus nurture /nur′chər/, a name given to a longstanding controversy as to the relative influences of genetics versus the environment in the development of personality. Nature is represented by instincts and genetic factors and nurture by social influences.

naturopath /nach′ərōpath′/ a person who practices naturopathy.

naturopathy /nach′ərop′əthē/ [L, *natura* + Gk, *pathos,* disease], a system of therapeutics based on natural foods, light, warmth, massage, fresh air, regular exercise, and the avoidance of medications. Advocates believe that illness can be healed by the natural processes of the body.

Nauheim bath /nou′hīm/ [Nauheim, Germany; AS, *baeth,* bath], a bath taken in water through which carbon dioxide is bubbled, followed by systematic exercises, used in the treatment of cardiac conditions. The procedure is named after the natural waters of Bad Nauheim, Germany. Also called **Nauheim treatment.**

nausea /nô′zē·ə, nô′zhə/ [Gk, *nausia,* seasickness], a sensation often leading to the urge to vomit. Common causes are seasickness and other motion sicknesses, early pregnancy, intense pain, emotional stress, gallbladder disease, food poisoning, and various enteroviruses. **–nauseate,** *v.,* **nauseous,** *adj.*

nausea and vomiting of pregnancy, a common condition of early pregnancy, characterized by recurrent or persistent nausea, often in the morning, that may result in vomiting, weight loss, anorexia, general weakness, and malaise. The causes of the condition are poorly understood. It usually does not begin before the sixth week after the last menstrual period and ends by the twelfth to the fourteenth week of pregnancy. Symptomatic relief is often obtained by eating small, easily digested meals frequently and by not allowing the stomach to be empty. In the past, antiemetic drugs were routinely prescribed for this complaint, but this practice is currently reserved for severe cases. Nausea and vomiting after the sixteenth week is an unusual complication of pregnancy, called persistent nausea and vomiting of pregnancy. If it is severe and intractable, hyperemesis gravidarum may ensue. Also called (nontechnical) **morning sickness.**

nauseous /nô'shəs, nô'zē·əs/ [Gk, nausia, seasickness], pertaining to feelings of nausea or reaction to things that may stimulate nausea.

Navane a trademark for a tranquilizer (thiothixene).

navel. See **umbilicus.**

navicular /navik'yələr/, boat-shaped; sunken.

navicular bone. See **scaphoid bone.**

navicular pads, tarsal supports for flat feet. They are inserted directly under the arch of the foot. Also called **shoe cookies.**

n.b., abbreviation for the Latin nota bene, 'note well'.

Nb, symbol for the element **niobium.**

NBRC, abbreviation for National Board for Respiratory Care.

NBS standard, (in nuclear medicine) a radioactive source standardized, or certified, or both, by the National Bureau of Standards.

nc, nC, abbreviation for **nanocurie.**

N-CAP, abbreviation for **Nurses' Coalition for Action in Politics.**

NCI, abbreviation for the National Cancer Institute. See **National Institutes of Health.**

NCLEX-RN abbreviation for **National Council Licensure Examination.**

Nd, abbreviation for the element **neodymium.**

N.D., abbreviation for Doctor of Naturopathy.

N.D.A., abbreviation for National Dental Association.

NE, abbreviation for **niacin equivalent.**

Ne, symbol for the element **neon.**

ne-, See **neo-.**

Neal-Robertson litter, a modified spine board for transporting trauma patients with spinal injuries.

near-death experience [ME, nere, deth; L, experientia, trial], the subjective observations of people who have either been close to clinical death or who may have recovered after having been declared dead. Many claim to have witnessed similar episodes of passing through a tunnel toward a bright light and encountering people who had preceded them in death.

near drowning [AS, near, almost; ME, drounen, to drown], a pathologic state in which the victim has survived exposure to circumstances that usually cause drowning. Cardiopulmonary resuscitation is performed immediately; hospitalization is always indicated. The return of consciousness does not necessarily assure recovery. Intensive supportive therapy may be required for up to several days. Compare **drowning.** See also **hypothermia.**

nearest neighbor analysis, (in molecular genetics) a bio-

chemical method used to estimate the frequency with which pairs of bases are located next to one another.

nearsightedness. See **myopia.**

nebula /neb'yələ/, pl. nebulae [L, cloud], **1.** a slight corneal opacity or scar that seldom obstructs vision and that can be seen only by oblique illumination. **2.** a murkiness in the urine. **3.** an oily concoction that is applied with an atomizer.

nebulization /neb'yəlīzā'shən/ [L, nebula, cloud; Gk, izein, to cause], a method of administering a drug by spraying it into the respiratory passages of the patient. The medication may be given with or without oxygen to help carry it into the lungs.

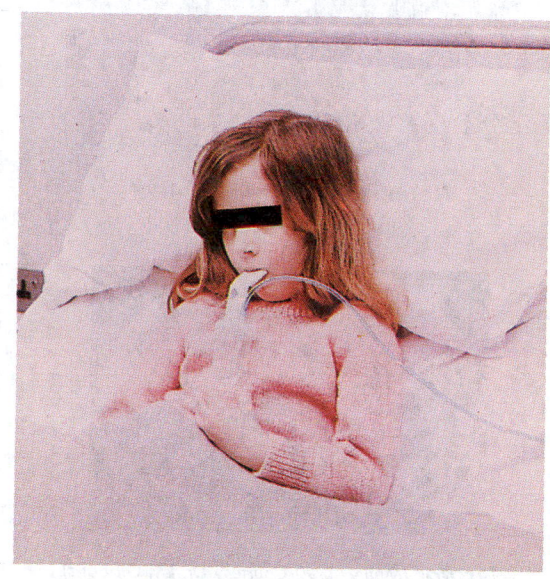

Drug administration via nebulization
(Turner-Warwick, 1993)

nebulize /neb'yəlīz/, to vaporize or disperse a liquid in a fine spray.

nebulizer /neb'yəlī'zər/, a device for producing a fine spray. Intranasal medications are often administered by a nebulizer. Also called **atomizer.**

NEC, abbreviation for **necrotizing enterocolitis.**

Necator /nekā'tər/ [L, necare, to kill], a genus of nematode that is an intestinal parasite and causes hookworm disease. See also Ancylostoma.

necatoriasis /nek'ətərī'əsis/ [L, necare, to kill; Gk, osis, condition], hookworm disease, specifically that caused by Necator americanus, the most common North American hookworm. The larvae live in the soil and reach the human digestive tract through contaminated food and water or through the skin of the feet and legs. Symptoms include diarrhea, nausea, abdominal pain, and anemia in the more severe cases. Treatment consists of first correcting the anemia if present and then anthelmintic therapy, usually with pyrantel pamoate or mebendazole. Prevention includes the elimination of soil pollution and the avoidance of skin contact with the soil. See also **ancylostomiasis, hookworm.**

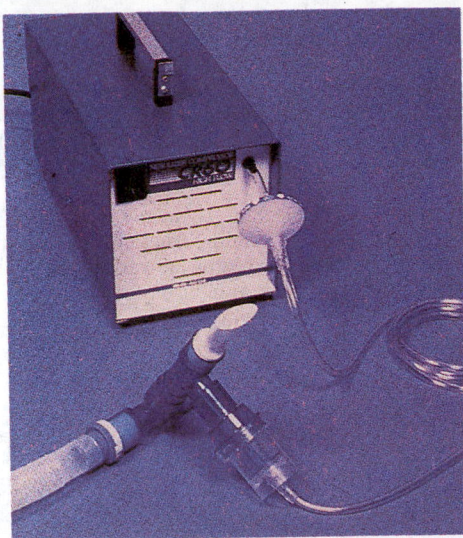

Nebulizer (Turner-Warwick, 1993)

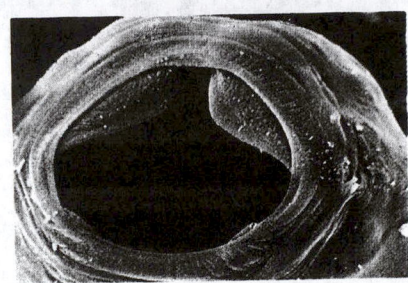

Necator (Muller, 1990/Courtesy Dr. LM Gibbons)

neck [AS, *hnecca*], a constricted section, such as the part of the body that connects the head with the trunk. Other such constrictions are the neck of the humerus and the neck of the femur.

neck dissection, surgical removal of the cervical lymph nodes, performed to prevent the spread of malignant tumors of the head and neck. Under general anesthesia, the cervical chain of lymph nodes with their lymphatic channels is removed in one mass to prevent the spread of cancer cells. After surgery, the patient is observed closely for signs of hemorrhage and difficulty in breathing. Compare **radical neck dissection.**

neck of femur [AS, *hnecca*; L, *femur*, thigh], the portion of the long bone of the thigh between the head and the greater and lesser trochanters.

neck righting reflex, 1. an involuntary response in newborns in which turning the head to one side while the infant is supine causes rotation of the shoulders and trunk in the same direction. The reflex enables the child to roll over from the supine to prone position. Absence of the reflex or persistence beyond about 10 months of age may indicate central nervous system damage. 2. any tonic reflex associated with the neck that maintains body orientation in relation to the head.

neck ring, a metal ring at the neck of a cervicothoracolumbosacral orthosis. It opens posteriorly for ease in putting on or removing the orthosis and is an attachment for a throat mold and occiput pads.

neck shaft angle, an angle created by the intersection of a line drawn through the femoral shaft and a line through the femoral head and neck.

neck sign. See **Brudzinki's sign.**

necro-, a combining form meaning 'of or pertaining to death or a corpse': *necronectomy, necrophilia, necrosis, necrotic.*

necrobiosis lipoidica /nek′rōbī·ō′sis lipoi′dikə/ [Gk, *nekros,* dead, *bios,* life; *lipos,* fat, *eidos,* form], a skin disease characterized by thin, shiny, yellow to red plaques on the shins or forearms. Telangiectases, crusting, and ulceration of these plaques may occur. Necrobiosis lipoidica is usually associated with diabetes mellitus and occurs most often in women. Treatment includes precise control of the diabetes and, possibly, intralesional application of corticosteroids.

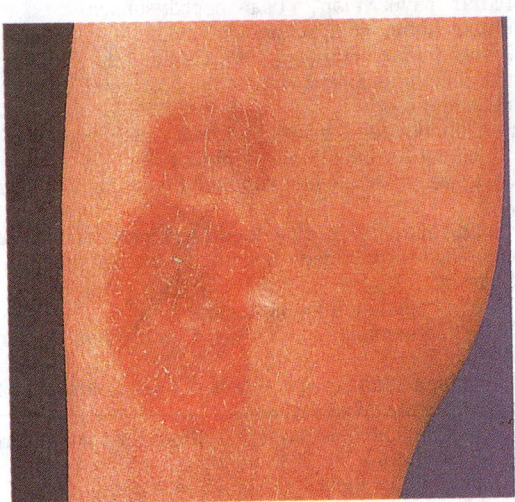

Necrobiosis lipoidica (McKee, 1993)

necrogenic /nek′rōjen′ik/ [Gk, *nekros,* dead; *genein,* to produce], 1. capable of causing death, as of cells or tissue. 2. originating or caused by infected dead matter. Also **necrogenous** /nekroj′ənəs/

necrology (necrol) /nekrol′əjē/ [Gk, *nekros,* dead; *logos,* science], the study of the causes of death, including the compilation and interpretation of mortality statistics.

necrolysis /nekrol′isis/ [Gk, *nekros* + *lysis,* loosening], disintegration or exfoliation of dead tissue. Compare **necrosis.** —**necrolytic,** *adj.*

necrophilia /nek′rōfil′yə/ [Gk, *nekros* + *philein,* to love], 1. a morbid liking for being with dead bodies. 2. a morbid desire to have sexual contact with a dead body, usually of men to perform a sexual act with a dead woman. —**necrophile, necrophiliac,** *n.*

necrophobia [Gk, *nekros,* death; *phobos,* fear], a morbid fear of death and dead bodies.

necropsy, necroscopy. See **autopsy.**

necrosis /nekrō′sis/ [Gk, *nekros* + *osis,* condition], localized tissue death that occurs in groups of cells in response to disease or injury. In **coagulation necrosis,** blood clots block the flow of blood, causing tissue ischemia distal to the clot; in **gangrenous necrosis,** ischemia combined with bacterial action causes putrefaction to set in. See also **gangrene.**

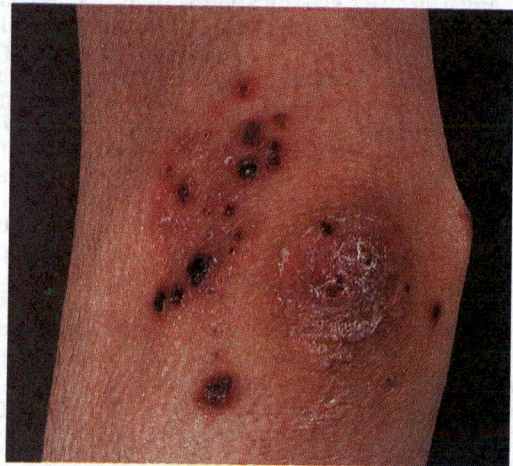

Tissue necrosis (du Vivier, 1993)

necrotic /nekrot′ik/,   pertaining to the death of tissue in response to disease or injury.

necrotizing /nek′rōtī′zing/ [Gk, *nekros*, death],   causing the death of tissues or organisms.

necrotizing angiitis.   See **periarteritis nodosa.**

necrotizing enteritis [Gk, *nekros* + *izein*, to cause, *enteron*, intestine, *itis*],   acute inflammation of the small and the large intestine by the bacterium *Clostridium perfringens,* characterized by severe abdominal pain, bloody diarrhea, and vomiting. Some people recover completely, some survive with chronic bowel obstruction, and some die of perforation of the intestine, dehydration, peritonitis, or septicemia.

necrotizing enterocolitis (NEC),   an acute inflammatory bowel disorder that occurs primarily in preterm or low-birthweight neonates. It is characterized by ischemic necrosis of the GI mucosa that may lead to perforation and peritonitis. The cause of the disorder is unknown, although it appears to be a defect in host defenses with infection resulting from normal GI flora rather than from invading organisms. Also called **pseudomembranous enterocolitis.** See also **enteritis.**

■ OBSERVATIONS: Significant predisposing factors of the condition include prematurity, hypovolemia, respiratory distress syndrome, sepsis, an indwelling umbilical catheter, exchange transfusion, and feeding with hyperosmolar or high-caloric formulas. The condition results from a reflex shunting of blood away from the GI tract, which leads to convulsive vasoconstriction of the mesenteric vessels supplying the intestines. The diminished blood supply interferes with the normal production of mucus and with other bowel functions and results in severe necrosis with bacterial invasion of the bowel wall. Bottle-fed infants are more susceptible to the disorder, possibly because formula lacks the im-

munoglobulin A antibodies and macrophages, found in breast milk, that may protect the GI mucosa from damage and bacterial invasion. Initial symptoms, which usually develop after several days of life, include temperature instability (usually hypothermia), lethargy, poor feeding, vomiting of bile, abdominal distention, blood in the stools, and decreased or absent bowel sounds. Signs of deterioration are apnea, pallor, hyperbilirubinemia, oliguria, abdominal tenderness, and erythema and edema of the anterior abdominal wall or palpable masses, with eventual respiratory failure leading to death. Diagnosis is confirmed by x-ray visualization of the intestine or by the presence of increased peritoneal fluid or pneumoperitoneum.

■ INTERVENTIONS: Treatment includes discontinuing oral feeding, beginning intravenous infusion, abdominal decompression by nasogastric suction, hydration, plasma or whole blood transfusion, and administration of broad-spectrum antibiotics (usually ampicillin, gentamicin, or kanamycin). With routine supportive management, improvement usually occurs within 48 to 72 hours. Oral feedings usually are not resumed for 10 days to 2 weeks. Total parenteral nutrition is necessary during that period. Surgical resection of the affected bowel segment may be necessary, especially if signs of intestinal perforation or peritonitis develop. If a large portion of bowel is affected, an ileostomy or colostomy may be necessary. Stenosis of the involved bowel segment may present later complications.

■ NURSING CONSIDERATIONS: The primary concern of the nurse is to observe high-risk, formula-fed infants for early symptoms of necrotizing enterocolitis, especially for difficulty in feeding, bile-stained regurgitation, bloody stools, temperature fluctuations, or a distended, shiny abdomen. After the diagnosis is confirmed, the nurse initiates nasogastric intubation for abdominal decompression and continues to monitor the baby constantly for dehydration and electrolyte balance. In addition to the ordered laboratory tests, daily weight is taken. Infants who are unable to take fluids by mouth require special oral care. A pacifier helps to meet the infant's need to suck. Parents are encouraged to visit and are helped to meet the emotional needs of the infant and to provide tactile, auditory, and visual stimulation. The nurse explains the usual course of the disease and the medical and nursing procedures, and keeps the parents informed of the infant's progress. Frequent visits to the care unit facilitate family-infant relationships and provide the nurse with an opportunity to teach proper care techniques before discharge.

necrotizing vasculitis,   an inflammatory condition of blood vessels, characterized by necrosis, fibrosis, and proliferation of the inner layer of the vascular wall, in some cases resulting in occlusion and infarction. Necrotizing vasculitis may occur in rheumatoid arthritis and is common in systemic lupus erythematosus, periarteritis nodosa, and progressive systemic sclerosis. The condition is usually treated with corticosteroids.

needle bath [AS, *naedl*, needle],   a shower in which fine jets of water are sprayed over the body.

needle biopsy,   the removal of a segment of living tissue for microscopic examination by inserting a hollow needle through the skin or the external surface of an organ or tumor and rotating it within the underlying cellular layers. See also **aspiration biopsy.**

needle filter,   a device, usually made of plastic, used for filtering medications that are drawn into a syringe before administration. Some syringe needles have built-in filters;

other filters are separate units that are attached to the needle before use. Manufacturers' instructions are usually supplied with such devices. Needle filters are commonly disposable items designed for one-time use.

needle holder, a surgical forceps used to hold and pass a suturing needle through tissue. Also called **suture forceps.**

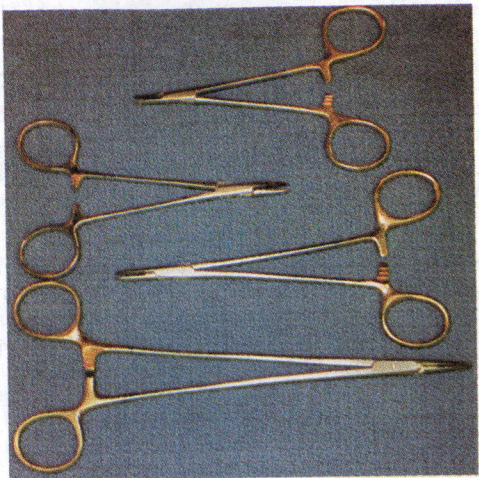

Needle holders *(Grossman, 1993)*

needle-stick injuries, accidental skin punctures resulting from contact with hypodermic syringe needles. The contact may occur accidentally during efforts to inject a patient or as a result of carelessly touching discarded medical waste. Such injuries can be dangerous, particularly if the needle

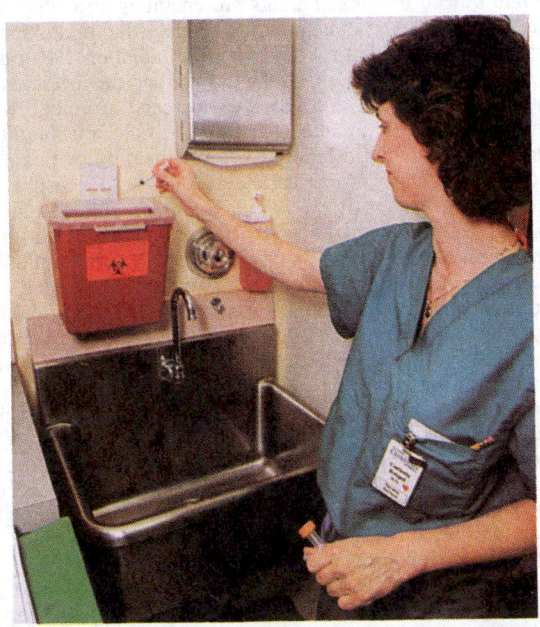

Prevention of needlestick injuries *(Wong, 1993)*

has been used in treatment of a patient with a severe blood-borne infection, such as AIDS. To prevent injuries, used needles are not capped or broken and are disposed of in a rigid, puncture-resistant container located near the site of use.

NEEP, abbreviation for **negative end-expiratory pressure.**

Neer and Horowitz classification system, a method of classifying proximal humeral fractures in children, based on the degree of separation of the epiphysis from the shaft.

Neer classification system, a method of classifying femoral supracondylar and intercondylar fractures. The system ranges from *type I* for minimal displacement through *type IIA* and *IIB* to *type III* for conjoined supracondylar and shaft fractures. The Neer system is also applied to humeral head and neck fractures.

negative (neg) /neg'ətiv/ [L, *negare*, to deny persistently], **1.** (of a laboratory test) indicating that a substance or a reaction is not present. **2.** (of a sign) indicating on physical examination that a finding is not present, often meaning that there is no pathologic change. **3.** (of a substance) tending to carry or carrying a negative chemical charge.

negative adaptation. See **habituation.**

negative anxiety, (in psychology) an emotional and psychologic condition in which anxiety prevents a person's normal functioning and interrupts the person's ability to perform the usual activities of daily living.

negative catalysis, a decrease in the rate of any chemical reaction caused by a substance that is not part of the process itself, not consumed and not affected by the reaction. Also called **inhibition.** Compare **catalysis.** See also **catalyst.**

negative electrode [L, *negare*, to deny; Gk, *elektron*, amber; *hodos*, way], a cathode, or the negative pole of an electric current or of a battery or dry cell.

negative end-expiratory pressure (NEEP), a technique used to counterbalance the increase in mean intrathoracic pressure caused by intermittent positive pressure breathing (IPPB) in an effort to return negative intrathoracic pressure for venous return to the right atrium. Generally, the negative pressure is applied to the circuit on exhalation by using a jet or Venturi system, and the resulting subatmospheric pressure is applied to the patient's airways.

negative feedback, **1.** (in physiology) a decrease in function in response to a stimulus; for example, the secretion of follicle-stimulating hormone decreases even as the amount of circulating estrogen increases. **2.** *informal.* a critical, de-

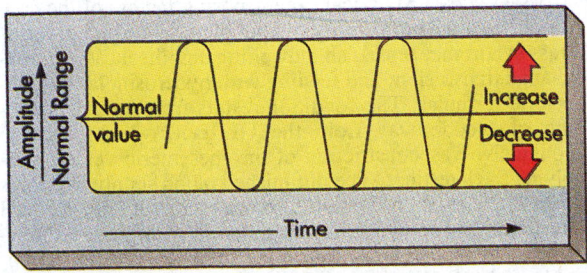

Negative feedback *(Seeley, 1992)*

rogatory, or otherwise negative response from one person to what another person has communicated.

negative identity, the assumption of a persona that is at odds with the accepted values and expectations of society.

negative pathognomonic symptom [L, *negare*, to deny; Gk, *pathos*, disease + *gnomen*, index + *symptoma*, that which happens], any symptom that is not usually found in a specific condition and if present would not be compatible with the diagnosis.

negative pi meson (pion), a form of electromagnetic radiation emitted from a proton linear accelerator.

negative pi meson (pion) radiotherapy, a form of radiotherapy using a negative pi meson (pion) beam emitted by a proton linear accelerator. In the treatment of certain tumors, negative pi meson particles are beamed at the tumor; the atomic nuclei of malignant cells take in the radioactive particles and explode, scattering intensely radioactive subatomic particles through the adjacent malignant tissue. Pion radiotherapy requires fewer rad and has a 60% greater biologic effect than conventional x-radiation techniques. It also may have less effect on normal tissue near the tumor. Some locally advanced neoplasms, especially those of the prostate, are destroyed. Gliomas and advanced cancers of the head and neck also may be well controlled with pion radiotherapy. Moderately acute toxicity occurs with treatment; chronic toxicity is minimal.

negative pressure, less than ambient atmospheric pressure, such as in a vacuum, at an altitude above sea level, or in a hypobaric chamber. Some ventilators have a negative cycle that may help stimulate or cycle exhalation in controlled ventilation in IPPB therapy.

negative punishment, a form of behavior modification in which the removal of something after an operant (behavior) decreases the probability of the operant's recurrence.

negative reinforcer, (in psychology) a stimulus that, when presented immediately after occurrence of a particular behavior, will decrease the rate of occurrence of the behavior.

negative relationship, (in research) an inverse relationship between two variables; as one variable increases, the other decreases. Also called **inverse relationship.** Compare **positive relationship.**

negativism /neg'ətiviz'əm/ [L, *negare*, to deny persistently], a behavioral attitude characterized by opposition, resistance, the refusal to cooperate with even the most reasonable request, and the tendency to act in a contrary manner. The resulting response may be passive, such as the immobile, rigid postures observed in catatonic schizophrenia, or active, such as in a belligerent, impulsive, or capricious act, such as lowering the arms when asked to raise them or sitting down when asked to stand.

NegGram, a trademark for an antibacterial (nalidixic acid).

neglect /nəglekt'/, a condition that occurs when a parent or guardian is unable to or fails to provide minimal physical and emotional care for a child or other dependent person.

negligence /neg'lijens/ [L, *negligentia*, carelessness], (in law) the commission of an act that a prudent person would not have done or the omission of a duty that a prudent person would have fulfilled, resulting in injury or harm to another person. In particular, in a malpractice suit, a professional person is negligent if harm to a client results from such an act or such failure to act, but it must be proved that other prudent members of the same profession would ordi-

narily have acted differently under the same circumstances. Thus negligence may be misfeasance, malfeasance, or nonfeasance.

negligence per se, (in law) a finding of negligence rendered in judgment of a professional action or inaction in violation of a statute or so at odds with common sense that beyond any doubt no prudent person would have been guilty of it.

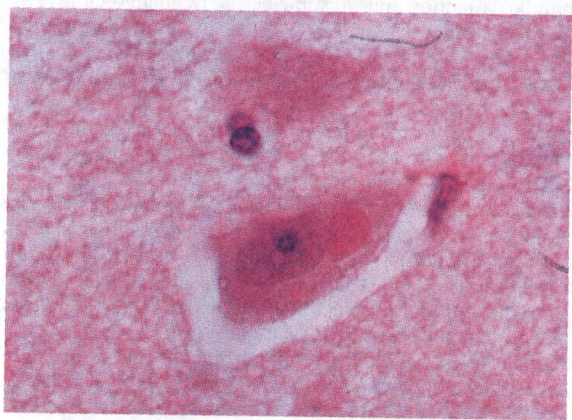

Negri bodies (Murray, 1990)

Negri bodies /nā'grē/ [Adelchi Negri, Italian physician, b. 1876; AS, *bodig*], intracytoplasmic inclusion bodies found in the brain and central nervous system cells of rabies victims.

NEI, abbreviation for **National Eye Institute.**

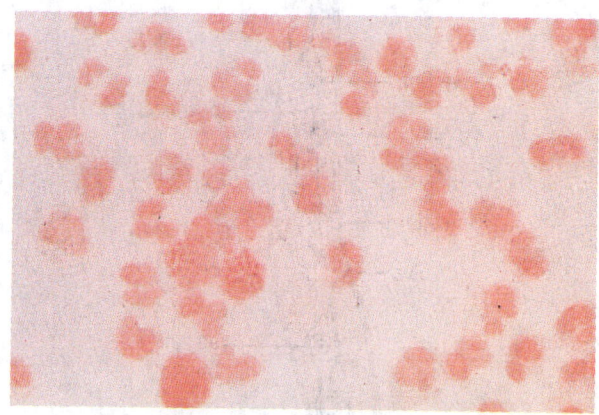

Neisseria gonorrhoeae (Murray, 1990)

Neisseria gonorrhoeae /nīser'ē·ə/ [Albert L. S. Neisser, Polish dermatologist, b. 1855; Gk, *gone*, seed, *rhoia*, flow], a gram-negative, nonmotile, diplococcal bacterium: usually seen microscopically as flattened pairs within the cytoplasm of neutrophils. It is the causative organism of gonorrhea. Also called **gonococcus.**

Neisseria meningitidis. See **meningococcus.**

NEJM, abbreviation for *New England Journal of Medicine.*

Nélaton's dislocation /nälätôNz'/ [Auguste Nélaton, French surgeon, b. 1807], a dislocation of the ankle in which the distal ends of the tibia and fibula are separated and the talus is forced upward between the tibia and fibula.

Nelson's syndrome [Donald H. Nelson, American physician, b. 1925], an endocrine disorder that may follow adrenalectomy for Cushing's disease. It is characterized by a marked increase in the secretion of ACTH and MSH by the pituitary gland. Treatment includes irradiation to decrease pituitary function and, in some cases, hypophysectomy. See also **Cushing's disease.**

nem, abbreviation for **Nahrungs-Einheit-Milch.**

nema-, a prefix meaning 'pertaining to a thread': *nematode, nematocide.*

-nema, a suffix meaning a 'threadlike stage in the development of chromosomes': *chromonema, plasmonema, uronema.*

nemato-, a combining form meaning 'pertaining to a nematode, or to a threadlike structure': *nematoblast, nematocide, nematodiasis.*

nematocides /nəmat'əsīdz/ [Gk, *nema*, thread, *eidos*, form; L, *caedere*, to kill], chemical pesticides that are employed to kill nematode worms.

nematocyst /nem'ətōsist'/ [Gk, *nema*, thread; *eidos*, form; *kystis*, bag], a barbed threadlike process on the surface of coelenterates and attached to a poison sac. The stinger, found on the Portuguese man-of-war and other types of jellyfish, can be ejected into the skin of a human or animal, causing painful and potentially fatal injury.

nematode /nem'ətōd/ [Gk, *nema* + *eidos*, form], a multicellular, parasitic animal of the phylum Nematoda. All roundworms belong to the phylum, including *Ancylostoma duodenale, Ascaris lumbricoides, Enterobius vermicularis, Necator americanus, Strongyloides stercoralis,* and several other species.

nematodiasis /nem'ətōdī'əsis/ [Gk, *nema*, thread; *eidos*, form; *osis*, condition], an infestation of nematode worms.

Nembutal, a trademark for a barbiturate (pentobarbital), used as an adjunct to anesthesia.

-nemia. See **-anemia.**

neo- /nē'ō-/, a prefix meaning 'new': *neobiogenesis, neocyte, neonatal.*

neoantigen /-an'tijən/ [Gk, *neos*, new, *anti*, against, *genein*, to produce], a new specific antigen that develops in a cell infected by oncogenic virus.

neobehaviorism /-bihā'vē·əriz'əm/ [Gk, *neos* + ME, *behaven*, behavior], a school of psychology based on the general principles of behaviorism but broader and more flexible in concept. It stresses experimental research and laboratory analyses in the study of overt behavior and in various subjective phenomena that cannot be directly observed and measured, such as fantasies, love, stress, empathy, trust, and personality. See also **behaviorism.**

neobehaviorist /-ist/, a disciple of the school of neobehaviorism.

neoblastic /-blas'tik/ [Gk, *neos* + *blastos*, germ], of or pertaining to a new tissue or development within a new tissue.

neocerebellum /-ser'əbell'əm/, those parts of the cerebellum that receive input via the corticopontocerebellar pathway.

neocortex /-kôr'teks/ [Gk, *neos*, new; L, *cortex*, bark], the most recently evolved part of the brain. In humans, the neocortex includes all of the cerebral cortex except for the hippocampal and piriform areas.

NeoDecadron, a trademark for a topical, fixed-combination drug containing a glucocorticoid (dexamethasone phosphate) and an antibacterial (neomycin sulfate).

neodymium (Nd) /-din'ē·əm/ [Gk, *neos* + *didymos*, twin], a rare earth element. Its atomic number is 60; its atomic weight is 144.27.

neoglottis /-glot'is/, a vibrating structure that replaces the glottis in alaryngeal speech, such as after a laryngectomy. Also called **pseudoglottis.**

neologism /nē·ol'əjiz'əm/ [Gk, *neos* + *logos*, word], **1.** a word or term newly coined or used with a new meaning. **2.** (in psychiatry) a word coined by a psychotic or delirious patient that is meaningful only to the patient.

neomycin sulfate /-mī'sin/, an aminoglycoside antibiotic.
■ INDICATIONS: It is prescribed in the treatment of infections of the intestine, in hepatic coma, and, topically, in the treatment of skin infections.
■ CONTRAINDICATIONS: Renal dysfunction, intestinal obstruction, or known hypersensitivity to this drug or to any aminoglycoside medication prohibits its use.
■ ADVERSE EFFECTS: Among the more serious adverse reactions are nausea, vomiting, diarrhea, malabsorption, or suprainfection. Prolonged treatment in patients with impaired renal function may result in the toxicities of systemic aminoglycosides. Hypersensitivity reactions may occur with topical administration of this drug.

neon (Ne) /nē'on/ [Gk, *neos*, new], a colorless, odorless gaseous element and one of the inert gases. Its atomic number is 10; its atomic weight is 20.2. Neon has no compounds and occurs in the atmosphere in the ratio of about 18 parts

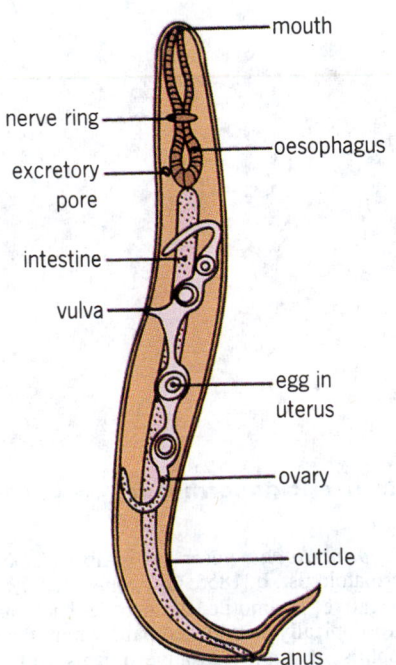

Principal features of adult female nematode
(Muller, 1990)

mouth
nerve ring
excretory pore
intestine
vulva
oesophagus
egg in uterus
ovary
cuticle
anus

per million. Some minerals and meteorites contain traces of this element. It is prepared commercially by the fractional distillation of liquefied air, and is one of the first components to boil off. Neon is an excellent conductor of electricity, which ionizes the gas and causes it to emit a reddish-orange glow; this characteristic makes neon useful in devices to warn against electric current overload.

neonatal /-nā′təl/ [Gk, *neos* + L, *natus*, born], the period of time covering the first 28 days after birth.

Neonatal Behavior Assessment Scale, a scale for evaluating and assessing an infant's alertness, motor maturity, irritability, consolability, and interaction with people. It is used as a tool for the evaluation of the neurologic condition and the behavior of a newborn infant. Using the scale, the individuality of an infant may be demonstrated for parents, and some researchers theorize that the quality of the parent-child relationship may be predicted.

neonatal breathing, respiration in newborn infants that begins when pulmonary fluid in the lungs is expelled by mechanic compression of the thorax during delivery and by resorption from the alveoli into the bloodstream and lymphatics. As air enters the lungs, the chest and lungs recoil to a resting position, but forceful inspirations are necessary to keep the lungs inflated. These forces come from changes in blood gas tension, strong Hering-Breuer reflexes, temperature, and tactile stimuli. Irregular fetal breathing movements, which occur during rapid eye movement sleep, may be observed as early as 13 weeks of gestation. At birth, the peripheral and central chemoreceptors are very active, and newborns are highly sensitive to carbon dioxide during the first weeks. However, control of rhythm is not fully developed at birth.

neonatal conjunctivitis. See **ophthalmia neonatorum.**

neonatal death, the death of a live-born infant during the first 28 days after birth. Early neonatal death is usually considered to be one that occurs during the first 7 days. Compare **infant death, perinatal death.**

neonatal developmental profile, an evaluation of the developmental status of a newborn infant based on three examinations: a gestational age inventory, a neurologic examination, and a Neonatal Behavior Assessment score.

neonatal hyperbilirubinemia. See **hyperbilirubinemia of the newborn.**

neonatal intensive care unit (NICU), a hospital unit containing a variety of sophisticated mechanic devices and special equipment for the management and care of premature and seriously ill newborn infants. The unit is staffed by a team of nurses and neonatologists who are highly trained in the pathophysiology of the newborn. See also **intensive care unit.**

neonatal jaundice. See **hyperbilirubinemia of the newborn.**

neonatal mortality, the statistic rate of infant death during the first 28 days after live birth, expressed as the number of such deaths per 1000 live births in a specific geographic area or institution in a given time.

neonatal period, the interval from birth to 28 days of age. It represents the time of the greatest risk to the infant; approximately 65% of all deaths that occur in the first year of life happen during this 4-week period.

neonatal pustular melanosis, a transient skin condition of the neonate characterized by vesicles present at birth that become pustular. The lesions contain neutrophils rather than

eosinophils as seen in erythema toxicum neonatorum, and they disappear within 72 hours, leaving dark spots that gradually fade by about 3 months of age.

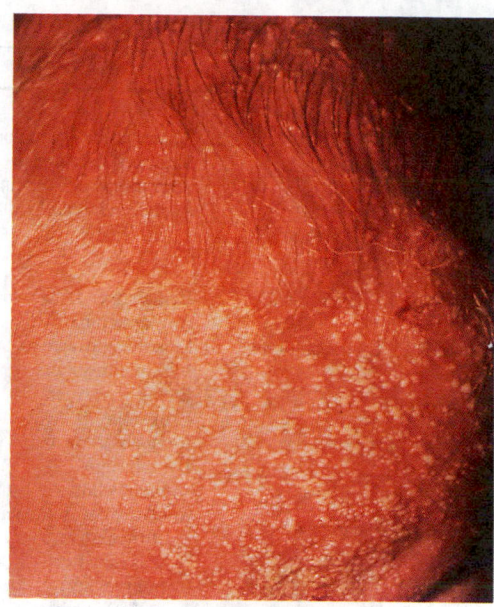

Neonatal pustular melanosis *(Zitelli, 1992)*

neonatal thermoregulation, the regulation of the body temperature of a newborn infant, which may be affected by evaporation, conduction, radiation, and convection.

■ METHOD: To prevent the loss of body heat through evaporation, the infant is patted dry with a warm towel immediately after birth. Loss of heat by conduction is prevented by wrapping the baby in a warm blanket or wrapping a warm blanket over the baby as the baby lies on the mother's skin and by warming all equipment that is to be used to touch, cover, or examine the infant. Loss of heat by radiation can be minimized by placing the baby under a radiant heater, on a warmed, padded surface, or in skin-to-skin contact with the mother. Loss of body heat by convection is prevented by avoiding drafts, air conditioning vents, and low ambient temperatures. Infant bassinets have high sides to prevent cross drafts.

■ INTERVENTIONS: The infant is kept covered and protected from any means of heat loss. Because the surface area of the head of a newborn is proportionately large when compared with the body, heat loss from the head may be great; therefore a cap or fold of blanket is placed around the head. Progressive family-centered maternity services, in which the practice after delivery is to place the infant skin-to-skin with the mother, often provide caps made of stockinet. An overhead radiant heater is rolled to the delivery bed to maintain a warm ambient temperature for the infant.

■ OUTCOME CRITERIA: The axillary temperature is normally between 36.5° C (97.5° F) and 37° C (98.6° F).

neonatal tyrosinemia. See **tyrosinemia.**

neonatal unit, a unit of a hospital that provides care and treatment of newborn infants through the age of 28 days, and longer if necessary.

neonate /nē′ənāt/, an infant from birth to 4 weeks of age.

neonatology /nē′ōnātol′əjē/ [Gk, *neos* + L, *natus*, born;

Classification of neoplasms

Parent tissue	Benign tumor	Malignant tumor
Epithelium		
Skin and	Papilloma	Squamous cell carcinoma
mucous	Polyp	Basal cell carcinoma
membrane		Transitional cell carcinoma
Glands	Adenoma	Adenocarcinoma
	Cystadenoma	
Endothelium		
Blood vessels	Hemangioma	Hemangioendothelioma
		Angiosarcoma
Lymph vessels	Lymphangioma	Lymphangiosarcoma
Bone marrow		Multiple myeloma
		Ewing's sarcoma
		Leukemia
		Lymphosarcoma
		Lymphangio-endothelioma
Lymphoid tissue		Reticular cell sarcoma (difficult to classify because of cell embryology)
		Lymphatic leukemia
Connective tissues		
Embryonic fibrous tissue	Myxoma	Myxosarcoma
Fibrous tissue	Fibroma	Fibrosarcoma
Adipose tissue	Lipoma	Liposarcoma
Cartilage	Chondroma	Chondrosarcoma
Bone	Osteoma	Osteogenic sarcoma
Synovial membrane	Synovioma	Synovial sarcoma
Muscle tissue		
Smooth muscle	Leiomyoma	Leiomyosarcoma
Striated muscle	Rhabdomyoma	Rhabdomyosarcoma
Nerve tissue		
Nerve fibers and sheaths	Neuroma	Neurogenic sarcoma
	Neurinoma (neurilemoma)	
	Neurofibroma	Neurofibrosarcoma
Ganglion cells	Ganglioneuroma	Neuroblastoma
Glial cells	Glioma	Glioblastoma
		Spongioblastoma
Meninges	Meningioma	
Pigmented neoplasms		
Melanoblasts	Pigmented nevus	Malignant melanoma
		Melanocarcinoma
Miscellaneous		
Placenta	Hydatidiform mole	Chorion-epithelioma (choriocarcinoma)
	Dermoid cyst	Embryonal carcinoma
		Embryonal sarcoma
		Teratocarcinoma

From Phipps WJ, Long BL, Woods NF, Cassmeyer VL: *Medical-surgical nursing: concepts and clinical practice*, ed 4, St Louis, 1991, Mosby.

Gk, *logos*, science], the branch of medicine that concentrates on the care of the neonate and specializes in the diagnosis and treatment of the disorders of the newborn infant. **–neonatologic, neonatological,** *adj.*, **neonatologist,** *n.*

neonatorum encephalitis /-nātôr′əm/ [Gk, *neos*, new; L, *natus*, born; Gk, *enkephalos*, brain; *itis*, inflammation], a brain inflammation that develops in the first four weeks of life. Also called **encephalitis neonatorum**.

neoplasia /nē′ōplā′zhə/ [Gk, *neos* + *plassein*, to mold], the new and abnormal development of cells that may be benign or malignant. **–neoplastic** /-plas′tik/, *adj.*

neoplasm /nē′ōplaz′əm/ [Gk *neos* + *plasma* formation], any abnormal growth of new tissue, benign or malignant. Also called **tumor.** See **benign, cancer, malignant. –neoplastic,** *adj.*

neoplastic /nē′ōplas′tik/ [Gk, *neos*, new; *plassein*, to mold], pertaining to **neoplasty.**

neoplastic fracture, a fracture resulting from a weakness in bone tissue caused by neoplasm or by a malignant growth. Also called **pathologic fracture.**

neoplastic pericarditis [Gk, *neos*, new + *plasma*, something formed + *peri*, around + *kardia*, heart + *itis*, inflammation], a pericardial inflammation, usually secondary to a malignant tumor within the area. Also called **carcinomatous pericarditis.**

neoplasty /nē′ōplas′tē/ [Gk, *neos*, new; *plassein*, to mold], a plastic surgery procedure to restore a part or add a new part.

Neosporin, a trademark for a topical, fixed-combination drug containing antibacterials (polymyxin B sulfate, neomycin sulfate, and bacitracin zinc).

neostigmine bromide /nē′ōstig′mēn/, a cholinergic.

■ INDICATION: It is prescribed in the treatment of myasthenia gravis.

■ CONTRAINDICATIONS: Bowel obstruction, urinary tract infection, or known hypersensitivity to this drug or to other bromides prohibits its use.

■ ADVERSE EFFECTS: Among the more serious adverse reactions are severe respiratory depression, ptyalism, and intestinal cramps.

Neo-Synephrine Hydrochloride, a trademark for a vasoconstrictor (phenylephrine hydrochloride).

neoteny /nē·ot′ənē/ [Gk, *neos*, new, *teinein*, to stretch], the attainment of sexual maturity during the larval stage of development, such as in certain amphibians, especially salamanders.

nephelometer /nef′əlom′ətər/ [Gk, *nephele*, cloud, *metron*, measure], a photometric apparatus used to determine the concentration of solids suspended in a liquid or a gas, such as may be used to determine the number of bacteria in a specimen. See also **nephelometry.**

nephelometry /nef′əlom′ətrē/, a technique of determining the concentration of solids suspended in a liquid or a gas by use of a nephelometer. **–nephelometric, nephelometrical,** *adj.*

nephr-. See **nephro-.**

nephrectomize /nəfrek′təmīz/ [Gk, *nephros*, kidney; *ektome*, cutting out], to perform a nephrectomy.

nephrectomy /-təmē/ [Gk, *nephros*, kidney, *ektome*, excision], the surgical removal of a kidney, performed to remove a tumor or otherwise diseased kidney. Before surgery, the fluid intake is increased to improve the excretion of waste products. The blood is typed and crossmatched for transfusion. During surgery, the kidney is approached through either a flank or a thoracoabdominal incision and is removed. If the thoracic cavity is opened, a chest tube is inserted and connected to water-seal drainage. The nurse observes carefully for rapid pulse, restlessness, sweating, and a drop in blood pressure. The urinary output is measured hourly, and fluid intake and body weight are closely monitored. Deep breathing is difficult because the incision is close to the diaphragm. The nurse reports at once any sudden shortness of breath, a sign of spontaneous pneumothorax that may occur if the pleura was accidentally nicked during surgery.

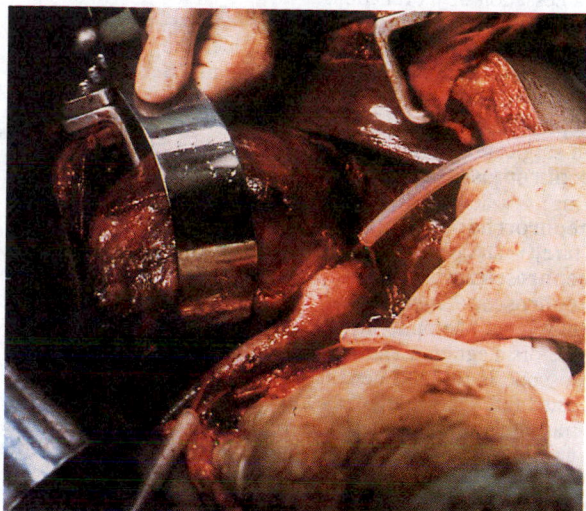

Radical nephrectomy (Weiss, 1988)

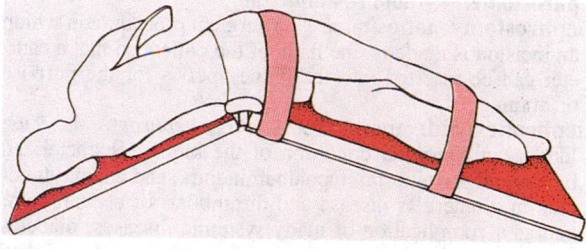

Positioning of patient for nephrectomy (Potter, 1993)

-nephric, a suffix meaning 'of or referring to the kidneys': *archinephric, cardionephric, splenonephric.*

nephritic /nəfrit'ik/ [Gk, *nephros,* kidney; *itis,* inflammation], pertaining to an inflammation of the kidney.

nephritic calculus. See **renal calculus.**

nephritic gingivitis [Gk, *nephros* + L, *icus,* like; *gingiva,* gum; Gk, *itis,* inflammation], a kind of stomatitis and gingivitis associated with kidney function failure, accompanied by pain, ammoniac odor, and increased salivation. Also called **uremic gingivitis.**

nephritis /nəfrī'tis/ [Gk, *nephros* + *itis,* inflammation],

any one of a large group of diseases of the kidney characterized by inflammation and abnormal function. Kinds of nephritis include **acute nephritis, glomerulonephritis, hereditary nephritis, interstitial nephritis, parenchymatous nephritis,** and **suppurative nephritis.**

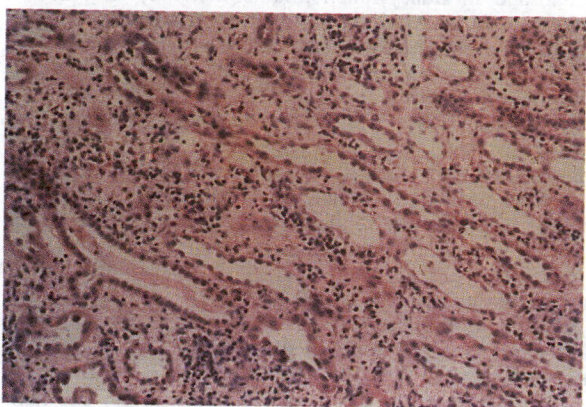

Acute interstitial nephritis (Brostoff, 1991)

nephro- /nef'rō-/, **nephr-,** a prefix meaning 'of or related to the kidneys': *nephroblastoma, nephrogram, nephrorrhagia.*

nephroangiosclerosis /nef'rō·an'jē·ō'sklerō'sis/ [Gk, *nephros* + *aggeion,* vessel, *skleros,* hard, *osis,* condition], necrosis of the renal arterioles, associated with hypertension. This condition is present in a small number of hypertensive individuals between 30 and 50 years of age. Early signs of the condition are headaches, blurring of vision, and a diastolic blood pressure greater than 120 mm Hg. Examination of the retina reveals hemorrhages, vascular exudates, and papilledema. The heart is usually enlarged, especially the left ventricle. Proteins and red blood cells are found in the urine. Heart failure and kidney failure may occur if the disease remains untreated. Treatment includes measures to lower blood pressure using diet and antihypertensive medications. Hemodialysis is used when preventive measures have failed. Also called **malignant hypertension.** See also **hypertension, renal failure.**

nephroblastoma. See **Wilms' tumor.**

nephrocalcinosis /nef'rōkal'sinō'sis/ [Gk, *nephros* + L, *calx,* lime; Gk, *osis,* condition], an abnormal condition of the kidneys in which deposits of calcium form in the parenchyma at the site of previous inflammation or degenerative change. Infection, hematuria, anal colic, and decreased function of the kidney may occur.

nephrogenic /nef'rōjen'ik/ [Gk, *nephros* + *genein,* to produce], **1.** generating kidney tissue. **2.** originating in the kidney.

nephrogenic ascites, the abnormal presence of fluid in the peritoneal cavity of patients undergoing hemodialysis for renal failure. The cause of this type of ascites is unknown. See also **ascites.**

nephrogenic cord, either of the paired longitudinal ridges of tissue that lie along the dorsal surface of the coelom in the early developing vertebrate embryo. It is formed from the fusion of the nephrotome tissue and gives rise to the structures making up the embryonic urogenital system. See also **mesonephros, metanephros, pronephros.**

nephrogenic diabetes insipidus, an abnormal condition in which the kidneys do not concentrate the urine, resulting in polyuria, polydipsia, and very dilute urine. The secretion of antidiuretic hormone (ADH) by the pituitary is normal, and all kidney function is normal except that there is no response to ADH. See also **diabetes insipidus.**

nephrogenous /nəfroj'ənəs/, of or pertaining to the formation and development of the kidneys.

nephrohypertrophy /-hīpur'trəfē/ [Gk, *nephros*, kidney; *hyper*, excessive; *trophe*, nourishment], enlargement of the kidney.

nephrolith /nef'rəlith/ [Gk, *nephros* + *lithos*, stone], a calculus formed in a kidney. **—nephrolithic,** *adj.*

nephrolithiasis /nef'rōlithī'əsis/, a disorder characterized by the presence of calculi in the kidney. See also **renal calculus.**

nephrology /nəfrol'əjē/ [Gk, *nephros* + *logos*, science], the study of the anatomy, physiology, and pathology of the kidney. **—nephrologic, nephrological,** *adj.*

nephrolytic /-lit'ik/ [Gk, *nephros* + *lysis*, loosening], of or pertaining to the destruction of the structure and function of a kidney.

-nephroma, a combining form meaning a 'tumor of the kidney or area of the kidney': *epinephroma, paranephroma.*

nephromere. See **nephrotome.**

nephron /nef'ron/ [Gk, *nephros*, kidney], a structural and functional unit of the kidney, resembling a microscopic funnel with a long stem and two convoluted sections. Each kid-

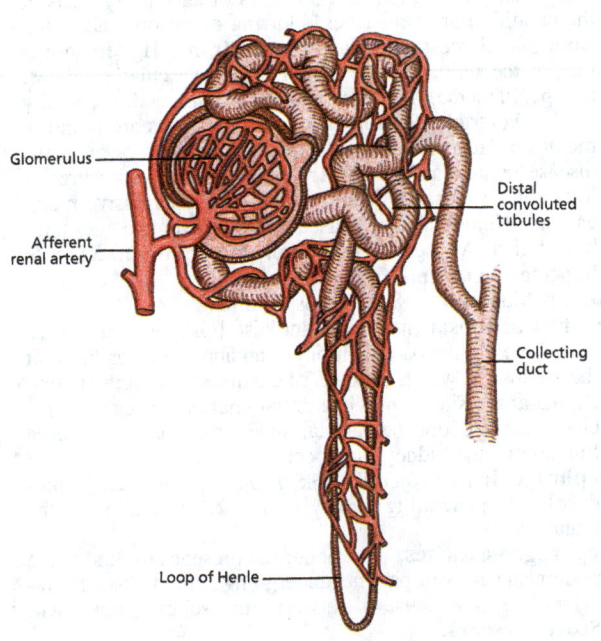

Nephron *(Potter, 1993)*

ney contains about 1.25 million nephrons, each consisting of the renal corpuscle, the loop of Henle, and the renal tubules. Each renal corpuscle consists of the glomerulus of renal capillaries enclosed within Bowman's capsule. The renal corpuscles and the convoluted portions of the renal tubules are located in the cortex of the kidney. The renal medulla contains the loops of Henle and the collecting tubules. Urine is formed in the renal corpuscles and in the renal tubules by filtration, reabsorption, and secretion. Also called **nephrone** /nef'rōn/. See also **kidney, malpighian corpuscle.**

nephronophthisis. See **medullary cystic disease.**

nephroparalysis /-pəral'isis/ [Gk, *nephros*, kidney; *paralyein*, to be palsied], a paralysis of the kidney resulting in a cessation of its functions.

nephropathy /nefrop'əthē/ [Gk, *nephros* + *pathos*, disease], any disorder of the kidney, including inflammatory, degenerative, and sclerotic conditions. See also **kidney disease.**

nephropexy /nef'rəpek'sē/ [Gk, *nephros* + *pexis*, fixation], a surgical operation to fixate a floating or ptotic kidney.

nephroptosis /nef'rəptō'sis/ [Gk, *nephros* + *ptosis*, falling], a downward displacement or dropping of a kidney.

nephrorrhaphy /nəfrôr'əfē/ [Gk, *nephros* + *rhaphe*, suture], an operation that sutures a floating kidney in place.

nephrosclerosis. See **nephroangiosclerosis.**

nephroscope /nef'rəskōp'/ [Gk, *nephros* + *skopein*, to look], a fiberoptic instrument that is used specifically for the disintegration and removal of renal calculi. The nephroscope is inserted percutaneously, and the calculi are located through use of x-ray films of the renal pelvis. An ultrasonic probe emitting high-frequency sound waves breaks up the calculi, which are removed by suction through the scope.

nephrosis. See **nephrotic syndrome.**

nephrostoma /-stō'mə/, *pl.* **nephrostomas, nephrostomata** [Gk, *nephros* + *stoma*, mouth], the funnel-shaped ciliated opening of the excretory tubules into the coelom of the early developing vertebrate embryo. Also called **nephrostome. —nephrostomic,** *adj.*

nephrostomy /nəfros'təmē/, a surgical procedure in which an incision is made on the flank of the patient so that a catheter can be inserted into the kidney pelvis for the purpose of drainage.

nephrotic syndrome /nəfrot'ik/ [Gk, *nephros* + L, *icus*, like], an abnormal condition of the kidney characterized by marked proteinuria, hypoalbuminemia, and edema. It occurs in glomerular disease and thrombosis of a renal vein, and as a complication of many systemic diseases, diabetes mellitus, amyloidosis, systemic lupus erythematosus, and multiple myeloma. The nephrotic syndrome occurs in a severe, primary form. The presenting symptoms include anorexia, weakness, proteinuria, hypoalbuminuria, and edema. Treatment and prognosis depend on the underlying cause of disease. Patients with primary nephrotic syndrome usually respond favorably to corticosteroids. Loop diuretics are used to control symptomatic edema, and dialysis may be necessary. Also called **nephrosis.—nephrotic** *adj.*

nephrotome /nef'rətom/ [Gk, *nephros* + *tome*, section], a zone of segmented mesodermal tissue in the developing vertebrate embryo lying along each side of the body dorsal to the abdominal cavity between the somite-forming dorsal mesoderm and the unsegmented lateral plate mesoderm. It is the primordial tissue for the urogenital system and gives

(figure labels:) Glomerulus · Afferent renal artery · Distal convoluted tubules · Collecting duct · Loop of Henle

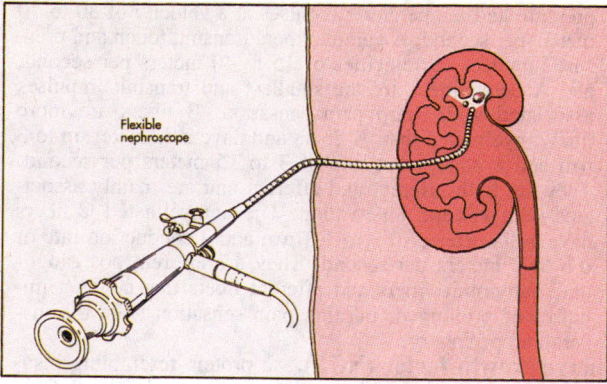

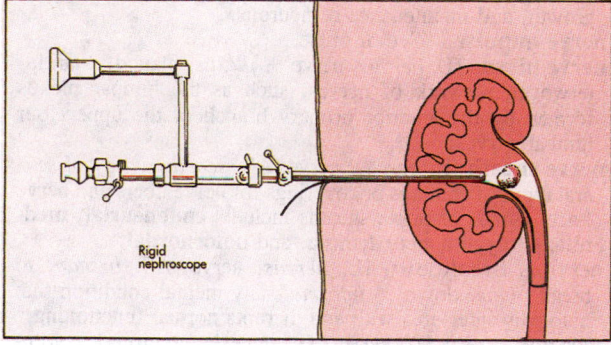

Nephroscopes (Brundage, 1992)

rise to the nephrogenic cord. Also called **intermediate cell mass, intermediate mesoderm, middle plate, nephromere.** See also **mesonephros, metanephros, pronephros.**

nephrotomography /-təmog'rəfē/ [Gk, *nephros* + *tome*, section, *graphein*, to record], sectional radiographic examination of the kidneys.

nephrotomy /nəfrot'əmē/ [Gk, *nephros* + *temnein*, to cut], a surgical procedure in which an incision is made in the kidney.

nephrotoxic /-tok'sik/ [Gk, *nephros* + *toxikon*, poison], toxic or destructive to a kidney.

nephrotoxin /-tok'sin/, a toxin with specific destructive properties for the kidneys.

nephroureterolithiasis /nef'rōyoo'tərōlithī'əsis/, the presence of calculi in the kidneys and ureters.

Neptazane, a trademark for a carbonic anhydrase inhibitor (methazolamide).

neptunium (Np) /nept(y)ōo'nē·əm/ [planet Neptune], a transuranic, metallic element. Its atomic number is 93; its atomic weight is 237. Although neptunium is considered a synthetic element, traces of natural neptunium have been found in uranium ores.

Nernst equation [Hermann W. Nernst, German physicist, b. 1864; L, *aequare*, to make equal], (in cardiology) an expression of the relationship between the electric potential across a membrane and the concentration ratio between permeable ions on either side of the membrane.

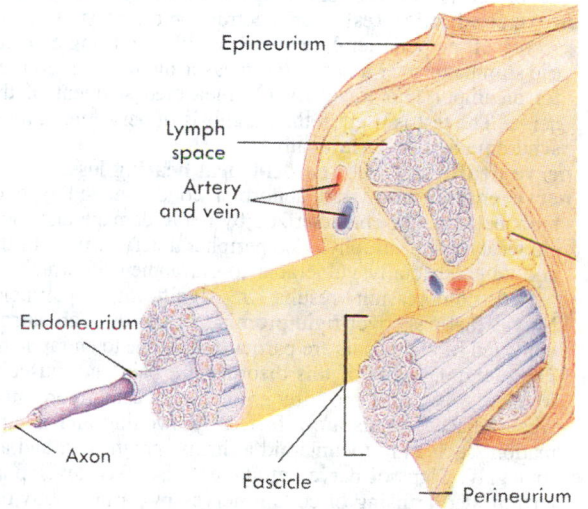

Cross-section of a nerve
(Thibodeau, 1993/Laurie O'Keefe/John Daugherty)

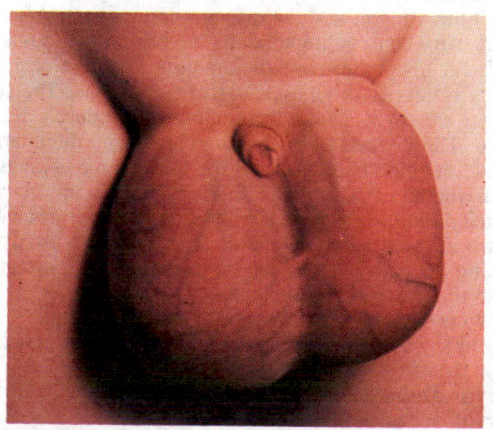

Scrotal edema in nephrotic syndrome (Zitelli, 1992)

nerve /nurv/ [L, *nervus*], one or more bundles of impulse-carrying fibers that connect the brain and the spinal cord with other parts of the body. Nerves transmit afferent impulses from receptor organs toward the brain and the spinal cord and efferent impulses peripherally to the effector organs. Each nerve consists of an epineurium enclosing fasciculi of nerve fibers, each fasciculus surrounded by its own sheath of connective tissue. Individual nerve fibers, which are microscopic, consist of formed elements within a matrix of protoplasm and are wrapped in a neurilemmal sheath.

Inside the neurilemma are nerve fibers, also enclosed in a myelin sheath, derived from the neurilemmal cells. See also **axon, dendrite, neuroglia, neuron.**

nerve accommodation, the ability of nerve tissue to adjust to a constant source and intensity of stimulation so that some change in either intensity or duration of the stimulus is necessary to elicit a response beyond the initial reaction. Accommodation is probably caused by reduced sodium ion permeability, which results in an increased threshold intensity and subsequent stabilization of the resting membrane potential.

nerve block anesthesia. See **conduction anesthesia.**

nerve cable graft, a multistrand free nerve graft, taken from elsewhere in the body, to bridge a large gap in one of the main nerves in the forearm.

nerve compression, a pathologic event that causes harmful pressure on one or more nerve trunks, resulting in nerve damage and muscle weakness or atrophy. Any nerve that passes over a rigid prominence is vulnerable, and the degree of damage depends on the magnitude and the duration of the compressive force. Various factors may contribute to susceptibility, such as inherited predisposition, malnutrition, trauma, and disease. Various activities associated with routine occupations may unduly compress especially vulnerablenerves, such as the median nerve, the radial nerve, the femoral nerve, and the plantar nerves. Rest and the cessation or modification of causative activities often heal nerve damage caused by compression. Surgery may be required to correct more severe cases. Compare **nerve entrapment.**

nerve conduction test, an electrodiagnostic test of the integrity of the peripheral nerves. It involves placing an electric stimulator over a nerve and measuring the time required for an impulse to travel over a measured segment of the nerve. The test is used in the diagnosis of nerve entrapment syndrome and polyneuropathies.

nerve deafness. See **sensorineural hearing loss.**

nerve entrapment, an abnormal condition and type of mononeuropathy, characterized by nerve damage and muscle weakness or atrophy. The peripheral nerve trunks of the body are especially vulnerable to entrapment in which repeated compression results in significant impairment. Nerves that pass over rigid prominences or through narrow bony and fascial canals are particularly prone to entrapment. The common signs of this disorder are pain and muscular weakness. Nerve damage by entrapment occurs more often when adjacent joints are affected by swelling and inflammation, such as in rheumatoid arthritis, pregnancy, and acromegaly. Signs of nerve entrapment also may develop after repeated bruising of certain nerves by various activities involving repeated motions, such as those associated with knitting and prolonged walking. One of the most common types of entrapment is **carpal tunnel syndrome.** Compare **nerve compression.**

nerve excitability [L, *nervus*, nerve; *excitare*, to rouse], the readiness of a nerve cell to respond to a stimulus. See also **all-or-none law.**

nerve fiber, a slender process of a neuron, usually the axon. Each fiber is classified as myelinated or unmyelinated. Myelinated fibers are further designated as A or B fibers; C fibers are unmyelinated. The A fibers are somatic and 1 to 20 μm in diameter and have a conduction velocity of 5 to 120 meters per second. The A alpha fibers are large fibers and transport impulses at a velocity of 60 to 100 meters per second; A beta fibers are smaller and transmit pressure and temperature impulses at a velocity of 30 to 70 meters per second; A gamma fibers transmit touch and pressure impulses at velocities of 15 to 40 meters per second; and A delta fibers are the smallest and transmit impulses associated with sharp pain sensation. B fibers are more finely myelinated than A fibers and have a diameter up to 3 μm, and a conduction rate of 3 to 15 meters per second. They are both afferent and efferent and are mainly associated with visceral innervation. The unmyelinated C fibers have a diameter of 0.3 to 1.3 μm and a conduction rate of 0.6 to 2 meters per second. They are efferent postganglionic autonomic fibers and afferent fibers that conduct impulses of prolonged, burning pain sensation from the viscera and periphery.

nerve growth factor (NGF), a protein resembling insulin whose hormonelike action affects differentiation, growth, and maintenance of neurons.

nerve impulse. See **impulse.**

nerve plexus [L, *nervus*, nerve + *plexus*, plaited], an interwoven network of nerves, such as the lumbar plexus formed by the anterior primary branch of the upper four lumbar nerves.

nerve sheath [L, *nervus*, nerve; AS, *scaeth*], any of several types of coatings or coverings for nerve fibers and nerve tracts. Kinds of nerve sheaths include: **endoneurial, medullary, myelin, neurilemma,** and **notochordal.**

nervous breakdown [L, *nervus*, nerve; AS, *brecan*, to break, *dune*, down], *informal.* any mental condition that markedly interferes with and disrupts normal functioning.

nervous emesis [L, *nervus*; Gk, *emesis*, vomiting], vomiting that is functional and psychogenic. The condition is most common among young women and is regarded as a psychological representation of a desire to reject something.

nervous prostration [L, *nervus* + *prosternere*, to throw down], a condition of irritable weakness and depression, which may be psychogenic or the result of a severe prolonged illness or exhausting experience.

nervous system [L, *nervus*, nerve; Gk, *system*], the extensive, intricate network of structures that activates, coordinates, and controls all the functions of the body. It is divided into the central nervous system, composed of the brain and the spinal cord, and the peripheral nervous system, which includes the cranial nerves and the spinal nerves. These morphologic subdivisions combine and communicate to innervate the somatic and the visceral parts of the body with the afferent and the efferent nerve fibers. Afferent fibers carry sensory impulses to the central nervous system; efferent fibers carry motor impulses from the central nervous system to the muscles and other organs. The somatic fibers are associated with the bones, the muscles, and the skin. The visceral fibers are associated with the internal organs, the blood vessels, and the mucous membranes. Various functions throughout the nervous system are coordinated through a vast complex of tiny structures, such as neurons, axons, dendrites, and ganglia. Compare **parasympathetic nervous system, sympathetic nervous system.** See also the Color Atlas of Human Anatomy.

nervous tachypnea [L, *nervus*; Gk, *tachys*, rapid + *pnoia*, breath], a neurotic symptom characterized by quick, shallow breathing.

nervus abducens. See **abducens nerve.**

nervus accessorius. See **accessory nerve.**

nervus facialis. See **facial nerve.**

nervus glossopharyngeus. See **glossopharyngeal nerve.**

nervus hypoglossus.   See **hypoglossal nerve.**

nervus oculomotorius.   See **oculomotor nerve.**

nervus olfactorius.   See **olfactory nerve.**

nervus opticus.   See **optic nerve.**

nervus terminalis.   See **terminal nerve.**

nervus trigeminus.   See **trigeminal nerve.**

nervus trochlearis.   See **trochlear nerve.**

nervus vagus.   See **vagus nerve.**

Nesacaine, a trademark for a long-acting local anesthetic (chloroprocaine), used in regional anesthetic block.

-ness, a suffix meaning 'a quality or state of being': *illness, painless.*

nested nails, in orthopedic surgery, a pair of nails placed side by side in the medullary canal of long bones.

Netromycin, a trademark for an antibiotic (netilmicin).

nettle rash [AS, *netele,* nettle; Fr, *rasche,* scurf], a fine, urticarial eruption resulting from skin contact with stinging nettle, a common weed with leaves containing histamine. It is characterized by stinging and itching that lasts from a few minutes to several hours.

network [AS, *net, wearc*], a system of interconnected computer terminals and peripheral equipment in which each user has some access to others using the system while sharing data, internal and external memories, and other capabilities.

networking,   **1.** (in psychiatric nursing) the process of developing a set of agencies and professional personnel who are able to create a system of communication and support for psychiatric patients, usually those newly discharged from inpatient psychiatric facilities. Kinds of networks include **natural network** and **professional network. 2.** a network of supportive contacts or services, such as the Women's Health Network.

net wt, abbreviation for *net weight.*

Neufeld nail /noi'felt/ [Alonzo J. Neufeld. American surgeon, b. 1906], an orthopedic nail with a V-shaped tip and shank used for fixating an intertrochanteric fracture. The nail is driven into the neck of the femur until it reaches a round metal plate screwed onto the side of the femur. The nail is secured to a receptacle on the plate. Also called **Neufeld angled nail.**

Neufeld roller traction, a traction device for a fractured femur, consisting of a cast for the calf and thigh hinged at the knee and suspended by a line to the anterior mid-thigh looped around a pulley and to a spring attached to the anterior midleg.

neur-.   See **neuro-.**

neural /nŏŏr'əl/ [Gk, *neuron,* nerve], of or pertaining to nerve cells and their processes.

-neural, -neuric, a suffix meaning 'of or relating to a nerve or nerves': *epineural, epithelioneural, myoneural.*

neural canal.   See **neurocoele.**

neural crest, the band of ectodermally derived cells that lies along the outer surface of each side of the neural tube in the early stages of embryonic development. The cells migrate laterally throughout the embryo and give rise to certain spinal, cranial, and sympathetic ganglia. Also called **ganglionic crest, ganglionic ridge.** See also **neural tube formation.**

neural ectoderm, the part of the embryonic ectoderm that develops into the neural tube. Also called **neuroderm.** See also **neural tube formation.**

neural fold, either of the paired longitudinal elevations resulting from the invagination of the neural plate in the early developing embryo. The folds unite to enclose the neural groove and form the neural tube. Also called **medullary fold.** See also **neural tube formation.**

neuralgia /nŏŏral'jə/ [Gk, *neuron + algos,* pain], an abnormal condition characterized by severe stabbing pain, caused by a variety of disorders affecting the nervous system. **–neuralgic,** *adj.*

neuralgic amytrophy /nŏŏral'jik/, a brachial plexus disorder characterized by sudden pain and muscle weakness in the upper limbs and possible muscular wasting or atrophy. The cause is unknown. Also called **Parsonage-Turner syndrome.**

neural groove, the longitudinal depression that occurs between the neural folds during the invagination of the neural plate to form the neural tube in the early stages of embryonic development. Also called **medullary groove.** See also **neural tube formation.**

neural impulse.   See **impulse.**

neural plate, a thick layer of ectodermal tissue that lies along the central longitudinal axis of the early developing embryo and gives rise to the neural tube and subsequently to the brain, spinal cord, and other tissues of the central nervous system. Also called **medullary plate.** See also **neural tube formation.**

neural tube, the longitudinal tube, lying along the central axis of the early developing embryo, that gives rise to the brain, spinal cord, and other neural tissue of the central nervous system. It consists of thick ectodermal tissue and is formed by the fusion of the neural folds, resulting from the invagination of the neural plate. Failure of the tube to close results in a number of congenital defects. Also called **cerebromedullary tube, medullary tube.** See also **neural tube defect, neural tube formation.**

neural tube defect, any of a group of congenital malformations involving defects in the skull and spinal column that are caused primarily by the failure of the neural tube to close during embryonic development. In some instances, the cleft results from an abnormal increase in cerebrospinal fluid pressure on the closed neural tube during the first trimester of development. The defect may occur at any point along the neural axis or extends the entire length of the spinal column, as in holorachischisis. The amount of deformity and disability depends on the degree of neural involvement, the most severe defect being complete cranioschisis, or the total absence of the skull and defective brain development. Other cerebral dysplasias resulting from the failure of the cranial end of the neural tube to fuse are meningoencephalocele and cranial meningocele. These defects, usually accompanied by severe mental and physical disorders, occur most often in the occipital region of the skull but may also occur in the frontal or basal regions. Most neural tube malformations are caused by incomplete fusion of one or more laminae of the vertebral column, with varying degrees of tissue protrusion and neural involvement. Such anomalies include rachischisis, spina bifida, myelocele, myelomeningocele, and meningocele. In all of these conditions there is constant risk of rupture of the saclike protrusion and danger of meningeal infection. Often, immediate surgical repair is necessary. Many of the major neural tube defects can be determined prenatally by ultrasonic scanning of the uterus and by the presence of elevated concentrations of alpha fetoprotein levels in the amniotic fluid. Such diagnostic tests are preferably performed during the fourteenth to sixteenth week of gestation so that termination of the pregnancy is possible. See also **anencephaly, Arnold-Chiari malformation, spina bifida cystica.**

neural tube formation, the various processes and stages involved in the embryonic development of the neural tube, which subsequently differentiates into the brain, the spinal cord, and other neural tissue of the central nervous system. The primitive tube originates from a flat, single layer of ectodermal tissue that extends longitudinally along the middorsal line of the embryonic disk from the area of the primitive streak forward to the cephalic extremity. This tissue, called the neural plate, grows rapidly and becomes striated and thickened. The rate of growth is greater along the midplane than at the margin, resulting in the invagination of the cells and formation of a hollow groove, the neural groove, bounded on either side by the elevated neural folds. With continued cell division the groove becomes deeper and the folds thicken so that they eventually meet and fuse, converting the neural groove into the neural tube. The closing of the neural tube occurs first at the midpoint and progresses toward both the caudal and the cephalic regions. At the cephalic end the tube expands into a large vesicle with three subdivisions that differentiate into the forebrain (prosencephalon), the midbrain (mesencephalon), and the hindbrain (rhombencephalon). The epithelium of the wall of the tube develops into the various tissues of the nervous system. The caudal portion of the tube subsequently forms the spinal cord. Along the outer surface of the neural tube is a thin layer of ectodermal cells that extends the entire length of the structure. These primordial cells migrate to other parts of the developing embryo and give rise to cranial and spinal ganglia and to certain cells of the autonomic nervous system. Failure of any part of the neural tube to close during early embryonic development results in a number of congenital defects. See also **neural tube defect.**

neurapraxia /nōōr′əprak′sē·ə/, the interruption of nerve conduction without loss of continuity of the axon.

neurasthenia /nōōr′əsthē′nē·ə/ [Gk, *neuron* + *a, sthenos,* not strength], **1.** an abnormal condition characterized by nervous exhaustion and a vague functional fatigue that often follows depression. **2.** (in psychiatry) a stage in the recovery from a schizophrenic experience, during which the patient is listless and apparently unable to cope with routine activities and relationships. **–neurasthenic,** *adj.*

neurasthenic /-əsthē′nik/ [Gk, *neuron,* nerve; *asthenia,* disability], pertaining to a disorder characterized by excessive fatigue, insomnia, weakness, anxiety,and mental and physical irritability.

-neure, -neuron, a combining form meaning a 'nerve cell': *ganglioneure, myoneure, sporadoneure.*

neurectomy /nōōek′təmē/ [Gk, *neuron,* nerve; *ektome,* cutting out], the surgical excision of a nerve segment.

neurenteric canal /nōōr′ənter′ik/ [Gk, *neuron* + *enteron,* intestine; L, *canalis,* channel], a tubular passage between the posterior part of the neural tube and the archenteron in the early embryonic development of lower animals. It corresponds to the notochordal canal of humans and the higher animals. Also called **archenteric canal, blastoporic canal, Braun's canal.**

neuresthenia. See **fatigue state.**

-neuria, a combining form meaning a '(specified) condition involving nerves': *acystineuria, ovariodysneuria.*

-neuric. See **-neural.**

neurilemma /nōōr′əlem′ə/ [Gk, *neuron* + *lemma,* sheath], a layer of cells composed of one or more Schwann cells that encloses the segmented myelin sheaths of peripheral nerve fibers. Each myelinated nerve fiber has a neurilemma cell for each internodal segment between the nodes of Ranvier. The cell nucleus is a flattened oval that lies in a small depression in the myelin. It is necessary for regeneration of peripheral nerves when they have been severed. The nerve fibers of the brain and the spinal cord are not enclosed by neurilemma. Also spelled **neurolemma.** Also called **sheath of Schwann.** **–neurilemmal, neurilemmatic, neurilemmatous,** *adj.*

neurilemoma. See **schwannoma.**

neurinoma /nōōr′inō′mə/, *pl.* **neurinomas, neurinomata** [Gk, *neuron* + *oma,* tumor], **1.** a tumor of the nerve sheath. It is usually benign but may undergo malignant change. A kind of neurinoma is **acoustic neurinoma.** See also **schwannoma. 2.** a neuroma.

neuritis /nōōrī′tis/, *pl.* **neuritides** [Gk, *neuron* + *itis,* inflammation], an abnormal condition characterized by inflammation of a nerve. Some of the signs of this condition are neuralgia, hyperthesia, anesthesia, paralysis, muscular atrophy, and defective reflexes.

neuro- /nōōr′ō-/, **neur-,** a combining form meaning 'of or pertaining to nerves': *neuroclonic, neurohormone, neuromast.*

neuroarthropathy /-ärthrop′əthē/ [Gk, *neuron* + *arthron,* joint, *pathos,* disease], a condition in which a disease of a joint is secondary to a disease of the nervous system.

neuroblast /nōōr′əblast/ [Gk, *neuron* + *blastos,* germ], any embryonic cell that develops into a functional neuron; an immature nerve cell. **–neuroblastic,** *adj.*

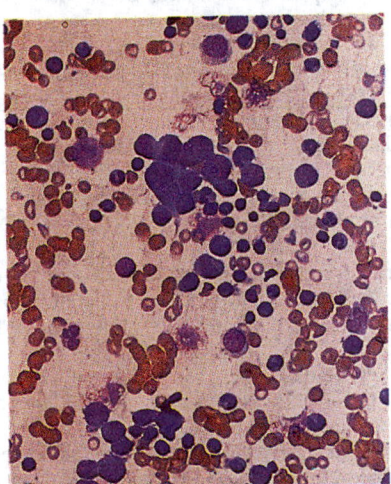

Neuroblastoma metastasized to the bone marrow
(Zitelli, 1992)

neuroblastoma /nōōr′ōblastō′mə/, *pl.* **neuroblastomas, neuroblastomata** [Gk, *neuron* + *blastos,* germ, *oma,* tumor], a highly malignant tumor composed of primitive ectodermal cells derived from the neural plate during embryonic life. The tumor may originate in any part of the sympathetic nervous system but is most common in the adrenal medulla. Neuroblastomas metastasize early and widely to lymph nodes, liver, lung, and bone. Symptoms may include an abdominal mass, respiratory distress, and anemia. Hormonally active adrenal lesions may cause irritability, flushing, sweating, hypertension, and tachycardia. Before metastasis, treatment with radical surgery, irradiation, and chemotherapy are often successful. Spontaneous remissions may occur with the tumor undergoing maturation and forming a benign ganglioneuroma. A kind of neuroblastoma is **Pepper's syndrome.**

neurocele. See **neurocoele**

neurocentral /-sen'trəl/ [Gk, *neuron* + *kentron*, center], pertaining to the centrum and the developing vertebrae in the early stages of embryology.

neurocentrum /-sen'trəm/ [Gk, *neuron* + L, *centrum*, center], the embryonic mesodermal tissue that subsequently gives rise to the vertebrae. See also **sclerotome.**

neuro check [Gk, *neuron* + ME, *chek*, stop], *nontechnical.* a brief neurologic assessment. The level of consciousness is evaluated as alert and oriented, lethargic, stuporous, or comatose. The movements of the extremities are determined to be voluntary or involuntary. The pupils of the eyes are observed for equality of dilatation, reactivity to light, and ability to accommodate.

neurocirculatory asthenia /-sur'kyələtôr'ē/ [Gk, *neuron* + L, *circulare*, to go around; Gk, *a, sthenos*, not strength], a psychosomatic disorder characterized by nervous and circulatory irregularities, including dyspnea, palpitation, giddiness, vertigo, tremor, precordial pain, and increased susceptibility to fatigue. The symptoms often result from or are associated with psychologic stress.

neurocoele /nŏŏr'əsēl/ [Gk, *neuron* + *koilos*, hollow], a system of cavities in the central nervous system of humans and other vertebrate animals. It consists of the ventricles of the brain and the central canal of the spinal cord, which originate from the neural tube during early embryonic development. Also spelled **neurocele, neurocoel.** Also called **neural canal.**

neurocytoma /nŏŏr'ōsītō'mə/ [Gk, *neuron* + *kytos*, cell, *oma*, tumor], a tumor composed of undifferentiated nerve cells that are usually ganglionic. Also called **neuroma.**

neuroderm. See **neuroectoderm.**

neurodermatitis /-dur'mətī'tis/ [Gk, *neuron* + *derma*, skin, *itis*, inflammation], a nonspecific, pruritic skin disorder seen in anxious, nervous individuals. Excoriations and lichenification are found on easily accessible, exposed areas of the body such as the forearms and forehead. Sometimes loosely (and incorrectly) applied to **atopic dermatitis.**

neurodevelopmental adaptation /-dəvel'əpmen'təl/, a type of therapy that emphasizes the inhibition/integration of primitive postural patterns and promotes the development of normal postural reactions and achievement of normal tone. The therapy is employed in the treatment of children with cerebral palsy.

neuroectoderm /nŏŏr'ō·ek'tədurm/ [Gk, *neuron* + *ektos*, outside, *derma*, skin], the part of the embryonic ectoderm that gives rise to the central and peripheral nervous systems, including some glial cells. **–neuroectodermal,** *adj.*

neuroendocrine /nŏŏr'ō·en'dəkrin/ [Gk, *neuron*, nerve; *endon*, within; *krinein*, to secrete], pertaining to or resembling the effects produced by endocrine glands strongly linked with the nervous system.

neuroepithelioma /nŏŏr'ō·ep'ithē'lē·ō'mə/ [Gk, *neuron* + *epi*, upon, *thele*, nipple, *oma*, tumor], an uncommon neoplasm of neuroepithelium in a sensory nerve. Also called **neuroepithelial tumor.**

neurofibroma /nŏŏr'ōfībrō'mə/, *pl.* **neurofibromas, neurofibromata** [Gk, *neuron* + L, *fibra*, fiber; Gk, *oma*, tumor], a fibrous tumor of nerve tissue resulting from the abnormal proliferation of Schwann cells. Multiple growths in the peripheral nervous system are often associated with abnormalities in other tissues. See also **neurofibromatosis.**

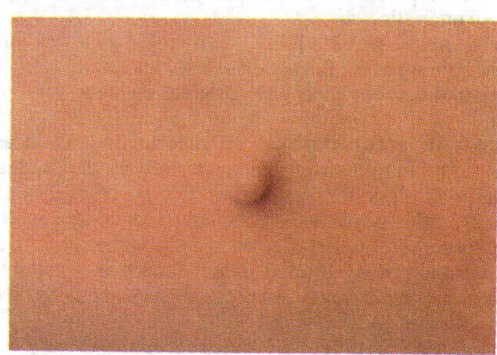

Neurofibroma (Weston, 1991)

neurofibromatosis /nŏŏr'ōfī'brōmətō'sis/ [Gk, *neuron* + *fibra*, fiber; Gk, *oma*, tumor, *osis*, condition], a congenital condition transmitted as an autosomal dominant trait, characterized by numerous neurofibromas of the nerves and skin, café-au-lait spots on the skin, and developmental anomalies of the muscles, bones, and viscera. Many large, pedunculated soft-tissue tumors may develop. Bone changes may result in skeletal deformities, especially curvature of the spine. Neurofibromas may develop in the alimentary tract, bladder, endocrine glands, and cranial nerves. Also called **multiple neuroma, neuromatosis, von Recklinghausen's disease.** (See Fig. p. 1064.)

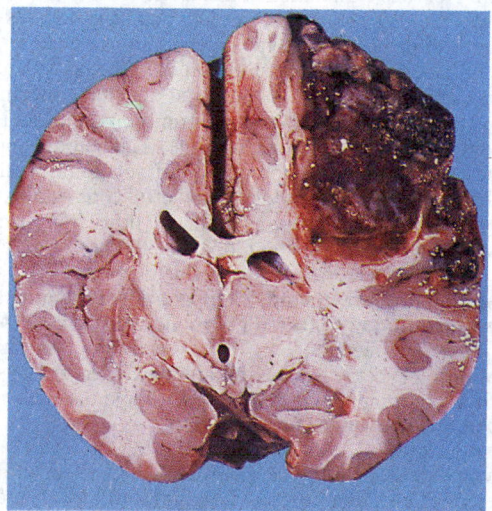

Neurocytoma of left frontal area
(Okazaki, 1988/by permission of Mayo Foundation)

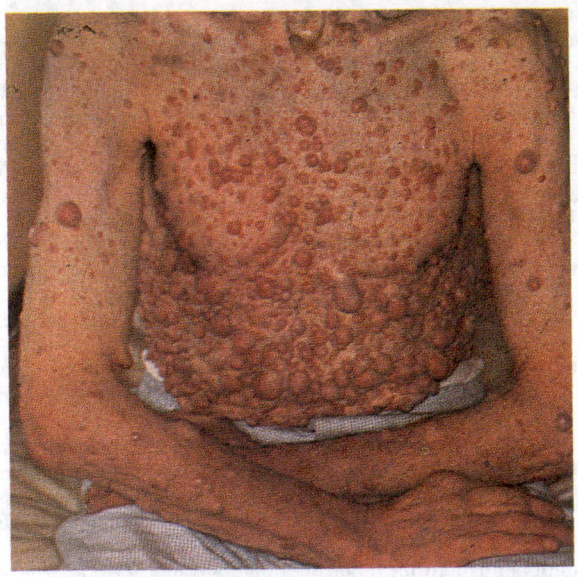

Neurofibromatosis *(Kamal, 1991)*

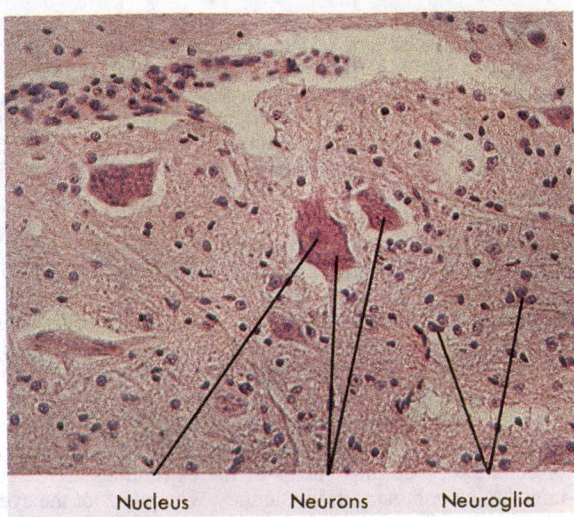

Nucleus   Neurons   Neuroglia

Neuroglia *(Seeley, 1992/Trent Stephens)*

neurogen /noōr'əjən/ [Gk, *neuron* + *genein*, to produce], a substance within the early developing embryo that stimulates the primary organizer to initiate the formation of the neural plate, which gives rise to the primary axis of the body. See also **neurotransmitter.**

neurogenesis /-jen'əsis/ [Gk, *neuron* + *genesis*, origin], the development of the tissue of the nervous system. **–neurogenetic,** *adj.*

neurogenic /-jen'ik/ [Gk, *neuron* + *genesis*, origin], **1.** pertaining to the formation of nervous tissue. **2.** the stimulation of nervous energy. **3.** originating in the nervous system.

neurogenic arthropathy, an abnormal condition associated with neural damage, characterized by the gradual and usually painless degeneration of a joint. One of the major causes of this condition is believed to be a minor injury that is disregarded by the affected individual because of a lack of sensation in the injured tissue. Inadequate rest and care aggravate such injuries and prevent proper healing. See also **neuropathic joint disease.**

neurogenic bladder, dysfunction of the urinary bladder caused by a lesion of the nervous system. Treatment is aimed at enabling the bladder to empty completely and regularly, preventing infection, controlling incontinence, and preserving kidney function. Kinds of neurogenic bladder are **spastic bladder, reflex bladder,** and **flaccid bladder.** Also called **neuropathic bladder.**

neurogenic fracture, a fracture associated with the destruction of the nerve supply to a specific bone.

neurogenic shock, a form of shock that results from peripheral vascular dilation.

neuroglia /noōrog'lē·ə/ [Gk, *neuron* + *glia*, glue], the supporting or connective tissue cells of the central nervous system. They perform the less specialized functions of the nerve network. Kinds of neuroglia include **astrocytes, oligodendroglia,** and **microglia.** Compare **neuron. –neuroglial,** *adj.*

neurography /noōrog'rəfē/, the study of the action potentials of the nerves.

neurohumor [Gk, *neuron* + L, *humor*, fluid], one of the chemical substances, formed and transmitted by a neuron, that is essential for the activity of adjacent neurons or nearby organs or muscles. Kinds of neurohumoral substances are **acetylcholine, dopamine, epinephrine, norepinephrine,** and **serotonin. –neurohumoral,** *adj.*

neurohypophyseal hormone /-hī'pōfiz'ē·əl/ [Gk, *neuron* + *hypo*, under, *phyein*, to grow], a hormone secreted by the posterior pituitary gland. Kinds of neurohypophyseal hormones are **oxytocin** and **vasopressin.** See also **pituitary gland.**

neurohypophysis /-hīpof'isis/ [Gk, *neuron* + *hypo*, under, *phyein*, to grow], the posterior lobe of the pituitary gland that is the source of antidiuretic hormone (ADH) and oxytocin. Nervous stimulation controls the release of both substances into the blood. The neurohypophysis releases ADH when stimulated by the hypothalamus by an increase in the osmotic pressure of extracellular fluid in the body. The hormone acts on the cells in the distal and the collecting tubules of the kidneys, making them more permeable to water and reducing the volume of urine. The neurohypophysis releases oxytocin under appropriate stimulation from the hypothalamus. Oxytocin produces powerful contractions of the pregnant uterus and causes milk to flow from lactating breasts. Stimulation of the nipples of the breast by a nursing infant triggers the release of this hormone. Also called **posterior pituitary gland.** Compare **adenohypophysis.**

neuroimmunology /noōr'ō·im'yoōnol'əjē/ [Gk, *neuron* + L, *immunis*, freedom; Gk, *logos*, science], the study of relationships between the immune and nervous systems, such as autoimmune activity in neurologic diseases.

neurol, abbreviation for **neurology.**

neurolemma. See **neurilemma.**

neurolepsis /-lep'sis/ [Gk, *neuron* + *lepsis*, seizure], an altered state of consciousness, as induced by a neuroleptic agent, characterized by quiescence, reduced motor activity, anxiety, and indifference to the surroundings. Sleep may occur, but usually the person can be aroused and can respond to commands. Drugs that produce neurolepsis may be administered with a narcotic analgesic to produce neurolept-analgesia, or with an anesthetic to produce neuroleptanesthesia.

neurolept. See **neuroleptic.**

neuroleptanalgesia /-lept′anəljē′zē·ə/ [Gk, *neuron* + *lepsis*, seizure, *a, algos*, not pain], a form of analgesia achieved by the concurrent administration of a neuroleptic and an analgesic. Anxiety, motor activity, and sensitivity to painful stimuli are reduced; the person is quiet and indifferent to the environment and surroundings. Sleep may or may not occur, but the patient is not unconscious and is able to respond to commands. If nitrous oxide with oxygen is also administered, neuroleptanalgesia can be converted to neuroleptanesthesia. Droperidol and fentanyl are often administered together to achieve neuroleptanesthesia.

neuroleptanesthesia /-lept′anəsthē′zhə/ [Gk, *neuron* + *lepsis*, seizure, *anaisthesia*, loss of feeling], a form of anesthesia achieved by the administration of a neuroleptic agent, a narcotic analgesic, and nitrous oxide with oxygen. Induction of anesthesia is slow, but consciousness returns quickly after the inhalation of nitrous oxide is stopped.

neuroleptic /-lep′tik/ [Gk, *neuron* + *lepsis*, seizure], **1.** of or pertaining to neurolepsis. **2.** also called **neurolept.** a drug that causes neurolepsis, such as the butyrophenone derivative, droperidol. See also **antipsychotic.**

neuroleptic anesthesia [Gk, *neuron*, nerve; *lepsis*, seizure; *anaisthesia*, lack of feeling], a form of anesthesia induced by an injection of a butyrophenone derivative with a narcotic analgesic.

neuroleptic malignant syndrome [Gk, *neuron*, nerve; *lepsis*, seizure; L, *malignus*, bad disposition; Gk, *syn*, together; *dromos*, course], a complication of psychotherapy with neuroleptic drugs given in therapeutic doses. It is characterized by hypertonicity, pallor, dyskinesia, hyperthermia, incontinence, unstable blood pressure, and pulmonary congestion.

neurolinguistic programing /-ling·gwis″tik/, a communication approach based on a conceptualization of levels of experience within the person and levels of the self. It involves both verbal and nonverbal messages, sensory experience, and awareness or perception through patterns of behavior that can be observed and perceived.

neurologic assessment /-loj′ik/ [Gk, *neuron* + *logos*, science; L, *icus*, like; *adsidere*, to approximate], an evaluation of the patient's neurologic status and symptoms.
■ METHOD: If alert and oriented, the patient is asked about instances of weakness, numbness, headaches, pain, tremors, nervousness, irritability, or drowsiness. Information is elicited regarding loss of memory, periods of confusion, hallucinations, and episodes of loss of consciousness. The patient's general appearance, facial expression, attention span, responses to verbal and painful stimuli, emotional status, coordination, balance, cognition, and ability to follow commands are noted. If the patient is disoriented, stuporous, or comatose, demonstrated signs of these states are recorded. Observations are made of the skin color and temperature; pupillary size, equality, dilatation, and reactions to light; the respiratory rate, rhythm, and quality; and chest movements and breath sounds. The pulse is checked; the ears and nose are examined for possible drainage; the strength of the handgrip is tested; and the extremities' sensations and voluntary and involuntary motions are assessed. The urinary output is determined for evidence of polyuria,

and the patient's speech is evaluated for signs of slurring and aphasia. Included in the record are concurrent diseases, such as hypertension, cancer, and coarctation of the aorta; past illnesses associated with head trauma; seizures, motor, sensory, or emotional disturbances; loss of consciousness; and neurologic, medical, or surgical procedures. Pertinent to the assessment are the patient's sleep pattern, medication, personality changes, relationships with family and friends, and a family history of seizures, stroke, mental illness, tumors, or sudden death. Diagnostic aids that may be required for a complete evaluation are a lumbar puncture, complete blood count, myelogram, echoencephalogram, brain scan, computerized tomogram, and determinations of glucose, fluid, and electrolyte levels.
■ NURSING INTERVENTION: The nurse may conduct the interview to obtain subjective data, examines the patient, and assembles the pertinent background information and the results of the diagnostic tests.
■ OUTCOME CRITERIA: A careful neurologic assessment is an important aid to the neurologist in establishing a diagnosis and the course of treatment.

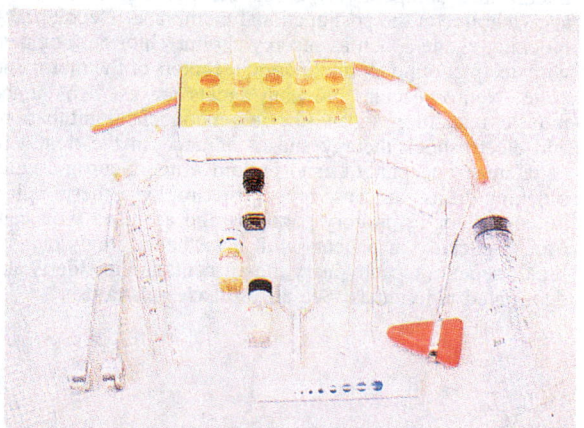

Equipment for neurologic assessment *(Chipps, 1992)*

neurologic examination, a systematic examination of the nervous system, including an assessment of mental status, of the function of each of the cranial nerves, of sensory and neuromuscular function, of the reflexes, and of proprioception and other cerebellar functions.

neurologist /noŏrol′əjist/, a physician who specializes in neurology.

neurology (neurol.) /noŏrol′əjē/ [Gk, *neuron* + *logos*, science], the field of medicine that deals with the nervous system and its disorders. **–neurologic, neurological,** *adj.* **neurologist,** *n.*

neuroma /noŏrō′mə/, *pl.* **neuromas, neuromata** [Gk, *neuron* + *oma*, tumor], a benign neoplasm composed chiefly of neurons and nerve fibers, usually arising from a nerve tissue. Pain radiating from the lesion to the periphery of the affected nerve is usually intermittent but may become continuous and severe.

-neuroma, a combining form meaning a 'tumor made up of nerve cells and fibers': *angiomyoneuroma, inoneuroma, myoneuroma.*

neuroma cutis,   a neoplasm in the skin that contains nerve tissue and may be extremely sensitive to painful stimuli.

neuroma telangiectodes.   See **nevoid neuroma.**

neuromatosis /nŏŏr′ōmətō′sis/ [Gk, *neuron* + *oma*, tumor, *osis*, condition],   a neoplastic disease characterized by numerous neuromas. Also called **multiple neuroma.** See also **neurofibromatosis.**

neuromodulator,   a substance that alters transmission of nerve impulses.

neuromotor /nŏŏr′ōmō′tər/ [Gk, *neuron*, nerve; L, *mover*, to move],   pertaining to both the nerves and muscles, or to nerve impulses transmitted to muscles.

neuromuscular /nŏŏr′ōmus′kyŏŏlər/ [Gk, *neuron* + L, *musculus*, muscle],   of or pertaining to the nerves and the muscles.

neuromuscular blockade,   the inhibition of a muscular contraction activated by the nervous system, possibly resulting in muscle weakness or paralysis.

neuromuscular blocking agent,   a chemical substance that interferes locally with the transmission or reception of impulses from motor nerves to skeletal muscles. Nondepolarizing agents, such as metocurine, pancuronium, and tubocurarine, competitively block the transmitter action of acetylcholine at the postjunctional membrane. Depolarizing blocking agents, such as succinylcholine chloride, compete with acetylcholine for cholinergic receptors of the motor end plate. Neuromuscular blocking agents are used to induce muscle relaxation in anesthesia, endotracheal intubation, and electroshock therapy and as adjuncts in the treatment of tetanus, encephalitis, and poliomyelitis. Neuromuscular blocking drugs can cause bronchospasm, hyperthermia, hypotension, or respiratory paralysis and are used with caution, especially in patients with myasthenia gravis or with renal, hepatic, or pulmonary impairment, and in elderly and debilitated individuals. See also **muscle relaxant.**

neuromuscular junction,   the area of contact between the ends of a large myelinated nerve fiber and a fiber of skeletal muscle. Also called **myoneural junction.** See also **motor end plate, myelin, nerve.**

neuromuscular spindle,   any one of a number of small bundles of delicate muscular fibers, enclosed by a capsule, in which sensory nerve fibers terminate. The spindles vary in length from 0.8 to 5 mm, accommodating as many as four large myelinated nerve fibers that pierce the capsule and lose their myelin sheaths. The nerve fibers end as naked axons encircling the intrafusal fibers with flattened expansions or ovoid disks.

neuromyal transmission /-mī′əl/ [Gk, *neuron* + *mys*, muscle; L, *transmittere*, to transmit],   the passage of excitation from a motor neuron to a muscle fiber at the myoneural junction.

neuromyelitis /nŏŏr′ōmī′əlī′tis/ [Gk, *neuron* + *myelos*, marrow, *itis*, inflammation],   an abnormal condition characterized by inflammation of the spinal cord and peripheral nerves.

neuron /nŏŏr′on/ [Gk, nerve],   the basic nerve cell of the nervous system, containing a nucleus within a cell body and extending one or more processes. Neurons are classified according to the direction in which they conduct impulses and according to the number of processes they extend. Sensory neurons transmit nerve impulses toward the spinal cord and the brain. Motor neurons transmit nerve impulses from the brain and the spinal cord to the muscles and the glandular tissue. Multipolar neurons, the bipolar neurons, and the unipolar neurons are classified according to the number of processes they extend to the different kinds of neurons. Multipolar neurons have one axon and several dendrites, as do most of the neurons in the brain and the spinal cord. Bipolar neurons, which are less numerous than the other types, have only one axon and one dendrite. Unipolar neurons are

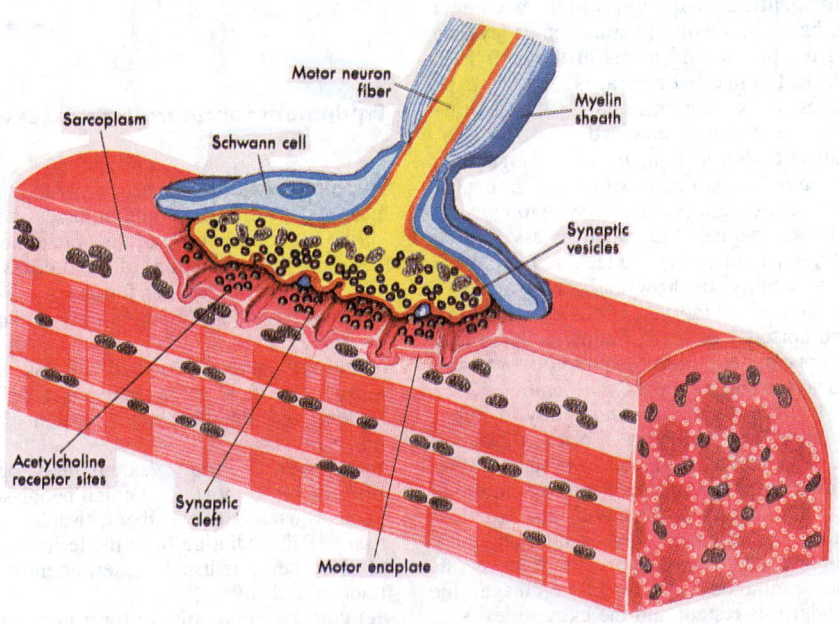

Neuromuscular junction *(Thibodeau, 1993/George Wassilchenko)*

embryonic structures that originate as bipolar bodies but fuse dendrites and axons into a single fiber that stretches for a short distance from the cell body before separating again into the two processes. All neurons have at least one axon and one or more dendrites and have a slightly gray color when clustered, as in the brain and the spinal cord. As the carriers of nerve impulses, neurons function according to electrochemical processes involving positively charged sodium and potassium ions and the changing electric potential of the extracellular and the intracellular fluid of the neuron. Also spelled **neurone.**

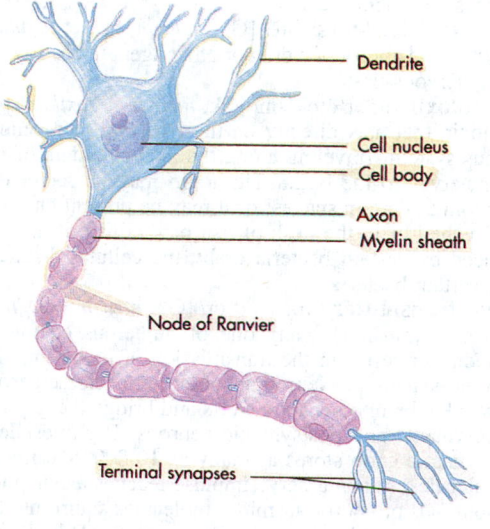

Dendrite

Cell nucleus

Cell body

Axon

Myelin sheath

Node of Ranvier

Terminal synapses

Neuron (Raven, 1992)

-neuron.   See **-neure.**

neuronal /nŏŏr′ənəl, nŏŏrō′nəl/ [Gk, *neuron*, nerve],   pertaining to or resembling a neuron.

neuronitis /nŏŏr′ənī′tis/ [Gk, *neuron* + *itis*, inflammation],   inflammation of a nerve or a nerve cell, especially the cells and the roots of the spinal nerves.

neuropathic bladder.   See **neurogenic bladder.**

neuropathic joint disease /-path′ik/ [Gk, *neuron* + *pathos*, disease],   a chronic, progressive, degenerative disease of one or more joints, characterized by swelling, instability of the joint, hemorrhage, heat, and atrophic and hypertrophic changes in the bone. Pain is usually less severe than would be expected by the appearance of the joint on an x-ray film. The disease is the result of an underlying neurologic disorder, such as tabes dorsalis from syphilis, diabetic neuropathy, leprosy, or congenital absence or depression of pain sensation. Early recognition of the disease and prophylactic protection of the joint may prevent further damage in some cases. Surgical reconstruction is not usually effective because healing is slow. Amputation may be necessary. Also called **Charcot's joint.**

neuropathy /nŏŏrop′əthē/ [Gk, *neuron* + *pathos*, disease],   inflammation or degeneration of the peripheral nerves, such as that associated with lead poisoning. **neuropathic,** *adj.*

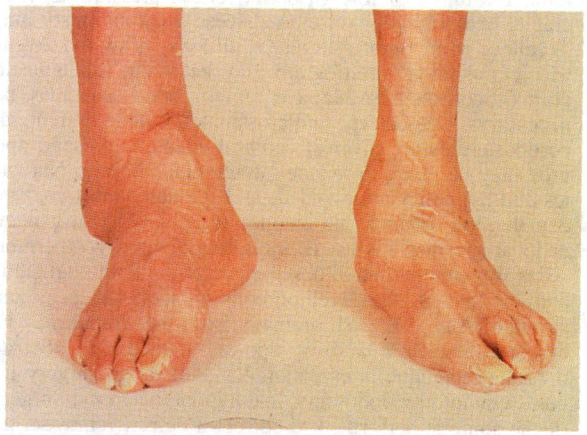

Neuropathic joint disease (Epstein, 1992)

neuroplasty /nŏŏr′əplas′tē/ [Gk, *neuron*, nerve; *plassein*, to mold],   plastic surgery to repair a nerve.

neuroplegia /nŏŏr′ōplē′jē·ə/ [Gk, *neuron* + *plege*, stroke],   nerve paralysis caused by disease, injury, or the effect of neuroleptic drugs, administered to achieve **neuroleptanalgesia** or **neuroleptanesthesia.** See also **lytic cocktail.**

neuropore /nŏŏr′opôr/ [Gk, *neuron* + *poros*, pore],   the opening at each end of the neural tube during early embryonic development. The closure of these apertures as the tube grows and differentiates occurs with such precision that they are used to indicate horizons XI and XII in the systematic anatomic charting of human embryonic development. Kinds of neuropores are **anterior neuropore** and **posterior neuropore.** See also **horizon, neural tube formation.**

neuropraxia /-prak′sē·ə/ [Gk, *neuron*, nerve; *prassein*, to do],   a condition where a nerve remains in place after a severe injury although it no longer transmits impulses.

neurorrhaphy /nŏŏrôr′əfē/ [Gk, *neuron*, nerve; *rhaphe*, suture],   a surgical procedure to suture a severed nerve.

neurosarcoma /-särkō′mə/ [Gk, *neuron* + *sarx*, flesh, *oma*, tumor],   a malignant neoplasm composed of nerve, connective, and vascular tissues. Also called **malignant neuroma.**

neuroscience /nŏŏr′ōsī′əns/ [Gk, *neuron*, nerve; L, *scientia*],   the study of neurology and related subjects, including neuroanatomy, neurophysiology, neuropharmacology, and neurosurgery.

neurosis /nŏŏrō′sis/ [Gk, *neuron* + *osis*, condition],   **1.** *obsolete.* any mental disorders characterized by various anxiety symptoms thought to be related to unresolved conflicts. **2.** *informal.* an emotional disturbance other than psychosis. See also **neurotic disorder.**

-neurosis,   a combining form meaning a 'disease of the nerves' or a 'mental disorder': *angioneurosis, psychoneurosis, synneurosis.*

neuroskeleton /-skel′ətən/ [Gk, *neuron*, nerve; *skeletos*, dried up],   the parts of the skeleton that surround or otherwise protect the nervous system, particularly the skull and vertebrae.

neurosurgery /-sur′jərē/ [Gk, *neuron* + *cheirourgos*, surgeon], any surgery involving the brain, spinal cord, or peripheral nerves. Brain surgery is performed to treat a wound, remove a tumor or foreign body, relieve pressure in intracranial hemorrhage, excise an abscess, treat parkinsonism, or relieve pain. Before surgery skull x-ray films and a ventriculogram or an arteriogram may be taken; a diagnostic electroencephalogram, lumbar tap, or brain scan may be necessary. A blood type and crossmatch is done. Parenteral corticosteroids are given if cerebral edema is present, and urea may be given to reduce intracranial pressure. Narcotics and hypnotics are avoided, and the nurse must confirm any that are ordered. No enemas are given. Light general or local anesthesia is used, occasionally with hypothermia. After surgery, the nurse observes carefully both vital signs and changes in the level of consciousness, speech, and strength. Any yellowish drainage from the wound may be cerebrospinal fluid and is reported immediately. Sterile dressing technique is essential. Kinds of brain surgery include craniotomy, lobotomy, and hypophysectomy. Surgery of the spine is performed to correct a defect, remove a tumor, repair a ruptured intervertebral disk, or relieve pain. Before surgery x-ray films are taken, and a blood type and crossmatch is done. General anesthesia or a spinal block is used. After surgery, the nurse keeps the bed flat and the patient's spine in good alignment. Return of sensation and motor function are monitored carefully. Kinds of spinal surgery include fusion and laminectomy. Surgery on the peripheral nerves is performed to remove a tumor, relieve pain, or reconnect a severed nerve. After surgery, the nurse observes closely the return of sensation to the area. One kind of nerve surgery is **sympathectomy.**

neurosyphilis /-sif′ilis/ [Gk, *neuron* + *sys*, hog, *philein*, to love], infection of the central nervous system by *Treponema pallidum*, the causative agent of syphilis, which may invade the meninges and cerebrovascular system. If the brain tissue is affected, general paresis may result; if the spinal cord is infected, tabes dorsalis may result. See also **syphilis,** *Treponema pallidum.* —**neurosyphilitic,** *adj.*

neurotendinous /-ten′dinəs/ [Gk, *neuron*, nerve; L, *tendo*, tendon], pertaining to both nerves and tendons.

neurotendinous spindle [Gk, *neuron* + L, *tendo*, tendon; AS, *spinel*, spindle], a capsule containing enlarged tendon fibers, found chiefly near the junctions of tendons and muscles. One or more nerve fibers pierce the side of the capsule and lose their medullary sheaths; the axons subdivide and terminate between the tendon fibers in irregular disks or varicosities. Also called **organ of Golgi.**

neurotic [Gk, *neuron* + *osis*, condition; L, *icus*, like], **1.** of or pertaining to neurosis or to a neurotic disorder. **2.** pertaining to the nerves. **3.** one who is afflicted with a neurosis. **4.** *informal.* an emotionally unstable person.

-neurotic, 1. a combining form meaning 'pertaining to a (specified) abnormal condition of the nerves': *angioneurotic, aponeurotic, vasoneurotic.* **2.** a combining form meaning 'pertaining to (psycho)neurosis': *hyperneurotic, psychoneurotic, unneurotic.*

neurotic depression. See **dysthemic disorder.**

neurotic disorder, any mental disorder characterized by a symptom or group of symptoms that a person finds distressing, unacceptable, and alien to the personality, such as severe anxiety, obsessional thoughts, and compulsive acts, and that produces psychologic pain or discomfort disproportionate to the reality of the situation.

neurotic personality [Gk, *neuron*, nerve + *osis*, condition; L, *personalis*, of a person], a personality characterized by traits and tendencies that increase the likelihood of a specific neurotic behavior. For example, the orderly, cautious, meticulous person may be prone to development of an obsessive-compulsive disorder.

neurotmesis /noor′otmē′sis/ [Gk, *neuron* + *tmesis*, cutting apart], a peripheral nerve injury in which the nerve is completely disrupted by laceration or traction. It requires surgical approximation, with unpredictable recovery.

neurotomy /noorot′əmē/, the surgical division of a nerve or nerves.

neurotoxic /noor′otok′sik/, having a poisonous effect on nerves and nerve cells, such as when ingested lead degenerates peripheral nerves.

neurotoxicity /-toksis′itē/ [Gk, *neuron*, nerve; *toxikon*, poison], the ability of a drug or other agent to destroy or damage nervous tissue.

neurotoxin /noor′otok′sin/ [Gk, *neuron* + *toxikon*, poison], a toxin that acts directly on the tissues of the central nervous system, traveling along the axis cylinders of the motor nerves to the brain. The toxin may be secreted in the venom of certain snakes, or it may be present on the spines of a shell or in the flesh of fish or shellfish; it may be produced by certain bacteria or by the cellular disintegration of certain bacteria.

neurotransmitter /-transmit′ər/ [Gk, *neuron* + L, *transmittere*, to transmit], any one of numerous chemicals that modify or result in the transmission of nerve impulses between synapses. Neurotransmitters are released from synaptic knobs into synaptic clefts and bridge the gap between presynaptic and postsynaptic neurons. Each vesicle within a synaptic knob stores as many as 10,000 neurotransmitter molecules. When a nerve impulse reaches a synaptic knob, thousands of neurotransmitter molecules squirt into the synaptic cleft and bind to specific receptors. This flow allows an associated diffusion of potassium and sodium ions that causes an action potential. Excitatory neurotransmitters decrease the negativity of postsynaptic membrane potentials; inhibitory neurotransmitters increase such potentials. Kinds of neurotransmitters include **acetylcholine, gamma-aminobutyric acid,** and **norepinephrine.**

neurotripsy /-trip′sē/, the surgical crushing of a nerve.

neurotropic viruses /-trop′ik/ [Gk, *neuron*, nerve + *tropein*, to turn; *virus*, poison], viruses with an unexplained attraction to nerve tissue. The predeliction also applies to certain toxic chemicals.

neurotropism /noorot′rəpiz′əm/ [Gk, *neuron*, nerve; *trepein*, to turn], **1.** the tendency for certain microorganisms, poisons, and nutrients to be attracted to nervous tissue. **2.** the tendency of basic dyes to be attracted to nervous tissue.

neurula /noor′ələ/, *pl.* **neurulas, neurulae** [Gk, *neuron*, nerve], an early embryo during the period of neurulation when the nervous system tissue begins to differentiate. The embryo at this level of growth represents a third stage in embryonic development, after the morula and blastocyst stages in humans and the higher animals and the blastula and gastrula stages in lower animals. In humans, the neurula stage occurs from about 19 to 26 days after fertilization.

neurulation /-ā′shən/ [Gk, *neuron* + L, *atus*, process], the development of the neural plate and the processes involved with its subsequent closure to form the neural tube during the early stages of embryonic development. See also **neural tube formation.**

neutral /n(y)oo'trəl/ [L, *neutralis*, neuter], the state exactly between two opposing values, qualities, or properties; for example, in electricity a neutral state is one in which there is neither a positive nor a negative charge, or in chemistry a neutral state is one in which a substance is neither acid nor alkaline. See also **acid, base, pH.**

neutralization /-īzā'shən/ [L, *neutralis* + Gk, *izein*, to cause], the interaction between an acid and a base that produces a solution that is neither acidic nor basic. The usual products of neutralization are a salt and water.

neutral rotation, the position of a limb that is turned neither toward nor away from the body's midline. When a person is supine and the leg is neutrally rotated, the toes should point straight up.

neutral thermal environment, an environment created by any method or apparatus to maintain the normal body temperature to minimize oxygen consumption and caloric expenditure, such as in an incubator or Isolette for a premature, sick, or low-birth-weight infant. See also **incubator, Isolette.**

neutron /n(y)oo'tron/ [L, *neuter*, neither; Gk, *elektron*, amber], (in physics) an elementary particle that is a constituent of the nuclei of all elements except hydrogen. It has no electric charge and is approximately the same size as a proton. Compare **electron, proton.** See also **atom.**

neutron activation analysis, the analysis of elements in a specimen, performed by exposing it to neutron irradiation to convert many elements to a radioactive form in which they can be identified by measuring their emissions of radiation. The method is applicable, to a limited extent, to human and animal studies.

neutropenia /noo'trōpē'nē·ə/ [L, *neuter*, neither; Gk, *penia*, poverty], an abnormal decrease in the number of neutrophils in the blood. The decrease may be relative or absolute. Neutropenia is associated with acute leukemia, infection, rheumatoid arthritis, vitamin B_{12} deficiency, and chronic splenomegaly. Compare **leukopenia.** See also **neutrophil.**

neutrophil /noo'trəfil/ [L, *neuter* + Gk, *philein*, to love], a polymorphonuclear, granular leukocyte that stains easily with neutral dyes. The nucleus stains dark blue and contains three to five lobes connected by slender threads of chromatin. The cytoplasm contains fine, inconspicuous granules. Neutrophils are the circulating white blood cells essential for phagocytosis and proteolysis by which bacteria, cellular debris, and solid particles are removed and destroyed. See also **basophil, eosinophil, granulocyte, polymorphonuclear leukocyte.**

neutrophil alkaline phosphatase. See **leukocyte alkaline phosphatase.**

neutrophilic leukemia. See **polymorphocytic leukemia.**

Neviaser procedure, the surgical transfer of a coracoacromial ligament to the clavicle for acromioclavicular separation.

nevoid amentia. See **Sturge-Weber syndrome.**

nevoid neuroma /nē'void/ [L, *naevus*, birthmark; Gk, *eidos*, form], a tumor of nerve tissue that contains numerous small blood vessels. Also called **neuroma telangiectodes.**

nevus /nē'vəs/ [L, *naevus*, birthmark], a pigmented, con-

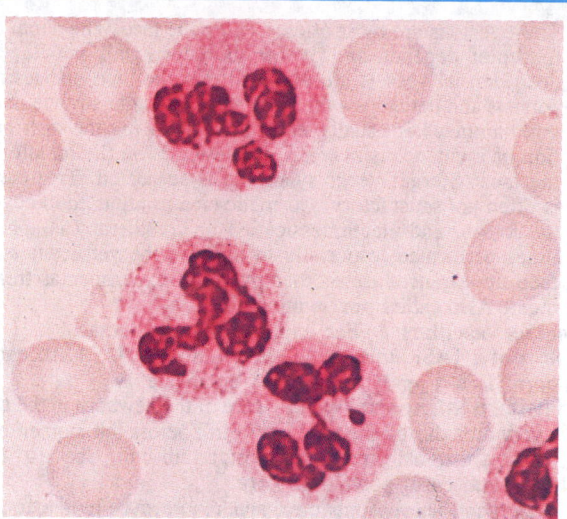

Neutrophils *(Hayhoe, 1992)*

genital skin blemish that is usually benign but may become cancerous. Any change in color, size, or texture or any bleeding or itching of a nevus merits investigation. Also called **birthmark, mole.** See also **blue nevus, junction nevus, nevus flammeus.**

nevus avaneus. See **spider telangiectasia.**

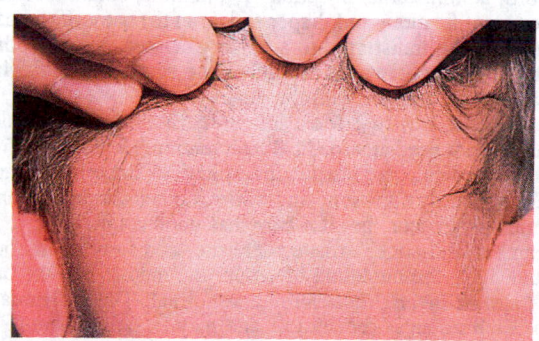

Nevus flammeus *(Zitelli, 1992)*

nevus flammeus /flam'ē·əs/, a flat capillary hemangioma that is present at birth and that varies in color from pale red to deep reddish purple. It is most commonly seen on the occiput and rarely causes any problems. If the lesion is on any other part of the body, it tends to be darker colored and, unlike the scalp lesions, does not regress spontaneously.

These lesions are most often seen on the face. The depth of the color depends on whether the superficial, middle, or deep dermal vessels are involved. On the face, the lesion persists and develops a thick verrucous nodular surface. Nevus flammeus is usually unilateral, following the distribution of a cutaneous nerve. If the lesion is on the middle of the face, Sturge-Weber syndrome is suspected. Treatment is often not satisfactory. Cosmetic creams are used to cover the lesion, and electrodessication or cryotherapy is sometimes performed, especially to improve the verrucous surface appearance. Laser therapy is an experimental treatment. Also called **port-wine stain.**

nevus vascularis. See **capillary hemangioma.**

newborn [AS, *niwe*, new, *boren*, to bear], **1.** recently born. **2.** a recently born infant; a neonate.

newborn intrapartal care, care of the newborn in the delivery area during the time after birth before the mother and infant are transferred to the postpartum unit. See also **intrapartal care, postpartal care.**

■ METHOD: The nasopharynx and mouth may be suctioned to remove excess mucus as the head is born. Depending on the preference and the condition of the mother and the policies of the maternity service, the baby may then be placed on the mother's abdomen and covered with a warm, dry blanket or taken by the nurse to an infant warmer. Apgar scores are assigned at 1 minute of age and at 5 minutes of age; less commonly, another is assigned at 10 minutes of age. The baby is handled gently and quietly; bright lights are often avoided, and maternal contact is encouraged.

■ NURSING INTERVENTION: The nurse is usually the first person to observe and examine the baby. Most newborns are healthy and normal; if abnormal function is observed, expert assistance may be summoned and emergency measures, including tracheal suction with a DeLee mucous trap attached to suction equipment and administration of oxygen by ventilator or mask, are initiated. If there are no problems, the nurse may instill erythromycin drops in the conjunctival sacs of the eyes, trim and clamp the umbilical cord, administer an injection of vitamin K, obtain footprints for identification, and diaper and wrap the baby. If the baby needs to be transferred to a nursery or special care facility, the nurse accompanies the infant and acts as the initial liaison for the mother with the nursery.

■ OUTCOME CRITERIA: Most infants born at term are healthy and do not need any medical intervention. Hemorrhage from the umbilical cord, difficult respiration, imperforate anus, endocrine dysfunction, and various other abnormal conditions may occur, but if a baby has good color, is alert, and can cry and suck, urinate, defecate, and respond to sound and light, the nurse may reassure the mother that the baby is almost invariably healthy and normal. The individuality of each infant is remarkable and may be pointed out to the mother.

new drug, a drug for which the Food and Drug Administration requires premarketing approval. A new drug is generally regarded as one for which safety and effectiveness have not yet been demonstrated for its prescribed use.

***New England Journal of Medicine (NEJM)*,** a weekly professional medical journal that publishes findings of medical research and articles about controversial political and ethical issues in the practice of medicine.

new growth, a neoplasm or tumor.

Newington orthosis, a bilateral orthosis similar to the **Toronto orthosis** except that flat bars are used and no joints are incorporated.

Newman, Margaret A., a nursing theorist who contributed to the study of nursing theories and models by defining three approaches to the discovery of nursing theory: "borrowing" of theories from related disciplines, analyzing nursing practice situations in search of conceptual relationships, and creating new conceptual systems from which theories can be derived.

newspaper sign. See **thumb sign.**

newton /n(y)o͞o′tən/ [Sir Isaac Newton, English scientist, b. 1642], a unit of force in the SI system that would impart an acceleration to one kilogram of mass of one meter per second per second.

new tuberculin [ME, *newe*; L, *tuber*, swelling], an extract of the tubercle bacillus from which all soluble material has been removed and glycerin added.

New World leishmaniasis. See **American leishmaniasis.**

New World typhus. See **murine typhus.**

Nezelof's syndrome /nez′əlofs/ [C. Nezelof, twentieth century French physician], an abnormal condition characterized by absent T cell function, deficient B cell function, fairly normal immunoglobulin levels, and little or no specific antibody production. The cause of Nezelof's syndrome is unknown. It affects both male and female siblings, indicating the possibility of a genetic disorder transmitted as an autosomal recessive trait. The disease may be caused by a cytogenic dysfunction of the stem cells, resulting in deficiencies of T cells and B cells. Another theory is that the disorder is caused by underdevelopment of the thymus gland and the consequent inhibition of T cell development. Still another holds that the disease results from the failure to produce or to secrete thymic humoral factors, especially thymosin.

■ OBSERVATIONS: Nezelof's syndrome causes progressively severe, recurrent, and eventually fatal infections. Signs that often appear in infants or in children up to 4 years of age include recurrent pneumonia, otitis media, chronic fungal infections, upper respiratory tract infections, diarrhea, and hepatosplenomegaly. The disease may enlarge the lymph nodes and the tonsils. These structures may be totally absent in infants with the disease. Involved patients may develop a tendency toward malignancy. Infection may cause sepsis, which is the usual cause of death. Symptoms that often suggest Nezelof's syndrome also include weight loss and poor eating habits. Definite diagnostic evidence of the disease includes defective B cell and T cell immunity despite a normal number of circulating B cells, a moderate to high rise in the number of T cells, a deficiency or an increase in one or more immunoglobulins, a nonreactive Schick test after DPT immunization, a reduced or an absent antibody reaction after specific antigen immunization, no thymus shadow on a chest x-ray film, thymus-dependent regions with abnormal lymphoid structure, and a decrease in the number of lymphocytes in the blood.

■ INTERVENTIONS: Initial supportive treatment of Nezelof's syndrome may include monthly injections of gamma globulin or monthly infusions of fresh frozen plasma and the heavy use of antibiotics to fight infection. The plasma infusions are especially beneficial if the patient cannot produce specific immunoglobulins. Cell-mediated immune function associated with T cells can usually be temporarily restored within weeks by a fetal thymus transplant. Repeated transplants are required to maintain the immunity. Cell-mediated immunity can be only partially restored with either transfer factor therapy or repeated injection of thymosin. Histocompatible bone marrow transplants have been used, but effective evaluation of this treatment method is incomplete.

■ NURSING CONSIDERATIONS: The nursing role in treating this disease is essentially supportive. The injection site for gamma globulin in a large muscle mass is massaged after the injection, and injection sites are rotated and recorded to prevent tissue damage. Gamma globulin doses greater than 1.5 ml are divided and injected into more than one site. The nursing role is also one of instruction and support for the parents of children affected by Nezelof's syndrome. Nurses commonly instruct parents on how to recognize the signs of infection and explain the dangers of allowing the affected child to become exposed to infection.

nF, abbreviation for *nanofarad.*

N.F., abbreviation for *National Formulary.*

NF1, a gene associated with neurofibromatosis. The gene is normally part of a family that helps regulate the timing of cell divisions. It may become defective, leading to neurofibromatosis expression, when an itinerant sequence of a DNA molecule becomes wedged in the NF1 gene. Other genetic disorders are believed to occur in a similar manner, by the dislocation of a "filler" sequence of a DNA molecule in a gene.

ng, abbreviation for **nanogram.**

NGF, abbreviation for **nerve growth factor.**

NG tube, abbreviation for **nasogastric tube.**

NGU, abbreviation for **nongonococcal urethritis.**

NHSC, abbreviation for **National Health Service Corps.**

Ni, symbol for the element **nickel.**

NIA, abbreviation for **National Institute on Aging.**

niacin /nī′əsin/, a white, crystalline, water-soluble vitamin of the B complex group usually occurring in various plant and animal tissues as nicotinamide. It functions as a coenzyme necessary for the breakdown and use of all major nutrients and is essential for a healthy skin, normal functioning of the GI tract, maintenance of the nervous system, and synthesis of the sex hormones. It also may be effective in improving circulation and reducing high blood cholesterol levels. Rich dietary sources of both niacin and its precursor tryptophan are meats, poultry, fish, liver, kidney, eggs, nuts, peanut butter, brewer's yeast, and wheat germ. Symptoms of deficiency include muscular weakness, general fatigue, loss of appetite, various skin eruptions, halitosis, stomatitis, insomnia, irritability, nausea, vomiting, recurring headaches, tender gums, tension, and depression. Severe deficiency results in pellagra. The vitamin is not stored in the body, and daily sources are needed. The recommended dietary allowance for adults is 15 to 20 NE (niacin equivalents) or mg of niacin. Also called **nicotinic acid.** See also **pellagra.**

niacinamide, /nī′əsin′əmīd/ a B complex vitamin. It is closely related to niacin but has no vasodilating action. Also called **nicotinamide.**

niacin equivalent (NE), an interconversion factor for estimating the contribution of tryptophan in the diet toward meeting the recommended daily allowance of niacin. The convention is to calculate 60 mg of tryptophan as the equivalent of 1 mg of niacin and to regard each as 1 niacin equivalent (NE).

N.I.B., abbreviation for *National Institute for the Blind.*

N.I.C.H.H.D., abbreviation for **National Institute of Child Health and Human Development.**

nick [ME *nyke* notch], (in molecular genetics) a fissure or split in a single strand of DNA that can be made with the enzyme deoxyribonuclease or with ethidium bromide.

nickel (Ni) [Ger *Kupfernickel* copper demon], a silvery-white metallic element. Its atomic number is 28; its atomic weight is 58.71. Large numbers of people are allergic to nickel. Nickel causes more cases of allergic contact dermatitis than all other metals combined. Many cases occur from exposure to jewelry, coins, buckles, and snaps and to continued use of 'carbonless' business forms. Nickel carbonyl, a volatile liquid, may produce serious lung damage if inhaled.

nickel dermatitis, an allergic contact dermatitis caused by the metal, nickel. Exposure comes usually from jewelry, wristwatches, metal clasps, and coins. Sweating increases the degree of rash. Treatment includes avoidance of exposure to nickel and reduction of perspiration. See also **contact dermatitis.**

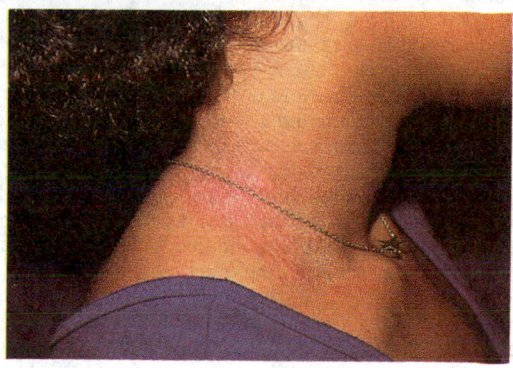

Nickel dermatitis (Weston, 1991)

nick translation, a method of labeling DNA in the laboratory by using the enzyme DNA polymerase.

Niclocide, a trademark for an anthelmintic (niclosamide).

niclosamide /niklō′səmīd/, an anthelmintic.

■ INDICATIONS: It is prescribed in the treatment of beef tapeworm and fish tapeworm infestations.

■ CONTRAINDICATIONS: Known sensitivity to this drug prohibits its use. Its safety in pregnant or nursing mothers or small children has not been established.

■ ADVERSE EFFECTS: Among the most serious adverse reactions are rectal bleeding, palpitations, alopecia, edema, nausea, and vomiting.

Nicobid, a trademark for two coenzymes (niacin and niacinamide), used as a vitamin supplement.

Nicola procedure, the surgical transfer of the long head of the biceps tendon through the humeral head for chronic anterior shoulder dislocation.

Nicholas procedure, a surgical procedure for repairing severe ligamentous injuries to the knee. It involves five procedures: a medial meniscectomy; a medial collateral ligament repair; a vastus medialis advancement; semitendinosus advancement, and a pes anserinus transfer. Also called **five-in-one repair.**

Nicorette, a trademark for a nicotine resin complex (nicotine polacrilex) used to aid patients trying to discontinue cigarette smoking.

nicotinamide. See **niacinamide.**

nicotine /nik'ətēn/ [Jean Nicot Villemain, French ambassador to Portugal, b. 1530], a colorless, rapidly acting toxic substance in tobacco that is one of the major contributors to the ill effects of smoking. It is used as an insecticide in agriculture and as a parasiticide in veterinary medicine. Ingestion of large amounts causes salivation, nausea, vomiting, diarrhea, headache, vertigo, slowing of the heartbeat, and, in acute cases, paralysis of respiratory muscles. Treatment depends on the symptoms. Pentobarbital is used to control convulsions, ephedrine for hypotension, and autonomic blocking agents to control visceral symptoms.

nicotine poisoning, poisoning from intake of nicotine. Nicotine poisoning is characterized by stimulation of the central and autonomic nervous systems followed by depression of these systems. In fatal cases, death occurs from respiratory failure.

nicotine polacrilex /pōlak'rileks/, a chewing gum (nicotine resin complex) source of nicotine as an adjunct for smoking cessation.

■ INDICATIONS: It may be prescribed as an aid for patients who are trying to quit cigarette smoking.

■ CONTRAINDICATIONS: Use by postmyocardial infarction patients, or those with severe or worsening angina pectoris or life-threatening dysrhythmias is prohibited. It should be used cautiously in patients with hyperthryroidism, hypertension, insulin-dependent diabetes, or peptic ulcers. Drug dosages may have to be adjusted in patients taking other drugs with effects that may be increased when cigarette smoking ceases. Patients should be monitored to ensure that they do not become dependent on the nicotine in the gum.

■ ADVERSE REACTIONS: The most serious adverse reactions include burning and soreness of the mouth, light-headedness, headache, hiccups, nausea, vomiting, and excessive salivation.

nicotinic acid. See **niacin.**

nicotinyl alcohol /nik'ətē'nil/, an alcohol used as a vasodilator, in the form of its tartrate salt, in the treatment of peripheral vascular disease, vascular spasm, varicose ulcers, decubital ulcers, chilblains, Méniére's disease, and vertigo.

NICU, abbreviation for **neonatal intensive care unit.**

nid-, a prefix meaning 'to nest': *nidal, nidus.*

NID, abbreviation for *National Institute for the Deaf.*

NIDA, abbreviation for **National Institute on Drug Abuse.**

nidation /nīdā'shən/ [L, *nidus,* nest], the process by which an embryo burrows into the endometrium of the uterus. Also called **implantation.** See also **placenta, uterus.**

-nidazole, a combining form for metronidazole-type antiprotozoal substances.

NIDDM, abbreviation for **non-insulin-dependent diabetes mellitus.**

nidus /nī'dəs/ [L, nest], a point or origin, focus, or nucleus of a disease process.

Niebauer prosthesis /nē'bou·ər/, a Silastic prosthesis for interphalangeal and thumb joint replacement.

Niemann-Pick disease /nē'monpik'/ [Albert Niemann, German pediatrician, b. 1880; Ludwig Pick, German pediatrician, b. 1868], an inherited disorder of lipid metabolism in which there are accumulations of sphingomyelin in the bone marrow, spleen, and lymph nodes. The disease, which in the United States and Canada is most common among Jewish people, begins in infancy or childhood and is characterized by enlargement of liver and spleen, anemia, lymphadenopathy, and progressive mental and physical deterioration. There is no effective treatment, and children with the disease usually die within a few years of the onset of symptoms. Also called **sphingomyelin lipoidosis.**

nifedipine /nifed'ipēn/, a calcium channel blocker.

■ INDICATIONS: It is prescribed for the treatment of vasospastic and effort-associated angina.

■ CONTRAINDICATION: Known hypersensitivity to this drug prohibits its use.

■ ADVERSE EFFECTS: Among the more serious adverse reactions are hypotension, peripheral edema, palpitations, dyspnea, nausea, dizziness, flushing, and headache.

nifur-, a combining form for 5-nitrofuran derivatives.

night blindness. See **nyctalopia.**

night guard. See **bite guard.**

Nightingale, Florence (1820–1910), considered the founder of modern nursing. After limited formal training in nursing in Germany and Paris, she became superintendent in 1853 of a small hospital in London. Her outstanding success in reorganizing the hospital led to a request by the British government to head a mission to the Crimea, where Britain was fighting a war with Russia. After her return to England, in 1856, she wrote *Notes on Hospitals* and *Notes on Nursing* and founded a training school for nurses at St. Thomas' Hospital, where she attracted well-educated, dedicated women. The graduates became matrons of the most important hospitals in Great Britain, thus raising the standards of nursing across the nation and eventually around the world. Although she was, by then, bedridden much of the time, she carried on her work on the sanitary reform of India, conducted a study of midwifery, helped establish visiting nurse services, and worked for the reform of the poor laws in which she proposed separate institutions for the sick, the insane, the incurable, and children. After Longfellow wrote *Santa Filomena,* she became known as "The Lady with The Lamp," and the Nightingale Pledge, named after her, embodies her ideals and has inspired thousands of young graduating nurses.

Nightingale ward, a kind of hospital ward, designed by Florence Nightingale, that revolutionized hospital design. The number of beds allowed in a ward of given size was limited to permit the circulation of air and for general cleanliness and the comfort of patients. Three sides of the ward were windowed to admit light and fresh air. Although multiple-bed wards are now obsolete in hospital design, the concerns and the benefits that impelled Miss Nightingale to create them remain central to hospital planning.

nightingalism /nī'ting·gā'lizəm/, an ideology emphasizing self-sacrifice on the part of a nurse whose primary concern is the welfare of the patient, with minimum personal attention to the needs of the nurse. See also **Nightingale, Florence.**

nightmare /nīt'mer/ [AS, *niht,* night, *mara,* incubus], a dream occurring during rapid eye movement sleep that arouses feelings of intense, inescapable fear, terror, distress, or extreme anxiety and that usually awakens the sleeper. Compare **pavor nocturnus, sleep terror disorder.**

night sight. See **hemeralopia.**

night splint, any splint or similar device used only at night.

nightstick fracture, an undisplaced fracture of the ulnar shaft caused by a direct blow.

night sweat [AS, *niht, swaetan*], sweating that occurs with a nocturnal fever, such as in a wasting disease like pulmonary tuberculosis.

night terrors [AS, *niht*; L, *terrour*],   a form of dissociated sleep, usually in children, in which there may be repeated episodes of abrupt awakening from sleep with signs of panic and anxiety. The subject may have only fragmentary dream images of a threatening nature. Also called **pavor nocturnus; sleep-terror disorder**.

night vision [AS, *niht*, night; L, *visio*, seeing],   a capacity to see dimly lit objects. It stems from a chemophysical phenomenon associated with the retinal rods. The rods contain the highly light-sensitive chemical rhodopsin, or visual purple, which is essential for the conduction of optic impulses in subdued light. Night vision is sharpest at the periphery of the retina because of the concentration of rods. Night vision may be diminished by a deficiency of vitamin A, an important component of rhodopsin.

nightwalking [AS, *niht*; ME, *walken*],   a disorder occurring during non-REM sleep in which the subject usually sits up in bed briefly, then gets up and walks around, opening doors, eating, and so on, and eventually returns to bed. The person has no memory of the event the next day. Also called **noctambulation, sleepwalking, somnambulism**.

nigr-,   a prefix meaning 'pertaining to black or a variation of the black color': *substantia nigra, nigrosin*.

nigrities linguae.   See **parasitic glossitis**.

N.I.H.,   abbreviation for **National Institutes of Health**.

nihilistic delusion /nī′hilis′tik/ [L, *nihil*, nothing, *icus*, form of; *deludere*, to deceive],   a persistent denial of the existence of particular things or of everything, including oneself, as seen in various forms of schizophrenia. A person who has such a delusion may believe that he lives in a shadow or limbo world or that he died several years ago and that only the spirit, in a vaporous form, really exists. See also **delusion**.

nikethamide /nīketh′əmīd/,   a central nervous system stimulant.

■ INDICATIONS: It is prescribed as an analeptic in the treatment of depression of the central nervous and respiratory systems.

■ CONTRAINDICATION: Known hypersensitivity to this drug prohibits its use.

■ ADVERSE EFFECTS: Among the most serious adverse reactions at high doses are tachycardia, hypertension, muscle spasm, and convulsions. Burning and itching are common.

Nikolsky's sign /nikol′skēz/ [Pyotr V. Nikolsky, Polish dermatologist, b. 1855],   easy separation of the stratum corneum layer of the epidermis from the basal cell layer by rubbing apparently normal skin areas; found in pemphigus and a few other bullous diseases.

Nilstat,   a trademark for an antifungal (nystatin).

NIMH,   abbreviation for *National Institute of Mental Health*.

90-90 traction.   See **traction, 90-90**.

ninth cranial nerve.   See **glossopharyngeal nerve**.

niobium (Nb) /nī·ō′bē·əm/ [Gk, *Niobe*, mythic daughter of Tantalus and Amphion],   a silver-gray metallic element. Its atomic number is 41; its atomic weight is 92.906. Formerly called **columbium**.

nipple [D, *knibbelen*, to nip],   a small cylindric, pigmented structure that projects just below the center of each breast. The tip of the nipple has about 20 tiny openings to the lactiferous ducts. The skin of the nipple is surrounded by the lighter pigmented skin of the areola. The depth of pigmentation of the nipple and areola in nulliparas varies from rosy pink to brown, depending on the complexion of the indi-

vidual. In pregnancy, the skin of the nipple darkens but loses some of its pigmentation when lactation is completed. Stimulation of the nipple in men and women causes the structure to become erect through the contraction of radiating smooth muscle bundles in the surrounding areola. In women the nipple enlarges somewhat and becomes more sensitive after puberty.

nipple cancer,   an inflammatory malignant neoplasm of the nipple and areola that is usually associated with carcinoma in deeper breast structures. It represents only a small percentage of breast cancers and usually begins in the nipple and spreads to the areola. Also called **Paget's disease of the nipple.**

nipple discharge,   spontaneous exudation of material from the nipple that may be normal, such as colostrum in pregnancy, or that may be a sign of endocrinologic, neoplastic, or infectious disease.

nipple shield,   a device to protect the nipples of a lactating woman. The shield is usually made of soft latex, is 4 or 5 cm wide, and has a tab on one side with which the mother may hold it. The baby nurses from a nipple at the center of the shield. It is most often used to allow sore or cracked nipples to heal while maintaining lactation. Also called **nipple protector.**

Nipride,   a trademark for a direct-acting vasodilator (sodium nitroprusside), used as an adjunct to anesthesia.

niridazole /nirid′əzōl/,   an antischistosomal. In the United States it is available from the Centers for Disease Control.

Nirschl procedure /nur′shəl/,   a surgical procedure for chronic epicondylitis. It involves excision of a hypercapsular tendon segment of the extensor carpi radialus brevis and decortication of the anterolateral condyle.

nirvanic state /nirvä′nik, nirvan′ik/,   (in Buddhist meditation) a state in which mental processes cease, often leading to a radical alteration of the personality.

NIS,   abbreviation for *Nursing Information System*.

Nissl body /nis′əl/ [Franz Nissl, German neurologist, b. 1860],   any one of the large granular structures in the cytoplasm of nerve cells that stains with basic dyes and contains ribonucleoprotein.

nit,   the egg of a parasitic insect, particularly a louse. It may be found attached to human or animal hair or to clothing fiber. See also **pediculosis.**

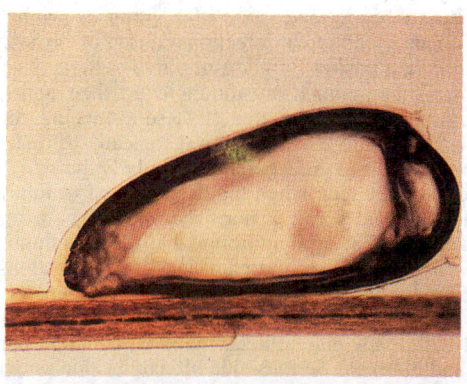

Microscopic view of a nit *(Zitelli, 1992)*

nitr, 1. abbreviation for **nitrocellulose.** 2. abbreviation for **nitroglycerine.**

nitr-, a prefix meaning 'related to nitrogen, nitrite, and nitrate.'

nitrazine paper /nī′trəzēn/, an absorbent strip of paper that turns specific colors when exposed to solutions of varied acidity or alkalinity. Also called **pH paper.**

nitric acid /nī′trik/ [Gk, *nitron*, soda; L, *acidus*, sour], a colorless, highly corrosive liquid that may give off suffocating brown fumes of nitrogen dioxide on exposure to air. Traces of nitric acid are found in rain water during a thunderstorm. Commercially prepared nitric acid is a powerful oxidizing agent used in photoengraving and metallurgy, in the manufacture of explosives, fertilizers, dyes, and drugs, and, occasionally, as a cauterizing agent for the removal of warts.

nitrite /nī′trīt/ [Gk, *nitron*, soda], an ester or salt of nitrous acid, used as a vasodilator and antispasmodic. Among the most widely used nitrites in medicine are amyl, ethyl, potassium, and sodium nitrite.

nitritoid reaction /nī′tritoid/, a group of adverse effects, including hypotension, flushing, lightheadedness, and fainting, produced by administration of arsenicals or gold. The reaction is similar to that caused by administration of nitrites.

nitro- /nī′trō-/, a combining form indicating presence of the group-NO$_2$: *nitrobenzol, nitrofuran, nitromethane.*

nitrobenzene poisoning /-ben′zēn/, a toxic condition caused by the absorption into the body of nitrobenzene, a pale yellow, oily liquid used in the manufacture of aniline, shoe dyes, soap, perfume, and artificial flavors. Nitrobenzene, especially its vapors, is extremely toxic. Exposure in industry is usually by inhalation of the fumes or by absorption through the skin. Symptoms of acute poisoning include headache, drowsiness, nausea, ataxia, cyanosis, and, in extreme cases, respiratory failure. Contaminated clothing is removed, and the skin is washed with vinegar, followed by soap and water. Oxygen, blood transfusion, and, in severe cases, hemodialysis may be required. Chronic exposure to nitrobenzene may cause headache, fatigue, loss of appetite, and anemia.

Nitro-Bid, a trademark for a coronary vasodilator (nitroglycerin), used as an antianginal agent.

nitrocellulose (nitr) /-sel′yəlōs/, a mixture of nitrate esters of cellulose made by treating cotton with nitric and sulfuric acids. Solutions in a mixture of ether and alcohol are used as "plastic skin" under the name of **collodion.** See also **pyroxylin.**

nitrofuran /-fyoo′ran/, one of a group of synthetic antimicrobials used to treat infections caused by protozoa or by certain gram-positive or gram-negative bacteria. The precise mechanism by which nitrofurans exert their antimicrobial effects is not known. Three of these agents are commonly prescribed. Nitrofurazone is used topically to treat superficial wounds and infections, particularly burns. Systemic toxicity is not seen when the drug is used in this way, although allergic skin reactions may occur. Furazolidone is used to treat bacterial and protozoal diarrhea and enteritis. Nitrofurantoin is used to treat urinary tract infections caused by *Escherichia coli* and other enteric pathogens of the urinary tract. Systemic administration of nitrofurans is associated with many side effects, the most common being nausea and diarrhea. Serious side effects include polyneuropathies and several hypersensitivity reactions, including pneu-

monitis and blood dyscrasias. Nitrofurans can cause hemolytic anemia in patients with glucose-6-phosphate dehydrogenase deficiency.

nitrofurantoin /nī′trōfyŏŏran′tō·in, -fyŏŏ′rəntō′in/, a urinary antibacterial.
■ INDICATIONS: It is prescribed in the treatment of certain urinary tract infections.
■ CONTRAINDICATIONS: Kidney dysfunction or known hypersensitivity to this drug prohibits its use. It is not given to children under 1 month of age or to pregnant or lactating women.
■ ADVERSE EFFECTS: Among the most serious adverse reactions is hypersensitivity pneumonitis, which can lead to fibrosis, neurotoxicity, and hemolytic anemia in patients with glucose-6-phosphate dehydrogenase deficiency. GI disturbances and fever are common.

nitrofurazone /-fyŏŏ′rəzōn/, a topical antibacterial.
■ INDICATIONS: It is prescribed in the prophylaxis and treatment of infection in second- and third-degree burns and in the treatment of infections of the skin and mucous membranes.
■ CONTRAINDICATION: Known hypersensitivity to this drug prohibits its use.
■ ADVERSE EFFECTS: Among the most serious adverse reactions are severe allergic reactions and suprainfections.

nitrogen (N) /nī′trəjən/ [Gk, *nitron*, soda, *genein*, to produce], a gaseous, nonmetallic element. Its atomic number is 7; its atomic weight is 14.008. Nitrogen constitutes approximately 78% of the atmosphere and is a component of all proteins and a major component of most organic substances. Nitrogen is found in mineral compounds, such as saltpeter, and is the seventeenth most abundant element in the earth's crust. Compounds of nitrogen are essential constituents of all living organisms, the proteins and the nucleic acids being especially basic to all life forms. Nitrogen forms a series of oxides and oxyacids, the most important of which is nitric acid. It also unites with hydrogen to form ammonia and with many metallic elements to form nitrides. Nitrogen is essential to the synthesis of proteins that the body must have, particularly nitrogen-containing compounds or amino acids derived directly or indirectly from plant food. Nitrogen follows a cycle from atmospheric gas into nitrogen-fixing bacteria, into green vascular plants, into humans and animals, and, by decay or in excreted nitrogenous wastes, as urea, back into the soil. Denitrifying bacteria in the soil break down nitrogenous compounds and release gaseous nitrogen. During a 24-hour period in a healthy individual the nitrogen excreted in the urine, feces, and perspiration, together with the nitrogen retained in dermal structures, such as the skin and hair, equals the nitrogen consumed in food and drink. The process of protein metabolism accounts for this nitrogen balance. When protein catabolism exceeds protein anabolism, the amount of nitrogen in the urine exceeds the amount of nitrogen consumed in foods, producing a negative nitrogen balance or a state of tissue wasting. A positive nitrogen balance exists in the body when the nitrogen intake in foods is greater than that excreted in urine. Conditions usually associated with positive nitrogen balance are those in which protein anabolism is proceeding faster than protein catabolism, such as in conditions associated with growth, pregnancy, and convalescence from a tissue-wasting illness. Nitrogen is a component of nitrous oxide, or laughing gas, which is sometimes used as an anesthetic. Nitrous oxide is a colorless, nonflammable, sweet-tasting gas. Three liters of nitrogen may be eliminated from the lungs and tissues in the first hour of anesthesia if a nitrous oxide-oxygen mixture is inspired. Precautions are taken to exhaust this nitrogen from the breathing circuit if high concentrations of both oxygen and nitrous oxide are desired. Nitrous oxide takes effect quickly and allows a fast recovery from anesthesia but is not considered suitable for prolonged surgery or for surgery requiring deep muscle relaxation. It must be administered with oxygen or air to prevent anoxia. Nitrogen is a component of nitrogen dioxide, which is irritating to the lungs and can cause pulmonary edema. Nitrogen dioxide can be released from silage and may produce symptoms of pulmonary damage in workers who perform ensilage tasks. Some studies indicate that measurable changes in pulmonary function occur when healthy individuals are exposed to nitrous oxide concentrations of two to three parts per million. Nitrogen is also a component of nitric and nitrous acids. Organic nitrates or polyol esters of nitric acid, such as nitroglycerin, and organic nitrites or esters of nitric acid, such as amyl nitrite, are effective vasodilators often used in relieving angina, but exactly how they function in dilating arterial and venous smooth muscle is not yet understood.

nitrogen balance, the relationship between the nitrogen taken into the body, usually as food, and the nitrogen excreted from the body in urine and feces. Most of the body's nitrogen is incorporated into protein. Positive nitrogen balance, which occurs when the intake of nitrogen is greater than its excretion, implies tissue formation. Negative nitrogen balance, which occurs when more nitrogen is excreted than is taken in, indicates wasting or destruction of tissue.

nitrogen cycle [Gk, *nitron,* nitre; *genein,* to produce; *kyklos,* circle], the circulation of nitrogen through natural processes in either of two ways: from the soil to plants and animals that excrete nitrogen products back into the soil or by bacterial fixation of atmospheric nitrogen through plants and animals that decay and release the element back into the atmosphere.

nitrogen fixation, the process by which free nitrogen in the atmosphere is converted by biologic or chemical means to ammonia and to other forms usable by plants and animals. Biologic nitrogen fixation is the more important process and is accomplished by microorganisms in the soil, either free living or in close association with root nodules of certain plants. In contrast, chemical nitrogen fixation, such as used in industry, requires extremely high temperatures and pressures.

nitrogen mustard. See **mechlorethamine hydrochloride.**

nitrogen narcosis, a condition of depressed central nervous system functions through high partial pressure of nitrogen. See also **decompression sickness.**

nitrogen washout curve, a graphic curve obtained by plotting the concentration of nitrogen in expired alveolar gas during oxygen breathing as a function of time. As a person begins to inhale pure oxygen after breathing ambient air, the nitrogen concentration decreases so that after 4 minutes healthy subjects have a nitrogen concentration in expired alveolar gas of less than 2%.

nitroglycerin (nitr) /-glis′ərin/, a coronary vasodilator.
■ INDICATION: It is prescribed for the prevention or relief of angina pectoris.
■ CONTRAINDICATION: Known hypersensitivity to this drug prohibits its use.

■ ADVERSE EFFECTS: Among the most serious adverse reactions are hypotension, flushing, headache, and syncope.

nitroglycerin tablets, tablets of glyceryl trinitrate, a volatile ester prepared by the action of nitric and sulfuric acids on glycerol. It is prescribed for the relief of heart symptoms. A potent smooth muscle relaxant and vasodilator, nitroglycerin is used in transdermal patches and an alcohol solution as well as in oral and sublingual tablets as a coronary vasodilator.

nitromersol, /-mur′sol/ an organic mercurial antiseptic that is not a highly effective germicide, sometimes used for the disinfecting of surgical instruments and as an antiseptic on the skin and mucous membranes.

nitroprusside sodium. See **sodium nitroprusside.**

nitrosamines /nīt′rəsam′ēn/, potentially carcinogenic compounds produced by reactions of nitrites with amines or amides normally present in the body. Nitrites are produced by bacteria in saliva, and in the intestine from nitrates normally present in vegetables and in nitrate-treated fish, poultry, and meats. More than 70% of ingested nitrates are from vegetables.

nitroso-, a combining form indicating presence of the group -N:O: *nitrosobacteria, nitrososubstitution.*

nitrosourea /nītrō′sōyo͝orē′ə/, one of a group of alkylating drugs used as an antineoplastic drug in the chemotherapy of brain tumors, multiple myeloma, Hodgkin's disease, adenocarcinomas, hepatomas, chronic leukemias, lymphomas, myelomas, and cancers of the breast and ovaries. They have been less successful in therapy for cancers of the lungs, head, neck, and GI tract. Like other alkylating agents, they have severe toxic effects, including bone marrow depression. Nausea and vomiting are almost always present. Safe use during pregnancy has not been established, and animal studies have generally shown teratogenicity and embryotoxicity. Carmustine and lomustine are typical examples of this group. See also **alkylating agent.**

Nitrospan, a trademark for a coronary vasodilator (nitroglycerin).

Nitrostat, a trademark for a coronary vasodilator (nitroglycerin).

nitrous oxide (N_2O) /nī′trəs/, a gas used as an anesthetic in dentistry, surgery, and childbirth. It provides light anesthesia and is delivered in various concentrations with oxygen. Nitrous oxide alone does not provide deep enough anesthesia for major surgery, for which it is supplemented with other anesthetic agents. It is often given for induction of anesthesia, preceded by the administration of a barbiturate or an analgesic narcotic. Nitrous oxide is neither explosive nor flammable, and recovery is rapid. It is not administered to patients with hypoxemia, respiratory disease, or intestinal occlusion.

Nix, a trademark for a topical pediculicide (permethrin).

Nizoral, a trademark for an antifungal agent (ketoconazole).

nl, abbreviation for *natural logarithm.*

NLN, abbreviation for **National League for Nursing.**

N-m, abbreviation for *newton meter.*

N/m^2, abbreviation for *newton per square meter.*

NMDP, abbreviation for **National Marrow Donor Program.**

NMNA, abbreviation for **National Male Nurses' Association.**

NMR, 1. abbreviation for **nuclear magnetic resonance.**

See **magnetic resonance. 2.** abbreviation for *nuclear magnetic resonance spectroscopy*.

NMR imaging. See **magnetic resonance imaging.**

No, symbol for the element **nobelium.**

N₂O, symbol for **nitrous oxide.**

nobelium (No) /nōbel'ē·əm/ [Alfred Nobel Institute, Stockholm, Sweden], a synthetic, transuranic metallic element. Its atomic number is 102. The atomic weight of its most stable isotope is 259.

noble gas. See **inert gas.**

Nocardia /nōkär'dē·ə/ [Edmund I. E. Nocard, French veterinarian, b. 1850], a genus of gram-positive aerobic bacteria, some species of which are pathogenic, such as *Nocardia asteroides*. See also **nocardiosis.**

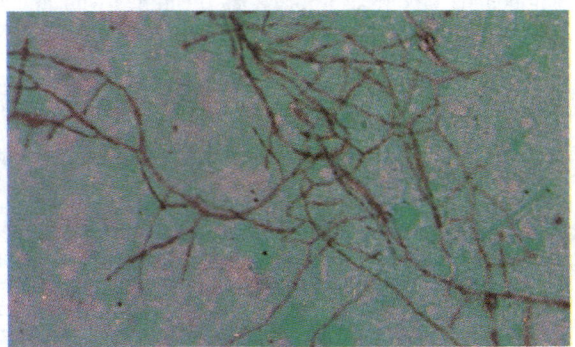

Nocardia *(Baron, 1990)*

nocardiosis /nōkär'dē·ō'sis/ [Edmund I. E. Nocard; Gk, *osis*, condition], infection with *Nocardia asteroides,* an aerobic gram-positive species of actinomycetes, characterized by pneumonia, often with cavitation, and by chronic abscesses in the brain and subcutaneous tissues. The organism enters via the respiratory tract and spreads by the bloodstream, especially in Cushing's syndrome. Surgical drainage of abscesses and sulfonamide therapy for 12 to 18 months cures between 50% and 60% of the cases treated.

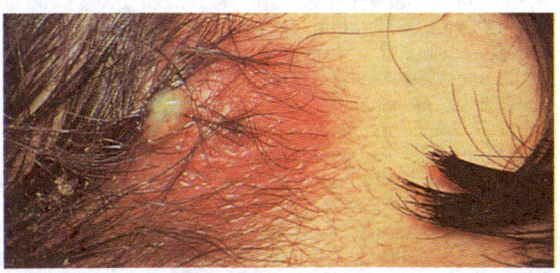

Nocardiosis *(Baran, 1991)*

noci-, a prefix meaning 'to cause harm, injury, or pain': *nociassociation, nociceptive, nociceptor.*

nociceptive /nō'sēsep'tiv/ [L, *nocere*, to injure, *capere*, to receive], pertaining to a neural receptor for painful stimuli.

nociceptive reflex [L, *nocere*, to injure + *capere*, to re-

ceive + *reflectere*, to bend back], a reflex caused by a painful stimulus.

nociceptive stimulus [L, *nocere*, to injure + *capere*, to receive + *stimulus*, goad], a painful, sometimes detrimental or injurious, stimulus.

nociceptor /nō'sēsep'tər/, somatic and visceral free nerve endings of thinly myelinated and unmyelinated fibers. They usually react to tissue injury but also may be excited by endogenous chemical substances.

no code [AS, *na*, not; L, *caudex*, book], a note written in the patient record and signed by a qualified, usually senior or attending physician, instructing the staff of the institution not to attempt to resuscitate a particular patient in the event of cardiac or respiratory failure. This instruction is usually given only when a patient is so gravely ill that death is imminent and inevitable. Also called **DNR** ("do not resuscitate") See also **code,** def. 5.

noct-, a prefix meaning 'pertaining to the night': *nocturia, nocturnal.*

noct., abbreviation for the Latin phrase, *nocte*, meaning 'at night.'

noctambulation. See **somnambulism.**

nocturia /noktŏŏr'ē·ə/ [L, *nocturnus*, by night; Gk, *ouron*, urine], urination, particularly excessive urination at night. Whereas it may be a symptom of renal disease, it may occur in the absence of disease in people who drink excessive amounts of fluids, particularly alcohol or coffee, before bedtime or in people with prostatic disease. It may occur in older patients, who may have excess fluids that are mobilized by lying down at night. Also called **nycturia.** Compare **enuresis.**

nocturnal /noktur'nəl/ [L, *nocturnus*, by night], **1.** pertaining to or occurring during the night. **2.** describing an individual or animal that is active at night and sleeps during the day.

nocturnal emission, involuntary emission of semen during sleep, usually in association with an erotic dream. Also called **wet dream.**

nocturnal enuresis [L, *nocturnus*, night; Gk, *enourein*], involuntary urination while asleep at night.

nocturnal paroxysmal dyspnea, an abnormal condition of the respiratory system, characterized by sudden attacks of shortness of breath, profuse sweating, tachycardia, and wheezing that awaken the person from sleep. The paroxysms may be induced by nightmares, noises, or coughing. The condition is usually associated with left ventricular failure or pulmonary edema. Characteristically, the attack is relieved by getting up and opening a window. See also **dyspnea.**

nocturnal penile tumescence (NPT) [L, *nocturnus*, night; *penile*, pertaining to the penis; *tumescere*, to begin to swell], a normal condition of penile erection that occurs during sleep throughout most of the lifetime of a male. The occurrence of NPT is important in the diagnosis of impotence, because it indicates that impotence may be psychogenic.

nod-, a combining form meaning 'knot': *nodal, nodose, nodulus.*

nodal bigeminy. See **junctional bigeminy.**

nodal event /nō'dəl/, an occurrence that may cause anxiety, such as birth, death, divorce, marriage, or a child leaving home.

nodal rhythm (NR) [L, *nodus*, knot; Gk, *rhythmos*], a cardiac rhythm that occurs when the atrioventricular node gains control of the heart beat, usually because of a defect in the function of the sinoatrial node. Also called **junctional rhythm**.

nodal tachycardia [L, *nodus*, knot; Gk, *tachys*, swift + *kardia*, heart], a rapid discharge of impulses from an ectopic focus in the area of the atrioventricular node.

node /nōd/ [L, *nodus*, knot], **1.** a small rounded mass. **2.** a lymph node. **3.** a single computer terminal in a network of terminals and computers.

nodular /nod′yələr/ [L, *nodus*, knot], (of a structure or mass) small, firm, and knotty. See also **node, nodule**.

nodular circumscribed lipomatosis, a condition in which circumscribed, encapsulated lipomas are distributed around the neck symmetrically, randomly, or like a collar. The adipose deposits may be painful and tender.

nodular cutaneous angiitis, an inflammatory condition of small arteries accompanied by lesions of the skin.

nodular fasciitis, an inflammation of the fascia that results in the formation of nodules.

nodular goiter [L, *nodus*, knot; Gk, *guttur*, throat], an enlarged goiter that contains nodules.

nodular melanoma, a melanoma that is uniformly pigmented, usually bluish-black and nodular and sometimes surrounded by an irregular halo of pale, unpigmented skin. The lesion is always raised and may be dome-shaped or polypoid. Most often the tumor is found in adults in middle age and occurs in 10% to 15% of patients with melanoma. See also **lentigo maligna melanoma, superficial spreading melanoma**.

nodule /nod′yōōl/ [L, *nodulus*, small knot], **1.** a small node. **2.** a small nodelike structure.

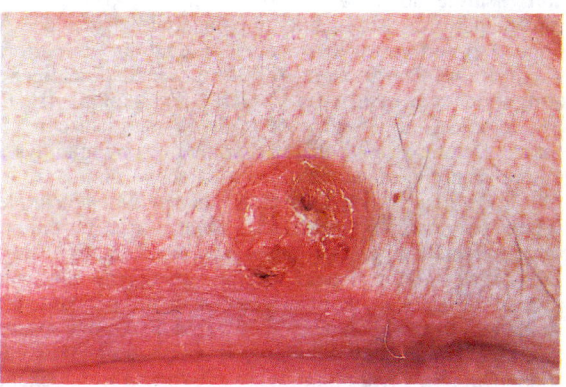

Nodule (du Vivier, 1993)

-noia, a suffix meaning '(condition of the) mind or will': *aponoia, hypernoia, hyponoia*.

noise, random signals or disturbances that interfere with the normal flow of data through pathways of computers and other electronic devices.

noise-induced hearing loss, a gradual loss of hearing caused by exposure to loud noise over an extended period of time, such as with an individual who works in a noisy environment. The hearing loss is sensorineural in nature and greatest in the higher frequencies. Although an early hearing loss may be temporary, it becomes permanent with increased exposure to noise. Compare **acoustic trauma**.

noise pollution, a noise level in an environment that is uncomfortable for the inhabitants.

nok, abbreviation for *next of kin*.

Noludar, a trademark for a sedative (methyprylon).

Nolvadex, a trademark for a nonsteroidal antiestrogen (tamoxifen).

noma /nō′mə/ [Gk, *nome*, distribution], an acute, necrotizing ulcerative process involving mucous membranes of mouth or genitalia. The condition is most commonly seen in children with poor nutrition and hygiene. There is rapid spreading and painless destruction of bone and soft tissue accompanied by a putrid odor. Fusospirochetal organisms have been implicated. Healing eventually occurs but often with disfiguring defects. Also called **acute necrotizing ulcerative mucositis, gangrenous stomatitis**.

-noma, a suffix meaning a 'spreading, invasive gangrene': *müllerianoma, pelidnoma*.

nomen-, a combining form meaning 'a name or pertaining to names': *nomenclature*.

nomenclature /nō′mənklā′chər, nōmen′-/ [L *nomen* name, *clamare* to call], a consistent, systematic method of naming used in a scientific discipline to denote classifications and to avoid ambiguities in names, such as binomial nomenclature in biology and chemical nomenclature in chemistry.

-nomia, a suffix meaning 'aphasia involving names or naming ability': *anomia, paranomia, dysnomia*.

Nomina Anatomica, the book of official international nomenclature for anatomy as designated by the International Congress of Anatomists.

nominal aphasia /nom′inəl/ [L, *nomen*; Gk, *a*, *phasis*, speech], a type of speech defect in which the person uses incorrect names in identifying objects. Minor episodes may be due to anxiety, fatigue, or senility, but severe cases can indicate a focal lesion on the left side of the brain. Also called **amnestic aphasia**.

nominal damages. See **damages**.

nomo-, a prefix meaning 'of or relating to usage or law': *nomogenesis, nomogram, nomotopic*.

nomogram /nom′əgram, nō′mə-/ [Gk, *nomos*, law, *gramma*, a record], **1.** a graphic representation, by any of various systems, of a numeric relationship. **2.** a graph on which a number of variables is plotted so that the value of a dependent variable can be read on the appropriate line when the values of the other variables are given.

-nomy, a combining form meaning 'received knowledge in a field': *pathonomy, physionomy, psychonomy*.

non- /non-/, a prefix meaning 'not': *noninvasive, noncompliant*.

nona-, noni-, a prefix meaning 'nine': *nonan, nonigravida, nonipara*.

nonabsorbable surgical sutures /-əbsôr′bəbəl/ [L, *non*, not + *absorbere*; Gk, *cheirourgos*, surgeon; L, *sutura*], sutures of silk, nylon, steel, or other materials that resist absorption. They are used mainly in deep tissues where it is important for them to remain *in situ*.

nonadherent dressing /-ədhir′ənt/ [L, *non, adhesio*, sticking to; OFr, *dresser*, to arrange], a dressing that usually does not stick to the dried secretions of a wound.

nonadhesive skin traction /-ədhē′siv/ [L, *non*, not, *adhesio*, sticking to], one of two kinds of skin traction in which the therapeutic pull of traction weights is applied with foam-backed traction straps that do not stick to the skin over the body structure involved. Nonadhesive skin traction straps

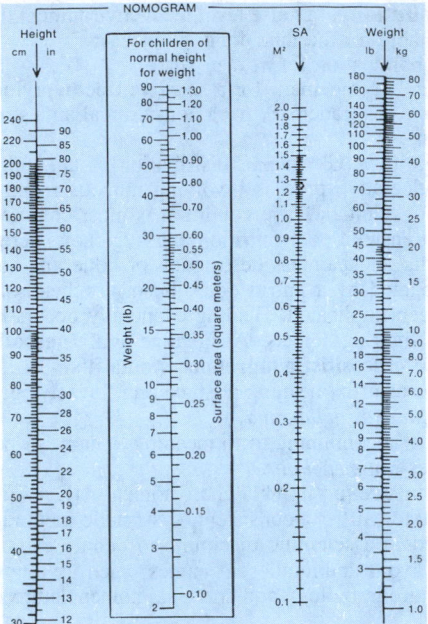

West nomogram

may be easily removed to facilitate skin care and are usually used when continuous traction is not required. The straps spread the traction pull over a wide area of skin surface, thus decreasing the vulnerability of the patient to skin breakdown. Compare **adhesive skin traction.**

non-A, non-B (NANB) hepatitis, See **hepatitis C.**

nonbacterial thrombic endocarditis /-baktir′ē-ə/ [L, *non,* + *bakerion,* small rod], one of the three main types of endocarditis, characterized by various kinds of lesions that affect the heart valves. Some studies indicate that this disease may be the first step in the development of bacterial endocarditis and that the lesions involved cause peripheral arterial embolisms resulting in death. This disease equally affects men and women between 18 and 90 years of age, causes heart murmurs in about 30% of the cases, and most often affects the valves on the left side of the heart. There is no successful treatment of nonbacterial thrombic endocarditis, but anticoagulation therapy may be employed to reduce the incidence of peripheral arterial embolism. See also **Libman-Sacks endocarditis.**

noncohesive gold foil /-kōhē′siv/ [L, *non* + *cohaerere,* to stick together], a thin sheet of pure gold, used for making dental restorations, such as crowns, that will not cohere at room temperature because of a protective surface coating.

noncommunicating hydrocephalus. See **hydrocephalus.**

noncompetitive inhibition /-kəmpet′itiv/, (in pharmacology) a form of inhibition in which a substance occupies a receptor and cannot be displaced from the receptor by increasing the numbers of other molecules through the principle of mass action.

noncompliance /-kəmpli′əns/ [L, *non* + *complere,* to complete], a nursing diagnosis accepted by the Fourth National Conference on the Classification of Nursing Diagnoses. The specific nature of the noncompliance is to be specified, such as 'noncompliance: medications.' It is defined as an informed decision on the part of the client not to adhere to a therapeutic suggestion because of a health belief, a cultural or spiritual value, or a problem in the relationship between the provider of the recommendation and the client. The critical defining characteristic, which must be present for the diagnosis to be made, is an observation of the client's failure to adhere to a recommendation or a statement by the client or knowledgeable other person that the recommendations are not being followed. Other defining characteristics include objective tests that show noncompliance, observation of physical or psychologic signs that demonstrate lack of compliance, or a failure to keep appointments. See also **nursing diagnosis.**

non compos mentis /non′ kom′pos men′tis/ [L, not of sound mind], a legal term applied to a person declared to be mentally incompetent.

nondirective therapy /-direk′tiv/ [L, *non* + *digere,* to direct], a psychotherapeutic approach in which the psychotherapist refrains from giving advice or interpretation as the client is helped to identify conflicts and to clarify and understand feelings and values. Compare **directive therapy.** See also **client-centered therapy.**

nondisjunction /-disjungk′chən/ [L, *non* + *disjungere,* to disjoint], failure of homologous pairs of chromosomes to separate during the first meiotic division or of the two chromatids of a chromosome to split during anaphase of mitosis or the second meiotic division. The result is an abnormal number of chromosomes in the daughter cells. Compare **disjunction.** See also **monosomy, trisomy.**

nonfat milk. See **skimmed milk.**

nonepileptic seizures. See **vasovagal seizures.**

nonfeasance /nonfē′zəns/ [L, *non* + *facere,* to do], a failure to perform a task, duty, or undertaking that one has agreed to perform or that one had a legal duty to perform. Compare **malfeasance, misfeasance.** See also **negligence.**

nongonococcal urethritis (NGU) /-gon′əkok′əl/ [L, *non* + Gk, *gone,* seed, *kokkos,* berry], an infectious condition of the urethra in males that is characterized by mild dysuria and a scanty to moderate amount of penile discharge. The discharge may be white or clear, thin or mucoid, or, less often, purulent. The infection is often caused by the obligate intracellular parasite *Chlamydia trachomatis.* The diagnosis of NGU is made by excluding a diagnosis of gonococcal urethritis by microscopic examination and bacteriologic culture of the exudate. Untreated NGU may result in urethral stricture, epididymitis, proctitis, and chronic inflammation of the urethra. Women exposed to the exudate during coitus may develop a hyperthropic erosion of the cervix and purulent cervical mucus. An infant in passing through the cervix and vagina of a mother infected with *C. trachomatis* may develop conjunctivitis and nasopharyngeal infection in the first few days after birth and pneumonia at 3 to 4 months. Most cases of NGU are successfully treated with tetracycline or erythromycin. Sexual contacts are treated whether or not they are symptomatic. Nearly 50% of all cases of urethritis are nongonococcal.

nonhemolytic jaundice /-hē′məlit′ik/ [L, *non,* Gk, *haima,* blood; *lysein,* to loosen; Fr, *jaune,* yellow], a form of jaundice that is due to a liver disease rather than the destruction of red blood cells.

non-Hodgkin's lymphoma /-hoj′kənz/, any kind of malignant lymphoma except Hodgkin's disease. Also called **lymphosarcoma.**

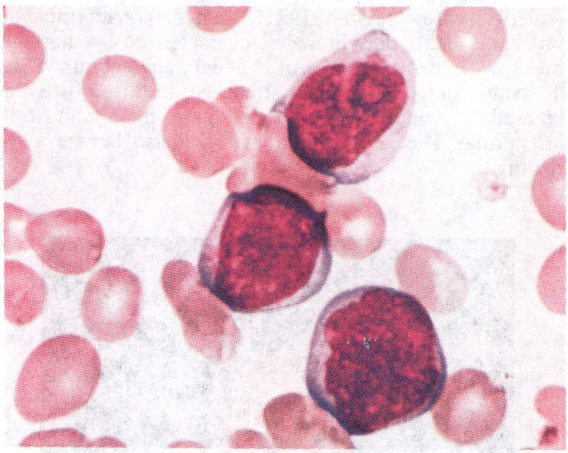

Non—Hodgkin's lymphoma (Hayhoe, 1992)

nonigravida /nō´nigrav´idə/ [L, *nonus*, nine; *gravida*, pregnant], indicating a woman pregnant for the ninth time.

nonimpact printer /-im´pakt/, a computer printer that produces an image on a medium, such as paper, by ink jet, or by thermal, electomagnetic, or xerographic means.

non-insulin-dependent diabetes mellitus (NIDDM), a type of diabetes mellitus in which patients are not insulin-dependent or ketosis prone although they may use insulin for correction of symptomatic or persistent hyperglycemia, and they can develop ketosis under special circumstances, such as infection or stress. Onset usually, after 40 years of age but can occur at any age. Two subclasses are presence or absence of obesity. About 60% to 90% are obese; in these patients glucose tolerance is often improved by weight loss. Hyperinsulemia and insulin resistance characterize some patients. There are probably multiple causes for the derangement of carbohydrate metabolism. Familial aggregation implies genetic factors, and this class includes diabetes presenting in childhood and adults in whom autosomal dominant inheritance is clearly established. Environmental factors superimposed on genetic susceptibility are probably involved in onset. Previously called adult-onset diabetes, ketosis-resistant diabetes, maturity-onset diabetes, maturity-onset type diabetes, MOD, stable diabetes. Also called **type II diabetes mellitus.** See also **diabetes mellitus.**

noninvasive /-invā´siv/ [L, *non* + *in*, into, *vadere*, to go], pertaining to a diagnostic or therapeutic technique that does not require the skin to be broken or a cavity or organ of the body to be entered, such as obtaining a blood pressure reading by auscultation with a stethoscope and sphygmomanometer.

nonionic /-ī·on´ik/, pertaining to compounds without a net negative or positive charge.

nonionizing radiation /-ī´əni´zing/ [L, *non* + Gk, *ion*, going, *izein*, to cause], radiation for which the mechanism of action in tissue does not directly ionize atomic or molecular systems through a single interaction.

nonipara /nōnip´ərə/ [L, *nonus*, nine; *parere*, to bear], a woman who has delivered nine offspring.

nonmedullated nerve fiber /-med´yəlā´tid/ [L, *non*, *medulla*, marrow; *nervus*, nerve; *fibra*, fiber], a nerve fiber that lacks the fatty myelin insulating sheath. Such fibers

form the gray matter of the nervous system, as distinguished from the white matter of medullated fibers.

nonmyelinated /-mī´əlinā´tid/ [L, *non*; Gk, *myelos*, marrow], pertaining to nerve fibers that lack a fatty myelin insulating sheath. See **nonmedullated nerve fiber**.

nonossifying fibroma /-os´ifī´ing/, a bone anomaly found in children as a sharply circumscribed, eccentrically located lesion in the metaphysis of long bones. A microscopic examination reveals whorl patterns of spindle cells, fibrous tissue, numerous xanthoma cells, and occasional giant cells.

nonosteogenic fibroma /non´ostē-əjen´ik/, a common bone lesion characterized by degeneration and proliferation of the medullary and cortical tissue, near the ends of the diaphyses of the large long bones of the lower extremities. Frequently the lesion causes no symptoms and is only discovered during x-ray examination of the skeleton for other reasons.

nonparametric test of significance /-per´əmet´rik/ [L, *non* + Gk, *para*, beside, *metron*, measure], (in statistics) one of several tests that use a qualitative approach to analyze rank order data and incidence data that cannot be assumed to have a normal distribution. Kinds of nonparametric tests of significance include **chi-square, Spearman's rho.**

nonparous /-per´əs/ [L, *non*, *parere*, to bear], indicating a woman who has never delivered a child. Also called **nulliparous.**

nonpenetrating wound /-pen´ətrā´ting/ [L, *non*, not + *penetrare*, to penetrate; AS, *wund*], a wound that does not break the surface of the skin.

nonpolar /-pō´lər/ [L, *non* + *polus*, pole], pertaining to molecules that have a hydrophobic affinity, are "water hating." Nonpolar substances tend to dissolve in nonpolar solvents.

nonproductive cough /-prəduk´tiv/ [L, *non* + *producere*, to produce], a sudden, noisy expulsion of air from the lungs that may be caused by irritation or inflammation and does not remove sputum from the respiratory tract. Expectorants, such as ammonium chloride, ammonium carbonate, sodium iodide, potassium iodide, ipecac, and terpin hydrate increase respiratory tract secretions and may result in productive coughing when administered to patients with respiratory infections. If suppression of coughing is required, antitussives that depress the cough reflex may be prescribed, including codeine or dextromethorphan. Intratracheal suctioning may be necessary when secretions cause severe respiratory difficulty and coughing is unproductive. Compare **productive cough.**

nonproprietary name /-prəprī´əter´ē/ [L, *non*, *proprietas*, owner; *nomen*, name], the chemical or generic name of a drug or device, as distinguished from a brand name or trademark. A nonproprietary name may be indicated by the letters, USAN, for United States Adopted Names. See **USAN.**

nonprotein nitrogen (NPN) /-prō´tēn/ [L, *non* + Gk, *proteios*, first rank; *nitron*, soda, *genein*, to produce], the nitrogen in the blood that is not a constituent of protein, such as the nitrogen associated with urea, uric acid, creatine, and polypeptides. Approximately one half of the nonprotein nitrogen in the blood is associated with urea. Measurement of NPN may aid assessment of kidney function. The normal concentrations in serum or plasma are 25 to 35 mg/dl; in whole blood, 25 to 50 mg/dl.

nonrapid eye movement. See **sleep.**

nonreflex bladder. See **flaccid bladder.**

nonreversible inhibitor /-rivur´sələl/ [L, *non* + *revertere*, to turn back; *inhibere*, to restrain], an effector substance that binds permanently to an active site of an enzyme, inhibiting the normal catalytic activity of the enzyme.

nonsecretor /-səkrē′tər/ [L, *non*, *secernere*, to separate], a person who does not secrete ABO blood group substances in mucous secretions of the saliva or gastric juice. The condition is genetically determined.

nonseg., abbreviation for *nonsegmented.*

nonsense mutation. See **amber mutation.**

nonsexual generation. See **asexual generation.**

nonshivering thermogenesis /-shiv′əring/, a natural method by which newborns can produce body heat by increasing their metabolic rate.

nonspecific urethritis (NSU) /-spəsif′ik/ [L, *non* + *species*, form], inflammation of the urethra not known to be caused by a specific organism. Onset of symptoms is often related to sexual intercourse. Its acute phase is seldom seen in women, but its chronic phase is a common urologic difficulty among them. The condition is noted by urethral discharge in men and by reddening of the urethral mucosa in women. Treatment with antibiotics is not always successful. See also **nongonococcal urethritis.**

nonspecific vaginitis [L, *non*, not + *species*, form + *facere*, to make + *vagina*, sheath; Gk, *itis*, inflammation], an obsolete term for a vaginal inflammation for which no specific pathogen can be found. Most cases of vaginitis today are found to be due to infections of *Garnerella vaginalis* in combination with anaerobic bacteria, although nearly one third of all cases are caused by a protozoa, *Trichomonas vaginalis.*

nonstress test (NST) /non′stres/, an evaluation of the fetal heart rate response to natural contractile activity or to an increase in fetal activity. Also called **fetal activity determination (FAD).**

nonsuppurative osteomyelitis /-sup′yərā′tiv/, tuberculosis of the bone.

nonthrombocytopenic purpura /-throm′bōsī′təpē′ik/, a disorder characterized by purplish or reddish skin areas. The condition does not involve a decrease in the number of platelets.

nontoxic /-tok′sik/, not poisonous. Also **atoxic.**

nontropical sprue /-trop′ikəl/ [L, *non*, not; Gk, *tropikos*, of the solstice; D, *sprouw*], a malabsorption syndrome resulting from an inborn inability to digest foods that contain gluten. See also **celiac disease.**

nonulcerative blepharitis /-ul′sərətiv′/ [L, *non* + *ilcus*, ulcer; Gk, *blepharon*, eyelid, *itis*, inflammation], a form of blepharitis characterized by greasy scales on the margins of the eyelids around the lashes and hyperemia and thickening of the skin. Nonulcerative blepharitis is often associated with seborrhea of the scalp, eyebrows, and the skin behind the ears.

nonunion /-yoo′nyən/, pertaining to a fractured bone that fails to heal properly.

nonverbal communication /-vur′bəl/, the transmission of a message without the use of words. It may involve any or all of the five senses. See also **body language**.

nonviable /vī′əbəl/ [L, *non*, *vita*, life], unable to exist independently after birth.

nonvital pulp [L, *non*, not + *vita*, life + *pulpa*, flesh], dead dental pulp in which the canal of the tooth has become necrotic because of a disease or trauma that interferes with the blood supply. Also called **dead pulp**.

Noonan's syndrome /noo′nənz/ [Jacqueline A. Noonan, American cardiologist, b. 1921], a hypergonadotropic disorder, occurring only in males, characterized by short stature, low-set ears, webbing of the neck, and cubitus valgus. Testicular function may be normal, but fertility is often decreased. The number and morphology of the chromosomes are normal. The cause is unknown. See also **Turner's syndrome.**

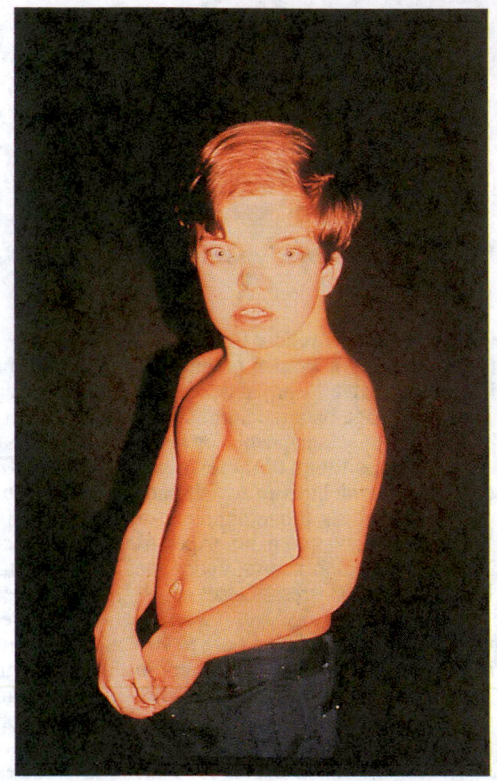

Noonan's syndrome *(Zitelli, 1992)*

Norcuron, a trademark for an intravenous neuromuscular blocking drug (vecuronium bromide).

norepinephrine /nôr′epinef′rin/, an adrenergic hormone that acts to increase blood pressure by vasoconstriction but does not affect cardiac output. It is synthesized naturally by the adrenal medulla and is available also as a drug, levarterenol, given to maintain the blood pressure in acute hypotension secondary to trauma, heart disease, or vascular collapse.

norepinephrine bitartrate, an adrenergic vasoconstrictor.

■ INDICATIONS: It is prescribed in the treatment of cardiac arrest and in certain acute hypotensive states.

■ CONTRAINDICATIONS: Hypovolemia, vascular thrombosis, or known hypersensitivity to this drug prohibits its use. It is not used in conjunction with cyclopropane or halothane anesthesia.

■ ADVERSE EFFECTS: Among the more serious adverse reactions are local tissue necrosis at the site of injection, bradycardia, headache, and hypertension.

no response (NR), the condition for which the maximum decrease in treated tumor volume is less than 50%.

norethindrone /nôreth'indrōn/, a progestin.

- INDICATIONS: It is prescribed in the treatment of abnormal uterine bleeding and endometriosis and is a component in oral contraceptive medications.

- CONTRAINDICATIONS: Thrombophlebitis, liver dysfunction, unusual vaginal bleeding, breast cancer, missed abortion, or known hypersensitivity to this drug prohibits its use. It is not recommended for use during pregnancy.

- ADVERSE EFFECTS: Among the more serious adverse reactions are breakthrough bleeding, amenorrhea, GI disturbances, breast changes, and masculinization of the female fetus.

norethindrone acetate and ethinyl estradiol, an oral contraceptive.

- INDICATIONS: It is prescribed for contraception, endometriosis, and hypermenorrhea.

- CONTRAINDICATIONS: Thrombophlebitis, cardiovascular disease, breast or reproductive organ cancer, unusual vaginal bleeding, gallbladder disease, liver tumor, or known hypersensitivity to this drug prohibits its use. It is not given to women over 40 years of age or during lactation, pregnancy, or suspected pregnancy. It is given with caution to women who smoke.

- ADVERSE EFFECTS: Among the more serious adverse reactions are thrombophlebitis, uterine fibroma, porphyria, embolism, jaundice, and cerebrovascular accident.

Norflex, a trademark for a skeletal muscle relaxant and antihistamine (orphenadrine citrate).

norfloxacin /nôrflok'səsin/, an oral antibacterial drug.

- INDICATIONS: It is prescribed for the treatment of urinary tract infections.

- CONTRAINDICATIONS: This product is not recommended for children or pregnant women. Concomitant use of nitrofurantoin drugs is not recommended.

- ADVERSE EFFECTS: Reported side effects include nausea, dizziness, and headache.

Norgesic Forte, a trademark for a fixed-combination drug containing a muscle relaxant with anticholinergic activity (orphenadrine citrate) and APC (aspirin, phenacetin, and caffeine), used for the relief of mild to moderate pain of acute musculoskeletal disorders.

norgestrel /nôrjes'trəl/, a progestin.

- INDICATIONS: It is prescribed alone or in combination with estrogen as a contraceptive.

- CONTRAINDICATIONS: Thrombophlebitis, liver dysfunction, unusual vaginal bleeding, breast cancer, missed abortion, or known hypersensitivity to this drug prohibits its use.

- ADVERSE EFFECTS: Among the more serious adverse reactions are amenorrhea, dysfunctional uterine bleeding, breast changes, and masculinization of a female fetus.

Norinyl, a trademark for an oral contraceptive containing a progestin (norethindrone) and an estrogen (mestranol).

Norisodrine Hydrochloride, a trademark for an adrenergic (isoproterenol hydrochloride).

Norlestrin, a trademark for an oral contraceptive containing an estrogen (ethinyl estradiol) and a progestin (norethindrone acetate).

Norlutin, a trademark for a progestin (norethindrone).

norm [L, *norma*, rule], **1.** a measure of a phenomenon generally accepted as the ideal standard performance against which other measures of the phenomenon may be measured. **2.** abbreviation for **normal**.

norma basalis /nôr'mə basā'lis/ [L, rule; Gk, *basis*, foundation], the inferior surface of the base of the skull with the mandible removed, formed by the palatine bones, the vomer, the pterygoid processes, and parts of the sphenoid and temporal bones.

normal (N) /nôr'məl/ [L, *norma*, rule], **1.** describing a standard, average, or typical example of a set of objects or values. **2.** describing a chemical solution in which 1 L contains 1 g of a substance or the equivalent in replaceable hydrogen ions. **3.** people in a nondiseased population. **4.** a gaussian distribution.

-normal, a combining form meaning 'relating to a norm': *centinormal, decanormal, prenormal.*

normal dental function, the correct and healthy action of opposing teeth during mastication.

normal diet. See **regular diet.**

normal dwarf. See **primordial dwarf.**

normal human plasma [L, *norma*, rule + *humanus*; Gk, *plassein*, to mold], sterile, disease-free human blood prepared from a pooled donor supply.

normal human serum albumin, an isotonic preparation of pooled human serum albumin for treating hypoproteinemia, hypovolemia, and threatened or existing shock.

normal hydrogen electrode (NHE), a reference electrode that is assigned a value of 0 volts.

normal last shoes, special orthopedic shoes for infants and children constructed with a normal sole, as opposed to a reverse or straight last shoe.

normal phase, a chromatographic mode in which the mobile phase is less polar than the stationary phase.

normal pressure hydrocephalus [L, *norma*, rule; *premere*, to press; Gk, *hydor*, water; *kephale*, head], a condition in which there is dilatation of the ventricles without an increase in intracranal pressure.

normal saline solution [L, *norma*, rule + *sal* + *solutus*, dissolved], a 0.9% w/v sterile solution of sodium chloride in water that is isotonic with blood and injectable intravenously.

normal sinus rhythm (NSR) [L, *norma*, rule + *sinus*, hollow; Gk, *rhythmos*], the normal heart beat produced when the pacemaker is in the sinoatrial node.

normal solution [L, *norma*, rule + *solutus*, dissolved], a solution that contains the gram-equivalent weight of a reagent per liter. It is denoted by the symbols N/l or N.

normal strain, a quantity described by the quotient of the change of length of a line and its original length.

normal stress, (in physics) a quantity described by the quotient of distributed force and area when the force is perpendicular to the area.

normal temperature [L, *norma*, rule + *temperatura*], for a normal person at rest, the normal oral clinical temperature is given as 98.6° F or 37.0° C, but actual "normal" temperatures may range a fraction of a degree or increments of a whole degree higher or lower because of effects of sleep, exercise, eating, sleeping, metabolism, and the ambient temperature. Rectal temperature also averages a fraction of a degree higher than oral temperatures, and axillary readings are lower than oral temperatures.

normo- /nôr'mə-/ [L, *norma*, the rule], a prefix meaning 'normal': *normocytic, normotensive.*

normoblast /nôr'məblast/ [L, *norma* + Gk, *blastos*, germ], a nucleated precursor cell in the bone marrow of the adult circulating erythrocyte. Developmental stages include the pronormoblast, the basophilic normoblast, the polychromatic normoblast, and the orthochromatic normoblast. After the extrusion of the nucleus of the normoblast, the young erythrocyte becomes known as a reticulocyte and enters the circulating blood. Compare **erythrocyte.** See also **reticulocyte.** **–normoblastic,** *adj.*

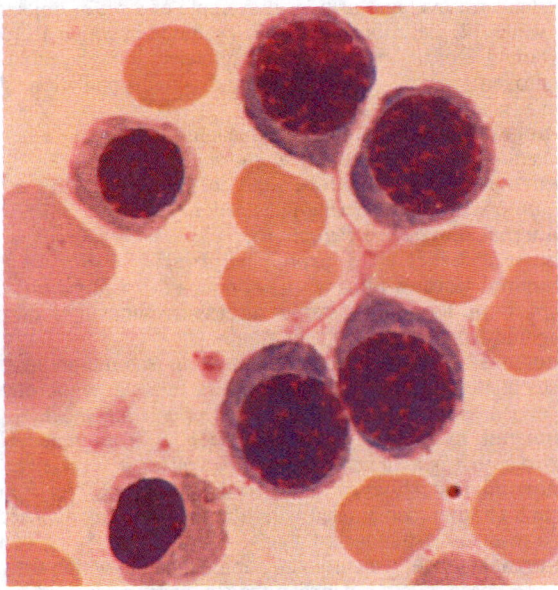

Normoblasts *(Hayhoe, 1992)*

normochromic /nôr′məkrō′mik/ [L, *norma* + Gk, *chroma*, color], pertaining to a blood cell having normal color caused by the presence of an adequate amount of hemoglobin. Compare **hypochromic.** See also **red cell indices.**

normocyte /nôr′məsīt/ [L, *norma* + Gk, *kytos*, cell], an ordinary, normal, adult red blood cell of average size having a diameter of 7 μ. Compare **macrocyte, microcyte.** **–normocytic,** *adj.*

Normodyne, a trademark for an antihypertensive drug (labetalol hydrochloride).

normoglycemic /-glīsē′mik/, pertaining to a normal blood glucose level.

normotensive /-ten′siv/, pertaining to the condition of having normal blood pressure. **–normotension,** *n.*

normoventilation /-ven′tilā′shən/, the alveolar ventilation rate that produces an alveolar carbon dioxide pressure of about 40 torr at any metabolic rate.

normoxia /nôrmok′sē·ə/, an ambient oxygen pressure of about 150 (plus or minus 10) torr, or the partial pressure of oxygen in atmospheric air at sea level.

Noroxin, a trademark for an oral antibacterial drug (norfloxacin).

Norpace, a trademark for an antidysrhythmic cardiac depressant (disopyramide phosphate).

Norplant; planned parenthood. See **contraception.**

Norplant System, a trademark for a method of implanting capsules of a contraceptive drug, levonorgestrel, beneath the skin of the upper arm of a woman. With the woman under local anesthesia, a set of six capsules, each 2.4 mm in diameter and 34 mm long, is inserted in a fan-shaped pattern through an incision about 10 cm above the elbow crease. The highly progestational drug diffuses through the walls of the capsules, maintaining a blood level of the progestin that can prevent pregnancy for up to 5 years, depending on individual differences in metabolism and body weight. The contraceptive effect can be interrupted by removing the capsules. The capsules are removed at the end of the fifth year, at which time a new set of capsules can be inserted if the woman wants to continue the protection.

Norpramin, a trademark for an antidepressant (desipramine hydrochloride).

Nor-QD, a trademark for an oral contraceptive containing a progestin (norethindrone), but no estrogen.

North American blastomycosis, an infection caused by inhaling the fungus *Blastomyces dermatitidis.* It may resemble bacterial pneumonia, and x-ray films of the chest may show cavities. Painless, well-demarcated, verrucous or ulcerated skin lesions occur on the face and hands. Occasionally, lesions of the oral mucous membrane may be mistaken for squamous cell carcinoma. The disease may progress to involve bones and the brain; many viscera are infected in fatal cases. Diagnosis is made by microscopic examination of body secretions. Treatment is ketoconazole/itraconazole or amphotericin B, given intravenously, depending on the severity, or, in severe cases, a combination of amphotericin B and sulfonamides. Also called **Gilchrist's disease.** Compare **paracoccidioidomycosis.**

North American Nursing Diagnosis Association (NANDA), a professional organization of registered nurses created in 1982. The purpose of the organization is 'to develop, refine, and promote a taxonomy of nursing diagnostic terminology of general use to the professional.'

North Asian tick-borne rickettsiosis, an infection, acquired in the Eastern Hemisphere, caused by *Rickettsia siberica,* transmitted by ticks, and resembling Rocky Mountain spotted fever. Usual findings include a generalized maculopapular rash involving palms and soles, fever, and lymph node enlargement. It is rarely fatal and responds quickly to treatment with chloramphenicol. No vaccine is available. See also **boutonneuse fever, relapsing fever.**

North Asian tick typhus. See **Siberian tick typhus.**

Northern blot test, an electrophoretic test for identifying the presence or absence of particular mRNA molecules and nucleic acid hybridization. See also **Southern blot test.**

nortriptyline hydrochloride /nôrtrip′tilēn/, a tricyclic antidepressant.

■ INDICATION: It is prescribed in the treatment of mental depression.

■ CONTRAINDICATIONS: Concomitant administration of monoamine oxidase inhibitors, recent myocardial infarction, or known hypersensitivity to this drug or to other tricyclic medications prohibits its use. It is used with caution in patients having a seizure disorder or a cardiovascular disease.

■ ADVERSE EFFECTS: Among the more serious adverse effects are sedation and GI, cardiovascular, and neurologic reactions. This drug interacts with many other drugs.

Norwegian scabies [Norway; L, *scabere,* to scratch], a severe infestation of human skin by an itch mite (*Sarcoptes scabiei*). The condition is associated with intense itching, crusting and scaling of the skin, and insect egg burrows that appear as discolored lines in the affected skin areas.

nose [AS, *nosu*], the structure that protrudes from the anterior portion of the skull and serves as a passageway for air to and from the lungs. The nose filters the air, warming, moistening, and chemically examining it for impurities that might irritate the mucous lining of the respiratory tract. The nose also contains the organ of smell, and it aids the faculty of speech. It consists of an internal portion and an external portion. The external portion, which protrudes from the face, is considerably smaller than the internal portion, which lies over the roof of the mouth. The hollow interior portion is separated into a right cavity and a left cavity by a septum. Each cavity is divided into the superior, middle, and inferior meati by the projection of nasal conchae. The external portion of the nose is perforated by two nostrils and the internal portion by two posterior nares. The pairs of sinuses that drain into the nose are the frontal, maxillary, ethmoidal, and sphenoidal sinuses. Ciliated mucous membrane lines the nose, closely adhering to the periosteum. The mucous membrane is continuous with the skin through the nares and with the mucous membrane of the nasal part of the pharynx through the choanae. The mucous membrane contains the olfactory cells that connect with the olfactory nerves.

nosebleed [AS, *nosu* + ME, *blod*, blood], abnormal hemorrhage from the nose. Emergency responses to nosebleed include seating the patient upright with the head thrust forward to prevent swallowing of blood. Pressure with both thumbs directly under the nostril and above the lips may block the main artery supplying blood to the nose. Alternatively, pressure with both forefingers on each side of the nostril often slows bleeding by blocking the main arteries and their branches. Continued bleeding may require the insertion of cotton or other absorbent material within the nostril and reapplication of pressure. Cold compresses on the nose, lips, and the back of the head may help control hemorrhage. Continued bleeding may require cautery. Also called **epistaxis.**

NOSIE, abbreviation for **nurses' observation scale for inpatient evaluation.**

noso-, a combining form meaning 'of or relating to disease': *nosochthonography, nosogeny, nosophobe.*

nosocomial /nos'əkō'mē·əl/ [Gk, *nosokomeian*, hospital], of or pertaining to a hospital.

nosocomial infection, an infection acquired at least 72 hours after hospitalization, often caused by *Candida albicans, Escherichia coli,* hepatitis viruses, herpes zoster virus, *Pseudomonas,* or *Staphylococcus.* Also called **hospital-acquired infection.**

nosology /nōsol'əjē/ [Gk, *nosos,* disease, *logos,* science], the science of classifying diseases. See also **nomenclature.**

nostrils. See **anterior nares.**

notch [Fr, *noche*], an indentation or a depression in a bone or other organ, such as the auricular notch or the cardiac notch.

nothing by mouth (NPO), [L, *nil per os,* nothing by mouth], a patient care instruction advising that the patient is prohibited from ingesting food, beverage, or medicine. It is usually posted above the bed of a patient who is about to undergo surgery or special diagnostic procedures requiring that the digestive tract be empty.

notifiable [L, *nota,* mark, *facere,* to make], pertaining to certain conditions, diseases, and events that must, by law, be reported to a governmental agency, such as birth, death, smallpox, certain other communicable diseases, and certain violations of public health regulations.

noto-, a combining form meaning 'of or related to the back': *notochord, notogenesis, notomyelitis.*

notochord /nō'tōkôrd/ [Gk, *noton,* back, *chorde,* cord],

an elongated strip of mesodermal tissue that originates from the primitive node and extends along the dorsal surface of the developing embryo beneath the neural tube, forming the primary longitudinal skeletal axis of the body of all chordates. In humans and other vertebrate animals, the structure is replaced by vertebrae, although a remnant of it remains as part of the nucleus pulposus of the intervertebral disks. See also **neural tube.** –**notochordal,** *adj.*

notochordal canal /no'tōkôr'dəl/ [Gk, *noton* + *chorde,* cord; L, *canalis,* channel], a tubular passage that extends from the primitive pit into the head process during the early stages of embryonic development in mammals. It perforates the splanchnopleure layer so that there is a temporary connection between the yolk sac and the amnion. Also called **chordal canal.**

notochordal plate. See **head process.**

notogenesis /nō'tōjen'əsis/ [Gk, *noton* + *genein,* to produce], the formation of the notochord. –**notogenetic,** *adj.*

notomelus /nətom'ələs/ [Gk, *noton* + *melos,* limb], a congenital malformation in which one or more accessory limbs are attached to the back.

nourish /nur'ish/ [L, *nutrire,* to suckle], to furnish or supply the essential foods or nutrients for maintaining life.

nourishment /nur'ishmənt/, **1.** the act or process of nourishing or being nourished. **2.** any substance that nourishes and supports the life and growth of living organisms.

Novahistine, a trademark for a fixed-combination drug containing an antihistamine (chlorpheniramine maleate) and an adrenergic decongestant (phenylpropanolamine).

Novocain, a trademark for a local anesthetic (procaine hydrochloride).

NOx, abbreviation for **nitrous oxide,** or any mixture of oxides of nitrogen.

noxious /nok'shəs/ [L, *noxius,* harm], harmful, injurious, or detrimental to health.

Noyes test /noiz/, an orthopedic knee test performed with the knee extended and the thigh relaxed. There is anterolateral tibial subluxation. The knee is gradually flexed with reduction of the subluxation occurring at about 30 degrees of flexion.

Np, symbol for the element **neptunium.**

NPH Iletin, a trademark for an insulin suspension (isophane).

NPH Insulin, a trademark for an insulin suspension (isophane).

NPN, abbreviation for **nonprotein nitrogen.**

NPO, abbreviation for nothing by mouth.

N-propyl alcohol /en'prō'pil/, a clear, colorless liquid used as a solvent for resins.

NPT, abbreviation for **nocturnal penile tumescence**.

NR, **1.** abbreviation for **no response. 2.** abbreviation for *nodal rhythm.*

NREM, abbreviation for *nonrapid eye movement.* See **sleep.**

NSAID, abbreviation for **nonsteroidal antiinflammatory drug.**

NSCCN, abbreviation for **National Society of Critical Care Nurses of Canada.**

n-s/m², abbreviation for *newton second per square meter.*

NSNA, abbreviation for **National Student Nurses Association.**

NSR, abbreviation for **normal sinus rhythm.**

NSU, abbreviation for **nonspecific urethritis.**

ntp, abbreviation for *normal temperature and pressure.*

nu /n(y)oo/, N, ν, the thirteenth letter of the Greek alphabet.

Nubain, a trademark for a synthetic analgesic (nalbuphine hydrochloride), used as an adjunct to anesthesia.

nuc, abbreviation for *nuclear.*

nucha-, a combining form meaning 'pertaining to the neck': *nuchal, subnuchal.*

nucha /noo'kə/, *pl.* **nuchae** [Fr, *nuque,* nape], the nape, or back of the neck. **–nuchal,** *adj.*

nuchal cord /noo'kəl/ [Fr, *nuque,* nape; Gk, *chorde*], an abnormal but common condition in which the umbilical cord is wrapped around the neck of the fetus in utero or of the baby as it is being born. It is usually possible to slip the loop or loops of cord gently over the child's head. Sometimes it is a single loose loop, and the shoulders may deliver through it. If it is tight, it may be clamped in two places and cut with sterile, blunt tipped scissors. The condition occurs in more than 25% of deliveries, more often with long cords than with short ones.

nuchal ligament, a large midline posterior ligament in the neck from the base of the skull to the seventh cervical vertebra.

nuchal rigidity, a resistance to flexion of the neck, a condition seen in patients with meningitis.

nuchocephalic reflex /noo'kəsefal'ik/, a test for diffuse cerebral dysfunction, such as in senility. When the shoulders are turned to the left or the right, the head fails to turn in the same direction within 1/2 second.

Nuck's canal, Nuck's diverticulum. See **processus vaginalis peritonei.**

nucle-. See **nucleo-.**

-nuclear, a combining form meaning 'of or referring to the nucleus': *circumnuclear, endonuclear, multinuclear.*

nuclear agenesis. See **Möbius' syndrome.**

nuclear family /n(y)oo'kle·ər/ [L, *nucleus,* nut kernal; *familia,* household], a family unit consisting of the biologic parents and their offspring. The nuclear family is a relatively recent product of Western society. Dissolution of a marriage results in dissolution of the nuclear family. The nuclear family unit is less efficient than an extended family unit in providing information and vital services to family members, as in child rearing, child care, and care of older family members. Because it is most often the kind of family from which doctors, nurses, social workers, teachers, and other professional people come, it is not surprising that the nuclear family is often regarded as the norm for family style. Allowances must be made for bias in a professional's attitude toward other kinds of family units that may answer the needs and expectations of other groups of people. Compare **extended family, matrifocal family.**

nuclear fission. See **fission.**

nuclear hyaloplasm. See **karyolymph.**

nuclear isomer, one of two or more nuclides with the same number of neutrons and protons in the nucleus (the same atomic number, or Z, and the same atomic mass, or A) but existing in different energy states.

nuclear magnetic resonance. See **magnetic resonance (MR).**

nuclear medicine, a medical discipline that uses radioactive isotopes in the diagnosis and treatment of disease. The major fields of nuclear medicine are physiologic function studies, radionuclide imaging, and therapeutic techniques.

nuclear medicine technologist, an allied health professional who specializes in the nuclear properties of radioactive and stable nuclides to make diagnostic evaluations of the anatomic or physiologic conditions of the body and to provide therapy with unsealed radioactive sources. Responsibilities include application of a special knowledge of radiation physics and safety regulations to limit radiation exposure; preparation and administration of radiopharmaceuticals; use of radiation detection devices and other kinds of laboratory equipment that measure the quantity and distribution of radionuclides deposited in a patient specimen; and performance of in-vivo and in-vitro diagnostic procedures.

nuclear problem, (in psychology) an underlying reason for an individual's reaction to a precipitating event.

nuclear sap. See **karyolymph.**

nuclear scanning, a diagnostic technique that employs an injected or ingested radioactive material and a scanning device for determining the size, shape, location, and function of various body parts. Also called **radionuclide organ imaging.**

nuclear spin, an intrinsic form of angular momentum possessed by atomic nuclei containing an odd number of nucleons (protons or neutrons).

nucleic acid /nookle'ik/ [L, *nucleus* + *acidus,* sour], a polymeric compound of high molecular weight composed of nucleotides, each consisting of a purine or pyrimidine base, a ribose or deoxyribose sugar, and a phosphate group. Nucleic acids are involved in energy storage and release and in the determination and transmission of genetic characteristics. Kinds of nucleic acid are **deoxyribonucleic acid** and **ribonucleic acid.** See also **nucleotide.**

nucleo- /n(y)oo'kle·ō-/, **nucle-,** a combining form meaning 'of or related to a nucleus': *nucleochylema, nucleokeratin, nucleolus.*

nucleocapsid /noo'kle·ōkap'sid/ [L, *nucleus* + *capsa,* box], a viral enclosure consisting of a capsid or protein coat that encloses nucleic acid. Some viruses consist solely of bare nucleocapsids; others have more complex enclosures.

nucleochylema /noo'kle·ō'kəlī'mə/ [L, *nucleus* + Gk, *chylos,* juice, *haima,* blood], the ground substance of the nucleus, as distinguished from that of the cytoplasm.

nucleochyme. See **karyolymph.**

nucleocytoplasmic /noo'kle·ōsī'tōplas'mik/ [L, *nucleus* + Gk, *kytos,* cell, *plasma,* something formed], of or relating to the nucleus and cytoplasm of a cell.

nucleocytoplasmic ratio, the ratio of the volume of a nucleus of a cell to the volume of the cytoplasm. The proportion is usually constant for a specific cell type, and an increase is indicative of malignant neoplasms. Also called **karyoplasmic ratio, nucleoplasmic ratio.**

nucleohistone /noo'kle·ōhis'tōn/ [L, *nucleus* + Gk, *histos,* tissue], a complex nucleoprotein that consists of deoxyribonucleic acid and a histone. It is the basic constituent of the chromatin in the cell nucleus.

nucleolar organizer /nookle'ələr/ [L, *nucleolus,* little nut kernel; Gk, *organon,* instrument, *izein,* to cause], a part of the nucleus of the cell, thought to consist of heterochromatin, that is responsible for the formation of the nucleolus. Also called **nucleolar zone, nucleolus organizer.**

nucleolus /nookle'ələs/, *pl.* **nucleoli** [L, little nut kernel], any one of the small, dense structures composed largely of ribonucleic acid and situated within the cytoplasm of cells. Nucleoli are essential in the formation of ribosomes that synthesize cell proteins.

nucleon /n(y)oo'kle·on/, a collective term applied to protons and neutrons within the nucleus.

nucleophilic /-fil'ik/, pertaining to some molecules, particularly nucleic acids and proteins, having electrons that can be shared and thus form bonds with alkylating agents.

nucleoplasm /nōo′klē·əplaz′əm/ [L, *nucleus* + Gk, *plasma*, something formed], the protoplasm of the nucleus as contrasted with that of the cell. Also called **karyoplasm.** Compare **cytoplasm.** **–nucleoplasmic,** *adj.*

nucleoplasmic ratio. See **nucleocytoplasmic ratio.**

nucleoprotein /-prō′tēn/ [L, *nucleus*, nut; Gk, *proteios*, first rank], a molecule in which protein is combined with nucleic acid in a cell nucleus.

nucleoside monophosphate kinase /nōo′klē·əsīd′/, a liver enzyme that catalyzes the transfer of a phosphate group from adenosine triphosphate, producing adenosine diphosphate and a nucleoside diphosphate.

nucleosome /nōo′klē·əsōm/ [L, *nucleus* + Gk, *soma*, body], any one of the repeating nucleoprotein units consisting of histones forming a complex with deoxyribonucleic acid that appear as the beadlike structures at distinct intervals along the chromosome.

5-nucleotidase /nōo′klē·ot′idās/, a nonlipid enzyme, elevated in some liver disorders and cancer of the pancreas. It is measured in the blood to distinguish between certain liver and bone diseases. The normal accumulations in serum are 0.1 to 6 units.

nucleotide /nōo′klē·ətīd′/, any one of the compounds into which nucleic acid is split by the action of nuclease. A nucleotide consists of a phosphate group, a pentose sugar, and a nitrogenous base. Chains of such structures form deoxyribonucleic acid molecules essential for life.

nucleus /n(y)ōo′klē·əs/ [L, nut kernel], **1.** the central controlling body within a living cell, usually a spheric unit enclosed in a membrane and containing genetic codes for maintaining life systems of the organism and for issuing commands for growth and reproduction. **2.** a group of nerve cells of the central nervous system having a common function, such as supporting the sense of hearing or smell. **3.** the center of an atom about which electrons rotate. **4.** the central element in an organic chemical compound or class of compounds. **–nuclear,** *adj.*

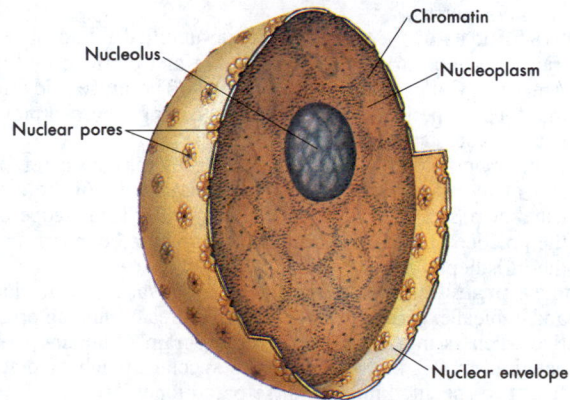

Nucleolus

Nuclear pores

Chromatin

Nucleoplasm

Nuclear envelope

Nucleus (*Thibodeau, 1993/William Ober*)

nucleus pulposus, the central portion of each intervertebral disk, consisting of a pulpy elastic substance that loses some of its resiliency with age. The nucleus pulposus may be suddenly compressed and squeeze out through the annu-

lar fibrocartilage, causing a herniated disk and extreme pain.

nuclide /nōo′klīd/ [L, *nucleus*, nut kernel], a species of atom characterized by the constitution of its nucleus, in particular by the number of protons and neutrons. Thus, Co-59 and Co-60 are both isotopes of cobalt and are each nuclides. Co-60 is a radionuclide because it undergoes radioactive decay.

nudge control, a prosthetic device with a mechanical unit that can be pressed by the chin to lock or unlock one or more joints of the apparatus.

NUG, abbreviation for **necrotizing ulcerative gingivitis.**

Nuhn's gland /noonz/ [Anton Nuhn, German anatomist, b. 1814], an anterior lingual gland in tissues on the inferior surface and near the apex and midline of the tongue.

null cell [L, *nullus*, not one, *cella*, storeroom], a lymphocyte that develops in the bone marrow and lacks the characteristic surface markers of the B and T lymphocytes. Null cells represent a small proportion of the lymphocyte population. Stimulated by the presence of antibody, null cells can attack certain cellular targets directly and are known as "natural killer," or NK cells. Compare **B cell, T cell.** See also **cytotoxin, immune gamma globulin.**

null hypothesis (H_0), (in research) a hypothesis that predicts that no difference or relationship exists among the variables studied that could not have occurred by chance alone.

nulli-, a prefix meaning 'none': nullipara, nulligravida.

nulligravida /nul′igrav′ədə/ a woman who has never been pregnant.

nullipara /nulip′ərə/, *pl.* **nulliparae** [L, *nullus*, not one, *parere*, to bear], a woman who has not been delivered of a viable infant. The designation "para 0" indicates nulliparity. Compare **multipara, primipara.**

nulliparity /nul′iper′itē/ [L, *nullus*, none; *parere*, to bear], the status of a woman who has never borne a child.

nulliparous /nulip′ərəs/ [L, *nullus*, none; *parere*, to bear], never having given birth.

num, abbreviation for *number.*

numbness /num′nəs/ [ME, *nomen*, loss of feeling], a partial or total lack of sensation in a part of the body, resulting from any factor that interrupts the transmission of impulses from the sensory nerve fibers. Numbness is often accompanied by tingling.

nummular dermatitis /num′yələr/ [L, *nummuli* petty cash; Gk, *derma*, skin, *itis*, inflammation], a skin disease characterized by coin-shaped, vesicular, or scaling eczema-like lesions on the forearms and the front of the calves. The cause is unknown.

Numorphan Hydrochloride, a trademark for a narcotic analgesic (oxymorphone hydrochloride).

Nupercainal, a trademark for a local anesthetic (dibucaine hydrochloride).

Nuremberg tribunal [Nuremberg, Germany; L, *tribunus*, platform for administration of justice], an international tribunal planned and implemented by the United Nations War Crimes Commission to detect, apprehend, try, and punish people accused of war crimes, establishing the **Nuremberg code.** In preparation for the prosecution of World War II criminals, the War Department of the United States assigned Andrew Ivy, M.D., to devise a set of principles to govern the participation of human beings in medical research. The principle and practice of informed consent was reinforced by the precedent set in the trials in which Nazi physicians were declared guilty of crimes against humanity in performing experiments on human beings who were not volunteers and did not consent. See also **Helsinki accords.**

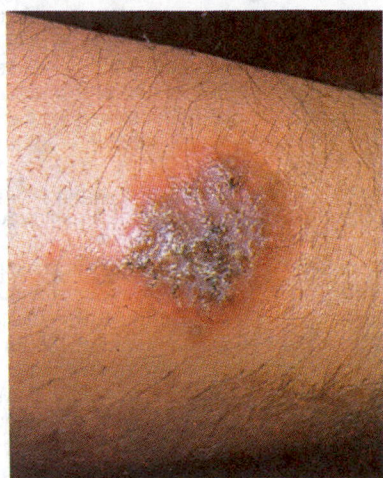

Nummular dermatitis (Cerio, 1992)

nurse [Ofr, *nurice*, from Late L, *nutricia*, from L, *nutrix*], **1.** a person educated and licensed in the practice of nursing; one who is concerned with 'the diagnosis and treatment of human responses to actual or potential health problems' (American Nurses' Association). The practice of the nurse includes data collection, diagnosis, planning, treatment, and evaluation within the framework of the nurse's singular concern with the patient's response to the problem, rather than to the problem itself. The concerns of the nurse are thus broader and less discrete and circumscribed than the traditional concerns of medicine. In a cooperative participatory relationship with the client or patient, the nurse acts to promote, maintain, or restore the health of the person; wellness is the goal. A collegial collaborative relationship with other health professionals who share a mission and a common data base furthers the practice of nursing. Guided by humanitarian, ethical principles, the nurse practices in a personal, nurturing, and protective manner that promotes health in all ways. The nurse may be a generalist or a specialist and, as a professional, is ethically and legally accountable for the nursing activities performed and for the actions of others to whom the nurse has delegated responsibility. **2.** to provide nursing care. See also **five-step nursing process, nursing, registered nurse.**

nurse anesthetist, a registered nurse qualified by advanced training in an accredited program in the speciality of nurse anesthesia to manage the care of the patient during the administration of anesthesia in selected surgical situations.

nurse-client interaction, any process in which a nurse and a client exchange or share information, verbally or nonverbally. It is fundamental to communication and is an essential component of the nursing assessment.

nurse-client relationship, a therapeutic relationship between a nurse and a client built on a series of interactions and developing over time. All interactions do not develop into relationships but may nonetheless be therapeutic. The relationship differs from a social relationship in that it is designed to meet the needs only of the client. Its structure varies with the context, the client's needs, and the goals of the nurse and the client. Its nature varies with the context, including the setting, the kind of nursing, and the needs of the client. The relationship is dynamic and uses cognitive and affective levels of interaction. It is time-limited and goal-oriented and has three phases. During the first phase, the phase of establishment, the nurse establishes the structure, purpose, timing, and context of the relationship and expresses an interest in discussing this initial structure with the client. Data collection for the nursing care plan continues, and basic goals for the relationship are stated. During the middle, developmental, phase of the relationship, the nurse and the client get to know each other better and test the structure of the relationship to be able to trust one another. The nurse is careful to assess correctly the degree of dependency that is necessary for the particular client. Plans may be devised for improved ways of coping with problems and achieving goals. The nurse is alert to the danger of losing objectivity during this phase. The last phase, termination, ideally occurs when the goals of the relationship have been accomplished, when both the client and the nurse feel a sense of resolution and satisfaction. Often this is not possible because the nurse is transferred or the client discharged; in either case both may be left with a feeling of frustration.

nurse clinician, a nurse who is prepared to identify and diagnose problems of clients by using increased knowledge and skills gained through advanced study in a specific area of nursing practice. The specialist may function independently within standing orders or protocols and collaborates with associates to implement a plan of care that is focused on the client.

nurse coordinator, a registered nurse who coordinates and manages the activities of nursing personnel engaged in specific nursing services, such as obstetrics or surgery, for two or more patient care units.

Nurse Corps, the branch within each of the armed services comprising the nurses within that service, such as the Army Nurse Corps. In each of the armed services, the members of the Nurse Corps have the rank, title, responsibilities, and status of commissioned officer.

nurse educator, a registered nurse whose primary area of interest, competence, and professional practice is the education of nurses.

nurse midwife, a registered nurse qualified by advanced training in obstetric and neonatal care and certified by the American College of Nurse Midwives. The nurse midwife manages the perinatal care of women having a normal pregnancy, labor, and childbirth.

nurse practice act, a statute enacted by the legislature of any of the states or by the appropriate officers of the districts or possessions. The act delineates the legal scope of the practice of nursing within the geographic boundaries of the jurisdiction.

nurse practitioner, a nurse who by advanced education and clinical experience in a specialized area of nursing practice, such as in a master's degree program in nursing, has acquired expert knowledge in the special branch of practice. See specific kinds of nurse practitioner.

nursery diarrhea /nur′sərē/ [L, *nutrix*, nurse; Gk, *dia*, through, *rhein*, to flow], diarrhea of the newborn. In nurseries, outbreaks of diarrhea caused by *Escherichia coli, Salmonella,* echoviruses, or adenoviruses are potentially life-threatening to the infant. The neonate may be infected at the time of birth by organisms from the mother's stool or infected later by organisms spread by the hands of hospital personnel. Fluid loss is the most serious aspect of the disease, leading to dehydration and electrolyte imbalance. Care includes maintaining fluid and electrolyte balance and administration of antibiotics, if appropriate. Good handwashing technique, use of disposable nursing bottles and nipples, and early isolation of infected infants reduce the possibility of such outbreaks.

nurse's aide, a person who is employed to carry out basic nonspecialized tasks in the care of a patient, such as bathing and feeding, making beds, and transporting patients, under the supervision and direction of a registered nurse. Many hospitals offer education and orientation programs for newly hired nurse's aides and in-service education for continued training.

Nurses' Association of the American College of Obstetrics and Gynecology (NAACOG), a national organization of nurses who work in obstetrics and gynecology. It functions in close association with the American College of Obstetrics and Gynecology.

Nurses' Coalition for Action in Politics (N-CAP), an organization that works in association with the American Nurses' Association. It raises funds for political contributions to candidates for public office at the state and national levels.

nurses' observation scale for inpatient evaluation (NOSIE), a systematic, objective behavioral rating scale that is applied by nurses to patient behavior.

nurses' registry, an employment agency or listing service for nurses who wish to work in a specific area of nursing, usually for a short period of time or on a per diem basis.

nurses' station, an area in a clinic, unit, or ward in a health care facility that serves as the administrative center for nursing care for a particular group of patients. It is usually centrally located and may be staffed by a ward secretary or clerk who assists with paperwork, telephone, and other communication. Before going on duty, nurses usually meet there to receive daily assignments, to review the patients' charts, and to update the files. In a critical care unit of a large teaching hospital, the nurses' station may also contain panels of visual display terminals that allow centralized monitoring of many patients and may also have computer terminals that allow access to information in the patients' records or to a data bank of clinical information. In other parts of a hospital, the nurses' station is equipped in any of various ways appropriate to the care of the patients in that area or unit.

nursing, 1. the practice in which a nurse assists "the individual, sick or well, in the performance of those activities contributing to health or its recovery (or to a peaceful death) that he would perform unaided if he had the necessary strength, will or knowledge. And to do this in such a way as to help him gain independence as rapidly as possible." (Virginia Henderson) 2. "the diagnosis and treatment of human responses to actual or potential health problems," (American Nurses' Association). There are four principal characteristics that further define nursing care: the phenomena that concern nurses; the use of theories to observe the need for nursing intervention and to plan nursing action; the nursing action taken; and an evaluation of the effects of the actions relative to the phenomena. This definition of nursing provides a framework for the nursing process including data collection, diagnosis, planning, treatment, and evaluation. The nursing process is supported by standards of nursing practice that are congruent with the definition and that

provide more specific guidelines for practice. These standards include systematic, continuous collection of data concerning the health status of the client in recorded form that is accessible and that may be communicated. A nursing diagnosis is derived from the data collected. A plan for nursing care incorporates goals derived from the nursing diagnosis and the priorities and approaches to achieve the goals as indicated by the nursing diagnosis. Nursing actions, which are selected and performed with the client's participation, provide for promotion, maintenance, or restoration of the health of the client and serve to maximize the health care abilities of the client. The progress or lack of progress toward the goal is mutually determined by the client and the nurse, resulting in reassessment, reordering of priorities, establishment of new goals, and revision of the plan for nursing care. Nursing touches on, intersects with, and complements other professional roles in health care, addressing itself to a wide range of health-related responses in people who are well and in those who are not. Nursing seeks to diagnose and treat the response to the problem; thus the concerns of nursing are less circumscribed and discrete than those of other health-related professions. These concerns include the following: limitations of the client's self-care ability; impaired ability to function in any fundamental area, such as sleeping, breathing, eating, maintaining circulation, pain; anxiety, fear, loneliness, grief, or other physical or emotional problems related to health, illness, or treatment; impaired social or intellectual processes; impaired ability to make decisions and choices; alteration of self-image as required by the change in health; dysfunctional perception of health or health care activities; extra demands posed by such normal life-processes as birth, growth, or death; and difficulty in affiliative relationships. Various concepts, principles, processes, and actions, developed and examined in nursing research, guide the steps in the nursing process, from initial observation and diagnosis through evaluation based on intrapersonal, interpersonal, and systems theories. The boundary for nursing practice is not static: It tends to move outward as the needs and capacities of society change. Collegial, collaborative practice with other health care professions further softens the boundaries of nursing practice. All health care professionals share a mission and a scientific data base, and to some degree their practices overlap. At its core, nursing is nurturative, generative, and protective; preventive care is a part of every nurse's practice. Nurses value independence and self-respect; they are guided by an ethical and humanitarian philosophy in which every human being deserves respect regardless of racial, social, cultural, sexual, economic, religious, or other factors. The nurse practices in the context of a relationship with the client, family, or group that is professional and yet close, in an interpersonal sense. The function of a nurse involves the physical intimacy of laying-on of hands; compassion and constant recognition of the person's dignity are essential. Nursing is practiced by specialists and by generalists; generalists provide most nursing care; specialists, having added to their knowledge of an organized and systematized body of knowledge and competencies, practice in specialized areas of nursing. Nursing care is given to people at all stages of life, in the home, hospital, place of employment, school, or other environment where nursing care is needed. Nurses are ethically and legally accountable for their practice and for delegation of responsibilities to others. 3. the professional practice of a nurse. 4. the process of acting as a nurse, of providing care that encourages and promotes the health of the person being served. See also **nursing process.**

nursing assessment, an identification by a nurse of the needs, preferences, and abilities of a patient. Assessment follows an interview with and observation of a patient by the nurse and considers the symptoms and signs of the condition, the patient's verbal and nonverbal communication, medical and social history, and any other information available. Among the physical aspects assessed are vital signs, skin color and condition, motor and sensory nerve function, nutrition, rest, sleep, activity, elimination, and consciousness. Among the social and emotional factors included in assessment are religion, occupation, attitude toward hospital and health care, mood, emotional tone, and family ties and responsibilities. Assessment is extremely important because it provides the scientific basis for a complete nursing care plan.

nursing assistant, *Canada.* a person trained in basic nursing techniques and direct patient care who practices under the supervision of a registered nurse. Also called **certified nursing assistant.**

nursing audit, a thorough investigation designed to identify, examine, or verify the performance of certain specified aspects of nursing care using established criteria. A **concurrent nursing audit** is performed during ongoing nursing care. A **retrospective nursing audit** is performed after discharge from the care facility, using the patient's record. Often, a nursing audit and a medical audit are performed collaboratively, resulting in a **joint audit.**

nursing bottle caries. See **baby bottle tooth decay**.

nursing care plan, a plan that is based on a nursing assessment and a nursing diagnosis, carried out by a nurse. It has four essential components: identification of the nursing care problems and statement of the nursing approach to solve those problems; statement of the expected benefit to the patient; statement of the specific actions by the nurse that reflect the nursing approach and achieve the goals specified; and evaluation of the patient's response to nursing care and readjustment of that care as required. The nursing care plan is begun when the patient is admitted to the health service, and, after the initial nursing assessment, a diagnosis is formulated and nursing orders are developed. The goal of the process is to ensure that nursing care is consistent with the patient's needs and progress toward self-care. A written nursing care plan should be a part of every patient's chart; an abbreviated form should be available for quick reference, such as in a Rand or Kardex file. See also **diagnosis, nursing assessment, nursing diagnosis, nursing orders, problem-solving approach to patient-centered care.**

nursing diagnosis, a statement of a health problem or of a potential problem in the client's health status that a nurse is licensed and competent to treat. Four steps are required in the formulation of a nursing diagnosis: A data base is established by collecting information from all available sources, including interviews with the client and the client's family, a review of any existing records of the client's health, observation of the response of the client to any alterations in health status, a physical assessment, and a conference or consultation with others concerned in the care of the client. The data base is continually updated. The second step includes analysis of the client's responses to the problems, healthy or unhealthy, and classification of those responses as psychologic, physiologic, spiritual, or socio-

logic. The third step is the organization of the data so that a tentative diagnostic statement can be made that summarizes the pattern of problems discovered. The last step is confirmation of the sufficiency and accuracy of the data base by evaluation of the appropriateness of the diagnosis to nursing intervention and by the assurance that, given the same information, most other qualified practitioners would arrive at the same nursing diagnosis. In use, each diagnostic category has three parts: the term that concisely describes the problem, the probable cause of the problem, and the defining characteristics of the problem. A number of nursing diagnoses have been identified and are listed as accepted by the North American Nursing Diagnosis Association (NANDA), and are updated and refined at periodic meetings of the group. The nursing diagnoses currently accepted by NANDA are listed in Appendix 19.

nursing differential, an allowance added to payments to hospitals for services rendered Medicaid patients in recognition of the cost of providing nursing services to such patients that is greater than the cost to the general patient population.

nursing ethics [L, *nutrix*, nurse; Gk, *ethikos*, character], the values or moral principles governing relationships between the nurse and patient, the patient's family, other members of the health professions, and the general public.

nursing goal, a general goal of nursing involving activities that are desirable but difficult to measure, such as self-care, good nutrition, and relaxation. Compare **nursing objective.**

nursing health history, data collected about a patient's level of wellness, changes in life patterns, sociocultural role, and mental and emotional reactions to illness.

nursing home. See **extended care facility.**

nursing intervention, any act by a nurse that implements the nursing care plan or any specific objective of that plan, such as turning a comatose patient to avoid the development of decubitus ulcers or teaching injection technique to a patient with diabetes before discharge from the hospital. The patient may require intervention in the form of support, limitation, medication, or treatment for the current condition or to prevent the development of further stress. As stress increases, the need to adapt and the need for nursing intervention increase. See also **adaptation, stress.**

nursing intervention model, (in nursing research) a conceptual framework used to determine appropriate nursing interventions. The model is a holistic representation of the client and the health care system. The client's physiologic, psychologic, sociocultural, and developmental status, the client's stressors and ability to react to them, and the levels and patterns of available health care are observed. The goal is to learn what nursing interventions would be most effective for the particular problem within the particular health care system.

nursing objective, a specific aim planned by a nurse to decrease a person's stress, or improve the ability to adapt, or both. A nursing objective may be physical, emotional, social, or cultural and may involve the person's family, friends, and other patients. It is the purpose of any specific nursing order or nursing intervention. Some common nursing objectives are adequate understanding by the patient of certain details of the condition, adequate and comfortable daily elimination, a certain amount of rest, a balanced diet, and participation in specific items of self-care. Compare **nursing goal.**

nursing observation, an objective, holistic evaluation

made by a nurse of the various aspects of a client's condition. It includes the person's general appearance, emotional affect, and nutritional status, habits, and preferences, as well as body temperature, skin condition, and any obvious abnormal processes, including those of which the client complains. The client's religious preference, ethnic background, and familial relationships are also noted. Compare **nursing assessment, nursing intervention.**

nursing orders, specific instructions for implementing the nursing care plan, including the patient's preferences, timing of activities, details of health education necessary for the particular patient, role of the family, and plans for care after discharge. Nursing orders must be signed by the professional nurse who writes them. They should not duplicate the orders of the medical staff or of other members of the health team.

nursing process, the process that serves as an organizational framework for the practice of nursing. It encompasses all of the steps taken by the nurse in caring for a patient: assessment, nursing diagnosis, planning, implementation, and evaluation. The rationale for each step is founded in nursing theory. The process requires a systematic approach to a nursing assessment of the person's situation, including an evaluation and reconciliation of the perceptions by the person, the person's family, and the nurse. A plan for the nursing actions to be taken may then be made, and, with the participation of the person and the person's family, the plan may be set. The plan developed with the person and the person's family is then implemented. The outcome is evaluated with the person and the person's family. The steps follow each other at the start of the process but may need to be taken concurrently in some situations. The process does not reach completion with evaluation; the steps are begun again, allowing recurrent evaluation of the assessment, plan, goals, and actions. See also **five-step nursing process, nursing.**

nursing process model, a conceptual framework in which the nurse-patient relationship is the basis of the nursing process. The nursing process is represented as dynamic and interpersonal, the nurse and the patient being affected by each other's behavior and by the environment around them. Each successful two-way communication is termed a "transaction" and can be analyzed to discover the factors that promote transactions. The constraints that the various systems in the environment (personal, interpersonal, and social) place on the development of the relationship are also examined. The nurse views the patient as a person with whom to communicate to have transactions that achieve defined adaptive objectives toward the goal of health.

nursing research, a detailed process in which a systematic study of a problem in the field of nursing is performed. One basic approach requires the following steps: identification of the problem; review of the literature; selection of a theoretical framework; statement of a hypothesis or hypotheses; definition of variables; determination of a method for weighting and counting variables; selection of a research design; choice of a population; plan for the analysis of the data; determination of interpretation; and plan for promulgation of the results. Nursing research is practice- or discipline-oriented and is essential for the continued development of the scientific base of professional nursing practice.

Nursing Research, a bimonthly refereed journal containing papers and other materials concerning nursing research. The goal of the journal is to stimulate research in nursing and disseminate research findings.

nursing rounds, chart rounds, walking rounds, teaching rounds, or grand rounds that are held specifically for nurses and that focus on nursing care problems. See also **rounds.**

nursing specialty, a nurse's selected professional field of practice, such as surgical, pediatric, obstetric, or psychiatric nursing. Compare **subspecialty.**

nursing supervisor, a nurse whose function is the administrative and clinical leadership of the nursing service of a division of a health care facility, such as a nursing supervisor of maternal and infant care nurses.

nursing theorist, a perosn who develops integrated concepts or frameworks of nursing roles, functions, objectives, and activities and their relationships to clients and the roles of other health professionals.

nursing theory, an organized framework of concepts and purposes designed to guide the practice of nursing.

nursology /nursol′əjē/ [L, *nutrix*, nurse; Gk, *logos*, science], a conceptual framework for the study and practice of nursing. It requires the nurse to interact with the patient in an 'authentic' way, without aloofness and the distance of professionalism; the nurse must take the risk of caring. The patient as a person is perceived as a 'subject' rather than an 'object'; the relationship is described as 'intersubjective,' and the parties to the relationship as 'nurse-nursed.' As a method, nursology requires that the nurse cut through the defenses and fears that prevent self-knowledge. The nurse tries to know the patient on an intuitive, subjective level and then, using reflection, on an objective, scientific level. The nurse recognizes that each person has an 'angular view' of the whole truth; comparison of the views of others is necessary for a perspective that allows a synthesis, often paradoxical but closer to the truth than any one person's angular view. The nurse must then struggle with the multiple views to arrive at a final synthesis. This process is called a progression from 'we to paradoxical one.' Nursology is intended to provide a model for nursing methods and for research. The nurse and the patient have the opportunity to grow, and the science of nursing may emerge from the 'angular' investigations and syntheses.

Nursoy, a trademark for a hypoallergenic nutritional supplement for infants.

nurture /nur′chər/, to feed, rear, foster, or care for, such as in the nourishment, care, and training of growing children.

nutation /nōōtā′shən/ [L, *nutare*, to nod], the act of nodding, especially involuntary nodding as occurs in some neurologic disorders.

nutcracker esophagus. See **symptomatic esophageal peristalsis.**

Nutramigen, a trademark for a milk-substitute formula that is prepared from a soy isolate base and is lactose free, prescribed for infants with galactosemia and as a protein supplement for people with lactose intolerance.

nutri-, a prefix meaning 'of or related to nourishment': *nutriceptor, nutrient, nutritorium.*

nutrient /nōō′trē·ənt/ [L, *nutriens*, nourishing], a substance that provides nourishment and affects the nutritive and metabolic processes of the body.

nutrient artery of the humerus, one of a pair of branches of the deep brachial arteries, arising near the middle of the arm and entering the nutrient canal of the humerus.

nutrient canal. See **interdental canal.**

nutrient enema [L, *nutriens*; Gk, *enienai*, injection], the introduction of saline or glucose into the body via the rectum. See also **artificial alimentation.**

nutriment /nōō'trimənt/ [L *nutriens* food that nourishes], any substance that nourishes and aids the growth and the development of the body. See also **food.**

nutrition /n(y)ōōtrish'ən/ [L *nutriens*], **1.** nourishment. **2.** the sum of the processes involved in the taking in of nutrients and in their assimilation and use for proper body functioning and maintenance of health. The successive stages include ingestion, digestion, absorption, assimilation, and excretion. **3.** the study of food and drink as related to the growth and maintenance of living organisms.

nutritional /n(y)ōōtrish'ənəl/ [L, *nutrire*, to nourish], pertaining to the quality of food or eating behavior that provides nourishment through assimilation of food to tissues.

nutritional alcoholic cerebellar degeneration. See **alcoholic nutritional cerebellar degeneration.**

nutritional anemia [L, *nutrire*, to nourish; Gk, *a, haima*, without blood], a disorder characterized by the inadequate production of hemoglobin or erythrocytes caused by a nutritional deficiency of iron, folic acid, or vitamin B_{12}, or other nutritional disorders. See also **iron deficiency anemia, megaloblastic anemia, pernicious anemia.**

nutritional care, the substances, procedures, and setting involved in assuring the proper intake and assimilation of nutriments, especially for the hospitalized patient.

■ METHOD: Depending on the patient's condition, nutritional requirements may be provided by regular meals with menus selected from the ordered diet, by tube feeding, or by parenteral hyperalimentation. Meals are served on attractive trays in an environment conducive to eating; distasteful procedures are avoided before and after mealtime. Patients who are unable to feed themselves are assisted, and abnormal intake of food is recorded and reported. Supplemental nourishment when indicated and fluids are offered between meals. The nutritional assessment includes observations of the patient's appetite, food preferences, allergies, height, intake and output, weight, measurements of the head, arms, abdomen, and skinfold thickness, the skin color and turgor, and the condition of the mouth, eyes, and hair. Any cutaneous lesions, thyroid enlargement, dental caries, loose teeth, ill-fitting dentures, gum problems, nausea, vomiting, dehydration, diarrhea, or constipation are noted.

■ INTERVENTIONS: The nurse sees that food is presented attractively, offers a washcloth and mouthwash before and after meals, and, when necessary, feeds the patient to maintain an adequate intake. If indicated, such as in obese patients or those with disorders requiring a highly restricted diet, the nurse restricts the intake of food as ordered. Tube feedings are administered as ordered.

■ OUTCOME CRITERIA: Obvious good health, a normal weight, and the absence of GI symptoms usually indicate that the individual's nutritional requirements are being fulfilled.

nutrition, altered: less than body requirements, a nursing diagnosis accepted by the Fourth National Conference on Nursing Diagnoses. It is defined as a state in which an individual experiences an intake of nutrients insufficient to meet metabolic needs. The defining characteristics of the condition may include loss of weight, reported intake of less food than is recommended, evidence or report of a lack of food, lack of interest in food, aversion to eating, alteration in the taste of food, feelings of fullness immediately after eating small quantities, abdominal pain with no other explanation, sores in the mouth, diarrhea or steatorrhea, pallor, weakness, and loss of hair. A related factor is an inability, based on psychologic, biologic, or economic factors, to ingest or to digest food or to absorb nutrients in sufficient quantity for the maintenance of normal health. See also **nursing diagnosis.**

nutrition, altered: more than body requirements, a nursing diagnosis accepted by the Fourth National Conference on Nursing Diagnoses. It is defined as a state in which an individual is experiencing an intake of nutrients that exceeds metabolic needs. The critical defining characteristics, one of which must be present for the diagnosis to be made, include weight gain of 20% greater than the ideal for the height and body build of the client, and triceps skin fold measurement greater than 15 mm in men and 25 mm in women. Other defining characteristics include a sedentary activity level and dysfunctional eating habits, including eating in response to internal cues other than hunger. A related factor is an excessive intake of food in relation to the body's metabolic needs. See also **nursing diagnosis.**

nutrition, altered: high risk for more than body requirements, a nursing diagnosis accepted by the Fourth National Conference on Nursing Diagnoses. It is defined as a state in which an individual is at risk of experiencing an intake of nutrients that exceeds metabolic needs. Risk factors include hereditary predisposition; excessive energy intake during late gestational life, early infancy, and adolescence; frequent, closely spaced pregnancies; dysfunctional psychologic conditioning in relationship to food; membership in a lower socioeconomic group; reported or observed obesity in one or both parents; rapid transition across growth percentiles in infants or children; reported use of solid food as a major food source before 5 months of age; observed use of food as reward or comfort measure; reported or observed higher baseline weight at beginning of each pregnancy; and dysfunctional eating patterns, including pairing food with other activities, concentrating food intake at the end of the day, eating in response to external cues (e.g., time of day or social situation), and eating in response to internal cues other than hunger (e.g., anxiety). See also **nursing diagnosis.**

nutritionist /n(y)ōōtrish'ənist/ [L *nutrire* to nourish], one who studies and applies the principles and science of nutrition.

Nutting, Mary Adelaide (1858–1947), a Canadianborn American nursing educator and reformer. As head of Johns Hopkins School of Nursing in Baltimore, beginning in 1894, she improved course content and teaching facilities, instituted the 6-months preparatory course, reduced the 12-hour day to 8 hours, and abolished the monthly payment system to students. At Teachers College, Columbia University, she created and developed the Department of Nursing and Health and became the first professor of nursing in the world. With Lavinia Dock, she wrote *History of Nursing*, a classic in nursing literature.

nux vomica /nuks' vom'ikə/ [L, *nux*, nut; *vomere*, to vomit], the dried ripe seeds of a small Asian tree, *Strychnos nux-vomica*, a source of the alkaloids strychnine and brucine. The seeds are powdered and the strychnine content reduced to a little more than one percent by the addition of lactose for use as a bitter tonic and nerve stimulant.

nvm, abbreviation for *nonvolatile matter.*

NVMA, abbreviation for *National Veterinary Medical Association.*

nyctalopia /nik'təlō'pē·ə/ [Gk, *nyx*, night, *alaos*, obscure, *ops*, eye], poor vision at night or in dim light resulting from decreased synthesis of rhodopsin, vitamin A deficiency, retinal degeneration, or a congenital defect. Also called **day sight, night blindness.** **—nyctalopic,** *adj.*

nycto-, a combining form meaning 'pertaining to night or darkness': *nyctohemeral, nyctophilia, nyctophobia.*

nyctophobia /nik'tō-/ [Gk, *nyx* + *phobos*, fear], an anxiety reaction characterized by an obsessive, irrational fear of darkness.

nycturia. See **nocturia.**

nylidrin hydrochloride /nil'idrin/, a peripheral vasodilator.

■ INDICATIONS: It is prescribed in the treatment of peripheral vascular disease and circulatory disturbances of the inner ear.

■ CONTRAINDICATIONS: Acute cardiac disease, paroxysmal tachycardia, thyrotoxicosis, progressive angina pectoris, or known hypersensitivity to this drug prohibits its use.

■ ADVERSE EFFECTS: The most serious adverse reaction is hypotension with dizziness, tachycardia, nausea, and weakness.

nympho-, a combining form meaning 'of or pertaining to the labia minora': *nymphocaruncular, nymphohymeneal, nymphoncus.*

nymphomania /nim'fəmā'nē·ə/ [Gk, *nymphe*, maiden, *mania*, madness], a psychosexual disorder of women characterized by an insatiable desire for sexual satisfaction, often resulting from an unconscious conflict concerning personal adequacy. Compare **satyriasis.** See also **psychosexual disorder.**

nymphomaniac /-mā'nē·ak/, **1.** a person with or displaying characteristics of nymphomania. **2.** of, pertaining to, or exhibiting nymphomania. **—nymphomaniacal** /nim'fəmənī'əkəl/, *adj.*

nystagmus /nīstag'məs/ [Gk, *nystagmos*, nodding], involuntary, rhythmic movements of the eyes; the oscillations may be horizontal, vertical, rotary, or mixed. Jerking nystagmus, characterized by faster movements in one direction than in the opposite direction, is more common than pendular nystagmus, in which the oscillations are approximately equal in rate in both directions. Jerking nystagmus occurs normally when an individual watches a moving object, but, on other occasions, it may be a sign of barbiturate intoxication or of labyrinthine vestibular, vascular, or neurologic disease. Labyrinthine vestibular nystagmus, most frequently rotary, is usually accompanied by vertigo and nausea. Vertical nystagmus is considered pathognomonic of disease of the brainstem's tegmentum, and nystagmus occurring only in the abducting eye is said to be a sign of multiple sclerosis. Seesaw nystagmus, in which one eye moves up and the other down, may be seen in bilateral hemianopia. Pendular nystagmus occurs in albinism, various diseases of the retina and refractive media, and in miners, after many years of working in darkness; in miners, the eye movements are very rapid, increase on upward gaze, and are often associated with vertigo, head tremor, and photophobia. **Electronystagmography,** used in testing for vestibular disease and in evaluating patients with vertigo, hearing loss, or tinnitus, records changes in the electric field around the eyes. Nystagmus is measured as the person gazes at various objects and is placed in various positions, and when cold or warm water or air is introduced into the external auditory canal. This final test causes nystagmus of equal intensity in normal individuals. In patients with an inner ear or neural disorder, nystagmus may be more intense, diminished, or absent. Also called **nystaxis.** **—nystagmic,** *adj.*

nystatin /nis'tətin/, an antifungal antibiotic.

■ INDICATIONS: It is prescribed in the treatment of fungal infections of the GI tract, vagina, and skin.

■ CONTRAINDICATION: Known hypersensitivity to this drug is the only contraindication.

■ ADVERSE EFFECTS: There are no known serious adverse reactions. Mild GI distress and mild skin reactions may occur.

nystaxis. See **nystagmus.**

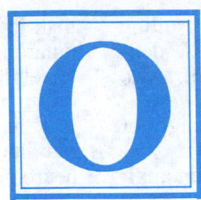

o, symbol for *ohm.*

O, symbol for the element **oxygen.**

O₂, symbol for *oxygen molecule.*

oario-. See **ovario-.**

OASDHI, abbreviation for **Old Age, Survivors, Disability and Health Insurance Program.**

oat cell carcinoma [AS, *ate*, oat; L, *cella*, storeroom; Gk, *karkinos*, crab, *oma*, tumor], a malignant, usually bronchogenic epithelial neoplasm consisting of small, tightly packed, round, oval, or spindle-shaped epithelial cells that stain darkly and contain neurosecretory granules and little or no cytoplasm. Tumors produced by these cells do not form bulky masses but usually spread along submucosal lymphatics. One third of all malignant tumors of the lung are of this type. Usually surgical resection is not possible, and chemotherapy and radiation therapy are not effective in treatment; thus the longterm prognosis is poor. Also called **small cell carcinoma.**

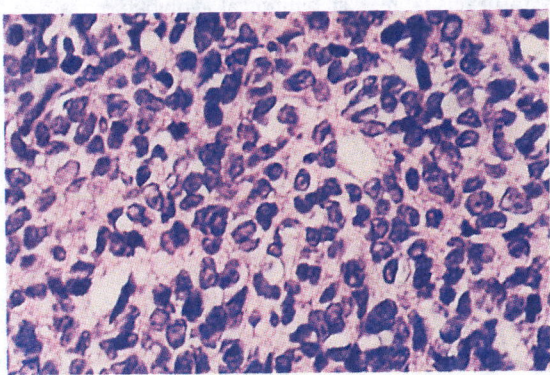

Oat cell carcinoma *(Skarin, 1991)*

OAWO, abbreviation for **opening abductory wedge osteotomy.**

ob., abreviation for the Latin word, *obit*, 'died.'

OB, *informal.* **1.** abbreviation for **obstetrician. 2.** abbreviation for **obstetrics.**

ob-, a prefix meaning 'against, in the way, oppose': *obdormition, obduction, obtuse.*

obduction /əbduk′shən/ [L, *obductio*, a covering], a forensic medical autopsy.

Ober and Barr procedure, a surgical method of treating weak biceps muscles by transfer of the brachioradialis.

Ober procedure, a method for treatment of paralyzed clubfeet by transfer of the posterior tibial tendon to the third cuneiform or metatarsal.

Ober test, an examination for tight tensor fascia lata. The patient lies on one side with the hip and knee flexed on the surface and the opposite hip extended while the knee is flexed. Inability to place the knee being tested on the table surface indicates a tight fascia lata.

obese /ōbēs′/ [L, *obesus*, swollen], pertaining to a corpulent or excessively heavy individual. Generally, a person is regarded as medically obese if the body weight is 20% above desirable body weight for the person's age, sex, height, and body build. Because the 'average' human body is approximately 25% fat, the proportion may be doubled for a medically defined obese person.

obesity /ōbē′sitē/ [L, *obesitas*, fatness], an abnormal increase in the proportion of fat cells, mainly in the viscera and subcutaneous tissues of the body. Obesity may be exogenous or endogenous. **Hyperplastic obesity** is caused by an increase in the number of fat cells in the increased adipose tissue mass. **Hypertrophic obesity** results from an increase in the size of the fat cells in the increased adipose tissue mass.

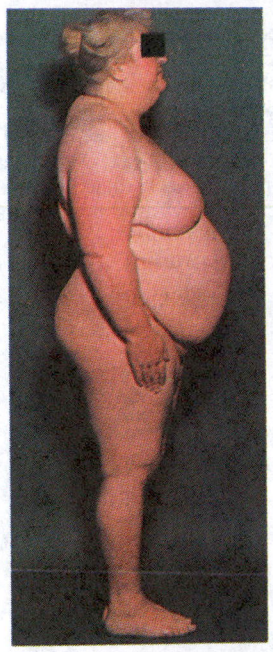

Obesity
(Forbes, 1993)

Obetrol, a trademark for a fixed-combination drug containing central nervous system stimulants (dextroamphetamine and amphetamine).

obfuscation /ob′fəskā′shən/ [L, *obfuscare*, to darken], the act of making something confused, clouded, or obscure.

OBG, abbreviation for *obstetrics and gynecology*.

OB-Gyn, *informal.* abbreviation for *obstetrics and gynecology*.

object /ob'jəkt/, (in psychology) something through which an instinct can achieve its goal. In psychoanalytic terms, a person other than self.

objective /əbjek'tiv/ [L, *objectare*, to set against], **1.** a goal. **2.** of or pertaining to a phenomenon or clinical finding that is observed; not subjective. An objective finding is often described in health care as a sign, as distinguished from a symptom, which is a subjective finding.

objective data collection, the process in which data relating to the client's problem are obtained by an observer through direct physical examination, including observation, palpation, and auscultation, and by laboratory analyses and radiologic and other studies. Compare **subjective data collection.**

objective lens, (in radiology) a lens that accepts light from the output phosphor of an image-intensifier tube and converts it into a parallel beam for recording the image on film.

objective sign [L, *objectum*, something cast before; *signum*, sign], a clinical observation that can be seen, heard, measured, or otherwise recorded by an examining physician or other health care provider.

objective symptom [L, *objectum*, something cast before; Gk, *symptoma*, that which happens], a symptom that is accompanied by signs that tend to confirm the patient's physical complaint and enables the examining physician to deduce the cause.

object permanence, a capacity to perceive that something exists even when it is not seen.

object relations, emotional bonds between one person and another, as contrasted with interest in and love for the self. It is usually described in terms of capacity for loving and reacting appropriately to others.

obligate /ob'ligit, -gāt/ [L, *obligare*, to bind], characterized by the ability to survive only in a particular set of environmental conditions, such as an obligate parasite, which

can survive only within the host organism. Compare **facultative.**

obligate aerobe, an organism that cannot grow in the absence of oxygen. Compare **facultative aerobe.** See also **aerobe.**

obligate anaerobe, an organism that cannot grow in the presence of oxygen, such as *Clostridium tetani, C. botulinum,* and *C. perfringens.* Compare **facultative anaerobe.** See also **anaerobe, anaerobic infection.**

obligate parasite. See **parasite.**

oblique /əblēk'/ [L, *obliquus*, slanted], a slanting direction or any variation from the perpendicular or the horizontal.

oblique bandage, a circular bandage applied spirally in slanting turns, usually to a limb.

oblique fiber, (in dentistry) any one of the collagenous fibers that is bundled together obliquely in the periodontal ligament, insert into the cementum, and extends more occlusally in the alveolus, composing approximately two thirds of the periodontal fibers.

oblique fissure of the lung, 1. the groove marking the division of the lower and the middle lobes in the right lung. **2.** the groove marking the division of the upper and the lower lobes in the left lung.

oblique fracture, a slanted fracture of the shaft on the long axis of a bone.

oblique illumination. See **illumination.**

oblique presentation [L, *obliquus*, slanting + *praesentare*, to show], a presentation in which the long axis of the fetus is oblique to the long axis of the mother.

obliquus externus abdominis /əblī'kə/ [L, slanted], one of a pair of muscles that is the largest and the most superficial of the five anterolateral muscles of the abdomen. A broad, thin, four-sided muscle that arises by eight fleshy digitations from the lower eight ribs and by the broad abdominal aponeurosis, it inserts in the iliac crest laterally and the linea alba. It is innervated by branches of the eighth through the twelfth intercostal nerves and by the iliohypogastric and ilioinguinal nerves. It acts to compress the con-

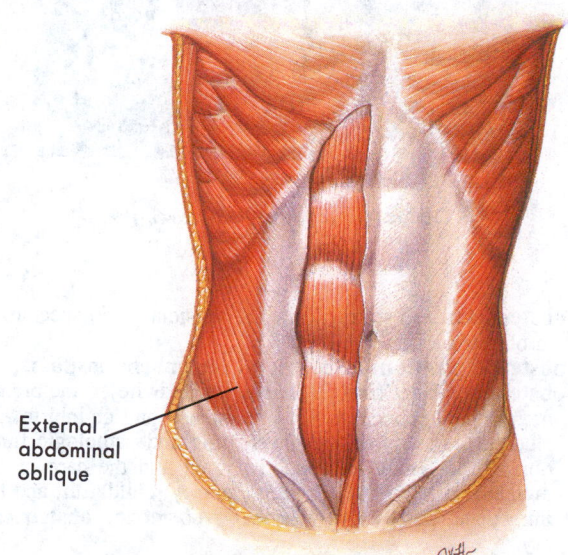

Obliquus externus abdominis
(Thibodeau, 1993/John V Hagen)

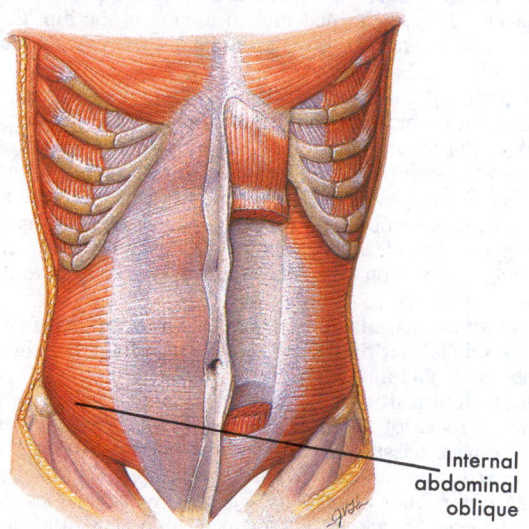

Obliquus internus abdominis
(Thibodeau, 1993/John V Hagen)

tents of the abdomen and assists in micturition, defecation, emesis, parturition, and forced expiration. Both sides acting together serve to flex the vertebral column, drawing the pubis toward the xiphoid process. One side alone functions to bend the vertebral column laterally and to rotate it, drawing the shoulder of the same side forward. Also called **descending oblique muscle, external oblique muscle.** Compare **obliquus internus abdominis, pyramidalis, rectus abdominis, transversus abdominis.**

obliquus internus abdominis, one of a pair of anterolateral muscles of the abdomen, lying under the obliquus externus abdominis in the lateral and ventral part of the abdominal wall. Smaller and thinner than the obliquus externus abdominis, it arises from the inguinal ligament, the iliac crest, and the lower portion of the lumbar aponeurosis. It inserts into the last three or four ribs and into the linea alba. The obliquus internus abdominis functions to compress the abdominal contents and assists in micturition, defecation, emesis, parturition, and forced expiration. Both sides acting together serve to flex the vertebral column, drawing the costal cartilages toward the pubis. One side acting alone acts to bend the vertebral column laterally and rotate it, drawing the shoulder of the opposite side downward. Also called **ascending oblique muscle, internal oblique muscle.** Compare **obliquus externus abdominis, pyramidalis, rectus abdominis, transversus abdominis.** (See Fig. p. 1093.)

obliteration /əblit′ərā′shən/ [L, *obliterare,* to efface], the removal or loss of function of a part of the body by surgery, disease, or degeneration.

obliterative phlebitis /əblit′ərətiv′/ [L, *obliterare,* to efface; Gk, *phleps,* vein + *itis,* inflammation], a form of phlebitis in which the inflammation results in permanent closure of the vessel. Also called **adhesive phlebitis.**

OBS, abbreviation for *organic brain syndrome.* See **organic mental disorder.**

observation [L, *observare,* to watch], **1.** the act of watching carefully and attentively. **2.** a report of what is seen or noticed, such as a nursing observation.

observation hip, a condition in which a patient experiences a limp, pain, and limited motion of the hip. Causes may include toxic synovitis, infection, or avascular necrosis.

obsession [L, *obsidere,* to haunt], a persistent thought or idea with which the mind is continually and involuntarily preoccupied and which suggests an irrational act.

obsessive-compulsive /əbses′iv/ [L, *obsidere,* to haunt; *compellere,* to impel], **1.** characterized by or relating to the tendency to perform repetitive acts or rituals, usually as a means of releasing tension or relieving anxiety. **2.** describing a person who has an obsessive-compulsive disorder.

obsessive-compulsive neurosis. See **compulsive ritual.**

obstetric /əbstet′rik/ [L, *obstetrix,* midwife], pertaining to obstetrics and midwifery.

obstetric anesthesia [L, *obstetrix,* midwife; Gk, *anaisthesia,* absence of feeling], any of various procedures used to provide anesthesia for childbirth. It includes local anesthesia for episiotomy or episiotomy repair, regional anesthesia for labor or delivery, such as by paracervical block or pudendal block, or, for a wider block—epidural, spinal, caudal, or saddle block. Anesthesia for cesarean section may be achieved with an epidural or spinal block or by general anesthesia.

obstetric forceps, forceps used to assist delivery of the fetal head. They vary in weight, length, shape, and mechanism of action, but all consist of a pair of instruments comprising a handle, a shank, and a blade. The blade is curved and, sometimes, fenestrated. The shank is long enough to allow the blade to reach the fetal head. The several styles of forceps are designed to assist in various clinical situations. The station of the fetus in the pelvis, the position of the head in relation to the pelvis, the size of the fetus, and the preference of the operator all affect the choice of forceps. Kinds of obstetric forceps include **Barton forceps, Elliot forceps, Kielland forceps,** and **Simpson forceps.** See also **forceps delivery.**

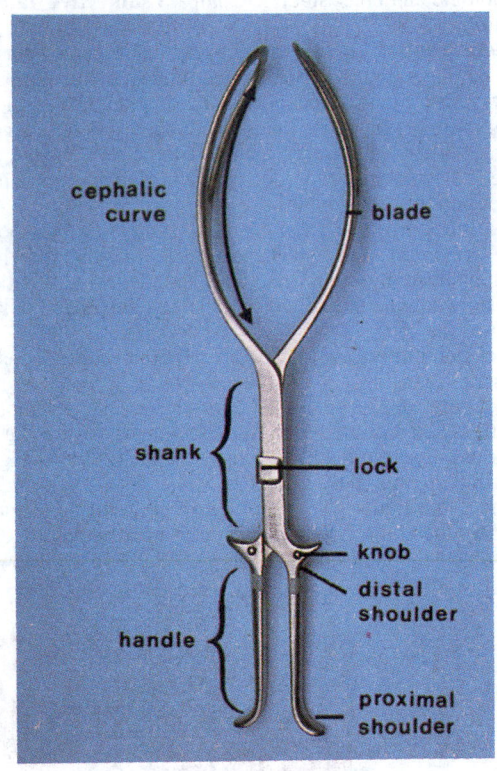

Obstetric forceps (Al-Azzawi, 1991)

obstetrician /ob′stətrish′ən/, a physician who specializes in obstetrics.

obstetric position. See **lateral recumbent position.**

obstetrics /əbstet′riks/ [L, *obstetrix,* midwife], the branch of medicine concerned with pregnancy and childbirth, including the study of the physiologic and pathologic function of the female reproductive tract and the care of the mother and fetus throughout pregnancy, childbirth, and the immediate postpartum period. —**obstetric, obstetrical,** *adj.*

obstetrix. See **midwife.**

obstipation /ob′stipē′shən/ [L, *obstipare,* to press], **1.** a condition of extreme and persistent constipation caused by obstruction in the intestinal or eliminatory system. See also **constipation. 2.** a process of blocking.   **—obstipant,** *n.,* **obstipate,** *v.*

obstruction /əbstruk'shən/ [L, *obstruere,* to build against], **1.** something that blocks or clogs. **2.** the act of blocking or preventing passage. **3.** the condition of being obstructed or clogged.   **—obstruct,** *v.,* **obstructive,** *adj.*

obstructive airways disease /əbstruk'tiv/, a classification of respiratory disease characterized by decreased airway size and increased airway secretions. It includes chronic bronchitis, abnormalities of the bronchi, and emphysema. See also **chronic obstructive pulmonary disease, cystic fibrosis.**

obstructive anuria [L, *obstruere,* to build against; Gk, *a, ouron,* without urine], an abnormal urologic condition characterized by an almost complete absence of urination and caused by an obstruction of the urinary tract. See also **obstructive uropathy.**

obstructive biliary cirrhosis [L, *obstruere,* to build against; *bilis,* bile; Gk, *kirrhos,* yellow; *osis,* condition], a form of secondary cirrhosis in which a stricture develops in the bile ducts. The condition may develop after cholecystectomy, gall stones, or a tumor.

obstructive constipation [L, *obstruere,* to build against; *constipare,* to crowd together], a condition in which feces are retained in the bowel because of a blockage in the lumen. Also called **alvine obstruction.**

obstructive jaundice.   See **cholestasis.**

obstructive sleep apnea, a form of sleep apnea involving a physical obstruction in the upper airways. The condition tends to affect mainly obese people, particularly those with secondary pulmonary insufficiency or a constitutional defect. A nonobese person with a congenital abnormality of the upper airways also may experience obstructive sleep apnea. The condition is usually marked by recurrent sleep interruptions, choking and gasping spells on awakening, and drowsiness caused by loss of normal sleep. Uncorrected, the disorder often leads to central sleep apnea, pulmonary failure, and cardiac abnormalities. See also **pickwickian syndrome.**

obstructive uropathy, any pathologic condition that results in obstruction of the flow of urine. The condition may lead to impairment of kidney function and an increased risk of urinary infection.

obtund /obtund'/ [L, *obtundere,* to blunt], **1.** to deaden pain. **2.** to render insensitive to unpleasant or painful stimuli by reducing the level of consciousness, such as by anesthesia or a strong narcotic analgesic.   **—obtundation, obtundity,** *n.,* **obtunded, obtundent,** *adj.*

obtundation /ob'tundā'shən/ [L, *obtundere,* to blunt, *atus,* process], the use of an agent that soothes and reduces irritation or pain by blocking sensibility at some level of the central nervous system, such as in the use of of narcotics to control pain and the giving of a tranquilizer as a calming agent.

obturator /ob'tərā'tər, ob'tyərā'tər/ [L, *obturare,* to close], **1.** a device used to block a passage or a canal or to fill in a space, such as a prosthesis implanted to bridge the gap in the roof of the mouth in a cleft palate. **2.** *nontechnical.* an obturator muscle or membrane. **3.** (in radiology) a device that is placed into a large bore cannula during insertion to prevent potential blockage by residual tissues.

obturator dislocation.   See **dislocation of hip.**

obturator externus, the flat, triangular muscle covering the outer surface of the anterior wall of the pelvis. It arises in several pelvic structures, including the rami of the pubis and the ramus of each ischium, and inserts into the trochanteric fossa of the femur. The obturator externus is innervated by a branch of the obturator nerve, which contains fibers of the third and the fourth lumbar nerves, and it functions to rotate the thigh laterally. Compare **obturator internus.**

obturator foramen, a large opening on each side of the lower portion of the hip bone, formed posteriorly by the ischium, superiorly by the illium, and anteriorly by the pubis.

obturator internus, a muscle that covers a large area of the inferior aspect of the lesser pelvis, where it surrounds the obturator foramen. It arises from the superior and the inferior rami of the pubis, the ischium, and the obturator membrane and inserts into the greater trochanter of the femur. It is innervated by a special nerve from the sacral plexus, which contains fibers from the lumbosacral trunk and the first and the second sacral nerves, and it functions to rotate the thigh laterally and to extend and abduct the thigh when it is flexed. Compare **obturator externus, piriformis.**

obturator membrane, a tough fibrous membrane that covers the obturator foramen of each side of the pelvis.

obturator muscles [L, *obturare,* to stop up; *musculus*], a pair of thigh muscles, the external and internal obturators. The external obturator flexes and rotates the thigh laterally, and the internal obturator abducts and rotates the thigh laterally.

obturator sign [L, *obturare,* to stop up; *signus,* sign], a sign of appendicitis. The internal rotation of the right leg with the leg flexed to 90° at the hip and knee with a resultant tightening of the internal obturator muscle may cause abdominal discomfort in appendicitis.

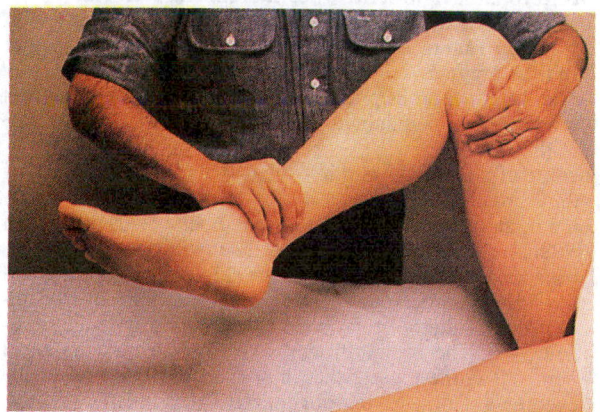

Obturator sign *(Seidel, 1991)*

obv, abbreviation for *obverse.*

oc-. See **ob-.**

O.C., abbreviation for **oral contraceptive.**

occ, abbreviation for **occipital.**

occipit, -occipito- [L, *occiput,* atlas], a prefix meaning 'relating to the back of the head': *occipital, occipitofrontal.*

occipital /oksip'itəl/, **1.** of or pertaining to the occiput.

2. situated near the occipital bone, such as the occipital lobe of the brain.

occipital artery, one of a pair of tortuous branches from the external carotid arteries that divides into six branches and supplies parts of the head and scalp. Each terminal portion at the vertex of the skull is accompanied by the greater occipital nerve.

occipital bone, the cuplike bone at the back of the skull, marked by a large opening, the foramen magnum, that communicates with the vertebral canal. Its inner surface is divided into four fossae. The occipital bone articulates with the two parietal bones, the two temporal bones, the sphenoid, and the atlas.

occipital lobe, one of the five lobes of each cerebral hemisphere, occupying a relatively small pyramidal portion of the occipital pole. The occipital lobe lies beneath the occipital bone and presents medial, lateral, and inferior surfaces. The medial surface is bounded anteriorly by the parietooccipital sulcus and the preoccipital notch and is divided by the posterior calcarine sulcus into the wedge-shaped cuneus and the lingual gyrus. The lateral surface of the lobe is divided by the lateral sulcus into the superior and the inferior occipital gyri. An imaginary transverse line across the preoccipital notch limits the inferior surface. Compare **central lobe, frontal lobe, parietal lobe, temporal lobe.**

occipital sinus, the smallest of the cranial sinuses and one of six posterior superior venous channels associated with the dura mater. It is located in the attached margin of the falx cerebelli, courses around the foramen magnum by several small channels, communicates with the posterior internal vertebral venous plexuses, and ends in the confluence of the sinuses. Compare **inferior sagittal sinus, straight sinus, superior sagittal sinus.**

occipito-. See **occipit-.**

occipitoaxial ligament. See **membrana tectoria.**

occipitobregmatic /oksip'itōbregmat'ik/ [L, *occiput* + Gk, *bregma,* front of the head], of or pertaining to the occiput and the bregma.

occipitofrontal /oksip'itōfrun'təl/ [L, *occiput* + *frons,* forehead], of or pertaining to the occiput and the frontal bone of the skull.

occipitofrontalis /oksip'itōfrəntal'is/, one of a pair of thin, broad muscles covering the top of the skull, consisting of an occipital belly and a frontal belly connected by an extensive aponeurosis. The frontal belly originates at the galea aponeurotica and inserts in the skin of the eyebrows and the nose. The occipital belly originates in the superior nuchal line of the occipital bone and inserts at the galea aponeurotica. The occipitofrontalis is innervated by the facial nerve. It is the muscle that draws the scalp and raises the eyebrows. Compare **temporoparietalis.**

occipitoparietal fissure. See **parietooccipital sulcus.**

occiput /ok'sipət/, *pl.* **occiputs, occipita** /oksip'itə/ ', the back part of the head. Also called **occiput cranii.**

occluded /əklōō'did/ [L, *occludere,* to shut up], closed, plugged, or obstructed.

occlusal /əklōō'səl/ [L, *occludere,* to close up], pertaining to a closure, such as the contact between the teeth of the upper and lower jaws.

occlusal adjustment, (in dentistry) the grinding of the occluding surfaces of teeth to improve the occlusion or relationship between opposing tooth surfaces, their supporting

structures, the muscles of mastication, and the temporomandibular joints.

occlusal contouring, the modification by grinding of irregularities of occlusal tooth forms, such as uneven marginal ridges, and extruded or malpositioned teeth.

occlusal form, the shape of the occluding surfaces of a tooth, a row of teeth, or any dentition.

occlusal harmony, a combination of healthy and nondisruptive occlusal relationships between the teeth and their supporting structures, the associated neuromuscular mechanisms, and the temporomandibular joints.

occlusal lug. See **occlusal rest.**

occlusal plane [L, *occludere,* to close up + *planum,* level ground], a plane passing through the occlusal surfaces of the teeth. It represents the mean of the curvature of the occlusal or biting surface.

occlusal radiograph, an intraoral radiograph made with the film placed on the occlusal surfaces of one of the arches. It shows the relationship of teeth to the underlying structures in the alveolar process, such as cysts and abscesses.

occlusal recontouring, the reshaping of an occlusal surface of a natural or artificial tooth.

occlusal relationship, the relationship of the mandibular teeth to the maxillary teeth when in a defined occlusal contact position.

occlusal rest, a support which is part of a removable partial denture and which is placed on the occlusal surface of a posterior tooth. Also called **occlusal lug.**

occlusal rest angle, (in dentistry) the angle formed by the occlusal rest with the upright minor connector. Also called **rest angle.**

occlusal spillway, a natural groove that crosses a cusp ridge or a marginal ridge of a tooth.

occlusal surface [L, *occludere,* to close up; *superficies,* surface], the surfaces of teeth in one arch that makes contact or near contact with the corresponding surfaces of the teeth in the opposing arch. Also called **masticatory surface.**

occlusal trauma, injury to a tooth and surrounding structures caused by malocclusive stresses, including trauma, temporomandibular joint dysfunction, and bruxism.

occlusion /əklōō'zhən/ [L, *occludere,* to shut up], **1.** (in anatomy) a blockage in a canal, vessel, or passage of the body. **2.** (in dentistry) any contact between the incising or masticating surfaces of the maxillary and mandibular teeth. **–occlude,** *v.,* **occlusive,** *adj.*

occlusion rim, an artificial dental structure with occluding surfaces attached to temporary or permanent denture bases, used for recording the relation of the maxilla to the mandible and for positioning the teeth. Also called **bite block.**

occlusive /əklōō'siv/, pertaining to something that effects an occlusion or closure, such as an occlusive dressing.

occlusive dressing, a dressing that prevents air from reaching a wound or lesion and that retains moisture, heat, body fluids, and medication. It may consist of a sheet of thin plastic affixed with transparent tape.

occlusometer. See **gnathodynamometer.**

occult /əkult'/ [L, *occultare,* to hide], hidden or difficult to observe directly, such as occult prolapse of the umbilical cord or occult blood.

occult blood, blood that is not apparent grossly appears from a nonspecific source, with obscure signs and symptoms. It may be detected by means of a chemical test or by

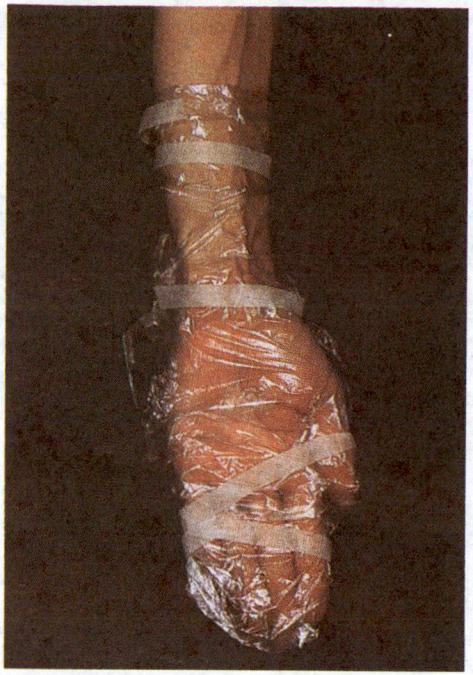

Occlusive dressing of the hand (Habif, 1990)

microscopic or spectroscopic examination. Occult blood is often present in the stools of patients with GI lesions.

occult blood test [L, *occultus*, hidden; AS, *blod*; L, *testum*, crucible], a test for the presence of microscopic amounts of blood in the feces secondary to bleeding in the digestive tract.

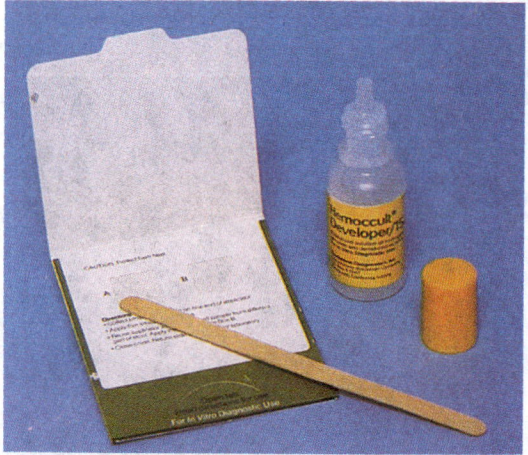

Supplies used in testing for occult blood in stool: cardboard Hemoccult slide, wooden applicator, and Hemoccult developing solution
(Potter, 1993)

occult carcinoma, a small carcinoma that does not cause overt symptoms. The carcinoma may remain localized, be discovered only incidentally at autopsy after death resulting from another cause, or metastasize and be discovered as a result of metastatic disease. Also called **latent carcinoma.**

occult fracture, a fracture that cannot be initially detected by radiographic examination but may be evident radiographically weeks later. The break is most likely to occur in the area of the ribs, tibia, metatarsals, or navicula. It is accompanied by the usual signs of pain and trauma and may produce soft tissue edema.

occupancy /ok'yəpənsē'/ [L, *occupare*, to seize], the ratio of average daily hospital census to the average number of beds maintained during the reporting period.

occupancy factor (T), the level of occupancy of an area adjacent to a source of radiation, used to determine the amount of shielding required in the walls. T is rated as full, for an office or laboratory next to an x-ray facility; partial, for corridors and restrooms; and occasional, for stairways, elevators, closets, and outside areas.

occupational accident /ok'yəpā'shənəl/ [L, *occupare*, to employ; *accidere*, to happen], an accidental injury to an employee that occurs in the workplace. Occupational accidents account for over 95% of occupational disabilities. In most cases the injured worker is eligible for compensation.

occupational asthma, an abnormal condition of the respiratory system resulting from exposure in the workplace to allergenic or other irritating substances. The condition is most common among people working with detergents, Western red cedar, cotton, flax, hemp, grain, flour, and stone. See also **asthma, byssinosis, occupational lung disease.**

occupational disability, a condition in which a worker is unable to perform the functions required to complete a job satisfactorily because of an occupational disease or an occupational accident.

occupational disease, a disease that results from a particular employment, usually from the effects of long-term exposure to specific substances or of continuous or repetitive physical acts.

occupational health, the ability of a worker to function at an optimum level of well-being at a worksite as reflected in terms of productivity, work attendance, disability compensation claims, and employment longevity.

occupational history, a portion of the health history in which questions are asked about the person's occupation, source of income, effects of the work on worker's health or the worker's health on the job, the duration of the job, and to what degree the occupation satisfies the person. Any adverse effects known to be associated with the work or the place of work are investigated by further questions by the interviewer; for example, a tennis player might be asked about musculoskeletal problems or a taxi driver about function of the urinary tract.

occupational lung disease, any one of a group of abnormal conditions of the lungs caused by the inhalation of dusts, fumes, gases, or vapors in an environment where a person works. See also **chronic obstructive pulmonary disease, metal fume fever, occupational asthma, silo fillers' disease.**

occupational medicine, a field of preventive medicine concerned with the medical problems and practices relating to occupations and especially to the health of workers in various industries.

occupational neurosis. See **occupational stress.**

occupational performance tasks, activities that can be used to measure the potential ability or actual proficiency in the handling of certain objects and use of skills related to a given occupation.

occupational socialization, the adaptation of an individual to a given set of job-related behaviors, particularly the expected behavior that accompanies a specific job.

occupational stress, a disorder associated with a job or work. The neurosis may be expressed in the form of extreme tension and anxiety, and the development of physical symptoms such as headache or cramps. Also called **occupational neurosis.** See also **burnout.**

occupational therapist (OT), an allied health professional who practices occupational therapy and who must be licensed, registered, certified, or otherwise regulated by law. The OT is concerned with the evaluation, diagnosis, and/or treatment of people whose ability to cope with activities of daily living is impaired by physical injury, illness, emotional disorder, congenital or developmental disability, or aging. Services include the design, fabrication, and application of orthoses; guidance in the selection and use of adaptive equipment; therapeutic activities to enhance functional performance; prevocational evaluation and training; and consultation concerning the adaptation of physical environment for the handicapped.

occupational therapy (OT), 'the use of purposeful activity with individuals who are limited by physical injury or illness, psychosocial dysfunction, developmental or learning disabilities, poverty and cultural differences, or the aging process to maximize independence, prevent disability, and maintain health. The practice encompasses evaluation, treatment, and consultation.' (American Occupational Therapy Association)

occupational therapy aid, a person who, under the supervision of an occupational therapist, performs clerical and related tasks necessary for the implementation of occupational therapy programs.

occupational therapy assistant. See **certified occupational therapy assistant.**

occurrence policy /əkurʹəns/ [L, *occurere*, to run; *politica*, pertaining to the state], a professional liability insurance policy that covers the holder during the period an alleged act of malpractice occurred. Occurrence policies are said to have a 'long tail,' because the statute of limitations on malpractice allegations is unlimited. Thus an individual could be sued years after an event took place. If the individual held an occurrence type of malpractice policy, there would be protection under that policy; under a claims-made policy there would not be protection unless the policy were current.

ochre mutation. See **amber mutation.**

ochronosis /ōʹkrənōʹsis/ [Gk, *ochros*, yellow, *osis*], an inherited error of protein metabolism characterized by an accumulation of homogentisic acid, resulting in degenerative arthritis and brown-black pigment deposited in connective tissue and cartilage, often caused by alkaptonuria or poisoning with phenol. Bluish macules may be noted on the sclera, fingers, ears, nose, genitalia, buccal mucosa, and axillae. The urine may be dark-colored. See also **alkaptonuria.**

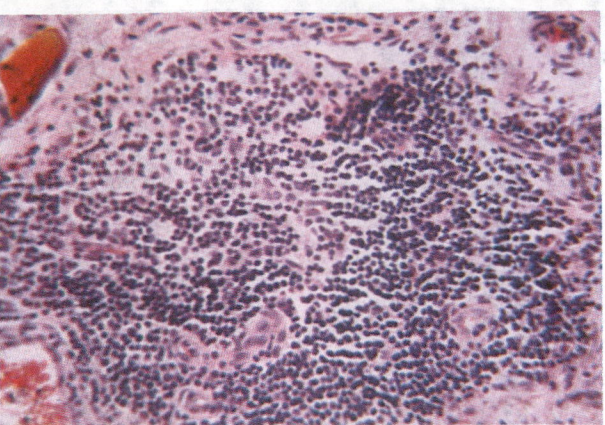

Ochronosis *(Schumacher, 1988)*

OCN, abbreviation for *Oncology Certified Nurse.*

ocontic pressure. See **colloid osmotic pressure.**

OCT, abbreviation for **oxytocin challenge test.**

octa-, octi-, octo-, a prefix meaning 'the number eight or series of eight': *octigravida, octapeptide, octagenarian.*

octaploid, octaploidic. See **polyploid.**

octigravida [L, *octo*, eight; *gravidare*, to impregnate], pertaining to a woman who is pregnant for the eighth time.

octo-, See **octa-.**

ocul., abbreviation for the Latin word *oculis,* 'pertaining to the eyes.'

ocular /okʹyələr/ [L, *oculus*, eye], **1.** of or pertaining to the eye. **2.** an eyepiece of an optic instrument.

ocular dysmetria, a visual disorder in which the eyes are unable to fix the gaze on an object or follow a moving object with accuracy.

ocular herpes [L, *oculus*, eye; Gk, *herpein*, to creep], a herpes virus infection of the eye. See also **herpes simplex keratitis; ophthalmic herpes zoster.**

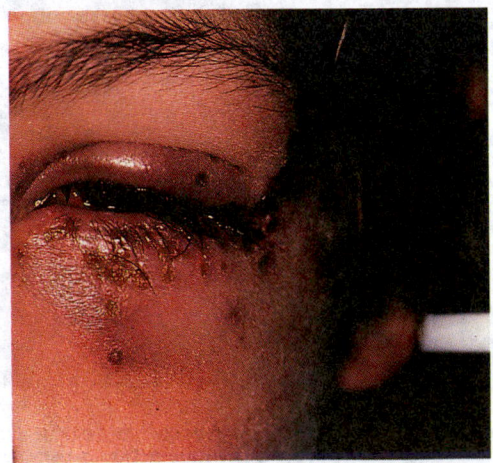

Ocular herpes *(Zitelli, 1992)*

ocular hypertelorism, a developmental defect involving the frontal region of the cranium, characterized by an abnormally widened bridge of the nose and increased distance between the eyes. The condition is often associated with other cranial and facial deformities and some degree of mental retardation. Also called **orbital hypertelorism.**

ocular hypotelorism, a developmental defect involving the frontal region of the cranium, characterized by a narrowing of the bridge of the nose and an abnormal decrease in the distance between the eyes, with resulting convergent strabismus. The condition is often associated with other cranial and facial deformities, primarily microcephaly and trigonocephaly, and some degree of mental retardation. Also called **orbital hypotelorism.**

ocular myopathy, slowly progressive weakness of ocular muscles, characterized by decreased mobility of the eye and drooping of the upper lid. The disorder may be unilateral or bilateral and may be caused by damage to the oculomotor nerve, an intracranial tumor, or a neuromuscular disease.

ocular refraction [L, *oculus,* eye + *refringere,* to break apart], the refraction of the eye.

oculo-, a combining form meaning 'of or pertaining to the eye': *oculofacial, oculomycosis, oculopathy.*

oculocephalic reflex /ok'yəlō'səfal'ik/ [L, *oculus* + Gk, *kephale,* head; L, *reflectere,* to bend backward], a test of the integrity of brainstem function. When the patient's head is quickly moved to one side and then to the other, the eyes will normally lag behind the head movement and then slowly assume the midline position. Failure of the eyes to either lag properly or revert back to the midline indicates a lesion on the ipsilateral side at the brainstem level. Also called **doll's eye maneuver.**

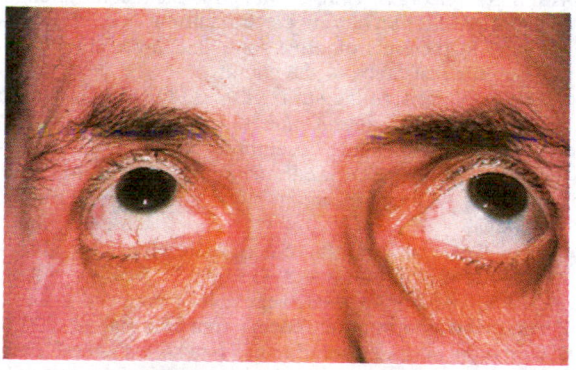

Oculogyric crisis *(Kamal, 1991)*

oculogyric crisis /ok'yo͞olōjī'rik/ [L, *oculus* + *gyrare,* to turn around], a paroxysm in which the eyes are held in a fixed position, usually up and sideways, for minutes or several hours, often occurring in postencephalitic patients with signs of parkinsonism. In some cases the eyes are held down or sideways and there may be spasm or closing of the lids. Oculogyric crises may be precipitated by emotional stress, and patients with the disorder frequently show psychiatric symptoms.

oculomotor /-mō'tər/ [L, *oculus,* eye; *motor,* mover], pertaining to movements of the eyeballs.

oculomotor nerve [L, *oculus* + *motor,* mover], either of a pair of cranial nerves essential for eye movements, supplying certain extrinsic and intrinsic eye muscles. They pass through the superior orbital fissure, connecting to the brain in nucleus III. Also called **nervus oculomotorius, third nerve.**

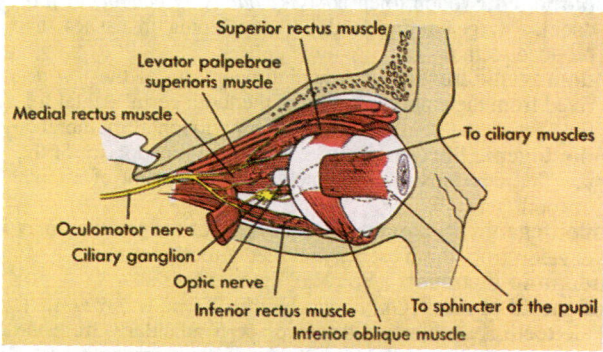

Oculomotor nerve *(Seeley, 1992/Michael Schenk)*

oculomotor nucleus [L, *oculus,* eye; *motor,* mover; *nucleus,* nut], a nucleus of a third cranial nerve arising in the midbrain.

Ocusert Pilo, a trademark for a cholinergic (pilocarpine).

OD, (*informal*). abbreviation for overdose.

O.D., 1. abbreviation for *oculus dexter,* a Latin phrase meaning 'right eye.' **2.** abbreviation for *Doctor of Optometry.*

OD'd /ōdēd'/ *slang.* overdosed, usually referring to a person who has suffered adverse effects from an excessively large dose of a drug of abuse.

Oddi's sphincter [Ruggero Oddi, Italian surgeon, b. 1864; Gk, *sphigkter,* binder], a band of circular muscle fibers around the lower part of the common bile duct and pancreatic duct, near the common duct junction of the duodenum.

-ode, a combining form meaning a 'type of pathway': *anode, cathode, electrode.*

odontalgia /ō'dontal'jə/ [Gk, *odous,* tooth; *algos,* pain], a toothache. Also called **odontodynia.**

odontectomy /ōdontek'təmē/ [Gk, *odous,* tooth, *ektome,* cut out], the extraction of a tooth.

odontia-. See **odonto-.**

odontiasis /ō'dontī'əsis/, the process of teething.

odontitis /ō'dontī'tis/ [Gk, *odous* + *itis,* inflammation], abnormal enlargement of a tooth, usually resulting from an inflammation of the odontoblasts (cells responsible for dentine formation) rather than of the mature, or erupted, tooth. It may be caused by infection, tumor, or trauma.

odonto- /ōdon'tō-/, **odont-, odontia-, odontic-,** meaning 'of or pertaining to the teeth': *odontoblast, odontopathy, periodontia, mesodontic.*

odontoblast /ōdon'təblast'/ [Gk, *odous,* tooth; *blastos,* germ], one of the connective tissue cells of the periphery of the dental pulp that develops into the primary and secondary dentin of a tooth.

odontodynia. See **odontalgia.**

odontodysplasia /-displā'zhə/ [Gk, *odous* + *dys,* bad, *plasis* forming], an abnormality in the development of the teeth, characterized by deficient formation of enamel and dentin. Also called **ghost teeth.** See also **shell teeth.**

odontogenesis /-jen′əsis/ [Gk, *odous*, tooth; *genein*, to produce], the origin and formation of developing teeth. Also called **odontogeny.** /ōdontoj′ənē/.

odontogenesis imperfecta. See **dentinogenesis imperfecta.**

odontogenic /ōdon′tōjen′ik/ [Gk, *odous* + *genein*, to produce], **1.** generating teeth. **2.** developing in tissues that produce teeth.

odontogenic fibroma, a benign neoplasm of the jaw derived from the embryonic part of the tooth germ, dental follicle, or dental papilla, or from the periodontal membrane.

odontogenic fibrosarcoma, a malignant neoplasm of the jaw that develops in a mesenchymal component of a tooth or tooth germ.

odontogenic myxoma, a rare tumor of the jaw that may develop from the mesenchyme of the tooth germ.

odontoid ligament. See **alar ligament.**

odontoid process [Gk, *odous* + *eidos*, form; L, *processus*], the toothlike projection that rises perpendicularly from the upper surface of the body of the second cervical vertebra or axis, which serves as a pivot point for the rotation of the atlas, or first cervical vertebra, enabling the head to turn.

odontoid vertebra. See **axis.**

odontology /ō′dontol′əjē/ [Gk, *odous* + *logos*, science], the scientific study of the anatomy and physiology of the teeth and of the surrounding structures of the oral cavity.

odontoma /ō′donto′mə/ [Gk, *odous* + *oma*, tumor], an anomaly of the teeth that resembles a hard tumor, such as dens in dente, enamel pearl, and complex or composite odontoma. It consists of cementum, dentin, enamel, and pulp tissue that may be arranged in the form of teeth. Also called **gestant anomaly.**

odor /ō′dər/ [L, a smell], a scent or smell. The sense of smell is activated when airborne molecules stimulate receptors of the first cranial nerve.

odoriferous /ō′dərif′ərəs/ [L, *odor*, smell; *ferre*, to bear], pertaining to something that produces a smell, particularly one that is strong or offensive.

odorous /ō′dərəs/ [L, *odor*, smell], pertaining to something that has an odor, smell, or fragrance.

ODTS, abbreviation for **organic dust toxic syndrome.**

-odyne, -odynia, odyno-, combining form meaning 'pertaining to pain': *anodyne, coccyodynia, odynolysis.*

odynophagia /od′inōfā′jə/ [Gk, *odyne*, pain, *phagein*, to swallow], a severe sensation of burning, squeezing pain while swallowing, caused by irritation of the mucosa or a muscular disorder of the esophagus, such as gastroesophageal reflux, bacterial or fungal infection, tumor, achalasia, or chemical irritation.

Oedipus complex /ed′ipəs, ē′dəpəs/ [Gk, *Oedipus*, mythic king who slew his father and married his mother], **1.** (in psychoanalysis) a child's desire for a sexual relationship with the parent of the opposite sex, usually with strong negative feelings for the parent of the same sex. **2.** a son's desire for a sexual relationship with his mother.

OEM, abbreviation for *optical electron microscope.*

OER, abbreviation for **oxygen enhancement ratio.**

o/f, symbol for *oxidation/fermentation.*

off-center grid, (in radiology) a focused grid that is perpendicular to the central-axis x-ray beam but shifted laterally, resulting in a cutoff across the entire grid.

off-focus radiation, (in radiology) x-ray artifacts caused by stray electrons that interact at positions on the anode at points other than the focal spot.

off-level grid, (in radiology) a grid that is not perpendicular to the central-axis x-ray beam. The cause is often a malpositioned x-ray tube rather than an improperly positioned grid.

off-line, access to computer information or equipment not part of an operating computer system, such as a drive not connected to the computer, a disk not connected to the computer, a disk not mounted on a drive, or a data printout sheet. Compare **on-line.**

ofloxacin /oflak′səsin/, an antibiotic of the carboxyfluoroquinolone type.

Ogden classification system, a system of categories for 17 different kinds of epiphyseal fractures.

Ogden plate, a long metal plate with slots designed to accept encircling bands. It is used for fixing long bone fractures associated with preexisting intramedullary devices such as rods or the stem of a prosthesis.

Ogen, a trademark for an estrogen (estropipate).

Ogsten line, a line drawn from the adduction tubercle to the intercondylar notch, used as a guide for transection of the condyle in osteotomy for knock-knee.

o.h., abbreviation for the Latin term, *omni hora,* 'hourly.'

OH, symbol for **hydroxyl.**

OHD, abbreviation for *organic heart disease.*

OHF, abbreviation for **Omsk hemorrhagic fever.**

ohm [Georg S. Ohm, German physicist, b. 1787], a unit of measurement of electric resistance. One ohm is the resistance of a conductor in which an electric potential of 1 V produces a current of 1 ampere. See also **ampere, Ohm's law, volt, watt.**

Ohm's law [Georg S. Ohm], the principle that the strength or intensity of an unvarying electric current is directly proportional to the electromotive force and inversely proportional to the resistance of the circuit.

-oi, -i, a plural-forming suffix in borrowings from Greek: *auloi, catanephroi, mesonephroi.*

-oid, **1.**a suffix meaning 'resembling or having the appearance of' something specified: *alkaloid, spheroid, trochoid.*

oiko-, eco-, a prefix meaning 'house': *oikofugic, oikology, oikophobia.*

oil [L *oleum*], any of a large number of greasy liquid substances not miscible in water. Oil may be fixed or volatile and is derived from animal, vegetable, or mineral matter.

oil retention enema, an enema containing about 200 to 250 ml of an oil-based solution given to soften a fecal mass.

ointment [L, *unguentum*, a salve], a semisolid, externally applied preparation, usually containing a drug. Various ointments are used as local analgesic, anesthetic, antiinfective, astringent, depigmenting, irritant, and keratolytic agents. Also called **salve, unction, unguent.**

-ol a suffix designating a member of the alcohol group: *ethanol, methanol, naphthol.*

-ol, -ole, a suffix meaning an 'oil': *benzol, furol, petrol, cholesterol.*

O.L., abbreviation for the Latin term *oculus laevus,* 'left eye.'

-ole, a suffix meaning a 'small or little example of the noun named': *arteriole.*

Old Age, Survivors, Disability and Health Insurance Program (OASDHI), a benefit program, administered by the Social Security Administration, that provides cash benefits to workers who are retired or disabled, their dependents, and survivors. This part of the program is commonly referred to as Social Security. The program also provides health insurance benefits for people over 65 and for disabled people under 65. This part of the program is commonly referred to as Medicare. See also **Medicare.**

old dislocation, a dislocation in which inflammatory changes have occurred.

old tuberculin [ME, *ald,* L, *tubercle*], the original formula for an extract of the tubercle bacillus used in the treatment of tuberculosis by Koch, using a glycerin-broth culture of *Mycobacterium tuberculosis* after filtration and concentration of the liquid.

Old World leishmaniasis. See **oriental sore.**

oleandomycin. See **troleandomycin.**

olecranon /ōlek′rənon/ [Gk, *olekranon,* tip of the elbow], a proximal projection of the ulna that forms the point of the elbow and fits into the olecranon fossa of the humerus when the forearm is extended. The anterior surface of the olecranon forms part of the trochlear notch that articulates with the humerus. Also called **olecranon process.**

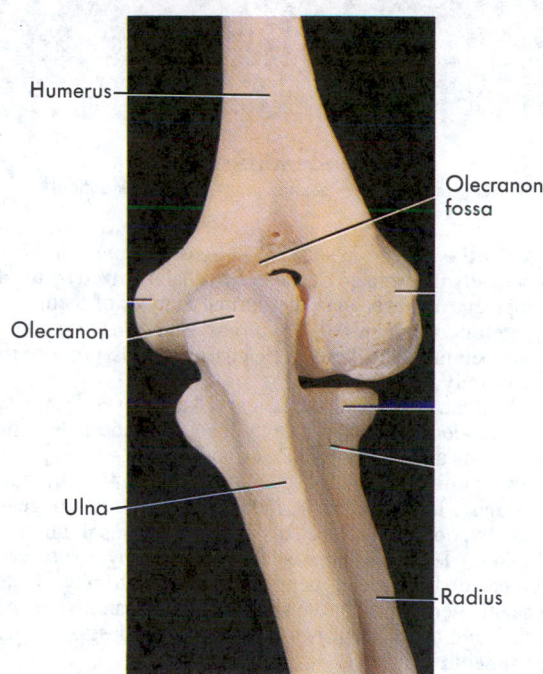

Olecranon and olecranon fossa *(Vidic, 1984)*

olecranon bursa, the bursa of the elbow.

olecranon fossa, the depression in the posterior surface of the humerus that receives the olecranon of the ulna when the forearm is extended. Compare **coronoid fossa.**

olecranon process. See **olecranon.**

olefiant gas. See **ethylene.**

olefin /ō′ləfin/ [L, *oleum,* oil, *facere,* to make], any of a group of unsaturated aliphatic hydrocarbons containing one or more double bonds in the carbon chain.

oleic acid /ōlē′ik/ [L, *oleum,* oil; *acidus,* sour], a colorless, liquid, monounsaturated fatty acid occurring in almost all natural fats. Commercial oleic acid is used in soaps, cosmetics, ointments, lubricants, and food additives.

oleo-, eleo-, a prefix meaning 'of or pertaining to oil': *oleocreosote, oleodistearin, oleoresin.*

oleovitamin /ō′lē·ōvī′təmin/, a preparation of fish-liver oil or edible vegetable oil that contains one or more of the fat-soluble vitamins or their derivatives.

oleovitamin A, an oily preparation, usually fish-liver oil or fish-liver oil diluted with an edible vegetable oil, containing the natural or synthetic form of vitamin A. See also **vitamin A.**

oelovitamin D$_2$. See **calciferol.**

olfaction /olfak′shən/ [L, *olfacere,* to smell], **1.** the act of smelling. **2.** the sense of smell.

olfactory /olfak′tərē/, of or pertaining to the sense of smell. –**olfaction,** *n.*

olfactory anesthesia. See **anosmia.**

olfactory bulb [L, *olfactus,* sense of smell; *bulbus,* swollen root], the area of the forebrain where the olfactory nerves terminate and the olfactory tracts arise.

olfactory center [L, *olfactare,* to smell at; Gk, *kentron*], the part of the brain responsible for the subjective appreciation of odors, a complex group of neurons located near the junction of the temporal and parietal lobes.

olfactory cortex [L, *olfactus,* sense of smell; *cortex,* bark], the part of the cerebral cortex, including the pyriform lobe and the hippocampus formation, that is concerned with the sense of smell. Also called **archeocortex.**

olfactory foramen, one of several openings in the cribriform plate of the ethmoid bone.

olfactory hallucination [L, *olfactus,* sense of smell; *alucinari,* wandering mind], a condition in which an individual has false perceptions of odors, which are usually repugnant or offensive. The hallucinations are sometimes associated with guilt feelings.

olfactory lobe [L, *olfactus,* sense of smell; Gk, *lobos,* lobe], a structure involved in the sense of smell in lower animals. Vestiges of the tissue are found in the cerebral hemispheres of humans.

olfactory nerve, one of a pair of nerves associated with the sense of smell. The olfactory nerve is cranial nerve I and is composed of numerous fine filaments that ramify in the mucous membrane of the olfactory area. The fibers of the olfactory nerve are nonmedullated and unite into fascic-

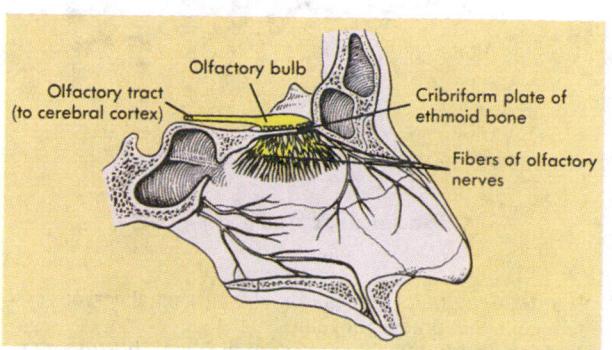

Olfactory nerve *(Seeley, 1992/Michael Schenk)*

uli that form a plexus under the mucous membrane and rise in grooves or canals in the ethmoid bone. The fibers pass into the skull and form synapses with the dendrites of the mitral cells. The area in which the olfactory nerves arise is situated in the most superior portion of the mucous membrane that covers the superior nasal concha. The olfactory sensory endings are modified epithelial cells and the least specialized of the special senses. The olfactory nerves connect with the olfactory bulb and the olfactory tract, which are components of the portion of the brain associated with the sense of smell.

olfactory receptors [L, *olfactus,* sense of smell + *recipere,* to receive], bipolar nerve cells located in the nasal epithelium. Axons of the cells become fibers of the olfactory nerve.

olig-. See **oligo-.**

oligemia /ol'ijē'mēə/ [Gk, *oligos,* little, *haima,* blood], a condition of hypovolemia or reduced circulating intravascular volume.

oligo- /ol'igō-/, **olig-,** a combining form meaning 'few, little': *oligocholia, oligodontia, oligosialia.*

oligoclonal banding /ol'igōklō'nəl/, a process by which cerebrospinal fluid IgG is distributed, after electrophoresis, in discrete bands. Approximately 90% of multiple sclerosis patients show oligoclonal banding.

oligodactyly /ol'igōdak'tilē/ [Gk, *oligos* + *dactylos,* finger], a congenital anomaly characterized by the absence of one or more of the fingers or toes. Also called **oligodactylia, oligodactylism.** **–oligodactylic,** *adj.*

oligodendroblastoma. See **oligodendroglioma.**

oligodendrocyte /ol'igōden'drəsīt/ [Gk, *oligos* + *dendron,* tree, *kytos,* cell], a type of neuroglial cell with dendritic projections that coil around axons of neural cells. The projections continue as myelin sheaths over the axons.

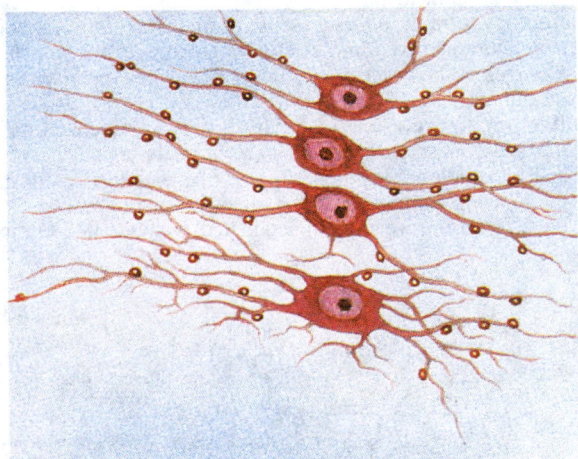

Oligodendrocytes (Chipps, 1992)

oligodendroglia /ol'igōdendrog'lē·ə/, central nervous system cells that produce myelin.

oligodendroglioma /ol'igōden'drōglī·ō'mə/, *pl.* **oligodendrogliomas, oligodendrogliomata** [Gk, *oligos* + *dendron,* tree, *glia,* glue, *oma,* tumor], an uncommon brain tumor composed of nonneural ectodermal cells that form part of the supporting connective tissue around nerve cells. The lesion, a firm, reddish-gray mass with calcified spots and a distinct margin, may be large. The tumor develops most often in frontal, parietal, and paraventricular sites but also may occur in the cerebellum. Also called **oligodendroblastoma.**

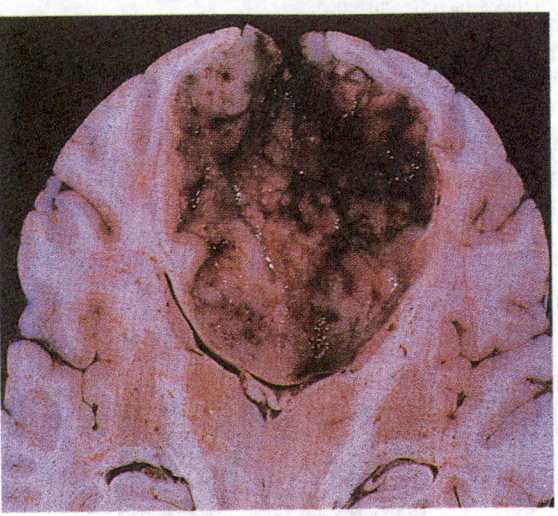

Oligodendroglioma
(Okazaki, 1988/by permission of Mayo Foundation)

oligodontia /ol'igōdon'shə/ [Gk, *oligos* + *odous,* tooth], a genetically determined dental defect characterized by the development of fewer than the normal number of teeth.

oligogenic /ol'igōjen'ik/ [Gk, *oligos* + *genein,* to produce], of or pertaining to hereditary characteristics produced by one or only a few genes.

oligohydramnios /-hidram'nē·əs/ [Gk, *oligos* + *hydor,* water, *amnion,* fetal membrane], an abnormally small amount or absence of amniotic fluid.

oligomeganephronia /ol'igōmeg'ənefrō'nē·ə/ [Gk, *oligos* + *megas,* large, *nephros,* kidney], a type of congenital renal hypoplasia associated with chronic renal failure in children. The condition is characterized by a decreased number of functioning nephrons and hypertrophy of other renal elements without the presence of aberrant tissue. Also called **oligomeganephronic renal hypoplasia.** **–oligomeganephronic,** *adj.*

oligomenorrhea /-men'ôrē'ə/ [Gk, *oligos* + L, *mensis,* month, *rhoia,* flow], abnormally light or infrequent menstruation. **–oligomenorrheic,** *adj.*

oligopnea, oligopnoea. See **bradypnea.**

oligospermia /ol'igōspur'mē·ə/ [Gk, *oligos* + *sperma,* seed], insufficient spermatozoa in the semen. Compare **azoospermia.**

oliguria /ol'igyŏor'ē·ə/ [Gk, *oligos* + *ouron,* urine], a diminished capacity to form and pass urine, less than 500 ml in every 24 hours, so that the end products of metabolism cannot be excreted efficiently. It is usually caused by imbalances in bodily fluids and electrolytes, by renal lesions, or by urinary tract obstruction. Also called **oliguresis.** Compare **anuria.** **-oliguric,** *adj.*

olisthetic /ōlisthet′ik/, pertaining to olisthy, or bone slippage.

olisthy /ōlis′thē/[Gk, *olisthanein*, to slip], the slippage of a bone from its normal anatomic site, as in the example of a 'slipped disk.'

olivary body /ol′iver′ē/ [L, *oliva*; AS, *bodig*], an olivary nucleus, part of an aggregate of small densely packed nerve cells, on the medula oblongata.

olivopontocerebellar /ol′ivōpon′tōsur′ibel′ər/ [L, *oliva*, olive, *pons*, bridge, *cerebellum*, small brain], of or pertaining to the olivae, the middle peduncles, and the cerebellum.

olivopontocerebellar atrophy (OPCA) /ol′ivōpon′tōsur′əbel′ər/, a group of hereditary ataxias characterized by mixed clinical features of pure cerebellar ataxia, dementia, parkinson-like symptoms, spasticity, choreoathetosis, retinal degeneration, myelopathy, and peripheral neuropathy. Various forms of OPCA are transmitted by autosomal dominant or recessive inheritance.

Ollier's disease. See **enchondromatosis.**

Ollier's dyschondroplasia /ol′ē·āz′/ [Louis X.E.L. Ollier, French surgeon, b. 1830; Gk, *dys*, bad, *chondros*, cartilage, *plasis*, formation], a rare disorder of bone development in which the epiphyseal tissue responsible for growth spreads through the bones, causing abnormal irregular growth and, eventually, deformity. The long bones and the ilia are most often affected. Orthopedic procedures to correct deformities may be necessary and helpful, but invalidism is the usual prognosis. A kind of dyschondroplasia is **hereditary multiple exostoses.** Also called **multiple enchondromatosis.**

-ology, a suffix meaning 'pertaining to the study or science of': *biology, pathology, physiology.*

-olol, a combining form meaning 'beta blocker.'

o.m., abbreviation for the Latin term *omni mane,* 'every morning.'

oma-. See **omo-.**

-oma, a suffix meaning a 'tumor': *capsuloma, lymphadenoma, neurinoma.*

omalgia /ōmal′jə/ [Gk, *omos*, shoulder, *algos*, pain], pain in the shoulder.

omarthritis /ō′märthrī′tis/, inflammation of the shoulder joint.

ombudsman /om′bədzmən/ [ONorse, *umbothsmathr*, commission man], a person who investigates and mediates patients' problems and complaints in relation to a hospital's services. Also called **patient representative.**

omega /ōmē′gə, ōmā′gə, om′əgə/, Ω, ω, the 24th letter of the Greek alphabet.

omental /ōmen′təl/ [L, *omentum*, membrane of the bowels], pertaining to the omentum.

omental bursa, a cavity in the peritoneum behind the stomach, the lesser omentum, and the lower border of the liver and in front of the pancreas and duodenum.

omentum /ōmen′təm/, *pl.* **omenta, omentums** [L, fatskin], an extension of the peritoneum that enfolds one or more adjacent organs with the stomach. See also **greater omentum, lesser omentum.** –**omental,** *adj.*

omicron /ōm′ikron/, O, o, the 15th letter of the Greek alphabet.

omission /ōmish′ən/ [L, *omittere*, to neglect], (in law) intentional or unintentional neglect to fulfill a duty required by law.

omni-, a combining form meaning 'all-powerful or all': *omnicide, omniform.*

omnifocal lens /om′nēfō′kəl/ [L, *omnis*, all; *focus*, hearth; *lentil*], an eyeglass lens designed for both near and far vision with the reading portion in a variable curve.

Omnipen, a trademark for an antibacterial (ampicillin).

omnipotence /omnip′ətəns/, (in psychology) an infantile perception that the outside world is part of the organism and within it, which leads to a primitive feeling of all-powerfulness.

omnivorous /omniv′ərəs/ [L, *omnis*, all; *vorare*, to devour], eating both plants and animal flesh.

omn.noct, abbreviation for the Latin term *omni nocte,* 'every night.'

omn.quad.hor., abbreviation for the Latin term *omni quadrante hora,* 'every quarter of an hour.'

omo-, oma-, a combining form meaning 'of or pertaining to the shoulder': *omoclavicular, omodynia, omohyoid.*

omophagia /om′ōfā′jē·ə/ [Gk, *omos*, raw; *phagein*, to eat], the eating of raw foods, particularly raw meat or fish.

omphal-. See **omphalo-.**

omphalic /omfal′ik/ [Gk, *omphalos*, navel], pertaining to the umbilicus.

omphalitis /om′fəlī′tis/, an inflammation of the umbilical stump, marked by redness, swelling, and purulent exudate in severe cases.

omphalo-, omphal-, a combining form meaning 'of or related to the navel': *omphalocele, omphaloma, omphalosite.*

omphaloangiopagus. See **allantoidoangiopagus.**

omphalocele /omʹfəlōsēl′/ [Gk, *omphalos* + *kele*, hernia], congenital herniation of intraabdominal viscera through a defect in the abdominal wall around the umbilicus. The defect is usually closed surgically soon after birth. Compare **gastroschisis.**

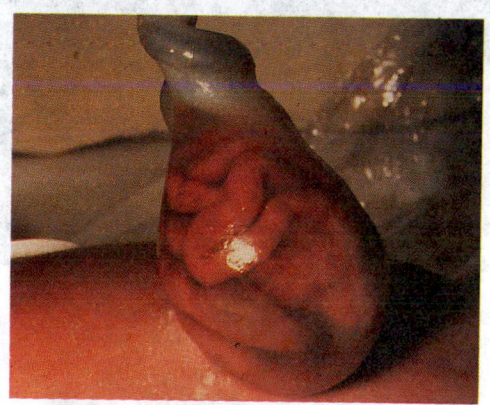

Omphalocele *(Zitelli, 1992)*

omphalodidymus. See **gastrodidymus.**

omphalogenesis /-jen′əsis/ [Gk, *omphalos* + *genesis*, origin], the formation of the umbilicus or yolk sac during embryonic development. –**omphalogenetic,** *adj.*

omphalomesenteric artery. See **vitelline artery.**

omphalomesenteric circulation. See **vitelline circulation.**

omphalomesenteric duct. See **yolk stalk.**

omphalomesenteric vein. See **vitelline vein.**

omphalopagus. See **monomphalus.**

omphalosite /om'falōsīt/ [Gk, *omphalos* + *sitos*, food], the underdeveloped parasitic member of unequal conjoined twins united by the vessels of the umbilical cord. The omphalosite has no heart, derives its blood supply from the placenta of the autosite, and is incapable of independent existence after birth. See also **allantoidoangiopagus.**

OMS, abbreviation for **Organisation Mondiale de la Santé.** See **World Health Organization.**

Omsk hemorrhagic fever (OHF) /ômsk/, an acute infection, seen in regions of the former U.S.S.R., caused by an arbovirus transmitted by the bite of an infected tick or by handling infected muskrats. The disease is characterized by fever, headache, epistaxis, GI and uterine bleeding, and other hemorrhagic manifestations. Treatment is supportive; recovery usually occurs.

-on, 1. a combining form meaning an 'elementary atomic particle': *electron, nucleon, proton.* **2.** a combining form meaning a 'unit': *magneton, photon.* **3.** a combining form meaning a '(nonmetallic) chemical element': *carbon, krypton, silicon.*

o.n., abbreviation for the Latin term *omni nocte*, 'every night.'

onanism. See **masturbation, withdrawal method.**

onchocerciasis /ong'kōsərkī'əsis/ [Gk, *onkos*, swelling, *kerkos*, tail, *osis*, condition], a form of filariasis common in Central and South America and in Africa, characterized by subcutaneous nodules, pruritic rash, and eye lesions. It is transmitted by the bites of black flies that deposit *Onchocerca volvulus* microfilariae under the skin. The microfilar-

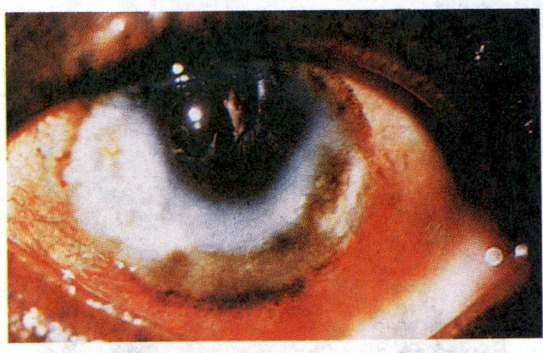

Eye lesion in onchoserciasis
(Muller, 1990/Courtesy Dr J Anderson)

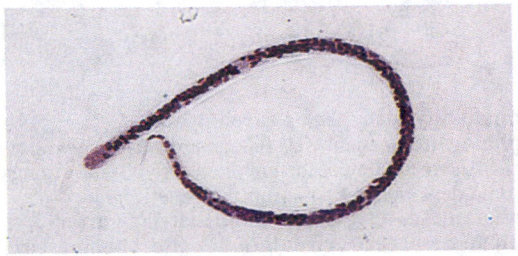

***Onchocerca volvulus* microfiliaria** *(Muller, 1990)*

iae migrate to the subcutaneous tissue and eyes, and fibrous nodules develop around the developing adult worms. Hypersensitive reactions to the dying microfilariae include extreme pruritus, a cellulitis-like rash, lichenification, depigmentation, and rarely, elephantiasis. Involvement of the eye may include keratitis, iridocyclitis, and, rarely, blindness from choroidoretinitis. Diagnosis is made by demonstrating microfilariae by skin biopsy or in the eye by slit lamp. Treatment is diethylcarbamazine for the microfilariae and surgical excision of nodules to remove adult worms. Protective clothing and control of black flies with DDT are the best preventives. Also called **river blindness.**

onco- /ong'kō-/, a combining form meaning 'relating to swelling, mass, or tumor': *oncology.*

oncofetal protein /-fē'təl/ [Gk, *onkos* + L, *fetus*, pregnant; Gk, *proteios*, first rank], a protein produced by or associated with a tumor cell, particularly an embryologic tumor.

oncogene /ong'kōjēn/ [Gk, *onkos* + *genein*, to produce], a potentially cancer-inducing gene. Under normal conditions, such genes play a role in the growth and proliferation of cells, but when altered in some way by a cancer-causing agent, such as radiation, a carcinogenic chemical, or an oncogenic virus, they may cause the cell to be transformed to a malignant state.

oncogenesis /ong'kōjen'əsis/ [Gk, *onkos* + *genesis*, origin], the process initiating and promoting the development of a neoplasm through the action of biologic, chemical, or physical agents. Compare **carcinogenesis, sarcomagenesis, tumorigenesis.**

oncogenic /ong'kōjen'ik/ [Gk, *ogkos*, swelling; *genein*, to produce], pertaining to the origin and development of tumors or cancer.

oncogenic virus, any one of over 100 viruses able to cause the development of a malignant neoplastic disease.

oncologist /ongkol'əjist/, a physician who specializes in the study and treatment of neoplastic diseases, particularly cancer.

oncology /ongkol'əjē/ [Gk, *onkos*, swelling, *logos*, science], **1.** the branch of medicine concerned with the study of malignancy. **2.** the study of cancerous malignancies.

Oncology Nursing Society (ONS), an organization of nurses interested or specializing in nursing of the patient with cancer. The national publication of the ONS is *Oncology Nursing Forum.*

oncotic /ongkot'ik/ [Gk, *ogkos*, a swelling], pertaining to or resulting from the presence of a tumor.

oncotic pressure [Gk, *ogkos*, swelling; L, *premere*, to press], the osmotic pressure of a colloid in solution, such as when there is a higher concentration of protein in the plasma on one side of a cell membrane than in the neighboring interstitial fluid. Also called **colloid osmotic pressure.**

oncotic pressure gradient, the pressure difference between the osmotic pressure of blood and that of tissue fluid or lymph. It is an important force in maintaining fluid balance between the vascular space and the interstitium.

Oncovin, a trademark for an antineoplastic (vincristine sulfate).

oncovirus /ong'kōvī'rəs/ [Gk, *onkos* + L, *virus*, poison], a member of a family of viruses associated with leukemia and sarcoma in animals and, possibly, in humans.

Ondine's curse /ondēnz'/ [L, *Undine*, mythic water nymph; ME, *curs*, invocation], apnea caused by loss of automatic control of respiration. The term refers to a syndrome in patients with decreased sensitivity to retained carbon dioxide.

A defect in the central chemoreceptor responsiveness to carbon dioxide leaves the patient with hypercapnia and hypoxemia, although fully able to breathe voluntarily. This condition may result in the pickwickian syndrome or the sleep-apnea syndrome, and it may be one cause of sudden infant death syndrome. Ondine's curse may occur as a result of drug overdose, such as with opioids; after bulbar poliomyelitis or encephalitis; or after surgery involving the brainstem or the higher segments of cervical cord, such as in cervical cordotomy for intractable pain.

-one, a combining form designating organic compounds: *acetone, ketone, quinone.*

one-and-a-half spica cast, an orthopedic cast used for immobilizing the trunk of the body cranially to the nipple line, one leg caudally as far as the toes, and the other leg caudally as far as the knee. For stability, a diagonal cross-bar connects the parts of the cast encasing the legs. This type of cast is used for immobilization during convalescence after healing of surgical hip repair or a fractured femur and for the correction and the maintenance of correction of a hip deformity. Compare **bilateral long leg spica cast, unilateral long leg spica cast.**

one-child sterility. See **acquired sterility.**

one-to-one care, a method of organizing nursing services in an inpatient care unit by which one registered nurse assumes responsibility for all nursing care provided one patient for the duration of one shift.

one-to-one relationship, a mutually defined, collaborative goal-directed client-therapist relationship for the purpose of psychotherapy.

oneiro-, a combining form meaning 'of or related to a dream': *oneirodynia, oneirology, oneiroscopy.*

-onide, a combining form for acetal-derived topical steroids.

-onium, a combining form for quaternary ammonium derivatives.

onlay [AS, *ana*, up, *licagan*, to lie], **1.** a cast type of metal restoration retained by friction and mechanical forces in a prepared tooth for restoring one or more cusps and adjoining occlusal surfaces of a tooth. **2.** an occlusal rest portion of a removable partial denture, extended to cover the entire occlusal surface of a tooth.

onlay graft, a bone graft in which the transplanted tissue is laid directly onto the surface of the recipient bone.

on-line, access to information or equipment that is part of an operating computer system linked to a central processing unit. Compare **off-line.**

ONS, abbreviation for **Oncology Nursing Society.**

onset of action, the time required after administration of a drug for a response to be observed.

onset of puberty [L, *pubertas*], a stage of development when genitalia reach maturity and secondary sex characteristics appear. The onset normally occurs in females between the ages of 11 and 13 with the development of breasts and during the phase of menarche. In males, puberty usually occurs between the ages of 12 and 14 and is characterized by the ejaculation of sperm. Also called **puberism.**

ontogenesis. See **ontogeny.**

ontogenetic /on'tōjənet'ik/, **1.** of, relating to, or acquired during ontogeny. **2.** an association based on visible morphologic characteristics and not necessarily indicative of a natural evolutionary relationship. Also called **ontogenic.**

ontogeny /ontoj'ənē/ [Gk, *ontos*, being, *genein*, to produce], the life history of one organism from a single-celled ovum

to the time of birth, including all phases of differentiation and growth. Compare **phylogeny.** See also **comparative anatomy.**

onych-. See **onycho-.**

onychia /ōnik'ē·ə/ [Gk, *onyx*, nail], inflammation of the nail bed. Compare **paronychia.**

-onychia, a combining form meaning a 'condition of the fingernails or toenails': *celonychia, melanonychia, pachyonychia.*

onycho-, onych-, a combining form meaning 'of or related to the nails': *onychogenic, onychohelcosis, onychopathology.*

onychodystrophy [Gk, *onyx*, nail; *dys*, bad; *trophe*, nourishment], a condition of malformed or discolored fingernails or toenails.

onychogryphosis /on'ikōgrifō'sis/ [Gk, *onyx* + *gryphein*, to curve, *osis*, condition], thickened, curved, clawlike overgrowth of fingernails or toenails.

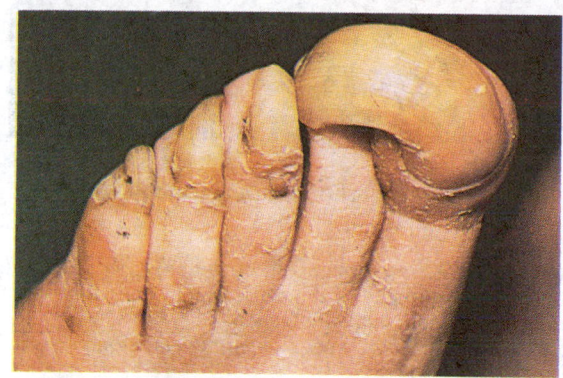

Onychogryphosis (Kamal, 1991)

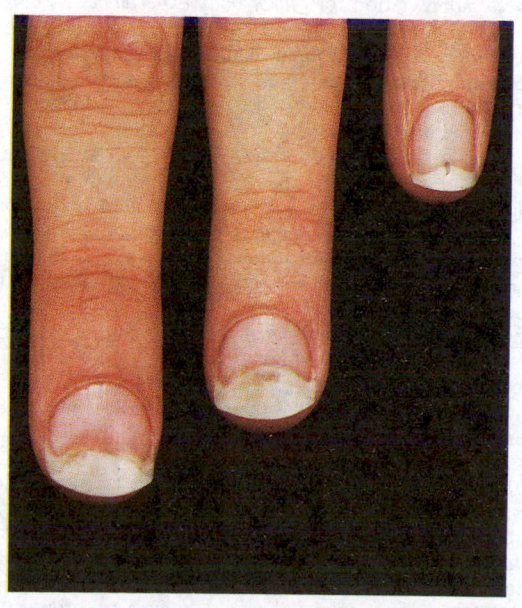

Onycholysis (du Vivier, 1993/Courtesy Institute of Dermatology)

onycholysis /on'ikol'isis/ [Gk, *onyx* + *lysein*, to loosen], separation of a nail from its bed, beginning at the free margin, associated with psoriasis, dermatitis of the hand, fungal infection, *Pseudomonas* infection, and many other conditions. (See Fig. p. 1105.)

onychomycosis /on'ikō'mīkō'sis/ [Gk, *onyx* + *mykes*, fungus, *osis*, condition], any fungus infection of the nails.

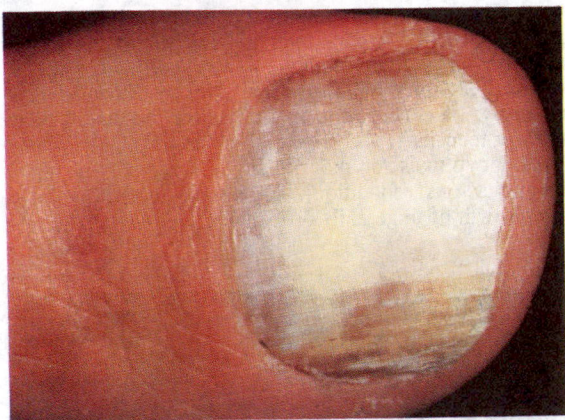

White superficial onychomycosis (Habif, 1990)

onychosis [Gk, *onyx*, nail; *osis*, condition], a condition of atrophy or dystrophy of the nails, usually caused by a dermatosis such as a fungal infection.

onychotomy /on'ikot'əmē/, a surgical incision into a nail bed.

oo- /ō'ə-/, a prefix meaning 'of or pertaining to an egg or ovum': *ooblast, oocytase, ootid.*

oob, abbreviation for *out of bed.*

oobe, abbreviation for *out of body experience.*

ooblast /ō'əblast/ [Gk, *oon*, egg, *blastos*, germ], the female germ cell from which the mature ovum is developed.

oocenter. See **ovocenter.**

oocyesis /ō'əsī·ē'sis/ [Gk, *oon* + *kyesis*, pregnancy], an ectopic ovarian pregnancy.

oocyst /ō'əsist/ [Gk, *oon* + *kystis*, bag], a stage in the development of any sporozoan in which after fertilization a zygote is produced that develops about itself an enclosing cyst wall. Oocysts of malarial parasites are found in the stomachs of infected mosquitoes. Oocysts of toxoplasma organisms are excreted in the feces of infected cats. Compare **oocyte.**

oocyte /ō'əsīt/ [Gk, *oon* + *kytos*, cell], a primordial or incompletely developed ovum.

oocytin /ō'əsī'tin/, the substance in a spermatozoon that stimulates the formation of the fertilization membrane after penetration of an ovum.

oogamy /ō·og'əmē/ [Gk, *oon* + *gamos*, marriage], **1.** sexual reproduction by the fertilization of a large, nonmotile female gamete by a smaller, actively motile male gamete, such as occurs in certain algae and the malarial parasite *Plasmodium.* **2.** heterogamy. Compare **isogamy.** **−oogamous,** *adj.*

oogenesis /ō'əjen'əsis/ [Gk, *oon* + *genesis*, origin], the process of the growth and maturation of the female gametes, or ova. Development begins during intrauterine life when the primordial germ cells within the epithelium of the fetal ovarian cortex give rise to precursor oogonia. By the time of birth, the oogonia have multiplied and developed into primary oocytes, each surrounded by a layer of epithelial cells that together form the primordial follicle. These have entered the prophase stage of the first meiotic division and remain suspended in this state until sexual maturity is reached. Then at monthly intervals one or sometimes two of the primary oocytes are stimulated simultaneously by the anterior pituitary hormones and the maturation of the follicle to continue meiotic division, forming a large secondary oocyte and a much smaller nonfunctional first polar body. The second meiotic division begins at about the time of ovulation and remains suspended in the prophase stage until fertilization stimulates the completion of the process, resulting in one large mature ovum, or ootid, and either one or three smaller secondary polar bodies that soon disintegrate. The ootid contains a pronucleus with the haploid number of maternal chromosomes that will fuse with the pronucleus of the spermatozoon to form the zygote. If fertilization does not occur, the ovum disintegrates and is discharged with the menses. The female infant is born with the entire number of primary oocytes that will function throughout reproductive life. Only a fraction of these survive until puberty and only a small percentage will be ovulated. Follicles containing the primary oocytes are found in varying stages of development in the ovary of the sexually mature woman. Egg and sperm formation differ considerably in the number and size of gametes resulting from gametogenesis, the total number of gametes produced in a lifetime, and the time sequence for the initiation of the meiotic divisions and the completion of the cycle. Also called **ovogenesis.** Compare **spermatogenesis.** See also **gametogenesis, meiosis, menstrual cycle, ovulation. −oogenetic,** *adj.*

oogonium /ō'əgō'nē·əm/, *pl.* **oogonia** [Gk, *oon* + *gonos*, offspring], the precursor cell from which an oocyte develops in the fetus during intrauterine life. It is derived from primordial germ cells, multiplies rapidly during gestation, and near the time of birth enters the prophase stage of the first meiotic division to form the primary oocyte. Also called **ovogonium.** See also **oogenesis.**

ookinesis /ō'əkinē'sis/ [Gk, *oon* + *kinesis*, movement], the mitotic phenomena occurring in the nucleus of the egg cell during maturation and fertilization. Also called **ookinesia.** See also **oogenesis. −ookinetic,** *adj.*

ookinete /ō'əkinēt'/ [Gk, *oon* + *kinein*, to move], the motile elongated zygote that is formed by the fertilization of the macrogamete during the sexual reproductive phase of the life cycle of a sporozoan, specifically the malarial parasite *Plasmodium.* It penetrates the lining of the stomach of the female *Anopheles* mosquito and attaches to the outer wall, where it forms an oocyst and gives rise to sporozoites.

oolemma. See **zona pellucida.**

oophor-. See **oophoro-.**

oophoralgia /ō'əfôral'jə/ [Gk, *oophoron*, ovary; *algos*, pain], a pain in an ovary.

oophorectomy /ō·əfərek'təmē/ [Gk, *oophoron*, ovary, *ektome*, excision], the surgical removal of one or both ovaries, performed to remove a cyst or tumor, excise an abscess, treat endometriosis, or, in breast cancer, remove the source of estrogen, which stimulates some kinds of cancer. If both ovaries are removed, sterility results and menopause is abruptly induced; in premenopausal women one ovary or a portion of one ovary may be left intact unless a malignancy is present. The operation often accompanies a hysterectomy. Regional or general anesthesia is used. Unless a malignancy is present, estrogen may be given to treat the unpleasant side effects of the abrupt onset of menopause. Also called **ovariectomy.**

oophoritis /ō′əferī′tis/,   an inflammatory condition of one or both ovaries, usually occurring with salpingitis.

oophoro-, oophor-, ootheco-,   a combining form meaning 'of or pertaining to the ovary': *oophorocytosis, oophorogenous, oophoroma.*

oophorosalpingectomy /ō′əfôr′əsal′pinjek′təmē/ [Gk, *oophoron* + *salpinx*, tube, *ektome*, excision],   the surgical removal of one or both ovaries and the corresponding oviducts, performed to remove a cyst or tumor, excise an abscess, or treat the condition of endometriosis. In a bilateral procedure the patient becomes sterile and menopause is induced. General anesthesia is used. Estrogen therapy may be started after bilateral surgery, unless a malignancy is present, to relieve the unpleasant side effects of the abrupt onset of menopause.

oophorosalpingitis /ō′əfôr′əsal′pinjī′tis/ [Gk, *oophoron*, ovary; *salpigx*, tube; *itis*, inflammation],   an inflammation involving both the ovary and the fallopian tube.

ooplasm /ō′əplaz′əm/ [Gk, *oon* + *plasma*, something formed],   the cytoplasm of the egg, or ovum, including the yolk in lower animals. Also called **ovoplasm.**

oosperm /ō′əspurm/ [Gk, *oon* + *sperma*, seed],   a fertilized ovum; the cell resulting from the union of the pronuclei of the spermatozoon and the ovum after fertilization; a zygote.

ootheco-.   See **oophoro-.**

ootid /ō′ətid/ [Gk, *ootidion*, small egg],   the mature ovum after penetration by the spermatozoon and completion of the second meiotic division but before the fusion of the pronuclei to form the zygote. It is one of the four cells resulting from oogenesis, the other three being nonfunctional secondary polar bodies, and corresponds to the four spermatid cells derived from spermatogenesis. See also **meiosis, oogenesis.**

OP,   **1.** abbreviation for *operative procedure.* **2.** abbreviation for **outpatient.**

opacity /ōpas′itē/ [L, *opacitus*, shadiness],   pertaining to an opaque quality of a substance or object, such as cataract opacity.

opaque /ōpāk′/ [L, *opacus*, obscure],   **1.** of or pertaining to a substance or surface that neither transmits nor allows the passage of light. **2.** neither transparent nor translucent.

OPD,   abbreviation for *Outpatient Department.*

-ope,   a combining form meaning a 'person having an eye defect': *asthenope, hyperope, protanope.*

open amputation [AS, *offan*, open; L, *amputare*, to cut away],   a kind of amputation in which a straight, guillotine cut is made without skin flaps. Open amputation is performed if an infection is probable or developing or has been recurrent. The cross section is left open for drainage, and skin traction is applied to prevent retraction. Antibiotic therapy is begun, and surgical closure is completed when the infection clears. Compare **closed amputation.** See also **gangrene.**

open-angle glaucoma.   See **glaucoma.**

open bite,   an abnormal dental condition in which the anterior teeth do not occlude in any mandibular position. Compare **closed bite.**

open charting,   a system of medical record keeping in which the patient has access to his chart. Open charting in

varying degrees is authorized in some mental health institutions.

open-circuit breathing system,   a type of breathing system used in cardiopulmonary therapy in which rebreathing does not occur. Gas is inspired through a breathing branch or limb that is connected to a gas source or open to the ambient atmosphere and then expired through a directional valve into a collecting reservoir or vented back into the ambient atmosphere.

open dislocation,   a dislocation in which the skin is broken, formerly called a **compound dislocation.**

open drainage.   See **drainage.**

open-drop anesthesia,   the oldest and simplest anesthetic technique, although it is not currently used in developed countries. A volatile liquid anesthetic agent is dripped, one drop at a time, onto a porous cloth or mask held over the patient's face. Chloroform and ether are the major general anesthetics adaptable to open-drop administration. Some psychologists believe that open-drop anesthesia can be a traumatic experience to a child and therefore consider this form of anesthesia ill-advised in pediatric use. It is not currently used in developed countries.

open fracture.   See **compound fracture.**

open fracture grading system,   a system of five categories of open fractures, ranging from a less than 1 cm clean wound that communicates to the fracture site to an open fracture requiring repair of arteries.

opening abductory wedge osteotomy (OAWO),   a procedure for treating a bunion deformity. It involves the use of a bone graft to open the wedge and bring the first metatarsal closer to the second.

opening pressure,   the amount of pressure measured in a manometer after insertion of a spinal needle into the subarachnoid space.

opening wedge osteotomy,   a bunion deformity treatment with a proximal cut in the metatarsal and reduction of the deformity. It is performed with or without tendon transfers.

open operation,   a surgical procedure that provides a full

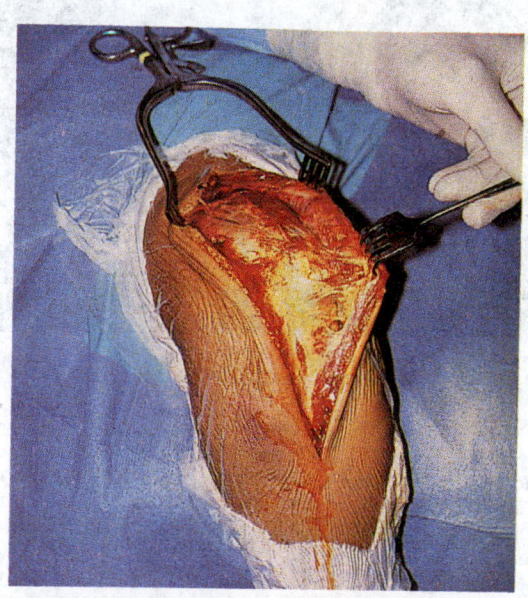

Open operation (Bray, 1993/Steve Young)

view of the structures or organs involved through membranous or cutaneous incisions.

open pneumothorax [AS, *open*; Gk, *pneuma*, air + *thorax*, chest], the presence of air or gas in the chest as a result of an open wound in the chest wall.

open reduction [AS, *open*; L, *reducere*, to lead back], a surgical procedure for reducing a fracture or dislocation by exposing the skeletal parts involved.

open system, a system that interacts with its environment.

open-wedge osteotomy, a straight cut made across a bone, creating angulation, leaving an open wedge-shaped gap.

open wound [AS, *open* + *wund*], a wound that disrupts the integrity of the skin.

operable /op′ərəbəl/ [L, *operari*, to work], susceptible to surgical intervention, as a disease or injury may be.

operant /op′ərənt/ [L, *operare*, to work], any act or response occurring without an identifiable stimulus. The result of the act or response determines whether or not it is repeated.

operant conditioning, a form of learning used in behavior therapy in which the person undergoing therapy is rewarded for the correct response and punished for the incorrect response. Also called **instrumental conditioning.**

operant level, the frequency or form of a performance under baseline conditions before any systematic conditioning procedures are introduced.

operating microscope /op′ərā′ting/ [L, *operari* + Gk, *mikros*, small, *skopein*, to look], a binocular microscope used in delicate surgery, especially surgery of the eye or ear. The standing type of operating microscope has a motorized zoom system operated by a foot pedal that quickly changes the magnification. The operating microscope that attaches to a surgeon's head has interchangeable oculars for different magnifications. Also called **surgical microscope.**

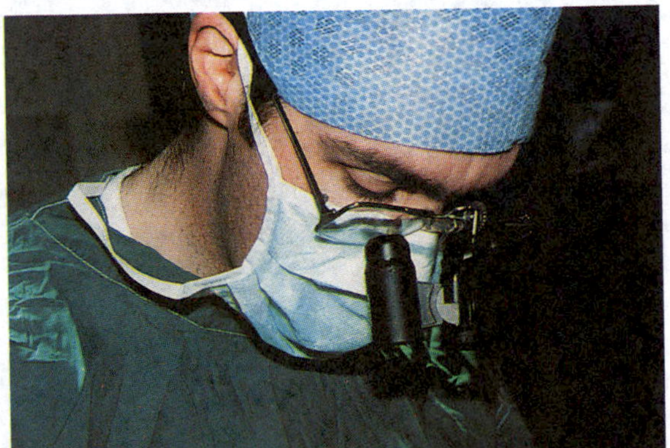

Operating telescope *(Eagling, 1986)*

operating room (OR, O.R.), **1.** a room in a health care facility in which surgical procedures requiring anesthesia are performed. **2.** *informal.* a suite of rooms or an area in a health care facility in which patients are prepared for surgery and undergo surgical procedures.

operating system (OS), the main system programs of a computer that manage the hardware and logical resources of a system, including inputøutput housekeeping system and data management.

operating telescope, a magnifying lens that gives low magnification and a wide field of vision.

operation /op′ərā′shən/, any surgical procedure, such as an appendectomy or a hysterectomy.

operationalization of behavior /op′ərā′shənal′īzāshən/, (in psychology) the stating of a patient's complaints or problems in specific, observable behavioral terms.

operative cholangiography /op′ərətiv′/ [L, *operari* + Gk, *chole*, bile, *aggeion*, vessel, *graphein*, to record], (in diagnostic radiology) a procedure for outlining the major bile ducts. It is performed during surgery by injecting a radiopaque contrast material directly into these ducts. It is usually performed to detect residual calculi in the biliary tract. See also **cholangiography.**

operative dental surgeon. See **dental surgeon.**

operator gene /op′ərā′tər/ [L, *operari* + Gk, *genein*, to produce], (in molecular genetics) a genetic unit that regulates the transcription of structural genes in its operon. The operator gene serves as the starting point in the coding sequence and interacts with a repressor protein in controlling the activity of structural genes.

operculum /ōpur′kyŏŏləm/, *pl.* **opercula, operculums** [L, a lid], a lid or covering, such as the mucous plug that blocks the cervix of the gravid uterus or the temporal operculum of the cerebral temporal hemisphere that overlaps the insula as an extension of the superior surface of the temporal lobe. **–opercular,** *adj.*

operon /op′əron/ [L, *operari*, to work], (in molecular biology) a segment of DNA consisting of an operator gene and one or more structural genes with related functions controlled by the operator gene in conjunction with a regulator gene. See also **operator gene, regulator gene.**

ophid-, a combining form meaning 'pertaining to a snake or snakelike': *ophidiophobia, ophidism, ophiasis.*

-ophidia, a combining form meaning 'venomous snakes': *thanatophidia, toxicophidia.*

ophth, abbreviation for **ophthalmology.**

ophthalm-. See **ophthalmo-.**

ophthalmia /ofthal′mē·ə/ [Gk, *ophthalmos*, eye], severe inflammation of the conjunctiva or of the deeper parts of the eye. Some kinds of ophthalmia are **ophthalmia neonatorum, sympathetic ophthalmia,** and **trachoma.**

-ophthalmia, a combining form meaning a 'pathologic or anatomic condition of the eye': *allophthalmia, echinophthalmia, polemophthalmia.*

ophthalmia neonatorum /nē′ōnətôr′əm/, a purulent conjunctivitis and keratitis of the newborn resulting from exposure of the eyes to chemical, chlamydial, bacterial, or viral agents. Chemical conjunctivitis usually occurs as a result of the instillation of silver nitrate in the eyes of a newborn to prevent a gonococcal infection. Also called **neonatal conjunctivitis.** See also **conjunctivitis.**

ophthalmic administration of medication /ofthal′mik/, the administration of a drug by instillation of a cream or ointment or by drops of a liquid preparation in the conjunctival sac. The correct strength and amount of the drug are selected, and the medication is instilled in the eye or eyes as directed. The order usually specifies O.D. for right eye, O.S. for left eye, or O.U. for each eye. Ophthalmic preparations are often refrigerated for storage but are given at room temperature. For administration, the patient is positioned comfortably, lying back on a bed or examining table

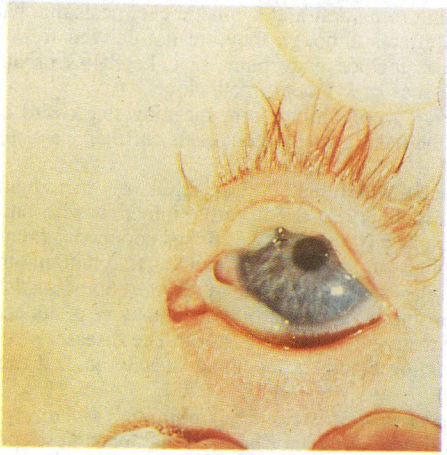

Ophthalmia neonatorum (Zitelli, 1992)

or sitting up with the neck hyperextended. The cul-de-sac of the conjunctival sac is exposed by gentle traction on the tissue just below the lower eyelid. The medication is placed in the sac as the patient is instructed to look away from the point of instillation. The dispenser is not allowed to touch the eye, and the medication is not placed directly on the cornea. The eyelid is slowly released, and the patient is asked to roll the eye around a few times to spread the medication over the entire surface of the eye.

ophthalmic herpes zoster. See **herpes zoster ophthalmicus.**

ophthalmic medical technician and technologist, an allied health professional who assists ophthalmologists by collecting data and administering treatment ordered by the ophthalmologist. These specialists are qualified to take medical histories, administer diagnostic tests, make anatomical and functional ocular measurements, test ocular functions, including visual acuity, visual fields, and sensorimotor functions, administer topical ophthalmic medications, and instruct the patient in home care and the use of contact lenses. Ophthalmic medical technologists perform all duties performed by technicians but are expected to do so at a higher level of expertise.

ophthalmic nerve [Gk, *ophthalmos*, eye; L, *nervus*, nerve], the first division of the trigeminal nerve (CN V), supplying the eyeball through the nasociliary branch. Branches also innervate the forehead, scalp, lacrimal gland, and dura mater.

ophthalmitis /of'thalmī'tis/ [Gk, *ophthalmos*, eye; *itis*, inflammation], an inflammation of the eye.

ophthalmo- /ofthal'mō-/, **ophthalm-,** a combining form meaning 'of or pertaining to the eye': *ophthalmodynia, ophthalmolith, ophthalmostat.*

ophthalmodynamometer /-din'əmom'ətər/ [Gk, *ophthalmos*, eye; *dynamis*, force; *metron*, measure], an instrument for measuring pressure on the sclera while the fundus is studied with an ophthalmoscope. It may be used to measure blood pressures in the ophthalmic artery.

ophthalmodynia /-din'ē·ə/ [Gk, *ophthalmos*, eye; *odyne*, pain], a pain in the eye.

ophthalmologist /of'thalmol'əjist/, a physician who specializes in ophthalmology.

ophthalmology (ophth) /of'thalmol'əjē/ [Gk, *ophthalmos*

+ *logos*, science], the branch of medicine concerned with the study of the physiology, anatomy, and pathology of the eye and the diagnosis and treatment of disorders of the eye. **–ophthalmologic, ophthalmological,** *adj.*

ophthalmoplasty /ofthal'mōplas'tē/ [Gk, *ophthalmos*, eye; *plassein*, to mold], plastic surgery of the eye or of the area around the eye.

ophthalmoplegia /ofthal'məplē'jē·ə/ [Gk, *ophthalmos* + *plege*, stroke], an abnormal condition characterized by paralysis of the motor nerves of the eye. Bilateral ophthalmoplegia of rapid onset is associated with acute myasthenia gravis, acute thiamin deficiency, botulism, and acute inflammatory cranial polyneuropathy. These diseases are potentially very destructive and require prompt attention. In some patients with myopathic ophthalmoplegia, structural abnormalities and biochemical disorders may be evident in limb muscles. Ophthalmoplegia is also associated with ocular dystrophy.

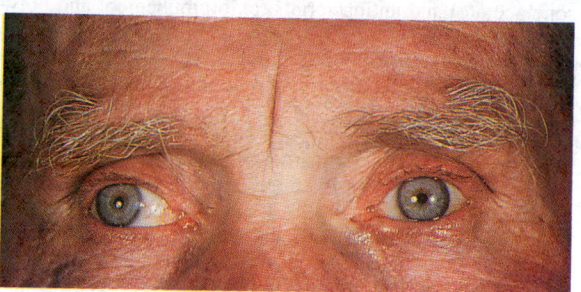

Ophthalmoplegia (Epstein, 1992)

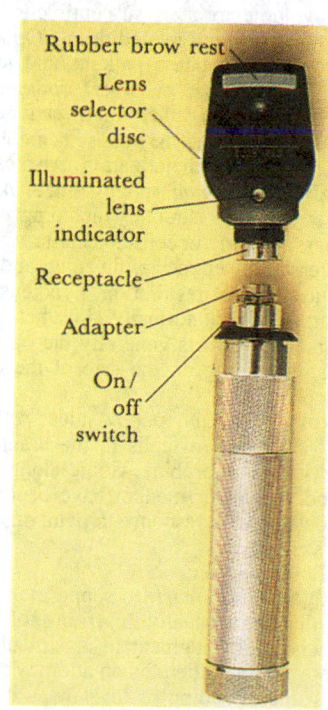

Rubber brow rest
Lens selector disc
Illuminated lens indicator
Receptacle
Adapter
On/off switch

Ophthalmoscope (Seidel, 1991)

ophthalmoscope /of′thalmol′əskōp/ [Gk, *ophthalmos* + *skopein*, to look], a device for examining the interior of the eye. It includes a light, a mirror with a single hole through which the examiner may look, and a dial holding several lenses of varying strengths. The lenses are selected to allow clear visualization of the structures of the eye at any depth. If the patient or the examiner ordinarily requires extensive correction of a refractive error, the examination may require that the corrective lenses normally worn be worn for the examination. (See Fig. p. 1109.)

ophthalmoscopy /of′thalmos′kəpē/, the technique of using an ophthalmoscope to examine the eye.

ophthalmospasm /ofthal′mōspaz′əm/ [Gk, *ophthalmos*, eye; *spasmos*], a sudden involuntary contraction of the eyeball.

Ophthochlor, a trademark for an ophthalmic preparation of an antibacterial and antirickettsial (chloramphenicol).

Ophthocort, a trademark for an ophthalmic, fixed-combination drug containing a glucocorticoid (hydrocortisone acetate) and antibacterials (chloramphenicol and polymyxin B sulfate).

-opia, -opic, -opical, -ops, -opsia, -opsy, -opy, a suffix meaning a '(specified) visual condition': *boopia, myopia, nonopia, senopia.*

opiate /ō′pē·it/ [Gk, *opion*, poppy sap], **1.** a narcotic drug that contains opium, derivatives of opium, or any of several semisynthetic or synthetic drugs with opium-like activity. **2.** *informal.* any soporific or narcotic drug. **3.** of or pertaining to a substance that causes sleep or relief of pain. Morphine and related opiates may produce unwanted side effects, such as nausea, vomiting, dizziness, and constipation. In rare instances a patient treated with an opiate may become delirious. Some patients also may develop increased sensitivity to pain after the opiate has worn off. Patients with reduced blood volume are more susceptible to the hypotensive effect of morphine and related drugs. Opiates are used with extreme caution in obese patients and in those with head injuries, emphysema, or other problems associated with decreased respiratory function. In patients with prostatic hypertrophy, morphine may cause acute urinary retention, requiring repeated catheterization. Also called **opioid.**

opiate poisoning [L, *opium*, poppy juice; *potio*, drink], toxic effects of a potent narcotic, including depression of the brain centers, causing unconsciousness. Acute intoxication is characterized by euphoria, flushing, and itching, followed by reduced rate of respiration, hypotension, lowered body temperature, and abnormally slow heart beat. Withdrawal is marked by effects generally the opposite of opiate poisoning, depending on the size of the dose and the duration of dependence.

opiate receptor [L, *opium*, poppy juice; *recipere*, to receive], any of a group of cells in the brain that bind to opiate drugs, such as morphine. Some along the aqueduct of Sylvius and the center median have been identified as receptors associated with response to pain; others have been found in the striatum.

-opic, -opical. See **-opia.**

opinion /əpin′yən/ [L, *opinari*, to suppose], **1.** (in law) a statement by the court, usually in writing, of the reasoning behind its decision or judgment in a particular case. **2.** a statement prepared for a client by an attorney that represents the attorney's understanding of the law as it pertains to a legal question posed by the client.

opioid /ō′pē·oid/ [L, *opium*, poppy juice; Gk, *eidos*, form], pertaining to natural and synthetic chemicals that have opiumlike effects although they are not derived from opium. Examples include endorphins or enkephalins produced by body tissues or synthetic methadone.

opistho-, a combining form meaning 'backward or relating to the back': *opisthognathism, opisthoporeia, opisthotonos.*

opisthorchiasis /ō′pisthôrkī′əsis/ [Gk, *opisthen*, behind, *orchis*, testicle, *osis*, condition], infection with one of the species of *Opisthorchis* liver flukes commonly found in the Philippines, India, Thailand, and Laos. Symptoms and signs are similar to those caused by *Clonorchis sinensis*. Carcinoma of the intrahepatic bile ducts may be a late complication. Treatment is unsatisfactory. The disease is prevented by avoiding eating raw or inadequately cooked freshwater fish.

Opisthorchis sinensis. See *Clonorchis sinensis.*

opisthotonos /ō′pisthot′ənəs/ [Gk, *opisthios*, posterior, *tonos*, straining], a prolonged severe spasm of the muscles causing the back to arch acutely, the head to bend back on the neck, the heels to bend back on the legs, and the arms and hands to flex rigidly at the joints.

opium /ō′pē·əm/ [Gk, *opion*, poppy sap], a milky exudate from the unripe capsules of *Papaver somniferum* and *Papaver album* yielding 9.5% or more of anhydrous morphine. It is a narcotic analgesic, a hypnotic, and an astringent. Opium contains several alkaloids, including codeine, morphine, and papaverine. See also **codeine, morphine sulfate, opium tincture, papaverine hydrochloride, paregoric.**

opium alkaloid, one of several alkaloids isolated from the milky exudate of the unripe seed pods of *Papaver somniferum*, a species of poppy indigenous to the Near East. Three of the alkaloids, codeine, papaverine, and morphine, are used clinically for the relief of pain, but their use entails the risk of physical or psychologic dependence. Morphine is the standard against which the analgesic effect of newer drugs for relief of pain is measured. The opium alkaloids and their semisynthetic derivatives, including heroin, act on the central nervous system, producing analgesia, change in mood, drowsiness, and mental slowness. The effects in a person who has pain are usually pleasant; euphoria and pain-free sleep are not uncommon, but nausea and vomiting sometimes occur. In usual doses the analgesic effects are achieved without loss of consciousness. The opium alkaloids have several other effects on the various systems of the body: Coughing is suppressed; the electric activity pattern of the brain resembles that of sleep; the pupils constrict; respiration is depressed in rate, minute volume, and tidal exchange; the secretory activity and motility of the GI tract are diminished; and biliary and pancreatic secretions are reduced. The use of morphine as an antidiarrheal preceded its use as an analgesic by hundreds of years. Prepared in a tincture, it remains the most effective constipating agent available.

opium tincture, an analgesic and antidiarrheal.
■ INDICATIONS: It is prescribed in the treatment of intestinal hyperactivity, cramping, and diarrhea.
■ CONTRAINDICATIONS: Drug dependence, the presence of toxic matter in the bowel, or known hypersensitivity to this drug prohibits its use.
■ ADVERSE EFFECTS: Among the more serious adverse reactions are drug dependence, toxic megacolon, and central nervous system depression.

opo-, a combining form meaning 'relating to juices or certain fluids, including hormones': *opsinuria.*

Oppenheim reflex /op'ənhīm/ [Herman Oppenheim, German neurologist, b. 1858], a variation of Babinski's reflex, elicited by firmly stroking downward on the anterior and medial surfaces of the tibia, characterized by extension of the great toe and fanning of other toes. It is a sign of pyramidal tract disease. Compare **Chaddock reflex, Gordon's reflex.** See also **Babinski's reflex.**

opportunistic infection [L, *opportunus*, convenient, *icus*, form], **1.** an infection caused by normally nonpathogenic organisms in a host whose resistance has been decreased by such disorders as diabetes mellitus, AIDS, or cancer, or by a surgical procedure, such as a cerebrospinal fluid shunt or a cardiac or urinary tract catheterization, or by immunosuppressive drugs. Long-term use of antibiotics or other drugs also may affect the immune system, creating opportunity for microorganisms not usually pathogenic to become pathogens. People with HIV are particularly susceptible to such infections. **2.** an unusual infection with a common pathogen, such as cellulitis, meningitis, or otitis media.

opposition [L, *opponere*, to oppose], the relation between the thumb and the other digits of the hand for the purpose of grasping objects between the thumb and fingers.

ops-, opto-, opti-, optico-, a prefix meaning 'visible, or pertaining to vision or sight': *optoblast, optometer, optostriate.*

opscan, abbreviation for *optical scanning.*

-ops,

-opsia. See **-opia.**

opsin, a protein that combines with retinal to form rhodopsin, or visual purple, in the rod photoreceptor cells of the retina.

opsonin /op'sənin/ [Gk, *opsonein*, to supply food], an antibody or complement split product that, on attaching to foreign material, microorganisms, or other antigens, enhances phagocytosis of that substance by leukocytes and other macrophages. **—opsonize,** *v.*

opsonization /op'sənizā'shən/ [Gk, *opsonein* + *izein*, to cause], the process by which opsonins render bacteria more susceptible to phagocytosis by leukocytes. Also called **opsonification.**

-opsy. See **-opia.**

-opter. See **ops-.**

opti-. See **ops-.**

optic [Gk, *optikos*, sight], of or pertaining to the eyes or to sight. Also **optical.**

-optic, -optical, a combining form meaning 'pertaining to vision': *bioptic, panoptic, preoptic.*

optical illusion [Gk, *optikos*, of sight; L, *illudere*, to mock], a false visual image derived from a misinterpretation of sensory stimuli caused by physical or psychological factors or both. A common optical illusion is the appearance of railroad tracks merging in the distance.

optical righting reflex [Gk, *optikos*, sight; AS, *riht*; L, *reflectere*, to bend back], a reflex that restores normal posture and head position with the help of visual clues.

optic angle. See **visual angle.**

optic atrophy /op'tik/, wasting of the optic disc resulting from degeneration of fibers of the optic nerve and optic tract. In primary optic atrophy the disc is white and sharply margined, the central depression (physiologic cup) is enlarged, and the optic foramen of the sclera is clearly seen. In secondary atrophy the disc is gray, its margins are blurred, the depression is filled in, and the foramen is difficult to detect. Optic atrophy may be caused by a congenital defect, inflammation, occlusion of the central retinal artery or internal carotid artery, alcohol, arsenic, lead, tobacco, or other toxic substances. Degeneration of the disc may accompany arteriosclerosis, diabetes, glaucoma, hydrocephalus, pernicious anemia, and various neurologic disorders.

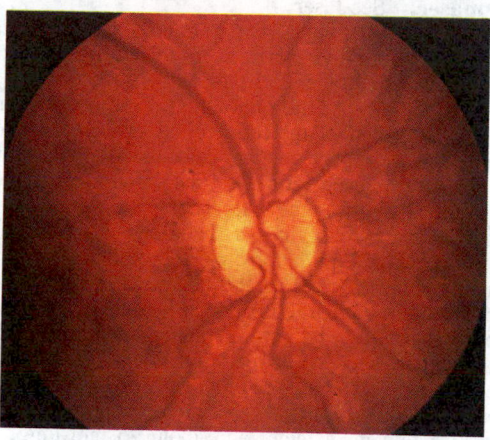

Optic atrophy (Zitelli, 1992)

optic chiasm [Gk, *optikos*, of sight; *chiasma*, crossed lines], a point near the thalamus and hypothalamus where portions of each optic nerve cross over.

optic coupling, a method of attaching the crystal window of a scintillator to the window of a photomultiplier tube so there is a minimum loss of light transmitted from the scintillator to the interior of the photomultiplier tube.

optic cup, a two-layered embryonic cavity that develops in early pregnancy. The optic cup is completed by the seventh week with the closing of the choroidal fissure. The cup initially develops from the infolding of the optic vesicle after the vesicle separates from the embryonic ectoderm. The cells of the optic cup differentiate to form the retina that first develops its layers of rods and cones in the central portion of the cup, growing as the layer gradually spreads toward the cup margin. The outer layer of the cup persists as the pigmented layer of the retina; the inner layer develops the nervous elements and the supporting fibers of the retina. Compare **optic stalk.**

optic density, a number describing the blackening of an x-ray film in any specified location. In general, the optic density is the logarithm of the ratio of incident to transmitted light through that area and is measured with a densitometer.

optic disc, the small blind spot on the surface of the retina, located about 3 mm to the nasal side of the macula. It is the only part of the retina that is insensitive to light. At its center the porus opticus marks the point of entrance of the central artery of the retina. Also called (*informal*) **blind spot, discus nervi optici.**

optic foramen [Gk, *optikos*, of sight; *foramen*, hole], an aperture in the root of the lesser wing of the sphenoid bone transmitting the optic nerve.

optic glioma, a slow-growing tumor on the optic nerve or in the chiasm. The tumor is composed of glial cells. Symptoms may include loss of vision, secondary strabismus, exophthalmos, and ocular paralysis.

optician /optish' ən/[Gk, *optikos*, sight], a person who grinds and fits eyeglasses and contact lenses by prescription. To become an optician, a person must graduate from high school and complete a 4- or 5-year apprenticeship. In some states licensure is required.

optic laser. See **laser.**

optic maser. See **laser.**

optic nerve, either of a pair of cranial nerves consisting mainly of coarse, myelinated fibers that arise in the retinal ganglionic layer, traverse the thalamus, and connect with the visual cortex. At the optic chiasm the fibers from the inner or nasal half of the retina cross to the optic tract of the opposite side. The remaining fibers from the temporal or outer half of each retina are uncrossed and pass to the visual cortex on the same side. The visual cortex functions in the perception of light and shade and in the perception of objects. Optic radiations conduct impulses from the geniculate bodies in the cerebral hemispheres to the visual cortices. The optic nerve is divided into portions within the bulb, orbit, optic canal, and cranial cavity. The intraocular portion of the nerve is about 1 mm long and contains unmyelinated fibers that become myelinated after passing through the lamina cribosa. The orbital portion of the nerve, about 3.5 mm in diameter and about 25 mm long, is invested by sheaths derived from the dura, the arachnoid, and the pia mater. The portion of the nerve within the optic canal lies superior to the ophthalmic artery, and the three sheaths are fused to each other, to the nerve, and to the periosteum of the bone, securing the nerve and preventing it from being forced back and forth in the foramen. The intracranial portion of the nerve rests on the anterior portion of the cranial sinus in close proximity to the internal carotid artery. The optic nerve is cranial nerve II and develops from a diverticulum of the lateral portion of the forebrain. The optic nerve fibers therefore correspond to a tract of fibers within the brain rather than to the other cranial nerves.

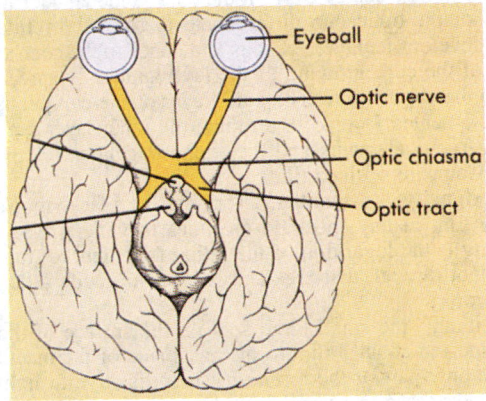

Optic nerve (Seeley, 1992)

- Eyeball
- Optic nerve
- Optic chiasma
- Optic tract

optic neuritis [Gk, *optikos*, of sight; *neuron*, nerve; *itis*, inflammation], inflammation, degeneration, or demyelinization of an optic nerve caused by a wide variety of diseases. Loss of vision is the cardinal symptom.

optic neuropathy [Gk, *optikos*, of sight; *neuron*, nerve; *pathos*, disease], a disease, generally noninflammatory, of the vision, characterized by dysfunction or destruction of the optic nerve tissues. Causes may include an interruption in the blood supply, compression by a tumor or aneurysm, a nutritional deficiency, and toxic effects of a chemical. The disorder, which can lead to blindness, usually affects only one eye.

optico-, See **ops-.**

opticokinetic. See **optokinetic.**

optic papilla. See **papilla.**

optic radiation [Gk, *optikos*, sight; L, *radiare*, to shine], a system of fibers from the lateral geniculate body of the thalamus that pass through the sublenticular portion of the internal capsule to the striate area.

optic righting, one of the five basic neuromuscular reactions that enable a person to change body positions. It involves a reflex that automatically orients the head to a new optical or visual fixation point, depending on the body position change.

optics /op'tiks/ [Gk, *optikos*, sight], **1.** (in physics) a field of study that deals with the electromagnetic radiation of wavelengths shorter than radio waves but longer than x-rays. **2.** (in physiology) a field of study that deals with vision and the process by which the functions of the eye and the brain are integrated in the perception of shapes, patterns, movements, spatial relationships, and color.

optic stalk, one of a pair of slender embryonic structures that become the optic nerve. In the embryo the optic stalk develops during the second week and attaches the optic vesicle to the wall of the brain. The stalk becomes complete during the seventh week of pregnancy when the choroidal fissure closes and is later converted into the optic nerve when nerve fibers fill the cavity of the stalk. Most of the fibers are centripetal and grow backward into the stalk from the nerve cells of the retina. A few fibers grow into the stalk from the brain. About the tenth week after birth, the fibers of the optic nerve receive their myelin sheaths. Compare **optic cup.**

optic system assessment, an evaluation of the patient's eyes, vision, and current and past disorders or injuries that may be responsible for abnormalities in the individual's optic system.

■ METHOD: The patient is interviewed to determine if vision is blurred, double, decreased, or absent in one or both eyes, or diminished peripherally at night or in bright light. The interviewer asks if halos or lights are seen and if the patient collides with unfamiliar objects, is unable to distinguish objects held too close or too far, if the eyes water, itch, or feel tender, painful, or fatigued, and if an injury to the eye, face, or head has occurred. Observations are made of the patient's general appearance, vital signs, kind of eyeglasses or contact lenses worn, the amount of tearing, ability to blink, tendency to rub the eyes, and visual acuity. Evidence is recorded of conjunctivitis, drainage, optic hemorrhage, edema or ptosis of the eyelids, exophthalmos, strabismus, nystagmus, scleral edema, chalazion, lacerations, contusions, or a foreign body in the eye. Carefully noted are signs of aging, glaucoma, cataract, retinal detachment, and the presence of multiple sclerosis, diabetes mellitus, myasthenia gravis, gonorrhea, thyroid dysfunction, sinus problems, or cerebral trauma or tumors. The patient's report of previous eye operations or treatments, head or face trauma, arteriosclerosis, glomerulonephritis, retinal degeneration, episodes of coma, therapy with oxygen, and drug misuse are investigated, as well as a family history of glaucoma or diabetes. Also explored are the possibility that the patient has a hazardous job or recreation (and note is made of any safety precautions taken), the individual's misuse of alcohol, and use of medication, especially antibiotics, antiemetics, miotics, mydriatics, and acetazolamide. Diagnostic aids for the evaluation include a test of visual fields, x-ray film of the orbit and skull, an ophthalmoscopic examination, tonometry, brain scan, and microscopic studies of conjunctival scrapings.

■ INTERVENTIONS: The nurse conducts the interview, makes the observations of the patient, and assembles the pertinent background data and the results of the diagnostic procedures.

■ OUTCOME CRITERIA: A careful assessment of the patient's eyes and vision and of certain aspects of the medical, family, and social history is a significant aid in establishing the diagnosis of an optic system disorder.

optic thermometer, a temperature-measuring device in which the properties of transmission and reflection of visible light are temperature dependent, the detection of which can be related to tissue temperature.

optic tract [Gk, *optikos,* sight; L, *tractus*], a flat band of nerve fibers running backward and laterally around each cerebral peduncle from the optic chiasma to the lateral geniculate body.

Optimine, a trademark for an antihistamine (azatadine maleate).

opto-. See **ops-.**

optokinetic /op′tōkinet′ik/ [Gk, *optikos,* of sight; *kinesis,* motion], pertaining to movement of the eyeballs in response to the movement of objects across the visual field, such as in optokinetic nystagmus. Also called **opticokinetic.**

optometrist /optom′ətrist/ [Gk, *optikos,* sight, *metron,* measure], a person who practices optometry. An optometrist is awarded the degree of Doctor of Optometry (O.D.) after completion of at least 2 years of college, followed by 4 years in an approved college of optometry. A state examination and license are also required. See also **optician, optometry.**

optometry /optom′ətrē/ [Gk, *optikos,* sight, *metron,* measure], the practice of testing the eyes for visual acuity, prescribing corrective lenses, and recommending eye exercises. See also **optician.**

OPV, abbreviation for **oral poliovirus vaccine.**

-opy. See **-opia.**

OR, O.R., abbreviation for **operating room.**

oral /ôr′əl/ [L, *oralis,* mouth], of or pertaining to the mouth. Compare **buccal, parenteral.**

oral administration of medication, the administration of a tablet, a capsule, an elixir, or a solution or other liquid form of medication by mouth. An adequate amount of water should be given to lubricate or dissolve the solid medications or to dilute the liquid forms for swallowing. Preparations with a disagreeable taste may be given with something of sufficient flavor to disguise the bad taste. Substances that are harmful to the teeth are given through a straw. People who have difficulty swallowing pills or capsules may find it easier to swallow the medication if they look up as they swallow. Looking up while swallowing opens the esophagus. Oral administration of medication includes **buccal administration of medication** and **sublingual administration of medication.**

oral airway, a curved tubular device of rubber, plastic, or

metal placed in the oropharynx during general anesthesia to maintain free passage of air and keep the tongue from obstructing the trachea. The artificial airway is not removed until the patient begins to awaken and regains pharyngeal, cough, and swallowing reflexes.

oral and maxillofacial surgeon. See **dental surgeon.**

oral cancer, a malignant neoplasm on the lip or in the mouth, occurring at an average age of 60 with a frequency eight times higher in men than in women. Predisposing factors in the cause of the disease are alcoholism, heavy use of tobacco, poor oral hygiene, ill-fitting dentures, syphilis, Plummer-Vinson syndrome, betel nut chewing, and, in lip cancer, overexposure to sun and wind and the smoking of pipes. Premalignant leukoplakia or erythroplasia or a painless nonhealing ulcer may be the first sign of oral cancer; localized pain usually appears later, but lymph nodes may be involved early in the course. Diagnostic measures include digital examination, biopsy, exfoliative cytology, x-ray film of the mandible, and chest films to detect metastatic lung lesions. Almost all oral tumors are epidermoid carcinomas; adenocarcinomas occur occasionally, whereas sarcomas and metastatic lesions from other sites are rare. Small primary lesions may be treated by excision or irradiation and more extensive oral tumors by surgery, with removal of involved lymph nodes and preoperative or postoperative radiotherapy. Among chemotherapeutic agents administered palliatively for inoperable or recurrent lesions are methotrexate, 5-fluorouracil, bleomycin, and adriamycin.

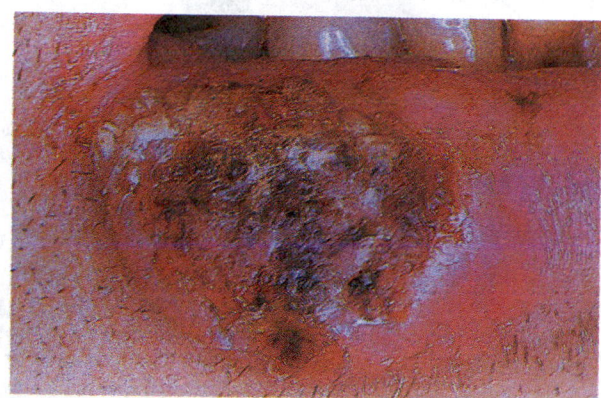

Oral cancer *(Cawson, 1987)*

oral cavity [L, *oralis,* pertaining to the mouth; *cavum,* cavity], the cavity of the mouth, including the tongue and teeth.

oral character, (in psychoanalysis) a kind of personality exhibiting patterns of behavior originating in the oral phase of infancy. This personality is characterized by optimism, self-confidence, and carefree generosity reflecting the pleasurable aspects of the stage, or pessimism, futility, anxiety, and sadism as manifestations of frustrations or conflicts occurring during the period. See also **oral eroticism, oral stage, psychosexual development.**

oral contraceptive, oral hormone medication for contraception. The two major hormones used are progestogen and a combination of progestogen and estrogen. The hormones act by inhibiting the productivity of gonadotropin-releasing hormone by the hypothalamus, and therefore the pituitary does not secrete gonadotropins to stimulate ovulation. This results in the endometrium of the uterus being thin and the cervical mucus being thick, thus preventing the penetration of sperm. Before oral contraceptives are prescribed, the woman receives a complete physical examination and a history is taken. While on the medication, she is reexamined after 3 months and then yearly. Combination hormones are given for 3 weeks with no medication in the fourth week to allow for withdrawal bleeding. If breakthrough bleeding occurs, the estrogen dose may need to be increased. If amenorrhea develops, the progestogen may need to be decreased. Contraindications to the medication include pregnancy, diabetes mellitus, liver disease, hyperlipidemia, thrombolic complications, coronary artery disease, and sickle cell disease. Patients with depression and migraine headaches and those who are heavy cigarette smokers need to be followed up more often. Amenorrhea often occurs in women who stop taking oral contraceptives and who have had a history of oligomenorrhea or amenorrhea. The pregnancy rate when oral contraceptives are used correctly is less than 0.2% a year. See also **contraception.**

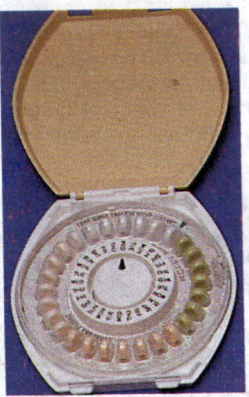

Oral contraceptives
(Edge, 1994)

oral dosage, the administration of a medicine by mouth.

oral eroticism, (in psychoanalysis) libidinal fixation at or regression to the oral stage of psychosexual development, often reflected in such personality traits as passivity, insecurity, and oversensitivity. Also called **oral erotism.** Compare **anal eroticism.** See also **oral character.**

oral examination [L, *oralis,* pertaining to the mouth; *examinatio,* to weigh], a clinical inspection and investigation of the hard and soft structures of the oral cavity for purposes of diagnosis, planning, treatment, and evaluation.

oral hairy leukoplakia. See **hairy leukoplakia.**

oral herpes. See **herpes simplex.**

oral hygiene, the condition or practice of maintaining the tissues and structures of the mouth. Oral hygiene includes brushing the teeth to remove food particles, bacteria, and plaque; massaging the gums with a toothbrush, dental floss, or water irrigator to stimulate circulation and remove foreign matter; and cleansing of dentures and ensuring their proper fit to prevent irritation. Dependent or unconscious patients are assisted in maintaining a healthy oral condition. Such care includes lubricating the lips and cleaning the inside of the cheeks, the roof of the mouth, and the tongue.

In addition, the nurse checks for loose teeth that might be swallowed or aspirated.

oral mucous membrane, altered, a nursing diagnosis accepted by the Seventh National Conference on the Classification of Nursing Diagnoses. The condition is defined as a state in which an individual experiences disruptions in the tissue layers of the oral cavity. Defining characteristics include oral pain or discomfort, coated tongue, xerostomia (dry mouth), stomatitis, oral lesions or ulcers, lack of or decreased salivation, leukoplakia, edema, hyperemia, oral plaque, desquamation, vesicles, hemorrhagic gingivitis, carious teeth, and halitosis. Related factors include pathologic condition of the oral cavity caused by radiation to head or neck, dehydration, chemical trauma (including acidic foods, drugs, noxious agents, and alcohol), mechanical trauma (such as ill-fitting dentures, braces, endotracheal or nasogastric tubes, and surgery in the oral cavity), taking nothing by mouth for more than 24 hours, ineffective oral hygiene, mouth breathing, malnutrition, infection, lack of or decreased salivation, and medication. See also **nursing diagnosis.**

oral pathology. See **dental pathology.**

oral poliovirus vaccine (OPV), an attenuated preparation of live poliovirus that confers immunity to poliomyelitis. Also called **Sabin vaccine.**

■ INDICATION: It is routinely prescribed for immunization against poliomyelitis.

■ CONTRAINDICATIONS: Immunosuppression, concomitant use of corticosteroids, cancer, immunoglobulin abnormalities, or acute infection prohibits its use.

■ ADVERSE EFFECTS: Adverse effects are uncommon. Cases of vaccine-induced paralytic disease have occurred but are very rare.

oral prophylaxis [L, *oralis,* pertaining to the mouth; Gk, *prophylax,* advance guard], the science and practice of preventing the onset of diseases of the teeth and adjoining mouth tissues.

oral rehydration solutions (ORS) [L, *oralis,* pertaining to the mouth; *re, hydor,* water; *solutus,* dissolved], solutions of electrolytes and glucose used in oral rehydration therapy. The recommended electrolytes include NaCl, KCl, and trisodium citrate.

oral rehydration therapy (ORT), the adjustment of water, glucose, and electrolyte balance in a dehydrated patient by giving fluids with measured amounts of essential ingredients by mouth.

oral sadism, (in psychoanalysis) a sadistic form of oral eroticism, manifested by such behavior as biting, chewing, and other aggressive impulses associated with eating habits. Compare **anal sadism.**

oral stage, (in psychoanalysis) the initial stage of psychosexual development, occurring in the first 12 to 18 months of life when the feeding experience and other oral activities are the predominant source of pleasurable stimulation.

oral surgeon. See **dental surgeon.**

oral surgery [L, *oralis,* pertaining to the mouth; Gk, *cheirourgos,* surgeon], a branch of surgery that is concerned primarily with operations on the jaws and surrounding soft tissues. Also called **maxillofacial surgery.** See also **dental surgeon.**

oral temperature [L, *oralis,* pertaining to the mouth + *temperatura*], the mean body temperature of a normal person as recorded by a clinical thermometer placed in the mouth. It is usually around 99° Fahrenheit or 37° Celsius, but may

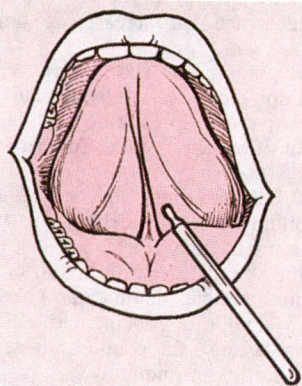

Placement of thermometer for oral temperature measurement
(Potter, 1993)

vary within a fraction of a degree depending on the individual and such factors as time of day, sleep, and exercise and whether measured before or after a meal. See also **normal temperature.**

Orap, a trademark for an oral neuroleptic drug for Tourette's disorder (pimozide).

orb /ôrb/ [L, *orbis,* circle], describing something spherical or globelike.

orbicular /ôbik′yələr/ [L, *orbiculus,* little disk], pertaining to something round.

orbicular bone [L, *orbiculus,* little disk; AS, *ban*], a knob on the end of the long process of the incus that articulates with the stapes.

orbicularis ciliaris /ôrbik′yo͞olär′is/ [L, *orbiculus,* little circle; *cilium,* eyelash], one of the two zones of the ciliary body of the eye, extending from the ora serrata of the retina to the ciliary processes at the margin of the iris. The orbicularis ciliaris is about 4 mm wide and increases in thickness as it approaches the ciliary processes.

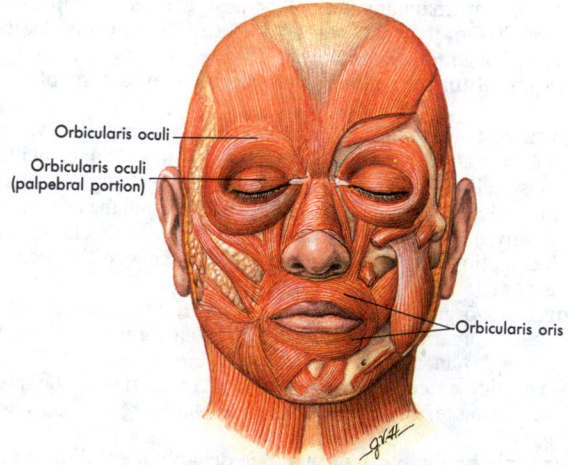

Orbicularis oculi
Orbicularis oculi (palpebral portion)
Orbicularis oris

Muscles of the face: orbicularis oculi and orbicularis oris
(Thibodeau, 1993/John V Hagen)

orbicularis oculi, the muscular body of the eyelid comprising the palpebral, orbital, and lacrimal muscles. It arises from the nasal part of the frontal bone, from the frontal process of the maxilla in front of the lacrimal groove, and from the anterior surface of the medial palpebral ligament. The palpebral muscle functions to close the eyelid gently; the orbital muscle functions to close it more energetically, such as in winking. Also called **orbicularis palpebrarum.** Compare **corrugator supercilii, levator palpebrae superioris.**

orbicularis oris, the muscle surrounding the mouth, consisting partly of fibers derived from other facial muscles, such as the buccinator, that are inserted into the lips, and partly of fibers proper to the lips. It is innervated by buccal branches of the facial nerve and serves to close and purse the lips.

orbicularis palpebrarum. See **orbicularis oculi.**

orbicularis pupillary reflex, a normal phenomenon elicited by forceful closure of the eyelids or attempting to close them while they are held apart, resulting first in constriction and then dilatation of the pupil.

orbit /ôr′bit/ [L, *orbita,* wheel rut], one of a pair of bony, conical cavities in the skull that accommodate the eyeballs and associated structures, such as the eye muscles, the nerves, and the blood vessels. The medial walls of the orbits are approximately parallel with each other and with the middle line, but the lateral walls diverge widely. The roof of each orbit is formed by the orbital plate of the frontal bone and the small wing of the sphenoid bones. The trochlear fovea of the orbital roof accommodates the cartilaginous pulley of the obliquus superior oculi, and the lacrimal fossa in the roof cradles the lacrimal gland. The superior orbital fissure between the roof and the lateral wall of the orbit admits various nerves, such as the oculomotor, trochlear, and ophthalmic division of the trigeminal and the abducent nerves. The openings that communicate with each orbit are the optic foramen, the superior and the inferior orbital fissures, the supraorbital foramen, the infraorbital canal, the anterior and the posterior ethmoidal foramina, the zygomatic foramen, and the canal for the nasolacrimal duct. —**orbital,** *adj.*

orbital aperture /ôr′bitəl/, an opening in the cranium to the orbit of the eye.

orbital fat, a semifluid cushion of fat that lines the bony orbit supporting the eye. Traumatic loss of the fat causes a sunken appearance of the eye. Replacement of the fat by tumor or abnormal tissue may be discovered on ophthalmologic examination. The examiner gently presses on the front of the eyes through the eyelids. Normally each eye may be displaced 0.5 cm into the socket.

orbital fissure [L, *orbita,* wheel track; *fissura,* cleft], the space between the floor and lateral wall of the orbit, serving as a conduit for nerves and blood vessels.

orbital hypertelorism. See **ocular hypertelorism.**

orbital hypotelorism. See **ocular hypotelorism.**

orbital pseudotumor, a specific inflammatory reaction of the orbital tissues of the eye, characterized by exophthalmos and edematous congestion of the eyelids.

orbitomeatal line /ô′bitō′mē·ā′təl/ [L, *orbita,* wheel rut, *meatus,* passage], a positioning line used in radiography of the skull that passes through the outer canthus of the eye and the center of the external auditory meatus.

orcheoplasty. See **orchioplasty.**

orchi-. See **orchio-.**

orchidectomy /ôr′kidek′təmē/ [Gk, *orchis,* testis, *ektome,* excision], a surgical procedure to remove one or both testes. It may be indicated for serious disease or injury to the testis or to control cancer of the prostate by removing a source of androgenic hormones. Also called **orchiectomy.**

orchiditis. See **orchitis.**

orchido-. See **orchio-.**

orchidoplasty. See **orchioplasty.**

orchiectomy. See **orchidectomy.**

orchio-, orchi-, orchido-, a combining form meaning 'of or pertaining to the testes': *orchiocatabasis, orchiopathy, orchioscirrhus.*

orchiopexy /ôr'kē·ōpek'sē/ [Gk, *orchis* + *pexis*, fixation], an operation to mobilize an undescended testis, bring it into the scrotum, and attach it so that it will not retract. Sometimes a suture is attached to the lower scrotum and taped to the inner thigh. The nurse must be careful not to disturb this tension attachment.

orchioplasty /ôr'kē·ōplas'tē/ [Gk, *orchis*, testis; *plassein*, to mold], a surgical procedure involving a testis. Also called **orcheoplasty, orchidoplasty.**

orchis. See **testis.**

orchitis /ôrkī'tis/ [Gk, *orchis* + *itis*, inflammation], inflammation of one or both of the testes, characterized by swelling and pain, often caused by mumps, syphilis, or tuberculosis. Symptomatic treatment includes support and elevation of the scrotum, cold packs, and analgesics. Also called **orchiditis.** –**orchitic,** *adj.*

orciprenaline sulfate. See **metaproterenol sulfate.**

ordered pairs [L, *ordo*, a series; *par*, equal], pertaining to graph coordinates in which the first number of the pair represents a distance along the x (horizontal) axis and the second number is plotted along the y (vertical) axis.

order of procedure, the sequence in which the required steps are taken to complete an operation, such as the preparation and filling of a tooth.

Orem, Dorthea E., author of the Self-Care Nursing Model, a nursing theory introduced in 1959. The Orem theory describes the role of the nurse in giving assistance to a person experiencing inabilities in self-care. The goal of the Orem system is to meet the patient's self-care demands until the family is capable of providing care. The process is divided into three categories: Universal, which consists of self-care to meet physiologic and psychosocial needs; Developmental, the self-care required when one goes through developmental stages; and Health Deviation, the self-care required when one has a deviation from a healthy status. Assessment is made of therapeutic self-care demand, the self-care agency, and self-care deficits in the areas of knowledge, skills, motivation, and orientation. There are three systems for meeting the patient's self-care deficits. They are Wholly Compensatory, in which the patient has no active role; Partly Compensatory, in which the patient and nurse have active roles, and Educative Development, in which patients can meet their need for self-care with some assistance from the nurse.

Oretic, a trademark for a diuretic (hydrochlorothiazide).

Oreticyl, a trademark for an antihypertensive, fixed-combination drug containing a diuretic (hydrochlorothiazide) and an antihypertensive (deserpidine).

Oreton Methyl, a trademark for an androgen (methyltestosterone).

-orexia, a combining form meaning '(condition of the) appetite': *cynorexia, dysorexia, anorexia.*

orexigenic /ôrek'sijen'ik/ [Gk, *orexis*, longing, *genein*, to produce], a substance that increases or stimulates the appetite.

oreximania /ôrek'simā'nē·ə/ [Gk, *orexis* + *mania*, madness], a condition characterized by a greatly increased appetite and excessive eating resulting from an unrealistic or exaggerated fear of becoming thin. Compare **anorexia nervosa.**

orexis /ôrek'sis/ [Gk, longing], 1. desire, appetite. 2. the aspect of the mind involving feeling and striving as contrasted with the intellectual aspect.

orf [AS], a viral skin disease acquired from sheep, characterized by painless vesicles that may progress to red, weeping nodules and, finally, to crusting and healing. Treatment is not necessary because the condition is self-limited, and active infection results in immunity.

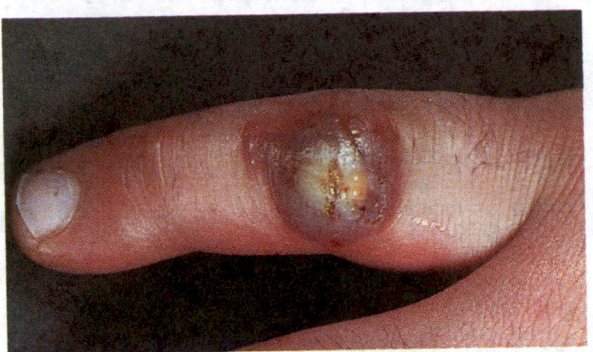

Orf *(du Vivier, 1993)*

organ [Gk, *organon*, instrument], a structural part of a system of the body that is composed of tissues and cells that enable it to perform a particular function, such as the liver, spleen, digestive organs, reproductive organs, or organs of special sense. Each one of the paired organs can function independently of the other. The liver, pancreas, spleen, and brain may maintain normal or near normal function with over 30% of the organ damaged, destroyed, or excised. Also called **organon, organum.**

organ albumin, albumin characteristic of a particular organ.

organelle /ôrgənel'/ [Gk, *organon*, instrument], 1. any one of various particles of living substance bound within most cells, such as the mitochondria, the Golgi complex, the endoplastic reticulum, the lysosomes, and the centrioles. 2. any one of the tiny organs of protozoa associated with locomotion, metabolism, and other processes. Also called **organella.**

organic /ôrgan'ik/ [Gk, *organikos*], 1. any chemical compound containing carbon. Compare **inorganic. 2.** of or pertaining to an organ.

-organic, a combining form meaning 'related to the internal organs of the body': *enorganic, homorganic, psychorganic.*

organic brain syndrome. See **organic mental disorder.**

organic chemistry, the branch of chemistry concerned with the composition, properties, and reactions of chemical compounds containing carbon.

organic disease [Gk, *organikos*; L, *dis*; Fr, *aise*, ease], any disease associated with detectable or observable changes in one or more body organs.

organic dust, dried particles of plants, animals, fungi, or bacteria that are fine enough to be windborne. Many kinds of organic dust cause various respiratory disorders if inhaled. See also **asthma, bagassosis, byssinosis, hay fever.**

organic dust toxic syndrome (ODTS), any nonallergic, noninfectious respiratory illness caused by inhalation of organic dust from moldy silage, hay, or other agricultural products. Symptoms include shaking chills or sweats, cough or shortness of breath, headache, anorexia, and myalgia. See also **farmer's lung, hypersensitivity pneumonitis.**

organic evolution, the theory that all existing forms of animal and plant life have descended with modification from previous, simpler forms or from a single cell; the origin and perpetuation of species.

organic foods, foods that have been produced and processed without the use of commercial chemicals such as fertilizers, pesticides, or synthetic substances that enhance color or flavor.

organic mental disorders (OMD), a class of disorders characterized by progressive deterioration of the mental processes, caused by permanent brain damage or temporary brain dysfunction. Also called **organic brain syndrome.**

organic motivation. See **physiological motivation.**

organic psychosis [Gk, *organikos* + *psyche*, mind + *osis*, condition], a condition characterized by a loss of contact with reality caused by an alteration in brain tissue function.

organic vertigo [Gk, *organikos*, L, *vertigo*, dizziness], vertigo that is associated with a central nervous system disorder, such as cerebellar lesions or tabes dorsalis.

Organisation Mondiale de la Santé. See **World Health Organization.**

organism /ôr′gəniz′əm/ [Gk, *organon*, instrument], an individual living animal or plant able to carry on life functions through mutually dependent organs or organelles.

organization center /ôr′gənīzā′shən/ [Gk, *organon* + *izein*, to cause], a focal point within the developing embryo from which the organism grows and differentiates. In vertebrates this point is the chordamesoderm of the dorsal lip of the blastopore.

organizer /ôr′gənī′zər/ [Gk, *organon* + *izein*, to cause], (in embryology) any part of the embryo that induces mor-

phologic differentiation in some other part. Those parts that are formed and in turn give rise to other parts are classified as organizers of the second degree, third degree, and so on as the embryo develops in complexity. Kinds of organizers include **nucleolar organizer, primary organizer.**

organo- /ôr′gənō-/, a combining form meaning 'of or pertaining to an organ or organs': *organofaction, organogenesis, organoleptic.*

organ of Corti [Gk, *organon*; Alfonso Corti, Italian anatomist, b. 1822], the true organ of hearing, a spiral structure within the cochlea containing hair cells that are stimulated by sound vibrations. The hair cells convert the vibrations into nerve impulses that are transmitted by the cochlear portion of the eighth cranial nerve to the brain. Also called **spiral organ of Corti.** See **basilar membrane.**

organ of Giraldès. See **paradidymis.**

organ of Golgi. See **neurotendinous spindle.**

organogenesis /-jen′əsis/ [Gk, *organon* + *genesis*, origin], (in embryology) the formation and differentiation of organs and organ systems during embryonic development. In humans the period extends from approximately the end of the second week through the eighth week of gestation. During this time the embryo undergoes rapid growth and differentiation and is extremely vulnerable to environmental hazards and toxic substances. Any interference with the sequential processes involved with organogenesis causes an arrest in development and results in one or more congenital anomalies. Also called **organogeny.** See also **embryologic development, prenatal development. –organogenetic,** *adj.*

organoid /ôr′gənoid/ [Gk, *organon* + *eidos*, form], **1.** resembling an organ. **2.** any structure that resembles an organ in appearance or function, specifically an abnormal tumor mass. **3.** See **organelle.**

organoid neoplasm, a growth that resembles a body organ. Compare **histoid neoplasm.**

organoid tumor. See **teratoma.**

organomegaly /-meg′əlē/ [Gk, *organon*, instrument; *megas*, large], abnormal enlargement of an organ, particularly an organ of the abdominal cavity.

organon. See **organ.**

organophosphates /-fos′fāts/, a class of anticholinesterase chemicals used in certain pesticides and medications.

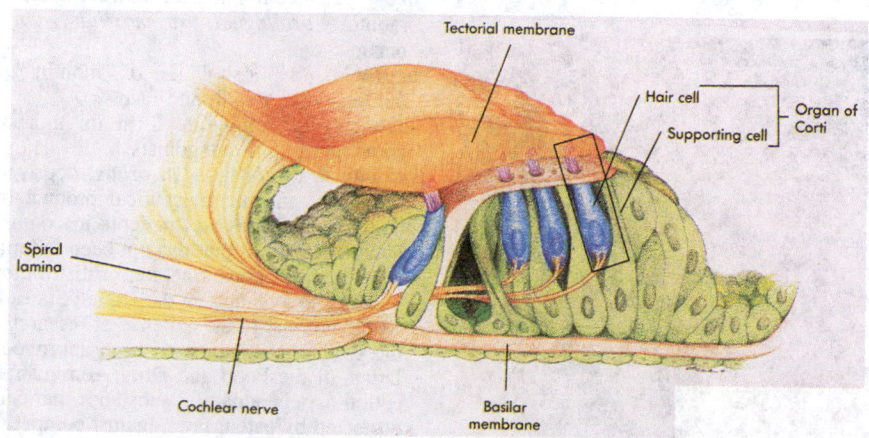

Organ of Corti (Seeley, 1992/Lisa Chuck/Michael Schenk)

They act by causing irreversible inhibition of cholinesterase.

organotherapy /-ther′əpē/ [Gk, *organon* + *therapeia*, treatment], the treatment of disease by administering animal endocrine glands or their extracts. Whole glands are no longer implanted, but substances derived from animal organs are widely used. Also called **Brown-Séquard's treatment.** –**organotherapeutic,** *adj.*

organotypic growth /ôr′gənōtip′ik/ [Gk, *organon* + *typos*, mark], the controlled reproduction of cells, such as occurs in the normal growth of tissues and organs. Compare **histiotypic growth.**

organ specificity, a substance or activity that is identified with a specific organ. The term is commonly applied to enzymes that function in particular organ systems.

organum. See **organ.**

orgasm /ôr′gasəm/ [Gk, *orgein*, to be lustful], the sexual climax, a series of strong, involuntary contractions of the muscles of the genitalia experienced as exceedingly pleasurable, set off by sexual excitation of critical intensity. –**orgasmic,** *adj.*

orgasmic maturity /ôrgas′mik/, the physiologic maturity of the reproductive system that enables the individual to complete the adult sexual response cycle.

orgasmic platform [Gk, *orgein;* Fr, *plate-forme,* a flat form], congestion of the lower vagina during sexual intercourse.

orient /ôr′ē·ənt/ [L, *oriens*, rising sun], 1. to make someone aware of new surroundings, including people and their roles, the layout of a facility, and its routines, rules, and services. New patients are oriented to a hospital as are new staff to a hospital unit. 2. to help a person become aware of a situation or simply of reality, such as when a patient recovers from anesthesia. –**orientation,** *n.,* **oriented,** *adj.*

oriental sore /ôr′ē·en′təl/ [L, *oriens* + AS, *sar*, painful], a dermatologic disease caused by the parasite *Leishmania tropica,* transmitted to humans by the bite of the sand fly. This form of leishmaniasis, characterized by ulcerative lesions, occurs primarily in Africa, Asia, and some Mediterranean countries. Oriental sore causes no systemic symptoms, but the sores are susceptible to secondary infections. Treatment options include infrared therapy and injection of

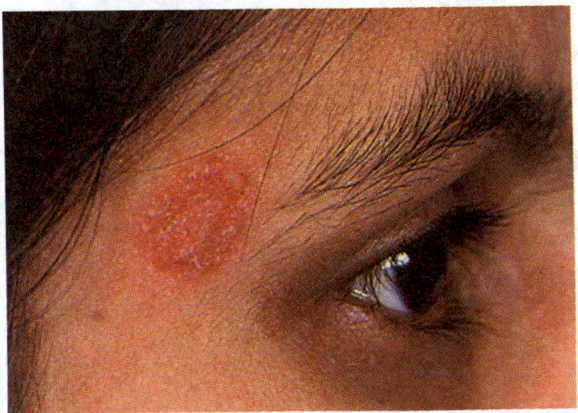

Oriental sore (Cerio, 1992)

ulcers with sodium antimony gluconate. Also called **Aleppo boil, cutaneous leishmaniasis, Delhi boil, Old World leishmaniasis, tropical sore.** See also **leishmaniasis.**

orientation /ôr′ē·əntā′shən/ [L, *oriens* + *itio*, process], 1. (in molecular genetics) the insertion of a fragment of genetic material into a vector so that the placement of the fragment is in the same direction as the genetic map of the vector (the n orientation) or in the opposite direction (the u orientation). 2. (in psychiatry) the awareness of one's physical environment with regard to time, place, and the identity of other people; the ability to adapt to such an existing or new environment. Disorientation is usually a symptom of organic brain disease and most psychoses.

orifice /ôr′ifis/ [L, *orificium*, opening], the entrance or the outlet of any cavity in the body. Also called **ostium.** –**orificial,** *adj.*

ori gene /ôr′ē/, (in molecular genetics) the site or region in which DNA replication starts.

origin /ôr′ijin/ [L, *origo*, source], the more fixed end of a muscle attachment. Compare **insertion.**

Orimune, a trademark for an active immunizing agent (live oral poliovirus vaccine).

Orinase, a trademark for an oral sulfanylurea antidiabetic (tolbutamide).

Ornade, a trademark for a fixed-combination drug containing an adrenergic decongestant (phenylpropanolamine hydrochloride), an antihistamine (chlorpheniramine maleate), and an anticholinergic (isopropamide iodide), used for the relief of symptoms of upper respiratory tract congestion.

ornithine /ôr′nithēn/, an amino acid, not a constituent of proteins, that is produced as an important intermediate substance in the urea cycle. It is formed by the hydrolization of arginine by arginase and is subsequently converted into citrulline. It decomposes by losing carbon dioxide, producing putrescine and a strong, foul odor characteristic of decaying animal tissue. Also called **diaminovaleric acid.**

ornithine carbamoyl transferase, an enzyme in the blood that increases in patients with liver and other diseases. Its normal concentrations in serum are 8 to 20 mIU/ml.

ornithine cycle. See **urea cycle.**

Ornithodoros /ôr′nithod′ərəs/ [Gk, *ornis*, bird, *doros*, leather bag], a genus of ticks, some species of which are vectors for the spirochetes of relapsing fevers.

ornithosis. See **psittacosis.**

oro-, 1. a combining form meaning 'of or pertaining to the mouth': *orolingual, oromaxillary, oropharynx.* 2. see **orrho-.**

orofacial /ôr′ōfā′shəl/ [L, *os*, mouth; *facies*, face], pertaining to the mouth and face.

-orphan, a combining form for morphinan-derived narcotic agonists or antagonists.

orphan drug /ôr′fən/ [L, *orbus*, deprived of parents; ME, *drogge*], any pharmaceutical product that may be available to physicians and patients in countries other than the United States but that has not been 'adopted' by a domestic pharmaceutical manufacturer or distributor. An orphan drug may not be available in the United States because total sales would not justify the expense of research and development, the product may not have been approved by the Bureau of Drugs of the Food and Drug Administration, or the medication may be a natural substance that cannot be effectively protected by patent laws against competition from a similar form of the product. Many orphan drugs are pharmaceutical products developed in Europe or Asia but were not available in the United States until several years later. The U.S. Orphan Drug Act of 1983 offers federal financial incentives to commercial and nonprofit organizations to develop and market drugs previously unavailable in the United States.

orphan virus [Gk, *orphanos,* without parents; L, *virus,* poison], a virus that has been isolated and identified although it has not been associated with any particular disease.

oropharynx /ôr′ōfer′ingks/ [L, *os,* mouth; Gk, *pharynx,* throat], one of the three anatomic divisions of the pharynx. It extends behind the mouth from the soft palate above to the level of the hyoid bone below and contains the palatine tonsils and the lingual tonsils. Compare **laryngopharynx, nasopharynx.** —**oropharyngeal,** *adj.*

Oroya fever. See **bartonellosis.**

orphenadrine citrate /ôrfen′ədrēn/, a skeletal muscle relaxant with anticholinergic and antihistaminic activity.

■ INDICATION: It is prescribed in the treatment of severe muscle strain.

■ CONTRAINDICATIONS: Myasthenia gravis, contraindications of anticholinergic agents, or known hypersensitivity to this drug prohibits its use.

■ ADVERSE EFFECTS: Among the most serious adverse reactions are those associated with anticholinergic activity, such as dry mouth and tachycardia, and allergic reactions.

orphenadrine hydrochloride, an anticholinergic and antihistaminic agent.

■ INDICATION: It is prescribed in the treatment of parkinsonism.

■ CONTRAINDICATIONS: Myasthenia gravis or another condition that contraindicates the use of anticholinergic agents or a known sensitivity to this drug prohibits its use.

■ ADVERSE EFFECTS: Among the most serious adverse reactions are anticholinergic side effects and allergic reactions.

-orrhagia, -rrhagia, -rrhage, a suffix meaning 'pertaining to excessive flow': *metrorrhagia, hemorrhage.*

-orrhea, -rrhea, a suffix meaning 'relating to flow or discharge': *rhinorrhea, galactorrhea.*

-orrhexis, -rrhexis, a suffix meaning 'to rupture': *angiorrhexis, enterorrexis.*

orrho-, oro-, a combining form meaning 'of or pertaining to blood serum': *orrhomeningitis, orrhoreaction, orrhorrhea.*

ORS, abbreviation for **oral rehydration solutions.**

ORT, abbreviation for **oral rehydration therapy.**

orthetist. See **orthotist.**

ortho, abbreviation for *orthopedic.*

ortho- /ôr′thə-/, a combining form meaning 'straight, normal, correct': *orthobiosis, orthodontist, orthotopic.*

orthoboric acid. See **boric acid.**

orthoclase ceramic feldspar /ôr′thəklās/ [Gk, *orthos,* straight, *klassis,* breaking; *keramikos,* pottery], a plentiful clay in the solid crust of the earth, used as a filler and to give body to fused dental porcelain. Compare **feldspar.**

Orthoclone OKT3, a trademark for an immunosuppressant drug (muromonab-CD3).

orthodontia. See **orthodontics.**

orthodontic appliance /-don′tik/ [Gk, *orthos* + *odous,* tooth], any device used to modify tooth position. Kinds of such appliances are fixed, movable, active, retaining, intraoral, and extraoral.

orthodontic band, a thin metal ring, usually made of stainless steel, fitted over a tooth for securing orthodontic attachments to a tooth.

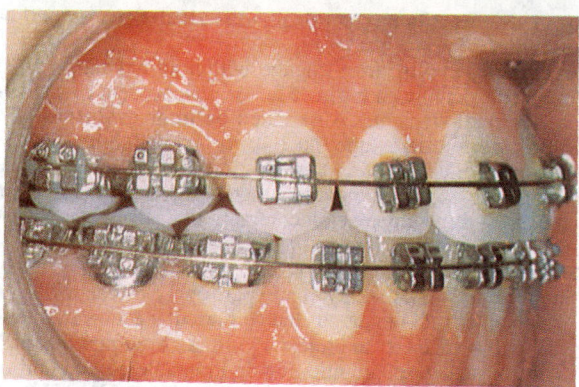

Fixed orthodontic appliance *(Bennett, 1993)*

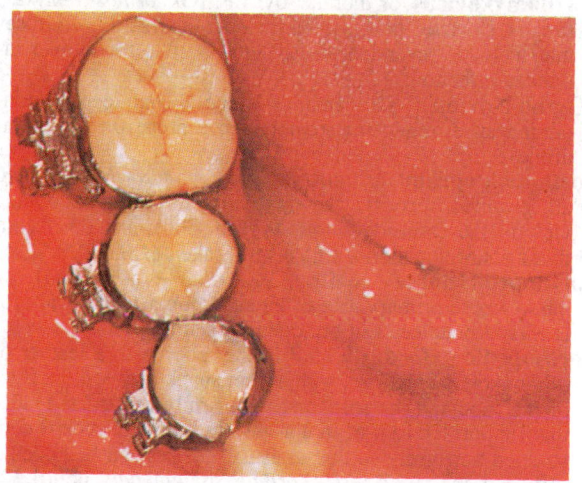

Orthodontic band *(Bennett, 1993)*

orthodontics /ôr′thədon′tiks/ [Gk, *orthos* + *odous,* tooth], the specialty of dentistry concerned with the diagnosis and treatment of malocclusion and irregularities of the teeth.

orthodontist /-don′tist/, a practitioner of the branch of dentistry that is concerned with the diagnosis, prevention, and correction of malocclusion of the teeth.

orthodromic conduction /ôr′thədrom′ik/ [Gk, *orthos* + *dromos,* course; L, *conducere,* to connect], the conduction of a neural impulse in the normal direction, from a synaptic junction or a receptor forward along an axon to its termination with depolarization. Compare **antidromic conduction.**

orthogenesis /ôr′thəjen′əsis/ [Gk, *orthos* + *genesis,* origin], the theory that evolution is controlled by intrinsic factors within the organism and progresses according to a predetermined course rather than in several directions as a result of natural selection and other environmental factors. —**orthogenetic,** *adj.*

orthogenic /-jen′ik/ [Gk, *orthos* + *genein,* to produce], **1.** of or pertaining to orthogenesis; orthogenetic. **2.** of or pertaining to the treatment and rehabilitation of children who are mentally or emotionally disturbed. See also **ortho-psychiatry.**

orthogenic evolution, change within an animal or plant induced solely by an intrinsic factor, independent of any environmental elements. Also called **bathmic evolution.**

orthokinetic cuff /-kinet'ik/ [Gk, *orthos,* straight; *kinesis,* movement; ME, *cuffe*], an elastic covering for a muscle to provide tactile stimulation that will induce contraction and at the same time restrict contraction of an opposing muscle.

orthokinetics /-kinet'iks/ [Gk, *orthos,* straight; *kinesis,* movement], **1.** therapy for hypertrophic osteoarthritis in which an effort is made to change muscular action from one group to another set to protect a joint. **2.** a therapy for spasticity by using an orthotic device to enable contraction of one muscle while inhibiting its antagonist. **3.** the effect of gravity on the brownian movement as manifested by the movement of particles in the same direction in sedimentation.

orthomyxovirus /ôr'thəmik'sōvī'rəs/ [Gk, *orthos* + *mykes,* fungus; L, *virus,* poison], a member of a family of viruses that includes several organisms responsible for human influenza infection.

Ortho-Novum, a trademark for an oral contraceptive containing an estrogen (mestranol) and a progestin (norethindrone).

orthopantogram /ôr'thəpan'təgram/ [Gk, *orthos* + *pan,* all, *gramma,* record], an x-ray film showing a panoramic view of the entire dentition, alveolar bone, and other contiguous structures on a single film, taken extraorally.

orthopedic nurse /-pē'dik/ [Gk, *orthos* + *pais* child], a nurse whose primary area of interest, competence, and professional practice is in orthopedic nursing.

orthopedic oxford, a hard leather shoe with a leather or rubber sole, sometimes with a steel shank between the floor of the shoe and the sole, and with firmly constructed sides that support the foot in an upright position. The shoe is constructed uniformly so that assistive devices can be added.

orthopedics /-pē'diks/ [Gk, *orthos,* straight; *pais,* child], a branch of medicine that is concerned with the prevention and correction of disorders of the locomotor system of the body, including the skeleton, muscles, joints, and related tissues.

orthopedic surgery [Gk, *orthos,* straight; *pais,* child; *cheirourgos,* surgeon], the branch of medicine that is concerned with the treatment of the musculoskeletal system mainly by manipulative and operative methods.

orthopedic traction, a procedure in which a patient is maintained in a device attached by ropes and pulleys to weights that exert a pulling force on an extremity or body part while countertraction is maintained. Traction is applied most often to reduce and immobilize fractures, but it also is used to overcome muscle spasm, to stretch adhesions, to correct certain deformities, and to help release arthritic contractures. Traction may be applied directly to the skin by attaching the rope-pulley-weight system to bands of adhesive, moleskin, or foam rubber or to a splint affixed to the affected limb; side arm traction is a kind of skin traction used to align a fractured humerus after open reduction. Skeletal traction is exerted directly on a bone in which a wire or pin is inserted under anesthesia in the open reduction of a fracture; the ends of the pin protruding through the skin on both sides of the bone are covered with corks and attached to a metal U-shaped spreader or bow, which in turn is attached to the traction rope. Skin or skeletal traction applied to a lower extremity by a balanced suspension apparatus, such as the Thomas splint and Pearson's attachment, permits the patient to move more freely in bed because the leg is balanced with countertraction and any slack in traction caused by the patient's movements is taken up by the suspension apparatus. Bryant's traction for treating fractures of the femur shaft in young children uses a suspension apparatus to hold the youngster's legs at right angles to the body. A girdle that fits over the iliac crests and pelvis is used in the application of traction to relieve low back pain, and a cervical halter is employed in applying traction to reduce neck pain; cervical traction also may be used when a fracture of the cervical spine is suspected. See specific devices and specific kinds of traction.

▪ METHOD: To maintain the required constant pull, the traction ropes are kept taut, free to ride over the pulleys, and securely tied to the weights that hang free—away from the bed and off the floor. Countertraction is maintained by elevating the patient's bed under the body part to which traction is applied and exerting a pull in the opposite direction; a chest restraint sheet may be applied to the patient in side arm traction for countertraction if necessary. During the initial stages of traction, the involved extremity is checked every 2 hours for quality of the distal pulse, color, warmth, motion, sensation, pain, and swelling. Blood pressure, temperature, pulse, and respirations are recorded every 4 hours until stable. Pain is controlled and the patient is positioned as ordered. If the patient is in balanced suspension, abduction of the leg and a 20-degree angle between the thigh and bed are maintained; the heel is kept free of the sling under the calf. A harness restraint is used to prevent a child in Bryant's traction from turning over, and the youngster's buttocks are raised slightly from the mattress. Bed linen is changed only as necessary, and an air mattress is used when required. Every 2 hours the patient is helped to cough and deep breathe; bony prominences are massaged, but vigorous rubbing is avoided. Lotion is applied to the skin, which is periodically inspected for signs of redness, abrasions, blisters, dryness, itching, excoriation, and pressure areas; special attention is given to the pin insertion sites of the patient in skeletal traction. The patient is observed every 4 hours for neurologic signs, such as tingling, numbness, and loss of sensation or motion; for thrombophlebitis in the involved extremity; and for evidence of a pulmonary blood clot or fat embolus, such as indicated by decreased breath sounds, fever, tachypnea, diaphoresis, anxiety, pallor, bloody or purulent sputum, and tachycardia. Oral hygiene is administered every 4 hours, and, unless contraindicated, a daily intake of 2500 to 3000 ml of fluids is encouraged. As the patient's condition improves, the position is changed every 4 hours; if the kind of traction permits and if the upper extremities are not involved, a trapeze is added to the bed. The patient is taught to perform range-of-motion exercises with the uninvolved extremities, dorsiflexion and plantar flexion of the ankles, and isometric exercises, such as gluteal and abdominal contraction. A high-protein, low-carbohydrate diet is served, and vitamin and iron therapy may be ordered. The immobilized patient uses a flat, fracture bedpan and usually requires stool softeners or a mild laxative.

▪ NURSING INTERVENTION: The patient in traction often needs extensive physical care and emotional support. The person is encouraged to verbalize feelings and concerns about prolonged hospitalization and absence from work or school. To the greatest degree possible, the nurse encourages the patient to participate in self-care and to engage in diversions, such as handicrafts, reading, watching television, and listening to the radio.

■ OUTCOME CRITERIA: The healthy young adult or adolescent in traction for the treatment of a fracture usually has an uneventful recovery, but diligent attention and nursing care are necessary to avoid the formation of decubitus ulcers, infection, constipation, kidney stones, and other sequelae of immobility.

orthopedist /-pēdist/, a specialist in orthopedics. Also called (informal) **orthopod.**

orthopnea /ôrthop′nē·ə/ [Gk, orthos + pnoia, breath]], an abnormal condition in which a person must sit or stand to breathe deeply or comfortably. It occurs in many disorders of the cardiac and respiratory systems, such as asthma, pulmonary edema, emphysema, pneumonia, and angina pectoris. See also **dyspnea.** **—orthopneic,** adj.

orthopneic position /ôr′thopnē′ik/ [Gk, orthos, straight; pnoia, breath; L, positio], a body position that enables a patient to breathe comfortably. Usually, it is one in which the patient is sitting up and is bent forward, with the arms supported on a table or chair arms. Also called **orthopnea posture.**

orthopod. See **orthopedist.**

orthopsychiatry /-sīkī′ətrē/ [Gk, orthos + psyche, mind, iatreia, treatment], the branch of psychiatry that specializes in correcting incipient and borderline mental and behavioral disorders, especially in children, and in developing preventive techniques to promote mental health and emotional growth and development. See also **mental hygiene.**

orthoptic /ôrthop′tik/ [Gk, orthos + ops, eye], **1.** of or pertaining to normal binocular vision. **2.** of or pertaining to a procedure or technique for correcting the visual axes of eyes improperly coordinated for binocular vision.

orthoptic examination, an ophthalmoscopic examination of the binocular function of the eyes. A stereoscopic instrument presents a slightly different picture to each eye. The examiner notes the degree to which the pictures are combined by the normal process of fusion. If the person has diplopia, separate pictures are seen. If the person has suppression amblyopia, only one picture is seen. Stereoscopic training may improve binocular vision in some conditions.

orthoptic training [Gk, orthos, straight; ops, eye; ME, trainen], a type of therapy for correction of squint or other ocular muscle disorders by the use of eye exercises.

orthoptist /ôrthop′tist/ [Gk, orthos + ops, eye], a person qualified by postsecondary training and successful completion of an examination by the American Orthoptist Council who, under the supervision of an ophthalmologist, tests eye muscles and teaches exercise programs designed to correct eye coordination defects.

orthoscopy /ôrthos′kəpē/ [Gk, orthos, straight; skopein, to view], the use of an **orthoscope** /ôr′thəskōp′/ for examining the fundus of the eye.

orthosis /ôrthō′sis/ [Gk, orthos, straight], a force system designed to control, correct, or compensate for a bone deformity, deforming forces, or forces absent from the body. Orthosis often involves the use of special braces. **—orthotic** /ôrthot′ik/, adj., n.

orthostatic /-stat′ik/ [Gk, orthos + statikos, standing], pertaining to an erect or standing position.

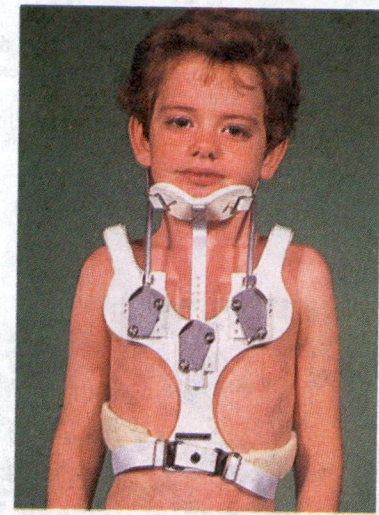

Orthosis (Houghton, 1989)

orthostatic albuminuria. See **orthostatic proteinuria.**

orthostatic hypotension, abnormally low blood pressure occurring when an individual assumes the standing posture. Also called **postural hypotension.**

orthostatic proteinuria, presence of protein in the urine of some people, especially teenagers who have been standing for a long period. It disappears when they recline and is of no pathologic significance. Also called **orthostatic albuminuria, postural albuminuria, postural proteinuria.**

orthotic /ôrthot′ik/ [Gk, orthos, straight], pertaining to **orthosis.**

orthotics /ôrthot′iks/ [Gk, orthos, straight], the design and use of external appliances to support a paralyzed muscle, promote a specific motion, or correct musculoskeletal deformities.

orthotist /ôr′thətist/ [Gk, orthos, straight], a person who designs, fabricates, and fits braces or other orthopedic appliances prescribed by physicians. A certified orthotist is one who successfully completed the examination of the American Orthotist and Prosthetic Association. Also spelled **orthetist.**

orthotonos /ôrthot′ənəs/ [Gk, orthos + tonos, tension], a straight, rigid posture of the body caused by a tetanic spasm, usually resulting from strychnine poisoning or tetanus infection. The neck and all other parts of the body are in a position of extension but not as severely as in opisthotonos. Compare **emprosthotonos.**

orthovoltage /-vōl′tij/ [Gk, orthos, straight; Count Alessandro Volta], the voltage range of 100 to 350 KeV supplied by some x-ray generators used for radiation therapy. They have been replaced in many hospitals and other health facilities by equipment that operates in the megavolt range.

Ortolani sign /ôr′təlä′nē/, an audible click heard in a test for a congenital dislocated hip. It is noted in infancy when the hip goes into the socket. Also called **Ortolani click.**

Ortolani's test [Marius Ortolani, twentieth century Italian surgeon; L, testum, crucible], a procedure used to evaluate the stability of the hip joints in newborns and infants. The baby is placed on his back, and the hips and knees are flexed at right angles and abducted until the lateral aspects of the knees are touching the table. The examiner's fingers are extended along the outside of the thighs, with the thumbs grasping the insides of the knees. Internal and external rotation are attempted, and symmetry of mobility is evaluated. A click or a popping sensation (Ortolani's sign) may be felt if the joint is unstable, because the head of the femur moves out of the acetabulum under pressure from the examiner's hands during rotation and abduction. See also **congenital dislocation of the hip.**

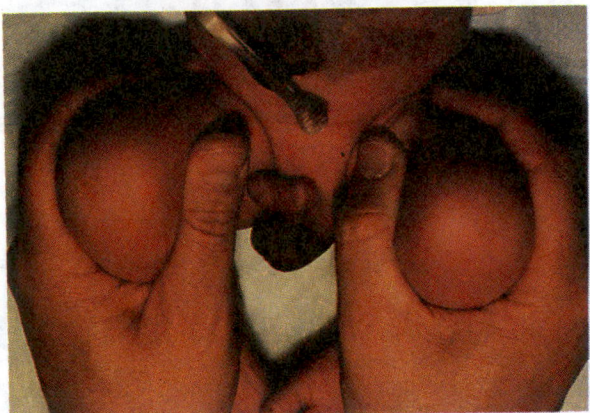

Ortolani's test *(Zitelli, 1992)*

Orudis, a trademark for a nonsteroidal antiinflammatory agent (ketoprofen).

-ory, a suffix that means 'pertaining to, function of, process of': *mammory, sensory.*

os. See **bone.**

Os, symbol for the element **osmium.**

OS, **1.** abbreviation for *oculus sinister,* a Latin phrase meaning 'left eye.' **2.** abbreviation for a computer **operating system.**

-os, a suffix signaling singular nouns: *biologos, hepatomphalos, megophthalmos.*

Osborne and Cotterill procedure, a surgical method of correcting a chronic dislocated elbow by the use of capsular reefing, the folding in or overlapping of soft tissue by surgical suture to make the structure tighter.

osc, **1.** abbreviation for **oscillator. 2.** abbreviation for **oscilloscope.**

os calcis. See **calcaneus.**

os capitatum. See **capitate bone.**

oscheo-, a combining form meaning 'of or pertaining to the scrotum': *oscheocele, oscheolith, oscheoma.*

oscillation /os'ilā'shən/ [L, *oscillare,* to swing], **1.** a back and forth motion. **2.** vibration or the effects of a mechanical or electrical vibrator.

oscillator (osc) /os'ilā'tər/ [L, *oscillare,* to swing], an electric or other device that produces oscillations, vibrations, or fluctuations, such as an alternating electric current generator.

oscilloscope (osc) /osil'əskōp/ [L, *oscillare,* to swing; Gk, *skopein,* to look], an instrument that displays a visual representation of electric variations on the fluorescent screen of a cathode ray tube. The graphic representation is produced by a beam of electrons on the screen. The beam is focused or directed by a magnetic field that is influenced in turn by a source such as an amplified current produced by heart contractions. As used in cardiology, the oscilloscope can function as a continuous electrocardiogram.

os coxae. See **innominate bone.**

os cuboideum. See **cuboid bone.**

-ose, **1.** a suffix meaning a 'carbohydrate': *cellulose, lactose, sucrose.* **2.** a suffix meaning a 'primary product of hydrolysis': *albumose, nucleose, myoproteose.*

Osgood osteotomy /oz'gŏŏd/, a surgical procedure for correction of malrotation of a femur.

Osgood-Schlatter disease /-shlat'ər/ [Robert B. Osgood, American surgeon, b. 1873; Carl Schlatter, Swiss surgeon, b. 1864], inflammation or partial separation of the tibial tubercle caused by chronic irritation, usually as a result of overuse of the quadriceps muscle. The condition is seen primarily in muscular, athletic adolescent boys and is characterized by swelling and tenderness over the tibial tubercle that increase with exercise or any activity that extends the leg. Treatment consists primarily of preventing further irritation during the healing process and may necessitate complete immobilization of the knee in a cast. Any residual nonunion of a proximal fragment after healing may require surgical excision. Also called **Osgood's disease, Schlatter-Osgood disease, Schlatter's disease.**

OSHA /ō'shä/, abbreviation for *Occupational Safety and Health Administration.*

os hamatum. See **hamate bone.**

os hyoideum. See **hyoid bone.**

-osis, **1.** a suffix meaning a '(specified) action, process, or result': *homeosis, narcosis, zygosis.* **2.** a suffix meaning 'increase in a pathologic condition': *calcicosis, psittacosis, varicosis.*

Osler's disease. See **Osler-Weber-Rendu syndrome, polycythemia.**

Osler's nodes /ōs'lərz/ [Sir William Osler, American-British physician, b. 1849], tender, reddish or purplish subcutaneous nodules of the soft tissue on the ends of fingers or toes, seen in subacute bacterial endocarditis and usually lasting only 1 or 2 days. The nodes represent bacterial embolisms from the infected heart valve.

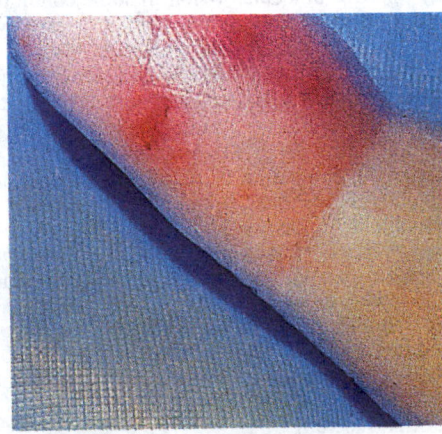

Osler nodes *(Zitelli, 1992; Courtesy Dr JF John, Jr)*

Osler-Weber-Rendu syndrome /ōs′lərweb′ərandōō′/ [Sir William Osler; Frederick P. Weber, British physician, b. 1863; Henri J.L.M. Rendu, French physician, b. 1844], a vascular anomaly, inherited as an autosomal dominant trait, characterized by hemorrhagic telangiectasia of skin and mucosa. Small red-to-violet lesions are found on the lips, the oral and nasal mucosa, the tongue, and the tips of fingers and toes. The thin, dilated vessels may bleed spontaneously or as a result of only minor trauma, and this condition becomes progressively severe. Bleeding from superficial lesions is often profuse and may result in severe anemia. No specific treatment is known, but accessible, bleeding lesions may be treated with pressure, styptics, and topical hemostatics. Transfusions may be indicated for acute hemorrhage, and iron deficiency anemia may require continuous treatment. Also called **hemorrhagic familial angiomatosis, hereditary hemorrhagic telangiectasia, Rendu-Osler-Weber syndrome.**

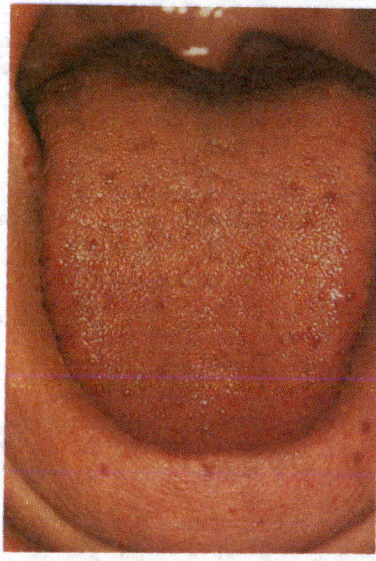

Osler-Weber-Rendu syndrome (Lamey, 1988)

os lunatum. See **lunate bone.**
osm, 1. abbreviation for **osmosis. 2.** abbreviation for **osmotic.**
os magnum. See **capitate bone.**
osmethesia /os′məthē′zhə/ [Gk, osme, smell, aisthesis, feeling], the ability to perceive and distinguish odors; the sense of smell.
-osmia, a suffix meaning '(condition of the) sense of smell': dysosmia, hemianosmia, merosmia.
osmium (Os) /oz′mē·əm/ [Gk, osme, smell], a hard, grayish, pungent-smelling metallic element. Its atomic number is 76; its atomic weight is 190.2. Used to produce alloys of extreme hardness, it is highly toxic.
osmo- /oz′mō-/, **1.** a prefix meaning 'of or pertaining to odors': osmoceptor, osmodysphoria, osmonosology. **2.** a combining form meaning 'pertaining to an impulse, or to osmosis': osmophilic, osmosology, osmotaxis.
osmoceptors /-sep′tərz/ [Gk, osme + L, recipere, to re-

ceive], receptors in the hypothalamus that respond to osmotic pressure, thereby regulating production of the antidiuretic hormone.
osmol. See **osmole.**
osmolal gap /ozmōl′əl/, a difference between the observed and calculated osmolalities in serum analysis. The calculated osmolar values include sodium concentration multiplied by 2, plus glucose and blood urea nitrogen.
osmolality /oz′mōlal′itē/, the osmotic pressure of a solution expressed in osmols or milliosmols per kilogram of water. Normal adult blood osmolality is 285 to 295 mOsm/kg H_2O. Compare **osmolarity.**
osmolar /osmō′lər/, of or pertaining to the osmotic characteristics of a solution of one or more molecular substances, ionic substances, or both, expressed in osmols or milliosmols.
osmolarity /oz′mōler′itē/, the osmotic pressure of a solution expressed in osmols or milliosmols per kilogram of the solution. Compare **osmolality.**
osmole /os′mōl/ [Gk, osmos, impulse, osis, condition + mole, (molecule)], the quantity of a substance in solution in the form of molecules, ions, or both (usually expressed in grams) that has the same osmotic pressure as one mole of an ideal nonelectrolyte. Also spelled **osmol.** **−osmolal,** adj.
osmology /ozmol′əjē/ [Gk, osme, odor; osmos, impulse; logos, science], **1.** the science of the sense of smell and the production and composition of odors. **2.** the branch of science that is concerned with osmosis.
osmometry /ozmom′ətrē/ [Gk, osmos, impulse, metron, measure], the field of study that deals with the phenomenon of osmosis and the measurement of osmotic forces. **−osmometric,** adj.
Osmone-Clarke procedure, a therapy for talipes valgus. It involves soft tissue release of the medial and lateral foot with peroneous brevis tendon transfer.
osmoreceptor /-risep′tər/ [Gk, osmos, impulse; L, recipere, to receive], **1.** a neuron in the hypothalamus that is sensitive to the fluid concentration in the blood plasma and regulates the secretion of antidiuretic hormone. **2.** a receptor of smell stimuli.
osmoregulation /-reg′yəlā′shən/ [Gk, osmos, impulse; L, regula, rule], the act of influencing or controlling the speed and extent of osmosis.

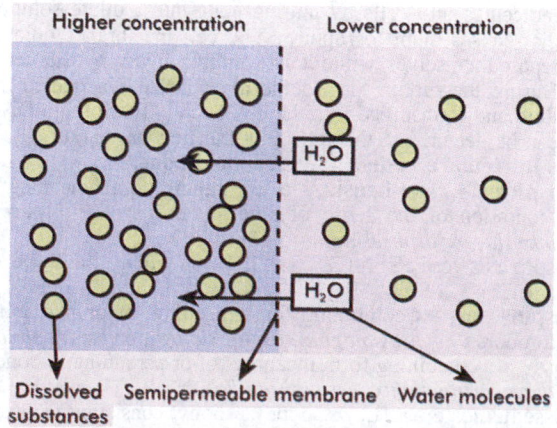

Higher concentration   Lower concentration

Dissolved substances   Semipermeable membrane   Water molecules

Osmosis (Potter, 1993)

osmosis (osm) /ozmō′sis, os-/ [Gk, *osmos*, impulse, *osis*, condition], the movement of a pure solvent, such as water, through a semipermeable membrane from a solution that has a lower solute concentration to one that has a higher solute concentration. The membrane is impermeable to the solute but is permeable to the solvent. The rate of osmosis depends on the concentration of solute, the temperature of the solution, the electric charge of the solute, and the difference between the osmotic pressures exerted by the solutions. Movement across the membrane continues until the concentrations of the solutions equalize. —**osmotic (osm)** /ozmot′ik/, *adj.*

osmotic diarrhea, a form of diarrhea associated with water retention in the bowel resulting from an accumulation of nonabsorbable water-soluble solutes. An excessive intake of hexitols, sorbitol, and mannitol (used as sugar substitutes in candies, chewing gum, and dietetic foods) can result in slow absorption and rapid small intestine motility, leading to osmotic diarrhea. The severity of the condition varies directly with the amount of such sugar substitutes consumed and diminishes when intake is reduced. Also called **chewing gum diarrhea, dietetic food diarrhea.**

osmotic diuresis, diuresis resulting from the presence of certain nonabsorbable substances in tubules of the kidney, such as mannitol, urea, or glucose.

osmotic fragility, a sensitivity to changes in osmotic pressure characteristic of red blood cells. Exposed to a hypotonic concentration of sodium in solution, red cells take in increasing quantities of water, swell until the capacity of the cell membrane is exceeded, and burst. Exposed to a hypertonic concentration of sodium in a solution, red cells give up intracellular fluid, shrink, and break up. Laboratory findings of exceptional fragility or resistance may be diagnostic of certain conditions. Hemolysis of normal cells begins in 0.39% to 0.45% salt solution and is complete in 0.30% to 0.33% salt solution in 24 hours at 37° C.

osmotic pressure, 1. the pressure exerted on a semipermeable membrane separating a solution from a solvent, the membrane being impermeable to the solutes in the solution and permeable only to the solvent. 2. the pressure exerted on a semipermeable membrane by a solution containing one or more solutes that cannot penetrate the membrane, which is permeable only by the solvent surrounding it. See also **osmosis.**

osmotic transfection, a method of inserting foreign DNA molecules into cells by putting cells into a dilute solution that causes them to rupture. The cell membranes quickly repair themselves without irreversible injury to the cells. During the rupture period the alien DNA is added to the fluid and is absorbed into the cell nuclei. The foreign DNA can be detected in the cells as a transfection marker.

os naviculare pedis. See **scaphoid bone.**

-osphresia, -osphrasia, a combining form meaning a 'condition of the sense of smell': *anosphresia, hyperosphresia, oxyosphresia.*

osphresis /osfrē′sis/ [Gk, smell], olfaction; the sense of smell.

osphresio-, a combining form meaning 'of or pertaining to odors': *osphresiolagnia, osphresiology, osphresiophilia.*

oss-, a combining form meaning 'of or pertaining to bone': *osseocartilaginous, ossicle, ossific.*

osseous /os′ē·əs/ [L, *os*, bone], bony; consisting of or resembling bone.

osseous labyrinth [L, *os*, bone; Gk, *labyrinthos*, maze], the bony portion of the internal ear, composed of three cavities: the vestibule, the semicircular canals, and the cochlea, transmitting sound vibrations from the middle ear to the eighth cranial nerve. All three cavities contain perilymph, in which a membranous labyrinth is suspended. Also called **labyrinthus osseus.** Compare **membranous labyrinth.**

ossicle /os′ikəl/ [L, *ossiculum*, little bone], a small bone, such as the malleus, the incus, or the stapes, which are ossicles of the middle ear. —**ossicular,** *adj.*

ossiferous /osif′ərəs/ [L, *os*, bone; *ferre*, to bear], pertaining to the formation of bone or bone tissue.

ossification /os′ifikā′shən/ [L, *os* + *facere*, to make], the development of bone. **Intramembranous ossification** is that preceded by membrane, such as in the process initially forming the roof and the sides of the skull. **Intracartilaginous ossification** is that preceded by rods of cartilage, such as that forming the bones of the limbs.

ossify /os′ifī/ [L, *os*, bone; *facere*, to make], to develop into bone.

ossifying fibroma /os′ifī′ing/ [L, *os* + *facere*, to make], a slow-growing, benign neoplasm, occurring most often in the jaws, especially the mandible. The tumor is composed of bone that develops within fibrous connective tissue.

oste- See **osteo-.**

ostealgia /os′tē·al′jə/ [Gk, *osteon* + *algos*, pain], any pain that is associated with an abnormal condition within a bone, such as osteomyelitis. —**ostealgic,** *adj.*

osteanagenesis. See **osteoanagenesis.**

osteitis /os′tē·ī′tis/ [Gk, *osteon* + *itis*, inflammation], an inflammation of bone, caused by infection, degeneration, or trauma. Swelling, tenderness, dull aching pain, and redness in the skin over the affected bone are characteristic of the condition. Some kinds of osteitis are **osteitis deformans** and **osteitis fibrosa cystica.** See also **osteomyelitis, Paget's disease.**

osteitis deformans. See **Paget's disease.**

osteitis fibrosa cystica, an inflammatory degenerative condition in which normal bone is replaced by cysts and fibrous tissue. It is usually associated with hyperparathyroidism.

osteitis fibrosa disseminata. See **Albright's syndrome.**

ostembryon. See **lithopedion.**

ostemia /ostē′mē·ə/, an abnormal congestion of blood in a bone.

ostempyesis /os′təmpī·ē′sis/, an accumulation of pus within a bone.

osteo /os′tē·ō/, 1. abbreviation for **osteopath.** 2. abbreviation for **osteopathy.**

osteo-, oste-, a prefix meaning 'of or pertaining to bone': *osteoanesthesia, osteocele, osteopathy.*

osteoanagenesis /os′tē·ō·an′əjen′əsis/ [Gk, *osteon* + *ana*, again, *genesis*, origin], the regeneration or formation of bone tissue. Also called **osteanagenesis.**

osteoaneurysm /-an′yəriz′əm/, an aneurysm within a bone.

osteoarthritis /os′tē·ō′ärthrī′tis/ [Gk, *osteon* + *arthron*, joint, *itis*, inflammation], a form of arthritis in which one or many joints undergo degenerative changes, including subchondral bony sclerosis, loss of articular cartilage, and proliferation of bone and cartilage in the joint, forming osteophytes. Inflammation of the synovial membrane of the joint is common late in the disease. The most common form of arthritis, its cause is unknown but may include chemical, mechanical, genetic, metabolic, and endocrine factors.

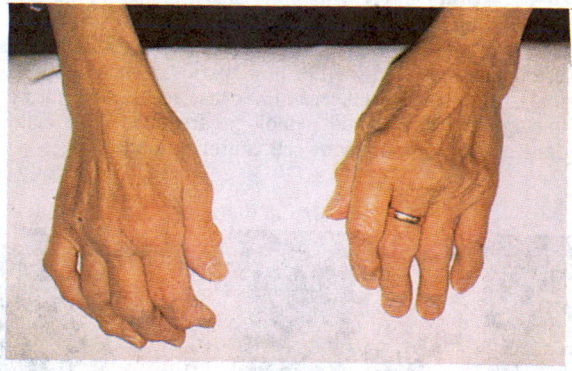

Osteoarthritis *(Kamal, 1991)*

Emotional stress often aggravates the condition. The condition usually begins with pain after exercise or use of the joint. Stiffness, tenderness to the touch, crepitus, and enlargement develop, and deformity, subluxation, and synovial effusion may eventually occur. Involvement of the hip, knee, or spine causes more disability than osteoarthritis of other areas. Treatment includes rest of the involved joints, heat, and antiinflammatory drugs. Systemic corticosteroids are contraindicated, but intraarticular injections of corticosteroids may give relief. Surgical treatment is sometimes necessary and may reduce pain and greatly improve the function of a joint. Hip replacement, joint debridement, fusion, and decompression laminectomy are some of the surgical procedures used in treating advanced osteoarthritis. Compare **rheumatoid arthritis.**

osteoarthritis deformans endemica.   See **Kashin-Bek disease.**

osteoarthropathy /-ärthrop′əthē/ [Gk, *osteon* + *arthron,* joint, *pathos,* disease], a disorder affecting bones and joints.

osteoarthrosis /-arthrō′sis/, a condition of chronic arthritis, usually mechanical, without inflammation.

osteoarticular /-artik′yələr/, pertaining to or affecting bones and joints.

osteoarticular graft, a transplant of bone tissue that contains an articular surface.

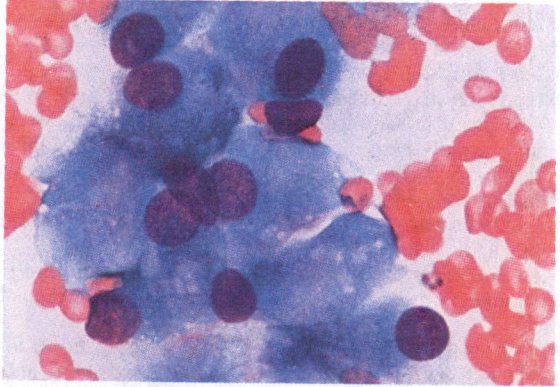

Osteoblasts in the bone marrow *(Hayhoe, 1992)*

osteoblast /os′tē·əblast′/ [Gk, *osteon* + *blastos,* germ], a cell that originates in the embryonic mesenchyme and, during the early development of the skeleton, differentiates from a fibroblast to function in the formation of bone tissue. Osteoblasts synthesize the collagen and glycoproteins to form the matrix and, with growth, develop into osteocytes. Also called **osteoplast.** See also **ossification.** —**osteoblastic,** *adj.*

osteoblastoma /-blastō′mə/, *pl.* **osteoblastomas, osteoblastomata,** a small, benign, fairly vascular tumor of poorly formed bone and fibrous tissue, occurring most frequently in the vertebrae, femur, tibia, or bones of the upper extremities in children and young adults. The tumor may cause pain, erosion, and resorption of native bone. Excision is the preferred treatment. Also called **osteoid osteoma.**

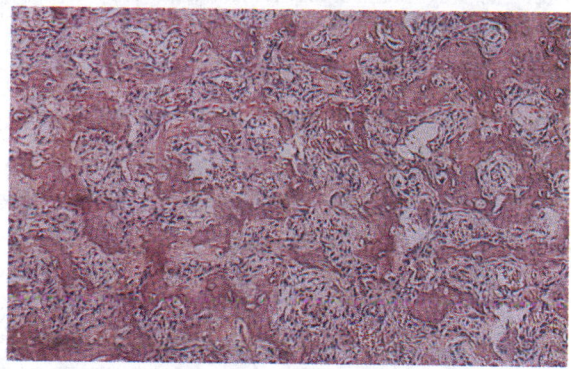

Osteoblastoma *(Bullough, 1988)*

osteocachexia /-kəkek′sē·ə/, a chronic disease that results in wasting of the bone, usually caused by malnutrition.

osteocarcinoma /-kär′sinō′mə/ [Gk, *osteon,* bone; *karkinos,* crab; *oma,* tumor], cancer of the bone.

osteochondral graft /-kon′drəl/, a transplant of tissue composed of both bone and cartilage.

osteochondritis /-kəndrī′tis/ [Gk, *osteon,* bone; *chondros,* cartilage; *itis,* inflammation], a disease of the epiphyses, or bone-forming centers of the skeleton, beginning with necrosis and fragmentation of the tissue, and followed by repair and regeneration. Types of the disorder include **osteochondritis deformans juvenilis, osteochondritis ischiopubica, osteochondritis juvenilis,** and **osteochondritis necroticans.**

osteochondritis dissecans [Gk, *osteon,* bone; *chondros,* cartilage; L, *dissecare,* to cut apart], a joint disorder in which a piece of cartilage and neighboring bone tissue become detached from the articular surface.

osteochondrodystrophy.   See **Morquio's disease.**

osteochondrofibroma /-kon′drōfībrō′mə/, a tumor containing tissues of osteoma, chondroma, and fibroma.

osteochondrolysis.   See **osteochondrosis dissecans.**

osteochondroma /os′tē·ōkondrō′mə/ [Gk, *osteon* + *chondros,* cartilage, *oma,* tumor], a benign tumor made of bone and cartilage.

osteochondromatosis /-kon′drōmətō′sis/, the transformation of synovial villi into bone and cartilage masses, causing loose bodies in the joints. It usually develops in joints affected by injury or degenerative diseases.

osteochondropathy /kəndrop′əthē/, a condition affecting both bone and cartilage and characterized by abnormal enchondral ossification.

osteochondrosarcoma /-kon′drōsärkō′mə/ [Gk, *osteon*, bone; *chondros*, cartilage; *karkinos*, crab; *oma*, tumor], a condition of sarcomatous tumors in the bone and cartilage.

osteochondrosis /-kondrō′sis/ [Gk, *osteon* + *chondros*, cartilage, *osis*, condition], a disease affecting the ossification centers of bone in children, initially characterized by degeneration and necrosis, followed by regeneration and recalcification. Kinds of osteochondrosis include **Legg-Calvé-Perthes disease, Osgood-Schlatter disease,** and **Scheuermann's disease.**

osteochondrosis dissecans /dis′əkənz/, the formation of a separate center of bone and cartilage on an epiphyseal surface. The stray fragment may remain in place, be absorbed, or break off and become a loose body.

osteoclasia /-klā′zhə/ [Gk, *osteon* + *klasis*, breaking], **1.** the destruction and absorption of bony tissue by osteoclasts, such as during growth or the healing of fractures. **2.** the degeneration of bone through disease. See also **osteolysis.**

osteoclasis /os′tē·ōk′ləsis/, the intentional surgical fracture of a bone to correct a deformity. Also called **osteoclasty. –osteoclastic,** *adj.*

osteoclast /os′tē·əklast′/ [Gk, *osteon* + *klasis*, breaking], **1.** also called **osteophage.** a large type of multinucleated bone cell that functions in the development and periods of growth or repair, such as the breakdown and resorption of osseous tissue. During bone healing of fractures, or during certain disease processes, osteoclasts excavate passages through the surrounding tissue by enzymatic action. Osteoclasts become activated in the presence of parathyroid hormone and also in a lymphokine substance produced by lym-

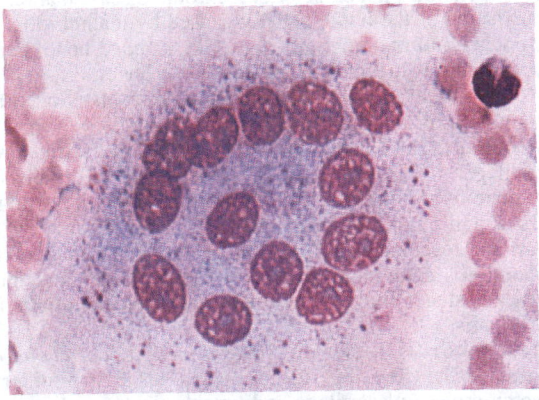

Osteoclasts in the bone marrow *(Hayhoe, 1992)*

phocytes in such diseases as multiple myeloma and malignant lymphomas. See also **ossification. 2.** a surgical instrument used in the fracturing or refracturing of bones for therapeutic purposes, such as correction of a deformity.

osteoclastic /-klas′tik/, **1.** pertaining to or of the nature of osteoclasts. **2.** destructive to bone.

osteoclastoma /os′tē·ōklastō′mə/, *pl.* **osteoclastomas,**

osteoclastomata [Gk, *osteon* + *klasis*, breaking, *oma*, tumor],a giant cell tumor of the bone that occurs most frequently at the end of a long bone and appears as a mass surrounded by a thin shell of new, periosteal bone. The lesion is often malignant and may cause local pain, loss of function, weakness, and pathologic fracture. Also called **giant cell myeloma, giant cell tumor of bone.**

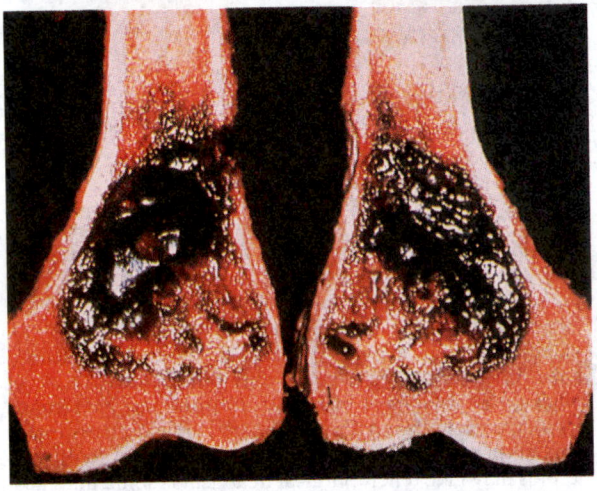

Osteoclastoma
(Fletcher, 1987/Courtesy Dr JC Macartney, Department of Histopathology, St. Thomas's Hospital Medical School, London)

osteoclasty. See **osteoclasis.**

osteocope /os′tē·əkōp/, a painful syphilitic bone disease.

osteocystoma /-sistō′mə/, a cystic tumor in a bone.

osteocyte /os′tē·əsīt/ [Gk, *osteon* + *kytos*, cell], a bone cell; a mature osteoblast that has become embedded in the bone matrix. It occupies a small cavity and sends out protoplasmic projections that anastomose with those of other osteoblasts to form a system of minute canals within the bone matrix. **–osteocytic,** *adj.*

osteodensitometer /den′sitom′ətər/ [Gk, *osteon*, bone; L, *densus*, thick; Gk, *metron*, measure], an apparatus for measuring the density of bone tissue.

osteodiastasis /-dī·as′təsis/, an abnormal separation of bones.

osteodynia /-din′ē·ə/, bone pain.

osteodystrophy /dis′trəfē/ [Gk, *osteon* + *dys*, bad, *trophe*, nourishment], any generalized defect in bone development, usually associated with disturbances in calcium and phosphorus metabolism and renal insufficiency, such as in renal osteodystrophy. Also called **osteodystrophia.**

osteoenchondroma /os′tē·ō·en′kəndrō′mə/, a benign bone and cartilage tumor within a bone.

osteofibrochondrosarcoma /-fī′brōkon′drōsärkō′mə/, a malignant tumor containing bone, cartilage, and fibrous tissues.

osteofibroma /-fībrō′mə/ [Gk, *osteon*, bone; L, *fibra*, fiber; Gk, *oma*, tumor], a tumor composed of both bony and fibrous tissues.

osteogenesis /-jen′əsis/ [Gk, *osteon* + *genesis*, origin], the origin and development of bone tissue. Also called **osteog-**

eny /os'tē·oj'ənē/. See also **ossification.** **–osteogenetic,**
osteogenic, *adj.*

osteogenesis imperfecta, a genetic disorder involving defective development of the connective tissue. It is inherited
as an autosomal dominant trait and is characterized by abnormally brittle and fragile bones that are easily fractured
by the slightest trauma. Also called **brittle bones, fragili-**
tas ossium, hypoplasia of the mesenchyme, osteopsathy-
rosis.

■ OBSERVATIONS: In its most severe form, the disease may be
apparent at birth, when it is known as **osteogenesis imper-**
fecta congenita. The newborn has multiple fractures that
have occurred in utero and is usually severely deformed,
because of imperfect formation and mineralization of bone.
Most infants die shortly after birth, although a few survive
as deformed dwarfs with normal mental development if no
head trauma has occurred. If the disease has a later onset,
it is called **osteogenesis imperfecta tarda** and usually runs
a milder course. Symptoms generally appear when the child
begins to walk, but they become less severe with age, and
the tendency to fracture decreases and often disappears after puberty. Other manifestations of the condition include
blue sclerae, translucent skin, hyperextensibility of ligaments, hypoplasia of the teeth, recurrent epistaxis, excess
diaphoresis, mild hyperpyrexia, and a tendency to bruise
easily and to develop otosclerosis with hearing loss. There
is a broad expressivity of the disease so that the number and
extent of pathologic features may range from minimal to severe involvement.

■ INTERVENTIONS: There is no known cure for the disease.
Treatment is predominantly supportive; extreme care must

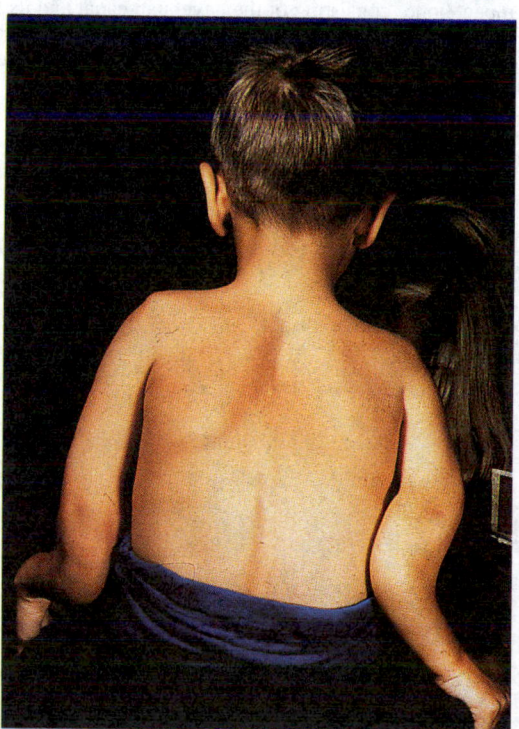

Osteogenesis imperfecta *(Bullough, 1988)*

be taken in handling patients, especially infants who are severely affected, to prevent fractures. In many children oral
administration of magnesium oxide may decrease the fracture rate, as well as the diaphoresis, hyperpyrexia, and constipation associated with the condition.

■ NURSING CONSIDERATIONS: The primary function of the nurse
is to educate the parents about the disease, especially the
extent of the child's limitations, and to help them plan suitable activities that will promote optimum growth and development and, at the same time, protect the child from
harm. Genetic counseling is also part of the goals of long-
term care.

osteogenic, composed of or originating from any tissue involved in the development, growth, or repair of bone. Also
osteogenous /os'tē·oj'ənəs/.

osteogenic sarcoma. See **osteosarcoma.**

osteogenous. See **osteogenic.**

osteogeny. See **osteogenesis.**

osteohalisteresis /-hal'istərē'sis/, a condition of soft bones
caused by a loss or deficiency of mineral elements.

osteoid /os'tē·oid/ [Gk, *osteon* + *eidos*, form], of, pertaining to, or resembling bone.

osteoid osteoma. See **osteoblastoma.**

osteolipochondroma /-līp'ōkəndrō'mə/, a cartilage tumor
with bone and fat elements.

osteolipoma /-līpō'mə/, a fatty tumor containing bone elements.

osteology /os'tē·ol'əgē/ [Gk, *osteon*, bone; *logos*, science],
the branch of medicine concerned with the development and
diseases of bone tissue.

osteolysis /os'tē·ol'isis/ [Gk, *osteon* + *lysis*, loosening],
the degeneration and dissolution of bone, caused by disease,
infection, or ischemia. The condition commonly affects the
terminal bones of the hands and feet, such as in acroosteolysis, and is seen in disorders involving blood vessels, such
as in Raynaud's disease, scleroderma, and systemic lupus
erythematosus. **–osteolytic,** *adj.*

osteoma /os'tē·ō'mə/, *pl.* **osteomas, osteomata,** a tumor
of bone tissue.

-osteoma, a combining form meaning a 'tumor composed
of bone tissue, usually benign': *endosteoma, myosteoma,*
periosteoma.

osteomalacia /-məlā'shə/ [Gk, *osteon* + *malakia*, soften-
ing], an abnormal condition of the lamellar bone, characterized by a loss of calcification of the matrix resulting in
softening of the bone, accompanied by weakness, fracture,
pain, anorexia, and weight loss. The condition is the result
of an inadequate amount of phosphorus and calcium available in the blood for mineralization of the bones. This deficiency may be caused by a diet lacking these minerals or
vitamin D, or by a lack of exposure to sunlight, hence an
inability to synthesize vitamin D, or by a metabolic disorder causing malabsorption. Osteomalacia results from and
also complicates many diseases and conditions. Treatment
usually includes the administration of the necessary vitamins
and minerals and therapy appropriate for the underlying disorder. See also **adult rickets, hyperparathyroidism,**
Paget's disease, rickets. (See Fig. p. 1128.)

osteomesopyknosis /-mez'ōpiknō'sis/, a genetic disorder
transmitted as an autosomal trait, characterized by osteosclerosis of the axial spine, the pelvis, and the proximal areas of long bones.

osteomyelitis /-mī·əlī'tis/ [Gk, *osteon* + *myelos*, marrow,
itis, inflammation], local or generalized infection of bone
and bone marrow, usually caused by bacteria introduced by

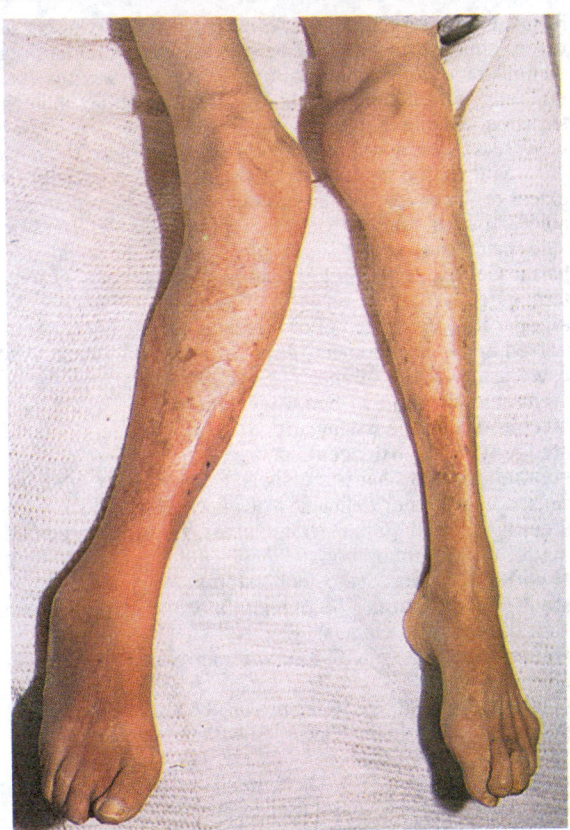

Osteomalacia (Kamal, 1991)

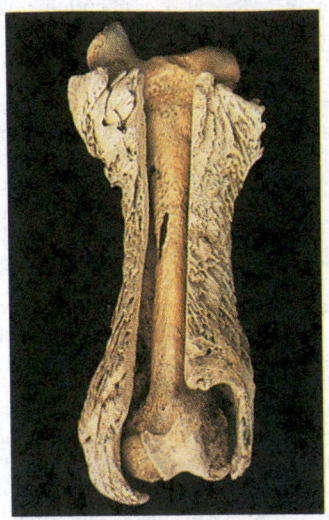

Chronic osteomyelitis
(Fletcher, 1987/Courtesy Professor PG Bullough, Cornell University Medical College, New York)

osteomyelodysplasia /os′tē·ōmī′əlō′displā′zhə/ [Gk, *osteon*, bone; *myelos*, marrow; *dys, plasis*, forming], a loss of bone tissue through absorption of minerals. The condition is usually associated with leukopenia and sometimes with fever, and may result from an excess of parathyroid hormone.

osteon /os′tē·on/ [Gk, bone], the basic structural unit of compact bone, consisting of the haversian canal and its concentric rings of 4 to 20 lamellae. Most of the units run with the long axis of the bone. Also called **Haversian system.**

trauma or surgery, by direct extension from a nearby infection, or via the bloodstream. Staphylococci are the most common causative agents.

■ OBSERVATIONS: The long bones in children and the vertebrae in adults are the commonest sites of infection as a result of hematogenous spread. Persistent, severe, and increasing bone pain, tenderness, guarding on movement, regional muscle spasm, and fever suggest this diagnosis. Draining sinus tracts may accompany posttraumatic osteomyelitis or osteomyelitis from a contiguous infection. Specific diagnosis and selection of therapy depend on bacterial examination of bone, tissue, or pus.

■ INTERVENTIONS: Treatment includes bed rest and parenteral antibiotics for several weeks. Surgery may be necessary to remove necrotic bone and tissue, to obliterate cavities, to remove infected prosthetic appliances, and to apply prostheses to stabilize affected parts. Chronic osteomyelitis may persist for years with exacerbations and remissions despite treatment.

■ NURSING CONSIDERATIONS: Any drainage is disposed of using unusual precautions. Absolute rest of the affected part may be necessary, with a careful positioning using pillows and sandbags for good alignment. During the early phase of infection, pain is extremely severe and extraordinary gentleness in moving and manipulating the infected part is essential. **—osteomyelitic,** *adj.*.

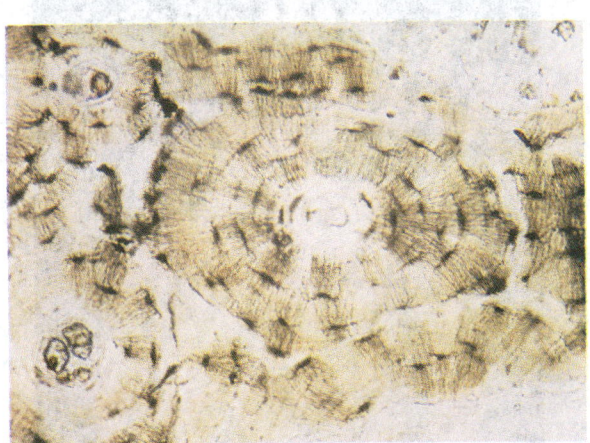

Osteon (Seeley, 1992/Trent Stephens)

-osteon, -osteum, a combining form meaning 'bone': *melacosteon, otosteon, pleurosteon.*

osteonal bone /os′tē·ō′nəl/, a microscopic description of bone tissue seen in mature adults. It is composed of tiny chalky tubes with an arteriole running down the middle and circular laminations of bone concentric with an artery.

osteonecrosis /os′tē·ō′nəkrō′sis/ [Gk, *osteon* + *nekros,* dead, *osis* condition], the destruction and death of bone tissue, such as from ischemia, infection, malignant neoplastic disease, or trauma. **–osteonecrotic,** *adj.*

osteopath (osteo) /os′tē·ōpath′/, a physician who specializes in osteopathy. Also called **osteopathist.**

osteopathic scoliosis See **congenital scoliosis.**

osteopathology /pathol′əjē/ [Gk, *osteon,* bone; *pathos,* disease; *logos,* science], the study of bone diseases.

osteopathy (osteo) /os′tē·op′əthē/ [Gk, *osteon* + *pathos,* disease], a therapeutic approach to the practice of medicine that uses all the usual forms of medical therapy and diagnosis, including drugs, surgery, and radiation, but that places greater emphasis on the influence of the relationship between the organs and the musculoskeletal system than is done in traditional medicine. Osteopathic physicians recognize and correct structural problems using manipulation. The process is important in both the diagnosis and the treatment of health problems. See also **physician. –osteopathic,** *adj.*

osteopedion. See **lithopedion.**

osteopenia /-pē′nē·ə/ [Gk, *osteon* + *penes,* poverty], a condition of subnormally mineralized bone, usually the result of a failure of the rate of bone matrix synthesis to compensate for the rate of bone lysis.

osteoperiosteal graft /-per′ē·os′tē·əl/, a bone graft that includes the periosteal membrane covering the bone.

osteopetrosis /os′tē·ōpētrō′sis/ [Gk, *osteon* + *petra,* stone, *osis* condition], an inherited disorder characterized by a generalized increase in bone density, probably caused by faulty bone resorption resulting from a deficiency of osteoclasts. In its most severe form, transmitted as an autosomal recessive condition, there is obliteration of the bone marrow cavity, causing severe anemia, marked deformities of the skull, and compression of the cranial nerves, which may result in deafness and blindness and lead to an early death. A milder, benign form, transmitted as an autosomal dominant trait, is characterized by short stature, fragile bones that fracture easily, and a tendency to develop osteomyelitis. Also called **ivory bones, marble bones, osteosclerosis fragilis.** See also **Albers-Schönberg disease. –osteopetrotic,** *adj.*

osteophage. See **osteoclast.**

osteophyte /os′tē·əfīt/, a bony outgrowth, usually found around the joint area.

osteoplast. See **osteoblast.**

osteoplastica /-plas′tikə/, a form of bone inflammation associated with cystic fibrosis.

osteoplasty /o′stē·əplastē/ [Gk, *osteon,* bone; *plassein,* to form], plastic surgery performed on bone tissue.

osteopoikilosis /os′tē·ōpoi′kilō′sis/ [Gk, *osteon* + *poikilos,* mottled, *osis,* condition], an inherited condition of the bones, transmitted as an autosomal dominant trait, characterized by multiple areas of dense calcification throughout the osseous tissue, producing a mottled appearance on x-ray examination. It is a benign condition, usually without symptoms, and of unknown cause. Also called **osteosclerosis fragilis congenita. –osteopoikilotic,** *adj.*

osteoporosis /os′tē·ōpərō′sis/ [Gk, *osteon* + *poros,* passage, *osis,* condition], a disorder characterized by abnormal rarefaction of bone, occurring most frequently in postmenopausal women, in sedentary or immobilized individuals, and in patients on long-term steroid therapy. The disorder may cause pain, especially in the lower back,

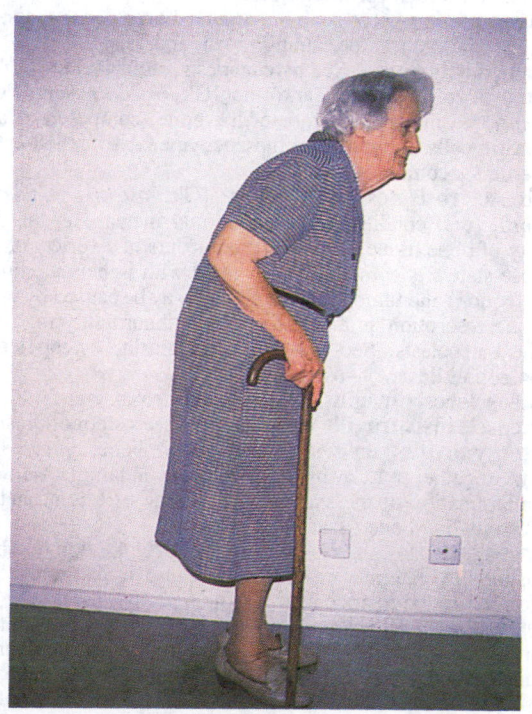

Extremely dense bone of osteopetrosis
(Bullough, 1988)

Typical posture seen in osteoporosis *(Shipley, 1993)*

pathologic fractures, loss of stature, and various deformities. Osteoporosis may be idiopathic or secondary to other disorders, such as thyrotoxicosis or the bone demineralization caused by hyperparathyroidism. Estrogen therapy is often used for the prevention and management of postmenopausal osteoporosis, but use of the hormone alone carries the risk of endometrial cancer.

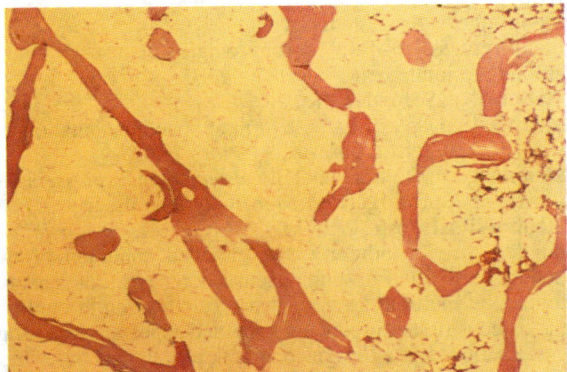

Photomicrograph of osteoporotic bone
(Christiansen, 1993)

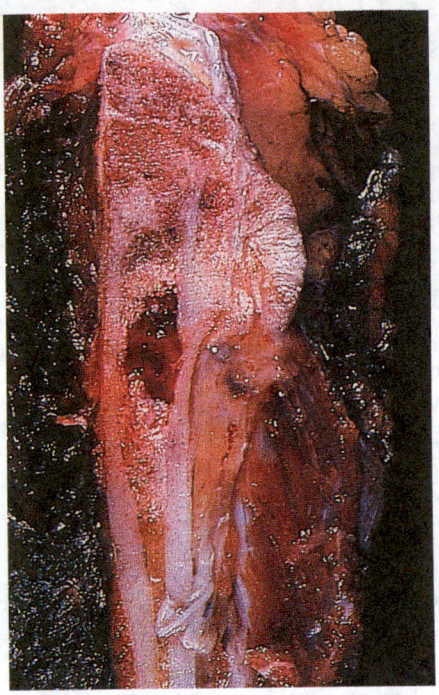

Osteosarcoma (Lewis MM, 1988)

osteoporosis of disuse [Gk, *osteon*, bone; *poros*, passage; *osis*, condition; L, *dis*, not; ME, *usen*, to act], a thinning of the bone mass that occurs in sedentary people or patients confined to bed for a long period.

osteoporotic /-pərot′ik/ [Gk, *osteon*, bone; *poros*, passage; *osis*, condition], pertaining to osteoporosis.

osteopsathyrosis. See **osteogenesis imperfecta.**

osteosarcoma /os′tē·ō′särkō′mə/ [Gk, *osteon* + *sarx*, flesh, *oma*], a malignant tumor of the bone, composed of anaplastic cells derived from mesenchyme. Also called **osteogenic sarcoma.**

osteosclerosis /os′tē·ōsklerō′sis/ [Gk, *osteon* + *skleros*, hard, *osis*, condition], an abnormal increase in the density of bone tissue. The condition occurs in a variety of disease states, is commonly associated with ischemia, chronic infection, and tumor formation, and may be caused by faulty bone resorption as a result of some abnormality involving the osteoclasts. See also **achondroplasia, osteopetrosis, osteopoikilosis.** **–osteosclerotic,** *adj.*

osteosclerosis fragilis. See **osteopetrosis.**

osteosclerosis fragilis congenita. See **osteopoikilosis.**

osteosynovitis /-sin′ōvī′tis/ [Gk, *osteon*, bone; *synovia* {Gk, *syn*, together + L, *ovum*, egg}; Gk, *itis*, inflammation], an inflammation of the synovial membrane of a joint and the surrounding bone tissue.

osteosynthesis /-sin′thəsis/, the surgical fixation of a bone using any internal mechanical means. It is usually performed in the treatment of fractures.

osteotabes /-tā′bēz/, a condition usually affecting infants in which bone marrow cells are destroyed and the marrow disappears.

osteotelangiectasia /-telan′jē·əktā′zhə/, a sarcoma of the bone characterized by dilated capillaries.

osteothrombophlebitis /-throm′bōfləbī′tis/, an inflam-

mation through intact bone by progressive thrombophlebitis of small venules.

osteothrombosis /-thrəmbō′sis/, a blockage of the blood vessels in the bone tissue.

osteotome /os′tē·ətōm′/ [Gk, *osteon* + *temnein*, to cut], a surgical instrument for cutting through bone.

osteotomy /os′tē·ot′əmē/ [Gk, *osteon* + *temnein*, to cut], the sawing or cutting of a bone. Kinds of osteotomy include block osteotomy, in which a section of bone is excised, cuneiform osteotomy to remove a bone wedge, and displacement osteotomy, in which a bone is redesigned surgically to alter the alignment or weightbearing stress areas.

osteotripsy /-trip′sē/, a method of treating callosities or any percutaneous reduction of a bony prominence.

-osteum. See **-osteon.**

ostium. See **orifice.**

ostium primum defect, ostium secundum defect. See **atrial septal defect.**

ostomate /os′təmāt/ [L, *ostium*, mouth], a person who has undergone an ostomy.

-ostomy, a suffix meaning to 'form a new opening or pertaining to a mouthlike opening': *colostomy*, *tracheostomy*.

ostomy /os′təmē/ [L, *ostium*, mouth], *informal.* a surgical procedure in which an opening is made to allow the passage of urine from the bladder or of intestinal contents from the bowel to an incision or stoma surgically created in the wall of the abdomen. An ostomy procedure may be performed to correct an anatomic defect, to relieve an obstruction in or to permit treatment of a severe infection or injury of the urinary or intestinal tract. Each procedure is named for the anatomic location of the ostomy, such as a colostomy, cecostomy, or cystostomy.

Comparison of ileostomy and colostomies

	Ileostomy	Ascending colostomy	Transverse colostomy	Descending or sigmoid colostomy
Location	Ileum	Ascending colon	Transverse colon	Sigmoid colon
Type of drainage	Liquid-to-paste consistency	Liquid-to-soft	Soft	Soft-to-formed
Bowel regulation	No	No	No	Only with irrigations
Fluid balance	Monitor for dehydration if high output diarrhea	Same as ileostomy	Dehydration may occur with bouts of diarrhea	Usually not a problem unless there were previous resections
Skin irritation	Occurs easily because of digestive enzymes	Same as ileostomy	Can occur from exposure to stool	Same as transverse colostomy
Other complications	Food blockage Prolapse of stoma Stricture Peristomal hernia	Prolapse Stricture Peristomal hernia	Prolapse Stricture Peristomal hernia	Prolapse Stricture Constipation Peristomal hernia

From Phipps WJ, Long BC, Woods NF, Cassmeyer VL: *Medical surgical nursing: concepts and clinical practice,* ed 4, St Louis, 1991, Mosby, p. 1338.

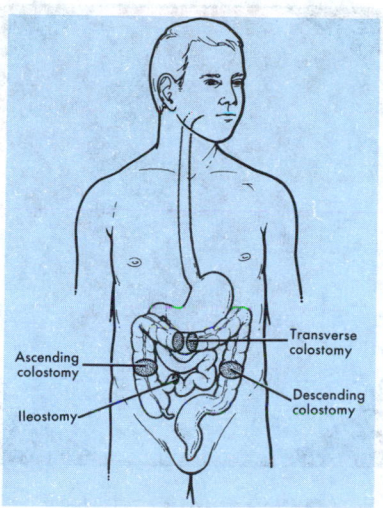

Ostomy sites

permits. Each time the temporary or permanent appliance is changed, the skin around the stoma is washed with soap and water, rinsed thoroughly, and patted dry with a clean towel. If the skin is irritated or excoriated, karaya powder, alone or mixed with an ointment, is spread over the area before the appliance is reinstalled. An adhesive substance may be used to maintain a tight seal with the appliance, and deodorant drops, aspirin, or various bismuth or chlorophyll preparations are added to the ostomy bag to control odor. The diet is planned according to the kind of ostomy; ileostomates require food high in sodium and potassium, such as bananas, citrus juices, molasses, and cola, and are advised to avoid fried, highly seasoned, and rich foods, nuts, raisins, raw fruits other than bananas, and anything that produces gas or causes diarrhea. Gas-producing foods, such as cabbage, beans, broccoli, cauliflower, and corn, foods causing disturbing odors, such as onions, eggs, and fish, and sharp condiments are contraindicated; a low-residue diet is ordered for most ostomates. The fluid intake is carefully maintained.

ostomy care, the management and support of a patient with a surgical opening created in the bladder, ileum, or colon for the temporary or permanent passage of urine or feces, necessitated by carcinoma, intestinal obstruction, trauma, or severe ulceration distal to the site of the incision. In most cases the opening is covered with a temporary disposable bag in the operating room.

■ METHOD: The patient with a colostomy or an ileostomy is helped to accept the stoma and the change in body image that frequently causes grief, or, in some instances, denial. Discussions of the person's feelings are encouraged, and questions regarding the procedure and possible changes in the person's lifestyle are answered in a positive manner. The disposable bag is changed whenever necessary, and the character, color, and amount of drainage are observed; mucous secretion from the stoma usually begins within 48 hours after the operation, fecal drainage within 72 hours. The stoma is inspected periodically for color, bleeding, stricture, retraction, and infection and is measured every other day to determine the size of the permanent appliance that is to be used as soon as the condition of the opening

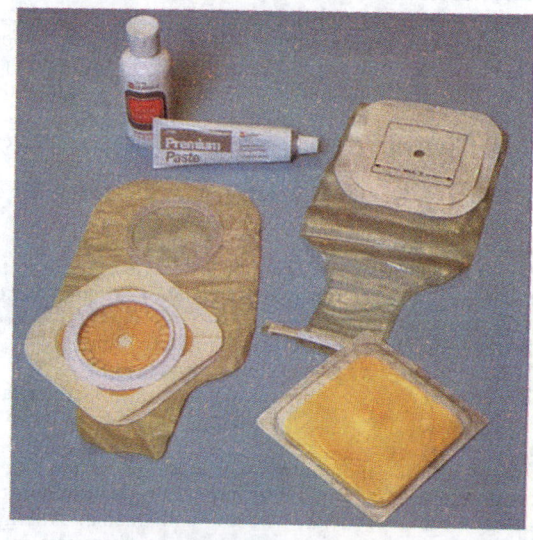

Ostomy pouches (Potter, 1993)

■ NURSING INTERVENTION: Before discharge, each step in the care of the stoma and surrounding skin is rehearsed with the patient, using the equipment that will be available at home. Appropriate diet instruction is provided, emphasizing the need to eat adequate meals regularly, to chew slowly, and to avoid extremely hot and very cold food. The patient is urged to establish a regular pattern of evacuation and to report any signs of wound infection or obstruction, such as nausea, vomiting, decreased drainage from the stoma, abdominal distention, and cramps. Normal daily activity is encouraged.

■ OUTCOME CRITERIA: The ability of the patient to adjust to the ostomy procedures and equipment is greatly affected by the nursing care received in the days after surgery. A positive, patient, and matter-of-fact approach, sensitive emotional support, and thorough teaching of self-care measures are essential aspects of ostomy nursing care.

ostomy irrigation, a procedure for cleansing, stimulating, and regulating evacuation of an artificially created orifice. Fluids used in irrigation include tap water and saline or medicated solutions. Necessary equipment includes properly sized irrigator tips, catheters, drainage bags that allow for insertion of the catheter, an irrigation container, and shields to prevent leakage. Loop and double-barrel colostomies require a sequential irrigation of the proximal loop, distal loop, and rectum to prevent the accumulation of discharge.

ostrac-, ostraco-, a combining form meaning 'like a hard shell': *astracosis, ostracod.*

os trapezium. See **trapezium.**

os trapezoideum. See **trapezoid bone.**

os trigonum /os'trigō'nəm/, a small foot bone just posterior to the talus. It is sometimes confused with a fracture of the posterior tubercle of the talus. Also called **Bardeleben's bone.**

os triquetrum. See **triangular bone.**

OT, 1. abbreviation for **occupational therapist. 2.** abbreviation for **occupational therapy.**

ot-. See **oto-.**

otalgia /ōtal'jə/, a pain in the ear. Also called **otodynia, otoneuralgia.**

OTC, abbreviation for **over the counter.**

Othello syndrome /ōthel'ō/ [Othello, jealous Shakespearean character], a psychopathologic condition characterized by suspicion of a spouse's infidelity and by morbid jealousy. This condition may be accompanied by rage and violence and is frequently associated with paranoia.

-otia, a combining form meaning '(condition of the) ear': *melotia, microtia, synotia.*

otic /ō'tik, ot'ik/ [Gk, *ous,* ear], of or pertaining to the ear. Also **auricular.**

-otic. See **oto-.**

otics /ō'tiks, ot'iks/, a group of drugs used locally to treat inflammation of the external ear canal or to remove excess cerumen.

otitic /ōtit'ik/ [Gk, *ous,* ear], pertaining to otitis.

otitic barotrauma. See **barotrauma.**

otitis /ōtī'tis/ [Gk, *ous* + *itis,* inflammation], inflammation or infection of the ear. Kinds of otitis are **otitis externa** and **otitis media.**

otitis externa, inflammation or infection of the external canal or the auricle of the external ear. Major causes are allergy, bacteria, fungi, viruses, and trauma. Allergy to nickel or chromium in earrings and to chemicals in hair sprays, cosmetics, hearing aids, and medications, particu-

larly sulfonamides and neomycin, is common. *Staphylococcus aureus, Pseudomonas aeruginosa,* and *Streptococcus pyogenes* are common bacterial causes. Herpes simplex and herpes zoster viruses are frequently implicated. Eczema, psoriasis, and seborrheic dermatitis also may affect the external ear. Abrasions of the ear canal may become infected, and excessive swimming may wash out protective cerumen, remove skin lipids, and lead to secondary infection. Otitis externa is more prevalent during hot, humid weather. Folliculitis is particularly painful in the external auditory meatus and is a common occupational hazard in nurses, caused by irritation from the earpieces of stethoscopes. Treatment includes oral analgesics, thorough local cleansing, topical antimicrobials to treat infection, or topical corticosteroids to reduce inflammation. Prevention includes measures to reduce maceration of the skin and to avoid trauma.

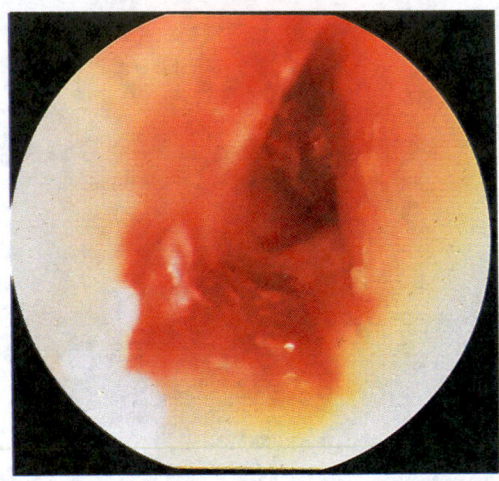

Otitis externa *(Zitelli, 1992)*

otitis interna. See **labyrinthitis.**

otitis mastoidea [Gk, *ous,* ear; *itis,* inflammation; *mastos,* breast; *eidos,* form], an inflammation of the inner ear associated with a mastoid infection.

otitis media, inflammation or infection of the middle ear, a common affliction of childhood. Acute otitis media is most often caused by *Haemophilus influenzae* or *Streptococcus pneumoniae.* Chronic otitis media is usually caused by gram-negative bacteria, such as *Proteus, Klebsiella,* and *Pseudomonas.* Allergy, *Mycoplasma,* and several viruses also may be causative factors. Otitis media is often preceded by an upper respiratory infection.

■ OBSERVATIONS: Organisms gain entry to the middle ear through the eustachian tube. The small diameter and horizontal orientation of the tube in infants predisposes them to infection. Obstruction of the eustachian tube and accumulation of exudate may increase pressure within the middle ear, forcing infection into the mastoid bone or rupturing the tympanic membrane. Symptoms of acute otitis media include a sense of fullness in the ear, diminished hearing, pain, and fever. Usually only one ear is affected. Squamous epithelium may grow in the middle ear through a rupture in the tympanic membrane, and development of a cholesteatoma and deafness may occur if repeated infections cause an opening to persist. Pneumococcal otitis media may spread to the meninges.

■ INTERVENTIONS: Accurate diagnosis of the causative microorganism is important for selection of effective antimicrobial therapy. Treatment also includes analgesics, local heat, nasal decongestants, needle aspiration of secretions collected behind the membrane, and myringotomy.

■ NURSING CONSIDERATIONS: Parents are taught to recognize and watch for early warning signs of otitis media. The use of vaporizers and decongestants is often recommended during an upper respiratory tract infection as prophylaxis against otitis media. Chronic otitis media may result in delays in speech development.

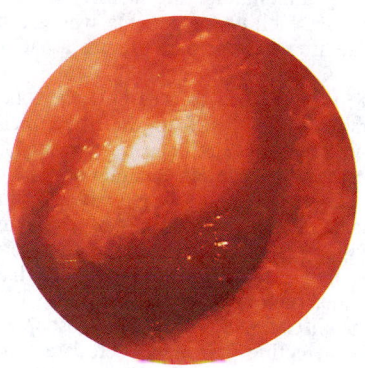

Otitis media *(Zitelli, 1992; Courtesy Dr. Michael Hawke)*

otitis sclerotica [Gk, *ous*, ear; *itis*, inflammation; *sclerosis*, hardening], a sclerosing type of inflammation of the middle ear.

oto- /ō'tō-/, **ot-, -otic,** a combining form meaning 'of or pertaining to the ear': *otoantritis, otoblennorrhea, otocyst, parotic, hematotic.*

otocephalus /ō'tōsef'ələs/, a fetus with otocephaly.

otocephaly /ō'tōsef'əlē/ [Gk, *ous* + *kephale*, head], a congenital malformation characterized by the absence of the lower jaw, defective formation of the mouth, and union or close approximation of the ears on the front of the neck. See also **agnathocephaly.** **–otocephalic, otocephalous,** *adj.*

otodynia. See **otalgia.**

otolaryngologist /-ler'ing·gol'əjist/ [Gk, *ous* + *larynx, logos,* science], a physician who specializes in the diagnosis and treatment of diseases and injuries of the ears, nose, and throat. Compare **otologist.**

otolaryngology /-ler'ing·gol'əjē/ [Gk, *ous* + *larynx, logos,* science], a branch of medicine dealing with the diagnosis and treatment of diseases and disorders of the ears, nose, throat, and adjacent structures of the head and neck.

otolith /ō'təlith/ [Gk, *ous,* ear; *lithos,* stone], **1.** a calculus in the middle ear. **2.** any of the crystals of calcium carbonate attached to the hair cells of the inner ear as gravity orientation receptors.

otolith righting reflex [Gk, *ous* + *lithos,* stone], an involuntary response in newborns in which tilting of the body

when the infant is in an erect position causes the head to return to the upright position. The reflex enables the infant to raise the head and is important for development of later gross motor skills. Absence of the reflex may indicate central nervous system damage.

otologist /ōtol'əjist/, a physician trained in the diagnosis and treatment of diseases and other disorders of the ear. Compare **otolaryngologist.**

otology /ōtol'əjē/ [Gk, *ous* + *logos,* science], the study of the ear, including the diagnosis and treatment of its diseases and disorders.

-otomy, a suffix meaning 'to make an incision or cut into': *phlebotomy, tracheotomy.*

otoneuralgia. See **otalgia.**

otoplasty /ō'təplas'tē/ [Gk, *ous* + *plassein,* to mold], a common procedure in reconstructive plastic surgery in which, for cosmetic reasons, some of the cartilage in the ears is removed to bring the auricle and pinna closer to the head.

otorrhea /ō'tərē'ə/ [Gk, *ous* + *rhoia,* flow], any discharge from the external ear. Otorrhea may be serous, sanguinous, or purulent, or contain cerebrospinal fluid. **–otorrheal, otorrheic, otorrhetic,** *adj.*

otosclerosis /ō'tōsklərō'sis/ [Gk, *ous* + *skleros,* hard, *osis,* condition], a hereditary condition of unknown cause in which irregular ossification in the bony labyrinth of the inner ear, especially of the stapes, occurs, causing tinnitus, then deafness. The deafness is usually first noticed between 11 and 30 years of age. Women are affected twice as often as men. The condition may worsen in pregnancy. Stapedectomy is usually successful in permanently restoring hearing. Also called **otospongiosis.**

otoscope /ō'təskōp'/ [Gk, *ous* + *skopein,* to look], an instrument used to examine the external ear, the eardrum, and, through the eardrum, the ossicles of the middle ear. It consists of a light, a magnifying lens, and a device for insufflation.

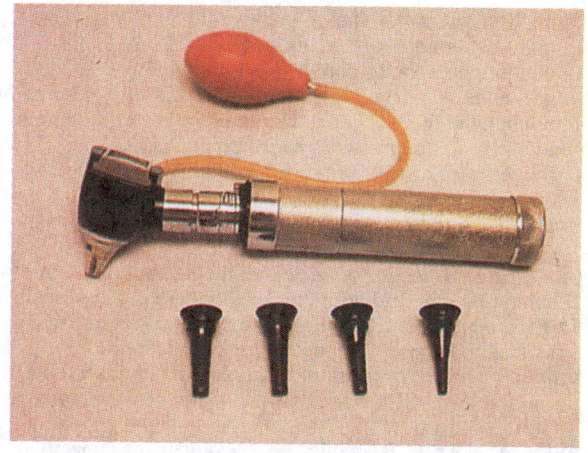

Otoscope with pneumatic attachments *(Seidel, 1991)*

otoscopy /ōtos'kəpē/ [Gk, *ous,* ear; *skopein,* to view], an inspection of the tympanic membrane and other parts of the outer ear with an otoscope.

otospongiosus. See **otosclerosis.**

ototoxic /ō'tōtok'sik/ [Gk, *ous* + *toxikon*, poison], (of a substance) having a harmful effect on the eighth cranial nerve or the organs of hearing and balance. Common ototoxic drugs include the aminoglycoside antibiotics, aspirin, furosemide, and quinine.

OTR, abbreviation for *occupational therapist, registered.* See **occupational therapist.**

Otrivin, a trademark for an adrenergic vasoconstrictor (xylometazoline hydrochloride), used as a nasal decongestant.

Otto pelvis /ot'ō/ [Adolph W. Otto, German surgeon, 1786-1845.], a type of hip dislocation in which there is a gradual central displacement of the femur. The cause is unknown.

OU, abbreviation for *oculus uterque,* a Latin phrase meaning 'each eye.'

Ouchterlony double diffusion [Orjan T.G. Ouchterlony, Swedish bacteriologist, b. 1914], a form of gel diffusion technique in which antigen and antibody in separate cells are allowed to diffuse toward each other.

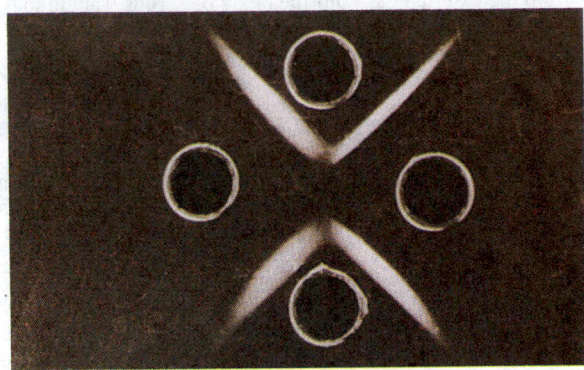

Ouchterlony double diffusion *(Baron, 1990)*

ounce (oz) /ouns/ [L, *uncia,* one twelfth], a unit of weight equal to ¹⁄₁₆ of a pound avoirdupois or 28.349 grams. Also called **ounce avoirdupois** /av'ərdəpoiz'/.

-ous, -eous, a combining form meaning an 'element or compound with a valence lower than the corresponding one ending in *-ic*': *cuprous, ferrous, hypochlorous.*

outbreeding [AS, *ut,* out, *bredan,* to breed], the production of offspring by the mating of unrelated individuals, organisms, or plants, which can lead to superior hybrid traits or strains. Compare **inbreeding.** See also **heterosis.**

outcome [AS, *ut* + *couman,* to come], the condition of a client at the end of therapy or of a disease process, including the degree of wellness and the need for continuing care, medication, support, counseling, or education.

outcome criteria, criteria that focus on observable or measurable results of nursing and other health service activities.

outcome data, data collected to evaluate the capacity of a client to function at a level described in the outcome statement of a nursing care plan or in standards for client care.

outcome measure, a measure of the quality of medical care, the standard against which the end result of the intervention is assessed.

outlet [AS, *ut* + *laetan,* to permit], an opening through which something can exit, such as the pelvic outlet.

outlet contraction. See **contraction.**

outlet contracture, an abnormally small pelvic outlet. It may be anteroposterior or transverse and is of significance in childbirth because it may impede or prevent the passage of a baby through the birth canal. Anteroposterior contracture caused by fixation of the coccyx may sometimes be overcome by the force of labor, freeing the bones and allowing them to move back. Significant narrowing of the space between the ischial tuberosities is unlikely to be overcome and is most commonly associated with a heavy, android type of pelvis.

outlet forceps. See **low forceps.**

outline form [AS, *ut* + *lin,* thread], the shape of the cavosurface of a prepared tooth cavity.

outpatient (OP), [AS, *ut* + L, *patientia,* endurance], **1.** a patient, not hospitalized, who is being treated in an office, clinic, or other ambulatory care facility. **2.** of or pertaining to a health care facility for patients who are not hospitalized or to the treatment or care of such a patient. Compare **inpatient.**

output [AS, *ut* + *putian,* to put], **1.** the total of any and all measurable liquids lost from the body, including urine, vomitus, diarrhea, and drainage from wounds, from fistulas, and removed by suction equipment. The output is recorded as a means of monitoring a patient's fluid and electrolyte balance. **2.** the end product of a system.

output device, any device that converts information from a computer into a form that is readable by humans or another machine, such as a printer or CRT.

ova and parasites test /ō'va/, a microscopic examination of feces for detecting parasites, such as amebas or worms and their ova, which are indicators of parasitic disorders.

ovale malaria. See **tertian malaria.**

ovalocytes /ō'vəlōsīts'/ [L, *ovalis,* egg-shaped; Gk, *kytos,* cell], oblong or oval-shaped red blood cells with pale centers that are found occasionally in patients with hemolytic anemias, thalassemias, and hereditary elliptocytosis. A genetic factor may be responsible for the presence of the abnormal blood cells. See also **elliptocytosis.**

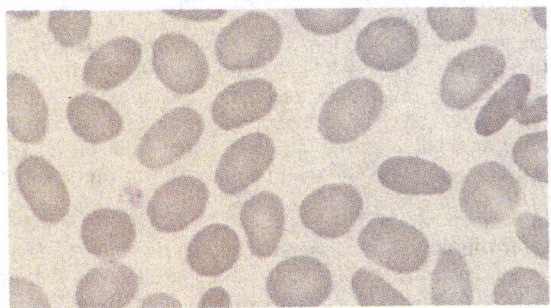

Ovalocytes *(Bain, 1989)*

ovalocytosis. See **elliptocytosis.**

oval window /ō'vəl/ [L, *ovum;* ME, *windoge*], an oval-shaped aperture in the wall of the middle ear, leading to the inner ear. The footplate of the stapes vibrates in the oval window, transmitting sound waves to the cochlea.

ovari-. See **ovario-.**

-ovaria, a combining form meaning '(condition of the)

ovary or ovarial activity': *anovaria, hyperovaria, hypoovaria.*

ovarian /ōver′ē·ən/ [L, *ovum*, egg], of or pertaining to the ovary.

ovarian artery, a slender branch of the abdominal aorta, arising caudal to the renal arteries, and supplying an ovary. Compare **testicular artery.**

ovarian cancer, See **ovarian carcinoma.**

ovarian carcinoma, a malignant neoplasm of the ovaries rarely detected in the early stage and usually far advanced when diagnosed. It occurs frequently in the fifth decade of life. The most common gynecologic tumor, ovarian cancer appears to be increasing in the United States. Risk factors of the disease are infertility, nulliparity or low parity, delayed childbearing, repeated spontaneous abortion, endometriosis, group A blood type, previous irradiation of pelvic organs, and exposure to chemical carcinogens, such as asbestos and talc. After an insidious onset and asymptomatic period, the tumor may become evident as a palpable abdominal or pelvic mass accompanied by irregular or excessive menses or postmenopausal bleeding. In advanced cases the patient may have ascites, edema of the legs, and pain in the abdomen and the backs of the legs. Regular yearly pelvic examinations after 40 years of age contribute significantly to early diagnosis and the possibility of curative treatment. Characteristic of the disease as it advances are abdominal swelling and discomfort, abnormal vaginal bleeding, weight loss, dysuria or abnormal frequency of urination, constipation, and a palpable ovarian mass, especially in postmenopausal women. A Pap smear may show malignant cells if the tumor is advanced; an ultrasonic examination can demonstrate an ovarian mass but does not distinguish between a benign and malignant lesion. A CT scan may be useful in detecting ovarian cancer, but a definitive diagnosis requires surgical exploration. Most ovarian carcinomas are papillary or serous, followed in frequency by mucinous, endometrial, and undifferentiated cancers. In many cases the cancer spreads over the surface of the peritoneum, and, early in the course of the lesion, tumor cells invade the lymphatic vessels under the diaphragm and the paraaortic nodes. Many kinds of tumors may arise in the ovary. About 85% are epithelial in origin, with papillary serous tumors the most common, followed by mucinous, endometrial, and undifferentiated solid cancers. The surgery rec-

ommended for ovarian cancer is total abdominal hysterectomy and bilateral salpingo-oophorectomy with omentectomy. Approximately one half of the tumors diagnosed are inoperable. Treatment of resectable lesions consists of total abdominal hysterectomy, removal of both ovaries and tubes, omentectomy, and biopsies of any suspicious sites, especially in the liver and diaphragm. Postoperative supervoltage irradiation of the pelvis and paraaortic lymph nodes is recommended; the instillation of radioisotopes is used in some cases. Chemotherapeutic agents that may be administered postoperatively include chlorambucil, cyclophosphamide, melphalean, and thiotepa.

ovarian cyst, a globular sac filled with fluid or semisolid material that develops in or on the ovary. It may be transient and physiologic or pathologic. Kinds of ovarian cysts include **chocolate cyst, corpus luteum cyst,** and **dermoid cyst.**

ovarian follicle [L, *ovum*; *folliculus,* small bag], a cavity or recess in an ovary containing a liquor that divides the follicular cells into layers and surrounds an ovum.

ovarian pregnancy, a rare type of ectopic pregnancy in which the conceptus is implanted within the ovary.

ovarian seminoma. See **dysgerminoma.**

ovarian varicocele, a varicose swelling of the veins of the uterine broad ligament. Also called **pelvic varicocele.**

ovarian vein, one of a pair of veins that emerge from convoluted plexuses in the broad ligament near the ovaries and the uterine tubes. The veins from each plexus ascend and unite to form single veins. The right ovarian vein opens into the inferior vena cava, and the left ovarian vein into the renal vein. In some individuals the ovarian veins contain valves and greatly enlarge during pregnancy. Compare **testicular vein.**

ovariectomy. See **oophorectomy.**

ovario-, ovari-, oario-, ootheco-, a combining form meaning 'of or pertaining to the ovary': *ovariocentesis, ovariosteresis, ovariotubal.*

ovary /ō′vərē/ [L, *ovum*, egg], one of the pair of female gonads found on each side of the lower abdomen, beside the uterus, in a fold of the broad ligament. At ovulation, an egg is extruded from a follicle on the surface of the ovary under the stimulation of the gonadotrophic hormones, follicle-stimulating hormone (FSH), and luteinizing hormone (LH). The mature ovarian follicle secretes the hormones estrogen and progesterone, which regulate the menstrual cycle by a negative-feedback system in which an increase in estrogen decreases the secretion of FSH by the pituitary gland and an increase in progesterone decreases the secretion of LH. Each ovary is normally firm and smooth and resembles an almond in size and shape. The ovaries are homologous to the testes.

Ovcon, a trademark for an oral contraceptive containing an estrogen (ethinyl estradiol) and a progestin (norethindrone acetate).

overbite /ō′vərbīt/ [AS, *ofer,* over, *bitan,* to bite], vertical overlapping of lower teeth by upper teeth, usually measured perpendicularly to the occlusal plane. Compare **overclosure, overjet.** (See Fig. p. 1136.)

overclosure /-klō′zhər/ [AS, *ofer* + L, *claudere,* to close], an abnormal condition in which the mandible rises too far before the teeth make contact, caused by the loss of occlusal vertical dimension.

overcompensation /-kom′pənsā′shən/ [AS, *ofer* + L, *compensare,* to weigh together], an exaggerated attempt to

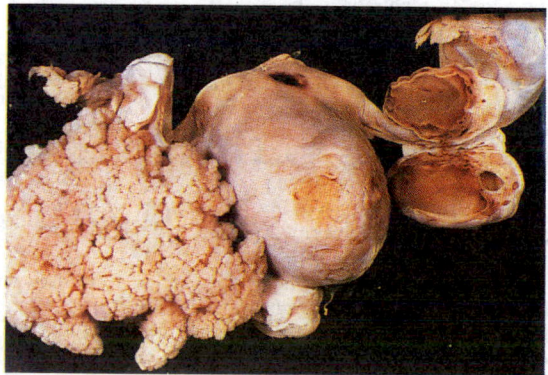

Ovarian carcinoma (Turk, 1986)

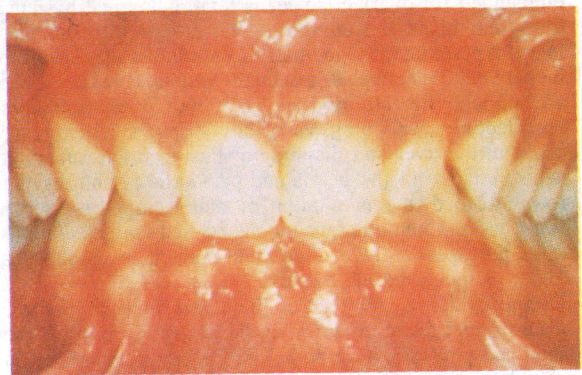

Overbite (Bennett, 1993)

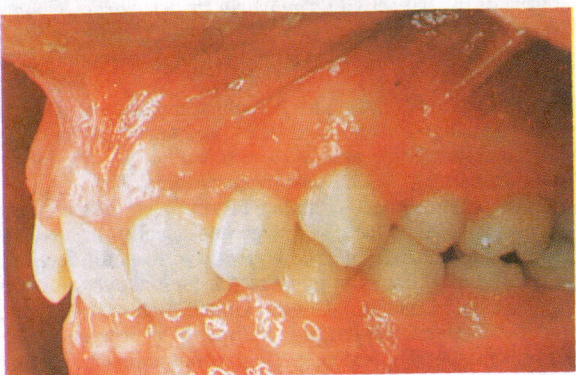

Overjet (Bennett, 1993)

overcome a real or imagined physical or psychologic deficit. The attempt may be conscious or unconscious. See also **compensation.**

overdenture /-den'cher/ [AS, *ofer* + L, *dens*, tooth], a complete or partial removable denture supported by retained roots to provide improved support, stability, and tactile and proprioceptive sensation and to reduce ridge resorption.

overdose (OD) /-dōs/, an excessive use of a drug, resulting in adverse reactions ranging from mania or hysteria to coma or death.

overdrive suppression /-drīv/ [AS, *ofer* + *drifan*, to drive], the inhibitory effect of a faster cardiac pacemaker on a slower one.

overflow /-flow/ [AS, *ofer* + *flowan*], the flooding or excessive discharge of a fluid, such as urine, saliva, or bile.

overflow incontinence [AS, *ofer* + *flowan*; L, *incontinentia*, inability to retain], an overflow of urine from a distended paralyzed bladder.

overgrowth [AS, *ofer*; ME, *growen*], an excessive growth, usually applied to organ or tissue development. Also called **hypertrophy.**

overhang /-hang/ [AS, *ofer* + *hangian*, to hang], an excess of dental filling material that projects beyond the margin of the associated tooth cavity.

overhydration /-hīdrā'shən/, an excess of water in the body.

overinclusiveness /-inkloo'sivnəs/ [AS, *ofer* + L, *includere*, to include], a type of association disorder observed in some schizophrenia patients. The individual is unable to think in a precise manner because of an inability to keep irrelevant elements outside perceptual boundaries.

overjet /-jet/ [AS, *ofer* + Fr, *jeter*, to throw], a horizontal projection of upper teeth beyond the lower teeth, usually measured parallel to the occlusal plane. Also called **horizontal overlap.** Compare **overbite, overclosure.**

overload /-lōd/, **1.** a burden greater than the capacity of the system designed to move or process it. **2.** (in physiology) any factor or influence that stresses the body beyond its natural limits and may impair its health.

overoxygenation /-ok'sijənā'shən/ [AS, *ofer* + Gk, *oxys*, sharp, *genein*, to produce; L, *atio*, process], an abnormal condition in which the oxygen concentration in the blood and other tissues of the body is greater than normal, and the carbon dioxide concentration is less than normal. The condition is characterized by a fall in blood pressure, de-

creased vital capacity, fatigue, errors in judgment, paresthesia of the hands and feet, anorexia, nausea and vomiting, and hyperemia.

overriding /-rīding/ [AS, *ofer* + *ridan*], the overlapping or telescoping of body parts, such as when one fragment of a fractured bone rests on another.

overripe cataract /-rīp/ [AS, *ofer*; OE, *reap*], a cataract in which a completely opaque lens solidifies and shrinks.

over the counter (OTC), (of a drug) available to the consumer without a prescription.

overweight /-wāt/ [AS, *ofer* + *gewiht*, weight], more than normal in body weight after adjustment for height, body build, and age, or 10 to 20 percent above the person's 'desirable' body weight.

ovi-, ovo-, a combining form meaning 'pertaining to an ovum or egg': *ovipara, oviposit, ovoplasm.*

oviduct. See **fallopian tube.**

oviferous /ōvif'ərəs/ [L, *ovum*, egg, *ferre*, to bear], bearing or capable of producing ova (egg cells).

oviparous /ōvip'ərəs/ [L, *ovum* + *parere*, to bring forth], giving birth to young by laying eggs. Compare **ovoviviparous, viviparous.**

oviposition /ō'vipəsish'ən/ [L, *ovum* + *ponere*, to place], the act of laying or depositing eggs by the female member of oviparous animals.

ovipositor /ō'vipos'itər/ [L, *ovum* + *ponere*, to place], a specialized organ, found primarily in insects, for depositing eggs on plants or in the soil.

ovo-. See **ovi-.**

ovocenter /ō'vəsen'tər/ [L, *ovum* + *centrum*, center], the centrosome of a fertilized ovum. Also called **oocenter** /ō'əsen'tər/.

ovoflavin /ō'vəflā'vin/ [L, *ovum* + *flavus*, yellow], a riboflavin derived from the yolk of eggs.

ovogenesis. See **oogenesis.**

ovoglobulin /ō'vəglob'yoōlin/ [L, *ovum* + *globulus*, small sphere], a globulin derived from the white of eggs.

ovogonium. See **oogonium.**

ovoid arch /ō'void/ [L, *ovum* + Gk, *eidos*, form; L, *arcus*, bow], a dental arch that curves smoothly from the molars on one side to those on the opposite side to form half an oval.

ovo-lacto-vegetarian. See **lacto-ovo-vegetarian.**

ovomucin /ō'vəmyoō'sin/ [L, *ovum* + *mucus*, slime], a glycoprotein derived from the white of eggs.

ovomucoid /ō′vəmyŏŏ′koid/ [L, *ovum* + *mucus*, slime; Gk, *eidos*, form], of or pertaining to a glycoprotein, similar to mucin, derived from the white of eggs.

ovoplasm. See **ooplasm.**

ovotestis /ō′vətes′tis/ [L, *ovum* + *testis*, testicle], a gonad that contains both ovarian and testicular tissue; a hermaphroditic gonad. **–ovotesticular,** *adj.*

ovovitellin. See **vitellin.**

ovoviviparous /ō′vəvivip′ərəs/ [L, *ovum* + *vivus*, living, *parere*, to bring forth], bearing young in eggs that are hatched within the body, such as some reptiles and fishes. Compare **oviparous, viviparous.**

Ovral, a trademark for an oral contraceptive containing a progestin (norgestrel) and an estrogen (ethinyl estradiol).

Ovrette, a trademark for an oral contraceptive containing a progestin (norgestrel).

ovulation /ov′yəlā′shən/ [L, *ovum* + *atio*, process], expulsion of an ovum from the ovary on spontaneous rupture of a mature follicle as a result of cyclic ovarian and pituitary endocrine function. It usually occurs on the fourteenth day after the first day of the last menstrual period and often causes brief, sharp lower abdominal pain on the side of the ovulating ovary. See also **oogenesis. –ovulate** /ov′yə′lāt/, *v.*

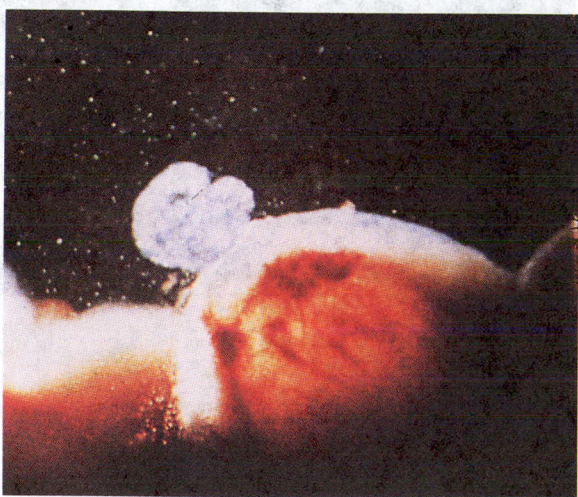

Ovulation *(Erlandsen, 1992)*

ovulation method of family planning, a natural method of family planning that uses observation of changes in the character and quantity of cervical mucus as a means of determining the time of ovulation during the menstrual cycle. Because pregnancy occurs with fertilization of an ovum extruded from the ovary at ovulation, the method is used to increase or decrease the woman's chance of becoming pregnant by causing or avoiding insemination by spontaneous or artificial means during the fertile period associated with ovulation. The cyclic changes in gonadotropic hormones, especially estrogen, cause changes in the quantity and character of cervical mucus. In the first days after menstruation, scant thick mucus is secreted by the cervix. These 'dry days' are 'safe days,' with ovulation several days away. The quantity of mucus then increases; it is pearly-white and sticky,

becoming clearer and less sticky as ovulation approaches; these 'wet days' are 'unsafe days.' During and just after ovulation the mucus is clear, slippery, and elastic; it resembles the uncooked white of an egg. The day on which this sign is most apparent is the 'peak day,' probably the day before ovulation. The 4 days after the 'peak day' are 'unsafe', fertilization might occur. By the end of the 4 days, the mucus becomes pearly-white and sticky again and progressively decreases in quantity until menstruation supervenes to begin a new cycle. Essential to the effectiveness of this method are thorough instruction by a family planning counselor and strong self-motivation in the couple. During the first cycle, abstinence may be necessary to allow observation of the mucus without the confusing addition of semen or contraceptive foam, cream, or jelly, if being used. Daily close monitoring of the mucus is necessary even after several cycles because the length of the 'safe' and 'unsafe' periods and the time of ovulation vary from cycle to cycle, as they do from woman to woman. Postpartally, and during lactation, the method is not effective until the menses have become regular. Effectiveness of the method in identifying the most fertile days of the cycle is augmented by using the basal body temperature method. This combined method is called the symptothermal method of planning. Proponents of the ovulation method claim the benefits of low cost, naturalness, and effectiveness. Detractors emphasize a limited public health application of the method, stating that it requires extensive teaching and self-motivation and that its effectiveness is limited by the ability of the user to observe correctly and diligently the changes in the cervical mucus. Abstinence may be necessary for up to 10 days by a woman whose menstrual cycles are long or are of irregular length. Also called **cervical mucus method of family planning.**

ovulatory /ov′yələtôr′ē/ [L, *ovum*], pertaining to ovulation.

Ovulen, a trademark for an oral contraceptive containing an estrogen (mestranol) and a progestin (ethynodiol diacetate).

ovum /ō′vəm/, *pl.* **ova** [L, egg], **1.** an egg. **2.** a female germ cell extruded from the ovary at ovulation.

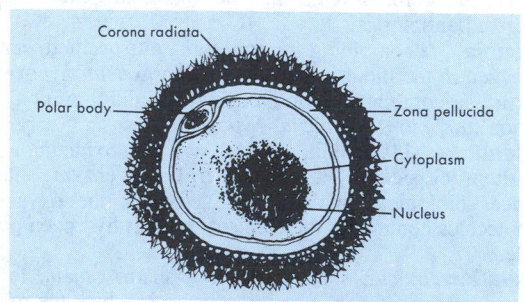

Ovum

ox-, oxi-, combining forms meaning 'pertaining to the presence of oxygen': *oxidize.*

oxacillin sodium /ok′səsil′in/, a penicillinase-resistant penicillin antibiotic.

■ INDICATION: It is prescribed in the treatment of severe infections caused by penicillinase-producing staphylococci.

■ CONTRAINDICATIONS: Known hypersensitivity to this drug or to any other penicillin prohibits its use.

■ ADVERSE EFFECTS: Among the most serious effects are anaphylaxis and other less severe allergic reactions, GI disturbances, and pruritus ani and vulvae.

-oxacin, a combining form for nalidixic acid-type antibacterial agents.

oxal-, oxalo-, combining forms indicating molecules derived from oxalic acid: *oxaloacetate, oxalic.*

oxaluric acid /ok'səloŏr'ik/, a compound derived from uric acid or from parabonic acid, which occurs in normal urine.

oxamniquine /oksam'nəkwēn/, an antischistosomal.

■ INDICATION: It is prescribed in the treatment of infection caused by *Schistosoma mansoni.*

■ CONTRAINDICATIONS: Renal failure, congestive heart failure, or known hypersensitivity to this drug prohibits its use.

■ ADVERSE EFFECTS: Among the more serious adverse reactions are dizziness, drowsiness, and convulsions, particularly in patients with a history of epilepsy.

-oxan, a combining form for benzodioxane-derived alpha-adrenoceptor antagonists.

oxandrolone /oksan'drəlōn/, an androgen.

■ INDICATIONS: It is prescribed in the treatment of testosterone deficiency, osteoporosis, and female breast cancer and for the stimulation of growth, weight gain, and red blood cell production.

■ CONTRAINDICATIONS: Cancer of the male breast or prostate, liver disease, pregnancy or suspected pregnancy, or known hypersensitivity to this drug prohibits its use.

■ ADVERSE EFFECTS: Among the more serious adverse reactions are hirsutism, acne, liver toxicity, electrolyte imbalances, and various endocrine effects in some patients.

oxazepam /oksā'zəpam/, a minor tranquilizer.

■ INDICATIONS: It is prescribed to relieve anxiety and nervous tension.

■ CONTRAINDICATIONS: Acute narrow-angle glaucoma, psychotic disorders, or known hypersensitivity to this drug prohibits its use.

■ ADVERSE EFFECTS: Among the more serious adverse reactions are withdrawal symptoms resulting from discontinuation of treatment. Dizziness and fatigue commonly occur.

-oxef, a combining form for oxacefalosporanic acid-derived antibiotics.

-oxemia, a combining form meaning a '(specified) state of oxygen in the blood': *anoxemia, hyperoxemia, hypoxemia.*

-oxia, a combining form meaning '(condition of) oxygenation': *anoxia, asthenoxia, hypoxia.*

oxidant /ok'sidənt/ [Gk, *oxys,* sharp], an oxidizing agent.

oxidase /ok'sidās/ [Gk, *oxys,* sharp], an enzyme that induces biological oxidation by activating the oxygen in molecules containing the element, such as hydrogen peroxide.

oxidation /ok'sidā'shən/ [Gk, *oxys,* sharp, *genein,* to produce, *atio,* process], **1.** any process in which the oxygen content of a compound is increased. **2.** any reaction in which the positive valence of a compound or a radical is increased because of a loss of electrons. **–oxidize,** *v.*

oxidation-reduction reaction, a chemical change in which electrons are removed (oxidation) from an atom or molecule, accompanied by a simultaneous transfer of electrons (reduction) to another. Also called **redux.**

oxidative phosphorylation, an ATP-generating process in which oxygen serves as the final electron acceptor. The process occurs in mitochondria and is the major source of

ATP generation in aerobic organisms. Also called **respirations**

oxidative water /ok'sidā'tiv/ [Gk, *oxys,* sharp, *genein,* to produce, *atus,* process], water produced by the oxidation of molecules of food substances, such as the conversion of glucose to water and carbon dioxide.

oxidize /ok'sidīz/ [Gk, *oxys,* sharp, *genein,* to produce, *izein,* to cause], (of an element or compound) to combine or cause to combine with oxygen, to remove hydrogen, or to increase the valence of an element through the loss of electrons. **–oxidation,** *n.,* **oxidizing,** *adj.*

oxidizing agent, a compound that readily gives up oxygen or attracts hydrogen or electrons from another compound. In chemical reactions an oxidizing agent acts as an acceptor of electrons, thereby increasing the valence of an element.

oxidoreductase /ok'sidō'riduk'tās/, an enzyme that catalyzes a reaction in which one substance is oxidized while another is reduced. An example is alcohol dehydrogenase.

oximeter /oksim'ətər/, any of several devices used to measure oxyhemoglobin in the blood.

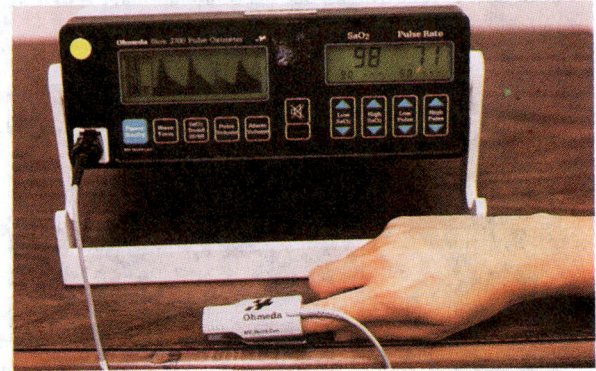

Pulse oximeter *(Wilson, 1991)*

Oxsoralen, a trademark for a pigmentation agent (methoxsalen).

oxtriphylline /oks'trəfil'ēn/, a bronchodilator.

■ INDICATIONS: It is prescribed in the treatment of bronchial asthma, bronchitis, and emphysema.

■ CONTRAINDICATIONS: Known hypersensitivity to this drug or other xanthine derivatives prohibits its use. It is used with caution in patients with ulcer or with coronary disease for whom cardiac stimulation might be harmful.

■ ADVERSE EFFECTS: Among the more common adverse reactions are GI distress, palpitations, nervousness, and insomnia.

oxy-, **1.** a combining form meaning 'sharp, quick, or sour': *oxyblepsia, oxycephalia, oxyecoia.* **2.** a combining form indicating the presence of oxygen in a compound: *oxyacanthine, oxycamphor, oxyquinoline.*

oxybenzene. See **carbolic acid.**

oxybutynin chloride /ok'siboŏ'tinin/, an anticholinergic.

■ INDICATION: It is prescribed in the treatment of neurogenic bladder.

■ CONTRAINDICATIONS: Glaucoma, obstruction of the GI or urinary tract, ulcerative colitis, paralytic ileus, toxic megacolon, or known hypersensitivity to this drug or to other anticholinergics prohibits its use.

■ ADVERSE EFFECTS: Among the more serious adverse effects are decreased sweating, urinary retention, blurred vision, tachycardia, and severe allergic reactions.

oxycephaly /okʹsisefʹəlē/ [Gk, *oxys* + *kephale*, head], a congenital malformation of the skull in which premature closure of the coronal and sagittal sutures results in accelerated upward growth of the head, giving it a long, narrow appearance with the top pointed or conic in shape. The cephalic index is over 75. Also called **acrocephaly, hypsicephaly, oxycephalia, steeple head, tower head, tower skull, turricephaly.** See also **craniostenosis.** −**oxycephalus,** *n.,* **oxycephalous,** *adj.*

oxycodone hydrochloride /okʹsikōdōn/, a narcotic analgesic.

■ INDICATION: It is used to treat moderate to severe pain.

■ CONTRAINDICATIONS: It is used with caution in many conditions, including head injuries, asthma, impaired renal or hepatic function, or unstable cardiovascular status. Known hypersensitivity to this drug prohibits its use.

■ ADVERSE EFFECTS: Among the most serious adverse reactions are drowsiness, dizziness, nausea, constipation, respiratory and circulatory depression, and drug addiction.

Oxy-5, a trademark for a keratolytic (benzoyl peroxide).

oxygen (O) /okʹsəjən/ [Gk, *oxys,* sharp, *genein,* to produce], a tasteless, odorless, colorless gas essential for human respiration. Its atomic weight is 15.9994; its atomic number is 8. In anesthesia, oxygen functions as a carrier gas for the delivery of anesthetic agents to the tissues of the body. It is given by mask at a rate of flow and concentration appropriate to the physical status of the patient, the surgical procedure, and the anesthetic agent being administered. In respiratory therapy, oxygen is administered to increase its amount and thus to decrease the amount of other gases circulating in the blood. Overdose of oxygen can cause irreversible toxicity in people with pulmonary abnormalities, especially when complicated by chronic carbon dioxide retention. Prolonged administration of high concentrations of oxygen may cause irreversible damage to infants' eyes. Because an oxygen-rich environment is favorable to fire and explosion, smoking, open flame, or electric spark must be avoided when oxygen is being administered. See also **oxygen toxicity.**

oxygenation /okʹsəjənāʹshən/, the process of combining or treating with oxygen. −**oxygenate,** *v.*

oxygen capacity of blood, the maximum amount of oxygen that can be made to combine chemically with hemoglobin in a unit of blood, excluding physically dissolved oxygen. Although 1 g of hemoglobin can theoretically bind a maximum of 1.34 ml (STPD) of oxygen, this value is never actually achieved in vivo because of such variable factors as the formation of carboxyhemoglobin and the presence of methemoglobin or other inactive hemoglobins.

oxygen concentration in blood, the concentration of oxygen in a blood sample, including both oxygen combined with hemoglobin and oxygen physically dissolved in blood.

oxygen consumption, the amount of oxygen in milliliters per minute required by the body for normal aerobic metabolism; normally about 250 ml/min.

oxygen cost of breathing, the rate at which the respiratory muscles consume oxygen as they ventilate the lungs.

oxygen debt, the quantity of oxygen taken up by the lungs during recovery from a period of exercise or apnea that is in excess of the quantity needed for resting metabolism during the preexercise period. Oxygen debt represents repayment of oxygen and energy stores that were depleted dur-

ing the time that oxygen uptake from the environment was inadequate for aerobic metabolism.

oxygen enhancement ratio (OER), a measure of tumor sensitivity to the presence or absence of oxygen, expressed as the ratio of radiation dose required to produce a given effect with no oxygen present to the dose required to produce the same effect in one atmosphere of air.

oxygen half-saturation pressure of hemoglobin, the oxygen pressure necessary for 50% saturation of hemoglobin at body temperature and at pH 7.4 or 40 torr carbon dioxide pressure. The value is commonly used as a measure of the affinity between oxygen and hemoglobin.

oxygen hood, a device placed over the head of neonatal patients to deliver high concentrations of oxygen.

oxygen mask, a device used to administer oxygen. It is shaped to fit snugly over the mouth and nose and may be secured in place with a strap or held with the hand. The mask has inspiratory and expiratory valves allowing oxygen to be inhaled or pumped into the respiratory tract and carbon dioxide to be exhaled into the environment. Oxygen flows at a prescribed rate through a catheter to the mask, often through a soft rubber bag that can be pumped by hand. See also **Ambu bag.**

oxygen radicals [Gk, *oxys,* sharp; L, *radix,* root], a substituent group of chemical elements rich in oxygen but incapable of prolonged existence in a free state. Oxygen radicals are used in some types of therapy.

oxygen saturation, the fraction of a total hemoglobin (HB) in the form of HbO_2 at a defined PO_2.

oxygen store, the total quantity of oxygen normally stored in the various body compartments, including the lungs, arterial and venous blood, and tissues. In a 70 kg human, blood contains about 800 ml oxygen as oxyhemoglobin, muscles contain about 150 ml as oxymyoglobin, alveolar gas contains a few hundred milliters, and about 50 ml is dissolved in the tissues.

oxygen tension, the force with which oxygen molecules that are physically dissolved in blood are constantly trying to escape, expressed as partial pressure (PO_2). The tension at any instant is related to the amount of oxygen physically dissolved in plasma; the larger amount carried in chemical combination with hemoglobin serves as a reservoir that releases oxygen molecules to physical solution when the tension decreases and that stores additional molecules of the gas when the tension increases.

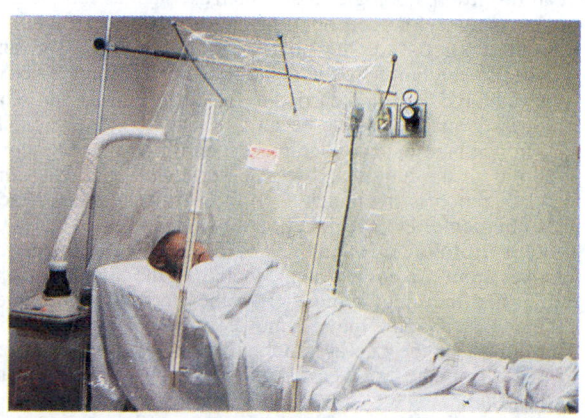

Oxygen tent *(Wilson, 1991)*

O-P

oxygen tent [Gk, *oxys,* sharp; ME, *tente*], a canopy that encloses the head and neck of a patient and contains a high oxygen tension.

oxygen therapy, any procedure in which oxygen is administered to a patient to relieve hypoxia.

■ METHOD: Of the many methods for providing oxygen therapy, the one selected depends on the condition of the patient and the cause of hypoxia. Low or moderate amounts of oxygen may be supplied to postoperative patients by a nasal catheter or cannula. Low concentrations, precisely measured, may be delivered by a Venturi mask to patients with chronic obstructive lung disease. If hypoxia is the result of impaired cardiac function, a high concentration of oxygen may be delivered by a nonrebreathing or partial rebreathing mask. Humidity and drugs in aerosol form may be given with oxygen using a variety of devices, such as an aerosol face mask, Croupette, or T-piece.

■ NURSING INTERVENTION: Thorough and careful observation of the patient's need for oxygen and response to therapy are important. The concentration of oxygen received by the patient must not be assumed by the rate and concentration at which it is delivered: A person whose respirations are rapid and shallow receives more oxygen than does a person breathing deeply and slowly. Many clinical situations require frequent laboratory evaluations of the levels of arterial blood gases. The adverse effects of oxygen therapy include respiratory depression, absorption atelectasis, alveolar collapse, alveolar edema, pulmonary congestion, intraalveolar hemorrhage, hyaline membrane formation, pain, retrolental fibroplasia, and disturbance of the central nervous system with seizures and, possibly, death. Thorough knowledge of the equipment used and of the condition being treated enables the nurse to care safely and effectively for the patient who requires oxygen.

■ OUTCOME CRITERIA: Oxygen therapy may be used in the treatment of any condition that results in hypoxia. Although there are several kinds of hypoxia, all result in hypoxemia. The administration of oxygen may relieve hypotension, cardiac dysrythmias, tachypnea, headache, disorientation, nausea, and agitation characteristic of hypoxia, as well as restore the ability of the cells of the body to carry on normal metabolic function.

oxygen tolerance, an increased capacity to withstand the toxic effects of hyperoxia as a result of any adaptive change occurring within an organism.

oxygen toxicity, a condition of oxygen overdosage that can result in pathologic tissue changes, such as retinopathy of prematurity or bronchopulmonary dysplasia.

oxygen transport, the process by which oxygen is absorbed in the lungs by the hemoglobin in circulating deoxygenated red cells and carried to the peripheral tissues. The process is made possible because hemoglobin has the ability to combine with oxygen present at a high concentration, such as in the lungs, and to release this oxygen when the concentration is low, such as in the peripheral tissues. See also **hemoglobin.**

oxygen uptake, the amount of oxygen an organism removes from the environment, including the amount of oxygen that the lungs remove from the ambient atmosphere, the amount that the blood removes from the alveolar gas in the lungs, or the rate at which an organ or tissue removes oxygen from the blood perfusing it. Also called **oxygen consumption.**

oxygen-utilization coefficient. See **coefficient.**

oxyhemoglobin /ok'sēhē'məglō'bin, -hem'-/ [Gk, *oxys* + *genein,* to produce, *haima,* blood; L, *globus,* ball], the product of combining hemoglobin with oxygen. The loosely bound complex dissociates easily when the concentration of oxygen is low.

oxyhemoglobin dissociation curve, a graphic expression of the affinity between oxygen and hemoglobin, or the amount of oxygen chemically bound at equilibrium to the hemoglobin in blood as a function of oxygen pressure. To define the curve completely, it should also include the pH, temperature, and carbon dioxide pressure.

oxyhemoglobin saturation, the amount of oxygen actually combined with hemoglobin, expressed as a percentage of the oxygen capacity of that hemoglobin.

Oxylone, a trademark for a glucocorticoid (fluorometholone).

oxymetazoline hydrochloride /ok'sēmətaz'əlēn/, a decongestant.

■ INDICATION: It is prescribed in the treatment of nasal congestion.

■ CONTRAINDICATIONS: Hyperthyroidism, diabetes, use of a monoamine oxidase inhibitor within 14 days, or known hypersensitivity to this drug prohibits its use.

■ ADVERSE EFFECTS: Among the more serious adverse reactions are rebound congestion, central nervous system stimulation, and, in children, a severe shocklike syndrome with coma, hypotension, and bradycardia.

oxymetholone /ok'sēmeth'əlōn/, an androgen.

■ INDICATIONS: It is prescribed in the treatment of testosterone deficiency, osteoporosis, and female breast cancer and for the stimulation of growth, weight gain, and red blood cell production.

■ CONTRAINDICATIONS: Cancer of the male breast or prostate, liver disease, pregnancy or suspected pregnancy, or known hypersensitivity to this drug prohibits its use.

■ ADVERSE EFFECTS: Among the more serious adverse reactions are hirsutism, acne, liver toxicity, electrolyte imbalances, and, depending on the age of the patient, various endocrine effects.

oxymorphone hydrochloride /ok'sēmôr'fōn/, a narcotic analgesic.

■ INDICATIONS: It is prescribed to reduce moderate to severe pain, as a preoperative medication, and to support anesthesia.

■ CONTRAINDICATION: Drug dependence or known hypersensitivity to this drug prohibits its use.

■ ADVERSE EFFECTS: Among the more serious adverse reactions are drug dependence, urinary retention, and respiratory or circulatory depression.

oxyopia /ok'sē·ō'pē·ə/ [Gk, *oxys* + *opsis* vision], unusual acuteness of vision. A person with normal (20/20) vision when standing 20 feet from the standard Snellen eye chart can read the seventh line of letters, each of which is an eighth of an inch high, while an individual with oxyopia can read smaller letters at that distance. Also called **oxyopy** /ok'sē·ō'pē/.

oxytetracycline /ok'sētet'rəsī'klēn/, a tetracycline antibiotic.

■ INDICATIONS: It is prescribed in the treatment of bacterial and rickettsial infections.

■ CONTRAINDICATIONS: Pregnancy, early childhood, or known hypersensitivity to this or to other tetracyclines prohibits its use. The drug is used with caution in patients who have renal or liver dysfunction.

■ ADVERSE EFFECTS: Among the more serious adverse reactions are GI disturbances, phototoxicity, potentially serious suprainfections, and various hypersensitivity reactions. Discoloration of teeth may occur in children exposed to the drug in utero or before 8 years of age.

oxytetracycline calcium,   a tetracycline antibiotic.

oxytocic /ok′sitō′sik/ [Gk, *oxys* + *tokos,* birth],   **1.** of or pertaining to a substance that is similar to the hormone oxytocin. **2.** any one of numerous drugs that stimulate the smooth muscle of the uterus to contract. The administration of an oxytocic can initiate and enhance rhythmic uterine contraction at any time, but relatively high doses are required for such responses in early pregnancy. These drugs are often used to initiate labor at term. Oxytocic agents commonly used include oxytocin, certain prostaglandins, and the ergot alkaloids. These drugs are used to induce or augment labor, control postpartum hemorrhage, correct postpartum uterine atony, produce uterine contractions after cesarean section or other uterine surgery, and induce therapeutic abortion. These drugs are used with extreme caution in parturients with severe hypotension and hypertension, partial placenta previa, cephalopelvic disproportion, or grand multiparity. The risk of using these agents is much higher in mothers who have undergone recent uterine surgery or who have suffered recent sepsis or trauma. The most serious adverse reaction is sustained tetanic contraction of the uterus resulting in fetal hypoxia or in rupture of the uterus.

oxytocin /ok′sitō′sin/,   an oxytocic.

■ INDICATIONS: It is prescribed to stimulate contractions in inducing or augmenting labor, and to contract the uterus to control postpartum bleeding.

■ CONTRAINDICATIONS: Cephalopelvic disproportion, unfavorable fetal position, or known hypersensitivity to this drug prohibits its use.

■ ADVERSE EFFECTS: Among the more serious adverse reactions are tetanic contraction, jaundice, uterine rupture, and fetal anoxia.

oxytocin challenge test,   a stress test for the assessment of intrauterine function of the fetus and the placenta. It is performed to evaluate the ability of the fetus to tolerate continuation of pregnancy or the anticipated stress of labor and delivery. A dilute intravenous infusion of oxytocin is begun, monitored by a meter or regulated by an infusion pump. The uterine activity is monitored with a tocodynamometer, and the fetal heart rate is monitored with an ultrasonic sensor as the uterus is stimulated to contract by the oxytocin. The amount of solution infused is increased as necessary to cause the uterus to contract for 30 to 40 seconds three times every 10 minutes. The fetal heart rate is observed for variability and for the timing of any marked variation from the normal in relation to uterine contractions.

Decelerations of the fetal heart rate in certain repeating patterns may indicate fetal distress. One quarter of the infants diagnosed by this method as being in distress are normal; therefore other tests of fetal well-being are recommended before performing an emergency cesarean section or induction of labor.

oxyuriasis.   See **enterobiasis.**

Oxyuris vermicularis.   See *Enterobius vermicularis.*

oz [L, *uncia*],   abbreviation for **ounce.**

oz ap [L, *uncia*],   abbreviation for *apothecary ounce,* a unit of weight equal to 31.1035 grams.

ozena /ōzē′nə/ [Gk, *ozein,* to have an odor],   a condition of the nose characterized by atrophy of the nasal chonchae and mucous membranes. Symptoms include crusting of nasal secretions, discharge, and, especially, a very offensive odor. Ozena may follow chronic inflammation of the nasal mucosa.

ozone [Gk, *ozein,* to have an odor],   a form of oxygen characterized by molecules having three atoms. Ozone is formed when oxygen is electrically charged, as might occur in a lightning storm. Ozone is used as a bleaching, cleaning, and oxidizing agent and has a faint, chlorinelike odor.

ozone shield,   the layer of ozone that hangs in the atmosphere from 20 to 40 miles above the surface of the earth and protects the earth from excessive ultraviolet radiation. Some experts claim that the manufacture of various chemicals, such as chlorofluorocarbons used as propellants in aerosol sprays, and the effects of high-flying jet aircraft are destroying this protective layer and allowing excessive amounts of ultraviolet radiation to penetrate the earth's atmosphere, thus subjecting humans to increased dangers of skin cancer and other health problems. Some chemistry experts and federal health officials also claim that an additional threat comes from nitrous oxide in nitrogenous fertilizers rising into the atmosphere and reacting unfavorably with the ozone shield. Other experts say the depletion of the ozone layer by chlorofluorocarbons may be offset by the release of carbon dioxide into the atmosphere from the combustion of fuels. One study indicates that ozone concentration has actually increased 6% since monitoring was begun more than 50 years ago. The ozone shield is implicated in certain health problems that affect some air travelers. See also **ozone sickness.**

ozone sickness,   an abnormal condition caused by the inhalation of ozone that may seep into jet aircraft at altitudes over 40,000 feet. It is characterized by headaches, chest pains, itchy eyes, and sleepiness. Exactly why and how ozone causes this condition is not known. It is more prevalent early in the year and occurs more often over the Pacific Ocean.

oz t [L, *uncia*],   abbreviation for *troy ounce,* a unit of weight equal to 31.103 grams.

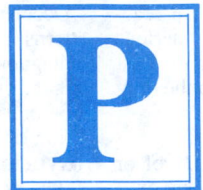

P

P, **1.** symbol for the element **phosphorus 2.** symbol for *gas partial pressure.* See **partial pressure. 3.** symbol for *after* or **post.**

p17, symbol for a protein that lines the interior of the HIV virus envelope.

p24, symbol for a protein that surrounds the RNA and reverse transcriptase of the HIV virus.

p-, symbol for **para-.**

P₂, symbol for *second pulmonic sound.*

P, **1.** (in genetics) symbol for *first parental generation.* **2.** symbol for *first pulmonic sound.*

P₅₀, the partial pressure of oxygen at which hemoglobin is half saturated with bound oxygen.

P1E1, P2E1, P3E1, P4E1, P6E1, trademarks for ophthalmic fixed-combination drugs containing a cholinergic (pilocarpine hydrochloride) and an adrenergic (epinephrine bitartrate). The numbers indicate the percentage of each ingredient in the solution; for example, P2E1 contains 2% pilocarpine HCl and 1% epinephrine bitartrate.

pA, symbol for *picoampere.*

Pa, **1.** symbol for *pascal.* **2.** symbol for the element **protactinium.**

PA, **1.** abbreviation for **physician's assistant. 2.** abbreviation for **pulmonary artery.**

P-A, p-a, abbreviation for **posteroanterior.**

P&A, **1.** abbreviation for *percussion and auscultation.* See **p** and **a. 2.** abbreviation for **posterior and anterior.**

PABA, abbreviation for **paraaminobenzoic acid,** a topical sunscreen.

pabulum /pab'yələm/ [L, food], any substance that is food or nutrient.

pac, abbreviation for *phenacetin-aspirin-caffeine.*

PAC, abbreviation for **premature atrial contraction.**

PA catheter, intravenous catheter that is inserted into the pulmonary artery.

PACE II, an interdisciplinary assessment and planning system that focuses on evaluation of the physical health of nursing home patients. It includes checklists of defined (diagnosed) conditions, abnormal laboratory or other findings, risk factors, and other impairments and disabilities.

pacemaker [L, *passus,* step; AS, *macian,* to make], **1.** the sinoatrial node of specialized nervous tissue located at the junction of the superior vena cava and the right atrium. It originates the contractions of the atria, which transmit the impulse on to the atrioventricular node, thereby initiating the contraction of the atria. An ectopic or indioventricular pacemaker may cause contractions in cases of abnormal heart functions. **2.** also called **cardiac pacemaker.** an electric apparatus used for maintaining a normal sinus rhythm of myocardial contraction by electrically stimulating the heart muscle. A pacemaker may be permanent or temporary, emit the stimulus at a constant and fixed rate, or it may fire only on demand, when the heart does not spontaneously contract at a minimum rate.

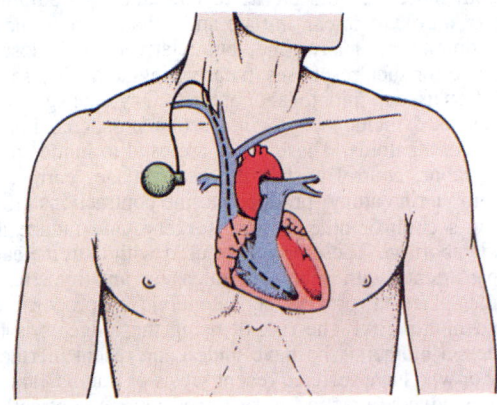

Pacemaker *(Thibodeau, 1993/George Wassilchenko)*

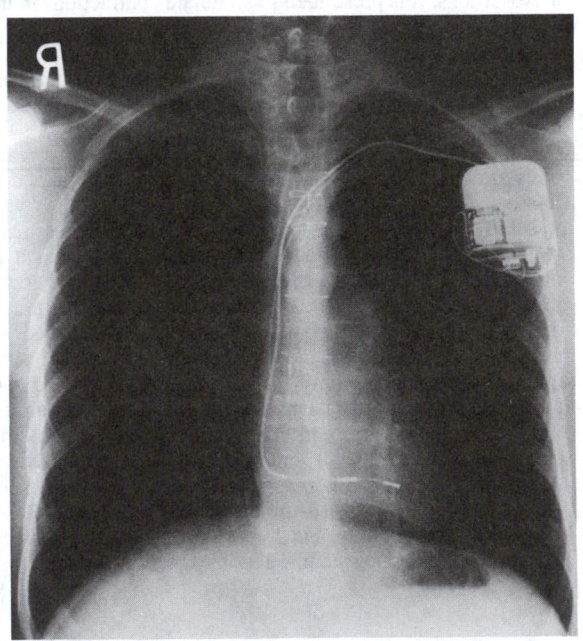

Pacemaker

pacemaker installation fluoroscopy, the fluoroscopic monitoring of the insertion of an artificial pacemaker, used as an aid for correct installation of the device.

pacer. See **pacemaker.**

pachometer. See **pachymeter.**

pachy- /pak'i-/, a combining form meaning 'thick': *pachyaria, pachycephaly, pachymucosa.*

pachycephaly /pak'ēsef'əlē/ [Gk, *pachy*, thick, *kephale*, head], an abnormal thickness of the skull, as in acromegaly. Also called **pachycephalia.** –**pachycephalic, pachycephalous,** *adj.*

pachydactyly /pak'ēdak'tilē/ [Gk, *pachy* + *daktylos*, finger], an abnormal thickening of the fingers or the toes. –**pachydactylic, pachydactylous,** *adj.*

pachyderma alba /-dur'mə/ [Gk, *pachy* + *derma*, skin; L, *albus*, white], an abnormal state of the buccal mucosa in which the appearance is suggestive of whitened elephant hide. Also called **pachyderma oralis.**

pachymeter /pakim'ətər/ [Gk, *pachy* + *metron*, measure], an instrument used to measure thickness, especially of thin structures, such as a membrane or a tissue. Also called **pachometer.**

pachynema /pak'inē'mə/ [Gk, *pachy* + *nema*, thread], the postsynaptic tetradic chromosome formation that occurs in the pachytene stage of the first meiotic prophase of gametogenesis.

pachyonychia congenita /pak'ē·ōnik'ē·ə/ [Gk, *pachy* + *onyx*, nail; L, *congenitus*, born with], a congenital deformity characterized by abnormal thickening and raising of the nails on the fingers and the toes, and hyperkeratosis of the palms of the hands and the soles of the feet. The papillae of the tongue also atrophy, causing a whitish coating over the lingual surface.

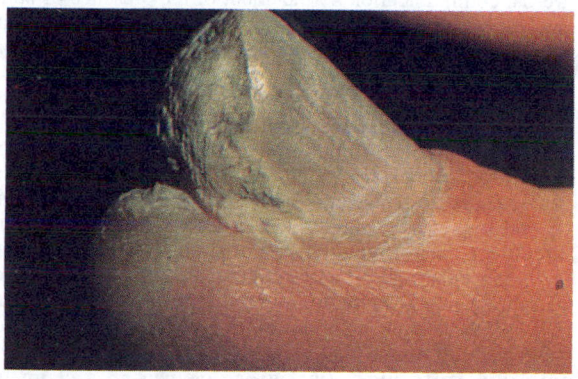

Pachyonychia congenita (Baran, 1991)

pachytene /pak'itēn/ [Gk, *pachy* + *tainia*, ribbon], the third stage in the first meiotic prophase of gametogenesis in which the paired homologous chromosomes form tetrads. The bivalent pairs become short and thick and intertwine so that four chromatids are visible. See also **diakinesis, diplotene, leptotene, zygotene.**

pacifier /pas'ifī'ər/ [L, *pacificare*, to bring peace], **1.** an agent that soothes or comforts. **2.** a nipple-shaped object used by infants and children for sucking. Such devices can be dangerous if they are too small or poorly constructed, because the entire object or part of it can be aspirated or lodged in the pharynx or trachea and obstruct the passage of air. The safest pacifiers are constructed in one piece, are large enough so that only the nipple fits into the mouth, and have a handle that can be easily grasped.

pacing [L, *passus*, step], the artificial electrical stimulation of a heart rhythm. Kinds of pacing include **atrial, coupled, endocardial, epicardial, programmed, AV sequential,** and **ventricular.** See also **programmable pacemaker.**

pacing wire [L, *passus*, step; AS, *wir*], an electrode of a pacemaker, a pacing catheter that is usually inserted into the patient's right ventricle.

Pacini's corpuscles /päsē'nēz/ [Filippo Pacini, Italian anatomist, b. 1812; L, *corpusculum*, little body], a number of special sensory end organs resembling tiny white bulbs, each attached to the end of a single nerve fiber in the subcutaneous, submucous, and subserous connective tissue of many parts of the body, especially the palm of the hand, sole of the foot, genital organs, joints, and pancreas. They average about 3 mm in diameter, are pressure sensitive, contain numerous concentric layers around a central core, and in cross section resemble an onion. Also called **pacinian corpuscles.** Compare **Golgi-Mazzoni corpuscles, Krause's corpuscles.**

pack [ME, *pakke*, bundle], **1.** a treatment in which the entire body or a portion of it is wrapped in wet or dry towels or in ice for various therapeutic purposes, as with cold packs for the reduction of high temperatures and swellings or for inducing hypothermia during certain surgical procedures, especially heart surgery and organ transplants. **2.** a tampon. **3.** the act of applying a dressing or dental cement to a surgical wound. **4.** a surgical dressing to cover a wound or to fill the cavity left from a tooth extraction, especially an extraction of a wisdom tooth.

package insert, a leaflet that, by order of the FDA, must be placed inside the package of every prescription drug. In it, the manufacturer is required to describe the drug, to state its generic name, and to give the applicable indications, contraindications, warnings, precautions, adverse effects, form, dosage, and administration.

packed cells [ME, *pakke*, bundle; L, *cella*, storeroom], a preparation of blood cells separated from liquid plasma, often administered in severe anemia to restore adequate levels of hemoglobin and red cells without overloading the vascular system with excess fluids. See also **bank blood, component therapy, pooled plasma.**

packed cell volume (PCV) [ME, *pakken*; L, *cella*, storeroom, *volumen*, papyrus, roll], a measured quantity of blood to which an anticoagulant has been added and the cells of which have been pressed together by the force of being centrifuged at 2000 rpm. Also called **hematocrit reading.**

packing [ME, *pakken*], **1.** material used to fill a wound or cavity. **2.** the act of inserting material into a wound or cavity.

PaCO_2, abbreviation for *partial pressure of carbon dioxide in arterial blood.*

pad [D, *paden*, a cushion], **1.** a mass of soft material used to cushion shock, prevent wear, or absorb moisture, such as the abdominal pads used to absorb discharges from abdominal wounds or to separate viscera and improve accessibility during abdominal surgery. **2.** (in anatomy) a mass of fat that cushions various structures, such as the infrapatellar pad lying below the patella between the patellar ligament, the head of the tibia, and the femoral condyles.

p.ae. [L, *partes, aequales*], symbol for *equal parts.*

paed-, paedo-. See **ped-, pedo-.**

paedogenesis. See **pedogenesis.**

Paget's disease /paj'əts/ [Sir James Paget, English surgeon, b. 1814], a common, nonmetabolic disease of bone of unknown cause, usually affecting middle-aged and elderly people, characterized by excessive bone destruction and unorganized bone repair.

- OBSERVATIONS: Most cases are asymptomatic or mild; however, bone pain may be the first symptom. Bowed tibias (saber shins), kyphosis, and frequent fractures are caused by the soft, abnormal bone in this condition. Enlargement of the head, headaches, and warmth over involved areas caused by increased vascularity are additional features. The serum alkaline phosphatase is often markedly elevated and there is increased urinary calcium and hydroxyproline. The x-ray picture of areas of decreased bone density adjacent to sites of increased density is characteristic. Radioactive bone scans help locate regions of active disease. Complications include fractures, kidney stones if the patient is immobilized, heart failure, deafness or blindness caused by pressure from bony overgrowth, and osteosarcoma.

- INTERVENTIONS: No treatment is necessary for mild cases. A high-protein, high-calcium diet, unless the patient is immobilized, is recommended. Parenteral synthetic salmon calcitonin may help the patient temporarily. Diphosphonates and mithramycin are also effective but require close monitoring for side effects.

- NURSING CONSIDERATIONS: Immobilization of the patient is avoided, if possible, to prevent hypercalcemia and kidney stones. Mild but regular exercise is recommended. Observation for neurologic signs and symptoms and prompt reporting of changes may help to avert irreversible nerve damage. Also called **osteitis deformans.**

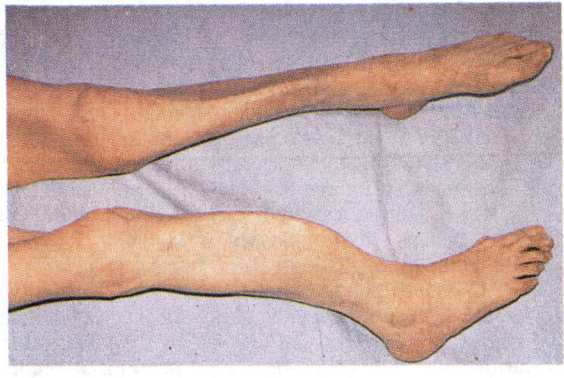

Paget's disease causing deformities in the legs
(Kamal, 1991)

Paget's disease of the nipple. See **nipple cancer.**

pagophagia /pā'gōfā'jē·ə/ [Gk, *pagos,* frost, *phagein,* to eat], an abnormal condition characterized by a craving to eat enormous quantities of ice. It is associated with a lack of nutrient iron. **–pagophagic, pagophagous,** *adj.*

-pagus, a suffix meaning 'conjoined twins': *craniopagus, pyropagus, thoracopagus.*

PAHA, abbreviation for **paraaminohippuric acid.**

PAHA sodium clearance test, a test for detecting kidney damage or certain muscle diseases. The test uses the sodium salt of paraaminohippuric acid for determining the rate at which the kidneys remove this salt from the blood and urine. The normal clearance rates in serum and 24-hour urine specimens are 600 to 750 ml/minute.

PAHO, abbreviation for *Pan American Health Organization.*

pain [L, *poena,* punishment], **1.** an unpleasant sensation caused by noxious stimulation of the sensory nerve endings. It is a subjective feeling and an individual response to the cause. Pain is a cardinal symptom of inflammation and is valuable in the diagnosis of many disorders and conditions. Pain may be mild or severe, chronic, acute, lancinating, burning, dull, or sharp, precisely or poorly localized, or referred. See also **referred pain. 2.** a nursing diagnosis accepted by the Fourth National Conference on the Classification of Nursing Diagnoses. As a symptom, pain is defined as a state in which an individual experiences and reports the presence of severe discomfort or an uncomfortable sensation. The defining characteristics are the verbal or nonverbal communication by the client of the presence of pain, including behavior that is self-protective; a narrowed focus that is indicated by an altered time perception, withdrawal from social contact, or impaired thought processes; distraction behavior, marked by moaning, crying, pacing, restlessness, or the seeking out of other people or activities; a facial mask of pain, recognized by eyes that appear dull and lusterless, a 'beaten' look, and fixed or scattered facial movements or grimace; alteration in muscle tone, ranging from listlessness to rigidity; and autonomic responses to increasing pain, including diaphoresis, changes in blood pressure and pulse rate, pupillary dilation, and an increased or decreased rate of respiration. Related factors include injury by biologic, chemical, physical, or psychologic agents. See also **nursing diagnosis.**

pain and suffering, (in law) an element in a claim for damages that allows recovery for the mental and physical pain, suffering, distress, and trauma that an individual has endured as a result of injury.

Characteristics of acute and chronic pain

Acute pain	Chronic pain	Chronic cancer pain
Identifiable cause	Cause hard to find	Usually identifiable cause
Short duration	Lasts longer than several months	Duration varies
Sudden onset	Begins gradually and persists	Onset varies
Well defined	May or may not be well defined	May or may not be well defined
Limited	Unlimited	Unlimited
Decreases with healing	Persists beyond healing time	May persist beyond healing
Reversible	Exhausting and useless	Exhausting and useless
Objective signs and symptoms	Objective signs absent	Objective signs absent
Anxiety	Depression and fatigue	Depression, fatigue, and anxiety

From Otto SE: *Oncology nursing,* St Louis, 1991, Mosby.

pain assessment, an evaluation of the reported pain and the factors that alleviate or exacerbate a patient's pain, used as an aid in the diagnosis and the treatment of disease and trauma. Responses to pain vary widely among individuals and depend on many different physical and psychologic factors, such as specific diseases and injuries and the health, pain threshold, fear and anxiety, and cultural background of the individual involved, as well as the way different individuals express their pain experiences. See also **pain intervention, pain mechanism.**

■ METHOD: The patient is asked to describe the cause of the pain, if known, its intensity, location, and duration, the events preceding it, and the pattern usually followed for handling pain. Severe pain causes pallor, cold perspiration, piloerection, dilated pupils, and increases in the pulse, respiratory rate, blood pressure, and muscle tension. When brief, intense pain subsides, the pulse may be slower and the blood pressure lower than before the pain began. If pain occurs frequently or is prolonged, the pulse rate and blood pressure may not increase markedly, and, if pain persists for many days, there may be an increased production of eosinophils and 17-ketosteroids and greater susceptibility to infections. The patient's statements regarding pain, the tone of voice, speed of speech, cries, groans, or other vocalizations, facial expressions, body movements, or tendency to withdraw are all noted. Pertinent background information in the assessment includes a record of the patient's chronic conditions, previous surgery, and any illnesses that caused pain, the patient's experiences with relatives and friends in pain, the role or position of the patient in the family structure, and the patient's use of alcohol and medications. Key aspects in evaluating pain intensity are the size of the pain area, the tenderness within the pain area, and the effects of movement and pressure on the pain. Duration of pain is considered in terms of hours, days, weeks, months, or years. Pain patterns are associated with various sensations such as burning, pricking, aching, rhythmic throbbing, and the effects on the sympathetic and the parasympathetic nervous systems. Evaluation includes the meanings the individual may attach to pain, such as a test of character, a penance, or a sign of worsening illness. Such interpretations may affect the intensity of pain and mask its significance.

■ NURSING INTERVENTION: The nurse establishes a relationship with the patient and uses individual counseling or group situations to teach the person about pain and how to modify the anxiety associated with it. Analgesics ordered for the patient are administered by the nurse before the pain becomes intense, for this increases their effectiveness. In addition to helping promote rest and relaxation, the nurse decreases noxious stimuli, provides other pleasant sensory input, and helps to distract the patient by using guided imagery, walking, watching television, or reading. If the patient believes that certain acceptable measures alleviate pain, the nurse uses them.

■ OUTCOME CRITERIA: Dramatic relief of intense or chronic pain is often difficult to accomplish, but the patient can be helped to learn to handle pain effectively and to function fairly normally.

pain, chronic, a nursing diagnosis accepted by the Seventh National Conference on the Classification of Nursing Diagnoses. Chronic pain is defined as a state in which the individual experiences pain that continues for more than 6 months. The defining characteristics include a verbal report or observed evidence of pain experienced for more than 6 months, fear of reinjury, altered ability to continue previous activities, anorexia, weight changes, changes in sleep patterns, facial mask, and guarded movements. Related factors include physical and psychosocial disability. See also **nursing diagnosis.**

pain intervention, the relief of the painful sensations experienced in suffering the physiologic and the psychologic effects of disease and trauma. Effective pain intervention depends on proper evaluation of the type of pain the patient is experiencing, the physical and the psychologic origins of the pain, and the behavioral patterns commonly associated with different kinds of pain. The most common method of pain intervention is the administration of narcotics, such as morphine, but many authorities believe that the exclusive use of pain-killing drugs without consideration and implementation of psychologic aids is too narrow an approach. There are few patients without a psychogenic overlay on the physical experience of pain, and comprehensive pain intervention employs methods and procedures that incorporate both psychologic and physical measures. Methods of pain intervention for acute pain are different from those for chronic pain. Acute pain, occurring in the first 24 to 48 hours after surgery, is often difficult to relieve, and narcotics seldom relieve all such pain. Some authorities believe that the individual who has undergone repeated surgical operations has a decreased tolerance for pain. The type of pain intervention usually depends on the description of the pain by the individual experiencing it. Mild pain may best be relieved by comfort measures and the distraction afforded by television, visitors, reading, and other passive activities. Moderate pain may best be relieved by a combination of comfort measures and drugs. Cognitive dissonance, often employed to dampen moderate pain, encourages the patient to reflect on pleasant experiences and describe them to health care personnel. Intervention to relieve severe pain often includes the administration of narcotics, purposeful interaction between the patient and attending hospital personnel, reduction of environmental stimuli, increased comfort measures, and 'waking imagined analgesia,' in which the patient is encouraged to concentrate on and become distracted by former pleasant experiences, such as relaxing on a beach surrounded by cool ocean water. In the alleviation of all types of pain, dampening or decreasing stimuli that create pain is the chief goal. Pain often increases in a cold room because the muscles of the patient tend to contract; but the local application of cold, such as with an ice pack, often alleviates pain by reducing swelling. Pain intervention seeks to reduce the effects of other factors that compound pain, such as fatigue and anxiety. Coping with pain becomes increasingly difficult as the patient becomes more tired. Sensory restriction may increase pain, because it blocks otherwise effective distraction; overstimulation may cause fatigue and anxiety, thus increasing pain. Religious beliefs may be effective in helping the patient to decrease pain or increase pain tolerance if the pain is viewed by the patient as requiring self-discipline or as a catharsis for past transgressions. Religious beliefs, however, may increase pain if the patient interprets the pain as punishment and relates the severity of the pain with the gravity of transgressions or faults. Pain intervention by the use of drugs includes the administration of mild nonnarcotic analgesics and of much more potent and potentially addictive opioids, such as morphine. Opioid analgesics administered for the relief of pain, cough, or diarrhea provide only symptomatic treatment and are used cautiously in the care of patients with acute or chronic diseases. Opioids may obscure the symptoms or the progress of the disease, and repeated daily administration of any opioid will eventually produce some tolerance to the therapeutic effects of the drug and some physical dependence on the dosage. The risk of developing psychologic and physical dependency on any drug is always present, especially with opioids. In usual doses, opioids relieve suffering by altering the emotional component of the painful experience and by effecting analgesia. Some care givers are so concerned about the addictive dangers of opioids that they tend to prescribe initial doses that are too low or too infrequent to alleviate pain. A typical dose of 10 mg of morphine relieves postoperative pain in only two thirds of patients. Some patients may require considerably more than the average dose of an opioid to experience adequate pain relief. Some other patients with more rapid metabolisms may require such drugs at shorter intervals. Many drugs are appropriate substitutes for the potent opioids morphine and codeine. Some of the effective semisynthetic substitutes are hydrocodone, dihydrocodeine, and meperidine. The narcotic analgesics act on the central nervous system, but the salicylates and other nonnarcotic drugs act at the site of origin of the pain. Some nonnarcotic drugs also have antiinflammatory and antipyretic activity, such as aspirin, indomethacin, ibuprofen, or naproxen. In patients who are sensitive to or are unable to take aspirin, acetaminophen is an acceptable substitute, as are the nonsteroidal antiinflammatory drugs. Pain intervention in the treatment of terminal illnesses employs numerous drugs that relieve pain and produce euphoria and tranquillity in patients who would otherwise suffer greatly. Analgesic mixtures of opioids and alcoholic solutions may be prescribed. Nerve block by the injection of alcohol, chordotomy, and other neurosurgical interventions may sometimes be employed. Other techniques include acupuncture, hypnosis, behavior modification, in which treatment consists of reducing medication and gradually increasing mobility through exercise and any other appropriate modality; biofeedback, and transcutaneous electric nerve stimulation. The latter technique is a noninvasive and nonaddictive method of modifying pain messages to the brain. See also **pain assessment.**

pain mechanism, the network that communicates unpleasant sensations and the perceptions of noxious stimuli throughout the body in association with physical disease and trauma involving tissue damage. The gate control theory of pain is an attempt to explain the role of the nervous system in the pain response. It states that pain signals reaching the nervous system excite a group of small neurons that form a 'pain pool.' When the total activity of these neurons reaches a minimum level, a theoretic gate opens up and allows the pain signals to proceed to higher brain centers. The areas in which the gates operate are considered to be in the spinal cord dorsal horn and the brainstem. The pattern theory holds that the intensity of a stimulus evokes a specific pattern, which is interpreted by the brain as pain. This perception is the result of the intensity and frequency of stimulation of a nonspecific end organ. Some authorities believe that bradykinin and histamine, two chemical substances produced by the body, cause pain. Recently discovered pain killers produced naturally by the body are the enkephalins and the endorphins. Some studies indicate that the enkephalins are 10 times as potent as morphine in reducing pain. It is known that after histamine and some other naturally oc-

curring chemical substances are released in the body, pain sensations travel along fast-conducting nerve fibers and slow-conducting nerve fibers. These pain-transmitting neuropathways communicate the pain sensation to the dorsal root ganglia of the spinal cord and synapse with certain neurons in the posterior horns of the gray matter. The pain sensation is then transmitted to the reticular formation and the thalamus by neurons that form the anterolateral spinothalamic tract. It is then conveyed to various areas of the brain, such as the cortex and the hypothalamus, by synapses at the thalamus. The immediate reaction to pain is transmitted over the reflex arc by sensory fibers in the dorsal horn of the spinal cord and by synapsing motor neurons in the anterior horn. This anatomic pattern of sensory and motor neurons allows the individual to move quickly at the touch of some harmful stimulus, such as extreme heat or cold. Nerve impulses alerting the individual to move away from such stimuli are simultaneously sent along efferent nerve fibers from the brain.

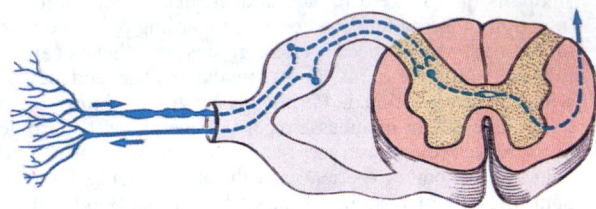

Pain reception pathway *(Potter, 1993)*

pain receptor, any one of the many free nerve endings throughout the body that warn of potentially harmful changes in the environment, such as excessive pressure or temperature. The free nerve endings constituting most of the pain receptors occur chiefly in the epidermis and in the epithelial covering of certain mucous membranes. They also appear in the stratified squamous epithelium of the cornea, in the root sheaths and in the papillae of the hairs, and around the bodies of sudoriferous glands. The terminal ends of pain receptors consist of unmyelinated nerve fibers that often anastomose into small knobs between the epithelial cells. Any kind of stimulus, if it is intense enough, can stimulate the pain receptors in the skin and the mucosa, but only radical changes in pressure and certain chemicals can stimulate the pain receptors in the viscera. Referred pain results only from stimulation of pain receptors located in deep structures, such as the viscera, the joints, and the skeletal muscles, and never from pain receptors in the skin.

paint [Fr, *peindre*], **1.** to apply a medicated solution to the skin, usually over a wide area. **2.** a medicated solution that is applied in this way. Kinds of paint include **antiseptics, germicides,** and **sporicides.**

pain threshold, the point at which a stimulus, usually one associated with pressure or temperature, activates pain receptors and produces a sensation of pain. Individuals with low pain thresholds experience pain much sooner and faster than individuals with higher pain thresholds; the reaction to stimulation of pain receptors varies with individuals.

PAL, abbreviation for *posterior axillary line.*

palatable /pal′ətəbəl/ [L, *palatum*, palate], pleasant to the taste, as food may be.

palatal /pal′ətəl/ [L, *palatum*, palate], **1.** of or pertaining to the palate. **2.** of or pertaining to the lingual surface of a maxillary tooth.

palate /pal′it/ [L, *palatum*], a structure that forms the roof of the mouth. It is divided into the hard palate and the soft palate. –**palatal, palatine** /pal′ətīn/, *adj.*

palatine /pal′ətin/ [L, *palatum*, palate], pertaining to or belonging to the palate.

palatine arch [L, *palatum; arcus*, bow], the vault-shaped muscular structure forming the soft palate between the mouth and the nasopharynx. An opening in the arch connects the mouth with the oropharynx; the uvula is suspended from the middle of the posterior border of the arch.

palatine bone, one of a pair of bones of the skull, forming the posterior part of the hard palate, part of the nasal cavity, and the floor of the orbit of the eye. It resembles a letter 'L' and consists of horizontal and vertical parts and three processes.

palatine ridge, any one of the four to six transverse ridges on the anterior surface of the hard palate.

palatine suture, one of a number of thin wavy lines marking the joining of the palatine processes that form the hard palate. See also **median palatine suture, transverse palatine suture.**

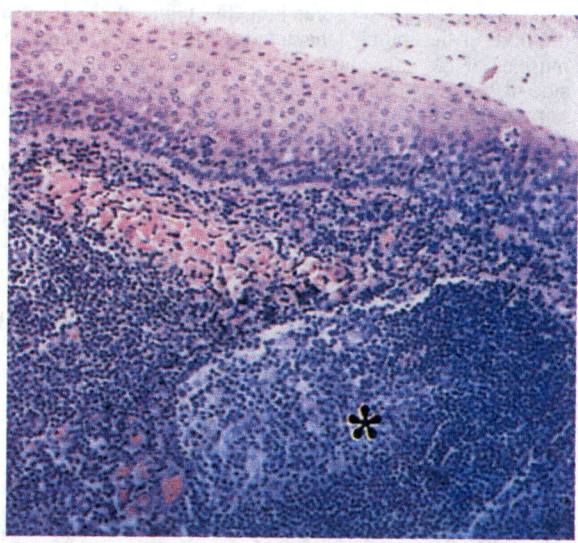

Histology of the palatine tonsil *(Erlandsen, 1992)*

palatine tonsil, one of a pair of almond-shaped masses of lymphoid tissue between the palatoglossal and the palatopharyngeal arches on each side of the fauces. They are covered with mucous membrane and contain numerous lymph follicles and various crypts.

palatitis, an inflammation of the hard palate.

palato- /pal′ətō-/, a combining form meaning 'of or pertaining to the palate': *palatoglossal, palatography, palatomaxillary.*

palatoglossal /-glos′əl/ [L, *palatum*, palate; Gk, *glossa*, tongue], pertaining to both the palate and the tongue.

palatomaxillary /-mak′siler′ē/ [L, *palatum* + *maxilla*, jaw], of or pertaining to the palate and the maxilla.

palatonasal /-nā′zəl/ [L, *palatum* + *nasus*, nose], of or pertaining to the palate and the nose.

pale infarct [L, *pallidus*, pallid; *infarcire*, to stuff], a wedge of dead tissue, white in color because of an absence of blood, causing an obstruction in an artery. Also called **anemic infarct.**

paleo-, a prefix meaning 'old': *paleocerebellar, paleogenesis, paleostriatum.*

paleogenesis. See **palingenesis.**

paleogenetic /-jənet′ik/ [Gk, *palaios*, long ago, *genesis*, origin], **1.** a trait or structure of an organism or species that originated in a previous generation. **2.** relating to the development of such a trait or structure.

paleontology. See **biology.**

pali-. See **palin-.**

palilalia /pal′ilā′lyə/ [Gk, *palin*, again, *lalein*, to babble], an abnormal condition characterized by the increasingly rapid repetition of the same word or phrase, usually at the end of a sentence.

palin-, pali-, a combining form meaning 'again': *palindromia, palinesthesia, palingenesis.*

palindrome /pal′indrōm′/ [Gk, *palin* + *dromos*, course], (in molecular genetics) a segment of DNA in which identical, or almost identical, sequences of bases run in opposite directions.

palingenesis /pal′injen′əsis/ [Gk, *palin* + *genesis*, origin], **1.** the regeneration of a lost part. **2.** the hereditary transmission of ancestral structural characteristics, especially abnormalities, in successive generations. Also called **paleogenesis.** Compare **cenogenesis.** –**palingenetic, palingenic,** *adj.*

palladium (Pd) /pəlā′dē·əm/ [Gk, *Pallas, Athena*, mythic goddess and protector of Troy], a hard, silvery metallic element. Its atomic number is 46; its atomic weight is 106.4. Highly resistant to tarnish and corrosion, palladium is used in high-grade surgical instruments and in dental inlays, bridgework, and orthodontic appliances.

palliate /pal′ē·āt/ [L, *palliare*, to cloak], to soothe or relieve. –**palliation,** *n.,* **palliative,** *adj.*

palliative treatment /pal′ē·ətiv′/ [L, *palliare*, to cloak, *tractare*, to handle], therapy designed to relieve or reduce intensity of uncomfortable symptoms but not to produce a cure. Some kinds of palliative treatment are the use of narcotics to relieve pain in a patient with advanced cancer, the creation of a colostomy to bypass an inoperable obstructing lesion of the bowel, and the debridement of necrotic tissue in a patient with metastatic malignancy. Compare **definitive treatment, expectant treatment.**

pallid /pal′id/ [L, *pallidus*, pale], lacking color.

pallidum. See **globus pallidus.**

pallium. See **cerebral cortex.**

pallor /pal′ər/ [L, paleness], an unnatural paleness or absence of color in the skin.

palm /päm/ [L, *palma*], the lower side of the hand, between the wrist and the bases of the fingers, when the hand is held horizontal with the thumb in medial position. –**palmar,** *adj.*

palm and sole system of identification, a method of

identifying individuals by the patterns of ridges in the skin of the palms of the hands and soles of the feet. Like fingerprints, the patterns are helpful in identification of infants and others.

palmar /pal'mər/ [L *palma*], pertaining to the palm.

palmar aponeurosis [L, *palma* + Gk, *apo*, from, *neuron*, nerve], fascia surrounding the muscles of the palm. Also called **palmar fascia.**

palmar crease, a normal groove across the palm of the hand.

palmar erythema, an inflammatory redness of the palms of the hands.

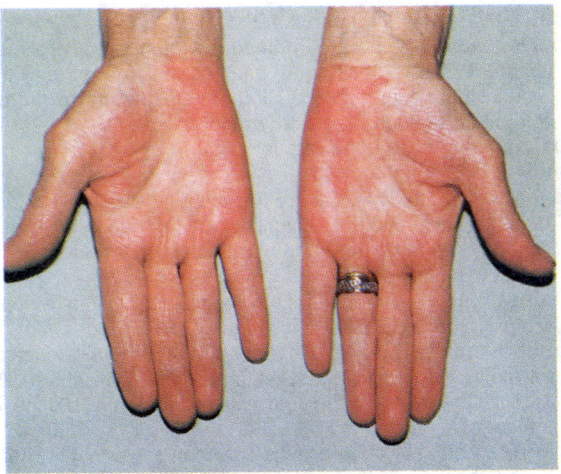

Palmar erythema
(Barrison, 1992/Courtesy Dr IN McNeil, Ealing Hospital, Uxbridge)

palmar fascia. See **palmar aponeurosis.**

palmar grasp reflex [L, *palma*, palm; ONor, *grapa*, grab], a flexion of the fingers caused by stimulation of the palm of the hand. The reflex is present at birth and usually disappears by the age of 6 months.

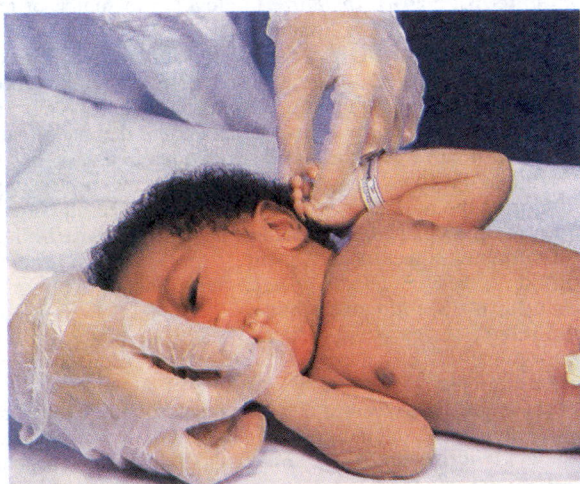

Palmar grasp reflex in the newborn *(Seidel, 1991)*

palmaris longus /pəlmer'is/, a long, slender, superficial, fusiform muscle of the forearm, lying on the medial side of the flexor carpi radialis. It arises from the medial epicondyle of the humerus by a tendon from the intermuscular septa between it and the adjacent muscles and from the antebrachial fascia. It inserts by a long, thin tendon into the flexor retinaculum and into the palmar aponeurosis. A tendinous slip of the muscle is often found extending to the thumb. The palmaris longus is innervated by a branch of the median nerve, which contains fibers from the sixth and the seventh cervical nerves, and it functions to flex the hand. Compare **flexor carpi radialis, flexor carpi ulnaris.**

palmar metacarpal artery, one of several arteries arising from the deep palmar arch, supplying the fingers.

palmar pinch, a thumbless grasp in which the tips of the other fingers are pressed against the palm of the hand. See also **pinch, tip pinch.**

palmar reflex, a reflex that curls the fingers when the palm of the hand is tickled.

palmature /pal'məchər/ [L, *palma*], an abnormal condition in which the fingers are webbed.

palm-chin reflex. See **palmomental reflex.**

palmitic acid /palmit'ik/ [L, *palma*], a saturated fatty acid that commonly occurs in animal and vegetable fats and oils. It is used in the manufacture of soaps and candles. Also called **hexadecanoic acid.**

palmityl alcohol. See **cetyl alcohol.**

palmomental reflex /pal'məmen'təl/ [L, *palma* + *mentum*, chin; *reflectere*, to bend backward], an abnormal neurologic sign, elicited by scratching the palm of the hand at the base of the thumb, characterized by contraction of the muscles of the chin and corner of the mouth on the same side of the body as the stimulus. It is occasionally seen in normal individuals, but an exaggerated reflex may be seen in pyramidal tract disease, latent tetany, increased intracranial pressure, and central facial paresis. Also called **palm-chin reflex.**

palpable /pal'pəbəl/ [L, *palpare*, to touch gently], perceivable by touch.

palpate /pal'pāt/, to use the hands or fingers to examine.

palpation /palpā'shən/ [L, *palpare*, to touch gently], a technique used in physical examination in which the examiner feels the texture, size, consistency, and location of certain parts of the body with the hands.

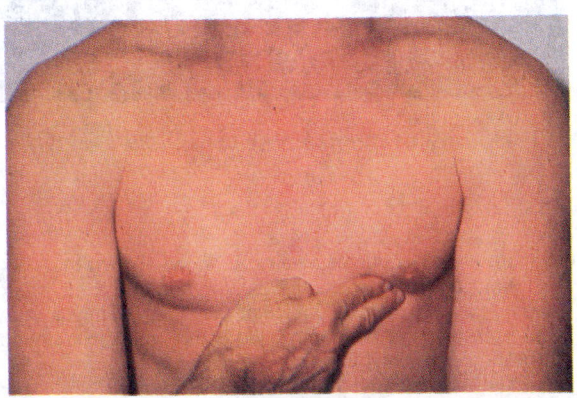

Palpation of apical pulse *(Seidel, 1991)*

palpatory percussion /pal'pətôr'ē/ [L, *palpare,* to touch gently; *percutere,* to strike hard], a technique in physical examination in which the vibrations produced by percussion are evaluated by using light pressure of the flat of the examiner's hand.

palpebra. See **eyelid.**

palpebral commissure. See **canthus.**

palpebral conjunctiva. See **conjunctiva.**

palpebral fissure /pal'pəbrəl/ [L, *palpebra,* eyelid; *fissura,* cleft], the opening between the margins of the upper and lower lids.

palpebral gland. See **meibomian gland.**

palpebra superior /pal'pəbrə/, *pl.* **palpebrae superiores,** the upper eyelid, larger and more movable than the lower eyelid and furnished with an elevator muscle.

palpebrate /pal'pəbrāt/, **1.** to wink or blink. **2.** having eyelids.

palpitate /pal'pitāt/ [L, *palpitare,* to flutter], to pulsate rapidly, as in the unusually fast beating of the heart under various conditions of stress and in patients with certain heart problems.

palpitation /pal'pitā'shən/ [L, *palpitare,* to flutter], a pounding or racing of the heart, associated with normal emotional responses or with heart disorders. Some people may complain of pounding hearts and display no evidence of heart disease, whereas others, with serious heart disorders, may not detect associated abnormal palpitations. Some patients complain of palpitations after receiving digitalis because it increases the force of heart contractions.

PALS, abbreviation for **pediatric advanced life support.**

palsy /pôl'zē/ [Gk, *para,* beyond, *lysis,* loosening], an abnormal condition characterized by paralysis. Some kinds of palsy are **Bell's palsy, cerebral palsy,** and **Erb's palsy.**

Paltauf's dwarf. See **pituitary dwarf.**

Paltauf's nanism /päl'toufs/ [Arnold Paltauf, Czechoslovakian physician, b. 1860; Gk, *nanos,* dwarf], dwarfism associated with excessive production or growth of lymphoid tissue.

-pamide, a suffix for sulfamoylbenzoic acid-derived diuretics.

-pamil, a suffix for verapamil-type coronary vasodilators.

Pamine, a trademark for an anticholinergic (methscopolamine bromide).

PAMP, abbreviation for *pulmonary arterial mean pressure.*

pampiniform /pampin'ifôrm/, having the shape of a tendril.

pampiniform body. See **epoophoron.**

pampiniform plexus [L, *pampinus,* vine tendril; *plexus,* plaited], a network of veins in the spermatic cord that drains the testes into the testicular vein in the lower abdomen.

pan- /pan-/, a combining form meaning 'all': *panacea, pancarditis, pandemic.*

panacea /pan'əsē'ə/ [Gk, *pan,* all, *akeia,* remedy], **1.** a universal remedy. **2.** an ancient name for an herb or a liquid potion with healing properties.

panacinar emphysema /panas'ənər/ [Gk, *pan* + L, *acinus,* grape; Gk, *en,* in, *physema,* blowing], a form of emphysema that affects all lung areas by causing dilation and atrophy of the alveoli and by destroying the vascular bed of the lung. Also called **panlobular emphysema.**

Panafil, a trademark for a topical, fixed-combination drug containing an enzyme (papain).

Panama fever. See **Chagres fever.**

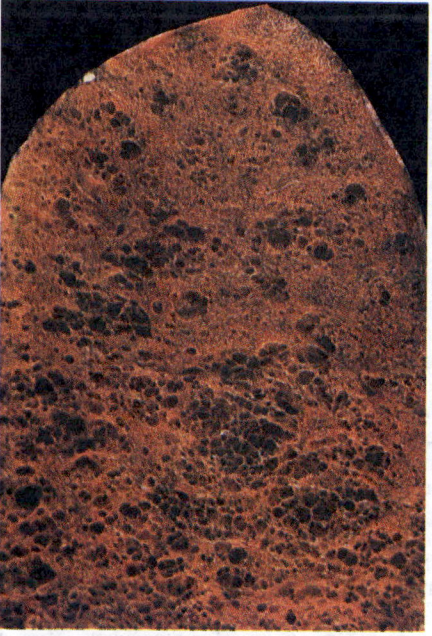

Panacinar emphysema *(Fletcher, 1987)*

panarteritis /-är'təri'tis/ [Gk, *pan,* all, *arteria,* artery, *itis* inflammation], an inflammation that involves all the tissue layers of an artery.

panarthritis /-ärthrī'tis/ [Gk, *pan* + *arthron* joint], an abnormal condition characterized by the inflammation of many joints of the body. **–panarthritic,** *adj.*

pancake kidney /pan'kāk/ [ME, *panne,* pan, *kaka,* cake; *kidnere*], a congenital anomaly in which the left and right kidneys are fused into a single mass in the pelvis. The fused kidney has two collecting systems and two ureters and frequently becomes obstructed because of its abnormal position.

pancarditis /-kärdī'tis/ [Gk, *pan* + *kardia,* heart, *itis,* inflammation], an abnormal condition characterized by inflammation of the entire heart, including the endocardium, myocardium, and pericardium.

Pancoast's syndrome /pan'cōsts/ [Henry K. Pancoast, American radiologist, b. 1875], **1.** a combination of signs associated with a tumor in the apex of the lung. The signs include neuritic pain in the arm, atrophy of the muscles of the arm and the hand, and Horner's syndrome and are caused by the damaging effects of the tumor on the brachial plexus. **2.** an abnormal condition caused by osteolysis in the posterior part of one or more ribs, sometimes involving associated vertebrae.

Pancoast's tumor. See **pulmonary sulcus tumor.**

pancolectomy /-kōlek'təmē/ [Gk, *pan* + *kolon,* colon, *ektome,* excision], the excision of the entire colon, requiring also an ileostomy.

pancreas /pan'krē·əs/ [Gk, *pan,* all, *kreas,* flesh], a fish-shaped, grayish pink nodular gland that stretches transversely across the posterior abdominal wall in the epigastric and hypochondriac regions of the body and secretes various substances, such as digestive enzymes, insulin, and glucagon. It is divided into a head, a body, and a tail. The head of the gland, divided from the body by a small constriction, is tucked into the curve of the duodenum. The tapered left extremity of the organ forms the tail. In adults, the pancreas is about 13 cm long and weighs more in a man than it does in a woman. A compound gland composed of exocrine and endocrine tissue, it contains a main duct that runs the length of the organ, draining smaller ducts and emptying into the duodenum at the major duodenal papilla, the same site that accommodates the entrance of the common bile duct. About 1 million endocrine cellular islets or islands of Langerhans are embedded between the exocrine units of the pancreas. Beta cells of the islands secrete insulin, which helps control carbohydrate metabolism. Alpha cells of the islets secrete glucagon that counters the action of insulin. The acinar units of the pancreas secrete digestive enzymes.

pancreas scan, an x-ray scan of the pancreas after the intravenous injection of a radioactive contrast medium, used for detecting various abnormalities, such as tumors, cysts, and infections.

pancreatectomy /pan′krē·ətek′təmē/ [Gk, *pan, kreas + ektome,* excision], the surgical removal of all or part of the pancreas, performed to remove a cyst or tumor, treat pancreatitis, or repair trauma. The resection is done using general anesthesia; the GI tract is reconstructed, usually with an anastomosis between the common bile duct and the upper jejunum. Drains are left in the wound. After surgery the patient is given a low-sugar, low-fat diet. If the entire pancreas is removed, a brittle type of diabetes develops, requiring precise management of both diet and insulin dosage. A frequent complication is the formation of a fistula in the pancreatic bile duct, allowing digestive enzymes to contact adjacent tissues.

-pancreat, a combining form meaning 'pertaining to the pancreas': *hepaticopancreatic, lienopancreatic, splenopancreatic.*

pancreatic /pan′krē·at′ik/ [Gk, *pan,* all, *kreas,* flesh], pertaining to the pancreas.

pancreatic cancer [Gk, *pan, kreas* + L, crab], a malignant neoplastic disease of the pancreas, characterized by anorexia, flatulence, weakness, dramatic weight loss, epigastric or back pain, jaundice, pruritus, a palpable abdominal mass, the recent onset of diabetes, and clay-colored stools if the pancreatic ducts are obstructed. Insulin-secreting tumors of islet cells cause hypoglycemia, especially in the morning. Nonfunctioning islet cell lesions produce gastrin, causing symptoms of peptic ulcer, or, in some cases, acute diarrhea and hypokalemia, and achlorhydria, the result of the lesion's elaboration of secretin. Diagnostic measures include barium x-ray studies of the stomach and duodenum, transhepatic cholangiography (ERCP), laboratory evaluation of liver function, celiac arteriography, and computerized axial tomography. Exploratory laparotomy is often required for a definitive diagnosis. About 90% of pancreatic tumors are adenocarcinomas; two thirds are in the head of the pancreas. Most tumors are not resectable at the time of diagnosis, but localized cancers in the pancreas may be treated by partial pancreatectomy with excision of the common bile duct, duodenum, and distal part of the stomach. Functioning islet cell lesions may be excised or treated with streptozotocin, an antibiotic toxic to beta cells of the pancreas. Total gastrectomy is recommended for nonfunctioning islet cell tumors that are accompanied by peptic ulcer disease. Radiotherapy or chemotherapy with 5-fluorouracil or mitomycin-C may offer temporary palliation, but cancer

of the pancreas has a poor prognosis: Few people live for more than 1 year after diagnosis. Pancreatic cancer occurs three to four times more often in men than in women. Though uncommon, it is increasing in incidence in the industrialized areas of the world. People who smoke more than 10 to 20 cigarettes a day, who have diabetes mellitus, or who have been exposed to polychlorinated biphenyl compounds are at increased risk of developing pancreatic cancer.

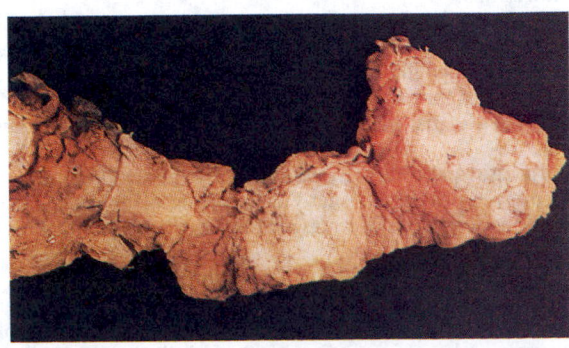

Pancreatic cancer (Fletcher, 1987)

pancreatic diabetes [Gk, *pan,* all, *kreas,* flesh, *diabainein,* to pass through], diabetes mellitus caused by a deficiency of insulin production by the islet cells of the pancreas. See also **diabetes mellitus.**

pancreatic diverticulum, one of a pair of membranous pouches arising from the embryonic duodenum. These two diverticula later form the pancreas and its ducts.

pancreatic dornase, an enzyme from beef pancreas that has been used as a mucolytic for upper respiratory infections and cystic fibrosis.

pancreatic duct, the primary secretory channel of the pancreas. Also called **duct of Wirsung.**

pancreatic enzyme, any one of the enzymes secreted by the pancreas in the process of digestion. The most important are trypsin, chymotrypsin, steapsin, and amylopsin. See also **pancreatic juice.**

pancreatic hormone, any one of several chemical compounds secreted by the pancreas, associated with the regulation of cellular metabolism. Major hormones secreted by the pancreas are insulin, glucagon, and pancreatic polypeptide. Insulin and glucagon are secreted by different types of cells within the alpha and beta cells of the islands of Langerhans; pancreatic polypeptide is secreted by a group of glandular cells arranged in a halo around each island of Langerhans.

pancreatic insufficiency, a condition characterized by inadequate production and secretion of pancreatic hormones or enzymes, usually occurring secondary to a disease process destructive of pancreatic tissue. Nutritional malabsorption, anorexia, poorly localized upper abdominal or epigastric pain, malaise, and severe weight loss often occur. Alcohol-induced pancreatitis is the most common form of the condition. Supportive care, specific treatment of the cause of the condition, and replacement or augmentation of the absent or lacking substances are usually recommended as therapy for pancreatic insufficiency.

pancreatic juice, the fluid secretion of the pancreas, produced by the stimulation of food in the duodenum. Pancreatic juice contains water, protein, inorganic salts, and enzymes. The juice is essential in breaking down proteins into their amino acid components, in reducing dietary fats to glycerol and fatty acids, and in converting starch to simple sugars.

pancreaticolienal node /panˈkrē·atˈikōˈlī·ēˈnəl/ [Gk, *pan, kreas* + L, *lien,* spleen, *nodus,* knot], a node in one of three groups of lymph glands associated with branches of the abdominal and the pelvic viscera that are supplied by branches of the celiac artery. The pancreaticolienal nodes accompany the splenic artery along the posterior surface and the upper border of the pancreas. Their afferents, which originate from the stomach, the spleen, and the pancreas, join the celiac group of preaortic nodes. Also called **splenic gland.** Compare **gastric node, hepatic node.**

pancreatin /panˈkrē·ətin′, -krēˈā′tin/, a concentrate of pancreatic enzymes from swine or beef cattle.

■ INDICATIONS: It is prescribed as an aid to digestion to replace endogenous pancreatic enzymes in cystic fibrosis and after pancreatectomy.

■ CONTRAINDICATIONS: Known hypersensitivity to this drug or to pork or beef protein prohibits its use.

■ ADVERSE EFFECTS: There are no known serious adverse reactions. High doses may cause nausea or diarrhea.

pancreatitis /panˈkrē·ətī′tis/ [Gk, *pan, kreas* + *itis,* inflammation], an inflammatory condition of the pancreas that may be acute or chronic. **Acute pancreatitis** is generally the result of damage to the biliary tract, such as by alcohol, trauma, infectious disease, or certain drugs. It is characterized by severe abdominal pain radiating to the back, fever, anorexia, nausea, and vomiting. There may be jaundice if the common bile duct is obstructed. The development of pseudocysts or abscesses in pancreatic tissue is a serious complication. Treatment includes nasogastric suction to re-move gastric secretions. To prevent any stimulation of the pancreas, nothing is given by mouth. Intravenous fluids and electrolytes are administered, and nonmorphine derivatives are given to relieve pain. The causes of **chronic pancreatitis** are similar to those of the acute form. When the cause is alcohol abuse, there may be calcification and scarring of the smaller pancreatic ducts. There is abdominal pain, nausea, and vomiting, as well as steatorrhea and creatorrhea, caused by the diminished output of pancreatic enzymes. Pancreatic insulin production may be diminished, and some patients develop diabetes mellitus. Treatment includes analgesics for pain and subtotal pancreatectomy when pain is intractable. A pancreatic extract is given orally to replace the missing enzymes; vitamin supplements are essential. Both forms of pancreatitis are diagnosed by history, physical examination, radiologic studies, endoscopy, and laboratory analysis of the amount of pancreatic enzymes in the blood.

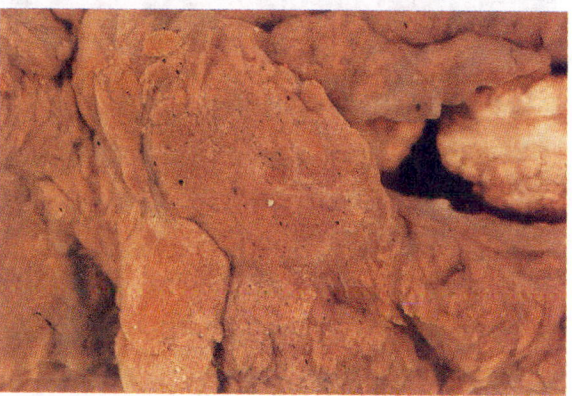

Chronic pancreatitis *(Fletcher, 1987)*

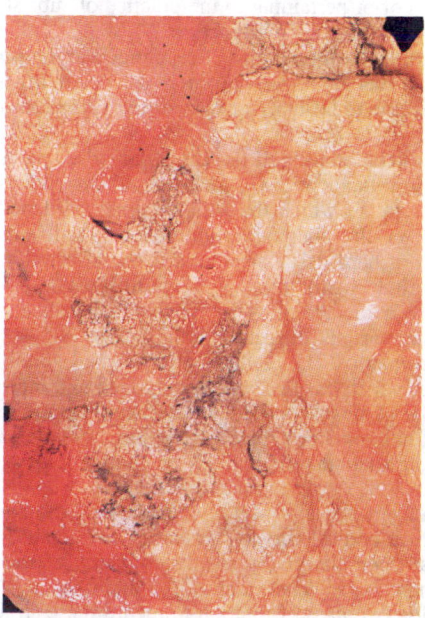

Acute pancreatitis *(Fletcher, 1987)*

pancreatoduodenectomy /panˈkrē·āˈtōdo͞oˈōdənek′-təmē/ [Gk, *pan, kreas* + L, *duoden,* twelve each; Gk, *ektome,* excision], a surgical procedure in which the head of the pancreas and the loop of duodenum that surrounds it are excised. The operation is performed to remove the periampullary masses occurring in certain forms of biliary tract cancer.

pancreatography /panˈkrē·ətogˈrəfē/ [Gk, *pan, kreas* + *graphein,* to record], visualization of the pancreas or its ducts by means of x-rays and contrast media injected into the ducts at surgery or via an endoscope, or by means of ultrasonography, computed tomography, or radionuclide imaging.

pancreatolith /-krē·atˈəlith/, a stone or calculus in the pancreas.

pancuronium bromide /-kyərōˈnē·əm/, a skeletal muscle relaxant.

■ INDICATIONS: It is prescribed as an adjunct to anesthesia and mechanical ventilation.

■ CONTRAINDICATIONS: It is used with caution in patients with myasthenia gravis and renal and hepatic disease and in pregnancy. Known hypersensitivity to this drug or to other bromides prohibits its use.

■ ADVERSE EFFECTS: The most serious adverse reaction is prolonged muscle relaxation and respiratory depression.

pancytopenia /panˈsītəpēˈnē·ə/ [Gk, *pan* + *kytos,* cell, *penia,* poverty], A marked reduction in the number of the red blood cells, white blood cells, and platelets. See also **anemia, aplasia.** –**pancytopenic,** *adj.*

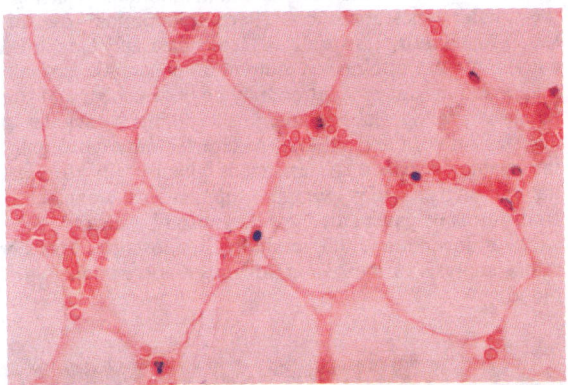

Blood marrow aspirate showing pancytopenia
(Hayhoe, 1992)

p and a, abbreviation for *percussion and auscultation,* as noted in the patient's chart after physical examination of the chest. See **auscultation, percussion.**

pandemia /-dēˈmē·ə/ [Gk, *pan,* all + *demos,* people], a disease epidemic that affects all or most of a population group.

pandemic /-dēˈmik/ [Gk, *pan* + *demos,* people], (of a disease) occurring throughout the population of a country, a people, or the world.

pandiastolic /-dīˈəstolˈik/ [Gk, *pan* + *dia,* through, *stellein,* to set], of or pertaining to the complete diastole. Also called **holodiastolic.**

panencephalitis /panˈəsefˈəlīˈtis/ [Gk, *pan* + *enkephale,* brain, *itis*], inflammation of the entire brain characterized by an insidious onset, a progressive course with deterioration of motor and mental functions, and evidence of a viral cause. Subacute sclerosing panencephalitis is an uncommon childhood disease thought to be caused by a 'slow' latent measles virus after recovery from a previous infection. Most of the patients are younger than 11 years of age, and many more boys than girls are affected. The disease results in ataxia, myoclonus, atrophy, cortical blindness, and mental deterioration. Antiviral drugs, immunosuppressants, and interferon inducers are sometimes administered, but the disease is usually unremitting and fatal.

panendoscope /-enˈdəskōp´/ [Gk, *pan* + *endon,* within, *skopein,* to look], a cystoscope that allows a wide view of the interior of the bladder.

panesthesia /-esthēˈzhə/ [Gk, *pan* + *aisthesis,* feeling], the total of all sensations experienced by an individual at one time. Compare **cenesthesia.**

pangenesis /-jenˈəsis/ [Gk, *pan* + *genesis,* origin], a darwinian theory that every cell and particle of a parent reproduces itself in progeny.

panhypopituitarism /ˌpanhīˈpōpitoō´itərizˈəm/ [Gk, *pan* + *hypo,* under, *pituita,* phlegm], generalized insufficiency of pituitary hormones, resulting from damage to or deficiency of the gland. **Prepubertal panhypopituitarism,** a

rare disorder usually associated with a suprasellar cyst or craniopharyngioma, is characterized by dwarfism with normal body proportions, subnormal sexual development, and insufficient thyroid and adrenal function. Diabetes insipidus is frequently present; there may be bitemporal hemianopia or complete blindness; skin is often yellow and wrinkled, but mentality is usually unimpaired. X-ray pictures show delayed fusion of the epiphyses, suprasellar calcification, and, frequently, destruction of the sella turcica. The condition is treated with cortisone, thyroid and sex hormones replacement, and human growth hormone. Postpubertal panhypopituitarism may be caused by postpartum pituitary necrosis, resulting from thrombosis of pituitary circulation during or after delivery. Characteristic signs of the disorder are failure to lactate, amenorrhea, weakness, cold intolerance, lethargy, and loss of libido and of axillary and pubic hair. There may be bradycardia or hypotension, and progression of the disorder leads to premature wrinkling of the skin and atrophy of the thyroid and adrenal glands. Treatment consists of the administration of ACTH, thyroid-stimulating hormone, and hormones of the target organs. Also called **hypophyseal cachexia, pituitary cachexia, Simmonds' disease.**

panhysterectomy /panˈhistərekˈtəmē/ [Gk, *pan* + *hystera,* uterus, *ektome,* excision], complete surgical removal of the uterus and cervix. See also **hysterectomy.**

panic /panˈik/, an intense, sudden, and overwhelming fear or feeling of anxiety that produces terror and immediate physiologic changes that result in paralyzed immobility or senseless, hysteric behavior.

panic attack [Gk, *panikos,* of the god Pan; Fr, *attaquer*], an episode of acute anxiety that occurs unpredictably with feelings of intense apprehension or terror, accompanied by dyspnea, dizziness, sweating, trembling, and chest pain or palpitations. The attack may last several minutes and may occur again in certain situations.

panic disorder. See **anxiety attack.**

panivorous /panivˈərəs/ [L, *panis,* bread, *vorare,* to devour], of or pertaining to the practice of subsisting exclusively on bread. –**panivore,** *n.*

panlobular emphysema. See **panacinar emphysema.**

Panner's disease, a rare form of osteochondrosis in which there is abnormal bony growth in the capitulum of the humerus.

panniculitis /pənikˈyəlīˈtis/ [L, *panniculus,* piece of cloth; Gk, *itis,* inflammation], a chronic inflammation of subcutaneous fat in which the skin becomes hardened, particularly over the abdomen and thorax. Small subcutaneous masses of hard tissue are found in the affected areas.

panniculus /pənikˈyələs/, *pl.* **panniculi** [L, small garment], a membranous layer, the many sheets of fascia covering various structures in the body.

pannus /panˈəs/ [L, cloth], an abnormal condition of the cornea, which has become vascularized and infiltrated with granular tissue just beneath the surface. Pannus may develop in the inflammatory stage of trachoma or after a detached retina, glaucoma, iridocyclitis, or another degenerative eye disease.

panography /pənogˈrəfē/, a method of tomography that visualizes bodies' curved surfaces at any depth. In dentistry this is accomplished by roentgenography of the maxillary and mandibular dental arches and the associated structures by using two axes of rotation to record these structures. An intensifying screened cassette with a 5- by 12-inch film rotates on a drum at the same time that the radiation unit ro-

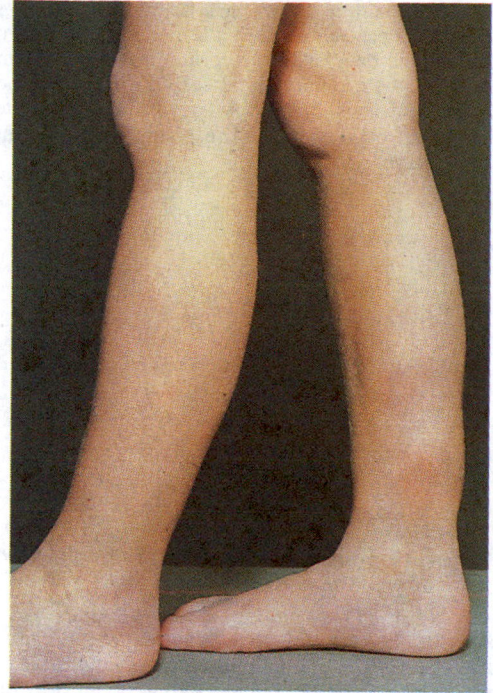

Panniculitis (Ansell, 1992)

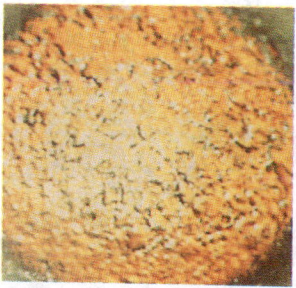

Reticular subepithelial pannus (Shingleton, 1991)

tates around the patient's head to record the structures before processing. See also **panoramic radiography.**

panophthalmitis /pan'ofthalmī'tis/ [Gk, *pan + ophthalmos,* eye, *itis*], an inflammation of the entire eye, usually caused by virulent pyogenic organisms, such as strains of meningococci, pneumococci, streptococci, anthrax bacilli, and clostridia. Initial symptoms are pain, fever, headache, drowsiness, edema, and swelling. As the infection progresses, the iris appears muddy and gray, the aqueous humor becomes turbid, and precipitates form on the posterior surface of the cornea. Treatment consists of intensive systemic and local antibiotic therapy; evisceration of the globe or excision of the eye may be required, but excision is contraindicated if surrounding tissues are infected.

panoramic radiograph /pan'ôram'ik/ [Gk, *pan + horama,* view; L, *radiare,* to shine; Gk, *graphein,* to record], a

method of tomography for visualization of curved body surfaces, such as the upper and lower jaws, on a single film. Also called **pantomography.**

PanOxyl, a trademark for a keratolytic (benzoyl peroxide).

panphobia /-fō'bē·ə/ [Gk, *pan + phobos,* fear], an anxiety disorder characterized by an irrational, vague fear or apprehension of some pervading or unknown evil; a generalized fear. Also called **panophobia, pantophobia. —panophobic,** *adj.*

pansystolic /-sistol'ik/, of or pertaining to the entire systole. Also **holosystolic.**

pansystolic murmur. See **systolic murmur.**

pant-. See **panto-.**

Panteric, a trademark for an enzyme (pancreatin).

panthenol /pan'thənôl/, an alcohol converted in the body to pantothenic acid, a vitamin in the B complex.

panting [Fr, *panteler,* to gasp], a ventilatory pattern characterized by rapid, shallow breathing with small tidal volume. Panting usually moves gas back and forth in the anatomic dead space at a high flow rate, which evaporates water, removes heat with little or no increase in alveolar ventilation rate, and avoids hypocapnia.

panto-, pant-, a combining form meaning 'all, the whole': *pantophobia, pantoscopic, pantosomatous.*

pantograph /pan'təgraf'/, **1.** a jointed device for copying a plane figure to any desired scale. **2.** a device that incorporates a pair of face bows fixed to the jaws, used for inscribing centrically related points and arcs leading to the points on segments relatable to the three craniofacial planes.

pantomography /-mog'əfē/ [Gk, *pan + graphein,* to record], panoramic radiography for obtaining radiographs of the maxillary and mandibular dental arches and related structures.

Pantopon, a trademark for a narcotic analgesic, fixed-combination drug containing hydrochlorides of opium alkaloids.

pantophobia. See **panphobia.**

pantothenic acid /pan'təthen'ik/, a member of the vitamin B complex. It is widely distributed in plant and animal tissues and may be an important element in human nutrition.

pantothenyl alcohol. See **panthenol.**

Panwarfin, a trademark for an anticoagulant (warfarin sodium).

Pao$_2$, symbol for **partial pressure of arterial oxygen.**

PA$_{O2}$, symbol for **alveolar oxygen concentration.**

P$_{AO2}$, symbol for *partial pressure of alveolar oxygen.*

papain /pəpā'ēn/, an enzyme from the fruit of *Carica papaya,* the tropic melon tree. It has been prescribed for enzymatic debridement of wounds and promotion of healing.

Papanicolaou test /pap'ənikəlou'/ [George N. Papanicolaou, American physician, b. 1883], a simple smear method of examining stained exfoliative cells. It is used most commonly to detect cancers of the cervix, but it may be used for tissue specimens from any organ. A smear, the **Pap smear,** is usually obtained during a routine pelvic examination. The technique permits early diagnosis of cancer and has contributed to a lower death rate from cervical cancer. The findings are usually reported descriptively and grouped into the following classes: Class I, only normal cells seen; Class II, atypical cells consistent with inflammation; Class III, mild dysplasia; Class IV, severe dysplasia, suspicious cells; Class V, carcinoma cells seen. Also called *(informal)* **Pap test.**

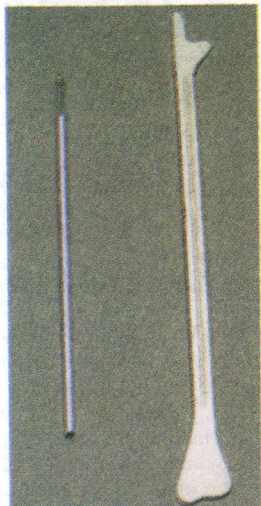

Implements used to obtain a Pap smear
(Seidel, 1991/Courtesy Cytobrush, Inc. Florida)

papilla /pəpil'ə/, *pl.* **papillae** [L, nipple],   **1.** a small nipple-shaped projection, such as the conoid papillae of the tongue and the papillae of the corium that extend from collagen fibers, the capillary blood vessels, and sometimes the nerves of the dermis. **2.** the optic papilla, a round white disc in the fundus oculi, which corresponds to the entrance of the optic nerve.

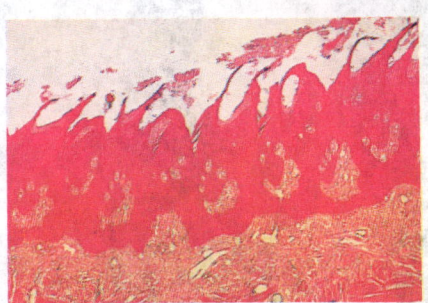

Filiform papillae of the tongue *(Berkovitz, 1992)*

papilla duodeni major.   See **hepatopancreatic ampulla.**
papilla of Vater.   See **hepatopancreatic ampulla.**
papillary /pap'əlerē/ [L, *papilla*, nipple],   of or pertaining to a papilla.
papillary adenocarcinoma,   a malignant neoplasm characterized by small papillae of vascular connective tissue covered by neoplastic epithelium that projects into follicles, glands, or cysts. The tumor is most common in the ovaries and thyroid gland. Also called **polyploid adenocarcinoma.**

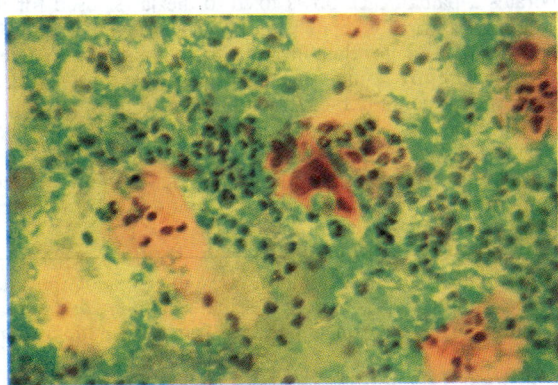

Positive Pap smear, indicative of cervical cancer
(Christiansen, 1993)

papaverine hydrochloride /papav'ərēn/,   a smooth muscle relaxant.
- INDICATIONS: It is prescribed in the treatment of cardiovascular or visceral spasms.
- CONTRAINDICATIONS: Complete atrioventricular heart block or known hypersensitivity to this drug prohibits its use.
- ADVERSE EFFECTS: The most serious adverse reactions include jaundice, increased blood pressure, and dysrhythmias.

paper chromatography [Gk, *papyros,* papyrus],   the separation of a mixture into its components by filtering it through a strip of special paper.
paper-doll fetus.   See **fetus papyraceus.**
paper radioimmunosorbent test (PRIST),   a technique for determining total IgE levels in patients with type I hypersensitivity reactions.
papill-,   a prefix meaning 'resembling a nipple': *papilledema, papillate, papilloma.*

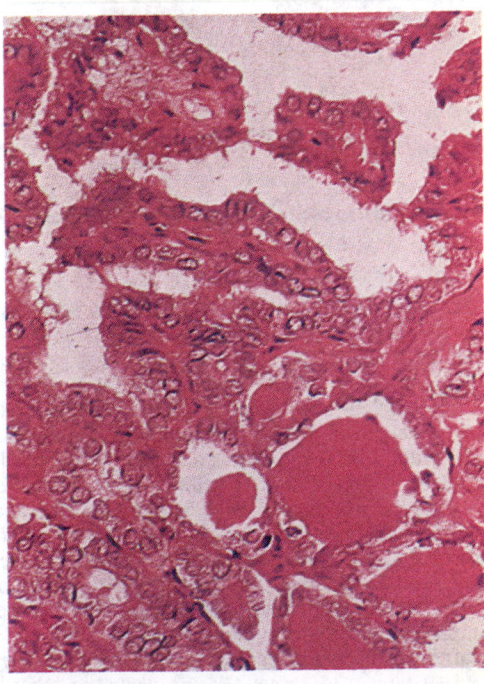

Papillary adenocarcinoma *(Skarin, 1991)*

papillary adenocystoma lymphomatosum, an unusual tumor, consisting of epithelial and lymphoid tissues, that develops in the area of the parotid and submaxillary glands. Also called **adenolymphoma, Warthin's tumor.**

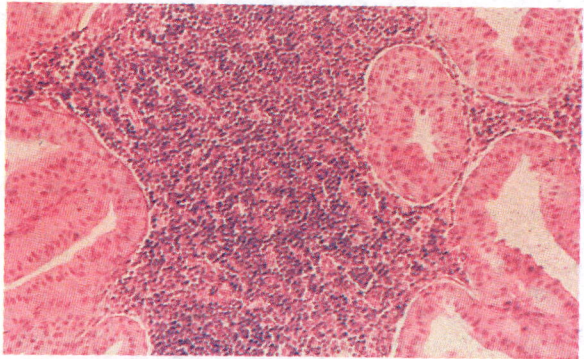

Papillary adenocystoma lymphomatosum
(Skarin, 1991)

papillary adenoma, a benign epithelial tumor in which the membrane lining the glandular tissue forms papillary processes that project into the alveoli or grow out of the surface of a cavity.

papillary carcinoma, a malignant neoplasm characterized by fingerlike projections.

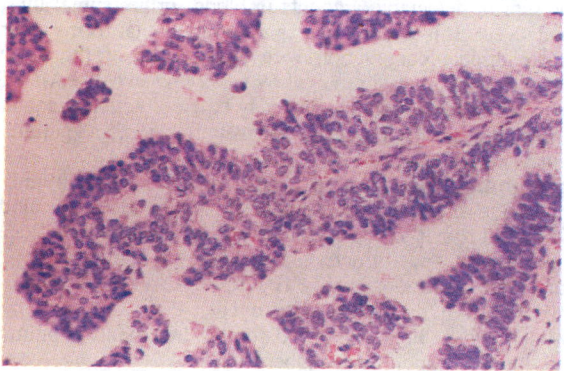

Papillary carcinoma in situ *(Skarin, 1991)*

papillary duct, any one of the thousands of straight collecting renal tubules that descend through the medulla of the kidney and join with others to form the common ducts opening into the renal papillae. Compare **Henle's loop.** See also **kidney.**

papillary muscle, any one of the rounded or conical muscular projections attached to the chordae tendineae in the ventricles of the heart. The papillary muscles vary in number, but the two main ones are the anterior papillary muscle and the posterior papillary muscle. The papillary muscles are associated with the atrioventricular valves that they help open and close. Compare **chorda tendinea, trabecula carnea.**

papillary tumor. See **papilloma.**

papillate /pap'ilit/, marked by papillae or nipplelike prominences.

papilledema /pap'ilədē'mə/, *pl.* **papilledemas, papilledemata** [L, *papilla* + Gk, *oidema*, swelling], swelling of the optic disc, visible on ophthalmoscopic examination of the fundus of the eye, caused by increased intracranial pressure. The meningeal sheaths that surround the optic nerves from the optic disc are continuous with the meninges of the brain; therefore increased intracranial pressure is transmitted forward from the brain to the optic disc in the eye to cause the swelling.

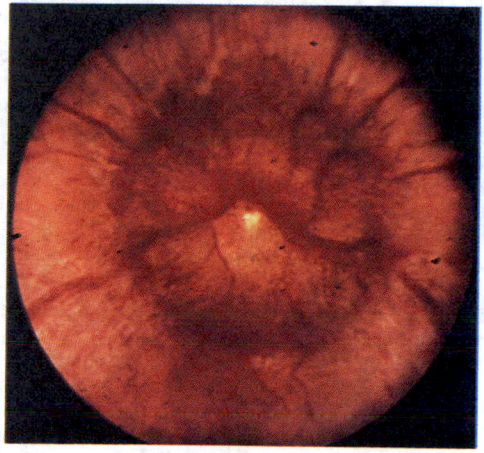

Papilledema *(Zitelli, 1992)*

papilliform /pəpil'ifôrm/, shaped like a papilla.

papillitis /pap'ilī'tis/ [L, *papilla* + Gk, *itis*, inflammation],
1. inflammation of a papilla, such as the lacrimal papilla.
2. inflammation of the optic disc.

papilloma /pap'ilō'mə/ [L, *papilla* + Gk, *oma*, tumor], a benign epithelial neoplasm characterized by a branching or lobular tumor. Also called **papillary tumor.**

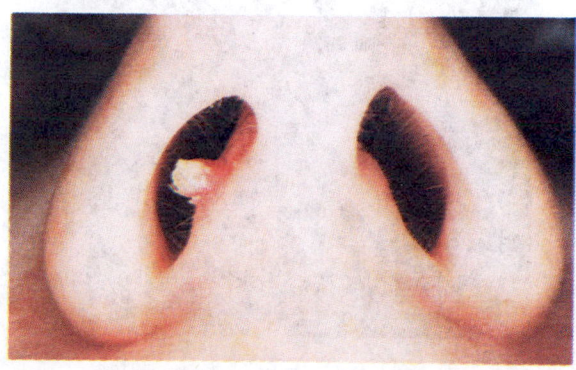

Papilloma *(Bingham, 1992)*

papillomacarcinoma /-kär'sinō'mə/ [L, *papilla*, nipple; Gk, *oma*, tumor, *karkinos*, crab, *oma*, tumor], a wartlike cancer that grows inward into a cavity or outward from a surface.

papillomatosis /pap'ilōmətō'sis/ [L, *papilla* + Gk, *oma*, tumor, *osis*, condition], an abnormal condition characterized by widespread development of nipplelike growths.

papillomatosis coronae penis. See **hirsutoid papilloma of the penis.**

papillomavirus /pap'ilō'məvī'rəs/ [L, *papilla* + Gk, *oma*, tumor; L, *virus*, poison], the virus that causes warts in humans.

papilloretinitis /pap'ilōret'inī'tis/ [L, *papilla* + *rete*, net; Gk, *itis*, inflammation], an inflammatory occlusion of a retinal vein.

papovavirus /pap'əvəvī'rəs/ [(acronym) *pa*pilloma, *po*lyoma, *va*cuolating, *virus*], one of a group of small DNA viruses, some of which may be potentially cancer-producing. The human wart is caused by a kind of papovavirus, but it very rarely undergoes malignant transformation. Kinds of papovaviruses are **papilloma papovavirus, polyoma papovavirus,** and **SV-40 papovavirus.**

pappataci fever. See **phlebotomus fever.**

pappus /pap'əs/ [Gk, *pappos*, down], the first growth of beard, characterized by downy hairs.

Pap smear. See **Papanicolaou test.**

Pap test. See **Papanicolaou test.**

papular /pap'yələr/ [L, *papula*, pimple], pertaining to or resembling papules.

papular scaling disease [L, *papula*, pimple; AS *scealu*], any of a group of skin disorders in which there are discrete, raised, dry, scaling lesions. Some kinds of papular scaling diseases are **lichen planus, pityriasis rosea,** and **psoriasis.** Also called **papulosquamous disease.**

papulation /pap'yəlā'shən/ [L, *papula*, pimple, *atus,* process], the development of papules.

papule /pap'yo͞ol/ [L, *papula*, pimple], a small, solid, raised skin lesion less than 1 cm in diameter, such as the lesions of lichen planus and nonpustular acne. Compare **macule.** –**papular,** *adj.*

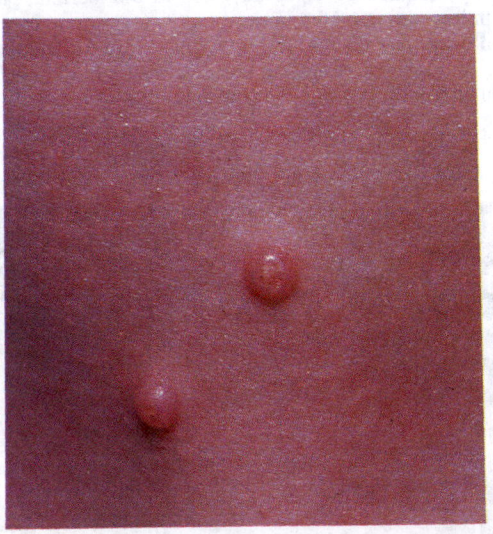

Papules *(du Vivier, 1993)*

papulo-, a combining form meaning 'relating to papules or pimples': *papular, papuliferous.*

papulosquamous /pap'yəlōskwä'məs/ [L, *papula*, pimple + *squama*, scale], pertaining to a skin eruption that is both papular and scaly.

papulosquamous disease. See **papular scaling disease.**

papyraceous /pap'irā'shəs/ [Gk, *papyros*, paper], having a paperlike quality.

papyraceous fetus. See **fetus papyraceus.**

Paquelin's cautery /pak'əlinz/ [Claude A. Paquelin, French physician, b. 1836; Gk, *kauterion*, branding iron], a cauterizing device consisting of a platinum loop through which a heated hydrocarbon is passed.

par, a pair, specifically a pair of cranial nerves, such as the par nonum or the ninth pair.

PAR, abbreviation for **pulmonary arteriolar resistance.**

par-, a combining form meaning 'aside, beyond, apart from, against': *parabacteria, parotid, parumbilical.*

para [L, *parere*, to bear], a woman who has produced an infant regardless of whether the child was alive or stillborn. The term is used with numerals to indicate the number of pregnancies carried to more than 20 weeks' gestation, such as para 2, indicating two pregnancies, regardless of the number of offspring produced in a single pregnancy. See also **nullipara, parity.**

para- /par'ə-/, **par-,** a prefix meaning 'similar, beside, beyond, supplementary to, disordered': *paramedical, parabiosis, paranoia, paraplegia.*

-para, -parous, a suffix meaning 'to bear or give birth': *primipara, ovovipara, pipipara.*

paraaminobenzoic acid (PABA) /per'ə·amē'nōbenzō'ik/, a substance often occurring in association with the vitamin B complex, found in cereals, eggs, milk, and meat and present in detectable amounts in blood, urine, spinal fluid, and sweat. It is widely used as a sunscreen that forms a partial chemical conjugation with constituents of the horny layer and that resists removal by water and sweat. PABA is a sulfonamide antagonist and may be an effective agent for the treatment of scleroderma, dermatomyositis, and pemphigus.

paraaminohippuric acid (PAHA, PHA) /per'ə·amē'-nōhipo͞or'ik/, the N-acetic acid of paraaminobenzoic acid. Its sodium salt is used for measuring the effective renal plasma flow and for determining kidney function.

paraaminosalicylic acid (PAS, PASA) /per'ə·amē'-nōsal'isil'ik/, a bacteriostatic agent.

■ INDICATIONS: It is prescribed for the treatment of pulmonary and extrapulmonary tuberculosis.

■ CONTRAINDICATIONS: Known hypersensitivity to this drug prohibits its use. It may interact with other drugs.

■ ADVERSE EFFECTS: Among the most serious reactions are nausea, vomiting, diarrhea, and abdominal pain. Fever, skin eruptions and other kinds of hypersensitivity reactions, goiter, hypokalemia, and acidosis may occur.

parabiotic syndrome /-bī·ot'ik/ [Gk, *para*, beside, *bios*, life; *syn*, together, *dromos*, course], a blood transfer condition that can occur between identical twin fetuses because of placental vascular anastomoses. One twin may become anemic and the other plethoric.

paracentesis /per'əsentē'sis/ [Gk, *para* + *kentesis*, puncturing], a procedure in which fluid is withdrawn from a cavity of the body. An incision is made in the skin, and a hollow trocar, cannula, or catheter is passed through the incision into the cavity to allow outflow of fluid into a collecting device. Paracentesis is most commonly performed to remove excessive accumulations of ascitic fluid from the abdomen. Stricts asepsis is followed. The paient is assessed for any adverse reaction.

paracentesis thoracis [Gk, *para* + *kentesis,* puncturing; *thorax,* chest], the aspiration of fluid or air, or both, through a needle inserted into the pleural cavity.

paracentral /-sen′trəl/ [Gk, *para* + *kentron*], close to a center or a central part.

paracervical /-sur′vikəl/ [Gk, *para* + L, *cervix,* neck], adjacent to the cervix.

paracervical block, a form of regional anesthesia in which a local anesthetic is injected into the area on each side of the uterine cervix that contains the plexus of nerves innervating the uterine cervix. Effective anesthesia for active labor is often achieved. The duration of the anesthetic effect depends on the agent used. Transient maternal hypotension or fetal bradycardia sometimes occurs after paracervical block, usually caused by inadvertent intravascular injection of the anesthetic.

paracetamol. See **acetaminophen.**

parachute reflex /per′əshoōt/, a variation of the **Moro reflex** or **startle reflex,** whereby an infant is tested for motor nerve development by suspending the infant in the prone position and then dropping the infant a short distance onto a soft surface. If the motor nerve development is normal, the infant at 9 months will extend the arms, hands, and fingers on both sides of the body in a protective movement.

several years of sulfonamides or, in severe cases, intravenous amphotericin B followed by oral sulfonamides. Also called **paracoccidioidal granuloma, South American blastomycosis.** Compare **North American blastomycosis.**

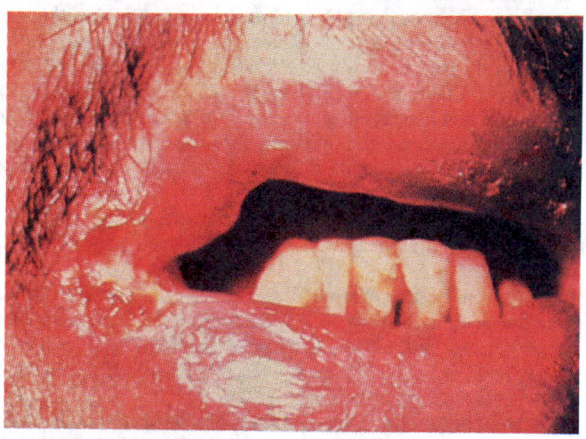

Paracoccidioidomycosis lesions around the lips
(Baron, 1990/Courtesy Upjohn Co.)

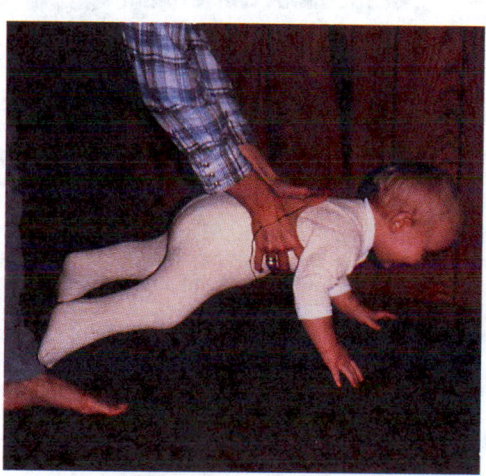

Parachute reflex *(Zitelli, 1992)*

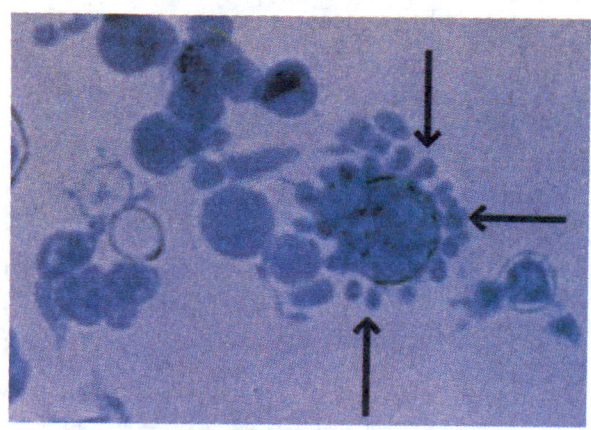

Paracoccidioides brasiliensis *(Baron, 1990)*

paracinesia. See **parakinesia.**

paracoccidioidomycosis /per′əkoksid′ē·oi′dōmīkō′sis/ [Gk, *para* + *kokkos,* berry, *eidos,* form, *mykes,* fungus, *osis,* condition], a chronic, occasionally fatal, fungal infection caused by *Paracoccidioides brasiliensis,* characterized by ulcers of the oral cavity, larynx, and nose. Other effects include large, draining lymph nodes, cough, dyspnea, weight loss, and skin, genital, and intestinal lesions. The disease occurs in Mexico and Central and South America and is acquired by inhalation of spores of the fungus. The diagnosis is made by microscopic examination of a smear prepared from a lesion. Treatment requires

paradichlorobenzene poisoning. See **naphthalene poisoning.**

paradidymal /-did′iməl/ [Gk, *para,* beside, *didymos,* twin], **1.** pertaining to the paradidymis. **2.** beside the testis.

paradidymis /per′ədid′imis/, *pl.* **paradidymides** /per′ədidim′idēz/ [Gk, *para* + *epi,* above, *didymos,* twin], a rudimentary structure in the male, situated on the spermatic cord of the epididymis, that consists of vestigial remains of the caudal part of the embryonic mesonephric tubules. A similar vestigial structure, the paroophoron, is found in the female. Also called **organ of Giraldes, parepididymis.** See also **appendix epididymis.**

paradigm /per′ədīm, -dim/, a pattern that may serve as a model or example.

Paradione, a trademark for an anticonvulsant (paramethadione).

paradoxic /-dok′sik/ [Gk, *paradoxos*, strange], pertaining to a person, situation, statement, or act that may appear to have inconsistent or contradictory qualities, or that may be true but that appears to be absurd or unbelievable. Also **paradoxical** /-dok′sikəl/.

paradoxical breathing [Gk, *paradoxos*; AS, *bræth*], a condition in which a part of the lung deflates during inspiration and inflates during expiration. The condition usually is associated with a chest trauma, such as an open chest wound or rib cage damage. In such cases, the paradoxical breathing that occurs spontaneously is sometimes called internal paradoxical breathing. External paradoxical breathing may be observed during deep general anesthesia.

paradoxical bronchospasm, a constriction of the airways after treatment with a sympathomimetic bronchodilator.

paradoxical incontinence. See **retention with overflow.**

paradoxical intention, a logotherapeutic technique that encourages a patient to do what he fears and if possible to exaggerate it to the point of humor. The technique is used in the treatment of phobias.

paradoxical pulse. See **pulsus paradoxus.**

paraffin /per′əfin/ [L, *paraum*, little + *affinis*, related], any of a group of hydrocarbons or hydrocarbon mixtures of the paraffin series as indicated by the formula, $C_nH_{(2n+2)}$. Examples include methane gas, kerosene, and paraffin wax.

paraffin bath [L, *parum*, too little, *affinis*, related], the application of heat to a specific area of the body through the use of paraffin. The part is quickly immersed in heated liquid wax and then withdrawn so that the wax solidifies to form an insulating layer. The procedure is repeated until the layer is 5 to 10 mm thick, and then the entire area is wrapped in an insulating fabric, such as a loose-fitting plastic bag or paper towels. The technique is effective for heating traumatized or inflamed areas, especially the hands, feet, and wrists, and is used primarily for patients with arthritis and rheumatism or any joint condition. Also called **wax bath.**

paraffin method, (in surgical pathology) a method used in preparing a selected portion of tissue for pathologic examination. The tissue is fixed, dehydrated, and infiltrated by and embedded in paraffin, forming a block that is cut with a microtome into slices 8 μm thick. This method, which is more commonly used than the frozen section method, is slower and therefore not used during surgery.

paraffin section [L, *parum*, little + *affinis*, related; *sectio*], a histologic section cut from tissue that has been embedded in paraffin wax.

Paraflex, a trademark for a skeletal muscle relaxant (chlorzoxazone).

parafollicular C cell /-folik′yələr/, a calcitonin-secreting cell located between follicles.

Parafon Forte, a trademark for a fixed-combination drug containing an analgesic-antipyretic (acetaminophen) and a skeletal muscle relaxant (chlorzoxazone), used for the relief of painful musculoskeletal conditions.

paraganglion /-gang′glē·on/, *pl.* **paraganglia** [Gk, *para* + *ganglion*, knot], any one of the small groups of chromaffin cells associated with the ganglia of the sympathetic nerve trunk and situated outside the adrenal medulla, most often near the sympathetic ganglia along the aorta and its branches. The paraganglia are also connected with the ganglia of the celiac, renal, suprarenal, aortic, and hypogastric plexuses. The paraganglia secrete the hormones epinephrine and norepinephrine. Also called **chromaffin body.** See also **chromaffin cell.**

paragonimiasis /per′əgon′imī′əsis/ [Gk, *para* + *gonimos*, generative, *osis*, condition], chronic infection with the lung fluke *Paragonimus westermani*, occurring most commonly in Asia. It is characterized by hemoptysis, bronchitis, and, occasionally, abdominal masses, pain and diarrhea, or cerebral involvement with paralysis, ocular pathologic conditions, or seizures. The disease is acquired by ingesting cysts in infected freshwater crabs or crayfish, the intermediate hosts. Adequate cooking of shellfish prevents the disease. Bithionol given orally is the usual treatment.

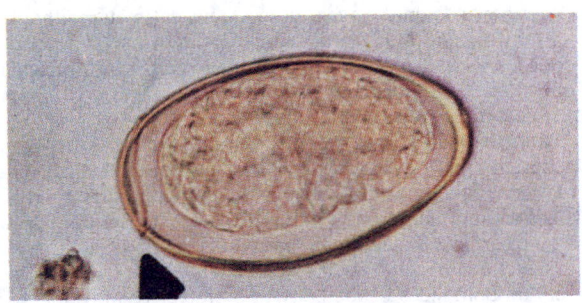

***Paragonimus westermani* egg**
(Murray, 1990/From Koneman EW, Allen SD, Dowell VR, and Sommers HM: Color Atlas and Textbook of Diagnostic Microbiology, ed 2, Philadelphia, 1979, Lippincott)

parahypnosis /-hipnō′sis/ [Gk, *para* + *hypnos*, sleep], a form of disordered sleep that is observed in hypnosis and narcosis.

parainfluenza virus /per′ə·in′flo͞o·en′zə/ [Gk, *para* + It, *influenza*, influence], a myxovirus with four serotypes, causing respiratory infections in infants and young children and, less commonly, in adults. Types 1 and 2 parainfluenza viruses may cause laryngotracheobronchitis or croup; type 3 is a cause of croup, tracheobronchitis, bronchiolitis, and bronchopneumonia in children; types 1, 3, and 4 are associated with pharyngitis and the common cold. Compare **influenza, rhinovirus.**

parakinesia /-kinē′zhə/ [Gk, *para* + *kinesis*, movement], an abnormality of movement resulting from a nerve disorder in a muscle, such as an irregularity of one of the ocular muscles. Also called **paracinesia** /-sinē′zhə/.

parakinesis. See **telekinesis.**

paraldehyde /peral′dəhīd/, a clear, colorless, strong-smelling liquid obtained by the polymerization of acetaldehyde with a small amount of sulfuric acid. Paraldehyde is used as a solvent and may be administered orally, intravenously, intramuscularly, or rectally to induce hypnotic states or sedation.

parallax /per′əlaks/ [Gk, *parallelos*, side-by-side], the apparent displacement of an object at different distances from the eyes when viewed by both eyes together. It is the basis of stereoscopic vision and depth perception.

parallel grid /per′əlel/ [Gk, *parallelos*, side-by-side; ME, *gredire*], (in radiography) an x-ray grid that has lead strips oriented parallel to each other.

parallelogram condenser /per′əlel′əgram′/ [Gk, *parallelos* + *gramma*, record; L, *condensare*, to make thick], (in dentistry) an instrument with a face shaped like a rectangle or parallelogram, used for compacting amalgams in filling teeth.

parallel play [Gk, *parallelos* + AS, *plegan*, to play], a form of play among a group of children, primarily toddlers, in which each one engages in an independent activity that is similar to but not influenced by or shared with the others. Compare **cooperative play.** See also **associative play, solitary play.**

parallel talk, a form of speech used during children's play therapy in which the clinician verbalizes activities of the child without requiring answers to questions. The parallel talk may take the form of 'I'm making a cake. You are making a cake, too.' The clinician repeats utterances of the child correctly and may parallel the child's actions.

Paralympics /per′əlim′piks/, [*paraplegic* + *Olympics*], an international competitive wheelchair sports event, usually held in association with the official quadrennial Olympic Games. Also called **Para Olympics.**

paralysis /pəral′isis/, *pl.* **paralyses** [Gk, *paralysein*, to paralyze], the loss of muscle function or the loss of sensation, or both. It may be caused by a variety of problems, such as trauma, disease, and poisoning. Paralyses may be classified according to cause, muscle tone, distribution, or the part of the body affected. See also **flaccid paralysis, spastic paralysis.** −**paralytic,** *adj.*

paralysis agitans. See **Parkinson's disease.**

paralytic /per′əlit′ik/ [Gk, *paralyein*, to be paralyzed], pertaining to the characteristics of paralysis.

paralytic dementia. See **paresis,** def. 2.

paralytic ileus [Gk, *paralyein*, to be paralyzed, *eilein*, to twist], a decrease in or absence of intestinal peristalsis that may occur after abdominal surgery or peritoneal injury or in connection with severe pyelonephritis, ureteral stone, fractured ribs, myocardial infarction, extensive intestinal ulceration, heavy metal poisoning, porphyria, retroperitoneal hematomas, especially those associated with fractured vertebrae, or any severe metabolic disease. The most common overall cause of intestinal obstruction, paralytic ileus is mediated by a hormonal component of the sympathoadrenal system. Also called **adynamic ileus.**

■ OBSERVATIONS: Paralytic ileus is characterized by abdominal tenderness and distention, absence of bowel sounds, lack of flatus, and nausea and vomiting. There may be fever, decreased urinary output, electrolyte imbalance, dehydration, and respiratory distress. The loss of fluids and electrolytes may be extreme, and, unless they are replaced, the condition may lead to hemoconcentration, hypovolemia, renal insufficiency, shock, and death.

■ INTERVENTIONS: The patient is kept in bed in a low Fowler's position, and nothing is given by mouth. An intestinal tube is inserted as a nasogastric tube into the duodenum and connected to intermittent suction and the patient is positioned to facilitate the advancement of the tube, which is checked every 30 to 60 minutes. The character of GI drainage is monitored every 2 to 4 hours, and any increase or decrease in the amount or changes in the color or consistency is reported. Bowel sounds, blood pressure, pulse, and respirations are checked every 2 to 4 hours and rectal temperature every 4 hours. Abdominal girth is measured every 2 hours, and report is made of any increase. Parenteral fluids with electrolytes and medication to promote peristalsis are administered as ordered; intake and output are measured, and if less than 30 ml of urine is excreted per hour, the physician is informed. The patient is helped to turn and deep breathe every 2 to 4 hours and is given oral hygiene every 1 to 2 hours. Active or passive range-of-motion exercises are performed every 4 hours. When intestinal output increases and bowel sounds return, the intestinal tube may be clamped and small amounts of warm tea or a carbonated beverage may be given. If pain, distention, or cramps do not recur, the intestinal tube may be removed, but a rectal tube or an enema may be ordered to relieve distention.

■ NURSING CONSIDERATIONS: The concerns of the nurse include monitoring and reporting the signs of paralytic ileus and its potential complications, ensuring that the patient is as comfortable as possible, and explaining to the patient the purpose of the intestinal tube. The nurse instructs the patient to avoid mouth breathing, because swallowed air can increase distention.

paralytic incontinence [Gk, *paralyein*, to be palsied; L, *incontinentia*, inability to retain], urinary or fecal incontinence resulting from loss of or impaired motor nerve control of the sphincter muscles.

paralytic mydriasis [Gk, *paralyein*, to be palsied; *mydriasis*, pupil enlargement], an area of depressed vision that is on the periphery of the field.

paralytic poliomyelitis [Gk, *paralyein*, to be palsied; *polios*, gray + *myelos*, marrow + *itis*, inflammation], a flaccid paralysis of the limbs resulting from damaged lower motor neurons. Progressive bulbar paralysis with respiratory and vasomotor failure may result when the brainstem nuclei are involved.

paralytic shellfish poisoning. See **shellfish poisoning.**

paralytic stroke [Gk, *paralyein*, to be palsied; AS, *strac*], a sudden attack of paralysis caused by disease or injury to the brain or spinal cord.

paralyze /per′əlīz/ [Gk, *paralyein*, to be palsied], **1.** to produce or enter into a state of paralysis. **2.** to cause loss of muscle power.

paramedic /-med′ik/ [Gk, *para* + L, *medicina*, art of healing], a person who acts as an assistant to a physician or in place of a physician, especially a person in the military, trained in emergency medical procedures. −**paramedical,** *adj.*

paramedical personnel, health care workers other than physicians, dentists, podiatrists, and nurses who have special training in the performance of supportive health care tasks. Paramedical personnel includes, for example, the **emergency medical technician, audiologist,** and **x-ray technologist.** Also called **allied health personnel.**

paramesonephric duct /per′əmēz′ōnef′rik/ [Gk, *para* + *mesos*, middle, *nephros*, kidney], one of a pair of embryonic ducts that develops into the uterus and the uterine tubes. Also called **müllerian duct.**

parameter /pəram′ətər/ [Gk, *para* + *metron*, measure], **1.** a value or constant used to describe or measure a set of data representing a physiologic function or system, as in the use of acid-base relationships of the blood as parameters for evaluating the function of a patient's respiratory system. **2.** a statistical value of a population group. **3.** *informal.* limits or boundary.

paramethadione /per′əmeth′ədī′ōn/, an anticonvulsant.
- INDICATION: It is prescribed for the prevention of seizures in petit mal epilepsy.
- CONTRAINDICATIONS: Blood dyscrasias, severe renal or hepatic impairment, or known hypersensitivity to this drug prohibits its use.
- ADVERSE EFFECTS: Among the more serious adverse reactions are exfoliative dermatitis, blood dyscrasias, and hepatitis. Sedation, hemeralopia, and moderate neutropenia may occur.

paramethasone acetate /-meth′əsōn/, a glucocorticoid.
- INDICATIONS: It is prescribed in the treatment of inflammatory and allergic conditions.
- CONTRAINDICATIONS: Systemic fungal infections or known hypersensitivity to this drug prohibits its use.
- ADVERSE EFFECTS: Among the more serious adverse reactions are GI, endocrine, and neurologic disturbances and fluid and electrolyte imbalance.

parametric imaging /-met′rik/ [Gk, *para* + *metron*, measure; L, *imago*, image], (in nuclear medicine) a diagnostic procedure in which an image of an administered radioactive tracer is derived according to a mathematical rule, such as by the division of one image by another.

parametric statistics, statistics that assume a population has a symmetric, such as gaussian or normal, distribution.

parametritis /per′əmetrī′tis/ [Gk, *para* + *metra*, womb, *itis*], an inflammatory condition of the tissue of the structures around the uterus. See also **pelvic inflammatory disease.**

parametrium /per′əmē′trē·əm/, *pl.* **parametria** [Gk, *para* + *metra*, womb], the lateral extension of the uterine subserous connective tissue into the broad ligament. Compare **endometrium, myometrium.**

paramitome. See **hyaloplasm.**

paramnesia /per′amnē′zhə/ [Gk, *para* + *amnesia*, forgetfulness], **1.** a perversion of memory in which one believes one remembers events and circumstances that never actually occurred. **2.** a condition in which words are remembered and used without the comprehension of their meaning. Compare **déjà vu.**

paramyxovirus /-mik′sōvī′rəs/ [Gk, *para* + *myxa*, mucus; L, *virus*, poison], a member of a family of viruses that includes the organisms that cause parainfluenza, mumps, and some respiratory infections.

paranasal /-nā′zəl/ [Gk, *para* + L, *nasus*, nose], situated near or alongside the nose, such as the paranasal sinuses.

paranasal sinus, one of the air cavities in various bones around the nose, such as the frontal sinus in the frontal bone lying deep to the medial part of the superciliary ridge and the maxillary sinus within the maxilla between the orbit, the nasal cavity, and the upper teeth. (Figure, p. 877) Compare **confluence of the sinuses, occipital sinus.**

paraneoplastic syndromes /-nē′əplas′tik/ [Gk, *para* + *neos*, new, *plassein*, to mold, *syn*, together, *dromos*, course], indirect effects of a tumor that occur distant to the tumor or metastatic site. They may result from the production of active proteins, polypeptides, or inactive hormones by the tumor.

parangi. See **yaws.**

paranoia /per′ənoi′ə/ [Gk, *para* + *nous*, mind], (in psychiatry) a disorder characterized by an elaborate overly suspicious system of thinking, with delusions of persecution and grandeur usually centered on one major theme, such as a financial matter, a job situation, an unfaithful spouse, or

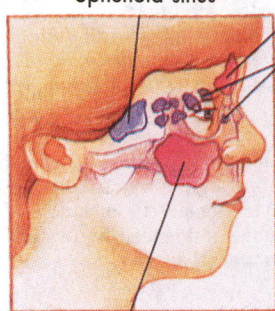

Paranasal sinuses *(Thibodeau, 1993/Margaret Gerrity)*

other problem. Also called **paranoea** /per′ənē′ə/. Compare **paranoid schizophrenia.**

paranoiac /per′ənoi′ak/, **1.** a person afflicted with or exhibiting characteristics of paranoia. **2.** of or pertaining to paranoia. Also **paranoeac.**

paranoid /per′ənoid/ [Gk, *para* + *nous*, mind, *eidos*, form], **1.** pertaining to or resembling paranoia. **2.** a person afflicted with a paranoid disorder. **3.** *informal.* a person, or pertaining to a person, who is overly suspicious or exhibits persecutory trends or attitudes.

paranoid disorder, any of a large group of mental disorders characterized by an impaired sense of reality and persistent delusions. Kinds of paranoid disorders include **acute paranoid disorder, paranoia,** and **shared paranoid disorder.**

paranoid ideation, an exaggerated, sometimes grandiose, belief or suspicion, usually not of a delusional nature, that one is being harassed, persecuted, or treated unfairly.

paranoid personality, a personality characterized by paranoia.

paranoid personality disorder, a disorder characterized by extreme suspiciousness and distrust of others to the degree that one blames them for one's mistakes and failures and goes to abnormal lengths to validate prejudices, attitudes, or biases.

paranoid reaction, a psychopathologic condition associated with aging and characterized by the gradual formation of delusions, usually of a persecutory nature and often accompanied by related hallucinations. Other manifestations of senile degeneration, such as memory loss and confusion, do not usually accompany the reaction, and the individual maintains orientation for time, place, and person.

paranoid schizophrenia, a form of schizophrenia characterized by persistent preoccupation with illogical, absurd, and changeable delusions, usually of a persecutory, grandiose, or jealous nature, accompanied by related hallucinations. The symptoms include extreme anxiety, exaggerated suspiciousness, aggressiveness, anger, argumentativeness, hostility, and violence. The condition occurs most frequently during middle age. Current therapy is not usually effective. Also called **heboid paranoia.** Compare **paranoia.** See also **schizophrenia.**

paranoid state, a transitory abnormal mental condition characterized by illogical thought processes and generalized suspicion and distrust, with a tendency toward persecutory ideas or delusions.

paranormal /-nôr′məl/ [Gk, *para* + L, *normalis*, rule], pertaining to phenomena that cannot be explained by normal scientific investigation.

paranuclear body. See **centrosome.**

ParaOlympics. See **Paralympics.**

paraoperative. See **perioperative.**

paraparesis /-pərē′sis/ [Gk, *para* + *paresis*, paralysis], a partial paralysis, usually affecting only the lower extremities.

paraperitoneal nephrectomy /-per′itənē′əl/ [Gk, *para* + *peri, tenein*, to stretch, *nephros*, kidney, *ektome*, cutting out], surgery to remove the kidney through an extra peritoneal incision.

parapertussis /per′əpərtus′is/ [Gk, *para* + L, *per*, very, *tussis*, cough], an acute bacterial respiratory infection caused by *Bordetella parapertussis*, having symptoms closely resembling those of pertussis. It is usually milder than pertussis, although it can be fatal. It is possible to be infected with both *B. parapertussis* and *B. pertussis* at the same time. A parapertussis vaccine is available and may be given in combination with pertussis vaccine.

parapharyngeal abscess /per′əfərin′jē·əl/ [Gk, *para* + *pharynx*, throat; L, *abscedere*, to go away], a suppurative infection of tissues adjacent to the pharynx, usually a complication of acute pharyngitis or tonsillitis. Infection may spread to the jugular vein, where it may cause thrombophlebitis and septic emboli. Systemic antibiotics and surgical drainage may be required. Also called **parapharyngeal space abscess.** Compare **peritonsillar abscess, retropharyngeal abscess.** See also **tonsillitis.**

paraphilia /per′əfil′yə/ [Gk, *para* + *philein*, to love], sexual perversion or deviation; a condition in which the sexual instinct is expressed in ways that are socially prohibited or unacceptable or are biologically undesirable, such as the use of an inanimate object for sexual arousal, sexual activity with another person that involves real or simulated suffering or humiliation, or sexual relations with a nonconsenting partner. Kinds of paraphilia include **exhibitionism, fetishism, pedophilia, transvestism, voyeurism,** and **zoophilia.** **–paraphiliac,** *adj., n.*

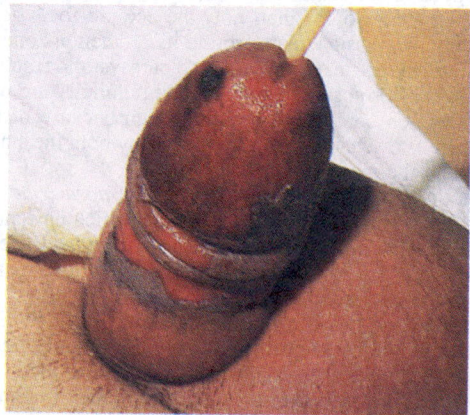

Paraphimosis
(Seidel, 1991/Courtesy Patrick C Walsh, MD, The Johns Hopkins University School of Medicine, Baltimore)

paraphimosis /per′əfīmō′sis/ [Gk, *para* + *phimoein*, to muzzle], a condition characterized by an inability to replace the foreskin in its normal position after it has been retracted behind the glans penis. Caused by a narrow or inflamed foreskin, the condition may lead to gangrene. Circumcision may be required. Compare **phimosis.**

paraphrasia /-frā′sē·ə/ [Gk, *para* + *phrasein*, to utter], speech that is incoherent, unintelligible, and apparently incomprehensible. However, the speech may be meaningful when carefully interpreted by a psychotherapist. Also called **jargon aphasia, word hash, word salad.**

paraplasm /per′əplaz′əm/ [Gk, *para* + *plassein*, to mold], any abnormal growth or malformation. Compare **hyaloplasm.** **–paraplasmic,** *adj.*

paraplastic /-plas′tik/ [Gk, *para* + *plassein*, to mold], **1.** misshapen or malformed. **2.** showing abnormal formative power; of the nature of a paraplasm.

paraplectic. See **paraplegic.**

paraplegia /per′əplē′jē·ə/ [Gk, *para* + *plege*, stroke], paralysis characterized by motor or sensory loss in the lower limbs and trunk. Approximately 11,000 spinal cord injuries reported each year in the United States involve paraplegia. Such injuries commonly occur as the result of automobile and motorcycle accidents, sporting accidents, falls, and gunshot wounds. Paraplegia less commonly results from nontraumatic lesions, such as scoliosis, spina bifida, or neoplasms. Compare **hemiplegia, quadriplegia.** **–paraplegic,** *adj., n.*

■ OBSERVATIONS: The signs and symptoms of paraplegia may develop immediately from trauma and include the loss of sensation, motion, and reflexes below the level of the lesion. Depending on the level of the lesion and whether damage to the spinal cord is complete or incomplete, the patient may lose bladder and bowel control and develop sexual dysfunctions. An incomplete spinal cord injury does not usually inhibit circumanal sensation, voluntary toe flexion, or sphincter control. A complete spinal cord injury destroys sensation and voluntary muscle control and usually causes the permanent loss of muscle function distal to the injury.

■ INTERVENTIONS: The treatment of paraplegia seeks to restore proper spine alignment, stabilize the injured spinal area, decompress any involved neurologic structures, and rehabilitate the patient as quickly as possible. At the accident scene, when spinal cord injury is suspected, the patient must not be moved until strapped and stabilized on a board. Such stabilization helps to prevent permanent damage to any injured spinal structures. Drugs such as baclofen may be administered to relieve any muscle spasms associated with dysfunction of the upper motor neurons.

■ NURSING CONSIDERATIONS: When the paraplegic patient progresses from bed rest to a wheelchair, the nurse is alert to any signs of orthostatic hypotension. Special binders and antiembolism hose are used to help the patient adjust to the transition from bed to wheelchair. Prevention of pressure sores is an important priority. Other treatment may include the administration of a high-bulk diet and suppositories to prevent constipation.

paraplegic /-plē′jik/ [Gk, *para* + *plege*, stroke], pertaining to a person affected by paraplegia or a condition resembling paraplegia. Also called **paraplectic.**

parapraxia /-prak′sē·ə/ [Gk, *para* + *praxis*, doing], **1.** the abnormal performance of purposive actions, such as one movement occurring in place of another intended movement. **2.** forgetfulness with a tendency to misplace things.

paraprotein /-prō'tēn/, any of the incomplete monoclonal immunoglobins that occur in plasma cell disorders.

parapsoriasis /per'əsərī'əsis/ [Gk, *para* + *psorian*, to itch], a group of chronic skin diseases resembling psoriasis, characterized by maculopapular, erythematous, scaly eruptions without systemic symptoms. Parapsoriasis is resistant to all treatment.

parapsychology /-sīkol'əjē/ [Gk, *para* + *psyche*, mind, *logos*, science], a branch of psychology concerned with the study of alleged psychic phenomena, such as clairvoyance, extrasensory perception, and telepathy.

paraquat poisoning /per'əkwot'/ [Gk, *para* + L, *quaterni*, four each, *potio*, drink], a toxic condition caused by the ingestion of paraquat dichloride, a highly poisonous pesticide. Characteristically, progressive pulmonary fibrosis and damage to the esophagus, kidneys, and liver develop several days after ingestion. After fibrosis begins, death is inevitable, usually within 3 weeks. The mechanism of action of the poison is unknown. Most often, poisoning results from accidental occupational exposure. There is considerable concern that the inhalation of the smoke of marijuana treated with the herbicide may cause intoxication, but no clinical syndrome resulting from such exposure has been documented.

parasacral /-sā'krəl/ [Gk, *para* + *sacrum*], pertaining to the area around the sacrum.

parasite /per'əsīt/ [Gk, *parasitos*, guest], **1.** an organism living in or on and obtaining nourishment from another organism. A **facultative parasite** may live on a host but is capable of living independently. An **obligate parasite** is one that depends entirely on its host for survival. **2.** See **parasitic fetus.** –**parasitic,** *adj.*

parasitemia /per'əsītē'mē·ə/ [Gk, *parasitos* + *haima*, blood], the presence of parasites in the blood. Compare **bacteremia, fungemia, viremia.**

parasitic fetus /-sit'ik/ [Gk, *parasitos* + L, *icus*, like, *fetus,* pregnant], the smaller, usually malformed member of conjoined, unequal, or asymmetric twins that is attached to and dependent on the more normal fetus for growth and development. Compare **autosite.**

parasitic fibroma, a pedunculated uterine fibroid deriving part of its blood supply from the omentum.

parasitic glossitis, a mycosis of the tongue, characterized by a black or brown furry patch on the posterior dorsal surface composed of hypertrophied filiform papillae that measure about 1 cm in length and are easily broken. The condition, caused by *Cryptococcus linguae-pilosasae* in symbiosis with *Nocardia lingualis,* produces no discomfort and may be treated with a simple mouthwash. The patch may disappear spontaneously and later reappear. Also called **anthracosis linguae, black hairy tongue, black tongue, glossitis parasitica, glossophytia, keratomycosis linguae, lingua villosa nigra, melanotrichia linguae, nigrities linguae.**

parasitic hemoptysis [Gk, *parasitos,* guest, *haima,* blood + *ptyein,* to spit], the spitting of bright red blood because of a parasitic infection. The condition usually involves lung flukes (*Paragonimus*) or tapeworms (*Echinococcus*).

parasitism /per'əsitiz'əm/ [Gk, *parasitos,* guest], an infestation or presence of parasites.

parasympathetic /-sim'pəthet'ik/ [Gk, *para* + *sympathein,* to feel with], of or pertaining to the craniosacral division of the autonomic nervous system, consisting of the oculomotor, facial, glossopharyngeal, vagus, and pelvic nerves.

The actions of the parasympathetic division are mediated by the release of acetylcholine and primarily involve the protection, conservation, and restoration of body resources. Preganglionic parasympathetic fibers, which emerge from the hypothalamus, other brain areas, and sacral segments of the spinal cord, form synapses in ganglia located near or in the walls of the organs to be innervated. Reactions to parasympathetic stimulation are highly localized and tend to counteract the adrenergic effects of sympathetic nerves. Parasympathetic fibers slow the heart, stimulate peristalsis, promote the secretion of lacrimal, salivary, and digestive glands, induce bile and insulin release, dilate peripheral and visceral blood vessels, constrict the pupils, esophagus, and bronchioles, and relax sphincters during micturition and defecation. Postganglionic parasympathetic fibers extend to the uterus, vagina, oviducts, and ovaries in females and to the prostate, seminal vesicles, and external genitalia in males, innervating blood vessels of pelvic organs in both sexes; stimulation of these nerves causes vasodilation in the clitoris and labia minora and erection of the penis.

parasympathetic ganglion [Gk, *para* + *sympathein,* to feel with, *gagglion,* knot], a cluster of nerve cell bodies of the parasympathetic division of the autonomic nervous system. The nerves are functionally antagonistic to those of the sympathetic division.

parasympathetic nervous system. See **autonomic nervous system.**

parasympatholytic, parasympatholytic drug. See **anticholinergic.**

parasympathomimetic /per'əsim'pəthō'mimet'ik/ [Gk, *para* + *sympathein,* to feel with, *mimesis,* imitation], **1.** of or pertaining to a substance producing effects similar to those caused by stimulation of a parasympathetic nerve. **2.** an agent whose effects mimic those resulting from stimulation of parasympathetic nerves, especially the effects produced by acetylcholine. Also called **cholinergic.**

parasympathomimetic drug. See **cholinergic.**

parasystole [Gk, *para* + *systole,* contraction], an independent ectopic rhythm whose pacemaker cannot be discharged by impulses of the dominant, usually sinus, rhythm because of an area of depressed conduction surrounding the parasystolic focus. In the classic parasystole, the interectopic intervals are exact multiples of a common denominator reflecting the protected status of the parasystolic focus. However, more often than not, the ectopic focus is influenced by the phasic events around its protection zone. Thus the sinus rhythm may modulate the parasystolic response so that criteria for absolute, undisturbed regularity are not fulfilled. Fusion beats are commonly seen because of the simultaneous discharge of the ventricles by both the sinus impulse and the parasystolic focus.

parataxic distortion /per'ətak'sik/ [Gk, *para* + *taxis,* arrangement], a defense mechanism in which current interpersonal relationships are perceived and judged according to a mode of reference established by an earlier experience. See also **transference.**

parataxic mode, a term introduced by H. S. Sullivan to identify a childhood perception of the physical and social environment as being illogical, disjointed, and inconsistent. The parataxic mode may persist into adulthood in some individuals.

Parathar, a trademark for a parathyroid diagnostic agent (teriparatide acetate).

parathion poisoning /per'əthī'on/ [Gk, *para* + *thio,* phosphate, *on;* L, *potio,* drink], a toxic condition caused by the ingestion, inhalation, or absorption through the skin of the highly toxic organophosphorus insecticide parathion. Symptoms include nausea, vomiting, abdominal cramps, confusion, headache, lack of muscular control, convulsions, and dyspnea. Treatment varies.

parathyroid-, parathyro-, a combining form meaning 'pertaining to the parathyroid glands': *parathyroidectomy.*

parathyroidectomy /-thī'roidek'təmē/ [Gk, *para* + *thyreos,* shield, *eidos,* form, *ektome,* cutting out], the surgical removal of the parathyroid gland.

parathyroid gland /-thī'roid/ [Gk, *para* + *thyreos,* shield, *eidos,* form; L, *glans,* acorn], one of several small structures, usually four in number, attached to the dorsal surfaces of the lateral lobes of the thyroid gland. The parathyroid glands secrete parathyroid hormone, which helps maintain the level of blood calcium concentration and ensures normal neuromuscular irritability, blood clotting, and cell membrane permeability. Each parathyroid gland has the appearance of an oval, brownish red disk and measures about 6 by 4 mm. The parathyroids are divided, according to their location, into the superior parathyroids and the inferior parathyroids. The superior parathyroids, usually two in number, are commonly situated, one on each side, on the caudal border of the cricoid cartilage beside the junction of the pharynx and the esophagus. The inferior parathyroids, also usually two in number, may be situated on the caudal edge of the lateral lobes of the thyroid gland, just caudal to the gland, or adjacent to one of the inferior thyroid veins. These glands are composed of intercommunicating columns of cells bound by connective tissue with a rich supply of capillaries. Parathyroid hypofunction usually causes tetany, which can be treated by the administration of calcium salts or parathyroid extracts.

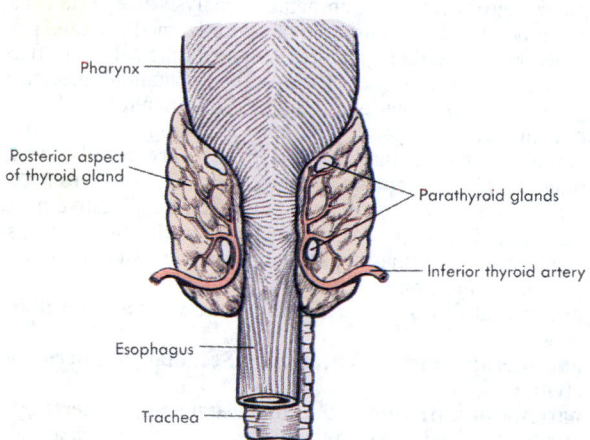

Parathyroid gland (Seeley, 1992/Andrew Grivas)

- Pharynx
- Posterior aspect of thyroid gland
- Parathyroid glands
- Inferior thyroid artery
- Esophagus
- Trachea

parathyroid hormone (PH), a hormone secreted by the parathyroid glands that acts to maintain a constant concentration of calcium in the extracellular fluid. The hormone regulates absorption of calcium from the GI tract, mobilization of calcium from the bones, deposition of calcium in the bones, and excretion of calcium in the breast milk, feces, sweat, and urine. Surgical removal of the parathyroid

glands, as may inadvertently occur in thyroidectomy, results in hypocalcemia, leading to anorexia, tetany, seizures, and death if not corrected. Normal parathyroid laboratory findings are less than 2000 pg/ml. See also **hypoparathyroidism.**

parathyroid injection, bovine parathyroid hormone.
- INDICATION: It is prescribed to regulate blood levels of calcium, especially in the treatment of hypoparathyroidism with tetany.
- CONTRAINDICATIONS: Hypercalcemia, tetany not caused by hypoparathyroidism, hypercalciuria, or known hypersensitivity to this drug prohibits its use.
- ADVERSE EFFECTS: Among the most serious adverse reactions are hypercalcemia and allergic reactions.

parathyroid tetany [Gk, *para* + *thyreos,* shield, *tetanos,* convulsive tension], a form of tetany that is caused by a deficiency of parathyroid secretion.

paratonia. See **gegenhalten.**

paratrooper fracture /-trōō'pər/ [Fr, *parasol, troupe,* company; L, *fractura,* break], a fracture of the distal tibia and its malleolus, commonly occurring when an individual jumps from an elevated platform, such as the back of a truck, or parachutes from an airplane and lands feet first on the ground, subjecting the ankles to extreme force.

paratyphoid fever /-tī'foid/ [Gk, *para* + *typhos,* stupor, *eidos,* form; L, *febris,* fever], a bacterial infection, caused by any *Salmonella* species other than *S. typhi,* characterized by symptoms resembling typhoid fever, although somewhat milder. See also **rose spots, Salmonella, salmonellosis, typhoid fever.**

paraurethral duct /per'əyŏorē'thrəl/ [Gk, *para* + *ourethra,* urethra; L, *ducere,* to lead], one of two ducts that drain the bulbourethral glands into the vestibule of the vagina. Also called **Skene's duct.**

paravaccinia virus /-vaksin'ē·ə/, a member of a subgroup of pox viruses that can infect humans through direct contact with infected livestock. It is related to the smallpox virus and is the cause of pseudocowpox, resulting in milker's nodules. See also **milker's nodule.**

paravertebral /-vur'təbrəl/ [Gk, *para* + L, *vertebra,* joint], pertaining to the area alongside the spinal column or near a vertebra.

paravertebral block [Gk, *para* + L, *vertebra,* OFr, *bloc*], **1.** the blocking of transmission of somatic impulses by the spinal nerves by injecting a local analgesic solution near the point of their emergence. **2.** the blocking of the paravertebral sympathetic chain of nerves anteriolateral to the vertebral bodies.

paraxial /perak'sē·əl/, pertaining to an organ or other structure located near the axis of the body.

parchment skin /pärch'mənt/ [Fr, *parchemin,* AS, *scinn*], thin, wrinkled or stretched atrophic skin.

Paredrine, a trademark for an adrenergic (hydroxyamphetamine hydrobromide).

paregoric /per'əgôr'ik/, a camphorated tincture of opium.
- INDICATIONS: It is prescribed in the treatment of diarrhea and as an analgesic.
- CONTRAINDICATIONS: Known hypersensitivity to this drug or to any opium derivative prohibits its use. It should not be used when diarrhea is caused by a toxic substance.
- ADVERSE EFFECTS: There are usually no adverse reactions. Occasionally, GI disturbances, including constipation, occur.

parenchyma /pəreng'kimə/ [Gk, *para* + *enchyma,* infusion], the tissue of an organ as distinguished from supporting or connective tissue.

parenchymal. See **parenchymatous.**

parenchymal cell /pəreng'kiməl/, any cell that is a functional element of an organ, such as a hepatocyte.

parenchymatous /per'əngkim'ətəs/ [Gk, *para* + *egchyma*, infusion], pertaining to or resembling the functional tissues of an organ or gland. Also called **parenchymal.**

parenchymatous neuritis [Gk, *para* + *enchyma*, infusion; L, *osus*, like], any inflammation affecting the substance, axons, or myelin of the nerve. Also called **axial neuritis, central neuritis.** See also **neuritis.**

parent [L, *parens*], a mother or father; one who bears offspring. **–parental,** *adj*.

parental generation (P₁) /pəren'təl/, the initial cross between two varieties in a genetic sequence; the parents of any individual, organism, or plant belonging to an F₁ generation.

parental grief, the behavioral reactions that characterize the grieving process and result in the resolution of the loss of a child from expected or unexpected death. All people who survive the loss of a loved one normally experience symptoms of both somatic and psychologic distress, such as feelings of guilt and hostility accompanied by changes in usual patterns of conduct. When the death of a child is expected from terminal illness, there is time for anticipatory grieving, so that parents can evaluate their relationship with the child, set priorities for the duration of time involved, and prepare for the actual death of the child. In such cases, parental grieving begins with the discovery of the diagnosis of a life-threatening condition. Parents' adjustment to the diagnosis involves a complete cycle of reactions that extends over an indefinite period of time, depending on the severity and nature of the disease. The immediate reaction is shock and disbelief, followed by acute grief at the anticipation of losing the child. Periods of depression, anger, hope, fear, and anxiety alternate during induction therapy, remission, and maintenance of the disease as parents learn to accept and cope with the situation. Heightened anticipatory grieving recurs during episodes of relapse, and the parents experience increased fear, depression, and the final acceptance of death during the terminal stages of the illness. Although families can prepare themselves for the expected loss, at the time of death there is a period of acute grief, during which parents need to express their deep sorrow and anger. An extended phase of mourning follows, with the eventual resolution of grief and integration into society. In sudden, unexpected death, parents are denied the advantages of anticipatory grief and, because of the lack of time to prepare, usually have extreme feelings of guilt and remorse. The nurse can especially help such parents to assess their feelings so that they can work through them and progress through the resolution of grief and the mourning process, which in unexpected death takes a much longer time. The function of the nurse during all phases of parental grief is primarily supportive, and the degree of intervention depends on the family's strengths and weaknesses in coping with the crisis. Nurses can act directly, or they can help to find other potential sources of support for the parents, such as extended family members, other parents who have lost children, or specific community services or agencies. A large part of the nursing support involves helping families explore new ways of coping, not only to meet the present crisis but to grow and change. Always an important

nursing consideration is the education of the parents about all aspects of the child's illness, especially in terminal conditions. See also **death, grief reaction.**

parental leave. See **family care leave.**

parental role conflict, a nursing diagnosis accepted by the Eighth National Conference on the Classification of Nursing Diagnoses. The condition is a state in which a parent experiences role confusion and conflict in response to a crisis. Among major defining characteristics is an expression by the parent or parents of concerns or feelings of inadequacy to provide for the child's physical and emotional needs during hospitalization or in the home. There is a demonstrated disruption in caretaking routines. The parent also expresses concerns about changes in parental role, family functioning, family communication, and family health. Minor characteristics include expressions of concern about perceived loss of control over decisions relating to the child and reluctance to participate in normal caretaking activities even with encouragement and support. Parents also verbalize or demonstrate feelings of guilt, anger, fear, anxiety, and frustration about the effect of the child's illness on the family process. Related factors include separation from the child caused by chronic illness; intimidation with invasive or restrictive modalities (such as isolation, intubation), specialized care centers, and policies; home care of a child with special needs (such as apnea monitoring, postural drainage, and hyperalimentation); and change in marital status; interruptions of family life caused by home care regimen (such as treatments, caregivers, and lack of respite). See also **nursing diagnosis.**

parent-child relationship. See **maternal-infant bonding.**

parent education, any educational experience geared toward the thoughtful conveyance of information enabling the parent to provide quality childrearing.

parent ego state, in transactional analysis an ego state that incorporates the feelings and behavior learned from the parents or other authority figures. A part of the self that offers advice like that of one's own parents, containing messages that emphasize what one 'ought to' or 'should not' do.

parenteral /pəren'tərəl/ [Gk, *para* + *enteron*, bowel], not in or through the digestive system. **–parenterally,** *adv*.

parenteral absorption, the taking up of substances within the body by structures other than the digestive tract.

parenteral dosage, pertaining to a medication administered by a route that bypasses the GI tract, such as a drug given by injection.

parenteral fluids. See **administration of parenteral fluids.**

parenteral hyperalimentation. See **total parenteral nutrition.**

parenteral nutrition, the administration of nutrients by a route other than through the alimentary canal, such as subcutaneously, intravenously, intramuscularly, or intradermally. The parenteral fluids usually consist of physiologic saline with glucose, amino acids, electrolytes, vitamins, and medications. They are not nutritionally complete but maintain fluid and electrolyte balance during the immediate postoperative period and in other conditions, such as shock, coma, malnutrition, and chronic renal and hepatic failures. See also **total parenteral nutrition.**

parent figure [L, *parens* + *figura*, form], **1.** a parent or a substitute parent or guardian who cares for a child, providing the physical, social, and emotional requirements necessary for normal growth and development. **2.** a person who symbolically represents an ideal parent, having those attributes that one conceptualizes as necessary for forming the perfect parent-child relationship.

parent image, a conscious and unconscious concept that a child forms concerning the roles and characteristics of the personality of the mother and father. See also **imago, primordial image.**

parenting, altered, a nursing diagnosis accepted by the Seventh National Conference on the Classification of Nursing Diagnoses. The diagnosis describes the changes in ability of nurturing figures to create an environment that promotes the optimum growth and development of another human being. The defining characteristics of the condition are multiple and may include constant complaints about the sex or the appearance of the new child, verbal self-assessment of inadequacy in the parental role, expressed disgust about the bodily functions of the child, failure to keep health care appointments for the child, inconsistent disciplinary practices, slow growth and development in the child, and an observed need on the part of the parent to receive approval from others. The critical defining characteristics, at least one of which must be present to make the diagnosis, include an observed lack of actions that demonstrate attachment to the child, inattentiveness to the needs of the child, inappropriate caretaking behavior, especially in toilet training and in sleep and feeding patterns, and a history of abuse or abandonment of the child. See also **nursing diagnosis.**

parenting, altered, high risk for, a nursing diagnosis accepted by the Seventh National Conference on the Classification of Nursing Diagnoses. The diagnosis is defined as the possibility of changes in ability of nurturing figures to create an environment that promotes the optimum growth and development of another human being. The cause of the problem may be complex and may involve several factors. Risk factors include lack of parental attachment behaviors; inappropriate visual, tactile, or auditory stimulation; negative identification or attachment of meanings to infant or child characteristics; verbalization of disappointment in or resentment toward the infant or child; noncompliance with health appointments; inappropriate caretaking behaviors; inappropriate or inconsistent discipline practices; history of child abuse or abandonment by primary caretaker; and multiple caretakers without consideration for the needs of the child. Related factors include lack of an available role model; lack of support; interruption of the process of bonding in the newborn period; unrealistic expectations for the self, the infant, or the partner; mental or physical illness; the presence of financial, legal, or cultural stressors; a lack of knowledge; limited cognitive ability; multiple pregnancies; and a recent crisis. See also **nursing diagnosis.**

Parents Anonymous, a self-help group for parents who have abused their children or who feel that they are prone to maltreat them. The organization offers support and guidance, provides a forum for discussing mutual problems, and furnishes distressed parents with a positive mechanism for coping with anger by talking to another member rather than by releasing their emotions on the child. See also **child abuse.**

Parents Without Partners, a self-help group for single parents, including those who are separated, divorced, or widowed.

parepididymis. See **paradidymis.**

paresis /pərē′sis, per′isis/ [Gk, *paralyein*, to be paralyzed],

1. motor weakness or partial paralysis related in some cases to local neuritis. **2.** also called **dementia paralytica, general paresis, paralytic dementia.** a late manifestation of neurosyphilis, characterized by generalized paralysis, tremulous incoordination, transient seizures, Argyll Robertson pupils, and progressive dementia caused by degeneration of cortical neurons. Paresis resulting from untreated syphilis usually develops in the third to fifth decades but may occur at an early age in patients with congenital syphilis. **—paretic,** *adj.*

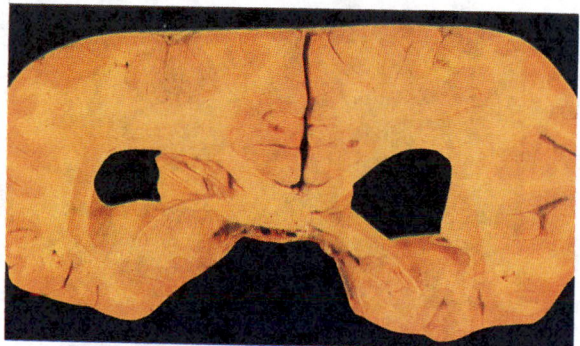

Cortical atrophy caused by paresis resulting from untreated syphylis
(Fletcher, 1987)

-paresis, a combining form meaning 'incomplete or partial paralysis': *hemiparesis.*

paresthesia /per′esthē′zhə/ [Gk, *para* + *erethizein*, to excite], any subjective sensation, experienced as numbness, tingling, or a 'pins and needles' feeling. Paresthesias often fluctuate according to such influences as posture, activity, rest, edema, congestion, or an underlying disease. When experienced in the extremities, it is sometimes identified as acroparesthesia.

paresthetic pain. See **paresthesia.**

paretic /peret′ik/ [Gk, *paresis,* paralysis], pertaining to or resembling partial paralysis.

paretic dementia. See **paresis.**

pareunia. See **coitus.**

pargyline hydrochloride /per′jəlēn/, a monoamine oxidase (MAO) inhibitor used as an antihypertensive.

■ INDICATION: It is prescribed in the treatment of moderate to severe hypertension.

■ CONTRAINDICATIONS: As with all MAO inhibitors, pheochromocytoma, malignant hypertension, hyperthyroidism, renal failure, concomitant use of sympathomimetic drugs, foods high in tyramine, alcoholic beverages, or hypersensitivity to this drug prohibits its use. It is not given to children under 12 years of age.

■ ADVERSE EFFECTS: Among the most serious adverse reactions are hepatotoxicity, orthostatic hypotension, hyperexcitability, constipation, and dry mouth. MAO inhibitors produce many adverse drug interactions.

paries /per′i·ēz/, *pl.* **parietes** /pərī′itēz/, the wall of an organ or cavity in the body.

parietal /pərī′ətəl/ [L, *paries,* wall], **1.** of or pertaining to the outer wall of a cavity or organ. **2.** of or pertaining to the parietal bone of the skull, or the parietal lobe of the brain.

parietal bone,   one of a pair of bones forming the sides of the cranium. Each parietal bone has two surfaces, four borders, and four angles and articulates with five bones: the opposite parietal, occipital, frontal, temporal, and sphenoid.

parietal cells [L, *paries,* wall, *cella,* storeroom],   the cells on the periphery of the gastric glands of the stomach. They are located on the basement membrane beneath the chief cells and secrete hydrochloric acid.

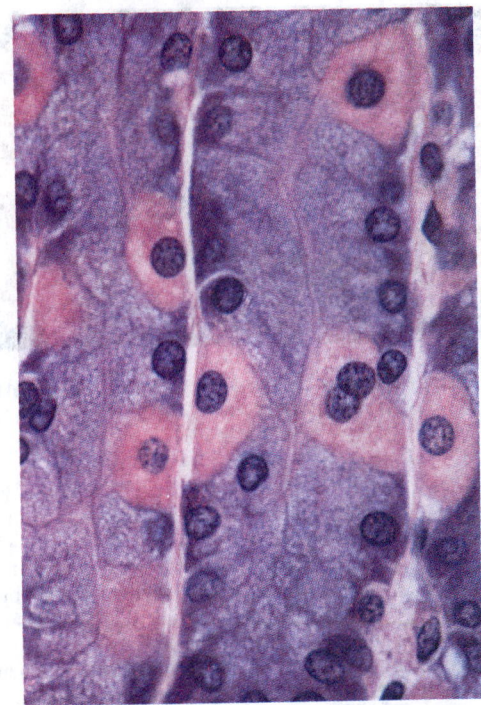

Parietal cells *(Mitros, 1988/Courtesy TH Kent, MD)*

parietal lobe,   a portion of each cerebral hemisphere that occupies the parts of the lateral and the medial surfaces that are covered by the parietal bone. On the lateral surface of the hemisphere the parietal lobe is separated from the frontal lobe by the central sulcus and from the temporal lobe by an imaginary line that extends from the posterior ramus of the lateral sulcus toward the occipital pole. On the parietal lobe the postcentral sulcus runs parallel with the central sulcus, so that the postcentral gyrus lies between them. The intraparietal sulcus extends posteriorly from the middle of the postcentral sulcus toward the occipital pole and joins the transverse occipital sulcus near the occipital pole. The part of the parietal lobe posterior to the postcentral sulcus is divided by the horizontal intraparietal sulcus into the superior and the inferior parietal lobules. On the medial surface of the hemisphere the parietooccipital sulcus separates the parietal and the occipital lobes. Compare **central lobe, frontal lobe, occipital lobe, temporal lobe.**

parietal lymph node,   one of the small oval glands that filter the lymph coursing through the lymphatic vessels in the walls of the thorax or through the lymphatic vessels associated with the larger blood vessels of the abdomen and the pelvis. The parietal lymph nodes of the thorax include the sternal nodes, intercostal nodes, and diaphragmatic nodes. The parietal lymph nodes of the abdomen and pelvis include the common iliac nodes, epigastric nodes, external iliac nodes, iliac circumflex nodes, internal iliac nodes, lumbar nodes, and sacral nodes. See also **lymph, lymphatic system, lymph node.**

parietal pain,   a sharp sensation of distress in the parietal pleura, aggravated by respiration and thoracic movements and caused by pneumonia, empyema, pneumothorax, asbestosis, tuberculosis, neoplasm, or the accumulation of fluid resulting from heart, liver, or kidney disease. Pain arising from the parietal pleura lining the chest wall is perceived over the involved area, but that arising from the central part of the diaphragm is referred to the posterior shoulder area; pain from the costal portions of the diaphragm is referred to the adjacent thoracic wall.

parietal pericardium [L, *paries,* wall; Gk, *peri + kardia,* heart],   an outer layer of the serous pericardium that is not in direct contact with the heart muscle.

parietal peritoneum,   the portion of the largest serous membrane in the body that lines the abdominal wall. Also called **parietal pleura.** Compare **visceral peritoneum.** See also **peritoneal cavity.**

parietal pleura.   See **parietal peritoneum.**

parietooccipital /pərī′ətō·oksip′itəl/ [L, *paries + occiput,* back of the head],   of or pertaining to the parietal and the occipital bones or lobes.

parietooccipital sulcus,   a groove on each cerebral hemisphere marking the division of the parietal and occipital lobes of the brain. Also called **occipitoparietal fissure.**

parietotemporal /-tem′pərəl/ [L, *paries,* wall, *tempus,* temple],   pertaining to the temporal and parietal bones of the cranium. Also **temporoparietal.**

-parin,   a combining form for heparin derivatives.

Parinaud's syndrome /per′ənōz/ [Henri Parinaud, French ophthalmologist, b. 1844],   a term often used to refer to conjunctivitis that is usually unilateral, follicular, and followed by enlargement of the preauricular lymph nodes and tenderness. The syndrome is frequently caused by infection with a species of the microorganism *Leptothrix.* It also may be associated with other infections, such as tularemia, cat-scratch fever, and lymphogranuloma venereum. Also called **Parinaud's oculoglandular syndrome, Parinaud's ophthalmoplegia.**

pari passu /per′ē pas′ōo/ [L, *par,* equal, *passus,* step],   at the same time or in equal proportions.

paritonsillar abscess.   See **parapharyngeal abscess.**

parity /per′itē/ [L, *parere,* to give birth],   **1.** (in obstetrics) the classification of a woman by the number of live-born children and stillbirths she has delivered at more than 28 weeks of gestation. Commonly, parity is noted with the total number of pregnancies and represented by the letter 'P' or the word 'para.' A para 4 (P4) gravida 5 (G5) has had four deliveries after 28 weeks and one abortion or miscarriage before 28 weeks. Currently, a more complete system is in use in which the total number of pregnancies is followed by the number of deliveries at term, the number of premature infants, the number of abortions or miscarriages before 28 weeks' gestation, and the number of children living at present. This system may be written as TPAL. **2.** (in epidemiology) the classification of a woman by the number of live-born children she has delivered. **3.** (in computer processing) the condition of a set of items, either even or odd in number, used as a means for checking errors, such as in the transmission of information between various elements of the same computer.

parkinsonian /pär'kinsō'nē·ən/ [James Parkinson, English physician, b. 1755],   pertaining to or resembling Parkinson's disease.

parkinsonian facies [Parkinson; L, *facies*, face],   a masklike and immobile facial expression, usually occuring with Parkinson's disease. Infrequent blinking also occurs.

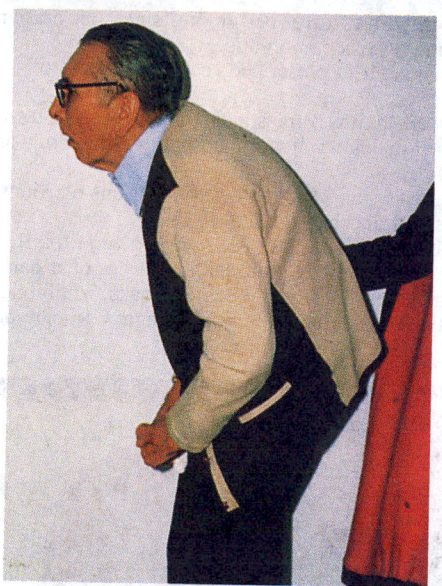

Typical posture of parkinsonism (Kamal, 1991)

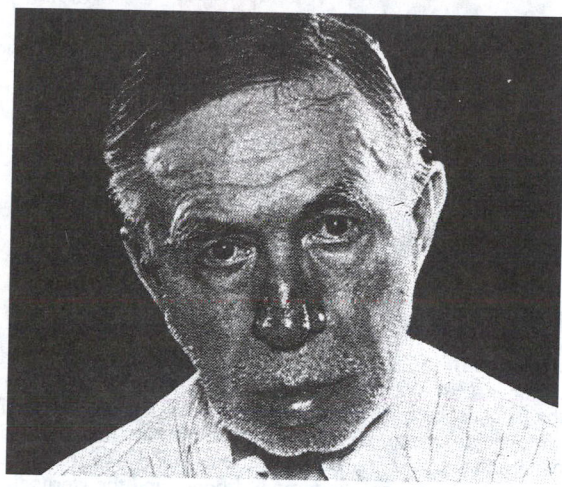

Parkinsonian facies

(Kamal, 1991/Courtesy Churchill Livingstone, Professor MS Pathy)

parkinsonian tremor [Parkinson; L, *tremor*, shaking],   a mild resting tremor with slow, regular oscillations of three to six per second, exacerbated by fatigue, cold, or emotions. The tremors usually, but not always, cease during voluntary movement of the affected part and during sleep.

parkinsonism /pär'kənsəniz'əm/ [James Parkinson],   a neurologic disorder characterized by tremor, muscle rigidity, hypokinesia, a slow shuffling gait, and difficulty in chewing, swallowing, and speaking, caused by various lesions in the extrapyramidal motor system. Signs and symptoms of parkinsonism resemble those of idiopathic Parkinson's disease and may develop during or after acute encephalitis and in syphilis, malaria, poliomyelitis, and carbon monoxide poisoning. Parkinsonism frequently occurs in patients treated with antipsychotic drugs, such as amitriptyline, chlorpromazine, fluphenazine, loxapine, thioridazine, and other phenothiazine derivatives. See also **Parkinson's disease.**

Parkinson's disease [James Parkinson],   a slowly progressive, degenerative, neurologic disorder characterized by resting tremor, pill rolling of the fingers, a masklike facies, shuffling gait, forward flexion of the trunk, loss of postural reflexes, and muscle rigidity and weakness. It is usually an idiopathic disease of people over 60 years of age, although it may occur in younger people, especially after acute encephalitis or carbon monoxide or metallic poisoning, particularly by reserpine or phenothiazine drugs. Typical pathologic changes are destruction of neurons in basal ganglia, loss of pigmented cells in the substantia nigra, and depletion of dopamine in the caudate nucleus, putamen, and pallidum, structures in the neostriatum that normally contain high levels of the neurotransmitter dopamine. Signs and symptoms of Parkinson's disease, which include resting tremor, bradykinesis, drooling, increased appetite, intolerance to heat, oily skin, emotional instability, and defective judgment, are increased by fatigue, excitement, and frustration. Palliative and symptomatic treatment of the disease focuses on correcting the imbalance between depleted dopamine and abundant acetylcholine in the striatum, because dopamine normally appears to inhibit excitatory cholinergic activity in this brain area. Levodopa, a dopamine precursor that crosses the blood-brain barrier, may be used, but many patients experience side effects, such as nausea, vomiting, insomnia, orthostatic hypotension, and mental confusion. Carbidopa-levodopa, which contains an inhibitor of the enzyme dopa decarboxylase, limits peripheral metabolism of levodopa and thus causes fewer side effects. Anticholinergic drugs, such as benztropine mesylate, biperiden, procyclidine, and trihexyphenidyl, may be used as therapeutic agents but often cause ataxia, blurred vision, constipation, dryness of the mouth, mental disturbances, slurred speech, and urinary urgency or retention. Amantadine hydrochloride, an antiviral drug with antiparkinsonian activity, promotes the accumulation of dopamine in extracellular or synaptic sites, but the therapeutic effectiveness may not last more than 3 months in some patients; side effects, such as mental confusion, visual disturbances, and seizures, occur infrequently. Also called **paralysis agitans.**

Parkinson's mask [Parkinson; Fr, *masque*],   an expressionless face with eyebrows raised, smoothing of facial muscles, but immobility of the facial muscles.

Parlodel,   a trademark for a dopamine receptor agonist (bromocriptine).

Parnate,   a trademark for an antidepressant (tranylcypromine sulfate).

paromomycin sulfate /per'əmōmī'sin/, an oral antiamebic aminoglycoside antibiotic.
- INDICATION: It is prescribed in the treatment of intestinal amebiasis.
- CONTRAINDICATIONS: Intestinal inflammation, intestinal obstruction, or known hypersensitivity to this drug prohibits its use.
- ADVERSE EFFECTS: Among the most serious reactions are GI distress and diarrhea.

paronychia /per'ənik'ē·ə/ [Gk, *para + onyx*, nail], an infection of the fold of skin at the margin of a nail. Treatment includes hot compresses or soaks, antibiotics, and, possibly, surgical incision and drainage. Compare **onychia.**

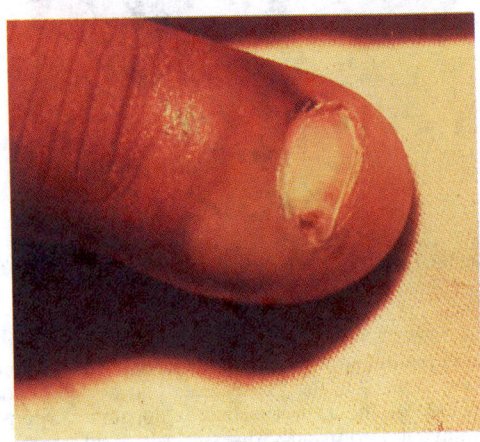

Paronychia
(Zitelli, 1992/Courtesy Dr Bernard Cohen, Children's Hospital of Pittsburgh)

paroophoritis /per'ō·of'ərī'tis/ [Gk, *para + oon*, egg, *pherein*, to bear, *itis*], **1.** inflammation of the paroophoron. **2.** inflammation of the tissues surrounding the ovary.

paroophoron /per'ō·of'əron/ [Gk, *para + oon*, egg, *pherein*, to bear], a small vestigial remnant of the mesonephros, consisting of a few rudimentary tubules lying in the broad ligament between the epoophoron and the uterus. It is most evident in very young girls. A similar vestigial structure, the aberrant ductule, is found in the male. Compare **epoophoron.**

parosmia /pəroz'mē·ə/ [Gk, *para + osme*, smell], any dysfunction or perversion concerning the sense of smell. See also **anosmia, cacosmia.**

parotid /pərot'id/ [Gk, *para + ous*, ear], near the ear.

parotid duct /pərot'id/ [Gk, *para + ous*, ear; L, *ducere*, to lead], a tubular canal, about 7 cm long, that extends from the anterior part of the parotid gland to the mouth. It crosses the masseter after leaving the parotid gland, pierces the buccinator, runs for a short distance obliquely forward between the buccinator and the mucous membrane of the mouth, and opens on the oral surface of the cheek through a small opening opposite the second upper molar tooth. As the parotid duct crosses the masseter, it receives the duct from the accessory portion of the parotid gland. The duct, which has a thick wall, is about 4 mm in diameter over most of its length but narrows considerably at the opening into the mouth. Also called **Stensen's duct.** See also **parotid gland.**

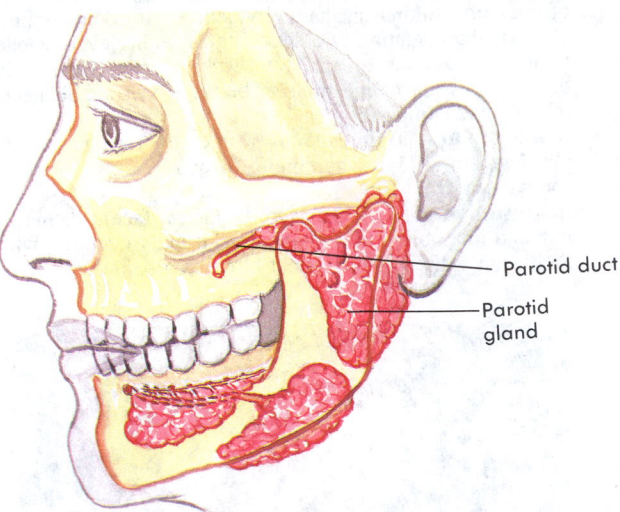

Parotid duct and parotid gland
(Thibodeau, 1993/Ernest W Beck)

parotidectomy /pərot'idek'təmē/ [Gk, *para + ous, ektome*, cutting out], the surgical removal of the parotid gland.

parotid gland [Gk, *para + ous*, ear; L, *glans*, acorn], one of the largest pairs of salivary glands that lie at the side of the face just below and in front of the external ear. The main part of the gland is superficial, somewhat flattened and quadrilateral, and lies between the ramus of the mandible, the mastoid process, the temporal bone, and the sternocleidomastoideus. It is wide superiorly and reaches nearly to the zygomatic arch, inferiorly tapering near the angle of the mandible. The rest of the gland is wedge-shaped and extends deeply toward the pharyngeal wall. It is enclosed in a capsule continuous with the deep cervical fascia. The parotid duct starts at the anterior part of the gland and opens on the inside of the cheek opposite the second upper molar. Compare **sublingual gland, submandibular gland.** See also **salivary gland.**

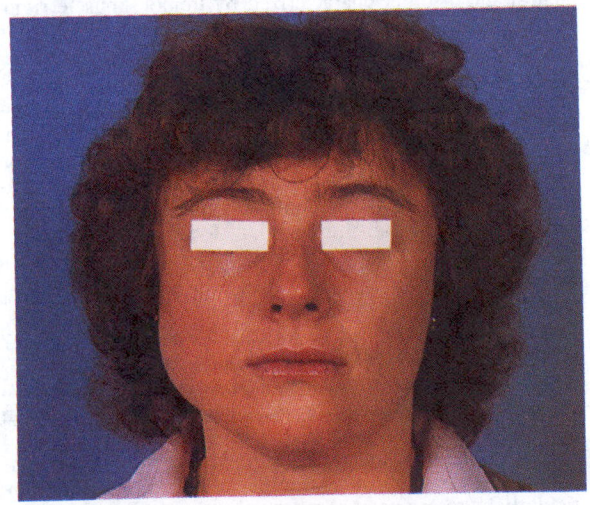

Acute parotitis *(Lamey, 1988)*

parotitis /per'ətī'tis/ [Gk, *para* + *ous*, ear, *itis*, inflammation], inflammation or infection of one or both parotid salivary glands. See also **mumps.**

parous /per'əs/, having borne 1 or more viable offspring.

-parous, a suffix meaning 'pertaining to the quantity of offspring produced simultaneously or to the method of gestation': *quadriparous, uniparous, viviparous.*

parovarian /per'ōver'ē·ən/ [Gk, *para* + L, *ovum*, egg], pertaining to residual tissues in the area near the fallopian tubes and the ovary.

parovarium. See **epoophoron.**

paroxysm /per'əksiz'əm/ [Gk, *paroxynein*, to stimulate], **1.** a marked, usually episodic increase in symptoms. **2.** a convulsion, fit, seizure, or spasm. –**paroxysmal,** *adj.*

paroxysmal atrial tachycardia [Gk, *paroxynein*, to stimulate], a period of vary rapid heart beats that begins and ends abruptly.

paroxysmal cold hemoglobinuria (PCH), a rare autoimmune disorder characterized by hemolysis and hematuria, associated with exposure to cold.

paroxysmal cough [Gk, *paroxysmos*, irritation; AS, *cohhetan*, cough], a severe attack of coughing, as may accompany whooping cough, bronchiectasis, or a lung injury.

paroxysmal hemoglobinuria, the sudden passage of hemoglobin in urine, occurring after local or general exposure to low temperatures, as in paroxysmal cold hemoglobinuria. See also **Marchiafava-Micheli disease.**

paroxysmal labyrinthine vertigo. See **Ménière's disease.**

paroxysmal nocturnal dyspnea (PND), a disorder characterized by sudden attacks of respiratory distress, usually occurring after several hours of sleep in a reclining position, most commonly caused by pulmonary edema resulting from congestive heart failure. The attacks are often accompanied by coughing, a feeling of suffocation, cold sweat, and tachycardia with a gallop rhythm. Sleeping with the head propped up on pillows may prevent dyspneic paroxysms at night, but treatment of the underlying cause is required to prevent fluid from accumulating in the lungs.

paroxysmal nocturnal hemoglobinuria (PNH), a disorder characterized by intravascular hemolysis and hemoglobinuria. It occurs in irregular episodes of several days' duration, especially at night. The basic defect in the red blood cell is an unusual sensitivity to lysis by complement or a deficiency or absence of acetylcholinesterase. The cause of the condition is unknown, but it is seen in association with abnormalities of the function of the bone marrow. Occurring predominantly in adults between 25 and 45 years of age, it is characterized by abdominal pain, back pain, and headache. Its course may be complicated by thrombotic episodes and by iron deficiency caused by excessive loss of hemoglobin. Therapy includes blood transfusion and the oral or parenteral administration of iron. Corticosteroids are sometimes employed and found useful; treatment of thromboses may require anticoagulant therapy.

paroxysmal nodal tachycardia [Gk, *paroxysmos*, irritation; L, *nodus*, knot; Gk, *tachys*, fast; *kardia*, heart], a sudden onset and termination of a rapid heart beat caused by a quick succession of discharges from an ectopic site in the area of the atrioventricular node.

paroxysmal supraventricular tachycardia, an ectopic rhythm in excess of 100 per minute and usually faster than 170 per minute that begins abruptly with a premature atrial or junctional beat and is supported by an AV nodal reentry mechanism or by an AV reentry mechanism involving an accessory pathway. Formerly called **paroxysmal atrial tachycardia** (PAT) or paroxysmal junctional tachycardia (PJT).

paroxysmal ventricular tachycardia [Gk, *paroxysmos,* irritation; L, *ventriculum,* small cavity; Gk, *tachys* + *kardia*], a sudden onset and termination of rapid heart beat caused by a quick succession of discharges from an ectopic site in the ventricle.

parrot fever. See **psittacosis.**

parry fracture. See **Monteggia's fracture.**

pars /pärs/ [L, part], a part, such as the pars abdominalis esophagi. See also **part.**

pars fetalis. See **fetal placenta.**

Parsidol, a trademark for an antiparkinsonian (ethopropazine hydrochloride).

Parsonage-Turner syndrome. See **neuralgic amytrophy.**

part [L, *pars*], a portion of a larger area, such as the condylar part of the occipital bone. See also **pars.**

part-, a combining form meaning 'of or related to childbirth': *parturient, parturifacient, parturiometer.*

part. aeq. abbreviation for the Latin phrase *partes aequales,* meaning 'in equal parts.'

parthenogenesis /pär'thənōjen'əsis/ [Gk, *parthenos*, virgin, *genesis*, origin], a type of nonsexual reproduction in which an organism develops from an unfertilized ovum, as in many lower animals. Initiation of the development of the unfertilized ovum may be artificially induced through mechanical or chemical stimulation. –**parthenogenetic, parthenogenic,** *adj.*

partial breech extraction. See **assisted breech.**

partial cleavage /pär'shəl/, mitotic division of only part of a fertilized ovum into blastomeres, usually the activated cytoplasmic portion surrounding the nucleus; restricted division. Compare **total cleavage.** See also **meroblastic.**

partial crown, a restoration that replaces surfaces of a tooth.

partial denture [L, *pars*, a part; *dens*, tooth], a dental prosthesis either fixed or removable used to replace one or more missing teeth. Kinds of partial dentures include **articulated, bridge, extension, fixed, fixed cantilever, removable, sectional,** and **unilateral.**

partial dislocation [L, *pars; dis* + *locare,* to place], the partial abnormal separation of the articular surface of a joint. Also called **incomplete dislocation; subluxation.**

partial hospitalization program, an organizational entity that provides therapeutic services to patients who use only day or night hospital services or adult day health services, rather than regular inpatient hospitalization services.

partial involution. See **uterine subinvolution.**

partially edentulous arch, a dental arch in which one or more but not all natural teeth are missing.

partial placenta previa, placenta previa in which the placenta is implanted in the lower uterine segment and partially covers the internal os of the uterine cervix. As the cervix dilates in labor, the portion of the placenta that lies over the cervix is separated, causing bleeding from the villous spaces of the uterine wall. Depending on the degree of separation, the bleeding may be scant or severe, resulting in hemorrhage that is life threatening to the mother and the baby. Treatment may require cesarean section if the pressure of the presenting part of the baby is not sufficient to tamponade the bleeding site, stopping the hemorrhage. Diagnosis of partial placenta previa may be made before bleeding occurs by ultrasonic visualization or digital palpation in the course of prenatal examination. See also **placenta previa.**

partial pressure, the pressure exerted by any one gas in a mixture of gases or in a liquid, with the pressure directly related to the concentration of that gas to the total pressure of the mixture. The concentration of oxygen in the atmosphere represents approximately 21% of the total atmospheric pressure, calculated at 760 mm Hg under standard conditions. Therefore, the partial pressure of atmospheric oxygen is about 160 mm Hg (760 × 0.21).

partial pressure of arterial oxygen (Pao₂), the part of total blood gas pressure exerted by oxygen gas. It is lower than normal in patients with asthma, obstructive lung disease, or certain blood diseases, and in healthy individuals during vigorous exercise. The normal partial pressure of oxygen in arterial blood is 95 to 100 mm Hg.

partial pressure of carbon dioxide, the portion of total blood gas pressure exerted by carbon dioxide. It decreases during heavy exercise, during rapid breathing, or in association with severe diarrhea, uncontrolled diabetes, or diseases of the liver or kidneys. It increases in people with chest injuries or respiratory disorders. The normal pressures of carbon dioxide in arterial blood are 35 to 45 mm Hg, and in venous blood, 40 to 45 mm Hg.

partial response, the condition in which the maximum decrease in treated tumor volume is at least 50% but less than 100%.

partial thromboplastin time (PTT), a test for detecting coagulation defects of the intrinsic system by adding activated partial thromboplastin to a sample of test plasma and to a control sample of normal plasma. The time required for the formation of a clot in test plasma is compared with that in the normal plasma. A delayed clotting time suggests an abnormality in one or more factors of the intrinsic system. If indicated, specific factor abnormalities can be identified by exposing the test plasma to a series of plasma samples with known factor deficiencies and observing for coagulation, which occurs only if the test plasma provides the missing clotting factors. Partial thromboplastin time is one of the basic tests used to measure specific factor activity and to detect hemophilias. It can also be used to monitor the activity of the anticoagulant, heparin. The normal PTT in plasma is 60 to 85 seconds after the addition to the plasma sample of partial thromboplastin reagent and ionized calcium. Compare **prothrombin time.** See also **hemostasis.**

particulate /pärtik′yəlit/, pertaining to a minute discrete particle or fragment of a substance or material.

-partite, a combining form meaning 'having the (specified) number of parts': *bipartite, tripartite, quadripartite.*

parts per million (PPM, ppm), the ratio of the concentration of one substance to the concentration of another, as a unit of solute dissolved in one million units of solvent. It may be further expressed in terms of weight-to-weight, volume-to-volume, or another relationship of units of measure.

parturient /pärt(y)ŏŏ′rē·ənt/ [L, *parturire,* to have labor pains], pertaining to the act of childbirth.

parturition /pär′t(y)ŏŏrish′ən/ [L, *parturire,* to desire to bring forth], the process of giving birth.

parulis. See **gumboil.**

PAS, PASA, abbreviation for **paraaminosalicylic acid.**

PASCAL /poskul′, paskal′/ [Blaise Pascal, French scientist,

b. 1623], a higher level computer compiler language, often used to teach programing.

Pascal's principle /poskuls′, paskals′/ [Blaise Pascal], (in physics) a law stating that a confined liquid transmits pressure applied to it from an external source equally in all directions. Pascal's principle provides the basis for all hydraulic devices.

passive [L *passivus*], pertaining to behavior that subordinates the individual's own interests to the demands of others.

passive-aggressive personality [L, *passivus + aggressus,* combative; *persona,* character], a personality characterized by passivity and aggression in which forceful actions or attitudes are expressed in an indirect, nonviolent manner, such as pouting, obstructionism, procrastination, inefficiency, stubbornness, and forgetfulness. Compare **aggressive personality, passive-dependent personality.** See also **passive-aggressive personality disorder.**

passive-aggressive personality disorder, a disorder characterized by the indirect expression of resistance to occupational or social demands, resulting in persistent, pervasive ineffectiveness, lack of self-confidence, poor interpersonal relationships, and pessimism that can lead, in severe cases, to major depression, alcoholism, or drug dependence. The behavior often reflects an unexpressed hostility or resentment stemming from a frustrating interpersonal or institutional relationship on which an individual is overdependent. Treatment may consist of behavior therapy or any of the various psychotherapeutic procedures, depending on the individual and the severity of the condition.

passive algolagnia. See **masochism.**

passive anaphylaxis. See **antiserum anaphylaxis.**

passive carrier [L, *passivus*; OFr, *carier*], **1.** a healthy person whose body carries the causal organisms of an infectious disease although the person has not contracted the disease and remains symptomless. **2.** a person who carries a gene associated with a hereditary trait although the trait is not expressed in the person. Also called **symptomless carrier.**

passive congestion [L, *passivus, congerere,* to heap together], an excessive amount of blood accumulation in an organ resulting from increased venous pressure.

passive-dependent personality [L, *passivus + Fr, dependre,* to depend; L, *persona,* character], a personality characterized by helplessness, indecisiveness, and a tendency to cling to and seek support from others. Compare **aggressive personality, passive-aggressive personality.**

passive euthanasia. See **euthanasia.**

passive exercise, repetitive movement of a part of the body as a result of an externally applied force or the voluntary effort of the muscles controlling another part of the body. Compare **active exercise.** See also **aerobic exercise, anaerobic exercise.**

passive expiration [L, *passivus, expirare,* to breathe out], normal expiration that occurs without direct muscular effort, as is the case in normal tidal breathing. The air is compressed from the lungs through recoil effect of elastic tissues of the chest and lungs.

passive immunity, a form of acquired immunity resulting from antibodies that are transmitted naturally through the placenta to a fetus or through the colostrum to an infant or artificially by injection of antiserum for treatment or prophylaxis. Passive immunity is not permanent and does not last as long as active immunity. See also **immune response.**

passive incontinence [L, *passivus, incomtinentia*], urine overflow that may occur when the bladder (musculus detrusor vesicae) is paralyzed and greatly distended.

passive lingual arch, an orthodontic appliance that may help maintain tooth space and dental arch length when bilateral primary molars are prematurely lost.

passive lung collapse [L, *passivus*; AS, *lungen*; L, *collabi*], a condition of dyspnea, cough, and hemoptysis with pigmented cells caused by an obstruction in blood flow from the lungs to the heart.

passive motion [L, *passivus, motio*], involuntary motion caused by an external force, differentiated from active, voluntary muscular effort.

passive movement, the moving of parts of the body by an outside force without voluntary action or resistance by the individual. Compare **active movement.**

passive play, play in which a person does not participate actively. For younger children such activity may include watching and listening to others, observing other children or animals, listening to stories, or looking at pictures. Older children are passively entertained by games and toys that require concentration and intellectual skill, such as chess, reading, listening to music, or watching television. Compare **active play.**

passive recoil, the normal, quiet act of exhalation caused by the rebound effect of elastic tissue of the lungs, aided by the force of surface tension.

passive sensitization [L, *passivus, sentire*, to feel], a temporary form of sensitization induced by injecting serum from a sensitized human or animal. See also **passive immunity.**

passive smoking, the inhalation by nonsmokers of the smoke from other people's cigarettes, pipes, and cigars. The amount of such ambient smoke inhaled by a nonsmoker is small compared with that inhaled by tobacco users, but research provides increasing evidence that passive smoking can aggravate respiratory illnesses and contribute to more serious illnesses, such as cancer, and can injure the health of nonsmoking spouses and of infants and unborn babies. Studies also show that individuals with chronic heart and lung diseases and allergies to tobacco can be adversely affected by passive smoking.

passive stretching, stretching that involves only noncontractile elements, such as ligaments, fascia, bursae, dura mater, and nerve roots. Examples include manipulation of a muscle, such as during therapeutic massage or during isometric exercises in which there is no range of motion of the body part involved.

passive symptom [L, *passivus*; Gk, *symptoma*, that which happens], a symptom that attracts little or no attention. Also called **static symptom.**

passive transfer test. See **Prausnitz-Küstner test.**

passive transport, the movement of small molecules across the membrane of a cell by diffusion. Passive transport occurs when the chemicals outside a cell become concentrated and start moving into the cell, changing the intracellular equilibrium. Passive transport is essential to various processes of metabolism, such as the intake of digestive products by the cells lining the intestines. Compare **active transport, osmosis.**

passive tremor, an involuntary trembling occurring when the person is at rest, one of the signs of Parkinson's disease. Also called **resting tremor.**

passivity /pəsif′itē/ [L, *passivus*], a mental state of being submissive, dependent, or inactive, as a form of maladaptation.

paste /pāst/, a topical semisolid formulation containing a pharmacologically active ingredient in a fatty base, a viscous or mucilaginous base, or a mixture of starch and petrolatum.

Pasteur effect /pasto͞or′, pästœr′/ [Louis Pasteur], the inhibiting effect of oxygen on carbohydrate fermentation by living cells.

Pasteurella /pas′tərel′ə/ [Louis Pasteur, French bacteriologist, b. 1822], a genus of gram-negative bacilli or coccobacilli, including species pathogenic to humans and domestic animals. *Pasteurella* infections may be transmitted to humans by animal bites. The plague bacillus, *Pasteurella pestis*, is now called *Yersinia pestis*; *P. tularensis*, which causes tularemia, has been reclassified as *Francisella tularensis*.

pasteurization /pas′tərīzā′shən/ [Louis Pasteur; Gk, *izein*, to cause], the process of applying heat, usually to milk or cheese, for a specified period of time for the purpose of killing or retarding the development of pathogenic bacteria. **–pasteurize,** *v.*

pasteurized milk /pas′tərīzd/ [Louis Pasteur; Gk, *izein*, to cause; AS, *moluc*, milk], milk that has been treated by heat to destroy pathogenic bacteria. By law, pasteurization requires a temperature of 145° to 150° F for not less than 30 minutes, followed by a temperature of 161° F for 15 seconds, followed by immediate cooling.

Pasteur, Louis (1822-1895), a French chemist who founded the 'germ theory' of infection and developed the 'pasteurization' process to kill pathogenic organisms in milk. Pasteur also developed several vaccines and pioneered in the development of stereochemistry by separating mirror image isomers.

Pasteur treatment [Louis Pasteur], a method of preventing rabies by daily injections of attenuated cultures of rabies virus cultured in the central nervous system tissues of rabbits. The treatment, developed by Pasteur, is no longer used. See **human diploid cell vaccine.**

past health [ME, *passen*, to pass; AS, *hoelth*, sound body], (in a health history) an overall summary of the person's general health to date, including past injuries, allergies, surgical procedures, immunizations, hospitalizations, and obstetric and psychiatric history. The past health history is obtained from the person or the person's family at the initial interview and becomes part of the permanent record.

pastoral counseling department /pas′tərəl/ [L, *pastor*, shepherd], the hospital chaplaincy service.

past pointing [OFr, *passer*; L, *punctus*, pricked], the inability to place a finger on another part of the body accurately, indicating a lack of coordination in voluntary movements.

Patau's syndrome. See **trisomy 13.**

patch [ME *pacche*], a small spot of surface tissue that differs from the surrounding area in color or texture or both and is not elevated above it.

patch test, a skin test for identifying allergens, especially those causing contact dermatitis. The suspected substance (food, pollen, animal fur) is applied to an adhesive patch that is placed on the patient's skin. Another patch, with nothing on it, serves as a control. After a certain period of time (usually 24 to 48 hours), both patches are removed. If the skin under the suspect patch is red and swollen and the control area is not, the test is said to be positive, and the

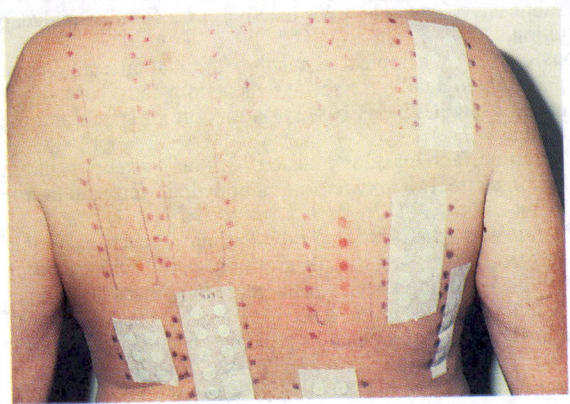

Patch testing (Holgate, 1993)

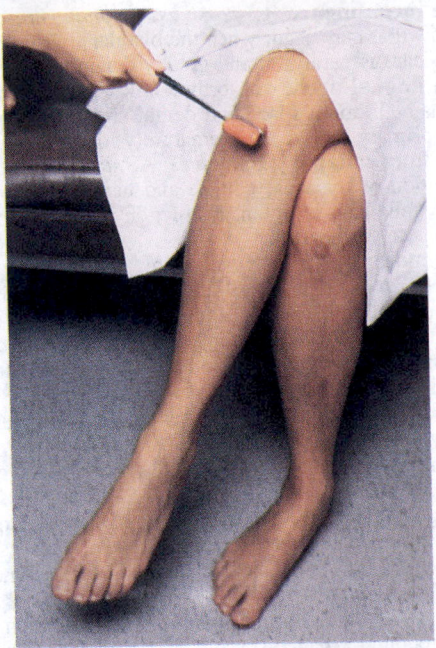

Elicitation of the patellar reflex (Belcher, 1992)

person is probably allergic to that substance. Compare **Prausnitz-Küstner test, radioallergosorbent test.**

patella /pətel'ə/ [L, small dish], a flat, triangular bone at the front of the knee joint, having a pointed apex that attaches to the ligamentum patellae. The convex, anterior surface of the bone is perforated for the passage of nutrient vessels and covered by an expansion from the tendon of the quadriceps femoris. Also called **knee cap.**

patellar /pətel'ər/ [L, *patella*, small disk], pertaining to the patella.

patellar bursa [L, *patella*, small disc; Gk, *byrsa*, wineskin], any of fluid-filled connective tissue sacs around the knee cap. Kinds of patellar bursae include: **infrapatellar, prepatellar,** and **suprapatella.**

patellar ligament [L, *patella + ligare*, to bind], the central portion of the common tendon of the quadriceps femoris. The ligament is a strong, flat, ligamentous band, about 8 cm long, attached proximally to the apex and the adjoining margins of the patella and distally to the tuberosity of the tibia. Its superficial fibers are continuous over the front of the patella with those of the tendon of the quadriceps femoris.

patellar reflex, a deep tendon reflex, elicited by a sharp tap on the tendon just distal to the patella, normally characterized by contraction of the quadriceps muscle and extension of the leg at the knee. The reflex is hyperactive in disease of the pyramidal tract above the level of the second lumbar vertebra. Also called **knee jerk reflex, quadriceps reflex.** See also **deep tendon reflex.**

patellar-tendon bearing prosthesis (PTB), an ankle-foot orthosis (AFO) that provides prolonged stretch to the posterior leg musculature and may create extension force at the knee joint.

patellar-tendon bearing supracondylar socket (PTB/ SC), a patellar-tendon bearing prosthesis with supracondylar (above a condyle) and suprapatellar (above the patella) suspension.

patellar-bearing supracondylar/suprapatellar socket (PTBSC/SP), a type of patellar-tendon below-the-knee (BK) bearing prosthesis with a socket that extends in front, medially, and laterally to accommodate both the patella and femoral condyles. The higher socket increases knee stability, and a suspension strap is not required.

patellectomy /pat'ələk'təmē/ [L, *patella*, small disc; Gk, *ektome*, cutting out], the surgical removal of the patella.

patency /pā'tənsē/ [L, *patens*, open], a state of being open or exposed.

patent /pā'tənt/ [L, *patens*, open], open and unblocked, such as a patent airway or a patent anus.

patent ductus arteriosus (PDA), an abnormal opening between the pulmonary artery and the aorta caused by fail-

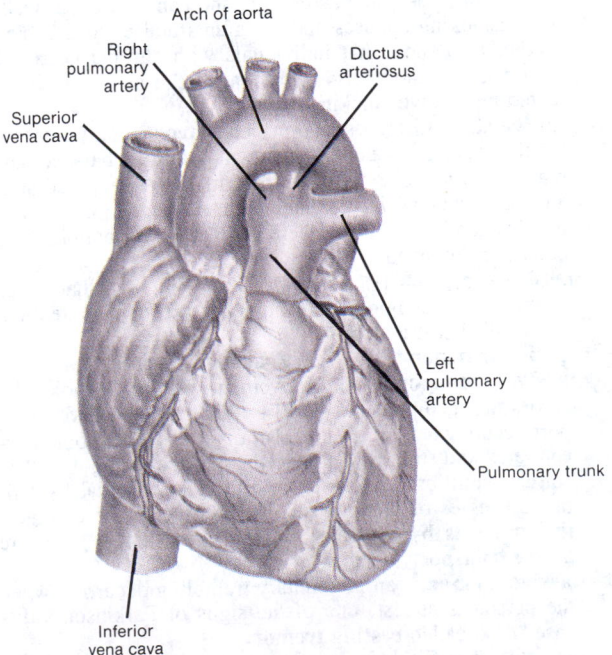

Patent ductus arteriosus (Canobbio, 1990)

Arch of aorta

Right pulmonary artery

Ductus arteriosus

Superior vena cava

Left pulmonary artery

Pulmonary trunk

Inferior vena cava

ure of the fetal ductus arteriosus to close after birth. The defect, which is seen primarily in premature infants, allows blood from the aorta to flow into the pulmonary artery and to recirculate through the lungs, where it is reoxygenated and returned to the left atrium and left ventricle, causing an increased workload on the left side of the heart and increased pulmonary vascular congestion and resistance. Clinical manifestations include cardiomegaly, especially of the left atrium and left ventricle, dilated ascending aorta, bounding pulses from increased systolic pressure, tachycardia, and a typical machinery-like murmur that is heard during all of systole and most of diastole. Characteristic auscultatory and radiologic findings are sufficient to confirm diagnosis so that cardiac catheterization is not necessary. Correction is delayed until the child is old enough to tolerate surgery and to allow time for spontaneous closure. Untreated complications include congestive heart failure, pulmonary vascular disease, calcification of the ductal site, and infective endocarditis. See also **congenital cardiac anomaly.**

patent medicine [L, *patens*, open, *medicina*], a nonprescription drug available to the general public without a prescription. The ingredients and contraindications are usually listed on the label or wrapper. Also called **OTC drug, proprietary drug.**

paternal /pətur′nəl/ [L, *pater*, father], pertaining to fatherhood, characteristic of a father, or related through a father.

paternal engrossment. See **bonding.**

paternity test /pətur′nitē/ [L, *pater, testum*, crucible], a test based on genetic blood groups and used mainly to exclude the possibility that a particular man could be the father of a specific child. For example, a man with group-AB blood could not be the father of a child with group-O blood, or vice versa.

Paterson-Kelly syndrome [Donald R. Paterson, Welsh physician, b. 1863; Adam B. Kelly, Scottish physician, b. 1865], a condition of the digestive system associated with iron deficiency anemia, characterized by the development of esophageal webs in the upper esophagus, making swallowing of solids difficult. The webs are easily ruptured during esophagoscopy and tube feeding and can produce hemorrhage. When the hemoglobin count is improved, the webs disappear. Also called **Plummer-Vinson syndrome.**

Paterson-Parker dosage system [James R. K. Paterson, English radiologist; H. M. Parker, twentieth century American-English physicist], a radiotherapy system that uses sources of specific relative loadings arranged according to defined rules, which lead to a homogenous dose in the implanted region.

path., **1.** abbreviation for **pathologic. 2.** abbreviation for **pathology.**

path-. See **patho-.**

-path, -pathic, -pathy, suffix meaning 'pertaining to disease or suffering': *cardiopath, naturopathic, osteopathy.*

-pathetic, -pathetical, a combining form meaning 'pertaining to emotions': *antipathetic, apopathetic, sympathetic.*

-pathic, See **-path.**

Pathilon, a trademark for an anticholinergic (tridihexethyl chloride).

patho- /path′ō-/, **path-,** a prefix meaning 'of or related to disease': *pathocrinia, pathoformic, pathography.*

pathodontia. See **dental pathology.**

pathogen /path′əjən/ [Gk, *pathos*, disease, *genein*, to produce], any microorganism capable of producing disease. –**pathogenic,** *adj.*

Modes of transmission of some common pathogens

Pathogen	*Common reservoir*
Gram-positive cocci	
Staphylococcus aureus	Contaminated objects, hands, and nasal tracts of health care workers, air, self
Group A *Streptococcus* organisms	Direct contact, air, hands, rarely objects
Enterococcus organisms	Self, hands of health care workers, environmental surfaces
Gram-negative rods	
Escherichia, Klebsiella, Enterobacter	Self, hands of health care workers, contaminated solutions
Proteus, Salmonella, Providencia, Serratia, Citrobacter	Contaminated food and water, hands of health care workers, self
Pseudomonas	Contaminated environment, hands, self
Anaerobic bacteria	
Clostridium, Bacteroides	Self, contaminated environment, hands
Fungal organisms	
Yeasts	Self, hands of health care workers
Fungi	Air, contaminated environment
Viruses	
Varicella	Air, direct contact
Herpes	Self, direct contact, air
Rubella	Direct contact, air
Hepatitis B	Contaminated instruments or injectables, direct contact

From Phipps WJ, Long BL, Woods NF, Cassmeyer VL: *Medical-surgical nursing: concepts and clinical practice,* ed 4, St Louis, 1991, Mosby.

pathogenesis /-jen′əsis/ [Gk, *pathos* + *genesis*, origin], the source or cause of an illness or abnormal condition.

pathogenic /-jen′ik/ [Gk, *pathos*, disease + *genein*, to produce], capable of causing or producing a disease. Also **pathogenetic.**

pathogenicity /-jənis′itē/, the ability of a pathogenic agent to produce a disease.

pathogenic occlusion, an abnormal closure of the teeth, capable of producing pathologic changes in the teeth, supporting tissues, and other components of the stomatognathic system.

pathognomonic /pəthog′nəmon′ik/ [Gk, *pathos* + *gnomon*, index], (of a sign or symptom) specific to a disease or condition, such as Koplik's spots on the buccal and lingual mucosa, which are indicative of measles.

pathognomonic symptom. See **symptom.**

pathologic (path.) /-loj′ik/ [Gk, *pathos* + *logos*, science], pertaining to a condition that is caused by or involves a disease process.

pathologic absorption, the taking up by the blood of an excretory or morbid substance.

pathologic amenorrhea [Gk, *pathos*, disease, *logos*, science, *a, men*, month, *rhoia*, to flow], a stoppage or absence of menstrual discharge from the uterus resulting from a disease.

pathologic anatomy, (in applied anatomy) the study of

the structure and morphology of the tissues and cells of the body as related to disease.

pathologic diagnosis, a diagnosis arrived at by an examination of the substance and function of the tissues of the body, especially of the abnormal developmental changes in the tissues by histologic techniques of tissue examination.

pathologic fracture. See **neoplastic fracture.**

pathologic histology [Gk, *pathos*, disease; *logos*, science; *histos*, tissue; *logos*, science], the specialized study of the effects of disease on minute structures, composition, and function of tissues.

pathologic microorganisms [Gk, *pathos*, disease + *logos*, science, *mikros*, small + *organon*, instrument, *ismos*, condition], any microscopic life form, from a virus to a nematode, that has the potential to cause disease.

pathologic mitosis, any cell division that is atypical, asymmetrical, or multipolar and results in the unequal number of chromosomes in the nuclei of the daughter cells. It is indicative of malignancy, as occurs in cancer and the genetic anomalies.

pathologic myopia, a type of progressive nearsightedness characterized by changes in the fundus of the eye, posterior staphyloma, and deficient corrected acuity.

pathologic physiology, **1.** the study of the physical and chemical processes involved in the functioning of diseased tissues. **2.** the study of the modification of the normal functioning processes of an organism caused by disease. Also called **morbid physiology.** See also **pathophysiology.**

pathologic reflex [Gk, *pathos*, disease + *logos*, science; L, *reflectere*, to bend back], any abnormal reflex that is caused by a lesion in or an organic disease of the nervous system.

pathologic retraction ring, a ridge that may form around the uterus at the junction of the upper and lower uterine segments during the prolonged second stage of an obstructed labor. The lower segment is abnormally distended and thin, and the upper segment is abnormally thick. The ring, which may be seen and felt abdominally, is a warning of impending uterine rupture. Also called **Bandl's ring.** Compare **physiologic retraction ring, constriction ring.**

pathologic sleep [Gk, *pathos*, disease + *logos*, science; AS, *slaep*], excessive sleep associated with a neurologic disorder such as encephalitis lethargica, or sleeping sickness.

pathologic triad, the combination of three respiratory disease conditions: bronchospasm, retained secretions, and mucosal edema. It is treated with bronchodilators, hydration and mucolytics, and decongestants.

pathologist /pəthol′əjist/, a physician who specializes in the study of disease, usually in a hospital, school of medicine, or research institute or laboratory. A pathologist usually specializes in autopsy or in clinical or surgical pathology.

pathology (path.) /pəthol′əjē/ [Gk, *pathos*, disease, *logos*, science], the study of the characteristics, causes, and effects of disease, as observed in the structure and function of the body. **Cellular pathology** is the study of cellular changes in disease. **Clinical pathology** is the study of disease by the use of laboratory tests and methods. **—pathologic,** *adj.*

pathomimicry. See **Munchausen's syndrome.**

pathophysiology /-fiz′ē·ol′əjē/ [Gk, *pathos*, disease, *physis*, nature, *logos*, science], the study of the biologic and physical manifestations of disease as they correlate with the underlying abnormalities and physiologic disturbances.

Pathophysiology does not deal directly with the treatment of disease; rather, it explains the processes within the body that result in the signs and symptoms of a disease. **—pathophysiologic,** *adj.*

pathosis, a disease condition.

pathway [AS, *paeth*, *weg*], **1.** a network of neurons that provides a transmission route for nerve impulses from any part of the body to the spinal cord and the cerebral cortex or from the central nervous system to the muscles and organs. Neural pathways in the body are the somatic sensory pathways and the somatic motor pathways. **2.** a chain of chemical reactions that produces various compounds in critical sequence, such as the Embden-Meyerhof pathway.

-pathy. See **-path.**

patient (pt.) /pā′shənt/ [L *pati* to suffer], **1.** a recipient of a health care service. **2.** a health care recipient who is ill or hospitalized. **3.** a client in a health care service.

patient advocate. See **ombudsman.**

patient care committee, a hospital staff organization, composed of medical, nursing, and other health professionals, with the assigned responsibility of monitoring all patient care practices to ensure that predetermined standards are met.

patient compensation fund, a fund usually established by state law and commonly financed by a surcharge on malpractice premiums and used to pay malpractice claims.

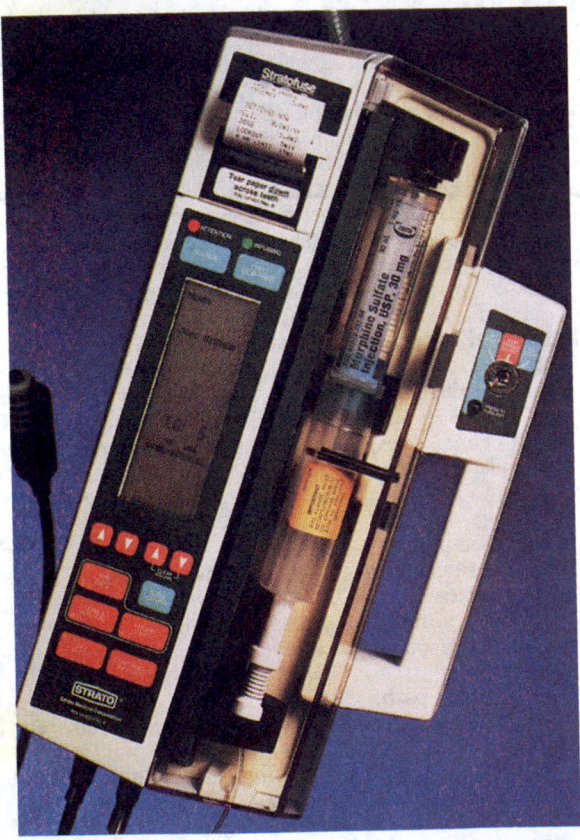

Patient-controlled analgesic device (Potter, 1993)

patient-controlled analgesia (PCA), a drug-delivery system that dispenses a preset IV dose of a narcotic analgesic into a patient when the patient pushes a switch on an electric cord. The device consists of a computerized pump with a chamber containing a syringe holding up to 60 ml of drug. The patient administers a dose of narcotic when the need for pain relief arises. A lockout interval device automatically inactivates the system if a patient tries to increase the amount of narcotic within a preset time period.

patient day (P.D.), a unit in a system of accounting used by health care facilities and health care planners. Each day represents a unit of time during which the services of the institution or facility were used by a patient; thus 50 patients in a hospital for 1 day would represent 50 patient days.

patient dumping, the premature discharge of Medicare or indigent patients from hospitals for economic reasons. A 1986 federal rule requires hospitals to advise Medicare patients on admission for treatment of their right to challenge what they consider as premature discharge after treatment. The regulation was adopted after initiation of a Medicare policy of paying hospitals according to a particular illness, regardless of the length of hospitalization, as an incentive for hospitals to reduce the period of inpatient care.

patient interview, a systematic interview of a patient, the purpose of which is to obtain information that can be used to develop an individualized plan for care. Also called **client interview.**

patient mix, **1.** the distribution of demographic variables in a patient population, often represented by the percentage of a given race, age, sex, or ethnic derivation. **2.** the distribution of indications for admission in a patient population, such as surgical, maternity, or trauma.

patient plan of care, a plan of care coordinated to include appropriate participation by each member of the health care team.

patient record, a collection of documents that provides a record of each episode in which a patient visited or sought treatment and received care or a referral for care from a health care facility. The record is confidential and is usually held by the facility, and the information in it is released only to the patient or with the patient's written permission. It contains the initial assessment of the patient's health status, the health history, laboratory reports of tests performed, notes by nurses and physicians regarding the daily condition of the patient and notes by consultants, as well as order sheets, medication sheets, admission records, discharge summaries, and other pertinent data. A problem-oriented medical record also contains a master problem list. The patient record is often a collection of papers held in a folder, but records may be computerized, making the record available on video display terminals or printouts.

patient representative. See **ombudsman.**

patient representative services, hospital services provided by designated staff members relating to the investigation and mediation of patients' complaints and the promotion and protection of patients' rights. See also **ombudsman.**

Patient's Bill of Rights, a list of the patient's rights promulgated by the American Hospital Association. It offers some guidance and protection to patients by stating the responsibilities that a hospital and its staff have toward patients and their families during hospitalization, but it is not a legally binding document. (See Table p. 1176.)

patterning /pat'ərning/ [ME *patron*], the method of treat-

ment or act of establishing a system or pattern of stimuli that will evoke a new set of responses. The process is commonly used to retrain people who have suffered a brain injury that disrupts normal sensory-motor activities.

pattern theory of pain. See **pain mechanism.**

patulous /pat'yələs/ [L, *patulus*, open], pertaining to something that is open or spread apart.

Paul-Bunnell test [John R. Paul, American physician, b. 1893; Walls W. Bunnell, American physician, b. 1902], a blood test for heterophil antibodies, used for confirming a diagnosis of infectious mononucleosis. See also **heterophil antibody test.**

Pautrier microabscess /pôtrēyā'/ [Lucien M. A. Pautrier, French dermatologist, b. 1876; Gk, *mikros*, small; L, *abscedere*, to go away], an accumulation of intensely staining mononuclear cells in the epidermis, characterizing malignant lymphoma of the skin, especially mycosis fungoides. See also **mycosis fungoides.**

Pauwels' fracture /pou'əlz/ [Friedrich Pauwels, twentieth century German surgeon; L, *fractura*, break], a fracture of the proximal femoral neck with varying degrees of angulation.

Pavabid, a trademark for a smooth muscle relaxant (papaverine hydrochloride).

pavement epithelium. See **squamous epithelium.**

Pavlov, Ivan Petrovich /pav'lôv, pä'vlôf/ (1849-1936), a Russian physiologist who discovered a pattern of conditioned stimulus-reflex learning, the manner in which the physiology of digestion is controlled by the nervous system, and a theory of the causes and treatment of human neuroses.

pavor /pā'vôr/ [L, quaking], a reaction to a frightening stimulus characterized by excessive terror.

pavor diurnus /dī·ur'nəs/, a sleep disorder occurring in children during daytime sleep in which they cry out in alarm and awaken in fear and panic. See also **sleep terror disorder.**

pavor nocturnus /noktur'nəs/, a sleep disorder occurring in children during nighttime sleep that causes them to cry out in alarm and awaken in fear and panic. See also **nightmare, sleep terror disorder.**

Pavulon, a trademark for a neuromuscular blocking agent (pancuronium bromide), used as an adjunct to anesthesia.

Payr's clamp /pī'ərz/ [Erwin Payr, German surgeon, b. 1871; AS, *clam*, fastener], a heavy clamp used in GI surgery.

Pb, symbol for the element **lead.**

PBI, abbreviation for **protein-bound iodine.**

PBL, abbreviation for *peripheral blood lymphocytes.*

p.c., abbreviation for the Latin, *post cibum,* after meals.

PC, abbreviation for *private corporation.*

PCB, abbreviation for **polychlorinated biphenyls.**

pcc, abbreviation for **precipitated calcium carbonate.**

PCH, abbreviation for **paroxysmal cold hemoglobinuria.**

PCIS, abbreviation for *Patient Care Information System,* an online computer system that contains full medical care data on all the residents or the patients in a facility.

Pco_2, symbol for **partial pressure of carbon dioxide.** See **partial pressure.**

PCP, **1.** abbreviation for **phencyclidine hydrochloride.** **2.** abbreviation for *Pneumocystis carinii pneumonia.*

PCR, abbreviation for **polymerase chain reaction.**

p.d., abbreviation for the Latin, *per diem,* by the day.

Pd, symbol for the element **palladium.**

A Patient's Bill of Rights*

The American Hospital Association Board of Trustees' Committee on Health Care for the Disadvantaged, which has been a consistent advocate on behalf of consumers of health care services, developed this bill of rights, which was approved by the AHA House of Delegates February 6, 1973. The following rights are affirmed:

1. The patient has the right to considerate and respectful care.

2. The patient has the right to obtain from his physician complete current information concerning his diagnosis, treatment, and prognosis in terms the patient can be reasonably expected to understand. When it is not medically advisable to give such information to the patient, the information should be made available to an appropriate person in his behalf. He has the right to know, by name, the physician responsible for coordinating his care.

3. The patient has the right to receive from his physician information necessary to give informed consent prior to the start of any procedure and/or treatment. Except in emergencies, such information for informed consent should include but not necessarily be limited to the specific procedure and/or treatment, the medically significant risks involved, and the probable duration of incapacitation. Where medically significant alternatives for care or treatment exist, or when the patient requests information concerning medical alternatives, the patient has the right to such information. The patient also has the right to know the name of the person responsible for the procedures and/or treatment.

4. The patient has the right to refuse treatment to the extent permitted by law, and to be informed of the medical consequences of his action.

5. The patient has the right to every consideration of his privacy concerning his own medical care program. Case discussion, consultation, examination, and treatment are confidential and should be conducted discreetly. Those not directly involved in his care must have the permission of the patient to be present.

6. The patient has the right to expect that all communications and records pertaining to his care should be treated as confidential.

7. The patient has the right to expect that within its capacity a hospital must make reasonable response to the request of a patient for services. The hospital must provide evaluation, service, and/or referral as indicated by the urgency of the case. When medically permissible a patient may be transferred to another facility only after he has received complete information and explanation concerning the needs for and alternatives to such a transfer. The institution to which the patient is to be transferred must first have accepted the patient for transfer.

8. The patient has the right to obtain information as to any relationship of his hospital to other health care and educational institutions insofar as his care is concerned. The patient has the right to obtain information as to the existence of any professional relationships among individuals, by name, who are treating him.

9. The patient has the right to be advised if the hospital proposes to engage in or perform human experimentation affecting his care or treatment. The patient has the right to refuse to participate in such research projects.

10. The patient has the right to expect reasonable continuity of care. He has the right to know in advance what appointment times and physicians are available and where. The patient has the right to expect that the hospital will provide a mechanism whereby he is informed by his physician or a delegate of the physician of the patient's continuing health care requirements following discharge.

11. The patient has the right to examine and receive an explanation of his bill regardless of source of payment.

12. The patient has the right to know what hospital rules and regulations apply to his conduct as a patient.

*Reprinted with the permission of the American Hospital Association, copyright 1972, *Nurs Outlook* 24:29.

P.D., PD,   1. abbreviation for **patient day. 2.** abbreviation for *Doctor of Pharmacy.* **3.** abbreviation for *prism diopter.* **4.** abbreviation for *pupil diameter.* **5.** abbreviation for *pupillary distance.* **6.** abbreviation for *pulse duration.*

PDA,   abbreviation for **patent ductus arteriosus.**

PDL,   abbreviation for **periodontal ligament.**

PDR,   abbreviation for *Physicians' Desk Reference.*

PE,   abbreviation for **pulmonary embolism.**

peak [ME, *pec*],   the amount of medication in the blood that represents the highest level during a drug administration cycle.

peak concentration,   the maximum amount of a substance or force, such as the highest concentration of a drug measured immediately after the drug has been administered.

peak height velocity,   a point in pubescence in which the tempo of growth is the greatest.

peak level,   the highest concentration, usually in the blood, that a substance reaches during the time period under consideration, after which the concentration declines, such as the highest blood glucose level attained during a glucose tolerance test.

peak method of dosing,   the administration of a drug dosage so that a specified maximum level is reached to produce a desired effect, such as lowering the blood pressure.

peak mucus sign,   a lubricative, cloudy to clear white cervical mucus that occurs during periods of high estrogen levels, particularly at the time of ovulation. See also **spinnbarkeit.**

Péan's forceps /pē·anz'/ [Jules E. Péan, French surgeon, b. 1830], *obsolete.*   a basic hemostatic clamp.

pearly penile papules.   See **hirsutoid papillomas of the penis.**

pearly tumor.   See **cholesteatoma.**

Pearson's product movement correlation [Karl Pearson, English mathematician, b. 1857],   (in statistics) a statistical test of the relationship between two variables measured in interval or ratio scales. Correlations computed fall between $+1.00$ and -1.00.

peau d'orange /pō'dôräNzh'/ [Fr, skin of orange],   a dimpling of the skin that gives it the appearance of the skin of an orange. It is common in advanced breast cancer.

pecilo-.   See **poikilo-.**

pectin /pek'tin/ [Gk, *pektos*, congealed],   a gelatinous carbohydrate substance found in fruits and succulent vegetables and used as the setting agent for jams and jellies and as an emulsifier and stabilizer in many foods. It also adds to the diet bulk necessary for proper GI functioning. See also **dietary fiber.**

pectineus /pektin'ē·əs/ [L, *pecten*, comb],   the most anterior of the five medial femoral muscles. It arises from the pectineal line and inserts in a rough line on the femur, extending distally and caudally from the lesser trochanter to

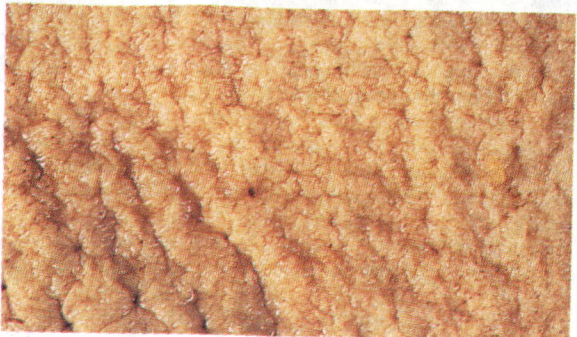

Peau d'orange *(Fletcher, 1987)*

the linea aspera. The muscle is innervated by a branch of the femoral nerve containing fibers from the second, the third, and the fourth lumbar nerves, and it functions to flex and adduct the thigh and to rotate it medially. Compare **adductor brevis, adductor longus, adductor magnus, gracilis.**

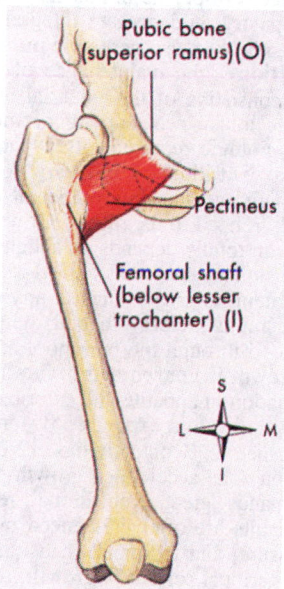

Pectineus muscle *(Thibodeau, 1993/Ernest W Beck)*

pector-, a prefix meaning 'of or pertaining to the breast': *pectoralgia, pectoriloquy, pectorophony.*

pectoral /pek′tərəl/ [L, *pectus*, breast], pertaining to the thorax or chest.

pectoralis major /pek′tərā′lis, pek′tərəlis/ [L, *pectus*, breast], a large muscle of the upper chest wall that acts on the joint of the shoulder. Thick and fan-shaped, it arises from the clavicle, the sternum, the cartilages of the second to the sixth ribs, and the aponeurosis of the obliquus externus abdominis. It inserts by a flat wide tendon into the crest of the greater tubercle of the humerus. The pectoralis major is innervated by the medial and lateral pectoral nerves

from the brachial plexus, which contain fibers from the fifth, sixth, seventh, and eighth cervical nerves, and by fibers from the first thoracic nerve. The pectoralis major serves to flex, adduct, and medially rotate the arm in the shoulder joint.

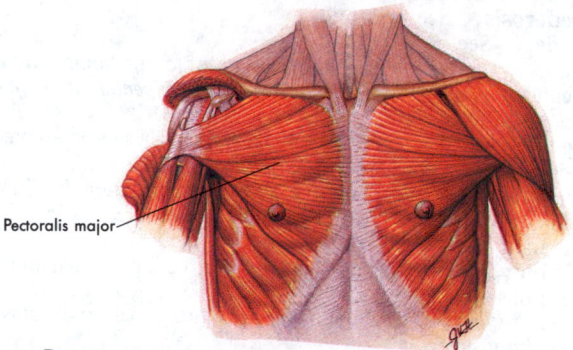

Pectoralis major *(Thibodeau, 1993/John V Hagen)*

pectoralis minor, a thin, triangular muscle of the upper chest wall beneath the pectoralis major. The base arises from the third, fourth, and fifth ribs on their upper, outer surfaces. It inserts as a flat tendon into the coracoid process of the scapula. The pectoralis minor is innervated by the medial pectoral nerve from the brachial plexus, which contains fibers from the eighth cervical and the first thoracic nerves, and it functions to rotate the scapula, to draw it down and forward, and to raise the third, the fourth, and the fifth ribs in forced inspiration. Compare **pectoralis major, subclavius.**

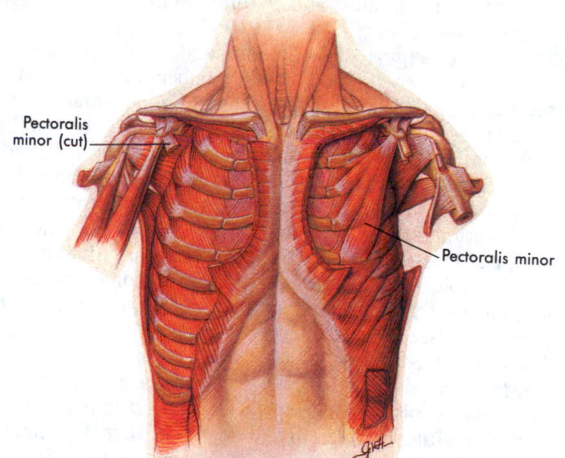

Pectoralis minor *(Thibodeau, 1993/John V Hagen)*

pectoriloquy /pek′təril′əkwē/, a phenomenon in which voice sounds, including whispers, are transmitted clearly through the pulmonary structures and are clearly audible through a stethoscope. It is often a sign of lung consolidation.

pectus excavatum. See **funnel chest.**

ped-. See **pedo-.**

-ped, -pede, a suffix meaning 'pertaining to foot or feet': *biped, taliped.*

pedagogy /ped′əgōj′ē/ [Gk, *pais,* child, *agogos,* leader], the art and science of teaching children, based on a belief that the purpose of education is the transmittal of knowledge.

pedal /ped′əl/ [L, *pes,* foot], pertaining to the foot.

-pedal. See **-pedic.**

pederosis. See **pedophilia.**

pedes. See **pes.**

pedia-, pedo-, a prefix meaning 'of or pertaining to a child': *pediatric, pediatrician, pediatrics, pedodontics, pedophilia.*

-pedia, -paedia, a suffix meaning 'to educate or a compendium of knowledge': *pharmacopedia, logopedia.*

Pediaflor, a trademark for a dental preparation (sodium fluoride), used as prophylaxis against dental caries in children.

Pedialyte, a trademark for a balanced solution containing various electrolytes.

Pediamycin, a trademark for an antibacterial (erythromycin ethylsuccinate).

pediatric /pē′dē·at′rik/ [Gk, *pais,* child + *iatreia,* treatment], pertaining to preventive and primary health care and treatment of children and the study of childhood diseases.

pediatric advanced life support (PALS), a system of critical care procedures and facilities, such as the intensive care nursery, for the basic and advanced treatment of seriously ill or injured infants and children. It includes the neonatal resuscitation program (NRP) as recommended by the American Academy of Pediatrics and the American Heart Association.

pediatric anesthesia [Gk, *pais,* child, *iatreia,* treatment], a subspecialty of anesthesiology dealing with the anesthesia of neonates, infants, and children up to 12 years of age.

pediatric dentistry. See **dentistry.**

pediatric dosage, the determination of the correct amount, frequency, and total number of doses of a medication to be administered to a child or infant. Such variables as the age, weight, body surface area, and ability of the child to absorb, metabolize, and excrete the medication must be considered, as well as the expected action of the drug, possible side effects, and potential toxicity. Various formulas have been devised to calculate pediatric dosage from a standard adult dose, although the most reliable method is to use the proportional amount of body surface area to body weight, based on one of the formulas. See also **Clark's rule, Cowling's rule, Young's rule.**

pediatric hospitalization, the confinement of a child or infant in a hospital for diagnostic testing or therapeutic treatment. Regardless of age or the degree of illness or injury, hospitalization constitutes a major crisis in the life of a child, and the emotional trauma elicits various behavioral reactions that the nurse must recognize and be prepared to cope with to facilitate recovery. The dominant factors influencing stress, which vary according to the child's developmental age, previous experience with illness, and the seriousness of the condition, include separation from the parents and familiar environment, disruption of routine patterns of daily life, loss of independence, and worry about bodily injury or painful experiences. The nurse can minimize stress by preparing the child and family through prehospital counseling; by encouraging active parental participation in the care of the child through rooming-in facilities or frequent visits; by maintaining as normal a daily routine as possible, especially with eating, sleeping, hygiene, and play activities; by explaining all hospital procedures and the immediate and long-term prognosis in terms that the child can easily understand; and by providing support and guidance for parents and siblings. The nurse also may use the hospital experience to foster an improved parent-child relationship and to teach other members of the family about proper health care. Emergency admission greatly in[001e]creases the emotional trauma of hospitalization, making the role of the nurse in counteracting negative reactions even more significant.

pediatrician /pē′dē·ətrish′ən/ [Gk, *pais,* child, *iatreia,* treatment], a physician who specializes in pediatrics. Also called **pediatrist** /pē′dē·at′rist/.

pediatric nurse practitioner (PNP), a nurse practitioner who, by advanced study and clinical practice, such as in a master's degree program or certificate program in pediatric nursing, has gained advanced knowledge in the nursing care of infants and children. See also **pediatric nursing.**

pediatric nursing, the branch of nursing concerned with the care of infants and children. Pediatric nursing requires knowledge of normal psychomotor, psychosocial, and cognitive growth and development, as well as of the health problems and needs of people in this age group. Preventive care and anticipatory guidance are integral to the practice of pediatric nursing. See also **pediatric nurse practitioner.**

pediatric nutrition, the maintenance of a proper, well-balanced diet, consisting of the essential nutrients and the adequate caloric intake necessary to promote growth and sustain the physiologic requirements at the various stages of development. Nutritional needs vary considerably with age, level of activity, and environmental conditions, and they are directly related to the rate of growth. In the prenatal period, growth totally depends on adequate maternal nutrition. During infancy the need for calories, especially in the form of protein, is greater than at any postnatal period because of the rapid increase in both height and weight. From toddlerhood through the preschool and middle childhood years, growth is uneven and occurs in spurts, with a resulting fluctuation in appetite and calorie consumption. In general, the average child expends 55% of energy on metabolic maintenance, 25% on activities, 12% on growth, and 8% on excretion. The accelerated growth phase during adolescence demands greater nutritional requirements, although food habits are often influenced by emotional factors, peer pressure, and fad diets. Inadequate nutrition, especially during critical periods of growth, results in retarded development or illness, such as anemia from deficiency of iron or scurvy from deficiency of vitamin C. An important function of the nurse is to give nutritional guidance and teach good eating habits. A special problem is overfeeding in the early childhood years, which may lead to obesity or hypervitaminosis. See also **dietary allowances,** and see specific vitamins.

pediatrics (peds) /pē′dē·at′triks/, a branch of medicine concerned with the development and care of children. Its specialties are the particular diseases of children and their treatment and prevention. Also called *(informal)* **peds.** —**pediatric,** *adj.*

pediatric surgery, the special preparation and care of the child undergoing surgical procedures for injuries, deformities, or disease. In addition to the usual fears and emotional trauma of illness and hospitalization, the child is especially concerned about being anesthetized. Younger children worry more about what will happen to them and how they will feel after awakening from anesthesia, whereas the older child fears the operation itself and possible death, the loss of control while under anesthesia, and any change in body image or mutilation of parts. The role of the nurse is to prepare the child psychologically and physically for the particular surgical procedure and any postoperative reactions, to offer support to the parents and involve them as much as possible in the care, both before and after surgery, and to explain immediate and long-term prognoses. See also **pediatric hospitalization.**

pediatrist.   See **pediatrician.**

-pedic, -paedic,   a suffix meaning 'of or pertaining to children or their treatment': *gymnopedic, orthopedic.*

-pedic, -pedal,   a suffix meaning 'referring or pertaining to the feet': *arthrosteopedic, talipedic, velocipedic.*

pedicle [L, *pediculus,* little foot],   a narrow stalk, stem, or tube of tissue attached to a tumor, skin flap, or organ.

pedicle clamp /ped′ikəl/ [L, *pediculus,* little foot; ME, *clam,* fastener],   a locking surgical forceps used for compressing blood vessels or pedicles of tumors during surgery. Also called **clamp forceps.**

pedicle flap operation,   a mucogingival surgical procedure for relocating or sliding gingival tissue from a donor site to an isolated defect, usually a tooth surface denuded of attached gingiva.

pediculicide /pədik′yoŏlisīd′/ [L, *pediculus,* louse, *caedere,* to kill],   any of a group of drugs that kill lice.

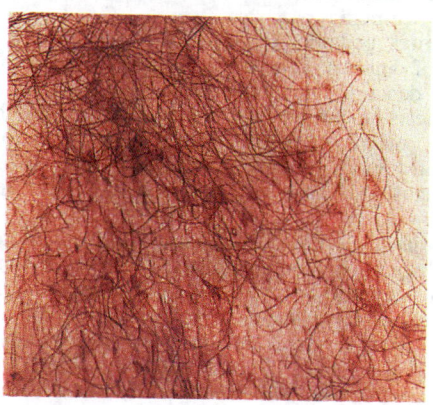

Pediculosis pubis *(du Vivier, 1993)*

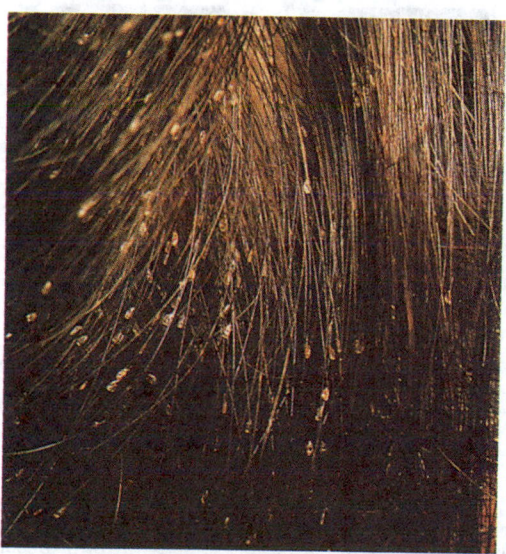

Pediculosis capitis *(Baran, 1991)*

pediculosis /pədik′yoŏlō′sis/ [L, *pediculosus,* lousy],   an infestation with bloodsucking lice. **Pediculosis capitis** is infestation of the scalp with lice. **Pediculosis corporis** is infestation of the skin of the body with lice. **Pediculosis palpebrarum** is infestation of the eyelids and eyelashes

with lice. **Pediculosis pubis** is infestation of the pubic hair region with lice. See also **crab louse, louse.**

■ OBSERVATIONS: Infestation with lice causes intense itching, often resulting in excoriation of the skin and secondary bacterial infection. Frequently, only the eggs of the lice may be seen. Body lice lay eggs in the seams of clothing; crab and head lice attach their eggs to hairs. Lice are spread by direct contact with infested clothing, people, or toilet seats. Body lice may transmit certain diseases, among them relapsing fever, typhus, and trench fever.

■ INTERVENTIONS: Treatment includes the topical use of 1% lindane as shampoo, lotion, or cream, or of permethrin (1.0% creme rinse). After the pediculicide is applied, the eggs are combed out of the hair with a fine-toothed comb. Lice and eggs on the eyelashes require topical treatment with an ophthalmic ointment containing 0.25% physostigmine. Infestation sometimes may be prevented by avoiding contact with the organism, by washing clothing or bedding in hot water, and by avoiding use of others' hats and combs.

pediculous /pədik′yələs/ [L, a little louse],   infested with sucking lice.

Pediculus humanus capitis,   a species of head lice.

Pediculus humanus corporis,   a species of body lice.

Pediculus pubis.   See **crab louse.**

pedigree /ped′əgrē/ [Fr, *pied de grue,* crane's foot pattern], **1.** line of descent; lineage; ancestry. **2.** (in genetics) a chart that shows the genetic makeup of a person's ancestors, used in the mendelian analysis of an inherited characteristic or disease in a particular family. Specific stylized symbols, usually plain and shaded or partially shaded squares and circles, are used, respectively, to designate normal males and females, those affected by the disease or trait, and those who are carriers. The generations are numbered with Roman numerals at the left with the most recent at the bottom, and members within each generation are designated by Arabic numerals from left to right according to age, the oldest at the left. The inquiry begins with the siblings of the affected person and proceeds to the parents and grandparents and any of their immediate relatives. See also **Punnett square.**

pedo-. See **pedia-.**

pedodontics /ped′ədon′tiks/ [Gk, *pais*, child, *odius*, tooth], a field of dentistry devoted to the diagnosis and the treatment of dental problems affecting children.

pedogenesis /pē′dōjen′əsis/ [Gk, *pais*, child, *genesis*, origin], the production of offspring by young or larval forms of animals, often by parthenogenesis, as in certain amphibians. Also spelled **paedogenesis.** **–pedogenetic,** *adj.*

pedophilia /ped′əfil′ē·ə/ [Gk, *pais*, child, *philein*, to love], **1.** an abnormal interest in children. **2.** (in psychiatry) a psychosexual disorder in which the fantasy or act of engaging in sexual activity with prepubertal children is the preferred or exclusive means of achieving sexual excitement and gratification. It may be heterosexual or homosexual. Also spelled **paedophilia.** Also called **pederosis.** See also **paraphilia.** **–pedophilic,** *adj.*

peds, *(informal)* abbreviation for **pediatrics.**

peduncle /pədung′kəl/ [L, *pes*, foot], a stemlike connecting part, such as the pineal peduncle or a peduncle graft. **–peduncular, pedunculate,** *adj..*

peduncular /pədung′kyələr/, pertaining to a pedicle or peduncle.

pedunculated /pədung′kyəlā′tid/ [L, *pes*, foot], pertaining to a structure with a stalk or peduncle.

pedunculus /pədung′kyələs/ [L, *pes*, foot], a stalk, stem, or any stalklike anatomical structure.

PEEP, abbreviation for **positive end expiratory pressure.**

Peeping Tom. See **voyeur.**

peer [L, *par*, equal], a person deemed an equal for the purpose at hand. It is usually an 'age mate,' or companion or associate on roughly the same level of age or mental endowment.

peer review, an appraisal by professional co-workers of equal status of the way an individual nurse or other health professional conducts practice, education, or research. The appraisal uses accepted standards as measures against which performance is weighed. See also **Professional Standards Review Organization.**

Peganone, a trademark for an anticonvulsant (ethotoin).

PEL, abbreviation for *permissible exposure limits.*

Pel-Ebstein fever /pel′eb′stēn/ [Pieter K. Pel, Dutch physician, b. 1852; Wilhelm Ebstein, German physician, b. 1836], a recurrent fever, occurring in cycles of several days or weeks, characteristic of Hodgkin's disease or malignant lymphoma. Also called **Murchison fever.**

Pelger-Huët anomaly /pel′gərhyo͞o′ət/ [Karel Pelger, Dutch physician, b. 1885; G. J. Huet, Dutch physician, b. 1879; Gk, *anomalia*, irregular], an inherited disorder characterized by granulocytes with unusually coarse nuclear material and dumbbell-shaped or peanut-shaped nuclei. Normal nuclear segmentation does not seem to occur, but there are no associated findings. See also **band.**

pell-, a prefix meaning 'of or pertaining to the skin': *pellagra, pellicle, pellicular.*

pellagra /pəlā′grə, pəlag′rə/ [It, *pelle*, skin, *agra*, rough], a disease resulting from a deficiency of niacin or tryptophan or a metabolic defect that interferes with the conversion of the precursor tryptophan to niacin. It is frequently seen in individuals whose diet consists primarily of maize, which is deficient in tryptophan. It is characterized by scaly dermatitis, especially of the skin exposed to the sun, glossitis,

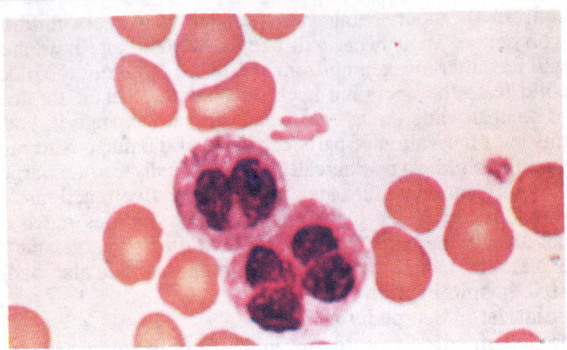

Pelger-Huët anomaly *(Hayhoe, 1992)*

inflammation of the mucous membranes, diarrhea, and mental disturbances, including depression, confusion, disorientation, hallucination, and delirium. Treatment and prophylaxis consist of administration of niacin and tryptophan, usually in conjunction with other vitamins, particularly thiamine and riboflavin, and a well-balanced diet containing foods rich in these nutrients, such as liver, eggs, milk, and meat. Kinds of pellagra are **pellagra sine pellagra** and **typhoid pellagra.** Compare **kwashiorkor.** **–pellagrous,** *adj.*

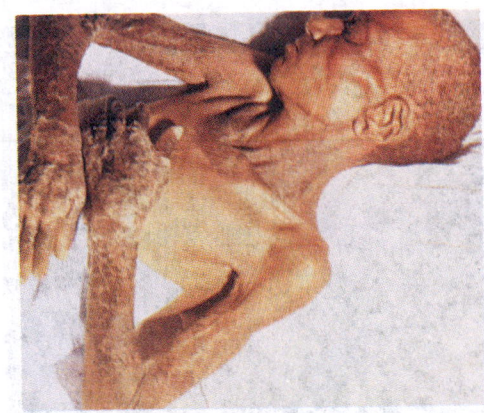

Dermatitis caused by pellagra *(McLaren, 1992)*

pellagra sine pellagra /sī′nē, sē′nə/, a form of pellagra in which the characteristic dermatitis is not present. See **pellagra.**

Pellegrini's disease /pel′əgrē′nēz/ [Augusto Pellegrini, Italian surgeon, b. 1877], ossification of the upper part of the medial collateral ligament, sometimes accompanied by bony growth at the internal condyle of the femur. The condition usually follows a leg injury. Also called **Pelligrini-Stieda disease.**

pelo-, a prefix meaning 'of or pertaining to mud': *pelohemia, pelology, pelotherapy.*

pelvi-,   a combining form meaning 'pertaining to the pelvis': *pelvimetry, pelvicophalometry.*

pelvic /pel'vik/ [L, *pelvis,* basin],   of or pertaining to the pelvis.

pelvic abscess [L, *pelvis,* basin; *abscedere,* to go away], a pus-producing lesion in the pelvic peritoneum, usually originating in the rectouterine pouch.

pelvic axis,   an imaginary curved line that passes through the centers of the various anteroposterior diameters of the pelvis.

pelvic bone [L, *pelvis,* basin; AS, *ban*],   a combination of the ilium, ischium, and pubis.

pelvic brim,   the curved top of the bones of the hip extending from the anterior superior iliac crest in front on one side around and past the sacrum to the crest on the other side. Below the brim is the pelvis.

pelvic cellulitis,   bacterial infection of the parametrium, occurring after childbirth or spontaneous therapeutic abortion. It represents an extension of infection via the blood vessels and lymphatics from a primary wound infection in the external genitalia, perineum, vagina, cervix, or uterus. It is characterized by fever, uterine subinvolution, chills and sweats, abdominal pain that spreads laterally and, if untreated, the formation of a large abscess and signs of peritonitis. It is seen most commonly between the third and the ninth days after delivery or abortion. Treatment includes an antibiotic, bed rest, intravenous fluids, and drainage of any abscess that forms. Oxytocics may be given to augment involution.

pelvic classification,   **1.** a process in which the anatomic and spatial relationships of the bones of the pelvis are evaluated, usually to assess the adequacy of the pelvic structures for vaginal delivery. Caldwell-Moloy's system of classification is the one most commonly used. **2.** one of the types in a classification system of the pelvis.

pelvic congestion syndrome,   an abnormal gynecologic condition characterized by chronic low back pain, dysuria, dysmenorrhea, vague lower abdominal pain, vaginal discharge, and dyspareunia. The cause of the symptoms is not understood; formerly it was thought that the vascular bed of the area was distended with blood, but this has not been demonstrated. Women between 25 and 45 years of age are most often affected.

pelvic diameter [L, *pelvis,* basin; Gk, *diametros,* measuring across],   **1.** at the rim of the pelvis, a line from the lumbosacral angle to the symphysis pubis. **2.** at the pelvic outlet, a line from the tip of the coccyx to the lower border of the symphysis pubis.

pelvic diaphragm,   the caudal aspect of the body wall, stretched like a hammock across the pelvic cavity and comprising the levator ani and the coccygeus muscles. It holds the abdominal contents, supports the pelvic viscera, and is pierced by the anal canal, the urethra, and the vagina. It is reinforced by fasciae and muscles associated with these structures and with the perineum.

pelvic examination,   a diagnostic procedure in which the external and internal genitalia are physically examined using inspection, palpation, percussion, and auscultation. It should be performed regularly throughout a woman's life. See also **female reproductive system assessment.**
■ METHOD: The woman empties her bladder, disrobes, and puts on an examining gown. Breast examination is often carried out before the pelvic examination. The woman is made as comfortable as possible in the dorsal lithotomy position,

her feet in stirrups and her buttocks at the very edge of the foot of the examining table, and is then draped. Particular attention is paid to the suprapubic area to detect any masses extending from the pelvis above the symphysis and to the groin to detect inguinal lymphadenopathy or hernia. If a mass is felt, percussion may be performed to delineate it. If pregnancy is suspected, palpation and percussion of the uterus and auscultation of fetal heart tones are attempted. The examiner then moves to the stool at the foot of the table between the patient's legs. The labia majora are spread apart to permit inspection of the clitoris, the urethral meatus, the labia minora, and the vaginal vestibule. Any swelling, discoloration, lesion, scar, cyst, discharge, or bleeding is noted. Skene's and Bartholin's glands and ducts are palpated and milked, and any secretions expressed are evaluated and a specimen is spread on culture media. The tone of the perineal and paravaginal musculature is assessed. Cystocele, rectocele, or varying degrees of uterine descensus may be observed as the woman is asked to bear down. Because lubricating jelly interferes with cytologic and bacteriologic studies, the speculum examination is usually performed without using the jelly. The speculum is warmed, lubricated with warm water, and introduced gradually. The examiner is careful to direct the speculum along the axis of the vagina, which is at an angle of approximately 45 degrees to the axis of the table if the woman is lying flat. The speculum may need to be moved lightly from side to side to slip it over the vaginal rugae. The woman is advised that she may feel a stretching sensation; the speculum is gently opened and its position is adjusted to hold the vaginal folds out of the way to reveal the cervix. The color and condition of the vaginal epithelium are observed, and the position, size, and quality of the superficial epithelium are evaluated. Specimens for bacteriologic study are obtained before the Pap test. For the Pap test, scrapings of the endocervix and the cervix and a sample of the vaginal secretions are secured on a Pap stick and an applicator and lightly spread on labeled glass slides. The slides are immediately sprayed with a fixative or dipped in it. The speculum is then closed, rotated slightly, removed from the vagina, and rinsed or placed directly in a germicidal solution. In the bimanual part of the examination, two gloved fingers are well lubricated and inserted slowly and gently into the vagina. The examiner uses the opposite hand to apply pressure to the lower abdomen in several positions and directions to bring the uterus, tubes, and ovaries into positions in which they may be felt. The size, shape, position, mobility, and consistency of the organs and tissues are evaluated, and any tenderness or discomfort is noted. Rectal or rectovaginal examination is then performed. Before the insertion of a finger in the anus, lateral pressure is applied to the sphincter, and the woman is urged to bear down lightly to relax the muscle and minimize discomfort.
■ NURSING INTERVENTION: Minor unthoughtfulness or inadvertent movement may cause tension and make the examination more difficult for the woman and for the examiner. Instruments, culture materials, a light, drapes, and a gown are all made ready beforehand. The table, instruments, and drapes are clean and warm. Materials from previous examinations are not in evidence. The woman is forewarned of what to expect at each step of the examination. Gentleness and quietness are exercised at all times. On completion of the examination, the woman is helped to slide well back on the table before sitting up. Syncope after pelvic examina-

tion is uncommon but not rare; there is risk of injury should the patient faint and fall from the examining table. The woman is observed briefly after sitting up before being left alone. She is then given tissues, a sanitary napkin or tampon, and a private area in which to dress.

■ OUTCOME CRITERIA: Pelvic examination may demonstrate many pelvic abnormalities and diseases. Cytologic and bacteriologic specimens are conveniently obtained. A pelvic examination cannot be satisfactorily performed without the cooperation of the woman being examined; inadequate relaxation, obesity, extensive scarring, pelvic tenderness, and heavy vaginal discharge also may preclude an adequate examination.

pelvic exenteration /eksen'tərā'shən/, the surgical removal of all reproductive organs and adjacent tissues.

pelvic floor, the soft tissues enclosing the pelvic outlet.

pelvic girdle [L, *pelvis*, basin; AS, *gyrdel*], a bony ring formed by the hip bones, the sacrum, and the coccyx.

pelvic inferior aperture. See **pelvic outlet.**

pelvic inflammatory disease (PID), any inflammatory condition of the female pelvic organs, especially one caused by bacterial infection. Characteristics of the condition include fever, foul-smelling vaginal discharge, pain in the lower abdomen, abnormal uterine bleeding, pain with coitus, and tenderness or pain in the uterus, affected ovary, or fallopian tube on bimanual pelvic examination. If an abscess has already developed, a soft, tender, fluid-filled mass may be palpated. Bed rest and antibiotics are usually prescribed, but surgical drainage of an abscess may be required. Severe, fulminating PID may necessitate hysterectomy to avoid fatal septicemia. If the cause is infection by gonococci or chlamydiae, the woman's sexual partners are also treated with antibiotics. Severe PID is usually very painful; the woman may be prostrate and require nacotic analgesia. Recurrent or severe PID often results in scarring of the fallopian tubes, obstruction, and infertility.

pelvic inlet, (in obstetrics) the inlet to the true pelvis, bounded by the sacral promontory, the horizontal rami of the pubic bones, and the top of the symphysis pubis. Because the infant must pass through the inlet to enter the true pelvis and to be born vaginally, the anteroposterior, transverse, and oblique dimensions of the inlet are important measurements to be made in assessing the pelvis in pregnancy. There are three anteroposterior diameters: the true conjugate, the obstetric conjugate, and the diagonal conjugate. The true conjugate can be measured only on x-ray films, because it extends from the sacral promontory to the top of the symphysis pubis. Its normal measurement is 11 cm or more. The obstetric conjugate is the shortest of the three, because it extends from the sacral promontory to the thickest part of the pubic bone. It measures 10 cm or more. The diagonal conjugate is the most easily and commonly assessed, because it extends from the lower border of the symphysis pubis to the sacral promontory. It normally measures 11.5 cm or more. The inlet is said to be contracted when any of these diameters is smaller than normal. The anteroposterior diameters are shorter than normal in the small gynecoid and platypelloid pelvis. The transverse diameter of the inlet is bounded by the inferior border of the walls of the iliac bones and is measured at the widest point. It is normally close to 13.5 cm but may be less in the small gynecoid pelvis and anthropoid pelvis. The oblique diameters of the pelvis extend from the juncture of the sacrum and ilium to the eminence on the ilium on the opposite side of the pelvis. Each oblique diameter measures nearly 13 cm.

This dimension is smaller than normal in the small gynecoid and platypelloid pelves. See also **android pelvis, anthropoid pelvis, gynecoid pelvis, platypelloid pelvis.**

pelvic kidney. See **ptotic kidney.**

pelvic minilaparotomy /min'ēlap'ərot'əmē/, a surgical operation in which the lower abdomen is entered through a small, suprapubic incision, performed most often for tubal sterilization but also for diagnosis and treatment of eccyesis, ovarian cyst, endometriosis, and infertility. It may be performed as an alternative to laparoscopy, often on an outpatient basis. General, regional, or local anesthesia is administered. The patient is placed in the supine position, and the abdomen is prepared with antiseptic solution and draped with sterile drapes. An incision a few centimeters long is made, usually transversely, in the suprapubic fold of skin in the midline, and is then carried down through the fat and fascia, between the rectus abdominis muscles, and into the peritoneal cavity. Bleeders are ligated, and a small self-retaining retractor is placed in the incision. A laparoscope may be used for visualization. The sterilization or other procedure is performed. After hemostasis is ensured, each tube is replaced in its anatomic position, and the incision is closed in layers. Because incisional pain in the postoperative period may mask the pain of intraperitoneal bleeding, vital signs are monitored frequently. Tachycardia and hypotension that are not alleviated by analgesia may be signs of hemorrhage or injury to the bowel. Before discharge, outpatients are carefully instructed in the postoperative danger signs and in the proper care of the incision at home. Arrangements are made for follow-up examination. Often, minilaparotomy may be performed faster and less expensively than laparoscopy. Though small, the minilaparotomy incision is considerably larger than is the usual laparoscopy incision. It is, therfore, less pleasing cosmetically, as well as more painful in the postoperative period. Compare **laparoscopy.**

pelvic outlet, the space surrounded by the bones of the lower portion of the true pelvis. In men, the shape of the pelvic outlet is narrower than in women, but this is of no clinical significance. In women, the shape and size of the pelvis vary and are of importance in childbirth. The shapes are classified by the length of the diameters as compared with each other and by the thickness of the bones. The diameters of the outlet are the anteroposterior, from the symphysis pubis to the coccyx, and the intertuberous, laterally from one to the other ischial tuberosity. See also **pelvic classification.**

pelvic pain, pain in the pelvis, as occurs in appendicitis, oophoritis, and endometritis. The character and onset of pelvic pain and any factors that alleviate or aggravate it are significant in making a diagnosis.

pelvic pole, the end of the axis at which the breech of the fetus is located.

pelvic presentation [L, *pelvis*, basin, *praesentare*, to show], a breech presentation.

pelvic rotation, one of the five major kinematic determinants of gait, involving the alternate rotation of the pelvis to the right and the left of the central axis of the body. The usual pelvic rotation occurring at each hip joint in most healthy individuals is approximately 4 degrees to each side of the central axis. Pelvic rotation occurs during the stance phase of gait and involves a medial to lateral circular motion. With normal locomotion or walking considered a progressive sinusoidal movement, pelvic rotation serves to minimize the vertical displacement of the center of gravity of the body during the act of walking. Analysis of pelvic ro-

correction of pathologic gaits. Compare **knee-ankle inter-action, knee-hip flexion, lateral pelvic displacement, pelvic tilt.**

pelvic rotunda [L, *pelvis,* basin, *rotundus,* wheel], a part of the ear appearing as a funnel-shaped depression of the tympanum above the fenestra cochlea.

pelvic tilt, one of the five major kinematic determinants of gait that lowers the pelvis on the side of the swinging lower limb during the walking cycle. Through the action of the hip joint the pelvis tilts laterally downward, adducting the lower limb in the stance phase of gait and abducting the opposite extremity in the swing phase of gait. The knee joint of the non-weight-bearing limb flexes during its swing phase to allow the pelvic tilt, which helps minimize the vertical displacement of the center of gravity of the body, thus conserving energy during walking. Pelvic tilt is often a factor in the diagnosis and treatment of various orthopedic diseases, deformities, and abnormal conditions and in the analysis and the correction of pathologic gaits. Compare **knee ankle interaction, knee hip flexion, lateral pelvic displacement, pelvic rotation.**

pelvic varicocele. See **ovarian varicocele.**

pelvifemoral /pel'vēfem'ərəl/ [L, *pelvis,* basin, *femur,* thigh], of or pertaining to the structures of the hip joint, especially the muscles and the area around the bony pelvis and the head of the femur that make up the pelvic girdle.

pelvifemoral muscular dystrophy. See **Leyden-Moebius muscular dystrophy.**

pelvimeter /pelvim'ətər/ [L, *pelvis,* basin; Gk, *metron,* measure], a device for measuring the diameter and capacity of the pelvis.

pelvimetry /pelvim'ətrē/, the act or process of determining the dimensions of the bony birth canal. Kinds of pelvimetry are **clinical pelvimetry** and **x-ray pelvimetry.**

pelvis /pel'viz/, *pl.* **pelves** [L, basin], the lower portion of the trunk of the body, composed of four bones, the two innominate bones laterally and ventrally and the sacrum and coccyx posteriorly. It is divided into the greater or false pelvis and the lesser or true pelvis by an oblique plane passing through the sacrum and the pubic symphysis. The greater pelvis is the expanded portion of the cavity situated cranially and ventral to the pelvic brim. The lesser pelvis is situated distal to the pelvic brim, and its bony walls are more complete than those of the greater pelvis. The inlet and outlet of the pelvis have three important diameters, anteroposterior, oblique, and transverse. The pelvis of a woman is usually less massive but wider and more circular than that of a man. **–pelvic,** *adj.*

pemoline /pem'əlēn/, a central nervous system stimulant.
■ INDICATIONS: It is prescribed in the treatment of minimal brain dysfunction and attention-deficit disorder in children.
■ CONTRAINDICATION: Known hypersensitivity to this drug prohibits its use.
■ ADVERSE EFFECTS: Some of the more serious adverse reactions are insomnia, GI disturbances, rash, convulsions, and hallucinations.

pemphigoid /pem'figoid/ [Gk, *pemphix,* bubble, *eidos,* form], a bullous disease resembling pemphigus, distinguished by thicker walled bullae arising from erythematous macules or urticarial bases. Oral lesions are uncommon. It may rarely be associated with an internal malignancy. Spontaneous remission occasionally occurs after several years. Treatment is usually with oral corticosteroids. Compare **pemphigus.**

pemphigus /pem'figəs, pemfī'gəs/ [Gk, *pemphix,* bubble], an uncommon, serious disease of the skin and mucous membranes, characterized by thin-walled bullae arising from apparently normal skin or mucous membrane. The bullae rupture easily, leaving raw patches. The person loses weight, becomes weak, and is subject to major infections. Treatment with corticosteroids and other immunosuppressive medications has changed the prognosis of this disease from

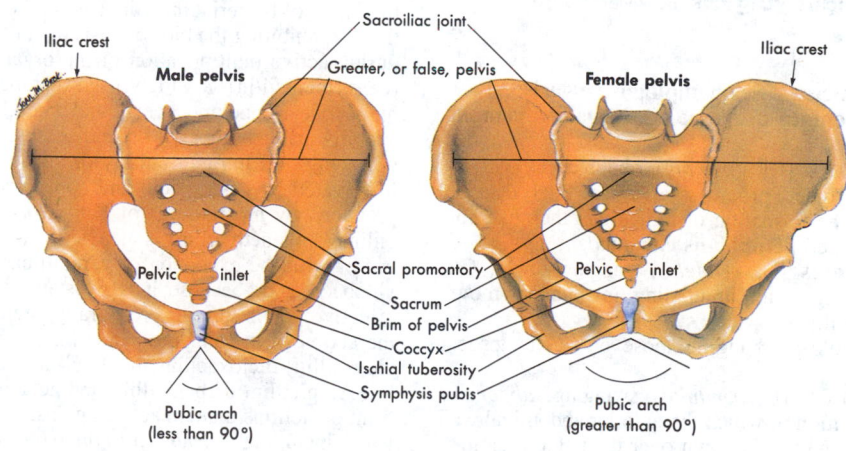

Comparison of male and female bony pelvis *(Thibodeau, 1993/Joan M Beck)*

an almost universally fatal one to a controllable problem compatible with a nearly normal life. The cause is unknown. Compare **pemphigoid.**

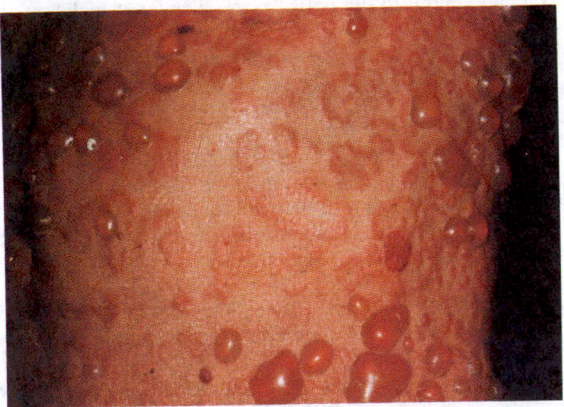

Bullous pemphigoid (Habif, 1990)

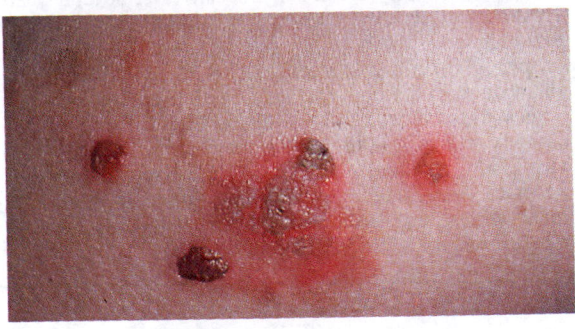

Pemphigus vulgaris (du Vivier, 1993)

pemphigus chronicus. See **pemphigus vulgaris.**
pemphigus erythematosus. See **erythematous pemphigus.**
pemphigus vulgaris [Gk, *pemphix*, bubble; L, *vulgus*, common], a chronic, progressive, often fatal disease, characterized by the formation of bullae on otherwise normal skin. Also called **pemphigus chronicus.**
pendular nystagmus [L, *pendulus*, hanging down; Gk, *nystagmos*, nodding], an undulating involuntary movement of the eyeball.
pendulous /pen'dələs/, hanging loose or lacking proper support.
pendulous abdomen [L, *pendulus*, swinging, *abdomen*] an abnormal condition in which the anterior abdominal wall becomes relaxed and hangs down over the pubic region.
-penem, a suffix for certain antibiotics, including analogues of penicillanic acid.
penetrance /pen'ətrəns/ [L, *penetrare*, to penetrate], (in genetics) a variable factor that modifies basic patterns of inheritance. It is the regularity with which an inherited trait is manifest in the person who carries the gene. If a gene always produces its effect on the phenotype, it is fully and

completely penetrant. Achondroplasia is caused by a fully penetrant gene; if the gene is present, achondroplasia results. If a gene produces its effect less frequently than 100% of the time, it is not fully penetrant. Retinoblastoma develops in 90% of the children carrying the gene; in 10% of children, the gene is nonpenetrant. **–penetrant,** *adj.*
penetrate /pen'ətrāt/ [L, *penetrare*], **1.** to enter or pierce a barrier. **2.** pertaining to the degree to which x-rays pass through matter.
penetrating wound /pen'ətrā'ting/ [L, *penetrare*; AS, *wund*], a wound that enters into a body area, organ, or cavity but does not pass through.
penfluridol /penfloo'ridol/, an antipsychotic drug, chemically similar to pimozide.
-penia, a suffix meaning a '(specified) deficiency': *glycopenia, lipopenia, thyropenia.*
penicillamine (D-penicillamine) /pen'isil'əmēn/, a chelating agent.
■ INDICATIONS: It is prescribed to bind with and remove metals from the blood in the treatment of heavy metal (especially lead) poisoning, in cystinuria, and in Wilson's disease. It is also prescribed as a palliative in the treatment of sclerosis and rheumatoid arthritis when other medications have failed.
■ CONTRAINDICATIONS: Known hypersensitivity to this drug or penicillamine-related aplastic anemia prohibits its use. It is not given during pregnancy or to patients who have kidney dysfunction.
■ ADVERSE EFFECTS: Among the more serious adverse reactions are fever, rashes, and blood dyscrasias. Severe bone marrow depression and immune disorders have been associated with long-term use of this drug. D-penicillamine is less toxic than the L form, and much of the reported toxicity is caused by the use of the L or DL forms.
penicillic acid /pen'isil'ik/, an antibiotic compound isolated from various species of the fungus *Penicillium.*
penicillin /pen'isil'in/ [L *penicillus* paintbrush], any one of a group of antibiotics derived from cultures of species of the fungus *Penicillium* or produced semisynthetically. Various penicillins administered orally or parenterally for the treatment of bacterial infections exert their antimicrobial action by inhibiting the biosynthesis of cell wall mucopeptides during active multiplication of the organisms. Penicillin G (benzylpenicillin), a widely used therapeutic agent for meningococcal, pneumococcal, and streptococcal infections, syphilis, and a number of other diseases, is rapidly absorbed when injected intramuscularly or subcutaneously, but it is inactivated by gastric acid and hydrolyzed by penicillinase produced by most strains of *Staphylococcus aureus.* Penicillin V (phenethicillin) is also active against gram-positive cocci, with the exception of penicillinase-producing staphylococci, and, because it is resistant to gastric acid, it is effective when administered orally. Penicillins resistant to the action of the enzyme penicillinase (beta-lactamase) are cloxacillin, dicloxacillin, methicillin, nafcillin, and oxacillin. Ampicillin, carbenicillin, and hetacillin are broad spectrum penicillins that are active against gram-negative organisms, including *Escherichia coli, Haemophilus influenzae, Neisseria gonorrhoeae, Proteus mirabilis,* and species of *Pseudomonas.* Hypersensitivity reactions are common in patients receiving penicillin and may appear in the absence of prior exposure to the drug, presumably because of unrecognized exposure to a food or other substance containing traces of the antibiotic. The most common hypersensitivity reactions are rash, fever, and bronchospasm, followed

in frequency by vasculitis, serum sickness, and exfoliative dermatitis. Some patients develop severe erythema multiforme accompanied by headache, fever, arthralgia, and conjunctivitis (Stevens-Johnson syndrome); the most frequent cause of anaphylactic shock is an injection of penicillin.

penicillinase /pen'əsil'ənās/, an enzyme elaborated by certain bacteria, including many strains of staphylococci, that inactivates penicillin and thereby promotes resistance to the antibiotic. A purified preparation of penicillinase, derived from cultures of saprophytic, spore-forming *Bacillus cereus*, is used in the treatment of adverse reactions to penicillin. Also called **beta-lactamase.**

penicillinase-producing staphylococci, strains of staphylococcal organisms that elaborate the penicillininactivating enzyme penicillinase (beta-lactamase) and thereby resist the bactericidal action of the antibiotic.

penicillinase-resistant antibiotic, an antimicrobial agent that is not rendered inactive by penicillinase, an enzyme produced by certain bacteria, especially by strains of staphylococci. The semisynthetic penicillins, cloxacillin sodium, dicloxacillin sodium, methicillin sodium, nafcillin sodium, and oxacillin sodium, resist the action of penicillinase and are used in treating infections caused by staphylococci that elaborate the enzyme.

penicillinase-resistant penicillin, one of the semisynthetic penicillins derived from *Penicillium*, a genus of mold. Among these drugs are cloxacillin sodium, dicloxacillin sodium, methicillin sodium, nafcillin sodium, and oxacillin sodium. They are not inactivated by the enzyme penicillinase (beta-lactamase), which is produced by certain strains of staphylococci. These resistant antibiotics are used in treating infections caused by organisms that elaborate the enzyme.

penicillin G benzathine, a long-acting, depot form of penicillin.

■ INDICATIONS: It is used in the treatment of group A beta-hemolytic streptococcal pharyngitis, group A beta-hemolytic streptococcal pyoderma, and syphilitic infection occurring outside the central nervous system. It is given by deep intramuscular injection to achieve steady concentrations in the plasma and to slow systemic absorption from the repository in the muscle over a period of 12 hours to several days.

■ CONTRAINDICATIONS: Hypersensitivity to this drug or to other penicillins prohibits its use.

■ ADVERSE EFFECTS: The most serious adverse reaction is anaphylaxis. The most common side effects are maculopapular rash, urticarial rash, fever, bronchospasm, vasculitis, serum sickness, and exfoliative dermatitis.

penicillin G potassium, an antibacterial.

■ INDICATIONS: It is prescribed in the treatment of many infections, including syphilis, rheumatic fever, and glomerulonephritis.

■ CONTRAINDICATIONS: Known hypersensitivity to this drug or to any penicillin prohibits its use.

■ ADVERSE EFFECTS: Among the more serious adverse effects are allergic reactions that vary from minor skin rashes to anaphylaxis. Nausea and diarrhea occur frequently.

penicillin phenoxymethyl. See **penicillin V.**

penicillin V, an antibacterial.

■ INDICATION: It is prescribed in the treatment of susceptible infections.

■ CONTRAINDICATIONS: Known hypersensitivity to this drug or to any penicillin prohibits its use.

■ ADVERSE EFFECTS: Among the more serious adverse reactions are anaphylaxis and urticaria.

penicilliosis /pen'isil'ē·ō'sis/ [L, *penicillum* + Gk, *osis*, condition], pulmonary infection caused by fungi of the genus *Penicillium*.

Penicillium /pen'isil'ē·əm/ [L, *penicillum*, paintbrush], a genus of fungi, some species of which have been tentatively linked to disease in humans. Penicillin G is obtained from *Penicillium chrysogenum* and *P. notatum*.

penile /pē'nīl/ [L, penis], pertaining to the penis.

penile cancer /pē'nīl/ [L, *penis*, penis, *cancer*, crab], a rare malignancy of the penis occurring in uncircumcised men and associated with genital herpesvirus infection and poor personal hygiene. Smegma may be a causative factor, but the specific substance and mechanism are unknown. Leukoplakia or the flat-topped papules of balanitis xerotica obliterans may be premalignant lesions, and the velvety, red, painful papules of Queyrat's erythroplasia are penile squamous cell carcinoma in situ. Cancer of the penis usually presents as a local mass or a bleeding ulcer and metastasizes early in its course. Surgical treatment involves partial or total amputation of the penis and excision of inguinal nodes and adjacent tissue when necessary. Radiotherapy is often used preoperatively and postoperatively. Methotrexate or bleomycin also may be administered, especially in metastatic disease.

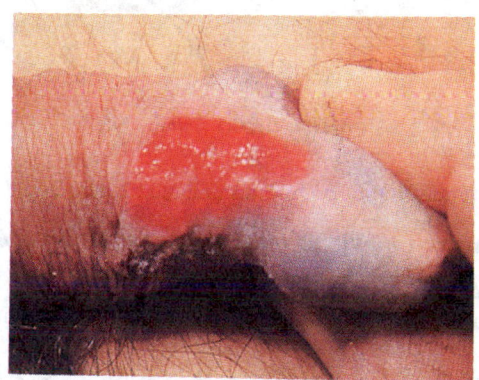

Penile cancer
(Seidel, 1991/Courtesy Patrick C Walsh, MD, The Johns Hopkins University School of Medicine, Baltimore)

penile prosthesis [L, *penis*; Gk, *prosthesis,* addition], a device that can be surgically implanted in the penis to treat impotence. Some such devices have mechanisms that control production of an erection. Penile implants may consist of inflatable plastic cavernosal cylinders attached to a fluid reservoir and a pump mechanism. The pump forces fluid into the cylinders to produce an erection.

penis /pē'nis/ [L, male sex organ], the external reproductive organ of a man, homologous with the clitoris of a woman. It is attached with ligaments to the front and sides of the pubic arch and is composed of three cylindrical masses of cavernous tissue covered with skin. The corpora cavernosa penis surrounds a median mass called the corpus spongiosum penis, which contains the greater part of the urethra. The subcutaneous fascia of the penis is directly continuous with that of the scrotum, which contains the testes.

penis envy, literally, female envy of the male penis, but generally a female wish for male attributes, position, and advantages. It is believed by some psychologists to be a significant factor in female personality development.

-pennate, a suffix meaning 'having feathers': *bipennate, pennate, unipennate.*

penniform /pen'ifôrm/ [L, *penna*, feather, *forma*, form], of or pertaining to the shape of a feather, especially the patterns of muscular fasciculi that correlate with the range of motion and the power of muscles. Penniform fasciculi converge on one side of certain tendons. Muscles with more fasciculi have greater power but less range of motion than muscles with fewer fasciculi. Compare **bipenniform, multipenniform.**

Penrose drain [Charles Bingham Penrose, American surgeon, b. 1862; AS, *draehen*, teardrop], a surgical drain device of gauze surrounded by rubber or other waterproof materials.

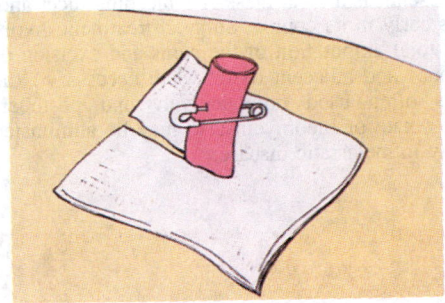

Penrose drain (Potter, 1993)

pent-, penta-, a prefix meaning 'five': *pentaploid, pentose, pentoside.*

pentadactyl /pen'tədak'til/ [Gk, *pente*, five, *daktylos*, fingers or toes], having five fingers per hand and five toes per foot.

pentaerythritol tetranitrate /pen'tə·erith'rətol/, a coronary vasodilator.

■ INDICATION: It is prescribed for the relief of angina pectoris.

■ CONTRAINDICATIONS: Known hypersensitivity to this drug prohibits its use. It is contraindicated in severe anemia, cerebral hemorrhage, and head injury.

■ ADVERSE EFFECTS: Among the most serious reactions are hypotension and allergic reactions. Headaches and flushing also may occur.

Pentam, a trademark for pentamidine isothionate, an antiprotozoal agent used in the treatment of pneumocystic pneumonia.

pentamidine, /pentam'idēn/, an antiprotozoal that is available only from the Centers for Disease Control. It is sometimes prescribed in the treatment of trypanosomiasis and leishmaniasis, but, because of its extreme toxicity, other agents are usually prescribed.

pentamidine isethionate a parenteral antiprotozoal drug.

■ INDICATIONS: It is prescribed in the treatment of pneumonia caused by *Pneumoncystis carinii*, particularly in patients who have AIDS.

■ CONTRAINDICATIONS: To reduce the risk of toxicity, the following tests must be carried out before, during, and after

therapy: BUN, serum creatinine, blood glucose, complete blood and platelet counts, liver function, serum calcium, and ECGs.

■ ADVERSE EFFECTS: Among adverse reactions are hypotension, hypoglycemia, leukopenia, thrombocytopenia, cardiac dysrhythmias, acute renal failure, hypocalcemia, Stevens-Johnson syndrome, elevated serum creatinine levels, elevated liver function results, pain or induration at the injection site, nausea, anorexia, fever, and rash.

Pentam 300, a trademark for a parenteral antiprotozoal drug used to treat pneumonia caused by *Pneumocystis carinii* (pentamidine isethionate).

pentaploid. See **polyploid.**

pentavalent /pəntav'ələnt/ [Gk, *pente*, five; L, *valere*, to have worth], **1.** a chemical radical or element that has a valency of five. **2.** pertaining to a body formed by the association of five chromosomes held together by chiasmata at the first division of meiosis.

pentazocine hydrochloride /pentā'zəsēn/, an agonist/antagonist narcotic analgesic.

■ INDICATION: It is prescribed for the relief of moderate to severe pain.

■ CONTRAINDICATIONS: Known hypersensitivity to this drug prohibits its use. It is administered with caution to patients with head injury or those with a history of drug abuse and dependency.

■ ADVERSE EFFECTS: Nausea and dizziness commonly occur. Other minor problems include constipation, hallucinations, euphoria, and drowsiness. High doses may cause respiratory and circulatory depression. This drug can precipitate acute withdrawal symptoms in narcotic-dependent individuals.

pentazocine lactate. See **pentazocine hydrochloride.**

Penthrane, a trademark for a general anesthetic (methoxyflurane).

Pentids, a trademark for an antibacterial (penicillin G potassium).

pentobarbital /pen'təbär'bitol/, a sedative and hypnotic.

■ INDICATIONS: It is prescribed as a preoperative sedative, in the treatment of insomnia, and in the control of acute convulsive disorders.

■ CONTRAINDICATIONS: Porphyria or known hypersensitivity to this drug or to other barbiturates prohibits its use. It is used with caution in patients having impaired respiratory or liver function or a history of dependence on sedative or hypnotic drugs.

■ ADVERSE EFFECTS: Among the more serious adverse reactions are respiratory or circulatory depression, paradoxical excitement, jaundice, or various hypersensitivity reactions. Nausea and hangover-like symptoms may be seen.

pentose /pen'tōs/ [Gk, *penta*, five; L, *osus*, having], a monosaccharide made of carbohydrate molecules, each containing five carbon atoms. It is produced by the body and is elevated after the ingestion of certain fruits, such as plums and cherries, and in certain rare diseases. It may be measured in the urine, where its normal concentrations after 24-hour collection are 2 to 5 mg/kg.

pentosuria /pen'təsŏŏr'ē·ə/ [Gk, *penta* + L, *osus*, having; Gk, *ouron*, urine], a rare condition in which pentose is found in the urine. Essential or idiopathic pentosuria is caused by a genetically transmitted error of metabolism.

Pentothal Sodium, a trademark for a barbiturate drug (thiopental sodium), used as a general anesthetic and as an anesthetic adjuvant.

pentoxifylline /pentok'sēfil'ēn/, an oral hemorrheologic drug.

■ INDICATIONS: It is prescribed for the treatment of intermittent claudication associated with chronic occlusive arterial limb disease.

■ CONTRAINDICATIONS: Patients with cardiovascular disorders should be closely monitored and their hypertensive dosage reduced if warranted. Patients on multiple drug regimens also should be closely monitored.

■ ADVERSE EFFECTS: Among the most serious adverse reactions are nausea, dyspepsia, dizziness, angina, dysrhythmias, and hypotension.

pentylenetetrazol /pen'tilē'nətet'rəzol/, a central nervous system stimulant.

■ INDICATIONS: It is prescribed as an analeptic to stimulate the respiratory, vagal, and vasomotor centers of the brain, to counter the effects of depressants, and to increase cerebral blood flow, especially in geriatric patients.

■ CONTRAINDICATIONS: Epilepsy and low convulsive threshold prohibit its use.

■ ADVERSE EFFECTS: Among the more serious adverse reactions are convulsion, confusion, and anorexia.

Pen-Vee K, a trademark for an antibacterial (penicillin V potassium).

Pepcid, a trademark for an antiulcer drug (famotidine).

Peplau, Hildegard E., a pioneer in nursing theory development and a proponent in the 1950s of the concept that nursing is an interpersonal process. Borrowing heavily from the knowledge base of psychology, Peplau proposed hypotheses based on the premise of the interpersonal process. From the early work evolved a nursing goal to foster the assumption that humans value, strive for, and have a right to independence. In a 1952 work, Peplau wrote that the nurse-patient relationship occurs in phases during which the nurse functions as a resource person, a counselor, and a surrogate. The four phases of the process were listed as orientation, identification, exploitation, and resolution. Thus the nurse assists in orientation when the patient with a need seeks help. Identification assures the patient that the nurse can understand the patient's situation. Exploitation begins when the patient uses the services available. Resolution is marked as old needs are met and newer ones emerge.

Pepper syndrome [William Pepper, American physician, b. 1874], a neuroblastoma of the adrenal glands that usually metastasizes to the liver.

pep pills, *slang.* amphetamines.

peps-, pept-, a prefix meaning 'of or pertaining to digestion': *pepsin, pepsiniferous, pepsitensin.*

-pepsia, -pepsy, -peptic, a suffix meaning 'pertaining to a state of the digestion': *anapepsia, colodyspepsia, oligopepsia, dyspeptic.*

pepsin /pep'sin/ [Gk, *pepsis,* digestion], an enzyme secreted in the stomach that catalyzes the hydrolysis of protein. Preparations of pepsin obtained from pork and beef stomachs are sometimes used as digestive aids. See also **enzyme, hydrolysis.**

pepsinogen /pəpsin'əjən/ [Gk, *pepsis + genein,* to produce], a zymogenic substance secreted by pyloric and gastric chief cells and converted to the enzyme pepsin in an acidic environment, as in the presence of hydrochloric acid produced in the stomach.

pepsinuria /pep'sinoōr'ē·ə/ [Gk, *pepsis,* digestion + *ouron,* urine], the presence of the pepsin enzyme in urine.

pept-. See **peps-.**

peptic [Gk, *peptein,* to digest], of or pertaining to digestion or to the enzymes and secretions essential to digestion.

-peptic, See **-pepsia.**

peptic ulcer /pep'tik/, a sharply circumscribed loss of the mucous membrane of the stomach, duodenum, or any other part of the GI system exposed to gastric juices containing acid and pepsin. Also called **gastric ulcer.**

■ OBSERVATIONS: Peptic ulcers may be acute or chronic. Acute lesions are almost always multiple and superficial. They may be totally asymptomatic and usually heal without scarring or other sequelae. Chronic ulcers are true ulcers: They are deep, single, persistent, and symptomatic; the muscular coat of the wall of the organ does not regenerate; a scar forms, marking the site, and the mucosa may heal completely. Peptic ulcers are caused by a combination of poorly understood factors, including an excessive secretion of gastric acid, inadequate protection of the mucous membrane, stress, heredity, and the taking of certain drugs, including the corticosteroids, certain antihypertensives, and antiinflammatory medications. Characteristically, ulcers cause a gnawing pain in the epigastrium that does not radiate to the back, is not aggravated by a change in position, and has a temporal pattern that mimics the diurnal rhythm of gastric acidity.

■ INTERVENTIONS: Symptomatic relief is provided with antacids and frequent, small, bland meals. The underlying cause is treated if known. Hemorrhage caused by perforation of the muscle and blood vessels may require surgical resection of the damaged area. The diagnosis and evaluation of peptic ulcers involve serial x-ray studies using a contrast medium, and endoscopy. A definitive diagnosis is important because the early signs of cancer of the stomach and duodenum are like those of peptic ulcers.

■ NURSING CONSIDERATIONS: The patient is reassured that in most cases the ulcers heal completely and that the pain may be controlled with simple measures. The nurse emphasizes the correct use of antacids and the other medications that have been prescribed. It is usually recommended that the patient eat frequent small meals consisting of foods known to be nonirritating. For many, but not all patients, fatty,

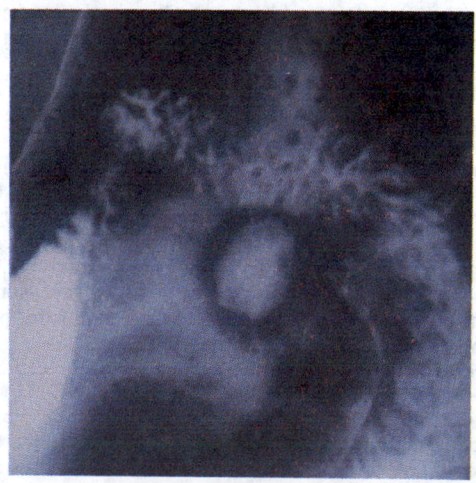

Peptic ulcer *(Mitros, 1988)*

highly spiced, heavy, or fibrous foods are likely to provoke pain. The use of tobacco and alcohol is discouraged.

peptidase /pep'tidās/ [Gk, *peptein*, to digest, *ase*, enzyme suffix], a protein-splitting enzyme that breaks peptides into amino acids. They occur naturally in plants, yeasts, certain microorganisms, and digestive juices.

peptide /pep'tīd/ [Gk, *peptein*, to digest], a molecular chain compound composed of two or more amino acids joined by peptide bonds. See also **amino acid, polypeptide, protein.**

peptone /pep'tōn/, a derived protein, which may be produced by hydrolysis of a native protein with an acid or enzyme.

per-, **1.** a prefix meaning 'throughout, or completely': *peracephalus, perfuse, permeable.* **2.** a prefix meaning 'a large amount (in chemical terms)' or to designate a combination of an element in its highest valence: *peracetate, peracid, perhydride.*

peracephalus /pur'əsef'ələs/, *pl.* **peracephali** [L, *per,* completely; Gk, *a, kephale,* not head], a fetus or individual with a malformed head.

per an., abbreviation for the Latin phrase *per annum,* 'yearly.'

perceived severity /pərsēvd'/ [L, *percipere,* to perceive; *severus,* serious], (in health belief model) a person's perception of the seriousness of the consequences of contracting a disease. Compare **perceived susceptibility.**

perceived susceptibility, (in health belief model) a person's perception of the likelihood of contracting a disease. Compare **perceived severity.**

percentage depth dose /pərsen'tij/ [L, *per,* completely, *centum,* hundred; ME, *dep,* deep; L, *dosis,* something given], (in radiotherapy) the amount of radiation delivered at a specified dose, expressed as a percentage of the skin dose.

percentile, the 100th part of a statistical distribution. A percentile rank of 80 indicates that 20% of the total number of cases scored above and 80% scored below in whatever characteristics were being studied.

percent solution, a relationship of a solute to a solvent, expressed in terms of weight of solute per weight of solution. An example of a true percent solution is 5 g of glucose dissolved in 95 g of water, forming 100 g of solution.

percent systole [L, *per, centum* + Gk, *systole,* contraction], an amount of time of each heartbeat that is devoted to the ejection of blood from the ventricle.

percept /pur'sept/ [L, *percipere,* to perceive], the mental impression of an object that is perceived through the use of the senses.

perception /pərsep'shən/ [L, *percipere,* to perceive], **1.** the conscious recognition and interpretation of sensory stimuli that serve as a basis for understanding, learning, and knowing or for the motivation of a particular action or reaction. **2.** the end result or product of the act of perceiving. Kinds of perception include **depth perception, extrasensory perception, facial perception,** and **stereognostic perception.** —**perceptive, perceptual,** *adj.*

perceptivity /pur'səptiv'itē/, the ability to receive sense impressions; perceptiveness.

perceptual constancy /pərsep'chōō·əl/ [L, *percipere,* to perceive; *cum,* together with, *stare,* to stand], in Gestalt psychology, the phenomenon in which an object is seen in the same way under varying circumstances.

perceptual defect, any of a broad group of disorders or dysfunctions of the central nervous system that interfere with the conscious mental recognition of sensory stimuli. Such conditions are caused by lesions at specific sites in the cerebral cortex that may result from any illness or trauma affecting the brain at any age or stage of development. Impairment of mental activity, cognitive processes, and emotional responses may be diffuse, as occurs in organic mental disorders, such as the psychoses, delirium, and dementia, and in attention deficit disorder, or they may be manifested focally, as in aphasia, apraxia, epilepsy, disorders of memory, cerebrovascular disorders, and various intercranial neoplasms.

perceptual deprivation, the absence of or decrease in meaningful groupings of stimuli, which may result from a constant background noise or constant inadequate illumination.

perceptual monotony, a mental state characterized by a lack of variety in the normal pattern of everyday stimuli.

perchloromethane. See **carbon tetrachloride.**

Percodan, a trademark for a central nervous system, fixed-combination drug containing narcotic analgesics (oxycodone hydrochloride and oxycodone terephthalate) and aspirin.

Percogesic, a trademark for a fixed-combination drug containing an antihistaminic (phenyltoloxamine citrate) and an analgesic (acetaminophen).

percolation /pur'kəlā'shən/ [L, *percolare,* to strain], **1.** the act of filtering any liquid through a porous medium. **2.** (in pharmacology) the removal of the soluble parts of a crude drug by passing a liquid solvent through it.

per con., abbreviation for the Latin phrase, *per contra,* 'the other side.'

Percorten, a trademark for an adrenocortical steroid (desoxycorticosterone acetate).

percuss /pərkus'/ [L, *percutere,* to strike through], to perform percussion by striking the thoracic or abdominal wall, thereby producing sound vibrations that aid in diagnosis.

percussion /pərkush'ən/ [L, *percutere,* to strike hard], a technique in physical examination of tapping the body with the fingertips to evaluate the size, borders, and consistency

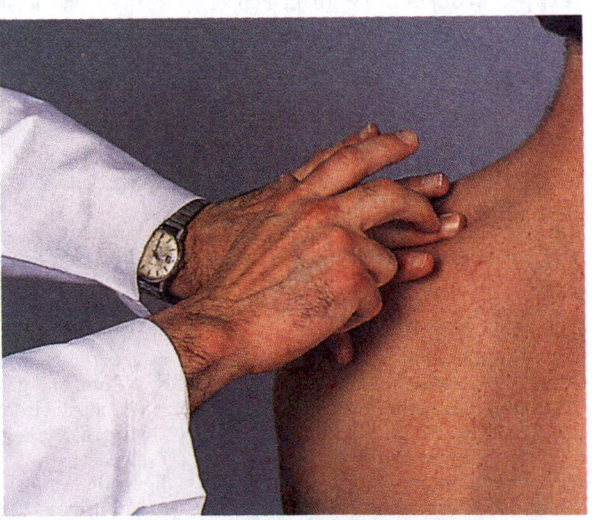

Indirect percussion technique *(Seidel, 1991)*

of some of the internal organs and to discover the presence and evaluate the amount of fluid in a cavity of the body. **Immediate** or **direct percussion** refers to percussion performed by striking the fingers directly on the body surface; **indirect, mediate,** or **finger percussion** involves striking a finger of one hand on a finger of the other hand as it is placed over the organ. See also **cupping and vibrating, percussor, pleximeter.** –**percuss,** v., **percussable,** adj.

percussor /pərkus'ər/ [L, a striker], a small, hammerlike diagnostic tool having a rubber head that is used to tap the body lightly in percussion. Also called **plexor.** See also **percussion.**

percutaneous /pur'kyōōtā'nē·əs/ [L, per + cutis, skin], performed through the skin, such as a biopsy, the aspiration of fluid from a space below the skin using a needle, catheter, and syringe, or the instillation of a fluid in a cavity or space by similar means.

graphic examination of the structure of the bile ducts. A needle is passed directly into a hepatic duct after which a contrast medium is injected.

percutaneous transluminal coronary angioplasty (PTCA), a technique in the treatment of atherosclerotic coronary heart disease and angina pectoris in which some plaques in the arteries of the heart are flattened against the arterial walls, resulting in improved circulation. The procedure involves threading a catheter through the vessel to the atherosclerotic plaque and inflating and deflating a small balloon at the tip of the catheter several times, then removing the catheter. The procedure is performed under x-ray or ultrasonic visualization. When it is successful, the plaques remain compressed and the symptoms of heart disease, including the pain of angina, are decreased. The alternative to this treatment is coronary bypass surgery, which is more expensive and dangerous and requires longer hospitalization.

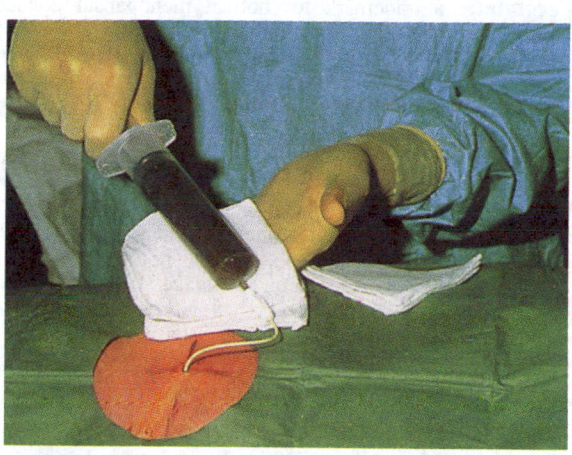

Percutaneous aspiration (Winawer, 1992)

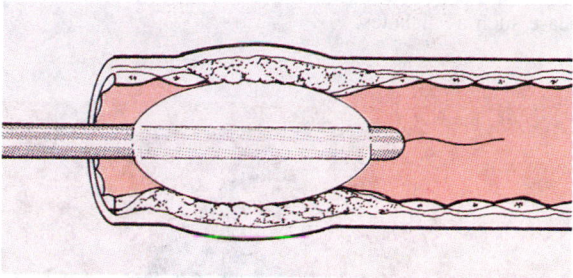

Percutaneous transluminal coronary angioplasty
(Canobbio, 1990)

percutaneous absorption, the process of absorption through the skin from topical application.

percutaneous catheter placement, (in arteriography) the technique in which an intracatheter is introduced through the skin into an artery and placed at the site or structure to be studied. The puncture site is infiltrated with a local anesthetic. A special needle is inserted into the artery, and a long, flexible spring guide is passed through the needle for approximately 15 cm. The needle is then removed, the catheter is advanced to the desired position, and the guide is withdrawn. Selective angiography and other diagnostic procedures are performed using this technique. The catheter is withdrawn at the end of the procedure.

percutaneous nephrolithotomy, a uroradiologic procedure performed to extract stones from within the kidney or proximal ureter by percutaneous surgery after the stones have been visualized radiologically.

percutaneous nephroscope, a thin fiberoptics probe that can be inserted into the kidney through an incision in the skin. Light transmitted along the fibers allows visualization of the inside of the kidney. The device is equipped with a tool that can be used to grasp and remove small stones.

percutaneous transhepatic cholangiography, a radio-

per diem rate /pər dē'əm, dī'əm/ [L, per diem, daily, ratus, reckoned], an established rate of payment for hospital services determined by dividing the total cost of providing routine inpatient services for a given period by the total number of inpatient days of care during the period.

Perez reflex /pərez', per'ez/ [Bernard Perez, French physician, b. 1836; L, reflectere, to bend backward], the normal response of an infant to cry, flex the limbs, and elevate the head and pelvis when supported in a prone position with a finger pressed along the spine from the sacrum to the neck. Persistence of the reflex beyond the age of 6 months may indicate brain damage.

perfectionism /pərfek'shəniz'əm/ [L, perficere, to complete], a subjective state in which a person pursues an impossibly high standard of performance and, in many cases, demands the same standards of others. Failure to attain the goals leads to feelings of defeat and other adverse psychologic consequences.

perfloxacin /pərflok'səsin/, an antibiotic of the carboxyfluoroquinolone type.

perfluorocarbons /pərflōōr'ōkär'bəns/, a group of chemicals somewhat capable of performing the function of hemoglobin in red blood cells by transporting oxygen through the circulatory system. They can be used for certain blood substitute purposes, regardless of the blood type of the patient, are stable at room temperatures, have a pH of 7.4, and are free of infectious pathogens. The blood substitute is an emulsion of perfluorodecalin and perfluorotripropylamine. Also called **artificial blood.**

perforans /pur'fôrənz/ [L, *perforare*, piercing through], penetrating. The term applies mainly to nerves, muscles, or other anatomic features that penetrate other structures, such as **perforans gasseri,** or nerves of the musculocutaneous tissues.

perforate [L, *perforare*, to pierce], **1.** /pur'fôrāt/ to pierce, punch, puncture, or otherwise make a hole. **2.** /pur'fôrit/ riddled with small holes. **3.** /pur'fôrit/ (of the anus) having a normal opening; not imperforate. **—perforation,** *n.*

perforating fracture, an open fracture caused by a projectile, making a small surface wound. See **Bezold's perforation.**

perforating ulcer /pur'fôrā'ting/ [L, *perforare*, to pierce through; *ilcus*], **1.** an ulcer that penetrates the thickness of a wall or membrane, such as a peptic ulcer of the digestive tract. **2.** a deep, painless ulcer, often on the sole of the foot, of a person whose skin is insensitive because of a disease such as diabetes.

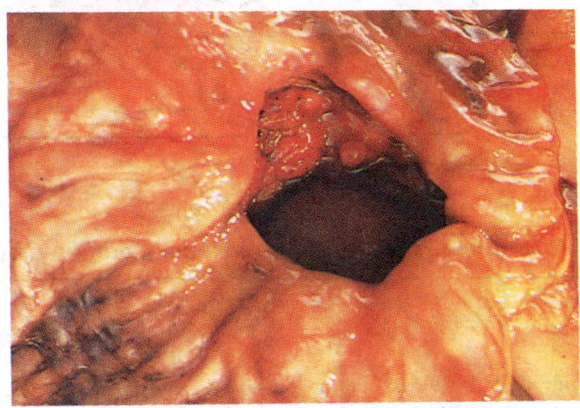

Perforating gastric ulcer *(Fletcher, 1987)*

perforation /pur'fôrā'shən/ [L, *perforare*, to pierce through], a hole or opening made through the entire thickness of a membrane or other tissue or material.

perforation of stomach or intestines, a condition in which disease or injury has resulted in a leakage of digestive tract contents into the peritoneal cavity. A common cause is a ruptured appendix or perforating peptic ulcer. Immediate surgical intervention is needed to prevent peritonitis.

perforation of the uterus, an accidental puncture of the uterus, as may occur with a curet or by an intrauterine contraceptive device.

perfusion /pərfyōō'zhən/ [L, *perfundere*, to pour over], **1.** the passage of a fluid through a specific organ or an area of the body. **2.** a therapeutic measure whereby a drug intended for an isolated part of the body is introduced via the bloodstream.

perfusionist /pərfyōō'zhənist/ [L, *perfundere*, to pour

over], an allied health professional who assists in performing procedures that involve extracorporeal circulation, such as during open-heart surgery, or hypothermia.

perfusion lung scan, a radiographic examination of the lungs and their function, performed after an intravenous injection of a contrast medium, such as radioactive albumin, and used to aid in the diagnosis of pulmonary embolism.

perfusion rate, the rate of blood flow through the capillaries per unit mass of tissue, expressed in ml/minute per 100 g.

perfusion scan. See **lung scan.**

perfusion technologist, a person who, under the supervision of a physician, operates a heart-lung machine used for cardiopulmonary bypass during surgery.

per gene, a segment of nucleic acid that is associated with circadian rhythms of some animal species. Mutations of the per gene locus result in alterations of their biorhythms. A similar DNA sequence occurs in human genes, but it is not known whether it affects human circadian rhythms.

Pergonal, a trademark for human menopausal gonadotropin used to treat anovulation and infertility.

peri- /per'i-/, a prefix meaning 'around': *periaxial, pericardial, pericolitis.*

Periactin, a trademark for an antihistaminic and antipruritic (cyproheptadine hydrochloride).

perianal /per'i·ā'nəl/ [Gk, *peri*, near + L, *anus*], located around the anus.

perianal abscess [Gk, *peri*, around; L, *anus, abscedere*, to go away], a focal, purulent, subcutaneous infection in the region of the anus. Treatment includes hot soaks, antibiotics, and, possibly, incision and drainage. If a rectal fistula or perianal space is found to be the cause of recurrent perianal abscesses, surgical excision is usually performed.

periaortic /per'i·ā·ôr'tik/ [Gk, *peri*, near + *aerein*, to raise], pertaining to the area around the aorta.

periapical /per'i·ap'ikəl/ [Gk, *peri* + L, *apex*, top], of or pertaining to the tissues around the apex of a tooth, including the periodontal membrane and the alveolar bone.

periapical abscess, an infection around the root of a tooth, usually a result of spread from dental caries. The abscess may extend into nearby bone, causing osteomyelitis, or, more often, it may spread to soft tissues, causing cellulitis and a swollen face, or it may perforate into the oral cavity or maxillary sinus. There may be associated fever, malaise, and nausea. Treatment includes drilling into the pulp of the tooth to establish drainage and relieve pain, followed by antibiotics and later root canal therapy or tooth extraction.

periapical cyst. See **radicular cyst.**

periapical fibroma, a mass of benign connective tissue that may form at the apex of a tooth with normal pulp.

periapical infection, infection surrounding the root of a tooth, often accompanied by toothache.

periapical radiograph, a dental x-ray used to detect changes in the bone support surrounding the roots of the teeth.

periappendicular /per'i·ap'əndik'yələr/ [Gk, *peri*, near + L, *appendere*, to hang upon], pertaining to the area around the appendix.

periarterial /per'i·ärtir'ē·əl/ [Gk, *peri*, near + *arteria*], pertaining to the area around an artery.

periarteritis /per'i·är'tərī'tis/ [Gk, *peri* + *arteria*, air pipe, *itis*], an inflammatory condition of the outer coat of one or more arteries and the tissue surrounding the vessel. Kinds of periarteritis are **periarteritis nodosa** and **syphilitic peri-arteritis.**

periarteritis gummosa.   See **syphilitic periarteritis.**

periarteritis nodosa,   a progressive, polymorphic disease of the connective tissue that is characterized by numerous large and palpable nodules or clusters of visible nodules along segments of middle-sized arteries, particularly near points of bifurcation. This process causes occlusion of vessels, resulting in regional ischemia, hemorrhage, necrosis, and pain. The early signs of the disease include tachycardia, fever, weight loss, and pain in the viscera. Kidney, lung, and intestinal involvement are common. Other systems and organs of the body also may be affected. Periarteritis nodosa is treated with corticosteroids and cytotoxic drugs.

periarticular /per'i·ärtik'yələr/ [Gk, *peri*, near + L, *articulus*, joint],   pertaining to the area around a joint.

peribronchiolar /-brong'kē·ō'lər/ [Gk, *peri*, near + *bronchiolus*],   pertaining to the area around the bronchioles.

pericardiac /-kär'dē·ak/ [Gk, *peri*, near + *kardia*, heart], **1.** pertaining to the pericardium. **2.** pertaining to the area around the heart. Also spelled **pericardial.**

pericardial adhesion /-kär'dē·əl/ [Gk, *peri*, near + *kardia*, heart; L, *adhesio*, sticking to],   an adhesion of the pericardium to the heart muscle, sometimes restricting action of the heart muscle. In some cases, a previous inflammation or surgery may result in dense fibrous adhesions that obliterate the pericardium. The condition may be general or localized and may involve adhesion between the two layers of pericardium, *internal adhesive pericarditis,* or between one layer and surrounding tissues, *external adhesive pericarditis.* Also called **adherent pericarditis.**

pericardial artery [Gk, *peri* + *kardia,* heart, *arteria,* air pipe],   one of several small vessels branching from the thoracic aorta, supplying the dorsal surface of the pericardium.

pericardial effusion [Gk, *peri,* near + *kardia,* heart; L, *effundere,* to pour out],   a collection of blood or other fluid into the pericardium.

pericardial friction rub [Gk, *peri,* near + *kardia,* heart; L, *fricare,* to rub; ME, *rubben*],   the rubbing together of inflamed membranes of the pericardium, as may occur in pericarditis, or after a myocardial infarction, producing a sound audible on auscultation.

pericardial rub.   See **pericardial friction rub.**

pericardial tamponade.   See **cardiac tamponade.**

pericardiocentesis /per'ikär'dē·ō'sintē'sis/ [Gk, *peri* + *kardia,* heart, *kentesis,* pricking],   a procedure for drawing fluid in the pericardial space between the serous membranes by surgical puncture and aspiration of the pericardial sac. Also called **pericardicentesis.**

pericarditis /per'ikärdī'tis/ [Gk, *peri* + *kardia,* heart, *itis*], an inflammation of the pericardium associated with trauma, malignant neoplastic disease, infection, uremia, myocardial infarction, collagen disease, or idiopathic causes.

■ OBSERVATIONS: Two stages are observed if treatment in the first stage does not halt progress of the condition to the extremely grave second stage. The first stage is characterized by fever, substernal chest pain that radiates to the shoulder or neck, dyspnea, and a dry, nonproductive cough. On examination a rapid and forcible pulse, a pericardial friction rub, and a muffled heartbeat over the apex are noted. The patient becomes increasingly anxious, tired, and orthopneic. During the second stage, a serofibrinous effusion develops within the pericardium, restricting cardiac activity; the heart

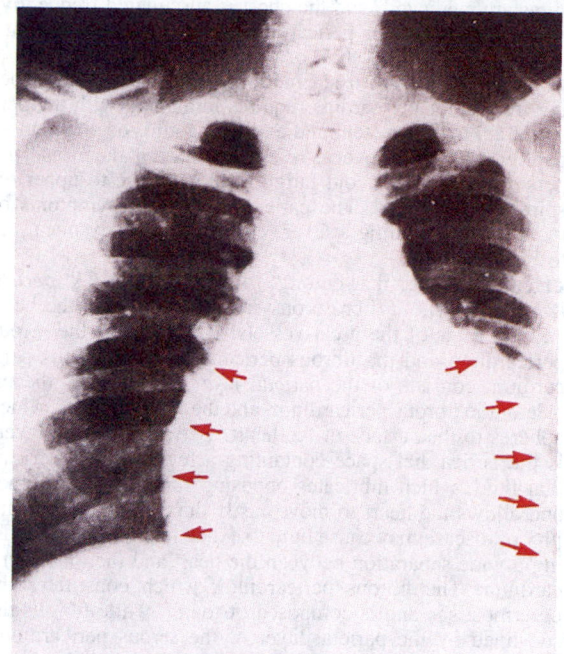

Pericardial effusion (*Guzzetta, 1992*)

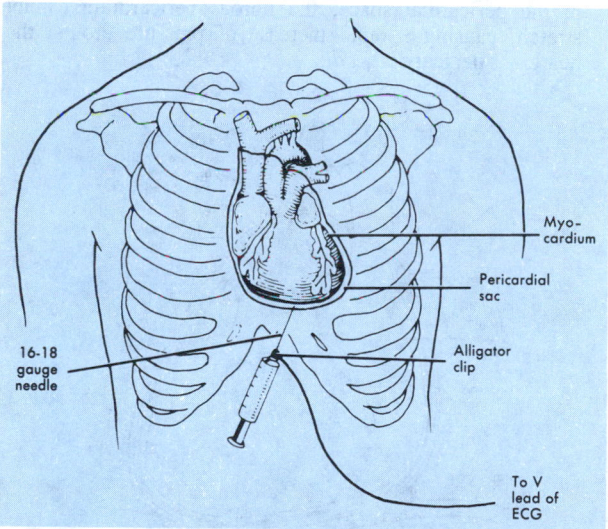

Pericardiocentesis

sounds become muffled, weak, and distant on auscultation. A bulge is visible on the chest over the precordial area. If the effusion is purulent, caused by bacterial infection, a high fever, sweat, chills, and prostration also occur.

■ INTERVENTIONS: The person is kept in bed, and the head of the bed is elevated 45 degrees to decrease dyspnea. Hypothermia treatment may be necessary to reduce the temperature. An antibiotic or antifungal and analgesic may be ordered. Oxygen and parenteral fluids are usually given, vital signs are evaluated, and the chest is auscultated frequently. Pericardiocentesis or pericardiotomy may be performed to remove accumulated fluid or to make a diagnosis.

■ NURSING CONSIDERATIONS: Emotional support of a patient being treated for pericarditis requires remaining with the person if anxiety is present and explaining all procedures thoroughly. During recovery, rest periods are planned and the person is urged to avoid fatigue and exposure to upper respiratory infections. The patient is told that symptoms of recurrence, including a fever, chest pain, and dyspnea, are to be reported.

pericardium /per′ikär′dē·əm/, *pl.* **pericardia** [Gk, *peri* + *kardia*, heart], a fibroserous sac that surrounds the heart and the roots of the great vessels. It consists of the serous pericardium and the fibrous pericardium. The serous pericardium consists of the parietal layer, which lines the inside of the fibrous pericardium, and the visceral layer, which adheres to the surface of the heart. Between the two layers is the pericardial space containing a few drops of pericardial fluid, which lubricates opposing surfaces of the space and allows the heart to move easily during contraction. Injury or disease may cause fluid to exude into the space, causing a wide separation between the heart and the outer pericardium. The fibrous pericardium, which constitutes the outermost sac and is composed of tough, white fibrous tissue lined by the parietal layer of the serous pericardium, fits loosely around the heart and attaches to large blood vessels emerging from the top of the heart but not to the heart itself. It is relatively inelastic and protects the heart and the serous membranes. If pericardial fluid or pus accumulates in the pericardial space, the fibrous pericardium cannot stretch, causing a rapid increase of pressure around the heart. **–pericardial,** *adj.*

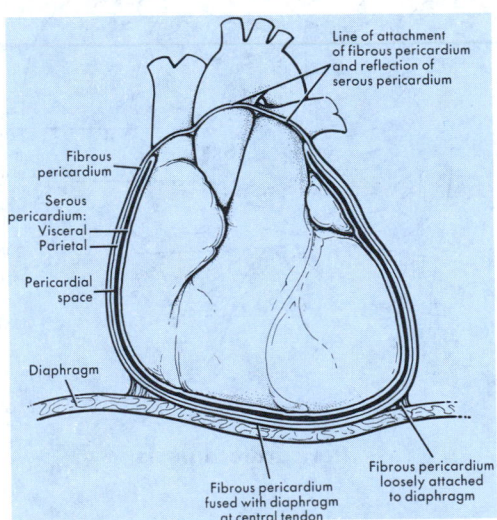

Pericardium

pericholangitis /per′əkō′lanjī′tis/ [Gk, *peri* + *chole*, bile, *aggeion*, vessel, *itis*, inflammation], an inflammatory condition of the tissues surrounding the bile ducts in the liver. Pericholangitis is a complication of ulcerative colitis and portal hypertension. Treatment of the ulcerative colitis has little effect on the liver disease. See also **ulcerative colitis.**

perichondrial bone /-kon′drē·əl/ [Gk, *peri*, near + *chondros*, cartilage; AS, *ban*], bone that forms in the perichondrium of the cartilaginous template. Also called **chondrial bone, periosteal bone.**

pericoronitis /-kôr′ənī′tis/, an inflammation of the gingival flap (gum tissue) around the crown of a tooth, usually associated with the eruption of a third molar. Treatment depends on the severity of the condition and may include the use of antibiotics or extraction of the tooth. In most cases the inflammation subsides after the tooth has fully erupted.

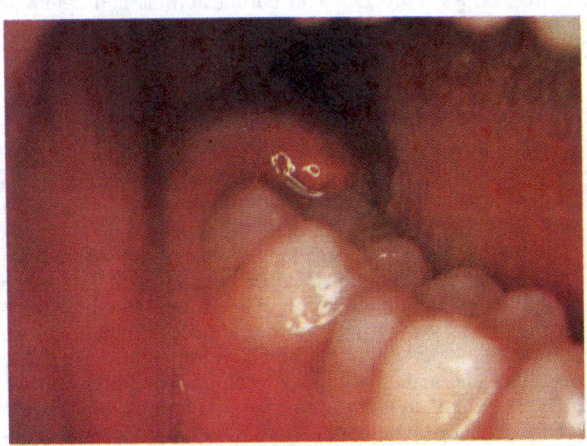

Pericoronitis (Lamey, 1988)

peridural anesthesia. See **epidural anesthesia.**

perifollicular /-folik′yələr/ [Gk, *peri*, near + L, *folliculus*, small bag], pertaining to the area around a follicle.

perifolliculitis /-folik′yəlī′tis/ [Gk, *peri* + L, *folliculus*, small bag; Gk, *itis*], inflammation of the tissue surrounding a hair follicle. Compare **folliculitis.**

perikaryon /per′iker′ē·on/ [Gk, *peri* + *karyon*, nut], the cytoplasm of a cell body exclusive of the nucleus and any processes, specifically the cell body of a neuron. **–perikaryontic,** *adj.*

perilymph /per′ilimf/ [Gk, *peri* + L, *lympha*, water], the clear fluid separating the osseous labyrinth from the membranous labyrinth in the internal ear. Compare **endolymph.**

perimeter /pərim′ətər/ [Gk, *peri*, near + *metron*, measure], **1.** the circumference, outer edge, or periphery of an object. **2.** an instrument for measuring visual fields. **3.** an instrument for measuring the circumference of teeth.

perimetrium /per′imē′trē·əm/ [Gk, *peri* + *metra*, womb], the serous membrane enveloping the uterus.

perinatal /per′inā′təl/ [Gk, *peri* + L, *natus*, birth], of or pertaining to the time and process of giving birth or being born.

perinatal AIDS, AIDS acquired by infants and children from their mothers during pregnancy, during delivery, or from ingesting infected breast milk. See **acquired immunodeficiency syndrome (AIDS).**

perinatal asphyxia. See **asphyxia neonatorum.**

perinatal death, **1.** the death of a fetus weighing more than 1000 g at 28 or more weeks of gestation. **2.** the death of an infant between birth and the end of the neonatal period.

perinatal mortality, the statistical rate of fetal and infant death, including stillbirths, from 28 weeks of gestation to the end of the neonatal period of 4 weeks after birth. Perinatal mortality is usually expressed as the number of deaths per 1000 live births in a specific geographic area or program in a given period of time.

perinatal period, a period extending approximately from the twenty-eighth week of gestation to the twenty-eighth day after birth.

perinatal physiology, the physiology of the process of giving birth or being born.

perinatologist /-nātol′əjəst/, a physician who specializes in the practice of perinatology.

perinatology /-nātol′əgē/ [Gk, *peri* + L, *natus,* birth; Gk, *logos,* science], a branch of medicine concerned with the study of the anatomy and physiology of the mother and her unborn and newborn infant and with the diagnosis and treatment of disorders occurring in them during pregnancy, childbirth, and the puerperium. **–perinatologic, perinatological,** *adj.*

perineal /per′inē′əl/ [Gk, *perineos,* perineum], pertaining to the perineum.

perineal body [Gk, *perineos,* perineum; AS, *bodig*], a mass of tissue composed of muscle and fascia between the vagina and rectum in females and between the urethra and rectum in males.

perineal care [Gk, *perineos,* perineum], a cleansing procedure prescribed for cleansing the perineum after various obstetric and gynecologic procedures. Sterile or clean perineal care may be prescribed.

■ METHOD: In the sterile procedure, the cleansing strokes always move from the vulva toward the anus and from the midline out. After each stroke, the disposable washcloth or pledget is discarded, and a new one is used for the next stroke. In sterile perineal care, a sterile basin, gloves, forceps, pledgets, and pitcher or measure containing solution are used. The draped patient is assisted into position on her back with a bedpan or a disposable pad beneath her buttocks, and 200 to 300 ml of solution is poured over the vulva. Then pledgets moistened with the solution are used to cleanse the area more thoroughly. The pledgets are held with sterile forceps or a sterile gloved hand. The area is dried using sterile pledgets, and the bedpan is removed. The patient then changes position and lies on her side for cleansing and drying of the posterior area; strokes should always move away from the perineal area. In providing clean perineal care, disposable washcloths, soap, and a basin or a squeeze bottle of warm water are used. A fresh, disposable washcloth is used for each stroke. The strokes are always from anterior to posterior. Soap may be used. A fresh pad or cloth is used to remove the soap and for each drying stroke. The patient then rolls to one side, and the posterior area is cleansed and dried in the same way.

■ NURSING INTERVENTION: Perineal care is given at prescribed intervals and after urination and defecation.

■ OUTCOME CRITERIA: Sterile and clean perineal care are practiced to remove secretions or dried blood from a wound and to avoid contaminating the urethral and vaginal areas or perineal wounds with fecal matter or urine.

perineal dislocation. See **dislocation of hip.**

perineal pad [Gk, *perineos,* perineum], a cushion of soft

material used to cover the perineum to absorb the menstrual flow or to protect a wound or incision.

perineo- [Gk, *perineos*], a combining form meaning 'related to the perineum': *perineostomy.*

perineorrhaphy /per′inē·ôr′əfē/ [Gk, *perineos* + *rhaphe,* suture], a surgical procedure in which an incision, tear, or defect in the perineum is repaired by suturing.

perineotomy /per′inē·ot′əmē/ [Gk, *perineos* + *temnein,* to cut], a surgical incision into the perineum. See also **episiotomy.**

perinephric abscess /-nef′rik/ [Gk, *peri,* near + *nephros,* kidney; L, *abscedere,* to go away], an abscess that develops in the fatty tissue around a kidney. It is usually secondary to an abscess originating earlier in the cortex of the organ. Also called **perinephritic abscess.**

perineum /per′inē′əm/ [Gk, *perineos*], the part of the body situated dorsal to the pubic arch and the arcuate ligaments, ventral to the tip of the coccyx, and lateral to the inferior rami of the pubis and the ischium and the sacrotuberous ligaments. The perineum supports and surrounds the distal portions of the urogenital and GI tracts of the body. In the female, the central fibrous perineal body is larger than in the male, and the bulbospongiosus, which is a sphincter around the orifice of the vagina and a cover over the clitoris, does not exist in the male perineum. In men and women, the muscles are innervated by the perineal branch of the pudendal nerve. **–perineal,** *adj.*

perinodal fibers /-nō′dəl/ [Gk, *peri* + L, *nodus,* knot], the atrial fibers surrounding the sinoatrial node.

period. See **menses.**

periodic /pir′ē·od′ik/ [Gk, *peri* + *hodos,* way], (of an event or phenomenon) recurring at regular or irregular intervals. **–periodicity,** *n.*

periodic apnea of the newborn, a normal condition in the full-term newborn infant characterized by an irregular pattern of rapid breathing followed by a brief period of apnea, usually associated with rapid eye movement (REM) sleep. Apnea in the newborn not associated with REM sleep or with periodic breathing is ominous because it is symptomatic of intracranial bleeding, seizure activity, infection, pneumonia, hypoglycemia, drug depression, or various cardiac defects. See also **sudden infant death syndrome.**

periodic breathing. See **Cheyne-Stokes respiration.**

periodic deep inspiration, (in respiratory therapy) periodic deep forced inspiration of compressed gas or air in controlled ventilation. Many ventilators can be set to provide a selected number of deep respirations each hour. The process helps prevent atelectasis. Also called **sigh.**

periodic fever [Gk, *peri,* near + *hodos,* way; L, *febris*], **1.** a hereditary illness affecting mainly Sephardic Jews, Armenians, and Arabs with intermittent episodes of fever accompanied by abdominal or pleuritic pain. Age of onset is between 10 and 20 years. Some cases are complicated by symptoms of arthritis, splenomegaly, and renal amyloidosis that may progress to a fatal kidney disorder. **2.** a common name for **familial Mediterranean fever.**

periodic hyperinflation, a normal phenomenon of an unconscious sighing or deep breathing. The involuntary act tends to occur most frequently during periods of physical inactivity. Because of the natural need for periodic hyperinflation of the lungs, an artificial sigh is often programmed into the mechanism of mechanical ventilators. See also **periodic deep inspiration.**

periodicity /pir′ē·ədis′itē/ [Gk, *periodikos,* periodical], events or episodes that tend to repeat at predictable intervals, such as filarial worms that appear in cutaneous blood vessels at night but not in daylight hours and types of malaria that cause paroxysms at 24-, 48-, or 72-hour intervals, depending on the species of pathogen.

periodic table, a systematic arrangement of the chemical elements, devised in 1869 by Dmitry Ivanovich Mendeleyev (Russian chemist, 1834-1907). By arranging the elements in order of their atomic weights, he was able to show relationships, such as valency, that occurred at regular intervals and was able to predict the properties of elements still undiscovered in the nineteenth century.

periodontal /per'ē·ōdon'təl/ [Gk, *peri* + *odous*, tooth], of or pertaining to the area around a tooth, such as the periodontium.

periodontal abscess [Gk, *peri*, near + *odous*, tooth; L, *abscedere*, to go away], a localized collection of inflammatory material, including pus, in the periodontal tissue. It is usually classified according to its location in the periodontal pocket, such as lateral alveolar, parietal, peridental, or lateral.

periodontal cyst, an epithelium-lined sac that contains fluid, most often occurring at the apex of a pulp-involved tooth. Periodontal cysts that occur lateral to a tooth root are less common.

periodontal disease, disease of the tissues around a tooth, such as an inflammation of the periodontal membrane or periodontal ligament.

periodontal ligament (PDL), the fibrous tissue that attaches the teeth to the alveoli, composed of many bundles of collagenous tissue arranged in groups between which is loose connective tissue interwoven with blood vessels, lymph vessels, and nerves. The periodontal ligament invests and supports the teeth.

periodontal pocket [Gk, *peri*, near + *odous*, tooth; Fr, *pochette*], a pathological increase in the depth of the gingival crevice or sulcus surrounding the tooth at the gingival margin. Kinds of periodontal pockets include: **gingival, infrabony, intrabony, intraalveolar, relative, simple, subcrestal, suprabony, supracrestal.**

periodontal probe [Gk, *peri*, near + *odous*, tooth; L, *probare*, to test], a slender instrument with identations spaced in millimeters designed for introduction into the gingival sulcus for the purpose of measuring its depth around the tooth.

periodontics /-don'tiks/ [Gk, *peri*, near + *odous*, tooth], a branch of dentistry concerned with the diagnosis, treatment, and prevention of diseases of the periodontium. Also called **periodontia, periodontology.**

periodontist /-don'tist/, a dentist who specializes in periodontics.

periodontitis /per'ē·ō'dontī'tis/, inflammation of the periodontium, which includes the periodontal ligament, the gingiva, and the alveolar bone. See also **periodontal, periodontal disease, periodontics.**

periodontoclasia [Gk, *peri* + *odous*, tooth, *klasis*, breaking], the loosening of permanent teeth because of breakdown and absorption of the supporting bone.

periodontology. See **periodontics.**

periodontosis /-dontō'sis/ [Gk, *peri* + *odous*, tooth, *osis*, condition], a rare disease that affects young people, especially women, and is characterized by idiopathic destruction of the periodontium.

perioperative /per'i·op'ərətiv/ [Gk, *peri*, near + L, oper-

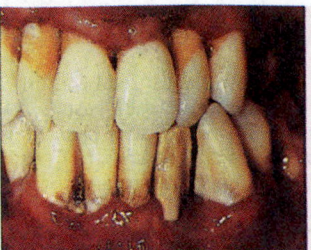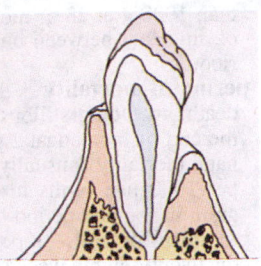

Advanced periodontitis *(Murray, 1990)*

ari, to work], pertaining to the time of the surgery. Also **paraoperative.**

perioperative nursing [Gk, *peri* + L, *operari*, to work, *nutrix*, nurse], nursing care provided surgery patients during the entire inpatient period, from admission to date of discharge.

periorbita /per'i·ôr'bitə/ [Gk, *peri* + L, *orbita*, wheel mark], the periosteum of the orbit of the eye. It is continuous with the dura mater and the sheath of the optic nerve and extends a process at the margin of the orbit to form the orbital septum. The periorbita is loosely connected to the bones of the orbit, from which it can be easily detached.

periorbital /per'i·ôr'bitəl/, pertaining to the area surrounding the socket of the eye.

periosteal /per'i·os'tē·əl/ [Gk, *peri* near + *osteon* bone], pertaining to the periosteum, the membrane covering the bone.

periosteal bone. See **perichondrial bone.**

periosteum /per'i·os'tē·əm/ [Gk, *peri* + *osteon*, bone], a fibrous vascular membrane covering the bones, except at their extremities. It consists of an outer layer of collagenous tissue containing a few fat cells and an inner layer of fine elastic fibers. Periosteum is permeated with the nerves and blood vessels that innervate and nourish underlying bone. The membrane is thick and markedly vascular over young bones but thinner and less vascular in later life. Bones that lose periosteum through injury or disease usually scale or die.

periostitis /per'i·ostī'tis/ [Gk, *peri* + *osteon*, bone, *itis*], inflammation of the periosteum. The condition is caused by chronic or acute infection or trauma and is characterized by tenderness and swelling of the bone affected, pain, fever, and chills. In severe cases blood or an albuminous serous exudate forms under the membrane. In syphilitic infections, periostitis may occur as an early symptom.

peripatetic /-pətet'ik/ [Gk, *peripatein*, to walk about], pertaining to an ambulatory patient.

peripheral /pərif'ərəl/ [Gk, *periphereia*, circumference], of or pertaining to the outside, surface, or surrounding area of an organ, other structure, or field of vision.

peripheral acrocyanosis of the newborn, a normal, transient condition of the newborn, characterized by pale cyanotic discoloration of the hands and feet, especially the fingers and toes. The blueness fades as the baby begins to breathe easily but returns if the baby is allowed to get chilled.

peripheral angiography [Gk, *peri*, around + *phereia*, boundary, *aggeion*, vessel, *graphein*, to record], the study of the peripheral blood vessels by radiography after an opaque dye has been injected into the circulation.

peripheral arteriovenography, an x-ray examination of the blood vessels in the peripheral parts of the body, such as the arms and legs, after the injection of a contrast medium into these vessels.

peripheral device, any hardware device aside from the central processing unit, such as a printer, CRT, or drive.

peripheral glioma. See **schwannoma.**

peripheral lesion [Gk, *perphereia*; L, *laesio,* hurting], an injury to any tissues distal to the main organ systems. A peripheral nerve lesion is usually traumatic and interrupts the flow of impulses between the site of the lesion and the nerve root or plexus.

peripheral motor neuron [Gk, *periphereia*; L, *motor,* mover; Gk, *neuron,* nerve], an effector neuron located outside the central nervous system, usually in a ganglion of a sympathetic or parasympathetic nervous system.

peripheral neurovascular dysfunction, high risk for, a nursing diagnosis accepted by the Tenth National Conference on the Classification of Nursing Diagnoses. High risk for peripheral neurovascular dysfunction is defined as a state in which an individual is at risk of experiencing a disruption in circulation, sensation, or motion of an extremity. Risk factors include fractures, mechanical compression (e.g., tourniquet, cast, brace, dressing, or restraint), orthopedic surgery, trauma, immobilization, burns, and vascular obstruction. See also **nursing diagnosis.**

peripheral nervous system, the motor and sensory nerves and ganglia outside the brain and spinal cord. The system consists of 12 pairs of cranial nerves, 31 pairs of spinal nerves, and their various branches in body organs. Sensory, or afferent, peripheral nerves transmitting information to the central nervous system and motor, or efferent, peripheral nerves carrying impulses from the brain usually travel together but separate at the cord level into a posterior sensory root and an anterior motor root. Fibers innervating the body wall are designated somatic; those supplying internal organs are termed visceral. The autonomic system includes the peripheral nerves involved in regulating cardiovascular, respiratory, endocrine, and other automatic body functions. Nerves in the sympathetic or thoracolumbar division of the autonomic system secrete norepinephrine and cause peripheral vasoconstriction, cardiac acceleration, coronary artery dilation, bronchodilation, and inhibition of peristalsis. Parasympathetic nerves, which constitute the craniosacral division of the autonomic system, secrete acetylcholine, cause peripheral vasodilation, cardiac inhibition, and bronchoconstriction, and stimulate peristalsis. Injury to a peripheral nerve results in loss of movement and sensation in the area innervated distal to the lesion.

peripheral neuropathy, any functional or organic disorder of the peripheral nervous system. A kind of peripheral neuropathy is **paresthesia.**

peripheral odontogenic fibroma, a fibrous connective tissue tumor associated with the gingival margin and believed to originate from the periodontium. It is a localized form of fibromatosis gingivae and commonly contains areas of calcification.

peripheral plasma cell myeloma. See **plasmacytoma.**

peripheral pulse [Gk, *periphereia*; L, *pulsare,* to beat], the series of waves of arterial pressure caused by left ventricle systoles as measured in the limbs.

peripheral resistance, a resistance to the flow of blood determined by the tone of the vascular musculature and the diameter of the blood vessels.

peripheral scotoma [Gk, *periphereia* + *skotos,* darkness, *oma* tumor], a lost area of the visual field that is located peripherally and does not involve the central region.

peripheral vascular disease, any abnormal condition that affects the blood vessels outside the heart and the lymphatic vessels. Different kinds and degrees of peripheral vascular disease are characterized by a variety of signs and symptoms, such as numbness, pain, pallor, elevated blood pressure, and impaired arterial pulsations. Various causative factors include obesity, cigarette smoking, stress, sedentary occupations, and numerous metabolic disorders. Peripheral vascular disease in association with bacterial endocarditis may involve emboli in terminal arterioles and produce gangrenous infarctions of various distal parts of the body, such as the tip of the nose, the pinna of the ear, the fingers, and the toes. Large emboli may occlude peripheral vessels and cause atherosclerotic occlusive disease. Treatment of severe cases may require amputation of gangrenous body parts. Less severe peripheral vascular problems may be treated by eliminating causative factors, especially cigarette smoking, and by the administration of various drugs, such as salicylates and anticoagulants. Some kinds of peripheral vascular disease are **arteriosclerosis** and **atherosclerosis.**

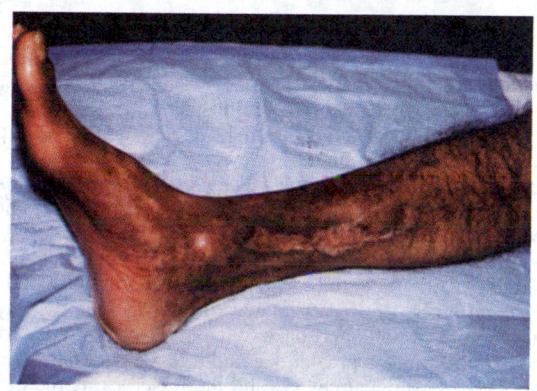

Peripheral vascular disease
(Bryant, 1992/Courtesy Abbott Northwestern Hospital, Minneapolis)

peripheral vision, a capacity to see objects that reflect light waves falling on areas of the retina distant from the macula.

periphery /pərif′ərē/ [Gk, *peri,* around, *phereia,* boundary], **1.** parts or areas near or outside a perimeter or boundary. **2.** the outer body parts, such as the skin or limbus.

perirectal /-rek′təl/ [Gk, *peri,* around + L, *rectus,* straight], pertaining to the area around the rectum.

perisinusitis /-sī′nəsī·tis/ [Gk, *peri,* around + L, *sinus,* hollow], an inflammation of the structures around a sinus.

peristalsis /-stal′sis, -stôl′sis/ [Gk, *peristellein,* to clasp], the coordinated, rhythmic, serial contraction of smooth muscle that forces food through the digestive tract, bile through the bile duct, and urine through the ureters. (See Fig. p. 1196.)

peristaltic /-stal′tik, -stôl′tik/ [Gk, *peristelein,* to clasp], pertaining to peristalsis.

peristomal /per′istō′məl/, pertaining to the area of skin

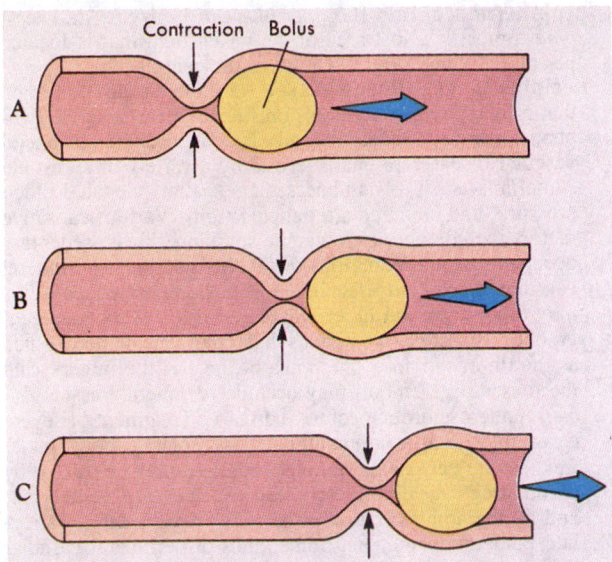

Peristalsis *(Thibodeau, 1993/Rolin Graphics)*

surrounding a stoma, or surgically created opening in the abdominal wall.

peritomeoscopy. See **abdominoscopy.**

peritoneal /-tənē′əl/ [Gk, *peri* + *tenein*, to stretch], pertaining to the peritoneum.

peritoneal abscess [Gk, *peri* + *tenein*; L, *abscedere*, to go away], an abscess in the peritoneal cavity, the result of peritonitis and usually complicated by adhesions.

peritoneal cavity /per′itōnē′əl/ [Gk, *peri* + *teinein*, to stretch], the potential space between the parietal and the visceral layers of the peritoneum. Normally, the two layers are in contact. The peritoneal cavity is divided by a narrow constriction into a greater sac and a lesser sac. The greater sac is the peritoneal cavity, and the lesser sac is the omental bursa. The omental bursa is associated with the dorsal surface of the stomach and the surrounding structures. See also **epiploic foramen.**

peritoneal dialysis, a dialysis procedure performed to correct an imbalance of fluid or of electrolytes in the blood or to remove toxins, drugs, or other wastes normally excreted by the kidney. The peritoneum is used as a diffusible membrane. Peritoneal dialysis may be performed nightly for chronically ill children while they sleep and also may be carried out regularly at home. It is contraindicated in patients with extensive intraabdominal adhesions, localized peritoneal infection, and gangrenous or perforated bowels, although peritonitis may itself sometimes be treated by peritoneal lavage and antibiotics, using peritoneal dialysis. ■ METHOD: Under local anesthesia, a many-eyed catheter is sutured in place in the peritoneum and a sterile dressing is applied. The catheter is connected to the inflow and outflow tubing with a 'Y' connector, and the air in the tubing is displaced by the dialysate to avoid introducing air into the peritoneal cavity. The amount and the kind of dialysate and the length of time for each exchange cycle vary with the age, size, and condition of the patient. There are three phases in each cycle. During inflow, the dialysate is introduced into the peritoneal cavity. During equilibration, the

dialysate remains in the peritoneal cavity; by means of osmosis, diffusion, and filtration, the needed electrolytes pass to the bloodstream via the vascular peritoneum to the blood vessels of the abdominal cavity, and the waste products pass from the blood vessels through the vascular peritoneum into the dialysate. During the third phase, (outflow), the dialysate is allowed to drain from the peritoneal cavity by gravity. ■ NURSING INTERVENTION: The fluid is warmed to body temperature before instillation, and heparin, antibiotics, or other additives may be added to the dialysate. The patient's fluid balance, respirations, pulse, blood pressure, temperature, and mental state are frequently evaluated, and blood glucose and electrolytes are tested regularly. The amount of fluid instilled and the amount and character of the fluid drained are noted. Bacteriologic cultures of the drainage are performed regularly, and a low-sodium, high-carbohydrate, high-fat, 20 to 40 g protein diet is usually given. Medication for pain may be necessary. The need for dialysis and the techniques, dangers, and advantages of peritoneal dialysis are explained to the patient and the patient's family. ■ OUTCOME CRITERIA: Peritoneal dialysis may result in several complications, including perforation of the bowel, peritonitis, atelectasis, pneumonia, pulmonary edema, hyperglycemia, hypovolemia, hypervolemia, and adhesions. Peritonitis, the most common problem, is usually caused by failure to use aseptic technique and is characterized by fever, cloudy dialysate, leukocytosis, and abdominal discomfort. Dialysis may usually be continued while the infection is treated with antibiotics, which are given systemically or intraperitoneally. Atelectasis and pneumonia may result from compression of the thoracic cavity, with decreased respiratory excursion and blood flow to the bases of the lungs caused by an excessive volume of dialysate in the peritoneal cavity. Dyspnea, tachypnea, rales, and tachycardia require reevaluation of the amount of dialysate, the raising of the head of the bed, and respiratory therapy to prevent atelectasis and pneumonia. Because patients with diabetes are at risk of developing hyperglycemia, serum and urine glucose levels are monitored, and, if necessary, sorbitol may be substituted for glucose in the dialysate. If dialysate fluid is retained in the peritoneal cavity, hypervolemia may occur, predisposing the patient to pulmonary edema and congestive failure. If the dialysate is removed too rapidly or if the dialysate used is a hypotonic glucose solution, hypovolemia may result. Adhesions often develop because of local irritation to the surrounding tissues caused by the intraperitoneal catheter.

peritoneal dialysis solution, a solution of electrolytes and other substances that is introduced into the peritoneum to remove toxic substances from the body.

peritoneal endometriosis [Gk, *peri* + *teinein*, to stretch, *endon*, within + *metra*, womb], ectopic endometrial tissue found in the pelvic cavity. See also **implantation endometriosis.**

peritoneal fluid, a naturally produced fluid in the abdominal cavity that lubricates surfaces, thereby preventing friction between the peritoneal membrane and internal organs.

peritoneo-, a combining form meaning 'pertaining to the peritoneum': *peritoneal, peritonitis.*

peritoneoscope. See **laparoscope.**

peritoneoscopy /-tō′nē·os′kəpē/ [Gk, *peri* + *teinein*, *skopein*, to view], the use of an endoscope to inspect the peritoneum through a stab incision in the abdominal wall.

peritoneum /per′itənē′əm/ [Gk, *peri* + *teinein*, to stretch], an extensive serous membrane that covers the entire abdominal wall of the body and is reflected over the contained viscera. It is divided into the parietal peritoneum and the visceral peritoneum. In men, the peritoneum is a closed membranous sac. In women, it is perforated by the free ends of the uterine tubes. The free surface of the peritoneum is smooth mesothelium, lubricated by serous fluid that permits the viscera to glide easily against the abdominal wall and against one another. The mesentery of the peritoneum fans out from the main membrane to suspend the small intestine. Other parts of the peritoneum are the transverse mesocolon, the greater omentum, and the lesser omentum. –**peritoneal,** *adj.*

peritonitis /per'itənī'tis/ [Gk, *peri* + *teinein,* to stretch, *itis*], an inflammation of the peritoneum produced by bacteria or irritating substances introduced into the abdominal cavity by a penetrating wound or perforation of an organ in the GI tract or the reproductive tract. Peritonitis is caused most commonly by rupture of the vermiform appendix but also occurs after perforations of intestinal diverticula, peptic ulcers, gangrenous gallbladders, gangrenous obstructions of the small bowel, or incarcerated hernias, as well as ruptures of the spleen, liver, ovarian cyst, or fallopian tube, especially in ectopic pregnancy. In some cases peritonitis is secondary to the release of pancreatic enzymes, bile, or digestive juices of the upper GI tract, and there are reports of postoperative peritonitis caused by cornstarch used to powder surgical gloves. The bacteria most frequently identified as causative agents in peritonitis are *Escherichia coli, Bacteroides, Fusobacterium,* and anaerobic and aerobic streptococci; *Klebsiella* and *Proteus* are uncommon, and *Clostridium, Staphylococcus aureus,* and gonococci are rare. Pneumococci occasionally found in peritonitis in girls are thought to enter the abdominal cavity via the vagina and fallopian tubes. See also **appendectomy, appendicitis.**
■ OBSERVATIONS: Characteristic signs and symptoms of peritonitis include abdominal distention, rigidity and pain, rebound tenderness, decreased or absent bowel sounds, nausea, vomiting, and tachycardia. The patient has chills and fever, breathes rapidly and shallowly, is anxious, dehydrated, and unable to defecate, and may vomit fecal material. Leukocytosis, an electrolyte imbalance, and hypovolemia are usually present, and shock and heart failure may ensue.
■ INTERVENTIONS: The patient is placed in bed in a semi-Fowler's position with the knees flexed to facilitate breathing and localize pus in the lower abdomen. Oxygen, parenteral fluids with electrolytes, antibiotics, and emetics are administered as ordered. A nasogastric or nasointestinal tube is passed for intermittent suctioning; an indwelling catheter is inserted, and a rectal tube may be used. Measurements are made of the intake and output of fluids, and the character, color, odor, and amount of drainage are noted. Blood pressure, apical pulse, and respiration are checked every 1 to 2 hours; at similar intervals the patient is turned and instructed in coughing and deep breathing. Rectal temperature, bowel sounds, and abdominal distention are checked every 2 to 4 hours. Pain is controlled with analgesia, and the dehydrated patient, whose lips tend to be dry and cracked, receives frequent mouth care. Paracentesis may be performed to withdraw ascitic fluid that is turbid or purulent in pyogenic peritonitis. Repair of the perforation or rupture responsible for the infection may be indicated, but surgery is usually delayed until the patient is stabilized. Pa-

tients who respond to antibiotic therapy receive a liquid diet when the nasogastric tube is removed and bowel sounds return and gradually progress to a diet appropriate for the disorder that caused the peritonitis.
■ NURSING CONSIDERATIONS: The patient acutely ill with peritonitis is usually very apprehensive and needs constant care.

peritonitis meconium [Gk, *peri* + *teinein, itis,* inflammation, *mekon,* poppy], a condition of peritonitis in a newborn resulting from rupture of the digestive tract. The inflammation is caused by leakage of meconium, or fetal contents, into the peritoneal cavity.

peritonsillar /-ton'silər/ [Gk, *peri* + L, *tonsilla*], pertaining to the area around a tonsil.

peritonsillar abscess [Gk, *peri* + L, *tonsilla,* tonsil, *abscedere,* to go away], an infection of tissue between the tonsil and pharynx, usually after acute follicular tonsillitis. The symptoms include dysphagia, pain radiating to the ear, and fever. Redness and swelling of the tonsil and adjacent soft palate are present. Treatment includes penicillin, warm saline irrigation, incision and drainage with suction if there is no spontaneous rupture of the abscess, and, sometimes, tonsillectomy. Also called **quinsy.** Compare **parapharyngeal abscess, retropharyngeal abscess.** See also **tonsillitis.**

Peritrate, a trademark for a vasodilator (pentaerythritol tetranitrate).

periumbilical /per'i·umbil'ikəl/ [Gk, *peri,* near + *umbilicus,* navel], pertaining to the area around the umbilicus.

periungual /per'i·ung'gwəl/ [Gk, *peri* + L, *unguis,* nail], of or pertaining to the area around the fingernails or the toenails.

perivascular goiter /per'ivas'kyo͞olər/ [Gk, *peri* + L, *vasculum,* little vessel; *guttur,* throat], an enlargement of the thyroid gland surrounding a large blood vessel.

perivascular spaces [Gk, *peri,* near; L, *vasculum,* little vessel, *spatium,* space], spaces that surround blood vessels as they enter the brain. They communicate with the subarachnoid space. Also called **Virchow-Robin spaces; Virchow's spaces.**

perivertebral /-var'təbəl/ [Gk, *peri,* near + *vertebra,* joint], pertaining to the area around a vertebra.

perivitelline /-vitel'ēn/ [Gk, *peri* + L, *vitellus,* yolk], surrounding the vitellus or yolk mass.

perivitelline space, the space between the ovum and the zona pellucida of mammals into which the polar bodies are released at the time of maturation. In some animals it is a fluid-filled space that separates the fertilization membrane from the vitelline membrane surrounding the ovum after the penetration of the spermatozoon.

perle /purl, perl/ [Fr. pearl], a soft capsule filled with medicine.

perlèche. See **cheilosis.**

perlingual /pərling'gwəl/ [L, *per, lingua,* tongue], pertaining to the administration of drugs through the tongue, which absorbs substances through its surface.

permanent dentition /pur'mənənt/ [L, *permanere,* to last], the eruption of the 32 permanent teeth, beginning with the appearance of the first permanent molars at about 6 years of age. The process is completed by 12 or 13 years of age except for the four wisdom teeth, which usually do not erupt until 18 to 25 years of age, or later. Also called **secondary dentition.** Compare **deciduous dentition, primary dentition.** (See Fig. p. 1198.)

permanent pacemaker [L, *permanere,* to remain, *passus,*

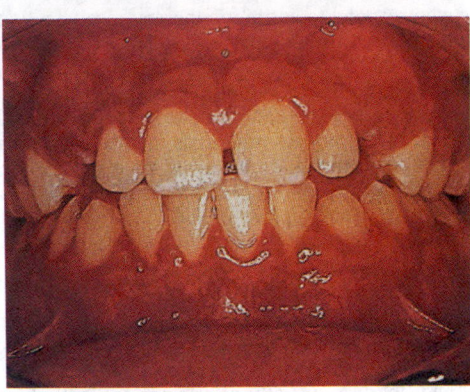

Early permanent dentition-eruption of 6-year molars and central incisors
(Zitelli, 1992)

step; ME, *maken*], any pacemaker implanted inside the body of a patient for permanent, long-term use.

permanent tooth, one of the set of 32 teeth that appear during and after childhood and usually last until old age. In each jaw they include four incisors, two canines, four premolars, and six molars. They are divided into the permanent teeth, which replace the 20 deciduous teeth of infancy, and the superadded teeth, which include 12 molars, three on each side of the upper and lower jaws. The permanent teeth start to develop in the ninth week of fetal life with the thickening of the epithelium along the line of the future jaw. They develop from the embryonic dental lamina and dental germ tissue. As the 10 permanent teeth develop in the fetus, they recede into the substance of the gum behind the deciduous teeth. The permanent teeth start to calcify soon after birth, the teeth in the lower jaw proceeding somewhat faster than those in the upper jaw. The permanent first molar in the lower jaw calcifies just after birth; the permanent incisors and the canines, approximately 6 months later; the premolars during the second year; the second molar at about the end of the second year; and the third molar at about the twelfth year. The permanent teeth erupt first in the lower jaw; the first molars in about the sixth year; the two central incisors about the seventh year; the two lateral incisors about the eighth year; the first premolars about the ninth year; the second premolars about the tenth year; the canines between the eleventh and the twelfth years; the second molars between the twelfth and the thirteenth years; and the third molars between the seventeenth and the twenty-fifth years. The eruption of each corresponding permanent tooth in the upper jaw lags only slightly behind that of the corresponding permanent tooth in the lower jaw. The third molars in many people are badly oriented or so deeply buried in bone that they must be surgically removed. In some individuals, one or all four of the third molars may not develop completely. Compare **deciduous tooth.** See also **tooth.**

permeability /pur′mē·əbil′itē/ [L, *permeare*, to pass through], the degree to which one substance allows another substance to pass through it. Kinds of permeability include: **capillary** and **magnetic.**

permeable /pur′mē·əbəl/ [L, *permeare*, to pass through], a condition of being pervious so that fluids and certain other substances can pass through, such as a permeable membrane. See also **osmosis.**

permethrin /pərməth′rin/, a topical pediculicide.

- INDICATIONS: It is used for the treatment of head lice and nits.
- CONTRAINDICATIONS: This product is contraindicated for patients who are allergic to pyrethrine, pyrethroids, or chrysanthemum flowers.
- ADVERSE EFFECTS: Among reported adverse reactions are itching, mild burning or stinging, numbness, discomfort, mild erythema, or scalp rash.

permissible dose /pərmis′ibəl/ [L, *permittere*, to permit, *dosis*, something given], (in radiotherapy) the amount of radiation that may be received by an individual in a specified period of time with the expectation of no significantly harmful results.

Permitil, a trademark for a tranquilizer (fluphenazine hydrochloride).

pernicious /pərnish′əs/ [L, *perniciosus*, dangerous], potentially injurious, destructive, or fatal unless treated, such as pernicious anemia.

pernicious anemia [L, *pernicosus*, destructive; Gk, *a*, *haima*, not blood], a progressive, megaloblastic, macrocytic anemia, affecting mainly older people, that results from a lack of intrinsic factor essential for the absorption of cyanocobalamin. The maturation of red blood cells in bone marrow becomes disordered, the posterior and lateral columns of the spinal cord deteriorate, the white blood cell count is reduced, and the polymorphonuclear leukocytes become multilobed. Extreme weakness, numbness and tingling in the extremities, fever, pallor, anorexia, and loss of weight may occur. The condition is usually treated with cyanocobalamin injection and with folic acid and iron therapy. See also **atrophic gastritis, intrinsic factor, nutritional anemia.**

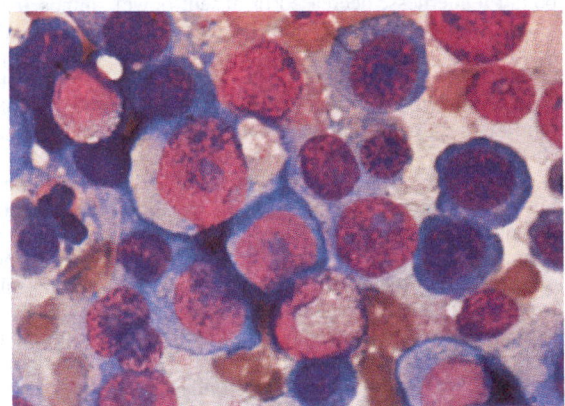

Pernicious anemia (Hayhoe, 1992)

pernicious vomiting [L, *perniciosus*, dangerous, *vomere*, to vomit], a severe, life-threatening episode of vomiting that may occur during pregnancy.

pernio. See **chilblain.**

pero- /pe′rō-, pir′ō-/, a combining form meaning 'maimed or deformed': *perobrachius, perodactylus, peromelus.*

perobrachius /pē′rōbrā′kē·əs/ [Gk, *peros,* damaged, *brachion,* arm], a fetus or individual with deformed arms.

perochirus /pē′rōkī′rəs/ [Gk, *peros* + *cheir,* hand], a fetus or individual with malformed hands.

perocormus. See **perosomus.**

perodactylus /pē′rōdak′tiləs/, a fetus or an individual with a deformity of the fingers or the toes, especially the absence of one or more digits.

perodactyly /pē′rōdak′tilē/ [Gk, *peros* + *daktylos,* finger], a congenital anomaly characterized by a deformity of the digits, primarily the complete or partial absence of one or more of the fingers or toes. Also called **perodactylia.**

peromelia /pē′rōmē′lyə/ [Gk, *peros* + *melos,* limb], a congenital anomaly characterized by the malformation of one or more of the limbs. Also called **peromely** /pərom′əlē/. –**peromelus,** *n.*

-perone, a suffix for certain neuroleptics or antianxiety agents.

peroneal /per′ənē′əl/ [Gk, *perone,* brooch], of or pertaining to the outer part of the leg, over the fibula and the peroneal nerve.

peroneal muscular atrophy, symmetric weakening or atrophy of the foot and the ankle muscles and hammertoes. This disease is a dominantly inherited condition and occurs in a hypertrophic neuropathy form or in a neuronal form. The hypertrophic neuropathy form results in demyelination of nerve fibers and characteristic onion bulb formations. Affected individuals usually have high plantar arches and an awkward gait, caused by weak ankle muscles. In the neuronal form, this condition usually starts in the second decade of life and causes muscle weaknesses similar to those associated with the hypertrophic neuronal form. Both forms of the disease also may involve mild sensory loss in the lower limbs. Affected individuals may be helped by corrective surgery and leg braces that stabilize weak ankle joints.

peroneo-, a combining form meaning 'related to the fibula or surrounding area': *peroneal.*

peroneus brevis /per′ənē′əs/ [Gk, *perone* + L, *brevis,* short], the smaller of the two lateral muscles of the leg, lying under the peroneus longus. The peroneus brevis arises from the fibula and inserts into the fifth metatarsal bone. Innervated by a branch of the superficial peroneal nerve, it contains fibers from the fourth and the fifth lumbar and the first sacral nerves. It pronates and plantar flexes the foot. Compare **peroneus longus.**

peroneus longus, the more superficial of the two lateral muscles of the leg. It arises from the head and the body of the fibula, converges to a long tendon that crosses the sole of the foot, and inserts into the first metatarsal bone and the medial cuneiform bone. The peroneus longus is innervated by a branch of the peroneal nerve, containing fibers from the fourth and the fifth lumbar and the first sacral nerves. The muscle pronates and plantar flexes the foot. Compare **peroneus brevis.**

peronia /pərō′nē·ə/ [Gk, *peros,* damaged], a congenital malformation or developmental anomaly.

peropus /pərō′pəs/ [Gk, *peros* + *pous,* foot], a fetus or individual with malformed feet, often in association with some defect of the legs.

per os /pər os′/ [L], by mouth.

perosomus /pē′rōsō′məs/ [Gk, *peros* + *soma,* body], a fetus or individual whose body, especially the trunk, is severely malformed. Also called **perocormus.**

perosplanchnia /pē′rōsplangk′nē·ə/ [Gk, *peros* + *splanch-* non, viscera], a congenital anomaly characterized by the malformation of the viscera.

peroxide. See **hydrogen peroxide.**

perphenazine /pərfen′əzēn/, an antipsychotic.

■ INDICATIONS: It is prescribed in the treatment of psychotic disorders and in the control of severe nausea and vomiting in adults.

■ CONTRAINDICATIONS: Parkinson's disease, the concurrent administration of central nervous system depressants, liver or renal dysfunction, severe hypotension, or known hypersensitivity to any phenothiazine prohibits its use.

■ ADVERSE EFFECTS: Among the more serious adverse reactions are hypotension, liver toxicity, a variety of extrapyramidal reactions, blood dyscrasias, and various hypersensitivity reactions.

per primam intentionem [L], by first intention.

per pro., abbreviation for the Latin term, *per procurationem,* 'on behalf of.'

per rectum [L], by rectum.

PERRLA /pur′lə/, abbreviation for *pupils equal, round, react to light, accommodation.* In the process of performing an assessment of the eyes, one evaluates the size and shape of the pupils, their reaction to light, and their ability to accommodate. If all findings are normal, the acronym is noted in the account of the physical examination.

Persa-Gel, a trademark for a keratolytic (benzoyl peroxide).

Persantine, a trademark for a coronary vasodilator (dipyridamole).

per se, by itself, or of itself.

per secundum intentionem [L], by second intention.

perseveration /pur′səvərā′shən/ [L, *persevero,* to persist], the involuntary and pathologic persistence of the same verbal response or motor activity regardless of the stimulus or its duration. The condition occurs primarily in patients with brain damage or organic mental disorders, although it may also appear in schizophrenia as an association disturbance.

persistent cloaca /pərsis′tənt/ [L, *persistere,* to persist, *cloaca,* sewer], a congenital anomaly in which the intestinal, urinary, and reproductive ducts open into a common cavity resulting from the failure of the urorectal septum to form during prenatal development. Also called **congenital cloaca.**

Persistin, a trademark for a central nervous system, fixed-combination drug containing analgesics (aspirin and salicylsalicylic acid).

persona /pərsō′nə/, *pl.* **personae** /-nē/ [L, mask], (in analytic psychology) the personality façade or role that a person assumes and presents to the outer world to satisfy the demands of the environment or society or as an expression of some intrapsychic conflict. The persona masks the person's inner being or unconscious self. Compare **anima.** See also **archetype.**

personal and social history /pur′sənəl/, (in a health history) an account of the personal and social details of a person's life that serves to identify the person. Place of birth, religion, race, marital status, number of children, military status, occupational history, and place of residence are the usual components of this part of the history, but it may often include other information, such as education, current living situation, and smoking, alcohol, and drug habits. The personal and social history is obtained at the initial interview and becomes a part of the permanent record.

personal assistance. See **custodial care.**

personal care services, the services performed by health care workers to assist patients in meeting the requirements of daily living.

personal identity disturbance, a nursing diagnosis accepted by the Seventh National Conference on the Classification of Nursing Diagnoses. The diagnosis is defined as the inability to distinguish between self and nonself. The defining characteristics and related factors are to be developed at a later conference. See also **nursing diagnosis.**

personality /pur'sənal'itē/ [L, *personalis*, role], **1.** the composite of the behavioral traits and attitudinal characteristics by which one is recognized as an individual. **2.** the pattern of behavior each person evolves, both consciously and unconsciously, as a means of adapting to a particular environment and its cultural, ethnic, national, and provincial standards.

personality disorder, a disruption in relatedness manifested in any of a large group of mental disorders characterized by rigid, inflexible, and maladaptive behavior patterns that impair a person's ability to function in society by severely limiting adaptive potential. Also called **character disorder.**

personality test, any of a variety of standardized tests used in the evaluation or assessment of various facets of personality structure, emotional status, and behavioral traits. Compare **achievement test, aptitude test, intelligence test, psychologic test.**

personal orientation, 1. a continually evolving process in which a person determines and evaluates the relationships that appear to exist between the person and other people. **2.** the assessment derived by a person regarding those relationships.

personal space, the area surrounding an individual that is perceived as private by the individual, who may regard a movement into the space by another person as intrusive. Personal space boundaries vary somewhat in different cultures, but in general it is regarded as a distance of about 1 meter (3 feet) around the individual.

personal unconscious, (in analytic psychology) the thoughts, ideas, emotions, and other mental phenomena acquired and repressed during one's lifetime. Compare **collective unconscious.**

personal zone, an individual protective zone in which the boundaries may contract or expand according to contextual characteristics, usually between 18 inches and 4 feet.

person year, a statistical measure representing one person at risk of developing a disease during a period of 1 year.

perspiration /pur'spirā'shən/ [L, *per* + *spirare*, to breath], **1.** the act or process of perspiring; the excretion of fluid by the sweat glands through pores in the skin. **2.** the fluid excreted by the sweat glands. It consists of water containing sodium chloride, phosphate, urea, ammonia, and other waste products. Perspiration serves as a mechanism for excretion and for regulating body temperature. Abnormal amounts of perspiration usually result from organic causes but may also be precipitated by severe emotional stress. Kinds of perspiration are **insensible perspiration** and **sensible perspiration.** See also **diaphoresis.**

perspire /pərspī'ər/ [L, *per spirare* to breathe], to sweat or excrete sweat.

per tertiam intentionem [L], by third intention.

Perthes' disease /per'tās/ [Georg C. Perthes, German surgeon, b. 1869], osteochondrosis of the head of the femur in children, characterized initially by epiphyseal necrosis or

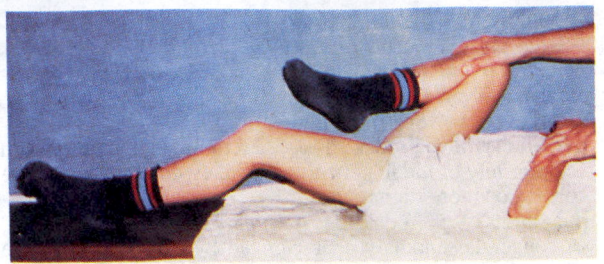

Perthes' disease (*Zitelli, 1992*)

degeneration followed by regeneration or recalcification. Also called **coxa plana, Legg-Calvé-Perthes disease, pseudocoxalgia, Waldenström's disease.**

Pertofrane, a trademark for an antidepressant (desipramine hydrochloride).

perturbation /pur'tərbā'shən/ [L, *per* + *tubare*, to disturb], a cause or a condition of disturbance, disorder, or confusion.

pertussis /pərtus'is/ [L, *per* + *tussis*, cough], an acute, highly contagious respiratory disease characterized by paroxysmal coughing that ends in a loud whooping inspiration. It occurs primarily in infants and in children less than 4 years of age who have not been immunized. The causative organism, *Bordetella pertussis*, is a small, nonmotile, gram-negative coccobacillus. A similar organism, *B. parapertussis*, causes a less severe form of the disease called parapertussis. Also called **whooping cough.**

■ OBSERVATIONS: Transmission occurs directly by contact or by inhalation of infectious particles, usually spread by coughing and sneezing, and indirectly through freshly contaminated articles. Diagnosis consists of positive identification of the organism in nasopharyngeal secretions. The initial stages of the disease are difficult to distinguish from bronchitis or influenza. A fluorescent antibody staining technique specific for the *B. pertussis* is an accurate means of early diagnosis. The incubation period averages 7 to 14 days, followed by 6 to 8 weeks of illness divided into three distinct stages: catarrhal, paroxysmal, and convalescent. Onset of the catarrhal stage is gradual, usually beginning with coryza, sneezing, a dry cough, a slight fever, listlessness, irritability, and anorexia. The cough becomes paroxysmal after 10 to 14 days and occurs as a series of short rapid bursts during expiration followed by the characteristic whoop, caused by a spasm of the epiglottis, a hurried, deep inhalation that has a high-pitched crowing sound. There is usually no fever, and the respiratory rate between paroxysms is normal. During the paroxysm there is marked facial redness or cyanosis and vein distention, the eyes may bulge, the tongue may protrude, and the facial expression usually indicates severe anxiety and distress. Large amounts of a viscid mucus may be expelled during or after paroxysms, which occur from four to five times a day in mild cases to as many as 40 to 50 times a day in severe cases. Vomiting frequently occurs after the paroxysms because of gagging or choking on the mucus. In infants, choking may be more common than the characteristic whoop. This stage lasts from 4 to 6 weeks, with the attacks being most frequent and severe during the first 1 to 2 weeks, then gradually declining and disappearing. During the convalescent stage, a simple persistent cough is usual. For a period of up to 2 years after the initial attack, paroxysmal coughing may accompany respiratory infections.

■ INTERVENTIONS: Routine treatment consists of bed rest, adequate nutritional intake, and adequate amounts of fluid. Erythromycin or another antibacterial may be prescribed to reduce transmission or to control secondary infection. Hospitalization may be necessary for infants and children with severe or prolonged paroxysms and for those with dehydration or other complications. Oxygen may be needed to relieve dyspnea and cyanosis; intravenous therapy may be necessary when prolonged vomiting interferes with adequate nutrition. Intubation is rarely necessary but may be lifesaving in infants if the thick mucus cannot be easily suctioned from the air passages. Pertussis immune globulin is available, but its efficacy has not been established and its use is not recommended. Active immunization is recommended with pertussis vaccine, usually in combination with diphtheria and tetanus toxoids in a series of three injections. One attack of the disease usually confers immunity, although some second, usually mild episodes have occurred.

■ NURSING CONSIDERATIONS: Severe paroxysms in an infant may require oxygen, suction, and intubation. The child needs to be kept calm and protected from respiratory irritants such as dirt, smoke, or dust. Overstimulation, noise, or excitement may precipitate paroxysms. Adequate nutrition and adequate fluids are encouraged through frequent, small feedings. Common complications of the disease include bronchopneumonia; atelectasis; bronchiectasis; emphysema; otitis media; convulsions; hemorrhage, including subarachnoid, subconjunctival, and epistaxis; weight loss; dehydration; hernia; prolapsed rectum; and asphyxia, especially in infants. Paroxysms can be fatal.

pertussis immune globulin, a passive immunizing agent against whooping cough. See also **pertussis.**

■ INDICATION: It is prescribed for immunization against whooping cough.

■ CONTRAINDICATION: Known hypersensitivity to this drug prohibits its use.

■ ADVERSE EFFECTS: Among the more serious adverse reactions is anaphylaxis.

pertussis vaccine, an active immunizing agent.

■ INDICATION: It is prescribed for immunization against pertussis when the administration of diphtheria, pertussis, and tetanus vaccine is contraindicated.

■ CONTRAINDICATIONS: Thrombocytopenia or known hypersensitivity to the vaccine prohibits its use.

■ ADVERSE EFFECTS: Among the most serious adverse reactions are severe allergic reactions, pain and induration at the site of injection, and fever.

per vaginam [L], via the vagina.

pervasive developmental disorder /pərvā′siv/ [L, *pervadere,* to go through], any of certain disorders of infancy and childhood that are characterized by severe impairment of relatedness and behavioral aberrations previously identified as childhood psychoses. The group of disorders includes infantile autism, childhood schizophrenia, and symbiotic psychosis.

perversion /pərvur′shən/ [L, *pervertere,* to turn about], 1. any deviation from what is considered normal or natural. 2. the act of causing a change from what is normal or natural. 3. *informal.* (in psychiatry) any of a number of sexual practices that deviate from what is considered normal adult behavior. See also **paraphilia.**

pervert /pur′vərt/ [L, *pervertere*], 1. *informal.* a person whose sexual pleasure is derived from stimuli almost universally regarded as unnatural, such as a fetishist or sadomasochist; a paraphiliac. 2. one whose sexual behavior deviates from a social or statistical norm but is not necessarily pathologic.

pes /pēz, pās/, *pl.* **pedes** /pē′dēz/ [L, foot], the foot or a footlike structure.

pes cavus, a deformity of the foot characterized by an excessively high arch with hyperextension of the toes at the metatarsophalangeal joints, flexion at the interphalangeal joints, and shortening of the Achilles tendon. The condition may be present at birth or appear later because of contractures or an imbalance of the muscles of the foot, as in neuromuscular diseases such as Friedreich's ataxia or peroneal muscular atrophy. Surgical treatment is indicated in severe cases, especially in children, although in milder forms the pain from the excessive pressure under the metatarsal heads can be relieved by sponge, rubber, or leather insoles fitted into the shoes. Also called **clawfoot, gampsodactyly, griffe des orteils** /grif′dezôrtä′i/, **talipes cavus.**

pes equinus [L, *pes* foot, *equinus,* pertaining to a horse], a foot deformity in which the toes are extremely flexed, walking is done on the dorsal surface, and the heel does not touch the ground. Also called **talipes equinus.**

pes planus, an abnormal but relatively common condition characterized by the flattening out of the arch of the foot. Also called **flatfoot.**

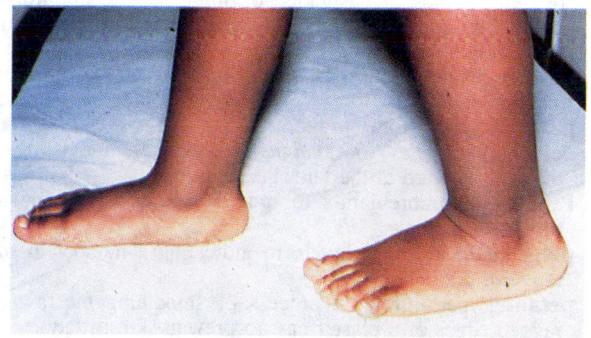

Pes planus (Zitelli, 1992)

pessary /pes′ərē/ [Gk, *pessos,* oval stone], a device inserted in the vagina to treat uterine prolapse, uterine retroversion, or cervical incompetence. It is employed in the treatment of women whose advanced age or poor general condition precludes surgical repair. Pessaries are also used in younger women in evaluating symptomatic uterine retroversion: If pelvic pain is relieved by anteversion of the uterus with the pessary in place and returns when retroversion recurs after the pessary is removed, retroversion is the cause of pain, and surgical uterine suspension can be expected to provide long-term relief. The pessary is also used in the management of cervical incompetence in pregnancy. It holds the uterus in a forward position in which intraabdominal and intrauterine pressure causes less stress on the neck of the womb. A pessary must be removed, usually daily, for cleaning. A **Smith-Hodge pessary** is a rubber- or vinyl-covered wire rectangle that fits between the pubic bone and the posterior vaginal fornix, supporting the uterus and holding the cervix in a posterior position. A **Gellhorn pessary** is an inflexible device made of Lucite in the form of a large collar button. It has a canal through the stem that allows drainage of vaginal secretions. The large end of the pessary is placed deep in the vagina, the small end of the stem protruding at the introitus. A **doughnut pessary** is a permanently inflated flexible rubber doughnut that is inserted to support the uterus by blocking the canal of the vagina. An **inflatable pessary** is a collapsible rubber doughnut to which is attached a flexible stem containing a rubber valve. The pessary is inserted collapsed, inflated with a bulb similar to that of a sphygmomanometer, and deflated for removal. A **Bee cell pessary** is a soft rubber cube; in each face of the cube is a conical depression that acts as a suction cup when the pessary is in the vagina. A **diaphragm pessary** is a contraceptive diaphragm used for uterovaginal support. A similar device of somewhat heavier construction is sometimes used. A **stem pessary** is a slim curved rod that can be fitted into the cervical canal for uterine positioning. It is rarely used today.

pessimism /pes'imiz'əm/ [L, *pessimus*, worst], the inclination to anticipate the worst possible results from any action or situation or to emphasize unfavorable conditions, even when progress or gain might reasonably be expected. –**pessimist**, *n.*

pesticide poisoning /pes'tisīd/ [L, *pestis*, plague, *caedere*, to kill; *potio*, drink], a toxic condition caused by the ingestion or inhalation of a substance used for the eradication of pests. Kinds of pesticide poisoning include **malathion poisoning** and **parathion poisoning.** See also **herbicide poisoning, rodenticide poisoning.**

pestilence /pes'tiləns/ [L, *pestilentia*, infectious disease], any epidemic of a virulent infectious or contagious disease.

pestis. See **bubonic plague.**

pes valgus [L, *pes*, foot, *valgus*, bowlegged], deviation of the foot outward at the talocalcanean joint.

PET /pet/, abbreviation for **positron emission tomography.**

peta- (P), a combining form indicating a number in the range of 10^{15}.

petaling /pet'əling/, a process of smoothing the raw or ragged edges of a plaster cast to prevent skin irritation.

petalo-, a combining form meaning 'of or related to a leaf': *petalobacteria, petalococcus.*

petechiae /pētē'kē·ē/, *sing.* **petechia** /-kē·ə/ [It, *petecchie*, flea-bite], tiny purple or red spots that appear on the skin

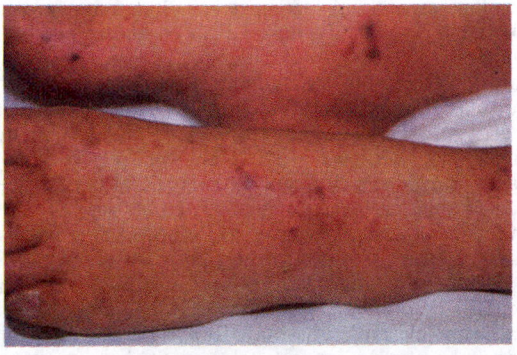

Petechiae *(Weston, 1991)*

as a result of minute hemorrhages within the dermal or submucosal layers. Petechiae range from pinpoint to pinhead size and are flush with the surface. Compare **ecchymosis.** –**petechial,** *adj.*

petechial [It, *petecchia*], pertaining to tiny red or purple spots caused by an extravasation of blood into the skin.

petechial fever /pitē'kē·əl/ [It, *petecchie* + L, *febris*, fever], any febrile illness accompanied by small petechiae on the skin, such as seen in the late stage of typhoid fever.

petechial hemorrhage [It, *petecchia*; Gk, *haima*, blood + *rhegnynei*, to gush], a small discrete hemorrhage under the skin.

pethidine. See **meperidine hydrochloride.**

petit mal seizure /pet'ē mal', ptē' mäl'/ [Fr, *petit*, small, *mal*, sickness, *saisir*, to seize], See **absence seizure.**

petit pas gait /pet'ē pä, ptē'pä/ a manner of walking with short, mincing steps and shuffling with loss of associated movements. It is seen in cases of parkinsonism as well as in patients with diffuse cerebral disease resulting from multiple small infarcts.

Petit's sinuses. See **aortic sinus.**

P.E.T.N., a trademark for a vasodilator (pentaerythritol tetranitrate).

petr-, petro- a prefix meaning 'of or pertaining to stone' or the petrous region of the temporal bone: *petrifaction, petroleum, petrous.*

Petren's gait /pet'rənz/, a hesitant form of walking in which a patient takes a few steps, halts, and then continues to take a few more steps. In some cases, the patient must be encouraged to begin the next brief period of walking. The condition is seen in elderly people and those with paretic disease.

Petri dish /pē'trē, pā'trē/ [Richard Julius Petri, German bacteriologist, b. 1852], a shallow circular glass dish used to hold solid culture media.

petrification /pet'rifikā'shən/, the process of becoming calcified or stonelike.

pétrissage /pā'trisäzh'/ [Fr, *petrir*, to knead], a technique in massage in which the skin is gently lifted and squeezed. Pétrissage promotes circulation and relaxes the muscles. Compare **effleurage, rolling effleurage.**

petrolatum /pet'rəlā'təm/ [L, *petra*, rock, *oleum*, oil], a purified mixture of semisolid hydrocarbons obtained from petroleum and commonly used as an ointment base or skin emollient.

petrolatum gauze /pet'rəlā'təm/, absorbent gauze permeated with white petrolatum.

petroleum distillate poisoning /pətrō'lē·əm/ [L, *petra*, *oleum* + *distillare*, to drop down; *potio*, drink], a toxic condition caused by the ingestion or inhalation of a petroleum distillate, such as fuel oil, lubricating oil, glue used in making model airplanes or the like, and various solvents. Nausea, vomiting, chest pain, dizziness, and severe depression of the central nervous system characterize the condition. Severe or fatal pneumonitis may occur if the substance is aspirated; therefore induced emesis is contraindicated. Gastric lavage may be indicated as well as other supportive therapy. See also **kerosene poisoning.**

petrosphenoidal fissure /pet'rōsfēnoi'dəl/ [Gk, *petros*, stone, *sphen*, wedge, *eidos*, form], a fissure on the floor of the cranial fossa between the posterior edge of the great wing of the sphenoid bone and the petrous part of the temporal bone.

petrous /pet'rəs/ [Gk, *petros*, stone], resembling a rock or stone.

Peutz-Jeghers syndrome /poits'jeg'ərz/ [J. L. A. Peutz, twentieth century Dutch physician; Harold J. Jeghers, American physician, b. 1904], an inherited disorder, transmitted as an autosomal dominant trait, characterized by multiple intestinal polyps, and abnormal mucocutaneous pigmentation, usually over the lips and buccal mucosa. If obstruction or bleeding occurs, surgical removal of the polyps may be indicated.

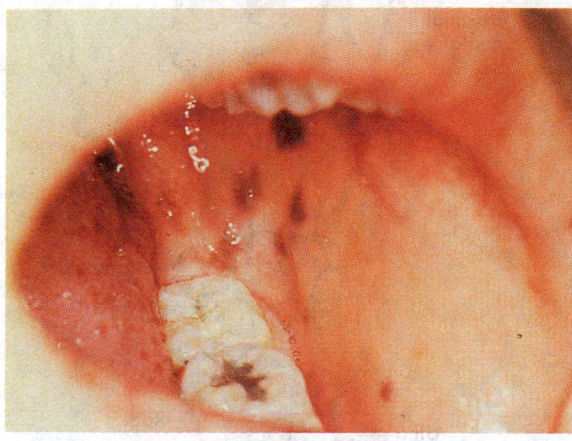

Peutz-Jeghers syndrome
(Epstein, 1992/Courtesy Joan Slack, Department of Clinical Genetics, Royal Free NHS Trust)

-pexis, -pexia, -pexy, a combining form meaning 'a fixation of' something specified: *glycopexis, hemopexis, splenopexis.*

Peyer's patches. See **intestinal tonsil.**

peyote /pā·ō'tē/ [Aztec, *peyotl*], **1.** a cactus from which a hallucinogenic drug, mescaline, is derived. **2.** mescaline.

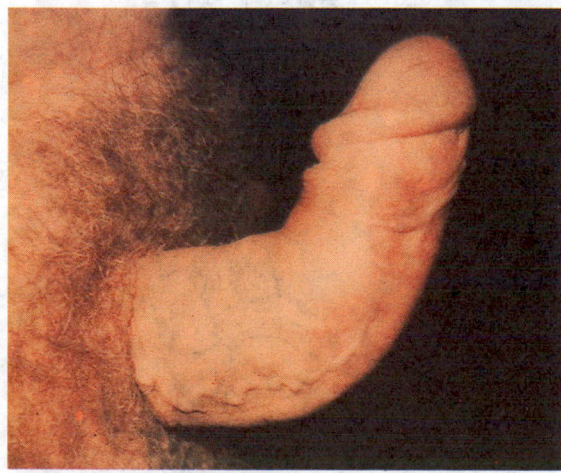

Peyronie disease
(Seidel, 1991/Courtesy Patrick C Walsh, MD, The Johns Hopkins University School of Medicine, Baltimore)

Peyronie's disease /pārōnēz'/ [François de la Peyronie, French physician, b. 1678], a disease of unknown cause resulting in fibrous induration of the corpora cavernosa of the penis. An association with Dupuytren's contracture of the palm has been recognized. The chief symptom of Peyronie's disease is painful erection. Palliative treatment includes radiation therapy and intralesional corticosteroid injections. There is no known cure.

pF, abbreviation for *picofarad.*

Pfizerpen-AS, a trademark for an antibacterial (penicillin G procaine).

PFT, abbreviation for **pulmonary function test.**

PG, abbreviation for **prostaglandin.**

PGI₂, abbreviation for **prostacyclin.**

PGY, abbreviation for *postgraduate year,* describing medical school graduates during their postgraduate training as interns (PGY-1, first year), residents (PGY-2, 3, 4), or fellows (PGY-4, 5).

pH, abbreviation for *potential hydrogen,* a scale representing the relative acidity (or alkalinity) of a solution, in which a value 7.0 is neutral, below 7.0 is acid, and above 7.0 is alkaline. The numeric pH value indicates the relative concentration of hydrogen atoms in the solution compared with that of a standard (one molar) solution; it is equal to the negative log of the hydrogen ion concentration expressed in moles per liter. See also **acid, acid-base balance.**

PH, abbreviation for **parathyroid hormone.**

Ph, symbol for **phenyl.**

Ph¹, symbol for **Philadelphia chromosome.**

PHA, 1. abbreviation for **paraaminohippuric acid. 2.** abbreviation for **phytohemagglutinin.**

phaco-, phako-, a prefix meaning 'of or related to a lens': *phacocele, phacocyst, phacoglaucoma.*

phacomalacia /fak'ōmǝlā'shǝ/ [Gk, *phalos,* lens, *malkia,* softness], an abnormal condition of the eye in which the lens of the eye becomes soft because of the presence of a soft cataract.

phacomatosis. See **phakomatosis.**

phage. See **bacteriophage, -phage.**

-phage, -phag, -phagia, -phagy, a suffix meaning to 'to eat or consume': *autophage, hemophage, mycophage, osteophage.*

phage typing /fāj/ [Gk, *phagein,* to eat; *typos,* mark], the identification of bacteria by testing their vulnerability to bacterial viruses.

-phagia, See **-phage.**

phago-, a prefix meaning 'of or pertaining to eating or ingestion': *phagocyte, phagokaryosis, phagology.*

phagocyte /fag'ǝsīt/ [Gk, *phagein* + *kytos,* cell], a cell that is able to surround, engulf, and digest microorganisms and cellular debris. **Fixed noncirculating phagocytes** include the fixed macrophages and the cells of the reticuloendothelial system. **Free circulating phagocytes** include the leukocytes. **–phagocytic,** *adj.*

phagocytic /-sit'ik/ [Gk, *phagein,* to eat + *kytos,* cell], pertaining to phagocytes or phagocytosis.

phagocytize /fag'ǝsitīz/ [Gk, *phagein,* to eat + *kytos,* cell], to engulf and destroy bacteria or other foreign materials. Also called **phagocytose.**

phagocytosis /fag'ǝsītō'sis/ [Gk, *phagein, kytos* + *osis,* condition], the process by which certain cells engulf and destroy microorganisms and cellular debris. The process includes five steps: (1) invagination, (2) engulfment, (3) internalization and formation of phagocyte vacuole, (4) fus-

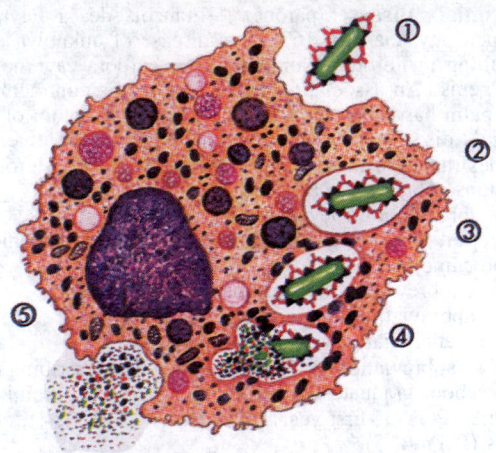

Phagocytosis *(Mudge-Grout, 1992)*

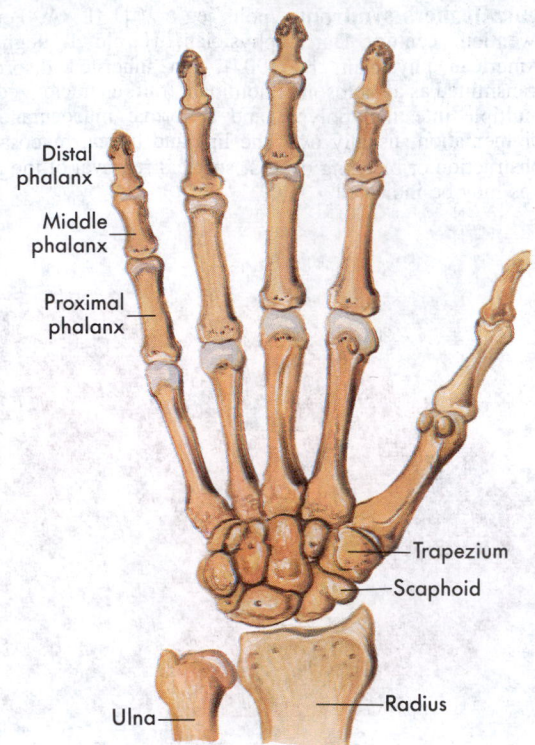

Phalanges of the hand *(Thibodeau, 1993/Ernest W Beck)*

ing of lysosomes to digest the phagocytosed material, and (5) release of digested microbial products.

-phagy. See **-phage**.

-phakia, a suffix meaning a 'lens': *aphakia, microphakia, pseudophakia*.

phako-. See **phaco-**.

phakomatosis /fak′ōmətō′sis/, *pl.* **phakomatoses** [Gk, *phako*, lens, *oma*, tumor, *osis*, condition], (in ophthalmology) any of several hereditary syndromes characterized by benign tumorlike nodules of the eye, skin, and brain. The four disorders designated phakomatoses are neurofibromatosis (Recklinghausen's disease), tuberous sclerosis (Bourneville's disease), encephalotrigeminal angiomatosis (Sturge-Weber syndrome), and cerebroretinal angiomatosis (von Hippel-Lindau disease). Also spelled **phacomatosis.**

phal, 1. abbreviation for **phalanges. 2.** abbreviation for **phalanx.**

phalangeal /fəlan′jē·al/ [Gk, *phalagx*, line of soldiers], pertaining to a phalanx.

phalanges. See **phalanx.**

-phalangia, a combining form meaning a 'condition of the bones of the fingers or toes': *bradyphalangia, symphalangia, triphalangia*.

phalanx (phal) /fā′langks/, *pl.* **phalanges (phal)** /fəlan′jēz/ [Gk, line of soldiers], any one of the 14 tapering bones composing the fingers of each hand and the toes of each foot. They are arranged in three rows at the distal end of the metacarpus and the metatarsus. The fingers each have three phalanges; the thumb has two. The toes each have three phalanges; the great toe has two. The phalanges of the foot are smaller and less flexible than those of the hand.

phall-. See **phallo-**.

phallic /fal′ik/ [Gk, *phallos*, penis], pertaining to the penis or penis-shaped.

phallic stage [L, *phallos*, penis, *stare*, to stand], (in psychoanalysis) the period in psychosexual development occurring between 3 and 6 years of age when emerging awareness and self-manipulation of the genitals are the predominant source of pleasurable experience. Fixation at this stage may lead to extreme aggressiveness in adulthood, or it may be a precipitating factor in the development of psychosexual disorders. See also **psychosexual development.**

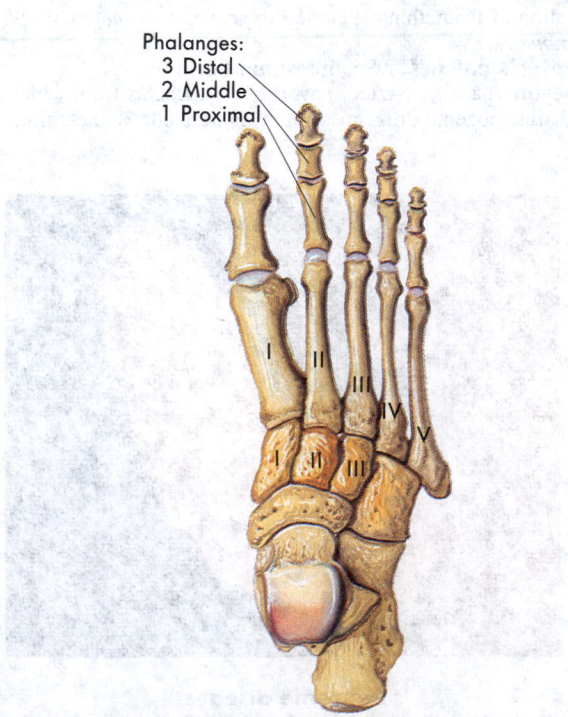

Phalanges of the foot *(Thibodeau, 1993/Ernest W Beck)*

phallic symbol [Gk, *phallos*, penis, *symbolon*, sign], in psychoanalysis, any object that may be thought to resemble a penis.

phallo-, phall-, a combining form meaning 'of or related to the penis': *phallocampsis, phallodynia, phalloplasty.*

phalloidine /faloi′din/, a poison present in the mushroom *Amanita phalloides.* Ingestion of phalloidine results in bloody diarrhea, vomiting, severe abdominal pain, kidney failure, and liver damage. Approximately 50% of phalloidine poisonings are fatal. Also spelled **phalloidin.**

phallus. See **penis.**

-phane, -phan, a suffix meaning a 'thing with a (specified) appearance': *diaphane, rhodophane, xanthophane.*

phanero-, a prefix meaning 'visible or apparent': *phanerogenetic, phaneromania, phaneroplasm.*

phantasm /fan′taz′əm/ [Gk, *phantasma*, vision], an illusory image, such as an optical illusion of something that does not exist.

phantom /fan′təm/ [Gk, *phantasma*, vision], a mass of material similar to human tissue used to investigate the interaction of radiation beams with human beings. Phantom materials can range from water to complex chemical mixtures that faithfully mimic the human body as it would interact with radiation.

phantom images, (in computed tomography) false images that appear but are not actually in the focal plane. They are created by the incomplete blurring or fusion of the blurred margins of some structures characteristic of the type of tomographic motion used.

phantom limb syndrome, a phenomenon common after amputation of a limb in which sensation or discomfort is experienced in the missing limb. In some people severe pain persists. See also **pseudesthesia.**

phantom tumor, a swelling resembling a tumor, usually caused by muscle contraction or gaseous distention of the intestines.

phao-. See **pheo-.**

phar, 1. abbreviation for **pharmacy. 2.** abbreviation for **pharmacology. 3.** abbreviation for **pharmaceutic.**

Phar.B., abbreviation for *Bachelor of Pharmacy.*

Phar.D., abbreviation for *Doctor of Pharmacy.*

pharmaceutic (phar) /fär′məso͞o′tik/ [Gk, *pharmakeuein,* to give drugs], **1.** of or pertaining to pharmacy or drugs. **2.** a drug.

pharmaceutical chemistry, the science dealing with the composition and preparation of chemical compounds used in medical diagnoses and therapies.

Pharm Chem, abbreviation for **pharmaceutical chemistry.**

pharmacist /fär′məsist/ [Gk, *pharmakon*], a person prepared to formulate and dispense drugs or medications through completion of a university program in pharmacy of at least four years' duration.

pharmaco- /fär′məkō-/, **pharmo-** a combining form meaning 'of or related to drugs or medicine': *pharmacochemistry, pharmacomania, pharmacosychosis.*

pharmacodynamics /-dīnam′iks/ [Gk, *pharmakon,* drug, *dynamis*, power], the study of how a drug acts on a living organism, including the pharmacologic response observed relative to the concentration of the drug at an active site in the organism.

pharmacogenetics /-jənet′iks/ [Gk, *pharmakon,* drug, *genesis,* origin], the study of the effect that the genetic factors belonging to a group or to an individual has on the response of the group or the individual to certain drugs.

pharmacokinetics /fär′məkōkinet′iks/ [Gk, *pharmakon* + *kinesis,* motion], (in pharmacology) the study of the action of drugs within the body, including the routes and mechanisms of absorption and excretion, the rate at which a drug's action begins and the duration of the effect, the biotransformation of the substance in the body, and the effects and routes of excretion of the metabolites of the drug.

pharmacologic agent /-loj′ik/, any oral, parenteral, or topical substance used to alleviate symptoms and treat or control a disease process or aid recovery from an injury.

pharmacologic treatment. See **treatment.**

pharmacologic vagotomy, the use of medications to curtail functions of the vagus nerve. Also called **medical vagotomy.**

pharmacologist /fär′məkol′əjist/, a specialist in pharmacology.

pharmacology (phar) /-kol′əjē/ [Gk, *pharmakon* + *logos,* science], the study of the preparation, properties, uses, and actions of drugs.

pharmacopoeia /fär′məkəpē′ə/ [Gk, *pharmakon* + *poiein,* to make], **1.** a compendium containing descriptions, recipes, strengths, standards of purity, and dosage forms for selected drugs. **2.** the available stock of drugs in a pharmacy. **3.** the total of all authorized drugs available within the jurisdiction of a given geographic or political area. Also spelled **pharmacopeia.** See also *British Pharmacopoeia, United States Pharmacopeia.*

pharmacotherapy /-ther′əpē/ [Gk, *pharmakon,* drug + *therapeia*], the use of drugs to treat diseases.

pharmacy (phar) /fär′məsē/ [Gk, *pharmakon*], **1.** the study of preparing and dispensing drugs. **2.** a place for preparing and dispensing drugs.

-pharmic, a combining form meaning 'related to drugs and medicinal remedies': *alexipharmic, antipharmic, polypharmic.*

pharmo-. See **pharmaco-.**

pharyng-. See **pharyngo-.**

pharyngeal /ferin′jē·əl/ [Gk, *pharynx*, throat], pertaining to the pharynx.

pharyngeal aponeurosis [Gk, *pharynx,* throat, *apo,* from, *neuron,* sinew], a sheet of connective tissue just beneath the mucosa of the pharynx.

pharyngeal bursa, a blind sac at the base of the pharyngeal tonsil.

pharyngeal reflex. See **gag reflex.**

pharyngeal tonsil, one of two masses of lymphatic tissue situated on the posterior wall of the nasopharynx behind the posterior nares. During childhood these masses often swell and block the passage of air from the nasal cavity into the pharynx, preventing the child from breathing through the nose. Also called **adenoid.**

pharynges. See **pharynx.**

pharyngitis /fer′injī′tis/ [Gk, *pharynx* + *itis*], inflammation or infection of the pharynx, usually causing symptoms of a sore throat. Some causes of pharyngitis are diphtheria, herpes simplex virus, infectious mononucleosis, and streptococcal infection. Specific treatment depends on the cause. Symptoms may be relieved by analgesic medication, drinking warm or cold liquids, or saline irrigation of the throat. See also **strep throat.**

pharyngo- /fəring′gō-/, **pharyng-,** a combining form meaning 'of or related to the pharynx': *pharyngocele, pharyngoglossus, pharyngorrhagia.*

pharyngoconjunctival fever /fəring′gōkon′jungktī′vəl/ [Gk, *pharynx* + L, *conjunctivus,* connecting; *febris,* fever], an adenovirus infection characterized by fever, sore throat, and conjunctivitis. An epidemic illness, particularly prevalent in summer, spread by droplet infection and direct contact. Contaminated water in lakes and swimming pools is a common source of infection. See also **adenovirus.**

pharyngoscope /fəring'gəskōp/ [Gk, *pharynx* + *skopein*, to view], an endoscopic device for examining the lining of the pharynx.

pharyngoscopy /fer'ing·gos'kəpē/ [Gk, *pharynx*, throat + *skopein*, to view], the examination of the throat with a pharyngoscope.

pharyngotonsillitis /-ton'silī'tis/ [Gk, *pharynx*; L, *tonsilla*; Gk, *itis*, inflammation], an inflammation involving the pharynx and the tonsils.

pharynx /fer'inks/ [Gk,], *pl.* **pharynxes, pharynges** the throat, a tubular structure about 13 cm long that extends from the base of the skull to the esophagus and is situated just in front of the cervical vertebrae. The pharynx serves as a passageway for the respiratory and digestive tracts and changes shape to allow the formation of various vowel sounds. The pharynx is composed of muscle, is lined with mucous membrane, and is divided into the nasopharynx, the oropharynx, and the laryngopharynx. It contains the openings of the right and the left auditory tubes, the openings of the two posterior nares, the fauces, the opening into the larynx, and the opening into the esophagus. It also contains the pharyngeal tonsils, the palatine tonsils, and the lingual tonsils. Also called **throat.** See also **larynx.**

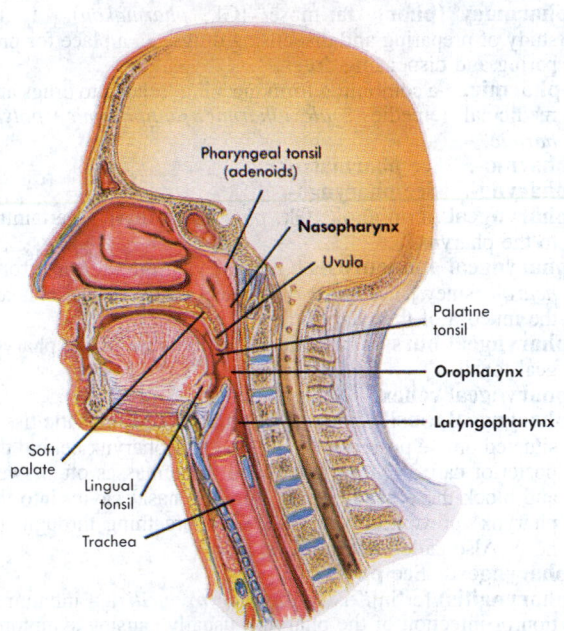

Pharyngeal tonsil
(adenoids)

Nasopharynx

Uvula

Palatine
tonsil

Oropharynx

Laryngopharynx

Soft
palate

Lingual
tonsil

Trachea

Pharynx *(Wilson, 1991)*

phase /fāz/ [Gk, *phasis*, appearance], in a periodic function, such as rotational or sinusoidal motion, the position relative to a particular part of the cycle.

phase 0, (in cardiology) the upstroke of the action potential.

phase 1, (in cardiology) the initial rapid repolarization phase of the action potential.

phase 2, (in cardiology) the plateau of the action potential; occurs during repolarization.

phase 3, (in cardiology) the terminal rapid repolarization phase of the action potential.

phase 4, (in cardiology) the period of electric diastole and the last of the four phases of cardiac action potential. A graph of phase 4 shows a gradual upward slope in a pacemaker cell, whereas phase 4 in a muscle cell is flat.

phase microscope, a microscope with a special condenser and objective containing a phase-shifting ring that allows the viewer to see small differences in refraction indexes as differences in image intensity or contrast. The phase microscope is used especially for examining transparent specimens, such as living or unstained cells and tissues.

phase of maximum slope, the time of rapid cervical dilation and rapid fetal descent in the active phase of labor. See **Friedman curve.**

phase one study, a clinical trial to assess the risk that might come from administering a new treatment modality. A **phase two study** evaluates the clinical effectiveness of the new modality, and a **phase three study** compares its effectiveness with the best existing treatment.

phasic /fā'zik/ [Gk, *phasis*], **1.** pertaining to a process proceeding in stages or phases. **2.** pertaining to a type of afferent or sensory nerve receptor of the proprioceptive system that responds to rate versus length changes in a muscle spindle. It is triggered by such stimuli as quick stretching, vibrations, and tapping.

-phasic. See **-phasia.**

-phasis, -phasia, -phasic, -phasy, a suffix meaning 'speech, utterance': *allophasis, heterophasis, paraphasis, aphasic.*

Ph.D., abbreviation for *Doctor of Philosophy.*

-phemia, a suffix meaning a '(specified) disorder of speech': *dysphemia, paraphemia, spasmophemia.*

phen-, a prefix indicating derivation from benzene: *phenacitin, phenicate, phenobarbitone.*

phenacemide /fənas'əmīd/, an anticonvulsant.
■ INDICATION: It is prescribed in the treatment of mixed seizures, particularly mixed forms of psychomotor seizures refractory to other drugs.
■ CONTRAINDICATIONS: Pregnancy, previous personality disturbances, or known hypersensitivity to this drug prohibits its use.
■ ADVERSE EFFECTS: Among the more serious adverse reactions are aplastic anemia, acute psychosis, paranoid and depressive reactions, nephritis, and hepatitis.

phenacetin /fənas'itin/, an analgesic.

Phenaphen, a trademark for an analgesic-antipyretic (acetaminophen and codeine).

phenazopyridine hydrochloride /fen'əzōpī'ridēn/, a urinary tract analgesic.
■ INDICATIONS: It is prescribed to reduce the pain of cystitis or other urinary tract infections.
■ CONTRAINDICATIONS: Renal insufficiency or known hypersensitivity to this drug prohibits its use.
■ ADVERSE EFFECTS: Among the more serious adverse reactions are headache and GI disturbances.

phencyclidine hydrochloride (PCP) /fensī'klidēn/, a piperidine derivative administered parenterally to achieve neuroleptic anesthesia. Because of its marked hallucinogenic properties, it is not used therapeutically in the United States. Its reported use as an abused substance has declined in recent years. Also called **angel dust.**

phendimetrazine tartrate /fen′dīmet′rəsēn/, a sympathomimetic amine used as an anorectic agent.

■ INDICATIONS: It is prescribed to decrease the appetite in the treatment of exogenous types of obesity.

■ CONTRAINDICATIONS: Cardiovascular disease, hypertension, hyperthyroidism, glaucoma, nervousness, a history of drug abuse, concomitant administration of central nervous system stimulants or monoamine oxidase inhibitors, or known hypersensitivity to this drug prohibits its use.

■ ADVERSE EFFECTS: Among the more serious adverse reactions are central nervous system stimulation, elevated blood pressure, insomnia, and dry mouth and tolerance to the drug.

-phene, -phen, a suffix denoting members of the phenol group: *camphene, phlobaphene, phosphene.*

phenelzine sulfate /fē′nəlzēn/, a monoamine oxidase (MAO) inhibitor.

■ INDICATIONS: It is prescribed in the treatment of endogenous and other types of depression.

■ CONTRAINDICATIONS: Liver dysfunction, congestive heart failure, pheochromocytoma, concomitant use of sympathomimetic drugs or foods high in tryptophan or tyramine, or known hypersensitivity to this drug prohibits its use.

■ ADVERSE EFFECTS: Among the most serious adverse reactions are orthostatic hypotension, vertigo, constipation, blurred vision, headache, overactivity, and dryness of the mouth. MAO inhibitors produce many adverse drug interactions.

Phenergan, a trademark for a phenothiazine derivative (promethazine), used as an adjunct to anesthesia.

phenformin /fen′fôrmin/, phenformin hydrochloride, an oral hypoglycemic. See also **non-insulin-dependent diabetes mellitus.**

phenic acid. See **carbolic acid.**

pheniramine maleate /fənir′əmēn, -min/, an antihistamine.

■ INDICATIONS: It is prescribed in the treatment of a variety of hypersensitivity reactions, including rhinitis, skin rash, and pruritus.

■ CONTRAINDICATIONS: Asthma or known hypersensitivity to this drug prohibits its use. It is not given to newborn infants or lactating mothers.

■ ADVERSE EFFECTS: Among the more serious adverse reactions are drowsiness, skin rash, and hypersensitivity reactions. Dry mouth and tachycardia commonly occur.

phenmetrazine hydrochloride /fənmet′rəzēn/, a sympathomimetic amine used as an anorectic agent.

■ INDICATIONS: It is prescribed to reduce the appetite and in the short-term treatment of exogenous obesity.

■ CONTRAINDICATIONS: Cardiovascular disease, hypertension, hyperthyroidism, glaucoma, history of drug abuse, concomitant use of a central nervous system stimulant or a monoamine oxidase inhibitor, or known hypersensitivity to this drug or other sympathomimetic drugs prohibits its use. It is not recommended for children under 12 years of age.

■ ADVERSE EFFECTS: Among the most serious adverse reactions are central nervous system stimulation, elevated blood pressure, insomnia, dry mouth, and others common to this class of drug.

phenobarbital /fē′nəbär′bital/, a barbiturate anticonvulsant and sedative-hypnotic.

■ INDICATIONS: It is prescribed in the treatment of a variety of seizure disorders and as a long-acting sedative.

■ CONTRAINDICATIONS: Porphyria, severe pain, respiratory problems, or known hypersensitivity to this drug or other barbiturates prohibits its use.

■ ADVERSE EFFECTS: Among the most serious adverse reactions are ataxia, porphyria, paradoxical excitement, drowsiness, occasional rashes, and, rarely, blood dyscrasias. It is involved in many drug interactions.

phenobarbital-phenytoin serum levels /-fen′itō′in/, the concentration of phenobarbital and phenytoin in the serum, monitored to maintain concentrations sufficient to control seizures but not high enough to cause toxic reactions. The control of seizures is commonly obtained in adults with plasma concentrations of phenobarbital that average 10 μg/ml per daily dose of 1 μg/kg; in children, 5 to 7 μg/ml per daily dose of 1 μg/kg. The control of seizures is commonly obtained with plasma concentrations of phenytoin that average 10 μg/ml, whereas toxic effects, such as nystagmus, typically develop with a concentration of 20 μg/ml. Ataxia may develop at a concentration of 30 μg/ml, and lethargy at a concentration of 40 μg/ml.

phenocopy /fē′nōkop′ē/ [Gk, *phainein,* to appear; L, *copia,* plenty], a phenotypic trait or condition that is induced by environmental factors but closely resembles a phenotype usually produced by a specific genotype. The trait is neither inherited nor transmitted to offspring. Such conditions as deafness, cretinism, mental retardation, and congenital cataracts are caused by mutant genes but also can result from a number of different agents, such as the rubella virus in the case of congenital cataracts. Phenocopies may present problems in genetic screening and genetic counseling so that all exogenous factors must be ruled out before any congenital trait or defect is labeled hereditary.

phenol /fē′nol/ [Gk, *phainein,* to appear; L, *oleum,* oil], **1.** a highly poisonous, caustic, crystalline chemical derived from coal tar or plant tar or manufactured synthetically. It has a distinctive, pungent odor and, in solution, is a powerful disinfectant, commonly called carbolic acid. **2.** Any of a large number and variety of chemical products closely related in structure to the alcohols and containing a hydroxyl group attached to a benzene ring. The phenols are components in dyes, plastics, disinfectants, antimicrobials, and other drugs, including salicylic acid.

phenol block, an injection of hydroxybenzene (phenol) into individual nerves, anesthetizing a selective block of those nerves. The technique is sometimes used to control spasticity in specific muscle groups or to block transmission of nerve impulses in conditions such as trigeminal neuralgia.

phenol camphor, an oily mixture of camphor and phenol, used as an antiseptic and toothache remedy.

phenol coefficient, a measure of the disinfectant activity of a given chemical in relation to carbolic acid. The activity is expressed as the ratio of a dilution of the chemical that kills in 10 minutes but not in 5 minutes to the 1:90 dilution of carbolic acid that kills in 10 minutes but not in 5 minutes.

phenolphthalein /fē′nolthal′ē·in, -thā′lēn/, **1.** a laxative that acts by stimulating the motor activity of the lower intestinal tract. **2.** an indicator of hydrogen ion in urine and gastric juice.

phenolphthalein laxative, a purgative that acts on the wall of the bowel.

■ INDICATIONS: It is prescribed in the treatment of chronic constipation and to prevent straining at the stool for postoperative patients and those with heart disease or hypertension.

■ CONTRAINDICATIONS: Symptoms of appendicitis, acute surgical abdomen, fecal impaction, intestinal obstruction or perforation, or known hypersensitivity to this drug prohibits its use.

■ ADVERSE EFFECTS: Among the most serious adverse reactions are abdominal cramping and pain, allergic reaction (particularly of the skin), dehydration, and laxative dependence.

phenol poisoning, corrosive poisoning caused by the ingestion of compounds containing phenol, such as carbolic acid, creosote, cresol, guaiacol, and naphthol. Characteristic of phenol poisoning are burns of the mucous membranes, weakness, pallor, pulmonary edema, convulsion, and respiratory, circulatory, cardiac, and renal failure. In treatment, the skin around the mouth and nose is washed, as are any external burns; the mouth, throat, esophagus, and stomach are lavaged with water and charcoal. Oxygen, intravenous fluids, electrolytes, and pain medication may be necessary. Rarely, esophageal stricture may develop as a complication of extensive tissue damage.

phenolsulfonphthalein /fē′nəlsul′fōnfthal′ē·in/, a bright red triphenylmethane dye soluble in water and used as an indicator at pH 7.7. Its sodium salt is injected intravenously and its rate of appearance in urine is used as a test for renal function. Also called **phenol red.**

phenomenon /finom′ənən/, *pl.* **phenomena** /finom′ənənl/ [Gk, *phainomenon,* something seen], a sign that is often associated with a specific illness or condition and is, therefore, diagnostically important.

phenothiazine /fē′nōthī′əzēn/, a yellow to green crystalline compound that is a source of dyes and is used in veterinary medicine to treat infestations of threadworms and roundworms. It is too toxic for humans, but derivatives of phenothiazine are used in tranquilizers and antihistamine medications. See also **phenothiazine derivatives.**

phenothiazine derivatives, any of a group of drugs that have a three ring structure in which two benzene rings are linked by a nitrogen and a sulfur. They represent the largest group of antipsychotic compounds in clinical medicine. Of the many phenothiazines and their congeners that are used as adjuncts to general anesthesia, antiemetics, major tranquilizers (antipsychotic agents), and antihistamines, the most widely used are the two prototypes, chlorpromazine and prochlorperazine; closely related are trimeprazine and triflupromazine. This group of drugs has largely revolutionized the practice of psychiatric medicine. Unlike the barbiturates, which act exclusively on the central nervous system (CNS), the phenothiazines exert significant influence on many organ systems of the body at once; for example, they exert antiadrenergic, anticholinergic, and antihistaminic activity. The effects on the CNS differ according to individual drug and patient status. All phenothiazine tranquilizers are withheld from patients with severe CNS depression or epilepsy and are given with caution to those with liver disease. These drugs are not recommended for use in pregnancy. See also specific drugs.

phenotype /fē′nətīp/ [Gk, *phainein,* to appear; *typos,* mark], **1.** the complete observable characteristics of an organism or group, including anatomic, physiologic, biochemical, and behavioral traits, as determined by the interaction of both genetic makeup and environmental factors. **2.** a group of organisms that resemble each other in appearance. Compare **genotype.** –**phenotypic,** *adj.*

phenoxy-, a combining form indicating the presence of a chemical group composed of phenyl and an atom of oxygen: *phenoxycaffeine*.

phenoxybenzamine hydrochloride /fēnok′sēben′zəmēn/, an antihypertensive.

■ INDICATIONS: It is prescribed in the control of hypertension and sweating in pheochromocytoma. If tachycardia is excessive, concomitant administration of propranolol may be necessary.

■ CONTRAINDICATIONS: Hypotension or known hypersensitivity to this drug prohibits its use.

■ ADVERSE EFFECTS: Among the more serious adverse reactions are severe hypotension, tachycardia, and GI irritation.

phenoxymethyl penicillin. See **penicillin V.**

phensuximide /fensuk′simīd/, an anticonvulsant.

■ INDICATIONS: It is prescribed to prevent and treat seizures in petit mal epilepsy.

■ CONTRAINDICATIONS: Known hypersensitivity to this drug or to any succinimide prohibits its use.

■ ADVERSE EFFECTS: Among the most serious adverse reactions are blood dyscrasias and a systemic lupuslike syndrome. Common reactions are GI disturbances and central nervous system depression with drowsiness or dizziness.

phentermine hydrochloride /fen′tərmēn/, a sympathomimetic amine used as an anorexic agent.

■ INDICATIONS: It is prescribed to decrease the appetite in the short-term treatment of exogenous obesity.

■ CONTRAINDICATIONS: Arteriosclerosis, cardiovascular disease, hypertension, glaucoma, hyperthyroidism, or known hypersensitivity to this drug or to other sympathomimetic drugs prohibits its use.

■ ADVERSE EFFECTS: Among the more serious adverse reactions are restlessness, insomnia, tachycardia, increased blood pressure, and dry mouth.

phentolamine /fentol′əmēn/, an antiadrenergic. It is administered as the hydrochloride form in tablets and as the mesylate form for injections.

■ INDICATIONS: It is prescribed in the control of symptoms of pheochromocytoma before and during surgery and for dermal necrosis and sloughing after extravasation of parenteral norepinephrine.

■ CONTRAINDICATIONS: History of myocardial infarction, angina, coronary artery disease, or known hypersensitivity to this drug prohibits its use.

■ ADVERSE EFFECTS: Among the more serious adverse reactions are tachycardia, cardiac dysrhythmias, anginal pain, and hypotension.

Phenurone, a trademark for an anticonvulsant (phenacemide).

phenyl (Ph) /fē′nil, fen′il/, a monovalent organic radical, C_6H_5, derived from benzene.

phenylacetic acid /fen′iləsē′tik/, a metabolite of phenylalanine excreted in urine in conjugation with glutamine.

phenylalanine (Phe) /fen′ilal′ənēn/, an essential amino acid necessary for the normal growth and development of infants and children and for normal protein metabolism throughout life. The normal value of this amino acid in the serum of adults is less than 3 mg/dl; in newborns, 1.2 to 3.5 mg/dl. It is abundant in milk, eggs, and other common foods. See also **amino acid, phenylketonuria, protein.**

phenylalaninemia /fen′ilaləninē′mē·ə/, the presence of phenylalanine in the blood. See also **hyperphenylalaninemia.**

phenylbutazone /-bōō′təzōn/, a nonsteroidal antiinflammatory agent.

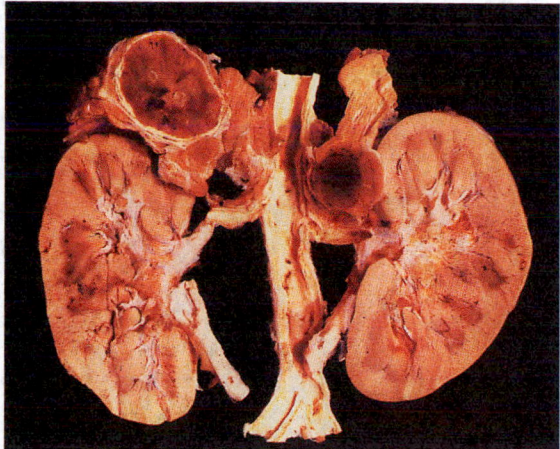

Chemical structure of phenylalanine (Seeley, 1992)

■ INDICATIONS: It is prescribed in the treatment of severe symptoms of arthritis, bursitis, and other inflammatory conditions.

■ CONTRAINDICATIONS: Impaired renal or hepatic function, a history of upper GI problems, blood dyscrasia, stomatitis caused by other drugs, hypertension, edema, or known hypersensitivity to this drug or to oxyphenbutazone prohibits its use. Caution is advised in administering this drug to children or elderly people.

■ ADVERSE EFFECTS: Among the more serious adverse reactions are fluid retention and potentially serious blood dyscrasias. GI irritation and nausea commonly occur. This drug interacts with many other drugs.

phenyl carbinol.   See **benzyl alcohol.**

phenylephrine hydrochloride /-ef′rēn/, an alpha-adrenergic agent.

■ INDICATIONS: It is prescribed to maintain blood pressure and is used locally as a nasal or ophthalmic vasoconstrictor.

■ CONTRAINDICATIONS: Narrow-angle glaucoma, concomitant administration of monoamine oxidase inhibitors, or known hypersensitivity to this drug prohibits its use.

■ ADVERSE EFFECTS: Among the more serious adverse reactions to the systemic administration of this drug are dysrhythmias and an excessive rise in blood pressure. Anxiety, congestion, and hypersensitivity reactions may occur from local administration of this drug.

phenylethyl alcohol /-eth′il/, a colorless, fragrant liquid with a burning taste, used as a bacteriostatic agent and preservative in medicinal solutions. Also called **benzyl carbonol.**

phenylic acid, phenylic alcohol.   See **carbolic acid.**

phenylketonuria (PKU) /fen′əlkē′tōnyŏŏr′ē·ə, fē′nəl-/, abnormal presence of phenylketone and other metabolites of phenylalanine in the urine, characteristic of an inborn metabolic disorder caused by the absence or a deficiency of phenylalanine hydroxylase, the enzyme responsible for the conversion of the amino acid phenylalanine into tyrosine. Accumulation of phenylalanine is toxic to brain tissue. Untreated individuals have very fair hair, eczema, a mousy odor of the urine and skin, and progressive mental retardation. Treatment consists of a diet low in phenylalanine. Phenylketonuria occurs approximately once in 16,000 births in the United States. Most states require a screening test for all newborns. See also **Guthrie test.** –**phenylketonuric,** *adj.*

phenyl methanol.   See **benzyl alcohol.**

phenylpropanolamine hydrochloride /fen′əlprō′pənol′-əmēn/, a sympathomimetic amine with vasoconstrictor action.

■ INDICATIONS: It is prescribed to relieve nasal congestion and related cold symptoms.

■ CONTRAINDICATIONS: Hypertension, coronary artery disease, concomitant administration of monoamine oxidase inhibitors, or known hypersensitivity to this drug prohibits its use.

■ ADVERSE EFFECTS: Among the more serious adverse reactions are nervousness, insomnia, anorexia, and increased blood pressure.

phenylpyruvic acid /fen′ilpīrōō′vik/, a product of the metabolism of phenylalanine. The presence of phenylpyruvic acid in the urine is indicative of phenylketonuria.

phenylpyruvic amentia.   See **phenylketonuria.**

phenyl salicylate, the salicylic ester of phenol. Also called **salol.** See also **salol camphor.**

phenyltoloxamine citrate /fen′iltəlok′səmēn/, an antihistamine usually used in a fixed-combination drug with an analgesic.

phenytoin /fen′ətō′in/, an anticonvulsant.

■ INDICATIONS: It is prescribed as an anticonvulsant in grand mal and psychomotor seizure disorders and as an antidysrhythmic agent, particularly in digitalis-induced dysrhythmias.

■ CONTRAINDICATIONS: Known hypersensitivity to this drug or to other hydantoins prohibits its use. It is used with caution in patients with a history of hepatic or hematologic abnormalities and in the presence of certain dysrhythmias.

■ ADVERSE EFFECTS: Among the more serious adverse reactions are ataxia, nystagmus, hypersensitivity reactions, and gingival hyperplasia. Rarely, a variety of severe reactions occur. This drug interacts with many other drugs.

pheo-, phao-, a combining form meaning 'dusky': *pheochrome, pheochromoblast, pheophytin.*

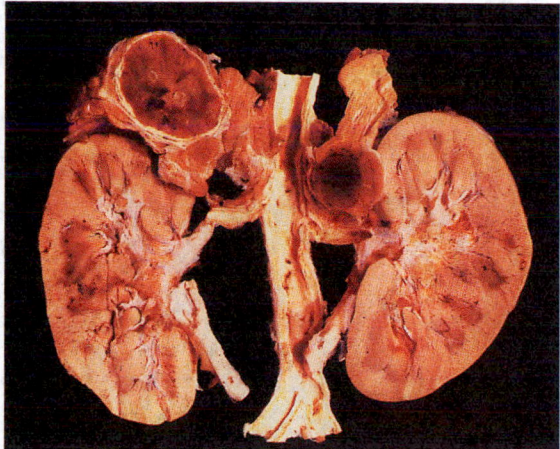

Adrenal pheochromocytoma (Turk, 1986)

pheochromocytoma /fē′ōkrō′mōsītō′mə/, *pl.* **pheochromocytomas, pheochromocytomata** [Gk, *phaios,* dark, *chroma,* color, *kytos,* cell, *oma,* tumor], a vascular tumor of chromaffin tissue of the adrenal medulla or sympathetic paraganglia, characterized by hypersecretion of epinephrine and norepinephrine, causing persistent or intermittent hypertension. Typical signs include headache, palpitation, sweating, nervousness, hyperglycemia, nausea, vomiting, and syncope. Weight loss, myocarditis, cardiac dysrhythmia, and heart failure may occur. The tumor occurs most frequently in young people, and only a small percentage of the lesions are malignant. The diagnosis may be established by laboratory assays showing increased catecholamines and their metabolites in urine and by pressor tests; intravenously injected histamine causes a sharp increase in blood pressure, and the administration of phentolamine produces a marked decrease. Surgical excision is the usual treatment; patients with nonresectable tumors may be treated with adrenergic blocking agents or with methyl tyrosine, a drug that reduces norepinephrine production.

pheresis. See **apheresis.**

pheromone /fer′əmōn′/ [Gk, *pherein,* to carry, *hormaein,* to stimulate], a hormonal substance secreted by an organism that elicits a particular response from another individual of the same species, but usually of the opposite sex.

phi /fī/, Π, π, the twenty-first letter of the Greek alphabet.

phil-, a prefix meaning 'having an affinity for or having a love for': *philanthropist, philocatalase, philoneism.*

-phil, -philic, -philous, a combining form meaning 'of that which has an attraction to or is stained by': *chromaphil, hydrophil, lipophil.*

-phile, **1.** a combining form meaning 'a lover or admirer' of somthing specified: *sarcophile.* **2.** a combining form meaning 'having an affinity for or being strongly attracted to a specified thing': *electrophile.*

Philadelphia chromosome (Ph¹) [Philadelphia, Pennsylvania], a translocation of the long arm of chromosome 22, often seen in the abnormal myeloblasts, erythroblasts, and megakaryoblasts of patients who have chronic myelocytic leukemia.

-philia, -phily, -philous-, a combining form meaning 'having a love, craving, affinity for': *cyanophilous, hydrophily, spasmophilia, necrophilia.*

-philous. See **-philia.**

philtrum /fil′trəm/, the vertical groove in the center of the upper lip.

-phily. See **-philia.**

phimosis /fimō′sis/ [Gk, muzzle], tightness of the prepuce of the penis that prevents the retraction of the foreskin over the glans. The condition is usually congenital but may be the result of infection. Circumcision is the usual treatment. An analogous condition of the clitoris occurs rarely. Compare **paraphimosis.** See also **phimosis vaginalis.**

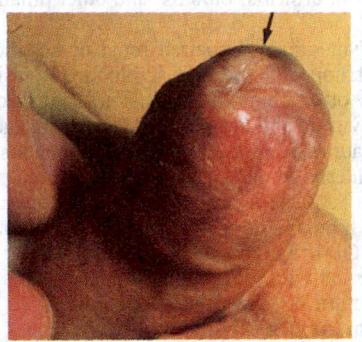

Phimosis *(Spitz, 1984)*

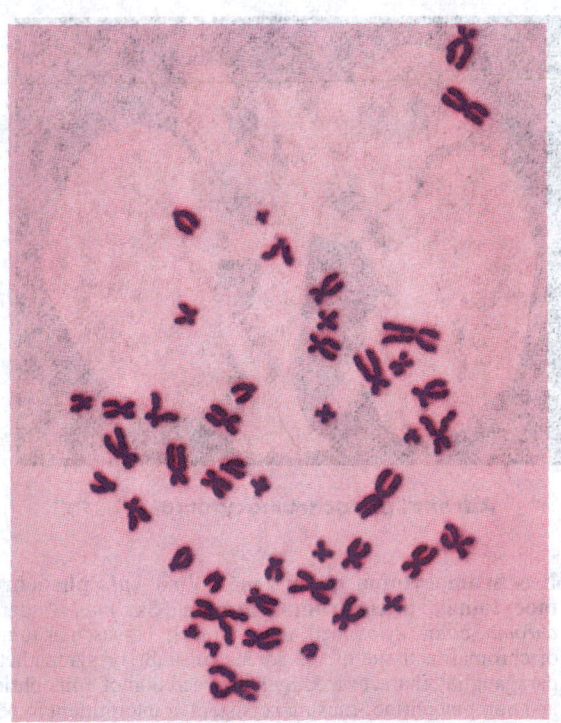

Philadelphia chromosome *(Hayhoe, 1992)*

phimosis vaginalis /vaj′inā′lis/, congenital narrowness or closure of the vaginal opening.

pHisoHex, a trademark for a detergent containing a topical antiinfective (hexachlorophene).

phleb-. See **phlebo-.**

phlebectomy /fləbot′əmē/ [Gk, *phleps,* vein + *ektome,* cutting out], the surgical removal of a vein or part of a vein.

phlebitis. See **thrombophlebitis.**

phlebo-, phleb- /fleb′ō-/, a combining form meaning 'of or related to a vein or veins': *phlebocarcinoma, phlebograph, phlebostenosis.*

phlebogram /fleb′əgram/ [Gk, *phleps,* vein, *gramma,* record], **1.** an x-ray film obtained by phlebography. **2.** a graphic representation of the venous pulse, obtained by phlebograph. Also called **venogram.**

phlebograph /fleb′əgraf′/, a device for producing a graphic record of the venous pulse.

phlebography /fləbog′rəfē/ [Gk, *phleps* + *graphein,* to record], **1.** the technique of preparing an x-ray image of veins injected with a radiopaque contrast medium. **2.** the technique of preparing a graphic record of the venous pulse by means of a phlebograph. Also called **venography.**

phlebostatic axis /-stat′ik/ [Gk, *phleps* + *stasis,* standing still], the approximate location of the right atrium, found by drawing an imaginary line from the fourth intercostal space at the right side of the sternum to an intersection with the midaxillary line.

phlebothrombosis /fleb′ōthrombō′sis/ [Gk, *phleps* + *thrombos,* lump, *osis,* condition], an abnormal venous condition in which a clot forms within a vein, usually caused by hemostasis, hypercoagulability, or occlusion. In contrast to thrombophlebitis, the wall of the vein is not inflamed.

phlebotomist /fləbot′əmist/ [Gk, *phleps*, vein + *ektome*], a physician or other individual with special training in the practice of opening veins to remove blood.

phlebotomize /fləbot′əmīz/ [Gk, *phleps*, vein + *ektome*, cutting out], to open a vein to remove blood.

phlebotomus fever /fləbot′əməs/ [Gk, *phleps* + *tomos*, cutting; L, *febris*, fever], an acute, mild infection, caused by one of five distinct arboviruses transmitted to humans by the bite of an infected sandfly, characterized by rapidly developing fever, headache, eye pain, conjunctivitis, myalgia, and, occasionally, a macular or urticarial rash. Aseptic meningitis also may occur. The disease is widespread in hot, dry areas where sandflies abound, and it has been seen in Panama and Brazil. Phlebotomus fever is self-limited, no fatalities have been recorded, and no specific therapy is available. Bed rest, fluids, and aspirin are recommended. A second attack may occur a few weeks after the first. Also called **pappataci fever, sandfly fever, three-day fever.**

phlebotomy /fləbot′əmē/ [Gk, *phleps* + *temnein*, to cut], the incision of a vein for the letting of blood, as in collecting blood from a donor. Phlebotomy is the chief treatment for polycythemia vera and may be performed every 6 months, or more frequently if required. The procedure is sometimes used to decrease the amount of circulating blood and pulmonary engorgement in acute pulmonary edema. At one time phlebotomy was practiced for almost every disorder. Also called **venesection.**

phleg-.   See **phlogo-.**

phlegm /flem/ [Gk, *phlegma*, mucus], thick mucus secreted by the tissues lining the airways of the lungs.

phlegmasia /flegmā′zhə/, *obsolete.*   an inflammation.

phlegmasia alba dolens [Gk, *phlegmone*, inflammation; L, *albus*, white; *dolens*, painful], thrombophlebitis of the femoral vein, resulting in edema of the leg and pain. It may occur after childbirth or after a severe febrile illness.

phlegmasia cerulea dolens, a severe form of thrombosis of a deep vein, usually the femoral vein. The condition is acute and fulminating and is usually accompanied by vast edema and cyanosis of the limb distal to the occluding thrombosis. Also called **blue phlebitis.**

phlegmatic /flegmat′ik/ [Gk, *phlegma*, sluggishness], pertaining to a person who is dull, apathetic, or not easily excitable.

phlegmon /fleg′mon/ [Gk, *phlegmone*, inflammation], an inflammation of connective tissue.

phlegmonous gastritis /fleg′mənsəs/ [Gk, *phlegmone* + *osis*, condition], a rare but severe form of gastritis, involving the connective tissue layer of the stomach wall. It occurs as a complication of systemic infection, peptic ulcer, cancer, surgery, or other severe stress and represents an acute abdominal emergency. Treatment includes surgery, antibiotics, and analgesics.

phlogo-, phleg-, a combining form meaning 'of or related to inflammation': *phlogocyte, phlogogen, phlogoxelotism.*

phlyctenular keratoconjunctivitis /flikten′yələr/ [Gk, *phlyktaina*, blister], an inflammatory condition of the cornea, characterized by tiny, ulcerating nodules, seen most often in children as a response to allergens found in tuberculin, gonococci, *Candida albicans,* or various parasites. Vitamin deficiency may be a factor. The condition responds to topical corticosteroids, but corneal scars may remain. Also called **phlyctenulosis, scrofulous keratitis.** See also **eczematous conjunctivitis.**

phob-, a combining form meaning 'of or pertaining to fear, panic, or morbid dread': *phobia, phobic, phobophobia.*

-phobe, -phobiac, -phobist, a suffix meaning 'one who fears' something specified: *dermatophobe, heliophobe, nosophobe.*

phobia /fō′bē·ə/ [Gk, *phobos*, fear], an anxiety disorder characterized by an obsessive, irrational, and intense fear of a specific object, such as an animal or dirt; of an activity, such as meeting strangers or leaving the familiar setting of the home; or of a physical situation, such as heights and open or closed spaces. Typical manifestations of phobia include faintness, fatigue, palpitations, perspiration, nausea, tremor, and panic. Some kinds of phobias are **agoraphobia, algophobia, claustrophobia, erythrophobia, gynephobia, laliophobia, mysophobia, nyctophobia, photophobia, xenophobia,** and **zoophobia.** Also called **phobic disorder, phobic neurosis, phobic reaction.** Compare **compulsion.** See also **simple phobia, social phobia.** **-phobic,** *adj.*

-phobia, a suffix meaning 'abnormal fear' of the object, experience, or place specified: *agoraphobia, claustrophobia, nyctophobia.*

phobiac /fō′bē·ak/, a person who exhibits or is afflicted with a phobia.

-phobiac.   See **-phobe.**

-phobic, -phobous, 1. a suffix meaning 'exhibiting or possessing an aversion for or fear of (something)': *Anglophobic, necrophobic, zoophobic.* **2.** a combining form meaning the 'absence of a strong affinity': *chromophobic, gentianophobic, osmiophobic.*

phobic /fō′bik/ [Gk, *phobos*, fear], pertaining to or resembling phobia.

phobic desensitization [Gk, *phobos*, fear; L, *de, sentire,* to feel], a method of resolving an ego dystonic or uncomfortable behavior pattern by reentry into the emotionally upsetting life situation in stages, first in fantasy and again in real life. It is similar to the psychotherapeutic techniques of **flooding** and **implosive therapy.**

phobic disorder.   See **anxiety disorders, phobia.**

phobic neurosis.   See **phobia.**

phobic state, a condition characterized by extreme anxiety resulting from the excessive, irrational fear of a particular object, situation, or activity. See also **phobia.**

-phobist.   See **-phobe.**

-phobous.   See **-phobic.**

phocomelia /fō′kəmē′lyə/ [Gk, *phoke,* seal, *melos,* limb], a developmental anomaly characterized by the absence of the upper portion of one or more of the limbs so that the feet or hands or both are attached to the trunk of the body by short, irregularly shaped stumps, resembling the fins of a seal. The condition, caused by interference with the embryonic development of the long bones, is rare and is seen primarily as a side effect of the drug thalidomide taken during early pregnancy. Also called **seal limbs.** Compare **amelia.** **-phocomelic,** *adj.*

phocomelic dwarf /fō′kəmē′lik/, a dwarf in whom the long bones of any or all of the extremities are abnormally short.

phocomelus /fōkom′ələs/, an individual who has phocomelia.

phon-.   See **phono-.**

phonation /fōnā′shən/ [Gk, *phone,* sound; L, *atio,* process], the production of speech sounds through the vibration of the vocal folds of the larynx.

-phone, a suffix meaning 'pertaining to sound or voice': *osteophone.*

phonetics /fōnet′iks/ [Gk, *phone,* voice], the science of speech sounds used in language.

-phonia. See **phony.**

phonic, of or pertaining to voice, sounds, or speech.

-phonic. See **-phony.**

phono-, phon- /fō′no-/, a prefix meaning 'of or related to sound, often specifically the sound of the voice': *phonocardiograph, phonopathy, phonopsia.*

phonocardiogram /-kär′dē·əgram′/, a graphic recording obtained from a phonocardiograph.

phonocardiograph /-kär′dē·əgraf′/ [Gk, *phone* + *kardia,* heart, *graphein,* to record], an electroacoustic device that produces graphic heart sound recordings, used in the diagnosis and monitoring of heart disorders. This instrument produces phonocardiograms by using a system of microphones and associated recording equipment. One microphone is usually placed on the chest near the base of the heart; another is positioned on the chest over the apex of the heart. The microphone placed over the base of the heart records the timing of the aortic and the pulmonary components of the second heart sound and the loudest murmurs. The microphone placed over the apex is connected to special filters that allow the recording of low-frequency sounds, such as those associated with atrial and ventricular gallops, as well as higher frequency sounds, such as those associated with mitral regurgitation and ventricular septal defect. To ensure an accurate recording, the examiner also uses audiophones to monitor the sounds and an oscilloscope to monitor cardiac impulses. **–phonocardiographic,** *adj.*

phonocardiography /-kär′dē·og′rəfē/ [Gk, *phone* + *kardia; graphein,* to record], the recording of heart sounds and murmurs by electromechanical apparatus.

phonology /fōnol′əjē/, the study of speech sounds, particularly the principles governing the way speech sounds are used in a given language.

phonophoresis /fō′nōfərē′sis/, an ultrasound therapeutic technique in which the high-frequency sound waves are used to force topical medicines into subcutaneous tissues. Continuous sonation for up to 10 minutes can drive a drug applied to the skin surface about 5 cm into muscle tissue. Drugs administered by phonophoresis include hydrocortisone, aspirin, and lidocaine. Because of the risk that the patient may be hypersensitive to the medication, the technique is used with caution.

phonoreceptor /-risep′tər/ [Gk, *phone,* voice; L, *recipere,* to receive], a device for receiving sound impulses.

-phony, -phonia, -phonic, a suffix meaning 'sound or to a type of speech': *autophony, egophony, organophonic.*

phor-, a prefix meaning 'bearing, carrying': *phoresis, phoroblast, phorology.*

-phore, -phor, a suffix meaning a 'bearer or possessor': *gluciphore, physaliphore, trochophore.*

-phoresis, a suffix meaning a 'movement in a (specified) manner or medium': *aphoresis, cataphoresis, diaphoresis.*

-phoria, **1.** a suffix meaning '(condition of the) visual axes of the eye': *anophoria, esophoria, exophoria.* **2.** a combining form meaning an 'emotional state': *adiaphoria, euphoria, ideaphoria.*

phosphatase /fos′fətāz/, an enzyme that acts as a catalyst

in chemical reactions involving phosphorus. See also **catalyst, enzyme.**

phosphate /fos′fāt/, a salt of phosphoric acid. Phosphates are extremely important in living cells, particularly in the storage and use of energy and the transmission of genetic information within a cell and from one cell to another. See also **adenosine diphosphate, adenosine triphosphate, phosphorus.**

phosphate-bond energy, the Gibbs energy for hydrolysis of a phosphate compound; a measure of relative phosphorylation power.

phosphatemia /fos′fātē′mē·ə/ [Gk, *phosphoros,* bringer of light; Gk, *haima,* blood], a condition of excessive phosphates in the blood.

phosphatide /fos′fətīd/, a phosphatidic acid from which the choline or colamine portion has been removed. It may occur as an intermediate in the biosynthesis of triglycerides and phospholipids. Also called **phosphotidate.**

phosphaturia /fos′fətŏŏr′ē·ə/ [Gk, *phosphoros,* bringer of light, *ouron* urine], a condition of excessive phosphates in the urine. Also called **phosphuria.**

phosphoglycerate kinase /fos′fōglis′ərāt/, an enzyme that catalyzes the reversible transfer of a phosphate group from adenosine triphosphate to D-3-phosphoglycerate, forming D-1,3-diphosphoglycerate. The reaction is one of the steps in glycolysis.

Phospholine Iodide, a trademark for a cholinergic (echothiophate iodide).

phospholipid /fos′fōlip′id/ [Gk, *phos,* light, *pherein,* to bear, *lipos* fat], one of a class of compounds, widely distributed in living cells, containing phosphoric acid, fatty acids, and a nitrogenous base. Two kinds of phospholipids are **lecithin** and **sphingomyelin.**

phosphomevalonate kinase /fos′fōməval′ənāt/, an enzyme that catalyzes the transfer of a phosphate group from adenosine triphosphate to produce adenosine diphosphate and 5-pyrophosphomevalonate.

phosphoresence /fos′fōres′əns/ [Gk, *phos,* light + *pherein,* to bear], **1.** a glow of yellow phosphorus caused by slow oxidation. **2.** the emission of visible light without accompanying heat as observed in phosphorus that has been exposed to radiation, continuing after radiation has ceased.

phosphoric acid /fosfôr′ik/, a clear, colorless, odorless liquid that is irritating to the skin and eyes and moderately toxic if ingested. It is used in the production of fertilizers, soaps, detergents, animal feeds, and certain drugs.

phosphorus (P) /fos′fərəs/ [Gk, *phos,* light, *pherein,* to bear], a nonmetallic chemical element occurring extensively in nature as a component of phosphate rock. Its atomic number is 15; its atomic weight is 30.975. Phosphorus forms a series of sulfides used commercially in the manufacture of matches. It can be prepared in yellow or white, red, and black allotropic forms. Phosphorus is essential for the metabolism of protein, calcium, and glucose. The body uses phosphorus in its combined forms, which are obtained from such nutritional sources as milk, cheese, meat, egg yolk, whole grains, legumes, and nuts. A nutritional deficiency of phosphorus can cause weight loss, anemia, and abnormal growth. Phosphorus is essential to the body for the production of adenosine triphosphate and for the process of glycolysis. Elemental white or yellow phosphorus is extremely poisonous and produces severe GI irritation. If ingested, it can produce hemorrhage, cardiovascular failure, and death. Chronic poisoning from phosphorus is characterized by anemia, cachexia, bronchitis, and necrosis of the mandible. Normal adult blood levels of phosphorus are 3.0 to 4.5 mg/dl or 0.97 to 1.45 mmol/L (SI units).

phosphorus poisoning, a toxic condition caused by the ingestion of white or yellow phosphorus, sometimes found in rat poisons, certain fertilizers, and fireworks. Intoxication is characterized initially by nausea, throat and stomach pain, vomiting, diarrhea, and an odor of garlic on the breath. After a few days of apparent recovery, nausea, vomiting, and diarrhea recur with renal and hepatic dysfunction. Treatment varies with manifestations. Physical contact with the vomitus and feces of the patient is avoided.

phosphorylase /fosfôr'iläs/ [Gk, *phosphoros,* bringer of light + *ase,* enzyme suffix], any of a group of physiologically important enzymes that catalyze reactions between phosphates and glycogen or other starch components, yielding glucose-1-phosphate.

phosphotidate. See **phosphatide.**

phosphuria. See **phosphaturia.**

phot-. See **photo-.**

photic /fō'tik/ [Gk, *phos,* light], pertaining to light.

-photic, a suffix meaning 'pertaining to the ability to see at a (specified) light level': *euryphotic, stenophotic, sthenophotic.*

photic epilepsy [Gk, *phos,* light, *epilepsia,* seizure], a condition in which epileptic attacks may be triggered by flickering light. Also called **photogenic epilepsy.**

photo- /fō'tō-/, **phot-,** a combining form meaning 'of or pertaining to light': *photoelectric, photoreceptor, phototropism.*

photoallergic /-əlur'gik/ [Gk, *photos,* light, *allos,* other, *ergein,* to work], exhibiting a delayed hypersensitivity reaction after exposure to light. Compare **phototoxic.** See also **photoallergic contact dermatitis.**

photoallergic contact dermatitis, a papulovesicular, eczematous, or exudative skin reaction occurring 24 to 48 hours after exposure to light in a previously sensitized person. The sensitizing substance concentrates in the skin and requires chemical alteration by light to become an active antigen. Among common photosensitizers are phenothiazines, hexachlorophene, oral hypoglycemic agents, and sulfanilamide. Prevention requires avoidance of the photosensitizer and of sunlight. Treatment is the same as that for any other inflammatory dermatitis.

photoallergy /-al'ərjē/ [Gk, *phos,* light, *allos,* other + *ergein,* to work], a sensitivity to light as a cause of allergic reactions.

photochemotherapy /-kē'mōther'əpē/ [Gk, *photos* + *chemeia,* alchemy, *therapeia,* treatment], a kind of chemotherapy in which the effect of the administered drug is enhanced by exposing the patient to light. Also called **photodynamic therapy.** See also **chemotherapy.**

photodisintegration /-disin'təgrā'shən/, (in radiology) the interaction of a high-energy x-ray photon with the nucleus of a target atom, resulting in the emission of a nucleon or other nuclear fragment. It may occur when a photon with energy greater than 10 MeV escapes interaction with the electron cloud or nuclear force field of an atom and is absorbed directly by the nucleus.

photodynamic therapy. See **photochemotherapy.**

photoelectron /-ilek'tron/ [Gk, *phos,* light + *elektron,* amber], any electron that is discharged when light strikes a metal surface.

photogenic epilepsy. See **photic epilepsy.**

photokinetic /-kinet'ik/ [Gk, *phos,* light, *kinesis,* movement], pertaining to any movement that is stimulated by light rays.

photometer /fōtom'ətər/ [Gk, *photos* + *metron,* 'measure], an instrument that measures light intensity. It usually is composed of a source of radiant energy, a filter for wavelength selection, a cuvette holder, a detector, and a readout device.

photomultiplier /-mul'tiplī'ər/ [Gk, *photos* + L, *multiplex,* many folds], a device used in many radiation detection applications that converts low levels of light into electric pulses. A bank of such tubes is used in gamma cameras to view the crystal.

photon /fō'ton/ [Gk, *photos*], the smallest quantity of electromagnetic energy. It has no mass and no charge but travels at the speed of light. Photons may occur in the form of x-rays, gamma rays, or a quantum of light. The energy (E) of a photon is expressed as the product of its frequency (v) and Planck's constant (h), as in the equation E = hv. X-ray photons occur in frequencies of from 10^{18} to 10^{21} Hz and energies that range upward from 1 KeV.

photophobia /-fō'bē·ə/ [Gk, *photos* + *phobos,* fear], **1.** abnormal sensitivity to light, especially by the eyes. The condition is prevalent in albinism and various diseases of the conjunctiva and cornea and may be a symptom of such disorders as measles, psittacosis, encephalitis, Rocky Mountain spotted fever, and Reiter's syndrome. **2.** (in psychiatry) a morbid fear of light with an irrational need to avoid light places. The anxiety disorder is seen more often in women than in men and is usually caused by a repressed intrapsychic conflict symbolically related to light. **—photophobic,** *adj.*

photopic eye. See **light-adapted eye.**

photopic vision /fōtop'ik/, daylight vision, which depends primarily on the function of the retinal cone cells.

photoprotective /-prətek'tiv/, protective against the potential adverse effects of ultraviolet light.

photoreaction /-rē·ak'shən/ [Gk, *phos* + L, *re, agere,* to act], any chemical reaction that is stimulated by the influence of light.

photoreceptor /-risep'tər/ [Gk, *phos,* light; L, *recipere,* to receive], a nerve cell that is receptive to light stimuli.

photorefractive keratectomy /-refrak'tiv/, a procedure for the treatment of near-sightedness in which a 30-second exposure to an excimer laser beam shaves a few layers of cells off the surface of the cornea. The laser flattens the cornea to reduce or eliminate myopia. Compare **radial keratotomy.**

photoscan /fō'tōskan'/, a radiograph that shows the distribution of a radiopharmaceutic in the body.

photosensitive /-sen'sitiv/ [Gk, *photos* + L, *sentire,* to feel], pertaining to increased reactivity of skin to sunlight caused by a disorder, such as albinism or porphyria, or more frequently resulting from the use of certain drugs. Relatively brief exposure to sunlight or to an ultraviolet lamp may cause edema, papules, urticaria, or acute burns in individuals with endogenous or acquired photosensitivity. Drugs inducing photosensitivity include phenothiazine tranquilizers, the antibiotic tetracycline, the antimycotic griseofulvin, the antibacterial nalidixic acid, oral hypoglycemic agents, the artificial sweetener calcium cyclamate, the oral contraceptive agents mestranol and norethynodrel, and halogenated salicylanides used in antifungal soaps. Treatment involves avoidance of exposure to sunlight or the photosensitizing agent. Methoxsalen and trioxsalen are potent photosensitizers sometimes used to enhance pigmentation or increase tolerance to sunlight, but overexposure or overdosage can cause severe reactions.

photosensitivity /-sen′sitiv″itē/, any abnormal response to exposure to light, specifically, a skin reaction requiring the presence of a sensitizing agent and exposure to sunlight or its equivalent. Photosensitivity includes photoallergic and phototoxic reactions and is common in systemic lupus erythematosis.

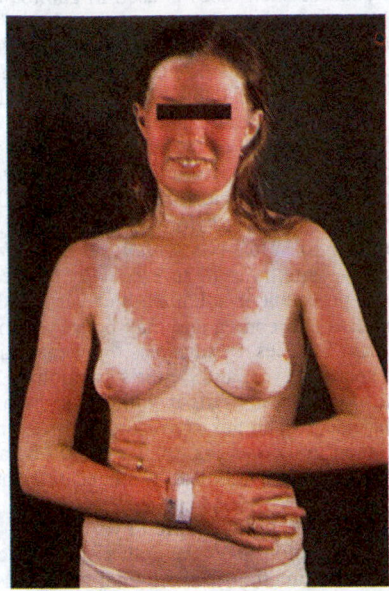

Typical photosensitive rash of SLE (Shipley, 1993)

photosensitization /-sen′sitizā′shən/ [Gk, *phos*, light + L, *sentire*, to feel], the process of rendering an organism sensitive to the effects of light rays.

photosynthesis /fōtōsin′thəsis/ [Gk, *photos* + *synthesis*, putting together], a process by which green plants containing chlorophyll synthesize chemical substances, chiefly carbohydrates, from atmospheric carbon dioxide and water, using light for energy and liberating oxygen in the process.

phototherapy /-ther′əpē/ [Gk, *photos* + *therapeia* treatment], the treatment of disorders by the use of light, especially ultraviolet light. Ultraviolet light may be employed in the therapy of acne, decubiti and other indolent ulcers, psoriasis, and hyperbilirubinemia. See also **photochemotherapy.** –**phototherapeutic,** *adj.*

phototherapy in the newborn, a treatment for hyperbilirubinemia and jaundice in the newborn that involves the exposure of an infant's bare skin to intense fluorescent light. The blue range of light accelerates the excretion of bilirubin in the skin, decomposing it by photooxidation.
■ METHOD: The infant is placed nude under the fluorescent lights with the eyes and genitalia covered. The baby is turned frequently, and the body temperature is monitored, using a skin thermistor. All vital signs are carefully noted, and details regarding position of the bulbs, time and duration of treatment, and the infant's response are charted. Ad-

verse effects of phototherapy include dehydration: An infant may need 25% more fluid during treatment. Loose stools and 'bronze baby' syndrome may occur.
■ INTERVENTIONS: The nurse performs phototherapy and may be responsible for collecting specimens for serial tests for bilirubin in the blood. The lights may scorch the nurse's hair and irritate the eyes; as protection, a cap and sunglasses may be worn. Breast feeding may be discontinued during treatment but often is not; additional water is always given. The family is encouraged to visit and to participate in caring for the infant. They may be told that the eyeshields are necessary but do not seem to bother the infant.
■ OUTCOME CRITERIA: Bilirubin levels usually decrease by 3 to 4 mg/dl in the first 8 to 12 hours of therapy; thus simple jaundice clears rapidly. Excess bilirubin and jaundice that are the result of hemolytic disease or infection may be controlled with phototherapy, but the underlying cause is treated separately. Recovery is usually complete. The long-term safety of phototherapy has not been established; short-term efficacy and practicality of use are certain.

phototoxic /-tok′sik/ [Gk, *photos* + *toxikon*, poison], characterized by a rapidly developing, nonimmunologic reaction of the skin when it is exposed to a photosensitizing substance and light. Compare **photoallergic.** See also **phototoxic contact dermatitis.**

phototoxic contact dermatitis, a rapidly appearing, sunburnlike response of areas of skin that have been exposed to the sun after contact with a photosensitizing substance. Hyperpigmentation may follow the acute reaction. Coal tar derivatives, oil of bergamot (often used in cosmetics and beverages), and many plants containing furocoumarin (cowslip, buttercup, carrot, parsnip, mustard, and yarrow) are known photosensitizing materials. Treatment includes Burow's solution, acid mantle cream, and topical corticosteroids.

pH paper. See **nitrazine paper**.

-phragma, -phragm, a combining form meaning a 'septum or musculomembranous barrier between cavities': *inophragma, mesophragma, telophragma.*

-phrasia, a combining form meaning an 'abnormal condition of speech': *aphrasia, echophrasia, embolophrasia.*

phren /fren/ [Gk, mind], **1.** the diaphragm. **2.** *obsolete.*

phrenetic /frənet′ik/ [Gk, *phren*], frenzied, delirious, maniacal.

phreni-, phrenico-, phreno-. a combining form meaning 'relating to the mind or the diaphragm': *phrenology, phrenalgia.*

-phrenia, a combining form meaning a 'disordered condition of mental activity': *hebephrenia, ideophrenia, kolyphrenia.*

phrenic /fren′ik/ [Gk, *phren*, mind], **1.** of or pertaining to the diaphragm. **2.** of or pertaining to the mind.

-phrenic, 1. a combining form meaning the 'diaphragm or adjacent regions of the body': *costophrenic, postphrenic, subphrenic.* **2.** a combining form meaning 'characteristic of a disorder of the mind': *hebephrenic, ideophrenic, schizophrenic.*

phrenic nerve, one of a pair of muscular branches of the cervical plexus, arising from the fourth cervical nerve. It contains about one half as many sensory as motor fibers and is generally known as the motor nerve to the diaphragm, although the lower thoracic nerves also help to innervate the diaphragm. The phrenic nerve lies on the ventral surface of the scalenus anterior, crossing from its lateral to its medial border. It continues with the scalenus anterior between the subclavian vein and the subclavian artery, enters the thorax, passes over the cupula of the pleura, continues along the lateral aspect of the pericardium, and reaches the diaphragm, where it divides into terminal branches. The right phrenic nerve is deeper and shorter than the left. The pleural branches of the phrenic nerve are very fine filaments supplying the mediastinal pleura. The pericardial branches are delicate filaments passing to the upper pericardium. The terminal branches diverge after passing separately through the diaphragm and are distributed on the abdominal surface of the diaphragm. On the right side, a branch near the inferior vena cava communicates with the phrenic plexus in association with a phrenic ganglion. There is no phrenic ganglion on the left side. Also called **internal respiratory nerve of Bell.** Compare **accessory phrenic nerve.**

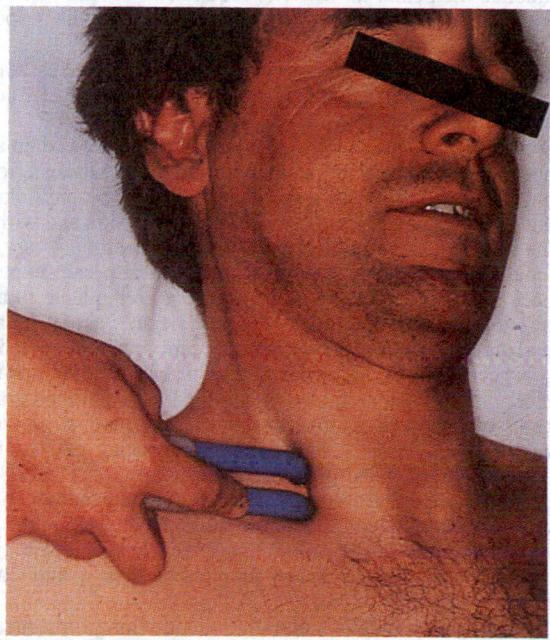

Evaluation of phrenic nerve function
(Turner-Warwick, 1993)

phrenico-, phreno-. See **phreni-.**
phthi-, a combining form meaning 'decay, wasting away': *phthisiogenesis, phthisiomania, phthisis.*
Phthirus /thī′rəs/ [Gk, *phtheir,* louse], a genus of bloodsucking lice that includes the species *Phthirus pubis,* the pubic louse, or crab.
phthisis /tis′is, thī′sis/ [Gk, *phthisis,* wasting away], any wasting disease involving all or part of the body, such as pulmonary tuberculosis.
-phthongia, a combining form meaning a 'condition of speech': *aphthongia, diphthongia, heterophthongia.*
phyco-, a combining form meaning 'of or pertaining to seaweed': *phycochrome, phycocyan, phycology.*
phycologist /fēkol′əjist/, a person who specializes in the study of algae. Also called **algologist.**
phycology /fēkol′əjē/ [Gk, *phykos,* seaweed, *logos,* sci-

ence], the branch of science that is concerned with algae. Also called **algology.**
phycomycosis /fī′kōmīkō′sis/ [Gk, *phykos* + *mykes,* fungus, *osis* condition], a fungal infection caused by a species of the order Phycomycetes. These organisms are common in the soil and are not usually pathogenic. Severe nosocomial pulmonary phycomycosis sometimes occurs with advanced diabetes mellitus that is untreated or out of control and complicated by ketoacidosis. See also **zygomycosis.**
phyl-, a combining form meaning 'guarding or preservation': *phylacagogic, phylactic, phylaxis.*
phylactic /filak′tik/ [Gk, *phylax,* guard], **1.** serving to protect. **2.** something that produces phylaxis.
-phylaxis, a combining form meaning 'protection': *anaphylaxis, prophylaxis.*
-phyll, -phyl, a combining form meaning a 'leaf': *chlorophyll, leukophyll.*
phyllo- /fil′ō-/, a combining form meaning 'of or pertaining to leaves': *phyllochlorin, phyllode, phyllosan.*
phylloquinone. See **vitamin K₁.**
phylo- /fī′lō-/, a combining form meaning 'type, kind, race, or tribe': *phylobiology, phylogenesis, phylogeny.*
phylogenesis. See **phylogeny.**
phylogenetic /fī′lōgənet′ik/ [Gk, *phylon,* tribe, *genesis,* origin], **1.** of, relating to, or acquired during phylogeny. **2.** based on a natural evolutionary relationship, such as a system of classification. Also called **phylogenic.**
phylogeny /filoj′ənē/ [Gk, *phylon* + *genesis*], the development of the structure of a particular race or species as it evolved from simpler forms of life. Compare **ontogeny.** See also **comparative anatomy.**
phylum /fī′ləm/ [Gk, *phylon,* tribe], a major classification category of the plant and animal kingdoms, representing one or more classes.
-phyma, a combining form meaning a 'swelling or tumor': *adenophyma, celiophyma, onychophyma.*
physi-. See **physio-.**
physiatrics /fiz′ē·at′riks/ [Gr, *physis,* nature + *iatrikos,* treatment], the diagnosis and treatment of disease by the use of physical agents such as heat, cold, light, water, electricity, and mechanical devices. Also called **physical medicine.**
physiatrist /fiz′ē·at′rist/, a physician specializing in physical medicine and rehabilitation who has been certified by the American Board of Physical Medicine and Rehabilitation after completing residency and other requirements.
-physical, a combining form meaning 'natural': *iatrophysical, medicophysical, psychophysical.*
physical abuse /fiz′ikəl/ [Gk, *physikos,* natural; L, *abuti,* to abuse], one or more episodes of aggressive behavior, usually resulting in physical injury with possible damage to internal organs, sense organs, the central nervous system, or the musculoskeletal system of another person.
physical allergy, an allergic response to physical factors, such as cold, heat, light, or trauma. Usually, specific antibodies are found in people having physical allergies. Common characteristics include pruritus, urticaria, and angioedema. There may be photosensitivity, caused by the use of certain cosmetics or drugs. Prophylaxis usually includes an attempt to remove the stimulus, and treatment involves the use of antihistamines or steroids. Compare **contact dermatitis.** See also **atopic.**
physical assessment, the part of the health assessment

representing a synthesis of the information obtained in a physical examination.

physical chemistry, the natural science dealing with the relationship between chemical and physical properties of matter.

physical diagnosis, the diagnostic process accomplished by the study of the physical manifestations of health and illness revealed in the physical examination, as guided by the patient's complete history and supported by various laboratory tests. Physical diagnosis is to medicine what the health assessment is to nursing.

physical examination, an investigation of the body to determine its state of health, using any or all of the techniques of inspection, palpation, percussion, auscultation, and smell. The physical examination, history, and initial laboratory tests constitute the data base on which a diagnosis is made and on which a plan of treatment is developed.

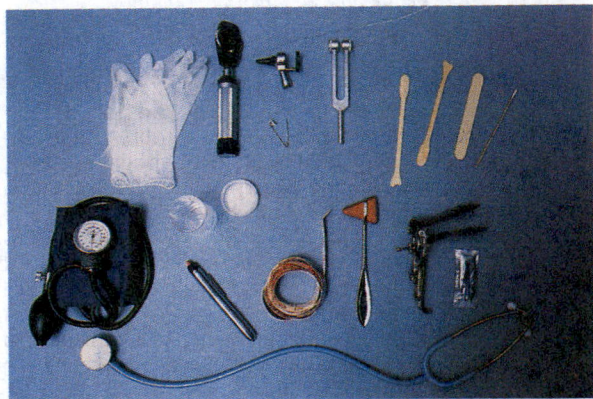

Equipment used during a physical examination
(Potter, 1993)

physical fitness, the ability to carry out daily tasks with alertness and vigor, without undue fatigue, and with enough energy reserve to meet emergencies or to enjoy leisure time pursuits.

physical medicine, the use of physical therapy techniques to return physically diseased or injured patients to a useful life. See also **rehabilitation.**

physical science, the study of the properties and behavior of nonliving matter. Some kinds of physical science are **chemistry, geology,** and **physics.** Compare **life science.**

physical sign [Gk, *physikos*, natural; L, *signum*], an objective indicator found during physical diagnosis or one detected by palpation, percussion, or auscultation.

physical therapist, a person who is licensed to assist in the examination, testing, and treatment of physically disabled or handicapped people through the use of special exercise, application of heat or cold, use of sonar waves, and other techniques. A physical therapist usually becomes qualified by taking a 4-year college course leading to a B.S. in physical therapy or a special 12-month certificate course after obtaining a bachelor's degree in a related field.

physical therapy, the treatment of disorders with physical agents and methods, such as massage, manipulation, therapeutic exercises, cold, heat (including shortwave, mi-

crowave, and ultrasonic diathermy), hydrotherapy, electric stimulation, and light to assist in rehabilitating patients and in restoring normal function after an illness or injury. Also called **physiotherapy.**

physical therapy aide, a person who, under the supervision of a licensed physical therapist, assists in carrying out patient treatment programs and performing related clerical tasks.

physician /fizish′ən/ [Gk, *physikos*, natural], a health professional who has earned a degree of Doctor of Medicine (M.D.) after completing an approved course of study at an approved medical school. Satisfactory completion of National Board Examinations, usually given during both the second and the final years of medical school and after graduation, is also required. An M.D. usually enters a hospital internship program for 1 year of postgraduate training before beginning practice or further training in a specialty. To practice medicine, an M.D. is required to obtain a license from the state in which professional services will be performed.

physician extender, a health care provider who is not a physician but who performs medical activities typically performed by a physician.

physician's assistant (PA), a person trained in certain aspects of the practice of medicine to provide assistance to a physician. A physician's assistant is trained by physicians and practices under the direction and supervision and within the legal license of a physician. Training programs vary in length from a few months to 2 years. Health care experience or academic preparation may be a prerequisite to admission to some programs. Most physician's assistants are prepared for the practice of primary care, but some practice subspecialties, including surgical assistance, dialysis, or radiology. National certification is available to qualified graduates of approved training programs. The national organization is the American Association of Physician's Assistants (AAPA). Also called **physician's associate.**

Physician's Desk Reference (PDR), a compendium compiled annually, containing information about drugs, primarily prescription drugs and products used in diagnostic procedures in the United States, supplied by their manufacturers.

physico- [Gr, *physikos*, natural], a combining form meaning 'natural or knowledge of nature': *physical, physiology.*

physics /fiz′iks/ [Gk, *physikos*, natural], the study of matter and energy, particularly as related to motion and force.

-physics, a combining form meaning the 'science of the nature of' something specified: *cytophysics, medicophysics, microphysics.*

physio-, physi-, a combining form meaning 'related to nature or to physiology': *physiochemical, physiognosis, physiotherapy.*

physiologic /fiz′ē·əloj′ik/ [Gk, *physis*, nature + *logos*, science], pertaining to physiology, particularly normal functions as opposed to the pathological.

physiological age [Gk, *physis*, nature, *logos*, science; L, *aetas*, age], the age of the body as determined by its stage of development or deterioration in terms of functional norms for various systems.

physiological albuminuria [Gk, *physis*, nature + *logos*, science; L, *albus*, white; Gk, *ouron*, urine], the presence of albumin in the urine in the absence of any disease usually associated with the condition.

physiological incompatibility, a condition in which substances, such as drugs, may have mutually antagonistic effects on the body.

physiological murmur [Gk, *physis* + *logos*; L, *murmur*, humming], a functional murmur produced by an alteration of function without evidence of heart damage or disease.

physiological salt solution, a normal saline solution, usually consisting of a sterile 0.9% w/v solution of sodium chloride in distilled water. It is isotonic with normal body fluids.

physiologic amenorrhea [Gk, *physis*, nature + *logos*, science; *a*, *men*, month, *rhoia*, to flow], an absence of menstruation for normal reasons, such as pregnancy, lactation, menopause, or prepuberty.

physiologic antidote [Gk, *physis* + *logos*; *anti*, *dotos*, that which is given], a drug that has the opposite effect on the body from that caused by a poisonous or toxic substance.

physiologic chemistry. See **biochemistry.**

physiologic contracture [Gk, *physikos* + *logos*, science; L, *contractio*, drawing together], a temporary condition in which muscles may contract and shorten for a considerable period of time. Drugs, extremes of temperature, and local accumulation of lactic acid are causes.

physiologic dead space. See **dead space.**

physiologic dwarf. See **primordial dwarf.**

physiologic flexion, an excessive amount of flexor tone that is normally present at birth because of the existing level of central nervous system maturation and fetal positioning in the uterus.

physiologic hypertrophy, a temporary increase in the size of an organ or part because of normal physiologic functions, such as occurs in the walls of the uterus and in the breasts during pregnancy.

physiologic jaundice [Gk, *physis*, nature + *logos*, science; Fr, *jaune*, yellow], a simple jaundice of newborn infants that involves the breaking down of the excessive number of red blood cells that may be present at birth.

physiologic motivation, a bodily need, such as for food or water, that initiates behavior directed toward satisfying the particular need. Also called **organic motivation.** Compare **social motivation.**

physiologic occlusion, 1. a closure of the teeth that complements and enhances the functions of the masticatory system. 2. a closure of the teeth that produces no pathologic effects on the stomatognathic system, normally dissipating the stresses placed on the teeth and creating a balance between the stresses and the adaptive capacity of the supporting tissues. 3. an acceptable occlusion in a healthy gnathic system.

physiologic psychology, the study of the interrelationship of physiologic and psychologic processes, especially the effects of a change from normal to abnormal.

physiologic retraction ring, a ridge around the inside of the uterus that forms during the second stage of normal labor at the junction of the thinned lower uterine segment and thickened upper segment as a result of progressive lengthening of the muscle fibers of the lower segment and concomitant shortening of the muscle fibers of the upper segment. Compare **constriction ring, pathologic retraction ring.**

physiologic saline. See **saline solution.**

physiologic third heart sound, a low-pitched extra heart sound heard early in diastole in a healthy child or young adult. It is of no clinical significance and usually disappears with age. The same sound, heard in an older person who

has heart disease, is an abnormal finding called a ventricular gallop. See also **gallop.**

physiologic tremor [Gk, *physis* + *logos*; L, *tremor*, shaking], any tremor caused by physiological factors, such as fatigue, fear, or cold.

physiologist /fiz′ē·ol′əjist/ [Gk, *physis*, nature + *logos*, science], a person who specializes in the science of living organisms.

physiology /fix′ē·ol′əjē/ [Gk, *physikos* + *logos*, science], 1. the study of the processes and function of the human body. 2. the study of the physical and chemical processes involved in the functioning of living organisms and their component parts. Kinds of physiology are **comparative physiology, developmental physiology, hominal physiology,** and **pathologic physiology.** Compare **anatomy.** See also the Appendix.

physiopathologic /fiz′ē·əpath′əloj′ik/ [Gk, *physis*, nature, *pathos*, disease, *logos*, science], pertaining to the physiological approach to disease.

physiotherapy. See **physical therapy.**

-physis, a combining form meaning a 'growth or growing': *metaphysis, onychophysis, zygapophysis.*

physo-, a combining form meaning 'of or pertaining to air or gas': *physocele, physocephaly, physometra.*

physostigmine /fī′sōstig′min/, a cholinergic acetylcholinesterase inhibitor.

■ INDICATIONS: It is prescribed in the treatment of some forms of glaucoma and to reverse effects of neuromuscular blocking agents.

■ CONTRAINDICATIONS: Narrow-angle glaucoma, iridocyclitis, or hypersensitivity to this drug prohibits its use.

■ ADVERSE EFFECTS: Among the more serious adverse reactions are bradycardia, dyspnea, bronchospasm, anorexia, and convulsions. Also called **eserine, eserine sulfate.**

physostigmine salicylate, an anticholinergic drug inhibitor.

■ INDICATIONS: It is prescribed in the treatment of central nervous system effects caused by drugs in clinical or toxic dosages capable of producing anticholinergic poisoning.

■ CONTRAINDICATIONS: Asthma, gangrene, diabetes, cardiovascular disease, or mechanical obstruction of the intestines or urinary tract prohibits its use. It is also not administered to patients in any vagotonic state and to those receiving choline esters or depolarizing neuromuscular blocking agents.

■ ADVERSE EFFECTS: Among the most serious adverse reactions are hypersalivation, bradycardia, convulsions, and hypertensive reactions.

phytanic acid storage disease /fītan′ik/, a rare genetic disorder of lipid metabolism in which there are accumulations of phytanic acid in the plasma and tissues. The condition is characterized by ataxia, peripheral neuropathy, retinitis pigmentosa, and abnormalities of the bone and skin. Also called **Refsum's syndrome.**

phyte-. See **phyto-.**

-phyte, a combining form meaning a 'plant that grows in or on or produces': *epiphyte, paraphyte, pteridophyte.*

phyto-, phyt-, a combining form meaning 'of or pertaining to a plant or plants': *phytobezoar, phytochemistry, phytoncide.*

phytogenesis /fī′tōjen′əsis/ [Gk, *phyton*, plant; *genein*, to produce], the origin and evolution of plant organisms.

phytogenous /fītoj′ənəs/ [Gk, *phyton*, plant, *genein*, to produce], pertaining to production by plant growth, origin in a plant, or the origin or formation of plant organisms.

phytohemagglutinin (PHA) /fī'tōhem'əglŏŏ'tinin/ [Gk, *phyton,* plant, *haima,* blood; L, *agglutinare,* to glue], a hemagglutinin that is derived from a plant, specifically the lectin obtained from the red kidney bean. Also called **phytolectin.**

phytohemagglutinin test, a test to identify genetic carriers of cystic fibrosis, performed by exposing white blood cells to phytohemagglutinin. A normal reaction involves a noticeable increase of cell protein.

phytolectin. See **phytohemagglutinin.**

phytonadione. See **vitamin K₁.**

pi /pī/, Π, π, the sixteenth letter of the Greek alphabet.

P.I., 1. (in patient records) abbreviation for *present illness.* **2.** abbreviation for *International Pharmacopeia.*

pia, abbreviation for **pia mater.**

piaarachnoid /pī'ə·arak'noid/ [L, *pia,* tender; Gk, *arachne,* spider; *eidos,* form], pertaining to both the pia mater and arachnoid layers of the meninges covering the brain and spinal cord.

pia mater (pia) /pē'ə mā'tər/ [L, *pia,* tender, *mater,* mother], the innermost of the three meninges covering the brain and the spinal cord. It is closely applied to both structures and carries a rich supply of blood vessels, which nourish the nervous tissue. The cranial pia mater covers the surface of the brain and dips deeply into the fissures and the sulci of the cerebral hemispheres. Extending into the transverse cerebral fissure, the cranial pia mater forms the tela choroidea of the third ventricle, combines with the ependyma to form the choroid plexuses of the third and the lateral ventricles, and passes over the roof of the fourth ventricle to form its tela choroidea and its choroid plexus. The spinal pia mater is thicker, firmer, and less vascular than the cranial pia mater and consists of two layers. The outer layer is composed of longitudinal collagenous fibers that are concentrated along the anterior median fissure as the linea splendens. The inner layer closely wraps the entire spinal cord and, at the end of the cord, is prolonged into the filum terminale. The pia mater also forms the denticulate ligament, which extends the entire length of the spinal cord on both sides between the dorsal and the ventral spinal nerve roots. Compare **arachnoid, dura mater.**

pian. See **yaws.**

pian bois. See **forest yaws.**

pica /pī'kə/ [L, *magpie*], a craving to eat substances that are not foods, such as dirt, clay, chalk, glue, ice, starch, or hair. The appetite disorder may occur with some nutritional deficiency states, with pregnancy, and in some forms of mental illness.

Pick's disease[1] [Arnold Pick, Czeck neurologist, b. 1851], a form of presenile dementia occurring in middle age. This disorder affects mainly the frontal and temporal lobes of the brain and characteristically produces neurotic behavior, slow disintegration of intellect, personality, and emotions, and degeneration of cognitive abilities. See also **dementia.**

Pick's disease[2] [Friedel Pick, Czech physician, b. 1867; L *dis,* Fr, *aise,* ease], a condition similar to polyserositis, with constrictive inflammation of the mediastinum and pericardium, leading to chronic venous congestion and cirrhosis. Also called **Pick's syndrome.**

Pick's disease[3] [Ludwig Pick, German physician, b. 1868; L *dis,* Fr, *aise,* ease], a rare chronic familial disease involving lipid metabolism, with large cells of the marrow, spleen, and glands filled with sphyngomyelin. Other char-

acteristics include anemia, digestive disorders, enlarged liver, and distended abdomen. Also called **Niemann-Pick disease.**

Pick's syndrome. See **Pick's disease**[2].

pickwickian syndrome /pikwik'ē·ən/ ['Pickwick Papers' by Charles Dickens], an abnormal condition characterized by obesity, decreased pulmonary function, somnolence, and polycythemia.

pico-, a combining form meaning 'one trillionth' (10^{-12}) of the unit designated: *picogram, picoliter, picometer.*

picogram pg /pī'kəgram/, a unit of measure equal to one trillionth of a gram, or 1×10^{-12} gram.

picornavirus /pīkôr'nəvī'rəs/ [It, *pico,* small, *RNA,* ribonucleic acid; L, *virus,* poison], a member of a group of small RNA viruses that are ether-resistant. The two main genera are *Enterovirus* and *Rhinovirus.* These viruses cause poliomyelitis, herpangina, aseptic meningitis, encephalomyocarditis, and foot-and-mouth disease.

picosecond (ps), a unit of measure equal to one trillionth of a second.

picro-, a combining form meaning 'bitter': *picroadonidin, picropyrine, picrotoxin.*

picrotoxin /pik'rōtok'sin/ [Gk, *pikros,* bitter, *toxikon,* poison], a central nervous system stimulant obtained from the seeds of *Anamirta cocculus,* formerly used as an antidote for acute barbiturate poisoning.

PID, abbreviation for **pelvic inflammatory disease.**

P.I.E., abbreviation for *pulmonary infiltrate with eosinophilia,* a hypersensitivity reaction, characterized by infiltration of alveoli with eosinophils and large mononuclear cells, edema, and inflammation of the lungs. Simple pulmonary eosinophilia, in which patchy, migratory infiltrates cause minimal symptoms, is a self-limited reaction that is elicited by helminthic infections and by certain drugs, such as paraaminosalicylic acid, sulfonamides, and chlorpropamide. A more prolonged illness, characterized by fever, night sweats, cough, dyspnea, weight loss, and more severe tissue reaction, occurs in certain drug allergies and bacterial, fungal, and parasitic infections. Tropical eosinophilia with paroxysmal nocturnal asthma, dyspnea, cough, low-grade fever, and malaise is related to filarial infection, and P.I.E. may occur in long-standing asthma and periarteritis nodosa. See also **Löffler's syndrome.**

piebald /pī'bôld/ [L, *pica,* magpie; ME, *balled,* smooth], having patches of white hair or skin because of an absence of melanocytes in those nonpigmented areas. It is a hereditary condition. Compare **albinism, vitiligo, piebaldism,** *n.*

Piedmont fracture /pēd'mənt/, an oblique fracture of the distal radius, with fragments of bone pulled into the ulna.

piedra. See **trichosporosis.**

Pierre Robin's syndrome /pyerob'inz, pyerōbaNs'/ [Pierre Robin, French histologist, b. 1867], a complex of congenital anomalies including a small mandible, cleft lip, cleft palate, other craniofacial abnormalities, and defects of the eyes and ears, including glaucoma. Intelligence is usually normal. Plastic surgery may achieve satisfactory cosmetic repair, but speech therapy, orthodontia, and psychologic counseling and support are often necessary.

-piesis, suffix for certain terms relating to pressure.

piez-, a combining form meaning 'of or related to pressure': *piezesthesia, piezallochromy, piezotherapy.*

piezochemistry /pī·ē'zōkem'istrē/ [Gk, *piezein,* to press upon, *chemeia* alchemy], a branch of chemistry concerned with reactions that occur under pressure.

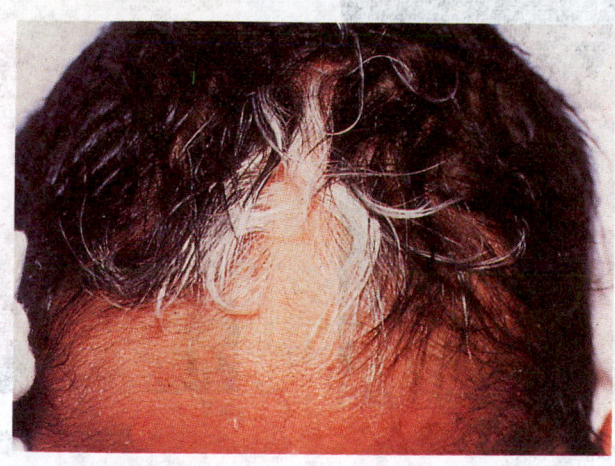

Piebaldism *(Zitelli, 1992)*

piezoelectric effect /pī·ē′zō·ilek′trik/ [Gk, *piezein,* to press, *elektron* amber; L *effectus*],   **1.** the generation of a voltage across a solid when a mechanical stress is applied. **2.** the dimensional change resulting from the application of a voltage. **3.** (in ultrasound) the conversion of one form of energy into another, such as the conversion of electrical energy into mechanical energy.

pigeon breast /pij′ən/ [L, *pipio,* young bird; AS, *broest,* breast],   a congenital structural defect characterized by a prominent anterior projection of the xiphoid and the lower part of the sternum and by a lengthening of the costal cartilages. It may cause cardiorespiratory complications but rarely warrants surgical correction. **–pigeon-breasted,** *adj.*

pigeon breeder's lung,   a respiratory disorder caused by acquired hypersensitivity to antigens in bird droppings. It is characterized by chills, fever, and breathing difficulty; the symptoms subside when exposure to the allergen ceases. Also called **bird breeder's lung, hen worker's lung.**

pigeon-toed.   See **metatarsus varus.**

piggyback port [AS, *piken,* pick; ME, *pakke,* pack; L, *portus,* haven],   a special coupling for the primary IV tubing that allows a supplementary, or piggyback, solution to run into the IV system. The piggyback port includes a backcheck valve that automatically prevents the primary IV solution from flowing while the piggyback solution is flowing. When the piggyback solution stops flowing, the backcheck valve starts the flow of the primary IV solution. Piggyback ports are part of piggyback IV sets, which are used solely for intermittent drug administration.

pigment [L, *pigmentum,* paint],   **1.** any organic coloring material produced in the body, such as melanin. **2.** any colored, paintlike, medicinal preparation applied to the skin surface. **–pigmentary, pigmented,** *adj.,* **pigmentation,** *n.*

pigmentary retinopathy /pig′mənter′ē/,   a disorder of the retina characterized by deposits of pigment and increasing loss of vision.

pigmented villonodular synovitis /pig′məntid/,   a dis-

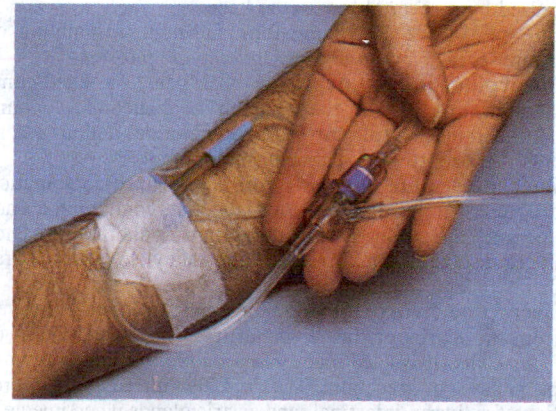

Piggyback port *(Potter, 1993)*

ease of the joints characterized by fingerlike proliferative growths of synovial tissue, with hemosiderin deposition within the synovial tissue. The cause of the disorder is unknown.

pigmy.   See **pygmy.**

pil,   abbreviation for the Latin, words *pilula,* pill, and *pilulae,* 'pills'.

pilar cyst /pī′lər/ [L, *pilus,* hair; Gk, *kystis,* bag],   an epidermoid cyst of the scalp. Its keratinized contents are firmer and less cheesy than the material in epidermoid cysts found elsewhere. The cyst originates from the middle portion of the epithelium of a hair follicle. Treatment is surgical excision. Also called **wen.** Compare **epidermoid cyst.** (See Fig. p. 1220.)

piles.   See **hemorrhoids.**

pili.   See **pilus.**

piliform /pī′lifôrm/ [L, *pilus,* hair],   the appearance of hair.

pi lines /pī′/,   x-ray film artifacts that occur as a result of dirt or chemical stains on a processing roller. They occur at intervals of 3.14 times the diameter of the roller.

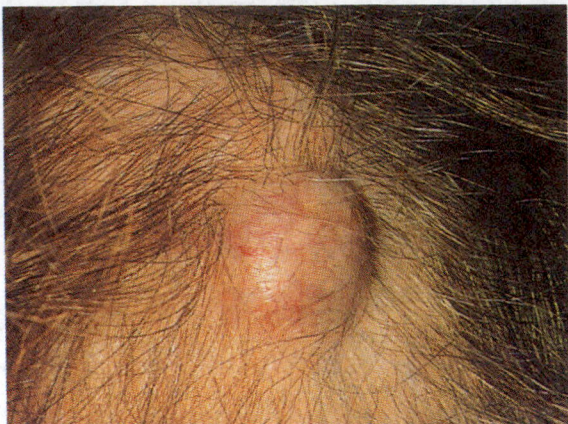

Pilar cyst (Baran, 1993)

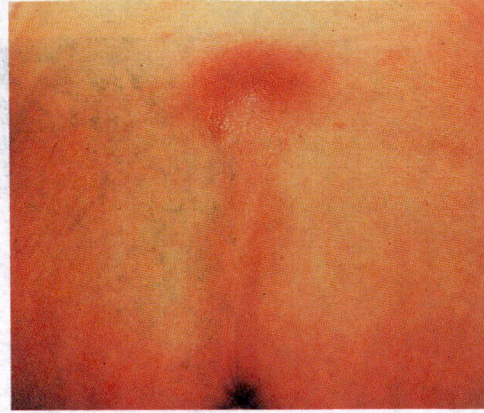

Pilondal cyst (Zitelli, 1992)

pill. See **tablet.**

pillion fracture /pil′yən/ [Gael, *pillean*, couch; L, *fractura*, break], a T-shaped fracture of the distal femur with displacement of the condyles posterior to the femoral shaft, caused by a severe blow to the knee.

pilo- /pī′lō-/, a combining form meaning 'resembling or composed of hair': *pilocystic, pilomotor, pilose.*

pilocarpine and epinephrine /-kär′pēn/, a fixed-combination drug used in the treatment of glaucoma, containing a cholinergic (pilocarpine hydrochloride) and an adrenergic vasoconstrictor (epinephrine bitartrate).

pilocarpine and physostigmine, a fixed-combination drug used in the treatment of glaucoma, containing a cholinergic (pilocarpine hydrochloride) and a short-acting cholinesterase inhibitor (physostigmine salicylate). Both ingredients reduce intraocular pressure.

pilocarpine hydrochloride, a cholinergic drug derived from the leaves of the jaborandi tree and other species of *Pilocarpus*. It is used mainly as a miotic to contract the pupil in cases of glaucoma. The drug also increases the secretion of salivary, intestinal, and gastric glands when injected, reduces the heartbeat, and constricts the bronchioles.

pilomotor reflex /pī′lōmō′tər/ [L, *pilus*, hair, *motor*, mover; *reflectere*, to bend backward], erection of the hairs of the skin in response to a chilly environment, emotional stimulus, or irritation of the skin. This normal reaction is abolished below the level of a transverse spinal cord lesion and may be exaggerated on the affected side in a patient with hemiplegia. Also called **gooseflesh, horripilation, piloerection.**

pilonidal /pī′lənī′dəl/ [L, *pilus*, hair + *nidus*, nest], a growth of hair in a cyst or other internal structure.

pilonidal cyst [L, *pilus* + *nidus*, nest], a cyst that often develops in the sacral region of the skin. Pilonidal cysts may sometimes be recognized at birth by a depression, sometimes a hairy dimple, in the midline of the back, in the sacrococcygeal area. Usually these cysts do not cause any problems, but occasionally a sinus or fistula develops in early adulthood that communicates with the skin, resulting in infection. A fistula also may develop to the spinal tract from a pilonidal cyst. If a cyst becomes infected or inflamed, it is excised, and the space is surgically closed after the infection or inflammation has been effectively treated.

pilonidal fistula, an abnormal channel containing a tuft of hair, situated most frequently over or close to the tip of the coccyx but also occurring in other regions of the body. Also called **pilonidal sinus.**

pilonidal sinus [L, *pilus* + *nidus*; *sinus*, curve], a cavity or sinus containing hair, such as the axilla or navel. In most instances, the hair originated in another area and became lodged in the sinus.

pilosebaceous /pī′lōsibā′shəs/ [L, *pilus* + *sebum*, fat], of or pertaining to a hair follicle and its oil gland.

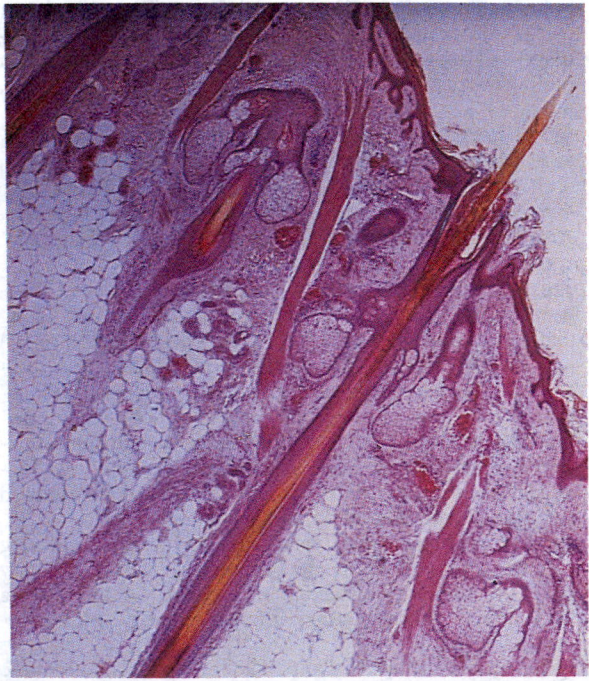

Pilosebaceous unit in the scalp
(du Vivier, 1993/Courtesy Dr. JS Dixon, University of Manchester)

PILOT /pī′lət/, a computer interpreter language, similar to BASIC, used in computer-assisted instruction.

pilus /pē′ləs/, *pl.* **pili** [L, hair], **1.** a hair or hairlike structure. **2.** (in microbiology) a fine, filamentous appendage found on certain bacteria and similar to flagellum except that it is shorter, straighter, and found in greater quantities in the organism. Pili consist solely of protein and are associated with antigenic properties of the cell surface.

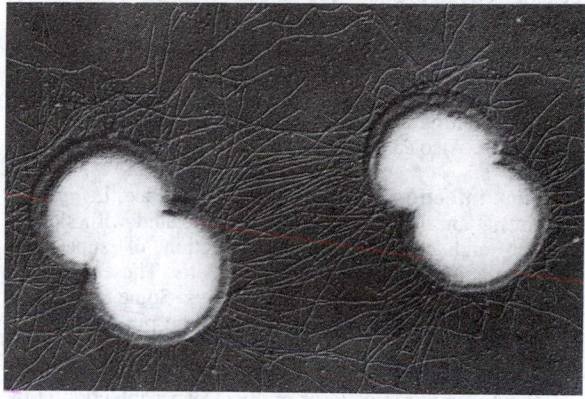

Pili extending from surface of
Neisseria gonorrhoeae
(Baron, 1990/Courtesy Chuen-mo To and C. C. Brinton, Jr.,
University of Pittsburgh)

Pima, a trademark for an expectorant (potassium iodide).
pimelo-, a combining form meaning 'of or related to fat': *pimeloma, pimelopterygium, pimelorrhea.*
pimozide /pim′əzīd/, an oral neuroleptic agent.
■ INDICATIONS: It is prescribed for the suppression of motor and phonic tics associated with Tourette's disorder.
■ CONTRAINDICATIONS: The drug may cause ECG changes, including a prolonged QT interval, and should not be given to patients with a congenital prolonged QT interval or a history of cardiac dysrhythmias. It also may lower the seizure threshold of patients also taking an anticonvulsant drug and should not be given to patients who may be taking a drug that may be the cause of Tourette's disorder symptoms.
■ ADVERSE EFFECTS: Among the more serious adverse reactions are extrapyramidal effects, persistent tardive dyskinesias, sedation, drowsiness, constipation, dry mouth, visual disturbances, and ECG changes.
pimple [ME, *pinple*], a small papule, pustule, or furuncle.
pin [AS, *pinn*], **1.** (in orthopedics) to secure and immobilize fragments of bone with a nail. **2.** See **nail,** def. 2. **3.** (in dentistry) a small metal rod or peg, used as a support in rebuilding a tooth.
pin and tube fixed orthodontic appliance, an orthodontic appliance for correcting and improving malocclusion. It employs a labial arch with vertical posts that insert into tubes attached to bands on the teeth.
pinch, a compression or squeezing of the end of the thumb in opposition to the end of one or more of the fingers. An example is the **pulp pinch,** a type of grasp in which the pulp, or fleshy mass at the end of the fingers, is pressed against the pulp at the end of the thumb. See also **lateral pinch, palmar pinch, tip pinch.**

pinch graft [Fr, *pince*; Gk, *graphion*, stylus], a small, circular deep graft of skin only a few millimeters in diameter. It is cut so that the center is of whole skin but the edges consist of only epidermis.
pinch grip. See **tip pinch.**
pinch meter, a type of dynamometer that measures the strength of a finger pinch.
pindolol /pin′dəlol/, a beta-adrenergic blocker with sympathomimetic activity.
■ INDICATIONS: It is prescribed in the treatment of hypertension, alone or concomitantly with a diuretic.
■ CONTRAINDICATIONS: Bronchial asthma, overt cardiac failure, cardiogenic shock, second- and third-degree heart block, or severe bradycardia prohibits its use. It must be used with caution in patients with diabetes.
■ ADVERSE EFFECTS: Among the most serious adverse reactions are bradycardia, hypotension, syncope, tachycardia, aggravation of bronchospasm, and GI disturbances.
pineal /pin′ē·əl/ [L, *pineus*, pine cone], **1.** pertaining to the pineal body. **2.** resembling a pine cone.
pineal body [L, *pineas*, pinecone; AS, *bodig*, body], a cone-shaped structure in the brain, situated between the superior colliculi, the pulvinar, and the splenium of the corpus callosum. Its precise function has not been established. It may secrete the hormone melatonin, which appears to inhibit the secretion of luteinizing hormone. Also called **epiphysis cerebri, pineal gland.**
pinealectomy /pin′ē·əlek′təme/ [L, *pineus* + Gk, *ektome*, cutting out], the surgical removal of the pineal body.
pineal gland. See **pineal body.**
pineal hyperplasia syndrome, an abnormal condition caused by overgrowth of the pineal gland. It is characterized by severe insulin resistance, dry skin, thick nails, hirsutism, early dentition, and sexual precocity. Although the teeth develop prematurely, they are malformed. External genitalia may reach adult size by the age of 4 years. Ketoacidosis may occur despite high levels of endogenous insulin. Similar abnormalities are associated with some pineal tumors.
pinealoma /pin′ē·əlō′mə/, *pl.* **pinealomas, pinealomata** [L, *pineas* + Gk, *oma*, tumor], a rare neoplasm of the pineal body in the brain, characterized by hydrocephalus, pupillary changes, gait disturbances, headache, nausea, and vomiting.
pineal peduncle [L, *pineus*, pine cone; *peduncle*, small foot], the stalk of the pineal body.
pineal tumor, a neoplasm of the pineal body. See also **pinealoma.**
pine tar [L, *pinus*, pine; AS, *teoru*, tar], a topical antieczematic and a rubefacient. It is a common ingredient in creams, soaps, and lotions used in the treatment of chronic skin conditions, such as eczema or psoriasis.
pinhole pupil [ME, *pyn* + *hol*; L, *pupilla*, little girl], a very small pupil, which may be congenital, an effect of the use of miotics, or the result of an inflamed iris.
pinhole retention [AS, *pinn*, pin, *hol*, hole; L, *retinere*, to hold], retention developed by drilling one or more holes, 2 to 3 mm in depth, in suitable areas of a cavity preparation to supplement resistance and retention form.
pinhole test, **1.** a test performed in examining a person who has diminished visual acuity to distinguish a refractive error from organic disease. A refractive error may be corrected with glasses and is not medically dangerous. Loss of visual acuity because of organic disease is serious because it may indicate a systemic, particularly a neurologic, dis-

ease and may signal the development of avoidable blindness. The test is simple to perform. Several pinholes, 0.5 to 2 mm in diameter, are punched in a card; the patient selects one and looks through it with one eye at a time, without wearing glasses. If visual acuity is improved, the defect is refractive; if not, it is organic. The pinhole effect results from blocking peripheral light waves, those most distorted by refractive error. **2.** (in radiology) a test to identify the size of the focal spot of the x-ray tube. Also, a tomography test used to trace the path of the tube movement.

Pin-Index Safety System (PISS), a system for identifying connectors for certain small cylinders of medical gases that have flush valve outlets rather than threaded outlets. The identifying code consists of a specific combination of two holes in the face of the valve into which connecting pins for a particular type of gas must fit in perfect alignment. For example, the index hole position for a cylinder of oxygen is 2-5, for nitrous oxide it is 3-5, and so on. See also **Diameter-Index Safety System (DISS)**.

pink disease. See **acrodynia**.

pinkeye. See **conjunctivitis**.

Pinkus' disease. See **lichen nitidus**.

pinna. See **auricle**.

pinocytic /pī′nəsit′ik/ [Gk, *pinein*, to drink, *kytos*, cell], pertaining to a pinocyte, particularly its ability to absorb liquids by phagocytosis in cellular metabolic processes.

pinocytosis /pī′nōsītō′sis/ [Gk, *pinein, kytos + osis*, condition], the process by which extracellular fluid is taken into a cell. The cell membrane develops a saccular indentation filled with extracellular fluid, then closes around it, forming a vesicle or a vacuole of fluid within the cell.

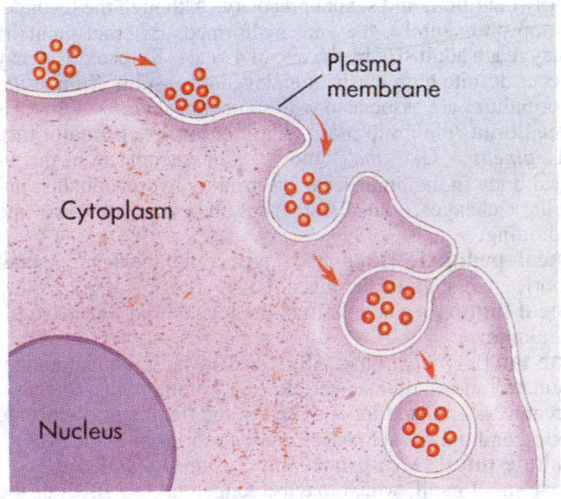

Pinocytosis *(Raven, 1992/Christy Krames)*

pinprick test, a test of a person's ability to detect a cutaneous pain sensation and to differentiate such sensations from pressure stimuli. The test is performed with a pin or needle gently applied to a skin area where it cannot be observed by the subject. The application of the pin or needle is alternated with a dull object pressed against the skin. Care

is taken to avoid penetration of the dermis, and the sharp object used should be sterilized or discarded after the test.

pinta /pēn′tə/ [Sp, spot], an infection of the skin caused by *Treponema carateum*, a common organism in South and Central America. The bacterium gains entry into the body through a break in the skin. Prolonged exposure and close contact appear to be necessary for transmission. The primary lesion is a slowly enlarging papule with regional lymph node enlargement, followed in 1 to 12 months by a generalized red to slate-blue macular rash. Eventually these lesions become depigmented. Diagnosis is based on serologic tests and darkfield microscopic examination of scrapings from skin lesions. Treatment with penicillin G is effective. The major complication of the disease is social ostracism resulting from the permanently disfiguring mottling of the skin. Also called **azula, carate, mal del pinto.** Compare **yaws**.

pin track infection [AS, *pinn;* ME, *trak*, trace; L, *inficere,* to taint], an abnormal condition associated with skeletal traction and characterized by infection of superficial, deeper, or soft tissues or by osteomyelitis. These infections may develop at skeletal traction pin sites. Some of the signs of pin track infection are erythema at the pin sites, drainage and odor, pin slippage, elevated temperature, and pain. Superficial infection at the pin site is treated with antibiotics administered topically or orally. Deeper infection at the pin sites usually requires removal of the pins and antibiotic therapy.

pinworm. See *Enterobius vermicularis*.

pio-, a combining form meaning 'of or pertaining to fat': *pionemia, piorthopnea, pioscope*.

PIo₂, the partial pressure of inspired oxygen.

pions /pī′onz/ [Gk, *pi*, 16th letter of Greek alphabet + *meson*, nuclear particle], a family of particles that can be created in nuclear reactions. Pions are unstable but can survive long enough to be formed into beams and used in certain types of medical therapy, such as the treatment of brain tumors. Pions of suitable energy can penetrate the skull, spare overlying normal tissue, and then deliver most of their energy into the tumor. See also **negative pi meson**.

Piper forceps. See **obstetric forceps**.

piperocaine hydrochloride /pī′pərōkān′/, a local anesthetic for the induction of spinal or caudal anesthesia.

pipette /pīpet′, pipet′/ [Fr, little pipe], **1.** a calibrated, transparent open-ended tube of glass or plastic used for measuring or transferring small quantities of a liquid or gas. **2.** using a pipette to dispense liquid.

Pipracel, a trademark for an antibiotic (piperacillin).

piriform /pir′ifôrm/ [L, *pirum*, pear + *forma*], pear-shaped.

piriform aperture [L, *pirum*, pear, *forma*, form; *apertura*, opening], the anterior nasal opening in the skull.

piriformis /pir′ifôr′mis/ [L, *pirum + forma*], a flat, pyramidal muscle lying almost parallel with the posterior margin of the gluteus medius. It is partly within the pelvis and partly at the back of the hip joint. It arises from the sacrum, the greater sciatic foramen, and the sacrotuberous ligament, and it inserts, by a rounded tendon, into the greater trochanter of the femur. The piriformis is innervated by branches of the first and the second sacral nerves and functions to rotate the thigh laterally and to abduct and to help extend it. Compare **obturator externus, obturator internus**.

Pirquet's test /pirkāz′/ [Clemens P. von Pirquet, Austrian physician, b. 1874], a tuberculin skin test that consists of scratching the tuberculin material onto the skin. Also called **von Pirquet's test.** See also **tuberculin test.**

pisiform /pī′sifôrm, pē′-/ [L, *pisum*, pea + *forma*], pea-shaped.

pisiform bone [L, *pisa*, pea, *forma*, form; AS, *ban*, bone], a small, spheroidal carpal bone in the proximal row of carpal bones. It articulates with the triangular bone and is attached to the flexor retinaculum, the flexor carpi ulnaris, and the abductor digiti minimi.

PISS, abbreviation for **Pin-Index Safety System.**

pistol-shot sound, a sharp, slapping sound heard by auscultation over the femoral pulse of a patient with aortic incompetence. It is caused by a large-volume pulse with a sharp rise in pressure.

pit and fissure cavity [AS, *pytt*; L, *fissura*, cleft; *cavum*, cavity], a cavity that starts in tiny faults in tooth enamel, usually on occlusal surfaces of molars and premolars.

pitch [ME, *picchen*], the quality of a tone or sound dependent on the relative rapidity of the vibrations by which it is produced.

pithing /pith′ing/ [AS, *pitha*], the destruction of the central nervous system of an experimental animal in preparation for physiologic research. It is usually done by inserting a blunt probe through a foramen.

Pitocin, a trademark for an oxytocic (oxytocin).

Pitressin, a trademark for an antidiuretic hormone (vasopressin).

pitting [AS, *pytt*], **1.** small, punctate indentations in fingernails or toenails, often a result of psoriasis. **2.** an indentation that remains for a short time after pressing edematous skin with a finger. **3.** small, depressed scars in the skin or other organ of the body. **4.** the removal by the spleen of material from within erythrocytes without damage to the cells.

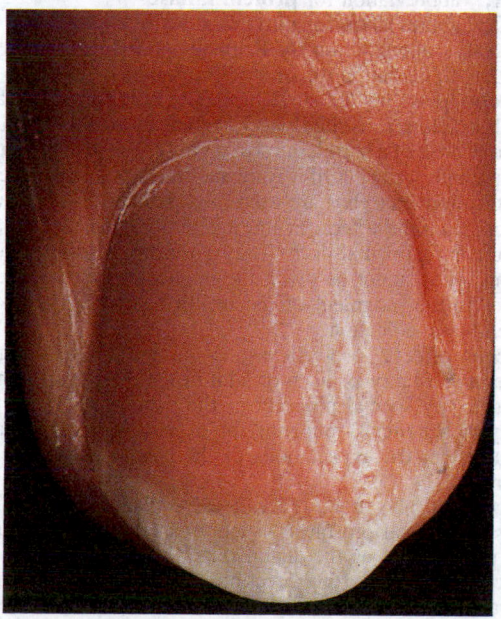

Pitting of the fingernails (*du Vivier, 1993*)

pitting edema [AS, *pytt*; Gk, *oidema*, swelling], an edema characterized by a condition in which a finger pressed into the skin over an accumulation of fluid will result in a temporary depression in the skin; normal skin and subcutaneous tissues quickly rebound when the pressure is released.

pituicyte /pit(y)ōō′isīt/ [L, *pituita*, phlegm; Gk, *kytos*, cell], a cell of the neurohypophysis.

pituit-, a combining form meaning 'of or related to phlegm': *pituita, pituitary, pituitous.*

pituitarism /pit(y)ōō′itəriz′əm/ [L, *pituita*, phlegm], any condition caused by a defect or failure of the pituitary gland.

pituitary. See **pituitary gland.**

pituitary adamantinoma. See **craniopharyngioma.**

pituitary cachexia. See **postpubertal panhypopituitarism.**

pituitary dwarf /pit(y)ōō′iter′ē/ [L, *pituita*, phlegm; AS, *dweorge*], a dwarf whose retarded development is caused by a deficiency of growth hormone resulting from hypofunction of the anterior lobe of the pituitary. In most cases the cause is unknown, and the defect is limited to a lack of somatotropin, although in some instances gonadotropins, adrenocorticotropic hormone, and thyroid stimulating hormone also may be deficient. The body is properly proportioned, with no facial or skeletal deformities, and there is normal mental and sexual development. The condition is usually diagnosed in childhood by radiographic examination of the bones and radioimmunoassay of levels of plasma growth hormone. Also called **hypophyseal dwarf, Lévi-Lorain dwarf, Paltauf's dwarf.**

pituitary gland [L, *pituita*, phlegm], an endocrine gland suspended beneath the brain in the pituitary fossa of the sphenoid bone, supplying numerous hormones that govern many vital processes. It is divided into an anterior adenohypophysis and a smaller posterior neurohypophysis. The anterior lobe of the gland is composed of polygonal cells related to the production of seven hormones. The hormones, controlled by hypothalamic releasing factors, include growth hormone (somatotropin), prolactin, thyroid-stimulating hormone, follicle-stimulating hormone (FSH), luteinizing hormone (LH), adrenocorticotropic hormone (ACTH), and melanocyte-stimulating hormone. The posterior lobe is morphologically an extension of the hypothalamus and the source of vasopressin (antidiuretic hormone) and oxytocin. Vasopressin inhibits diuresis and raises blood pressure. Oxytocin stimulates the contraction of smooth muscle, especially in the uterus. The pituitary gland is larger in a woman than in a man and becomes further enlarged during pregnancy. Also called **hypophysis, hypohysis cerebri.** See also **adenohypophysis, neurohypophysis.**

pituitary myxedema [L, *piuita*; Gk, *myxa*, mucus + *oidema*, swelling], a type of hypothyroid condition secondary to an anterior pituitary disease.

pituitary nanism, a type of dwarfism associated with hypophyseal infantilism. See also **pituitary dwarf.**

pituitary snuff lung, a type of hypersensitivity pneumonitis that sometimes occurs among takers of pituitary snuff. The antigens to which the hypersensitivity reaction occurs are found in serum proteins of cows and pigs and in pituitary tissue. Symptoms of the acute form of the disease include chills, cough, fever, dyspnea, anorexia, nausea, and vomiting. The chronic form of the disease is characterized by fatigue, chronic cough, weight loss, and dyspnea on exercise. Also called **pituitary snuff takers' disease.**

pituitary stalk, a structure that connects the pituitary gland with the hypothalamus.

pit viper [AS, *pytt;* L, *vipera,* snake], any one of a family of venomous snakes found in the Western Hemisphere and Asia, characterized by a heat-sensitive pit between the eye and nostril on each side of the head and hollow, perforated fangs that are usually folded back in the roof of the mouth. With the exception of coral snakes, all indigenous poisonous snakes in the United States are pit vipers. See also **copperhead, cottonmouth, rattlesnake.**

pityriasis /pitərī′əsis/ [Gk, *pityron,* bran], any of a number of skin diseases that have in common lesions that resemble dandrufflike scales without obvious signs of inflammation.

pityriasis alba [Gk, *pityron,* bran; L, *albus,* white], a common idiopathic dermatosis characterized by round or oval, finely scaling patches of hypopigmentation, usually on the cheeks. The lesions are sharply demarcated and occasionally pruritic and are found primarily in children and adolescents. The condition may recur, but spontaneous clearing is the usual prognosis. Treatment includes lubricating creams, topical corticosteroids, and less commonly, coal tar creams. Compare **pityriasis rosea.**

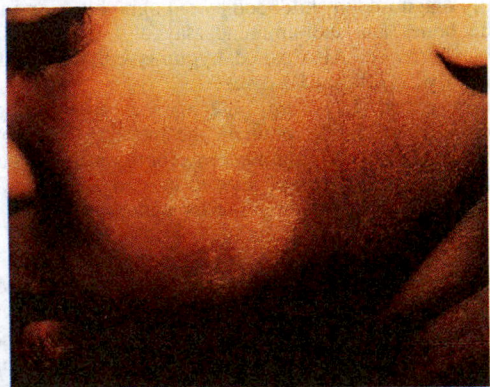

Pityriasis alba (*Zitelli, 1992*)

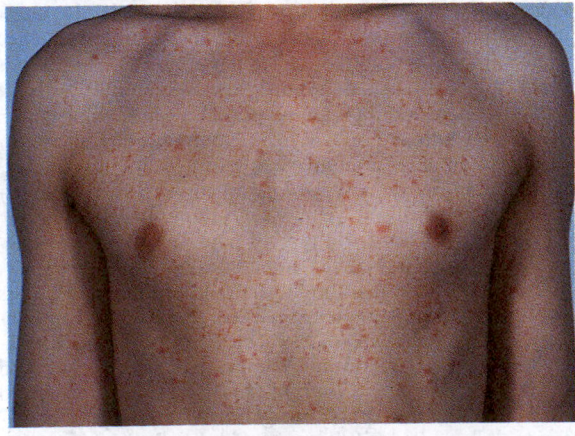

Pityriasis rosea (*du Vivier, 1993*)

pityriasis rosea, a self-limited skin disease in which a slightly scaling, pink, macular rash spreads over the trunk and other unexposed areas of the body. A characteristic feature is the **herald patch,** a larger, more scaly lesion that precedes the diffuse rash by several days. The smaller lesions tend to line up with the long axis parallel to normal lines of cleavage of the skin. Mild itching is the only symptom. The disease lasts 4 to 8 weeks and rarely recurs. It is unusual and apparently not contagious, and its cause is unknown. Compare **pituriasis alba.**

Pityrosporum. See *Malassezia.*

pivot joint /piv′ət/ [Fr, hinge; L, *jungere,* to join], a synovial joint in which movement is limited to rotation. The joint is formed by a pivotlike process that may turn within a ring composed partly of bone and partly of ligament. The proximal radioulnar articulation is a pivot joint in which the head of the radius rotates within the ring formed by the radial notch of the ulna and the annular ligament. Also called **trochoid joint.** Compare **ball and socket joint, condyloid joint, gliding joint, hinge joint, saddle joint.**

pivot transfer, the movement of a person from one site to another, such as from a bed to a wheelchair, when there is a loss of control of one side of the body. The person is helped to a position on the strong side of the body, either left or right, with both feet on the floor, heels behind the knees, and knees lower than the hips. The person stands with the weight on the strong leg and pivots on it, and carefully lowers the body into the wheelchair.

pixels, abbreviation for *picture elements,* small cells of information that make up the matrix of a digital image; a two-dimensional representation of the voxel or volume element.

PJC, abbreviation for **premature junctional complex.**

PK, abbreviation for **psychokinesis.**

pK$_a$, the negative logarithm of the ionization constant of an acid. A measure of the strength of an acid.

PKA, abbreviation for **protein kinase.**

PKD, abbreviation for **polycystic kidney disease.**

PK test, abbreviation for **Prausnitz-Küstner test.**

PKU, abbreviation for **phenylketonuria.**

placebo /pləsē′bō/ [L, shall please], an inactive substance, such as saline, distilled water, or sugar, or a less than effective dose of a harmless substance, such as a water-soluble vitamin prescribed as if it were an effective dose of a needed medication. Placebos are used in experimental drug studies to compare the effects of the inactive substance with those of the experimental drug. They are also prescribed for patients who cannot be given the medication they request or who, in the judgment of the health care provider, do not need that medication.

placebo effect, a physical or emotional change occurring after a substance is taken or administered that is not the result of any special property of the substance. The change may be beneficial, reflecting the expectations of the patient and, often, the expectations of the person giving the substance.

placement /plās′mənt/ [Fr, *placer,* to place], the positioning of a dental prosthesis, such as a removable denture in its planned site on the dental arch.

placement path, the direction of placement and removal of a removable partial denture on its supporting oral structures. The path can be varied by altering the plane to which the guiding abutment surfaces of the denture are made parallel. The choice of a placement path is considered a compromise that best fulfills five requirements: minimal torque for abutment teeth; minimal interference; maximum retention; the establishment of adequate guide plane surfaces; and acceptable esthetics.

placent-, a combining form meaning 'a cakelike mass': *placenta, placentapepton, placentogenesis.*

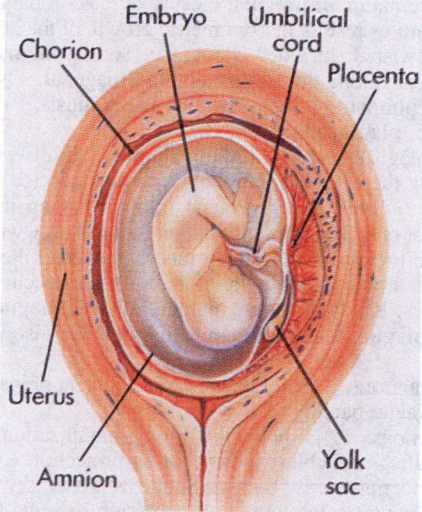

Placenta *(Raven, 1992/Nadine Sokol)*

Labels on figure: Chorion, Embryo, Umbilical cord, Placenta, Uterus, Amnion, Yolk sac

placenta /pləsen'tə/ [L, cake], a highly vascular fetal organ through which the fetus absorbs oxygen, nutrients, and other substances and excretes carbon dioxide and other wastes. It begins to form on approximately the eighth day of gestation when the blastocyst touches the wall of the uterus and adheres to it. The blastocyst becomes surrounded by an outer layer of syncytiotrophoblast and an inner layer of cytotrophoblast. The trophoblast is able to digest cells of the endometrium, causing a small erosion on the uterine wall in which an embryo nidates. Under the influence of increasing amounts of progesterone, secreted by the corpus luteum of the ovary, the embryo and the placenta continue to develop. A hormone, chorionic gonadotropin, is secreted by the developing placenta and is present in the maternal blood and urine. The trophoblastic layer continues to infiltrate the maternal tissues with fingerlike projections, called chorionic villi. Separating the villi are lakes of blood in the eroded tissue. The maternal blood flows into the lakes surrounding the villi, allowing nutrients, gases, and other substances to pass into the fetal circulation by diffusion, hydrostatic pressure, and osmosis. The placenta is able to secrete large amounts of progesterone by the third month of pregnancy, enough to relieve the corpus luteum of that function. At term the normal placenta weighs one seventh to one fifth of the weight of the infant. The maternal surface is lobulated and divided into cotyledons. It has a dark red, rough, liverlike appearance. The fetal surface is smooth and shiny, covered with the fetal membranes, and marked by the large white blood vessels beneath the membranes that fan out from the centrally inserted umbilical cord. The time between the delivery of the infant and the expulsion of the placenta is the third and last stage of labor.

-placenta, a combining form meaning an 'organ shaped like a flat cake': *ectoplacenta, hemiplacenta, subplacenta.*

placenta abruptio. See **abruptio placentae.**

placenta accreta, a placenta that invades the uterine muscle, making separation from the muscle difficult.

placenta battledore, a condition in which the umbilical cord is inserted into the margin of the placenta.

placenta bipartitia. See **bilobate placenta.**

placental /pləsen'təl/ [L, *placenta,* cake], pertaining to the placenta.

placental bruit [L, *placenta,* flat cake; Fr, *bruit,* noise], a humming noise caused by fetal circulation, heard in the pregnant uterus. It is synchronized with the mother's pulse.

placental dysfunction. See **placental insufficiency.**

placental dystocia, a prolonged or otherwise difficult delivery of the placenta. See also **dystocia.**

placental hormone, one of the several hormones produced by the placenta, including human placental lactogen, chorionic gonadotropin, estrogen, progesterone, and a thyrotropin-like hormone.

placental infarct, a localized ischemic, hard area on the fetal or maternal side of the placenta.

placental insufficiency, an abnormal condition of pregnancy, manifested clinically by retardation of the rate of fetal and uterine growth. One or more placental abnormalities cause dysfunction of maternal-placental or fetal-placental circulation sufficient to compromise fetal nutrition and oxygenation. Some of the abnormalities that can result in placental insufficiency are abnormal implantation of the placenta, multiple pregnancy, abnormal attachments of the umbilical cord or anomalies of the cord itself, and abnormalities of the placental membranes. Histopathologic abnormalities that can cause placental insufficiency include intravillous thrombi, placental infarction, and breaks in the placental membrane that result in fetal bleeding into the maternal circulation. Placental insufficiency also may result from placental senescence in postmaturity, from systemic diseases, such as erythroblastosis fetalis and diabetes mellitus, or from bacterial, viral, parasitic, or fungal infections. Also called **placental dysfunction.** See also **intrauterine growth retardation, postmature infant.**

placental presentation [L, *placenta,* flat cake; *presentare,* to show], a complication of childbirth in which the placenta is located in or near the lower uterine segment. Also called **placenta previa.**

placental scan, a scan of the uterus of a pregnant woman, performed after an intravenous injection of a contrast medium, used for locating the fetus and placenta and for detecting intrauterine bleeding.

placental sinus. See **marginal sinus.**

placental stage of labor, the third stage of labor when the placenta and membranes are expelled from the uterus after birth of the child.

placental thrombosis [L, *placenta,* flat cake; Gk, *thrombos,* lump + *osis,* condition], intravascular coagulation that occurs in the placenta and veins of the uterus.

placental transmission [L, *placenta,* flat cake, L, *transmittere,* to transmit], the transference of a drug or other substance across the placenta.

placenta previa /prē'vē·ə/, a condition of pregnancy in which the placenta is implanted abnormally in the uterus so that it impinges on or covers the internal os of the uterine cervix. It is the most common cause of painless bleeding in the third trimester of pregnancy. Its cause is unknown. The

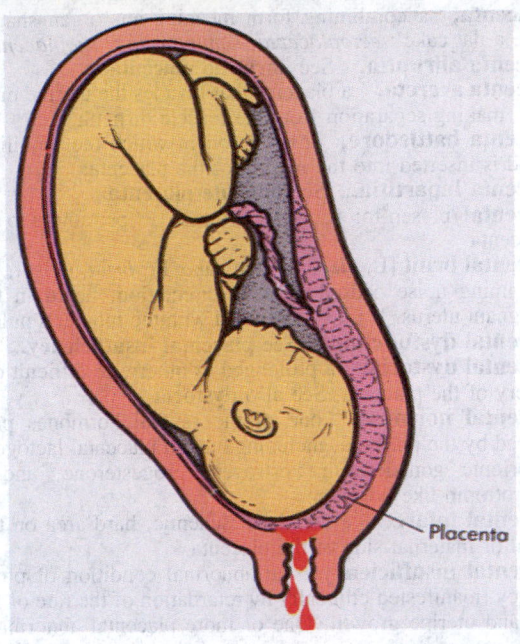

Placenta previa (Raven, 1992/Marcia Williams)

incidence of the condition increases with increased parity from approximately 1 in 1500 primiparas to approximately 1 in 20 grand multiparas. Even slight dilatation of the internal os can cause enough local separation of an abnormally implanted placenta to result in bleeding. If severe hemorrhage occurs, immediate cesarean section is usually required to stop the bleeding and to save the mother's life; it is performed regardless of the stage of fetal maturity. Before hemorrhage, placenta previa may be diagnosed by ultrasonography and treated with complete bed rest under close observation. Even at rest, sudden massive hemorrhage can occur without warning. Vaginal examination is usually contraindicated if placenta previa is present or suspected because palpation can cause local placental separation and precipitate hemorrhage. Cautious and very gentle intracervical palpation may be performed to determine the existence and exact extent of previa. Before this examination, an intravenous infusion is begun, the woman's blood is typed and crossmatched, and preparations for immediate cesarean section are made. If the placenta is next to or near, rather than touching or covering, the cervical os, labor and vaginal delivery may be attempted. **Complete previa** refers to a placenta that has grown to completely cover the internal cervical os; **low-lying placenta** identifies a placenta that is just within the lower uterine segment, and **partial** or **marginal previa** is a condition in which the placenta partially covers the internal cervical os. See also **central placenta previa, marginal placenta previa,** and **partial placenta previa.** Also called *(informal)* **previa.** Compare **abruptio placentae.**

placenta previa partialis, a placenta that partially obstructs the internal cervical os.

placenta souffle [L, *placenta*, flat cake; Fr, *souffle*, puff],

a soft blowing or humming sound produced by fetal circulation at the placenta.

placenta succenturiata, an accessory placenta.

Placidyl, a trademark for a sedative (ethchlorvynol).

Plafon fracture, a fracture that involves the buttress portion of the malleolus of a bone.

plagiocephaly /plā′jē·ōsef′əlē/ [Gk, *plagios,* askew, *kephale,* head], a congenital malformation of the skull in which premature or irregular closure of the coronal or lambdoidal sutures results in asymmetric growth of the head, giving it a twisted, lopsided appearance so that the maximum length is not along the midline but on a diagonal. Also called **plagiocephalism.** See also **craniostenosis. –plagiocephalic, plagiocephalous,** *adj.*

plague /plāg/ [L, *plaga,* blow], an infectious disease transmitted by the bite of a flea from a rodent infected with the bacillus *Yersinia pestis.* Plague is primarily an infectious disease of rats: The rat fleas feed on humans only when their preferred rodent hosts, usually rats, have been killed by the plague in a rat epizootic; therefore epidemics occur after rat epizootics. Kinds of plague include **bubonic plague, pneumonic plague,** and **septicemic plague.** See also *Yersinia pestis.*

plague vaccine, an active immunizing agent prepared with killed plague bacilli.

■ INDICATIONS: It is prescribed for immunization against plague after probable exposure or as protection for travelers in endemic areas, such as Southeast Asia.

■ CONTRAINDICATIONS: Immunosuppression or acute infection prohibits its use.

■ ADVERSE EFFECTS: Among the most serious adverse reactions are allergic reactions, inflammation at the site of injection, headache, and malaise.

plaintiff /plān′tif/ [ME, *plaintif,* one who complains], (in law) a person who files a lawsuit initiating a legal action. The plaintiff complains or sues for remedial relief and names a complainant in various civil actions. In criminal actions, the prosecution is the plaintiff, acting in behalf of the people of the jurisdiction.

-plakia, a combining form meaning 'a plate or flat plane, usually on a mucous membrane': *leukoplakia, malacoplakia, melanoplakia.*

planar xanthoma /plā′nər/ [L, *planum,* level; Gk, *xanthos,* yellow, *oma* tumor], a yellow or orange flat macule or slightly raised papule containing foam cells and occurring in clusters in localized areas, such as the eyelids. These lesions may be widely distributed over the body. Also called **plane xanthoma, xanthoma planum.** See also **xanthelasmatosis.**

Planck's constant /plangks/ [Max Planck, German physicist, b. 1858], a fundamental physical constant that relates the energy of radiation to its frequency. It is expressed as 6.63×10^{-27} erg-seconds or 6.63×10^{-34} joule-seconds. See also **photon.**

plane [L, *planum,* level], **1.** a flat surface determined by three points in space. **2.** an extension of a longitudinal section through an axis, such as the coronal, horizontal, transverse, frontal, and the sagittal planes used to identify the position of various parts of the body in the study of anatomy. **3.** the act of paring or of rubbing away. **4.** a superficial incision in the wall of a cavity or between tissue layers, especially in plastic surgery. **–planar,** *adj.*

planes of anesthesia. See **Guedel's signs.**

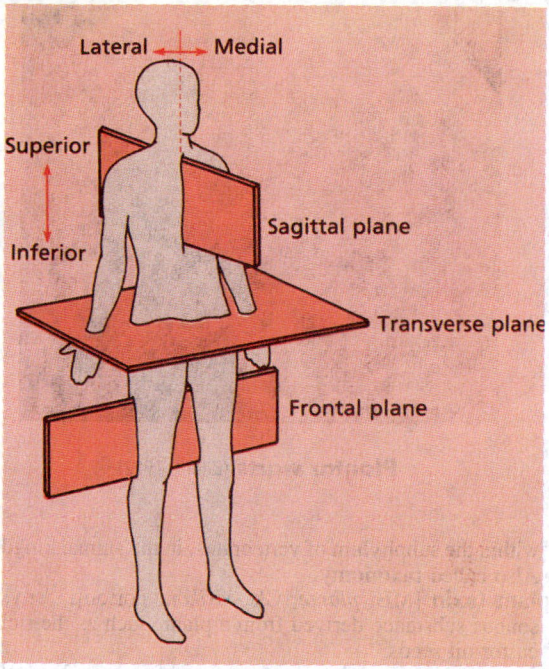

Planes of the body (Potter, 1993)

-plania, a combining form meaning the 'deviation from its normal location': *choloplania, pyoplania, spiloplania.*

planigraphic principle /plan′igraf′ik/, a rule of tomography in which the fulcrum or axis of rotation is raised or lowered to alter the level of the focal plane but the tabletop height remains constant.

plankton /plangk′tən/ [Gk, *planktos,* wandering], nearly microscopic bits of plant and animal life that swarms in lakes and oceans and provides the basic food for aquatic animals.

planned change, an alteration of the status quo by means of a carefully formulated program that follows four steps: unfreezing the present level, establishing a change relationship, moving to a new level, and freezing at the new level. The program can be implemented by collaborative, coercive, or emulative means.

planned parenthood, a philosophic framework central to the development of contraceptive methods, contraceptive counseling, and family planning programs and clinics. Advocates hold that it is the right of each woman to decide when to conceive and bear children and that contraceptive and gynecologic care and information should be available to her to help her become or avoid becoming pregnant. See also **contraception.**

planning [L, *planum*], (in five-step nursing process) a category of nursing behavior in which a strategy is designed for the achievement of the goals of care for an individual patient, as established in assessing and analyzing. Planning includes developing and modifying a care plan for the patient, cooperating with other personnel, and recording relevant information. To develop the plan, the nurse anticipates the patient's needs according to established priorities; in-

volves the patient and the patient's family and significant others in designing the plan; uses all information necessary for managing care of the patient, including recorded information from other health professionals, and the age, sex, culture, ethnicity, and religion; plans for the patient's comfort, activity, and function; and chooses nursing measures that are necessary to deliver care as planned. With the cooperation of other health personnel, the nurse coordinates care for the benefit of the patient and identifies resources in the hospital or community for social or health assistance as needed by the client or the patient's family. All information relevant to the management of the patient's care plan is recorded. Planning follows analyzing and precedes implementing in the five-step nursing process. See also **analyzing, assessing, evaluating, implementing, nursing process.**

plano-, a combining form meaning 'wandering': *planocyte, planotopokinesia.*

plantago seed /plantā′gō/, a bulk-forming laxative derived from *Plantago psyllium* seeds.

■ INDICATIONS: It is prescribed in the treatment of constipation and nonspecific diarrhea.

■ CONTRAINDICATIONS: Symptoms of appendicitis, intestinal obstruction, or GI ulceration prohibit its use.

■ ADVERSE EFFECTS: Among the more serious adverse effects are intestinal obstruction and allergic reactions.

plantar /plan′tər/ [L, *planta,* sole], of or pertaining to the sole of the foot. Also called **volar.**

plantar aponeurosis, the tough fascia surrounding the muscles of the soles of the feet. Also called **plantar fascia.**

plantar arch [L, *planta,* sole + *arcus,* bow], the arterial arch in the sole of the foot, over the metatarsal bone.

plantar flexion [L, *planta,* sole + *flectere,* to bend], a toe-down motion of the foot at the ankle. It is measured in degrees from the 0-degree position of the foot at rest on the ground in a standing position.

plantar grasp reflex, a reflex characterized by the flexion of the toes when the sole of the foot is stroked gently. It is present in babies at birth but should disappear after 6 weeks.

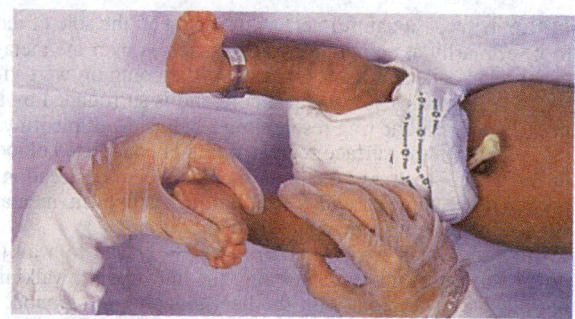

Plantar grasp reflex in the newborn (Seidel, 1991)

plantaris /planter′is/ /plantä′ris/ [L, *planta*], one of three superficial muscles at the back of the leg, between the soleus and the gastrocnemius. The plantaris is a small muscle that arises from the distal part of the linea aspera of the femur and from the oblique popliteal ligament of the knee joint. It has a small fusiform belly, ending in a long, slender tendon that inserts into the calcaneus. The plantaris is innervated by a branch of the tibial nerve, containing fibers from the fourth and the fifth lumbar and the first sacral nerves. It flexes the foot and the leg. Compare **gastrocnemius, soleus.**

plantar neuroma, a neuroma of the sole of the foot.

plantar reflex, the normal response, elicited by firmly stroking the outer surface of the sole from heel to toes, characterized by flexion of the toes. Compare **Babinski's reflex.**

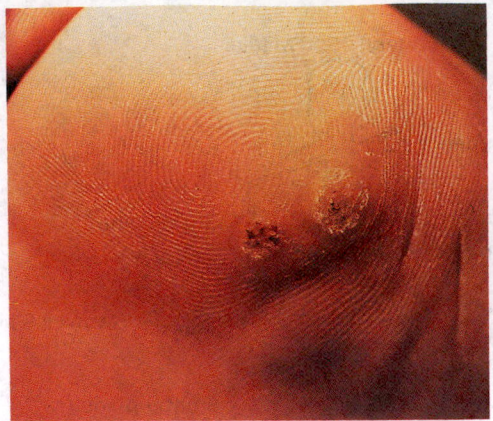

Plantar warts *(Zitelli, 1992)*

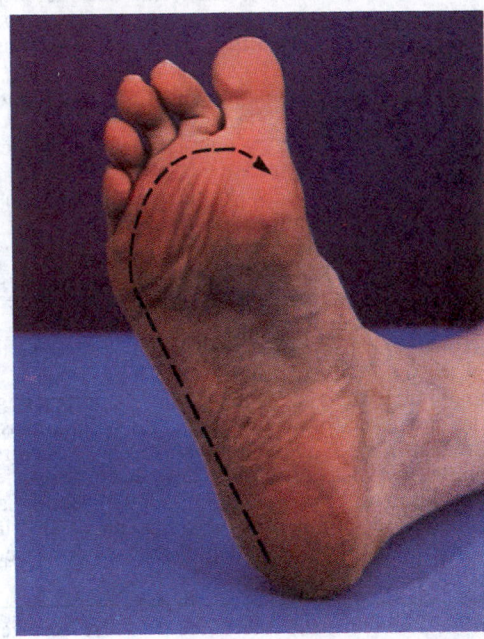

Plantar reflex *(Seidel, 1991)*

plantar wart, a painful verrucous lesion on the sole of the foot, primarily at points of pressure, such as over the metatarsal heads and the heel. Caused by the common wart virus, it appears as a soft, central core and is surrounded by a firm, hyperkeratotic ring resembling a callus. Multiple, tiny, black spots on the surface represent bits of coagulated blood in the wart. Treatment methods include electrodesiccation, cryotherapy, topical acids, cantharidin, and even mental suggestion. See also **mosaic wart.**

plantigrade /plan'tigrād'/ [L, *planta* + *gradi,* to walk], of, pertaining to, or characterizing the human gait; walking on the sole of the foot with the heel touching the ground.

plant or animal classification, the system of identification of organisms according to their natural relationships based on such common factors as embryology, structure, or physiological chemistry. In the system for plants, the descending order of categories is: kingdom, division, class, order, genus, species. For animals, the categories are: kingdom, phylum, class, order, family, genus, species. Humans are members of a species, *Homo sapiens,* of the genus *Homo,* in a family of hominidae, which are two-legged members of the order of primates, in a class of mammals,

within the subphylum of vertebrates, in the animal kingdom. Also called **taxonomy.**

plant toxin [ME, *plante*; Gk, *toxikon,* poison], any poisonous substance derived from a plant, such as the ricin of castor-oil seeds.

plaque /plak/ [Fr, plate], **1.** a flat, often raised, patch on the skin or any other organ of the body. **2.** a patch of atherosclerosis. **3.** also called **dental plaque.** a thin film on the teeth made up of mucin and colloidal material found in saliva and often secondarily invaded by bacteria.

Plaquenil Sulfate, a trademark for an antimalarial, antiarthritic, and lupus erythematosus suppressant (hydroxychloroquine sulfate).

-plasia, -plastia, a combining form meaning '(condition of) formation or development': *alloplasia, anosteoplasia, cacoplasia.*

-plasm, -plasma, a combining form meaning 'cell or tissue substance': *deutoplasm, mitoplasm, phytoplasm.* See also **-plasma.**

plasma /plaz'mə/ [Gk, something formed], the watery, straw-colored, fluid portion of the lymph and the blood in which the leukocytes, erythrocytes, and platelets are suspended. Plasma is made up of water, electrolytes, proteins, glucose, fats, bilirubin, and gases and is essential for carrying the cellular elements of the blood through the circulation, transporting nutrients, maintaining the acid-base balance of the body, and transporting wastes from the tissues. Plasma and interstitial fluid correspond closely in content and concentration of proteins; therefore plasma is important in maintaining the osmotic pressure and the exchange of fluids and electrolytes between the capillaries and the tissues. Compare **serum.**

-plasma-, a combining form meaning 'the liquid portion of the blood': *plasmablast, plasmacyte, plasmapheresis, ectoplasma, hydroplasma, ovoplasma.* See also **-plasm.**

plasma cell, a lymphoid or lymphocyte-like cell found in the bone marrow, connective tissue, and, sometimes, the blood. It contains an eccentric nucleus with deeply staining chromatin material arranged in a pattern like the spokes of a wheel or a clock face. Plasma cells are involved in the immunologic mechanism and are formed in large numbers in multiple myeloma. See also **B cell, multiple myeloma.**

plasma cell leukemia, an unusual neoplasm of blood-

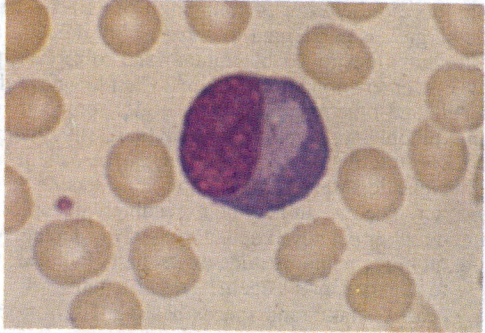

Plasma cell *(Powers, 1989)*

forming tissues in which the predominant cells are plasmacytes. The disease may develop with multiple myeloma or arise independently. Bence Jones proteinuria, abnormal serum globulins, hepatomegaly, and splenomegaly are usual in plasma cell leukemia. In most cases plasma cell leukemia is fatal, but some patients respond to treatment with alkylating agents and glucocorticoids.

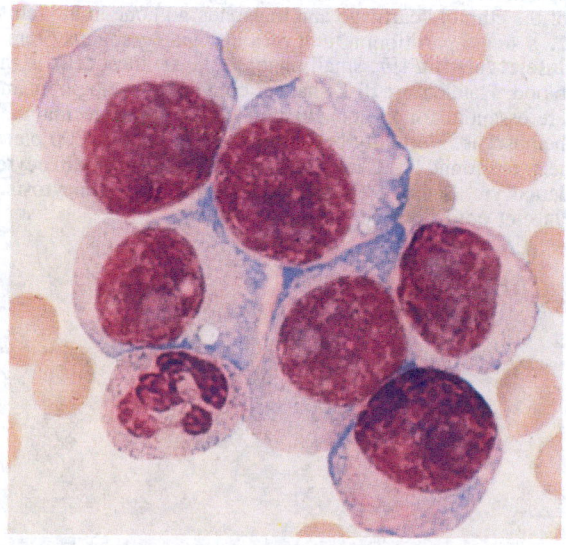

Plasma cell leukemia *(Hayhoe, 1992)*

plasma cell myeloma.   See **multiple myeloma.**
plasmacytoma /plaz′məsītō′mə/, *pl.* **plasmacytomas, plasmacytomata,**   a focal neoplasm containing plasma cells that may develop in the bone marrow, as in multiple myeloma, or outside the bone marrow, as in tumors of the viscera and the mucosa of the nasal, oral, and pharyngeal areas. Also called **peripheral plasma cell myeloma, plasma cell tumor.**
plasma exchange therapy [Gk, *plassein,* to mold; L, *ex, cambire,* to change; Gk, *therapeia,* treatment],   a method of treating certain diseases by removing a portion of plasma from the blood supply of a patient and replacing it with plasma from a disease-free person.

plasma expander,   a substance, usually a high molecular weight dextran, that is administered intravenously to increase the oncotic pressure of a patient.
plasma membrane.   See **cell membrane.**
plasmapheresis /plaz′məfərē′sis/,   the removal of plasma from withdrawn blood by centrifugation, the reconstitution of the cellular elements in an isotonic solution, and the reinfusion of this solution into the donor. Compare **leukapheresis, plateletpheresis.**
plasma protein,   any proteins, including albumin, fibrinogen, prothrombin, and the gamma globulins, that constitute about 6% to 7% of the blood plasma in the body. These substances help maintain water balance affecting osmotic pressure, increase blood viscosity, and help maintain blood pressure. All the plasma proteins except the gamma globulins are synthesized in the liver. See also **antibody, serum.**
plasma renin activity,   the action of the enzyme renin, measured in plasma to aid in the diagnosis of adrenal disease associated with hypertension. The normal value in plasma is 0.2 to 4 ng/ml/hour, depending on salt intake and the length of time the patient is in an upright postion before a renin activity test.
plasma thromboplastin antecedent.   See **factor XI.**
plasma thromboplastin component deficiency.   See **hemophilia.**
plasmasome.   See **plasmosome.**
plasma volume,   the total volume of plasma in the body, elevated in diseases of the liver and spleen and in vitamin C deficiency, lowered in Addison's disease, dehydration, and shock. The normal plasma volume in males is 39 ml/kg of body weight; in females, 40 ml/kg.
plasma volume extender [Gk, *plassein;* L, *volumen,* roll of papyrus; *extendere,* to stretch out],   an intravenous solution of dextran, proteins, or other substances used to treat shock caused by blood volume loss.
plasmid /plaz′mid/ [Gk, *plasma,* something formed],   (in bacteriology) any type of intracellular inclusion considered to have a genetic function, especially a molecule of DNA separate from the bacterial chromosome that determines traits not essential for the viability of the organism but that in some way changes the organism's ability to adapt. R (resistance) factor is an example: A bacterium containing the factor is able to resist many antibacterial drugs that act in many different ways. Plasmid may be passed from one bacterium to another, and it is replicated in later generations of any bacterium carrying it.
plasmidotrophoblast.   See **syncytiotrophoblast.**
plasmin.   See **fibrinolysin.**
plasminogen.   See **fibrinogen.**
plasmo-,   a combining form meaning 'of or related to plasma, or to the substance of a cell': *plasmocyte, plasmodium, plasmosome.*
Plasmodium /plazmō′dē·əm/ [Gk, *plasma* + *eidos,* form],   a genus of protozoa, several species of which cause malaria, transmitted to humans by the bite of an infected *Anopheles* mosquito. **Plasmodium falciparum** causes falciparum malaria, the most severe form of the disease; **P. malariae** causes quartan malaria; **P. ovale** causes mild tertian malaria with oval red blood cells; and **P. vivax** causes common tertian malaria. See also **Anopheles, blackwater fever, malaria.** (See Fig. p. 1230.)
plasmosome /plaz′məsōm/ [Gk, *plasma* + *soma* body],   the true nucleolus of a cell as distinguished from the karyosomes in the nucleus. Also spelled **plasmasome.**

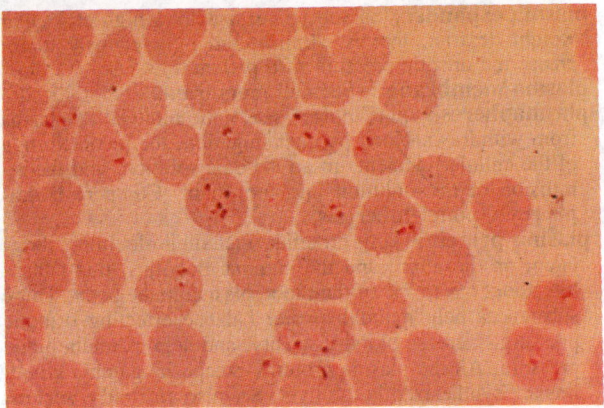

Plasmodium falciparum *(Murray, 1990)*

plast-, a combining form meaning 'to form, mold, or develop': *plastidogenetic, plastodynamia, plastogamy.*

-plast, -plastia, -plasia, -plastic, a combining form meaning 'pertaining to the formation or development of a': *anaplastic, hemoplastic.*

plaster [Gk, *emplastron*], **1.** any composition of a liquid and a powder that hardens when it dries, used in shaping a cast to support a fractured bone as it heals, such as plaster of paris. **2.** a home remedy consisting of a semisolid mixture applied to a part of the body as a counterirritant or for other therapeutic reasons, such as a mustard plaster.

plaster cast [Gk, *emplastron*, plaster; ONorse, *kasta*], a traditional cast designed to encase and immobilize a part of the body in a circumferentially wrapped plaster-of-paris—impregnated gauze roll that has been dipped in warm water. Modern casts are often made of materials such as glass fibers or plastic instead of plaster of paris.

plaster of paris [Gk, *plassein*, originated in Paris, France], a white powder, calcium sulfate hemihydate, which is mixed with water to make a paste that can be molded to encase a body part.

-plastia. See **-plasia. -plastic.** See **-plast.**

plasticity /plastis′itē/ [Gk, *plassein*, to mold], the quality of being plastic or formative.

plastic surgery [Gk, *plassein*, to mold; *cheirourgos*, surgery], the alteration, replacement, or restoration of visible portions of the body, performed to correct a structural or cosmetic defect. In performing corrective plastic surgery, the surgeon may use tissue from the patient or from another person or an inert material that is nonirritating, has a consistency appropriate to the use, and is able to hold its shape and form indefinitely. Implants are commonly used in mammoplasty for breast augmentation. Skin grafting is the most common procedure in plastic surgery. Z-plasty and Y-plasty are simpler techniques often performed instead of a graft in areas of the body covered by skin that is loose and elastic, such as the neck, axilla, throat, and inner aspect of the elbow. Dermabrasion is used to remove pockmarks, scars from acne, or signs of traumatic skin damage. Chemical peeling is another technique in corrective plastic surgery; it is used primarily for removing fine wrinkles on the face. Tattooing, in which a pigment is tattooed into the skin of a graft, is performed to change the color of the graft to re-

semble more closely the surrounding skin. Reconstructive plastic surgery is performed to correct birth defects, to repair structures destroyed by trauma, and to replace tissue removed in other surgical procedures. Cleft lip and cleft palate repair and other maxillofacial surgical procedures, including rhinoplasty, otoplasty, and rhytidoplasty, are among these reconstructive procedures. Care of the patient before and after plastic surgery may require considerable sensitivity and tact. The patient may be exceedingly uncomfortable about the real or perceived appearance of the defect. An accepting, nonjudgmental attitude on the part of all staff members is to the patient's benefit. Optimal nutritional status helps a graft to 'take' and speeds healing. Each procedure and technique involves particular kinds of care in the preoperative and postoperative periods. Instructions and assistance in self-care activities are also specific to the various procedures. Success of most of the procedures depends greatly on the patient's cooperation and fastidious nursing care. The correction of a visible abnormality may be of inestimable benefit to the patient's assurance, self-esteem, and function in society. See also specific procedures.

-plasty, a suffix meaning 'molding, formation, or surgical repair on a (specified) body part or by (specified) means': *bronchoplasty, cervicoplasty, uveoplasty.*

plate [Fr, *plat*, flat dish], **1.** a flat structure or layer, such as a thin layer of bone or the frontal plate between the sides of the ethmoid cartilage and the sphenoid bone in the fetus. **2.** a single partitioning unit of a chromatographic system.

platelet /plat′lit/ [Fr, small plate], the smallest cells in the blood. Platelets are disk-shaped, contain no hemoglobin and are essential for the coagulation of blood and to maintain hemostasis. Normally between 200,000 and 300,000 platelets are found in 1 ml^3 of blood. Compare **erythrocyte, leucocyte.** See also **thrombocytopenia, thrombocytosis.**

Platelet count. See **count.**

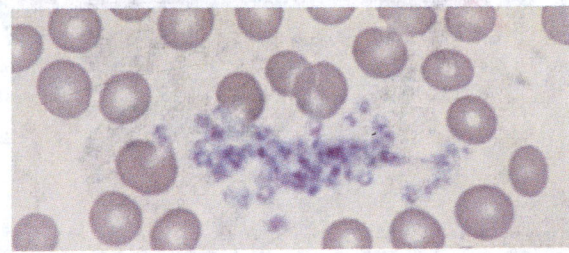

Platelets *(Bain, 1989)*

plateletpheresis /plat′litfer′əsis/ [Fr, *platelet* + Gk, *aphairesis*, to carry away], the removal of platelets from withdrawn blood, the remainder of the blood being reinfused into the donor. Also called **thrombapheresis, thrombotapheresis.** Compare **leukapheresis, plasmapheresis.**

-platin, a combining form for platinum-based antineoplastics.

platinized gold foil /plat′inīzd/ [Sp, *plata*, silver; AS, *geolu*, gold; L, *folium*, leaf], a thin sheet rolled or hammered from platinum sandwiched between two sheets of gold, used for making portions of dental restorations requiring greater hardness than that obtained by using other materials, such as copper amalgam.

Platinol, a trademark for an antineoplastic (cisplatin).

platinum (Pt) /plat′ənəm/ [Sp, *plata*, silver], a silvery-white, soft metallic element. Its atomic number is 78; its atomic weight is 195.09. Platinum is used in dentistry, jewelry, and the manufacture of chemical apparatus that must withstand high temperatures.

platinum foil, a very thin sheet of rolled pure platinum that has a high fusing point, making it an ideal matrix in various soldering procedures for fabricating orthodontic appliances and dentures. It is also commonly used as the internal form of porcelain dental restorations during fabrication.

platy-, a combining form meaning 'broad or flat': *platy-basia, platycephalous, platycnemic*.

Platyhelminthes /plat′ihelmin′thēz/ [Gk, *platys*, flat, *helmins*, worm], a phylum of parasitic flatworms that includes the Cestoda subclass of tapeworms and Trematoda class of flukes.

platypelloid pelvis /plat′əpel′oid/ [Gk, *platys*, wide, *pella*, bowl, *eidos*, form; L, *pelvis*, basin], a rare type of pelvis in which the inlet is round like the gynecoid type in the anterior section, but the posterior section is foreshortened by its flat and heavy border. The sacrum is hollow and inclines posteriorly, and the sidewalls are convergent. In the midplane, the transverse diameter is much wider than the narrowed anteroposterior diameter. Vaginal delivery is not usually possible in women who have platypelloid pelves. This type of pelvis is present in 3% of women.

platysma /plətiz′mə/ [Gk, *platys*, flat], one of a pair of wide muscles at the side of the neck. It arises from the fascia covering the superior parts of the pectoralis major and the deltoideus, crosses the clavicle, and rises obliquely and medially along the side of the neck. The anterior fibers of the platysma interlace, inferior and posterior to the symphysis menti, with the fibers of the muscle of the opposite side. The posterior fibers of the platysma cross the mandible, some inserting into the bone below the oblique line, others into the skin and the subcutaneous tissue of the lower part of the face. Many of the fibers blend with the muscles at the angle and the lower part of the mouth. The platysma covers the external jugular vein as the vein descends from the angle of the mandible to the clavicle. The platysma is innervated by the cervical branch of the facial nerve and serves to draw down the lower lip and the corner of the mouth. When the platysma fully contracts, the skin over the clavicle is drawn toward the mandible, increasing the diameter of the neck.

play [AS, *plegan*, sport], any spontaneous or organized activity that provides enjoyment, entertainment, amusement, or diversion. It is essential in childhood for the development of a normal personality and as a means for developing physically, intellectually, and socially. Play provides an outlet for releasing tension and stress, as well as a means for testing and experimenting with new or fearful roles or situations. It is an indispensable part of the nursing care of children, especially in the hospital. It helps relieve the tension and anxiety of being in unfamiliar surroundings and separated from parents, and it gives the child a sense of security and a means of expressing fears and fantasies. Play also offers the nurse one of the most effective methods of communicating with and gaining the trust of the child and helping the child to understand treatments and procedures. Kinds of play include **active play, associative play, coop-**erative play, dramatic play, parallel play, passive play, skill play, and solitary play. See also **play therapy.**

play therapy, a form of psychotherapy in which a child plays in a protected and structured environment with games and toys provided by a therapist, who observes the behavior, affect, and conversation of the child to gain insight into thoughts, feelings, and fantasies. As conflicts are discovered, the therapist often helps the child understand and work through them.

pleasure principle /plezh′ər/ [Fr, *plaisir*, pleasure; L, *principium*], (in psychoanalysis) the need for immediate gratification of instinctual drives. Compare **reality principle.**

pledget /plej′ət/, a small, flat compress made of cotton gauze, or a tuft of cotton wool, lint, or a similar synthetic material, used to wipe the skin, absorb drainage, or clean a small surface.

-plegia, -plegic, a combining form meaning 'a (specified) paralysis': *cycloplegia, paraplegic*.

Plegine, a trademark for an anorexiant (phendimetrazine tartrate).

pleiades /plē′ədēz/ [*Pleiades* star cluster in constellation Taurus], *obsolete.* a mass of enlarged lymph nodes.

pleio-. See **pleo-.**

pleiotropic gene /plī′ətrop′ik/, a gene that produces a complex of unrelated phenotypic effects.

pleiotropy /plī·ot′rəpē/ [Gk, *pleion*, more, *trepein* to turn], (in genetics) the production by a single gene of a multiple, different, and apparently unrelated manifestation of a particular disorder, such as the cluster of symptoms in Marfan's syndrome, aortic aneurysm, dislocation of the optic lens, skeletal deformities, and arachnodactyly, any or all of which may be present.

pleo-, pleio-, a prefix meaning 'more': *pleochromatic, pleomastia, pleomorphism*.

plessimeter. See **pleximeter.**

plethora /pleth′ərə/ [Gk, *plethore*, fullness], a term applied to the beefy red coloration of a newborn. The 'boiled lobster' hue of the infant's skin is caused by an unusually high proportion of erythrocytes per volume of blood. The term formerly was used to describe any red-faced person. **–plethoric,** *adj.*

plethysmogram /pləthiz′məgram′/ [Gk, *plethynein*, to increase, *gramma*, to record], a tracing produced by a plethysmograph.

plethysmograph /pləthiz′məgraf′/, an instrument for measuring and recording changes in the sizes and volumes of extremities and organs by measuring changes in their blood volumes. **–plethysmographic,** *adj.,* **plethysmography,** *n.*

plethysmography /pleth′izmog′rəfē/ [Gk, *plethynein*, to increase + *graphein*, to record], the measurment of changes in the volume of organs or other body parts, particularly those changes resulting from blood flow.

pleur-. See **pleuro-.**

pleura /ploor′ə/, *pl.* **pleurae** [Gk, rib], a delicate serous membrane enclosing the lung, composed of a single layer of flattened mesothelial cells resting on a delicate membrane of connective tissue. Beneath the membrane is a stroma of collagenous tissue containing yellow elastic fibers. The pleura divides into the visceral pleura, which covers the lung, dipping into the fissures between the lobes, and the parietal pleura, which lines the chest wall, covers the diaphragm, and reflects over the structures in the mediastinum. The parietal and visceral pleurae are separated from each other by a small amount of fluid that acts as a lubricant as the lungs expand and contract during respiration. See also **pleural cavity, pleural space.** **–pleural,** *adj.*

pleural [Gk, *pleura* rib],   pertaining to the pleura.

pleural cavity /plŏŏr′əl/ [Gk, *pleura*, rib; L, *cavum*, cavity],   the cavity within the thorax that contains the lungs. Between the ribs and the lungs are the visceral and parietal pleurae.

pleural effusion,   an abnormal accumulation of fluid in the intrapleural spaces of the lungs, characterized by fever, chest pain, dyspnea, and nonproductive cough. The fluid involved is an exudate or a transudate from inflamed pleural surfaces. A transudate that accumulates in pulmonary edema is commonly aspirated. An exudate may result from pulmonary infarction, trauma, tumor, or infection, such as tuberculosis. The specific cause of the exudate is treated, and the exudate may be aspirated or surgically drained. Other treatment may include the administration of corticosteroids, diuretics, and vasodilators, oxygen therapy, and intermittent positive pressure breathing.

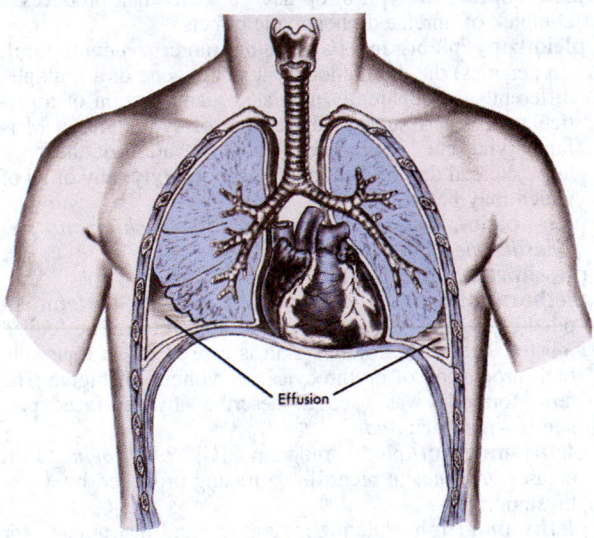

Pleural effusion (Wilson, 1990)

pleural friction rub [Gk, *pleura*, rib; L, *fricare*, to rub; ME, *rubben*],   a rubbing, grating sound that occurs with pleurisy as one layer of the pleural membrane slides over the other during breathing.

pleural space,   the potential space between the visceral and parietal layers of the pleurae. The space contains a small amount of fluid that acts as a lubricant, allowing the pleurae to slide smoothly over each other as the lungs expand and contract with respiration.

pleura pulmonalis [Gk, *pleura*, rib; L, *pulmo*, lung],   the portion of the pleural membrane that covers the lungs, as distinguished from the parietal layer of pleura that lines the inner aspect of the thoracic cavity.

pleurisy /plŏŏr′əsē/ [Gk, *pleura* + *itis*, inflammation],   inflammation of the parietal pleura of the lungs, character-

ized by dyspnea and stabbing pain, leading to restriction of ordinary breathing with spasm of the chest on the affected side. A pleural friction rub may be heard on auscultation. Simple pleurisy with undetectable exudate is called fibrinous or dry; pleural effusion indicates extensive inflammation with considerable amounts of exudate in the pleural spaces. Common causes of pleurisy include bronchial carcinoma, lung or chest wall abscess, pneumonia, pulmonary infarction, and tuberculosis. The condition may result in permanent adhesions between the pleura and adjacent surfaces. Treatment consists of relief of pain and therapy for the primary disease. See also **pleural effusion, pleurodynia, pulmonary edema.**

pleurisy with effusion [Gk, *pleuritis*; L, *effundere*, to pour out],   pleurisy in which inflammation has progressed to an effusion into the intrapleural space, characterized by fluid with a high specific gravity caused by a high concentration of fibrin and clots.

pleuritic /plŏŏri′tik/ [Gk, *pleura*, rib],   pertaining to a condition of pleurisy.

pleuritis.   See **pleurisy.**

pleuro- /plŏŏr′ō-/, **pleur-,**   a combining form meaning 'of or pertaining to the pleura, to a side, or to a rib': *pleurocentrum, pleurography, pleuropulmonary.*

pleurodynia /plŏŏr′ōdin′ē·ə/ [Gk, *pleura* + *odyne*, pain],   acute inflammation of the intercostal muscles and the muscular attachment of the diaphragm to the chest wall. It is characterized by sudden severe pain and tenderness, fever, headache, and anorexia. These symptoms are aggravated by movement and breathing. The lungs are not affected, and characteristically there is no cough or pleural effusion. See also **epidemic pleurodynia.**

pleuropericardial rub /-per′ikär′dē·əl/ [Gk, *pleura* + *peri*, around, *kardia*, heart; ME, *rubben*, to scrape],   an abnormal coarse friction sound heard on auscultation of the lungs during late inspiration and early expiration. It is caused by the visceral and parietal pleural surfaces rubbing against each other. The sound is not affected by coughing. A pleural rub indicates primary inflammatory, neoplastic, or traumatic pleural disease, or inflammation secondary to infection or neoplasm. Also called **pleural friction rub.** See also **breath sound, Kussmaul breathing, rale, rhonchi, wheeze.**

pleuroperitoneal cavity.   See **splanchnocoele.**

pleuropneumonia /plŏŏr′ōnŏŏmō′nē·ə/ [Gk, *pleura* + *pneumon*, lung],   **1.** a combination of pleurisy and pneumonia. **2.** an infection of cattle resulting in inflammation of both the pleura and lungs, caused by microorganisms of the *Mycoplasma* group. See also **Mycoplasma, pleuropneumonia-like organism.**

pleuropneumonia-like organism (PPLO),   a group of filterable organisms of the genus *Mycoplasma* similar to *M. mycoides*, the cause of pleuropneumonia in cattle.

pleurothotonos /plŏŏr′əthot′ənəs/ [Gk, *pleurothen*, side of the body, *tonos*, tension],   an involuntary, severe, prolonged contraction of the muscles of one side of the body, resulting in an acute arch to that side. It is usually associated with tetanus infection or strychnine poisoning. Compare **emprosthotonos, opisthotonos, orthotonos.** **–pleurothotonic,** *adj.*

plex-,   a prefix meaning 'a stroke or to strike': *plexalgia, pleximeter, plexor.*

-plex, -plexus,   a suffix meaning 'a braid or pertaining to a nerve, a network': *brachiplex, cerviplex, veniplex.*

-plexia, -plexy, a combining form meaning '(condition resulting from a crippling or serious occurrence': *apoplexia, pagoplexia, selenoplexia.*

plexiform neuroma /plek'sifôrm/ [L, *plexus,* braided, *forma,* form; Gk, *neuron,* nerve, *oma,* tumor], a neoplasm composed of twisted bundles of nerves. Also called **Verneuil's neuroma.**

pleximeter /pleksim'ətər/ [Gk, *plessein,* to strike, *metron,* measure], a mediating device, such as a percussor or finger, used to receive light taps in percussion. Also called **plessimeter.** See also **percussion.**

plexor. See **percussor.**

plexus /plek'səs/, *pl.* **plexuses** [L, braided], a network of intersecting nerves and blood vessels or of lymphatic vessels. The body contains many plexuses, such as the brachial plexus, the cardiac plexus, the cervical plexus, and the solar plexus.

-plexus. See **-plex.**

-plexy. See **-plexia.**

plic-, a prefix meaning a 'fold or ridge': *plicadentin, plication, plicotomy.*

plica /plī'kə/, *pl.* **plicae** /plī'sē/ [L, plicare, to fold], a fold of tissue within the body, such as the plicae transversales of the rectum and the plicae circulares of the small intestine. –**plical,** *adj.*

plica circularis. See **circular fold.**

plicae transversales recti /plī'sē/, semilunar, transverse folds in the rectum that support the weight of feces. Also called **Houston's valves.** See also **rectum.**

plicamycin /plī'kəmī'sin/, an antineoplastic agent. Previously called **mithramycin.**

■ INDICATIONS: It is prescribed primarily in the treatment of malignant tumors of the testis. It is also prescribed in the treatment of hypercalcemia and hypercalciuria associated with cancer.

■ CONTRAINDICATIONS: Clotting disorders, thrombocytopenia, kidney or liver dysfunction, bone marrow depression, or known hypersensitivity to this drug prohibits its use.

■ ADVERSE EFFECTS: Among the more serious adverse reactions are thrombocytopenia and clotting defects. Nausea and stomatitis commonly occur.

plica semilunaris, the semilunar fold of the conjunctiva that extends laterally from the lacrimal caruncle. It has a concave free border directed toward the cornea. In some individuals it contains smooth muscular fibers.

plication /plīkā'shən/, any operation that involves folding, shortening, or decreasing the size of a muscle or hollow organ, such as the stomach, by taking in tucks.

plication of stomach [L, *plicare,* to fold; Gk, *stomakhos,* gullet], a surgical treatment for obesity in which tucks are created in the wall of the stomach.

plica umbilicalis lateralis. See **lateral umbilical fold.**

plica umbilicalis mediana. See **middle umbilical fold.**

Plimmer's bodies [Henry G. Plimmer, English biologist, b. 1856], small, round, encapsulated bodies found in cancers and once thought to be the causative parasites. Also called **Behla's bodies.**

-ploid, -ploidy a combining form meaning 'having a (specified) number of chromosome sets': *heptaploid, octaploid, polyploid.*

ploidy /ploi'dē/, [Gk, *eidos,* form], the status of a cell nucleus in regard to the number of complete chromosome sets it contains.

plug [D, *plugge,* stopper], a mass of tissue cells, mucus, or other matter that blocks a normal opening or passage of the body, such as a cervical plug.

plumbism /plum'izəm/ [L, *plumbum,* lead], a chronic form of lead poisoning caused by absorption of lead or lead salts.

Plummer's disease [Henry S. Plummer, American physician, b. 1874], goiter characterized by a hyperfunctioning nodule or adenoma and thyrotoxicosis. Also called **toxic nodular goiter.**

Plummer-Vinson syndrome /plum'ərvin'sən/ [Henry S. Plummer; Porter P. Vinson, American physician, b. 1890], a rare disorder associated with severe and chronic iron deficiency anemia, characterized glossitis, koilonychia, and by dysphagia caused by esophageal webs at the level of the cricoid cartilage. Also called **sideropenic dysphagia.** Compare **Paterson-Kelly syndrome.**

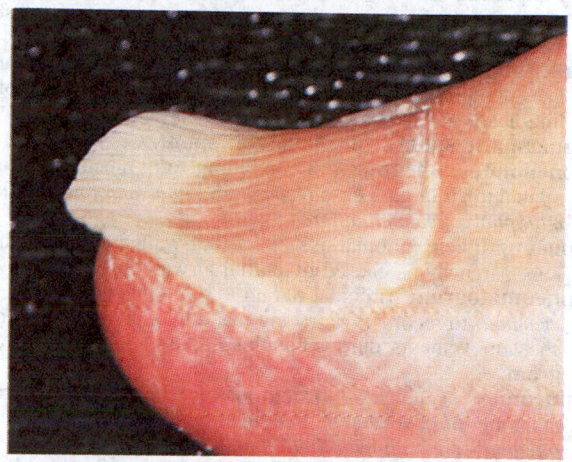

Koilonychia, commonly seen in Plummer-Vinson syndrome
(Baran, 1991)

plunging goiter. See **diving goiter.**

pluri-, a prefix meaning 'more': *pluriceptor, plurimenorrhea, pluritissular.*

pluricentric blastoma. See **blastoma.**

pluripara /plŏŏrip'ərə/ [L, *plus,* more + *parere,* to bear], a woman who has borne several children.

pluripolar mitosis. See **multipolar mitosis.**

plutonium (Pu) /plŏŏtō'nē·əm/ [planet, *Pluto*], a synthetic transuranic metallic element. Its atomic number is 94; its atomic weight is 242. A highly toxic waste product of nuclear power plants, plutonium was used in the assembly of early nuclear weapons.

pm, abbreviation for *picometer.*

Pm, symbol for the element **promethium.**

P.M.D., abbreviation for *private medical doctor.* Also called **L.M.D.**

pmh, abbreviation for *past medical history.*

PMI, abbreviation for **point of maximum impulse.**

PMN, abbreviation for **polymorphonuclear cell.**

PMS, pms, abbreviation for **premenstrual syndrome.**

PMT, abbreviation for *premenstrual tension.* See **premenstrual syndrome.**

PND, 1. abbreviation for **paroxysmal nocturnal dyspnea. 2.** abbreviation for **postnasal drip.**

-pnea, -pnoea, pneo-, a combining form meaning 'breath or breathing': *brachypnea, dyspnea, pneoscope.*

pneopneic reflex /nē'ōnē'ik/ [Gk, *pnoe,* breath; L, *reflectere,* to bend back], a change in the normal rhythm of breathing when an irritating gas is introduced into the lungs.

pneuma-. See **pneumato-.**

pneumatic /nōōmat'ik/ [Gk, *pneuma* air], pertaining to air or gas.

pneumatic condenser [Gk, *pneuma,* air; L, *condensare,* to thicken], (in dentistry) a pneumatic device, developed by George M. Hollenback, to deliver a compacting force to restorative material used in filling tooth cavities. The force is delivered by controlled pneumatic pressure and develops compacting blows that can be varied in intensity. The frequency of the blows may be up to 360 strokes/minute. Also called **Hollenback condenser.**

pneumatic heart driver, a mechanical device that regulates compressed air delivery to an artificial heart, controlling heart rate, percent systole, and delay in systole.

pneumatic splint. See **inflatable splint.**

pneumato-, pneuma-, a combining form meaning 'of or related to air or gas, or to respiration': *pneumatology, pneumatophore, pneumatothorax.*

pneumatocele /nōōmat'əsēl'/, a thin-walled cavity in the lung parenchyma caused by partial airway obstruction.

pneumatogram /nōōmat'əgram'/ [Gk, *pneuma,* air + *gramma,* to record], a tracing made by a pneumograph of chest movements during breathing. Also called **pneumogram**.

pneumo- /n(y)ōō'mō-/, **pneumono-,** a combining form meaning 'of or related to the lungs, to air, or to the breath': *pneumobacillin, pneumocele, pneumolith.*

pneumobelt /nōō'mōbelt/, a corset with an inflatable bladder that fits over the abdominal area. The bladder is connected by a hose to a ventilator that delivers positive pressure at an adjustable rate and pressure. It is used to assist in the respiratory rehabilitation of patients with high cervical injuries so that neck muscle effort can be spared for other activities.

pneumocentesis /-sentē'sis/ [Gk, *pneumon* + *kentesis,* pricking], a procedure in which a lung is punctured to drain fluid contents.

pneumococcal /nōō'mōkok'əl/ [Gk, *pneumon,* lung, *kokkos,* berry], of or pertaining to bacteria of the genus *Pneumococcus.*

pneumococcal meningitis [Gk, *pneumon,* lung + *kokkos,* berry, *menigx,* membrane, *itis,* inflammation], meningitis caused by pneumococcal infection. Also called **streptococcus pneumoniae.**

pneumococcal vaccine, an active immunizing agent containing antigens of the 14 types of *Pneumococcus* associated with 80% of the cases of pneumococcal pneumonia.

■ INDICATIONS: It is prescribed for people over 2 years of age who are at high risk of developing severe pneumococcal pneumonia.

■ CONTRAINDICATIONS: Pregnancy, early childhood (under 2 years of age), or known hypersensitivity to the vaccine prohibits its use.

■ ADVERSE EFFECTS: Among the more serious adverse reactions are inflammation at the site of injection, fever, and hypersensitivity reactions.

pneumococcus /nōō'mōkok'əs/, *pl.* **pneumococci** /'kok'sī/ [Gk, pneumon + *kokkos,* berry], a gram-positive diplococcal bacterium of the species *Streptococcus pneumoniae,* the most common cause of bacterial pneumonia. More than 85 subtypes of this organism are known. A vaccine protective against 35 serotypes has been developed and is recommended for those over 65 years of age, those with a chronic lung disease, or patients who have HIV infection. See also **lobar pneumonia, pneumonia.**

pneumoconiosis /nōō·mōkō'nē·ō'sis/ [Gk, *pneumon* + *konis,* dust, *osis,* condition], any disease of the lung caused by chronic inhalation of dust, usually mineral dusts of occupational or environmental origin. Some kinds of pneumoconioses are **anthracosis, asbestosis, silicosis.**

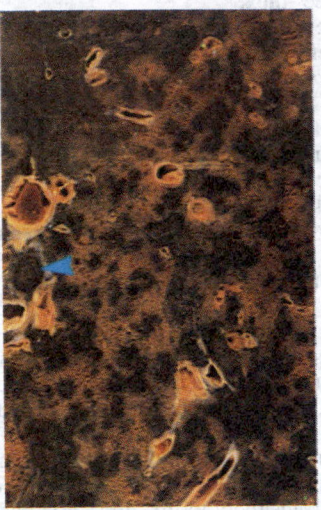

Coal worker's pneumoconiosis *(Fletcher, 1987)*

pneumoconstriction /nōō'mōkənstrik'shən/, an area of collapsed lung tissue that results from mechanical stimulation of an exposed portion of the lung. It is produced by local reflex muscular closure of alveolar ducts and alveoli.

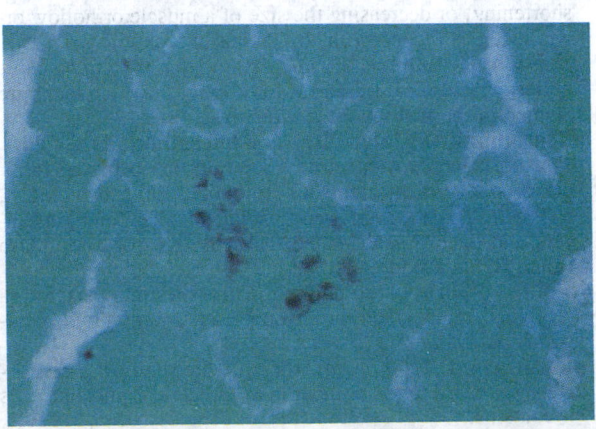

Pneumocystis carinii pneumonia *(Murray, 1990)*

Pneumocystis carinii /nōō′mōsis′tis kərin′ē·ī/, a microorganism that causes pneumocystosis, a type of interstitial cell pneumonitis.

pneumocystis pneumonia [Gk, *pneuma*, air + *kystis*, bag; *pneumon*, lung], a type of interstitial plasma cell pneumonia in which the alveoli become honeycombed with an acidophilic material. The patients may or may not be febrile but usually are weak, dyspneic, and cyanotic.

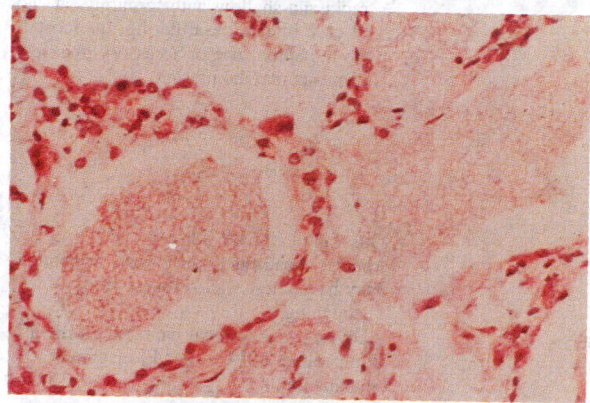

Pneumocystis pneumonia (Turner-Warwick, 1993)

pneumocystosis /nōō′mōsistō′sis/ [Gk, *pneumon* + *kystis*, bag, *osis*, condition], infection with the parasite *Pneumocystis carinii*, usually seen in patients with AIDS, infants, or debilitated or immunosuppressed people, particularly those with lymphomas, and characterized by fever, cough, tachypnea, and, frequently, cyanosis. The diagnosis is difficult to make and usually requires bronchoscopy and special staining techniques. Mortality nears 100% in untreated patients. Treatment with pentamidine isethionate or a combination of trimethoprim and sulfamethoxazole is effective. Patients at risk should receive prophylaxis against acute infection. Also called **interstitial plasma cell pneumonia.**

pneumoencephalogram /nōō′mō·ensef′əlōgram′/, a radiograph of the brain made during pneumoencephalography.

pneumoencephalography /nōō′mō·ensef′əlog′rəfē/ [Gk, *pneuma*, air, *enkephalos*, brain, *graphein*, to record], a procedure for the radiographic visualization of the ventricular space, basal cisterns, and subarachnoid space overlying the cerebral hemispheres of the brain. Air, helium, or oxygen is injected into the lumbar subarachnoid space after the intermittent removal of the cerebrospinal fluid by lumbar puncture. See also **encephalography, ventriculography.** –**pneumoencephalographic,** *adj.*

pneumogastric nerve. See **vagus nerve.**

pneumogram. See **pneumatogram.**

pneumograph /nōō′məgraf/, a device that records breathing movements by means of an inflated coil around the chest. It measures mainly the ventilatory cycle rather than the amplitude of breathing movements.

pneumohemopericardium, See **hemopneumopericardium.**

pneumohemothorax /-hem′ōthôr′aks/ [Gk, *pneuma*, air + *haima*, blood + *thorax*, chest], an accumulation of air and blood in the pleural cavity.

pneumomediastinum /nōō′mōmē′dē·əstī′nəm/ [Gk, *pneuma*, air, *mediastinus*, midway], the presence of air or gas in the mediastinal tissues, which in infants may lead to pneumothorax or pneumopericardium, especially in those with respiratory distress syndrome or aspiration pneumonitis. In older children the condition may result from bronchitis, acute asthma, pertussis, cystic fibrosis, or bronchial rupture from cough or trauma.

pneumonectomy /nōō′mənek′təmē/ [Gk, *pneumon*, lung, *ektome*, excision], the surgical removal of all or part of a lung.

pneumonia /nōōmō′nē·ə/ [Gk, *pneumon*, lung], an acute inflammation of the lungs, usually caused by inhaled pneumococci of the species *Streptococcus pneumoniae*. The alveoli and bronchioles of the lungs become plugged with a fibrous exudate. Pneumonia may be caused by other bacteria, as well as by viruses, rickettsiae, and fungi. Kinds of pneumonia are **aspiration pneumonia, bronchopneumonia, eosinophilic pneumonia, interstitial pneumonia, lobar pneumonia, mycoplasma pneumonia,** and **viral pneumonia.**

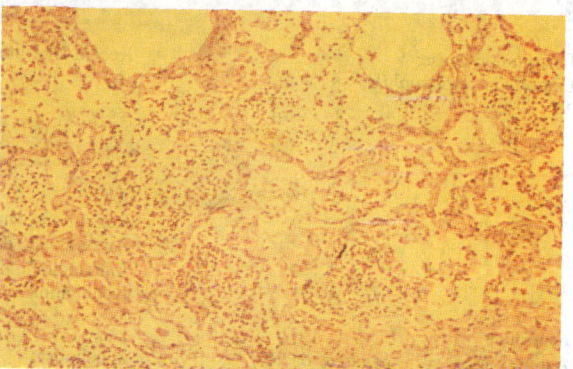

Photomicrograph of pneumonia (Christiansen, 1993)

■ OBSERVATIONS: Characteristic of pneumonia are severe chills, a high fever (which may reach 105° F), headache, cough, and chest pain. Inflammation of the lower lobe of the right lung may produce a pain suggesting appendicitis. An effusion of red blood cells into the alveolar spaces, resulting from histolytic damage by the microorganism, causes a rust-colored sputum that may be a diagnostic sign of pneumococcal infection. As the disease progresses, sputum may become thicker and more purulent, and the person may experience painful attacks of coughing. Respiration usually becomes more difficult, painful, shallow, and rapid. The pulse increases in rapidity, often measuring 120 or more beats a minute. Other signs may include profuse sweating and cyanosis. GI disorders and an outbreak of herpes simplex about the face also may occur. In children, pneumonia may be accompanied by convulsion. As the alveoli become filled with exudate, the affected area of a lobe becomes increasingly firm and consolidated. A distinctive kind of rale is heard on auscultation. X-ray films are taken to evaluate consolidation; laboratory analysis of sputum and cultures of the blood help in identifying the causative organism.

■ INTERVENTIONS: The treatment of pneumonia includes bed rest, fluids, antibiotics, analgesics, and, if necessary, oxygen. The antibiotic prescribed is specific for the bacterium identified in the laboratory analysis of sputum or blood. Pen

Etiology, risk factors, and signs and symptoms of pneumonia

Etiology	Risk factors	Signs and symptoms
Typical syndrome S. pneumoniae, uncomplicated	Sickle-cell disease; hypogammaglobulinemia; multiple myeloma	Sudden onset with shaking chill; fever (39° to 40° C; 102.2° to 104° F), pleuritic chest pain, productive cough; sputum—green and purulent and may be blood tinged, 'rusty'; respirations—rapid and shallow with 'grunting' at end of each breath; nasal flaring, intercostal rib retraction, use of accessory muscles, cyanosis may be present
Streptococcus, complicated (empyema, metastatic infection) H. influenzae S. aureus	Advanced age COPD Alcoholism Recent influenza	
Atypical syndrome Common causes: mycoplasma pneumonia, viral pathogens	Childhood Young adults	Onset gradual over 3-5 days Malaise, headache, sore throat, dry cough May have chest wall soreness from coughing
Uncommon cause: Legionella pneumophila	Recent URI influenza	Above plus abdominal pain and diarrhea Temperature 40° C (104° F) or greater Shaking chills Respiratory distress Renal failure, hyponatremia, hypophosphatemia, elevated creatine phosphokinase
P. carinii	Renal transplantation Autoimmune disease Immunologic deficiency Debilitation	Rapid or gradual onset with increasing dyspnea, dry cough, tachypnea, hypoxemia X-ray—diffuse interstitial involvement
Aspiration Aspiration of: gram-negative bacilli; *Klebsiella, Pseudomonas, Serratia, Enterobacter, Escherichia, Proteus;* gram-positive bacilli	Alcoholism Debilitation Hospitalization, nosocomial infection	*Mixed anaerobic:* At first gradual onset Low-grade fever, cough Sputum—increased production, musty smelling Chest x-ray—interstitial involvement in dependent portion of lung
Staphylococcus Gastric acid aspiration	Altered consciousness	*Gram-negative or gram-positive infection:* May also present same clinical picture as classic pneumonia; sudden onset of respiratory distress, severe dyspnea, cyanosis, coughing, hypoxemia, followed by signs and symptoms of secondary infection
Aspiration of inert substances, water, barium, nutritional supplements		
Hematogenous Occurs when pathogens are spread to lungs via bloodstream, *Staphylococcus, E. coli,* enteric anerobes	Infected intravascular catheter Endocarditis IV drug abuse Intraabdominal abscess Pyonephrosis Empyema of gallbladder	Pulmonary symptoms minimal compared with the symptoms of septicemia; most common complaints—nonproductive cough and pleuritic pain similar to that seen in *pulmonary embolism*

Adapted from Phipps WJ, Long BL, Woods NF, Cassmeyer VL: *Medical-surgical nursing: concepts and clinical practice,* ed 4, St Louis, 1991, Mosby.

icillin G is usually prescribed for pneumococcal pneumonia. The antibiotic is administered intramuscularly until the patient's temperature is normal for 2 days. Analgesics are given as needed for relief of chest pain. Oxygen is administered by tent, mask, or catheter to patients who are cyanotic, very weak, or delirious; the amount of oxygen to be given is determined through serial laboratory analyses of blood gases. Expectorants, postural drainage, and aspiration of the bronchi are often prescribed. Chest x-ray films are advised during the acute phase, after therapy has been completed, and on a follow-up examination 4 to 6 weeks later. Mild pneumonia is often treated without hospitalization.

■ NURSING CONSIDERATIONS: Fluid and electrolytes are often lost during prolonged high fever; intravenous replacement is often required. Ice packs or cold, wet compresses may be needed to reduce the fever. Fever, loss of fluids, and breathing through the mouth result in a need for care of the mouth and the nares, where herpes lesions frequently develop. The nurse collects samples of sputum for laboratory analysis, administers antibiotics and other medications, and notes the temperature, pulse, and respiration as often as necessary.

-pneumonia, a combining form meaning an 'inflammation of the lungs': *necropneumonia, splenopneumonia, typhopneumonia.*

-pneumonic, 1. a combining form meaning 'related to pneumonia': *bronchopneumonic, peripneumonic, pleuropneumonic.* **2.** a combining form meaning 'related to the lungs': *gastropneumonic, hepatopneumonic.*

pneumonic plague /noomon'ik/ [Gk, *pneumon,* lung; L, *plaga,* stroke], a highly virulent and rapidly fatal form of plague characterized by bronchopneumonia. There are two forms: **Primary pneumonic plague** results from involvement of the lungs in the course of bubonic plague; **secondary pneumonic plague** results from the inhalation of infected particles of sputum from a person having pneumonic plague. Compare **bubonic plague, septicemic plague.** See also **plague, Yersinia pestis.**

pneumonitis /noo'mənī'tis/, *pl.* **pneumonitides** [Gk, *pneumon + itis*], inflammation of the lung. Pneumonitis may be caused by a virus or may be a hypersensitivity reaction to chemicals or organic dusts, such as bacteria, bird droppings, or molds. It is usually an interstitial, granulomatous, fibrosing inflammation of the lung, especially of the bronchioles and alveoli. Dry cough is a common symptom. Treatment depends on the cause but includes removal of any offending agents and the administration of corticosteroids to reduce inflammation. Compare **pneumonia.**

pneumono-. See **pneumo-.**

pneumoperitoneum /-per'itōnē'əm/ [Gk, *pneuma,* air, *peri,* around, *teinein,* to stretch], the presence of air or gas within the peritoneal cavity of the abdomen. It may be spontaneous, such as from rupture of a hollow gas-containing organ, or induced for diagnostic or therapeutic purposes.

pneumotachometer /-takom'ətər/, a device that measures the flow of respiratory gases. The pressure gradient is directly related to flow, thus allowing a computer to derive a flow curve measured in liters per minute.

pneumothorax /noo'mōthôr'aks/ [Gk, *pneuma,* air, *thorax,* chest], a collection of air or gas in the pleural space causing the lung to collapse. Pneumothorax may be the result of an open chest wound that permits the entrance of air, the rupture of an emphysematous vesicle on the surface of the lung, or a severe bout of coughing, or it may occur spontaneously without apparent cause.

■ OBSERVATIONS: The onset of pneumothorax is accompanied by a sudden, sharp chest pain, followed by difficult, rapid breathing, cessation of normal chest movements on the affected side, tachycardia, a weak pulse, hypotension, diaphoresis, an elevated temperature, pallor, dizziness, and anxiety.

■ INTERVENTIONS: The patient is assured that the condition can be treated, is urged to remain quiet, and is placed in bed in Fowler's position. Oxygen is administered through a nasal cannula, unless contraindicated, and the air is immediately aspirated from the pleural space. A chest tube is inserted

and attached to a water seal drainage system; the tube is not removed until air is no longer expelled through the underwater drainage system and an x-ray examination shows that the lung is completely expanded. Pain may be controlled by administering appropriate analgesics, but the use of respiratory depressants is avoided. Intermittent positive pressure breathing may be administered, and the patient is taught how to turn, cough, breathe deeply, and perform passive exercises and is told to avoid stretching, reaching, or making sudden movements.

■ NURSING CONSIDERATIONS: The patient is advised not to smoke but to drink fluids copiously, to exercise, to avoid fatigue and strenuous activity, and to report any symptoms of recurrence to the physician, such as chest pain, difficult breathing, fever, or respiratory infection.

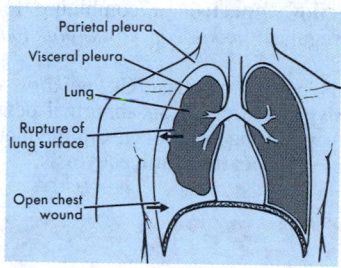

Pneumothorax (Wilson, 1990)

PNF, abbreviation for **proprioceptive neuromuscular facilitation.**

PNH, abbreviation for **paroxysmal nocturnal hemoglobinuria.**

-pnoea. See **-pnea.**

PNP, abbreviation for **pediatric nurse practitioner.**

p.o., an abbreviation for the Latin phrase *per os,* 'by mouth'; a route for administration of medications.

Po, symbol for the element **polonium.**

Po₂, symbol for *partial pressure of oxygen.* See **partial pressure.**

pockmark [AS, *pocc, meark*], a pitted scar on the skin, usually the result of a smallpox pustule at the site.

pod-. See **podo-.**

podagra. See **agoraphobia.**

podalic /pōdal'ik/ [Gk, *pous,* foot], pertaining to the feet.

podalic version, the shifting of the position of a fetus so as to bring the feet to the outlet during labor.

podiatrist, a health professional who diagnoses and treats disorders of the feet. Podiatrists complete a 4-year postgraduate educational program leading to a degree of Doctor of Podiatric Medicine (DPM). Also called *(obsolete)* **chiropodist.**

podiatry /pədī'ətrē/ [Gk, *pous + iatros,* healer], the diagnosis and treatment of diseases and other disorders of the feet. Formerly called **chiropody.**

-podium, a combining form meaning 'something footlike': *axiopodium, phyllopodium, pseudopodium.*

podo-, pod-, a combining form meaning 'of or related to the foot': *podogram, podology, podotrochilitis.*

podophyllotoxin /pō'dōfil'ətok'sin/ [Gk, *pous + phyllon,* leaf, *toxikon,* poison], any one of a group of substances derived from the roots of *Podophyllum peltatum,* a common plant species known as mayapple, or American mandrake. Podophyllin, a resinous preparation of podophyllotoxin, is prescribed in the topical treatment of condyloma acuminatum and other types of warts. Several podophyllotoxin derivatives have been used as purgatives and studied for their antineoplastic effects, including the inhibition of mitosis. Podophyllotoxins are not recommended for use in early pregnancy.

podophyllum /pod′əfil′əm/ [Gk, *pous* + *phyllon* leaf], the dried rhizome and roots of *Podophyllum peltatum*, from which a caustic resin is derived for use in removing certain warts.

poecil-. See **poikilo-.**

-poetic, -poietic, a suffix meaning 'referring to production of something specified': *cholepoetic, oenopoetic, uropoetic.*

-poesis, -poiesis. a suffix meaning 'formation or production of': *cholanopoiesis, erythropoiesis, hemopoiesis.*

-poietic. See **-poetic.**

poikilo-, pecilo-, poecil-, a combining form meaning 'varied or irregular': *poikilocarynosis, poikiloderma, poikilothymia.*

poikilocytosis /poi′kilō′sītō′sis/ [Gk, *poikilos,* variation, *kytos,* cell, *osis,* condition], an abnormal degree of variation in the shape of the erythrocytes in the blood. Compare **anisocytosis, macrocytosis, microcytosis.**

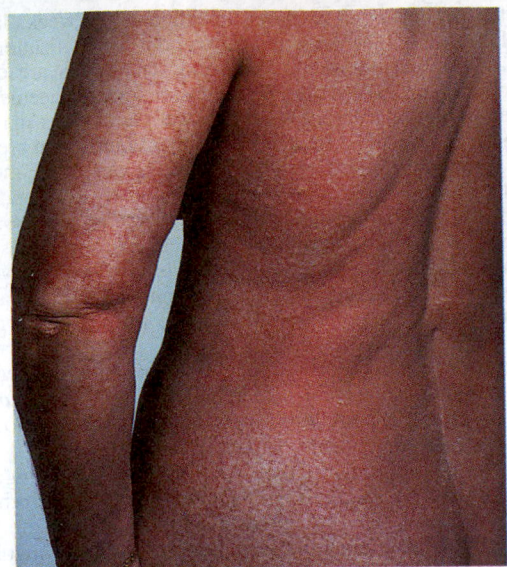

Poikiloderma atrophicans vasculare
(du Vivier, 1993/Courtesy St. Mary's Hospital)

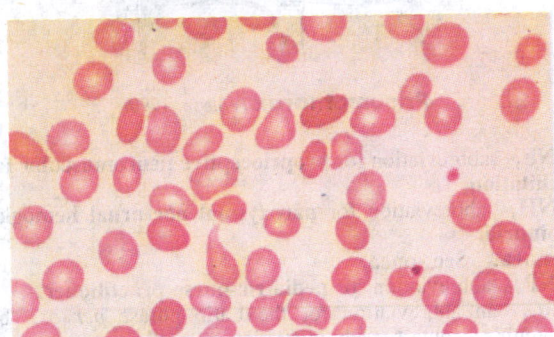

Poikilocytosis *(Hayhoe, 1992)*

poikiloderma atrophicans vasculare /-dur′mə/ [Gk, *poikilos,* variation, *derma,* skin, *a, trophe,* not nourishment; L, *vasculum,* little vessel], an abnormal skin condition characterized by hyperpigmentation or hypopigmentation, telangiectasia, and atrophy of the epidermis. It may be symmetric or patchy, localized or widespread. It tends to be permanent.

poikiloderma of Civatte, a common benign, progressive dermatitis characterized by erythematous patches on the face and neck that become dry and scaly. As the condition progresses, pigment is deposited around the hair follicles extending down the lateral aspects of the neck. Photosensitivity is sometimes associated with this dermatitis. Also called **reticulated pigmented poikiloderma.**

poikilothermic. See **cold blooded.**

point [L, *punctus,* pricked], a small spot or designated area.

point behavior [L, *punctus,* pricked; AS, *bihabban,* to behave], the orientation of body parts in a certain direction within a quantum of space.

point forceps, a dental instrument used in filling root canals. It holds the filling cones during their placement.

point lesion, a disruption of single chemical bonds caused

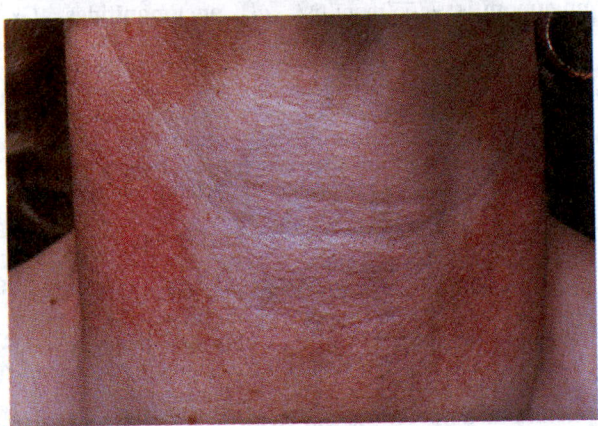

Poikiloderma of Civatte *(du Vivier, 1993)*

by effects of ionizing radiation on a macromolecule. Also called **molecular lesion.**

point mutation [L, *punctus,* pricked + *mutare,* to change], a mutation in which only a single base-pair of DNA is changed.

point of maximum impulse (PMI), the place where the apical pulse is palpated as strongest, often in the fifth intercostal space of the thorax, just medial to the left midclavicular line.

poise /poiz/ [Jean L. M. Poiseuille, French physiologist, b. 1799], a unit of liquid or gas (fluid) viscosity expressed in terms of gm × cm^{-1} × sec^{-1}. The centipoise, or 1/100 of a poise, is more commonly used.

poison /poi′zən/ [L, *potio,* drink], any substance that impairs health or destroys life when ingested, inhaled, or absorbed by the body in relatively small amounts. Some toxicologists suggest that, depending on dosages, all substances are poisons. Many experts state that it is impossible to categorize any chemical as either safe or toxic and that the real concern is the risk or hazard associated with the use of any substance. Clinically, all poisons are divided into those that respond to specific treatments or antidotes and those for which there is no specific treatment. Research continues to develop effective antitoxins for poisons, but there are relatively few effective antidotes, and the treatment of poisoned individuals is based mainly on eliminating the toxic agent from the body before it can be absorbed. Maintaining respiration and circulation is the most important aspect of such treatment. See also **poisoning treatment.** **–poisonous,** *adj.*

poison control center, one of a nearly worldwide network of facilities that provide information regarding all aspects of poisoning or intoxication, maintain records of their occurrence, and refer patients to treatment centers.

poisoning, 1. the act of administering a toxic substance. 2. the condition or physical state produced by the ingestion of, injection of, inhalation of, or exposure to a poisonous substance. Identification of the poison and the presentation of a container label are critical to expeditious diagnosis and treatment.

poisoning, high risk for, a nursing diagnosis accepted by the Seventh National Conference on the Classification of Nursing Diagnoses. The diagnosis describes the accentuated risk of accidental exposure to or ingestion of drugs or dangerous products in doses sufficient to cause poisoning. The risk factors may be internal (individual) or external (environmental). Internal risk factors include reduced vision, verbalization of occupational setting without adequate safeguards, lack of safety or drug education, lack of proper precautions, cognitive or emotional difficulties, and insufficient finances. External risk factors include large supplies of drugs in the house; medicines or dangerous products stored in unlocked cabinets accessible to children or confused people; availability of illicit drugs potentially contaminated by poisonous additives; flaking, peeling paint or plaster in the presence of young children; chemical contamination of food and water; unprotected contact with heavy metals or chemicals; paint or lacquer in poorly ventilated areas or without effective protection; presence of poisonous vegetation; and presence of atmospheric pollutants. See also **nursing diagnosis.**

poisoning treatment, the symptomatic and supportive care given a patient who has been exposed to or who has ingested a toxic drug, commercial chemical, or other dangerous substance. In the case of oral poisoning, a primary effort should be directed toward recovery of the toxic substance before it can be absorbed into the body tissues. If vomiting does not occur spontaneously, it should be induced after first identifying the poison, if possible. If the poison is a petroleum distillate, such as kerosene, or a caustic or corrosive substance, vomiting should *not* be induced. Before any attempt to induce emesis, the victim, if conscious, should be given one or two glasses of milk or water. A carbonated beverage should never be given an oral poisoning patient. Because of the danger of hypernatremia, the patient, and particularly a child, should not be given water containing salt or mustard. Syrup of ipecac can be given, if available, to induce vomiting, and the dosage can be repeated one time. But if the ipecac fails to induce vomiting, vomiting should be encouraged by stimulating the patient's gag

Actions in selected situations with a conscious victim who has ingested poison*

Corrosive or caustic substances
Do not attempt to neutralize the substance.
Do not induce vomiting.
Offer the victim a glass of milk or water.

Noncorrosive substances
The decision of whether to induce vomiting depends on the substance ingested, the amount ingested, and the physical condition of the victim. In general, when pure petroleum distillates are ingested, vomiting is *not* indicated.
For other materials, vomiting may be induced. The Regional Poison Center can help in this evaluation.

Methods of inducing vomiting
1. Give 1 tbsp (15 ml) syrup of ipecac followed by 1 glass of water. (Dose can be repeated once only if vomiting does not occur within 15 to 20 minutes.) Do not allow emetic to remain in stomach.
2. Physician's order: Apomorphine hydrochloride 0.03 mg/lb subcutaneously. (Contraindicated if respiratory depression is present or patient is comatose.) Apomorphine is rarely used. Can be reversed by the administration of naloxone.

*Information supplied by the American Association of Poison Control Centers, University of California Medical Center, San Diego.

reflex at the back of the throat. Ipecac, which can be a GI irritant, should not be allowed to remain in the stomach. Ipecac also should not be given with milk or charcoal, both of which can interfere with its action. In certain cases, an antidote may be administered to render the poison inert or to prevent its absorption, as by giving a mild solution of vinegar or citrus juice to neutralize an alkali. A physician should be summoned to take charge of the case. If a physician is not available, the nearest poison control center should be contacted immediately for expert guidance.

poison ivy, any of several species of climbing vine of the genus *Rhus,* characterized by shiny, three-pointed leaves. It is common in North America and causes severe allergic contact dermatitis in many people. Localized vesicular eruption with itching and burning results and may be treated with

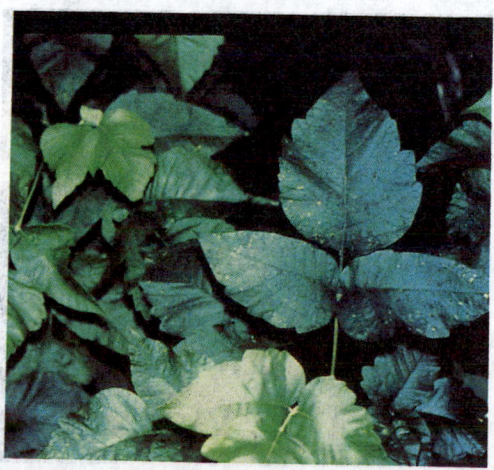

Poison ivy (*Zitelli, 1992*)

antipruritic lotions, cool compresses, or topical corticosteroid ointment or cream. Severe cases may require corticosteroids given intramuscularly or orally. See also **rhus dermatitis, urushiol.**

poison ivy dermatitis [L, *potio*, drink; ME, *ivi*; Gk, *derma*, skin + *itis*, inflammation], a type of skin eruption caused by exposure to a nonvolatile oil, toxicodendrol, present in the leaves and other plant parts of poison ivy, a member of the *Rhus toxicodendron* genus. Other *Rhus* species producing the same kind of contact dermatitis are poison oak and poison sumac. Also called **rhus dermatitis.**

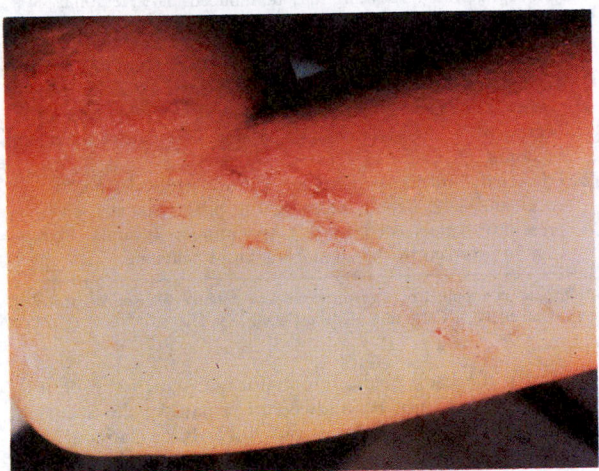

Poison ivy dermatitis *(Zitelli, 1992)*

poison oak, any of several species of shrub of the genus *Rhus,* common in North America. Skin contact results in allergic dermatitis in many people. The characteristics and the treatment of the condition are similar to those of poison ivy. See also **rhus dermatitis, urushiol.**

poison sumac /sŏŏ'mak/, a shrub of the genus *Rhus,* common in North America. Skin contact results in allergic der-

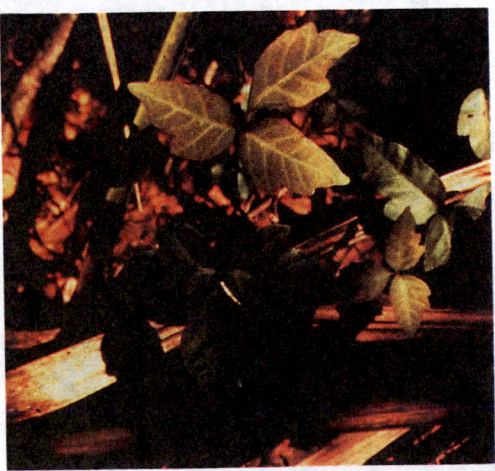

Poison oak *(Zitelli, 1992/Courtesy Dr. Mary Jelks)*

matitis in many people. The characteristics and the treatment of the condition are similar to those of poison ivy. See also **rhus dermatitis, urushiol.**

poker spine. See **bamboo spine.**

polar [L, *polus*, pole], pertaining to molecules that are hydrophilic, or 'water-loving.' Polar substances tend to dissolve in polar solvents. See also **pole, polus.**

Polaramine, a trademark for an antihistaminic (dexchlorpheniramine maleate).

polar body, one of the small cells produced during the two meiotic divisions in the maturation process of female gametes, or ova. It is nonfunctional and incapable of being fertilized. See also **oogenesis.**

polarity /pōler'itē/ [L, *polus*], **1.** the existence or manifestation of opposing qualities, tendencies, or emotions, such as pleasure and pain, love and hate, strength and weakness, dependence and independence, masculinity and femininity. The concept is central to various psychotherapeutic approaches, such as client-centered therapy, in which the key to self-actualization lies in accepting polarity within oneself. **2.** (in physics) the distinction between a negative and a positive electric charge.

polarity therapy, a technique of massage based on the theory that the body has positive and negative energy patterns that must be balanced to establish physical harmony.

polarization /pōlərīzā'shən/ [L, *polus* + Gk, *izein*, to cause], the concentration within a population or group of members' interests, beliefs, and allegiances around two conflicting positions.

polarization microscope [L, *polus,* pole; Gk, *mikros,* small, *skopein* to view], a microscope that uses polarized light for special diagnostic purposes, such as examining crystals of chemicals found in patients with gout and related disorders.

polarized light /po'lərīzd/ [L, *polus*; AS, *leoht*], light that is propagated in such a way that the radiation waves occur in only one direction in the vibration plane and not at random.

polarographic oxygen analyzer /pō'lərōgraf'ik/, an electrochemical device used to analyze the proportion of oxygen molecules in respiratory care systems. The oxygen is measured in terms of an electron current produced after it acquires electrons from a negative electrode in a hydroxide bath. Batteries are used to polarize the electrodes in the bath.

pole [L, *polus*], **1.** (in biology) an end of an imaginary axis drawn through the symmetrically arranged parts of a cell, organ, ovum, or nucleus. **2.** (in anatomy) the point on a nerve cell at which a dendrite originates. **–polar,** *adj.*

poles of kidney, either end of an axis through the length of a kidney. They are designated as the **upper pole of the kidney (extremitas superior renis)** and the **inferior pole of the kidney (extremitas inferior renis).**

pol gene, a segment of a retrovirus, such as the human T cell leukemia virus (HTLV), that encodes its reverse transcriptase enzyme.

policy /pol'isē/ [L, *politia*, the state], a principle or guideline that governs an activity and that employees or members of an institution or organization are expected to follow.

polio /pōlē·ō/. See **poliomyelitis.**

polio-, a combining form meaning 'of or related to gray matter in the nervous system': *polioclastic, polioencephalitis, poliomyelitis.*

polioencephalitis /pō′lē·ō′ensef′əlī′tis/ [Gk, *polios,* gray, *enkephalos,* brain, *itis*], an inflammation of the gray matter of the brain caused by infection of the brain by a poliovirus.

polioencephalomeningomyelitis /pō′lē·ō′ensef′əlō′ məning′gōm′īəlī′tis/ [Gk, *polios,* gray + *egkephalos,* brain + *menigx,* membrane + *myelos,* marrow + *itis,* inflammation], an inflammation that involves the gray matter of the brain and spinal cord and also the meninges.

polioencephalomyelitis /pō′lē·ō′ensef′əlōmī′əlī′tis/ [Gk, *polios, enkephalos* + *myelos,* marrow, *itis*], inflammation of the gray matter of the brain and the spinal cord, caused by infection by a poliovirus.

poliomyelitis /pō′lē·ōmī′əlī′tis/ [Gk, *polios* + *myelos,* marrow, *itis*], an infectious disease caused by one of the three polioviruses. Asymptomatic, mild, and paralytic forms of the disease occur. Several factors influence susceptibility to the virus and the course of the disease: More boys than girls are severely affected, stress increases susceptibility, more pregnant than nonpregnant women acquire the paralytic form of the disease, and the severity of the infection increases with age. It is transmitted from person to person through fecal contamination or oropharyngeal secretions. Also called *(informal)* **polio.** See also **poliovirus.**

■ OBSERVATIONS: Asymptomatic infection has no clinical features, but it confers immunity. Abortive poliomyelitis lasts only a few hours and is characterized by minor illness with fever, malaise, headache, nausea, vomiting, and slight abdominal discomfort. Nonparalytic poliomyelitis is longer lasting and is marked by meningeal irritation with pain and stiffness in the back and by all the signs of abortive poliomyelitis. Paralytic poliomyelitis begins as abortive poliomyelitis. The symptoms abate, and for several days the person seems well. Malaise, headache, and fever recur; pain, weakness, and paralysis develop. The peak of paralysis is reached within the first week. In spinal poliomyelitis, viral replication occurs in the anterior horn cells of the spine, causing inflammation, swelling, and, if severe, destruction of the neurons. The large proximal muscles of the limbs are most often affected. Bulbar poliomyelitis results from viral multiplication in the brainstem. Bulbar and spinal poliomyelitis often occur together.

■ INTERVENTIONS: Treatment of the abortive and nonparalytic forms of the disease is symptomatic, consisting of bed rest, good nutrition, and avoidance, for at least 2 weeks, of overexertion, stress, and fatigue. Treatment of the paralytic form includes hospitalization with observation for advance of the disease, the application of hot packs and the giving of baths, range-of-motion exercise, and assisted ventilation when necessary. As soon as the acute febrile stage is over, active, comprehensive rehabilitation is promptly begun.

■ NURSING CONSIDERATIONS: The more quickly function returns, the better the outcome. The pain and muscle spasm of the acute period cause the person to want to remain immobile. Such immobility enhances the tendency to deformity, and the nurse may be of great help in encouraging the person to exercise and to participate actively in the rehabilitative program. Poliomyelitis, which has not been eradicated, may be prevented by immunization. Families are encouraged to obtain the complete series for all family members, particularly before traveling in countries where the disease is endemic. Formerly, when epidemic, poliomyelitis was seen chiefly in the summer. Now the few cases occurring are sporadic rather than seasonal.

poliomyelitis vaccine. See **poliovirus vaccine.**

poliosis /pō′lē·ō′sis/ [Gk, *polios + osis,* condition], depigmentation of the hair on the scalp, eyebrows, eyelashes, mustache, beard, or body. The condition may be inherited and generalized or acquired and localized in patches. Acquired localized poliosis often occurs in alopecia areata.

poliovirus /-vī′rəs/ [Gk, *polios* + L, *virus,* poison], the causative organism of poliomyelitis. There are three serologically distinct types of this very small RNA virus. Infection or immunization with one type does not protect against the others.

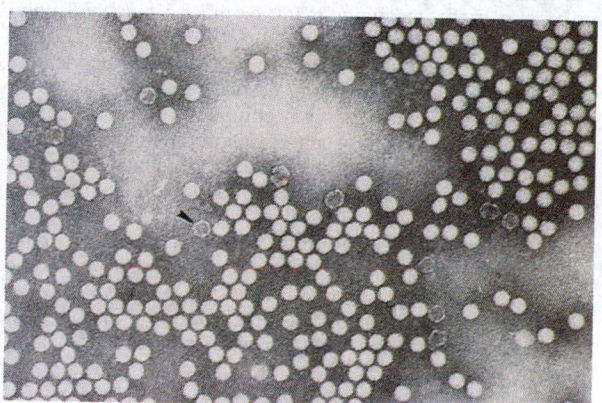

Electron micrograph of poliovirus
(Murray, 1990/Courtesy Centers for Disease Control, Atlanta)

poliovirus vaccine, a vaccine prepared from poliovirus to confer immunity to it. TOPV, the trivalent live oral form of vaccine, is recommended for all children under 18 years of age who have no specific contraindications. The inactivated poliovirus vaccine (IPV) is recommended for infants and children who are immunodeficient and for unvaccinated adults. TOPV is called Sabin vaccine; IPV is called Salk vaccine. IPV is given subcutaneously. Rarely, vaccine-associated paralysis occurs after administration of TOPV; this reaction has not occurred with IPV.

polishing [L, *polire,* to make smooth], a tendency of patients with right temporal lobe lesions to deny dysphoric affect and minimize socially disapproved behavior while exaggerating other qualities.

political nursing /pəlit′ikəl/ [L, *politia,* the state; *nutrix,* nurse], the use of knowledge about power processes and strategies to influence the nature and direction of health care and professional nursing. The constituency of political nursing is patients, both diagnosed and potential, as communities, groups, or individuals.

pollakiuria /pol′əkēyoor′ē·ə/ [Gk, *pollache,* frequent, *ouron,* urine], an abnormal condition characterized by unduly frequent passage of urine.

pollen coryza /pol′ən/ [L, dust; Gk, *koryza,* runny nose], acute seasonal rhinitis caused by exposure to an allergenic. Also called **hay fever.**

pollex /pol′eks/, *pl.* **pollices** [L], the thumb; also, the big toe.

pollinosis. See **hay fever.**

pollutant /pəloo′tənt/ [L, *polluere,* to defoul], an un wanted substance that occurs in the environment, usually with health-threatening effects. Pollutants may exist in the atmosphere as gases or fine particles that may be irritating to the lungs, eyes, and skin, as dissolved or suspended substances in drinking water, and as carcinogens or mutagens in foods or beverages.

polonium (Po) /pəlō′nē·əm/ [Polonia, Poland], a radioactive element that is one of the disintegration products of uranium. Its atomic number is 84; its atomic weight is approximately 210.

polus /pō′ləs/, *pl.* **poli** [L, pole], either of the opposite ends of any axis; the official anatomic designation for the extremity of an organ. See also **pole.** —**polar,** *adj.*

poly-, a prefix meaning 'many or much': *polyacid, polycholia, polydactylia.*

polyacrylamide /-akril′əmīd/, a polymer of acrylamide and usually some crosslinking derivative.

polyamine /pol′ē·am′ēn/, any compound that contains two or more amine groups, such as spermidine and spermine, which are normally occurring tissue constituents in humans. Many polyamines function as essential growth factors in microorganisms.

polyanionic /pol′ē·an′ī·on′ik/ [Gk, *polys,* many, *ana,* again, *ion,* going], pertaining to multiple negative electric charges.

polyarteritis /pol′ē·är′tərī′tis/ [Gk, *polys* + *arteria,* air pipe, *itis* inflammation, an abnormal inflammatory condition of several arteries.

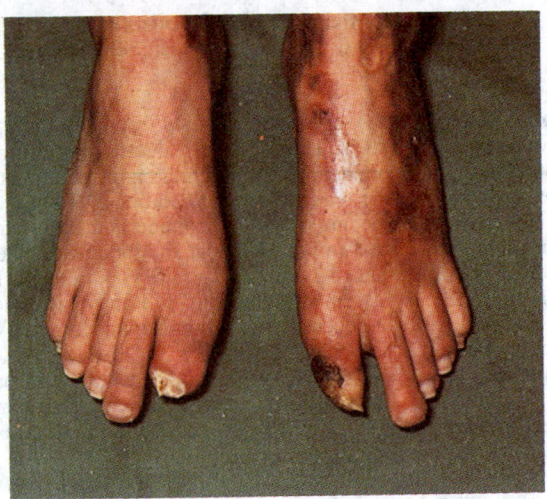

Polyarteritis nodosa (Swales, 1991)

polyarteritis nodosa, a severe and poorly understood collagen vascular disease in which there is widespread inflammation and necrosis of small and medium-sized arteries and ischemia of the tissues they serve. Any organ or organ system may be affected. The disease attacks men and women between 20 and 50 years of age. Its cause is unknown, although immunologic factors are suspected. Polyarteritis nodosa may be acute and rapidly fatal, or chronic and wasting. It is characterized by fever, abdominal pain, weight loss, neuropathy, and, if the kidneys are affected, hypertension, edema, and uremia. Some symptoms may mimic GI or cardiac disorders. Diagnosis is based on the clinical

signs, laboratory tests, and biopsy of sites affected by the disease. Mortality in polyarteritis nodosa is high, especially if there is kidney involvement. Aggressive treatment includes massive doses of corticosteroids. Immunosuppressive drugs have been used experimentally with some success. Physical therapy helps the patient to maintain muscle tone and prevents or slows the development of disability.

polyarthritis /-ärthrī′tis/, an inflammation that involves more than one joint. The inflammation may migrate from one joint to another, or there may be simultaneous involvement of two or more joints.

polyarticular /-ärtik′yələr/ [Gk, *polys,* many; *articulus,* joint], pertaining to many joints.

polychlorinated biphenyls (PCBs) /-klôr′inā′tid/, a group of more than 30 isomers and compounds used in plastics, insulation, and flame retardants and varying in physical form from oily liquids to crystals and resins. All are potentially toxic and carcinogenic. The toxicity varies with the type of PCB and concurrent exposure to other substances, such as carbon tetrachloride. Mild exposure may cause chloracne; severe exposure may result in hepatic damage.

polychromasia. See **polychromatophilia.**

polychromatic /-krōmatik/ [Gk, *polys* + *chroma,* color], a light of many colors or wavelengths. The term is usually applied to white light although it may also refer to a defined portion of the spectrum.

polychromatophil /pol′ēkrōmat′fl′yə/, any cell that may be stained by several different dyes.

polychromatophilia /pol′ēkrō′matəfil′yə/ [Gk, *polys, chroma* + *philein,* to love], an abnormal tendency of a cell, particularly an erythrocyte, to be dyed by a variety of laboratory stains. Also called **polychromasia.**

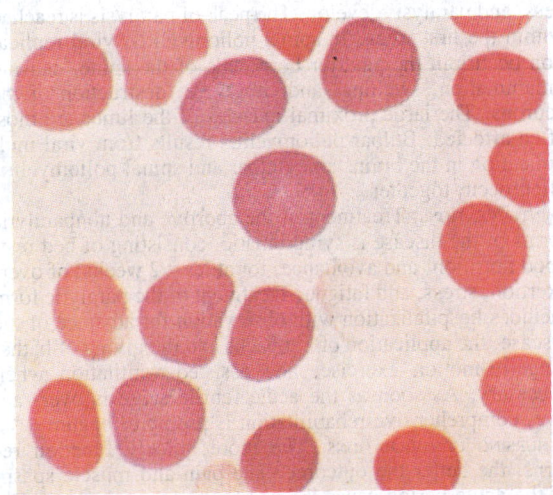

Polychromatophilia (Hayhoe, 1992)

Polycillin, a trademark for an antibacterial (ampicillin).

polyclonal /pol′ēklō′nəl/ [Gk, *polys* + *klon,* cutting], **1.** of, pertaining to, or designating a group of identical cells or organisms derived from several identical cells. **2.** of, pertaining to, or designating several groups of identical cells or organisms (clones) derived from a single cell.

polyclonal gammopathy. See **gammopathy.**

Polycose, a trademark for a nutritional supplement containing glucose polymers derived from cornstarch.

polycystic /-sis'tik/ [Gk, *polys* + *kystis*, bag], characterized by the presence of many cysts.

polycystic kidney disease (PKD), an abnormal condition in which the kidneys are enlarged and contain many cysts. There are three forms of the disease. **Childhood polycystic disease (CPD)** is uncommon and may be differentiated from adult or congenital polycystic disease by genetic, morphologic, and clinical facets. Death usually occurs within a few years as the result of portal hypertension and liver and kidney failure. A portacaval shunt may prolong life into the twenties. **Adult polycystic disease (APD)** may be unilateral, bilateral, acquired, or congenital. The condition is characterized by flank pain and high blood pressure. Kidney failure eventually develops, progressing to uremia and death. **Congenital polycystic disease (CPD)** is a rare congenital aplasia of the kidney involving all or only a small segment of one or both kidneys. Severe bilateral aplasia results in death shortly after birth. Minor aplasia may cause no dysfunction and may never be diagnosed.

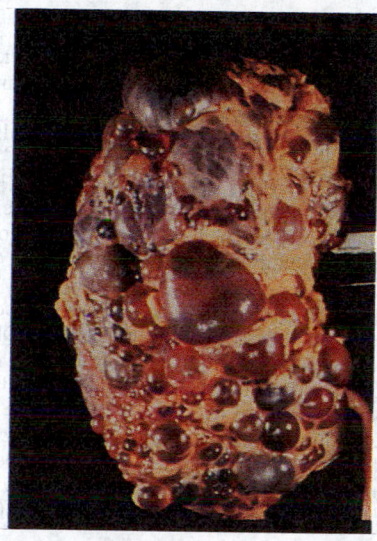

Adult polycystic kidney disease *(Weiss, 1988)*

polycystic ovary syndrome, an abnormal condition characterized by anovulation, amenorrhea, hirsutism, and infertility. It is caused by an endocrine imbalance with increased levels of testosterone, estrogen, and luteinizing hormone (LH) and decreased secretion of follicle stimulating hormone (FSH). The increased level of LH associated with this disorder may be the result of an increased sensitivity of the pituitary to stimulation by releasing hormone or of excessive stimulation by the adrenal gland. Polycystic ovary may also be associated with a variety of problems in the hypothalamic-pituitary-ovarian axis, with extragonadal sources of androgens, or with androgen-producing tumors. This condition is transmitted as an X-linked dominant or autosomal dominant trait. The depressed but continuous production of FSH associated with this disorder causes continuous partial development of ovarian follicles. Numerous follicular cysts, 2 to 6 mm in diameter, may develop. The affected ovary commonly doubles in size and is invested by a

smooth, pearly-white capsule. The increased level of estrogen associated with this abnormality raises the risk of cancers of the breast and the endometrium. Depending on the severity of symptoms and whether the patient wants to become pregnant, treatment involves suppression of hormonal stimulation of the ovary, usually using female hormones or resection of part of one or both ovaries.

polycythemia /pol'ēsīthē'mē·ə/ [Gk, *polys* + *kytos*, cell, *haima* blood], an increase in the number of erythrocytes in the blood that may be primary or secondary to pulmonary disease, heart disease, or prolonged exposure to high altitudes, or idiopathic. Also called **Osler's disease, polycythemia vera.** Compare **hypoplastic anemia, leukemia.** See also **altitude sickness, erythrocytosis.**

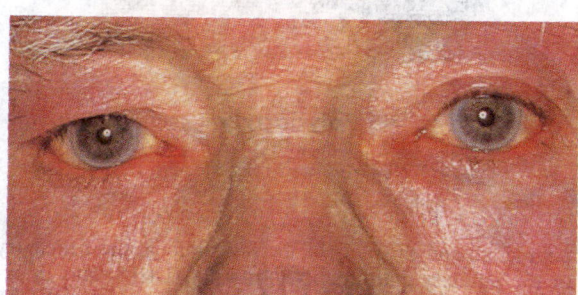

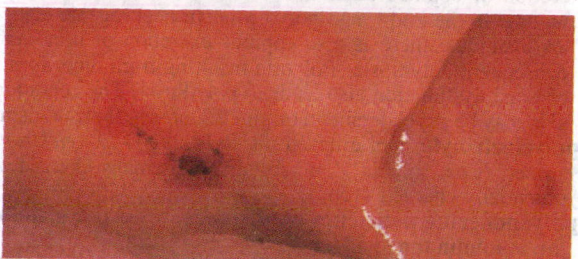

Polycythemia rubra vera—dark color of skin and mucous membranes
(Lamey, 1988)

polycythemia rubra vera (PV) [Gk, *polys*, many + *kytos*, cell + *haima*, blood], a condition of unknown cause characterized by a marked increase in the red blood cell count, packed cell volume, cellular hemoglobin, leukocytes, platelets, and total blood volume. The skin and mucous membranes acquire a maroon or plum color and the patient develops hepatomegaly, splenomegaly, hypertension, and neurological symptoms. The condition is associated with an F chromosome defect. Also called **primary polycythemia; Vaquez disease.**

polydactyly /-dak'tilē/ [Gk, *polys* + *daktylos*, finger], a congenital anomaly characterized by the presence of more than the normal number of fingers or toes. The condition is usually inherited as an autosomal dominant characteristic and can usually be corrected by surgery shortly after birth. Also called **polydactylia, polydactylism, hyperdactyly.** (See Fig. p. 1244.)

polydipsia /pol'ēdip'sē·ə/ [Gk, *polys* + *dipsa*, thirst], **1.** excessive thirst characteristic of several different conditions, including diabetes mellitus in which an excessive concentration of glucose in the blood osmotically increases the excretion of fluid via increased urination, which leads to hy-

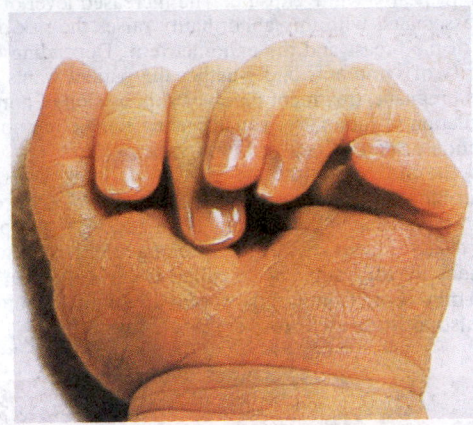

Polydactyly
(Zitelli, 1992/Courtesy Dr. Christine L Williams, New York Medical College)

povolemia and thirst. In diabetes insipidus, the deficiency of the pituitary antidiuretic hormone (ADH) results in excretion of copious amounts of dilute urine, reduced fluid volume in the body, and polydipsia. In nephrogenic diabetes insipidus, there is also copious excretion of urine and consequent polydipsia. Polyuria resulting from other forms of renal dysfunction also leads to polydipsia. The condition also may be psychogenic in origin. **2.** *informal*. alcoholism.

polyelectrolyte /pol′ē·ilek′trəlīt/ [Gk, *polys* + *elektron*, amber, *lytos*, soluble], a substance with many charged or potentially charged groups.

polyendocrine deficiency syndromes. See **polyglandular autoimmune syndromes**.

polyesthesia /pol′ē·esthē′zhə/ [Gk, *polys* + *aisthesis*, feeling], a sensory disorder involving the sense of touch in which a stimulus to one area of the skin is felt at other sites in addition to the one stimulated.

polyestradiol phosphate /-es′tradī′ôl/, an antineoplastic estrogen compound.

■ INDICATIONS: It is prescribed for cancer of the prostate and postmenopausal breast cancer.

■ CONTRAINDICATIONS: Male breast cancer, estrogen-dependent neoplasia, thrombophlebitis, or known hypersensitivity to this drug prohibits its use.

■ ADVERSE EFFECTS: Among the more serious adverse reactions are loss of libido, impotence, gynecomastia, fluid retention and edema, and, rarely, cholestatic jaundice.

polygene /pol′ējēn′/ [Gk, *polys* + *genein*, to produce], any of a group of nonallelic genes that individually exert a small effect but together interact in a cumulative manner to produce a particular characteristic within an individual, usually of a quantitative nature, such as size, weight, skin pigmentation, or degree of intelligence. Also called **cumulative gene, multiple factor, multiple gene.** See also **multifactorial inheritance.** –**polygenic,** *adj*.

polygenic inheritance. See **multifactorial inheritance**.

polyglandular autoimmune syndromes, disorders of subnormal functioning of more than one endocrine gland. Type I is characterized by the appearance of mucocutaneous candidiasis, often occurring in childhood, and is associated with hypoparathyroidism and adrenal insufficiency.

Type I condition occurs in siblings, without involvement of other generations in the family. Type II involves primary adrenal insufficiency and primary thyroid failure occurring in the same patient for unclear reasons. It has been demonstrated that many of these patients have an autoimmune disorder, with formation of antibodies against cellular fractions of many endocrine glands. Also called **polyendocrine deficiency syndromes**.

polyglucosan /-gloo′kəsan/ [Gk, *polys* + *glykys*, sweet], a large molecule consisting of many anhydrous polysaccharides.

polyhybrid /-hī′brid/ [Gk, *polys* + L, *hybrida*, offspring of mixed parents], (in genetics) pertaining to or describing an individual, organism, or strain that is heterozygous for more than three specific traits, that is the offspring of parents differing in more than three specific gene pairs, or that is heterozygous for more than three particular characteristics or gene loci being followed.

polyhybrid cross, (in genetics) the mating of two individuals, organisms, or strains that have different gene pairs that determine more than three specific traits or in which more than three particular characteristics or gene loci are being followed.

polyhydramnios. See **hydramnios**.

polyleptic /pol′ēlep′tik/ [Gk, *polys* + *lambanein*, to seize], describing any disease or condition marked by numerous remissions and exacerbations.

polyleptic fever, a fever occurring paroxysmally, such as smallpox and relapsing fever.

polymer /pol′imər/ [Gk, *polys* + *meros*, part], a compound formed by combining or linking a number of monomers, or small molecules. A polymer may be composed of a variety of different monomers or of many units of the same monomer.

polymerase chain reaction (PCR) /pol′ēmer′ās, polim′ərās/, a process whereby a strand of DNA can be cloned millions of times within a few hours. The process can be used to make prenatal diagnoses of genetic diseases and to identify an individual by analysis of a single tissue cell.

polymerize /pol′əmərīz/ [Gk, *polys*, many + *meros*, parts], to convert two or more molecules into a polymer.

polymicrobial /-mīkrō′bē·əl/ [Gk, *polys*, many + *mikros*, small + *bios*, life], pertaining to a number of species of microbes.

polymicrobic infections /-mīkrō′bik/ [Gk, *polys*, many + *mikros*, small + *bios*, life; L, *inficere*, to stain], an infection involving more than one species of pathogens. Also called **mixed infection**.

polymicrogyria. See **microgyria**.

polymorphic /-môr′fik/ [Gk, *polys*, many + *morphe*, form], pertaining to the ability to assume two or more distinct forms, such as the existence of two or more forms of chromosomes or hemoglobins in a population.

polymorphism /pol′ēmôr′fizəm/ [Gk, *polys* + *morphe*, form], **1.** the state or quality of existing or occurring in several different forms. **2.** the state or quality of appearing in different forms at different stages of development. Kinds of polymorphism are **balanced polymorphism** and **genetic polymorphism.** –**polymorphic,** *adj*.

polymorphocytic leukemia /pol′ēmôr′fəsit′ik/ [Gk, *polys*, *morphe* + *kytos*, cell; *leukos*, white, *haima*, blood], a neoplasm of blood-forming tissues in which mature, segmented granulocytes are predominant. Also called **mature cell leukemia, neutrophilic leukemia**.

polymorphonuclear /pol′ēmôr′fōnoo′klē·ər/ [Gk, *polys*,

morphe + L, *nucleus,* nut],   having a nucleus with a number of lobules or segments connected by a fine thread.

polymorphonuclear cell (PMN), a leukocyte with a multilobed nucleus, such as a neutrophil.

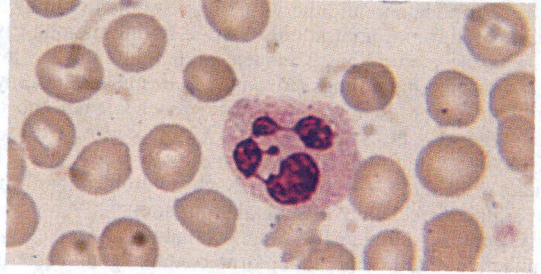

Polymorphonuclear cell (Bain, 1989)

polymorphonuclear leukocyte,   a white blood cell containing a segmented lobular nucleus; an eosinophil, basophil, or neutrophil. See also **granulocyte.**

polymorphous /pol'ēmôr'fəs/ [Gk, *polys* + *morphe,* form], occurring in many varying forms, possibly changing in structure or appearance at different stages.

polymorphous light eruption,   a common, recurrent, superficial vascular reaction to sunlight or ultraviolet light in susceptible individuals. Within 1 to 4 days after exposure to the light, small, erythematous papules and vesicles appear on otherwise normal skin, then disappear within 2 weeks. A delayed allergic response is a possible cause. Tanning reduces the severity of the reaction.

Polymox,   a trademark for an antibiotic (amoxicillin).

polymyalgia rheumatica /-mī·al'jə/ [Gk, *polys* + *mys,* muscle, *algos,* pain; *rheuma,* flux],   a chronic, episodic, inflammatory disease of the large arteries that usually develops in people over 60 years of age. Polymyalgia rheumatica and temporal arteritis are believed to represent the same disease process with slightly different symptoms. Polymyalgia rheumatica primarily affects the muscles, and it is characterized by pain and stiffness of the back, shoulder, or neck, usually becoming more severe on rising in the morning. There may also be a cranial headache, as in temporal arteritis, which affects the temporal and occipital arteries, causing a severe, throbbing headache. Serious complications of arterial inflammation include arterial insufficiency, coronary occlusion, stroke, or blindness. Usually, patients with polymyalgia rheumatica or temporal arteritis have marked elevations of the erythrocyte sedimentation rate. Both forms of the disease may follow a self-limited course; however, adrenocorticosteroids have proven highly effective in reducing inflammation and in speeding recovery. Both forms are probably autoimmune conditions. Also called **polymyalgia arteritica, temporal arteritis.**

polymyositis /pol'ēmī'ōsī'tis/ [Gk, *polys* + *mys,* muscle, *itis*],   inflammation of many muscles, usually accompanied by deformity, edema, insomnia, pain, sweating, and tension. Some forms of polymyositis are associated with malignancy. See also **dermatomyositis.**

polymyxin /-mik'sin/,   an antibiotic.

■ INDICATIONS: It is used topically and systemically in the treatment of gram-negative bacterial infections, including meningitis, corneal ulcerations, and otitis media.

■ CONTRAINDICATIONS: Hypersensitivity to this drug prohibits its use. It is used with great caution in patients with impaired renal function.

■ ADVERSE EFFECTS: Among the more serious adverse reactions when this drug is used systemically are nephrotoxicity and various neurologic alterations, including blockade of neuromuscular junction. Pain or phlebitis at the site of injection also may occur. When this drug is applied locally, irritation and allergic reactions of the skin or mucosa are sometimes seen.

polymyxin B sulfate,   an antibiotic.

■ INDICATIONS: It is prescribed for infections caused by microorganisms sensitive to this drug, including urinary tract infections, septicemia, and conjunctivitis.

■ CONTRAINDICATIONS: Known hypersensitivity to this drug prohibits its use. Extreme caution is necessary when it is given systemically to people with impaired renal function.

■ ADVERSE EFFECTS: Among the more serious adverse reactions when given systemically are nephrotoxicity, neurotoxicity, and drug fever. When given topically allergies are the most common problem.

polyneuralgia /-nŏŏral'jə/ [Gk, *polys,* many + *neuron,* nerve + *algos,* pain],   a type of neuralgia that affects several nerves at the same time.

polyneuritic psychosis.   See **Korsakoff's psychosis.**

polyneuritis /-nŏŏrī'tis/ [Gk, *polys,* many + *neuron,* nerve + *itis* inflammation],   an inflammation involving many nerves.

polyneuropathy /-nŏŏrop'əthē/ [Gk, *polys,* many + *neuron,* nerve + *pathos,* disease],   a condition in which many peripheral nerves are afflicted with a disorder.

polyoma papovavirus.   See **papillomacarcinoma.**

polyopia /pol'ē·ō'pē·ə/ [Gk, *polys* + *ops,* eye],   a defect of sight in which one object is perceived as many images; multiple vision. The condition can occur in one or both eyes. See also **diplopia.**

polyp /pol'ip/ [Gk, *polys* + *pous,* foot],   a small tumorlike growth that projects from a mucous membrane surface.

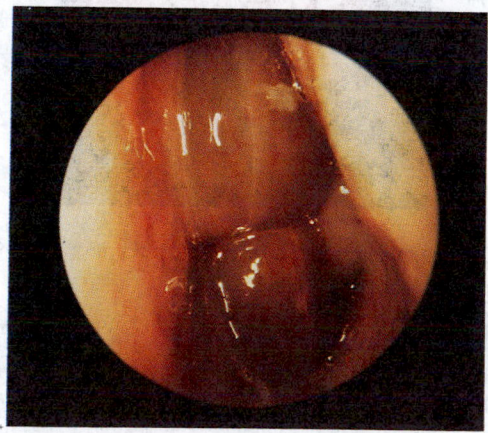

Nasal polyp (Zitelli, 1992)

polypapilloma /-pap'ilō'mə/ [Gk, *polys,* many; L, *papilla,* nipple; Gk, *oma*],   multiple papillomas or stalked tumors.

polypeptide /pol'ēpep'tīd/,   a chain of amino acids joined by peptide bonds. A polypeptide has a larger molecular weight than a peptide but a smaller molecular weight than a protein. Polypeptides are formed by partial hydrolysis of proteins or by synthesis of amino acids into chains.

polyphagia /pol´ēfā´jē·ə/ [Gk, *polys* + *phagein*, to eat], eating to the point of gluttony. See also **bulimia.**

polypharmacy /-fär´məsē/, the use of a number of different drugs by a patient who may have one or several health problems.

polyploid /pol´əploid/ [Gk, *polys* + *plous*, times], **1.** of or pertaining to an individual, organism, strain, or cell that has more than the two complete sets of chromosomes normal for the somatic cell. The multiple of the haploid number characteristic of the species is denoted by the appropriate prefix, as in triploid, tetraploid, pentaploid, hexaploid, heptaploid, octaploid, and so on. Polyploidy is rare in animals, producing organisms that are abnormal in appearance and usually infertile, but it is common in plants; such plants are generally larger, have larger cells, and are more hardy than those with the normal diploid number. **2.** such an individual, organism, strain, or cell. Also called **polyploidic.** Compare **aneuploid.**

polyploid adenocarcinoma. See **papillary adenocarcinoma.**

polyploidy /pol´iploi´dē/ /pol´əploi´dē/, the state or condition of having more than two complete sets of chromosomes.

polypoid [Gk, *polys*, many + *pous*, foot, *eidos*, form], like a polyp or tumor on a stalk.

polyposis /-pōsis/ [Gk, *polys* + *pous*, foot, *osis*, condition], an abnormal condition characterized by the presence of numerous polyps on a part. See also **familial polyposis.**

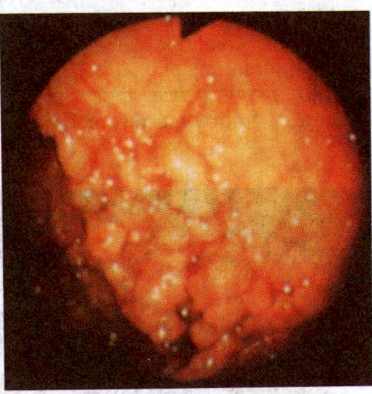

Familiar adenomatous polyposis (Barrison, 1992)

polyposis coli [Gk, *polys*, many + *pous*, foot, *osis*, condition; *kolikos* colon], a condition of multiple polyps in the large intestine.

polyradiculitis /pol´ērədik´yōōlī´tis/ [Gk, *polys* + L, *radicula*, rootlet; Gk, *itis*], inflammation of many nerve roots, such as found in Guillain-Barré syndrome.

polyribosome. See **polysome.**

polysaccharide /-sak´ərīd/ [Gk, *polys* + *sakcharon*, sugar], a carbohydrate that contains three or more molecules of simple carbohydrates. Examples of polysaccharides are dextrins, starches, glycogens, celluloses, gums, inulin, and pentose.

polysome /pol´isōm/ [Gk, *polys* + *soma*, body], (in genetics) a group of ribosomes joined together by a molecule of messenger RNA containing the genetic code. The structure is found in the cytoplasm during protein synthesis. Also called **ergosome, polyribosome.** See also **translation.**

polysomy /pol´isō´mē/, the presence of a chromosome in at least triplicate in an otherwise diploid somatic cell as the result of chromosomal nondisjunction during meiotic division in the maturation of gametes. The chromosome may be duplicated three times (trisomy), four times (tetrasomy), or more times. In males with Klinefelter's syndrome the genotype may be XXXY or XXXXY instead of the usual XXY associated with the syndrome; among polysomic females with three, four, or five X chromosomes there may be a higher frequency of mental retardation.

Polysporin, a trademark for an ophthalmic and topical, antiinfective, fixed-combination drug containing antibacterials (polymyxin B sulfate and bacitracin).

polysynaptic /-sinap´tik/ [Gk, *polys*, many + *synaptein*, to join], pertaining to nerve cells that end in synapses.

polysyndactyly /-sindak´tilē/ [Gk, *polys*, many, *syn*, together, *daktylos*, finger or toe], multiple webbing or fusion between fingers or toes.

polytene chromosome /pol´itēn/ [Gk, *polys* + *tainia*, band], an excessively large type of chromosome consisting of bundles of unseparated chromonemata filaments. It is found primarily in the saliva of certain insects. See also **giant chromosome.**

polythiazide /-thī·az´īd/, a diuretic and antihypertensive.
- INDICATIONS: It is prescribed in the treatment of hypertension and edema.
- CONTRAINDICATIONS: Anuria or known hypersensitivity to this drug, other thiazides, or sulfonamide derivatives prohibits its use.
- ADVERSE EFFECTS: Among the more serious adverse reactions are hypokalemia, hyperglycemia, hyperuricemia, and various hypersensitivity reactions.

polyunsaturated /-unsach´ərā´tid/ [Gk, *polys*, many; AS, *un*, not; L, *saturare*, to fill], pertaining to a chemical compound containing double or triple valency bonds that can be opened to accept more atoms in the molecule, thereby becoming saturated. A polyunsaturated fatty acid is one in which there are two or more links in the chain of carbon atoms that can be opened to accept hydrogen atoms.

polyunsaturated fatty acid. See **unsaturated fatty acid.**

polyuria /pol´ēyōōr´ē·ə/ [Gk, *polys* + *ouron*, urine], the excretion of an abnormally large quantity of urine. Some causes of polyuria are diabetes insipidus, diabetes mellitus, diuretics, excessive fluid intake, and hypercalcemia.

polyvalent antiserum. See **antiserum.**

polyvalent vaccine /-vā´lənt/ [Gk, *polys*, many; L, *valere*, worth, *vaccinus*, cow], a vaccine prepared from several different antigenic types of a species. Also called **multivalent vaccine.**

Poly-Vi-Flor, a trademark for an oral, pediatric, fixed-combination drug containing several vitamins and sodium fluoride.

polyvinyl chloride (PVC) /-vī´nil/, a common synthetic thermoplastic material that releases hydrochloric acid when burned and that may contain carcinogenic vinyl chloride molecules as a contaminant.

POMP /pomp/, an abbreviation for a combination drug regimen used in the treatment of cancer, containing three antineoplastics, Purinethol (mercaptopurine), Oncovin (vincristine sulfate), methotrexate, and prednisone (a glucocorticoid).

Pompe's disease [J. C. Pompe, twentieth century Dutch physician; L, *dis,* opposite of; Fr, *aise,* ease], a form of muscle glycogen storage disease in which there is a generalized accumulation of glycogen, resulting from a deficiency of acid maltase (alpha-1, 4-glucosidase). It is usually fatal in infants, caused by cardiac or respiratory failure. Children with Pompe's disease appear mentally retarded and hypotonic, seldom living beyond 20 years of age. In adults muscle weakness is progressive, but the disease is not fatal. Also called **glycogen storage disease, type II.** See also **glycogen storage disease.**

pompholyx. See **dyshidrosis.**

POMR, abbreviation for **problem-oriented medical record.**

Pondimin, a trademark for an anorexiant (fenfluramine hydrochloride).

pono-, a prefix meaning 'of or related to pain': *ponograph, ponopalmosis, ponophobia.*

ponos. See **kala-azar.**

pons /ponz/, *pl.* **pontes** /pon′tēz/ [L, bridge], **1.** any slip of tissue connecting two parts of a structure or an organ of the body. **2.** a prominence on the ventral surface of the brainstem, between the medulla oblongata and the cerebral peduncles of the midbrain. The pons consists of white matter and a few nuclei and is divided into a ventral portion and a dorsal portion. The ventral portion consists of transverse fibers separated by longitudinal bundles and small nuclei. The dorsal portion comprises the tegmentum, which is a continuation of the reticular formation of the medulla. The tegmentum contains the nucleus of the abducens nerve, the nucleus of the facial nerve, the motor nucleus of the trigeminal nerve, the sensory nuclei of the trigeminal nerve, the nucleus of the cochlear division of the eighth nerve, the superior olive, and the nuclei of the vestibular division of the eighth nerve. Also called **bridge of Varolius.**

Ponstel, a trademark for an antiinflammatory and analgesic (mefenamic acid).

pont-, a prefix meaning 'bridge': *pontic, ponticulus, pontimeter.*

Pontiac fever. See **Legionnaires' disease.**

pontic /pon′tik/ [L, *pons,* bridge], the suspended member of a removable partial denture or fixed ridge, such as an artificial tooth, usually occupying the space previously occupied by the natural tooth crown.

pontine /pon′tīn/ [L, *pons,* bridge], pertaining to the pons. Also spelled **pontile.**

pontine center. See **apneustic center.**

pontine nucleus [L, *pons,* bridge, *nucleus,* nut], nerve cells in the basilar part of the pons where impulses are relayed between the cerebrum and cerebellum.

Pontocaine Hydrochloride, a trademark for a local anesthetic (tetracaine hydrochloride).

pooled plasma [AS, *pol;* Gk, *plasma,* something formed], a liquid component of whole blood, collected and pooled to prepare various plasma products or to use directly as a plasma expander when whole blood is unavailable or is contraindicated. It is useful in surgery and in the treatment of hypovolemia because of its stability and availability in freeze-dried form. It is collected from blood banks or prepared directly from donors by plasmapheresis. It is thin and colorless or slightly yellow. Of the total volume of normal blood, 55% to 65% is plasma. See also **bank blood, component therapy, packed cells.**

poorly differentiated lymphocytic malignant lymphoma, a lymphoid neoplasm containing cells resembling lymphoblasts that have a fine nuclear structure and one or more nucleoli. Also called **lymphoblastic lymphoma, lymphoblastic lymphosarcoma, lymphoblastoma.**

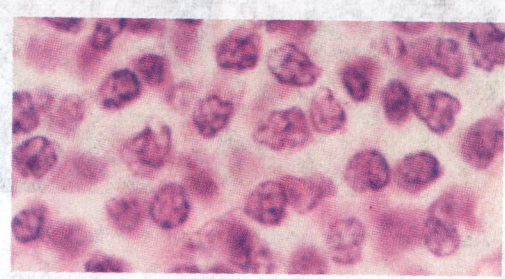

Poorly differentiated lymphocytic malignant lymphoma
(Skarin, 1991)

popliteal /poplit′ē·əl, pop′litē′əl/ [L, *poples,* hollow of the knee], pertaining to the area behind the knee.

popliteal artery /pop′litē′əl/ [L, *poples,* the ham; Gk, *arteria,* air pipe], a continuation of the femoral artery, extending from the opening in the abductor magnus, passing through the popliteal fossa at the knee, dividing into eight branches, and supplying various muscles of the thigh, leg, and foot. Its branches are the superior muscular, sural, cutaneous, medial superior genicular, lateral superior genicular, middle genicular, medial inferior genicular, and lateral inferior genicular.

popliteal node, a node in one of the groups of lymph glands in the leg. Approximately seven small popliteal nodes are imbedded in the fat of the popliteal fossa at the back of the knee. One node is near the terminal section of the saphenous vein and drains the area around the vein. Another node lying between the popliteal artery and the posterior surface of the knee joint drains that region. The other popliteal nodes lie along the popliteal vessels and receive the afferent trunks accompanying the anterior and posterior tibial vessels. Most of the efferents of the popliteal nodes course along the femoral vessels to the deep inguinal nodes. Compare **anterior tibial node, inguinal node.**

popliteal pulse, the pulse of the popliteal artery, palpated behind the knee of a person lying prone with the knee flexed. (See Fig. p. 1248.)

population /pop′yəlā′shən/ [L, *populus,* the people], **1.** (in genetics) an interbreeding group of individuals, organisms, or plants characterized by genetic continuity through several generations. **2.** a group of individuals collectively occupying a particular geographic locale. **3.** any group that is distinguished by a particular trait or situation. **4.** any group measured for some variable characteristic from which samples may be taken for statistical purposes.

population at risk, a group of people who share a characteristic that causes each member to be vulnerable to a particular event, such as nonimmunized children who are exposed to poliovirus or immunosuppressed people who are exposed to herpesvirus. Also called **vulnerable population.**

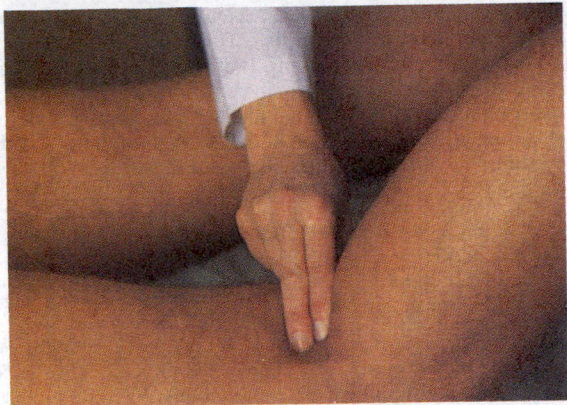

Assessment of popliteal pulse (Potter, 1993)

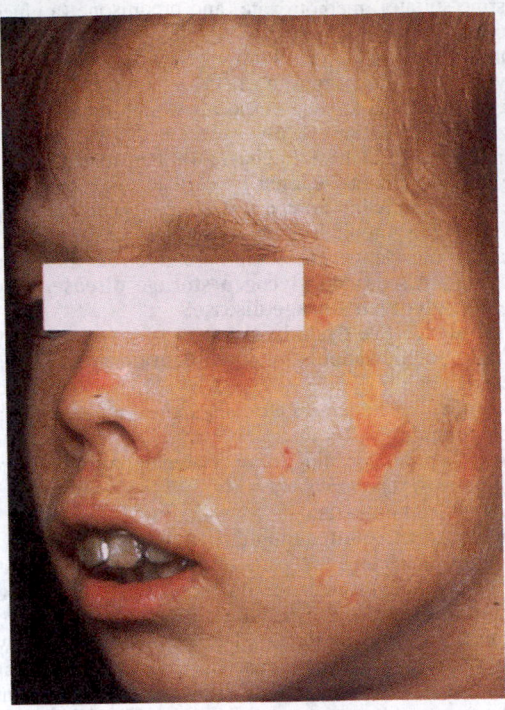

Photosensitivity seen in erythropoietic porphyria
(McKee, 1993/Courtesy Dr. G Murphy, Institute of Dermatology, London)

population genetics, a branch of genetics that applies mendelian inheritance to groups and studies the frequency of alleles and genotypes in breeding populations. See also **Hardy-Weinberg equilibrium principle.**

por-, poro-, a prefix meaning 'a cavity, opening, passage or pore': *porencephalia, porion, porotomy.*

porcine /pôr'sīn/ [L, *porcinus,* pork], obtained from or related to hogs, such as porcine insulin.

porcine graft [L, *porcinus,* pig-like; Gk, *graphion,* plant stylus], a temporary biologic heterograft made from the skin of a pig.

-pore, a suffix meaning an 'opening or passageway': *metapore, myelopore, neuropore.*

poriomania /pôr'ē·ōmā'nē·ə/, a tendency to leave home impulsively or to be a vagabond.

pork tapeworm. See *Taenia solium.*

pork tapeworm infection [L, *porcus,* pig, hog (male); AS, *taeppe,* tape, *wyrm,* worm; L, *inficere,* to taint], an infection of the intestine or other tissues, caused by adult and larval forms of the tapeworm *Taenia solium.* The pork tapeworm is unique in that it can use humans as both intermediate hosts for larvae and definitive hosts for the adult worm. Humans are usually infected with the adult worm after eating contaminated, undercooked pork. The infection is rare in the United States but relatively common in South America, Asia, and Russia. See also **cysticercosis, tapeworm infection.**

poro-, See **por-.**

porosis /pərō'sis/ [Gk *poros* passage], a condition of thinning bone tissue, particularly its supporting connective tissue, such as in osteoporosis.

porous /pôr'əs/ [Gk, *poros,* passage], pertaining to something with pores or openings.

porphobilinogen /pôr'fōbilin'əjən/, a chromogen substance that is an intermediate in the biosynthesis of heme and porphyrins. It appears in the urine of people with porphyria, representing an error of metabolism. See also **heme, porphyria.**

porphyria /pôrfir'ē·ə/ [Gk, *porphyros,* purple], a group of inherited disorders in which there is abnormally increased production of substances called porphyrins. Two major classifications of porphyria are **erythropoietic porphyria,** characterized by the production of large quantities of porphyrins in the blood-forming tissue of the bone marrow, and **hepatic porphyria,** in which large amounts of porphyrins

are produced in the liver. Clinical signs common to both classifications of porphyria are photosensitivity, abdominal pain, and neuropathy.

porphyrin /pôr'fərin/ [Gk, *porphyros*], any iron- or magnesium-free pyrrole derivative occurring in many plant and animal tissues. Normal findings of porphyrins in urine are 50 to 300 mg/24 hr.

portability /pôr'təbil'itē/ [L, *portare,* to carry], a property of computer software that permits its use in a variety of compatible operating systems.

portacaval shunt /pôr'təkā'vəl/ [L, *porta,* gateway, *cavus,* cavity; ME, *shunten*], a shunt created surgically to increase the flow of blood from the portal circulation by carrying it into the vena cava.

Portagen, a trademark for a nutritional supplement containing protein, carbohydrate, and fat.

porta hepatitis. See **portal fissure.**

portal /pôr'təl/ [L, *portalis,* gate], **1.** an entrance. **2.** pertaining to the porta hepatis, or portal vein.

portal circulation [L, *portalis,* gate, *circulare,* to go around], the pathway of blood flow from the gastrointestinal tract and spleen to the liver via the portal vein and its tributaries.

portal fissure [L, *porta* + *fissura,* cleft], a fissure on the visceral surface of the liver along which the portal vein, the hepatic artery, and the hepatic ducts pass. Also called **porta hepatis.**

portal hypertension, an increased venous pressure in the portal circulation caused by compression or by occlusion in the portal or hepatic vascular system. It results in splenomegaly, large collateral veins, ascites, and, in severe cases, systemic hypertension and esophageal varices. Portal hypertension is frequently associated with cirrhosis.

portal of entry, the route by which an infectious agent enters the body.

portal system, the network of veins that drains the blood from the abdominal portion of the digestive tract, the spleen, the pancreas, and the gallbladder and conveys blood from these viscera to the liver.

portal systemic encephalopathy. See **hepatic coma.**

portal vein, a vein that ramifies like an artery in the liver and ends in capillary-like sinusoids that convey the blood to the inferior vena cava through the hepatic veins. In the adult, the portal vein has no valves; but in the fetus and during a brief postnatal period the tributaries of the portal vein contain valves that soon atrophy and disappear. In some individuals, the valves persist as degenerate structures. About 8 cm long, the portal vein is formed at the level of the second lumbar vertebra by the junction of the superior mesenteric and the splenic veins. The portal vein passes behind the duodenum and ascends through the lesser omentum to the porta hepatis, where it divides into the right and the left branches. The vein is surrounded by the hepatic plexus of nerves and is accompanied by numerous lymphatic vessels and some lymph nodes. Accompanied by corresponding branches of the hepatic artery, the right branch of the portal vein enters the right lobe of the liver and the left branch enters the left lobe. The tributaries of the portal vein are the lienal vein, the superior mesenteric vein, the coronary vein, the pyloric vein, the cystic vein, and the paraumbilical vein.

portal venous shunt. See **postcaval shunt.**

Porter-Silber reaction [Curt C. Porter, American biochemist, b. 1914; Robert H. Silber, American biochemist, b. 1915], a reaction, visible as a change in color to yellow, that indicates the amount of adrenal steroids (the 17-hydroxycorticosteroids) excreted per day in the urine. The test is used to evaluate adrenocortical function.

portoenterostomy /pôr′tō·en′tərəs′təmē/ [L, *porta* + Gk, *enteron*, bowel, *stoma*, mouth, *temnein*, to cut], a procedure to correct biliary atresia in which the jejunum is anastomosed by a Roux-en-Y loop to the portal fissure region to establish bile flow from the bile ducts to the intestine. The operation is successful in most cases, but late mortality in a significant number of patients occurs because of chronic medical problems. Without the operation, biliary cirrhosis develops with an attendant early death. Also called **Kasai operation.**

port-wine stain. See **nevus flammeus.**

position /pəzish′ən/ [L, *positio*], **1.** any one of many postures of the body, such as the anatomic position, lateral recumbent position, or semi-Fowler's position. See specific positions. **2.** (in obstetrics) the relationship of an arbitrarily chosen fetal reference point, such as the occiput, sacrum, chin, or scapula, on the presenting part of the fetus, to its location in the maternal pelvis.

-position, a combining form meaning the 'putting or setting in place': *electrodeposition, juxtaposition, reposition.*

positional behavior /pəzish′ənəl/, the orientation of the body regions to claim a quantum of space. Positional behavior involves four body regions: head and neck, upper torso, pelvis and thighs, and lower legs and feet.

positive /poz′itiv/ [L, *positivus*,], **1.** (of a laboratory test) indicating that a substance or a reaction is present. **2.** (of a sign) indicating on physical examination that a finding is present, often meaning that there is pathologic change.

3. (of a substance) tending to carry or carrying a positive chemical charge.

positive end expiratory pressure (PEEP), (in respiratory therapy) the addition of positive airway pressure at the end of the exhalation phase. Each successive breath begins from a new baseline. Ventilation is controlled by a flow of air delivered in cycles of constant pressure through the respiratory cycle. The patient is usually but not always intubated, and a ventilator cycles the air through an endotracheal tube. PEEP is used for the relief of respiratory distress secondary to prematurity, pancreatitis, shock, pulmonary edema, trauma, surgery, or other conditions in which spontaneous respiratory efforts are inadequate and arterial levels of oxygen are deficient. During PEEP therapy close observation is necessary; PEEP may decrease venous return to the heart. Blood gases and vital signs are monitored closely. If PEEP does not significantly improve the patient's condition, its level is increased or it may be discontinued. Compare **continuous positive airway pressure.**

positive feedback, **1.** (in physiology) an increase in function in response to a stimulus; for example, micturition increases after the flow of urine has started, or the uterus contracts more frequently and with greater strength after it has begun to contract in labor. **2.** *informal.* an encouraging, favorable, or otherwise positive response from one person to what another person has communicated.

positive identification, the unconscious modeling of one's personality on that of another who is admired and esteemed. See also **identification.**

positive pressure, **1.** a greater than ambient atmospheric pressure. **2.** (in respiratory therapy) any technique in which compressed gas or air is delivered to the airways at greater than ambient pressure. Positive pressure techniques in respiratory therapy require a flow-regulating device and a delivery system, such as a cannula, mouthpiece, endotracheal tube, or tracheostomy tube.

positive pressure breathing unit. See **IPPB unit.**

positive relationship, (in research) a direct relationship between two variables; as one increases, the other can be expected to increase. Also called **direct relationship.** Compare **negative relationship.**

positive signs of pregnancy, three unmistakable signs of pregnancy: fetal heart tones, heard on auscultation; fetal skeleton, seen on x-ray film or ultrasonogram; and fetal parts, felt on palpation.

positron /pos′itron/, a positive electron, or positively charged particle emitted from neutron-deficient radioactive nuclei.

positron emission topography (PET) [L, *positivus* + Gk, *elektron*, amber; L, *emittere*, to send out; Gk, *tome*, section, *graphein* to record], a computerized radiographic technique that employs radioactive substances to examine the metabolic activity of various body structures. In PET studies the patient either inhales or is injected with a biochemical, such as glucose, carrying a radioactive substance that emits positively charged particles, or positrons, that combine with negatively charged electrons normally found in the cells of the body. When the positrons combine with these electrons, gamma rays are emitted. The electronic circuitry and computers of the PET device detect the gamma rays and convert them into color-coded images that indicate the intensity of the metabolic activity of the organ involved. The radioactive substances used in the PET technique are very short-lived, so that patients undergoing a PET scan are exposed to very small amounts of radiation. Researchers use

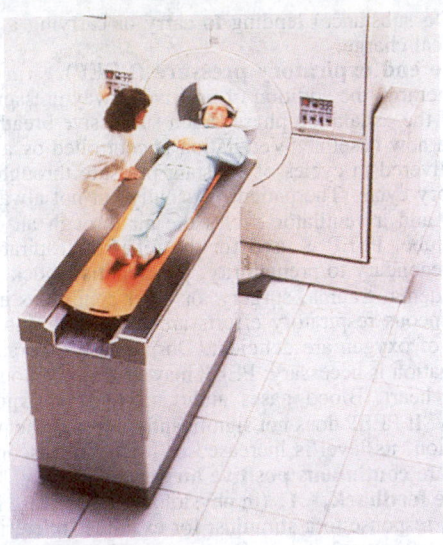

Positioning of patient for PET scan (Chipps, 1992)

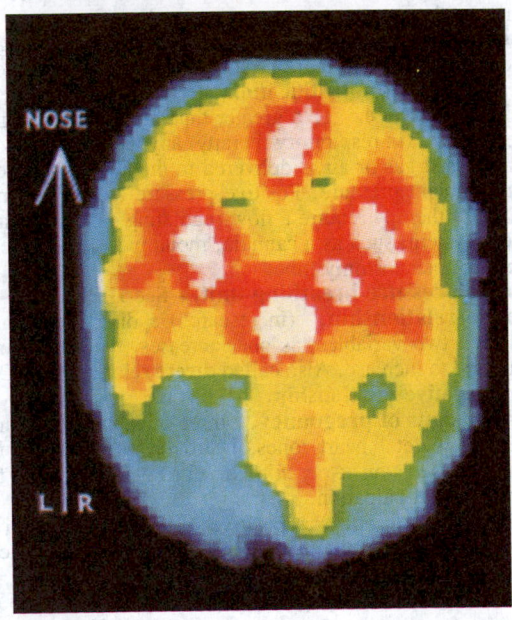

NOSE

L R

Image produced by PET scan
(Perkin, 1986/Drs L Henriksen, OB Paulson, NA Lassen, Department
of Neuromedicine, Rigshospitalet, Copenhagen, Denmark)

PET to study blood flow and the metabolism of the heart
and the blood vessels. There is also a growing application
of the technique in the study and diagnosis of cancer and in
studies of the biochemical activity of the brain.

Posner-Schlossman syndrome. See **glaucomatocyclitic
crisis.**

post-, a prefix meaning 'after or behind': *postabortal, post-
cerebellar, postdiastolic.*

postcaval shunt /-kā'vəl/ [L, *post,* after, *vena cava*; ME,
shunten], any of several surgical anastomoses of the por-

tal and systemic circulations to relieve symptoms of portal
hypertension. Also called **portacaval shunt; portal venous
shunt.**

postcentral gyrus /-sen'trəl/ [L, *post,* after; Gk, *kentron,*
center, *gyros,* turn], a convolution of the brain immediately posterior to the central sulcus of the cerebrum.

postcoital /-kō'itəl/ [L, *post,* after + *coire,* to come to-
gether], after sexual intercourse.

postcommissurotomy syndrome /-kəmis'yərot'əmē/ [L,
post, after, *commissura,* a union; Gk, *temnein,* to cut], a
condition of unknown cause occurring within the first few
weeks after cardiac valvular surgery, characterized by intermittent episodes of pain and fever, which may last weeks
or months and then resolve spontaneously.

postconcussional syndrome /-kənkush'ənəl/ [L, *post* +
concussio, shake violently], a condition after head trauma,
characterized by dizziness, poor concentration, headache,
hypersensitivity, and anxiety. It usually resolves itself without treatment. Also called **posttraumatic syndrome.**

postdate pregnancy /-dāt'/ [L, *post,* after; *data; praegnans,* bearing child], a pregnancy that lasts more than 42
weeks. Also called **postterm pregnancy.**

posterior /postir'ē·ər/ [L, behind], **1.** in the back part of
a structure, such as of the dorsal surface of the human body.
2. the back part of something. **3.** toward the back. Compare **anterior.**

posterior Achilles bursitis, a painful heel condition
caused by inflammation of the bursa between the Achilles
tendon and the calcaneus. It is commonly associated with
Haglund's deformity.

posterior asynclitism. See **asynclitism.**

posterior atlantoaxial ligament, one of five ligaments
connecting the atlas to the axis. It is broad, thin, and fixed
to the inferior border of the anterior arch of the atlas and to
the ventral surface of the body of the axis. Compare **anterior atlantoaxial ligament.**

posterior atlantooccipital membrane, one of a pair of
thin, broad fibrous sheets that form part of the atlantooccipital joint between the atlas and the occipital bone and
contain an opening for the vertebral artery and the suboccipital nerve. Also called **posterior atlantooccipital ligament.** Compare **anterior atlantooccipital membrane.**

posterior auricular artery, one of a pair of small
branches from the external carotid arteries, dividing into auricular and occipital branches and supplying parts of the ear,
scalp, and other structures in the head.

posterior column [L, *posterus,* coming after, *columna*],
the posterior horns of the gray matter in the spinal cord.
Also called **gray column, posterior; columna posterior.**

posterior common ligament. See **posterior longitudinal
ligament.**

posterior costotransverse ligament, one of the five ligaments of each costotransverse joint, comprising a fibrous
band passing from the neck of each rib to the base of the vertebra above. Compare **superior costotransverse ligament.**

posterior drawer sign, an orthopedic test in which the
patient is positioned with hips at 45 degrees and knees
flexed at 90 degrees while the examiner sits on the foot and
pushes the tibia backward. Also, with both the hips and
knees flexed at 90 degrees, the heels are held together and
the knees are observed for comparison of relative posterior
sag of the tibia.

posterior fontanel, a small triangular area between the
occipital and parietal bones at the junction of the sagittal
and lambdoidal sutures. See also **fontanel.**

posterior fossa, a depression on the posterior surface of the humerus, above the trochlea, that lodges the olecranon of the ulna when the elbow is extended.

posterior horn [L, *posterior,* behind, *cornu,* horn], the horn-shaped projections of gray matter in the posterior region of the spinal cord. Also called **cornu posterioris.**

posterior longitudinal ligament, a thick, strong ligament attached to the dorsal surfaces of the vertebral bodies, extending from the occipital bone to the coccyx. Also called **posterior common ligament.** Compare **anterior longitudinal ligament.**

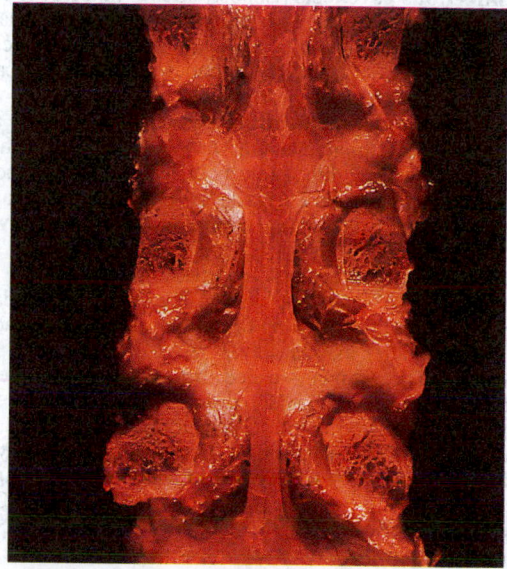

Posterior logitudinal ligament *(Bullough, 1988)*

posterior mediastinal node, a node in one of three groups of thoracic visceral nodes, connected to the part of the lymphatic system that serves the esophagus, pericardium, diaphragm, and convex surface of the liver. Most of the efferents of the posterior mediastinal nodes end in the thoracic duct, but some join the tracheobronchial nodes. Compare **anterior mediastinal node.**

posterior mediastinum, the irregularly shaped caudal portion of the mediastinum, parallel with the vertebral column. It is bounded ventrally by the pericardium, caudally by the diaphragm, dorsally by the vertebral column from the fourth to the twelfth thoracic vertebra, and laterally by the mediastinal pleurae. It contains the bifurcation of the trachea, two primary bronchi, esophagus, thoracic duct, many large lymph nodes, and various vessels, such as the thoracic portion of the aortic arch. Compare **anterior mediastinum, middle mediastinum, superior mediastinum.**

posterior nares, a pair of posterior openings in the nasal cavity that connect the nasal cavity with the nasopharynx and allow the inhalation and the exhalation of air. Each is an oval aperture that measures about 2.5 cm vertically and is about 1.5 cm in diameter. Also called **choana.** Compare **anterior nares.**

posterior neuropore, the opening at the caudal end of the embryonic neural tube. It closes at about the 25 somite stage, which indicates the end of horizon XII in the numeric anatomic charting of human embryonic development. Compare **anterior neuropore.** See also **horizon.**

posterior palatal seal area, the area of soft tissues along the junction of the hard and soft palates on which displacement, within the physiologic tolerance of the tissues, can be applied by a denture to aid its retention.

posterior pituitary, posterior pituitary gland. See **neurohypophysis.**

posterior rhizotomy [L, *posterior,* behind; Gk, *rhiza,* root + *temnein,* to cut], a surgical procedure for cutting the posterior, or sensory, nerve root for the relief of intractable pain.

posterior tibial artery, one of the divisions of the popliteal artery, starting at the distal border of the popliteus muscle, passing behind the tibia, dividing into eight branches, and supplying various muscles of the lower leg, foot, and toes. Its eight branches are the peroneal, nutrient (tibial), muscular, posterior medial malleolar, communicating, medial calcaneal, medial plantar, and lateral plantar. Compare **anterior tibial artery.**

posterior tibialis pulse, the pulse of the posterior tibialis artery palpated on the medial aspect of the ankle, just posterior to the prominence of the ankle bone.

posterior tooth, any of the maxillary and mandibular premolars and molars of the primary or permanent dentition, or of prostheses.

posterior vein of left ventricle, one of the five tributaries of the coronary sinus that drains blood from the capillary bed of the myocardium. It courses along the diaphragmatic surface of the left ventricle, accompanying the circumflex branch of the left coronary artery. In some individuals, it ends in the great cardiac vein. Compare **great cardiac vein, middle cardiac vein, small cardiac vein.**

postero- /pos'tərō-/, a prefix meaning 'of or related to the posterior part': *posteroanterior, posteromedian, posterosuperior.*

posteroanterior /-antir'ē·ər/ [L, *posterus,* coming after, *anterior,* before], the direction from back to front.

posteroinferior /-infir'ē·ər/ [L, *posterus,* coming after + *inferior,* lower], pertaining to a position that is both lower and behind.

posterolateral /-lat'ərəl/ [L, *posterus,* coming after + *latus,* side], pertaining to a position behind and to the side.

posterolateral thoracotomy /pos'tərōlat'ərəl/, a chest surgery technique in which an incision is made in the submammary fold, below the tip of the scapula. The incision is continued posteriorly along the course of the ribs and upward as far as the spine of the scapula. It requires division of the trapezius, rhomboideus, latissimus dorsi, and serratus anterior muscles. Compare **anterolateral thoracotomy, median sternotomy.** See also **thoracotomy.**

postganglionic /-gang'glē·on'ik/ [L, *post,* after; Gk, *gagglion,* knot], distal to a ganglion.

postganglionic neuron [L, *post,* after; Gk, *gagglion,* knot, *neuron,* nerve], a neuron that is distal to or beyond a ganglion.

postgastrectomy care /-gastrek'təmē/ [L, *post* + Gk, *gaster,* stomach, *ektome* excision], nursing care after the removal of all or part of the stomach. Drainage of the nasogastric tube normally changes from bright red to dark in the first 24 hours. If the tube becomes blocked, this fact is reported at once, because gastric distention strains the suture lines. Adequate medication for pain allows deeper breathing and coughing, because the incision is close to the diaphragm. When bowel sounds reappear and a small amount of water given by the ounce is retained, the naso-gastric tube is removed. Small, bland meals are offered hourly as tolerated. An increase in temperature or dyspnea indicates a leakage of oral fluids around the anastomosis. The diet is changed slowly to a regular diet, with five or six dry small feedings daily. Fluids are given hourly between meals. The most common complication of gastrectomy is the dumping syndrome, with fullness and discomfort, including vertigo, sweating, palpitation, and nausea occurring 5 to 30 minutes after eating, as food enters the small bowel. Small, dry meals, eaten lying down, along with sedatives and antispasmodics, may prevent the symptoms, although they may persist up to 1 year after surgery. Other possible complications include marginal peptic ulcer, in which gastric acids come into contact with a suture line; afferent loop syndrome, in which the duodenal loop is blocked and pancreatic juices and bile flow back into the stomach; vitamin B_{12} and folic acid deficiency; reduced absorption of calcium and vitamin D; and functional hyperinsulinism, in which carbohydrates now passing directly into the small bowel cause an outpouring of insulin into the bloodstream and a resultant hypoglycemia within 2 hours.

posthepatic cirrhosis. See **cirrhosis.**

posthepatic jaundice /pōst'hepat'ik/ [L, *post,* after; Gk, *hepar,* liver; Fr, *jaune,* yellow], jaundice caused by obstruction of the bile ducts.

posthumous /pos'chəməs/ [L, *post,* after + *humare,* to bury], after a person's death.

posthypnotic suggestion /-hipnot'ik/ [L, *post,* after; Gk, *hypnos,* sleep; L, *suggerere,* to suggest], an action suggested to a hypnotized subject during a trance and carried out upon awakening from the trance. The action is in response to a cue and the subject usually does not know why he or she is performing the act.

postictal /pōst'iktəl/ [L, *post* + Gk, *ikteros,* jaundice], after a convulsion. **–postictus,** *n.*

postinfectious /-infek'shəs/ [L, *post* + *inficere,* to taint], after an infection.

postinfectious encephalitis. See **encephalitis.**

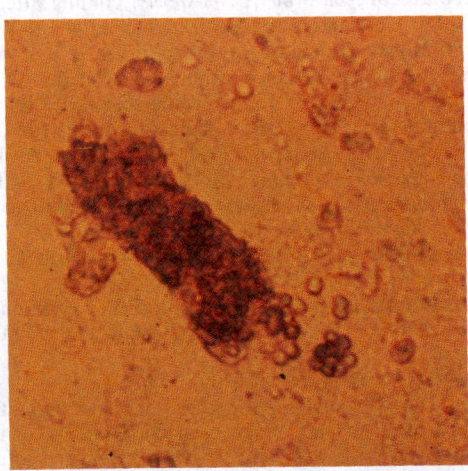

Red blood cell cast from patient with postinfectious glomerulonephritis
(Zitelli, 1992)

postinfectious glomerulonephritis, the acute form of glomerulonephritis, which may follow 1 to 6 weeks after a streptococcal infection, most often in childhood. Characteristics of the disease are hematuria, oliguria, edema, and proteinuria, especially in the form of granular casts. There may be slight impairment of renal function in adults, but most patients recover fully in 1 to 3 months. There is no specific treatment for this form of glomerulonephritis; the dietary restriction of protein and the prescription of diuretics may be necessary until kidney function returns to normal. See also **chronic glomerulonephritis, subacute glomerulonephritis.**

postinfectious psychosis [L, *post,* after + *inficere,* to stain; Gk, *psyche,* mind + *osis,* condition], psychotic behavior that follows a serious infection such as pneumonia, scarlet fever, malaria, uremia, or typhoid fever. Also called **infectious-exhaustive syndrome.**

postlumbar puncture headache /-lum'bar/ [L, *post,* after + *lumbus,* loin, *punctura*; AS, *heafod* + *acan*], a headache that occurs within a few hours of a lumbar puncture and usually lasts 1 or 2 days to several weeks. It may be accompanied by nausea and vomiting and improves when the patient lies down.

postmastectomy exercises /-məstek'təmē/ [L, *post* + Gk, *mastos,* breast, *ektome,* excision], exercises essential to the prevention of shortening of the muscles and contracture of the joints after mastectomy.

■ METHOD: The woman is asked to flex and extend the fingers of the affected arm and to pronate and supinate the forearm immediately on return to her room after recovery from anesthesia and surgery. On the first postoperative day she is asked to squeeze a rubber ball in her hand. Brushing her teeth and hair is encouraged as effective exercises. Other exercises are usually taught, including four that are called climbing the wall, arm swinging, rope pulling, and elbow spreading. They are performed as follows:

Climbing the wall: The patient stands facing a wall, toes close to the wall. The elbows are bent and the palms of the hands are placed on the wall at shoulder height. The hands are moved up the wall together until the woman feels pain or pulling on the incision, then returned to the starting position.

Arm swinging: While standing, the patient bends forward from the waist, allowing both arms to relax and hang naturally. The arms are swung together from the shoulders from left to right and then in circles parallel to the floor, clockwise and counterclockwise. She straightens up slowly.

Rope pulling: A rope is attached over a shower rod or a hook. Each end of the rope is grasped, and the patient alternately pulls each end, raising one arm after the other to the height at which incisional pain or pulling is felt. The rope is shortened until the affected arm is raised almost directly overhead.

Elbow spreading: The hands are clasped behind the neck, and the elbows are slowly raised to chin level while the head is held erect. Gradually, the elbows are spread apart to the point at which incisional pain or pulling is felt.

■ INTERVENTIONS: Specific exercises may be ordered. The patient is shown how to do them and is encouraged to continue them at home.

■ OUTCOME CRITERIA: With proper exercise, full range of motion returns; both arms can be extended fully and equally high over the head. The woman benefits from having something active to do to help herself during the difficult period of adjustment after mastectomy. Many activities of daily life provide good exercise, such as reaching high shelves, hanging clothes, and gardening.

postmature /-məchoor'/ [L, *post* + *maturare*, to become ripe], **1.** overly developed or matured. **2.** of or pertaining to a postmature infant. See also **dysmaturity**. –**postmaturity**, *n.*

postmature infant, an infant born after the end of the forty-second week of gestation, bearing the physical signs of placental insufficiency. Characteristically, the baby has dry, peeling skin, long fingernails and toenails, and folds of skin on the thighs and, sometimes, on the arms and buttocks. Hypoglycemia and hypokalemia are common. Postmature infants often look as if they have lost weight in utero. The newborn is fed early, and the calcium and potassium levels in the blood are monitored and corrected, if necessary, to avoid seizures and neurologic damage. To avoid the syndrome, labor may be induced as gestation approaches 42 weeks. To anticipate the problems associated with the syndrome, the fetus and the mother may be electronically monitored through labor.

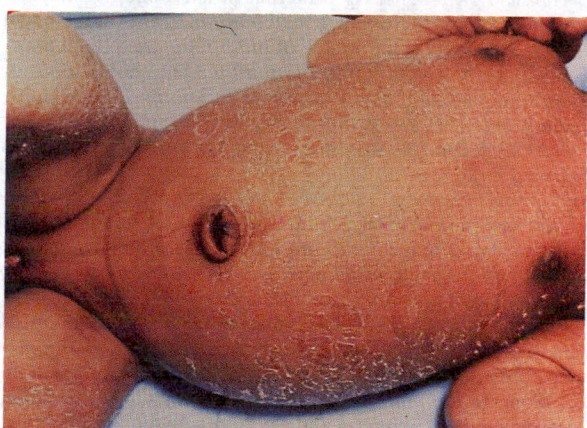

Dry skin of postmature infant (Zitelli, 1992)

postmaturity /-məchoo'ritē/ [L, *post*, after + *maturare*, to make ripe], beyond the normal date for maturity.

postmenopausal /-men'əpô'səl/ [L, *post* + *mensis*, month; Gk, *pauien*, to cease], of or pertaining to the period of life after the menopause.

postmenopausal vaginitis [L, *post*, after + *mensis*, month; Gk, *pauein*, to cease; L, *vagina*, sheath; Gk, *itis*, inflammation], an inflammation caused by degenerative changes in the vaginal mucosa after menopause. Also called **atrophic vaginitis.**

postmortem /-môr'təm/ [L, *post* + *mors*, death], **1.** after death. **2.** *informal.* **postmortem examination.**

postmortem cesarean section [L, *post*, after + *mors*, death; *secare*, to cut; *sectio*], delivery of a fetus by incision into the uterus after death of a woman.

postmortem delivery. See **postmortem cesarean section.**

postmortem examination [L, *post*, after + *mors*, death; *examinatio*], an examination of a body after death by a person trained in pathology. Also called **autopsy,** (*informal*) **postmortem.**

postmortem graft [L, *post*, after + *mors*, death; Gk, *graphion*, stylus], the transplanting of a cornea, artery, or other body part from a dead individual to repair a defect in a living body. Also called **cadaver graft.**

postmyocardial infarction syndrome /-mī·əkär'dē·əl/ [L, *post* + Gk, *mys*, muscle, *kardia*, heart; L, *infarcire*, to stuff], a condition that may occur days or weeks after an acute myocardial infarction. It is characterized by fever, pericarditis with a friction rub, pleurisy, pleural effusion, and joint pain. It tends to recur and often provokes severe anxiety, depression, and fear that it is another heart attack. Treatment includes aspirin, reassurance, and a short course of corticosteroids. Nursing care includes close observation and emotional support, especially when debilitating anxiety and depression are present.

postnasal /-nā'zəl/ [L, *post*, after + *nasus*, nose], pertaining to the region behind the nose, or the posterior part of the nasal fossae.

postnasal drip (PND) [L, *post* + *nasus*, nose; AS, *dryppan*], a drop-by-drop discharge of nasal mucus into the posterior pharynx, often accompanied by a feeling of obstruction, an unpleasant taste, and fetid breath, caused by rhinitis, chronic sinusitis, or hypersecretion by the nasopharyngeal mucosa. Methods of treatment include the application of drops or sprays of phenylephrine or ephedrine sulfate to constrict blood vessels and reduce hyperemia, sinus irrigation to improve drainage, and the use of appropriate antibiotics. Therapy for allergies may be indicated in some cases, and surgery may be required if the nasal passages are obstructed by polyps or a deviated septum.

postnecrotic cirrhosis /-nekrot'ik/ [L, *post* + Gk, *nekros*, dead; *kirrhos*, yellowish, *osis*, condition], a nodular form of cirrhosis that may follow hepatitis or other inflammation of the liver. Also called **posthepatic cirrhosis.** See also **cirrhosis.**

postoperative /-op'ərətiv'/ [L, *post* + *operari*, to work], of or pertaining to the period of time after surgery. It begins with the patient's emergence from anesthesia and continues through the time required for the acute effects of the anesthetic or surgical procedures to abate.

postoperative atelectasis, a form of atelectasis in which collapse of lung tissue is caused by the depressant effects of anesthetic drugs. Deep breathing and coughing are encouraged at frequent intervals postoperatively to prevent this condition.

postoperative bed, a bed prepared for a patient who is weak or unconscious, as when recovering from anesthesia. The bed is in the flat position. The bottom sheet may be covered with a cotton bath blanket that is tucked tightly beneath the mattress. The top linen is fan-folded to the far side of the bed and not tucked in. The bed is made in this way to simplify transferring a patient from a stretcher into the bed.

postoperative care, the management of a patient after surgery. See also **preoperative care.**

■ METHOD: On the patient's discharge from the operating room, the surgical drapes, ground plate, and restraints are removed and a sterile dressing is applied to the incision. The patency and connections of all drainage tubes and the flow rate of parenteral infusions are checked. The patient's cleanliness and dryness are given attention, and the gown is changed, avoiding exposing the individual. Four people transfer the patient slowly and cautiously to a recovery room bed, maintaining body alignment and protecting the limbs. When indicated, an oral or nasal airway is inserted or a pre viously inserted endotracheal tube is suctioned; respiration may be supported with a pulmonator or intermittent positive pressure breathing (IPPB); if respiration remains impaired, the anesthetist is notified. The blood pressure, pulse, and respirations are initially reported to the anesthetist and are then checked every 15 minutes or as ordered. At similar intervals, the level of consciousness, reflexes, and movements of extremities are observed, and the incision, drainage tubes, and intravenous infusion site are inspected. Nothing is given orally; medication, blood or blood components, oxygen, and IPPB are administered as ordered, and fluid intake and output are measured. Pain is controlled by administration of analgesics. The patient is kept warm, dry, and positioned for optimal ventilation and comfort. At the first sign of vomiting, the head is turned to one side and suction is applied. Oral hygiene is administered every 1 to 2 hours to keep the mouth and tongue moist. The chest is auscultated for breath sounds every 30 minutes, and the patient, when reactive, is helped to turn, cough, and deep breathe every 1 to 2 hours. The rectal or axillary temperature is taken every 1 to 4 hours. When completely awake and able to move the extremities well, and after having exhibited stable vital signs, the patient may be transferred to the assigned room, provided the drainage tubes are functioning, the dressings show no bleeding or excessive drainage, and the anesthesiologist approves the move. The family is informed of the patient's progress and expectations in the postoperative period. The airway patency; rate, depth, and character of respirations; pulse; blood pressure; temperature; skin color; level of consciousness; and condition of dressings and drainage tubes are assessed. If respirations are noisy, the patient is assisted in coughing. A rapid, weak, thready pulse may indicate increased bleeding and is reported, especially if other signs of impending shock, such as hypotension or decreased consciousness, are evident. The dressing is examined at frequent intervals, and excessive drainage is reported immediately. The patient is positioned for comfort and good ventilation with the side rails of the bed raised for safety and the head slightly elevated, unless contraindicated. A cardiac monitor may be connected. Parenteral fluids and medication for pain are administered as ordered. Fluid intake and output are measured; range-of-motion exercises to extremities are performed, and ambulation, when ordered, is assisted.

■ NURSING INTERVENTION: The recovery room nurse performs the immediate postoperative procedures, and the clinical unit nurse provides ongoing care, emotional support, and instructions for the patient and family. Special attention is given to preventing trauma postoperatively, as may occur when confused or elderly patients fall getting out of bed. Falls by postoperative patients are second to errors in medication as the most common incidents reported by hospitals.

■ OUTCOME CRITERIA: Meticulous postoperative care prevents falls, infections, and other complications and promotes the healing of the incision and restoration of the patient to health.

postoperative cholangiography, (in diagnostic radiology) a procedure for outlining the major bile ducts. A radiopaque contrast material is injected into the common bile duct via a T-tube inserted during surgery. It is usually performed after a cholecystectomy to discover any residual calculi. See also **cholangiography.**

postoperative ileus [L, *post* + *operari,* to work; Gk, *eilein,*

to twist], an obstruction to normal intestinal function caused by a loss of peristaltic muscular action of the ileus after surgery.

postparalytic /-per′əlit′ik/ [L, *post;* Gk, *paralyein,* to be palsied], pertaining to something that occurred after paralysis.

postpartal care /-pär′təl/ [L, *post* + *partus,* bringing forth], care of the mother and her newborn baby during the first few days of the puerperium. See also **antepartal care, intrapartal care, newborn intrapartal care.**

■ METHOD: The physical and physiologic changes of involution in the mother are observed for deviation from the normal. The uterus contracts after delivery, causing bleeding from the site of placental implantation to diminish. It is the size of a softball; the fundus is below the umbilicus. The lochia changes color and consistency during the first few days. Lochia rubra flows for up to 1 week, followed by straw-colored lochia serosa, and, finally, by clear, sticky lochia alba. The abdominal wall is soft, but muscle tone returns with time and exercise. On the third day the milk usually begins to fill the breasts.

■ NURSING INTERVENTION: Maternal-infant bonding may be augmented by increased contact between the mother and baby. The nurse is the source of most of the teaching that occurs in the postpartum phase. Breast feeding, bottle feeding, nutrition, care of the umbilical and diaper areas, baby baths, safety practices and accident prevention, and exercises for physical reconditioning are taught during the postpartum phase.

■ OUTCOME CRITERIA: During the first hours and days after delivery the nurse encourages frequent mother-infant contact. The mother's nuturing abilities are fostered and developed; many new mothers need time and contact with the baby to acquire skills of infant care and to develop feelings of love. As the mother gives to the baby, she gains satisfaction. If the baby is prevented from taking, or the mother from giving, both become frustrated. Toxemia, hemorrhage, and infection are the chief medical problems of the puerperium, but they are not common and are largely avoidable. Fatigue, breast engorgement, psychologic depression, and superficial thrombophlebitis are more common, but not usual.

postpartum /pōstpär′təm/, after childbirth.

postpartum blues [L, *post,* after; *parturire,* labor pains; ME, *bleu*], an emotional effect of childbirth experienced by mothers, consisting mainly of transient feelings of depression for a period of about 72 hours. If the depression persists for a longer period, it may be due to lack of interest in the infant or a reaction to the physical and mental stress of pregnancy. The condition may require psychotherapy or antidepressant medications.

postpartum depression [L, *post* + *partus; deprimere,* to press down], an abnormal psychiatric condition that occurs after childbirth, typically from 3 days to 6 weeks postpartum. It is characterized by symptoms that range from mild 'postpartum blues' to an intense, suicidal, depressive psychosis. Severe postpartum depression occurs approximately once in every 2000 to 3000 pregnancies. The cause is not proven; neurochemical and psychologic influences have been implicated. Approximately one third of patients are found to have had some degree of psychiatric abnormality predating the pregnancy. The disorder recurs in subsequent pregnancies in 25% of cases. Some women at risk for postpartum depression may be identified during the prenatal period by their having made no preparations for the expected baby, by their expressing unrealistic plans for post-partum work or travel, or by their denying the reality of the responsibilities of parenthood. Depending on the severity of the disorder, psychoactive medication or psychiatric hospitalization may be necessary.

postpartum hemorrhage [L, *post*, after + *parturire*, labor pains; Gk, *haima*, blood, *rhegnynei*, to gush], excessive bleeding (a loss of more than 500 ml of blood) after childbirth.

postpartum iliofemoral thrombophlebitis [L, *post*, after + *parturire*, labor pains, *ilia*, flank, *femur*, thigh; Gk, *thrombos*, lump, *phleps*, vein, *itis*, inflammation], a condition of thrombophlebitis involving the iliofemoral artery after childbirth.

postpartum pituitary necrosis [L, *post* + *parturire*, *pituita*, phlegm; GK, *nekros*, dead, *osis*, condition], a condition of hypopituitarism resulting from hypovolemia and shock in the immediate postpartum period. The patient may not develop lactation, pubic and axillary hair may be lost, and symptoms of hypoglycemia and amenorrhea are experienced. See **Sheehan's syndrome**.

postpartum psychosis [L, *post*, after + *parturire*, labor pains; Gk, *psyche*, mind], an episode of psychosis, either depressive or schizophrenic, after childbirth. Because the condition usually tends to develop in the month after childbirth, it is believed that endocrinologic factors are a cause.

postperfusion syndrome /-pərfyoo′zhən/ [L, *post* + *perfundere*, to pour over], a cytomegalovirus (CMV) infection, occurring between 2 and 4 weeks after the transfusion of fresh blood containing CMV. It is characterized by prolonged fever, hepatitis, rash, atypical lymphocytosis, and, occasionally, jaundice. No specific treatment is yet available.

postpericardiotomy syndrome /pōst′perikär′dē·ot′əmē/ [L, *post* + Gk, *peri*, around, *kardia*, heart, *temnein*, to cut], a condition that sometimes occurs days or weeks after pericardiotomy, characterized by symptoms of pericarditis, often without any fever. It appears to be an autoimmune response to damaged muscle cells of the myocardium and pericardium. See also **pericarditis**.

postpill amenorrhea /-pill′/ [L, *post* + *pilla*, ball; Gk, *a* not, *men*, month, *rhoia*, flow], failure of normal menstrual cycles to resume within 3 months after discontinuation of oral contraception. The pathophysiology of this uncommon condition is poorly understood. Postpill amenorrhea is rarely permanent. See also **amenorrhea**.

postpoliomyelitis muscular atrophy (PPMA) /-pō′lē·ōmī′əlī′tis/ [L, *post*, after; Gk, *polios*, gray; *myelos*, marrow + *itis*, inflammation; L, *musculus*; Gk, *a*, *trophe*, nourishment], a recurrence of neuromusclar symptoms in people who had recovered from acute paralytic polio many years earlier. The chief symptom is muscular weakness and the condition may affect the same muscles as before or muscles that were not damaged in the earlier polio attack.

postpolycythemic myeloid metaplasia /-pol′isīthē′mik/ [L, *post* + Gk, *polys*, many, *kytos*, cell, *haima*, blood; *myelos*, marrow, *eidos*, form; *meta*, with, *plassein*, to mold], a late development in polycythemia vera, characterized by anemia caused by sclerosis of the bone marrow. The production of red blood cells occurs only in the liver and spleen. This condition is frequently complicated by leukemia, especially if the patient has been treated with ionizing radiation. See also **myeloid metaplasia, polycythemia**.

postprandial,   after a meal.

postprandial pain [L, *post*, after + *prandium*, lunch; *poena*, penalty], pain that occurs after a meal.

postpubertal, postpubertal,   See **postpuberty**.

postpubertal panhypopituitarism /-pyoo′bərtəl/ [L, *post* + *pubertas*, maturation; Gk, *pan*, all, *hypo*, below, *pituita*, phlegm], insufficiency of pituitary hormones, caused by postpartum pituitary necrosis resulting from thrombosis of the circulation of the gland during or after delivery. The disorder, characterized initially by weakness, lethargy, failure to lactate, amenorrhea, loss of libido, and intolerance to cold, leads to loss of axillary and pubic hair, bradycardia, hypotension, premature wrinkling of the skin, and atrophy of the thyroid and adrenal glands. Treatment consists of the administration of ACTH, thyroid stimulating hormone, or thyroid, adrenal, and sex hormones. Also called **Simmonds' disease, hypophyseal cachexia, pituitary cachexia**.

postpuberty /-pyoo′bərtē/ [L, *post* + *pubertas*], a period of approximately 1 to 2 years after puberty during which skeletal growth slows and the physiologic functions of the reproductive years are established. Also called **postpubescence. –postpuberal, postpubertal, postpubescent,** *adj*.

postrenal anuria /-rē′nəl/ [L, *post* + *renes*, kidney; Gk, *a*, *ouron*, not urine] cessation of urine production caused by obstruction in the ureters.

postresection filling.   See **retrograde filling**.

postsynaptic /-sinap′tik/ [L, *post* + Gk, *synaptein*, to join], **1.** situated after a synapse. **2.** occurring after a synapse has been crossed.

postterm infant.   See **postmature infant**.

postterm pregnancy.   See **postdate pregnancy**.

posttransfusion syndrome /-transfyoo′zhən/ [L, *post*, after + *transfundere*, to pour through; Gk, *syn*, together + *dromos*, course], a complex of adverse reactions that may accompany or follow IV administration of blood or blood components. Reactions may include hemolytic effects, headache and back pain, allergies to an unknown component in donor blood, circulatory overloading, effects of cold blood that chill the patient's cardiovascular system, and effects of microaggregates in stored blood.

posttrauma response /-trô′mə/, a nursing diagnosis accepted by the Seventh National Conference on the Classification of Nursing Diagnoses. The condition is defined as the state of an individual experiencing a sustained painful response to unexpected extraordinary life events. Critical defining characteristics include reexperience of the traumatic event, which may be identified in cognitive, affective, or sensory motor activities (flashbacks, intrusive thoughts, repetitive dreams or nightmares, excessive verbalization of the traumatic event, or verbalization of survival guilt or guilt about behavior required by survival). Among minor defining characteristics is psychic or emotional numbness, such as impaired interpretation of reality, confusion, dissociation or amnesia, vagueness about the traumatic event, or constricted affect. Another characteristic is an altered lifestyle with self-destructiveness, including substance abuse, suicide attempt, or other acting-out behavior, difficulty with interpersonal relationships, development of a phobia regarding the trauma, poor impulse control or irritability, and explosiveness. Related factors include disasters, wars, epidemics, rape, assault, torture, catastrophic illness, or accident. See also **nursing diagnosis**.

posttraumatic /pōst′trômat′ik/ [L, *post*, after, Gk, *trauma*, wounded], pertaining to any emotional, mental or physiological consequences after a major illness or injury.

posttraumatic amnesia [L, *post* + Gk, *trauma*, wound], a period of amnesia between a brain injury resulting in memory loss and the point at which the functions concerned with memory are restored.

posttraumatic epilepsy. See **traumatic epilepsy.**

posttraumatic osteoporosis /-trômat′ik/ [L, *post*, after; Gk, *trauma*, wound, *osteon*, bone + *poros*, passage + *osis*, condition], osteoporosis that develops after an injury or other severe health episode.

posttraumatic spondylitis. See **Kümmell's disease.**

posttraumatic stress disorder (PTSD), an anxiety disorder characterized by an acute emotional response to a traumatic event or situation involving severe environmental stress, such as a natural disaster, airplane crash, serious automobile accident, military combat, and physical torture.

posttraumatic syndrome. See **postconcussional syndrome.**

postulate /pos′chəlāt/ [L, *postulare*, to demand], a hypothesis that is offered as true without proof or as a basis for argument or debate.

postural albuminuria. See **orthostatic proteinuria.**

postural background movements /pos′chərəl/ [L, *ponere*, to place], the spontaneous body adjustments, requiring vestibular and proprioceptive integration, that maintain the center of gravity, keep the head and body in alignment, and stabilize body parts, such as the shoulder girdle when the hand reaches for a distant object.

postural drainage, the use of positioning to drain secretions from specific segments of the bronchi and the lungs into the trachea. Coughing normally expels secretions from the trachea.

■ METHOD: Positions are selected that promote drainage from the affected parts of the lungs. Pillows and raised sections of the hospital bed are used to support or elevate parts of the body. The procedure is begun with the patient level, and the head is gradually lowered to a full Trendelenburg position. Inhalation through the nose and exhalation through the mouth is encouraged. Simultaneously the nurse may use cupping and vibration over the affected area of the lungs to dislodge and mobilize secretions. The person is then helped to a position conducive to coughing and is asked to breathe deeply at least three times and to cough at least twice. See also **cupping and vibrating.**

■ NURSING INTERVENTION: A patient who is dyspneic, or who has hemoptysis or signs of cerebral hemorrhage, increased intracerebral pressure, or lung abscess is not placed in a head-down position without caution and a specific medical order.

Suction is kept available in all cases in which the patient might not be able to expel the secretions that have drained into the trachea. The patient's tolerance for the procedure and the position is carefully observed; fatigue is avoided.

■ OUTCOME CRITERIA: Effectiveness of the procedure depends on positioning that allows drainage by gravity and on liquefaction, ciliary action, and effective breathing. As the secretions are cleared, the patient becomes better able to breathe, is more comfortable, and may move about more freely; thus the respiratory passages may remain freer of obstructing secretions and regain their normal function.

postural hypotension. See **orthostatic hypotension.**

postural proteinuria. See **orthostatic proteinuria.**

postural reflex [L, *ponere*, to place; *reflectere*, to turn backward], any of several reflexes associated with the maintenance of normal body posture.

postural vertigo. See **cupulolithiasis.**

posture /pos′chər/ [L, *ponere*, to place], the position of the body with respect to the surrounding space. A posture is determined and maintained by coordination of the various muscles that move the limbs, by proprioception, and by the sense of balance.

postvaccinal encephalitis /-vak′sinəl/ [L, *post*, after, *vaccinus*, of a cow; Gk, *enkephalos*, brain + *itis*, inflammation], acute encephalitis after vaccination.

postvaccinal encephalomyelitis [L, *post*, after; *vaccinus*, of a cow; Gk, *enkephalos*, brain, *myelos*, marrow, *itis*, inflammation], acute encephalomyelitis after vaccination.

postviral fatigue syndrome /-vīrəl/ [L, *post*, after, *virus*, poison; *fatigare*, to tire; Gk, *syn*, together + *dromos*, course], a condition of chronic muscle fatigue unrelieved by rest after a viral infection. Other symptoms may include visual and hearing difficulties, low-grade fever, stiff neck, urinary frequency, and insomnia. Also called **benign myalgic encephalomyelitis, Iceland disease, Royal Free disease.**

pot-, a combining form meaning 'of or related to drinking': *potable, potocytosis, potomania.*

potable /pō′təbəl/ [L *potare* to drink], fit for drinking.

potassemia /pōt′əsē′meiə/ [Du, *potasschen*; Gk, *haima*, blood], an excess of potassium in the blood.

potassium (K) /pətas′ē·əm/ [D, *potasschen*, potash], an alkali metal element, the seventh most abundant element in the earth's crust. Its atomic number is 19; its atomic weight is 39.1. Potassium salts are necessary to the life of all plants and animals. Potassium in the body constitutes the predominant intracellular cation, helping to regulate neuromuscular excitability and muscle contraction. Sources of potassium in the diet are whole grains, meat, legumes, fruit, and vegetables. The average adequate daily intake for most adults is 2 to 4 g. Potassium is important in glycogen formation, protein synthesis, and the correction of imbalances of acid-base metabolism, especially in association with the action of sodium and hydrogen ions. Potassium salts are very important as therapeutic agents but are extremely dangerous if used improperly. The kidneys play an important role in controlling its secretion and absorption. Aldosterone stimulates sodium reabsorption and potassium secretion by the kidneys; the major extrarenal adaptation to this process involves the absorption of potassium by the body tissues, especially the tissues of the muscles and the liver. The intracellular concentrations of potassium and hydrogen are higher than those of the extracellular fluid of the body, and when the extracellular hydrogen ion concentration increases, as in acidosis, potassium ions move from the cells into the extracellular fluid. When the extracellular hydrogen ion decreases, as in alkalosis, potassium ions move from the extracellular fluid into the cells. Extracellular acidosis produces hyperkalemia. Extracellular alkalosis produces hypokalemia. Potassium is most commonly depleted in the body by an increased rate of excretion by the kidneys or the GI tract or, more rarely, by the skin. Normal adult levels of blood potassium are 3.5 to 5.0 mEq/L or 3.5 to 5.0 mmol/L (SI units). Increased renal excretion may be caused by diuretic therapy, large doses of anionic drugs, or renal disorders. Increased GI secretion of potassium may occur with the loss of GI fluid through vomiting, diarrhea, surgical drainage, or the chronic use of laxatives. Potassium loss through the skin is rare but can result from perspiring during excessive exercise in a hot environment.

potassium chloride (KCl), a white crystalline salt used

Positions for postural drainage (From Potter PA and Perry AG Fundamentals of Nursing, ed. 3. St. Louis, Mosby, 1993.)

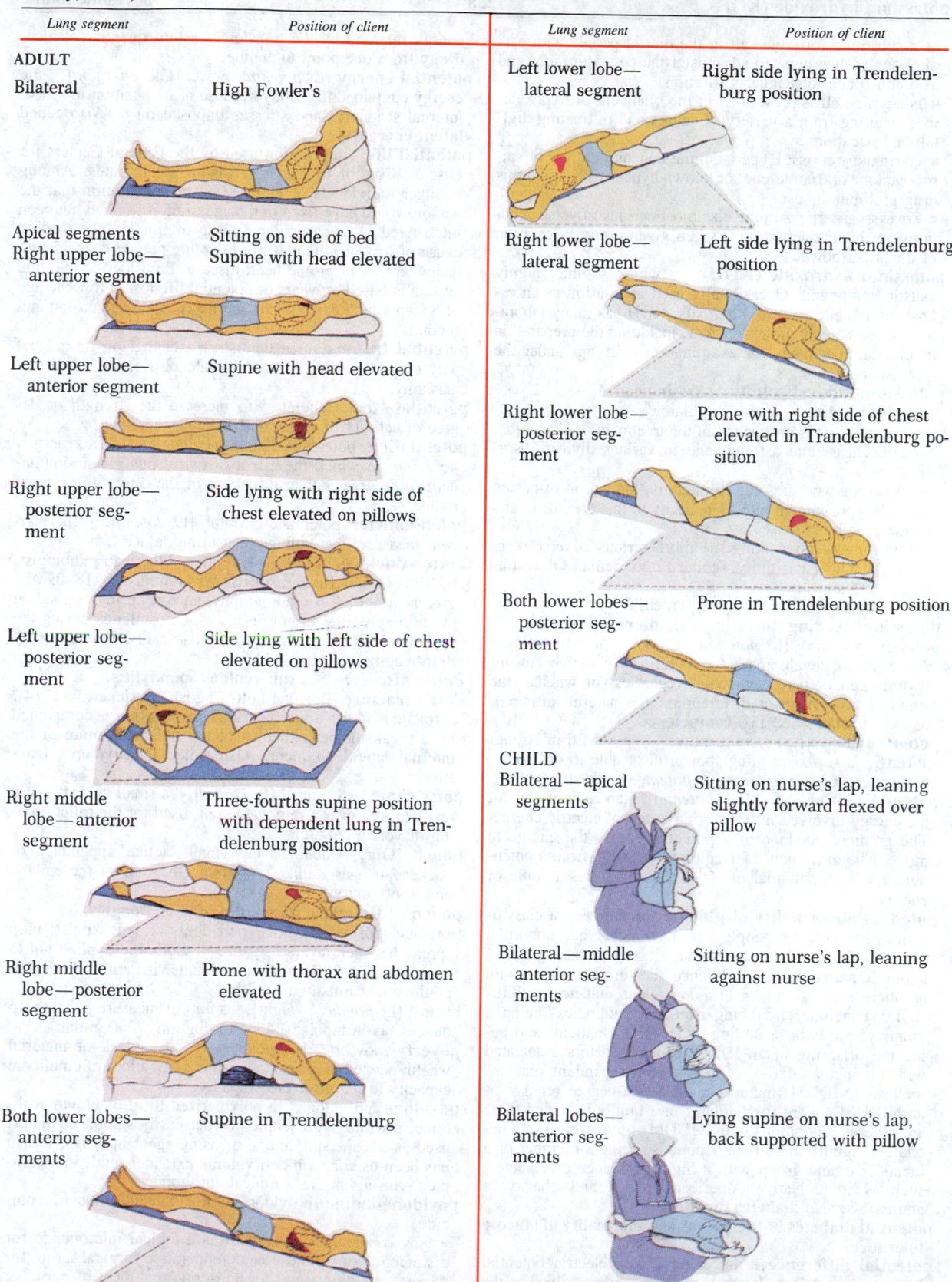

Lung segment	Position of client	Lung segment	Position of client

ADULT

Bilateral — High Fowler's

Apical segments Right upper lobe—anterior segment — Sitting on side of bed Supine with head elevated

Left upper lobe—anterior segment — Supine with head elevated

Right upper lobe—posterior segment — Side lying with right side of chest elevated on pillows

Left upper lobe—posterior segment — Side lying with left side of chest elevated on pillows

Right middle lobe—anterior segment — Three-fourths supine position with dependent lung in Trendelenburg position

Right middle lobe—posterior segment — Prone with thorax and abdomen elevated

Both lower lobes—anterior segments — Supine in Trendelenburg

Left lower lobe—lateral segment — Right side lying in Trendelenburg position

Right lower lobe—lateral segment — Left side lying in Trendelenburg position

Right lower lobe—posterior segment — Prone with right side of chest elevated in Trandelenburg position

Both lower lobes—posterior segment — Prone in Trendelenburg position

CHILD

Bilateral—apical segments — Sitting on nurse's lap, leaning slightly forward flexed over pillow

Bilateral—middle anterior segments — Sitting on nurse's lap, leaning against nurse

Bilateral lobes—anterior segments — Lying supine on nurse's lap, back supported with pillow

as a substitute for table salt in the diet of people with cardiovascular disorders, to administer the potassium ion, and as a constituent of Ringer's solution.

■ INDICATIONS: It is prescribed in the treatment of hypokalemia resulting from a variety of causes and in treating digitalis intoxication.

■ CONTRAINDICATIONS: Hyperkalemia, concomitant use of spironolactone or triamterene, or known hypersensitivity to this drug prohibits its use.

■ ADVERSE EFFECTS: Among the most serious adverse reactions are hyperkalemia and, when given orally, ulceration of the small bowel.

potassium hydroxide (KOH), a white, soluble, highly caustic compound. Occasionally used in solution as an escharotic for bites of rabid animals, KOH has many laboratory uses as an alkalinizing agent, including the preparation of clinical specimens for examination for fungi under the microscope.

potassium indoxyl sulfate. See **indican.**

potassium iodide, a bronchodilator.

■ INDICATIONS: It is prescribed in the treatment of bronchitis, bronchiectasis, and asthma, and in various thyroid disorders.

■ CONTRAINDICATIONS: Acute bronchitis, known or suspected pregnancy, or known hypersensitivity to this drug or to any iodide prohibits its use.

■ ADVERSE EFFECTS: Among the more serious adverse reactions are hypersensitivity, goiter, myxedema, GI disturbance, and skin lesions.

potassium penicillin V. See **penicillin V.**

potassium-sparing diuretic. See **diuretic.**

potency /pō′tənsē/ [L, *potentia*, power], (in embryology) the range of developmental possibilities of which an embryonic cell or part is capable, regardless of whether the stimulus for growth or differentiation is natural, artificial, or experimental. See also **competence.**

potent /pō′tənt/ [L, *potentia*, power], powerful or strong.

-potent, a suffix meaning 'powerful or able to do' something specified: *pluripotent, unipotent, viripotent.*

potential /pəten′shəl/ [L, *potentia*], an expression of the energy involved in transfering a unit of electric charge. The gradient or slope of a potential causes the charge to move. The movement of 1 colomb of charge from a potential of V to a potential of $V - 1$ volts requires 1 joule of energy.

potential abnormality of glucose tolerance, a classification that includes people who have never had abnormal glucose tolerance but who have an increased risk of diabetes or impaired glucose tolerance. Factors associated with an increased risk of insulin-dependent diabetes mellitus (IDDM) include circulating islet cell antibodies, being a monozygotic twin or sibling of an IDDM patient, and being the offspring of an IDDM patient. Factors associated with an increased risk of non-insulin-dependent diabetes mellitus (NIDDM) include being a first-degree relative of an NIDDM patient (particularly in a family in which there are several generations with NIDDM), giving birth to a neonate weighing more than 9 pounds, being a member of a racial or ethnic group with a high prevalence of diabetes, such as some Native American groups, and obesity in adults. See also **diabetes mellitus.**

potential diabetes. See **potential abnormality of glucose tolerance.**

potential difference, the difference in electric potential between two points. It represents the work involved in the

energy released by the transfer of a unit quantity of electricity from one point to another.

potential energy [L, *potentia*, power; Gk, *energeia*], the energy contained in a body because of its position in space, internal structure, and stresses imposed on it. Also called **latent energy.**

potential life, a criterion used by the Federal Centers for Disease Control to gauge premature death rates. Among younger individuals, it is based on an assumption that the person would have lived to the age of 65 if life had not been interrupted by a particular disease or injury. The leading cause of loss of potential life in young people is accidents, followed by cancer and heart disease. For older people, the system is based on years of potential life lost before the age of 85, in which case cancer and heart disease rank first and second.

potential trauma, (in dentistry) a change in tissue that may occur because of existing malocclusion or dental disharmony.

potentiate /pōten′shē·āt/, to increase the strength or degree of activity of something.

potentiation /pōten′shē·ā′shən/ [L, *potentia*], a synergistic action in which the effect of two drugs given simultaneously is greater than the effect of the drugs given separately.

potentiometer /pōten′shē·om′ətər/ [L, *potentia* + Gk, *metron*, measure], a voltage-measuring device.

Potter-Bucky grid [Hollis E. Potter, American radiologist, b. 1880; Gustav Bucky, American radiologist, b. 1880; ME, *gredire*, grate], (in radiography) an x-ray grid designed on the principle of a moving grid, which oscillates during the exposure of a radiographic film. Also called **Potter-Bucky diaphragm.** See also **grid.**

Pott's disease. See **tuberculous spondylitis.**

Pott's fracture [Percival Pott, English physician, b. 1714], a fracture of the fibula near the ankle, often accompanied by a break of the malleolus of the tibia or rupture of the internal lateral ligament. Also called **Dupuytren's fracture.**

potty chair [AS, *pott*; ME, *chaire*], a small chair that has an open seat over a removable pot, used for the toilet training of young children.

pouch [OFr, *pouche*], any small saclike appendage or pocket, such as Rathke's pouch in the roof of the embryonic roof cavity.

pouch of Douglas. See **cul-de-sac of Douglas.**

poultice /pōl′tis/ [L, *puls*, porridge], a soft, moist, pulp spread between layers of gauze or cloth and applied hot to a surface to provide heat or to counter irritation. A kind of poultice is a **mustard poultice.**

pound [L, *pondus*, weight], a unit of measure equal to 16 ounces, avoirdupois: 0.45359 kilogram; 7000 grains.

poverty /pov′ərtē/ [L, *paupertas*], **1.** a lack of material wealth needed to maintain existence. **2.** a loss of emotional capacity to feel love or sympathy.

povidone /pō′vidōn/, a polymerized form of vinylpyrrolidone, a white hygroscopic powder easily soluble in water, used as a dispersing and suspensing agent in drugs. It also has been used as a blood volume extender, and, in a complex with iodine, as a topical antiseptic.

povidone-iodine /pō′vidōnī′ədīn/, an antiseptic microbicide.

■ INDICATIONS: It is prescribed as a topical microbicide for disinfection of wounds, as a preoperative surgical scrub, for vaginal infections, and for antiseptic treatment of burns.

■ CONTRAINDICATIONS: Known hypersensitivity to this drug or to iodine prohibits its use.

■ ADVERSE EFFECTS: Among the more serious adverse reactions are local skin irritation, redness, and swelling.

Powassan virus infection [Powassan, Ontario], an uncommon form of encephalitis caused by a tick-borne arbovirus found in eastern Canada and the northern United States.

powder bed [L, *pulvis*, dust; AS, *bedd*], a treatment in which large areas of a patient's body are kept in contact with a powdered medication for a certain length of time. It is usually repeated three times a day, as necessary. An already made bed is prepared by placing a full-sized sheet lengthwise over the linen. The powder is spread on the sheet from a shaker. The patient lies supine on the powdered sheet. Areas of skin that are apposed are separated with gauze, and powder is shaken over the patient's body. The powdered sheet is then wrapped around the limbs and the trunk from the side to keep the powder in contact with the body. The patient is virtually helpless during treatment and requires close attention from the nurse.

powdered gold [L, *pulvis* + AS, *geolu*, yellow], a fine granulation of pure gold, produced by atomizing the molten metal or by chemical precipitation. It is used in some dental restorations, such as prepared tooth cavities, and is available as clusters of granules or as pellets of gold powder contained in an envelope of gold foil.

powerlessness /pow'ərləsnes'/ [Fr, *pouvoir*, to have power; AS, *loes*, limited, *nes*, condition], a nursing diagnosis accepted by the Fifth National Conference on the Classification of Nursing Diagnoses. Powerlessness is defined as a perceived lack of control over a current health-related situation or problem and the client's perception that any action he or she takes will not affect the outcome of the particular situation. The defining characteristics may be of a severe, moderate, or passive nature. Severe characteristics include the client's verbal expression of having no control or influence over self-care, the particular situation, or its outcome; apathy; or depression over physical deterioration that occurs despite compliance with regimens. Moderate characteristics include the client's nonparticipation in or lack of interest in the mode of care, in decision making regarding regimens, or in monitoring progress; the client's verbal expression of dissatisfaction and frustration regarding the inability to perform previous activities; the reluctance to express true feelings, fearing alienation of others; general irritability or passivity; and expressions of resentment, anger, guilt, or doubt regarding role performance. Passive characteristics involve expressions of uncertainty about fluctuating energy levels. Related factors include the health care environment, a regimen related to the illness, or a generalized lifestyle of helplessness. See also **nursing diagnosis.**

power of attorney [Fr, *pouvoir* + OFr, *atorne*, legal agent], a document authorizing one person to take legal actions in behalf of another, who acts as an agent for the grantor. The legality of a power of attorney may be challenged if the grantor can be found to have been mentally incompetent at the time the authority was granted.

power stroke, a working stroke with a dental scaling instrument, used for splitting or dislodging calculus from the surface of a tooth or tooth root.

pox [ME, *pokkes*, pustules], **1.** any of several vesicular or pustular exanthematous diseases. **2.** the pitlike scars of smallpox. **3.** *archaic.* syphilis.

poxvirus /poksvī'rəs/ [ME, *pokkes* + L, *virus*, poison], a

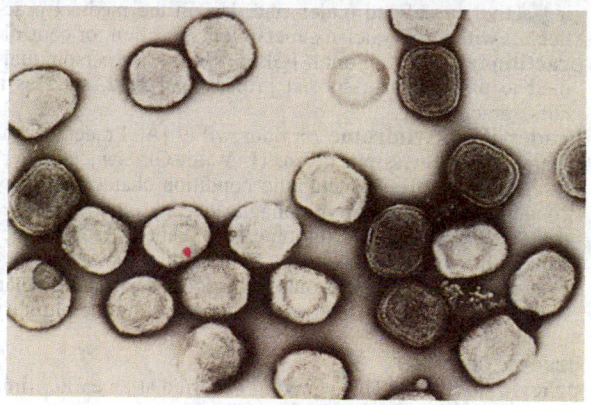

Poxvirus
(Murray, 1990/Courtesy Centers for Disease Control, Atlanta)

member of a family of viruses that includes the organisms that cause molluscum contagiosum, smallpox, and vaccinia.

PPD, abbreviation for **purified protein derivative.**

PPLO, abbreviation for **pleuropneumonia-like organism.** See *Mycoplasma.*

ppm, PPM abbreviation for **parts per million.**

PPMA, abbreviation for **postpoliomyelitis muscular atrophy**.

PPO, abbreviation for **preferred provider organization.**

PPS, abbreviation for **prospective payment system.**

PPV, abbreviation for *positive pressure ventilation.* See **positive pressure,** def. 2.

Pr, symbol for the element **praseodymium.**

practical anatomy. See **applied anatomy.**

practical nurse. See **licensed practical nurse.**

practice guideline, a detailed description of a process of patient care management that will facilitate improvement or maintenance of health status or slow the decline in health status in certain chronic clinical conditions. The purpose of a practice guideline is to assist health care providers to identify preferred treatment by providing linkages among diagnoses, treatments, and outcomes, and by describing alternatives available for each patient. Practice guidelines provide a basis for evaluation of care and allocation of resources.

practice models /prak'tis/ [Gk, *praktikos*, practical], the different patterns in delivery of health care services by means of which health care is made available to diverse groups of people in different settings.

practice setting, the context or environment within which nursing care is given.

practice theory, (in nursing research) a theory that describes, explains, and prescribes nursing practice in general. It serves as the basis for specific items in the curriculum of nursing education and for the development of theories in the administration of nursing and nursing education.

practicing /prak'tising/, the second subphase of the separation-individuation phase in Mahler's system of preoedipal development, when the child is able to move away from the mother and return to her. The child may feel elation in response to this investigation of the environment and through practicing locomotor skills.

practicing medicine without a license, (in law) practicing activities defined under state law in the medical practice act without physician supervision, direction, or control.

practitioner /praktish′ənər/ [Gk, *praktikos*], a person qualified to practice in a special professional field, such as a nurse practitioner.

Prader-Willi syndrome /prä′dər wil′ē/ [A. Prader, twentieth century Swiss physician; H. Willi; Gk, *syn*, together, *dromos,* course], a metabolic condition characterized by congenital hypotonia, hyperphagia, obesity, and mental retardation. When the development of diabetes mellitus occurs with the other symptoms, the condition is called Royer's syndrome. The syndrome is associated with a less than normal secretion of gonadotropic hormones by the pituitary gland.

prae-. See **pre-.**

praevia /prē′vē·ə/, [L], having occurred at an earlier time or in front of a place. Also **praevius.**

praecox [L, premature], pertaining to something that occurred at at earlier stage of life or development.

-pragia, a combining form meaning 'quality of action': *bradypragia, dyspragia, tachypragia.*

Pragmatar, a trademark for a topical, fixed-combination drug containing an antieczematic (cetyl alcohol–coal tar distillate), a keratolytic (salicylic acid), and a scabicide (precipitated sulfur).

pragmatic /pragmat′ik/, pertaining to a belief that ideas are valuable only in terms of their consequences.

pragmatism /prag′mətizəm/ [Gk, *pragma*, deed], a philosophy concerned with actual practice and practical results as opposed to theory and speculation.

pralidoxime chloride /pral′ədok′sēm/, a cholinesterase reactivator.

■ INDICATIONS: It is prescribed as an antidote for organophosphate poisoning and drug overdosage in the treatment of myasthenia gravis.

■ CONTRAINDICATION: Known hypersensitivity to this drug prohibits its use. It is contraindicated in poisoning by carbamate insecticides that react with pralidoxime.

■ ADVERSE EFFECTS: Among the most serious adverse reactions are dizziness, tachycardia, hyperventilation, and muscle weakness. These reactions are most common when the drug is injected too rapidly.

-pramine, a combining form for imipramine-type compounds.

Pramosone, a trademark for a topical, fixed-combination drug containing a glucocorticoid (hydrocortisone acetate) and a topical anesthetic (pramoxine hydrochloride).

pramoxine hydrochloride /prəmok′sēn/, a local anesthetic for the relief of pain and itching associated with dermatoses, anogenital pruritus, hemorrhoids, anal fissure, and minor burns.

prandial /pran′dē·əl/ [L, *prandium,* lunch], pertaining to a meal. The term is used in relation to timing, such as postprandial or preprandial. **–prandiality,** *n.*

praseodymium (Pr) /prä′sē·ōdīm′ē·əm/ [Gk, *prasaios,* light-green, *didymos,* twin], a rare earth metallic element. Its atomic number is 59; its atomic weight is 140.91.

Prausnitz-Küstner (PK) test /prous′nitskist′nər/ [Otto C. W. Prausnitz, Polish bacteriologist, b. 1876; Heinz Küstner, Polish gynecologist, b. 1897], a skin test in which an allergic response is transferred to a nonallergic person who acts as a surrogate to permit identification of the allergen. After the allergic patient is screened for hepatitis and other serum-borne diseases, a small amount of the patient's serum is injected intradermally into several sites on a nonallergic person (usually a relative). After 24 to 48 hours, suspected antigens are applied to these sites on the nonallergic person. A sensitive skin response (wheal and flare reaction) indicates that the suspect antigen is indeed causing hypersensitivity in the allergic patient. The Prausnitz-Küstner test is performed only when skin sensitivity testing cannot be performed directly on the allergic patient. Also called **passive transfer test, PK test.** Compare **patch test, radioallergosorbent test.** See also **anaphylaxis.**

-praxia, a combining form meaning 'to achieve or to do (perform)': *dyspraxia, eupraxia, hypopraxia.*

praxis [Gk, action], a concept that deals with actions and overt behavior, or the performance of an action to the exclusion of metaphysical thought.

-praxis /prak′sis/, a combining form meaning 'to achieve, doing, an act, or treatment based on theory': *actinopraxis, echopraxis, parapraxis.*

prazepam /praz′əpam/, an antianxiety agent derived from benzodiazepine.

■ INDICATIONS: It is prescribed for the treatment of anxiety disorders or the short-term relief of symptoms of anxiety.

■ CONTRAINDICATIONS: Acute narrow-angle glaucoma or known sensitivity to this drug or other benzodiazepines prohibits its use.

■ ADVERSE EFFECTS: Among the more serious, but rare, adverse reactions are confusion, tremor, palpitations, and diaphoresis.

-prazole, a combining form for antiulcerative benzimidazole derivatives.

prazosin hydrochloride /prä′zəsin/, an antihypertensive.

■ INDICATIONS: It is prescribed in the treatment of hypertension and to decrease afterload in congestive heart disease.

■ CONTRAINDICATIONS: Known hypersensitivity to this drug prohibits its use. Concomitant use with beta blockers may result in loss of consciousness.

■ ADVERSE EFFECTS: Among the more serious adverse reactions are tachycardia, fainting, drowsiness, angina, and a sudden drop in blood pressure after the initial dose.

pre-, prae-, a prefix meaning 'before or in front of': *preataxic, precritical, pregenital.*

preadmission certification /prē′ədmish′ən/, a system whereby physicians are required to obtain advance approval for nonemergency admission of Medicare patients to hospitals. The system is intended to determine whether the patient can be treated as an outpatient or in another, less expensive manner than hospitalization. Emergency admissions require post hoc approval.

preagonal ascites /prē·ag′ənəl/ [L, *prae,* before; Gk, *agon,* struggle; *askos,* bag], a rapid accumulation of fluid within the peritoneal cavity, representing the transudation of serum from the circulatory system. Preagonal ascites immediately precedes death in some cases. See also **ascites.**

preanesthetic medication. See **premedication.**

preaortic node /prē′ā·ôr′tik/ [L, *prae* + Gk, *aerein,* to raise; L *nodus* knot], a node in one of the three sets of lumbar lymph nodes that serve various abdominal viscera supplied by the celiac, superior mesenteric, and inferior mesenteric arteries. The preaortic nodes lie ventral to the aorta and are divided into the celiac nodes, superior mesenteric nodes, and inferior mesenteric nodes. Most of the efferent vessels from the preaortic nodes unite to form the lymphatic intestinal trunk that enters the cisterna chyli. Compare **lateral aortic node, retroaortic node.**

precancerous /-kan'sərəs/ [L, *pre* + *cancer*, crab], pertaining to a stage of abnormal tissue growth that is likely to develop into a malignant tumor.

precancerous dermatitis. See **intraepidermal carcinoma.**

precedent /pres'ədənt/ [L, *praecedere*, to go before], a previously adjudged decision that serves as an authority in a similar case.

Precef, a trademark for a cephalosporin-type antibiotic (ceforanide).

precentral gyrus /-sen'trəl/ [L, *pre*; Gk, *kentron*, center, *gyros*, turn], a convolution of the cerebral hemisphere immediately anterior to the central sulcus of the cerebrum in each hemisphere. It is the location of the motor strip that controls voluntary movements of the contralateral side of the body.

preceptorship /-sep'tərship'/ [L, *prae* + *capere*, to take up], the position of teacher or instructor, also a nurse who serves as a preceptor for a new graduate.

precession /-sesh'ən/ [L, *praecedere*, to go before], a comparatively slow gyration of the axis of a spinning body, so as to trace out a cone, caused by the application of a torque. The magnetic moment of a nucleus with spin will experience such a torque when inclined at an angle to the magnetic field, resulting in precession at the Larmor frequency.

precipitant /-sip'ətənt/ [L, *praecipitare*, to throw down], a substance that causes another substance to settle, separate, or deposit from a solution, such as a reagent that causes certain metals to precipitate.

precipitate /prəsip'itāt, -it/ [L, *praecipitare*, to cast down], **1.** to cause a substance to separate or to settle out of solution. **2.** a substance that has separated from or settled out of a solution. **3.** occurring hastily or unexpectedly.

precipitate delivery /-sip'itit/, childbirth that occurs with such speed or in such a situation that the usual preparations cannot be made. See also **emergency childbirth.**

precipitating factor /-sip'itā'ting/, an element that causes or contributes to the occurrence of a disorder.

precipitation /-sip'itā'shən/ [L, *praecipitare*, to throw down], a process whereby solid particles are made to settle out of a solution so they can be separated from other dissolved substances.

precipitin /prəsip'itin/ [L, *praecipitare* + Gk, *anti*, against; AS *bodig* body; Gk, *genein* to produce], an antibody that causes formation of an insoluble complex when combined with a specific soluble antigen. Compare **agglutinin.** See also **agglutination, antiglobulin.**

precision rest /prisish'ən/ [L, *praecidere*, to cut short; AS, *rest*], a rigid denture support consisting of two tightly fitting parts, the insert of which rests firmly against the gingival portion of the device.

preclinical /-klin'ikəl/ [L, *pre*; Gk, *kline*, bed], a stage in a disease when a specific diagnosis cannot be made because adequate signs and symptoms have not yet developed.

precocious /-kō'shəs/ [L, *praecoquere*, to mature early], pertaining to the early, often premature, development of physical or mental qualities.

precocious carrier. See **amebic carrier state.**

precocious dentition, the abnormal acceleration of the eruption of the deciduous or permanent teeth, usually associated with an endocrine imbalance, such as excess pituitary growth hormone or hyperthyroidism. Compare **retarded dentition.**

precocious puberty [L, *praecoquere*, early ripening; *pubertas*], abnormally early development of sexual maturity. It is usually marked by ovulation in girls before the age of 8 and the production of mature sperm in a boy before the age of 10.

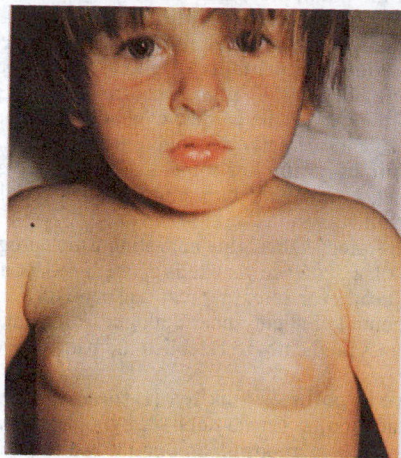

Precocious puberty (Dynski-Klien, 1986)

precognition /-kognish'ən/, the alleged intuitive foreknowledge of events. Compare **premonition.**

preconscious /-kon'shəs/ [L, *prae*, before, *conscire*, to be aware], **1.** before the development of self-consciousness and self-awareness. **2.** (in psychiatry) the mental function in which thoughts, ideas, emotions, or memories not in immediate awareness can be brought into the consciousness, usually through associations, without encountering any intrapsychic resistance or repression. **3.** the mental phenomena capable of being recalled, although not present in the conscious mind.

precordia /prekôr'dē·ə/ [L, *pre* + *cor*, heart], pertaining to the front area of the thorax that lies over the heart.

precordial /prēkôr'dē·əl/ [L, *prae* + *cor*, heart], of or pertaining to the precordium, which forms the region over the heart and the lower part of the thorax.

precordial lead /lēd/ [L, *pre*, before + *cor*, heart; AS *laedan*], an electrocardiographic lead from the chest wall over the heart. Also called **chest lead.**

precordial movement, any motion of the anterior wall of the thorax localized in the area over the heart. Kinds of precordial movements include **apical impulse, left ventricular thrust,** and **right ventricular thrust.**

precordial pain [L, *pre*, before + *cor*, heart; *poena*, penalty], a pain in the chest wall area over the heart.

precordium /-kôr'dē·əm/ [L, *pre*, before + *cor*, heart], the part of the front of the chest wall that overlays the heart and the epigastrium.

precursor /-kur'sər/ [L, *prae* + *currere*, to run], a prognostic characteristic or feature of a patient's health data, such as an x-ray or laboratory finding, that is associated with a higher or lower risk of death than the average.

precursor therapy, a type of treatment involving the use of nutrients that may influence neurologic clinical conditions. An example is the use of choline, a B complex vitamin precursor of acetylcholine, in the treatment of tardive dyskinesia.

-pred, pred-, a combining form for prednisone or prednisolone derivatives.

predeciduous dentition /-disid′yoo·əs/ [L, *prae* + *decidere*, to fall off], the epithelial structures found in the mouth of the infant preceding the eruption of the deciduous teeth. See also **deciduous dentition, teething.**

prediabetes. See **potential abnormality of glucose tolerance, previous abnormality of glucose tolerance.**

prediastole /-dī·as′təlē/ [L, *pre*, before; Gk, *dia* + *stellein*, to set], the part of the cardiac cycle between the late systolic phase and the early diastolic phase.

prediastolic murmur /-dī·əstol′ik/ [L, *pre*; Gk, *dia* + *stellein*, to set; L, *murmur*, humming], a murmur heard during the cardiac systole.

predicate /pred′ikāt/, (in neurolinguistic programming) the part of a sentence that tells something about the subject. Predicates can refer to direct sensory experience or they can be neutral. Patient-nurse dialogues often make use of the patient's predicates to establish the patient's sensory experience.

predictive hypothesis /-dik′tiv/ [L, *prae* + *dicere*, to say; Gk, foundation], (in research) a hypothesis that predicts the nature of a relationship among the variables to be studied.

predictive validity, validity of a test or a measurement tool that is established by demonstrating its ability to predict the results of an analysis of the same data using another test instrument or measurement ool. See also **validity.**

predictor variable. See **independent variable.**

predisposing cause /-dispō′sing/ [L, *pre* + *disponere*, to arrange, *causa*], any condition that enhances the specific cause of a disease, such as being susceptible because of hereditary or lifestyle factors.

predisposing factor [L, *prae* + *disponere*, to dispose], any conditioning factor that influences both the type and amount of resources that the individual can elicit to cope with stress. It may be biologic, psychologic, or sociocultural in nature.

predisposition /-dis′pəzish′ən/ [L, *pre* + *disponere*, to arrange], a state of being particularly susceptible.

prednisolone /prednis′əlōn/, a glucocorticoid.
- INDICATIONS: It is prescribed as treatment for inflammation of the skin, conjunctiva, and cornea, and for immunosuppression.
- CONTRAINDICATIONS: Fungal infections or known hypersensitivity to this drug prohibits its systemic use. Viral or fungal infections of the skin, impaired circulation, or known hypersensitivity to this drug prohibits its topical use.
- ADVERSE EFFECTS: Among the more serious adverse reactions to the systemic administration of this drug are GI, endocrine, neurologic, fluid, and electrolyte disturbances. A variety of skin reactions may occur from topical administration of this drug.

prednisone /pred′nisōn/, a glucocorticoid.
- INDICATIONS: It is prescribed in severe inflammation and immunosuppression.
- CONTRAINDICATIONS: Viral or fungal infections of the skin, impaired circulation, or known hypersensitivity to this drug prohibits its use.
- ADVERSE EFFECTS: Among the more serious adverse reactions to the systemic administration of the drug are GI, endocrine, neurologic, fluid, and electrolyte disturbances. A

variety of skin reactions may occur from topical administration of this drug.

preeclampsia /prē′iklamp′sē·ə/ [L, *prae* + Gk, *ek*, out, *lampein*, to flash], an abnormal condition of pregnancy characterized by the onset of acute hypertension after the twenty-fourth week of gestation. The classic triad of preeclampsia is hypertension, proteinuria, and edema. The cause of the disease remains unknown despite 100 years of research by thousands of investigators. It occurs in 5% to 7% of pregnancies, most often in primigravidas, and is more common in some areas of the world than others; the incidence is particularly high in the southeastern portion of the United States. The incidence increases with increasing gestational age, and it is more common with multiple gestation, hydatidiform mole, or hydramnios. A typical lesion in the kidneys, glomeruloendotheliosis, is pathognomonic. Termination of the pregnancy results in resolution of the signs and symptoms of the disease and in healing of the renal lesion. Preeclampsia is classified as mild or severe. Mild preeclampsia is diagnosed if one or more of the following signs develop after the twenty-fourth week of gestation: systolic blood pressure of 140 mm Hg or more or a rise of 30 mm or more above the woman's usual systolic blood pressure; diastolic blood pressure of 90 mm Hg or more or a rise of 15 mm or more above the woman's usual diastolic blood pressure; proteinuria, and edema. Severe preeclampsia is diagnosed if one or more of the following is present: systolic blood pressure of 160 mm Hg or more or a diastolic blood pressure of 110 mm Hg or more on two occasions 6 hours apart with the woman at bed rest; proteinuria of 5 g or more in 24 hours; oliguria of less than 400 ml in 24 hours; ocular or cerebral vascular disorders, and cyanosis or pulmonary edema. Preeclampsia commonly causes abnormal metabolic function, including negative nitrogen balance, increased central nervous system irritability, hyperactive reflexes, compromised renal function, hemoconcentration, and alterations of fluid and electrolyte balance. Complications include premature separation of the placenta, hypofibrinogenemia, hemolysis, cerebral hemorrhage, ophthalmologic damage, pulmonary edema, hepatocellular

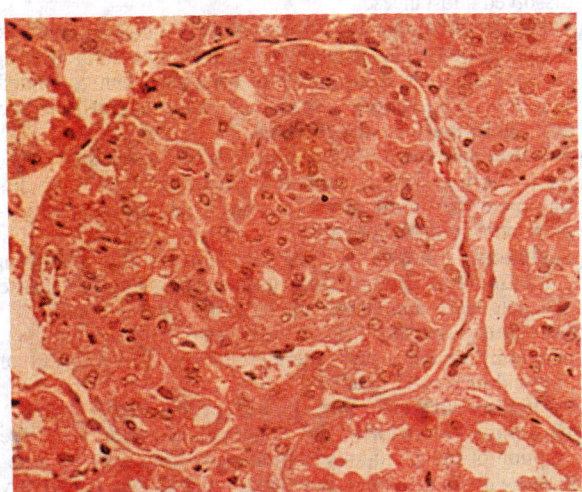

Renal changes in preeclampsia
(*Swales, 1991/Courtesy Professor P Kincaid-Smith*)

changes, fetal malnutrition, and lowered birth weight. The most serious complication is eclampsia, which can result in maternal and fetal death. Healthy living conditions, including a diet high in protein, calories, and essential nutritional elements, and rest and exercise are associated with a decreased incidence of preeclampsia. Treatment includes rest, sedation, magnesium sulfate, and antihypertensives. Ultimately, if eclampsia threatens, delivery by induction of labor or cesarean section may be necessary. See also **eclampsia.** Also called **toxemia of pregnancy.**

preemie. See **premature infant.**

preexcitation /prē′eksitā′shən/ [L, *prae* + *excitare,* to arouse], activation of part of the ventricular myocardium earlier than would be expected if the activating impulses traveled only down the normal routes or had experienced a normal delay within the AV node. This may be a result of either an AV accessory (Wolff-Parkinson-White syndrome), which is reflected on the electrocardiogram by a short PR and broad QRS, or an excessively fast intranodal pathway (Lown-Ganong-Levine syndrome), which manifests with a short PR and a normal QRS. The degree of preexcitation is determined by how fast the impulse traverses the atrial tissue and the accessory pathway or the AV node. See also **accessory pathway.**

preexisting condition /prē′iksis′ting/ [L, *pre* + *existere,* to have reality, *conditio*], any injury, disease, or disability that may have occurred at some time in the past and might predispose an individual to limited health in the future.

preferential anosmia /pref′əren′shəl/ [L, *praeferens,* being preferred; Gk, *a, osme,* not smell], the inability to smell certain odors. The condition is often caused by psychologic factors concerning either a particular smell or the situation in which the smell occurs.

preferred provider organization (PPO) /-furd′/ [L, *praeferre,* to put before], an organization of physicians, hospitals, and pharmacists whose members discount their health care services to subscriber patients. A PPO may be organized by a group of physicians, an outside entrepreneur, an insurance company, or a company with a self-insurance plan. See also **health maintenance organization.**

preformation /-fôrmā′shən/ [L, *prae* + *formatio,* formation], an early theory in embryology in which the organism is contained in minute and complete form within the germ cell and after fertilization grows from microscopic to normal size. Compare **epigenesis.**

preformed water /-fôrmd′/ [L, *prae* + *forma,* form; AS, *waeter*], the water that is contained in foods.

prefrontal lobotomy /-frôn′təl/ [L, *prae* + *frons,* forehead; Gk, *lobos,* lobe, *temnein,* to cut], a surgical procedure in which connecting fibers between the prefrontal lobes of the brain and the thalamus are severed. An archaic technique, it is rarely used today but formerly was an accepted procedure for treating schizophrenic patients with uncontrollable, destructive behavior. After surgery, patients were often apathetic, docile, and lacking social graces. If only the white fibers are severed, the procedure is called a prefrontal leucotomy.

preg. abbreviation for **pregnancy.**

preganglionic neuron /-gang′glē·on′·ik/ [L, *pre*; Gk, *gagglion,* knot, *neurom,* nerve], a neuron whose axon terminates in contact with another nerve cell located in a peripheral ganglion.

Pregestimil, a trademark for a hypoallergenic, nutritional supplement for infants.

pregnancy (preg) /preg′nənsē/ [L, *praegnans* pregnant],

the gestational process, comprising the growth and development within a woman of a new individual from conception through the embryonic and fetal periods to birth. Pregnancy lasts approximately 266 days (38 weeks) from the day of fertilization, but it is clinically considered to last 280 days (40 weeks; 10 lunar months; 91/3 calendar months) from the first day of the last menstrual period. The expected date of delivery (EDD) is calculated on the latter basis even if a woman's periods are irregular. If a woman is certain that coitus occurred only once during the month of conception and if she knows the date on which coitus occurred, the EDC may be calculated as 266 days from that date. Pregnancy begins after coitus at or near the time of ovulation (usually about 14 days before a woman's next expected menstrual period). Of the millions of ejaculated sperm cells, thousands reach the female ovum in the outer end of the fallopian tube, but usually only one penetrates the egg for union of the male and female pronuclei and conception. The zygote, genetically a unique entity, begins cell division as it is transported to the uterine cavity, where it implants in the uterine wall. Maternal and embryologic elements together form the beginnings of the placenta, which grows into the substance of the uterus. The placenta functions in maternal-fetal exchange of nutrients and waste products, although the maternal and fetal bloods do not normally mix. The conceptus is, in some aspects, like a foreign graft or transplant in the mother. Although the mother normally does not activate an immune response, all of her tissues and organs undergo change, many of them profound and some of them permanent.

■ PSYCHOLOGIC CHANGES: The emotional experiences of pregnancy, as reported by pregnant women, are normal and healthy, but extraordinary. A pregnant woman is 'herself,' but in a very unfamiliar way. She has a sense of heightened function and expectancy. Being keenly aware of the rapid and inevitable changes her body is undergoing, she is more intensely interested in herself. Her concern for the perfection of her baby, her anticipation of the exertion of labor, and her contemplation of the new or expanded responsibilities of motherhood all serve to intensify her emotional tone.

■ CARDIOVASCULAR CHANGES: Cardiac output increases 30% to 50% in pregnancy. The increase begins at about the sixth week, reaches a maximum about the sixteenth week, declines slightly after the thirtieth week, and rapidly falls off after delivery. It returns to prepregnancy level about the sixth week postpartum. The stroke volume of the heart increases, and the pulse rate becomes more rapid: Normal pulse rate in pregnancy is approximately 80 to 90 beats per minute. Blood pressure may drop slightly after the twelfth week of gestation and return to its usual level after the twenty-sixth week. The circulation of blood to the pregnant uterus near term is about one liter per minute, requiring about 20% of the total cardiac output. Total blood volume also increases in pregnancy; plasma volume increases more than red cell volume, and this results in a drop in the hematocrit, caused by dilution. The white blood cells increase: The normal WBC count in pregnancy is often over 15,000/ml.

■ PULMONARY CHANGES: Although vital capacity and Po$_2$ remain the same in pregnancy, respiratory rate, tidal and minute volumes, and plasma pH increase. Inspiratory and expiratory reserves, residual volume and residual capacity, and plasma Pco$_2$ diminish.

■ RENAL CHANGES: The glomerular filtration rate (GFR) and

the renal plasma flow increase approximately 30% to 50% in pregnancy; the pattern of change closely parallels that of cardiac function. A marked dilatation of the excretory tract often occurs and is called hydronephrosis of pregnancy. It is the result of the pressure exerted on the ureters by the enlarging uterus and by the influence of the hormone progesterone. Blood urea nitrogen (BUN) normally increases as much as 10 mg/dl, and blood creatinine drops to approximately 0.7 mg/dl. Positional influences on renal function are more marked in pregnancy because of the pressure of the uterus on the great vessels. Renal function is better in the recumbent position than in the standing position and is better in the left lateral recumbent position than in the supine position.

■ GASTROINTESTINAL CHANGES: Progesterone, which is increased in pregnancy, causes some relaxation of GI smooth muscle. Heartburn may result from delayed gastric emptying and relaxation of the sphincter at the gastroesophageal junction. Decreased colonic motility and pressure on the rectum and sigmoid colon from the enlarging uterus may result in constipation. Nausea and vomiting may occur, usually early in pregnancy, probably caused by the effect of human chorionic gonadotropin. The incidence of gallbladder disease is slightly increased.

■ ENDOCRINE CHANGES: Protein binding is increased in pregnancy. Because most hormones are circulated in protein-bound forms, the function of most endocrine glands is altered. Thyroid function changes markedly in a way that mimics hyperthyroidism as indicated by a thyroid test. Adrenal hormone levels are increased and are probably responsible for striae gravidarum, which are similar to the striae of hyperadrenalism. Sugar metabolism is altered by estrogen, progesterone, and glucocorticoids; the need for insulin is increased. The placenta produces four hormones: human chorionic gonadotropin (HCG), progesterone, estrogen, and human placental lactogen (HPL). HCG prolongs the life of the corpus luteum early in pregnancy. Progesterone functions to support the modified endometrium of the uterus, called the decidua, and to stimulate the development of the breast acini. Estrogen stimulates uterine and breast growth. HPL stimulates the growth and development of breast tissue in preparation for lactation; it also has an antiinsulin effect for the sparing of maternal glucose for the benefit of the fetus.

■ BREAST CHANGES: The breasts become firm and tender early in pregnancy. This tenderness constitutes a subjective symptom of pregnancy. As the breasts enlarge and soften, the tenderness disappears. The areola around the nipple becomes more deeply pigmented, and the areolar glands become prominent. As the tubules and acini of the mammary glands develop, a clear or whitish watery material, called colostrum, begins to issue from the nipple.

■ SKIN CHANGES: Perspiration increases. Erythema of the thenar and hypothenar eminences of the palms becomes apparent. Hair growth may be stimulated. Telangiectasias are extremely common. Striae over the abdomen, breasts, and buttocks appear in some women. New deposits of the pigment melanin cause freckles to intensify; the linea nigra in the midline of the lower abdomen becomes darker and may extend nearly to the xiphoid process. There may be a darkening of the skin of the face over the nose across the malar eminences and above the eyebrows. This is called chloasma, or the 'mask of pregnancy.'

■ WEIGHT CHANGES: Normal weight gain may vary within wide limits in pregnancy. Average weight gain is 25 to 30 pounds, but greater increases are common without ill effects.

■ NUTRITIONAL CHANGES: Requirements for dietary iron, protein, and calcium increase out of proportion to the need for an overall increase in intake of calories and other nutrients.

pregnancy gingivitis, an enlargement or hyperplasia of the gingivae caused by hormonal imbalance during pregnancy. It is usually limited to the interdental papillae.

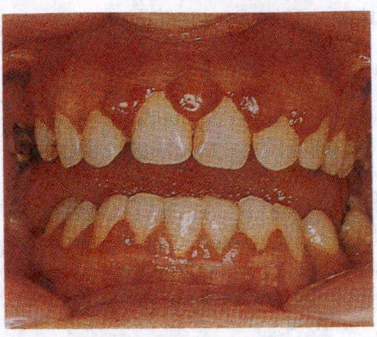

Pregnancy gingivitis (Lamey, 1988)

pregnancy luteoma. See **luteoma.**

pregnancy rate, (in statistics) the ratio of pregnancies per 100 woman-years, calculated as the product of the number of pregnancies in the women observed multiplied by 12 (months), divided by the product of the number of women observed multiplied by the number of months observed. For example, if 50 women used one contraceptive method for 12 months and 5 of them became pregnant, the pregnancy rate would be 10 per 100 woman-years.

pregnancy test. See **HCG radioreceptor assay.**

pregnanediol /pregnān′dē·ol/, a crystalline, biologically inactive compound found in the urine of women during pregnancy or the secretory phase of the menstrual cycle. A dihydroxy derivative of the saturated steroid pregnane, pregnanediol is formed by the reduction of progesterone.

pregnant /preg′nənt/ [L, *praegnans*], gravid, with child.

prehensile /-hen′sil/ [L, *prehendre*, to seize], able to grasp.

prehension /-hen′shən/, the use of the hands and fingers to grasp or pick up objects.

prehospital care, any initial medical care given an ill or injured patient by a paramedic or other person before the patient reaches the hospital emergency department.

preinvasive carcinoma. See **carcinoma in situ.**

preload /prē′lōd/ [L, *prae* + AS, *lad*], the stretch of myocardial fiber at end diastole. The ventricular end diastolic pressure and volume reflect this parameter.

preload filling pressure, the load on the ventricular muscle fibers at the end of diastole or just before contraction. The preload on the heart is estimated by the left ventricular filling pressure. Cardiac performance increases with preload to a point.

Preludin, a trademark for an anorexiant (phenmetrazine hydrochloride).

premalignant fibroepithelioma /-məlig′nənt/ [L, *prae* + *malignus*, bad disposition, *fibra*, fiber; Gk, *epi*, above, *thele,* nipple, *oma,* tumor], an elevated Caucasian-flesh-colored sessile neoplasm formed of interlacing ribbons of epithelial cells on a hyperplastic mesodermal stroma. The tumor occurs most often on the lower trunk of older people and may be found in association with or develop into superficial basal cell carcinoma.

Premarin, a trademark for conjugated estrogens.

Premarin with Methyltestosterone, a trademark for a hormonal, fixed-combination drug containing Premarin and an androgen (methyltestosterone).

premarket approval (P.M.A.) /-mâr′kit/, permission given by the federal government to equipment manufacturers to sell their devices to the medical profession.

premature /-məcho̅o̅r′/ [L, *prae* + *maturare,* to ripen], **1.** not fully developed or mature. **2.** occurring before the appropriate or usual time. **–prematurity,** *n.*

premature alopecia [L, *praematurus,* too soon; Gk, *alopex,* fox mange], acquired baldness in a person who is not old.

premature atrial complex, a cardiac dysrhythmia characterized by an atrial depolarization occurring earlier than expected, indicated electrocardiographically as an early P wave. Premature atrial complexes may occur occasionally, or in a regular pattern, or several may occur in sequence. The dysrhythmia may be the result of atrial enlargement or ischemia, or may be increased by stress, caffeine, or nicotine. Isolated premature atrial beats usually have no significance, but their frequent occurrence may lead to atrial tachycardia or fibrillation and to decreased cardiac output. Also called **atrial premature beat.**

premature beat [L, *praematurus,* too soon; AS, *beatan*], a heart contraction, usually ectopic, that occurs earlier than expected in the ongoing rhythm pattern.

premature contraction, any contraction of either the ventricle or atrium that occurs early with respect to the dominant rhythm.

premature ejaculation, uncontrollable, untimely ejaculation of semen often caused by anxiety during sexual intercourse. Behavioral techniques can be learned by the man and his partner to extend the length of time between erection and ejaculation. See also **ejaculation, erection.**

premature impulse, any impulse that occurs early with respect to a dominant rhythm.

premature infant, any neonate, regardless of birth weight, born before 37 weeks of gestation. Because exact gestational age is often difficult to determine, low birth weight is a significant criterion for identifying the high-risk infant with incomplete organ system development. Predisposing factors associated with prematurity include multiple pregnancy, toxemia, chronic disease, acute infection, sensitization to blood incompatibility, and any severe trauma that may interfere with normal fetal development. In most instances the cause is unknown. The incidence of prematurity is highest among women from low socioeconomic circumstances for whom poor nutrition and lack of prenatal medical care are often precipitating factors. The premature infant usually appears small and scrawny, with a large head in relation to body size, and weighs less than 2500 g. The skin is bright pink, smooth, shiny, and translucent with the underlying vessels clearly visible. The arms and legs are extended, not flexed, as in the full-term infant. There is little subcutaneous fat, sparse hair, few creases on the soles and palms, and poorly developed ear cartilage. In boys, the scrotum has few rugae and the testes may be undescended; in girls, the labia gape and the clitoris is prominent. Among the common problems of the premature infant are variations in thermoregulation, chilling, apnea, respiratory distress, sepsis, poor sucking and swallowing reflexes, small stomach capacity, lowered tolerance of the alimentary tract that may lead to necrotizing enterocolitis, immature renal function, hepatic dysfunction often associated with hyperbilirubinemia, incomplete enzyme systems, and susceptibility to various metabolic upsets, such as hypoglycemia, hyperglycemia, and hypocalcemia. The degree of complications and the rate of survival of premature infants are directly related to the state of physiologic and anatomic maturity of the various organ systems at the time of birth, the condition of the infant other than prematurity, and the quality of postnatal care. With treatment in a neonatal intensive care unit, survival rates improve yearly. Increasing numbers of very small babies develop normally, and those who do not have seizures or apneic spells in the first few days will not suffer neurologic or physical sequelae of their prematurity. Of primary concern for the nurse caring for the premature infant is the stabilization of body temperature by maintaining a neutral thermal environment, the maintenance of respiration, the prevention of infection, the provision of adequate nutrition and hydration, and the conservation of energy. Important functions of the nurse are to involve the parents in the care of the infant, to explain therapeutic procedures, and to facilitate attachment between the infant and family. Also called **(informal) preemie, preterm infant.** Compare **postmature infant.** (See Figs. p. 1266.)

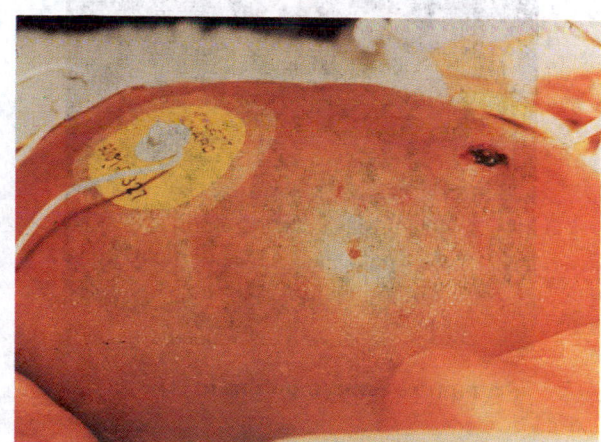

Skin of premature infant (*Zitelli, 1992*)

premature labor, labor that occurs earlier in pregnancy than normal, either before the fetus has reached a weight of 2000 to 2500 g or before the thirty-seventh or thirty-eighth week of gestation. No single measure of fetal weight or gestational age is used universally to designate premature birth; local or institutional policy dictates which of several standards is applied. Prematurity is a concomitant of 75% of births that result in neonatal mortality. It may occur spontaneously, or it may be brought about iatrogenically. The incidence of premature labor increases in inverse proportion to maternal age, weight, and socioeconomic status. Incidence is higher for black women, for women who have not

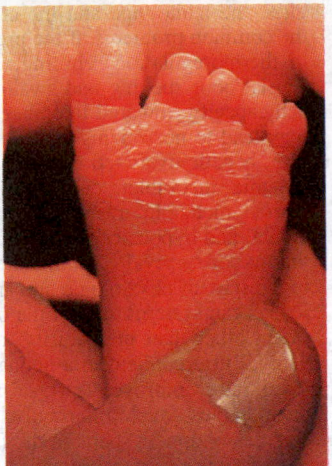
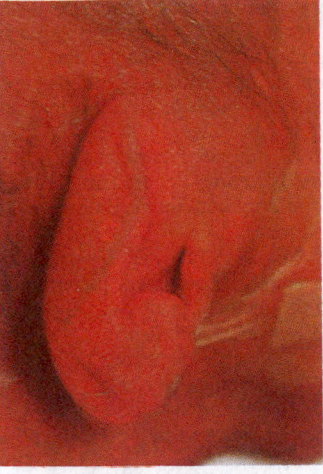

Sole creases and ear cartilage of premature infant
(Zitelli, 1992)

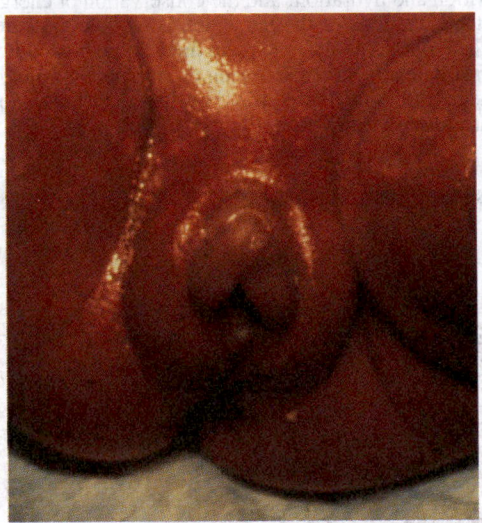

Premature female genitalia *(Zitelli, 1992)*

had adequate prenatal care or whose obstetric history is abnormal, and for women who smoke or whose diets are deficient in protein or calories. Predisposing conditions include maternal infection, low weight gain, uterine bleeding, multiple gestation, polyhydramnios, uterine abnormalities, incompetent cervix, premature rupture of membranes, and intrauterine fetal growth retardation. The cause of premature labor is poorly understood; in some cases, there may be several contributing causes. In some pregnancies, premature labor may be homeostatic, resulting in the best possible outcome under the particular, abnormal conditions. If premature labor itself constitutes a threat to the fetus, the outcome of pregnancy may be improved if labor can be inhibited. Determining accurately which pregnancies are likely to benefit from the inhibition of labor and which are not is difficult. Medications used to stop labor are not al-

ways effective. Misdiagnosis of gestational age and fetal condition may lead to induction of labor that is inadvertently premature; premature babies whose births have been brought about inappropriately early account for 15% of admissions to newborn intensive care nurseries. Also called **preterm labor.** See also **small for gestational age infant.**
premature rupture of membranes, the spontaneous rupture of the amniotic sac before the onset of labor.
premature systole [L, *praematurus;* Gk, *systole,* contraction], a systole that occurs too early as a result of a discharge of an ectopic focus in the atria, atrioventricular junction, or ventricle.
premature thelarche. See **thelarche.**
premature ventricular contraction (PVC), a cardiac sinus conducted dysrhythmia characterized by ventricular depolarization occurring earlier than expected, shown on the electrocardiogram as an early, wide QRS complex without a preceding related P wave. Premature ventricular complexes may occur occasionally, in a regular pattern, or as several in sequence. They may be caused by stress, acidosis, electrolyte imbalance, hypoxemia, hypercapnia, ventricular enlargement, or a toxic reaction to drugs. Isolated PVCs are not clinically significant in healthy individuals, but they may produce decreased cardiac output in people with heart disease, and frequent PVCs may be a precursor of ventricular tachycardia or fibrillation.
prematurity /-məchoo′ritē/ [L, *praematurus,* too early], pertaining to a happening before the usual or expected time, such as a premature birth.
premed /-med′/, abbreviation for *premedical student.*
premedication /-med′ikā′shən/ [L, *prae + medicare,* to heal], **1.** any sedative, tranquilizer, hypnotic, or anticholinergic medication administered before anesthesia. The choice of drug depends on such variables as the patient's age and physical condition and the specific operative procedure. **2.** the administration of such medications. **—premedicate,** *v.*
premenarchal /-mənär′kəl/ [L, *pre,* before + *mensis,* month; Gk, *archaios* from the beginning], before the start of the first menstrual period.

premenopausal /-men′əpô′səl/ [L, *prae* + *mensis*, month; Gk, *pauein* to cease], before the start of menopause.

premenstrual /-men′stroo·əl/ [L, *pre*, before + *menstrualis*, monthly], before the start of menstruation, each month.

premenstrual syndrome (PMS) [L, *prae* + *menstrualis*, monthly, *tendere*, to stretch], a syndrome of nervous tension, irritability, weight gain, edema, headache, mastalgia, dysphoria, and lack of coordination occurring during the last few days of the menstrual cycle before the onset of menstruation. There are several theories that attempt to explain the cause of the syndrome, including nutritional deficiency, stress, hormonal imbalance, and various emotional disorders.

premise /prem′is/ [L, *prae* + *mittere*, to send], a proposition that is laid down as the base of an argument, and which is usually established beforehand.

premolar /prēmō′lər/ [L, *prae* + *mola*, mill], one of eight teeth, four in each dental arch, located lateral to and posterior to the canine teeth. The premolars appear during childhood and are usually first and secondary primary molars. The term refers to a position in front of the molars. They are smaller and shorter than the canine teeth. The crown of each premolar is compressed anteroposteriorly and surmounted by two cusps. The neck of the premolar is oval; the root is usually single and compressed, except for the upper first premolars, which usually have two roots. Also, there is usually an anterior and a posterior groove. The upper premolars are larger than the lower premolars. Also called **bicuspid.** Compare **canine tooth, incisor, molar.**

premonition /-mənish′ən/, a sense of an impending event without prior knowledge of it.

premonitory /-mon′iter′ē/ [L, *prae* + *monere*, to warn], an early symptom or sign of a disease. The term is commonly used to describe minor symptoms that precede a major health problem.

premorbid personality /-môr′bid/, a personality characterized by early signs or symptoms of a mental disorder. The specific defects may indicate whether the condition will progress toward schizophrenia, a bipolar disorder, or another type of condition.

prenatal /-nā′təl/ [L, *prae* + *natus*, birth], prior to birth; occurring or existing before birth, referring to both the care of the woman during pregnancy and the growth and development of the fetus. Also called **antenatal.** See also **antepartal care.**

prenatal care [L, *pre*, before + *natus*, birth; ME, *caru*, sorrow], the health care provided the mother and fetus before childbirth.

prenatal development, the entire process of growth, maturation, differentiation, and development that occurs between conception and birth. On approximately the fourteenth day before the next expected menstrual period, ovulation usually occurs. If the egg is fertilized, it immediately begins the course to fetal maturity and birth. During the first 14 days the fertilized ovum undergoes cell division several times, becoming a morula and then a blastocyst that is able to implant in the uterine wall. From the beginning of the third to the end of the seventh week of embryonic development, implantation deepens and completes. Primitive uteroplacental circulation originates between the enlarging trophoblast and the maternal endometrial tissue of the uterus. The amniotic cavity appears as an opening between the inner cell mass and the invading trophoblast. A thin lining in the cavity becomes the amnion. At this point the embryo is a two-layered embryonic disk composed of an ectoderm and an endoderm. As the disk thickens in the middle, giving rise to the third cell layer, or mesoderm, the basic structural systems of the body begin to form. The neural tube develops as a precursor of the central nervous system in the midline of the cranial portion of the ectoderm. Primitive blood vessels and blood cells, a heart tube, and umbilical vessels are formed and begin to function. Arm and leg buds may be seen, and rudimentary gut, lungs, and kidneys form. By the fifth week, the brain has begun to grow rapidly, the heart tube is divided into chambers, the palate and the upper lip are forming, and the urogenital system is developing. By the end of the seventh week, all essential systems are present. The period of time from the eighth week to birth is called the fetal stage. From the eighth to the tenth week the fetus continues to grow and develop rapidly. The head is almost one half of its total length, and arms, legs, and face are clearly recognizable. The fetus floats in the amniotic fluid of the amniotic sac within the uterus; the umbilical vessels in the cord extend to a rapidly growing placenta. By the twelfth week the features of the face are formed and the eyelids are present but not yet closed, because they have not divided into upper and lower eyelids. The palate is fusing, there is a neck between the large head and the body, and tooth buds and nail beds have begun to form. Identification of the external genitalia is possible for the first time. From the thirteenth to the sixteenth weeks, the arms, legs, and trunk grow rapidly, and the fetus is active. Scalp hair develops. The skeleton of the fetus is calcified and may be seen on an x-ray film. Respiratory movements may sometimes be detected by a sonogram. Between the seventeenth and the twentieth weeks of pregnancy, the mother usually first feels the baby move. The fetus looks like a very small baby at this time. There are eyebrows and tiny nipples; during fetoscopic examination, the fetus has been seen and photographed sucking its thumb and grasping its own umbilical cord. At the twenty-fourth week the external ears are smooth and soft and the skin is wrinkled and translucent. The body is covered with lanugo and vernix and weighs a little more than 1 pound. At 28 weeks subcutaneous fat begins to develop, fingernails and toenails are present, the eyelids are separate, the eyes may open, scalp hair is well developed, and, in males, the testes are at the internal inguinal ring or below. In a modern neonatal intensive care unit most of the babies born at 28 weeks survive. By the thirty-second week, the fetus weighs between 3 and 4 pounds. The hair is fine and woolly, the fingernails and toenails have grown to the tips of the fingers and toes and there are one or two creases on the anterior part of the soles of the feet. The areolae of the breasts are visible, but flat. In females, the clitoris is prominent and the labia majora are small and separated. At 36 weeks, the body and the limbs are fuller and more rounded, creases involve the anterior two thirds of the soles, and the skin is thicker and less translucent. As the fetus reaches term, between 38 and 42 weeks, the vernix decreases, and the ear cartilage is developed. In males, the testes are in the scrotum; in females, the labia majora meet in the midline and cover the labia minora and the clitoris. At 40 weeks, the average fetus weighs 7¼ pounds and is between 19 and 22 inches long. Prenatal development may be adversely affected by several factors. Between 2 and 14 weeks of gestation, ionizing radiation and some drugs may have profound effects on morphologic and functional development. During the first 10 days of development any damage usually kills the conceptus. Various viruses, malnutrition, trauma, or maternal disease also may affect the morphologic development of a rapidly differentiating structure or organ during the embryologic or early fetal stage. After 14 weeks, when all of the organs, systems, and parts of the body have formed, any adverse effects are largely functional; major morphologic damage does not occur. (Figure, pp. 958-959)

prenatal diagnosis, any of various diagnostic techniques to determine whether a developing fetus in the uterus is affected with a genetic disorder or other abnormality. Such

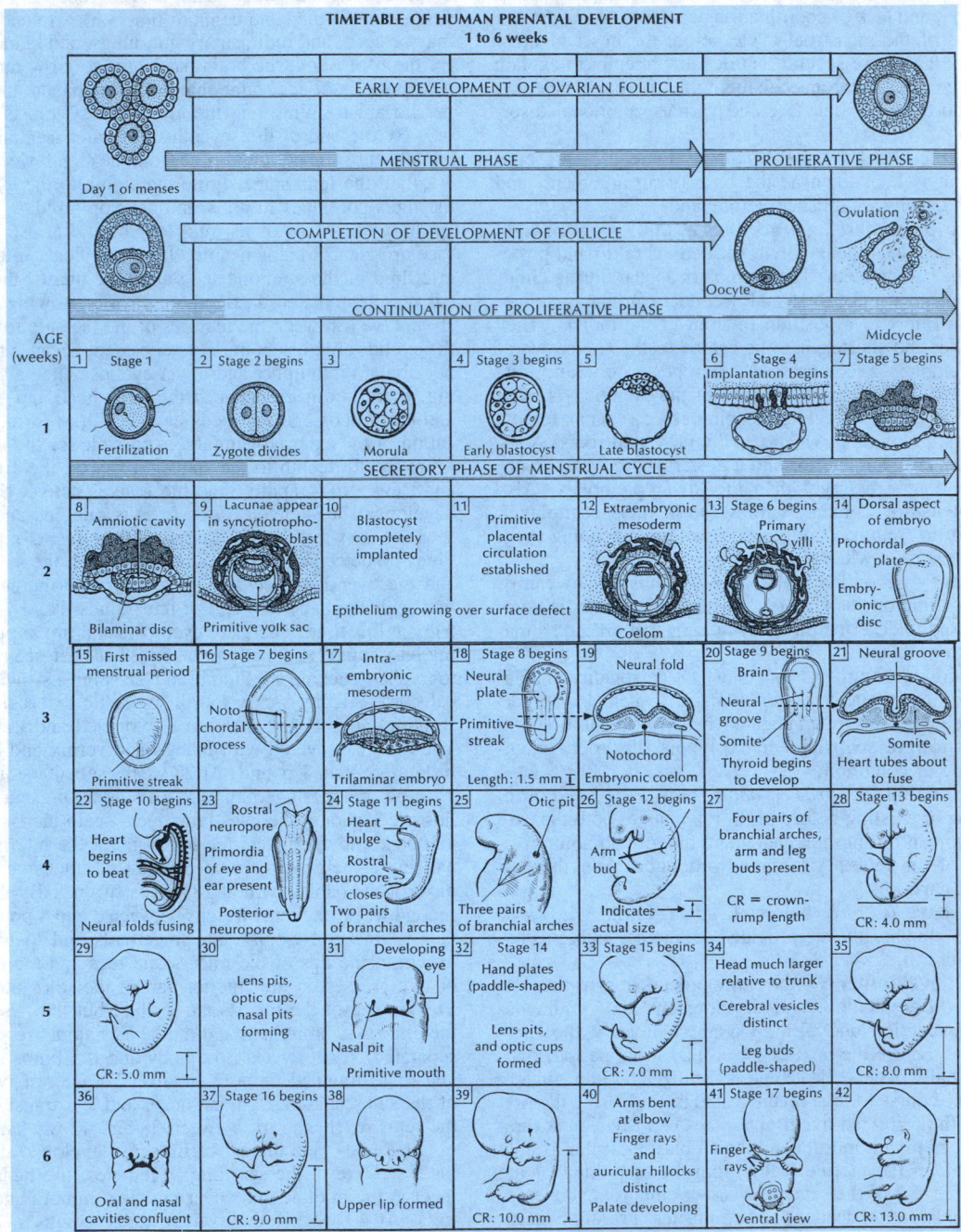

Timetable of prenatal development
(From Moore, KL: The developing human, ed 3, Philadelphia, 1983, WB Saunders Co.)

procedures as x-ray examination and ultrasound scanning can be used to follow fetal growth and detect structural abnormalities; amniocentesis enables fetal cells to be obtained from the amniotic fluid for culture and biochemical assay to detect metabolic disorders and for chromosomal analysis; fetoscopy enables fetal blood to be withdrawn from a blood vessel of the placenta and examined for disorders, such as thalassemia, sickle cell anemia, and Duchenne's muscular dystrophy. If any of the tests are positive and the child is likely to be born with a severe defect or disease, the parents need support and advice from genetic counselors on whether to terminate the pregnancy. If the parents decide to have the baby, the nurse can help to educate them about the specific disorder and to prepare them for the spe-

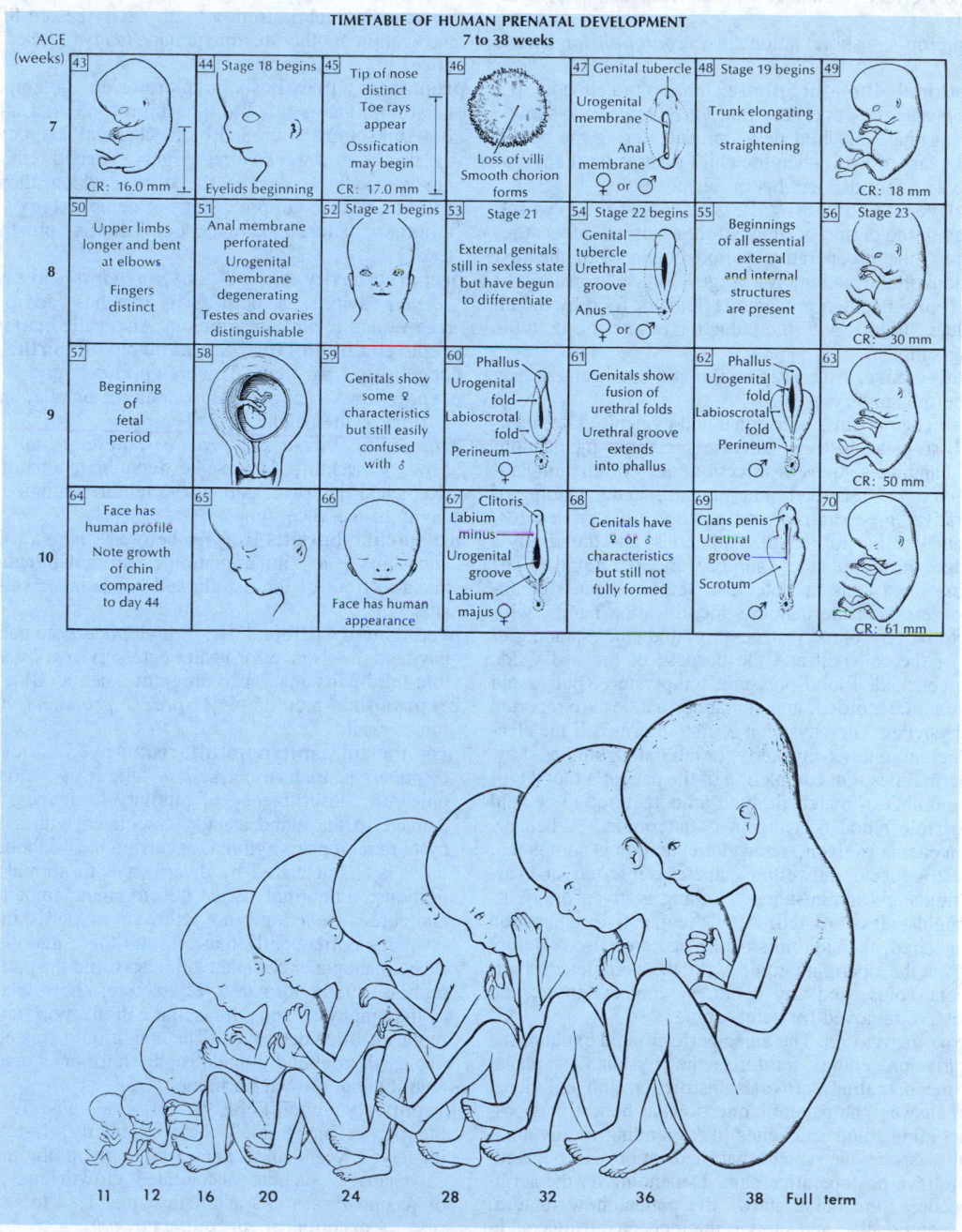

Timetable of prenatal development
(From Moore, KL: The developing human, ed 3, Philadelphia, 1983, WB Saunders Co.)

cial care required of a handicapped or genetically defective child. Also called **antenatal diagnosis.** See also **genetic counseling, genetic screening.**

prenatal surgery, any surgical procedure that is performed on a fetus. The technique has been used to correct hydrocephalus and obstructions of the urinary tract.

preoccupation /prē·ok'yəpā'shən/, a state of being self-absorbed or engrossed in one's own thoughts to a degree that hinders effective contact with or relationship to external reality.

pre-op /prē·op'/, abbreviation for *preparation for operation.*

preoperational thought phase /prē·op'ərā'shənəl/ [L, *prae* + *operari,* to work; AS, *thot;* Gk, *phainein,* to show], a piagetian phase of child development, during the period of 2 to 7 years of age, when the child focuses on the use of language as a tool to meet his or her needs.

preoperative /prē·op'ərətiv'/ [L, *prae* + *operari,* to work], pertaining to the period of time before a surgical procedure. Commonly, the preoperative period begins with the first preparation of the patient for surgery, such as when, 12 hours before scheduled procedure, fluids or food by mouth is forbidden. It ends with the induction of anesthesia in the operating suite.

preoperative care, the preparation and management of a patient before surgery.
■ METHOD: The patient's nutritional and hygienic state, medical and surgical history, allergies, current medication, physical handicaps, signs of infection, and elimination habits are noted and recorded. The patient's understanding of the operative, preoperative, and postoperative procedures, the patient's ability to verbalize anxieties, and the family's knowledge of the planned surgery are ascertained. The signed informed consent statement, the physician's preoperative orders, and the patient's identification bands, willingness to receive blood if necessary, and understanding of the use of the call bell and the purpose of the bed's side rails are checked. Blood pressure, temperature, pulse, and respiration are recorded, and any abnormalities are reported to the physician. The physician is also informed if the electrocardiogram, chest x-ray study, or laboratory studies show any abnormalities. On completion of the patient's blood typing, the number of matched blood units required to be held for a possible blood transfusion is determined. When ordered, an enema is given, a bowel preparation is completed, a nasogastric tube or indwelling catheter is inserted, and parenteral fluids are administered. Nothing is given orally after midnight unless ordered. After preoperative medication is administered, the side rails of the bed are raised. Before leaving for the operating room with the completed chart, the patient voids, and any dentures, contact lenses, and valuables are removed for safekeeping.
■ NURSING INTERVENTION: The nurse performs and explains the preoperative procedures, reinforces the physician's explanation of the operation, provides instruction and emotional support, answers the patient's questions as honestly as possible, avoiding standard clichés in responding to any anxiety, and reassures the patient that medication will be available to relieve postoperative pain. Depending on the surgical procedure, the nurse shows the patient how to turn, cough, deep breathe, and support the incision during coughing. The nurse informs the patient and the patient's family about the postoperative period in the recovery room or the intensive care unit, if indicated.

■ OUTCOME CRITERIA: The patient who is carefully prepared for an operation, psychologically and physically, experiences less anxiety and is more likely to make an uneventful recovery.

prep, 1. abbreviation for *prepare* **2.** abbreviation for **preparation,** particularly when referring to preparation for surgery.

preparation (prep) /prep'ərā'shən/ [L, *praeparare,* to make ready], **1.** making a site ready for a procedure, such as removing debris from a tooth cavity before filling. **2.** a medication or other treatment made ready for use. **3.** a specimen.

preparatory prosthesis /prep'ərətôr'ē/, a temporary artificial limb that is fitted to the stump soon after amputation. It permits ambulation and biomechanical adaptation during the first several weeks after surgery. A rigid removal dressing is usually applied to the stump, which allows for inspection of the stump for signs of hemorrhage or tissue deterioration before a permanent or definitive prosthesis is fitted.

prepared cavity /priperd'/ [L, *praeparare,* to make ready; *cavum,* cavity], a tooth cavity that has been prepared to receive and retain a restoration. Also called **cavity prep.**

prepared childbirth. See **natural childbirth.**

prepartum /-pär'təm/, before child delivery.

prepatellar /-pətel'ər/ [L, *pre,* before, *patella,* small disk], in front of the patella.

prepatellar bursa [L, *prae* + *patella,* small dish; Gk, *byrsa,* wineskin], a bursa between the tendon of the quadriceps and the lower part of the femur continuous with the cavity of the knee joint.

prepatellar bursitis [L, *pre,* before + *patella*; Gk, *byrsa,* wineskin + *itis* inflammation], an inflammation of the bursa in front of the patella and beneath the skin over the site.

prepayment /-pā'mənt/ [L, *prae* + *pacere,* to pacify], the payment in advance for health care services, by subscribers to a third-party insurance program, such as Blue Cross.

preprandial /-pran'dē·əl/ [L, *prae* + *prandium,* lunch], before a meal.

prepubertal panhypopituitarism /-pyōō'bərtəl/ [L, *prae,* + *pubertas,* maturity; Gk, *pan,* all, *hypo,* under, *pituita,* phlegm], insufficiency of pituitary hormones, caused by damage to the gland usually associated with a suprasellar cyst or craniopharyngioma, occurring in childhood. The disorder is characterized by dwarfism with normal body proportions, subnormal sexual development, impaired thyroid and adrenal function, and yellow, wrinkled skin. Diabetes insipidus is frequently present, and there may be bitemporal hemianopia or complete blindness, but the patient's mentality is usually normal. X-ray pictures show delayed fusion of the epiphyses and suprasellar calcification, and the sella turcica is often destroyed. The condition is treated with cortisone, thyroid and gonadotrophic hormones, and, if available, human growth hormone.

prepuberty /-pyōō'bərtē/ [L, *prae* + *pubertas,* maturity], the period immediately before puberty, lasting approximately 2 years and characterized by preliminary physical changes, such as accelerated growth and appearance of secondary sex characteristics, that lead to sexual maturity. **–prepuberal, prepubertal,** *adj.*

prepubescence /prē'pyōōbes'əns/, the state of being prepubertal. **–prepubescent,** *adj.*

prepubescent /-pyōōbes'ənt/ [L, *pre,* before + *pubescere,* hairy], the period of time immediately before the emergence of puberty.

prepuce /prē'pyo͞os/ [L, *praeputium*, foreskin], a fold of skin that forms a retractable cover, such as the foreskin of the penis or the fold around the clitoris. **–prepucial, preputial,** *adj.*

prerenal /-rē'nəl/ [L, *pre*, before + *ren*, kidney], **1.** located in front of the kidney. **2.** occurring before reaching the kidney.

prerenal anuria [L, *prae* + *renes*, kidneys; Gk, *a, ouron*, not urine], cessation of urine production caused by the blood pressure in the kidney being too low to maintain glomerular filtration pressure.

prerenal uremia [L, *pre*, before + *ren*, kidney; Gk, *ouron*, urine + *haima*, blood], a condition of kidney failure in which the primary cause may be outside the kidney, as in some severe cases of alkalosis.

presby- /prez'bē/, a combining form 'pertaining to aging or being elderly': *presbyopia, presbyacusia, presbyatrics.*

presbycardia /prez'bēkär'dē·ə/ [Gk, *presbys*, old man, *kardia*, heart], an abnormal cardiac condition, especially affecting elderly individuals and associated with heart failure in the presence of other complications, such as heart disease, fever, anemia, mild hyperthyroidism, and excess fluid administration. Presbycardia may be associated with decreased elasticity of the musculature of the heart and with mild fibrotic changes of the heart valves, but the basis for these changes and the associated pigmentation of the heart is not known. Some authorities believe that presbycardia only rarely produces heart failure but that the condition does decrease the adaptive capacity of the heart and predisposes elderly patients to heart failure in the presence of other illnesses.

presbycusis /-ko͞o'sis/ [Gk, *presbys* + *akousis*, hearing], loss of hearing sensitivity and speech intelligibility, associated with aging.

presbyopia /prez'bē·ō'pē·ə/ [Gk, *presbys* + *ops*, eye], farsightedness resulting from a loss of elasticity of the lens of the eye. The condition commonly develops with advancing age. Compare **visual accommodation. –presbyopic,** *adj.*

presbyopic /prez'bē·op'ik/ [Gk, *presby*, old man, *ops*, eye], pertaining to a decrease in accommodation of the lens as one grows older, and usually resulting in hyperopia or farsightedness.

preschizophrenic state /prēskit'səfren'ik, prē'-/ [L, *prae* + Gk, *schizein*, to split, *phren* mind], a period before psychosis is evident when the patient deviates from normal behavior but does not demonstrate psychotic symptoms of delusions, hallucinations, or stupor.

prescreen /-skrēn/ [L, *prae* + ME, *screen*], **1.** to evaluate a patient or a group of patients to identify those who are at greater risk of developing a particular condition to select those who are in particular need of special diagnostic procedures or health care. **2.** *informal.* a rapid, superficial examination of a person who does not appear to be acutely ill. It may include taking a medical history.

prescribe /priskrīb'/ [L, *prae* + *scribere* to write], **1.** to write an order for a drug, treatment, or procedure. **2.** to recommend or encourage a course of action.

prescription /priskrip'shən/, an order for medication, therapy, or a therapeutic device given by a properly authorized person to a person properly authorized to dispense or perform the order. A prescription is usually in written form and includes the name and address of the patient, the date, the [4]+ symbol (superscription), the medication prescribed (inscription), directions to the pharmacist or other dispenser (subscription), directions to the patient that must appear on the label, the prescriber's signature, and, in some instances, an identifying number.

prescription drug [L, *prae* + *scribere*; Fr, *drogue*], a drug that can be dispensed to the public only with a prescription. The designation of a drug as a prescription drug is made by the Food and Drug Administration.

prescriptive intervention mode /priskrip'tiv/ [L, *praescriptus*, prescribed, *intervenire*, to come between, *modus*, measure], a therapeutic situation in which the health professional tells the patient explicitly how to solve a problem, so that less collaboration between the consultant and patient is needed.

prescriptive theory, a theory that comprises a description of a specific activity, a statement of the goal of the activity, and an analysis of the elements of the activity that, together, constitute a prescription for reaching the goal.

presence /prez'əns/ a mode of being available in a situation with the wholeness of one's individual being; a gift of self that can be given freely, invoked or evoked.

presenile /-sē'nīl/ [L, *pre*, before + *senex*, aged], pertaining to a condition in which a person manifests signs of aging in early or middle life.

presenile dementia. See **Alzheimer's disease.**

presentation. See **fetal presentation.**

presentation of the cord. See **funic presentation.**

present health [L, *praesentare*, to show; AS, *haelth*], (in a health history) a chronologic, succinct account of any recent changes in the health of the patient and of the circumstances or symptoms that prompted the person to seek health care.

presenting part /prəsen'ting/ [L, *praesentare* + *pars*, part], the part of the fetus that lies closest to the internal os of the cervix.

presenting symptom. See **symptom.**

preservative /prisur'vətiv/ [L, *praeservare*, to keep], a chemical or other agent that reduces the rate of decomposition of a substance.

presomite embryo /prēsō'mīt/ [L, *prae* + Gk, *soma*, body, *en* in, *bryein* to grow], an embryo in any stage of development before the appearance of the first pair of somites, which, in humans, usually occurs around 19 to 21 days after fertilization of the ovum.

-pressin, a combining form for vasoconstrictors, particularly vasopressin derivatives.

pressor /pres'ər/ [L, *premere*, to press], describing a substance that tends to cause a rise in blood pressure.

pressoreceptor /pres'ōrisep'tər/ [L, *premere*, to press + *recipere*, to receive], a nerve ending that is sensitive to changes in blood pressure.

pressure /presh'ər/ [L, *premere*, to press], a force, or stress, applied to a surface by a fluid or an object, usually measured in units of mass per unit of area, such as pounds per square inch.

pressure acupuncture, a system of acupuncture involving the application of pressure, such as by the tip of a finger, to certain specified points of the body. See also **acupuncture.**

pressure area, an oral area that is subject to excessive displacement of soft tissue by a prosthesis.

pressure bandage, a bandage applied to stop bleeding, prevent edema, or provide support for varicose veins.

pressure dressing, a dressing firmly applied to exert pressure, usually on a wound for hemostasis.

pressure edema, 1. edema of the lower extremities caused by pressure of a pregnant uterus against the large veins of the area. **2.** edema of the fetal scalp after cephalic presentation.

pressure necrosis. See **decubitus ulcer.**

pressure point, 1. a point over an artery where the pulse may be felt. Pressure on the point may be helpful in stopping the flow of blood from a wound distal to the point. **2.** a site that is extremely sensitive to pressure, such as the phrenic pressure point along the phrenic nerve between the sternocleidomastoid and the scalenus anticus on the right side; pressure at this site may be symptomatic of gallbladder dysfunction.

pressure-sensitive adhesive, a drug-delivery device that uses polymers that are permanently tacky at room temperature and will adhere to the skin when slight pressure is applied.

pressure sore. See **decubitus ulcer.**

pressure support ventilation (PSV), the augmentation for spontaneous breathing effort with a specific amount of positive airway pressure. The patient initiates the inspiratory flow, generating his or her own V_t and frequencies.

pressure ventilator, a ventilator in which gas delivery is limited by a predetermined pressure.

pressure ulcer. See **decubitus ulcer.**

presumptive signs /-sump'tiv/ [L, *praesumere,* to take beforehand; *signum,* mark], manifestations that indicate a pregnancy although they are not necessarily positive. Presumptive signs may include cessation of menses and morning sickness. See also **Chadwick's sign.**

preswing stance stage /prē'swing/ [L, *prae* + AS, *swingan,* to fling; L, *stare,* to stand; OFr, *estage,* stage], one of the five stages in the stance phase of walking or gait, involving a brief transitional period of double limb support during which one leg of the body is rapidly relieved of body-bearing weight and prepared for the swing forward. The type of preswing used by an individual is a factor in the diagnoses of many abnormal orthopedic conditions. Compare **initial contact stance stage, loading response stance stage, midstance, terminal stance.** See also **swing phase of gait.**

presymptomatic disease /-simp'təmat'ik/ [L, *prae* + Gk, *symptoma,* a happening], an early stage of disease when physiologic changes have begun although no signs or symptoms are observed.

presynaptic /-sinap'tik/ [L, *prae* + *synaptein,* to join], **1.** situated near or before a synapse. **2.** before a synapse is crossed.

presystole /-sis'təlē/ [L, *pre,* before; Gk, *systole,* contraction], an interval in the cardiac cycle immediately before systole.

presystolic /-sistol'ik/ [L, *prae* + Gk, *systole,* contraction], of or pertaining to the period preceding systole.

presystolic murmur [L, *pre,* before; Gk, *systole*; L, *murmur,* humming], a heart mumur in cases of mitral stenosis, before diastole.

preterm /prē'turm'/ [L, *pre,* before; Gk, *terma,* limit], **1.** events before a specific date. **2.** pertaining to a shorter than normal period of gestation.

preterm birth, any birth that occurs before the thirty-seventh week of gestation. See also **premature infant.**

preterm infant. See **premature infant.**

preterm labor. See **premature labor.**

pretibial /prētib'ē·əl/ [L, *prae* + *tibia,* shinbone], of or pertaining to the area of the leg in front of the tibia.

pretibial fever, an acute infection caused by *Leptospira autumnalis,* characterized by headache, chills, fever, enlarged spleen, myalgia, low white blood cell count, and a rash on the anterior surface of the legs. Also called **Fort Bragg fever.**

pretrial discovery. See **discovery.**

prevalence /prev'ələns/ [L, *praevalentia,* a powerful force], (in epidemiology) the number of all new and old cases of a disease or occurrences of an event during a particular period of time. Prevalence is expressed as a ratio in which the number of events is the numerator and the population at risk is the denominator. See also **rate.**

prevention /-ven'shən/ [L, *praevenire,* to anticipate], (in nursing care) any action directed toward preventing illness and promoting health to avoid the need for secondary or tertiary health care. Prevention includes such nursing actions as assessment; application of prescribed measures, such as immunization; health teaching; early diagnosis and treatment; and recognition of disability limitations and rehabilitation potential. In acute care nursing, many interventions are simultaneously therapeutic and preventive.

preventive /-ven'tiv/ [L, *praevenire,* to anticipate], tending to slow, stop, or interrupt the course of an illness or to decrease the incidence of a disease.

preventive care, a pattern of nursing and medical care that focuses on the prevention of disease and health maintenance and includes early diagnosis of disease, discovery and identification of people at risk of developing specific problems, counseling, and other intervention to avert a health problem. Screening tests, health education, and immunization programs are common examples of preventive care. Also called **primary nursing.**

preventive dentistry [L, *praevenire,* to anticipate + *dens,* tooth], the science of the prevention of disease affecting the teeth.

preventive health care. See **preventive care.**

preventive medicine [L, *praevenire,* to anticipate + *medicina*], the branch of medicine that is concerned with the prevention of disease and methods for increasing the power of the patient and community to resist disease and prolong life.

preventive nursing [L, *praevenire,* to anticipate + *nutrix,* nurse], the branch of nursing that is concerned with general health promotion, teaching of early recognition and treatment of disease, encouraging lifestyle modification, and prevention of further deterioration of the disabled.

preventive psychiatry, the use of theoretical knowledge and skills to plan and implement programs designed to achieve primary, secondary, and tertiary prevention.

preventive treatment, a procedure, measure, substance, or program designed to prevent a disease from occurring or a mild disorder from becoming more severe. Various diseases are prevented by immunizations with vaccines, antiseptic measures, the avoidance of smoking, regular exercise, a prudent diet, adequate rest, the correction of congenital anomalies, and screening programs for the detection of preclinical signs of disorders. Also called **prophylactic treatment.**

previa. See **placenta previa.**

previllous embryo /prēvil'əs/ [L, *prae* + *villus,* hairy; Gk, *en* in, *bryein,* to grow], an embryo of a placental mammal at any stage before the development of the chorionic villi, which, in humans, begin to form between the first and second months after fertilization of the ovum.

previous abnormality of glucose tolerance /prē′vē·əs/, a classification that includes people who previously had diabetic hyperglycemia or impaired glucose tolerance but whose fasting plasma glucose levels have returned to normal. Included in this category are people who had gestational diabetes but whose plasma levels returned to normal after parturition and obese people whose plasma levels returned to normal after they lost weight. Previously called latent diabetes, prediabetes. See also **diabetes mellitus.**

previtamin. See **provitamin.**

prevocational evaluation /-vōkā′shənəl/, an evaluation of the abilities and limitations of a patient undergoing rehabilitation from a disabling disorder. The goal is to find eventual employment in a sheltered workshop or in the general community. The evaluation usually leads to selective placement of the patient in an appropriate business or industry.

prevocational training, a rehabilitation program designed to prepare a patient for the performance of useful, paid work in a sheltered setting or community. It may involve training in basic work skills and counseling as required for a typical employment setting.

priapism /prī′əpiz′əm/ [Gk, *priapos,* phallus], an abnormal condition of prolonged or constant penile erection, often painful and seldom associated with sexual arousal. It may result from urinary calculi or a lesion within the penis or the central nervous system. It sometimes occurs in men who have acute leukemia.

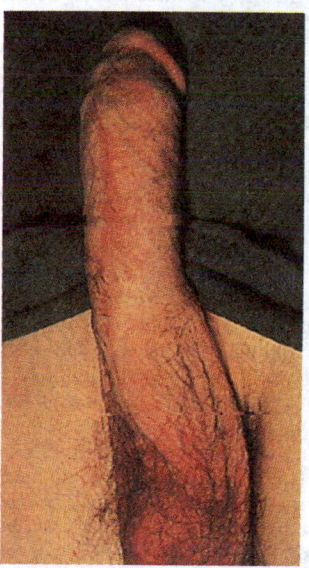

Priapism *(Lloyd-Davies, 1983)*

priapitis /prī′əpī′tis/, inflammation of the penis.
priapus. See **penis.**
prickle cell layer. See **stratum spinosum.**
prickly heat. See **miliaria.**
-pride, a combining form for sulpiride derivatives.
-pril, a combining form for captopril-type antihypertensive agents. See **amide-compound local anesthetic.**

prilocaine hydrochloride /pril′ōkān/, a local anesthetic agent of the amide family, used for nerve block, epidural, and regional anesthesia. It is not used for spinal or topical anesthesia. Prilocaine hydrochloride is about one half as toxic as lidocaine, but because methemoglobinemia is a possible reaction, prilocaine hydrochloride is not used for patients with hypoxic conditions of any kind.

prim-, primi-, a prefix meaning 'first': *primerite, primigravida, primitiae.*

-prim, a combining form for trimethoprim-type antibacterials.

Primacor, a trademark for a phosphodiesterase inhibitor (milrinone).

prima facie rights /prī′mə fā′shē·ə/, rights on the surface, or face, that may be overridden by stronger conflicting rights or by other values.

primal scream therapy /prī′məl/, a form of psychotherapy developed by Arthur Janov that focuses on repressed pain of infancy or childhood. The goal of the therapy is for the patient to surrender his or her neurotic defenses and 'become real.'

primaquine phosphate /prī′məkwin/, an antimalarial.
■ INDICATIONS: It is prescribed in the treatment of malaria and prevention of relapse during recovery from the disease.
■ CONTRAINDICATIONS: Lupus erythematosus, rheumatoid arthritis, concomitant use of bone marrow depressants or hemolytic drugs, or known hypersensitivity to this drug prohibits its use.
■ ADVERSE EFFECTS: Among the more serious adverse reactions are hemolytic anemia, agranulocytosis, and abdominal distress.

primary /prī′mərē/ [L, *primus,* first], **1.** first in order of time, place, development, or importance. **2.** not derived from any other source or cause, specifically the original condition or set of symptoms in disease processes, such as a primary infection or a primary tumor. **3.** (in chemistry) noting the first and most simple compound in a related series, formed by the substitution of one of two or more atoms or of a group in a molecule, such as in amine or carboxyl radicals. Compare **secondary, tertiary.**

primary abscess [L, *primus + abscedere,* to go away], an abscess that develops at the original point of infection by a pus-producing microorganism.

primary afferent fiber. See **gamma efferent fiber.**

primary amenorrhea. See **amenorrhea.**

primary amputation, amputation performed after severe trauma, after the patient has recovered from shock, and before infection has set in. Compare **secondary amputation.**

primary amyloidosis. See **amyloidosis.**

primary anesthesia [L, *primus,* first; Gk, *anaisthesia,* lack of feeling], any anesthetic or analgesic given a surgical patient before the administration of chemical agents that produce reversible unconsciousness.

primary apnea, a self-limited condition characterized by an absence of respiration. It may follow a blow to the head and is common immediately after birth in the newborn who breathes spontaneously when the carbon dioxide in the circulation reaches a certain level. Reflexes are present, and the heart is beating, but the skin color may be pale or blue and muscle tone is diminished. No treatment is necessary, but careful observation, maintenance of body temperature, and oral pharyngeal aspiration are usually performed. Within seconds the baby usually begins breathing, becomes pinker, moves the arms and legs, and cries. Compare **periodic apnea of the newborn, secondary apnea.**

primary atelectasis, failure of the lungs to expand fully at birth, most commonly seen in premature infants or those narcotized by maternal anesthesia. The infant is usually cared for in an incubator in which the temperature and humidity may be closely monitored. Nursing care includes frequent changes of position of the infant to assist respiration, suctioning to remove bronchial secretions, and very slow feedings to avoid abdominal distention.

primary atypical pneumonia. See **mycoplasma pneumonia.**

primary biliary cirrhosis, a chronic inflammatory condition of the liver. It is characterized by generalized pruritus, enlargement and hardening of the liver, weight loss, and diarrhea with pale, bulky stools. Petechiae, epistaxis, or hemorrhage resulting from hypoprothrombinemia may also be evident. Pathologic fractures and collapsed vertebrae may develop as the result of the associated malabsorption of vitamin D and calcium. Xanthomas commonly develop when the serum cholesterol level exceeds 450 mg/dl. The cause of primary biliary cirrhosis is unknown, although it is associated with autoimmune disorders. The condition most often affects women 40 to 60 years of age. The diagnosis is confirmed by liver biopsy and cholangiography. Antibody is nearly always present. Jaundice, dark urine, pale stools, and cutaneous xanthosis may occur in the later stages of this disease. Treatment commonly includes the administration of fat-soluble vitamins A, D, E, and K to prevent and correct deficiencies caused by malabsorption. Life expectancy is about 5 years for symptomatic patients after the onset of jaundice. Compare **secondary biliary cirrhosis.**

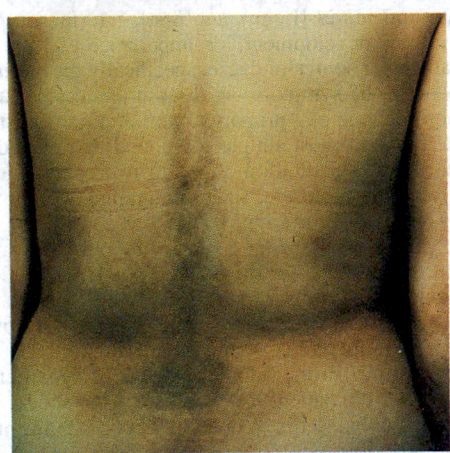

Skin changes in primary biliary cirrhosis
(Epstein, 1992)

primary bronchus, one of the two main air passages that branch from the trachea and convey air to the lungs as part of the respiratory system. The right primary bronchus is about 2.5 cm long and wider and shorter than the left primary bronchus, and enters the right lung nearly opposite the fifth thoracic vertebra. The left primary bronchus is about 5 cm long, passes under the aortic arch, and courses ventral to the esophagus, the thoracic duct, and the descending aorta before dividing into bronchi for the superior and the anterior lobes of the lung. The bronchi, like the trachea, are composed of rings of hyaline cartilage, fibrous tissue, mucous membrane, and glands. The carina at the bottom of the trachea separates the two primary bronchi and is situated to the left of the midline so that the right primary bronchus is a more direct extension of the trachea than the left. Hence foreign objects entering the trachea usually drop into the right bronchus rather than the left.

primary carcinoma, a neoplasm at the site of origin.

primary care, the first contact in a given episode of illness that leads to a decision regarding a course of action to resolve the health problem. Primary care usually is provided by a physician, but some primary care functions are also handled by nurses.

primary care physician [L, *primus*; ME, *caru,* sorrow; Gk, *physikos,* natural], a physician who usually is the first health professional to examine a patient and who recommends secondary care physicians, medical or surgical specialists with expertise in the patient's specific health problem, if further treatment is needed.

primary caries. See **dental caries.**

primary constriction. See **centromere.**

primary cutaneous melanoma, the site of origin for melanoma on the skin.

primary degenerative dementia. See **senile psychosis.**

primary dementia [L, *primus* + *de, mens,* mind], a gradual progressive deterioration of memory, cognition, judgment, abstract thought, and behavior that may develop in a person around age 65.

primary dental caries, dental caries developing in the enamel of a tooth that was previously unaffected. See also **incipient carious lesion.**

primary dentition. See **deciduous dentition.**

primary dermatitis [L, *primus*; Gk, *derma,* skin + *itis,* inflammation], skin eruption caused by a substance that can produce cell damage on initial contact, instead of dermatitis that develops as a sensitivity reaction to an allergen.

primary distal RTA. See **distal-renal tubular acidosis (distal RTA).**

primary drive. See **drive.**

primary dysmenorrhea. See **dysmenorrhea.**

primary endometriosis [L, *primus*; Gk, *endon,* within, *metra,* womb, *osis,* condition], an ingrowth of the muscle walls of the uterus by the mucous membrane lining of the organ. Also called **adenomyosis; endometriosis interna.**

primary enuresis [L, *primus*; Gk, *enourein,* to urinate], involuntary voiding of urine in a child who has not been toilet trained.

primary fissure, a fissure that marks the division of the anterior and posterior lobes of the cerebellum.

primary gain, a benefit, primarily relief from emotional conflict and freedom from anxiety, attained through the use of a defense mechanism or other psychologic process. Compare **secondary gain.**

primary gangrene [L, *primus*; Gk, *gaggraina*], a form of gangrene that occurs without preceding inflammation.

primary health care, a basic level of health care that includes programs directed at the promotion of health, early diagnosis of disease or disability, and prevention of disease. Primary health care is provided in an ambulatory facility to limited numbers of people, often those living in a particular geographic area. It includes continuing health care, as provided by a family nurse practitioner.

primary hemorrhage [L, *primus*; Gk, *haima,* blood; *rhegnynei,* to gush], a hemorrhage immediately after an injury.

primary host. See **definitive host.**

primary hypertension. See **essential hypertension.**

primary iritis [L, *primus*; Gk, *iris*, rainbow + *itis*, inflammation], an inflammation of the iris that results from a source within the body, such as a systemic disease. Also called **endogenous iritis.**

primary lesion [L, *primus* + *laesio*, hurting], a sore or wound that develops at the point of inoculation of the disease, usually applied to a syphilis chancre. Also called **initial lesion.**

primary nurse, a nurse who is responsible for the planning, implementation, and evaluation of the nursing care of one or more clients 24 hours a day for the duration of the hospital stay. See also **primary nursing.**

primary nursing, a system for the distribution of nursing care in which care of one patient is managed for the entire 24-hour day by one nurse who directs and coordinates nurses and other personnel, schedules all tests, procedures, and daily activities for that patient, and cares for that patient personally when on duty. In an acute care situation, the primary care nurse might be responsible for only one patient; in an intermediate care situation, the primary care nurse might be responsible for three or more patients. Nurse midwives and other nurse practitioners practice primary nursing, and many hospital nursing services are replacing team nursing with primary nursing. Some advantages are continuity of care for the patient, accountability of the nurse for that care, patient-centered care that is comprehensive, individualized, and coordinated, and the professional satisfaction of the nurse. Compare **team nursing.**

primary organizer, the part of the dorsal lip of the blastopore that is self-differentiating and induces the formation of the neural plate that gives rise to the main axis of the embryo.

primary physician, 1. the physician who usually takes care of a patient; the physician who first sees a patient for the care of a given health problem. 2. a family practice physician or general practitioner. See also **family medicine.**

primary pneumonic plague. See **pneumonic plague.**

primary polycythemia. See **polycythemia vera.**

primary prevention, a program of activities directed toward improvement of the general well-being while also involving specific protection for selected diseases, such as immunization against measles.

primary processes, unconscious processes, originating in the id, that obey laws different from those of the ego. These processes are seen in the least disguised form in infancy and in the dreams of the adult.

primary proximal renal tubular acidosis. See **proximal renal tubular acidosis.**

primary relationships, relationships with intimates, close friends, and family.

primary sensation, a feeling or impression resulting directly from a particular stimulus. See **sensation,** def. 1.

primary sequestrum, a piece of dead bone that completely separates from sound bone during the process of necrosis. Compare **secondary sequestrum.**

primary shock, a state of physical collapse comparable to fainting. It may be the result of slight pain, such as that produced by venipuncture, or may be caused by fright. Primary shock is usually mild, self-limited, and of short duration. Severe injury may prolong and merge primary shock with secondary shock. Compare **hemorrhagic shock.**

primary sterility [L, *primus* + *sterilis*, barren], the inability to produce an offspring because of a functional failure of the ovaries or the testes.

primary tooth. See **deciduous tooth.**

primary triad, in Beck's theory of depression, the three major cognitive patterns that force the individual to view self, environment, and future in a negativistic manner.

primary tuberculosis, the childhood form of tuberculosis, most commonly occurring in the lungs, the posterior pharynx, or, rarely, the skin. Infants lack resistance to the disease, being easily infected and especially vulnerable to rapid and extensive spread of the infection through their bodies. In childhood, the disease is usually brief and benign, characterized by regional lymphadenopathy, calcification of the tubercles, and residual immunity. The disease may reactivate later in life. The tuberculin test will be positive for life. See also **tuberculosis.**

primate /prī'māt, prī'mit/ [L, *primus*, first], a member of the biological order of animals of the chordate class Mammalia. The primate order includes lemurs, monkeys, apes, and humans. Most primates have large brains, stereoscopic vision, and hands and feet developed for grasping.

Primaxin, a trademark for a broad-spectrum parenteral antibiotic (imipenem/cilastatin sodium).

prime mover /prīm/ [L, *primus* + *movere*, to move], a muscle that acts directly to produce a desired movement amid other muscles acting simultaneously to produce indirectly the same movement. Most movements of the body require the combined action of numerous muscles. Compare **antagonist, fixation muscle, synergist.**

primidone /prī'mədōn/, an anticonvulsant.

■ INDICATIONS: It is prescribed in the treatment of seizure disorders, including grand mal, psychomotor, and focal epilepsy-like seizures.

■ CONTRAINDICATIONS: Porphyria or known hypersensitivity to this drug or to phenobarbital, a metabolite of primidone, prohibits its use.

■ ADVERSE EFFECTS: The most serious adverse reaction, seen on rare occasions, is megaloblastic anemia. Drowsiness, ataxia, and dizziness are common. Other adverse effects of phenobarbital may be seen.

primigravida /prim'igrav'idə/ [L, *primus* + *gravidus*, pregnant], a woman pregnant for the first time. Also called **gravida 1.** Compare **multigravida, primipara.** **—primigravid,** *adj.*

primipara /primip'ərə/, *pl.* **primiparae** [L, *primus* + *parere*, to bear], a woman who has given birth to one viable infant, indicated by 'para 1' on the patient's chart. Compare **multipara, nullipara, primigravida.**

primiparity /prim'iper'itē/ [L, *primus* + *parere*, to bear], the condition of having borne one child.

primiparous /primip'ərəs/ [L, *primus* + *parere*, to bear], pertaining to a woman who has borne one child.

primitive /prim'itiv/ [L, *primivus*], 1. undeveloped; undifferentiated; rudimentary; showing little or no evolution. 2. embryonic; formed early in the course of development; existing in an early or simple form. Compare **definitive.**

primitive fold. See **primitive ridge.**

primitive groove, a furrow in the posterior region of the embryonic disk that indicates the cephalocaudal axis resulting from the active involution of cells forming the primitive streak.

primitive gut. See **archenteron.**

primitive line. See **primitive streak.**

primitive node, a knoblike accumulation of cells at the cephalic end of the primitive streak in the early stages of embryonic development in humans and the higher animals. It consists of mesoderm cells that give rise to the notochord, and it corresponds to the dorsal lip of the blastopore in lower animals. Also called **Hensen's knot, Hensen's node.**

primitive pit, a minute indentation at the anterior end of the primitive groove in the early developing embryo. It lies posterior to the primitive node and probably functions as an opening into the notochordal canal in humans and the higher animals and into the neurenteric canal in the lower animals.

primitive reflex, any reflex normal in an infant or fetus. Its presence in an adult usually indicates serious neurologic disease. Some kinds of primitive reflexes are **grasp reflex, Moro reflex,** and **sucking reflex.**

primitive ridge, a ridge that bounds the primitive groove in the early stages of embryonic development. Also called **primitive fold.** See also **primitive streak.**

primitive streak, a dense area on the central posterior region of the embryonic disk, formed by the morphogenetic movement of a rapidly proliferating mass of cells that spreads between the ectoderm and endoderm, giving rise to the mesoderm layer. This seamlike elongation indicates the cephalocaudal axis along which the embryo develops, and it corresponds to the blastopore of lower animal groups. Also called **primitive line.**

primordial /primôr′dē·əl/ [L, *primordium,* origin], **1.** characteristic of the most undeveloped or primitive state, specifically those cells or tissues that are formed in the early stages of embryonic development. **2.** first or original; primitive.

primordial cyst, a follicular cyst, consisting of an epithelium-lined sac that contains fluid and appears radiographically as a light area in the affected jaw. It develops from a dental enamel organ before the formation of hard tissue.

primordial dwarf, a person of extremely short stature who is otherwise perfectly formed, with the usual proportions of body parts and normal mental and sexual development. The condition may be genetically related, involving some defect in the ability to use growth hormone, or it may occur sporadically within a particular population. Also called **hypoplastic dwarf, normal dwarf, physiologic dwarf, pure dwarf, true dwarf.** See also **pituitary dwarf, pygmy.**

primordial germ cell, any of the large spheric diploid cells that are formed in the early stages of embryonic development and are precursors of the oogonia and spermatogonia. They are formed outside of the gonads and migrate to the embryonic ovaries and testes for maturation. See also **oogenesis, spermatogenesis.**

primordial image, (in analytic psychology) the archetype or original parent, representing the source of all life. It occurs in the memory as a stage preceding the differentiation of the actual mother and father. See also **collective unconscious.**

primordium /primôr′dē·əm/, *pl.* **primordia** [L, origin], the first recognizable stage in the embryonic development and differentiation of a particular organ, tissue, or structure. Also called **anlage** /un′lägə/, **rudiment.**

principal /prin′sipəl/ [L, *principalis,* first in rank], first in authority or importance.

principal cell. See **chief cell.**

Principen, a trademark for an antibacterial (ampicillin).

principle /prin′sipəl/ [L, *principium,* foundation], **1.** a general truth or settled rule of action. **2.** a prime source or element from which anything proceeds. **3.** a law on which others are founded or from which others are derived.

principles of instrumentation, in dentistry, the six principles for the use of mirrors and other hand and motor-driven devices: 1. grasp; 2. fulcrum; 3. insertion; 4. adaptation and angulation; 5. activation (lateral pressure and working stroke); 6. rest.

Prinivil, a trademark for an angiotensin-converting enzyme (ACE) inhibitor (lisinopril).

P-R interval, in electrocardiography, the interval measured from the beginning of the P wave to the beginning of the QRS complex, representing the atrioventricular conduction time.

printout, a printed copy of information produced by a computer's printer.

Prinzmetal's angina [Myron Prinzmetal, American cardiologist, b. 1908], a variation of angina pectoris in that chest pain is experienced at rest, rather than in relation to effort. The pain tends to occur at night, and there is an electrocardiographic S-T segment elevation instead of depression. It is associated with proximal high-grade coronary artery obstructive lesions or coronary spasm or both. Also called **variant angina.**

priority /prī·ôr′itē/ [L, *prius,* previously], actions established in order of importance or urgency to the welfare or purposes of the organization, patient, or other person at a given time.

Priscoline Hydrochloride, a trademark for a peripheral vasodilator (tolazoline hydrochloride).

prism /priz′əm/ [Gk, *prisma* that which is sawn through], **1.** a solid figure, with a triangular or polygonal crosssection, bounded by parallelograms. **2.** enamel prism, or calcified rods, surrounded by organic prism cuticle joined together to form tooth enamel. **3.** an adverse prism or verger prism used to test and train ocular muscles.

privacy /prī′vəsē/, a culturally specific concept defining the degree of one's personal responsibility to others in regulating behavior that is regarded as intrusive. Some privacy-regulating mechanisms are physical barriers (closed doors or drawn curtains, such as around a hospital bed) and interpersonal types (lowered voices or not smoking).

-privia, a suffix meaning a '(specified) condition of loss or deprivation': *calciprivia, hormonoprivia, paraprivia.*

privileged communication /priv′ilijd/, a legal term employed in court-related proceedings concerning the right to reveal information that belongs to the person who spoke. It may prevent the listener from disclosing the information without the permission of the speaker. Privileged communication may exist between a patient and a health professional only if the law specifically establishes it.

privileges /priv′ilij′əs/ [L, *privilegium,* private law], authority granted to a physician or dentist by a hospital governing board to provide patient care in the hospital. Clinical privileges are limited to the individual's professional license, experience, and competence. Emergency privileges may be granted by a hospital governing board or chief executive officer in an emergency situation and without regard to the physician or dentist's regular service assignment or status. Temporary privileges may be granted a physician or dentist to provide health care to patients for a limited period or to a specific patient.

Privine Hydrochloride, a trademark for an adrenergic (naphazoline hydrochloride).

PRL, abbreviation for **prolactin.**

prn, (in prescriptions) abbreviation for **pro re nata,** a Latin phrase meaning 'as needed.' The times of administration are determined by the needs of the patient. Also **p.r.n.**

Pro, abbreviation for the amino acid **proline.**

pro- /prō-, prə-/, a prefix meaning 'first, or in front of': *procallus, procheilon, progravid.*

proaccelerin. See **factor V.**

probability /prob'əbil'itē/ [L, *probabilitas*], **1.** a measure of the increased likelihood that something will occur. **2.** a mathematic ratio of the number of times something will occur to the total number of possible occurrences.

probable signs /prob'əbəl/ [L, *probabalis,* credible; *signum,* mark], clinical signs that there is a definite likelihood of pregnancy. Examples include enlargement of the abdomen, Goodell's sign, Hegar's sign, Braxton Hicks' sign, and positive hormonal test results. Compare **presumptive signs.**

proband. See **propositus.**

Pro-Banthine, a trademark for an anticholinergic (propantheline bromide).

probenecid /prōben'əsid/, a uricosuric and adjunct to antibiotics.

■ INDICATIONS: It is prescribed in the treatment of gout and as an adjunct prolonging the activity of penicillin or cephalosporins in some infections, such as gonorrhea.

■ CONTRAINDICATIONS: Uric acid kidney stones, blood dyscrasias, or known hypersensitivity to this drug prohibits its use. It is not initiated during acute attack of gout but is continued if an attack intervenes during treatment. It is not given to children under 2 years of age. Concomitant administration of salicylates decreases the effect of probenecid.

■ ADVERSE EFFECTS: Among the most serious adverse reactions are hemolytic anemia, GI disturbances, headache, urinary frequency, and minor allergic reactions. It is involved in many drug interactions, particularly salicylate drugs.

problem /prob'ləm/ [Gk, *proballein,* to throw forward], any health care condition that requires diagnostic, therapeutic, or educational action. An active problem requires immediate action, whereas an inactive problem is one of the past. A subjective problem is one reported by the patient, whereas one noted by an observer is regarded as an objective problem.

problem-oriented medical record (POMR), a method of recording data about the health status of a patient in a problem-solving system. The POMR preserves the data in an easily accessible way that encourages ongoing assessment and revision of the health care plan by all members of the health care team. The particular format of the system used varies from setting to setting, but the components of the method are similar. A data base is collected before beginning the process of identifying the patient's problems. The data base consists of all information available that contributes to this end, such as information collected in an interview with the patient and family or others, information from a health assessment or physical examination of the patient, and information from various laboratory tests. It is recommended that the data base be as complete as possible, limited only by potential hazard, pain or discomfort to the patient, or excessive expense of the diagnostic procedure. The interview, augmented by prior records, provides the patient's history, including the reason for contact, an identifying statement that is a descriptive profile of the person, a family illness history, a history of the current illness, a history of past illness, an account of the patient's current health practices, and a review of systems. The physical examination or health assessment makes up the second major

part of the data base. The extent and depth of the examination vary from setting to setting and depend on the services offered and the condition of the patient. The next section of the POMR is the master problem list. The formulation of the problems on the list is similar to the assessment phase of the nursing process. Each problem as identified represents a conclusion or a decision resulting from examination, investigation, and analysis of the data base. A problem is defined as anything that causes concern to the patient or to the care giver, including physical abnormalities, psychologic disturbance, and socioeconomic problems. The master problem list usually includes active, inactive, temporary, and potential problems. The list serves as an index to the rest of the record and is arranged in five columns: a chronologic list of problems, the date of onset, the action taken, the outcome of the problem (often its resolution), and its date. Problems may be added, and intervention or plans for intervention may be changed; thus the status of each problem is available for the information of all members of the various professions involved in caring for the patient. The third major section of the POMR is the initial plan, in which each separate problem is named and described, usually written on the progress note in a SOAP format: S stands for the subjective data from the patient's point of view; O stands for the objective data acquired by inspection, percussion, auscultation, and palpation and from laboratory tests; A is an assessment of the problem that is an analysis of the subjective and objective data; and P is the plan, including further diagnostic work, therapy, and education or counseling. After an initial plan for each problem is formulated and recorded, the problems are followed in the progress notes by narrative notes in the SOAP format or by flow sheets showing the significant data in a tabular manner. A discharge summary is formulated and written, relating the overall assessment of progress during treatment and the plans for follow-up or referral. The summary allows a review of all the problems initially identified and encourages continuity of care for the patient.

problem-solving approach to patient-centered care, (in nursing) a conceptual framework that incorporates the overt physical needs of a patient with covert psychologic, emotional, and social needs. It provides a model for caring for the whole person as an individual, not as an example of a disease or a medical diagnosis. Nursing is defined within this model as a problem-solving process. The patient is viewed as a person who is in an impaired state, less than usually able to perform self-care activities. Nursing problems are conditions experienced by the patient or the patient's family in which the nurse may provide professional service. The nurse makes a nursing diagnosis that identifies the impaired state and determines the care needed to augment the patients' ability to perform self-care. The requirements for care are classified in four levels. Care given to sustain life is sustenal care; care given to assist the patient in self-care is remedial care; care that helps the patient to develop new skills and goals in self-care is restorative care; and care given to guide the patient to a level of self-help beyond the normal level is preventive care. The approach identifies 21 nursing problems and sorts them into four groups: problems relating to comfort, hygiene, and safety; physiologic balance; psychologic and social factors; and sociologic and community factors. See also **nursing care plan.**

probucol /prōbyoo'kəl/, an anticholesteremic.

■ INDICATIONS: It is prescribed in the treatment of primary

hypercholesterolemia in patients who have not responded to diet, weight control, or other therapies.

■ CONTRAINDICATION: Known sensitivity to this drug prohibits its use.

■ ADVERSE EFFECTS: Among the most serious adverse reactions are a prolongation of the QT interval on an electrocardiogram, diarrhea, palpitations, syncope, dizziness, paresthesia, and eosinophilia.

procainamide hydrochloride /prōkān′əmīd/, an antidysrhythmic agent.

■ INDICATIONS: It is prescribed in the treatment of a variety of cardiac dysrhythmias, including premature ventricular contractions, ventricular tachycardia, and atrial fibrillation.

■ CONTRAINDICATIONS: Myasthenia gravis, heart block, or known hypersensitivity to this drug, to procaine, or to related local anesthetics prohibits its use.

■ ADVERSE EFFECTS: Among the more serious adverse reactions are GI disturbances, hypersensitivity reactions, agranulocytosis, and a syndrome resembling lupus erythematosus.

procaine hydrochloride /prō′kān/, a local anesthetic of the ester family.

■ INDICATIONS: Procaine is administered for local anesthesia by infiltration and injection and for caudal, epidural, and other regional anesthetic procedures. It is not used for topical anesthesia.

■ CONTRAINDICATIONS: Known hypersensitivity to anesthetics of the ester group prohibits its use. It is not injected into inflamed or infected tissue, and large doses are not given to patients with heart block.

■ ADVERSE EFFECTS: Among the most serious adverse reactions are potentially serious neurologic and cardiovascular reactions that result from inadvertent intravascular administration. Allergic reactions also may occur.

procarbazine hydrochloride /prōkär′bəzēn/, an antineoplastic.

■ INDICATIONS: It is prescribed in the treatment of a variety of neoplasms, including Hodgkin's disease and lymphomas.

■ CONTRAINDICATIONS: Bone marrow depression or known hypersensitivity to this drug prohibits its use.

■ ADVERSE EFFECTS: Among the most serious adverse reactions are bone marrow depression and GI disturbances, particularly nausea and vomiting.

Procardia, a trademark for a calcium channel blocker (nifedipine).

procaryocyte. See **prokaryocyte.**

procaryon. See **prokaryon.**

procaryosis. See **prokaryosis.**

Procaryotae /prōker′ē·ō′tē/, (in bacteriology) a kingdom of bacteria, viruses, and blue-green algae that includes all microorganisms in which the nucleoplasm has no basic protein and is not surrounded by a nuclear membrane. The kingdom has two divisions, cyanobacteria, which includes the blue-green bacteria, and bacteria. Also called **Monera.** See also **procaryosyte.**

procaryote. See **prokaryote.**

procedure /prəsē′jər/ [L, *procedere,* to proceed], the sequence of steps to be followed in establishing some course of action.

procerus /prəsir′əs/ [L, stretched], one of three muscles of the nose. Arising from the fascia of the nasal bone and the lateral nasal cartilage and inserting into the skin over the lower part of the forehead between the eyebrows, it is a

small pyramidal muscle, innervated by buccal branches of the facial nerve. The procerus functions to draw down the eyebrows and wrinkle the nose. Compare **depressor septi, nasalis.**

process /pros′əs/ [L, *processus*], **1.** a series of related events that follow in sequence from a particular state or condition to a conclusion or resolution. **2.** a natural growth that projects from a bone or other part. **3.** to put through a particular series of interdependent steps, as in preparing a chemical compound.

process criteria, criteria identified by the American Nurses Association Division on Psychiatric and Mental Health Nursing Practice that focus on nursing activities.

processor. See **central processing unit.**

process recording, (in nursing education) a system used for teaching nursing students to understand and analyze verbal and nonverbal interaction. The conversation between nurse and patient is written on special forms or in a special format. The student nurse is instructed to record observations, perceptions, thoughts, and feelings, as well as the words exchanged. The process recording is then studied by the nursing instructor to discover and to help the student nurse identify patterns of difficulty in communicating with the patient.

processus vaginalis peritonei /prəses′əs/ [L, *processus,* process; *vagina,* sheath; Gk, *peri,* around, *tenein,* to stretch], a diverticulum of the peritoneal membrane that during embryonic development extends through the inguinal canal. In males it descends into the scrotum to form the processus vaginalis testis; in females it is usually completely obliterated. Also called **Nuck's canal, Nuck's diverticulum.**

prochlorperazine /-klôrper′əzēn/, a phenothiazine antipsychotic and antiemetic.

■ INDICATIONS: It is prescribed in the treatment of psychotic disorders and for the control of nausea and vomiting.

■ CONTRAINDICATIONS: Parkinson's disease, the concurrent administration of central nervous system depressants, liver or renal dysfunction, severe hypotension, or known hypersensitivity to any phenothiazine prohibits its use.

■ ADVERSE EFFECTS: Among the more serious adverse effects are hypotension, liver toxicity, extrapyramidal reactions, blood dyscrasias, and hypersensitivity reactions.

prochlorperazine maleate. See **prochlorperazine.**

prochromosome. See **karyosome.**

procidentia /-siden′shə/ [L, *procidere,* to fall forward], the prolapse of an organ. The term is usually applied to a prolapsed uterus.

procoagulant /-ko·ag′yələnt/, a precursor or other agent that mediates the coagulation of blood. Examples include fibrinogen and prothrombin.

proconvertin. See **factor VII.**

procreate /prō′krē·āt/ [L, *procreare,* to beget], to produce offspring.

procreation /-krē·ā′shən/ [L, *procreare,* to create], the entire reproductive process of producing offspring. —**procreate,** *v.*

proct-. See **procto-.**

proctalgia /proktal′jə/ [Gk, *proktos,* anus + *algos,* pain], a neurologic pain in the anus or lower rectum.

proctalgia fugax [Gk, *proktos* + *algos,* pain; L, *fugax,* fleeting], periodic pain in the anus, possibly muscular in origin, that follows a pattern and is sometimes relieved by food and drink.

-proctia, a combining form meaning 'pertaining to the anus or rectum': *ankyloproctia, cacoproctia, coloproctia*.

proctitis /prokti′tis/ [Gk, *proktos*, anus, *itis*], inflammation of the rectum and anus caused by infection, trauma, drugs, allergy, or radiation injury. Acute or chronic, it is accompanied by rectal discomfort and the repeated urge to pass feces with the inability to do so. Pus, blood, or mucus may be present in the stools, and tenesmus may be present. Also called **rectitis**.

procto- /prok′tō-/, **proct-,** a combining form meaning 'of or pertaining to anus or rectum': *proctocele, proctorrhea, proctoscopy*.

proctocele. See **rectocele.**

proctocolectomy /prok′tōkəlek′təmē/, a surgical procedure in which the anus, rectum, and colon are removed. An ileostomy is established for the removal of digestive tract wastes. The procedure is a common treatment for severe, intractable ulcerative colitis. See also **ileoanal anastomosis**.

Proctocort, a trademark for a glucocorticoid (hydrocortisone).

proctodeum proktō′dē·əm/, *pl.* **proctodea** [Gk, *proktos* + *hodiaos*, a route], an invagination of the ectoderm, behind the urorectal septum of the developing embryo, that forms the anus and anal canal when the cloacal membrane ruptures. Also spelled **proctodaeum** (*pl.* **proctodaea**). Compare **stomodeum**. **–proctodeal, proctodaeal,** *adj.*

proctodynia /-din′ē·ə/ [Gk, *proktos* + *odyne*, pain], pain in or around the anus.

proctologist /proktol′əjist/, a physician who specializes in proctology.

proctology /proktol′əjē/ [Gk, *proktos* + *logos*, science], the branch of medicine concerned with treating disorders of the colon, rectum, and anus.

proctoplasty /prok′təplas′tē/ [Gk, *proktos*, anus + *plassein*, to mold], a plastic surgery procedure on the anus and rectum.

proctoscope /prok′təskōp′/ [Gk, *proktos* + *skopein*, to look], an instrument used to examine the rectum and the distal portion of the colon. It consists of a light mounted on a tube or speculum. Compare **sigmoidoscope.**

proctoscopy /proktos′kəpē/, the examination of the rectum with an endoscope inserted through the anus.

proctosigmoidoscopy /prok′tōsig′moidos′kəpē/ [Gk, *proktos* + *sigmoid* + *skopein*, to view], the use of a sigmoidoscope to examine the rectum and pelvic colon.

procyclidine hydrochloride /prōsī′klədēn/, an anticholinergic.

■ INDICATIONS: It is prescribed in the treatment of parkinsonism, and to relieve extrapyramidal dysfunctions and to control sialorrhea that are side effects of other medications.

■ CONTRAINDICATIONS: Narrow-angle glaucoma, asthma, obstruction of the genitourinary or GI tract, severe ulcerative colitis, or known hypersensitivity to this drug prohibits its use.

■ ADVERSE EFFECTS: Among the more serious adverse effects are confusion, disorientation, blurred vision, central nervous system effects, tachycardia, dry mouth, decreased sweating, and hypersensitivity reactions.

prodromal /-drō′məl/ [Gk, *pro,* before + *dromos,* course], pertaining to early symptoms that may mark the onset of a disease.

prodromal labor [Gk, *prodromos,* running before; L, *labor,* work], the early period in parturition before uterine contractions become forceful and frequent enough to result in progressive dilatation of the uterine cervix.

prodromal phase, a clear deterioration in function before the active phase of a mental disturbance that is not caused by a disorder in mood or a psychoactive substance and includes some residual phase symptoms.

prodromal symptom [Gk, *pro* + *dromos,* course; *symptoma,* that which happens], a symptom that may be the first indication of the onset of a disease.

prodrome /prō′drōm/ [Gk, *prodromos,* running before], **1.** an early sign of a developing condition or disease. **2.** the earliest phase of a developing condition or disease. **–prodromal,** *adj.*

prodrug /prō′drug/, an inactive or partially active drug that is metabolically changed in the body to an active drug.

product evaluation committee /prod′əkt/, a hospital committee composed of medical, nursing, purchasing, and administrative staff members whose purpose is to evaluate health-care-related products and advise on their procurement.

productive cough /prəduk′tiv/ [L, *producere* + AS, *cohhetan,* to cough], a sudden, noisy expulsion of air from the lungs that effectively removes sputum from the respiratory tract and helps clear the airways, permitting oxygen to reach the alveoli. Coughing is stimulated by irritation or by inflammation of the respiratory tract caused most frequently by infection. Deep breathing, with contraction of the diaphragm and intercostal muscles and forceful exhalation, promotes productive coughing in patients with respiratory infections. Mucolytic agents liquefy mucus in the respiratory tract so that it can be raised and expectorated more easily. Anticholinergic drugs, such as atropine, decrease pulmonary secretions. See also **nonproductive cough.**

-profen, a combining form for ibuprofen-type antiinflammatory or analgesic substances.

professional corporation (PC) /prəfesh′ənəl/ [L, *professio,* profession], a corporation formed according to the law of a particular state for the purpose of delivering a professional service. In some states, corporations may not practice law, medicine, surgery, or dentistry, but in some states nurses may form or be partners in a professional corporation. According to the laws of the various states, professional corporations may offer legal and tax benefits to the members of the corporation.

professional liability, the legal obligation of health care professionals, or their insurers, to compensate patients for injury or suffering caused by acts of omission or commission by the professionals. Professional liability better describes the responsibility of all professionals to their clients than does the concept of malpractice, but the idea of professional liability is central to malpractice.

professional network, (in psychiatric nursing) the network of professional resources available to support the psychiatric outpatient in the community. The network may include a therapist, a hospital day treatment program, social work agency, and other agencies.

professional organization, an organization whose members share a professional status, created to deal with issues of concern to the professional group or groups involved.

Professional Standards Review Organization (PSRO), an organization formed under Social Security Act Amendments of 1972 to review the services provided under Medicare, Medicaid, and Maternal Child Health programs. Review is conducted by physicians to ascertain the need for the program and to ensure that it is carried out in accord with certain criteria, norms, and standards, and, in institutional situations, in a proper setting. The PSRO requires that regional organizations be formed to conduct these reviews throughout the nation.

profibrinolysin. See **fibrinogen.**

profile /prō'fīl/ [L, *profilare*, to outline], a short sketch, diagram, or summary relating to a person or thing.

profunda /prōfun'də/ [L, *profundus*, deep], pertaining to structures, mainly blood vessels, that are deeply embedded in tissues.

profuse sweat /prəfyoōs'/ [L, *profundere*, to pour out; AS, *swaetan*], excessive perspiration. Also called **diaphoresis.**

progenitive /-jen'itiv/ [Gk, *pro*, before, *genein*, to produce], capable of producing offspring; reproductive.

progenitor /-jen'itər/ [Gk, *pro + genein*], 1. a parent or ancestor. 2. someone or something that begets or creates.

progeny /proj'ənē/ [L, *progenies*], 1. offspring; an individual or organism resulting from a particular mating. 2. the descendants of a known or common ancestor.

progeria /prōjir'ē·ə/ [Gk, *pro + geras*, old age], an abnormal congenital condition characterized by premature aging, the appearance in childhood of gray hair and wrinkled skin, small stature, absence of pubic and facial hair, and the posture and habitus of an aged person. Death usually occurs before 20 years of age. Compare **infantilism.**

progestagen. See **progestogen.**

Progestasert, a trademark for a progestin (progesterone).

progestational /prō'jestā'shənəl/ [Gk, *pro* + L, *gestare*, to bear], of or pertaining to a drug with effects similar to those of progesterone, the hormone produced by the corpus luteum and adrenal cortex during the luteal phase of the menstrual cycle that prepares the uterus for reception of the fertilized ovum. Natural and synthetic preparations of progesterone and its derivative medroxyprogesterone acetate are used in the treatment of secondary amenorrhea and abnormal uterine bleeding. Progestational compounds, such as norethindrone and norgestrel, are constituents of oral contraceptives. The use of progestins to prevent habitual or threatened abortion is no longer recommended.

progestational agent [L, *pro + gestare*, to bear, *agere*, to do], any chemical having the same action as progesterone produced by the corpus luteum and the placenta.

progestational phase. See **secretory phase.**

progesterone /prəjes'tərōn/, a natural progestational hormone.

■ INDICATIONS: It is prescribed in the treatment of various menstrual disorders, infertility associated with luteal phase dysfunction, and repeated spontaneous abortion.

■ CONTRAINDICATIONS: Thrombophlebitis, liver dysfunction, breast cancer, missed abortion, or hypersensitivity to this drug prohibits its use.

■ ADVERSE EFFECTS: Among the more serious adverse reactions are pain at the site of injection, catabolic effects, and electrolyte disturbances.

progestin /-jes'tin/ 1. progesterone. 2. any of a group of hormones, natural or synthetic, secreted by the corpus luteum, placenta, or adrenal cortex that have a progesterone-like effect on the uterine endometrial lining to prepare it for implantation of the blastocyst.

progestogen /-jes'təjən/, any natural or synthetic progestational hormone. Also spelled **progestagen.** Also called **progestin.**

proglottid /prōglot'id/ [Gk, *pro + glossa*, tongue], a sex-

ual segment of an adult tapeworm, containing both male and female reproductive organs. Each mature segment is shed and produces additional tapeworms.

prognathism /prog'nəthiz'əm/ [Gk, *pro + gnathos*, jaw], an abnormal facial configuration in which one or both jaws project forward. It is considered real or imaginary, depending on anatomic and developmental factors involved. Real prognathism may exist when both the mandible and the maxilla increase in length or when the length of the maxilla is normal and the mandibular length increases excessively. Imaginary prognathism may exist when the maxilla is underdeveloped and the mandibular length is normal. **–prognathic,** adj.

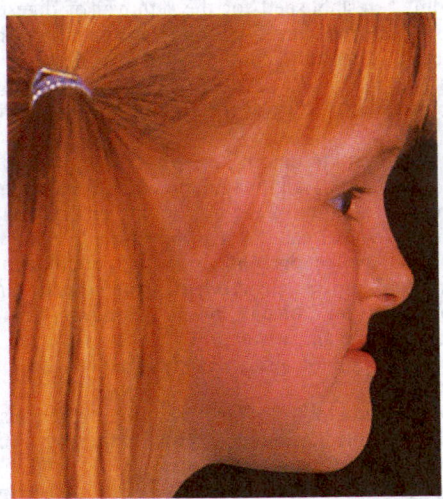

Prognathic mandible *(Salyer, 1989)*

prognosis /prognō'sis/ [Gk, *pro + gnosis*, knowledge], a prediction of the probable outcome of a disease based on the condition of the person and the usual course of the disease as observed in similar situations.

prognostic /prognos'tik/ [Gk, *pro + gnosis*, knowledge], pertaining to signs and symptoms that may indicate the outcome of a disease or injury.

program /prō'grəm/ [Gk, *pro + gramma*, record], a sequence of instructions, written in computer programming language, that controls the functions of a computer.

program documentation. See **documentation.**

programmable pacemaker /-gram'əbəl/ [Gk, *pro + graphein*, to write; L, *passus*, step; ME, *maken*], an electronic pacemaker with multiple settings that can be changed after implantation.

programmed pacing. See **pacing.**

programmer /prō'grəmər/, a person skilled in writing or coding computer programs.

programming language. See **language.**

progravid /-gravid/ [L, *pro + gravid*, pregnant], before pregnancy.

progression /-gresh'ən/, a carcinogenic process whereby cells altered by initiators undergo a second genetic mutation that allows uncontrollable growth. They progress to malignant cells.

progressive /-gres'iv/ [L, *progredi*, to advance], describing the course of a disease or condition in which the characteristic signs and symptoms become more prominent and severe, such as progressive muscular atrophy.

progressive assistive exercise, an exercise designed to progressively improve the strength of a muscle group by gradually increasing resistance against contractions with the assistance of a therapist.

progressive bulbar paralysis [L, *progredi,* to advance, *bulbus,* swollen root; Gk, *paralyein* to be paralyzed], a motor neuron disease characterized by weakness of the laryngeal, pharyngeal, tongue, and facial muscles. The patient experiences progressive dysarthria and dysphagia. Also called **Duchenne's paralysis.** See **association paralysis.**

progressive interstitial hypertrophic neuropathy. See **Déjérine-Sottas disease.**

progressive myonecrosis. See **myonecrosis.**

progressive myopia [L, *progredi;* Gk, *myops,* nearsighted], a condition in which myopia increases at a more rapid rate than normal, often continuing into adulthood.

progressive ophthalmoplegia [L, *progredi*], a form of ocular muscle paralysis that usually begins with ptosis and gradually involves all of the extraocular muscles.

progressive patient care, a system of care in which patients are placed in units on the basis of their needs for care as determined by the degree of illness rather than in units based on a medical specialty. The usual levels or stages of progressive patient care are intensive care, intermediate care, and minimal care.

progressive relaxation, a technique for combating tension and anxiety by systematically tensing and relaxing muscle groups.

progressive resistance exercise, a method of increasing the strength of a weak or injured muscle by gradually increasing the resistance against which the muscle works, such as by using graduated weights over a period of time. Also called **graduated resistance exercise.** See also **active resistance exercise.**

progressive spinal muscular atrophy of infants. See **Werdnig-Hoffmann disease.**

progressive subcortical encephalopathy. See **Schilder's disease.**

progressive supranuclear palsy [L, *supra,* above; *nucleus,* nut; Gk, *paralyein*], a mild form of paralysis involving muscles innervated by the cranial nerves and affecting primarily the face, throat, and tongue.

progressive systemic sclerosis (PSS), the most common form of scleroderma.

progress notes [L, *progredi* + *nota,* mark], (in the patient record) notes made by a nurse and physician that describe the patient's condition and the treatments given or planned. Progress notes may follow the problem-oriented medical record format. The physician's progress notes usually focus on the medical or therapeutic aspects of the patient's condition and care; the nurse's progress notes, although recording the medical conditions of the patient, usually focus on the objectives stated in the nursing care plan. These objectives might include responses to prescribed treatments, the person's ability to perform activities of daily living, and acceptance or understanding of a particular condition or treatment. Progress notes in an in-hospital setting are recorded daily; progress notes in a clinic or office setting are usually preceded by an episodic or interval history and are written as an account of each visit.

proinsulin /prō·in′s(y)əlin/ [L, *pro* + *insula,* island], a single-chain protein molecule that is a precursor of insulin.

projectile vomiting /-jek′til/, expulsive vomiting that is extremely forceful.

projection /-jek′shən/ [L, *projectio,* thrown forward], **1.** a protuberance; anything that thrusts or juts outward. **2.** the act of perceiving an idea or thought as an objective reality. **3.** (in psychology) an unconscious defense mechanism by which an individual attributes his or her own unacceptable traits, ideas, or impulses to another.

projection reconstruction imaging, the techniques used in NMR imaging to obtain a cross-sectional image of an object. Such an image is computer reconstructed from a series of projections, NMR profiles, recorded all around the object by rotating the direction of the gradient field superimposed on the static magnetic field.

projective test /-jek′tiv/ [L, *projectio,* thrown forward], a kind of diagnostic, psychologic, or personality test that uses unstructured or ambiguous stimuli, such as inkblots, a series of pictures, abstract patterns, or incomplete sentences, to elicit responses that reflect a projection of various aspects of the individual's personality. See also **Rorschach test.**

prokaryocyte /prōker′ē·əsīt′/ [Gk, *protos,* first, *karyon,* nut, *kytos,* cell], a cell without a true nucleus and with nuclear material scattered throughout the cytoplasm. Prokaryocytic organisms (**Procaryotae**) include bacteria, viruses, rickettsiae, chlamydiae, mycoplasmas, actinomycetes, and certain algae. Also spelled **procaryocyte.** Compare **eukaryocyte.**

prokaryon /prōker′ē·on/ [Gk, *protos* + *karyon,* nut], **1.** nuclear elements that are not bound by a membrane but are spread throughout the cytoplasm. **2.** an organism containing such unbound nuclear elements. Also spelled **procaryon.** Compare **eukaryon.**

prokaryosis /-ker′ē·ō′sis/ [Gk, *protos, karyon* + *osis,* condition], the condition of not containing a true nucleus surrounded by a nuclear membrane. Also spelled **procaryosis.** Compare **eukaryosis.**

prokaryote /prōker′ē·ōt/ [Gk, *protos* + *karyon*], an organism that does not contain a true nucleus surrounded by a nuclear membrane, characteristic of lower forms, such as bacteria, viruses, and blue-green bacteria. Division occurs through simple fission. Also spelled **procaryote.** Compare **eukaryote. –prokaryotic,** *adj.*

prolactin (PRL) /prōlak′tin/ [Gk, *pro,* before, *lac,* milk], a hormone produced and secreted into the bloodstream by the anterior pituitary. Prolactin, acting with estrogen, progesterone, thyroxine, insulin, growth hormone, glucocorticoids, and human placental lactogen, stimulates the development and growth of the mammary glands. After parturition, prolactin together with glucocorticoids is essential for the initiation and maintenance of milk production. Prolactin synthesis and release from the pituitary is mediated by the central nervous system in response to suckling by the infant. When suckling or its mechanical equivalent ceases, prolactin secretion slows and milk production ceases. Prolactin is similar to growth hormone in its chemical structure. Prolactin excess is seen in the presence of prolactin-secreting pituitary tumors in both sexes. Also called **lactogenic hormone, luteotropin.**

prolapse /prō′laps, prōlaps′/ [L, *prolapsus,* falling], the falling, sinking, or sliding of an organ from its normal position or location in the body, such as a prolapsed uterus.

prolapsed cord /prōlapst′/, an umbilical cord that protrudes beside or ahead of the presenting part of the fetus.

prolapsed hemorrhoid [L, *prolapsus,* falling; Gk, *haimorrhois,* a vein that loses blood], internal hemorrhoids that protrude through the anal orifice.

prolapse of anus [L, *prolapsus,* falling, *anus*] the protrusion of the mucous membrane of the anus through the external sphincter.

prolapse of rectum [L, *prolapsus*, falling, *rectus*, straight], a protrusion of the mucous membrane of the lower portion of the rectum through the anal orifice.

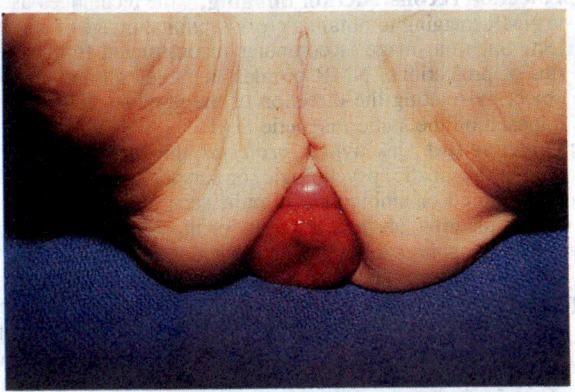

Prolapse of rectum (Zitelli, 1992)

prolapse of uterus [L, *prolapsus*, falling, *uterus*, womb], the descent of the uterine cervix into the vagina, partly into the vagina, or outside the vagina.

Prolastin, a trademark for an inherited protein-deficiency disorder leading to emphysema (alpha₁-proteinase inhibitor, human).

proliferate /-lif'ərāt/ [L, *proles*, offspring + *ferre*, to bear], to grow by multiplication of cells, parts, or organisms.

proliferation /-lif'ərā'shən/ [L, *proles*, offspring, *ferre*, to bear], the reproduction or multiplication of similar forms. The term is usually applied to increases of cells or cysts.

proliferative phase /-lif'ərətiv/, the phase of the menstrual cycle after menstruation. Under the influence of follicle stimulating hormone from the pituitary, the ovary produces increasing amounts of estrogen, causing the lining of the uterus to become dense and richly vascular. The phase is terminated by rupture of a mature follicle and subsequent ovulation. Compare **menstrual phase, secretory phase.**

prolific /lif'ik/ [L, *proles*, offspring + *ferre*, to bear], highly productive.

proline (Pro) /prō'lēn/, a nonessential amino acid found in many proteins of the body, particularly collagen. See also **amino acid, protein.**

Proloid, a trademark for a thyroid hormone preparation (thyroglobulin).

prolonged gestation /-longd'/ [L, *prolongare*, to lengthen + *gestare*, to bear], a pregnancy that lasts longer than the usual time of 41 weeks.

prolonged release [Gk, *pro*, before, *longus*, long], a term applied to a drug that is designed to deliver a dose of a medication over an extended period of time. The most common device for this purpose is a soft, soluble capsule containing minute pellets of the drug for release at different rates in the GI tract, depending on the thickness and nature of the oil, fat, wax, or resin coating on the pellets. Another system consists of a porous plastic carrier impregnated with the drug and a surfactant to facilitate the entry of GI fluids that slowly leach out the drug. Ion exchange resins that bind to drugs and liquids containing suspensions of slow-release drug granules are also used to provide medication over an extended period. Various mechanisms and vehicles have also been developed to prolong the release of drugs after injection.

Proloprim, a trademark for an antibacterial (trimethoprim).

promethazine hydrochloride /-meth'əzēn/, a phenothiazine antiemetic, antihistamine, and sedative.
- ■ INDICATIONS: It is prescribed in the treatment of motion sickness, nausea, rhinitis, itching, and skin rash.
- ■ CONTRAINDICATIONS: Known hypersensitivity to this drug or to other phenothiazines prohibits its use.
- ■ ADVERSE EFFECTS: Drowsiness, hypotension, and dry mouth are the most common adverse reactions.

promethium (Pm) /-mē'thē·əm/ [L, *Prometheus*, mythic character who brought fire to earth], a radioactive, rare earth, metallic element. Its atomic number is 61; its atomic weight is 145.

prominence /prom'inəns [L, *prominentia*, sticking out], any elevation or projection of a structural feature.

promontory of the sacrum /prom'əntôr'ē/ [L, *promontorium*, headland], the superior projecting part of the sacrum at its junction with the L5 vertebra.

promoter /-mō'tər/ [L, *promovere*, to move forward], **1.** (in molecular genetics) a DNA sequence that initiates RNA transcription of the genetic code. **2.** a cocarcinogenic factor that encourages cells altered by initiators to reproduce at a faster than normal rate, increasing the probability of malignant transformation. Examples include DDT, phenobarbital, saccharin, sunlight, and some chemicals in cigarette smoke. Effects of promoters are sometimes reversible.

prompt insulin zinc suspension [L, *promptus*, ready], a fast-acting noncrystalline semilente insulin prescribed in the treatment of diabetes mellitus when a prompt, intense, and short-acting response is desired. It is only slightly slower to act than insulin injection. See also **fast-acting insulin.**

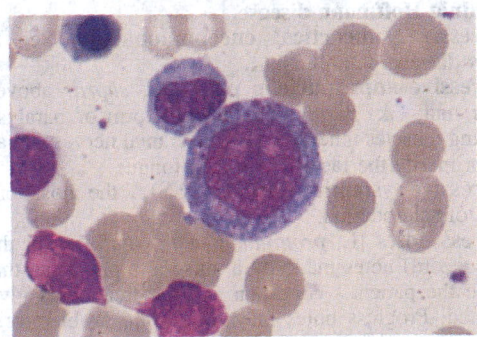

Promyelocyte (Powers, 1989)

promyelocyte /prōmī'ələsīt'/, a large mononuclear blood cell that contains a single, regular, symmetric nucleus and a few undifferentiated cytoplasmic granules. As an intermediate stage in development between a myeloblast and a myelocyte, promyelocytes in the circulating blood are indicative of leukemia.

pronate /prō'nāt/ [L, *pronare*, to bend forward], to place in a prone position of lying flat with the face forward.

pronation /prōnā'shən/ [L, *pronare*, to bend forward], **1.** assumption of a prone position, one in which the ventral surface of the body faces downward. **2.** (of the arm) the rotation of the forearm so that the palm of the hand faces downward and backward. **3.** (of the foot) the lowering of the medial edge of the foot by turning it outward and through abduction movements in the tarsal and metatarsal joints. **–pronate,** *v.*

pronator reflex /prōnā′tər/ [L, *pronare* + *reflectere*, to bend backward], a reflex elicited by holding the patient's hand vertically and tapping the distal end of the radius or ulna, resulting in pronation of the forearm. Hyperactivity of the reflex may be seen with lesions of the pyramidal system above the level of the sixth cervical nerve root. Also called **ulnar reflex.**

pronator syndrome [L, *pronare*, to bend forward; Gk, *syn*, together + *dromos*, course], the compression of the median nerve between the two heads of the pronator teres muscle.

pronator teres, /ter′əs/, a superficial muscle of the forearm, arising from a humeral and an ulnar head. The humeral head is the larger and more superficial, originating near the medial epicondyle, from the tendon common to the superficial muscles of the forearm, from certain intermuscular septa, and from the antebrachial fascia. The ulnar head originates in the coronoid process of the ulna. Fibers from both portions of the muscle pass obliquely across the forearm, ending in a flat tendon that inserts into the radius. The pronator teres is innervated by a branch of the median nerve, which contains fibers from the sixth and the seventh cervical nerves, and it functions to pronate the hand. Compare **flexor carpi radialis, flexor carpi ulnaris, flexor digitorum superficialis, palmaris longus**.

prone /prōn/ [L, *pronus*, inclined forward], **1.** having a tendency or inclination. **2.** (of the body) being in horizontal position when lying face downward. Compare **supine.**

Pronemia, a trademark for a hematinic, fixed-combination drug containing iron, vitamin B_{12}, intrinsic factor concentrate, vitamin C, and folic acid.

proneness profile /prōn′nəs/ [L, *pronus* + *profilare*, to outline], a screening process that evaluates the probability of developmental problems occurring in the early years of a child's life. Screening ideally begins in the course of prenatal care and continues after birth. Several of the variables in the proneness profile that appear to be significant in selecting the infants who are at risk are the perinatal health status of the mother and infant, especially complications of pregnancy, delivery, the neonatal period, and the puerperium; characteristics of the mother, especially her temperament, educational level, perception of the life situation, and perception of the infant; characteristics of the infant, including alertness, activity pattern, and responsiveness; and the behaviors of the infant and care giver as they interact. The proneness profile is followed by a developmental profile that assesses the current status of the infant and care giver. Three areas to be considered are characteristics of the infant, including adaptation and response to the environment, the ability to give interpretable cues, and the developmental progress as compared with established norms; characteristics of the care giver, including adaptation to the new infant, sensitivity to cues from the infant, and techniques for relieving distress; and the healthful quality of the environment, including health, safety, comfort, and stimulation.

prone-on-elbows, a body position in which the person rests the upper part of the body on the elbows while lying face down. The position is used as an initial rehabilitation exercise in training a person with a cerebellar dysfunction to achieve ambulation. From prone-on-elbows the person can practice weight shifting through the hips to a quadruped position without the risk of falling from a standing position.

pronephric duct /-nef′rik/ [Gk, *pro*, before, *nephros*, kidney; L, *ducere*, to lead], one of the paired ducts that connect the tubules of each of the pronephros with the cloaca in the early developing vertebrate embryo. They later become the functional mesonephric ducts. Also called **archinephric canal, archinephric duct.**

pronephric tubule, any of the segmentally arranged excretory units of the pronephros in the early developing vertebrate embryo. The tubules open into the pronephric duct and communicate with the coelom through a nephrostoma. In humans and the higher vertebrates the tubules are present only in vestigial form; in lower animals, they are functional.

pronephros /-nef′rəs/, *pl.* **pronephroi** [Gk, *pro* + *nephros*, kidney], the primordial excretory organ in the developing vertebrate embryo. It consists of a series of pronephric tubules that arise along the anterior portion of the nephrotome and empty into the cloaca by way of the pronephric duct. In humans and other mammals the structure is nonfunctional, representing the first of three excretory systems that are formed one after the other in an anterior to posterior sequence and that disappear with the formation of the mesonephros. The organ is functional in certain primitive fishes, such as lampreys, and serves as a provisional kidney in some fishes and amphibians. Also called **pronephron** (*pl.* **pronephra**), **archinephron, head kidney.** See also **mesonephros, metanephros.** **–pronephric,** *adj.*

prone position [L, *pronare*, to bend forward + *positio*], a postural position of facing downward while lying flat.

prone posture [L, *pronare*, to bend forward + *ponere*, to place], a posture assumed by lying flat with the face forward during certain disorders of the spine or viscera.

Pronestyl, a trademark for a cardiac depressant (procainamide hydrochloride).

pronucleus /-nōō′klē-əs/, *pl.* **pronuclei** [Gk, *pro* + L, *nucleus*, nut], the nucleus of the ovum or the spermatozoon after fertilization but before the fusion of the chromosomes to form the nucleus of the zygote. Each contains the haploid number of chromosomes, is larger than the normal nucleus, and is diffuse in appearance. The female pronucleus of the mature ovum is formed only after penetration by the sperm and the completion of the second mitotic division and polar body formation. The nucleus then loses its nuclear envelope to release the chromosomes so that synapsis can occur with the chromosomes of the male pronucleus, which is contained in the head of the spermatozoon. Also called **germinal nucleus, germ nucleus.** See also **oogenesis, spermatogenesis.**

propagation /prop′əgā′shən/ [L, *propagare*, to generate], the process of increasing or causing to increase.

propantheline bromide /-pan′thəlēn/, an anticholinergic.
■ INDICATION: It is prescribed as an adjunct in peptic ulcer therapy.
■ CONTRAINDICATIONS: Narrow-angle glaucoma, asthma, obstruction of the genitourinary or GI tract, severe ulcerative colitis, or known hypersensitivity to this drug prohibits its use.
■ ADVERSE EFFECTS: Among the more serious adverse reactions are blurred vision, central nervous system effects, tachycardia, dry mouth, decreased sweating, and hypersensitivity reactions.

proparacaine hydrochloride /prōper′əkān/, a rapid-acting, topical anesthetic of the amide family used for ophthalmologic procedures. It is used for tonometry, gonioscopy, removal of foreign objects from the eye, and other minor optic procedures, and preoperatively for major eye surgery. One drop gives 15 minutes of optic anesthesia. Prolonged use may injure the eye. Proparacaine hydrochloride is not administered to individuals with cardiac disease, hyperthyroidism, or multiple allergies. People given the drug should be warned not to touch their eyes until the anesthetic has worn off. Adverse optic reactions may occur with proparacaine, but systemic reactions are rare. Also called **proxymetacaine.**

properidin system. See **alternative pathway of complement activation.**

prophase /prō′fāz/ [Gk, *pro* + *phasis,* appearance], the first of four stages of nuclear division in mitosis and in each of the two divisions of meiosis. In mitosis, the chromosomes progressively shorten and thicken to form individually recognizable elongated double structures composed of two chromatids held together by a centromere; the nucleolus and nuclear membrane disappear, the spindle and polar bodies are formed, and the chromosomes begin to migrate toward the midplane of the developing spindle. In the first meiotic division, prophase is complex and subdivided into five stages: leptotene, zygotene, pachytene, diplotene, and diakinesis. In the second meiotic division, the same processes occur as in mitotic prophase. See also **anaphase, interphase, meiosis, metaphase, mitosis, telophase.**

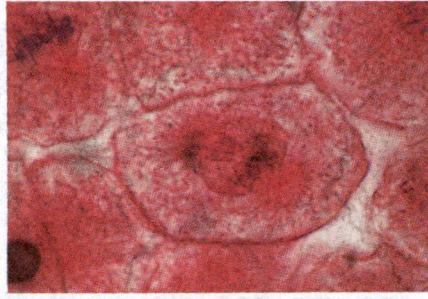

Prophase
(Seeley, 1992/Ed Reschke/Michael Abbey, Science Source)

prophylactic /prō′filak′tik/ [Gk, *prophylax,* advance guard], **1.** preventing the spread of disease. **2.** an agent that prevents the spread of disease. **3.** See **condom. –prophylactically,** *adv.*

prophylactic forceps. See **low forceps.**

prophylactic odontomy, (in dentistry) the surgical removal of harmful pits and fissures in the posterior primary and permanent molars to prevent and preclude the formation of caries in those areas.

prophylactic treatment. See **preventive treatment.**

prophylaxis /prō′filak′sis/ [Gk, *prophylax*], prevention of or protection against disease, often involving the use of a biologic, chemical, or mechanical agent to destroy or prevent the entry of infectious organisms.

Propionibacterium /prō′pē·on′ēbaktir′ē·əm/ [Gk, *pro* + *pion,* fat, *bacterion* small rod], a genus of nonmotile, anaerobic, gram-positive bacteria found on the skin of humans, in the intestinal tract of humans and animals, and in

dairy products. **P. acnes** is common in acne pustules (formerly called **Corynebacterium acnes).**

propionicacidemia /prō′pē·on′ikas′idē′mē·ə/ [Gk, *pro* + *pion;* L, *acidus,* sour; Gk, *haima,* blood], a rare inherited metabolic defect caused by the failure of the body to metabolize the amino acids threonine, isoleucine, and methionone, characterized by lethargy and mental and physical retardation. Acidosis occurs as a result of the accumulation of propionic acid in the body. A diet low in these amino acids is difficult to achieve but is the only treatment. **–propionicacidemic,** *adj.*

propionic fermentation /prō′pē·on′ik/ [Gk, *pro* + *pion;* L, *fermentare,* to cause to ferment], the production of propionic acid by the action of certain bacteria on sugars or lactic acid.

Proplex, a trademark for human clotting factor IX.

proportional gas detector /-pôr′shənəl/ a device for measuring alpha and beta forms of radioactivity.

proportional mortality [L, *pro* + *portio,* part; *mortalis,* subject to death], a statistical method of relating the number of deaths from a particular condition to all deaths within the same population group for the same time period.

proposition /prop′əzish′ən/ [L, *proponere,* to place forward], **1.** a statement of a truth to be demonstrated or an operation to be performed. **2.** to bring forward or offer for consideration, acceptance, or adoption.

propositus /prōpoz′itəs/ [L, *proponere,* to place forward], a person from whom a genealogic lineage is traced, as is done to discover the pattern of inheritance of a familial disease or a physical trait.

propoxyphene /prōpok′səfēn/, a mild centrally acting narcotic analgesic.

■ INDICATION: It is prescribed to relieve mild to moderate pain.

■ CONTRAINDICATIONS: Concurrent administration of tranquilizers or antidepressant drugs, current alcohol or drug abuse, or known hypersensitivity to this drug prohibits its use. It is not recommended for use by people who are suicidal or prone to alcohol or drug addiction or by women who are pregnant, because neonatal withdrawal symptoms have been observed.

■ ADVERSE EFFECTS: Among the more serious reactions are hepatic dysfunction and severe depression of the central nervous system occurring with overdose or drug interaction. A small number of people may experience nausea, dizziness, sedation, or vomiting when correctly taking a usual, prescribed dosage.

propoxyphene hydrochloride, an analgesic.

■ INDICATION: It is prescribed for the relief of mild to moderate pain.

■ CONTRAINDICATIONS: Known hypersensitivity to this drug or known narcotic addiction prohibits its use.

■ ADVERSE EFFECTS: Among the more serious adverse reactions are respiratory depression, paradoxical excitement, and convulsions.

propranolol hydrochloride /-pran′əlol/, a beta-adrenergic blocking agent.

■ INDICATIONS: It is prescribed in the treatment of angina pectoris, cardiac dysrhythmias, and hypertension.

■ CONTRAINDICATIONS: Asthma, certain dysrhythmias, congestive heart failure, concomitant use of monamine oxidase inhibitors, or known hypersensitivity to this drug prohibits its use.

■ ADVERSE EFFECTS: Among the more serious adverse reac-

tions are heart failure, heart block, increased airway resistance, augmentation of hypoglycemic response, GI disturbances, and hypersensitivity reactions. Withdrawal syndrome has been observed in some patients.

proprietary /-prī'əterē/ [L, *proprietas,* a property], **1.** of or pertaining to an institution or other organization that is operated for profit. **2.** of or pertaining to a product, such as a drug or device, that is made for profit.

proprietary hospital, a hospital operated as a profit-making organization. Many proprietary hospitals are owned by physicians who operate the hospital primarily for their own patients but also accept patients from other physicians. Some proprietary hospitals are owned by investor groups or large corporations.

proprietary medicine, any pharmaceutic preparation or medicinal substance that is protected from commercial competition because its ingredients or method of manufacture is kept secret or is protected by trademark or copyright.

proprioception /prō'prē·əsep'shən/ [L, *proprius,* one's own, *capere,* to take], sensation pertaining to stimuli originating from within the body regarding spatial position and muscular activity or to the sensory receptors that they activate. Compare **exteroceptive, interoceptive.** See also **autotopagnosia.**

proprioceptive /-prē·ə·sep'tiv/ [L, *proprius,* one's own + *capere,* to take], pertaining to the sensations of body movements, and awareness of posture, enabling the body to orient itself in space without visual clues.

proprioceptive neuromuscular facilitation (PNF), an activity, such as a therapeutic technique, that helps initiate a proprioceptive response in a person. An example is a slow rocking movement that relaxes an anxious person by stimulating vestibular and proprioceptive nerve receptors. Techniques are used to facilitate total body responses or selective postural extensors.

proprioceptive receptors [L, *propius,* one's own + *capere,* to take; *recipere,* to receive], sensory nerve terminals, found in muscles, joints, tendons, and the inner ear, that are sensitive to body position and movement.

proprioceptive reflex [L, *proprius* + *capere,* to take; *reflectere,* to bend backward], any reflex initiated by stimulation of proprioceptive receptors, such as the increase in respiratory rate and volume induced by impulses arising from muscles and joints during exercise.

proprioceptive sensation [L, *propius* + *capere; sentire,* to feel], the feelings of body movement and position, including motion of the arms and legs, resulting from stimuli received by special sense organs in the muscles, tendons, joints, and labyrinth of the ear. The stimuli may be produced by changes in muscle tension or stretching and reaction to the pull of gravity on the body.

proprioceptor /prō'prē·əsep'tər/ [L, *proprius* + *capere*], any sensory nerve ending, such as those located in muscles, tendons, joints, and the vestibular apparatus, that responds to stimuli originating from within the body regarding movement and spatial position. Compare **exteroceptor, interoceptor.** See also **mechanoreceptor.**

proptosis /proptō'sis/ [L, *prop* + *ptosis,* falling], bulging, protrusion, or forward displacement of a body organ or area.

propulsion /-pul'shən/ [L, *propellere,* to drive forward], **1.** the process of pushing forward. **2.** the tendency of some patients, particularly those afflicted with nervous disorders, to push or fall forward while walking as their center of gravity is displaced.

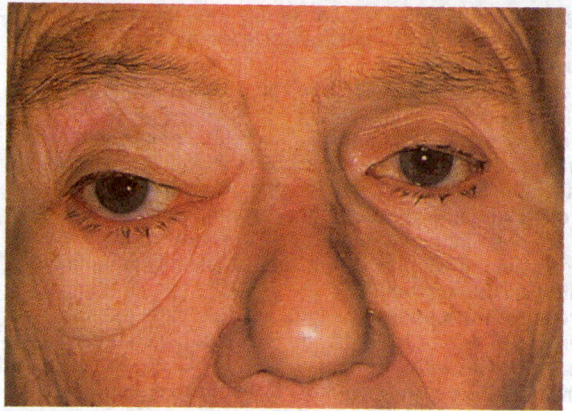

Proptosis of the left eye *(Kamal, 1991)*

propylene glycol /prop'ilēn/, a colorless viscous liquid used as a solvent in the preparation of certain medications. It also inhibits the growth of fungi and microorganisms and is used commercially as an antifreeze.

propylformic acid. See **butyric acid.**

propylthiouracil /prō'pilthī'əyŏŏr'əsil/, an inhibitor of thyroid hormone biosynthesis.

■ INDICATIONS: It is prescribed in the treatment of hyperthyroidism and thyrotoxic crisis, and in preparation for thyroidectomy.

■ CONTRAINDICATIONS: Mental depression, cold intolerance, or known hypersensitivity to this drug prohibits its use. Caution is recommended in pregnancy.

■ ADVERSE EFFECTS: Among the more serious adverse reactions are GI distress, pruritus, and rashes. Rarely, blood dyscrasia occurs.

pro re nata . See **prn.**

pros-. See **proso-.**

proscribe /prōskrīb'/, to forbid. **–proscriptive,** *adj.*

prosector /-sek'tər/ [L, *prosecare,* to cut off], a person who, under the supervision of a pathologist, performs gross dissections and prepares autopsy specimens for pathologic examination.

prosencephalon /pros'ensef'əlon/ [Gk, *pro* + *enkephalon,* brain], the portion of the brain that includes the diencephalon and the telencephalon. It develops from the anterior of the three primary vesicles of the embryonic neural tube and contains various structures, such as the thalamus and hypothalamus, that control important body functions and affect the consciousness, the appetite, and the emotions. Also called **forebrain.** Compare **mesencephalon. –prosencephalic,** *adj.*

proso-, pros-, a prefix meaning 'forward, or anterior': *prosocoele, prosodemic, prosogaster.*

Pro Sobee, a trademark for a commercial milk-substitute formula that is prepared from a soy isolate base and is lactose free, prescribed for infants with galactosemia and people with lactose intolerance. It is supplemented with other nutrients, is fortified with vitamins and minerals, and is available in both powder and liquid forms. See also **Nutramigen.**

prosopalgia. See **trigeminal neuralgia.**

-prosopia, a combining form meaning '(condition of the) face': *ateloprosopia, lipoprosopia, schizoprosopia.*

prosopo- /pros'əpō-/,   a combining form meaning 'of or related to the face': *prosopoanoschisis, prosopodiplegia, prosoponeuralgia.*

prosopopilary virilism /pros'əpōpī'lərē/,   a heavy growth of facial hair.

prosopospasm /pros'əpōspaz'əm/ [Gk, *prosopon,* face + *spasmos*],   a spasm of the facial muscles, such as may occur in tetanus.

prosoposternodidymus /pros'əpōstur'nədid'əməs/ [Gk, *prosopon,* face, *sternon,* chest, *didymos,* twin],   a fetus consisting of conjoined twins united laterally from the head through the sternum.

prosopothoracopagus /pros'əpōthôr'əkop'əgəs/ [Gk, *prosopon* + *thorax,* chest, *pagos,* fixed],   conjoined symmetric twins who are united laterally in the frontal plane from the thorax through most of the head region.

prospective medicine /-spek'tiv/ [L, *proscipere,* to look forward; *medicina,* art of healing],   the early identification of pathologic or potentially pathologic processes and the prescription of intervention to stop the processes.

prospective payment system (PPS),   a payment mechanism for reimbursing hospitals for inpatient health care services in which a predetermined rate is set for treatment of specific illnesses. The system was originally developed by the federal government for use with Medicare recipients. See also **diagnosis related group.**

prospective reimbursement,   a method of payment to an agency for health care services to be delivered based on predictions of what the agency's costs will be for the coming year.

prospective study,   a study designed to determine the relationship between a condition and a characteristic shared by some members of a group. The population selected is healthy at the beginning of the study. Some of the members of the group share a particular characteristic, such as cigarette smoking. The researcher follows the population group over a period of time, noting the rate at which a condition, such as lung cancer, occurs in the smokers and in the nonsmokers. A prospective study may involve many variables or only two; it may seek to demonstrate a relationship that is an association or one that is causal. The kinds of data collected, the numbers of people studied, and other details of the design of the study affect the kind of analysis and the interpretation of the data. Compare **retrospective study.**

prost-, -prost,   a combining form for prostaglandin derivatives.

prostacyclin (PGI₂) /pros'təsī'klin/,   a prostaglandin. It is a biologically active product of arachidonic acid metabolism in human vascular walls and is a potent inhibitor of platelet aggregation. It inhibits the vasoconstrictor effect of angiotensin and stimulates renin release.

prostaglandin (PG) /pros'təglan'din/ [Gk, *prostates,* standing before; L, *glans,* acorn],   one of several potent hormonelike unsaturated fatty acids that act in exceedingly low concentrations on local target organs. They are produced in small amounts and have a large array of significant effects. Prostaglandins given by nebulizer, in tablets, or in solutions for oral or intravenous use effect changes in vasomotor tone, capillary permeability, smooth muscle tone, aggregation of platelets, endocrine and exocrine functions, and the autonomic and central nervous systems. Some of the pharmacologic uses of the prostaglandins are termination of pregnancy and treatment of asthma and gastric hyperacidity.

prostanoic acid /pros'tənō'ik/,   a 20-carbon aliphatic acid

that is the basic framework for prostaglandin molecules, which differ according to the location of hydroxyl and keto substitutions at various positions along the molecule.

Prostaphlin,   a trademark for an antibacterial (oxacillin sodium).

prostate-,   a combining form meaning 'pertaining to the prostate': *prostatectomy, prostatitis, prostalgia.*

prostate /pros'tāt/ [Gk, *prostates,* standing before],   a gland in men that surrounds the neck of the bladder and the urethra and produces a secretion that liquefies coagulated semen. It is a firm structure about the size of a chestnut, composed of muscular and glandular tissue. It is located in the pelvic cavity, below the caudal part of the symphysis pubis and ventral to the rectum, through which it can be felt, especially when enlarged. A depression on its cranial border accommodates the entry of the two ejaculatory ducts and divides the posterior surface of the gland into the middle lobe above, and a larger, lower portion below. A sinus about 6 mm long runs upward and backward in the gland behind the middle lobe and is part of the urethra. The prominent lateral surfaces of the prostate are covered by a plexus of veins and by the ventral portions of the levator ani. The portion of the gland in front of the urethra is composed of dense muscular tissue. In most men the urethra lies along the junction of the anterior portion and the middle third of the prostate. The ejaculatory ducts pass obliquely through the posterior part of the gland. The prostatic secretion consists of alkaline phosphatase, citric acid, and various proteolytic enzymes. It contracts during ejaculation of seminal fluid.

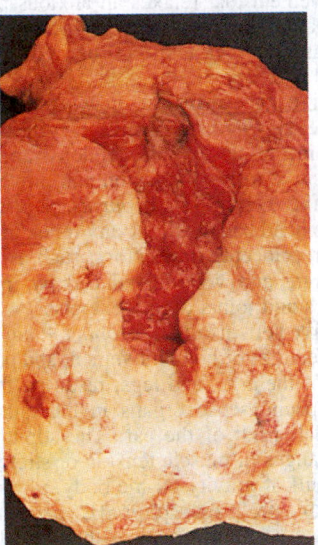

Prostate cancer *(Fletcher, 1987)*

prostate cancer,   a slowly progressive adenocarcinoma of the prostate gland that affects an increasing proportion of American males after the age of 50. It is the third leading cause of cancer deaths with more than 120,000 new cases reported in the United States each year. The cause is unknown, but it is believed to be hormone-related. The disease may cause no direct symptoms but can be detected in the course of diagnosing bladder or uretal obstruction, hematuria, or pyuria. The cancer can spread to cause bone pain in the pelvis, ribs, or vertebrae. It is commonly detected by digital rectal examination followed by core-needle biopsy. Treatment is by surgery, radiation therapy, and hormones, depending on the age of the patient, extent of the disease, and other individual factors.

prostatectomy /pros′tətek′təmē/ [Gk, *prostates* + *ektome,* excision], surgical removal of a portion of the prostate gland, such as performed for benign prostatic hypertrophy, or the total excision of the gland, as performed for malignancy. An indwelling urinary catheter is inserted, and a type and crossmatch of blood is done to prepare for possible transfusion. Either a general or a spinal anesthetic is used. Kinds of approaches include transurethral, the most common, in which a resectoscope is inserted and through it shavings of prostatic tissue are cut off at the bladder opening. The perineal approach is used for biopsy when early cancer is suspected or for the removal of calculi. In a suprapubic approach, a large catheter is positioned into the bladder through the abdomen. Wound drains are left in place in both the perineal and the suprapubic types. After surgery, hematuria is expected for several days; on the first day the bleeding is frank and usually venous, and may be controlled by increasing the pressure in the balloon end of the urethral catheter. If arterial in nature, the bleeding will be bright red with numerous clots and increased viscosity and may lead to hemorrhagic shock, requiring transfusion and surgical intervention. The catheters are connected to a closed system of either constant or intermittent drainage. Meticulous aseptic technique is required to prevent infection when tending catheters, tubings, and collection bags, as well as when changing the dressing. Catheter patency is ensured, and pain is assessed, because blockage or kinking of the drainage tubes may be the cause. Accidental removal or dislodging of catheters is avoided. Bladder spasm may occur if a catheter becomes blocked or from the irritation of the balloon of the catheter in the bladder. Antispasmodic drugs may prevent spasm but are not given in severe cardiac disease or if glaucoma is present. The nurse also assesses the patient's ability to void in adequate amounts when the urethral catheter is removed. Complications of prostatectomy include urethral stricture, especially with the transurethral approach, urinary incontinence, and impotence.

prostate-specific antigen (PSA), a protein produced by the prostate gland that may be present at elevated levels in patients with cancer or other diseases of the prostate.

prostatic /prostat′ik/, pertaining to the prostate gland.

prostatic calculus [Gk, *prostates,* one standing before; L, *calculus,* pebble], a solid pathological concretion formed in the prostate, usually of calcium carbonate and/or calcium phosphate.

prostatic catheter, a catheter that is approximately 16 inches long and has an angled tip. It is used in male catheterization to pass an enlarged prostate gland obstructing the urethra.

prostatic ductule /duk′tyool/ [Gk, *prostates* + L, *ductulus,* little duct], any one of 12 to 20 tiny excretory tubes that convey the alkaline secretion of the prostate gland and open into the floor of the prostatic portion of the urethra. The ductules are joined together by areolar tissue, supported by extensions of the fibrous capsule of the prostate and its muscular stroma, and wrapped in a delicate network of capillaries.

prostatic hypertrophy. See **prostatomegaly.**

prostatic syncope [Gk, *prostates,* one standing before; *syn,*

together + *koptein,* to cut], a temporary loss of consciousness because of restricted cerebral blood flow that may occur during a prostate examination.

prostatic utricle, the portion of the urethra in men that forms a cul-de-sac about 6 mm long behind the middle lobe of the prostate. It is composed of fibrous tissue, muscular fibers, and mucous membrane; numerous small glands open on its inner surface. It is derived from the atrophied paramesonephric ducts and is homologous with the uterus in women. Also called **uterus masculinis.** See also **prostate.**

prostatism /pros′tətiz′əm/ [Gk, *prostates,* one standing before], an abnormal condition of the prostate gland, particularly an enlargement of the gland resulting in an obstruction to the urinary flow.

prostatitis /pros′təti′tis/ [Gk, *prostates* + *itis,* inflammation], acute or chronic inflammation of the prostate gland, usually the result of infection. The patient complains of burning, frequency, and urgency. Treatment consists of administration of antibiotics, sitz baths, bed rest, and fluids. Compare **benign prostatic hypertrophy.**

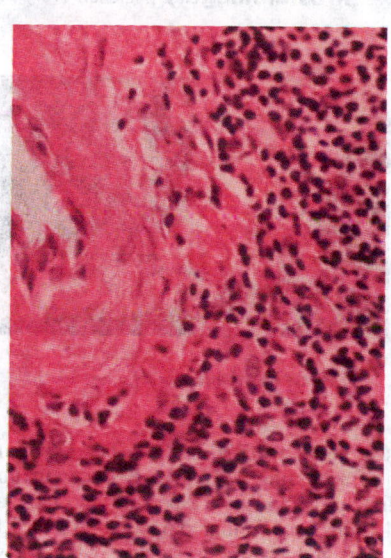

Chronic prostatitis *(Weiss, 1988)*

prostatomegaly /pros′tətōmeg′əlē/ [Gk, *prostates* + *megas,* large], the hypertrophy or enlargement of the prostate gland. (See Fig. p. 1288.)

prosthesis /prosthē′sis/, *pl.* **prostheses** [Gk, addition], **1.** an artificial replacement for a missing part of the body, such as an artificial limb or total joint replacement. **2.** a device designed and applied to improve function, such as a hearing aid. See also **maxillofacial prosthesis, Starr-Edwards prosthesis.**

prosthetic heart valve /prosthet′ik/ [Gk, *prosthesis,* addition; AS, *hoerte;* L, *valva* door, leaf], an artificial heart valve.

prosthetic restoration. See **restoration.**

prosthetics /prosthet′iks/ [Gk, *prosthesis,* addition], the branch of surgery concerned with the design, construction,

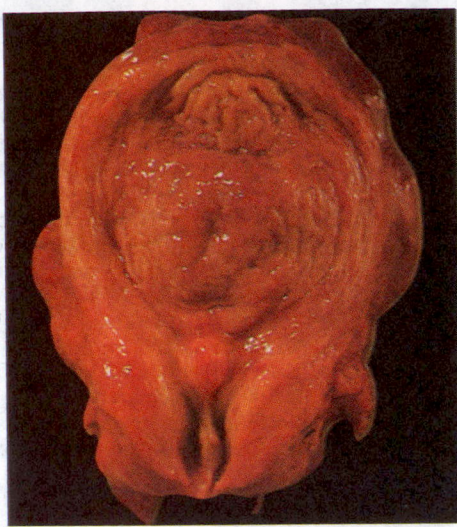

Prostatomegaly *(Fletcher, 1987)*

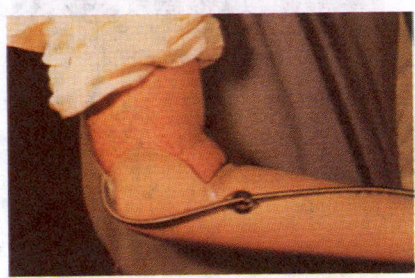

Prosthetic limb *(Hunter, 1990)*

and attachment of artificial limbs or other systems to replace function of a missing body part. See also **orthotics**.

prosthetist /pros'thətist/, a person who fabricates and fits artificial limbs and similar devices prescribed by a physician. A certified prosthetist is one who has successfully completed the examination of the American Orthotic and Prosthetic Association.

prosthodontics /pros'thədon'tiks/ [Gk, *prosthesis* + *odous,* tooth], a branch of dentistry devoted to the construction of artificial appliances that replace missing teeth or restore parts of the face.

Prostigmin, a trademark for a neuromuscular blocking agent (neostigmine) used as an adjunct to anesthesia.

Prostin F2 Alpha, a trademark for a prostaglandin abortifacient (dinoprost tromethamine).

Prostin VR Pediatric, a trademark for a proprietary form of prostaglandin (alprostadil).

prostration /prostrā'shən/ [L, *prosternere,* to throw down], a condition of extreme exhaustion and inability to exert oneself further, as in heat prostration or nervous prostration. —**prostrate,** *adj.*

prot-. See **proto-.**

protactinium (Pa) /-taktin'ē·əm/ [Gk, *protos,* first, *aktis,* ray], a radioactive element. Its atomic number is 91; its atomic weight is 231. The most long-lived isotope of protactinium is p 231, which has a half life of 34,000 years and is produced as an intermediate in the radioactive decay of uranium 235. Its own decay products are actinium and an alpha particle.

protamine sulfate /prō'təmēn/, a heparin antagonist derived from fish sperm.

■ INDICATION: It is prescribed to diminish or reverse the anticoagulant effect of heparin, particularly in cases of heparin overdosage.

■ CONTRAINDICATIONS: Pregnancy, allergy to fish, or known hypersensitivity to this drug prohibits its use.

■ ADVERSE EFFECTS: Among the more serious adverse reactions are hypotension, dyspnea, and bradycardia. Dosage greater than needed to neutralize heparin causes the toxic and anticoagulant effects of protamine itself.

protamine zinc insulin (P2I) suspension, a long-acting insulin that is absorbed slowly at a steady rate. Some patients can be treated with only one injection daily, but combination therapy with regular insulin may be necessary for adequate control.

protanopia /-tənō'pē·ə/, a form of color blindness in which the person is unable to distinguish shades of red. Also called **red blindness.**

protaxic mode of experience /-tak'sik/ (in psychology) a type of primitive experience characterized by sensations, feelings, and fragmented images of short duration that are not logically connected.

protease /prō'tē·ās/, an enzyme that is a catalyst in the breakdown of protein. See also **proteolytic.**

protection, altered, a nursing diagnosis accepted by the Ninth National Conference on the Classification of Nursing Diagnoses. Altered protection is defined as a state in which an individual experiences a decrease in the ability to guard the self from internal or external threats, such as illness or injury. The defining characteristics are deficient immunity, impaired healing, altered clotting, maladaptive stress response, neurosensory alterations, chilling, perspiring, dyspnea, cough, itching, restlessness, insomnia, fatigue, anorexia, weakness, immobility, disorientation, and pressure sores. Related factors are extremes of age, inadequate nutrition, alcohol abuse, abnormal blood profiles (leukopenia, thrombocytopenia, anemia, coagulation), drug therapies (antineoplastic, corticosteroid, immune, anticoagulant, thrombolytic), treatments (surgery, radiation), and diseases such as cancer and immune disorders. See also **nursing diagnosis.**

protective /-tek'tiv/ [L, *protegere,* to cover], guarding another person from danger or injury and providing a safe environment.

protective apron. see **lead apron.**

protective isolation [L, *protegere,* to cover in front; It, *isolare* detached], 1. the practice of confining a patient with a virulent infectious disease in a separate area so that contact with other people can be minimized. 2. the practice of placing a highly susceptible person, such as an immunodeficient patient, in a separate area where the risk of contact with pathogenic microorganisms can be controlled.

protein /prō'tē·in, prō'tēn/ [Gk, *proteios*], any of a large group of naturally occurring, complex, organic nitrogenous compounds. Each is composed of large combinations of amino acids containing the elements carbon, hydrogen, nitrogen, oxygen, usually sulfur, and occasionally phosphorus, iron, iodine, or other essential constituents of living cells. Twenty-two amino acids have been identified as vital for proper growth, development, and maintenance of health. The body can synthesize 14 of these amino acids, called nonessential, whereas the remaining eight must be obtained from dietary sources and are termed essential. Protein is the major source of building material for muscles, blood, skin, hair, nails, and the internal organs. It is necessary for the formation of hormones, enzymes, and antibodies and may act as a source of heat and energy, and it functions as an essential element in proper elimination of waste materials. Rich dietary sources are meat, poultry, fish, eggs, milk, and cheese, which are classified as complete proteins because they contain the eight essential amino acids. Nuts and legumes, including navy beans, chick-peas, soybeans, and split peas, are also good sources but are incomplete proteins, because they do not contain all the essential amino acids. Protein deficiency causes abnormal growth and tissue development in children, leading to kwashiorkor and marasmus, whereas in adults it results in lack of vigor and stamina, weakness, mental depression, poor resistance to infection, impaired healing of wounds, and slow recovery from disease. Excessive intake of protein may in some conditions result in fluid imbalance. Normal adult findings of total blood protein are 6 to 8 g/dl.

proteinase /prō'tē· inās/ [Gk, *proteios*, first rank, *ase*, enzyme suffix], a proteolytic enzyme that splits protein molecules at central linkages.

protein-bound iodine (PBI), iodine that is firmly bound to protein in serum, the measurement of which indirectly indicates the concentration of circulating thyroxine (T_4). A PBI of less than the normal range of 4 to 8 [mu]/ml of serum is indicative of hypothyroidism, and a PBI of more than the normal values indicates hyperthyroidism. The test is currently used less frequently because of the availability of more sensitive measurements of T_4.

protein calorie malnutrition. See **energy protein malnutrition.**

proteinemia /prōtē·inē'mē·ə/ [Gk, *proteios*, first rank + *haima*, blood], an excessive level of protein in the blood. Also called **hyperproteinemia**.

protein hydrolysate injection, a fluid and nutrient replenisher.

■ INDICATIONS: It is prescribed to correct a negative nitrogen balance and in other clinical situations requiring parenteral nutrition.

■ CONTRAINDICATIONS: Renal failure, anuria, severe liver disease, hepatic coma, or known hypersensitivity to one or more of the amino acids prohibits the use of this drug.

■ ADVERSE EFFECTS: Among the more serious adverse reactions are hypotension, abdominal pain, convulsions, phlebitis, thrombosis, and edema.

protein kinase, a protein that catalyzes the transfer of a phosphate group from adenosine triphosphate to produce a phosphoprotein.

protein metabolism, the processes whereby protein foodstuffs are used by the body to make tissue proteins, together with the processes of breakdown of tissue proteins in the production of energy. Food proteins are first broken down into amino acids, then absorbed into the bloodstream, and finally used in body cells to form new proteins. Amino acids in excess of the body's needs may be converted by liver enzymes into keto acids and urea. The keto acids may be used as sources of energy via the Krebs citric acid cycle, or they may be converted into glucose or fat for storage. Urea

is excreted in urine and sweat. Growth hormones and androgens stimulate protein formation, and adrenal cortical hormones tend to cause breakdown of body proteins. Diseases affecting protein metabolism include homocystinuria, liver disease, maple sugar urine disease, and phenylketonuria.

protein sensitization [Gk, *proteios*, first rank, L, *sentire*, to feel], a reaction that follows parenteral introduction of a foreign protein into the body. Symptoms of varying severity, including serum sickness, occur when the same foreign protein is reintroduced into the body at a later date.

proteinuria /prō'tēnyŏŏr'ē·ə/ [Gk, *proteios* + *ouron*, urine], the presence in the urine of abnormally large quantities of protein, usually albumin. Healthy adults excrete less than 250 mg of protein per day. Persistent proteinuria is usually a sign of renal disease or renal complications of another disease, such as hypertension or heart failure. However, proteinuria can result from heavy exercise or fever. Also called **albuminuria.**

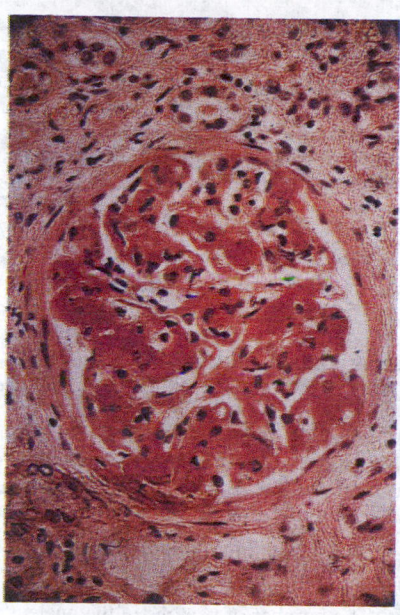

Proteinuria *(Williams, 1993)*

proteo-, a combining form meaning 'of or pertaining to protein': *proteocrasis, proteolysis, proteopepsis.*

proteolipid /prō'tē·ōlip'id/ [Gk, *proteios*; *lipos*, fat], a type of lipoprotein in which lipid material forms more than one half of the molecule. It is insoluble in water and occurs primarily in the brain.

proteolysis /prō'tē·ol'isis/ [Gk, *proteios* + *lysis*, loosening], a process in which water added to the peptide bonds of proteins breaks down the protein molecule. Numerous enzymes may catalyze this process. The action of mineral acids and heat also may induce proteolysis.

proteolytic /prō'tē·əlit'ik/, of or pertaining to any substance that promotes the breakdown of protein.

Proteus /prō'tē·əs/ [Gk, *Proteus*, mythic god who changed shapes], a genus of motile, gram-negative bacilli often associated with nosocomial infections, normally found in feces, water, and soil. *Proteus* may cause urinary tract infections, pyelonephritis, wound infections, diarrhea, bacteremia, and endotoxic shock. Some species are sensitive to penicillin; most respond to the aminoglycoside antibiotics and cephalosporins.

Proteus mirabilis   a species of anaerobic, motile, rod-shaped bacteria found in putrid meat, abscesses, and fecal material. It is a leading cause of urinary tract infections.

Proteus morgani,   a species of bacteria associated with infectious diarrhea in infants.

Proteus vulgaris,   a species of bacteria that is a frequent cause of urinary tract infections. The bacteria are found in feces, water, and soil.

prothrombin /prōthrom'bin/ [L, *pro* before; Gk, *thrombos*, lump], a plasma protein precursor of thrombin. It is synthesized in the liver if adequate vitamin K is present. Also called **factor II.** See also **blood clotting.**

prothrombinemia /-ē'mē·ə/ [L, *pro*, before; Gk, *thrombos*, lump; *haima* blood], the presence of prothrombin in the blood.

prothrombin time (PT),   a one-stage test for detecting certain plasma coagulation defects caused by a deficiency of factors V, VII, or X. Thromboplastin and calcium are added to a sample of the patient's plasma and, simultaneously, to a sample from a normal control. The amount of time required for clot formation in both samples is observed. Thrombin is formed from prothrombin in the presence of adequate calcium, thromboplastin, and the essential tissue coagulation factors. A prolonged PT therefore indicates deficiency in one of the factors, as in liver disease, vitamin K deficiency, or anticoagulation therapy with the drug coumarin. Normal findings of prothrombin time are 11 to 12.5 seconds; 85% to 100%. Compare **partial thromboplastin time.** See also **blood clotting.**

proto-, prot-,   a prefix meaning 'first': *protoblast, protoxin, protopathic.*

protocol /prō'təkôl/ [Gk, *protos*, first, *kolla*, glued page], a written plan specifying the procedures to be followed in giving a particular examination, in conducting research, or in providing care for a particular condition. See also **standing orders.**

proton /prō'ton/ [Gk, *protos*, first], a positively charged particle that is a fundamental component of the nucleus of all atoms. The number of protons in the nucleus of an atom equals the atomic number of the element. Compare **electron, neutron.** See also **atomic weight.**

proton density,   a measure of proton concentration, or the number of atomic nuclei per given volume. It is one of the major determinants of magnetic resonance signal strength in hydrogen imaging.

Protopam Chloride,   a trademark for a cholinesterase reactivator (pralidoxime chloride).

protopathic /prō'topath'ik/, pertaining to the somatic sensations of fast localized pain; slow, poorly localized pain; and temperature.

protoplasm /prō'təplaz'əm/ [Gk, *protos* + *plasma*, something formed], the living substance of a cell, usually composed of myriad molecules of water, minerals, and organic compounds.

protoplasmic /-plaz'mik/ [Gk, *protos*, first + *plasma*, something formed], pertaining to or composed of protoplasm.

protoplast /prō'təplast/ [Gk, *protos* + *plassein*, to mold], 1. (in biology) the protoplasm of a cell without its contain-

ing membrane. 2. a first entity or an original. **–protoplastic,** *adj.*

protoporphyria /prō'tōpôrfir'ē·ə/ [Gk, *protos* + *porphyros*, purple, *haima*, blood], increased levels of protoporphyrin in the blood and feces.

protoporphyrin /prō'tōpôr'firin/ [Gk, *protos* + *porphyros*], a kind of porphyrin that combines with iron and protein to form a variety of important organic molecules, including catalase, hemoglobin, and myoglobin. See also **heme.**

protostoma.   See **blastopore.**

prototaxic mode /prō'tətak'sik/ [Gk, *protos* + *taxis*, arrangement; *modus*, measure], a stage in infancy, according to a Sullivanian theory, characterized by a lack of differentiation between the self and the environment.

prototype /prō'tətīp/ [Gk, *protos*, first + *typos*, mark], the primary or original form of an object or organism.

protozoa /prō'təzō'ə/, *sing.* **protozoon** [Gk, *protos* + *zoon*, animal], single-celled microorganisms of the class Protozoa, the lowest form of animal life. Protozoa are more complex than bacteria, forming a self-contained unit with organelles that carry on such functions as locomotion, nutrition, excretion, respiration, and attachment to other objects or organisms. Approximately 30 protozoa are pathogenic to humans. **–protozoal, protozoan,** *adj.*

protozoal infection /-zō'əl/, any disease caused by single-celled organisms of the class Protozoa. Some kinds of protozoal infections are **amebic dysentery, kala-azar, malaria,** and **trichomonas vaginitis.**

protozoan /-zō'ən/ [Gk, *protos*, first + *zoon*, animal], pertaining to or caused by protozoa.

protracted dose /prōtrak'tid/ [L, *pro*, before, *trahere*, to draw, *dosis*, something given], (in radiotherapy) a low amount of radiation delivered continuously over a relatively long period of time.

protriptyline hydrochloride /-trip'tilēn/, a tricyclic antidepressant.

■ INDICATIONS: It is prescribed in the treatment of endogenous depression marked by withdrawal and anergy.

■ CONTRAINDICATIONS: Concomitant administration of monoamine oxidase inhibitors, recent myocardial infarction, or known hypersensitivity to any tricyclic medication prohibits its use. It is used with caution where anticholinergics are contraindicated, in seizure disorders, and in patients with cardiovascular disease.

■ ADVERSE EFFECTS: Among the more serious adverse reactions are sedation and anticholinergic side effects. A variety of GI, cardiovascular, and neurologic reactions may occur. This drug interacts with many other drugs.

Protropin,   a trademark for a synthetic human growth hormone (somatrem) used to increase the growth rate of children with hypopituitary dwarfism.

protrusio bulbi.   See **exophthalmia.**

protrusion /-trŌŌ'zhən/ [L, *protrudere*, to push forward], a state or condition of being forward or projecting.

protrusive incisal guide angle /-trŌŌ'siv/, (in dentistry) the inclination of the incisal guide in the sagittal plane.

protrypsin.   See **trypsinogen.**

protuberance /-t(y)ŌŌ'bərəns/ [L, *pro* + *tuberare*, to swell], an anatomic landmark that appears as a blunt projection or swelling, such as the chin, buttock, or bulge of the frontal bone above the eyebrow.

proud flesh [AS, *prud, flaesc*], excessive granulation tissue. See also **cicatrix, keloid, scar.**

Proventil,   a trademark for a bronchodilator (albuterol).

Provera, a trademark for a progestin (medroxyprogesterone acetate).

provider, a hospital, clinic, health care professional, or group of health care professionals who provide a service to patients.

Provincial/Territorial Nurses Association (PTNA), an association of Canadian nurses organized at the provincial or territorial level. The Canadian Nurses' Association is a federation of the 11 PTNAs.

provirus /-vī'rəs/, a stage of viral replication in which the viral genetic information has been integrated into the genome of the host cell. It may be activated spontaneously or by a specific stimulus to progress to a complete virus.

provitamin /prōvī'təmin/, a precursor of a vitamin; a substance found in certain foods that in the body may be converted into a vitamin. Also called **previtamin.**

provocative diagnosis /-vok'ətiv/ [L, *provocare,* to call forth; Gk, *dia,* through, *gnosis,* knowledge], a diagnosis in which the identity and cause of an illness are discovered by inducing an episode of the condition; for example, in immunology an allergen causing an allergic response is shown to be an etiologic factor in the patient's allergic condition.

prox, abbreviation for **proximal.**

proxemics /proksē'miks/ [L, *proximus,* nearest], the study of spatial distances between people and their effect on interpersonal behavior, especially in relation to density of population, placement of people within an area, territoriality, personal space, and the opportunity for privacy.

proximal /prok'siməl/ [L, *proximus*], nearer to a point of reference, usually the trunk of the body, than other parts of the body. Proximal interphalangeal joints are those closest to the hand.

proximal cavity, a cavity that occurs on the mesial or distal surface of a tooth.

proximal contact [L, *proximus,* nearest + *contingere,* to touch], the contact between the distal surface of one tooth and the mesial surface of an adjacent tooth.

proximal contour, the shape or form of the medial or the distal surface of a tooth.

proximal dental caries, decay that may occur in the mesial or distal surface of a tooth.

proximal radioulnar articulation, the pivot joint between the circumference of the head of the radius and the ring formed by the radial notch of the ulna and the annular ligament. The joint allows the rotary movements of the head of the radius in pronation and supination. Also called **superior radioulnar joint.** Compare **distal radioulnar articulation.**

proximal renal tubular acidosis (proximal RTA), an abnormal condition characterized by excessive acid accumulation and bicarbonate excretion. It is caused by the defective reabsorption of bicarbonate in the proximal tubules of the kidney and the resulting flow of excessive bicarbonate into the distal tubules, which normally secrete hydrogen ions. This disruption impedes the formation of titratable acids and ammonium for excretion and ultimately leads to metabolic acidosis. Treatment is as for renal tubular acidosis. In **primary proximal RTA** the defective reabsorption of bicarbonate is the sole causative factor. In **secondary proximal RTA** the reabsorptive defect is one of several causative factors and may result from tubular cell damage produced by various disorders, such as Fanconi's syndrome. Compare **distal renal tubular acidosis.**

proximate /prok'simit/ [L, *proximus,* nearest], the nearest to a point of origin or attachment. Compare **distal.**

proximate cause [L, *proximare,* to approach], a legal concept of cause and effect relationships in determining, for example, whether an injury would have resulted from a particular cause.

proximity principle /proksim'itē/ [L, *proximus + principium,* origin], a rule that when two or more objects are close to each other, they may be seen as a perceptual unit.

proximo-, a combining form meaning 'near or opposite of distal, central, or a point of attachment': *proximity, proximal, proximolabial.*

proxymetacaine. See **proparacaine hydrochloride.**

Prozac, a trademark for an oral antidepressant (fluoxetine hydrochloride).

PrP, abbreviation for *prion protein,* a viruslike infectious agent associated with Creutzfeldt-Jakob disease.

prurigo /prōōrī'gō/ [L, an itch], any of a group of chronic inflammatory conditions of the skin characterized by severe itching and multiple, dome-shaped, small papules capped by tiny vesicles. Later (as a result of repeated scratching), crusting and lichenification may occur. Some causes of prurigo are allergies, drugs, endocrine abnormalities, malignancies, and parasites. Specific treatment depends on the cause. Symptomatic therapy is the same as for pruritus. A mild form of the disease is called **prurigo mitis,** and a more severe form, **prurigo agria** or **prurigo ferox.** See also **pruritus.** **–pruriginous,** *adj.*

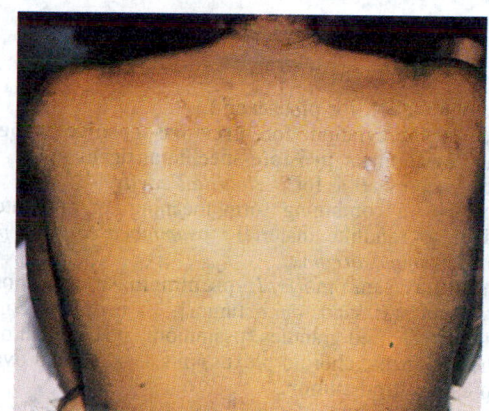

Prurigo *(Parkin, 1991)*

pruritus /prōōrī'təs/ [L, *prurire,* to itch], the symptom of itching, an uncomfortable sensation leading to the urge to scratch. Scratching often results in secondary infection. Some causes of pruritus are allergy, infection, jaundice, lymphoma, and skin irritation. Treatment is best directed at the cause; symptomatic relief may be obtained by antihistamines, starch baths, topical corticosteroids, cool water, or alcohol applications. **–pruritic,** *adj.*

pruritus ani, a common chronic condition of itching of the skin around the anus. Some causes are candidal infection, contact dermatitis, external hemorrhoids, pinworms, psoriasis, and psychogenic illness. Treatment is best directed at the specific cause; however, symptomatic relief may be obtained by careful cleansing, soothing creams or lotions, topical corticosteroids, antihistamines, and tranquilizers.

pruritus vulvae, itching of the external genitalia of a female. The condition may become chronic and result in lichenification, atrophy, and occasionally malignancy. Some causes of pruritus vulvae are contact dermatitis, lichen sclerosus et atrophicus, psychogenic pruritus, trichomoniasis, and vaginal candidiasis. Treatment of the condition depends on its cause.

Prussian blue /prush'ən/ [Prussia, Germany; ME, *blew*], a chemical stain used on microscopic preparations. It demonstrates the presence of copper by developing a bright blue color.

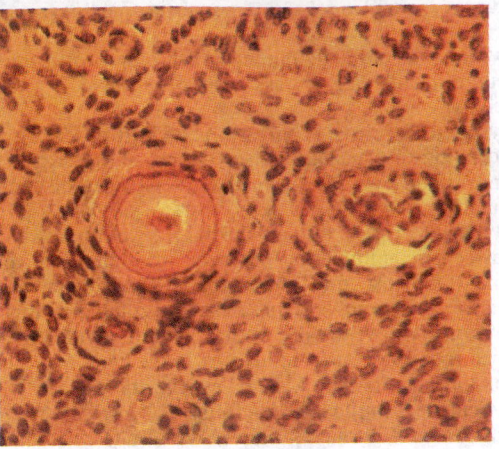

Psammoma body
(Perkin, 1986/Dr RO Barnard, Department of Neuropathology, Maida Vale Hospital, London, UK)

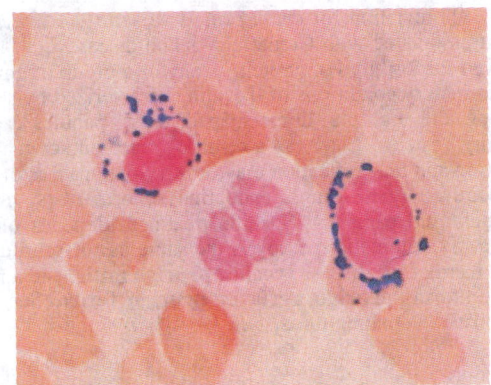

Prussian blue stain *(Hayhoe, 1992)*

ps, abbreviation for **picosecond.**

PSA, 1. abbreviation for **pressure-sensitive adhesive.** **2.** abbreviation for **prostate-specific antigen.**

P sac, abbreviation for *pericardial cavity.*

psammo-, a combining form meaning 'of or related to sand or to sandlike material': *psammocarcinoma, psammoma, psammosarcoma.*

psammoma /samō'mə/, *pl.* **psammomas, psammomata** [Gk, *psammos,* sand, *oma,* tumor], a neoplasm containing small calcified granules (psammoma bodies) that occurs in the meninges, choroid plexus, pineal body, and ovaries. Also called **sand tumor.**

psammoma body, a round, layered mass of calcareous material occurring in benign and malignant epithelial and connective tissue neoplasms and in some chronically inflamed tissue.

-pselaphesia, -pselaphesis, a combining form meaning '(condition of the) tactile sense': *apselaphesia, hyperpselaphesia, hypopselaphesia.*

pseud- See **pseudo-.**

pseudarthritis /sōo'därthrī'tis/ [Gk, *pseudes,* false + *arthron,* joint + *itis,* inflammation], musculoskeletal pain that does not involve the joints.

pseudesthesia /sōo'desthē'zhə/ [Gk, *pseudes,* false, *aisthesis,* feeling], a sensation experienced without an external stimulus or a sensation that does not correspond to the causative stimulus, such as phantom limb pain.

pseudo- /sōo'dō-/, **pseud-,** a prefix meaning 'false': *pseudoangina, pseudocyst, pseudorubella.*

pseudoallele /-əlēl'/ [Gk, *pseudes + allelon,* of one another], (in genetics) one of two or more closely linked genes on a chromosome that appear to function as a single member of an allelic pair but occupy distinct, nearly correspond-ing loci on homologous chromosomes. Such gene pairs produce a mutant effect in the diploid state when located on homologous chromosomes but are capable of being separated by crossing over during meiosis to produce a wild-type effect when recombined on either of the homologues. **—pseudoallelic,** *adj.,* **pseudoallelism,** *n.*

pseudoankylosis /-ang'kilō'sis/ [Gk, *pseudes,* false + *agkylosis,* joint stiffness], fibrous ankylosis, or false ankylosis caused by inflexibility of body structures outside the joint.

pseudoanorexia /-an'ərek'sē·ə/ [Gk, *pseudes + a, orexis,* not appetite], a condition in which an individual eats secretly while claiming a lack of appetite and inability to eat. Also called **false anorexia.**

pseudoarthrosis. See **false joint.**

pseudoataxia /-ətak'sē·ə/ [Gk, *pseudes,* false + *ataxia,* lack of order], a loss of control over voluntary movements that does not involve an organic lesion.

pseudobulbar paralysis /-bul'bər/ [Gk, *pseudes,* false; L, *bulbus,* swollen root; *paralyein,* to be palsied], a condition resembling progressive bulbar paralysis, with dysarthria and dysphagia, but in which weakness of the bulbar muscles is of the upper motor neuron type and which may result from multiple bilateral infarcts of the cerebral cortex in some cases.

pseudochylous ascites /sōo'dōkī'ləs/ [Gk, *pseudes + chylos,* juice; *askos,* bag], the abnormal accumulation in the peritoneal cavity of a milky fluid that resembles chyle. The turbidity of the fluid is caused by cellular debris in the fluid. Pseudochylous ascites is indicative of an abdominal tumor or infection. Compare **chylous ascites.** See also **ascites.**

pseudocoxalgia. See **Perthes' disease.**

pseudocyesis /sōo'dōsī·ē'sis/ [Gk, *pseudes + kyesis,* pregnancy], a condition in which a woman believes she is pregnant when she is not. Certain signs and symptoms suggest pregnancy, such as the absence of the menses, although conception has not occurred and therefore there is no embryonic development. The condition may be psychogenic in origin or caused by a tumor or endocrine dysfunction. Also called **false pregnancy, pseudopregnancy, spurious pregnancy.**

pseudocyst /soo'dəsist/ [Gk, *pseudes* + *kystis*, bag], a space or cavity containing gas or liquid but without a lining membrane. Pseudocysts commonly occur after pancreatitis when digestive juices break through the normal ducts of the pancreas and collect in spaces lined by fibroblasts and surfaces of adjacent organs. Symptoms are caused by displacement of abdominal structures or fluid or by atelectasis at the base of the left lung. Ultrasound and computerized tomography are useful in diagnosis; surgical drainage is the best therapy. See also **pancreatitis.**

pseudodementia /-dimen'shə/, affective disorders, particularly depression, that mimic the signs and symptoms of dementia.

pseudoephedrine hydrochloride /-ef'ədrēn/, an adrenergic that acts as a vasoconstrictor and bronchodilator.
■ INDICATIONS: It is prescribed for the relief of nasal congestion and eustachian tube congestion.
■ CONTRAINDICATIONS: Known hypersensitivity to sympathomimetic drugs prohibits its use. Interaction with monoamine oxidase inhibitors may cause hypertensive crisis. It is prescribed with caution in patients who have hypertension, glaucoma, heart disease, diabetes, or urinary retention.
■ ADVERSE EFFECTS: Among the more serious adverse reactions are central nervous system stimulation, headache, and tachycardia.

pseudoephedrine sulfate. See **pseudoephedrine hydrochloride.**

pseudofracture /-frak'shər/ [Gk, *pseudes*, false; L, *fractura*], radiologic evidence of a thickened periosteum and new bone formation over what looks like an incomplete fracture.

pseudogene /soo'dōjēn'/ [Gk, *pseudes* + *genein*, to produce], (in molecular genetics) a sequence of nucleotides that resembles a gene and may be derived from one but lacks a genetic function.

pseudoglottis. See **neoglottis.**

pseudogout. See **chondrocalcinosis.**

pseudohermaphrodite /-hərmaf'redīt/ [Gk, *pseudes*, false; *Hermaphroditos*, son of Hermes and Aphrodite], a congenital condition in which a person has either male or female gonads but external genitalia of the opposite sex, or both.

pseudohermaphroditism /-hərmaf'rəditiz'əm/ [Gk, *pseudes* + *Hermaphroditos*, mythic son of Hermes and Aphrodite], a condition in which a person exhibits the somatic characteristics of both sexes though possessing the physical characteristics of either males (testes) or females (ovaries). Also spelled **pseudohermaphrodism.** See also **feminization,** def. 2, **hermaphroditism.**

pseudohypertrophic muscular dystrophy. See **Duchenne's muscular dystrophy.**

pseudojaundice /-jôn'dis/ [Gk, *pseudes* + Fr, *jaune*, yellow], a yellow discoloration of the skin that is not caused by hyperbilirubinemia. The excessive ingestion of carotene results in a form of pseudojaundice.

pseudomembrane /-mem'brān/ [Gk, *pseudes*, false; L, *membrana*], a membrane consisting of coagulated fibrin, bacteria, and leukocytes that forms in the throats of diphtheria patients.

pseudomembranous colitis /-mem'brənəs/ [Gk, *pseudes* + L, *membrana*, thin skin], a diarrheal disease frequently found in hospitalized patients who have received antibiotics that caused overgrowth of the anaerobic, spore-forming toxin producing *Clostridium difficile.* Patients have profuse watery diarrhea, fever, and cramping, and are found to have exudates of the colon on endoscopy. Diagnosis is made by identifying the offending toxin in the stool of the affected patient. Antidiarrheals are strictly contraindicated as a life-threatening dilatation of the bowel called toxic megacolon may result. The bacterium is passed from patient to patient by healthcare workers who fail to adequately wash their hands. Strict isolation of infected stools is necessary to prevent outbreaks of epidemics. Treatment with oral vancomycin or parenteral metronidazole usually will result in abatement of symptoms within 3 to 5 days.

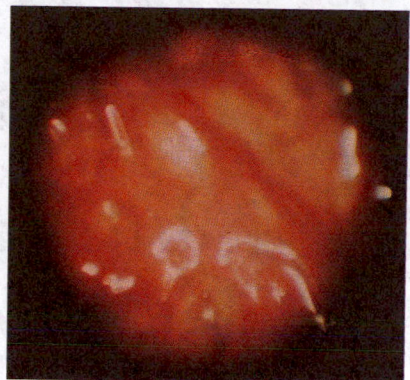

Pseudomembranous colitis—endoscopic veiw
(Mitros, 1988)

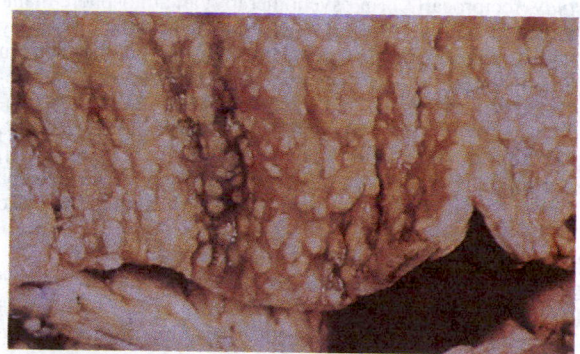

Pseudomembranous colitis—autopsy specimen
(Baron, 1990)

pseudomembranous enterocolitis. See **necrotizing enterocolitis.**

pseudomembranous stomatitis, a severe inflammation of the mouth that produces a membranelike exudate. The inflammation may be caused by a variety of bacteria or by chemical irritants. It may produce dysphagia, pain, fever, and swelling of the lymph glands, or it may remain localized and mild.

pseudomonad /soo'dōmō'nad, soōdom'ənad/, a bacterium of the genus *Pseudomonas.*

Pseudomonas /soōdom'ənas/ [Gk, *pseudes* + *monas*, unit], a genus of gram-negative bacteria that includes several free-living species of soil and water and some opportunistic pathogens, such as *Pseudomonas aeruginosa*, isolated from wounds, burns, and infections of the urinary tract. Pseudomonads are notable for their fluorescent pigments and their resistance to disinfectants and antibiotics.

Pseudomonas aeruginosa [Gk, *pseudes,* false, *monas,* unity], a species of gram-negative nonsporing motile bacilli that may cause various human diseases ranging from purulent meningitis to nosocomial infected wounds. Also called **Pseudomonas pyocyanea**.

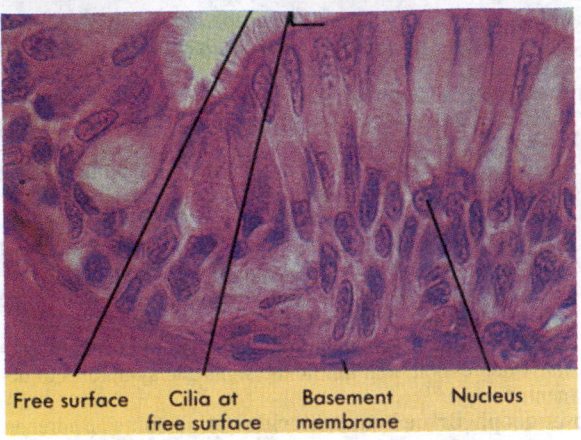

Pseudostratified columnar epithelium
(Seeley, 1992/Ed Reschke)

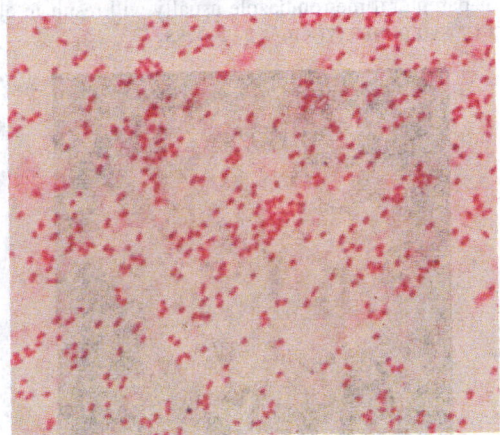

Pseudomonas aeruginosa (Turner-Warwick, 1993)

pseudomutuality /-mōō′tyōō·al′itē/ [Gk, *pseudes* + L, *mutuus,* reciprocal], (in psychotherapy) an atmosphere maintained by family members in which there is surface harmony and a high degree of agreement with one another, but in which the atmosphere of agreement covers deep and destructive intrapsychic and interpersonal conflicts. The family acts 'as if' it is close and happy, when in fact it is not.

pseudopod /sōō′dəpod/ [Gk, *pseudes,* false + *pous,* foot], a temporary protoplasmic limblike process of an amoeba that can be extended to propel itself or to engulf food. Also called **pseudopodium**.

pseudopregnancy. See **pseudocyesis.**

pseudorabies. See **infectious bulbar paralysis.**

pseudorubella. See **roseola infantum.**

pseudosclerema. See **adiponecrosis subcutanea neonatorum.**

pseudostratified /-strā′tifīd/ [Gk, *pseudes,* false, *stratum,* cover], pertaining to a type of columnar epithelium in which the nuclei of adjacent cells are at different levels.

pseudotumor /-t(y)ōō′mər/ [Gk, *pseudes* + L, *tumor,* swelling], a false tumor.

pseudotumor cerebri, a condition characterized by increased intracranial pressure, headache, blurring of the optic disc margins, vomiting, and papilledema without neurologic signs, except palsy of the sixth cranial nerve. Also called **benign intracranial hypertension, meningeal hydrops.**

pseudoxanthoma elasticum. See **Grönblad-Strandberg syndrome.**

psi /sī/, Ψ, ψ, the twenty-third letter of the Greek alphabet.

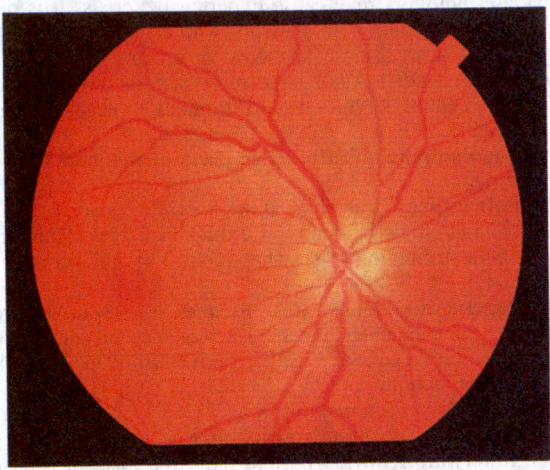

Blurring of disk margins in pseudotumor cerebri
(Greenberger, 1993)

p.s.i., abbreviation for **pounds per square inch**.

psia, abbreviation for *pounds per square inch, absolute.*

psig, abbreviation for *pounds per square inch, gauge.*

psilocin /sī′ləsin/, one of several indole-derived psychomimetic drugs. It is related chemically to psilocybin.

psilocybin /sī′lōsī′bin,-sib′in/, a psychedelic drug and an active ingredient of various Mexican hallucinogenic mushrooms of the genus *Psilocybe mexicana.* It can produce altered states of mood and consciousness and has no acceptable medical use in the United States. Psilocybin is controlled under Schedule I of the Comprehensive Drug Abuse Prevention and Control Act of 1970, which bans the prescription of psilocybin and numerous other drugs and allows their procurement and use only for special research projects authorized by the Drug Enforcement Administration of the U.S. Department of Justice.

psittacosis /sit′əkō′sis/ [Gk, *psittakos,* parrot], an infectious illness caused by the bacterium *Chlamydia psittaci,* characterized by respiratory, pneumonia-like symptoms and transmitted to humans by infected birds, especially parrots. The clinical manifestations of the disease are extremely variable and resemble a great number of infectious diseases, but fever, cough, anorexia, and severe headache are almost always present. A history of exposure to birds is highly suggestive, because all chlamydiae are difficult to isolate and culture. A demonstrated rise in antibody titer confirms a diagnosis. Tetracycline is usually used to treat psittacosis and is continued for 10 to 14 days after the fever subsides. Isolation is advised. Also called **ornithosis, parrot fever.** See also *Chlamydia.*

psm, abbreviation for **presystolic murmur**.

psoas major /sō'əs/ [Gk, *psoa*, loin], a long muscle originating from the transverse processes of the lumbar vertebrae and the fibrocartilages and sides of the vertebral bodies of the lower thoracic vertebrae and the lumbar vertebrae. It joins the iliacus to form the iliopsoas deep in the pelvis as it passes under the inguinal ligament and inserts in the lesser trochanter. It acts to flex and laterally rotate the thigh and to flex and laterally bend the spine. Compare **psoas minor.**

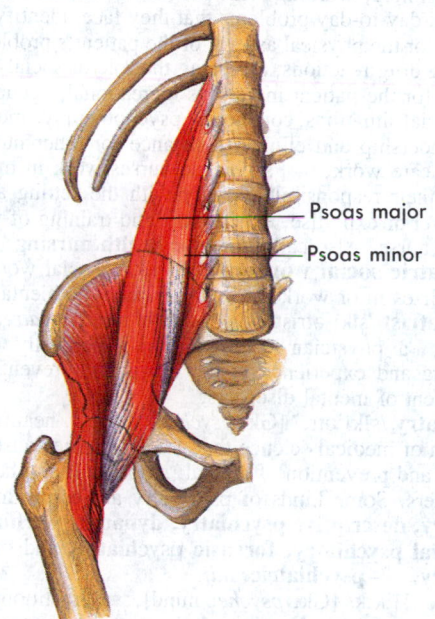

Psoas major and minor (Thibodeau, 1993/Ernest W Beck)

psoas minor, a long, slender muscle of the pelvis, ventral to the psoas major. Many individuals do not have this muscle. It arises from the bodies of the twelfth thoracic and the first lumbar vertebrae and from the disk between them and ends in a long, flat tendon that inserts into the pectineal line of the pelvis and into the iliac fascia. The psoas minor is innervated by a branch of the first lumbar nerve and functions to flex the spine. Compare **psoas major.**

psor-, a combining form meaning 'of or related to itching': *psora, psorocomium, psorous.*

psoralen-type photosensitizer /sôr'ələn/, any one chemical compound that contains photosensitizing psoralen and

that reacts on exposure to ultraviolet light to increase the melanin in the skin. Naturally occurring psoralen photosynthesizers, such as 5- and 8-methoxypsoralen, are found in buttercups, carrot greens, celery, clover, cockleburs, dill, figs, limes, parsley, and meadow grass. Some psoralen-type photosensitizers produced as pharmaceutics are methoxsalen and trioxalen; both are used to enhance skin pigmentation or tanning in the treatment of skin diseases, such as psoriasis and vitiligo. Such drugs are carefully administered to avoid oversensitization of the skin and other complications. Psoralen-type photosensitizers are also used in the manufacture of some perfumes, colognes, and pomades. Such chemicals cause unique skin reactions, such as berlock dermatitis, in some individuals. Oil of bergamot, extracted from the peels of small oranges grown in southern France and Italy, is a photosensitizing psoralen used as a tea flavoring and in perfumes.

psoriasis /sərī'əsis/ [Gk, itch], a common, chronic skin disorder characterized by circumscribed red patches covered by thick, dry, silvery, adherent scales that are the result of excessive development of epithelial cells. Exacerbations and remissions are typical. Lesions may be anywhere on the body but are more common on extensor surfaces, bony prominences, scalp, ears, genitalia, and the perianal area. An arthritis, particularly of distal small joints, may accompany the skin disease. Treatment includes topical and intralesional corticosteroids, ultraviolet light, tar solution baths, creams and shampoos, methotrexate, and photochemotherapy. Subcategories of psoriasis include **guttate psoriasis, nummular psoriasis,** and **pustular psoriasis.** See also **psoriatic arthritis.** −psoriatic /sôr'ē·at'ik/, *adj.*

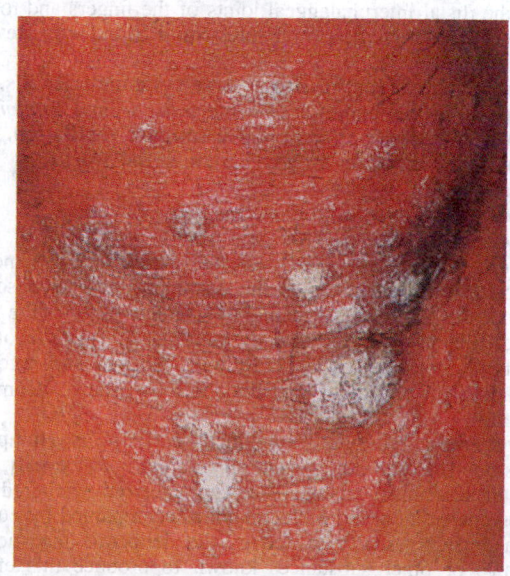

Psoriasis (Habif, 1990)

psoriasis universalis [Gk, *psoriasis,* itch; L, *universus,* on the whole], a severe attack of psoriasis in which most or all of the skin is involved.

psoriatic arthritis /sôr'ī·at'ik/, a form of arthritis associ-

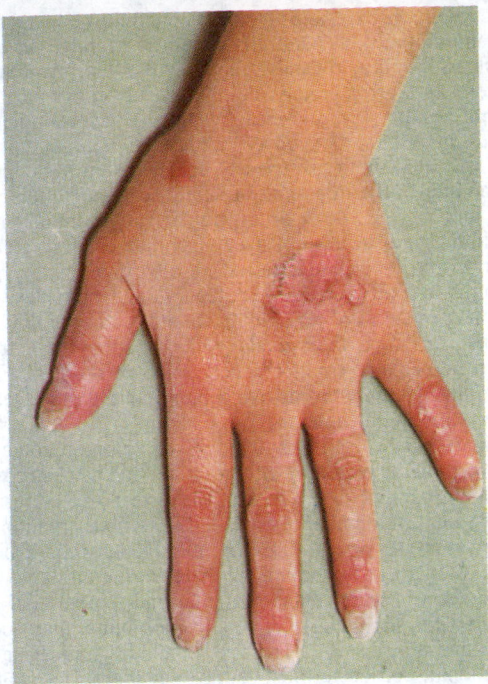

Psoriatic arthritis (Shipley, 1993)

ated with psoriatic lesions of the skin and nails, particularly at the distal interphalangeal joints of the fingers and toes.

PSRO, abbreviation for **Professional Standards Review Organization.**

PSS, abbreviation for **progressive systemic sclerosis.**

PSSO, abbreviation for *peer specialist second opinion.*

PSV, abbreviation for **pressure support ventilation.**

PSW, abbreviation for **psychiatric social worker.**

psych-. See **psycho-.**

psych, abbreviation for **psychology.**

psychalgia. See **psychic pain.**

psyche /sī′kē/ [Gk, mind], **1.** the aspect of one's mental faculty that encompasses the conscious and unconscious processes. **2.** the vital mental or spiritual entity of the individual as opposed to the body or soma. **3.** (in psychoanalysis) the total components of the id, ego, and superego, including all conscious and unconscious aspects. Compare **soma.**

psychedelic /sī′kədel′ik/ [coined in 1956 by Humphrey Osmond from Gk, *psyche* + *deloun*, to reveal], **1.** of or describing a mental state characterized by altered sensory perception and hallucination, accompanied by euphoria or fear, usually caused by the deliberate ingestion of drugs or other substances known to produce this effect. **2.** of or describing any drug or substance that causes this state, such as mescaline or psilocybin.

psychiatric /sī′kē·at′rik/ [Gk, *psyche*, mind + *iatreia*, treatment], pertaining to psychiatry.

psychiatric disorder. See **mental disorder.**

psychiatric emergency service [Gk, *psyche* + *iatreia*, healing], a hospital service that provides immediate initial evaluation and treatment to acutely disturbed mental patients on a 24-hour-a-day basis.

psychiatric foster care, a service for discharged psychiatric patients who receive observation and care in an approved foster home.

psychiatric home care, a service whereby a discharged psychiatric patient is provided observation and care in his or her place of residence.

psychiatric hospital, a health care facility providing inpatient and outpatient therapeutic services to clients with behavioral or emotional illnesses.

psychiatric inpatient unit, a hospital ward or similar area used for the treatment of inpatients who require psychiatric care.

psychiatric nurse practitioner, a nurse practitioner who, by advanced study and clinical practice, such as in a master's program in psychiatric nursing, has gained expert knowledge in the care and prevention of mental disorders. See also **psychiatric nursing.**

psychiatric nursing, the branch of nursing concerned with the prevention and cure of mental disorders and their sequelae. It employs theories of human behavior as its scientific framework and requires the use of the self as its art or expression in nursing practice. Some of the activities of the psychiatric nurse include the provision of a safe therapeutic milieu; working with patients or clients concerning the real day-to-day problems that they face; identifying and caring for the physical aspects of the patient's problems, including drug reactions; assuming the role of social agent or parent for the patient in various recreational, occupational, and social situations; conducting psychotherapy; and providing leadership and clinical assistance for other nurses and health care workers. Psychiatric nurses work in many settings; their responsibilities vary with the setting and with the level of expertise, experience, and training of the individual nurse. Also called **mental health nursing.**

psychiatric social worker (PSW), a social worker who specializes in or works exclusively with the mentally ill.

psychiatrist /sīkī′ətrist/ [Gk, *psyche*, mind + *iatreia*, treatment], a physician with additional medically qualified training and experience in the diagnosis, prevention, and treatment of mental disorders.

psychiatry /sīkī′ətrē/ [Gk, *psyche* + *iatreia*, healing], the branch of medical science that deals with the causes, treatment, and prevention of mental, emotional, and behavioral disorders. Some kinds of psychiatry are **community psychiatry, descriptive psychiatry, dynamic psychiatry, existential psychiatry, forensic psychiatry,** and **orthopsychiatry.** —**psychiatric,** *adj.*

psychic /sī′kik/ [Gk, *psyche*, mind], a practitioner of the systematic study of parapsychology, a category of usually alleged psychologic phenomena that cannot be explained by scientific thinking.

-psychic, a combining form meaning 'relating to the relation between mind and body': *allopsychic, biopsychic, physiopsychic.*

psychic blindness [Gk, *psyche*, mind; AS, *blind*], a somatoform disorder that is manifested by the total or partial loss of vision in eyes that are organically normal. Despite the symptoms claimed, the patient usually reacts to light and avoids objects that might cause injury. The condition is frequently the result of an inner conflict or psychologic stress, such as an unconscious effort to avoid a threatening or guilt situation. Also called **hysterical blindness.**

psychic contagion. See **psychic infection.**

psychic deafness [Gk, *psyche*; AS, *deaf*], an obsolete term for loss of hearing that develops unconsciously in response to severe emotional stress. Also called **hysterical deafness**.

psychic energy, body energy such as thinking, perceiving, and remembering. See also **libido**.

psychic impotence [Gk, *psyche*, mind; L, *in*, *potentia*, power], a functional disorder of the male who is unable to perform sexual intercourse despite normal genitalia and sexual desire. The term is generally applied to an inability to achieve and maintain an erection, but may be manifested in other forms such as premature ejaculation or the need for certain conditions.

psychic infection, [Gk, *psyche* + L, *inficere*, to taint], the spread of psychic effects or influences on others on a small scale, as in folie á deux, or on a large scale, as in the dance and witch manias of the Middle Ages or the spread of hysteric or panic reactions in a crowd. Also called **psychic contagion.** See also **sympathy**.

psychic pain [Gk, *psyche*, mind; L, *poena*, penalty], a functional pain that, in the absence of any organic cause, is usually associated with feelings of acute anxiety. In some cases, the person may experience hallucinations or obsessions. Also called **psychalgia**.

psychic suicide, the termination of one's own life without the use of physical means or agents, such as by an older person, widowed after many years of marriage, who becomes sufficiently depressed to lose 'the will to live.'

psychic trauma, an emotional shock or injury or a distressful situation that produces a lasting impression, especially on the subconscious mind. Some causes of psychic trauma may include abuse or neglect in childhood, rape, and loss of a loved one. Psychotherapeutic sessions in which the injured person can ventilate feelings can help alleviate psychic trauma.

psycho- /sī´kō-, sī´kə-/, **psych-,** a combining form meaning 'of or related to the mind': *psychoauditory*, *psychodynamics*, *psychedelic*.

psychoactive /-ak´tiv/ [Gk, *psyche*, mind; L, *activus*], pertaining to a drug or other agent that affects such normal mental functioning as mood, behavior, or thinking processes. Examples include stimulants, sedatives, or hallucinogens.

psychoanalysis /-ənal´isis/ [Gk, *psyche* + *analyein*, to separate parts], a branch of psychiatry founded by Sigmund Freud devoted to the study of the psychology of human development and behavior. From its systematized method for investigating the processes of the mind evolved a system of psychotherapy based on the concepts of a dynamic unconscious, using such techniques as free association, dream interpretation, and the analysis of defense mechanisms, especially resistance and transference. Through these devices, emotions and behavior are traced to the influence of repressed instinctual drives in the unconscious. Treatment consists of helping the individual become aware of the existence of repressed emotional conflicts, analyzing their origin, and through the process of insight bringing them into the consciousness so that irrational and maladaptive behavior can be altered. See also **psychosexual development**.

psychoanalyst /-an´əlist/, a psychotherapist, usually a psychiatrist, who has had special training in psychoanalysis and who applies the techniques of psychoanalytic theory.

psychoanalytic /-an´əlit´ik/, **1.** of or pertaining to psychoanalysis. **2.** using the techniques or principles of psychoanalysis.

psychobiologic resilience /-bī·əloj´ik/, a concept that proposes a recurrent human need to weather periods of stress and change throughout life. The ability to weather each period of disruption and reintegration successfully leaves the person better able to deal with the next change.

psychobiology /-bī´ol´əjē/ [Gk, *psyche* + *bios*, life, *logos*, science], **1.** the study of biochemical foundations of thought, mood, emotion, affect, and behavior. **2.** personality development and functioning in terms of the interaction of the body and the mind. **3.** a school of psychiatric thought introduced by Adolf Meyer that stresses total life experience, including biologic, emotional, and sociocultural factors in assessing the psychologic makeup or mental status of an individual.

psychocatharsis. See **catharsis**.

psychodiagnosis /-dī´agnō´sis/ [Gk, *psyche*, mind; *dia* + *gnosis*, knowledge], the study of a personality through observations of behavior and mannerisms, combined with various tests.

psychodrama /-dram´ə/, a form of group psychotherapy, originated by J. L. Moreno, in which people act out their emotional problems through improvisational dramatizations. Also called **role playing therapy**.

psychodynamics /-dīnam´iks/ [Gk, *psyche* + *dynamis*, power], the study of the forces that motivate behavior. It may include the influence of past experiences on present behavior and the influence of mental forces on development and behavior.

psychogenesis /sī´kōjen´əsis/ [Gk, *psyche* + *genesis*, origin], **1.** the development of the mind or of a mental function or process. **2.** the development or production of a physical symptom or disease from mental or psychic origins rather than organic factors. **3.** the development of emotional states, either normal or abnormal, from the interaction of conscious and unconscious psychologic forces. Compare **somatogenesis**.

psychogenic /sī´kōjen´ik/ [Gk, *psyche* + *genein*, to produce], **1.** originating within the mind. **2.** referring to any physical symptom, disease process, or emotional state that is of psychologic rather than physical origin. Also **psychogenetic.** See also **psychosomatic**.

psychogenic pain [Gk, *psyche*, mind; L, *poena*, penalty], a functional pain that does not have any organic cause.

psychogenic pain disorder, a disorder characterized by persistent and severe pain for which there is no apparent organic cause. The condition is often accompanied by other sensory or motor dysfunction, such as paresthesia or muscle spasm. The cause may be one or many unresolved needs or conflicts.

psychokinesia /sī´kōkinē´zhə, -kīnē´zhə/ [Gk, *psyche* + *kinesis*, motion], **1.** impulsive, maniacal behavior resulting from deficient or defective inhibitions. **2.** (in parapsychology) psychokinesis.

psychokinesis (PK) /sī´kōkinē´sis, -kīnē´sis/ [Gk, *psyche* + *kinesis*, motion], the alleged direct influence of the mind or will on matter that would result in the production of motion in objects without the intervention of the physical senses or a physical force.

psychokinetics /sī´kōkinet´iks, -kīnet´iks/, the study of psychokinesis.

psychologic /sī´kəloj´ik/ [Gk, *psyche*, mind + *logos*, science], pertaining to or involving psychology. Also **psychological**.

psychologic miscarriage, an absence or deficiency of a mother's love for her infant.

psychologic test [Gk, *psyche* + *logos*, science; L, *testum*, crucible], any of a group of standardized tests designed to measure or ascertain such characteristics of an individual as intellectual capacity, motivation, perception, role behavior, values, level of anxiety or depression, coping mechanisms, and general personality integration. Compare **achievement test, aptitude test, intelligence test, personality test.**

psychologist /sīkol'əjist/, a person who specializes in the study of the structure and function of the brain and related mental processes of animals and humans. A clinical psychologist is one who is qualified by graduate degree in psychology and training in clinical psychology and who provides testing and counseling services to patients with mental and emotional disorders.

psychology (psych) /sīkol'əjē/ [Gk, *psyche* + *logos*, science], **1.** the study of behavior and of the functions and processes of the mind, especially as related to the social and physical environment. **2.** a profession that involves the practical applications of knowledge, skills, and techniques in the understanding of, prevention of, or solution to individual or social problems, especially in regard to the interaction between the individual and the physical and social environment. **3.** the mental, motivational, and behavioral characteristics and attitudes of an individual or group of individuals. Kinds of psychology include **analytic psychology, animal psychology, behaviorism, clinical psychology, cognitive psychology, experimental psychology, humanistic psychology,** and **social psychology. –psychologic, psychological,** *adj.,* **psychologically,** *adv.*

psychometrician /-mətrish'ən/ [Gk, *psyche*, mind + *metron*, measure], a specialist who performs quantitative estimation or measurement of personality and intelligence.

psychometrics /sī'kōmet'riks/ [Gk, *psyche* + *metron*, measure], the development, administration, or interpretation of psychologic and intelligence tests. Also called **psychometry** /sīkom'ətrē/.

psychomotor /-mō'tər/ [Gk, *psyche* + L, *motare*, to move about], pertaining to or causing voluntary movements usually associated with neural activity.

psychomotor and physical development of infants, a branch of pediatric psychiatry that is concerned with the development of skills requiring coordination of sensory processes and motor activities, including infant reflexes, developmental timetables, and emotional and behavioral disorders.

psychomotor development, the progressive attainment by the child of skills that involve both mental and muscular activity, such as the ability of the infant to turn over, sit, or crawl at will and of the toddler to walk, talk, control bladder and bowel functions, and begin solving cognitive problems. The mean chronologic ages at which certain psychomotor skills are attained by most children follow.

12 weeks	Looks at own hand
20 weeks	Able to grasp objects voluntarily.
24 weeks	Able to roll from back to front at will.
44 weeks	Creeps with abdomen off the floor and imitates speech sounds.
15 months	Able to walk without help.
24 months	Has a vocabulary of 300 or more words and uses pronouns.
30 months	Able to jump with both feet.
3 years	Able to ride a tricycle and to feed self well.
4 years	Able to hop and skip on one foot, catch and throw a ball; is independent, boasts, tattles, and shows off.
5 years	Able to tie shoelaces, cut with scissors, tries to please, interested in facts about world, gets along more easily with parents.

psychomotor domain, the area of observable performance of skills that require some degree of neuromuscular coordination.

psychomotor epilepsy. See **psychomotor seizure.**

psychomotor learning, the acquisition of ability to perform motor skills.

psychomotor retardation, a slowing of motor activity related to a state of severe depression.

psychomotor seizure, a temporary impairment of consciousness, often associated with temporal lobe disease and characterized by psychic symptoms, loss of judgment, automatic behavior, and abnormal acts. No apparent convulsions occur, but there may be loss of consciousness or amnesia for the episode. During the seizure the individual may appear drowsy, intoxicated, or violent; asocial acts or crimes may be committed, but normal activities, such as driving a car, typing, or eating, may continue at an automatic level. Psychic symptoms, including visual and auditory hallucinations, a sense of unreality, and déja[gv] vu may be present and may be accompanied by visceral symptoms, such as chest pain, transient respiratory arrest, tachycardia, and GI discomfort, and by abnormal sensations of smell and taste. Also called **psychomotor epilepsy.**

psychoneuroimmunology /-nŏŏr'ō·imyŏŏnol'əjē/, a discipline that studies the relationships between psychologic states and the immune response.

psychoneurosis. See **neurosis.**

psychoneurotic. See **neurotic.**

psychoneurotic disorder. See **neurotic disorder.**

psychopath /sī'kōpath/ [Gk, *psyche* + *pathos*, disease], a person who has an antisocial personality disorder. Also called **sociopath.** See also **antisocial personality, antisocial personality disorder. —psychopathic** /sī'kōpath'ik/, adj.

psychopathia. See **psychopathy.**

psychopathia sexualis /sī'kōpā'thē·ə sek'shŏŏ·al'is/ [Gk, *psyche* + *pathos*, disease; L, *sexus*, male or female], a mental disease characterized by sexual perversion.

psychopathic. See **psychopath.**

psychopathic personality. See **antisocial personality.**

psychopathologist /-pəthol'əjist/, one who specializes in the study and treatment of mental disorders.

psychopathology /-pəthol'əjē/, **1.** the study of the causes, processes, and manifestations of mental disorders. **2.** the behavioral manifestation of any mental disorder.

psychopathy /sīkop'əthē/, any disease of the mind, congenital or acquired, not necessarily associated with subnormal intelligence. Also called **psychopathia.**

psychopharmacology /-far̄məkol'əjē/ [Gk, *psyche* + *pharmakon*, drug, *logos*, science], the scientific study of the effects of drugs on behavior and normal and abnormal mental functions.

psychophylaxis. See **mental hygiene.**

psychophysical preparation for childbirth /-fiz'ikəl/, a program that prepares women for giving birth by teaching them the physiology of the process, exercises to improve muscle tone and physical stamina, and various techniques of breathing and relaxation to promote control and comfort during labor and delivery. There are several methods of psychophysical preparation for childbirth. Among the goals of all of the methods are a decrease in the mother's fear and pain, a decrease in or elimination of the use of analgesia and anesthesia in childbirth, and an increase in the mother's participation and cooperation, with a resulting reduced need for obstetric intervention. Methods of psychophysical preparation for childbirth include **Bradley method, Lamaze method,** and **Read method.**

psychophysics /-fiz'iks/ [Gk, *psyche* + *physikos,* natural], the branch of psychology concerned with the relationships between physical stimuli and sensory responses.

psychophysiologic /-fiz'ē·əloj'ik/ [Gk, *psyche* + *physikos,* natural], having physical symptoms resulting from psychogenic origins; psychosomatic.

psychophysiologic disorder, any of a large group of mental disorders characterized by the dysfunction of an organ or organ system controlled by the autonomic nervous system, such as a peptic ulcer, which may be caused or aggravated by emotional factors. The disorders are named and classified according to the organ system involved, such as cardiovascular, respiratory, musculoskeletal, and GI. Also called **psychosomatic illness, psychosomatic reaction.**

psychophysiology /-fiz'ē·ol'əjē/, **1.** the study of physiology as it relates to various aspects of psychologic or behavioral function. See also **psychophysiologic disorder. 2.** the study of mental activity by physical examination and observation.

psychoprophylactic preparation for childbirth /-prō'filak'tik/, a system of prenatal education for giving birth using the Lamaze method of natural childbirth. See also **psychophysical preparation for childbirth.**

psychosexual /-sek'shoo·əl/ [Gk, *psyche* + L, *sexus,* male or female], of or pertaining to the psychologic and emotional aspects of sex. See also **psychosexual development, psychosexual disorder. –psychosexuality,** *n.*

psychosexual development, (in psychoanalysis) the emergence of the personality through a series of stages from infancy to adulthood. Each stage is relatively fixed in time and characterized by a dominant mode of achieving libidinal pleasure through the interaction of the person's biologic drives and the restraints of the environment.

psychosexual disorder, any condition characterized by abnormal sexual attitudes, desires, or activities resulting from psychologic rather than organic causes. See also **gender identity disorder, paraphilia, psychosexual dysfunction.**

psychosexual dysfunction, any of a large group of sexual maladjustments or disorders caused by an emotional or psychologic problem.

psychosis /sīkō'sis/, *pl.* **psychoses** [Gk, *psyche* + *osis,* condition], any major mental disorder of organic or emotional origin characterized by a gross impairment in reality testing, whereby the individual incorrectly evaluates the accuracy of his or her perceptions and thoughts and makes incorrect references about external reality, even in the face of contrary evidence.

-psychosis, a combining form meaning a 'serious mental disorder': *autopsychosis, encephalopsychosis, pharmacopsychosis.*

psychosocial /-sō'shəl/, [Gr, *psyche* + L, *socialis,* partners], pertaining to a combination of psychologic and social factors.

psychosocial assessment, an evaluation of a person's mental health, social status, and functional capacity within the community.

psychosocial development, (in child development) a description devised by Erik Erikson of the normal serial development of trust, autonomy, identity, and intimacy; the

development begins in infancy and progresses as the infantile ego interacts with the environment. For the child to reach a new stage, the preceding one must be fully realized. The sequence and chronology of the stages coincide with the psychosexual stages of development as described by Freud.

psychosomatic /sī'kōsəmat'ik/ [Gk, *psyche* + *soma,* body], **1.** of or pertaining to psychosomatic medicine. **2.** relating to, characterized by, or resulting from the interaction of the mind or psyche and the body. **3.** the expression of an emotional conflict through physical symptoms. See also **conversion disorder, psychogenic, psychophysiologic disorder.**

psychosomatic approach, the interdisciplinary or holistic study of physical and mental disease from a biologic, psychosocial, and sociocultural point of view.

psychosomatic illness. See **psychophysiologic disorder.**

psychosomatic medicine, the branch of medicine concerned with the interrelationships between mental and emotional reactions and somatic processes, in particular the manner in which intrapsychic conflicts influence physical symptoms. It maintains that the body and mind are one inseparable entity and that both physiologic and psychologic techniques should be applied in the study and treatment of illness. Also called **psychosomatics.**

psychosomatic pain [Gk, *psyche,* mind + *soma,* body; L, *poena,* penalty], pain that is caused in part by a psychogenic problem.

psychosomatic reaction. See **psychophysiologic disorder.**

psychosomatics. See **psychosomatic medicine.**

psychosomatogenic /-sōmat'əjen'ik/, pertaining to factors that cause or lead to the development of psychophysiologic coping measures as learned responses to stressors.

psychosurgery /-sur'jərē/ [Gk, *psyche* + *cheirourgos*], surgical interruption of certain nerve pathways in the brain, performed to treat selected cases of chronic, unremitting anxiety, agitation, or obsessional neuroses. Psychosurgery is performed when the condition is severe and when alternative treatments, such as psychotherapy, drugs, and electroshock, have proven ineffective. The procedure may be a limited prefrontal lobotomy, in which connecting fibers in the frontal region are cut, or a modified bifrontal tractotomy, in which nerve tracts of the brainstem are severed. Light general anesthesia is given. Postoperative nursing care includes observation for signs of leakage of cerebrospinal fluid. A marked alteration of personality is unavoidable. Various cognitive and affective functions also are affected, depending on the location of the induced lesion, the extent of destruction of nerve tissue, and the age, sex, and condition of the patient. Modern psychotherapeutic drugs have replaced psychosurgery in most cases.

psychosynthesis /-sin'thəsis/, a form of psychotherapy that focuses on three levels of the unconscious—lower, middle, and higher unconscious, or superconscious. The goal of the treatment is the recreation or integration of the personality.

psychotherapeutic drugs /-ther'əp(y)oo'tik/ [Gk, *psyche,* mind, *therapeutike,* medical practice; Fr, *drogue*], drugs that are prescribed for their effects in relieving symptoms of anxiety, depression, or other mental disorders.

psychotherapeutics /-tiks/ [Gk, *psyche* + *therapeia,* treatment], the treatment of personality disorders by means of psychotherapy.

psychotherapist /-ther'ə pist/, one who practices psychotherapy, including psychiatrists, licensed psychologists, psychiatric nurses, psychiatric social workers, and individuals trained in counseling. The specific requirements for education and training differ markedly in content, breadth, and duration, depending on the form of psychotherapy practiced. Licensing procedures and definitions of practice vary from state to state. Compare **psychoanalyst.**

psychotherapy /-ther′əpē/ [Gk, *psyche* + *therapeia*, treatment], any of a large number of related methods of treating mental and emotional disorders by psychologic techniques rather than by physical means.

psychotic /sīkot′ik/ [Gk, *psyche* + *osis*, condition], **1.** of or pertaining to psychosis. **2.** a person exhibiting the characteristics of a psychosis.

psychotic disorder. See **psychosis.**

psychotic insight, a stage in the development of a psychosis that follows an initial experience of confusion, bizarreness, and apprehension. At this point, an insight is reached that enables the patient to interpret the external world in terms of a delusional system of thinking. With the new insight, the factors that had previously been confusing become a part of the systematized pattern of the delusion, which, although irrational to an observer, is perceived by the patient as the attainment of exceptionally lucid thinking.

psychotic reaction. See **psychosis.**

psychotomimetic /sīkot′ōmimet′ik/, a drug or other substance whose effects mimic the symptoms of psychosis, such as hallucinations.

psychotropic /-trop′ik/ [Gk, *psyche* + *trepein*, to turn], exerting an effect on the mind or modifying mental activity.

psychotropic drugs, drugs that affect the psychic functions, behavior, or experience of a person using them.

psychro-, a combining form meaning 'of or pertaining to cold': *psychrometer, psychrophilic, psychrophore.*

psyllium seed. See **plantago seed.**

pt., 1. abbreviation for *pint.* **2.** abbreviation for **patient.**

Pt, symbol for the element **platinum.**

PT, 1. abbreviation for **physical therapist 2.** abbreviation for **physical therapy. 3.** abbreviation for **prothrombin time.**

PTA, abbreviation for **plasma thromboplastin antecedent.**

PTB, abbreviation for **patellar-tendon bearing prosthesis.**

PTB/SC, abbreviation for **patellar-tendon bearing supracondylar socket.**

PTCA, abbreviation for **percutaneous transluminal coronary angioplasty.**

pteroylglutamic acid. See **folic acid.**

pterygium /tərij′ē·əm/ [Gk, *pterygion*, wing], a thick, triangular bit of pale tissue that extends medially from the nasal border of the cornea to the inner canthus of the eye.

-pterygium, a suffix meaning a '(specified) abnormality of the conjunctiva': *loxopterygium, pimelopterygium, symblepharopterygium.*

pterygoid /ter′igoid/ [Gk, *pteryx*, wing + *eidos*, form], pertaining to a winglike structure.

pterygoideus lateralis /ter′igoi′dē·əs/ [Gk, *pteryx*, wing, *eidos*, form], one of the four muscles of mastication. Extending almost horizontally from the infratemporal fossa and the condyle of the mandible, it is a short, thick, somewhat conical muscle, arising by two heads from the great wing of the sphenoid, the infratemporal crest, and the lateral pterygoid plate. It inserts into the condyle of the

mandible and into the articular disk of the temporomandibular articulation. The pterygoideus lateralis is innervated by the lateral pterygoid nerve and functions to open the jaws, protrude the mandible, and move the mandible from side to side. Also called **external pterygoid muscle.** Compare **masseter, pterygoideus medialis, temporalis.**

pterygoideus medialis, one of the four muscles of mastication. Arising from the pyramidal process of the palatine bone and from the tuberosity of the maxilla and inserting into the medial surface of the ramus of the mandible, it is innervated by the medial pterygoid nerve and acts to close the jaws. Also called **internal pterygoid muscle.** Compare **masseter, pterygoideus lateralis, temporalis.**

pterygoid plexus, one of a pair of extensive networks of veins between the temporalis and the pterygoideus lateralis, extending between surrounding structures in the infratemporal fossa. The plexus receives deoxygenated blood from various tributaries that correspond with branches of the maxillary artery; it communicates with the cavernous sinus through the foramen of Vesalius and with the facial vein through the deep facial and angular veins. Compare **maxillary vein.**

pterygoid process [Gk, *pteryx*, wing + *eidos*, form; L, *processus*], one of the processes of the sphenoid bone.

pterygomandibular /ter′igōmandib′yələr/ [Gk, *pteryx*, wing + *eidos*, form; L, *mandere*, to chew], pertaining to the pterygoid process and the mandible.

pterygomaxillary /-mak′silerē/ [Gk, *pteryx*, wing + *eidos*, form; L, *maxilla*, jaw], pertaining to the sphenoid bone and the maxilla.

pterygomaxillary notch, a fissure at the junction of the maxilla and the pterygoid process of the sphenoid bone. See **hamular notch.**

PTH, abbreviation for **parathyroid hormone**.

PTNA, abbreviation for **Provincial/Territorial Nurses Association.**

ptoma- /tō′mə-/, a combining form meaning 'of or related to a corpse': *ptomaine, ptomatopsia, ptomatopsy.*

ptomaine /tō′mān/ [Gk, *ptoma*, corpse], an imprecise term introduced in the nineteenth century to identify a group of nitrogenous substances found in putrefied proteins. Because injection of the substances produced toxic reactions, theamines were once regarded as poisonous. Later studies showed the same substances were produced by the normal digestion of proteins in the human intestine without toxic effects.

ptosis /-ō′sis/ [Gk, falling], an abnormal condition of one or both upper eyelids in which the eyelid droops because of a congenital or acquired weakness of the levator muscle or paralysis of the third cranial nerve. Partial ptosis and a small pupil may be caused by an unusual hematologic disorder of the sympathetic portion of the autonomic nervous system. The condition may be treated surgically by shortening the levator muscle.

-ptosis /-tō′sis/ a suffix meaning a 'falling, dropping, or prolapse of an organ': *esophagoptosis, hepatoptosis, uvulaptosis.*

ptotic kidney /tō′tik/, a kidney that is abnormally situated in the pelvis, usually over the sacral promontory behind the peritoneum. The condition of having a ptotic kidney may be either congenital or secondary to trauma. It is usually asymptomatic, but pregnancy may result in obstruction of the flow of urine from the kidney.

PTT. See **partial thromboplastin time.**

ptyalin /tī′əlin/ [Gk, *ptyalon*, spittle], a starch-digesting enzyme present in saliva. Also called **amylase.**

ptyalism /tī′əliz′əm/ [Gk, *ptyalon*, spittle], excessive salivation, such as sometimes occurs in the early months of pregnancy. It is also a clinical sign of mercury poisoning. Also called **hyperptyalism.** See also **sialorrhea.**

ptyalo-, /tī′əlō/, a combining form meaning 'of or related to the saliva': *ptyalocele, ptyalogenic, ptyalography.*

-ptysis, a combining form meaning a 'spitting of matter': *albuminoptysis, hemoptysis, plasmoptysis.*

Pu, symbol for the element **plutonium.**

pub-, pubo-, a combining form meaning 'grown up or adult': *puberal, puberty, pubescence.*

pubarche /pyo̅o̅bär′kē, pyo̅o̅′bärkē/ [L, *puber*, maturity, *arch*, beginning], onset of puberty, marked by the beginning of the development of secondary sexual characteristics.

puberism. See **onset of puberty.**

pubertal /p(y)o̅o̅′bərtəl/ [L, *pubertas*, age of maturity], pertaining to puberty.

puberty /p(y)o̅o̅′bərtē/ [L, *pubertas*, age of maturity], the period of life at which the ability to reproduce begins.

puberulic acid /pyo̅o̅ber′yo̅o̅lik/, an antibiotic isolated from the mold *Penicillium puberulum* that prevents the replication of gram-positive bacteria.

pubescent /p(y)o̅o̅bes′ənt/ [L, *pubescere*, to reach puberty], pertaining to the beginning of puberty.

pubescent uterus [L, *pubescere*, to reach puberty; *uterus*, womb], a uterus in which the cervix and body remain of equal length, the premenstruation state, in adult life.

pubic /p(y)o̅o̅′bik/ [L, *pubis*], pertaining to or involving the region of the pubic symphysis.

-pubic, a combining form meaning 'of, referring to, or relating to the frontal part of the pelvis': *iliopubic, retropubic, vesicopubic.*

pubic bone. See **pubis.**

pubic dislocation. See **dislocation of hip.**

pubic hair /p(y)o̅o̅′bik/ [L, *pubis*; AS, *haer*], hair of the pubic region.

pubic region [L, *pubes*, signs of maturity; *Regio*, to rule], the most inferior part of the abdomen in the lower zone between the right and left inguinal regions and below the umbilical region. Also called **hypogastric region, hypogastrium.** See also **abdominal regions.**

pubic symphysis, the slightly movable interpubic joint of the pelvis, consisting of two pubic bones separated by a disk of fibrocartilage and connected by two ligaments. Also called **symphysis pubis.**

pubis /pyo̅o̅′bis/, *pl.* **pubes** [L, *pubes*], one of a pair of pubic bones that, with the ischium and the ilium, form the hip bone and join the pubic bone from the opposite side at the pubic symphysis. The pubis forms one fifth of the acetabulum and is divisible into the body, the superior ramus, and the inferior ramus. The external surface of the pubis is rough and serves as the origin of the adductor longus, the obturator externus, the adductor brevis, and the proximal part of the gracilis. The internal surface of the pubis is smooth; it forms part of the anterior wall of the pelvis, giving origin to the levator ani and the obturator internus, and attachment to the puboprostatic ligaments and a few muscular fibers from the bladder. The pubic crest affords attachment to the rectus abdominis, the pyramidalis, and the inguinal falx. The lateral portion of the superior ramus of the pubis presents the superior, the inferior, and the dorsal surfaces. The superior surface presents the iliopectineal line, and the inferior ramus gives origin to the gracilis, a portion

of the obturator externus, the adductor brevis, the adductor magnus, the obturator internus, and the constrictor urethrae. Compare **ilium, ischium.**

public health [L, *publicus*, of the people; AS, *haelth*], a field of medicine that deals with the physical and mental health of the community, particularly in such areas as water supply, waste disposal, air pollution, and food safety. In the United States, there are more than 3000 state, county, or city public health agencies. The U.S. Public Health Service was organized originally in 1798 to provide hospital care for American merchant seamen. Subsequent legislation has expanded the role of the federal agency to include such services as the Food and Drug Administration, the National Library of Medicine, health care for Native Americans and Alaska Natives, protection against impure and unsafe foods, drugs, cosmetics, and medical devices, control of alcohol and drug abuse, and protection against unsafe radiation-producing projects.

public health dentistry. See **dentistry.**

public health nursing, a field of nursing that is concerned with the health needs of the community as a whole. Public health nurses may work with families in the home, in schools, at the workplace, in government agencies, and at major health facilities. A home care nursing service is provided by nurses who have special training in public health and are employed by such voluntary agencies as the Visiting Nurses Association or Visiting Nurse Service. Public health nurses enter practice through a baccalaureate program accredited by the National League for Nursing, which prepares the nurse to work as a generalist. Additional recognition is offered through a certification program sponsored by the Division of Community Health Nursing of the American Nurses' Association (ANA).

publish or perish [L, *publicare*, to make public; *perire*, to come to naught], *informal.* a practice followed in many academic institutions in which a contract for employment is renewed at the same rank only if a candidate has demonstrated scholarship and professional status by having had work published in a book or in a reputable, refereed, professional or scientific journal. This work is in addition to whatever obligations for teaching or professional practice are entailed in the position.

pubo-. See **pub-.**

pubococcygeal /p(y)o̅o̅′bōkoksīje̅·əl/ [L, *pubis*; Gk, *kokkyx*, cuckoo's beak], pertaining to the pubis and the coccyx.

pubococcygeus exercises /pyo̅o̅′bōkoksij′e̅·əs/ [L, *pubes* + Gk, *kokkyx*, cuckoo's beak; L, *exercere*, to make strong], a regimen of isometric exercises in which a woman executes a series of voluntary contractions of the muscles of her pelvic diaphragm and perineum in an effort to increase the contractility of her vaginal introitus or to improve her retention of urine. Also called **Kegel exercises.**

■ METHOD: The exercise involves the familiar muscular squeezing action that is required to stop the urinary stream while voiding; that action is performed in an intensive, repetitive, and systematic way throughout each day.

■ NURSING INTERVENTION: The woman is instructed in how to duplicate the squeezing, pulling-up action. A woman whose muscles are particularly attenuated may have difficulty understanding or feeling the muscular action involved. It is often helpful for her to be told that the action is exactly the same as that required to stop the flow of urine. When the woman can effect the contraction required, she is asked to hold the contraction for 6 to 10 seconds, allowing the muscles to relax completely between contractions. She is then advised to perform four to six repetitions of the contraction in a series and to repeat the series three to four times each day. She is further advised that the physiology of muscular exercise is such that weakened muscles may make gains in strength during the early phases of an exercise program, and that, with diligence, she can expect to notice significant improvement in control that will continue as she maintains the regimen of exercise.

■ OUTCOME CRITERIA: Laxity and weakness of the pubococcygeus muscles, often a result of childbirth, may predispose certain women to looseness of the vaginal introitus and to stress incontinence. These problems may be ameliorated as the strength and tone of the muscles are increased through exercise. The rapidity with which a woman can, during voiding, close off the urinary stream is taken as a measure of the strength and tone of her pubococcygeus muscles. Ideally, she should be able to perform the action completely and almost instantly.

pudenda, pudendal. See **pudendum.**

pudendal block /p(y)ōōden′təl/ [L, *pudendus,* shameful, scandalous; Fr, *bloc,* lump], a form of regional anesthetic block administered to relieve the discomfort of the expulsive second stage of labor. The pudendal nerves are anesthetized by the injection of a local anesthetic near the trunk of each nerve as it passes over the sacrospinous ligament, just below the ischial spine. A 10 ml syringe, a long needle, and a guide are used in the procedure. The injection is most easily performed transvaginally; the transperitoneal approach is technically more difficult and is more uncomfortable for the woman. Pudendal block anesthetizes the perineum, vulva, clitoris, labia majora, and perirectal area without affecting the muscular contractions of the uterus. When the block is properly administered, the risk is minimal.

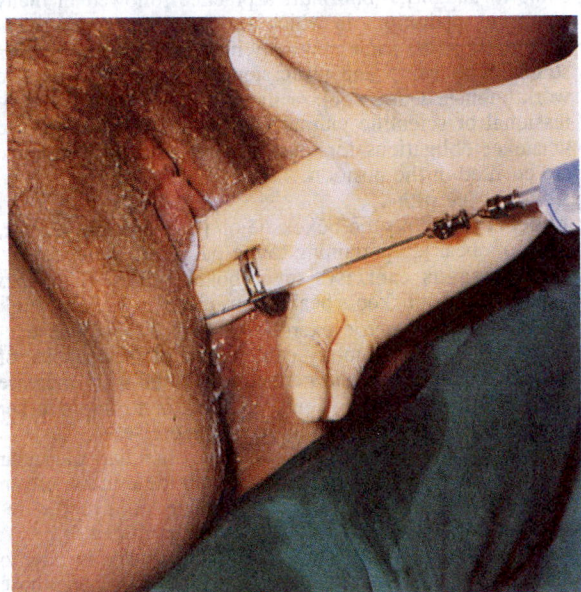

Administration of pudendal block (Al-Azzawi, 1991)

pudendal canal. See **Alcock's canal.**
pudendal nerve, one of the branches of the pudendal plexus that arises from the second, third, and fourth sacral nerves, passes between the piriformis and coccygeus, and leaves the pelvis through the greater sciatic foramen. It crosses the spine of the ischium and reenters the pelvis through the lesser sciatic foramen. It accompanies the internal pudendal vessels through a fascial tunnel along the lateral wall of the ischiorectal fossa and divides into two terminal branches near the urogenital diaphragm. The branches of the pudendal nerve are the inferior rectal nerve, perineal nerve, and dorsal nerve of the penis or of the clitoris. See also **pudendal plexus.**

pudendal plexus, a network of motor and sensory nerves formed by the anterior branches of the second, the third, and all of the fourth sacral nerves. It is often considered part of the sacral plexus. The pudendal plexus lies in the posterior hollow of the pelvis, on the ventral surface of the piriformis. The branches of the plexus are the visceral branches, the muscular branches, and the pudendal nerve. The visceral branches arise from the second, third, and fourth sacral nerves and supply the bladder, prostate, seminal vesicles, uterus, external genitalia, and some of the intestinal tract. The muscular branches arise from the fourth, and, sometimes, the third and fifth sacral nerves and supply the levator ani, sphincter ani, and coccygeus. The pudendal nerve arises from the second, third, and fourth sacral nerves and divides into five branches supplying the genital structures and the pelvic region. Compare **lumbar plexus, sacral plexus.**

pudendum /p(y)ōōden′dəm/, *pl.* **pudenda** [L, *pudens,* modest], the external genitalia, especially of women. In a woman it comprises the mons veneris, the labia majora, the labia minora, the vestibule of the vagina, and the vestibular glands. In a man it comprises the penis, scrotum, and testes. –**pudendal,** *adj.*

puer-, a combining form meaning 'child': *puericulture, puerilism, puerperium, puerperal.*

puericulture /pyōō′ərikul′chər/ [L, *pueri,* children, *colere,* to cultivate], the rearing and training of children. –**puericulturist,** *n.*

puerile /pyōō′əril, -īl/ [L, *puerilis,* childish], of or pertaining to children or childhood; juvenile. –**puerility,** *n.*

puerilism /pyōō′əriliz′əm/ [L, *puerilis,* childish], childishness, particularly when manifested in an older adult.

puerpera /pyōō·er′pərə/ [L, *puerpus,* childbirth], a woman who has just given birth or is in labor.

puerperal /pyōō·er′pərəl/ [L, *puerpus,* childbirth], **1.** of or pertaining to the period immediately after childbirth. **2.** of or pertaining to a woman (a puerpera) who has just given birth to an infant.

puerperal eclampsia [L, *puerpus,* childbirth; Gk, *ek,* out, *lampein* to flash], a condition of coma and convulsive seizures caused by toxins that develop during pregnancy or labor.

puerperal endometritis. See **puerperal fever.**

puerperal fever, a syndrome associated with systemic bacterial infection and septicemia that occurs after childbirth, usually as a result of unsterile obstetric technique. It is characterized by endometritis, fever, tachycardia, uterine tenderness, and foul lochia; if untreated, prostration, renal failure, bacteremic shock, and death may occur. The causative organism is most often one of the hemolytic streptococci. Puerperal fever was little known before hospital childbirth became common, early in the nineteenth century; but then it became an endemic and frequently epidemic scourge that resulted in the deaths of many thousands of mothers and infants. Maternal mortality rates of 20% and higher were common in parts of the world where childbirth occurred in hospitals. Ignaz Philipp Semmelweis, in Vienna, noted that women attended by midwives were much less likely to contract the disease than those attended by physicians and medical students. Midwives did not perform frequent vaginal examinations during labor and did not participate in autopsies. Although the germ theory of disease had not yet been elaborated, Semmelweis deduced that the causative agent of the disease was being transmitted by doctors and students from the infected cadavers in the autopsy room to women in labor on the maternity wards. By instituting a policy requiring that the hands and instruments of obstetric attendants be disinfected, maternal mortality in his clinic dropped dramatically. His work was widely ignored or discredited for almost half a century because physicians were unwilling to believe that they were the agents of transmission. Late in the nineteenth century, after Pasteur's discovery of microbes, Semmelweis was posthumously vindicated. Sterile techniques were gradually instituted, but not until the fourth decade of the twentieth century did puerperal fever cease to be the leading cause of maternal death. Postpartum uterine infection is common but is effectively treated with massive parenteral doses of antibiotics before it becomes a systemic illness. Also called **childbed fever, puerperal sepsis.**

puerperal mania, a rare, acute mood disorder that sometimes occurs in women after childbirth, characterized by a severe manic reaction. See also **mania.** Compare **postpartum depression, postpartum psychosis.**

puerperal mastitis [L, *puerpus*, childbirth; Gk, *mastos*, breast + *itis*, inflammation], a form of acute mastitis in a nursing mother.

puerperal metritis. See **puerperal fever.**

puerperal phlebitis [L, *puerpus*, childbirth; Gk, *phleps*, vein + *itis*, inflammation], an inflammation that begins in a uterine vein after childbirth and spreads to other veins, particularly the iliac and femoral veins.

puerperal psychosis. See **postpartum psychosis.**

puerperal sepsis, an infection acquired during the puerperium.

puerperium /pyoo'ərpir'ē·əm/ [L, *puerperus*], the time after childbirth, lasting approximately 6 weeks, during which the anatomic and physiologic changes brought about by pregnancy resolve and a woman adjusts to the new or expanded responsibilities of motherhood and nonpregnant life.

PUFA, abbreviation for **polyunsaturated fatty acid.**

puff [ME *puf*] a short, soft, blowing sound heard on auscultation.

Pulex /pyoo'leks/ [L, flea], a genus of fleas some species of which transmit arthropod-borne infections, such as plague and epidemic typhus.

pulmo-, pulmon-, a combining form meaning 'of or pertaining to the lungs': *pulmogram, pulmolith, pulmometer.*

pulmonary /pool'məner'ē/ [L, *pulmoneus*], of or pertaining to the lungs or the respiratory system. Also **pulmonic** /poolmon'ik/.

pulmonary acid aspiration syndrome. See **Mendelson's syndrome.**

pulmonary alveolar proteinosis [L, *pulmoneus*, lungs; *alveolus*, little hollow; Gk, *proteios*, first rank + *osis*, condition], a condition in which the air sacs of the lungs become filled with protein and lipids. The cause is unknown, and the disease progresses to respiratory failure.

pulmonary alveolus, one of the numerous terminal air sacs in the lungs in which oxygen and carbon dioxide are exchanged.

pulmonary angiography [L, *pulmonous*, lungs; Gk, *aggeion*, vessel, *graphein*, to record], the radiographic study of the blood vessels of the lungs after the injection of an opaque contrast medium into the pulmonary circulation.

pulmonary anthrax. See **woolsorter's disease.**

pulmonary arteriolar resistance (PAR), pressure loss per unit of blood flow from the pulmonary artery to a pulmonary vein.

pulmonary artery [L, *pulmoneous*, relating to the lungs; Gk, *arteria*, windpipe], either the left pulmonary artery supplying the left lung or the right pulmonary artery supplying the right lung. The lobar branches are named according to the lobe they supply, such as apical (*ramus apicalis*).

pulmonary artery catheter [L, *pulmoneus*, lungs; Gk, *rteria*; *katheter*, a thing lowered], a catheter inserted into a pulmonary artery to measure cardiac output, pulmonary arterial pressure, and capillary wedge pressure.

pulmonary artery wedge pressure [L, *pulmoneus*; Gk, *arteria*; ME, *wegge*; L, *premere*, to press], the blood pressure as measured by a transducer when a catheter is wedged into a distal branch of the pulmonary artery. The pressure measured is that of the pulmonary vein and, indirectly, that of the left atrium and the left ventricle during diastole.

pulmonary atresia [L, *pulmoneous*, lungs; Gk, *a, tresis,* boring], a congenital heart defect of the right ventricular outflow tract. In one form there is an intact ventricular septum with an interatrial communication and a persistent patent ductus arteriosus. A more extreme form is the four-defect **tetralogy of Fallot.**

pulmonary atrium, any of the spaces at the end of an alveolar duct into which alveoli open.

pulmonary carcinosis. See **alveolar cell carcinoma.**

pulmonary circulation [L, *pulmoneus*, lungs + *circulare*], the blood flow through a network of vessels between the heart and the lungs for the oxygenation of blood and removal of carbon dioxide. (See Fig. p. 1304.)

pulmonary compliance, a measure of the elasticity or expansibility of the lungs.

pulmonary congestion [L, *pulmoneus*, lungs; *congerere*, to heap together], an excessive accumulation of fluid in the lungs, usually associated with either an inflammation or congestive heart failure.

pulmonary disease, an abnormal condition of the respiratory system, characterized by cough, chest pain, dyspnea, hemoptysis, sputum production, stridor, and wheezing. Less common symptoms may be anxiety, arm and shoulder pain, tenderness in the calf of the leg, erythema nodosum, swelling of the face, headache, hoarseness, pain in the joints, and somnolence. Diagnostic procedures used for pulmonary diseases include bronchoscopy, cytologic, serologic, and biochemical examination of bronchial secretions, laryngoscopy, pulmonary function tests, and radiography. Pulmonary diseases are either obstructive or restrictive. Obstructive respiratory diseases are the result of an obstacle in the airway that impedes the flow of air. Such obstructions may be bronchospasm, edema of the bronchial mucosa, loss of lung elasticity, or thick bronchial secretions. Obstructive diseases are characterized by reduced expiratory flow rates

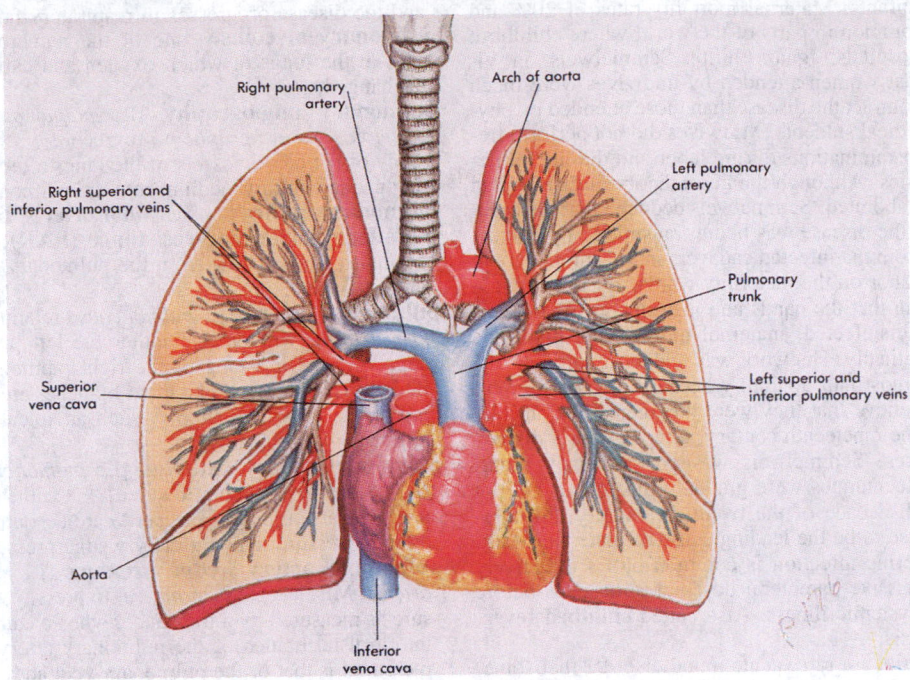

Pulmonary circulation *(Wilson, 1990)*

and increased total lung capacities. Acute obstructive respiratory diseases include asthma, bronchitis, and bronchiectasis; chronic conditions may be combinations of emphysema and bronchitis. Patients with obstructive diseases may have acute respiratory failure from any respiratory stress, such as infections or general anesthesia. Restrictive respiratory diseases are caused by conditions that limit lung expansion through an actual reduction in the volume of inspired air, such as fibrothorax, a neuromuscular disorder, kyphosis, scoliosis, spondylitis, or surgical removal of lung tissue. Characteristic features of restrictive respiratory diseases are decreased forced vital capacity and total lung capacity, with increased work of breathing and inefficient exchange of gases. Acute restrictive conditions are the most common pulmonary cause of acute respiratory failure.

pulmonary edema, the accumulation of extravascular fluid in lung tissues and alveoli, caused most commonly by congestive heart failure and also occurring in barbiturate and opiate poisoning, diffuse infections, hemorrhagic pancreatitis, renal failure, and after a stroke, skull fracture, near drowning, inhalation of irritating gases, and rapid administration of whole blood, plasma, serum albumin, or intravenous fluids. In congestive heart disease serous fluid is pushed back through the pulmonary capillaries into alveoli and quickly enters bronchioles and bronchi.
■ OBSERVATIONS: The patient with pulmonary edema breathes rapidly and shallowly with difficulty, is usually restless, apprehensive, hoarse, pale, or cyanotic, and may cough up frothy, pink sputum. The peripheral and neck veins are usually engorged; the blood pressure and heart rate are increased; and the pulse may be full and pounding or weak and thready. There may be edema of the extremities, crack-

les in the lungs, respiratory acidosis, and profuse diaphoresis.
■ INTERVENTIONS: Acute pulmonary edema is an emergency requiring prompt treatment. The patient is placed in bed in a high Fowler's position, and the immediate administration of intravenous morphine sulfate is usually ordered to relieve pain, to quiet breathing, and to allay apprehension. A cardiotonic, such as digitalis, a fast-acting diuretic, such as furosemide or ethacrynic acid, and a bronchodilator, such as aminophylline, may be given, and oxygen may be ordered. While the patient is acutely ill, the blood pressure, respira-

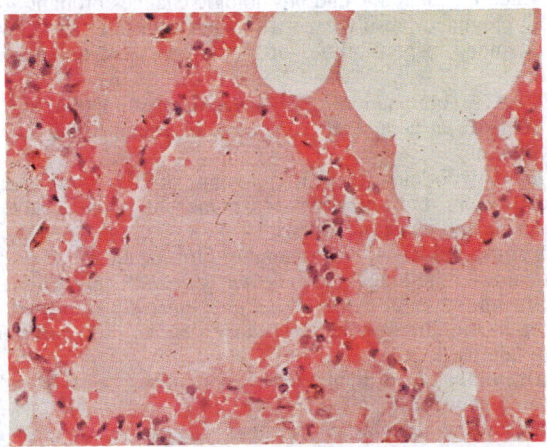

Pulmonary edema *(Swales, 1991)*

tion, apical pulse, and breath sounds are checked every hour or continually monitored. Parenteral fluids, if indicated, are infused slowly in limited quantities; a low-sodium diet is served; and the patient's intake and output of fluids are measured. The patient is weighed daily, and any sudden gain is noted and reported.

■ NURSING CONSIDERATIONS: In addition to receiving continued care and emotional support, the patient exercises to tolerance, plans frequent rest periods, reports any symptoms, avoids smoking, and follows the regimen ordered for medication, diet, and return checkups.

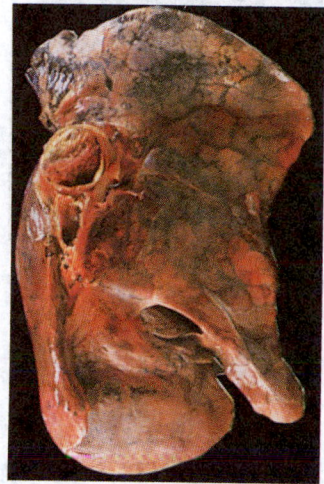

Pulmonary embolism (Fletcher, 1987)

pulmonary embolism (PE),　the blockage of a pulmonary artery by foreign matter such as fat, air, tumor tissue, or a thrombus that usually arises from a peripheral vein. Predisposing factors include an alteration of blood constituents with increased coagulation, damage to blood vessel walls, and stagnation or immobilization, especially when associated with childbirth, congestive heart failure, polycythemia vera, or surgery. Pulmonary embolism is difficult to distinguish from myocardial infarction and pneumonia. It is characterized by dyspnea, sudden chest pain, shock, and cyanosis. Pulmonary infarction, which often occurs within 6 to 24 hours after the formation of a pulmonary embolus, is further characterized by pleural effusion, hemoptysis, leukocytosis, fever, tachycardia and atrial dysrhythmias, and a striking distention of the neck veins. Analysis of blood gases reveals arterial hypoxia and reduced arterial carbon dioxide tension. Pulmonary embolism is detected by chest x-ray films, pulmonary angiography, and radioscanning of the lung fields. Two thirds of patients with a massive pulmonary embolus die within 2 hours. Initial resuscitative measures include external cardiac massage, oxygen, vasopressor drugs, embolectomy, and correction of acidosis. The formation of further emboli is prevented by the use of anticoagulants, and, sometimes, streptokinase or urokinase. Ambulation, exercise, and electric stimulation of the calf muscles also are recommended.

pulmonary emphysema,　a chronic obstructive disease of the lungs, marked by an overdistention of the alveoli and destruction of the supporting alveolar structure.

pulmonary fibrosis.　See fibrosis of the lungs.

pulmonary function laboratory,　an area of a hospital or other health facility used for examination and evaluation of patients' respiratory functions.

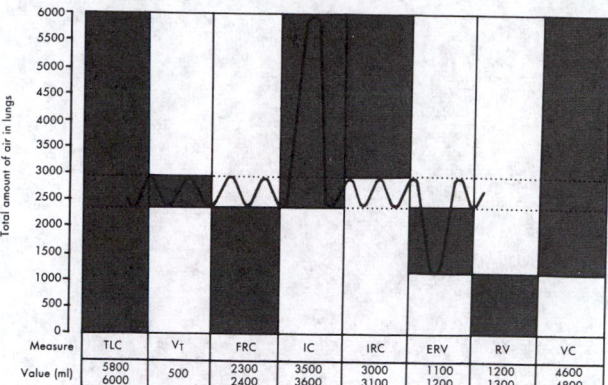

Measure	TLC	VT	FRC	IC	IRC	ERV	RV	VC
Value (ml)	5800 6000	500	2300 2400	3500 3600	3000 3100	1100 1200	1200 1300	4600 4800

Pulmonary function tests (Thompson, 1993)

pulmonary function test (PFT),　a procedure for determining the capacity of the lungs to exchange oxygen and carbon dioxide efficiently. There are two general kinds of respiratory function tests. One measures ventilation, or the ability of the bellows action of the chest and lungs to move gas in and out of alveoli; the other kind measures the diffusion of gas across the alveolar capillary membrane and the perfusion of the lungs by blood. Efficient gas exchange in the lungs requires a balanced ventilation-perfusion ratio, with areas receiving ventilation well perfused and areas receiving blood flow capable of ventilation. Basic ventilation studies are performed with a spirometer and recording device as the patient breathes through a mouthpiece and connecting tube; a nose clip prevents nasal breathing. Measurements or calculations are made of the tidal volume (TV), or gas inspired and expired in a normal breath; the inspiratory reserve volume (IRV), or the maximal volume that can be inspired after a normal respiration; the expiratory reserve volume (ERV), or the maximal volume that can be expired forcefully after a normal expiration; the residual volume (RV), or the gas remaining in the lungs after maximal expiration; and the minute volume, or the gas inspired and expired in 1 minute of normal breathing. The vital capacity of the lungs is equal to TV + IRV + ERV, and the total lung capacity to TV + IRV + ERV + RV. The forced expiratory volume (FEV), or the amount of air forcibly expelled in the first second after a maximal inspiration, and the maximal breathing capacity (MBC), or the amount of gas exchanged per minute with maximal rate and depth of respiration, have special clinical significance. Bronchospirometric measurements of the ventilation and oxygen consumption of each lung separately are performed using a specially constructed double-lumen catheter with two balloons; one balloon is inflated to seal off the contralateral lung when the other lung is tested. Arterial blood gas studies, including determinations of the acidity, partial pressure of carbon dioxide and of oxygen, and the oxyhemoglobin saturation, provide information on the diffusion of gas across the alveolar capillary membrane and the adequacy of oxygenation of tissues.

pulmonary hypertension, a condition of abnormally high pressure within the pulmonary circulation.

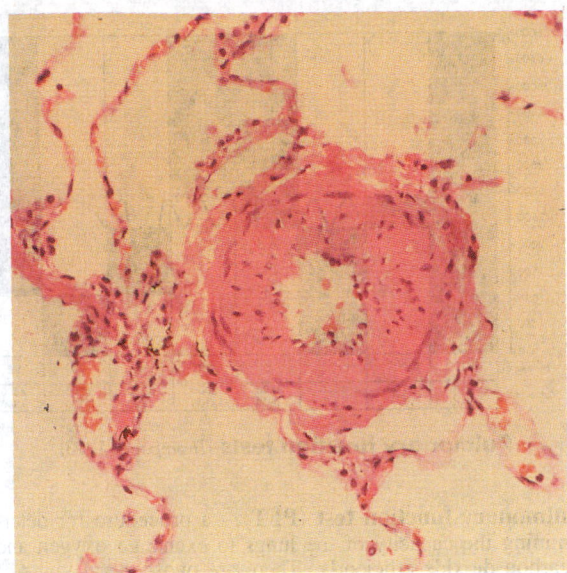

Pathology of pulmonary hypertension
(Turner-Warwick, 1993)

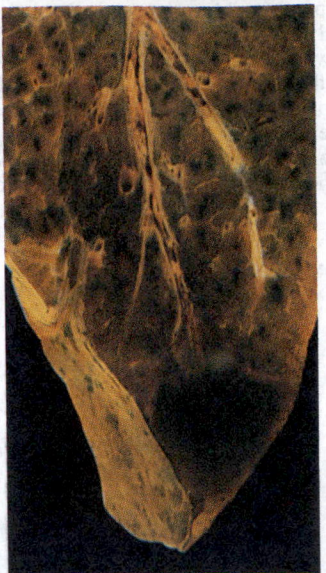

Pulmonary infarction *(Fletcher, 1987)*

pulmonary infarction (PI) [L, *pulmoneus*, lungs + *infarcire*, to stuff], an obstruction in a branch of a pulmonary artery resulting from a thrombus that may have originated in a leg or pelvic vein. After it is released into the venous circulation, the thromboembolus is carried in the bloodstream to one of the lungs, where it is filtered by the pulmonary vascular system.

pulmonary infiltrate with eosinophilia. See **P.I.E.**

pulmonary insufficiency [L, *pulmoneus*, lungs + *in, sufficere*, to suffice], a failure of the pulmonary valve to close properly.

pulmonary oxygen toxicity [L, *pulmoneus*, lungs; Gk, *toxikon*, poison], a form of oxygen poisoning caused by breathing high partial pressures of oxygen. Pathophysiologic effects include pulmonary capillary endothelial damage and alveolar epithelial cell destruction. Clinical manifestations include cough, substernal pain, nausea, vomiting, and atelectasis.

pulmonary stenosis, an abnormal cardiac condition, generally characterized by concentric hypertrophy of the right ventricle with relatively little increase in diastolic volume. When the ventricular septum is intact, this condition may be caused by valvular stenosis, by infundibular stenosis, or by both; it produces a pressure difference during systole between the right ventricular cavity and the pulmonary artery. Pulmonary stenosis is most often congenital but also may be produced after birth by any of a number of types of lesions. Severe pulmonary stenosis may result in heart failure and death, but mild to moderate forms of this disorder are relatively well tolerated. Also called **pulmonic steno-**

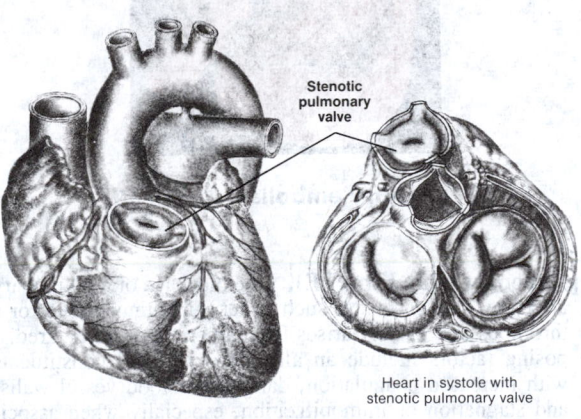

Stenotic pulmonary valve

Heart in systole with stenotic pulmonary valve

Pulmonary stenosis *(Canobbio, 1990)*

sis. See also **congenital cardiac anomaly, valvular heart disease, valvular stenosis.**

pulmonary sulcus tumor, a destructive, invasive neoplasm that develops at the apex of the lung and infiltrates the ribs, vertebrae, and brachial plexus. Also called **Pancoast's tumor.**

pulmonary surfactant, a surfactant agent found in the lungs that functions to reduce the surface tension of the fluid on the surface of the cells of the lower respiratory system, enhancing the elasticity of the alveoli and bronchioles and thus the exchange of gases in the lungs.

pulmonary trunk, the short, wide vessel that conveys venous blood from the right ventricle of the heart to the lungs. It is approximately 5 cm long and 3 cm in diameter, and it ascends obliquely, dividing into right and left branches.

pulmonary tuberculosis. See **tuberculosis.**

pulmonary valve, a cardiac structure composed of three

semilunar cusps that close during each heartbeat to prevent blood from flowing back into the right ventricle from the pulmonary artery. The cusps are separated by sinuses that resemble tiny buckets when they are closed and filled with blood. These flaps grow from the lining of the pulmonary artery and, when they collapse from the inflow of ventricular blood, open the valve and allow deoxygenated blood to flow through the pulmonary artery and on to the lungs. Compare **aortic valve, mitral valve, tricuspid valve.**

pulmonary vascular resistance (PVR), the resistance in the pulmonary vascular bed against which the right ventricle must eject blood.

pulmonary vein, one of a pair of large vessels that return oxygenated blood from each lung to the left atrium of the heart. The right pulmonary veins pass dorsal to the right atrium and the superior vena cava. The left pulmonary veins pass ventral to the descending thoracic aorta. Compare **pulmonary trunk.**

pulmonary ventilation [L, *pulmoneus,* lungs + *ventilate,* to wave], the process of inhaling and exhaling air through the lungs.

pulmonary wedge pressure (PWP), the pressure produced by an inflated latex balloon against a pulmonary artery, as part of a procedure used in the diagnosis of congestive heart failure, myocardial infarction, and other conditions. A Swan-Ganz catheter, or similar balloon-tipped catheter, is inserted through a subclavian, jugular, or femoral vein to the vena cava and on through the right atrium and ventricle to the pulmonary artery. When the balloon is inflated, it can continuously measure pulmonary pressure, which is recorded by bedside instruments.

pulmonary Wegener's granulomatosis, a rare, fatal disease of young or middle-aged men, characterized by granulomatous lesions of the respiratory tract, focal necrotizing arteritis, and, finally, widespread inflammation of body organs. Pulmonary infarction and glomerulonephritis may occur.

pulmonic. See **pulmonary.**

-pulmonic. a combining form meaning 'relating to the lungs': *apulmonic, gastropulmonic, intrapulmonic.*

pulmonic stenosis. See **pulmonary stenosis.**

pulp [L, *pulpa,* flesh], any soft, spongy tissue, such as that contained within the spleen, the pulp chamber of the tooth, or the distal phalanges of the fingers and the toes. **–pulpy,** *adj.*

pulp abscess [L, *pulpa,* flesh + *abscedere,* to go away], a pus-producing abscess that develops in the pulp of a tooth.

pulp canal, the space occupied by the pulp in the radicular portion of the tooth. Also called **root canal.**

pulp cavity, the space in a tooth bounded by the dentin and containing the dental pulp. It is divided into the pulp chamber and the pulp or root canal.

pulpectomy /pulpek'təmē/ [L, *pulpa,* flesh; Gk, *ektome,* excision], the surgical removal, either complete or partial, of the pulp from a tooth. See also **surgical endodontics.**

pulpitis /pulpī'tis/, infection or inflammation of the dental pulp. See also **caries.**

pulpless tooth /pulp'ləs/, a tooth in which the dental pulp is necrotic or has been removed. Also called **devital tooth, nonvital tooth.**

pulp stone. See **denticle.**

pulsate /pul'sāt/ [L, *pulsare,* to beat], to throb or vibrate rhythmically, such as the expansion and contraction rhythm of the heart.

pulsatile /pul'sətil/ [L, *pulsatio,* beating], pertaining to an activity characterized by a rhythmic pulsation.

pulsatile assist device (PAD), a flexible valveless balloon conduit contained within a rigid plastic cylinder that is inserted into the arterial circulation to provide pulsatile cardiopulmonary bypass perfusion.

pulsating exophthalmos /pul'sāting/ [L, *pulsare,* to beat; Gk, *ex, ophthalmos,* eye], an eye disorder characterized by a bulging, pulsating eyeball. The cause is an arteriovenous aneurysm involving the internal carotid artery and the cavernous sinus of the orbit.

pulse [L, *pulsare,* to beat], **1.** a rhythmic beating or vibrating movement. **2.** a brief electromagnetic wave. **3.** the regular, recurrent expansion and contraction of an artery produced by waves of pressure caused by the ejection of blood from the left ventricle of the heart as it contracts. The phenomenon is easily detected on superficial arteries, such as the radial and carotid arteries, and corresponds to each beat of the heart. The normal number of pulse beats per minute in the average adult varies from 60 to 80, with fluctuations occurring with exercise, injury, illness, and emotional reactions. The average pulse rate for a newborn is 120 beats per minute, which slows throughout childhood and adolescence. Girls, beginning about 12 years of age, and women have a higher rate than boys and men.

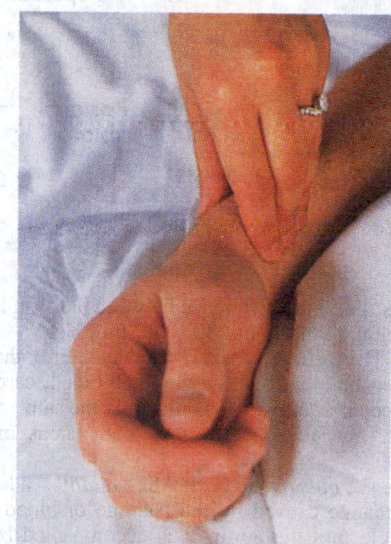

Pulse assessment *(Potter, 1993)*

pulse deficit, a condition that exists when the radial pulse is less than the ventricular rate as auscultated at the apex or seen on the electrocardiogram. The condition indicates a lack of peripheral perfusion.

pulse height analyzer, (in radiology) a device that accepts or rejects electronic pulses according to their amplitude or energy. It is commonly used to select certain gamma radiation energies.

pulseless disease. See **Takayasu's arteritis.**

pulse MR, MR techniques that use radiofrequency pulses and Fourier transformation of the MR signal. Pulse MR has largely replaced the older continuous wave techniques.

pulse point, any one of the sites on the surface of the body where arterial pulsations can be easily palpated. The most commonly used pulse point is over the radial artery at the wrist. Other pulse points include the temporal artery in front of the ear, the common carotid artery at the lower level of the thyroid cartilage, the facial artery at the lower margin of the jaw, and the femoral, popliteal, and dorsalis pedis points.

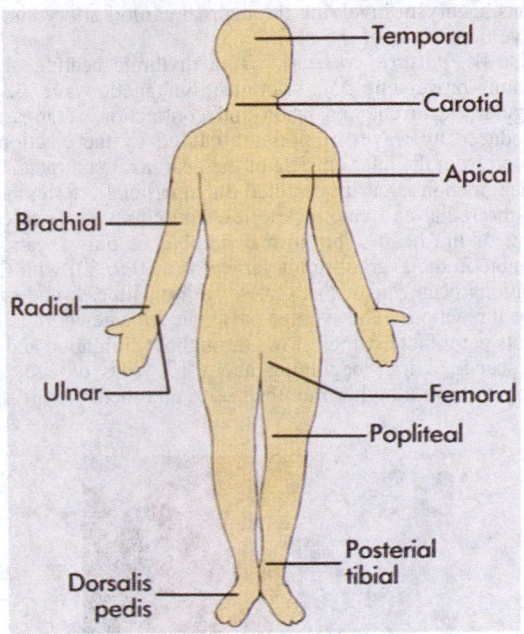

Pulse points (Potter, 1993)

pulse pressure, the difference between the systolic and diastolic pressures, normally 30 to 40 mm Hg.

pulse rate [L, *pulsare* + *reri*, to calculate], the number of beats per minute as measured on the radial, carotid, femoral, and pedal arteries. Normally, it is the same rate as the heart beat, but pulses in various body areas may differ slightly.

pulse wave [L, *pulsare*, to beat; AS, *wafian*], a local blood pressure change caused by the passage of blood from the left ventricle into the aorta. It is accompanied by a wave action through the artery.

-pulsion, a combining form meaning the 'action or condition of pushing forward': *compulsion, lateropulsion, retropulsion.*

pulsus alternans /pul′səs ôl′tərnanz/ [L, *pulsare* + *alternare*, to alternate], a pulse characterized by a regular alternation of weak and strong beats without changes in the length of the cycle. Also called **alternating pulse.**

pulsus magnus. See **full pulse.**

pulsus paradoxus, an abnormal decrease in systolic pressure and pulse wave amplitude during inspiration. The normal fall in pressure is less than 10 mm Hg, and an excessive decline may be a sign of tamponade, adhesive pericarditis, severe lung disease, advanced heart failure, and other conditions. Also called **paradoxical pulse.**

pulsus parvus et tardus [L, *pulsus*, beat + *parvus*, small

+ *tardus*, slow], a small pulse with low pressure that rises and falls slowly. The condition occurs in aortic stenosis.

pulsus tardus [L, *pulsare*, to beat + *tardus*, slow], a pulse with a gradual rise and fall in amplitude.

pulvule /pul′vyo͞ol/ [L, *pulvis*, dust], a proprietary capsule containing a dose of a drug in powder form.

pumice /pum′is/ [L, *pumex*], a very finely divided volcanic rock, used in powdered or solid form for smoothing or polishing surfaces.

pump [ME, *pumpe*], **1.** an apparatus used to move fluids or gases by suction or by positive pressure, such as an infusion pump or stomach pump. **2.** a physiologic mechanism by which a substance is moved, usually by active transport across a cell membrane, such as a sodium pump. **3.** to move a liquid or gas by suction or positive pressure.

pump lung. See **congestive atelectasis.**

pump oxygenator [ME, *pumpe*; Gk, *oxys*, sharp + *genein*, to produce], a device that pumps oxygenated blood through the body during cardiopulmonary surgery.

punch biopsy [L, *pungere*, to prick; Gk, *bios*, life, *opsis*, view], the removal of living tissue for microscopic examination, usually bone marrow aspirates from the sternum, by means of a punch.

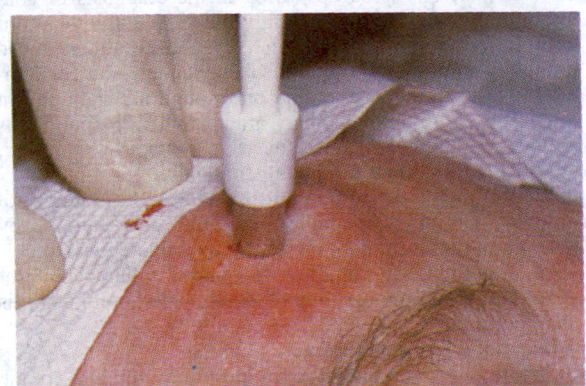

Punch biopsy (Stone, 1989)

punch forceps, a surgical instrument used to cut out a disk of dense or resistant tissue, such as bone and cartilage. The ends of the blades of the punch forceps are perforated to grip the involved tissue. There are several varieties of this instrument, with blades and tips specially designed for different surgical needs.

punct-, a prefix meaning 'a point, or like a point': *punctate, punctiform, punctograph.*

punctum lacrimale /pungk′təm/, *pl.* **puncta lacrimalia** [L, *punctum*, prick; *lacrima*, tear], a tiny aperture in the margin of each eyelid that opens into the lacrimal duct. The puncta release the tears that travel from the lacrimal glands through the lacrimal ducts to the conjunctiva. Puncta clogged with mucus or dirt cause irritation and discomfort.

puncture /pungk′chər/ [L, *punctura*], **1.** to prick or pierce a surface, as with a needle or knife. **2.** a wound or opening made by piercing.

puncture of the antrum [L, *punctura*; Gk, *antron*, cave], a cavity or hollow, as is made in piercing the wall of the maxillary sinus to drain pus.

puncture wound [L, *punctura;* AS, *wund*], a traumatic injury caused by the penetration of the skin by a narrow object, such as a knife, nail, or slender fragment of metal, wood, glass, or other material. In such an injury to the eye, a lung, or a visceral organ, the object or implement is not removed until the person has been transported to a medical facility. Minor puncture wounds are treated with thorough cleansing. If a puncture wound is allowed to close at the skin before deeper healing has occurred, suppuration often results. A tetanus booster inoculation is usually given for such wounds.

punitive damages. See **damages.**

Punnett square [Reginald C. Punnett, twentieth century English geneticist; OFr, *esquarre*], a checkerboard, graphlike diagram, used in charting genetic ratios, that shows all of the possible combinations of male and female gametes when one or more pairs of independent alleles are crossed. Letters representing the male gametes are placed along the Y-axis and those of the female along the X-axis, with the results of the various crossings occupying the squares in a geometric pattern. See also **pedigree.**

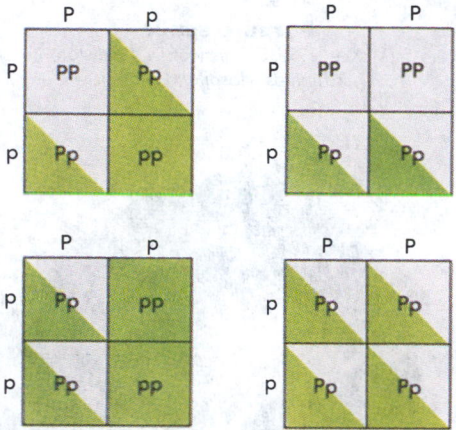

Punnett square *(Thibodeau, 1993/Rolin Graphics)*

P.U.O., abbreviation for *pyrexia of unknown origin.*

pupa /pyoo′pə/ [L, doll], a second stage in the life cycle of certain (*endopterytgote*) insects between a larva and adult. It shows the basic external features of the adult form but without expanded wings.

pupil /pyoo′pəl/ [L, *pupa,* doll], a circular opening in the iris of the eye, located slightly to the nasal side of the center of the iris. The pupil lies behind the anterior chamber of the eye and the cornea and in front of the lens. Its diameter changes with contraction and relaxation of the muscular fibers of the iris as the eye responds to changes in light, emotional states, and other kinds of stimulation. The pupil is the window of the eye through which light passes to the lens and the retina. See also **dilatator pupillae, sphincter pupillae.** –**pupillary,** *adj.*

pupil-. See **pupillo-.**

pupilla /pyoo̅opil′ə/ [L], the pupil of the eye.

pupillary /pyoo̅o′pilerē/ [L, *pupilla*] pertaining to the pupil.

pupillary reflex. See **accommodation reflex, light reflex.**

pupillary skin reflex. See **ciliospinal reflex.**

pupillo-, pupill-, a combining form meaning 'of or pertaining to the pupil': *pupillometer, pupilloplegia, pupillostatometer.*

PUPs, abbreviation for *previously untreated patients,* usually infants participating in clinical trials.

pur-, a combining form meaning 'of or related to pus': *puric, puriform, purohepatitis.*

pure dwarf. See **primordial dwarf.**

pure science. See **science.**

pure tone audiometry. See **audiometry.**

pure vegetarian. See **strict vegetarian.**

purgation. See **catharsis.**

purgative /pur′gətiv/ [L, *purgare,* to purge], a strong medication usually administered by mouth to promote evacuation of the bowel or several bowel movements.

purge /purj/ [L, *purgare*], **1.** to evacuate the bowels, as with a cathartic. **2.** a cathartic. **3.** to make free of an unwanted substance. –**purgative,** *n., adj.*

purified protein derivative (PPD) /pyoo̅o′rifīd/, a dried form of tuberculin used in testing for past or present infection with tubercle bacilli. This product is usually introduced into the skin during such tests and may produce a tuberculin reaction within 48 to 72 hours. Also called **PPD of Seibert, PPD-S.** See also **Mantoux test, tine test, tuberculin test, tuberculosis.**

purine /pyoo̅o′rēn/ [L, *purus,* pure, *urina,* urine], any one of a large group of nitrogenous compounds. Purines are produced as end products in the digestion of certain proteins in the diet, but some are synthesized in the body. Purines are also present in many medications and other substances, including caffeine, theophylline, and various diuretics, muscle relaxants, and myocardial stimulants. Hyperuricemia may develop in some people as a result of an inability to metabolize and excrete purines. A low-purine diet or a purine-free diet may be required. Foods that are high in purines include anchovies and sardines; sweetbreads, liver, kidneys, and other organ meats; legumes; and poultry. The foods lowest in purine content include eggs, fruit, cheese, nuts, sugar, gelatin, and vegetables other than legumes.

purine base [L, *purus,* pure], any of the purine derivatives found in animal waste products. They include hypoxanthine, xanthine, and uric acid.

purine-free diet, a diet that excludes foods that are rich sources of purines, end products of digestion of certain proteins. Foods high in purines include particularly organ meats, such as liver, kidney, and sweetbreads, as well as red meats, poultry, and fish. Those items can be replaced by milk, eggs, cheese, and some vegetable sources of protein.

purine-low diet, a diet that excludes some foods rich in purines, such as certain meat products, fish, and poultry, and particularly anchovies, meat extracts, sardines, and organ meats. Also called **low-purine diet.**

Purinethol, a trademark for an antineoplastic (mercaptopurine).

Purkinje cells /pərkin′jə/ [Johannes E. Purkinje, Polish physiologist, b. 1787], large neurons that provide the only output from the cerebellar cortex after the cortex processes sensory and motor impulses from the rest of the nervous system.

Purkinje's fibers, myocardial fibers that are a continuation of the bundle branches and extend into the muscle walls of the ventricles. See also **Purkinje's network.**

Purkinje's network /pərkin′jēz, pur′kinjēz, -jāz/,   a complex network of muscle fibers that spread through the right and the left ventricles of the heart and carry the impulses that contract those chambers almost simultaneously. Purkinje's fibers ramify from cardiac muscle fibers spreading into the right ventricle and are continuous with the muscle of the right ventricle. The fibers that connect with Purkinje's fibers start in the atrioventricular (AV) node in the right atrium of the heart, along the lower part of the interatrial septum. Impulses generated in the sinoatrial (SA) node travel swiftly through the muscle fibers of both atria of the heart, starting atrial contraction. As the impulse enters the AV node from the right atrium, it slows and allows both atria to contract completely before traveling into the ventricles. The velocity of the impulse increases after the impulse leaves the AV node and spreads via the bundle of His to Purkinje's fibers. Purkinje's fibers, which can be identified only with the aid of a microscope, are larger in diameter than ordinary cardiac muscle fibers and contain relatively few peripheral myofibrillae. They have abundant sarcoplasm and larger central nuclei than ordinary cardiac muscle. See also **cardiac cycle, intraventricular block.**

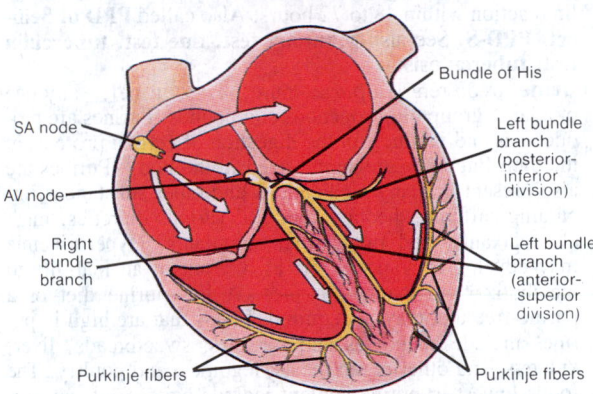

Purkinje's network (Canobbio, 1990)

purposeful activity /pur′pəsfool/,   activity that depends on consciously planned and directed involvement of the person. It is believed that conscious involvement in body movements enhances the development of sensorimotor control and coordination during therapeutic or rehabilitative exercises.

purpur-,   a combining form meaning 'purple': *purpuriferous, purpuriparous, purpurogenous.*

purpura /pur′pyərə/ /pur′pyoorə/ [L, purple],   any of several bleeding disorders characterized by hemorrhage into the tissues, particularly beneath the skin or mucous membranes, producing ecchymoses or petechiae. The two major kinds of purpura are **thrombocytopenic purpura** and **nonthrombocytopenic purpura.** **–purpuric,** *adj.*

purpura rheumatica [L, *purpura,* purple; Gk, *rheum,* flow],   a distinctive clinical sign associated with hemorrhages of the skin and other tissues. The lesions are red or purple and do not blanche on pressure. Purpura is either related to a disorder of the blood or an abnormality affecting the blood vessels.

purpura senile /senē′lā/ [L, *purpura,* purple; *senilis,* aged],   a skin condition affecting older people and characterized by fragile blood vessel walls that rupture on minimal trauma.

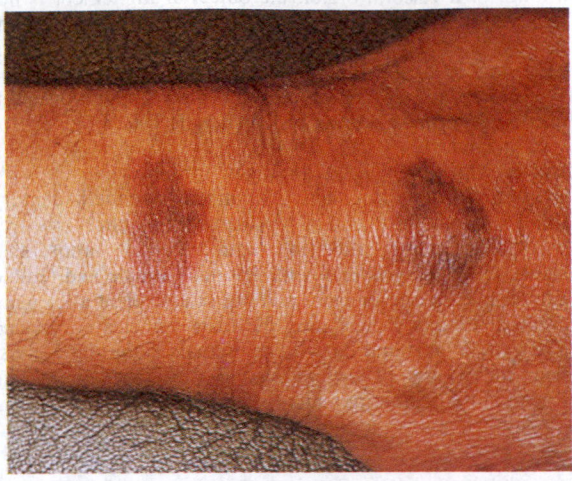

Purpura senile
(McKee, 1993/Courtesy of Dr J Newton, St Thomas' Hospital, London)

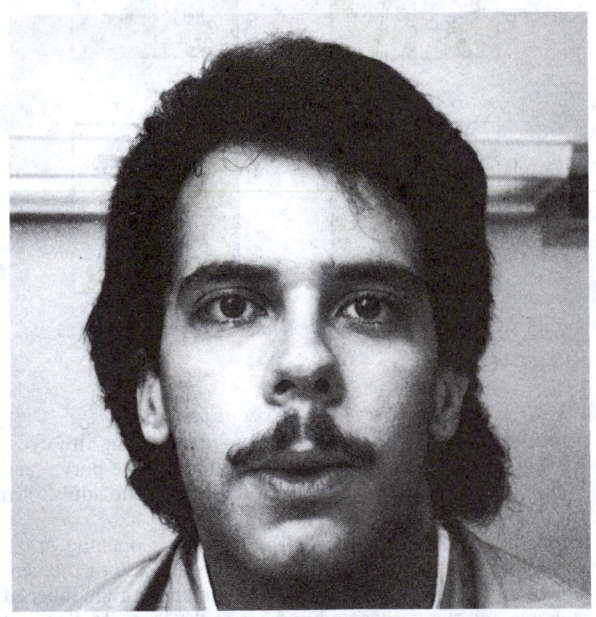

Pursed lip breathing (Wilson, 1991)

pursed-lip breathing /purst-/,   respiration characterized by deep inspirations followed by prolonged expirations through pursed lips.

purse-string suture [L, *sutura*],   a continuous suture inserted in a circle about a round wound. The opening is closed by tightly drawing the ends of the suture together.

purulence /pyoor′(y)ələns/ [L, *purulentus,* pus formation], the condition of producing or discharging pus. Also called **purulency.**

purulent /pyŏŏr′(y)ələnt/ [L, containing pus], producing or containing pus.

purulent conjunctivitis [L, *purulentus*, pus formation + *conjunctivus*, connecting; Gk, *itis*, inflammation], an inflammation of the conjunctiva caused by suppurative microorganisms, including species of streptococci, gonococci, and pneumococci.

purulent diarrhea [L, *purulentus*, pus formation; Gk, *dia*, *rhein*, to flow], diarrhea in which stools contain pus, a sign of a purulent gastrointestinal tract infection.

purulent inflammation [L, *purulentus*, pus formation + *inflammare*, to set afire], an inflammation that is accompanied by the formation of pus.

purulent iritis [L, *purulentus*, pus formation; Gk, *iris*, rainbow + *itis*, inflammation], an inflammation of the iris accompanied by the formation of pus.

purulent keratitis [L, *purulentus*, pus formation; Gk, *keras*, horn + *itis*, inflammation], a severe form of keratitis leading to disintegration of the cornea if untreated. The condition commonly begins with a bacterial infection of the lacrimal sac, occurs frequently in elderly patients who have poor nutrition, and spreads into a pus-producing ulcer.

purulent pancreatitis [L, *purulentus*, pus formation; Gk, *pan*, all + *kreas*, flesh + *itis*, inflammation], inflammation of the pancreas accompanied by pus formation.

purulent rhinitis [L, *purulentus*, pus formation; Gk, *rhis*, nose + *itis*, inflammation], an infection of the nasal mucosa that is accompanied by pus formation. The condition is often secondary to a systemic infection, such as measles.

purulent synovitis [L, *purulentus*, pus formation; Gk, *syn*, together; L, *ovum*, egg], an inflammation of the synovial membrane of a joint with pus formation in the cavity.

pus [L, corrupt matter], a creamy, viscous, pale yellow or yellow-green fluid exudate that is the result of fluid remains of liquefactive necrosis of tissues. Its main constituent is an abundance of polymorphonuclear leukocytes. Bacterial infection is its most common cause. The character of the pus, including its color, consistency, quantity, or odor, may be of diagnostic significance.

pus in urine [L, *pus*; Gk, *ouron*, urine], the presence of pus in a urine sample, indicating a urinary tract infection anywhere from the kidneys to the urethra. Cloudiness in urine may be caused by either pus or chemicals, a difference determined by simple laboratory tests.

pustular /pus′chələr/ [L, *pustula*, blister], pertaining to or resembling pustules.

pustular psoriasis [L, *pustula*, blister; Gk, *psoriasis*, itch], a severe form of psoriasis consisting of bright red patches and sterile pustules all over the body. Crops of lesions lasting 4 to 7 days occur every few days in cycles over weeks or months. Recurrences are inevitable. Fever, leukocytosis, and hypoalbuminemia are associated. In rare cases, hypovolemia and kidney failure occur. Hospitalization may be necessary for fluid replacement, steroid therapy, and sedation. Compare **guttate psoriasis.** See also **psoriasis.**

pustule /pus′chŏŏl/ /pus′chōōl/ [L, *pustula*], a small, circumscribed elevation of the skin containing fluid that is usually purulent. **–pustular,** *adj.*

putamen /pyŏŏtā′mən/ [L, *putamen*, husk], a part of the lentiform nucleus that is lateral to the globus pallidus. It is

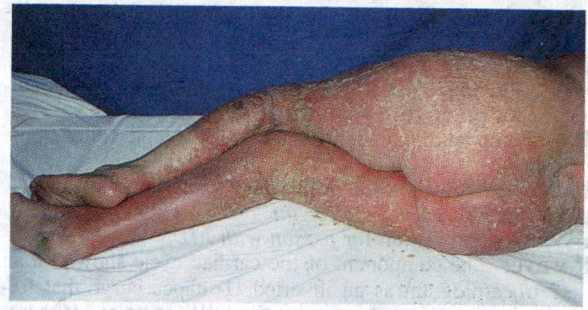

Pustular psoriasis *(McKee, 1993)*

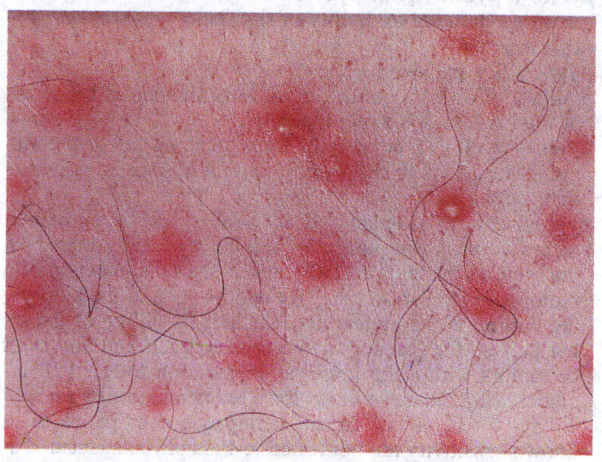

Pustule *(du Vivier, 1993)*

associated with the corpus striatum and receives connections from the suppressor centers of the cortex.

putrefaction /pyŏŏ′trəfak′shən/ [L, *puter*, rotten, *facere*, to make], the decay of enzymes, especially proteins, that produces foul-smelling compounds, such as ammonia, hydrogen sulfide, and mercaptans. **–putrefactive,** *adj.*

putrefactive /-fak′tiv/ [L, *puter*, rotten + *facere*, to make], causing, promoting, or relating to putrefaction.

putrefy /pyŏŏ′trəfī/ [L, *puter*, rotten, *facere*, to make], to decay, with the production of foul-smelling substances, especially putrescine and mercaptans associated with the decomposition of animal tissues and proteins.

putrescine /pyŏŏ′tresēn/, a foul-smelling, toxic ptomaine produced by the decomposition of the amino acid ornithine during the decay of animal tissues, bacillus cultures, and fecal bacteria.

putrid /pyŏŏ′trid/ [L, *putridus*, rotten], decomposed.

putromaine /pyŏŏtrō′mān/, any toxin produced by the decay of food within a living body.

P value, (in research) the statistical probability attached to the occurrence of a given finding by chance alone in comparison with the known distribution of possible findings, considering the kinds of data, the technique of analysis, and the number of observations. The P value may be noted as a decimal: p < .01 means that the likelihood of the phenomena tested occurring by chance alone is less than 1%.

PVB. See **VBP.**

PVC, **1.** abbreviation for **polyvinyl chloride. 2.** abbreviation for **premature ventricular contraction.**

P.V. Carpine, a trademark for a cholinergic (pilocarpine nitrate).

PVR, abbreviation for **pulmonary vascular resistance.**

pW, abbreviation for *picowatt.*

PWA, abbreviation for *person with AIDS.*

P wave, the component of the cardiac cycle shown on an electrocardiogram as an inverted U-shaped curve that follows the T wave and precedes the QRS complex. It represents atrial depolarization.

P' wave (P prime wave), a P wave that is generated from other than the sinus node; an ectopic P wave.

PWP, abbreviation for **pulmonary wedge pressure.**

pycno-, pykno- [Gk, *pyknos,* thick], a combining form meaning 'relating to density or thickness': *pyknometer, pyknophrasia.*

pyel-. See **pyelo-.**

pyelitis /pī′əlī′tis/, *obsolete.* an inflammation of the pelvis of the kidney. See **pyelonephritis.**

pyelo-, pyel-, a combining form meaning 'of or pertaining to the pelvis or the kidney': *pyelocaliectasis, pyelocystitis, pyelograph.*

pyelogram /pī′əlōgram′/ [Gk, *pyekos,* pelvis, *gramma,* record], an x-ray picture of the kidneys and ureters. An intravenous pyelogram (IVP), taken after the injection of a radiopaque dye, shows the size and location of the kidneys, the outline of the ureters and bladder, the filling of the renal pelves, the patency of the urinary tract, and any cysts or tumors within the kidneys. Preparation for an IVP includes withholding of fluids for 8 hours and testing for sensitivity to the iodine in the radiopaque dye; people with known sensitivity are not tested lest anaphylaxis occur. Patients able to tolerate the dye may feel warm and experience a salty taste when the material is injected. Retrograde pyelograms, which demonstrate filling of the renal collecting structures, are taken after the contrast medium is injected into the ureters by means of catheters in a cystoscope introduced through the urethra into the bladder. Also called **urogram.**

pyelography. See **intravenous pyelography.**

pyelolithotomy /pī′əlō′lithot′əmē/, a surgical procedure in which renal calculi are removed from the pelvis of the ureter.

pyelonephritis /pī′əlōnəfrī′tis/ [Gk, *pyelos* + *nephros,* kidney, *itis,* inflammation], a diffuse pyogenic infection of the pelvis and parenchyma of the kidney. **Acute pyelonephritis** is usually the result of an infection that ascends from the lower urinary tract to the kidney. *Escherichia coli* contamination of the urethral meatus is a common cause in females. Infection may spread to the kidney from other locations in the body. The onset of acute pyelonephritis is rapid, characterized by fever, chills, pain in the flank, nausea, and urinary frequency. A urinalysis reveals the presence of bacteria and white blood cells. Antimicrobial treatment is continued for 10 days to 2 weeks. Relapse or reinfection is common. **Chronic pyelonephritis** develops slowly after bacterial infection of the kidney and may progress to renal failure. Most cases are associated with some form of obstruction, such as a stone or a stricture of the ureter.

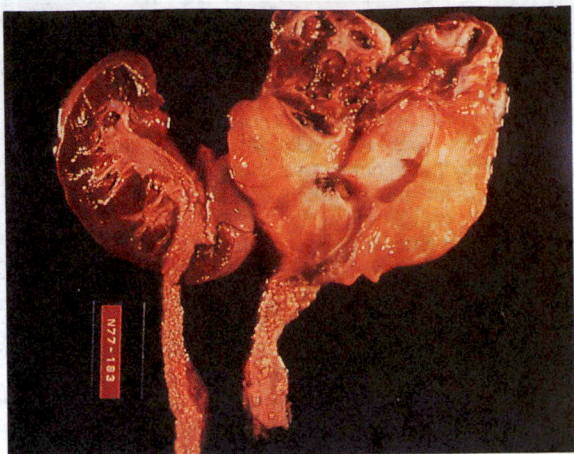

Chronic pyelonephritis (Weiss, 1988)

Treatment includes removal of the cause of obstruction and long-term antimicrobial therapy.

pyemic embolism /pī·ē′mik/ [Gk, *pyon,* pus + *haima,* blood + *embolos,* plug], an infective embolus producing an abscess. Also spelled *pyaemic embolism.*

pygmalianism /pigmā′lē·əniz′əm/ [Gk, *Pygmalion,* mythic, sculptor who fell in love with his statue], a psychosexual abnormality in which the individual directs erotic fantasies toward an object that he or she has created.

pygmy /pig′mē/ [L, *pygmaeus,* dwarf], an extremely small person whose bodily parts are proportioned accordingly; a primordial dwarf. Also spelled **pigmy.**

pygo- /pī′gō-/, a combining form meaning 'of or pertaining to the buttocks': *pygoamorphus, pygodidymus, pygopagus.*

pygoamorphus /pī′gō·əmôr′fəs/ [Gk, *pyge,* buttocks, *a, morphe,* not form], asymmetric, conjoined twins in which the parasitic member is represented by an undifferentiated amorphous mass attached to the autosite in the sacral region.

pygodidymus /pī′gōdid′əməs/ [Gk, *pyge* + *didymos,* twin], **1.** a malformed fetus that has a double pelvis and hips. **2.** conjoined twins who are fused in the cephalothoracic region but separated at the pelvis.

pygomelus /pīgom′ələs/ [Gk, *pyge* + *melos,* limb], a malformed fetus that has an extra limb or limbs attached to the buttock. Also called **epipygus.**

pygopagus /pīgop′əgəs/ [Gk, *pyge* + *pegos,* fixed], conjoined twins consisting of two fully formed or nearly formed fetuses united in the sacral region so that they are back to back.

pyknic /pik′nik/ [Gk, *pyknos,* thick], describing a body structure characterized by short, round limbs, a full face, a short neck, stockiness, and a tendency toward obesity. Compare **asthenic habitus, athletic habitus.** See also **endomorph.**

pykno-. See **pycno-.**

pyle-, a prefix meaning 'of or related to the portal vein': *pylemphraxis, pylephlebectasis, pylephlebitis.*

pylon /pī′lon/ [Gk, gate], an artificial lower limb, often a narrow vertical support consisting of a socket with wooden side-supports and a rubber-clad peg end. It may be used as a temporary prosthesis.

pyloric /pīlôr′ik/ [Gk, *pyle,* gate + *ouros,* guard], pertaining to the pylorus.

pyloric obstruction and dilation /pīlôr′ik/ [Gk, *pyle,* gate + *ouros,* guard; L, *obstruere,* to build against, *dilatare,* to widen], a reaction of the stomach to pyloric obstruction, which increases the resistance to the expulsion of partly digested food from the stomach. As a result, the stomach may become hypertrophied, then dilated. Excessive consumption of food and beverages contributes to the condition.

pyloric orifice [Gk, *pyle,* gate, *ouros,* guard; L, *orificium,* opening], the opening of the stomach into the duodenum lying to the right of the middle line at the level of the cranial border of the first lumbar vertebra. The orifice is usually indicated on the surface of the stomach by the circular, duodenopyloric constriction.

pyloric spasm. See **pylorospasm.**

pyloric sphincter, a thickened muscular ring in the stomach, separating the pylorus from the duodenum. Also called **pyloric valve.**

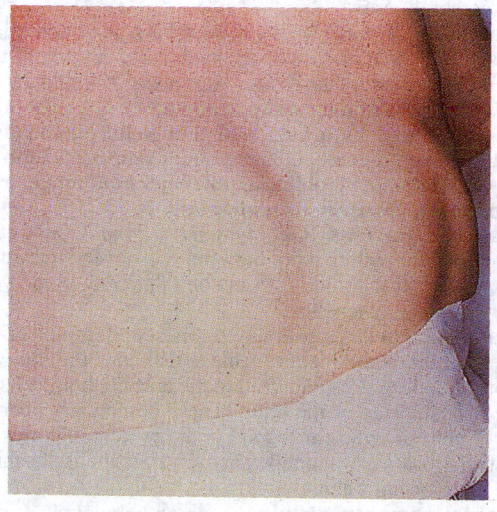

Pyloric stenosis causing giant gastric waves after a feeding
(Zitelli, 1992)

pyloric stenosis, a narrowing of the pyloric sphincter at the outlet of the stomach, causing an obstruction that blocks the flow of food into the small intestine. The condition occurs as a congenital defect in one of 200 newborns and, occasionally, in older adults secondary to an ulcer or fibrosis at the outlet. Diagnosis is made in infants by the presence of forceful projectile vomiting and palpation of a hard, prominent pylorus, and in infants and adults by x-ray examinations after a barium meal. Surgical correction is done using light general anesthesia, after the stomach is emptied.

The muscle fibers of the outlet are cut, without severing the mucosa, to widen the opening. After surgery in adults, a stomach tube remains in place and observation is maintained for signs of hemorrhage or of blockage of the tube. See also **pyloromyotomy.**

pyloric ulcer. See **peptic ulcer.**

pyloric valve. See **pyloric sphincter.**

pyloro-, a combining form meaning 'of or related to the pylorus': *pylorodilator, pyloroplasty, pyloroptosis.*

pyloromyotomy /pīlôr′ōmī·ot′əmē/ [Gk, *pyle, ouros* + *mys,* muscle, *temnein,* to cut], the incision of the longitudinal and circular muscle of the pylorus, which leaves the mucosa intact but separates the incised muscle fibers. It is the treatment of choice for hypertrophic pyloric stenosis. Also called **Fredet-Ramstedt operation.** See also **pyloric stenosis.**

pyloroplasty /pīlôr′əplas′tē/ [Gk, *pyle, ouros* + *plassein,* to mold], a surgical procedure performed to relieve pyloric stenosis. Before surgery, any electrolyte imbalances or fluid deficiencies are corrected; sodium chloride and potassium chloride solutions may be given to correct ion losses from vomiting, which is characteristic of the condition. With the patient under anesthesia, the passageway is dilated. As treatment for the duodenal ulcer, the operation allows the alkaline secretions of the duodenum to flow back into the stomach. Branches of the vagus nerve that supply the acid-secreting portion of the stomach may be cut, reducing the acidity of the stomach contents. Diarrhea is a common postoperative complication.

pylorospasm /pīlôr′əspaz′əm/ [Gk, *pyle, ouros* + *spasmos*], a spasm of the pyloric sphincter of the stomach, as occurs in pyloric stenosis.

pylorotomy /pī′lôrot′əmē/ [Gk, *pyle,* gate + *ouros,* guard, + *temnein,* to cut], a surgical incision of the pylorus, usually performed to remove an obstruction.

pylorus /pīlôr′əs/, *pl.* **pylori, pyloruses** [Gk, *pyle,* gate, *ouros,* guard], a tubular portion of the stomach that angles to the right from the body of the stomach toward the duodenum. The most common position of the pylorus is about 3 cm to the right of the sagittal axis. It is distinctively marked by the thickening of the pyloric sphincter, and its lining is composed of an intestinal kind of epithelium rather than the gastric kind common to the body of the stomach. **–pyloric,** *adj.*

pyo- /pī′ō-/, a combining form meaning 'of or related to pus': *pyocalyx, pyocele, pyocyte.*

Pyocidin Otic, a trademark for an otic, fixed-combination drug containing a glucocorticoid (hydrocortisone) and an antibacterial (polymyxin B sulfate).

pyocyst /pī′əsist/ [Gk, *pyon,* pus + *kytos,* cell], a pus-filled cyst.

pyoderma /pī′ōdur′mə/ [Gk, *pyon,* pus, *derma,* skin], any purulent skin disease, such as impetigo. Also called **pyodermia.** (See Fig. p. 1314.)

pyogenic /pī′əjen′ik/ [Gk, *pyon* + *genein,* to produce], pus-producing.

pyogenic granuloma, a small, nonmalignant mass of excessive granulation tissue, usually found at the site of an injury. Most often a dull red color, it contains numerous capillaries, bleeds easily, and is very tender; it may be attached by a narrow stalk. Treatment is with electrocautery or topical silver nitrate. Also called **telangiectatic granuloma.** See also **granuloma.** (See Fig. p. 1314.)

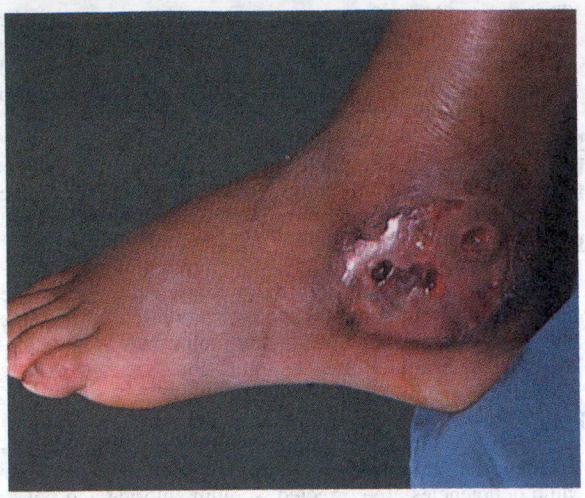

Pyoderma gangrenosum *(Shipley, 1993)*

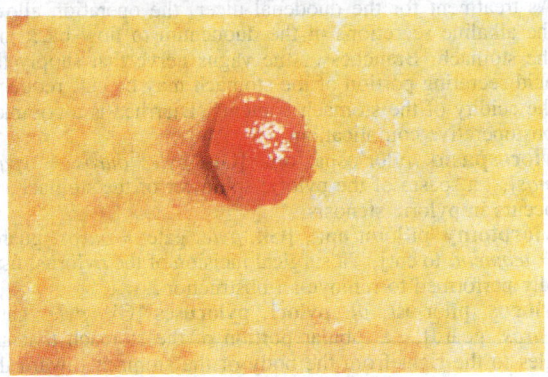

Pyogenic granuloma *(Goldstein, 1992/Courtesy of Beverly Sanders, MD)*

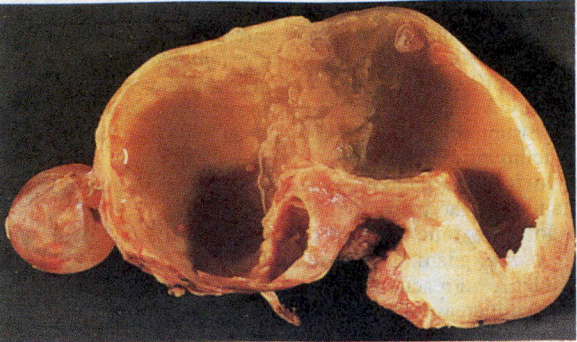

Pyosalpinx *(Fletcher, 1987)*

pyogenic infection [Gk, *pyon*, pus + *genein*, to produce; L, *inficere*, to stain], any infection that results in pus production.

pyogenic microorganisms [Gk, *pyon*, pus + *genein*, to produce + *mikros*, small + *organon*, instrument], microorganisms that produce pus. They include species of bacilli, clostridia, gonococci, meningococci, pseudomonas, staphylococci, and streptococci.

pyohemothorax /-hem′ōthôr′aks/ [Gk, *pyon*, pus + *haima*, blood + *thorax*, chest], an accumulation of blood and pus in the pleural cavity.

pyophylactic /-filak′tik/ [Gk, *pyon*, pus + *phylax*, protector], providing protection against purulent infections, such as with taking an antibiotic before the onset of an infection.

pyorrhea /pī′ərē′ə/ [Gk, *pyon* + *rhoia*, flow], **1.** a discharge of pus. **2.** a purulent inflammation of the tissues surrounding the teeth. **–pyorrheal,** *adj.*

pyorrhea-, a combining form meaning 'the flowing or discharge of pus':*ophthalmopyorrhea, otopyorrhea.*

pyosalpinx /pī′ōsal′pingks/ [Gk, *pyon* + *salpinx*, tube], an accumulation of pus in a fallopian tube. See also **salpingitis.**

pyramid /pir′əmid/ [Gr, *pyramis*], a mass of tissue rising to an apex, such as the pyramids of the cerebellum and kidneys.

pyramidal /piram′idəl/ [Gk, *pyramis*], of or pertaining to the shape of a pyramid.

pyramidal cell [Gk, *pyramis*; L, *cella*, storeroom], a neuron with a pyramid-shaped cell body in the gray matter of the cerebral cortex.

pyramidalis /piram′idā′lis/, one of a pair of anterolateral muscles of the abdomen, contained in the lower end of the sheath of the rectus abdominis. It is a small, triangular muscle that arises from the pubis and inserts into the linea alba. It is innervated by a branch of the twelfth thoracic nerve and functions to tense the linea alba. Compare **obliquus externus abdominis, obliquus internus abdominis, rectus abdominis, transversus abdominis.**

pyramidal nucleus [Gk, *pyramis*; L, *nucleus*, nut], a band of gray matter lying between the olivary nucleus and the midline that projects fibers contralaterally to the vermis of part of the cerebellum.

pyramidal tract, a pathway composed of groups of nerve fibers in the white matter of the spinal cord through which motor impulses are conducted to the anterior horn cells on the opposite side of the brain. These descending fibers, the nerve cells of which are found in the precentral cortex, regulate the voluntary and reflex activity of the muscles through the anterior horn cells.

pyrantel pamoate /pīran′təl/, an anthelmintic.
■ INDICATIONS: It is prescribed in the treatment of infestation by roundworms or pinworms.
■ CONTRAINDICATION: Known hypersensitivity to this drug prohibits its use. Caution should be used in anemia or severe malnutrition.
■ ADVERSE EFFECTS: Among the more serious adverse reactions are nausea, abdominal cramps, diarrhea, dizziness, and skin rash.

pyrazinamide /pī′rəzin′əmīd/, an antimycobacterial.
■ INDICATIONS: It is prescribed in combination chemotherapy in the treatment of tuberculosis of hospitalized patients who fail to respond to other medications.
■ CONTRAINDICATIONS: Severe liver damage or known hypersensitivity to this drug prohibits its use.
■ ADVERSE EFFECTS: Among the more serious adverse reactions are hepatotoxicity and hyperuricemia.

pyrectic /pīrek'tik/ [Gk, *pyretos* fever], pertaining to or characterized by fever. Also called *pyretic*.

pyrethrin and piperonyl butoxide /pī'rəthrin, piper'ənil/, a fixed-combination scabicide and pediculicide.

■ INDICATIONS: It is prescribed in the treatment of infestations of head, body, and pubic lice.

■ CONTRAINDICATIONS: Known hypersensitivity to ragweed or to this drug prohibits its use.

■ ADVERSE EFFECTS: Among the more serious adverse reactions are irritation of the skin and the mucous membranes.

pyreto-, a combining form meaning 'of or pertaining to fever': *pyretogen, pyretography, pyretotherapy.*

pyretogenic /pī'rətojen'ik/ [Gk, *pyretos*, fever + *genein*, to produce], inducing, causing, or resulting from a fever.

pyrexia. See **fever.**

-pyrexia, a combining form meaning a 'febrile condition': *apyrexia, electropyrexia, physiopyrexia.*

Pyridium, a trademark for an analgesic (phenazopyridine hydrochloride).

pyridostigmine bromide /pir'idōstig'mēn/, a cholinergic.

■ INDICATIONS: It is prescribed in the treatment of myasthenia gravis and is used as an antagonist to nondepolarizing muscle relaxants, such as curare.

■ CONTRAINDICATIONS: Intestinal or urinary obstruction, bradycardia, hypotension, or known hypersensitivity to this drug or to other anticholinesterases prohibits its use.

■ ADVERSE EFFECTS: Among the more serious adverse reactions are nausea, diarrhea, abdominal cramps, muscle cramps, and weakness.

pyridoxal phosphate /pir'ədok'səl/, an enzyme in the body that acts with pyridoxamine phosphate and transaminase to catalyze the reversible transfer of an amino group from an alpha-amino acid to an alpha-keto acid, especially alpha-ketoglutaric acid. Such processes are essential to metabolism.

pyridoxamine phosphate /pir'ədok'səmēn/, an enzyme that participates with pyridoxal phosphate and transaminase in the reversible transfer of an amino group from an alpha-amino acid to an alpha-keto acid.

pyridoxine /pir'ədok'sēn/, a water-soluble, white, crystalline vitamin that is part of the B complex group, derived from pyridine, and converted in the body to pyridoxal and pyridoxamine for synthesis. It functions as a coenzyme essential for the synthesis and breakdown of amino acids, the conversion of tryptophan to niacin, the breakdown of glycogen to glucose 1-phosphate, the production of antibodies, the formation of heme in hemoglobin, the formation of hormones important in brain function, the proper absorption of vitamin B_{12}, the production of hydrochloric acid and magnesium, and the maintenance of the balance of sodium and potassium, which regulates body fluids and the functioning of the nervous and musculoskeletal systems. Rich dietary sources are meats, especially organ meats, whole-grain cereals, soybeans, peanuts, wheat germ, and brewer's yeast; milk and green vegetables supply smaller amounts. The most common symptoms of deficiency are seborrheic dermatitis about the eyes, nose, and mouth and behind the use ears; cheilosis; glossitis and stomatitis; nervousness; depression; peripheral neuropathy; and lymphopenia, leading to convulsions in infants and anemia in adults. Treatment and prophylaxis consist of administration of the vitamin and a diet rich in foods containing it. Several drugs interfere with the use of pyridoxine, notably isoniazid and penicillamine, and supplements of the vitamin are recommended with the of these drugs. The need for increased amounts of pyridoxine occurs during pregnancy, lactation, exposure to radiation, cardiac failure, aging, and use of oral contraceptives. The RDA for pyridoxine is 2.0 mg/day for men and 1.6 mg/day for women. Also called **vitamin B_6.**

pyridoxine hydrochloride. See **pyridoxine.**

pyriform /pir'ifôrm/ [L, *pirum*, pear + *forma*], pear-shaped.

pyrilamine maleate /piril'əmēn/, an antihistamine.

■ INDICATIONS: It is prescribed in the treatment of a variety of hypersensitivity reactions, including rhinitis, skin rash, and pruritus.

■ CONTRAINDICATIONS: Asthma or known hypersensitivity to this drug prohibits its use. It is not given to newborn infants or lactating mothers.

■ ADVERSE EFFECTS: Drowsiness, skin rash, hypersensitivity reactions, dry mouth, and tachycardia commonly occur.

pyrimethamine /pir'imeth'əmēn/ an antimalarial.

■ INDICATIONS: It is prescribed in the treatment of malaria and toxoplasmosis.

■ CONTRAINDICATIONS: Use in chloroguanide-resistant malaria is contraindicated. Caution is recommended in use of the drug to treat toxoplasmosis because dosages needed may be at toxic level.

■ ADVERSE EFFECTS: Among the more serious adverse reactions, primarily with large doses, are megaloblastic anemia, atrophic glossitis, leukopenia, and convulsions.

pyrimethamine and sulfadoxine, /sulfədok'sēn/ an antimalarial fixed-combination drug.

■ INDICATIONS: It is prescribed for prophylaxis and attacks of malaria.

■ CONTRAINDICATIONS: Megaloblastic anemia, infant age of less than 2 months, pregnancy at term and during the nursing period, or hypersensitivity to pyrimethamine or the sulfonamides prohibits its use.

■ ADVERSE EFFECTS: The most serious adverse reactions are hypersensitivity reactions, pancreatitis, mental depression, convulsions, hallucinations, and several blood dyscrasias.

pyrimidine /pərim'ədēn/, an organic compound of heterocyclic nitrogen found in nucleic acids and in many drugs, including the antiviral drugs acyclovir, ribavirin, and trifluridine.

pyro- /pī'rō-/, a prefix meaning 'of or related to fire or heat, or produced by heating': *pyrocatechin, pyrodextrin, pyromania.*

pyrogen /pī'rəjən/ [Gk, *pyr*, fire, *genein*, to produce], any substance or agent that tends to cause a rise in body temperature, such as some bacterial toxins. See also **fever.** –**pyrogenic,** *adj.*

pyrolagnia /pī'rōlag'nē·ə/ [Gk, *pyr* + *lagneia*, lust], sexual stimulation or gratification from watching or setting fires.

pyromania /pī'rōmā'nē·ə/ [Gk, *pyr* + *mania*, madness], an impulse-control disorder characterized by an uncontrollable urge to set fires.

pyromaniac /pī'rōmā'nē·ak/, **1.** a person with or displaying characteristics of pyromania. **2.** of, pertaining to, or exhibiting pyromania. –**pyromaniacal,** *adj.*

pyrosis. See **heartburn.**

pyroxylin. See **nitrocellulose.**

pyrrole /pirōl', pir'ōl/ [Gk, *pyrrhos*, red], a heterocyclic-substance occurring naturally in many compounds in the body. Heme and porphyrin are pyrrole derivatives.

Pyrroxate, a trademark for a respiratory, fixed-combination drug containing an adrenergic (methoxyphenamine hydrochloride), an antihistaminic (chlorpheniramine maleate), analgesics (aspirin and phenacetin), and a stimulant (caffeine).

pyruvate kinase /pī′rəvāt/, an enzyme essential for anaerobic glycolysis in red blood cells. It catalyzes the transfer of a phosphate group from adenosine triphosphate to produce adenosine diphosphate.

pyruvate kinase deficiency, a congenital hemolytic disorder transmitted as an autosomal recessive trait. The homozygous condition is characterized by severe chronic hemolysis. The heterozygous form is usually asymptomatic and of no clinical significance, although mild to severe anemia may occur.

pyruvic acid /pīrōō′vik/, a compound formed as an end product of glycolysis, the anaerobic stage of glucose metabolism. Exposed to oxygen and acetylcoenzyme A at the entrance to the Krebs cycle, the compound is converted to lactic acid that accumulates in muscle tissue.

pyuria /pīyōōr′ē·ə/, the presence of white blood cells in the urine, usually a sign of an infection in the urinary tract. The presence of one to four leukocytes per high-power field count during a laboratory urine examination is considered to be within the normal range for a male or female patient. Excessive leukocytes suggest a bacterial or other infection. A bacterial pyuria usually is caused by a viral infection of the bladder and urethra. Miliary pyuria is characterized by the presence of blood cells, pus cells, and epithelial cells, in addition to bacteria. See also **bacteriuria**.

PZI, abbreviation for **protamine zinc insulin**. See **protamine zinc insulin suspension.**

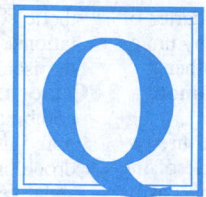

Q, 1. symbol for *blood volume*. **2.** symbol for *quantity*. **3.** symbol for *coulomb*.

Q·, symbol for *rate of blood flow*.

QA, abbreviation for **quality assurance.**

Q angle, the angle of incidence of the quadriceps muscle relative to the patella. The Q angle determines the tracking of the patella through the trochlea of the femur. As the angle increases, the chance of patellar compression problems increases.

QAP, abbreviation for **quality assurance program.**

q.d., 1. (in prescriptions) abbreviation for *quaque die* /dē′ā/, a Latin phrase meaning 'every day.' Also called **quotid. 2.** abbreviation for *quartile deviation*.

q diem, See **q.d.**

qdrnt, abbreviation for **quadrant**.

Q fever [L, *febris*], an acute febrile illness, usually respiratory, caused by the rickettsia *Coxiella burnetii* (*Rickettsia burnetii*). The disease is spread through contact with infected domestic animals, by inhaling the rickettsiae from their hides, drinking their contaminated milk, or being bitten by a tick harboring the organism. Onset is abrupt, and high fever may persist for 3 weeks or more. The illness is especially common among those who work with sheep, goats, and cattle. Treatment with tetracycline is usually effective in 36 to 48 hours. People who are regularly exposed to domestic animals can be vaccinated against Q fever. Also called **Australian Q fever.** Compare **scrub typhus.**

q.h., (in prescriptions) abbreviation for *quaque hora*, a Latin phrase meaning 'every hour.'

q.2h., (in prescriptions) abbreviation for *quaque secunda hora*, a Latin phrase meaning 'every 2 hours.'

q.3h., (in prescriptions) abbreviation for *quaque tertia hora*, a Latin phrase meaning 'every 3 hours.'

q.4h., (in prescriptions) abbreviation for *quaque quarta hora*, a Latin phrase meaning 'every 4 hours.'

q.6h., (in prescriptions) abbreviation for *quaque sex hora*, a Latin phrase meaning 'every 6 hours.'

q.8h., (in prescriptions) abbreviation for *quaque octa hora*, a Latin phrase meaning 'every 8 hours.'

q.i.d., (in prescriptions) abbreviation for *quater in die* /dē′ā/, a Latin phrase meaning 'four times a day.'

q.l., abbreviation for the Latin *quantum libet*, a Latin phrase meaning 'as much as one pleases.'

qli, abbreviation for *quality of life index*.

QRS complex, a series of wave forms on an electrocardiogram that represent depolarization of ventricular muscle cells. The term, 'QRS complex,' is assigned by convention to describe both normal and abnormal ventricular depolarization. The variable morphologies of the QRS complex are described in detail by labelling each deflection above and below the baseline as Q,R, or S wave; upper and lower case letters are used to describe the amplitude of each waveform. In the QRS complex, a Q wave is the negative deflection preceding an R wave; an R wave is the first positive deflec-

tion, and an S wave is the negative deflection following an R wave. If there is no R wave, a totally negative complex is designated QS. Some variations of the QRS complex are rS, qR, RS, rSR′, qRs, and QR.

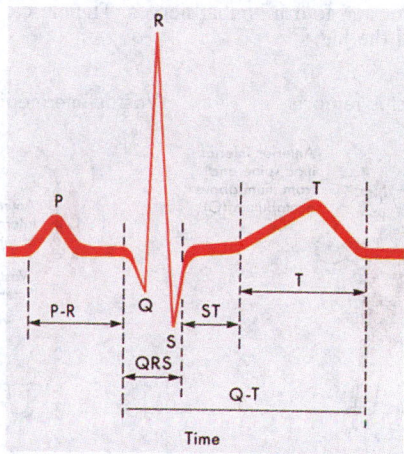

Normal ECG waveform showing QRS complex and Q-T interval
(Berne, 1988)

QRST complex [L, *complexus*], components of an electrocardiogram, consisting of the QRS complex, the S-T segment, the Q-T interval, the T wave, and the U wave. It represents depolarization and repolarization of the ventricles.

QRST interval [L, *intervallum* space between ramparts], the electrocardiographic period of ventricular electrical activity.

q.s., (in prescriptions) abbreviation for *quantum sufficit*, a Latin phrase meaning 'quantity required.'

Q's test. See **Queckenstedt's test.**

qt, abbreviation for **quart.**

Q-T interval, the portion on an electrocardiogram from the beginning of the QRS complex to the end of the T wave, reflecting the length of the refractory period of the heart. A long Q-T interval is associated with the life-threatening ventricular tachycardia known as torsades des pointes.

Quaalude, a trademark for a sedative-hypnotic (methaqualone). It is no longer distributed in the United States.

quack. See **charlatan.**

quad, 1. abbreviation for *quadriceps*, **2.** abbreviation for *quadrilateral*, **3.** abbreviation for **quadrant**, **4.** abbreviation for **quadriplegia.**

quadr-, quadri-, a prefix meaning 'four': *quadrangular, quadribasic, quadrivalent.*

quadrant (gdrnt,) quad. /kwod′rənt/ [L, *quadrans* a

fourth part],   **1.** one quarter of a circle. **2.** one quarter of an anatomic area formed by the division of the area by imaginary vertical and horizontal lines bisecting each other.

quadratus labii superioris.   See **zygomaticus minor.**

quadr-.   See **quodr-.**

quadriceps femoris /kwod′riseps/ [L, *quattuor*, four, *caput*, head; *femur*, thigh],   the great extensor muscle of the anterior thigh, composed of the rectus femoris, the vastus lateralis, the vastus medialis, and the vastus intermedius. The quadriceps forms a large dense mass covering the front and sides of the femur. Tendons of the four parts of the muscle unite at the distal part of the thigh, forming a single strong tendon that embeds the patella and inserts onto the tibial tuberosity. The quadriceps is innervated by branches of the femoral nerve, which contains fibers from the second, third, and fourth lumbar nerves. The muscle functions to extend the leg.

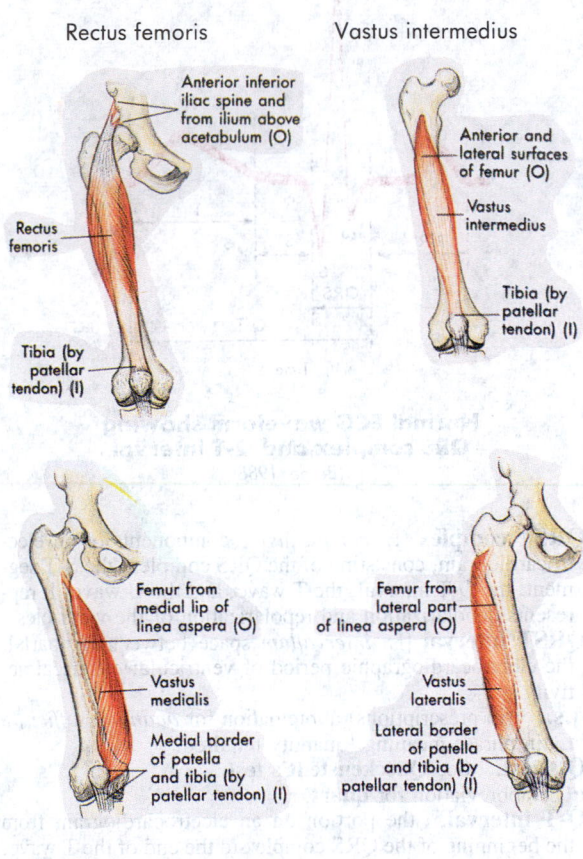

Quadriceps femoris group of thigh muscles:
(Thibodeau, 1993/Ernest W. Beck)

quadriceps reflex.   See **patellar reflex.**

quadrigeminal /kwod′rijem′inəl/ [L, *quadrigeminum*, fourfold],   **1.** in four parts. **2.** a fourfold increase in size or frequency. **3.** having four symmetrical parts.

quadrigeminal pulse,   a pulse in which a pause occurs after every fourth beat.

quadrilateral socket /kwod′rilat′ərəl/,   a four-sided pros-

thetic socket design for people with above-the-knee amputations. The posterior brim is designed to fit directly beneath the ischial tuberosity so that the person literally sits on it.

Quadrinal,   a trademark for a respiratory, fixed-combination drug containing a smooth muscle relaxant (theophylline calcium salicylate), an adrenergic (ephedrine hydrochloride), an expectorant (potassium iodide), and a sedative-hypnotic (phenobarbital).

quadripedal extensor reflex.   See **Brain's reflex.**

quadriplegia (quad.) /kwod′rəple′jē·ə/ [L, *quattuor*, four; Gk, *plege*, stroke],   an abnormal condition characterized by paralysis of the arms, the legs, and the trunk of the body below the level of an associated injury to the spinal cord. This disorder is usually caused by spinal cord injury, especially in the area of the fifth to the seventh vertebrae. Automobile accidents and sporting mishaps are common causes. This condition affects about 150,000 Americans, the majority of whom are men between 20 and 40 years of age. Signs and symptoms commonly include flaccidity of the arms and the legs and the loss of power and sensation below the level of the injury. Cardiovascular complications also may develop from any injury that damages the spinal cord above the fifth cervical vertebra because of an associated block of the sympathetic nervous system. A major cause of death from such injury is respiratory failure. Other symptoms may include low body temperature, bradycardia, impaired peristalsis, and autonomic dysreflexia. Diagnosis is based on a complete physical and neurologic examination with x-ray pictures of the head, chest, and abdomen to rule out underlying injuries. Spinal x-ray examinations and myelography show any fractures and spinal cord blockages. Treatment starts at the accident scene, where the neck and the spine of the patient are immobilized. Additional immobilization at the hospital commonly includes the use of halo traction. Diuretics and steroids are administered to decrease spinal cord edema. After an appropriate period of therapy, surgery is commonly performed to fuse unstable spinal sections and remove bone fragments. Nursing considerations include maintaining adequate respiration and the integrity of the GI system and preventing complications such as hypothermia, bradycardia, catheter obstruction, and fecal impaction. A quadriplegic patient who suffers hypothermia is wrapped in blankets instead of being warmed with hot water bottles or electromechanic devices because such devices can burn the skin of the patient experiencing severe sensory loss. Abdominal binders and antiembolism hose are used when the patient is placed in an upright position. Patients who develop bradycardia are commonly connected to a cardiac monitor and intravenously administered an antimuscarinic drug, such as atropine. Fecal impaction may cause hypertension and is always a possible complication. Throughout the therapy for quadriplegia, constant psychologic support from attending nurses benefits the patient and family and encourages healthy communication. Compare **hemiplegia, paraplegia.**

quadruped /kwod′rŏŏped′/ [L, *quattuor*, four, *pes*, foot],   **1.** any four-footed animal. **2.** a human whose body weight is supported by both arms as well as both legs. See also **prone-on-elbows.**

quadruplet /kwod′rŏŏplit, kwodrŏŏ′plit/ [L, *quadruplex* fourfold],   any one of four offspring born of the same gestation period during a single pregnancy. See also **Hellin's law.**

qual anal,   abbreviation for **qualitative analysis.**

quale /kwā′lē/, *pl.* **qualia** /kwā′lē·ə/ [L, *qualis*, what kind of], **1.** the quality of a particular thing. **2.** a quality considered as an independent entity. **3.** (in psychology) a feeling, sensation, or other conscious process that has its unique, particular quality regardless of its external meaning or frame of reference.

qualified /kwol′ifīd/ [L, *qualis*], pertaining to a health professional or health facility that is formally recognized by an appropriate agency or organization as meeting certain standards of performance related to the professional competence of an individual or the eligibility of an institution to participate in an approved health care program.

qualitative /kwol′itā′tiv/ [L, *qualis*], of or pertaining to the quality, value, or nature of something.

qualitative analysis [L, *qualis*, what kind; Gk, *analysis* a loosening] **1.** (in chemistry) the study of a sample of material to determine what chemical substances are present. **2.** (in research) analysis and interpretation of data that cannot be analyzed by statistical methods.

qualitative melanin test, a test for detecting melanin in the urine of patients with malignant melanomas.

qualitative test, a test that determines the presence or absence of a substance.

quality /kwol′itē/ [L, *qualis*], (in radiotherapy) a descriptive specification of the penetrating nature cf the x-ray beam as influenced by kilovoltage and filtration. Kilovoltage produces more penetration. Filtration removes the 'softer' wavelengths and 'hardens' the beam.

quality assessment measures, formal, systematic, organizational evaluation of overall patterns or programs of care, including clinical, consumer, and systems evaluation.

quality assurance (QA), (in health care) any evaluation of services provided and the results achieved as compared with accepted standards. In one form of quality assurance, various attributes of health care, such as cost, place, accessibility, treatment, and benefits, are scored in a two-part process. First, the actual results are compared with standard results; then, any deficiencies noted or identified serve to prompt recommendations for improvement.

quality assurance program (QAP), a system of review of selected hospital medical/nursing records by medical/nursing staff members, performed for the purposes of evaluating the quality and effectiveness of medical/nursing care in relation to accepted standards.

quality factor, (in radiotherapy) evaluation of the biologic damage that radiation can produce. It is observed that identical doses of different types of radiation can produce differing levels of damage. In the field of radiation protection, biologically equivalent doses are set equal to one another by multiplying the actual absorbed dose by a number called the quality factor. The resulting quantity is called dose equivalent, measured in sieverts or rems.

quality of life [L, *qualis*, what kind; AS, *lif*], a measure of the optimum energy or force that endows a person with the power to cope successfully with the full range of challenges encountered in the real world. The term applies to all individuals, regardless of illness or handicap, on the job, at home, or in leisure activities. Quality enrichment methods can include activities that reduce boredom and allow a maximum amount of freedom in choosing and performing various tasks.

quantitative /kwon′titā′tiv/ [L, *quantus*, how much], capable of being measured.

quantitative analysis [L, *quantum*, how much; Gk, *anal-*ysis, a loosening], **1.** (in chemistry) the determination of the amounts of constituents in a sample of material. Kinds of quantitative analysis include **gravimetric analysis, volumetric analysis,** and **spectrophotometric analysis. 2.** (in research) the use of statistical methods to analyze data.

quantitative inheritance. See **multifactorial inheritance.**

quantitative test [L, *quantum*, how much; *testum*, crucible], a test that determines the amount of a substance per unit volume or unit weight.

quantum mechanics. See **quantum theory.**

quantum mottle. See **mottle.**

quantum theory /kwon′təm/ [L, *quantus* + Gk, *theoria*, speculation], (in physics) the theory dealing with the interaction of matter and electromagnetic radiation, particularly at the atomic and subatomic levels, according to which radiation consists of small units of energy called quanta. Radiation can be absorbed only in whole quanta, and the energy content of a quantum is inversely proportional to its wavelength. Energy and frequency are expressed as $E = hv$; photon energy is inversely proportional to photon wavelength, $E = hc/v$. Also called **quantum mechanics.**

quarantine /kwor′əntēn/ [It, *quarantina*, forty], **1.** isolation of people with communicable disease or of those exposed to communicable disease during the contagious period in an attempt to prevent spread of the illness. **2.** the practice of detaining travelers or vessels coming from places of epidemic disease, originally for 40 days, for the purpose of inspection or disinfection.

quart (qt) /kwôrt/ [L, *quartus*, one-fourth], a unit of volume fluid measure equivalent to one-fourth gallon, two pints, 32 ounces, or 946.24 milliliters. The British Imperial quart is equal to 1.136 liters, and the American quart for dry measure is 1.101 liters.

quartan /kwôr′tən/ [L, *quartanus*, relating to the fourth], recurring on the fourth day, or at about 72-hour intervals. See also **quartan malaria.**

quartan malaria, a form of malaria, caused by the protozoan *Plasmodium malariae*, characterized by febrile paroxysms that occur every 72 hours. Also called **quartan fever.** Compare **falciparum malaria, tertian malaria.** See also **malaria.**

quaternary /kwot′əner′ē, kwətur′nərē/ [L, *quattuor*, four], pertaining to a chemical compound in which four atoms or groups of elements are bonded to one atom, such as a quaternary ammonium compound in which four organic radicals are substituted for the four hydrogen molecules on an ammonium ion.

quaternary ammonium derivative, a substance whose chemical structure has four carbon groups attached to a nitrogen atom. It is usually a strong base, highly water soluble but relatively insoluble in lipids.

quarti-, a prefix meaning 'fourth': *quartipara, quartisect, quartisternal*.

quartile /kwôr′təl, kwôr′tīl/ [L, *quartus*, one fourth], one-fourth of the distribution of scores. The first quartile would be the lowest 25 percent of scores, the second quartile would represent the 26 to 50 percent range of scores, and so on.

quartz silicosis. See **silicosis.**

Queckenstedt's test /kwek′ənstets/ [Hans H. G. Queckenstedt, German physician, b. 1876], a test for an obstruction in the spinal canal in which the jugular veins on each side of the neck are compressed alternately. The pressure of the spinal fluid is measured by a manometer connected to a lumbar puncture needle or catheter. Normally, occlusion of the veins of the neck causes an immediate rise in spinal fluid pressure; if the vertebral canal is blocked, no rise occurs. If increased intracranial pressure is suspected, this test should not be performed. See also **spinal canal.**

Queensland tick typhus, an infection caused by *Rickettsia australis,* occurring in Australia, transmitted by ticks, and resembling mild Rocky Mountain spotted fever. Treatment includes the administration of chloramphenicol or tetracycline. Prevention depends on avoiding tick bites and on the prompt removal of attached ticks. Compare **boutonneuse fever, North Asian tick-borne rickettsiosis, Rocky Mountain spotted fever.**

Quelidrine, a trademark for a respiratory, fixed-combination drug containing adrenergics (phenylephrine hydrochloride and ephedrine hydrochloride), an antihistaminic (chlorpheniramine maleate), an antitussive (dextromethorphan hydrobromide), and an expectorant (ammonium chloride).

quellung reaction /kwel'ung/ [Ger, *Quellung,* swelling; L, *re,* again, *agere,* to act], the swelling of the capsule of a bacterium, seen in the laboratory when the organism is exposed to specific antisera. This phenomenon is used to identify the genera, species, or subspecies of the bacteria causing a disease, including *Haemophilus influenzae, Neisseria meningitides,* and many kinds of streptococci. Also called **Neufeld capsular swelling test.**

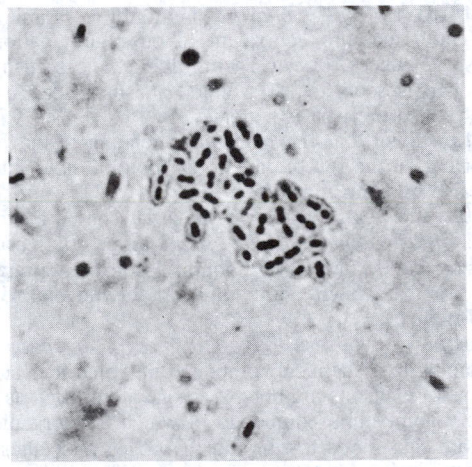

Quellung reaction with *S. pneumoniae* (Baron, 1990)

Quengle cast /kwen'gəl/, a two-section, hinged orthopedic cast for immobilizing the lower extremities from the foot or ankle to below the knee and the upper thigh to a level just above the knee. The two parts of the cast are connected by special hinges at knee level, medially and laterally. The Quengle cast is used for the gradual correction of knee contractures.

quercetin /kwur'sitin/, a yellow, crystalline, flavonoid pigment found in oak bark, the juice of lemons, asparagus, and other plants. It is used to reduce abnormal capillary fragility.

querulous paranoia /kwer'(y)ələs/ [L, *queri,* to complain; Gk, *para,* beside, *nous,* mind], a form of paranoia characterized by extreme discontent and habitual complaining, usually about imagined slights by others. Also called **paranoia querulans.**

Quervain's disease /kervänz', kerveNz'/ [Fritz de Quervain, Swiss surgeon, b. 1868; L, *dis*; Fr, *aise,* ease], chronic tenosynovitis of the abductor pollicis longus and extensor pollicis brevis muscles of the thumb.

Questran, a trademark for an ion exchange resin used to lower blood cholesterol levels (cholestyramine resin).

Quibron, a trademark for a respiratory, fixed-combination drug containing a smooth muscle relaxant (theophylline) and an expectorant (guaifenesin).

quick connect [ME, *quic,* living; L, *connectere,* to bind], a plastic or similar connecting device that is attached to or implanted in a patient who will be joined to an electromechanical or other apparatus. A patient whose circulatory system is supported by an artificial heart, for example, may have a push-fit connector sewn to the natural atria, aorta, and pulmonary artery; a plastic lip on the artificial ventricle then can be securely snapped onto the quick-connect device.

quickening /kwik'(ə)ning/ [ME, *quic,* living], the first feeling by a pregnant woman of movement of her baby in utero, usually occurring between 16 and 20 weeks of gestation.

Quick's test [Armand J. Quick, American physician, b. 1894], **1.** a test for jaundice. The patient is given an oral dose of sodium benzoate, which is conjugated in the liver with glycine to form hippuric acid. The amount of hippuric acid excreted in the urine is inversely proportional to the degree of liver damage. **2.** a test for hemophilia. A solution of thromboplastin is added to oxalated blood plasma and calcium chloride. The amount of time required for formation of a firm clot is inversely proportional to the amount of prothrombin in the plasma.

Quigley traction /kwig'lē/, a type of traction for lateral malleolar and trimalleolar fractures in which a stockinette is placed around the leg and ankle and is attached to an overhead frame, thus suspending the leg by the ankle.

quin-, a combining form meaning 'of or related to quinine': *quiniretin, quinometry, quinotoxin.*

-quin, -quine, a combining form naming antimalarial medicinal compounds from quinine: *aminoquin, diodoquin, Floraquin.*

quinacrine hydrochloride /kī'nəkrēn/, an anthelmintic and an antimalarial.

■ INDICATIONS: It is prescribed in the treatment of giardiasis and cestodiasis and in the treatment and suppression of malaria.

■ CONTRAINDICATIONS: Pregnancy, concomitant administration of primaquine, or known hypersensitivity to this drug prohibits its use. It is used with caution in patients having a history of psychosis and in patients over 60 years of age.

■ ADVERSE EFFECTS: Among the more serious adverse reactions are severe psoriasis, aplastic anemia, acute hepatic necrosis, nausea, vomiting, and jaundice.

Quinaglute, a trademark for a cardiac depressant (quinidine gluconate).

Quincke's disease [Heinrich Iraenaeus Quincke, German physician, b. 1842; L, *dis*; Fr, *aise,* ease], angioneurotic edema, a potentially fatal chronic condition of subcutaneous edema, abdominal pain, urticaria, and laryngeal edema. Also called **angioedema, Quinke's edema.**

Quincke's pulse /kwing'kēz/ [Heinrich I. Quincke, German physician, b. 1842], an abnormal alternate blanching and reddening of the skin that may be observed in several ways, such as by pressing the front edge of the fingernail and watching the blood in the nail bed recede and return. This pulsation is characteristic of aortic insufficiency and other abnormal conditions but also may occur in otherwise normal individuals. Formerly, it was thought to be caused by pulsation of the capillaries, but study has shown it is caused by pulsation of subpapillary arteriolar and venous plexuses. Also called **capillary pulse.**

quinethazone /kwəneth′əzōn/, a diuretic and antihypertensive.

- INDICATIONS: It is prescribed in the treatment of hypertension and edema.
- CONTRAINDICATIONS: Known hypersensitivity to this drug, to other thiazide medication, or to sulfonamide derivatives prohibits its use.
- ADVERSE EFFECTS: Among the more serious adverse effects are hypokalemia, hyperglycemia, hyperuricemia, and hypersensitivity reactions.

Quinidex, a trademark for a cardiac depressant (quinidine sulfate).

quinidine /kwin′ədēn, -din/, an antidysrhythmic agent used as a bisulfate, gluconate, polygalacturonate, or sulfate.

- INDICATIONS: It is prescribed in the treatment of atrial flutter, atrial fibrillation, premature ventricular contractions, and tachycardias.
- CONTRAINDICATIONS: Known hypersensitivity to this drug prohibits its use. It is contraindicated in some dysrhythmias, particularly those associated with heart block.
- ADVERSE EFFECTS: Among the most serious adverse reactions are cardiac dysrhythmia, hypertension, and cinchonism. Rare, but potentially fatal, hypersensitivity reactions, such as anaphylaxis and thrombocytopenia, may occur. Diarrhea, nausea, and vomiting are common.

quinidine gluconate. See **quinidine.**

quinine /kwī′nīn/ [Sp, *quina*, bark], a white, bitter crystalline alkaloid, made from cinchona bark, used in antimalarial medications.

quinine dihydrochloride, an antimalarial. See **quinine sulfate.**

quinine sulfate, an antimalarial with antipyretic, analgesic, and muscle relaxant activity.

- INDICATIONS: It is prescribed in the treatment of malaria, particularly malaria caused by *Plasmodium falciparum,* and nocturnal leg cramps.
- CONTRAINDICATIONS: Glucose 6-phosphate dehydrogenase deficiency and certain cardiac disorders prohibit its use.
- ADVERSE EFFECTS: Among the more serious adverse reactions are symptoms of cinchonism or known hypersensitivity to this drug, including tinnitus, headache, and visual, hearing, and GI disturbances. Hemolysis, blood dyscrasia, and various hypersensitivity reactions also may occur.

quinolone /kwin′əlōn/, any of a class of antibiotics that act by interrupting the replication of DNA molecules in bacteria. The action involves inhibition of the bacteria's gyrase so that daughter segments of DNA cannot acquire the proper twist needed to divide. An example is nalidixic acid.

Quinora, a trademark for a cardiac depressant (quinidine sulfate).

quinque-, a prefix meaning 'five': *quinquecuspid, quinquetubercular, quinquevalent.*

quinsy. See **peritonsillar abscess.**

quint-, a prefix meaning 'fifth or fivefold': *quintessence, quintipara, quintuplet.*

quintan /kwin′tən/ [L, *quintanus,* relating to the fifth], recurring on the fifth day, or at about 96-hour intervals. See also **trench fever.**

quintana fever. See **trench fever.**

quintessence /kwintes′əns/ [L, *quinta, essentia,* the fifth essence], **1.** a highly concentrated extract of any substance. **2.** a tincture or extract containing the most essential components of plant materials.

quintuplet /kwin′tōōplit, kwintōō′plit/ [L, *quintuplex,* fivefold], any one of five offspring born of the same gestation period during a single pregnancy. See also **Hellin's law.**

quotid. See **q.d.**

q.v., 1. abbreviation for the Latin phrase, *quantum vis,* 'as much as you please.' **2.** abbreviation for the Latin phrase *quod vide,* 'which see.'

Q wave, the component of the QRS complex shown on an electrocardiogram as a short downward deflection preceding an R wave. See also **QRS complex.**

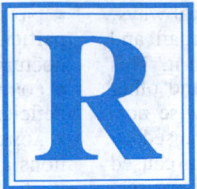

r, **1.** abbreviation for *right*. **2.** symbol for *resistance ohm*.

R, **1.** abbreviation for **metabolic respiratory quotient.** **2.** abbreviation for **resolution. 3.** abbreviation for **respiratory exchange ratio. 4.** abbreviation for **roentgen. 5.** symbol for **gas constant.**

R$_f$, symbol for a ratio used in paper chromatography and thin-layer chromatography, representing the distance from the origin to the center of the separated zone divided by the distance from the origin to the solvent front. **2.** abbreviation for **radiofrequency.**

R$_i$, symbol for *inhibitory receptor* molecule.

R$_s$, symbol for *stimulatory receptor* molecule.

R$_x$, symbol for the Latin phrase, *recipe,* 'take.'

Ra, symbol for the element **radium.**

RA, **1.** abbreviation for **rheumatoid arthritis; 2.** abbreviation for *right atrium*.

rabbit fever. See **tularemia.**

rabbit test. See **Friedman's test.**

rabid /rab′id/ [L, *rabidus,* raving], pertaining to or suffering from rabies, displaying signs of madness, agitation, delirium, hallucinations, and bizarre behavior.

rabies /rā′bēz/ [L, *rabere,* to rave], an acute, usually fatal viral disease of the central nervous system of animals. It is transmitted from animals to people by infected blood, tissue, or, most commonly, saliva. Also called *(obsolete)* **hydrophobia.** –**rabid** /rab′id/, *adj.*

■ OBSERVATIONS: The reservoir of the virus is chiefly wild animals, including skunks, bats, foxes, dogs, raccoons, and cats. After introduction into the human body, often by a bite of an infected animal, the virus travels along nerve pathways to the brain and, later, to other organs. An incubation period ranges from 10 days to 1 year and is followed by a prodromal period characterized by fever, malaise, headache, paresthesia, and myalgia. After several days, severe encephalitis, delirium, agonizingly painful muscular spasms, seizures, paralysis, coma, and death ensue.

■ INTERVENTIONS: Few nonfatal cases have been documented in humans; survival in those cases has been the result of intensive supportive nursing and medical care. There is no treatment once the virus has reached the tissue of the nervous system. Local treatment of wounds inflicted by rabid animals may prevent the disease. The wound is cleansed with soap, water, and a disinfectant. A deep wound may be cauterized and rabies immune globulin (RIG) injected directly into the base of the wound. For active immunization, a series of five intramuscular injections with a human diploid cell rabies vaccine (HDCV) or duck embryo vaccine is begun. If HDCV is administered, the injections are given on the day of exposure and on days 3, 7, 14, 28, and 90. Great effort is made to locate and examine the animal. The animal that is suspected of being rabid is not immediately killed but put in isolation and carefully observed. If the animal is well in 10 days, there is little danger of rabies de-

veloping from the bite. Tissue from the animal's brain may be examined microscopically or by fluorescent antibody screening techniques.

■ NURSING CONSIDERATIONS: Rabies virus infection can be eradicated from most communities by prophylactic immunization of domestic animals, stringent measures for the control of domestic animals, and the elimination of any wild animals acting as reservoirs of infection. The nurse and other health workers may encourage compliance with such efforts and teach the necessity of avoiding direct contact with wild animals and the importance of immediate first aid for any animal bite.

rabies immune globulin (RIG), a solution of antirabies immune globulin.

■ INDICATIONS: It is used in conjunction with rabies duck embryo vaccine for possible protection against rabies in persons suspected of exposure to rabies.

■ CONTRAINDICATIONS: Previous administration of this preparation or known hypersensitivity to this solution, to gamma globulin, or to thimerosal prohibits its use.

■ ADVERSE EFFECTS: Among the more serious adverse reactions are soreness at the site of injection, fever, and hypersensitivity reactions.

rabies vaccine (DEV), a sterile suspension of killed rabies virus prepared from duck embryo.

■ INDICATIONS: It is prescribed for immunization and postexposure prophylaxis against rabies.

■ CONTRAINDICATIONS: A history of allergic reaction to chicken or duck eggs or to protein prohibits its use.

■ ADVERSE EFFECTS: Among the most serious adverse reactions are severe hypersensitivity reactions and pain and inflammation at the site of injection.

rabies virus group [L, *rabere,* to rave + *virus,* poison; It, *gruppo,* knot], the genus of viruses that includes the organism that causes rabies in humans, the *lyssa* virus. See also **Rhabdovirus.**

race [It, *razza*], **1.** a vague, unscientific term for a group of genetically related people who share certain physical characteristics. **2.** a distinct ethnic group characterized by traits that are transmitted through their offspring.

racemic /rāsē′mik/ [L, *racemus,* bunch of grapes], pertaining to a compound made up of levorotatory isomers, rendering it optically inactive under polarized light.

racemic epinephrine, a mixture of two isomers of epinephrine. It is a less potent form of epinephrine, with fewer side effects, and is used as an aerosol in the treatment of acute croup.

racemose /ras′əmōs′/ [L, *racemus*], like a bunch of grapes. The term is used in describing a structure in which many branches terminate in nodular, cystlike forms, such as pulmonary alveoli.

racemose aneurysm, a pronounced dilatation of lengthened and tortuous blood vessels, that may form a tumor. Also called **cirsoid aneurysm.**

-racetam, a combining form for piracetam-type nootrope substances.

rachial /rā′kē·əl/ [Gk, *rhachis*, backbone], pertaining to spinal column. Also **rachidial** /rākid′ē·əl/.

rachio-, rachi-, rhachi-, a prefix meaning 'of or related to the spine': *rachiocampsis, rachiotome, rachiotomy.*

rachiopagus /rā′kē·op′əgəs/ [Gk, *rachis*, backbone, *pagos,* fixed], conjoined symmetric twins united back to back along the spinal column. Also called **rachipagus.**

rachischisis /rəkis′kəsis/ [Gk, *rachis + schizein,* to split], a congenital fissure of one or more vertebrae. See also **neural tube defect, spina bifida.**

rachischisis totalis. See **complete rachischisis.**

rachitic /rəkit′ik/, **1.** of or pertaining to rickets. **2.** resembling or suggesting the condition of one afflicted with rickets.

rachitic dwarf, a person whose retarded growth is caused by rickets. See also **Fanconi's syndrome.**

rachitis /rəkī′tis/ [Gk, *rachis + itis,* inflammation], **1.** rickets. **2.** an inflammatory disease of the vertebral column.

rachitis fetalis annularis, congenital enlargement of the epiphyses of the long bones.

rachitis fetalis micromelia, congenital shortening of the long bones.

racial immunity /rā′shəl/ [It, *razza;* L *immunis,* free], a form of natural immunity shared by most of the members of a genetically related population. Compare **individual immunity, species immunity.**

racial unconscious. See **collective unconscious.**

rad /rad/, abbreviation for *radiation absorbed dose;* the basic unit of absorbed dose of ionizing radiation. One rad is equal to the absorption of 100 ergs of radiation energy per gram of matter, and therefore differs from the roentgen. See also **absorbed dose, rem.**

radarkymography /rā′därkĭmog′rəfē/ [radar + Gk, *kyma,* wave, *graphein,* to record], a radar (radio detection and ranging) technique for showing the size and outline of the heart, using a radar tracking device and a fluoroscopic screen to display images produced by electric impulses passed over the chest surface.

Radford nomogram, a mathematical chart device used in respiratory therapy to estimate combined tidal volumes and rates for mechanical ventilation. It is based on three parameters of body weight, sex, and respiratory rate.

radi-, a combining form meaning 'root': *radiciform, radicotomy, radiectomy.*

radial /rā′dē·əl/ [L, *radius,* ray], pertaining to the radius.

radial artery [L, *radius,* ray], an artery in the forearm, starting at the bifurcation of the brachial artery and passing in 12 branches to the forearm, wrist, and hand. In the forearm, it extends from the neck of the radius to the forepart of the styloid process; in the wrist, from the styloid process to the carpus; in the hand, from the carpus, across the palm, to the little finger. In the forearm, the branches of the radial artery are the radial recurrent, muscular, palmar carpal, and superficial palmar; in the wrist, the branches are the dorsal carpal and the first dorsal metacarpal. In the hand, the branches are the princeps pollicis, radialis indicis, deep palmar arch, palmar metacarpal, perforating, and recurrent.

radial keratotomy, a surgical procedure in which a series of tiny shallow incisions are made on the cornea, causing it to bulge slightly to correct for nearsightedness. The operation is performed using local anesthesia and requires

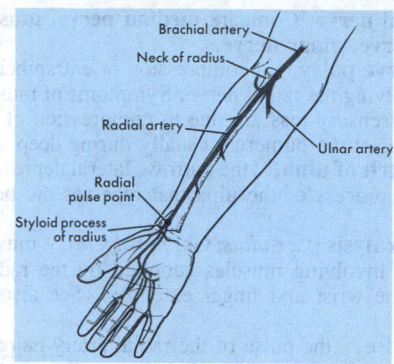

Radial artery

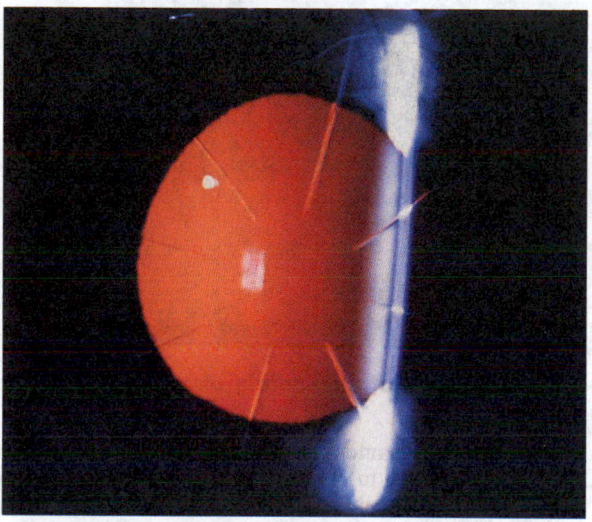

Postoperative appearance of incisions in radial keratotomy
(Jaffe, 1990)

only 10 minutes. Hospitalization is not necessary. Radial keratotomy usually corrects mild to moderate myopia.

radial nerve, the largest branch of the brachial plexus, arising on each side as a continuation of the posterior cord. It supplies the skin of the arm and forearm and their extensor muscles. It crosses the tendon of the latissimus dorsi beneath the axillary artery, passes the inferior border of the teres major, and winds around the medial side of the humerus to enter the triceps between the medial and the long heads of that muscle. It spirals down the arm close to the humerus in the groove separating the origins of the medial and the long heads of the triceps, accompanied by the deep brachial artery. On the lateral side of the arm it pierces the lateral intermuscular septum, runs between the brachialis and the brachioradialis, and divides into the superficial and the deep branches. The branches of the radial nerve are the medial muscular branches, the posterior brachial cutaneous nerve, the posterior muscular branches, the posterior antebrachial cutaneous nerve, the lateral muscular branches, the superficial branch, and the deep branch. Also called **mus-**

culospiral nerve. Compare **median nerve, musculocutaneous nerve, ulnar nerve.**

radial nerve palsy, a compression or entrapment neuropathy involving the radial nerve. Symptoms of muscle weakness and sensory loss are due to compression of the radial nerve against the humerus, usually during deep sleep.

radial notch of ulna, the narrow, lateral depression in the coronoid process of the ulna that receives the head of the radius.

radial paralysis [L, *radius*; Gk, *paralyein*], musculospiral paralysis involving muscles supplied by the radial nerve, mainly the wrist and finger extensors. See also **dropped wrist.**

radial pulse, the pulse of the radial artery palpated at the wrist over the radius. The radial pulse is the one most often taken, because of the ease with which it is palpated.

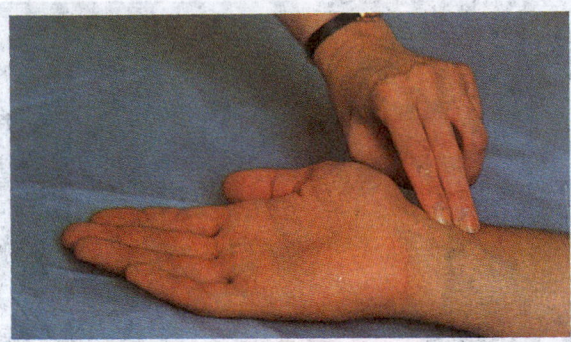

Palpation of the radial pulse (Potter, 1993)

radial recurrent artery, a branch of the radial artery, arising just distal to the elbow, ascending between the branches of the radial nerve, and supplying several muscles of the arm and the elbow.

radial reflex, a normal reflex elicited by tapping over the distal radius, with the response being flexion of the forearm. Flexion of the fingers may also occur if the reflex is hyperactive.

radiant /rā′dē·ənt/ [L, *radiare*, to shine], pertaining to any object that emits rays or is the center of rays that spread outward.

radiant energy [L *radiare* to emit rays; Gk *energeia*], energy emitted as electromagnetic radiation, such as radio waves, infrared radiation, visible light, ultraviolet light, x-rays, and gamma rays.

radiate /rā′dē·āt/ [L, *radiare*, to emit rays], to diverge or spread from a common point.

radiate ligament, a ligament that connects the head of a rib with a vertebra and an associated intervertebral disk. Each of the 24 radiate ligaments consists of three flat fasciculi attached to the head of a rib. The superior fasciculus connects with the vertebra above, the inferior fasciculus connects with the vertebra below, and the middle fasciculus connects to the disk between the two vertebrae. Radiate ligaments to the tenth, eleventh, and twelfth ribs have only two fasciculi.

radiation /rā′dē·ā′shən/ [L, *radiatio*], **1.** the emission of energy, rays, or waves. **2.** (in medicine) the use of a radioactive substance in the diagnosis or treatment of disease.

radiation absorbed dose (rad), a unit of absorbed dose of ionizing radiation. One rad is equal to 0.01 J/kg, or 100 ergs of ionizing radiation per gram of tissue or other substance.

radiation burn, a burn resulting from exposure to radiant energy in the form of sunlight, x-rays, or nuclear emissions or explosion. Ionizing radiation can produce tissue damage directly by striking a vital molecule such as DNA.

radiation caries, a morbid increase in tooth decay caused by ionizing radiation of the oral and maxillary structure. Radiation caries is often a side effect of treatment for oral malignancies. See also **dental caries.**

radiation cataract [L, *radiare*, to shine; Gk, *katarrhaktes*, portcullis], a cataract that is caused by excessive exposure of the eye to x-rays or other types of radiation that cause a change in the protein molecules of the lens.

radiation dermatitis [L, *radiare*, to shine; Gk, *derma*, skin + *itis*, inflammation], an acute or chronic inflammation of the skin due to exposure to ionizing radiation, as in cancer radiation therapy. Symptoms, which may not appear until three weeks after exposure, include redness, blistering, and sloughing of the skin. In severe cases, the condition can progress to scarring, fibrosis, and atrophy. There may also be changes in skin pigmentation.

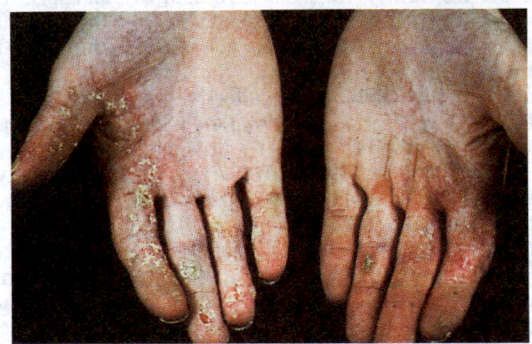

Radiation dermatitis
*(du Vivier, 1993; Courtesy Dr. A Warin,
St. John's Hospital for Diseases of the Skin)*

radiation detector, a device for converting radiant energy to an observable form, used for detecting the presence and sometimes the amount of radiation. A Geiger-Müller detector counts and registers the number of particles reaching it from a radioactive source and can be designed with sufficient sensitivity to detect cosmic radiation. An ionization chamber detects exposure to radiation by collecting the ion pairs formed by the passage of radiation through the device.

Radiation Effects Research Foundation (RERF), an organization that studies the long-term effects of survivors of atomic bombings of Hiroshima and Nagasaki during World War II. The studies have focused on the incidence of leukemia, which reached a plateau around 1950, then began declining, and the varied effects related to the different types of radiation produced by the two bombs, one fueled with uranium and the other with plutonium. The RERF is successor to the Atomic Bomb Casualty Commission.

radiation exposure, a measure of the ionization produced in air by x-rays or gamma rays. It is the sum of the electric charges on all ions of one sign that are produced when all electrons liberated by photons in a volume of air are completely stopped, divided by the mass of air in the volume element. The unit of exposure is the roentgen. See also **acute radiation exposure.**

radiation hygiene, the art and science of protecting human beings from injury by radiation by seeking to reduce clinical exposure from external radiation through protective barriers of radiation-absorbing material, ensuring safe distances between people and radiation sources, reducing radiation exposure times, or employing combinations of all these measures. To protect against the dangers of internal radiation, precautions seek to restrict inhalation, ingestion, and other modes of entry of radioactive substances into the body.

radiation oncologist, a physician with special training in the use of ionizing radiation in the treatment of cancers.

radiation oncology, the study of the treatment of cancer using ionizing radiation.

radiation protection, employment of devices, equipment, distance, and barriers to reduce the risk of exposure to ionizing radiation in a health care facility, research center, or industrial site where radiation-emitting devices are used. The risk also varies with the type and intensity of radiation.

radiation sensitivity, a measure of the response of tissue to ionizing radiation.

radiation sickness, an abnormal condition resulting from exposure to ionizing radiation. The severity of the condition is determined by the volume of radiation, the length of time of exposure, and the area of the body affected. Moderate exposure may cause headache, nausea, vomiting, anorexia, and diarrhea; long-term exposure may result in sterility, damage to the fetus in pregnant women, leukemia or other forms of cancer, alopecia, and cataracts.

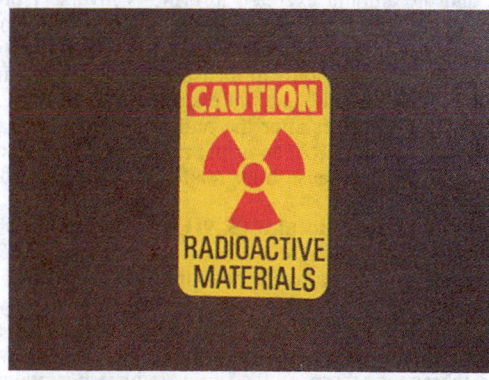

Radiation symbol *(Judd, 1988)*

radiation symbol, a universal symbol consisting of a 'purple propeller' pattern of three fan-shaped images arranged at positions 120° apart as if radiating from a solid dark circle on a yellow background. The symbol is intended to identify sources or containers of radioactive materials and areas of potential radiation rxposure.

radiation syndrome. See **radiation sickness.**

radiation therapy. See **radiotherapy.**

radiation therapy technologist, an allied health profes-

sional who administers radiation therapy services to patients, observing patients during treatment, and maintaining records. Duties may include tumor localization, dosimetry, patient follow-up, and patient education.

radical /rad′ikəl/ [L, *radix,* root], **1.** a group of atoms that acts together and forms a component of a compound. The group tends to remain bound together when a chemical reaction removes it from a compound and attaches it to another. A radical does not exist freely in nature. **2.** pertaining to drastic therapy, such as the surgical removal of an organ, limb, or other part of the body.

radical dissection, the surgical removal of tissue in an extensive area surrounding the operative site. Most often it is performed to identify and excise all tissue that may possibly be malignant to decrease the chance of recurrence.

radical mastectomy, surgical removal of an entire breast, pectoral muscles, axillary lymph nodes, and all fat, fascia, and adjacent tissues. It is performed in the treatment of cancer of the breast. Preoperatively, in addition to giving usual preoperative care, the staff encourages verbalization of the patient's fears of the disease, of the surgery, and of the loss of her breast. Her self-image is usually severely threatened, and she characteristically grieves in anticipation of a loss of femininity. The postoperative period is physically and emotionally painful; the woman is best warned by supportive but realistic explanations before surgery. Edema of the arm on the affected side is the rule, because the axillary lymphatic structures that drain the lymph from the arm are removed during surgery. Atelectasis may develop if deep breathing and coughing are not regularly performed. The incision is painful but may be expected to become less so during the first few days; it should not become more inflamed or painfully swollen. A pressure dressing is usually applied and left in place until bleeding and drainage have decreased. A drain is usually left in the wound for several days. The woman may be anxious, depressed, angry, or withdrawn, or she may reflect hopelessness. In addition to the usual postoperative measures, the nurse elevates the affected arm above the level of the right atrium; checks the color, sensation, and motion of the fingers; checks the graft site if a graft was performed; and applies reinforcement to the pressure dressing as necessary. Later in the postoperative period, the patient is assisted in range of motion exercises for all extremities and is taught, with assistance, to perform gradually increasing arm and shoulder exercises. In discussion and in providing physical care, the loss of the breast is dealt with frankly; to avoid the fact is not helpful to the patient. Slowly the patient is involved in caring for herself more completely, a process that continues as she gradually resumes her normal daily activities. On discharge, she is encouraged to shower daily, to apply an emollient, like cocoa butter, to the incision, and to examine the remaining breast monthly. Reach to Recovery may be involved in counseling and support before and after a mastectomy. Chemotherapy and radiation therapy may continue after surgery. The woman is told never to allow blood to be drawn from the affected arm; intravenous injection is also to be avoided in that arm. Blood pressure measurement, vaccination, and other injections are best performed on the other arm. Compare **modified radical mastectomy, simple mastectomy.** See also **lumpectomy, mastectomy.**

radical neck dissection, dissection and removal of all lymph nodes and removable tissues under the skin of the neck, performed to prevent the spread of malignant tumors of the head and neck that have a reasonable chance of being controlled. Before surgery, thorough mouth hygiene is given and antibiotics are begun. Under general anesthesia, a tracheostomy is done; the tumor, surrounding tissues, and the lymph nodes on the affected side are then removed in one mass from the angle of the jaw to the clavicle, forward to midline, and back to the angle of the jaw. A total laryngectomy may be done as part of the surgery. After surgery, the nurse suctions the tracheostomy as necessary and observes vital signs for indications of hemorrhage or difficulty in breathing. A humidifier or vaporizer will ease coughing and production of mucus. IV fluids are continued in the arm not used for writing. Extensive work with a speech pathologist may be necessary to learn esophageal speech. Radiation of the tumor site may be begun, and chemotherapy may continue. Compare **neck dissection.**

radical surgery [L, *radix*, root; Gk, *cheirourgos*, surgeon], surgery that is usually extensive and complex and intended to correct a severe health threat such as a rapidly growing cancer.

radical therapy,   **1.** a treatment intended to cure, not palliate. **2.** a definitive, extreme treatment; not conservative, such as radical mastectomy rather than simple or partial mastectomy.

radical vulvectomy.   See **vulvectomy.**

radicular /rədik′yələr/ [L, *radix*, root], pertaining to a root, such as a spinal nerve root.

radicular cyst [L, *radicula*, small root; Gk, *kystis*. bag], (in dentistry) a cyst with a wall of fibrous connective tissue and a lining of stratified squamous epithelium that is attached to the apex of the root of a tooth with dead pulp or a defective root canal filling.

radicular retainer,   a type of retainer that lies within the body of a tooth, usually in the root portion, such as a dowel crown. The retention or resistance to displacement and shear is developed by extending an attached dowel into the root canal of the tooth involved. See **radicular retention.**

radicular retention,   retention developed by placing metal projections into the root canals of pulpless teeth. See **radicular retainer.**

radiculitis /rədik′yəlī′tis/ [L, *radix*, root; Gk, *itis*, inflammation], an inflammation involving a spinal nerve root, resulting in pain and hyperesthesia.

radiculopathy /rədik′yəlop′əthē/ [L, *radix*, root; Gk, *pathos*, disease], a disease involving a spinal nerve root.

radii.   See **radius.**

radio- /rā′dē·ō-/,   a combining form meaning 'of or related to radiation,' sometimes specifically to emission of radiant energy, to radium, or to the radius: *radioactive, radiobiology, radiohumeral.*

radioactive /-ak′tiv/ [L, *radius*, ray, *activus*, active], giving off radiation as the result of the disintegration of the nucleus of an atom.

radioactive contamination,   the undesirable addition of radioactive material to the body or part of the environment, such as clothing or equipment. Beta radiation contamination of the body of health care personnel is only possible through the ingestion, inhalation, or absorption of the source, as when the skin is contaminated with a beta emitter contained in an absorbable chemical form. Instruments, drapes, surgical gloves, and clothing that come in contact with serous fluids, blood, and urine of patients containing beta or gamma radiation emitters may be contaminated. The severity of the contamination is directly related to the

elapsed time between the administration of the isotope and surgery; on completion of the procedure, possibly contaminated material is isolated and checked; if found to be contaminated, it is disposed of according to institutional or federal standards for the disposal of radioactive waste.

radioactive contrast media,   a solution or colloid containing material of high atomic number, used for visualizing soft tissue structures. Radiopharmaceutics indicate their positions or distribution in the body by their gamma ray emissions.

radioactive decay,   the disintegration of the nucleus of an unstable nuclide by the spontaneous emission of charged particles, photons, or both.

radioactive element,   an element subject to spontaneous degeneration of its nucleus accompanied by the emission of alpha particles, beta particles, or gamma rays. All elements with atomic numbers greater than 83 are radioactive. Several radioactive elements not found in nature have been produced by the bombardment of stable elements with atomic particles in a cyclotron. Some kinds of radioactive elements are radium, thorium, uranium. Compare **stable element.** See also **radioactivity.**

radioactive half-life.   See **half-life.**

radioactive iodine (RAI),   a radioactive isotope of iodine, used as a tracer in biology and medicine.

radioactive iodine excretion,   the elimination by the body of radioactive iodine (RAI) administered in a test of thyroid function and in the treatment of hyperthyroidism. Most RAI is excreted in urine, but small amounts may be found in sputum, perspiration, feces, and vomitus.

radioactive iodine excretion test,   a method of evaluating thyroid function by measuring the amount of radioactive iodine (RAI) in urine after the patient is given an oral tracer dose of the radioisotope 131I. Normally, 5% to 35% of the dose is absorbed by the thyroid, but absorption is increased in hyperthyroidism and decreased in hypothyroidism, and the amount excreted in urine is inversely proportional to the uptake of RAI. After administration of the tracer, a scintillation detector is placed over the patient's neck at 2, 6, and 24 hours to measure the RAI accumulated by the thyroid, and the amount excreted is assayed in urine collected for 24 hours after the oral dose. Diarrhea can result in low values of RAI in urine; renal failure, by decreasing excretion, can cause high readings. See also **radioactive iodine uptake.**

radioactive iodine uptake (RAIU),   the absorption and incorporation by the thyroid of radioactive iodine (RAI), administered orally as a tracer dose in a test of thyroid function and as larger doses for the treatment of hyperthyroidism. The radioisotope 131I is rapidly absorbed in the stomach and is concentrated in the thyroid. Patients receiving a large therapeutic dose of RAI may require hospitalization for several days. Normal findings of radioactive iodine uptake are: 2 hours, 4%-12% absorbed; 6 hours, 6%-15% absorbed; 24 hours, 8%-30% absorbed. See also **radioactive iodine excretion test.**

radioactive tracer,   a molecule to which a radioactive atom, or tag, has been attached so that it can be followed through a physiologic system with radiation detectors.

radioactivity /-activ′itē/,   the emission of corpuscular α or β or electromagnetic γ radiations as a consequence of nuclear disintegration. Natural radioactivity is a property exhibited by all chemical elements with an atomic number greater than 83; artificial or induced radioactivity is created through the bombardment of naturally occurring isotopes with subatomic particles or high levels of gamma or x-radiation.

radioallergosorbent test (RAST) /rā′dē·ō′alur′gōsôr′bənt/ [L, *radius* + Gk, *allos,* other, *ergein,* to work; L, *absorbere,* to swallow],   a test in which a technique of radioimmunoassay is used to identify and quantify IgE in serum that has been mixed with any of 45 known allergens. If an atopic allergy to a substance exists, an antigen-antibody reaction occurs with characteristic conjugation and clumping. The test is an in vitro method of demonstrating allergic reactions. Compare **patch test, Prausnitz-Küstner test.**

radiobiology /-bī·ol′əjē/ [L, *radius* + *bios,* life, *logos,* science],   the branch of the natural sciences dealing with the effects of radiation on biologic systems.   **–radiobiologic, radiobiological,** *adj.*

radiocarpal articulation /-kär′pəl/ [L, *radius* + Gk, *karpos,* wrist],   the condyloid joint at the wrist that connects the radius and distal surface of an articular disk with the scaphoid, the lunate, and the triangular bones. The joint involves four ligaments and allows all movements but rotation. Also called **wrist joint.**

radiochemistry /-kem′istrē/ [L, *radius* + Gk, *chemiea,* alchemy],   the branch of chemistry that deals with the properties and behavior of radioactive materials and the use of radionuclides in the study of chemical and biologic problems.

radiocurable /-kyōō′rəbəl/,   pertaining to the susceptibility of tumor cells to destruction by ionizing radiation.

radiofrequency /-frē′kwənsē/ **(rf)** [L, *radius* + *frequens*], the portion of the electromagnetic spectrum with frequencies lower than about 1010 Hz, used to produce magnetic resonance images.

radio frequency ablation,   unmodulated high frequency alternating current flow that is applied to tissue to cause heat and cell injury for the purpose of destroying troublesome areas and pathways to the heart. The technique has replaced surgical ablation.

radiograph /rā′dē·əgraf′/,   an x-ray image. Also called **radiogram.**

radiographer /rā′dē·og′rəfər/,   an allied health professional who provides patient services using radiographic imaging modalities as directed by a physician. Duties may include processing of film, evaluating radiologic equipment, managing a radiographic quality assurance program, and providing patient education relevant to specific imaging procedures.

-radiographic.   See **radiography.**

radiographic contrast medium.   See **radiopaque dye.**

radiographic grid /-graf′ik/,   a device used to reduce the amout of scatter radiation reaching the radiographic film. Grids are fabricated using parallel strips of radiopaque materials with alternating strips of radiolucent materials. See also **grid.**

radiographic magnification,   a radiographic procedure used to improve visualization of fine blood vessels and small bony structures. Magnification is achieved by increasing the distance of the object from the radiographic image receptor.

radiography /rā′dē·og′rəfē/ [L, *radius* + Gk, *graphein,* to record],   the production of shadow images on photographic emulsion through the action of ionizing radiation. The image is the result of the differential attenuation of the radiation in its passage through the object being radiographed.   **–radiographic,** *adj.*

radioimmunoassay (RIA) /rā′dē·ō·im′yənō·os′ā/imyōō′nō·as′ā/ [L, *radius* + *immunis.* free; Fr, *essayer,* to try],   a technique in radiology used to determine the concentration of an antigen, antibody, or other protein in the serum. A radioactively labeled substance known to react in a certain way with the suspected protein is injected, and any reaction is monitored.

radioimmunosorbent assay test /rā′dē·ō·im′yənōsôr′bənt/ [L, *radius, immunis* + *absorbere,* to swallow],   a test that uses serum immunoglobulin E to detect allergies to various substances, such as certain cosmetics, animal fur, dust, and grasses.

radioiodine /rā′dē·ō·ī′ədīn/ [L, *radius* + Gk, *ioeides,* violet],   a radioactive isotope of iodine used in nuclear medicine and radiotherapy. It is used especially in the treatment of some thyroid conditions and in diagnostic radiology by various scanning techniques. A common form of radioiodine is 131I.

radioisotope /rā′dē·ō·ī′sətōp/ [L, *radius* + Gk, *isos,* equal, *topos* place],   a radioactive isotope of an element, used for therapeutic and diagnostic purposes.

radioisotope scan,   a two-dimensional representation of the gamma rays emitted by a radioisotope, showing its concentration in a body site, such as the thyroid gland, brain, or kidney. Radioisotopes used in diagnostic scanning may be administered intravenously or orally.

-radiologic.   See **radiology.**

-radiological.   See **radiology.**

radiologic anatomy /-loj′ik/ [L, *radius* + Gk, *logos,* science],   (in applied anatomy) the study of the structure and morphology of the tissues and organs of the body based on their x-ray visualization.

radiologic technologist,   a person who, under the supervision of a physician radiologist, operates radiologic equipment and assists radiologists and other health professionals, and whose competence has been tested and approved by the American Registry of Radiologic Technologists. Also called **x-ray technician.**

radiologist /rā′dē·ol′əjist/,   a physician who specializes in radiology. A certified radiologist is one whose competence has been tested and approved by the American Board of Radiology.

radiology /-ol′əjē/ [L, *radius* + *logos,* science],   the

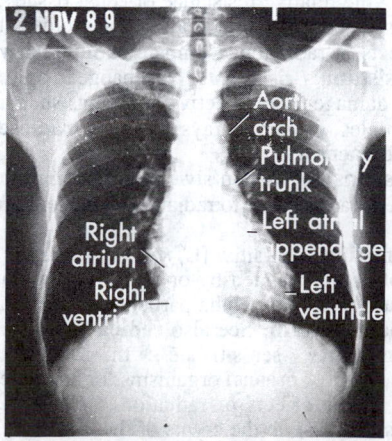

Normal radiograph of the chest (Canobbio, 1990)

branch of medicine concerned with radioactive substances and, using various techniques of visualization, with the diagnosis and treatment of disease using any of the various sources of radiant energy. Three subbranches of radiology are **diagnostic radiology,** which concerns itself with imaging using external sources of radiation; **nuclear medicine,** which is involved with imaging radioactive materials that are placed into body organs; and **therapeutic radiology,** which is concerned with the treatment of cancer using radiation. **–radiologic, radiological,** *adj.*

radiolucent /-loo′sənt/ [L, *radiare,* to shine + *lucere,* to shine], pertaining to materials that allow x-rays to penetrate with a minimum of absorption.

radiolucency /-loo′sənsē/ [L, *radius* + *lucere,* to shine], a characteristic of materials of relatively low atomic number that have low attenuation characteristics, allowing most x-rays to pass through them, producing relatively dark images. **–radiolucent,** *adj.*

radionecrosis /-nəkrō′sis/, tissue death caused by radiation.

radionuclide /-noo′klīd/ [L, *radius* + *nucleus,* nut kernel], **1.** an isotope (or nuclide) that undergoes radioactive decay. **2.** any of the radioactive isotopes of cobalt, iodine, phosphorus, strontium, and other elements, used in nuclear medicine for treatment of tumors and cancers and for nuclear imaging of internal parts of the body. See also **nuclear scanning.**

radionuclide angiocardiography, the radiographic examination of cardiac blood vessels after an intravenous injection of a radiopharmaceutic.

radionuclide imaging, the noninvasive examination of various parts of the body, especially the heart, using a radiopharmaceutic, such as thallium 201, and a detection device, such as a gamma camera, rectilinear scanner, or positron camera. See also **cardiac radionuclide imaging.**

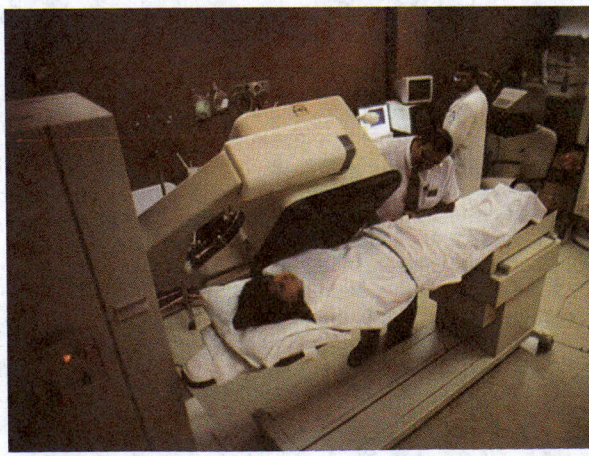

Equipment for radionuclide imaging (Gray, 1992)

radionuclide organ imaging. See **nuclear scanning.**

radiopacity /-pas′itē/ [L, *radiare,* to shine + *opacus,* obscure], the quality of being radiopaque, or having the ability to stop or reduce the passage of x-radiation.

radiopaque /-pāk′/ [L, *radius* + *opacus,* obscure], not

permitting the passage of x-rays or other radiant energy. Bones are relatively radiopaque and therefore show as white areas on an exposed x-ray film. Lead is markedly radiopaque and therefore is widely used to shield x-ray equipment and atomic power sources. See also **radioactive element, radioactivity, radiopaque dye.** **–radiopacity,** *n.*

radiopaque dye, a chemical substance that does not permit the passage of x-rays. Various radiopaque compounds are used to outline the interior of hollow organs such as heart chambers, blood vessels, respiratory passages, and the biliary tract in x-ray or fluoroscopic pictures. Also called **radiographic contrast medium.** Compare **radiolucency.**

radiopharmaceutical /-fär′məsoo′tik/ [L *radius* + Gk *pharmakeuein* to give a drug], a drug that contains radioactive atoms. Kinds of radiopharmaceuticals are **diagnostic radiopharmaceutic, research radiopharmaceutical,** and **therapeutic radiopharmaceutical.**

radiopharmacist /-fär′məsist/, a trained professional responsible for the formulation and dispensing of prescribed radioactive tracers and for the clinical aspects of radiopharmacy. Radiopharmacists are required to receive training in radioactive tracer techniques, in the safe handling of radioactive materials, in the preparation and quality control of drugs for administration to humans, and in the basic principles of nuclear medicine. Some states require that radioactive drugs be dispensed by licensed pharmacists only; others recognize radiopharmaceutic specialists who are not necessarily graduates of a school of pharmacy.

radiopharmacy /-fär′məsē/ [L, *radius* + Gk, *pharmakeuein,* to give a drug], a facility for the preparation and dispensing of radioactive drugs and for the storage of radioactive materials, inventory records, and prescriptions of radioactive substances. The radiopharmacy is usually the correlation point for radioactive wastes, the unit responsible for waste disposal or storage, and a center for clinical investigations employing radioactive tracers. It may also be a center for research and for the training of students and residents in radiology and nuclear medicine.

radioprotective drugs /-prətek′tiv/ [L, *radiare,* to shine + *protegere,* to cover; Fr, drogue], pharmaceuticals that protect the body against ionizing radiation. An example is Lugol's solution, an aqueous solution of iodine used to supply iodine internally, thereby blocking the uptake of radioactive iodine.

radioresistance /-risis′təns/ [L, *radius* + *resistare,* to withstand], the relative resistance of cells, tissues, organs, organisms, chemical compounds, or any other substances to the effects of radiation. Compare **radiosensitivity.**

radioresistant /-risis′tənt/, unchanged by or protected against damage by radioactive emissions such as x-rays, alpha particles, or gamma rays. Compare **radiosensitive.** See also **radioactivity.**

radioresponsive /-rispon′siv/, pertaining to the sensitivity of a chemical or tissue to radiation, whether harmful or beneficial.

radiosensitive /-sen′sitiv/ [L, *radius* + *sentire,* to feel], capable of being changed by or reacting to radioactive emissions such as x-rays, alpha particles, or gamma rays. Compare **radioresistant.** See also **radioactivity.**

radiosensitivity /-sen′sitiv′itē/, the relative susceptibility of cells, tissues, organs, organisms, or any other living substances to the effects of radiation. Cells of self-renewing systems, as those in the crypts of the intestine, are the most radiosensitive. Cells that divide regularly but mature between divisions, such as spermatogonia and spermatocytes, are next in radiosusceptibility. Long-lived cells that usually do not undergo mitosis unless there is a suitable stimulus include the less radiosensitive liver, kidney, and thyroid cells. Least sensitive are fixed postmitotic cells that have lost the ability to divide, such as neurons. Connective tissue and blood vessels are intermediate in radiosensitivity; parenchymal cells are affected by moderate doses of radiation that do not damage connective tissue.

radiosensitizers /-sen′sitī′zərs/ [L, *radius*, *sentire* + Gk, *izein*, to cause], drugs that enhance the killing effect of radiation on cells.

radiotherapy /-ther′əpē/ [Gk, *radius* + Gk, *therapeia*, treatment], the treatment of neoplastic disease by using x-rays or gamma rays, usually from a cobalt source, to deter the proliferation of malignant cells by decreasing the rate of mitosis or impairing DNA synthesis.

■ METHOD: Before radiotherapy, the procedure, its purpose, duration, painlessness, and the need to remain completely still during irradiation are explained to the patient. Potential sequelae, such as erythema, edema, desquamation, hyperpigmentation, atrophy, pruritus or skin pain, altered taste, anorexia, nausea, vomiting, headache, hair loss, malaise, tachycardia, and increased susceptibility to infection may be discussed in response to specific questions raised by the patient. A preliminary visit to the radiology department may be arranged so that the equipment and the room in which the patient will be positioned on a table can be seen. From this position the patient is able to communicate with the radiotherapist who is in an adjoining booth. Daily hygiene measures are completed before treatment; on returning from irradiation, the patient is placed in a noninfectious environment or, if necessary, in protective isolation; friends, family, other patients and staff members with infections, especially upper respiratory tract infections, are not permitted to visit. Skin care is administered after irradiation and every 4 hours thereafter, but the ink markings placed by the radiologist on the skin to mark the focus of treatment are not removed between treatments, and the treated area is not washed with water; sterile mineral oil, lanolin, or petroleum jelly may be applied if the radiologist approves. The patient wears loose garments and rests on an air mattress, foam or gel pad, or sheepskin; a footboard or bed cradle is used to elevate the top sheet and blanket. Cosmetics are avoided, and underarm deodorants or antiperspirants are contraindicated if the axillary area is irradiated. If hair loss occurs, the patient may wear a wig, scarf, cap, or toupee. High-protein supplements, soothing gelatins, and ice cream are provided, and other food is served when desired by the patient; six small, bland feedings may be tolerated more easily than regular meals. Quiet periods are maintained before and after meals. Antiemetics and vitamins are administered as ordered, and tube feedings or total parenteral nutrition may be indicated if the patient's food intake is severely decreased. Oral hygiene, using a soft-bristled brush and dilute mouthwash, or, if needed, foam or sponge swabs and a saline rinse, is administered whenever required, and a fluid intake of 2000 to 3000 ml daily is maintained unless contraindicated. In preparation for discharge, the patient is instructed to follow the hospital practices for skin care, oral hygiene, fluid intake, and a high-protein, nutritious diet but to avoid eating immediately before and after irradiation. The patient is told to avoid tight clothing, extremes of temperature, exposure to sunlight, tub

Potential side effects of radiation therapy

External	Internal implants
Abdomen: gastritis; nausea and vomiting	Bleeding
Fatigue	Infection
Gonads: amenorrhea; sexual dysfunction	Fever, redness, and drainage at insertion site
Pelvis: diarrhea; cystitis	Sexual dysfunction
Skin: erythema, dry to wet desquamation; areas of perineum, groin, and gluteal fold have increased risk for breakdown due to moisture, warmth, and lack of air circulation	**Intracavitary**
	Bleeding; infection; sexual dysfunction
	Intraoperative
	Anorexia; nausea and vomiting

From Otto SE: *Oncology nursing*, St Louis, 1991, Mosby.

baths or showers until ordered, and persons with infections and to report to the physician any symptom of infection, inability to eat, severe diarrhea, increasing headache, and fatigue, or increasing redness, swelling, itching, or pain at the site of therapy.

■ NURSING INTERVENTION: The nurse offers thorough explanation of the radiotherapy, provides care after treatment, and prepares the patient for discharge and, if indicated, continued therapy on an outpatient basis.

■ OUTCOME CRITERIA: Radiotherapy can control or arrest the development of a number of forms of cancer and provide palliation in some inoperable tumors; the maintenance of adequate nutrition and meticulous care of the skin may allow the person to avoid the most serious and unpleasant side effects of radiotherapy.

radioulnar articulation /-ul′nər/ [L, *radius* + *ulna*, elbow], the articulation of the radius and the ulna, consisting of a proximal articulation, a distal articulation, and three sets of ligaments.

radium (Ra) /rā′dē·əm/ [L, *radius*, ray], a radioactive metallic element of the alkaline earth group. Its atomic number is 88. Four radium isotopes occur naturally and have different atomic weights: 223, 224, 226, and 228. The isotope with atomic weight 226 is the most abundant. It is formed by the disintegration of uranium 238, has a half-life of 1620 years, and decays by alpha emission to form radon 222. Radium occurs in the uranium minerals carnotite and pitchblende, which contain about 3×10^{-7} g of radium per g of uranium. Radium salts have been used extensively as radiation sources in the treatment of cancer but are gradually being replaced in such therapy by cobalt and cesium.

radium insertion, the introduction of metallic radium (Ra) into a body cavity, such as the uterus or cervix, to treat cancer.

radium therapy [L, *radius*, ray; Gk, *therapeia*, treatment], the use of radium and its radioactive emissions to treat disease.

radium 226, a radioactive substance used for most of this century to fill the needles and tubes required for brachytherapy. Radium use is now being replaced by cesium 137 and cobalt 60, which have similar energy characteristics and are not subject to hazardous leakage as radium sources sometimes are.

radius /rā′dē·əs/, *pl.* **radii** /rā′dē·ī/ [L, ray], one of the bones of the forearm, lying parallel to the ulna. Its proximal end is small and forms a part of the elbow joint. The distal end is large and forms a part of the wrist joint. The radius receives the insertions of various muscles and articulates with the humerus, ulna, scaphoid, lunate and triangular bones.

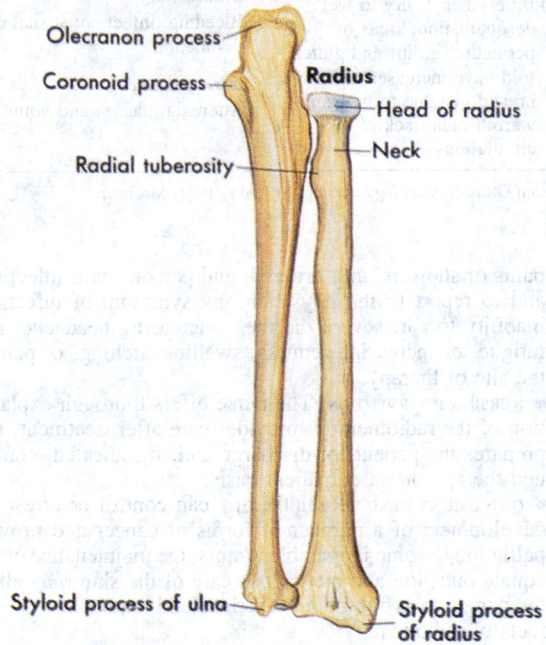

Olecranon process
Coronoid process
Radius
Head of radius
Neck
Radial tuberosity
Styloid process of ulna
Styloid process of radius

Radius and ulna (Thibodeau, 1993/Ernest W Beck)

radix. See **root.**

radon (Rn) /rā'don/ [L, *radiare*, to emit rays], a radioactive, inert, gaseous, nonmetallic element. Its atomic number is 86; its atomic weight is 222. Radon, a decay product of radium, is used in radiation cancer therapy.

radon daughters, electrically charged ions that are decay products of radon gas. Radon daughters are regarded as a potential health hazard by the Environmental Protection Agency (EPA) because they tend to adhere to surfaces, such as alveoli of the lungs, where they can cause ionizing radiation damage. Radon is released by rocks, soil, and groundwater and is a common source of background radiation, with an intensity that varies in different geographic areas.

radon seed, a small sealed tube of glass or gold containing radon, and visible radiographically, for insertion into body tissues in the treatment of malignancies.

radon 222, the radioactive daughter of radium 226 that has been used to fill seeds for permanent implantation into tumors. This material is being replaced by the more manageable radionuclide iodine 125.

RAI, abbreviation for **radioactive iodine.**

RAIU, abbreviation for **radioactive iodine uptake.**

RA latex test, abbreviation for *rheumatoid arthritis latex test*. See **latex fixation test.**

rale /rāl, ral, räl/ [Fr, *râle* rattle], a common abnormal respiratory sound heard on auscultation of the chest during inspiration, characterized by discontinuous bubbling noises. Fine rales have a crackling sound produced by air entering distal bronchioles or alveoli that contain serous secretions, as in congestive heart failure, pneumonia, or early tuberculosis. Coarse rales originate in the larger bronchi or trachea and have a lower pitch. Kinds of rales are **sibilant rale** and **sonorous rale.** Although the term **rale** is commonly used the American Thoracic Society now prefers **crackle,** as this term is more descriptive of the actual sound heard. Compare **rhonchus, wheeze.**

RAM. See **random-access memory.**

rami-, a combining form meaning 'branch': *ramicotomy, ramification, ramisection.*

ramification /ram'ifikā'shən/ [L, *ramus*, branch + *facere*, to make], a branching, distribution.

ramify. See **ramus.**

Ramsay Hunt's syndrome [James Ramsay Hunt, American neurologist, b. 1874], a neurologic condition resulting from invasion of the seventh nerve ganglia and the geniculate ganglion by varicella zoster virus, characterized by severe ear pain, facial nerve paralysis, vertigo, hearing loss, and, often, mild, generalized encephalitis. The vertigo may last days or weeks but usually resolves itself. The facial paralysis may be permanent, and the hearing loss, which is rarely permanent, may be partial or total. Treatment usually includes the prescription of corticosteroid drugs. Also called **herpes zoster oticus.**

ramus /rā'məs/, *pl.* **rami** [L, branch], a small, branchlike structure extending from a larger one or dividing into two or more parts, such as a branch of a nerve or artery or one of the rami of the pubis. **–ramification,** *n.* **ramify,** *v.*

random-access memory (RAM) /ran'dəm/, the part of a computer's memory available to execute programs and temporarily store data. The memory to which the operator has random access usually can be used for both reading and writing. RAM data is automatically erased when the computer is turned off unless the file has been saved. See also **direct-access memory.**

random controlled trial [ME, *randoun*, run violently; Fr, *contrôle*, check + *trier*, to grind], a study plan for a proposed new treatment in which subjects are assigned on a random basis to participate either in an experimental group receiving the new treatment or in a control group that does not.

random genetic drift. See **genetic drift.**

randomization [ME, *randoun*, run violently], the process of assigning subjects or objects to a control or experimental group on a random basis.

random mating [ME, *randoun*, run violently + *gemate*], a pairing of subjects when each individual has an equal chance of mating with those of other genetic backgrounds.

random sampling [ME, *randoun*, run violently; L, *exemplum*], a method of sampling for a study in which each individual has the same chance of being selected and the choice of a particular individual does not affect the chances of the others.

random selection, a method of choosing subjects for a research study in which all members of a particular group have an equal chance of being selected.

random voided specimen, a voided urine specimen obtained at any point of a 24-hour period.

range /rānj/ [OFr, *ranger*, to arrange in a row], the interval between the lowest and the highest values in a series of data.

range of accommodation [OFr, *ranger*; L, *accommoda-tio*], the distance between the farthest point that an object can be seen clearly with accommodation fully relaxed and the nearest distance that an object can be seen with full accommodation, measured in inches or centimeters.

range of motion (ROM) [OFr, *ranger*; L, *motio*], the range of movement of a joint, from maximum extension to maximum flexion, as measured in degrees of a circle.

range of motion exercise [Fr, *rang*, rank; L, *motio*, movement], any body action involving the muscles, the joints, and natural directional movements, such as abduction, extension, flexion, pronation, and rotation. Such exercises are usually applied actively or passively in the prevention and treatment of orthopedic deformities, in the assessment of injuries and deformities, and in athletic conditioning.

ranitidine /ranit′idēn/, a histamine H_2 receptor antagonist.
- INDICATIONS: It is prescribed in the treatment of duodenal and gastric ulcers and gastric hypersecretory conditions.
- CONTRAINDICATIONS: Known sensitivity to this drug prohibits its use. The drug should be used in pregnancy only if clearly needed.
- ADVERSE EFFECTS: Among the most serious adverse reactions are headaches and rashes.

Rankine scale [William J. M. Rankine, Scottish physicist, b. 1820], an absolute temperature scale calculated in degrees Fahrenheit. Absolute zero on the Rankine scale is −460° F, equivalent to −273° C. See also **Kelvin scale.**

ranula /ran′yŏŏlə/, *pl.* **ranulae** [L, *rana,* frog], a large mucocele in the floor of the mouth, usually caused by obstruction of the ducts of the sublingual salivary glands and less commonly caused by obstruction of the ducts of the submandibular salivary glands.

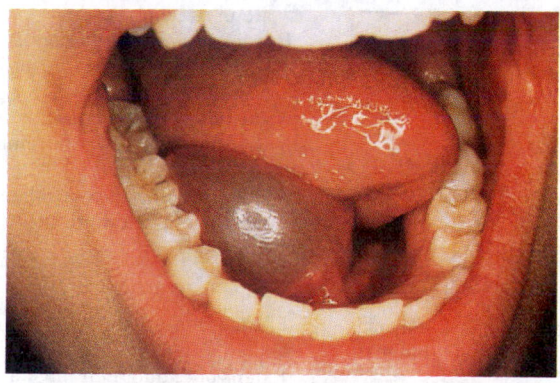

Ranula (Bingham, 1992)

Ranvier's nodes /ränvē·āz′, räN-/ [Louis A. Ranvier, French pathologist, b. 1835], constrictions in the medullary substance of a nerve fiber at more or less regular intervals.

rape [L, *rapere,* to seize], a sexual assault, homosexual or heterosexual, the legal definitions for which vary from state to state. Rape is a crime of violence or one committed under the threat of violence, and its victims are treated for medical and psychologic trauma. See also **statutory rape.**
- OBSERVATIONS: Characteristically, the victim is frightened and feels vulnerable, humiliated, and personally violated.

Rape preventive measures

Prevention of attack

Set house lights to go on and off by timer
Keep light on at all entrances
Place safety locks on windows and doors
Have key ready before reaching door of house or car
Look in car before entering
Insist on identification before letting a stranger in house; check identification with agency if suspicious
Do not list first name on mailbox or in telephone directory
Make arrangements with neighbor for needed assistance
Be alert when walking in street; walk in lighted areas
Walk down center of street if possible
Avoid lonely or enclosed areas

If attacked

Run toward a lighted house; yell "Fire"
Spit in rapist's face; act bizarre; vomit
Rip off rapist's glasses
Step hard on his foot (instep)
Aim at eyes—try to gouge eyes, scrape face
Hit throat at Adam's apple (larynx)
Use fighting and screaming with caution; this may scare some rapists, encourage others
Try talking to avoid rape
If powerless, make close observations about rapist, car, location

From Phipps WJ, Long BL, Woods NF, Cassmeyer VL: *Medical-surgical nursing: concepts and clinical practice,* ed 4, St Louis, 1991, Mosby.

General physical examination may reveal cuts, bruises, and other injuries. Pelvic or genital examination may show traumatic injury to the internal or external genitalia or anus.
- INTERVENTIONS: Careful physical examination should be conducted by specially trained health-care personnel and a detailed history obtained. Specimens are obtained as indicated. Ideally, counseling is available and offered immediately to all victims of rape. In the case of a woman who has been raped by a man, a pregnancy test may be performed and specific injuries treated. If the test is positive, prophylaxis against conception may be administered. Usually, antibiotics are given to prevent the development of venereal disease. Arrangements for ongoing emotional support are made.
- NURSING CONSIDERATIONS: A trained, empathetic nurse of the same sex is assigned to stay with the victim. Privacy for the history, examination, and police interview is ensured. The victim may or may not choose to talk to the police, but the police must be informed in every case. The victim must sign a special form to allow specimens to be released to a law enforcement agency. In general, it is the role of the nurse and other specially trained medical workers to examine, to treat, and to collect specimens as necessary, not to decide that rape has occurred. Before discharge, it should be ascertained that someone can be with the victim, since depression, anger, guilt, and fear may occur after rape.

rape counseling, counseling by a trained person provided to a victim of rape. Rape counseling ideally begins at the time the crime is first reported, as in an emergency room. Initially, the counselor offers sensitive support for the victim by accepting the victim in a nonprejudicial, noncritical way. The victim's response to the trauma of the assault is empathetically elicited, and three basic statements are made: The counselor is sorry that the rape happened, is glad that

Body Part	Type of Joint	Type of Movement	Body Part	Type of Joint	Type of Movement
Neck, cervical spine	Pivotal	Flexion: bring chin to rest on chest Extension: return head to erect position Hyperextension: bend head back as far as possible			Circumduction: move arm in full circle (Circumduction is combination of all movements of ball-and-socket joint.)
		Lateral flexion: tilt head as far as possible toward each shoulder	Elbow	Hinge	Flexion: bend elbow so that lower arm moves toward its shoulder joint and hand is level with shoulder Extension: straighten elbow by lowering hand
		Rotation: turn head as far as possible in circular movement	Forearm	Pivotal	Supination: turn lower arm and hand so that palm is up Pronation: turn lower arm so that palm is down
Shoulder	Ball and socket	Flexion: raise arm from side position forward to position above head Extension: return arm to position at side of body Hyperextension: move arm behind body, keeping elbow straight	Wrist	Condyloid	Flexion: move palm toward inner aspect of forearm Extension: move fingers so that fingers, hands, and forearm are in same plane Hyperextension: bring dorsal surface of hand back as far as possible Abduction (radial flexion): bend wrist medially toward thumb
		Abduction: raise arm to side to position above head with palm away from head Adduction: lower arm sideways and across body as far as possible			Adduction (ulnar flexion): bend wrist laterally toward fifth finger
		Internal rotation: with elbow flexed, rotate shoulder by moving arm until thumb is turned inward and toward back External rotation: with elbow flexed, move arm until thumb is upward and lateral to head	Fingers	Condyloid hinge	Flexion: make fist Extension: straighten fingers Hyperextension: bend fingers back as far as possible
					Abduction: spread fingers apart Adduction: bring fingers together

From Potter and Perry AG *Fundamentals of Nursing: Concepts, Process, and Practice, ed. 3.* St. Louis, 1993, Mosby–Year Book, Inc.

Body Part	Type of Joint	Type of Movement
Thumb	Saddle	Flexion: move thumb across palmar surface of hand Extension: move thumb straight away from hand Abduction: extend thumb laterally (usually done when placing fingers in abduction and adduction) Adduction: move thumb back toward hand Opposition: touch thumb to each finger of same hand
Hip	Ball and socket	Flexion: move leg forward and up Extension: move back beside other leg
		Hyperextension: move leg behind body
		Abduction: move leg laterally away from body Adduction: move leg back toward medial position and beyond if possible Internal rotation: turn foot and leg toward other leg External rotation: turn foot and leg away from other leg

Body Part	Type of Joint	Type of Movement
		Circumduction: move leg in circle
Knee	Hinge	Flexion: bring heel back toward back of thigh Extension: return leg to the floor
Ankle	Hinge	Dorsal flexion: move foot so that toes are pointed upward Plantar flexion: move foot so that toes are pointed downward
Foot	Gliding	Inversion: turn sole of foot medially Eversion: turn sole of foot laterally
Toes	Condyloid	Flexion: curl toes downward Extension: straighten toes Abduction: spread toes apart Adduction: bring toes together

the injuries are not worse, and does not think that the victim was wrong or did anything wrong. Counseling personnel may provide supportive services and advocacy and liaison between the victim and medical, legal, and law enforcement authorities. This involves staying with the victim during medical examination, police or district attorney's questioning, and throughout the criminal justice process.

rape-trauma syndrome, a nursing diagnosis accepted by the Fourth National Conference on the Classification of Nursing Diagnoses. The syndrome results from the experience of being raped, which is defined as forced, violent sexual penetration against the victim's will and consent. The trauma syndrome that develops from this attack includes an acute phase of disorganization and a longer phase of reorganization in the victim's life. The defining characteristics are divided into three subcomponents: **rape trauma, compound reaction,** and **silent reaction.** The defining characteristics of **rape trauma** in the acute phase are emotional reactions of anger, guilt, and embarrassment, fear of physical violence and death, humiliation, wish for revenge, and multiple physical complaints, including GI distress, genitourinary discomfort, tension, and disturbance of the normal patterns of sleep, activity, and rest. The long-term phase of rape trauma is characterized by changes in the usual patterns of daily life (even a change in residence), nightmares and phobias, and a need for support from friends and family. The **compound reaction** is characterized by all of the defining characteristics of rape trauma, reliance on alcohol or drugs, or the recurrence of the symptoms of previous conditions, including psychiatric illness. The **silent reaction** sometimes occurs in place of the rape trauma or compound reaction. The defining characteristics of the silent reaction are an abrupt change in the victim's usual sexual relationships, an increase in nightmares, an increasing anxiety during the interview about the rape incident, a marked change in sexual behavior, denial of the rape or refusal to discuss it, and the sudden development of phobic reactions. See also **nursing diagnosis.**

raphe /rā'fē/ [Gk, *rhaphe,* seam], a line of union of the halves of various symmetric parts, such as the abdominal raphe of the linea alba or the raphe penis, which appears as a narrow, dark streak on the inferior surface of the penis. Also spelled **rhaphe.**

raphe of tongue [Gk, *rhaphe,* seam; AS, *tunge*], a fibrous wall that forms a line of union between the right and left sides of the tongue.

rapid-acting insulin. See **short-acting insulin.**

rapid eye movement. See **sleep.**

rapid pulse /rap'id/ [L, *rapidus,* rush + *pulsare,* to beat], a pulse faster than normal.

rapport /rapôr'/ [Fr, agreement], a sense of mutuality and understanding; harmony, accord, confidence, and respect underlying a relationship between two persons, an essential bond between a therapist and patient.

rapprochement /räprôshmäN'/ [Fr, *rapprocher,* to bring together], (in psychology) the third subphase of the separation-individuation phase of Mahler's system of preoedipal development. This subphase occurs from approximately 14 months to 2 years or more. This stage is characterized by a rediscovery of mother after the initial separation of the practicing subphase. The narcissistic inflation of the practicing subphase is replaced by a realization of separation and vulnerability.

raptus /rap'təs/ [L, *rapere,* to seize], **1.** a state of intense

emotional or mental excitement, often characterized by uncontrollable activity or behavior resulting from an irresistible impulse; ecstasy; rapture. **2.** any sudden or violent seizure or attack.

rare earth element [L, *rarus,* thin; AS, *earthe;* L, *elementum*], a metallic element having an atomic number between 57 to 71, inclusively. These closely related substances are classified in three groups: the cerium metals are lanthanum, cerium, praseodymium, neodymium, promethium, and samarium; the terbium metals are europium, gadolinium, and terbium; the yttrium metals are dysprosium, holmium, erbium, thulium, yttrium, ytterbium, and lutetium. Also called **rare earth metal.**

rare earth screen, a fluorescent material, such as calcium tungstate, used as the basis of x-ray intensifying screens. In recent years, new materials including the rare earths yttrium and gadolinium also have found application in such devices. These rare earths enable lower radiation doses to be used while producing acceptable film densities.

RAS, abbreviation for **reticular activating system.**

rash [OFr, *rasche,* scurf], a skin eruption. Kinds of rashes are **butterfly rash, diaper rash, drug rash,** and **heat rash.**

Rashkind procedure /rash'kind/ [William J. Rashkind, American physician, b. 1922; L, *procedere,* to go forth], the enlargement of an opening in the cardiac septum between the right and left atria, performed to relieve congestive heart failure in newborns with certain congenital heart defects by improving the oxygenation of the blood. The procedure allows more mixing between oxygenated blood from the lungs and systemic blood without the risk of surgery, sustaining life until the infant is 2 to 3 years of age and a shunt can be created to carry systemic blood to the lungs. Preoperatively, a cardiac catheterization is done to pinpoint the defect. Under light general anesthesia, a deflated balloon is passed pervenously through the foramen ovale into the left atrium. The balloon is inflated and pulled across the septum to enlarge the opening. Postoperatively, the infant is observed carefully for respiratory difficulty, signs of hypoxia, or decreasing cardiac output. Humidified oxygen is administered. Fluids and electrolytes are closely monitored. Also called **balloon septostomy.**

Rasmussen's. See **aneurysm.**

RAST. See **radioallergosorbent test.**

rat-bite fever [AS, *raet; bitan,* to bite], either of two distinct infections transmitted to humans by the bite of a rat or mouse, characterized by fever, headache, malaise, nausea, vomiting, and rash. In the United States, the disease is more commonly caused by *Streptobacillus moniliformis,* and its unique features are rash on palms and soles, painful joints, prompt healing of the wound, and a duration of 2 weeks. In the Far East, rat-bite fever is usually caused by *Spirillum minus* and is associated with an asymmetric rash on the extremities, no joint symptoms, a relapsing fever, swelling at the site of the wound, regional lymphadenopathy, and a duration of from 4 to 8 weeks. Relapse is common. Penicillin administered intramuscularly is effective in treating either form of the disease. Rat-bite fever resulting from infection caused by *Streptobacillus moniliformis* is also called **Haverhill fever;** infection caused by *Spirillum minus* is also called **sodoku.**

rate [L, *ratus,* reckoned], a numeric ratio, often used in the compilation of data concerning the prevalence and incidence of events, in which the number of actual occurrences appears as the numerator and the number of possible occurrences appears as the denominator, as when 1 person in 15 fails an examination the failure rate is said to be 1/15 (or 'one in fifteen'). Standard rates are stated in conventional units of population, such as neonatal mortality per 1000 or maternal mortality per 100,000.

rate-pressure product, the heart rate multiplied by the systolic blood pressure. It is a clinical indicator of myocardial oxygen demand.

Rathke's pouch /rät'kēz/ [Martin Heinrich Rathke, German anatomist, b. 1793; OFr, *pouche*], a depression that forms in the roof of the mouth of an embryo, anterior to the buccopharyngeal membrane, around the fourth week of gestation. The walls of the diverticulum develop into the anterior lobe of the pituitary gland.

Rathke's pouch tumor. See **craniopharyngioma.**

ratio /rā'shō/ [L, a reckoning], the relationship of one quantity to one or more other quantities expressed as a proportion of one to the others, and written either as a fraction (8/3) or linearly (8:3).

rational /rash'ənəl/ [L, *rationalis,* reasonable], **1.** of or pertaining to a measure, method, or procedure based on reason. **2.** of or pertaining to a therapeutic method based on an understanding of the cause and mechanisms of a specific disease and the potential effects of the drugs or procedures used in treating the disorder. **3.** sane; capable of normal reasoning or behavior.

rationale /rash'ənal'/ [L, *rationalis*], a system of reasoning or a statement of the reasons used in explaining data or phenomena.

rational emotive therapy (RET), a form of cognitive therapy, originated by Albert Ellis, that emphasizes a reorganization of one's cognitive and emotional functions, a redefinition of one's problems, and a change in one's attitudes to develop more effective and suitable patterns of behavior. RET is conducted with individuals and with groups.

rationalization /rash'ənal'īzā'shən/, the most commonly used defense mechanism in which an individual justifies ideas, actions, or feelings with seemingly acceptable reasons or explanations. It is often used to preserve self-respect, reduce guilt feelings, or to obtain social approval or acceptance.

rational treatment. See **treatment.**

ratio solution, the relationship of a solute to a solvent expressed as a proportion, such as 1:100, or parts per thousand.

rattle [ME, *ratelen*], an abnormal sound heard by auscultation of the lungs in some forms of pulmonary disease. It consists of a coarse vibration caused by the movement of moisture and the separation of the walls of small air passages during respiration.

rattlesnake [ME, *ratelen* + AS, *snacan,* to creep], a poisonous pit viper with a series of loosely connected, horny segments at the end of the tail that make a noise like a rattle when shaken. More than 25 species of rattlesnakes are found in the Americas, including many parts of the United States. They have a hematoxin in their venom, and they are responsible for most of the poisonous snake bites in the United States. See **snakebite.**

rat typhus. See **murine typhus.**

Raudixin, a trademark for an antihypertensive (purified *Rauwolfia serpentina*).

Rauwiloid, a trademark for an antihypertensive (alseroxylon).

rauwolfia /rôwol'fē·ə, rou-, rä-/ [Leonhard Rauwolf, 16th century German botanist], the dried roots of *Rauwolfia serpentina* that provide the extracts for hypotensive agents and tranquilizing alkaloid drugs, like reserpine.

rauwolfia alkaloid, any one of more than 20 alkaloids derived from the root of a climbing shrub, *Rauwolfia serpentina,* indigenous to India and the surrounding area. Formerly used as an antipsychotic agent, it is today confined to the treatment of hypertension. Numerous trademark formulations of the principal alkaloid reserpine are available.

rauwolfia serpentina, the dried root from *Rauwolfia serpentina,* used as an antihypertensive.

■ INDICATIONS: It is prescribed in the treatment of mild hypertension and hypertensive emergencies.

■ CONTRAINDICATIONS: Mental depression, peptic ulcer, ulcerative colitis, electroconvulsive therapy, or known hypersensitivity to this drug prohibits its use. It can interact adversely with monoamine oxidase inhibitors.

■ ADVERSE EFFECTS: Among the more serious adverse reactions are symptoms resembling parkinsonism, glaucoma, cardiac arrhythmias, and GI bleeding.

Rauzide, a trademark for a cardiovascular, fixed-combination drug containing a diuretic (bendroflumethiazide) and an antihypertensive (rauwolfia serpentina).

raw data, (in magnetic resonance imaging) the information obtained by radio reception of the MR signal as stored by a computer. Specific computer manipulation of these data is required to construct an image from it.

ray [L, *radius*], a beam of radiation, such as heat or light, moving away from a source.

Raynaud's phenomenon /rānōz'/ [Maurice Raynaud, French physician, b. 1834], intermittent attacks of ischemia of the extremities of the body, especially the fingers, toes, ears, and nose, caused by exposure to cold or by emotional stimuli. The attacks are characterized by severe blanching of the extremities, followed by cyanosis, then redness; they are usually accompanied by numbness, tingling, burning, and often pain. Normal color and sensation are restored by heat. The attacks usually occur secondary to such conditions as scleroderma, rheumatoid arthritis, systemic lupus erythematosus, thoracic outlet syndrome, drug

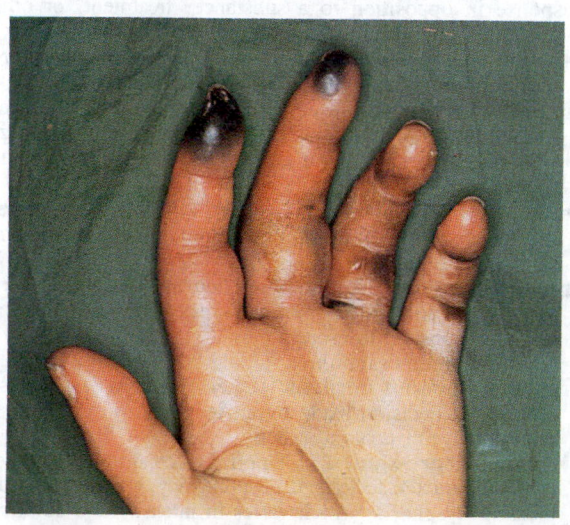

Raynaud's phenomenon *(Kamal, 1991)*

intoxications, dysproteinemia, myxedema, primary pulmonary hypertension, and trauma. The condition is called **Raynaud's disease** when there is a history of symptoms for at least 2 years with no progression of symptoms and no evidence of an underlying cause. Therapy for the secondary form depends on recognition and treatment of the underlying disease. Idiopathic forms, which occur most frequently in young women 18 to 30 years of age, may be controlled by protecting the body and extremities from the cold and by the use of mild sedatives and vasodilators.

Raynaud's sign. See **acrocyanosis.**

Rb, symbol for the element **rubidium.**

RBBB, abbreviation for **right bundle branch block.**

RBC, abbreviation for *red blood cell.* See **erythrocyte.**

RBE, abbreviation for **relative biologic effectiveness.**

R.C.P., abbreviation for **Royal College of Physicians.**

RCPSC, abbreviation for **Royal College of Physicians and Surgeons of Canada.**

R.C.S., abbreviation for **Royal College of Surgeons.**

RD, abbreviation for *registered dietician.*

RDA, abbreviation for **recommended dietary allowance.**

rdi, abbreviation for *recommended daily intake.*

RDS, abbreviation for *respiratory distress syndrome.* See **respiratory distress syndrome of the newborn.**

Re, symbol for the element **rhenium.**

re-, a prefix meaning 'back, again, contrary': *reaction, recombination, recurrent.*

reabsorption /rē'əbsôrp'shən/, the process of something being absorbed again, such as the removal of calcium from the bone back into the blood.

reacher /rē'chər/, a pair of extended tongs that can be used by persons with upper extremity disabilities to grasp objects on shelves and similar areas beyond their usual reach. Also called **extended arm.**

Reach to Recovery [AS, *reacan,* to reach; ME, *recoveren,* to get back], a national volunteer organization that offers counseling and support to women who have breast cancer and to their families. Many of the members have had mastectomies themselves.

reaction /rē·ak'shən/ [L, *re,* again, *agere,* to act], a response in opposition to a substance, treatment, or other stimulus, such as an antigen-antibody reaction in immunology, a hypersensitivity reaction in allergy, or an adverse reaction in pharmacology. **—react,** *v.,* **reactive,** *adj.*

reaction formation, a defense mechanism in which a person expresses toward another person or situation feelings, attitudes, or behavior that are the opposite of what would normally be expected.

reaction time [L, *re-, agere,* to act; AS, *tima*], the interval between the application of a stimulus and the beginning of a response.

reactivate /rē·ak'tivāt/ [L, *re- + activus*], to make active again, as in adding fresh serum to restore the potency of an original supply of the serum.

-reactive. See **reaction.**

reactive decision /rē·ak'tiv/ [L, *re + activus*], (in psychology) a decision made by an individual in response to the influence or goals of others.

reactive depression, an emotional condition characterized by an acute feeling of despondency, sadness, and depressive dysphoria, which varies in intensity and duration. The condition is caused in response to some identifiable external situation or environmental stress and is relieved when the circumstance is altered or the conflict understood and resolved. Also called **exogenous depression, situational depression.** Compare **endogenous depression.** See also **depression.**

reactive inflammation [L, *re- + activus + inflammare,* to set afire], an inflammation that develops as a reaction to an antigen.

reactive schizophrenia, a form of schizophrenia caused by environmental factors rather than by organic changes in the brain. The onset of the disease is usually rapid; symptoms are of brief duration, and the affected individual appears well immediately before and after the schizophrenic episode. See also **schizophrenia, schizophreniform disorder.**

reactor /rē·ak'tər/, **1.** (in psychology) a family therapist who lets a family in therapy take the lead and then follows in that direction. **2.** (in radiology) a cubicle in which radioisotopes are artificially produced.

read [AS, *raedan,* to advise], (of a computer) to retrieve or transfer data from some storage location or medium, such as a disk.

reading [AS, *raedan*], (in molecular genetics) the linear process in which the genetic information contained in a nucleotide sequence is decoded, as in the translation of the messenger RNA directives for the sequence of the amino acids in a polypeptide.

reading disorders, a language disorder in which a one's reading ability is significantly below intellectual capacity. Tests show the problem does not involve mental retardation, chronological age, or inadequate schooling, but is marked by faulty oral reading, slow reading, and reduced comprehension.

Read method, a method of psychophysical preparation for childbirth designed by Dr. Grantly Dick-Read. It was the first 'natural childbirth' program, a term coined by Dr. Read. Basically, Read held that childbirth is a normal, physiologic procedure and that the pain of labor and delivery is of psychologic origin—the fear tension pain syndrome. He countered women's fears with education about the physiologic process, encouraged a positive, welcoming attitude, corrected false information, and led tours of the hospital before birth. To decrease tension, he developed a series of breathing exercises for use during the various stages of labor. To foster relaxation and optimal physical function in labor and in recovery after delivery, he incorporated a series of physical exercises to be performed regularly in classes and in practice at home during pregnancy. The woman is helped to manage labor and delivery using the Read method in the following way: During the early and mid-first stage of labor, before cervical dilatation has reached 7 cm, contractions are 2 to 5 minutes apart and last for 30 to 40 seconds. The mother lies on her back with her knees bent. Abdominal breathing is used during contractions. Her hands are placed over her lower abdomen, fingers touching. She breathes deeply and slowly—in through her nose and out through her mouth. The abdominal wall rises with each inhalation, which she can feel with her hands. The rate of breathing is no more than six breaths in 30 seconds, or 12 to 18 in one contraction. During the late part of the first stage of labor, after 7 cm of cervical dilatation, the contractions are 1 ½ to 2 minutes apart and last for 40 to 60 seconds. Costal or diaphragmatic breathing is used during contractions. Her hands are placed on her sides, over the ribs. She breathes in more shallowly, feeling her ribs move sideways against her hands. Each breath is drawn in through her nose and exhaled through her mouth. The abdominal wall does not rise and fall with this kind of breathing. The rate of breathing is no more than six breaths in 30 seconds, or 12 to 18 in one contraction. At the end of the first stage of labor, near full dilatation, contractions may be very strong, occurring every 1 ½ to 2 minutes and lasting 60 to 90 seconds. The mother lies on her back with her knees bent. Panting respirations are used during the contractions. The mother holds one of her hands on her sternum, which rises and falls as she pants lightly and rapidly through her mouth. Panting continues through the end of the first stage to full dilatation as the urge to push grows. Panting helps the woman to avoid pushing. During the second, or expulsive, stage of labor after full dilatation of the cervix, the contractions occur every 1 ½ to 2 minutes, last 60 to 90 seconds, and are accompanied with an urge to bear down and push. The woman lies back, head and shoulders supported in a semisitting position. She is helped to draw her legs up, holding them with her hands behind the lower thighs, thighs on her abdomen and spread apart. As each contraction begins, she raises her head, takes a deep breath, tucks her chin on her chest, blocks the escape of air from her lungs, and bears down. During each contraction she may need to blow the air out, refill her lungs and push again two or three times. Throughout labor she is helped to understand what is occurring and to participate and accept the experience in anticipation of the birth of the baby. Currently, many authorities who advocate use of other aspects of the Read method strongly recommend that a woman in labor not lie on her back. Supine hypotension is frequently the result of this position, because the uterus can fall back, occluding the vena cava and decreasing the volume of blood returned to the heart, thus reducing the volume of the cardiac output. Maternal hypotension follows, resulting in decreased placental perfusion and an inadequate supply of oxygen to the fetus. Today, the woman using the Read method spends most of labor lying on her side or in a semisitting position with her knees, back, and head well supported. Compare **Bradley method, Lamaze method.**

read-only memory (ROM),   the portion of a computer's memory where information is permanently stored. The operator has random access to the memory, but only for purposes of reading the contents. Special equipment is required to write or erase a read-only memory.

readthrough [AS, *raedan + thurh,* through],   (in molecular genetics) transcription of RNA beyond the normal termination sequence in the DNA template, caused by the occasional failure of RNA polymerase to respond to the endpoint signal.

reagent /rē·ā′jənt/ [L, *re,* again, *agere,* to act],   a chemical substance known to react in a specific way. A reagent is used to detect or synthesize another substance in a chemical reaction.

reagin /rē′ājin/ [L, *re + agere*],   **1.** an antibody associated with human atopy, such as asthma and hay fever. It attaches to mast cells and basophils and sensitizes the skin and other tissues. In antigen-antibody reactions it triggers the release of histamine and other mediators that cause atopic symptoms. **2.** a nonspecific, nontreponemal antibody-like substance found in the serum of individuals with syphilis. It can combine with an antigen prepared as a lipid extract of normal tissue, a phenomenon that constitutes the basis of the serologic tests for syphilis. **–reaginic,** *adj.*

reaginic antibody /rē′əgin′ik/,   an IgE immunoglobulin

that is elevated in hypersensitive individuals. See also **reagin, reagin-mediated disorder.**

reagin-mediated disorder,   a hypersensitivity reaction, such as hay fever or an allergic response to an insect sting, produced by reaginic antibodies (IgE immunoglobulins), causing degranulation and the release of histamine, bradykinin, serotonin, and other vasoactive amines. An initial sensitizing dose of the antigen induces the formation of specific IgE antibodies, and their attachment to mast cells and basophils results in hypersensitivity to a subsequent challenging dose of the antigen. Reactions range from a simple wheal and flare on the skin to life-threatening anaphylactic shock, depending on the amount and route of entrance of the sensitizing dose and challenging dose, the amount and distribution of IgE antibodies, the responsiveness of the host, the timing of exposure to the allergen, and the tissues in which the antigen-antibody reaction occurs. The abundance of mast cells in the skin, nose, and lungs makes those areas susceptible to IgE-mediated reactions. Allergens that commonly cause these reactions include plant spores, pollens, animal danders, stings, serum proteins, foods, and certain drugs. See also **allergy, generalized anaphylaxis, hay fever.**

reality /rē·al′itē/ [L, *res,* factual],   the culturally constructed world of perception, meaning, and behavior that members of a culture regard as an absolute.

reality orientation,   a formal activity that uses specific approaches to assist confused or disoriented persons toward an awareness of reality, or the 'here and now' as by emphasizing the hour, day, month, and weather.

reality principle,   an awareness of the demands of the environment and the need for an adjustment of behavior to meet those demands, expressed primarily by the renunciation of immediate gratification of instinctual pleasures to obtain long-term and future goals. In psychoanalysis, this function is held to be performed by the ego. Compare **pleasure principle.**

reality testing,   an ego function that enables one to differentiate between external reality and any inner imaginative world and to behave in a manner that exhibits an awareness of accepted norms and customs. Impairment of reality testing is indicative of a disturbance in ego functioning that may lead to psychosis.

reality therapy,   a form of psychotherapy developed by William Glassner in which the aims are to help define and assess basic values within the framework of a current situation and to evaluate the person's present behavior and future plans in relation to those values. The emphasis in treatment is on the present rather than the past; it focuses on responsible behavior as a means of personal fulfillment. The focus is on behavior rather than feelings.

real time [L, *res,* factual; AS, *tid,* tide],   an application of computerized equipment that allows data to be processed with relation to ongoing external events, so that the operators can make immediate diagnostic or other decisions based on the current data output. Ultrasound scanning uses real time control systems, making results available almost simultaneously with the generation of the input data.

real-time imaging,   See **dynamic imaging.**

real-time scanning,   the scanning or imaging of an entire object, or a cross-sectional slice of the object, at a single moment. To produce such a 'snapshot' image, scanning data must be recorded quickly over a very short time rather than by accumulation over a longer period.

reamer [AS, *ryman,* to make room],   **1.** a tool with a straight or spiral cutting edge, used in a rotating motion to enlarge a hole or clear an opening. **2.** (in dentistry) an instrument with a tapered and loosely spiraled metal shaft, used for enlarging and cleaning root canals.

reapproximate /rē'əprok'simāt/ [L, *re*, again, *approximare*, to come near], to rejoin tissues separated by surgery or trauma so that their anatomic relationship is restored. **–reapproximation,** *n.*

reasonable care /rē'zənəbəl/ [L, *rationalis*], the degree of skill and knowledge used by a competent health practitioner in treating and caring for the sick and injured.

reasonable person, (in law) a hypothetical person who possesses the qualities that are used as an objective standard on which to judge a defendant's action in a negligence suit. In such suits, it must be decided whether or not a reasonable person, under the same circumstances, would have acted in the same way as the defendant.

reasonably prudent person doctrine /rē'zənəblē'/, a concept that a person of ordinary sense will use ordinary care and skill in meeting the health care needs of a patient.

reattachment /rē'ətach'mənt/ [L, *re-*; OFr, *attachier*], **1.** the rejoining of accidentally severed body parts. **2.** the rejoining of periodontal membrane fibers to the cementum of a tooth and the alveolar bone to restore a loosened tooth.

rebase /rēbās'/ [L, *re*, again, *basis*, base], a process of refitting a denture by replacing or adding to its base material without changing the occlusal relationships of the teeth.

rebirthing /rēbur'thing/, a form of psychotherapy developed by Leonard Orr that focuses on the breath and breathing apparatus. Orr believes the premature severing of the umbilical cord deprives the newborn of oxygen and forces him or her to suddenly learn to breathe through fluid-filled lungs, resulting in panic and terror with every breath taken. The goal of treatment is to overcome the trauma of the birth-damaged breathing apparatus so the person is able to use the breath as a supportive and creative part of life.

rebound /rēbound'/ [Fr, *rebondir*, to bounce], **1.** recovery from illness. **2.** a sudden contraction of muscle after a period of relaxation, often seen in conditions in which inhibitory reflexes are lost.

rebound congestion, swelling and congestion of the nasal mucosa that follows the vasodilator effects of decongestant medications.

rebound phenomenon [OFr, *rebondir*; Gk, *phainomenon*, anything seen], a renewal of reflex activity after the stimulus that triggered the original action has been removed. It may be indicative of a lesion of the cerebellum.

rebound tenderness, a sign of inflammation of the peritoneum in which pain is elicited by the sudden release of a hand pressing on the abdomen. See also **appendicitis, peritonitis.**

rebreathing /rēbrē'thing/ [L, *re* + AS, *braeth*, breath], breathing into a closed system. Exhaled gas mixes with the gas in the closed system, and some of this mixture is then reinhaled. Rebreathing, which may result in progressively decreasing concentrations of oxygen and progressively increasing concentrations of carbon dioxide, can occur in poorly ventilated environments.

rebreathing bag, (in anesthesia) a flexible bag attached to a mask. The rebreathing bag may function as a reservoir for anesthetic gases during surgery or for oxygen during resuscitation. It may be squeezed to pump the gas or air into the lungs.

recalcification /rēkal'sifikā'shən/ [L, *re-*, + *calx*, lime + *facere*, to make], the replacement of lost calcium salts in the body needed for normal neuromuscular excitability, excitation-coupling contraction in cardiac and smooth muscle stimulus-secretion coupling, maintenance of tight junctions between cells, blood clotting, and compressional strength of bone.

recannulate /rēkan'yəlāt/ [L, *re* + *cannula*, small reed], to make a new opening through an organ or tissue, such as opening a passage through an occluded blood vessel.

recapitulation theory /rē'kəpit'yəlā'shən/ [L, *re* + *capitulum*, small head], the theory, formulated by German naturalist Ernst Heinrich Haeckel, that an organism during the course of embryonic development passes through stages that resemble the structural form of several ancestral types of the species as it evolved from a lower to a higher form of life. It is summarized by the statement 'Ontogeny recapitulates phylogeny.' Also called **biogenetic law, Haeckel's law.**

receiver /risē'vər/ [L, *recipere*, to receive], (in communication theory) the person or persons to whom a message is sent.

receptive aphasia /risep'tiv/, a form of sensory aphasia marked by impaired comprehension of language. Also called **Wernicke's aphasia.**

receptor /risep'tər/ [L, *recipere*, to receive], **1.** a chemical structure usually of protein/carbohydrate on the surface of a cell that combines with an antigen to produce a discrete immunologic component. **2.** a sensory nerve ending that responds to various kinds of stimulation. **3.** a specific cellular protein that must first bind a hormone before cellular response can be elicited. The protein may be in the cytoplasm or in the cell membrane.

receptor site [L, *recipere*, to receive + *situs*], a location on a cell surface where certain molecules, such as enzymes, neurotransmitters, or viruses, attach to interact with cellular components.

receptor theory of drug action, the concept that certain drugs produce their effects by acting discretely at some specific receptor site on a cell or molecule within the cell or its membrane.

recess /rē'ses, rises'/ [L, *recedere*, to retreat], a small hollow cavity, such as the epitympanic recess in the tympanic cavity of the inner ear or the retrocecal recess extending as a small pocket behind the cecum.

recessive /rises'iv/ [L, *recedere*], of, pertaining to, or describing a gene the effect of which is masked or hidden if there is a dominant gene at the same locus. If both genes are recessive and produce the same trait, the trait is expressed in the individual. See also **autosomal-recessive inheritance, dominance.**

recessive gene, the member of a pair of genes that lacks the ability to express itself in the presence of its more dominant allele; it is expressed only in the homozygous state. Compare **dominant gene.**

recessive trait, a genetically determined characteristic that is expressed only when present in the homozygotic state.

recidivism (recid) /risid'iviz'əm/ [L, *recidivus*, falling back], a tendency by an ill person to relapse or return to a hospital.

recipient /risip'ē·ənt/ [L, *recipere*, to receive], the person who receives a blood transfusion or tissue graft, or organ.

reciprocal /rəsip'rəkəl/ [L, *reciprocare*, to move backward], pertaining to a type of body movement that aids in communication, such as body language that indicates affiliation between people.

reciprocal beat, an atrial or ventricular complex resulting from a return of an impulse to its chamber of origin. Also called **echo beat.**

reciprocal changes, the changes seen in EKG leads facing the opposite wall to a myocardial infarction. The changes were formerly thought to be purely electrical but are now considered a sign of more extensive myocardial damage.

reciprocal gene. See **complementary gene.**

reciprocal inhibition, the theory in behavior therapy that if an anxiety-producing stimulus occurs simultaneously with a response that diminishes anxiety, the stimulus may cause less anxiety, as deep chest or abdominal breathing and relaxation of the deep muscles appear to diminish anxiety and pain in childbirth. See also **systemic desensitization.**

reciprocal roentgens, (in radiology) the measure of x-ray film speed, used in the formula speed = 1/number of roentgens needed to produce a density of 1.

reciprocal translocation, the mutual exchange of genetic material between two nonhomologous chromosomes. Also called **interchange.** Compare **balanced translocation, robertsonian translocation.**

reciprocity /res′ipros′itē/ [Fr, *réciprocité*], a mutual agreement to exchange privileges, dependence, or relationships, as an agreement between two governing bodies to accept the medical credentials of physicians licensed in either community.

Recklinghausen's canal /rek′linghou′sənz/ [Friedrich D. von Recklinghausen, German pathologist, b. 1833], the small lymph space in the connective tissues of the body.

Recklinghausen's disease. See **neurofibromatosis.**

Recklinghausen's tumor [Friedrich D. von Recklinghausen], a benign tumor, derived from smooth muscle containing connective tissue and epithelial elements. The tumor that occurs in the wall of the oviduct or posterior uterine wall. Also called **adenomyosis of the uterus.**

reclining /riklī′ning/, leaning backward. —**recline,** *v.*

reclining position. See **jackknife position.**

recluse spider. See **brown spider.**

recombinant /rēkom′binənt/ [L, *re*, again, *combinare*, to combine], **1.** the cell or organism that results from the recombination of genes within the DNA molecule, regardless of whether naturally or artificially induced. **2.** of or pertaining to such an organism or cell. See also **recombinant DNA.**

recombinant blood factor VIII. See **FVIII.**

recombinant DNA, a DNA molecule in which rearrangement of the genes has been artificially induced. Enzymes are used to break isolated DNA molecules into fragments that are then rearranged in the desired sequence. Portions of DNA material from another organism of the same or a different species may also be introduced into the molecule, which is then replicated, resulting in both genotypic and phenotypic alterations in the organism. See also **genetic engineering.**

recombinant tPA, See **tissue plasminogen activator.**

recombination /rē′kombinā′shən/ [L, *re* + *combinare*], **1.** (in genetics) the formation of new combinations and arrangements of genes within the chromosome as a result of independent assortment of unlinked genes, crossing over of linked genes, or intracistronic crossing over of nucleotides. See also **recombinant DNA. 2.** a method of measurement of radiation by ionimetric techniques in which it is necessary to collect the liberated charges to arrive at a value of total charge per unit mass of air. Recombination of ions will lower the value collected and will cause an underestimation

of dose, particularly in intense fields. A technique for determining the magnitude of ionic recombination is routinely applied in accurate dosimetry.

Recombivax HB, a trademark for a hepatitis B vaccine (recombinant).

recommended dietary allowance (RDA) /rek′əmen′did/ [L, *re* + *commendere*, to commend], the amount of nutrients, particularly kilocalories, protein, vitamins and minerals, recommended as a necessary part of one's daily food intake to maintain normal health.

recon /rē′kon/ [L, *re* + *combinare* + Gk, *ion*, going], (in molecular genetics) the smallest genetic unit that is capable of recombination, thought to be a triplet of nucleotides.

reconstitution /rē′konstit(y)oo′shən/ [L, *re* + *constituere*, to establish], the continuous repair of tissue damage.

reconstruction time /rē′kənstruk′shən/, (in computed tomography) the period between the end of a scan and the appearance of an image.

record /ricôrd′/, a written form of communication that permanently documents information relevant to the care of a patient.

Recovery /rikuv′əry/, a self-help group that provides support for persons discharged from inpatient psychiatric hospitals.

recovery room (RR, R.R.) [ME, *recoveren;* AS *rum*], an area adjoining the operating room to which surgical patients are taken while still under anesthesia, before being returned to their rooms. It is also identified as the post-anesthesia recovery area (PAR). Vital signs and adequacy of ventilation are carefully observed as the patient recovers conciousness. The recovery room has equipment and a specially trained nursing staff with a nurse anesthetist or anesthesiologist available. See also **postoperative care.**

recreational drug, any substance with pharmacologic effects that is taken voluntarily for personal pleasure or satisfaction rather than for medicinal purposes. The term is generally applied to alcohol, barbiturates, amphetamines, THC, PCP, cocaine, and heroin, but also includes caffeine in coffee and cola beverages.

recreational therapy /rē′krē·ā′shənəl/ [L, *recreare*, to renew], a form of adjunctive treatment in which games or other group activities are used as a means of modifying maladaptive behavior, awakening social interests, or improving the ability to communicate in depressed, withdrawn people.

recrudescence /rē′kroōdes′əns/ [L, *re* + *crudescere*, to become hard], a return of symptoms of a disease during a period of recovery.

recrudescent /-ənt/ [L, *recrudescere*, to break out again], the return of disease symptoms after a period of remission.

recrudescent hepatitis, a form of acute viral hepatitis marked by a relapse during the period of recovery. A minority of patients experience it, and the prognosis for ultimate recovery is rarely affected.

recrudescent typhus. See **Brill-Zinsser disease.**

recruitment /rikroōt′mənt/, **1.** the perception of a rapid growth of loudness, commonly seen in sensorineural hearing losses that are cochlear in nature. The impaired ear cannot hear faint sounds, but hears intense sounds as loudly as a normal ear. **2.** in muscle contractions, the ability to recruit additional motor units into action as the need to overcome resistance increases.

rect-, a prefix meaning 'pertaining to the rectum': *rectal, rectalgia, rectorrhea.*

recta. See **rectum.**

-rectal. See **rectum.**

rectal abscess /rek′təl/ [L, *rectus*, straight + *abscedere*, to go away], an abscess in the perianal area.

rectal alimentation [L, *rectus*, straight + *alimentum*, nourishment], the delivery of nourishment in concentrated form by injection or installation through the rectum.

rectal anesthesia [L, *rectus*, straight], general anesthesia achieved by the insertion, injection, or infusion of an anesthetic agent into the rectum; this procedure is performed rarely because of the unpredictability of absorption of the drug into the blood.

rectal cancer. See **colorectal cancer.**

rectal instillation of medication, the instillation of a medicated suppository, cream, or gel into the rectum. Some conditions treated by this method are constipation, pruritus ani, and hemorrhoids. The patient lies on the side, with the lower leg extended and the upper leg flexed. The nurse or physician unwraps the suppository and, wearing a glove, raises the upper buttock, exposing the anus. The suppository may be self-lubricating, or it may need to be lubricated with a water-soluble lubricant. The suppository is then gently inserted past the anal sphincter. Occasionally, a drug may be given in a medicated enema. See also **enema.**

rectal reflex, the normal response (defecation) to the presence of an accumulation of feces in the rectum. Also called **defecation reflex.**

rectal temperature [L, *rectus*, straight + *temperatura*], temperature as measured in the rectum. Rectal temperatures average 0.3 to 0.4° C or 0.5 to 0.75° F higher than oral temperatures.

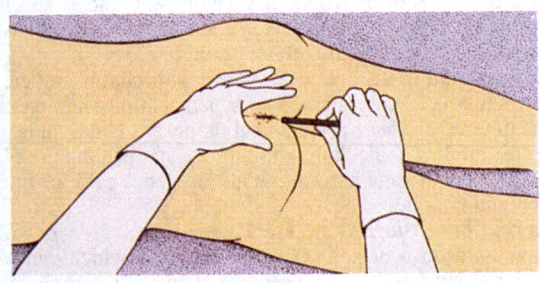

Placement of thermometer for rectal temperature assessment
(Potter, 1993)

rectal thermometer [L, *rectus*; Gk, *therme*, heat + *metron*, measure], a clinical thermometer suitable for measuring body temperature rectally.

rectal tube, a flexible tube inserted into the rectum to assist in the relief of flatus.

rectifier /rek′tifī′ər/, an electrical device that converts alternating current (AC) into pulsating direct current (DC). Rectifiers are used to power x-ray tubes, which require a DC electrical source.

rectilinear scanner /rek′tilin′ē·ər/, (in nuclear medicine) a device that generates an image of an anatomical structure by detecting radioactivity within the structure.

rectitis. See **proctitis.**

recto- /rek′tō-, rek′tə-/, a prefix meaning 'straight or pertaining to the rectum': *rectoscope, rectosigmoidoscopy.*

rectocele /rek′təsēl′/ [L, *rectus* + Gk, *koilos*, hollow], a protrusion of the rectum and the posterior wall of the vagina into the vagina. The condition, which occurs after the muscles of the vagina and pelvic floor have been weakened by childbearing, old age, or surgery, may reflect a congenital weakness in the wall and may, if severe, result in dyspareunia and difficulty in evacuating the bowel. Reconstructive surgery is often helpful and is combined with any other necessary perineal, pelvic, or vaginal repair. Also called **proctocele.** Compare **cystocele.**

rectocolitis. See **coloproctitis.**

rectosigmoid /-sig′moid/ [L, *rectus* + Gk, *sigma*, S-shaped, *eidos* form], pertaining to the portion of the large intestine that includes the lower portion of the sigmoid and the upper portion of the rectum.

rectosigmoidoscopy /-sig′moidəs′kəpē/ [L, *rectus*, straight; Gk, *sigma*, S-shaped + *eidos*, form + *skopein*, to view], the examination of the rectum and pelvic colon with a sigmoidoscope.

rectouterine excavation, rectouterine pouch. See **cul-de-sac of Douglas.**

rectovaginal fistula /-vaj′ənəl/ [L, *rectus*, straight + *vagina*, sheath + *fistula*, pipe], an abnormal passage or opening between the rectum and the vagina.

rectovaginal ligament, one of the four main uterine support ligaments. It helps hold the uterus in position by maintaining traction on the cervix. Also called **posterior ligament.**

rectovesical /-ves′ikəl/ [L, *rectus*, straight + *vesica*, bladder], pertaining to the rectum and bladder.

rectum /rek′təm/, *pl.* **rectums, recta** [L, *rectus*], the portion of the large intestine, about 12 cm long, continuous with the descending sigmoid colon, just proximal to the anal canal. It follows the sacrococcygeal curve, ends in the anal canal, and usually contains three transverse semilunar folds: one situated proximally on the right side, a second one extending inward from the left side, and the third and largest fold projecting caudally. Each fold is about 12 mm wide. The folds overlap when the intestine is empty. **—rectal,** *adj.*

rectus abdominis /rek′təs/, one of a pair of anterolateral muscles of the abdomen, extending the whole length of the ventral aspect of the abdomen. The pair is separated by the

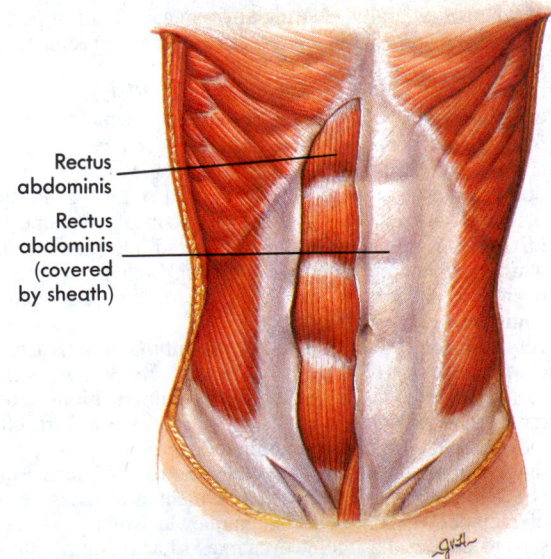

Rectus abdominis

Rectus abdominis (covered by sheath)

Rectus abdominus muscles
(Thibodeau, 1993/John V Hagen)

linea alba. Each rectus arises in a lateral tendon from the crest of the pubis and is interlaced by a medial tendon with that of the opposite side. The rectus abdominis inserts into the fifth, the sixth, and the seventh ribs. It is innervated by branches of the seventh through the twelfth intercostal nerves and functions to flex the vertebral column, tense the anterior abdominal wall, and assist in compressing the abdominal contents. Compare **obliquus externus abdominis, obliquus internus abdominis, pyramidalis, transversus abdominis.**

rectus capitis anterior. See **rectus muscle.**

rectus capitis lateralis. See **rectus muscle.**

rectus femoris, a fusiform muscle of the anterior thigh, one of the four parts of the quadriceps femoris. It arises in an anterior tendon originating in the iliac spine and in a posterior tendon originating in the brim of the acetabulum. The two tendons unite and spread into a broad, thick aponeurosis that extends downward over the thigh in the center of the quadriceps femoris. The aponeurosis narrows into a flattened tendon, one portion inserting into the base of the patella and the other portion inserting into the tibial tuberosity. The rectus femoris is innervated by branches of the femoral nerve, which contain fibers from the second, third, and fourth lumbar nerves, and it functions to flex the leg. Compare **vastus intermedius, vastus lateralis, vastus medialis.** See also **quadriceps femoris.**

rectus muscle [L, straight; *musculus*], a muscle of the body that has a relatively straight form. Some rectus muscles are **rectus abdominis, rectus capitis anterior,** and **rectus capitis lateralis.**

recumbency /rikum′bənsē/ [L, *recumbere,* to lie down], the state of lying down or leaning against something.

recumbent /rikum′bənt/ [L *recumbere* to lie down], lying down or leaning backward. See also **reclining.** **–recumbency,** *n.*

recuperate /rikōō′pərāt/ [L, *recupare,* to regain], to recover one's health and strength.

recuperation /rikōō′pərā′shən/ [L, *recupare,* to regain], the process of recovering health and strength.

recurrence /rikur′əns/ [L, *recurrere,* to run back], the reappearance of a sign or symptom of a disease after a period of remission.

recurrent /rikur′ənt/ [L, *recurrere,* to run back], a disease sign or symptom that returns periodically.

recurrent bandage [L, *recurrere,* to run back], a bandage that is wrapped several times around itself, usually applied to the head or an amputated stump.

recurrent fever. See **relapsing fever.**

recurrent inhibition. See **Renshaw cells.**

recurvatum /rē′kərvā′təm/ [L, *recurvare,* to bend back], backward thrust of the knee caused by weakness of the quadriceps or a joint disorder.

red blindness. See **protanopia.**

red blood cell. See **erythrocyte.**

red blood cell count [AS, *read, blod;* L, *cella,* storeroom; Fr, *conter,* to count], a count of the erythrocytes in a specimen of whole blood, commonly made with an electronic counting device. The normal concentrations of red blood cells in the whole blood of males are 4.6 to 6.2 million/mm^3; in females, the concentrations are 4.2 to 5.4 million/mm^3.

Red Book of the American Academy of Pediatrics, a book published by the American Academy of Pediatrics, Inc., that serves as the standard reference source of immunization procedures for children and adults.

red bug. See **chigger.**

red cell. See **erythrocyte.**

red cell indexes, a series of relationships that characterize the red cell population in terms of size, hemoglobin content, and hemoglobin concentration. Derived mathematically from the red cell count and the hemoglobin and hematocrit values, the indexes are useful in making differential diagnoses of several kinds of anemia. The values reported are the mean corpuscular hemoglobin (MCH), the mean corpuscular hemoglobin concentration (MCHC), and the mean corpuscular volume (MCV). Also called **red cell indices.** See also **iron deficiency anemia.**

red corpuscle. See **erythrocyte.**

Red Cross. See **American Red Cross, International Red Cross Society.**

red fever. See **dengue fever.**

red hepatization. See **hepatization.**

red infarct [AS, *read;* L, *infarcire,* to stuff], a pathologic change that occurs in brain tissue that has been rendered ischemic by lack of blood. With restricted blood flow, diapedesis of red blood cells occurs into the parenchyma of the brain without actually producing a well-formed hematoma but only infiltration of erythrocytes.

red marrow [AS, *read;* AS, *mearh,* marrow], the red vascular substance consisting of connective tissue and blood vessels containing primitive blood cells, macrophages, megakaryocytes, and fat cells. It is found in the cavities of many bones, including the flat and the short bones, the bodies of the vertebrae, the sternum, the ribs, and the articulating ends of the long bones. Red marrow manufactures and releases leukocytes and erythrocytes into the bloodstream. Compare **yellow marrow.**

red mite. See **chigger.**

redon /rē′don/, the smallest unit of the DNA molecule capable of recombination; it may be as small as one deoxyribonucleotide pair. Compare **cistron, muton.**

redox, an abbreviation for *reduction-oxidation* (reaction). See **oxidation-reduction reaction.**

red phenol. See **phenolsulfonphthalein.**

red tide. See **shellfish poisoning.**

reduce /rid(y)ōōs′/ [L, *reducere,* to draw backward], **1.** (in surgery) the restoration of a part to its original position after displacement, as in the reduction of a fractured bone by bringing ends or fragments back into alignment or of a hernia by returning the bowel to its normal position. A fracture may be reduced using local or general anesthesia. If performed by outside manipulation alone, the reduction is said to be closed; if surgery is necessary, it is said to be open. See also **fracture, hernia, invagination, traction. 2.** to decrease the amount, size, extent, or number of something, as of body weight.

reducible hernia /rid(y)ōō′səbəl/ [L, *reducere,* to lead back + *hernia,* rupture], a hernia in which the protruding tissues can be manipulated into a normal position.

reducing agent /rid(y)ōō′sing/ [L, *reducere,* to lead back + *agere,* to do], a substance that donates electrons to another substance in a chemical reaction.

reducing diet. See **reduction diet.**

reduction /riduk′shən/ [L, *reducere*], **1.** also called **hydrogenation.** the addition of hydrogen to a substance. **2.** the removal of oxygen from a substance. **3.** the decrease in the valence of the electronegative part of a compound. **4.** the addition of one or more electrons to a molecule or atom of a substance. **5.** the correction of a fracture, hernia, or luxation. **6.** the reduction of data, as in converting interval data to an ordinal or nominal scale of measurement.

reduction diet, a diet that is low in calories, used for reduction of body weight. The diet must supply fewer calories than the individual expends each day while supplying all the essential nutrients for maintaining health. A diet of this type may provide 1200 calories per day from the basic food groups. Meats are usually broiled, roasted, stewed, or sautéed; vegetables are steamed or eaten raw; starches and fats are limited; and fresh fruits replace desserts. Foods to be avoided are sweetened carbonated beverages, fried foods, pastries, and most snack foods. Vitamin and mineral deficiencies may result if such a diet is not carefully planned. Also called **low-caloric diet, reducing diet.**

reduction division. See **meiosis.**

reductionism /riduk'shəniz'əm/, an approach that tries to explain a form of behavior or an event in terms of a specific category of phenomena, such as biologic, psychologic, or cultural, negating the possibility of an interrelation of causal phenomena.

Reed-Sternberg cell [Dorothy M. Reed, American pathologist, b. 1874; Karl Sternberg, Austrian pathologist, b. 1872], one of a number of large, abnormal, multinucleated reticuloendothelial cells in the lymphatic system found in Hodgkin's disease. The number and proportion of Reed-Sternberg cells identified are the basis for the histopathologic classification of Hodgkin's disease.

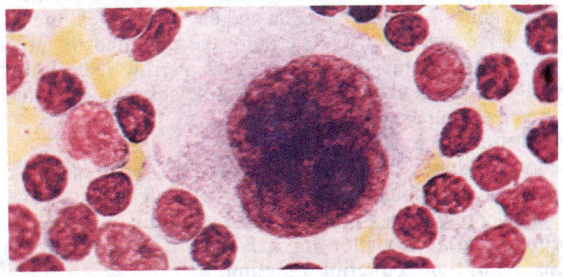

Reed-Sternberg cell (Hayhoe, 1992)

reefer. See **cannabis.**

reentry /rē·en'trē/ [L, re, again; Fr, entree], (in cardiology) the reactivation of myocardial tissue for the second or subsequent time by the same impulse. Reentry is one of the most common arrhythmogenic mechanisms. It is the mechanism of paroxysmal supraventricular tachycardia caused by SA nodal reentry, AV nodal reentry, and AV reentry using the AV node and an accessory pathway, as well as some forms of ventricular tachycardia and extrasystoles. An atrial microreentry circuit is also thought to be the mechanism of atrial flutter. AV and AV nodal mechanisms can be terminated by a vagal maneuver.

refereed journal /ref'ərēd'/ [L, referre, to bring back; diunalis, daily record], a professional or literary journal in which articles or papers are selected for publication by a panel of referees who are experts in the field. They read and evaluate each of the articles submitted for publication. The important national professional journals in medicine and nursing are refereed.

reference electrode /ref'ərəns/ [L, referre + Gk, elektron, amber, hodos, way], an electrode that has an established potential and is used as a reference against which other potentials may be measured.

reference group, a group with which a person identifies or wishes to belong.

referential idea. See **idea of reference.**

referential index deletions /ref'əren'shəl/, a neurolinguistic programing term that pertains to the omission of the specific person being discussed.

referral /rifur'əl/ [L, referre, to bring back], a process whereby a patient or the patient's family is introduced to additional health resources in the community, as in helping a patient find an appropriate community health nurse after discharge from a hospital.

referred pain /rifurd'/ [L, referre + poena, pain], pain felt at a site different from that of an injured or diseased organ or part of the body. Angina, the pain of coronary artery insufficiency, may be felt in the left shoulder, arm, or jaw. In disease of the gallbladder, pain may be felt in the right shoulder or scapular region.

referred sensation, a feeling or impression that occurs at a site other than at which the stimulus is initiated. Also called **reflex sensation.** See also **sensation,** def. 1.

refined birth rate /rifīnd/ [L, re + finire, to finish], the ratio of total births to the total female population, considered during a period of 1 year. Compare **birth rate, crude birth rate, true birth rate.**

refl, abbreviation for reflexive.

reflecting /riflek'ting/, a communication technique in which the listener picks up the feeling tone of the patient's message and repeats it back to the patient. It encourages the patient to continue with clarifying comments.

reflection /riflek'shən/ [L, reflectere, to bend backward], 1. (in cardiology) a form of reentry in which, after encountering delay in one fiber, an impulse enters a parallel fiber and returns retrogradely to its source. 2. (in ultrasonography) the return or reentry of acoustic energy where there is a discontinuity in the characteristic acoustic impedance along the propagation path. The intensity of the reflection is related to the ratio of the characteristic acoustic impedance across the interface.

reflective layer /riflek'tiv/, (in radiology) a thin layer of magnesium oxide or titanium oxide between the phosphor and the base of an intensifying screen. Its function is to intercept and redirect isotropically emitted light from the phosphor to the x-ray film.

reflex /rē'fleks/ [L, reflectere, to bend backward], 1. a backward or return flow of energy or of an image, as a reflection. 2. a reflected action, particularly an involuntary action or movement.

reflex action, the involuntary functioning or movement of any organ or part of the body in response to a particular stimulus. The function or action occurs immediately, without the involvement of the will or consciousness.

reflex apnea, involuntary cessation of respiration caused by irritating, noxious vapors or gases.

reflex arc [L, reflectere, to bend back + arcus, bow], a simple neurologic unit of a sensory neuron that carries a stimulus impulse to the spinal cord where it connects with a motor neuron that carries the reflex impulse back to an appropriate muscle or gland.

reflex bladder. See **spastic bladder.**

reflex center [L, reflectere, to bend back; Gk, kentron], any part of the nervous system in which reception of afferent impulses results in a discharge of efferent impulses leading to some change in a muscle or gland.

reflex dyspepsia, an abnormal condition characterized by

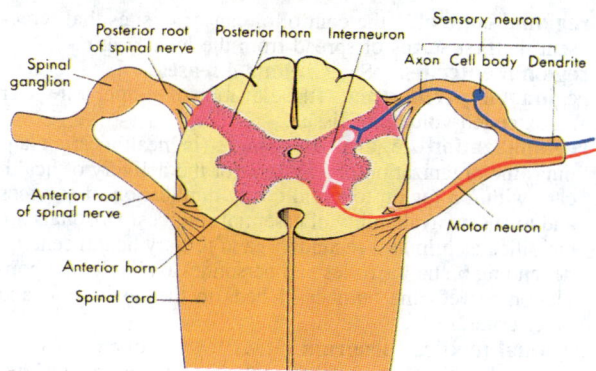

Reflex arc (Chipps, 1992)

impaired digestion associated with the disease of an organ not directly involved with digestion. See also **dyspepsia.**

reflex emesis [L, *reflectere,* to bend back; Gk, *emesis,* vomiting], vomiting or gagging that is induced by touching the mucous membrane of the throat or as a result of other noxious stimuli. Also called **gag reflex, vomiting reflex.**

reflex hammer [L, *reflectere,* to bend back; AS, *hamer*], a percussion mallet with a rubber head used to tap tendons, nerves, or muscles to elicit reflex reactions.

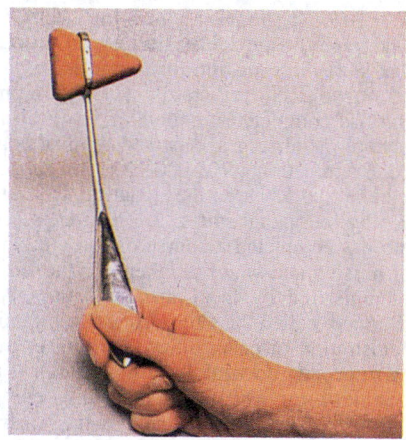

Reflex hammer (Seidel, 1991)

reflex inhibiting pattern (RIP), a conscious set of neuromuscular actions directed toward inhibition of a natural reflex. Examples include actions taken to suppress a sneeze and the learned inhibitions of toilet training.

reflexology /rē'fleksol'əjē/, a system of treating certain disorders by massaging the soles of the feet, using principles similar to those of acupuncture.

reflex sensation. See **referred sensation.**

reflex tachycardia [L, *reflectere,* to bend back; Gk, *tachys,* fast + *kardia,* heart], a rapid heart sinus rhythm caused by a variety of autonomic nervous system effects, such as blood pressure changes, fever, or emotional stress.

reflex vasodilatation [L, *reflectere,* to bend back + *vas,* vessel + *dilatare,* to spread out], any blood vessel dilata-

tion that results from stimulation of vasodilator nerves or inhibition of vasoconstrictors of the sympathetic nervous system, including epinephrine-type drugs.

reflux /rē'fluks/ [L, *refluere,* to flow back], an abnormal backward or return flow of a fluid. Kinds of reflux include **gastroesophageal reflux, hepatojugular reflux,** and **vesicoureteral reflux.**

reflux esophagitis, esophageal irritation and inflammation that results from reflux of the stomach contents into the esophagus.

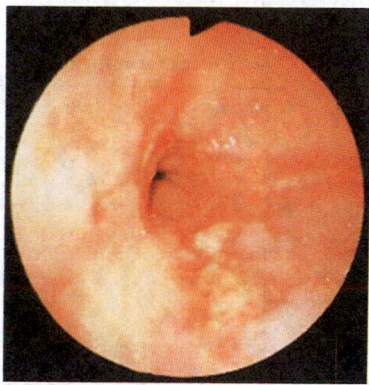

Reflux esophagitis (Winawer, 1992)

refracting angle. See **angle of refraction.**

refracting medium. See **medium.**

refraction /rifrak'shən/ [L, *refringere,* to break up], **1.** the change of direction of energy as it passes from one medium to another of different density. **2.** an examination to determine and to correct refractive errors of the eye. **3.** (in ultrasonography) the phenomenon of bending wave fronts as the acoustic energy propagates from the medium of one acoustic velocity to a second medium of differing acoustic velocity.

refraction of eye [L, *refringere,* to break apart; AS, *éage*], the deflection of light from a straight path through the eye by various ocular tissues, including the cornea, lens, aqueous humor, and vitreous body.

refractive error /rifrak'tiv/, a defect in the ability of the lens of the eye to focus an image accurately, as occurs in nearsightedness and farsightedness.

refractive index, a numeric expression of the refractive power of a medium, as compared with that of air, which has a refractive index value of 1. The refractive index is related to the number, charge, and mass of vibrating particles in the material through which light is passing and may be used as a measure of the total solids in a solution.

refractometer /rē'frəktom'ətər/ [L, *refringere* + Gk, *metron,* measure], an instrument for measuring the refractive index of a substance and used primarily for measuring the refractivity of solutions.

refractoriness /rifrak'tôrines'/, the property of excitable tissue that determines how closely together two action potentials can occur.

refractory /rifrak'tərē/ [L, *refringere*], pertaining to a disorder that is resistant to treatment.

refractory period, the time from phase 0 to the end of

phase 3 of the action potential, divided into effective and relative. In pacing terminology, the period during which a pulse generator is unresponsive to an input signal of specified amplitude. The effective refractory period is from phase 0 to approximately -60 mV during phase 3 of the action potential, a time during which it is impossible for the myocardium to respond with a propagated action potential, or even to a strong stimulus. The **relative refractory period** is from approximately -60 mV during phase 3 to the end of phase 3 of the action potential, the time during which a depressed response is possible to a strong stimulus. Also called **refractory state; refractory phase.**

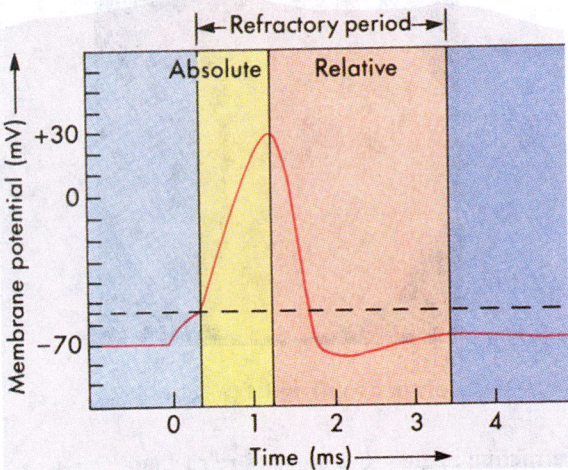

Refractory period *(Thibodeau, 1993/Rolin Graphics)*

reframing /rēfrā'ming/, changing the conceptual and/or emotional viewpoint in relation to which a situation is experienced and placing it in a different frame that fits the "facts" of a concrete situation equally well, thereby changing its entire meaning.

Refsum's syndrome /ref'sŏŏmz/ [Sigvald Refsum, Norwegian physician, b. 1907], a rare, hereditary disorder of lipid metabolism in which phytanic acid cannot be broken down. The syndrome is characterized by ataxia, abnormalities of the bones and skin, peripheral neuropathy, and retinitis pigmentosa. Foods containing phytanic acid must be avoided to prevent progressive deterioration. Also called **phytanic acid storage disease.**

regimen /rej'imən/ [L, guidance], a strictly regulated therapeutic program, such as a diet or exercise schedule.

regional /rē'jənəl/ [L, *regio*, direction], of or pertaining to a geographic area, such as a regional medical facility, or to a part of the body, such as regional anesthesia.

regional anatomy, the study of the structural relationships within the organs and the parts of the body. Kinds of regional anatomy are **surface anatomy** and **cross-sectional anatomy.**

regional anesthesia, anesthesia of an area of the body by injecting a local anesthetic to block a group of sensory nerve fibers. Kinds of regional anesthesia include **brachial plexus anesthesia, caudal anesthesia, epidural anesthesia, intercostal anesthesia, paracervical block, pudendal block,** and **spinal anesthesia.** Compare **general anesthesia, local anesthesia, topical anesthesia.** See also **anesthesia.**

regional control, the control of cancer in sites that represent the first stages of spread from the local origin.

regional enteritis. See **Crohn's disease.**

regional hyperthermia, the elevation of temperature over an extended volume of tissue.

regionalization /rē'jənal'īzā'shən/, (in health care planning) the organization of a system for the delivery of health care within a region to avoid costly duplication of services and to ensure availability of essential services. Hospitals are classified as primary, secondary, and tertiary health centers, depending on the facilities and personnel available, the population served, the number of beds in the institution, and other criteria.

regional medical program (RMP), a program of community health planning that includes all the medical resources available in a region that may be mobilized to meet a specific medical objective. The RMP was authorized by the Health, Disease, Cancer and Stroke Amendments passed by the U.S. Congress in 1965. See also **regionalization.**

region of interest (ROI), (in positron emission tomography) an area that circumscribes a desired anatomic location. Image processing systems permit drawing of ROIs on images. The average parametric value is computed for all pixels within the ROI and returned to the operator.

region of recombination, the first stage of amplitude of an electric signal in a gas-filled radiation detector, when the voltage is very low. No electrons are attracted to the central electrode, and ion pairs produced in the chamber will recombine.

register /rej'istər/ [L, *regerere*, to bring back], (in computed tomography) a device in the central processing unit (CPU) that stores information for future use.

registered nurse (RN) /rej'istərd/, **1.** *U.S.* a professional nurse who has completed a course of study at a state approved school of nursing and passed the National Council Licensure Examination (NCLEX-RN). A registered nurse may use the initials RN after the signature. RNs are licensed to practice by individual states. **2.** *Canada.* a professional nurse who has completed a course of study at an approved school of nursing and who has taken and passed an examination administered by the Canadian Nurses Association Testing Service, called the Comprehensive Examination for Nurse Registration Licensure. See also **nurse, nursing.**

registered record administrator (RRA), a medical record administrator who has successfully completed the credentialing examination conducted by the American Medical Record Association.

registered respiratory therapist (RRT), an allied health professional who has successfully completed the registry examination of the National Board for Respiratory Care (NBRC) and who specializes in scientific knowledge and theory of clinical problems of respiratory care. Usually a 2-year or 4-year college affiliation leading to an associate or bachelor's degree is required. Duties include the collection and evaluation of patient data to determine an appropriate care plan, selection and assembly of equipment, conducting therapeutic procedures and modifying prescribed plans to achieve one or more specific objectives.

registered technologist (R.T.), a title awarded by the American Registry of Radiologic Technologists as certification of qualification to act as an x-ray technologist. See also **radiologic technologist.**

registrar /rej'isträr/, an administrative officer whose responsibility is to maintain the records of an institution.

registration /rej'istrā'shən/ [L, *registratio*], **1.** a learning or memory recording made in the central nervous system of an impression resulting from a stimulus. **2.** the recording of vital personal information, such as health data. **3.** the recording of professional qualification information relevant to government licensing regulations.

registry /rej'istrē/ [L, *regerere*, to bring back], **1.** an office or agency in which lists of nurses and records pertaining to nurses seeking employment are maintained. **2.** (in epidemiology) a listing service for incidence data pertaining to the occurrence of specific diseases or disorders, such as a tumor registry.

Regitine, a trademark for an alpha-adrenergic blocking agent (phentolamine hydrochloride).

Regonol, a trademark for a neuromuscular blocking agent (pyridostigmine), used as an adjunct to anesthesia.

regression /rigresh'ən/ [L, *regredi*, to go back], **1.** a retreat or backward movement in conditions, signs, or symptoms. **2.** a return to an earlier, more primitive form of behavior. **3.** a tendency in physical development to become more typical of the population than of the parents, such as a child who attains a height closer to the average than that of tall or short parents. **–regress,** *v.*

Regroton, a trademark for a cardiovascular, fixed-combination drug containing a diuretic (chlorthalidone) and an antihypertensive (reserpine).

regular diet /reg'yələr/ [L, *regula*, rule], a full, well-balanced diet containing all of the essential nutrients needed for optimal growth, repair of the tissues, and normal functioning of the organs. Such a diet contains foods rich in proteins, carbohydrates, fats, minerals, and vitamins in proportions that meet the specific caloric requirements of the individual. Also called **full diet, normal diet.**

regular insulin, a fast-acting, insulin prescribed in the treatment of diabetes mellitus when the desired action is prompt, intense, and short-acting. Regular insulin prepared from zinc insulin crystals is slightly longer-acting than the amorphous noncrystalline form of this type of insulin preparation. Regular insulin injection is the only form of insulin suitable for intramuscular administration.

regulative cleavage. See **indeterminate cleavage.**

regulative development /reg'yələ'tiv/ [L, *regula*, rule], a type of embryonic development in which the fertilized ovum undergoes indeterminate cleavage, producing blastomeres that have similar developmental potencies and are each capable of giving rise to a single embryo. Determination of the particular organs and parts of the embryo occurs during later stages of development and is influenced by inductors and intercellular interaction. Damage or destruction of various cells during the early stages of development results in readjustments and substitutions so that a normal organism is formed. Compare **mosaic development.**

regulator gene /reg'yələ'tər/, (in molecular genetics) a genetic unit that regulates or suppresses the activity of one or more structural genes. Also called **repressor gene.**

regulatory sequence /reg'yələtôr'ē/ [L, *regula* + *sequi,* to follow], (in molecular genetics) a series of DNA nucleotides that regulate the expression of a gene.

regurgitant menstruation. See **retrograde menstruation.**

regurgitant murmur /rigur'jitənt/ [L, *re-, gurgitare,* to flow back + *murmur,* humming], a heart murmur caused by a defective valve as blood flows backwards through the partly closed valve cusps. Kinds of regurgitant murmurs include diastolic, pansystolic, and systolic.

regurgitation [L, *re,* again, *gurgitare,* to flood], **1.** the

backward flow from the normal direction, as the return of swallowed food into the mouth. **2.** the backward flow of blood through a defective heart valve, named for the affected valve, as in **aortic regurgitation.** See also **reflux.**

regurgitation jaundice /rēgur'jitā'shən/ [L, *re-, gurgitare,* to flow back; Fr, *jaune,* yellow], jaundice caused by bile pigment entering the blood and lymphatic systems as a result of biliary obstruction.

rehabilitation (rehab) /rē'habilitā'shən/ [L, *re + habitalas,* aptitude], the restoration of an individual or a part to normal or near normal function after a disabling disease, injury, addiction, or incarceration. **–rehabilitate,** *v.*

rehabilitation center, a facility providing therapy and training for rehabilitation. The center may offer occupational therapy, physical therapy, vocational training, and special training, such as speech therapy. See also **rehabilitation.**

Rehfuss stomach tube /rā'fəs/ [Martin E. Rehfuss, American physician, b.1887], a specially designed gastric tube with a graduated syringe, used for withdrawing specimens of the contents of the stomach for study after a test meal.

rehydration /rē'hīdrā'shən/ [L, *re-;* Gk, *hydor,* water], restoration of normal water balance in a patient by giving fluids orally or intravenously.

Reid's base line [Robert W. Reid, Scottish anatomist, b. 1851], the base line of the skull, a hypothetic line extending from the infraorbital point to the superior border of the external auditory meatus. Also called **anthropologic base line, Frankfurt line.**

Reifenstein's syndrome /rī'fənstīnz/ [Edward C. Reifenstein, Jr., American physician, b. 1908], male hypogonadism of unknown origin, marked by azoospermia, undescended testes, gynecomastia, testosterone deficiency, and elevated gonadotropin titers. The condition appears to be inherited as an x-linked recessive trait, but no chromosomal abnormality has been identified.

reimbursement /rē'imburs'mənt/ [L, *re + im,* in; Fr, *bourse,* purse], a method of payment, usually by a third-party payer, for medical treatment or hospital costs. Cost-based reimbursement covers payment for all allowable costs incurred in the provision of services to patients included in a contract. Prospective reimbursement provides for additional payment by which costs incurred in providing services to patients are based on actual costs determined at the end of a fiscal period.

reinforcement /rē'infôrs'mənt/ [L, *re +* Fr, *enforcir,* to strengthen], (in psychology) a process in which a response is strengthened by the fear of punishment or the anticipation of reward.

reinforcement-extinction, a process of socialization in which one learns to engage in certain behaviors (reinforcement) or to avoid certain behaviors (extinction). The anticipated result is that the reinforced behaviors become habitual and those that undergo extinction disappear.

reinforcer /rē'infôr'sər/, (in psychology) a consequence that increases the probability that an operant will recur.

Reiter's syndrome /rī'tərz/ [Hans Reiter, German physician, b. 1862], an arthritic disorder of adult males, believed to result from a myxovirus or *Mycoplasma* infection. The syndrome most often affects the ankles, feet, and sacroiliac joints and is usually associated with conjunctivitis and urethritis. The onset may be marked by unexplained diarrhea and low-grade fever, followed in 2 to 4 weeks by conjunctivitis. Lesions that become superficial ulcers may form on the palms and the soles. Arthritis usually persists after the conjunctivitis and urethritis subside, but it may become episodic. Treatment includes a short course of tetracycline to treat the infection and phenylbutazone to relieve pain and inflammation in the joint. Recovery is expected, but recurrent arthritic symptoms may continue for several years.

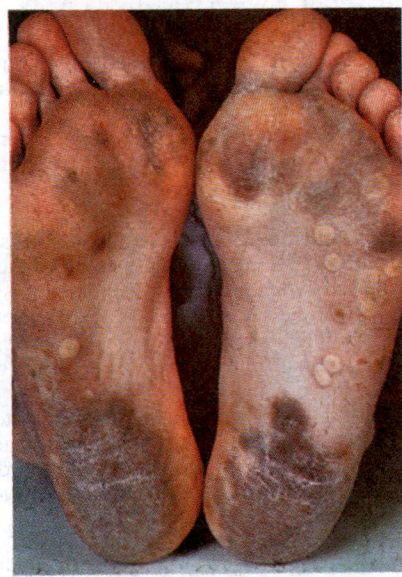

Lesions on the feet in Reiter's syndrome
(Boyle, 1981)

reject analysis /rē′jekt/, (in radiology) the study of repeated radiographs to determine the cause for their being discarded.

rejection /rijek′shən/ [L, *re + jacere*, to throw], **1.** (in medicine) an immunologic response to organisms or substances that the system recognizes as foreign, including grafts or transplants. **2.** (in psychiatry) the act of excluding or denying affection to another person.

rejunctive /rijungk′tiv/, (in contextual psychotherapy,) pertaining to a relationship that is characterized by moves toward trustworthy relatedness.

rejuvenation /rējōō′vənā′shən/ [L, *re-, juvenis,* youth], the restoration of youthful health and vitality.

Rela, a trademark for a skeletal muscle relaxant (carisoprodol).

relapse /rilaps′/ [L, *relabi,* to slide back], **1.** to exhibit again the symptoms of a disease from which a patient appears to have recovered. **2.** the recurrence of a disease after apparent recovery.

relapsing [L, *relabi,* to fall back], pertaining to the return of disease after a period of apparent recovery.

relapsing fever, any one of several acute infectious diseases, marked by recurrent febrile episodes, caused by various strains of the spirochete *Borrelia.* The disease is transmitted by both lice and ticks and is often seen during wars and famines. It has occurred in several western states of the United States but is more commonly found in South America, Asia, and Africa. The first episode usually starts with a sudden high fever (104° to 105° F), accompanied by chills, headache, neuromuscular pains, and nausea. A rash may appear over the trunk and extremities, and jaundice is common during the later stages. Each attack lasts 2 or 3 days and culminates in a crisis of high fever, profuse sweating, and a rise in heart and respiratory rate. This is followed by an abrupt drop in temperature and a return to normal blood pressure. People typically relapse after 7 to 10 days of normal temperature and eventually recover completely. In louse-borne disease, there is usually only a single relapse; in tick-borne disease, several successively milder relapses may occur. For a diagnosis to be made, the spirochete must be seen on a blood smear obtained during an attack. Treatment is with a long-acting penicillin, tetracycline, or chloramphenicol. Antimicrobial therapy may induce a Herxheimer reaction, therefore treatment is withheld during a febrile crisis. Bed rest, sponge baths, and aspirin alleviate the symptoms. Disinfection of clothing and bedding is necessary to destroy any lice or ticks. Also called **African tick fever, famine fever, recurrent fever, spirillum fever, tick fever.**

relapsing polychondritis, a rare disease of unknown cause resulting in inflammation and destruction of cartilage with replacement by fibrous tissue. Autoimmunity may be involved in this condition. Most commonly the ears and noses of middle-aged people are affected with episodes of tender swelling, often accompanied by fever, arthralgias, and episcleritis. Consequences include floppy ears, collapsed nose, hearing loss, or hoarseness and airway obstruction because of laryngeal and tracheal cartilage involvement. Corticosteroids suppress the activity of the disease.

relation searching /rilā′shən/ [L, *relatio*], (in nursing research) a study design used to discover and describe relationships between and among variables. It may be used to describe various nursing situations to examine the efficacy of certain aspects of nursing care.

relationship therapy /rilā′shənship′/ [L, *relatio* + AS, *scieppan,* to shape], a therapy that is based on a totality of client-therapist relationship and encourages the growth of self in the client. It has been described as "an experience in living that takes place within a relationship with another person."

relative biologic effectiveness (RBE) /rel′ətiv/ [L, *relatio*], (in radiotherapy) a measure of the cell-killing ability of a particular radiation compared with a reference radiation. The reference is 250 keV x-rays. The ratio of cells killed with the test radiation over that of the 250 keV radiation is the RBE.

relative centrifugal force (RCF), a method of comparing the force generated by various centrifuges based on the speeds of rotation and distances from the center of rotation.

relative cephalopelvic disproportion. See **cephalopelvic disproportion.**

relative growth, the comparison of the various increases in size of similar organisms, tissues, or structures at different time intervals.

relative humidity, the amount of moisture in the air compared with the maximum the air could contain at the same temperature.

relative periodontal pocket. See **periodontal pocket.**

relative refractory period. See **refractory period.**

relative risk, the ratio of the frequency of a certain disorder in groups exposed and groups not exposed to a particular hereditary or environmental factor, such as cigarette smoking or inhaling of cigarette smoke by nonsmokers. In many cases, the relative risk is modified by the duration or intensity of exposure to the causative factors.

relative sterility [L, *relatio* + *sterilis,* barren], a condition of infertility in which one or more factors tend to reduce the chances of becoming pregnant. See also **sterility.**

relative value unit, a comparable service measure used by hospitals to permit comparison of the amounts of resources required to perform various services within a single department or between departments. It is determined by assigning weight to such factors as personnel time, level of skill, and sophistication of equipment required to render patient services.

relativism. See **cultural relativism.**

relax /rilaks′/ [L, *relaxare,* to ease], to reduce tension.

relaxant /rilak′sənt/ [L, *relaxare,* to ease], a drug or other agent that tends to reduce tension, as a muscle relaxant or bowel relaxant.

relaxation /rē′laksā′shən/ [L, *relaxare,* to ease], **1.** a reducing of tension, as when a muscle relaxes between contractions. **2.** (in magnetic resonance imaging) the return of excited nuclei to their normal unexcited state by the release of energy.

relaxation oven, (in mammography) a part of the xerographic plate conditioner system used to eliminate ghost images. The plate is heated in the oven so that any residual electrostatic charge on the surface will be removed.

relaxation response, a protective mechanism against stress that brings about decreased heart rate, lower metabolism, and decreased respiratory rate. It is the physiologic opposite of the 'fight or flight,' or stress, response.

relaxation therapy, treatment in which patients are taught to perform breathing and relaxation exercises and to concentrate on a pleasant situation. An integral part of the Lamaze method of childbirth, relaxation therapy is also used to relieve various kinds of pain and physical manifestations of stress. Various yoga exercises and aspects of hypnotherapy may be included in the treatment program, and biofeedback techniques may be used to demonstrate actions that induce relaxation. Some patients learn through relaxation therapy to relax taut muscles at will, to abort migraine attacks, or to reduce their blood pressure. See also **Lamaze method.**

relaxation time, (in MRI) the characteristic time it takes for a sample of atoms, whose nuclei have first been aligned along a static magnetic field and then excited to a higher energy (MR) state by a radiofrequency signal, to return to a lower energy equilibrium state. Two time parameters are used to describe the return, or relaxation, to the equilibrium state once the rf source is turned off. T_1 describes the relaxation of the system of spins into a condition of thermal equilibrium with its surroundings, whereas T_2 describes the relaxation of the energy that is traded within the system itself. Maps or 'images' of the values of T_1 or T_2 as a function of position in the cross-sectional view can be made.

relaxin /rilak′sin/, a hormone obtained from the corpora lutea of swine and used to relax the pelvic ligaments and dilate the cervix during labor. The medication has also been used to treat dysmenorrhea.

release therapy /rilēs/ [ME, *relesen,* to release], a type of pediatric psychotherapy used to treat children with stress and anxiety related to a specific, recent event.

releasing hormone (RH), one of several peptides produced by the hypothalamus and secreted directly into the anterior pituitary via a connecting vein. Each of the releas-ing hormones stimulates the pituitary to secrete a specific tropic hormone; thus, corticotropic releasing hormone stimulates the pituitary to secrete adrenocorticotropic hormone, whereas growth hormone releasing hormone stimulates the secretion of growth hormone. Also called **releasing factor.**

releasing stimulus, (in psychology) an action or behavior by one individual that serves as a cue to trigger a response in others. An example is yawning by one person, which results in yawning by others in the group.

reliability /rilī′əbil′itē/ [L, *religare,* to fasten behind], (in research) the extent to which a test measurement or a device produces the same results with different investigators, observers, or administration of the test over time. If repeated use of the same measurement tool on the same sample produces the same consistent results, the measurement is considered reliable.

relief area [L, *relevare,* to lighten], the portion of the tissue surface under prosthesis on which pressures are reduced or eliminated.

relieving factor /rilē′ving/, an agent that alleviates a symptom.

religiosity /rilij′ē·os′itē/ [L, *religiosus,*], a psychiatric symptom characterized by the demonstration of excessive or affected piety.

-relin, a combining form for prehormones or hormone-release stimulating peptides.

reline /rēlīn/ [L, *re* + *linea*], the resurfacing of the tissue side of a denture with new base material.

-relix, a combining form for hormone-release inhibiting peptides.

relocation stress syndrome /rē′lōkā′shən/, a nursing diagnosis accepted by the Tenth National Conference on the Classification of Nursing Diagnoses. It is defined as physiologic and/or psychosocial disturbances as a result of a transfer from one environment to another. The major defining characteristics are a change in environment or location, anxiety, apprehension, increased confusion (elderly population), depression, and loneliness. The minor defining characteristics are a verbalization of unwillingness to relocate, sleep disturbance, change in eating habits, dependency, GI disturbances, increased verbalization of needs, insecurity, lack of trust, restlessness, sad affect, unfavorable comparison of post/pretransfer staff, verbalization of being concerned or upset about the transfer, vigilance, weight change, and withdrawal. Related factors include past, concurrent, and recent losses, losses involved with decision to move, feeling of powerlessness, lack of adequate support system, little or no preparation for the impending move, moderate to high degree of environmental change, history and types of previous transfers, impaired psychosocial health status, and decreased physical health status. See also **nursing diagnosis.**

rem /rem, är′ē′em′/, abbreviation for *roentgen equivalent man.* A dose of ionizing radiation that produces in humans the same effect as one roentgen of x-radiation or gamma radiation. See also **sievert.**

REM /rem, är′ē′em′/, abbreviation for **rapid eye movement.** See also **sleep.**

remasking /rēmas′king/, (in digital fluoroscopy) the production of one or more additional mask images if the first is inadequate due to patient motion, noise, or other factors. See also **mask image.**

remedial /rimē′dē·əl/ [L, *remediare,* to cure], designed to improve or cure.

reminiscence /rem′inis′əns/ [L, *reminisci,* to remember], the recollection of past personal experiences and significant events.

reminiscence therapy, a psychotherapeutic technique in which self-esteem and personal satisfaction are restored, particularly in older persons, by encouraging patients to review past experiences of a pleasant nature.

remission /rimish′ən/ [L, *remittere,* to abate], the partial or complete disappearance of the clinical and subjective characteristics of a chronic or malignant disease. Remission may be spontaneous or the result of therapy. In some cases remission is permanent and the disease is cured. Compare **cure.**

remittent fever /rimit′ənt/ [L, *remittere + febris,* fever], diurnal variations of an elevated temperature with exacerbations and remissions but never a return to normal.

remnant radiation /rem′nənt/ [L, *remanere,* to remain], the measurable radiation that passes through an object and can produce an image on radiographic film.

remodeling /rēmod′əling/ [L, *re- + modus,* to copy again], the process of changing a body part or area, as in reconstructive surgery.

remote afterloading /rimōt′/ [L, *removere,* to remove], (in radiotherapy) a technique in which an applicator, such as an acrylic mold of an area to be irradiated, is placed in or on the patient and then loaded from a safe source with a high-activity radioisotope. The mold or applicator contains grooves for the insertion of nylon tubes into which the radioactive material can be introduced. Remote afterloading is used in the treatment of head, neck, vaginal, and cervical tumors.

remotivation /rē′mōtivā′shən/ [L, *re + motus,* movement], the use of special techniques that stimulate patients to become motivated to learn and interact.

remotivation group, a treatment group that is organized with the purpose of stimulating the interest, awareness, and communication of withdrawn and institutionalized mental patients.

removable lingual arch /rimōō′vəbəl/ [L, *removere,* to remove], an orthodontic arch wire designed to fit the lingual surface of the teeth and aid orthodontic movement of the dentition involved. Two posts soldered to each end of the wire fit snugly into the vertical tubes of the associated molar anchor bands.

removable orthodontic appliance, a device placed inside the mouth to correct or alleviate malocclusion and designed to be removed or replaced by the patient.

removable partial denture. See **partial denture.**

removable rigid dressing, a dressing similar to a cast used to encase the stump of an amputated limb. It is usually applied to permit the fitting of a temporary prosthesis so that ambulation can begin soon after surgery.

ren-, a combining form meaning 'of or pertaining to the kidneys': *renicardiac, reniform, renocortical.*

renal /rē′nəl/ [L, *ren,* kidney], of or pertaining to the kidney.

renal acidosis [L, *ren,* kidney + *acidus,* sour; Gk, *osis,* condition], an excessive increase in the H⁺ ions in body fluids because of impaired kidney function. The acidosis can result from excessive loss of bicarbonate or from the inability to excrete phosphoric and sulfuric acid.

renal adenocarcinoma. See **renal cell carcinoma.**

renal angiography, a radiographic examination of the renal artery and associated blood vessels, after the injection of a contrast medium.

renal anuria, cessation of urine production caused by intrinsic renal disease.

renal artery, one of a pair of large, visceral branches of the abdominal aorta, arising caudal to the superior mesenteric artery at the level of the disk between the first and second lumbar vertebrae. The left renal artery is somewhat more cranial than the right. Before reaching the kidney, each divides into four branches. The renal arteries supply the kidneys, suprarenal glands, and the ureters.

renal biopsy, the removal of kidney tissue for microscopic examination, conducted to establish the diagnosis of a renal disorder and to aid in determining the stage of the disease, the appropriate therapy, and the prognosis. An open biopsy involves an incision, permits better visualization of the kidney, and carries a lower risk of hemorrhage; a closed or percutaneous biopsy performed by aspirating a specimen of tissue with a needle requires a shorter period of recovery and is less likely to cause infection.

■ METHOD: Before biopsy, the procedure is explained and the patient is medically evaluated and tested for bleeding or coagulation time. The patient's blood is usually typed and crossmatched with two units of donor blood that are held for a possible transfusion until there is no threat of bleeding after the procedure. An open biopsy is generally carried out in the operating room, but the percutaneous procedure may be performed in the radiology department or in the patient's room. The location of the kidney, determined by a plain x-ray film, dye contrast study, or fluoroscopic examination, is marked on the patient's skin in ink for a needle biopsy. The patient is then placed prone over a sandbag and soft pillow with the body bent at the level of the diaphragm, the shoulders on the bed, and the spine in straight alignment. A local anesthetic is injected, and the physician inserts the biopsy needle in the lower pole of the kidney, because this area contains the smallest number of large renal vessels. The needle is quickly withdrawn, and, after pressure is applied to the site for 20 minutes, a pressure bandage is applied; the patient is turned and kept supine and motionless for the next 4 hours. The dressing, blood pressure, and pulse are checked every 15 to 60 minutes for 2 hours, the temperature every 4 hours for 24 hours; excessive drainage, decreased blood pressure, tachycardia, or elevated temperature is reported to the physician. Fluids are forced to the maximum allotted for the patient's condition; the amount and character of urinary output are noted, and the physician is informed if hematuria occurs. The patient is kept in bed for at least 24 hours and is cautioned not to lift any heavy objects for 10 days.

■ NURSING INTERVENTION: The nurse offers an explanation of the procedure, prepares and positions the patient for the percutaneous procedure, and, on its completion, provides care and emotional support.

■ OUTCOME CRITERIA: A biopsy is the most accurate measure for determining the nature and stage of a renal pathologic condition.

renal calculus, a concretion occurring in the kidney. If the stone is large enough to block the ureter and stop the flow of urine from the kidney, it must be removed by either major surgical or radiologic fluoroscopy procedures. Also called **kidney stone, nephritic calculus.** See also **nephroscope.**

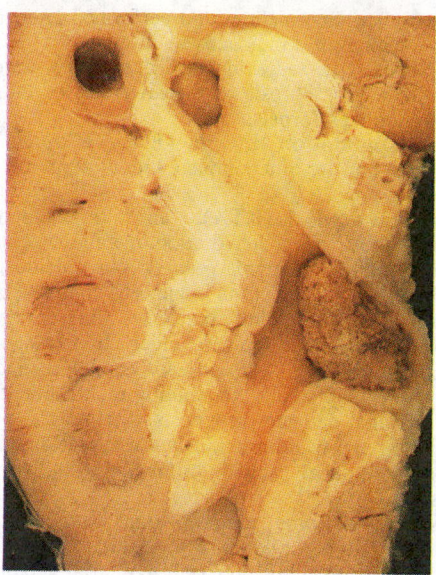

Renal calculus (Fletcher, 1987)

renal calyx, the first unit in the system of ducts in the kidney carrying urine from the renal pyramid of the cortex to the renal pelvis for excretion through the ureters. There are two divisions: The **minor calyx,** with several others, drains into a larger **major calyx,** which in turn joins other major calyces to form the renal pelvis.

renal capsule [L, *ren,* kidney + *capsula,* little box], a protective connective tissue capsule surrounding the kidney.

renal cell carcinoma, a malignant neoplasm of the kidney, composed predominantly of large cells with clear cytoplasm that originate in tubular epithelium. The tumor may develop in any part of the kidney, becoming a large mass that may grow into the tributaries of the renal vein. Hematuria and pain are usually present. Metastasis, especially to the lungs and bones, may occur early in the course of development. Treatment includes surgery and radiotherapy. Also called **adenocarcinoma of the kidney, clear cell carcinoma of the kidney.** See also **Wilms' tumor.**

renal colic, sharp, severe pain in the lower back over the kidney, radiating forward into the groin. Renal colic usually accompanies forcible dilatation of a ureter followed by spasm as a stone is lodged or passed through it. See also **urinary calculus.**

renal corpuscle. See **malpighian corpuscle.**

renal cortex, the soft, granular, outer layer of the kidney, containing approximately 1.25 million glomeruli, which remove body wastes in the form of urine.

renal dialysis [L, *ren,* kidney; Gk, *dia,* + *lysis,* loosening], a process of diffusing blood across a semipermeable membrane to remove substances that a normal kidney would eliminate, including poisons, drugs, urea, uric acid, and creatinine. Renal dialysis may restore electrolytes and acid-base imbalances. See also **continuous ambulatory peritoneal dialysis, hemodialysis.**

renal diet, a diet prescribed in chronic renal failure and designed to control the intake of protein, potassium, sodium, phosphorus, and fluids, depending on individual conditions. Carbohydrates and fats are the principal sources of energy. Protein is limited; the amount is determined by the patient's condition and is usually supplied from milk, eggs, and meat. Cereals, bread, rice, and pasta are the primary sources of calories. Some vegetables and fruits are included, depending on the degree of restriction of potassium and phosphorus. Special commercial flours and breads have been developed that are protein-free and low in potassium and sodium. The low potassium level of the diet also makes it useful in hyperkalemia. The diet is nutritionally inadequate and should be supplemented with vitamins and electrolytes. See also **Giordano-Giovannetti diet.**

renal dwarf, a dwarf whose retarded growth is caused by renal failure.

renal failure, inability of the kidneys to excrete wastes, concentrate urine, and conserve electrolytes. The condition may be acute or chronic. **Acute renal failure** is characterized by oliguria and by the rapid accumulation of nitrogenous wastes in the blood. It is caused by hemorrhage, trauma, burn, toxic injury to the kidney, acute pyelonephritis or glomerulonephritis, or lower urinary tract obstruction. Many forms of acute renal failure are reversible after the underlying cause has been identified. Treatment includes restricted intake of fluids and of all substances that require excretion by the kidney. Antibiotics and diuretics are also used. **Chronic renal failure** may result from many other diseases. The early signs include sluggishness, fatigue, and mental dullness. Later, anuria, convulsions, GI bleeding, malnutrition, and various neuropathies may occur. The skin may turn yellow-brown and become covered with uremic frost. Congestive heart failure and hypertension are frequent complications, the results of hypervolemia. Urinalysis reveals greater than normal amounts of urea and creatinine, waxy casts, and a constant volume of urine regardless of variations in water intake. Anemia frequently occurs. The prognosis depends on the underlying cause. Treatment usually includes restricted water and protein intake and the use of diuretics. When medical measures have been exhausted,

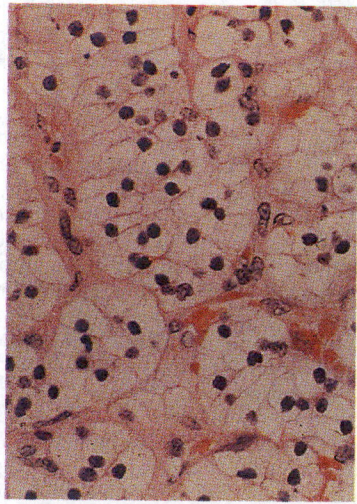

Renal cell carcinoma (Weiss, 1988)

long-term hemodialysis is often begun, and kidney transplantation is considered.

renal glycosuria [L, *ren*, kidney; Gk, *glykys*, sweet + *ouron*, urine], a familial condition characterized by lowered renal threshold to sugar. Blood sugar levels may be normal although sugar is excreted in the urine.

renal hematuria [L, *ren*, kidney; Gk, *haima*, blood + *ouron*, urine], presence of blood in the urine because of a kidney disorder.

renal hypertension, hypertension resulting from kidney disease, including chronic glomerulonephritis, chronic pyelonephritis, renal carcinoma, and renal calculi. Analgesic abuse and certain drug reactions may also result in renal hypertension. Therapy depends on the cause and may include administration of antibiotics or diuretics or surgery. Untreated renal hypertension is likely to result in kidney damage and cardiovascular disease.

renal insufficiency [L, *ren*, kidney + *in*, + *sufficere,* to suffice], partial kidney function failure characterized by less than normal urine excretion.

renal nanism, dwarfism associated with infantile renal osteodystrophy.

renal osteodystrophy, a condition resulting from chronic renal failure and characterized by uneven bone growth and demineralization. See also **renal nanism, renal rickets.**

renal papilla. See **papilla.**

renal pelvis [L, *ren,* + *pelvis,* basin], a funnel-shaped dilatation that drains urine from the kidney into the ureter.

renal pyramid [L, *ren,* kidney; Gk, *pyramis*], one of the conical masses of tissue that form the kidney medulla. The base of each pyramid adjoins the kidney's cortex. The pyramids consist of the loops of Henle and the collecting tubules of the nephrons.

renal rickets, a condition characterized by rachitic changes in the skeleton and caused by chronic nephritis. See also **renal osteodystrophy.**

renal scan, a scan of the kidneys to determine their size, shape, and exact position, used to aid in the diagnosis of a

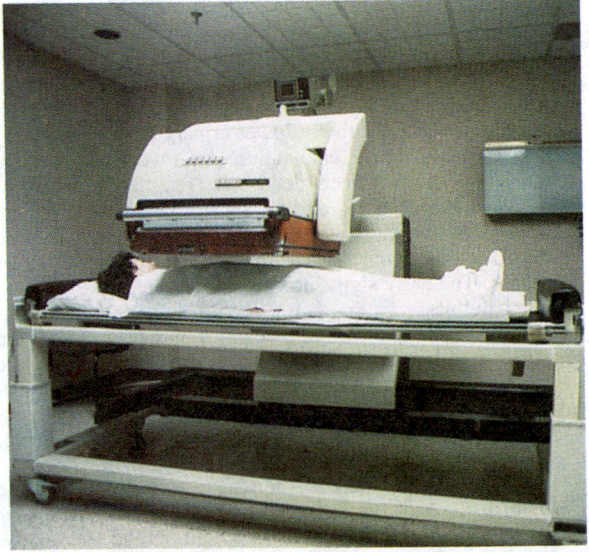

Equipment for renal scan (Brundage, 1992)

tumor or other abnormalities and performed after the intravenous injection of a radioactive substance.

renal sclerosis [L, *ren*, kidney; Gk, *skerosis*, hardening], arteriosclerosis or fibrosis of the arterioles of the kidney. See also **nephrosclerosis.**

renal transplantation [L, *ren*, kidney + *transplantare*], the surgical transfer of a complete kidney from a donor to a recipient.

renal tubular acidosis (RTA), an abnormal condition associated with persistent dehydration, metabolic acidosis, hypokalemia, hyperchloremia, and nephrocalcinosis. It is caused by the inability of the kidneys to conserve bicarbonate and to adequately acidify the urine. Some forms of RTA are more prevalent in women, older children, and young adults. Prolonged RTA can cause hypercalciuria and the formation of kidney stones. Depending on treatment and the extent of renal damage, prognosis is usually good. Compare **distal renal tubular acidosis, ketoacidosis, metabolic acidosis, proximal renal tubular acidosis, respiratory acidosis.**

■ OBSERVATIONS: Some common signs and symptoms of RTA, especially in children, may include anorexia, vomiting, constipation, retarded growth, polyuria, nephrocalcinosis, and rickets. In children and adults RTA can also cause urinary tract infections and pyelonephritis. Confirming diagnosis of distal RTA is based on laboratory tests that show impaired urine acidification in association with systemic metabolic acidosis. Confirming diagnosis of proximal RTA is based on tests that show bicarbonate wasting as a result of impaired reabsorption. Other significant laboratory findings may show decreased sodium bicarbonate, pH, potassium, and phosphorus; increased serum chloride, alkaline phosphatase, urinary bicarbonate, and potassium; and urine with low specific gravity.

■ INTERVENTIONS: Treatment seeks to replace excessively secreted substances, especially bicarbonate, and may include the administration of sodium bicarbonate tablets, potassium to counter low potassium levels, vitamin D to preserve calcium metabolism, and antibiotics to counter pyelonephritis. Surgery may be required to excise renal calculi.

■ NURSING CONSIDERATIONS: The nurse carefully monitors all laboratory tests, especially those involving potassium levels and urine pH. The urine of the patient is strained to capture any kidney stones for analysis, and the nurse is alert to any signs of hematuria. Patients with low potassium levels are usually advised to eat potassium-rich foods, such as bananas, oranges, and baked potatoes. The patient and family also benefit from advice and encouragement in seeking genetic counseling and RTA screening.

renal tubule [L, *ren*, kidney + *tubulus*, small tube], the part of the kidney's nephron that leads from the glomerulus to the collecting tubules. It consists of a looping segment and two convoluted sections. These are reabsorptive canals that secrete, collect, and conduct urine.

Rendu-Osler-Weber syndrome. See **Osler-Weber-Rendu syndrome.**

Renese, a trademark for a diuretic and antihypertensive (polythiazide).

renin /rē′nin/ [L, *ren,* kidney], a proteolytic enzyme, produced by and stored in the juxtaglomerular apparatus that surrounds each arteriole as it enters a glomerulus. The enzyme affects the blood pressure by catalyzing the change of angiotensinogen to angiotensin, a strong pressor. Normal findings of adult plasma renin, measured in an upright position and sodium depleted, are 2.9-10.8 ng/ml/hr. Compare **rennin.**

renin test. See **plasma renin activity.**

rennin /ren'in/ [ME, *rennen,* to run], a milk-curdling enzyme that occurs in the gastric juices of infants and is also contained in the rennet produced in the stomach of calves and other ruminants. It is an endopeptidase that converts casein to paracasein and was formerly used extensively as a curdling agent by the cheese industry. An artificially produced microbial rennet, rather than the enzyme extracted from rennet in calves, is used in one half of the cheese produced in the United States today. Compare **renin.**

renogram /rē'nəgram/, a graphic image made by a radiographic scan of the kidneys after injection of a radiopharmaceutic. It represents radioactivity versus time and is used to assess renal function.

-renone, a combining form for spironolactone-type aldosterone antagonists.

Renshaw cells /ren'shô/ [B. Renshaw, American neurologist, b. 1911; L, *cella,* storeroom], small cells that reduce motor neuron discharge through a feedback circuit involving axon collaterals that excite interneurons. The system prevents rapid repeated firing of motor neurons.

reovirus /rē'ōvī'rəs/ [*respiratory enteric orphan* + L, *virus*], any one of three ubiquitous, double-stranded RNA viruses found in the respiratory and alimentary tracts in healthy and in sick people. Reoviruses have been implicated in some cases of upper respiratory tract disease and infantile gastroenteritis.

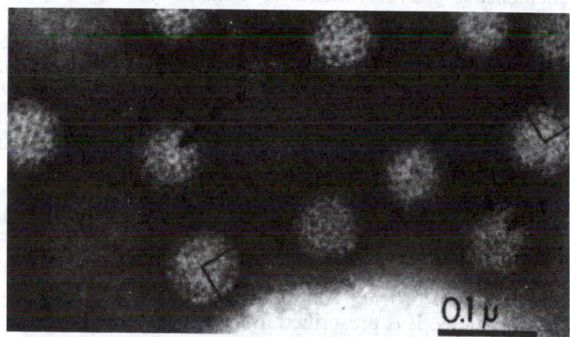

Reovirus structure
(Murray, 1990; From Luftig RB et al: Virology 48:170, 1972)

repercussion /rē'pərkush'ən/ [L, *repercussio,* rebounding], **1.** (in obstetrics) ballottement. **2.** being driven back by a powerful resistance. **3.** the reduction of a swelling or tumor.

repetition compulsion [L, *repetere,* to repeat], an unconscious need to revert to and repeat earlier situations, patterns of behavior, and acts to experience previously felt emotions or relationships. See also **compulsion.**

replacement /riplās'mənt/ [Fr, *replacer,* to put in place again], the substitution of a missing part or substance with a similar structure or substance, such as the replacement of an amputated limb with a prosthesis or the replacement of lost blood with donor blood.

replacement therapy, **1.** the use of a medicinal product to replace a natural hormone or enzyme that the body is no longer able to produce in sufficient amounts. **2.** a psychotherapeutic technique of replacing abnormal behavior with healthy, constructive activities.

replacement transfusion, the removal of all or most of a patient's diseased blood and its simultaneous replacement with an equal volume of normal blood.

replication /rep'likā'shən/ [L, *replicare,* to fold back], **1.** a process of duplicating, reproducing, or copying; literally, a folding back of a part to form a duplicate. **2.** (in research) the exact repetition of an experiment performed to confirm the initial findings. **3.** (in genetics) the duplication of the polynucleotide strands of DNA or the synthesis of DNA. The process involves the unwinding of the double helix molecule to form two single strands, each of which acts as a template for the synthesis of a complementary strand. The two resulting molecules of DNA each contain one new and one parental strand, which coil to form the double helix. **–replicate,** *v.*

replicator /rep'likā'tər/ [L, *replicare*], (in genetics) the segment of the DNA molecule that initiates and controls the replication of the polynucleotide strands.

replicon /rep'ləkon/ [L, *replicare*], (in genetics) a replication unit; the segment of the DNA molecule that is undergoing replication. The unit is regulated by a section of the molecule called the regulator, which controls replication and coordinates it with cell division.

Repligen, trademark for an HIV vaccine that contains a gp120 V3 loop. The V3 loop generates neutralizing antibodies that block the HIV virus from infecting helper T cells.

repolarization /rēpō'lərīzā'shən/ [L, *re + polus,* pole; Gk, *izein* to cause], (in cardiology) the process by which the cell is restored to its resting potential. The repolarization process begins after phase 0 of the action potential and is completed by the end of phase 3. It encompasses the effective and the relative refractory periods and correlates with the QT interval on th ECG. See also **phase 0, phase 1, phase 2, phase 3.**

report /ripôrt'/ [L, *re + portare,* to carry], (in nursing) the transfer of information from the nurses on one shift to the nurses on the following shift. Report is given systematically at the time of change of shift. The head nurse, team leader, or primary nurse conducts the report, summarizing the progress and status of each patient, for the nurses who will next assume responsibility for the care. The provider of the information is said to 'give report' and the oncoming staff to 'take report.' Report may be given to the assembled oncoming staff, or it may be tape recorded so that staff members can listen to it individually or in a group on their own schedule. The Kardex and medcard of each patient are updated before report, and staff members are informed of the changes during report.

reportable diseases /ripôr'təbəl/, diseases that must be reported by the physician to public health authorities, given their contagious nature. They include but are not limited to malaria, influenza, poliomyelitis, relapsing fever, typhus, yellow fever, cholera, and bubonic plague.

repositioning /rē'pəzish'əning/ [L, *reponere,* to put back], the restoration of an organ or body part to its natural position, as reposing an inverted uterus or changing the position of the jaws.

representative group /rep'rəsen'tətiv/, a group of individuals whose members represent all the various sectors of a community.

repression /ripresh'ən/ [L, *reprimere*, to press back], **1.** the act of restraining, inhibiting, or suppressing. **2.** (in psychoanalysis) an unconscious defense mechanism whereby unacceptable thoughts, feelings, ideas, impulses, or memories, especially those concerning some traumatic past event, are pushed from the consciousness because of their painful guilt association or disagreeable content and are submerged in the unconscious, where they remain dormant but operant and dynamic. Such repressed emotional conflicts are the source of anxiety that may lead to any of the anxiety disorders. Compare **suppression.** −**repress,** *v,* **repressive,** *adj.*

repressive-inspirational approach /ripres'iv/, a psychotherapeutic approach used in some groups to discourage the breaking down of defense mechanisms. Members are encouraged to focus on positive feelings and group strengths. This approach is commonly used in groups of patients with chronic mental illness.

repressor /ripres'ər/ [L, *reprimere*, to press back], (in molecular genetics) a protein produced by the regulator gene. It binds to a sequence of nucleotides in the operator gene, which regulates the structural gene. The repressor, when bound, blocks the transcription of the gene.

repressor gene. See **regulator gene.**

reproduction /rē'prəduk'shən/ [L, *re + producere,* to produce], **1.** the process by which animals and plants give rise to offspring; procreation; the sum total of the cellular and genetic phenomena involved in the transmission of organic life from one organism to successive generations similar to the parents so that the perpetuation and continuity of the species is maintained. In humans, the germ cells, the spermatozoa in the male and the ova in the female, which are produced by the testes and ovaries, unite during fertilization to form the new individual. Kinds of reproduction include **asexual reproduction, cytogenic reproduction, sexual reproduction, somatic reproduction,** and **unisexual reproduction.** See also **fertilization, oogenesis, pregnancy, spermatogenesis. 2.** the creation of a similar structure, situation, or phenomenon; duplication; replication. **3.** (in psychology) the recalling of a former idea, impression, or something previously learned. −**reproductive,** *adj.*

reproductive /rē'prəduk'tiv/ [L, *re-, producere,* to produce], pertaining to the process of reproduction.

reproductive endocrinology, the study of the maternal female hormone system, including the activities of the hypothalamus, pituitary, and ovaries from puberty through menopause.

reproductive system, the male and female gonads, associated ducts and glands, and the external genitalia that function in the procreation of offspring. In women these include the ovaries, fallopian tubes, uterus, vagina, clitoris, and vulva. In men these include the testes, epididymis, vas deferens, seminal vesicles, ejaculatory duct, prostate, and penis. Also called **genital tract, genitourinary system, urogenital system.** See also the Color Atlas of Human Anatomy.

repulsion /ripul'shən/ [L, *repellere,* to drive away], **1.** the act of repelling, disjoining. **2.** a force that separates two bodies or things. **3.** (in genetics) the situation in linked inheritance in which the alleles of two or more mutant genes are located on homologous chromosomes so that each chromosome of the pair carries one or more mutant and wild-

type genes, which are located close enough to be inherited together. Compare **coupling.** See also **transconfiguration.**

request for proposal (RFP) /rikwest/ [L, *requaerere,* to require; *propronere,* to propound], a solicitation by a funding agency for proposals to accomplish a particular goal. The RFP lists the requirements a project must meet in order to receive funding.

required arch length /rikwī'ərd/ [L, *requaerere,* to require], the sum of the mesiodistal widths of all the natural teeth in a dental arch.

RES, abbreviation for **reticuloendothelial system.**

rescinnamine /risin'əmin/, an alkaloid antihypertensive and sedative.

■ INDICATIONS: It is prescribed in the treatment of mild hypertension involving the cardiovascular or central nervous system, or both.

■ CONTRAINDICATIONS: Mental depression, electroconvulsive therapy, or known hypersensitivity to this drug prohibits its use.

■ ADVERSE EFFECTS: Among the more serious adverse reactions are GI, cardiovascular, and central nervous system disturbances.

research /risurch', rē'surch/ [Fr, *rechercher,* to investigate], the diligent inquiry or examination of data, reports, and observations in a search for facts or principles.

research instrument, a testing device for measuring a given phenomenon, such as a paper and pencil test, a questionnaire, an interview, or a set of guidelines for observation.

research measurement, an evaluation of the quantity or incidence of a given variable as obtained by using a research instrument.

research radiopharmaceutical, a drug that is labeled with a small quantity of a radioactive tracer to allow its biodistribution to be studied; it may later be used in a nonradioactive form.

resect /risekt'/ [L, *re + secare,* to cut], to remove tissue from the body by surgery.

resection /risek'shən/, the cutting out of a significant portion of an organ or structure. Resection of an organ may be partial or complete. One type of resection is a **wedge resection.**

reserpine /res'ərpēn/, an antihypertensive.

■ INDICATIONS: It is prescribed in the treatment of high blood pressure and certain neuropsychiatric disorders.

■ CONTRAINDICATIONS: Mental depression, peptic ulcer, ulcerative colitis, or known hypersensitivity to this drug prohibits its use.

■ ADVERSE EFFECTS: Among the more serious adverse reactions are mental depression, extrapyramidal reactions, impotence, aggravation of peptic ulcer, and paradoxical excitement.

reserve /rizurv'/ [L, *reservare,* to save], a potential capacity to maintain the vital functions of the body in homeostasis by adjusting to increased need, such as cardiac reserve, pulmonary reserve, and alkali reserve. See also **homeostasis.**

reserve capacity [L, *reservare,* to save; Gk, *aer*], the volume of air that can be exhaled with maximum effort after completion of a normal expiration. Also called **reserve air.**

reserve cell carcinoma. See **oat cell carcinoma.**

reservoir /rez'əvwär/ [Fr, réservoir], a chamber or receptacle for holding or storing a fluid.

reservoir bag, a component of an anesthesia machine in which gas accumulates, forming a reserve supply of gas for use when the quantity of flow is inadequate. This component also permits 'bagging,' or manual control of ventilation, and serves as a visible monitor of machine function.

reservoir host, a nonhuman host that serves as a means of sustaining an infectious organism as a potential source of human infection. Wild monkeys are reservoir hosts for the yellow fever virus, which can spread from the jungle to infect humans.

reservoir of infection, a continuous source of infectious disease. People, animals, and plants may be reservoirs of infection.

resident /rez′idənt/ [L, *residere*, to remain], a physician in one of the postgraduate years of clinical training after the first, or internship, year. The length of residency varies according to the specialty. See also **PGY.**

resident bacteria, bacteria living in a specific area of the body.

residential care facility /rez′iden′shəl/, a facility that provides custodial care to persons who, because of physical, mental, or emotional disorders, are not able to live independently.

residual /rizij′ōō·əl/ [L, *residuum*, remainder], pertaining to the portion of something that remains after an activity that removes the bulk of the substance.

residual cyst, an odontogenic cyst that remains in the jaw after the removal of a tooth.

residual dental caries, any decayed material left in a prepared tooth cavity.

residual function [L, *residuum*, remainder + *functio*, performance], the remaining ability to function after a serious illness or injury.

residual ridge, the portion of the dental ridge that remains after the alveolar process has disappeared after extraction of the teeth.

residual urine, urine that remains in the bladder after urination.

residual volume [L, *residuum*, remainder + *volumen*, papyrus roll], the amount of air remaining in the lungs at the end of a maximum expiration.

residue-free diet /rez′id(y)ōō/ [L, *residuum*, remainder; AS, *freo;* Gk, *diaita*, lifestyle], a diet free of nondigestible cellulose or fiber, such as found in semisolid bland food.

residue schizophrenia [L, *residuum*], a form of schizophrenia in which the essential features include the presence of residual symptoms without evidence of delusions, hallucinations, incoherence, or gross disorganization. See also **schizophrenia.**

resilience /rizil′yənt/ [L, *resilere*, to spring back], the ability of a body to return to its original form after being stretched or compressed.

res ipsa loquitur /rās′ ip′sə lok′witōōr/ [L, the thing speaks for itself], a legal concept that is important in many malpractice suits, describing a situation in which an injury occurred when the defendant was solely and exclusively in control and in which the injury would not have occurred had due care been exercised. Classic examples of res ipsa loquitur are a sponge left in the abdomen after abdominal surgery or the amputation of the wrong extremity.

resistance /rizis′təns/ [L, *resistere*, to withstand], **1.** an opposition to a force, such as the resistance offered by the constriction of peripheral vessels to the blood flow in the circulatory system. **2.** the frictional force that opposes the flow of an electric charge, as measured in ohms. **3.** (in respiratory therapy) the process or power of acting against a force placed on it, pertaining to thoracic resistance, tissue resistance, and airway resistance.

resistance form, the shape given to a prepared tooth cavity to impart strength and durability to the restoration and remaining tooth structure.

resistance to flow, (in respiratory therapy) the pressure differential required to produce a unit flow change.

resistance transfer factor. See **R factor.**

resistance vessels, the blood vessels, including small arteries, arterioles, and metarterioles that form the major portion of the total peripheral resistance to blood flow.

resistive magnet /resis′tiv/, a simple electromagnet in which electricity passing through coils of wire produces a magnetic field.

resocialization /rēsō′shəlīzā′shən/ [L, *re* + *socialis*, partners; Gk, *izein*, to cause], the reintegration of a client into family and community life after critical or long-term hospitalization.

resolution [L, *re* + *solvere*, to solve], **1.** the ability of an imaging process to distinguish adjacent structures in the object, and an important measure of image quality. **2.** the state of having made a firm determination or decision on a course of action. **3.** the ability of a chromatographic system to separate two adjacent peaks, the degree of separation between two components being abbreviated as **R.**

resolving power /rizol′ving/, **1.** the ability to separate closely migrating substances, as in electrophoresis. **2.** the ability to distinguish closely positioned objects as distinct entities.

resolving time, (in radiology) the minimum time between ionization that can be detected by a Geiger-Müller-type scintillation device.

resonance /rez′ənəns/ [L, *resonare*, to sound again], **1.** an echo or other sound produced by percussion of an organ or cavity of the body during a physical examination. **2.** the process of energy absorption by an object that is tuned to absorb energy of a specific frequency only. Other frequencies do not affect the object. An example is the effect of the vibration of a tuning fork of a particular frequency, causing only other tuning forks of the same frequency to vibrate also. **–resonant,** *adj.*

resonant /rez′ənənt/ [L, *resonare*, to sound again], pertaining to a sound that vibrates on percussion or is amplified by sympathetic vibrations in another medium.

resonating /rez′ənā′ting/ [L, *resonare*, to sound again], pertaining to vibrations or pulsations that are synchronous with a source of sound waves or electromagnetic oscillations.

resorb /risôrb′/ [L, *resorbere*], to absorb again.

resorbent /risôr′bənt/ [L, *resorbere*], a material or agent that is used to absorb blood or other substances.

resorcinated camphor /rizôr′sinā′tid/, a mixture of camphor and resorcinol, used for the treatment of pediculosis and itching.

resorcinol /rizôr′sinol/, an antiseptic substance used as a keratolytic agent in the dermatoses. It is also used in dyes and pharmaceuticals and as a chemical intermediate.

resorcinol test. See **Boas' test.**

resorption /risôrp′shən/ [L, *resorbere*, to swallow again],

1. the loss of substance or bone by physiologic or pathologic means, such as the reduction of the volume and size of the residual ridge of the mandible or maxillae. **2.** the ce-

Respiratory patterns

Type/pattern	Rate (breaths per minute)	Clinical significance
Eupnea	16-20	Normal

Tachypnea	>35	Respiratory failure Response to fever Anxiety Shortness of breath Respiratory infection

Bradypnea	<10	Sleep Respiratory depression Drug overdose Central nervous system (CNS) lesion

Apnea	Periods of no respiration lasting >15 seconds	May be intermittent such as in sleep apnea Respiratory arrest

Hyperpnea	16-20	Can result from anxiety or response to pain Can cause marked respiratory alkalosis, paresthesia, tetany, confusion

Kussmaul's	Usually >35, may be slow or normal	Tachypnea pattern associated with diabetic ketoacidosis, metabolic acidosis, or renal failure

Cheyne-Stokes	Variable	Crescendo-decrescendo pattern caused by alterations in acid base status. Underlying metabolic problem or neurocerebral insult

Biot's	Variable	Periods of apnea and shallow breathing caused by CNS disorder; found in some healthy clients

Apneustic	Increased	Increased inspiratory time with short grunting expiratory time; seen in CNS lesions of the respiratory center

From Weilitz PB: *Pocket guide to respiratory care*, St Louis, 1991, Mosby.

mentoclastic and dentinoclastic action that may occur on a tooth root.

Respbid, a trademark for a smooth muscle relaxant (theophylline).

Res. Phys., abbreviation for *resident physician*.

respiration /res′pirā′shən/ [L, *respirare*, to breathe], the process of the molecular exchange of oxygen and carbon dioxide within the body's tissues, from the lungs to cellular oxidation processes. The rate varies with the age and condition of the person. Certain types of breathing patterns commonly referred to as 'respiration' are **Biot's respiration, Cheyne-Stokes respiration,** and **Kussmaul's respiration.**

respiration of infants [L, *respirare*, to breathe + *infans*, unable to speak], a rate of breathing that averages 40 to 50 breaths per minute at birth and declines to 15 to 20 breaths per minute at puberty.

respiration rate [L, *respirare*, to breathe + *ratum*, rate], the number of inspirations per minute, ranging from a rapid 40 to 50 bpm for newborns, through 20 to 25 bpm for older children, and 15 to 20 bpm for most teenagers and adults. An adult rate of 25 breaths per minute may be regarded as accelerated while a rate of less than 12 breaths per minute is abnormally slow.

respirator /res′pirā′tər/ [L, *respirare*], an apparatus used to modify air for inspiration or to improve pulmonary ventilation. See also **nebulizer, IPPB unit.**

respiratory /res′pərətôr′ē, rispī′rətôr′ē/ [L, *respirare*], of or pertaining to respiration.

respiratory acidosis, an abnormal condition characterized by increased arterial PCO_2, excess carbonic acid, and increased plasma hydrogen ion concentration. It is caused by reduced alveolar ventilation, which can result from various disorders, such as airway obstruction, medullary trauma, neuromuscular disease, chest injuries, pneumonia, pulmonary edema, emphysema, and cardiopulmonary arrest. It may also be caused by the suppression of respiratory reflexes with narcotics, sedatives, hypnotics, or anesthetics. The hypoventilation associated with this condition inhibits the excretion of carbon dioxide, which consequently combines with water in the body to produce excessive carbonic acid and thus reduces blood pH. Also called **carbon dioxide acidosis.** Compare **metabolic acidosis.** See also **metabolic alkalosis, respiratory alkalosis.**

■ OBSERVATIONS: Some common signs and symptoms of respiratory acidosis are headache, dyspnea, fine tremors, tachycardia, hypertension, and vasodilatation. Confirming diagnosis is usually based on arterial blood gas values for PCO_2 over the normal 45 mm Hg and on pH values below 7.35. Ineffective treatment of acute respiratory acidosis can lead to coma and death.

■ INTERVENTIONS: Treatment of this condition seeks to remove or to inhibit the underlying causes of associated hypoventilation. Any airway obstructions are immediately removed. Treatment may include mechanical ventilation, oxygen therapy and the intravenous administration of bronchodilators and sodium bicarbonate.

■ NURSING CONSIDERATIONS: The patient with respiratory acidosis is carefully monitored for any changes in respiratory, cardiovascular, and central nervous system functions, arterial blood gas pressures, and electrolyte concentrations. In patients requiring mechanic ventilation, patent airways are maintained and tracheal tubes are suctioned as needed. Adequate hydration is also important.

respiratory alkalosis, an abnormal condition characterized by decreased PCO_2, decreased hydrogen ion concentration, and increased blood pH. It is caused by pulmonary and nonpulmonary problems. Some pulmonary causes are acute asthma, pulmonary vascular disease, and pneumonia. Some nonpulmonary causes are aspirin toxicity, anxiety, fever, metabolic acidosis, inflammation of the central nervous system, gram-negative septicemia, and hepatic failure. The hyperventilation associated with respiratory alkalosis most commonly stems from extreme anxiety. Compare **metabolic alkalosis.** See also **metabolic acidosis, respiratory acidosis.**

■ OBSERVATIONS: Deep and rapid breathing at rates as high as 40 respirations per minute is a major sign of respiratory alkalosis. Other symptoms are light-headedness, dizziness, peripheral paresthesia, tingling of the hands and the feet, muscle weakness, tetany, and cardiac arrhythmia. Confirming diagnosis is often based on PCO_2 levels below 35 mm Hg, but the measurement of blood pH is critical in differentiating between metabolic acidosis and respiratory alkalosis. In the acute stage, blood pH rises in proportion to the fall in PCO_2, but in the chronic stage it remains within the normal range of 7.35 to 7.45. The carbonic acid concentration is normal in the acute stage of this condition but below normal in the chronic stage.

■ INTERVENTIONS: Treatment of respiratory alkalosis concentrates on removing the underlying causes. Severe cases, especially those caused by extreme anxiety, may be treated by having the patient breathe into a paper bag and inhale exhaled carbon dioxide to compensate for the deficit being created by hyperventilation. Sedatives may also be administered to decrease the ventilation rate.

■ NURSING CONSIDERATIONS: The nurse monitors neurologic, neuromuscular, and cardiovascular functions, arterial blood gases, and serum electrolytes. The patient benefits from explanations about laboratory tests and treatment.

respiratory arrest, the cessation of breathing.

respiratory assessment, an evaluation of the condition and function of a person's respiratory system.

■ METHOD: The nurse asks if the person coughs, wheezes, is short of breath, tires easily, or experiences chest or abdominal pain, chills, fever, excessive sweating, dizziness, or swelling of feet and hands. Signs of confusion, anxiety, restlessness, flaring nostrils, cyanotic lips, gums, earlobes, or nails, clubbing of extremities, fever, anorexia, and a tendency to sit upright are noted if present. The person's breathing is closely observed for evidence of slow, rapid, irregular, shallow, or Cheyne-Stokes respiration, hyperventilation, a long expiratory phase or periods of apnea, and for retractions in the suprasternal, supraclavicular, substernal, or intercostal areas during breathing. The presence of tachycardia, bradycardia, or sinus arrhythmia or evidence of congestive heart failure, such as rales, rhonchi, edema, hepatosplenomegaly, abdominal distention, or pain, is recorded. The thorax is examined for scoliosis, kyphosis, funnel or barrel chest, or unequal shoulder height and is palpated for indications of thoracic expansion, tracheal deviation, crepitations, or fremitus. Percussion is performed to evaluate resonance, hyperresonance, tympany, and dull or flat sounds and rales, rhonchi, wheezing, friction rubs, the transmission of spoken words through the chest wall, and decreased or absent breath sounds are detected by auscultation. Background information pertinent to the evaluation includes allergies, recent exposure to infection, immunizations, exposure to environmental irritants, previous respiratory disorders and operations, preexisting chronic conditions, medication currently taken, the person's smoking habits, and the family history. Valuable diagnostic aids are a chest x-ray examination, complete blood count, electrocardiogram, pulmonary function tests, bronchoscopy, determinations of blood gases and electrolytes, studies of sputum, throat, or nasopharyngeal cultures, and gastric washings, lung scans, and biopsies.

■ NURSING INTERVENTION: The nurse collects the background information and the results of diagnostic tests and may perform the examination. In a respiratory care unit, a nurse clinician or practitioner may have greatly expanded responsibilities, such as interpreting data from electrocardiographic tracings, setting up and adjusting a respirator, titrating medications, and obtaining specimens for blood gas determination.

■ OUTCOME CRITERIA: An accurate and thorough assessment of respiratory function is an essential component of the physical examination and is vital to the diagnosis or ongoing care of a respiratory illness.

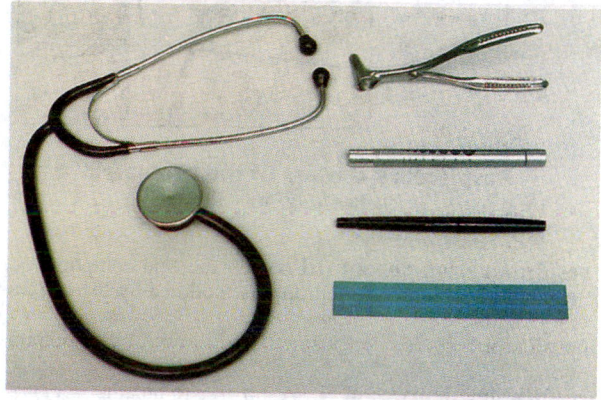

Equipment for respiratory system assessment
(Wilson, 1991)

respiratory bronchiole. See **bronchiole.**

respiratory burn, tissue damage to the respiratory system resulting from the inhalation of a hot gas or burning particles, as may occur in a fire or explosion. Immediate hospitalization and oxygen therapy are recommended. Compare **smoke inhalation.**

respiratory care practitioner, a health professional with special training and experience in the treatment and rehabilitation of patients with respiratory disordees. The respiratory care practitioner typically does not diagnose but must be competent with patient assessment skills in a variety of clinical settings.

respiratory center, a group of nerve cells in the pons and medulla of the brain that control the rhythm of breathing in response to changes in levels of oxygen and carbon dioxide in the blood and cerebrospinal fluid. Change in the concentration of oxygen and carbon dioxide or hydrogen ion levels in the arterial circulation and in cerebrospinal fluid activate central and peripheral chemoreceptors; these send impulses to the respiratory center, increasing or decreasing the breathing rate. This response is essential for normal breathing. In patients with retention of carbon dioxide, as in chronic bronchitis or emphysema, the respiratory center becomes insensitive to carbon dioxide, and the main stimulus to ventilation is then hypoxemia. If such patients inhale gases with a high oxygen content, breathing is depressed, leading to a further rise of blood carbon dioxide. The respiratory center is inhibited by barbiturates, anesthetics, tranquilizing agents, and morphine. See also **hyperventilation, hypoventilation, hypoxia.**

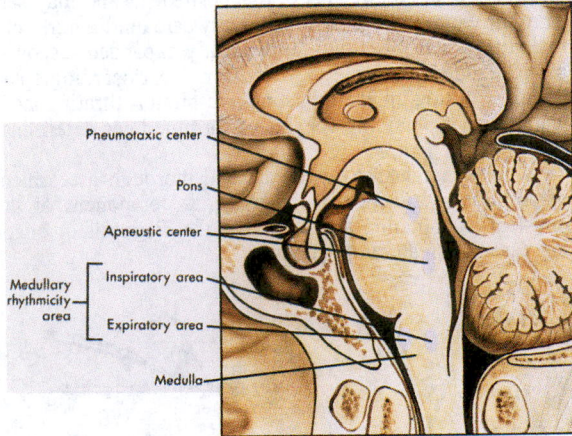

Respiratory centers of the brainstem
(Thibodeau, 1993/Bill Ober)

respiratory component (αPco_2),   the acid component of an acid-base control system that is modified by the respiratory status.

respiratory cycle,   an inspiration followed by an expiration.

respiratory depressant [L, *respirare*, to breathe + *depremere*, to press down],   a drug or other agent that diminishes normal breathing functions. Most respiratory depressants, such as alcohol and opiates, act by depressing the central nervous system.

respiratory depression [L, *respirare*, to breathe + *depremere*, to press down],   respiration that is slow, below 12 inspirations per minute, or feeble, failing to provide full ventilation and perfusion of the lungs.

respiratory distress syndrome of the newborn (RDS), an acute lung disease of the newborn, characterized by airless alveoli, inelastic lungs, more than 60 respirations a minute, nasal flaring, intercostal and subcostal retractions, grunting on expiration, and peripheral edema. The condition occurs most often in premature babies. It is caused by a deficiency of pulmonary surfactant, resulting in overdistended alveoli and, at times, hyaline membrane formation, alveolar hemorrhage, severe right-to-left shunting of blood, increased pulmonary resistance, decreased cardiac output, and severe hypoxemia. The disease is self-limited; the infant dies in 3 to 5 days or completely recovers with no aftereffects. Treatment includes measures to correct shock, acidosis, and hypoxemia and use of continuous positive airway pressure to prevent alveolar collapse. Also called **hyaline membrane disease.** Compare **adult respiratory distress syndrome.**

respiratory exchange ratio (R),   the ratio of carbon dioxide product to that of oxygen consumption or uptake, expressed by the formula $\dot{V}CO_2/\dot{V}O_2$.

respiratory failure,   the inability of the cardiac and pulmonary systems to maintain an adequate exchange of oxygen and carbon dioxide in the lungs. Respiratory failure may be oxygenation or hypercapniac. Oxygenation failure is characterized by hyperventilation and occurs in diseases that affect the alveoli or interstitial tissues of the lobes of the lungs, such as alveolar edema, emphysema, fungal infections, leukemia, lobar pneumonia, lung carcinoma, various pneumoconioses, pulmonary eosinophilia, sarcoidosis, or tuberculosis. Ventilatory failure, characterized by increased arterial tension of carbon dioxide, occurs in acute conditions in which retained pulmonary secretions cause increased airway resistance and decreased lung compliance, as in bronchitis and emphysema. Ventilation may also be reduced by depression of the respiratory center by barbiturates or opiates, hypoxia, hypercarbia, intracranial diseases, trauma, or lesions of the neuromuscular system or thoracic cage. Respiratory failure in preexisting chronic lung diseases may be precipitated by added stress, as with cardiac failure, surgery, anesthesia, or upper respiratory tract infections. Treatment of respiratory failure includes clearing the airways by suction, bronchodilators, or tracheostomy, antibiotics for infections usually present, anticoagulants for pulmonary thromboemboli, and electrolyte replacement in fluid imbalance. Oxygen may be administered in some cases; in others it may further decrease the respiratory reflex by removing the stimulus of a decreased elevated level of oxygen. Chronic respiratory failure may result in cor pulmonale with congestive heart failure and respiratory acidosis. See also **airway obstruction, carbon dioxide, hypercapnia, hyperventilation, hypoxemia, hypoxia, respiratory acidosis.**

respiratory insufficiency [L, *respirare*, to breathe; *in, sufficere*, to suffice],   a failure of the respiratory system to maintain adequate ventilation and perfusion of the lungs.

respiratory muscles,   the muscles that produce volume changes of the thorax during breathing. The inspiratory muscles include the hemidiaphragms, external intercostals, scaleni, sternomastoids, trapezius, pectoralis major, pectoralis minor, subclavius, latissimus dorsi, serratus anterior, and muscles that extend the back. The expiratory muscles are the internal intercostals, abdominals, and the muscles that flex the back.

respiratory quotient (RQ),   the body's total exchange of oxygen for carbon dioxide, expressed as the ratio of the volume of carbon dioxide produced to the volume of oxygen consumed per unit of time at steady state conditions. Depending on the net metabolic needs of all parts of the body at a given moment, the ratio ranges from 0.7 to 1.0 and averages around 0.8.

respiratory rate,   the normal rate of breathing at rest, about 12 to 20 inspirations per minute. The hydrogen ion concentration in the cerebrospinal fluid controls the rate of respiration. The rate may be more rapid in fever, acute pulmonary infection, diffuse pulmonary fibrosis, gas gangrene, left ventricular failure, thyrotoxicosis, and states of tension. Slower breathing rates may result from head injury, coma, or narcotic overdose. See also **bradypnea, hyperpnea, hypopnea.**

respiratory rhythm,   a regular oscillating cycle of inspiration and expiration, controlled by neuronal impulses transmitted between the muscles of inspiration in the chest and the respiratory centers in the brain. The normal breathing pattern may be altered by a prolonged expiratory phase in obstructive diseases of the airway, such as asthma, chronic bronchitis, and emphysema, or by Cheyne-Stokes respiration in patients with raised intracranial pressure or heart failure. See also **apnea, Biot's respiration, Hering-Breuer reflexes, hyperventilation, hypoventilation, tachypnea.**

respiratory syncytial virus (RSV, RS virus), a member of a subgroup of myxoviruses that in tissue culture causes formation of giant cells or syncytia. It is a common cause of epidemics of acute bronchiolitis, bronchopneumonia, and the common cold in young children and sporadic acute bronchitis and mild upper respiratory tract infections in adults. Symptoms of infection with this virus include fever, cough, and severe malaise. Occasional fatalities occur in infants. Systemic invasion by the virus does not happen, and secondary bacterial invasion is uncommon. Treatment includes rest and the administration of aspirin and nasal decongestants. No effective vaccine for prevention is available. Compare **rhinovirus.** See also **bronchiolitis, bronchitis, bronchopneumonia, cold.**

respiratory system. See **respiratory tract.**

respiratory therapist, a graduate of a school approved by the American Medical Association designed to qualify the person for the registry examination of the National Board of Respiratory Care (NBRC). See also **registered respiratory therapist.**

respiratory therapy (RT), 1. any treatment that maintains or improves the ventilatory function of the respiratory tract. **2.** *informal.* the department in a health care facility that provides respiratory therapy for the clients of the facility.

respiratory therapy technician, a graduate of an AMA-approved school designed to qualify the person for technician certification examination of the National Board for Respiratory Care (NBRC). It usually requires a 1-year hospital-based program combining a special curriculum of basic sciences with supervised clinical experience.

respiratory therapy technician, certified (CRTT), an allied health professional who administers general respiratory care. Duties can include collection and review of clinical data, examination of the patient by inspection, palpation, percussion, and auscultation, and assembling and maintaining equipment used in respiratory care.

respiratory tract, the complex of organs and structures that performs the pulmonary ventilation of the body and the exchange of oxygen and carbon dioxide between the ambient air and the blood circulating through the lungs. It also warms the air passing into the body and assists in the speech function by providing air for the larynx and the vocal cords. Every 24 hours about 500 cubic feet of air passes through the respiratory tract of the average adult, who breathes in and out between 12 and 18 times a minute. The respiratory tract is divided into the upper respiratory tract and the lower respiratory tract. Also called **respiratory system.** See also the Color Atlas of Human Anatomy.

respiratory tract infection, any infectious disease of the upper or lower respiratory tract. **Upper respiratory tract infections** include the common cold, laryngitis, pharyngitis, rhinitis, sinusitis, and tonsillitis. **Lower respiratory tract infections** include bronchitis, bronchiolitis, pneumonia, and tracheitis.

respiratory zone, the terminal air units where gas ex-

change actually occurs, usually below the seventeenth division of bronchi.

respirometer /res'pirom'ətər/ [L, *respirare*, to breath; Gk, *metron*, measure], an instrument used to analyze the quality of a patient's respirations.

respite care /res'pit/ [L, *respicere*, to look back], **1.** short-term health services to the dependent older adult, either at home or in an institutional setting. **2.** the provision of temporary care for a patient who requires specialized or intensive care or supervision that is normally provided by his or her family at home. Respite care provides the family with relief from demands of the patient's care.

respite time /res'pit/, relief time from responsibilities for the care of a patient.

respondeat superior /respon'dē·at/ [L, let the master answer], the concept that an employer may be held liable for torts committed by employees acting within the scope of their employment.

respondent conditioning. See **classic conditioning.**

responder /rispon'dər/ [L, *respondere*, to promise in return], a person whose tumor shrinks in volume by at least 50% as a result of chemotherapy, radiation, or other treatment.

response /rispons'/ [L, *responsum*, reply], (in psychology) a cost category of negative punishment in which the reinforcer is lost or withdrawn after an operant.

response time, 1. the period between the input of information into a computer and the response or output. **2.** the period between the application of a stimulus and the response of a cell or cells.

rest [AS, *restan*, to rest], an extension from a prosthesis that affords vertical support for a dental restoration.

rest angle. See **occlusal rest angle.**

rest area, a surface prepared on a tooth or fixed restoration into which the rest fits, providing support for a removable partial denture.

resting cell, a cell that is not undergoing division. See also **interphase.**

resting membrane potential, the transmembrane voltage that exists when the heart muscle is at rest.

resting potential [AS, *rest*; L, *potentia*, power], the electrical potential across a nerve cell membrane before it is stimulated to release the charge. The resting potential for a neuron is between 50 and 100 millivolts, with the excess of negatively charged ions inside the cell membrane.

resting tremor. See **tremor.**

restitution /res'tit(y)oo'shən/, the spontaneous turning of the fetal head to the right or left after it has extended through the vulva.

rest jaw relation, (in dentistry) the postural relation of the mandible to the maxillae when the patient is resting comfortably in the upright position. The condyles are in a neutral, unstrained position in the glenoid fossae, and the mandibular musculature is in a state of minimum tonic contraction to maintain posture.

rest joint position, the position of a joint where the joint surfaces are relatively incongruent and the support structures are relatively lax. The position is used extensively in passive mobilization procedures.

restless legs syndrome [AS, *restlaes*; ONorse, *leggr*], a benign condition of unknown origin characterized by an irritating sensation of uneasiness, tiredness, and itching deep within the muscles of the leg, especially the lower part of the limb, accompanied by twitching and, sometimes, by pain. The only relief is walking or moving the legs. The condition may be associated with various psychiatric disorders, probably as a form of extrapyramidal hyperkinesis. Also called **anxietas tibiarum, Ekbom syndrome, Wittmaack-Ekbom syndrome.**

restoration /res′tôrā′shən/ [L, *restaurare*, to restore], any tooth filling, inlay, crown, partial or complete denture, or prosthesis that restores or replaces lost tooth structure, teeth, or oral tissues. Also called **prosthetic restoration.**

restoration contour, the profile of the surfaces of teeth that have been restored.

restoration of cusps, a reduction and inclusion of tooth cusps within a tooth cavity preparation and their restoration to functional occlusion with an artificial dental material.

restorative /ristôr′ətiv/ [L, *restaurare*], pertaining to the power or ability to restore or renew a person to a normal state of health or consciousness.

Restoril, a trademark for a hypnotic agent (temazepam).

restraint /ristrānt′/ [L, *restringere*, to confine], any one of numerous devices used in aiding the immobilization of patients, especially children in traction. Some kinds of restraints are specially designed slings, jackets, or diapers. Restraints often involve a certain amount of emotional trauma for the patient and are carefully employed. They are most effective when used consistently. Restraints that are too tight may cause skin irritation; those that fit too loosely do not serve their purpose. During the course of any therapy, restraints are usually removed every 4 hours or more frequently to assess skin integrity and provide skin care, often a massage of the area involved and an alcohol rub.

restraint in bed [L, *restringere*, to confine; AS, *bedd*], the confinement of a person to bed rest by the use of mechanical or physical or chemical means, if needed.

restraint of trade, an illegal act that interferes with free competition in a commercial or business transaction so as to restrict the production of a product or the provision of a service, affect the cost of a product or a service, or control the market in any way to the detriment of the consumers or purchasers of the service or product. The Clayton Act and the Sherman Antitrust Act are federal statutes that embody the basic concepts of the definition and of the illegal nature of restraint of trade.

restriction endonuclease /ristrik′shən en′dōnoo′klē-ās/ [L, *restringere*, + Gk, *endon*, within; L, *nucleus* nut; Fr, *diastase*, enzyme], (in molecular genetics) an enzyme that cleaves DNA at a specific site. Each of the many different endonucleases isolated from various bacteria acts at a species-specific cleav age site, making it possible for researchers to divide DNA into discrete segments.

restriction fragment, a fragment of viral or cellular nucleic acid produced by cleavage of the DNA molecule by specific endonucleases.

restriction fragment length polymorphism (RFLP), a marker for a DNA segment of a chromosome that is associated with a hereditary disease. RFLPs are used in the detection of sequence variations in human genomic DNA segments. They are believed to be inherited according to Mendelian laws. RFLPs have been used to detect genes associated with several inherited disorders, including Huntington's disease.

restrictive cardiomyopathy /ristrik′tiv/ [L, *restringere,* to confine; Gk, *kardia*, heart + *mys*, muscle + *pathos*, disease], a form of heart disease characterized by diastolic non compliance or poor compliance of the ventricles as in

constrictive pericarditis. Also called **constrictive cardiomyopathy.**

restrictive disease, a respiratory disorder characterized by restriction of expansion of the lungs or chest wall, resulting in diminished lung volumes and capacities.

rest seat. See **rest area.**

résumé, resume. See **curriculum vitae.**

resuscitation /risus′itā′shən/ [L, *resuscitare*, to revive], the process of sustaining the vital functions of a person in respiratory or cardiac failure while reviving him or her, using techniques of artificial respiration and cardiac massage, correcting acid-base imbalance, and treating the cause of failure. See also **cardiopulmonary resuscitation.** −**resuscitate,** *v.*

resuscitator /risus′itā′tər/, an apparatus for pumping air into the lungs. It consists of a mask snugly applied over the mouth and nose, a reservoir for air, and a manually or electrically powered pump. Often oxygen may be added to the air in the reservoir.

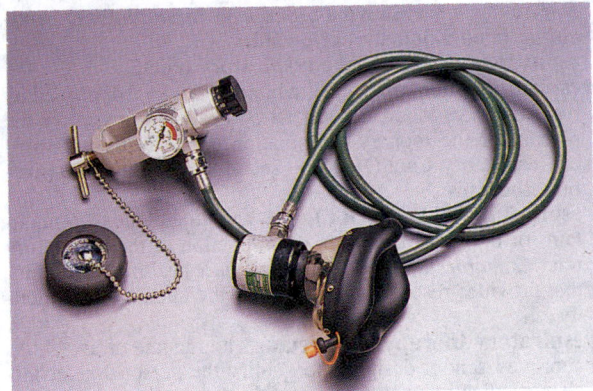

Manually controlled oxygen powered resuscitator
(Judd, 1988)

RET, abbreviation for **rational emotive therapy.**

retail dentistry /rē′təl/ [ME, *retailen*, to divide into pieces], the practice of fee-for-service dentistry in an exclusively retail environment, such as a shopping center or a department store, with the specific intention of attracting the customers of such retail centers and by using the marketing techniques of the retailers involved.

-retain. See **retention.**

retained placenta /ritānd′/ [L, *retinere*, to hold + *placenta*, flat cake], the failure of the placenta to be delivered during an appropriate period, usually 30 minutes, following birth of the infant.

retainer [L, *retinere*, to hold], **1.** the part of a dental prosthesis that connects an abutment tooth with the suspended portion of a bridge. It may be an inlay, a partial crown, or a complete crown. **2.** an appliance for maintaining teeth and jaw positions gained by orthodontic procedures. **3.** the portion of a fixed prosthesis that attaches a pontic to the abutment teeth. **4.** any clasp, attachment, or device for fixing or stabilizing a dental prosthesis.

retaining orthodontic appliance, an orthodontic device for holding the teeth in place, following orthodontic tooth movement, until the occlusion is stabilized.

-retard. See **retarded.**

retardation /rē'tärdā'shən/ [L, *retardare*, to check], the slowing down of any mental or physical activity or failure of intellectual abilities to develop normally. Psychomotor retardation may occur in depression and a conditioned response to an unconditioned stimulus may be retarded in appearance.

retarded /ritär'did/, [L, *retarder*, to slow down], (of physical, intellectual, social, or emotional development) abnormally slow. **—retard** /ritärd'/, *v.*

retarded dentition, the abnormal delay of the eruption of the deciduous or permanent teeth resulting from malnutrition, malposition of the teeth, a hereditary factor, or a metabolic imbalance, such as hypothyroidism. Compare **precocious dentition.**

retarded depression, the depressive phase of bipolar disorder.

retarded ejaculation, the inability of a male to ejaculate after having achieved an erection. This often accompanies the aging process.

retch [AS, *hraecan*, to spit], a strong attempt to vomit without bringing up anything. Compare **eructation, vomit.**

rete /rē'tē/ [L, net], a network, especially of arteries or veins. **—retial** /rē'tē·əl/, *adj.*

rete arteriosum [L, *rete*, net: Gk, *arteria*], an anastomotic network of small arteries at a point before they branch into arterioles and capillaries. Also called **arterial network.**

retention /riten'shən/, **1.** a resistance to movement or displacement. **2.** the ability of the digestive system to hold food and fluid. **3.** the inability to urinate or defecate. **4.** the ability of the mind to remember information acquired from reading, observation, or other processes. **5.** the inherent property of a dental restoration to maintain its position without displacement under axial stress. **6.** a characteristic of proper tooth cavity preparation in which provision is made for preventing vertical displacement of the cavity filling. **7.** a period of treatment during which an individual wears an appliance to maintain teeth in positions to which they have been moved by orthodontic procedures. **—retain,** *v.*

retention enema [L, *retinere*, to hold; Gk, *enema*, clyster], a medicinal or nutrient enema specially formulated so it will remain in the bowel without stimulating the nerve endings that would ordinarily result in evacuation.

retention form, the provision made in a prepared tooth cavity to enhance retention of a restoration and to prevent its displacement.

retention groove, a depression formed by the opposing vertical constrictions in the preparation of a tooth, which improves the retention of a restoration.

retention of urine, an abnormal, involuntary accumulation of urine in the bladder as a result of a loss of muscle tone in the bladder, neurologic dysfunction or damage to the bladder, obstruction of the urethra, or the administration of a narcotic analgesic, especially morphine.

retention pin, a small metal projection that extends from a dental metal casting into the dentin of a tooth to improve the retention of a tooth restoration.

retention procedure, a method established by state laws or mental health codes for committing a person to a psychiatric institution. Most states recognize four types of retention: emergency, informal, involuntary, and voluntary.

retention time (t_a), **1.** (in chromatography) the amount of time elapsed from the injection of a sample into the chromatographic system to the recording of the peak (band) maximum of the component in the chromatogram. **2.** the length of time a compound is retained on a chromatography column.

retention with overflow [L, *retinere*, to hold; AS, *ofer* + *flowan*], a complication of urinary incontinence in which the pressure of retained urine after a voiding results in dribbling. Also called **paradoxical incontinence.**

rete peg. See **epithelial peg.**

-retial. See rete.

reticul-, a combining form meaning 'netlike': *recticulation, reticulocyte, reticulopod.*

reticular /ritik'yələr/ [L, *reticulum*, little net], (of a tissue or surface) having a netlike pattern or structure of veins.

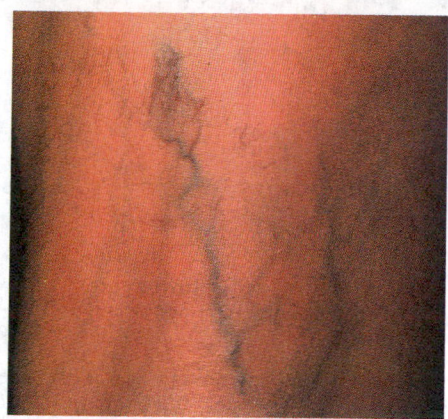

Reticular vein (Goldman, 1992)

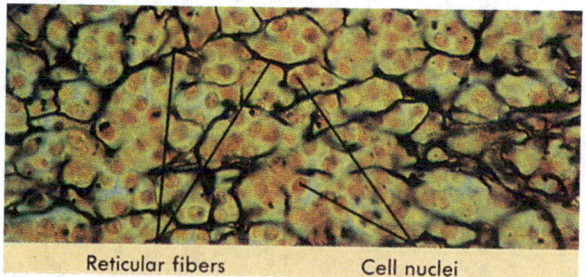

Reticular fibers   Cell nuclei

Reticular tissue (Seeley, 1992/Ed Reschke)

reticular activating system (RAS), a functional (rather than a morphologic) system in the brain essential for wakefulness, attention, concentration, and introspection. A network of nerve fibers in the thalamus, hypothalamus, brainstem, and cerebral cortex contribute to the system. (See Fig. p. 1360.)

reticular formation, a small, thick cluster of neurons, nestled within the brainstem, that controls breathing, the heartbeat, the blood pressure, the level of consciousness, and other vital functions of the body. The reticular formation constantly monitors the state of the body through connections with the sensory and the motor tracts. Certain nerve cells in the formation regulate the flow of hydrochloric acid in the stomach; other cells regulate swallowing, tongue movements, and movements of the face, eyes, and tongue.

reticulation film fault /ritik'yəlā'shən/ [L, *reticulum* + *atio*, process], a defect in a radiograph or developed photographic film that appears as a network of corrugations. It is usually caused by film development with an excessive

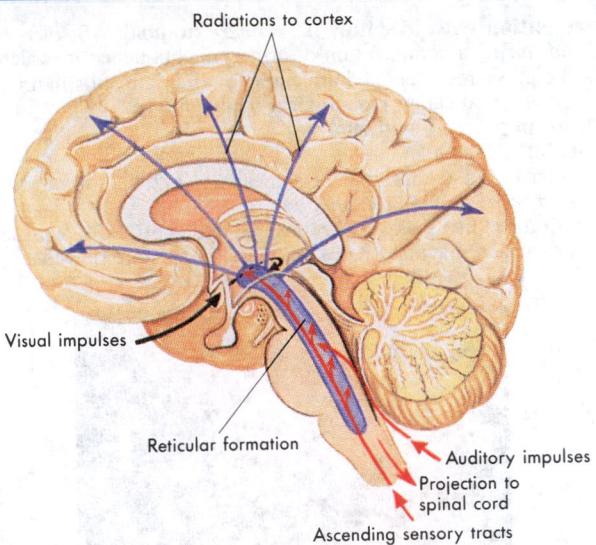

Reticular activating system
(Thibodeau, 1993/Ernest W Beck)

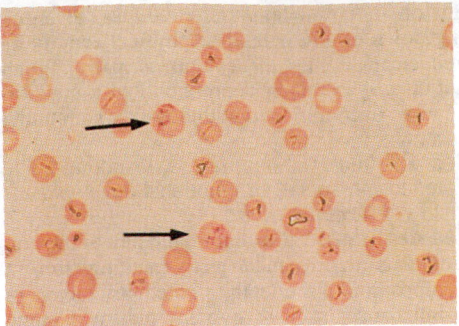

Reticulocytes (Powers, 1989)

temperature difference between any two of the three darkroom solutions: the developer, the fixer, and the clearing
agent.
reticulin /ritik′yəlin/ [L, *reticulum*,], an albuminoid substance found in the connective fibers of reticular tissue.

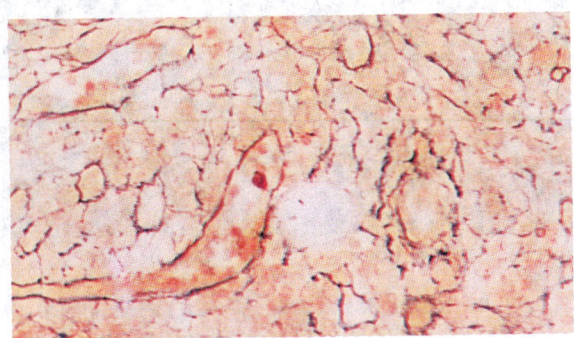

**Reticulin fibers in the bone marrow of a patient
with angioimmunoblastic lymphadenopathy**
(Hayhoe, 1992)

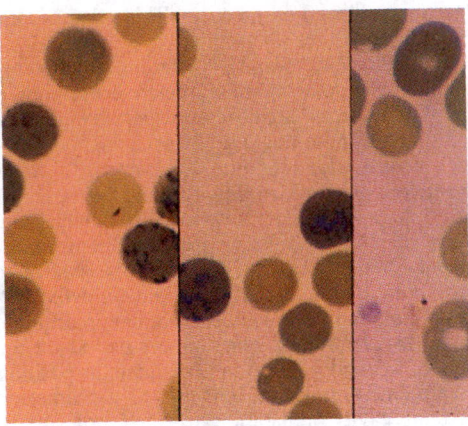

**Reticulocyte count (left to right):
high, normal, and low**
(Zitelli, 1987)

reticulocyte /ritik′yələsīt′/ [L, *reticulum* + Gk, *kytos*, cell],
an immature erythrocyte characterized by a meshlike pattern of threads and particles at the former site of the nucleus. Reticulocytes normally account for less than 2% of
the circulating erythrocytes; a greater proportion reflects an
increased rate of erythropoiesis. Compare **erythrocyte.** See
also **normoblast.**
reticulocyte count, a count of the number of reticulocytes
in a whole blood specimen, used in determining bone marrow activity. The reticulocyte count is lowered in hemolytic
diseases; it is elevated after hemorrhage or during recovery
from anemia. The normal concentration of reticulocytes in
whole blood is 25,000 to 75,000 cells/μL.

reticulocytopenia /ritik′yələsī′təpē′nē·ə/ [L, *reticulum* +
Gk, *kytos*, cell, *penia*, poverty], a decrease below the normal range of 0.5% to 1.5% in the number of reticulocytes
in a blood sample.
reticulocytosis /-sītō′sis/, an increase in the number of reticulocytes in the circulating blood that may represent a normal increase in activity of the bone marrow in response to
blood loss, acclimatization to living at a higher altitude, or
therapy for anemia.
reticuloendothelial cells /ritik′yəlō·en′dōthē′lē·əl/ [L,
reticulum + Gk, *endon,* within, *thele,* nipple], cells lining vascular and lymph vessels capable of phagocytosing
bacteria, viruses, and colloidal particles or of forming immune bodies against foreign particles.
reticuloendothelial system (RES), a functional, rather
than anatomic, system of the body involved primarily in defense against infection and in disposal of the products of
the breakdown of cells. It is made up of macrophages, the
Kupffer cells of the liver, and the reticulum cells of the
lungs, bone marrow, spleen, and lymph nodes. Disorders
of this system include **eosinophilic granuloma, Gaucher's
disease, Hand-Schüller-Christian syndrome,** and
Niemann-Pick disease.
reticuloendotheliosis /ritik′yəlō·en′dōthē′lē·ō′sis/, an
abnormal condition characterized by increased growth and

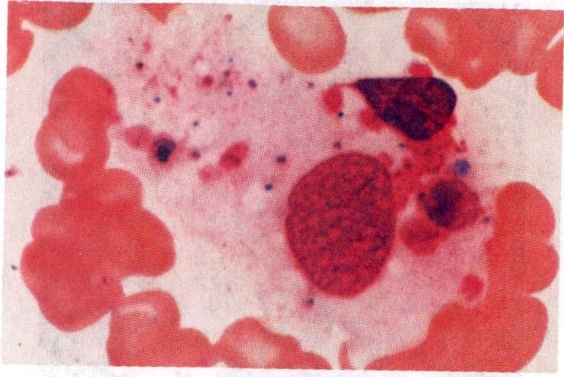

Reticuloendothelial cell (Hayhoe, 1992)

proliferation of the cells of the reticuloendothelial system. See **reticuloendothelial system.**

reticulogranular /-gran'yələr/ [L, *reticulum* + *granulum*, little grain], pertaining to a cloudy appearance of the lungs on a chest radiograph of a patient with respiratory distress syndrome.

reticulosarcoma. See **undifferentiated malignant lymphoma.**

reticulum cell sarcoma. See **histiocytic malignant lymphoma.**

-retin, a combining form for retinol derivatives.

retin-, a combining form meaning 'pertaining to the retina': *retinol, retinopathy.*

retina /ret'inə/ [L, *rete*, net], a 10-layered, delicate nervous tissue membrane of the eye, continuous with the optic nerve, that receives images of external objects and transmits visual impulses through the optic nerve to the brain. The retina is soft, semitransparent, and contains rhodopsin, which gives it a purple tint. The retina becomes clouded and opaque if exposed to direct sunlight. It develops from the embryonic optic cup in the eighth month of pregnancy and consists of the outer pigmented layer and the nine-layered retina proper. These nine layers, starting with the most internal, are the internal limiting membrane, the stratum opticum, the ganglion cell layer, the inner plexiform

layer, the inner nuclear layer, the outer plexiform layer, the outer nuclear layer, the external limiting membrane, and the layer of rods and cones. The outer surface of the retina is in contact with the choroid; the inner surface with the vitreous body. The retina is thinner anteriorly, where it extends nearly as far as the ciliary body, and thicker posteriorly, except for a thin spot in the exact center of the posterior surface where focus is best. The nervous fibers end anteriorly in the jagged ora serrata at the ciliary body, but the membrane of the retina extends over the back of the ciliary processes and the iris. See also **Jacob's membrane, macula, optic disc.**

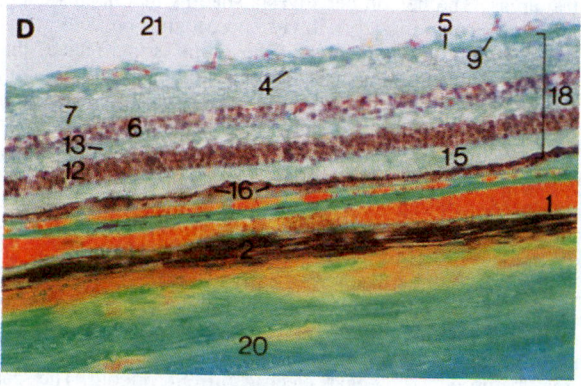

Structure of the retina (England, 1992)
4: ganglion cell layer, 5: inner limiting membrane, 6: inner nuclear layer, 7: inner plexiform layer, 11: outer limiting membrane, 12: outer nuclear layer, 13: outer plexiform layer, 15: layer of rods and cones

Retin-A, a trademark for a keratolytic (tretinoin).

retinaculum /ret'inak'yələm/, *pl.* **retinacula** [L, halter], **1.** a structure that retains an organ or tissue. **2.** an instrument for retracting tissues during surgery.

retinaculum extensorum manus, the thick band of antebrachial fascia that wraps tendons of the extensor muscles of the forearm at the distal ends of the radius and the ulna. Also called **dorsal carpal ligament, extensor retinaculum of the hand.** Compare **retinaculum flexorum manus.**

retinaculum flexorum manus, the thick, fibrous band of antebrachial fascia that wraps the carpal canal surrounding the tendons of flexor muscles of the forearm at the distal ends of the radius and the ulna. Also called **flexor retinaculum of the hand, volar ligament.**

retinal /ret'inəl, ret'inal'/ [L, *rete*], **1.** an aldehyde precursor of vitamin A produced by the enzymatic dehydration of retinol. It is the active form of the vitamin necessary for night, day, and color vision. See also **retinene, vitamin A. 2.** pertaining to the retina.

retinal detachment, a separation of the retina from the choroid in the back of the eye, usually resulting from a hole in the retina that allows the vitreous humor to leak between the choroid and the retina. Severe trauma to the eye, such as a contusion or penetrating wound, may be the proximate cause, but in the great majority of cases retinal detachment is the result of internal changes in the vitreous chamber as-

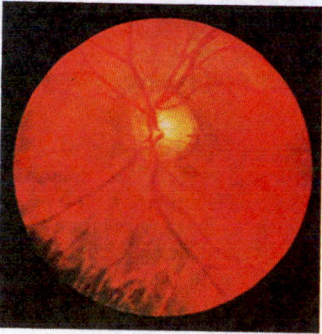

Normal retina—ophthalmoscopic view
(from *Selected topics in Ophthalmology*, Medcom Clinical Lecture Guides, Garden Grove, California, 1973, Medcom, Inc.)

sociated with aging, or, less frequently, with inflammation of the interior of the eye.

■ OBSERVATIONS: In most cases retinal detachment develops slowly. The first symptom is often the sudden appearance of a large number of floating spots loosely suspended in front of the affected eye. The person may not seek help, because the number of spots tends to decrease during the days and weeks after the detachment. The person may also notice a curious sensation of flashing lights as the eye is moved. Because the retina does not contain sensory nerves that relay sensations of pain, the condition is painless. Detachment usually begins at the thin peripheral edge of the retina and extends gradually beneath the thicker, more central areas. The person perceives a shadow that begins laterally and grows in size, slowly encroaching on central vision. As long as the center of the retina is unaffected, the vision, when the person is looking straight ahead, is normal; when the center becomes affected, the eyesight is distorted, wavy, and indistinct. If the process of detachment is not halted, total blindness of the eye ultimately results. The condition does not spontaneously resolve itself.

■ INTERVENTIONS: Surgery is usually required to repair the hole and prevent the leakage of vitreous humor that separates the retina from its source of nourishment, the choroid. If the condition is discovered early, when the hole is small and the volume of vitreous humor lost is not large, the retinal hole may be closed by causing a scar to form on the choroid and to adhere to the retina around the hole. The scar may be produced by heat, electric current, or cold. The scar is held against the retina by local pressure achieved by a variety of surgical techniques.

■ NURSING CONSIDERATIONS: Retinal detachment requires treatment. The degree of restoration of sight depends on the extent and duration of separation; maximum vision is achieved within 3 months after surgery. Unless replaced, a detached retina slowly dies after several years of detachment. Blindness resulting from retinal detachment is irreversible.

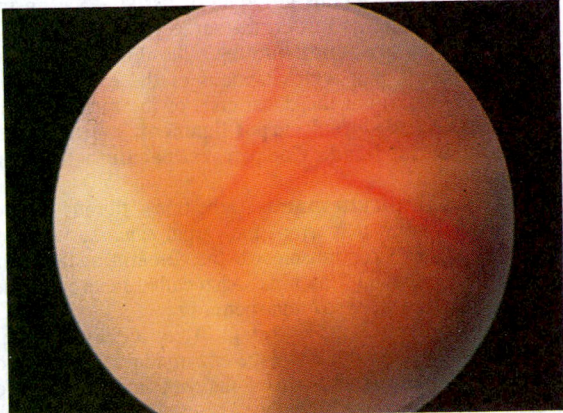

Retinal detachment (*Schumacher, 1988*)

retinene /ret′inin/ [L, *rete*], either of the two carotenoid pigments found in the rods of the retina that are precursors of vitamin A and are activated by light. See also **retinal, retinol.**

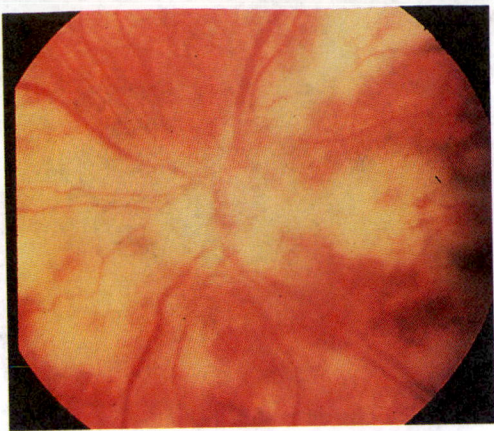

Retinitis secondary to CMV infection (*Zitelli, 1992*)

retinitis /ret′inī′tis/ [L, *rete*, net; Gk, *itis*, inflammation], an inflammation of the retina.

retinitis pigmentosa [L, *rete*, net; Gk, *itis*, inflammation; L, *pigmentum*, paint], a group of diseases, often hereditary, characterized by bilateral primary degeneration of the retina, beginning in childhood and progressing to blindness by middle age. Clinical signs include night blindness, reduced visual fields, and pigmentation of the retina, macular degeneration, and eventually, total loss of vision.

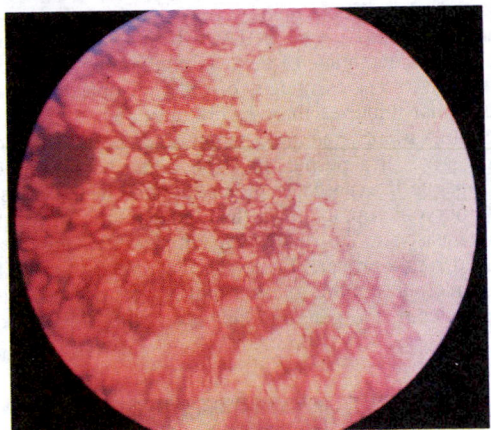

Retinitis pigmentosa (*Zitelli, 1992*)

retinoblastoma /ret′inōblastō′mə/, *pl.* **retinoblastomas, retinoblastomata** [L, *rete* + Gk, *blastos*, germ, *oma*, tumor], a congenital, hereditary neoplasm developing from retinal germ cells. Characteristic signs are diminished vision, strabismus, retinal detachment, and an abnormal pupillary reflex. The rapidly growing tumor may invade the brain and metastasize to distant sites. Treatment includes removal of the eye and as much of the optic nerve as possible, followed by radiation and chemotherapy. It is bilateral in about 30% of the cases; the more affected eye is enucleated, and the other eye is treated with radiation, antibiotics, cryotherapy, or photocoagulation, singly or in combi-

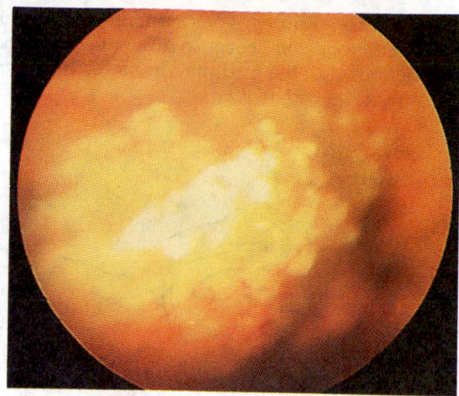

Retinoblastoma (Zitelli, 1992)

nation. Because nearly 20% of the cases are transmitted as an autosomal dominant trait with incomplete penetration, genetic counseling is advisable.

retinocerebral angiomatosis. See **cerebroretinal angiomatosis.**

retinochoroiditis /-kôr′oidī′tis/ [L, *rete*, net; Gk, *chorion*, skin + *itis*, inflammation], an inflammation of the retina and choroid coat of the eye. Also called *choroidoretinitis.*

retinodialysis /ret′inō′dī·al′isis/ [L, *rete* + Gk, *dia*, through, *lysis* loosening], a separation or tear in the retina in its anterior part, in the area of the ora serrata, just behind the ciliary body.

retinoid /ret′inoid/, [L, *rete*, net; Gk, *eidos*, form], resembling the retina.

retinol /ret′inol/ [L, *rete*], the cis-trans form of vitamin A. It is found in the retinas of mammals. Also called **vitamin A₁.**

retinopathy /ret′inop′əthē/ [L, *rete* + Gk, *pathos*, disease], a noninflammatory eye disorder resulting from changes in the retinal blood vessels.

retinoscope /ret′inəskōp′/ [L, *rete*, net; Gk, *skopein*, to view], an instrument used in retinoscopy to determine errors of refraction.

retinoscopy /ret′inos′kəpē/ [L, *rete*, net; Gk, *skopein*, to view], a procedure for examining the eyes for possible errors of refraction. The examiner shines a light into the eyeball and notes the movements of reflex from the fundus. This indicates the types of lenses needed to neutralize the refractive errors.

retirement center /ritī′ərmənt/ [Fr, *retirer*, to withdraw; Gk, *kentron*, center], a facility or organized program to provide social services and activities for senior citizens who generally do not require ongoing health care.

retract /ritrakt/ [L, *retractare*, to draw back], to shrink, make shorter, or pull back.

retracted nipple [L, *retractare*, to draw back; ME, *neb*], a nipple drawn inward. as the result of cancer, adhesions below the skin surface or a natural condition present at birth.

retraction /ritrak′shən/ [L, *retractare*, to draw back], **1.** the displacement of tissues to expose a part or structure of the body. **2.** a distal movement of the teeth. **3.** a distal or retrusive position of the teeth, dental arch, or jaw.

retraction of the chest, the visible sinking-in of the soft tissues of the chest between and around the firmer tissue of the cartilaginous and bony ribs, as occurs with increased inspiratory effort. Retraction begins in the intercostal spaces. If increased effort is needed to fill the lungs, supraclavicular and infraclavicular retraction may be seen. In infants, sternal retraction occurs with only slight increase in respiratory effort, caused by the pliability of their chests. Compare **intercostal bulging.**

retractor /ritrak′tər/ [L, *retractare*], an instrument for holding back the edges of tissues and organs to maintain exposure of the underlying anatomic parts, particularly during surgery, such as an army retractor or a double-ended Richardson retractor.

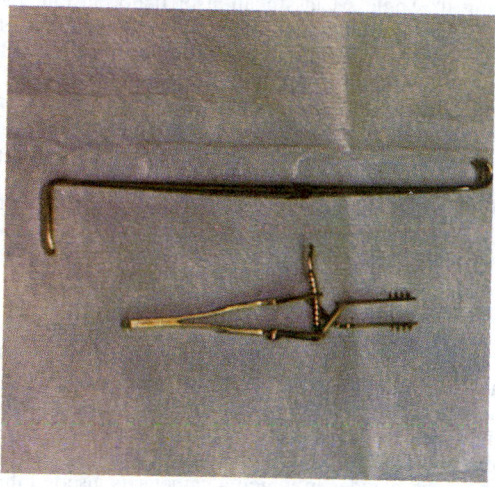

Retractors (Grossman, 1993)

retro-, a prefix meaning 'backward, or located behind': *retronasal, retroperitoneal, retroversion.*

retroanterograde amnesia /-anter′ōgrād/ [L, *retro*, backwards + *antero*, foremost + *gradus*, step; Gk, *amnesia*, forgetfulness], a memory disorder in which current events may be assigned to the past and past events may be regarded as current.

retroaortic node /re′trō·ā·ôr′tik/ [L, *retro*, backward; Gk, *aerein*, to raise], a node in one of three sets of lumbar lymph nodes that serve various structures in the abdomen and the pelvis. They lie below the cisterna chyli on the bodies of the third and the fourth lumbar vertebrae and receive the lymphatic trunks from the lateral aortic nodes and preaortic nodes. The efferents from the retroaortic nodes end in the cisterna chyli. Compare **lateral aortic node, preaortic node.**

retroauricular /-ôrik′yələr/ [L, *retro*, backward + *auricula*, little ear], pertaining to a location behind the ear.

retrobulbar /-bul′bər/ [L, *retro*, backward + *bulbus*, swollen root], **1.** pertaining to the area behind the pons. **2.** pertaining to the area behind the eyeball.

retrobulbar neuritis [L, *retro*, backward + *bulbus*, swollen root; Gk, *neuron* + *itis*, inflammation], a form of neuritis that involves the optic nerve or the optic disc. Also called **optic neuritis.**

retrocecal /-sē′kəl/ [L, *retro*, backward + *caecus*, blind], pertaining to the region behind the cecum.

retroclusion /ret′roklōō′zhən/, a method of controlling hemorrhage from an artery by compressing it between tissues on either side. A needle is inserted through the tissues above the bleeding vessel, then turned around and down so it also passes through the tissues beneath the artery.

retroflexion /-flek′shən/ [L, *retro* + *flectere*, to bend], an abnormal position of an organ in which the organ is tilted back acutely, folded over on itself.

retroflexion of the uterus, a condition in which the body of the uterus is bent backward at an angle with the cervix, whose position usually remains unchanged.

retrognathia /ret′rōnā′thē·ə/ [L, *retro*, backward; Gk, *gnathos*, jaw], a condition in which either or both jaws recede with respect to the frontal plane of the forehead. According to Angle's Classification of malocclusion, the facial profile of a person with Class II or distoclusion is retrognathic. Also called **mandibular (or maxillary) retroposition; mandibular (or maxillary) retrusion.**

retrognathism /ret′rōnā′this′əm/ [L, *retro* + Gk, *gnathos*, jaw], a facial abnormality in which one or both jaws, usually the mandible, are posterior to their normal facial positions. Also called **bird-face retrognathism.**

retrograde /ret′rəgrād/ [L, *retro* + *gradus*, step], **1.** moving backward; moving in the opposite direction to that which is considered normal. **2.** degenerating; reverting to an earlier state or worse condition. **3.** catabolic.

retrograde amnesia, the loss of memory for events occurring before a particular time in a person's life, usually before the event that precipitated the amnesia. The condition may result from disease, brain injury or damage, or a traumatic emotional incident. Compare **anterograde amnesia.**

retrograde cystoscopy, a technique in radiology for examining the bladder in which a catheter is inserted through the urethra into the bladder, allowing the urine present in the bladder to pass through the catheter. A radiopaque medium is introduced, filling the bladder, and the contour of the bladder is observed, using serial x-ray films or fluoroscopy, as the contrast medium is voided. See also **cystogram, retrograde pyelography.**

retrograde ejaculation [L, *retro*, backward + *gradus*, step + *ejaculari*, to throw out], an ejaculation of semen in a reverse direction, into the urinary bladder. The effect is sometimes the result of prostate surgery or a congenital condition.

retrograde filling, a filling placed in the apical portion of a tooth root to seal the apical portion of the root canal. Also called **postresection filling.**

retrograde flow [L, *retro*, backward; AS, *flowan*], the flow of fluid in a direction other than normal, as in regurgitation.

retrograde infantilism. See **acromegalic eunuchoidism.**

retrograde infection, an infection that spreads along a tubule or duct against the flow of secretions or excretions, as in the urinary and lymphatic systems.

retrograde menstruation, a backflow of menstrual discharge through the uterine cavity and the fallopian tubes into the peritoneal cavity. Fragments of endometrium may attach to the ovaries or other organs, causing endometriosis. Also called **regurgitant menstruation.**

retrograde pyelography, a radiologic technique for examining the structures of the collecting system of the kidneys that is especially useful in locating a urinary tract obstruction. A radiopaque contrast medium is injected through a urinary catheter into the ureters and the calyces of the pel-

ves of the kidneys. Rarely, severe anaphylactoid reaction to the medium may occur, because of a patient's hypersensitivity to the iodine in the medium, and infection or trauma may result from the catheterization.

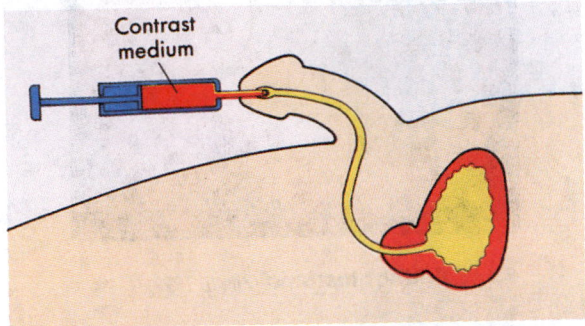

Technique for retrograde pyelography (Gray, 1992)

retrograde urography. See **retrograde pyelography.**

retrograde Wenckebach, a progressively lengthening conduction of impulses from the ventricles or AV junction to the atria until an impulse fails to reach the atria.

retrogression /-gresh′ən/ [L, *retro* + *gradi*, to step], a return to a less complex state, condition, or behavioral adaptation; degeneration; deterioration. See also **regression.**

retrolental fibroplasia /-len′təl/ [L, *retro* + *lentil*, lens; *fibra*, fiber; Gk, *plassein*, to mold], a formation of fibrous tissue behind the lens of the eye, resulting in blindness. The disorder is caused by administration of excessive concentrations of oxygen to premature infants.

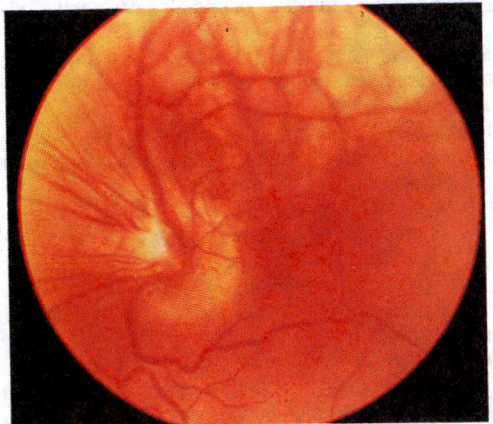

Retrolental fibroplasia (Zitelli, 1992)

retromolar pad /-mō′lər/ [L, *retro* + *mola*, mill; D, *paden*, cushion], a mass of soft tissue, usually pear-shaped, that marks the distal termination of the mandibular residual ridge. It is composed of fibers of the buccinator muscle, the pterygomandibular raphe, the superior constrictor muscle, the temporal tendon, and mucous glands.

retromylohyoid space /ret′rōmī′lōhī′oid/ [L, *retro* + Gk, *myle*, mill, *hyoeides*, upsilon-shaped; L, *spatium*], the part of the alveolingual sulcus that is distal to the distal end of the mylohyoid ridge.

retroperitoneal /-per'tənē'əl/ [L, *retro* + Gk, *peri*, around, *teinein*, to stretch], of or pertaining to organs closely attached to the abdominal wall and partly covered by peritoneum, rather than suspended by that membrane.

retroperitoneal fibrosis, a chronic inflammatory process, usually of unknown cause, in which fibrous tissue surrounds the large blood vessels in the lower lumbar area. It frequently causes constriction of the midportion of the ureters, which may lead to hydronephrosis and azotemia. Occasionally the fibrosis spreads upward to involve the duodenum, bile ducts, and superior vena cava. Symptoms include low-back and abdominal pain, weakness, weight loss, fever, and, with urinary tract involvement, frequency of urination, hematuria, polyuria, or anuria. Methysergide, taken to prevent migraine headaches, is one known cause of this condition. Treatment includes stopping methysergide and instituting surgical release of the ureters from the fibrosis with transplantation laterally or intraperitoneally.

retroperitoneal lymph node dissection, surgical removal of lymph nodes behind the peritoneum, usually performed in an attempt to eliminate sites of lymphoma or metastases from malignancies originating in pelvic organs or genitalia.

retroperitoneum /-per'itənē'əm/ [L, *retro*, backward; Gk, *peri*, *teinein*, to stretch], the space behind the peritoneum.

retropharyngeal abscess /-fərin'jē-əl/ [L, *retro* + Gk, *pharynx*, throat], a collection of pus in the tissues behind the pharynx accompanied by difficulty in swallowing, fever, and pain. Occasionally, the airway becomes obstructed. Treatment includes appropriate parenteral antibiotics and surgical drainage. Tracheostomy may be necessary. Compare **parapharyngeal abscess, peritonsillar abscess.**

retroplacental /-pləsen'təl/, behind the placenta.

retrospective chart audit /-spek'tiv/ [L, *retro* + *spicere*, to look], a format for an audit developed by the Joint Commission on the Accreditation of Hospitals. The audit involves several steps that outline a procedure for evaluating the effectiveness of the care given at a particular institution and for correcting any deficiencies found by reviewing the patient's records after discharge and comparing the data with standards held to be adequate by the Commission.

retrospective nursing audit. See **nursing audit.**

retrospective study, a study in which a search is made for a relationship between one (usually current) phenomenon or condition and another that occurred in the past, such as a study of the family histories of young women diagnosed as having clear cell adenomas of the vagina, which yielded a relationship between the administration of diethylstilbestrol to the mothers of the women during pregnancy and the development of the condition in the daughters.

retrosternal /-stur'nəl/ [L, *retro*, backward; Gk, *sternon*, chest], pertaining to the area behind the sternum.

retrouterine /re'trōyoo'tərin/, behind the uterus.

retroversion /-vur'zhən/ [L, *retro* + *vertere*, to turn], **1.** a common condition in which an organ is tipped backward, usually without flexion or other distortion. The uterus may be retroverted in as many as one fourth of normal women. Uterine retroversion is measured as first-, second-, or third-degree, depending on the angle of tilt with respect to the vagina. Compare **anteversion.** See also **anteflexion, retroflexion. 2.** an abnormal condition in which the teeth or other maxillary and mandibular structures are posterior to

their normal positions. Also called **retrusion.** −**retrovert,** *v.*

Retrovir, trademark for a brand of antiretroviral drug, **zidovudine.**

retrovirus /-vī'rəs/ [L, *retro* + *virus*], any of a family of RNA viruses containing reverse transcriptase in the virion. During replication the viral DNA becomes integrated into the DNA of the host cell. Retroviruses are enveloped and assemble their capsids in the cytoplasm of the host cell. The HIV, which causes AIDS, is a retrovirus.

retrusion. See **retroversion.**

revascularization /rēvas'kyələr'īzā'shən/ [L, *re* + *vasculum*, small vessel; Gk, *izein*, to cause], the restoration by surgical means of blood flow to an organ or a tissue being replaced, as in bypass surgery.

reverberation /rivur'bərā'shən/, the phenomenon of multiple reflections within a closed system.

Reverdin's needle /'reverdaNz'/ [Albert Reverdin, Swiss surgeon, b. 1881], a surgical needle with an eye that can be opened and closed with a slide.

reversal film /rivur'səl/, (in radiology) a reverse-tone duplicate of an x-ray image, showing black changed to white and white to black. It is produced by exposing single-emulsion film through a standard x-ray film. Also called **diapositive, positive mask.**

reverse anaphylaxis. See **inverse anaphylaxis.**

reverse Barton's fracture /rivurs'/ [L, *revertere*, to turn back; John R. Barton, American surgeon, b. 1794], a fracture of the volar articular surface of the radius with associated displacement of the carpal bones and radius.

reverse bevel. See **contra bevel.**

reverse curve, (in dentistry) a convex curve of occlusion, as viewed in the frontal plane.

reversed bandage /rivurst'/, a roller bandage that is reversed on itself with a half twist so that it lies smoothly, conforming to the contour of the extremity. See also **roller bandage.**

reversed coarctation. See **Takayasu's arteritis.**

reversed phase, a chromatographic mode in which the mobile phase is more polar than the stationary phase.

reverse isolation, isolation procedures designed to protect a patient from infectious organisms that might be carried by the staff, other patients, or visitors or on droplets in the air or on equipment or materials. Absolute reverse isolation is rarely necessary and requires elaborate specialized equipment. Protective modified reverse isolation is less restrictive but is not prolonged needlessly, because the patient usually comes to feel lonely and sensorily deprived. Handwashing, gowning, gloving, sterilization or disinfection of materials brought into the area, and other details of housekeeping vary with the reason for the isolation and the usual practices of the hospital.

reverse peristalsis [L, *revertere*, to turn back; Gk, *peristellein*, to clasp], peristalsis that propels the contents in a direction opposite to the normal outward direction.

reverse transcriptase (RT), an enzyme that is present in the virion of retroviruses. Reverse transcriptase occurs in leukoviruses and RNA tumor viruses of eukaryotic cells. Also called **RNA-dependent DNA polymerase.** See also **retrovirus.**

reverse Trendelenburg, a position in which the lower extremities are lower than the body and head, which are elevated on an inclined plane.

reversible brain syndrome, any of a group of acute brain disorders characterized by a disruption of cognition, as in delirium. The disorder is related to a variety of biologic stressors, and recovery is possible.

review of systems (ROS) /rivyo͞o/ [Fr, *revoir*, to see again], (in a health history) a system-by-system review of the functions of the body. The ROS is begun during the initial interview with the patient and completed during the physical examination, as physical findings prompt further questions. One outline of the systems and some of the signs and symptoms that might be noted or reported are as follows:

■ SKIN: bruising, discoloration, pruritus, birthmarks, moles, ulcers, decubiti, changes in the hair or nails.

■ HEMATOPOIETIC: spontaneous or excessive bleeding, fatigue, enlarged or tender lymph nodes, pallor, history of anemia.

■ HEAD AND FACE: pain, traumatic injury, ptosis.

■ EARS: ringing in the ears, change in hearing, running or discharge from the ears, deafness, dizziness.

■ EYES: change in vision, pain, inflammation, infections, double vision, scotomata, blurring, tearing.

■ MOUTH AND THROAT: dental problems, hoarseness, dysphagia, bleeding gums, sore throat, ulcers or sores in the mouth.

■ NOSE AND SINUSES: discharge, epistaxis, sinus pain, obstruction.

■ BREASTS: pain, change in contour or skin color, lumps, discharge from the nipple.

■ RESPIRATORY TRACT: cough, sputum, change in sputum, night sweats, nocturnal dyspnea, wheezing.

■ CARDIOVASCULAR SYSTEM: chest pain, dyspnea, palpitations, weakness, intolerance of exercise, varicosities, swelling of extremities, known murmur, high blood pressure, asystole.

■ GASTROINTESTINAL SYSTEM: nausea, vomiting, diarrhea, constipation, quality of appetite, change in appetite, dysphagia, gas, heartburn, melena, change in bowel habits, use of laxatives or other drugs to alter the function of the GI tract.

■ URINARY TRACT: dysuria, change in color of urine, change in frequency of urination, pain with urgency, incontinence, edema, retention.

■ GENITAL TRACT (FEMALE): menstrual history, obstetric history, contraceptive use, discharge, pain or discomfort, pruritus, history of venereal disease.

■ GENITAL TRACT (MALE): penile discharge, pain or discomfort, pruritus, skin lesions, hematuria, history of venereal disease.

■ SKELETAL SYSTEM: heat, redness, swelling, limitation of function, deformity, crepitation; pain in a joint or an extremity, the neck, or back, especially with movement.

■ NERVOUS SYSTEM: dizziness, tremor, ataxia, difficulty in speaking, change in speech, paresthesia, loss of sensation, seizures, syncope.

■ ENDOCRINE SYSTEM: tremor, palpitations, intolerance of heat or cold, polyuria, polydipsia, polyphagia, diaphoresis, exophthalmos, goiter.

■ PSYCHOLOGIC STATUS: nervousness, instability, depression, phobia, sexual disturbances, criminal behavior, insomnia, night terrors, mania, memory loss, perseveration, disorientation.

Reye's syndrome /rāz′/ [Ralph D. K. Reye, 20th century Australian pathologist], a combination of acute encephalopathy and fatty infiltration of the internal organs that may follow acute viral infections. This syndrome has been associated with influenza B, chickenpox (varicella), the enteroviruses, and the Epstein-Barr virus. It usually affects people under 18 years of age, characteristically causing an exanthematous rash, vomiting, and confusion about 1 week after the onset of a viral illness. In the late stage, there may be extreme disorientation followed by coma, seizures, and respiratory arrest. Laboratory tests reveal greater than normal amounts of SGOT and SGPT, bilirubin, and ammonia in the blood. A specimen obtained by liver biopsy shows fatty degeneration and confirms the diagnosis. Mortality varies between 20% and 80%, depending on the severity of symptoms. The cause of Reye's syndrome is unknown; however, there appears to be an association with the administration of aspirin. Therefore, aspirin should not be given in cases of chickenpox or suspected influenza. No specific treatment is available. Insulin, antibiotics, and mannitol may be given. Blood gases, blood pH, and blood pressure are monitored frequently. Intensive, supportive nursing care with meticulous monitoring of all vital functions and prompt correction of any imbalance are of extreme significance in the outcome of this syndrome.

rf, 1. abbreviation for **radiofrequency.** 2. abbreviation for **rheumatic fever.**

RF, abbreviation for **rheumatoid factor.**

R factor, an episome in bacteria that is responsible for drug resistance and is transmissible to progeny and to other bacterial cells by conjugation. The portion of the episome involved in replication and transmission is called **resistance transfer factor.**

RFP, abbreviation for **request for proposal.**

RF test. See **latex fixation test.**

Rh, 1. abbreviation for *rhesus*. See **Rh factor.** 2. symbol for the chemical element **rhodium.**

-rh-. For combining forms containing -rh-, see -(r)rh . . .; for example, -(r)rhachia, -(r)rhage.

r/h, 1. abbreviation for **relative humidity.** 2. abbreviation for *roentgens per hour*.

rhabdo-, rhabdi-, a combining form meaning 'rod-shaped' or 'of or pertaining to a rod': *rhabdocyte, rhabdomyoma, rhabdosarcoma.*

rhabdomyo-, a combining form meaning 'striated or skeletal muscle': *rhabdomyolysis, rhabdomyoma.*

rhabdomyoma /rab′dōmī·ō′mə/, *pl.* **rhabdomyomas, rhabdomyomata** [Gk, *rhabdos*, rod, *mys*, muscle, *oma*], a tumor of striated muscle that may occur in the uterus, vagina, pharynx, or tongue, or in the heart. Also called **myoma striocellulare.**

rhabdomyosarcoma /rab′dōmī′ō·särkō′mə/, *pl.* **rhabdomyosarcomas, rhabdomyosarcomata** [Gk, *rhabdos* + *mys*, muscle, *sarx*, flesh, *oma*], a highly malignant tumor, derived from primitive striated muscle cells, that occurs most frequently in the head and neck and is also found in the genitourinary tract, extremities, body wall, and retroperitoneum. In some cases, the onset is associated with trauma. The initial symptoms depend on the site of tumor development and indicate local tissue or organ destruction, such as dysphagia, vaginal bleeding, hematuria, or obstruction of the flow of urine. Diagnostic measures may include barium x-ray studies, angiography, or tomography. Embryonal rhabdomyosarcoma occurs in the head, neck, or trunk of young children; alveolar rhabdomyosarcoma is usually seen in the extremities of adolescents; and the pleomorphic form is most common in the legs of adults. Surgical excision is rarely possible, because the tumor is poorly encapsulated and tends to spread. Amputation of an affected limb or extremity may be curative. Radiotherapy and chemother-

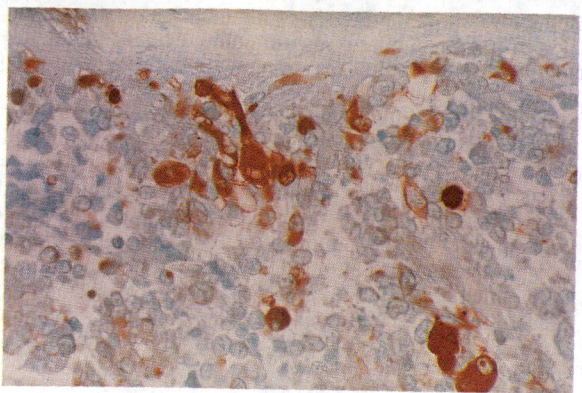

Rhabdomyosarcoma *(Skarin, 1991)*

apy with combinations of actinomycin D, adriamycin, cyclophosphamide, and vincristine may greatly increase the length of survival. Also called **rhabdosarcoma.**

rhabdovirus /rab'dōvī'rəs/ [Gk, *rhabdos* + L, *virus*, poison], a member of a family of viruses that includes the organism causing rabies.

-(r) rhachia. See **-rh-.**

-(r) rhage. See **-rh-.**

rhachi-. See **rachio-.**

rhagades /rag'ədēz/ [Gk, chinks], cracks or fissures in skin that has lost its elasticity, especially common around the mouth. See also **cheilosis.**

-rhage, -rrhage, -rhagia, -rrhagia a combining form meaning 'excessive flow': *metrorrhagia, hemorrhage.*

Rh antiserum [Rh, rhesus; Gk, *anti*, L, *serum*, whey], a serum that contains Rh antibodies.

rhaphe. See **raphe.**

-rhaphy, -rrhaphy, a suffix meaning 'suturing in place': *colporrhaphy, gastrorrhaphy.*

Rh blood group. See **Rh factor.**

rhd, 1. abbreviation for *radioactive health data*. **2.** abbreviation for **rheumatic heart disease.**

Rh$_o$(D) immune globulin, a passive immunizing agent.

■ INDICATIONS: It is prescribed to prevent Rh sensitization after abortion, miscarriage, ectopic pregnancy, or normal birth to an Rh-negative mother of an Rh-positive infant or fetus.

■ CONTRAINDICATIONS: It is not given to an Rh$_o$(D)- positive patient or to the infant or those previously immunized.

■ ADVERSE EFFECTS: The most serious adverse reaction is anaphylaxis.

-rhea, -rrhea, a suffix meaning 'flow or discharge': *rhinorrhea, galactorrhea.*

rhenium (Re) /rē'nē·əm/ [L, *Rhenus*, Rhine], a hard, brittle metallic element. Its atomic number is 75; its atomic weight is 186.2. Rhenium has a high melting point and is used in x-ray tube anodes and in thermometers for measuring high temperatures.

rheo-, a combining form meaning 'of or pertaining to electric current, stream, or to a flow': *rheobase, rheoscope, rheotaxis, rheostosis.*

Rheomacrodex, a trademark for a plasma expander (dextran 40).

rheostat /rē'əstat/ [Gk, *rheos*, current + *statikos*, causing to stand], a variable resistance electrical device that can be adjusted to control the strength of a current.

Rhesus factor. See **Rh factor.**

rheumatic /rōomat'ik/ [Gk, *rheuma*, flux], of or pertaining to rheumatism.

-rheumatic, a suffix meaning 'relating to or exhibiting traits of rheumatism': *postrheumatic, prerheumatic, pseudorheumatic.*

rheumatic aortitis, an inflammatory condition of the aorta, occurring in rheumatic fever and characterized by disseminated focal lesions that may progressively form patches of fibrosis.

rheumatic arteritis, a complication of rheumatic fever characterized by generalized inflammation of arteries and arterioles. Fibrin, mixed with cellular debris, may invade, thicken, and stiffen the vessel wall, and the vessel may be surrounded by hemorrhage and exudate.

rheumatic carditis [Gk, *rheumat* + *kardia*, heart + *itis*, inflammation], the pericarditis, myocarditis, and endocarditis that may be associated with acute rheumatic fever.

rheumatic chorea. See **Sydenham's chorea.**

rheumatic endocarditis [Gk, *rheumatismos*, that which flows + *endon*, within + *kardia*, heart + *itis*, inflammation], an inflammation of the endocardium in association with acute rheumatic fever.

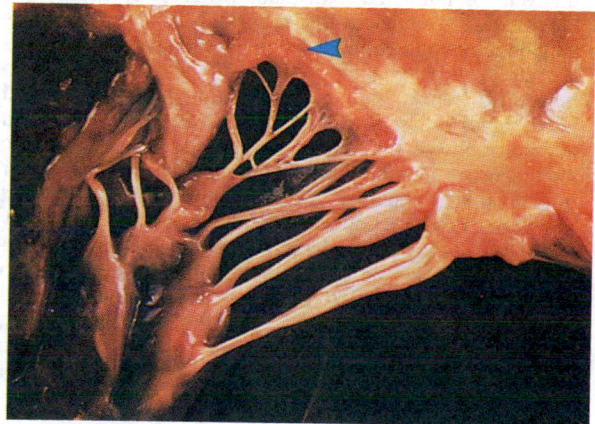

Rheumatic endocarditis *(Fletcher, 1987)*

rheumatic fever, an inflammatory disease that may develop as a delayed reaction to inadequately treated Group A beta-hemolytic streptococcal infection of the upper respiratory tract. This disorder usually occurs in young school-age children and may affect the brain, heart, joints, skin, or subcutaneous tissues. See also **rheumatic heart disease.**

■ OBSERVATIONS: The onset of rheumatic fever is usually sudden, often occurring in from 1 to 5 symptom-free weeks after recovery from a sore throat or from scarlet fever. Early symptoms usually include fever, joint pains, nose bleeds, abdominal pain, and vomiting. The major manifestations of this disease include migratory polyarthritis affecting numerous joints and carditis, which causes palpitations, chest pain, and, in severe cases, symptoms of cardiac failure. Sydenham's chorea, which may develop, is usually the sole, late sign of rheumatic fever and may initially be manifested as an increased awkwardness and an associated tendency to

drop objects. As the chorea progresses, irregular body movements may become extensive, occasionally involving the tongue and the facial muscles, resulting in incapacitation of the affected individual. Other developments may include transient erythema marginatum with circular lesions and subcutaneous rheumatic nodules on various joints and tendons, the spine, and the back of the head. There is no specific diagnostic test for rheumatic fever. The development of serum antibodies to streptococcal antigens is a positive diagnostic sign. Affected individuals may also develop leukocytosis, moderate anemia, and proteinuria. C-reactive protein, evaluated in a specimen of blood, is abnormally high. Recurrences of rheumatic fever are common. Except for carditis, all the manifestations of this disease usually subside without any permanent effects. Mild cases may last 3 to 4 weeks. Severe cases with associated arthritis and carditis may last 2 to 3 months.
■ INTERVENTIONS: Management of this disease includes bed rest and severe restriction of normal activity. Penicillin is often administered, even if throat cultures are negative, and steroids or salicylates may be used, depending on the severity of any associated carditis and arthritis.
■ NURSING CONSIDERATIONS: The nurse is alert to signs of toxicity associated with salicylate and steroid therapies. Symptoms largely determine the type of nursing care. Large volumes of fluids are usually administered, and the nurse routinely helps minimize joint pains by properly positioning the patient. Throughout the course of the disease the patient benefits from emotional support and appropriate diversions.

rheumatic heart disease, damage to heart muscle and heart valves caused by episodes of rheumatic fever. When a susceptible person acquires a group A beta-hemolytic streptococcal infection, an autoimmune reaction may occur in heart tissue, resulting in permanent deformities of heart valves or chordae tendineae. Involvement of the heart may be evident during acute rheumatic fever, or it may be discovered long after the acute disease has subsided. See also **aortic stenosis, mitral stenosis, rheumatic fever.**

rheumatic nodules [Gk, *rheumatismos*, that which flows; L, *nodulus*, small knot], aggregations of fibroblasts and lymphoid cells that may accumulate in soft tissues and over bony prominences of patients afflicted with rheumatoid arthritis and rheumatic fever.

rheumatic scoliosis [Gk, *rheumatismos*, that which flows + *skoliosis*, curvature], a form of scoliosis associated with muscle spasms and acute inflammation. Also called **inflammatory scoliosis.**

rheumatid /rōō′mətid/ [Gk, *rheumatismos*, that which flows], a skin eruption that sometimes occurs with rheumatic disorders.

rheumatism /rōō′mətiz′əm/ [Gk, *rheumatismos*, that which flows], *nontechnical.* **1.** any of a large number of inflammatory conditions of the bursae, joints, ligaments, or muscles characterized by pain, limitation of movement, and structural degeneration of single or multiple parts of the musculoskeletal system. **2.** the syndrome of pain, limitation of movement, and structural degeneration of elements in the musculoskeletal system as may occur in gout, rheumatoid arthritis, systemic lupus erythematosus, ankylosing spondylitis, and many other diseases. **–rheumatic, rheumatoid,** *adj.*

rheumatoid arteritis /rōō′mətoid/ [Gk, *rheumatismos*, that which flows + *arteria*, artery + *itis*, inflammation], inflammation of the arterial walls associated with a rheumatic disorder. See also **rheumatoid coronary arteritis.**

rheumatoid arthritis [Gk, *rheumatismos* + *eidos*, form; *arthron*, joint, *itis*, inflammation], a chronic, destructive, sometimes deforming, collagen disease that has an autoimmune component. Rheumatoid arthritis is characterized by symmetric inflammation of the synovium and increased synovial exudate, leading to thickening of the synovium and swelling of the joint. Rheumatoid arthritis usually first appears in early middle age, between 36 and 50 years of age, and most commonly in women. The course of the disease is variable but is most frequently marked by remissions and exacerbation. Also called **arthritis deformans, atrophic arthritis.** See also **ankylosing spondylitis, juvenile rheumatoid arthritis.**

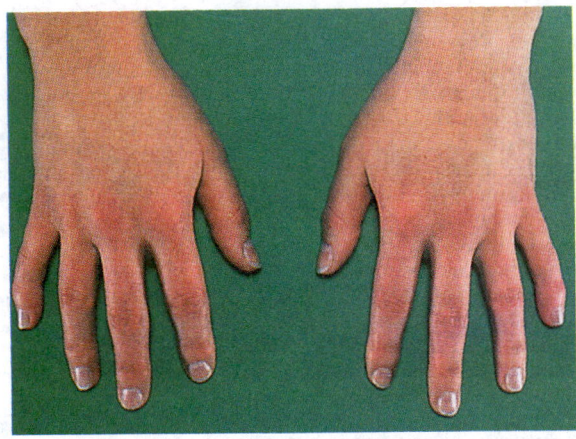

Early rheumatoid arthritis of the hands
(Shipley, 1993)

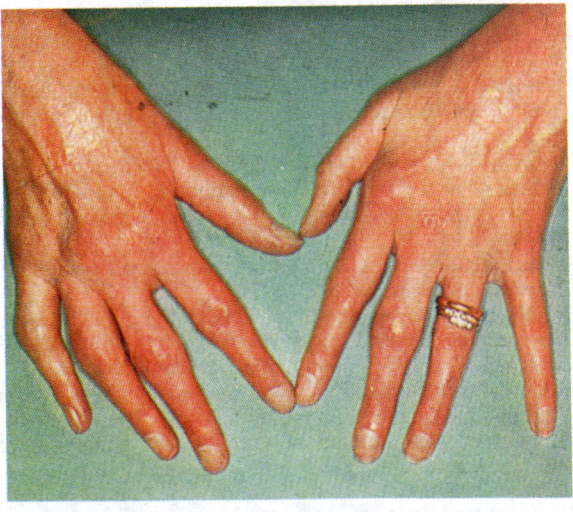

Advanced rheumatoid arthritis of the hands
(Shipley, 1993)

Rheumatoid arthritis

Clinical stages	*Functional classification*
Stage I, early 1. X-ray films show no evidence of destructive changes. 2. X-ray films may show evidence of osteoporosis.	**Class I** No loss of functional capacity.
Stage II, moderate 1. X-ray films show evidence of osteoporosis, possibly with slight destruction of cartilage or subchondral bone. 2. Joints are not deformed, but mobility may be limited. 3. Adjacent muscles are atrophied. 4. Extraarticular soft-tissue lesions (as nodules and tenovaginitis) may be present.	**Class II** Functional capacity impaired but sufficient normal activities despite joint pain or limited mobility.
Stage III, severe 1. X-ray films show cartilage and bone destruction, as well as osteoporosis. 2. Joint deformity (such as subluxation, ulnar deviation, or hyperextension) exists but not fibrous or bony ankylosis. 3. Muscle atrophy is extensive. 4. Extraarticular soft-tissue lesions (such as nodules and tenovaginitis) are often present.	**Class III** Functional capacity adequate to perform few if any occupational or self-care tasks. **Class IV** Patient confined to bed or wheelchair and capable of little or no self-care.
Stage IV, terminal 1. Fibrous or bony ankylosis exists in addition to all criteria listed for stage III.	

From Billings DM, Stokes LG: *Medical surgical nursing: common health problems of adults and children across the life span*, ed 2, St Louis, 1987, Mosby.

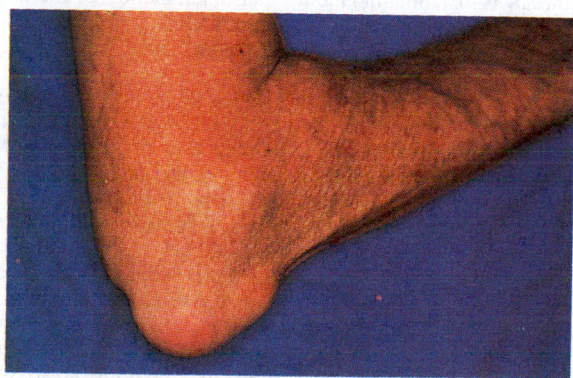

Rheumatoid nodule of the elbow
(Kamal, 1991/Courtesy Dr. JP Miller)

classified on the basis of functional capacity: Class I, no loss of function; Class II, minor impairment of functional capacity with some pain and immobility; Class III, capacity limited to a few tasks; and Class IV, in which the patient is confined to bed or a wheelchair.

Rheumatoid arthritis may first be present with constitutional symptoms, including fatigue, weakness, and poor appetite. Other early signs include low-grade fever, anemia, and an increased erythrocyte sedimentation rate. The symptoms listed by the American Rheumatism Association include morning stiffness, joint pain or tenderness, swelling of at least two joints, subcutaneous nodules (called arthritic nodules and usually found at pressure points, such as the elbows), structural changes in the joint seen on x-ray film, a positive rheumatoid factor agglutination test, decreased precipitation of mucin from synovial fluid, and characteristic histologic changes on pathologic examination of the fluid. Immune complexes are characteristically present in both the blood serum and the synovial fluid. Rheumatoid factor (RF) is present in serum and joint fluid of most persons with rheumatoid arthritis, and higher titers of rheumatoid factor are correlated with more severe forms of the disease, in particular forms with extraarticular manifestations. Antinuclear antibodies and special rheumatoid precipitins are also occasionally present. Extraarticular manifestations may include cardiac involvement, vasculitis, pulmonary disease, and proteinuria. There may also be a thickening of the synovium, called pannus formation. In long-term, severe, chronic rheumatoid arthritis, Felty's syndrome may be present.

■ **INTERVENTIONS:** The basic principles of treatment include sufficient rest, exercise to maintain joint function, medication for the relief of pain and the reduction of inflammation, orthopedic intervention to prevent or correct deformities, and excellent nutrition—with weight loss, if neces-

■ **OBSERVATIONS:** The medical diagnosis and prognosis of a case are based on a variety of clinical and laboratory findings. Clinical data, using mainly x-ray studies and physical examination, classify the progress of rheumatoid arthritis into four stages. Stage I, representing early effects, is based on x-ray films showing the onset of bone changes. Stage II, moderate rheumatoid arthritis, is assigned cases in which there is evidence of some muscle atrophy and loss of mobility, in addition to x-ray findings. Stage III, severe rheumatoid arthritis, is marked by joint deformity, extensive muscle atrophy, and soft tissue lesions, as well as definite bone and cartilage destruction. Stage IV, the terminal category, includes all the Stage III clinical signs plus fibrous or bony ankylosis. Rheumatoid arthritis cases may also be

sary. Salicylates are usually given. If improvement is not achieved, other antiinflammatories, such as indomethacin, phenylbutazone, antimalarials, gold salts, or some antineoplastic drugs may be used. Corticosteroids are prescribed with caution because of side effects, including gastric ulcer, adrenal suppression, and osteoporosis. Other treatments, including diathermy, ultrasound, warm paraffin applications, exercise under water, and applications of heat, are occasionally used.

■ NURSING CONSIDERATIONS: Rheumatoid arthritis is not always progressive, deforming, or debilitating. The nurse can play an important role by monitoring drug treatment so that adequate medication is taken, by noting side effects, and by adjusting treatment. Most people who have rheumatoid arthritis may continue in their jobs. The nurse encourages the person to get sufficient sleep and to rest both the small joints and weight-bearing joints. Suggestions about the most effective use of heat or cold, instruction in muscle-strengthening exercise and methods for easing pain and preventing deformities, such as the proper use of pillows, splints, or molds, as well as emotional support are often given by the nurse. Because stress often precedes exacerbation of the condition, the person is counseled to avoid situations known to cause anxiety, worry, fatigue, infection, and other stressors.

rheumatoid coronary arteritis,   an abnormal condition, characterized by a thickening of the tunica intima of the coronary arteries, which may produce coronary insufficiency. Rheumatoid coronary arteritis is a collagen disease that affects the connective tissue by inflammation and fibrinoid degeneration. It is commonly treated with glucocorticoids.

rheumatoid factor (RF),   antiglobulin antibodies often found in the serum of patients with a clinical diagnosis of rheumatoid arthritis. Rheumatoid factors are present in about 70% of such cases, but they may also be found in such widely divergent diseases as tuberculosis, parasitic infections, leukemia, and connective tissue disorders. See also **latex fixation test.**

rheumatologist /roo′mətol′ə′jist/,   a specialist in rheumatology.

rheumatology /-ol′əjē/ [Gk, *rheuma*, flux, *logos*, science], the study of disorders characterized by inflammation, degeneration, or metabolic derangement of connective tissue and related structures of the body. These disorders are sometimes referred to collectively as rheumatism.

Rh factor,   an antigenic substance present in the erythrocytes of 85% of the people. A person having the factor is Rh+ (Rh positive); a person lacking the factor is Rh− (Rh negative). If an Rh− person receives Rh+ blood, hemolysis and anemia occur. Rh+ infants may be exposed to antibodies to the factor produced in the Rh− mother's blood, resulting in red cell destruction and erythroblastosis fetalis. Transfusion, blood typing, and cross-matching depend on Rh+ and ABO classification. The Rh factor was first identified in the blood of a rhesus (Rh) monkey. See also **erythroblastosis fetalis, Rh$_o$(D) immune globulin.**

Rh genes [Rh, rhesus; Gk, *genein*, to produce],   a series of allelic genes that account for the various Rh blood groups. The four variations of the Rh$^+$ gene are identified as R^o, R^1, R^2, and R^z, whereas the four types of Rh-gene are designated as r, r′, r″, and r$_y$.

rhigo-,   a combining form meaning 'shivering or cold': *rhigolene, rhigosis, rhigotic.*

Rh immune globulin [Rh, rhesus; L, *immunis*, free from + *globulus*],   an immune globulin that is administered to

all Rh- mothers after every abortion or delivery unless the infant is Rh- or unless the mother's serum already contains anti-Rh$_o$(D) reagent.

rhin-.   See **rhino-.**

Rh incompatibility,   (in hematology) a lack of compatibility between two groups of blood cells that are antigenically different because of the presence of the Rh factor in one group and absence of the Rh factor in the other. See also **Rh factor.**

rhinencephalon /rī′nensef′ələn/, *pl.* **rhinencephala** [Gk, *rhis*, nose, *encephalon*, brain],   a portion of each cerebral hemisphere that contains the limbic system, which is associated with the emotions. The rhinencephalon develops in the embryo from a longitudinal ridge at the rostral extremity of the cerebral hemisphere. The rostral part of the ridge becomes the primitive olfactory lobe; the caudal part becomes the piriform lobe. In an adult, the caudal part of the piriform lobe is absorbed into the gyrus hippocampus. See also **limbic system. –rhinencephalic,** *adj.*

rhinitis /rīnī′tis/ [Gk, *rhis* + *itis*, inflammation], inflammation of the mucous membranes of the nose, usually accompanied by swelling of the mucosa and a nasal discharge. It may be complicated by sinusitis. Rhinitis may be acute, allergic, atrophic, or vasomotor. Also called **coryza.**

rhino- /rī′nō-/, **rhin-,**   a combining form meaning 'of or pertaining to the nose or to a noselike structure': *rhinocephalia, rhinolalia, rhinoplasty.*

rhinolaryngitis /-ler′injī′tis/ [Gk, *rhis*, nose + *larynx*, throat + *itis*, inflammation],   an inflammation of the mucous membranes of the nose and throat.

rhinopathy /rīnop′əthē/ [Gk, *rhis* + *pathos*, disease],   any disease or malformation of the nose.

rhinophycomycosis /rī′nōfī′kōmīkō′sis/,   an infection of the nasal and paranasal sinuses caused by the phycomycete *Entomophthora coronata.* The infection often spreads to surrounding tissues, including the eye and brain.

rhinophyma /rī′nōfī′mə/ [Gk, *rhis* + *phyma*, tumor],   a form of rosacea in which there is sebaceous hyperplasia, redness, prominent vascularity, swelling, and distortion of the skin of the nose. Treatment includes dermabrasion, electrosurgery, and plastic surgery. See also **rosacea.**

rhinoplasty /rī′nəplas′tē/ [Gk, *rhis* + *plassein*, to mold],   a procedure in plastic surgery in which the structure of the nose is changed. Bone or cartilage may be removed, tissue grafted from another part of the body, or synthetic material implanted to alter the shape. Under local anesthesia intranasal incisions are made and the nose is reshaped. Postoperatively, any respiratory difficulty is reported immediately and the patient is kept in mid-Fowler's position. Frequent oral care is given, and ice compresses are applied to decrease the pain and edema that usually occur. Edema and discoloration around the eyes is expected to last for several days. The procedure is most frequently performed for cosmetic reasons.

rhinorrhagia /rī′nôrā′jə/ [Gk, *rhis*, nose + *rhegnynein*, to gush forth],   a profuse nosebleed.

rhinorrhea /rī′nôrē′ə/ [Gk, *rhis* + *rhoia*, flow],   **1.** the free discharge of a thin watery nasal fluid. **2.** the flow of cerebrospinal fluid from the nose after an injury to the head.

rhinoscope /rī′nəskōp/,   an instrument for examining the nasal passages through the anterior nares or through the nasopharynx.

rhinoscopy /rīnos′kəpē/ [Gk, *rhis* + *skopein*, to look],   an examination of the nasal passages to inspect the mucosa and detect inflammation, deformities, or asymmetry, as in de-

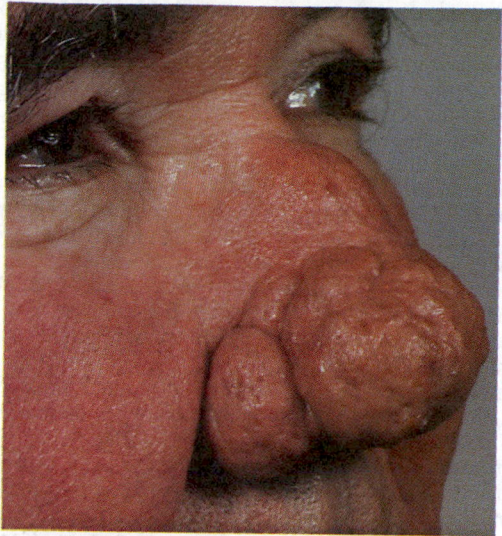

Rhinophyma *(du Vivier, 1993)*

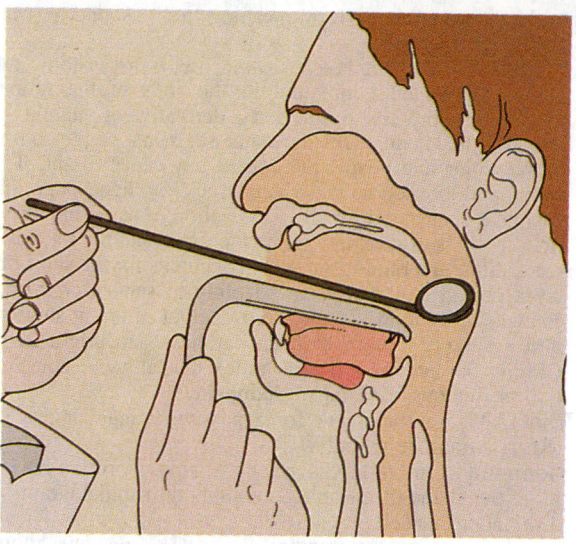

Anterior rhinoscopy *(Epstein, 1992)*

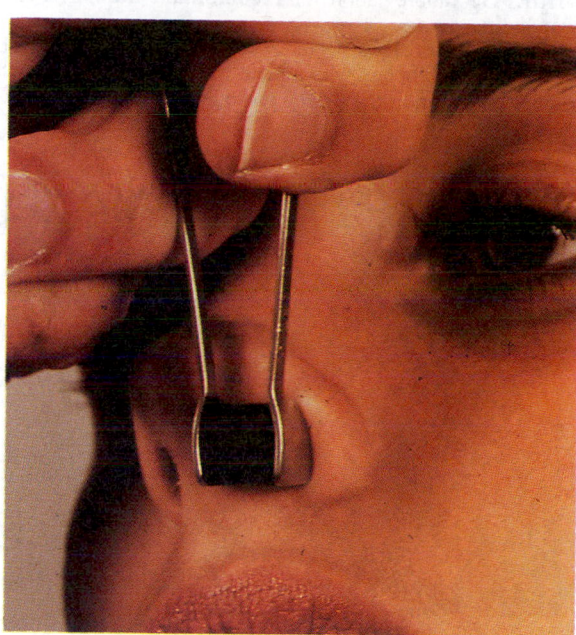

Posterior rhinoscopy *(Epstein, 1992)*

viation of the septum. The nasal passages may be examined anteriorly, by introducing a speculum into the anterior nares, or posteriorly, by introducing a rhinoscope through the nasopharynx. **—rhinoscopic,** *adj.*

rhinosporidiosis /rī′nōspərid′ē·ō′sis/ [Gk, *rhis* + *sporo,* seed, *osis,* condition], an infection caused by the fungus *Rhinosporidium seeberi,* characterized by fleshy red polyps on mucous membranes of nose, conjunctiva, nasopharynx, and soft palate. The disease may be acquired by swimming or bathing in infected water. The most effective treatment is electrocautery.

rhinotomy /rīnot′əmē/ [Gk, *rhis* + *temnein,* to cut], a surgical procedure in which an incision is made along one side of the nose, performed to drain accumulated pus from an abscess or a sinus infection. Under local anesthesia, the flap of skin and lining of the nose are turned back to provide a full view of the nasal passages for radical sinus surgery.

rhinovirus /rī′nōvī′rəs/ [Gk, *rhis* + L, *virus,* poison], any of about 100 serologically distinct, small RNA viruses that cause about 40% of acute respiratory illnesses. Infection is characterized by dry, scratchy throat, nasal congestion, malaise, and headache. Fever is minimal. Nasal discharge lasts 2 or 3 days. Children may also develop a cough. Type-specific antibodies may last for 2 to 4 years. The treatment is nonspecific and may include rest, analgesics, antihistamines, and nasal decongestants. Complete recovery is usual. Compare **adenovirus, parainfluenza virus, respiratory syncytial virus.** See also **cold.**

rhitid-. See **rhytid-.**

rhitidoplasty. See **rhytidoplasty.**

rhitidosis /rit′idō′sis/ [Gk, *rhytis,* wrinkle, *osis,* condition], a wrinkling, especially of the cornea. Also spelled **rhytidosis.**

rhizo-, a combining form meaning 'of or related to a root': *rhizodontropy, rhizome, rhizotomist.*

rhizomelic /rī′zəmel′ik/ [Gk, *rhizo,* root, *melos,* limb], pertaining to the hip and shoulder joints.

rhizotomy /rīzot′əmē/, the surgical resection of the dorsal root of a spinal nerve, performed to relieve pain.

Rh negative. See **Rh factor.**

rho /rō/, P, ρ, the seventeenth letter of the Greek alphabet.

Rhodesian trypanosomiasis /rōdē′zhən/, an acute form of African trypanosomiasis, caused by the parasite *Trypanosoma brucei rhodesiense.* The disease may progress rapidly, causing encephalitis, coma, and death in only a few weeks. Also called **kaodzera.** Compare **Gambian trypanosomiasis.** See also **African trypanosomiasis.**

rhodium (Rh) /rō′dē·əm/ [Gk, *rhodon,* rose], a grayish-white metallic element. Its atomic number is 45; its atomic weight is 102.91. Rhodium is used for providing a hard lustrous coating on other metals and in the making of mirrors.

rhodo-, a combining form meaning 'red': *rhodocyte, rhodopsin, rhodotoxin.*

rhodopsin /rōdop′sin/ [Gk, *rhodon*, rose, *opsis*, vision], the purple pigmented compound in the rods of the retina, formed by a protein, opsin, and a derivative of vitamin A, retinal. Rhodopsin gives the outer segments of the rods a purple color and adapts the eye to low-density light. The compound breaks down when struck by light, and this chemical change triggers the conduction of nerve impulses. Brief periods of darkness allow the opsin and the retinal to reconstitute the rhodopsin, which accounts for the short delay a person experiences in adapting to sudden or drastic changes in lighting, as when moving out of bright sunlight into a darkened room or from darkness into bright light. Closing the eyes is a natural reflex that allows reconstitution of rhodopsin. Compare **iodopsin.**

RhoGAM, a trademark for a passive immunizing agent (Rh₀(D) immune globulin).

rhomboid /rom′boid/ [Gk, *rhomb* + *eidos*, form], resembling the shape of an oblique equilateral parallelogram, as a rhomboid muscle.

rhomboideus major /romboi′dē·əs/ [Gk, *rhombos*, rhombus, *eidos*, form], a muscle of the upper back below and parallel to the rhomboideus minor. Arising from the spinous processes of the third, fourth, and fifth thoracic vertebrae and inserting into the lower half of the medial border of the scapula, it is innervated by the dorsal scapular nerve from the brachial plexus and, with the rhomboideus minor, functions to draw the scapula toward the vertebral column while supporting it and drawing it slightly upward. Compare **latissimus dorsi, levator scapulae, rhomboideus minor, trapezius.**

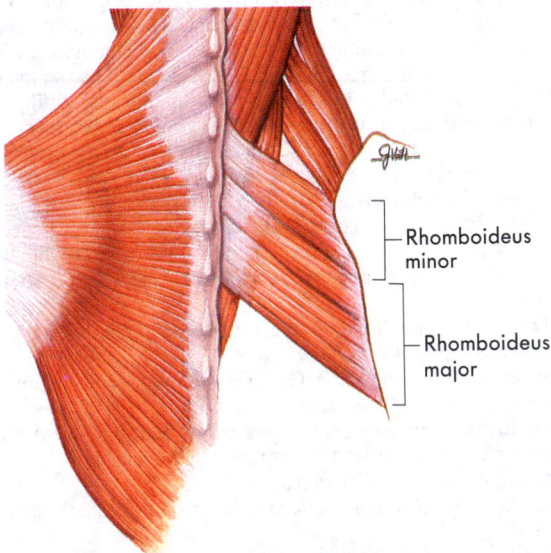

Rhomboideus major and Rhomboideus minor
(Thibodeau, 1993/John V Hagen)

rhomboideus minor, a muscle of the upper back, above and parallel to the rhomboideus major. It arises from the ligamentum nuchae and from the spinous processes of the seventh cervical and first thoracic vertebrae. It inserts into the upper part of the medial border at the root of the spine

of the scapula. It is innervated by the dorsal scapular nerve from the brachial plexus, which contains fibers from the fifth cervical nerve and, with the rhomboideus major, acts to draw the scapula toward the vertebral column while supporting the scapula and drawing it slightly upward. Compare **latissimus dorsi, levator scapulae, rhomboideus major, trapezius.**

rhomboid glossitis. See **median rhomboid glossitis.**

rhonchi /rong′kī/, *sing.* **rhonchus** /rong′kəs/ [Gk, *rhonchos*, snore], abnormal sounds heard on auscultation of an airway obstructed by thick secretions, muscular spasm, neoplasm, or external pressure. The continuous rumbling sounds are more pronounced during expiration, and they characteristically clear on coughing, which gurgles do not. Also called **rale, wheeze.**

rhonchus [Gk, *rhogchos*, snore], the sound produced by air moving into and out of the bronchi when there is a partial obstruction.

rhotacism /rō′təsiz′əm/ [Gk, *rho*, letter R], a speech disorder characterized by a defective pronunciation of words containing the sound /r/, or by the excessive use of the sound /r/, or by the substitution of another sound for /r/. Compare **lallation, lambdacism.**

Rh positive. See **Rh factor.**

r-HuEPO, abbreviation for **recombinant human erythropoietin.**

rhus dermatitis /rōōs/, [Gk, *rhous*, sumac], a skin rash resulting from contact with a plant of the genus *Rhus*, such as poison ivy, poison oak, or poison sumac. See also **contact dermatitis.**

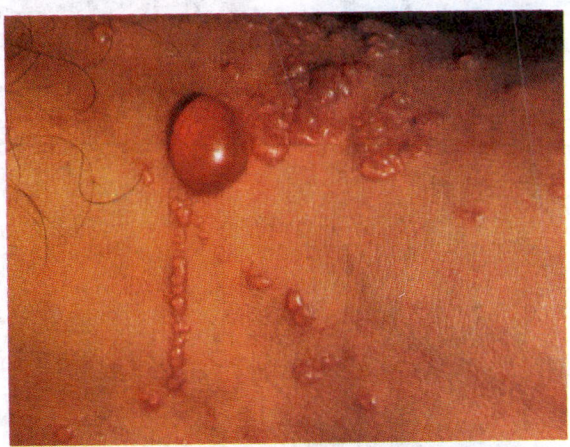

Rhus dermatitis *(Habif, 1990)*

rhyp-, a prefix meaning 'of or pertaining to filth': *rhyparia, rhypophagy, rhypophobia.*

rhythm /rith′əm/ [Gk, *rhythmos*], the relationship of one impulse to neighboring impulses as measured in time, movement, or regularity of action.

rhythmic nystagmus /rith′mik/ See **nystagmus.**

rhythm method. See **natural family planning method.**

rhytid-, rhitid-, a prefix meaning 'wrinkle, or wrinkled': *rhytidectomy, rhytidosis.*

rhytidoplasty /ritid′ōplas′tē/ [Gk, *rhytis*, wrinkle, *plassein*, to mold], a procedure in reconstructive plastic surgery in which the skin of the face is tightened, wrinkles are removed, and the skin is made to appear firm and smooth. An incision is made at the hairline, and excess skin is separated from the supporting tissue and excised. The edges of the remaining skin are pulled up and back and sutured at the hairline. A pressure dressing is applied and left in place for 24 to 48 hours. Postoperative medication for pain is often necessary. The sutures are removed several days after discharge in an outpatient facility or in the surgeon's office. Also spelled **rhitidoplasty.**

rhytidosis.   See **rhitidosis.**

RIA.   See **radioimmunoassay.**

rib [AS, roof],   one of the 12 pairs of elastic arches of bone forming a large part of the thoracic skeleton. The first seven ribs on each side are called **true ribs** because they articulate directly with the sternum and the vertebrae. The remaining five ribs are called **false ribs,** the first three attaching ventrally to ribs above; the last two ribs are free at their ventral extremities and are called **floating ribs.**

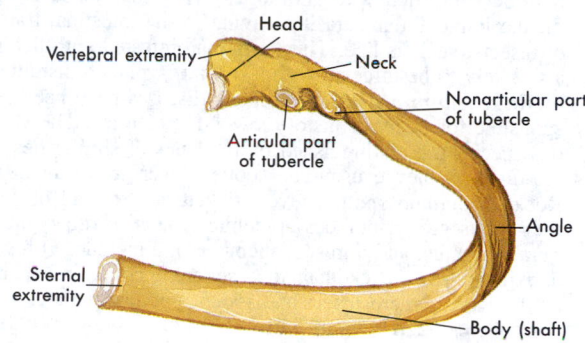

Labels: Head, Neck, Nonarticular part of tubercle, Vertebral extremity, Articular part of tubercle, Angle, Sternal extremity, Body (shaft)

Rib (Thibodeau, 1993/Ernest W Beck)

ribavirin /rī′bəvir′in/,   an aerosol antiviral drug.
■ INDICATIONS: It is prescribed for the treatment of respiratory synctial virus (RSV) infections for the lower respiratory tract in infants and small children.
■ CONTRAINDICATIONS: It is not recommended for infants requiring assisted ventilation.
■ ADVERSE EFFECTS: Reported side effects include bacterial pneumonia, pneumothorax, apnea, hypotension, and cardiac arrest, conditions which also may have resulted from the patient's underlying disease; deteriorated respiratory function, rash, conjunctivitis, and reticulocytosis.

rib fracture,   a break in a bone of the thoracic skeleton caused by a blow or crushing injury or by violent coughing or sneezing. The ribs most commonly broken are the fourth to eighth, and, if the bone is splintered or the fracture is displaced, sharp fragments may pierce the lung, causing hemothorax or pneumothorax.
■ OBSERVATIONS: The patient with a fractured rib suffers pain, especially on inspiration, and usually breathes rapidly and shallowly. The site of the break is generally very tender to the touch, and the crackling of bone fragments rubbing together may be heard on auscultation. Breath sounds may be absent, decreased, or accompanied by rales and rhonchi. The location and nature of the fracture are determined by chest x-ray studies, and the patient is observed for signs of hemoptysis, hemothorax, flail chest, atelectasis, pneumothorax, and pneumonia.
■ INTERVENTIONS: Fractured ribs may be splinted with an elastic belt, an Ace bandage, or adhesive strapping; to prevent

irritation, the area may be shaved and painted with tincture of benzoin before the adhesive tape is applied. If hospitalization is required, the patient is placed in a semi-Fowler's position, and the blood pressure, pulse, temperature, respirations, and breath sounds are checked every 2 to 4 hours. An analgesic may be ordered, but morphine sulfate is avoided. The patient is assisted in turning and is instructed in how to deep breathe, to cough, and to perform range of motion exercises of extremities. If strapping and analgesic medication fail to relieve pain, the physician may perform a regional nerve block by infiltrating the intercostal spaces above and below the fracture site with 1% procaine.
■ NURSING CONSIDERATIONS: The nurse assists in splinting the chest, administers the ordered medication, and helps the patient to turn.

riboflavin /ri′bōflā′vin/ [ribose + L, flavus, yellow],   a yellow crystalline, water-soluble pigment, one of the heat-stable components of the B vitamin complex. It combines with specific flavoproteins and functions as a coenzyme in the oxidative processes of carbohydrates, fats, and proteins. It is also important in the prevention of some visual disorders, especially cataracts. Small amounts of riboflavin are found in the liver and kidneys, but it is not stored to any great degree in the body and must be supplied regularly in the diet. Common sources are organ meats, milk, cheese, eggs, green leafy vegetables, meat, whole grains, and legumes. Deficiency of riboflavin produces cheilosis, local inflammation, desquamation, encrustation, glossitis, photophobia, corneal opacities, proliferation of corneal vessels, seborrheic dermatitis about the nose, mouth, forehead, ears, and scrotum, trembling, sluggishness, dizziness, edema, inability to urinate, and vaginal itching. Also called **vitamin B$_2$.** See also **ariboflavinosis.**

ribonuclear protein /rī′bōnōō′klē·ər/ [ribose; L, nucleus, nut] Gk, proteios, first rank],   a conjugated protein consisting of a protein molecule and nucleic acid.

ribonuclease /-nōō′klē·ās/,   a class of endonucleases that hydrolyze ribonucleic acids.

ribonucleic acid (RNA) /rī′bōnōōklē′ik/ [ribose + L, nucleus, nut; acidus, sour],   a nucleic acid, found in both the nucleus and cytoplasm of cells, that transmits genetic instructions from the nucleus to the cytoplasm. In the cytoplasm, RNA functions in the assembly of proteins. See also **deoxyribonucleic acid.**

ribonucleotide /-nōō′klē·ətīd′/,   a class of nucleotides in which the pentose is D-ribose.

ribose /rī′bōs/,   a 5-carbon sugar that occurs as a component of ribonucleic acid.

ribosome /rī′bəsōm/ [ribose + Gk, soma, body],   a cytoplasmic organelle composed of ribonucleic acid and protein that functions in the synthesis of protein. Ribosomes interact with messenger RNA and transfer RNA to join together amino acid units into a polypeptide chain according to the sequence determined by the genetic code. The structures appear singly or in clusters as polysomes, or they may be attached to endoplasmic reticulum. See also **translation.**

rib shaking,   a procedure in physiotherapy involving constant downward pressure with an intermittent shaking motion of the hands on the rib cage over the area being drained. It is done with the flat part of the palm of the hand over the lung segment being drained during 4 to 12 prolonged exhalations by the patient through pursed lips.

rib vibration,   a procedure in physiotherapy, similar to rib shaking, but done with a downward vibrating pressure with the flat part of the palm during exhalations.

RICE, abbreviation for *rest, ice, compression, elevation,* referring to the treatment for sprains and strains.

rice diet [Gk, *oryza*, rice, *diaita*, lifetstyle], a diet consisting only of rice, fruit, fruit juices, and sugar, supplemented with vitamins and iron. Salt is strictly forbidden. It is prescribed for the treatment of hypertension, chronic renal disease, and obesity. The diet is somewhat modified after blood pressure is lowered and other symptoms are alleviated. It should not be followed for any length of time, because the severe dietary restrictions may lead to nutritional deficiencies or imbalance. Also called **Duke diet, Kempner rice-fruit diet.**

Richards, Linda (1841–1930), a nurse considered to be the first American-trained nurse, being graduated in the first class of the New England Hospital for Women and Children. She then studied at the Nightingale Training School in London and, in 1873, organized the Massachusetts General Hospital Training School. In 1885, she was sent to Japan to develop a training school at the Charity Hospital. In 1891, she took charge of the Philadelphia Visiting Nurse Society. She is credited with being the first to keep written records on patients, a practice she started when she worked as night superintendent at Bellevue Hospital in New York under Sister Helen.

Richet's aneurysm. See **fusiform aneurysm.**

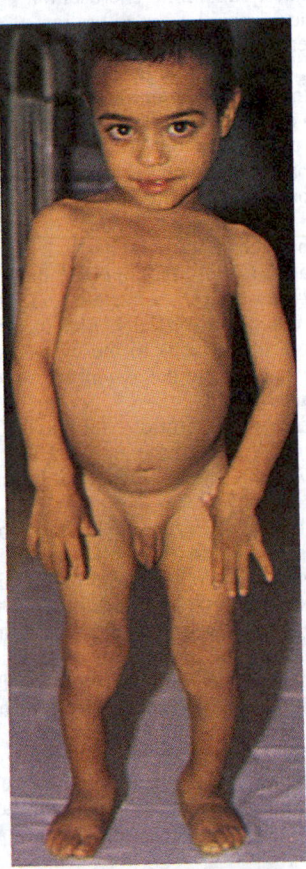

Rickets *(McLaren, 1992)*

rickets /rik′əts/ [Gk, *rachis*, backbone, *itis*, inflammation], a condition caused by the deficiency of vitamin D, seen primarily in infancy and childhood, and characterized by abnormal bone formation. Symptoms include soft pliable bones causing such deformities as bowlegs and knock-knees, nodular enlargements on the ends and sides of the bones, muscle pain, enlarged skull, chest deformities, spinal curvature, enlargement of the liver and spleen, profuse sweating, and general tenderness of the body when touched. Prophylaxis and treatment include a diet rich in calcium, phosphorus, and vitamin D and adequate exposure to sunlight. Kinds of rickets include **adult rickets, celiac rickets, renal rickets,** and **vitamin D resistant rickets.** See also **osteodystrophy, osteomalacia, vitamin D.**

Rickettsia /riket′sē-ə/ [Howard Taylor Ricketts, American pathologist, b. 1871], a genus of microorganisms that combine aspects of both bacteria and viruses. They can be observed with a light microscope, divide by fission, and may be controlled with antibiotics. They also exist as viruslike intracellular parasites, living in the intestinal tracts of insects, such as lice. Thus, a human infested with lice is also likely to be infected with a form of typhus transmitted by *Rickettsia prowazeki.* Rickettsial diseases have been responsible for many of history's worst epidemics. The various species are distinguished on the basis of similarities in the diseases they cause: The spotted fever group includes Rocky Mountain spotted fever, rickettsialpox, and others; the typhus group includes epidemic typhus, scrub typhus, murine typhus; and a miscellaneous group includes Q fever and trench fever. Rickettsial diseases are uncommon in parts of the world where insect and rodent populations are well controlled. **–rickettsial,** *adj.*

rickettsial disease [*Rickettsia*; L, *dis,* Fr, *aise*, ease], an infection caused by a species of *Rickettsia.* Examples include Rocky Mountain spotted fever and typhus.

rickettsialpox /riket′sē-əlpoks′/ [Howard T. Ricketts; ME, *pokkes*, pustules], a mild, acute infectious disease caused by *Rickettsia akari* and transmitted from mice to humans by mites. It is characterized by an asymptomatic, crusted primary lesion, chills, fever, headache, malaise, myalgia, and a rash resembling chickenpox. About 1 week after onset of symptoms, small, discrete, maculopapular lesions appear on any part of the body, but rarely on palms or soles. These lesions become vesicular and dry and form scabs. Eventually the scabs fall off, leaving no scars. Chloramphenicol or tetracycline will hasten recovery. Prevention involves the elimination of house mice. Also called **Kew Gardens spotted fever.** Compare **Rocky Mountain spotted fever.** See also *Rickettsia.*

rickettsiosis /riket′sē-ō′sis/, *pl.* **rickettsioses** [Howard T. Ricketts; Gk, *osis*, condition], any of a group of infectious diseases caused by microorganisms of the genus *Rickettsia.* Kinds of rickettsioses include a spotted fever group (**boutonneuse fever, rickettsialpox, Rocky Mountain spotted fever**), a typhus group (**epidemic typhus, murine typhus, scrub typhus**), and a miscellaneous group (**Q fever, trench fever**). See also **rickettsia.**

rider's bone [AS, *ridan*, to ride, *ban*, bone], a bony deposit that sometimes develops in horseback riders on the inner side of the lower end of the tendon of the adductor muscle of the thigh. Also called **cavalry bone.**

riders' sprain [OFr, *espreindre*, to force out], a sprain of the adductor muscles of the thigh resulting from horseback riding.

ridge /rij/ [AS, *hyrcg*], a projection or projecting structure, such as the gastrocnemial ridge on the posterior surface of the femur, giving attachment to the gastrocnemius muscle.

ridge extension, an intraoral surgical operation for deepening the labial, buccal, or lingual sulci.

ridge lap, the part of an artificial tooth that is adjacent to or laps the residual ridge.

Ridura, a trademark for an oral antiarthritic drug (auranofin).

Riedel's struma, Riedel's thyroiditis. See **fibrous thyroiditis.**

Rieder's cell leukemia /rē'dərz/ [Hermann Rieder, German physician, b. 1858], a malignant neoplasm of blood-forming tissues, characterized by the presence in blood of large numbers of atypical myeloblasts with immature cytoplasm and relatively mature lobulated, indented nuclei.

RIF, abbreviation for *resistance-inducing factor.*

rifa-, a combining form for rifamycin-derived antibiotics.

Rifadin, a trademark for an antibacterial (rifampin).

rifampin /rif'ampin/, an antibacterial.
- INDICATIONS: It is prescribed in the treatment of tuberculosis, in meningococcal prophylaxis, and as an antileprotic.
- CONTRAINDICATIONS: Liver dysfunction or disease or known hypersensitivity to this drug or to rifamycin prohibits its use.
- ADVERSE EFFECTS: Among the more serious adverse reactions are liver toxicity and a syndrome resembling influenza. GI distress, aches and cramps, discoloration of urine, saliva, and sweat commonly occur. This drug interacts with many other drugs.

Rift Valley fever, an arbovirus infection of Egypt and east Africa spread by mosquitoes or by handling infected sheep and cattle. It is characterized by abrupt fever, chills, headache, and generalized aching, followed by epigastric pain, anorexia, loss of taste, and photophobia. The disease is of short duration, and recovery is usually complete. There is no specific treatment. A killed virus vaccine that provides protection for 2 years is available for those at risk, such as laboratory workers and veterinarians.

RIG, abbreviation for **rabies immune globulin.**

Riga-Fede disease /rē'gä fā'dā/ [Antonio Riga, Italian physician, b. 1832; Francesco Fede, Italian pediatrician, b. 1832], an ulceration of the lingual frenum in some infants, caused by abrasion of the frenum by natal or neonatal teeth. Also called **Fede's disease.**

right atrial catheter, an indwelling intravenous catheter inserted centrally or peripherally and threaded into the superior vena cava and right atrium.

right atrioventricular valve. See **tricuspid valve.**

right brachiocephalic vein [AS, *riht;* Gk, *brachion,* arm, *kephale,* head], a vessel, about 2.5 cm long, that starts in the root of the neck at the junction of the internal jugular and the subclavian veins on the right side and descends vertically from behind the sternal end of the clavicle to join the left brachiocephalic vein and form the superior vena cava. The right brachiocephalic vein, like the left, receives various tributaries, such as the vertebral vein, the internal thoracic vein, and the inferior thyroid vein. Compare **left brachiocephalic vein.**

right bundle branch block, an abnormal cardiac condition characterized by impaired transmission of an electrical impulse down the right bundle branch of fibers that transmit impulses from the bundle of His to the right ventricle. This dysfunction may be a complete or an incomplete block of impulses and may be caused by a lesion in the right bun-

dle branch or a small focal lesion in the AV bundle. A right bundle branch block is often associated with right ventricular hypertrophy, especially in individuals under 40 years of age. In older individuals a right bundle branch block is commonly caused by coronary artery disease. A complete right bundle branch block commonly occurs after surgical closure of a ventricular septal defect.

right common carotid artery, the shorter of the two common carotid arteries, arising from the brachiocephalic trunk, passing obliquely from the level of the sternoclavicular articulation to the cranial border of the thyroid cartilage, and dividing into the right carotid arteries. Compare **left common carotid artery.**

right coronary artery, one of a pair of branches of the ascending aorta, arising in the right posterior aortic sinus, passing along the right side of the coronary sulcus, dividing into the right interventricular artery and a large marginal branch, supplying both ventricles, the right atrium, and the sinoatrial node. Compare **left coronary artery.**

right coronary vein. See **small cardiac vein.**

right-handedness, a natural tendency to favor the use of the right hand. Also called **dextrality.** See also **cerebral dominance, handedness.**

right-hand rule, a principle of physics in which the direction of current flow in a wire is related to the position of the imaginary lines of force of the magnetic field about the wire. Thus, if the fingers of the right hand are flexed to represent the magnetic field and the thumb is extended, the thumb points in the direction of current flow.

right-heart failure, an abnormal cardiac condition characterized by the impairment of the right side of the heart and congestion and elevated pressure in the systemic veins and capillaries. Right-heart failure is often related to left-heart failure because both sides of the heart are part of a circuit and what affects one side will eventually affect the other. The most common cause of right-heart failure is left-heart failure, but right ventricular infarction, pulmonic stenosis, and pulmonary hypertension can also result in right-heart failure. In failure associated with either side of the heart, cardiac output is usually decreased. Compare **left-heart failure.**

right hepatic duct, the duct that drains bile from the right lobe of the liver into the common bile duct.

righting reflex [AS, *riht;* L, *refectere,* to bend backward], any reflex that tends to return an animal to its normal body position in space when it has been moved from the normal position and that adjusts head to body position or vice versa. The head and trunk are thus kept in alignment. These reflexes involve a number of sensory receptors including the eyes, labyrinth, and muscles. See also **body righting reflex.**

right interventricular artery. See **dorsal interventricular artery.**

right lymphatic duct, a vessel that conveys lymph from the right upper quadrant of the body into the blood-stream in the neck at the junction of the right internal jugular and the right subclavian veins. About 1.25 cm long, the duct courses over the medial border of the scalenus anterior. At its orifice are two semilunar valves that prevent venous blood from flowing backward into the duct. Lymph drains into the right lymphatic duct from numerous capillaries and vessels and from three lymphatic trunks in the right quadrant. Compare **thoracic duct.** See also **lymphatic system.**

right-to-know laws, laws that require employers to inform workers regarding health effects of materials they must handle, including toxic chemicals and radioactive substances. Under the authority of the U.S. Occupational Safety and Health Act of 1970, the National Institute for Occupational Safety and Health (NIOSH) periodically revises recommendations or limits of exposure to potentially hazardous substances in the workplace. It also recommends appropriate preventive measures designed to reduce or eliminate adverse health effects of these hazards and publishes its recommendations in a variety of public documents.

right-to-left shunt [ME, *shunten*], a venoarterial shunt in which unoxygenated venous blood passes directly into the arterial system, bypassing the lungs as in the tetralogy of Fallot and other conditions.

right pulmonary artery, the longer and slightly larger of the two arteries conveying venous blood from the heart to the lungs, rising from the pulmonary trunk, bending to the right behind the aorta, and dividing into two branches at the root of the right lung. Compare **left pulmonary artery.**

right-sided failure. See **right-heart failure.**

right subclavian artery, a large artery that arises from the brachiocephalic artery. It has several important branches: the axillary, vertebral thoracic, and internal thoracic arteries and the cervical and costocervical trunks, perfusing the right side of the upper body.

right ventricle, the relatively thin-walled chamber of the heart that pumps blood received from the right atrium into the pulmonary arteries to the lungs for oxygenation. The right ventricle is shorter and rounder than the long, conical left ventricle. The chordae tendineae of the tricuspid valve of the right ventricle are finer than the coarse strands of the chordae tendineae of the left ventricle. See also **heart.**

rigidity /rijid′itē/ [L, *rigere*, to be stiff], a condition of hardness, stiffness, or inflexibility. **–rigid,** *adj.*

rigidus /rij′idəs/ [L, stiff], a deformity characterized by limited motion, especially dorsiflexion of the great toe. This condition causes pain and may ultimately produce degenerative changes of involved joints.

rigor /rig′ər/ [L, stiffness], **1.** a rigid condition of the tissues of the body, as in rigor mortis. **2.** a violent attack of shivering that may be associated with chills and fever.

rigor mortis /môr′tis/, the rigid stiffening of skeletal and cardiac muscle shortly after death.

rim [OE, *rima*, edge], an outer edge, which may be curved or circular, as on an occluding surface built on a temporary or permanent denture base.

Rimactane, a trademark for an antibacterial (rifampin).

rima glottidis. See **glottis.**

Rimso-50, a trademark for an antiinflammatory agent (dimethyl sulfoxide), used in the treatment of interstitial cystitis.

ring chromosome [AS, *hring*], a circular chromosome formed by the fusion of the two ends. It is the primary type of chromosome found in bacteria.

Ringer's lactate solution, a fluid and electrolyte replenisher.
- ■ INDICATIONS: It is prescribed for correction of extracellular volume and electrolyte depletion.
- ■ CONTRAINDICATIONS: Kidney failure, congestive heart failure, or hypoproteinemia prohibits its use.
- ■ ADVERSE EFFECTS: Among the more serious adverse reactions are sodium excess and fluid overload, which may lead to pulmonary and peripheral edema.

ring removal from swollen finger, a technique for re-

moving a ring from a swollen finger. It consists of slipping a string under the ring while moving the ring toward the hand. The string is then wound around the swollen part of the finger a number of times, after which the string is unwound from the hand side, gradually easing the ring toward the free end of the finger. The process may need to be repeated to complete the removal.

ringworm. See **tinea.**

Rinne tuning fork test /rin′ē/ [Heinrich A. Rinne, German otologist, b. 1819], a method of distinguishing conductive from sensorineural hearing loss. The test is performed with tuning forks of 256, 512, and 1024 cycles, placed one-half inch from the external auditory meatus and again with the vibrating stem placed over the mastoid bone. While one ear is tested, the other is masked. In sensorineural loss the sound is heard longer by air conduction, while in conductive hearing loss the sound is heard longer by bone conduction.

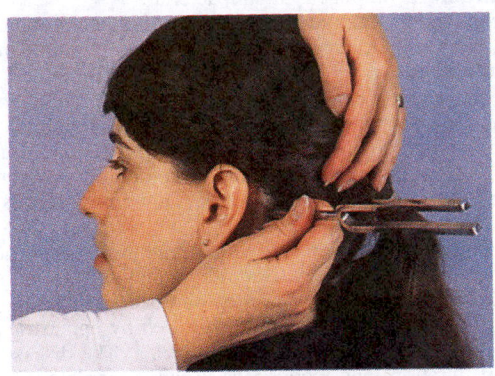

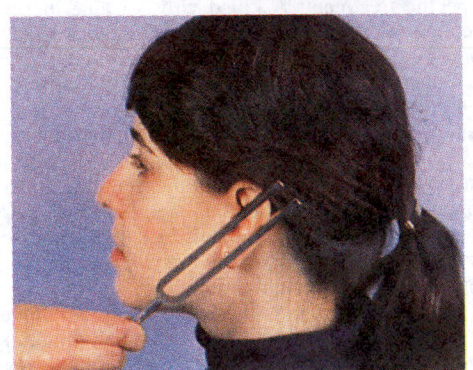

Rinne tuning fork test *(Seidel, 1991)*

-rinone, a combining form for amrinone-type cardiotonic agents.

Rio Grande fever. See **abortus fever.**

Riopan, a trademark for an antacid (magaldrate).

RIP, abbreviation for **reflex inhibiting pattern.**

ripe cataract [OE, *ripan*; Gk, *katarrhaktes*, portcullis], a mature cataract that produces swelling and opacity of the entire lens. Also called **mature cataract.**

risk-benefit analysis, the consideration as to whether a medical or surgical procedure, particularly a radical approach, is worth the risk to the patient as compared to possible benefits if the procedure is successful.

risk factor [Fr, *risque,* hazard; L, *factor,* maker], a factor that causes a person or a group of people to be particularly vulnerable to an unwanted, unpleasant, or unhealthful event, such as immunosuppression, which increases the incidence and severity of infection, or cigarette smoking, which increases the risk of developing a respiratory or cardiovascular disease.

risk management, a function of administration of a hospital or other health facility directed toward identification, evaluation, and correction of potential risks that could lead to injury to patients, staff members, or visitors and in property loss or damage.

risorius /risôr′ē·əs/ [L, *ridere,* to laugh], one of the 12 muscles of the mouth. Arising in the fascia over the masseter and inserting into the skin at the corner of the mouth, it is innervated by mandibular and buccal branches of the facial nerve and acts to retract the angle of the mouth, as in a smile.

Risser cast /ris′ər/ [Joseph C. Risser, American surgeon, b. 1892], an orthopedic device for encasing the entire trunk of the body, extending over the cervical area to the chin. In rare cases it extends over the hips to the knees. The Risser cast is of plaster of paris or fiberglass and is used to immobilize the trunk of the body in the treatment of scoliosis and in the preoperative or the postoperative correction or the maintenance of correction of scoliosis. Compare **body jacket, turnbuckle cast.**

risus sardonicus /rē′səs särdon′ikəs/ [L, laughter; Gk, *sardonius,* mocking], a wry, masklike grin caused by spasm of the facial muscles, as seen in tetanus.

Ritalin Hydrochloride, a trademark for a central nervous system stimulant (methylphenidate hydrochloride) used to treat narcolepsy and attention deficit disorder.

Ritgen maneuver, an obstetric procedure used to control delivery of the head. It involves applying upward pressure from the coccygeal region to extend the head during actual delivery, thereby protecting the musculature of the perineum.

ritodrine hydrochloride /rit′ədrēn/, a beta-sympathomimetic amine agent.
■ INDICATION: It is prescribed in pregnancy management to stop the uterus from contracting in preterm labor.
■ CONTRAINDICATIONS: It is not given before the twentieth week of gestation. Known hypersensitivity to this drug prohibits its use.
■ ADVERSE EFFECTS: Among the more serious adverse reactions are tachycardia, palpitations, headache, nausea, and alterations in blood pressure. Pulmonary edema and death have occurred when it has been given concomitantly with corticosteroids to prevent the development of respiratory distress syndrome in the premature neonate.

Ritter's disease [Gottfried Ritter von Rittershain, Czech pediatrician, b. 1820], a rare, staphylococcal infection of newborns that begins with red spots about the mouth and chin, gradually spreading over the entire body and followed by generalized exfoliation. Vesicles and yellow crusts may also be present. Ritter's disease is usually fatal unless treated with antibiotics, which should be selected on the basis of bacterial sensitivity tests. Also called **dermatitis exfoliativa neonatorum.** Compare **toxic epidermal necrolysis.**

river blindness. See **onchocerciasis.**

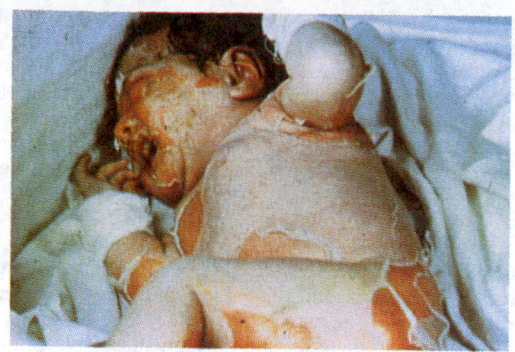

Ritter's disease *(Weston, 1991)*

Rivinus′ notch /rēvē′nəs/ [Augustus Q. Rivinus, German anatomist, b. 1652], a deficiency in the tympanic sulcus of the ear that forms an attachment for the flaccid part of the tympanic membrane and the mallear folds.

R.L.E., abbreviation for *right lower extremity.*

R.L.L., abbreviation for *right lower lobe of lung.*

r-loop, (in molecular genetics) a distinctive loop formation seen under an electron microscope. It is composed of a single helical strand of DNA, wound with a hybrid strand containing another single strand of DNA with a strand of RNA.

R.L.Q., abbreviation for *right lower quadrant.*

R.M.P., abbreviation for *right mentoposterior presentation* of fetal face.

RMSF, abbreviation for **Rocky Mountain spotted fever.**

R.M.T., abbreviation for *right mentotransverse* fetal position.

Rn, symbol for the element **radon.**

RN, abbreviation for **registered nurse.**

RNA, abbreviation for **ribonucleic acid.**

RNA polymerase, (in molecular genetics) an enzyme that catalyzes the assembly of ribonucleoside triphosphates into RNA, with single-stranded DNA serving as the template. Also called **RNA nucleotidyltransferase.**

RNase, abbreviation for **ribonuclease.**

RNA splicing, (in molecular genetics) the process by which base pairs that interrupt the continuity of genetic information in DNA are removed from the precursors of messenger RNA.

RN, C, abbreviation for *registered nurse, certified.*

RN, CNA, abbreviation for *registered nurse, certified in Nursing Administration.*

RN, CNAA, abbreviation for *registered nurse, certified in Nursing Administration, Advanced.*

RN, CS, abbreviation for *registered nurse, certified Specialist.*

R.O.A., abbreviation for *right occipitoanterior* fetal position.

Robaxin, a trademark for a skeletal muscle relaxant (methocarbamol).

Robb, Isabel Hampton (1860–1910), a Canadian-born American nursing educator and writer. She was the first to institute a systematic, step-by-step course for nursing students that integrated clinical experience and classwork and the first educator to arrange for the affiliation of her students at other hospitals for specialized training. She also helped establish university affiliation for nursing education and for postgraduate courses. When the Johns Hopkins School of Nursing was established in Baltimore, in 1889, she became its first director, establishing the high standards for both the practical and theoretic aspects of nursing education that became the base from which she worked to establish national standards. She was one of the founders of *The American Journal of Nursing* and of the forerunner of the American Nurses' Association.

robertsonian translocation /rob'ərtsō'nē·ən/, the exchange of entire chromosome arms, with the break occurring at the centromere, usually between two nonhomologous acrocentric chromosomes, to form one large metacentric chromosome and one extremely small chromosome that carries little genetic material and through successive cell divisions may be lost, leading to a reduction in total chromosome number. Compare **balanced translocation, reciprocal translocation.**

Robinul, a trademark for an anticholinergic (glycopyrrolate).

Robitussin, a trademark for an expectorant (guaifenesin), available in various fixed-combination preparations with an antihistamine, a decongestant with a cough suppressant.

Rocaltrol, a trademark for a regulator of calcium (calcitriol).

Rocephin, a trademark for a cephalosporin antibiotic (ceftriaxone sodium).

rocker knife, a knife that cuts with a rocking motion, designed for patients who have the use of only one hand.

rock fever. See **brucellosis.**

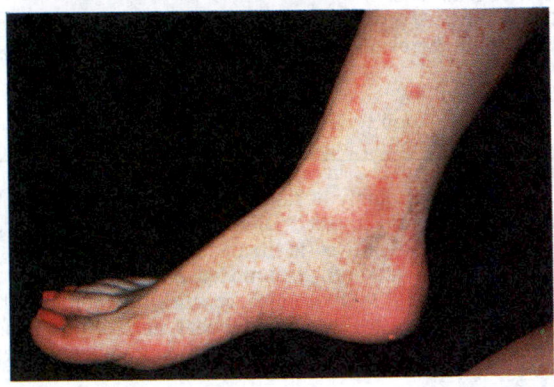

Rash typical of Rocky Mountain spotted fever
(Goldstein, 1992/Courtesy Medical College of Georgia,
Department of Dermatology)

Rocky Mountain spotted fever (RMSF), a serious tickborne infectious disease occurring throughout the temperate zones of North and South America, caused by *Rickettsia rickettsii* and characterized by chills, fever, severe headache, myalgia, mental confusion, and rash. Erythematous macules first appear on wrists and ankles, spreading rapidly over the extremities, trunk, face, and, usually, on the palms and soles. Hemorrhagic lesions, constipation, and abdominal distention are also common. The diagnosis is based on clinical examination and is confirmed by laboratory analyses, including immunofluorescent antibody screens, complement fixation test, and Weil-Felix test. Early treatment with chloramphenicol or tetracycline is important, because

more than 20% of untreated patients die from shock and renal failure. A diet high in protein is important to avoid hypoproteinemia. Nursing care is especially important to avoid decubitus ulcers and hypostatic or aspiration pneumonia. Immunity follows recovery. Prevention includes the use of insect repellents, the wearing of protective clothing, frequent inspection of the body and careful removal of wood or dog ticks, and immunization with killed vaccine for those frequently exposed to ticks. Care must be taken not to crush ticks, because infection may be acquired through skin abrasions. Also called **mountain fever, mountain tick fever, spotted fever.** Compare **murine typhus, rickettsialpox.** See also **boutonneuse fever, scrub typhus, typhus.**

rod [AS, *rodd*], **1.** a straight cylindric structure. **2.** one of the tiny cylindric elements arranged perpendicular to the surface of the retina. Rods contain the chemical rhodopsin, which adapts the eye to detect low-intensity light and gives the rods a purple color. Each rod is 40 to 60 μ in length and about 2 μ thick and consists of a slender, reactive outer segment and an inner granular segment. When bright light strikes a rod, rhodopsin rapidly breaks down; it reforms gradually in low-intensity light. Compare **cone.** See also **iodopsin, Jacob's membrane, rhodopsin.**

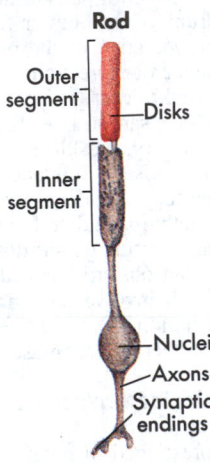

Rod
Outer segment — Disks
Inner segment
Nuclei
Axons
Synaptic endings

Rod (Thibodeau, 1993/Marsha J Dohrmann)

rodenticide poisoning /rōden'tisīd/ [L, *rodere*, to gnaw, *caedere*, to kill; *potio*, drink], a toxic condition caused by the ingestion of a substance intended for the control of rodent populations. See also **phosphorus poisoning, thallium poisoning, warfarin poisoning.**

rodent ulcer /rō'dənt/ [L, *rodere*, to gnaw; *ilcus*, ulcer], a slowly developing serpiginous ulceration of a basal cell carcinoma of the skin. See also **basal cell carcinoma.**

rods and cones [AS, *rodd*; Gk, *konos*], the light-sensitive cells of the retina. The rods, under the visual purple pigment epithelium, are located mainly around the periphery of the retina. The cones receive color stimuli.

roentgen (R) /rent'gən, ren'jən/ [William K. Roentgen, German physicist, b. 1845], the quantity of x- or gamma radiation that creates 1 electrostatic unit of ions in 1 ml of air at 0° C and 760 mm of pressure. In radiotherapy or radiodiagnosis, the roentgen is the unit of the emitted dose. See also **rad, rem.**

roentgen fetometry, the use of radiographic techniques to measure the fetus in utero.

roentgenology /rent′gənol′əjē/ [Roentgen; Gk, *logos,* science], Obsolete. The study of the diagnostic and therapeutic uses of x-rays. See also **radiology, roentgen, x-ray.**

roentgen ray. Obsolete. See **x-ray.**

Roferon-A, a trademark for a parenteral antineoplastic (interferon-alfa-2a).

Rogers, Martha, a nurse theorist who developed the Science of Unitary Man, a nursing theory introduced in 1970. The Rogers theory has strong ties to the general systems theory with elements of a developmental model. It considers four "building blocks": Energy Fields, Universe of Open Systems, Pattern and Organization, and Four Dimensionality. Energy Fields refers to conceptualization of humans and their environment as matter or energy evidenced by wave patterns. Open Systems refers to views of persons as open systems who interact continuously with the environment. Pattern and Organization describes the way Energy Fields emerge, characterized by wave patterns. Four Dimensionality has been interpreted as a form of clairvoyance in which there is a "transcendence of time-space interaction," or an ability to transcend time to see into the future.

Rohrer's constants, the constants in an empiric equation for airway resistance. It is expressed as $R = K_1 + K_2V$, where R is resistance, V is instantaneous volumetric flow rate, K_1 is a constant representing gas viscosity and airway geometry, and K_2 is a constant representing gas density and airway geometry.

Rokitansky's disease. See **Budd-Chiari syndrome.**

Rolando's fissure [Luigi Rolando, Italian anatomist, b. 1773; L, *fissura,* cleft], the central sulcus of the cerebrum.

Rolando's fracture /rōlan′dōz/ [Luigi Rolando, Italian anatomist, b. 1773], a fracture of the base of the first metacarpal.

role [Fr, rôle], a socially expected behavior pattern associated with an individual's function in various social groups. Roles provide a means for social participation and a way to test identities for consensual validation by significant others.

role ambiguity. See **role strain.**

role blurring, the tendency for professional roles to overlap and become indistinct, where there is a shared body of knowledge among and between disciplines.

role change, a situation in which status is retained while role expectations change, as when a nurse moves from the role of a primary caregiver to that of administrator.

role clarification, gaining the knowledge, information, and cues needed to perform a role.

role conflict, the presence of contradictory and often competing role expectations.

role incongruence. See **role strain.**

role model [Fr, rôle, stage roll; L, *modus,* small copy], a person who inspires others to imitate his or her persona. The role model may be a real person, as a parent, or a symbolic character as depicted in movies or television programs.

role overload, a condition in which there is insufficient time in which to carry out all of the expected role functions.

role overqualification. See **role strain.**

role performance, altered, a nursing diagnosis accepted by the Seventh National Conference on the Classification of Nursing Diagnoses. Altered role performance is a disruption in the way one perceives one's role performance. The defining characteristics include a change in self-

perception of one's role, denial of the role, a change in others' perception of one's role, conflict in roles, a change in physical capacity to resume one's role, lack of knowledge of role, and change in usual patterns of responsibility. See also **nursing diagnosis.**

role playing, a psychotherapeutic technique in which a person acts out a real or simulated situation as a means of understanding intrapsychic conflicts.

role playing therapy. See **psychodrama.**

role reversal, the act of assuming the role of another person to appreciate how the person feels, perceives, and behaves in relation to himself and others.

role strain, stress associated with expected roles or positions, experienced as frustration. **Role ambiguity** is a type of role strain that occurs when shared specifications set for an expected role are incomplete or insufficient to tell the involved individual what is desired and how to do it. **Role incongruence** is role stress that occurs when an individual undergoes role transitions requiring a significant modification in attitudes and values. **Role overqualification** is a type of role stress that occurs when a role does not require full use of a person's resources.

Rolfing. See **structural integration.**

roll [OFr, *rolle*], intrinsic joint movements on an axis parallel to the articulating surface. The axis can remain stationary or move in a plane parallel to the joint surface.

roller bandage, a long, tightly wound strip of material that may vary in width. It is generally applied as a circular bandage.

roller clamp, a device, usually made of plastic, equipped with a small roller that may be rolled counterclockwise to close off primary intravenous tubing or clockwise to open it. The roller clamp may also be manipulated to increase and decrease the flow of the intravenous solution and is easily moved with the thumb, thus making it a one-handed convenience in the administration of intravenous therapy. Compare **screw clamp, slide clamp.**

rolling effleurage, a circular rubbing stroke used in massage to promote circulation and muscle relaxation, especially on the shoulder and buttocks. It is performed with the hand flat, the palm and closely held fingers acting as a unit. Compare **effleurage, pétrissage.**

ROM, 1. abbreviation for *range of motion.* 2. abbreviation for *read-only memory.*

Romberg sign /rom′bərg/ [Moritz H. Romberg, German physician, b. 1795; L, *signum,* mark], an indication of loss of the sense of position in which the patient loses balance when standing erect, feet together, and eyes closed. Also called **Romberg test.** (See Fig. p. 1380.)

Rondec-DM, a trademark for a fixed-combination drug containing an antihistamine (carbinoxamine maleate), an antitussive (dextromethorphan hydrobromide), and an adrenergic decongestant and bronchodilator (pseudoephedrine hydrochloride).

Rondomycin, a trademark for an antibiotic (methacycline hydrochloride).

rongeur forceps /rônzhur′, rôNzhœr′/ [Fr, *ronger,* to gnaw; L, *forceps,* pair of tongs], a kind of biting forceps that is strong and heavy, used for cutting bone. Also called **rongeur.**

R-on-T phenomenon, a cardiac event in which a stimulus causes premature depolarization of cells that have not completed the repolarization process. It is noted on the electrocardiogram as a QRS complex falling somewhere within

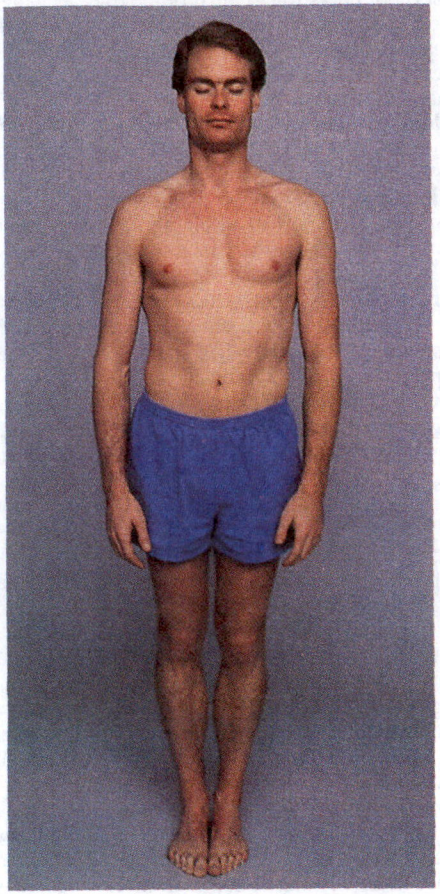

Evaluation of the Romberg sign *(Seidel, 1991)*

surface of a tooth to remove accretions and induce the development of healthy gingival tissues.

root end cyst. See **radicular cyst.**

root furcation, 1. the anatomical area at which the roots of a multi-rooted tooth divide. 2. abnormal resorption of bone in multirooted teeth, resulting from periodontal disease.

rooting reflex, a normal response in newborns when the cheek is touched or stroked along the side of the mouth to turn the head toward the stimulated side and to begin to suck. The reflex disappears by 3 to 4 months of age but in some infants may persist until 12 months of age.

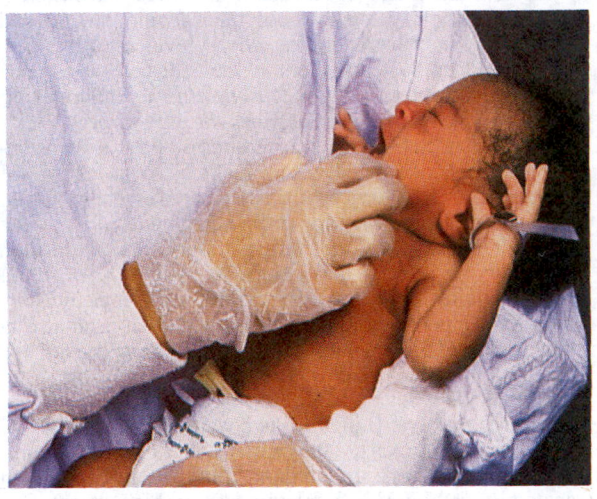

Elicitation of the rooting reflex *(Seidel, 1991)*

the T wave of the preceding beat. The R-on-T phenomenon may resuly in ventricular tachycardia or ventricular fibrillation.

room [AS, *rum*], any area surrounded by four walls within a building, especially one in which a patient is housed, treated, or cared for.

rooming-in, (in a hospital) a practice that allows mothers and new babies to share accommodations, remaining together in the hospital as they would at home rather than being separated.

room temperature [AS, *rúm*; L, *temperatura*], the air temperature as measured in a specific part of a room.

root /rōot, rŏot/ [AS, *rot*], the lowest part of an organ or a structure by which something is firmly attached, such as the anatomic root of the tooth, which is covered by cementum. Also called (*Latin*) **radix** /rā′diks/ (*pl.* **radices**).

root amputation. See **apicoectomy.**

root canal. See **pulp canal.**

root canal file, a small metal hand instrument with tightly spiraled blades, used for cleaning and shaping a root canal.

root canal filling, a material placed in the root canal system of a tooth to seal the space previously occupied by the dental pulp.

root curettage, the debridement and planing of the root

root resection. See **apicoectomy.**

root resorption of teeth [AS, *rot*; L, *resorbere*, to suck back; AS, *toth*], destruction of the cementum or dentin, or bone, by cementoclastic or osteoclastic activity. If only the apex is dissolved, it may result in a short, blunted root. When resorption occurs in the middle of the root, it generally results in penetration of the pulp canal.

root retention, a technique that removes the crown of a root canal treated tooth and retains enough of the root and gingival attachment to support a removable prosthesis.

root submersion, a root retention in which the tooth structure is reduced below the level of the alveolar crest and the soft tissue is allowed to heal over it. This technique is used for minimizing residual ridge resorption.

R.O.P., abbreviation for *right occipitotransverse fetal position.*

Rorschach test /rôr′shäk, rôr′shokh/ [Hermann Rorschach, Swiss psychiatrist, b. 1884], a projective personality assessment test developed by the Swiss psychiatrist Hermann Rorschach. It consists of 10 pictures of inkblots, five in black and white, three in black and red, and two multicolored, to which the subject responds by telling, in as many interpretations as is desired, what images and emotions each design evokes. Replies are evaluated according to whether the response is to the entire or only part of the image; whether color, shading, shape, or location of individual elements is significant; whether movement is seen; and the degree of complexity to which each interpretation is given. Scoring is primarily subjective and is based on both the subject's responses and the general reaction to the circumstances under which the test is administered. The test is designed to assess the degree to which intellectual and emotional factors are integrated in the subject's perception of the environment. See also **Holtzman inkblot technique.**

ROS, abbreviation for **review of systems.**

rosacea /rōzā′shē·ə/ [L, *rosaceus,* rosy], a chronic form of acne seen in adults of all ages and associated with telangiectasia, especially of the nose, forehead, and cheeks. Also called **acne rosacea.** See also **rhinophyma.**

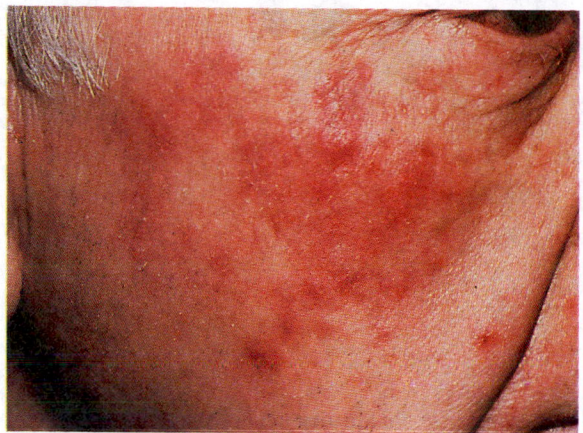

Rosacea (du Vivier, 1986/Courtesy King's College Hospital)

rose fever [L, *rosa; febris,* fever], a common misnomer for seasonal allergic rhinitis caused by pollen, most frequently of grasses, that is airborne at the time roses are in bloom. Roses are not the cause of common spring and summer allergic reactions; their pollen is not dispersed by the wind but is carried from flower to flower by insects.

Rosenmüller's organ. See **epoophoron.**

Rosenthal's syndrome. See **hemophilia C.**

roseo- a combining form meaning rose colored, as a roseola rash.

roseola /rōzē′ələ/ [L, *roseus*], any rose-colored rash. See also **roseola infantum.**

roseola infantum, a benign, viral, endemic illness of infants and young children, attributed to a parvovirus and characterized by abrupt, high sustained or spiking fever, mild pharyngitis, and lymph node enlargement. Febrile convulsions may occur. After 4 or 5 days the fever suddenly drops to normal, and a faint, pink, maculopapular rash appears on the neck, trunk, and thighs. The rash may last a few hours to 2 days. Diagnosis is based on high fever with rather mild illness and the rash. Sequelae may occur as a result of the convulsions. There is no specific therapy or vaccine. Aspirin or acetaminophen are often used to try to control fever. Anticonvulsive medication may be indicated. Also called **exanthem subitum, sixth disease, Zahorsky's disease.**

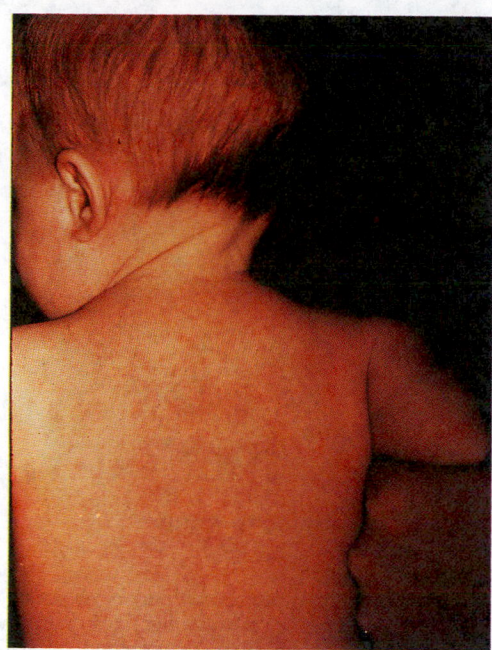

Macular rash of roseola infantum (Zitelli, 1992)

rose spots [L, *rosa* + ME, *spotte*], small erythematous macules occurring on the upper abdomen and anterior thorax and lasting 2 or 3 days, characteristic of typhoid and paratyphoid fevers.

Rose-Waaler test. See **sheep cell agglutination test.**

rost-, a prefix meaning 'of or pertaining to a beak': *rostellum, rostrad, rostriform.*

rostral /ros′trəl/, beak-shaped. **–rostrum,** *n.*

rostrum /ros′trəm/ [L, beak], a beaklike projection, as the rostrum of the sphenoid bone.

rot-, a combining form meaning 'turned, or to turn': *rotate, rotatory, rotexion.*

R.O.T., abbreviation for *right occipitotrasverse* fetal position.

rotameter /rōtam′ətər/ [L, *rota,* wheel; Gk, *metron,* measure], a device operated by a needle valve in an anesthetic gas machine that measures gases by speed of flow, according to their viscosity and density. Also called **flowmeter.**

rotary nystagmus /rō′tərē/ [L, *rotare,* to rotate; Gk, *nystagmos,* nodding], a form of nystagmus in which the eyeball makes rotary motions, around an axis.

rotating tourniquet /rō′tāting/ [L, *rotare,* to rotate; Fr, *tourniquet,* garrote], one of four constricting devices used in a rotating order to pool blood in the extremities to relieve congestion in the lungs in the treatment of acute pulmonary edema. Use of the rotating touriquet has declined in recent years due to the development of vasodilating drugs and diuretics. (See Fig. p. 1382.)

rotation /rōtā′shən/ [L, *rotare*], **1.** a turning around an axis. **2.** one of the four basic kinds of motion allowed by various joints: the rotation of a bone around its central axis, which may lie in a separate bone, as in the pivot formed by the dens of the axis around which the atlas turns. A bone, such as the humerus, may also rotate around its own longi

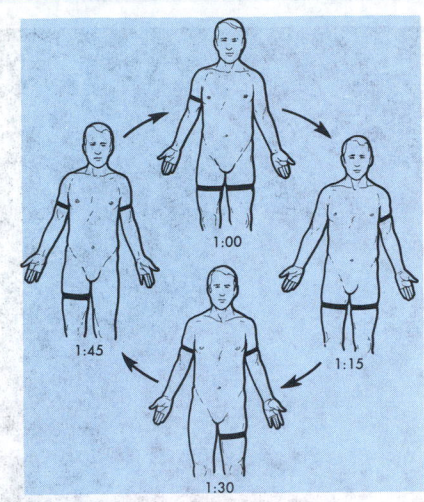

Rotating tourniquets

tudinal axis, or the axis of rotation may not be quite parallel to the long axis of the rotating bone, as in movement of
the radius on the ulna during pronation and supination of
the hand. Compare **angular movement, circumduction,
gliding. 3.** (in obstetrics) the turning of the fetal head to
descend through the pelvis.
rotator /rō′tātər/ [L, *rotare*, to rotate],   a muscle that rotates on an axis, as the cervical, thoracic, and lumbar mus-
culi rotatores, which function to extend and rotate the vertebral column toward the opposite side.

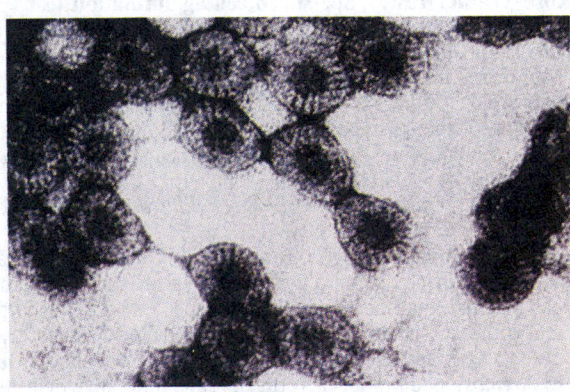

Rotavirus (Baron, 1990)

rotavirus /rō′təvī′rəs/,   a double-stranded RNA molecule
that appears as a tiny wheel, with a clearly defined outer
layer, or rim, and an inner layer of spokes. The organism
replicates in the epithelial cells of the intestine and is a cause
of acute gastroenteritis with diarrhea, particularly in infants.
Various strains also infect domestic and wild animals. Human infections tend to peak during the winter months. See
also **adult rotavirus (ADRV).**
Rotokinetic treatment table /rō′tōkinet′ik/,   a special bed
equipped with an automatic turning device that completely

immobilizes patients while rotating them from 90 to 270 degrees around a horizontal axis.
Rotor syndrome /rō′tər/,   a rare condition of the liver inherited as an autosomal recessive trait. It is similar to Dubin-
Johnson syndrome but can be distinguished by the normal
functioning of the gallbladder and normal pigmentation of
the liver. See also **Dubin-Johnson syndrome, hyperbilirubinemia of the newborn.**
rotula.   See **troche.**
roughage.   See **dietary fiber.**
rouleaux /rōōlō′/, *sing.* **rouleau** [Fr, cylinder],   an aggregation of red cells that may be caused by abnormal proteins,
as in multiple myeloma or macroglobulinemia, but is most
often a microscopic artifact. Compare **hemagglutination.**
See also **erythrocyte sedimentation rate.**

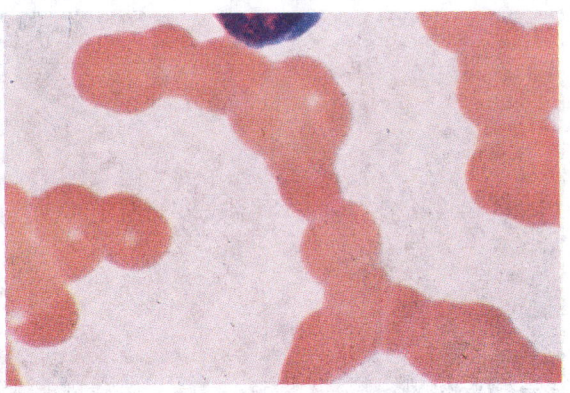

Rouleaux (Hayhoe, 1992)

round ligament [L, *rotundus*, round; *ligare*, to bind],   **1.** a
curved fibrous band that is attached at one end to the fovea
of the head of the femur and at the other to the transverse
ligament of the acetabulum. **2.** a fibrous cord extending
from the umbilicus to the anterior part of the liver. It is the
remnant of the umbilical vein. **3.** in the female, a fibromuscular band that extends from the anterior surface of the
uterus through the inguinal canal to the labium majus. The
structure is homologous to the spermatic cord in the male.
rounds,   *informal.* a teaching conference or a meeting in
which the clinical problems encountered in the practice of
nursing, medicine, or other service are discussed. Kinds of
rounds include **grand rounds, nursing rounds, teaching
rounds,** and **walking rounds.**
round window [OFr, *rund;* ONorse, *vindauga*],   a round
opening in the medial wall of the middle ear leading into
the cochlea and covered by a secondary tympanic membrane. Also called **fenestra cochleae; fenestra rotunda.**
roundworm,   any worm of the class Nematoda, including
*Ancylostoma duodenale, Ascaris lumbricoides, Enterobius
vermicularis,* and *Strongyloides stercoralis.*
route of administration /rōōt, rout/ [Fr, *route,* course; L,
administrare, to serve],   (of a drug) any one of the ways
in which a drug may be administered, such as intramuscularly, intranasally, intravenously, orally, rectally, subcutaneously, sublingually, topically, or vaginally. Some medications can be given only by one route because absorption
or maximum effectiveness occurs by that route only or be-

cause the specific substance is toxic or damaging when given by another route.

Roux-en-Y /roo'enwī', roo'änēgrek'/ [César Roux, Swiss surgeon, b. 1857], an anastomosis of the small intestine in the shape of the letter Y. The proximal end of the divided intestine is anastomosed end-to-side to the distal loop and a portion of the distal loop is anastomosed to another part of the digestive tract, such as the esophagus.

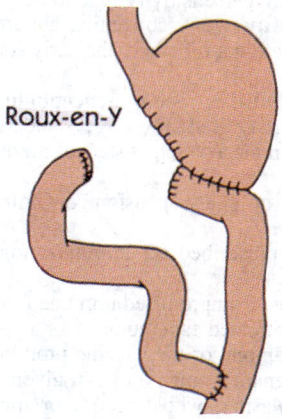

Roux-en-Y (Winawer, 1992)

Rovsing's sign /rov'singz/ [Nils T. Rovsing, Danish surgeon, b. 1862], an indication of acute appendicitis in which pressure on the left lower quadrant of the abdomen causes pain in the right lower quadrant. See also **appendicitis.**

Royal College of Physicians (R.C.P.), a professional organization of physicians in the United Kingdom.

Royal College of Physicians and Surgeons of Canada (RCPSC), a national Canadian organization that recognizes and confers membership on certain qualified physicians and surgeons.

Royal College of Surgeons (R.C.S.), a professional organization of surgeons in the United Kingdom.

Royal free disease. See **postviral fatigue syndrome.**

Roy, Sister Callista, a nursing theorist who introduced the Adaptation Model of Nursing in 1970 as a conceptual framework for nursing curricula, practice, and research. In the Roy model, the human is viewed as an adaptive system. Changes occur in the system in response to stimuli. If the change promotes the integrity of the individual, it is an adaptive response. Otherwise, it is a maladaptive response. The theory provides two mechanisms for coping or adapting. One, a Regulator Mechanism, is concerned with neural, endocrine, and perception-psychomotor processes. The other, a Cognator Mechanism, is concerned with perception, learning, judgment, and emotion. Four modes for effecting adaptation of a system are physiologic needs, self-concept, role function, and interdependence. The nurse achieves the goal of promoting the patient's adaptation in situations of health and sickness by manipulating stimuli. Nursing intervention is required when the coping mechanism of the patient loses effectiveness in illness.

RPF, abbreviation for *renal plasma flow.*

rpm, abbreviation for *revolutions per minute.*

RQ, abbreviation for *respiratory quotient.*

RR, R.R., abbreviation for **recovery room.**

R.R.A., abbreviation for **registered record administrator.**

-(r)rhage, a suffix meaning a 'rupture, an excessive fluid discharge': *hemorrhage, lymphorrhage, phleborrhage.*

-(r)rhagia, a suffix meaning a 'fluid discharge of excessive quantity': *lymphorrhagia, meningorrhagia, tracheorrhagia.*

-(r)rhagic, a suffix meaning 'of, pertaining, or referring to a kind or condition of excessive fluid discharge': *haemorrhagic, lymphorrhagic, serohemorrhagic.*

-(r)rhaphy, -(r)rhaphia, a suffix meaning a 'suturing in place': *cysticorrhaphy, meningeorrhaphy, osteorrhaphy.*

-(r)rhea, -(r)rhoea, -(r)rhoeica, a suffix meaning 'fluid discharge, flow': *anarrhea, cystirrhea, laryngorrhea.*

-(r)rheic, -(r)rheal, -(r)rhetic, -(r)rhoeic, a suffix meaning 'pertaining to a fluid discharge': *cryptorrheic, diarrheic, pyorrheic.*

-(r)rhexis, a suffix meaning a 'rupture of a (specified) body part': *arteriorrhexis, cardiorrhexis, plasmarrhexis.*

-(r)rhine, a suffix meaning 'having a (specified sort of) nose': *leptorrhine, mesorrhine, platyrrhine.*

-(r)rhinia, a suffix meaning '(condition of the) nose': *arrhinia, birrhinia, microrrhinia.*

-(r)rhoeica, -(r)rhoea. See **-(r)rhea.**

-(r)rhythmia, a combining form meaning 'regularly occurring involuntary behavior or actions': *bradyrrhythmia, dysrrhythmia, tachyrrhythmia.*

R-R interval, the interval from the peak of one QRS complex to the peak of the next as shown on an electrocardiogram. It is used to assess the ventricular rate. See also **cardiac cycle.**

rRNA, abbreviation for *ribosomal RNA.*

RRT, abbreviation for **registered respiratory therapist.**

RSV, RS virus, abbreviation for **respiratory syncytial virus.**

RT, abbreviation for **respiratory therapy.**

R.T., abbreviation for **registered technologist.**

RTA, abbreviation for **renal tubular acidosis.**

r.t.c., abbreviation for *return to clinic,* noted on the chart, usually followed by a date on which a subsequent appointment has been made for the patient.

Ru, symbol for the element **ruthenium.**

rub [ME, *rubben,* to tear out], the movement of one surface moving over another, thereby producing friction, as when pleural membranes produce friction rub.

rub-, rube-, a prefix meaning 'red': *rubedo, ruber, rubor.*

rubber. See **condom.**

rubber-band ligation, a method of treating hemorrhoids by placing a rubber band around the hemorrhoidal portion of the blood vessel, causing it to slough off after a period of time. The technique is employed in some cases as an alternative to surgery. See also **ligation.**

rubber dam [ME, *rubben,* to scrape; AS, *demman,* to dam up], a thin sheet of latex rubber for isolating one or more teeth during a dental procedure.

rubber dam clamps forceps, (in dentistry) a type of forceps with beaks designed to engage holes in a rubber dam clamp to facilitate its placement.

rubbing alcohol [ME, *rubben,* to scrape; Ar, *alkohl,* essence], a disinfectant for skin and instruments. It contains 70% isopropyl alcohol by volume, the remainder consisting of water and denaturants, with or without color or perfume. It may cause dryness of the skin. Rubbing alcohol is for external use only and is flammable.

rubefacient /rōō′bəfā′shənt/ [L, *ruber*, red, *facere*, to make], **1.** a substance or agent that increases the reddish coloration of the skin. **2.** increasing the reddish coloration of the skin.

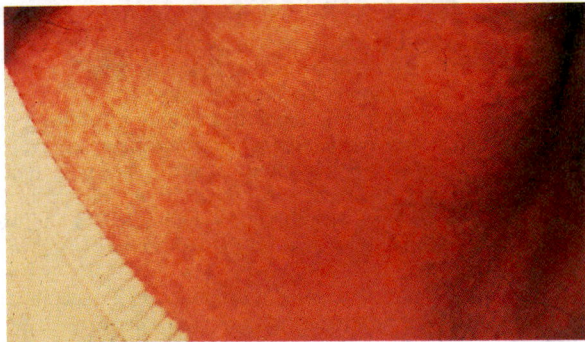

Rubella *(Zitelli, 1992/Courtesy Dr. Michael Sherlock)*

rubella /rōōbel′ə/ [L, *rubellus*, somewhat red], a contagious viral disease characterized by fever, symptoms of a mild upper respiratory tract infection, lymph node enlargement, arthralgia, and a diffuse, fine, red, maculopapular rash. The virus is spread by droplet infection, and the incubation time is from 12 to 23 days. Also called **German measles, three-day measles.** Compare **measles, scarlet fever.**

■ OBSERVATIONS: The symptoms usually last only 2 or 3 days except for arthralgia, which may persist longer or recur. One attack confers lifelong immunity. If a woman acquires rubella in the first trimester of pregnancy, fetal anomalies may result, including heart defects, cataracts, deafness, and mental retardation. An infant exposed to the virus in utero at any time during gestation may shed the virus for up to 30 months after birth. Complications of postnatal rubella are rare.

■ INTERVENTIONS: The illness itself is mild and needs no special treatment. Live attenuated rubella vaccine is advised for all children to reduce chances of an epidemic and thus to protect pregnant women. The vaccine is not given to women already pregnant, and it is recommended that pregnancy be avoided for 3 months after the administration of rubella vaccine. Spread of the virus from a recently vaccinated individual rarely occurs. Immune serum globulin containing rubella antibodies may help prevent fetal infection in exposed susceptible pregnant women, but ordinary gamma globulin will not protect the fetus.

■ NURSING CONSIDERATIONS: Temporary arthralgia is common after vaccination. Women of childbearing age working with children may be tested for immunity to rubella and vaccinated if not immune. The only proof of immunity is the laboratory demonstration of antibodies to the rubella virus. The rash and malaise of rubella resemble those of scarlet fever, some cases of mononucleosis, and allergic drug reactions, leading some people to think they have had rubella when they have not.

rubella and mumps virus vaccine, a suspension containing live attenuated mumps and rubella viruses.

■ INDICATIONS: It is prescribed for immunization against rubella and mumps.

■ CONTRAINDICATIONS: Acute infection or known hypersensitivity to avian proteins prohibits its use. It is not given to a patient whose immune function is compromised or to a pregnant woman. It is not given for 3 months after the use of plasma, whole blood, or an immune serum globulin. Pregnancy is avoided for 3 months after immunization.

■ ADVERSE EFFECTS: Among the more serious adverse effects are mild to severe hypersensitivity reactions.

rubella embryopathy, any congenital abnormality in an infant caused by maternal rubella in the early stages of pregnancy.

rubella panencephalitis. See **panencephalitis.**

rubella titer [L, *ruber,* red; Fr, *titre,* standard], a serological test to determine a patient's state of immunity against rubella.

rubella virus vaccine, a suspension containing live attenuated rubella virus.

■ INDICATION: It is prescribed for immunization against rubella.

■ CONTRAINDICATIONS: Compromised immune function, fever, acute infection, untreated tuberculosis, or hypersensitivity to proteins of the animal of the vaccine prohibits its use. It is not given to pregnant women, nor is it given for 3 months after the use of plasma, whole blood, or immune serum globulin. Pregnancy should be avoided for 3 months after immunization.

■ ADVERSE EFFECTS: Among the most serious adverse reactions are severe hypersensitivity reactions and local pain.

rubeola. See **measles.**

ruber /rōō′bər/, (L), red.

rubescent /rōōbes′ənt/, reddening.

-rubicin, a combining form for daunorubicin-type antineoplastic antibiotics.

rubidium (Rb) /rōōbid′ē·əm/ [L, *rubidus,* reddish], a soft metallic element of the alkali metals group. Its atomic number is 37; its atomic weight is 85.47. Slightly radioactive, it is used in radioisotope scanning.

Rubin's test [Isador C. Rubin, American gynecologist, b. 1883], a test performed in the process of evaluating the cause of infertility by assessing the patency of the fallopian tubes. Carbon dioxide gas (CO_2) is introduced into the tubes under pressure through a cannula inserted into the cervix. The CO_2 is passed through from a syringe connected to a manometer at pressures of up to 200 mm Hg. If the tubes are open, the gas enters the abdominal cavity and the recorded pressure falls below 180 mm Hg. A high-pitched bubbling can be heard through the abdominal wall with the stethoscope as the gas escapes from the tubes. The patient may complain of shoulder pain from diaphragmatic irritation; an x-ray film will show free gas under the diaphragm. If the tubes are blocked, gas cannot escape from the tubes into the abdominal cavity; the pressure recorded on the manometer remains at 200 mm Hg. A tracing may be made to show tubal peristalsis, any leakage in the system, tubal spasm, or partial obstruction. After the test, the patient rests for a 3-hour period. Crampy pain, dizziness, nausea, and vomiting may occur; positioning with the pelvis higher than the head, in genupectoral position or in Trendelenburg's position, allows the gas to stay in the pelvis and give some relief by avoiding diaphragmatic irritation.

rubivirus /rōō′bēvī′rəs/, a member of the togavirus family, which includes the rubella virus.

rubor /rōō'bôr/, redness, especially when accompanying inflammation.

rubricyte /rōō'brisīt/ [L, *ruber*, red; Gk, *kytos*, cell], a nucleated red blood cell; the marrow stage in the normal development of an erythrocyte.

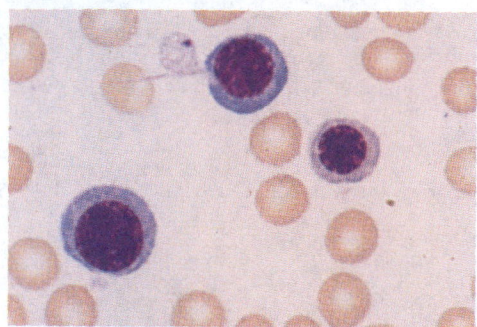

Rubricytes *(Powers, 1989)*

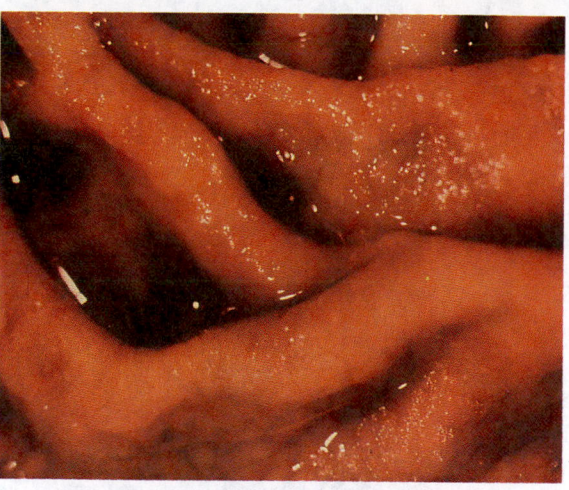

Rugae of stomach *(Mitros, 1988)*

ructus. See **eructation.**

rudiment /rōō'dimənt/ [L, *rudimentum*, beginning], an organ or tissue that is incompletely developed or nonfunctional. –**rudimentary,** *adj.*

rudimentary /rōō'dimen'tərē/, [L, *rudimentum*, beginning], pertaining to something either vestigial or embryonic.

Ruffini's corpuscles /rōōfē'nēz/ [Angelo Ruffini, Italian histologist, b. 1864], a variety of oval-shaped nerve endings in the subcutaneous tissue, located principally at the junction of the dermis and the subcutaneous tissue. Ruffini's corpuscles consist of strong connective tissue sheaths enclosing nerve fibers with many branches that end in small knobs. Compare **Golgi-Mazzoni corpuscles, Pacini's corpuscles.**

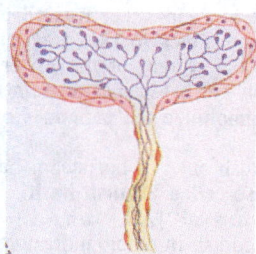

Ruffini's corpuscles *(Thibodeau, 1993/Rolin Graphics)*

RU486, a drug that can end a pregnancy when administered as a one-dose pill within the first 6 weeks after conception. It acts by interfering with the role of progesterone in implantation of the fertilized egg. Two days after taking RU486, the woman receives injection of another drug that causes the uterus to contract and expel the lining.

ruga /rōō'gə/, *pl.* **rugae** /rōō'jē/ [L, wrinkle], a ridge or fold, such as the rugae of the stomach, which presents large folds in the mucous membrane of that organ.

rugae of vagina, [L, *ruga*, ridge + *vagina*, sheath], the transverse ridges on the mucous membrane lining the vagina, which allow the vagina to stretch during childbirth.

R.U.L., abbreviation for *right upper lobe* of lung.

rule of bigeminy [L, *regula*, model; *bis*, double, *geminus*, twin], (in cardiology) the tendency of a lengthened ventricular cycle to precipitate a ventricular premature complex.

rule of confidentiality, a principle that personal information about others, particularly patients, should not be revealed to persons not authorized to receive such information.

rule of co-occurrence /kō'əkur'əns/, a mandate that a person use the same level of lexical and syntactic structure when speaking.

rule of nines, a formula for estimating the amount of body surface covered by burns by assigning 9% to the head and each arm, twice 9% (18%) to each leg, and the anterior and posterior trunk, and 1% to the perineum. This is modified in infants and children because of the different body proportions.

rule of three, (in respiratory therapy) an arterial oxygen tension that is three times the value of the inspired oxygen concentration. It is regarded as an empirical guide to a temporarily acceptable minimal oxygenation or expression of clinical observation and has no scientific basis.

ruminant /rōō'minənt/ [L, *ruminare*, to chew again], pertaining to animals that chew their cud and to human infants that may regurgitate and reswallow a meal.

rumination /rōō'minā'shən/ [L, *ruminare*, to chew again], habitual regurgitation of small amounts of undigested food with little force after every feeding, a condition commonly seen in infants. It may be a symptom of overfeeding, of eating too fast, or of swallowing air. It has little or no clinical significance. More copious and forceful regurgitation may indicate a more serious condition, such as an allergic intestinal reaction, an infectious disease, an obstruction of the intestinal tract, or a metabolic disorder. See also **vomit.**

runner's high, a feeling of euphoria experienced by some crosscountry runners and joggers as they near the end of a run. The feeling of elation is believed to be associated with the body's production of endorphins during physical stress.

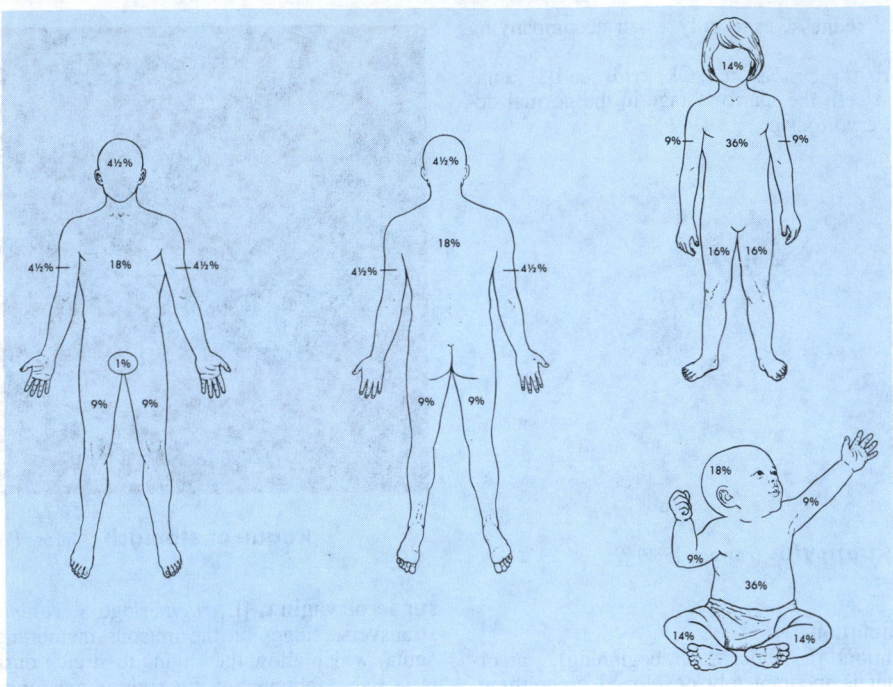

Rule of nines

rupture /rup′chər/ [L, *rumpere*, to break], **1.** a tear or break in the continuity or configuration of an organ or body tissue, including those instances when other tissue protrudes through the opening. See also **hernia. 2.** to cause a break or tear.

ruptured intervertebral disk. See **herniated disk.**

rupture of membranes [L, *rumpere*, to break + *membrana*], the rupture of the amniotic sac, usually at the start of labor.

rupture of uterus in pregnancy, a tear or break in the uterus because of trauma or other causes, possibly accompanied by displacement of the fetus and amniotic sac into the peritoneal cavity. The patient may experience acute pain because of tissue damage and irritation of the peritoneal tissues. Excessive loss of blood may be marked by hypotension, fluid volume deficit, and altered cardiac output.

RUQ, abbreviation for *right upper quadrant.*

Rural Clinics Assistance Act /rōō′rəl/, an act of Congress that permitted the establishment of clinics in certain areas designated rural and underserved and in some inner cities. The clinics are designed to provide primary care through teams of physicians and nurse practitioners. The act is significant to nursing by being the first federal legislation to allow third-party reimbursement directly to nurses practicing in expanded roles.

Russell dwarf [Alexander Russell, 20th century Scottish physician; AS, *dweorge*], a person affected with **Russell's syndrome,** a congenital disorder in which short stature is associated with various anomalies of the head, face, and skeleton and with varying degrees of mental retardation.

Russell's bodies [William Russell, Scottish physician, b. 1852; AS, *bodig,* body], the mucoprotein inclusions found in globular plasma cells in cancer and inflammations. The bodies contain surface gamma globulins, derived from the condensation of internal cellular secretions. Also called **cancer bodies, fuchsin bodies.**

Russell's syndrome. See **Russell dwarf.**

Russell traction [R. Hamilton Russell, 20th century Australian surgeon; L, *trahere,* to pull along], a unilateral or a bilateral orthopedic mechanism that combines suspension and traction to immobilize, position, and align the lower extremities in the treatment of fractured femurs and hip and knee contractures and in the treatment of disease processes of the hip and knee. Russell traction is applied as adhesive or nonadhesive skin traction and employs a sling to relieve the weight of the lower extremities subjected to traction pull. A jacket restraint is often incorporated to help immobilize the patient. Compare **split Russell traction.**

Russian bath /rush′ən/, a hot steam bath followed by a cold plunge. Also called **Finnish bath.**

rusty sputum /rus′tē/ [AS, *rust;* L, *sputum,* spittle], sputum that is reddish in color, indicative of blood.

ruthenium (Ru) /rōōthē′nē·əm/ [Ruthenia, region of western Ukraine], a hard, brittle, metallic element. Its atomic number is 44; its atomic weight is 101.07.

rutherfordium(Rf). See **element 104.**

rutin /rōō′tin/, a bioflavonoid obtained from buckwheat and used in the treatment of capillary fragility.

RV, abbreviation for **residual volume.**

RVC, abbreviation for *responds to verbal commands.*

R wave. See **QRS complex.**

rxn, RXN, symbol for drug reaction.

s, **1.** abbreviation for **steady state. 2.** abbreviation for the Latin word *sinister,* 'left'.

s̄, s, symbol for the Latin word, *sine,* 'without'.

S, **1.** symbol for **sulfur. 2.** symbol for *saturation of hemoglobin.*

S₁, the first heart sound in the cardiac cycle occurring at the outset of ventricular systole. It is associated with closure of the mitral and tricuspid valves and is synchronous with the apical pulse. Auscultated at the apex, it is louder, longer, and lower than the second sound (S₂), which follows it.

S₂, the second heart sound in the cardiac cycle. It is associated with closure of the aortic and pulmonic valves at the outset of ventricular diastole. Auscultated at the base of the heart, the second sound is louder than the first.

S₃, the third heart sound in the cardiac cycle. Normally, it is audible only in children and physically active young adults. In older people, it is an abnormal finding and usually indicates myocardial failure. It is heard with the bell of a stethoscope placed lightly over the apex of the heart with the patient lying down, tipped to the left.

S₄, the fourth heart sound in the cardiac cycle. It occurs late in diastole on contraction of the atria. Rarely heard in normal subjects, it indicates an abnormally increased resistance to ventricular filling, as in hypertensive cardiovascular disease, coronary artery disease, cardiomyopathy, and aortic stenosis.

S1, S2, . . ., symbols for sacral nerves.

SA, **1.** abbreviation for *sinoatrial (S-A node).* **2.** abbreviation for **surface area. 3.** abbreviation for **surgeon's assistant.**

Sabin-Feldman dye test /sā′binfeld′mən/ [Albert B. Sabin, American virologist, b. 1906; H. A. Feldman; AS, *deag;* L, *testum,* crucible], a diagnostic test for toxoplasmosis that depends on the presence of specific antibodies that block the uptake of methylene blue dye by the cytoplasm of the *Toxoplasma* organisms.

Sabin vaccine. See **oral poliovirus vaccine.**

sac /sak/ [Gk, *sakkos,* sack], a pouch or a baglike organ, such as the abdominal sac of the embryo that develops into the abdominal cavity.

saccade /sakād′/ [Fr, *saccader,* to jerk], pertaining to something jerky, broken, or abrupt, such as rapid shifts of eye movement or a staccato voice.

saccadic eye movement /sakad′ik/, an extremely fast voluntary movement of the eyes, allowing the eyes to accurately fix on a still object in the visual field as the person moves or the head turns.

sacchari-. See **saccharo-.**

saccharide /sak′ərīd′/, any of a large group of carbohydrates, including all sugars and starches. Almost all carbohydrates are saccharides. See also **carbohydrate, sugar.**

saccharin /sak′ərin/ [Gk, *sakcharon,* sugar], **1.** a white, crystalline, synthetic sweetening agent derived from coal tar. Although it is up to 500 times as sweet as sugar, it has no food value. **2.** having a sweet taste, especially cloyingly sweet. Also called **saccharine** /-rīn, -rin/.

saccharo-, sacchari-, a combining form meaning 'of or pertaining to sugar': *saccharobiose, saccharorrhea, saccharosuria.*

Saccharomyces /sak′ərōmī′sēz/ [Gk, *sakcharon* + *mykes,* fungus], a genus of yeast fungi, including brewer's and baker's yeast, as well as some pathogenic fungi, that cause such diseases as bronchitis, moniliasis, and pharyngitis.

saccharomycosis /sak′ərōmīkō′sis/ [Gk, *sakcharon, mykes,* + *osis,* condition], **1.** infection with yeast fungi, such as the genera *Candida* or *Cryptococcus.* **2.** *obsolete.* cryptococcosis or European blastomycosis.

saccular /sak′yələr/ [L, *sacculus*], pertaining to a pouch, or shaped like a sac.

saccular aneurysm, a localized dilatation of an artery in which only a small area of the vessel, not the entire circumference, is distended, forming a saclike swelling or protrusion. It is usually caused by trauma. Also called **ampullary aneurysm, sacculated aneurysm.** Compare **fusiform aneurysm.**

sacculated /sak′yəlā′tid/ [L, *sacculus,* small sack], a condition of small sacs, pouches, or saclike dilatations.

sacculated aneurysm. See **saccular aneurysm.**

saccule /sak′yool/ [L, *sacculus*], a small bag or sac, such as the air saccules of the lungs. See also **sacculus.** **—saccular,** *adj.*

sacculus /sak′yoolǝs/, *pl.* **sacculi** ′, a little sac or bag, especially the smaller of the two divisions of the membranous labyrinth of the vestibule, which communicates with the cochlear duct through the ductus reuniens in the inner ear. See also **saccule.**

Sachs' disease. See **Tay-Sachs disease.**

SA conduction time, the conduction time for an impulse from the sinus node to the atrial musculature, measured from the SA deflection in the SA nodal electrocardiogram to the beginning of the P wave in a bipolar record, or to the beginning of the high right atrial electrogram in a unipolar record.

sacral /sā′krəl, sak′rəl/ [L, *sacer,* sacred], of or pertaining to the sacrum.

sacral bone, a composite bone formed by the fusion during maturation of five sacral vertebrae that were separate at birth. The sacrum forms the back of the pelvis.

sacral canal, an extension of the vertebral canal through the sacrum.

sacral foramen, one of several openings between the fused segments of the sacral vertebrae in the sacrum through which the sacral nerves pass.

sacral nerves, the five segmental nerves from the sacral portion of the spinal cord, the first four emerging through the anterior sacral foramina and the fifth from between the sacral foramen and the coccyx.

sacral node, a node in one of the seven groups of parietal lymph nodes of the abdomen and the pelvis, situated within the sacrum. The sacral nodes are located in relation to the middle and the lateral sacral arteries and receive lymphatics from the rectum and the posterior wall of the pelvis. Compare **lumbar node.** See also **lymph, lymphatic system, lymph node.**

sacral plexus, a network of motor and sensory nerves formed by the lumbosacral trunk from the fourth and fifth lumbar, and by the first, second, and third sacral nerves. They converge toward the caudal portion of the greater sciatic foramen and unite to become a large, flattened band, most of which continues into the thigh as the sciatic nerve. The plexus lies against the posterior, lateral wall of the pelvis between the piriformis and the internal iliac vessels embedded in the pelvic subserous fascia. The nerves of the plexus, except for the third sacral nerve, divide into ventral and dorsal portions. Branches from these divisions are the nerve to the quadratus femoris and the gemellus inferior, the nerve to the obturator internus and the gemellus superior, the nerve to the piriformis, the superior gluteal nerve, the inferior gluteal nerve, the posterior femoral cutaneous nerve, the perforating cutaneous nerve, the sciatic nerve, and the pudendal nerve. Compare **lumbar plexus.**

sacral vertebra, one of the five segments of the vertebral column that fuse in the adult to form the sacrum. The ventral border of the first sacral vertebra projects into the pelvis. The bodies of the other sacral vertebrae are smaller than that of the first and are flattened and curved ventrally, forming the convex, anterior surface of the sacrum. The rudimentary spinous processes of the first several sacral vertebrae surmount the middle sacral crest, and the transverse processes of the sacral vertebrae form the lateral sacral crests. The sacral hiatus at the caudal end of the sacral canal develops from the incomplete growth of the spinous processes of the last two sacral vertebrae. The resultant widened aperture is used by anesthesiologists for the insertion of a needle to administer caudal analgesia. Compare **cervical vertebra, coccygeal vertebra, lumbar vertebra, thoracic vertebra.** See also **sacrum, vertebra.**

sacro- /sā′krō-/, a prefix meaning 'of or pertaining to the sacrum': *sacrococcyx, sacroiliac, sacrolumbalis.*

sacrococcygeal /-koksij′ē·əl/ [L, *sacer,* sacred; Gk, *kokkyx,* cuckoo's beak], pertaining to the sacrum and the coccyx.

sacroiliac /sā′krō·il′ē·ak/ [L, *sacer + ilium,* flank], pertaining to the part of the skeletal system that includes the sacrum and the ilium bones of the pelvis.

sacroiliac articulation, an immovable joint in the pelvis formed by the articulation of each side of the sacrum with an iliac bone.

sacroiliac joint, an irregular synovial joint between the sacrum and the ilium on either side.

sacrospinalis /sak′rōspinal′is/ [L, *sacer + spina,* backbone], a large, fleshy muscle of the back that divides into a lateral iliocostalis column, an intermediate longissimus column, and a medial spinalis column. Each column consists of three parts. The sacrospinalis is sheathed in the fascia thoracolumbalis and arises in a broad, thick tendon from the sacrum, the ilium, and the lumbar vertebrae. It inserts into the ribs and into certain cervical vertebrae and is innervated by the branches of the dorsal primary divisions of the spinal nerves. It extends and flexes the vertebral column and the head, and it draws the ribs downward. Also called **erector spinae.**

sacrum /sā′krəm, sak′rəm/ [L, *sacer,* sacred], the large,

triangular bone at the dorsal part of the pelvis, inserted like a wedge between the two hip bones. The base of the sacrum articulates with the last lumbar vertebra, and its apex articulates with the coccyx; various muscles attach to its spinal crest. The sacrum is shorter and wider in women than in men. **−sacral,** *adj.*

SAD, abbreviation for **seasonal affective disorder.**

saddleback nose. See **saddle nose.**

saddle block anesthesia [AS, *sadol;* Fr, *bloc;* Gk, *anaisthesia,* lack of feeling], a form of regional nerve block in which the parts of the body anesthetized are those that would touch a saddle, were the patient sitting astride one. It is performed by injecting a local anesthetic into the spinal cavity as the patient sits with the head on the chest, back curved, and legs down. Saddle block anesthesia is common in some centers for anesthesia during childbirth. See also **obstetric anesthesia.**

saddle joint, a synovial joint in which surfaces of contiguous bones are reciprocally concavoconvex. A saddle joint permits no axial rotation but allows flexion, extension, adduction, and abduction, as in the carpometacarpal joint of the thumb. Also called **articulatio sellaris.** Compare **condyloid joint, pivot joint.**

saddle nose [AS, *sadol + nosu*], a sunken nasal bridge caused by injury or disease and resulting in damage to the nasal septum. Also called **saddleback nose.**

sadism /sā′dizəm, sad′izəm/ [Marquis Donatien A. F. de Sade, French writer, b. 1740], **1.** abnormal pleasure derived from inflicting physical or psychologic pain or abuse on others; cruelty. **2.** also called **active algolagnia.** (in psychiatry) a psychosexual disorder characterized by the infliction of physical or psychologic pain or humiliation on another person, either a consenting or nonconsenting partner, to achieve sexual excitement or gratification. The condition is usually chronic in form, is seen predominantly in men, may result from conscious or unconscious motivations or desires, and, in severe cases, can lead to rape, torture, and murder. Kinds of sadism are **anal sadism** and **oral sadism.** Compare **masochism.** See also **algolagnia, sadomasochism. −sadistic,** *adj.*

sadist /sā′dist/, a person who is afflicted with or practices sadism.

sadistic. See **sadism.**

sadomasochism /sā′dōmas′əkiz′əm/ [Marquis de Sade; Leopold von Sacher-Masoch, Austrian author, b. 1836], a personality disorder characterized by traits of sadism and masochism. See also **algolagnia, masochism, sadism.**

sadomasochist /sā′dōmas′əkist/ [Comte de Sade; Sacher-Masoch], a person who practices sadomasochism.

safe period. See **natural family planning method.**

safe sex, intimate sexual practices between nonpromiscuous partners who use condoms or other methods to prevent the exchange of sexually related diseases. Although perfect safety is virtually impossible without abstinence, the known risks of infections by HIV viruses or other organisms transmitted through sexual contact can be reduced by safe sex practices.

safety director /sāf′tē/ [Fr, *sauver,* to save, *directeur,* manager], a member of a hospital staff whose activities are related to safety functions, such as fire prevention, environmental safety, and disaster planning activities.

sagittal /saj′ətəl/ [L, *sagitta,* arrow], (in anatomy) of or pertaining to a suture or an imaginary line extending from the front to the back in the midline of the body or a part of the body.

Safer sexual practices to reduce the risk of HIV transmission

Safe

Mutual masturbation
Dry (social) kissing
Massage
Hugging
Fantasy
Nonshared sex toys

Lower to moderate risk

French (wet) kissing
Urine contact
Cunnilingus
Vaginal intercourse with latex condom
Fisting (manual-anal intercourse)
Fellatio with semen ingested
Anal intercourse with latex condom
Analingus or rimming (oral-anal contact)

Highest risk

Unprotected anal intercourse
Unprotected vaginal intercourse

From Price SA, Wilson LM: *Pathophysiology: clinical concepts of disease processes*, ed 4, St Louis, 1992, Mosby.

sagittal axis, a hypothetical line through the mandibular condyle that serves as an axis for rotation movements of the mandible.

sagittal fontanel, a soft area located in the sagittal suture, halfway between the anterior and posterior fontanels. It may be found in some normal newborns and also some with Down's syndrome.

sagittal plane, the anteriorposterior plane or the section parallel to the median plane of the body. Compare **frontal plane, median plane, transverse plane.**

sagittal sinus [L, *sagitta,* arrow + *sinus,* hollow], either of two venous sinuses of the dura mater. The superior venous sinus begins near the crista galli and drains backward to empty into a confluence of sinuses near the occipital area. The inferior venous sinus begins in the lower margin of the cerebral falx and follows the superior venous sinus, emptying into the straight sinus.

sagittal suture, the serrated connection between the two parietal bones of the skull, coursing down the midline from the coronal suture to the upper part of the lambdoidal suture.

SaH, SAH, abbreviation for **subarachnoid hemorrhage.**

SAIN, abbreviation for **Society for Advancement in Nursing.**

Saint Vitus' dance /sāntvī′təs/, a motor nerve disorder characterized by irregular, involuntary jerky movements of the limbs and facial muscles. Historically, the condition was once confused with symptoms of a dance mania that reportedly was cured by a pilgrimmage to the shrine of Saint Vitus. Also called **Saint Modestus' disease, Saint Vitus' disease.** See also **Sydenham's chorea.**

sal-, -sal, a prefix for salicylic acid derivatives.

salaam convulsion /säläm′/ [L, *convulsio,* cramp], a violent muscle spasm of the sternomastoid muscles marked by head bobbing or bowing. Also called **West's syndrome.**

salbutamol. See **albuterol.**

salicylanilide /sal′isilan′ilīd/, a topical antifungal prescribed in the treatment of tinea capitis caused by *Microsporum audouinii.* It is applied to the scalp in a 3% to 5% ointment; stronger concentrations cause skin irritation.

salicylate /səlis′əlāt/ [Gk, *salix,* willow, *hyle,* matter], any of several widely prescribed drugs derived from salicylic acid. Salicylates exert analgesic, antipyretic, and antiinflammatory actions. The most important is acetylsalicylic acid, or aspirin. Sodium salicylate also has been used systemically, and it exerts similar effects. Many of the actions of aspirin appear to result from its ability to inhibit cyclooxygenase, a rate-limiting enzyme in prostaglandin biosynthesis. Aspirin is used in a wide variety of conditions, and, in the usual analgesic dosage, it causes only mild adverse effects. Severe occult GI bleeding or gastric ulcers may occur with frequent use. Large doses taken over a long period can cause significant impairment of hemostasis. Occasionally, an asthmalike reaction is produced in hypersensitive individuals. Because of the ready availability of aspirin, accidental and intentional overdosage is common. Symptoms of salicylate intoxication include tinnitus, GI disturbances, abnormal respiration, acid-base imbalance, and central nervous system disturbances. Fatalities have occurred from ingestion of as little as 10 grains of aspirin in adults or as little as 4 ml of methyl salicylate (oil of wintergreen) in children. In addition to aspirin and sodium salicylate, which are used systemically, methyl salicylate is used topically as a counterirritant in ointments and liniments. Methyl salicylate can be absorbed through the skin in amounts capable of causing systemic toxicity. Another salicylate, salicylic acid, is too irritating to be used systemically and is used topically as a keratolytic agent, for example, for removing warts.

salicylated /səlis′ilā′tid/ [Gk, *salix,* willow + *hyle,* matter], pertaining to a chemical formed as a salt or ester of salicylic acid.

salicylate poisoning, a toxic condition caused by the ingestion of salicylate, most often in aspirin or oil of wintergreen. Intoxication is characterized by rapid breathing, vomiting, headache, irritability, ketosis, hypoglycemia, and, in severe cases, convulsions and respiratory failure. Treatment may include prompt induced emesis or gastric lavage with activated charcoal, the administration of a saline cathartic, a parenteral infusion of sodium bicarbonate, injection of vitamin K if bleeding is present, and correction of dehydration, hypoglycemia, and hypokalemia. Sodium bicarbonate by mouth is contraindicated.

salicylazosulfapyridine. See **sulfasalazine.**

salicylic acid /sal′isil′ik/, a keratolytic agent.

■ INDICATIONS: It is prescribed in the treatment of hyperkeratotic skin conditions and as an adjunct in fungal infections.

■ CONTRAINDICATIONS: Diabetes, impaired circulation, or known hypersensitivity to this drug prohibits its use.

■ ADVERSE EFFECTS: Among the more serious adverse reactions are skin inflammation and salicylism.

salicylism /sal′isil′izəm/ [Gk, *salix,* willow, *hyle,* matter, *ismos,* practice], a syndrome of salicylate toxicity.

saline /sā′līn/ [L, *sal,* salt], **1.** pertaining to a substance that contains a salt of an alkali metal or earth. **2.** pertaining to something that is salty or has the characteristics of common table salt.

saline cathartic [L, *sal,* salt; Gk, *katharsis,* cleansing], one of a large group of cathartics administered to achieve prompt, complete evacuation of the bowel. A watery semifluid evacuation usually occurs within 3 to 4 hours. The most common indication for the administration of any of these agents is preparation of the bowel for diagnostic examination. Various preparations, including magnesium sulfate, sodium phosphate, sodium sulfate, and several naturally occurring mineral waters, may be used to achieve catharsis. The palatability, cost, and adverse systemic reactions of the saline cathartics depend on the particular agent used and the dose of the agent given.

saline enema [L, *sal*, salt; Gk, *enienai*, to send in], a salt-water enema. Hypertonic saline enemas are used to treat worm infestations, by inducing peristalsis and evacuation. It may require two teaspoons of salt per 0.5 liter of warm water, sometimes with magnesium sulfate added, instilled slowly, and retained as long as possible. A normal saline enema of one teaspoonful of salt per 0.5 liter of water is instilled slowly and retained as long as possible to combat shock or replace lost fluids.

saline infusion, the therapeutic introduction of a physiologic salt solution into a vein.

saline irrigation, the washing out of a body cavity or wound with a stream of salt solution, usually an isotonic aqueous solution of sodium chloride.

saline solution, a solution containing sodium chloride. Depending on the use, it may be hypotonic, isotonic, or hypertonic with body fluids.

saliva /səlī′və/ [L, spittle], the clear, viscous fluid secreted by the salivary and mucous glands in the mouth. Saliva contains water, mucin, organic salts, and the digestive enzyme ptyalin. It serves to moisten the oral cavity, to initiate the digestion of starches, and to aid in the chewing and swallowing of food.

salivary /sal′iver′ē/ [L, saliva], of or pertaining to saliva or to the formation of saliva.

salivary duct, any one of the ducts through which saliva passes. Kinds of salivary ducts are **Bartholin's duct, duct of Rivinus, parotid duct,** and **submandibular duct.**

salivary fistula, an abnormal communication from a salivary gland or duct to an opening in the mouth or on the skin of the face or neck.

salivary gland, one of the three pairs of glands secreting into the mouth, thus aiding the digestive process. The salivary glands are the parotid, the submandibular, and the sublingual glands. They are racemose structures consisting of numerous lobes subdivided into smaller lobules connected by dense areolar tissue, vessels, and ducts. The ducts ramify inside each lobule, ending in alveoli. One kind of alveolus secretes a viscid fluid containing mucin. The other kind secretes serous fluid. The sublingual gland secretes mucus; the parotid gland, serous fluid; the submandibular gland, both mucus and serous fluid. The lobules of the salivary glands are richly supplied with blood vessels and fine plexuses of nerves. The hilum of the submandibular gland contains Langley's ganglion of nerve cells.

salivary gland cancer, a malignant neoplastic disease of a salivary gland, occurring most frequently in a parotid gland. About 75% of tumors that develop in the salivary glands are benign, characteristically slow-growing, painless, mobile masses that are cystic or rubbery in consistency. In contrast, malignant tumors are rapid-growing, hard, lumpy, fixed, and frequently tender. Pain, trismus, and facial palsy may occur. Diagnostic measures include x-ray studies, with sialographic studies and mandibular and chest films to detect metastases, and cytologic studies of saliva from Stensen's duct. Direct biopsies are not recommended. The most common malignant neoplasms are mucoepidermoid, adenoid cystic, solid, and squamous cell carcinomas. Treatment usually consists of the surgical removal of the lobe containing a benign tumor and total parotidectomy with a radical neck dissection if the lesion is advanced. Radiotherapy is administered for residual, recurrent, or inoperable cancers, and chemotherapy may be palliative.

saliva substitute. See **artificial saliva.**

salivation /sal′ivā′shən/, the process of saliva secretion by the salivary glands.

salivatory /sal′ivətôr′ē/ [L, *saliva*, spittle], stimulating the production of saliva. Also **sialogenous.**

Salk vaccine. See **poliovirus vaccine.**

sallow /sal′ō/ [ME, *salou*, dirty-gray], sickly in complexion.

salmon calcitonin. See **calcitonin.**

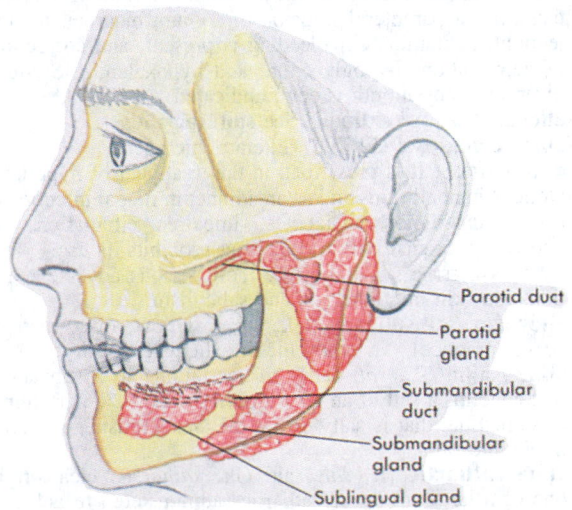

Salivary glands *(Thibodeau, 1993/Ernest W Beck)*

Parotid duct
Parotid gland
Submandibular duct
Submandibular gland
Sublingual gland

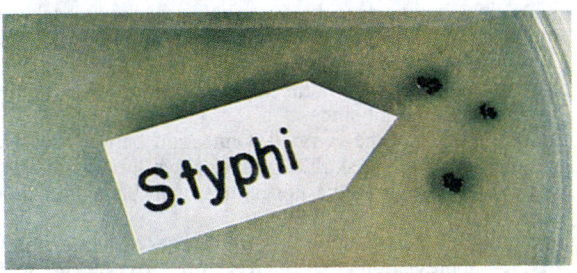

Colonies of *salmonella typhi* on bismuth sulfite agar
(Baron, 1990)

Salmonella /sal′mənel′ə/ [Daniel E. Salmon, American pathologist, b. 1850], a genus of motile, gram-negative, rod-shaped bacteria that includes species causing typhoid fever, paratyphoid fever, and some forms of gastroenteritis. See also **salmonellosis.**

Salmonella enteritidis [Daniel E. Salmon; Gk, *enteron*, intestine], a species of *Salmonella* causing food poisoning and gastroenteritis in humans.

salmonellosis /sal′mənəlō′sis/ [Daniel E. Salmon; Gk, *osis*, condition], a form of gastroenteritis, caused by ingestion of food contaminated with a species of *Salmonella*, characterized by an incubation period of 6 to 48 hours followed by sudden, colicky abdominal pain, fever, and bloody, watery diarrhea. Nausea and vomiting are common, and abdominal signs may resemble acute appendicitis or cholecystitis. Symptoms usually last from 2 to 5 days, but diarrhea and fever may persist for up to 2 weeks. Dehydration may occur. There is no specific treatment. Antibiotics may prolong the excretion of *Salmonella* in stools and are usually not indicated. Adequate cooking, good refrigeration, and careful handwashing may reduce the frequency of outbreaks. See also **food poisoning.**

salol. See **phenyl salicylate.**

salol camphor /sal′ol/, a clear, oily mixture of two parts of camphor and three parts of phenyl salicylate, used as a local antiseptic.

Salonica fever. See **trench fever.**

salpingectomy /sal′pinjek′təmē/ [Gk, *salpinx*, tube, *ektome*, excision], surgical removal of one or both fallopian tubes, performed to remove a cyst or tumor, excise an abscess, or, if both tubes are removed, as a sterilization procedure or for tubal pregnancy. Often the operation is done with a hysterectomy or an oophorectomy. Either spinal block or general anesthesia may be given. Postoperatively, the patient is instructed to avoid sharply flexing the thighs or the knees. Persistent low back pain or the presence of bloody or scanty urine indicates a ureter may have been injured during surgery.

salpinges. See **salpinx.**

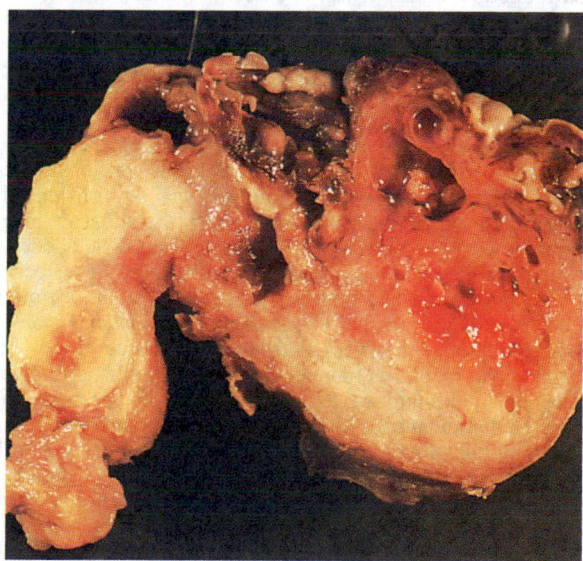

Chronic salpingitis (Fletcher, 1987)

salpingian. See **salpinx.**

salpingitis /sal′pinjī′tis/ [Gk, *salpinx* + *itis*, inflammation], an inflammation or infection of the fallopian tube. See also **pelvic inflammatory disease.**

salpingo- /salping′gō-/, a combining form meaning 'of or

pertaining to a eustachian or a fallopian tube': *salpingocele, salpingolysis, salpingoplasty.*

salpingo-oophorectomy /-ō′əfôrek′təmē/, the surgical removal of a fallopian tube and an ovary.

salpingo-oophoritis /-ō′əfôrī′tis/ [Gk, *salpinx*, tube + *oophoron*, ovary + *itis*, inflammation], an inflammation of a fallopian tube and associated ovary.

salpingostomy /sal′ping·gos′təmē/ [Gk, *salpinx* + *stoma*, mouth], the formation of an artificial opening in a fallopian tube. The procedure is performed to restore patency in a tube whose fimbriated opening has been closed by infection or by chronic inflammation or to drain an abscess or an accumulation of fluid. Either regional or general anesthesia is used. A prosthesis may be inserted to maintain the patency of the fallopian tube and to direct the route of the ova to assist fertilization. Postoperatively, the nurse cautions the patient against sharply flexing the thighs or the knees. Low back pain or scanty or bloody urine may indicate that a ureter has been injured during the procedure, requiring surgical intervention.

salpinx /sal′pingks/, *pl.* **salpinges** /salpin′jēz/ [Gk, tube], a tube, such as the *salpinx auditiva* or the *salpinx uterina.* **–salpingian,** *adj.*

salt /sôlt/ [AS, *sealt*], **1.** a compound formed by the chemical reaction of an acid and a base. Salts are usually composed of a metal and a nonmetal and may behave chemically as metals or nonmetals. **2.** sodium chloride (common table salt). **3.** a substance, such as magnesium sulfate (Epsom salt), used as a purgative.

saltation /saltā′shən/ [L, *saltare*, to dance], (in genetics) a mutation causing a significant difference in appearance between parent and offspring or an abrupt variation in the characteristics of the species. **–saltatorial, saltatoric, saltatory** /sal′tətôr′ē/, *adj.*

saltatory conduction /sal′tətôr′ē/ [L, *saltare* + *conducere*, to lead together], impulse transmission that skips from node to node. (See Fig. p. 1392.)

saltatory evolution, the appearance of a sudden, abrupt change within a species, caused by mutation; the progression of a species by sudden major changes rather than by the gradual accumulation of minor changes. The phenomenon occurs predominantly in plants as a result of polyploidy. See also **emergent evolution.**

salt cake, sodium sulfate anhydrous; a technical grade of sodium sulfate used in detergents, dyes, soaps, and other industrial products. See also **sodium sulfate.**

salt depletion, the loss of salt from the body through excessive elimination of body fluids by perspiration, diarrhea, vomiting, or urination, without corresponding replacement. See also **electrolyte balance, heat exhaustion.**

Salter fracture. See **epiphyseal fracture.**

salt-free diet. See **low-sodium diet.**

saltpeter /sôlt′pē′tər/ [L, *sal*, salt + *petra*, rock], common name for potassium nitrate, KNO_3, used in gunpowder, pickling, and medicines.

salt-poor diet [Gk *diaita* life-style], a diet providing 500 mg or less of sodium chloride daily. To ensure that the maximum intake of salt does not exceed the limit, it is necessary to record the amount of dietary sodium chloride, including amounts contained in medications taken by a patient. Note: some 'salt-free' diets may contain as much as 1000 mg of sodium chloride per day.

Saluron, a trademark for an antihypertensive and diuretic (hydroflumethiazide).

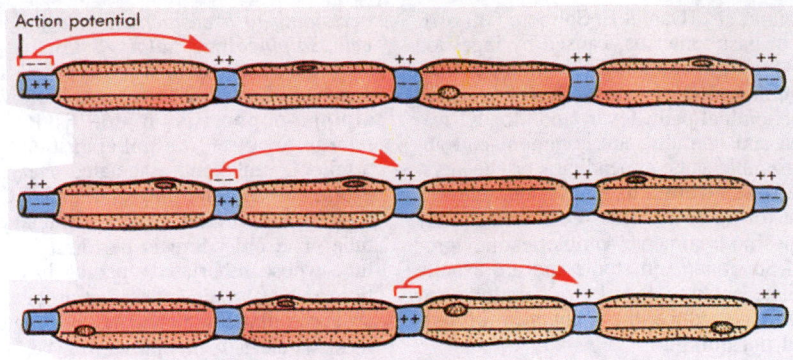

Saltatory conduction (Seeley, 1992/Scott Bodell)

salvage therapy /sal'vij/ [Fr, *sauver*, to save; Gk, *thera-peia*, treatment], therapy administered to sites at which previous therapies have failed and the disease has recurred.

salve. See **ointment.**

samarium (Sm) /səmer'ē·əm/ [Colonel Samarski, 19th century Russian mine official], a rare earth, metallic element. Its atomic number is 62; its atomic weight is 150.35.

sample [L, *exemplum*], in research, a group or portion of the whole that can be used to demonstrate characteristics of the whole. Kinds of samples include **cluster, convenience, random,** and **stratified.**

sanatorium. See **sanitarium.**

sand bath, the application of warm, dry sand or of damp sand to the body.

sand flea. See **chigoe,** def. 1.

sandfly fever. See **phlebotomus fever.**

Sandhoff's disease, a variant of Tay-Sachs disease that includes defects in both the enzymes hexosaminidase A and B. It is characterized by a progressively more rapid course and is found in the general population, not restricted as is Tay-Sachs disease. Also called **gangliosidosis type II.** See also **Tay-Sachs disease.**

Sandoz Clinical Assessment—Geriatric, an examination of psychologic function that is administered to elderly people to assist in the diagnostic process.

sand tumor. See **psammoma.**

sangui-, a combining form meaning 'of or pertaining to blood': *sanguicolous, sanguiferous, sanguinolent.*

sanguine /sang'gwin/ [L, *sanguis*, blood], pertaining to an abundant and active blood circulation, ruddy complexion, and an attitude full of vitality and confidence.

sanguineous /sang·gwin'ē·əs/ [L, *sanguis*, blood], pertaining to blood or containing blood, such as full-blooded. Also **sanguinous** /sang'gwinəs/.

sanita-, a combining form meaning 'of or pertaining to health': *sanitarium, sanitas, sanitation.*

sanitarium /san'iter'ē·əm/ [L, *sanare*], to restore health], a facility for the treatment of patients suffering from chronic mental or physical diseases, or the recuperation of convalescent patients. Also called **sanatorium.**

sanitary landfill /san'iterē/ [L, *sanitas*, health; AS, *land, fyllan*, to fill], a solid waste disposal site, usually a swamp area, ravine, or canyon where the waste is compacted by heavy machines and covered with earth.

sanitation /san'itā'shən/ [L, *sanitas*, health], the science of maintaining a healthful, disease-free and hazard-free, environment.

sanitize /san'itīz/ [L, *sanitas*, health], to take action needed to clean the environment or a part of it, removing or reducing pathogenic microorganisms and their habitats.

San Joaquin fever /san'wôkēn'/ [San Joaquin Valley, California; L, *febris*, fever], the primary stage of coccidioidomycosis.

SA node. See **sinoatrial node.**

Sanorex, a trademark for an anorexiant (mazindol).

Sansert, a trademark for a vasoconstrictor (methysergide maleate).

Santyl, a trademark for an enzyme (collagenase).

SaO$_2$, symbol for the percent of oxygen *saturation of arterial blood*.

saphenous [Gk, *saphenes*, manifest], pertaining to certain anatomic structures in the leg, such as arteries, veins, or nerves.

saphenous nerve /səfē'nəs/ [Gk, *saphenes* manifest; L, *nervus*, nerve], the largest and longest branch of the femoral nerve, supplying the skin of the medial side of the leg. It courses deep to the sartorius, accompanied by the femoral artery posteriorly, and crosses from the lateral to the medial side of the sartorius, within the fascial cover of the adductor canal. At the tendinous arch in the adductor magnus, it leaves the artery, pierces the fascia of the adductor canal, descends along the medial side of the knee, penetrates the fascia lata between the tendons of the sartorius and the gracilis, and becomes subcutaneous. It accompanies the great saphenous vein along the medial side of the leg, and at the medial border of the tibia in the distal third of the leg divides into two terminal branches. One branch joins the medial cutaneous and the obturator nerves to form the subsartorial plexus. A large infrapatellar branch passes to the skin over the patella and on the lateral side of the knee joins with branches of the lateral femoral cutaneous nerve to form the patellar plexus. One branch of the saphenous nerve below the knee supplies the ankle. Another branch below the knee supplies the medial side of the foot. See also **femoral nerve.**

saphenous vein. See **great saphenous vein.**

sapo-, a combining form meaning 'of or pertaining to soap': *sapogenin, saponaceous, sapotoxin.*

saponaceous /sap'ənā'shəs/ [L, *sapo*, soap], pertaining to soap.

saponification /sapon'ifikā'shən/ [L, *sapo*, soap + *facere*, to make], the production of soap.

saponified, pertaining to a substance chemically hydrolized into soaps or acid salts and glycerol by heating with an alkali.

saponin /sap'ənin/ [L, *sapo*, soap], a soapy material found in some plants, especially soapwort (Bouncing Bet) and certain lilies. It is used in demulcent medications to provide a sudsy quality. Natural saponins, which can be hemolytic toxins, have largely been replaced by synthetic preparations.

sapro-, a combining form meaning 'relating to decay or putrefaction': *saprophytes, saprophagus, saprolite.*

saprophyte /sap'rəfit/ [Gk, *sapros*, rotten, *phyton*, plant], an organism that lives on dead organic matter. **—saprophytic,** *adj.*

SAR, abbreviation for **structure-activity relationship.**

saralasin, a competitive antagonist of angiotensin. It is administered by intravenous injection to assess the role of the renin-angiotensin system in the maintenance of blood pressure.

-sarc, a combining form meaning '(specified type of) flesh': *ectosarc, endosarc, perisarc.*

sarco- /sär'kō-/, a combining form meaning 'of or related to the flesh': *sarcoadenoma, sarcode, sarcolyte.*

sarcoadenoma /-ad'ənō'mə/ [Gk, *sarx*, flesh + *aden*, gland + *oma*, tumor], a mixed tumor containing both glandular and connective tissue characteristics. Also called **adenosarcoma.**

sarcocarcinoma /-kär'sinō'mə/ [Gk, *sarx*, flesh + *karkinos*, crab + *oma*, tumor], a mixed tumor with characteristics of both sarcomas and carcinomas.

sarcodina. See **protozoa.**

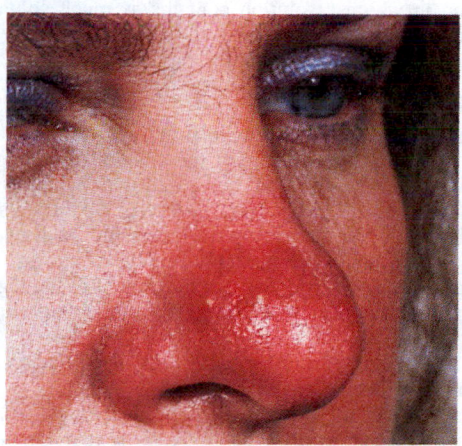

Sarcoidosis eruption affecting the nose
(du Vivier, 1993)

sarcoidosis /sär'koidō'sis/ [Gk, *sarx*, flesh, *eidos*, form, *osis*, condition], a chronic disorder of unknown origin characterized by the formation of tubercles of nonnecrotizing epithelioid tissue. Common sites are the lungs, spleen, liver, skin, mucous membranes, and lacrimal and salivary glands, usually with involvement of the lymph glands. Diminished reactivity to tuberculin frequently accompanies the disorder. The lesions usually disappear over a period of months or years but progress to widespread granulomatous inflammation and fibrosis. Also called **sarcoid of Boeck.**

sarcoidosis cordis, a form of sarcoidosis in which granulomatous lesions develop in the myocardium. Mild cases with few infiltrates are asymptomatic. In severe cases, car-

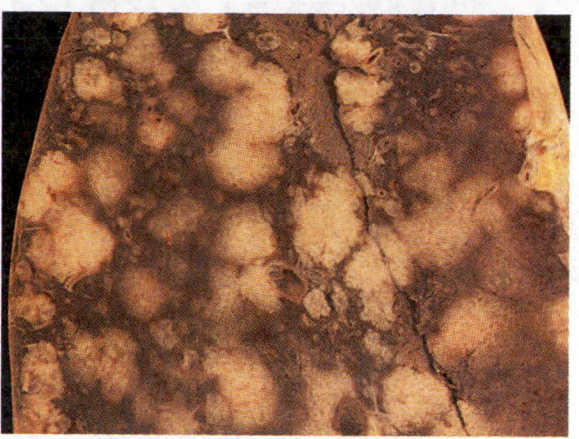

Sarcoidosis affecting the spleen *(Fletcher, 1987)*

diac failure may result. See also **sarcoidosis.**

sarcolemma /-lem'ə/ [Gk, *sarx*, flesh + *lemma*, sheath], a membrane that covers smooth, striated, and cardiac muscle fibers.

sarcoma /särkō'mə/, *pl.* **sarcomas, sarcomata** [Gk, *sarx*, + *oma*, tumor], a malignant neoplasm of the soft tissues arising in fibrous, fatty, muscular, synovial, vascular, or neural tissue, usually first presenting as a painless swelling. About 40% of sarcomas occur in the lower extremities, 20% in the upper extremities, 20% in the trunk, and the rest in the head, neck, or retroperineum. The tumor, composed of closely packed cells in a fibrillar or homogeneous matrix, tends to be vascular and is usually highly invasive. Trauma probably does not play a role in the cause, but sarcomas may arise in burn or radiation scars. Small tumors may be managed by local excision and postoperative radiotherapy, but bulky sarcomas of the extremities may require amputation followed by irradiation for local control and combination chemotherapy to eliminate small foci or neoplastic cells. See specific sarcomas. (See Figs. p. 1394.)

-sarcoma, a combining form meaning a 'malignant tumor from connective tissue': *angiosarcoma, hemangiosarcoma, myelosarcoma.*

sarcoma botryoides /bot'rē·oi'dēz/, a tumor derived from primitive striated muscle cells, occurring most frequently in young children and characterized by a painful, edematous, polypoid grapelike mass in the upper vagina or on the uterine cervix or the neck of the urinary bladder. See also **rhabdomyosarcoma.**

sarcomagenesis /särkō'məjen'əsis/ [Gk, *sarx*, *oma* + *genesis*, origin], the process of initiating and promoting the development of a sarcoma. Compare **carcinogenesis, oncogenesis, tumorigenesis. —sarcomagenetic,** *adj.*

sarcomas. See **sarcoma.**

sarcomata. See **sarcoma.**

sarcomere /sär'kōmir/ [Gk, *sarx* + *meros*, part], the smallest functional unit of a myofibril. Sarcomeres occur as repeating units along the length of a myofibril, occupying the region between Z disks of the myofibril.

sarcoplasm /sär'kōplaz'əm/ [Gk, *sarx*, flesh + *plassein*, to mold], the semifluid cytoplasm of muscle cells.

sarcoplasmic reticulum /-plas'tik/ [Gk, *sarx* + *plassein*, to mold; L, *reticulum*, little net], a network of tubules and sacs in skeletal muscles that plays an important role in mus-

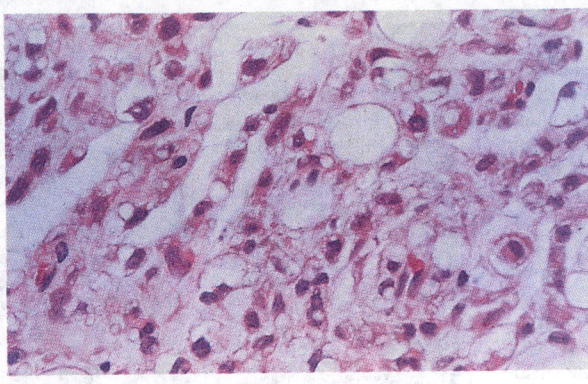 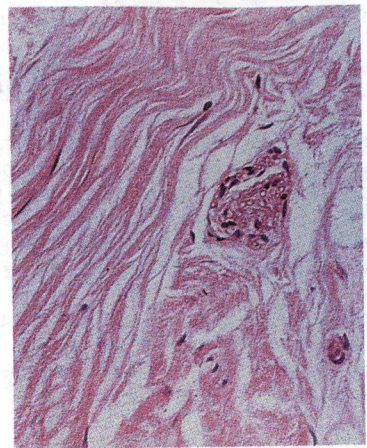

Sarcomas—liposarcoma (left) and neurofibrosarcoma (right) *(Bullough, 1984)*

cle contraction and relaxation by releasing and storing calcium ions. This network is analogous, but not identical, to the endoplasmic reticulum of other cells.

Sarcoptes scabiei /särkop′tēz skā′bē·ī/ [Gk, *sarx* + *koptein*, to cut; L *scabere* to scratch], the genus of itch mite that causes scabies.

sartorius /särtôr′ē·əs/ [L, *sartor*, tailor], the longest muscle in the body, extending from the pelvis to the calf of the leg. It is a narrow muscle that arises from the anterior superior iliac spine, passes obliquely across the proximal anterior part of the thigh from the lateral to the medial side, and inserts, by a tendon and an aponeurosis, into the tibia. It is innervated by branches of the femoral nerve. It acts to flex the thigh and rotate it laterally and to flex the leg and rotate it medially. Compare **quadriceps femoris.**

satellite cells /sat′əlīt/[L, *satelles*, attendant + *cella*, storeroom], glial cells that form around damaged nerve cells.

satellite clinic [L, *satelles* attendant; Gk, *kline*, bed], a health care facility usually operated under the auspices of a large institution but situated in a location some distance from the larger health center.

satiety /sətī′ətē/, the satisfied feeling of being full after eating.

saturated /sach′ərā′tid/ [L, *saturare*, to fill], **1.** having absorbed or dissolved the maximum amount of a given substance, such as a solution in which no more of the solute can be dissolved. **2.** also called **saturated hydrocarbon.** an organic compound that contains the maximum number of hydrogen atoms so that only single valence bonds exist in the carbon chain, such as in saturated fatty acids. Compare **unsaturated.**

saturated calomel electrode (SCE), a reference electrode commonly used in polarography.

saturated fatty acid, any of a number of glyceryl esters of certain organic acids in which all the atoms are joined by single bonds. These fats are chiefly of animal origin and include beef, lamb, pork, veal, whole-milk products, butter, most cheeses, and a few plant fats such as cocoa butter, coconut oil, and palm oil. Ordinary oleomargarine and hydrogenated shortenings also contain saturated fatty acids. A diet high in saturated fatty acids may contribute to a high serum cholesterol level and, in some studies of some pop-

ulation groups, is associated with an increased incidence of coronary heart disease. Compare **unsaturated fatty acid.**

saturated hydrocarbon. See **saturated.**

saturated solution, a solution in which the solvent contains the maximum amount of solute it can take up. See also **solute, solvent.**

saturation /sach′ərā′shən/ [L, *saturare*, to fill], **1.** a condition in which a solution contains as much solute as can remain dissolved. **2.** a measure of the degree to which oxygen is bound to hemoglobin, expressed as a percentage of the possible limit. **3.** a chemical compound in which all the valency bonds have been filled.

saturation index of hemoglobin [L, *saturare*, to fill + *index*, pointer], a measure of the amount of hemoglobin in a given amount of blood, compared with normal.

Saturday night palsy [Gk, *paralyein*, to be palsied], a radial nerve paralysis caused by pressure on the arm after the person has fallen asleep, usually during an alcoholic binge. A similar type of palsy may result in the legs during alcoholic slumber on a sofa. Also called **Saturday night paralysis.**

saturn-, a combining form meaning 'lead' /led/: *saturnine, saturnism, saturnotherapy.*

satyriasis /sat′irī′əsis/ [Gk, *satyros*, lecherous, *osis*, condition], excessive or uncontrollable sexual desire in the male. Also called **satyromania.** Compare **nymphomania.**

sauna bath /sô′nə/ [Finn, *sauna;* AS, *baeth*, a bath in which hot vapor is used to induce sweating, followed by rubbing of the body, and ending with a cold shower. Also called **Finnish bath, Russian bath.**

saur-, a combining form meaning 'lizard, or reptile': *sauriasis, sauriderma, sauroid.*

Sayre's jacket /serz/ [Lewis A. Sayre, American surgeon, b. 1820; ME, *jaket*], a cast applied for support and immobilization in the treatment of certain abnormalities of the spinal column.

Sb, symbol for the element **antimony.**

SBE, 1. abbreviation for **self-breast examination. 2.** abbreviation for **subacute bacterial endocarditis.**

sc, 1. abbreviation for *sine correctione,* a Latin phrase meaning "without correction." **2.** abbreviation for **subcutaneously.**

Sc, symbol for the element **scandium.**

scab. See **eschar.**

scabicide /skab′isīd/ [L, *scabere,* to scratch, *caedere,* to kill], any one of a large group of drugs that destroy the itch mite, *Sarcoptes scabiei.* These drugs are applied topically in a lotion or cream-based preparation. All are potentially toxic and irritating to the skin. They are used with caution in treating children. Kinds of scabicides include **crotamiton, lindane.**

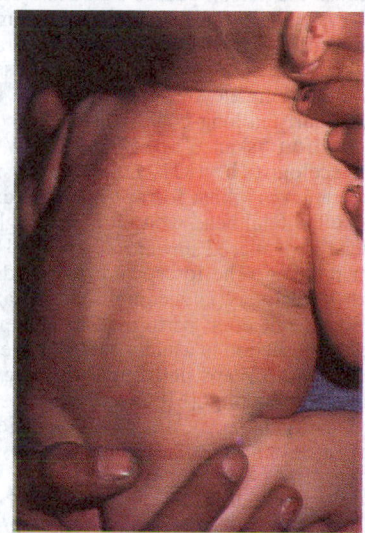

Scabies rash on infant (Weston, 1991)

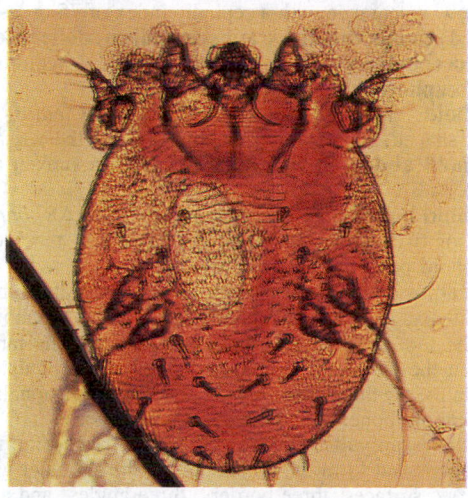

Adult scabies mite (Zitelli, 1992)

scabies /skā′bēz/ [L, *scabere,* to scratch], a contagious disease caused by *Sarcoptes scabiei,* the itch mite, characterized by intense itching of the skin and excoriation from scratching. The mite, transmitted by close contact with infected humans or domestic animals, burrows into outer layers of the skin, where the female lays eggs. Two to 4 months after the first infection, sensitization to the mites and their products begins, resulting in a pruritic papular rash most common on the webs of fingers, flexor surfaces of wrists, and thighs. Secondary bacterial infection may occur. Diagnosis may be made by microscopic identification of adult mites, larvae, or eggs in scrapings of the burrows. All contacts are treated simultaneously with lindane (1%), crotamiton (10%), or other scabicide applied locally. Oral antihistamines and salicylates reduce itching.

scabietic /skā′bē·et′ik/ [L, *scabere,* to scratch], pertaining to scabies.

scag, *slang.* heroin.

scald /skôld/ [L, *calidus,* hot], a burn caused by exposure of the skin to a hot liquid or vapor.

scalded skin syndrome. See **toxic epidermal necrolysis.**

scale [OFr *escale* husk], **1.** a small, thin flake of keratinized epithelium. **2.** to remove incrusted material from the surface of a tooth.

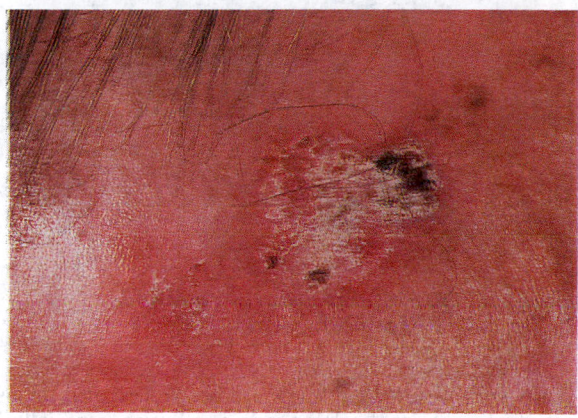

Scale of lupus erythematosus (du Vivier, 1993)

scalene /skā′lēn/ [Gk, *skalenos,* uneven], pertaining to one of the scalenous muscles.

scalenus /skālē′nəs/ [Gk, *skalenos*], one of a group of four muscles arising from the cervical vertebrae with insertions on the first or second rib.

scalenus anticus syndrome. See **Nafziger's syndrome.**

scalp [ME], the skin covering the head, not including the face and ears.

scalpel /skal′pəl/ [L, *scalprum,* knife], a small, pointed knife with a convex edge. Some scalpels use interchangeable blades for specific surgical procedures, such as operating and amputating. (See Fig. p. 1396.)

scalp medication, 1. a cream, ointment, lotion, or shampoo used to treat dermatologic conditions of the scalp. **2.** the application of a medication to the scalp. If a cream, ointment, or lotion is to be applied, a shampoo is usually given first. The hair is dried, combed, and parted in the middle, and the medication is spread with the fingertips. After treatment, the medication may need to be washed off the scalp and hair with an alkaline shampoo.

scalp tourniquet [ME, *skalp;* OFr *tunicle*], a bandage applied to the scalp to restrict blood flow during administration of antineoplastic drugs. The tourniquet controls the hair loss that commonly accompanies use of cancer-suppressing drugs.

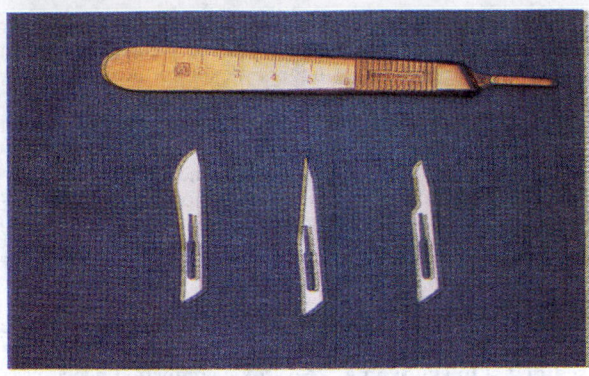

Scalpel handle with three blades (Grossman, 1993)

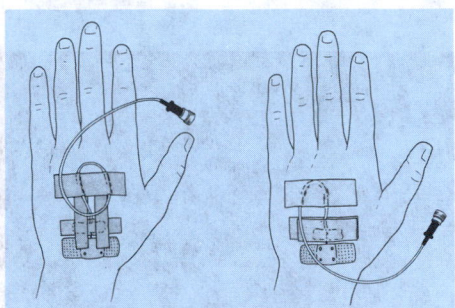

**Acceptable securing methods
for scalp vein needles**

scalp vein needle, a thin-gauge needle designed for use on the veins of the scalp or other small veins, especially in children.

scamping speech [ONorse, *skammr,* scant; ME, *speche*], abnormal speech in which consonants or whole syllables are left out of words because of the person's inability to shape the sounds. Also called **clipped speech.**

scan. See **scanning.**

scandium (Sc) /skan'dē·əm/ [Scandinavia], a grayish metallic element. Its atomic number is 21; its atomic weight is 44.956.

scanning [L, *scandere,* to climb], a technique for carefully studying an area, organ, or system of the body by recording and displaying an image of the area. A concentration of a radioactive substance that has an affinity for a specific tissue may be administered by IV to enhance the image. The liver, brain, and thyroid can be examined, tumors can be located, and function can be evaluated by various scanning techniques. See specific scanning techniques. **−scan,** *n., v.*

scanning electron microscope (SEM), an instrument similar to an electron microscope in that a beam of electrons instead of visible light is used to scan the surface of a specimen. The beam is moved in a point-to-point manner over the surface of the specimen. The number of electrons emerging from the sample is proportionate to the shape, density, and other properties of the sample. These electrons are deflected, collected, accelerated, and directed against a scintillator. The large number of photons thus created are converted into an electric signal that, in turn, modulates the beam scanning the surface of the specimen. The image produced is of less magnification than that produced by an electron microscope, but it appears to be three-dimensional and lifelike. Compare **electron microscope, transmission scanning electron microscope.**

scanning electron microscopy, the technique using a scanning electron microscope on an electrically conducting sample.

scanning speech, abnormal speech characterized by a staccato-like articulation in which the words are clipped and broken because the person pauses between syllables.

scanography /skanog'rəfē/ [L, *scandere,* to climb; Gk, *graphein,* to record], a method of producing a radiogram of an internal body organ or structure by using a series of parallel beams that eliminate size distortion. The technique is applied particularly in long-bone radiography.

Scanzoni rotation /skanzō'nē/ [Friedrich W. Scanzoni, German gynecologist, b. 1821; L, *rotare,* to rotate], an obstetric operation in which forceps having a curved shank are applied to the fetal head while it is still high in the pelvis. The head is displaced upward and rotated to the occiput anterior position. The forceps are removed and repositioned, and the delivery is accomplished by axis traction. The operation is not often performed in modern obstetrics because cesarean section is usually safer for the mother and the baby. See also **forceps delivery, obstetric forceps.**

scapegoating /skāp'gōting/ [ME, *escapen,* to escape; *goot*], the projection of blame, hostility, or suspicion onto one member of a group by other members to avoid self-confrontation.

scapho-, a combining form meaning 'boat-shaped': *scaphocephaly, scaphohydrocephaly, scaphoid.*

scaphocephaly /skaf'ōsef'əlē/ [Gk, *skaphe,* skiff, *kephale,* head], a congenital malformation of the skull in which premature closure of the sagittal suture results in restricted lateral growth of the head, giving it an abnormally long, narrow appearance with a cephalic index of 75 or less. Also called **scaphocephalis, scaphocephalism, dolichocephaly, mecocephaly.** See also **craniostenosis. −scaphocephalic, scaphocephalous,** *adj.*

scaphoid /skaf'oid/ [Gk, *skaphe,* skiff + *eidos,* form], boat-shaped, such as the scaphoid bone of the wrist.

scaphoid abdomen, an abdomen with a sunken anterior wall.

scaphoid bone [Gk, *skaphe* + *eidos,* form; AS, *ban*], either of two similar bones of the hand and the foot. The scaphoid bone of the hand is slanted at the radial side of the carpus and articulates with the radius, trapezium, trapezoideum, capitate, and lunate bones. The scaphoid bone of the foot is located at the medial side of the tarsus between the talus and cuneiform bones and articulates with the talus, the three cuneiform bones, and, occasionally, with the cuboid bone. Also called **navicular bone.**

scapula /skap'yələ/, one of the pair of large, flat, triangular bones that form the dorsal part of the shoulder girdle. It has two surfaces, three borders, three angles, and a prominent dorsal spine. The acromion of the scapula forms the summit of the shoulder. The coracoid process, resembling a raven's beak, accommodates the attachment of various muscles, including the pectoralis minor, and ligaments, including the trapezoid. Also called **shoulder blade.**

-scapula, a combining form meaning a 'shoulder blade or a part of it': *mesoscapula, prescapula, proscapula.*

scapular line /skap'yələr/, an imaginary vertical line drawn through the inferior angle of the scapula.

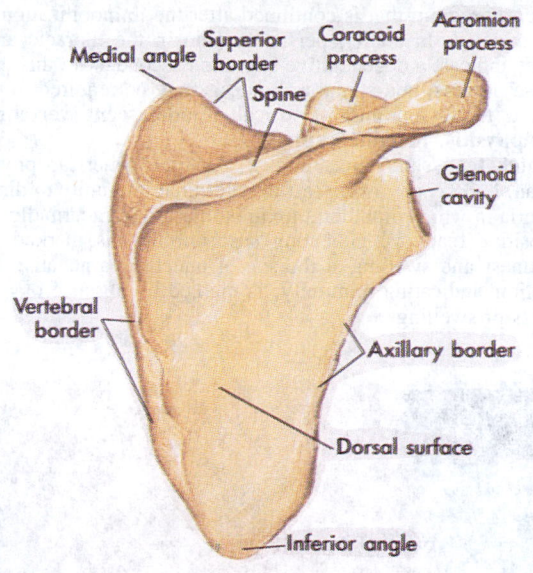

Scapula (Thibodeau, 1993)

Labels on scapula diagram: Medial angle, Superior border, Spine, Coracoid process, Acromion process, Glenoid cavity, Vertebral border, Axillary border, Dorsal surface, Inferior angle

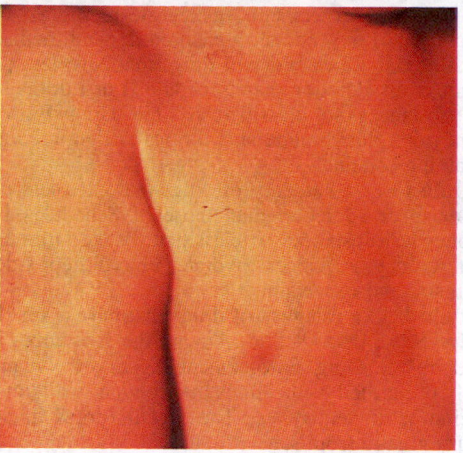

Scarlet fever (Zitelli, 1992/Courtesy Dr. Michael Sherlock)

scapulo- /skap′yəlō-/ [L, *scapulae*, shoulder blades], a combining form meaning 'relating to the scapula, or shoulder blade': *scapulodynia, scapulopexy.*

scapulohumeral /-hyo͞o′mərəl/ [L, *scapula* + *humerus*, shoulder], of or pertaining to the structures of muscles and the area around the scapula and humerus that make up the shoulder girdle.

scapulohumeral muscular dystrophy. See **Erb's muscular dystrophy.**

scapulohumeral reflex, a normal response to tapping the vertebral border of the scapula, resulting in adduction of the arm. Absence of the reflex may indicate a lesion in the region of the fifth cervical segment of the spinal cord.

scapus /skā′pəs/ [Gk, *skapos*, rod], a stem or shaft, such as the scapus penis.

scar. See **cicatrix.**

scarification /sker′ifikā′shən/ [L, *scarifare*, to scratch open], multiple superficial scratches or incisions in the skin, such as those made for the introduction of a vaccine. The term is erroneously used to mean "producing a scar."

scarify /sker′əfī/ [L, *scarifare*], to make multiple superficial incisions into the skin; to scratch. Vaccination against smallpox is achieved by scarifying the skin under a drop of vaccine. See also **scarification.**

scarlatina. See **scarlet fever.**

scarlatiniform /skär′lətē′nifôrm/ [It, *scarlattina*; L, *forma*, form], resembling the rash of **scarlet fever.**

scarlet fever /skär′lit/ [OFr, *escarlate*; L, *febris*, fever], an acute contagious disease of childhood caused by an erythrotoxin-producing strain of group A hemolytic *Streptococcus.* The infection is characterized by sore throat, fever, enlarged lymph nodes in the neck, prostration, and a diffuse bright red rash. Also called **scarlatina.**

scarlet rash [OFr, *escarlate* + *rasche*, scurf], any scarlitini or rosy skin eruption that accompanies an infection, such as scarlet fever or German measles.

scarlet red, an azo dye that has been used to impart color to pharmaceutic preparations.

scato-, skato-, a combining form meaning 'of or related to dung or to fecal matter': *scatophagy, scatophilia, scatoscopy.*

scatologic /skatəloj′ik/, pertaining to **scatology.**

scatology /skatol′əjē/ [Gk, *skatos*, dung + *logos*, science], the science of feces. Also called **coprology.**

scattered radiation /skat′ərd/ [ME, *scateren*, to throw away; L *radiare* to shine], radiation that travels in a direction other than that of its source energy, such as secondary radiation and stray radiation. Also called **backscatter radiation.**

scattergram /skat′ərgram′/ [ME, *scateren* + Gk, *gramma*, record], a graph representing the distribution of two variables in a sample population. One variable is plotted on the vertical axis; the second on the horizontal axis. The scores or values of each sample unit are usually represented by dots. A scattergram demonstrates the degree or tendency to which the variables occur in association with each other.

scattering [ME, *scateren*], (in radiology) an effect produced by the interaction of low-energy x-rays with matter. The incident photon interacts with a target atom, causing it to become excited and release the excess energy as a secondary or scattered photon. The net result is a secondary photon with the same energy and wavelength as the incident photon, but a change in direction. Also called **Thompson scattering.** See also **Compton scatter.**

scavenger cell /skav′ənjər/ [ME, *scavager*; L, *cella*, storeroom], a phagocytic cell that removes tissue debris and some invading pathogens. It may or may not be mobile.

scavenging system. See **gas scavenging system.**

Sc.D., abbreviation for *Doctor of Science.*

SCE, abbreviation for saturated **calomel electrode.**

scel-, a combining form meaning 'leg': *scelalgia, scelotyrbe.*

-scelia, a combining form meaning '(condition of the) legs': *macroscelia, polyscelia, rhaeboscelia.*

Schedule I, a category of drugs not considered legitimate for medical use. Among the substances so classified by the Drug Enforcement Agency are mescaline, LSD, heroin, and marijuana. Special licensing procedures must be followed to use these or other Schedule I substances.

Schedule II, a category of drugs considered to have a strong potential for abuse or addiction, but which have legitimate medical use. Among the substances so classified by the Drug Enforcement Agency are morphine, cocaine, pentobarbital, oxycodone, alphaprodine, and methadone.

Schedule III, a category of drugs that have less potential for abuse or addiction than Schedule II or I drugs. Among the substances so classified by the Drug Enforcement Agency are glutethimide and various analgesic compounds containing codeine.

Schedule IV, a category of drugs that have less potential for abuse or addiction than those of Schedules I to III. Among the substances so classified by the Drug Enforcement Agency are chloral hydrate, chlordiazepoxide, meprobamate, and oxazepam.

Schedule V, a category of drugs that have a small potential for abuse or addiction. Among the substances so classified by the Drug Enforcement Agency are many commonly prescribed medications that contain small amounts of codeine or diphenoxylate. The specific drugs in Schedule V vary greatly from state to state.

Schedule of Drugs [L, *scheda,* sheet of paper; Fr, *drogue*], a classification system that categorizes drugs by their potential for abuse. The schedule is divided into five groups: Schedules I to V. The assignment of drugs to the categories varies from state to state. All substances in Schedules II to V require a written prescription signed by a physician. Schedule I substances are not approved for medical use. Specific regulations for dispensing these substances vary from state to state and from institution to institution. See also **controlled substance, Controlled Substance Act,** and specific schedules.

schema /skē′mə/, an innate knowledge structure that allows a child to organize in his or her mind ways to behave in his or her environment.

Scheuermann's disease /shoi′ərmonz/ [Holger W. Scheuermann, Danish surgeon, b. 1877], an abnormal skeletal condition characterized by a fixed kyphosis that develops at puberty and is caused by wedge-shaped deformities of one or several vertebrae. The cause of the disease is unknown, but authorities have speculated that it may result from infection, inflammatory processes, aseptic necrosis, disk deterioration, mechanical influences, inadequate circulation during rapid growth, or disturbances of epiphyseal growth resulting from protrusion of the intervertebral disk through deficient or defective cartilaginous plates. The most striking pathologic feature of Scheuermann's disease is the presence of wedge-shaped vertebral bodies, seen on radiographic examination, that create an excessive curvature. Scheuermann's disease occurs most frequently in children between 12 and 16 years of age, with the onset at puberty, and the incidence is greater in girls than in boys. The onset is insidious and often associated with a history of unusual physical activity or participation in sports. The most frequent symptom is poor posture with accompanying symptoms of fatigue and pain in the involved area. Tenderness and stiffness also may affect the area involved or may affect the entire spinal column. In most affected individuals the kyphosis is within the thoracic vertebrae. If the disease is diagnosed at the onset, the associated posture may be corrected actively and passively. Otherwise, the associated posture becomes fixed within a period of 6 to 9 months. The most effective treatment of Scheuermann's disease is immobilization with a plaster cast or with a Milwaukee brace. The immobilization is continuous for 10 to 12 months, with additional immobilization at night for about the same length of time. Immobilization is usually supplemented with an exercise program that is continued after the immobilization is terminated. In adults, persistent pain in the thoracic area may indicate a degenerative alteration secondary to this disease process, and spinal arthrodesis may be required to relieve the symptoms. Also called **adolescent vertebral epiphysitis, juvenile kyphosis.**

Schick test /shik/ [Bela Schick, Austrian-American physician, b. 1877], a skin test to determine immunity to diphtheria in which diphtheria toxin is injected intradermally. A positive reaction, indicating susceptibility, is marked by redness and swelling at the site of injection; a negative reaction, indicating immunity, is marked by absence of redness or swelling.

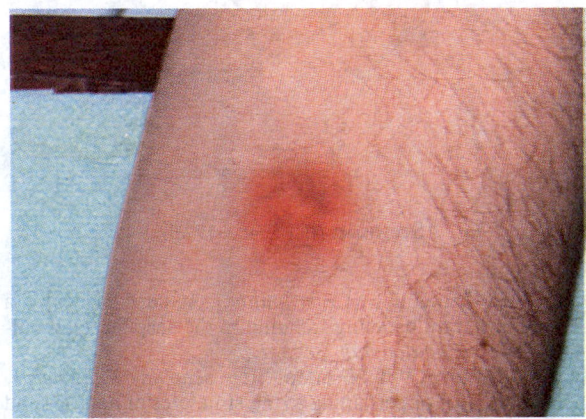

Positive Schick test (Hart, 1992)

Schick test control [Bela Schick, Austrian-American physician, b. 1877; L, *testum,* crucible; Fr, *contrôle,* check], a preparation used in carrying out the Schick test for diphtheria immunization.

Schilder's disease /shil′dərz/ [Paul F. Schilder, American neurologist, b. 1886], a group of progressive, severe, neurologic diseases beginning in childhood. All are characterized by demyelination of the white matter of the brain with muscle spasticity, optic neuritis, aphasia, deafness, adrenal insufficiency, and dementia. Many of the signs resemble those of multiple sclerosis. There is no known treatment. The cause may be viral or genetic. Also called **Schilder's encephalitis, encephalitis periaxialis diffusa, Flatau-Schilder disease, progressive subcortical encephalopathy.** See also **adrenoleukodystrophy.**

Schiller's test /shil′ərz/ [Walter Schiller, American pathologist, b. 1887], a procedure for indicating areas of abnormal epithelium in the vagina or on the cervix of the uterus as a guide in selecting biopsy sites for cancer detection. A potassium iodide or aqueous iodine solution is painted on the vaginal walls and cervix under direct visualization. Normal epithelium contains glycogen and stains a deep brown color; abnormal epithelium, containing no glycogen, will not stain, and nonstaining sites may then be included in tissue biopsies. The test is not specific for malignancy, because inflammation, ulceration, and keratotic lesions also may not accept the iodine stain.

Schilling's leukemia. See **monocytic leukemia.**

Schilling test /shil′ing/ [Robert Schilling, American physician, b. 1919], a diagnostic test for pernicious anemia in which vitamin B_{12} tagged with radioactive cobalt is administered orally, and GI absorption is measured by determining the radioactivity of urine samples collected over a 24-hour period. Normal findings show excretion of 8% to 40% of radioactive vitamin B_{12} within 24 hours. In people with pernicious anemia, the ability to absorb vitamin B_{12} is reduced, so that excretion of radioactive material in the urine is reduced.

schindylesis /skin′dilē′sis/ [Gk, splintering], an articulation of certain bones of the skull in which a thin plate of one bone enters a cleft formed by the separation of two layers of another bone, such as the insertion of the vomer bone into the fissure between the maxillae and the palatine bones.

Schiötz′ tonometer /shē·ets′/ [Hjalmar Schiötz, Norwegian ophthalmologist, b. 1850; Gk, *tonos*, stretching, *metron*, measure], a tonometer used to measure intraocular pressure by observing the depth of indentation of the cornea made by the weighted plunger on the device after a topical anesthetic is applied.

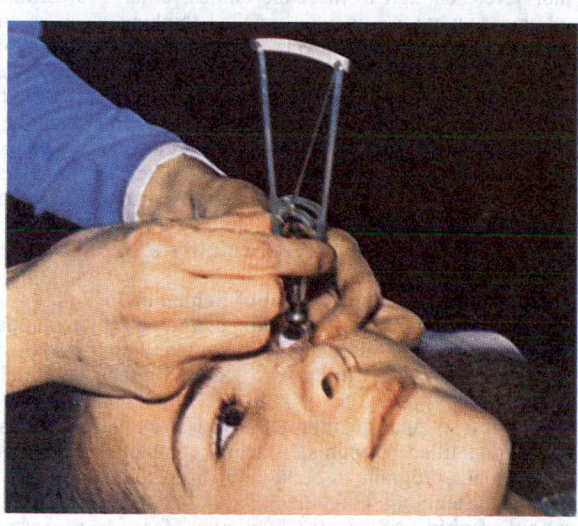

Schiötz′ tonometer *(Bedford, 1986)*

Schirmer's test. See **test for lacrimation.**

schisto-, a combining form meaning 'split, or cleft': *schistocelia, schistocephalus, schistomelia.*

schistocyte /shis′tōsīt/ [Gk, *schistos*, cleft, *kytos*, cell], an erythrocyte cell fragment characteristic of hemolysis or cell fragmentation associated with severe burns and intravascular coagulation.

Schistosoma /shis′təsō′mə/ [Gk, *schistos*, cleft, *soma*, body], a genus of blood flukes that may cause urinary, GI, or liver disease in humans and that requires freshwater snails as intermediate hosts. *Schistosoma hematobium*, found chiefly in Africa and the Middle East, affects the bladder and pelvic organs, causing painful, frequent urination and hematuria. *S. japonicum*, found in Japan, the Philippines, and Eastern Asia, causes GI ulcerations and fibrosis of the liver. *S. mansoni*, found in Africa, the Middle East, the Car-

ibbean, and tropical America, causes symptoms similar to those caused by *S. japonicum*. Also called **Bilharzia** /bilhär′zē·ə/. See also **schistosomiasis.**

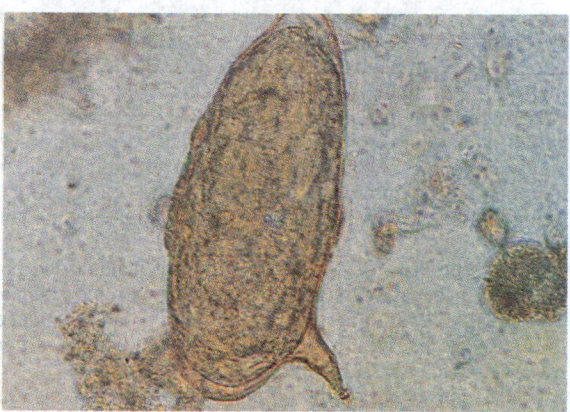

***Schistosoma mansoni* egg** *(Murray, 1990)*

schistosomiasis /shis′təsōmī′əsis/ [Gk, *schistos, soma* + *osis,* condition], a parasitic infection caused by a species of fluke of the genus *Schistosoma,* transmitted to humans, the definitive host, by contact with fresh water contaminated by human feces. A single fluke may live in one part of the body, depositing eggs frequently, for up to 20 years. The eggs are irritating to mucous membrane, causing it to thicken and become papillomatous. Symptoms depend on the part of the body infected. *Schistosoma* may be found in the bladder, rectum, liver, lungs, spleen, intestines, and portal venous system. Pain, obstruction, dysfunction of the affected organ, and anemia may result. Diagnosis requires morphologic identification of the ova or the parasite. Treatment is difficult; antimony drugs may be effective but are so toxic they seldom can be given. Inoculation with a small dose of *Klebsiella pneumoniae* has been effective experimentally in killing some species of *Schistosoma.* Prevention is more effective. Proper disposal of human waste, chlorination of water, and eradication of the intermediate host, the freshwater snail *Australorbis glabratus,* are totally effective. Second only to malaria in the number of people affected, schistosomiasis is particularly prevalent in the tropics and in the Orient. Also called **bilharziasis.** See also **blood fluke, Schistosoma.**

schistosomicide /shis′təsō′məsīd/ [Gk, *schistos, soma* + L *caedere,* to kill], a drug destructive to schistosomes, blood flukes transmitted by snails to human hosts in many parts of Africa, Brazil, and Asia. Niridazole, metrifonate, oxamniquine hycanthone hydrochloride, and various salts of antimony, including stibophen, are potent antischistosomal agents. **−schistosomicidal,** *adj.*

schizo- /skit′sə-, skiz′ə-/, a combining form meaning 'divided, or related to division': *schizocephalia, schizogenesis, schizophrenia.*

schizoaffective disorder /skit′sō·afek′tiv/ [Gk, *schizein,* to split; L, *affectus,* state of mind; *dis,* opposite of, *ordo,* rank], a condition that includes characteristics of schizophrenia and a mood disorder but fails to meet the DSM-III-R criteria for either diagnosis.

schizogenesis /skit′səjen′əsis/ [Gk, *schizein* + *genesis,* origin], reproduction by fission. **—schizogenetic, schizogenic, schizogenous,** *adj.*

schizogony /skitsog′ənē/ [Gk, *schizein* + *genein,* to produce], **1.** reproduction by multiple fission. **2.** the asexual reproductive stage of sporozoans, specifically the portion of the life cycle of the malarial parasite that occurs in the erythrocytes or liver cells. See also *Plasmodium,* **—schizogonic, schizogonous,** *adj.*

schizoid /skit′soid, skiz′oid/ [Gk, *schizein* + (*phren,* mind), *eidos,* form], **1.** characteristic of or resembling schizophrenia; schizophrenic. **2.** a person, not necessarily a schizophrenic, who exhibits the traits of a schizoid personality.

schizoid personality, a functioning but maladjusted person whose behavior is characterized by extreme shyness, oversensitivity, introversion, seclusiveness, and avoidance of close interpersonal relationships. See also **schizoid personality disorder, schizophrenia.**

schizoid personality disorder, a personality disorder (DSM-III-R) characterized by a defect in the ability to form social relationships, as shown by emotional coldness and aloofness, withdrawn and seclusive behavior, and indifference to praise, criticism, and the feelings of others. The person is unable to express hostility and ordinary aggressive feelings and reacts to disturbing experiences with apparent detachment.

schizont /skit′sont/ [Gk, *schizein* + *on,* being], the multinucleated cell stage during the sexual reproductive phase in the life cycle of a sporozoan, such as the malarial parasite *Plasmodium.* It is produced by the multiple fission of the trophozoite in a cell of the vertebrate host and subsequently segments into merozoites. Also called **agamont.** Compare **sporont.** See also **schizogony.**

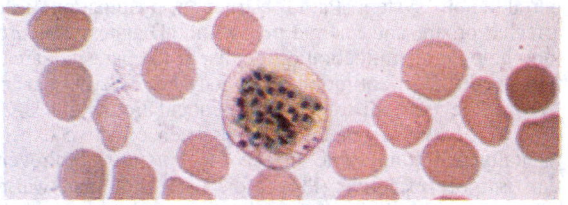

Schizont *(Hayhoe, 1992)*

schizonticide /skitson′təsīd/ [Gk, *schizein* + *on,* being; L, *caedere,* to kill], a substance that destroys schizonts. **—schizonticidal,** *adj.*

schizophasia /skit′səfā′zhə, skiz′ə-/ [Gk, *schizein* + *phasis,* speech], the disordered, incomprehensible speech characteristic of some forms of schizophrenia. See also **word salad.**

schizophrene /skit′səfrēn′, skiz′ə-/ [Gk, *schizein,* to split, *phren* mind], a person afflicted with schizophrenia.

schizophrenia /skit′səfrē′nē·ə, skiz′ə-/ [Gk, *schizein,* to split, *phren,* mind], any one of a large group of psychotic disorders characterized by gross distortion of reality, disturbances of language and communication, withdrawal from social interaction, and the disorganization and fragmentation of thought, perception, and emotional reaction. Apa-

thy and confusion; delusions and hallucinations; rambling or stylized patterns of speech, such as evasiveness, incoherence, and echolalia; withdrawn, regressive, and bizarre behavior; and emotional lability often occur. The condition may be mild or require prolonged hospitalization. No single cause of the disease is known; genetic, biochemical, psychologic, interpersonal, and sociocultural factors are usually involved.

schizophrenic /skit′səfren′ik, skiz′ə-/, **1.** of or pertaining to schizophrenia. **2.** a person with schizophrenia.

schizophreniform disorder /-fren′ifôrm/ [Gk, *schizein, phren* + L, *forma,* form], a condition exhibiting the same symptoms as schizophrenia but characterized by an acute onset with resolution in 2 weeks to 6 months.

schizophrenogenic /skit′səfren′əjen′ik, skiz′ə-/ [Gk, *schizein, phren* + *genein,* to produce], tending to cause or produce schizophrenia.

Schizotrypanum cruzi. See **Chagas' disease.**

schizotypal personality disorder /skit′sōtī′pəl/ [Gk, *schizein* + *typos,* mark; L, *personalis,* character; *dis,* opposite of, *ordo,* rank], a condition characterized by oddities of thought, perception, speech, and behavior that are not severe enough to meet the clinical criteria for schizophrenia. Symptoms include magical thinking, such as superstitiousness, belief in clairvoyance and telepathy, and bizarre fantasies; ideas of reference; recurrent illusions, such as sensing the presence of a force or person not actually present; social isolation; peculiar speech patterns, including ideas expressed unclearly or words used deviantly; and exaggerated anxiety or hypersensitivity to real or imagined criticism. See also **schizoid personality disorder, schizophrenia.**

Schlatter-Osgood disease, Schlatter's disease. See **Osgood-Schlatter disease.**

Schlemm's canal. See **canal of Schlemm.**

Schneiderian carcinoma /shnīdir′ē·ən/, an epithelial malignancy of the nasal mucosa and paranasal sinuses.

Schönlein-Henoch purpura. See **Henoch-Schönlein purpura.**

school nurse practitioner (S.N.P.), a registered nurse who is qualified through satisfactory completion of a nurse practitioner program to serve as a nurse practitioner in a school system.

school phobia [AS, *scol;* Gk, *phobos,* fear], an extreme separation anxiety disorder of children, usually in the elementary grades, characterized by a persistent, irrational fear of going to school or being in a school-like atmosphere. Such children are usually oversensitive, shy, timid, nervous, and emotionally immature and have pervasive feelings of inadequacy. They typically try to cope with their fears by becoming overdependent on others, especially the parents.

Schüffner's dots, coarse pink or red granules seen in the red blood cells of patients with tertiary malaria. They are signs of *Plasmodium vivax* or *P. ovale* and are absent in blood cells of patients infected with other types of malaria.

Schultz-Charlton phenomenon [Werner Schultz, German physician, b. 1878; Willy Charlton, German physician, b. 1889], a cutaneous reaction to the intradermal injection of scarlatina antiserum in a person who has a scarlatiniform rash. The rash blanches.

Schultze's mechanism, the delivery of a placenta with the fetal surfaces presenting.

Schwann cells /shwon/ [Friedrich T. Schwann, German

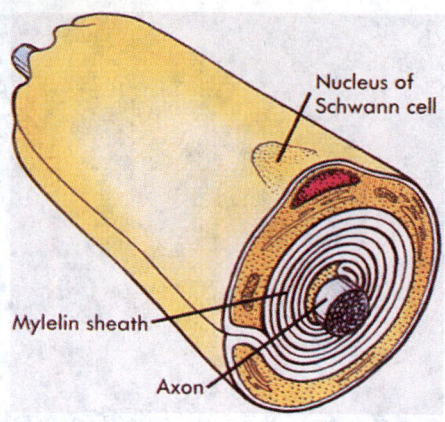

Schwann cell forming a myelin sheath
(Seeley, 1992/Scott Bodell)

anatomist, b. 1810],   cells of ectodermal origin that make up the neurilemma.

schwannoma /shwonō′mə/, *pl.* **schwannomas, schwannomata** [Friedrich Schwann; Gk, *oma*, tumor],   a benign, solitary, encapsulated tumor arising in the neurilemma (Schwann's sheath) of peripheral, cranial, or autonomic nerves. Also called **Schwann cell tumor, neurilemoma.**

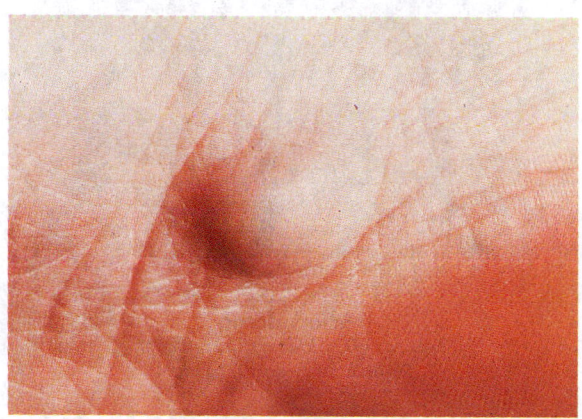

Schwannoma on the sole of the foot *(du Vivier, 1993)*

schwannosis /shwonō′sis/ [Friedrich Schwann, German anatomist, b. 1810; Gk, *osis*, condition],   a condition of overgrowth of the neurilemma or sheath of Schwann.

Schwann's sheath.   See **neurilemma.**

Schwann's white substance /shwons/ [Friedrich T. Schwann; AS, *hwit;* L, *substantia*],   an obsolete term for the myelin of a medullated nerve fiber.

Schwartz bed.   See **hyperextension bed.**

Schwartzman-Sanarelli phenomenon /shvorts′man san′ərel′ē/ [Gregory Schwartzman, American physician, b. 1896; Guiseppe Sanarelli, Italian physician, b. 1864],   a phenomenon induced experimentally in the investigation of the role of coagulation in renal disease. Animals injected twice with a bacterial endotoxin develop massive disseminated intravascular coagulation with thrombosis of the blood vessels in the kidneys. Also called **Schwartzman phenomenon.**

scia-.   See **skia-.**

sciatic /sī·at′ik/ [Gk, *ischiadikos*, hip joint],   near the ischium, such as the sciatic nerve or the sciatic vein.

sciatica /sī·at′ikə/,   an inflammation of the sciatic nerve, usually marked by pain and tenderness along the course of the nerve through the thigh and leg. It may result in a wasting of the muscles of the lower leg.

sciatic dislocation.   See **dislocation of hip.**

sciatic nerve,   a long nerve originating in the sacral plexus and extending through the muscles of the thigh, leg, and foot, with numerous branches.

SCID,   abbreviation for **severe combined immunodeficiency disease.**

science /sī′əns/ [L, *scientia*, knowledge],   a systematic attempt to establish theories to explain observed phenomena and the knowledge obtained through these efforts. **Pure science** is concerned with the gathering of information solely for the sake of obtaining new knowledge. **Applied science** is the practical application of scientific theory and laws. See also **hypothesis, law, scientific method, theory.**

Science of Unitary Human Beings   a conceptual model and theory of nursing proposed by Martha Rogers in 1970. Its four basic concepts focus on the nature and direction of 'unitary human development.' They include: (1) human and environmental energy fields, (2) complete and continuous openess of the energy fields, (3) human energy fields perceived as single waves that give identity to a field, and (4) 'pandimensionality,' a nonlinear domain without spatial or temporal attributes.

scientific method /sī′əntif′ik/,   a systematic, ordered approach to the gathering of data and the solving of problems. The basic approach is the statement of the problem followed by the statement of a hypothesis. An experimental method is established to help prove or disprove the hypothesis. The results of the experiment are observed, and conclusions are drawn from observed results. The conclusions may tend to uphold or to refute the hypothesis.

scientific rationale,   a reason, based on supporting scientific evidence, why a particular action is chosen.

scintigram /sin′tigram′/ [L, *scintillare*, to sparkle; Gk *gramma* record],   in nuclear medicine, a recording of the radioactivity emitted by a tracer in an organism or organ system.

scintigraph /sin′tigraf′/,   a photographic recording produced by an imaging device showing the distribution and intensity of radioactivity in various tissues and organs after the administration of a radiopharmaceutical.

scintillating scotoma /sin′tilā·ting/ [L, *scintillatio*, sparkling; Gk *skotos* dark + *oma* tumor],   an abnormal area of the visual field that is positive and luminous, sometimes becoming hemianopic and appearing in a migraine aura.

scintillation detector /sin′tilā′shən/ [L, *scintillatio*, sparkling],   **1.** a device that relies on the emission of light or ultraviolet radiation from a crystal subjected to ionizing radiation. The light is detected by a photomultiplier tube and converted to an electric signal that can be processed further. An array of scintillation detectors is used in a gamma camera. **2.** a device used to measure the amount of radioactivity in an area of the body.

scintiscan /sin′tiscan′/, a photographic display of the distribution of a radiopharmaceutical within the body.

scirrho-, a combining form meaning 'hard, or related to a hard cancer or scirrhus': *scirrhoid, scirrhoma, scirrhosarca.*

scirrhous carcinoma /skir′əs/ [Gk, *skirrhos*, hard; *karkinos*, crab, *oma*, tumor], a hard, fibrous, particularly invasive tumor in which the malignant cells occur singly or in small clusters or strands in dense connective tissue. Also called **carcinoma fibrosum.** See also **breast cancer.**

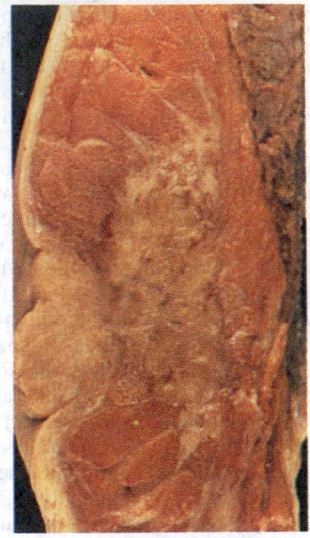

Scirrhous carcinoma of the breast (Fletcher, 1987)

scissor gait /siz′ər/ [L, *scindere*, to cut; ONorse, *gata*, way], a manner of walking cross-legged, as observed in spastic paraplegia.

scissor legs [L, *scindere*, to cut; ONorse, *leggr*, legs that are crossed because of a disorder of the adductor muscles of the thigh or a deformity of the hip.

scissors [L, *scindere*, to cut], a sharp instrument composed of two opposing cutting blades, held together by a central pin on which the blades pivot. The most common dissecting scissors are the straight **Mayo,** for cutting sutures; the **Snowden-Pencer,** for deep, delicate tissue; the long, curved **Mayo,** for deep, heavy, or tough tissue; the short, curved **Metzenbaum,** for superficial, delicate tissue; and the long, blunt, curved **Metzenbaum,** for deep, delicate tissue.

SCL, abbreviation for *soft contact lens.*

scler-. See **sclero-.**

sclera /sklir′ə/ [Gk, *skleros*, hard], the tough, inelastic, opaque membrane covering the posterior five sixths of the eyebulb. It maintains the size and form of the bulb and attaches to muscles that move the bulb. Posteriorly, it is pierced by the optic nerve and, with the transparent cornea, makes up the outermost of three tunics covering the eyebulb.

scleredema /sklir′ədē′mə/ [Gk, *skleros* + *oidema*, swelling], an idiopathic skin disease characterized by nonpitting induration beginning on the face or neck and spreading downward over the body, sparing the hands and feet. There also may be swelling of the tongue, restriction of the move-

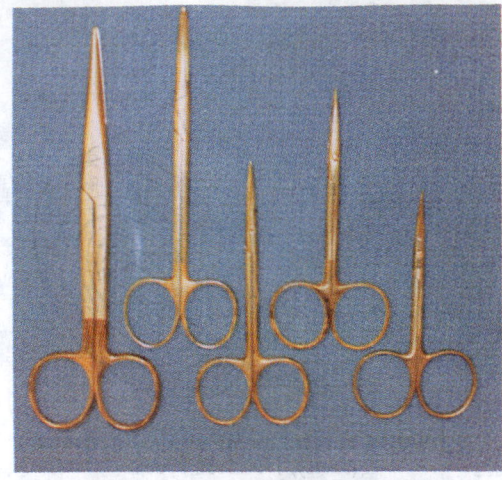

Scissors: Mayo, curved Metzenbaum, baby Metzenbaum, sharp- sharp, and iris
(Grossman, 1993)

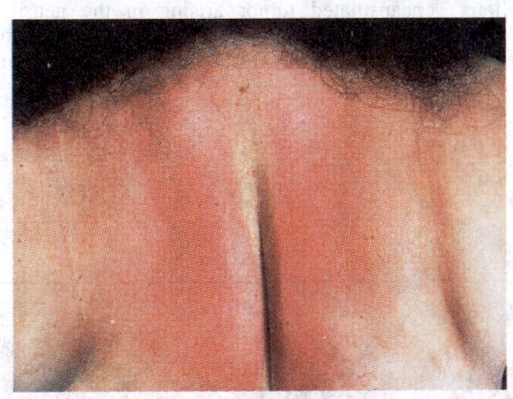

Scleredema
(McKee, 1993/Courtesy Dr. C Stephens,
St. Thomas' Hospital, London)

ments of the eyes, and pericardial, pleural, and peritoneal effusions. Resolution occurs after several months, but recurrences are common. The condition often follows a streptococcal infection or an exanthem of childhood. There is no specific treatment. Compare **scleroderma.**

sclerema neonatorum /sklirē′mə/ [Gk, *skleros* + *neos*, new; L, *natus*, birth], a progressive generalized hardening of the skin and subcutaneous tissue of the newborn. It is usually a fatal condition that occurs as a result of severe cold stress in severely ill premature infants subject to such life-threatening conditions as metabolic acidosis, hypoglycemia, GI or respiratory infection, or gross malformation. Also called **scleredema neonatorum, sclerema adiposum.**

scleritis /sklirī′tis/ [Gk, *skleros*, hard + *itis*, inflammation], an inflammation of the sclera.

sclero-, scler- /sklir′ō-, skler′ō-/, a combining form meaning 'hard,' often used to show relationship to the sclera: *scleroadipose, sclerocorneal, sclerodesmia.*

sclerodactyly /sklir'ōdak'tilē/ [Gk, *skleros* + *daktylos,* finger], a musculoskeletal deformity affecting the hands of people with scleroderma. The fingers are fixed in a semi-flexed position, with tightened skin to the wrist. The fingertips may be ulcerated.

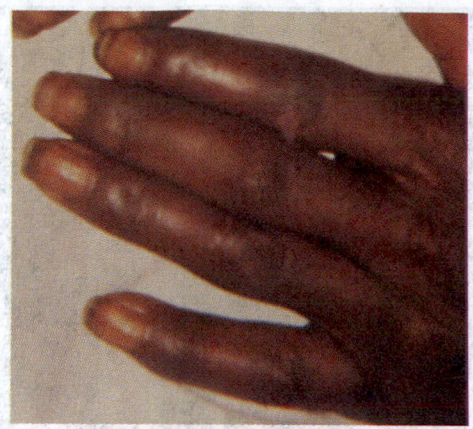

Sclerodactyly *(Zitelli, 1992)*

scleroderma /sklir'ōdur'mə/ [Gk, *skleros* + *derma,* skin], a relatively rare autoimmune disease affecting the blood vessels and connective tissue. The disease is characterized by fibrous degeneration of the connective tissue of the skin, lungs, and internal organs, especially the esophagus, digestive tract, and kidneys. Scleroderma is most common in middle-aged women. Also called **progressive systemic sclerosis (PSS).**
■ OBSERVATIONS: The most common initial complaints are changes in the skin of the face and fingers. Raynaud's phenomenon occurs with a gradual hardening of the skin and swelling of the distal extremities. In the early stages, the disease may be confused with rheumatoid arthritis or Raynaud's disease. As the disease progresses, there is deformity of the joints and pain on movement. Skin changes include edema, then pallor; then the skin becomes firm; finally, it becomes slightly pigmented and fixed to the underlying tissues. At this stage the skin of the face is taut, shiny, and masklike, and the patient may have difficulty in chewing and swallowing. Scleroderma may occur in a mild form with the person living 30 to 50 years, or there may be early death because of cardiac, renal, pulmonary, or intestinal involvement. Localized forms of scleroderma may occur; these cases are benign and occur only as small circumscribed patches on the skin. A biopsy of the lesion may be done to diagnose the condition. X-ray examination of the lungs and GI tract may be diagnostic in the systemic form of the disease. Blood tests may reveal antinuclear antibodies.
■ INTERVENTIONS: There is no specific drug prescribed to cure scleroderma; however, corticosteroids may be useful in treating the symptoms of the disease, and salicylates and mild analgesics are given to ease pain in the joints. Physical therapy slows the development of muscle contracture and resultant deformity and debility.
■ NURSING CONSIDERATIONS: Severe renal disease is a major

cause of death, although death may result from the involvement of other organs. The usual indication that renal disease is present is the abrupt onset of severe arterial hypertension that does not respond to medication. Nephrectomy or renal transplant may be performed. In the advanced stages of scleroderma, patients often require help to eat, and mouth and skin care is particularly important. As the patient becomes more helpless, there is a need for considerable emotional support.

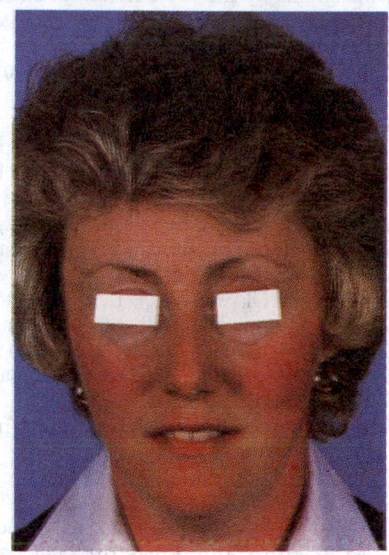

Scleroderma *(Lamey, 1988)*

scleroderma neonatorum, See **sclerema neonatorum.**
-scleroma, a combining form meaning an 'induration, a hardening of the tissues': *laryngoscleroma, pharyngoscleroma, rhinoscleroma.*
scleromalacia perforans /sklir'ōmələ'shə/ [Gk, *skleros* + *malakia,* softening; L *perforare* to pierce], a condition of the eyes in which devitalization and sloughing of the sclera occur as a complication of rheumatoid arthritis. The pig-

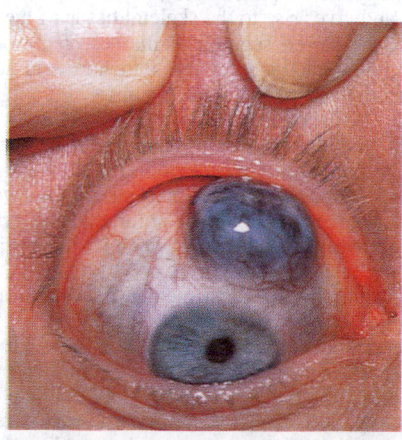

Scleromalacia perforans *(Schumacher, 1988)*

mented uvea becomes exposed, and glaucoma, cataract formation, and detachment of the retina may result.

sclerose /sklərōz'/ [Gk, *skleros*], to harden or to cause hardening. **−sclerotic**, *adj.*

sclerosing /sklirō'zing/ [Gk, *skleros*, hard], pertaining to the tissue changes or other factors involved in the progress of sclerosis.

sclerosing hemangioma [Gk, *skleros* + *haima*, blood, *aggeion* vessel, *oma* tumor], a solid, cellular tumorlike nodule of the skin or a mass of histiocytes, thought to arise from a hemangioma by the proliferation of endothelial and connective tissue cells.

sclerosing keratitis [Gk, *skleros*, hard + *keras*, horn + *itis*, inflammation], **1.** a form of corneal inflammation in which nodular infiltrates appear near the margin of the cornea in association with a ring of anterior scleritis. **2.** a form of corneal inflammation characterized by an opaque triangle in the deep layers of the cornea, with the base of the triangle near the sclerosing area.

sclerosing phlebitis [Gk, *skleros*, hard + *phleps*, vein + *itis*, inflammation], an inflammation of a vein that has become hardened and obstructed.

sclerosing solution [Gk, *skleros* + L, *solvere*, to dissolve], a liquid containing an irritant that causes inflammation and resulting fibrosis of tissues. It may be used in cauterizing ulcers, arresting hemorrhage, and treating hemangiomas.

sclerosis /sklirō'sis/ [Gk, *sklirosis*, hardening], a condition characterized by hardening of tissue resulting from any of several causes, including inflammation, the deposit of mineral salts, and infiltration of connective tissue fibers. **−sclerotic**, *adj.*

-sclerosis, a suffix meaning 'an abnormal hardening of the tissue': *atherosclerosis, arteriosclerosis, phleboscerosis.*

sclerotherapy /-ther'əpē/ [Gk, *skleros*, hard + *therapeia*, treatment], the use of sclerosing chemicals to treat varicosities such as hemorrhoids or esophageal varices. The agent produces inflammation and later fibrosis and obliteration of the lumen.

sclerotic /sklirot'ik/ [Gk, *skleros*, hard], pertaining to induration or hardening.

sclerotomal pain distribution /-tō'məl/, the referral of pain from pain-sensitive tissues covering the axial skeleton along a sclerotomal segment.

sclerotome /sklir'ətōm/ [Gk, *skleros* + *temnein*, to cut], (in embryology) the part of the segmented mesoderm layer in the early developing embryo that originates from the somites and gives rise to the skeletal tissue of the body, specifically, the paired segmented masses of mesodermal tissue that lie on each side of the notochord and develop into the vertebrae and ribs. See also **somite.**

scoleces. See **scolex.**

scoleco-, a combining form meaning 'of or pertaining to a worm': *scolecoid, scolecoidectomy, scolecology.*

scolex /skō'leks/, *pl.* **scoleces** /skō'ləsēz/ [Gk, worm], the headlike segment or organ of an adult tapeworm that has hooks, grooves, or suckers by which it attaches itself to the wall of the intestine.

scolio-, a combining form meaning 'twisted or crooked': *scoliodontic, scoliokyphosis, scoliosiometry.*

scoliometer /skō'lē·om'ətər/ [Gk, *skoliosis*, curvature], a device for measuring the amount of abnormal curvature in the spine.

scoliosis /skō'lē·ō'sis/ [Gk, *skoliosis*, curvature], lateral curvature of the spine, a common abnormality of childhood. Causes include congenital malformations of the spine, po-

liomyelitis, skeletal dysplasias, spastic paralysis, and unequal leg length. Unequal heights of hips or shoulders may be a sign of this condition. Early recognition and orthopedic treatment may prevent progression of the curvature. Treatment includes braces, casts, exercises, and corrective surgery. See also **congenital scoliosis, kyphoscoliosis, kyphosis, lordosis, spinal curvature.**

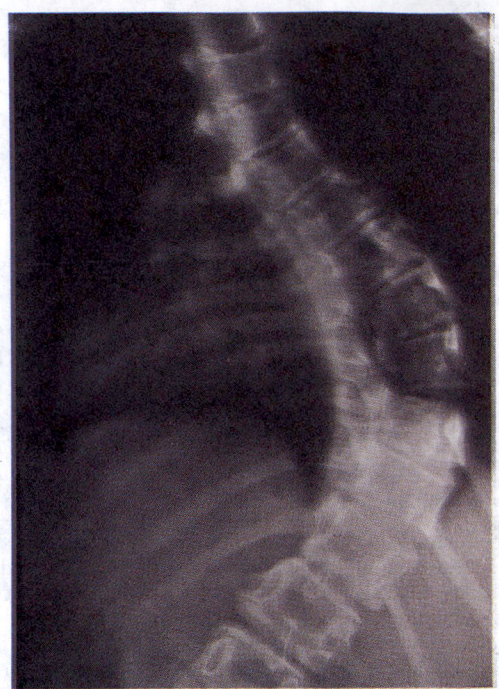

Radiograph of the spine in scoliosis *(Zitelli, 1992)*

scoliotic pelvis /skō'lē·ot'ik/ [Gk, *skoliosis*, curvature; L, *pelvis*, basin], an abnormal pelvic area caused by the effects of scoliosis bending the sacrum to one side.

scombroid /skom'broid/ [Gk, *scombros*, mackerel + *eidos*, form], pertaining to fish of the spiny-finned percoid *Scombridae* and *Scomberescidae* families, which include skipjack, mackerel, bonito, and tuna.

scombroid poisoning, toxic effects of eating scombroid types of fish that have begun bacterial decomposition after being caught. Scombroid fish contain large amounts of free hitidine in the muscle tissue, which gives rise to toxic levels of histamine under conditions of histidine decarboxylation by any of a dozen species of bacteria. Scombroid poisoning is not limited to consumption of fresh fish; the problem also may affect commercially canned tuna. Symptoms, which usually last no more than 24 hours, include nausea, vomiting, diarrhea, epigastric pain, and urticaria. Treatment is symptomatic.

scop-, a combining form meaning 'to examine, observe': *scopograph, scopometer, scopophilia.*

-scope, a suffix meaning an 'instrument for observation or a visual examination': *ciliariscope, episcope, pelviscope.*

scopolamine /skōpol'əmēn/ [Giovanni A. Scopoli, Italian naturalist, b. 1723], an anticholinergic alkaloid obtained from the leaves and seeds of several solanaceous plants. It is a central nervous system depressant and is used to prevent motion sickness and as an antiemetic, a sedative in obstetrics, and a cycloplegic and mydriatic. Also called **hyoscine.**

scopolamine hydrobromide,   an anticholinergic.

■ INDICATIONS: It is prescribed in the treatment of nausea and vomiting, as a sedative and preanesthetic medication, and as a cycloplegic and mydriatic medication in ophthalmic procedures.

■ CONTRAINDICATIONS: Narrow-angle glaucoma, asthma, obstruction of the genitourinary or GI tracts, severe ulcerative colitis, or known hypersensitivity to this drug prohibits its use.

■ ADVERSE EFFECTS: Among the more serious adverse reactions are blurred vision, central nervous system effects, tachycardia, dry mouth, decreased sweating, and hypersensitivity reaction.

scopophilia /skō′pəfil′ē·ə, skop′-/ [Gk, *skopein,* to look, *philein,* to love],   **1.** sexual pleasure derived from looking at sexually stimulating scenes or at another person's genitals; voyeurism. **2.** a morbid desire to be seen; exhibitionism. Also called **scotophilia. –scopophiliac, scopophilic, scoptophiliac, scoptophilic.** *adj., n.*

scopophobia /skō′pə-/ [Gk, *skopein + phobos,* fear],   an anxiety disorder characterized by a morbid fear of being seen or stared at by others. The condition is commonly seen in schizophrenia. See also **phobia.**

scoptophilic.   See **scopophilia.**

-scopy,   a suffix meaning 'observation or a visual examination': *bioscopy, stomachoscopy, thoracoscopy.*

-scorbic,   a suffix meaning 'of or referring to the prevention or treatment of scurvy': *antiscorbic, ascorbic, glucoascorbic.*

-scorbutic, -scorbic, -scorbutical,   a suffix meaning 'pertaining to scurvy': *antiscorbutic, postscorbutic, scorbutic.*

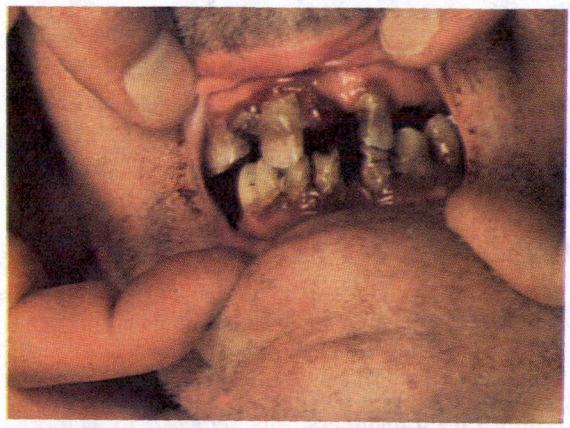

Scorbutic gingivitis *(McLaren, 1992/Courtesy Dr RW Vilter)*

scorbutic gingivitis /skôrbyōō′tik/ [Fr, *scorbutique,* scurvy; L, *gingiva,* gum; Gk, *itis,* inflammation],   an abnormal condition, characterized by inflamed or bleeding gums and caused by vitamin C deficiency.

scorbutic pose,   the characteristic posture of a child with scurvy, with thighs and legs semiflexed and hips rotated outward. The child usually lies motionless without voluntary movements of the extremities because of the pain that accompanies any motion. See also **scurvy.**

scorbutus.   See **scurvy.**

scorpion sting /skôr′pē·on/ [Gk, *skorpios;* AS, *stingan*],   a painful wound produced by a scorpion, an arachnid with a hollow stinger in its tail. The stings of many species are only slightly toxic, but some, including *Centruroides sculpturatus* of the southwestern United States, may inflict fatal injury, especially in small children. Initial pain is followed within several hours by numbness, nausea, muscle spasm, dyspnea, and convulsion. Treatment includes ice applied to the wound and intravenous calcium gluconate to control muscle spasm, if necessary. Severe cases may require oxygen and respiratory assistance. Narcotic analgesia is contraindicated. An antivenin is available in some areas.

scoto-,   a combining form meaning 'of or related to darkness': *scotodinia, scotogram, scotographic.*

scotoma /skōtō′mə/, *pl.* **scotomas, scotomata** [Gk, *skotos,* darkness, *oma,* tumor],   a defect of vision in a defined area in one or both eyes. A common prodromal symptom is a shimmering film appearing as an island in the visual field.

scotophilia.   See **scopophilia.**

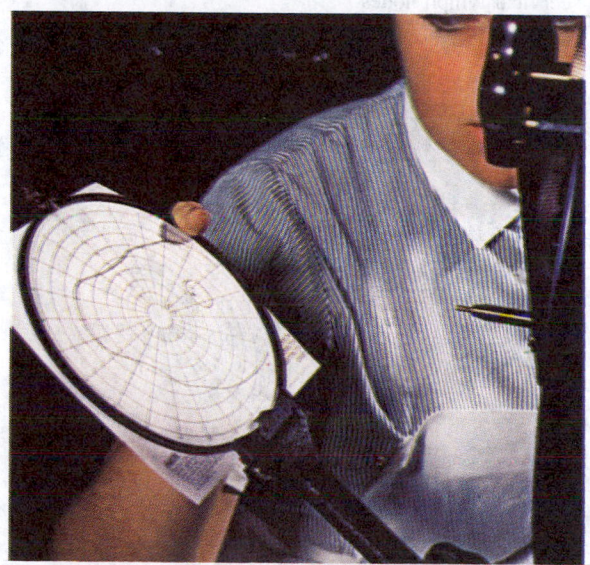

Chart used for scotoma test *(Bedford, 1986)*

scotopic vision /skōtop′ik/ [Gk, *skotos,* dark; L, *visio,* seeing],   the ability of the eye to adjust for vision in darkness or dim light. Also called **night vision.**

scratch test [ME, *scratten;* L, *testum,* crucible],   a skin test for identifying an allergen, performed by placing a small quantity of a solution containing a suspected allergen on a lightly scratched area of the skin. If a wheal forms within 15 minutes, allergy to the substance is indicated.

screamer's nodule.   See **vocal cord nodule.**

screening [ME, *scren*],   **1.** a preliminary procedure, such as a test or examination, to detect the most characteristic sign or signs of a disorder that may require further investigation. **2.** the examination of a large sample of a population to detect a specific disease or disorder, such as hypertension.

screen memory [ME, *scren;* L, *memoria*], a consciously tolerable memory that replaces one that is emotionally painful to recall.

screw clamp [OFr, *escroe,* screw; AS, *clam,* fastener], a device, usually made of plastic, equipped with a screw that can be manipulated to close and open the primary IV tubing for regulating the flow of intravenous solution. Turning the screw clockwise closes the tubing; turning it counterclockwise opens the tubing. Different positions of the screw between the open and the closed positions allow the intravenous fluid to flow at different rates. Compare **roller clamp, slide clamp.**

scrib-, script-, a combining form meaning 'write': *scribble, scribomania, prescription.*

Scribner shunt [Belding S. Scribner, American physician, b. 1921], a type of arteriovenous bypass, used in hemodialysis, consisting of a special tube connection outside the body.

scripting /skrip'ting/, a technique of family therapy involving the development of new family transactional patterns.

scrofula /skrof'yələ/ [L, *scrofa,* brood sow], *archaic.* primary tuberculosis with abscess formation, usually of the cervical lymph nodes.

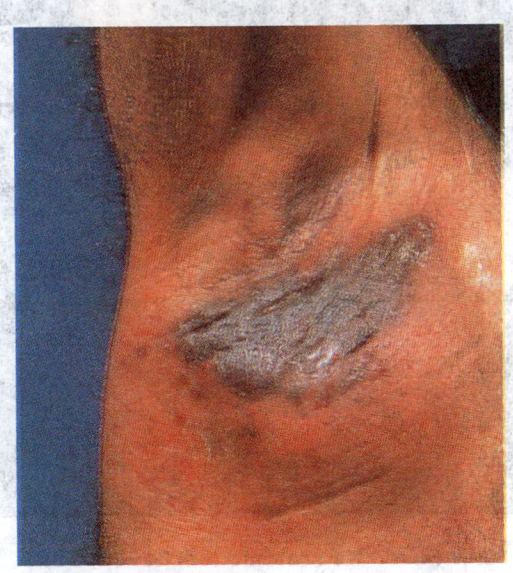

Scrofula (McKee, 1993)

scrotal /skrō'təl/ [related to L, *scrupus,* (sharp) stone], pertaining to the scrotum.

scrotal cancer [related to L, *scrupus,* (sharp) stone], an epidermoid malignancy of the scrotum, characterized initially by a small sore that may ulcerate. The lesion occurs most frequently in elderly men who have been exposed to soot, pitch, crude oil, mineral oils, polycyclic hydrocarbons, or arsenic fumes from copper smelting. Treatment involves wide surgical excision of the tumor and resection of inguinal nodes. In the eighteenth century, Sir Percival Pott associated scrotal cancer in chimney sweeps with exposure to soot. It is the first malignancy shown to be caused by an environmental carcinogen. Also called **chimney-sweeps' cancer, soot wart.**

scrotal raphe, a line of union of the two halves of the scrotum. It is generally more highly pigmented than the surrounding tissue.

scrotal tongue, a nonpathologic condition in which the tongue is deeply furrowed and resembles the surface of the scrotum.

scrotum /skrō'təm/ the pouch of skin containing the testes and parts of the spermatic cords. It is divided on the surface into two lateral portions by a ridge that continues ventrally to the undersurface of the penis and dorsally along the middle line of the perineum to the anus. In young, robust individuals the scrotum is short and corrugated, and closely wraps the testes. In older people and debilitated individuals, and in warm environments, the scrotum becomes elongated and flaccid. The lateral left portion of the scrotum usually hangs lower than the right, corresponding with the longer length of the left spermatic cord. The two layers of the scrotum are the skin and the dartos tunic. The skin is very thin, has a brownish color, and is usually wrinkled. It is supplied with sebaceous follicles that secrete a substance with a characteristic odor and has thinly scattered, kinky hairs with roots that are visible through the skin. The dartos tunic is composed of a thin layer of unstriated muscular fibers around the base of the scrotum, continuous with the two layers of the superficial fascia of the groin and the perineum. The tunic projects an internal septum that divides the pouch into two cavities for the testes, extending between the scrotal ridge and the root of the penis. The tunic is closely united to the skin but separated from subjacent parts by a distinct fascial cleft on which it glides. The scrotum is highly vascular and contains no fat. See also **testis.** —**scrotal,** *adj.*

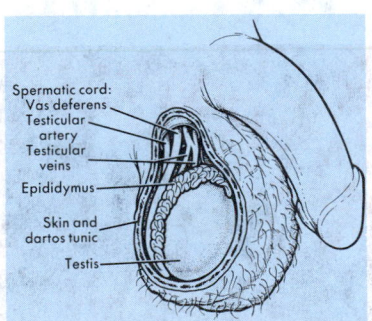

Spermatic cord:
Vas deferens
Testicular artery
Testicular veins
Epididymus
Skin and dartos tunic
Testis

Scrotum

scrub. See **surgical scrub.**

scrubbed team members [ME, *scrobben,* to scrub], the surgeons, physicians, nurses, and technicians who are scrubbed for surgical procedures in a sterile environment.

scrub itch. See **Leeuwenhoekia australiensis.**

scrub nurse, a registered nurse or operating room technician who assists surgeons during operations.

scrub room, a special hospital area where surgeons and surgical teams use disposable sterile brushes and bactericidal soaps to wash and scrub their fingernails, hands, and forearms before performing or assisting in surgical operations. Scrub rooms and meticulous washing techniques improve the sterile environment of the operating room and reduce the risk of bacterial infection.

scrub typhus, an acute, febrile disease of Asia, India, northern Australia, and the western Pacific islands, caused by several strains of the genus *Rickettsia tsutsugamushi* and transmitted from infected rodents to humans by mites. The clinical course ranges from mild to severe and is characterized by a necrotic papule or black eschar at the site of the lesion caused by the bite of the small arachnid. Tender, enlarged regional lymph nodes, fever, severe headache, eye pain, muscle aches, and a generalized rash usually occur. In severe cases, the myocardium and the central nervous system may be involved. The Weil-Felix reaction and indirect fluorescent antibody tests are useful in diagnosis. Treatment with broad spectrum antibiotics, such as chloramphenicol, doxycycline, or tetracycline, has reduced mortality to nearly zero. Person-to-person transmission is not known to occur. No effective vaccine is available, and second attacks are common because of antigenic differences in various strains of rickettsiae. Prevention includes avoiding mite-infested terrain, reducing the rodent population, destroying scrub vegetation, and using insect repellents. Also called **Japanese flood fever, Japanese river fever, mite typhus, tsutsugamushi disease.** Compare **Q fever, Rocky Mountain spotted fever, typhus.**

scruple /skrōō′pəl/ [L, *scrupulus,* small stone], a measure of weight in the apothecaries' system, equal to 20 grains or 1.296 g. See also **apothecaries' weight, metric system.**

sculpting /skulp′ting/, a technique of family therapy involving construction of a live family portrait that depicts family alliances and conflicts.

scultetus bandage /skəltē′təs/ [Johann Schultes, German surgeon, b. 1595], a many-tailed bandage with an attached central piece. The tails are overlapped; the last two, tied or pinned, act to secure the others. A scultetus bandage may be opened or removed without moving the bandaged part of the body.

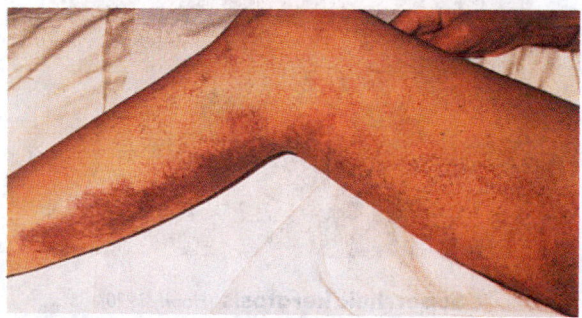

Scurvy—mucocutaneous hemorrhages in the legs
(Kamal, 1991/Courtesy Dr RH MacDonald)

scurvy /skur′vē/ [Scan, *scurfa,* scabby], a condition resulting from lack of ascorbic acid in the diet. It is characterized by weakness, anemia, edema, spongy gums, often with ulceration and loosening of the teeth, a tendency to mucocutaneous hemorrhages, and induration of the muscles of the legs. Treatment and prophylaxis of the disease consist of administration of ascorbic acid and the inclusion of fresh vegetables and fruits in the diet. Also called **scorbutus.** See

also **ascorbic acid, citric acid, infantile scurvy, scorbutic pose.**

scut work [L, *scutella,* kitchen maid; AS, *werc*], a derogatory, colloquial term for menial tasks, usually of a nontherapeutic nature, that are a necessary part of the work routine performed by the staff of a health care facility.

scypho-, a combining form meaning 'a cup-shaped part': *scyphozoan, scyphus, scyphistoma.*

SD, abbreviation for **standard deviation.**

SDMS, abbreviation for *Society of Diagnostic Medical Sonographers.*

Se, symbol for the element **selenium.**

S.E., abbreviation for **standard error.**

sealed source [ME, *seel,* mark; Fr, *sourdre,* to spring], (in radiotherapy) a source of radiant energy in which the radioactive material is permanently encased in a container or bonding material in a manner to prevent leakage. Sealed sources, such as seeds, needles, and specially designed applicators, are used in the implantation of cesium 137, iodine 125, iridium 192, radium 226, and other radionuclides for the treatment of various malignant tumors.

sealer cement, a compound used in filling a root canal. It is applied as a plastic that solidifies after insertion and fills depressions in the surface of the canal.

seal limbs. See **phocomelia.**

seasickness. See **motion sickness.**

seasonal affective disorder (SAD) /sē′zənəl/, a mood disorder associated with the shorter days and longer nights of autumn and winter. Symptoms include lethargy, depression, social withdrawal, and work difficulties. The patients also consume excess amounts of carbohydrates, gaining weight. The symptoms recede in the spring when days become longer. The condition is associated with the effect of light on melatonin secretion and is treated with exposure to bright light for 5 to 6 hours per day.

Seattle Foot /sē·at′əl/, a trademark for a stored-energy foot prosthesis that contains a rodlike piece of plastic, a keel, that extends from the toe to the heel where it turns upward toward the ankle. See also **keel, stored-energy foot.**

seatworm. See *Enterobius vermicularis.*

sea urchin sting /ur′chin/ [AS, *sae, herichon,* hedgehog], an injury inflicted by any of a variety of sea urchins, in which the skin is punctured and, in some species, venom released. A venomous sting is characterized by pain, muscular weakness, numbness around the mouth, and dyspnea. Immediate removal of the spines is necessary and may require the use of a local anesthetic. An antiseptic and a dressing are applied until the wound is healed. In all cases the broken spines cause local pain and irritation. Infection may result. See also **stingray.**

seawater bath [AS, *sae, waeter*], a bath taken in warm seawater or in saline solution.

sebaceous /sibā′shəs/ [L, *sebum,* sweat], fatty, oily, or greasy, usually referring to the oil-secreting glands of the skin or to their secretions.

sebaceous cyst, a misnomer for epidermoid cyst or pilar cyst.

sebaceous follicle [L, *sebum,* sweat + *folliculus,* small bag], a sebaceous gland that opens into a hair follicle.

sebaceous gland, one of the many small sacculated organs in the dermis. They are located throughout the body in close association with all types of body hair but are especially abundant in the scalp, the face, the anus, the nose, the mouth, and the external ear. They are rare in the palms of the hands and the soles of the feet. Each gland consists of a single duct that emerges from a cluster of oval alveoli. Each alveolus is composed of a transparent basement membrane enclosing epithelial cells. The outer cells are small and polyhedral and continuous with the cells lining the duct. The remainder of the alveolus is composed of larger cells containing lipid, except in the center, where disintegrated cells leave a cavity filled with their debris and a mass of sebum cutaneum. The ducts from most sebaceous glands open into the hair follicles, but some open onto the surface of the skin, as in the labia minora and the free margin of the lips. The sebum secreted by the glands oils the hair and the surrounding skin, helps prevent evaporation of sweat, and aids in the retention of body heat. The sebaceous glands in the nose and face are large and lobulated, and often swell with accumulated secretion. Compare **sudoriferous gland.**

seborrhea /seb′ərē′ə/ [L, *sebum* + Gk, *rhoia*, flow], any of several common skin conditions in which there is an overproduction of sebum resulting in excessive oiliness or dry scales. See also **seborrheic blepharitis, seborrheic dermatitis.** —**seborrheic** /seb′ərē′ik/, *adj.*

seborrhea capitis [L, *sebum*, sweat; Gk, *rhoia*, flow; L, *caput*, the head], seborrhea of the scalp.

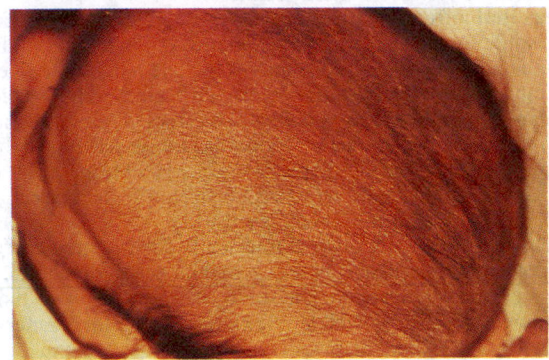

Seborrhea capitis (cradle cap) (Zitelli, 1992/Courtesy Dr. Michael Sherlock)

seborrhea congestiva [L, *sebum*, sweat; Gk, *rhoia*, flow; L, *congerere* to heap together], an obsolete term for lupus erythematodes.

seborrheic /seb′ərē′ik/ [L, *sebum*, sweat], pertaining to or resembling seborrhea.

seborrheic blepharitis, a form of seborrheic dermatitis in which the eyelids are erythematous and the margins are covered with a granular crust.

seborrheic dermatitis, a common, chronic, inflammatory skin disease characterized by dry or moist, greasy scales and yellowish crusts. Common sites are the scalp, eyelids, face, external surfaces of the ears, axillae, breasts, groin, and gluteal folds. In acute stages there may be exudate and infection resulting in secondary furunculosis. Occasionally generalized exfoliation results. In some people seborrheic dermatitis is associated with paralysis agitans, diabetes mellitus, malabsorption disorders, epilepsy, or an allergic reaction to gold or arsenic. Treatment includes selenium sulfide shampoos, topical and oral corticosteroids, topical antibiotics, proper therapy for any underlying systemic

disorder, and avoidance of sweating and external irritants. Kinds of seborrheic dermatitis include **cradle cap, dandruff,** and **seborrheic blepharitis.**

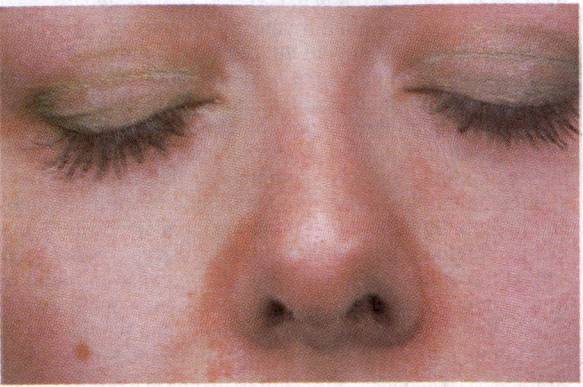

Seborrheic dermatitis (McKee, 1993/Courtesy Dr. MM Black, St. Thomas' Hospital, London)

seborrheic keratosis, a benign, well-circumscribed, slightly raised, tan to black, warty lesion of the skin of the face, neck, chest, or upper back. The macules are loosely covered with a greasy crust that leaves a raw pulpy base when removed. Itching is common. Treatment includes curettage, electrodesiccation, or cryotherapy using local anesthesia. Also called **seborrheic wart.**

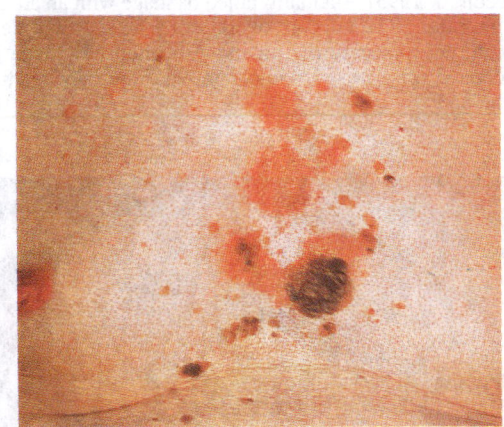

Seborrheic keratosis (Habif, 1990)

seb-, a combining form meaning 'sebum': *sebiferous, sebaceous, sebiparous.*

sebum /sē′bəm/ [L, grease], the oily secretion of the sebaceous glands of the skin, composed of keratin, fat, and cellular debris. Combined with sweat, sebum forms a moist, oily, acidic film that is mildly antibacterial and antifungal and protects the skin against drying.

Seckel's syndrome. See **bird-headed dwarf.**

seclusion /siklōō′zhən/ [L, *secludere*, to isolate], (in psychiatric nursing) the isolation of a patient in a special room to decrease stimuli that might be causing or exacerbating the patient's emotional distress.

secobarbital /sek′obär′bital/, a sedative and hypnotic.
- INDICATIONS: It is prescribed in the treatment of insomnia and agitation, and as an anticonvulsant and preoperative sedative.
- CONTRAINDICATIONS: Impaired liver function or known hypersensitivity to this drug or to any barbiturate prohibits its use.
- ADVERSE EFFECTS: Among the more serious adverse reactions are central nervous system and respiratory depression, hypersensitivity reactions, and paradoxical excitement. Kidney damage may result from the polyethylene glycol that is used as a diluent in injectable preparations of the drug.

Seconal, a trademark for a sedative-hypnotic (secobarbital).

secondary /sek′ənder′ē/ [L, *secundus,* second], second in importance or in incidence or belonging to the second order of sophistication or development, such as a secondary health care facility or secondary education.

secondary amenorrhea. See **amenorrhea.**

secondary amputation, amputation performed after suppuration has begun after severe trauma. An area is left open for drainage, and antibiotics are given. Compare **primary amputation.**

secondary amyloidosis. See **amyloidosis.**

secondary analysis, the study of a problem using previously compiled data.

secondary apnea, an abnormal condition in which respiration is absent and will not begin again spontaneously. Resuscitation is initiated immediately with artificial respiration; oxygen, cardiac massage, analysis of blood gases, and other treatment and medication specific to the underlying cause may be necessary. Secondary apnea may result from any event that severely impedes the absorption of oxygen into the bloodstream. Compare **primary apnea.**

secondary areola, a second ring appearing around the areola of the breast during pregnancy that is more pigmented than the areola before pregnancy.

secondary biliary cirrhosis, an abnormal hepatic condition characterized by obstruction of the bile duct with or without infection. It involves periportal inflammation with progressive fibrosis, destruction of parenchymal cells, and nodular degeneration. Compare **primary biliary cirrhosis.**

secondary bronchus, See **bronchus, primary bronchus.**

secondary care, 1. the provision of a specialized medical service by a physician specialist or a hospital on referral by a primary care physician. 2. the retardation of an existing illness or other pathologic condition.

secondary caries. See **dental caries.**

secondary dementia, dementia resulting from another, concurrent form of psychosis. See also **dementia.**

secondary dental caries, dental caries developing in a tooth already affected by the condition; often a new cavity forms adjacent to or beneath the restorative filling of an old cavity.

secondary dentition. See **permanent dentition.**

secondary distal RTA. See **distal renal tubular acidosis (distal RTA).**

secondary drive. See **drive.**

secondary dysmenorrhea. See **inflammatory dysmenorrhea.**

secondary enuresis [L, *secundus,* second; Gk, *enourein,* to urinate], enuresis in an older child who has demon-

strated bedtime control for a year or more. It is typically the result of psychological stress, but it also may be an early sign of an organic disorder, such as diabetes mellitus.

secondary fissure, a fissure between the uvula and the pyramid of the cerebellum.

secondary fracture. See **neoplastic fracture.**

secondary gain, an indirect benefit, usually obtained through an illness or debility. Such gains may include monetary and disability benefits, personal attentions, or escape from unpleasant situations and responsibilities. Compare **primary gain.**

secondary gangrene [L, *secundus,* second; Gk, *gaggraina*], a form of gangrene in which putrefaction follows the primary tissue necrosis, resulting in malodorous and toxic products.

secondary gestation [L, *secundus,* second + *gestare,* to bear], a pregnancy in which the ovum becomes displaced from its original site of implantation but continues development at a different location.

secondary health care, an intermediate level of health care that includes diagnosis and treatment, performed in a hospital having specialized equipment and laboratory facilities. Secondary health care is provided to a larger group of people from a larger geographic area than those served by primary care.

secondary hemorrhage [L, *secundus,* second; Gk, *haima,* blood + *rhegnynei,* to gush], a hemorrhage that develops 24 hours or more after the original injury or surgery. It is often caused by an infection.

secondary host. See **intermediate host.**

secondary hydrocephalus [L, *secundus,* second; Gk, *hydor,* water + *kephale,* head], hydrocephalus that develops after an injury or infection, such as syphilis or meningitis.

secondary hypertension, elevated blood pressure associated with several primary diseases, such as renal, pulmonary, endocrine, and vascular diseases. See also **hypertension.**

secondary hypertrophic osteoarthropathy. See **clubbing.**

secondary infection, an infection by a microorganism that follows an initial infection by another kind of organism.

secondary iritis [L, *secundus,* second; Gk, *iris,* rainbow + *itis,* inflammation], an inflammation of the iris that follows an infection or other disorder in a neighboring part of the eye, such as the cornea.

secondary nutrient, a substance that acts as a stimulant to activate the flora of the GI tract to synthesize other nutrients.

secondary occlusal traumatism, occlusal stress that affects previously weakened periodontal structures. The stress may not be excessive for normal tissues but can be damaging to the weakened structures.

secondary peritonitis [L, *secundus,* second; Gk, *peri tenein,* to stretch + *itis,* inflammation], inflammation of the peritoneum caused by the spread of infection from neighboring tissue.

secondary pneumonia [L, *secundus,* second; Gk, *pneumon,* lung], pneumonia that develops during the course of another disease, such as diphtheria or tularemia.

secondary polycythemia [L, *secundus,* second; Gk, *polys,* many + *kytos,* cell + *haima,* blood], a form of polycythemia that develops as a result of another disorder, such as a pulmonary disease.

secondary port, a control device for regulating the flow of a primary and a secondary intravenous solution. It consists of a Y-shaped plastic apparatus that attaches to the primary IV tubing and allows the primary and secondary IV solutions to flow separately or to flow simultaneously. Compare **piggyback port.**

secondary prevention, a level of preventive medicine that focuses on early diagnosis, use of referral services, and rapid initiation of treatment to stop the progress of disease processes or a handicapping disability.

secondary proximal renal tubular acidosis. See **proximal renal tubular acidosis.**

secondary radiation, radiation that results from the scattering of primary x-rays. Secondary radiation often accounts for fogging of x-ray film.

secondary relationships, relationships with those who provide or accept services, or with acquaintances and friends, as distinguished from family members and intimate friends.

secondary sequestrum, a piece of dead bone that partially separates from sound bone during the process of necrosis but may be pushed back into position. Compare **primary sequestrum.**

secondary sex characteristic, any of the external physical characteristics of sexual maturity secondary to hormonal stimulation that develops in the maturing individual. These characteristics include the adult distribution of hair and the development of the penis or breasts and the labia.

secondary shock, a state of physical collapse and prostration caused by numerous traumatic and pathologic conditions. It develops over a period of time after severe tissue damage and may merge with primary shock, accompanied by various signs, such as weakness, restlessness, low body temperature, low blood pressure, cold sweat, and reduced urinary output. Blood pressure drops progressively in this state, and death may occur within a relatively short time after onset unless appropriate treatment intervenes. Secondary shock is often associated with heat stroke, crushing injuries, myocardial infarction, poisoning, fulminating infections, burns, and other life-threatening conditions. The pathology of this state reflects changes in the capillaries, which become dilated and engorged with blood. Petechial hemorrhages develop in the serous membranes, edema swells the soft tissues, and the vital organs undergo degenerative changes. Compare **hemorrhagic shock, primary shock.**

secondary symptom. See **symptom.**

secondary syphilis. See **syphilis.**

secondary teeth. See **permanent teeth.**

secondary thrombocytosis. See **thrombocytosis.**

second cranial nerve. See **optic nerve.**

second cuneiform bone. See **intermediate cuneiform bone.**

second filial generation. See **F₂.**

second intention. See **intention.**

second messenger, a chemical substance inside a cell that carries information further along the signal pathway from the internal portion of a membrane-spanning receptor embedded in the cell membrane. It may be in the form of an enzyme's product or ion fluxes.

second opinion [L, *secundus* + *opinari,* to suppose], a patient privilege of requesting an examination and evaluation of a health condition by a second physician to verify or challenge the diagnosis by a first physician. The

situation is most likely to arise when an examination by a first physician results in a recommendation for surgery.

second-order change, a change that changes the system itself.

second-order kinetics, a chemical reaction in which the rate of the reaction is determined by the concentration of two chemical entities involved. Also called **second-order reaction.** See also **kinetics.**

second sight. See **senopia.**

second stage of labor [L, *secundus,* second; OFr, *estage;* L, *labor,* work], the period of childbirth from full dilatation of the cervix to delivery of the fetus.

secrete /sikrēt'/ [L, *secernere,* to separate], to discharge a substance into a cavity, vessel, or organ or onto the surface of the skin, as by a gland. **—secretion,** *n.*

secretin /sikrē'tin/ [L, *secernere*], a digestive hormone that is produced by certain cells lining the duodenum and jejunum when fatty acids of partially digested food enter the intestine from the stomach. It stimulates the pancreas to produce a fluid high in salts but low in enzymes. Secretin has a limited stimulating effect on the production of bile. See also **pancreas.**

secretin test, a test of pancreatic function after stimulation with a hormone, secretin. The test measures the volume and bicarbonate concentration of pancreatic secretions. Normal volume findings are 2 to 4 ml/kg body weight HCO⁻³ (bicarbonate): 90 to 130 mEq/L. A lower than normal volume suggests an obstructing malignancy. Reduced bicarbonate and amylase concentration is usually diagnostic of chronic pancreatitis.

secretion /sikrē'shən/ [L, *secernere,* to separate], **1.** the release of chemical substances manufactured by cells of glandular organs. **2.** a substance released.

secretoinhibitory /sikrē'tō·inhib'itôr'ē/ [L, *secernere,* to separate + *inhibere,* to restrain], pertaining to a function of inhibiting secretion.

secretory /sikrē'tərē/ [L, *secernere,* to separate], pertaining to or contributing to the function of secretion.

secretory duct [L, *secernere*], (of a gland) a small duct that has a secretory function and joins with an excretory duct.

secretory phase, the phase of the menstrual cycle after the release of an ovum from a mature ovarian follicle. The corpus luteum, stimulated by luteinizing hormone (LH), develops from the ruptured follicle. It secretes progesterone, which stimulates the development of the glands and arteries of the endometrium, causing it to become thick and spongy. In a negative-feedback response to the increased level of progesterone in the blood, the secretion of LH from the pituitary decreases. In the absence of an embryo and its secretion of chorionic gonadotropin, the secretory phase ends. The corpus luteum involutes, progesterone levels fall, and menstruation occurs. Also called **luteal phase, progestational phase.** Compare **menstrual phase, proliferative phase.**

secretory piece, a polypeptide chain attached to an IgA molecule. The secretory piece is necessary for secretion of the immunoglobulin molecule into mucosal spaces.

sect-, -sect, a combining form meaning 'to cut': *section, sector, dissect.*

section /sek'shən/ [L, *sectio*], **1.** a cut surface or slice of tissue. **2.** the act of cutting tissue.

sectional arch wire /sek'shənəl/ [L, *sectio,* a cutting; *arcus* bow; AS, *wir*], a wire attached to only a few teeth, usually on one side of a dental arch or in the anterior segment of the arch to cause or guide orthodontic tooth movement.

sectional denture. See **partial denture.**

Sectral, a trademark for a beta-adrenergic blocking agent (acebutolol).

secund-, a combining form meaning 'second, or following': *secundigravida, secundina, secundine.*

secundigravida /səkund'dəgrav'idə/ [L, *secundus,* second, *gravidus,* pregnancy], a woman who is pregnant for the second time. Also called **gravida 2. –secundigravid,** *adj.*

secundines /səkun'dīnz/ [L, *secundus*], the placenta, umbilical cord, and membranes of afterbirth.

secundipara /sek'əndip'ərə/ [L, *secundus + parere,* to give birth], a woman who has borne two viable children in separate pregnancies.

SED, abbreviation for **skin erythemadose.** See **threshold dose.**

sedation /sidā'shən/ [L, *sedatio,* soothing], an induced state of quiet, calmness, or sleep, as by means of a sedative or hypnotic medication.

sedative /sed'ətiv/ [L, *sedatus*], **1.** of or pertaining to a substance, procedure, or measure that has a calming effect. **2.** an agent that decreases functional activity, diminishes irritability, and allays excitement. Some sedatives have a general effect on all organs; others affect principally the activities of the heart, stomach, intestines, nerve trunks, respiratory system, or vasomotor system. Barbiturates, benzodiazepines, and nonbarbiturate sedatives, such as chloral hydrate, furazepam, glutethimide, and various minor tranquilizers, are used to induce sleep, reduce pain, facilitate the induction of anesthesia, and treat convulsive conditions, anxiety states, and irritable bowel syndrome. See also **sedative-hypnotic.**

sedative bath, the immersion of the body in water for a prolonged period of time, used especially as a calming procedure for agitated patients.

sedative-hypnotic, a drug that reversibly depresses the activity of the central nervous system, used chiefly to induce sleep and to allay anxiety. Barbiturates and many nonbarbiturate sedative-hypnotics with diverse chemical and pharmacologic properties share the ability to depress the activity of all excitable tissue, but the arousal center in the brainstem is especially sensitive to their effects. Various sedative-hypnotics and minor tranquilizers with similar effects are used in the treatment of insomnia, acute convulsive conditions, and anxiety states, and to facilitate the induction of anesthesia. Although sedative-hypnotics have a soporific effect, they may interfere with rapid eye movement (REM) sleep associated with dreaming and, when administered to patients with fever, may act paradoxically and cause excitement rather than relaxation. Sedative-hypnotics may interfere with temperature regulation, depress oxygen consumption in various tissues, and produce nausea and skin rashes; and, in elderly patients, may cause dizziness, confusion, and ataxia. Drugs in this group have a high potential for abuse that often results in physical and psychologic dependence; treatment of dependence involves gradual reduction of the dosage, because abrupt withdrawal frequently causes serious disorders, including convulsions. Acute reactions to an overdose of a sedative-hypnotic may be treated with an emetic, activated charcoal, gastric lavage, and measures to maintain airway patency. Among nonbarbiturate sedative-hypnotics are chloral hydrate, eth-

chlorvynol, ethinamate, glutethimide, paraldehyde, triclofos sodium, minor tranquilizers (chlordiazepoxide, flurazepam, diazepam), diphenhydramine, and meprobamate. See also **barbiturate.**

sedentary /sed'ənter'ē/ [L, *sedentarius,* sitting], pertaining to a condition of inaction, such as work or recreation that can be performed in the sitting posture.

sedentary living [L, *sedentarius;* AS, *lif*], a pattern of daily living that requires a minimum amount of physical effort.

sediment /sed'imənt/ [L, *sedimentum,* settling], a deposit of relatively insoluble material that settles to the bottom of a container of liquid.

sedimentation /sed'imäntā'shən/ [L, *sedimentum,* settling], the deposition of insoluble materials to the bottom of a liquid. The process may be accelerated by centrifugation.

sedimentation rate (SR) [L, *sedimentum + ratum,* rate], the speed of settling of red blood cells in a vertical glass column of citrated plasma. It is used to monitor inflammatory or malignant disease and to aid in the detection and diagnosis of occult diseases, such as tuberculosis. See also **erythrocyte sedimentation rate.**

sed. rate, *informal.* erythrocyte sedimentation rate.

Seeing Eye dog. See **guide dog.**

segment /seg'mənt/ [L, *segmentum,* that which is cut off], a component, portion, or part of a structure, such as a lobe of the liver or part of the intestine.

segmental bronchus /segmen'təl/ [L, *segmentum,* piece cut off], a secondary bronchus branching from a primary bronchus to a tertiary bronchus.

segmental fracture, a bone break in which several large bone fragments separate from the main body of a fractured bone. The ends of such fragments may pierce the skin, as in an open fracture, or may be contained within the skin, as in a closed fracture.

segmental reflex [L, *segmentum + reflectere,* to bend back], a reflex that involves a pathway through only a single segment of the spinal cord.

segmental resection, a surgical procedure in which a part of an organ, gland, or other part of the body is excised, such as a segmental resection of a part of an ovary performed to diminish the hormonal secretion of the gland by decreasing the amount of secretory tissue in the gland.

segmentation /seg'məntā'shən/ [L, *segmentum + atio,* process], **1.** the repetition of structured parts or the process of dividing into segments or similar parts, such as the formation of somites or metameres. **2.** the division of the zygote into blastomeres; cleavage.

segmentation cavity. See **blastocoele.**

segmentation cell. See **blastomere.**

segmentation method, a technique for filling tooth root canals in which a preselected gutta-percha cone is cut into segments and the tip section sealed into the apex of a root. The other sections are usually warmed and condensed against the first piece with a plugger. More cone segments are then added until the canal is filled.

segmentation nucleus, the nucleus of the zygote resulting from the fusion of the male and female pronuclei in the fertilized ovum. It is the final stage in fertilization and initiates the first cleavage of the zygote. Also called **cleavage nucleus.**

segmented hyalinizing vasculitis /segmen'tid/, a chronic, relapsing inflammatory condition of the blood vessels of the lower legs associated with nodular or purpuric skin lesions that may become ulcerated and leave scars. Also called **livedo vasculitis.**

segmented neutrophil, a neutrophil with a filament between the lobes of its nucleus.

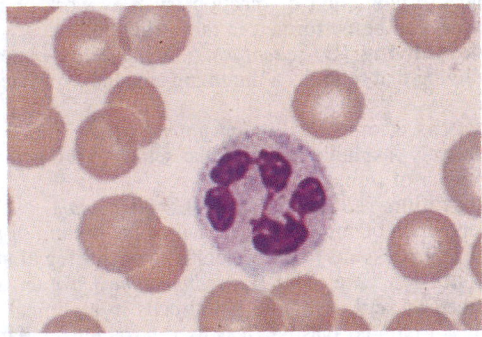

Segmented neutrophil (Powers, 1989)

segregation /seg'rəgā'shən/ [L, *segregare,* to separate], (in genetics) a principle stating that the pairs of chromosomes bearing genes derived from both parents are separated during meiosis. Chance alone determines which gene, maternal or paternal, will travel to which gamete. See also **dominance, independent assortment.**

seizure /sē'zhər/ [Fr, *saisir,* to seize], a hyperexcitation of neurons in the brain leading to a sudden, violent involuntary series of contractions of a group of muscles that may be paroxysmal and episodic, as in a seizure disorder, or transient and acute, as after a head concussion. A seizure may be clonic or tonic, focal, unilateral, or bilateral. Also called **convulsion.**

seizure threshold, the amount of stimulus necessary to produce a convulsive seizure. All humans can have seizures if the provocation is sufficient. Those who have spontaneous convulsions are said to have a "low seizure threshold."

Seldane, a trademark for an oral antihistamine (terfenadine).

selection /silek'shən/ [L, *seligere,* to choose], **1.** the act or product of choosing. **2.** (in genetics) the process by which various factors or mechanisms determine and modify the reproductive ability of a genotype within a specific population, thus influencing evolutionary change. Kinds of selection are **artificial selection, natural selection,** and **sexual selection.**

selective absorption. See **differential absorption.**

selective abstraction /silek'tiv/ [L, *seligere,* to choose], a type of cognitive distortion in which focus on one aspect of an event negates all other aspects.

selective angiography, a graphic procedure that allows selective visualization of the aorta, the major arterial systems, or a particular vessel. It is performed using a percutaneous catheter. A few milliliters of a radiopaque substance are injected when the catheter is in place. The patient is observed for signs of sensitivity to the radiopaque medium, including chills, tremor, or shortness of breath. After the procedure, the catheter is withdrawn, and pressure is placed on the puncture site to prevent bleeding. Blood pressure is checked every 15 minutes for 2 hours.

selective grinding, any modification of the occlusal forms of the teeth, produced by corrective grinding at selected places to improve occlusion and tooth function.

selective inattention, the screening out of unwanted stimuli, particularly the part of a message the listener does not want to hear.

selectively permeable. See **semipermeable.**

selectivity /silektiv'itē/ [L, *seligere*], the capacity factor ratios of two substances measured under identical chromatographic conditions. Also called **chromatographic selectivity, separation factor.**

selectivity coefficient, the degree to which an ion-selective electrode (ISE) responds to a particular ion with respect to a reference ion.

selenium (Se) /silē'nē·əm/ [Gk, *selene,* moon], a metalloid element of the sulfur group. Its atomic number is 34; its atomic weight is 78.96. Selenium occurs mainly in iron, copper, lead, and nickel ores and in the form of metallic selenides. One of the chief sources commercially is the flue dust produced by the burning of pyrites to make sulfuric acid. Selenium occurs as a trace element in foods, and research continues to determine the most effective daily allowances for different age groups. Dietary experts say that the estimated safe, adequate intake of selenium for infants 6 months of age is 0.04 mg, for adults 0.05 to 0.2 mg. Although selenium deficiency can result in liver problems and degeneration of muscles in some animals, in humans its need has not yet been clearly defined. Authorities stress that all intakes of selenium and other trace elements in foods are considered safe and effective within recommended ranges, but consumption of greater amounts or smaller amounts over extended periods of time will increase the risk of marginal toxicity or marginal deficiency, respectively. The bright orange, insoluble powder selenium sulfide is used externally in the control of seborrheic dermatitis, dandruff, and other forms of dermatosis. Selenium sulfide, employed as a lotion, is used in some therapeutic shampoos containing 2.5% of selenium sulfide in a detergent vehicle; it is sold without prescription as a 1% detergent suspension in a scented detergent vehicle. Adverse effects may include conjunctivitis if the preparation enters the eyes, increased oiliness or dryness of the hair, and orange tinting of gray hair. The antidandruff effectiveness of selenium sulfide is thought to stem from its antimitotic activity and its residual adherence to the hair after shampooing. Normal skin absorbs very little of the drug, but inflamed or damaged skin absorbs it readily. Selenium is used in the nuclear medicine compound selenomethionine for diagnosing parathyroid tumors. The element is also used as a photoconductive layer of xeroradiographic plates. Burns and dermatitis venenata may result from prolonged skin contact.

selenium sulfide, an antifungal and antiseborrheic. See also **selenium.**

■ INDICATIONS: It is prescribed for dandruff and for seborrheic dermatitis of the scalp.

■ CONTRAINDICATIONS: Acute scalp inflammation or known hypersensitivity to this drug prohibits its use.

■ ADVERSE EFFECTS: Among the more serious adverse reactions are dermatitis after prolonged skin contact or keratitis after accidental conjunctival contact.

self, *pl.* **selves** /selvz/ [AS], **1.** the total essence or being of a person; the individual. **2.** those affective, cognitive, and spiritual qualities that distinguish one person from another; individuality. **3.** a person's awareness of his own being or identity; consciousness; ego. See also **personality.**

self-acceptance [AS, *self;* L, *accipere,* to take], the recognition and acceptance of one's own qualities and limitations.

self-actualization, (in humanistic psychology) the fundamental tendency toward the maximum realization and fulfillment of one's human potential.

self-alien. See **ego-dystonic.**

self-alienation. See **depersonalization.**

self-anesthesia, the self-administered inhalational anesthesia in which whiffs of anesthetic gas are inhaled from a handheld breathing device controlled by the patient. This form of anesthesia is most common in England.

self-breast examination (SBE), a procedure in which a woman examines her breasts and their accessory structures for evidence of change that could indicate a malignant process. The SBE is usually performed 1 week to 10 days after the first day of the menstrual cycle, when the breasts are smallest and cyclic nodularity is least apparent. Self-examination is encouraged during all phases of a woman's

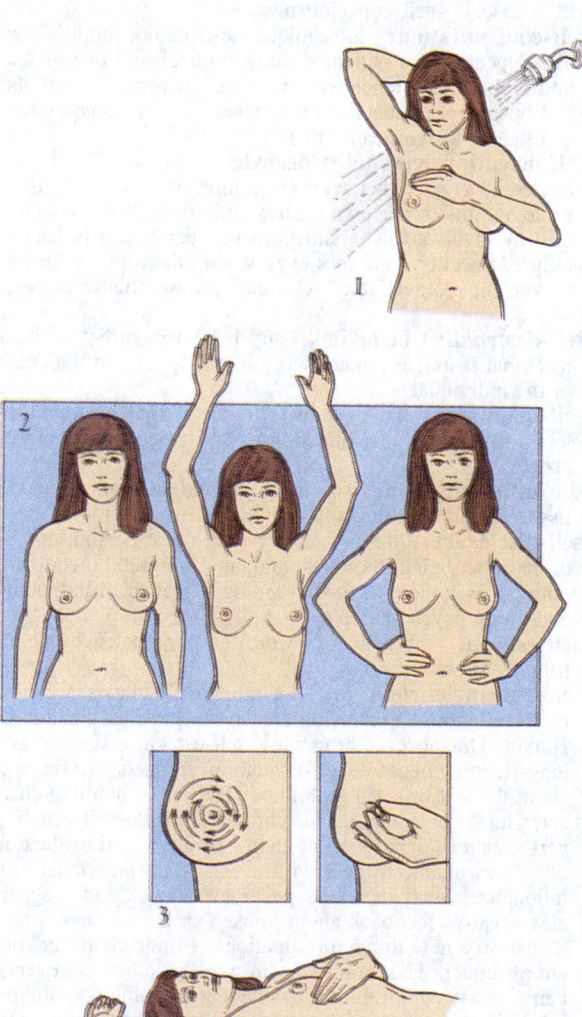

Self-breast examination *(Payne, 1989)*

adult life; a woman who regularly and carefully performs the examination is better able to detect small abnormalities than is a woman who is not familiar with her own breasts. The techniques are similar to those of the examination of the breast as performed in the health assessment or physical examination. Also called **breast self-examination (BSE).** See also **breast examination.**

self-care, **1.** the personal and medical care performed by the patient, usually in collaboration with and after instruction by a health professional. The need of a patient for assistance and the ability to develop a higher level of self-care must be evaluated in forming any nursing care plan. Maximal self-care appropriate to the condition and to the patient is often the ultimate goal of nursing care. Occupational therapy services also help restore, develop, or maintain the skills necessary to permit physically and mentally disabled people to perform the daily living tasks of self-care. **2.** the health care by laypeople of their families, friends, and themselves, including identification and evaluation of symptoms, medication, and treatment. Self-care is self-limited, voluntary, and wholly outside professional health care systems but may include consultation with a physician or other health care professional as a resource. **3.** personal care accomplished without technical assistance, such as eating, washing, dressing, using the telephone, and attending to one's own elimination, appearance, and hygiene. The goal of rehabilitation medicine is maximal personal self-care.

self-care deficit, bathing/hygiene, a nursing diagnosis accepted by the Fourth National Conference on the Classification of Nursing Diagnoses. The condition is defined as a state in which the individual experiences impaired ability to perform or complete bathing and hygiene activities for himself or herself. The deficit is separated into functional categories and is graded from 0 (functions independently) to 4 (requires total assistance). The major defining characteristics of the deficit include inability to wash the body or parts of the body, inability to get or get to water for bathing, and inability to regulate water temperature or flow. Related factors include intolerance for activity because of decreased strength and endurance, pain or discomfort, perceptual or cognitive impairment, neuromuscular impairment, musculoskeletal impairment, and depression or severe anxiety. See also **nursing diagnosis.**

self-care deficit, dressing/grooming, a nursing diagnosis accepted by the Fourth National Conference on the Classification of Nursing Diagnoses. It is defined as a state in which the individual experiences impaired ability to perform or complete dressing and grooming activities for himself or herself. The deficit is separated into functional categories and is graded from 0 (functions independently) to 4 (requires total assistance). The major defining characteristics of a deficit in self-dressing or self-grooming include impaired ability to don or to remove necessary items of clothing, to fasten clothing, to obtain or replace articles of clothing, and to maintain a satisfactory appearance. Related factors include intolerance for activity because of decreased strength or endurance, pain or discomfort, impairment of cognitive or perceptual function, neuromuscular impairment, musculoskeletal impairment, and depression or marked anxiety. See also **nursing diagnosis.**

self-care deficit, feeding, a nursing diagnosis accepted by the Fourth National Conference on the Classification of Nursing Diagnoses. The condition is defined as a state in which the individual experiences impaired ability to perform or complete feeding activities for himself or herself. The deficit is separated into functional categories and is graded from 0 (functions independently) to 4 (requires total assistance). The major defining characteristic is an inability to bring food from a receptacle to the mouth. Related factors include intolerance for activity because of decreased strength or endurance, pain or discomfort, impairment of cognitive or perceptual function, neuromuscular impairment, musculoskeletal impairment, and depression or marked anxiety. See also **nursing diagnosis.**

self-care deficit, toileting, a nursing diagnosis accepted by the Fourth National Conference on the Classification of Nursing Diagnoses. The condition is defined as a state in which the individual experiences impaired ability to perform or complete toileting activities for himself or herself. The deficit is separated into functional categories and is graded from 0 (functions independently) to 4 (requires total assistance). The major defining characteristics of a self-toileting deficit include inability to get to the toilet or to the commode, to sit down on or to arise from the toilet or commode, to get the necessary clothing on or off, and to perform the proper toilet hygiene. In addition, the person may not be able to flush the toilet or to empty the commode. Related factors include impaired transfer ability, impaired mobility status, intolerance for activity because of decreased strength or endurance, pain or discomfort, impairment of cognitive or perceptual function, neuromuscular impairment, musculoskeletal impairment, and depression or severe anxiety. See also **nursing diagnosis.**

self-care theory, a model, central to Dorothea Orem's concept of nursing, used to provide a conceptual framework for nursing care directed toward self-care by the client to the greatest degree possible. The model requires an assessment of the client's capability for self-care and need for care. The need for care includes biophysical and psychosocial needs and the specific needs that are the result of the illness.

self-catheterization, a procedure performed by a patient to empty the bladder and prevent it from becoming overdistended with urine. The patient who cannot empty the bladder completely but can retain urine for 2 to 4 hours at a time can be taught self-catheterization if he or she is willing to learn and has some manual dexterity and the ability to palpate the bladder.

■ METHOD: Necessary equipment consists of a pan or toilet, two 14 French catheters, a water-soluble lubricant, soap, water, and a clean washcloth and towel; women usually require a magnifying mirror initially to identify the urethral meatus, and men may prefer to perform the procedure sitting on a low stool rather than on a toilet. Women are taught to perform self-catheterization initially in a semi-Fowler's position, using a pan, but later they generally can carry out the procedure sitting on or standing over a toilet. The patient is instructed to clean the urinary meatus and labia or glans penis with soap and water, to grasp the catheter 3 or 4 inches from the tip, and to lubricate the tip before it is gently inserted in the meatus: Women insert 3 to 5 cm of the catheter, and men insert 20 cm. Urine is allowed to flow into the pan or toilet until the bladder is empty. The catheter is then removed, washed in soap and water, thoroughly rinsed, dried by rolling it in a clean towel, and placed in a clean plastic or paper bag for the next self-catheterization.

■ NURSING INTERVENTIONS: The nurse teaches the procedure and ensures that the patient understands its purpose and the need to perform it at designated times, and the importance of forcing fluids up to 3000 ml daily, unless contraindicated. The nurse makes certain that the patient is able to identify the urinary meatus.

■ OUTCOME CRITERIA: Regular self-catheterization by the patient who cannot empty the bladder allows the person to work and participate in the normal activities of daily living and to prevent kidney infection and other renal pathology.

self-concept, the composite of ideas, feelings, and attitudes that a person has about his or her own identity, worth, capabilities, and limitations. Such factors as the values and opinions of others, especially in the formative years of early childhood, play an important part in the development of the self-concept.

self-conscious, **1.** the state of being aware of oneself as an individual entity that experiences, desires, and acts. **2.** a heightened awareness of oneself and one's actions as reflected by the observations and reactions of others; socially ill at ease. —**self-consciousness,** *n.*

self-confrontation, a technique for behavior modification that depends on a patient's recognition of and dissatisfaction with inconsistencies in his or her own values, beliefs, and behaviors, or between his or her own personal system and that of a significant other.

self-defeating personality disorder a personality characterized by a type of behavior that inhibits the individual from achieving his or her own desires and goals. It is characterized by involvement in situations that continuously lead to failure, rejection, and loss even when other options for involvement are available. Also called **masochistic personality.**

self-destructive behavior, any behavior, direct or indirect, that if uninterrupted, will ultimately lead to the death of the individual.

self-diagnosis, the diagnosis of one's own health problems, usually without direction or assistance from a physician.

self-differentiation, specialization and diversification of a tissue or part resulting solely from intrinsic factors.

self-disclosure, the process by which one person lets his or her inner being, thoughts, and emotions be known to another. It is important for psychologic growth in individual and group psychotherapy.

self-esteem, the degree of worth and competence one attributes to oneself.

self-esteem, chronic low, a nursing diagnosis accepted by the Eighth National Conference on the Classification of Nursing Diagnoses. Chronic low self-esteem is defined as a long-standing negative self-evaluation and negative feelings about the self or self-capabilities. The major defining characteristics (long-standing or chronic) include self-negating verbalization, expression of shame or guilt, and evaluation of self as unable to deal with events. The individual also rationalizes away or rejects positive feedback and exaggerates negative feedback about himself or herself and is hesitant to try new things or situations. Minor characteristics are a frequent lack of success in work or other life events; being overly conforming and dependent on others' opinions; a lack of eye contact with others; being nonassertive, passive, or indecisive; and excessively seeking reassurance. See also **nursing diagnosis.**

self-esteem disturbance, a nursing diagnosis accepted by the Eighth National Conference on the Classification of

Nursing Diagnoses. The condition is defined as a negative self-evaluation and negative feelings about the self or self-capabilities, which may be directly or indirectly expressed. The defining characteristics include self-negating verbalization, expressions of shame or guilt, evaluation of self as unable to deal with events, rationalization or rejection of positive feedback and exaggeration of negative feedback about himself or herself, and hesitancy to try new things or situations. The individual with a self-esteem disturbance also may deny problems obvious to others, project blame or responsibility for problems on others, rationalize personal failures, be hypersensitive to slight or criticism, and show grandiosity. See also **nursing diagnosis.**

self-esteem, situational low, a nursing diagnosis accepted by the Eighth National Conference on the Classification of Nursing Diagnoses. Situational low self-esteem is defined as a negative self-evaluation with feelings about the self that develop in response to a loss or change in an individual who previously had a positive self-evaluation. The major defining characteristics are an episodic occurrence of negative self-appraisal in response to life events and verbalization of negative feelings about the self, such as helplessness or uselessness. Minor characteristics of the condition are self-negating verbalizations, expression of shame or guilt, evaluation of oneself as unable to handle situations or events, and difficulty in making decisions. See also **nursing diagnosis.**

self-fulfilling prophecy, a principle that states that a belief in or the expectation of a particular resolution is a factor that contributes to its fulfillment.

self-help group, a group of people who meet to improve their health through discussion and special activities. Characteristically, self-help groups are not led by a professional. A women's self-help group may be primarily supportive or it may be concerned with learning to perform basic tests, such as a Pap test, or with identification and treatment of common gynecologic problems, such as vaginal infections. Compare **group therapy.**

self-hypnosis [AS, *self;* Gk, *hypnos,* sleep], the process of putting oneself into a trancelike state by autosuggestion, such as concentration on a single thought or object. Some subjects are more susceptible than others.

self-ideal, a perception of how one should behave based on certain personal standards. The standard may be either a carefully constructed image of the kind of person one would like to be or merely a number of aspirations, goals, or values one would like to achieve.

self-image, the total concept, idea, or mental image one has of oneself and of one's role in society; the person one believes oneself to be.

self-imposed guilt, a restrictive type of guilt of which the individual is aware and from which he or she is unable to break free.

self-insurance, a system whereby hospitals or health professionals may, in lieu of commercial insurance, assume financial responsibility for their liability.

self-limited, (of a disease or condition) tending to end without treatment.

self-limited disease [AS, *self;* L, *limes,* boundary + *dis,* not; Fr, *aise,* ease], a disease restricted in duration by its own pattern of characteristics and not by other influences.

self-management approach, a treatment approach in which patients assume responsibility for their behavior, changing their environment, and planning their future.

self-mutilation, high risk for a nursing diagnosis accepted by the Tenth National Conference on the Classification of Nursing Diagnoses. It is defined as a state in which an individual is at high risk to injure but not kill himself or herself, and that produces tissue damage and tension relief. Risk factors include being a member of an at-risk group, inability to cope with increased psychologic/physiological tension in a healthy manner, feelings of depression, rejection, self-hatred, separation anxiety, guilt, and depersonalization, fluctuating emotions, command hallucinations, need for sensory stimuli, parental emotional deprivation, and a dysfunctional family. Groups at risk include clients with borderline personality disorder, especially females 16 to 25 years of age, clients in a psychotic state (frequently males in young adulthood), emotionally disturbed and/or battered children, mentally retarded and autistic children, clients with a history of self-injury, and clients with a history of physical, emotional, or sexual abuse. See also **nursing diagnosis.**

self-other, a concept that characterizes people who believe that sources of power are within the self as opposed to those who believe the source of power is in others.

self-radiolysis, a process in which a compound is damaged by radioactive decay products originating in an atom within the compound.

self-responsibility, a concept of holistic health by which individuals assume responsibility for their own health.

self-retaining catheter, an indwelling urinary catheter that has a double lumen. One channel allows urine to drain from the bladder into a collecting bag; the other channel has a balloon at the bladder end and a diaphragm at the other end. Several centimeters of air or sterile water are injected through the diaphragm to fill the balloon in the bladder and hold the catheter in place. To remove the catheter, the air or water is withdrawn through the diaphragm. Also called **Foley catheter.**

self-system, the organization of experiences that acts as a protective mechanism against anxiety.

self-theory, a personality theory that uses one's self-concept in integrating the function and organization of the personality. See also **humanistic psychology.**

self-threading pin, a threaded pin screwed into a hole drilled in tooth dentin to improve retention of a restoration.

self-transcendence, the ability to focus attention on doing something for the sake of others, as opposed to self-actualization, in which doing something for oneself is an end goal.

sella turcica /sel′ə tur′sikə/ [L, *sella,* seat; *turcica,* Turkish], a transverse depression crossing the midline on the superior surface of the body of the sphenoid bone and containing the pituitary gland.

Sellick's maneuver. See **crocoid pressure.**

Selsun, a trademark for an antifungal and antiseborrheic (selenium sulfide), used as a shampoo.

SEM, abbreviation for **scanning electron microscope.**

semantics /siman′tiks/ [Gk, *semantikos,* significant], the study of language with special concern for the meanings of words or other symbols.

-seme, a combining form meaning '(one) having an orbital (cephalometric) index of less than 84, more than 89, or in between' as specified by the prefix: *megaseme, mesoseme, microseme.*

semeio-, a combining form meaning 'sign or symptom': *semeiography, semeiology, semeiotic.*

semen /sē'mən/ [L, seed], the thick, whitish secretion of the male reproductive organs discharged from the urethra on ejaculation. It contains various constituents, including spermatozoa in their nutrient plasma and secretions of the prostate, seminal vesicles, and various other glands. Also called **seminal fluid, sperm.** –**seminal,** *adj.*

semi- /sem'ē-/, a prefix meaning 'one half': *semicoma, semisupination, semivalent.*

semicircular canal /-sur'kyələr/ [L, *semi*, half, *circulare*, to go around; *canalis*, channel], any of three bony, fluid-filled loops in the osseous labyrinth of the internal ear, associated with the sense of balance. The posterior, superior, and lateral canals, each about 0.8 mm in diameter and perpendicular to each other, open into the cochlea. The posterior canal is the longest.

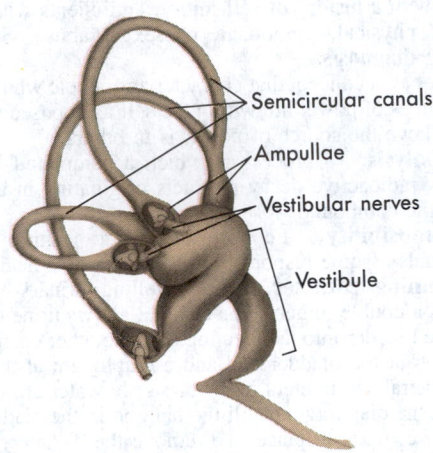

Semicircular canals *(Thibodeau, 1993/Marsha J Dohrmann)*

semicircular duct, one of three ducts that make up the membranous labyrinth of the inner ear. See also **membranous labyrinth.**

semicoma. See **coma.**

semicomatose /-kō'mətōs/ [L, *semi*, half; Gk, *koma*, deep sleep], pertaining to a condition of semicoma, from which a patient can be aroused. See also **coma, Glasgow Coma Scale.**

semiconductor /-kənduk'tər/, a solid crystalline substance whose electrical conductivity is intermediate between that of a conductor and an insulator. An **n-type semiconductor** has loosely bound electrons that are relatively free to move about inside the material. A **p-type semiconductor** is one with holes, or positive traps, in which electrons may be bound. The holes may be free to migrate through the material.

semiconscious /-kon'shəs/, an impaired state of consciousness, characterized by obtundation, stupor, or hypersomnia, from which a patient can be aroused only by energetic stimulation.

semi-Fowler's position /-fon'lərz/ [L, *semi*; George R. Fowler], placement of the patient in an inclined position, with the upper half of the body raised by elevating the head of the bed approximately 30 degrees.

semilente insulin. See **intermediate-acting insulin.**

semilunar bone. See **lunate bone.**

semilunar valve /-lŌŌ'nər/ [L, *semi* + *luna*, moon; *valva*, folding door], **1.** a valve with half-moon-shaped cusps, such as the aortic valve and the pulmonary valve. **2.** any one of the cusps constituting such a valve. See also **heart valve, mitral (bicuspid) valve, tricuspid valve.**

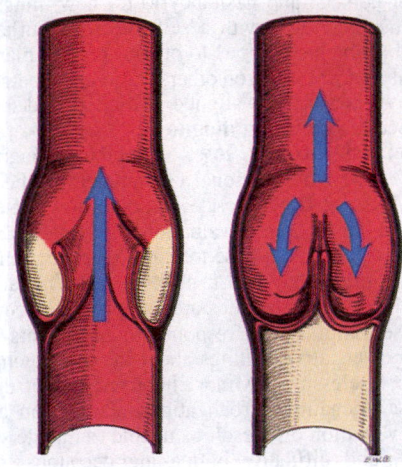

Semilunar valves *(Thibodeau, 1993/Ernest W Beck)*

semimembranosus /-ēmem'brənō'səs/ [L, *semi* + *membrana*, membrane], one of three posterior femoral muscles. Situated at the back and medial side of the thigh, it originates in a thick tendon attached to the tuberosity of the ischium and inserts into the horizontal groove on the medial condyle of the tibia. The tendon of insertion passes some fibers laterally and upward to insert on the lateral condyle of the femur and form part of the oblique popliteal ligament behind the knee. The tendon of insertion forms one

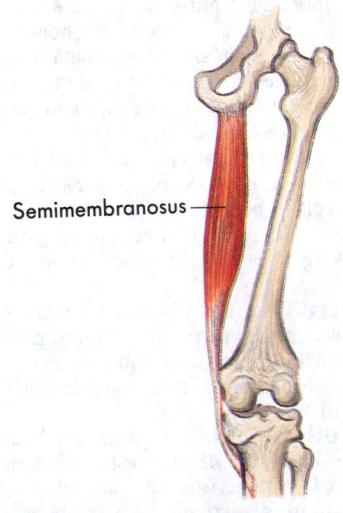

Semimembranosus

Semimembranosis muscle
(Thibodeau, 1993/Ernest W Beck)

of the two medial hamstrings. The muscle is innervated by several branches of the tibial portion of the sciatic nerve, containing fibers from the fifth lumbar and the first two sacral nerves, and functions to flex the leg, to rotate it medially after flexion, and to extend the thigh. Compare **biceps femoris, hamstring muscle, semitendinosus.**

semimembranous /-men'brənəs/ [L, *semi* half + *membrana*], pertaining to a muscle or other tissue that is partly membrane or fascia, such as the semimembranous hamstring muscle.

seminal. See **semen.**

seminal duct /sem'inəl/ [L, *semen* + *ducere*, to lead], any duct through which semen passes, such as the vas deferens or the ejaculatory duct.

seminal emission [L, *semen*, seed + *emittere*, to send out], a discharge of semen.

seminal fluid. See **semen.**

seminal fluid test, any of several tests of semen to detect abnormalities in a male reproductive system and to determine fertility. Some common factors considered are seminal fluid liquefaction time and spermatic quantity, morphology, motility, volume, and pH. Normal values in some of these tests are: sperm count, 60 million to 150 million/ml of seminal fluid; pH, more than 7 (7.7 average); ejaculation volume, 1.5 to 5.0 ml; motility, 60% of sperm.

seminal vesicle, either of the paired, saclike glandular structures behind the urinary bladder in the male and functioning as part of the reproductive system. Each sac is pyramidal in shape and convoluted in appearance, and at the anterior extremity becomes constricted into a narrow, straight duct that joins the vas deferens to form the ejaculatory duct. The seminal vesicles produce a fluid that is added to the secretion of the testes and other glands to form the semen.

seminal vesiculitis, inflammation of a seminal vesicle.

seminarcosis. See **twilight sleep.**

semination /sem'inā'shən/, the introduction of semen into the female genital tract.

seminiferous /sem'inif'ərəs/ [L, *semen* + *ferre*, to bear], transporting or producing semen, such as the tubules of the testis.

seminiferous tubules [L, *semen*, seed + *ferre*, to bear + *tubulus*], long threadlike tubes packed in areolar tissue in the lobes of the testes.

seminoma /sem'inō'mə/, *pl.* **seminomas, seminomata** [L, *semen* + *oma*, tumor], a malignant tumor of the testis. It is the most common testicular tumor and is believed to arise from the seminiferous epithelium of the mature or maturing testis. The two types are classic, or typical, and spermatocytic, with anaplastic being a variant of classic. Compare **dysgerminoma.**

semipermeable /-pur'mē·əbəl/ [L, *semi*, half + *permeare*, to pass through], pertaining to a membrane that allows the passage of some molecules but prevents the passage of others. Also **selectively permeable.**

semipermeable membrane [L, *semi* + *permeare*, to pass through], a membrane barrier to the passage of substances above a specific size, but which allows the movement through the membrane of substances below that size.

semiprone /-prōn'/ [L, *semi*, half + *pronus*, leaning forward], lying on one's side, with the thigh on the upper side flexed against the abdomen, and the arm on the lower side extended back. See also **Sims' position.**

semiprone side position. See **Sims' position.**

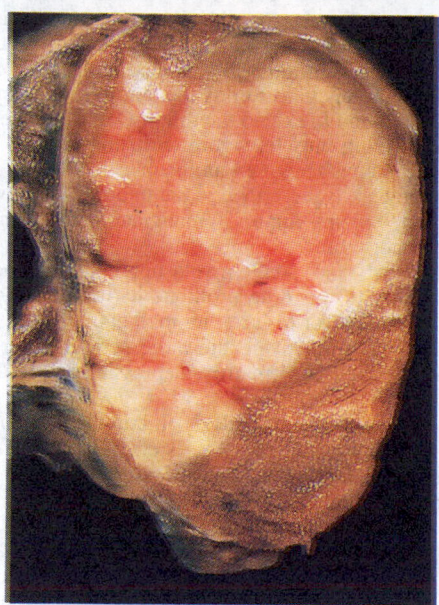

Seminoma *(Fletcher, 1987)*

semirecumbent /-rikum'bənt/, in a reclining position.

semisynthetic /-sinthet'ik/ [L, *semi*, half; Gk, *synthesis*, putting together], pertaining to a natural substance that has been partially altered by chemical manipulation.

semitendinosus /sem'iten'dinō'səs/ [L, *semi* + *tendere*, to stretch], one of three posterior femoral muscles of the thigh, remarkable for the great length of its tendon of insertion. It is a fusiform muscle located in the posterior and medial portion of the thigh, arising from the tuberosity of the ischium. It ends just distal to the middle of the thigh in a long, round tendon that crosses the semitendinosus and curves around the medial condyle of the tibia and inserts

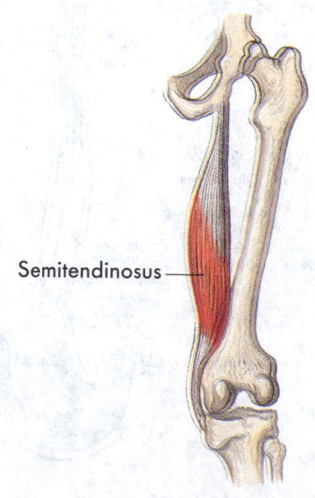

Semitendinosus

Semitendinosus *(Thibodeau, 1993/Ernest W Beck)*

into the medial surface of the tibia. The muscle is innervated by branches of the tibial portion of the sciatic nerve, containing fibers from the fifth lumbar and the first two sacral nerves. It functions to flex the leg, to rotate it medially after flexion, and to extend the thigh. Compare **biceps femoris, hamstring muscle, semimembranosus.**

semustine /səmus′tēn/, an antineoplastic.

- INDICATIONS: It is prescribed in the treatment of Lewis lung carcinoma, brain tumors, malignant melanoma, and Hodgkin's disease.

- CONTRAINDICATIONS: Acute myelosuppression or known hypersensitivity to this drug prohibits its use. It is not given during pregnancy or to lactating mothers.

- ADVERSE EFFECTS: Among the more serious adverse reactions are delayed bone marrow depression and thrombocytopenia.

sender [AS, *sendan,* to send], (in communication theory) the person by whom a message is encoded and sent.

senescence /sənes′əns/ [L, *senescere,* to grow old], growing old.

senescent /sənes′ənt/ [L, *senescere,* to grow old], aging or growing old. See also **senile. −senescence,** *n.*

Sengstaken-Blakemore tube [Robert W. Sengstaken, American neurosurgeon, b. 1923; Arthur H. Blakemore, American surgeon, b. 1897], a thick catheter having a triple lumen and two balloons, used to produce pressure by balloon tamponade to arrest hemorrhaging from esophageal varices. Attached to a tube, one balloon is inflated in the stomach and exerts pressure against the upper orifice. Similarly attached, another longer and narrower balloon exerts pressure on the walls of the esophagus. The third tube is used for withdrawing gastric contents. Also called **Blakemore-Sengstaken tube.** See also **tube.**

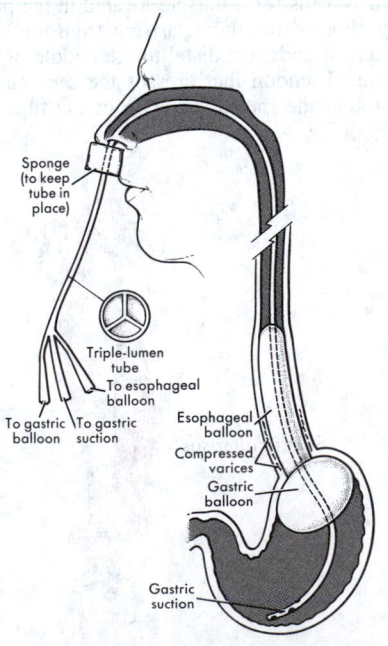

Sengstaken-Blakemore tube

senile /sē′nīl/ [L, *senilis,* old], pertaining to or characteristic of old age or the process of aging, especially the physical or mental deterioration accompanying aging. See also **aging. −senescent,** *adj.,* **senility,** *n.*

senile angioma. See **cherry angioma.**

senile cataract, a kind of cataract, associated with aging, in which a hard opacity forms in the nucleus of the lens of the eye.

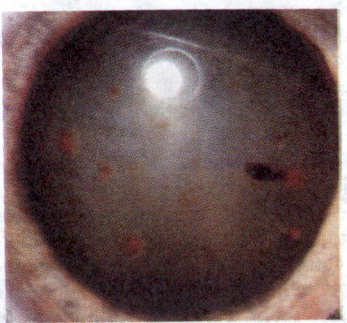

Senile cataract *(Donaldson, 1976)*

senile delirium, disorientation and mental feebleness associated with extreme age and characterized by restlessness, insomnia, aimless wandering, and less commonly, hallucination. See also **delirium, senile psychosis.**

senile dementia. See **senile psychosis.**

senile dental caries, tooth decay occurring at an advanced age. Senile dental caries is usually characterized by cavity formation in or around the cementum layer and root surfaces. See also **dental caries.**

senile endometritis, *obsolete.* endometritis in a postmenopausal woman.

senile involution, a pattern of retrograde changes occurring with advancing age and resulting in the progressive shrinking and degeneration of tissues and organs.

senile keratosis. See **actinic keratosis.**

senile memory. See **anterograde memory.**

senile nanism, dwarfism associated with progeria.

senile psychosis, an organic mental disorder of the aged, resulting from the generalized atrophy of the brain with no evidence of cerebrovascular disease. Symptoms include loss of memory, impaired judgment, decreased moral and esthetic values, inability to think abstractly, and periods of confusion, confabulation, and irritability, all of which may range from mild to severe.

senile tremor [L, *senilis,* aged + *tremor,* shaking], a tremor associated with aging.

senile vaginitis [L, *senilis,* aged + *vagina,* sheath + *itis,* inflammation], a condition of atrophy of the vagina resulting from the postmenopausal loss of estrogen secretion.

senile wart. See **actinic keratosis.**

senility /sinil′itē/ [L, *senilis,* aged], the general state of reduced mental and physical vigor associated with aging.

senna /sen′ə/ [Ar, *sana*], the dried leaflets or pods of *Cassia acutifolia* or *Cassia augustifolia,* used as a cathartic.

senopia /senō′pē·ə/ [L, *senex,* old man, *opsis,* vision], an improvement in the near vision of the aged caused by the myopia associated with increasing lenticular nuclear sclerosis. This type of sclerosis commonly leads to the development of nuclear cataracts. Also called **genontopia, second sight.**

sens-, a combining form meaning 'perception or feeling': *sensation, sensimeter, sensitinogen.*

sensate focus technique /sen′sāt/, a therapeutic program for the treatment of erectile dysfunction in males.

sensation /sensā′shən/ [L, *sentire*, to feel], **1.** a feeling, impression, or awareness of a bodily state or condition that results from the stimulation of a sensory receptor site and transmission of the nerve impulse along an afferent fiber to the brain. Kinds of sensation include **delayed sensation, epigastric sensation, primary sensation, referred sensation,** and **subjective sensation. 2.** a feeling or an awareness of a mental or emotional state, which may or may not result in response to an external stimulus.

sense [L, *sentire*], **1.** the faculty by which stimuli are perceived and conditions outside of and within the body are distinguished and evaluated. The major senses are sight, hearing, smell, taste, touch, and pressure. Other senses include hunger, thirst, pain, temperature, proprioception, and spatial, time, and visceral sensations. **2.** the ability to feel; a sensation. **3.** the capacity to understand; normal mental ability. **4.** to perceive through a sense organ.

sensible perspiration /sen′sibəl/ [L, *sensibilis*, perceptible], loss of fluid from the body through the secretory activity of the sweat glands in a quantity sufficient to be observed. Compare **insensible perspiration.**

sensitive /sen′sitiv/ [L, *sentire*, to feel], **1.** able to perceive and transmit a sensation or stimulus. **2.** affected by low concentrations of antimicrobial drugs, said of microorganisms. **3.** abnormally susceptible to a subject, such as a drug or foreign protein.

sensitive volume [L, *sentire* + *volumen*, paper roll], (in NMR imaging) the region of the object from which an NMR signal will preferentially be acquired because of strong magnetic field inhomogeneity elsewhere. The effect can be enhanced by use of a shaped rf (radio frequency) field that is strongest in the sensitive region.

sensitivity /sen′sitiv′itē/ [L, *sentire*], **1.** capacity to feel, transmit, or react to a stimulus. **2.** susceptibility to a substance, such as a drug or an antigen. See also **allergy, hypersensitivity. –sensitive,** *adj.*

sensitivity test, a laboratory method for testing the effectiveness of antibiotics. It is usually done on organisms known to be potentially resistant to antibiotic therapy in vitro. A report of 'resistant' means the antibiotic is not effective in inhibiting the growth of a pathogen, whereas use of an effective antibiotic results in a 'sensitive' report.

sensitivity training group, a group that offers members a supportive atmosphere in which to experiment with and alter behavioral patterns and interpersonal reactions. The focus of sensitivity training is on learning what occurs during group interactions, testing and refining new behavioral responses in light of the reactions they evoke, and applying those responses to situations outside the group setting. Also called **T group.** See also **encounter group, psychotherapy.**

sensitization /sen′sitīzā′shən/ [L, *sentire* + Gk, *izein*, to cause], **1.** an acquired reaction in which specific antibodies develop in response to an antigen. This is deliberately caused in immunization by injecting a disease-causing or-

ganism that has been altered in such a way that it is no longer infectious yet remains able to cause the production of antibodies to fight the disease. Allergic reactions are hypersensitivity reactions that result from excess sensitization to a foreign protein. **2.** a photodynamic method of destroying microorganisms by inserting into a solution substances, such as fluorescing dyes, that absorb visible light and emit energy at wavelengths destructive to the organism. **3.** *nontechnical.* anaphylaxis. **–sensitize,** *v.*

sensitized /sen′sitīzd/, pertaining to tissues that have been made susceptible to antigenic substances. See also **allergy.**

sensitized vaccine [L, *sentire*, to feel + *vaccinus*, of a cow], a vaccine that is prepared by suspending microorganisms in their own homologous immune serum.

sensorimotor /sen′sərēmō′tər/ [L, *sentire*, to feel + *mover*], pertaining to both sensory and motor nerve functions.

sensorimotor phase [L, *sentire* + *motor*, mover], the developmental phase of childhood, encompassing the period from birth to 2 years of age, according to piagetian psychology.

sensorimotor therapy, therapy that is designed to enhance the integration of reflex phenomena and the emergence of voluntary motor behaviors concerned with posture and locomotion.

sensorineural /sen′sərēnoor′əl/ [L, *sentire*, to feel; Gk, *neuron*], pertaining to sensory nerves.

sensorineural hearing loss [L, *sentire* + Gk, *neuron*, nerve], a form of hearing loss in which sound is conducted normally through the external and middle ear but a defect in the inner ear or auditory nerve results in hearing loss. Sound discrimination may or may not be affected. Amplification of the sound with a hearing aid will help many people with sensorineural hearing loss, but others have an intolerance to loud noises, and thus hearing aids must be adjusted properly to avoid discomfort. Compare **conductive hearing loss.**

sensorium /sensôr′ē·əm/, (in psychology) the part of the consciousness that includes the special sensory perceptive powers and their central correlation and integration in the brain. A clear sensorium conveys the presence of a reasonably accurate memory together with a correct orientation for time, place, and person.

sensory /sen′sərē/ [L, *sentire* to feel], **1.** pertaining to sensation. **2.** pertaining to a part or all of the body's sensory nerve network.

sensory apraxia. See **ideational apraxia.**

sensory area [L, *sentire*, to feel + *area*, space], the regions of the cerebral cortex that receive impulses from sensory nerves, including thalamic, nucleic, and parietal lobes.

sensory-based language, the use of nonverbal behavior in neurolinguistic communication. Examples include puzzled expressions, scowling, and finger-pointing.

sensory deficit, a defect in the function of one or more of the senses.

sensory deprivation [L, *sentire* + ME, *depriven*, to deprive; L, *atio*, process], an involuntary loss of physical awareness caused by detachment from external sensory stimuli. Such deprivation often results in psychologic disorders, such as panic, mental confusion, depression, and hallucinations. Sensory deprivation may be associated with various handicaps and conditions, such as blindness, heavy sedation, and prolonged isolation.

sensory end organ [L, *sentire,* to feel; AS, *ende;* Gk, *organon,* instrument], any of the specialized nerve endings devoted to detection of specific environmental stimuli, such as smell, sight, hearing, temperature, or touch.

sensory integration, the organization of sensory input for use, a perception of the body or environment, an adaptive response, a learning process, or the development of some neural function.

sensory integrative dysfunction, a disorder or irregularity in brain function that makes sensory integration difficult. Many, but not all, learning disorders stem from sensory integrative dysfunctions.

sensory integrative therapy, therapy that involves sensory stimulation and adaptive responses to it according to a child's neurologic needs. Treatment usually involves full body movements that provide vestibular, proprioceptive, and tactile stimulation. It usually does not include desk activities, speech training, reading lessons, or training in specific perceptual or motor skills. The goal is to improve the brain's ability to process and organize sensations.

sensory nerve, a nerve consisting of afferent fibers that conduct sensory impulses from the periphery of the body to the brain or spinal cord via the dorsal spinal roots.

sensory nucleus of trigeminal nerve, a collection of nerve cells in the pons that serve as the main nucleus for reception of tactile fibers of the trigeminal area.

sensory overload, a condition in which the central nervous system receives much more sound, visual, or other environmental stimuli per time frame than can be processed effectively. A person in a modern urban environment is more likely to experience this condition, and it has been suggested that the defensive personality of some urbanites reflects an unconscious effort to screen out excessive sensory inputs.

sensory pathway [L, *sentire,* to feel; AS, *paeth* + *weg*], the route followed by a sensory nerve impulse from an end organ to a reflex center in the brain or spinal cord.

sensory/perceptual alterations (visual, auditory, kinesthetic, gustatory, tactile, olfactory) /pərsep′choo·əl/, a nursing diagnosis accepted by the Fourth National Conference on the Classification of Nursing Diagnoses. It is defined as a state in which an individual experiences a change in the amount or patterning of incoming stimuli accompanied by a diminished, exaggerated, distorted, or impaired response to such stimuli. The defining characteristics of the disturbance include disorientation; change in the ability to abstract, conceptualize, or solve problems; change in behavior and in sensory acuity; restlessness; irritability; inappropriate response to stimuli; lack of concentration; rapid mood changes; exaggerated emotional responses; noncompliance; motor incoordination; and hallucination. Other possible defining characteristics are complaints of fatigue, changes in posture and muscular tension, and inappropriate responses. Related factors include excessive or insufficient environmental stimulation, involving therapeutic restrictions, such as isolation, intensive care, or traction; those socially related, such as institutionalization, excess age, mental illness, or mental retardation; changes in the reception, transmission, or integration of stimuli, because of neurologic disease or trauma, altered status of the sense organs, the inability to communicate, sleep deprivation, or pain; endogenous or exogenous chemical alteration in the perception of stimuli; or psychologic stress or disturbance. See also **nursing diagnosis.**

sensory-perceptual overload, a state in which the volume and intensity of various stimuli overcome the ability of the individual to discriminate among the varying stimuli. See also **sensory-perceptual alterations.**

sensory receptor [L, *sentire,* to feel + *recipere,* to receive], a specialized nerve ending that, when stimulated, initiates an afferent or sensory nerve impulse.

sensory root [L, *sentire,* to feel], the proximal end of a dorsal afferent nerve as it is attached to the spinal cord.

sensory threshold [L, *sentire,* to feel; AS, *therscold*], the point at which increasing stimuli trigger the start of an afferent nerve impulse. Absolute threshold is the lowest point at which response to a stimulus can be perceived.

sensual /sen′shoo·əl/ [L, *sensualis*], pertaining to a great interest in sex, food, or other sensory satisfying activities.

sentient /sen′shənt/ [L, *sentire,* to feel], possessing sensitivity or powers of sensation and perception.

sentinel gland /sen′tinəl/ [Fr, *sentinelle;* L, *glans,* acorn], a node or growth that is associated with the presence of a nearby tumor or ulcer. An example is a supraclavicular node with cancer cells that have metastasized from an undiscovered primary cancer.

sentinel node. See **Virchow's node.**

SEP, abbreviation for **somatosensory evoked potential.**

s-EPO, abbreviation for *serum erythropoietin.*

separation anxiety /sep′ərā′shən/ [L, *separare,* to separate, *atio,* process], fear and apprehension caused by separation from familiar surroundings and significant people. The syndrome occurs commonly in an infant when separated from its mother or from its mothering figure or when it is approached by a stranger. In a separation crisis, the child goes through three distinct states. The protest stage is marked by loud cries, which can last for several days and during which the child is inconsolable. In the second phase, the child stops crying and becomes depressed, a result of increasing hopelessness, grief, and mourning. The third stage is one of detachment or denial in which the child outwardly appears to have adjusted but actually has become resigned.

separation factor. See **selectivity.**

separator /sep′ərā′ter/ [L, *separare,* to separate], an instrument for wedging teeth apart, used in the examination of proximal tooth surfaces and in finishing proximal restorations. It is stabilized against the teeth with modeling compound to prevent tissue damage.

seps-, a prefix meaning 'of or pertaining to decay': *sepsin, sepsis, sepsometer.*

sepsis /sep′sis/ [Gk, *sepein,* to become putrid], infection, contamination. Compare **asepsis.** **–septic,** *adj.*

-sepsis, a suffix meaning 'decay caused by a (specified) cause or of a (specified) sort': *colisepsis, endosepsis, typhosepsis.*

sept-, 1. a prefix meaning 'of or pertaining to the nasal septum': *septectomy, septometer, septotomy.* 2. a prefix meaning 'seven': *septigravida, septipara, septivalent.*

septa. See **septum.**

septal /sep′təl/ [L, *saeptum,* fence], pertaining to a septum.

septal cartilage. See **nasal cartilage.**

septal defect [L, *saeptum,* enclosure; *defectus,* failure], an abnormal, usually congenital defect in the wall separating two chambers of the heart. Depending on the size and the site of the defect, various amounts of oxygenated and deoxygenated blood mix, causing a decrease in the amount of oxygen carried in the blood to the peripheral tissues. Kinds of septal defects are **atrial septal defect** and **ventricular septal defect.**

septate /sep′tāt/, pertaining to a structure divided by a septum.

septic /sep′tik/ [Gk, *septikos,* putrid], pertaining to an infection with pyogenic microorganisms.

-septic, a suffix meaning 'referring to decay of a sort or associated with a (specified) cause': *aseptic, colyseptic, uroseptic.*

septic abortion [Gk, *septikos,* to become putrid], spontaneous or induced termination of a pregnancy in which the life of the mother may be threatened because of the invasion of germs into the endometrium, myometrium, and beyond, requiring immediate and intensive care, massive antibiotic therapy, evacuation of the uterus, and, often, emergency hysterectomy to prevent death from overwhelming infection and septic shock. Compare **infected abortion.** See also **criminal abortion, induced abortion.**

septic arthritis, an acute form of arthritis, characterized by bacterial inflammation of a joint caused by the spread of bacteria through the bloodstream from an infection elsewhere in the body or by contamination of a joint during trauma or surgery. The joint is stiff, painful, tender, warm, and swollen. The diagnosis is confirmed by bacteriologic identification of an organism in a specimen obtained by aspiration of the joint. Parenteral antibiotics are given to prevent destruction of the joint and are continued for several weeks after inflammation has resolved. Repeated aspiration of the joint or surgical incision and drainage may be performed to relieve pressure on the joint. Physical therapy as the joint heals is helpful to restore it to full range of motion. Also called **acute bacterial arthritis.**

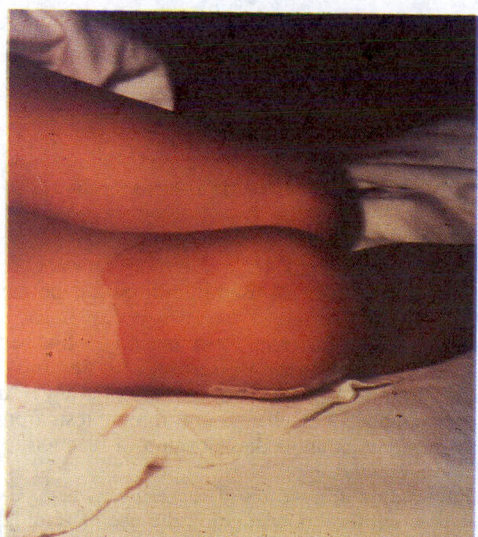

Septic arthritis *(Zitelli, 1992)*

septicemia /sep′tisē′mē·ə/ [Gk, *sepein + haima,* blood], systemic infection in which pathogens are present in the circulating bloodstream, having spread from an infection in any part of the body. It is diagnosed by culture of the blood and is vigorously treated with antibiotics. Characteristically, septicemia causes fever, chill, prostration, pain, headache, nausea, or diarrhea. Also called **blood poisoning.** Compare **bacteremia.** See also **septic shock.** −**septicemic,** *adj.*

-septicemia, -septicaemia, a combining form meaning '(condition of the) blood caused by virulent microorganisms': *pyosepticemia, streptosepticemia.*

septicemic. See **septicemia.**

septicemic plague /sep′tisē′mik/, a rapidly fatal form of bubonic plague in which septicemia with meningitis occurs before buboes have had time to form. Compare **bubonic plague, pneumonic plague.** See also **plague, Yersinia pestis.**

septic fever, an elevation of body temperature associated with infection by pathogenic microorganisms or in response to a toxin secreted by a microorganism.

septic infarct [Gk, *septikos,* putrid; L, *infarcire,* to stuff], an infected segment of dead tissue.

septic shock, a form of shock that occurs in septicemia when endotoxins or exotoxins are released from certain bacteria in the bloodstream. These toxins cause decreased vascular resistance, resulting in a drastic fall in the blood pressure. Fever, tachycardia, increased respirations, and confusion or coma also may occur. Septic shock is usually preceded by signs of severe infection, often of the genitourinary or GI system. The causative organism is most frequently gram-negative. Antibiotics, vasopressors, and intravenous fluids and volume expanders are usually given. In some cases, treatment with monoclonal antibodies may be considered. Kinds of septic shock include **toxic shock syndrome** and **bacteremic shock.** See also **shock.**

septic sore throat [Gk, *septikos,* putrid; AS, *sar, + throte*], a severe throat infection, usually caused by a streptococcus strain, resulting in fever and marked exhaustion.

septostomy /septos′təmē/, the creation of an opening in a septum by surgery.

Septra, a trademark for the antibacterial, co-trimoxazole (a 1:5 mixture of the antibacterials trimethoprim and sulfamethoxazole.)

septum /sep′təm/, *pl.* **septa** [L, *saeptum,* enclosure], a partition or wall, such as the interatrial septum that separates the atria of the heart.

septuplet /septup′lit/ [L, *septuplum,* group of seven], any one of seven children born of a single pregnancy.

sequela /sikwē′lə/, *pl.* **sequelae** [L, *sequi,* to follow], any abnormal condition that follows and is the result of a disease, treatment, or injury, such as paralysis after poliomyelitis, deafness after treatment with an ototoxic drug, or a scar after a laceration.

sequence /sē′kwəns/ [L, *sequi,* to follow], an order of arrangement of objects or events, as the sequence of peptides in a protein molecule.

sequential imaging, (in nuclear medicine) a diagnostic procedure in which a series of closely timed images of the rapidly changing distribution of an administered radioactive tracer is used to determine a physiologic process or processes within the body.

sequential line imaging, (in MR imaging) techniques in which the image is built up from successive lines through the object.

sequential multiple analysis (SMA), the biochemical examination of various substances in the blood, such as albumin, alkaline phosphatase, bilirubin, calcium, cholesterol, and others, using a computerized laboratory analyzer that produces a printout showing measured values of the substances tested. These analyses are commonly designated as **SMA-6, SMA-12,** or **SMA-18,** according to the number of blood constituents tested.

sequential pacing. See **pacing.**

sequential plane imaging, (in MR imaging) a technique in which the image of an object is built up from successive planes in the object. In various schemes, the planes are selected by oscillating gradient magnetic fields or selective excitation.

sequential point imaging, (in MR imaging) techniques in which the image is built from successive point positions in the object.

sequester /sikwes'tər/ [L, *sequestare*, to lay aside], to detach, separate, or isolate, such as a patient sequestered to prevent the spread of an infection.

sequestered antigens theory, a theory of autoimmunity, stressing the relationship between antigen exposure, immunogenic cells, and body cells, maintaining that immunologic tolerance depends on a certain degree of contact between immunologic cells and body cells and on a certain degree of antigen exposure. The theory holds that certain sequestered antigens in the brain, the lenses of the eye, and spermatozoa are isolated from the circulations of the blood and the lymph and do not contact the immune system. When body tissues are damaged, the sequestered antigens are suddenly exposed to the immune system but are not recognized as such by the body, and an autoimmune reaction results. Compare **forbidden clone theory.**

sequestered edema, edema localized in the tissues surrounding a newly created surgical wound.

sequestra. See **sequestrum.**

sequestration /sēkwestrā'shən/ [L, *sequestare*, to lay aside], **1.** the isolation of a patient or group of patients. **2.** a method of controlling hemorrhage of the head or trunk by isolating fluid in the arms and legs from the general circulation. **3.** allowing blood from the systemic circulation to perfuse a nonfunctioning part of a lung.

sequestrum /sikwes'trəm/, *pl.* **sequestra** [L, a deposit], a fragment of dead bone that is partially or entirely detached from the surrounding or adjacent healthy bone.

sequestrum forceps, a forceps with small, powerful teeth used for extracting necrotic or sharp fragments of bone from surrounding tissue.

sequoiasis /sikwoi'əsis/ [sequoia (tree) + Gk, *osis*, condition], a type of hypersensitivity pneumonitis common among workers in sawmills where redwood is processed. The antigens are the fungus *Pullularia pullulans* and species of the genus *Graphium,* found in moldy redwood sawdust. Characteristics of the acute disease include chills, fever, cough, dyspnea, anorexia, nausea, and vomiting. Symptoms of the chronic disease include productive cough, dyspnea on exertion, fatigue, and weight loss.

Ser, abbreviation for the amino acid **serine.**

Sera. See **Serum.**

Ser-Ap-Es, a trademark for an antihypertensive, fixed-combination drug containing a diuretic (hydrochlorothiazide) and antihypertensives (reserpine and hydralazine hydrochloride).

Serax, a trademark for a tranquilizer (oxazepam).

serendipity /ser'əndip'itē/ [Serendip, author Horace Walpole's mythic land of pleasant surprises], the act of accidental discovery. A number of important medications have evolved through serendipity, such as the discovery of antidepressant activity in a drug originally developed to treat tuberculosis.

Serentil, a trademark for a phenothiazine tranquilizer (mesoridazine).

serial /sir'ē·əl/ [L, *series,* in a row], pertaining to a succession, arrangement, or order of items.

serial determination [L, *series,* in a row; *determinare,* to limit], a laboratory test that is repeated at stated intervals, as in a series of repeated tests for cardiac enzymes in blood samples taken from a suspected myocardial infarction patient.

serial dilution, a laboratory technique in which a substance, such as blood serum, is decreased in concentration in a series of proportional amounts. In antibody analysis, for example, a serum sample may be distributed in a series of tubes so that each has one half of the amount of the previous tube in the series, resulting in titers of 1:5, 1:10, 1:20, and so on.

serial extraction, the extraction of selected primary teeth over a period of years, frequently ending with the removal of the first premolar teeth, to relieve crowding of the dental arches during eruption of the lateral incisors, canines, and premolars.

serial section [L, *series,* row + *sectio*], one of a number of consecutive slices of tissue.

serial speech, overlearned speech involving a series of words, such as counting or reciting days of the week.

series /sir'ēs/, *pl.* **series** /sir'ēs/ [L, in a row], a chain of objects or events arranged in a predictable order, such as the series of stages through which a mature blood cell develops.

serine (Ser) /ser'ēn/, a nonessential amino acid found in many proteins in the body. It is a precursor of the amino acids, glycine and cysteine. See also **amino acid, protein.**

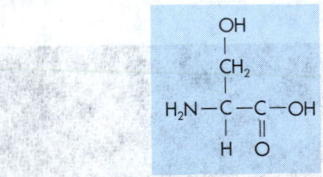

Chemical structure of serine (Seeley, 1992)

Sernylan, a trademark for a veterinary anesthetic (phencyclidine hydrochloride), used illicitly as a euphoric called **PCP.**

sero- /sir'ō-/, a combining form meaning 'of or pertaining to blood serum': *seroculture, serogenesis, serolin.*

seroconversion /-kənvur'zhən/ [L, *serum,* whey + *conversio,* turned about], a change in serologic tests from negative to positive as antibodies develop in reaction to an infection or vaccine.

serodiagnosis /-dī'əgnō'sis/ [L, *serum,* whey; Gk, *dia,* through + *gnosis,* knowledge], the use of serologic tests in the diagnosis of disease.

serofibrinous pericarditis /-fī'brinəs/ [L, *serum,* whey + *fibra,* fibrin; Gk, *peri,* near + *kardia,* heart + *itis,* inflammation], a form of fibrinous pericarditis marked by a serous exudate.

serologic /-loj'ik/ [L, *serum,* whey; Gk, *logos,* science], pertaining to the branch of medicine concerned with the study of blood sera. Also **serological.**

serological. See **serology.**

serologic diagnosis /siroloj′ik/ [L, *serum*, whey; Gk, *dia*, through, *gnosis*, knowledge], a diagnosis that is made through laboratory examination of antigen-antibody reactions in the serum. Also called **immunodiagnosis, serum diagnosis.**

serologic test [L, *serum*, whey + *testum*, crucible], any diagnostic test made with serum.

serologist /sirol′əjist/ [L, *serum*, + Gk, *logos*, science], a bacteriologist or medical technologist who prepares or supervises the preparation of serums used to diagnose and treat diseases and to immunize people against infectious diseases.

serology /sirol′əjē/ [L, *serum* + Gk, *logos*, science], the branch of laboratory medicine that studies blood serum for evidence of infection by evaluating antigen-antibody reactions in vitro. —**serologic, serological,** *adj.*

Seromycin, a trademark for a tuberculostatic (cycloserine).

seronegative /-neg′ətiv/ [L, *serum*, whey + *negare*, to deny], a serological test with negative results.

seropositive /-pos′itiv/ [L, *serum*, whey + *positivus*], a serological test with positive results.

seroprevalence /-prev′ələns/, the overall occurrence of a blood-borne disease within a defined population at one point in time. An example is HIV seroprevalence.

serosa /sirō′sə/ [L, *serum*], any serous membrane, such as the tunica serosa that lines the walls of body cavities and secretes a watery exudate.

serosanguineous /sir′ōsang·gwin′ē·əs/, (of a discharge) thin and red; composed of serum and blood. Also **serosanguinous** /sir′ōsang′gwinəs/.

serotonin /ser′ətō′nin, sir′-/ [L, *serum* + Gk, *tonos*, tone], a naturally occurring derivative of tryptophan found in platelets and in cells of the brain and the intestine. Serotonin is released from platelets on damage to the blood vessel walls. It acts as a potent vasoconstrictor. Serotonin in intestinal tissue stimulates the smooth muscle to contract. In the central nervous system, it acts as a neurotransmitter. Lysergic acid diethylamide interferes with the action of serotonin in the brain. The normal concentrations of serotonin in the urine are 0.05 to 0.2 μg/ml. Also called **5-hydroxytryptamine.**

serous [L, *serum*, whey], pertaining to, resembling, or producing serum.

serous fluid /sir′əs/ [L, *serum* + *fluere*, to flow], a fluid that has the characteristics of serum.

serous membrane, one of the many thin sheets of tissue that line closed cavities of the body, such as the pleura lining the thoracic cavity, the peritoneum lining the abdominal cavity, and the pericardium lining the sac that encloses the heart. Between the visceral layer of serous membrane covering various organs and the parietal layer lining the cavity containing such organs is a potential space moistened by serous fluid. The fluid reduces the friction of the structures covered by the serous membrane, such as the lungs, which move against the thoracic walls in respiration. Compare **mucous membrane, skin, synovial membrane.**

Serpasil, a trademark for an antihypertensive (reserpine).

Serpasil-Apresoline, a trademark for a fixed-combination drug containing two antihypertensives (reserpine and hydralazine hydrochloride).

Serpasil-Esidrix, a trademark for an antihypertensive fixed-combination drug containing a diuretic (hydrochlorothiazide) and an antihypertensive (reserpine).

serpent ulcer /sur′pənt/ [L, *serpens*, snake], an ulceration of the skin that heals in one area while extending to another. Also called **serpiginous ulcer.**

-serpine, a combining form for *Rauwolfia alkaloid* derivatives.

Serratia /serā′shə/ [L, *serra*, saw teeth], a genus of motile, gram-negative bacilli capable of causing infection in humans, including bacteremia, pneumonia, and urinary tract infections. *Serratia* organisms are frequently acquired in hospitals. See also **nosocomial infection.**

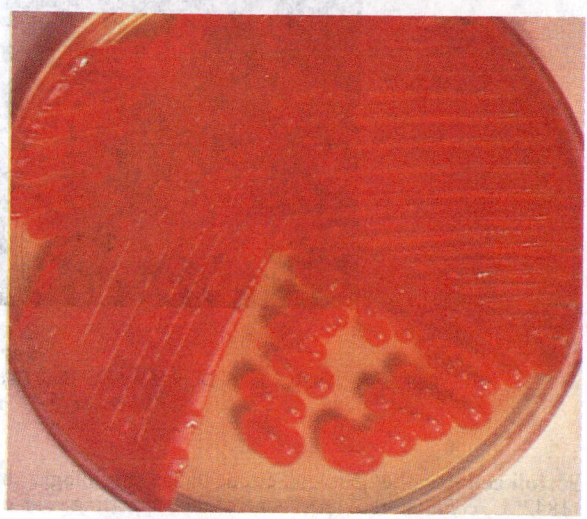

Serratia marcescens (Baron, 1990)

serratus anterior /serā′təs/ [L, *serra*, saw teeth], a thin muscle of the chest wall extending from the ribs under the arm to the scapula. Arising from the outer surface and upper border of the first eight or nine ribs, it inserts into the medial angle, the vertebral border, and the inferior angle of the scapula. It is innervated by the long thoracic nerve of the brachial plexus that contains fibers of the fifth, the sixth, and the seventh cervical nerves. It acts to rotate the scapula and to raise the shoulder, as in full flexion and abduction of the arm. Compare **pectoralis major, pectoralis minor, subclavius.**

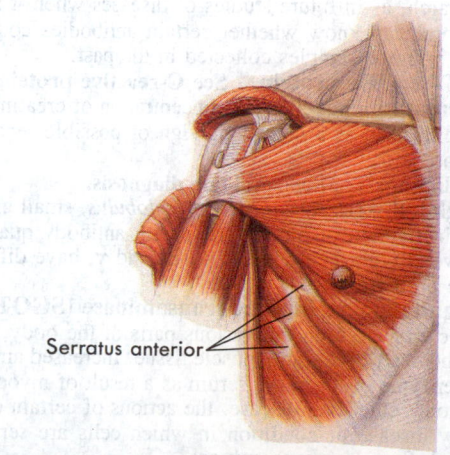

Serratus anterior

Serratus anterior (Thibodeau, 1993/John V Hagen)

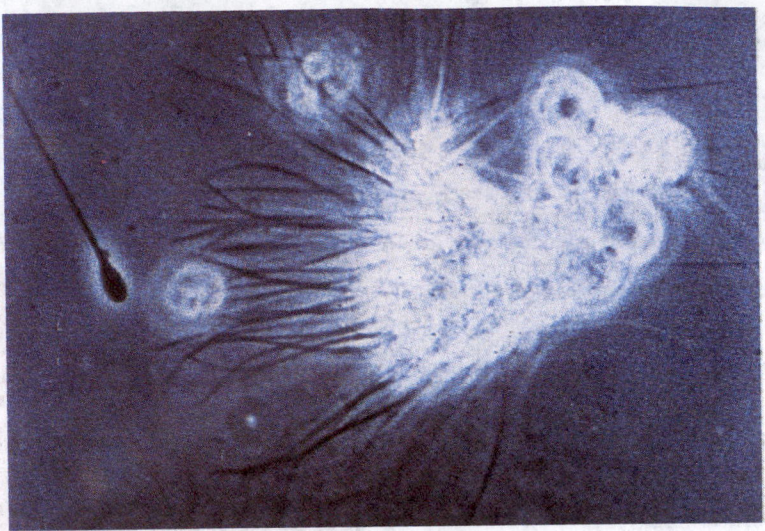

Sertoli cell
(Erlandsen, 1992/Courtesy Dr. Richard Blandau, Department of Biological Structure, University of Washington School of Medicine, Seattle, Washington)

Sertoli cell /sertō′lē/ [Enrico Sertoli, Italian physiologist, b. 1842; L, *cella*, storeroom], one of the supporting cells of the seminiferous tubules of the testes. The cytoplasm of the cells contain spermatids.

Sertoli-Leydig cell tumor. See **arrhenoblastoma.**

serum /sir′əm/, *pl.* **sera** [L, whey], **1.** also called **blood serum.** any serous fluid that moistens the surfaces of serous membranes. **2.** any clear, watery fluid that has been separated from its more solid elements, such as the exudate from a blister. **3.** the clear, thin, and sticky fluid portion of the blood that remains after coagulation. Serum contains no blood cells, platelets, or fibrinogen. **4.** a vaccine or toxoid prepared from the serum of a hyperimmune donor for prophylaxis against a particular infection or poison.

serum albumin, a major protein in blood plasma, important in maintaining the osmotic pressure of the blood.

serum bank, a facility for the storage of frozen samples of blood serum. The specimens are used mainly for medical research, as in future studies of diseases when it might be important to know whether certain antibodies could be present in blood samples collected in the past.

serum C-reactive protein. See **C-reactive protein.**

serum creatinine level, the concentration of creatinine in the serum, used as a diagnostic sign of possible renal impairment.

serum diagnosis. See **serologic diagnosis.**

serum globulin [L, *serum*, whey + *globulus*, small globe], a protein fraction of blood serum with antibody qualities. The several types of fractions, α, β, and γ, have different specific properties.

serum glutamic oxaloacetic transaminase (SGOT), a catalytic enzyme found in various parts of the body, especially the heart, liver, and muscle tissue. Increased amounts of the enzyme occur in the serum as a result of myocardial infarction, acute liver disease, the actions of certain drugs, and any disease or condition in which cells are seriously damaged. See also **transaminase.**

serum glutamic pyruvic transaminase (SGPT), a catalytic enzyme normally found in high concentration in the liver. Greater than normal amounts in the serum indicate liver damage. See also **transaminase.**

serum hepatitis. See **hepatitis B.**

serum osmolality [L, *serum*, whey; Gk, *osmos*, impulse], pertaining to the osmotic concentration of blood serum, expressed in terms of ions of solute per unit of solution.

serum protein [L, *serum*, whey; Gk, *proteios*, first rank], any of the proteins in blood serum. See also **serum globulin.**

serum sickness, an immunologic disorder that may occur 2 to 3 weeks after the administration of an antiserum. Caused by an antibody reaction to an antigen in the donor serum, the condition is characterized by fever, splenomegaly, swollen lymph nodes, skin rash, and joint pain. Treatment is symptomatic and supportive and may include corticosteroids. See also **angioneurotic edema, antigen-antibody reaction, Arthus reaction.**

serum urea nitrogen. See **urea nitrogen.**

service of process /sur′vis/ [L, *servus*, a slave; *processus*, going forth], (in law) the delivery of a writ, summons, or complaint to a defendant. Once delivered or left with the party for whom it is intended, it is said to have been served. The original of the document is shown; a copy is served. Service of process gives reasonable notice to allow the person to appear, testify, and be heard in court.

sesamoid /ses′əmoid/ [Gk, *sesamon* + *eidos*, form], nodular objects having the shape and size of sesame seeds. See **sesamoid bone.**

sesamoid bone [Gk, *sesamon*, sesame, *eidos* form], any one of numerous small, round, bony masses embedded in certain tendons that may be subjected to compression and tension. The largest sesamoid bone is the patella, which is embedded in the tendon of the quadriceps femoris at the knee.

sesqui-, a combining form meaning 'one and one half': *sesquibasic, sesquibo, sesquihora.*

sessile /ses'əl/ [L, *sessilis,* sitting], **1.** (in biology) attached by a base rather than by a stalk or a peduncle, such as a leaf that is attached directly to its stem. **2.** permanently connected.

set, a predisposition to behave in a certain way.

set-, a combining form meaning 'of or related to a bristle': *setaceous, setiferous, seton.*

settlement [AS, *setlan,* to put in place], (in law) an agreement made between parties to a suit before a judgment is rendered by a court.

setup [AS, *settan,* to set, *up,* on high], **1.** an arrangement of artificial teeth on a trial denture base. **2.** a laboratory procedure in which teeth are removed from a plaster cast and repositioned in wax, used as a diagnostic procedure or to produce a mold for a positioner appliance.

seventh cranial nerve. See **facial nerve.**

severe combined immunodeficiency disease (SCID) /sivēr'/ [L, *servus,* slave], an abnormal condition characterized by the complete absence or by the marked deficiency of B cells and T cells with the consequent lack of humoral immunity and cell-mediated immunity. This disease occurs as an X-linked recessive disorder affecting only males and as an autosomal recessive disorder affecting both males and females. It results in a pronounced susceptibility to infection and is usually fatal. The precise cause of SCID is not known, but research indicates it may be caused by a cytogenic dysfunction of the embryonic stem cells in differentiating B cells and T cells. The affected individual consequently has a very small thymus and little or no protection against infection.

■ OBSERVATIONS: Pronounced susceptibility to infection usually becomes obvious in affected individuals 3 to 6 months after birth, when maternal immunoglobulin reserves are diminishing. Diagnosis is difficult because B cell immunity dysfunction is hard to detect in any individual until 5 months after birth, when immunoglobulin levels should be 1% of normal. Infants with SCID commonly fail to thrive and develop a variety of complications, such as sepsis, watery diarrhea, persistent pulmonary infections, and common viral infections that are often fatal. Some infants with SCID develop mild infections and low-grade fevers that last for several months, while the infant uses maternal immunoglobulin stores, and then flare into serious, fatal conditions when maternal antibodies are totally depleted, usually within 1 year. Some of the more obvious symptoms after the infant has used most of the maternal immunoglobulin stores are cyanosis, rapid respirations, and normal chest sounds with an abnormal chest x-ray picture. Maternal IgG is persistent, and gram-negative infections in the infant usually do not appear until after the sixth month of life. Normal infants less than 5 months of age have very small amounts of IgM and IgA, and normal IgG levels only reflect maternal IgG. The combination of several symptoms may confirm the diagnosis of SCID. Such symptoms include the absence or the severe reduction of T cell and B cell immunity, a lymph node biopsy that shows no lymphocytes, plasma cells, or lymphoid follicles, and no skin reaction to swabbing with dinitrochlorobenzene. Most infants with SCID die from severe infection within 1 year after birth.

■ INTERVENTIONS: Treatment of SCID seeks to develop the immune system and to prevent infection. The only satisfactory treatment available to correct immunodeficiency is his-tocompatible bone marrow transplant, but such a procedure may cause a graft-versus-host reaction, thus increasing the risk of infection and fatal consequences. Placing the infant with SCID in a completely sterile environment for a long time is a method of treatment that has prolonged the lives of some affected individuals, but this option does not prove successful if the infant involved has already had recurring infections.

■ NURSING CONSIDERATIONS: Supportive treatment is the primary approach in caring for the SCID patient. Nurses commonly try to promote an encouraging atmosphere of growth and development while providing the parents of SCID infants with spiritual and psychologic support in the face of the nearly inevitable early death of the patient. The infant must remain in strict protective isolation and benefits from frequent parental visits, gifts of toys, and frequent nursing attention. Toys brought to an infant in protective isolation should be the kind that can be easily sterilized.

Sever's disease. See **calcaneal epiphysitis.**

Sevin, a trademark for carbaryl, a widely used carbamate insecticide that causes reversible inhibition of cholinesterase. Although less toxic than parathion, carbaryl, when concentrated, may produce skin irritation and systemic poisoning characterized by nausea, vomiting, cramps, diarrhea, diaphoresis, excessive salivation, dyspnea, weakness, loss of coordination, and slurred speech; large doses may cause coma and death. Carbaryl on the skin is promptly removed by washing with water. Treatment of systemic poisoning includes the immediate intravenous or intramuscular injection of 1 to 4 mg of atropine sulfate, the administration of artificial respiration and oxygen, gastric lavage, and intravenous isotonic saline to correct dehydration.

sex [L, *sexus,* sex], **1.** a classification of male or female based on many criteria, among them anatomic and chromosomal characteristics. **2.** coitus. Compare **gender.**

sex-, a prefix meaning 'six': *sexdigitate, sexivalent, sextan.*

sex chromatin, a densely staining mass within the nucleus of all nondividing cells of normal mammalian females. It represents the facultative heterochromatin of the inactivated X chromosome. Examination of cells obtained by amniocentesis for the presence or absence of sex chromatin is a technique used for determining the sex of a baby before birth. Sex chromatin is also found as a drumsticklike mass attached to one of the nuclear lobes in polymorphonuclear leukocytes in normal females. Also called **Barr body.** See also **Lyon hypothesis.**

sex chromosome, a chromosome that is responsible for the sex determination of offspring; it carries genes that transmit sex-linked traits and conditions. In humans and other mammals there are two distinct sex chromosomes, the X and the Y chromosomes, which are unequally paired and appear in females in the XX combination and in males as XY. Compare **autosome.**

sex chromosome mosaic, an individual or organism whose cells contain variant chromosomal numbers involving the X or Y chromosomes. Such variations are found in most of the syndromes associated with sex chromosome aberrations, primarily Turner's syndrome, and may be caused by nondisjunction of the chromosomes during the second meiotic division of gametogenesis or by some error in chromosome distribution during cell division of the fertilized ovum. Sex chromosome mosaics often have sexual abnormalities, but because of the sex hormones the overall phenotype is uniform and not mosaic in external characteristics, as in certain animals and insects. See also **intersexuality.**

sex-controlled.   See **sex-influenced.**

sex determination [L, *sexus*, sex + *determinare*],   an examination of the cellular differences between male and female organisms, to find the XY chromosome combination in genetic male or the Barr body in genetic female chromosomes. Whole body differences include secondary sexual characteristics and skeletal variations.

sex factor.   See **F factor.**

sex-influenced,   of or pertaining to an autosomal genetic trait or condition, such as patterned baldness or gout, that in one sex is expressed phenotypically in both homozygotes and heterozygotes, whereas in the other sex a phenotypic effect is produced in homozygotes only. Also called **sex-controlled.**

sexism /sek'sizəm/,   a belief that one sex is superior to the other and that the superior sex has endowments, rights, prerogatives, and status greater than those of the inferior sex. Sexism results in discrimination in all areas of life and acts as a limiting factor in educational, professional, and psychologic development. **–sexist,** *n., adj.*

sex-limited,   of or pertaining to an autosomal genetic trait or condition that is expressed phenotypically in only one sex, although the genes for it may be carried by both sexes. Such traits or conditions are typically influenced by hormonal or environmental conditions.

sex-linked,   pertaining to genes or to the normal or abnormal characteristics or conditions they transmit. The genes are carried on the sex chromosomes, particularly the X chromosome. See also **sex-linked disorder, X-linked inheritance, Y-linked.** **–sex linkage,** *n.*

sex-linked disorder,   any disease or abnormal condition that is determined by the sex chromosomes or a defective gene on a sex chromosome. These may involve a deviation in the number of either the X or Y chromosomes, as occurs in Turner's syndrome and Klinefelter's syndrome, most occurrences of which are a result of nondisjunction during meiosis. Such aberrations in the number of sex chromosomes do not produce the severe clinical effects that are associated with autosomal aberrations, although some degree of mental deficiency is usually apparent. Other sex-linked disorders are transmitted by single gene defects carried on the X chromosome. X-linked dominant mutants, such as hypophosphatemic vitamin D resistant rickets, are rare, and males are more seriously affected than females. In inheritance patterns, X-linked dominant conditions are transmitted by affected males to all of their daughters but none of their sons, by affected heterozygous females to one half of their children regardless of sex, and by affected homozygous females to all of their children. X-linked recessive mutants are more common and are responsible for such traits and disorders as color blindness, ocular albinism, the Xg blood types, hemophilia, Duchenne muscular dystrophy, and inborn errors of metabolism. Such conditions are always transmitted by females so that those predominantly affected are males, because they have only one X chromosome and all genes, whether recessive or dominant, are expressed. Affected males never transmit the condition to their sons, but all of their daughters will be carriers; they, in turn, will transmit the trait to one half of their sons. Occasionally, heterozygous females for X-linked recessive disorders show varying degrees of expression, but never as severe as those of the affected male. There are no known clinically significant traits or conditions associated with the genes on the Y

chromosome; its only known function is triggering the development of male characteristics.

sex-linked ichthyosis,   a congenital skin disorder characterized by large, thick, dry scales that are dark in color and that cover the neck, scalp, ears, face, trunk, and flexor surfaces of the body, such as the folds of the arms and the backs of the knees. It is transmitted by females as an X-linked recessive trait and appears only in males. The condition is managed by topical applications of emollients and the use of keratolytic agents to facilitate removal of the scales. Also called **X-linked ichthyosis.** See also **ichthyosis.**

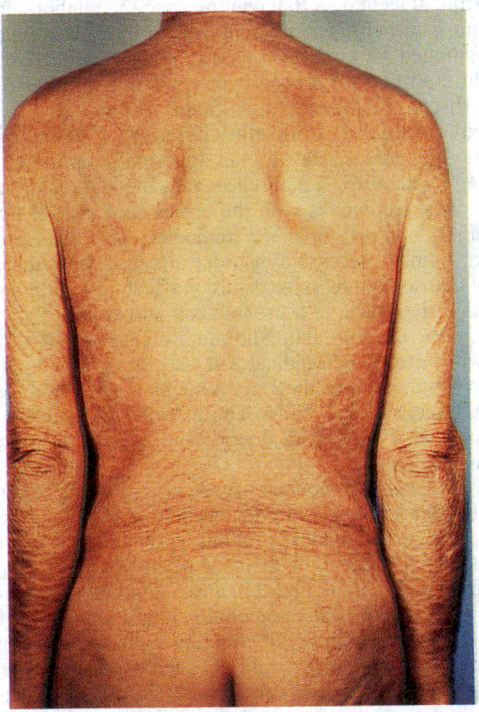

Sex-linked ichthyosis *(Zitelli, 1992)*

sex mosaic.   See **sex chromosome mosaic.**

sex role,   the expectations held by society regarding what behavior is appropriate or inappropriate for each sex.

sex surrogate [L, *sexus* + *surrogare*, substitute],   in sex therapy, a professional substitute trained to help the patient overcome inhibitions. Also called **surrogate partner.**

sextuplet /seks'tup'lit/ [L, *sextus*, six],   one of six children born of a single pregnancy.

sexual /sek'shŌŌ·əl/,   of or pertaining to sex.

sexual abuse,   the sexual mistreatment of another person by fondling, rape, or forced participation in unnatural sex acts or other perverted behavior. Victims tend to experience a traumatic feeling of loss of control of themselves.

sexual assault,   the forcible perpetration of an act of sexual contact on the body of another person, male or female, without his or her consent. Legal criteria vary among different communities.

sexual aversion disorder,   a persistent or extreme aversion to or avoidance of all or nearly all genital sexual contact with a partner.

sexual dwarf, an adult dwarf whose genital organs are normally developed.

sexual dysfunction, a nursing diagnosis accepted by the Fourth National Conference on the Classification of Nursing Diagnoses. It is defined as the state in which an individual experiences a change in sexual function that is viewed as unsatisfying, unrewarding, or inadequate. The defining characteristics of the condition include a statement by the client of the perceived dysfunction, a physical alteration or limitation imposed by disease or treatment, a reported inability to achieve sexual satisfaction, an alteration in the sexual relationship with the partner, and a change in interest in oneself or in others. Related factors include a biologic, psychologic, or social alteration in sexuality caused by an ineffectual or absent role model, physical abuse, psychosocial abuse, as in a harmful relationship, misinformation or lack of information, a conflict in values, a lack of privacy, or an alteration in body structure or function, as may result from pregnancy, recent childbirth, drugs, surgery, congenital anomalies, or trauma. See also **female sexual dysfunction, male sexual dysfunction, nursing diagnosis.**

sexual fantasy, mental images of an erotic nature that can lead to sexual arousal.

sexual generation, reproduction by the union of male and female gametes.

sexual harassment, an aggressive, sexually motivated act of physical or verbal violation of a person over whom the aggressor has some power. Sexual harassment of women in the workplace is against the law, because it represents an abridgment of the victim's right to equal opportunity, privacy, and freedom from assault. Sexual harassment may be heterosexual or, as is common in prison, homosexual.

sexual health [L, *sexus;* AS, *haelth*], a condition defined by the World Health Organization as freedom from sexual diseases or disorders and a capacity to enjoy and control sexual behavior without fear, shame, or guilt.

sexual history, (in a patient record) the portion of the patient's personal history concerned with sexual function and dysfunction. A sexual history is particularly important in gathering data from a patient who has a disease of the reproductive tract, who experiences sexual dysfunction, or who requests contraception, abortion, or sterilization. The extent of the history varies with the patient's age and condition and the reason for securing the history. A short sexual history is recommended as part of every complete physical examination. The therapist needs a detailed sexual history to understand the patient's complaint and to plan treatment. It may include age at onset of sexual intercourse, the kind and frequency of sexual activity, and the satisfaction derived from it.

sexual hormones, chemical substances produced in the body that cause specific regulatory effects on the activity of organs of the reproductive system.

sexual intercourse. See **coitus.**

sexuality /sek′shoo·al′itē/, 1. the sum of the physical, functional, and psychologic attributes that are expressed by one's gender identity and sexual behavior, whether or not related to the sex organs or to procreation. 2. the genital characteristics that distinguish male from female.

sexuality patterns, altered, a nursing diagnosis accepted by the Seventh National Conference on the Classification of Nursing Diagnoses. The diagnosis describes the state in which an individual expresses concern regarding his or her sexuality. The major defining characteristics include reported difficulties, limitations, or changes in sexual behaviors or activities. Related factors include a knowledge or skill deficit about alternative responses to health-related transitions or altered body functions or structure (illness or medical); lack of privacy; lack of a significant other; ineffective or absent role model; conflicts with sexual orientation or variant preferences; fear of pregnancy or of acquiring sexually transmitted disease; and an impaired relationship with a significant other. See also **nursing diagnosis.**

sexually deviant personality /sek′shoo·əlē/, a sexual behavior that differs significantly from what is considered normal for a society. Either the quality or object of the sexual drives may be at variance with the accepted cultural norms for adults.

sexually transmitted disease (STD), a contagious disease usually acquired by sexual intercourse or genital contact. These diseases are the most common communicable diseases, and the incidence has risen over the past 2 decades despite improved methods of diagnosis and treatment. Historically, the five venereal diseases were gonorrhea, syphilis, chancroid, granuloma inguinale, and lymphogranuloma venereum. To these have been added scabies, herpes genitalis and anorectal herpes and warts, pediculosis, trichomoniasis, genital candidiasis, molluscum contagiosum, nonspecific urethritis, chlamydial infections, cytomegalovirus, and AIDS. Also called **venereal disease.** See also specific diseases.

sexual mores, socially acceptable sexual behavior, usually based on fixed, morally binding customs governing sexual behaviors that are harmful to others or the group, such as rape, incest, and sexual abuse of children.

sexual orientation, the clear, persistent desire of a person for affiliation with one sex rather than the other. See also **homosexuality, heterosexuality.**

sexual psychopath, an individual whose sexual behavior is openly perverted, antisocial, and criminal. See also **antisocial personality disorder.**

sexual reassignment, a change in the gender identity of a person by legal, surgical, hormonal, or social means.

sexual reflex, (in males) a reflex in which tactile or cerebral stimulation results in penile erection, priapism, or ejaculation. Also called **genital reflex.**

sexual reproduction [L, *sexus,* sex + *re, producere,* to produce], replication of an organism by the formation of gametes. Generally, this requires the fusion of male spermatozoa and female ova, but parthenogenesis is an exception.

sexual response cycle, the four phases of biologic sexual response: excitement, plateau, orgasm, and resolution.

sexual sadism. See **sadism.**

sexual selection, the theory that mates are chosen according to the attraction of or preference for certain characteristics, such as coloration or behavior patterns, so that eventually only those particular traits appear in succeeding generations. The theory explains the wide variety of sexual characteristics among the various species.

sexual tasks, specific skills learned in various phases of development in the life cycle continuum to allow an adult to function normally in the sexual realm.

sexual therapist, a health-care professional with specialized knowledge, skill, and competence in assisting individuals who experience sexual difficulties.

sexual therapy, a type of counseling that aids in the resolution of pathologic conditions so that a healthy sexuality can be maintained.

sfc, abbreviation for *spinal fluid count.*

SFD, abbreviation for **small for dates.** See **small for gestational age infant.**

SGA, abbreviation for **small for gestational age.** See **small for gestational age infant.**

SGOT, abbreviation for **serum glutamic oxaloacetic transaminase.**

SGPT, abbreviation for **serum glutamic pyruvic transaminase.**

shadow /shad′ō/ [AS, *sceadu*], (in psychology) an archetype that represents the unacceptable aspects and components of behavior.

shadow cells. See **ghost cells.**

shaken baby syndrome, a condition of whiplash-type injuries, ranging from bruises on the arms and trunk to retinal hemorrhages, coma, or convulsions, as observed in infants and children who have been violently shaken. This form of child abuse often results in intracranial bleeding from tearing of cerebral blood vessels. Physicians are required by law to report cases of suspected child abuse and are granted immunity from liability for filing such reports.

shared governance, an organized, systematic approach to decision making that enables all levels of nurses to participate in the resolution of clinical, professional, and administrative practice issues.

shared paranoid disorder [AS, *scearan*, to shear], a psychopathologic condition characterized by identical manifestations of the same mental disorder, usually ideas, in two closely associated or related people. Also called **folie à deux** /fôlē′ädœ′, -dā′, -dōo′/.

shared services, administrative, clinical, or other service functions that are common to two or more hospitals or other health care facilities and that are used jointly or cooperatively by them.

shark skin. See **dyssebacea.**

Sharpey's fiber [William Sharpey, English anatomist, b. 1802], (in dentistry) any one of the many collagenous bundles of fibers of the periodontal ligament that have become embedded in the cementum during its formation.

sharps, any needles, scalpels, or other articles that could cause wounds or punctures to personnel handling them. See also **needle-stick injuries.**

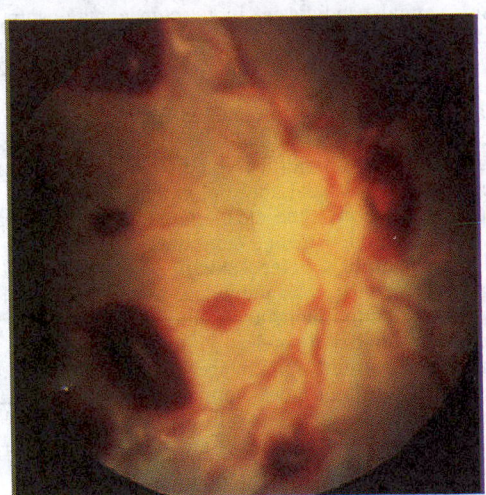

Retinal hemorrhages seen in shaken baby syndrome
(Zitelli, 1992/Courtesy Dr. Stephen Lusdwig, Children's Hospital of Philadelphia)

shake test, a "foam" test for fetal lung maturity. It is more rapid than determination of the L/S ratio.

shaking palsy. See **parkinsonism.**

shallow breathing /shal′ō/ [ME, *schalowe*, little depth], a respiration pattern marked by slow, shallow, and generally ineffective inspirations and expirations. It is usually caused by drugs and indicates depression of the medullary respiratory centers.

shaping [AS, *scieppan*, to shape], a procedure used for conditioning a person undergoing behavior therapy to develop new behavioral responses. Initially, any act remotely resembling the desired behavior is reinforced; gradually, the criterion is made more stringent until the desired response is attained.

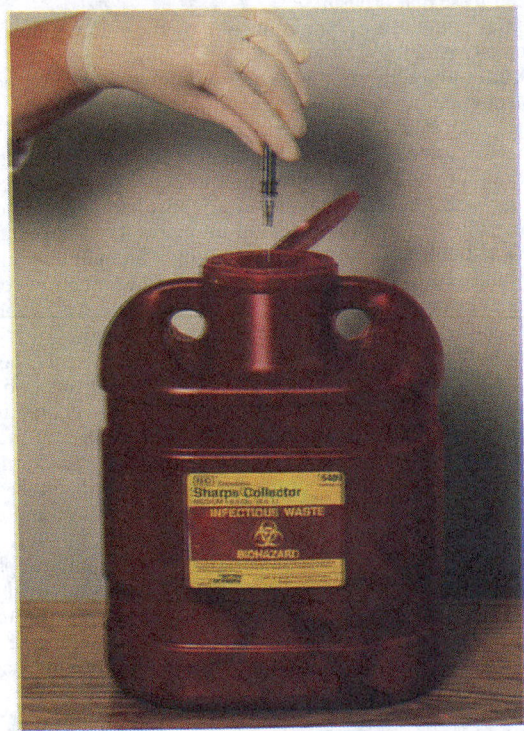

Sharps container (Potter, 1993)

shaving stroke [AS, *scafan*, to shave; *strican*, to stroke], a phase of the working stroke of a periodontal curet, used for smoothing or planing a tooth or tooth root surface.

SHCC, abbreviation for **Statewide Health Coordinating Committee.**

shear /shir/ [AS, *scearan*, to cut], an applied force or pressure exerted against the surface and layers of the skin as tissues slide in opposite but parallel planes.

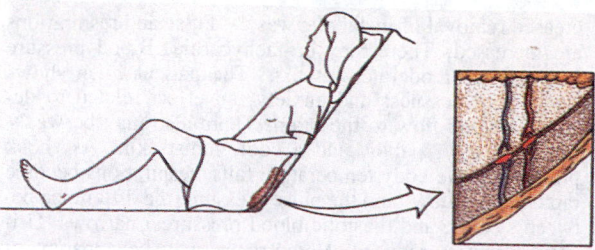

Shearing force (Potter, 1993)

shearling /shir'ling/, a sheepskin placed on a bed to help prevent decubitus ulcers.

sheath /shēth/ [AS, *scaeth*], a tubular structure that surrounds an organ or any other part of the body, such as the sheath of the rectus abdominis muscle or the sheath of Schwann, which covers various nerve fibers.

sheath of Schwann [AS, *scaeth;* Friedrich Theodor Schwann, German anatomist, b. 1810], a neurilemma sheath of nucleated cells enclosing a nerve fiber.

Sheehan's syndrome [Harold L. Sheehan, English pathologist, b. 1900], a postpartum condition of pituitary necrosis and hypopituitarism after circulatory collapse resulting from uterine hemorrhaging.

sheep cell agglutination test (SCAT), a test for the presence of the rheumatoid factor in blood serum, using red blood cells of sheep that have been sensitized with rabbit antisheep erythrocyte immune globulin. The globulin will be agglutinated if the serum contains the rheumatoid factor. Also called **Paul-Bunnell test; Rose-Waaler test; sheep red-cell agglutination test.**

sheep cell test [AS, *sceap;* L, *cella,* storeroom; *testum,* crucible], a method that mixes human blood cells with the red blood cells of sheep to determine the absence or the deficiency of human T-lymphocytes. When mixed with human blood cells, the red blood cells of sheep cluster around the human T-lymphocytes and form characteristic rosettes. An electron microscope is used to identify the rosettes. An absence or a decrease in the number of rosettes indicates a deficiency or absence of T cells. The sheep cell test is used to diagnose several diseases, such as DiGeorge's syndrome, that decrease or destroy the cellular immunity provided by T cells.

sheet bath [AS, *scete, baeth*], the application of wet sheets to the body, used primarily as an antipyretic procedure.

sheet wadding, stretchable sheets of cotton padding used to cover the skin before a cast is applied. The stretching allows for some extremity edema without the cast becoming too tight.

shellfish poisoning [AS, *scell, fisc*], a toxic, neurologic condition that results from eating clams, oysters, or mussels that have ingested the poisonous protozoa commonly called the 'red tide.' The characteristic symptoms appear within a few minutes and include nausea, light-headedness, vomiting, and tingling or numbness around the mouth, followed by paralysis of the extremities and, possibly, respiratory paralysis. Saxitoxin, the causative agent, is not destroyed by cooking; however, the severity of the illness is diminished if the water used in cooking is not consumed. Treatment includes an intravenous injection of a weak so-

lution of prostigmin methylsulfate and the administration of oxygen and artificial respiration. See also **venerupin poisoning.**

shell shock [AS, *scell;* Fr, *choc*], any of a number of mental disorders, ranging from extreme fear to dementia, commonly attributed to the noise and concussion of exploding shells or bombs but actually resulting from a traumatic reaction to the stress of combat. See also **combat fatigue, posttraumatic stress disorder.**

shell teeth, a type of dental dysplasia characterized by large pulp chambers, insufficient coronal dentin, and, usually, no roots.

sheltered workshop [ME, *sheltrun,* body of guards; AS, *werc, sceoppa,* stall], a facility or program, either for outpatients or for residents of an institution, that provides vocational experience in a controlled working environment. The workshop also offers related vocational rehabilitation services, such as job interview training, to people with physical or mental disabilities.

shield [AS, *scild*], (in radiation technology) a material for preventing or reducing the passage of charged particles or radiation. A shield may be designated by the radiation it is intended to absorb, such as a gamma ray shield, or according to the kind of protection it is intended to give, such as a background, biologic, or thermal shield. Lucite and aluminum can be used for beta-radiation shields, but lead is required for gamma ray shields. The amount of material needed to provide shielding is expressed as the half-value layer, which is the quantity required to reduce the radiation intensity at a point in space by one half.

shift [AS, *sciftan,* to divide], **1.** (in nursing) the particular hours of the day during which a nurse is scheduled to work. The day shift is usually 7:00 AM to 3:00 PM or 8:00 AM to 4:00 PM. The evening shift is usually 3:00 PM to 11:00 PM or 4:00 PM to 12:00 midnight, and the night shift the remaining hours. The evening shift is also called "relief," presumably because nurses originally worked 12-hour shifts and the evening and night shift was thought to be relief for the day nurse. Many innovations in staffing practice currently allow variations on the traditional 5-day, 40-hour week, such as a nurse electing to work a shorter week, preferring longer hours for fewer days. **2.** an abrupt change in an analytic system that continues at the new level.

shift to the left, (in hematology) a predominance of immature leukocytes, noted in a differential white blood cell count. It is usually indicative of an infection or inflammation. The term derives from a graph of blood components in which immature cell frequencies appear on the left side of the graph.

shift to the right, (in hematology) a preponderance of polymorphonuclear neutrophils having three or more lobes, indicating maturity of the cell. The phenomenon is common in severe liver disease and advanced pernicious anemia. It indicates a relative lack of blood-forming activity.

Shigella /shigel'ə/ [Kiyoshi Shiga, Japanese bacteriologist, b. 1870], a genus of gram-negative pathogenic bacteria that causes gastroenteritis and bacterial dysentery, such as *Shigella dysenteriae.* It is also associated with hemolytic-uremic syndromes. See also **shigellosis.**

Shigella dysenteriae, a species of the bacterial family *Enterobacteriaceae* that causes a severe form of dysentery in humans. The *dysenteriae* subgroup of *Shigella* is most common in Asia and is particularly virulent. Also called *Shigella shigae.*

shigellosis /shig′əlō′sis/ [Kiyoshi Shiga + Gk, *osis*, condition], an acute bacterial infection of the bowel, characterized by diarrhea, abdominal pain, and fever, that is transmitted by hand-to-mouth contact with the feces of individuals infected with bacteria of a pathogenic species of the genus *Shigella*. These organisms may be carried in the stools of asymptomatic people for up to several months and may be spread through contact with contaminated objects, food, or flies, especially in poor, crowded areas. The disease occurs in isolated outbreaks in the United States but is endemic in underdeveloped areas of the world. It is especially common and usually most severe in children. Diagnosis is made by isolating and identifying *Shigella* in a specimen of stool. The likelihood of encountering or engendering antibiotic-resistant organisms is very high; therefore the preferred treatment for shigellosis is supportive and the major goal is to prevent dehydration. Antimicrobials are given if the disease is severe or if the likelihood of further transmission is great. Isolation and strict handwashing precautions are instituted. Shigellosis infections must be reported to the public health department. Also called **bacillary dysentery.**

shin bone. See **tibia.**

shingles. See **herpes zoster.**

shin splints [AS, *scinu*, shin; ME, *splinte*], a painful condition of the lower leg caused by strain of the long flexor muscle of the toes after strenuous athletic activity, such as running. In many instances it is the result of inadequate training. Treatment usually involves rest and exercise therapy. Surgery is sometimes necessary.

shipyard eye. See **epidemic keratoconjunctivitis.**

Shirodkar's operation /shir′odkärz′/, a surgical procedure called a cerclage in which the cervical canal is closed by a purse-string suture embedded in the uterine cervix encircling the canal. It is performed to correct an incompetent cervix that has failed to retain previous pregnancies. Under spinal block or general anesthesia, a 5 mm wide band of nonabsorbable material is buried beneath the mucosa of the cervix and pulled in a purse-string manner to close the cervix. The band may be left in place permanently, in which case subsequent deliveries are by cesarean section. Occasionally, a temporary cerclage is done, sewing in the band and leaving the ends exposed in the vagina. The band is then removed before labor and vaginal delivery. Postoperatively, infection or vaginal fistula may occur. If labor begins with the suture in place, the suture is removed promptly or the infant is delivered by cesarean section, before rupture of the uterus occurs.

shock [Fr, *choc*], an abnormal condition of inadequate blood flow to the body's peripheral tissues, with life-threatening cellular dysfunction, hypotension, and oliguria. The condition is usually associated with inadequate cardiac output, changes in peripheral blood flow resistance and distribution, and tissue damage. Causal factors include hemorrhage, vomiting, diarrhea, inadequate fluid intake, or excessive renal loss, resulting in hypovolemia. Kinds of shock include **anaphylactic shock, septic shock, cardiogenic shock, diabetic shock, electric shock, hypovolemic shock,** and **neurogenic shock.**

■ OBSERVATIONS: The signs and symptoms of different kinds of shock are similar and are related to the condition of hypovolemia. There is decreased blood flow with a resulting reduction in the delivery of oxygen, nutrients, hormones, and electrolytes to the body's tissues and a concomitant de-

creased removal of metabolic wastes. Pulse and respirations are increased. There may be tachycardia. Blood pressure may decline moderately at first. The patient often shows signs of restlessness and anxiety, an effect related to decreased blood flow to the brain. There also may be weakness, lethargy, pallor, and a cool, moist skin. As shock progresses, the body temperature falls, respirations become rapid and shallow, and the pulse pressure (the difference between systolic and diastolic blood pressures) narrows. Urinary output is reduced. Hemorrhage may be apparent or concealed, although other factors, such as vomiting or diarrhea, may account for the deficiency of body fluids.

■ INTERVENTIONS: Blood volume must be restored quickly so that there can be a rapid return of oxygenated blood to the perfusion-deprived tissues. Blood volume is expanded with intravenous fluids, such as a lactated Ringer's solution or a 5% dextrose in normal saline solution. Whole blood, plasma, and plasma substitutes also may be given. Nothing should be given by mouth, and sedatives, tranquilizers, or narcotics should not be administered, with the exception that morphine may be given intravenously in cases of severe pain. However, respiratory depression must be avoided because hypoventilation and hypoxemia with acidosis can lead to death. Metabolic acidosis may occur.

■ NURSING CONSIDERATIONS: After vital functions are restored and diagnosis has been carried out, the patient in shock must be monitored continuously until recovery is assured. The patient should remain flat in bed, but if there are no head injuries, the lower extremities can be raised slightly to improve venous return. The Trendelenburg position should be avoided because it tends to push the abdominal organs against the diaphragm, reducing effectiveness of the heart and lung functions. Position changes should be made slowly and gently. The patient must be kept warm, but external heat should be avoided. If shivering occurs, just enough covering should be added to control the shivering. Vasoactive drugs may be ordered when the blood volume is adequate. In some instances, extreme vasoconstriction may result in pain requiring analgesic medications. The patient's skin color, temperature, intravenous and oral fluid intakes, urinary output, and level of consciousness should be checked at frequent intervals and recorded. Individualized use of nursing process is critical.

shock lung. See **acute respiratory distress syndrome.**

shock therapy [Fr, *choc*; GK, *therapeia*], a psychotherapeutic procedure for treating depression and other severe disorders by producing an epileptiform convulsion in the patient. The shock is induced by delivering an electric current through the brain.

shock treatment. See **shock therapy.**

shock trousers, pneumatic trousers designed to counteract hypotension associated with internal or external bleeding, and hypovolemia. Shock trousers may be contraindicated in patients with pulmonary edema, cardiogenic shock, increased intracranial pressure, or eviscerations.

■ METHOD: The shock trousers are required when the patient loses consciousness, has a decreased or falling blood pressure, and shows signs of respiratory distress, such as dyspnea, rapid breathing, a cough, and pink, frothy sputum. The leg pulses may be diminished or absent, and the feet may appear pale, mottled, and cold. Before the pressurized trousers are applied, they are checked for tears or leaks and the proper functioning of their valves; any kinks or twists in the tubes connecting the trousers to the pneumatic pump are removed. The patient is placed in a flat, supine position over the open trousers, and the leg sections and portion that encircles the abdomen just below the rib cage are firmly secured in place by closing the Velcro straps or zippers. The exact times at which the trousers' sections are inflated are recorded, and the inflated sections are checked every 15 minutes. The patient's blood pressure, respiration, and apical and peripheral pulses also are checked every 15 minutes, and chest sounds are auscultated hourly. Parenteral fluids, whole blood, plasma protein fractions, and other plasma volume expanders are administered as ordered; the flow rate of expanders is adjusted according to central venous pressure readings. An indwelling urethral catheter is connected to a closed gravity drainage system, and fluid intake and output are measured hourly; if less than 30 ml of urine per hour is excreted, renal failure may occur. Monitoring of blood gases and intermittent suctioning through a nasogastric tube may be ordered. The trousers are not deflated or removed until the blood volume replacement is stable and the patient's physician is in attendance. As each section of the trousers, starting with the abdominal section, is gradually deflated, the patient's blood pressure, respiration, and apical pulse are checked every 5 to 10 minutes; if the blood pressure drops 4 to 6 mm Hg, deflation is stopped.

■ INTERVENTIONS: The nurse checks, applies, and inflates the shock trousers and remains with the patient during the entire procedure. The vital signs are monitored at frequent intervals, parenteral fluids and plasma volume expanders are given, measures of the intake and output are taken and recorded, and emotional support is provided.

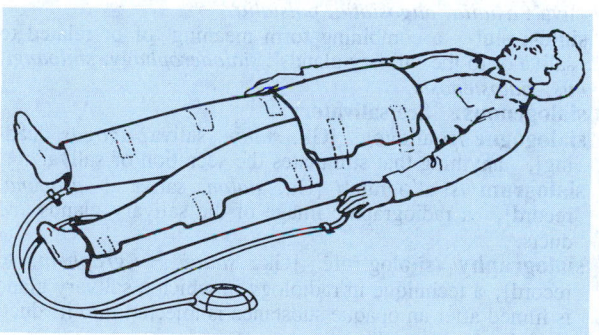

Shock trousers

shoe cookies. See **navicular pads.**
short-acting [AS, *short;* L, *agere,* to do], pertaining to or characterizing a therapeutic agent, usually a drug, with a brief period of effectiveness, generally beginning soon after the substance or measure is administered.
short-acting insulin, an aqueous preparation of the antidiabetic principle of beef pancreas or pork pancreas that begins to act within 1 hour of injection and reaches a peak of action in 2 to 4 hours. The duration of action of regular insulin is 4 to 6 hours and of crystalline zinc insulin 5 to 8 hours. Also called **rapid-acting insulin.** See also **insulin.** Compare **intermediate-acting insulin, long-acting insulin.**
shortage area /shôr'tij/ [AS, *sceort;* L, *acticum,* process], a geographic area, county as a census tract, or area designated by the federal government as being undersupplied with certain kinds of health care services, hence possibly

eligible for aid under certain federal programs, including the National Health Service Corps or the Rural Clinics Assistance Act.
short-arm cast, an orthopedic cast applied to immobilize the hand or the wrist. The short-arm cast incorporates the hand below the wrist; it is used in treating fractures, for postoperative positioning, and for correction or maintenance of correction of deformities of the hand and the wrist. Compare **long-arm cast.**
short bones, bones that occur in clusters and usually permit movement of the extremities, such as the carpals and tarsals.
short-bowel syndrome [AS, *sceort;* OFr, *boel;* Gk, *syn,* together + *dromos,* course], a loss of intestinal surface for absorption of nutrients caused by the surgical removal of a section of bowel.
short course tuberculosis chemotherapy, a 6-month treatment regimen for patients with tuberculosis who would otherwise continue to receive medications for at least 18 to 24 months after sputum has become negative for tubercle bacilli. The short course requires a combination of four drugs, isoniazid (INH), rifampin (RMP), pyrazinamide (PZA), and either ethambutol (EMB), or streptomycin.
short-gut syndrome, a congenital disorder in which an infant's intestine is too short or underdeveloped to allow normal food digestion. The child is maintained on parenteral nutrition until the intestine grows or develops further or is replaced by surgical transplant. A small child who becomes dependent on parenteral feeding may have to be taught chewing and swallowing processes when the short-gut syndrome is eventually corrected.
shorting [AS, *sceort*], the fraudulent practice of dispensing a quantity of drug less than that called for in the prescription and of charging for the quantity specified in the prescription. See also **kiting.**
short-leg cast, an orthopedic cast used for immobilizing fractures in the lower extremities from the toes to the knee. The short-leg cast is also used in severe sprains and torn soft tissue of the ankle, for postoperative positioning and immobilization of the foot and the ankle, and for correction or maintenance of correction of a deformity of the foot or the ankle. Compare **long-leg cast.**
short-leg cast with walker, an orthopedic cast with rubber walkers on the bottom. It immobilizes the leg from the toes to the knee and allows the patient to walk.
Short Portable Mental Status Questionnaire, a 10-item questionnaire used to screen older adults for cognitive impairment. It tests orientation, remote and recent memory, practical skills, and mathematical ability.
short-PR-normal-QRS syndrome. See **Lown-Ganong-Levine syndrome.**
short sightedness. See **myopia, nearsightedness.**
short stature [AS, *sceort* short; L, *statura,* man's height], a body height that is less than 70% of the average for a population of the same age, culture, and gender, and other peer factors.
short sight. See **myopia.**
short-term memory, memory of recent events.
short-wave diathermy [AS, *sceort* + *wafian;* Gk, *dia therme,* heat], a method of providing heat deep in the body by short-wave electrical currents. The high-frequency short-wave uses wavelengths of from 3 to 30 meters. It is used to treat chronic arthritis, bursitis, sinusitis, and other conditions.

shotgun therapy [AS, *scot;* ME, *gonne;* Gk, *therapeia,* treatment], *informal.* any treatment that has a wide range of effect and that therefore can be expected to correct the abnormal condition even though the particular cause is unknown. Shotgun therapy may cause more than an acceptable rate of side effects and is rarely desirable or necessary.

shoulder [AS, *sculder*], the junction of the clavicle, scapula, and humerus where the arm attaches to the trunk of the body. See also the Color Atlas of Human Anatomy.

shoulder blade. See **scapula.**

shoulder girdle [AS, *sculder* + *gyrdel*], a partial arch at the top of the trunk formed by the scapula and clavicle.

shoulder-hand syndrome, a neuromuscular condition characterized by pain and stiffness in the shoulder and arm, limited joint motion, swelling of the hand, muscle atrophy, and decalcification of the underlying bones. The condition occurs most commonly after myocardial infarction but may be associated with other known or unknown causes.

shoulder joint, the ball and socket articulation of the humerus with the scapula. The joint includes eight bursae and five ligaments, including the glenoidal labrum that deepens the articular cavity and protects the edges of articulating bones. Also called **humeral articulation.**

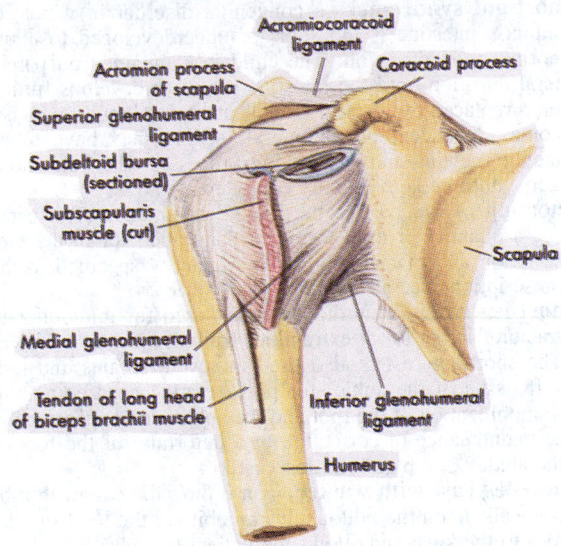

Shoulder joint (Thibodeau, 1993/Ernest W Beck)

shoulder presentation [AS, *sculder;* L, *praesentare,* to show], the part of the fetus that occupies the center of the birth canal when the presentation is associated with a transverse or oblique lie.

shoulder spica cast, an orthopedic cast applied to immobilize the trunk of the body to the hips, the wrist, and the hand. It incorporates a diagonal shoulder support between the hip and arm portions. The shoulder spica cast is used in the treatment of shoulder dislocations and injuries or in the positioning and immobilization of the shoulder after surgery.

shoulder subluxation, the separation of the humeral head from the glenoid cavity, resulting in strain on the soft tissues surrounding the joint.

show. See **vaginal bleeding.**

shreds [AS, *screade,* piece cut off], glossy filaments of mucus in the urine, indicating inflammation in the urinary tract. Also called **mucous shreds.**

shunt [ME, *shunten*], **1.** to redirect the flow of a body fluid from one cavity or vessel to another. **2.** a tube or device implanted in the body to redirect a body fluid from one cavity or vessel to another.

shunt, left to right, a diversion of blood from the left side of the heart to the right, such as through a septal defect, or from the systemic to the pulmonary circulation, such as from a patent ductus arteriosus.

Shy-Drager syndrome /shī′drā′gər/ [G. Milton Shy, American neurologist, b. 1919; Glenn A. Drager, American physician, b. 1917], a rare, progressive neurologic disorder of young and middle-aged adults. It is characterized by orthostatic hypotension, bladder and bowel incontinence, atrophy of the iris, anhidrosis, tremor, rigidity, incoordination, ataxia, and muscle wasting. Treatment includes drug therapy to control motor symptoms and to maintain an adequate blood pressure. Antigravity stockings may prevent pooling of blood in the lower extremities. See also **orthostatic hypotension.**

Si, symbol for the element **silicon.**

SI, abbreviation for *Systme International d'Unités,* the French name for the **International System of Units.**

SIADH, abbreviation for **syndrome of inappropriate antidiuretic hormone secretion.**

sial-. See **sialo-.**

sialadenitis /sī′əlad′ənī′tis/, any inflammation of one or more of the salivary glands.

-sialia, a combining form meaning '(condition of the) saliva': *asialia, oligosialia, polsialia.*

sialo-, sial- a combining form meaning 'of or related to saliva or to the salivary glands': *sialoaerophagy, sialoangitis, sialostenosis.*

sialogenous. See **salivatory.**

sialogogue /sī·al′əgog′/ [Gk, *sialon,* saliva, *agogos,* leading], anything that stimulates the secretion of saliva.

sialogram /sī·al′əgram′/ [Gk, *sialon,* saliva + *gramma,* record], a radiographic image of the salivary glands and ducts.

sialography /sī·əlog′rəfē/ [Gk, *sialon* + *graphein,* to record], a technique in radiology in which a salivary gland is filmed after an opaque substance is injected into its duct. —**sialographic,** *adj.*

sialolith /sī·al′əlith/ [Gk, *sialon* + *lithos,* stone], a calculus formed in a salivary gland or duct.

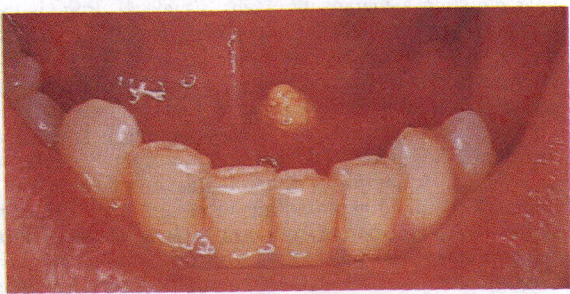

Sialolith (Lamey, 1988)

sialolithiasis /-lithī′əsis/, a pathologic condition in which one or more calculi or stones are formed in a salivary gland.

sialorrhea /sī·al′ərē′ə/ [Gk, *sialon* + *rhoia*, flow], an excessive flow of saliva that may be associated with a variety of conditions, such as acute inflammation of the mouth, mental retardation, mercurialism, pregnancy, teething, alcoholism, or malnutrition. Also called **hypersalivation, ptyalism.**

Siamese twins /sī′əmēz/ [Chang and Eng, conjoined twins born in Siam (now Thailand) in 1811], conjoined, equally developed twin fetuses that were produced from the same ovum. The severity of the condition ranges from superficial fusion, such as of the umbilical vessels, to that in which the heads or complete torsos are united and several internal organs are shared. With modern surgical techniques, most Siamese twins can be successfully separated. See also **conjoined twins.**

sib [AS *sibb*], pertaining to a close blood relationship. See also **sibling.**

Siberian tick typhus /sībir′ē·ən/ [Siberia], a mild, acute febrile illness seen in north, central, and east Asia, caused by *Rickettsia siberica*, transmitted by ticks, and characterized by a diffuse maculopapular rash, headache, conjunctival inflammation, and a small ulcer or eschar at the site of the tick bite. Treatment with chloramphenicol or tetracycline is associated with an excellent prognosis. Also called **North Asian tick-borne rickettsiosis.** See also **rickettsia, typhus.**

sibilant /sib′īlənt/ [L, *sibilare*, to hiss], a hissing sound or one in which the predominant sound is that of "S".

sibilant rale [L, *sibalare*, to hiss], an abnormal whistling sound that may emanate from the lungs of an individual with a respiratory disorder or disease. It is caused by the passage of air through a lumen narrowed by the accumulation of mucus or other viscid fluid.

Siblin, a trademark for a bulk laxative containing psyllium seed.

sibling /sib′ling/ [AS, *sibb*, kin], **1.** also called *(informal)* **sib.** one of two or more children who have both parents in common; a brother or sister. The number, age differences, sex, and birth order of siblings can greatly affect the childhood environment and relationships within a family, which also may include step-siblings and half-siblings. Sibling rivalry and jealousy are common in first-born children, especially when there is a 2- to 4-year difference in age. In general, sibling relationships help teach the child important social patterns and moral values, such as competitiveness, loyalty, and sharing. **2.** of or pertaining to a brother or sister.

sibship /sib′ship/ [AS *sibb* kin, *scieppan* to shape], **1.** the state of being related by blood. **2.** a group of people descended from a common ancestor who are used as a basis for genetic studies. **3.** brothers and sisters considered as a group.

sic [L], thus.

sicc-, a combining form meaning 'dry': *siccative, siccolabile, siccostabile.*

sickle cell [AS, *sicol*, crescent; L., *cella*, storeroom], an abnormal, crescent-shaped red blood cell containing hemoglobin S, characteristic of sickle cell anemia.

sickle cell anemia, a severe, chronic, incurable, hemoglobinopathic, anemic condition that occurs in people homozygous for hemoglobin S (Hb S). The abnormal hemoglobin results in distortion and fragility of the erythrocytes. Sickle cell anemia is characterized by crises of joint pain, throm-

bosis, and fever and by chronic anemia, with splenomegaly, lethargy, and weakness. See also **congenital nonspherocytic hemolytic anemia, elliptocytosis, hemoglobin S, sickle cell crisis.**

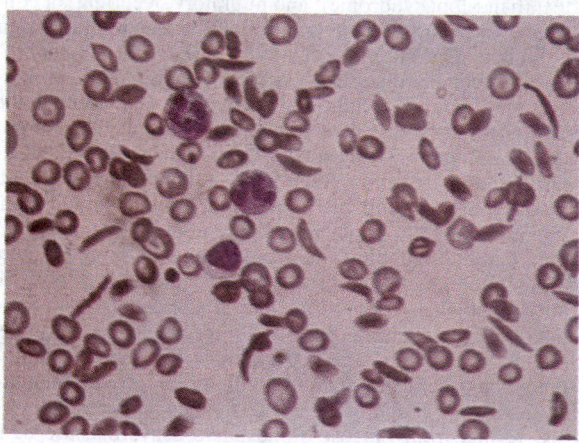

Sickle cell anemia *(Hart, 1992)*

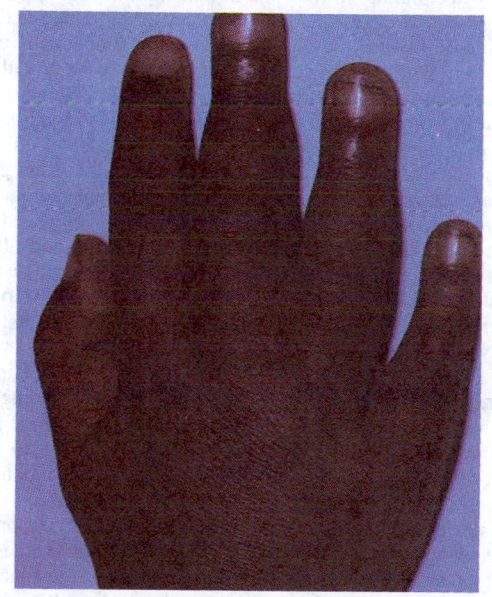

Sickle cell dactylitis *(Zitelli, 1992)*

sickle cell crisis, an acute, episodic condition that occurs in children with sickle cell anemia. The crisis may be vasoocclusive, resulting from the aggregation of misshapen erythrocytes, or anemic, resulting from bone marrow aplasia, increased hemolysis, folate deficiency, or splenic sequestration of erythrocytes. See also **hemoglobin S, sickle cell anemia.**

■ OBSERVATIONS: Painful vasoocclusive crisis is the most common of the sickle cell crises. It is usually preceded by an upper respiratory or GI infection without an exacerbation of anemia. The clumps of sickled erythrocytes obstruct blood vessels, resulting in occlusion, ischemia, and infarction of adjacent tissue. Characteristics of this kind of crisis are leukocytosis, acute abdominal pain from visceral hypoxia, painful swelling of the soft tissue of the hands and feet (hand-foot syndrome), and migratory, recurrent, or constant joint pain, often so severe that movement of the joint is limited. Persistent headache, dizziness, convulsions, visual or auditory disturbances, facial nerve palsies, coughing, shortness of breath, and tachypnea may occur if the central nervous system or lungs are affected. Other problems associated with vasoocclusion include priapism, hematuria, and retinopathy. Anemic crisis is characterized by a dramatic, rapid drop in hemoglobin levels resulting from various causes. Aplastic crisis resulting in severe anemia occurs because red blood cell production is diminished by acute viral, bacterial, or fungal infection. Megaloblastic anemia (another form of anemic crisis) results from folic acid deficiency during periods of accelerated erythropoiesis. Severe anemia between crises is not common unless there is a generalized state of malnutrition. Hyperhemolytic crisis, characterized by anemia, jaundice, and reticulocytosis, results from glucose-6-phosphate dehydrogenase deficiency or in reaction to multiple transfusions. Acute sequestration crisis, which occurs in young children 6 months to 5 years of age, results when large quantities of blood suddenly accumulate in the spleen, causing massive splenic enlargement, severe anemia, shock, and, ultimately, death. Susceptibility to infection is a common problem of young children with sickle cell anemia and may be greatly increased during periods of crisis. Systemic infection and septicemia from pneumococcus or *Haemophilus influenzae* are not uncommon and may be rapidly fatal. In older children, local infection, especially osteomyelitis, rather than generalized septicemia is frequently a complicating factor.

■ INTERVENTIONS: Therapy consists of immediate transfusion of packed red cells in the acute anemic crisis and alleviation of severe abdominal and joint pain with analgesics or narcotics as needed in vasoocclusive crisis. Short-term oxygen therapy, hydration by oral or intravenous means, electrolyte replacement to counteract metabolic acidosis resulting from hypoxia, and antibiotics to treat any existing infection may be necessary. Pneumococcal and meningococcal vaccine is recommended for children between 2 and 5 years of age because they are highly susceptible to infection. Partial exchange transfusions are often mandatory in life-threatening crises, such as when sickling occurs in the vessels of the brain or lungs, and may be used as a preventive technique, although multiple transfusions increase the risk of hepatitis, hemosiderosis, and transfusion reactions. Oral anticoagulants have been used to relieve the pain of vasoocclusion, but these increase the risk of bleeding. Priapism, a painful condition frequently seen in vasoocclusive crisis, may be treated by aspirating the corpora cavernosa. In children with recurrent splenic sequestration, splenectomy may be a life-saving procedure. The process is not routinely recommended because surgery increases the risk of acidosis and hypoxia from anesthesia, and, in time, the spleen usually atrophies through progressive fibrotic changes. Infarction of tissue in any organ is a potential hazard in sickle cell crisis, and special management and treatment are warranted by the specific site of damage. Typical complications include uremia (requiring renal transplantation or hemodialysis), chronic functional pulmonary impair-

ment, aseptic necrosis of the hip, and microvascular occlusion that may lead to venous thrombosis.

■ NURSING CONSIDERATIONS: The primary concern of the nurse during a crisis is to initiate procedures that reduce sickling. Foremost is prevention of tissue deoxygenation and resulting hypoxia by maintaining bed rest to minimize energy expenditure and oxygen use, although some exercise is necessary to promote circulation. Hydration and electrolyte balance are essential. A complete record of fluid intake and output is maintained, and adequate therapy is calculated accordingly. Serum sodium is monitored closely to avoid hyponatremia. Oxygen is given in severe anoxia, although prolonged administration depresses bone marrow activity and thus aggravates anemia. Management of pain in vasoocclusion is often difficult and may require experimentation with various drugs and schedules before adequate relief is achieved. The application of warmth is often soothing; cold is contraindicated, because it enhances vasoconstriction and sickling. The nurse constantly monitors the child's condition for splenomegaly, infection, evidence of shock or cerebrovascular accident, hypervolemia, transfusion reaction, or increasing anemia. An important aspect of nursing care is the continued emotional support for parents whose child has a chronic illness that is potentially fatal.

sickle cell dactylitis [AS, *sicol;* L, *cella,* storeroom; Gk, *daktylos,* finger + *itis,* inflammation], a painful inflammation of one or more fingers caused by an attack of sickle cell anemia.

sickle cell thalassemia, a heterozygous blood disorder in which the genes for sickle cell and for thalassemia are both inherited. A mild form and a severe form may be identified, depending on the degree of suppression of beta-chain synthesis by the thalassemia gene. In the mild form synthesis is only partially suppressed, and the red cell may contain from 25% to 35% normal hemoglobin A along with a greater concentration of hemoglobin S. The clinical course is relatively mild. In the severe form, beta-chain synthesis is completely suppressed and only hemoglobin S appears in the red cells. The clinical course is generally as severe as in homozygous sickle cell anemia. See also **hemoglobinopathy, hemoglobin S, hemoglobin S-C disease.**

sickle cell trait, the heterozygous form of sickle cell anemia, characterized by the presence of both hemoglobin S and hemoglobin A in the red blood cells. Anemia and the other signs of sickle cell anemia do not occur. People who have the trait are informed and counseled regarding the possibility of having an infant with sickle cell disease if both parents have the trait. See **hemoglobin S.**

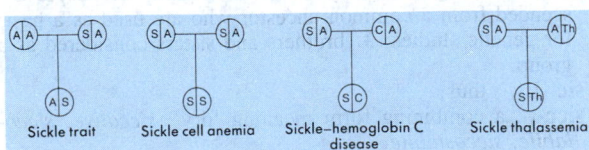

Sickle cell inheritance pattern

sick role [AS, *seoc;* Fr, character], a pattern of behavior in which a person adopts the symptoms of a physical or mental disorder to be cared for, sympathized with, and protected from the demands and stresses of life.

sick sinus syndrome (SSS) [AS, *seoc;* L, *sinus,* hollow], a complex of syndromes associated with sinus node dysfunction. The condition may result from a variety of cardiac diseases, ranging from cardiomyopathies to inflammatory myocardial disease, but is most commonly related to either intermittent sinoatrial block or inadequate sinoatrial conduction. It is characterized by severe sinus bradycardia alone, sinus bradycardia alternating with tachycardia, or sinus bradycardia with atrioventricular block. The most common symptoms are lethargy, weakness, light-headedness, dizziness, and episodes of near syncope to actual loss of consciousness. The severity of symptoms is related to the duration of the asystolic period. Although many patients may be symptomatic, especially elderly patients with episodes of near syncope associated with a prior history of palpitations, accurate diagnosis can be made only with electrocardiographic documentation of sinoatrial block. At present the only treatment is by the implantation of a permanent demand pacemaker.

SICU, abbreviation for *surgical intensive care unit.*

side effect [AS, *side;* L, *effectus*], any reaction or consequence that results from a medication or therapy. This can be an effect carried beyond the desired limit, such as hemorrhaging from an anticoagulant, or a reaction unrelated to the primary object of the therapy, such as an anaphylactic reaction to an antibiotic. Usually, although not necessarily, the effect is undesirable and may manifest itself as nausea, dry mouth, dizziness, blood dyscrasias, blurred vision, discolored urine, or tinnitus.

sidero- /sid'ərō-/, a combining form meaning 'of or pertaining to iron': *siderocyte, siderofibrous, sideropenic.*

sideroblast /sid'ərōblast'/ [Gk, *sideros,* iron, + *blastos,* germ cell], an iron-rich, nucleated red blood cell in the bone marrow.

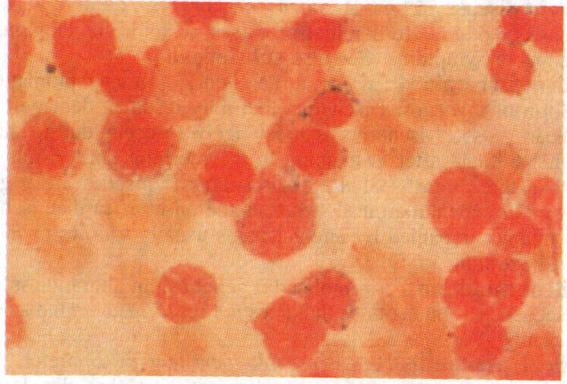

Sideroblast in the bone marrow (Kamal, 1991)

sideroblastic anemia /sid'ərōblas'tik/ [Gk, *sideros,* iron, *blastos,* germ], a heterogenous group of chronic hematologic disorders characterized by normocytic or slightly macrocytic anemia, hypochromic and normochromic red blood cells, and decreased erythropoiesis and hemoglobin synthesis. The red blood cells contain a perinuclear ring of iron-stained granules. The condition may be acquired or hereditary, and primary or secondary to another condition. The cause of the disease is not understood. Treatment may in-

clude extract of liver, pyridoxine, folic acid, and blood transfusion. Compare **iron deficiency anemia, siderosis.**

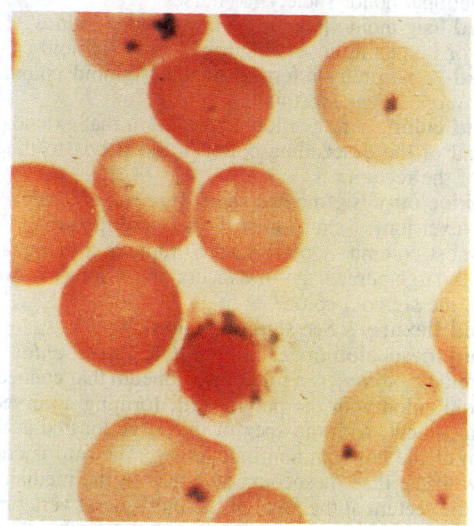

Sideroblastic anemia (Zitelli, 1992)

siderocyte /sid'ərosīt'/ [Gk, *sideros,* iron, *kytos,* cell], an abnormal erythrocyte in which particles of nonhemoglobin iron are visible.

sideropenic dysphagia. See **Plummer-Vinson syndrome.**

siderosis /sid'ərō'sis/ [Gk, *sideros* + *osis,* condition], **1.** a variety of pneumoconiosis caused by the inhalation of iron dust or particles. **2.** the introduction of color in any tissue caused by the presence of excess iron. **3.** an increase in the amounts of iron in the blood. See also **hemochromatosis, hemosiderosis, sideroblastic anemia.**

siderotic granules /sid'ərot'ik/, inclusion bodies seen in the red blood cells of splenectomy patients and in cases of hemoglobin synthesis and hemolytic anemia. The granules contain iron, which takes a Prussian blue stain.

side-to-side anastomosis. See **anastomosis.**

SIDS, abbreviation for **sudden infant death syndrome.**

SIECUS /sē'kəs/, abbreviation for *Sex Information and Education Council of the United States.*

sievert (Sv) /sē'vərt/ [R. M. Sievert, 20th century Swedish physicist], a unit-dose-equivalent radiation. The sievert has identical units to the gray and is determined by multiplying the absorbed dose by the quality factor, a number that has been determined to accurately compare the health consequences of that type of radiation with x-rays. The rem bears the same relationship to the rad as the sievert does to the gray.

sig., abbreviation for the Latin *signetur,* phrase 'let it be labeled (according to prescription).'

sigh, a deep breath that may be 1.5 times the normal V_t. It plays a role in pumonary hygiene. See **periodic deep inspiration.**

sight /sīt/ [AS, *gesiht*], **1.** the special sense that enables the shape, size, position, and color of objects to be perceived; the faculty of vision. It is the principal function of the eye. **2.** that which is seen.

Sigma, /sig'məl/, Σ, σ and s, the eighteenth letter of the Greek alphabet.

Sigma Theta Tau International /sig'mə thā'tə tou'/, an international honor society for nurses.

sigmoid /sig'moid/ [Gk, *sigma,* S-shaped, *eidos,* form], **1.** of or pertaining to an S shape. **2.** the sigmoid colon.

sigmoid-, a prefix referring to the 'sigmoid colon': *sigmoidoscope, sigmoidectomy.*

sigmoid colon, the portion of the colon that extends from the end of the descending colon in the pelvis to the juncture of the rectum.

sigmoidectomy /sig'moidek'təmē/ [Gk, *sigma, eidos* + *ektome,* excision], excision of the sigmoid flexure of the colon, most commonly performed to remove a malignant tumor. A large percentage of cancers of the lower bowel occur in the sigmoid colon.

sigmoid flexure. See **sigmoid colon.**

sigmoid mesocolon /mez'ōkō'lən/ [Gk, *sigma, eidos* + *mesos,* middle, *kolon*], a fold of peritoneum that connects the sigmoid colon with the pelvic wall, forming a curved line of attachment, with the apex of the curve located at the division of the left common iliac artery. The fold is continuous with the iliac mesocolon and ends in the median plane over the rectum at the level of the third sacral vertebra. Between the two layers of the fold are the sigmoid and the superior rectal vessels. Compare **mesentery proper, transverse mesocolon.**

sigmoid notch, a concavity on the superior surface of the mandibular ramus between the coronoid and condyloid processes.

sigmoidoscope /sigmoi'dəskōp'/ [Gk, *sigma, eidos* + *skopein,* to look], an instrument used to examine the lumen of the sigmoid colon. It consists of a tube and a light, allowing direct visualization of the mucous membrane lining the colon. Compare **proctoscope.**

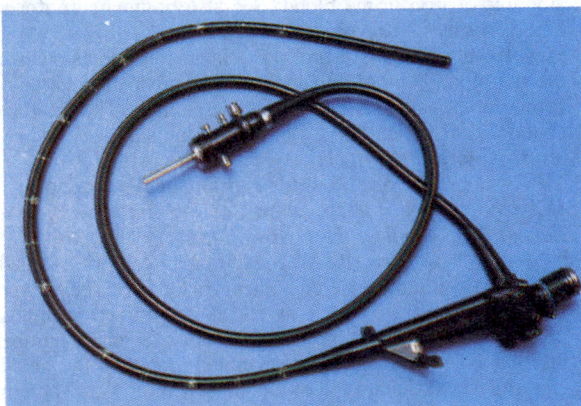

Flexible sigmoidoscope *(Doughty, 1993)*

sigmoidoscopy /sig'moidos'kəpē/, the inspection of the rectum and sigmoid colon by the aid of a sigmoidoscope.

sign /sīn/ [L, *signum,* mark], an objective finding as perceived by an examiner, such as a fever, a rash, the whisper heard over the chest in pleural effusion, or the light band of hair seen in children after recovery from kwashiorkor.

Many signs accompany symptoms; for example, erythema and a maculopapular rash are often seen when a patient complains of pruritus. Compare **symptom.**

signal molecule /sig'nəl/ [L, *signum,* mark], a hormone, neurotransmitter, or other agent that transfers information from one cell or organ to another. Examples include steroid hormones, insulin, and growth factors. A photon may have a similar effect on a retinal receptor.

signal node. See **Virchow's node.**

signal symptom. See **symptom.**

signal-to-noise ratio (SNR), the number used to describe the relative contributions to a detected signal of the true signal and random superimposed signals or 'noise.'

signe de journal. See **thumb sign.**

significance /signif'ikəns/ [L, *significare,* to signify], **1.** (in research) the statistical probability that a given finding is very unlikely to have occurred by chance alone. The conventional standard for attributing significance is a finding that occurs fewer than 5 times in 100 by chance alone ($p < .05$). **2.** the importance of a study in developing a practice or theory, as in nursing practice.

significant other /signif'ikənt/, a person who is considered by an individual as being special and as having an effect on that individual.

sign language [L, *signum* + *lingua,* tongue], a form of communication often used with and among deaf people consisting of hand and body movements. Many variations exist, including American Sign Language, Signed English, and finger spelling.

sign-off, a procedure for terminating interaction between a user and a computer. **–sign off,** *v.*

sign-on, a procedure for initiating interaction between a user and a computer. **–sign on,** *v.*

silanization /sil'əniza'shən/, (in chromatography) the chemical process of converting the SiOH moieties of a stationary form to the ester form.

silent disease /sī'lənt/ [L, *silens, dis;* Fr, *aise,* ease], a disease or other disorder that produces no clinically obvious signs or symptoms. See also **subclinical.**

silent ischemia [L, *silere,* to be silent], an asymptomatic form of myocardial ischemia that may result in damage to heart muscle. Ischemia is most likely to occur during the first 6 hours after awakening in the morning, and in more than three fourths of the cases studied, episodes are triggered by mental arousal, whereas the onset of cardiac ischemia accompanied by anginal pains usually follows physical exertion.

silent mutation, (in molecular genetics) an alteration in a sequence of nucleotides that does not result in an amino acid change.

silent peritonitis [L, *silens;* Gk, *peri tenein,* to stretch + *itis,* inflammation], a case of peritonitis that develops without clinical signs or symptoms.

silhouette sign /sil'ōō·et'/, an x-ray artifact caused by an infiltrate that obscures the demarcating line between lung segments.

silicate dental cement /sil'ikāt/ [L, *silex,* flint], a relatively hard, translucent material used primarily to restore anterior teeth. Like other dental cements, it is prepared by mixing a liquid and a powder. The powder of silicate cement is acid-soluble glass prepared by fusing oxides of calcium, silicon, aluminum, and other ingredients with a fluoride flux. The liquid is a buffered phosphoric acid solution.

silico-, a combining form meaning 'pertaining to silica or quartz': *silicosis, silicosiderosis, silicotuberculosis.*

silicon (Si) /sil′ikon/ [L, *silex,* flint], a nonmetallic element, second to oxygen as the most abundant of the elements. Its atomic number is 14; its atomic weight is 28. It occurs in nature as silicon dioxide and in silicates. The silicates are used as detergents, corrosion inhibitors, adhesives, and sealants. Elemental silicon is used in metallurgy and in transistors and other electronic components. About 60% of the rocks in the earth's crust contain silicon, and silica dusts are associated with many mining operations. Protracted inhalation of silica dusts can cause silicosis, which increases the susceptibility to other pulmonary diseases.

silicone /sil′ikōn/ [L, *silex,* flint], any organic silicon polymer compound used in medicine, as an adhesive, a lubricant, or a substitute for rubber, especially in prosthetic devices.

silicone septum, a vascular access device used in intravenous therapy. It consists of a silicone partition that covers the port chamber housed in the metal or plastic body of an implanted infusion port.

silicosis /sil′ikō′sis/, a lung disorder caused by continued, long-term inhalation of the dust of an inorganic compound, silicon dioxide, which is found in sands, quartzes, flints, and many other stones. Silicosis is characterized by the development of nodular fibrosis in the lungs. In advanced cases, severe dyspnea may develop. The incidence of silicosis is highest among industrial workers exposed to silica powder in manufacturing processes; in those who work with ceramics, sand, or stone; and in those who mine silica. Also called **grinder's disease, quartz silicosis.** See also **chronic obstructive pulmonary disease, inorganic dust.**

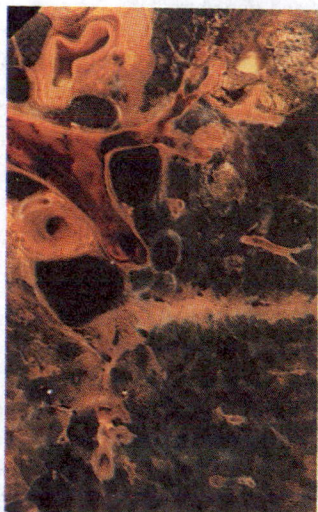

Silicosis *(Fletcher, 1987)*

silk suture [AS, *seolc;* L, *sutura,* seam], a braided, fine, black suture material, usually used to close incisions, wounds, and cuts in the skin. It is not absorbed by the body and is removed after approximately 7 days.

silo filler's disease /sī′lō/ [Fr, *ensilotage,* ensilage; AS, *fyllan,* to fill], a rare, acute, respiratory condition seen in agricultural workers who have inhaled nitrogen oxide as they work with fermented fodder in closed, poorly ventilated areas such as silos. Characteristically, symptoms of respiratory distress and pulmonary edema occur several hours after exposure. Loss of consciousness may occur. Observation in the hospital and respiratory assistance often are required. The condition is rarely fatal.

Silvadene, a trademark for an antibacterial (sulfadiazine silver).

silver (Ag) [AS, *seolfor*], a whitish precious metal occurring mainly as a sulfide. Its atomic number is 47; its atomic weight is 107.88. It is quite soft and is usually alloyed with small amounts of copper to increase its durability. Silver dissolves readily in nitric acid and is used extensively to produce silver halides used in photographic emulsions. It is frequently associated in small amounts with the ores of zinc, copper, and lead and is used extensively as a component of amalgams of dental fillings and in many medications, especially antiseptics and astringents. Some antiseptics containing silver are mild silver protein and strong silver protein, preparations that render silver colloidal in the presence of protein. Mild silver protein contains not less than 19% and not more than 23% silver. Strong silver protein contains not less than 7.5% and not more than 8.5% silver. Both preparations are used externally as antiseptics and do not have irritating properties. Silver nitrate is also used externally as an antiseptic and astringent, especially in the prevention of ophthalmia neonatorum. It is also used as a lubricant on the bearings of x-ray tubes, and silver halides are used in x-ray films. Silver picrate, the ionizable salt of silver, is used in the treatment of trichomoniasis and in the treatment of moniliasis of the vagina.

silver amalgam [AS, *seolfor;* Gk, *malagma*], an alloy of silver, tin, copper, mercury, and zinc used in dentistry to fill prepared tooth cavities.

silver cone method, a technique for filling tooth root canals. A prefitted silver cone is sealed into the apex of a root canal, and any remaining canal space is filled with gutta-percha or sealer.

Silver dwarf [Henry K. Silver, American pediatrician, b. 1918], a person who has **Silver's syndrome,** a congenital disorder in which short stature is associated with lateral asymmetry, various anomalies of the head, face, and skeleton, and precocious puberty.

silver-fork fracture. See **Colles' fracture.**

Silverman-Anderson score, a system of assessing the degree of respiratory distress.

silver nitrate, a topical antiinfective.

■ INDICATIONS: A 1% solution is prescribed for the prevention of gonococcal ophthalmia in newborns and stronger concentrations for use on wet dressings.

■ CONTRAINDICATIONS: Known sensitivity to this drug prohibits its use. It should not be used with bacitracin, which inactivates silver nitrate.

■ ADVERSE EFFECTS: Among the more serious adverse reactions are severe local inflammation, burns, and argyria.

silver salts poisoning, a toxic condition caused by the ingestion of silver nitrate, characterized by discoloration of the lips, vomiting, abdominal pain, dizziness, and convulsions. Treatment includes gastric lavage with salt water, followed by demulcents and fluid therapy. Anticonvulsant and antihypotensive therapy may be necessary.

Silver's syndrome.   See **Silver dwarf.**

silver sulfadiazine,   a topical antimicrobial.

■ INDICATIONS: It is prescribed to prevent or treat infection in second- and third-degree burns.

■ CONTRAINDICATIONS: Known hypersensitivity to this drug, to silver, or to sulfonamides prohibits its use. It is not given in the last weeks of pregnancy or to newborn or premature infants.

■ ADVERSE EFFECTS: Among the most serious adverse reactions are rashes, fungal infections, neutropenia, and kernicterus.

simethicone /simeth′ikōn/,   an antiflatulent.

■ INDICATION: It is prescribed to decrease excess gas in the GI tract.

■ CONTRAINDICATIONS: There are no significant contraindications.

■ ADVERSE EFFECTS: Adverse reactions include belching and rectal flatus.

simian crease /sim′ē·ən/ [L, *simia*, ape; ME, *creste*, crest], a single crease across the palm produced from the fusion of proximal and distal palmar creases, seen in congenital disorders, such as Down syndrome. Also called **simian line.**

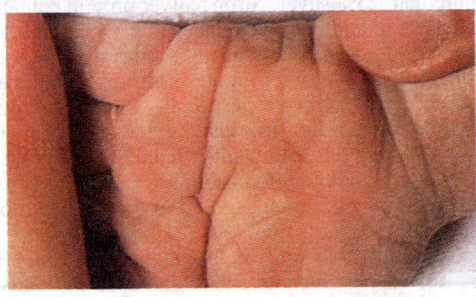

Simian crease (Zitelli, 1992)

simian virus 40,   a vacuolating virus isolated from the kidney tissue of rhesus monkeys.

simil-,   a combining form meaning 'like': *Similac, similimum.*

Similac preparations,   a trademark for a group of commercial modified milk products that are prepared especially for infant feeding. They are made from a nonfat base of cow's milk supplemented with such substances as lactose, coconut and soy oils, and monosaccharides and disaccharides and fortified with vitamins and minerals. The ratio of the various nutrients, such as iron or one of the other minerals, is altered in the different preparations to accommodate infants with particular nutritional requirements or nutritional problems, such as nephrogenic diabetes insipidus. The formulas are packaged in both powder and liquid form.

Simmonds' disease.   See **postpubertal panhypopituitarism.**

simplate bleeding time test,   a blood test for determining how quickly platelets form a plug when exposed to air. Platelet plug formation is the first step in clotting and, if slower than 8 minutes, indicates platelet deficiency or the effect of a drug, such as aspirin.

simple angioma [L, *simplex*, not mixed],   a tumor consisting of a network of small vessels or distended capillaries surrounded by connective tissue.

simple astigmatism [L, *simplex*, not mixed; Gk, *a, stigma* point],   **1.** simple myopic astigmatism in which one principal meridian is in focus on the retina and the other in front of it. **2.** simple hyperopic astigmatism in which one meridian is focused on the retina and the other behind it.

simple cavity,   a cavity that involves only one surface of a tooth.

simple diarrhea [L, *simplex*, not mixed; Gk, *dia, rhein*, to flow],   a form of diarrhea in which the loose stools contain normal feces.

simple dislocation [L, *simplex*, not mixed + *dis, locare*, to place],   dislocation without a penetrating wound.

simple figure-of-eight roller arm sling,   a sling prepared by placing the patient in a supine or sitting position with the affected arm flexed adjacent to the chest. The open sling should fit under the arm and over the chest. The bandage is fixed with a single turn toward the uninjured side around the arm and chest, crossing the elbow above the external epicondyle. In the next step, the bandage is brought forward under the tip of the elbow, after making a second turn that overlaps two thirds of the first. Then the bandage is brought upward along the flexed arm to the base of the neck on the uninjured side. Finally, the bandage is brought down over the scapula and across the chest and arm, overlapping and continuing in a figure-of-eight pattern.

simple fission.   See **binary fission.**

simple fracture,   an uncomplicated, closed fracture in which the bone does not break the skin. Compare **compound fracture.**

simple glaucoma [L, *simplex*, unmixed; Gk, *glaucoma*, cataract],   chronic open-angle glaucoma in which the angle is open when the intraocular fluid pressure is increased but with associated lowered outflow of fluid. There may be visual field loss and optic atrophy.

simple goiter [L, *simplex*, not mixed + *guttur*, sore throat],   a goiter not accompanied by signs or symptoms of hyperthyroidism.

simple mastectomy,   a surgical procedure in which a breast is completely removed and the underlying muscles and adjacent lymph nodes are left intact. The procedure may be performed to remove small malignant neoplasms of the breast, or it may be done as a palliative measure to remove an ulcerated carcinoma in advanced breast cancer. Postoperatively, the process of recovery from a simple mastectomy is less uncomfortable and faster than from a radical or modified radical mastectomy, but nursing care is similar. Compare **modified radical mastectomy, radical mastectomy.** See also **mastectomy.**

simple meningitis.   See **sterile meningitis.**

simple periodontal pocket.   See **periodontal pocket.**

simple phobia,   an anxiety disorder characterized by a persistent, irrational fear of specific things, such as animals, dirt, light, or darkness. Compare **social phobia.** See also **phobia.**

simple protein,   a protein that yields amino acids as the only or chief product on hydrolysis. The class includes albumins, globulins, glutelins, alcohol-soluble proteins, albuminoids, histones, and protamines. See also **complex protein.**

simple reflex [L, *simplex*, not mixed + *reflectere*, to bend back],   a reflex with a motor nerve component that involves only one muscle.

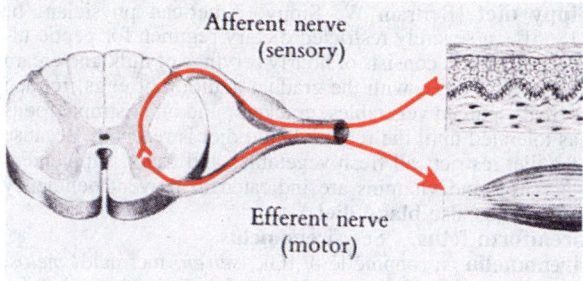

Simple reflex arc *(Rudy, 1984)*

simple stomatitis [L, *simplex*; Gk, *stoma*, mouth + *itis*, inflammation], a simple inflammation of the mucous membranes of the mouth with redness, swelling, and an excess of mucus. Also called **catarrhal stomatitis.**

simple sugar, a monosaccharide, such as glucose.

simple tubular gland, one of the many multicellular glands with only one tube-shaped duct, such as various glands within the epithelium of the intestine.

simple vulvectomy. See **vulvectomy.**

Simpson forceps. See **obstetric forceps.**

Sims' position [James M. Sims, American gynecologist, b. 1813], a position in which the patient lies on the left side with the right knee and thigh drawn upward toward the chest. The chest and abdomen are allowed to fall forward. It is the position of choice for administering enemas or conducting rectal examinations.

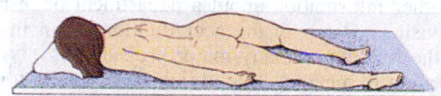

Sims' position *(Potter, 1993)*

simulation /sim'yəlā'shən/ [L, *simulare*, to imitate], a mode of computer-assisted instruction in which a student receives basic information about a topic and then must interact with the computer to gain deeper understanding of the information and topic. Simulation enables the student to explore situations that might be too expensive, dangerous, or time consuming in real life.

sin-, sinus-, a combining form meaning 'hollow, cavity, or to curve': *sinography, sinus, sinusotomy.*

sinap-, a combining form meaning 'of or related to mustard': *sinapine, sinapiscopy, sinapism.*

sinciput /sin'siput/ [L, half a head], the anterior or upper part of the head. See also **bregma.**

Sinemet, a trademark for a central nervous system fixed-combination drug containing a decarboxylase inhibitor (carbidopa) and an antiparkinsonian (levodopa).

Sinequan, a trademark for a tricyclic antidepressant (doxepin hydrochloride).

sinew /sin'yōō/ [ME, *sinewe*], the tendon of a muscle, such as the thick, flattened tendon attached to the short head of the biceps brachii. See also **tendon.**

singer's nodule. See **vocal cord nodule.**

single-blind study [L, *singulus*, one by one; AS, *blind*; L, *studere*, to be busy], an experiment in which the person

collecting data knows whether the subject is in the control group or the experimental group, but subjects do not. See also **double-blind study.**

single component insulin [L, *singulus* + *componere*, to bring together + *insula*, island of Langerhans], any highly purified insulin with less than 10 ppm of proinsulin.

single footling breech. See **footling breech.**

single monster, a fetus with a single body and head but severely malformed or duplicated parts or organs.

single-parent family, a family consisting of only the mother or the father and one or more dependent children.

single-photon emission computed tomography (SPECT), a variation of computed tomography (CT) scanning in which the ray sum is defined by the collimator holes on the gamma-ray detector rotating around the patient. SPECT units usually consist of large crystal gamma cameras mounted on a gantry that permits rotation of the camera around the patient. Multiple detectors are used to reduce the imaging time.

single room occupant (SRO), a single person, usually an elderly individual, who lives alone in a single room of a low-cost hotel or apartment building.

singultus. See **hiccup.**

sinister /sin'istər/ [L, *left*], left, at the left side, at the left hand.

sinistral /sinis'trəl,/ [L, *sinister*, left], relating to the left side.

sinistrality. See **left-handedness.**

sinistro-, a combining form meaning 'left, or related to the left side': *sinistrocardia, sinistrophobia, sinistrotorsion.*

sinoatrial [L *sinus* + *atrium* hall], pertaining to the sinus node and atrium.

sinoatrial (SA) block /sī'nō·ā'trē·əl/ [L, *sinus*, hollow, *atrium*, hall; Fr, *bloc*], a conduction disturbance in the heart during which an impulse formed within the SA node is blocked from depolarizing the atria. The condition is indicated on the electrocardiogram by the absence of some P waves. Causes include excessive vagal stimulation, acute infections, and atherosclerosis. SA block also may be an adverse reaction to quinidine or digitalis. Treatment for symptomatic SA block includes the use of atropine and isoproterenol, and, if these are not effective, regulation of the heart with an electronic pacemaker. See also **atrioventricular block, heart block, intraatrial block, intraventricular block.**

sinoatrial (SA) node, a cluster of hundreds of cells located in the right atrial wall of the heart, near the opening of the superior vena cava. It comprises a knot of modified heart muscle that generates impulses that travel swiftly throughout the muscle fibers of both atria, causing them to contract. Specialized pacemaker cells in the node have an intrinsic rhythm that is independent of any stimulation by nerve impulses from the brain and the spinal cord. Slender fusiform cells making up the sinoatrial node are largely filled with sarcoplasm but contain a few striated fibrillae. The cells are irregularly grouped together and, at the edge of the node, merge with the atrial musculature. The sinoatrial node will normally "fire" at a rhythmic rate of 70 to 75 beats per minute. If the node fails to generate an impulse, pacemaker function will shift to another excitable component of the cardiac conduction system, such as the atrioventricular node or Purkinje's fibers. Certain hormones and various autonomic impulses can affect the sinoatrial node and cause it to "fire" faster, such as during strenuous physical activity. During a lifetime of 70 years the node generates about 2 billion impulses. Surgical implantation of an artificial pacemaker is a common procedure for individuals suffering from a defective sinoatrial node. Also called **Keith-Flack node, pacemaker.** Compare **atrioventricular node, Purkinje's network.**

sinus /sī′nəs/ [L, hollow], a cavity or channel, such as a cavity within a bone, a dilated channel for venous blood, or one permitting the escape of purulent material.

sinus-, See **sin-.**

sinus bradycardia. See **bradycardia.**

sinus dysrhythmia, an irregular heart rhythm characterized by alternate speeding up and slowing down of the heart rate. It is often associated with the vagal effects of respiration.

sinuses of morgagni. See **aortic sinus.**

sinuses of valsalva. See **aortic sinus.**

sinusitis /sīnəsī′tis/ [L, sinus + Gk, itis, inflammation], an inflammation of one or more paranasal sinuses. It may be a complication of an upper respiratory infection, dental infection, allergy, a change in atmosphere, as in air travel or underwater swimming, or a structural defect of the nose. With swelling of nasal mucous membranes the openings from sinuses to the nose may be obstructed, resulting in an accumulation of sinus secretions, causing pressure, pain, headache, fever, and local tenderness. Complications include cavernous sinus thrombosis and spread of infection to bone, brain, or meninges. Treatment includes steam inhalations, nasal decongestants, analgesics, and, if infection is present, antibiotics. Surgery to improve drainage may be performed in the treatment of chronic sinusitis.

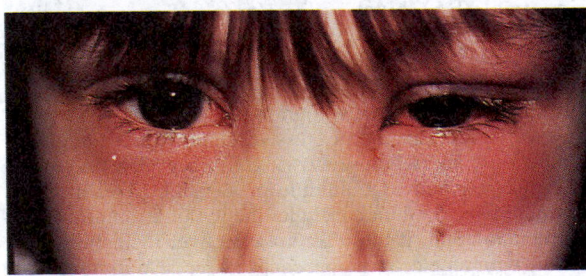

Child with sinusitis
(Zitelli, 1992/Courtesy Dr Ellen Wald, Children's Hospital of Pittsburgh)

sinus node, an area of specialized heart tissue near the entrance of the superior vena cava that generates the cardiac impulse and is in turn controlled by the autonomic nervous system. Also called **SA node.**

sinusoid /sī′nəsoid/ [L, sinus + Gk, eidos, form], an anastomosing blood vessel, somewhat larger than a capillary, lined with reticuloendothelial cells.

sinus pacemaker. See **sinus node.**

sinus rhythm, a cardiac rhythm stimulated by the sinus (sinoatrial) node.

sinus tachycardia [L, sinus, hollow; Gk, tachys, fast + kardia, heart], a rapid heartbeat generated by stimulation of the sinoatrial pacemaker. The rate is generally between 100 and 160 beats per minute.

sinus venosus defect. See **atrial septal defect.**

si op. sit (in prescriptions), abbreviation for the Latin phrase *si opus sita*, 'if necessary.'

Sippy diet [Bertram W. Sippy, American physician, b. 1866], a severely restricted dietary regimen for peptic ulcer patients. It consists of hourly servings of milk and cream for several days, with the gradual addition of eggs, refined cereals, puréed vegetables, crackers, and other simple foods as tolerated until the regular bland diet is reached. Because the diet restricts all fresh vegetables and fruits, supplementary iron and vitamins are indicated to prevent deficiency states. See also **bland diet.**

sireniform fetus. See **sirenomelus.**

sirenomelia /sī′rənəmē′lē·ə/ [Gk, seiren, mermaid, melos, limb], a congenital anomaly in which there is complete fusion of the lower extremities and no feet. Also called **apodial symmelia.**

sirenomelus /sī′rənom′ələs/, an infant who has sirenomelia. Also called **sireniform fetus, sympus apus.**

siriasis /sirī′əsis/ [Gk, sieros, scorching], sunstroke. See also **heat hyperpyrexia.**

-sis, a suffix meaning an 'action, process, condition, state, or result of': *centesis, genesis, stasis.*

Sister Kenny's treatment [Elizabeth Kenny, Australian nurse, b. 1886; Fr *traitement*], poliomyelitis therapy in which the patient's limbs and back are wrapped in warm, moist woolen cloths and, after the pain subsides, the patient is taught to exercise affected muscles, especially by swimming. Equally important is passive movement of affected limbs with simultaneous stimulation at the site of muscle origins, carried out after hot packs.

site [L, situs, location], **1.** location. See also **situs. 2.** a quantum of space occupied and defined by a cluster of people.

site visit, a visit made by designated officials to evaluate or to gather information about a department or institution. A site visit is a step in the accreditation of an institution and in the funding of many major projects.

-sitia, a suffix meaning '(condition of) appetite for food': *apositia, asitia, eusitia.*

sito-, sitio-, a combining form meaning 'of or pertaining to food': *sitomania, sitotherapy, sitiophobia.*

sitosterol /sītos′tərôl/ [Gk, sitos, food, stereos, solid; Ar, alkohl, essence], a mixture of sterols derived from plants, such as wheat germ, used for treating hyperbetalipoproteinemia and hypercholesterolemia that are unresponsive to dietary measures. Its use is controversial, for a dispersing action in the mixture tends to cause loose bowel movements and may leads to diarrhea or interfere with the absorption of concomitantly administered medications. Use in pregnancy is not recommended.

situational anxiety /sich′oo·ā′shənəl/ [L, situs, location], a state of apprehension, discomfort, and anxiety precipitated by the experience of new or changed situations or events. Situational anxiety is not abnormal and requires no treatment; it usually disappears as the person adjusts to the new experiences. See also **anxiety, anxiety neurosis.**

situational crisis, (in psychiatry) a crisis that arises suddenly in response to an external event or a conflict concerning a specific circumstance. The symptoms are transient, and the episode is usually brief.

situational depression, (in psychiatry) an episode of emotional and psychologic depression that occurs in response to a specific set of external conditions or circumstances. See **major mood disorders.**

situational loss, the loss of a person, thing, or quality, resulting from a change in a life situation, including changes related to illness, body image, environment, and death.

situational psychosis, (in psychiatry) a psychotic episode that results from a specific set of external circumstances.

situational supports, people who are available and can be depended on to help a patient solve problems.

situational theory, a leadership theory in which the manager chooses a leadership style to match the particular situation.

situational therapy, (in psychiatry) a kind of psychotherapy in which the milieu is part of the treatment program. See also **milieu therapy.**

situation relating /sich'ōō·ā'shən/, (in nursing research) a study design used to explain or predict phenomena in nursing practice in which a relationship is thought to exist among certain practices or characteristics of the population being studied.

situation therapy. See **milieu therapy.**

situs /sī'təs/ [L, location], the normal position or location of an organ or part of the body.

situs inversus viscerum, the transposition of the abdominal and thoracic organs to opposite sides of the body.

sitz bath /sits, zits/ [Ger, *Sitz,* seat; AS, *bæth*], a bath in which only the hips and buttocks are immersed in water or saline solution. The procedure is used for patients who have had rectal or perineal surgery. Also called **hip bath.**

SI units, the international units of physical amounts. Examples of these units are the volume of a liter, the length of a meter, or the precise amount of time in a minute. A group of scientists (Comité International des Poids et Mesures) meets regularly to define the units.

sixth disease. See **roseola infantum.**

sixth cranial nerve. See **abducens nerve.**

Sjögren-Larsson syndrome /shō'grenlär'sən/ [Torsten Sjögren, Swedish pediatrician, b. 1859; T. Larsson, twentieth century Swedish pediatrician], a congenital condition, inherited as an autosomal recessive trait, characterized by ichthyosis, mental deficiency, and spastic paralysis.

Sjögren's syndrome [Henrik S. C. Sjögren, Swedish ophthalmologist, b. 1899], an immunologic disorder characterized by deficient moisture production of the lacrimal, salivary, and other glands and resulting in abnormal dryness of the mouth, eyes, and other mucous membranes. The

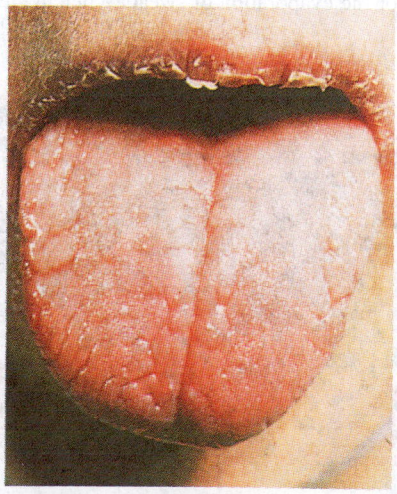

Sjögren's syndrome *(Shipley, 1993)*

symptoms affect primarily women over the age of 40. In some people the condition affects only the eyes or mouth, whereas in others nearly any body system may be involved. Atrophy of the lacrimal glands can lead to desiccation of the cornea and conjunctiva with damage to the tissues. Atrophy of the salivary glands results in dental disorders and loss of taste and odor sensations. When the lungs are affected, the dryness increases susceptibility to pneumonia and other respiratory infections. Sjögren's syndrome is frequently associated with Raynaud's phenomenon, rheumatoid arthritis, Waldenström's macroglobulinemia, and lymphoma. Treatment includes application of artificial tears and the use of soft contact lenses that can be moistened often, sipping fluids frequently to prevent mouth dryness, and avoiding use of medications that tend to deplete body fluids. See **dry eye syndrome, keratoconjunctiva sicca.**

SK, abbreviation for **streptokinase.**

SK-Ampicillin, a trademark for an antibacterial (ampicillin).

skato-. See **scato-.**

SK-Bamate, a trademark for a sedative (meprobamate).

skeletal. See **skeleton.**

skeletal enchondromatosis. See **enchondromatosis.**

skeletal fixation /skel'ətəl/ [Gk, *skeletos,* dried up; L, *figere,* to fasten], any method of holding together the fragments of a fractured bone by the attaching of wires, screws, plates, or nails. See also **external pin fixation.**

skeletal muscle. See **striated muscle.**

skeletal system, all of the bones and cartilage of the body that collectively provide the supporting framework for the muscles and organs. See also the Color Atlas of Human Anatomy.

skeletal traction, one of the two basic kinds of traction used in orthopedics for the treatment of fractured bones and the correction of orthopedic abnormalities. Skeletal traction is applied to the affected structure by a metal pin or wire inserted in the tissue of the structure and attached to traction ropes. Skeletal traction is often used when continuous traction is desired to immobilize, position, and align a fractured bone properly during the healing process. Infection of the pin tract is one of the complications that may develop with skeletal traction, and careful scrutiny of pin sites is an important precaution. Some common signs of infection of the pin tracts are erythema, drainage, noxious odor, pin slippage, temperature elevation, and pain. Superficial infection of pin tracts is often treated with antibiotic therapy. Deeper infections usually require pin removal and antibiotic therapy. Compare **skin traction.** See also **Dunlop skeletal traction.**

skeleto-, a combining form meaning 'relating to the skeleton': *skeletogenous, skeletonic.*

skeleton /skel'ətən/ [Gk, *skeletos,* dried up], the supporting framework for the body, comprising 206 bones that protect delicate structures, provide attachments for muscles, allow body movement, serve as major reservoirs of blood, and produce red blood cells. The skeleton is divided into the axial skeleton, which has 74 bones, the appendicular skeleton with 126 bones, and the 6 auditory ossicles. The skeleton is derived from the mesoderm that grows from the primitive streak as skeletal cells multiply, change, and migrate into various regions and form the membranous skeleton. Most of the membranous skeleton changes to cartilaginous skeleton in which ossification centers spread to form the bony skeleton. The four types of bones composing the skeleton are the long bones, including the humerus, the ulna, the femur, the tibia, the fibula, and the phalanges of the fingers and the toes; the short bones, including the carpals and the tarsals; the flat bones, including the frontal bone and the parietal bone of the cranium, the ribs, and the shoulder bones; and the irregular bones, including the vertebrae, the bones of the sacrum, the bones of the coccyx, and certain bones of the skull, such as the sphenoid, the ethmoid, and the mandible. The skeleton changes throughout life as bone formation and bone destruction proceed concurrently. During childhood and adolescence, bone formation proceeds faster than bone destruction. Between 35 and 40 years of age, bone destruction proceeds faster than bone formation. In advanced age bone destruction increases, bones become thin and brittle, vertebrae may collapse, and height decreases. See also **bone,** and see the Color Atlas of Human Anatomy. **–skeletal,** *adj*.

Skene's duct. See **paraurethral duct.**

Skene's glands /skēnz/ [Alexander J. C. Skene, American gynecologist, b. 1838], the largest of the glands opening into the urethra of women. They contain ducts that open just within the urethral orifice.

skew /skyōō/ [ME, *skewen*, to escape], a deviation from a line or symmetric pattern, such as data in a research study that do not follow the expected statistical curve of distribution because of the unwitting introduction of another variable.

skia-, scia-, a combining form meaning 'of or related to shadows, especially of internal structures as produced by roentgen rays': *skiabaryt, skiagenol, skiagraph.*

skilled nursing facility (SNF) [ME, *skil,* distinction], an institution or part of an institution that meets criteria for accreditation established by the sections of the Social Security Act that determine the basis for Medicaid and Medicare reimbursement for skilled nursing care, including rehabilitation and various medical and nursing procedures. Written policies and protocols are formulated with appropriate professional consultation. Law requires that these policies designate which level of caregiver is responsible for implementation of each policy, that the care of every patient be under the supervision of a physician, that a physician be available on an emergency basis, that records be maintained regarding the condition and care of every patient, that nursing service be available 24 hours a day, and that at least one full-time registered nurse be employed. Other criteria stipulate that the facility have appropriate facilities for storing and dispensing drugs and biologics, that it maintain a use review plan, that all licensing requirements of the state in which it is located be met, and that an overall budget be maintained.

Skillern's fracture /skil'ərnz/ [Penn G. Skillern, American surgeon, b. 1882], an open fracture of the distal radius associated with a greenstick fracture of the distal ulna.

skill play [ME, *skil + plega,* sport], a form of play in which a child persistently repeats an action or activity until it has been mastered, such as throwing or catching a ball.

skills training, the teaching of specific verbal and nonverbal behaviors and the practicing of these behaviors by the patient.

skimmed milk [Dan, *skumme,* scum removal; AS, *meolc*], milk from which the fat has been removed. Most of the vitamin A is removed with the cream, although all other nutrients remain. It is available as fluid skimmed milk, fortified skimmed milk, nonfat dry milk, and a form of buttermilk. Also called **nonfat milk, skim milk.**

skimming [Dan, *skumme*], a practice, sometimes employed by health programs that receive their income on a prepaid or capitation basis, of seeking to enroll only relatively healthy individuals as a means of increasing profits by decreasing costs. See also **skimping.**

skimping [Swed, *skrympa,* to shrink], a practice, sometimes employed by health programs that receive their income on a prepaid or capitation basis, of delaying or denying services to enrolled members of the program as a means of increasing profits by decreasing costs. See also **skimming.**

skin [AS, *scinn*], the tough, supple cutaneous membrane that covers the entire surface of the body. It is the largest organ of the body and is composed of five layers of cells. Each layer is named for its unique function, texture, or position. The deepest layer is the stratum basale. It anchors the more superficial layers to the underlying tissues, and it provides new cells to maintain the cells lost by abrasion from the outermost layer. The cells of each layer migrate upward as they mature. Above the stratum basale lies the stratum spinosum. The cells in this layer are polygonal with tiny spines on their surfaces. As the cells migrate to the next layer, the stratum granulosum, they become flat, lying parallel with the surface of the skin. Over this layer lies a clear, thin band of homogenous tissue called the stratum lucidum. The boundaries of the cells are not visible in this layer. The outermost layer, the stratum corneum, is composed of scaly, squamous plaques of dead cells that contain keratin. This horny layer is thick over areas of the body subject to abrasion, such as the palms of the hands, and thin over other more protected areas. The color of the skin varies according to the amount of melanin in the epidermis. Genetic differences determine the amount of melanin. The ultraviolet rays of the sun stimulate the production of melanin, which absorbs the rays and simultaneously darkens the skin. Modified skin continues into various parts of the body, such as mucous membrane, as in the lining of the vagina, the bladder, the lungs, the intestines, the nose, and the mouth. Mucous membrane lacks the heavily keratinized layer of the outside skin. It secretes the mucus that lubricates and protects associated structures. The skin helps to cool the body when the temperature rises by radiating the heat of increased blood flow in expanded blood vessels and by providing a surface for the evaporation of sweat. When the temperature

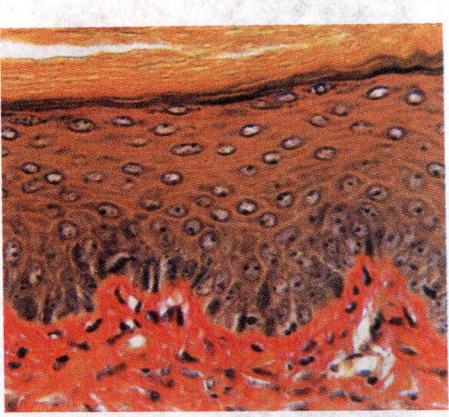

Photomicrograph of the skin (*Thibodeau, 1993*)

Skin color variations

Color	Condition	Causes	Assessment locations
Bluish (cyanosis)	Increased amount of deoxygenated hemoglobin (associated with hypoxia)	Heart or lung disease, cold environment	Nail beds, lips, mouth, skin (severe cases)
Pallor (decrease in color)	Reduced amount of oxyhemoglobin	Anemia	Face, conjunctivae, nail beds, palms of hands
	Reduced visibility of oxyhemoglobin resulting from decreased blood flow	Shock	Skin, nail beds, conjunctivae, lips
	Vitiligo	Congenital or autoimmune condition causing lack of pigment	Patchy areas on skin over face, hands, arms
Yellow-orange (jaundice)	Increased deposit of bilirubin in tissues	Liver disease, destruction of red blood cells	Sclera, mucous membranes, skin
Red (erythema)	Increased visibility of oxyhemoglobin caused by dilation or increased blood flow	Fever, direct trauma, blushing, alcohol intake	Face, area of trauma, sacrum, shoulders, other common sites for pressure ulcers
Tan-brown	Increased amount of melanin	Suntan, pregnancy	Areas exposed to sun: face, arms; areola, nipples

From Potter PA, Perry AG: *Fundamentals of nursing: concepts, process, and practice*, ed 3, St Louis, 1993, Mosby.

drops, the blood vessels constrict and the production of sweat diminishes. Also called **cutaneous membrane, integument.**

skin barrier, an artificial layer of skin, usually made of plastic, applied to skin before the application of tape or ostomy drainage bags. It protects the real skin from chronic irritation.

skin button, a plastic and fabric device that covers the drivelines of an artificial heart at their exit point from the skin. Its purpose is to eliminate the transmission of pumping pressure to the surrounding tissues.

skin cancer, a cutaneous neoplasm caused by ionizing radiation, certain genetic defects, or chemical carcinogens, including arsenics, petroleum, tar products, and fumes from some molten metals, or by overexposure to the sun or other sources of ultraviolet light. Skin cancers, the most common and most curable malignancies, are also the most frequent secondary lesions in patients with cancer in other sites. Risk factors are a fair complexion, xeroderma pigmentosa, vitiligo, senile and seborrheic keratitis, Bowen's disease, radiation dermatitis, and hereditary basal cell nevus syndrome. The most common skin cancers are basal cell carcinomas and squamous cell carcinomas. Tumors of the sebaceous glands or sweat glands occur infrequently and are adenocarcinomas. Basal cell carcinomas, typically raised, hard, reddish lesions with a pearly surface, do not metastasize, in contrast to scaly, slightly elevated squamous cell tumors that may become exophytic, friable growths with extensive ulceration and a nonhealing scab. A definitive diagnosis may be established by incisional biopsy or by excisional biopsy, which may be the only treatment required for small lesions. Surgery is usually indicated if the lesion is large, if bone or cartilage is invaded, or if lymph nodes are involved. Radiotherapy may be preferable for some smaller facial lesions and is commonly recommended for the treatment of skin tumors without distinct margins. Because of the possibility of recurrence of cancer, surgery is favored for the treatment of younger patients. Topical zinc chloride may be used in treating fairly common recurrent skin cancers; topical 5-fluorouracil is recommended for refractory premalignant actinic keratosis and for superficial basal cell carcinomas. An immunotherapeutic method is based on the induction of delayed hypersensitivity and consists of painting the lesions with a cream containing dinitrochlorobenzene (DNCB) and triethylene-immuno-benzoquinone (TEIB). Despite the curability of skin cancer, it causes many deaths because people fail to obtain treatment. Lesions caused by actinic rays may be prevented by applying a sunscreen containing paraaminobenzoic acid (PABA).

skin erythema dose. See **threshold dose.**

skin flap [AS, *scinn*; ME, *flappe*], a layer of skin, usually separated by dissection from deeper layers of tissue.

skinfold calipers, an instrument used to measure the breadth of a fold of skin, usually on the posterior aspect of the upper arm or over the lower ribs of the chest.

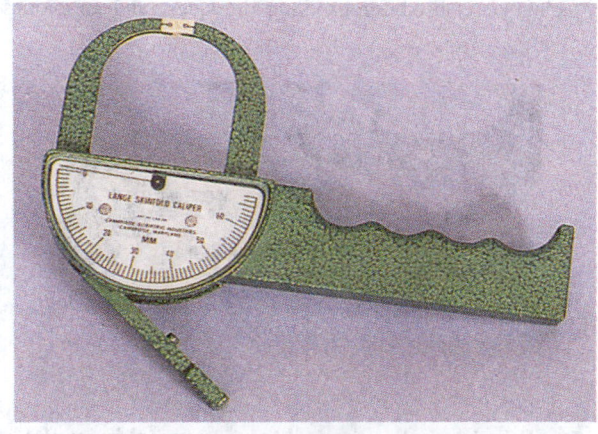

Skinfold calipers (Seidel, 1991)

skinfold thickness [AS, *scinn,* + *fealden,* + *thicce*], a measure of the amount of subcutaneous fat, obtained by inserting a fold of skin into the jaws of a caliper. The skinfolds are usually measured on the upper arm, thigh, or upper abdomen, and the caliper measurements are later compared with precalibrated standard tables to indirectly assess the body fat content of an individual.

skin graft, a portion of skin implanted to cover areas where skin has been lost through burns or injury or by surgical removal of diseased tissue. To prevent tissue rejection of permanent grafts, the graft is taken from the patient's own body or from the body of an identical twin. Skin from another person or animal can be used as a temporary cover for large burned areas to decrease fluid loss. The area from which the graft is taken is called the donor site; that on which it is placed is called the recipient site. Various techniques are used, including pinch, split-thickness, full-thickness, pedicle, and mesh grafts. In pinch grafting, ¼-inch pieces of skin are placed as small islands on the recipient site that they will grow to cover. These will grow even in areas of poor blood supply and are resistant to infection. The split-thickness graft consists of sheets of superficial and some deep layers of skin. Grafts of up to 4 inches wide and 10 to 12 inches long are removed from a flat surface—abdomen, thigh, or back—with an instrument called a dermatome. The grafts are sutured into place; compression dressings may be applied for firm contact, or the area may be left exposed to the air. A split-thickness graft cannot be used for weight-bearing parts of the body or to cover those subject to friction, such as the hand or foot. A full-thickness graft contains all of the layers of skin and is more durable and effective for weight-bearing and friction-prone areas. A pedicle graft is one in which a portion remains attached to the donor site whereas the remainder is transferred to the recipient site. Its own blood supply remains intact, and it is not detached until the new blood supply has fully developed. This type is often used on the face, neck, or hand. A mesh graft is composed of multiple slices of new skin. A successful new graft of any type is well established in about 72 hours and can be expected to survive unless a severe infection or trauma occurs. The procedure may be done with local anesthesia. Preoperatively, both the donor and the recipient site must be free of infection and the recipient site must have a good blood supply. Postoperatively, stretching or motion of the recipient site is prevented. Strict sterile technique is used for handling dressings, and antibiotics

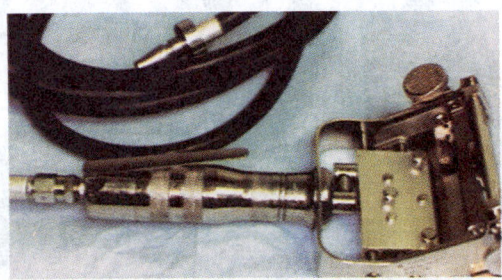

Stryker dermatome used to prepare skin grafts
(Grossman, 1993)

may be given prophylactically to prevent infection. Good nutrition with a high-protein, high-calorie diet is essential. The nurse may roll the surface of the graft regularly with a sterile applicator to express accumulated fluid to the edge of the graft, allowing better adhesion. See also **graft.**

skin integrity, impaired, a nursing diagnosis accepted by the Fourth National Conference on the Classification of Nursing Diagnoses. It is defined as a state in which an individual's skin is adversely altered. The defining characteristics of the problem are disruption of the surface of the skin, destruction of cell layers of the skin, and invasion of structures of the body through the skin. Risk factors may be environmental (external) or somatic (internal). Environmental factors that may affect the development of impaired skin integrity include heat, cold, or chemical substances; mechanical factors, such as a shearing force or pressure, restraint, or laceration; radiation; physical immobilization; and humidity. Somatic factors include drugs, obesity or emaciation, malnutrition, metabolic disturbance, circulatory disturbance, altered sensation or pigmentation, developmental factors, immunologic deficit, a disturbance in excretions or secretions, psychogenic factors, edema, or change in the turgor of the skin. See also **nursing diagnosis.**

skin integrity, impaired, high risk for, a nursing diagnosis accepted by the Fourth National Conference on the Classification of Nursing Diagnoses. It is defined as a state in which an individual's skin is at risk of being adversely altered. Risk factors may be environmental (external) or somatic (internal). Environmental factors include hypothermia or hyperthermia; presence of an injurious chemical substance; shearing force or pressure, restraint, or laceration; radiation; physical immobilization; presence on the skin of excretions or secretions; and an abnormally high humidity. Somatic factors include reaction to some medications; obesity or emaciation; an abnormal metabolic state; alteration in circulation, sensory function, or pigmentation; bony prominences; adverse developmental factors; decrease in normal skin turgor; and psychogenic or immunologic abnormalities. See also **nursing diagnosis.**

Skinner box [Burrhus F. Skinner, American psychologist, b. 1904; L, *buxus,* boxwood], a boxlike laboratory apparatus used in operant conditioning in animals, usually containing a lever or other device that when pressed reinforces by either giving a reward, such as food or an escape outlet, or removing a punishment, such as an electric shock. Also called **standard environmental chamber.** See also **operant conditioning.**

skin pigment [AS, *scinn;* L, *pigmentum,* paint], any skin coloring caused by melanin deposits in skin and hair. The coloring may be modified by substances in the blood, such as the several blood pigments, bile, or malarial parasites.

skin prep, a procedure for cleansing the skin with an antiseptic before surgery or venipuncture. Skin preps are performed to kill bacteria and pathologic organisms and to reduce the risk of infection. Various skin prep devices are available for this procedure. Such devices are commonly constructed of plastic, filled with a specific antiseptic, and equipped with an applicator. The antiseptic is applied by rubbing the device in a circular motion over the skin. Some of the most common antiseptics contained in skin prep devices are iodine, povidone-iodine, and ethyl alcohol. Each antiseptic has associated advantages and disadvantages. The iodine skin prep kills bacteria, fungi, viruses, protozoa, and yeasts and is an inexpensive and reliable device. The disadvantages of iodine, in addition to its discoloring of the skin, are that it may burn or chap the skin and may cause an allergic reaction. Povidone-iodine, which consists of water-soluble complexes of iodine and organic compounds, is less irritating than iodine tinctures or solutions and does not stain the skin as much as iodine. However, povidone-iodine is less effective than regular iodine solutions, may be absorbed through the skin during prolonged use, and may cause an allergic reaction. Ethyl alcohol, which is not effective against spore-forming organisms, viruses, and tubercle bacilli, is effective as a fat solvent and a germicidal when used in concentrations of 70% to 80% and may be used as a substitute skin prep antiseptic when the patient is allergic to iodine. Some disadvantages of ethyl alcohol are that it evaporates quickly, is highly flammable, and dries the skin excessively. Most skin prep devices are prepackaged and are disposable items for one-time use. To prep the skin with such a device before a venipuncture, the device is moved in a circular motion with the applicator rubbing the skin at the intended venipuncture site. The venipuncture site is swabbed with the antiseptic for about 1 minute. The antiseptic is spread over an area about 2 inches in diameter with the venipuncture site at the center.

skin tag, See **cutaneous papilloma.**

skin test, a test to determine the reaction of the body to a substance by observing the results of injecting the substance intradermally or of applying it topically to the skin. Skin tests are used to detect allergens, to determine immunity, and to diagnose disease. Kinds of skin tests include **patch test, Schick test,** and **tuberculin test.**

skin traction, one of the two basic types of traction used in orthopedics for the treatment of fractured bones and the correction of orthopedic abnormalities. Skin traction applies pull to an affected body structure by straps attached to the skin surrounding the structure. Kinds of skin traction are **adhesive skin traction** and **nonadhesive skin traction.** Compare **skeletal traction.** See also **Dunlop skin traction.**

skin turgor [AS, *scinn*; L, *turgere*, to swell], the resilience of the normal skin when subjected to physical distortion, such as by pinching or pressing. The relative speed with which the skin resumes its normal appearance after stretching or compression is an indicator of skin hydration. Turgor is slower in older people.

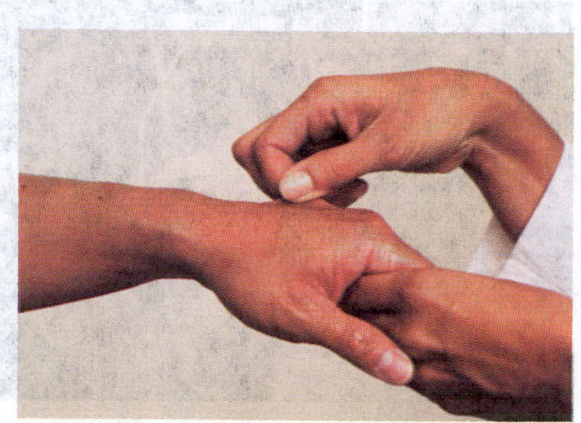

Assessment of skin turgor (Canobbio, 1990)

sklero-. See **sclero-.**

SK-Penicillin VK, a trademark for an antibacterial (penicillin V potassium).

SK-Pramine, a trademark for a tricyclic antidepressant (imipramine hydrochloride).

SK-65 Compound, a trademark for a fixed-combination drug containing analgesics (propoxyphene hydrochloride, aspirin, and phenacetin) and a stimulant (caffeine).

SK-Tetracycline, a trademark for an antibiotic (tetracycline).

skull [ME, *skulle*, shell], the bony structure of the head, consisting of the cranium and the skeleton of the face. The cranium, which contains and protects the brain, consists of eight bones. The skeleton of the face is composed of 14 bones.

SL, abbreviation for **soda lime.**

slander [Fr, *esclandre*, scandal], any words spoken with malice that are untrue and prejudicial to the reputation, professional practice, commercial trade, office, or business of another person. Formerly, slander included published defamation, but at present it is limited to spoken accusation. To bring legal action in slander, the slandered person must be able to demonstrate real temporal damages—except for cases in which the defamation relates to the person's business or profession or in which the malicious words question the person's chastity or accuse the person of being a criminal or of having a loathsome disease. Compare **libel.**

slant of occlusal plane [ME *slenten* to slope], (in dentistry) the inclination measured by the angle between the extended occlusal plane and the axis-orbital plane.

SLE, abbreviation for **systemic lupus erythematosus.**

sleep [AS, *slaepan*, to sleep], a state marked by reduced consciousness, diminished activity of the skeletal muscles, and depressed metabolism. People normally experience sleep in patterns that follow four observable, progressive stages. A device such as an encephalograph is used to record the recurrent pattern of brain waves during the stages: During stage 1, the brain waves are of the theta type, followed in stage 2 by the appearance of distinctive sleep spindles; during stages 3 and 4, the theta waves are replaced by delta waves. These four stages represent three fourths of a period of typical sleep and collectively are called **nonrapid eye movement (NREM)** sleep. The remaining time is usually occupied with **rapid eye movement (REM)** sleep, which can be detected with electrodes placed on the skin around the eyes so that tiny electric discharges from contractions of the eye muscles are transmitted to recording equipment. The REM sleep periods, lasting from a few minutes to half an hour, alternate with the NREM periods. Dreaming occurs during REM time. Individual sleep patterns normally change throughout life because daily requirements for sleep gradually diminish from as much as 20 hours a day in infancy to as little as 6 hours a day in old age. Infants tend to begin a sleep period with REM sleep, whereas REM activity usually follows the four stages of NREM sleep in adults.

sleep apnea, a sleep disorder characterized by periods of an absence of attempts to breathe. The person is momentarily unable to move respiratory muscles or maintain airflow through the nose and mouth. See also **apnea.**

sleeping pill, 1. *informal.* a sedative taken for insomnia or for postoperative sedation. 2. an over-the-counter pill, classified pharmaceutically as an aid to sleeping. Antihistamines, such as pyrilamine maleate and doxylamine succinate, depend for sedative action on side effects, which may disappear with continued use of such agents. The use of all drugs that depress the central nervous system is contraindicated for pregnant and lactating women and for patients with asthma, glaucoma, or prostatic hypertrophy.

sleeping sickness. See **African trypanosomiasis.**

sleep pattern disturbance, a nursing diagnosis accepted by the Fourth National Conference on the Classification of Nursing Diagnoses. It is defined as disruption of sleep time that causes discomfort or interferes with desired lifestyle. The critical defining characteristics, at least one of which must be present to make the diagnosis, are difficulty in falling asleep, wakening earlier than usual, interruption of the night's sleep by periods of wakefulness, or not feeling rested after sleep. Other defining characteristics are changes in behavior and performance, including increasing irritability, restlessness, disorientation, lethargy, and listlessness; physical signs, such as mild, fleeting nystagmus, slight hand tremor, ptosis of the eyelid, and expressionless face; thick speech with mispronunciation and incorrect words; dark circles under the eyes; frequent yawning; and changes in posture. Related factors are sensory factors, which may be either internal (illness or psychological stress) or external (environmental changes or social cues). See also **nursing diagnosis.**

sleep terror disorder [AS, *slaepan;* L, *terrere,* to frighten], a condition occurring during stages 3 or 4 of nonrapid eye movement sleep that is characterized by repeated episodes of abrupt awakening, usually with a panicky scream, accompanied by intense anxiety, confusion, agitation, disorientation, unresponsiveness, marked motor movements, and total amnesia concerning the event. The disorder is seen usually in children, is more common in boys than in girls, and is extremely variable in frequency but is more likely to occur if the individual is fatigued or under stress, or has been given a tricyclic antidepressant or neuroleptic at bedtime. Compare **nightmare.** See also **pavor nocturnus.**

sleepwalking. See **somnambulism.**

slide clamp [AS, *slidan; clam,* fastener], a device, usually constructed of plastic, employed to regulate the flow of intravenous solution. The slide clamp has a graduated opening through which the intravenous tubing passes. Pushing the tube into the narrow end of the opening constricts the tube and reduces the flow rate of the intravenous solution. Sliding the wide end of the opening over the tube increases the flow rate. Compare **roller clamp, screw clamp.**

sliding filaments [AS, *slidan;* L, *filamentum,* thread], interdigitated thick and thin filaments of a sarcomere. In muscle contraction, they slide past each other so that the sarcomere becomes shorter although the filament lengths do not change. The action of the sliding filaments contributes to the increased thickness of a muscle in contraction.

sliding transfer, the movement of a person in a sitting position from one site to another, such as from a bed to a wheelchair, by sliding the person along a transfer board.

sling [ME, *slingen,* to hurl], a bandage or device used to support an injured part of the body.

sling restraint, a therapeutic device, usually constructed of felt, used to assist in the immobilization of patients, especially orthopedic patients in traction. The sling is placed over the pelvis to reduce pelvic motion with lower extremity traction or over the abdominal area as countertraction with Dunlop traction. With lower extremity tractions, the sling restraint is attached to both sides of the bedspring frame. With Dunlop traction the sling restraint is attached to the opposite side of the bedspring frame. If the Dunlop traction is used in association with a Bradford frame, the sling restraint is attached under the frame. The sling restraint is rarely used with balanced suspension and is not usually used with Cotrel traction, halo-femoral traction, halo-pelvic traction, or suspension for elevation. Compare **diaper restraint, jacket restraint.**

slip-on blood pump [ME, *slippen,* slippery; *on*], a plastic mesh device with an attached squeeze bulb, rubber tubing, and pressure gauge, used to help administer large amounts of blood quickly. The plastic mesh slips over the blood bag and applies pressure to the bag when the bulb is squeezed. The pressure gauge displays a danger zone, usually marked in red, and indicates pressure limits for safe blood administration. Forcing blood into the veins at excessive pressure may damage the red blood cells or may disconnect the primary intravenous line.

slipped disk. See **herniated disk.**

slipped femoral epiphysis, a failure of the femoral epiphyseal plate that tends to occur primarily in overweight adolescents as a result of hormonal changes. Clinical features include hip stiffness and pain, with difficulty in walking. There also may be knee pain and external rotation of the affected leg. The condition is treated by orthopedic surgery.

slipping patella [ME, *slippen;* L, *patella,* small disc], a patella that undergoes recurrent dislocation.

slipping rib, a chest pain caused by a loose ligament that allows slippage of one of the lower five ribs. One of the ribs may slip inside or outside an adjacent rib, causing pain or discomfort that may mimic a disorder of the pancreas, gallbladder, or other upper abdominal organ.

slit lamp [AS, *slitan;* Gk, *lampein,* to shine], an instrument used in ophthalmology for examining the conjunctiva, lens, vitreous humor, iris, and cornea. A high-intensity beam of light is projected through a narrow slit, and a cross section of the illuminated part of the eye is examined through a magnifying lens.

slit lamp microscope, a microscope for ophthalmic examination. It permits the viewer to examine the endothelium of the posterior surface of the cornea in a projected band of light that is shaped like a slit.

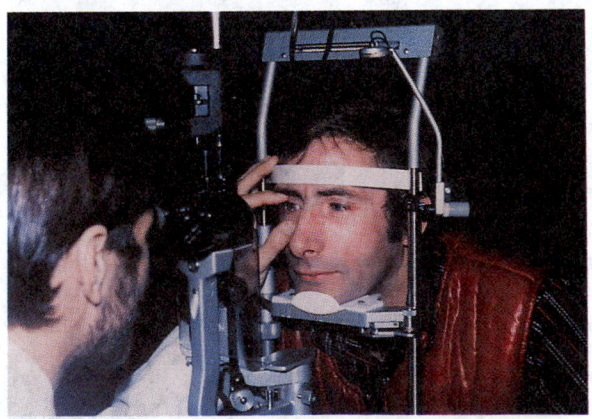

Slit lamp microscope *(Eagling, 1986)*

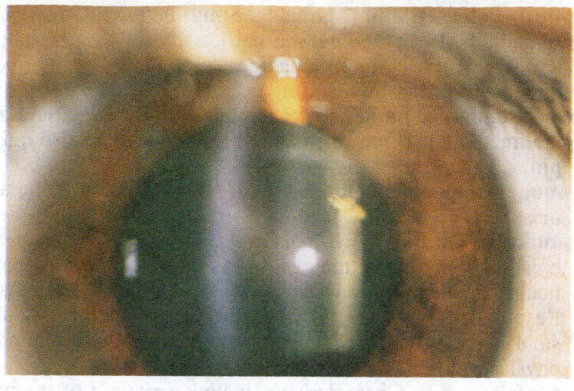

Image seen through a slit lamp microscope
(Spalton, 1984)

slit scan radiography, a technique for producing x-rays of body structures without length distortion by scanning a fan-shaped beam through a narrow slit collimator. The beam divergence perpendicular to the scan results in some distortion of width.

slit tongue. See **forked tongue.**

Slo-Phyllin, a trademark for a bronchodilator (theophylline).

slough /sluf/ [ME, *sluh,* husk], **1.** to shed or cast off dead tissue cells of the endometrium, which are shed during menstruation. **2.** the tissue that has been shed.

slow-acting insulin. See **long-acting insulin.**

slow diastolic depolarization [AS, *slaw,* dull], the slow loss of negativity that occurs during phase 4 of the action potential in cardiac cells having automaticity.

Slow-K, a trademark for a slow-release tablet of an electrolyte replacement (potassium chloride).

slow pulse [ME, *slowe;* L, *pulsare,* to beat], a pulse rate of less than 60 beats per minute. The rate is commonly found among older people, conditioned athletes, and patients receiving beta blocker medications.

slow-reacting substance of anaphylaxis (SRS-A), a group of active substances, including histamine and leukotrienes, that are released during an anaphylactic reaction. They cause the smooth muscle contraction and vascular dilation that mark the signs and symptoms of anaphylaxis.

slow response action potential, (in cardiology) an action potential produced when none of the fast sodium channels is available for depolarization and the fiber is activated via slow calcium channels, producing an action potential with a slow upstroke velocity, low amplitude, and consequent slow conduction.

slow-twitch (ST) fiber, a muscle fiber that develops less tension more slowly than a fast-twitch fiber. The ST fiber is usually fatigue resistant and has adequate oxygen and enzyme activity. Studies indicate that world-class endurance runners apparently have high percentages of ST fibers. See also **fast-twitch (FT) fiber.**

slow virus, a virus that remains dormant in the body after initial infection. Years may elapse before symptoms occur. Several degenerative diseases of the central nervous system are believed to be caused by slow viruses, including subacute sclerosing panencephalitis and kuru.

slurred speech /slurd/ [D, *sleuren,* to drag; ME, *speche*], abnormal speech in which words are not enunciated clearly or completely but are run together or partially eliminated. The condition may be caused by weakness of the muscles of articulation, damage to a motor neuron, cerebellar disease, drug usage, or carelessness.

Sm, symbol for the element **samarium.**

SMA, 1. a trademark for a nutritional supplement for infants. **2.** abbreviation for **sequential multiple analysis.**

SMA-6, SMA-12, SMA-18. See **sequential multiple analysis.**

SMA 12, SMA 24, a trademark for a system that uses a small computer to perform 12 or 24 different blood chemistry tests from a single blood sample.

smack, *slang.* heroin.

small calorie. See **calorie.**

small cardiac vein [AS, *smael*], one of the five tributaries of the coronary sinus that drains blood from the myocardium. It runs through the coronary sulcus between the right atrium and the right ventricle and opens into the right side of the coronary sinus. It conveys blood from the back of the right atrium and the right ventricle and, in some individuals, is joined by the right marginal vein. Also called **right coronary vein.** Compare **great cardiac vein, middle cardiac vein, posterior vein of left ventricle.**

small cell carcinoma. See **oat cell carcinoma.**

smallest cardiac vein, one of the tiny vessels that drain deoxygenated blood from the myocardium into the atria. A few of these vessels end in the ventricles. Also called **vein of Thebesius.** Compare **anterior cardiac vein.** See also **coronary vein.**

small for gestational age (SGA) infant, an infant whose weight and size at birth fall below the tenth percentile of appropriate for gestational age infants, whether delivered at term or earlier or later than term. Factors associated with smallness or retardation of intrauterine growth other than genetic influences include any disorder causing short stature, such as dwarfism; malnutrition caused by placental insufficiency; and certain infectious agents, including cytomegalovirus, rubella virus, and *Toxoplasma gondii.* Other factors associated with the smallness of an SGA infant include cigarette smoking by the mother during pregnancy, her addiction to alcohol or heroin, and her having received methadone treatment. Asphyxia may be a significant risk for the SGA infant during labor and delivery if the condition is the result of placental insufficiency. Such an infant has a low Apgar score, becomes acidotic in labor and at birth, and is likely to develop hypoglycemia within the first hours or days of life. Given adequate nutrition and caloric intake, some SGA infants show phenomenal catch-up growth. Also called **small for dates (SFD) infant.** Compare **large for gestational age infant.** See also **dysmaturity.**

small intestine, the longest portion of the digestive tract, extending for about 7 m from the pylorus of the stomach to the iliocecal junction. It is divided into the duodenum, jejunum, and ileum. Decreasing in diameter from beginning to end, it is situated in the central and caudal part of the abdominal cavity, surrounded by large intestine. Compare **large intestine.** (See Fig. p. 1448.)

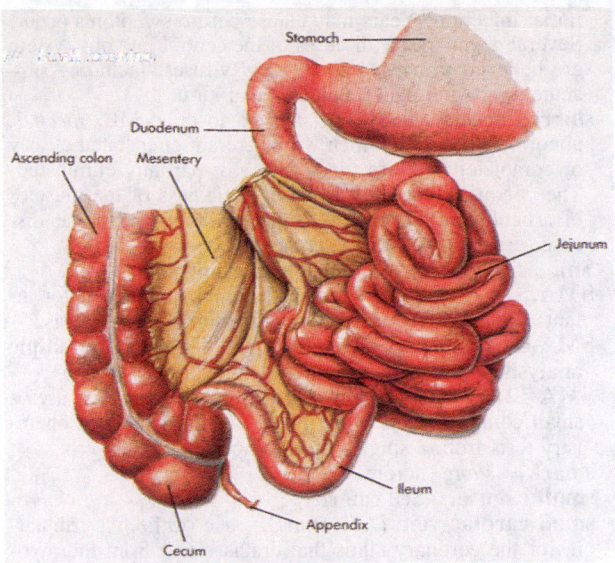

Small intestine *(Seeley, 1992/John Daugherty)*

small omentum.   See **lesser omentum.**

smallpox /smôl′poks/ [AS, *smael, pocc*], a highly contagious viral disease characterized by fever, prostration, and a vesicular, pustular rash. It is caused by one of two species of poxvirus, variola minor (alastrim) or variola major. Because human beings are the only reservoir for the virus, worldwide vaccination with vaccinia, a related poxvirus, has been effective in eradicating smallpox. For several years no natural case of the disease has been known to occur. Also called **variola.**

smallpox vaccine, a vaccine prepared from dried smallpox virus. It is indicated only for laboratory workers exposed to pox viruses.

small sciatic nerve [AS, *smael*; Gk, *ischiadikos*, of the hip joint; L, *nervus*], the posterior femoral cutaneous nerve, which pierces the fascia and subdivides into filaments, supplying the skin from the level of the greater trochanter to the middle of the thigh.

smear [AS, *smeoru*, grease], a laboratory specimen for microscopic examination prepared by spreading a thin film of tissue on a glass slide. A dye, stain, reagent, diluent, or lysing agent may be applied to the specimen, depending on the purpose of the examination.

smegma /smeg′mə/ [Gk, soap], a secretion of sebaceous glands, especially the cheesy, foul-smelling secretion sometimes found under the foreskin of the penis and at the base of the labia minora near the glans clitoris.

smell [ME, *smellen*, to detect odors], **1.** the special sense that enables odors to be perceived through the stimulation of the olfactory nerves; olfaction. See also **anosmia. 2.** any odor, pleasant or unpleasant.

smelling salt [ME, *smellen*; AS, *sealt*], aromatized ammonium carbonate to which may be added ammonia. It is used as a stimulant to arouse a person who has fainted.

Smith fracture [Robert W. Smith, Irish surgeon, b. 1807], a reverse Colles' fracture of the wrist, involving volar displacement and angulation of a distal bone fragment.

Smith-Hodge pessary.   See **pessary.**

Smith-Petersen nail [Marius N. Smith-Petersen, American surgeon, b. 1886; AS, *naegel*, nail], a three-flanged stainless steel nail used in orthopedic surgery to anchor the fractured neck of the femur to its head. It is introduced below the prominence of the greater trochanter and passed through the fractured part into the head of the femur. See also **nail, pin.**

smog, a polluting combination of smoke and fog in the atmosphere.

smoke inhalation [AS, *smoca*; L, *in*, within, *halare*, to breathe], the inhalation of noxious fumes or irritating particulate matter that may cause severe pulmonary damage. Respiratory burns are difficult to distinguish from simple smoke inhalation. Chemical pneumonitis, asphyxiation, and physical trauma to the respiratory passages may occur.

■ OBSERVATIONS: Characteristics include irritation of the upper respiratory tract, singed nasal hairs, dyspnea, hypoxia, dusty gray sputum, rhonchi, rales, restlessness, anxiety, cough, and hoarseness. Pulmonary edema may develop up to 48 hours after exposure.

■ INTERVENTIONS: Respiration is assisted by means of an airway and humidified oxygen, administered as necessary. Intravenous fluids, endotracheal intubation or tracheostomy, nasogastric tube, and bronchodilators may be ordered. Arterial blood gases are monitored, and corticosteroids may be given.

■ NURSING CONSIDERATIONS: The characteristics of smoke inhalation and its treatment vary with the nature of the fumes or matter inhaled and the extent of exposure; it is therefore important to know the circumstances, nature, period of exposure, and whether the person has a history of chronic respiratory or cardiac disease. Observation for at least several hours is usual; if pulmonary edema is anticipated, observation may be required for up to 48 hours.

smokeless tobacco [ME, *smoca*; Sp, *tabaco*], **1.** chewing tobacco or tobacco powder that allows the stimulating components of tobacco to be absorbed through the digestive tract, or through the mucus membrane in the case of snuff. **2.** a transdermal nicotine patch that can be affixed to the upper part of the body to satisfy the person's craving for nicotine.

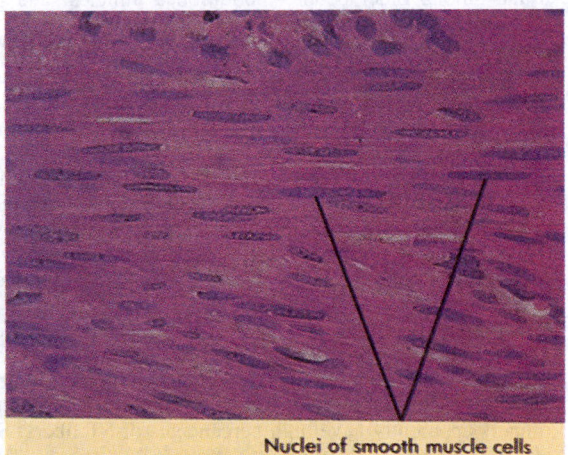

Smooth muscle *(Seeley, 1992/Ed Reschke)*

smooth muscle [AS, *smoth*], one of two kinds of muscle, composed of elongated, spindle-shaped cells in muscles not under voluntary control, such as the smooth muscle of the intestines, stomach, and other visceral organs. The heart muscle is an exception because it is a striated involuntary muscle. The nucleated cells of smooth muscle are arranged parallel to one another and to the long axis of the muscle they form. Smooth muscle fibers are shorter than striated muscle fibers, have only one nucleus per fiber, and are smooth in appearance. Biofeedback devices may help many people gain partial control of contractions of involuntary smooth muscles. Also called **involuntary muscle, unstriated muscle.** Compare **striated muscle, cardiac muscle.**

smooth pursuit eye movement, the tracking by the eyes of a slowly moving object at a steady coordinated velocity, rather than in saccades.

smooth surface cavity, a cavity formed by decay that starts on surfaces of teeth without pits, fissures, or enamel faults.

SMR, abbreviation for **submucous resection.**

smudge cell [ME, *sogen*, to soil], a degenerated leukocyte as seen in blood smears from patients with chronic lymphatic leukemia.

Sn, symbol for the element **tin.**

S.N., abbreviation for *student nurse*, used in signing nursing notes.

SNA, abbreviation for **State Nurses' Association.**

snail [AS, *snagel*, slug], an invertebrate of the order Gastropoda, several species of which are intermediate hosts of the blood flukes that cause schistosomiasis in humans. See also *Schistosoma*, **schistosomiasis.**

snakebite [AS, *snacan*, to creep, *bitan*], a wound resulting from penetration of the flesh by the fangs of a snake. Bites by snakes known to be nonvenomous are treated as puncture wounds; those produced by an unidentified or poisonous snake require immediate attention. The person is kept still, the wound is washed with soap and water, and a partially constrictive tourniquet is applied to retard the absorption of the venom; the tourinquet is released after 10 minutes. Incision of the skin through the bite marks is made and suction applied to assist bleeding and in removing the toxin. To avoid cutting muscles, nerves, or blood vessels, the incision should be only skin deep. An appropriate antivenin may be given that protects against the venom of most pit vipers, including the rattlesnakes, copperheads, and cottonmouths that are responsible for 98% of the poisonous snakebites in the United States. Bites of pit vipers are characterized by pain, redness, and edema; followed by weakness, dizziness, profuse perspiration, nausea, vomiting, or weak pulse; subcutaneous hemorrhage; and, in severe cases, shock. Treatment includes the use of analgesics and sedatives, antibiotics, and antitetanus prophylaxis to prevent infections from pathogens found in the mouths of snakes. Patients sensitive to horse serum in antivenin may require cortisone for the control of hives, urticaria, and other allergic reactions. Coral snakes rarely bite, but their venom contains a neurotoxin that can cause respiratory paralysis.

snake venom [AS, *snacan*; L, *venenum*], a poison produced in glands of certain snakes and injected through fangs into a victim's flesh. The exact composition of snake venoms vary with different species, but generally they are complex mixtures of neurotoxins, proteolytic enzymes, and phosphatases. About 20 of more than 100 North American species of snakes are venomous, accounting for about 8000 snake venom poisonings a year. A venomous snake bite is considered a medical emergency.

snapping hip [ME, *snappen*; AS, *hype*], a condition in which a tendon slips over the greater trochanter when the hip is moved, possibly producing a loud snapping sound.

snare /sner/ [AS, *sneare*, noose], a device designed for holding a wire noose, used in removing small pedunculated growths. The operator tightens the wire around the peduncle, thus removing the growth.

sneeze [AS, *snesen*, to sneeze], a sudden, forceful, involuntary expulsion of air through the nose and mouth occurring as a result of irritation to the mucous membranes of the upper respiratory tract, such as by dust, pollen, or viral inflammation. Also called **sternutation.**

Snellen chart [Hermann Snellen, Dutch ophthalmologist, b. 1834], one of several charts used in testing visual acuity. Letters, numbers, or symbols are arranged on the chart in decreasing size from top to bottom.

Snellen test, a test of visual acuity using a Snellen chart. The person being tested stands 20 feet from the chart and reads as many of the symbols as possible, reading each line and proceeding downward from the top. A score is assigned in the form of a ratio, comparing the subject's performance to that of a statistically normal subject's performance. A person who can read at 20 feet what the average person can read at this distance has 20/20 vision.

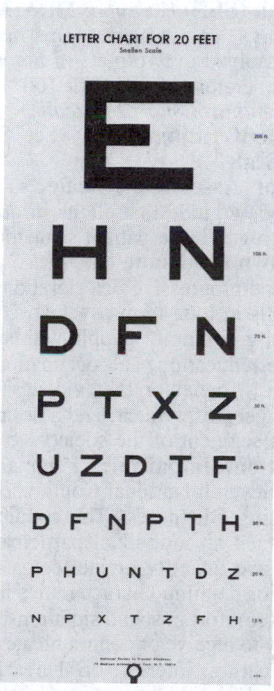

Snellen chart
Reproduced with permission of the National Society to Prevent Blindness.

SNF, abbreviation for **skilled nursing facility.**

snout reflex [ME, *snoute*, muzzle], an abnormal sign elicited by tapping the nose, resulting in a marked facial grimace. It usually indicates bilateral corticopontine lesions.

snow blindness [AS, *snaw* + *blind*], a condition of photophobia, sometimes accompanied by conjunctivitis, as a result of overexposure of the eyes to the glare of sun on snow.

Snowden-Pencer scissors. See **scissors.**

SNP, abbreviation for **sodium nitroprusside.**

S.N.P., abbreviation for **school nurse practitioner.**

snuff dipping, the practice of extracting juices from moist, fine-cut chewing tobacco placed in the mucobuccal fold of the mouth. The practice has been associated with an increased incidence of leukoplakia, tooth and gum diseases, and possible oral cancer.

snuffles [D, *snuffelen,* to sniff], a nasal discharge in infancy characteristic of congenital syphilis. See also **syphilis.**

soap [L, *sapo*], **1.** a compound of fatty acids and an alkali. Soap cleanses because molecules of fat are attracted to molecules of soap in a water solution and are pulled off the dirty surface into the water. **2.** a metallic salt of any salt produced from an acid. Compare **detergent.**

SOAP /sōp′, es′ō′ā′pē′/, (in a problem-oriented medical record) abbreviation for *subjective, objective, assessment, and plan,* the four parts of a written account of the health problem. In taking and charting the patient history and physical examination, a SOAP statement is made for each syndrome, problem, symptom, or diagnosis. Charting by this is said to be 'soaped,' and charts produced using it are called 'soap charts.' See also **problem-oriented medical record (POMR).**

soapsuds enema (SSE) [L, *sapo*; MDu, *sudse,* marsh water; Gk, *enienai*], an evacuent enema made of one ounce of soft soap dissolved in two pints of hot water and administered at a temperature of 38° C or 100° F.

SOB, abbreviation for *short of breath.*

social adjustment rating scale. See **Social Readjustment Rating Scale.**

Social Behavior Assessment Scale /sō′shəl/, a semistructured interview guide that elicits information from significant others regarding a patient's functioning.

social breakdown syndrome [L, *socius,* partner; AS, *brecan, dune*], the progressive deterioration of social and interpersonal skills in long-term psychiatric patients.

social class, a grouping of people with similar values, interests, income, education, and occupations.

social deviance, behavior that violates social standards, engendering anger, resentment, and a desire for punishment in a significant segment of the society.

social interaction, impaired, a nursing diagnosis accepted by the Seventh National Conference on the Classification of Nursing Diagnoses. The condition is defined as the state in which an individual participates in an insufficient or excessive quantity or ineffective quality of social exchange. Major defining characteristics include verbalized or observed discomfort in social situations; verbalized or observed inability to receive or communicate a satisfying sense of belonging, caring, interest, or shared history; observed use of unsuccessful social interaction behaviors; and dysfunctional interaction with peers, family, and/or others. A family report of change of style or pattern of interaction is also a characteristic. Related factors include a knowledge or skill deficit about ways to enhance mutuality, communication barriers, self-concept disturbance, absence of available significant others or peers, limited physical mobility, therapeutic isolation, sociocultural dissonance, environmental barriers, and altered thought processes. See also **nursing diagnosis.**

social isolation, a nursing diagnosis accepted by the Fifth National Conference on the Classification of Nursing Diagnoses. The diagnosis defines a condition in which a feeling of aloneness is experienced that the client acknowledges as a negative or threatening state imposed by others. The defining characteristics may be objective, subjective, or both. Objective characteristics include the absence of family and friends; the absence of a supportive or significant personal relationship with another person; the client's withdrawal and preoccupation with his or her own thoughts and interests; meaningless actions or interests and activities inappropriate to the client's developmental age; a physical or mental handicap or illness; or unacceptable social behavior. Subjective characteristics include verbal expression of feeling different from and rejected by others, acknowledgment of values unacceptable to the dominant cultural group, absence of a significant purpose in life, inability to meet the expectations of others, and the expressed feeling of insecurity in social situations. Related factors are those that lead to unsatisfactory personal relationships, such as unaccepted social behavior or social values, the inability to engage in social situations, immature interests or attitudes inappropriate for the developmental age of the client, alterations in physical appearance or mental status, or illness. See also **nursing diagnosis.**

socialization /sō′shəlīzā′shən/, **1.** the process by which an individual learns to live in accordance with the expectations and standards of a group or society, acquiring the beliefs, habits, values, and accepted modes of behavior primarily through imitation, family interaction, and educational systems; the procedure by which society integrates the individual. **2.** (in psychoanalysis) the process of adjustment that begins in early childhood by which the individual becomes aware of the need to accommodate inner drives to the demands of external realty. See also **internalization.**

socialized medicine /sō′shəlīzd/, a system for the delivery of health care in which the expense of care is borne by a governmental agency supported by taxation rather than being paid directly by the client on a fee-for-service or contract basis.

social learning theory, a concept that the impulse to behave aggressively is subject to the influence of learning, socialization, and experience. Social learning theorists believe aggression is learned under voluntary control, by observation of aggressive behavior in others, and by direct experience.

social margin, the sum total of all resources (material, personal, and interpersonal) available to assist an individual in coping with stress.

social medicine, an approach to the prevention and treatment of disease that is based on the study of human heredity, environment, social structures, and cultural values.

social mobility, the process of moving upward or downward in the social hierarchy.

social motivation, an incentive or drive resulting from a sociocultural influence that initiates behavior toward a particular goal. Compare **achievement motivation, physiologic motivation.**

social network, an interconnected group of cooperating significant others, who may or may not be related, with whom a person interacts.

social network therapy, the gathering together of patient, family, and other social contacts into group sessions for the purpose of problem solving.

social order, the manner in which a society is organized and the rules and standards required to maintain that organization.

social phobia, an anxiety disorder characterized by a compelling desire for the avoidance of and a persistent, irrational fear of situations in which the individual may be exposed to scrutiny by others, such as speaking, eating, or performing in public, or using public lavatories or transportation. Compare **simple phobia.** See also **phobia.**

social psychiatry, a branch of psychiatry based on the study of social influences on the development and course of mental diseases. In treatment, social psychiatry favors the use of milieu or other situational approaches to therapy.

social psychology, the study of the effects of group membership on the behavior, attitudes, and beliefs of the individual.

social readjustment rating scale, a scale of 43 common life events associated with some degree of disruption of an individual's life. The scale was developed by psychologists T. J. Holmes and R. Rahe, who found that a number of serious physical disorders, such as myocardial infarction, peptic ulcer, and infections, and a variety of psychiatric disorders were associated with an accumulation of 200 or more points on the rating scale within a period of 1 year. Most disruptive on one's life, according to the psychologists, was the death of a spouse, an event that warranted 100 points. The lowest rated event was a minor law violation, rated at 11 points.

social sanctions, the measures used by a society to enforce its rules of acceptable behavior.

Social Security Act, a U.S. federal statute that provides for a national system of old age assistance, survivors' and old age insurance benefits, unemployment insurance and compensation, and other public welfare programs, including Medicare and Medicaid.

social worker, a person with advanced education in dealing with social, emotional, and environmental problems associated with an illness or disability. A **medical social worker** usually has completed a master's degree program that includes experience in counseling patients and their families in a hospital setting. A **psychiatric social worker** may specialize in counseling individuals and families in dealing with social, emotional, or environmental problems pertaining to mental illness.

society /səsī'ətē/, a nation, community, or broad group of people who establish particular aims, beliefs, or standards of living and conduct.

Society for Advancement in Nursing (SAIN), a group established for advancement of the profession of nursing through higher education.

sociobiology /sō'sē·ō'bī·ol·əjē/ [L, *socius,* companion; Gk, *bios,* life + *logos,* science], the systematic study of biology as a basis for human behavior. Proponents contend that disease, stress, and aggression are natural pressures for maintaining an optimal level of population.

socioeconomic status /sō'sē·ō·ik'ənom'ik/ [L, *socius,* companion + *oeconomicus,* methodical + *status,* state], the position of an individual on a social-economic scale that measures such factors as education, income, type of occupation, place of residence, and in some populations, heritage and religion.

sociogenic /-jen'ik/ [L, *socius* + Gk, *genesis,* origin], pertaining to personal or group activities that are motivated by social values and constraints.

sociolinguistics /-ling·gwis'tiks/, the study of the relation-

Social readjustment rating scale

	Life event	Mean value
1.	Death of spouse	100
2.	Divorce	73
3.	Marital separation	65
4.	Jail term	63
5.	Death of close family member	63
6.	Personal injury or illness	53
7.	Marriage	50
8.	Fired at work	47
9.	Marital reconciliation	45
10.	Retirement	45
11.	Change in health of family member	44
12.	Pregnancy	40
13.	Sex difficulties	39
14.	Gain of new family member	39
15.	Business readjustment	39
16.	Change in financial state	38
17.	Death of close friend	37
18.	Change to different line of work	36
19.	Change in number of arguments with spouse	35
20.	Mortgage or loan for major purchase (home, etc.)	31
21.	Foreclosure of mortgage or loan	30
22.	Change in responsibilities at work	29
23.	Son or daughter leaving home	29
24.	Trouble with in-laws	29
25.	Outstanding personal achievement	28
26.	Spouse begins or stops work	26
27.	Begin or end school	26
28.	Change in living conditions	25
29.	Revision of personal habits	24
30.	Trouble with boss	23
31.	Change in work hours or conditions	20
32.	Change in residence	20
33.	Change in schools	20
34.	Change in recreation	19
35.	Change in church activities	19
36.	Change in social activities	18
37.	Mortgage or loan for lesser purchase (car, TV, etc.)	17
38.	Change in sleeping habits	16
39.	Change in number of family get-togethers	15
40.	Change in eating habits	15
41.	Vacation	13
42.	Christmas	12
43.	Minor violations of the law	11

Reprinted with permission from Holmes TH, Rahe RH: *J Psychosom Res* 11:213-218, 1967, Pergamon Press.

ship between language and the social context in which it occurs.

sociology /sō'sē·ol'əjē/ [L, *socius* + Gk, *logos,* science], the study of group behavior within a society.

sociopath. See **psychopath.**

sociopathic. See **psychopathic.**

sociopathic personality. See **antisocial personality.**

sociopathy /sō'sē·op'əthē/ [L, *socius,* companion; Gk, *pathos,* disease], a personality disorder characterized by a lack of social responsibility and failure to adapt to ethical and social standards of the community.

socket, the part of a prosthesis into which the stump of the remaining limb fits. Most modern prosthetic sockets are made of plastic materials, which are lighter and easier to clean than traditional leather sockets and odorless. Also called **bucket.**

soda [It, *sodo,* solid], a compound of sodium, particularly sodium bicarbonate, sodium carbonate, or sodium hydroxide.

soda lime (SL), a mixture of sodium and calcium hydroxides used to absorb exhaled carbon dioxide in an anesthesia rebreathing system.

sodium (Na) /sō'dē·əm/ [soda + L, *ium* (coined by Sir Humphry Davy, English chemist, b. 1778)], a soft, grayish metal of the alkaline metals group. Its atomic number is 11; its atomic weight is 22.99. Sodium is one of the most important elements in the body. Sodium ions are involved in acid-base balance, water balance, the transmission of nerve impulses, and the contraction of muscles. The recommended daily intake of sodium is 250 to 750 mg for infants 6 months to 1 year of age, 900 to 2700 mg for children 11 years of age or older, and 1100 to 3300 mg for adults. Sodium is an important component of more than 8 L of secretions produced by the body every day. These secretions include saliva, gastric and intestinal secretions, bile, and pancreatic fluid. The total daily secretion of sodium into these alimentary tract fluids averages between 1200 and 1400 mEq. A 154-pound adult has a total body pool of 2800 to 3000 mEq. Sodium is also linked to chlorine, which is the most important extracellular anion in the body. Sodium is the chief electrolyte in interstitial fluid, and its interaction with potassium as the main intracellular electrolyte is critical to survival. A decrease in the sodium concentration of the interstitial fluid immediately decreases osmotic pressure, making it hypotonic to intracellular fluid osmotic pressure. The kidney is the chief regulator of sodium levels in body fluids and will excrete sodium-free urine when the body needs to conserve sodium. In high temperatures, such as those associated with fever, the body loses sodium through sweat, further diluting sodium reserves with additional water drunk by the affected individual. To avoid serious complications, depleted sodium must be replaced. Sodium salts, such as sodium bicarbonate, are widely used in medications. Sodium bicarbonate has an immediate and rapid antacid action on the stomach, but any excess rapidly enters the intestine so that the substance has a shorter action than other antacids. Sodium bicarbonate, which is very effective in rendering the urine alkaline, is an ingredient in many solutions used as douches, mouthwashes, and enemas. Sodium is also important in the transport of sodium and potassium ions through the cytoplasmic membrane.

sodium acid glutamate. See **sodium glutamate.**

sodium arsenite poisoning, a toxic condition caused by the ingestion of sodium arsenite, an insecticide and weedkiller. The characteristic symptoms of arsenite poisoning are similar to those of arsenic poisoning, as is the treatment. See also **arsenic poisoning.**

sodium barbital, the sodium salt of 5,5-diethylbarbituric acid, a hypnotic and sedative drug.

sodium bicarbonate, an antacid, electrolyte, and urinary alkalinizing agent.
■ INDICATIONS: It is prescribed in the treatment of acidosis, gastric acidity, peptic ulcer, and indigestion.
■ CONTRAINDICATIONS: Pyloric obstruction, renal disease, congestive heart failure, or bleeding ulcer prohibits its use.
■ ADVERSE EFFECTS: Among the more serious adverse reactions are gastric distention, acid rebound, bicarbonate-induced alkalosis, hypernatremia, and hyperkalemia.

sodium chloride, common table salt (NaCl), used as a fluid and electrolyte replenisher, isotonic vehicle, irrigating solution, and enema.

sodium chloride and dextrose. See **dextrose and sodium chloride injection.**

sodium etidronate. See **etidronate disodium.**

sodium fluoride poisoning, a chronic condition of fluorine poisoning that occurs in some communities where the fluorine concentration in the water supply exceeds 1 ppm. Signs of the condition include mottling of tooth enamel and severe osteosclerosis. Also called **fluorosis.**

sodium glutamate, a salt of glutamic acid used for the treatment of hepatic coma and the enhancement of the flavor of foods. Also called **monosodium glutamate (MSG), sodium acid glutamate.**

sodium hypochlorite solution, a 5% aqueous solution of NaOCl used as a disinfectant for utensils not harmed by its bleaching action.

sodium iodide, an iodine supplement.
■ INDICATIONS: It is prescribed in the treatment of thyrotoxic crisis and neonatal thyrotoxicosis, and in the management of hyperthyroidism before thyroidectomy.
■ CONTRAINDICATIONS: Hyperkalemia or known hypersensitivity to this drug prohibits its use.
■ ADVERSE EFFECTS: Among the more serious adverse reactions are salivary gland swelling, metallic taste, rashes, and GI disturbances. Acute poisoning may result in angioedema and pulmonary edema.

sodium lactate injection, an electrolyte replenisher that has been prescribed for metabolic acidosis.

sodium nitroprusside (SNP), a vasodilator.
■ INDICATIONS: It is prescribed primarily in the emergency treatment of hypertensive crises and in heart failure.
■ CONTRAINDICATIONS: Certain compensatory forms of hypertension, such as coarctation of the aorta or impaired cerebral circulation, or known hypersensitivity to the drug prohibits its use.
■ ADVERSE EFFECTS: Among the most serious adverse reactions are a rapid fall in blood pressure or symptoms of cyanide poisoning (cyanide is produced by the metabolism of nitroprusside). Muscle spasms also may occur.

sodium perborate, an oxygen-liberating antiseptic ($NaBO_2.H_2O_2.3H_2O$) that may be used in the treatment of necrotizing ulcerative gingivitis and other kinds of gingival inflammation and for bleaching pulpless teeth. Prolonged or indiscriminate use of the compound may cause burns of the oral mucosa and blacken the tongue.

sodium phenobarbital, the sodium salt of phenylethylbarbituric acid, a long-acting sedative and hypnotic. It can be administered orally or parenterally and is used in the therapeutic management of seizure disorders.

sodium phosphate, a saline cathartic.
■ INDICATIONS: It is prescribed to achieve prompt, thorough evacuation of the bowel and, in lower dosage, for laxative effect.
■ CONTRAINDICATIONS: Congestive heart failure, abdominal pain, edema, megacolon, hypovolemia, salt-restricted diet, or hypersensitivity to this drug prohibits its use. Frequent administration in any dosage is not recommended.
■ ADVERSE EFFECTS: Among the more severe adverse reactions are dehydration, hypovolemia, abdominal cramping, and electrolyte imbalance.

sodium phosphate P32, an antineoplastic, antipolycythemic, radioactive agent.

■ INDICATIONS: It is prescribed for polycythemia vera, for neoplasms, including myelocytic leukemia, and for localizing tumors of the eye.

■ CONTRAINDICATIONS: Polycythemia vera with leukopenia or decreased platelet count, chronic myelocytic leukemia with leukopenia or erythrocytopenia, concurrent administration of other alkalating agents, or hypersensitivity to this drug prohibits its use.

■ ADVERSE EFFECT: The most serious adverse reaction is radiation sickness.

sodium pump, a mechanism for transporting sodium ions across cell membranes against an opposing concentration gradient. Sodium is normally moved from a region of low concentration within a cell to the extracellular fluid that contains a much higher concentration. Energy for this transport system is obtained from the hydrolysis of adenosine triphosphate by special enzymes. See also **calcium pump, electrolyte balance.**

sodium-restricted diet. See **low-sodium diet.**

sodium salicylate, an analgesic, antipyretic, and antirheumatic.

■ INDICATIONS: It is prescribed to relieve pain and fever.

■ CONTRAINDICATIONS: GI ulceration or bleeding or known hypersensitivity to this drug or to other salicylates prohibits its use. It is not given to a newborn infant.

■ ADVERSE EFFECTS: Among the most serious adverse reactions are GI bleeding and salicylate poisoning caused by overdose. Abdominal pain, nausea, and vomiting also may occur.

sodium stibocaptate, an investigational parasiticide for certain schistosomal infections. It is available from the Centers for Disease Control. Also called **stibocaptate.**

sodium sulfate, a saline cathartic for habitual constipation caused by peristaltic disorders.

■ INDICATIONS: It is prescribed to achieve prompt, thorough evacuation of the bowel and, in lower dosage, for laxative effect.

■ CONTRAINDICATIONS: Congestive heart failure, hypovolemia, or hypersensitivity to this drug prohibits its use. Frequent administration, in any dosage, is not recommended.

■ ADVERSE EFFECTS: Among the more severe adverse reactions are dehydration, hypovolemia, and electrolyte imbalance.

sodium sulfate anhydrous. See **salt cake.**

Sodium Versenate, a trademark for a metal chelating agent (edetate disodium).

sodoku. See **rat-bite fever.**

sodomist /sod′əmist/ [Sodom, Biblical city in ancient Palestine], a person who practices sodomy. Also called **sodomite** /sod′əmīt/.

sodomy /sod′əmē/ [Sodom, Biblical city in ancient Palestine], **1.** anal intercourse. **2.** intercourse with an animal. **3.** a vague term for "unnatural" sexual intercourse. **sodomize,** *v.*

soft chancre [AS, *softe;* Fr, *canker*], a usually painless local genital ulcer that follows an infection by *Haemophilus ducreyi* and is accompanied by suppuration of the inguinal lymphatic nodes, or inguinal buboes. Complications may include phimosis, urethral stricture or fistula, and marked tissue destruction. Also called **chancroid.**

soft contact lens [AS, *softe;* L, *contingere* + *lentil*], a contact lens made of a flexible plastic material that can be shaped more easily to fit the eyeball. Disadvantages are that soft lenses are more easily damaged, do not provide vision

as sharp as alternative methods, and must be disinfected periodically because they tend to harbor bacteria.

soft data [AS, *softe;* L, *datum,* something given], health information that is mainly subjective as provided by the patient and the patient's family, including pain or other sensations, lifestyle habits, and family health history.

soft diet, a diet that is soft in texture, low in residue, easily digested, and well tolerated. It provides the essential nutrients in the form of liquids and semisolid foods, such as milk, fruit juices, eggs, cheese, custards, tapioca and puddings, strained soups and vegetables, rice, ground beef and lamb, fowl, fish; mashed, boiled, or baked potatoes; wheat, corn, or rice cereals; and breads. Omitted are raw fruits and vegetables, coarse breads and cereals, rich desserts, strong spices, all fried foods, veal, pork, nuts, and raisins. It is commonly recommended for people who have GI disturbances or acute infections, or for anyone unable to tolerate a normal diet.

softening of bones /sô′fəning, sof′əning/ [AS, *softe* + *ban*], any disease that results in a loss of the mineral content of the bones. See also **osteomalacia.**

soft fibroma, a fibroma that contains many cells. Also called **fibroma molle** /mol′ē/.

soft money, *informal.* (in a university, school, or agency) income from unstable sources, such as grants or contracts.

soft neurologic sign, a mild or slight neurologic abnormality that is difficult to detect or interpret.

soft palate, the structure composed of mucous membrane, muscular fibers, and mucous glands, suspended from the posterior border of the hard palate forming the roof of the mouth. When the soft palate rises, as in swallowing and in sucking, it separates the nasal cavity and the nasopharynx from the posterior part of the oral cavity and the oral portion of the pharynx. The posterior border of the soft palate hangs like a curtain between the mouth and the pharynx. Suspended from the posterior border is the conical, pendulous, palatine uvula. Arching laterally from the base of the uvula are the two curved, musculomembranous pillars of the fauces. Compare **hard palate.**

soft radiation, a relatively long wavelength with less penetrating radiation than short wavelength radiation.

soft tissue rheumatism. See **fibrositis.**

software, the programs that control a computer and cause it to perform specific functions. Compare **hardware.**

software bug. See **bug.**

soft water [AS, *softe* + *waeter*], a water that does not contain salts of calcium or magnesium, which precipitate soap solutions.

sol, a colloidal state in which a solid is suspended throughout a liquid, such as a soap or starch in water. The fluidity of cytoplasm depends on its sol/gel balance.

sol., abbreviation for **solution.**

-sol, a suffix meaning a 'colloidal solution': *electrosol, nitromersol, plastisol.*

solar-, a prefix meaning 'of or pertaining to the sun': *solarium, solarization, solarize.*

solar fever. See **dengue fever, sunstroke.**

solarium /sōler′ē·əm/ [L, terrace exposed to sun], a large, sunny room serving as a lounge for ambulatory patients in a hospital.

solar keratosis. See **actinic keratosis.**

solar plexus /sō′lər/ [L, *sol,* sun; *plexus,* network], a dense network of nerve fibers and ganglia that surrounds the roots of the celiac and the superior mesenteric arteries at the level of the first lumbar vertebra. It is one of the great autonomic plexuses of the body in which the nerve fibers of the sympathetic system and the parasympathetic system combine. The denser part of the solar plexus lies between the suprarenal glands, on the ventral surface of the crura of the diaphragm and on the abdominal aorta. The preganglionic parasympathetic fibers reach the plexus through the anterior and the posterior vagi on the stomach. The preganglionic sympathetic fibers reach the plexus through the greater and the lesser splanchnic nerves. Secondary plexuses emerging from the solar plexus are the abdominal aortic plexus, the hepatic plexus, the inferior mesenteric plexus, the phrenic plexus, the renal plexus, the spermatic plexus, the superior gastric plexus, the splenic plexus, the superior hypogastric plexus, the superior mesenteric plexus, and the suprarenal plexus. Also called **celiac plexus.**

solar radiation, the emission and diffusion of actinic rays from the sun. Overexposure may result in sunburn, keratosis, skin cancer, or lesions associated with photosensitivity.

solar sneeze reflex [L, *sol*, sun; ME, *snesen*; L, *reflectere*, to bend back], a sneeze that may be caused by exposure to bright sunlight.

solar therapy [L, *sol*, sun; Gk, *therapeia*, treatment], the therapeutic use of sunlight. Also called **heliotherapy.**

Solatene, a trademark for an ultraviolet screen (beta-carotene), used in the treatment of erythropoietic protoporphyria.

sole [L, *solea*], the plantar surface of the foot.

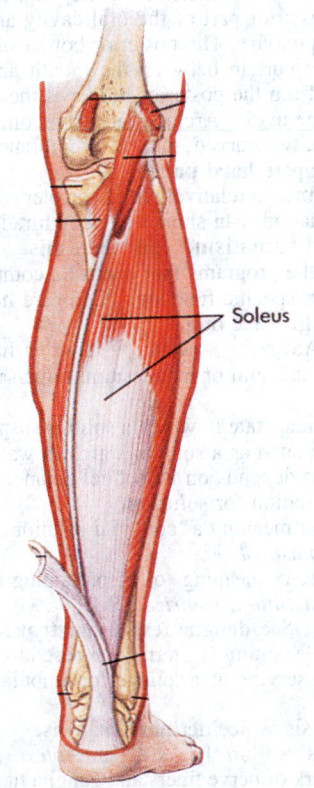

/ — Soleus

Soleus (*Seeley, 1992/John V Hagen*)

soleus /sō'lē·əs/ [L, *solea*, sole of foot], one of three superficial posterior muscles of the leg. It is a broad flat muscle lying just under the gastrocnemius and arising by tendinous fibers from the head of the fibula, from the popliteal line, and from the medial border of the tibia. The fibers of the soleus merge near the middle of the leg with those of the gastrocnemius to form the tendo calcaneus, which inserts into the calcaneus of the foot. The soleus is innervated by a branch of the tibialis nerve, containing fibers from the first and the second sacral nerves. The soleus plantar flexes the foot. Compare **gastrocnemius, plantaris.**

Solfoton, a trademark for an anticonvulsant and sedative-hypnotic (phenobarbital).

Solganal, a trademark for a gold salt antirheumatic (aurothioglucose).

solid /sol'id/ [L, *solidus*], **1.** a dense body, figure, structure, or substance that has length, breadth, and thickness, is not a liquid or a gas, contains no significant cavity or hollowness, and has no breaks or openings on its surface. **2.** describing such a body, figure, structure, or substance.

solitary coin lesion /sol'iter·ē/ [L, *solitarius*, standing alone; *cuneus*, wedge; *laesus*, injury], a nodule identified on a chest x-ray film by clear normal lung tissue surrounding it. A coin lesion is usually between 1 and 6 cm in size and often malignant.

solitary play, a form of play among a group of children within the same room or area in which each child engages in an independent activity using toys that are different from the others', concentrating solely on the particular activity, and showing no interest in joining in or interfering with the play of others. Compare **cooperative play.** See also **associative play, parallel play.**

solubility /sol'yəbil'itē/ [L, *solubilis*, able to dissolve], **1.** the maximum amount of a solute that can dissolve in a specific solvent under a given set of conditions. **2.** the concentration of a solute in a solvent at its saturation point.

solubility coefficient. See **coefficient.**

-soluble, a suffix meaning 'able to be dissolved': *acetosoluble, hydrosoluble, liposoluble.*

Solu-Cortef, a trademark for a glucocorticoid (hydrocortisone sodium succinate).

Solu-Medrol, a trademark for a glucocorticoid (methylprednisolone sodium succinate).

solute /sol'yo͞ot, sō'lo͞ot/ [L, *solutus*, dissolved], a substance dissolved in a solution.

solution (Sol.) /səlo͞o'shən/ [L, *solutus*], a mixture of one or more substances dissolved in another substance. The molecules of each of the substances disperse homogenously and do not change chemically. A solution may be a gas, a liquid, or a solid. Compare **colloid, suspension.** See also **solute, solvent.**

-solve, a combining form meaning 'to loosen': *dissolve, resolve.*

solvent /sol'vənt/ [L, *solvere*, to dissolve], **1.** any liquid in which another substance can be dissolved. **2.** *informal.* an organic liquid, such as benzene, carbon tetrachloride, and other volatile petroleum distillate, that when inhaled can cause intoxication as well as damage to mucous membranes of the nose and throat and the tissues of the kidney, liver, and brain. Repeated, prolonged exposure can result in addiction, brain damage, blindness, and other serious consequences, some of them fatal. See also **benzene poisoning, carbon tetrachloride, glue sniffing, petroleum distillate poisoning.**

som-, a combining form for growth hormone derivatives.

soma /sō'mə/, *pl.* **somas, somata** [Gk, body], **1.** the body, as distinguished from the mind or psyche. **2.** the body, excluding germ cells. **3.** the body of a cell. **—somatic** /sōmat'ik/, **somal,** *adj.*

Soma, a trademark for a skeletal muscle relaxant (carisoprodol).

soma-. See **somato-.**

somal. See **soma.**

somata. See **soma.**

-soma, -somus, a suffix meaning a 'body or portion of a body': *hystersoma, microsoma, prosoma, pleurosomus, hemisomus.*

-somatia, -somatic, a suffix meaning 'pertaining to the body': *diplosomatia, exsomatic, macrosomatia, microsomatia.*

somatic. See **soma, psychosomatic.**

-somatic. See **somatia.**

somatic cavity. See **coelom.**

somatic cell /sōmat'ik/, any of the cells of body tissue that have the diploid number of chromosomes, as distinguished from germ cells, which contain the haploid number. Compare **germ cell.**

somatic chromosome, any chromosome in a diploid or somatic cell, as contrasted with those in a haploid or gametic cell; an autosome.

somatic delusion, a false notion or belief concerning body image or body function. See also **delusion.**

somatic mutation [Gk, *soma*, body; L, *mutare*, to change], a sudden change in the chromosomal material in somatic cell nuclei affecting derived cells but not offspring.

somatic therapy, a form of treatment that affects one's physiologic functioning.

somatist /sō'mətist/, a psychotherapist or other health professional who believes that every neurosis and psychosis has an organic cause.

somatization /sō'mətīzā'shən/ [Gk, *soma*, body], a process whereby a mental event is expressed in a body disorder or physical symptom. Examples include peptic ulcers and asthma. See also **conversion.**

somatization disorder [Gk, *soma* + *izein*, to cause], a disorder characterized by recurrent, multiple, physical complaints and symptoms for which there is no organic cause. The condition typically occurs in adolescence or in the early adult years and is rarely seen in men. The symptoms vary according to the individual and the underlying emotional conflict. Some common symptoms are GI dysfunction, paralysis, temporary blindness, cardiopulmonary distress, painful or irregular menstruation, sexual indifference, and pain during intercourse. Hypochondriasis may develop if the condition is untreated. Also called **Briquet's syndrome.**

somato-, /sō'mətō-, sōmat'o-/ **soma-,** a combining form meaning 'of or pertaining to the body': *somatoceptor, somatogenic, somatopleural.*

somatoform disorder /sōmat'əfôrm, sō'mətōfôrm'/ [Gk, *soma* + L, *forma*, form], any of a group of neurotic disorders, characterized by symptoms suggesting physical illness or disease, for which there are no demonstrable organic causes or physiologic dysfunctions. The symptoms are usually the physical manifestations of some unresolved intrapsychic factor or conflict. Kinds of somatoform disorders are **conversion disorder, hypochondriasis, psychogenic pain disorder,** and **somatization disorder.**

somatogenesis /sō'mətəjen'əsis/ [Gk, *soma* + *genein*, to produce], **1.** (in embryology) the development of the body from the germ plasm. **2.** the development of a phys-

ical disease or of symptoms from an organic pathophysiologic cause. Compare **psychogenesis.** **—somatogenic, somatogenetic,** *adj.*

somatoliberin. See **growth hormone releasing factor.**

somatomedin. See **growth hormone.**

somatomegaly /sō'mətōmeg'əlē/ [Gk, *soma* + *megas*, large], a condition in which the body is abnormally large because of an excessive secretion of somatotropin or an inadequate secretion of somatostatin.

somatoplasm /sô'mətōplaz'əm/ [Gk, *soma* + *plasma*, something formed], the nonreproductive protoplasmic material of the body cells, as distinguished from the reproductive material of the germ cells. Compare **germ plasm.**

somatopleure /sô'mətōplŏŏr'/ [Gk, *soma* + *pleura*, side], the tissue layer that forms the body wall of the early developing embryo. Consisting of an outer layer of ectoderm lined with somatic mesoderm, it continues as the amnion and chorion external to the embryo. Compare **splanchnopleure.** **—somatopleural,** *adj.*

somatosensory evoked potential (SEP) /-sen'sərē/ [Gk, *soma* + L, *sentire*, to feel], evoked potential elicited by repeated stimulation of the pain and touch systems. It is the least reliable of the evoked potentials studied as monitors of neurologic function during surgery.

somatosplanchnic /-splangk'nik/ [Gk, *soma* + *splanchna*, viscera], of or pertaining to the trunk of the body and the visceral organs.

somatostatin /sō'mətōstat'in/, a hormone produced in the hypothalamus that inhibits the factor that stimulates release of somatotropin from the anterior pituitary gland. It also inhibits the release of certain hormones, including thyrotropin, adrenocorticotropic hormone, glucagon, insulin, and cholecystokinin, and of some enzymes, including pepsin, renin, secretin, and gastrin. Also called **growth hormone release inhibiting hormone.**

somatotherapy /-ther'əpē/, the treatment of physical disorders, as distinguished from psychotherapy.

somatotropic /-trop'ik/ [[Gk, *soma*, body + *trope*, a turn], pertaining to an agent that influences the body or body cells.

somatotropic hormone, somatotropin. See **growth hormone.**

somatotype /sō'mətōtīp'/ [Gk, *soma* + *typos*, mark],

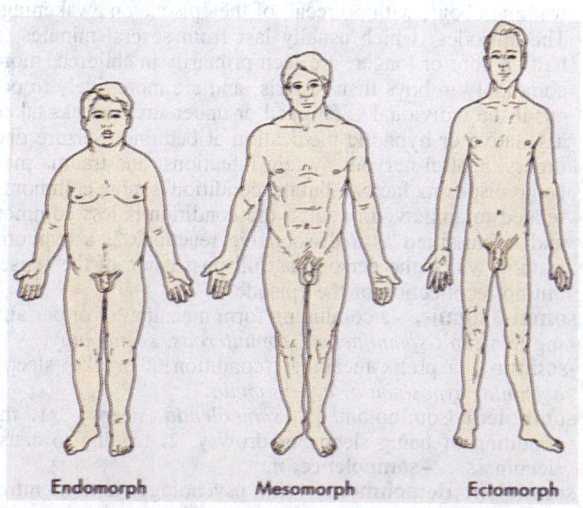

Somatotype *(Thibodeau, 1993/Joan M Beck)*

Endomorph   Mesomorph   Ectomorph

1. body build or physique. **2.** the classification of individuals according to body build based on certain physical characteristics. The primary types are **ectomorph, endomorph,** and **mesomorph.**

somatrem /sō'mətrem/, a synthetic polypeptide growth hormone produced by recombinant DNA technology.
- INDICATIONS: It is prescribed for patients who fail to grow because of limited endogenous growth hormone secretion.
- CONTRAINDICATIONS: This product is contraindicated for patients with closed epiphyses or who show evidence of underlying intracranial lesions. Concurrent use with a glucocorticoid may inhibit the effects of somatrem. The hormone may produce insulin resistance in some patients.
- ADVERSE EFFECTS: Among reported adverse reactions are insulin resistance and hypothyroidism.

-some, a combining form meaning 'a body' of a specified sort: *chromosome, microsome, sarcosome.*

-somia, a combining form meaning '(condition of) possessing body': *agenosomia, diplosomia, microsomia.*

somite /sō'mīt/ [Gk, *soma*], any of the paired, segmented masses of mesodermal tissue that form along the length of the neural tube during the early stage of embryonic development in vertebrates. These structures give rise to the vertebrae and differentiate into various tissues of the body, including the voluntary muscle, bones, connective tissue, and dermal layers of the skin. The first somite to appear is in the future occipital region, and the formation of new somites continues in a caudal direction until 36 to 38 have developed.

somite embryo, an embryo in any stage of development between the formation of the first and the last pairs of somites, which in humans occurs in the third and fourth weeks after fertilization of the ovum.

somn-. See **somni-.**

Somnafac, a trademark for a sedative-hypnotic (methaqualone hydrochloride).

somnambulance. See **somnambulism.**

somnambulism /somnam'byəliz'əm/ [L *somnus* sleep, *ambulare* to walk], **1.** also called **noctambulation, sleepwalking.** a condition occurring during stages 3 or 4 of nonrapid eye movement sleep that is characterized by complex motor activity, usually culminating in leaving the bed and walking about, with no recall of the episode on awakening. The episodes, which usually last from several minutes to half an hour or longer, are seen primarily in children, more commonly in boys than in girls, and are more likely to occur if the individual is fatigued or under stress or has taken a sedative or hypnotic medication at bedtime. Seizure disorders, central nervous system infections, and trauma may be predisposing factors, but the condition is more commonly related to anxiety. In adults, the condition is less common and is classified as a dissociative reaction. **2.** a hypnotic state in which the person has full possession of the senses but no recollection of the episode.

somni-, somn-, a combining form meaning 'of or pertaining to sleep': *somnifacient, somniferous, somnipathy.*

-somnia, a prefix meaning '(condition of or like) sleep': *asomnia, hyposomnia, hypersomnia.*

somnolent /som'nələnt/ [L, *somnolentia*, sleepy], **1.** the condition of being sleepy or drowsy. **2.** tending to cause sleepiness. −**somnolence,** *n.*

somnolent detachment, (in, psychology) a term introduced by Sullivan for a type of security operation in which a person falls asleep when confronted by a highly threatening, anxiety-producing experience. The mechanism originates in infancy.

Somogyi phenomenon [Michael Somogyi, American biochemist, b. 1883; Gk, *phainomenon*], a diabetes mellitus rebound effect in which an overdose of insulin induces hypoglycemia. This starts the release of hormones that stimulate lipolysis, gluconeogenesis, and glycogenolysis, leading to hyperglycemia and ketosis. Treatment involves gradually lowering the insulin dose to achieve an optimum level.

Somophyllin, a trademark for a bronchodilator (theophylline).

-somus. See **-soma.**

son-, a prefix meaning 'of or pertaining to sound': *sonitus, sonometer, sonotone.*

sonogram, sonography. See **ultrasonography.**

sonographer /sōnog'rəfər/, an allied health professional with special training in the use of ultrasound equipment for diagnostic and therapeutic purposes. Also called **diagnostic medical sonographer, medical donographer, ultrasonographer.**

sonorous rale /sənô'əs/ [L, *sonor*, noise], a snoring sound that may be produced by the vibration of a mass of thick secretion lodged in a bronchus. This sound is associated with various lung or respiratory disorders.

soot wart. See **scrotal cancer.**

sopor /sō'pər/ [L, deep sleep], a sleep that is as deep or sound as the state of stupor.

soporiferous /sop'ərif'ərəs/ [L *sopor*, deep sleep + *ferre*, to bear], tending to cause deep sleep, such as an agent that induces deep sleep.

soporific /sop'ərif'ik/ [L, *sopor*, deep sleep, *facere*, to make], **1.** of or pertaining to a substance, condition, or procedure that causes sleep. **2.** a soporific drug. See also **hypnotic, sedative.**

sorbent /sôr'bənt/ [L, *sorbere*, to swallow], the property of a substance that allows it to interact with another compound, usually to make it bind.

sorbic acid /sôr'bik/, a compound occurring naturally in berries of the mountain ash. Commercial sorbic acid derived from acetaldehyde is used in fungicides, food preservatives, lubricants, and plasticizers.

Sorbitrate, a trademark for an antianginal (isosorbide dinitrate).

sordes /sôr'dēz/, *pl.* **sordes** [L, *sordere*, to be dirty], dirt or debris, especially the crusts consisting of food, microorganisms, and epithelial cells that accumulate on teeth and lips during a febrile illness or one in which the patient takes nothing by mouth. Sordes gastricae is undigested food and mucus in the stomach.

sore /sôr, sōr/ [AS, *sar*], **1.** a wound, ulcer, or lesion. **2.** tender or painful.

sore throat [AS, *sar* + *throte*], any inflammation of the larynx, pharynx, or tonsils.

Sorrin's operation, a surgical technique for treating a periodontal abscess, used especially when the marginal gingiva appears healthy and provides no access to the abscess. A semilunar incision is made below the abscess area in the attached gingiva, leaving the gingival margin undisturbed. The tissue flap produced by the incision is raised, accessing the abscessed area for curettage, after which the wound is sutured.

s.o.s., abbreviation for the Latin phrase *si opus sit,* 'if necessary.'

Soto's syndrome. See **cerebral gigantism.**

souffle /soo'fəl/ [Fr, breath], a soft murmur heard through a stethoscope. When detected over the uterus in a pregnant woman, it is coincident with the maternal pulse and is caused by blood circulating in the large uterine arteries.

soul food [AS, *sawel*, *foda*], food linked with cultural or traditional origins, especially African-American, that contributes emotional significance and personal satisfaction to an individual.

sound [L, *sonus*], an instrument used to locate the opening of a cavity or canal, to test the patency of a canal, to ascertain the depth of a cavity, or to reveal the contents of a canal or cavity. A sound is used to determine the depth of the uterus, to detect stones in the bladder, and, less commonly, to assist in correctly inserting a urinary catheter in the urethra through the urinary meatus.

source-image receptor distance /sôrs, sōrs/ [OFr, *sourse*, origin; L, *imago*, likeness], the distance between the focus of an x-ray beam and the x-ray film as measured along the beam. Also called **focal film distance.**

South African genetic porphyria. See **variegate porphyria.**

South American blastomycosis. See **paracoccidioidomycosis.**

South American trypanosomiasis. See **Chagas' disease.**

Southern blot test /suth′ərn/, a gene analysis method used to identify specific DNA fragments and in the diagnosis of cancers and hemoglobinopathies. It involves the placement of a nitrocellulose film on agaraose gel surfaces with dry blotting material on the film. Liquid is then transported from a reservoir beneath the gel through the gel and nitrocellulose layer. The film adsorbs the DNA fragments. The fragments are then analyzed for rearrangements in immunoglobulin or cell receptor genes, chromosomal translocations, oncogene amplifications, and point mutations within oncogenes. Immunoglobulins and T cell receptor genes bear signatures that identify various leukemias and lymphomas. See also **Northern blot test.**

Southey's tube /sou′thēz/ [Reginald Southey, English physician, b. 1835], *obsolete.* a small, very thin cannula introduced into edematous tissue to withdraw fluid, especially from the legs or feet, to relieve the edema of congestive heart failure. Also called **Southey-Leech tube.** See also **cannula, tube.**

Sp, *pl.* **sp., spp.,** abbreviation for **species.**

space [L, *spatium*], an actual or a potential cavity of the body, such as the complemental spaces in the pleural cavity that are not occupied by lung tissue and the lymph spaces occupied by lymph.

space maintainer, a fixed or movable appliance for preserving the space created by the premature loss of one or more teeth.

space medicine, a branch of medicine concerned with the effects of travel in space, beyond the atmosphere and pull of gravity, including weightlessness, motion sickness, and restricted physical activity.

space obtainer, an appliance for increasing the space between adjoining teeth.

space regainer, a fixed or removable appliance for moving a displaced permanent tooth into its normal position in a dental arch.

space sickness. See **air sickness; motion sickness.**

Spanish fly. See **cantharis.**

spano-, a combining form meaning 'scanty or scarce': *spanogyny, spanomenorrhea, spanopnea.*

sparganosis /spär′gənō′sis/ [Gk, *sparganon*, swaddling

clothes, *osis*, condition], an infection with larvae of the fish tapeworm of the pseudogenus Sparganum, characterized by painful subcutaneous swellings or swelling and destruction of the eye. It is acquired by ingesting larvae in contaminated water or in inadequately cooked, infected frog flesh. Treatment includes surgery and local injection of ethyl alcohol to kill the larvae.

Sparine, a trademark for a phenothiazine antipsychotic and antiemetic (promazine hydrochloride).

sparteine sulfate, an alkaloid salt used to treat cardiac disorders and formerly used as an oxytocic to reduce uterine bleeding during the third stage of labor.

spasm /spaz′əm/ [Gk, *spasmos*], **1.** an involuntary muscle contraction of sudden onset, such as habit spasms, hiccups, stuttering, or a tic. **2.** a convulsion or seizure. **3.** a sudden, transient constriction of a blood vessel, bronchus, esophagus, pylorus, ureter, or other hollow organ. Compare **stricture.** See also **bronchospasm, pylorospasm.**

-spasm, a combining form meaning 'twitching or involuntary contraction' of a specified sort: *gastrospasm, neurospasm, vasospasm.*

spasmatic asthma /spazmat′ik/ [Gk, *spasmos* + *asthma*, panting], an airway obstruction characterized by paroxysms of wheezing and coughing caused by spasms of the bronchioles and inflammation of the bronchial mucosa.

spasmatic croup See **laryngismus.**

spasmo-, a combining form meaning 'of or pertaining to spasm(s)': *spasmodermia, spasmophemia, spasmophilia.*

-spasmodic, -spasmodical, a combining form meaning 'of, pertaining, or referring to a convulsion': *angiospasmodic, antispasmodic, postspasmodic.*

spasmodic croup. See **laryngismus.**

spasmodic dysphonia /spazmod′ik/ [Gk, *spasmodes*, spasms; *dys*, bad, *phone*, voice], a speech disorder in which phonation is intermittently blocked by spasms of the larynx. The cause is unknown. Also called **spastic dysphonia.**

spasmodic stricture [Gk, *spasmodes*; L, *strictura*, compression], a narrowing of a passage in which there is no organic change but there are merely muscle spasms.

spasmodic tic [Gk, *spasmodes*; Fr, *tic*], any repetitive movement in which spasmodic muscle group contractions occur at variable intervals.

spasmodic torticollis [Gk, *spasmodes*; L, *tortus*, twisted + *collum*, neck], a form of torticollis characterized by episodes of spasms of the neck muscles. The condition is often transient in nature, and examination seldom reveals a physical cause. In some cases, severe stress and muscular spasm may be the cause.

spasmogen /spaz′məjən/, any substance that can produce smooth muscle contractions, as in the bronchioles; examples are histamine, bradykinin, and serotonin.

spastic /spas′tik/ [Gk, *spastikos*, drawing in], of or pertaining to spasms or other uncontrolled contractions of the skeletal muscles. See also **cerebral palsy. −spasticity,** *n.*

spastic aphonia, a condition in which a person is unable to speak because of spasmodic contraction of the abductor muscles of the throat.

spastic bladder, a form of neurogenic bladder caused by a lesion of the spinal cord above the voiding reflex center. It is marked by loss of bladder control and bladder sensation, incontinence, and automatic, interrupted, incomplete voiding. It is most often caused by trauma, but may be a result of tumor or multiple sclerosis. Also called **reflex bladder, automatic bladder.** Compare **flaccid bladder.**

spastic colon. See **irritable bowel syndrome.**

spastic constipation [Gk, *spasmos*, spasm; L, *constipare*, to crowd together], a form of constipation associated with neurasthenia and constrictive spasms in part of the intestine. The condition may be a sign of lead poisoning.

spastic dysphonia. See **spasmodic dysphonia.**

spastic entropion. See **ectropion, entropion.**

spastic gait [Gk, *spasmos*, spasm; ONorse, *gata*], a pattern of walking in which the legs are stiff, the feet plantarflexed, and movements made by circumduction. The steps also may be accompanied by toe dragging.

spastic hemiplegia, paralysis of one side of the body with increased tendon reflexes and uncontrolled contraction occurring in the affected muscles.

spastic ileus [Gk, *spasmos*, spasm + *eilein*, to twist], a form of intestinal obstruction caused by bowel spasms.

spasticity /spastis′itē/ [Gk, *spastikos*, drawing in], a form of muscular hypertonicity with increased resistance to stretch. It usually involves the flexors of the arms and the extensors of the legs. The hypertonicity is often associated with weakness, increased deep reflexes, and diminished superficial reflexes. Moderate spasticity is characterized by movements that require great effort and lack of normal coordination. Slight spasticity may be marked by gross movements that are coordinated smoothly, but combined selective movement patterns are incoordinated or impossible.

spastic paralysis, an abnormal condition characterized by the involuntary contraction of one or more muscles with associated loss of muscular function. Compare **flaccid paralysis.**

spastic paraplegia [Gk, *spasmos*, spasm + *para* + *plege*, stroke], a form of partial paralysis affecting mainly older people. It is accompanied by irritability and spastic contractions of the leg muscles.

spastic pseudoparalysis. See **Creutzfeldt-Jakob disease.**

spastic pseudosclerosis. See **Creutzfeldt-Jakob disease.**

spastic strabismus [Gk, *spasmos* + *strabismos*, squint], squint caused by spasmodic contractions of ocular muscles.

spatial dance /spā′shəl/ [L, *spatium*, space; ME, *dauncen*, to drag along], the body shifts or movements used by individuals as they try to adjust the distance between themselves and other individuals. See also **spatial zones.**

spatial relationships, 1. orientation in space; the ability to locate objects in the three-dimensional external world using visual or tactile recognition and make a spatial analysis of the observed information. Spatial orientation normally is a function of the right hemisphere of the brain. 2. the relative locations of various personnel and equipment in an operating room with particular emphasis on what is sterile, clean, or contaminated. The operating room nurse must maintain an awareness of the arrangement of people, the height of personnel in relation to each other and to table level, and the proximity of sterile to nonsterile areas.

spatial summation. See **summation,** def. 2.

spatial zones, the areas of personal space in which most people interact. Four basic spatial zones are the intimate zone, in which distance between individuals is less than 18 inches; the personal zone, between 18 inches and 4 feet; the social zone, extending between 4 and 12 feet; and the public zone, beyond 12 feet.

SPE, abbreviation for **sucrose polyester.**

Spearman's rho /spir′mənz rō′/ [Charles E. Spearman, English psychologist, b. 1863; *rho* 17th letter in the Greek alphabet], a statistical test for correlation between two rank-ordered scales. It yields a statement of the degree of interdependence of the scores of the two scales.

special care unit /spesh′əl/ [L, *specialis*, individual], a hospital unit with the necessary specialized equipment and personnel for handling critically ill or injured patients, such as an intensive care unit, burn unit, or cardiac care unit.

special gene system, a plasmid, transposon, or other genetic fragment that is able to transfer genetic information from one cell to another.

specialing /spesh′əling/, *informal.* 1. (in psychiatric nursing) the constant attendance of a professional staff member to a disturbed patient to protect the patient from harming the self or others and to observe the patient's behavior. The patient so "specialed" is accompanied in all activities by the staff member. 2. (in nursing) the giving of nursing care to only one person, such as when acting as a private duty nurse or when caring for a patient whose needs are so great that a nurse is required at all times.

specialist /spesh′əlist/, a health care professional who practices a specialty. A specialist usually has advanced clinical training and may have a postgraduate academic degree.

specialist in blood bank technology. See **blood bank technology specialist.**

special sense, the sense of sight, smell, taste, touch, or hearing.

specialty /spesh′əltē/ [L, *specialis*], a branch of medicine or nursing in which the professional is specially qualified to practice by having attended an advanced program of study, by having passed an examination given by an organization of the members of the specialty, or by having gained experience by extensive practice in the specialty.

specialty care, specialized medical services provided by a physician specialist.

species (Sp) /spē′sēz, spē′shēz/, *pl.* **species (sp., spp.)** /spē′sēz, spē′shēz/ [L, form], the category of living things below genus in rank. A species includes individuals of the same genus who are similar in structure and chemical composition and who can interbreed. See also **genus.**

species immunity, a form of natural immunity shared by all members of a species. Compare **individual immunity, racial immunity.**

species-specific [L, *specere*, to see + *facere*, to make], 1. pertaining to the characteristics of a particular species. 2. having a characteristic effect on, or interaction with, cells, tissues, or membranes of a particular species; said of an antigen, drug, or infective agent.

species specificity. See **specificity.**

specific absorption rate (SAR) /spisif′ik/ [L, *species*, form], (in hyperthermia treatment) the rate of absorption of heat energy (W) per unit mass of tissue in units of W/kg.

specific activity, 1. (in nuclear medicine) the radioactivity of a radioisotope per unit mass of the element or compound, expressed in microcuries per millimole or disintegrations per second per milligram. 2. the relative activity per unit mass, expressed as counts per minute per milligram. The specific activity of potassium in the human body is the same as that of the environment or diet, and, because potassium is associated chiefly with muscle tissue, a whole body count of 40K, after administration of the radioisotope, can be used to distinguish lean body mass from total body mass.

specific gravity, the ratio of the density of a substance to the density of another substance accepted as a standard. The usual standard for liquids and solids is water. Thus a liquid or solid with a specific gravity of 4 is four times as dense as water. Hydrogen is the usual standard for gases. See also **density, mass.**

specific immune globulin, a special preparation obtained from human blood that is preselected for its high antibody count against a specific disease, such as varicella zoster immune globulin.

specificity /spes′əfis′itē/ [L, *species*, form + *facere*, to make], the quality of being distinctive. Kinds of specificity may include **group, species,** and **type.**

specificity of association, the uniqueness of a relationship between a causal factor and the occurrence of a disease.

specific rates, statistical rates in which both the events in both the numerator and the denominator are restricted to a specific subgroup of a population.

specific treatment. See **treatment.**

specific ulcer [L, *species* + *facere*, to make + *ilcus*], ulcer associated with a specific disease, as a syphilitic ulcer.

specific viscosity [L, *species* + *facere*, to make + *viscosus*, sticky], the internal friction of a fluid, which may be measured by comparing the rate of flow of the fluid through a tube with the rate of a standard liquid under standard conditions.

specimen /spes′imən/ *pl.* **specimens** [L, *specere*, to look], a small sample of something, intended to show the nature of the whole, such as a urine specimen.

SPECT, abbreviation for *single-photon emission computed tomography.*

SPECTamine, a trademark for a lipid-soluble brain-imaging agent (iofetamine hydrochloride I123).

spectator ions /spek′tātər/, ions that are not involved in a chemical reaction. They may be deleted in writing of the equation ionically.

Spectazole, a trademark for an antifungal (econazole nitrate).

spectinomycin hydrochloride /spek′tinōmī′sin/, an antibiotic.

■ INDICATIONS: It is prescribed in the treatment of gonorrhea and certain infections in penicillin-allergic patients.

■ CONTRAINDICATION: Known hypersensitivity to this drug prohibits its use.

■ ADVERSE EFFECTS: The more serious adverse reactions are oliguria, urticaria, chills, fever, dizziness, and nausea.

spectr-, a combining form meaning 'image': *spectrograph, spectrophobia, spectrum.*

spectra. See **spectrum.**

Spectrobid, a trademark for a semisynthetic penicillin (bacampicillin).

Spectrocin, a trademark for a topical, fixed-combination drug containing antibacterials (neomycin sulfate and gramicidin).

spectrometer /spektrom′ətər/ [L, *spectrum*, image; Gk, *metron*, measure], an instrument for measuring wavelengths of rays of the spectrum, the deviation of refracted rays, and the angles between faces of a prism. Kinds of spectrometers are **mass spectrometer** and **Mössbauer spectrometer.**

spectrometry /spektrom′ətrē/, the procedure of measuring wavelengths of light and other electromagnetic waves. See also **spectrometer.** **–spectrometric,** *adj.*

spectrophotometric. See **spectrophotometry.**

spectrophotometric analysis. See **quantitative analysis.**

spectrophotometry /spek′trōfətom′ətrē/, the measurement of color in a solution by determining the amount of

light absorbed in the ultraviolet, infrared, or visible spectrum, widely used in clinical chemistry to calculate the concentration of substances in solution. **–spectrophotometric,** *adj.*

spectrum /spek′trəm/, *pl.* **spectra** [L, image], **1.** a range of phenomena or properties occurring in increasing or decreasing magnitude. Radiant or electromagnetic energy is arranged on the basis of wavelength and frequency. Electromagnetic radiation includes spectra of radio waves, infrared waves, visible light, ultraviolet waves, x-rays, and gamma rays. **2.** the range of effectiveness of an antibiotic. A broad-spectrum antibiotic is effective against a wide range of microorganisms. See also **antibiotic, electromagnetic radiation, wave.**

speculum /spek′yələm/ [L, mirror], a retractor used to separate the walls of a cavity to make examination possible, such as an ear speculum, an eye speculum, a nasal speculum, or a vaginal speculum.

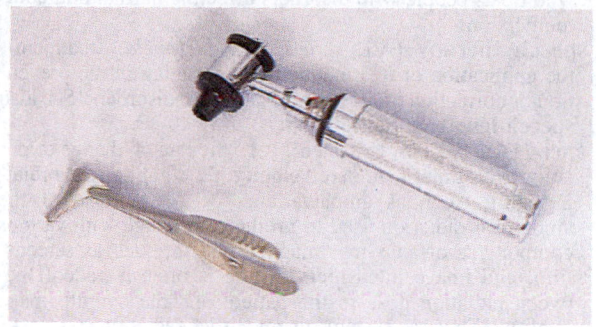

Nasal specula (Seidel, 1991)

speech [ME, *speche*], **1.** the utterance of articulate vocal sounds that form words to give expression to one's thoughts or ideas. **2.** communication by means of spoken words. **3.** the faculty of language production, which involves the complex coordination of the muscles and nerves of the organs of articulation. Any neurologic or muscular injury or defect involving these organs results in various speech impediments or dysfunctions. Kinds of dysfunctions include **ataxic speech, explosive speech, mirror speech, scamping speech, scanning speech, slurred speech,** and **staccato speech.** See also **speech dysfunction.**

speech abnormalities. See **speech dysfunction.**

speech audiometry. See **audiometry.**

speech center [AS, *spaec*; Gk, *kentron*], a unilateral area in the posterior part of the inferior frontal gyrus and usually on the side contralateral to the dominant hand. Also associated with articulate speech are Brodmann's areas 44 and 45.

speech dysfunction, any defect or abnormality of speech, including aphasia, alexia, stammering, stuttering, aphonia, and slurring. Speech problems may develop from any of a variety of causes, among them neurologic injury to the cerebral cortex, muscular paralysis caused by trauma, disease, or cerebrovascular accident; structural abnormality of the organs of speech; emotional or psychologic tension, strain, or depression; hysteria; and severe mental retardation. See also **speech.**

speech-language pathologist, an individual with graduate professional training in human communication, its development, and disorders. The person specializes in the measurement and evaluation of language abilities, auditory processes and speech production, clinical treatment of children and adults with speech and language disorders, and research methods in the study of communication processes. See also **speech therapist.**

speech pathology,   **1.** the study of abnormalities of speech or of the organs of speech. **2.** the diagnosis and treatment of abnormalities of speech as practiced by a speech pathologist or a speech therapist.

speech reading, [ME, *reden,* to explain],   a method of verbal communication in which one uses the visual clues of the speaker's lip and facial movements, along with residual hearing. Gestures and 'body language' also are observed. Also called **lip reading.**

speech synthesizer [AS, *spaec*; Gk, *synthesis,* placing together],   an electronic apparatus with a keyboard that produces sounds that imitate the human voice.

speech therapist,   a person trained in speech pathology who treats people with disorders affecting normal oral communication.

speech therapy [AS, *spaec*; Gk, *therapeia,* treatment],   the application of treatments and counseling in the prevention or correction of speech and language disorders. See also **speech-language pathologist.**

speed [AS, *spedan,* to hasten],   **1.** the rate of change of position with time. Compare **velocity. 2.** *slang.* any stimulating drug, such as amphetamine. **3.** a reciprocal of the amount of radiation used to produce an image with various components of an x-ray imaging system, such as screens, film, and image intensifiers. There is often a tradeoff between radiation dose to the patient and the overall image quality. Thus a system using little radiation is 'fast,' whereas one requiring more radiation is 'slow.' **4.** the amount of exposure of film to light or x-rays needed to produce a desired image. X-ray film speed usually is indicated as the reciprocal of the exposure in roentgens necessary to produce a density of 1 above the base and fog levels.

speed shock,   a sudden adverse physiologic reaction of a patient to intravenous medications or drugs that are administered too quickly. Some signs of speed shock are a flushed face, headache, a tight feeling in the chest, irregular pulse, loss of consciousness, and cardiac arrest.

sPEEP,   abbreviation for **spontaneous PEEP.**

spell of illness [ME, *spel, illr,* bad],   a period regarded by Medicare rules as the number of days between the admission of an insured patient to a hospital and the day that marks the end of a period during which the insured has not been an inpatient in a hospital or a skilled nursing facility.

sperm.   See **semen, spermatozoon.**

-sperm,   a combining form meaning a 'seed': *gymnosperm, oosperm, zygosperm.*

spermatic cord /spərmat′ik/ [Gk, *sperma,* seed; *chorde,* string],   a structure extending from the deep inguinal ring in the abdomen to the testis, descending nearly vertically into the scrotum. The left spermatic cord is usually longer than the right; consequently the left testis usually hangs lower than the right. Each cord comprises arteries, veins, lymphatics, nerves, and the vas deferens of the testis.

spermatic duct.   See **vas deferens.**

spermatic fistula,   an abnormal passage communicating with a testis or a seminal duct.

spermatid /spur′mətid, spəmat′id/ [Gk, *sperma,* seed],   a male germ cell that arises from a spermatocyte and that be-

comes a mature spermatozoon in the last phase of the continual process of spermatogenesis.

spermato- /spur′mətō-, spərmat′ō-/ **spermo-,**   a combining form meaning 'of or pertaining to seed, specifically to the male generative element': *spermatoblast, spermatocyst, spermatogenesis.*

spermatocele /spərmat′əsēl′, spur′-/ [Gk, *sperma* + *kele,* tumor],   a cystic swelling, either of the epididymis or of the rete testis, that contains spermatozoa. It lies above, behind, and separate from the testis; it is usually painless and requires no therapy.

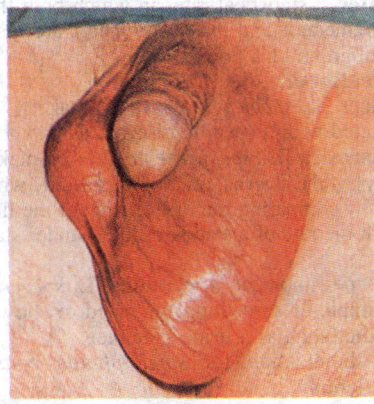

Spermatocele *(Lloyd-Davies, 1983)*

spermatocide /spərmat′əsīd, spur′-/ [Gk, *sperma* + L, *caedere,* to kill],   a chemical substance that kills spermatozoa by reducing their surface tension, causing the cell wall to break down by a bactericidal effect or by creating a highly acidic environment. Among many spermatocidal agents used in various contraceptive creams are lactic acid, phenylmercuric acetate, chloramine polyethylene glycol, benzethonium chloride, and certain quinine compounds. Also called **spermicide.**

spermatocyte /spur′mətōsīt′/ [Gk, *sperma* + *kytos,* cell],   a male germ cell that arises from a spermatogonium. Each spermatocyte gives rise to two haploid secondary spermatocytes that become spermatids.

spermatocytogenesis.   See **spermatogenesis.**

spermatogenesis /spərmat′əjen′əsis, spur′-/ [Gk, *sperma* + *genesis,* origin],   the process of development of spermatozoa, including the first stage, called spermatogenesis, in which spermatogonia become spermatocytes that develop into spermatids, and the second stage, called spermiogenesis, in which the spermatids become spermatozoa. **—spermatogenic, spermatogenous** /spur′mətoj′ənəs/, *adj.*

spermatogonia, *pl.* **spermatogonia** /-gō′nē·əm/ [Gk, *sperma* + *gone,* generation],   a male germ cell that gives rise to a spermatocyte early in spermatogenesis.

spermatopathia /-path′ē·ə/ [Gk, *sperma,* seed + *pathos,* disease],   pertaining to diseased sperm or their associated organs. Also called **spermopathy** /spərmop′əthē/.

spermatozoa.   See **spermatozoon.**

spermatozoon /spur′mətəzō′ən, spərmat′-/, *pl.* **spermatozoa** /-zō′ə/ [Gk, *sperma* + *zoon,* animal],   a mature male germ cell that develops in the seminiferous tubules of the testes. Resembling a tadpole, it is about 50 μm (1/500 inch) long and has a head with a nucleus, a neck, and a tail that provides propulsion. Developed in vast numbers after puberty, it is the generative component of the semen, impregnating the ovum and resulting in fertilization. See **spermatogenesis.**

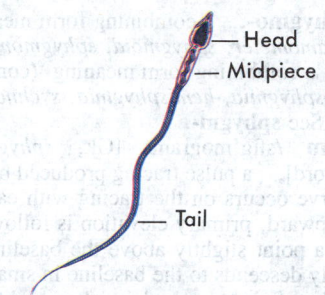

Spermatozoon (Thibodeau, 1993/William Ober)

sperm bank /spurm/ [Gk, *sperma,* seed; It, *banca,* bench], a facility for storage of semen to be used for artificial insemination.

-spermia, -spermy, a combining form meaning '(condition of) possessing or producing seed': *aspermia, asthenospermia, necrospermia.*

spermicidal /spur′misī′dəl/, destructive to spermatozoa.

spermicide. See **spermatocide.**

spermiogenesis. See **spermatogenesis.**

spermo-. See **spermato-.**

spermopathy. See **spermatopathia.**

-spermy. See **-spermia.**

SPF, abbreviation for **sunscreen protective factor index.**

sp.gr., abbreviation for **specific gravity.**

sphacel-, a combining form meaning 'of or pertaining to gangrene': *sphaceloderma, sphacelotoxin, sphacelus.*

-sphaera, -sphaere. See **-sphere.**

sphaero-. See **sphero-.**

S-phase, the phase of a cell reproductive cycle in which DNA is synthesized before mitosis.

spheno-, a combining form meaning 'of or pertaining to the sphenoid bone or to a wedge': *sphenocephaly, sphenoidotomy, sphenotemporal.*

sphenoethmoid recess /sfē′nō·eth′moid/ [Gk, *sphen,* wedge + *eidos,* form; L, *recedere,* to retreat], a narrow opening in the lateral wall of the nasal cavity bounded above by the cribriform plate of the ethmoid and the body of the sphenoid and below by the superior nasal concha. It opens into the sphenoidal sinus of the skull.

sphenoid /sfē′noid/ [Gk, *sphen,* wedge + *eidos,* form], **1.** wedge-shaped. **2.** See **sphenoid bone.**

sphenoidal fissure /sfēnoi′dəl/ [Gk *sphen* wedge, *eidos* form], a cleft between the great and small wings of the sphenoid bone.

sphenoidal sinus, one of a pair of cavities in the sphenoid bone of the skull, lined with mucous membrane that is continuous with that of the nasal cavity. Each sinus is approximately spheroidal, with a diameter of about 2 cm, but its shape and size vary from person to person. A large sphenoidal sinus may extend into the roots of the pterygoid processes, into the great wings, or into the occipital bone. The cavities are very small at birth and develop largely after pu-

berty. Compare **ethmoidal air cells, frontal sinus, maxillary sinus.**

sphenoid bone, the bone at the base of the skull, anterior to the temporal bones and the basilar part of the occipital bone. It resembles a bat with its wings extended. Also called **sphenoid.**

sphenoid fontanel, an anterolateral fontanel that is usually not palpable. See also **fontanel.**

sphenoiditis /sfē′noidī′tis/ [Gk, *sphen,* wedge + *eidos,* form + *itis,* inflammation], an inflammation of the sphenoidal sinus.

sphenomandibular ligament /sfē′nōmandib′yələr/ [Gk, *sphen, eidos* + L, *mandere,* to chew], one of a pair of flat, thin ligaments comprising part of the temporomandibular joint between the mandible of the jaw and the temporal bone of the skull. It is attached to the spine of the sphenoid bone and becomes broader as it descends to the lingula of the mandibular foramen.

sphere /sfir/ a globe-shaped object, theoretically generated by a circle revolving on a diameter as its axis.

-sphere /sfir/, **-sphaera, -sphaere,** **1.** a suffix meaning a 'spheric body': *chondriosphere, oncosphere, somosphere.* **2.** a combining form meaning a 'realm that supports life': *biosphere, vivosphere, zoosphere.*

sphero-, sphaero-, a combining form meaning 'round or pertaining to a sphere': *spherocyte, spherolith, spherometer.*

spherocyte /sfir′əsīt/ [Gk, *sphaira,* sphere, *kytos,* cell], an abnormal spheric red cell that contains more than the normal amount of hemoglobin. Spherocytes can be identified under the microscope on stained blood specimens. Osmotic fragility of the red blood cells increases in the presence of increased numbers of spherocytes. **–spherocytic,** *adj.*

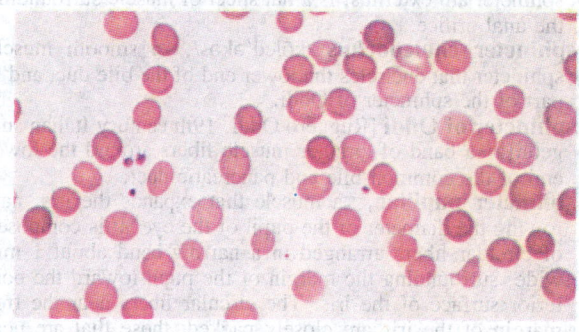

Spherocytes (Hayhoe, 1992)

spherocytic anemia /sfir′əsit′ik/, a hematologic disorder inherited as an autosomal dominant trait and characterized by hemolytic anemia caused by the presence of red blood cells that are spheric rather than round and biconcave. The cells are fragile and tend to hemolyze in the oxygen-poor peripheral circulatory system. Episodic crises of abdominal pain, fever, jaundice, and splenomegaly occur. Because repeated transfusions are often needed to treat the anemia, siderosis may develop. Splenectomy may then be necessary. Compare **congenital nonspherocytic hemolytic anemia.** See also **elliptocytosis.**

spherocytosis /sfir′ōsītō′sis/, the abnormal presence of spherocytes in the blood. Compare **elliptocytosis.** (See Fig. p. 1462.)

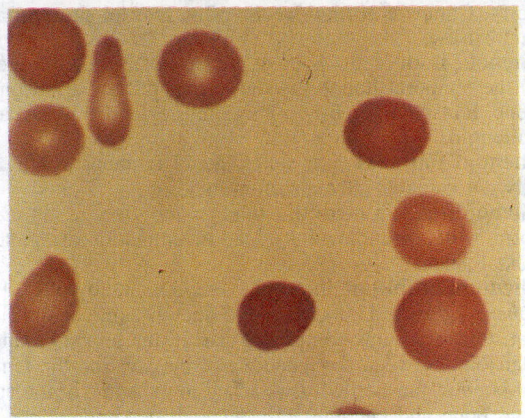

Spherocytosis *(Zitelli, 1992)*

spheroidea. See **ball and socket joint.**

spherule /sfer′yōōl/ [Gk, *sphaira*, ball], a small ball.

sphincter /sfingk′tər/ [Gk, *sphingein*, to bind], a circular band of muscle fibers that constricts a passage or closes a natural opening in the body, such as the hepatic sphincter in the muscular coat of the hepatic veins near their union with the superior vena cava, and the external anal sphincter, which closes the anus.

sphincter-, a combining form pertaining to a 'band' or to a 'sphincter': *sphincteric, sphincterectomy, sphincteral.*

sphincter ani, a double set of circular muscles at the opening of the anus. One, the sphincter ani internus, consists of a thickened inner circular coat of the bowel; the other, the sphincter ani externus, is a flat sheet of muscle surrounding the anal orifice.

sphincter choledochus /kōled′əkəs/, a smooth muscle sphincter that encircles the lower end of the bile duct and is part of the sphincter of Oddi.

sphincter of Oddi [Ruggero Oddi, 19th century Italian surgeon], a band of circular muscle fibers around the lower end of the common bile and pancreatic duct.

sphincter pupillae, a muscle that expands the iris, narrowing the diameter of the pupil of the eye. It is composed of circular fibers arranged in a narrow band about 1 mm wide, surrounding the margin of the pupil toward the posterior surface of the iris. The circular fibers near the free margin of the iris are closely packed; those that are near the periphery of the band are more separated and form incomplete circles. The fibers of the sphincter pupillae blend with the fibers of the dilatator pupillae near the margin of the pupil and are innervated by a motor root of the ciliary ganglion from the oculomotor nerve. Compare **dilatator pupillae.**

sphincter virginae. See **bulbocavernosus.**

sphingolipid /sfing′gōlip′id/ [Gk, *sphingein*, to bind, *lipos*, fat], a compound that consists of a lipid and a sphingosine. It is found in high concentrations in the brain and other tissues of the nervous system, especially membranes.

sphingomyelin /sfing′gōmī′əlin/ [Gk, *sphingein* + *myelos*, marrow], any of a group of sphingolipids containing phosphorus. It occurs primarily in the tissue of the nervous system, generally in membranes, and in the lipids in the blood.

sphingomyelin lipidosis, any of a group of diseases characterized by an abnormality in the ability of the body to store sphingolipids. Kinds of sphingomyelin lipidosis include **Gaucher's disease, Niemann-Pick disease,** and **Tay-Sachs disease.** See also **angiokeratoma corporis diffusum.**

sphingosine /sfing′gōsēn/, a long-chain unsaturated amino alcohol, a major constituent of sphingolipids and sphingomyelin.

sphygm-, sphygmo-, a combining form meaning 'pulse': *sphygmodynamometer, sphygmoid, sphygmomanometer.*

-sphygmia, a combining form meaning '(condition of the) pulse': *anisosphygmia, hemisphygmia, sychnosphygmia.*

sphygmo-. See **sphygm-.**

sphygmogram /sfig′məgram/ [Gk, *sphygmos*, pulse, *gramma*, record], a pulse tracing produced by a sphygmograph. A curve occurs on the tracing with each atrial pulsation. An upward, primary elevation is followed by a sudden drop to a point slightly above the baseline. The curve then gradually descends to the baseline in small decrements of amplitude. Sphygmographic abnormalities of rate, rhythm, and form may be diagnostically useful in an assessment of cardiovascular function.

sphygmograph /sfig′məgraf/, an instrument that records the force of the arterial pulse on a tracing called a sphygmogram. **–sphygmographic,** *adj.*

sphygmoid /sfig′moid/ [Gk, *sphygmos*, pulse + *eidos*, form], pertaining to or resembling the pulse.

sphygmomanometer /sfig′mōmənom′ətər/ [Gk, *sphygmos*

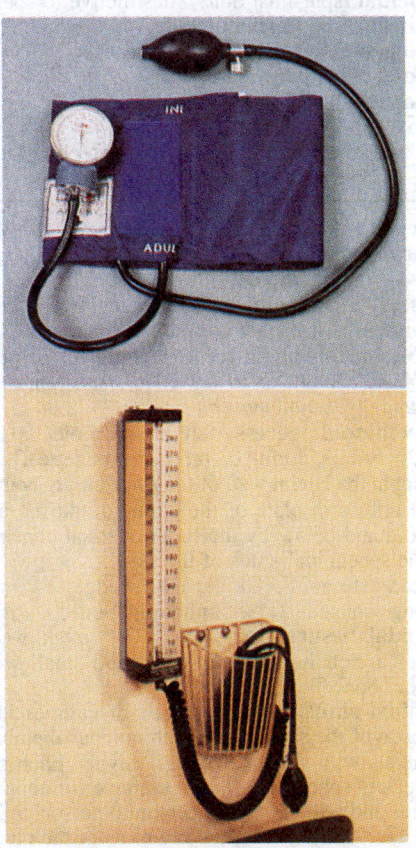

Sphygmomanometers: aneroid and mercury
(Sorrentino, 1992)

+ *manos*, thin, *metron*, measure], an instrument for indirect measurement of blood pressure. It consists of an inflatable cuff that fits around the arm, a bulb for controlling air pressure within the cuff, and a mercury or aneroid manometer. Pressure in the brachial artery is estimated by the column of mercury it balances when the cuff is inflated. See also **blood pressure, manometer.**

sphygmoplethysmograph /-pləthis′məgraf′/ [Gk, *sphygmos*, pulse + *plethysmos*, increase + *graphein*, to record], an instrument for measuring and recording the arterial pulse curve and blood flow in a limb.

spica [L, spike, or ear of wheat], a figure-of-eight bandage that, when applied to a joint, resembles the head of a stalk of wheat.

spica bandage /spī′kə/ [L, *spica*, spike of wheat; Fr, *bande*, strip], a figure-of-eight bandage in which each turn generally overlaps the previous to form a succession of V-like designs. It may be used to give support, to apply pressure, or to hold a dressing in place on the chest, limbs, thighs, or pelvis.

spica cast, an orthopedic cast applied to immobilize part or all of the trunk of the body and part or all of one or more extremities. It is used to treat various fractures, such as of the hip and the femur, and in correcting or maintaining the correction of hip deformities. Kinds of spica casts are **bilateral long-leg spica cast, one-and-a-half spica cast, shoulder spica cast,** and **unilateral long-leg spica cast.**

spicule /spik′yo͞ol/ [L, *spiculus*, sharp point], a sharp body with a needlelike point.

spider angioma [ME, *spithre*; Gk, *aggeion*, vessel, *oma*, tumor], a form of telangiectasis characterized by a central, elevated, red dot the size of a pinhead from which small blood vessels radiate. Spider angiomas are often associated with elevated estrogen levels, such as occur in pregnancy or when the liver is diseased and unable to detoxify estrogens. Also called **spider nevus.** See also **telangiectasia.**

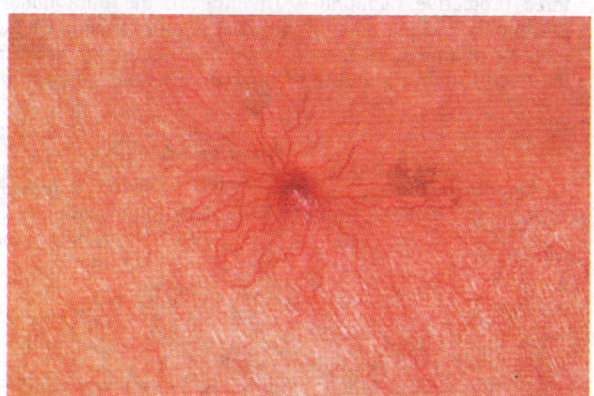

Spider angioma *(Kamal, 1991/Courtesy Dr. Derek Martin)*

spider antivenin. See **black widow spider antivenin.**

spider bite [ME, *spithre*; AS, *bitan*; L, *potio*, drink], a puncture wound produced by the bite by any of nearly 60 species of venomous spiders found in North America. Most spiders have fangs that are too short or fragile to penetrate the skin, but some are dangerous to humans. These include the black widow, *Lactrodectus mactans;* the brown recluse, *Loxosceles reclusa;* and species of jumping spiders and ta-

rantulas. Spider venom may contain enzymatic proteins, including peptides that may affect neuromuscular transmission or cardiovascular function. Signs and symptoms include local burning followed by radiating pain. Loss of consciousness, convulsions, and death may occur.

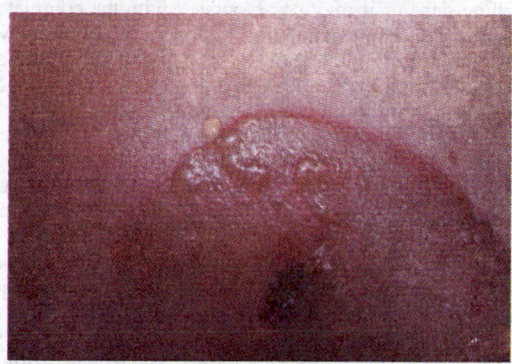

Brown recluse spider bite *(Weston, 1991)*

spider nevus. See **spider angioma.**

spider telangiectasia [ME, *spithre*; Gk, *telos*, end + *aggeion*, vessel + *ektasis*, dilatation], a branched group of dilated capillary blood vessels forming a spiderlike image on the skin. Also called **nevus araneus.**

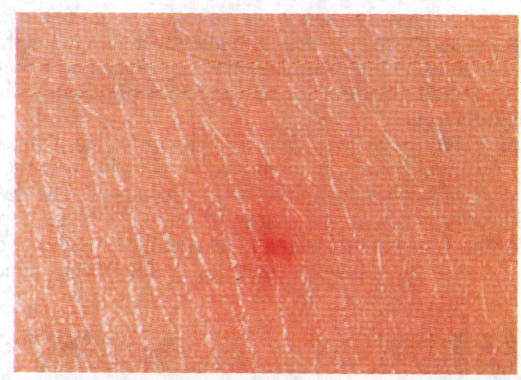

Spider telangiectasia *(McKee, 1993)*

spikeboard /spīk′bôrd/, a device that enables people with upper extremity handicaps to stabilize foods when only one hand is available for meal preparation.

spillway [AS, *spillan*, to destroy, *weg*, wagon track], a channel or passageway through which food normally escapes from the occlusal surfaces of the teeth during mastication.

spin [AS, *spinnan*, to draw threads], **1.** the intrinsic angular momentum of an elementary particle or a nucleus of an atom. **2.** intrinsic joint movements about an axis perpendicular to the articular surface.

spina /spī′nə/, *pl.* **spinae** [L, backbone], **1.** the spinal column. **2.** a spine or a thornlike projection, such as the bony projection on the anterior border of the ilium, forming the anterior end of the iliac crest.

spina bifida /bif'ədə, bī'fədə/, congenital neural tube defect characterized by a developmental anomaly in the posterior vertebral arch. Spina bifida is relatively common, occurring approximately 10 to 20 times per 1000 births. It may occur with only a small deformed lamina separated by a midline gap, or it may be associated with the complete absence of laminae surrounding a large area. In cases where the separation is wide enough, contents of the spinal canal protrude posteriorly, and a myelomeningocele is evident. This more serious deformity is associated with gross deficits not normally manifested in spina bifida. Neurologic deficits do not usually accompany the anomalies involving only bony deformity. Direct signs and symptoms are rarely noted in spina bifida, which is frequently diagnosed accidentally during radiographic examinations required for other reasons. Spina bifida that does not involve herniation of the meninges or the contents of the spinal canal rarely requires treatment. Also called **spinal dysrhaphis.**

spina bifida anterior, incomplete closure along the anterior surface of the vertebral column. The defect is often associated with developmental anomalies of the abdominal and thoracic viscera.

spina bifida cystica, a developmental defect of the central nervous system in which a hernial cyst containing meninges (meningocele), spinal cord (myelocele), or both (myelomeningocele) protrudes through a congenital cleft in the vertebral column. The protruding sac is encased in a layer of skin or a fine membrane that can easily rupture, causing the leakage of cerebrospinal fluid and an increased risk of meningeal infection. The severity of neurologic dysfunction and associated defects depends directly on the degree of nerve involvement. The most severe type is lumbosacral myelomeningocele, which is frequently associated with hydrocephalus and the Arnold-Chiari malformation. Compare **spina bifida occulta.** See also **myelomeningocele, neural tube defect.**

spina bifida occulta, defective closure of the laminae of the vertebral column in the lumbosacral region without hernial protrusion of the spinal cord or meninges. The defect, which is quite common, occurs in about 5% of the population and is identified externally by a skin depression or dimple, dark tufts of hair, telangiectasis, or soft, subcutaneous

lipomas at the site. Because the neural tube has closed, there are usually no neurologic impairments associated with the defect. However, any abnormal adhesion of the spinal cord to the area of the malformation may lead to neuromuscular disturbances, usually problems with gait and foot weakness and with the bowel and bladder sphincters. Compare **spina bifida cystica.**

spinea. See **spina.**

spinal /spī'nəl/ [L, *spina*], **1.** of or pertaining to a spine, especially the spinal column. **2.** *informal.* spinal anesthesia, such as saddle block or caudal anesthesia.

spinal accessory nerve. See **accessory nerve.**

spinal anesthesia [L, *spina*, backbone; Gk, *anaisthesia*, lack of feeling], a state of insensitivity to pain in the lower part of the body produced by injection of an analgesic drug or anesthetic drug into the subarachnoid space of the spinal cord. Also called **subarachnoid block anesthesia.**

spinal aperture, a large opening formed by the body of a vertebra and its arch.

spinal arachnoid. See **arachnoidea spinalis.**

spinal block [L, *spina*, backbone; OFr, *bloc*], an obstruction of cerebrospinal fluid circulation. See also **subarachnoid block anesthesia.**

spinal canal, the cavity within the vertebral column.

spinal caries. See **tuberculous spondylitis.**

spinal column. See **vertebral column.**

spinal cord, a long, nearly cylindric structure lodged in the vertebral canal and extending from the foramen magnum at the base of the skull to the upper part of the lumbar region. A major component of the central nervous system, the adult cord is approximately 1 cm in diameter, with an average length of 42 to 45 cm and a weight of 30 g. The cord conducts sensory and motor impulses to and from the brain and controls many reflexes. Thirty-one spinal nerves originate from the cord: 8 cervical, 12 thoracic, 5 lumbar, 5 sacral, and 1 coccygeal. It has an inner core of gray material consisting mainly of nerve cells and is enclosed by three protective membranes (meninges): the dura mater, arachnoid, and pia mater. The cord is an extension of the medulla oblongata of the brain and ends caudally between the twelfth thoracic and third lumbar vertebrae, often at or

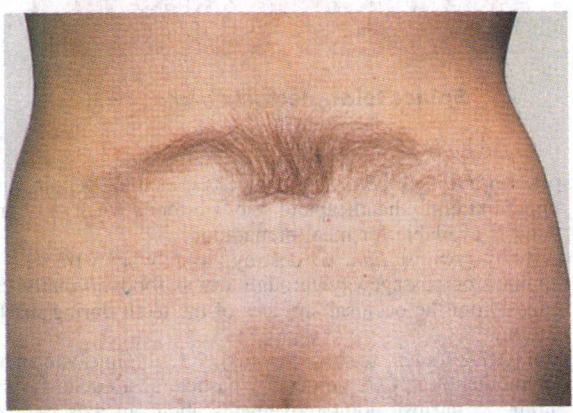

Spina bifida occulta *(Forbes, 1993)*

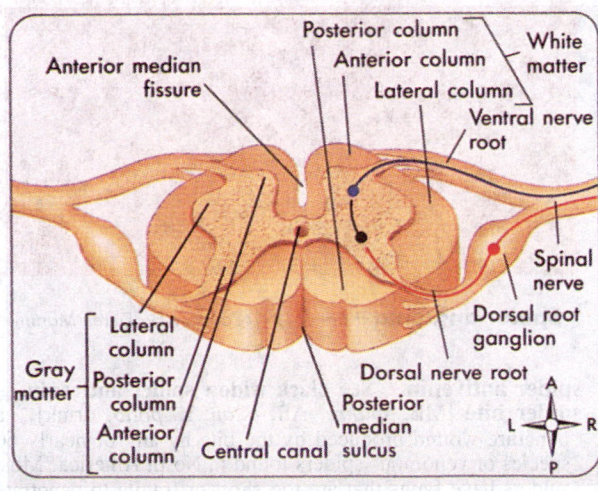

Cross-section of the spinal cord
(Thibodeau 1993/Rolin Graphics)

adjacent to the disk between the first and second lumbar vertebrae. Until the third month of fetal life, the cord occupies the entire length of the vertebral canal. Thereafter, the canal lengthens faster than the cord. By the sixth fetal month, the caudal end of the cord reaches only as far as the upper sacrum. At birth it is on a level with the third lumbar vertebra. Originating in the ectoderm, like the entire nervous system, the cord develops from the caudal portion of the embryonic neural plate. Also called **chorda spinalis, medulla spinalis.** See also **spinal nerves.**

spinal cord compression, an abnormal and often serious condition resulting from pressure on the spinal cord. The symptoms range from temporary numbness of an extremity to permanent quadriplegia, depending on the cause, severity, and location of the pressure. Causes include spinal fracture, vertebral dislocation, tumor, hemorrhage, and edema associated with contusion. See also **herniated disk, spondylolisthesis.**

spinal cord injury, any one of the traumatic disruptions of the spinal cord, often associated with extensive musculoskeletal involvement. Common spinal cord injuries are vertebral fractures and dislocations, such as those commonly suffered by individuals involved in car accidents, airplane crashes, or other violent impacts. Such trauma may cause varying degrees of paraplegia and quadriplegia. Injuries to spinal structures below the first thoracic vertebra may produce paraplegia. Injuries to the spine above the first thoracic vertebra may cause quadriplegia. Injuries that completely transect the spinal cord cause permanent loss of motor and sensory functions activated by neurons below the level of the lesions involved. Spinal cord injuries produce a state of spinal shock, characterized by flaccid paralysis, and complete loss of skin sensation at the time of the injury. Within a few weeks the muscles affected may become spastic, and the skin sensation may return to a slight degree. The motor and the sensory losses that prevail a few weeks after the injury are usually permanent. Musculoskeletal complications are associated with the neurologic involvement of spinal cord injuries, and prevention of decubitis ulcers and the treatment of any loss of bladder and bowel control are continuing concerns. Treatment of spinal cord injuries varies considerably and involves numerous approaches, such as orthopedic exercises, ambulatory techniques, and special physical and psychologic therapy.

spinal cord tumor, a neoplasm of the spinal cord of which more than 50% are extramedullary, about 25% are intramedullary, and the rest are extradural. Symptoms usually develop slowly and may progress from unilateral paresthesia and a dull ache to lancinating pain, weakness in one or both legs, abnormal deep tendon reflexes, and, in advanced cases, monoplegia, hemiplegia, or paraplegia. Function of the autonomic nervous system is sometimes disturbed, causing areas of dry, cold, bluish pink skin or profuse sweating of the lower extremities. The diagnosis is made by x-ray and myelographic examination. About 30% of spinal cord tumors are circumscribed, encapsulated meningiomas, and 25% are schwannomas; these two kinds are found chiefly in the thoracic region. Some 20% are gliomas, and the others consist of congenital lipomas, epidermoids, and metastatic lesions. The dura is resistant to invasion, but many extradural tumors are metastatic lesions from primary cancers in the prostate, lung, breast, thyroid, and GI tract. Most extramedullary and nonmetastatic extradural tumors are surgically removed; intermedullary lesions are enucleated, whenever possible; and inoperable tumors are treated with radiotherapy and chemotherapy. Tumors of the spinal cord may arise at any age but appear most frequently in the third decade of life and are one fourth as common as brain neoplasms.

spinal curvature, any persistent, abnormal deviation of the vertebral column from its normal position. Kinds of spinal curvature are **kyphoscoliosis, kyphosis, lordosis,** and **scoliosis.**

spinal dysrhaphis. See **spina bifida.**

spinal fasciculi. See **spinal tract.**

spinal fluid. See **cerebrospinal fluid.**

spinal fusion, the fixation of an unstable segment of the spine, accomplished by skeletal traction or immobilization of the patient in a body cast but most frequently by a surgical procedure. Operative ankylosis may be performed in the treatment of spinal fractures or after discectomy or laminectomy for the correction of a herniated vertebral disk. Surgical fusion involves the stabilization of a spinal section with a bone graft or synthetic device introduced through a posterior incision in the lumbar region; in the less frequently fused cervical region the incision may be anterior or posterior. Also called **spondylosyndesis.**

spinal headache, a headache occurring after spinal anesthesia or lumbar puncture, caused by a loss of cerebrospinal fluid (CSF) from the subarachnoid space, resulting in traction of the meninges on the pressure-sensitive intracranial structures. Severe spinal headache may be accompanied by diminished aural and visual acuity. Treatment usually includes keeping the patient flat in bed to relieve the meningeal irritation, encouraging an increased fluid intake to increase the intravascular volume and increase the production and volume of cerebrospinal fluid, and administering analgesics to reduce pain. If severe headache persists, an autologous blood patch procedure may be performed in which 10 cca of the patient's blood is injected over the leaking puncture site in the dura to prevent further loss of CSF. Meningeal irritation and backache may persist for several days. The incidence of spinal headache is greatest when a large-bore needle is used for the initial anesthetic or diagnostic procedure.

spinal manipulation, the forced passive flexion, extension, and rotation of vertebral segments, carrying the elements of articulation beyond the usual range of movement to the limit of anatomic range. Spinal manipulation may be used effectively in physiotherapy for the treatment of vertebral and sacroiliac dislocations, sprains, and adhesions.

spinal muscular atrophy. See **Duchenne's disease.**

spinal nerves, the 31 pairs of nerves without special names that are connected to the spinal cord and numbered according to the level of the cord at which they emerge. There are 8 cervical, 12 thoracic, 5 lumbar, and 5 sacral pairs, and 1 coccygeal pair. The first cervical pair of nerves emerges from the spinal cord in the space between the first cervical vertebra and the occipital bone. The rest of the cervical pairs and all the thoracic pairs emerge horizontally through the intervertebral foramen of their respective vertebrae, such as the second cervical pair, which emerges through the foramina above the second cervical vertebra. The lumbar, the sacral, and the coccygeal nerve pairs descend from their points of origin at the lower end of the cord before reaching the intervertebral foramina of their respective vertebrae. Each spinal nerve attaches to the spinal cord by an anterior root and a posterior root. The posterior

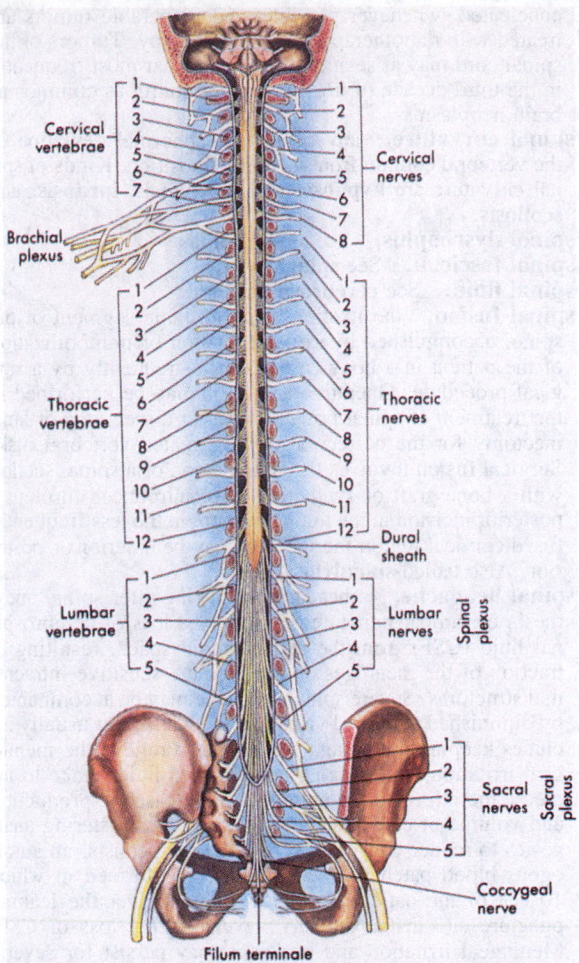

Spinal column and spinal nerves (Chipps, 1992)

roots accompany a distended spinal ganglion within the vertebral foramina. Emerging from the cord, each spinal nerve divides into the anterior, the posterior, and the white rami, with the anterior and the posterior rami serving the voluntary nervous system, and the white rami serving the autonomic nervous system. The posterior rami subdivide into lesser nerves that extend into the muscles and the skin of the posterior surface of the head, the neck, and the trunk. The anterior rami, except for those of the thoracic nerves, subdivide and pass fibers to the skeletal muscles and the skin of the extremities. Subdivisions of the anterior rami form complex plexuses, such as the brachial plexus, from which smaller nerves emerge to innervate the hand and most of the arm. A broken neck may damage the right and the left phrenic nerves that come from the third, fourth, and fifth cervical nerves. Such damage may prevent nerve impulses from reaching the phrenic nerves, which supply the diaphragm, and thus stop respiration. The sacral plexus in the pelvic cavity comprises certain spinal nerve fibers from the lumbar and the sacral regions and gives rise to the great sciatic nerve in the back of the thigh. See also **spinal cord.**

spinal puncture. See **lumbar puncture.**

spinal reflex [L, *spina* + *reflectere*, to bend back], any reflex with a pathway through the spinal cord but not the brain.

spinal shock, a form of shock associated with acute injury to the spinal cord. See also **shock.**

spinal tract, any one of the ascending (sensory) and descending (motor) pathways for sensory or motor nerve impulses that is found in the white matter of the spinal cord. Twenty-one different tracts lie within the dorsal, the ventral, and the lateral funiculi of the white substance. Ascending tracts conduct impulses up the spinal cord to the brain; descending tracts conduct impulses down the cord from the brain. The four major ascending tracts are the lateral spinothalamic, the ventral spinothalamic, the fasciculi gracilis and cuneatus, and the spinocerebellar. The four major descending tracts are the lateral corticospinal, the ventral corticospinal, the lateral reticulospinal, and the medial reticulospinal. Touch, pressure, proprioception, temperature, and pain are sensory stimuli transmitted via the spinal tracts. Reflex and voluntary motor activity are regulated by motor nerve stimulation from the brain and brainstem to the motor neurons of the spinal cord.

spin density, (in nuclear magnetic resonance imaging) a measure of the hydrogen concentration. It is a quantity proportional to the number of hydrogen nuclei precessing at the Larmor frequency and contributing to the NMR signal. See also **Larmor frequency.**

spindle [AS, *spinel*, to spin], 1. the fusiform figure of achromatin in the cell nucleus during the late prophase and the metaphase of mitosis. It consists of tiny fibers radiating out from the centrosomes and connecting them with one another. 2. a type of brain wave, consisting of a short series of changes in electric potential with a frequency of 14 per second. 3. any one of the special receptor organs comprising the neurotendinous and the neuromuscular spindles distributed throughout the body. These kinds of spindles serve as special receptor organs that detect the degree of stretch in a muscle or at the junction of a muscle with its tendon and are essential in maintaining muscle tone.

spindle cell carcinoma, a rapidly growing neoplasm composed of fusiform squamous cells.

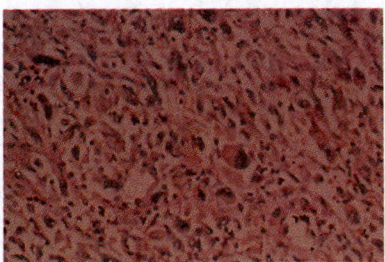

Spindle cell carcinoma (Weiss, 1988)

spindle cell nevus. See **benign juvenile melanoma.**
spine, the vertebral column, or backbone.
spine of scapula [L, *spina*, backbone + *scapulae*, shoulder blades], a sharp-edged plate of bone projecting backward from the flattened scapula base.
spin-lattice relaxation time. See **relaxation time.**

spinnbarkeit /spin′bärkīt, shpin′-/ [Ger, threadability], the clear, slippery, elastic consistency characteristic of cervical mucus during ovulation. It has the consistency of an uncooked egg white, and it is a valuable sign of the peak fertile period in a woman's menstrual cycle. Observation of spinnbarkeit is useful in natural methods of family planning, in the clinical evaluation of infertility, and in discovering the optimum time for artificial insemination. Spinnbarkeit may be evaluated by the length to which a string of mucus can be drawn between the fingers before breaking. See also **ovulation method of family planning.**

spino-, a combining form meaning 'of or pertaining to the spine': *spinocain, spinoglenoid, spinotransversarius.*

spinocerebellar /spī′nōser′əbel′ər/ [L, *spina* + *cerebellum,* small brain], of or pertaining to the spinal cord and the cerebellum.

spinocerebellar disorder, an inherited disorder characterized by a progressive degeneration of the spinal cord and cerebellum, often involving other parts of the nervous system as well. These disorders tend to occur within families and can be inherited as dominant or recessive traits. Onset is usually early, during childhood or adolescence. No effective treatment is known. Some kinds of spinocerebellar degeneration are **ataxia telangiectasia, Charcot-Marie-Tooth disease, Dejerine-Sottas disease, Friedreich's ataxia, olivopontocerebellar atrophy,** and **Refsum's syndrome.**

spinofallopian tube shunt. See **ventriculofallopian tube shunt.**

spinous /spī′nəs/ [L, *spina,* backbone], pertaining to an object that has the shape of a spine or thorn.

spinous process [L, *spina,* backbone + *processus*], a spinelike projection of bony tissue, such as the spinous process of a vertebra.

spinous process of vertebrae, the bony projection extending posteriorly from a vertebral arch.

spin-spin relaxation time. See **relaxation time.**

spinth-, a combining form meaning 'spark': *spinthariscope, spintherometer, spintheropia.*

spir-, **1.** a combining form meaning 'a coil, or coiled': *spiradenitis, spireme, spirillum.* **2.** a combining form meaning 'of or pertaining to the breath or to breathing': *spiracle, spirogram, spirophore.*

spiral bandage /spī′rəl/ [Gk, *speira,* coil; Fr, *bande,* strip], any roller bandage applied around a limb that ascends the body part with each turn overlapping the previous one by half to two thirds of a bandage width.

spiral fracture [Gk, *speira,* coil], a bone break in which the disruption of bone tissue is spiral, oblique, or transverse to the long axis of the fractured bone.

spiral organ of Corti. See **organ of Corti.**

spiral reverse bandage, a spiral bandage that is turned and folded back on itself as necessary to make it fit the contour of the body more securely.

spirillary rat-bite fever, spirillum fever. See **rat-bite fever.**

spirit /spir′it/ [L, *spiritus,* breath], **1.** any volatile liquid, particularly one that has been distilled. **2.** a volatile substance dissolved in alcohol. See also **volatile.**

spirit of ammonia [L, *spiritus,* breath; *Ammon,* temple in Libya], a solution of 3% ammonium carbonate in alcohol with flavorings added. It is mixed with water for use as a stimulant and carminative.

spiritual distress (distress of the human spirit) /spir′ichoo·əl/, a nursing diagnosis accepted by the Fourth National Conference on the Classification of Nursing Diagnoses. It is defined as disruption in the life principle that pervades a person's entire being and that integrates and transcends one's biological and psychosocial nature. The defining characteristics include stated anger against the deity or questions about the meaning of the suffering being experienced. The client may joke in a macabre fashion, regard the illness as punishment, have nightmares, cry, act in a hostile or apathetic manner, express self-blame or deny all responsibility for the problem, express anger or resentment against religious figures, and cease participation in religious practices. Related factors include separation from religious or cultural ties, a change in beliefs or value system, intense suffering, severe stress, or prolonged treatment. See also **nursing diagnosis.**

spiritual therapy [L, *spiritus,* breath + Gk, *therapeia,* treatment], psychotherapy that involves moral and religious influences on behavior and physical health.

Spirochaeta pallida /spī′rəkē′tə/ [Gk, *speira,* coil + *chaite,* hair; L, *pallidus,* pale], a species of flexible, spiral, motile microorganisms that is the cause of human syphilis. Also called ***Treponema pallidum.***

spirochete /spī′rəkēt′/ [Gk, *speira,* coil, *chaite,* hair], any bacterium of the genus *Spirochaeta* that is motile and spiral-shaped with flexible filaments. Kinds of spirochetes include the organisms responsible for leptospirosis, relapsing fever, syphilis, and yaws. Compare **bacillus, coccus, vibrio.** –**spirochetal,** *adj.*

spirochetemia /spī′rōkətē′mē·ə/ [Gk, *speira,* coil + *chaite,* + *haima,* blood], the presence of spirochetal organisms in the blood. See also **spirochete.**

spirogram /spī′rōgram/ [Gk, *speira* + *gramma,* record], a visual record of respiratory movements made by a spirometer, used in the assessment of pulmonary function and capacity.

spirograph /spī′rəgraf/ [Gk, *speira* + *graphein,* to record], a device for recording respiratory movements. See also **spirometer.** –**spirographic,** *adj.*

spirometer /spīrom′ətər/ [Gk, *speira* + *metron,* measure], an instrument that measures and records the volume of inhaled and exhaled air, used to assess pulmonary function. Volumetric information is recorded on a chart, called a spirogram. –**spirometric,** *adj.*

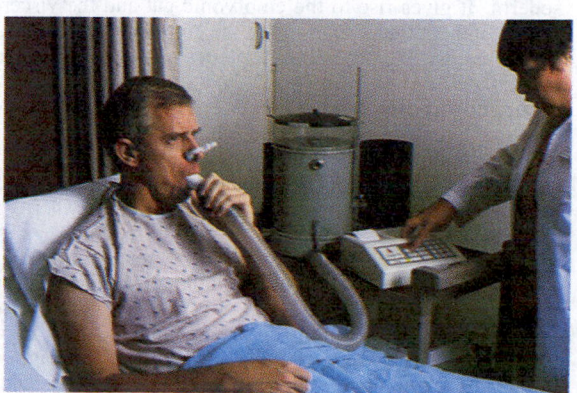

Spirometer *(Wilson, 1990)*

spirometry /spīrom'ətrē/, laboratory evaluation of the air capacity of the lungs by means of a spirometer. Compare **blood gas determination.** **−spirometric,** *adj.*

spironolactone /spī'rənəlak'tōn/, a potassium-sparing aldosterone antagonist diuretic.

■ INDICATIONS: It is prescribed in the treatment of primary hyperaldosteronism, edema of congestive heart failure, cirrhosis of the liver accompanied by edema, the nephrotic syndrome, essential hypertension, and hypokalemia.

■ CONTRAINDICATIONS: Anuria, acute renal insufficiency, significant impairment of renal function, or hyperkalemia prohibits its use.

■ ADVERSE EFFECTS: Among the most serious adverse reactions are hyperkalemia, gynecomastia, mental confusion, ataxia, impotence, amenorrhea, hirsutism, and urticaria.

spittle [AS, *spittan,* spew], saliva.

Spitz nevus. See **benign juvenile melanoma.**

SPL. See **Staphage Lysate.**

splanchn-. See **splanchno-.**

splanchnic /splangk'nik/, of or pertaining to the internal organs; visceral.

-splanchnic, a combining form meaning 'viscera, entrails': *somaticosplanchnic, trisplanchnic, vagosplanchnic.*

splanchnic engorgement, the excessive filling or pooling of blood within the visceral vasculature after the removal of pressure from the abdomen, such as in the excision of a large tumor, birth of a child, or drainage of a large quantity of urine from the bladder.

splanchnic nerves [Gk, *splagchna,* viscera; *nervus*], a network of nerves, mainly preganglionic fibers, with filaments innervating the penis and clitoris, as well as the uterus, rectum, and other structures of the abdominal cavity.

splanchno-, splanchn-, a combining form meaning 'of or pertaining to a viscus or to the splanchnic nerve': *splanchnocele, splanchnography, splanchnoptosis.*

splanchnocele /splangk'nōsēl'/ [Gk, *splanchna,* viscera, *kele,* hernia], hernial protrusion of any abdominal viscera. See also **splanchnocoele.**

splanchnocoele /splangk'nōsēl'/ [Gk, *splanchna,* viscera, *koilos,* hollow], a part of the embryonic body cavity, or coelom, that gives rise to the abdominal, pericardial, and pleural cavities. Also called **pleuroperitoneal cavity.**

splanchnopleure /splangk'nōploor'/ [Gk, *splanchna* + *pleura,* side], a layer of tissue in the early developing embryo, formed by the union of endoderm and splanchnic mesoderm. It gives rise to the embryonic gut and the visceral organs and continues external to the embryo as the yolk sac and allantois. Compare **somatopleure.** **−splanchnopleural,** *adj.*

splanchnosomatic reaction. See **viscerosomatic reaction.**

S-plasty /es'plas'tē/, a technique of plastic surgery in which an S-shaped instead of a straight line incision is made to reduce tension and improve healing in areas where the skin is loose.

splayfoot [ME, *splaien;* AS, *fot*], a foot that is flat and extremely everted, away from the midline. See also **talipes valgus.**

spleen [Gk, *splen*], a soft, highly vascular, roughly ovoid organ situated between the stomach and the diaphragm in the left hypochondriac region of the body. It is considered part of the lymphatic system because it contains lymphatic nodules. It has a dark purple color and varies in shape in different individuals and within the same individual at different times. The precise function of the spleen has baffled physiologists for more than 100 years, but the most recent research indicates it performs various tasks, such as defense, hemopoiesis, blood storage, and the destruction of red blood cells and platelets. Macrophages lining the sinuses of the spleen destroy microorganisms by phagocytosis. The spleen also produces leukocytes, monocytes, lymphocytes, and plasma cells. It produces red cells before birth and is believed to produce red cells after birth only in extreme and hemolytic anemia. If the body suffers severe hemorrhage, the spleen can increase the blood volume from 350 ml to 550 ml in less than 60 seconds. In the adult the spleen is usually about 12 cm long, 7 cm wide, and 3 cm thick. Its weight increases from 17 g or less in the first year to about 170 g at 20 years of age, then slowly decreases to about 122 g at 75 to 80 years of age. The variation in the weight of adult spleens is 100 to 250 g and, in extreme cases, 50 to 400 g. The size of the spleen increases during and after digestion and often increases during illness. It can weigh as much as 9 kg in a victim of malarial fever. The splenic nerves are derived from the celiac plexus and are mostly unmyelinated, distributing to the blood vessels of the organ and to the smooth muscle of the splenic capsule and trabeculae. Compare **thymus.** **−splenic** /splen'ik/, *adj.*

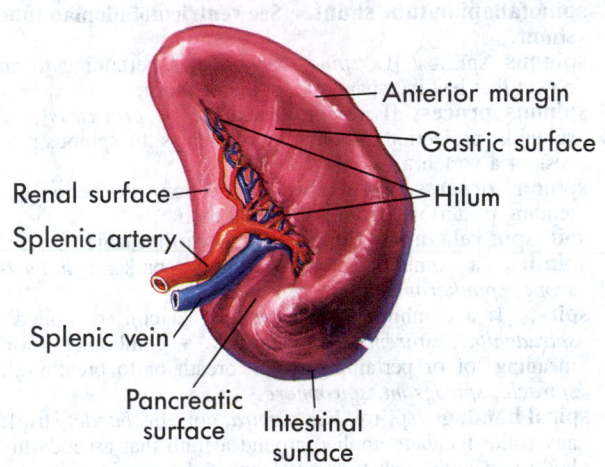

Anterior margin
Gastric surface
Renal surface
Hilum
Splenic artery
Splenic vein
Pancreatic surface
Intestinal surface

Spleen (*Thibodeau, 1993/David J Mascaro*)

spleen scan, the scan of the spleen after the injection of radioactive red blood cells, performed to detect a tumor, damage, or other problem.

splen-. See **spleno-.**

splenectomy /splənek'təmē/ [Gk, *splen* + *ektome,* excision], the surgical excision of the spleen.

-splenia, a combining form meaning 'condition of the spleen': *asplenia, eusplenia, microsplenia.*

splenic. See **spleen.**

splenic flexure /splen'ik/ [Gk, *splen,* spleen; L, *flectere,* to bend], the left flexure of the colon, as it bends at the junction of the transverse and descending segments of the colon, near the spleen.

splenic flexure syndrome [Gk, *splen* + L, *flectere,* to bend], a recurrent pain and abdominal distention in the left upper quadrant of the abdomen caused by a pocket of gas trapped in the large intestine below the spleen, at the flexure of the transverse and descending colon. The symptoms are relieved by defecation or passing flatus.

splenic gland. See **pancreaticolienal node.**

splenic vein. See **lienal vein.**

splenius capitis /splē′nē·əs/ [Gk, *splenion*, bandage; L, *caput*, head], one of a pair of deep muscles of the back. Arising from the ligamentum nuchae, the seventh cervical vertebra, and the first three or four thoracic vertebrae, it inserts in the occipital bone and the mastoid process of the temporal bone. The muscle is innervated by the lateral branches of the dorsal primary divisions of the middle and the lower cervical nerves and acts to rotate, extend, and bend the head.

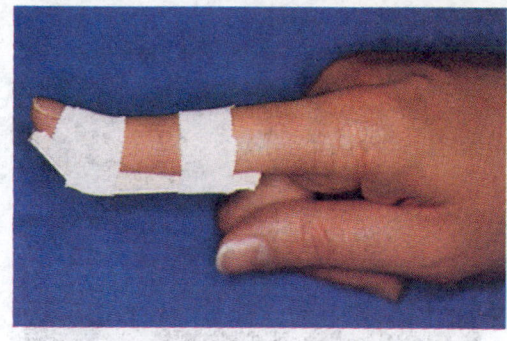

Splinting of finger *(Grossman, 1993)*

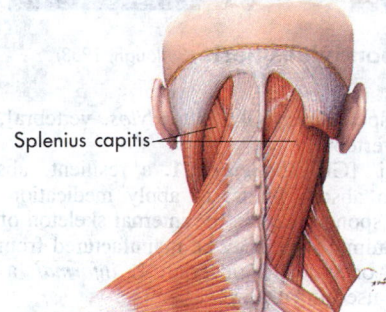

Splenius capitis

Splenius capitis muscle *(Thibodeau, 1993/John V Hagen)*

splenius cervicis, one of a pair of deep muscles of the back. Arising from a narrow tendinous band from the spinous processes of the third through the sixth thoracic vertebrae, it inserts into the transverse processes of the upper two or three cervical vertebrae. The muscle is innervated by the lateral branches of the dorsal primary divisions of the middle and the lower cervical nerves. The splenius cervicis acts to rotate, bend, and extend the head and neck. Also called **splenius colli.**

spleno-, splen-, a combining form meaning 'of or pertaining to the spleen': *splenocele, splenodiagnosis, splenomalacia.*

splenohepatomegaly /splē′nōhep′ətōmeg′əlē/ [Gk, *splen,* spleen + *hepar,* liver + *megas,* great], an abnormal simultaneous increase in the sizes of the liver and spleen.

splenomedullary leukemia. See **acute myelocytic leukemia, chronic myelocytic leukemia.**

splenomegaly /splē′nōmeg′əlē, splen′-/ [Gk, *splen* + *megas,* large], an abnormal enlargement of the spleen, as is associated with portal hypertension, hemolytic anemia, Niemann-Pick disease, or malaria.

splenomyelogenous leukemia. See **acute myelocytic leukemia, chronic myelocytic leukemia.**

splint [D, *splinte,* piece of wood], **1.** an orthopedic device for immobilization, restraint, or support of any part of the body. It may be rigid (of metal, plaster, or wood) or flexible (of felt or leather). **2.** (in dentistry) a device for anchoring the teeth or modifying the bite. Compare **brace, cast.**

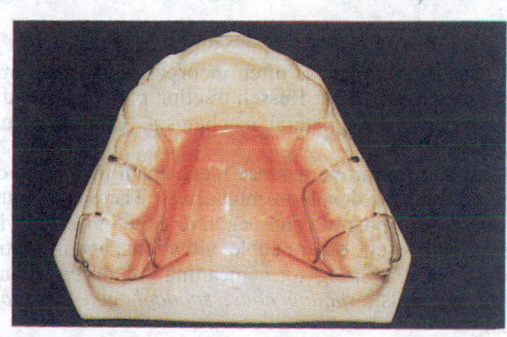

Dental splint
(Witzig, 1991/Courtesy of the Ohlendorf Co., St. Louis)

splinter [D, *splinte*], a sharp pointed piece of bone or other substance.

splinter fracture [D, *splinte*], a comminuted fracture with thin, sharp bone fragments.

splinter hemorrhage, linear bleeding under a fingernail or toenail, resembling a splinter. It is seen after trauma and in patients with bacterial endocarditis. (See Fig. p. 1470.)

splinting, the process of immobilizing, restraining, or supporting a body part.

split gene [D, *splitten,* to split], (in molecular genetics) a genetic unit whose continuity is interrupted.

split personality. See **multiple personality.**

split Russell traction, an orthopedic mechanism that combines suspension and traction to immobilize, position, and align the lower extremities in the treatment of congenital hip dislocation and hip and knee contractures, and in the correction of orthopedic deformities. Split Russell traction, usually applied as adhesive or nonadhesive skin traction, employs a sling to relieve the weight of the lower extremities. The traction weights are suspended from pulley and rope systems at the foot and the head of the patient's

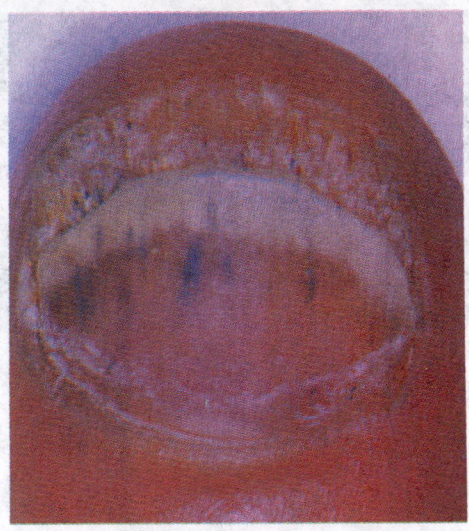

Splinter hemorrhage *(Baran, 1991)*

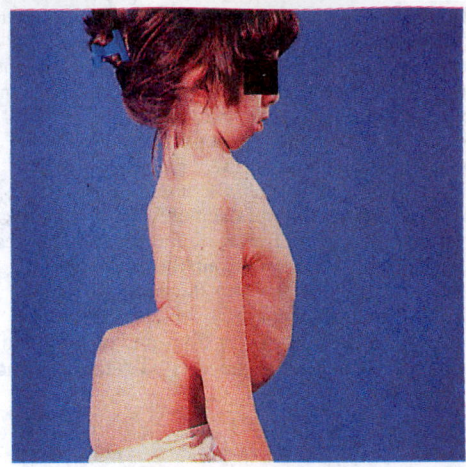

Spondylolisthesis *(Bullough, 1988)*

bed; a jacket restraint is often incorporated to help immobilize the patient. Split Russell traction may be applied as a unilateral or as a bilateral mechanism. Compare **Russell traction.**

splitting, a primitive defense mechanism that when overused represents a developmental arrest. There is a failure to synthesize the positive and negative experiences and ideas one has of oneself, other people, situations, and institutions.

spodo-, a combining form meaning 'of or pertaining to waste materials': *spodogenous, spodophagous, spodophorous.*

spondyl-, a combining form meaning 'pertaining to a physiologic condition or changes of the vertebrae': *spondylopathy, spondylosis.*

-spondylic /spondil'ik/, a combining form meaning 'referring to the vertebrae': *cyclospondylic, monospondylic, tectospondylic.*

spondylitic [Gk, *sphondylos,* vertebra], pertaining to a person afflicted with spondylitis.

spondylitis /spon'dəlī'tis/ [Gk, *sphondylos,* vertebra, *itis*], an inflammation of any of the spinal vertebrae, usually characterized by stiffness and pain. The condition may follow traumatic injury to the spine, or it may be the result of infection or rheumatoid disease. See also **ankylosing spondylitis.**

spondylitis ankylopoietica. See **Strümpell-Marie disease.**

spondylo-, a combining form meaning 'of or pertaining to a vertebra or to the spinal column': *spondylocace, spondylodidymia, spondylolysis.*

spondylolisthesis /spon'dilō'listhē'sis/ [Gk, *sphondylos* + *olisthanein,* to slip], the partial forward dislocation of one vertebra over the one below it, most commonly the fifth lumbar vertebra over the first sacral vertebra. See also **spinal cord compression.**

spondylosis /spon'dilō'sis/ [Gk, *sphondylos* + *osis*], a condition of the spine characterized by fixation or stiffness of a vertebral joint. See also **ankylosing spondylitis, spondylitis.**

spondylosyndesis. See **spinal fusion.**

spondylous /spon'diləs/ [Gk, *sphondylos,* vertebra], pertaining to a vertebra.

sponge /spunj/ [Gk, *spongia*], **1.** a resilient, absorbent mass used to absorb fluids, to apply medication, or to cleanse. The sponge may be the internal skeleton of a certain marine animal, or it may be manufactured from cellulose, rubber, or synthetic material. **2.** *informal.* a folded gauze square used in surgery.

sponge bath, the procedure of washing the patient with a damp washcloth or sponge, used when a full bath is not necessary or as a method of reducing body temperature.

sponge contraceptive. See **vaginal sponge.**

sponge gold. See **mat gold.**

spongio-, a combining form meaning 'like a sponge or related to a sponge': *spongioblast, spongiopilin, spongiosis.*

spongioblastoma /spun'jē·ōblastō'mə/, *pl.* **spongioblastomas, spongioblastomata** [Gk, *spongia* + *blastos,* germ, *oma,* tumor], a neoplasm composed of spongioblasts, embryonic epithelial cells that develop around the neural tube and transform into cells of the supporting connective tissue of nerve cells or cells of lining membranes of the ventricles and the spinal cord canal. Also called **glioblastoma, gliosarcoma, spongiocytoma.**

spongioblastoma multiforme. See **glioblastoma multiforme.**

spongioblastomas. See **spongioblastoma.**

spongioblastomata. See **spongioblastoma.**

spongioblastoma unipolare, a rare neoplasm composed of parallel spongioblasts. The tumor may occur near the third ventricle, in the pons and brainstem, in basal ganglia, or in the terminal filament of the spinal cord.

spongiocytoma. See **spongioblastoma.**

spongy /spun'jē/ [Gk, *spoggia*], pertaining to or resembling a sponge.

spongy bone [Gk, *spoggia;* AS, *ban*], a latticelike arrangement of bony plates and trabeculae occuring at the ends of the long bones. Also called **cancellous bone.**

spontaneous /spontā'nē·əs/ [L, *sponte,* willingly], occurring naturally and without apparent cause, such as spontaneous remission.

spontaneous abortion, a termination of pregnancy before the twentieth week of gestation as a result of abnormalities of the conceptus or maternal environment. More than 10%

of pregnancies end as spontaneous abortions, almost all caused by blighted ova that have congenital defects incompatible with life. Also called **miscarriage.** Compare **induced abortion.**

spontaneous delivery, a vaginal birth occurring without the mechanical assistance of obstetric forceps or vacuum aspirator.

spontaneous evolution, the unassisted delivery of a fetus in the transverse position. See also **Denman's spontaneous evolution.**

spontaneous fracture. See **neoplastic fracture.**

spontaneous generation, the theoretical origin of living organisms from inanimate matter; abiogenesis.

spontaneous labor, a labor beginning and progressing without mechanical or pharmacologic stimulation.

spontaneous PEEP (sPEEP), a spontaneous breathing system with end-expiratory pressure.

spontaneous phagocytosis [L, *sponte*, free will; Gk, *phagein*, to eat + *kytos*, cell + *osis*, condition], ingestion of antigenic particles by phagocytes of the reticuloendothelial system.

spontaneous pneumothorax [L, *sponte*, free will; Gk, *pneuma*, air + *thorax*, chest], the presence of air or gas in the intrapleural space as a result of a rupture of the lung parenchyma and visceral pleura with no demonstrable cause.

spontaneous ventilation, normal breathing, unassisted, in which the patient creates the pressure gradient through muscle and chest wall movements that move the air into and out of the lungs.

spontaneous version [L, *sponte*, free will + *vertere*, to turn], a change in the lie of a fetus that occurs without manipulation.

spoon nail [AS, *spon* + *naegel*], a nail of the finger or toe that is thin and concave.

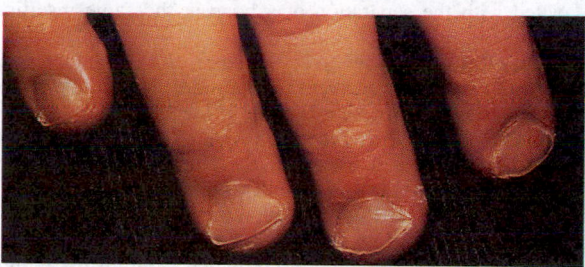

Spooning of nails (*Zitelli, 1992*)

spor-. See **sporo-.**

sporadic /spôrat′ik/ [Gk, *sporaden*, scattered], (of a number of events) occurring at scattered, intermittent, and apparently random intervals.

-sporangium, a combining form meaning an 'encasement of spores': *haplosporangium, oosporangium, sporangium.*

spore [Gk, *sporos*, seed], 1. a reproductive unit of some genera of fungi or protozoa. 2. a form assumed by some bacteria that is resistant to heat, drying, and chemicals. Under proper environmental conditions the spore may revert to the actively multiplying form of the bacterium. Diseases caused by spore-forming bacteria include anthrax, botulism, gas gangrene, and tetanus.

-spore, a suffix meaning a 'reproductive element': *archespore, chlamydospore, hemispore.*

sporicidal /spôr′isī′dəl/ [Gk, *sporos*, seed; L, *caedere*, to kill], spore-killing, as are certain chemicals or other agents.

sporicide /spôr′isīd/ [Gk, *sporos* + L, *caedere*, to kill], any agent effective in destroying spores, such as compounds of chlorine and formaldehyde, and the gluteraldehydes.

sporiferous /spôrif′ərəs/, producing or bearing spores.

spork, a spoonlike food utensil with fork tines specially designed for people with upper extremity disabilities.

sporo-, spor-, a combining form meaning 'of or pertaining to a spore': *sporocyst, sporogenesis, sporogeny.*

sporoblast /spôr′əblast′/ [Gk, *sporos* + *blastos*, germ], any cell that gives rise to a sporozoite or spore during the sexual reproductive phase of the life cycle of a sporozoan, specifically the cells resulting from the multiple fission of the encysted zygote of the malarial parasite *Plasmodium,* from which the sporozoites develop.

sporocyst /spôr′əsist/ [Gk, *sporos* + *kystis*, bag], 1. any structure containing spores or reproductive cells. 2. a saclike structure, or oocyst, secreted by the zygote of certain protozoa before sporozoite formation. 3. the second larval stage in the life cycle of parasitic flukes. The saclike organism develops from the miracidium, or first larval stage, in the body of a freshwater snail host and contains germinal cells that give rise either to daughter sporocysts that develop into cercariae or to rediae. See also **fluke.**

sporogenesis /spôr′ōjen′əsis/ [Gk, *sporos* + *genesis*, origin], 1. also called **sporogeny** /spôroj′ənē/. the formation of spores. 2. reproduction by means of spores. **—sporogenic,** adj.

sporogenous /spôroj′ənəs/ [Gk, *sporos* + *genein*, to produce], describing an animal or plant that reproduces by spores.

sporogeny. See **sporogenesis.**

sporogony /spôrog′ənē/ [Gk, *sporos* + *genesis*, origin], reproduction by means of spores, specifically the formation of sporozoites during the sexual stage of the life cycle of a sporozoan, primarily the malarial parasite *Plasmodium.* Fusion of the sex cells occurs in the body of the invertebrate host, the female *Anopheles* mosquito in the case of *Plasmodium,* where the encysted zygote undergoes multiple division, giving rise to the sporozoites. Compare **schizogony.**

sporont /spôr′ont/ [Gk, *sporos* + *on*, being], a mature protozoan parasite in the sexual reproductive stage of its life cycle. It undergoes conjugation to form a zygote, which produces sporozoites by multiple fission. Compare **schizont.** See also **sporogony.**

sporonticide /spôron′tisīd/ [Gk, *sporos, on* + L, *caedere*, to kill], any substance that destroys sporonts, such as chloroquine and other antimalarial drugs. **—sporonticidal,** adj.

sporophore /spôr′əfôr/ [Gk, *sporos* + *pherein*, to bear], the part of an organism or plant that produces spores.

sporophyte /spôr′əfīt/ [Gk, *sporos* + *phyton*, plant], the asexual, spore-bearing stage in plants that reproduce by alternation of generations.

sporotrichosis /spôr′ōtrikō′sis/ [Gk, *sporos* + *thrix*, hair, *osis*, condition], a common, chronic fungal infection caused by the species *Sporothrix schenckii,* usually characterized by skin ulcers and subcutaneous nodules along lymphatic channels. It rarely spreads to involve bones, lungs, joints, or muscles. The fungus is found in soil and decaying vegetation and usually enters the skin by accidental injury. Treatment may include amphotericin B or itraconazole.

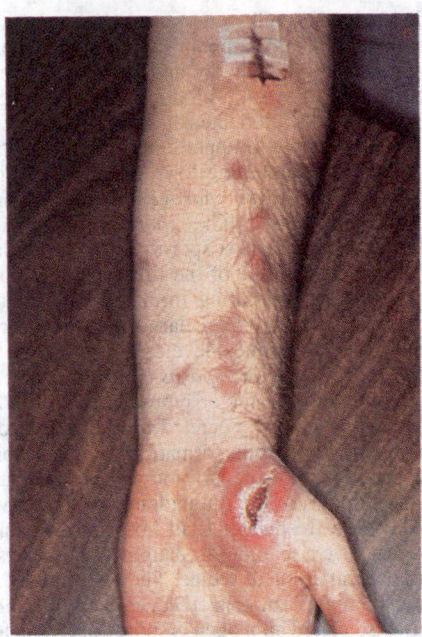

Lymphocutaneous sporotrichosis (Murray, 1990)

Sporotrichum /spôrot′rikəm/ [Gk, *sporos* + *thrix*, hair], a genus of soil-inhabiting fungi formerly thought to cause sporotrichosis.

Sporozoa /spôr′əzō′ə/ [Gk, *sporos* + *zoon*, animal], a class of parasite in the phylum Protozoa that is characterized by the absence of any external organs of locomotion. Included in this class are the genera *Toxoplasma* and *Plasmodium.*

sporozoite /spôr′əzō′īt/ [Gk, *sporos* + *zoon*, animal], any of the cells resulting from the sexual union of spores during the life cycle of a sporozoan. It refers specifically to the elongated nucleated cells produced by the multiple fission of the zygote contained in the oocyst in the female *Anopheles* mosquito during the sexual reproductive stage of the life cycle of the malarial parasite *Plasmodium.* On release from the oocyst, the sporozoites migrate to the salivary glands of the mosquito, where they are transmitted to humans and develop within the parenchymal cells of the liver as merozoites. Also called **falciform body.** See also **malaria, Plasmodium.**

sport [ME, *disporten*, to amuse], **1.** an individual or organism that differs drastically from its parents or others of its type because of genetic mutation; a mutant. **2.** a genetic mutation. **3.** See **lusus naturae.**

sports medicine, a branch of medicine that specializes in the prevention and treatment of injuries resulting from training and participation in athletic events. More than 1 million people are treated for sports injuries each year in the United States alone. Most sports injuries involve muscle sprains, strains, and tears, which frequently result from in-

adequate preliminary 'warm-up' exercises. Among the most common sports injuries are shin splints, runner's knee, pulled hamstring muscles, Achilles tendonitis, ankle sprain, arch sprain, charley horse, tennis elbow, baseball finger, dislocations, muscle cramps, bursitis, myofascitis, costochondritis, hernia, and 'Little League elbow.'

sporulation /spôr′yəlā′shən/ [Gk, *sporos* + L, *atus,* process], **1.** a type of reproduction that occurs in lower plants and animals, such as fungi, algae, and protozoa, and involves the formation of spores by the spontaneous division of the cell into four or more daughter cells, each of which contains a portion of the original nucleus. **2.** the formation of a refractile body, or resting spore, within certain bacteria that makes the cell resistant to unfavorable environmental conditions. The cell regains its viability when the conditions become favorable. See also **spore.**

spot [ME, blot], (in psychotherapy) a small quantum of space that becomes the territorial object and extension of point behavior.

spot film, a radiograph made instantly during fluoroscopy. The technique may be used to make a permanent record of a transiently observed effect or to record with definition and detail a small anatomic area.

spotted fever. See **Rocky Mountain spotted fever.**

spotting [ME, *spot,* different color], the appearance of a blood-stained discharge from the vagina between menstrual periods, during pregnancy, or at the beginning of labor.

sprain [origin unknown], a traumatic injury to the tendons, muscles, or ligaments around a joint, characterized by pain, swelling, and discoloration of the skin over the joint. The duration and severity of the symptoms vary with the extent of damage to the supporting tissues. Treatment requires support, rest, and alternating cold and heat. Ultrasound therapy may speed recovery. X-ray pictures are often indicated to be certain that no fracture has occurred.

sprain fracture, a fracture that results from the separation of a tendon or ligament at the point of insertion, associated with the separation of a bone at the same insertion site.

sprain of ankle or foot [AS, *ancleow* + *fot*], sudden traction on a muscle, ligament, or capsule. The injury is not severe enough to cause a rupture of the tissue.

sprain of back [AS, *baec*], a sudden traction injury to muscles and related tissues of the back. The tissues may have undergone traumatic strain without being ruptured.

spreader bar /spred′ər/, a metal bar with curved hoop areas for attaching hooks or pins for traction.

spreadsheet /spred′shēt/, a computer program that simulates a business or scientific worksheet and performs the necessary calculations when data is changed.

spring forceps [AS, *springan,* to jump], a kind of forceps that includes a spring mechanism, used for grasping an artery to arrest or prevent hemorrhage. Also called **bulldog forceps.**

spring lancet, a lancet with a spring-triggered blade. It may be used for collecting small specimens of blood for laboratory tests. See also **lancet.**

sprinter's fracture [Swed, *sprinta,* to spurt; L, *fractura,* to break], a fracture of the anterior superior or the anterior inferior spine of the ilium, caused by a fragment of bone being forcibly pulled by a violent muscle spasm.

sprue /sprōō/ [D, *sprouw,* kind of tumor], a chronic disorder resulting from malabsorption of nutrients from the small intestine and characterized by a broad range of symptoms, including diarrhea, weakness, weight loss, poor appetite, pallor, muscle cramps, bone pain, ulceration of the mucous membrane lining the digestive tract, and a smooth, shiny tongue. It occurs in both tropical and nontropical forms and affects both children and adults. Also called **catarrhal dysentery.** See also **malabsorption syndrome, nontropical sprue, tropical sprue.**

SPRX, a trademark for an anorexiant (phendimetrazine tartrate).

SPSS, (in statistics) abbreviation for *Statistical Package for the Social Sciences,* a computer program often used in research in clinical nursing for the analysis of complex data from large samples.

spur [AS, *spura*], a projection of bone or metal from a body structure or appliance. See also **exostosis.**

spurious pregnancy. See **pseudocyesis.**

sputum /spyoo′təm/ [L, spittle], material coughed up from the lungs and expectorated through the mouth. It contains mucus, cellular debris, or microorganisms, and it also may contain blood or pus. The amount, color, and constituents of the sputum are important in the diagnosis of many illnesses, including tuberculosis, pneumonia, cancer of the lung, and the pneumoconioses.

sputum specimen [L, *spuo*, to spit out + *specere, to look],* a sample of material expelled from the respiratory passages taken for laboratory analysis to determine the presence of pathogens.

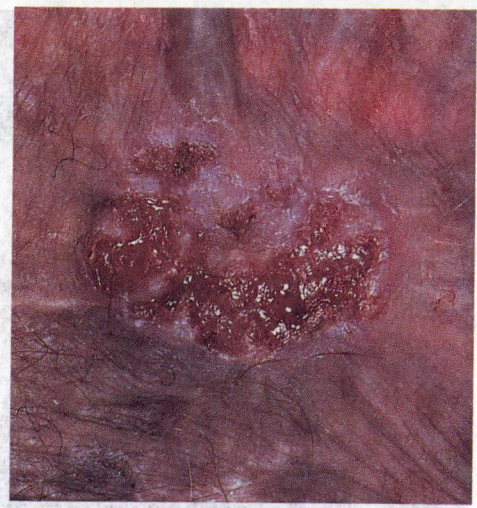
Squamous cell carcinoma *(du Vivier, 1993)*

squamous epithelium [L, *squama,* scale; Gk, *epi,* above, *thele,* nipple], a sheet of flattened scalelike cells, attached together at the edges. Also called **pavement epithelium.**

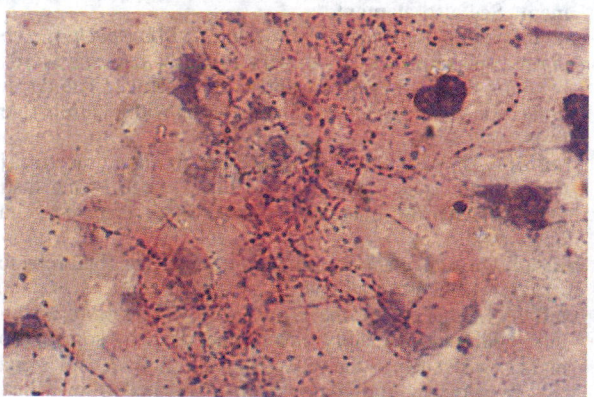
Sputum specimen (acid-fast stain) *(Murray, 1990)*

squam-, a combining form meaning 'of or pertaining to scales': *squamatization, squamocellular, squamopetrosal.*

squama /skwā′mə/, *pl.* **squamae, 1.** a flattened scale from the epidermis. **2.** the thin, expanded part of a bone, especially in the cranial wall.

squamous [L, *squama,* scale], platelike, scaly, or covered with scales.

squamous cell /skwā′məs/ [L, *squama,* scale; *cella,* storeroom], a flat, scalelike epithelial cell.

squamous cell carcinoma, a slow-growing, malignant tumor of squamous epithelium, frequently found in the lungs and skin and occurring also in the anus, cervix, larynx, nose, and bladder. The neoplastic cells characteristically resemble prickle cells and form keratin pearls on the surface of lesions. Also called **epidermoid carcinoma.**

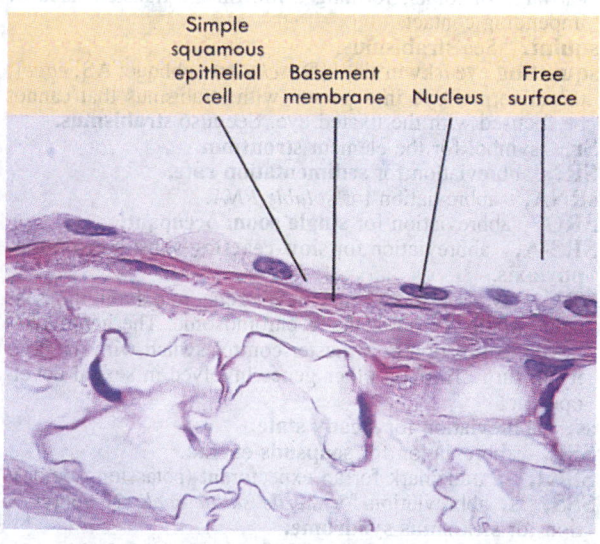
Simple squamous epithelium *(Seeley, 1992/Ed Reschke)*

Labels: Simple squamous epithelial cell / Basement membrane / Nucleus / Free surface

square centimeter (cm^2) /skwer/, a unit of area measurement equivalent to one centimeter in length multiplied by one centimeter in width where one centimeter equals 0.3937 inch or 0.03281 foot.

square window [OFr, *esquarre;* ME, *windowe,* wind-eye], an angle of the wrist between the hypothenar prominence and forearm. It is used as a reference point for estimating the gestational age of a newborn infant. (See Fig. p. 1474.)

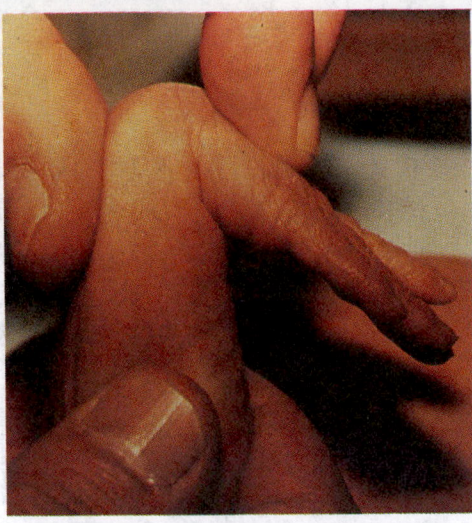

Square window test (Zitelli, 1992)

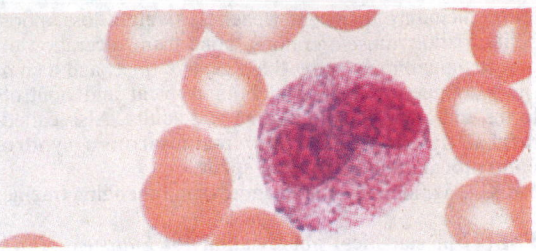

Stab cell (Hayhoe, 1992)

squeeze dynamometer /skwēz/ [AS, *cwesan,* to press tightly; Gk, *dynamis,* force, *metron,* measure], a dynamometer for measuring the muscular strength of the grip of the hand.

squeeze-film lubrication, the exudation of fluid from the cartilage of joints, forming a film in the transient area of impending contact.

squint. See **strabismus.**

squinting eye /skwin′ting/ [D, *schuinte,* oblique; AS, *eage*], the abnormal eye in a person with strabismus that cannot be focused with the fixated eye. See also **strabismus.**

Sr, symbol for the element **strontium.**

SR, abbreviation for **sedimentation rate.**

sRNA, abbreviation for *soluble RNA.*

SRO, abbreviation for **single room occupant.**

SRS-A, abbreviation for **slow-reacting substance of anaphylaxis.**

SRY, symbol for a 'maleness' gene found on the sex-determining region of the Y chromosome. The gene is believed to function as a master control switch with the ability to turn off or on other genes involved in sexual development.

ss, abbreviation for **steady state.**

SSE, abbreviation for **soapsuds enema.**

SSKI, a trademark for an expectorant (potassium iodide).

SSS, **1.** abbreviation for *sterile saline soak.* **2.** abbreviation for **sick sinus syndrome.**

SSSS, abbreviation for **staphylococcal scalded skin syndrome.**

S's test. See **Sulkowitch's test.**

ST, abbreviation for **slow-twitch.** See **slow-twitch fiber.**

stab [Swed *stabbe* thick stick], a nonsegmented neutrophil.

stab culture [ME, *stabbe,* piercing wound; L, *colere,* to cultivate], a culture made by dipping a needle into an inoculum and then into a transparent gelatin or agar medium.

stab form. See **band.**

-stabile, a combining form meaning 'stable, resistant to change': *coctostabile, hydrostabile, tempostabile.*

stabile diabetes. See **non-insulin-dependent diabetes mellitus.**

stabilization /stab′ilīzā′shən/ [L, *stabilis,* firm, *atus,* process], **1.** the physiologic and metabolic process of attaining homeostasis. **2.** the seating of a fixed or removable denture so that it will not tilt or be displaced under pressure. **3.** the control of induced stress loads and the development of measures to counteract such forces so that the movement of the teeth or of a prosthesis does not irritate surrounding tissues.

stable /stā′bəl/ [L, *stabilis,* firm], remaining unchanged.

stable condition, a state of health in which the prognosis indicates little if any immediate change.

stable element [L, *stabilis,* firm; *elementum*], a nonradioactive element, one not subject to spontaneous nuclear degeneration. Some kinds of stable elements are calcium, iron, lead, potassium, and sodium. Compare **radioactive element.** See also **element.**

staccato speech /stəkä′tō/ [It, detached; ME, *speche*], abnormal speech in which the person pauses between words, breaking the rhythm of the phrase or sentence. The condition is sometimes observed in association with multiple sclerosis.

stadium /stā′dē·əm/, *pl.* **stadia** [Gk, *stadion,* racetrack], a significant stage in a fever or illness, such as the fastigium of a febrile illness or the prodromal stage of a viral infection.

Stadol, a trademark for an opioid analgesic (butorphanol tartrate), used as an adjunct to anesthesia.

staff [AS, *staef*], **1.** the people who work toward a common goal and are employed or supervised by someone of higher rank, such as the nurses in a hospital. **2.** a designation by which a staff nurse is distinguished from a head nurse or other nurse. **3.** (in nursing education) the nonprofessional employees of the institution, such as librarians, technicians, secretaries, and clerks. **4.** (in nursing service administration) the units of the organization that provide service to the 'line,' or administratively defined hierarchy; for example, the personnel office is 'staff' to the director of nursing and the nursing service administration.

staff development, (in nursing) a process that assists individual nurses in an agency or organization in attaining new skills and knowledge, gaining increasing levels of competence, and growing professionally. Various resources outside the agency employing the nurse may be used. The process may include such programs as orientation, in-service education, and continuing education. Many fields outside of nursing also develop and use programs for staff development that are specific to their needs.

staffing, the process of assigning people to fill the roles designed for an organizational structure through recruitment, selection, and placement. Centralized staffing involves a system whereby a master plan is developed at the top level of the organization. Cyclical staffing is a system in which workdays and time off for personnel are repeated in regular cycles, such as every 6 weeks.

staffing pattern, (in hospital or nursing administration) the number and types or categories of staff assigned to the particular units and departments of a hospital or other health care facility. Staffing patterns vary with the unit, department, and shift.

staff of Æsculapius, a staff carried by Æsculapius, the Greek god of medicine. It is used as the traditional symbol of the physician. A single serpent entwines the staff of Æsculapius. It is often confused with the caduceus, a staff with two serpents (which is the staff of Hermes, the Greek god of commerce and travel), symbolizing (because of this misunderstanding) the U.S. Army Medical Corps. See **Æsculapius.**

stage [OFr, *estage*], **1.** a platform. **2.** a period or phase.
-stage, a combining form meaning a '(specified) phase': *aecidiostage, multistage, uredostage.*

stages of anesthesia. See **Guedel's signs.**

stages of dying [OFr, *estage*, stage; ME, *dyen*, to lose life], the five emotional and behavioral stages that may occur after a person first learns of approaching death. The stages, identified and described by Elisabeth Kübler-Ross, are denial and shock, anger, bargaining, depression, and acceptance. The stages may occur in sequence or they may recur, as the person moves forward and backward—especially between denial, anger, and bargaining. Caring for a dying person requires sensitivity to the signs of each stage. At first, shock may be accompanied by signs of panic. The person may refuse care and deny the diagnosis and prognosis. Denial serves as a defense against the shock. Anger often follows this stage. It is characterized by abusive language, refusal to perform basic self-care responsibilities, negative criticism of anyone who wants to help, and other kinds of angry behavior. The third stage, bargaining, reflects the need of the person for time to accept the situation. A common observation of this period is the patient's attempt to make a bargain, "If I could live until Christmas, …" Commonly, the person goes back and forth from anger to bargaining: sometimes silent, sometimes grieving, and sometimes apathetic, depressed, insomniac, and distant. The fourth stage is a time of depression in which the person goes through a period of grieving before death, mourning over past experiences and anticipating impending losses. The final stage, acceptance, is one of inner peace and resolution that death is a certainty. The person may show his or her acceptance by being disinterested in present or future events, being preoccupied with past events, preferring few visitors, and wanting quiet and solitude. Nursing care includes administering adequate pain relief, ensuring privacy and dignity, and giving sensitive, honest emotional support to both patient and family. See also **emotional care of the dying patient, hospice.**

stagnant anoxia /stag′nənt/ [L, *stagnum*, standing water; Gk, *a*, without, *oxys*, sharp, *genein*, to produce], a condition in which there is inadequate blood flow in the capillaries, causing low tissue oxygen tension and reduced oxygen exchange. This state is associated with shock, cardiac standstill, and thrombosis.

stain [OFr, *desteindre*, to dye], **1.** a pigment, dye, or substance used to impart color to microscopic objects or tissues to facilitate their examination and identification. Kinds of stains include **acid-fast stain, Gram's stain,** and **Wright's stain. 2.** to apply pigment to a substance or tissue to examine it under a microscope. **3.** an area of discoloration.

stained film fault, a defect in a radiograph or developed photographic film that appears as a streaky discoloration or abnormal opacity. It is usually caused by contaminated development solutions, improper rinsing, exhausted solutions, inadequate washing, or damage to the film emulsion during processing.

-stalsis, a suffix meaning a 'contraction in the alimentary canal': *antistalsis, catastalsis, retrostalsis.*

stammering [AS, *stamerian,* to stutter], a speech dysfunction characterized by spasmodic pauses, hesitations, and faltering utterances, such as mispronunciation or transposition of letters within a word. The term is frequently used synonymously with stuttering, especially in Great Britain.

stamp cusp [ME, *stampen;* L, *cuspis,* point], a cusp that works in a fossa, such as any of the maxillary lingual cusps.

stance phase of gait [L, *stare,* to stand; Gk, *phainein,* to show; ME, *gate,* a way], the first phase of the normal gait cycle that begins with the strike of the heel on the ground and ends with the lift of the toe at the beginning of the swing phase of gait: the brief period in which both feet are on the ground.

standard [OFr, *estandart*], **1.** an evaluation that serves as a basis for comparison for evaluating similar phenomena or substances, such as a standard for the preparation of a pharmaceutic substance, or a standard for the practice of a profession. **2.** a pharmaceutic preparation or a chemical substance of known quantity, ingredients, and strength that is used to determine the constituents or the strength of another preparation. **3.** of known value, strength, quality, or ingredients. **4.** predetermined criteria used to provide guidance in the operation of a health care facility to ensure quality performance by the personnel. −**standardize,** *v.,* **standardization,** *n.*

standard air chamber, a radiation measuring device used by national and international calibration laboratories to provide exposure calibrations of ion chambers for use in the diagnostic or orthovoltage energy range. Secondary ion chambers are intercompared with a standard chamber to provide a calibration factor for the field instrument, which will make its readings traceable to the standardization laboratory.

standard bicarbonate, the bicarbonate ion concentration of plasma separated anaerobically from whole blood that has been saturated with oxygen and equilibrated at carbon dioxide pressure of 40 torr at 38° C. It is a measure of the metabolic disturbance of acid-base balance in a sample of blood after any respiratory disturbance present has been corrected.

standard of care, a written statement describing the rules, actions, or conditions that direct patient care. Standards of care guide practice and can be used to evaluate performance.

standard death certificate, a form for a death certificate that is commonly used throughout the United States. It is the preferred form of the United States Census Bureau.

standard deviation (SD), (in statistics) a mathematic statement of the dispersion of a set of values or scores from the mean. Each sample value is subtracted from the sample mean and squared, and the squares are summed. The square root of the summed squares gives a mathematically standardized value so that sample deviations can be compared.

standard environmental chamber. See **Skinner box.**

standard error (S.E.), (in statistics) the variability in scores that can be expected if measurements are made on random samples of the same size from the same universe of population, phenomena, or observations. The standard error provides a framework within which a determination of the difference between groups may be made. It is an element used in determining statistic significance by means of a wide variety of formulas and methods.

standardization. See **standard.**

standardize. See **standard.**

standardized death rate, the number of deaths per 1000 people of a specified population during 1 year. This rate is adjusted to avoid distortion by the age composition of the population. A standard population is used for determining this rate. Also called **adjusted death rate.**

standards of nursing practice, a set of guidelines for providing quality nursing care and a criteria for evaluating care. Such guidelines help assure patients that they are receiving high-quality care. The standards are important if a legal dispute arises over the quality of care provided a patient.

standing orders [L, *stare*, to stand; *ordo*, rank], a written document containing rules, policies, procedures, regulations, and orders for the conduct of patient care in various stipulated clinical situations. The standing orders are usually formulated collectively by the professional members of a department in a hospital or other health care facility. Standing orders usually name the condition and prescribe the action to be taken in caring for the patient, including the dosage and route of administration for a drug or the schedule for the administration of a therapeutic procedure.

stann-, a combining form meaning 'of or pertaining to tin': *stanniferous, stanniform, stannoxyl.*

stannous fluoride /stan'əs/ [L, *stannum*, tin + *fluere*, to flow], a salt of fluorine and tin used in oral hygiene products to reduce caries activity.

stanozolol /stənō'zəlol, /, an androgenic anabolic steroid.
■ INDICATIONS: It is prescribed in the treatment of aplastic anemia and osteoporosis.
■ CONTRAINDICATIONS: Cancer of the breast or prostate, nephrosis, pregnancy, or known hypersensitivity to this drug prohibits its use.
■ ADVERSE EFFECTS: Among the most serious adverse reactions are various androgenic effects in males and females, hypoestrogenic effects in females, and allergic reactions. GI disturbances also may occur.

St. Anthony's fire. See **ergot poisoning.**

stape-, a combining form referring to the 'stapes': *stapedial, stapedectomy.*

stapedectomy /stā'pədek'təmē/ [L, *stapes*, stirrup; Gk, *ektome*, excision], removal of the stapes of the middle ear and insertion of a graft and prosthesis, performed to restore hearing in the treatment of otosclerosis. The stapes that has become fixed is replaced so that vibrations again transmit sound waves through the oval window to the fluid of the inner ear. Under local anesthesia, the stapes is removed and the opening into the inner ear is covered with a graft of body tissue. One end of a small plastic tube or piece of stainless steel wire is attached to the graft; the other end is attached to the two remaining bones of the middle ear, the malleus and the incus. Headache and dizziness are expected early in the postoperative period. The patient's hearing does not improve until the edema subsides and the packing is re-

moved. Possible complications include infection of the outer, middle, or inner ear, displacement or rejection of the graft or the prosthesis, and leaking of perilymph around the prosthesis into the middle ear, with ringing in the ear and dizziness. Compare **incudectomy.**

stapedius /stəpē'dē·əs/, a small muscle on the wall of the tympanic cavity of the middle ear. It pulls the head of the stapes posteriorly, tilting the baseplate, and, with the tensor tympani, acts reflexively in response to loud sounds to reduce excessive vibrations that could injure the internal ear.

stapes /stā'pēz/ [L, stirrup], one of the three ossicles in the middle ear, resembling a tiny stirrup. It transmits sound vibrations from the incus to the internal ear. Compare **incus, malleus.** See also **middle ear.**

Staphage Lysate (SPL), a trademark for an active immunizing agent (staphylococcal antigen phage lysed), used in staphylococcal infection.

Staphcillin, a trademark for an antibacterial (methicillin sodium).

staphyl-, staphylo- /staf'əlo-/, a combining form meaning "grapelike clusters" and pertaining to conditions of the uvula: *staphyloplasty, staphyloncus;* or a micrococcal infection: *staphylolysin, staphyloderm.*

staphylococcal /-kok'əl/ [Gk, *staphyle*, bunch of grapes + *kokkos*, berry], pertaining to a genus of facultatively anaerobic gram-positive cocci.

staphylococcal antigen phage lysed. See **Staphage Lysate.**

staphylococcal infection [Gk, *staphyle* bunch of grapes, *kokkos*, berry; L, *inficere*, to taint], an infection caused by any one of several pathogenic species of *Staphylococcus*, commonly characterized by the formation of abscesses of the skin or other organs. Staphylococcal infections of the skin include carbuncles, folliculitis, furuncles, and hidradenitis suppurativa. Bacteremia is common and may result in endocarditis, meningitis, or osteomyelitis. Staphylococcal pneumonia often follows influenza or other viral disease and may be associated with chronic or debilitating illness. Acute gastroenteritis may result from an enterotoxin produced by certain species of staphylococci in contaminated food. Treatment usually includes bed rest, analgesics, and an antimicrobial drug that is resistant to penicillinase, an enzyme secreted by many species of *Staphylococcus*. Surgical drainage, especially of deep abscesses, is often necessary.

staphylococcal pneumonia [Gk, *staphyle* + *kokkos* + *pneumon*, lung], pneumonia caused by a staphylococcus infection.

staphylococcal scalded skin syndrome (SSSS), an abnormal skin condition characterized by epidermal erythema, peeling, and necrosis that gives the skin a scalded appearance. This disorder affects primarily infants 1 to 3 months of age and other children, but it also may affect adults. It is caused by strains of *Staphylococcus aureus*, especially group II phage types. Deficient immune functions and renal insufficiency may predispose individuals to the disease. SSSS is more common in the newborn infant because of undeveloped immunity and renal systems.
■ OBSERVATIONS: A prodromal upper respiratory tract infection with concomitant purulent conjunctivitis is commonly associated with SSSS. Epidermal complications develop in the erythemal stage, the exfoliation stage, and the desquamation stage. Erythema often spreads around the mouth and other orifices and may extend over the entire body in wide

circles as the skin becomes tender and the superficial layer of the skin sloughs from friction. The exfoliation stage follows the erythema stage by 24 to 48 hours and is commonly manifested by slight crusting and erosion, which may spread from around the orifices to wider skin areas. More severe forms of SSSS may cause large, soft bullae to erupt and extend over wide skin areas. The eventual rupture of these bullae reveals areas of denuded skin. The desquamation stage of SSSS occurs after the exfoliation stage, and is characterized by the drying up of affected areas and the formation of powdery scales. Normal skin replaces the scales within 5 to 7 days. Diagnosis is based on close observation of the development of SSSS through its three characteristic stages. Erythema multiforme and drug-induced toxic epidermal necrolysis are similar to SSSS but may be ruled out in differential diagnosis by exfoliative cytology and biopsy. Confirming diagnosis is usually made on the basis of isolation of group II *Staphylococcus aureus* in cultures of skin lesions. The mortality in SSSS is 2% to 3%, death usually being caused by complications of fluid and electrolyte loss, sepsis, and involvement of other body systems. ▪ INTERVENTIONS: Treatment of SSSS commonly includes the administration of systemic antibiotics to prevent secondary infections and the replacement of body fluids to maintain fluid and electrolyte balance. ▪ NURSING CONSIDERATIONS: The nursing role in the treatment of this disorder focuses on special care for the neonate, such as maintenance of body temperature by placing the infant in an incubator, careful monitoring of intake and output, administration of IV fluids, maintenance of skin integrity, and careful, regular checks of vital signs. Nurses caring for SSSS patients should be especially alert for any sudden rise in temperature, which could indicate sepsis and the immediate need for aggressive treatment. A strict aseptic technique is needed to prevent any secondary infection. The aseptic technique is especially important during the exfoli-

ation stage, during which open lesions increase the risk of infection. The patient is loosely clothed and covered to minimize friction, which sloughs off the affected skin. Cotton is inserted between the affected fingers and toes to prevent webbing. During the recovery period, warm baths and soaks aid the healing, and gentle debridement of exfoliated areas hastens the healing process. Helpful to parents is the justifiable assurance from the nurse that complications and residual scars from SSSS rarely occur.

Staphylococcus /staf′ilōkok′əs/, *pl.* **staphylococci** [Gk, *staphyle* + *kokkos*, berry], a genus of nonmotile, spheric, gram-positive bacteria. Some species are normally found on the skin and in the throat; certain species cause severe, purulent infections or produce an enterotoxin, which may cause nausea, vomiting, and diarrhea. Life-threatening staphylococcal infections may arise within hospitals. *Staphylococcus aureus* is a species frequently responsible for abscesses, endocarditis, impetigo, osteomyelitis, pneumonia, and septicemia. *S. epidermidis,* formerly called *S. albus,* occasionally causes endocarditis in the presence of intracardiac prostheses. See also **staphylococcal infection.** −**staphylococcal,** *adj.*

Staphylococcus aureus [Gk, *staphyle* + *kokkos*; L, *aurum,* gold], a species of *Staphylococcus* that produces a golden pigment with some color variations. It is also responsible for a number of pyogenic infections, such as boils, carbuncles, and abscesses.

staphylokinase /staf′ilōkī′nās/, an enzyme, produced by certain strains of staphylococci, that catalyzes the conversion of plasminogen to plasmin in various animal hosts of the microorganism.

staple /stā′pəl/, a piece of stainless steel wire used to close certain surgical wounds.

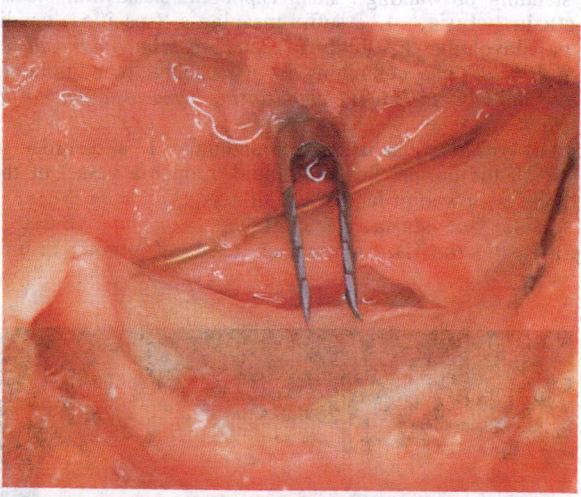

Staple *(Johnson, 1993)*

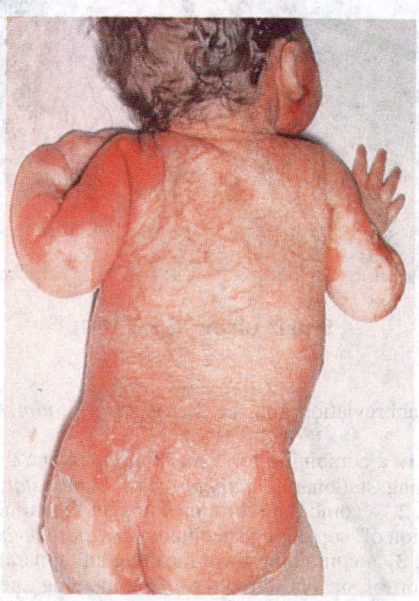

Staphylococcal scalded skin syndrome *(Hart, 1992)*

stapling [ME, *stapel*, stake], a method of fastening tissues together at the end of surgery by using a U-shaped piece of wire as a suture. The ends of the wire are bent toward the center to close the staple.

starch [AS, *stearc*, strong], the principal molecule used for the storage of food in plants. Starch is a polysaccharide and is composed of long chains of glucose subunits. In animals, excess glucose is stored as glycogen. The molecular structure of glycogen is similar to that of starch. See also **carbohydrate, glucose, glycogen.**

Starling's law of the heart [Ernest H. Starling, English physiologist, b. 1866; AS, *lagu*, law, *heorte*, heart], a rule that the force of the heartbeat is determined by the length of the fibers composing the myocardial walls.

Starr-Edwards prosthesis [A. Starr, 20th century American physician; M. L. Edwards, 20th century American physician; Gk, *prosthesis*, attachment], an artificial cardiac valve. A caged-ball form of device, it obstructs the valve opening and prevents the backward flow of blood. See also **prosthesis.**

start codon. See **initiation codon.**

startle reflex /stär′təl/ [ME, *stertlen*, to rush; Gk, *syn*, together + *dromos*, course], a reflex response to a sudden, unexpected stimulus. The reaction may be accompanied by physiologic effects including increased heartbeat and respiration, closing of the eyes, and flexion of trunk muscles. The reaction is rapid, pervasive, and uncontrollable, regardless of the unexpected stimulus, which may be as simple as a touch. However, premature and immature infants may not show the reaction. Also called **startle reaction; startle syndrome.** See also **Moro reflex.**

start point [ME, *sterte;* L, *punctum*, prick], (in molecular genetics) the initial nucleotide transcribed from the DNA template in the formation of messenger RNA.

starvation /stärvā′shən/ [ME, *sterven*, to die], **1.** a condition resulting from the lack of essential nutrients over a long period of time and characterized by multiple physiologic and metabolic dysfunctions. **2.** the act or state of starving or being starved. See also **malnutrition.**

stas-, a combining form meaning 'stopped, or relation to standing or walking': *stasibasiphobia, stasidynic, stasis.*

-stasia, -stasis, 1. a suffix meaning a '(specified) condition involving the ability to stand': *astasia, ananastasia, dysstasia.* **2.** a combining form meaning '(condition of) stoppage or inhibition': *cholestasia, hemostasia, menostasia.*

stasis /stā′sis, stas′is/ [Gk, standing], **1.** a disorder in which the normal flow of a fluid through a vessel of the body is slowed or halted. **2.** stillness.

-stasis. See **-stasia.**

stasis dermatitis, a common result of venous insuffi-

ciency of the legs beginning with ankle edema and progressing to tan pigmentation, patchy erythema, petechiae, and induration. Ultimately, there may be atrophy and fibrosis of the skin and subcutaneous tissue, with ulcerations that are slow to heal. The tan pigment is hemosiderin from blood leaking through capillary walls under elevated venous pressure. The involved skin is very easily irritated or sensitized to topical medications. The underlying venous insufficiency must be treated. The dermatitis is often treated by bed rest, Burow's solution for oozing lesions, antibiotics for infection, and corticosteroids to reduce inflammation. Also called **venous stasis dermatitis.** See also **stasis ulcer.**

stasis ulcer, a necrotic craterlike lesion of the skin of the lower leg caused by chronic venous congestion. The ulcer is often associated with stasis dermatitis and varicose veins. Healing is slow, and good nursing care to prevent irritation and infection is essential. Potentially sensitizing agents should not be used. Bed rest, elevation, and pressure bandages are usually ordered, and appropriate antibiotics, Burow's solution compresses, Unna's paste boot, pinch grafts, and surgery to improve venous flow are useful in treatment. Also called **varicose ulcer.** See also **stasis dermatitis.**

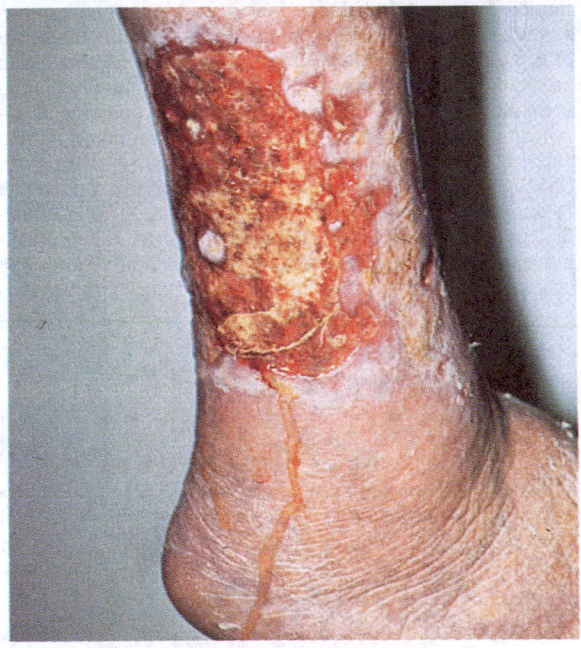

Stasis ulcer *(Kamal, 1991)*

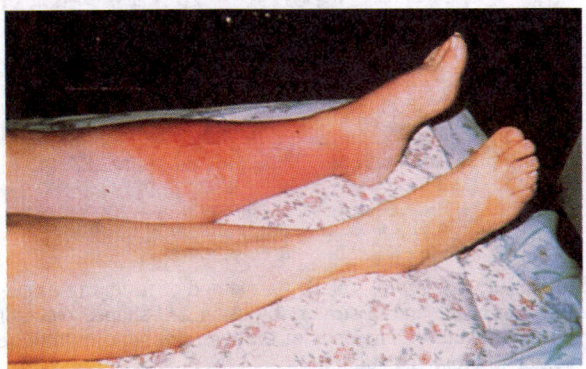

Stasis dermatitis *(Christiansen, 1993)*

stat., abbreviation for the Latin word *statim*, 'immediately.'

-stat, 1. a combining form meaning a 'device for keeping something stationary': *catheterostat, hysterostat, ophthalmostat.* **2.** a combining form meaning an 'instrument for the regulation of' something specified: *hemostat, rheostat, thermostat.* **3.** a combining form meaning an 'apparatus for the reflection of, in one direction of' something specified: *siderostat.* **4.** a combining form meaning a 'device for studying in a state of rest': *hydrostat, orbitostat, microstat.* **5.** a combining form meaning an 'agent for stopping the growth of': *bacteriostat, fungistat, mycostat.*

state /stāt/ [L, *status,* condition], the circumstances or qualities that characterize a person, thing, or way of being at a particular time.

-state, a combining form meaning the 'result of a (specified) process': *anastate, catastate, mesostate.*

State Board Test Pool Examination (SBTPE), revised and retitled in 1982 as the NCLEX-RN, an examination prepared by the National Council of State Boards of Nursing for testing the competency of a person to perform safely as a newly licensed registered nurse. Each jurisdiction within the United States and its territories regulates entry into the practice of nursing; each requires the candidate to pass the examination. The content of the examination is planned to test the candidates' knowledge of the nursing process as applied to the broad areas of nursing practice, including maternal and child health, medical and surgical nursing, and psychiatric nursing. The process includes five steps: assessing, analyzing, planning, implementing, and evaluating. Knowledge, comprehension, application, and analysis of the nursing process are tested as they apply to decision-making situations.

state medicine. See **socialized medicine.**

State Nurses' Association (SNA), an association of nurses at the state level. The various State Nurses' Associations are constituent units of the American Nurses' Association.

Statewide Health Coordinating Committee (SHCC), a component of the national network of Health Systems Agencies.

static /stat'ik/ [Gk, *statikos,* causing to stand], without motion, at rest, in equilibrium. Compare **dynamic.**

static cardiac work, the energy transfer that occurs during the development and maintenance of ventricular pressure immediately before the opening of the aortic valve.

static electricity film fault, a defect in a radiograph or a developed photographic film, which appears as lightning-like streaks. It is caused by too rapid opening of the film packet or transfer of static electricity from the user to the film.

static equilibrium, the ability of an individual to adjust to displacements of his or her center of gravity while maintaining a constant base of support.

static imaging, (in nuclear medicine) a diagnostic procedure in which a radioactive substance is administered to a patient to visualize an internal organ or body compartment. An image or set of images is made of the fixed or slowly changing distribution of the radioactivity.

static pressure [Gk, *statikos,* causing to stand; L, *premere,* to press], a condition of equalized blood pressure throughout the body when the heart beat is stopped. A nonmoving fluid exerts a uniform pressure in all directions.

static reflex [Gk, *statikos,* causing to stand; L, *reflectrere,* to bend, back], a reflex that helps one maintain normal posture and muscle tone when the body is at rest.

static scoliosis [Gk, *statikos,* causing to stand + *skoliosis,* curvature], a form of scoliosis resulting from a difference in the length of the legs.

static symptom. See **passive symptom.**

station /stā'shən/ [L, *stare,* to stand], the level of the biparietal plane of the fetal head relative to the level of the ischial spines of the maternal pelvis. An imaginary plane at the level of the spines is designated 'zero station.' Higher and lower stations are numbered at intervals of 1 cm and labeled as minus above and plus below. For example, 'station minus three' is 3 cm above the spines, and 'station plus two' is 2 cm below the spines. In breech presentation, the bitrochanteric diameter of the breech is used to determine station. See also **dilatation, effacement, labor.**

stationary grid /stā'shəner'ē/ [L, *stare* + ME, *gridere,* gridiron], (in radiography) an x-ray grid that does not move or oscillate during the exposure of a radiographic film. The image of the lead strips that compose the grid appear on the radiograph.

stationary lingual arch, an orthodontic arch wire that is designed to fit the lingual surface of the teeth and is soldered to the associated anchor bands.

statistic /stetis'tik/ [L, *status,* condition], a number that describes a property of a set of data or other numbers.

Statistical Package for the Social Sciences. See **SPSS.**

statistical significance [L, *status,* condition + *significare,* to signify], an interpretation of statistical data that indicates an occurrence was probably the result of a causative factor and not simply a chance result. Statistical significance at the 1% level indicates a 1 in 100 chance that a result can be ascribed to chance.

statistics /stətis'tiks/, a mathematical science concerned with measuring, classifying, and analyzing objective information.

statotonic reflex. See **attitudinal reflex.**

status /stā'təs, stat'əs/ [L, condition], **1.** a specified state or condition, such as emotional status. **2.** an unremitting state or condition, such as status asthmaticus.

status asthmaticus, an acute, severe, and prolonged asthma attack. Hypoxia, cyanosis, and unconsciousness may follow. Treatment includes bronchodilators given intravenously or by aerosol inhalation, corticosteroids, controlled positive pressure ventilation, sedation, frequent therapy, and emotional support. A bronchodilator may be given by aerosol inhalation from a ventilator. See also **allergic asthma, asthma.**

status dysraphicus. See **dysraphia.**

status epilepticus, a medical emergency characterized by continual seizures occurring without interruptions. Status epilepticus can be precipitated by the sudden withdrawal of anticonvulsant drugs, inadequate body levels of glucose, a brain tumor, a head injury, a high fever, or poisoning. Therapy includes intravenous administration of anticonvulsant drugs, nutrients, and electrolytes. An adequate airway is usually maintained with an oral pharyngeal or endotracheal tube.

statute of limitations /stach'o͞ot/ [L, *statuere,* to place; *limes,* boundary, (in law) a statute that sets a limit of time during which a suit may be brought or criminal charges may be made. In a malpractice suit, dispute may arise as to whether the time set by the particular statute of limitations begins to run at the time of the injury or at the time of the discovery of the injury.

statutory rape /stach'ətôr'ē/ [L, *statuere,* to place; *rapere,* to seize], (in law) sexual intercourse with a female below the age of consent, which varies from state to state. See also **rape.**

STD, abbreviation for **sexually transmitted disease.**

steady state (s, ss) /sted'ē/ [AS, *stedefast,* firm in its place; L *status* condition], a basic physiologic concept implying that the various forces and processes of life are in a state of homeostasis. Living organisms are in constant flux, working to balance the internal and external environments in an effort to avoid a deficiency or an excess that might cause illness. Steady state is a complete state of well-being involving total adaptation.

steam sterilization [ME, *steme*, vapor; L, *sterilis*, barren], the destruction of all forms of microbial life on an object by exposing the object to moist heat for 15 minutes at 121°.

steap-, stear-. See **stearo-**.

-stearic, a combining form meaning '(specified) fat or fat derivatives': *aleostearic, ketostearic, neurostearic*.

Stearns' alcoholic amentia /sturnz/ [A. Warren Stearns, American physician, b. 1885; Ar, *alkohl*, essence; L, *ab*, from, *mens*, mind], a form of insanity brought on by alcohol, characterized by an emotional disturbance of a less severe nature than that of delirium tremens but of longer duration and with greater mental clouding and amnesia.

stearo-, steap-, stear-, steato-, a combining form meaning 'of or pertaining to fat': *stearoconotum, stearodermia, stearopten*.

stearrhea [Gk, *stear*, fat + *rhoia*, flow], excessive secretion of fat.

stearyl alcohol, a solid substance, prepared by the catalytic hydrogenation of stearic acid, used in various ointments.

steato-. See **stearo-**.

steatorrhea /stē'ətərē'ə/ [Gk, *stear*, fat, *rhoia*, flow], greater than normal amounts of fat in the feces, characterized by frothy, foul-smelling fecal matter that floats, as in celiac disease, some malabsorption syndromes, and any condition in which fats are poorly absorbed by the small intestine.

steatorrhea simplex, See **seborrhea**.

Steele-Richardson-Olszewski syndrome [John C. Steele; J. Clifford Richardson; Jerzy Olszewski; 20th century Canadian neurologists], a rare, progressive, neurologic disorder of unknown cause, occurring in middle age, more often in men. It is characterized by paralysis of eye muscles, ataxia, neck and trunk rigidity, pseudobulbar palsy, and parkinsonian facies. Dementia and inappropriate emotional responses also are common. Treatment usually includes the antiparkinsonian drug levodopa for control of extrapyramidal symptoms. Also called **progressive supranuclear palsy.** See also **Parkinson's disease**.

steeple head. See **oxycephaly**.

Steinert's disease. See **myotonic muscular dystrophy**.

Stein-Leventhal syndrome. See **polycystic ovary syndrome**.

Steinmann pin /stīn'mən/ [Fritz Steinmann, Swiss surgeon, b. 1872; AS, *pinn*], a wide diameter pin used for heavy skeletal traction, as in the tibia or femur.

Stelazine, a trademark for a phenothiazine tranquilizer (trifluoperazine).

stell-, a combining form meaning 'of or pertaining to a star': *stellate, stellectomy, stellula*.

stellate /stel'it, -āt/ [L, *stella*, star], star-shaped or arranged in the pattern of a star.

stellate fracture, a fracture that involves the central point of impact or injury and radiates numerous fissures throughout surrounding bone tissue.

stellate ganglion [L, *stella*, star; Gk, *gagglion*, knot], a large irregular ganglion on the lowest part of the cervical sympathetic trunk fused with the first thoracic ganglion. Its branches communicate with the seventh and eighth cervical nerves.

stem cell [AS, *stemm*, tree, trunk; L, *cella*, storeroom], a formative cell; a cell whose daughter cells may give rise to other cell types. A **pluripotential stem cell** is one that has the potential to develop into several different types of mature cells, including lymphocytes, granulocytes, thrombocytes, and erythrocytes.

stem cell leukemia, a neoplasm of blood-forming organs in which the predominant malignant cell is too immature to classify. The acute disease has a rapid, relentless course. Also called **embryonal leukemia, hemoblastic leukemia, hemocytoblastic leukemia, lymphoidocytic leukemia, undifferentiated cell leukemia.**

stem cell lymphoma. See **undifferentiated malignant lymphoma**.

stem pessary. See **pessary**.

steno-, a prefix meaning 'short, contracted, or narrow': *stenobregmate, stenocephaly, stenothorax*.

stenosis /stinō'sis/ [Gk, *stenos*, narrow, *osis*, condition], an abnormal condition characterized by the constriction or narrowing of an opening or passageway in a body structure. Kinds of stenosis include **aortic stenosis** and **pyloric stenosis**. **–stenotic,** *adj.*

-stenosis, a suffix meaning 'narrowed or constricted': *angiostenosis, aortostenosis*.

stenotic [Gk, *stenos*, narrow], pertaining to a structure that is narrowed or strictured.

Stensen's duct. See **parotid duct**.

stent [Charles R. Stent, nineteenth century English dentist], **1.** a compound used in making dental impressions and medical molds. **2.** a mold or device made of stent, used in anchoring skin grafts and for supporting body openings and cavities during grafting or vessels and tubes of the body during surgical anastomosis.

step-care therapy, a therapeutic program that begins with a simple, conservative type of treatment but may advance to more complex stages as needed to achieve control of a disease or disorder. An example is step-care therapy of hypertension, in which the first step is limited to nonpharmacologic treatments such as weight control, low-salt diet, and exercise for the patient. If the first step fails to produce results, the next step may be the prescription of diuretics, followed by the use of beta blockers, ACE inhibitors, or other drugs, until an effective form of treatment is found.

steppage gait /step'ij/ [AS, *staepe*; ONorse, *gata*, way], a gait in which the legs are raised abnormally high, as in cases of drop foot.

step reflex. See **dance reflex**.

stepping reflex. See **dance reflex**.

stepwedge /step'wej/, an aluminum device that, when exposed to x-rays, displays a range of exposure intensities on a radiograph. These exposure 'steps' are analyzed to determine the speed characteristics of the radiographic film. Also called **penetrometer.**

Sterane, a trademark for a glucocorticoid (prednisolone).

Sterapred, a trademark for a glucocorticoid (prednisone).

sterco-, a combining form meaning 'of or pertaining to feces': *stercobilin, stercolith, stercoremia*.

stereo- /stir'ē'·ō-/, a combining form meaning 'solid, three dimensional, or firmly established': *stereoblastula, stereograph, stereopsis*.

stereognosis /stir'·ē·ōgnō'sis/ [Gk, *stereos*, solid, *gnosis*, knowledge], **1.** the faculty of perceiving and understanding the form and nature of objects by the sense of touch. **2.** perception by the senses of the solidity of objects. **–stereognostic,** *adj.*

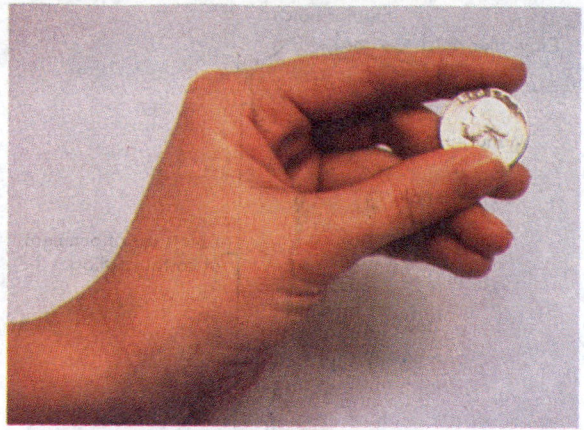

Assessment of stereognosis *(Seidel, 1991)*

stereognostic perception /stir′ē·ōgnos′tik/ [Gk, *stereos,* solid, *gnosis,* knowledge], the ability to recognize objects by the sense of touch.

stereoisomer /stir′ē·ō·ī′səmər/ [Gk, *stereos,* solid + *isos,* equal + *meros,* part], one of two or more chemical compounds that contain the same atoms linked in the same way but are organized differently in space. For example, one may be the mirror-image of the other.

stereoisomeric specificity /-ī′səmer′ik/ [Gk, *stereos* + *isos,* equal, *meros,* part], specificity of an enzyme for one enantiomer of a racemic mix.

stereoophthalmoscope /stir·ē·ō′ofthal′məskōp/, an ophthalmoscope fitted with two eyepieces so the examiner can view a three-dimensional interior of the eye.

stereopsis, the quality of visual fusion.

stereoradiography /-rā′dē·og′rəfē/ [Gk, *stereos* + L, *radiare,* to shine; Gk, *graphein,* to record], a technique for producing radiographs that give a three-dimensional view of an internal body structure. The stereoradiographs are produced by combining two separate x-ray films, each made from a slightly different angle without movement of the body part being x-rayed. The developed films are then viewed through a stereoscope.

stereoscopic microscope /-skop′ik/ [Gk, *stereos* + *skopein,* to look], a microscope that produces three-dimensional images through the use of double eyepieces and double objectives. The three-dimensional image is created because the double optic systems have independent light paths. Also called **Greenough microscope.**

stereoscopic parallax. See **binocular parallax.**

stereoscopic radiograph, a composite of two radiographs, made by shifting the position of the x-ray tube a few centimeters between each of two exposures. The result is a three-dimensional presentation of the radiograph when viewed through steroscopic lenses.

stereotaxic neuroradiography /-tak′sik/ [Gk, *stereos* + *taxis,* arrangement; *neuron,* nerve; L, *radiare,* to shine; Gk, *graphein,* to record], an x-ray procedure commonly performed during neurosurgery to guide the insertion of a needle into a specific area of the brain.

stereotype /stir′ē·ətīp/ [Gk, *stereos* + *typos,* mark], a generalization about a form of behavior, an individual, or a group.

stereotypical. See **stereotypy.**

stereotypic behavior /stir′ē·ōtip′ik/, a pattern of body movements that has autistic and symbolic meaning for an individual.

stereotypy /ster′ē·ətī′pē/ [Gk, *stereos* + *typos,* mark], the persistent, inappropriate, mechanical repetition of actions, body postures, or speech patterns, usually occurring with a lack of variation in thought processes or ideas. It is often seen in patients with schizophrenia. −**stereotypical,** *adj.*

sterile /ster′il/ [L, *sterilis,* barren], **1.** free from living microorganisms. **2.** barren; unable to produce children because of a physical abnormality, often the absence of spermatogenesis in a man or blockage of the fallopian tubes in a woman. Compare **impotence. 3.** aseptic. −**sterility,** *n.*

sterile field, 1. a specified area, such as within a tray or on a sterile towel, that is considered free of microorganisms. **2.** an area immediately around a patient that has been prepared for a surgical procedure. The sterile field includes the scrubbed team members, who are properly attired, and all furniture and fixtures in the area.

sterile meningitis [L, *sterilis,* barren; Gk, *menigx,* membrane + *itis,* inflammation], a form of meningitis, usually involving a viral infection, in which there is primarily a lymphocytic response in the cerebrospinal fluid. Also called **benign lymphocytic meningitis, simple meningitis.**

sterility /stəril′itē/ [L, *sterilis,* barren], a condition of being unable to conceive or reproduce the species.

sterilization /ster′ilīzā′shən/ [L, *sterilis* + Gk, *izein,* to cause], **1.** a process or act that renders a person unable to produce children. See also **hysterectomy, tubal ligation, vasectomy. 2.** a technique for destroying microorganisms using heat, water, chemicals, or gases. −**sterilize,** *v.*

sterilize /ster′ilīz/ [L, *sterilis,* barren], **1.** to make powerless to reproduce, such as by surgery. **2.** to destroy all living organisms and viruses in a material.

sternal /stur′nəl/ [Gk, *sternon,* chest], pertaining to the sternum.

-sternal, a suffix meaning 'pertaining to the sternum': *adsternal, presternal, suprasternal.*

sternal node [Gk, *sternon,* chest; L, *nodus,* knot], a node in one of the three groups of thoracic parietal lymph nodes. They are situated at the anterior ends of the intercostal spaces, adjacent to the internal thoracic artery. The afferent vessels of the sternal nodes drain the lymph from the breast, the diaphragmatic surface of the liver, and the deep, ventral thoracic wall. The efferent vessels of the sternal nodes usually form a single lymphatic trunk on each side. The trunk may open directly into the junction of the internal jugular and the subclavian veins; or the trunk on the right side may join the right lymphatic subclavian trunk, and the trunk on the left side may join the thoracic duct. Also called **internal mammary node.** Compare **diaphragmatic node, intercostal node.** See also **lymphatic system, lymph node.**

sternal puncture [Gk, *sternon,* chest; L, *punctura*], a diagnostic procedure in which a needle is inserted into the marrow of the sternum to remove blood samples for diagnosis.

Sternheimer-Malbin stain /sturn′hīmərmal′bin/, a crystal violet and safranin stain used in urinalyses to provide additional contrast for certain casts and cells.

-sternia, a combining form meaning '(condition of the) sternum': *asternia, koilosternia, schistosternia.*

sterno- /stur′nō-/, a combining form meaning 'of or pertaining to the sternum': *sternocleidal, sternocostal, sternopagus.*

sternoclavicular /-klavik′yələr/ [Gk, *sternon*, chest; L, *clavicula*, little key],   pertaining to the sternum and clavicle.

sternoclavicular articulation [Gk, *sternon* + L, *clavicula*, little key],   the double gliding joint between the sternum and the clavicle. It involves the sternal end of the clavicle, the superior and lateral part of the manubrium, the cartilage of the first rib, and six ligaments.

sternocleidomastoid /-klī′dōmas′toid/ [Gk, *sternon*, chest + *kleis*, key + *mastos*, breast + *eidos*, form],   a muscle of the neck that is attached to the mastoid process and superior nuchal line and by separate heads to the sternum and clavicle. Also called **sternomastoid.**

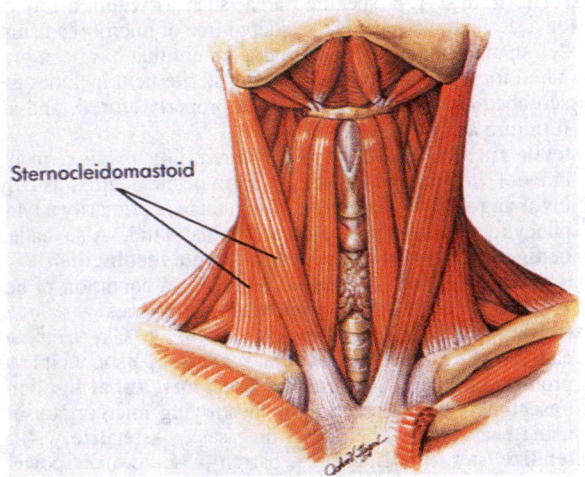

Sternocleidomastoid muscle of the neck
(Seeley, 1992/John V Hagen)

sternocostal articulation /-kos′təl/ [Gk, *sternon* + L, *costa*, rib],   the gliding articulation of the cartilage of each true rib and the sternum, except for the articulation of the first rib in which the cartilage is directly united with the sternum to form a synchondrosis. Each sternocostal articulation also involves five ligaments.

sternohyoideus /stur′nōhī·oi′dē·əs/ [Gk, *sternon* + *hyoeides*, upsilon-shaped],   one of the four infrahyoid muscles. Arising from the medial end of the clavicle, the posterior sternoclavicular ligament, and the manubrium sterni and inserting into the inferior border of the hyoid bone, it is a thin, narrow muscle innervated by fibers from the first, second, and third cervical nerves. It acts to depress the hyoid bone. Also called **sternohyoid muscle.** Compare **sternothyroideus.**

sternomastoid.   See **sternocleidomastoid.**

sternothyroideus /stur′nōthīroi′de·əs/ [Gk, *sternon* + *thyreos*, shield, *eidos*, form],   one of the four infrahyoid muscles. Arising from the dorsal surface of the manubrium sterni and inserting into the thyroid cartilage, it is innervated by fibers from the first, second, and third cervical nerves, through the ansa cervicalis. It acts to depress the thyroid cartilage. Also called **sternothyroid muscle.** Compare **sternohyoideus.**

sternum /stur′nəm/ [Gk, *sternon*],   the elongated, flattened bone forming the middle portion of the thorax. It supports the clavicles, articulates directly with the first seven pairs of ribs, and comprises the manubrium, the gladiolus (body),

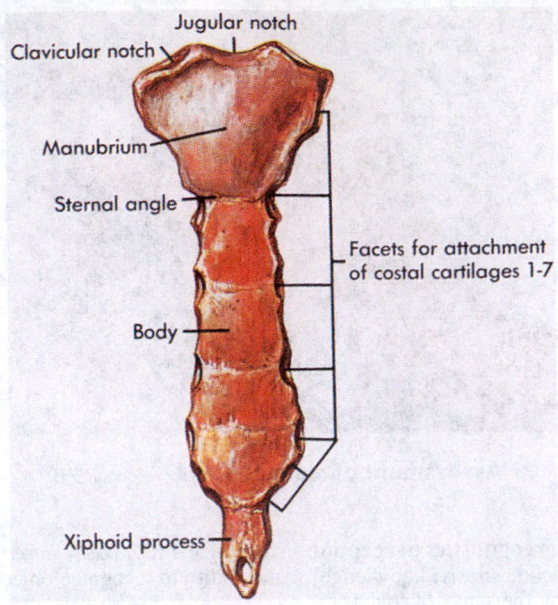

Sternum *(Seeley, 1992/David J Mascaro & Associates)*

and the xiphoid process. It is composed of highly vascular tissue covered by a thin layer of bone. The sternum is longer in men than in women.

sternutation.   See **sneeze.**

steroid /stir′oid/ [Gk, *stereos* + *eidos*, form],   any of a large number of hormonal substances with a similar basic chemical structure, produced mainly in the adrenal cortex and gonads.

steroid acne [Gk, *stereos*, solid; L, *oleum*, oil; Gk, *eidos*, form + *akme*, point],   a form of acne caused by the use of corticosteroids.

steroid hormones [Gk, *stereos*, solid; L, *oleum*, oil; Gk, *eidos*, form + *hormaein*, to set in motion],   any of the ductless gland secretions that contain the basic steroid nucleus in their chemical formulae. The natural steroid hormones include the androgens, estrogens, and adrenal cortex secretions.

steroid hormone therapy [Gk, *stereos*; L, *oleum*, oil; Gk, *eidos*, form + *hormaein*, to set in motion + *therapeia*, treatment],   treatment with any of the steroid hormones, such as the use of estrogen to reduce symptoms of postmenopausal disorders.

sterol /stir′ôl/ [Gk, *stereos* + Ar, *alkohl*, essence],   a large subgroup of steroids containing an OH group at position 3 and a branched aliphatic side chain of eight or more carbon atoms at position 17. Kinds of sterols include **cholesterol** and **ergosterol.**

stertorous /stur′tərəs/ [L, *stertere*, to snore],   pertaining to a respiratory effort that is strenuous or struggling; having a snoring sound.

stetho-, steth-,   a combining form meaning 'of or pertaining to the chest': *stethometer, stethomyitis, stethospasm.*

stethomimetic /steth′ōmimet′ik/,   pertaining to any condition causing or associated with a reduction of chest volume below its normal value. The condition may be congenital, temporary, or permanent.

stethoscope /steth′əskōp/ [Gk, *stethos*, chest, *skopein*, to look], an instrument, used in mediate auscultation, consisting of two earpieces connected by means of flexible tubing to a diaphragm, which is placed against the skin of the patient's chest or back to hear heart and lung sounds.

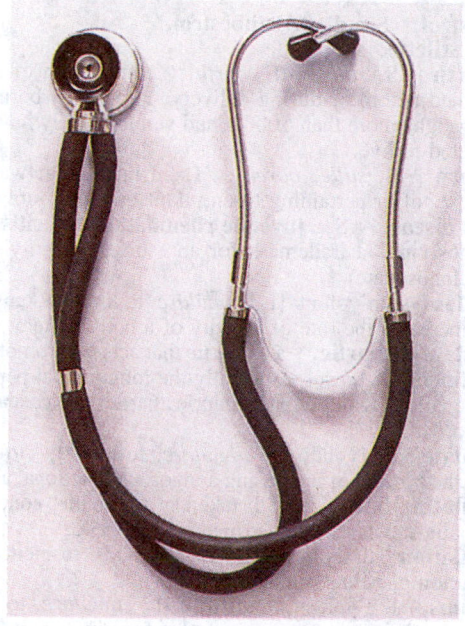

Stethoscope *(Seidel, 1991)*

Stevens-Johnson syndrome [Albert M. Stevens, American pediatrician, b. 1884; F. C. Johnson, American physician, b. 1894], a serious, sometimes fatal inflammatory disease affecting children and young adults. It is characterized by the acute onset of fever, bullae on the skin, and ulcers on the mucous membranes of the lips, eyes, mouth, nasal passage, and genitalia. Pneumonia, pain in the joints, and prostration are common. A complication may be perforation of the cornea. The syndrome may be an allergic reaction to certain drugs, or it may follow pregnancy, herpesvirus I, or other infection. It is seen rarely in association with malignancy or with radiation therapy. Treatment includes bed rest, antibiotics for pneumonia, glucocorticoids, analgesics, mouthwashes, and sedatives. See also **erythema multiforme.** (See Fig. p. 1484.)

Stewart, Isabel Maitland (1878–1963), a Canadian-born American nursing educator and writer. The first nurse to receive a master's degree from Columbia University in New York, she succeeded Mary Adelaide Nutting as Professor of Nursing at Teachers College at that university. She was instrumental in upgrading the nursing curriculum and in directing educational policies and became an important figure in international nursing affairs.

STH, abbreviation for **somatotropic hormone.**

sthen-. See **stheno-.**

-sthenia, a combining form meaning 'power or strength': *angiosthenia, eusthenia, hyposthenia.*

sthenic fever /sthen′ik/ [Gk, *sthenos,* power; L, *febris,* fever], high body temperature associated with thirst, dry skin, and, often, delirium.

stheno-, sthen-, a combining form meaning 'of or pertaining to strength': *sthenometer, sthenoplastic, sthenopyra.*

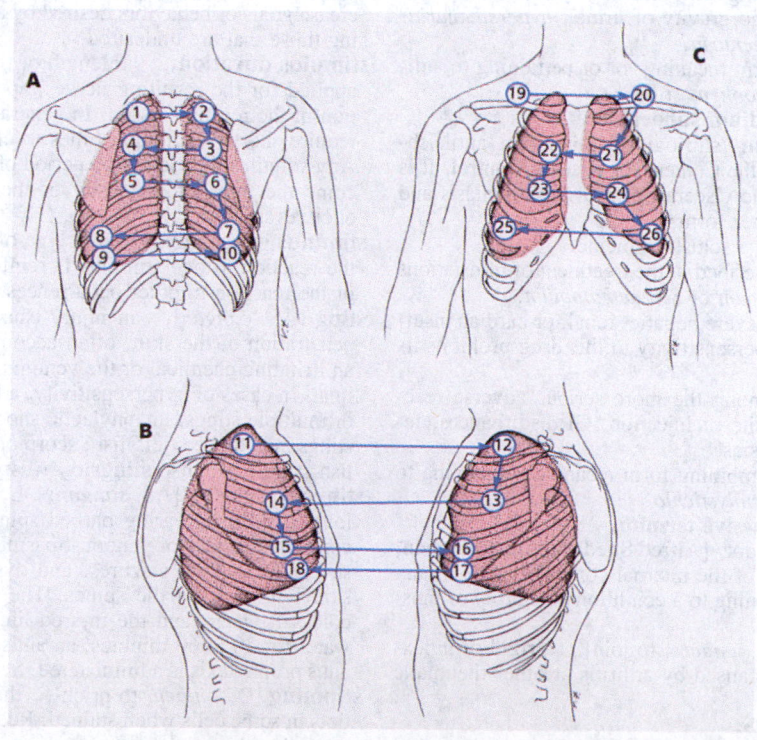

Stethoscope placement *(Potter, 1993)*

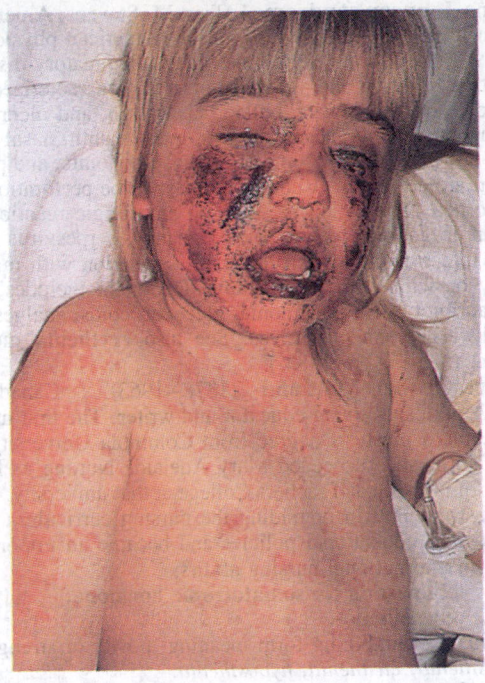

Stevens-Johnson syndrome *(Zitelli, 1992)*

-sthenuria, a combining form meaning '(condition of) urination or of the specific gravity of urine': *hypersthenuria, isosthenuria, normosthenuria.*

stib-, a combining form meaning 'of or pertaining to antimony': *stibamine, stibophen, stiburea.*

stibocaptate. See **sodium stibocaptate.**

stibogluconate sodium /stib′ōgloō′kənāt/, an antileishmanial available from the Centers for Disease Control. It is a drug of choice for the visceral form of leishmaniasis and has some effect on other forms.

stibophen /stib′əfin/, a schistosomicide.
■ INDICATIONS: It is prescribed in the treatment of infestations of *Schistosoma japonicum* or *S. haematobium.*
■ CONTRAINDICATIONS: Severe hepatic, renal, or cardiac insufficiency or known hypersensitivity to this drug prohibits its use.
■ ADVERSE EFFECTS: Among the more serious adverse reactions are pain at the site of injection, GI disturbances, fever, and blood dyscrasias.

stich-, -stichia, a combining form meaning 'pertaining to rows': *stichochrome, polystichia.*

sticky ends. See **cohesive termini.**

Stieda's fracture /stē′dəz/ [Alfred Stieda, German surgeon, b. 1869], a fracture of the internal condyle of the femur.

stiff [OE, *stif*], pertaining to a condition of rigidity or muscular inflexibility.

stiff joint [OE, *stif;* L, *jungere*, to join], a rigid or inflexible joint, as may be caused by arthritis or other rheumatic disorders.

stiff lung. See **ARDS.**

stigma /stig′mə/, *pl.* **stigmas, stigmata** [Gk, brand], **1.** a moral or physical blemish. **2.** a mental or physical characteristic that serves to identify a disease or a condition.

stigmatism /stig′mətiz′əm/ [Gk, *stigma*, brand], **1.** normal visual accommodation and refraction whereby light rays fall onto the retina. **2.** a condition of abnormal skin markings.

stilbestrol. See **diethylstilbestrol.**

stilet, stilette. See **stylet.**

stillbirth [AS, *stille;* ME, *burth*], **1.** the birth of a fetus that died before or during delivery. **2.** a fetus, born dead, that weighs more than 1000 g and would usually have been expected to live.

stillborn [AS, *stille, boren*], **1.** an infant that was born dead. **2.** of or pertaining to an infant that was born dead.

Still's disease. See **juvenile rheumatoid arthritis.**

Stilphostrol, a trademark for an estrogen (diethylstilbestrol diphosphate).

stimulant /stim′yələnt/ [L, *stimulare*, to incite], any agent that increases the rate of activity of a body system.

stimulant cathartic, a cathartic that acts by promoting the motility of the bowel, especially the longitudinal peristalsis of the colon. Kinds of stimulant cathartics are **cascara** and **senna.**

stimulate /stim′yəlāt/ [L, *stimulare*, to incite], to excite, as in the process of increasing a vigorous functional activity.

stimulating bath, a bath taken in water that contains an aromatic substance, an astringent, or a tonic.

stimulation /stim′yəlā′shən/ [L, *stimulare*, to incite], the condition of being stimulated.

stimulus, /stim′yələs/ *pl.* **stimuli** [L, *stimulare*, to incite], anything that excites or incites an organism or part to function, become active, or respond. **–stimulate,** *v.*

stimulus control, a strategy for self-modification that depends on manipulating the antecedents of behavior to increase goals or behaviors desired by a patient while decreasing those that are undesired.

stimulus duration, the length of time a stimulus must be applied for the resulting nerve impulse to produce excitation in the receptor tissue. In general, more intense stimuli require shorter excitation times to effect cellular response. Any stimulus that acts for a period of time too brief to overcome the threshold intensity of the receptor cell will not elicit a response.

stimulus generalization, a type of conditioning in which the reaction to one stimulus is reinforced to allow transfer of the reaction to other occurrences.

sting [AS, *stingan*], an injury caused by a sharp, painful penetration of the skin, often accompanied by exposure to an irritating chemical or the venom of an insect or other animal. In cases of hypersensitivity, a highly venomous sting, or multiple stings, anaphylactic shock may occur. Kinds of stings include bee, jellyfish, scorpion, sea urchin, and shellfish stings. See also **stingray, wasp.**

stingray /sting′rā/ [AS, *stingan* + L, *raia*, ray-fish], a flat, long-tailed fish bearing barbed spines on its back that are connected to sacs of venom. Spasm of the skeletal muscles, severe local pain, seizures, and dyspnea may occur if the skin is broken by the spines. The wound is washed with cold salt water, and the injured limb is placed in very hot water for 30 to 60 minutes; an antiseptic is applied and tetanus prophylaxis is administered. See also **sea urchin sting.**

stippling [D, *stippen*, to prick], the appearance of colored dots in some cells when stained. Red stippling in blood cells stained with eosinhematoxylin is a sign of malaria.

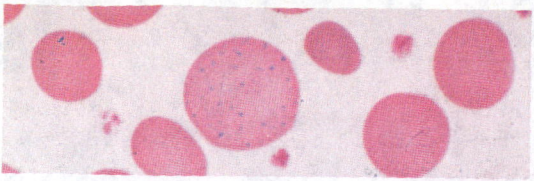

Basophilic stippling (Hayhoe, 1992)

stitch [ME, *stiche*], **1.** a suture. **2.** a sudden sharp pain.

stitch abscess [ME, *stiche*; L, *abscedere*, to go away], an abscess that develops around a suture.

St. Louis encephalitis /sāntloo'is/ [St. Louis, Missouri; Gk, *enkephalon*, brain, *itis*, inflammation], an arbovirus infection of the brain transmitted from birds to humans by the bite of an infected mosquito. It occurs most commonly in the central and southern portions of the United States and is characterized by headache, malaise, fever, stiff neck, delirium, and convulsions. Sequelae may include visual and speech disturbances, difficulty in walking, and personality changes. Convalescence may be prolonged, and death may result. Compare **California encephalitis, equine encephalitis.** See also **encephalitis.**

stocking aid, a device that enables a handicapped person to pull on a pair of stockings. One type consists of a dowel with a cuphook on the end.

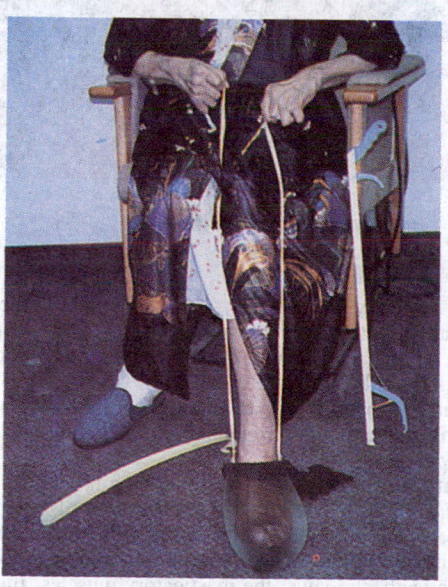

Stocking aid (Shipley, 1993)

stoker's cramp. See **heat cramp.**

Stokes-Adams syndrome. See **Adams-Stokes syndrome.**

-stole, a suffix referring to the contraction, retraction, or dilation of various organs: *anastole, diastole, peristole*.

stoma /stō'mə/, *pl.* **stomas, stomata** [Gk, mouth], **1.** a pore, orifice, or opening on a surface. **2.** an artificial opening of an internal organ on the surface of the body, created surgically, such as for a colostomy, ileostomy, or tracheostomy. **3.** a new opening created surgically, between two body structures, such as for a gastroenterostomy, pancreaticogastrostomy, pancreatoduodenostomy, or pyeloureterostomy.

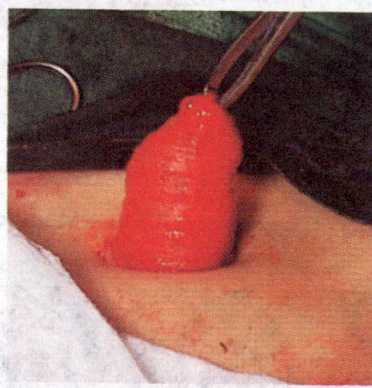

Normal ileostomy stoma
(Barrison, 1992/Courtesy Mr JA Williams)

-stoma, -stome, a suffix meaning a 'mouth or opening': *hypostoma, metastoma, tetrastoma*.

stomach /stum'ək/ [Gk, *stomakhos*, gullet], the major organ of digestion, located in the right upper quadrant of the abdomen and divided into a body and a pylorus. It receives and partially processed food and drink funneled from the mouth through the esophagus and moves nutritional bulk into the intestines. The stomach lies in the epigastric and left hypogastric regions bounded by the anterior abdominal wall and the diaphragm between the liver and the spleen. The shape of the stomach is modified by the amount of contents, stage of digestion, development of gastric musculature, and condition of the intestines. It is lined with a mucous coat, a submucous coat, a muscular coat, and a serous coat, all richly supplied with blood vessels and nerves, and contains fundic, cardiac, and pyloric gastric glands. Also called **gaster.** (See Fig. p. 1486.)

stomach ache [Gk, *stomakhos*, gullet; ME, *aken*, pain], pain in the stomach area. Also called **gastralgia, gastrodynia, stomachalgia.**

stomach cancer [Gk, *stomakhos*, gullet + *karkinos*, crab], a malignant neoplasm of the stomach lining. Most stomach cancers are carcinomas. The remainder are classified as lymphomas and leiomyosarcomas. Commonly associated with gastritis and intestinal metaplasia, the cause is unknown. The worldwide incidence varies: In Japan, stomach cancer is the most common malignancy, but in the United States it ranks as the seventh most common cause of cancer deaths. No specific symptoms are present with early stages. Complaints such as anemia, fatigability, weight loss, and epigastric distress may suggest peptic ulcer, dysphagia, or other digestive disorders.

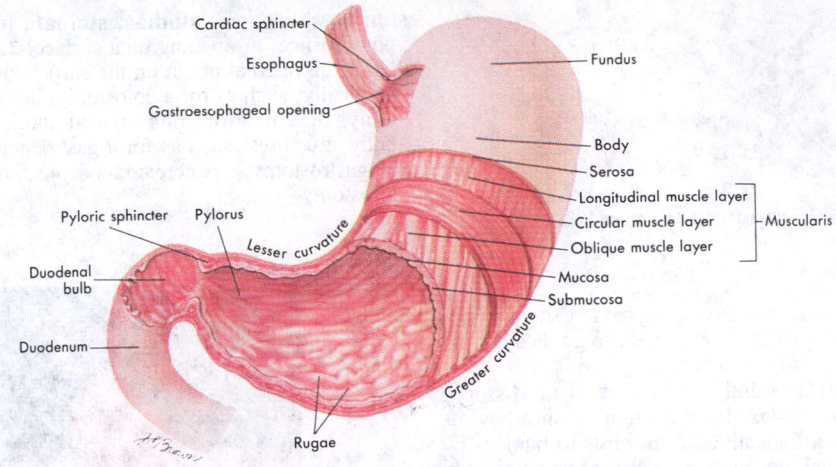

Stomach (Thibodeau, 1993/G David Brown)

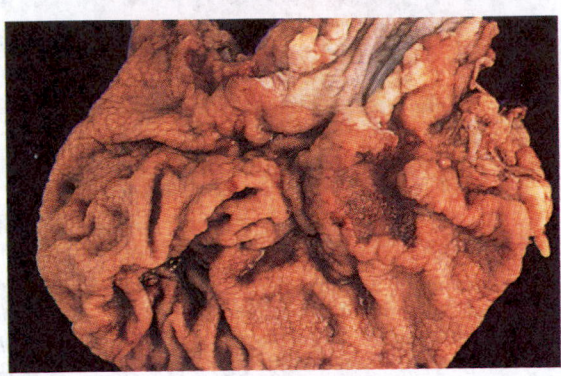

Adenocarcinoma of the stomach
(Fletcher, 1987)

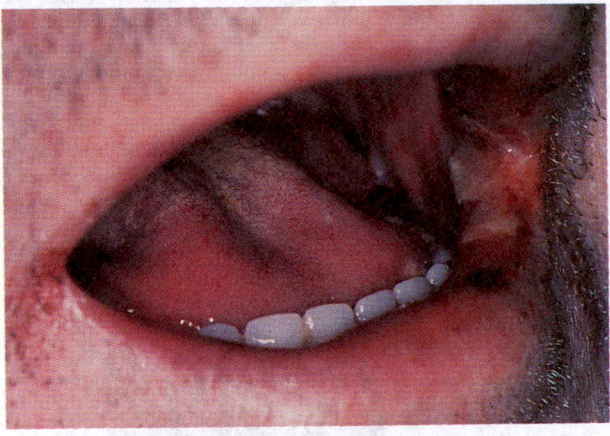

Uremic stomatitis (Lamey, 1988)

stomach pump, a pump for withdrawing the contents of the stomach through a tube passed through the mouth or nose into the stomach.

stomach tube, a tube used to introduce nutrients into the stomach, remove fluids and ingested poisons, or decompress the stomach. Also called **gastrostomy tube; G tube.**

stomadeal. See **stomodeum.**

stomadaeum, stomadeum. See **stomodeum.**

stomal /stō'məl/ [Gk, mouth], pertaining to one or more stomata or mouthlike openings. Also **stomatal** /stō'mətəl/.

stomal peptic ulcer, a marginal peptic ulcer. See also **peptic ulcer.**

stomata. See **stoma.**

stomatal. See **stomal.**

stomatitis /stō'mətī'tis/ [Gk, *stoma + itis,* inflammation], any inflammatory condition of the mouth. It may result from infection by bacteria, viruses, or fungi, from exposure to certain chemicals or drugs, from vitamin deficiency, or from a systemic inflammatory disease. Kinds of stomatitis include **aphthous stomatitis, pseudomembranous stomatitis, thrush,** and **Vincent's infection.**

stomatitis parasitica [Gk, *stoma,* mouth + *itis,* inflammation + *parasitos,* guest], an inflammation of the mucous membranes of the mouth by a yeast fungus, *Candida albi-*cans, typically expressed by a white coating on the tongue. It may affect infants or immunosuppressed people with HIV, or appear as an outgrowth secondary to antibiotic therapy. Also called **thrush.**

stomato-, stomo-, a combining form meaning 'of or pertaining to the mouth': *stomatodysodia, stomatogastric, stomatopathy.*

stomatognathic system /stō'mətōnath'ik/ [Gk, *stoma + gnathos,* jaw; *systema*], the combination of organs, structures, and nerves involved in speech and reception, mastication, and deglutition of food. This system is composed of the teeth, the jaws, the masticatory muscles, the tongue, the lips, surrounding tissues, and the nerves that control these structures.

stomatology /stō'mətol'əjē/ [Gk, *stoma + logos,* science], the study of the morphology, structure, function, and diseases of the oral cavity. —**stomatologist,** *n.,* **stomatologic, stomatological,** *adj.*

-stome, See **-stoma.**

-stomia, a suffix meaning '(condition of the) mouth': *atelostomia, atretostomia, hygrostomia.*

stomion /stō′mē·on/ [Gk, *stoma*], the median point of the oral slit when the mouth is closed.

stomo-. See **stomato-.**

stomodeum /stom′ədē′əm/, *pl.* **stomodeums, stomodea** [Gk, *stoma* + *odaios*, a way], an invagination in the ectoderm located in the foregut of the developing embryo that forms the mouth. Also spelled **stomodaeum, stomadeum, stomadaeum.** Compare **proctodeum.** – **stomodeal, stomodaeal, stomadeal,** *adj.*

-stomy, a suffix meaning 'surgical opening': *gastrostomy, lobostomy, tracheostomy.*

stone. See **calculus.**

-stone, a combining form meaning a 'calculus in a human organ or duct': *bilestone, gallstone, wombstone.*

stool. See **feces.**

stool softener. See **fecal softener.**

stopcock, a valve that controls the flow of fluid or air through a tube.

stop needle [AS, *stoppian*, to stop; *naedel*], a needle with a shoulder flange that prevents it from penetrating beyond a certain distance.

storage capacity /stôr′ij/, the amount of data that can be stored on a computer disk or tape, usually expressed in kilobytes, megabytes, gigabytes, or terabytes (one trillion bytes).

stored-energy foot, a lower-limb prosthesis designed to imitate the springlike action of a natural foot and leg. A device stores energy when weight is put on the artificial leg. When the weight is shifted to the other leg, the stored energy is released, returning the prosthesis to its original shape.

storing fermentation [L, *staurare*, to store; *fermentum*, leaven], the rapid, gaseous clotting of milk caused by *Clostridium perfringens.*

stork bite. See **telangiectatic nevus.**

Stoxil, a trademark for an antiviral (idoxuridine).

STP, *slang.* a psychedelic agent, dimethoxy-4-methylamphetamine (DOM). STP is an abbreviation for *serenity, tranquillity, and peace.*

STPD, abbreviation for *standard temperature, standard pressure, dry.*

STPD conditions of a volume of gas, the conditions of a volume of gas at 0° C and 760 torr, and containing no water vapor. It should contain a calculable number of moles of a particular gas.

Str., abbreviation for *Streptococcus.*

strab-, a combining form meaning 'squinting': *strabismometer, strabometry, strabotomy.*

strabismal /strabiz′məl/ [Gk, *strabismos*, squint], pertaining to the condition of strabismus.

strabismus /strəbiz′məs/ [Gk, *strabismos*, squint], an abnormal ocular condition in which the eyes are crossed. There are two kinds of strabismus, paralytic and nonparalytic. Paralytic strabismus results from the inability of the ocular muscles to move the eye because of neurologic deficit or muscular dysfunction. The muscle that is dysfunctional may be identified by watching as the patient attempts to move the eyes to each of the cardinal positions of gaze. If the affected eye cannot be directed to a position, the examiner infers that the associated ocular muscle is the dysfunctional one. Because this kind of strabismus may be caused by tumor, infection, or injury to the brain or the eye, an ophthalmologic examination is recommended. Nonparalytic strabismus is a defect in the position of the two eyes in relation to each other. The condition is inherited. The person cannot use the two eyes together but has to fix with one or the other. The eye that looks straight at a given time is the fixing eye. Some people have alternating strabismus, using one eye and then the other; some have monocular strabismus, affecting only one eye. Visual acuity diminishes with diminished use of an eye, and suppression amblyopia may develop. Nonparalytic strabismus and suppression amblyopia are treated most successfully in early childhood. Treatment consists mainly of covering the fixing eye, forcing the child to use the deviating eye. The earlier it is begun, the more rapid and effective the treatment. By 6 years of age, a deviating eye has usually become so suppressed that treatment is not effective and permanent visual loss has occurred. The eyes might be straightened by surgery, but suppression amblyopia will not be corrected. Also called **squint.** – **strabismal, strabismic, strabismical,** *adj.*

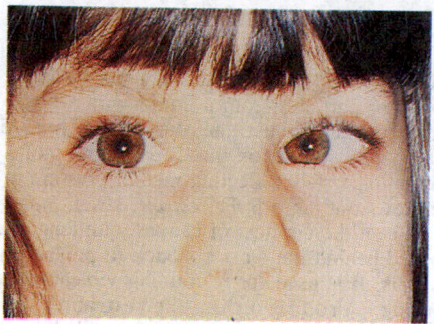

Strabismus (Zitelli, 1992)

straight line blood set /strāt/ [ME, *streght*], a common device, composed of plastic components, for delivering blood infusions. It includes the plastic tubing, the clamp, the drip chamber, and the filter. Some kinds of straight-line blood sets contain filters within drip chambers; others have separate filters. The latter kind can be filled by squeezing the attached drip chamber but must not be squeezed itself or it may rupture. The former kind can be filled by squeezing the section of the blood set that contains the filter and the drip chamber. Before infusion, the filter of either kind is tapped with the fingers to dislodge any trapped air bubbles. Compare **component drip set, component syringe set, microaggregate recipient set, Y-set.**

straight sinus [ME, *streght* + L, *sinus*, hollow], one of the six posterior-superior venous channels of the dura mater, draining blood from the brain into the internal jugular vein. It has no valves and is located at the junction of the falx cerebri with the tentorium cerebelli. It is triangular in section and increases in size as it runs posteriorly from the end of the inferior sagittal sinus to the transverse sinus of the opposite side. It receives the inferior sagittal sinus, the great cerebral vein, and the superior cerebellar veins. Compare **inferior sagittal sinus, superior sagittal sinus, transverse sinus.**

straight wire fixed orthodontic appliance, an orthodontic appliance used for correcting and improving malocclusion. It is a variation of the edgewise fixed orthodontic appliance and is designed to decrease arch wire adjustments by reorienting arch wire slots. (See Fig. p. 1488.)

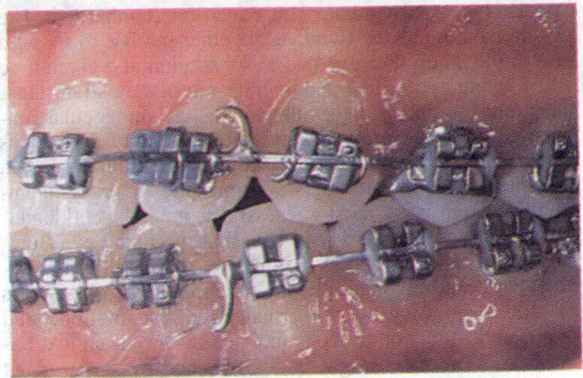

Straight wire fixed orthodontic appliance
(Bennett, 1993)

strain [ME, *streinen*], **1.** to exert physical force in a manner that may result in injury, usually muscular. **2.** to separate solids or particles from a liquid with a filter or sieve. **3.** damage, usually muscular, that results from excessive physical effort. **4.** a taxon that is a subgroup of a species. **5.** an emotional state reflecting mental pressure or fatigue.

straitjacket /strāt′jakit/ [OFr, *estreit*, strict, *jaquette*, short coat], a coatlike garment of canvas with long sleeves that can be tied behind the wearer's back to prevent movement of the arms. It is used for restraining violent or uncontrollable people. Also called **camisole restraint.**

strangle /strang′gəl/ [L, *strangulare*, to choke], to cause an interruption of breathing by conpressing or constricting the trachea. Also **strangulate.**

strangulated /strang′gyəlā′tid/ [L, *strangulare*, to choke], pertaining to a constriction or compression of the trachea or other upper airway structure that interrupts the normal flow of air.

strangulated hemorrhoids [L, *strangulare*, to choke; Gk, *haimorrhoise*, vein that discharges blood], prolapsed hemorrhoids that have become trapped by the anal sphincter, causing the blood supply to become occluded by the sphincter's constricting action.

strangulated hernia [L, *strangulare*, to choke + *hernia*, rupture], a hernia in which the blood vessels have become constricted by the neck of the hernial sac, resulting in ischemia and possible gangrene if blood circulation is not quickly restored.

strangulation /strang′gyəlā′shən/ [L, *strangulare*, to choke], the constriction of a tubular structure of the body, such as the trachea, a segment of bowel, or the blood vessels of a limb, that prevents function or impedes circulation. See also **intestinal strangulation.**

strap [AS, *stropp*], **1.** a band, such as that made of adhesive plaster, that is used to hold dressings in place or to attach one thing to another. **2.** to bind securely.

strapping, the application of overlapping strips of adhesive tape to an extremity or body area to exert pressure and hold a structure in place, performed in the treatment of strains, sprains, dislocations, and certain fractures.

strata. See **stratum.**

strati-, a combining form meaning 'layer': *stratification, stratiform, stratigraphy.*

stratified /strat′ifid/ [L, *stratum* + *facere*, to make], arranged in layers.

stratified epithelium [L, *stratum* + *facere*; Gk, *epi*, above + *thele*, nipple], closely packed sheets of epithelial cells arranged in layers over the external surface of the body and lining most of the hollow structures. The layers may include stratified squamous, stratified columnar, or stratified columnar ciliated types of cells.

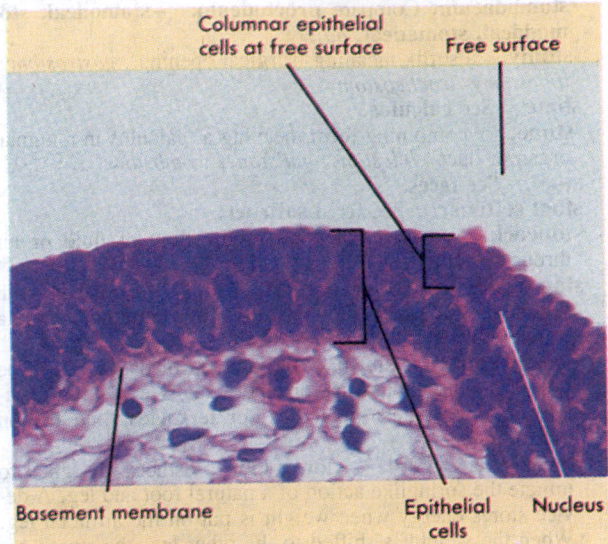

Stratified columnar epithelium
(Seeley, 1992/Ed Reschke)

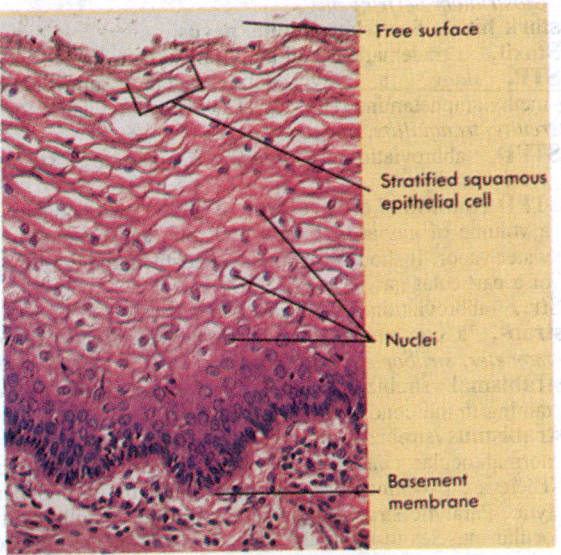

Stratified squamous epithelium
(Seeley, 1992/Ed Reschke)

stratified sample. See **sample.**

stratiform cartilage. See **fibrocartilage.**

stratiform fibrocartilage /strat′ifôrm/ [L, *stratum*, layer, *forma*, form; *fibra*, fiber, *cartilago*, cartilage], a structure made of fibrocartilage that forms a thin coating of osseous grooves through which tendons of certain muscles glide. Small masses of stratified fibrocartilage also develop in the tendons of some muscles that glide over bones, as in the tendons of the peroneus longus and the tibialis posterior. Compare **circumferential fibrocartilage, connecting fibrocartilage, interarticular fibrocartilage.**

stratum /strā′təm, strat′əm/, *pl.* **strata** [L, layer], a uniformly thick sheet or layer, usually associated with other layers, such as the stratum basale of the epidermis.

stratum basale, **1.** also called **basal layer, stratum germinativum.** the deepest of the five layers of the skin, composed of tall cylindric cells. This layer provides new cells by mitotic cell division. Compare **stratum corneum, stratum granulosum, stratum lucidum, stratum spinosum.** See also **skin. 2.** the deepest layers of the uterine decidua, containing uterine gland terminals.

stratum corneum, the horny, outermost layer of the skin, composed of dead cells converted to keratin that continually flakes away. The thickness of the layer is correlated with the normal wear of the area it covers. The stratum corneum is thick on the palms of the hands and the soles of the feet but thin over some protected areas. Also called **horny layer.** Compare **stratum basale, stratum granulosum, stratum lucidum, stratum spinosum.** See also **skin.**

stratum germinativum. See **stratum basale.**

stratum granulosum, one of the layers of the epidermis, situated just below the stratum corneum except in the palms of the hands and the soles of the feet, where it lies just under the stratum lucidum. The stratum granulosum contains visible granules in the cytoplasm of its cells, which die, become keratinized, move to the surface, and flake away. Compare **stratum basale, stratum corneum, stratum lucidum, stratum spinosum.** See also **skin.**

stratum lucidum, one of the layers of the epidermis, situated just beneath the stratum corneum and present only in the thick skin of the palms of the hands and the soles of the feet. It contains translucent eleidin that forms keratin. Also called **clear cell layer.** Compare **stratum basale, stratum corneum, stratum granulosum, stratum spinosum.** See also **skin.**

stratum spinosum, one of the layers of the epidermis, composed of several layers of polygonal cells. It lies on top of the stratum basale and beneath the stratum granulosum and contains tiny fibrils within its cellular cytoplasm. When the cells of the stratum spinosum are pulled apart, they present minute spines at their surfaces. Also called **prickle cell layer.** Compare **stratum basale, stratum corneum, stratum granulosum, stratum lucidum.** See also **skin.**

stratum spongiosum, one of the three layers of the endometrium of the uterus, containing tortuous, dilated uterine glands and a small amount of interglandular tissue. With the stratum compactum it forms the functional part of the endometrium during pregnancy. Compare **stratum basale.** See also **decidua, placenta.**

strawberry gallbladder /strô′berē/ [AS, *streawberig;* ME, *gal,* gall; AS, *blaedre*], a tiny, yellow gallbladder spotted with deposits on the red mucous membrane, characteristic of cholesterolosis.

strawberry hemangioma, strawberry mark. See **capillary hemangioma.**

strawberry tongue, a strawberry-like coloration of the inflamed tongue papillae. It is a clinical sign of scarlet fever and is also seen in Kawasaki syndrome.

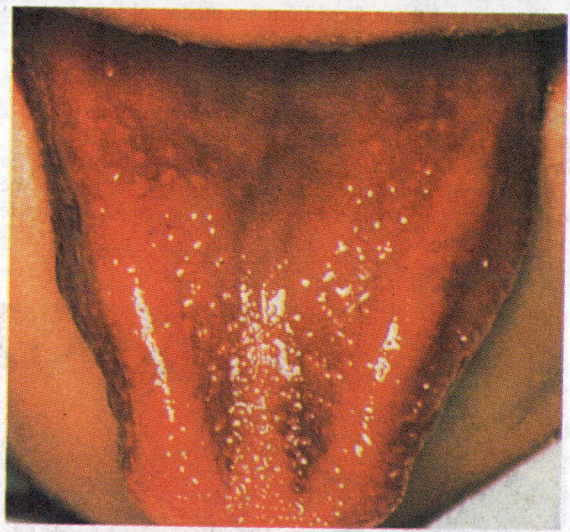

Strawberry tongue *(Ansell, 1992)*

stray light [OFr, *estraier,* to wander; AS, *leoht,* illumination], radiant energy that reaches a photodetector and that consists of wavelengths other than those defined by the filter or monochromator.

stray radiation. See **leakage radiation.**

streak [AS, *strican,* to stroke], a line or a stripe, such as the primitive streak at the caudal end of the embryonic disk.

strength [AS, *strengou*], the ability of a muscle to produce or resist a physical force.

strength of association, the degree of relationship between a causal factor and the occurrence of a disease, usually expressed in terms of a relative risk ratio.

strepho-, streph-, a combining form meaning 'twisted': *strephopodia, strephosymbolia, strephotome.*

strep throat [*Streptococcus* + AS, *throte*], *informal.* an infection of the oral pharynx and tonsils caused by a hemolytic species of *Streptococcus,* usually belonging to group A. The infection is characterized by sore throat, chills, fever, swollen lymph nodes in the neck, and, sometimes, nausea and vomiting. The symptoms usually begin abruptly a few days after exposure to the organism in airborne droplets or after direct contact with an infected person. Also called **streptococcal sore throat.**

■ OBSERVATIONS: The throat is diffusely red, and tonsils often are covered with a yellow or white exudate. Diagnosis is confirmed by bacteriologic culture and identification of the streptococcal bacteria in a specimen taken from the throat. Complications of strep throat are otitis media, scarlet fever, and sinusitis; other complications include acute glomerulonephritis and acute rheumatic fever.

■ INTERVENTIONS: Treatment usually includes intramuscular injection of benzathine penicillin G or the administration of penicillin for 10 days. Erythromycin may be given to people allergic to penicillin. For recurrent infections, tonsillectomy may be recommended.

■ NURSING CONSIDERATIONS: Analgesics and throat irrigation with warm saline solution may give relief from pain. Family members and other contacts are observed for signs of infection, and those for whom streptococcal infection presents a special risk are treated prophylactically.

strepticemia.   See **streptococcemia.**

strepto- /strep'tō-/,   a combining form meaning 'twisted': *streptobacilli, streptococcal, streptomicrodactyly.*

streptobacillary rat-bite fever.   See **Haverhill fever.**

Streptobacillus moniliformis [Gk, *streptos*, curved; L, *bacillum*, small rod; *monile*, necklace, *forma*, form],   a species of necklace-shaped bacteria that can cause rat-bite fever in humans.

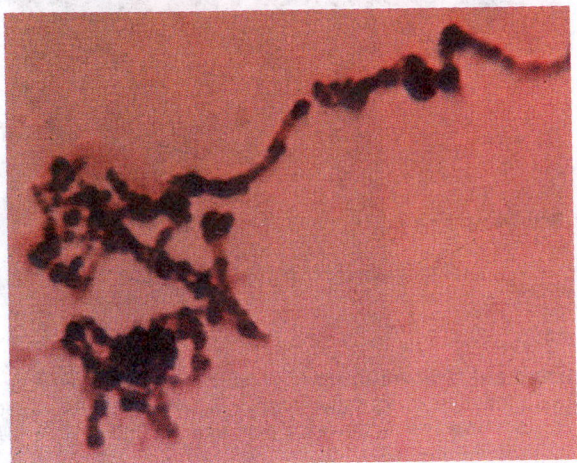

Streptobacillus moniliformis (Baron, 1990)

streptococcal [Gk, *streptos*, curved + *kokkos*, berry],   pertaining to any of the species of streptococcus.

streptococcal angina /strep'təkok'əl/ [Gk, *streptos* + *kokkos*, berry; L *angina*, quinsy],   a condition in which feelings of choking, suffocation, and pain occur as the result of a streptococcal infection.

streptococcal infection,   an infection caused by pathogenic bacteria of one of several species of the genus *Streptococcus* or their toxins. Almost any organ of the body may be involved. The infections occur in many forms, including cellulitis, endocarditis, erysipelas, impetigo, meningitis, pneumonia, scarlet fever, tonsillitis, and urinary tract infection. See also **strep throat.**

streptococcal sore throat.   See **strep throat.**

streptococcemia /-koksē'mē·ə/ [Gk, *streptos*, curved + *kokkos*, berry],   a condition of streptococci bacteria in the blood. Also called **strepticemia.**

Streptococcus (Str.) /strep'təkok'əs/ [Gk, *streptos* + *kokkos*, berry],   a genus of nonmotile, gram-positive cocci classified by serologic types (Lancefield groups A through T), by hemolytic action (alpha, beta, gamma) when grown on blood agar, and by reaction to bacterial viruses (phage types 1 to 86). The various species occur in pairs, short chains, and chains. Some are facultative aerobes, and some are anaerobic. Some species also are hemolytic, and others are nonhemolytic. Many species cause disease in humans. *Streptococcus faecalis*, a penicillin-resistant, group D enterococcus and normal inhabitant of the GI tract, may cause infection of the urinary tract or endocardium. *S. pneumoniae* (formerly *Diplococcus pneumoniae*) causes a majority

of the cases of bacterial pneumonia in the United States. *S. pyogenes* belongs to group A and may cause tonsillitis and respiratory, urinary, or skin infections. Some beta-hemolytic strains may lead to rheumatic fever or to glomerulonephritis. *S. viridans*, a member of the normal flora of the mouth, is the most common cause of bacterial endocarditis, especially when introduced into the bloodstream during dental procedures.

Streptococcus pneumoniae [Gk, *streptos*, curved + *kokkos*, berry + *pneumon*, lung],   any of 70 antigenic types of pneumococci that cause pneumonia and other diseases in humans.

Streptococcus pyogenes [Gk, *streptos*, curved + *kokkos*, berry + *pyon*, pus + *genein*, to produce],   a species of streptococcus with many strains that are pathogenic to humans, including the β-hemolytics in Lancefield Group A. It causes suppurative diseases, such as scarlet fever and strep throat.

Streptococcus viridans [Gk, *streptos*, curved + *kokkos*, berry],   a species of streptococcus similar to *pyogens* strains. It produces α-hemolysis in cultures and is a common cause of subacute bacterial endocarditis and other infections in humans.

streptokinase /strep'təkī'nās/ [Gk, *streptos*, + *kinesis*, motion; (ase) enzyme],   a fibrinolytic activator that enhances the conversion of plasminogen to the fibrinolytic enzyme plasmin. It is used in the treatment of certain cases of pulmonary and coronary embolism.

streptokinase-streptodornase /-strep'tōdôr'nās/,   two enzymes derived from a strain of *Streptococcus hemolyticus.*
- INDICATIONS: It is prescribed for debridement of purulent exudates, clotted blood, radiation necrosis, or fibrinous deposits resulting from trauma or infection.
- CONTRAINDICATIONS: Active hemorrhage, acute cellulitis, or danger of reopening bronchopleural fistulas prohibits its use.
- ADVERSE EFFECTS: Among the more serious adverse reactions are pyrogenic reactions and irritation.

streptolysin /streptol'isis/ [Gk, *streptos* + *lysein*, to loosen],   a filterable substance, produced by streptococci, that liberates hemoglobin from red blood cells.

streptomycin sulfate /strep'təmī'sin/,   an aminoglycoside antibiotic.
- INDICATIONS: It is prescribed in the treatment of tuberculosis, endocarditis, and certain other infections.
- CONTRAINDICATIONS: Labyrinthine disease or known hypersensitivity to this drug prohibits its use. It must be used with caution in impaired renal function and in the elderly.
- ADVERSE EFFECTS: Among the most serious adverse reactions are ototoxicity, nephrotoxicity, muscle weakness, and allergic reactions.

streptozocin /strep'təzō'sin/,   an investigational antineoplastic used in the treatment of a variety of neoplasms, including metastatic islet cell tumors of the pancreas. It is an antibiotic substance from *Streptomyces acromogenes.*

stress [OFr, *estrecier*, to tighten],   any emotional, physical, social, economic, or other factor that requires a response or change, such as dehydration, which can cause an increase in body temperature, or a separation from parents, which can cause a young child to cry. Stress also may be applied therapeutically to promote change, such as implosive therapy for phobic patients, in which the patient is given support while being exposed to the situation that produces anxiety and is thereby gradually desensitized. The nature and degree of stress observed in a patient are frequently evaluated by the nurse as part of the ongoing holistic nursing assessment. See also **general adaptation syndrome.**

stress-adaptation theory, a concept that stress depletes the reserve capacity of individuals, thereby increasing their vulnerability to health problems.

stress amenorrhea [OFr, *estrecier;* GK, *a + men,* month *+ rhoia,* to flow], a cessation in menstruation because of physical or mental stress.

stress-bearing area. See **basal seat area.**

stress behavior, a change from a person's normal behavior in response to a stressor.

stress fracture, a fracture, especially of one or more of the metatarsal bones, caused by repeated, prolonged, or abnormal stress.

stress incontinence. See **incontinence.**

stress inoculation, a procedure useful in helping patients control anxiety by substituting positive coping statements for statements that bring about anxiety.

stress kinesic, a type of behavioral characteristic of personal conversation, such as the use of body shifts or movements, that marks the flow of speech and generally coincides with linguistic stress patterns.

stress management, methods of controlling factors that require a response or change within a person by identifying the stressors, eliminating negative stressors, and developing effective coping mechanisms to counteract the response constructively. Examples include progressive muscular relaxation, guided imagery, biofeedback, breathing techniques, and active problem solving.

stressor /stres′ər/ [OFr, *estrecier,* to tighten], anything that causes wear and tear on the body's physical or mental resources. See also **general adaptation syndrome.**

stress reaction. See **general adaptation syndrome, posttraumatic stress disorder.**

stress response syndrome. See **posttraumatic stress disorder.**

stress test, a test that measures the function of a system of the body when subjected to carefully controlled amounts of physiological stress. The data produced allow the examiner to evaluate the condition of the system being tested. Cardiopulmonary function, respiratory function, and intrauterine fetal placental function are tested with stress tests. See **exercise electrocardiogram, oxytocin challenge test.**

stress ulcer, a gastric or duodenal ulcer that develops in previously unaffected individuals subjected to severe stress, such as a severe burn. See also **Curling's ulcer.**

stretching of contractures [AS, *streccan;* L, *contractura,* drawing together], procedures for release of muscle that has been shortened because of paralysis, spasm, or fibrosis. The procedures may include tissue grafts, scar tissue removal, tendon transfer, and incision of a joint capsule.

stretch mark. See **stria.**

stretch receptors [AS, *streccan;* L, *recipere,* to receive], specialized sensory nerve endings in muscle spindles or tendons that are stimulated by stretching movements.

stretch reflex [AS, *streccan;* L, *reflectere,* to bend back], a reflex muscle contraction after it is stretched as a result of stimulation of proprioceptive receptors in the muscle. Tendon reflexes function in a similar manner. Also called **myotatic reflex.**

stri-, a combining form meaning 'line, stripe, or streak': *striation, striocellular, striomuscular.*

stria /strī′ə/, *pl.* **striae** [L, furrow], a streak or a linear scar that often results from rapidly developing tension in the

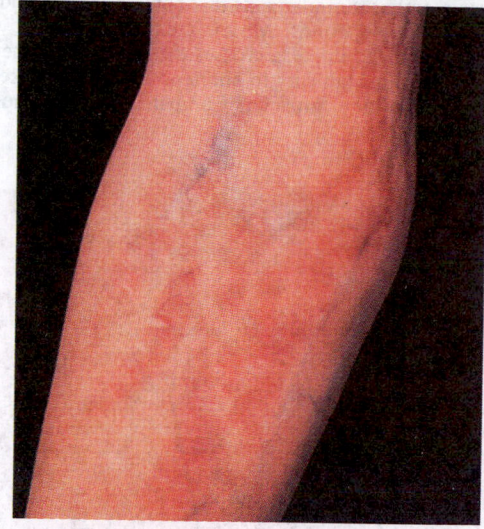

Stria *(Stone, 1989)*

skin, such as seen on the abdomen after pregnancy. Purplish striae are one of the classic findings in hyperadrenocorticism. Also called **stretch mark.**

stria atrophica. See **linea alba.**

striae. See **stria.**

stria gravidarum, irregular depressions with red to purple colorations that appear in the skin of the abdomen, thighs, and buttocks of pregnant women.

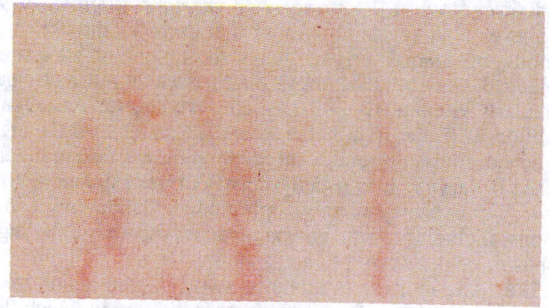

Striae gravidarum *(Epstein, 1992)*

striatal /strī·ā′təl, strī′ətəl/ [L, *striatus,* striped], pertaining to the corpus striatum.

striate /strī′āt/ [L, *striatus,* striped], identifying something that is striped, is marked by parallel lines, or has structural lines. Also **striated.**

striated muscle /strī′ātid/ [L, *stria + musculus,* muscle], muscle tissue, including all the skeletal muscles, that appears microscopically to consist of striped myofibrils. Striated muscles are composed of bundles of parallel, striated fibers under voluntary control; the heart, a striated involuntary muscle, is an exception. Each striated muscle is covered by a thin connective epimysium and divided into bundles of sheathed fibers containing smaller myofibrils. Each myofibril comprises thick filaments that consist of molecules of myosin and of thin filaments that consist of actin and two other protein compounds. Muscle contraction occurs when an electrochemical impulse crosses the myoneural junction, causing the thin filaments to shorten. Also called **skeletal muscle, voluntary muscle.** Compare **cardiac muscle, smooth muscle.**

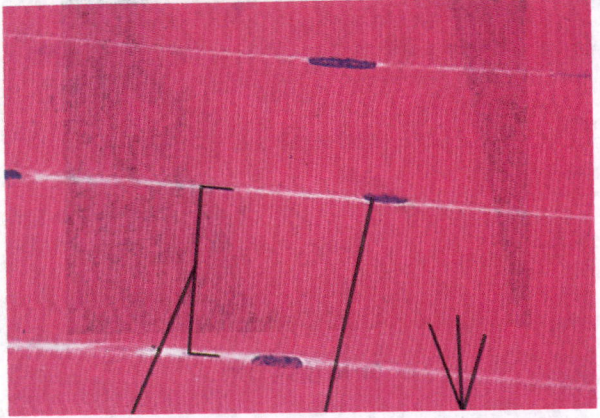

Striated muscle (Seeley, 1992/Ed Reschke)

stricture /strik'chər/ [L, *stringere*, to tighten], an abnormal temporary or permanent narrowing of the lumen of a hollow organ, such as the esophagus, pylorus of the stomach, ureter, or urethra, caused by inflammation, external pressure, or scarring. Treatment varies depending on the cause. Compare **spasm.**

strict vegetarian [L, *stringere* + *vegetare*, to grow, *arius*, believer], a vegetarian whose diet excludes the use of all foods of animal origin. Such diets, unless adequately planned, may be deficient in many essential nutrients, particularly vitamin B_{12}. Also called **pure vegetarian, vegan.**

stridor /strī'dôr/ [L, harsh sound], an abnormal, high-pitched, musical sound, caused by an obstruction in the trachea or larynx. It is usually heard during inspiration. Stridor may indicate several neoplastic or inflammatory conditions, including glottic edema, asthma, diphtheria, laryngospasm, or papilloma.

strike [AS, *strican*, to advance swiftly], an action taken by the employees of a company or institution in which they stop reporting for work in an effort to cause the employer to accede to certain demands. A strike usually follows unsuccessful negotiations between representatives of the union and management.

string carcinoma [AS, *strenge*, cord; Gk, *karkinos*, cancer, *oma*, tumor], a malignancy of the large intestine, usually the ascending or transverse colon. On radiologic visualization, it causes the intestine to appear to be tied in segments like a string of large beads.

strip membranes [Ger, *strippe*, strap; L, *membrana*, thin skin], (in obstetrics) a procedure in which an examiner digitally frees the membranes of the amniotic sac from the wall of the lower segment of the uterus in the small area around the cervical os. It is done to stimulate labor, but, because infection or hemorrhage may result, it is not recommended.

stripping, 1. *nontechnical*. a surgical procedure for the re-

moval of the long and the short saphenous veins of the legs. See also **milking, varicose veins. 2.** the mechanical removal of a very small amount of enamel from the mesial or distal surfaces of teeth to alleviate crowding.

stroke. See **cerebrovascular accident.**

stroke prone profile [AS, *strac*], a predictive index using a complex of risk factors that indicate susceptibility of a person to cerebrovascular accident (CVA). The factors include advanced age, hypertension, a history of transient ischemic attacks, cigarette smoking, heart disorders, associated embolism, family hisory of CVA, use of oral contraceptives, diabetes mellitus, physical inactivity, obesity, hypercholesteremia, and hyperlipidemia.

stroke volume, the amount of blood ejected by the ventricle during a ventricle contraction.

stroke volume index, the stroke volume divided by the body surface area.

stroma /strō'mə/, *pl.* **stromas, stromata** [Gk, covering], the supporting tissue or the matrix of an organ, as distinguished from its parenchyma. Some kinds of stromata are the vitreous stroma, which encloses the vitreous humor of the eye, and Rollet's stroma, which contains the hemoglobin of a red blood cell. **–stromatic,** *adj.*

stroma-, a prefix meaning 'connective tissue forming framelike support for an organ': *stromatin, stromatogenous, stromatosis.*

-stroma, a suffix meaning 'supporting tissue of an organ': *blastostroma, mesostroma, myostroma.*

stromata. See **stroma.**

stromatic. See **stroma.**

Strongyloides /stron'jiloi'dēz/ [Gk, *strongylos*, round, *eidos*, form], a genus of parasitic intestinal nematode. A species of *Strongyloides*, *S. stercoralis*, causes strongyloidiasis.

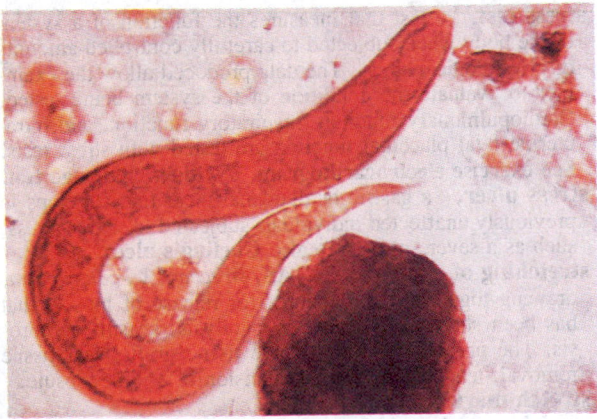

***Strongyloides stercoralis* larvae** (Murray, 1990)

strongyloidiasis /stron'jəloidī'əsis/, infection of the small intestine by the roundworm *Strongyloides stercoralis*, acquired when larvae from the soil penetrate intact skin, incidentally causing a pruritic rash. The larvae pass to the lungs via the bloodstream, sometimes causing pneumonia. Larvae then migrate up the air passages to the pharynx, are swallowed, and develop into adult worms in the small intestine. Bloody diarrhea and intestinal malabsorption may result.

Rarely, fatal disseminated strongyloidiasis occurs. Diagnosis depends on finding larvae in freshly passed feces. Treatment often includes administration of thiabendazole. Proper sanitary methods for the disposal of excrement could eliminate the disease. Wearing shoes prevents contagion from contaminated soil. Also called **threadworm infection.**

strontium (Sr) /stron´sh(ē)əm/ [Strontian, Scotland], a metallic element. Its atomic number is 38; its atomic weight is 87.62. Chemically similar to calcium, it is found in bone tissue. Isotopes of strontium are used in radioisotope scanning procedures of bone. Strontium 85 (85Sr) and strontium 87 (87Sr) mimic calcium metabolism and are used in studies of bone physiology and disorders. These radionuclides can be counted with any standard detector or imaged at a very early stage in bone disease, whereas x-ray films of bone without the use of a radioactive tracer can show decreased density only after approximately 50% of bone is decalcified. Most 85Sr or 87Sr is deposited in bone within 1 hour after injection; increased deposition of these radionuclides is strongly linked to osteoblastic activity and new bone formation. In addition to four naturally occurring isotopes (88Sr, 87Sr, 86Sr, and 84Sr), 12 artificial strontium isotopes are produced by nuclear reactions. Strontium 90, the longest-lived, is the most dangerous constituent of fallout from atomic bomb tests. It can replace some of the calcium in food, become concentrated in teeth and bones, and continue to emit electrons that can cause death in the host. Cows concentrate strontium 90 in their milk.

-strophe, -strophy, a suffix meaning 'turning or twisting': *cardianastrophe, enstrophe, phallanastrophe.*

stropho-, a combining form meaning 'twisted': *strophocephalus, strophosomus.*

-strophy. See **-strophe.**

structural /struk´chərəl/ [L, *structura,* arrangement], pertaining to the arrangement or pattern of component parts of an object or organism.

structural chemistry [L, *structura,* arrangement], the science dealing with the molecular structure of chemical substances.

structural gene, (in molecular genetics) a unit of genetic information that specifies the amino acid sequence of a polypeptide.

structural integration, a technique of deep massage intended to help in the realignment of the body by altering the length and tone of myofascial tissues. The basis of the practice is the belief that misalignment of myofascial tissues, occurring as a result of improper posture and emotional and physical traumas, may have an overall detrimental effect on a person's energy level, self-image, muscular efficiency, perceptions, and general health. Also called **Rolfing.**

structural model, a model of family therapy that views the family as an open system and identifies subsystems within the family that carry out specific family functions. When faced with demands for change, individual family members, family subsystems, or the family as a whole may respond with growth behaviors or with maladaptive behaviors. The goal of family therapy is to help family members learn new scripts or transactional patterns.

structure /struk´chər/ [L, *structura*], a part of the body, such as the heart, a bone, a gland, a cell, or a limb.

structure-activity relationship (SAR), the relationship between the chemical structure of a drug and its activity.

strum-, a combining form meaning 'of or pertaining to a goiter, or to scrofula': *strumectomy, strumiform, strumitis.*

struma [L, a scrofulous tumor], an obsolete term for goiter and for a tuberculous swelling of the lymph glands.

struma lymphomatosa. See **Hashimoto's disease.**

Strümpell-Marie disease /strim´pəlmärē´/ [Ernst Adolf Gustav Gottfried von Strümpell, German neurologist, b. 1853; Pierre Marie, French neurologist, b. 1853; L, *dis* Fr, *aise,* ease], ankylosing spondylitis. Also called **rheumatoid spondylitis; Marie-Strümpell arthritis, spondylitis ankylopoietica.**

strychnine /strik´nin, strik´nīn/ [Gr, *strychnos,* nightshade], a white crystalline alkaloid obtained from the leaves of the *Strychnos nux-vomica* plant. It is extremely toxic to the central nervous system, producing as a classic strychnine poisoning symptom an arched back.

strychnine poisoning [Gk, *strychnos;* L, *potio,* a drink], toxic effects of ingesting strychnine, a central nervous system stimulant. Symptoms include restlessness and hyperacuity of hearing and vision. Minor stimuli may produce convulsions, but there may be complete muscle relaxation between convulsions. One classic sign of strychnine poisoning is an arched back.

Stryker wedge frame /strī´kər/, an orthopedic bed that allows the patient to be rotated as required to either the supine or prone position. Like the Foster bed, the Stryker wedge frame is used in the immobilization of patients with unstable spines, postoperative management of multilevel spinal fusions, and management of severe burn patients. Use of the Stryker wedge frame is not recommended if hyperextension of the spine is required or if lower extremity traction is needed. The Stryker wedge frame comes in only one size, the only accommodation to different body builds being an adjustable crossbar on the anterior circle of the frame. If the crossbar is properly adapted, the patient is held firmly between the frames without the addition of pillows or extra padding. The elevation lock of the wedge is useful for elevating the head end of the anterior frame when the patient is prone. In the immediate postoperative period it is also

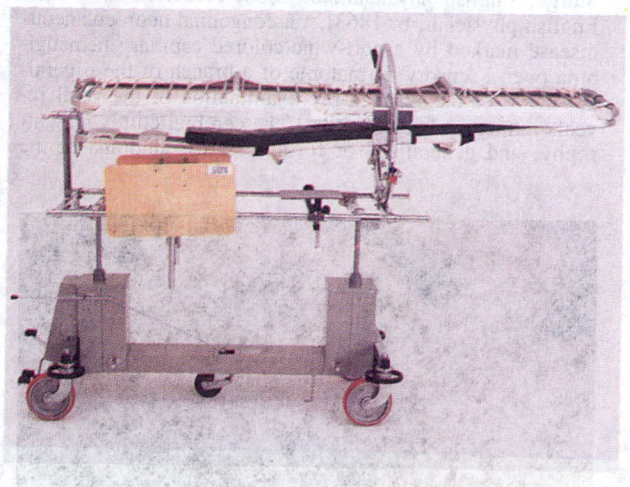

Stryker wedge frame
(Sorrentino, 1992/Courtesy The Stryker Corporation, Kalamazoo, Michigan)

useful for increasing pulmonary expansion by decreasing visceral pressure on the diaphragm. When a patient is in halo or tong cervical traction, the elevation lock provides countertraction up to a maximum of 7 inches. Most hospitals provide the nursing staff with charts to determine the elevation needed for countertraction according to the weight of the patient and the pull forces of traction weights. Compare **CircOlectric bed, Foster bed, hyperextension bed.**

S-T interval [L, *intervallum,* space between ramparts], the component of the cardiac cycle shown on an electrocardiogram as an isoelectric line after the QRS complex, before the ascent of the T wave. It represents phase 2 of the action potential. Elevation or depression of the S-T interval is the hallmark of myocardial ischemia or injury and coronary artery disease. Also called **S-T segment.**

Stuartnatal 1 + 1, a trademark for an oral, prenatal, fixed-combination drug containing vitamins and minerals.

Stuart-Power factor. See **factor X.**

stump [ME, *stumpe*], the part of a limb after amputation that is proximal to the portion amputated.

stump hallucination, the sensation of the continued presence of an amputated limb. See also **hallucination, phantom limb syndrome.**

stunned myocardium, impaired myocardial contractile function, cellular biochemistry, and microvasculature function in the absence of gross myocardial necrosis for minutes to days caused by ischemia of short duration.

stupefacient /st(y)o͞o′pəfā′shənt/ [L, *stupere,* to stun + *facere,* to make], a narcotic or other agent that has the effect of making a person stuporous.

stupor /st(y)o͞o′pər/ [L, senselessness], a state of lethargy and unresponsiveness in which a person seems unaware of the surroundings. The condition occurs in neurologic and psychiatric disorders. The person may be totally or almost totally immobile and unresponsive, even to painful stimuli. Kinds of stupor are **anergic stupor, benign stupor, delusion stupor,** and **epileptic stupor.**

stuporous /st(y)o͞o′pərəs/ [L, *stupere,* to stun], in a state of reduced consciousness and diminished spontaneous movement.

Sturge-Weber syndrome /sturj′web′ər/ [William A. Sturge, English physician, b. 1850; Frederick P. Weber, English physician, b. 1863], a congenital neurocutaneous disease marked by a port-wine-colored capillary hemangioma over a sensory dermatome of a branch of the trigeminal nerve of the face. X-ray examination of the skull reveals intracranial calcification. The cerebral cortex may atrophy, and generalized or focal seizures, angioma of the choroid, secondary glaucoma, optic atrophy, and new cutaneous hemangiomas may develop. There is no known cure. Treatment is supportive and includes anticonvulsive medication. Also called **encephalotrigeminal angiomatosis.**

stuttering [D, *stotteren*], a speech dysfunction characterized by spasmodic enunciation of words, involving excessive hesitations, stumbling, repetition of the same syllables, and prolongation of sounds. The condition may result from a cerebellar disease or a neuromuscular defect or injury of the organs of articulation, but in most cases the cause is emotional or psychologic. Hesitancy and lack of fluency in speech are normal characteristics of language development during the preschool years, when a child's mental ability and level of comprehension exceed muscular coordination and vocabulary acquisition. However, if undue emphasis or stress is placed on this pattern, the child becomes conscious of the difficulties associated with acquisition and may develop a fear of speaking. Stuttering usually can be reversed until about 7 years of age. Prevention must begin early in childhood, and the nurse or physician can help parents by making them aware of the normal patterns in a child's speech and by suggesting ways that can encourage a child's speech development. If stuttering persists, treatment by a speech therapist may be necessary. See also **stammering.**

sty [ME *styanye* eyelid tumor], a purulent infection of a meibomian or sebaceous gland of the eyelid, often caused by a staphylococcal organism. Also spelled **stye.** Also called **hordeolum.**

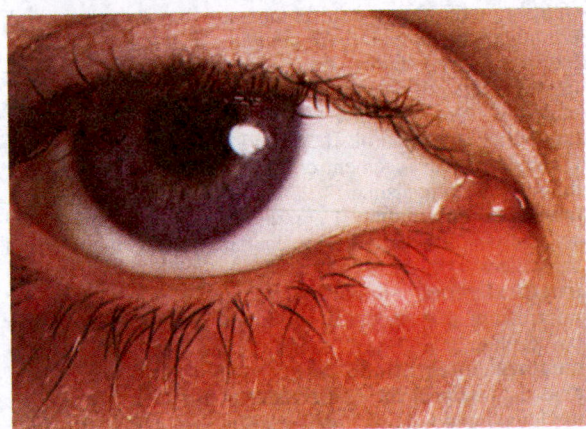

Sty (Bedford, 1986)

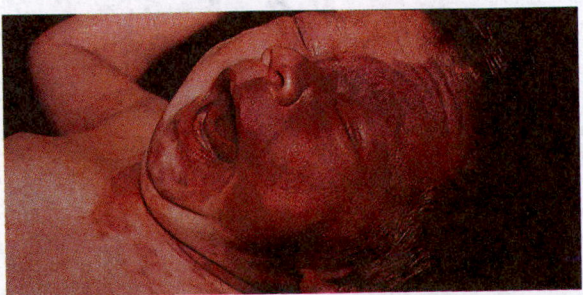

Sturge-Weber syndrome (Zitelli, 1992)

-style, a combining form meaning a 'bone attached to an internal structure': *cephalostyle, sarcostyle, zygostyle.*

stylet /stī′lət, stīlet′/ [It, *stiletto,* dagger], a thin metal probe for inserting into or passing through a needle, tube, or catheter to clean the hollow bore or for inserting in a soft, flexible catheter to make it stiff as the catheter is placed in a vein or passed through an orifice of the body. Also spelled **stilet, stilette.**

stylo-, a combining form meaning 'like a pillar, stake, or pole,': *stylomastoid, stylomyloid, stylostixis, styloid.*

stylohyoideus /stī′lōhī·oi′dē·əs/ [Gk, *stylos,* pillar, *hyoeides,* upsilon-shaped], one of four suprahyoid muscles, lying anterior and superior to the posterior belly of the digastricus. It is a slender muscle that arises from the styloid process and inserts into the hyoid bone. It is pierced near its insertion by the tendon of the digastricus. It is innervated by fibers of the mandibular branch of the facial nerve, and it serves to draw the hyoid bone up and back. Also called **stylohyoid bone.** Compare **digastricus, geniohyoideus, mylohyoideus.**

stylohyoid ligament /stī'lōhī'oid/, the ligament attached to the tip of the styloid process of the temporal bone and to the lesser cornu of the hyoid bone. It frequently contains a small cartilage in its center and is often partially ossified.

styloid /stī'loid/ [Gk, *stylos,* pillar + *eidos,* form], long and tapered, like a pen or stylus.

styloid process [Gk, *stylos* + *eidos;* L, *processus*], any of several projections of bone tissue, particularly a projection on the temporal bone.

stylomandibular ligament /stī'lōmandib'yələr/ [Gk, *stylos* + L, *mandere,* to chew, *ligare,* to bind], one of a pair of specialized bands of cervical fascia, forming an accessory part of the temporomandibular joint. It extends from the styloid process of the temporal bone to the ramus of the mandible between the masseter and pterygoideus muscles and separates the parotid gland from the submandibular gland. Compare **sphenomandibular ligament.**

styptic /stip'tik/ [Gk, *styptikos,* astringent], **1.** a substance used as an astringent, often to control bleeding. A chemical styptic induces coagulation of blood. A cotton pledget used as a compress to control bleeding is a mechanical styptic. **2.** acting as an astringent or agent to control bleeding.

sub-, suf-, sup-, a prefix meaning 'under, below, down, near, almost, or moderately': *subacid, subdental.*

subacromial /-əkrō'mē·əl/ [L, *sub,* beneath; Gk, *akron,* extremity + *omos.* shoulder], below the acromion.

subacromial bursa [L, *sub,* under; Gk, *akron,* extremity, *omos,* shoulder; *byrsa,* wineskin], the bursa separating the acromion and deltoid muscle from the insertion of the supraspinatus muscle and the greater tubercle of the humerus.

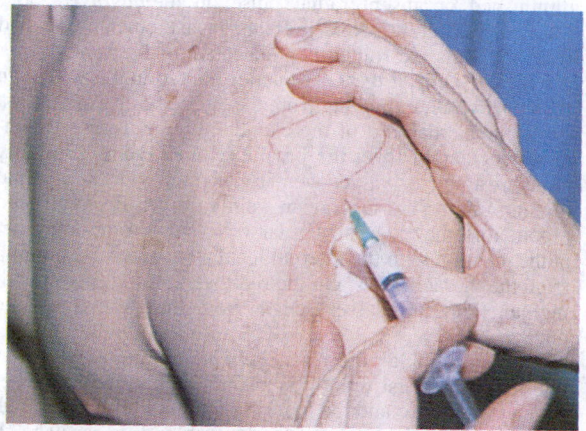

Injection of the subacromial bursa (Shipley, 1993)

subacute /-əkyo͞ot'/ [L, *sub* + *acutus,* sharp], **1.** less than acute. **2.** of or pertaining to a disease or other abnormal condition present in a person who appears to be clinically well. The condition may be identified or discovered by means of a laboratory test or by radiologic examination.

subacute bacterial endocarditis (SBE), a chronic bacterial infection of the valves of the heart, characterized by

a slow, quiet onset with fever, heart murmur, splenomegaly, and the development of clumps of abnormal tissue, called vegetations, around an intracardiac prosthesis or on the cusps of a valve. Various species of *Streptococcus* or *Staphylococcus* are commonly the cause of SBE. Dental procedures are associated with infection by *Streptococcus viridans,* surgical procedures with *Streptococcus faecalis,* and self-infection (especially by drug abusers) with *Staphylococcus aureus*. See also **bacterial endocarditis, endocarditis, Janeway lesions.**

■ OBSERVATIONS: The infected vegetations may separate from the valve or prosthesis and form emboli. Osler's nodes, petechiae, Roth's spots, and splinter hemorrhages under the fingernails are common manifestations of blood-borne metastases of these emboli. Bacteriologic examination of cultures of the blood may allow specific diagnosis and treatment.

■ INTERVENTIONS: Treatment requires prolonged and regular administration of an antibiotic that is known to be effective against the causative organism. If a prosthesis has become infected, it is usually removed. Before surgery or a dental procedure, prophylactic antibiotics are given. During the acute phase of illness, the fever is treated with antipyretic medication and bed rest; adequate high-protein diet and fluids are encouraged.

■ NURSING CONSIDERATIONS: Bed rest and hospitalization may be necessary for several weeks. Emotional and psychologic support may help the patient adjust to the necessary inactivity and to understand that SBE is a chronic illness.

subacute combined degeneration of the spinal cord. See **combined system disease.**

subacute glomerulonephritis, an uncommon noninfectious disease of the glomerulus of the kidney characterized by proteinuria, hematuria, decreased production of urine, and edema. Of unknown cause, the disease may progress rapidly, and renal failure may occur. Kidney transplantation and dialysis are the only treatments available. See also **chronic glomerulonephritis, postinfectious glomerulonephritis, uremia.**

subacute infection [L, *sub,* beneath + *acutus,* sharp + *inficere,* to stain], a disease condition that is not chronic and that runs a rapid and severe, but less than acute, course.

subacute myelooptic neuropathy (SMON), a condition of muscular pain and weakness, usually below the T12 vertebra, painful dysesthesia of the limbs, and, in some cases, optic atrophy. The patient usually experiences a significant alteration of gait.

subacute sclerosing panencephalitis, an uncommon, slow virus infection caused by the measles virus and characterized by diffuse inflammation of brain tissue, personality change, seizures, blindness, dementia, fever, and death. The condition occurs in children and in adolescents who have had measles at a very early age. No effective therapy is known. See also **slow virus.** (See Fig. p. 1496.)

subacute thyroiditis. See **de Quervain's thyroiditis.**

subaortic /-ā·ôr'tik/ [L, *sub* + Gk, *aerein,* to rise], pertaining to the area of the body below the aorta.

subaortic stenosis [L, *sub,* beneath; Gk, *aerein,* to raise + *stenos* narrow + *osis* condition], a narrowing of the left ventricle outflow tract below the aortic valve. Also called **aortic valvar stenosis.**

subaponeurotic /-ap'ōno͞orot'ik/ [L, *sub,* beneath; Gk, *apo,* from + *neuron* nerve; L *tendo*], beneath an aponeurosis.

subarachnoid /sub'ərak'noid/ [L, *sub* + Gk, *arachne,* spi-

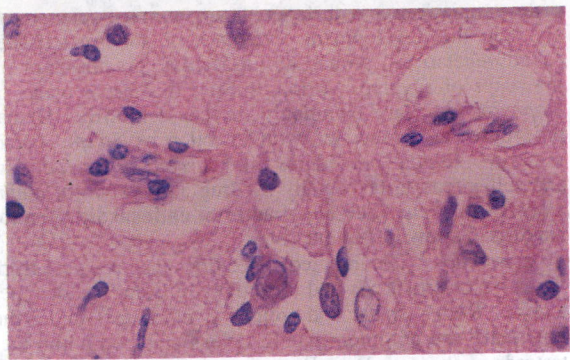

**Inflammation of brain cells in subacute
sclerosing panencephalitis**
(Okazaki, 1988/by permission of Mayo Foundation.)

der, *eidos* form], situated under the arachnoid membrane
and above the pia mater.

subarachnoid block anesthesia, a form of spinal anesthesia involving the injection of an anesthetic into the space
between the arachnoidea and pia mater. This procedure is
an especially effective form of rapid spinal anesthesia but
one requiring great skill to avoid contamination or neurologic trauma. See also **obstetric anesthesia.**

subarachnoid hemorrhage (SaH, SAH), an intracranial
hemorrhage into the cerebrospinal fluid –filled space between the arachnoid and pial membranes on the surface of
the brain. The hemorrhage may extend into the brain if the
force of the bleeding from the broken vessel is sudden and
severe. The cause may be trauma, rupture of an aneurysm,
or an arteriovenous anomaly.

■ OBSERVATIONS: The first symptom of a subarachnoid hemorrhage is a sudden extremely severe headache that begins
in one localized area and then spreads, becoming dull and
throbbing. The localized pain results from vascular distortion and injury. The generalized ache is the result of meningeal irritation from blood in the subarachnoid space. Other
characteristics of subarachnoid hemorrhage can include diz-

ziness, rigidity of the neck, pupillary inequality, vomiting,
seizures, drowsiness, sweating and chills, stupor, and loss
of consciousness. A brief period of unconsciousness immediately after the rupture is common; severe hemorrhage may
result in continued unconsciousness, coma, and death. Delirium and confusion often persist through the first weeks
of recovery, and permanent brain damage is common.

subarachnoid space, the space between the arachnoid
and pia mater membranes.

subatomic /-ətom′ik/ [L, *sub*, beneath; Gk, *atmos*, indivis-
ible], pertaining to the particles and phenomena that are
within an atom.

subaxillary /-ak′siler′ē/ [L, *sub*, beneath + *axilla*, wing],
beneath the axilla.

subcapital fracture /-kap′itəl/ [L, *sub*, + *caput*, head], a
fracture of tissue just below the head of a bone that pivots
in a ball and socket joint, such as the head of the femur.

subcapsular /-kap′s(y)ələr/ [L, *sub*, beneath + *capsula*, little box], below a capsule.

subcapsular cataract [L, *sub* + *capsula*, little box], a
condition marked by opacity or cloudiness beneath the anterior or posterior capsule of the lens of the eye.

subclavian /səbklā′vē·ən/ [L, *sub* + *clavicula*, little key],
situated under the clavicle, such as the subclavian vein.

subclavian artery, one of a pair of arteries that vary in
origin, course, and the height to which they rise in the neck
but having six similar main branches supplying the vertebral column, spinal cord, ear, and brain. See also **left subclavian artery, right subclavian artery.**

subclavian steal syndrome, a vascular syndrome caused
by an occlusion in the subclavian artery proximal to the origin of the vertebral artery. The block results in a reversal
of the normal blood pressure gradient in the vertebral artery and decreased blood flow distal to the occlusion. This
condition is characterized by episodes of flaccid paralysis
of the arm, pain in the mastoid and occipital areas, and a
diminished or absent radial pulse on the involved side.
Markedly different blood pressure measurements obtained
from the arms are sometimes indicative of the condition.

subclavian vein, the continuation of the axillary vein in
the upper body, extending from the lateral border of the first
rib to the sternal end of the clavicle, where it joins the internal jugular to form the brachiocephalic vein. It usually
contains a pair of valves near its junction with the internal
jugular vein. The subclavian vein receives deoxygenated
blood from the external jugular vein and, on the left side,
at the junction with the internal jugular vein, receives lymph
from the thoracic duct. On the right side, at the corresponding junction, it receives lymph from the right lymphatic
duct.

subclavius /səbklā′vē·əs/ [L, *sub* + *clavicula*], a short
muscle of the chest wall. It is a small, cylindric muscle between the clavicle and the first rib and arises in a short, thick
tendon from the junction of the first rib and its cartilage. It
inserts into the groove on the inferior surface of the clavicle between the costoclavicular and the conoid ligaments.
The subclavius is innervated by a special nerve from the
lateral trunk of the brachial plexus, which contains fibers
from the fifth and sixth cervical nerves, and it acts to draw
the shoulder down and forward. Compare **pectoralis major, pectoralis minor, serratus anterior.**

subclinical /-klin′ikəl/ [L, *sub* + Gk, *kline*, bed], of or
pertaining to a disease or abnormal condition that is so mild
it produces no symptoms.

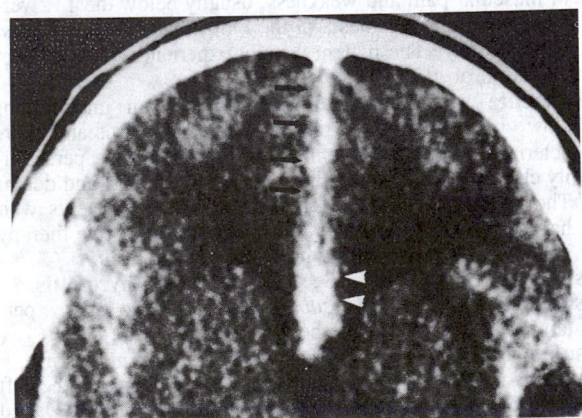

**Uncontrasted CT scan of
subarachnoid hemorrhage**
(Latchaw, 1991)

subclinical diabetes. See **impaired glucose tolerance.**

subcollateral gyrus /-kəlal′ərəl/ [L, *sub* + *con* + *lateralis;* Gk *gyros* turn], below the collateral fissure or sulcus of the cerebrum.

subconscious /-kon′shəs/ [L, *sub* + *conscire,* to be aware], **1.** imperfectly or partially conscious. **2.** *obsolete.* (in psychiatry) the preconscious and the unconscious. **—subconsciousness,** *n.*

subconscious memory, a thought, sensation, or feeling that is not immediately available for recall to the conscious mind.

subconsciousness. See **subconscious.**

subcrepitant rale /-krep′itənt/ [L, *sub,* beneath + *crepitus,* crackling; Fr, *râle,* rattle], a rale that is only faintly crepitant.

subcrestral periodontal pocket. See **periodontal pocket.**

subculture /sub′kulchər/ [L, *sub* + *colere,* to cultivate], an ethnic, regional, economic, or social group with characteristic patterns of behavior and ideals that distinguish it from the rest of a culture or society.

subcutaneous /sub′kyo̅o̅tā′nē·əs/ [L, *sub* + *cutis,* skin], beneath the skin.

subcutaneous adipose tissue [L, *sub,* beneath + *cutis,* skin + *adeps,* fat; OFr, *tissu*], fat deposits beneath the skin.

subcutaneous emphysema, the presence of free air or gas in the subcutaneous tissues. The air or gas may originate in the rupture of an airway or alveoli and migrate through the subpleural spaces to the mediastinum and neck. The face, neck, and chest may appear swollen. Skin tissues can be painful and may produce a "crackling" sound as air moves under them. The patient may experience dyspnea and appear cyanotic if the air leak is severe. Treatment may require an incision to release the trapped air. Also called **aerodermectasia.**

subcutaneous fascia, a continuous layer of connective tissue over the entire body between the skin and the deep fascial investment of the specialized structures of the body, such as the muscles. It comprises an outer, normally fatty layer and an inner, thin elastic layer. Between the two layers lie superficial blood vessels, nerves, lymphatics, the mammary glands, most of the facial muscles, and the platysma. Also called **subcutaneous layer.** Compare **deep fascia, subserous fascia.**

subcutaneous fat necrosis. See **adiponecrosis subcutanea neonatorum.**

subcutaneous infusion. See **hypodermoclysis.**

subcutaneous injection, the introduction of a hypodermic needle into the subcutaneous tissue beneath the skin, usually on the upper arm, thigh, or abdomen. A 24- or 25-gauge needle 2 cm long is used. The drug is prepared and drawn into the syringe. The cleansed area of skin is held by the thumb and forefinger to tense and steady the injection site. The needle is inserted at an angle of 45 to 60 degrees, piercing the skin quickly and advancing steadily to minimize the pain. The barrel or plunger is withdrawn slightly to ascertain whether the syringe of the needle has inadvertently entered a blood vessel. If no blood is aspirated, the drug is injected slowly, the needle is withdrawn, and the skin is massaged gently with a sterile alcohol sponge. Certain drugs that are extremely irritating to the skin are injected into the deep subcutaneous tissues using a variation of the technique. The skin tissue overlying the injection site is grasped with the thumb and forefinger but elevated in a roll, rather than

tensed and flattened. The angle of injection may be as great as 90 degrees to the skin. Heparin, insulin, and emetine are injected in this way. If subcutaneous injections are repeated, each is performed at least 5 cm from the previous site. A diagram of a plan for the rotation of injection sites helps to avoid overuse of one area of skin.

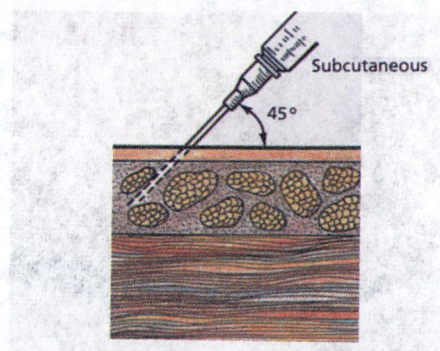

Insertion of needle for subcutaneous injection
(Potter, 1993)

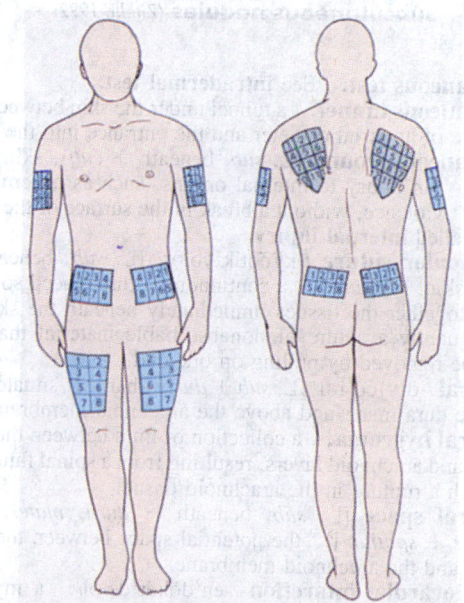

Rotation of sites for subcutaneous injections
(Potter, 1993)

subcutaneous layer. See **subcutaneous fascia.**

subcutaneous mastectomy, a surgical procedure in which all the breast tissue of one or both breasts is removed, leaving the skin, areola, and nipple intact. The adjacent lymph nodes, pectoralis major, and pectoralis minor are not removed. It may be performed on women who are at great risk of developing breast cancer. Reconstruction of the breasts is performed, with the assistance of a plastic surgeon, through the insertion of prostheses to return the normal contour to the breasts.

subcutaneous nodule, a small, solid boss, or node, beneath the skin that can be detected by touch. Subcutaneous nodules consisting chiefly of Aschoff bodies are found in patients with rheumatic fever. Minute subcutaneous nodules formed by the perivascular infiltration of mononuclear cells occur in typhus.

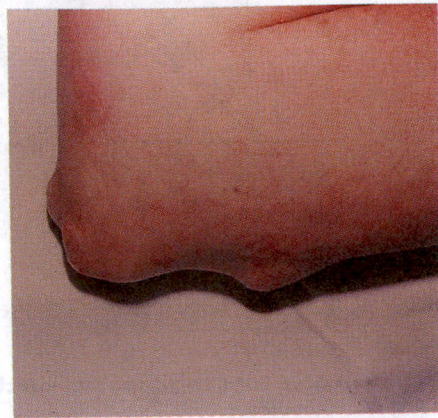

Subcutaneous nodules (Zitelli, 1992)

subcutaneous test. See **intradermal test.**

subcutaneous tunnel, a tunnel under the skin between the exit site of an atrial catheter and the entrance into the vein.

subcutaneous wound [L, *sub*, beneath + *cutis*, skin; AS, *wund*], an injury to internal organs, such as by crushing or other violence, without a break in the surface of the skin. Also called **internal injury.**

subcuticular suture /-kyo͞otik′yələr/ [L, *sub*, beneath + *cutis*, skin + *sutura*], a continuous suture placed so as to bring together the tissues immediately beneath the skin. It is frequently a suture of nonabsorbable material that can later be removed by pulling on one end.

subdural /-d(y)o͞o′rəl/ [L, *sub* + *durus*, hard], situated under the dura mater and above the arachnoid membrane.

subdural hygroma, a collection of fluid between the dura mater and arachnoid layers, resulting from a spinal fluid leak through a rupture in the arachnoid tissue.

subdural space [L, *sub*, beneath + *dura*, *mater*, hard mother + *spatium*], the potential space between the dura mater and the arachnoid membrane.

subendocardial infarction /-en′dōkär′dē·əl/, a myocardial infarction that involves only the innermost layer of the myocardium, and in some cases portions of the middle layer of tissue, but does not extend to the epicardial region.

subepidermal /-ep′idur′məl/ [L, *sub*, beneath; Gk, *epi*, above + *derma*, skin], beneath the epidermis.

subgerminal cavity. See **blastocoele.**

subgingival calculus /-jinjī′vəl/ [L, *sub* + *gingiva*, gum], a deposit of various mineral salts, such as calcium phosphate and calcium carbonate, that accumulates with organic matter and oral debris on the teeth or within the gingival crevice, the gingival pocket, or the periodontal pocket. It is usually darker, more pigmented, and denser than supragingival calculus.

subgingival curettage, the debridement of an ulcerated epithelial attachment and subjacent gingival corium to eliminate inflammation and shrink and restore gingival tissue.

subintentional suicide. See **benign suicide.**

subintimal /-in′timəl/ [L, *sub* + *intimus*, innermost], the area beneath the intima or membrane lining a blood vessel, usually a large artery.

subinvolution /-in′vəlo͞o′shən/ [L, *sub* + *involere*, to roll up], delayed or absent involution of the uterus during the postpartum period. The causes of subinvolution include retained fragments of placenta, uterine fibromyomas, and infection. Regardless of the cause of the condition, it is characterized by longer and heavier bleeding after childbirth and, on pelvic examination, a larger and softer uterus than would be expected at that time. Treatment includes ergonovine given by mouth for 2 or 3 days, and, if an infection is present, an antibiotic. The hemoglobin or hematocrit is also evaluated, and iron is given if necessary. A follow-up examination is performed 2 weeks later.

subinvolution of the uterus [L, *sub*, beneath + *involere*, to roll up + *uterus*, womb], an incomplete involution of the uterus after labor.

subjective /-jek′tiv/ [L, *subicere*, to expose], **1.** pertaining to the essential nature of an object as perceived in the mind rather than to a thing in itself. **2.** existing only in the mind. **3.** that which arises within or is perceived by the individual, as contrasted with something that is modified by external circumstances or something that may be evaluated by objective standards. **4.** pertaining to a person who places excessive importance on his own moods, attitudes, or opinions; egocentric.

subjective data collection, the process in which data relating to the patient's problem are elicited from the patient. The interviewer encourages a full description of the onset, the course, and the character of the problem and any factors that aggravate or ameliorate it. Compare **objective data collection.**

subjective sensation, a feeling or impression that is not associated with or does not directly result from any external stimulus. See also **sensation,** def. 1.

subjective symptoms [L, *subicere*, to expose; Gk, *symptoma*], symptoms that are observed only by the patient and cannot be objectively confirmed.

subjects /sub′jekts/, people, animals, or events selected for a study to examine a particular variable or condition, such as the effects of a new medication or therapy.

sublethal dose /-lē′thəl/ [L, *sub*, beneath + *letum*, death; Gk, *dosis*, giving], a dose of a potentially lethal substance that is not large enough to cause death.

sublethal gene [L, *sub* + *lethum*, death; Gk, *genein*, to produce], a gene whose presence causes abnormalities or impairs the functioning of an organism but does not cause its death. Compare **lethal gene.**

subleukemic leukemia. See **aleukemic leukemia.**

sublimate /sub′limāt/ [L, *sublimare*, to lift up], to refine or divert instinctual impulses and energy from their immediate goal to one that can be expressed in a social, moral, or aesthetic manner acceptable to the person and to society.

sublimation /-limā′shən/ [L, *sublimare*], **1.** a defense mechanism by which an unacceptable instinctive drive is unconsciously diverted to and expressed through a personally approved, socially accepted means. **2.** (in psychoanalysis) the process of diverting certain components of the sex drive to a socially acceptable, nonsexual goal. Compare **displacement.**

Sublimaze Citrate, a trademark for a narcotic analgesic (fentanyl citrate).

subliminal /-lim′inəl/ [L, *sub* + *limen*, threshold], taking place below the threshold of sensory perception or outside the range of conscious awareness.

subliminal self [L, *sub*, beneath + *limen*, threshold; AS, *self*], a level of mental activity at which an individual under normal waking conditions may function without consciousness. See also **preconscious; unconscious.**

sublingual /səbling'gwəl/ [L, *sub* + *lingua*, tongue], beneath the tongue.

sublingual administration of a medication, the administration of a drug, such as nitroglycerin, usually in tablet form, by placing it beneath the tongue until the tablet dissolves.

sublingual caruncle [L, *sub*, beneath + *lingua*, tongue + *caruncula*, small piece of flesh], a small fleshy growth under the tongue.

sublingual duct. See **Bartholin's duct, duct of Rivinus.**

sublingual gland, one of a pair of small salivary glands situated under the mucous membrane of the floor of the mouth, beneath the tongue. It is a narrow, almond-shaped structure, and weighs about 2 g. It is in relationship, inferiorly, with the mylohyoideus; posteriorly, with the submandibular gland; laterally, with the mandible; and medially, with the genioglossus from which it is separated by the lingual nerve and the submandibular duct. It has from 8 to 20 ducts, some of which join to form the sublingual duct. The sublingual gland secretes mucus produced by its alveoli. Compare **parotid gland, submandibular gland.**

subluxation. See **incomplete dislocation.**

submandibular /məndib'yələr/ [L, *sub* + *mandible*], below the mandible, or lower jaw.

submandibular duct [L, *sub* + *mandere*, to chew], a duct through which a submandibular gland secretes saliva. Also called **submaxillary duct.**

submandibular gland, one of a pair of round, walnut-sized salivary glands in the submandibular triangle, reaching anteriorly to the anterior belly of the digastricus and posteriorly to the stylomandibular ligament. The ligament lies between the submandibular gland and the parotid gland. The submandibular gland extends superiorly under the inferior border of the mandible and extends a deep process anteriorly above the mylohyoideus muscle. The upper portion of the superficial surface of the gland lies partly against the submandibular depression on the inner surface of the mandible and partly on the pterygoideus medialis. The lower part is covered by skin, superficial fascia, platysma, and deep cervical fascia. The submandibular duct is about 5 cm long, starts at the deep surface of the gland, runs between the sublingual gland and the genioglossus, and opens on a small papilla at the side of the frenulum linguae. The gland secretes both mucus and a thinner serous fluid, which aid the digestive process. Compare **sublingual gland, parotid gland.** See also **salivary gland.**

submaxillary /-mak'siler'ē/ [L, *sub* + *maxilla*], below the maxilla, or upper jaw.

submaxillary duct. See **submandibular duct.**

submeatal /-mē·ā'təl/ [*sub*, beneath + *meatus*, passage], pertaining to tissues beneath a meatus, such as the mastoid air cells under the acoustic meatus or the hard palate beneath the nasal meatus.

submental /-men'təl/ [L, *sub* + *mentum*, chin], beneath the chin.

submentovertex /-men'tōvur'teks/ [L, *sub* + *mentum*, chin, *vertex* peak], a reference point at the base of the skull used in preparing radiographic projections of the skull and its associated structures.

submetacentric /sub'metəsen'trik/ [L, *sub* + Gk, *meta*, besides, *kentron*, center], pertaining to a chromosome in which the centromere is located approximately equidistant between the center and one end so that the arms of the chromatids are not equal in length. Compare **acrocentric, metacentric, telocentric.**

submucous /m(y)ō͞o'kəs/, beneath a mucous membrane.

submucous resection (SMR) [L, *sub* + *mucous* + *re* + *secare*, to cut], a surgical procedure for correcting a deviated nasal septum, leaving the mucous membrane of the septum intact.

suboccipitobregmatic /-aksip'itō'bregmat'ik/ [L, *sub* + *occiput*, back of the head; Gk, *bregma*, front of the head], pertaining to the smallest anteroposterior diameter of an infant's head when it is well flexed during labor.

subperiosteal fracture /sub'perē·os'tē·əl/ [L, *sub* + Gk, *peri*, around, *osteon*, bone], a fracture in a bone beneath the periosteum that does not disrupt the periosteal covering.

subphrenic /-fren'ik/ [L, *sub* + Gk, *phren*, diaphragm], pertaining to the area beneath or under the diaphragm.

subphrenic abscess [L, *sub*, beneath; Gk, *phren*, diaphragm; L, *abscedere*, to go away], an abscess that develops on or near the undersurface of the diaphragm, usually as a result of peritonitis or from another visceral site.

subpoena /-pē'nə/ [L, *sub* + *poena*, penalty], (in law) a document from a court commanding that a person appear at a certain time and place to testify on a specific matter. Subpoenas are governed by federal rules for criminal procedure or for civil procedure.

subpoena duces tecum, (in law) a subpoena commanding a person to bring books, papers, records, or other items to the court.

subpubic dislocation. See **dislocation of hip.**

subsartorial canal. See **abductor canal.**

subscapularis /-skap'yələr'is/ [L, *sub*, beneath + *scapulae*, shoulder blades], the muscle arising from the subscapular fossa with insertion in the humerus. (See Fig. p. 1500.)

subserous fascia /-sir'əs/ [L, *sub* + *serum*, whey; *fascia*, band], one of three kinds of fascia, lying between the internal layer of deep fascia and the serous membranes lining the body cavities in much the same manner as the subcutaneous fascia lies between the skin and the deep fascia. It is thin in some areas, such as between the pleura and the chest wall, and thick in other areas, where it forms a pad of adipose tissue. Compare **deep fascia, subcutaneous fascia.**

subsistence /-sis'təns/ [L, *subsistere*, to stand still], the state of being sustained or remaining alive with a minimum of life essentials.

subspecialty /-spesh'əltē/ [L, *sub* + *specialis*, individual], (in nursing) a nurse's particular professional and highly specialized field of practice, such as nursing in dialysis, oncology, neurology, or newborn intensive care. Compare **specialty.**

substance /sub'stəns/ [L, *substantia*, essence], **1.** any drug, chemical, or biologic entity. **2.** any material capable of being self-administered or abused because of its physiologic or psychologic effects.

substance abuse, the overindulgence in and dependence on a stimulant, depressant, or other chemical substance, leading to effects that are detrimental to the individual's physical or mental health, or the welfare of others.

substance P, a polypeptide neurotransmitting substance that is synthesized by the body and acts to stimulate vasodilation and contraction of intestinal and other smooth mus-

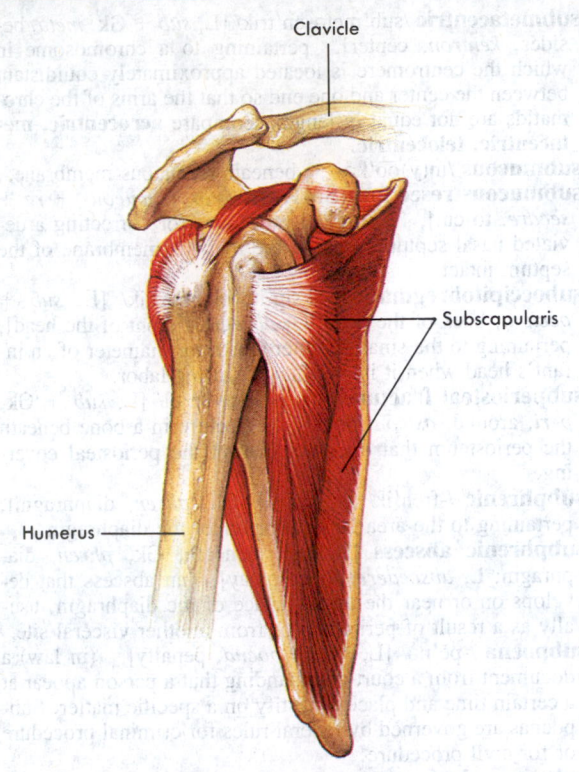

Clavicle

Subscapularis

Humerus

Subscapularis muscle (Thibodeau, 1993/John V Hagen)

cles. It also plays a part in salivary secretion, diuresis, and natriuresis, and it affects the function of the peripheral and central nervous systems. It has been isolated from certain cells of the GI and biliary tracts.

substandard /-stan'dərd/ [L, sub, beneath; OFr, estandart], below the predetermined model or measure.

substantia alba /-stan'shə/ [L, substantia, essence + albus, white], the portion of the central nervous system that is enclosed in myelin sheaths. The myelin contributes a white coloring to otherwise gray nerve tissue.

substantia nigra [L, substantia, essence + niger, black], a dark band of gray matter lying between the tegmentum of the midbrain and the crus cerebri. Also called locus niger.

substantive epidemiology /sub'stəntiv/ [L, subtantia + Gk, epi, upon, demos, people, logos, science], the body of knowledge derived from epidemiologic studies, including for each disease the natural history of the disorder, patterns of occurrence, and risk factors for developing the disease.

substantivity /-stantiv'itē/, the property of continuing therapeutic action despite removal of the vehicle, such as applied to certain shampoos.

substernal /-stur'nəl/ [L, sub; Gk, sternon, chest], beneath the sternum.

substernal goiter [L, sub + Gk, sternon, chest; L, guttur, throat], an enlargement of the thyroid gland, a portion of which is beneath the sternum.

substitution /-stit(y)oo'shən/, a mental defense mechanism, operating unconsciously, by which an unattainable or unacceptable goal, emotion, or object is replaced by one that is more attainable or acceptable.

substitutive therapy /-stit(y)oo'tiv/ [L, substituere, to put in place of; Gk, therapeia, treatment], a treatment that effects a condition incompatible with or antagonistic to the condition being treated. Also called **allopathy.**

substrate /sub'strāt/ [L, sub + stratum, layer], a substance acted on and changed by an enzyme in any chemical reaction.

substrate depletion phase, a period during an enzyme assay when the concentration of substrate is falling and the assay is not following zero-order kinetics.

substratum /-strā'təm/ [L, sub + stratum, layer], any underlying layer; a foundation.

subsystem /-sub'sistəm/, a smaller component of a large system composed of individuals or dyads, formed by generation, gender, interest, or function.

subthalamus /-thal'əməs/ [L, sub + Gk, thalamos, chamber], a portion of the diencephalon that serves as a correlation center for optic and vestibular impulses relayed to the globus pallidus. It is a transition zone between the thalamus and the tegmentum mesencephali, squeezed between the cerebral peduncle and the mammillary area. It accommodates prolongations of the red nucleus and the substantia nigra and contains fibrous masses of the fields of Forel. Compare **epithalamus, hypothalamus, metathalamus, thalamus.** –**subthalamic,** adj.

subtle /sut'əl/ [L, subtilis,], having a low intensity; not severe and having no serious sequelae, such as a mild infection or inflammation.

subtotal /sub'tōtəl/ [L, sub, beneath + totus, whole], less than complete.

subtotal hysterectomy [L, sub + totus; Gk, hystera, womb + extome, excision], the surgical removal of the body of the uterus without removing the cervix.

subtrochanteric osteotomy /-trō'kənter'ik/ [L, sub; Gk, trochanter, runner + osteon, bone + temnein, to cut], a surgical procedure that divides the shaft of the femur below the lesser trochanter to correct ankylosis of the hip joint.

subungual /səbung'gwəl/ [L, sub + unguis, nail], under a fingernail or toenail.

subungual hematoma, a collection of blood beneath a nail that usually results from trauma. The pain accompanying this condition may be quickly alleviated by burning or drilling a small hole through the nail to release the blood.

succ-, a combining form meaning 'of or pertaining to a juice': succagogue, succorrhea, succus.

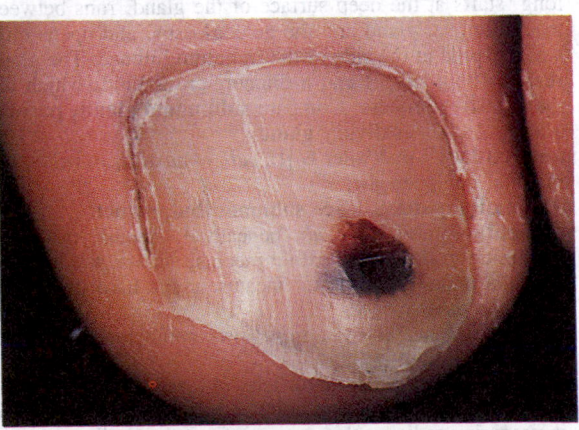

Subungual hematoma (du Vivier, 1993)

succagogue. See **-agogue, -agog.**

succenturiate placenta. See **accessory placenta.**

succi. See **succus.**

succinic acid /suksin′ik/, a compound found in certain hydatid cysts and in lichens, amber, and fossils. Commercial succinic acid, produced by the fermentation of ammonium tartrate, is used in lacquer and dyes. Succinic acid was formerly used in the treatment of diabetic ketoacidosis.

succinylcholine chloride /suk′sinilkō′lēn/, a skeletal muscle relaxant.

■ INDICATIONS: It is prescribed as an adjunct to anesthesia, to reduce muscle contractions during surgery or mechanical ventilation, and to facilitate endotracheal intubation.

■ CONTRAINDICATIONS: Known hypersensitivity to this drug prohibits its use. Caution is used in administering this drug to patients with low pseudocholinesterase levels and in patients with myasthenia gravis or renal failure.

■ ADVERSE EFFECTS: Among the more serious adverse reactions are cardiac dysrhythmia and severe respiratory depression.

succus /suk′əs/, *pl.* **succi** /suk′sī/ [L, juice], a juice or fluid, usually one secreted by an organ, such as succus prostaticus of the prostate.

succussion splash /səkush′ən/ [L, *succutere,* to shake up; ME, *plasche,* puddle], the sound elicited by shaking the body of an individual who has free fluid and air or gas in a hollow organ or body cavity. This sound may be present over a normal stomach but also may be heard with hydropneumothorax, large hiatal hernia, or intestinal or pyloric obstruction.

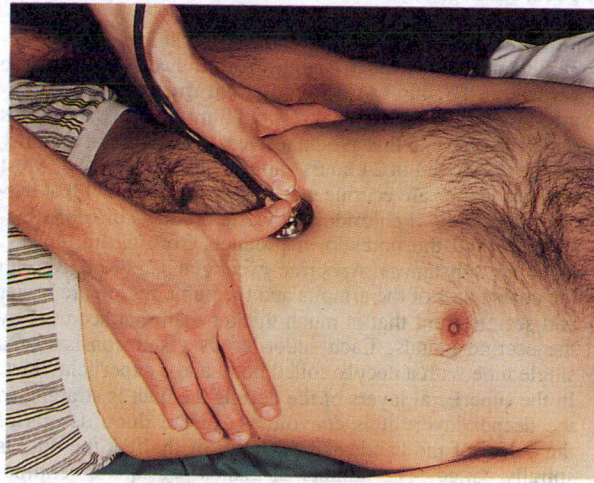

Testing for succussion splash (Epstein, 1992)

suck [L, *sugere,* to suck], **1.** to draw a liquid or semiliquid into the mouth by creating a partial vacuum through motions of the lips and tongue. **2.** to hold on the tongue and dissolve by the movements of the mouth and action of the saliva. **3.** to draw fluid into the mouth, specifically to draw milk from the breast or nursing bottle.

sucking blisters, the pale, soft pads on the upper and lower lips of a baby that look like blisters but are not. They form as soon as the baby begins to suck well, at the breast or on a bottle. They seem to augment the seal of the lips

around the nipple or breast. Some babies are born with them, having sucked on their own fingers, hand, or arm before birth.

sucking reflex, involuntary sucking movements of the circumoral area in newborns in response to stimulation. The reflex continues throughout infancy and often occurs without stimulation, such as during sleep. Compare **rooting reflex.**

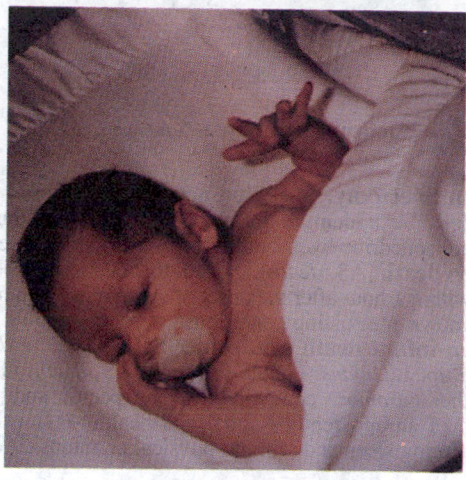

Sucking reflex (Zitelli, 1992)

suckle [L, *sugere*], **1.** to provide nourishment, specifically to breast feed. **2.** to take in nourishment, especially by feeding from the breast.

suckling, an infant that has not been weaned.

Sucostrin, a trademark for a depolarizing agent (succinylcholine), used as an adjunct to anesthesia.

sucrose /sōō′krōs/ [Fr, *sucre,* sugar], sugar derived from sugar cane, sugar beets, and sorghum.

sucrose polyester (SPE), a synthetic, nonabsorbable fat that, when added to the diet, reduces plasma cholesterol levels by increasing the excretion of cholesterol in the feces. It is formulated to have the characteristic texture, taste, and consistency of regular margarine or vegetable oil and adds no calories to the diet.

suction /suk′shən/ [L, *sugere,* to suck], the aspiration of a gas or fluid by reducing air pressure over its surface, usually by mechanical means.

suction biopsy [L, *sugere,* to suck; Gk, *bios,* life, *opsis,* view], a procedure for obtaining tissue or fluid samples from lymph nodes or a deep lesion by using suction and a trochar or cannula. Also called **aspiration biopsy.**

suction curettage, a method of curettage in which a specimen of the endometrium or the products of conception are removed by aspiration. Under local or light general anesthesia, the cervix is dilated, a catheter is introduced into the uterus, and suction is applied. Postoperative care includes monitoring vital signs for symptoms of blood loss. Also called **vacuum aspiration.** Compare **dilatation and curettage.**

suction drainage. See **drainage.**

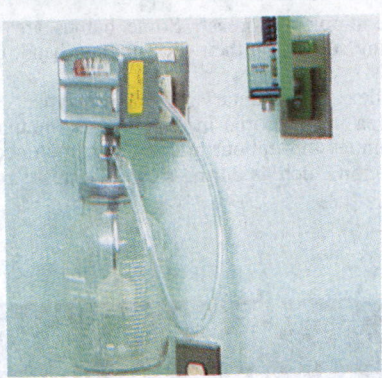

Suction apparatus (Sorrentino, 1992)

suction lipectomy. See **liposuction.**

Sudafed, a trademark for an adrenergic vasoconstrictor (pseudoephedrine hydrochloride), used as a decongestant.

sudden death [AS, *déath*], death that occurs unexpectedly and within 1 hour after the onset of symptoms, with or without known preexisting conditions.

sudden infant death syndrome (SIDS) [ME, *sodain,* to come up; L, *infans,* unable to speak; AS, *death;* Gk, *syn,* together, *dromos,* course], the unexpected and sudden death of an apparently normal and healthy infant that occurs during sleep and with no physical or autopsic evidence

Epidemiology of SIDS

Factors	Occurrence
Incidence	1.4:1000 live births
Peak age	2 to 4 months; 90% occur by 6 months
Sex	Higher percentage of males affected
Time of death	During sleep
Time of year	Increased incidence in winter; peak in January
Racial	Greater incidence in Native Americans and blacks, followed by whites; lower incidence in Chinese
Socioeconomic	Increased occurrence in lower socioeconomic class
Birth	Higher incidence in:
	Premature infants, especially infants of low birth weight
	Multiple births*
	Neonates with low Apgar scores
	Infants with central nervous system disturbances and respiratory disorders such as bronchopulmonary dysplasia
	Increasing birth order (subsequent siblings as opposed to firstborn child)
Sleep habits	Prone position
	Use of polystyrene-filled cushions
	Overheating
Feeding habits	Lower incidence in breast-fed infants
Siblings	May have greater incidence
Maternal	Younger age
	Cigarette smoking, including antenatal
	Drug addiction (heroin, methadone, and possibly cocaine)

From Wong DL, Whaley LF: *Essentials of pediatric nursing,* ed 4, St Louis, 1993, Mosby.
*Although a rare event, simultaneous death of twins from SIDS can occur.

of disease. It is the most common cause of death in children between 2 weeks and 1 year of age, with an incidence rate of 1 in every 300 to 350 live births. The origin is unknown, but multiple causes have been proposed, including lack of biotin in the diet, abnormality of the endogenous-opioid system, mechanical suffocation, a defect in respiratory mucosal defense, prolonged apnea, an unknown virus, anatomic abnormality of the larynx, and immunoglobulin abnormalities. It is known that the condition occurs more often in infants 10 to 14 weeks of age, especially those born prematurely, in boys more often than in girls, and during the winter months; and that it is seen more often among babies who have recently had a minor illness such as upper respiratory infection, or in infants born to women less than 20 years of age who have had at least one previous child, who begin prenatal care in the third trimester, or who smoke or are anemic or drug dependent. The syndrome is neither contagious nor hereditary, although there is a greater than average risk of its occurrence within the same family, which may indicate the influence of polygenic factors. Nursing considerations consist predominantly of support and counseling, such as assessing how the parents feel about the death to help them through the resolution of grief, learning what they know about the syndrome, supplying them with whatever information and literature they need, and finding out how they are coping with any guilt feelings and how the siblings, if any, are coping with the death. The nurse also can supply information about local groups of parents who have lost a child from SIDS. Also called **cot death, crib death.** See also **parental grief.**

sudo-, a combining form meaning 'of or pertaining to sweat': *sudogram, sudokeratosis, sudorrhea.*

sudor /sōō′dôr/ [L, *sweat*], perspiration.

sudoriferous duct /sōō′dərif′ərəs/ [L, *sudor,* sweat, *facere,* to make], a duct leading from a sweat gland to the surface of the skin. Also called **sweat duct.**

sudoriferous gland, one of about 3 million tiny structures within the dermis that produce sweat. The average quantity of sweat secreted in 24 hours varies from 700 to 900 g. Most of these glands are eccrine glands, producing sweat that carries away sodium chloride, the waste products urea and lactic acid, and the breakdown products from garlic, spices, and other substances. Apocrine sweat glands associated with the coarse hair of the armpits and the pubic region are larger and secrete fluid that is much thicker than that secreted by the eccrine glands. Each sudoriferous gland consists of a single tube with a deeply coiled body and a superficial duct. In the superficial layers of the dermis the duct is straight; in the deeper layers it is convoluted. In the thick dermis of the palms of the hands and the soles of the feet the duct is spirally coiled. The number of glands per square centimeter of skin varies in different parts of the body, the sudoriferous glands being very plentiful on the palms of the hands and on the soles of the feet and least numerous in the neck and the back; they are completely absent in the deeper portions of the external auditory meatus, the prepuce, and the glans penis, and are more numerous in the fingers of Asians and African-Americans than in the fingers of Europeans. Also called **sweat gland.** Compare **sebaceous gland.**

sudorific /sōō′dərif′ik/ [L, *sudor,* sweat, *facere,* to make], **1.** of or pertaining to a substance or condition, such as heat or emotional tension, that promotes sweating. **2.** a sudorific agent. Sweat glands are stimulated by cholinergic drugs. The alkaloid pilocarpine is a potent sudorific drug, but it is rarely used for that purpose in modern medicine. Also called **diaphoretic.**

suf-. See **sub-.**

Sufenta, a trademark for an intravenous analgesic-anesthetic (sufentanil citrate).

sufentanil citrate /sufen'tənil/, an intravenous analgesic and anesthetic.

■ INDICATIONS: It is used as an adjunct to general anesthesia and as a primary anesthetic with 100% oxygen.

■ CONTRAINDICATIONS: Sufentanil can cause respiratory depression and musculoskeletal rigidity; readily available drugs and equipment are required to reduce such adverse effects. Sufentanil is a Schedule II controlled substance.

■ ADVERSE EFFECTS: Among the more serious adverse reactions are hypotension, hypertension, bradycardia, and chest wall rigidity.

suffocation /suf'əkā'shən/ [L, *suffocare*, to choke], an interruption in breathing with oxygen deprivation, usually caused by an obstruction in the airways. The condition may be accidental, intentional, or the result of disease or inadequate levels of respirable gases in the atmosphere.

suffocation, high risk for, a nursing diagnosis accepted by the Seventh National Conference on the Classification of Nursing Diagnoses. The diagnosis is defined as the accentuated risk of accidental suffocation (inadequate air available for inhalation). The risk factors may be internal (individual) or external (environmental). Internal risk factors include reduced olfactory sensation, reduced motor abilities, lack of safety education, lack of safety precautions, cognitive or emotional difficulties, and disease or injury processes. External risk factors include a pillow or a propped bottle placed in an infant's crib, a vehicle warming in a closed garage, children playing with plastic bags or inserting small objects into their mouths or noses, discarded or unused refrigerators or freezers without removed doors, unattended children in bathtubs or pools, household gas leaks, smoking in bed, eating too large mouthfuls of food, use of fuel-burning heaters not vented to outside, low-strung clothesline, and a pacifier hung around infant's neck. See also **nursing diagnosis.**

suffocative goiter /suf'əkā'tiv/ [L, *suffocare*, to choke; *guttur*, throat], an enlargement of the thyroid gland causing a sensation of suffocation on pressure.

sugar /shŏŏg'ər/ [Gk, *sakcharon*], any of several water-soluble carbohydrates. The two principal categories of sugars are monosaccharides and disaccharides. A monosaccharide is a single sugar, such as glucose, fructose, or galactose. A disaccharide is a double sugar, such as sucrose (table sugar) or lactose. See also **carbohydrate, fructose, galactose, glucose, saccharide, sucrose.**

sugar alcohol, an alcohol produced by the reduction of an aldehyde or ketone of a sugar.

suggestibility /səjəs'tibil'itē/, pertaining to a person's susceptibility to having his or her ideas or actions changed by the influence of others.

suggestion /səjəs'chən/ [L, *suggerere*, to propose], **1.** the process by which one thought or idea leads to another, as in the association of ideas. **2.** the use of persuasion, exhortation, or another device to implant an idea, thought, attitude, or belief in the mind of another as a means of influencing or altering behavior or states of mind. See also **hypnosis. 3.** an idea, belief, or attitude implanted in the mind of another. Compare **autosuggestion.**

suicidal /sŏŏ'isī'dəl/ [L, *sui*, of oneself, *caedere*, to kill], of, relating to, or tending toward self-destruction.

suicidal melancholia, *obsolete.* a state of severe depression in which suicidal tendencies are prominent.

suicide /sŏŏ'isīd/ [L, *sui*, of oneself, *caedere*, to kill], **1.** the intentional taking of one's own life. **2.** *informal.* the ruin or destruction of one's own interests. **3.** a person who commits or attempts self-destruction. Early signs of suicidal intent include depression; expressions of guilt, tension, and agitation; insomnia; loss of weight and appetite; neglect of personal appearance; and direct or indirect threats to commit suicide.

suicide gesture, (in psychiatric nursing) an apparent attempt by a patient to cause self-injury without lethal consequences and generally without actual intent to commit suicide. A suicide gesture serves to attract attention to the patient's disturbed emotional status but is not as serious as a suicide attempt.

suicide prevention center, a crisis-intervention facility dealing primarily with people preoccupied with suicidal thoughts. Such facilities are usually operated by professional social workers with special training in counseling possible suicide victims in person or by telephone.

suicidology /sŏŏ'isīdol'əjē/ [L, *sui, caedere* + Gk, *logos,* science], the study of the prevention and the causes of suicide. **−suicidologist,** *n.*

Suladyne, a trademark for an antiinfective, fixed-combination drug containing antibacterials (sulfamethizole and sulfadiazine) and a urinary antiseptic (phenazopyridine hydrochloride).

sulcate. See **sulcus.**

sulci. See **sulcus.**

sulcoplasty. See **vestibuloplasty.**

sulculus /sul'kyələs/ [L, *sulcus*], a small sulcus.

sulcus /sul'kəs/, *pl.* **sulci** /sul'sī/ [L, furrow], a shallow groove, a depression, or a furrow on the surface of an organ, such as a sulcus that separates the convolutions of the cerebral hemisphere. A sulcus is usually not as deep as a fissure but, in the terminology of anatomy, sulcus and fissure are often used interchangeably. **−sulcate,** *adj.*

sulcus centralis cerebri. See **central sulcus.**

sulcus pulmonalis, a depression on each side of the vertebral bodies that accommodates the posterior portion of the lung.

sulfa-, a combining form for sulfonamide antimicrobials.

sulfacetamide /sul'fəset'əmīd/, a topical antibacterial.

■ INDICATIONS: It is most commonly prescribed for the prophylaxis of infection after injury to the cornea and in the treatment of bacterial conjunctivitis and urinary tract infections.

■ CONTRAINDICATIONS: Known hypersensitivity to the drug or to other sulfonamides or impaired kidney function prohibits its use.

■ ADVERSE EFFECTS: Among known adverse reactions are local pain, overgrowth of nonsusceptible pathogens, and hypersensitivity reaction to the drug.

Sulfacet-R, a trademark for a topical, fixed-combination drug containing a scabicide (sulfur), an antibacterial (sulfacetamide sodium), and an antiseptic and astringent (zinc oxide).

sulfachlorpyridazine /sul'fəklôr'pirid'əzēn/, a sulfonamide antibacterial.

■ INDICATION: It is prescribed in the treatment of infection, particularly of the urinary tract.

■ CONTRAINDICATIONS: Porphyria, urinary tract obstruction, or known hypersensitivity to this or to other sulfonamides prohibits its use.

■ ADVERSE EFFECTS: Among the more serious adverse reac-

tions are crystalluria, severe allergic reactions, photosensitivity, and blood dyscrasias.

sulfacytine /sulfas'itēn/, a sulfonamide antibacterial.
- INDICATIONS: It is prescribed in the treatment of infection, particularly primary pyelonephritis, and cystitis.
- CONTRAINDICATIONS: Porphyria, urinary tract obstruction, or known hypersensitivity to sulfonamides prohibits its use.
- ADVERSE EFFECTS: Among the more serious adverse reactions are crystalluria, photosensitivity, severe allergic reactions, and blood dyscrasias.

sulfadiazine /sul'fədī'əzēn/, a sulfonamide antibacterial.
- INDICATIONS: It is prescribed in the treatment of infection, particularly of the urinary tract, and as a rheumatic fever prophylaxis.
- CONTRAINDICATIONS: Porphyria, urinary tract obstruction, or known hypersensitivity to sulfonamides prohibits its use.
- ADVERSE EFFECTS: Among the more serious adverse effects are crystalluria, photosensitivity, severe allergic reactions, and blood dyscrasias.

sulfa drugs /sul'fə/, a group of bacteriostatic agents that inhibit the biosynthesis of folic acid.

sulfamethizole /sul'fəmeth'izōl/, a sulfonamide antibacterial.
- INDICATIONS: It is prescribed in the treatment of infection, particularly pyelonephritis, pyelitis, and cystitis.
- CONTRAINDICATIONS: Porphyria, urinary tract obstruction, or known hypersensitivity to sulfonamides prohibits its use.
- ADVERSE EFFECTS: Among the more serious adverse reactions are crystalluria, photosensitivity, blood dyscrasias, and severe allergic reactions.

sulfamethoxazole /sul'fəmethok'səzōl/, a sulfonamide antibacterial.
- INDICATIONS: It is prescribed in the treatment of otitis media, bronchitis, and certain urinary tract infections.
- CONTRAINDICATIONS: It is not given during the last trimester of pregnancy, during lactation, or to children under 2 months of age. Known hypersensitivity to this drug or other sulfonamides prohibits its use.
- ADVERSE EFFECTS: Among the more serious adverse reactions are crystalluria and rash, fever, and other allergic reactions.

sulfamethoxazole and trimethoprim /trīmeth'əprim/, a fixed-combination antibacterial.
- INDICATIONS: It is prescribed in the treatment of urinary tract infections, otitis media, and shigellosis.
- CONTRAINDICATIONS: It is used with caution in patients with impaired renal or hepatic function, with possible folate deficiency, or with known hypersensitivity to either drug or to sulfonamides. It is not recommended for use in infants under 2 months of age or in the third trimester of pregnancy.
- ADVERSE EFFECTS: Among the more serious adverse reactions are crystalluria and rashes, fever, and other allergic reactions.

Sulfamylon, a trademark for a topical antiinfective (mafenide acetate).

sulfanilic acid /sul'fənil'ik/, a red-tinged, white crystalline compound used in the synthesis of sulfonamides and as a reagent in tests for phenol, fecal matter in water, albumin, aldehydes, and glucose. Also called **paraaminobenzenesulfonic acid.**

sulfasalazine /sul'fəsalaz'ēn/, a sulfonamide; salicylazosulfapyridine.
- INDICATIONS: It is prescribed in the treatment of mild to moderate ulcerative colitis and as adjunctive therapy in severe cases.

- CONTRAINDICATIONS: Urinary obstruction, porphyria, or known hypersensitivity to this drug, to other sulfonamide medications, or to salicylates prohibits its use. It is not given during the last trimester of pregnancy.
- ADVERSE EFFECTS: Among the more serious adverse reactions are crystalluria, blood dyscrasias, and severe hypersensitivity reactions. GI symptoms and anorexia commonly occur.

sulfate /sul'fāt/, a salt of sulfuric acid. A sulfate is usually a combination of a metal with sulfuric acid. Natural sulfates, such as sodium sulfate, calcium sulfate, and potassium sulfate, are plentiful in the body.

sulfathiazole /sul'fəthī'əzōl/, a sulfonamide antibacterial no longer commonly used.

sulfatide lipidosis /sul'fətīd/, an inherited lipid metabolism disorder of childhood caused by a deficiency of cerebroside sulfatase enzyme. It results in an accumulation of metachromatic lipids in tissues of the central nervous system, kidney, spleen, and other organs, leading to dementia, paralysis, and death by the age of 10 years. Also called **metachromatic leukodystrophy.** See also **lipidosis.**

sulfhemoglobin /sulfhem'əglō'bin/, a form of hemoglobin found in the blood in trace amounts that contains an irreversibly bound sulfur molecule that prevents normal oxygen binding.

sulfhemoglobinemia /-ē'mē·ə/, the presence of abnormal sulfur-containing hemoglobin circulating in the blood.

sulfinpyrazone /sul'finpir'əzōn/, a uricosuric.
- INDICATIONS: It is prescribed in the treatment of chronic gout and intermittent gouty arthritis.
- CONTRAINDICATIONS: Peptic ulcer, ulcerative colitis, renal dysfunction, or known hypersensitivity to this drug or to phenylbutazone prohibits its use. It is not usually given during an acute attack of gout.
- ADVERSE EFFECTS: Among the more serious adverse reactions are GI ulcers, blood dyscrasias, and dermatitis.

sulfisoxazole /sul'fisok'səzōl/, a sulfonamide antibacterial.
- INDICATIONS: It is prescribed in the treatment of conjunctivitis and urinary tract infections, including vaginitis, cystitis, and pyelonephritis.
- CONTRAINDICATIONS: Porphyria, urinary tract obstruction, or known hypersensitivity to this drug or to sulfonamide medications prohibits its use. It is not given during the last trimester of pregnancy or to children under 2 months of age.
- ADVERSE EFFECTS: Among the more serious adverse reactions are crystalluria, blood dyscrasias, and severe hypersensitivity reactions.

sulfiting agents /sul'fīting/, food preservatives composed of potassium or sodium bisulfite or potassium metabisulfite. Sulfiting agents are used in processing of beer, wine, baked goods, soup mixes, and some imported seafoods and by restaurants to impart a 'fresh' appearance to salad fruits and vegetables. The chemicals can cause a severe allergic reaction in people who are hypersensitive to sulfites. The reactions are marked by flushing, faintness, hives, headache, GI distress, breathing difficulty, and, in extreme cases, loss of consciousness and death.

sulfo- /sul'fō-, sul'fə-/, a combining form naming chemical compounds, showing presence of divalent sulfur or of the group SO$_2$OH: *sulfonamide, sulfomethane, sulfophenol.*

sulfobromophthalein /sul'fəbrō'məfthal'ēn, -ē·in/, a substance used in its disodium salt form for evaluating the function of the liver. See also **bromsulphalein test.**

sulfonamide /səlfon'əmīd/, one of a large group of synthetic, bacteriostatic drugs that are effective in treating infections caused by many gram-negative and gram-positive microorganisms. They are bacteriostatic rather than bactericidal. Some sulfonamides are short acting, some are intermediate acting, and some are long acting, depending on the speed with which they are excreted. They are used in treating many urinary tract infections. Some people are hypersensitive to the drugs. Sulfonamides are given with caution to people who have impaired liver or kidney function, and they are not given in the last trimester of pregnancy or to young infants, because mental retardation sometimes occurs. Hemolytic anemia, agranulocytosis, thrombocytopenia, or aplastic anemia, drug fever, and jaundice may occur, particularly with long-acting sulfonamides given for more than 10 days. Most sulfonamides are given orally.

sulfonates /sul'fənāts/, a class of anticholinesterase compounds used as insecticides.

sulfonylurea /sul'fənilyŏŏr'ē·ə/, an oral antidiabetic agent that stimulates the pancreatic production of insulin. Hypersensitivity to sulfonamides is a contraindication for using such agents, and ethanol consumption is incompatible with all sulfonylureas. The safety of these drugs for use in pregnant women has not been established, making insulin the preferred drug in treating diabetes in pregnancy. Aspirin or other salicylates taken with any sulfonylurea may intensify the hypoglycemic effect.

sulfosalicylic acid /sul'fōsalisil'ik/, a white or faintly pink crystalline substance that is highly water-soluble, used as a reagent in tests for albumin and as an intermediate compound in the manufacture of dyes and surfactants.

sulfoxone sodium /sulfok'sōn/, a bacteriostatic sulfone derivative.

- INDICATIONS: It is prescribed in the treatment of leprosy and dermatitis herpetiformis.
- CONTRAINDICATIONS: Advanced renal amyloidosis or known sensitivity to this drug prohibits its use.
- ADVERSE EFFECTS: Among the most serious adverse reactions are hemolysis, hemolytic anemia, toxic epidermal necrolysis, and several blood dyscrasias.

Sulfoxyl, a trademark for a topical fixed-combination drug containing a disinfectant (benzoyl peroxide) and a scabicide (sulfur).

sulfur (S) /sul'fər/ [L], a nonmetallic, multivalent, tasteless, odorless chemical element that occurs abundantly in yellow crystalline form or in masses, especially in volcanic areas. Its atomic number is 16; its atomic weight is 32.06. It is used to produce sulfuric acid and used commercially in metallurgy, rubber vulcanization, petroleum refining, and many other industrial processes. Sulfur has been used in the treatment of gout, rheumatism, and bronchitis and as a mild laxative. The sulfonamides, or sulfa drugs, are used in the treatment of various bacterial infections. Also spelled **sulphur.**

-sulfuric, -sulphuric, a combining form meaning 'compounds containing sulfur, especially in its highest valences': *hydrosulfuric, persulfuric, thiosulfuric.*

sulfuric acid /sulf(y)ŏŏ'rik/, a clear, colorless, oily, highly corrosive liquid that generates great heat when mixed with water. An extremely toxic substance, sulfuric acid causes severe skin burns, blindness on contact with the eyes, serious lung damage if the vapors are inhaled, and death if it is ingested. In industry, sulfuric acid is used in the manufacture of fertilizers, dyes, glue, and other acids, in the purifying of petroleum, and in the pickling of metals. Weak solutions of sulfuric acid are used in the treatment of gas-

tric hypoacidity and serous diarrhea. It was formerly called **oil of vitriol.**

sulfurous acid /sul'fərəs/, a weak inorganic acid used as a chemical reducing and bleaching agent. It has been used in medicine in skin lotions and nasal and throat sprays. Sulfites formed by the acid may be used in antiseptics, antifermentatives, and antizymotics.

sulindac /sulin'dek/, an antiinflammatory agent.

- INDICATIONS: It is prescribed in the treatment of osteoarthritis, rheumatoid arthritis, and ankylosing spondylitis.
- CONTRAINDICATIONS: Pregnancy, lactation, or known hypersensitivity to this drug, to aspirin, or to nonsteroidal antiinflammatory drugs prohibits its use. It is used with caution in patients who have upper GI tract disease or impaired renal function.
- ADVERSE EFFECTS: Among the more serious adverse reactions are GI upset, peptic ulcer, dizziness, tinnitus, and skin rash. This drug interacts with many other drugs.

Sulkowitch's test /sul'kəwichs/ [Hirsh W. Sulkowitch, American physician, b. 1906], an examination of the urine for the presence of calcium. A reagent, containing oxalic acid, ammonium oxalate, and glacial acetic acid, mixed with urine, causes calcium to precipitate out of the urine. Also called **S's test.** See also **hypercalciuria.**

sulphur. See **sulfur.**

Sultrin, a trademark for a vaginal fixed-combination drug containing antibacterials (sulfathiazole, sulfacetamide, and sulfabenzamide).

sumac [Ar, *summaq*], any of a number of species of trees and shrubs in the *Anacardiaceae* family, including the *Rhus* varieties, which have poisonous properties. See **poison ivy, poison oak, poison sumac, rhus dermatitis.**

summary judgment [L, *summa*, total; *jus*, law, *dicere*, to state], (in law) a judgment requested by any party to a civil action to end the action when it is believed that there is no genuine issue or material fact in dispute. Summary judgment may be directed toward part or all of a claim or defense and may be based on the proceedings in court or on affidavits or other outside materials.

summation [L, *summa*, total], **1.** an accumulative effect or action; a total aggregate; totality. **2.** (in neurology), the concentration of a neurotransmitter at a synapse, either by increasing the frequency of nerve impulses in each fiber (temporal summation) or by increasing the number of fibers stimulated (spatial summation), so that the threshold of the postsynaptic neuron is overcome and an impulse is transmitted. See also **facilitation,** def. 2.

summons /sum'əns/ [OFr, *somondre*, to remind secretly], (in law) a document issued by a clerk of the court on the filing of a complaint. A sheriff, marshal, or other appointed person serves the summons, notifying a person that an action has been begun against him or her. See also **service of process.**

Sumycin, a trademark for an antibiotic (tetracycline hydrochloride).

sunbath [AS, *sunne, baeth*], the exposure of the naked body to the sun.

sunDare, a trademark for an ultraviolet screen (cinoxate).

sundowning /sun'douning/ [AS, *sunne + ofdune,* off the hill], a condition in which elderly people tend to become confused or disoriented at the end of the day. Many of them have diminished visual acuity and varying degrees of sensorineural and conduction hearing loss. With less light, they lose visual cues that help them to compensate for their sensory impairments.

sunrise syndrome, a condition of unstable cognitive ability on arising in the morning. Compare **sundowning.**

sunscreen protective factor index (SPF), a system of evaluating the effectiveness of various formulations for protecting the skin from actinic rays of the sun. Protective agents are rated from 1 to 50 by the FDA. A sun protective factor of 15 means that the sunscreen provides 15 times the protection of unprotected skin. Among the most highly rated sunscreen lotions are nonopaque combinations of PABA ester and benzophenone.

sunstroke [AS, *sunne* + *strac*, stroke], a morbid condition caused by overexposure to the sun and characterized by a high fever, convulsions, and coma. See also **heat hyperpyrexia.**

sup-. See **sub-.**

Supen, a trademark for an antibacterial (ampicillin).

super- /sōo′pər-/, a prefix meaning 'above, or implying excess': *superduct, superfunction, supernumerary.*

superego /-ē′gō/ [L, *super*, over; Gk, *ego*, I], (in psychoanalysis) that part of the psyche, functioning mostly in the unconscious, that develops when the standards of the parents and of society are incorporated into the ego. The superego has two parts, the conscience and the ego ideal. See also **ego, ego ideal, id.**

superfecundation /-fekəndā′shən/ [L, *super* + *fecundare*, to be fruitful], the fertilization of two or more ova released during one menstrual cycle by spermatozoa from the same or different males during separate acts of sexual intercourse.

superfetation /-fētā′shən/ [L, *super* + *fetus*, pregnancy], the fertilization of a second ovum after the onset of pregnancy, resulting in the presence of two fetuses of different degrees of maturity developing within the uterus simultaneously. Also called **superimpregnation.**

superficial /-fish′əl/ [L, *superficies*, surface], **1.** of or pertaining to the skin or another surface. **2.** not grave or dangerous.

superficial abscess [L, *superficialis* + *abscedere*, to go away], an abscess that develops above the fascia layer.

superficial fading infantile hemangioma, a superficial, temporary, salmon-colored patch in the center of the forehead, face, or occiput of many newborns. It fades during the first 2 years of life, but it may temporarily deepen in color if the child becomes flushed or angry.

superficial implantation, (in embryology) the partial embedding of the blastocyst within the uterine wall so that it and, later, the chorionic sac protrude into the uterine cavity. Also called **central implantation, circumferential implantation.**

superficial inguinal node, a node in one of the two groups of inguinal lymph glands in the upper femoral triangle of the thigh. The nodes form a chain distal to the inguinal ligament and receive afferents from the skin of the penis, scrotum, perineum, buttocks, and abdominal wall below the level of the umbilicus. Compare **anterior tibial node, popliteal node.**

superficial reflex, any neural reflex initiated by stimulation of the skin. Kinds of superficial reflexes are **abdominal reflex, anal reflex,** and **cremasteric reflex.** Compare **deep tendon reflex.**

superficial sensation, the awareness or perception of feelings in the superficial layers of the skin in response to touch, pressure, temperature, and pain. Such sensations are conveyed to the brain via the spinothalamic system. Compare **deep sensation.**

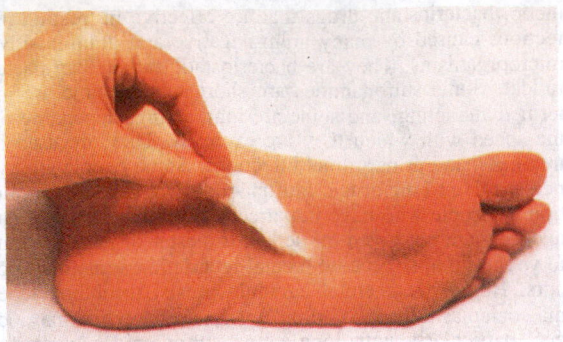

Superficial tactile sensation (Seidel, 1991)

superficial spreading melanoma, the most common melanoma that grows outward, spreading over the surface of the affected organ or tissue. It occurs most commonly on the lower legs of women and the torso of men. The lesion is raised and palpable, unevenly pigmented, and irregularly shaped, and has an unclear border. See also **lentigo-maligna melanoma, nodular melanoma.**

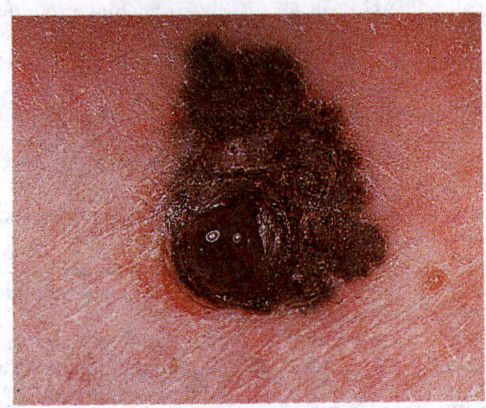

Superficial spreading melanoma (du Vivier, 1993)

superficial temporal artery, an artery at each side of the head that can be easily felt in front of the ear and is often used for taking the pulse. It is the smaller of the two terminal branches of the external carotid and arises in the substance of the parotid gland. It crosses the zygomatic process of the temporal bone and about 5 cm above the process divides into the frontal branch and the parietal branch. Compare **deep temporal artery, middle temporal artery.**

superficial vein, one of the many veins between the subcutaneous fascia just under the skin. Compare **deep vein.**

superimpregnation. See **superfetation.**

superinfection /-infek′shən/ [L, *super* + *inficere*, to taint], an infection occurring during antimicrobial treatment for another infection. It is usually a result of change in the normal tissue flora favoring replication of some organisms by diminishing the vitality and then the number of competing organisms, as yeast microbes flourish during penicillin therapy prescribed to cure a bacterial infection.

superior /səpir′ē·ər/ [L, higher], situated above or oriented toward a higher place, as the head is superior to the torso. Compare **inferior.**

superior aperture of minor pelvis, an opening bounded by the crest and pecten of the pubic bones, the arch-shaped lines of the ilia, and the anterior margin of the base of the sacrum.

superior aperture of thorax, an elliptic opening at the summit of the thorax bounded by the first thoracic vertebra, the first ribs, and the upper margin of the sternum.

superior carotid triangle [L, *superior,* higher; Gk, *karos,* heavy sleep; L, *triangulus,*], a triangle bounded by the sternocleidomastoid muscle, in front and below by the omohyoid muscle, and above by the stylohyoid and digastric muscles.

superior conjunctival fornix, the space in the fold of the conjunctiva created by the reflection of the conjunctiva covering the eyeball and the lining of the upper lid. Compare **inferior conjunctival fornix.**

superior costotransverse ligament, one of five ligaments associated with each costotransverse joint, except that of the first rib. It passes from the neck of each rib to the transverse process of the vertebra immediately above and is associated with the intercostal vessels and the intercostal nerves. The first rib has no superior costotransverse ligament. Compare **posterior costotransverse ligament.**

superior gastric node, a node in one of two sets of gastric lymph glands, accompanying the left gastric artery. The node is divided into the upper group of nodes on the stem of the artery, the lower group of nodes accompanying branches of the artery along the cardiac half of the lesser curvature of the stomach, and the paracardial group of nodes around the neck of the stomach. The superior gastric nodes receive their afferent vessels from the stomach and pass their efferent vessels to the celiac group of preaortic nodes. Compare **inferior gastric node.**

superior hemorrhagic polioencephalitis. See **Wernicke's encephalopathy.**

superior mediastinum, the cranial portion of the mediastinum in the middle of the thorax, containing the trachea, the esophagus, the aortic arch, and the origins of the sternohyoidei and the sternothyroidei. The superior mediastinum is bounded by the superior aperture of the thorax, the plane of the superior limit of the pericardium, the manubrium, the upper four thoracic vertebrae, and laterally the mediastinal aspect of the parietal pleurae of the lungs. Compare **anterior mediastinum, middle mediastinum, posterior mediastinum.**

superior mesenteric artery, a visceral branch of the abdominal aorta, arising caudal to the celiac artery, dividing into five branches, and supplying most of the small intestine and parts of the colon. The branches are the inferior pancreaticoduodenal, intestinal, ileocolic, right colic, and middle colic.

superior mesenteric node, a node in one of the three groups of visceral lymph nodes that serve the viscera of the abdomen and the pelvis. The superior mesenteric nodes are associated with branches of the superior mesenteric artery and are divided into mesenteric nodes, iliocolic nodes, and mesocolic nodes. Compare **gastric node, inferior mesenteric node.**

superior mesenteric vein, a tributary of the portal vein that drains the blood from the small intestine, the cecum, and the ascending and the transverse colons. It begins in the right iliac fossa, ascends between the two mesenteric layers to the right of the superior mesenteric artery, and joins the lienal vein to form the portal vein, dorsal to the neck of the pancreas. The tributaries of the superior mesenteric vein are the intestinal vein, the ileocolic vein, the right colic vein, the middle colic vein, the gastroepiploic vein, and the pancreaticoduodenal vein. See also **portal vein.**

superior olivary nucleus [L, *supurus* + *oliva* + nut], a collection of nerve cells appearing as a clump of gray matter in the pons. The nucleus receives fibers from the cochlear nerve receptors on the same and opposite sides through the trapezoid body. It assists in the localization of sound by comparing the time difference between sounds received by the left and right ears.

superior profunda artery. See **deep brachial artery.**

superior radioulnar joint. See **proximal radioulnar articulation.**

superior sagittal sinus, one of the six venous channels in the posterior of the dura mater, draining blood from the brain into the internal jugular vein. It has no valves and presents a triangular section as the sinus courses posteriorly through a groove in the frontal bone and passes along the convex margin of the falx cerebri to the occipital protuberance, usually continuing as the right transverse sinus. The superior sagittal sinus receives the superior cerebral veins, veins from the diploe, and, near the posterior extremity of the sagittal suture, the anastomosing emissary veins from the pericranium and the veins from the dura mater. It also anastomoses with veins of the nose, the scalp, and the diploe. Compare **inferior sagittal sinus, straight sinus, transverse sinus.**

superior subscapular nerve /səbskap′yələr/, one of two small nerves on opposite sides of the body that arise from the posterior cord of the brachial plexus. It supplies the superior part of the subscapularis. Compare **inferior subscapular nerve.**

superior thyroid artery, one of a pair of arteries in the neck, usually rising from the external carotid artery, that supplies the thyroid gland and several muscles in the head.

superior ulnar collateral artery, a long, slender division of the brachial artery, arising just distal to the middle of the arm, descending to the elbow, and anastomosing with the posterior ulnar recurrent and inferior ulnar collateral arteries.

superior vena cava, the second largest vein of the body, returning deoxygenated blood from the upper half of the body to the right atrium. It is about 2 cm in diameter and 7 cm long and is formed by the junction of the two brachiocephalic veins at the level of the first intercostal space behind the sternum on the right side. The section of the superior vena cava closest to the heart composes about one half of the vessel's length and is within the pericardial sac, covered by the serous pericardium. It has no valves and just before it enters the pericardium receives the azygous vein and several small pericardial veins. Compare **inferior vena cava.**

supernatant /-nā′tənt/ [L, *super* + *natare,* to swim], the clear upper portion of any mixture after it has been centrifuged.

supernormal excitability /-nôr′məl/, the ability of the myocardium to respond to a stimulus that would be ineffective earlier or later in the cardiac cycle.

supernormal period, a period at the end of phase 3 of

the cardiac cycle when activation can be initiated with less stimulus than is required at maximal repolarization.

supernumerary nipples /-nōō′mərer′ē/ [L, *super* + *numerus*, number; ME, *neb*, beak], an excessive number of nipples, which are usually not associated with underlying glandular tissue. They may vary in size from small pink dots to that of normal nipples.

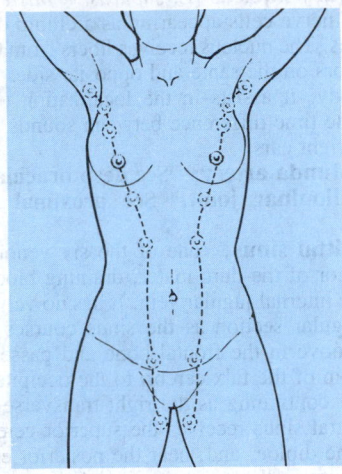

supernumerary nipples

supernumerary tooth [L, *super*, above + *numerus*, number; AS, *toth*], any tooth in addition to the normal 32 teeth in permanent dentition or the 20 teeth in deciduous dentition.

superoxide /-ok′sīd/, a common reactive form of oxygen that is formed when molecular oxygen gains a single electron. Superoxide radicals can attack susceptible biologic targets, including lipids, proteins, and nucleic acids.

superoxide dismutase (SOD), an enzyme composed of metal-containing proteins that converts superoxide radicals into less toxic agents. It is the main enzymatic mechanism for clearing superoxide radicals from the body.

supersaturate /-sach′ərāt/ [L, *super*, above + *saturare*, to fill], a solution that contains solute above the saturation point at a given temperature. Also called **metastable solution.**

supervision /-vizh′ən/, (in psychology) a process whereby a therapist is helped to become a more effective clinician through the direction of a supervisor who provides theoretical knowledge and therapeutic techniques and supports the working through of transference and countertransference reactions.

supervisor /sōō′pərvī′zər/ [L, *super* + *videre*, to see], (in hospital or public health nursing) the midlevel management position between the director of nursing and head nurses of a division or of several units. In many hospitals "clinical director" is the preferred term. The supervisor's responsibilities are primarily administrative, although they may include clinical leadership for the nurses working in a group of units, wards, or divisions.

supervitaminosis /-vī′təminō′sis/ [L, *super*, above + *vita* + *amine*; Gk, *osis*, condition], a condition of ingesting an excessive amount of vitamins. Signs and symptoms vary with specific vitamin excesses. See also **hypervitaminosis.**

supinate /sōō′pənāt/, pertaining to a supine position or turning the palm upward.

supination /sōō′pinā′shən/ [L, *supinus*, lying on the back], **1.** one of the kinds of rotation allowed by certain skeletal joints, such as the elbow and the wrist joints, which allow the palm of the hand to turn up. **2.** the position of lying on the back, face up. See also **supine.** Compare **pronation.** –**supinate,** *v.*

supinator jerk reflex. See **supinator longus reflex.**

supinator longus. See **brachioradialis.**

supinator longus reflex /sōō′pinā′tər/ [L, *reflectere*, to bend back], a contraction of the brachioradialis muscle, causing flexion at the elbow joint, on tapping the point of insertion of the supinator longus muscle at the lower end of the radius. Also called **radial reflex, supinator jerk reflex.**

supine /səpīn′, sōō′pīn/ [L, *supinus*], lying horizontally on the back. Also called **dorsal decubitus position.** Compare **prone.** See also **body position.**

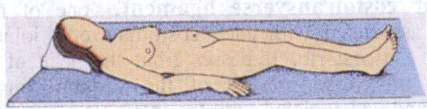

Supine position (Potter, 1993)

supine hypotension, a fall in blood pressure that occurs when a pregnant woman is lying on her back. It is caused by impaired venous return that results from pressure of the gravid uterus on the vena cava. Also called **vena caval syndrome.**

supplemental air. See **reserve air.**

supplemental inheritance /sup′ləmen′təl/ [L, *supplere*, to complete; *in*, in, *hereditare*, hereditary], the acquisition or expression of a genetic trait or condition from the presence of two independent pairs of nonallelic genes that interact in such a way that one gene supplements the action of the other.

supplementary gene /sup′ləmen′tərē/ [L, *supplere* + Gk, *genein*, to produce], one of two pairs of nonallelic genes that interact in such a way that one pair needs the presence of the other to be expressed, whereas the second pair can produce an effect independent of the first.

support /səpôrt′/ [L, *supportare*, to bring up], **1.** to sustain, hold up, or maintain in a desired position or condition, as in physically supporting the abdominal muscles with a scultetus binder or emotionally supporting a client under stress. **2.** the assistance given to this end, such as physical support, emotional support, or life support.

supporting area [L, *supportare* + *area*, space], any of the areas of maxillary or mandibular edentulous ridges that are considered best suited to bear the forces of mastication with functioning dentures.

supportive psychotherapy /səpôr′tiv/, a form of psychotherapy that concentrates on creating an effective means of communication with an emotionally disturbed person rather than on trying to produce psychologic insight into the underlying conflicts. Through such supportive measures as reassurance, reinforcement of the person's defenses, direction, suggestion, and persuasion, the therapist participates directly in the solution of specific problems. Compare **nondirective therapy.**

supportive treatment. See **treatment.**

suppository /səpoz′ətôr′ē/ [L, *sub*, under, *ponere*, to place], an easily melted medicated mass for insertion in the rectum, urethra, or vagina. Theobroma oil, glycerinated gelatin, and high-molecular-weight polyethylene glycols are common vehicles for drugs in suppositories that are cone- or spindle-shaped for insertion in the rectum, globular or egg-shaped for use in the vagina, and pencil-shaped for insertion in the urethra. Drugs administered by rectal suppository are absorbed systemically, and this route is especially useful in babies, in uncooperative patients, and in cases of vomiting or certain digestive disorders.

suppressant /səpres'ənt/ [L, *supprimere*, to press down], an agent that suppresses or diminishes a physical or mental activity, such as a medication that reduces hyperkinetic behavior or the excretory or secretory activity of a gland.

suppressed menstruation /səprest'/ [L, *supprimere*, to press down + *menstruare*], a failure of menstruation to occur when expected, as in amenorrhea.

suppression /səpresh'ən/ [L, *supprimere*], (in psychoanalysis) the conscious inhibition of or effort to conceal unacceptable or painful thoughts, desires, impulses, feelings, or acts. Compare **repression.**

suppression amblyopia, a partial loss of vision, usually in one eye, caused by cortical suppression of central vision to avoid diplopia. It occurs commonly in strabismus in the eye that deviates and does not fixate. Early recognition of strabismus and amblyopia is essential, because occlusive therapy that forces use of the bad eye may dramatically improve the child's vision if begun early. It is ineffective after 6 years of age, and near blindness in the affected eye may result.

suppression of menses. See **suppressed menstruation.**

suppressor gene /səpres'ər/, (in molecular genetics) a genetic unit that is able to reverse the effect of a specific kind of mutation in other genes.

suppressor mutation, (in molecular genetics) a mutation that partially or completely restores a function lost by a primary mutation occurring in a different genetic site.

suppressor T cell. See **T cell.**

suppurate /sup'yərāt/ [L, *suppurare*, to form pus], to produce purulent matter. **–suppuration,** *n.,* **suppurative** /sup'yərā'tiv/, *adj.*

suppuration /sup'yərā'shən/ [L, *suppurare*, to form pus], the production and exudation of pus.

suppurative /sup'yərətiv'/ [L, *suppurare*, to form pus], pus-forming.

suppurative fever [L, *suppurare*, to form pus + *febris*, fever], a fever accompanied by pus formation.

suppurative pancreatitis [L, *suppurare*, to form pus; Gk, *pan*, all + *kreas*, flesh + *itis*, inflammation], a form of pancreas inflammation accompanied by the appearance of small abscesses.

suppurative phlebitis [L, *suppurare*, to form pus; Gk, *phleps*, vein + *itis*, inflammation], a vein inflammation as a result of septicemia or a nearby pyogenic infection.

supra- /sŏō'prə-/, a prefix meaning 'above or over': *suprabuccal, supradural, suprarenalism.*

suprabony periodontal pocket. See **periodontal pocket.**

supracallosus gyrus /-kəlō'ses/ [L, *supra,* above + *callosus,* hard; Gk, *gyros,* turn], the gray matter covering the corpus callosum of the brain.

supracervical hysterectomy /-sur'vikəl/ [L, *supra,* above + *cervix,* neck; Gk, *hystera,* womb + *ektome,* excision], a subtotal hysterectomy in which the body of the uterus is removed, leaving the cervix.

supraclavicular /-kləvik'yələr/ [L, *supra,* above, *clavicula,* little key], above the clavicle, or collar bone.

supraclavicular nerve, one of a pair of cutaneous branches of the cervical plexus, arising from the third and the fourth cervical nerves, mostly from the fourth nerve. It emerges from the posterior border of the sternocleidomastoideus and crosses the posterior triangle of the neck under the deep fascia. Near the clavicle it pierces the fascia and the platysma in the anterior, the middle, and the posterior groups. The anterior group supplies the skin of the infraclavicular region, the middle group supplies the skin over the pectoralis major and the deltoideus, and the posterior group supplies the skin of the cranial and the dorsal parts of the shoulder.

supraclavicular triangle [L, *supra,* above + *clavicula,* little key + *triangulus*], the lower and anterior areas of the neck, bounded by the omohyoid muscle above, the sternocleidomastoid muscle in front, and the clavicle below. The first rib is in the base of the triangle.

supracondylar /-kon'dilər/ [L, *supra,* above; Gk, *kondylos,* knuckle], above a condyle.

supracondylar fracture /sŏō'prəkon'dilər/ [L, *supra* + *kondylos,* knuckle], a fracture involving the area between the condyles of the humerus or the femur.

supracrestal periodontal pocket. See **periodontal pocket.**

supragingival calculus /-jinjī'vəl/ [L, *supra* + *gingiva,* gum], a deposit composed of various mineral salts, such as calcium phosphate, and calcium carbonate, which accumulates with organic matter and oral debris on the teeth occlusal or coronal to the gingival crest.

suprainfection /-infek'shən/ [L, *supra* + *inficere,* to taint], a secondary infection usually caused by an opportunistic pathogen, such as a fungal infection after the antibiotic treatment of another infection or pneumonia in a patient debilitated by another illness.

supraoptic nucleus /-op'tik/ [L, *supra,* above; Gk, *optikos;* L, *nucleus,* nut], a hypothalamic nucleus that lies in the optic chiasma with fibers extending to the posterior lobe of the pituitary.

suprapatellar /-pətel'ər/ [L, *supra,* above + *patella,* small disc], above the patella.

suprapubic /-p(y)ŏō'bik/ [L, *supra* + *pubes,* signs of maturity], located above the symphysis pubis.

suprapubic catheter [L, *supra* + *pubis;* Gk, *katheter,* a thing lowered into], a urinary bladder catheter that is inserted through the skin about one inch above the symphysis pubis. The device is installed under a general or local anesthetic and may be left in place for a time, sutured to the abdominal skin.

suprarenal /-rē'nəl/ [L, *supra* + *ren,* kidney], above the kidney, such as the suprarenal gland.

suprascapular ligament /-skap'yələr/ [L, *supra,* above + *scapulae,* shoulder blades + *ligare,* to bind], a ligament that extends from the base of the coracoid process to the medial end of the suprascapular notch.

suprascapular nerve /sŏō'prəskap'yələr/ [L, *supra* + *scapula,* shoulderblade], one of a pair of branches from the cords of the brachial plexus. It arises from the superior trunk, passes to the scapular notch, and, in the supraspinatous fossa, branches to the supraspinatus, the shoulder joint, the infraspinatus, and the scapula.

suprasellar cyst. See **craniopharyngioma.**

supraspinal /-spī'nəl/ [L, *supra,* above + *spina,* backbone], above the spine.

supraspinal ligament [L, *supra* + *spina*, backbone], the ligament that connects the apices of the spinous processes from the seventh cervical vertebra to the sacrum. Between the spinous processes it is continuous with the interspinal ligaments; from the seventh cervical vertebrae it continues upward to the external occipital protuberance and the medial nuchal line as the ligamentum nuchae.

supraspinous fossa /-spī′nəs/ [L, *supra*, above + *spina*, backbone + *fossa*, ditch], a depressed area on the dorsal surface of the scapula, above the spine.

suprasternal /-stur′nəl/, above the sternum, adjacent to the neck.

supratentorial /-tentôr′ē·əl/ [L, *supra*, above + *tentorium*, tent], above a tentorium.

supravaginal hysterectomy /-vaj′inəl/ [L, *supra*, above + *vagina*, sheath; Gk, *hystera*, womb + *ektome*, excision], a subtotal hysterectomy in which the body of the uterus is removed but the cervix remains.

supraventricular tachycardia (SVT) /-ventrik′yələr/ [L, *supra* + *ventriculus*, belly], any cardiac rhythm exceeding 100 beats per minute that originates above the ventricles, in the SA node, atria, or AV junction.

suprofen /səprō′fən/, an oral nonsteroidal antiinflammatory analgesic.

■ INDICATIONS: It is used in the treatment of mild to moderate pain and primary dysmenorrhea.

■ CONTRAINDICATIONS: This drug is contraindicated for patients who experience asthma, rhinitis, urticaria, or other allergic reactions from the use of aspirin or other nonsteroidal antiinflammatory drugs. It is not recommended for patients with a history of peptic ulcers or risk of other types of gastrointestinal bleeding.

■ ADVERSE EFFECTS: Reported side effects include severe flank pain, nausea, vomiting, dyspepsia, abdominal pain, diarrhea, constipation, flatulence, headache, dizziness, sedation, and sleep disturbances.

Suprol, a trademark for an oral nonsteroidal antiinflammatory analgesic (suprofen).

suramin sodium /sōō′rəmin/, an antitrypanosomal and an antifilarial available from the Centers for Disease Control. It is used primarily for treatment and prophylaxis of African trypanosomiasis and onchocerciasis.

Surfacaine, a trademark for a local anesthetic agent (cyclomethycaine sulfate).

surface anatomy /sur′fəs/ [L, *superficies* surface], the study of the structural relationships of the external features of the body to the internal organs and parts. Compare **cross-sectional anatomy.**

surface anesthesia. See **topical anesthesia.**

surface area (SA), the total area exposed to the outside environment. The surface area of an object increases with the square of the object's linear dimensions; volume increases as the cube of the object's linear dimensions. Thus the larger of two objects of the same shape will have less surface area per unit volume than the smaller object. Most loss of body heat takes place from the body surface.

surface biopsy, the removal of living tissue for microscopic examination by scraping the surface of a lesion. The procedure is used primarily to diagnose cancer of the uterine cervix. See also **exfoliative cytology.**

surface tension, the tendency of a liquid to minimize the area of its surface by contracting. This property causes liquids to rise in a capillary tube, affects the exchange of gases in the pulmonary alveoli, and alters the ability of various liquids to wet another surface.

surface therapy, a form of radiotherapy administered by placing one or more radioactive sources on or near an area of body surface. The resulting array of sources is called a surface mold, surface applicator, or plaque.

surface thermometer, a device that detects and indicates the temperature of the surface of any part of the body.

surfactant /sərfak′tənt/ [L, *superficies*], **1.** an agent, such as soap or detergent, dissolved in water to reduce its surface tension or the tension at the interface between the water and another liquid. **2.** certain lipoproteins that reduce the surface tension of pulmonary fluids, allowing the exchange of gases in the alveoli of the lungs and contributing to the elasticity of pulmonary tissue. See also **alveolus, atelectasis, surface tension.**

Surfadil, a trademark for a topical fixed-combination drug containing an antihistaminic (methapyrilene hydrochloride) and a topical anesthetic (cyclomethycaine sulfate).

Surfak, a trademark for a stool softener (docusate calcium).

surfer's nodules [ME, *suffe*, rush; L, *nodus*, knot], nodules on the skin of the knees, ankles, feet, or toes of a surfer caused by repeated contact of the skin with an abrasive, sandy surfboard. The nodules slowly diminish in size and disappear if surfing is discontinued. When treatment is necessary, injection of corticosteroids is usually effective.

surgeon's assistant (SA) /sur′jənz/ [Gk, *cheirourgos*, surgeon; L, *assistere*, to cause to stand], a medical professional trained to assist in surgery and in the preoperative and postoperative periods under the supervision of a licensed physician qualified to practice surgery.

surgery /sur′jərē/ [Gk, *cheirourgos*], the branch of medicine concerned with diseases and trauma requiring operative procedures. –**surgical,** *adj.*

-surgery, -chirurgia, a combining form meaning the 'treatment of illness or deformity': *cardiosurgery, chemosurgery, radiosurgery.*

surgical /sur′jikəl/ [Gk, *cheirourgos*], pertaining to the treatment of disease by manipulative and operative methods.

surgical abdomen. See **acute abdomen.**

surgical anatomy, (in applied anatomy) the study of the structure and morphology of the tissues and organs of the body as they relate to surgery.

surgical anesthesia, the third stage of general anesthesia. See also **general anesthesia, Guedel's signs.**

surgical diathermy. See **electrocoagulation.**

surgical fever [Gk, *cheirourgos;* L, *febris*], a fever that develops after surgery. Under modern aseptic techniques, fever is unlikely to accompany an operation.

surgical induction of labor. See **induction of labor.**

surgical ligature, the exposure of an unerupted tooth by placing a metal ligature around its cervix. The free ends of the ligature are fixed to a fine precious metal chain attached to an orthodontic appliance. These components act together to produce traction on the unerupted tooth and force it through the gum tissues.

surgical menopause [Gk, *cheirourgos*, surgeon; L, *mensis*, month; Gk, *pauein*, to cease], the creation of a menopausal state by surgical termination of menstrual function.

surgical microscope. See **operating microscope.**

surgical neck of humerus [Gk, *cheirourgos*, surgeon; AS, *hnecca;* L, *humerus*, shoulder], the shaft of the humerus distal to the tuberosities. It is a region particularly vulnerable to fracture and surgical correction.

surgical pathology, the study of disease by the study of tissue specimens obtained during surgery. The surgical pathologist often examines specimens during surgery to determine how the operation should be modified or completed. Various techniques are used. The appearance of the specimen is first noted; then slices of the tissue are prepared by the paraffin or frozen section method and microscopically examined by a physician trained in pathology.

surgical scrub, **1.** a bactericidal soap or solution used by surgeons and surgical nurses before performing or assisting in surgery. **2.** the act of washing the fingernails, hands, and forearms in a prescribed manner for a specific period of time, with a bactericidal soap or solution before a surgical procedure.

surgical sectioning, an oral surgery procedure for dividing a tooth to facilitate its removal. A variety of instruments is used for surgical sectioning, such as osteotomes and power-driven burs.

surgical shock [Gk, *cheirourgos*, surgeon; Fr, *choc*], a condition of shock that may follow surgery, with signs of low blood volume, failure of peripheral circulation, sweating, thirst, restlessness, and cyanosis of the extremities.

surgical suite, a group of one or more operating rooms and adjunct facilities, such as sterile storage area, scrub room, and recovery room.

surgical technologist, an allied health professional who prepares the operating room by selecting and opening sterile supplies; assembles, adjusts, and checks nonsterile equipment to ensure it is in good working order; and operates sterilizers, lights, suction machines, electrosurgical units, and diagnostic equipment. Surgical technologists have primary responsibility for maintaining the sterile field and being constantly vigilant that all members of the surgical team adhere to aseptic technique.

surgical treatment. See **treatment.**

Surital Sodium, a trademark for a barbiturate (thiamylal sodium), used as a general anesthetic.

Surmontil, a trademark for an antidepressant (trimipramine maleate).

surrogate /sur′əgāt/ [L, *surrogare*, to substitute], **1.** a substitute; a person or thing that replaces another. **2.** (in psychoanalysis) a substitute parental figure, a symbolic image or representation of another, as may occur in a dream. The identity of the person represented often remains in the unconscious.

surrogate parenting, a form of artificial insemination in which a fertile woman who is not the wife of the sperm donor agrees to be impregnated by the husband and to carry the child to term, at which time the offspring is surrendered to the care of the infertile wife. The surrogate mother usually receives a fee for bearing the child.

surrogate partner. See **sex surrogate.**

sursum-, a combining form meaning 'upward': *sursumduction, sursumvergence, sursumversion.*

surveillance /sərvā′ləns/ [Fr, *surveiller*, to watch over], supervising or observing a patient or a health condition.

surveyed height of contour /sərvād′/ [OFr, *surveir*, to survey; AS, *heah*, high; It, *contornare*, to surround], a line, scribed or marked on a cast, that designates the greatest convexity relative to a selected path of denture placement and removal.

survival curve /sərvī′vəl/ [Fr, *survivre*, to survive; L, *curvus*, bent], a curve obtained by plotting the number or percentage of organisms surviving at different intervals against doses of radiation.

survivor guilt /sərvī′vər/ [OFr, *survivre*; ME, *gilt*, sin], feelings of guilt for surviving a tragedy in which others died. In some cases, the person may believe the tragedy occurred because he or she 'did something bad'; in others, the person may feel guilty for not taking proper steps to avert the tragedy. Also called **survival guilt.**

susceptible /səsep′tibəl/ [L, *suscipere*, to undertake], being predisposed, liable, or sensitive to effects of an infectious disease, allergen, or other pathogenic agent; lacking immunity or resistance.

susceptibility /səsep′tibil′itē/ [L, *suscipere*, to undertake], the condition of being more than normally vulnerable to a disease or disorder.

suspension /səspen′shən/ [L, *suspendere*, to hang], **1.** a liquid in which small particles of a solid are dispersed, but not dissolved, and in which the dispersal is maintained by stirring or shaking the mixture. If left standing, the solid particles settle at the bottom of the container. See also **colloid, solution. 2.** a treatment, used primarily in spinal disorders, consisting of suspending the patient by the chin and shoulders. **3.** a temporary cessation of pain or of a vital process.

suspension sling, a sling usually made of muslin or lightweight canvas and employed primarily to provide support, such as against the gravitational pull on an injured arm. An example is a common triangular sling.

suspensory ligament /səspen′sərē/ [L, *suspendere*, to hang + *ligare*, to bind], any of a number of ligaments that help support an organ or body structure, such as the suspensory ligaments inside the eye that hold the lens in tension.

suspensory ligament of the lens. See **zonula ciliaris.**

sustained release. See **prolonged release.**

sustenance /sus′tənəns/ [L, *sustenare*, to sustain], **1.** the act or process of supporting or maintaining life or health. **2.** the food or nutrients essential for maintaining life.

susto /sōōs′tō/, a culture-bound syndrome found in Central American populations. It is related to stress engendered by a self-perceived failure to fulfill sex-role expectations.

sutilains /sōō′tilānz/, a proteolytic enzyme.
- INDICATIONS: It is prescribed for debridement of certain wounds, ulcers, and second- and third-degree burns.
- CONTRAINDICATIONS: Wounds communicating with major body cavities, wounds containing exposed major nerves or nervous tissue, or fungating neoplastic ulcers prohibit its use. It is not given during pregnancy.
- ADVERSE EFFECTS: Among the more serious adverse reactions are bleeding, paresthesias, and dermatitis.

sutura /sōōchōō′rə/, *pl.* **suturae** [L, suture], an immovable, fibrous joint in which certain bones of the skull are connected by a thin layer of fibrous tissue. Compare **gomphosis, syndesmosis.**

sutura dentata, an immovable fibrous joint that is one kind of true suture in which toothlike processes interlock along the margins of connecting bones of the skull. Compare **sutura limbosa, sutura serrata.**

sutura limbosa, an immovable fibrous joint that is one kind of true suture in which beveled and serrated edges of certain connecting bones of the skull, such as the parietal and temporal bones, overlap and interlock. Compare **sutura dentata, sutura serrata.**

sutura plana, a fibrous joint that is one kind of false suture in which rough, contiguous edges of certain bones of the skull, such as the maxillae, form a connection. Compare **sutura squamosa.**

sutura serrata, an immovable fibrous joint that is one kind of true suture in which connecting bones interlock along serrated edges that resemble fine-toothed saws. Compare **sutura dentata, sutura limbosa.**

sutura squamosa, an immovable fibrous joint that is one kind of false suture in which overlapping, beveled edges unite certain bones of the skull, such as the temporal and the parietal bone. Compare **sutura plana.**

suture /sōō'chər/ [L, *sutura*], **1.** a border or a joint, such as between the bones of the cranium. **2.** to stitch together cut or torn edges of tissue with suture material. **3.** a surgical stitch taken to repair an incision, tear, or wound. **4.** material used for surgical stitches, such as absorbable or nonabsorbable silk, catgut, wire, or synthetic material.

suture forceps. See **needle holder.**

Sv, abbreviation for **sievert.**

SV40, abbreviation for **simian virus 40.**

SvO₂, symbol for the percent of oxygen saturation of mixed venous blood.

SVR, abbreviation for systemic **vascular resistance.**

swab /swob/ [D, *swabber*, ship's drudge], a stick or clamp for holding absorbent gauze or cotton, used for washing, cleansing, or drying a body surface, for collecting a specimen for laboratory examinations, or for applying a topical medication.

swaddling /swod'ling/ [OE, *swethel*, swaddling band], **1.** long narrow bands of cloth once used to wrap a newborn. **2.** a method of wrapping a newborn, especially a premature or at risk newborn, that provides maximal comfort.

swallowing /swol'ō·ing/ [AS, *swelgan*], the process that usually involves movement of food from the mouth to the stomach via the esophagus. Coordination of muscles is needed from the tongue to the esophageal sphincter. See **swallowing reflex.**

swallowing, impaired, a nursing diagnosis accepted by the Seventh National Conference on the Classification of Nursing Diagnoses. It is defined as the state in which an individual has decreased ability to voluntarily pass fluids and/or solids from the mouth to the stomach. The major defining characteristic is observed evidence of difficulty in swallowing, such as stasis of food in the oral cavity, coughing, or choking. Evidence of aspiration is also a characteristic. Among related factors are neuromuscular impairment, such as decreased or absent gag reflex, and decreased strength or excursion of muscles involved in mastication. Other factors are perceptual impairment, facial paralysis, mechanical obstruction (such as edema, tracheostomy tube, or tumor), tumor, fatigue, limited awareness, and an irritated oropharyngeal cavity. See also **nursing diagnosis.**

swallowing reflex [AS, *swelgan*; L, *reflectere*, to bend back], a sequence of reflexes that begins when a bolus of food is manipulated by the tongue and other oral cavity muscles to the palate or the pharynx.

swamp fever. See **leptospirosis, malaria.**

Swan-Ganz catheter /swän'ganz'/ [Harold J. C. Swan, American physician, b. 1922; William Ganz, American cardiologist, b. 1919; Gk, *katheter*, something lowered], a long, thin cardiac catheter with a tiny balloon at the tip. It is used during anesthesia to determine left ventricular function by measuring pulmonary arterial wedge pressure.

swan neck deformity /swän/ [D, *zwaan*; AS, *hnecca*, neck; L, *deformis*, misshapen], **1.** an abnormal condition of the finger characterized by flexion of the distal interphalangeal joint and hyperextension of the proximal interphalangeal joint. It is caused by a taut profundus tendon in the presence of a weakened distal interphalangeal joint, and may

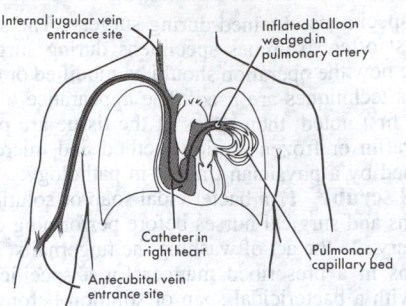

Swan-Ganz catheter

be combined with a volar plate rupture. The condition is seen most often in rheumatoid arthritis. Also called **zig-zag. 2.** a structural abnormality of the kidney tubules associated with rickets. The kidney tubule connecting the glomerulus with the convoluted portion of the tubule is narrowed into a configuration referred to as 'swan neck.' There is also a thinning and atrophy of the distal tubule and a shortening of the convoluted portion.

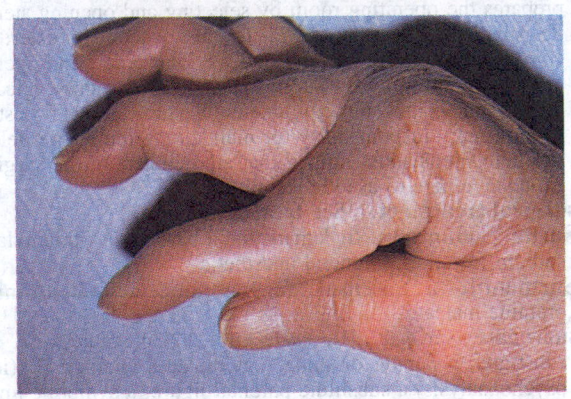

Swan neck deformity *(Kamal, 1991)*

S wave, the component of the cardiac cycle shown on an electrocardiogram as a line slanting downward sharply from the peak of the R wave to the beginning of the upward curve of the T wave. It represents the final phase of the QRS complex.

sweat. See **perspiration.**

sweat bath, a bath given to induce sweating.

sweat duct [AS, *swaetan*, to sweat; L, *ducere*, to lead], any one of the tiny tubules conveying sweat to the surface of the skin from about 2 million sweat glands throughout the body. Each sweat duct is the most superficial part of a coiled tube that forms the body of each sweat gland and opens onto the surface through a funnel-shaped opening. The sweat ducts in the armpits and in the groin are larger than in other parts of the body. Ducts and sweat glands abound on the palms of the hands and the soles of the feet. There are about 370 sweat ducts rising from a corresponding number of sweat glands per square centimeter on each palm. Each duct is composed of a basement membrane with two or three layers of polyhedral cells and is lined with a thin cuticle.

sweat gland. See **sudoriferous gland.**

sweating. See **diaphoresis.**

sweat test, a method for evaluating sodium and chloride excretion from the sweat glands, often the first test performed in the diagnosis of cystic fibrosis. The sweat glands are stimulated with a drug, such as pilocarpine, and the perspiration produced is analyzed. The eccrine glands of patients with cystic fibrosis produce sodium and chloride concentrations that are three to six times those of the normal. Chloride levels above 60 mEq/L and sodium levels above 90 mEq/L are considered diagnostic for the disease. The test is very reliable, and although it may be useful at any age, it is usually performed on infants from 2 weeks to 1 year of age. See also **cystic fibrosis.**

Swedish massage /swē′dish/ [Fr, *masser*], a regimen of massage combined with physical exercises.

Sweet localization method, a radiographic technique for locating a foreign body in the eye by making two x-ray films of the eye while the patient's head is immobilized. A small metal ball and a cone are placed at precise distances from the center of the cornea as register marks while lateral and perpendicular x-ray views of the eye are made. A three-dimensional view of the eye is constructed from the two x-ray films, and, guided by the positions of the ball and cone, the location of the foreign body in the eye is plotted from the intersection of lines through the ball and cone.

Swift's disease. See **acrodynia.**

swimmer's ear [AS, *swimman*, to swim; *eare*], *informal.* otitis externa resulting from infection transmitted in the water of a swimming pool.

swimmer's itch, an allergic dermatitis caused by sensitivity to schistosome cercarias that die under the skin, leading to erythema, urticaria, and a papular rash lasting 1 or 2 days. Treatment usually includes oral antihistamines and antipruritic lotions. See also **schistosomiasis.**

swing phase of gait [AS, *swingan* + Gk, *phasis*, appearance; ME, *gate* a way], one of the two phases in the rhythmic process of walking. The swing phase of gait follows the stance phase and is divided into the initial swing, the midswing, and the terminal swing stages.

swoon [OE, *geswogen*, unconscious], a fainting spell.

sy-. See **syn-.**

sycosis barbae /sikō′sis/ [Gk, *sycon*, fig, *osis*, condition; L, *barba*, beard], an inflammation of hair follicles of skin that has been shaved. Treatment includes light and infrequent shaving, topical and systemic antibiotics, and daily plucking of infected hairs. Also called **barber's itch, sycosis vulgaris.**

Sydenham's chorea /sid′ənhamz/ [Thomas Sydenham, English physician, b. 1624; Gk, *choreia*, dance], a form of chorea associated with rheumatic fever, usually occurring during childhood. The cause is a streptococcal infection of the vascular and perivascular tissues of the brain. The choreic movements increase over the first 2 weeks, reach a plateau, and then diminish. The child is usually well within 10 weeks. With undue exertion or emotional strain, the condition may recur. Also called **chorea minor, rheumatic chorea.**

syl-. See **syn-.**

sylvatic plague /silvat′ik/ [L, *sylva*, forest; *plaga*, stroke], an endemic disease of wild rodents caused by *Yersinia pestis* and transmissable to humans by the bite of an infected

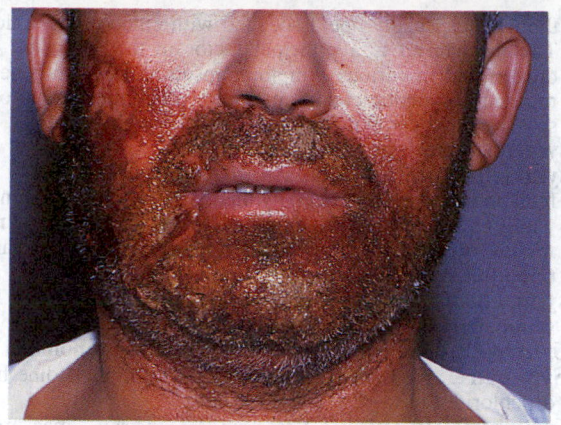

Sycosis barbae *(du Vivier, 1993)*

flea. It is found on every continent except Australia. See also **bubonic plague.**

sylvian aqueduct /sil′vē·ən/ [Franciscus Sylvius, Dutch anatomist, b. 1614], L, *aquaductus,* canal], a canal from the third to the fourth ventricle of the midbrain. Also called **Sylvius' aqueduct.**

sylvian fissure [Franciscus Sylvius; L, *fissura,* cleft], the lateral sulcus of the cerebral hemisphere. Also called **Sylvian sulcus.**

Sylvius' aqueduct. See **Sylvian aqueduct.**

sym-. See **syn-.**

symbiosis /sim′bē·ō′sis/ [Gk, *syn,* together, *bios,* life], **1.** (in biology) a mode of living characterized by close association between organisms of different species, usually in a mutually beneficial relationship. **2.** (in psychiatry) a state in which two mentally disturbed people are emotionally dependent on each other. **3.** pathologic inability of a child to separate from its mother emotionally and, sometimes, physically.

symbiotic /sim′bē·ot′ik/ [Gk, *syn,* together + *bios,* life], characterized by or concerned with symbiosis or living together.

symbiotic phase, in Mahler's system of preoedipal development, the stage between 1 and 5 months when the infant participates in a 'symbiotic orbit' with the mother. All parts of the mother, including voice, gestures, clothing, and space in which she moves, are joined with the infant.

symbol /sim′bəl/ [Gk, *symbolon,* sign], **1.** an image, object, action, or other stimulus that represents something else by reason of conscious association, convention, or other relationship. **2.** an object, mode of behavior, or feeling that disguises a repressed emotional conflict through an unconscious association rather than through an objective relationship, as in dreams and neuroses.

-symbolia, a suffix meaning '(condition involving) the ability to interpret symbols': *asymbolia, dyssymbolia, strephosymbolia.*

symbolism /sim′bəlizəm/, **1.** the representation or evocation of one idea, action, or object by the use of another, as in systems of writing, poetic language, or dream metaphor. **2.** (in psychiatry) an unconscious mental mechanism characteristic of all human thinking in which a mental image stands for but disguises some other object, person, or thought, especially one associated with emotional conflict. The mechanism is a principal factor in the formation of dreams and in various symptoms resulting from such neurotic and psychotic conditions as conversion reactions, obsessions, and compulsions. Also called **symbolization.**

symelus.   See **symmelus.**

symmelia /simē'lyə/ [Gk, *syn*, together, *melos*, limb], a fetal anomaly characterized by the fusion of the lower limbs with or without feet. Kinds of symmelia are **apodial symmelia, dipodial symmelia, monopodial symmelia,** and **tripodial symmelia.**

symmelus /sim'ələs/, a malformed fetus characterized by symmelia. Also spelled **symelus.**

Symmer's disease.   See **giant follicular lymphoma.**

Symmetrel, a trademark for an antiviral (amantadine hydrochloride).

symmetric /simet'rik/ [Gk, *syn* + *metron*, measure], (of the body or parts of the body) equal in size or shape; very similar in relative placement or arrangement about an axis. Also **symmetrical.** Compare **asymmetric.** –**symmetry,** *n.*

symmetric lipomatosis.   See **nodular circumscribed lipomatosis.**

symmetric tonic neck reflex, a normal response in infants to assume the crawl position by extending the arms and bending the knees when the head and neck are extended. The reflex disappears when neurologic and muscular development enables independent limb movement for actual crawling. Also called **crawling reflex.** See also **tonic neck reflex.**

symmetry /sim'ətrē/ [Gk, *syn*, together + *metron*, measure], in anatomy, the correspondence of parts on opposite sides of the body, or equality of parts on both sides of a dividing line.

sympathectomize /sim'pəthek'təmiz/, *v.* [Gk, *sympathein*, to feel with + *ektome*, excision], to interrupt the conduction of nerve impulses along part of the sympathetic trunk by surgery or drugs.

sympathectomy /sim'pəthek'təmē/ [Gk, *sympathein*, to feel with, *ektome*, excision], a surgical interruption of part of the sympathetic nerve pathways, performed for the relief of chronic pain or to promote vasodilation in vascular diseases, such as arteriosclerosis, claudication, Buerger's disease, and Raynaud's phenomenon. The sheath around an artery carries the sympathetic nerve fibers that control constriction of the vessel. Removal of the sheath causes the vessel to relax and expand and allows more blood to pass through it. The operation also may be done with a vascular graft, to increase the blood flow through the graft area. Preoperatively the physician may assess the effect of surgery by injecting sympathetic ganglia with a local anesthesia to interrupt temporarily the sympathetic nerve impulses. The nerves lie along the spinal column and are approached through the back or the neck, using local anesthesia. Postoperatively, the adequacy of circulation in the affected extremity is monitored. An arteriogram shows a widened pathway.

sympathetic /sim'pəthet'ik/ [Gk, *sympathein*, to feel with], **1.** displaying of compassion for another's grief. **2.** pertaining to a division of the autonomic nervous system.

sympathetic amine, a drug that produces effects resembling those manifested by stimulation of the sympathetic nervous system.

sympathetic eye.   See **sympathizing eye.**

sympathetic ganglion [Gk, *sympathein*, to feel with + *ganglion*, knot], a collection of multipolar nerve cells along the course of the sympathetic trunk. Nearly two dozen of the ganglia serve as 'cell stations' on efferent pathways between the cervical and sacral parts of the sympathetic trunk.

sympathetic imbalance [Gk, *sympathein*, to feel with; L, *in balance*], pertaining to vagotony or vagus nerve tension and hyperexcitability of the parasympathetic nervous system as opposed to the sympathetic nervous system. Also called **vagotonia.**

sympathetic irritation [Gk, *sypathein*, to feel with; L, *irritare*, to tease], inflammation of one organ after inflammation of a related organ, such as when trauma to an eye is followed by similar symptoms in the uninjured eye.

sympathetic nerve [Gk, *sympathein*, to feel with; L, *nervus*], any nerve of the sympathetic branch of the autonomic nervous system.

sympathetic nervous system.   See **autonomic nervous system.**

sympathetic ophthalmia, a granulomatous inflammation of the uveal tract of both eyes occurring after an injury to the uveal tract of one eye. Corticosteroids may be helpful in treatment, but surgical enucleation of the originally injured eye may be necessary to preserve vision in the uninjured eye. Also called **metastatic ophthalmia, migratory ophthalmia.**

sympathetic symptom [Gk, *sympathein*, to feel with + *symptoma*, that which occurs], a symptom occurring in one body area when the causative lesion is actually in another area. See also **referred pain.**

sympathetic trunk, one of a pair of chains of ganglia extending along the side of the vertebral column from the base of the skull to the coccyx. Each trunk is part of the sympathetic nervous system and consists of a series of ganglia connected by cords containing various types of fibers. The cranial end of the trunk is formed by the superior cervical ganglion from the internal carotid nerve of the head. In some individuals the caudal ends of both trunks merge into a single ganglion at the coccyx. Interconnection of the trunks is common but rarely occurs above the fifth lumbar nerve. In addition to the ganglia, the trunks contain the preganglionic fibers, which are small and myelinated, the postganglionic fibers, which are mostly unmyelinated, some myelinated afferent fibers, and some unmyelinated afferent fibers. The central ganglia of each trunk are irregularly shaped structures with diameters ranging from 1 to 10 mm. Each sympathetic trunk distributes branches with postganglionic fibers to the autonomic plexuses, the cranial nerves, the individual organs, the nerves accompanying arteries, and the spinal nerves.

sympathizing eye /sim'pəthī'zing/, (in sympathetic ophthalmia) the uninfected eye that becomes infected by lymphatic or blood-borne metastasis of the microorganism. Also called **sympathetic eye.**

sympathize.   See **sympathy.**

sympatholytic, sympatholytic agent.   See **antiadrenergic.**

sympathomimetic /sim'pəthō'mimet'ik/ [Gk, *sympathein* + *mimesis*, imitation], denoting a pharmacologic agent that mimics the effects of stimulation of organs and structures by the sympathetic nervous system by occupying adrenergic receptor sites and acting as an agonist or by increasing the release of the neurotransmitter norepinephrine at postganglionic nerve endings. Various sympathomimetic agents are used as decongestants of nasal and ocular mucosa, such as bronchodilators in the treatment of asthma, bronchitis, bronchiectasis, and emphysema; and vasopressors and cardiac stimulants in the treatment of acute hypotension and shock; they are also used for maintaining normal blood pressure during operations using spinal anesthesia. Drugs in this group include cyclopentamine, dobutamine, dopamine, ephedrine, isoproterenol, metaproterenol, metaraminol, mephentermine, methoxamine, methoxyphenamine, naphazoline, norepinephrine, phenylephrine, phenylpropanolamine, propylhexedrine, protokylol, pseudoephedrine, terbutaline sulfate, tetrahydrozoline, tuaminoheptane, xylmetazoline, and epinephrine, a synthetic isomer of the hormone secreted by the adrenal medulla. Adverse effects of sympathomimetic drugs may be nervousness, severe headache, anxiety, vertigo, nausea, vomiting, dilated pupils, glycosuria, and dysuria. Also **adrenergic.**

sympathomimetic amine. See **adrenergic.**

sympathomimetic bronchodilator, a medication that reduces bronchial muscle spasm because of action that mimics the sympathetic nervous system in producing smooth muscle relaxation.

sympathy /sim′pəthē/ [Gk, *sympathein*], **1.** an expressed interest or concern regarding the problems, emotions, or states of mind of another. Compare **empathy. 2.** the relation that exists between the mind and body causing the one to be affected by the other. **3.** mental contagion or the influence exerted by one individual or group on another and the effects produced, such as the spread of panic, uncontrollable laughter, or yawning. **4.** the physiologic or pathologic relationship between two organs, systems, or parts of the body. **—sympathetic,** *adj.,* **sympathize,** *v.*

symphalangia /sim′fəlan′jē·ə/ [Gk, *syn*, together, *phalanx*, finger], **1.** a condition, usually inherited, characterized by ankylosis of the fingers or toes. **2.** a congenital anomaly in which webbing of the fingers or toes occurs in varying degrees, often in conjunction with other defects of the hands or feet. Also called **symphalangism.** See also **syndactyly.**

symphocephalus /sim′fōsef′ələs/ [Gk, *symphes*, growing together, *kephale*, head], twin fetuses joined at the head. The term is often used as a general designation for fetuses with varying degrees of the anomaly. See also **cephalothoracopagus, craniopagus, syncephalus.**

symphyseal angle /simfiz′ē·əl/ [Gk, *symphysis*, growing together; L, *angulus*, corner], (in dentistry) the angle of the chin, which may be protruding, straight, or receding, according to type.

symphyses. See **symphysis.**

symphysic. See **symphysis.**

symphysic teratism /simfiz′ik/, a congenital anomaly in which there is a fusion of normally separated parts or organs, such as a horseshoe kidney, or in which parts close prematurely, such as the skull bones in craniostenosis.

symphysis /sim′fəsis/, *pl.* **symphyses** [Gk, growing, together], **1.** also called **fibrocartilaginous joint.** a line of union, especially a cartilaginous joint in which adjacent bony surfaces are firmly united by fibrocartilage. **2.** *informal.* symphysis pubis. **—symphysic,** *adj.*

symphysis pubis. See **pubic symphysis.**

sympodia /simpō′dē·ə/ [Gk, *syn*, together, *pous*, foot], a congenital developmental anomaly characterized by fusion of the lower extremities. See also **sirenomelus, sympus.**

symptom /simp′təm/ [Gk, *symptoma*, that which happens], a subjective indication of a disease or a change in condition as perceived by the patient. The halo symptom of glaucoma is the seeing by the patient of colored rings around a single light source. Many symptoms are accompanied by objective signs, such as pruritus, which is often reported with erythema and a maculopapular eruption on the skin. Some symptoms may be objectively confirmed, such as numbness of a body part, which may be confirmed by absence of response to a pin prick. **Primary symptoms** are symptoms that are intrinsically associated with the disease process. **Secondary symptoms** are a consequence of the disease process. Compare **sign.**

symptomatic /simp′təmat′ik/ [Gk, *symptoma*, that which happens], having characteristics of a symptom or indications of a specific disease.

symptomatic esophageal peristalsis, a condition in which peristaltic progression in the body of the esophagus is normal but contractions in the distal esophagus are of increased amplitude and duration. Also called **esophageal spasm, nutcracker esophagus.**

symptomatic impotence [Gk, *symptoma*, that which happens; L, *in*, *potentia*, power], impotence that is the result of poor health or the use of medications.

symptomatic nanism, dwarfism associated with defects in bone growth, tooth formation, and sexual development.

symptomatic neuralgia [[Gk, *symptoma*, that which happens + *neuron*, nerve + *algos*, pain], nerve pain that is secondary to a disease condition.

symptomatic torticollis [Gk, *symptoma*; L, *tortus*, twisted + *collum*, neck], stiff neck caused by a disease in the neck, such as rheumatoid torticollis or myogenic torticollis.

symptomatic treatment. See **treatment.**

symptomatology /simp′təmətol′əjē/ [Gk, *symptoma* + *logos*, science], the science of symptoms of disease in general or of the symptoms of a specific disease.

symptom-bearer, (in psychology) a family member frequently seen as the patient who is functioning poorly because family dynamics interfere with functioning at a higher level.

symptom complex, See **syndrome.**

symptomless carrier. See **passive carrier.**

symptothermal method of family planning /simp′təthur′məl/ [Gk, *symptoma* + *therme*, heat], a natural method of family planning that incorporates the ovulation and basal body temperature methods of family planning. It is more effective than either method used alone and requires fewer days of abstinence, because it enables the fertile period of the menstrual cycle to be more precisely identified.

sympus /sim′pəs/ [Gk, *syn*, together, *pous*, foot], a malformed fetus in which the lower extremities are completely fused or rotated and the pelvis and genitalia are defective. Kinds of sympuses are **sirenomelus, sympus dipus,** and **sympus monopus.** See also **symmelus.**

sympus apus. See **sirenomelus.**

sympus dipus /dē′pəs/, a malformed fetus in which the lower extremities are fused and both feet are formed.

sympus monopus /mon′əpəs/, a malformed fetus in which the lower extremities are fused and one foot is formed. Also called **monopodial symmelia, uromelus.**

syn-, sy-, syl-, sym-, a prefix meaning 'union, or association': *synalgia, syncephalus, synchronous.*

synadelphus /sin′ədel′fəs/, *pl.* **synadelphi** [Gk, *syn* + *adelphos*, brother], a conjoined twin fetal monster with a single head and trunk and eight limbs. Also called **syndelphus, cephalothoracoiliopagus.**

Synalar, a trademark for a glucocorticoid (fluocinolone acetonide).

Synanon, a residential center that provides a therapeutic community approach to rehabilitation for drug abusers.

synapse /sin′aps, sinaps′/ [Gk, *synaptein*, to join], **1.** the region surrounding the point of contact between two neurons or between a neuron and an effector organ, across which nerve impulses are transmitted through the action of a neurotransmitter, such as acetylcholine or norepinephrine. When an impulse reaches the terminal point of one neuron, it causes the release of the neurotransmitter, which diffuses across the gap between the two cells to bind with receptors in the other neuron, muscle, or gland, triggering electric changes that either inhibit or continue the transmission of the impulse. Synapses are polarized so that nerve impulses normally travel in only one direction; they are also subject to fatigue, oxygen deficiency, anesthetics, and other chemical agents. Kinds of synapses include **axoaxonic synapse, axodendritic synapse, axodendrosomatic synapse, axosomatic synapse,** and **dendrodendritic synapse.** Compare **ephapse. 2.** to form a synapse or connection between neurons. **3.** (in genetics) to form a synaptic fusion between homologous chromosomes during meiosis. −**synaptic,** *adj.*

synapsis /sinap′sis/, *pl.* **synapses,** the pairing of homologous chromosomes during the early meiotic prophase stage in gametogenesis to form double or bivalent chromosomes.

synaptic /sinap′tik/ [Gk, *synaptein*, to join], pertaining to or resembling a synapse.

synaptic cleft, the microscopic, extracellular space at the synapse that separates the membrane of the terminal nerve endings of a presynaptic neuron and the membrane of a postsynaptic cell. Nerve impulses are transmitted across this cleft by means of a neurotransmitter. See also **neuromuscular junction.** Also called **synaptic gap.**

synaptic junction, the membranes of both the presynaptic neuron and the postsynaptic receptor cell together with the synaptic cleft. See also **synapse.**

synaptic transmission, the passage of a neural impulse across a synapse from one nerve fiber to another by means of a neurotransmitter. Compare **ephaptic transmission.**

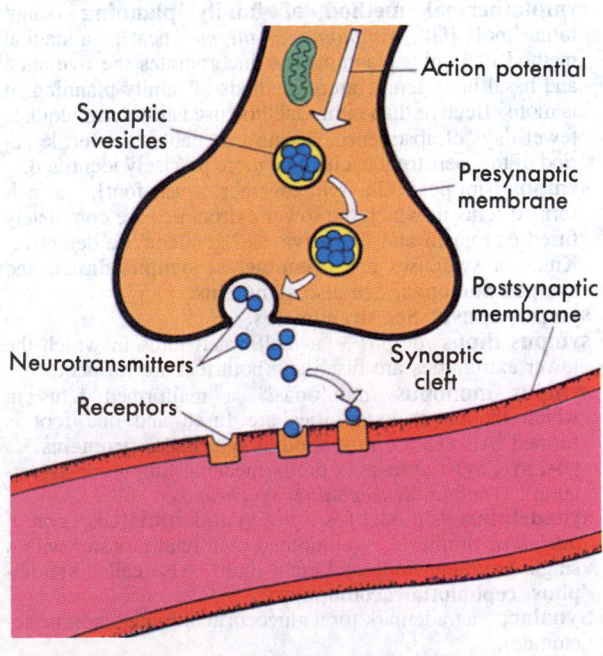

Synaptic transmission (*Chipps, 1992*)

synarthrosis. See **fibrous joint.**
syncheilia. See **synchilia.**
syncephalus /sinsef′ələs/ [Gk, *syn* + *kephale*, head], a conjoined twin monster having a single head and two bodies. Also called **monocephalus.**
synchilia /singkē′lyə/ /singkē′lē·ə/ [Gk, *syn* + *cheilos*, lip], a congenital anomaly in which there is complete or partial fusion of the lips; atresia of the mouth. Also spelled **syncheilia.**
synchondrosis /sing′kondrō′sis/, *pl.* **synchondroses** [Gk, *syn* + *chondros*, cartilage], a cartilaginous joint between two immovable bones, such as the synchondroses of the cranium, the pubic symphysis, the sternum, and the manubrium.
synchorial /singkôr′ē·əl/ [Gk, *syn* + *chorion*, skin], pertaining to multiple fetuses that share a common placenta, as in monozygosity.
synchronized intermittent mandatory ventilation (SIMV) /sing′krənīzd/, periodic assisted mechanical breaths occurring at preset intervals when the patient makes an inspiratory effort that is sensed by the ventilator. Spontaneous breathing by the patient occurs between the assisted mechanical breaths. The machine will provide a mechanical breath if the patient fails to do so within the set time interval.
synchronous /sing′krənəs/, occurring at the same time.
synclitism /sing′klitiz′əm/ [Gk, *syn* + *klinein*, to lean], **1.** (in obstetrics) a condition in which the sagittal suture of the fetal head is in line with the transverse diameter of the inlet, equidistant from the maternal symphysis pubis and sacrum. This position is usually found on examination either late in pregnancy or early in labor, as the fetal head descends into the pelvic inlet. As labor progresses, posterior asynclitism develops, and, as the head descends further, anterior asynclitism is evident because of the shape of the true pelvis below the inlet. **2.** (in hematology) the normal condition in which the nucleus and the cytoplasm of the blood cells mature simultaneously and at the same rate.
syncope /sing′kəpē/ [Gk, *synkoptein*, to cut short], a brief lapse in consciousness caused by transient cerebral hypoxia. It is usually preceded by a sensation of light-headedness and often may be prevented by lying down or by sitting with the head between the knees. It may be caused by many different factors, including emotional stress, vagal stimulation, vascular pooling in the legs, diaphoresis, or sudden change in environmental temperature or body position.
syncretic thinking /singkret′ik/ [Gk, *synkretismos*, combined beliefs; AS, *thencan*, to think], a stage in the development of the cognitive thought processes of the child. During this phase thought is based purely on what is perceived and experienced. The child is incapable of reasoning beyond the observable or of making deductions or generalizations. Through imaginative play, questioning, interaction with others, and the increasing use of language and symbols to represent objects, the child begins to learn to make associations between ideas and to elaborate concepts. In Piaget's classification, this stage occurs between 2 and 7 years of age and is preceded by the sensorimotor stage of development, when the child progresses from reflex activity to repetitive and imitative behavior. Compare **abstract thinking, concrete thinking.** −**syncresis,** *n.*
syncytia. See **syncytium.**
syncytial /sinsish′əl/, pertaining to a syncytium.
syncytial virus a virus that induces the formation of syn-

Diagram labels:
- Action potential
- Synaptic vesicles
- Presynaptic membrane
- Postsynaptic membrane
- Neurotransmitters
- Synaptic cleft
- Receptors

cytia, particularly in cell cultures. Syncytial viruses are members of the spumavirinae subfamily of retroviridae and tend to cause a foamy appearance in syncytial cells.

syncytiotrophoblast /sinsish′ē·ōtrof′əblast′/ [Gk, *syn* + *kytos,* cell, *trophe,* nutrition, *blastos,* germ], the outer syncytial layer of the trophoblast of the early mammalian embryo that erodes the uterine wall during implantation and gives rise to the villi of the placenta. Also called **plasmidotrophoblast, syncytial trophoblast, syntrophoblast.** Compare **cytotrophoblast.** –**syncytiotrophoblastic,** *adj.*

syncytium /sinsit′ē·əm/, *pl.* **syncytia** [Gk, *syn* + *kytos,* cell], a group of cells in which the protoplasm of one cell is continuous with that of adjoining cells.

syndactyl. See **syndactyly.**

syndactylia. See **syndactyly.**

syndactylism /sindak′tiliz′ən/ [Gk, *syn,* together + *daktylos,* finger or toe], a condition in which two or more fingers or toes are fused.

syndactylous. See **syndactyly.**

syndactylus /sindak′tiləs/, a person with webbed fingers or toes.

syndactyly /sindak′təlē/ [Gk, *syn* + *daktylos,* finger], a congenital anomaly characterized by the fusion of the fingers or toes. It varies in degree of severity from incomplete webbing of the skin of two digits to complete union of digits and fusion of the bones and nails. Also called **syndactylia, syndactylism.** –**syndactyl, syndactylous,** *adj.*

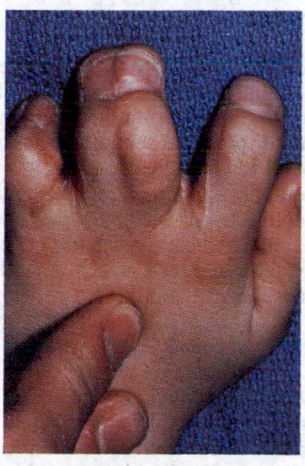

Syndactyly *(Lewis, 1989)*

syndelphus. See **synadelphus.**

syndesis /sin′dəsis/ [Gk, *syn,* together + *dein,* to bind], surgical fixation of a joint. Also called **arthrodesis.**

syndesmo-, a combining form meaning 'of or pertaining to the connective tissue or particularly the ligaments': *syndesmochorial, syndesmography, syndesmoma.*

syndesmosis /sin′desmō′sis/, *pl.* **syndesmoses** [Gk, *syndesmos,* ligament], a fibrous articulation in which two bones are connected by interosseous ligaments, such as the anterior and the posterior ligaments in the tibiofibular articulation. Compare **gomphosis, sutura.**

syndrome /sin′drəm/ [Gk, *syn,* together, *dromos,* course], a complex of signs and symptoms resulting from a common cause or appearing, in combination, to present a clin-

ical picture of a disease or inherited abnormality. See also specific syndromes. Also called **symptom complex.**

syndrome of inappropriate antidiuretic hormone secretion (SIADH), an abnormal condition characterized by the excessive release of antidiuretic hormone (ADH) that upsets the fluid and electrolytic balances of the body. It results from various malfunctions, such as the inability of the body to produce and secrete dilute urine, water retention, increased extracellular fluid volume, and hyponatremia. SIADH develops in association with diseases that affect the osmoreceptors of the hypothalamus. Oat cell carcinoma of the lung is the most common cause, affecting about 80% of involved patients. Less common causes are disorders that affect the central nervous system, such as brain tumors and lupus erythematosus; pulmonary diseases, such as pneumonia; cancers of the pancreas and the prostate; and pathologic reactions to various drugs, such as chlorpropamide, vincristine sulfate, carbamazepine, and clofibrate. Prognosis depends on the underlying disease and the response of the patient to treatment.

■ OBSERVATIONS: Common signs and symptoms of SIADH are weight gain despite anorexia, vomiting, nausea, muscle weakness, and irritability. In some patients SIADH may produce coma and convulsions. Most of the free water associated with this syndrome is intracellular, and associated edema is rare unless excess water volume exceeds 4 mOsm. Confirming diagnosis is based on urine osmolality that exceeds 150 mOsm/kg of water and serum osmolality of less than 280 mOsm/kg of water. Normal urine osmolality is 1.5 times serum osmolality. Other significant results include less than normal concentrations of blood urea nitrogen, serum creatinine, and albumin and a concentration of sodium in the urine higher than normal.

■ INTERVENTIONS: Treatment of SIADH commonly includes restriction of water intake and may require administration of normal saline to raise the serum sodium level if water intoxication is severe. Furosemide may be administered to block circulatory overload, and drugs, such as demeclocycline hydrochloride and lithium, may be administered to block renal response to ADH. Surgery and chemotherapy are other alternatives to remove or destroy neoplasms that may be the underlying causes of this syndrome.

■ NURSING CONSIDERATIONS: Nurses monitor the SIADH patient for any signs of hyponatremia, weight change, and fluid imbalance. The patient is carefully advised on the importance of restricted water intake to prevent water intoxication and is closely observed for any indications of restlessness, congestive heart failure, and convulsions.

synechia /sinek′ē·ə/, *pl.* **synechiae** [Gk, continuity], an adhesion, especially of the iris to the cornea or lens of the eye. It may develop from glaucoma, cataracts, uveitis, or keratitis or as a complication of surgery or trauma to the eye. Synechiae prevent or impede flow of aqueous fluid between the anterior and posterior chambers of the eye and may lead rapidly to blindness. Immediate treatment consists of dilating the pupils with a mydriatic agent, followed by treatment of the underlying cause.

Synemol, a trademark for a glucocorticoid (fluocinolone acetonide).

syneresis /siner′əsis/ [Gk, *syn* + *hairein,* to draw], the drawing together or coagulation of particles of a gel with separation from the medium in which the particles were suspended, such as occurs in blood clot retraction.

synergic. See **synergistic.**

synergism. See **synergy.**

synergist /sin'ərjist/ [Gk, *syn* + *ergein*, to work], an organ, agent, or substance that augments the activity of another organ, agent, or substance.

synergistic /sin'ərjis'tik/ [Gk, *syn*, together + *ergein*, to work], pertaining to the acting or working together of a number of components, as when groups of muscles function in a coordinated manner. Also **synergic** /sinūr'jik/.

synergistic agent, a substance that augments or adds to the activity of another substance or agent.

synergistic muscles, groups of muscles that contract together to accomplish the same body movement.

synergy /sin'ərjē/ [Gk, *syn* + *ergein*, to work], **1.** the process in which two organs, substances, or agents work simultaneously to enhance the function and effect of one another. **2.** the coordinated action of a set of muscles that work together to produce a specific movement, as in a reflex action. **3.** a combined action of different parts of the autonomic nervous system, as in the sympathetic and parasympathetic innervation of secreting cells of the salivary glands, with both systems having a secretory effect. **4.** the interaction of two or more drugs to produce a certain effect, as in the exaggerated response to tyramine in a person who is treated with a monoamine oxidase inhibitor. Also called **synergism.**

syngeneic /sin'jənē'ik/ [Gk, *syn* + *genesis*, origin], **1.** (in genetics) denoting an individual or cell type that has the same genotype as another individual or cell. **2.** (in transplantation biology) denoting tissues that are antigenically similar. Also **isogeneic.** Compare **allogeneic, xenogeneic.**

Synkayvite, a trademark for a brand of menadione, synthetic vitamin K₃.

synkinesis /sin'kinē'sis/ [Gk, *syn*, together + *kinesis*, movement], an involuntary movement by one part of the body when an intentional movement is made by another part. In imitative synkinesis, movement may be detected in paralyzed muscles when normal muscles are moved and vice versa.

synophthalmia. See **cyclopia.**

Synophylate, a trademark for a bronchodilator (theophylline sodium glycinate).

synopsis /sinop'sis/ [Gk, *syn*, together + *opsis*, vision], a brief review, condensation, summary, or abridgement.

synostosis /sin'ostō'sis/ [Gk, *syn*, together + *osteon*, bone], the joining of two bones by the ossification of connecting tissues. It occurs normally in the fusion of cranial bones to form the skull.

synostotic joint /sin'ostot'ik/ [Gk, *syn* + *osteon*, bone], a joint in which bones are joined to bones and there is no movement between them, as in the bones of the adult sacrum or skull.

synotia /sīnō'shə/ [Gk, *syn* + *ous*, ear], a congenital malformation characterized by the union or approximation of the ears in front of the neck, often accompanied by the absence or defective development of the lower jaw. Compare **agnathia.** See also **otocephaly.**

synotus /sīnō'təs/, a fetus with synotia.

synovectomy /sin'ōvek'təmē/ [Gk, *syn* + L, *ovum*, egg; Gk, *ektome*, excision], the excision of a synovial membrane of a joint.

synovia /sīnō'vē·ə/ [Gk, *syn* + L, *ovum*], a transparent, viscous fluid, resembling the white of an egg, secreted by synovial membranes and acting as a lubricant for many joints, bursae, and tendons. It contains mucin, albumin, fat, and mineral salts. Also called **synovial fluid.**

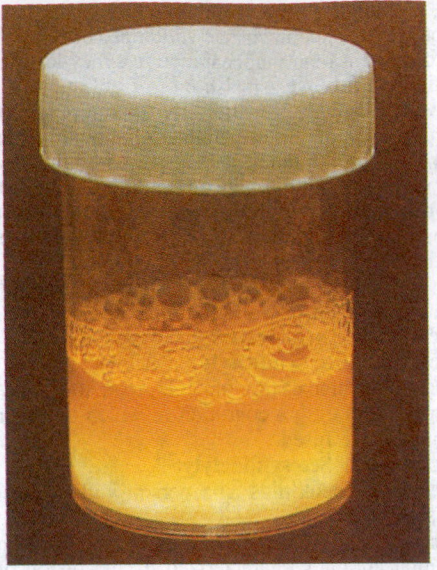

Inflammatory synovial fluid (Shipley, 1993)

synovial /sīnō've·əl/ [Gk, *syn*, together; L, *ovum*, (egg white)], pertaining to, consisting of, or secreting synovia, the lubricating fluid of the joints, bursae and tendon sheaths.

synovial bursa, one of the many closed sacs filled with synovial fluid in the connective tissue between the muscles, the tendons, the ligaments, and the bones. The synovial bursae facilitate the gliding of muscles and tendons over bony and ligamentous prominences. Compare **synovial membrane, synovial tendon sheath.**

synovial chondroma, a rare cartilaginous growth developing in the connective tissue below the synovial membrane of the joints, tendon sheaths, or bursa. Foci on the surface may develop stalks and then detach, resulting in numerous loose bodies within the joint. Also called **synovial chondromatosis.**

synovial crypt, a pouch in the synovial membrane of a joint.

synovial fluid. See **synovia.**

synovial joint, a freely movable joint in which contiguous bony surfaces are covered by articular cartilage and connected by ligaments lined with synovial membrane. Kinds of synovial joints are **ball and socket joint, condyloid joint, gliding joint, hinge joint, pivot joint, saddle joint,** and **uniaxial joint.** Also called **diarthrosis.** Compare **cartilaginous joint, fibrous joint.**

synovial membrane, the inner layer of an articular capsule surrounding a freely movable joint. The synovial membrane is loosely attached to the external fibrous capsule. It secretes into the joint a thick fluid that normally lubricates the joint but that may accumulate in painful amounts when the joint is injured. Compare **synovial bursa, synovial tendon sheath.**

synovial sarcoma, a malignant tumor, composed of synovioblasts, that begins as a soft swelling and often metastasizes through the bloodstream to the lung before it is discovered.

synovial sheath, any one of the membranous sacs enclosing a tendon of a muscle and facilitating the gliding of a tendon through a fibrous or a bony tunnel, such as that under the flexor retinaculum of the wrist.

synovial tendon sheath, one of the many membranous sacs enclosing various tendons that glide through fibrous and bony tunnels in the body, such as those under the flexor retinaculum of the wrist. One layer of the synovial sheath lines the tunnel; the other covers the tendon. The sheath secretes synovial fluid, which lubricates the tendon. Compare **synovial bursa, synovial membrane.**

synovitis /sin′əvī′tis/ [Gk, *syn* + L, *ovum;* Gk, *itis*], an inflammatory condition of the synovial membrane of a joint as the result of an aseptic wound or a traumatic injury, such as a sprain or severe strain. The knee is most commonly affected. Fluid accumulates around the capsule; the joint is swollen, tender, and painful; and motion is restricted. In most cases, the inflammation subsides, and the fluid is resorbed without medical or surgical intervention.

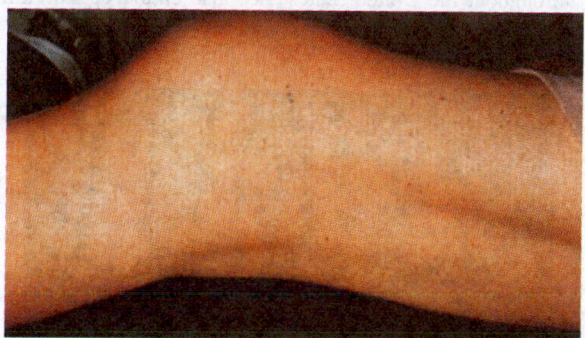

Synovitis of the knee (Shipley, 1993)

synovium /sinō′vē·əm/ [Gk, *syn,* together; L, *ovum,* (egg white)], a synovial membrane.

syntactic aphasia /sintak′tik/ [Gk, *syn,* together + *taxis,* arrangement + *a phasis,* speech], an inability to arrange words in a logical sequence, with the result that what is spoken is not understood.

syntax /sin′taks/ [Gk, *syn* + *taxis,* arrangement], a property of language involving structural cues for the arrangement of words as elements in a phrase, clause, or sentence.

syntaxic mode /sintaks′ik/, the ability to perceive whole, logical, coherent pictures as they occur in reality, according to the Sullivan theory of psychology.

synteny /sin′tənē/ [Gk, *syn* + *taina,* ribbon], (in genetics) the presence on the same chromosome of two or more genes that may or may not be transmitted as a linkage group but that appear to be able to undergo independent assortment during meiosis. The term is used primarily in human genetics where linked inheritance patterns are more difficult to determine. See also **linkage.**

synthesis /sin′thəsis/ [Gk, *synthenai,* to put together], a level of cognitive learning in which the individual puts together the elements of previous learning levels to create a unified whole.

-synthesis, a combining form meaning 'putting together or formation of': *narcosynthesis, psychosynthesis, velosynthesis.*

synthesize /sin′thəsīz/ [Gk, *synthesis,* putting together], to

form by building, as in forming complex chemical compounds such as proteins from simpler units of amino acids.

synthetic /sinthet′ik/, of or pertaining to a substance that is produced by an artificial rather than a natural process or material.

synthetic chemistry, the science dealing with the formation of more complex chemical compounds from simpler substances.

synthetic human growth hormone, a synthetic form of somatotropin produced by recombinant DNA techniques from a strain of *E. coli* bacteria. The polypeptide hormone consists of 191 amino acid residues in a sequence identical to that of natural human growth hormone.

synthetic insulin [Gk, *synthesis,* putting together; L, *insula,* island (of Langerhans)], a form of insulin synthesized in a non-disease-producing strain of *E. coli* bacteria or in yeast cells that has been genetically altered by the addition of the human gene for insulin production.

synthetic oleovitamin D. See **viosterol.**

synthetic saliva. See **artificial saliva.**

Synthroid, a trademark for a thyroid hormone (levothyroxine sodium).

Syntocinon, a trademark for an oxytocic (oxytocin).

syntrophoblast. See **syncytiotrophoblast.**

syphilis /sif′ilis/ [from the name of a literary figure (1530) who was thus infected (literally, 'lover of swine,' from GK *sys,* pig + *philos,* loving)], a sexually transmitted disease caused by the spirochete, *Treponema pallidum,* characterized by distinct stages of effects over a period of years. Any organ system may become involved. The spirochete is able to pass through the human placenta, producing congenital syphilis. Also called **leus.**

■ OBSERVATIONS: The first stage (**primary syphilis**) is marked by the appearance of a small, painless, red pustule on the skin or mucous membrane between 10 and 90 days after exposure. The lesion may appear anywhere on the body where contact with a lesion on an infected person has occurred, but is seen most often in the anogenital region. It quickly erodes, forming a painless, bloodless ulcer, called a chancre, exuding a fluid that swarms with spirochetes. The chancre may not be noticed by the patient, and many people may become infected. It heals spontaneously within 10 to 40 days, often creating the mistaken impression that the sore was not a serious event. The second stage (**secondary syphilis**) occurs about 2 months later, after the spirochetes have increased in number and spread throughout the body. This stage is characterized by general malaise, anorexia, nausea, fever, headache, alopecia, bone and joint pain, or the appearance of a morbilliform rash that does not itch, flat white sores in the mouth and throat, or condylomata lata papules on the moist areas of the skin. The disease remains highly contagious at this stage and can be spread by kissing. The symptoms usually continue for from 3 weeks to 3 months but may be recurrent over a period of 2 years. The third stage (**tertiary syphilis**) may not develop for 3 to 15 or more years. It is characterized by the appearance of soft, rubbery tumors, called gummas, that ulcerate and heal by scarring. Gummas may develop anywhere on the surface of the body and in the eye, liver, lungs, stomach, or reproductive organs. Tertiary syphilis may be painless, unnoticed except for gummas, or it may be accompanied by deep, burrowing pain. The ulceration of the gummas may result in punched-out areas of the palate, nasal septum, or larynx. Various tissues and structures of the body, including the central nervous system, myocardium, and the valves of the heart, may be damaged or destroyed, leading to mental or physical disability and premature death. **Congenital syphilis** resulting from prenatal infection may result in the birth of a deformed or blind infant. In some cases, the infant appears to be well until, at several weeks of age, snuffles, sometimes with a blood-stained or mucopurulent discharge, and skin lesions, particularly on the palms and soles or in the genital region are observed. Such children also may have visual or hearing defects, and progeria and poor health may develop. Diagnosis of syphilis is made by darkfield microscopy of fluid from primary or secondary stage lesions, by bacteriologic study of blood samples, and by an examination of cerebrospinal fluid. Because of the slow development of the disease during the early stages, the various serologic tests, including the obsolete Wassermann, may not be accurate until months after exposure. Repeated tests and crosschecking with more than one test may be required in some cases. The report by a person that exposure to syphilis has occurred is often the only evidence available to the clinician.

■ INTERVENTIONS: Patients with primary or secondary syphilis are usually given benzathine penicillin or an equivalent in a single dose of 2.4 million units. The objective is to maintain penicillin in the bloodstream for a number of days, because *Treponema pallidum* divides at an average rate of once every 33 hours, and the antibiotic is most effective during the stage of cell division. Larger doses of penicillin, 7.2 million units total, are administered in 3 doses 1 week apart for tertiary syphilis. Infants and small children with congenital syphilis are usually given 50,000 units/kg intramuscularly. Treatment of an infected mother with penicillin during the first 4 months of pregnancy usually prevents the development of congenital syphilis in the fetus. Treating the mother with antibiotics later in the pregnancy usually eliminates the infection but may not protect the fetus. Patients should be reexamined clinically and serologically 3 months and 6 months after treatment. HIV-infected patients (also infected with syphilis) should be seen at 1, 2, 3, 6, 9, and 12 months for follow-up.

■ NURSING CONSIDERATIONS: Special care and aseptic precautions are taken while handling the highly contagious fluid from syphilitic lesions used in diagnostic testing, because the infection may be acquired through a cut or break in the skin. The nurse must discuss the disease course, its treatment, and ways of preventing future infections with the patient. The extremely contagious nature of the infection is explained, and the importance of treatment for all who may have been exposed is emphasized. Tact, patience, and understanding are required to reassure the patient, and to secure the patient's cooperation in accepting treatment and in assisting in the identification and location of others needing treatment. Active, serologically documented cases of syphilis must, by law, be reported to local Departments of Health throughout the United States. See also **chancre, Hutchinson's teeth, Hutchinson's triad, snuffles.**

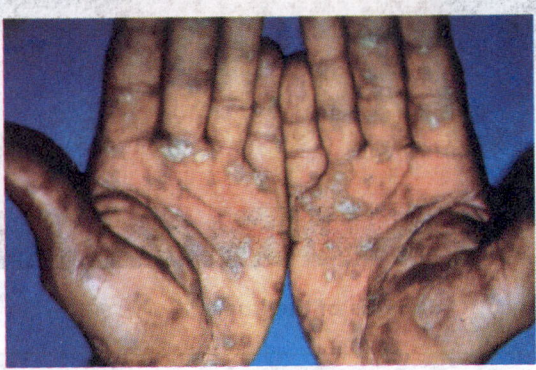

Secondary syphilis (Goldstein, 1992)

syphilitic /sif′ilit′ik/, pertaining to, resembling, or infected with syphilis. Also **luetic** /lōō·et′ik/.

syphilitic aortitis, an inflammatory condition of the aorta, occurring in tertiary syphilis and characterized by diffuse dilatation with gray, wheal-like plaques containing calcium on the inner coat and scars and wrinkles on the outer coat. The middle layer of the vascular wall is usually infiltrated with plasma cells and contains fragments of damaged elastic tissue and many newly formed blood vessels. There may be damage to the aortic valves, narrowing of the mouths of the coronary arteries, and the formation of thrombi. Cerebral embolism may result. Signs of syphilitic aortitis are substernal pain, dyspnea, bounding pulse, and high systolic blood pressure. Penicillin may slow the course of the disease, but it cannot reverse the structural damage to the vessels and the heart. Also called **Döhle-Heller disease, luetic aortitis.**

syphilitic dementia [L, *de, mens* mind], a general mental deterioration disorder resulting from a syphilis infection. Specific symptoms may vary from memory impairment to personality changes and are severe enough to interfere with social and occupational activities. If untreated, the disease may progress to dementia paralytica, paralysis, and death.

Primary syphilis
(Greenberger, 1993/Courtesy Dr WS Royster, US Public Health Service, Kansas City, Missouri)

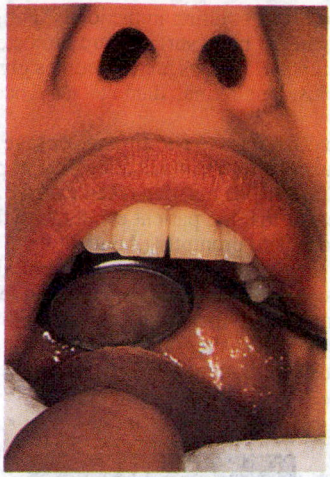

Syphilitic aortitis (Fletcher, 1987)

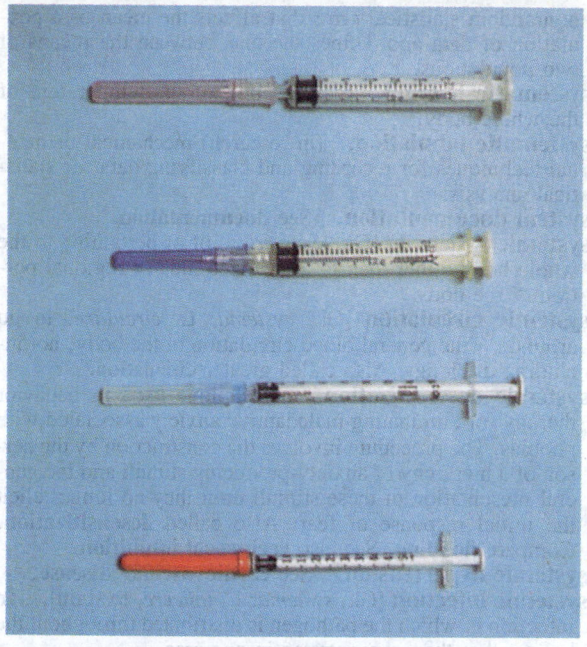

Syringes (Potter, 1993)

syphilitic endocarditis [*endon*, within + *kardia*, heart + *itis*, inflammation], a thickening and stretching of the cusps of the aortic valve, with aortic valve incompetence, caused by a syphilis infection of the aorta.

syphilitic fever [L, *febris*], pyrexia that is due to a syphilis infection.

syphilitic heart disease. See **cardiovascular disease.**

syphilitic meningoencephalitis. See **general paresis.**

syphilitic periarteritis, an inflammatory condition of the outer coat of one or more arteries occurring in tertiary syphilis and characterized by soft gummatous perivascular lesions infiltrated with lymphocytes and plasma cells. Also called **periarteritis gummosa.** See also **syphilitic aortitis.**

syphilitic retinopathy [L, *rete*, net; Gk, *pathos*, disease], an invasion of the retina and optic nerve by a spreading syphilis infection. Primary retinal lesions are associated with the blood vessels, and the choroid layer is often affected first. There may be occlusion of the retinal vessels.

syr., The Latin work syrupus, 'syrup.'

syring-. See **syringo-.**

syringe /sərinj′, sir′inj/ [Gk, *syrinx*, tube], a device for withdrawing, injecting, or instilling fluids. A syringe for the injection of medication usually consists of a calibrated glass or plastic cylindric barrel having a close-fitting plunger at one end and a small opening at the other to which the head of a hollow-bore needle is fitted. Medication of the desired amount may be pulled up into the barrel by suction as the plunger is withdrawn and injected by pushing the plunger back into the barrel, forcing the liquid out through the needle. A syringe for irrigating a wound or body cavity or for extracting mucus or another body fluid from an orifice or body cavity is usually larger than the kind used for injection. It often has a rubber bulb at one end and a blunt, soft-tipped, flexible tube with an opening at the other end. The bulb is squeezed to eject a fluid and is released to withdraw one. Kinds of syringe include **Asepto syringe, bulb syringe, hypodermic syringe, Luer-Lok syringe,** and **tuberculin syringe.**

syringectomy /sir′injek′təmē/ [Gk, *syrinx*, tube + *ektome*, excision], a surgical procedure for excising the walls of a fistula.

syringo-, syring- /siring′gō-/, a combining form meaning 'of or pertaining to a tube or a fistula': *syringobulbia, syringocystoma, syringomyelitis*.

syringomeningocele /-məning′gōsēl′/ [Gk, *syrinx*, tube + *meningx*, membrane + *kele*, tumor], a meningocele that is connected to the central canal of the spinal cord. See also **spina bifida.**

syringomyelia /-mī·ē′lyə/ [Gk, *syrinx*, tube + *myelos*, marrow], a chronic progressive disease of the spinal cord, marked by elongated central fluid-containing cavities, surrounded by gliosis or a proliferation of neurological tissue. Symptoms begin early in adulthood, usually involving the cervical region with muscular wasting in the upper limbs. It is more common in males.

syringomyelocele /siring′gōmī′əlōsēl′/ [Gk, *syrinx* + *myelos*, marrow, *kele*, hernia], a hernial protrusion of the spinal cord through a congenital defect in the vertebral column in which the cerebrospinal fluid within the central cavities of the cord is greatly increased so that the cord tissue forms a thin-walled sac that lies close to the membrane of the cavity. See also **myelomeningocele, neural tube defect, spina bifida.**

syrup of ipecac /sir′əp/, an emetic preparation of ipecac fluid extract, glycerin, and syrup used to treat certain types of poisonings and drug overdoses. See also **ipecac.**

system /sis′təm/ [Gk, *systema*], **1.** a collection or assemblage of parts that, unified, make a whole. Physiologic systems, such as the cardiovascular or reproductive systems, are made up of structures specifically able to engage in processes that are essential for a vital function in the body. **2.** a set of computer programs and hardware that work together for some specific purpose.

systematic /sis′təmat′ik/ [Gk, *systema*], pertaining to a system.

systematic error [Gk, *systema*; L, *errare*, to wander], a nonrandom statistical error that affects the mean of a population of data and defines the bias between the means of two populations.

systematic heating, the elevation of the temperature of the whole body.

systematic tabulation, (in research) mechanical or manual techniques for recording and classifying data for statistical analysis.

system documentation. See **documentation.**

systemic /sistem'ik/ [Gk, *systema*], of or pertaining to the whole body rather than to a localized area or regional portion of the body.

systemic circulation [Gk, *systema;* L, *circulare,* to go around], the general blood circulation of the body, not including the lungs. Also called greater circulation.

systemic desensitization, a technique used in behavior therapy for eliminating maladaptive anxiety associated with phobias. The procedure involves the construction by the person of a hierarchy of anxiety-producing stimuli and the general presentation of these stimuli until they no longer elicit the initial response of fear. Also called **desensitization.** Compare **flooding.** See also **reciprocal inhibition.**

systemic hypertension. See **cardiovascular disease.**

systemic infection [Gk, *systema;* L, *inficere,* to stain], an infection in which the pathogen is distributed throughout the body rather than concentrated in one area.

systemic lesion [Gk, *systema;* L, *laesio,* attack], a pathological disturbance that involves a system of tissues with a common function.

systemic lupus erythematosus (SLE), a chronic inflammatory disease affecting many systems of the body. The pathophysiology of the disease includes severe vasculitis, renal involvement, and lesions of the skin and nervous system. The primary cause of the disease has not been determined; viral infection or dysfunction of the immune system has been suggested. Adverse reaction to certain drugs also may cause a lupuslike syndrome. Four times more women than men have SLE. Also called **disseminated lupus erythematosus, lupus erythematosus.**

■ OBSERVATIONS: The initial manifestation is often arthritis. An erythematous rash over the nose and malar eminences, weakness, fatigue, and weight loss also are frequently seen early in the disease. Photosensitivity, fever, skin lesions on the neck, and alopecia where the skin lesions extend beyond the hairline may occur. The skin lesions may spread to the mucous membranes and other tissues of the body. They do not ulcerate but cause degeneration of the tissues affected. Depending on the organs involved, the patient also may have glomerulonephritis, pleuritis, pericarditis, peritonitis, neuritis, or anemia. Renal failure and severe neurologic abnormalities are among the most serious manifestations of the disease. Diagnosis of SLE is made by subjective and objective findings based on physical examination and laboratory findings, including antinuclear antibody in the cerebrospinal fluid and a positive lupus erythematosus (LE) cell reaction in a lupus erythematosus preparation (LE prep). Other laboratory examinations may be useful, depending on the organs, tissues, and systems affected by the disease.

■ INTERVENTIONS: In many cases SLE may be controlled with corticosteroid medication administered systemically. Care and treatment vary with the severity and nature of the disease and the body systems that are affected. Topical steroids may be applied to the rash; salicylates may be given to alleviate pain and swelling in the joints. Fatigue and stress are avoided, and all body surfaces are protected from direct sunlight. Antimalarial drugs are sometimes given to treat cutaneous lesions, but retinal damage may occur with prolonged use.

■ NURSING CONSIDERATIONS: The timing, dosage, side effects, and toxic reactions to the medications are explained before discharge. The steroids must be taken exactly as prescribed, and, in the event that the patient cannot take them, the doctor is to be consulted promptly. An identification card is carried bearing the patient's diagnosis, a list of all medications and their dosage, and the doctor's name and telephone number. As in any disease marked by chronic remission and exacerbation of many distressing symptoms, the patient may require extensive emotional and psychologic support.

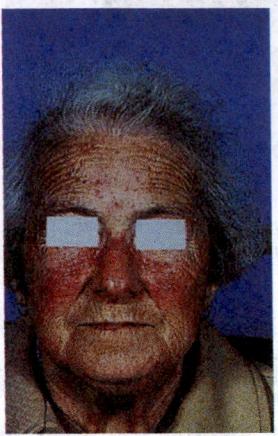

"Butterfly rash" of systemic lupus erythematosus
(Lamey, 1988)

systemic mycosis [Gks, *systema,* + *mykess* fungus + *osiss* condition], a fungal infection that involves more than one body system or area.

systemic oxygen consumption, the amount of oxygen consumed by the body's tissues as measured during a period of 60 seconds.

systemic remedy, a medicinal substance that is given orally, parenterally, or rectally to be absorbed into the circulation for treatment of a health problem. Many remedies or medications administered locally or regionally are to some degree absorbed systemically. Medication administered systemically may have various local effects, but the intent is to treat the whole body.

systemic vascular resistance (SVR), the resistance against which the left ventricle must eject to force out its stroke volume with each beat. As the peripheral vessels constrict, the SVR increases.

systemic vein, one of a number of veins that drain deoxygenated blood from most of the body. Systemic veins arise in tiny plexuses that receive blood from the billions of capillaries lacing the body tissues and converge into trunks that increase in size as they pass toward the heart. They are larger and more numerous than the arteries, have thinner walls, and collapse when they are empty. Kinds of systemic veins are identified according to location, such as deep veins, superficial veins, and venous sinuses. Groups of systemic veins include the coronary veins, the superior vena cava and its tributaries in the upper body, and the inferior vena cava and its tributaries in the lower body.

system of care /sis′təm/, a framework within which health care is provided, comprising health care professionals; recipients, consumers, or patients; energy resources or dynamics; organizational and political contexts or frameworks; and processes or procedures. Current theory recognizes that an analysis of the provision of health care requires knowledge of the systems of care.

system overload, an inability to cope with messages and expectations from a number of sources within a given time limit.

systems software a group of computer utilities programs that control the execution of applications programs.

systems theory, a holistic medical concept in which the human patient is viewed as an integrated complex of open systems rather than as semiindependent parts. The health care approach in this theory requires the incorporation of family, community, and cultural factors as influences to be considered in the diagnosis and treatment of the patient.

systole /sis′təlē/ [Gk, *systole*, contraction], the contraction of the heart, driving blood into the aorta and pulmonary arteries. The occurrence of systole is indicated by the first heart sound heard on auscultation, by the palpable apex beat, and by the peripheral pulse.

-systole, a suffix referring to 'types and locations of the higher blood pressure measurement': *dyssystole, hysterosystole, tachysystole*.

systolic /sistol′ik/ [Gk, *systole*, contraction], pertaining to or resulting from a heart contraction.

systolic click [Gk, *systole,* contraction; Fr, *cliqueter* to click], an extra sound having a clicklike quality heard in mid- or late systole, and believed to originate from the abnormal motion of the mitral valve. The most frequent cause of systolic clicks is prolapse of a mitral valve leaflet, in which case there may be an associated late systolic regurgitant murmur sometimes called the click syndrome.

systolic dysfunction a loss of cardiac muscle with volume overload and decreased contractility.

systolic ejection period, the amount of time spent in systole per minute.

systolic gradient, the difference in pressure in the left atrium and left ventricle during systole.

systolic murmur, cardiac murmur occurring during systole. Systolic murmurs include ejection murmurs often heard in pregnancy or in people with anemia, thyrotoxicosis, or aortic or pulmonary stenosis; pansystolic murmurs heard in people with incompetence of the mitral or tricuspid valve; and late systolic murmurs, also caused by mitral valve incompetence.

systolic pressure, the blood pressure measured during the period of ventricular contraction (systole). In blood pressure readings, it is normally the higher of the two measurements.

T, **1.** symbol for **temperature. 2.** abbreviation for *tumor.*
See **cancer staging.**

T₁, T₂. See **relaxation time.**

T₃, symbol for **triiodothyronine.**

T₄, symbol for **thyroxine.**

Ta, symbol for the element **tantalum.**

TA, abbreviation for **transactional analysis.**

ta-. See **tono-.**

tabardillo. See **Mexican typhus.**

tabe-, a combining form meaning 'of or pertaining to wasting (away)': *tabefaction, tabescent, tabetiform.*

tabes /tā′bēz/ [L, *tabes,* wasting], a gradual, progressive wasting of the body in any chronic disease.

tabes dorsalis [L, *tabes,* wasting; *dorsum,* the back], an abnormal condition characterized by the slow degeneration of all or part of the body and the progressive loss of deep tendon reflexes. This disease involves the posterior columns and the posterior roots of the spinal cord and destroys the large joints of affected limbs in some individuals. A wide-base ataxic gait is usually present. It is often accompanied by incontinence and impotence and severe flashing pains in the abdomen and the extremities. The cause of tabes dorsalis is syphilitic.

tabetic crisis /tābet′ik/ [L, *tabes,* wasting; Gk, *krisis,* turning point], an exacerbation of pain in tabes dorsalis because of syphilis.

tabetic gait [L, *tabes,* wasting; ONorse, *gata,* a way], a high-steppage gait associated with the tertiary form of tabes. The condition results from degeneration of the dorsal columns of the spinal cord and of sensory nerve trunks. See **tabes dorsalis.**

tabetic neuritis [L, *tabes,* wasting; Gk, *neuron,* nerve + *itis,* inflammation], a form of neuritis that accompanies a syphilitic infection or tabes dorsalis, involving the dorsal posterior column spinal pathways.

tablet /tab′lit/ [Fr, *tablette,* lozenge], a small, solid dosage form of a medication. It may be compressed or molded in its manufacture, and it may be of almost any size, shape, weight, and color. Most tablets are intended to be swallowed whole, but some may be dissolved in the mouth, chewed, or dissolved in liquid before swallowing; some may be placed in a body cavity.

taboo /təboo′/, something that is forbidden by a society as unacceptable or improper. Incest is a taboo common to many societies.

taboparesis /tā′bōpəre′sis/ [L, *tabes,* wasting; Gk, *paralyein,* to be palsied], a form of paralysis associated with cerebral syphilis. Also called **taboparalysis.**

tabula rasa /tā′boolä rä′sä, tab′yəle rā′sə/, a term used to describe a child's mind at birth as a receptive 'blank slate.'

Tacaryl, a trademark for an antihistamine (methdilazine).

TACE, a trademark for an estrogen (chlorotrianisene).

tache laiteuse. See **macula albidae.**

tache noire /täshnô·är′/ [Fr, black spot], a local ulcerous lesion marking the point of infection in certain rickettsial diseases, such as African tick typhus and scrub typhus.

tacho-, a combining form meaning 'of or pertaining to speed': *tachogram, tachography, tachometer.*

tachy- /tak′ē-/, a combining form meaning 'swift or rapid': *tachycardia, tachyphrenia, tachysystole.*

tachycardia /tak′ikär′dē·ə/ [Gk, *tachys,* fast, *kardia,* heart], a condition in which the myocardium contracts at a rate greater than 100 beats per minute. The heart rate normally accelerates in response to fever, exercise, or nervous excitement. Pathologic tachycardia accompanies anoxia, such as caused by anemia, congestive heart failure, hemorrhage, or shock. Tachycardia acts to increase the amount of oxygen delivered to the cells of the body by increasing the amount of blood circulated through the vessels.

tachycardiac /-kär′dē·ak/ [Gk, *tachys,* fast + *kardia,* heart], pertaining to or affected by tachycardia.

tachydysrythmia /tak′ē·ərith′mē·ə/ [Gk, *tachys* fast + *a, rhythmos,* rhythm], an abnormally rapid heart beat.

tachykinin. See **substance P.**

tachyphylaxis /tak′əfəlak′sis/ [Gk, *tachys,* + *phylax,* guard], **1.** (in pharmacology) a phenomenon in which the repeated administration of some drugs results in a marked decrease in effectiveness. **2.** also called **mithridatism.** (in immunology) rapidly developing immunity to a toxin because of previous exposure, such as from previous injection of small amounts of the toxin.

tachypnea /tak′ipnē′ə/ [Gk, *tachys* + *pnoia,* breathing], an abnormally rapid rate of breathing, such as seen with hyperpyrexia. See also **pulmonary ventilation.**

tack, the degree of stickiness of an adhesive required to affix a therapeutic foreign substance, such as a transdermal delivery device, to the skin.

tact-, a prefix meaning 'of or pertaining to touch': *tactile, tactilogical, taction.*

-tactic, -tactical, -taxic, **1.** a suffix meaning 'exhibiting agent-controlled orientation or movement': *chemotactic, eosinotactic, thermotactic.* **2.** a suffix combining form meaning 'having an arrangement of something': *cytotactic, leukotactic, phyllotactic.*

tactile /tak′təl/, tak′tīl/ [L, *tactus,* touch], of or pertaining to the sense of touch.

tactile amnesia [L, *tactus;* Gk, *amnesia,* forgetfulness], a loss of the ability to determine the shape of objects through the sense of touch. See also **astereognosis.**

tactile anesthesia, the absence or lack of the sense of touch in the fingers, possibly resulting from injury or disease. This condition can be congenital or psychosomatic and may cause the patient to incur severe burns, serious cuts, contusions, or abrasions. See also **traumatic anesthesia.**

tactile corpuscle, any one of many small, oval end organs associated with the sense of touch, widely distributed throughout the body in peripheral areas, such as the papillae of the corium of the hand and foot, front of the forehead, skin of the lips, mucous membrane of the tongue, palpebral conjunctivae, and skin of the mammary papillae. Each corpuscle consists of a tiny round structure surrounded by a capsule penetrated by a nerve fiber that spirals through the interior of the capsule and ends in globular enlargements. Also called **Meissner's corpuscle.**

tactile corpuscle of Meissner. See **Wagner-Meissner corpuscle.**

tactile defensiveness, a sensory integrative dysfunction characterized by tactile sensations that cause excessive emotional reactions, hyperactivity, or other behavior problems.

tactile discrimination [L, *tactus* + *discrimen* division], the ability to discriminate among objects by the sense of touch.

tactile fremitus, a tremulous vibration of the chest wall during breathing that is palpable on physical examination. It may indicate inflammation, infection, congestion, or consolidation of a lung or a part of a lung.

tactile hair [L, *tactus*; AS, *haer*], a hair shaft that is sensitive to the sensation of touch.

tactile hallucination [L, *tactus* + *alucinare,* wandering mind], a subjective experience of touch in the absence of tactile stimulation.

tactile hyperesthesia [L, *tactus*; Gk, *hyper,* excessive + *aesthesis,* sensitivity], an abnormal increase in the sense of touch.

tactile image, a mental concept of an object as perceived through the sense of touch. See also **image.**

tactile localization [L, *tactus* + *locus,* place], the ability to identify, without looking, the exact point on the body that a tactile stimulus is applied. The localization test is applied in sensory evaluation tests.

tactile sensation [L, *tactus* + *sentire,* to feel], the sensation of touch.

tactile system [L, *tactus*; Gk, *systema*], the part of the nervous system that is concerned with the sense of touch.

Taenia /tē′nē·ə/ [Gk, *tainia,* ribbon], a genus of large, parasitic, intestinal flatworm of the family Taeniidae, class Cestoda, having an armed scolex and a series of segments in a chain. Taeniae are among the most common parasites infecting humans and include *Taenia saginata,* the beef tapeworm, and *T. solium,* the pork tapeworm.

taenia-. See **tenia-.**

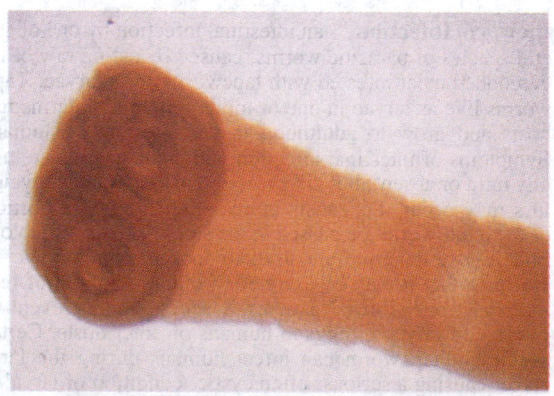

Taenia saginata scolex (Muller, 1990)

Taenia saginata, a species of tapeworm that inhabits the tissues of cattle during its larval stage and infects the intestine of humans in its adult form. *Taenia saginata* may grow to a length of between 12 and 25 feet and is the tapeworm species that most often infects humans. Also called **beef tapeworm.** See also **tapeworm, tapeworm infection.**

taeniasis /tēnī′əsis/ [Gk, *tainia* + *osis,* condition], an infection with a tapeworm of the genus *Taenia.* See also **tapeworm infection.**

Taenia solium, a species of tapeworm that most commonly inhabits the tissues of pigs during its larval stage and infects the intestine of humans in its adult form. Infrequently, humans will serve as the intermediate hosts for this tapeworm, and larval infestation of the muscle and brain tissue may occur. Also called **pork tapeworm.** See also **cysticercosis, tapeworm, tapeworm infection.**

TAF, abbreviation for **tumor angiogenesis factor**.

TAG, abbreviation for 3,4,6-tri-O-acetyl-D-glucal.

Tagamet, a trademark for a histamine H_2 receptor antagonist (cimetidine).

tail bud. See **end bud.**

tail fold [AS, *taegel; fealdan,* to fold], a curved ridge formed at the caudal end of the early developing embryo. It consists of the tail bud, which in lower animals gives rise to the caudal appendage and in humans forms the hindgut.

tail of Spence, the upper outer tail of breast tissue that extends into the axilla.

tailor's bottom. See **weaver's bottom.**

tailor's bunion. See **bunionette.**

Takayasu's arteritis /tä′kəyä′sōōz/ [Michishige Takayasu, Japanese physician, b. 1871], an inflammatory disorder of the aorta, its major branches, and the pulmonary artery. It is characterized by progressive occlusion of the innominate and the left subclavian and left common carotid arteries above their origin in the aortic arch. Signs of the disorder are absence of a pulse in both arms and in the carotid arteries, transient paraplegia, transient blindness, and atrophy of facial muscles. Also called **aortic arch syndrome, brachiocephalic arteritis, pulseless disease.**

talbutal /tal′byōōtə/, a barbiturate sedative-hypnotic.

■ INDICATION: It is prescribed as a hypnotic in the treatment of insomnia.

■ CONTRAINDICATIONS: Previous addiction to sedative-hypnotics, porphyria, impaired hepatic function, or known hypersensitivity to this drug or to other barbiturates prohibits its use.

■ ADVERSE EFFECTS: Among the more serious adverse effects are respiratory depression, drug hangover, allergic reactions, porphyria, and physical dependence.

talip-, a combining form meaning 'a nontraumatic (usually congenital) twisting defect or clubfooted': *taliped, talipes, talipomanus.*

talipes /tal′ipēz/ [L, *talus,* ankle, *pes,* foot], a deformity of the foot, usually congenital, in which the foot is twisted and relatively fixed in an abnormal position. Talipes refers to deformities that involve the foot and ankle, whereas pes refers only to a deformity of the foot. Kinds of talipes include **talipes calcaneovalgus, talipes calcaneovarus,** and **talipes equinovarus.** See also **pes cavus, pes planus.**

talipes calcaneovalgus. See **clubfoot.**

talipes cavus. See **pes cavus.**

talipes equinovarus. See **clubfoot.**

talo-, a prefix meaning 'of or pertaining to the ankle': *talocalcaneal, talocrural, talofibular.*

talonavicular /tā'lōnəvik'yələr/ [L, *talon*, bird claw + *naviculus*, scaphoid], pertaining to the talus and the navicular bones.

talus /tā'ləs/, *pl.* **tali** [L, ankle], the second largest tarsal bone. It supports the tibia, rests on the calcaneus, and articulates with the malleoli and with the navicular bones. It consists of a body, neck, and head. Also called **ankle bone, astragalus.**

Talwin, a trademark for an antagonist/agonist analgesic (pentazocine).

Tambocor, a trademark for an oral antidysrhythmic drug (flecainide acetate).

Tamm-Horsfall protein (THP), a mucoprotein found in the matrix of renal tubular casts. THP is secreted in the loop of Henle.

tamoxifen /təmok'səfin/, a nonsteroidal antiestrogen used in the palliative treatment of advanced breast cancer in premenopausal and postmenopausal women whose tumors are estrogen-dependent.

tampon /tam'pon/ [Fr, plug], a pack of cotton, a sponge, or other material for checking bleeding or absorbing secretions in cavities or canals or for holding displaced organs in position.

tamponade /tam'pənād'/ [Fr, *tamponner*, to plug up], stoppage of the flow of blood to an organ or a part of the body by pressure, such as by a tampon or a pressure dressing applied to stop a hemorrhage or by the compression of a part by an accumulation of fluid, such as in cardiac tamponade.

tangentiality /tanjen'chē·al'itē/ [L, *tangere*, to touch], expressions or responses characterized by a tendency to digress from an original topic of conversation. Tangentiality can destroy or seriously hamper the ability of people to communicate effectively.

tangible elements /tan'jibəl/ [L, *tangere* + *elementum*, first principle], objects that can be seen or touched, as distinguished from emotions, knowledge, or abstractions.

Tangier disease /tanjir'/ [Tangier Island, Virginia], a rare familial deficiency of high-density lipoproteins, characterized by low blood cholesterol and an abnormal orange or yellow discoloration of the tonsils and pharynx. There also may be enlarged lymph nodes, liver, and spleen; muscle atrophy; and peripheral neuropathy. No specific treatment is known.

tannic acid /tan'ik/ [Celt, *tann*, oak; L, *acidus*, sour], a substance obtained from the bark and fruit of various trees and shrubs, particularly the nutgalls of oak trees. The acid is used as an astringent and protein precipitant. Also called **tannin.**

tanning [Fr, *tanner*, to tan], a process in which the pigmentation of the skin deepens as a result of exposure to ultraviolet light. Skin cells containing melanin darken immediately. New melanin is formed within 2 to 3 days and moves upward rapidly, allowing the darkening process to continue.

tantalum (Ta) /tan'tələm/ [Gk, *Tantalus*, mythic king of Phrygia], a silvery metallic element. Its atomic number is 73; its atomic weight is 180.95. Relatively inert chemically, tantalum is used in prosthetic devices such as skull plates and wire sutures.

tantrum /tan'trəm/, a sudden outburst or violent display of rage, frustration, and bad temper, usually occurring in a maladjusted child and certain emotionally disturbed people. The activity is usually not directed at anyone or anything specific but toward the environment in general and is used primarily as a device for attempting to control others and the surroundings. Also called **temper tantrum.**

TAO, a trademark for an antibacterial (troleandomycin).

tapering arch /tā'pəring/ [AS, *tapor*, slender; *arcus*, bow], a dental arch that converges from the molars to the central incisors to such a degree that lines passing through the central grooves of the molars and premolars intersect within 1 inch (2.5 cm) anterior to the central incisors.

tapeworm /tāp'wurm/ [AS, *taeppe*, *wyrm*], a parasitic, intestinal worm belonging to the class Cestoda and having a scolex and a ribbon-shaped body composed of segments in a chain. Humans usually acquire tapeworms by eating the undercooked meat of intermediate hosts contaminated by the cysticerus or larval form of the tapeworm. In the human alimentary canal the worm develops into an adult with an attaching head, or scolex, and numerous hermaphroditic segments, or proglottids, each of which is capable of producing eggs. Kinds of tapeworm include **Diphyllobothrium latum, Taenia saginata,** and **Taenia solium.** Also called **cestode.**

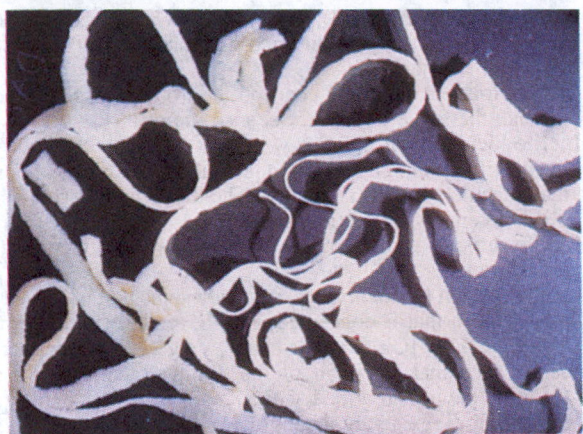

Tapeworm
(Hart, 1992/Courtesy Liverpool School of Tropical Medicine)

tapeworm infection, an intestinal infection by one of several species of parasitic worms, caused by eating raw or undercooked meat infested with tapeworm or its larvae. Tapeworms live as larvae in one or more vertebrate intermediate hosts and grow to adulthood in the intestine of humans. Symptoms of intestinal infection with adult worms are usually mild or absent, but diarrhea, epigastric pain, and weight loss may occur. Diagnosis is made when eggs or portions of the adult worm are passed in the stool. The drugs niclosamide and quinacrine are used to loosen and dissolve the worm so that it may be excreted. Sanitary disposal of fecal material from affected patients is necessary to prevent the passage of larvae or eggs to humans or other hosts. Certain species of tapeworm can infect humans during the larval stage, causing a serious, often cystic, condition of larval infestation. Also called **cestodiasis.** See also **cysticercosis, tapeworm.**

tapho-,   a combining form meaning 'of or pertaining to the grave': *taphophilia, taphophobia.*

tapotement /täpôtmäN′/ [Fr, *tapoter,* to pat],   a type of massage in which the body is tapped in a rhythmic manner with the tips of the fingers or the sides of the hands, using short, rapid, repetitive movements. The procedure is often used on the chest wall of patients with bronchitis to help loosen the mucus in the air passages. See also **massage.**

Taractan,   a trademark for a tranquilizer (chlorprothixene).

tardive dyskinesia /tär′div/ [L, *tardus,* late; Gk, *dys,* difficult, *kinesis* movement],   an abnormal condition characterized by involuntary, repetitious movements of the muscles of the face, the limbs, and the trunk. This disorder most commonly affects older people who have been treated for extended periods with phenothiazine. The involuntary movements associated with the condition may slacken or disappear after weeks or months and have been significantly reduced in some individuals by the administration of cholinergic drugs. See also **antiparkinsonian.**

tardy peroneal nerve palsy [L, *tardus;* Gk, *perone,* brooch; L *nervus; paralyein* to lose control],   an abnormal condition and a type of mononeuropathy in which the peroneal nerve is excessively compressed where it crosses the head of the fibula. Such compression may occur when an individual falls asleep with the legs crossed.

tardy ulnar nerve palsy,   an abnormal condition characterized by atrophy of the first dorsal interosseous muscle and difficulty in the performance of fine manipulations. It may be caused by injury of the ulnar nerve at the elbow and commonly affects individuals with a shallow ulnar groove or those who persistently rest their weight on their elbows. Signs and symptoms of this disorder may include numbness of the small finger, of the contiguous half of the proximal and the middle phalanges of the ring finger, and of the ulnar border of the hand. Treatment of this condition concentrates on the prevention of further injury of the ulnar nerve. Therapy may include the use of a doughnut cushion for the elbow to relieve the pressure on the ulnar nerve. Severe cases of this disorder may be corrected by surgical procedures that mobilize and transplant the nerve to a site in front of the medial epicondyle.

target /tär′git/ [OFr, *targuete,* small shield],   **1.** (in radiotherapy) any object area subjected to bombardment by radioactive particles or another form of diagnostic or therapeutic radiation. **2.** a device used to contain stable materials and subsequent radioactive materials during bombardment by high-energy nuclei from a cyclotron or other particle accelerator.

target cell, 1. also called **leptocyte.** an abnormal red blood cell characterized by a densely stained center surrounded by a pale unstained ring circled by a dark, irregular band. Target cells occur in the blood after splenectomy, in anemia, in hemoglobin C disease, and in thalassemia. Compare **discocyte, spherocyte. 2.** any cell having a specific receptor that reacts with a specific hormone, antigen, antibody, antibiotic, sensitized T cell, or other substance.

target organ, 1. (in radiotherapy) an organ intended to receive a therapeutic dose of irradiation, such as the kidney when high-energy x-rays or gamma rays are beamed to the renal area for the treatment of a tumor. **2.** (in nuclear medicine) an organ intended to receive the greatest concentration of a diagnostic radioactive tracer, such as the liver, which accumulates 99Tc sulfur colloid when it is injected intravenously to detect hepatic lesions. **3.** (in endocrinol-

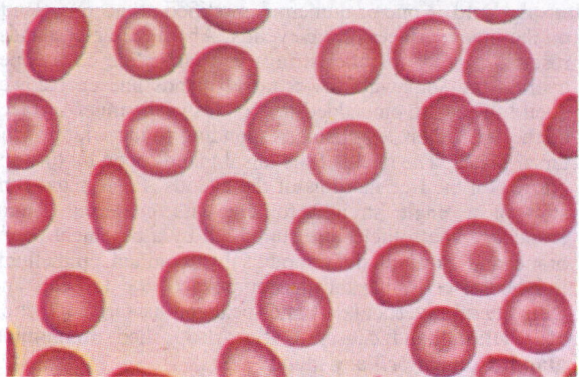

Target cells *(Hayhoe, 1992)*

ogy) an organ most affected by a specific hormone, such as the thyroid gland, which is the target organ of thyroid stimulating hormone secreted by the anterior pituitary gland.

target symptoms,   symptoms of an illness that are most likely to respond to a specific treatment, such as a particular psychopharmacologic drug.

tarsal /tär′səl/ [L, *tarsalis,* eyelid or instep],   of or pertaining to the tarsus, or ankle bone.

tarsal arches [Gk, *tarsos,* flat surface; L, *arcus,* rainbow], the superior and inferior branches of the palpebral artery supplying the eyelid.

tarsal bone,   any one of seven bones making up the tarsus of the foot, consisting of the talus, calcaneus, cuboid, navicular, and the three cuneiforms.

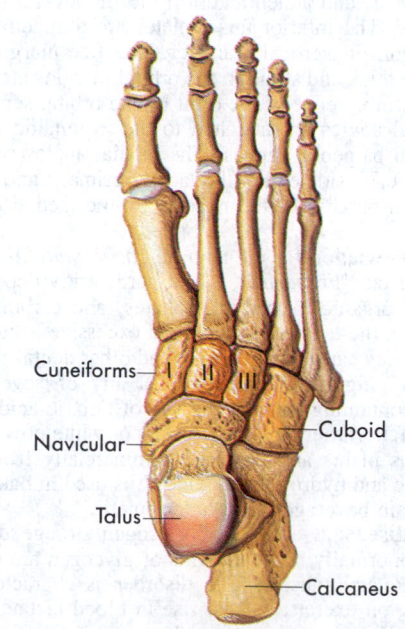

Tarsal bones *(Thibodeau, 1993/Ernest W Beck)*

tarsal gland, one of numerous modified sebaceous glands on the inner surfaces of the eyelids. About 30 tarsal glands, resembling tiny, parallel strings of pearls, line each upper eyelid, and somewhat fewer tarsal glands line each lower eyelid. They are embedded in grooves in the inner surfaces of the tarsi, their lengths corresponding to the width of the tarsal plates. The ducts of the tarsal glands open by tiny apertures on the free margins of the eyelids. Each gland consists of a single straight follicle with numerous lateral branches. The follicles are supported by a basement membrane and lined at their mouths by stratified epithelium. Polyhedral cells line the deeper parts of the follicles and their lateral diverticula. Acute localized bacterial infection of a tarsal gland causes a sty. Also called **meibomian gland.** Compare **ciliary gland.**

tarsal plate. See **tarsus.**

tarsal tunnel syndrome, an abnormal condition and a kind of mononeuropathy, characterized by pain and numbness in the sole of the foot. This disorder may be caused by fractures of the ankle that compress the posterior tibial nerve and may be corrected by appropriate orthopedic therapy or by surgery.

tarso-, a prefix meaning 'of or pertaining to the instep of the foot or to the edge of the eyelid': *tarsoclasis, tarsomalacia, tarsometatarsal.*

tarsometatarsal /tär′sōmet′ətär′səl/ [Gk, *tarsos,* flat surface, *meta,* beyond, *tarsos*], of or pertaining to the metatarsal bones and the tarsus of the foot, especially the articulations of the metatarsal bones with the cuneiform and cuboid bones at the instep of the foot.

tarsus /tär′səs/, *pl.* **tarsi** [Gk, *tarsos,* flat surface], **1.** the area of articulation between the foot and the leg. **2.** also called **tarsal plate.** any one of the plates of cartilage about 2.5 cm long that form the eyelids. One tarsal plate shapes each eyelid. The superior tarsal plates form the upper eyelids. The inferior tarsal plates form the lower eyelids. The superior tarsal plates are semilunar and about 10 mm wide at the center, and attach anteriorly to the levator palpebrae superioris. The inferior tarsal plates are thin, elliptic, and about 5 mm in vertical diameter. The free margins of the plates are thick and straight, the orbital margins are attached to the circumference of the orbit by the orbital septum, and the lateral angles are attached to the zygomatic bones by the lateral palpebral raphes. The medial angles of the two plates on each side end at the lacus lacrimalis and attach to the frontal process of the maxilla by the medial palpebral ligament.

tart, abbreviation for the *tartrate carboxylate anion.*

tartar /tär′tär/ [Fr, *tartre*], **1.** a hard, gritty deposit composed of organic matter, phosphates, and carbonates that collects on the teeth and gums. An excessive accumulation of tartar may cause gum disease and other dental problems. See also **gingivitis, pyorrhea. 2.** any of several compounds containing tartrate, the salt of tartaric acid.

tartaric acid /tärter′ik/, a colorless or white powder found in various plants and prepared commercially from maleic anhydride and hydrogen peroxide. It is used in baking powder, certain beverages, and tartar emetic.

Tarui's disease, a form of glycogen storage disease in which abnormally large amounts of glycogen are deposited in the skeletal muscle. The disorder is characterized by cramping on exercise but no rise in blood lactate, and hemolysis. Biopsy of the affected organ reveals the absence of the enzyme phosphofructokinase. Also called **glycogen storage disease type VII.** See also **glycogen storage disease.**

-tas, a noun-forming combining form: *fragilitas, graviditas, infertilitas.*

task functions, behaviors that focus or direct activities toward movements with work or labor overtones.

task group, a group in which structured verbal or nonverbal exercises are used to help a person gain emotional, physical, and other personal awareness.

task-oriented behavior, actions involving a person's cognitive abilities in an attempt to solve problems, resolve conflicts, and gratify the person's needs to reduce or avoid distress.

taste [ME, *tasten*], the sense of perceiving different flavors in soluble substances that contact the tongue and trigger nerve impulses to special taste centers in the cortex and the thalamus of the brain. The four basic traditional tastes are sweet, salty, sour, and bitter. The front of the tongue is most sensitive to salty and sweet substances; the sides of the tongue are most sensitive to sour substances; and the back of the tongue is most sensitive to bitter substances. The middle of the tongue produces virtually no taste sensation. Chemoreceptor cells in the taste buds of the tongue detect different substances. Adults have about 9000 taste buds, most of them situated on the upper surface of the tongue. The sense of taste is intricately linked with the sense of smell, and taste discrimination is very complex. Many experts believe the capacity to perceive different tastes involves a synthesis of chemoreactive nerve impulses and coordinating brain processes, still not completely understood.

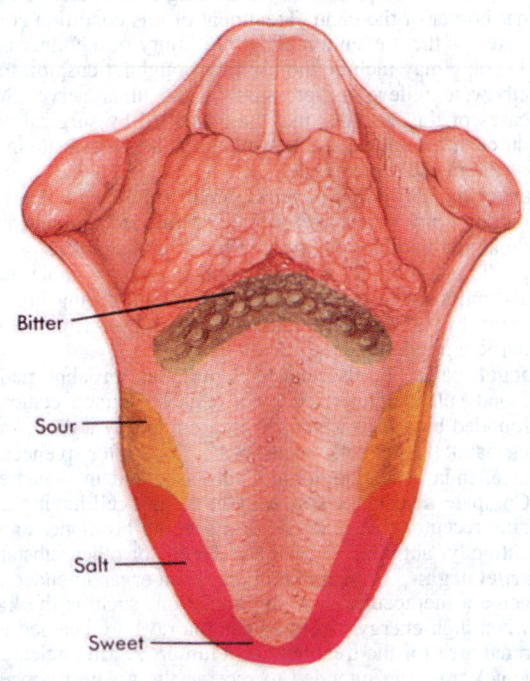

Taste regions of the tongue
(Seeley, 1992/Marsha J Dohrmann)

taste bud, any one of many peripheral taste organs distributed over the tongue and the roof of the mouth. The four basic taste sensations registered by chemical stimulation of the taste buds are sweet, sour, bitter, and salty. All other tastes perceived are combinations of these four basic flavors. Each taste bud rests in a spheric pocket, which extends through the epithelium. Gustatory cells and supporting cells form each bud, which has a surface opening and an opening in the basement membrane. Also called **gustatory organ.**

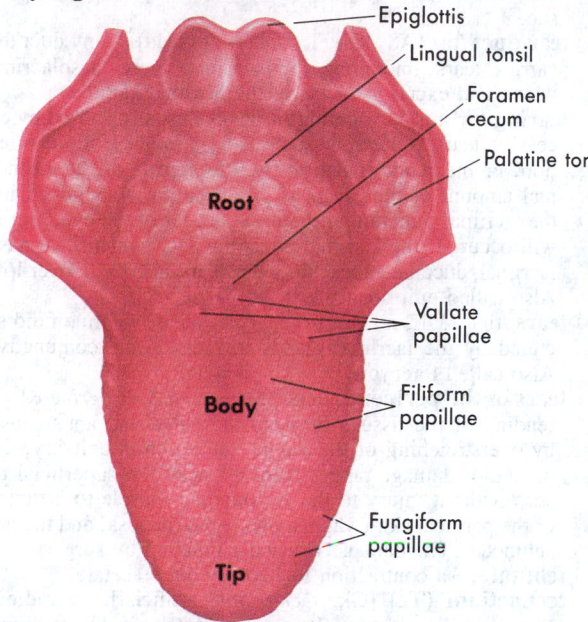

Taste bud (Thibodeau, 1992)

Labels: Epiglottis — Lingual tonsil — Foramen cecum — Palatine tonsil — Root — Vallate papillae — Body — Filiform papillae — Fungiform papillae — Tip

taste papilla [OFr, *taster;* L, *papilla,* nipple], small nipplelike elevations on the tongue. They contain sense organs that are sensitive to the chemicals identified with tastes, which vary with their location on the tongue.

TAT, abbreviation for **tetanus antitoxin.**

tattoo /tatōō'/ [Tahitian, *tatau,* marks], a permanent coloration of the skin by the introduction of foreign pigment. A tattoo may accidentally occur when a bit of graphite from a broken pencil point is embedded in the skin. Small tattoos can be removed by surgical excision. Dermabrasion is preferred for removal of extensive areas of pigment. **–tattoo,** *v.*

tau /tou,tō'/, T, τ, the nineteenth letter of the Greek alphabet.

tauto-, a prefix meaning 'same': *tautomenial, tautomeral, tautomerism.*

tautomer /tôtəmir/, structural isomers that differ only in the position of a hydrogen atom, or proton. Because tautomers can be rapidly interconverted by proton transfer in aqueous solutions, they are usually in equilibrium with one another. Keto and enol isomers are common examples of tautomers.

Tavist, a trademark for an antihistaminic agent (clemastine).

tax-, a combining form meaning 'order or arrangement': *taxis, taxology, taxonomy.*

-taxia, -taxis, -taxy, a combining form meaning '(condition of) internal ordering or arrangement': *acrotaxia, diataxia,cataxia, heterotaxia, prostaxia.* See also **-taxis.**

-taxic. See **-tactic.**

-taxis, -taxia, -taxy, **1.** a combining form meaning a '(specified) arrangement': *biotaxis, heterotaxis, homotaxis.* **2.** a combining form meaning a 'movement of an organism in response to a stimulus': *aerotaxis, electrotaxis, geotaxis.* See also **-taxia.**

taxol /tak'sol/, an anticancer drug derived from the bark of the rare, slow-growing Pacific yew tree. It is used in the treatment of ovarian cancer. Taxol prevents cancer cells from dividing; it arrests cell division by attaching to microtubules that regulate the formation of spindles necessary for cell division. Taxol's anticancer effect was discovered by the National Cancer Institute in 1963 during a routine investigation of thousands of plant compounds. It takes about 60 pounds of yew bark to produce enough taxol to treat a single patient for several weeks.

taxonomic /tak'sənom'ik/ [Gk, *taxis,* arrangement + *nomos,* law], pertaining to the orderly classification of organisms into appropriate groups, or taxa, on the basis of interrelationships, with the use of suitable names.

taxonomy /takson'əmē/ [Gk, *taxis,* arrangement, *nomos,* rule], a system for classifying organisms on the basis of natural relationships and assigning them appropriate names. **–taxonomic,** *adj.*

-taxy. See **-taxia, -taxis.**

Taylor, Effie J. (1874–1970), a Canadian-born American nurse who was graduated from Johns Hopkins School of Nursing. After graduation she continued at Johns Hopkins at the Phipps Psychiatric Institute, served as a nurse in World War I, and went to Yale University School of Nursing in 1923, succeeding Annie Goodrich as dean in 1934. She served as president of the International Council of Nurses during World War II.

Taylor brace [Charles F. Taylor, American surgeon, b. 1827], a padded steel brace used to support the spine. Also called **Taylor splint.**

Tay-Sachs disease /tā'saks'/ [Warren Tay, English ophthalmologist, b. 1843; Bernard Sachs, American neurologist, b. 1858], an inherited, neurodegenerative disorder of lipid metabolism caused by a deficiency of the enzyme hexosaminidase A, which results in the accumulation of sphingolipids in the brain. The condition, which is transmitted as an autosomal recessive trait, occurs predominantly in families of Eastern European Jewish origin, specifically the Ashkenazic Jews, and is characterized by progressive mental and physical retardation and early death. Symptoms first appear by 6 months of age, after which no new skills are learned and there is progressive loss of those skills already acquired. Convulsions and atrophy of the optic nerve head occur after 1 year, followed by blindness, with a cherry-red spot on each retina, spasticity, dementia, and paralysis. Most children die between 2 and 4 years of age. There is no specific therapy for the condition, and intervention is purely symptomatic and supportive. The disease can be diagnosed in utero through amniocentesis. Also called **amaurotic familial idiocy, gangliosidosis type I, infantile cerebral sphingolipidosis, Sachs' disease.** See also **Sandhoff's disease.**

Tay's spot. See **cherry-red spot.**

Tazicef, a trademark for a cephalosporin antibiotic (ceftazidime).

Tb, symbol for the element **terbium.**

TB, 1. abbreviation for **tuberculosis.** 2. abbreviation for *tubercle bacillus.*

T bandage, a bandage in the shape of the letter T. It is used for the perineum and sometimes for the head. Also called **crucial bandage, Heliodorus' bandage.**

TBP, 1. abbreviation for **bithionol.** 2. abbreviation for *total bypass.*

Tbs., tbsp., abbreviation for *tablespoon.*

TBT, abbreviation for **tracheobronchial tree.**

TBW, abbreviation for **total body water.**

TBZ, abbreviation for *tetrabenazine,* an anesthetic adjuvant.

t.c., abbreviation for *telephone call.*

Tc, symbol for the element **technetium.**

TC, abbreviation for **therapeutic community.**

TCDD (2, 3, 7, 8-tetrachlorodibenzopara-dioxin). See **dioxin.**

T cell, a small circulating lymphocyte produced in the bone marrow that matures in the thymus. T cells primarily mediate cellular immune responses, such as graft rejection and delayed hypersensitivity. One kind of T cell, the **helper cell,** affects the production of antibodies by B cells; a **suppressor T cell** suppresses B cell activity. Compare **B cell.** See also **antibody, immune response.**

T-4 cell, a thymus-derived lymphocyte of the body's immune system with a role of destroying or neutralizing cells or substances identified as "nonself." T-4 cells are 'helper/inducer' cells that secrete a substance, interleukin-2, which in turn stimulates the activity of natural killer cells, gamma interferon, and suppressor T-8 cells. The human immunodeficiency virus (HIV) commonly targets the T-4 cells with the result that the body's immune defenses are severely damaged and opportunistic infections are allowed to flourish.

Td, abbreviation for **tetanus and diphtheria toxoids.**

TD, abbreviation for **toxic dose.**

TD50. See **median toxic dose.**

TDD, abbreviation for *transdermal drug delivery.*

tDNA, abbreviation for **transfer DNA.**

t.d.s. abbreviation for Latin phrase, '(*ter die sumendum,* to be taken) three times a day.

Te, symbol for the elemen **tellurium.**

tea. See **cannabis.**

teacher's nodule. See **vocal cord nodule.**

teaching hospital [AS, *taecan,* to show how], a hospital associated with a university that has accredited programs in various specialties of medical practice.

teaching rounds, informal conferences held regularly, often at the beginning of the day. Various members of the department and staff may attend, including nurses, residents, interns, students, attending physicians, and faculty. Specific problems in the care of current patients are discussed. See also **nursing rounds.**

team nursing [AS, *team,* family; L, *nutrix,* nourishment], a decentralized system in which the care of a patient is distributed among the members of a team. The charge nurse delegates authority to a team leader who must be a professional nurse. This nurse leads the team—usually of 4 to 6 members—in the care of between 15 and 25 patients. The team leader assigns tasks, schedules care, and instructs team members in details of care. A conference is held at the beginning and at the end of each shift to allow team members to exchange information and the team leader to make changes in the nursing care plan for any patient. Compare **primary nursing.**

team practice, professional practice by a group of professionals that may include physicians, nurses, and others, such as a social worker, nutritionist, or physical therapist, who manage the care of a specified number of patients as a team, usually in an outpatient setting.

tear /ter/ [ME *teren* to rend], to rip, rend, or pull apart by force.

teardrop fracture /tir′drop/ [AS, *tear, dropa;* L, *fractura,* break], an avulsion fracture of one of the short bones, such as a vertebra, causing a tear-shaped disruption of bone tissue.

tear duct /tir/ [AS, *tear;* L, *ducere,* to lead], any duct that carries tears, including the lacrimal ducts, nasolacrimal ducts, and excretory ducts of the lacrimal glands.

tearing /tir′ing/, watering of the eye usually caused by excessive tear production, such as by strong emotion, infection, or mechanic irritation by a foreign body. If the normal amount of fluid tears is produced but not drained into the lacrimal punctum at the nasal border of the eye, tearing will occur. If the lacrimal punctum, sac, cuniculi, or nasolacrimal duct becomes blocked, tears also will overflow. Also called **epiphora.**

tears /tirs/ [ME, *tere*], a watery saline or alkaline fluid secreted by the lacrimal glands to moisten the conjunctiva. Also called **dacryon.**

tears of the perineum /ters/ [ME, *teren;* Gk, *perineos*], a rending of the tissues between the vulva and anus caused by overstretching of the vagina during child delivery. The degree of damage ranges from a tear of the superficial tissues without injury to the surrounding muscle to a rupture of the perineal skin, vaginal and rectal mucosa, and the anal sphincter. The damage is usually repaired by surgery.

tebutate, a contraction for tertiary butyl acetate.

technetium (Tc) [Gk, *technectos,* artificial], a radioactive, metallic element. Its atomic number is 43; its atomic weight is 99. The first synthetic element, technetium also occurs in nature. Isotopes of technetium are used in radioisotope scanning procedures of internal organs, such as the liver and spleen. Formerly called **masurium.**

technetium 99, the radionuclide most commonly used to image the body in nuclear medicine scans. It is preferred because of its short half-life and because the emitted photon has an appropriate energy for normal imaging techniques. The "m" indicates that this radionuclide is generated on-site from a molybdenum source.

technic. See **technique.**

-technic, -technics, -technique, technology, techny, a suffix referring 'to the skillful way or the mechanics of doing something:' *mnemotechnics, zymo-technique.*

technician /teknishm′ən/ [Gk, *technikos,* skillful], a person with special training and experience in some form of technical procedures, usually those involving mechanical adjustments, such as maintaining and operating radiologic equipment.

-technics. See **technic.**

technique /teknēk′/ [Gk, *technikos,* skillful], the method and details followed in performing a procedure, such as those used in conducting a laboratory test, a physical examination, a psychiatric interview, a surgical operation, or any process requiring certain skills or an ordered sequence of actions. Also spelled **technic.**

-technique. See **technic.**

techno-, a combining form meaning 'art': *technopsychology, technocausis, technology.*

technologist /teknol′əjist/ [Gk, *techne,* art + *logos,* science], a person who studies the application of processes for making natural resources beneficial for humans. A medical technologist may work under the supervision of a physician in general clinical laboratory procedures.

-technology, -techny. See **technic.**

tecto-, a prefix meaning 'rooflike': *tectocephalic, tectorial, tectum.*

Tedral, a trademark for a respiratory fixed-combination drug containing a bronchodilator (theophylline), an adrenergic (ephedrine hydrochloride), and a sedative-hypnotic (phenobarbital).

teenager. See **adolescent.**

teether /tē′ther/, an object, such as a teething ring, on which an infant can bite or chew during the teething process.

teething /tē′thing/ [AS, *toth*], the physiologic process of the eruption of the deciduous teeth through the gums. It normally begins around the sixth month of life and occurs periodically until the complete set of 20 teeth has appeared at about 30 to 36 months. Discomfort and inflammation result from the pressure exerted against the periodontal tissue as the crown of the tooth breaks through the membranes. General signs of teething include excessive drooling, biting on hard objects, irritability, difficulty in sleeping, and refusal of food. Fever or diarrhea often occurs during teething but is indicative of illness rather than of teething. The pain and inflammation usually may be soothed by cold, such as with a frozen teething ring, cold metal spoon, or ice wrapped in a washcloth. Use of teething powders and procedures, such as rubbing or cutting the gums, are discouraged because of the possibility of infection or complications from ingestion of the medication. **– teethe,** *v.*

teething ring, a circular device, usually made of plastic or rubber, on which an infant may chew or bite during the teething process.

Teflon, a trademark for a substance (polytetrafluoroethylene) used for the construction of surgical implants in restorative surgery.

teg-, a combining form meaning 'of or pertaining to a cover': *tegmen, tegmental, tegument.*

Tegison, a trademark for an antipsoriatic vitamin A derivative (etretinate).

Tegopen, a trademark for an antibacterial (cloxacillin sodium).

Tegretol, a trademark for an analgesic and anticonvulsant (carbamazepine).

TEIB, abbreviation for *triethylene-immunobenzoquinone.*

tela-, a combining form meaning 'a web or weblike structure': *telalgia, telangiectasia, telangitis.*

-tela, a combining form meaning a 'weblike membrane': *aulatela, epitela, metatela.*

telangiectasia /təlan′jē·ektā′zhə/ [Gk, *telos,* end, *aggeion,* vessel, *ektasis,* dilatation], permanent dilatation of groups of superficial capillaries and venules. Common causes are actinic damage, atrophy-producing dermatoses, rosacea, elevated estrogen levels, and collagen vascular diseases. See also **Osler-Weber-Rendu syndrome, spider angioma.**

telangiectasia lymphatica [Gk, *telos,* end + *aggeion,* vessel + *ektasis,* dilatation; L, *lympha,* water], a congenital or acquired condition of obstructed, dilated lymphatic vessels, resulting in lymphangiomata.

telangiectatic epulis /təlan′jē·ektat′ik/, a benign red tu-

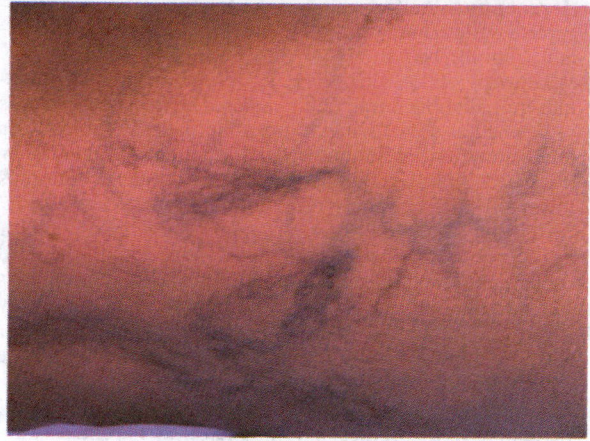

Telangiectasia *(Goldman, 1991)*

mor of the gingiva, containing prominent blood vessels. Low-grade or chronic irritation is a risk factor.

telangiectatic fibroma. See **angiofibroma.**

telangiectatic glioma, a tumor composed of glial cells and a network of blood vessels, which give the mass a vivid pink appearance.

telangiectatic granuloma. See **pyogenic granuloma.**

telangiectatic lipoma. See **angiolipoma.**

telangiectatic nevus, a common skin condition of neonates, characterized by flat, deep-pink localized areas of capillary dilatation that occur predominantly on the back of the neck, lower occiput, upper eyelids, upper lip, and bridge of the nose. The areas disappear permanently by about 2 years of age. Also called **capillary flames, stork bite.**

telangiectatic sarcoma, a malignant tumor of mesodermal cells with an unusually rich vascular network.

tele-, teleo-, a combining form meaning 'relating to the end or occurring at a distance': *telalgia, telosynapsis.*

telediagnosis /tel′ədī′əgnō′sis/ [Gk, *tele,* far off + *dia,* through + *gnosis,* knowledge], a process whereby a disease diagnosis, or prognosis, is made by the electronic transmission of data between distant medical facilities.

telekinesis /tel′əkinē′sis/ [Gk, *tele,* far off + *kinesis,* movement], a concept of parapsychology that one can control external events, such as the movement of a solid object, by the powers of the mind. For example, practitioners of telekinesis may believe it possible, by thought processes alone, to influence the roll of dice. Also called **parakinesis; psychokinesis.**

telemetry /telem′ətrē/ [Gk, *tele,* far off + *metron,* measure], the electronic transmission of data between distant points.

telencephalon /tel′ensef′əlon/ [Gk, *telos,* end + *egekephalos,* brain], the paired brain vesicles or endbrain from which the cerebral hemispheres are derived.

teleo-. See **tele-.**

telepathist /təlep′əthist/, **1.** a person who believes in telepathy. **2.** a person who claims to have telepathic powers.

telepathy /təlep′əthē/ [Gk, *tele,* afar, *pathos,* feeling], the alleged communication of thought from one person to another by means other than the physical senses. Also called **thought transference.** See also **extrasensory perception, parapsychology. – telepathic,** *adj.,* **telepathize,** *v.*

telereceptive /tel'ərisep'tiv/, pertaining to the exteroceptors of hearing, sight, and smell that detect stimuli distant from the body.

teletherapy /tel'əther'əpē/ [Gk, *tele* + *therapeia*, treatment], radiation therapy administered by a machine that is positioned at some distance from the patient. Typically, a teletherapy unit can rotate around a patient and thus allow use of multiple beams that intersect at the tumor and thus lower the dose to surrounding normal tissue.

tellurium (Te) /teloo'rē·əm/ [L, *tellus*, earth, ground, soil], an element exhibiting metallic and nonmetallic chemical properties. Its atomic number is 52; its atomic weight is 127.60. Inhaling vapors of tellurium results in a garlicky breath.

telo-, a combining form meaning 'of or pertaining to the end': *telobiosis, telodendron, telosynapsis.*

telocentric /tel'əsen'trik/ [Gk, *telos,* end, *kentron,* center], pertaining to a chromosome in which the centromere is located at the end, so that the chromatids appear as straight filaments. Compare **acrocentric, metacentric, submetacentric.**

telogen. See **hair.**

telophase /tel'əfāz/ [Gk, *telos* + *phasis,* appearance], the final of the four stages of nuclear division in mitosis and in each of the two divisions in meiosis. The newly produced daughter chromosomes from the preceding anaphase stage assemble at the poles of the division spindle and become long and slender, the nuclear membrane forms around them, the nucleolus reappears, and the cytoplasm begins to divide. See also **anaphase, interphase, meiosis, metaphase, mitosis, prophase.**

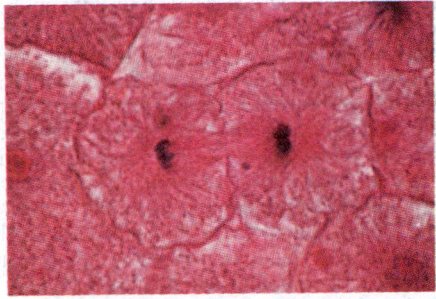

Telophase
(Seeley, 1992/Ed Reschke/Michael Abbey, Science Source)

Temaril, a trademark for an antihistamine (trimeprazine tartrate).

temazepam /temaz'əpam/, a benzodiazepine hypnotic agent.
■ INDICATIONS: It is prescribed for the relief of transient and intermittent insomnia.
■ CONTRAINDICATIONS: Pregnancy or lactation prohibits its use. It is not recommended for patients under 18 years of age. Patients should avoid use of alcohol while also using temazepam.
■ ADVERSE EFFECTS: The most serious adverse reactions are confusion, euphoria, anorexia, ataxia, palpitations, hallucinations, horizontal nystagmus, and paradoxical reactions.

Temovate, a trademark for a topical corticosteroid (clobetasol propionate).

temper [L, *temperare,* to moderate], **1.** to moderate or soften the effects. **2.** a state of mind regarding calmness or anger.

temperament /temp'(ə)rəmənt/ [L, *temperamentum,* mixture in proper proportions], the features of a persona that reflect an individual's emotional disposition, the way he or she behaves, feels, and thinks.

temperate phage /tem'pərit/ [L, *temperare,* to temper; Gk, *phagein,* to eat], a bacteriophage whose genome is incorporated into the host bacterium. It persists through many cell divisions of the bacterium without destroying the host, in contrast to a virulent phage that lyses and kills its host.

temperature /tem'pə(r)chər/ [L, *temperies,* mildness], **1.** a relative measure of sensible heat or cold. **2.** (in physiology) a measure of sensible heat associated with the metabolism of the human body, normally maintained at a constant level of 98.6° F (37° C) by the thermotaxic nerve mechanism that balances heat gains and heat losses. **3.** *informal.* a fever.

temperature of infant [L, *temperatura* + *infans,* infant], the neonatal temperature, which normally ranges from 35.5° to 37.5° C (96° to 99.5° F). It is unstable because of immature physiologic mechanisms.

temperature sense. See **thermic sense.**

temper tantrum. See **tantrum.**

template /tem'plit/ [L, *templum,* section], (in genetics) the strand of DNA that acts as a mold for the synthesis of messenger RNA. This messenger RNA contains the same sequence of nucleic acids as the DNA strand and carries the code to the ribosomes, which are located in the cytoplasm, for the synthesis of proteins.

tempo-, **1.** a prefix meaning 'of or pertaining to time': *tempolabile, temporal, tempostabile.* **2.** a prefix meaning 'of or pertaining to the temples, in the lateral regions of the head': *temporal, temporalis, temporomandibular.*

temporal /tem'pərəl/ [L, *tempus,* temple], **1.** pertaining to a limited time. **2.** pertaining to the temporal bone of the skull.

temporal arteritis [L, *temporalis,* temporary, *arteria,* air pipe, *itis,* inflammation], a progressive inflammatory disorder of cranial blood vessels, principally the temporal artery, occurring most frequently in women over 70 years of age. Characteristic changes in the involved vessels include granulomatous disruption of the elastic layer and engulfment of fiber fragments by giant cells in the intimal and medial layers. The temporal artery is typically tender, swollen, and pulseless, but may be clinically normal. Symptoms are intractable headache, difficulty in chewing, weakness, rheumatic pains, and loss of vision if the central retinal artery becomes occluded. Also called **cranial arteritis, giant cell arteritis, Horton's arteritis.**

temporal artery, any one of three arteries on each side of the head: the superficial temporal artery, the middle temporal artery, and the deep temporal artery.

temporal bone, one of a pair of large bones forming part of the lower cranium and containing various cavities and recesses associated with the ear, such as the tympanic cavity and the auditory tube. Each temporal bone consists of four portions: the mastoid, the squama, the petrous, and the tympanic.

temporal bone fracture, a break of the temporal bone of the skull, sometimes characterized by bleeding from the ear. Diminished hearing, facial paralysis, or infection of the tympanic cavity leading to meningitis may occur.

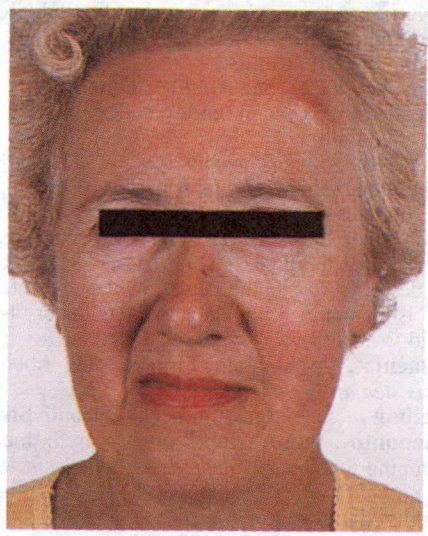

Temporal arteritis—note swollen temporal artery
(Shipley, 1993)

temporal gyrus [L, *tempus*; Gk, *gyros*, turn], any of three convolutions, inferior, middle, or superior, on the lateral surface of the temporal lobe of the brain.

temporalis /tem′pəral′is/ [L, temporary], one of the four muscles of mastication. It is a broad radiating muscle that arises from the whole of the temporal fossa and the surface of the temporal fascia. It inserts into the ramus of the mandible near the last molar tooth, and it is innervated by the anterior and the posterior temporal nerves. The temporalis acts to close the jaws and retract the mandible. Also called **temporal muscle.** Compare **masseter, pterygoideus lateralis, pterygoideus medialis.**

temporal lobe, the lateral region of the cerebrum, below the lateral fissure. Within the temporal lobe of the brain is the center for smell, some association areas for memory and learning, and a region where choice is made of thoughts to express. Compare **frontal lobe, occipital lobe, parietal lobe.**

temporal lobe epilepsy. See **psychomotor seizure.**

temporal muscle. See **temporalis.**

temporal subtraction, the subtraction of two or more digitized x-ray images that were acquired at different times. The subtraction process eliminates information in the image that was static. If during the intervening period contrast material is introduced into the organ, the subtracted image will contain only the space filled with the contrast material.

temporal summation. See **summation,** def. 2.

temporary base. See **baseplate.**

temporary pacemaker /tem′pərer′ē/ [L, *temporarius,* not permanent + *passus,* step; ME, *maken*], an artificial electronic heart pacemaker attached outside the patient's body and connected to a transvenous probe located within the heart. It is an interim procedure used when the heart rate is excessively slow.

temporary removable splint [L, *temporarius,* not permanent + *removere;* Du, *splinte],* any of a variety of dental

appliances, including occlusal splints, used when limited stability of the teeth is required. It may be placed on or removed from teeth at will. Examples include Hawley's orthodontic appliance and Elbrecht's cast metal splint.

temporary stopping [L, *temporalis* + AS, *stoppian,* to stop up], a mixture of gutta-percha, zinc oxide, white wax, and coloring, used for temporarily sealing dressings in tooth cavities. It softens on heating and rehardens at room temperature but is not hard enough to be used effectively in tooth areas under occlusal stress.

temporary tooth. See **deciduous tooth.**

temporomandibular /tem′pərō′mandib′yələr/ [L, *temporal* + *mandere,* to chew], pertaining to the articulation between the temporal bone and the condyle of the mandible.

temporomandibular joint (TMJ), [L, *temporalis* + *mandere,* to chew; *jungere,* to join], one of two joints connecting the mandible of the jaw to the temporal bone of the skull. It is a combined hinge and gliding joint, formed by the anterior parts of the mandibular fossae of the temporal bone, the articular tubercles, the condyles of the mandible, and five ligaments.

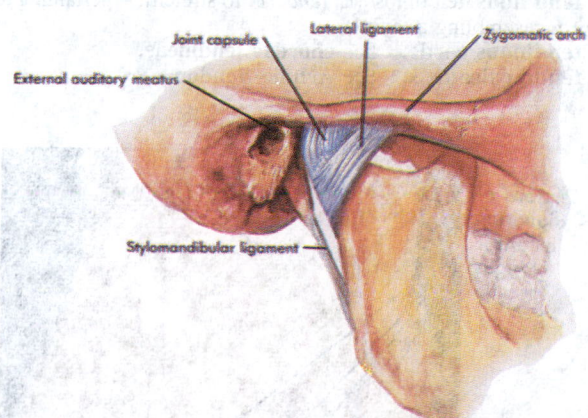

Temporomandibular joint *(Seeley, 1992/David J Mascaro & Associates)*

temporomandibular joint pain dysfunction syndrome (TMJ), an abnormal condition characterized by facial pain and by mandibular dysfunction, apparently caused by a defective or dislocated temporomandibular joint. Some common indications of this syndrome are the clicking of the joint when the jaws move, limitation of jaw movement, subluxation, and temporomandibular dislocation.

temporomandibular ligament [L, *temporalis* + *mandere,* to chew + *ligare,* to bind], an oblique band of tissue that extends downward and backward from the zygomatic process to the neck of the mandible.

temporoparietal. See **parietotemporal.**

temporoparietalis /tem′pərōpərī′ətal′is/ [L, *temporalis* + *paries,* wall], one of a pair of broad, thin muscles of the scalp, divided into three parts, which fan out over the temporal fascia and insert into the galea aponeurotica. The three parts include an anterior temporal portion, a superior parietal portion, and a triangular portion in between. The temporoparietalis was formerly considered part of the superior and the inferior auricularis. On both sides, it acts in combination with the occipitofrontalis to wrinkle the forehead, to widen the eyes, and to raise the ears. It is innervated by branches of the facial nerve. Compare **occipitofrontalis.**

TEN, abbreviation for **toxic epidermal necrolysis.**

tenacious /tenā′shəs/ [L, *tenax,* holding fast], pertaining to secretions that are sticky or adhesive or otherwise tend to hold together, such as mucus and sputum.

tenacity /tenas′itē/ [L, *tenax,* holding fast], the ability to be persistent or remain attached.

tenaculum /tənak′yələm/, *pl.* **tenacula** [L, holder], a clip or clamp with long handles used to grasp, immobilize, and hold an organ or a piece of tissue. Kinds of tenacula include the **abdominal tenaculum,** which has long arms and small hooks, the **forceps tenaculum,** which has long hooks and is used in gynecologic surgery, and the **uterine** or **cervical tenaculum,** which has short hooks or open, eye-shaped clamps used to hold the cervix.

tendinitis /ten′dənī′tis/ [L, *tendere,* to stretch; Gk, *itis,* inflammation], an inflammatory condition of a tendon, usually resulting from strain. Treatment may include rest, corticosteroid injections, and support. Also spelled **tendonitis.**

tendino-. See **teno-.**

tendinous /ten′dinəs/ [L, *tendere,* to stretch], pertaining to or resembling a tendon.

tendinous cords. See **chordae tendineae.**

tendo calcaneus. See **Achilles tendon.**

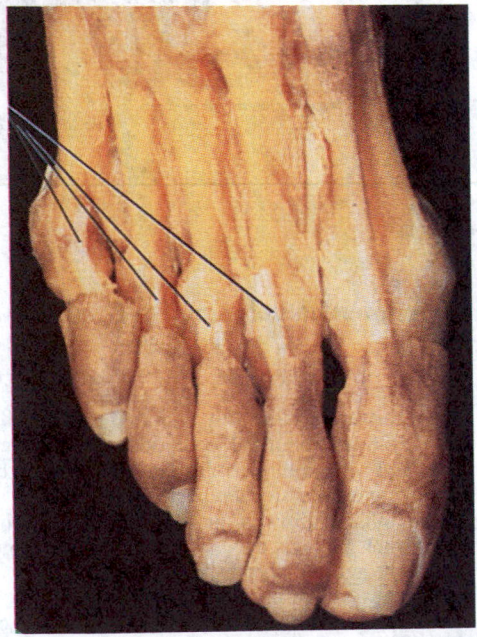

Tendons (Thibodeau, 1993)

Tendons of digitorum extensor longus muscle

tendon /ten′dən/ [L, *tendo*], one of many white, glistening fibrous bands of tissue that attach muscle to bone. Except at points of attachment, tendons are sheathed in delicate fibroelastic connective tissue. Larger tendons contain a thin internal septum, a few blood vessels, and specialized sterognostic nerves. Tendons are extremely strong, flexible, and inelastic, and occur in various lengths and thicknesses. Compare **ligament.** –**tendinous,** *adj.*

tendonitis. See **tendinitis.**

tendon of Achilles. See **Achilles tendon.**

tendon reflex. See **deep tendon reflex.**

tendo-. See **teno.**

tendosynovitis. See **tenosynovitis.**

tenesmic /tənez′mik/ [Gk, *teinesmos,* straining], pertaining to or resembling tenesmus.

tenesmus /tənez′məs/ [Gk, *tendere,* to stretch], persistent, ineffectual spasms of the rectum or bladder, accompanied by the desire to empty the bowel or bladder. Intestinal tenesmus is a common complaint in inflammatory bowel disease and irritable bowel syndrome.

tenia-, taenia-, a combining form meaning 'ribbon, band': *taeniasis, teniafuge, taenidium.*

tennis elbow. See **lateral humeral epicondylitis.**

teno-, tenonto-, tendo-, tendino-, a prefix meaning 'of or pertaining to a tendon': *tenodesis, tenodynia, tenomyotomy.*

tenofibril. See **tonofibril.**

Tenon's capsule. See **fascia bulbi.**

tenonto-. See **teno-.**

Tenormin, a trademark for a beta-blocker (atenolol).

tenosynovitis /ten′ōsin′əvī′tis/ [Gk, *tenon,* tendon, *syn,* together; L, *ovum,* egg; Gk, *itis*], inflammation of a tendon sheath caused by calcium deposits, repeated strain or trauma, high levels of blood cholesterol, rheumatoid arthritis, gout, or gonorrhea. In some instances movement yields crackling noise over the tendon. Most cases not associated with systemic disease respond to rest. Local injections of adrenocorticosteroids may provide relief; surgery is indicated if the condition persists. Also called **tendosynovitis.**

tenotomy /tənot′əmē/ [Gk, *tenon,* tendon, *temnein,* to cut], the total or partial severing of a tendon, performed to correct a muscle imbalance, such as in the correction of strabismus of the eye or in clubfoot.

TENS, abbreviation for **transcutaneous electric nerve stimulation.**

Tensilon, a trademark for a cholinesterase reactivator (edrophonium), used as a curare antagonist and as a diagnostic aid in myasthenia gravis.

tensiometer /ten′sē·om′ətər/ [L, *tendere,* to stretch; Gk, *metron,* measure], a device for measuring the surface tension of a liquid.

tension /ten′shən/ [L, *tendere,* to stretch], **1.** the act of pulling or straining until taut. **2.** the condition of being taut, tense, or under pressure. **3.** a state or condition resulting from the psychologic and physiologic reaction to a stressful situation, characterized physically by a general increase in muscle tonus, heart rate, respiration rate, and alertness and psychologically by feelings of strain, uneasiness, irritability, and anxiety. See also **stress.**

-tension. See **-tention.**

tension headache, a pain that affects the head as the result of overwork or emotional strain, and involving tension in the muscles of the neck, face, and shoulder.

tension pneumothorax [L, *tendere,* to stretch; Gk, *pneuma,* air + *thorax*], a condition of air in the intrapleural space of the thorax caused by a rupture through the chest wall or lung parenchyma associated with the valvular opening. Air passes through the valve during coughing but cannot escape on exhalation.

tensor /ten′sər/ [L, *tendere,* to stretch], any one of the muscles of the body that tenses a structure, such as the tensor fasciae latae of the thigh. Compare **abductor, adductor, depressor, sphincter.**

tensor fasciae latae, one of the 10 muscles of the gluteal region, arising from the outer lip of the iliac crest, the iliac spine, and the deep fascia lata. It inserts between the two layers of fascia lata in the proximal third of the thigh. The tensor fasciae latae is innervated by a branch of the superior gluteal nerve, which contains fibers from the fourth and fifth lumbar and the first sacral nerves, and it functions to flex the thigh and to rotate it slightly medially. Also called **tensor fasciae femoris.**

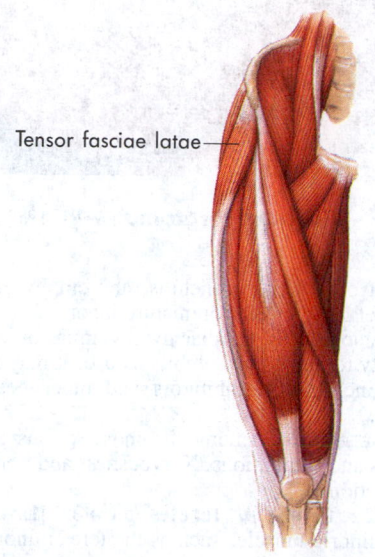

Tensor fasciae latae—

Tensor fasciae latae (*Thibodeau, 1993/John V Hagen*)

tent [ME, *tente*], **1.** a transparent cover, usually of plastic, supported over the upper part of a patient by a frame. Used in the treatment of respiratory conditions, it provides a controlled environment into which steam, oxygen, vaporized medication, or droplets of cool water may be sprayed, such as an oxygen tent. **2.** a cone made of various materials inserted into a cavity or orifice of the body to dilate its opening, such as a laminaria tent. **3.** a pack placed in a wound to hold it open to ensure that healing progresses from the base of the wound upward to the skin.

tentative /ten′tətiv/ [L, *tentare,* to touch], not final or definite, such as an experimental finding that has not been validated.

tenth cranial nerve. See **vagus nerve.**

tenth-value layer (TVL) [ME, *tenpe;* L, *valere,* to be worth; AS *lecgan* to lie], the thickness of material required to attenuate a beam of radiation to one tenth of its original intensity. See also **half-value layer.**

-tention, a suffix meaning the 'condition of being held': *historetention, retention.*

-tention, -tension, a suffix meaning 'condition of being stretched or strained, or in which pressure is exerted': *attention, distention, intention.*

tentorial herniation /tentôr′ē·əl/ [L, *tentorium,* a tent; *hernia,* rupture], the protrusion of brain tissue into the tento-

rial notch, caused by increased intracranial pressure resulting from edema, hemorrhage, or a tumor. Characteristic signs are severe headache, fever, flushing, sweating, abnormal pupillary reflex, drowsiness, hypotension, and loss of consciousness. Also called **transtentorial herniation.**

tentorial notch [L, *tentorium,* tent; OFr, *enochier*], an area occupied by the midbrain and enclosed by the free border of the tentorium cerebelli and the sphenoid bone.

tentorium /tentôr′ē·əm/, *pl.* **tentoria** [L, a tent], any part of the body that resembles a tent, such as the tentorium of the hypophysis that covers the hypophyseal fossa.

tentorium cerebelli, one of the three extensions of the dura mater that separates the cerebellum from the occipital lobe of the cerebrum. Compare **falx cerebelli, falx cerebri.**

Tenuate, a trademark for an anorexiant (diethylpropion hydrochloride).

tenure /ten′yər/ [L, *tenere,* to hold], (in a university) a faculty appointment with few limits on the number of years it may be held; a permanent appointment usually awarded to a person who has advanced to the rank of professor and who demonstrates scholarship and excellence in a specific field of study.

-tepa, a combining form for antineoplastic thiotepa derivatives.

Tepanil, a trademark for an anorexiant (diethylpropion hydrochloride).

tephr-, a prefix meaning 'gray or ash-colored': *tephromalacia, tephromyelitis, tephrylometer.*

tepid, moderately warm to the touch.

tera-, a prefix meaning 'one trillion': *terabyte, terahertz.*

teramorphous [Gk, *teras,* monster, *morphe,* form], of the nature of or characteristic of a monster.

teras /ter′əs/, *pl.* **terata** [Gk, monster], a severely deformed fetus; a monster. **—teratic,** *adj.*

teratism /ter′ətiz′əm/, any congenital or developmental anomaly that is produced by inherited or environmental factors, or by a combination of the two; any condition in which a severely malformed fetus is produced. Kinds of teratism include **atresic teratism, ceasmic teratism, ectopic teratism, ectrogenic teratism, hypergenetic teratism,** and **symphysic teratism.** Also called **teratosis.**

terato-, a combining form meaning 'of or related to a monster': *teratoblastoma, teratogenesis, teratoma.*

teratogen /ter′ətəjen′/ [Gk, *teras* + *genein,* to produce], any substance, agent, or process that interferes with normal prenatal development, causing the formation of one or more developmental abnormalities in the fetus. Teratogens act directly on the developing organism or indirectly, affecting such supplemental structures as the placenta or some maternal system. The type and extent of the defect are determined by the specific kind of teratogen, its mode of action, the embryonic process affected, genetic predisposition, and the stage of development at the time the exposure occurred. The period of highest vulnerability in the developing embryo is from about the third through the twelfth week of gestation, when differentiation of the major organs and systems occurs. Susceptibility to teratogenic influence decreases rapidly in the later periods of development, which are characterized by growth and elaboration. Among the known teratogens are chemical agents, including such drugs as thalidomide, alkylating agents, and alcohol; infectious agents, especially the rubella virus and cytomegalovirus; ionizing radiation, particularly x-rays; and environmental

Human teratogens

Drugs and chemicals	Infections
Alcohol	Cytomegalovirus
Androgens	Rubella
Anticoagulants (warfarin and	Syphilis
dicumarol)	Toxoplasmosis
Antithyroid drugs	Varicella
(propylthiouracil, iodide,	
and methimazole)	**Exposures** (e.g., radiation)
Chemotherapeutic drugs	
(methotrexate and	**Maternal conditions**
aminopterin)	Diabetes mellitus
Diethylstilbestrol (DES)	Phenylketonuria
Lead	
Lithium	
Organic mercury	
Phenytoin	
Polychlorinated biphenyls	
(PCBs)	
Isoretinoin*	
Streptomycin	
Tetracycline	
Thalidomide	
Trimethadione	
paramethadione	
Valproic acid	

From Reed GB, Claireaux AE, Bain AD, editors: *Diseases of the fetus and newborn: pathology, radiology, and genetics,* St Louis, 1989, Mosby.
*Trade name: Accutane, a synthetic derivative of vitamin A.

factors, such as the age and general health of the mother or any intrauterine trauma that may affect the fetus, especially during the later stages of pregnancy. Compare **mutagen. –teratogenic,** *adj.*

teratogenesis /ter′ətōjen′əsis/, the development of physical defects in the embryo. Also called **teratogeny** /ter′ətoj′ēnē/. **–teratogenetic,** *adj.*

teratogenic agent. See **teratogen.**

teratogenous /ter′ətoj′ənəs/ [Gk, *teras,* monster + *genein,* to produce], developed from fetal membranes.

teratogeny. See **teratogenesis.**

teratoid /ter′ətoid/ [Gk, *teras* + *eidos,* form], of or pertaining to abnormal physical development; resembling a monster.

teratoid tumor. See **dermoid cyst.**

teratologist /ter′ətol′əjist/, one who specializes in the science of teratology.

teratology /-tol′əgē/ [Gk, *teras* + *logos,* science], the study of the causes and effects of congenital malformations and developmental abnormalities. **–teratologic, teratological,** *adj.*

teratoma /ter′ətō′mə/, *pl.* **teratomas, teratomata,** a tumor composed of different kinds of tissue, none of which normally occur together or at the site of the tumor. Teratomas are most common in the ovaries or testes.

teratocis. See **teratism.**

terbium (Tb) /tur′bē·əm/ [Yterby, Sweden], a rare earth metallic element. Its atomic number is 65; its atomic weight is 158.294.

terbutaline sulfate /terbyoo′təlēn/, a beta-adrenergic stimulant.
■ INDICATIONS: It is prescribed as a bronchodilator in the

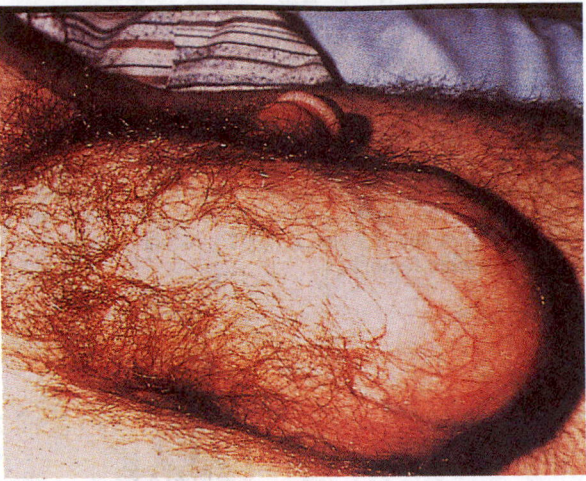

Testicular teratoma *(Weiss, 1988)*

treatment of asthma, bronchitis, and emphysema and as a uterine relaxant to treat premature labor.
■ CONTRAINDICATIONS: Cardiac dysrhythmias or known hypersensitivity to this drug prohibits its use. It may interact with monoamine oxidase inhibitors and other beta-adrenergic blockers.
■ ADVERSE EFFECTS: Among the most serious reactions are dizziness and palpitations. Nervousness and tremor are common reactions.

teres /tir′ēz, ter′ēz/, *pl.* **teretes** /ter′ətēz/ [L, rounded], a long, cylindric muscle, such as the teres minor or the teres major. **–teres,** *adj.*

teres major, a thick, flat muscle of the shoulder. Arising from the dorsal surface of the scapula and from the fibrous septa between the teres major, the teres minor, and the infraspinatus, it is innervated by a branch of the lower subscapular nerve from the brachial plexus, which contains fibers from the fifth and the sixth cervical nerves, and it functions to adduct, extend, and rotate the arm medially. Compare **teres minor.**

teres minor, a cylindric, elongated muscle of the shoulder. Arising from the dorsal surface of the scapula and from two aponeurotic laminae, one of which separates it from the teres major, the other from the infraspinatus, it is inserted into the humerus and is innervated by a branch of the axillary nerve, which contains fibers from the fifth cervical nerve. The teres minor functions to rotate the arm laterally, weakly adduct the arm, and draw the humerus toward the glenoid fossa of the scapula, strengthening the shoulder joint. Compare **teres major.**

terfenadine /terfen′ədēn/, a histamine H$_1$-receptor antagonist.
■ INDICATIONS: It is used to relieve symptoms of seasonal allergic rhinitis.
■ CONTRAINDICATIONS: It should not be used by patients who have a known sensitivity to terfenadine or related products.
■ ADVERSE EFFECTS: The most commonly reported side effects are dry mouth and throat.

terminal /tur′minəl/ [L, *terminus,* boundary], **1.** (of a

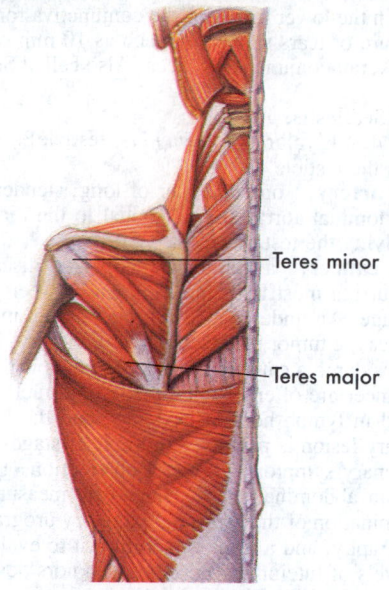

Teres major and teres minor
(Thibodeau, 1993/John V Hagen)

structure or process) near or approaching its end, such as a terminal bronchiole or a terminal disease. **2.** an input/output (I/O) device that has two-way communication capability with a computer. A terminal usually has a keyboard and a cathode-ray or video display screen, or a text printing facility.
—**terminate,** *v.,* **terminus,** *n.*

terminal arteriole [L, *terminus,* boundary + *arteriola,* little artery], an arteriole that divides into capillaries.

terminal bronchiole. See **bronchiole.**

terminal cancer [L, *terminalis* + *cancer,* a crab], an advanced stage of a cancer with death as the inevitable prognosis.

terminal disinfection, the process of cleaning equipment and airing of a room after the release of a patient who has been treated for an infectious disease.

terminal drop, a rapid decline in cognitive function and coping ability that occurs 1 to 5 years before death.

terminal illness [L, *terminalis;* ME, *yfel,* evil], an advanced stage of a disease with an unfavorable prognosis and no known cure.

terminal nerve, a small nerve originating in the cerebral hemisphere in the region of the olfactory trigone, classified by most anatomists as part of the olfactory, or first cranial, nerve. The terminal nerve courses anteriorly along the olfactory tract and passes through the ethmoid bone. Most filaments of the nerve form a single strand that passes to the membrane near the anterior superior border of the nasal septum and communicates in the nasal cavity with the ophthalmic division of the trigeminal nerve. The central connections of the terminal nerve end in the septal nuclei, the olfactory lobe, and the posterior commissural and supraoptic regions of the brain.

terminal stance, one of the five stages in the stance phase of a walking gait, directly associated with the continuation of single limb support or the period during which the body

moves forward on the supporting foot. Double limb support is initiated during the latter part of terminal stance, which is often a factor in the analysis of many abnormal orthopedic conditions and the diagnosis of weaknesses that may develop in certain muscles used in walking, such as the quadriceps femoris and the gluteus maximus. Compare **initial contact stance stage, loading response stance stage, midstance, preswing stance stage.** See also **swing phase of gait.**

terminal sulcus of right atrium, a shallow channel on the external surface of the right atrium between the superior and inferior venae cavae.

termination codon /tur'minā'shən/, (in molecular genetics) a unit in the genetic code that specifies the end of the sequence of amino acids in a polypeptide.

termination phase, the last stage of a therapeutic relationship when attained goals are evaluated and outcomes achieved. During this stage practioners also may help patients establish networks of support, other than the therapist-patient relationship, that may help in coping with future problems.

termination sequence, (in molecular genetics) a DNA segment at the end of a unit that is transcribed to messenger RNA from the DNA template.

term infant [Gk, *terma,* limit], any neonate, regardless of birth weight, born after the end of the thirty-seventh and before the beginning of the forty-third week of gestation. Infants delivered at term usually measure from 48 to 53 cm from head to heel and weigh between 2700 and 4000 g.

terpin hydrate and codeine elixir /tur'pin/, a preparation of the expectorant terpin hydrate, with sweet orange peel tincture, benzaldehyde, glycerin, alcohol, syrup, water, and the antitussive narcotic codeine. Terpin hydrate diminishes secretions and promotes healing of the mucous membrane, and codeine depresses the cough center in the medulla oblongata; prolonged use may lead to addiction.

Terra-Cortril, a trademark for a topical fixed-combination drug containing a glucocorticoid (hydrocortisone) and an antibiotic (oxytetracycline).

Terramycin, a trademark for an antibiotic (oxytetracycline).

tertiary syphilis /tur'sharē/ [L, *tertius,* third], the most advanced stage of syphilis, resulting in infections of the cardiovascular and neurological systems and marked by destructive lesions involving many tissues and organs. Late-stage syphilis is symptomatic but not contagious.

territorial /ter'ətôr'ē·əl/ [L, *territorium,* district], a type of body movement that aids in communication. A territorial will frame an interaction and define an individual's "territory." See also **territoriality.**

territoriality /ter'itôr'ē·al'itē/, an emotional attachment to and defense of certain areas related to one's existence. Humans and animals generally establish a claim to or occupy a defined or undefined area over which they can maintain some degree of control.

terti-, a combining form meaning 'third': *tertiary, tertigravida, tertipara.*

tertian /tur'shən/ [L, *tertius,* third], occurring every 48 hours or third day, including the first day of occurrence, such as vivax or tertian malaria, in which fever occurs every third day. Compare **quartan.** See also **malaria.**

tertian malaria, a form of malaria, caused by the protozoan *Plasmodium vivax* or *Plasmodium ovale,* characterized by febrile paroxysms that occur every 48 hours. **Vivax ma-**

laria, caused by *Plasmodium vivax,* is the most common form of malaria, and although it is rarely fatal, it is the most difficult form to cure. Relapses are common. **Ovale malaria,** caused by *Plasmodium ovale,* is usually milder and causes only a few short attacks. Both types of tertian malaria are treated with chloroquine. Compare **falciparum malaria, quartan malaria.** See also **malaria.**

tertiary /tur'shē-ə-rē, tursh'ərē/ [L, *tertius,* third], third in frequency or in order of use; belonging to the third level of sophistication of development, such as a tertiary health care facility.

tertiary health care, a specialized, highly technical level of health care that includes diagnosis and treatment of disease and disability in sophisticated, large research and teaching hospitals. Specialized intensive care units, advanced diagnostic support services, and highly specialized personnel are usually characteristic of tertiary health care. It offers a highly centralized care to the population of a large region; in some cases, to the world.

tertiary prevention, a level of preventive medicine that deals with the rehabilitation and return of a patient to a status of maximum usefulness with a minimum risk of recurrence of a physical or mental disorder.

tesla /tes'lə/ [Nikola Tesla, American engineer, b. 1856], a unit of magnetic flux density, defined by the International System of Units as 1 weber per square meter, the equivalent of 1 volt/second per square meter, or 10,000 gauss.

Teslac, a trademark for an antineoplastic (testolactone).

Tessalon, a trademark for a local anesthetic agent (benzonatate).

test [L, *testum,* crucible], **1.** an examination or trial intended to establish a principle or determine a value. **2.** a chemical reaction or reagent that has clinical significance. **3.** to detect, identify, or conduct a trial. See also **laboratory test.**

test-, a combining form meaning 'of or pertaining to the testicles': *testicond, testitoxicosis, testosterone.*

testamentary capacity /tes'təmen'tərē/, a person's competency to make a will, including the requirement that he or she be aware that a will is being made, of the nature and extent of the property covered by the will, and of the identities of the beneficiaries.

testcross [L, *testum* + *crux,* cross], **1.** (in genetics) the cross of a dominant phenotype with a recessive phenotype to determine either the degree of genetic linkage or whether the dominant phenotype is homozygous or heterozygous. **2.** the subject undergoing such a test.

testes, See **testis.**

testes determining factor (TDF) /tes'tēz/, a Y-chromosome gene that is believed to determine male sexual development. Studies indicate that individuals with the normal female (XX) sex chromosome combination may develop as males if the TDF gene has migrated to one of the X chromosomes. Also, an individual with the normal male (XY) chromosome pair may develop as a female if the TDF gene is missing from the Y chromosome.

test for acetone in urine, a part of routine urinalysis. Normal findings are negative, as acetone and other ketones are not normally present in urine. Exceptions include such cases as poorly controlled diabetic patients, alcoholics, and people who may be fasting or on special high-protein diets.

test for lacrimation, a test for possible keratoconjunctivitis sicca conducted by placing a 35 mm long piece of filter paper in the lower fornix of the conjunctiva for five minutes. Failure of tears to wet as much as 10 mm of the strip indicates keratoconjunctivitis sicca. Also called **Schirmer's test.**

testicle. See **testis.**

testicular /testik'yələr/ [L, *testiculus,* testicle], of or pertaining to the testicle.

testicular artery, one of a pair of long, slender branches of the abdominal aorta, arising caudal to the renal arteries and supplying the testis.

testicular cancer, a malignant neoplastic disease of the testis occurring most frequently in men between 20 and 35 years of age. An undescended testicle is often involved. In many cases the tumor is detected after an injury, but trauma is not considered a causative factor. Patients with early testicular cancer are often asymptomatic, and metastases may be seeded in lymph nodes, the lungs, and the liver before the primary lesion is palpable. In the later stages there may be pulmonary symptoms, ureteral obstruction, gynecomastia, and an abdominal mass. Diagnostic measures include transillumination of the scrotum, excretory urography, lymphangiography, and a urine or serum test to evaluate circulating levels of luteinizing hormone. Tumors develop more often in the right than in the left testis. Seminomas are the most curable lesions and the most common, representing 40% of all testicular tumors. Embryonal carcinomas are more highly malignant and represent 15% to 20% of these tumors. Teratocarcinomas and choriocarcinomas also occur. Radiotherapy and surgical excision are usually recommended to treat seminoma. Chemotherapy using combinations of drugs is recommended for nonseminomatous tumors. Chemotherapeutic agents, used in various combinations, are increasing the survival of patients with testicular cancer. Some of these drugs are actinomycin D, bleomycin, cis-platinum, cyclophosphamide, methotrexate, and vincristine.

testicular duct. See **vas deferens.**

testicular feminization. See **feminization.**

testicular self-examination (TSE), a recommended (National Health Institute) procedure for detecting tumors or other abnormalities in the male testes. TSE should be performed once a month, usually after a warm bath or shower because the heat causes scrotal skin to relax, thereby increasing the chances of detecting any tissue abnormality. The TSE is conducted in four simple steps, starting with standing in front of a mirror and looking for any swelling on the skin of the scrotum. One testicle may appear larger than the other and one may hang lower, which is usually normal. Next, each testicle is examined with both hands, placing the fingers under the testicle while the thumbs are placed on top. The testicle is then rolled gently between the thumbs and fingers. In the next step, the epididymis, a normal cordlike structure on the top and back of each testicle, should be found. A small pea-sized lump is felt for on the front or side of a testicle. The lump is usually painless. Testicular cancer almost always occurs in only one testicle. It is highly curable when detected at an early stage.

testicular vein, one of a pair of veins emerging from convoluted venous plexuses, forming the greater mass of the spermatic cords. Veins from each plexus start from small veins at the back of the testes, ascend along the spermatic cords, anterior to the ductus deferens, pass through the deep inguinal ring, and unite to form a single vein. The right tes-

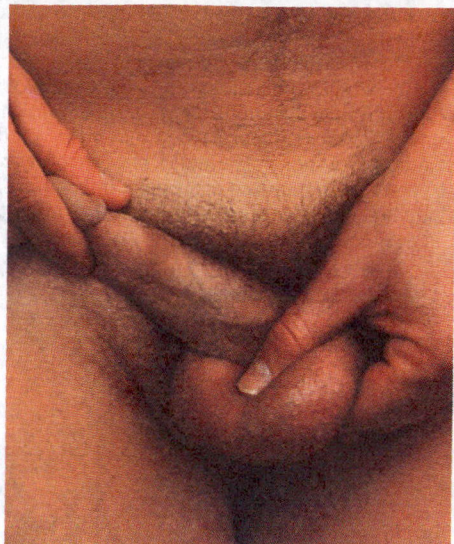

Testicular self-examination (Seidel, 1991)

ticular vein opens into the inferior vena cava; the left testicular vein into the left renal vein. Both testicular veins contain valves. Compare **ovarian vein**.

testimony /tes´timō´nē/ [L, *testimonium*, evidence], the statement of a witness, usually made orally and given under oath, such as at a court trial.

testis /tes´tis/, *pl.* **testes** /tes´tēz/, [L], one of the pair of male gonads that produce semen. The adult testes are suspended in the scrotum by the spermatic cords; in early fetal life they are contained in the abdominal cavity behind the peritoneum. Before birth they normally descend into the scrotum and during development are covered with layers of tissue derived from the serous, the muscular, and the fibrous layers of the abdominal parietes. The coverings of the testes are the skin and the dartos tunic of the scrotum, the external spermatic fascia, the cremasteric layer, the internal spermatic fascia, and the tunica vaginalis. Each testis is a laterally compressed oval body about 4 cm long and 2.5 cm wide, and weighs about 12 g. It is positioned obliquely in the scrotum, with the cranial extremity directed ventrally and slightly laterally, and the caudal end directed dorsally and slightly medially. The anterior border, the lateral surfaces, and the extremities of the organ are convex, free, smooth, and covered by the tunica vaginalis. The convoluted epididymis lying on the posterior border of the testis is about 20 feet long and connects with the vas deferens through which spermatozoa pass during ejaculation. Each testis consists of several hundred conical lobules containing the tiny coiled seminiferous tubules, each about 75 mm long, in which spermatozoa develop. In early life the tubules are pale in color but in old age become invested with yellow fatty matter. The tubules converge to form the rete testis, which is drained by the efferent ducts into the head of the epididymis. The testis, developed in the lumbar region, may be retained in the abdomen, the deep inguinal ring, or the inguinal canal. A man with both testes undescended is sterile but may not be impotent. The testes are

supplied with blood by the two internal spermatic arteries that arise from the aorta, are served by the testicular veins that form the pampiniform plexuses constituting the greater part of the spermatic cords, and are innervated by the spermatic plexuses of nerves from the celiac plexuses of the autonomic nervous system. Compare **ovary**. See also **scrotum**.

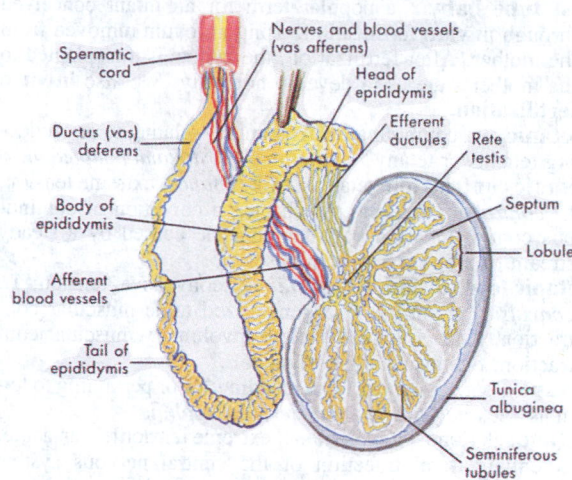

Testis (Thibodeau, 1993/Ernest W Beck)

test method, a method chosen for experimental testing or study by means of method evaluation.

test of patency of tear duct, a procedure in which drops of a weak sugar solution are placed in the eye. If the patient then detects a sweet taste the tear duct is assumed open.

testolactone /tes´təlak´tōn/, an antineoplastic androgen analog.

■ INDICATIONS: It is prescribed in the treatment of postmenopausal breast cancer and in premenopausal women whose ovarian function has been terminated.

■ CONTRAINDICATIONS: Pregnancy, lactation, or known hypersensitivity to this drug prohibits its use. It is not given to men.

■ ADVERSE EFFECTS: Among the more serious adverse reactions are hypercalcemia and peripheral neuropathies with numbness or tingling.

testosterone /testos´tərōn/, a naturally occurring androgenic hormone.

■ INDICATIONS: It is prescribed for androgen deficiency, for female breast cancer, and for stimulation of growth, weight gain, and red blood cell production.

■ CONTRAINDICATIONS: Cancer of the male breast or prostate, liver disease, pregnancy or suspected pregnancy, or known hypersensitivity to this drug prohibits its use.

■ ADVERSE EFFECTS: Among the more serious adverse reactions are fluid retention, masculinization, acne, and erythrocythemia.

testosterone cyclopentylpropionate. See **testosterone cypionate**.

testosterone cypionate, a long-acting form of testosterone.

testosterone derivative. See **anabolic steroid**.

testosterone enanthate, a long-acting form of testosterone.

testosterone propionate, an androgen given intramuscularly. See also **testosterone.**

test tube, a tube made of transparent material having one open end. It is used in the growth of bacteriologic specimens, in the analysis of some chemical functions, and in many other common laboratory functions. See also **tube.**

test tube baby, a popular term for an infant conceived through in vitro fertilization, using an ovum removed from the mother. After fertilization, the zygote is transplanted to the mother's uterus to develop normally. See also **in-vitro fertilization.**

-tetanic, a combining form meaning 'relating to or producing tetanus or tetany': *antitetanic, posttetanic, subtetanic.*

tetanic contraction /tetan′ik/ [Gk, *tetanos,* extreme tension; L, *contractio,* drawing together], a condition of continuous contraction in a voluntary muscle caused by a steady stream of efferent nerve impulses.

tetanic convulsion [Gk, *tetanos,* convulsive tension; L, *convulsio,* cramp], **1.** a generalized tonic muscular contraction. **2.** a prolonged violent involuntary muscular contraction. See also **tonic convulsion**.

tetano-, a combining form meaning 'of or pertaining to tetanus': *tetanolysin, tetanometer, tetanophilic.*

tetanus /tet′ənəs/ [Gk, *tetanos,* extreme tension], an acute, potentially fatal infection of the central nervous system caused by an exotoxin, tetanospasmin, elaborated by an anaerobic bacillus, *Clostridium tetani.* More than 50,000 people a year die of tetanus infection worldwide. The toxin is a neurotoxin and is one of the most lethal poisons known. *C. tetani* infects only wounds that contain dead tissue. The bacillus is a common resident of the superficial layers of the soil and a normal inhabitant of the intestinal tracts of cows and horses; therefore barnyards and fields fertilized with manure are heavily contaminated.

■ OBSERVATIONS: The bacillus may enter the body through a puncture wound, abrasion, laceration, or burn, via the uterus into the bloodstream in septic abortion or postpartum sepsis, or through the stump of the umbilical cord of the newborn. The dead tissue of the area is low in oxygen; this is the environment essential for the replication of *C. tetani.* The infection occurs in two clinical forms: one with an abrupt onset, high mortality, and a short incubation period (3 to 21 days); the other with less severe symptoms, a lower mortality, and a longer incubation period (4 to 5 weeks). Wounds of the face, head, and neck are the ones most likely to result in fatal infection, because the bacillus may travel rapidly to the brain. The disease is characterized by irritability, headache, fever, and painful spasms of the muscles resulting in lockjaw, risus sardonicus, opisthotonos, and laryngeal spasm; eventually, every muscle of the body is in tonic spasm. The motor nerves transmit the impulses from the infected central nervous system to the muscles. There is no lesion; even at autopsy no organic lesion is seen and the cerebrospinal fluid is clear and normal.

■ INTERVENTIONS: Prompt and thorough cleansing and debridement of the wound are essential for prophylaxis. A booster shot of tetanus toxoid is given to previously immunized people; tetanus immune globulin and a series of three injections of tetanus toxoid are given to those not immunized. People who are known to have been adequately immunized within 5 years do not usually require immunization. The treatment of people who have the infection includes maintenance of an airway, giving of an antitoxin as soon as possible, sedation, control of the muscle spasms, and assurance of a normal fluid balance. The room is kept quiet, and benzodiazepines may be given to reduce hypertonicity; penicillin G is administered for infection; and a tracheostomy is performed and oxygen given for ventilation.

■ NURSING CONSIDERATIONS: The nurse may encourage everyone to be actively immunized against the infection. The vaccine is safe and effective. Immunization more often than required is not recommended.

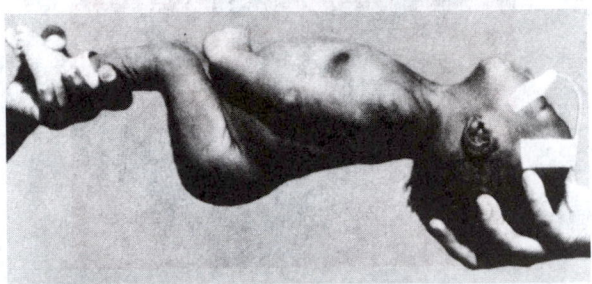

Infant with tetanus and characteristic muscle spasms *(Lambert, 1982)*

tetanus and diphtheria toxoids (Td), an active immunizing agent containing detoxified tetanus and diphtheria toxoids that slowly produce an antigenic response to the diseases.

■ INDICATIONS: It is prescribed for immunization against tetanus and diphtheria in children under 7 years of age when pertussis vaccine present in the usual diphtheria, pertussis, and tetanus trivalent vaccine is contraindicated.

■ CONTRAINDICATIONS: Immunosuppression, concomitant use of corticosteroids, or acute infection prohibits its use.

■ ADVERSE EFFECTS: Among the most serious adverse reactions are allergic reactions and stinging at the site of injection.

tetanus antitoxin (TAT), a tetanus immune serum that neutralizes exotoxins in tetanus infection.

■ INDICATIONS: It is prescribed for short-term immunization against tetanus after possible exposure to the organism and in tetanus treatment.

■ CONTRAINDICATIONS: It is not given if the more effective tetanus immune globulin is available or if there is a known sensitivity to equine serum.

■ ADVERSE EFFECTS: Among the most serious adverse reactions are allergic reactions and pain and inflammation at the site of injection.

tetanus immune globulin (TIG), an injectable solution prepared from the globulin of an immune human. It is effective and much safer than tetanus antitoxin.

■ INDICATIONS: It is prescribed for short-term immunization against tetanus after possible exposure to the organism and tetanus treatment.

■ CONTRAINDICATIONS: Known hypersensitivity to this drug prohibits its use. It should not be substituted for tetanus toxoid.

■ ADVERSE EFFECTS: The most serious adverse reaction is anaphylaxis. Fever and pain and inflammation at the site of injection may occur.

tetanus toxoid, an active immunizing agent prepared from detoxified tetanus toxin that produces an antigenic response in the body, conferring permanent immunity to tetanus infection.

- INDICATION: It is prescribed for primary active immunization against tetanus.
- CONTRAINDICATIONS: Immunosuppression or immunoglobulin abnormalities, acute infection, or illness prohibits its use.
- ADVERSE EFFECTS: The most serious adverse reaction is hypersensitivity. Pain and inflammation at the site of injection may occur.

tetany /tet'ənē/ [Gk, *tetanos,* extreme tension], a condition characterized by cramps, convulsions, twitching of the muscles, and sharp flexion of the wrist and ankle joints. These symptoms are sometimes accompanied by attacks of stridor. Tetany is a manifestation of an abnormality in calcium metabolism, which can occur in association with vitamin D deficiency, hypoparathyroidism, alkalosis, or the ingestion of alkaline salts. Kinds of tetany are **duration tetany, gastric tetany, hyperventilation tetany,** and **hypocalcemic tetany.**

tetart-, a combining form meaning 'fourth': *tetartanopia, tetartocone, tetartoconoid.*

tetra- /tet'rə/, **tetro-** /tet'rə/, a combining form meaning 'four': *tetracycline, tetrahydric, tetranopsia.*

tetrachlormethane. See **carbon tetrachloride.**

tetracycline /tet'rəsī'klēn/, a broad spectrum antibiotic.

- INDICATIONS: It is prescribed for the treatment of many bacterial and rickettsial infections.
- CONTRAINDICATIONS: Significantly impaired liver or renal function or known hypersensitivity to this drug prohibits its use. Because it may cause permanent discoloration of the teeth, its use is contraindicated in the last half of pregnancy and during a child's first 8 years of life.
- ADVERSE EFFECTS: Among the more serious adverse reactions are renal toxicity, hepatotoxicity, severe GI disturbances, enterocolitis, inflammatory lesions with monilial overgrowth in the anogenital area, hemolytic anemia, thrombocytopenia, eosinophilia, and rashes.

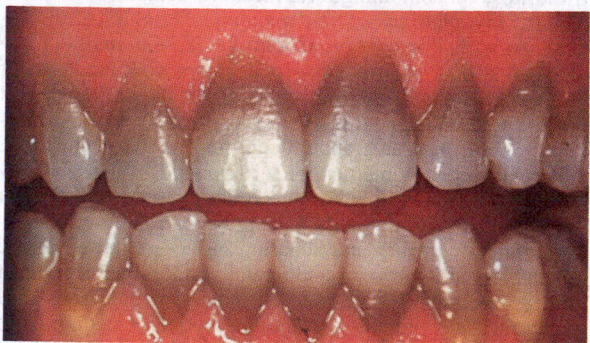

Severe discoloration of the teeth caused by tetracycline (Jordan, 1993)

tetracycline hydrochloride, a tetracycline antibiotic.

- INDICATIONS: It is prescribed in the treatment of a variety of infections.
- CONTRAINDICATIONS: Known hypersensitivity to this drug or to other tetracyclines prohibits its use. Use during pregnancy or in children under 8 years of age may result in discolor-

ation of the child's teeth. It is to be administered with caution with renal or liver impairment.

- ADVERSE EFFECTS: Among the most serious reactions are potentially serious suprainfections, various allergic reactions, phototoxicity, and GI disturbances.

tetrad /tet'rad/ [Gk, *tetras,* quadrant], (in genetics) a group of four chromatids of a synapsed pair of homologous chromosomes during the first meiotic prophase stage of gametogenesis. The group is formed in preparation for the two meiotic divisions in the maturation process of gametes. —**tetradic,** *adj.*

tetradactyly /-dak'tilē/ [Gk, *tetra* + *dactylos*], the presence of only four fingers on each hand or four toes on each foot.

tetrahydrocannabinol (THC) /-hi'drōkənab'inol/, the active principle, occurring as two psychomimetic isomers, in the hemp plant *Cannabis sativa,* used in the preparation of marijuana, hashish, bhang, and ganja. THC, a rapidly metabolized beta-adrenergic agonist, increases pulse rate, causes conjunctival reddening and a feeling of euphoria, and has variable effects on blood pressure, respiratory rate, and pupil size. The drug affects memory, cognition, and the sensorium, decreases motor coordination, and increases appetite. Propranolol blocks the peripheral effects of THC but not the psychic effects. Overdoses of THC may be treated by 'talking down' the patient and administering sedative barbiturates or diazepam parenterally. Nonintoxicating doses of THC are used experimentally in the treatment of glaucoma and to relieve nausea and increase the appetite in patients receiving cancer chemotherapy. See also **cannabis.**

tetrahydrozoline hydrochloride /-hīdroz'əlēn/, an adrenergic vasoconstrictor.

- INDICATIONS: It is prescribed for the treatment of nasal and nasopharangeal congestion and as an ophthalmic vasoconstrictor.
- CONTRAINDICATIONS: Glaucoma or known hypersensitivity to this drug or to other vasoconstrictors prohibits its use. It is used with caution in patients who have cardiovascular disease.
- ADVERSE EFFECTS: Among the more serious adverse reactions are irritation to mucosa, rebound nasal congestion, and effects associated with systemic absorption, including sedation and alterations in cardiovascular function.

tetraiodothyronine. See **thyroxine.**

tetralogy /tetrol'əjē/ [Gk, *tetra,* four + *logos,* word], any group of four writings, symptoms, or other related factors. See **tetralogy of Fallot.**

tetralogy of Fallot /falō'/ [Gk, *tetra,* four, *logos,* word; Etienne-Louis A. Fallot, French physician, b. 1850], a congenital cardiac anomaly that consists of four defects: pulmonic stenosis, ventricular septal defect, malposition of the aorta so that it arises from the septal defect or the right ventricle, and right ventricular hypertrophy. The primary symptoms in the infant are cyanosis and hypoxia, difficulty in feeding, failure to gain weight, and poor development. In older children a typical squatting position and clubbing of the fingers and toes are evident. A pansystolic murmur is usually heard, and the second heart sound is faint or absent. Diagnosis of the condition is primarily based on the history and physical symptoms, although cardiac catheterization is performed to evaluate the severity of the defects. Treatment consists mainly of supportive measures and palliative surgical procedures, primarily systemic to pulmonary anastomoses, to decrease tissue hypoxia and prevent com-

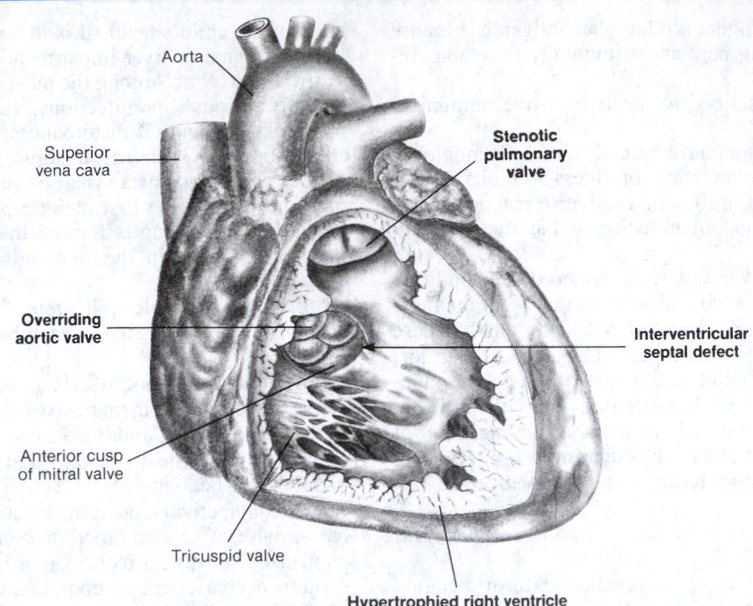

Aorta

Superior
vena cava

Stenotic
pulmonary
valve

Overriding
aortic valve

Interventricular
septal defect

Anterior cusp
of mitral valve

Tricuspid valve

Hypertrophied right ventricle

Tetralogy of Fallot *(Cannobio, 1990)*

plications until the child is old enough to tolerate total corrective surgery. The optimal age for surgical repair is approximately 1 year. Also called **Fallot's syndrome.** See also **blue baby, trilogy of Fallot.**

tetramer /tet′rəmer/ [Gk, *tetra* + *meros*, part], something that is composed of four parts, such as a protein composed of four polypeptide subunits.

tetraplegia /-plē′jə/ [Gk, *tetra,* four + *plege,* stroke], paralysis of both arms and both legs.Also called **quadriplegia.**

tetraploid (4n) /tet′rəploid/ [Gk, *tetraploos,* fourfold, *eidos,* form], **1.** also **tetraploidic.** of or pertaining to an individual, organism, strain, or cell that has four complete sets of chromosomes, quadruple the normal haploid number characteristic of the species. In humans, the tetraploid number is 92 and is extremely rare, found only occasionally in abortuses and stillborn fetuses. **2.** such an individual, organism, strain, or cell. Compare **diploid, haploid, triploid.** See also **polyploid.**

tetraploidy /tet′rəploi[L]dē/, the state or condition of having four complete sets of chromosomes.

Tetrex, a trademark for an antibiotic (tetracycline phosphate complex.)

tetro-. See **tetra-.**

TFIIE, a general transcription factor involved in complementary DNA encoding. TFIIE consists of two subunits, TFIIE-alpha and TFIIE-beta.

T fracture /tē′frakchər/, an intercondylar fracture in which the fracture lines are T-shaped.

TGF, abbreviation for **transforming growth factor.**

T group. See **sensitivity training group.**

Th, symbol for the element **thorium.**

thalamic /thalam′ik/ [Gk, *thalamos,* chamber], pertaining to the thalamus.

thalamic peduncle [Gk, *thalamos,* chamber; L, *pes,* foot],

a group of fibers linking the thalamus with the hypothalamus.

thalamic syndrome [Gk, *thalamos* + *syn,* together + *dromos,* course], a vascular disorder involving the ventral and posterolateral nuclei of the thalamus and related nerve fibers causing disturbances of sensation and partial or complete paralysis of one side of the body. A major effect is an increased threshold to all stimuli on the opposite side of the body so that any stimuli may cause an exaggerated response. Also called **Déjérine-Roussy syndrome.**

thalamo-, a combining form meaning 'relating to the thalamus,: *thalamocortical, thalamotomy.*

thalamus /thal′əməs/, *pl.* **thalami** [Gk, *thalamos,* chamber], one of a pair of large oval organs forming most of the lateral walls of the third ventricle of the brain and part of the diencephalon. It relays sensory impulses to the cerebral cortex, measures about 4 cm long and 1.5 cm wide, and consists of numerous nuclei arranged in anterior, lateral, intralaminar, medial, and posterior groups. On each side the thalamus extends caudally beyond the third ventricle, with its medial and superior surfaces exposed in the ventricle and its inferior and lateral surfaces buried against other structures. It is composed mainly of gray substance and translates impulses from appropriate receptors into crude sensations of pain, temperature, and touch. It also participates in associating sensory impulses with pleasant and unpleasant feelings, in the arousal mechanisms of the body, and in the mechanisms that produce complex reflex movements. Compare **epithalamus, hypothalamus, subthalamus. –thalamic,** *adj.*

thalassemia /thal′əsē′mē·ə/ [Gk, *thalassa,* sea, *a, haima,* not blood], a hemolytic hemoglobinopathy anemia characterized by microcytic, hypochromic, and short-lived red blood cells caused by deficient hemoglobin synthesis. People of Mediterranean origin are more often affected than others. Transmitted as an autosomal recessive gene, the disease occurs in two forms. **Thalassemia major (Cooley's anemia),** the homozygous form, evident in infancy, is recognized by anemia, fever, failure to thrive, and splenomegaly, and is confirmed by characteristic changes in the red blood cells on microscopic examination. Frequent transfusions are necessary to maintain oxygen-carrying capacity of the blood. Red cells are rapidly destroyed, freeing large amounts of iron to be deposited in the skin, which becomes bronzed and freckled. The iron is also deposited in the heart, liver, and pancreas, which become fibrotic and dysfunctional. The spleen may become so enlarged that respiratory excursion is impeded and the abdominal organs are crowded. Headache, abdominal pain, fatigue, and anorexia often occur. No cure exists. The nurse is aware that the child is uncomfortable and that growth and sexual development are usually retarded. Rarely, a child with thalassemia major is able to function without transfusions, thereby avoiding the massive ill effects of accumulated iron deposits. **Thalassemia minor,** the heterozygous form, is characterized only by a mild anemia and minimal red blood cell changes. Thalassemia minima is a form that lacks clinical symptoms, although patients show hematologic evidence of the disease. Nursing considerations in the care of thalassemia patients and their families should include observation for ill effects of transfusion, education and counseling about the disease, and referral for genetic counseling. See also **hemochromatosis, hemosiderosis.**

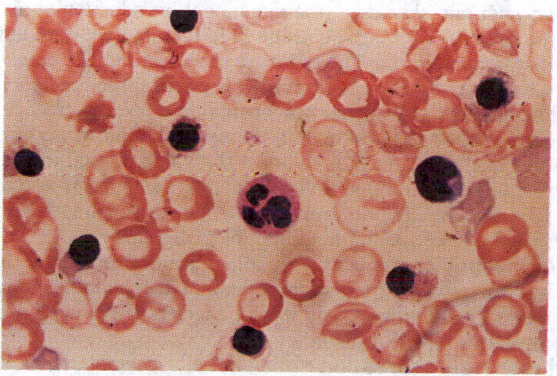

Thalassemia major—characteristic abnormal red blood cells
(Zitelli, 1992)

thalasso-, a combining form meaning 'of or pertaining to the sea': *thalassophobia, thalassotherapy.*

thalidomide /thalid′əmīd/, a sedative-hypnotic, withdrawn from general use because of its potential for teratogenic effects, particularly phocomelia, when taken during pregnancy. It is sometimes prescribed for treatment of leprosy.

thallium (Tl) /thal′ē·əm/ [Gk, *thallos,* green line], a soft, bluish-white metallic element that exhibits some nonmetallic chemical properties. Its atomic number is 81; its atomic weight is 204.37. Many of its compounds are highly toxic. Thallium sulfate is widely used as a rat poison.

thallium poisoning, a toxic condition caused by the ingestion or the absorption through the skin of thallium salts, especially thallium sulfate. Characteristic of the condition are abdominal pain, vomiting, bloody diarrhea, tremor, delirium, and alopecia. Treatment varies with the symptoms. Anticonvulsant and antihypotensive medication may be necessary. Thallium has been used in insect and rodent poisons, fireworks, and some cosmetic hair removers, but this extremely toxic and cumulative poison was banned for use in household products in 1965.

thanato-, a combining form meaning 'of or pertaining to death': *thanatobiologic, thanatognomonic, thanatology.*

thanatology /than′ətol′əjē/ [Gk, *thanatos,* death, *logos,* science], the study of death and dying. **—thanatologist,** *n.*

thanatophoric dwarf /than′ətōfôr′ik/ [Gk, *thanatos* + *phoros,* bearer; AS, *dweorge*], an infant with severe micromelia, the limbs usually extending straight out from the trunk, an extremely narrow chest, and flattened vertebral bodies with wide intervertebral spaces. Death usually occurs from respiratory complications shortly after birth.

Thanatos /than′ətəs/ [Gk, death], a freudian term for the death instinct.

thanotopsy. See **autopsy.**

thaumato-, a combining form meaning 'pertaining to marvel or miracles': *thaumatology, thaumaturgic, thaumaturgy.*

THC, abbreviation for **tetrahydrocannabinol.**

the blues, *informal.* a designation for Blue Cross (an insurance system that pays the costs of treatment by a hospital or clinic) and Blue Shield (an insurance system that pays the costs of treatment by a professional).

thec-, a prefix meaning 'of or pertaining to a sheath, such as of a tendon': *thecal, thecitis, thecodont.*

theca /thē′kə/, *pl.* **thecae** /thē′sē/, a sheath or capsule, such as the theca cordis or pericardium.

theca cell tumor [Gk, *theke,* sheath; L, *cella,* storeroom; *tumor,* swelling], an uncommon benign fibroid tumor of the ovary, composed of theca cells and usually containing granulosa (follicular) cells. Characteristically solid masses with yellow fatty streaks, these tumors are frequently associated with excessive estrogen production and tend to develop cystic degeneration. Also called **fibroma thecocellulare xanthomatodes, thecoma.**

thecal /thē′kəl/ [Gk, *theke,* sheath], pertaining to a theca or sheath.

-thecium, a combining form meaning a 'sack or container': *bdellepithecium, epithecium, perithecium.*

thecocellulare xanthomatodes, thecoma. See **theca cell tumor.**

Theden's bandage /tā′dənz/ [Johann C. A. Theden, German surgeon, b. 1714], a roller bandage applied below the injury and continued upward over a compress, used to stop bleeding. Also called **Genga's bandage.**

thel-, a combining form meaning 'of or pertaining to the nipple': *thelalgia, theleplasty, thelitis.*

thelarche /thilär′kē/ [Gk, *thele,* nipple, *archaios,* beginning], the beginning of female pubertal breast development normally occuring between 9 and 13 years of age, thelarche is before puberty at the beginning of the phase of rapid growth. **Premature thelarche** is precocious breast development in a female without other evidence of sexual maturation. Compare **menarche.**

-thelia, a suffix meaning '(condition of the) nipples': *epithelia, hyperthelia, microthelia.*

-thelioma, a suffix meaning a 'tumor in a cellular tissue': *celiothelioma, hemendothelioma, perithelioma.*

-thelium, a suffix meaning a 'layer of (specified kind of) cellular tissue': *desmepithelium, mesothelium.*

thely-, a combining form meaning 'female': *thelyblast, thelygenic, thelyplasty.*

thenar /thē'när/ [Gk, palm of the hand], **1.** the ball of the thumb. **2.** of or pertaining to the thumb side of the palm.

thenar eminence [Gk, *thenar*, palm of the hand; L, *eminentia*, projection], a raised rounded area on the palm of the hand near the base of the thumb.

theo-, a combining form meaning 'of or pertaining to a god': *theomania, theophobia, theotherapy.*

Theobid, a trademark for a smooth muscle relaxant (theophylline).

theobromine /thē'əbrō'min/, a substance (methylxanthine) that is related chemically to caffeine and theophylline and differs from them by the number and distribution of methyl groups. Theobromine occurs naturally in cocoa, cola nuts, and tea. It acts as a diuretic, vasodilator, cardiac stimulant, and smooth muscle relaxant.

Theo-Dur, a trademark for a bronchodilator (theophylline).

Theolair, a trademark for a bronchodilator (theophylline) used for the relief of acute bronchial asthma.

theophylline /thē·əfil'ēn/ [L, *thea*, tea; Gk, *phyllon*, leaf], a bronchodilator.
■ INDICATIONS: It is prescribed to relax the smooth muscle of the bronchial passages in the treatment of bronchospasm in bronchial asthma, bronchitis, and emphysema.
■ CONTRAINDICATIONS: Hypertension, cardiac disease, liver disease, renal disease, or concurrent treatment with other xanthines may prohibit its use.
■ ADVERSE EFFECT: Among the most serious adverse reactions are hypersensitivity, GI bleeding, palpitations, and seizures.

theorem /thē'ərəm/ [Gk, *theorein*, to look at], **1.** a proposition to be proved by a chain of reasoning and analysis. **2.** a rule expressed by symbols or formulae.

theoretic effectiveness /thē·əret'ik/ [Gk, *theorein* + L, *efficere*, to do], (of a contraceptive method) the effectiveness of a medication, device, or method in preventing pregnancy if used consistently and exactly as intended, without error. Compare **use effectiveness.**

theoretic plate number (N), a number defining the efficiency of a chromatographic column.

theory /thē'ərē/ [Gk, *theorein*, to look at], an abstract statement formulated to predict, explain, or describe the relationships among concepts, constructs, or events. Theory is developed and tested by observation and research, using factual data.

theotherapy /thē'ōther'əpē/ [Gk, *theos*, god, *therapeia*, treatment], a therapeutic approach to the prevention, diagnosis, and treatment of disease and dysfunction based on religious or spiritual beliefs.

Theovent, a trademark for a smooth muscle relaxant (theophylline).

therapeutic /ther'əpyoo'tik/ [Gk, *therapeuein*, to treat], **1.** beneficial. **2.** pertaining to a treatment.

-therapeutic, -therapeutics, a suffix meaning 'pertaining to medical treatment by (specified) techniques': *kinetotherapeutic, orthotherapeutic, radiotherapeutics.*

therapeutic abortion, 1. a termination of early pregnancy deemed necessary by a physician. **2.** *informal.* any legal induced abortion. Compare **elective abortion.** See also **induced abortion.**

therapeutic communication, a process in which the nurse consciously influences a client or helps the client to a better understanding through verbal or nonverbal communication.

therapeutic community (TC), (in mental health) a treatment facility in which the entire milieu is part of the treatment. The physical environment, the other clients, the staff, and the policies of the facility influence the function of the individual in the activities of daily living in the community. The concept of a therapeutic community is integral to milieu therapy.

therapeutic dose [Gk, *therapeia*, treatment + *dosis*, giving], the dose that may be required to produce a desired effect.

therapeutic equivalent, a drug that has essentially the same effect in the treatment of a disease or condition as one or more other drugs. A drug that is a therapeutic equivalent may or may not be chemically equivalent, bioequivalent, or generically equivalent. See also **bioequivalent, chemical equivalent, generic equivalent.**

therapeutic exercise, any exercise planned and performed to attain a specific physical benefit, such as maintenance of the range of motion, strengthening of weakened muscles, increased flexibility of a joint, or improved cardiovascular and respiratory function.

therapeutic gain, the ratio of the biologic effect of a therapy on a tumor compared with the effect on surrounding normal tissue. Higher therapeutic gains mean lower complications of therapy.

therapeutic index, the difference between the minimum therapeutic and minimum toxic concentrations of a drug.

therapeutic pneumothorax [Gk, *therapeia*, treatment + *pneuma*, air; *thorax*], the intentional introduction of air in the intrapleural space, causing partial collapse of the lung. It was used in the 1940s for treatment of certain cases of tuberculosis. Also called **artificial pneumothorax.**

therapeutic radiopharmaceutical, a radioactive drug administered to a patient to deliver radiation to body tissues internally, such as iodide 131, which is used to ablate thyroid tissue in hyperthyroid patients, cesium 137, iridium 192, radium 226, or strontium 90, which is implanted in a sealed source for the treatment of malignancies.

therapeutic recreation, an allied health category, staffed by people with expertise in organizing and supervising recreational activities designed to accelerate recovery from mental or physical disorders.

therapeutic recreation specialist, a person who assists patients in their recovery or rehabilitation after physical or emotional illness or disability by planning and supervising recreation programs.

therapeutics /ther'əpyoo'tiks/ [Gk, *therapeia*, treatment], a branch of health care that is concerned with the treatment of disease, seeking to relieve symptoms or to produce a cure.

-therapeutics. See **therapeutic.**

therapeutic temperature, in hyperthermia treatment, temperatures between 42° and 45° C (107° and 113° F).

-therapia, -therapy, a suffix meaning 'a specific type of medical care': *balneotherapia, odontotherapia, hypnotherapy.*

therapist /ther'əpist/, a person with special skills, obtained through education and experience, in one or more areas of health care.

therapy /ther'əpē/ [Gk, *therapeia*], the treatment of any disease or a pathologic condition, such as inhalation therapy, which administers various medicines for patients suffering from diseases of the respiratory tract.

-therapy,   See **-therapia.**

therio-,   a combining form meaning 'of or pertaining to beasts': *theriomimicry, theriotherapy, theriotomy.*

therm-.   See **thermo-.**

-therm, -thermia, -thermy,   a suffix meaning 'pertaining to a state of heat: *allotherm, azothermia, hypothermia, poikilotherm.*

thermal /thur′məl/ [Gk, *therme,* heat],   of or pertaining to the production, application, or maintenance of heat. Also **thermic.**

thermal burn,   tissue injury, usually of the skin, caused by exposure to extreme heat. See also **burn.**

thermal dilution,   See **thermodilution.**

thermal field size,   the area over which therapeutic heating is likely to be produced.

thermalgesia /thur′məljē′zē·ə/[Gk, *therme,* heat + *algos,* pain],   pain caused by exposure to high temperatures.

thermal radiation [Gk, *therme,* heat; L, *radiare,* to shine],   the emission of energy in the form of heat.

-thermia.   See **-therm.**

thermic fever /thur′mik/.   See **heat hyperpyrexia.**

thermic sense [Gk, *therme,* heat; L, *sentire,* to feel],   the network of sense organs and connecting pathways that allow an appreciation of temperature changes. Also called **temperature sense.**

thermistor /thərmis′tər/ [Gk, *therme* + L, *resistere,* to withstand],   a kind of thermometer for measuring minute changes in temperature. The resistance of a thermistor varies with the ambient temperature, thereby enabling accurate measurements of small temperature changes. See also **temperature, thermometer.**

thermo-, /thur′mō-/,   **therm-** a combining form meaning 'of or pertaining to heat': *thermochemistry, thermogenesis, thermopalpation.*

thermocautery /thur′mōkô′tərē/ [Gk, *therme* + *kauterion,* branding iron],   the use of a needle or snare heated by direct flame, a heated hydrocarbon vapor, or an electric current in the destruction of tissue. See also **Paquelin's cautery.**

thermochemistry /-kem′istrē/ [Gk, *therme,* heat + *chemia,* alchemy],   a branch of chemistry that is concerned with the heat changes involved in chemical reactions.

thermocoagulation /-kō·ag′yəlā′shən/ [Gk, *therme,* heat; L, *coagulare*],   the use of high-frequency electric currents to destroy tissue through heat coagulation.

thermocouple /thur′məkup′əl/ [Gk, *therme* + Fr, *couple,* pair],   a temperature-measuring device that relies on the production of a temperature-dependent voltage at the junction of two dissimilar metals.

thermodilution /-dilyōō′zhən/,   a method of cardiac output determination. A bolus of solution of known volume and temperature is added to the bloodstream, and the resultant cooling of blood temperature is detected by a thermistor previously placed in the pulmonary artery with a catheter.

thermodynamics /-dīnam′iks/ [Gk, *therme,* heat + *dynamis,* power],   the science of the interconversion of heat and work.

thermogenesis /thur′mōjen′əsis/ [Gk, *therme* + *genesis,* origin],   production of heat, especially by the cells of the body.   **–thermogenetic,** *adj.*

thermogenic center.   See **thermoregulatory centers.**

thermograph /thur′məgraf′/ [Gk, *therme* + *graphein,* to record],   **1.** a photographic record of the amount of heat radiated from the surface of the body, revealing 'hot spots' of potential tumors or other disorders. **2.** a device consisting of a thermometer, inked stylus, and chart for continuous recording of the ambient temperature.

thermography /thərmog′rəfē/,   a technique for sensing and recording on film hot and cold areas of the body by means of an infrared detector that reacts to blood flow. Disease states that manifest increased or decreased blood flow present thermographic patterns that can be distinguished from those of normal areas.   **–thermographic,** *adj.*

thermoinhibitory center.   See **thermoregulatory centers.**

thermolabile /thur′məlā′bəl/ [Gk, *therme* + L, *labilis,* slipping],   easily destroyed or altered by heat. Also called **heat labile.** Compare **thermostable.**

thermoluminescent dosimetry /-lōō′mines′ənt/   [Gk, *therme* + L, *lumen,* light; Gk, *dosis,* giving something, *metron,* measure],   a method of measuring the ionizing radiation to which a person is exposed by a device that stores the radiant energy and releases it later as ultraviolet or visible light. The device contains a crystalline material that is altered in structure by the radiation. It stores the radiation's energy, which is later released by heating the material. The light emitted is detected by a photomultiplier tube that generates an electric signal of a magnitude that reflects the amount of ionizing radiation originally received.

thermometer /thermom′ətər/ [Gk, *therme* + *metron,* measure],   an instrument for measuring temperature. It usually consists of a sealed glass tube, marked in degrees of Celsius or Fahrenheit, and containing liquid, such as mercury or alcohol. The liquid rises or falls as it expands or contracts according to changes in temperature. Some kinds of thermometers are **clinical thermometer, digital thermometer, electronic thermometer,** and **tympanic membrane thermometer.**

thermoneutral environment /-nōō′trəl/ [Gk, *therme* + L, *neutralis,* neutral; ME, *environ,* around],   **1.** an environment that keeps body temperature at an optimum point at which the least amount of oxygen is consumed for metabolism. **2.** an environment that enables a neonate to maintain a body temperature of 36.5° C (97.7° F) with a minimal requirement of energy and oxygen.

thermonuclear /-nōō′klē·ər/ [Gk, *therme,* heat; L, *nucleus,* nut],   pertaining to a reaction in which isotopes of hydrogen (protium, deuterium, or tritium) can be fused at temperatures of nearly 100,000,000° C into heavier nuclei of helium atoms. The process is the source of energy of the sun and is used in the explosion of thermonuclear weapons.

thermopenetration /-pen′ətrā′shən/ [Gk, *therme* + L, *penetrale,* passing through],   the use of diathermic techniques to produce warmth within the body tissues for therapeutic purposes. Also called **transthermia.**

thermophilic /-fil′ik/ [Gk, *therme,* heat + *philein,* to love],   pertaining to organisms that thrive in warmth of up to 70° C, well above normal human body temperature of 37° C.

thermoradiotherapy /-rā′dē·ōther′əpē/,   a therapeutic process that applies ionizing radiation to any part of the body in which the temperature has been raised by artificial means. Thermoradiography seeks to increase the radiosensitivity of the body part being treated.

thermoreceptor /-risep′tər/ [Gk, *therme,* heat; L, *recipere,* to receive],   nerve endings that are sensitive to heat or a rise in body temperature.

thermoregulation /-reg′yəlā′shən/ [Gk, *therme* + L, *regula,* rule],   the control of heat production and heat loss, specifically the maintenance of body temperature through physiologic mechanisms activated by the hypothalamus.

thermoregulation, ineffective, a nursing diagnosis accepted by the Seventh National Conference on the Classification of Nursing Diagnoses. Ineffective thermoregulation is defined as the state in which an individual's temperature fluctuates between hypothermia and hyperthermia. The critical defining characteristic is the fluctuation in body temperature above or below the normal range. Related factors include trauma or illness, immaturity, aging, and fluctuating environmental temperature. See also **nursing diagnosis.**

thermoregulatory centers /reg′yələtôr′ē/ [Gk, *therme,* heat; L, *regula,* rule; Gk, *kentron,* center], centers located in the hypothalamus concerned mainly with the regulation of heat production, heat inhibition, and heat conservation to maintain a normal body temperature. Kinds of thermoregulatory centers include: **thermogenic center, thermoinhibitory center, thermotaxic center.**

thermostable /-stā′bəl/, unaffected by or resistant to change by an increase in temperature. Compare **thermolabile.**

thermostat /thur′məstat/ [Gk, *therme* + *statos,* standing], a device for the automatic control of a heating or cooling system. **–thermostatic,** *adj.*

thermotoxic center. See **thermoregulatory centers.**

thermotaxis /-tak′sis/ [Gk, *therme* + *taxis,* arrangement], **1.** the normal adjustment and regulation of body temperature. **2.** the movement of an organism in response to heat, either toward the stimulus (positive thermotaxis) or away from the stimulus (negative thermotaxis). Also called **thermotropism.**

thermotherapeutic penetration /-ther′əpyoo′tik/, the depth to which heating to therapeutic temperatures is likely to extend.

thermotherapy /-ther′əpē/ [Gk, *therme* + *therapeia,* treatment], the treatment of disease by the application of heat. Thermotherapy may be administered as dry heat with heat lamps, diathermy machines, electric pads, or hot water bottles or as moist heat with warm compresses or immersion in warm water. Warm soaks or compresses may be used to treat local infections, to relax muscles and relieve pain in patients with motor problems, and to promote circulation in peripheral vascular disorders, such as thrombophlebitis. **–thermotherapeutic,** *adj.*

thermotropism. See **thermotaxis.**

-thermy. See **-therm.**

theta /thē′tə, thā′tə/, Θ, θ, the eight letter of the Greek alphabet.

theta wave [Gk, *theta,* eighth letter of Greek alphabet; AS, *wafian*], one of the several types of brain waves, characterized by a relatively low frequency of 4 to 7 Hz and a low amplitude of 10 [Grk m]V. Theta waves are the 'drowsy waves' of the temporal lobes of the brain and are observed in electroencephalograms when the individual is awake but relaxed and sleepy. Also called **theta rhythm.** Compare **alpha wave, beta wave, delta wave.**

-thetic, -thetical, a suffix meaning 'to put, place, set': *metathetic, prosthetic, synthetic.*

thiabendazole /thī·əben′dəzōl/, an anthelmintic.

■ INDICATIONS: It is prescribed in the treatment of a variety of worm infestations, including hookworms, roundworms, and pinworms.

■ CONTRAINDICATIONS: Erythema multiforme, Stevens-

Johnson syndrome, or known hypersensitivity to this drug prohibits its use.

■ ADVERSE EFFECTS: Among the more serious adverse reactions are anorexia, central nervous system effects, severe GI disturbances, dizziness, and hypotension.

thiamine /thī′əmin/ [Gk, *theion,* containing sulfur + *amine,* ammonia], a water-soluble, crystalline compound of the B complex vitamin group, essential for normal metabolism and for the health of the cardiovascular and nervous systems. Thiamine plays a key role in the metabolic breakdown of glucose to yield energy in body tissues. Rich sources of thiamine are pork, organ meats, green leafy vegetables, legumes, sweet corn, egg yolk, corn meal, brown rice, yeast, the germ and husks of grains, berries, and nuts. It is not stored in the body and must be supplied daily. A deficiency of thiamine affects chiefly the nervous system, the circulation, and the GI tract. Symptoms include irritability, emotional disturbances, loss of appetite, multiple neuritis, increased pulse rate, dyspnea, reduced intestinal motility, and heart irregularities. Severe deficiency causes beriberi. Also spelled **thiamin.** Also called **antiberiberi factor, antineuritic vitamin, vitamin B_1.**

thiazide diuretic. See **diuretic.**

thiethylperazine /thī·eth′ilper′əzēn/, a phenothiazine antiemetic.

■ INDICATIONS: It is prescribed to control nausea and vomiting.

■ CONTRAINDICATIONS: Parkinson's disease, central nervous system disorders, liver or renal dysfunction, severe hypotension, or known hypersensitivity to phenothiazine medications prohibits its use.

■ ADVERSE EFFECTS: Among the more serious adverse effects are hypotension, liver toxicity, a variety of extrapyramidal reactions, blood dyscrasias, and hypersensitivity reactions.

thigh [AS *theoh*], the section of the lower limb between the hip and the knee.

thigh bone. See **femur.**

thigm-, a suffix meaning 'of or pertaining to touch': *thigmesthesia, thigmocyte, thigmotropic.*

thinking [AS, *thencan,* to think], **1.** the cognitive process of forming mental images or concepts. **2.** the process of cognitive problem solving through the sorting, organizing, and classification of facts. Kinds of thinking include **abstract thinking, concrete thinking,** and **syncretic thinking.** See also **imagination.**

thin-layer chromatography (TLC), a method of separating two or more chemical compounds in a solution through their differential migrations across a thin layer of adsorbent spread over a glass or plastic plate.

thio- /thī′ō-/, a prefix designating the presence of sulfur: *thioarsenite, theocarbamide, thiocyanate.*

thioamide derivative /thī′ō·am′īd/, one of a group of antithyroid drugs prescribed in the treatment of hyperthyroidism. Thioamide drugs act by inhibiting the synthesis of thyroid hormone. The principal thioamides are propylthiouricil, methimazole, methylthiouricil, and carbamizole. Adverse reactions include agranulocytosis, hypersensitivity, and a mild transient pruritus. Because agranulocytosis may occur very rapidly, serial white blood cell counts are not useful in diagnosing that complication of treatment. Instead, the patient is requested to report immediately instances of sore throat and fever, which often herald the onset of agranulocytosis. Prompt discontinuation of the drug, before serious depletion of granulocytic white cells develops, usually results in complete recovery. Use of antithyroid medications in pregnancy may result in fetal hypothyroidism, goiter, and cretinism.

thioctic acid /thī·ok′tik/, a pyruvate oxidation factor found in liver and yeast, used in bacterial culture media.

thioester /thī′ō·es′tər/, an important group of biologic chemicals formed by the hydrosulfides and carboxylic acids and identified by an ester bond involving the -SH radical. Examples include the coenzyme A thioesters.

thioguanine /thī′ōgwä′nēn/, an antineoplastic.
- INDICATIONS: It is prescribed in the treatment of a variety of malignant neoplastic diseases, including the acute leukemias.
- CONTRAINDICATIONS: Known hypersensitivity or resistance to this drug prohibits its use. It is not given to pregnant women.
- ADVERSE EFFECTS: Among the most serious adverse reactions are bone marrow depression, GI distress, and stomatitis.

thiopental sodium /-pen′təl/, a potent ultrashort-acting barbiturate, used as a general anesthetic for surgical procedures that are expected to require 15 minutes or less, as an induction agent for other general anesthetics, as a hypnotic component in balanced anesthesia, and as an adjunct to regional anesthesia. It is administered intravenously in adults; in children it is occasionally given rectally. By depressing the central nervous system, thiopental sodium induces hypnotic sleep in less than 1 minute after infusion. It has no analgesic properties and therefore must be supplemented by analgesics. It is a powerful respiratory and myocardial depressant and may be habit-forming. See also **barbiturate.**

thioridazine hydrochloride /-rid′əzēn/, a phenothiazine antipsychotic.
- INDICATIONS: It is prescribed in the treatment of childhood behavioral disorders, geriatric mental disorders, depression, and alcohol withdrawal.
- CONTRAINDICATIONS: Parkinson's disease, concurrent administration of central nervous system depressants, hepatic or renal dysfunction, severe hypotension, or known hypersensitivity to this drug or to other phenothiazine medications prohibits its use.
- ADVERSE EFFECTS: Among the more serious adverse reactions are hypotension, hepatotoxicity, a variety of extrapyramidal reactions, blood dyscrasias, and hypersensitivity reactions.

Thiosulfil, a trademark for a sulfonamide antibacterial (sulfamethizole).

thiotepa /thī′ōtep′ə/, an antineoplastic alkylating agent.
- INDICATIONS: It is prescribed in the treatment of a variety of malignant neoplastic diseases, including adenocarcinoma of the breast and ovary, and urinary bladder carcinomas.
- CONTRAINDICATIONS: Bone marrow depression, pregnancy, liver or kidney dysfunction, or known hypersensitivity to this drug prohibits its use.
- ADVERSE EFFECTS: Among the most serious adverse reactions are bone marrow depression, anorexia, nausea, and headache.

thiothixene /-thī′ksēn/, a thioxanthene antipsychotic.
- INDICATIONS: It is prescribed in the treatment of acute agitation and mild to severe psychotic disorders.
- CONTRAINDICATIONS: Parkinson's disease, concurrent administration of central nervous system depressants, hepatic or renal dysfunction, severe hypotension, or known hyper-

sensitivity to this drug or to phenothiazine medications prohibits its use. It is not recommended for children under 12 years of age.
- ADVERSE EFFECTS: Among the more serious adverse reactions are hypotension, hepatotoxicity, a variety of extrapyramidal reactions, blood dyscrasias, and hypersensitivity reactions.

thiouracil /thī′ōyŏōr′əsil/ [Gk, *theion,* sulfur + *ouron,* urine], a chemical compound derived from thiourea that inhibits the formation of thyroxine in the thyroid gland and is used to treat hyperthyroidism.

thioxanthene derivative /thī·oksan′thēn/, any one of a group of antipsychotic drugs, each of which is similar to the phenothiazenes in indication, action, and adverse effects.

third cranial nerve. See **oculomotor nerve.**

third cuneiform bone. See **lateral cuneiform bone.**

third-party reimbursement, reimbursement for services rendered to a person in which an entity other than the receiver of the service is responsible for the payment. Third-party reimbursement for the cost of a subscriber's health care is commonly paid in full or in part by a health insurance plan, such as Blue Shield or Blue Cross.

third stage of labor, the expulsion of the placenta, membranes, and a small amount of blood and amniotic fluid, occurring within 5 to 30 minutes after delivery of the fetus.

third ventricle [Gk, *tritos,* below second rank; L, *ventriculum*], a cavity of the brain bounded on each side by a thalamus and the hypothalamus. It communicates anteriorly with the lateral ventricles and posteriorly with the aqueduct of the midbrain.

third ventriculostomy /ventrik′yəlos′təmē/ [L, *tertius,* three; *ventriculum,* little belly; Gk, *stoma,* mouth], a surgical procedure for draining cerebrospinal fluid into the cisterna chiasmatis of the subarachnoid space in hydrocephalus, usually in the newborn. The procedure is not commonly performed and is used chiefly when the cisterna magna is not available for Torkildsen's operation. The third ventriculostomy makes an opening on the anterior wall of the floor of the third ventricle into the interpeduncular cistern and is performed to correct an obstructive type of hydrocephalus.

thirst /thurst/ [AS, *thurst*], a perceived desire for water or other fluid. The sensation of thirst is usually referred to the mouth and throat.

Thiry-Vella fistula /thī′rēvel′ə/ [Ludwig Thiry, Austrian physiologist, b. 1817; Luigi Vella, Italian physiologist, b. 1825], an artificial passage from the abdominal surface of an experimental animal to an isolated intestinal loop, created surgically for the study of intestinal secretions. The continuity of the animal's gut is restored by anastomosis of the severed sections, and the isolated loop's vascular connections and mesenteric attachment are preserved. The ends of the isolated segment are attached to two openings in the skin of the abdomen to form a closed internal loop.

thixo-, a combining form meaning 'of or pertaining to touch': *thixolabile, thixotropic, thixotropy.*

Thomas' splint [Hugh Owen Thomas, English surgeon, b. 1834], **1.** a rigid splint constructed of steel bars that are curved to fit the involved limb and held in place by a cast or a rigid bandage. It is used in the treatment of chronic joint diseases. **2.** also called **Thomas' ring splint.** A rigid metal splint that extends from a ring at the hip to beyond the foot. It is used in the treatment of a fractured leg and, in conjunction with various traction and suspension devices, to immobilize and position a fractured femur of the preoperative or the postoperative patient.

Thompson scattering. See **scattering.**

Thomsen's disease. See **myotonia congenita.**

thoracentesis. See **thoracocentesis.**

thoracic /thôras′ik/, of or pertaining to the thorax.

-thoracic, a combining form meaning 'of, referring, or relating to the chest': *abdominothoracic, extrathoracic, intrathoracic.*

thoracic actinomycocis. See **actinomycosis.**

thoracic aorta [Gk, *thorax* chest; *aerein,* to raise], the large upper portion of the descending aorta, starting at the caudal border of the fourth thoracic vertebra, dividing into seven branches, and supplying many parts of the body, such as the heart, ribs, chest muscles, and stomach. Its seven branches are the pericardial, bronchial, esophageal, mediastinal, posterior intercostal, subcostal, and superior phrenic. See also **descending aorta.** Compare **abdominal aorta.**

thoracic cage [Gk, *thorax,* chest; L, *cavus,* hollow], the bony framework that surrounds the organs and soft tissues of the chest. It consists of 12 thoracic vertebrae, 12 pairs of ribs, and the sternum.

thoracic cavity [Gk, *thorax,* chest; L, *cavum*], the cavity enclosed by the ribs, the thoracic portion of the vertebral column, the sternum, the diaphragm, and associated muscles.

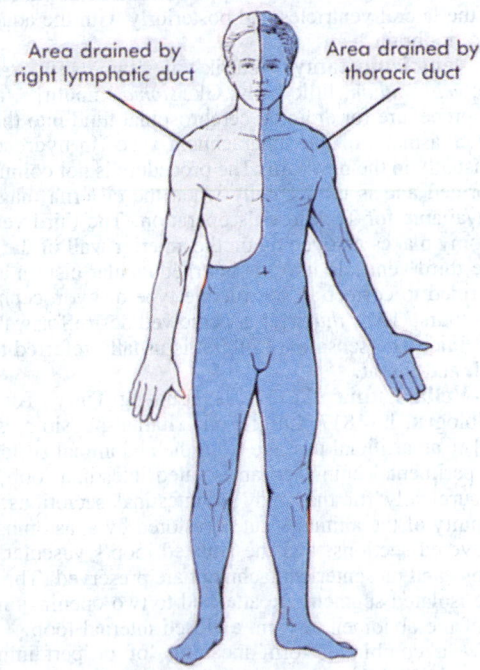

Area drained by right lymphatic duct

Area drained by thoracic duct

Thoracic duct drainage (colored area)
(Seeley, 1992/G David Brown)

thoracic duct, the common trunk of all the lymphatic vessels in the body, except those on the right side of the head, the neck, and the thorax, the right upper limb, the right lung, the right side of the heart, and the diaphragmatic surface of the liver. In the adult it is 38 to 45 cm long and 3 to 5 mm in diameter. It begins high in the abdomen at the cisterna chyli, ventral to the second lumbar vertebra, enters the thorax through the aortic hiatus of the diaphragm, and ascends into the neck through the posterior mediastinum, between the aorta and the azygous vein. In the neck it arches over the clavicle and opens into the junction of the left internal jugular and the left subclavian veins. The thoracic duct contains various valves, including two at this orifice that prevent venous blood from flowing into the lymphatic system. Compare **right lymphatic duct.** See also **lymphatic system.**

thoracic fistula, an abnormal opening in the chest wall that ends blindly or that communicates with the thoracic cavity.

thoracic medicine, the branch of medicine concerned with the diagnosis and treatment of disorders of the structures and organs of the chest, especially the lungs.

thoracic nerves, the 12 spinal nerves on each side of the thorax, including 11 intercostal nerves and one subcostal nerve. They are distributed mainly to the walls of the thorax and the abdomen. The thoracic nerves do not enter a plexus but follow independent courses, making them different from other spinal nerves. The first two intercostal nerves innervate the upper limb and the thorax; the next four supply only the thorax; and the lower five supply the walls of the thorax and the abdomen. Each subcostal thoracic nerve innervates the abdominal wall and the skin of a buttock. The thoracic portion of the sympathetic trunk contains a series of ganglia often coalesced in a single mass that, when independent, corresponds approximately to the thoracic spinal nerves. The roots of the ganglia are supplied by each thoracic nerve. The first thoracic ganglion, larger than the rest, is elongated, lying in the medial end of the first intercostal space, and usually combined with the inferior cervical ganglion into a stellate ganglion. The second to the tenth ganglia lie opposite the intervertebral disk associated with but slightly lower than the corresponding thoracic nerve. In most individuals the last thoracic ganglion lies on the body of the twelfth thoracic vertebra and, by its connection to both the eleventh and the twelfth thoracic nerves, serves a dual role as a single ganglion. See also **autonomic nervous system.**

thoracic outlet syndrome, an abnormal condition and a type of mononeuropathy characterized by paresthesia. It may be caused by a nerve root compression by a cervical disk.

thoracic parietal node, one of the lymph glands in the thorax, associated with various lymphatic vessels and divided into sternal nodes, intercostal nodes, and diaphragmatic nodes. See also **lymphatic system, lymph node.**

thoracic surgery [Gk, *thorax,* chest + *cheirourgos,* surgeon], the branch of medicine that deals with disease and injuries of the thoracic area by manipulative and operative methods.

thoracic vertebra, one of the 12 bony segments of the spinal column of the upper back designated T1 to T12. T1 is just below the seventh cervical vertebra (C7), and T12 is just above the first lumbar vertebra (L1). The thoracic portion of the spine is flexible and has a concave ventral curvature. Each vertebra has a broad, thick lamina; long, obliquely directed spinous processes; and thick, strong articular facets. The vertebrae are separated from each other by intervertebral disks. The vertebrae become thicker and heavier in descending order from T1 to T12. Compare **cervical vertebra, lumbar vertebra, sacral vertebra.**

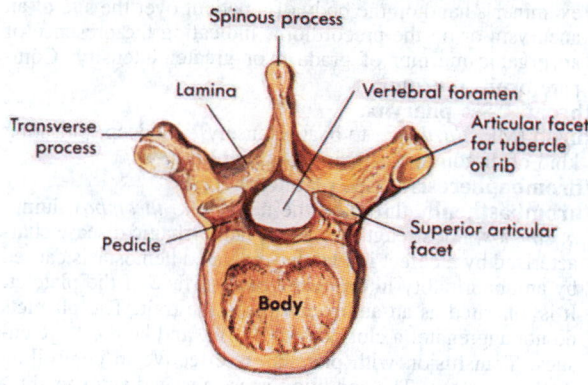

Thoracic vertebra
(Seeley, 1992/David J. Mascaro & Associates)

of orthovoltage x-ray beams to improve the penetrating ability.

thorax /thôr′aks/, *pl.* **thoraxes, thoraces** [Gk, chest], the cage of bone and cartilage containing the principal organs of respiration and circulation and covering part of the abdominal organs. It is formed ventrally by the sternum and costal cartilages and dorsally by the 12 thoracic vertebrae and the dorsal parts of the 12 ribs. The thorax of women has less capacity, a shorter sternum, and more movable upper ribs than that of men. Also called **chest.**

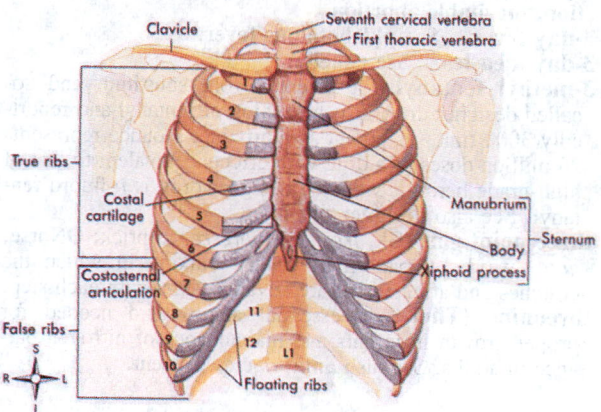

Thorax *(Thibodeau, 1993/David J Mascaro & Associates)*

thoracic visceral node, a node in the three groups of lymph nodes connected to the part of the lymphatic system that serves certain structures within the thorax, such as the thymus, pericardium, esophagus, trachea, lungs, and bronchi. The thoracic visceral nodes include the anterior mediastinal nodes, the posterior mediastinal nodes, and the tracheobronchial nodes. Compare **thoracic parietal node.** See also **lymph, lymphatic system, lymph node.**

thoraco- /thôr′əkō-/, a combining form meaning 'of or pertaining to the chest': *thoracobronchotomy, thoracocentesis, thoracomyodynia.*

thoracocentesis /thôr′əkō′sentē′sis/ [Gk, *thorax* + *kentesis,* puncture], the surgical perforation of the chest wall and pleural space with a needle for the aspiration of fluid for diagnostic or therapeutic purposes or for the removal of a specimen for biopsy. The procedure is usually performed using local anesthesia, with the patient in an upright position. Thoracocentesis may be used in the treatment of pleural effusion, as may occur in bronchogenic carcinoma. Fluid samples may be examined for erythrocyte, leukocyte, and differential white cell counts, and protein, glucose, and amylase concentrations, and may be cultured for studies of microorganisms that may be present. Also called **thoracentesis.**

thoracodorsal nerve /thôr′əkōdôr′səl/ [Gk, *thorax* + L, *dorsum,* back], a branch of the brachial plexus, usually arising between the two subscapular nerves. It courses along the posterior wall of the axilla and terminates in branches that supply the latissimus dorsi.

thoracodynia /-din′ē·ə/ [Gk, *thorax,* chest + *odyne,* pain], chest pain.

thoracolumbar fascia /thôr′əkōlum′bər/, a noncontractile structure that functions in a manner similar to a ligament in the lumbar area. It extends from the iliac crest and sacrum to the thoracic cage and envelops the paravertebral musculature.

thoracostomy /thôr′əkos′təmē/ [Gk, *thorax* + *stoma,* mouth], an incision made into the chest wall to provide an opening for the purpose of drainage.

thoracotomy /thôr′əkot′əmē/ [Gk, *thorax* + *temnein,* to cut], a surgical opening into the thoracic cavity.

Thoraeus filters /thôrē′əs/, combinations of metals, usually tin, copper, and aluminum, used to modify the quality

Thorazine, a trademark for a phenothiazine (chlorpromazine) used as an antiemetic and tranquilizer.

thorium (Th) /thôr′ē·əm/ [ONorse, *Thor,* god of thunder], a heavy, grayish, radioactive, metallic element. Its atomic number is 90; its atomic weight is 232.04. Thorium is used in nuclear medicine and in radiation therapy.

thought broadcasting /thôt/ [AS, *thot*], a symptom of psychosis in which the patient believes that his or her thoughts are "broadcast" beyond the head so that other people can hear them.

thought insertion, a belief by some mentally ill patients that thoughts of other people can be inserted into their own minds.

thought processes, altered, a nursing diagnosis accepted by the Fourth National Conference on the Classification of Nursing Diagnoses. It is defined as the state in which an individual experiences a disruption in cognitive operations and activities. The defining characteristics of the problem include distraction, egocentrism, abnormal cognitive function, abnormal interpretations of the environment; decreased ability to grasp ideas; impaired ability to reason, solve problems, calculate, conceptualize, or make decisions; disorientation; inappropriate social behavior; altered sleep patterns; delusions or hallucinations; and attention to environmental cues that is more or less acute than might normally be expected. Another possible defining characteristic is thinking based on inappropriate concepts or unreal situations. Related factors include physiologic changes, psychologic conflicts, loss of memory, impaired judgment, or sleep deprivation. See also **nursing diagnosis.**

thought transference. See telepathy.

Thr, abbreviation for **threonine.**

threadworm. See Enterobius vermicularis.

threadworm infection. See **strongyloidiasis.**

thready pulse /thred'ē/ [AS, *thraed;* L, *pulsare,* to beat], an abnormal pulse that is weak and often fairly rapid; the artery does not feel full, and the rate may be difficult to count. It is characteristic of hypovolemia, such as occurs with severe hemorrhage.

threatened abortion /thret'ənd/ [AS, *threat,* coercion; L, *ab,* away, *oriri,* to be born], a condition in pregnancy before the twentieth week of gestation characterized by uterine bleeding and cramping sufficient to suggest that miscarriage may result. A threatened abortion is generally managed with rest and observation. Compare **incomplete abortion, inevitable abortion.**

3-day fever. See **phlebotomus fever.**

3-day measles. See **rubella.**

3-methyl fentanyl, a potent heroin substitute and so-called designer drug. It is an analog of fentanyl and reportedly 3000 times as potent as morphine; 1 ounce represents 25 million doses of a drug with effects equivalent to that of high-grade heroin. A related designer drug is *p*-fluoro fentanyl. See also **designer drugs.**

three-point gait [Gk, *treis;* L, *pungere,* to prick; ONorse, *gata,* way], a pattern of crutch walking in which the crutches and affected leg are advanced first with each step.

threonine (Thr), an essential amino acid needed for proper growth in infants and maintenance of nitrogen balance in adults. See also **amino acid, protein.**

Chemical structure of threonine *(Seeley, 1992)*

threp-, a combining form meaning 'of or pertaining to nutrition': *threpsis, threpology, threptic.*

threshold /thresh'ōld/ [AS, *therscold*], the point at which a stimulus is great enough to produce an effect; for example, a pain threshold is the point at which a person becomes aware of pain.

threshold dose [AS, *therscold;* Gk, *dosis,* giving], a measure of a dose of radiation exposure defined in terms of conditions needed to produce a visible erythema in a given proportion of people exposed. Also called **minimal erythema dose (MED), skin erythema dose (SED), threshold erythema dose (TED).**

threshold limit values, the maximum concentration of a chemical to which workers can be exposed for a fixed period, such as 8 hours per day, without developing a physical impairment.

threshold of consciousness [AS, *therscold;* L, *conscire,* to be aware], the lowest limit of perception of a stimulus.

threshold stimulus [AS, *therscold;* L, *stimulare,* to incite], a stimulus that is just sufficient to produce a response. Below that level, no action or response is likely without additional intensity of the stimulus. Also called **limen; liminal stimulus.**

thrill [AS, *thyrlian,* to pierce], a fine vibration, felt by an examiner's hand on the body of a patient over the site of an aneurysm or on the precordium, indicating the presence of an organic murmur of grade 4 or greater intensity. Compare **bruit, murmur.**

throat. See **pharynx.**

throb [ME, *throbben,* to beat intensely], a deep, pulsating kind of discomfort or pain. **–throbbing,** *adj., n.*

thrombapheresis. See **plateletpheresis.**

thrombasthenia /throm'basthē'nē·ə/ [Gk, *thrombos,* lump, *a, sthenos,* not strength], a rare hemorrhagic disease characterized by a defect in platelet-mediated hemostasis caused by an abnormality in the membrane surface of the platelet. It is inherited as an autosomal recessive trait. The platelets do not aggregate, a clot does not form, and hemorrhage ensues. Transfusion with platelets is effective in controlling the hemorrhage. The condition is an inherited autosomal recessive trait.

thrombectomy /thrombek'təmē/ [Gk, *thrombos* + *ektome,* excision], the removal of a thrombus from a blood vessel, performed as emergency surgery to restore circulation to the affected part. Before surgery, anticoagulant therapy is begun, and an arteriogram is done to locate the thrombus. During surgery, a longitudinal incision is made into the blood vessel and the clot is removed. Postoperatively, the blood pressure is maintained close to its preoperative level because a decrease would predispose to further clotting. Compare **embolectomy.**

thrombi See **thrombus.**

thrombin /throm'bin/, an enzyme formed from prothrombin, calcium, and thromboplastin in plasma during the clotting process. Thrombin causes fibrinogen to change to fibrin, which is essential in the formation of a clot. See also **blood clot.**

thrombo- /throm'bō-/, a combining form meaning 'of or pertaining to a clot or thrombosis': *thromboarteritis, thrombocystis, thrombolysis.*

thromboangiitis obliterans /throm'bō·an'jē·ī'tis/ [Gk, *thrombos* + *aggeion,* vessel, *itis,* inflammation; L, *obliterare,* to cancel], an occlusive vascular condition, usually of a leg or a foot, in which the small and medium-sized arteries become inflamed and thrombotic. Early signs of the condition are burning, numbness, and tingling of the foot or leg distal to the lesion. Phlebitis and gangrene may develop as the disease progresses. Pulsation in the limb below the damaged blood vessels is often absent. The goal of therapy is to avoid all factors that decrease the blood supply to the extremity, such as cigarette smoking, and to use all means possible to increase the supply. Amputation may be necessary if the condition progresses to gangrene with chronic infection and extensive tissue destruction. Men are affected more often than women; most of the affected men smoke and are between 20 and 40 years of age. Also called **Buerger's disease.**

thrombocytapheresis. See **plateletpheresis.**

thrombocyt-, a combining form meaning 'pertaining to a thrombocyte or platelet': *thrombocytopenia, thrombocytosis.*

thrombocyte. See **platelet.**

thrombocytopathy /throm'bōsītop'əthē/ [Gk, *thrombos* + *kytos,* cell, *pathos,* disease], any disorder of the blood coagulation mechanism caused by an abnormality or dysfunction of platelets. Kinds of thrombocytopathies include **thrombocytopenia** and **thrombocytosis. –thrombocytopathic,** *adj.*

thrombocytopenia /throm'bōsī'təpē'nē·ə/ [Gk, *thrombos,* *kytos* + *penia,* poverty], an abnormal hematologic condition in which the number of platelets is reduced. There may be a decreased production of platelets, decreased survival of platelets and increased consumption of platelets or splenomegaly. Thrombocytopenia is the most common cause of bleeding disorders. Bleeding is usually from small capillaries. Treatment requires a specific diagnosis of the cause. All drugs are stopped because nearly any drug may cause the condition. Adrenal corticosteroids and transfusion may be necessary.

thrombocytopenic purpura /-sī′təpē′nik/ [Gk, *thrombos* + *kytos,* cell + *penia,* poverty; L, *purpura,* purple], a bleeding disorder characterized by a marked decrease in the number of platelets, resulting in multiple bruises, petechiae, and hemorrhage into the tissues. Etiologies include infection and drug sensitivity and toxicity. A diagnosis is reached only by the exclusion of other causes. Considered to be a manifestation of an autoimmune response, two distinct entities, acute and chronic thrombocytopenia, can be differentiated on clinical manifestations alone. The acute form usually occurs in children between 2 and 6 years of age and is benign, with complete recovery usually apparent within 6 weeks. The chronic form usually occurs in adults between 20 and 50 years of age. Recovery is rarely spontaneous and often requires adrenocortical steroids or splenectomy. Compare **disseminated intravascular coagulation.** See also **idiopathic thrombocytopenic purpura, hemophilia, hemorrhagic diathesis, thrombasthenia.**

thrombocytosis /throm′bōsītō′sis/ [Gk, *thrombos, kytos* + *osis,* condition], an abnormal increase in the number of platelets in the blood. **Benign thrombocytosis,** or **secondary thrombocytosis,** is asymptomatic and usually occurs after splenectomy, inflammatory disease, hemolytic anemia, hemorrhage, or iron deficiency; as a response to exercise; or after treatment with vincristine, in advanced carcinoma, Hodgkin's disease, or other lymphomas. **Essential thrombocythemia** is characterized by episodes of spontaneous bleeding alternating with thrombotic episodes. The platelets may reach levels exceeding 1,000,000/μL. Compare **thrombocytopenia.** See also **polycythemia.**

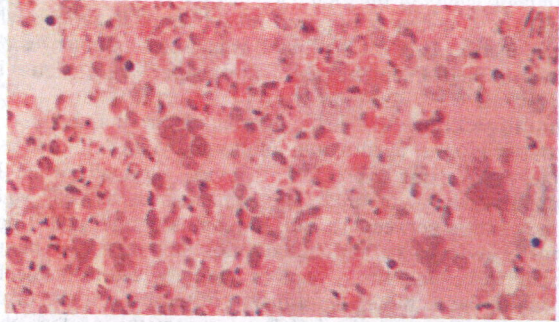

Thrombocytosis *(Hayhoe, 1992)*

thromboembolism /-em′bəliz′əm/ [Gk, *thrombos* + *embolos,* plug], a condition in which a blood vessel is blocked by an embolus carried in the bloodstream from the site of formation of the clot. The area supplied by an obstructed artery may tingle and become cold, numb, and cyanotic. Treatment includes quiet bed rest, warm wet packs, and anticoagulants to prevent the formation of additional thrombi.

Embolectomy may be indicated, especially if the aorta or common iliac artery is obstructed. An embolus in the lungs causes a sudden, sharp thoracic or upper abdominal pain, dyspnea, cough, fever, and hemoptysis. Obstruction of the pulmonary artery or one of its main branches may be fatal. Emboli are diagnosed by x-ray films and other radiologic techniques, including lung scans and angiography.

thrombogenic /-jen′ik/ [Gk, *thrombos* + *genein,* to produce], pertaining to a thrombus or a factor causing a thrombus or clot.

thrombolytic /-lit′ik/ [Gk, *thrombos* + *lysis,* a loosening], pertaining to a drug or other agent that dissolves thrombi.

thrombopenia /-pē′nē·ə/ [Gk, *thrombos,* lump + *penia,* poverty], See **thrombocytopenia.**

thrombopenic purpura. See **hemorrhagic purpura.**

thrombophlebitis /-fləbī′tis/ [Gk, *thrombos* + *phleps,* vein, *itis*], inflammation of a vein, often accompanied by formation of a clot. It occurs most commonly as the result of trauma to the vessel wall, hypercoagulability of the blood, infection, chemical irritation, postoperative venous stasis, prolonged sitting, standing, or immobilization, or a long period of intravenous catheterization. Also called **phlebitis.**

■ OBSERVATIONS: Thrombophlebitis of a superficial vein is generally evident; the vessel feels hard and thready or cordlike and is extremely sensitive to pressure; the surrounding area may be erythematous and warm to the touch, and the entire limb may be pale, cold, and swollen. Deep vein thrombophlebitis is characterized by aching or cramping pain, especially in the calf when the patient walks or dorsiflexes the foot (Homan's sign).

■ INTERVENTIONS: Thrombophlebitis of a vein of the arm or hand caused by the irritation of an intravenous catheter is usually treated by removing the catheter, elevating the arm, and applying moist heat. When the condition occurs in a vein of the leg, the person is maintained on complete bed rest in a comfortable position that does not restrict venous return. The legs are elevated, if ordered, but pillows are not used and the knees are never bent unless the foot of the bed is raised. Anticoagulant therapy and streptokinase may be administered, and moist heat is applied to the affected area; intense heat, which may burn edematous skin, is avoided. Every 4 hours the blood pressure, temperature, pulse, respiration, circulation of the affected extremity, skin condition, and pulses in all the extremities are checked; a Doppler ultrasonic sensing device may be used. Observation for signs of pulmonary embolism, myocardial infarction, cardiovascular accident, or decreased renal function is constant. The affected limb is covered with a bed cradle, is not washed or massaged, and is measured daily, with the size recorded. Active and passive range-of-motion exercises are performed with the unaffected extremities. As inflammation subsides, the use of support or antiembolic stockings is demonstrated, and an exercise program is initiated.

thrombophlebitis migrans. See **migratory thrombophlebitis.**

thrombophlebitis purulenta, an inflammation of a vein associated with the formation of a soft purulent thrombus that infiltrates the wall of the vessel.

thromboplastin /-plas′tin/ [Gk, *thrombos* + *plassein,* to mold], a complex substance that initiates the clotting process by converting prothrombin to thrombin in the presence of calcium ion. It is found in most tissue cells, red cells, and leukocytes. This substance functions as factor III in blood coagulation. See also **blood clotting.**

thrombosis /thrombō'sis/, *pl.* **thromboses,** an abnormal vascular condition in which thrombus develops within a blood vessel of the body. See also **blood clotting.**

thrombotic /thrombot'ik/ [Gk, *thrombos,* lump], caused or characterized by thrombosis.

thrombotic phlegmasia. See **phlegmasia alba dolens.**

thrombotic thrombocytopenic purpura (TTP) [Gk, *thrombos,* lump; *thrombos, kytos,* cell, *penia,* poverty; L, *purpura,* purple], a disorder characterized by thrombocytopenia, hemolytic anemia, and neurologic abnormalities. It is accompanied by a generalized purpura with the deposition of microthrombi within the capillaries and smaller arterioles. It includes a chronic form and an acute fulminating form that may be fatal in weeks. Therapy includes corticosteroids, splenectomy, and therapeutic plasma exchange. Compare **disseminated intravascular coagulation.** See also **thrombocytopenic purpura.**

thrombus /throm'bəs/, *pl.* **thrombi** [Gk, *thrombos,* lump], an aggregation of platelets, fibrin, clotting factors, and the cellular elements of the blood attached to the interior wall of a vein or artery, sometimes occluding the lumen of the vessel. Kinds of thrombi include **agonal thrombus, hyaline thrombus, laminated thrombus,** and **white thrombus.** Also called **blood clot.** Compare **embolus.**

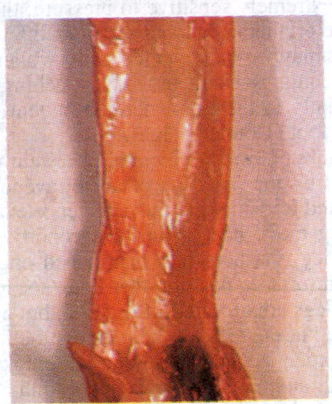

Thrombus adherent to carotid artery (Perkin, 1986)

through-and-through drainage /thrŏ̄o/ [ME, *thurgh;* AS, *drachen,* tear drop], a method of irrigating a body organ by inserting two tubes, one to introduce the fluid and another to drain the fluid that accumulates within the organ.

through transmission, (in ultrasonography) the process of imaging by transmitting the sound field through a specimen and picking up the transmitted energy on a far surface or a receiving transducer.

thrush [Dan, *troeske,* dryness], candidiasis of the tissues of the mouth.

thulium (Tm) /thŏ̄o'lē·əm/ [L, *Thule,* northern island], a rare earth metallic element. Its atomic number is 69; its atomic weight is 168.93. Thulium that has been irradiated in a nuclear reactor gives off gamma radiation.

thumb /thum/ [AS *thuma*], the first and shortest digit of the hand, classified by some anatomists as one of the fingers because its metacarpal bone ossifies in the same manner as those of the phalanges. Other anatomists classify the thumb separately, regarding it as composed of one metacarpal bone and only two phalanges. The metacarpal bone

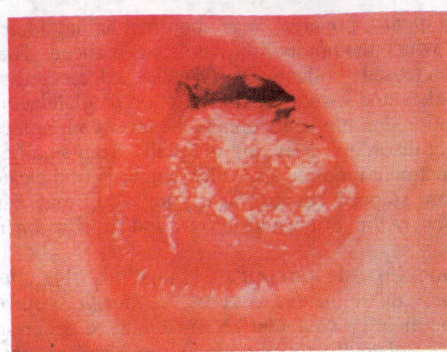

Thrush (Seidel, 1991/Mead Johnson & Co.)

of the thumb articulates with the trapezium of the carpus and is controlled by the thenar muscles, which occupy the radial side of the hand, and by the abductor pollicis longus, the extensor pollicis brevis, and the extensor pollicis longus. The thenar muscles include the abductor pollicis longus, the opponens pollicis, the flexor pollicis brevis, and the adductor pollicis. The nerves that innervate the various muscles controlling the thumb include branches of the radial nerve, the deep palmar branch of the ulnar nerve, and a branch of the median nerve. The metacarpal bone of the thumb, like the metacarpals of the other digits, ossifies from a center in the body of the bone and from a center at the distal end. Ossification begins in the middle of the eighth or ninth week of fetal life. About the third year of life the base extremity of the metacarpal of the thumb starts to ossify, uniting with the body of the metacarpal about the twentieth year of life. The phalanges of the thumb ossify from centers in the bodies of the phalanges and from centers at their proximal extremities. Ossification of the phalangeal body begins about the eighth week of fetal life.

thumb forceps, a surgical instrument used to grasp soft tissue, especially while suturing.

thumb sign [AS, *thuma;* L, *signum*], the flexing of the terminal phalanx of the thumb against the flexed index finger, as in holding a piece of paper. It is observed in patients who are unable to adduct the thumb because of an ulnar lesion. Also called **Froment sign, newspaper sign, signe de journal.**

thumbsucking, the habit of sucking the thumb for oral gratification. It is normal in infants and young children as a pleasure-seeking or comforting device, especially when the child is hungry or tired. The habit reaches its peak when the child is between 18 and 20 months of age, and it normally disappears as the child develops and matures. Thumbsucking beyond 4 to 6 years of age may lead to malocclusion of the teeth and deformation of the bony tissue of the thumb. Excessive thumbsucking, especially in older children, may be indicative of some emotional problem.

thymi. See **thymus.**

-thymia, a combining form meaning '(condition of the) mind or will': *amphithymia, barythymia, poikilothymia.*

thymic /thī'mik/, of or pertaining to the thymus gland.

thymic hypoplasia, thymic parathyroid aplasia. See **DiGeorge's syndrome.**

thymine /thī'mīn/, a major pyrimidine base found in nucleotides, and a fundamental constituent of DNA. See also **cytosine, uracil.**

thymo-,   **1.** a combining form meaning 'of or pertaining to the thymus gland': *thymocyte, thymolysis, thymoma.* **2.** a combining form meaning 'of or pertaining to the spirit or mind': *thymogenic, thymopathy, thymopsyche.*

thymol /thī'mol/,   a synthetic or natural thyme oil, used as an antibacterial and antifungal, that is an ingredient in some over-the-counter preparations for the treatment of hemorrhoids, acne, and tinea pedis. It is also used as a stabilizer in various pharmaceutical preparations.

thymoma /thīmō'mə/, *pl.* **thymomas, thymomata** [Gk, *thymos,* thyme, flowers, *oma* tumor],   a usually benign tumor of the thymus gland that may be associated with myasthenia gravis or an immune deficiency disorder.

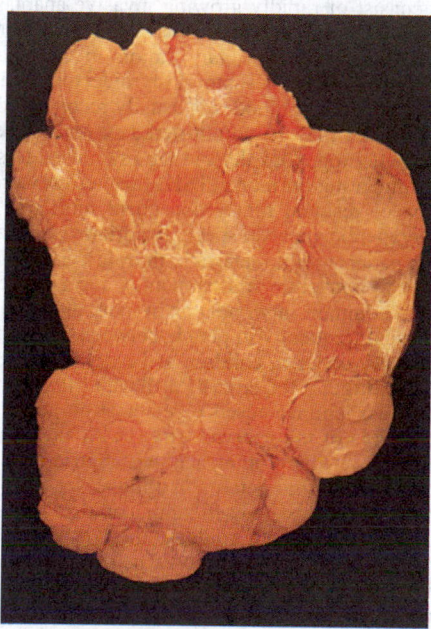

Thymoma *(Fletcher, 1987)*

thymosin /thī'məsin/,   **1.** a naturally occurring immunologic hormone secreted by the thymus gland. It is present in greatest amounts in young children and decreases in amount throughout life. **2.** an investigational drug derived from bovine thymus extracts and prescribed as an immunomodulator in experimental treatments for certain diseases, such as systemic lupus erythematosus or rheumatoid arthritis.

thymus /thī'məs/, *pl.* **thymuses, thymi** [Gk, *thymos,* thyme, flowers],   a single unpaired gland that is located in the mediastinum, extending superiorly into the neck to the lower edge of the thyroid gland and inferiorly as far as the fourth costal cartilage. It was once considered a minor vestigial structure, because of the fact that it decreases with age. Research has established, however, that the thymus is the primary central gland of the lymphatic system. The endocrine activity of the thymus is believed to depend on the hormone thymosin, which is composed of biologically active peptides critical to the maturation and the development of the immune system. The T cells of the cell-mediated immune response develop in this gland before migrating to the lymph nodes and the spleen. The gland consists of two lateral lobes closely bound by connective tissue, which also encloses the entire organ in a capsule. Superficial to the gland is the sternum. Lying deep to the thymus are the great vessels and the cranial portion of the pericardium. The two lobes of the gland differ in size, and, in many individuals, the right lobe overlaps the left lobe. The thymus is about 5 cm long, 4 cm wide, and 6 mm thick. The lobes are composed of numerous lobules, which vary from 0.5 to 2 mm in diameter. The lobules are separated by delicate connective tissue. Each lobule is composed of a dense cellular cortex and an inner, less dense medulla. The cortices are composed almost entirely of small lymphocytes secured by reticular tissue with relatively few reticular cells. The medullae contain far fewer lymphocytes than the cortices and are composed of reticular tissue that contains more reticular cells. The thymus develops in the embryo from the third branchial pouch and increases in size until attaining a weight of 12 to 14 g before birth. The size of the organ relative to the rest of the body is largest when the individual is about 2 years of age. The thymus usually attains its greatest absolute size at puberty, when it weighs about 35 g. After puberty, the organ undergoes involution as the small lymphocytes of the cortices disappear and the reticular tissue is compressed. Adipose tissue often replaces the receding thymic tissue, but the connective tissue capsule of the gland may persist. With aging, the gland may change in color from pinkish-gray to yellow, and in the elderly individual may appear as small islands of thymic tissue covered with fat and surrounded by the yellowish capsule. The normal involution of the thymus may be superseded by rapid accidental involution caused by starvation or by acute disease. The gland is supplied by arteries derived from the internal thoracic and from the superior and the inferior thyroids. The veins of the gland end in the left brachiocephalic vein and in the thyroid veins. The lymphatics of the thymus end in the anterior mediastinal, the tracheobronchial, and the sternal nodes. The gland is innervated by tiny nerves derived from the vagi and the sympathetic. Branches from the descendens hypoglossi and the phrenic nerve reach the thymic capsule but do not penetrate the glandular tissue. Compare **spleen.**

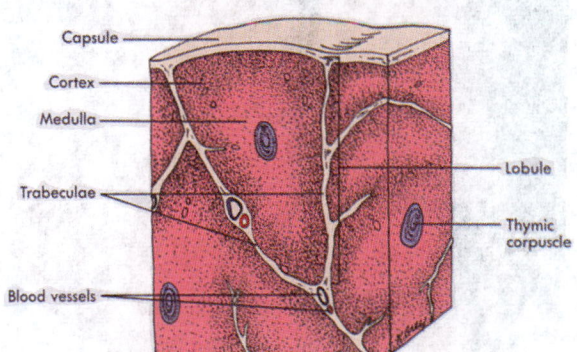

Thymus: cross-section of lobule
(Seeley, 1992/Kathy Mitchell Grey)

Thypinone,   a trademark for the synthetic thyrotropin releasing hormone (protirelin), used as an adjunctive agent in the diagnostic assessment of thyroid function.

Thyrar,   a trademark for thyroid hormone.

-thyrea, -thyreosis, -thyroidism,   a combining form

meaning a 'condition of the thyroid gland': *athyrea, hypothyrea, hyperthyrea.*

thyro- /thī'rō-/, **thyroido-, thyreo-,** a combining form meaning 'a shield or pertaining to the thyroid gland': *thyroactive, thyroidectomy, thyroiditis.*

thyrocalcitonin. See **calcitonin.**

thyrocervical trunk /-sur'vikəl/ [Gk, *thyreos,* shield, *eidos,* form; L, *cervix,* neck; *truncus*], one of a pair of short, thick arterial branches, arising from the first portion of the subclavian arteries, close to the medial border of the scalenus anterior, supplying numerous muscles and bones in the head, neck, and back. Each is divided into three branches: the inferior thyroid, suprascapular, and transverse cervical.

thyrocricotomy /-krīkot'əmē/ [Gk, *thyreos,* shield + *eidos,* form + *krikos,* ring + *temnein,* to cut], a tracheotomy procedure in which the cricovocal membrane is divided.

thyrogenic /-jen'ik/ [Gk, *thyreos,* shield + *eidos,* form + *genein,* to produce], pertaining to an origin in the thyroid gland. Also **thyrogenous** /thīroj'ənəs/.

thyroglobulin /-glōb'yəlin/, a purified extract of porcine thyroid. See also **thyroid hormone.**

■ INDICATIONS: It is prescribed in the treatment of cretinism, myxedema, goiter, and other hypothyroid states.

■ CONTRAINDICATIONS: Cardiovascular disease, hypopituitarism, or known hypersensitivity to this drug may prohibit its use.

■ ADVERSE EFFECTS: Among the more serious adverse reactions are tremors, nervousness, palpitation and tachycardia, and dysrythmias when given in excessive doses.

thyroid. See **thyroid gland, thyroid hormone.**

thyroid acropathy /thī'roid/ [Gk, *thyreos,* shield, *eidos,* form; *akron,* extremity, *pathos,* disease], swelling of subcutaneous tissue of the extremities and clubbing of the digits, occurring rarely in patients with thyroid disease and usually associated with pretibial myxedema or exophthalmos.

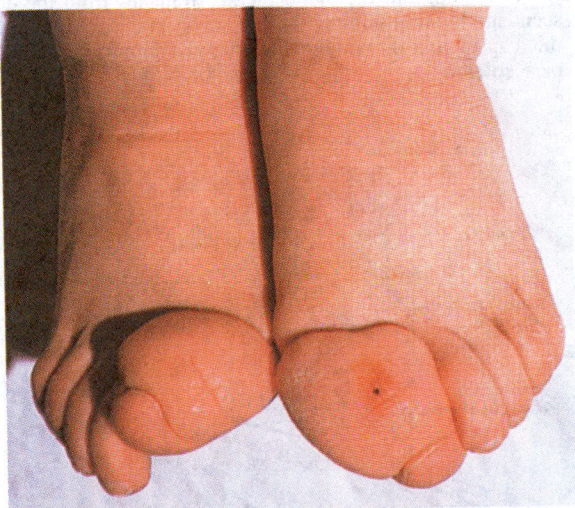

Thyroid acropathy (Schumacher, 1988)

thyroid cancer, a neoplasm of the thyroid gland, usually characterized by slow growth and a slower and more prolonged clinical course than that of other malignancies. A significant carcinogenic effect of exposure to ionizing radiation is demonstrated by the high rate of thyroid cancer in survivors of exposure to atomic bomb explosions and in individuals who have been treated with radiotherapy for an enlarged thymus in infancy or for acne or other skin disorders in adolescence. Nontoxic colloid goiters and follicular adenomas may be precursors of malignant thyroid tumors. The first sign of cancer may be an increase in size of the thyroid gland, a palpable nodule, hoarseness, dysphagia, dyspnea, or pain on pressure. Diagnostic measures include x-ray examination, transillumination of the gland, radioisotope scanning, needle biopsy, and ultrasonic examination. More than one half of thyroid malignancies are papillary carcinomas, about one third are follicular carcinomas, and the rest consist of rapidly growing invasive anaplastic carcinomas, medullary carcinomas that secrete calcitonin, and metastatic lesions from primary tumors in the breast, kidneys, or lungs. Total or subtotal thyroidectomy with excision of involved lymph nodes is usually recommended. Radioactive iodine may be administered postoperatively, and high doses of exogenous thyroid are often used to suppress thyroid stimulating hormone (TSH) in an effort to cause the regression of residual tumor dependent on TSH. Various chemotherapeutic agents, especially adriamycin, may be effective in patients with metastatic thyroid cancer that is unresponsive to conventional treatment. Cancer of the thyroid is twice as common in women as in men; although it is diagnosed most frequently in people between 30 and 50 years of age, it may occur in children and elderly individuals.

thyroid cartilage, the largest cartilage of the larynx, consisting of two laminae fused together at an acute angle in the middle line of the neck to form the Adam's apple. Immediately above this prominence the laminae are separated by the superior thyroid notch. An oblique line runs caudally from the outer surface of each lamina and serves for the attachment of the sternothyroideus, the thyrohyoideus, and the constrictor pharyngis inferior. The cranial border of the thyroid cartilage secures the thyrohyoid membrane; the caudal border holds the cricoid cartilage, and the dorsal border receives insertions of the stylopharyngeus and the pharyngopalatinus. Compare **cricoid.**

thyroid crisis [Gk, *thyreos,* shield + *eidos,* form + *krisis,* turning point], a sudden exacerbation of symptoms of thyrotoxicosis characterized by fever, sweating, tachycardia, extreme nervous excitability, and pulmonary edema. It usually occurs in a patient whose thyrotoxicosis treatment is inadequate, and the paroxysm is triggered by a stressful infection or injury. If untreated, the crisis is often fatal. Also called **thyroid storm, thyrotoxic crisis.** See also **Graves' disease.**

thyroid dermoid cyst, a tumor derived from embryonal tissues that is believed to have developed in the thyroid gland or in the thyrolingual duct.

thyroidectomized /thī'roidek'təmīzd/ [Gk, *thyreos,* shield + *eidos,* form + *ektome,* excision], pertaining to a patient or condition in which the thyroid gland has been removed.

thyroidectomy /thī'roidek'təmē/ [Gk, *thyreos* + *eidos,* form, *ektome,* excision], the surgical removal of the thyroid gland, performed for colloid goiter, tumors, or hyperthyroidism that does not respond to iodine therapy and antithyroid drugs. All but 5% to 10% of the gland is removed; regrowth usually begins shortly after surgery, and thyroid function may return to normal. For cancer of the thyroid, the entire gland is removed, along with surrounding structures from neck to collarbone, in a radical neck dissection. Before surgery, the basal metabolism rate is lowered to normal by giving iodine and antithyroid drugs. If a tumor is present, a frozen section of the affected tissue is examined by a pathologist. If malignant cells are found, most or all of the gland is removed. After surgery the patient is most comfortable in semi-Fowler's position with continuous mist inhalation administered to liquefy oral secretions. Oral suctioning may be necessary. A tracheotomy set and oxygen are kept in the room. Postoperatively, the patient is observed for signs of hemorrhage, respiratory difficulty caused by edema of the glottis, and the muscular twitching of tetany from accidental removal of a parathyroid gland.

thyroid function test,   any of several laboratory tests performed to evaluate the function of the thyroid gland. Often several of the tests are performed simultaneously. Thyroid function tests include protein-bound iodine, butanol-extractable iodine, T_3, T_4, free thyroxine index, thyroxin-binding globulin, thyroid stimulating hormone, long-acting thyroid stimulator, radioactive iodine uptake, and radioactive iodine excretion.

Thyroid gland *(Seeley, 1992/Andrew Grivas)*

thyroid gland [Gk, *thyreos,* shield, *eidos,* form], a highly vascular organ at the front of the neck, usually weighing about 30 g, consisting of bilateral lobes connected in the middle by a narrow isthmus. It is slightly heavier in women than in men and enlarges during pregnancy. The thyroid gland secretes the hormone thyroxin directly into the blood and is part of the endocrine system of ductless glands. It is essential to normal body growth in infancy and childhood, and its removal greatly reduces the oxidative processes of the body, producing a lower metabolic rate characteristic of hypothyroidism. The apices of the conic lobes of the gland are directed cranially and laterally as far as the lower middle of the thyroid cartilage. The bases of the lobes are on the level with the fifth or the sixth tracheal ring. Each lobe is about 5 cm long, a maximum of 3 cm wide, and usually about 2 cm thick. The lateral surface is convex and covered by the skin, the sternocleidomastoideus, the omohyoi-

deus, the sternohyoideus, and the sternothyroideus. The deep fascia forms a capsule for the gland. The thyroid is activated by the pituitary thyrotrophic hormone and requires iodine to elaborate thyroxine. The arteries of the thyroid are remarkably large and form numerous anastomoses. Compare **parathyroid gland.**

thyroid hormone, an iodine-containing compound secreted by the thyroid gland, predominantly as thyroxine (T_4) and in smaller amounts as four-times-more-potent triiodothyronine (T_3). These hormones increase the rate of metabolism; affect body temperature; regulate protein, fat, and carbohydrate catabolism in all cells; maintain growth hormone secretion, skeletal maturation, and the cardiac rate, force, and output; promote central nervous system development; stimulate the synthesis of many enzymes; and are necessary for muscle tone and vigor. Derivatives of thyronine, T_4 and T_3, are synthesized in the thyroid gland by a complex process involving the uptake, oxidation, and incorporation of iodide and the production of thyroglobulin, the form in which the hormones apparently are stored in thyroid follicular colloid. After the proteolysis of thyroglobulin, T_4 and T_3 are released and transported in the blood in strong, but noncovalent, association with certain plasma proteins; T_4 accounts for approximately 90% of iodine in circulation and T_3 for 5%. All phases of the production and the release of T_4 and T_3 are regulated by the thyroid stimulating hormone (TSH) secreted by the anterior pituitary gland. The production of thyroid hormones is excessive in Graves' disease and toxic nodular goiter (Plummer's disease), diminished in myxedema, and absent in cretinism. T_4's normal 6-to-7-day half-life in blood is reduced to 3 or 4 days in hyperthyroidism and extended to 9 or 10 days in myxedema. T_3 has a normal half-life of 2 days or less and, like T_4, is metabolized most actively in the liver. Pharmaceutic preparations of thyroid hormones extracted from animal glands and the synthetic compounds, levothyroxine sodium and liothyronine sodium, are used as replacement therapy in patients with hypothyroidism. The dosage is initially low and is gradually increased to the optimal level based on the patient's clinical response and tests of the findings on thyroid function studies. Overdosage or a rapid increase in the dosage may result in signs of hyperthyroidism, such as nervousness, tremor, tachycardia, cardiac dysrhythmia, and menstrual irregularity.

-thyroidism. See **-thyrea.**

thyroiditis /thī'roidī'tis/, inflammation of the thyroid gland. Acute thyroiditis, caused by staphylococcal, streptococcal, or other infections, is characterized by suppuration and abscess formation and may progress to subacute diffuse disease of the gland. Subacute thyroiditis is marked by fever, weakness, sore throat, and a painfully enlarged gland containing granulomas composed of colloid masses surrounded by giant cells and mononuclear cells. Chronic lymphocytic thyroiditis (Hashimoto's disease), characterized by lymphocyte and plasma cell infiltration of the gland and by diffuse enlargement, seems to be transmitted as a dominant trait and may be associated with various autoimmune disorders. Another chronic form of thyroiditis is Riedel's struma, a rare progressive fibrosis, usually of one lobe of the gland but sometimes involving both lobes, the trachea, and surrounding muscles, nerves, and blood vessels. Radiation thyroiditis occasionally occurs 7 to 10 days after the treatment of hyperthyroidism with radioactive iodine 131.

thyroido-. See **thyro.**

thyroid releasing hormone. See **thyrotropin releasing hormone.**

thyroid stimulating hormone (TSH), a substance, secreted by the anterior lobe of the pituitary gland, that controls the release of thyroid hormone and is necessary for the growth and function of the thyroid gland. The secretion of TSH is regulated by thyrotropin releasing factor, elaborated in the median eminence of the hypothalamus. Normal adult blood levels are 2 to 10 mU/L (SI units). Also called **thyrotropin.** See also **thyroid hormone.**

thyroid storm, a crisis in uncontrolled hyperthyroidism caused by the release into the bloodstream of increased amounts of thyroid hormones. The storm may occur spontaneously or be precipitated by infection, stress, or a thyroidectomy performed on a patient who is inadequately prepared with antithyroid drugs. Characteristic signs are fever that may reach 106° F, a rapid pulse, acute respiratory distress, apprehension, restlessness, irritability, and prostration. The patient may become delirious, lapse into a coma, and die of heart failure.

Thyrolar, a trademark for a thyroid hormone (liotrix).

thyromegaly /-meg'əlē/ [Gk, *thyreos*, shield + *eidos*, form + *megas*, large], enlargement of the thyroid gland.

thyrotonine (T3) triiodothyronine. See **thyroid hormone.**

thyrotoxic crisis. See **thyroid crisis.**

thyrotoxicosis. See **Graves' disease.**

thyrotrophic /-trof'ik/ [Gk, *thyreos*, shield + *eidos*, form + *trophe*, nutrition], influencing the thyroid gland, such as the thyroid stimulating hormone (TSH). Also **thyrotropic.**

thyrotropic hormone. See **thyroid stimulating hormone.**

thyrotropin. See **thyroid stimulating hormone.**

thyrotropin (systemic) /-trō'pin/, a preparation of bovine thyroid stimulating hormone that increases the uptake of radioactive iodine in the thyroid and the secretion of thyroxine by the thyroid.

■ INDICATIONS: It is prescribed in diagnostic tests and to enhance uptake of 131I in the treatment of thyroid cancer.

■ CONTRAINDICATIONS: Coronary thrombosis or known hypersensitivity to this drug prohibits its use. It should not be given in untreated Addison's disease or after myocardial infarction.

■ ADVERSE EFFECTS: Among the most serious adverse reactions are symptoms of hyperthyroidism, allergic reactions, hypotension, and dysrhythmias.

thyrotropin releasing hormone, a substance elaborated in the median eminence of the hypothalamus that stimulates the release of thyrotropin (thyroid stimulating hormone) from the anterior pituitary gland. Also called **thyrotropin releasing factor (TRF), TSH releasing factor.**

thyroxine (T₄) /thīrok'sēn/, a hormone of the thyroid gland, derived from tyrosine, that influences metabolic rate. Also called **tetraiodothyronine.**

thyroxine-binding globulin, a plasma protein that binds with and transports thyroxine in the blood.

Thytropar, a trademark for bovine thyrotropin.

Ti, symbol for the element **titanium.**

TI, abbreviation for *therapeutic index.*

TIA, abbreviation for **transient ischemic attack.**

tibia-, a combining form meaning 'pertaining to the tibia': *tibial, tibialis, tibiafemoral.*

tibia /tib'ē·ə/ [L, shin bone], the second longest bone of the skeleton, located at the medial side of the leg. It articulates with the fibula laterally, the talus distally, and the femur proximally, forming part of the knee joint. It attaches to the ligament of the patella and to various muscles, including the popliteus and the flexor digitorum longus. Also called **shin bone.**

tibial /tib'ē·əl/ [L, *tibia*, shin bone], pertaining to the largest long bone of the lower leg.

tibialis anterior /tib'ē·ā'lis/ [L, *tibia* + *anticus*, in front], one of the anterior crural muscles of the leg, situated on the lateral side of the tibia. It is a thick, fleshy muscle proximally and tendinous distally, arising from various origins, such as the lateral side of the tibia, and inserting into the first cuneiform bone and the first metatarsal bone. It is innervated by a branch of the deep peroneal nerve, in which there are fibers from the fourth and the fifth lumbar and the first sacral nerves, and dorsiflexes and supinates the foot. Also called **tibialis anticus.** Compare **extensor digitorum longus.**

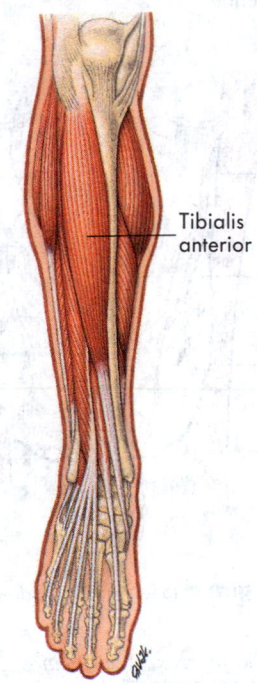

Tibialis anterior

Tibialis anterior *(Thibodeau, 1993/John V Hagen)*

tibial torsion [L, *tibia* + *torquere*, to twist], a lateral or a medial twisting rotation of the tibia on its longitudinal axis, as in the pronation of the hand because of the contraction of the pronator teres and the pronator quadratus, or the supination of the hand, caused by the contraction of the supinator muscle. Compare **femoral torsion.**

tibia valga [L, *tibia*, shinbone; *valgus*, bowlegged], a bowed tibia with the convex surface toward the outside of the leg.

tic. See **mimic spasm.**

Ticar, a trademark for an antibiotic (ticarcillin).

ticarcillin /tik'ärsil'in/, an antibiotic.

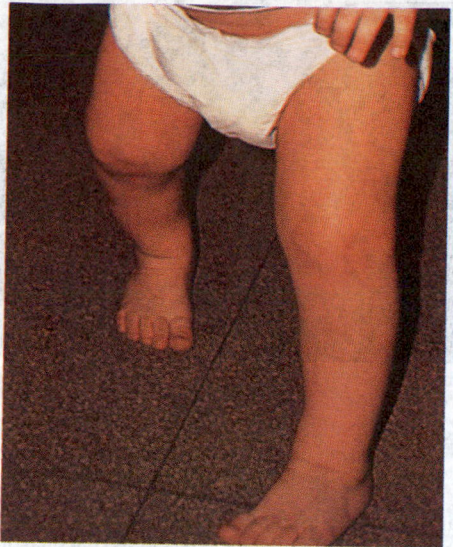

Tibial torsion (internal) *(Zitelli, 1992)*

■ INDICATIONS: It is prescribed in the treatment of bacterial septicemia, and skin, soft tissue, and respiratory infections caused by both gram-negative and gram-positive organisms.
■ CONTRAINDICATION: A history of allergic reaction to any of the penicillins prohibits its use.
■ ADVERSE EFFECTS: Among the most serious adverse reactions are anaphylactic reactions, thrombocytopenia, leukopenia, neutropenia, eosinophilia, vein irritation, and phlebitis.

tic douloureux /tikdo͞olo͞oroeʹ/ [Fr, painful spasm], a brief extremely painful attack of trigeminal neuralgia. It is unilateral and limited to the distribution of the trigeminal, fifth cranial, nerve. An attack is easily and unexpectedly provoked by any stimulus of the facial muscles, from touching to speaking, and may occur repetitively. See also **trigeminal neuralgia.**

-tic, a suffix meaning 'pertaining to': *paralytic, therapeutic.*

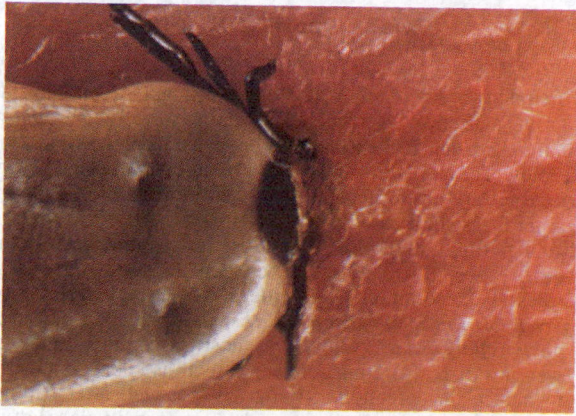

Tick bite *(Habif, 1990)*

tick bite [ME, *tike;* AS, *bitan,* to bite], a puncture wound produced by the toothed beak of a bloodsucking tick, a small, tough-skinned, arachnid. Ticks transmit several diseases to humans, and a few species carry a neurotoxin in their saliva that may cause ascending paralysis beginning in the legs. Nervousness, loss of appetite, tingling and headache, followed by muscle pain, and, in extreme cases, respiratory failure may occur. Symptoms often disappear when the attached tick is carefully removed with forceps. Placing a drop of alcohol or ether on the tick or coating it with petrolatum or nail polish facilitates removal. See also **Lyme disease, Q fever, relapsing fever, Rocky Mountain spotted fever, tularemia.**

tick-borne rickettsiosis [ME, *tike + beren; Rickettsia,* Gk, *osis,* condition], any disease transmitted by Ixodid ticks carrying the *Rickettsia* pathogens, microorganisms smaller than bacteria but larger than viruses. A common infectious species in North America is *Rickettsia rickettsii,* the cause of Rocky Mountain spotted fever.

tick fever. See **relapsing fever.**

tick paralysis, a rare, progressive, reversible disorder caused by several species of ticks that release a neurotoxin that causes weakness, incoordination, and paralysis. The tick must feed on the host for several days before the symptoms appear, and removal of the tick leads to rapid recovery. Because respiratory or bulbar paralysis can cause death, it is important to search for ticks, frequently hidden in scalp hair, on a patient with these symptoms.

t.i.d., (in prescriptions) abbreviation for the Latin phrase *ter in die* /deʹaⁿ/, 'three times a day.'

tidal /tiʹdəl/ [AS, *tid,* time] pertaining to an alternating process, such as a rise-and-fall, ebb-and-flow, or periodic lapse of time.

tidal drainage. See **drainage.**

tidal volume (TV) [AS, *tid,* time; L, *volumen,* paper roll], the amount of air inhaled and exhaled during normal ventilation. Inspiratory reserve volume, expiratory reserve volume, and tidal volume make up vital capacity. See also **pulmonary function test.**

tide [AS, *tid*], a variation, increase or decrease, in the concentration of a particular component of body fluids, such as acid tide, fat tide. **–tidal,** *adj.*

tidemark, a transitional zone, appearing as a wavy line, that marks the junction between calcified and uncalcified cartilage.

Tietze's syndrome /tētʹsēz/, **1.** a disorder characterized by nonsuppurative swellings of one or more costal cartilages causing pain that may radiate to the neck, shoulder, or arm and mimic the pain of coronary artery disease. The syndrome may accompany chronic respiratory infections, and, if the costal swellings are extremely painful, infiltration with procaine and hydrocortisone may provide relief. **2.** albinism, except for normal eye pigment, accompanied by deaf mutism and hypoplasia of the eyebrows.

TIG, abbreviation for **tetanus immune globulin.**

Tigan, a trademark for an antiemetic (trimethobenzamide hydrochloride).

tight junction /tīt/ [ME, *thight,* strong; L, *jungere,* to join], the zonula occludens of the junctional complex between cells in which the plasma membranes of adjacent cells are in direct contact and where there is no intercellular space.

tilt table [AS, *tealt,* unsteady; Fr, *tablette*], an examining table that can be rocked back and forth, seesaw fashion, during study of the response of a patient's circulatory system to gravitational forces.

timbre /tim′bər/ [Fr], **1.** a characteristic sound quality of a voice or musical instrument, as determined by harmonics of the sound and distinguished from intensity and pitch. **2.** a second metallic sound hear in aortic dilation.

timed collection, the collection of a specimen, such as a urine or stool sample, for a specific period of time.

timed release. See **prolonged release.**

timed vital capacity [AS, *tima*; L, *vita*, life + *capacitas*], a diagnostic test of certain lung disorders, determined by the percentage of predicted vital capacity that adults can expire forcefully for at least 3 seconds after a maximal inspiration.

time-sharing, performing two or more tasks with a computer at the same time. The computer actually processes a small portion of one task at a time, switching from one to another in a commutative manner, but it can handle so many data in brief time segments that the operator or operators are not aware of the computer switching.

timolol maleate /tim′əlol/, a beta-adrenergic receptor blocking agent.
- INDICATIONS: It is prescribed for reducing intraocular pressure in chronic open-angle, aphakic, and secondary glaucoma.
- CONTRAINDICATIONS: Bronchial asthma, COPD, sinus bradycardia, or known hypersensitivity to this drug prohibits its use. It is used with caution in patients with contraindications to systemic use of beta-adrenergic receptor blocking agents.
- ADVERSE EFFECTS: The most serious adverse reaction is blurring of vision. Mild eye irritation also may occur.

Timoptic, a trademark for a beta-adrenergic receptor blocking agent (timolol maleate).

tin (Sn) [AS], a whitish metallic element. Its atomic number is 50; its atomic weight is 118.69. Tin oxide is used in dentistry as a polishing agent for teeth and in some restorative procedures.

Tinactin, a trademark for an antifungal (tolnaftate).

tincturetinct. /tingk′chər/, a substance in a solution that is diluted with alcohol.

tincture of iodine [L, *tinctura*; Gk, *ioeides*, violet], a mixture of sodium iodide in an alcohol-water solution, used as a skin disinfectant. The term is no longer in official use.

Tindal, a trademark for a phenothiazine (acetophenazine maleate), used as a tranquilizer.

tine, a sharp, projecting point, as a prong of a fork.

tinea /tin′ē·ə/ [L, worm], a group of fungal skin diseases caused by dermatophytes of several kinds, characterized by itching, scaling, and, sometimes, painful lesions. Tinea is a general term that refers to infections of various causes, which are seen on several sites; the specific type is usually designated by a modifying term. Diagnosis is made by demonstrating fungus on smear or by culture. Also called, loosely, **ringworm.**

tinea capitis, a superficial fungal infection of the scalp, most common in children. Most infections are caused by species of *Trichophyton*. The infection may lead to hair loss and may become secondarily infected with bacteria, causing a severe inflammation. Symptoms include severe itching and scaling of the scalp. Treatment with topical fungicidal agents is usually sufficient. Also called **ringworm.**

tinea corporis, a superficial fungal infection of the non-hairy skin of the body, most prevalent in hot, humid cli-

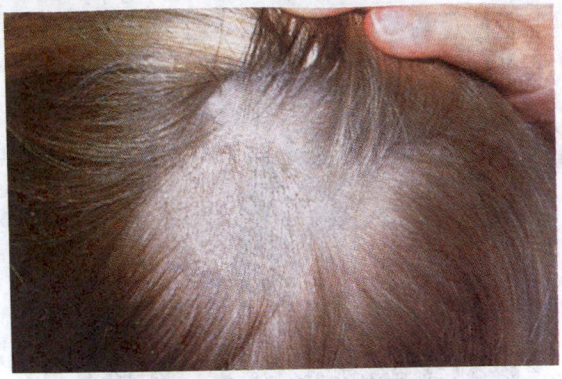

Tinea capitis
(Goldstein, 1992/Courtesy Department of Dermatology, University of North Carolina at Chapel Hill)

mates and usually caused by species of *Trichophyton* or *Microsporum*. Topical fungicides, such as miconazole, are used for moderate cases; severe infection calls for griseofulvin.

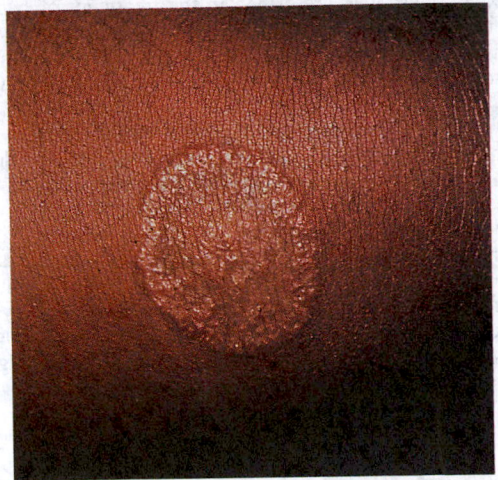

Tinea corporis *(Zitelli, 1992)*

tinea cruris /krōō′ris/, a superficial fungal infection of the groin, caused by species of *Trichophyton* or *Epidermophyton floccosum*. It is most common in the tropics and among males. Topical antifungals, such as miconazole and clotrimazole, are often prescribed. Griseofulvin is used only for severe, resistant cases. Also called **jock itch.**

tinea pedis, a chronic superficial fungal infection of the foot, especially of the skin between the toes and on the soles. It is common worldwide and is usually caused by *Trichophyton mentagrophytes*, *T. rubrum*, and *Epidermophyton floccosum*. Adults are most susceptible, and the wearing of constricting footwear, such as sneakers, seems to induce the infection. Drying the feet well after bathing and applying powder between the toes help prevent it. Griseofulvin is the most effective treatment, but miconazole

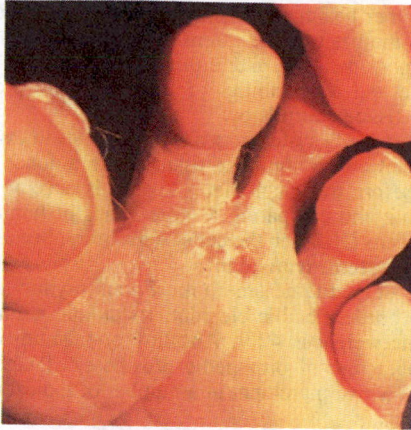

Tinea pedis
*(Greenberger, 1993/Courtesy Loren H Amundson,
University of South Dakota, Sioux Falls)*

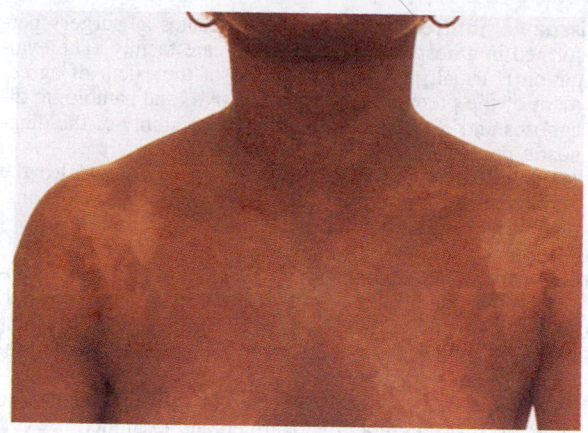

Tinea versicolor
*(McKee, 1993/Courtesy Dr. MM Black,
St. Thomas' Hospital, London)*

and tolnaftate are also used. Recurrence is common. Also called **athlete's foot**.

tinea unguium /un'gwē·əm/,   a superficial fungal infection of the nails caused by various species of *Trichophyton* and, occasionally, by *Candida albicans*. It is more common on the toes than the fingers and can cause complete crumbling and destruction of the nails. Griseofulvin is the drug of choice, but it must be continued until the nail has regrown completely.

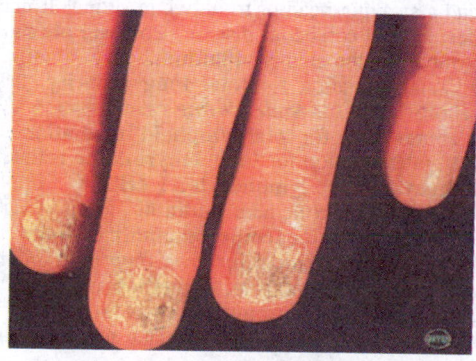

Tinea unguium
(Seidel, 1991/Courtesy American Academy of Dermatology)

tinea versicolor,   a fungal infection of the skin caused by *Malassezia furfur* and characterized by finely desquamating, pale tan patches on the upper trunk and upper arms that may itch and do not tan. In dark-skinned people the lesions may be depigmented. The fungus fluoresces under Wood's light and may be easily identified in scrapings viewed under a microscope. Treatment usually includes a single application of selenium sulfide left on overnight and rinsed off by thorough showering in the morning. The pale patches may persist for up to 1 year after successful treatment.

Tinel's sign /tinelz'/ [Jules Tinel, French neurosurgeon, b. 1879],   an indication of irritability of a nerve, resulting in

a distal tingling sensation on percussion of a damaged nerve. The sign is often present in the carpal tunnel syndrome and is produced by tapping over the median nerve on the volar aspect of the wrist.

tine test /tīn/ [ME, *tind*, rake tooth; L, *testum*, crucible],   a tuberculin skin test in which a small disposable disk with multiple tines bearing tuberculin antigen is used to puncture the skin. The method is widely used to test for sensitivity to the tuberculin antigen. Induration around the puncture site indicates previous exposure or active disease, requiring further testing. See also **tuberculin test.**

tingling [ME, *tinklen*, to tinkle],   a prickly sensation in the skin or a part of the body, accompanied by diminished sensitivity to stimulation of the sensory nerves, felt by a person as the area is numbed by local anesthetic, by exposure to the cold, or as it 'goes to sleep' from pressure on a nerve.

tinnitus /tinī'təs/ [L, *tinnire*, to tinkle],   a subjective noise sensation heard in one or both ears. It may be a sign of acoustic trauma, Ménière's disease, otosclerosis, presbycusis, or an accumulation of cerumen impinging on the eardrum or occluding the external auditory canal. It occasionally occurs for no apparent reason.

tinnitus aurium   See **tinnitus.**

tinted denture base,   a denture base that simulates the coloring of natural oral tissue.

-tion,   a suffix meaning 'act of, process of, result of': *elongation, irritation.*

tipped uterus /tipt/ [ME, *tipen*, upset; L, *uterus*, womb],   a uterus that is displaced from its normal position. See **uterine anteflexion, uterine anteversion, uterine retroflexion, uterine retroversion.**

tip pinch,   a grasp in which the tip of the thumb is pressed against any or each of the tips of the other fingers. Also called **pinch grip.** See also **palmar pinch, pinch.**

tip seal,   the closure of an ampule accomplished by melting a bead of glass at the neck of the ampule.

tissue /tish'ōo/ [Fr, *tissu*, fabric],   a collection of similar cells acting together to perform a particular function.

tissue activator.   See **fibrinokinase.**

tissue-base relationship,   (in dentistry) the relationship of the base of a removable prosthesis to subjacent structures.

tissue committee, a group that evaluates all surgery performed in a hospital or other health care facility. The evaluation is usually made on the basis of the extent of agreement of the preoperative, postoperative, and pathologic diagnoses and on the relevance and acceptability of the diagnostic procedures. See also **tissue review.**

tissue culture [OFr, *tissu*; L, *colere*, to cultivate], the maintenance of growth in vitro, under artificial conditions, of tissue or organ specimens.

tissue dextrin. See **glycogen.**

tissue dose, (in radiotherapy) the amount of radiation absorbed by tissue in the region of interest, expressed in rad.

tissue fixation, a process in which a tissue specimen is placed in a fluid that preserves the cells as nearly as is possible in their natural state.

tissue fixative, a fluid that preserves cells in their natural state, so that they may be identified and examined.

tissue integrity, impaired, a nursing diagnosis accepted by the Seventh National Conference on the Classification of Nursing Diagnoses. Impaired tissue integrity is defined as a state in which an individual experiences damage to mucous membrane, corneal, integumentary, or subcutaneous tissue. The principal characteristic is damaged or destroyed tissue. Related factors are altered circulation, nutritional deficit or excess, knowledge deficit, and impaired physical mobility. Other factors are irritants, such as chemical (including body excretions, secretions, and medications), thermal (temperature extremes), mechanical (pressure, shear, friction), and radiation (including therapeutic radiation). See also **nursing diagnosis.**

tissue kinase. See **fibrinokinase.**

tissue macrophage [OFr, *tissu*;, Gk, *makros*, large, *phagein*, to eat], a large, mobile, highly phagocytic cell derived from monocytes. These cells become mobile when stimulated by inflammation, migrating to the affected area.

tissue perfusion, altered (renal, cerebral, cardiopulmonary, gastrointestinal, peripheral), a nursing diagnosis accepted by the Fourth National Conference on the Classification of Nursing Diagnoses. It is defined as a state in which an individual experiences a decrease in nutrition and oxygenation at the cellular level caused by a deficit in capillary blood supply. The defining characteristics of the condition include coldness of the affected extremity, paleness on elevation of the extremity, diminished arterial pulses, and changes in the arterial blood pressure when measured in the affected extremity. Claudication, gangrene, brittle nails, slowly healing ulcers or wounds, shiny skin, and lack of hair are also commonly seen. Related factors include interruption of the venous or arterial circulation to the affected part of the body, hypovolemia or hypervolemia, or a condition that causes abnormal exchange of fluids and nutrients to or from the cells to or from the circulation. See also **nursing diagnosis.**

tissue plasminogen activator (TPA), a clot-dissolving substance produced naturally by cells in the walls of blood vessels. It is also manufactured synthetically by genetic engineering techniques. TPA activates plasminogen to dissolve clots and has been used therapeutically to remove blood clots blocking coronary arteries.

tissue response, any reaction or change in living cellular tissue when it is acted on by disease, toxin, or other external stimulus. Some kinds of tissue responses are **immune response, inflammation,** and **necrosis.**

tissue review, a review of the surgery performed in a hospital or other health care facility. The evaluation is usually made on the basis of the extent of agreement of the preoperative, postoperative, and pathologic diagnoses and on the relevance and acceptability of the diagnostic procedures. See also **tissue committee.**

tissue typing, a systematized series of tests to evaluate the intraspecies compatibility of tissues from a donor and a recipient before transplantation. Typing is accomplished by identifying and comparing a large series of human leukocyte antigens (HLA) in the cells of the body. See also **HLA, immune system, transplant.**

titanium (Ti) /tītā'nē·əm/ [Gk, *Titan*, mythic giant], a grayish, brittle metallic element. Its atomic number is 22; its atomic weight is 47.9. An alloy of titanium is used in the manufacture of orthopedic prostheses. Titanium dioxide is the active ingredient in a number of topical ointments and lotions.

titer /tī'tər/ [Fr, *titre*, to make a standard] **1.** the normality of a solution or substance, determined by titration to find the equivalence of two reactants. **2.** the extent to which an antibody can be diluted before losing its power to react with a specific antigen. **3.** the highest dilution of a serum that causes clumping of bacteria.

titillation /tit'ilā'shən/ [L, *titillare*, to tickle], tickling.

Title [L, *titulus*, title], a section of the Social Security Act that provides for the establishment, funding, and regulation of a service to a specific segment of the population, such as Title XIX, which includes medical coverage under Medicaid, and Title X, which awards lump-sum grants for family planning programs.

titre. See **titer.**

titubation /tich'əbā'shən/ b [L, *titubare*, to stagger], unsteady posture characterized by a staggering or stumbling gait and a swaying head or trunk while sitting. It may be a manifestation of cerebellar disease. Compare **ataxia.**

Tl, symbol for the element **thallium.**

TLC, **1.** abbreviation for **total lung capacity. 2.** *informal.* abbreviation for *tender loving care.*

TLI, abbreviation for **total lymphoid irradiation.**

T.L.R., abbreviation for **tonic labyrinthine reflex.**

T lymphocyte. See **lymphocyte, T cell.**

Tm, symbol for the element **thulium.**

TMJ, abbreviation for **temporomandibular joint.**

TMP/SMX, abbreviation for *trimethoprim sulfamethoxazole.* See **sulfamethoxazole, trimethoprim.**

TNF, abbreviation for **tumor necrosis factor.**

TNM, a system for staging malignant neoplastic disease. See also **cancer staging.**

t.n.t.c., abbreviation for *too numerous to count,* usually applied to organisms or cells viewed on a slide under a microscope.

t.o., abbreviation for *telephone order.*

toadstool poisoning /tōd'stool/ [AS, *tadige, stol*; L, *potio,* drink], a toxic condition caused by ingestion of certain varieties of poisonous mushrooms. See **mushroom poisoning.**

tobacco /təbak'ō/ [Sp, *tabaco*], a plant whose leaves are dried and used for smoking and chewing, and in snuff. See also **nicotine.**

tobacco withdrawal syndrome, a change in mood or performance associated with the cessation of or reduction in exposure to nicotine. Symptoms may range from lack of concentration to anxiety and temper outbursts.

TOBEC, abbreviation for **total body electric conductivity.**

tobramycin sulfate /tō'brəmī'sin/, an aminoglycoside antibiotic.

- INDICATIONS: It is prescribed in the treatment of external occular infection, septicemia, and lower respiratory tract and central nervous system infections.
- CONTRAINDICATIONS: Kidney dysfunction, use of potent diuretics, or known hypersensitivity to this or other aminoglycosides prohibits its use.
- ADVERSE EFFECTS: Among the more serious adverse reactions are ototoxicity and nephrotoxicity.

Tobruk plaster /tō'brŏŏk/, a plaster cast splint with tapes for skin traction coming through openings in the plaster and connected with Thomas' splint. It covers and immobilizes the leg from foot to groin. Also called **Tobruk splint.**

tocainide hydrochloride /tōkā'nīd/, an oral lidocaine-type antidysrhythmic drug.

- INDICATIONS: It is prescribed for the suppression of symptomatic ventricular dysrhythmias.
- CONTRAINDICATIONS: Tocainide may cause adverse cardiovascular effects, such as worsened dysrhythmias and hypotension. It should not be given to patients with second- or third-degree AV block who do not also have an artificial ventricular pacemaker. It should not be administered to a patient with an uncorrected potassium deficit, and it may interact with beta-blockers, particularly in patients with known heart failure.
- ADVERSE EFFECTS: Among the most serious adverse reactions are hypotension, dysrhythmias, dizziness, paresthesias, numbness, tremor, nausea, vomiting, rash, and headache.

-tocia, **1.** a combining form meaning 'conditions of labor': *mogitocia, omotocia, tomotocia.* **2.** a combining form meaning the 'product of parturition': *deuterotocia, dystrophiadystocia, odontocia.*

-tocin, a combining form for oxytocin derivatives.

toco-, toko- /tō'kō-/, a prefix meaning 'pertaining to childbirth or labor': *tocodynamometer, tocography, tocomania.*

tocodynamometer /tō'kōdī'nəmom'ətər/ [Gk, *tokos,* birth, *dynamis,* force, *metron,* measure], an electronic device for monitoring and recording uterine contractions in labor. It consists of a pressure transducer that is applied to the fundus of the uterus by means of a belt, which is connected to a machine that records the duration of the contractions and the interval between them on graph paper. The relative intensity of the contractions is also indicated but cannot be quantified. The tocodynamometer is a component of external monitoring in childbirth. Also spelled **tokodynamometer.** See also **electronic fetal monitor.**

tocolytic drug /-lit'ik/, any drug used to suppress premature labor.

tocopherol. See **vitamin E.**

tocotransducer /-transd(y)ōō'sər/ [Gk, *tokos* + L, *trans,* through, *ducer,* to lead], an electronic device used to measure uterine contractions. See also **tocodynamometer.**

toddler [ME, *toteren,* to walk unsteadily], a child between 12 and 36 months of age. During this period of development the child acquires a sense of autonomy and independence through the mastery of various specialized tasks, such as control of bodily functions, refinement of motor and language skills, and acquisition of socially acceptable behavior, especially toleration of delayed gratification and acceptance of separation from the mother or parents. The period is characterized by exploration of the environment and by rapid cognitive development as the child strives for self-assertion and personal interaction with others while struggling with parental discipline and sibling rivalry. Of primary importance for the nurse is an understanding of the dynamics of the growth and development of the toddler to help parents deal effectively with appropriate nutrition, toilet training, temper tantrums, prevention of accidental injury (primarily from falls, poisoning, and burns), and childhood fears, especially anxiety as a result of separation from the parents.

toddlerhood /tod'lərhŏŏd'/, the state or condition of being a toddler.

Todd's paralysis [Robert Bentley Todd, English physician, b. 1809; Gk, *paralyein,* to be palsied], a transient postepileptic paralysis of an arm or leg.

toe, any one of the digits of the feet.

toe clonus [AS, *tá;* Gk, *klonos*], an increased reflex activity in the large toe caused by a sudden extension of the first phalanx.

toe drop [AS, *tá + dropa*], a condition in which the toes droop and cannot be lifted because of paralysis of the tibial muscles.

toeing in. See **metatarsus varus.**

toeing out. See **metatarsus valgus.**

toenail [AS, *ta, naegel*], one of the heavy ungual structures covering the terminal phalanges of the toes. Also called **unguis** /ung'gwis/.

Tofranil, a trademark for a tricyclic antidepressant (imipramine hydrochloride).

togaviruses /tō'gəvī'rəsəs/ [L, *toga,* cloak, *virus,* poison], a family of arboviruses that includes the organisms causing encephalitis, dengue, yellow fever, and rubella.

toilet training, the process of teaching a child to control the functions of the bladder and bowel. Training programs vary, but all emphasize a positive, consistent, nonpunitive, and nonpressured approach, and each program is individualized, depending on the mental and physical age and state of the child, the parent-child relationship, and readiness of the child to learn. Training often begins around 24 months of age, when voluntary control of the anal and urethral sphincters is achieved by most children. When the child has mastered some motor skills, is aware of his or her ability to control the body, and can communicate adequately, training is likely to be easy. Resistance occurs if the parents try to train the child before the child is physiologically and psychologically ready. Bowel training is usually accomplished before bladder training because the urge to evacuate the bowel is stronger than the urge to empty the bladder, and the need is less frequent and more regular. Nighttime bladder control may not be achieved until the child is 4 or 5 years of age or older. Behavior modification, using a system of rewards for each of the various phases of the training, has been successful with both normal and mentally retarded children. A major nursing function is to identify the readiness of the child to learn and to work with the parents, advising them in a nonauthoritarian way of the various techniques.

-toin, a combining form for hydantoin derivative antiepileptics.

token economy [AS, *tacen,* to show; Gk, *oikonomia,* household, management], a technique of reinforcement used in behavior therapy in the management of a group of people, such as in hospitals, institutions, or classrooms. Individuals are rewarded for specific activities or behavior with tokens they can exchange for desired objects or privileges.

toko-. See **toco-.**

tokodynamometer. See **tocodynamometer.**

tolazamide /tolaz′əmid/, an oral sulfonylurea antidiabetic.

■ INDICATIONS: It is prescribed in the treatment of stable or non-insulin-dependent diabetes mellitus and for some patients sensitive to other types of sulfonylureas or who have failed to respond to other similar drugs.

■ CONTRAINDICATIONS: Unstable diabetes, serious impairment of renal, hepatic, or thyroid function, pregnancy, or known hypersensitivity to this drug or to other sulfonylurea medications prohibits its use.

■ ADVERSE EFFECTS: Among the more serious adverse effects are hypoglycemia and skin reactions. Blood dyscrasias may occur.

tolazoline hydrochloride /tolaz′əlēn/, a peripheral vasodilator.

■ INDICATIONS: It is prescribed in the treatment of spastic peripheral vascular disorders, including Buerger's disease, Raynaud's disease, and scleroderma.

■ CONTRAINDICATIONS: Coronary artery disease, cerebrovascular accident, or known hypersensitivity to this drug prohibits its use.

■ ADVERSE EFFECTS: Among the more serious adverse reactions are cardiac dysrhythmia, hypertension, exacerbation of peptic ulcer, and a paradoxical response in seriously damaged limbs.

tolbutamide /tolbōō′təmīd/, an oral sulfonylurea antidiabetic.

■ INDICATIONS: It is prescribed in the treatment of stable non-insulin-dependent diabetes mellitus uncontrolled by diet alone and for some patients changing from insulin to oral therapy.

■ CONTRAINDICATIONS: Unstable diabetes, serious impairment of renal, hepatic, or thyroid function, pregnancy, or known hypersensitivity to this drug or to other sulfonylurea medications prohibits its use.

■ ADVERSE EFFECTS: Among the more serious adverse reactions are hypoglycemia and skin reactions. Blood dyscrasias may occur.

Tolectin, a trademark for a nonsteroidal antiinflammatory agent (tolmetin sodium).

tolerance /tol′ərəns/ [L, tolerare, to endure], the ability to endure hardship, pain, or ordinarily injurious substances, such as drugs, without apparent physiologic or psychologic injury. A kind of tolerance is **work tolerance.**

tolerance dose. See **maximum permissible dose.**

Tolinase, a trademark for an antidiabetic (tolazamide).

tolmetin sodium /tol′mətin/, a nonsteroidal antiinflammatory agent.

■ INDICATIONS: It is prescribed primarily in the treatment of rheumatoid arthritis, juvenile rheumatoid arthritis, and osteoarthritis.

■ CONTRAINDICATIONS: Impaired renal function, GI disease, or known hypersensitivity to this drug, to aspirin, or to nonsteroidal antiinflammatory medications prohibits its use.

■ ADVERSE EFFECTS: Among the more serious adverse reactions are peptic ulcer and GI distress. Dizziness, skin rash, and tinnitus commonly occur. This drug interacts with many other drugs.

tolnaftate /tolnaf′tāt/, an antifungal.

■ INDICATIONS: It is prescribed in the treatment of superficial fungus infections of the skin, including tinea pedis, tinea cruris, and tinea versicolor.

■ CONTRAINDICATION: Known hypersensitivity to this drug prohibits its use.

■ ADVERSE EFFECTS: Among the more common adverse reactions are hypersensitivity reactions and mild irritation of the skin.

-tome, **1.** a combining form meaning a 'cutting instrument': labiotome, neurotome, thyrotome. **2.** a combining form meaning a '(specified) segment or region': dermomyotome, pleurotome, viscerotome.

-tomic, -tomical, a suffix meaning 'related to incisions or sections of tissue': dermatomic, phlebotomic, somatomic.

tomo-, a combining form meaning 'preparation of a section or layer': tomograph.

tomogram /tō′məgram′/ [Gk, tome, section + gramma, record], a radiograph produced by tomography.

tomographic DSA /-graf′ik/, the visualization of blood vessels in the body in three dimensions. See also **digital subtraction angiography (DSA).**

tomography /təmog′rəfē/ [Gk, tome + graphein, to record], an x-ray technique that produces a film representing a detailed cross section of tissue structure at a predetermined depth. It is a valuable diagnostic tool for the discovery and identification of space-occupying lesions, such as might be found in the brain, liver, pancreas, and gallbladder. See also **computed tomography, position emission tomography.**

-tomy, a suffix meaning a 'surgical incision': cystotomy, oncotomy, phlebotomy.

tone. See **tonus.**

tone deafness [Gk, tonos, stretching; AS, déaf], an inability to detect the pitch or changing pitch of a musical note or a voice change.

tongue /tung/ [AS, tunge], the principal organ of the sense of taste that also assists in the mastication and the deglutition of food. It is located in the floor of the mouth within

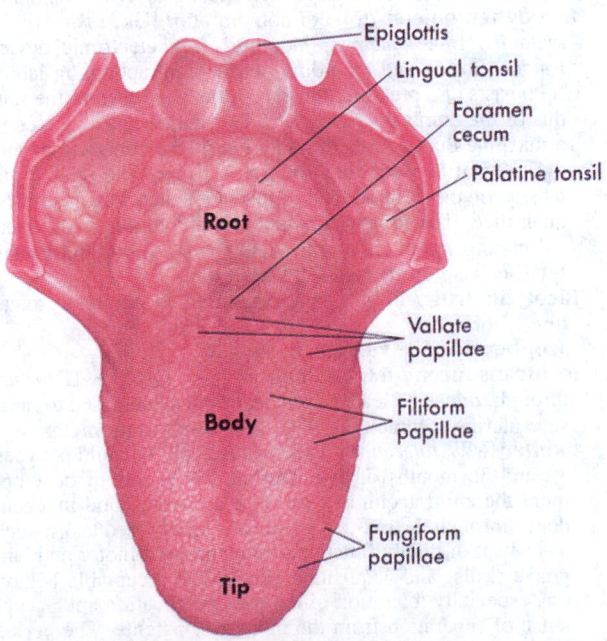

Tongue (Thibodeau, 1993 Rolin Graphics)

the curve of the mandible. Its root is connected to the hyoid bone posteriorly by the hypoglossi and the genioglossi muscles. It is also connected to the epiglottis by three folds of mucous membrane, to the soft palate by the glossopalatine arches, and to the pharynx by the constrictores pharyngis superiores and by the mucous membrane. The apex of the tongue rests anteriorly against the lingual surfaces of the lower incisors. The mucous membrane connecting the tongue to the mandible reflects over the floor of the mouth to the lingual surface of the gingiva and in the midline of the floor is raised into a vertical fold. The dorsum of the tongue is divided into symmetric halves by a median sulcus, which ends posteriorly in the foramen cecum. A shallow sulcus terminalis runs from this foramen laterally and forward on either side to the margin of the organ. From the sulcus, the anterior two thirds of the tongue are covered with papillae. The posterior third is smoother and contains numerous mucous glands and lymph follicles. The use of the tongue as an organ of speech is not anatomic but a secondary acquired characteristic. Also called **lingua.**

tongue-thrust swallow, an immature form of swallowing in which the tongue is projected forward instead of retracted during the act of swallowing. It may result in forward displacement of the maxilla with consequent malocclusion of the teeth.

tongue-tie. See **ankyloglossia.**

-tonia, -tony, a suffix meaning '(condition or degree of) muscle tension': *angiotonia, hemotonia, neurotony, vagotony, vasotonia.*

tonic /ton'ik/, pertaining to a type of afferent or sensory nerve receptor that responds to length changes placed on the noncontractile portion of a muscle spindle. It may be triggered by a mechanical external force such as positioning, or by an internal stretch caused by intrafusal muscle contraction.

-tonic, **1.** a combining form meaning the 'quality of muscle contraction or tonus': *hypertonic, myatonic, normotonic.* **2.** a combining form meaning a 'solution with a comparative concentration': *hypertonic, hypotonic, isotonic.*

tonic convulsion [Gk, *tonos,* stretching; L, *convulsio,* cramp], a prolonged generalized contraction of the skeletal muscles.

tonicity /tōnis'itē/ [Gk, *tonikos,* stretching], the quality of possessing tone, or tonus.

tonic labyrinthine reflex [Gk, *tonikos* + *labyrinthos,* maze; L, *reflectere,* to bend backward], a normal postural reflex in animals, abnormally accentuated in decerebrate humans, characterized by extension of all four limbs when the head is positioned in space at an angle above the horizontal in quadripeds or in the neutral, erect position in humans. Also called **decerebrate rigidity.**

tonic neck reflex, a normal response in newborns to extend the arm and the leg on the side of the body to which the head is quickly turned while the infant is supine and to flex the limbs of the opposite side. The reflex, which prevents the infant from rolling over until adequate neurologic and motor development occurs, disappears by 3 to 4 months of age to be replaced by symmetric positioning of both sides of the body. Absence or persistence of the reflex may indicate central nervous system damage. Also called **asymmetric tonic neck reflex.** See also **symmetric tonic neck reflex.**

tonic spasm [Gk, *tonos,* stretching + *spasmos*], a sustained contraction of a muscle as distinguished from a transient clonic contraction.

tono-, a combining form meaning 'pertaining to tone or tension': *tonoclonic, tonoscillograph, tonoplast.*

Tonocard, a trademark for a lidocaine-type oral antidysrhythmic drug (tocainide hydrochloride).

tonoclonic /ton'əklon'ik/ [Gk, *tonos,* stretching + *klonos,* tumult], pertaining to muscular spasms that are tonic and then clonic.

tonofibril /ton'əfī'bril/ [Gk, *tonos,* tension, *fibrilla,* small fiber], a bundle of fine filaments found in the cytoplasm of epithelial cells. The individual strands, or **tonofilaments,** spread throughout the cytoplasm and extend into the intercellular bridge to converge at the desmosome. The system of fibers functions as a supportive element within the cytoskeleton. In keratinizing epithelium, the strands are the main precursor of keratin. Also called **epitheliofibril, tenofibril.** See also **keratohyalin.**

tonometer /tōnom'ətər/ [Gk, *tonos* + *metron,* measure], an instrument used in measuring tension or pressure, especially intraocular pressure.

tonometry /tōnom'ətrē/, the measuring of intraocular pressure by determining the resistance of the eyeball to indentation by an applied force. Several kinds of tonometers are used. The air-puff tonometer, which does not touch the eye, records deflections of the cornea from a puff of pressurized air. The Schiötz impression and the aplanation tonometers record the pressure needed to indent or flatten the corneal surface.

tonsil /ton'səl/ [L, *tonsilla*], a small rounded mass of tissue, especially lymphoid tissue, such as that composing the palatine tonsils in the oropharynx. Compare **intestinal tonsil, lingual tonsil, palatine tonsil, pharyngeal tonsil.**

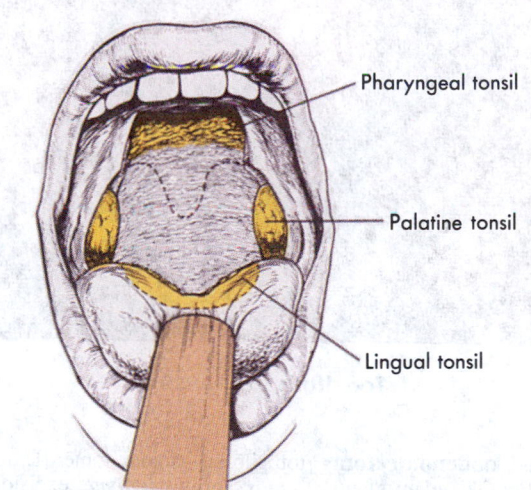

Tonsils *(Seeley, 1992/David J Mascaro & Associates)*

tonsill-, a prefix meaning 'pertaining to the tonsils': *tonsillectomy, tonsillith, tonsillitis.*

tonsillar /ton'silər/ [L, *tonsilla*] pertaining to the palatine tonsil.

tonsillar crypt [L, *tonsilla;* Gk, *kryptos,* hidden], a small tubular invagination on the surface of a palatine or pharyngeal tonsil.

tonsillar fossa. See **amygdaloid fossa.**

tonsillar herniation [L, *tonsilla* + *hernia,* rupture], the herniation of tonsils of the cerebellum through the foramen magnum of the skull. It may occur as a result of intracranial pressure from an injury or tumor.

tonsillectomy /ton′silek′təmē/ [L, *tonsilla* + Gk, *ektome*, excision], the surgical excision of the palatine tonsils, performed to prevent recurrent tonsillitis. Before surgery, several laboratory tests, including a bleeding and clotting time, complete blood count, and urinalysis are done. Tonsillar tissue is dissected and removed, usually using general anesthesia, and bleeding areas are sutured or cauterized. An airway remains in place until swallowing returns. An increase in pulse rate, falling blood pressure, restlessness, or frequent swallowing warns of possible hemorrhage. On recovery from anesthesia, ice chips or clear liquids without a drinking straw may be offered. Tonsillectomy is often combined with adenoidectomy.

tonsillitis /-ī′tis/, an infection or inflammation of a tonsil. Acute tonsillitis, frequently caused by streptococcus infection, is characterized by severe sore throat, fever, headache, malaise, difficulty in swallowing, earache, and enlarged, tender lymph nodes in the neck. Acute tonsillitis may accompany scarlet fever. Treatment includes systemic antibiotics, analgesics, and warm irrigations of the throat. Soft foods and ample fluids are given. Tonsillectomy is sometimes performed for recurrent tonsillitis or tonsillar abscess. See also **peritonsillar abscess, scarlet fever, strep throat.**

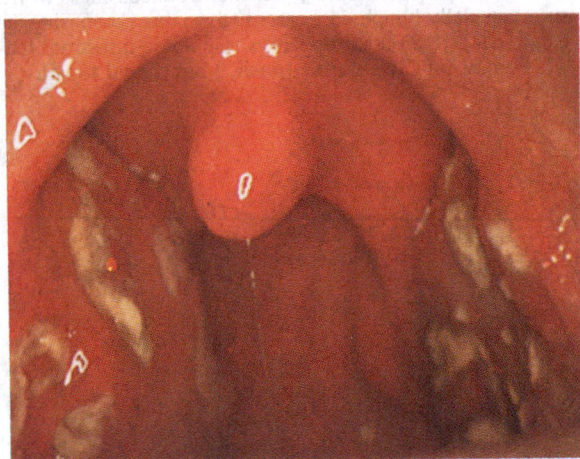

Tonsillitis (Forbes, 1993)

tonsilloadenoidectomy /ton′silō·ad′ənoidek′təmē/ [L, *tonsilla*; Gk, *aden*, gland + *eidos*, form + *ektome*, excision], the surgical removal of tonsil and adenoid tissues.

tonus /tō′nəs/ [Gk, *tonos*, tension], **1.** the normal state of balanced tension in the tissues of the body, especially the muscles. Partial contraction or alternate contraction and relaxation of neighboring fibers of a group of muscles hold the organ or the part of the body in a neutral, functional position without fatigue. Tone is essential for many normal body functions, such as holding the spine erect, the eyes open, and the jaw closed. **2.** the state of the tissues of the body being strong and fit. Also called **tone.**

-tony. See **-tonia.**

tooth, *pl.* **teeth** [AS, *toth*], one of numerous dental structures that develop in the jaws as part of the digestive system and are used to cut, grind, and process food in the mouth for ingestion. Each tooth consists of a crown, which projects above the gum; two to four roots, embedded in the alveolus; and a neck, which stretches between the crown and the root. Each tooth also contains a cavity filled with pulp, richly supplied with blood vessels and nerves that enter the cavity through a small aperture at the base of each root. The solid portion of the tooth consists of dentin, enamel, and a thin layer of bone on the surface of the root. The dentin composes the bulk of the tooth. The enamel covers the exposed portion of the crown. Two sets of teeth appear at different periods of life: the 20 deciduous teeth appear during infancy, the 32 permanent teeth during childhood and early adulthood. See also **deciduous tooth, permanent tooth.**

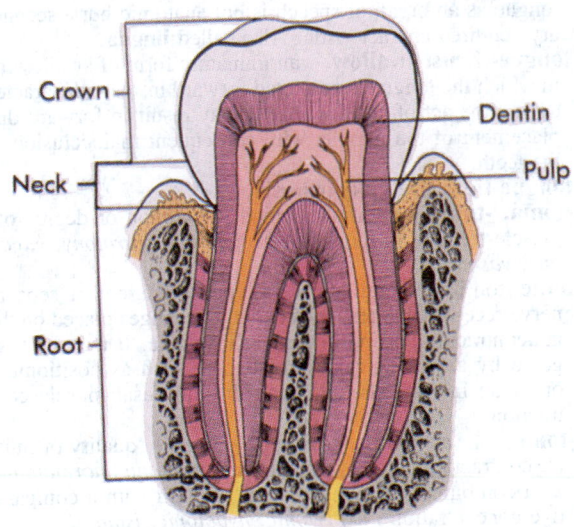

Tooth (Potter, 1993)

tooth abscess [AS, *toth*; L, *abscedere*, to go away], a collection of pus, usually close to the root of a tooth and often the result of an untreated cavity. If untreated, the pressure of the abscess may destroy the alveolar bone and adjoining soft tissues. Also called **dental abscess.**

toothache /tōō′thāk/ [AS, *toth* + *aeca*], a pain in a tooth, usually caused by caries that have extended into the dentin or pulp, or by traumatic occlusion. See also **pulpitis.**

tooth alignment, the arrangement of the teeth in relation to their supporting bone or alveolar process, adjacent teeth, and opposing dentitions.

tooth-borne, describing a dental prosthesis or part of a prosthesis that depends entirely on abutment teeth for support.

tooth-borne base, a denture base restoring an edentulous area that has abutment teeth at each end for support. The tissue that it covers is not used for support of the base.

toothbrush, an implement of various design, with bristles fixed to a head at the end of a handle, used for brushing and cleaning the teeth and gingivae and for massaging the gingival tissues.

tooth form, the identifying curves, lines, angles, and contours of a tooth that differentiate it from other teeth.

tooth fulcrum, axis of movement of a tooth subjected to lateral forces, considered to be at the middle third of the portion of the tooth root embedded in the alveolus.

tooth germ, a primitive cell in the embryo that is the precursor of a tooth.

tooth inclination, the angle of slope of a tooth or teeth from the vertical plane, such as mesially, distally, lingually, buccally, or labially inclined.

tooth rotation [AS, *toth*; L, *rotare*, to rotate], **1.** the malposition of a tooth that has turned around its longitudinal axis, or that has been turned by an orthodontic appliance to a normal position. **2.** the process by which the tooth is turned.

top-, topo-, a combining form meaning 'relating to place or location': *topesthesia, topalgia, topognosia.*

tophaceous /tōfā′shəs/, pertaining to the presence of tophi.

tophaceous gout [L, *tufa*], a form of purine metabolism disorder characterized by formation of chalky deposits of sodium biurate under the skin and in the joints. If untreated, the deposits may eventually destroy the involved joints.

tophus /tō′fəs/, *pl.* **tophi** [L, *tufa*, porous rock], a calculus, containing sodium urate deposits, that develops in periarticular fibrous tissue, typically in patients with gout.

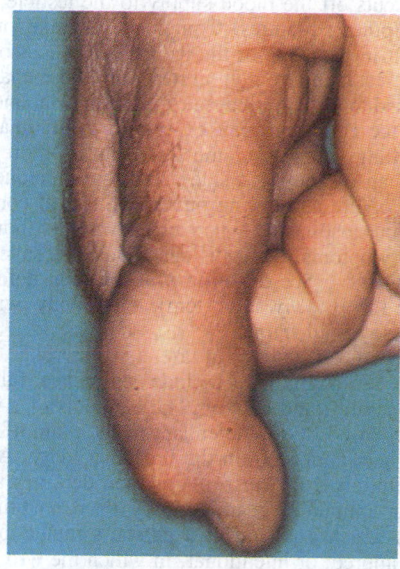

Tophus (Shipley, 1993)

-topia, -topy, a combining form meaning '(condition of) placement of organs in the body': *heterotopia, normotopia, skeletopia.*

topical /top′ikəl/ [Gk, *topos*, place], **1.** of or pertaining to the surface of a part of the body. **2.** of or pertaining to a drug or treatment applied topically.

topical anesthesia, surface analgesia produced by application of a topical anesthetic in the form of a solution, gel, or ointment to the skin, mucous membrane, or cornea. The most common ingredients include benzocaine, butamben, cyclomethycaine, dibucaine, dimethisoquin, diperodon, dy-

clonine, lidocaine, piperocaine, pramoxine, hexylcaine, and tetracaine. Cocaine may be applied in solution to the mucous membranes of the nasal passages in certain otolaryngeal or maxillofacial procedures. Also called **surface anesthesia.** Compare **general anesthesia, local anesthesia, regional anesthesia.**

Topicort, a trademark for a topical glucocorticoid (desoximetasone).

topo-. See **top-.**

topognosis /top′ognō′sis/ [Gk, *topos* + *gnosis*, recognition], the ability to recognize tactile stimuli.

topographic /top′əgraf′ik/, (in psychiatry) pertaining to a freudian conceptualization of the layers of human consciousness.

topographic anatomy [Gk, *topos*, place + *graphein*, to record + *ana* + *temnein*, to cut], the study of a specific region of a body structure, such as a lower leg, including all of the systems in the part and their relationship to each other. Also called **regional anatomy.**

topographic disorientation, a form of disorientation based on Freud's topographic model of the mental apparatus, consisting of conscious, preconscious, and unconscious sytems for interpreting perceptions of the outside world and internal perceptions. Under certain conditions, such as frustration or sleep, psychic energy reanimates unconscious memories, resulting in hallucinations in mental disorders.

topography /təpog′refē/ [Gk, *topos*, place + *graphein*, to record], the anatomic description of a body part in terms of the region in which it is located.

TOPV, abbreviation for *trivalent oral polio vaccine.*

TORCH /tôrch/, an abbreviation for *toxoplasmosis, other, rubella virus, cytomegalovirus, and herpes simplex viruses,* a group of agents that can infect the fetus or the newborn infant, causing a constellation of morbid effects called the TORCH syndrome.

TORCH syndrome, infection of the fetus or newborn by one of the TORCH agents. The outcome of a pregnancy complicated by a TORCH agent may be abortion, stillbirth, intrauterine growth retardation, or premature delivery.

■ OBSERVATIONS: At delivery and during the first days after birth an infant infected with any one of the organisms may demonstrate various clinical manifestations, such as fever, lethargy, poor feeding, petechiae on the skin, purpura, pneumonia, hepatosplenomegaly, jaundice, hemolytic and other anemias, encephalitis, microcephaly, hydrocephalus, intracranial calcifications, hearing deficits, chorioretinitis, and microophthalmia. In addition, each of the agents is associated with several other abnormal clinical findings involving abnormal immune response, cataracts, glaucoma, vesicles, ulcers, and congenital cardiac defects.

■ INTERVENTIONS: Before pregnancy women may be tested for susceptibility to the rubella virus and inoculated against it if not immune. There are currently no vaccines that confer immunity to the other TORCH agents, but the mother may be serologically tested for antibody levels to them. During pregnancy toxoplasmosis is asymptomatic in about 90% of cases, making diagnosis unlikely. If infection is suspected, serial paired serologic tests are performed: A high, rising titer indicates recent infection. Transplacental infection occurs in 35% of mothers infected during pregnancy. If it is contracted in the first trimester, before the placenta is fully developed, the infant may not become infected; if the infection is contracted, severe congenital manifestations of the syndrome usually occur. If the fetus is infected after the first trimester, the baby is usually born with asymptomatic or mild disease; the infection may be spread from the baby during the newborn period. Sulfadiazone, pyrimethamine, and folinic acid are sometimes given to treat the infection.

Primary cytomegalovirus infection during pregnancy is usually asymptomatic. If the infection is suspected, serologic testing may be performed to demonstrate primary infection, because infants born to mothers infected for the first time during pregnancy are much more likely to develop severe congenital anomalies than if the infection is a reactivation of previous cytomegalovirus infection. There is no specific treatment. The child is considered to be infectious, but contagion among newborns from a congenitally infected infant has not been proven.

Transplacental rubella virus infection in pregnancy during the first 8 weeks is likely to cause infection in 50% of fetuses and to result in demonstrable defects in 85% of those infected. The risk becomes less as gestation increases to 24 weeks, after which time infection has not been known to result in defects. Rubella is the only TORCH virus that is usually symptomatic, and therefore it is often recognized. Many mothers infected during the first trimester choose to abort the pregnancy. There is no treatment for the infection, but screening and immunization before pregnancy could prevent virtually all cases of congenital rubella.

Herpesvirus infection (HSV) in pregnancy is rarely transplacentally transmitted to the fetus. Primary infection during pregnancy sometimes results in spontaneous abortion or premature delivery. In the newborn the infection is usually systemic and life threatening. The fetus is most apt to become infected by the virus shed from an active genital lesion during vaginal delivery or as the result of vaginal examination or the placement of an intrauterine catheter or a fetal scalp electrode during labor. There is no treatment: If the mother has active genital herpesvirus lesions, intrapartal internal monitoring is contraindicated, vaginal examinations are often omitted, regional anesthetic techniques are avoided, and the infant is delivered by cesarean section. The TORCH infections caused by other agents are asymptomatic in pregnancy, revealing themselves by the syndrome after birth. The congenital effects are not amenable to change or to amelioration by any known treatment.

■ NURSING CONSIDERATIONS: Newborn infants who are infected with a TORCH agent or who bear the stigmata of TORCH syndrome are considered to be potential sources of neonatal spread of infection. Rubella screening and vaccination are encouraged. Only 10% of the cases of TORCH syndrome are proven to be associated with a known agent (toxoplasmosis, rubella virus, cytomegalovirus, or herpesvirus); 90% are the result of 'other' infections; therefore pregnant women are instructed to avoid contact with people ill with infectious diseases to the greatest extent possible.

Torecan, a trademark for a phenothiazine antiemetic (thiethylperazine maleate).

Torkildsen's procedure. See **ventriculocisternostomy.**

Tornalate, a trademark for an orally inhaled bronchodilator (bitolterol mesylate).

torque /tôrk/ [L, *torquere*, to twist], **1.** a twisting force produced by contraction of the medial femoral muscles that tend to rotate the thigh medially. **2.** (in dentistry) a force applied to a tooth to rotate it on a mesiodistal or buccolingual axis. **3.** a rotary force applied to a denture base. Compare **torsion.**

torr /tôr/ [Evangelista Torricelli, Italian physicist, b. 1608], a unit of pressure equal to 1333.22 dynes/cm2, or 1.33322

millibars. One torr is the pressure required to support a column of mercury 1 mm high when the mercury is of standard density and subjected to standard acceleration. These standard conditions are 0° C and 45° latitude, where the acceleration of gravity is 980.6 cm/sec2. In reading a mercury barometer at other temperatures and latitudes, corrections commonly exceeding 2 torr may be required to compensate for the thermal expansion of the measuring scale used.

tors-, a combining form meaning 'twisted': *torsiometer, torsive, torsiversion.*

torsades de pointes /tôrsäd′ depô·aNt′, tôr′säd dəpoint′/ [Fr, *torsader*, to twist together, *pointes*, tips], a type of ventricular tachycardia with a spiral-like appearance ("twisting of the points") and complexes that at first look positive and then negative on an electrocardiogram. It is precipitated by a long QT interval, which often is drug induced (quinidine, procainamide, or disopyramide), but which may be the result of hypokalemia or profound bradycardia.

torsion /tôr′shən/ [L, *torquere*, to twist], **1.** the process of twisting in a positive (clockwise) or negative (counterclockwise) direction. **2.** the state of being turned. **3.** (in dentistry) the twisting of a tooth on its long axis.

torsion dystonia. See **dystonia musculorum deformans.**

torsion fracture, a spiral fracture, usually caused by a torsion injury.

torsion of the testis, the axial rotation of the spermatic cord that cuts off the blood supply to the testicle, epididymis, and other structures. Complete ischemia for 6 hours may result in gangrene of the testis. Partial loss of circulation may result in atrophy. Certain testes are anatomically predisposed to torsion because of inadequate connective tissue, but the condition may be caused by trauma with severe swelling. Torsion of the testis occurs more often on the left than on the right side and is most frequent in the first year of life and during puberty. Surgical correction is required in most cases; if performed within 5 hours of the onset of symptoms, the testis can usually be saved.

torsion spasm. See **dystonia musculorum deformans.**

torso /tôr′sō/ [L, *thyrsus*, stem], the body without the limbs. Also called **trunk.**

tort [L, *tortus*, twisted], (in law) a civil wrong, other than a breach of contract. Torts include negligence, false imprisonment, assault, and battery. The elements of a tort are: a legal duty owed by the defendant to the plaintiff, a breach of duty, and damage from the breach of duty. A tort may be constitutional, in which one person deprives another of a right or immunity guaranteed by the Constitution; personal, in which a person or a person's reputation or feelings are injured; or intentional, in which the wrong is a deliberate act that is unlawful. Many other kinds of torts exist. **−tortious,** *adj.*

torticollis /tôr′tikol′is/ [L, *tortus*, twisted, *collum*, neck], an abnormal condition in which the head is inclined to one side as a result of the contraction of the muscles on that side of the neck. It may be congenital or acquired. Treatment may include surgery, heat, support, or immobilization, depending on the cause and the severity of the condition. Also called **wryneck.** See also **spasmodic torticollis.**

tortipelvis /-pel′vis/ [L, *tortus,* twisted + *pelvis,* basin], a form of muscular dystonia resulting in a distortion of the pelvis, or spine and hips.

tortuous /tôr′choo·əs/ [L, *tortus,* twisted], having or making twists and turns.

Torula histolytica. See *Cryptococcus neoformans.*

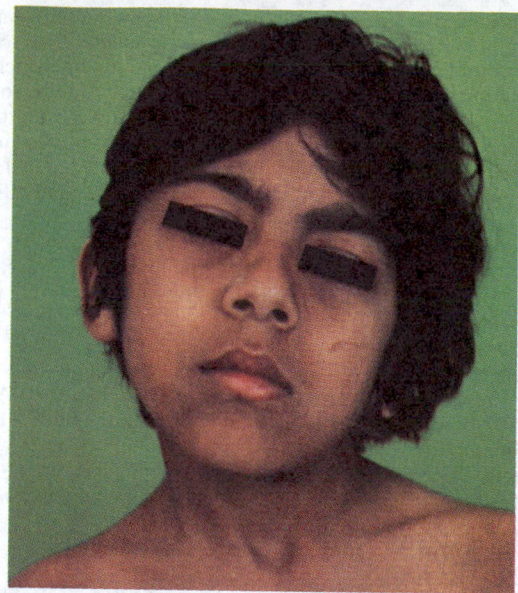

Torticollis (Bingham, 1992)

torulopsosis /tôr′yəlopsō′sis, tôr′yo͞olop′səsis/ [L, *torulus,* small swelling; Gk, *opsis,* appearance, *osis,* condition], an infection with the yeast *Torulopsis glabrata,* a normal inhabitant of the oropharynx, GI tract, and skin that causes disease in severely debilitated patients, in those with impaired immune function, or, sometimes, in patients having prolonged urinary catheterization. Systemic infection is usually treated with amphotericin B.

torulosis. See **cryptococcosis.**

torus fracture. See **lead pipe fracture.**

torus palatinus [L, *torus,* swelling + *palatum,* palate], a bony ridge along the hard palate at the line of fusion of the left and right jawbone segments. It is a hereditary feature.

total anomalous venous return [L, *totus,* whole; Gk, *anomalos,* uneven; L, *vena,* vein; ME, *retournen,* to turn back], a rare congenital cardiac anomaly in which the pulmonary veins attach directly to the right atrium or to various veins draining into the right atrium rather than directing flow to the left atrium. Clinical manifestations include cyanosis, pulmonary congestion, and heart failure. Other cardiac defects also may be present, such as atrial septal defect, which shunts unoxygenated systemic blood to the left side of the heart and helps decompress the right atrium. Corrective surgery is indicated, usually after 1 year of age, but may be necessary at an earlier age if pulmonary venous obstruction or severe congestive heart failure is present. See also **congenital cardiac anomaly.**

total body electric conductivity (TOBEC), a method of measuring body composition by the differences in electrical conductivity of fat, bone, and muscle. It is used for monitoring fitness of athletes; in clinical studies of weight control in which physicians want to determine if weight loss is due to fat, water, or other tissues; and in measurement of fat content of dietary meats. See also **bioelectrical impedance analysis (BIA).**

total body radiation, radiation that exposes the entire body so that, theoretically, all cells in the body receive the same radiation.

total body water (TBW), all the water within the body, including intracellular and extracellular water plus the water in the GI and urinary tracts.

total cleavage, mitotic division of the fertilized ovum into blastomeres. Compare **partial cleavage.**

total color blindness. See **color blindness.**

total communication, the combined use of oral language and manual communication by a person with hearing loss.

total hip replacement, a surgical procedure to correct a hip joint damaged by degenerative disease, often arthritis. The head of the femur and the acetabulum are replaced with metal components. The acetabulum is plastic coated to avoid metal-to-metal articulating surfaces.

total iron, the total iron concentration in the blood. The normal concentrations in serum are 50 to 150 [Grk m]g/dl.

total joint replacement, a surgical procedure for the treatment of severe arthritis and other disorders in which the normal articulating surfaces are replaced by metal and plastic prostheses. The operation most commonly involves replacement of the hip joint with a metallic femur head and a plastic-coated metal acetabulum, such as in the Charnley low-friction arthroplasty procedure. Similar methods are used to restore function to the knee or other joints.

total lung capacity (TLC), the volume of gas in the lungs at the end of a maximum inspiration. It equals the vital capacity plus the residual capacity.

total lymphoid irradiation (TLI), a method of inducing a strong immunosuppresive effect in patients undergoing bone marrow transplants, treatment of certain lymphomas, or other therapies requiring immunosuppression. TLI involves exposing all lymph nodes, the thymus, and spleen to a total of 2000 rad in 100 rad doses from a linear accelerator before graft implantation.

total macroglobulins, the heavy serum macroglobulins that are elevated in various diseases, such as cancer, and infections. The normal concentrations in serum are 70 to 430 mg/dl.

total nitrogen, the nitrogen content of the feces, measured to detect various disorders, such as pancreatic insufficiency and impaired protein digestion. The normal amount in a 24-hour fecal specimen is 10% of intake, or 1 to 2 g.

total parenteral nutrition (TPN), the administration of a nutritionally adequate hypertonic solution consisting of glucose, protein hydrolysates, minerals, and vitamins through an indwelling catheter into the superior vena cava. The high rate of blood flow results in rapid dilution of the solution, and full nutritional requirements can be met indefinitely. The procedure is used in prolonged coma, severe uncontrolled malabsorption, extensive burns, GI fistulas, and other conditions in which feeding by mouth cannot provide adequate amounts of the essential nutrients. In infants and children it is used when feeding by way of the GI tract is impossible, inadequate, or hazardous, such as in chronic intestinal obstruction from peritoneal sepsis or adhesions, inadequate intestinal length, or chronic nonremitting severe diarrhea. The hyperalimentation solution is infused through conventional tubing with an intravenous filter attached to remove any contaminates. In adults the catheter is placed directly into the subclavian vein and threaded through the right innominate vein into the superior vena cava. In infants and small children the catheter is usually threaded to the central venous location by way of the jugular vein, which is entered through a subcutaneous tunnel beneath the scalp. Strict asepsis must be maintained because infection is a grave and present danger of this therapy. Other solutions are never in-

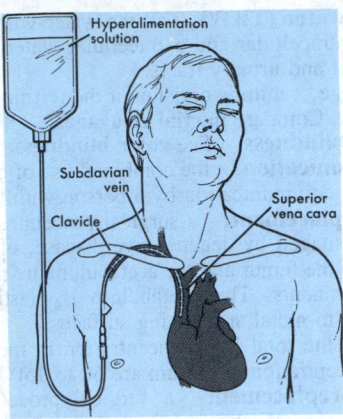

Total parenteral nutrition (adult)

stilled through this catheter. Also called **hyperalimentation, intravenous alimentation, parenteral hyperalimentation, total parenteral alimentation.**

total peripheral resistance, the maximum degree of resistance to blood flow caused by constriction of the systemic blood vessels.

total renal blood flow (TRBF), the total volume of blood that flows into the renal arteries. The average TRBF in a normal adult is 1200 ml per minute.

touch /tuch/ [Fr, *toucher,* to touch], **1.** the ability to feel objects and to distinguish their various characteristics; the tactile sense. **2.** the ability to perceive pressure when it is exerted on the skin or the mucosa of the body. **3.** to palpate or examine with the hand, such as the digital examination of the abdomen, rectum, or vagina.

touch deprivation, a lack of tactile stimulation, especially in early infancy, which if continued for a sufficient length of time may lead to serious developmental and emotional disturbances, such as stunted growth, personality disorders, and social regression. In severe cases, a child who is deprived of adequate physical handling and emotional stimulation may not survive infancy. See also **hospitalism.**

touch receptors [Fr, *toucher;* L, *recipere,* to receive], specialized sensory nerve endings that are sensitive to tactile stimuli.

Tourette's syndrome. See **Gilles de la Tourette's syndrome.**

tourniquet /tur′nikit, toŏr′-/ [Fr, turnstile], a device used in controlling hemorrhage, consisting of a wide constricting band applied to the limb proximal to the site of bleeding. The use of a tourniquet is a drastic measure and is to be employed only if the hemorrhage is life threatening and if other safer measures have proved ineffective. See also **hemorrhage.**

tourniquet infusion method, a technique of intraarterial regional chemotherapy used in the treatment of osteogenic sarcoma. The technique uses one or two external tourniquets, depending on the location of the tumor, that slow or interrupt the blood flow to a limb temporarily while an anticancer drug, such as adriamycin, is infused into the area. The method increases the concentration of an antineoplastic drug by as much as 100 times as compared with an alternative technique of injecting the drug into the circulation

without application of a tourniquet, which results in rapid dilution of the drug by the normal blood volume.

tourniquet test, a test of capillary fragility, in which a blood pressure cuff is applied for 5 minutes to a person's arm and is inflated to a pressure halfway between the diastolic and systolic blood pressure. The number of petechiae within a circumscribed area of the skin may be counted, or the results may be reported in a range from negative (no petechiae) to +4 positive (confluent petechiae).

tower head, tower skull. See **oxycephaly.**

tox-, toxi-, toxico-, toxo- [Gk, *toxikon,* poison], a combining form meaning 'relating to toxins or poisons': *toxin, toxicology.*

-toxaemia. See **-toxemia.**

toxemia /toksē′mē·ə/ [Gk, *toxikon,* poison, *haima,* blood], the presence of bacterial toxins in the bloodstream. Also called **blood poisoning.** See also **preeclampsia.** **–toxemic,** *adj.*

-toxemia, -toxaemia, a suffix meaning a '(specified) toxic substance in the blood': *ectotoxemia, gonotoxemia, ophiotoxemia.*

toxemia of pregnancy. See **preeclampsia.**

toxi-. See **tox-.**

-toxia, a combining form meaning 'condition resulting from a poison in a (specified) region of the body': *neurotoxia, thyrotoxia, urotoxia.*

toxic /tok′sik/ [Gk, *toxikon*], **1.** of or pertaining to a poison. **2.** (of a disease or condition) severe and progressive.

-toxic, -toxical, a combining form meaning 'pertaining to poison': *cardiotoxic, hematoxic, spermatoxic.*

toxic albuminuria [Gk, *toxikon,* poison; L, *albus,* white; Gk, *ouron,* urine], a condition of serum albumin in the urine caused by the presence of toxic substances in the body.

toxic allergic syndrome. See **Löffler syndrome, P.I.E.**

toxic amblyopia, partial loss of vision because of retrooptic bulbar neuritis, caused by poisoning with quinine, lead, wood alcohol, nicotine, arsenic, or certain other poisons.

toxic delirium [Gk, *toxikon,* poison; L, *delirare,* to rave], a symptom of disordered mental status as a result of poisoning.

toxic dementia, dementia resulting from excessive use of or exposure to a poisonous substance. See also **dementia.**

toxic dilatation of colon [Gk, *toxikon,* poison; L, *dilatare,* to widen; Gk, *kolon*], a condition of transverse colon dilatation as a complication of amebic colitis, ulcerative colitis, or other bowel disease. Symptoms may include cramping, fever, rapid heart beat, and mental confusion.

toxic dose (TD), (in toxicology) the amount of a substance that may be expected to produce a toxic effect. See also **median toxic dose.**

toxic encephalitis [Gk, *toxikon,* poison + *enkephalos,* brain + *itis,* inflammation], encephalitis caused by heavy metal poisoning. It is characterized by convulsions and cerebral edema.

toxic epidermal necrolysis (TEN), a rare skin disease, characterized by epidermal erythema, superficial necrosis, and skin erosions. This condition, which affects mainly adults, makes the skin appear scalded, often leaving scars. The cause of TEN is unknown, but it may result from toxic or hypersensitive reactions. It is commonly associated with drug reactions, such as those associated with butazones, sulfonamides, penicillins, barbiturates, and hydantoins. Other drugs may be involved, and the disease also has been associated with airborne toxins, such as carbon monoxide. TEN also may indicate an immune response, or it may be associated with severe physiologic stress. A similar skin disorder may be the result of a staphylococcal infection.

■ OBSERVATIONS: Early signs of the condition include inflammation of the mucous membranes, fever, malaise, a burning sensation in the conjunctivae, and pervasive tenderness of the skin. The first phase of TEN is manifested by diffuse erythema. The second phase involves vesiculation and blistering. The third phase is marked by extensive epidermal necrolysis and desquamation. As the disease progresses, large flaccid bullae develop and rupture, exposing wide expanses of denuded skin. Tissue fluids and electrolytes are consequently lost, resulting in extensive systemic complications, such as pulmonary edema, bronchopneumonia, GI and esophageal hemorrhage, sepsis, shock, renal failure, and disseminated intravascular coagulation. These extreme conditions contribute to the high mortality associated with TEN, which is about 30%, especially among the infirm and the elderly. Confirming diagnosis is based on symptoms in the third phase of the disease, such as skin denuded by even slight friction, affecting the areas of erythema. Diagnosis is commonly supported by bacteriologic culture and Gram's stains of lesions to determine whether infection exists. The presence of leukocytosis, fluid and electrolyte imbalances, albuminuria, and elevated transaminase levels are characteristic and help confirm the diagnosis. Erythema multiforme and exfoliative dermatitis may be ruled out by exfoliative biopsy and cytology.

■ INTERVENTIONS: Treatment of TEN commonly involves the administration of IV fluids to replace body fluids and maintain electrolyte balance. Frequent laboratory analyses are necessary to monitor hematocrit and hemoglobin, serum proteins, electrolytes, and blood gases.

■ NURSING CONSIDERATIONS: Nursing care of patients with TEN requires meticulous monitoring of vital signs, central venous pressure, and urinary output. Any signs of renal failure, such as decreased urinary output, and of bleeding are of immediate concern. It is important to detect and quickly treat any septic infection. Temperature elevations are reported immediately, and all laboratory work, such as blood cultures and sensitivity tests, are performed promptly. Ocular lesions are common with TEN, and frequent eye care is often needed to remove exudate. Protective isolation and prophylactic antibiotic therapy may be required to prevent secondary infection. Nurses also make sure that the TEN patient does not wear tight clothing and is covered loosely to minimize the friction that causes skin sloughing. A Stryker frame or a CircOlectric bed may be helpful in caring for the patient. Analgesics are administered as needed, and cool sterile compresses may be applied to relieve discomfort. Psychologic and emotional support for the patient and the family is also a key nursing concern.

toxic erythema [Gk, *toxikon* poison + *erythema* redness], an inexact term sometimes applied to reddish skin eruptions of undetermined origin.

toxic erythema of the newborn. See **erythema neonatorum.**

toxic gastritis. See **corrosive gastritis.**

toxic goiter, an enlargement of the thyroid gland associated with exophthalmia and systemic disease. See also **Graves' disease.**

toxic hemoglobinuria. See **hemoglobinuria.**

toxicity /toksis'itē/ [Gk, *toxikon*], **1.** the degree to which something is poisonous. **2.** a condition that results from ex-

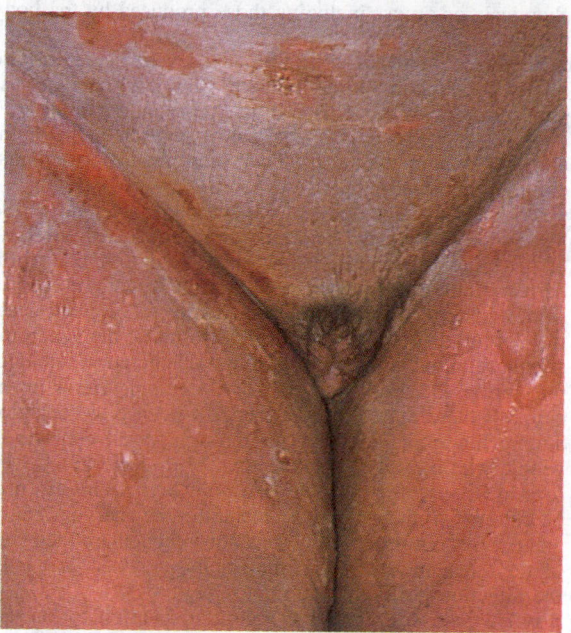

Toxic epidermal necrolysis (McKee, 1993)

posure to a toxin or to toxic amounts of a substance that does not cause adverse effects in smaller amounts.

toxic neuritis [Gk, *toxikon*, poison + *neuron*, nerve + *itis*, inflammation], a painful nerve inflammation caused by a metallic, bacterial, or other poison.

toxic nodular goiter, an enlarged thyroid gland characterized by numerous discrete nodules and hypersecretion of thyroid hormones, occurring most frequently in elderly individuals. Typical signs of thyrotoxicosis, such as nervousness, tremor, weakness, fatigue, weight loss, and irritability, are usually present, but exophthalmia is rare; anorexia is more common than hyperphagia, and cardiac dysrhythmia or congestive heart failure may be a predominant manifestation. When clinical findings suggest thyrotoxicosis, a therapeutic trial of antithyroid drugs, such as propylthiouracil or methimazole, is indicated, but after the diagnosis is established, radioactive iodine is considered the treatment of choice, and large doses are usually required.

toxico-. See **tox-.**

toxicokinetics /tok'sikō'kinet'iks/, the passage through the body system of a toxic agent or its metabolites, usually in an action similar to that of pharmacokinetics.

toxicologist /tok'sikol'əjist/, a specialist in toxicology.

toxicology /-ol'əjē/, the scientific study of poisons, their detection, their effects, and methods of treatment for conditions they produce. –**toxicologic, toxicological,** *adj.*

toxic or drug-induced hepatitis, hepatitis resulting from a chemical, parasitic, or metabolic poison.

toxicosis /tok'sikō'sis/ [Gk, *toxikon*, poison + *osis*, condition], a disease condition caused by the absorption of metabolic or bacterial poisons.

toxic substance [Gk, *toxikon*, poison; L, *substantia*, essence], any poison.

toxic psychosis, psychosis that results from the effects of chemicals or drugs, including those produced by the body itself.

toxic shock syndrome (TSS), a severe acute disease caused by infection with strains of *Staphylococcus aureus,* phage group I, that produces a unique toxin, enterotoxin F. It is most common in menstruating women using high-absorbency tampons but has been seen in newborn infants, children, and men.

■ OBSERVATIONS: The onset of the syndrome is characterized by sudden high fever, headache, sore throat with swelling of the mucous membranes, diarrhea, nausea, and erythroderma. Acute renal failure, abnormal liver function, confusion, and refractory hypotension usually follow, and death may occur. It is probable that mild forms of the syndrome are not reported and therefore are not diagnosed. There does not appear to be any seasonal or geographic factor in the cause of the disease, and there is no evidence of contagion among household members or through sexual contacts of people who have TSS. Bacteremia, or discernible local infection, is absent in most cases. *Staphylococcus aureus* may be cultured from many sites, including the pharynx, nares, and cervix, but the drastic effects of infection are the result of the toxin released from the organism rather than from the infection itself.

■ INTERVENTIONS: Aggressive volume expansion by the administration of large amounts of intravenous fluid, assisted ventilation, and administration of vasopressors may be necessary in treating severe TSS. Early recognition and active supportive treatment greatly improve the survival rates and decrease both prolonged morbidity and recurrence.

■ NURSING CONSIDERATIONS: The use of highly absorbent tampons is associated with a greater incidence of the disease than the use of regular tampons, but a few cases have occurred in women who have never used tampons. The nurse counsels women to avoid the high-absorbency tampons and to report any illness occurring during the menses that is accompanied by nausea, diarrhea, and fever. Recurrence is likely; a mild undiagnosed episode during a preceding menstrual period is often reported when severe TSS is diagnosed. Women who have had TSS are usually advised to avoid using any kind of tampons for at least several months.

toxin /tok′sin/, a poison, usually one produced by or occurring in a plant or microorganism. See also **endotoxin, exotoxin.**

-toxin, a combining form meaning 'poison': *cynotoxin, hypnotoxin, zootoxin.*

toxin-antitoxin [Gk, *toxikon,* poison; *anti,* against; *toxikon*], a mixture of toxin and antitoxin. Diphtheria toxin-antitoxin was formerly used for active immunization.

toxo-. See **tox-.**

toxocariasis /tok′sōkərī′əsis/ [Gk, *toxo,* bow, *kara,* head, *osis,* condition], infection with the larvae of *Toxocara canis,* the common roundworm of dogs and cats. Ingestion of viable eggs, commonly found in soil, leads to the spread of tiny larvae throughout the body, resulting in respiratory symptoms, enlarged liver, skin rashes, eosinophilia, and delayed ocular lesions. Children who eat dirt are particularly subject to this disease. Specific drug therapy is not very useful; the outcome is usually good without therapy. Regular worming of pets helps prevent infection. Also called **visceral larva migrans.**

toxoid /tok′soid/ [Gk, *toxikon,* poison, *eidos,* form], a toxin that has been treated with chemicals or with heat to decrease its toxic effect but that retains its antigenic power.

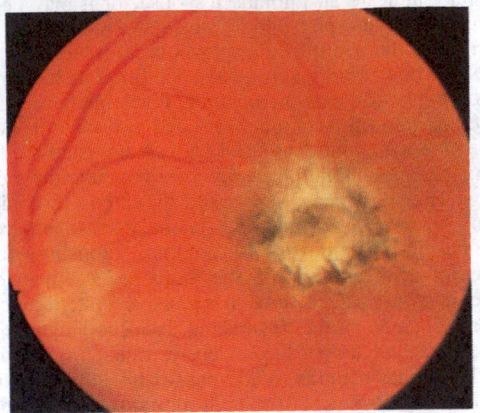

Toxocariasis: histology of an infected eye
(Zitelli, 1992)

It is given to produce immunity by stimulating the creation of antibodies. See also **toxin, vaccine.**

Toxoplasma /tok′sōplaz′mə/ [Gk, *toxikon* + *plasma,* something formed], a genus of protozoa with only one known species, *Toxoplasma gondii,* an intracellular parasite of cats and other hosts that causes toxoplasmosis in humans.

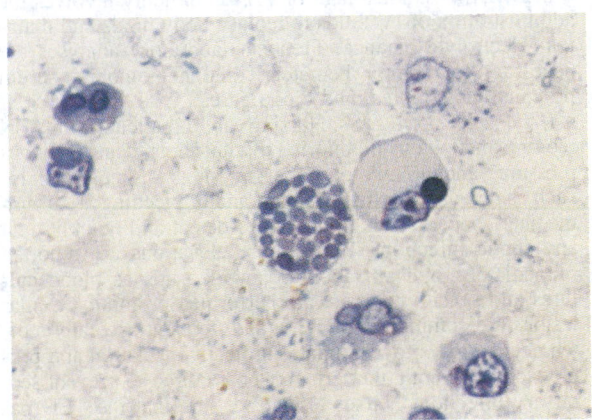

Toxoplasma: *Toxoplasma gondii* cysts in brain section
(Tilton, 1992)

toxoplasmosis /tok′sōplazmō′sis/ [Gk, *toxikon, plasma* + *osis,* condition], a common infection with the protozoan intracellular parasite *Toxoplasma gondii,* characterized in the congenital form by liver and brain involvement with cerebral calcification, convulsions, blindness, microcephaly or hydrocephaly, and mental retardation. The acquired form is characterized by rash, lymphadenopathy, fever, malaise, central nervous system disorders, myocarditis, and pneumonitis.

■ OBSERVATIONS: Cats acquire the organism by eating infected birds and mice. Cysts of the organism are transmitted from cat feces to humans or by human ingestion of inadequately cooked meat containing the cysts. Transplacental transmission occurs only during acute infection of the mother, but the disease is very serious in the fetus and in those with AIDS or other immunosuppressive conditions or impaired immune system. Diagnosis is made by demonstrating rising antibody titers or by immunofluorescent antibody tests. Infection confers immunity.

■ INTERVENTIONS: Combinations of sulfonamides with pyrimethamine are recommended as treatment, possibly reducing the severity of the illness in the fetus.

■ NURSING CONSIDERATIONS: All meat should be heated to at least 140° F (60° C) throughout to kill this parasite. Pregnant women who are not immune are advised not to handle cats, cat feces, or litter boxes.

TPA, abbreviation for **tissue plasminogen activator.**

TPAL. See **parity.**

TPN, abbreviation for **total parenteral nutrition.**

TPR, abbreviation for *temperature, pulse, respiration.*

trabecula carnea /trəbek′yələ/, *pl.* **trabeculae carneae** [L, little beam; *carneus* flesh], any one of the irregular bands and bundles of muscle projecting from the inner surfaces of the ventricles, except in the arterial cone of the right ventricle. Some of these trabeculae are ridges of muscle along the ventricular walls; others are short projections into the ventricular cavities; still others form the ventricular papillary muscles. Compare **chordae tendineae.** See also **heart, left ventricle, right ventricle.**

trabeculae, (in ophthalmology) the portion of the eye in front of the canal of Schlemm and within the angle created by the iris and the cornea.

trabecula septomarginalis. See **moderator band.**

trabeculectomy /trəbek′yələk′təmē/ [L, *trabecula* + Gk, *ektome*, excision], the surgical removal of a section of corneoscleral tissue to increase the outflow of aqueous humor in patients with severe glaucoma. The procedure usually involves removal of the canal of Schlemm and the trabecular meshwork.

trabeculoplasty trabek′yələplśtē, a plastic surgery procedure used in the treatment of glaucoma. An argon laser beam is used to blanch the trabecular network of the eye, thereby permitting drainage of the excess fluid causing increased pressure within the eyeball.

trabeculotomy /-ot′əmē/, a surgical opening in an orbital trabecula to increase the outflow of aqueous humor.

trace element [L, *trahere*, to draw; *elementum* first principle], an element essential to nutrition or physiologic processes, found in such minute quantities that analysis yields a presence of virtually zero amounts.

trace gas, a gas or vapor that escapes into the atmosphere during an anesthetic procedure. Because these substances may have adverse effects on the health of personnel exposed to them, scavenging equipment is often installed in operating rooms to clean the air. See also **gas scavenging system.**

tracer [L, *trahere*, to draw], **1.** see also **radioisotope scan.** a radioactive isotope that is used in diagnostic x-ray techniques to allow a biologic process to be seen. The tracer, which is introduced into the body, binds with a specific substance and is followed with a scanner or fluoroscope as it passes through various organs or systems in the body. Kinds of tracers include **radioactive iodine (131^I)** and **radioactive carbon (^{14}C). 2.** a mechanical device that graphically records the outline or movements of an object or part of the body. **3.** a dissecting instrument that is used to isolate vessels and nerves. **–trace,** *v.*

tracer depot method, (in nuclear medicine) a technique used to determine local skin or muscle blood flow, based on the rate at which a radioactive tracer deposited in a tissue is removed by diffusion into the capillaries and washed out by the local blood supply. If blood flow is diminished or absent, as in dead skin, the deposited tracer does not wash out.

trachea /trā′kē·ə/ [Gk, *tracheia*, rough artery], a nearly cylindric tube in the neck, composed of cartilage and membrane, that extends from the larynx at the level of the sixth cervical vertebra to the fifth thoracic vertebra, where it divides into two bronchi. The trachea conveys air to the lungs; it is about 11 cm long and 2 cm wide. The ventral surface of the tube is covered in the neck by the isthmus of the thyroid gland and various other structures, such as the sternothyroideus and the sternohyoideus. Dorsally, the trachea is in contact with the esophagus. Also called **windpipe.** See also **primary bronchus. –tracheal,** *adj.*

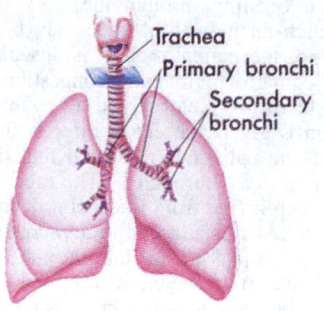

Trachea (Thibodeau, 1993/Lisa Shoemaker, Joan M Beck)

tracheal /trā′kē·əl/ [Gk, *tracheia*, rough artery], pertaining to the trachea.

tracheal breath sound, a normal breath sound heard in auscultation of the trachea. Inspiration and expiration are equally loud, the expiratory sound being heard during the greater part of expiration, whereas the inspiratory sound stops abruptly at the height of inspiration, with a pause before the sound of expiration is heard. Compare **vesicular breath sound.**

tracheal tugging [Gk, *tracheia*, rough artery; ME, *toggen*], an effect of an aortic aneurysm in which the trachea is tugged downward with each heart contraction.

tracheitis /trā′kē·ī′tis/, any inflammatory condition of the trachea. It may be acute or chronic, resulting from infection, allergy, or physical irritation. Also called **trachitis.**

trachelagra. See **agoraphobia.**

trachelo-, a combining form meaning 'pertaining to the neck or a necklike structure': *trachelobregmatic, trachelocystitis, tracheloschisis.*

trachelodynia. See **cervicodynia.**

tracheo- /trā′kē·ō-/, a combining form meaning 'pertaining to the trachea': *tracheobronchial, tracheomalacia, tracheorrhaphy.*

tracheobronchial tree (TBT) /-brong′kē·əl/ [Gk, *tracheia, + bronchos*, windpipe], an anatomic complex that includes the trachea, the bronchi, and the bronchial tubes. It conveys air to and from the lungs and is a primary structure in respiration. See also **bronchial tree.**

tracheobronchitis /trā′kē·ōbrongkī′tis/, inflammation of the trachea and bronchi, a common form of pulmonary infection.

tracheobronchomegaly /-brong'kōmeg'əlē/, an abnormally large upper airway, in which the trachea may be as wide as the spinal column.

tracheoesophageal fistula /trā'kē·ō·ē·ē'səfā'jē·əl/, [Gk, *tracheia + oisophagos*, gullet], a congenital malformation in which there is an abnormal tubelike passage between the trachea and the esophagus.

tracheoesophageal shunt, a surgical procedure enabling a laryngectomee to speak by constructing a passageway between the trachea and the esophagus. The operation results in an ability to produce esophageal speech with normal respiration as a source of air and without the need to belch to produce voice sounds.

tracheomalacia /trā'kē·ōmələ'shə/, an eroding of the trachea, usually caused by excessive pressure from a cuffed endotracheal tube.

tracheostomy /trā'kē·os'təmē/ [Gk, *tracheia + stoma,* mouth], an opening through the neck into the trachea through which an indwelling tube may be inserted. After tracheostomy, the patient's chest is auscultated for breath sounds indicative of pulmonary congestion, mucous membranes and fingertips are observed for cyanosis, and humidified oxygen is given via tent or directly into the tracheostomy tube. The patient is reassured that the tube is open and that air can pass through it. The tube is suctioned frequently to keep it free from tracheobronchial secretions using a suction catheter attached to a Y-connector. The catheter is inserted 6 to 8 inches into the tube. The catheter is rotated, and intermittent suction is applied for no longer than 5 seconds. The patient is taught to cough to move secretions up and out of the bronchi. The nurse holds the tube stable during intense coughing to prevent its displacement. Should the outer tube be expelled, the nurse uses a dilator or hemostat to hold the trachea open until another tube can be inserted. A fluid intake of 3000 ml per day is recommended. The dressing is changed as necessary, the area is kept dry and clean, and frequent oral care is given. Pen and paper or a magic slate is kept available for communication because the patient cannot speak. Complications of tracheostomy include pneumothorax, respiratory insufficiency, obstruction of the tracheostomy tube or its displacement from the lumen of the trachea, pulmonary infection, atelectasis, tracheoesophageal fistula, hemorrhage, and mediastinal emphysema. If the procedure was done as an emergency, the tracheostomy is closed after normal breathing is restored. If the tracheostomy is permanent, such as with a laryngectomy, the patient is taught self-care. Compare **tracheotomy.**

tracheostomy care [Gk, *tracheia,* rough artery + *stoma,* mouth], care of the tracheostomy patient, consisting of maintenance of a patent airway, adequate humidification, aseptic wound care, and sterile tracheal aspiration. Complications can include injury to the vocal cords, gastric distention and regurgitation, occlusion of the endotrachial tube, and an increased risk of infection.

tracheotomy /trā'kē·ot'əmē/ [Gk, *tracheia + temnein,* to cut], an incision made into the trachea through the neck below the larynx, performed to gain access to the airway below a blockage with a foreign body, tumor, or edema of the glottis. The opening may be made as an emergency measure at an accident site, at a hospitalized patient's bedside, or in the operating room. Local or general anesthesia may be used, if available. The patient's neck is hyperextended,

and an incision is made through the skin through the second, third, or fourth tracheal ring. A small hole is made in the fibrous tissue of the trachea, and the opening is then dilated to allow the intake of air. In an emergency any available instrument may be used as a dilator, even the barrel of a ballpoint pen with the inner portion removed. If the blockage persists, a tracheostomy tube is inserted; if not, the incision is closed after normal respirations are established. After surgery the patient is observed for recurrent respiratory difficulty or cyanosis. Compare **tracheostomy.**

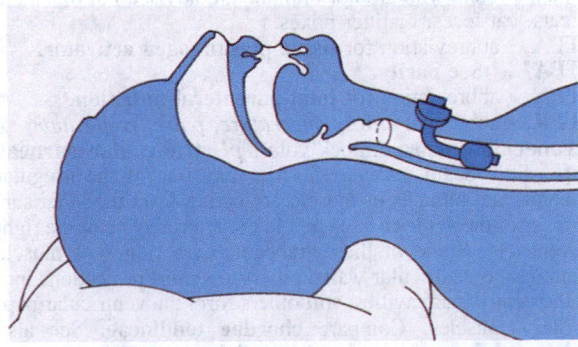

Tracheostomy *(Wilson, 1990)*

tracheotomy tube [Gk, *tracheia,* rough artery + *temnein,* to cut; L, *tubus*], a curved hollow tube of rubber, metal, or plastic, surgically inserted in the trachea to relieve a breathing obstruction.

trachitis, See **tracheitis**.

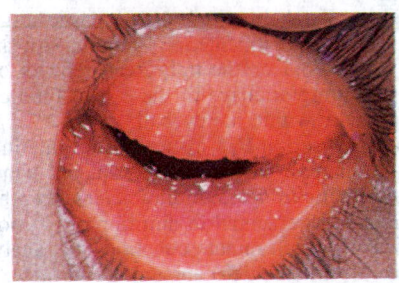

Trachoma *(Forbes, 1993)*

trachoma /trəkō'mə/ [Gk, roughness], a chronic infectious disease of the eye caused by the bacterium *Chlamydia trachomatis,* characterized initially by inflammation, pain, photophobia, and lacrimation. If untreated, follicles form on the upper eyelids and grow larger until the granulations invade the cornea, eventually causing blindness. Tetracycline, erythromycin, and topical sulfonamides usually provide effective treatment. Scarred eyelids may be surgically repaired. Trachoma is a significant cause of blindness and is endemic to hot, dry, poverty-ridden areas. In the United States, it is found in the Southwest. Teaching an affected population about the spread of trachoma and having an adequate water supply for washing hands, towels, and handkerchiefs are important factors in eliminating the disease.

Also called **Egyptian ophthalmia, granular conjunctivitis.**

tracing [L, *trahere*, to draw], a graphic record of a physical event, such as an electrocardiograph tracing made by pens on a moving sheet of paper while recording the electric impulses of heart muscle contractions.

tract [L, *tractus*, trail], **1.** an elongate group of tissues and structures that function together as a pathway, such as the digestive tract or the respiratory tract. **2.** (in neurology) the neuronal axons that are grouped together to form a pathway.

traction /trak′shən/ [L, *trahere*, to draw], **1.** (in orthopedics) the process of putting a limb, bone, or group of muscles under tension by means of weights and pulleys to align or to immobilize the part or to relieve pressure on it. See also **orthopedic traction. 2.** the process of pulling a part of the body along, through, or out of its socket or cavity, such as axis traction with obstetric forceps in delivering an infant. Kinds of traction include **Bryant's traction, Buck's traction, Russell traction, skeletal traction, skin traction,** and **split Russell traction.**

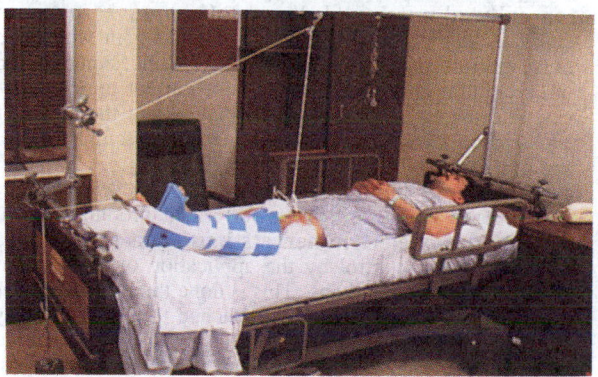

Traction (Thompson, 1989)

traction frame, an orthopedic apparatus that supports the pulleys, the ropes, and the weights by which traction is applied to various parts of the body or by which various parts of the body are suspended. Traction frames are used in the treatment of bone fractures and dislocations, and disease processes of the musculoskeletal system; in the correction of various orthopedic deformities; and in the general immobilization of specific areas of the body. The main components of a traction frame are metal uprights that attach to the bed and support an overhead metal bar. In addition to traction equipment, traction frames are often rigged with trapeze bars that the patient can grasp to help in changing positions and to exercise the muscles of the arms and the trunk. The components of a traction frame are securely clamped together when in use but can be easily disassembled and reassembled. Compare **IV-type traction frame, claw-type traction frame, Balkan traction frame.**

traction, 90-90 an orthopedic mechanism, used especially in pediatrics, that combines skeletal traction and suspension with a short-leg cast or a splint to immobilize and position the lower extremity in the treatment of a displaced fractured femur. This type of traction is usually unilateral with the opposite leg in Buck's traction or in split Russell traction

for immobilization. The pin used in this kind of skeletal traction is inserted into bone in the knee area and attached to a riser running through a pulley on an overhead traction frame to a pulley and weight system fitted over the foot of the bed. The pulley and weight system at the foot of the bed also accommodates additional attachments to the short-leg cast or splint of the involved lower limb. Application of 90-90 traction also may incorporate a jacket restraint to help immobilize the patient. A variation of this type of traction is often used with adults in the treatment of low back pain.

traction response, the response to traction applied to the spine. Alterations of certain signs and symptoms of a musculoskeletal disorder may be revealed by traction tests. For example, if traction relieves a symptom, it may indicate impingement of a nerve root. Traction also may be used therapeutically to increase joint range, overcome muscle spasms, shorten soft tissues, or neutralize pressure and relieve pain in various joints.

trademark, a word, symbol, or device assigned to a product by its manufacturer, registered or not registered, as a part of its identity. See also **generic name.**

tragal /trā′gəl/ [Gk, *tragos*, goat], pertaining to the tragus.

tragophony. See **egophony.**

tragus /trā′gəs/, *pl.* **tragi** /trā′jī/ [Gk, *tragos*, goat], a small extension of the auricular cartilage of the ear, anterior to the external meatus.

trainable /trā′nəbəl/ [L, *trahere*, to draw], pertaining to a mentally retarded person who is capable of some degree of self-care and social adjustment in a supervised setting but would not benefit from formal education.

trained reflex. See **conditioned response.**

traineeship /trānē′ship/ [L, *trahere*, to draw; AS, *scieppan*, to shape], a grant of money allocated to an individual for advanced study in a given field. In nursing, many graduate students have been awarded federal traineeships that provide funds for tuition and living expenses.

training effect, a rehabilitation influence effect for heart patients that can be measured by changes in cardiac function.

training grant, a grant of money or other resources to provide training in a particular field. Many schools of nursing receive federal or state grants to provide specific educational programs. Funds may be allocated for faculty salaries, student aid, or other expenses.

trait [Fr, trace], **1.** a characteristic mode of behavior or any mannerism or physical feature that distinguishes one individual or culture from another. **2.** any characteristic quality or condition that is genetically determined and inherited as a specific genotype. A trait is expressed in the phenotype as dominant or recessive for the particular characteristic; it is inherited in the genotype as homozygous dominant, homozygous recessive, or heterozygous in the ratio of 1:2:1. In medicine, the term *trait* is used specifically to denote the heterozygous state of a recessive disorder, such as the sickle cell trait. See also **dominance, gene, Mendel's laws, recessive.**

Tral, a trademark for an anticholinergic (hexocyclium methylsulfate).

trance [L, *transire*, to be pass], **1.** a sleeplike state characterized by the complete or partial suspension of consciousness and loss or diminution of motor activity, as seen in hypnosis, the dissociative form of hysteria, and various cataleptic and ecstatic states. **2.** a dazed or bewildered condition; stupor. **3.** a state of detachment from one's immediate surroundings, such as in deep concentration or day-dreaming. Kinds of trances are **alcoholic trance, death trance, hypnotic trance,** and **induced trance.**

Trancopal, a trademark for an antianxiety agent (chlormezanone).

Trandate, a trademark for an antihypertensive drug (labetalol hydrochloride).

tranquilizer /trang′kwilĭ′zər/ [L, *tranquillus,* calm], a drug prescribed to calm anxious or agitated people, ideally without decreasing their consciousness. Major tranquilizers, such as derivatives of phenothiazine, butyrophenone, and thioxanthene, are generally used in the treatment of psychoses. Minor tranquilizers usually prescribed for the treatment of anxiety, irritability, tension, or psychoneurosis include chlordiazepoxide, diazepam, and hydroxyzine. Tranquilizers tend to induce drowsiness and have the potential for causing physical and psychologic dependence. See also **antipsychotic.**

trans- /trans-,tranz-/, a prefix meaning 'across, through, over': *transabdominal, transferase, transplacental.*

transabdominal /-abdom′inəl/ [L, *trans,* across + *abdomen,* belly], pertaining to a procedure through the abdominal wall.

transactional analysis (TA) /-ak′shənəl/ [L, *transigere,* to drive through; Gk, *analyein,* to loosen], a form of psychotherapy developed by Eric Berne, based on a theory that three different, coherent, organized egos exist throughout life simultaneously in every person, representing the child, the adult, and the parent. Interactions between people are transactions, originating from a person in one of the ego states, and received by another person who may be in a complementary or a crossed ego state. Transactions are motivated by a need for recognition and contact called 'strokes.' Transactions occur in six kinds of 'time structure': withdrawal, rituals, pastimes, games, activities, and intimacy. The way in which a person structures time reflects internal conflicts and patterns adopted to cope with those conflicts. The goal of transactional analysis is to enable clients to communicate from the ego state appropriate to the situation and the responses of the individuals, thereby decreasing conflict.

transaminase /transam′inās/ [L, *trans,* across, *amine,* ammonia; Fr, *diastase,* enzyme], an enzyme that catalyzes the transfer of an amino group from an alpha-amino acid to an alpha-keto acid, with pyridoxal phosphate and pyridoxamine phosphate acting as coenzymes. Glutamic-oxaloacetic transaminase (GOT), normally present in serum and various tissues, especially in the heart and liver, is released by damaged cells, and, as a result, a high serum level of GOT may be diagnostic in myocardial infarction or hepatic disease. Glutamic-pyruvic transaminase (GPT), a normal constituent of serum and various tissues, especially in the liver, is released by injured tissue and may be present in high concentrations in the sera of patients with acute liver disease. Also called **aminotransferase.**

transaortic /-ā·ôr′tik/ [L, *trans,* across; Gk, *aerein,* to raise], pertaining to a procedure through the aorta.

transcellular water /-sel′yələr/ [L, *trans* + *cella,* storeroom], the portion of extracellular water that is enclosed by an epithelial membrane and whose volume and composition are determined by the cellular activity of that membrane.

transcendence /transen′dəns/ [L, *trans* + *scandere,* to climb], the rising above one's previously perceived limits or restrictions.

transcervical fracture /transur′vikəl/ [L, *trans,* across +

cervix, neck + *fractura*], a fracture through the neck of the femur.

transcondylar fracture /transkon′dilər/ [L, *trans* + Gk, *kondylos* condyle], a fracture that occurs transversally and distal to the epicondyles of any one of the long bones.

transconfiguration /-kənfig′yərā′shən/ [L, *trans* + *configurare,* to form from], **1.** (in genetics) the presence of the dominant allele of one pair of genes and the recessive allele of another pair on the same chromosome. **2.** the presence of at least one mutant gene and one wild-type gene of a pair of pseudoalleles on each chromosome of a homologous pair. Also called **transarrangement, transposition.** Compare **cis configuration.**

transcortical apraxia. See **ideomotor apraxia.**

transcortin /-kôr′tin/, a diglobulin protein that binds a majority of cortisol in the plasma. Also called **corticosteroid-binding globulin.**

transcriptase /transkrip′tās/, an enzyme that induces transcription.

transcription /transkrip′shən/ [L, *trans* + *scribere,* to write], (in molecular genetics) the process by which RNA is formed from a DNA template in the process of manufacturing a protein. See also **anticodon, genetic code.**

transcultural nursing /-kul′chərəl/ [L, *trans* + *colere,* to cultivate; *nutrix,* nurse], a field of nursing in which the nurse transcends ethnocentricity and practices nursing in other cultural environments. Because current nursing process and theory are not culturally bound and the needs of each person are considered individually, transcultural nursing is a part of all nursing practice.

transcutaneous /-k(y)o͞otā′nē·əs/ [L, *trans* + *cutis,* skin], pertaining to a procedure that is performed through the skin.

transcutaneous electric nerve stimulation (TENS), a method of pain control by the application of electric impulses to the nerve endings. This is done through electrodes that are placed on the skin and attached to a stimulator by flexible wires. The electric impulses generated are similar to those of the body, but different enough to block transmission of pain signals to the brain. TENS is noninvasive and nonaddictive, with no known side effects. It is contraindicated in patients with a demand-type cardiac pacemaker.

transcutaneous nerve stimulation. See **transcutaneous electric nerve stimulation.**

transcutaneous oxygen/carbon dioxide monitoring, a method of measuring the oxygen or carbon dioxide in the blood by attaching electrodes to the skin. Oxygen is commonly measured through an oximeter, which contains heating coils to raise the skin temperature and increase blood flow at the surface. Oxygen content is calculated in terms of light absorption at various wavelengths. Transcutaneous carbon dioxide electrodes are similar to blood gas electrodes, with a Teflon membrane tip that is permeable to gases.

transdermal delivery system /-dur′məl/ [L, *trans* + Gk, *derma,* skin], a method of applying a drug to unbroken skin. The drug is absorbed continuously through the skin and enters the systemic system. It is used particularly for the administration of nitroglycerin and scopolamine.

transducer /-d(y)o͞o′sər/ [L, *trans* + *ducere* to lead], (in ultrasound) a hand-held device that sends and receives a soundwave signal. It changes electrical impulses into soundwaves, receives the reflected soundwave, and converts it back into electrical energy.

transduction /-duk′shən/, (in molecular genetics) a method of genetic recombination by which DNA is trans-

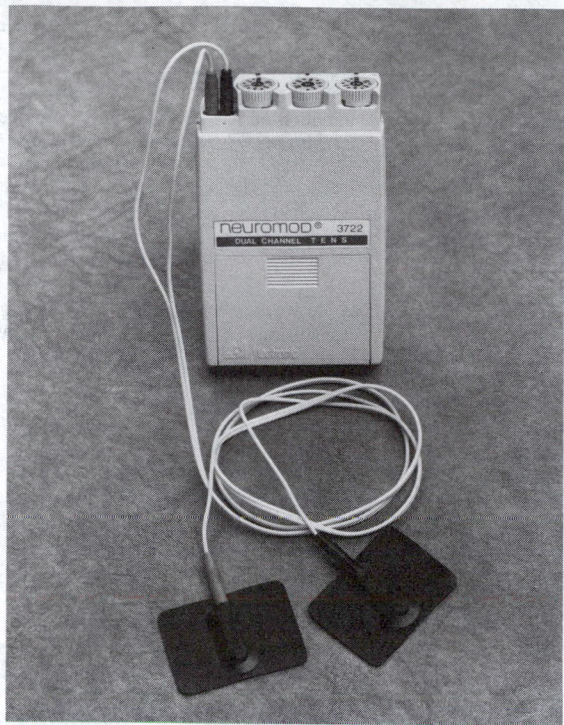

TENS

ferred from one cell to another by a viral vector. Various bacteriophages transduce genetic material from one species of bacteria to another.

transect /transekt′/ [L, *trans* + *secare*, to cut], to sever or cut across, as in preparing a cross section of tissue.

transection. See **transsection.**

transfection /-fek′shən/ [L, *trans* + *inficere*, to taint], (in molecular genetics) the process by which a bacterial cell is infected with purified DNA or RNA isolated from a virus or a viral vector, following a specific pretreatment. Acute transfection is short-term infection.

transfer agreement /trans′fur/ [L, *transferre*, to carry over; *ad*, toward, *gratus*, pleasure], a written hospital agreement between two health care institutions for the transfer of patients from one to another and for the orderly exchange of pertinent clinical information on the patients transferred.

transferase /trans′fərās/ [L, *transferre* + Fr, *diastase*, enzyme], any of a group of enzymes that catalyzes the transfer of a chemical group or radical, such as the phosphate, methyl, amine, or keto groups, from one molecule to another.

transfer DNA (tDNA), (in molecular genetics) DNA transferred from its original source and present in transformed cells.

transference /fur′əns/ [L, *transferre*], **1.** the shifting of symptoms from one part of the body to another, as occurs in conversion disorder. **2.** (in psychiatry) an unconscious defense mechanism whereby feelings and attitudes originally associated with important people and events in one's early life are attributed to others in current interpersonal situations. **3.** (in psychoanalysis and psychotherapy) the feelings of a patient for the analyst to whom the patient has

attributed or assigned the qualities, attitudes, and feelings of a person or people significant in his or her emotional development, usually a figure from childhood. The phenomenon is used as a tool in understanding the emotional problems of the patient and their origins. See also **countertransference, parataxic distortion.**

transfer factor, a leukocyte extract that transfers delayed hypersensitivity from one person to another. Transfer factor has been studied for its possible use in the treatment of chronic mucocutaneous candidiasis and Wiskott-Aldrich syndrome and as a means of transferring antitumor immunity to patients with various types of cancer.

transfer factor of lungs. See **diffusing capacity.**

transferrin /transfer′in/, a trace protein present in the blood that is essential in the transport of iron from the intestine into the bloodstream, making it available to the normoblasts in the bone marrow. It also may take part in a slower exchange with ferritin, hemosiderin, and other iron forms in the tissues. See also **hemosiderin, iron transport.**

transferring /-fur′ing/ [L, *trans*, across + *ferre*, to bring], relocating a person in need from one location to another.

transfer RNA (tRNA), (in molecular genetics) a kind of RNA that transfers the genetic code from messenger RNA for the production of a specific amino acid. There are at least 20 different kinds of tRNA, each of which is able to combine covalently with a specific amino acid and to bond with at least one messenger RNA nucleotide triplet. Also called **adaptor RNA.**

transformation /-fôrmā′shən/ [L, *transformare*, to change shape], (in molecular genetics) the process in which exogenous genes are integrated into chromosomes in a form that is recognized by the replicative and transcriptional apparatus of the host cell. Transformation occurs rarely in most cell populations.

transformer /-fôr′mər/ [L, *transformare*, to change shape], an electrical apparatus that changes alternating current of one voltage into a different voltage of the same frequency.

transforming growth factor (TGF), a group of proteins produced by the cells of a tumor that, when inoculated into a normal cell culture, causes a disorderly increase in the number of cells in the culture.

transfusion /-f(y)o͞o′zhən/ [L, *trans* + *fundere*, to pour], the introduction into the bloodstream of whole blood or blood components, such as plasma, platelets, or packed red cells. Whole blood may be infused into the recipient directly from a donor matched for the ABO blood group and antigenic subgroups, but more frequently the donor's blood is collected and stored by a blood bank. See also **blood transfusion.**

transfusion reaction, a systemic response by the body to the administration of blood incompatible with that of the recipient. The causes include red cell incompatibility, and allergic sensitivity to the leukocytes, platelets, plasma protein components of the transfused blood, or potassium or citrate preservatives in the banked blood. See also **hemolysis.**

■ OBSERVATIONS: Fever is the most common transfusion reaction; urticaria is a relatively common allergic response. Asthma, vascular collapse, and renal failure occur less commonly. A hemolytic reaction from red cell incompatibility is serious and must be diagnosed and treated promptly. Symptoms develop shortly after beginning the transfusion, before 50 ml have been given, and include a throbbing headache, sudden, deep, and severe lumbar pain, precordial pain, dyspnea, and restlessness. Objective signs include

Immunologic reactions to blood transfusions

Reaction	Cause	Mechanism	Symptoms	Occurrence	Action
Acute hemolytic	Recipient antibody incompatible with transfused red cells	RBCs agglutinate, rapid hemolysis Capillary plugging (type II hypersensitivity)	Lumbar pain Constriction of chest Pain in vein Fever, chills Hemoglobinuria Signs of shock	Shortly after initiation of transfusion	Stop transfusion Continue IV saline Blood unit and blood sample from patient sent to lab for immediate testing Treat for shock and renal failure
Delayed hemolytic	Anamnestic immune response	Slow hemolysis	Jaundice Anemia	Days to weeks after transfusion	Monitor adequacy of urinary output and degree of anemia
Allergic	Transfer of an antigen or a reaginic antibody from donor to recipient	Immune sensitivity to foreign serum protein (type I hypersensitivity)	Urticaria Anaphylaxis (wheezing, dyspnea, shock)	Within 30 min after initiation of transfusion	Mild: give antihistamine, continue transfusion Severe: give aqueous epinephrine (0.5 ml of 1:1000 solution)
Febrile	Reaction of antigen on WBC or platelets Bacterial contamination	Leukocyte agglutination Bacterial pyrogens	Fever, chills	Within 30 to 90 min after initiation of transfusion	Stop transfusion Continue IV saline Antipyretics after ruling out hemolytic reaction Transfuse with leukocyte-poor blood or washed RBCs
Graft-versus-host disease	Immunodeficient person receives lymphocytes	Engraftment of donor lymphocytes that are then "rejected"	Dermatitis Stomatitis Diarrhea Liver dysfunction	Delayed	Steroids Azathioprine Symptomatic therapy
Noncardiac pulmonary edema	Donor antibodies react with recipient HLA antigen	Infiltration of pulmonary bed by microaggregates that block blood flow	Fever, chills Urticaria Cough Orthopnea Cyanosis Shock	During transfusion or shortly thereafter	Continue IV saline Give oxygen as needed Steroids Furosemide

From Phipps WJ, Long BL, Woods NF, Cassmeyer VL: *Medical-surgical nursing: concepts and clinical practice,* ed 4, St Louis, 1991, Mosby.

ruddy facial flushing followed by cyanosis and distended neck veins, rapid, thready pulse, diaphoresis, and cold, clammy skin. Profound shock may occur within 1 hour. ■ INTERVENTIONS: When a hemolytic reaction is suspected, the transfusion is promptly terminated and the infusion line kept open with a normal solution of intravenous fluid. The remaining bank blood is saved for a repeat type and crossmatch against a fresh sample of blood from the recipient. Direct and indirect antiglobulin tests are usually ordered to detect hemolytic antibodies, and a sample of urine is examined for free hemoglobin. Immediate treatment may include IV mannitol and a solution of 5% dextrose in water to maintain urine flow of more than 100 ml per hour. In the presence of oliguria, the possibility of acute renal failure is evaluated and the patient is managed accordingly. Hypovolemia is corrected with saline or plasma expanders, but the administration of more whole blood is avoided, if possible. ■ NURSING CONSIDERATIONS: The need for exceptional care to ensure that typed and crossmatched blood conforms to compatibility standards is emphasized. The identifying information on the container of blood is always checked against the transfusion records and the patient's ID on the band. Questioning the patient about previous transfusions may elicit warning indications of possible adverse reactions. After the transfusion is started, the patient is watched for objective signs of a transfusion reaction and is questioned for subjective symptoms. Routine temperature checks are done to detect febrile reactions that can be controlled by antipyretic drugs.

transient /tran'shənt, tran'zē·ənt/ [L, *transire,* to go through], pertaining to a condition that is temporary, such as transient ischemic attack.

transient global amnesia (TGA) [L, *transire,* to go through + *globus,* ball; Gk, *amnesia,* forgetfulness], a temporary, short-term memory loss followed by full recovery. The disorder tends to affect middle-aged adults and may be attributed to cerebral ischemia. It is usually not accompanied by other mental deficiences.

transient ischemic attack (TIA), an episode of cerebrovascular insufficiency, usually associated with a partial occlusion of an artery by an atherosclerotic plaque or an embolism. The symptoms vary with the site and the degree of occlusion. Disturbance of normal vision in one or in both eyes, dizziness, weakness, dysphasia, numbness, or unconsciousness may occur. The attack is usually brief, lasting a few minutes; rarely, symptoms continue for several hours.

transient myopia [L, *transire,* to go through; Gk, *myops,* nearsighted], a temporary change in visual accommodation secondary to trauma, high blood sugar level, sulfanilamide therapy, and other conditions.

transillumination /-iloo'minā'shən/ [L, *trans,* through, *illuminare,* to light up], **1.** the passage of light through a solid or liquid substance. **2.** the passage of light through body tissues for the purpose of examining a structure interposed between the observer and the light source. A diaphanoscope is an instrument introduced into a body cavity to transilluminate tissues.

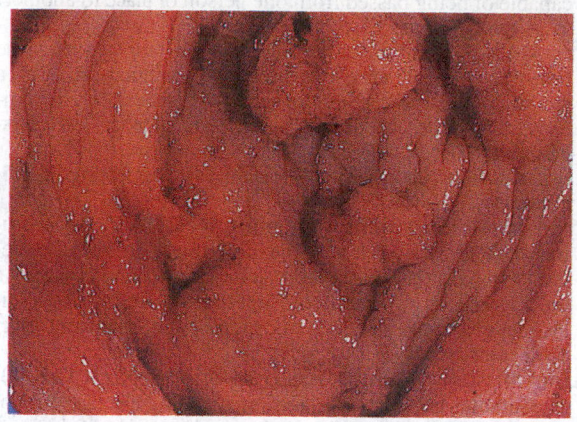

**Transition cell carcinoma:
3 large papillary tumors**
(Weiss, 1988)

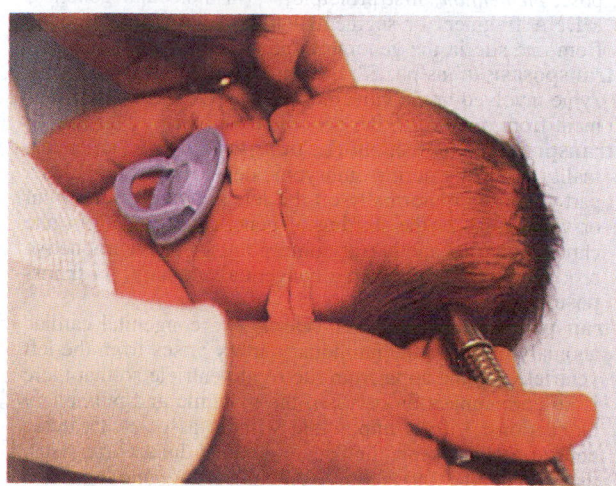

Transillumination of an infant's scalp *(Seidel, 1991)*

transition /tranzish'ən/ [L, *transire,* to go through], the last phase of the first stage of labor, sometimes indicated by cervical dilation of 8 to 10 cm.

transitional /tranzish'ənəl/ [L, *transire,* to go through], between a previous and a succeeding state, or in a state of becoming something else.

transitional cell carcinoma, a malignant, usually papillary tumor derived from transitional stratified epithelium, occurring most frequently in the bladder, ureter, urethra, or renal pelvis. The majority of tumors in the collecting system of the kidney are of this kind. They have a better prognosis than squamous cell carcinomas in the same site.

transitional dentition. See **mixed dentition.**

transitional object, an object used by a child to provide comfort and security while he or she is away from a secure base, such as mother or home.

transitional zone [L, *transire,* to go through; Gk, *zone,* belt], a part of the crystalline lens of the eye where epithelial-capsule cells change into lens fibers.

transitory mania /tran'sitôr'ē/ [L, *transire,* to go through; Gk *mania* madness], a mood disorder characterized by the sudden onset of manic reactions that are of short duration, usually lasting from 1 hour to a few days. See also **mania.**

translation /-lā'shən/ [L, *translatio,* handing over], (in molecular genetics) the process in which the genetic information carried by nucleotides in messenger RNA directs the amino acid sequence in the synthesis of a specific polypeptide. See also **anticodon, genetic code.**

translocation /-lōkā'shən/ [L, *trans + locus,* place], (in genetics) the rearrangement of genetic material within the same chromosome or the transfer of a segment of one chromosome to another nonhomologous one. In simple translocations, one end segment of one chromosome is transferred onto the end of another nonhomologous one, involving a single break in only one of the chromosomes. Translocations in which material from the middle of one chromosome is shifted to the middle of another one are more complex and involve at least three breaks in the participating chromosomes. Such shifting of genetic material can result in serious disorders, such as Down syndrome, which is caused by a 14/21 translocation, and chronic granulocytic leukemia, in which part of the long arm of chromosome 22 is translocated to the short arm of chromosome 9. Kinds of translocations are **balanced translocation, reciprocal translocation,** and **robertsonian translocation.**

translucent /-loo'sənt/ [L, *trans,* across + *lucens,* shining], pertaining to a medium through which light can pass in a diffused manner so that a field is illuminated but objects cannot be seen distinctly. Compare **transparent.**

transmigration /-mīgrā'shən/ [L, *trans + migrare,* to migrate], a movement from one side to another, from inside to outside, or from outside to inside.

transmissible /-mis'ibəl/ [L, *transmittere,* to transmit], capable of being passed from one person or place to another, as in the transmission of a disease.

transmission /-mish'ən/ [L, *transmittere*, to transmit], the transfer or conveyance of a thing or condition, such as a neural impulse, infectious or genetic disease, or a hereditary trait, from one person or place to another. **—transmissible,** *adj.*

transmission electron microscopy. See **electron microscopy.**

transmission scanning electron microscope, an instrument that transmits a highly magnified, well-resolved, three-dimensional image on a television screen, thus combining the advantages of the electron and the scanning electron microscopes. Compare **electron microscope, scanning electron microscope.**

transmission scanning electron microscopy (TSEM), a technique using a transmission scanning electron microscope in which the atomic number of the portion of the sample being scanned is determined and used to modulate a beam of electrons in a cathode-ray tube and in the beam scanning the sample. The image produced is clear, three-dimensional, and highly magnified. Compare **electron microscopy, scanning electron microscopy.**

transmitted light [L, *transmittere*, to transmit; AS, *leoht*], light that has been transmitted through a transparent medium.

transmitter substance. See **neurotransmitter.**

transmural /-m(y)ŏŏ'rəl/ [L, *trans + murus*, wall], pertaining to the entire thickness of the wall of an organ, such as a transmural myocardial infarction.

transmural infarction, the death of myocardial tissue that extends from the endocardium to the epicardium as a result of a myocardial infarction.

transmutation /-m(y)ŏŏtā'shən/ [L, *transmutare*, to change], **1.** a mutation, as when a significant species change occurs during evolution. **2.** the conversion of one chemical element into another by radioactive bombardment.

transovarial transmission /-ōver'ē·əl/ [L, *trans + ovum*, egg], the transfer of pathogens to succeeding generations through invasion of the ovary and infection of the egg, such as occurs in arthropods, primarily ticks and mites.

transparent /-per'ənt/ [L, *trans*, across, *parere*, to appear], pertaining to a clear medium that allows for the transmission of light so that objects on the other side are distinguishable. Compare **translucent.**

transplacental /trans'pləsen'təl/ [L, *trans + placenta*, cake], across or through the placenta, specifically in reference to the exchange of nutrients, waste products, and other material between the developing fetus and the mother.

transplant /trans'plant, transplant'/ [L, *transplantare*], **1.** to transfer an organ or tissue from one person to another or from one body part to another to replace a diseased structure, to restore function, or to change appearance. Skin and kidneys are the most frequently transplanted structures; others include cartilage, bone, corneal tissue, portions of blood vessels and tendons, and, recently, hearts and livers. Preferred donors are identical twins or people having the same blood type and immunologic characteristics. Success of the transplant depends on overcoming the rejection of the donor tissue by the immune system of the recipient. Under local or general anesthesia, the recipient site is prepared and the donor structure is grafted in place; its oxygenation and blood supply are preserved during the procedure until the circulation can be restored at the new site. After surgery,

circulation in the area is observed for signs of impairment. Antilymphocytic serum may be given, with steroids, to suppress the production of antibodies to the foreign tissue proteins. Signs of rejection reaction include fever, pain, and loss of function, usually occurring in the first 4 to 10 days after transplantation. An abscess may form if the reaction is not subdued promptly. The grafted structure may require several weeks to become established. Late rejection may occur several months or even 1 year later. **2.** any tissue or organ that is transplanted. **3.** of or pertaining to a tissue or organ that is transplanted, to a recipient of a donated tissue or organ or to a phenomenon associated with the procedure. Also called **graft, transplantation.**

transplantation /-plantā'shən/ [L, *transplantare*, to transplant], the transfer of tissue from one site to another or from one person or organism to another.

transplantation endometriosis [L, *transplantare*, to transplant; Gk, *endon*, within + *metra*, womb + *osis*, condition], endometrial tissue that is accidentally transplanted to the incision wound during pelvic surgery.

transport /trans'pôrt/ [L, *trans*, across + *portare*, carry], the movement or transference of biochemical substances from one site to another. Active transport involves an expenditure of energy whereas passive transport allows movement down a gradient without an energy expenditure.

transposable element /-pō'zəbəl/ [L, *transponere*, to transpose; *elementum*, first principle], (in molecular genetics) a DNA fragment or segment that can move or be moved from one site in the genome to another.

transposase /trans'pəzās/, (in molecular genetics) an enzyme involved in the movement of a DNA fragment or segment from one site in the genome to another.

transposition /-pəsish'ən/ [L, *transponere*], **1.** an abnormality occurring during embryonic development in which a part of the body normally on the left is found on the right or vice versa. **2.** the shifting of genetic material from one chromosome to another at some point in the reproductive process, often resulting in a congenital anomaly. **—transpose,** *v.*

transposition of the great vessels, a congenital cardiac anomaly in which the pulmonary artery arises from the left ventricle and the aorta from the right ventricle so that there is no communication between the systemic and pulmonary circulations. Life is impossible without associated cardiac defects, such as septal defects or a patent ductus arteriosus, that enable the mixing of oxygenated and unoxygenated blood. The severity of the condition depends on the type and size of the associated defect. The primary symptoms are cyanosis and hypoxia, especially in infants with small septal defects, although cardiomegaly is usually evident a few weeks after birth. Signs of congestive heart failure develop rapidly, especially in infants with large ventricular septal defects. Definitive diagnosis is based on cardiac catheterization. Surgical correction of the defect is postponed, if possible, until after 6 months of age, when the infant can better tolerate the procedure. Immediate palliative surgical procedures, such as balloon septostomy, may be performed to decrease pulmonary vascular resistance and prevent congestive heart failure. See also **blue baby.**

transposon /transpō'sən/ [L, *transponere + on*], a gene or a group of genes that are mobile and, like plasmids, act to transfer genetic instructions from one place to another. Transposons travel piggyback from virus to virus on bacteriophages. The genetic material is incorporated into the vi-

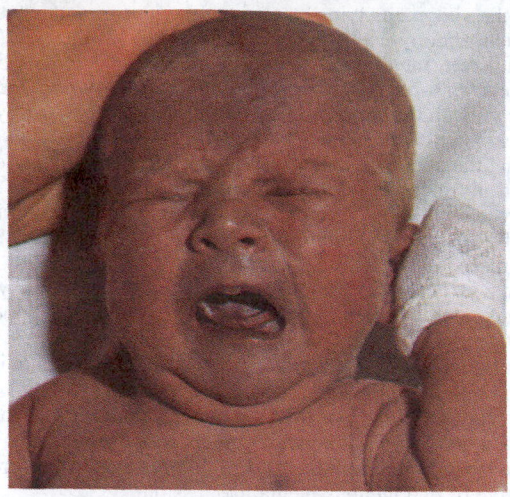

Transposition of the great vessels: characteristic blue appearance (Forbes, 1993)

rus when the virus infects a bacterial cell. As the bacteria replicates itself, it also copies the genetic instructions brought by the transposon.

transpulmonary pressure /-pul'mǝner'ē/, the difference between intraalveolar and intrapleural pressure, or the pressure acting across the lung from the intrapleural space to the alveoli.

transsect.   See **transect.**

transsection /transek'shǝn/ [L, *trans*, across + *sectio*], a crosssection of a biological specimen or a cut across the long axis. Also spelled **transection.**

transseptal fiber /transep'tǝl/ [L, *trans* + *saeptum*, wall], (in dentistry) any one of the many fibers of the gingival fiber system that extends horizontally from the supraalveolar cementum of a tooth, through the interdental attached gingiva above the septum of the alveolar bone, to the cementum of an adjacent tooth.

transsexual /transek'cho͞o·ǝl/, a person whose gender identity is opposite his or her biologic sex.

transsexualism /-iz'ǝm/, a condition in which a person has an intense desire to discard one's biologic sex and live as a member of the opposite sex. It is considered a psychiatric disorder if the condition continues for more than 2 years. Some transsexual individuals crossdress and seek medical or surgical help to change their physical sex characteristics.

transtentorial herniation /trans'tentôr'ē·ǝl/ [L, *trans* + *tentorium*, tent; *hernia*, rupture], a bulge of brain tissue out of the cranium through the tentorial notch, caused by increased intracranial pressure. See also **tentorial herniation.**

transthermia.   See **thermopenetration.**

transthoracic pacemaker /-thôras'ik/ [L, *trans*, across; Gk, *thorax*, chest; L, *passus*, step; ME, *maken*], a permanent heart pacemaker with the pulse generator located in the abdominal wall and the pacing wires attached directly to the epicardium.

transtracheal oxygen /-trā'kē·ǝl/ [L, *trans*, across; Gk, *tracheia*, rough artery + *oxys*, sharp + *genein*, to produce], a method of administering oxygen to a patient requiring ox-

ygen therapy by establishing a low-flow catheter route directly into the trachea. It is a sometimes preferred alternative to the administration of oxygen through a nasal canula.

transtrochanteric osteotomy /-trō'kǝnter'ik/ [L, *trans* across; Gk, *trochanter*, runner + *osteon* + *temnein*, to cut], a surgical division of the upper end of the femur through the area of the trochanters.

transudate /trans'yǝdāt/ [L, *trans* + *sudare*, to sweat], a fluid passed through a membrane or squeezed through a tissue or into the space between the cells of a tissue. It is thin and watery and contains few blood cells or other large proteins. See also **edema.**

transudation /-yǝdā'shǝn/, **1.** the passage of a substance through a membrane as a result of a difference in hydrostatic pressure. **2.** the passage of a fluid through a membrane with nearly all the solutes of the fluid remaining in solution or suspension.

transudative ascites /transyo͞o'dǝtiv/, an abnormal accumulation in the peritoneal cavity of a fluid that characteristically contains scant amounts of protein and cells. Ascitic fluids with protein counts of less than 2.5 g/ml are considered to be transudates. Transudative ascites is indicative of cirrhosis or congestive heart failure rather than infection, inflammation, or the presence of a tumor.

transurethral resection (TUR) /trans'yo͞orē'thrǝl/ [L, *trans*, + Gk, *ourethra*, urethra; L, *re*, again, *secare*, to cut], a surgical procedure through the urethra, such as in transurethral prostatectomy. Compare **suprapubic.**

transverse /-vurs'/ [L, *transversus*, oblique], at right angles to the long axis of any common part, such as the planes that cut the long axis of the body into upper and lower portions and are at right angles to the sagittal and frontal planes.

transverse colon, the segment of the colon that extends from the end of the ascending colon at the hepatic flexure on the right side across the midabdomen to the beginning of the descending colon at the splenic flexure on the left side.

transverse fissure, a fissure dividing the dorsal surface of the diencephalon and the ventral surface of the cerebral hemisphere. Also called **fissure of Bichat.**

transverse foramen [L, *transversus* + *foramen*, hole], an opening through the transverse process of a cervical vertebra.

transverse fracture, a fracture that occurs at right angles to the longitudinal axis of the bone involved.

transverse lie, abnormal presentation of a fetus in which the long axis of the baby's body is across the long axis of the mother's body; unless the baby turns spontaneously or is turned by means of external or internal version, vaginal delivery is impossible.

transverse ligament of the atlas, a thick, strong ligament stretched across the ring of the atlas, holding the dens against the anterior arch. As it crosses the dens, it arches cranially and caudally, forming the cruciate ligament of the atlas. The transverse ligament divides the circular opening of the atlas into posterior and anterior parts. The posterior part transmits the spinal cord and its membranes; the anterior part contains the dens.

transverse mesocolon /mez'ōkō'lǝn/, a broad fold of the peritoneum connecting the transverse colon to the dorsal wall of the abdomen. It is continuous with the greater omentum along the ventral surface of the transverse colon and contains between its layers the vessels that supply the transverse colon. Its two layers diverge along the anterior border of the pancreas. Compare **mesentery proper, sigmoid mesocolon.**

transverse myelitis [L, *transversus;* Gk, *myelos,* marrow + *itis,* inflammation], an acute attack of spinal cord inflammation involving both sides of the cord.

transverse palatine suture, the line of junction between the processes of the maxilla and the horizontal portions of the palatine bones that form the hard palate.

transverse plane, any one of the planes cutting across the body perpendicular to the sagittal and the frontal planes, dividing the body into caudal and cranial portions. Also called **cardinal horizontal plane.** Compare **frontal plane, median plane, sagittal plane.**

transverse presentation [L, *transversus + praesentare,* to show], a presentation of the fetal body in an oblique or transverse position across the birth canal.

transverse relaxation time. See **relaxation time.**

transverse sinus, one of a pair of large venous channels in the posterior superior group of sinuses serving the dura mater. Each transverse sinus starts at the internal occipital protuberance and one, usually the right, is a direct continuation of the superior sagittal sinus; the other is a continuation of the straight sinus. Each transverse sinus curves slightly to the base of the petrous portion of the temporal bone and within the margin of the tentorium. It leaves the tentorium and becomes the sigmoid sinus, which curves inferiorly and medially to the jugular foramen and ends in the internal jugular vein. The transverse sinuses are often of different size, the larger one usually formed by the superior sagittal sinus. Each transverse sinus receives the blood from the superior petrosal sinus at the base of the temporal bone; each anastomoses with the veins of the pericranium through the mastoid and the condyloid emissary veins; and each receives some of the inferior cerebral and the inferior cerebellar veins and some of the veins from the diploe. Compare **confluence of the sinuses, inferior sagittal sinus, occipital sinus, straight sinus, superior sagittal sinus.**

transversus abdominis /-vur′səs/, one of a pair of transverse abdominal muscles that are the anterolateral muscles of the abdomen, lying immediately under the obliquus internus abdominis. Arising from the inguinal ligament, the iliac crest, the thoracolumbar fascia, and the last six ribs, it inserts into the linea alba. It is innervated by branches of the seventh through the twelfth intercostal nerves and by the iliohypogastric and the ilioinguinal nerves. It serves to constrict the abdomen and, by compressing the contents, to assist in micturition, defecation, emesis, parturition, and forced expiration. Compare **obliquus externus abdominis, obliquus internus abdominis, pyramidalis, rectus abdominis.**

transvestism /-ves′tizəm/, a tendency to achieve psychic and sexual relief by dressing in the clothing of the opposite sex.

Tranxene, a trademark for a benzodiazepine tranquilizer (chlorazepate dipotassium).

tranylcypromine sulfate /tran′əlsip′rəmēn/, a monoamine oxidase inhibitor that acts as an antidepressant.

■ INDICATIONS: It is prescribed in the treatment of severe reactive or endogenous mental depression.

■ CONTRAINDICATIONS: Cerebrovascular or cardiovascular diseases, paranoid schizophrenia, liver dysfunction, alcoholism, pheochromocytoma, or known hypersensitivity to this drug prohibits its use. It is not given to children under 16 years of age.

■ ADVERSE EFFECTS: Among the most serious adverse reactions are severe hypertensive episodes that can be precipitated by ingestion of foods rich in tyramine or by concurrent administration of many sympathomimetic drugs. Common side effects include headache, vertigo, dry mouth, blurred vision, and orthostatic hypotension.

trapezium /trəpē′zē·əm/, *pl.* **trapeziums, trapezia** [Gk, *trapezion,* small table], a carpal bone in the distal row of carpal bones. It has a deep groove on the palmar surface between the scaphoid and first metacarpal bones. The lateral surface is broad and rough for the attachment of ligaments. A deep groove in its palmar surface transmits the tendon of the flexor carpi radialis. The opponens pollicis and the abductor brevis originate on the palmar surface. The trapezium articulates with the scaphoid proximally, the first metacarpal distally, and the trapezoideum and the second metacarpal medially. Also called **greater multangular, os trapezium.**

trapezius /trəpē′zē·əs/ [Gk, *trapezion,* small table], a large, flat triangular muscle of the shoulder and upper back. It arises from the occipital bone, the ligamentum nuchae, and the spinous processes of the seventh cervical and all the thoracic vertebrae. It is innervated by the third and fourth cervical nerves and by the spinal accessory nerve. It acts to rotate the scapula, raise the shoulder, and abduct and flex the arm.

trapezoid /trap′əzoid/ [Gk, *trapezion,* a small table + *eidos,* form], having the shape of a trapeze, an irregular four-sided figure with one set of parallel sides.

trapezoidal arch /trap′əzoidəl/ [Gk, *trapezion + eidos,* form; L, *arcus,* bow], a dental arch that has slightly less convergence than that of a tapering arch. The anterior teeth in the arch are somewhat square or abruptly rounded from tip to tip of the canines, which are at the corners of the arch.

trapezoid bone [Gk, *trapezion, eidos* + AS, *ban*], the smallest carpal bone, located in the distal row of carpal bones between the trapezium and the capitate. It resembles a wedge, with the broad end at the dorsal surface, the narrow end at the palmar surface. The trapezoid articulates with the scaphoid proximally, the second metacarpal distally, the

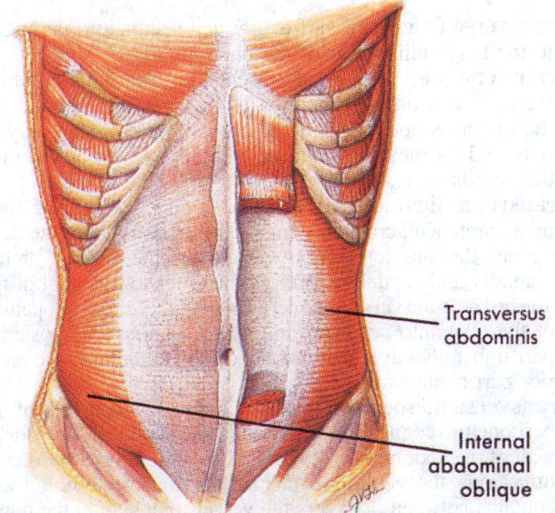

Transverse abdominis *(Thibodeau, 1993/John V Hagen)*

Transversus abdominis

Internal abdominal oblique

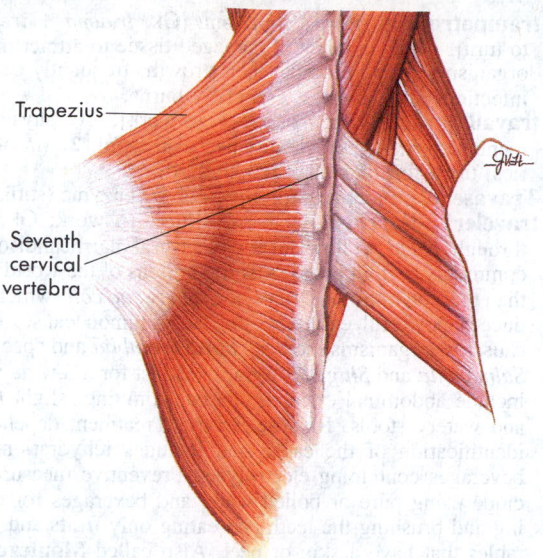

Trapezius (Thibodeau, 1993/John V Hagen)

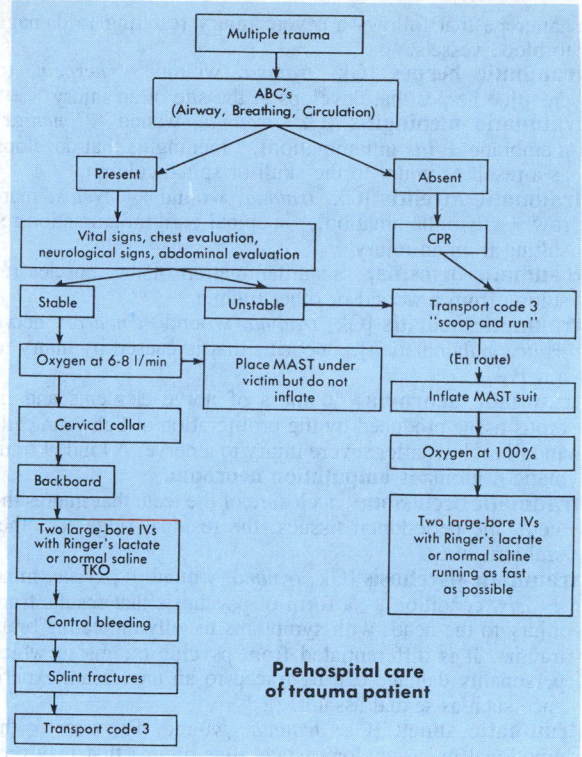

Prehospital care of trauma patient

trapezium laterally, and the capitate medially. Also called **lesser multangular bone, os trapezoideum.**

trauma /trou'mə, trô'mə/ [Gk, wound], **1.** physical injury caused by violent or disruptive action, or by the introduction into the body of a toxic substance. **2.** psychic injury resulting from a severe emotional shock. —**traumatic,** *adj.,* **traumatize,** *v.*

-trauma, a combining form meaning a 'wound or injury, psychic or physical': *arthrotrauma, barotrauma, neurotrauma.*

trauma center, a service providing emergency and specialized intensive care to critically ill and injured patients.

trauma, high risk for, a nursing diagnosis accepted by the Seventh National Conference on the Classification of Nursing Diagnoses. It is defined as the accentuated risk of accidental tissue injury, such as a wound, burn, or fracture. The risk factors may be internal (individual) or external (environmental). Internal risk factors include weakness; poor vision; balancing difficulties; reduced temperature or tactile sensation; reduced muscle or eye-hand coordination; lack of safety education, precautions, or equipment; cognitive or emotional difficulties; and history of previous trauma. External risk factors include slippery floors, stairs, or walkways (such as highly waxed, wet, or icy); a bathtub without hand grip or antislip equipment; unsteady chairs or ladders; defective electric wires or appliances; obstructed passageways; potential igniting gas leaks; unscreened fires or heaters; inadequately stored combustibles or corrosives; contact with intense cold or heat (such as very hot water); overexposure to sun, sunlamps, or radiotherapy; and exposure to dangerous machinery. Others include unsafe driving (drunk driving, excessive speeds, absent visual aids), nonuse or misuse of seat restraints, nonuse of headgear for motorized cyclists, and unsafe road or road-crossing conditions. Some external risk factors affecting children are a lack of safe stair rails or safety gates, unsafe window protection, highly flammable children's toys or clothing, and children playing with matches or fireworks. See also **nursing diagnosis.**

trauma registry, a repository of data on the incidence, diagnosis, and treatment of acute trauma victims treated by emergency service personnel.

Trauma Score, a system of combining cardiopulmonary assessment with the Glasgow Coma Scale in estimating the degree of injury and the prognosis in a patient who has suffered a head injury. Cardiopulmonary factors include respiratory rate and chest expansion, systolic blood pressure, and capillary refill. The neurologic factors are eye opening, verbal response, and motor response.

traumatic /trômat'ik/ [Gk, *trauma,* wound], pertaining to an injury, usually a serious and unexpected injury.

traumatic anesthesia [Gk, *trauma* + *anaisthesia,* loss of feeling], a total lack of normal sensation in a part of the body, resulting from injury, destruction of nerves, or interruption of nerve pathways. See also **tactile anesthesia.**

traumatic delirium, delirium after severe head injury, characterized by alertness and consciousness with disorientation, confabulation, and amnesia apparent. See also **delirium.**

traumatic dislocation [Gk, *trauma,* wound; L, *dis, locare*], a dislocation caused by an injury.

traumatic epilepsy [Gk, *trauma,* wound + *epilepsia,* seizure], a form of epilepsy caused by an injury. Also called **posttraumatic epilepsy.**

traumatic fever, an elevation in body temperature secondary to mechanic trauma, particularly a crushing injury. Such fevers may last 1 or 2 days. The increased body temperature may help provide resistance to subsequent infection, and increased wound temperature may accelerate local healing.

traumatic gangrene [Gk, *trauma,* wound + *gaggraina*],

gangrene that follows a severe injury resulting in damage to blood vessels.

traumatic herpes [Gk, *trauma*, wound + *herpein*, to creep], herpes that develops at the site of an injury.

traumatic meningitis [Gk, *trauma*, wound + *menigx*, membrane + *itis* inflammation], meningitis that develops as a result of injury to the skull or spinal column.

traumatic myelitis [Gk, *trauma*, wound + *myelos*, marrow + *itis*, inflammation], a spinal cord inflammation resulting from an injury.

traumatic myositis, an inflammation of the muscles resulting from a wound or other trauma.

traumatic neuritis [Gk, *trauma*, wound + *neuron*, nerve + *itis*, inflammation], neuritis that is caused by injury to a nerve.

traumatic neuroma, a mass of nerve elements and fibrous tissue produced by the proliferation of Schwann cells and fibroblasts after severe injury to a nerve. A kind of traumatic neuroma is **amputation neuroma.**

traumatic occlusion, a closure of the teeth that injures the teeth, the periodontal tissues, the residual ridge, or other oral structures.

traumatic psychosis [Gk, *trauma*, wound + *psyche*, mind + *osis*, condition], a form of psychosis that results from injury to the head, with symptoms usually indicating brain trauma. It is differentiated from psychic trauma in which personality damage can be traced to an unpleasant experience such as sexual assault.

traumatic shock [Gk, *trauma*, wound; Fr, *choc*], the emotional or psychologic state after trauma that may produce abnormal behavior. The most common types are hypovolemic shock from blood loss and neurogenic shock, from a disruption of the integrity of the spinal cord.

traumatic spondylopathy. See **Kümmell's disease.**

traumatic thrombosis [Gk, *trauma*, wound + *thrombos*, lump + *osis*, condition], intravascular coagulation of a vein or other blood vessel after injury or irritation. The condition may develop as an adverse effect of an intravenous injection that damages the wall of a vein.

traumato-, a combining form meaning 'pertaining to trauma, or to an injury or wound': *traumatogenic, traumatopnea, traumatopyra.*

traumatology /trôʹmətolʹəjē/ [Gk, *trauma* + *logos*, science], **1.** the study of wounds and injuries. **2.** a surgical specialty dealing with the treatment of wounds, injuries, and resulting disabilities. **–traumatologic, traumatological,** *adj.*

traumatopathy /trôʹmətopʹəthē/ [Gk, *trauma* + *pathos*, disease], a pathologic condition resulting from a wound or injury. **–traumatopathic,** *adj.*

traumatophilia /trôʹmətōfilʹē·ə/ [Gk, *trauma* + *philein*, to love], a psychologic state in which the individual derives unconscious pleasure from injuries and surgical operations. **–traumatophiliac,** *n.*, **traumatophilic,** *adj.*

traumatopnea /trôʹmətopʹnē·ə/ [Gk, *trauma* + *pnein*, to breathe], partial asphyxia with collapse of the patient, caused by a penetrating thoracic wound permitting air to enter the pleural space and compress the lungs.

traumatopyra /trôʹmətōpīʹrə/ [Gk, *trauma* + *pyr*, fire], an elevated temperature resulting from a wound or injury.

traumatotherapy /-therʹəpē/ [Gk, *trauma* + *therapeia*, treatment], the medical, surgical, and psychologic treatment of wounds, injuries, and disabilities resulting from trauma. **–traumatotherapeutic,** *adj.*

traumatropism /trômatʹrəpizʹəm/ [Gk, *trauma* + *trepein*, to turn], the tendency of damaged tissue to attract microorganisms and to promote their growth, frequently causing infections after injuries, especially burns.

travail /trəvālʹ/ [OFr, *travaillier*, to work], **1.** physical or mental exertion, especially when distressful. **2.** (in obstetrics) the effort of labor and childbirth.

Travase, a trademark for a proteolytic enzyme (sutilains).

traveler's diarrhea [OFr, *travaillier*, to work; Gk, *dia*, through, *rhein*, to flow], any of several diarrheal disorders commonly seen in people visiting regions of the world other than their own. Some strains of *Escherichia coli*, which produce a powerful exotoxin, are the common cause. Other causative organisms include *Giardia lamblia* and species of *Salmonella* and *Shigella*. Symptoms last for a few days and include abdominal cramps, nausea, vomiting, slight fever, and watery stools. Relapse is rare. Treatment depends on identification of the cause and includes rehydration with beverages containing electrolytes. Preventive measures include using pure or boiled water and beverages for drinking and brushing the teeth and eating only fruits and vegetables that have a skin or peel. Also called **Montezuma's revenge, turista.**

TRBF, abbreviation for **total renal blood flow.**

Treacher Collins' syndrome, an inherited disorder, characterized by mandibulofacial dysostosis. See also **Pierre Robin's syndrome.**

treatment [Fr, *traitement*], **1.** the care and management of a patient to combat, ameliorate, or prevent a disease, disorder, or injury. **2.** a method of combating, ameliorating, or preventing a disease, disorder, or injury. Active or curative treatment is designed to cure; palliative treatment is directed to relieve pain and distress; prophylactic treatment is for the prevention of a disease or disorder; causal treatment focuses on the cause of a disorder; conservative treatment avoids radical measures and procedures; empiric treatment employs methods shown to be beneficial by experience; rational treatment is based on a knowledge of a disease process and the action of the measures used. Treatment may be pharmacologic, using drugs; surgical, involving operative procedures; or supportive, building the patient's strength. It may be specific for the disorder, or symptomatic to relieve symptoms without effecting a cure.

treatment guardian, a person who is appointed by the court for the purpose of consenting to or refusing medical treatment for a patient.

treatment plan [Fr, *traitement*; L, *planta*], (in dentistry) a schedule of procedures and appointments designed to restore, step by step, the oral health of a patient. The plan contains the advantages, disadvantages, costs, alternatives, and sequelae of treatment. It must be presented to the patient for approval.

treatment room, a room in a patient care unit, usually in a hospital, in which various treatments or procedures requiring special equipment are performed, such as removing sutures, draining a hematoma, packing a wound, or performing an examination.

Trecator-SC, a trademark for a tuberculostatic (ethionamide).

Trechona /trikonʹə/, a genus of spiders, family Dipluridae, the bite of which is toxic and irritating to humans.

tree [AS, *treow*], **1.** (in anatomy) an anatomic structure with branches that spread out like those of a tree, such as the bronchial tree and the tracheobronchial tree. **2.** a pattern of searching for information in a computer data base, following a series of branching options from a general category to reach specific desired items while eliminating unwanted possibilities. MEDLINE and other computer data bases are organized in a 'logic tree' pattern.

-trema, 1. a combining form meaning a 'hole, orifice, opening': *gonotrema, helicotrema, peritrema.* 2. a combining form meaning 'creatures possessing an opening': *Eurytrema, Monotrema, Troglotrema.*

trematode /trem'ətōd/ [Gk, *trematodes,* pierced], any species of flatworm of the class Trematoda, some of which are parasitic to humans, infecting the liver, the lungs, and the intestines. Kinds of trematodes include the organisms causing **clonorchiasis, fascioliasis, paragonimiasis,** and **schistosomiasis.** Also called **fluke.**

tremor /trem'ər, trē'mər/ [L, shaking], rhythmic, purposeless, quivering movements resulting from the involuntary alternating contraction and relaxation of opposing groups of skeletal muscles, occurring in some elderly individuals, in certain families, and in patients with various neurodegenerative disorders. Senile tremor is characterized by fine, quick movements, especially of the hands, rhythmic head nodding, and increased trembling during purposeful movements. Familial tremor, which may be hereditary, and the tremor occurring in multiple sclerosis also increase during voluntary movement and may be intensified by anxiety, excitement, and self-consciousness. The tremors of Graves' disease, alcoholism, mercury poisoning, and other toxicoses are usually less rhythmic, and the tremor in lead poisoning often affects the lips. The fine, quick, continuous tremor present in Parkinson's disease sometimes disappears during purposeful movements. Kinds of tremors are **resting tremor** and **intention tremor.**

tremulous /trem'yələs/ [L, *tremulare,* to tremble], pertaining to tremors, or involuntary muscular contractions.

tremulous pulse [L, *tremulare,* to tremble + *pulsare,* to beat], a feeble, fluttering pulse.

trench fever [OFr *trenchier* to carve; L, *febris,* fever], a self-limited infection, caused by *Rochalimaea quintana,* a rickettsial organism transmitted by body lice, characterized by weakness, fever, rash, and leg pains. It was common during World War I but is now rare. Also called **quintana fever.**

trench foot [OFr, *trenchier,* to cut off; AS, *fot*], a condition of moist gangrene of the foot caused by the freezing of wet skin.

trench mouth. See **acute necrotizing gingivitis.**

Trendelenburg gait /trendel'ənbərg, tren'd(e)lənburg'/ [Friederich Trendelenburg, German surgeon, b. 1844], an abnormal gait associated with a weakness of the gluteus medius. The Trendelenburg gait is characterized by the dropping of the pelvis on the unaffected side of the body at the moment of heelstrike on the affected side. In this deviation, the pelvic drop during the walking cycle lasts until heelstrike on the unaffected side and is accompanied by an apparent lateral protrusion of the affected hip. The person with a Trendelenburg gait also shortens the step on the unaffected side and displays a lateral deviation of the entire trunk and the affected side during the stance phase of the affected lower limb. The Trendelenburg gait is one of the more common gait deviations. Also called **uncompensated gluteal gait.** Compare **compensated gluteal gait.**

Trendelenburg's operation, the ligation of varicose veins whose valves are ineffective, performed to remove

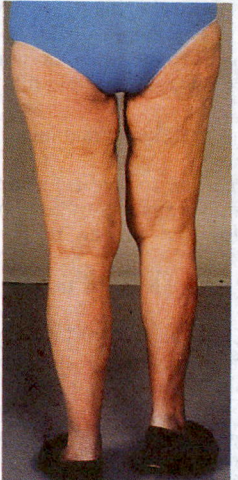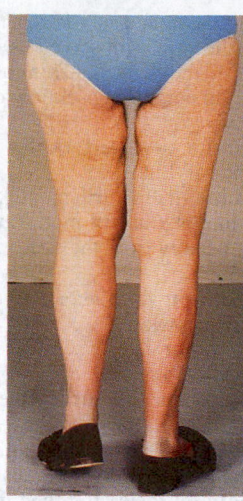

Trendelenburg gait: pelvis tilts to left when patient stands on normal left leg (A), but pelvis fails to tilt to the right when patient stands on affected right leg (B)
(Dieppe, 1986)

weakened portions of veins and pockets in which thrombi might lodge. During sugery, the saphenous vein is ligated at the groin, where it joins the femoral vein. A wire device, called a stripper, is threaded through the lumen of the vein from groin to ankle; the wire and the vein are then pulled from the groin incision. Incisions may be made at several sites along the leg. Bleeding is minimal. After surgery a pressure bandage is applied from foot to thigh, and the foot of the bed is elevated 6 to 9 inches raising the legs above the level of the heart. The patient is encouraged to walk but discouraged from standing or sitting. Cyanosis of the toes indicates possible constriction by the dressings. Elastic bandages remain in place until the seventh day after surgery, when the sutures are usually removed. Possible complications include hemorrhage, infection, nerve damage, and thrombosis.

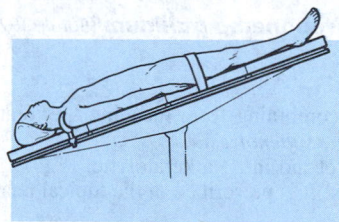

Trendelenburg's position

Trendelenburg's position, a position in which the head is low and the body and legs are on an inclined plane. It is sometimes used in pelvic surgery to displace the abdominal organs upward, out of the pelvis, or to increase the flow of blood to the brain in hypotension and shock.

Trendelenburg's test, a simple test for incompetent valves in a person who has varicose veins. The person lies down and elevates the leg to empty the vein, then stands, and the vein is observed as it fills. If the valves are incompetent, the vein fills from above; if the valves are normal, they do not allow backflow of blood, and the vein fills from below.

Trental, a trademark for an oral hemorrheologic drug (pentoxifylline).

trephine /trifīn′, trifēn′/ [Gk, *trypan*, to bore], a circular, sawlike instrument used in removing pieces of bone or tissue, usually from the skull. Also called **trepan** /trē′pan, tripan′/.

trepidation /trep′idā·shən/ [L, *trepidare*, to tremble], a state of anxiety.

Treponema /trep′ənē′mə/ [Gk, *trepein*, to turn, *nema*, thread], a genus of spirochetes, including some pathogenic to humans, such as the organisms causing bejel, pinta, syphilis, and yaws.

Treponema pallidum, an actively motile, slender spirochetal organism that causes syphilis.

treponematosis /trep′ənē′mətō′sis/, *pl.* **treponematoses** [Gk, *trepein, nema + osis,* condition], any disease caused by spirochetes of the genus *Treponema*. All these infections are effectively treated with penicillin; often one dose, given intramuscularly, results in cure. Kinds of treponematoses are **bejel, pinta, syphilis,** and **yaws.**

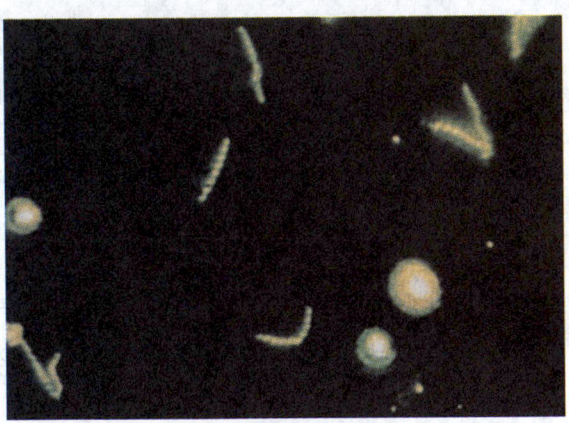

Treponema pallidum *(Baron, 1990)*

-tresia, a combining form meaning 'perforation': *atresia, proctotresia, sphenotresia.*

tretinoin /tret′inō′in/, a keratolytic.
- INDICATION: It is prescribed in the topical treatment of acne vulgaris.
- CONTRAINDICATION: Known hypersensitivity to this drug prohibits its use.
- ADVERSE EFFECTS: Among the more serious adverse reactions are red, edematous, blistered, or crusted skin.

Trexan, a trademark for an oral opioid antagonist (naltrexone hydrochloride).

-trexate, a suffix for folic acid analogues used as antimetabolites.

TRF, abbreviation for **thyrotropin releasing factor.** See **thyrotropin releasing hormone.**

TRH, abbreviation for **thyrotropin releasing hormone.**

Triage rating systems

Five-tier system (used in military triage)
Dead or will die
Life-threatening—readily correctable
Urgent—must be treated within 1 to 2 hours
Delayed—noncritical or ambulatory
No injury—no treatment necessary

Four-tier system
Immediate—seriously injured, reasonable chance of survival
Delayed—can wait for care after simple first aid
Expectant—extremely critical, moribund
Minimal—no impairment of function, can either treat self or be treated by a nonprofessional

Three-tier system
Life-threatening—readily correctable
Urgent—must be treated within 1 to 2 hours
Delayed—no injury, noncritical, or ambulatory

Two-tier system
Immediate versus delayed
Immediate—life-threatening injuries that are readily correctable on scene and those that are urgent
Delayed—no injury, noncritical injuries, ambulatory victims, moribund, or dead

tri-, a prefix meaning 'three or thrice': *triage, tribrachia, tridermoma.*

triacetin /trī·as′itin/, an antifungal.
- INDICATIONS: It is prescribed in the treatment of superficial fungus infections of the skin, including athlete's foot.
- CONTRAINDICATIONS: There are no known contraindications.
- ADVERSE EFFECTS: There are no known serious adverse effects.

triacetyloleandomycin. See **troleandomycin.**

triad /trī′əd/ [Gk, *trias*, three], a combination of three, such as two parents and a child.

triage /trē·äzh′/ [Fr, *trier*, to sort out], **1.** (in military medicine) a classification of casualties of war and other disasters according to the gravity of injuries, urgency of treatment, and place for treatment. **2.** a process in which a group of patients is sorted according to their need for care. The kind of illness or injury, the severity of the problem, and the facilities available govern the process, as in the emergency room of a hospital. **3.** (in disaster medicine) a process in which a large group of patients is sorted so that care can be concentrated on those who are likely to survive.

trial forceps /trī′əl/ [Fr, *trier*, to sort out], an obstetric operation consisting of an attempt to deliver an infant with obstetric forceps. The forceps are applied to the baby's head, and moderate traction is applied. The delivery is continued only if the trial indicates that delivery can be accomplished safely. The procedure is abandoned if proper application of the forceps or rotation of the baby's head is not possible or if the trial indicates that completion of the delivery with forceps will require inordinately heavy traction likely to be more traumatic to mother or baby than cesarean section. Trial forceps is usually performed with a double setup so that cesarean section can be carried out immediately if necessary. Compare **failed forceps.** See also **double setup.**

trial of labor [L, *terere*, to thresh grain + *labor* work], child delivery in which there is doubt as to whether the head of the fetus will pass through the pelvic brim and the situation must be monitored and assessed carefully to avoid fetal or maternal distress.

triamcinolone /trī′amsin′əlōn/,   a glucocorticoid.

■ INDICATIONS: It is prescribed as an antiinflammatory agent in the treatment of dermatoses, stomatitis, and lichen planus lesions.

■ CONTRAINDICATIONS: Fungal infections or known hypersensitivity to this drug prohibits its systemic use. Viral or fungal infections of the skin, impaired circulation, or known hypersensitivity to this drug prohibits its topical use.

■ ADVERSE EFFECTS: Among the more serious adverse reactions to the systemic administration of the drug are GI, endocrine, neurologic, fluid, and electrolyte disturbances. A variety of skin reactions may occur from topical administration of this drug.

triamterene /trī·am′tərēn/,   a potassium-sparing diuretic.

■ INDICATIONS: It is usually prescribed alone or with another diuretic in the treatment of edema, hypertension, and congestive heart failure.

■ CONTRAINDICATIONS: Anuria, severe liver or kidney dysfunction, hyperkalemia, or known hypersensitivity to this drug prohibits its use.

■ ADVERSE EFFECTS: Among the most serious adverse reactions are electrolyte disturbances, particularly hyperkalemia. GI disturbances also may occur.

triangle [L, *triangulus* three-cornered],   a predictable emotional process that takes place when there is difficulty in a relationship. Triangles represent dysfunctional efforts to reduce fusion or conflict in a relationship. The three corners of a triangle can be composed of three people or two people and an object, group, or issue.

triangular bandage /trī·ang′gyələr/,   a square of cloth folded or cut into the shape of a triangle. It may be used as a sling, a cover, or a thick pad to control bleeding.

triangular bone,   the pyramidal carpal bone in the proximal row on the ulnar side of the wrist. It articulates with the lunate bone laterally, the pisiform anteriorly, the hamate distally, and the triangular articular disk that separates it from the lower end of the ulna. Also called **cuneiform bone, os triquetrum.**

triangular dullness.   See **Koranyi's sign.**

Triavil,   a trademark for a central nervous system fixed-combination drug containing a phenothiazine tranquilizer (perphenazine) and a tricyclic antidepressant (amitriptyline hydrochloride).

triazolam /tri·az′əlam/,   a benzodiazepine hypnotic agent.

■ INDICATIONS: It is prescribed in the short-term treatment of insomnia.

■ CONTRAINDICATIONS: Known sensitivity to this drug or other benzodiazepines prohibits its use. It is not given to pregnant women, nursing mothers, or patients younger than 18 years.

■ ADVERSE EFFECTS: Among the most serious adverse reactions are anterograde amnesia, paradoxical reactions, tachycardia, depression, confusion or memory impairment, and visual disturbances.

tribe [L, *tribus*],   a taxonomic division of organisms, subordinate to a family and superior to a genus, or subtribe.

-tribe,   a suffix meaning a 'surgical instrument used to crush a body part': *cephalotribe, sphenotribe, vasotribe.*

tribology /tribol′əjē/ [Gk, *tribo,* to rub + *logos,* science],   the study of friction, wear, and lubrication of articulating surfaces.

TRIC /trik/,   abbreviation for *trachoma inclusion conjunc-*

tivitis agent, which refers to *Chlamydia trachomatis,* the organism that causes both inclusion conjunctivitis and trachoma. See also **Chlamydia.**

tricarboxylic acid cycle.   See **citric acid cycle, Krebs cycle.**

triceps brachii /trī′seps brak′ē·ī/ [L, three-headed; *brachium,* arm],   a large muscle that extends the entire length of the dorsal surface of the humerus. Proximally, it has a long head, a lateral head, and a medial head. The long head arises in a flattened tendon originating on the scapula; the lateral head arises from the posterior surface of the humerus, the lateral border of the humerus, and the lateral intermuscular septum; the medial head arises from the posterior body of the humerus, the medial body of the humerus, and the whole length of the medial intermuscular septum. The three portions of the muscle converge in a long tendon and insert in the posterior aspect of the olecranon. The triceps brachii is innervated by branches of the radial nerve, contains fibers from the seventh and the eighth cervical nerves, and functions to extend the forearm and to adduct the arm. Also called **triceps, triceps extensor cubiti.** Compare **biceps brachii.**

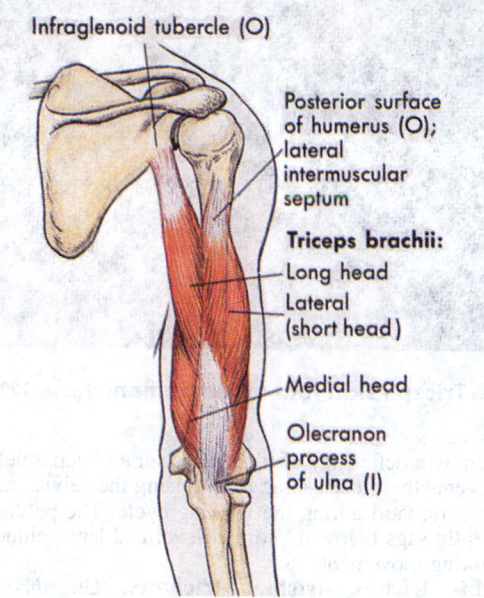

Infraglenoid tubercle (O)

Posterior surface of humerus (O); lateral intermuscular septum

Triceps brachii:

Long head

Lateral (short head)

Medial head

Olecranon process of ulna (I)

Triceps brachii *(Thibodeau, 1993/Ernest W Beck)*

triceps reflex,   a deep tendon reflex elicited by tapping sharply the triceps tendon proximal to the elbow with the forearm in a relaxed position. The response is a definite extension movement of the forearm. The reflex is accentuated by lesions of the pyramidal tract above the level of the seventh or eighth vertebra. See also **deep tendon reflex.** (See Fig. p. 1586.)

triceps skinfold,   the thickness of a fold of skin around the triceps muscle. It is measured primarily to estimate the amount of subcutaneous fat.

triceps surae limp,   an abnormal action in the walking or gait cycle, associated with a deficiency in the elevating and the propulsive factors on the affected side of the body, es-

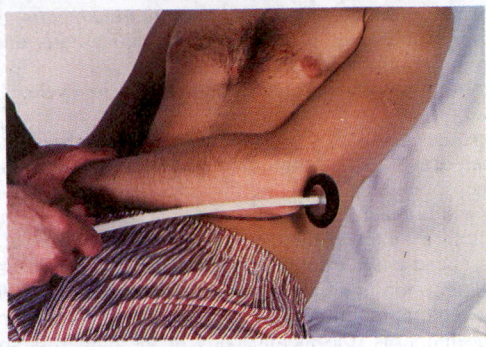

Triceps reflex test *(Epstein, 1992)*

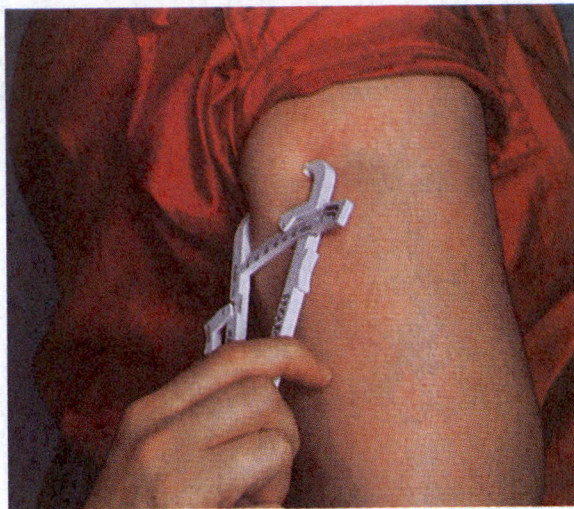

Triceps skin fold measurement *(Potter, 1993)*

pecially a deficiency of the triceps surae. Such a deficiency prevents the triceps surae from raising the pelvis and carrying it forward during the walking cycle. The pelvis consequently sags below its normal level and lags behind in the walking movement.

trichi-, tricho-, -trichia, -trichosis, [Gk, *thrix*, hair], combining forms meaning 'relating to hair', *trichinosis, trichophagia, glossotrichia.*

trichiasis /trikī'əsis/ [Gk, *thrix*, hair, *osis*, condition], an abnormal inversion of the eyelashes that irritates the eyeball. It usually follows infection or inflammation. Compare **ectropion.**

trichinosis /trik'inō'sis/ [Gk, *thrix* + *osis*, condition], infestation with the parasitic roundworm *Trichinella spiralis*, transmitted by eating raw or undercooked pork or bear meat. Early symptoms of infection include abdominal pain, nausea, fever, and diarrhea; later, muscle pain, tenderness, fatigue, and eosinophilia are observed. Light infections may be asymptomatic. Also called **trichinellosis, trichiniasis.**

■ OBSERVATIONS: Encysted larvae in improperly cooked pork mature in the intestines of the host, with mature worms depositing their larvae in the intestinal wall. The larvae penetrate the intestinal mucosa and move to other parts of the body through the blood and lymphatic systems, ultimately invading skeletal muscles, especially the diaphragm and the chest muscles, where they encyst. Larval penetration of the brain or the heart may result in death. Serologic tests, skin sensitivity tests, and microscopic examination of specimens of infested muscle obtained by a biopsy often contribute to the diagnosis.

■ INTERVENTIONS: There is no specific treatment. Analgesics, thiabendazole, and corticosteroids may relieve symptoms. Bed rest is recommended to prevent relapse and possible death. After 2 or 3 months, the organisms are completely encysted and cause no further symptoms.

■ NURSING CONSIDERATIONS: Prevention requires cooking pork or wild game at 350° F (176° C) for 35 minutes a pound. Freezing at 10° F (−12° C) for 20 days also kills the larvae. Pork or pork products should never be eaten raw, and even smoked or salted meat may still harbor viable larvae. Routine inspection of carcasses for trichinella organisms is not performed in the United States, where the disease is on the decline.

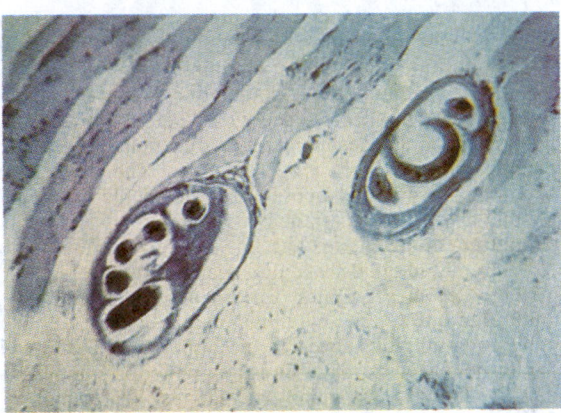

Trichinosis is caused by *Trichinella spiralis* shown here as encysted larva in biopsied muscle
(Finegold, 1986)

trichlormethiazide /trī'klôrməthī'əzīd/, a thiazide diuretic and antihypertensive.

■ INDICATIONS: It is prescribed in the treatment of hypertension and edema.

■ CONTRAINDICATIONS: Anuria or known hypersensitivity to this drug, to thiazide medications, or to sulfonamide derivatives prohibits its use.

■ ADVERSE EFFECTS: Among the more serious adverse effects are hypokalemia, hyperglycemia, hyperuricemia, and various hypersensitivity reactions.

trichloroethylene /trīklôr'ō·eth'ilēn/, a general anesthetic, administered by mask with N_2O, for dentistry, minor surgery, and the first stages of labor. It is too cardiotoxic for deep anesthesia; even in light planes of anesthesia, dysrhythmias may occur but may be reversed by administering oxygen and discontinuing the anesthesia. Trichloroethylene must not be given by rebreathing circuits using soda lime, because highly toxic gases may result. Its safety for use in early pregnancy has not been documented. It is contraindicated in severe cardiac disease of any kind, eclampsia, or preeclampsia and should not be combined with epinephrine.

tricho-. See **trichi-.**

trichobasalioma hyalinicum. See **cylindroma,** def. 2.

trichoepithelioma /trik′ō·ep′ithē′lē·ō′mə/, *pl.* **trichoepitheliomas, trichoepitheliomata** [Gk, *thrix* + *epi*, above, *thele* nipple, *oma* tumor], a cutaneous tumor derived from the basal cells of the follicles of fine body hair. One form of trichoepithelioma is an inherited condition and usually occurs as multiple growths. Also called **acanthoma adenoides cysticum, epithelioma adenoides cysticum.**

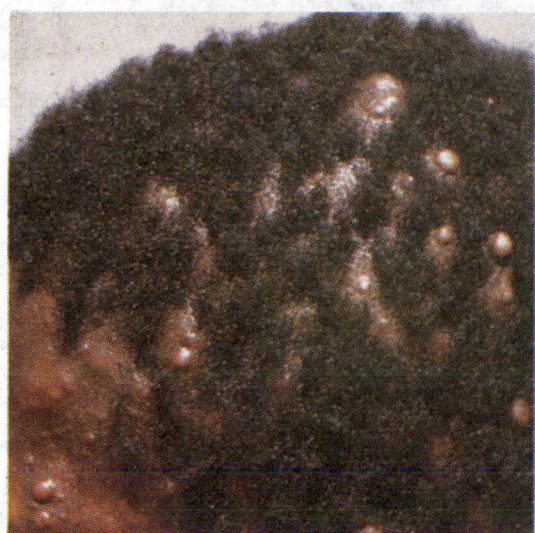

Trichoepithelioma
(McKee, 1993/Courtesy Dr. D McGibbon/
St. Thomas Hospital, London)

trichoid /trik′oid/, resembling a hair.

trichologia /trik′əlō′jē·ə/ [Gk, *thrix* + *legein*, to pull], an abnormal condition in which a person pulls out his or her own hair, usually seen only in delirium.

trichomatous /trikom′ətəs/ [Gk, *trichoma*, hairy, growth], **1.** pertaining to an introversion of the margin of the eyelid. **2.** pertaining to matted hair or ingrowing hair.

trichomonacide /trik′ōmon′əsīd/ [Gk, *thrix* + *monas*, unit; L, *caedere*, to kill], an agent destructive to *Trichomonas vaginalis*, a parasitic protozoan flagellate that causes a refractory type of vaginitis, cystitis, and urethritis. Metronidazole is used in the treatment of women with trichomoniasis and their asymptomatic partners. **—trichomonacidal,** *adj.*

Trichomonas vaginalis /trik′əmon′əs/ [Gk, *thrix*, *monas* + L, *vagina*, sheath], a motile protozoan parasite that causes vaginitis with a copious malodorous discharge and pruritus. See also **trichomoniasis.**

trichomoniasis /trik′əmənī′əsis/ [Gk, *thrix*, *monas* + *osis*, condition], a vaginal infection caused by the protozoan *Trichomonas vaginalis*, characterized by itching, burning, and frothy, pale yellow to green, malodorous vaginal discharge. With chronic infection all symptoms may disappear, although the organisms are still present. In men, infection is usually asymptomatic but may be evidenced by a persistent or recurrent urethritis. Infection is transmitted by sexual intercourse, rarely by moist washcloths, or, in newborns, by passage through the birth canal. Diagnosis is by microscopic examination of fresh vaginal secretions. Treatment is by oral metronidazole. Reinfection is common if sexual partners are not treated simultaneously.

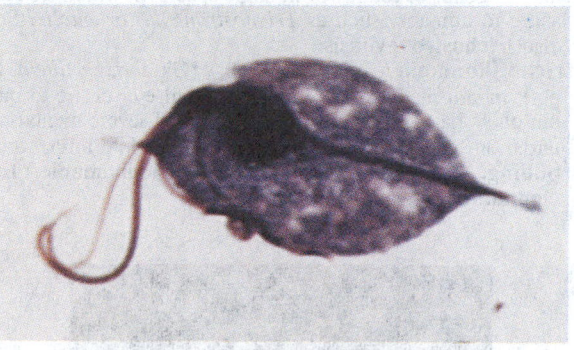

***Trichomonas vaginalis* trophozite**
(Murray, 1990/Reproduced with permission from LR Ash and TC Orihel: Atlas of human parasitology, ed 2, 1984 by the American Society of Clinical Pathologists Press, Chicago)

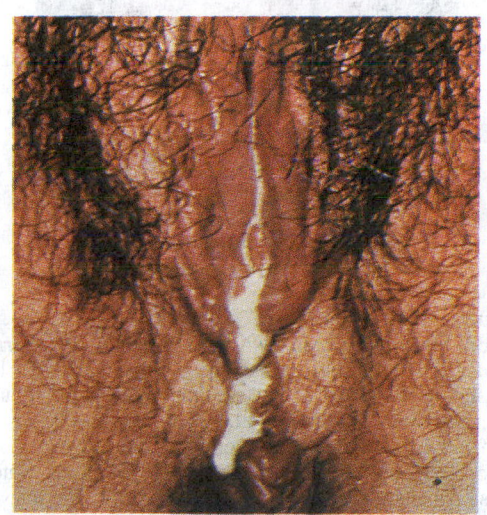

Trichomoniasis *(Zitelli, 1992/Courtesy Dr. E Wald)*

tricopathy /trikop′əthē/ [Gk, *thrix*, hair + *pathos*, disease], any disease condition involving the hair.

trichophytic granuloma. See **Majocchi's granuloma.**

Trichophyton /trikof′iton/ [Gk, *thrix* + *phyton*, plant], a genus of fungi that infects skin, hair, and nails. See also **dermatomycosis, dermatophyte.**

trichosis /trikō′sis/ [Gk, *thrix*, hair + *osis*, condition], any abnormal condition of hair growth, including alopecia, excessive female hair growth, or abnormal hair color.

-trichosis. See **trichi-.**

trichosporosis [Gk, *thrix*, hair + *spora*, seed + *osis*, condition], a fungus disease of the hair shaft, giving the hair a metallic appearance and caused by *Trichosporon*. Also called **piedra**.

trichostrongyliasis /trik'ōstron'jəlī'əsis/ [Gk, *thrix* + *strongylos*, round, *osis*, condition], infestation with *Trichostrongylus*, a genus of nematode worm. Also called **trichostrongylosis**. See also **nematode**.

Trichostrongylus /trik'ōstron'jiləs/ [Gk, *thrix* + *strongylos*], a genus of roundworm, some species of which are parasitic to humans, such as *Trichostrongylus orientalis*. See also **trichostrongyliasis**.

trichotillomania /trik'ōtil'ōmā'nē·ə/ [Gk, *thrix* + *tillein*, to pull, *mania* madness], a morbid impulse or desire to pull out one's hair, frequently seen in cases of severe mental retardation and delirium. Also called **trichomania, hair pulling**. See also **trichologia**. −**trichotillomanic, trichomanic**, *adj*.

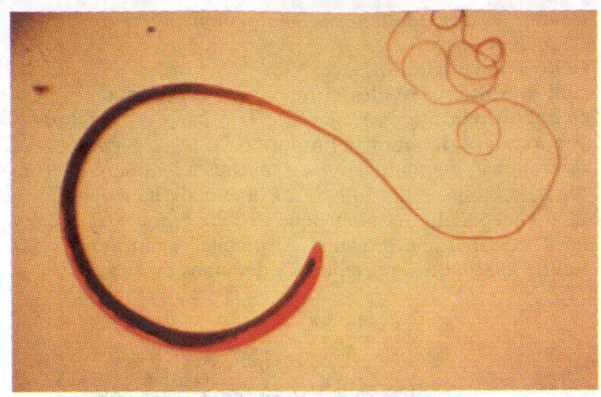

Trichuris trichiura (Hart, 1992/Courtesy Liverpool School of Tropical Medicine)

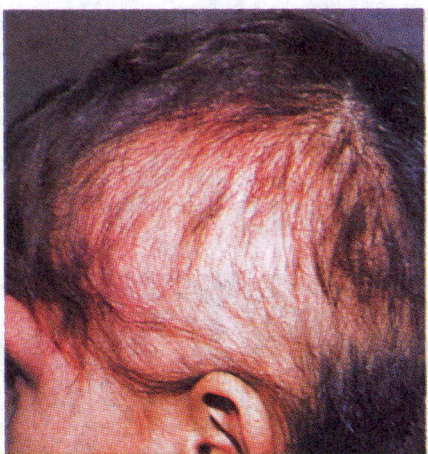

Trichotillomania (Habif, 1990)

trichuriasis /trik'yŏŏrī'əsis/ [Gk, *thrix* + *oura*, tail, *osis*, condition], infestation with the roundworm *Trichuris trichiura*. The condition is usually asymptomatic, but heavy infestation may cause nausea, abdominal pain, diarrhea, and, occasionally, anemia and rectal prolapse. It is common in tropical areas with poor sanitation. Eggs are passed in feces. Contamination of the hands, food, and water results in ingestion of the eggs, which hatch in the intestines, where the adult worms embed two thirds of their length in the intestinal mucosa. The worms may live 15 to 20 years. Treatment is with mebendazole; prevention includes proper disposal of feces and good personal hygiene. Also called **trichiuriasis** /trik'ē-/.

Trichuris /trikyŏŏr'is/ [Gk, *thrix* + *oura*] a genus of parasitic roundworms of which the species *Trichuris trichiura* infects the intestinal tract. Adult worms, which are 30 to 50 mm long, resemble a whip, with a threadlike anterior and a thicker posterior. Also called **whipworm**. See also **trichuriasis**.

trick knee. See **locked knee**.

tricrotic pulse /trīkrot'ik/, an abnormal pulse that has three peaks of elevation on a sphygmogram, representing the pressure wave from the heart in systole followed by two pressure waves in diastole.

tricuspal. See **tricuspid tooth**.

tricuspid /trīkus'pid/ [Gk, *tri*, three; L, *cuspis*, point], **1.** of or pertaining to three points or cusps. **2.** of or pertaining to the tricuspid valve of the heart.

tricuspid area [Gk, *treis*, three; L, *cuspis*, point], a region of the chest, near the left lower sternum and opposite the fourth and fifth costal cartilages, where sounds of the tricuspid heart valve are best heard by auscultation. Also called **tricuspid-valve area**.

tricuspid atresia, a congenital cardiac anomaly characterized by the absence of the tricuspid valve so that there is no opening between the right atrium and right ventricle. Other cardiac defects, such as atrial and ventricular septal defects, are usually present, allowing some shunting of blood into the lungs. Clinical manifestations include severe cyanosis, dyspnea, anoxia, and signs of right-sided heart failure. Definitive diagnosis is made by cardiac catheterization, although radiographic studies usually reveal a small, underdeveloped right ventricle and large atria, giving the heart a round shape, and decreased pulmonary vascularity. Immediate palliative treatment includes pulmonary artery anastomoses to increase blood flow to the lungs and atrial septostomy if the atrial septal defect is small. Total corrective surgery has been successful in a limited number of older children.

tricuspid murmur [Gk, *treis*, three; L, *cuspis* point + *murmur*, humming], one of the heart murmurs caused by a defective tricuspid valve. The tricuspid diastolic and systolic murmurs resemble mitral valve diastolic and systolic murmurs.

tricuspid stenosis, narrowing or stricture of the tricuspid valve. It is relatively uncommon and usually associated with lesions of other valves caused by rheumatic fever. Clinical characteristics include diastolic pressure gradient between the right atrium and ventricle, jugular vein distention, pulmonary congestion, and in severe cases, hepatic congestion and splenomegaly.

tricuspid tooth [Gk, *treis*, three; L, *cuspis*, point; AS, *toth*], a tooth with three cusps, rare in humans. Also called **tricuspal**.

tricuspid valve, a valve with three main cusps situated between the right atrium and the right ventricle of the heart. The cusps of the tricuspid valve include the ventral, dorsal, and medial cusps. The ventral cusp is the largest, the pos-

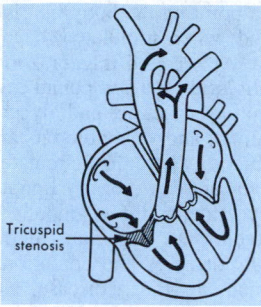

Tricuspid stenosis

terior cusp the smallest. The cusps are composed of strong fibrous tissue and are anchored to the papillary muscles of the right ventricle by several tendons. As the right and the left ventricles relax during the diastole phase of the heart beat, the tricuspid valve opens, allowing blood to flow into the ventricle. In the systole phase of the heartbeat both blood-filled ventricles contract, pumping out their contents, while the tricuspid and mitral valves close to prevent any backflow. Also called **right atrioventricular valve.** Compare **aortic valve, mitral valve, pulmonary valve, semilunar valve.** See also **atrioventricular valve, heart valve.**

tricuspid-valve area.   See **tricuspid area.**

tricyclic antidepressant.   See **antidepressant.**

tricyclic compound /trīsik′lik/ [Gk, *tri* + *kyklos,* circle; L, *componere,* to put together], a chemical substance containing three rings in the molecular structure, especially a tricyclic antidepressant drug, such as imipramine, amitriptyline, doxepin, and nortriptyline, used in the treatment of reactive or endogenous depression. These drugs also have anticonvulsant, antihistaminic, anticholinergic, hypotensive, and sedative effects. See also **antidepressant.**

trident /trī′dənt/ [Gk, *treis,* three; L, *dens,* tooth], a tooth with three points or cusps. Also called **tridentate.** See also **tricuspid.**

Tridesilon, a trademark for a glucocorticoid (desonide).

tridihexethyl chloride /trī′dīhek′səthil/, an anticholinergic.

■ INDICATIONS: It is prescribed in the treatment of GI muscle spasm and to reduce gastric secretion and GI motility.

■ CONTRAINDICATIONS: Narrow-angle glaucoma, asthma, obstruction of the genitourinary or GI tract, severe ulcerative colitis, or known hypersensitivity to this drug prohibits its use.

■ ADVERSE EFFECTS: Among the more serious adverse effects are blurred vision, tachycardia, dry mouth, decreased sweating, and hypersensitivity reactions. It may cause prostatic hypertrophy in elderly men.

Tridione, a trademark for an anticonvulsant (trimethadione).

trientine hydrochloride /trī·en′tēn/, an oral medication for treatment of an inherited defect in copper metabolism.

■ INDICATIONS: It is prescribed for the relief of symptoms of Wilson's disease.

■ CONTRAINDICATIONS: Known hypersensitivity to this drug prohibits its use.

■ ADVERSE EFFECTS: The most serious side effects are possible iron deficiency and hypersensitivity reactions.

triethanolamine polypeptide oleate-condensate /trī·eth′ənol′əmēn/, a ceruminolytic agent prescribed to reduce excessive earwax, used as a solution in propylene glycol. A possible serious adverse effect is severe contact dermatitis.

trifacial nerve.   See **trigeminal nerve.**

trifluoperazine hydrochloride /trī′flo͞o·ōper′əzēn/, a phenothiazine tranquilizer.

■ INDICATIONS: It is prescribed in the treatment of anxiety, schizophrenia, and other psychotic disorders, and as an antiemetic.

■ CONTRAINDICATIONS: Parkinson's disease, concurrent administration of central nervous system depressants, hepatic or renal dysfunction, severe hypotension, or known hypersensitivity to this drug prohibits its use.

■ ADVERSE EFFECTS: Among the more serious adverse effects are hypotension, hepatotoxicity, a variety of extrapyramidal reactions, blood dyscrasias, and hypersensitivity reactions.

trifluorothymidine /trīflo͞or′ōthī′mədēn/, an antiviral. Also called **trifluridine.**

■ INDICATIONS: It is prescribed in the treatment of keratoconjunctivitis, herpetic keratitis, and other forms of keratitis caused by herpes simplex virus.

■ CONTRAINDICATIONS: Known hypersensitivity to this drug prohibits its use. Ocular toxicity may result from continued use beyond 21 days.

■ ADVERSE EFFECTS: Among the more serious adverse effects are hypersensitivity reactions, stromal edema, and increased ocular pressure.

triflupromazine hydrochloride /trī′flupro̅′məzēn/, a phenothiazine tranquilizer.

■ INDICATIONS: It is prescribed in the treatment of severe agitation and other psychotic disorders and for the control of severe vomiting.

■ CONTRAINDICATIONS: Parkinson's disease, concurrent administration of central nervous system depressants, liver or renal dysfunction, severe hypotension, or known hypersensitivity to this drug or to other phenothiazine medications prohibits its use.

■ ADVERSE EFFECTS: Among the more serious adverse effects are hypotension, liver toxicity, a variety of extrapyramidal reactions, blood dyscrasias, and hypersensitivity reactions.

trifluridine.   See **trifluorothymidine.**

trifocal lens /trīfō′kəl/ [Gk, *treis,* three; L, *focus,* hearth + *lens,* lentil], an eyeglass lens ground for viewing objects at three different distances—near, intermediate, and far.

trifurcation /-furkā′shən/ [Gk, *treis,* three; L, *furca,* fork], pertaining to a vessel or other structure with three branches.

trigeminal /trījem′inəl/ [Gk, *treis,* three; L, *geminus,* twins], pertaining to the three-branch trigeminal (fifth cranial) nerve innervating the face, eyes, nose, mouth, and jaws.

trigeminal nerve [Gk, *tri* + geminus, twin], either of the largest pair of cranial nerves, essential for the act of chewing, general sensibility of the face, and muscular sensibility of the obliquus superior. The trigeminal nerves have sensory, motor, and intermediate roots and connect to three areas in the brain. Also called **fifth cranial nerve, nervus trigeminus, trifacial nerve.** (See Fig. p. 1590.)

trigeminal neuralgia, a neurologic condition of the trigeminal facial nerve, characterized by paroxysms of flashing, stablike pain radiating along the course of a branch of the nerve from the angle of the jaw. It is caused by degeneration of the nerve or by pressure on it. Any or all of the

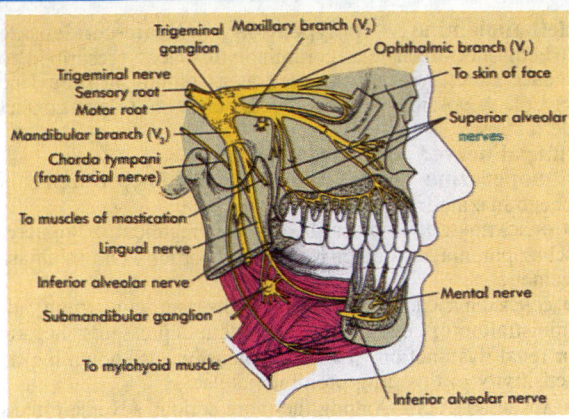

Trigeminal nerve
(Seeley, 1992/David J Mascaro & Associates)

three branches of the nerve may be affected. Neuralgia of the first branch results in pain around the eyes and over the forehead; of the second branch, in pain in the upper lip, nose, and cheek; of the third branch, in pain on the side of the tongue and the lower lip. The momentary bursts of pain recur in clusters lasting many seconds; paroxysmal episodes of the pains may last for hours. Also called **prosopalgia, tic douloureux.**

trigeminal pulse, an abnormal pulse in which every third beat is absent. See also **bigeminal pulse, trigeminy.**

trigeminy /trījem′inē/ [Gk, *tri* + L, *geminus*, twin], **1.** a grouping in threes. **2.** a cardiac dysrhythmia characterized by the occurrence of three heartbeats, two normal beats followed by an ectopic beat in a repeating pattern. **−trigeminal,** *adj.*

trigger [Du, *trekker*], a substance, object, or agent that initiates or stimulates an action.

triggered activity [D, *trekker* that which pulls; L, *activus*], rhythmic cardiac activity that results when a series of afterdepolarizations reach threshold potential.

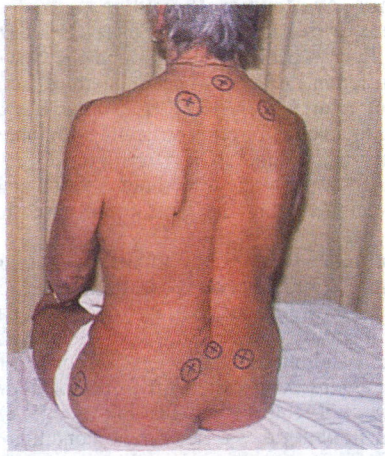

Trigger points in the cervical and lumbar regions
(Shipley, 1993)

trigger point, a point on the body that is particularly sensitive to touch and, when stimulated, becomes the site of a painful neuralgia. Also called **trigger zone.**

triglyceride /trīglis′ərīd/, a compound consisting of a fatty acid (oleic, palmitic, or stearic) and glycerol. Triglycerides make up most animal and vegetable fats and are the principal lipids in the blood, where they circulate, bound to a protein, forming high- and low-density lipoproteins. The total amount of triglyceride and the amount, proportion, and kinds of lipoproteins are important in the diagnosis and treatment of many diseases and conditions, including diabetes, hypertension, and heart disease. Normally the total amount of triglyceride in the blood does not exceed 200 mg to 300 mg/dl.

trigone /trī′gōn/ [Gk, *trigonos*, three-cornered, **1.** a triangle. **2.** the first three dominant cusps, considered collectively, of an upper molar.

trigone of the bladder. See **trigonum vesicae.**

trigonitis /trī′gənī′tis/, inflammation of the trigone of the bladder, which often accompanies urethritis.

trigonum vesicae /trīgō′nəm/, a triangular area of the bladder between the opening of the ureters and the orifice of the urethra. Also called **trigone of the bladder.**

trihexyphenidyl hydrochloride /trīhex′ifen′idil/, an anticholinergic agent.
■ INDICATIONS: It is prescribed in the treatment of Parkinson's disease and to control drug-induced extrapyramidal reactions.
■ CONTRAINDICATIONS: Narrow-angle glaucoma, asthma, obstruction of the genitourinary or GI tract, severe ulcerative colitis, or known hypersensitivity to this drug prohibits its use.
■ ADVERSE EFFECTS: Among the more serious adverse effects are blurred vision, central nervous system effects, tachycardia, dry mouth, decreased sweating, and hypersensitivity reactions.

trihybrid /trīhī′brid/ [Gk, *tri* + *hybrida*, mixed offspring], (in genetics) pertaining to or describing an individual, organism, or strain that is heterozygous for three specific traits, that is the offspring of parents differing in three specific gene pairs, or that is heterozygous for three particular characteristics or gene loci being followed.

trihybrid cross, (in genetics) the mating of two individuals, organisms, or strains that have different gene pairs that determine three specific traits or in which three particular characteristics or gene loci are being followed.

trihydric alcohol /trīhid′rik/, an alcohol containing three hydroxyl groups.

triiodothyronine (T₃) /trī′ī·ō′dōthī′rənēn/, a hormone that helps regulate growth and development, helps control metabolism and body temperature, and, by a negative-feedback system, acts to inhibit the secretion of thyrotropin by the pituitary. Triiodothyronine is produced mainly from the metabolism of thyroxine in the peripheral tissues but is also synthesized by and stored in the thyroid gland as an amino acid residue of the protein thyroglobulin. Triiodothyronine circulates in the plasma, where it is bound mainly to thyroxine-binding globulin and thyroxine-binding prealbumin, proteins that protect the hormone from metabolism and excretion during its half-life of 2 days or less before it is degraded in the liver. The hormone acts principally by complementing thyroxine in the control of protein synthesis. It is a component of various drugs, such as liotrix and liothyronine sodium, used in the treatment of hypothyroidism and simple goiter. Normal adult blood levels are 110 to 230 ng/dl. See also **thyroid hormone.**

Trilafon, a trademark for a phenothiazine tranquilizer (perphenazine).

trilaminar blastoderm /trīlam'inər/ [Gk, *tri* + L, *lamina,* plate; Gk, *blastos,* germ, *derma,* skin], the stage of embryonic development in which all three of the primary germ layers, the ectoderm, mesoderm, and entoderm, have formed. Compare **bilaminar blastoderm.**

trill [It, *trillare* to make a ringing sound], a vibratory, quavering, warbling sound, as produced by human voice, birds, insects, or musical instruments.

trilogy of Fallot /tril'əjē, falō'/ [Gk, *tri* + *logos,* word; Etienne-Louis A. Fallot, French physician, b. 1850], a congenital cardiac anomaly consisting of the combination of pulmonic stenosis, interatrial septal defect, and right ventricular hypertrophy. For discussion of diagnosis and treatment, see **tetralogy of Fallot.**

trilostane /tril'əstān/, a synthetic steroid that inhibits the synthesis of adrenal steroids.
■ INDICATIONS: It is prescribed for the treatment of Cushing's syndrome.
■ CONTRAINDICATIONS: Trilostane is contraindicated for pregnant women or for patients with severe kidney or liver impairment or adrenal insufficiency. Its use may result in adrenal cortical hypofunction, especially under conditions of surgical stress, trauma, acute illness, or concurrent use of aminoglutethimide or mitotane.
■ ADVERSE EFFECTS: Among adverse reactions of trilostane use are nausea, flatulence, abdominal cramps, diarrhea, bloating, headache, and burning of the oral or nasal membranes.

trimalleolar fracture. See **Cotton's fracture.**

trimeprazine tartrate /trīmep'rəzēn/, an antipruritic.
■ INDICATIONS: It is prescribed in the treatment of pruritus and hypersensitivity reactions of the skin.
■ CONTRAINDICATIONS: Coma, bone marrow depression, lactation, or known hypersensitivity to this drug prohibits its use. It is not given to children under 6 months of age or to patients receiving large amounts of central nervous system depressants.
■ ADVERSE EFFECTS: Among the more serious reactions are paradoxical excitement, parkinson-like problems, hepatitis, and GI disturbance.

trimester /trīmes'tər, trī'-/ [L, *trimestris,* three months], one of the three periods of approximately 3 months into which pregnancy is divided. The first trimester includes the time from the first day of the last menstrual period to the end of 12 weeks. The second trimester, closer to 4 months in length than 3, extends from the twelfth to the twenty-eighth week of gestation. The third trimester begins at the twenty-eighth week and extends to the time of delivery.

trimethadione /trī'methədī'ōn/, an anticonvulsant.
■ INDICATIONS: It is prescribed to prevent seizures in petit mal epilepsy, particularly seizures that are resistant to other therapies.
■ CONTRAINDICATIONS: Severe renal or hepatic impairment, blood dyscrasias, or known hypersensitivity to this drug prohibits its use.
■ ADVERSE EFFECTS: Among the more serious adverse reactions are exfoliative dermatitis, blood dyscrasias, and aplastic anemia. Sedation and hemeralopia may occur.

trimethaphan camsylate /trīmeth'əfan/, a ganglionic blocking agent.
■ INDICATIONS: It is prescribed to produce controlled hypo-

tension during surgery and to lower blood pressure in hypertensive emergencies.
■ CONTRAINDICATIONS: It is not used where hypotension places a patient in undue risk or when hypersensitivity to this drug prohibits its use.
■ ADVERSE EFFECTS: The most serious adverse reaction is severe hypotension.

trimethobenzamide hydrochloride /trīmeth'ōben'zəmid/, an antiemetic.
■ INDICATION: It is prescribed for the relief of nausea and vomiting.
■ CONTRAINDICATIONS: Reye's syndrome or known hypersensitivity to this drug prohibits its use.
■ ADVERSE EFFECTS: Among the most serious adverse reactions with high doses are drowsiness, diarrhea, allergic reactions, and extrapyramidal reactions. Adverse reactions are rare at usual dosages.

trimethoprim /trīmeth'əprim/, an antibacterial.
■ INDICATIONS: It is prescribed in the treatment of various infections, particularly of the urinary tract, middle ear, and bronchi.
■ CONTRAINDICATIONS: Known hypersensitivity to this drug prohibits its use. It should not be used to treat streptococcal pharyngitis.
■ ADVERSE EFFECTS: Among the more serious adverse reactions are blood dyscrasias and allergic, GI, and central nervous system disorders.

trimethoprim and sulfamethoxazole. See **sulfamethoxazole and trimethoprim.**

trimethylene. See **cyclopropane.**

trimipramine maleate /trimip'rəmēn/, an antidepressant.
■ INDICATIONS: It is prescribed in the treatment of anxiety, depression, and insomnia.
■ CONTRAINDICATIONS: Concomitant use of a monoamine oxidase inhibitor within 14 days or known hypersensitivity to this drug prohibits its use. It is not given during recovery from myocardial infarction or to schizophrenic patients. It is not recommended for children.
■ ADVERSE EFFECTS: Among the more serious adverse reactions are tachycardia, seizures, parkinsonism, blurred vision, hypotension, and aggravation of glaucoma.

Trimox, a trademark for an antibiotic (amoxicillin trihydrate).

Trimpex, a trademark for an antibacterial (trimethoprim).

Trinalin Retabs, a trademark for an antihistamine (azatadine maleate).

Trinsicon, a trademark for a hematinic fixed-combination drug containing iron, vitamin B_{12}, and intrinsic factor concentrate.

trioxsalen /trī·ok'sələn/, a melanizing agent.
■ INDICATIONS: It is prescribed to enhance pigmentation, for repigmentation of the skin in idiopathic vitiligo, and to increase tolerance to sunlight.
■ CONTRAINDICATIONS: Diseases associated with photosensitivity, such as porphyria, acute lupus erythematosus, or leukoderma of infectious origin, or the concomitant use of drugs having any photosensitizing activity prohibits its use.
■ ADVERSE EFFECTS: Among the most serious adverse reactions are severe burns from excessive exposure to ultraviolet light. Gastric irritation and nausea also may occur.

tripelennamine citrate. See **tripelennamine hydrochloride.**

tripelennamine hydrochloride /trī'pelen'əmēn/, an antihistamine.

- INDICATIONS: It is prescribed in the treatment of rhinitis and hypersensitivity reactions of the skin.
- CONTRAINDICATIONS: Asthma, glaucoma, difficulty in emptying the bladder, concomitant administration of a monoamine oxidase inhibitor, or known hypersensitivity to this drug prohibits its use. It is not given to premature or newborn infants or to lactating mothers.
- ADVERSE EFFECTS: Among the more serious adverse reactions are sedation, tachycardia, and GI upset.

triphasic /trīfā'zik/ [Gk, *treis*, three + *phasis*, appearance], having three phases or stages.

triple-dye treatment, a therapy for burns in which three dyes, 6% gentian violet, 1% brilliant green, and 0.1% acriflavin base, are applied.

triplegia /trīplē'jə/ [Gk, *treis*, three + *plege*, stroke], a condition of paralysis on one side of the body plus paralysis of an arm or leg on the opposite side.

triple lumen catheter [L, *triplus*, triple; L, *lumen*, light; Gk, *katheter*, a thing lowered into], any catheter with three separate passages. In a triple-lumen urinary catheter, one passage is for irrigation, one for drainage, and one for air.

triple point, a situation in which a given substance may exist in solid, liquid, and vapor forms at the same time. Every substance has a theoretical triple point, which depends on ideal conditions of temperature and pressure.

triple response, a triad of phenomena that occur in sequence after the intradermal injection of histamine. First, a red spot develops, spreading outward for a few millimeters, reaching its maximal size within 1 minute and then turning bluish. Next, a brighter red flush of color spreads slowly in an irregular flare around the original red spot. Finally, a wheal, filled with fluid, forms over the original spot. Also called **triple response of Lewis.**

triple sugar iron reaction, any one of several reactions seen in certain bacterial cultures growing on triple sugar iron agar, a culture medium used to aid in the identification of *Escherichia coli, Proteus, Salmonella, Shigella,* and other pathogenic enteric bacteria.

triple sulfonamides. See **trisulfapyrimidines.**

triplet /trip'lit/ [L, triplus], 1. any one of three offspring born of the same gestation period during a single pregnancy. See also **Hellin's law.** 2. (in genetics) the unit of three consecutive bases in one polynucleotide chain of DNA or RNA that codes for a specific amino acid. See also **codon, genetic code.**

triple X syndrome. See **XXX syndrome.**

triploid (3n) /trip'loid/ [L, *triplus + eidos*], 1. also **triploidic.** of or pertaining to an individual, organism, strain, or cell that has three complete sets of chromosomes, triple the normal haploid number characteristic of the species. In humans, the triploid number is 69, found in rare cases of aborted or stillborn fetuses. Of those triploid fetuses born alive, all are characterized by gross and multiple malformations; they live only for a few hours. 2. such an individual, organism, strain, or cell. Compare **diploid, haploid, tetraploid.** See also **polyploid.**

triploidy /trip'loidē/, the state or condition of having three complete sets of chromosomes.

tripod /trī'pod/ [Gk, *tri*, three + *pous*, foot], any object with three legs or three feet.

tripodial symmelia /trīpō'dē·əl/ [Gk, *tri*, three, *pous*, foot; *syn*, together, *melos*, limb], a fetal anomaly characterized by the fusion of the lower extremities and the presence of three feet.

triprolidine hydrochloride /trī·prol'idēn/, an antihistamine.

- INDICATIONS: It is prescribed in the treatment of a variety of hypersensitivity reactions, including rhinitis, skin rash, and pruritus.
- CONTRAINDICATIONS: Asthma or known hypersensitivity to this drug prohibits its use. It is not given to newborn infants or lactating mothers. Adverse reactions may occur in elderly patients.
- ADVERSE EFFECTS: Drowsiness, skin rash, hypersensitivity reactions, dry mouth, and tachycardia may occur.

tripsis /trip'sis/ [Gk rubbing], 1. massage. 2. the process of reducing the particle size of a substance by grinding it with a mortar and pestle. Also called **trituration.**

-tripsis, a combining form meaning 'to crush, break, or pulverize': *anatripsis, entripsis, syntripsis.*

-tripsy, a combining form meaning 'to crush, break, or pulverize': *basiotripsy, lithotripsy, sarcotripsy.*

trisaccharide /trīsak'ərīd/ [Gk, *treis*, three + *sakcharon*, sugar], a carbohydrate composed of three monosaccharide units linked together.

trismus /triz'məs/ [Gk, *trismos* gnashing], a prolonged tonic spasm of the muscles of the jaw. Also called (*informal*) **lockjaw.** See also **tetanus.**

trisomy /trī'səmē/ [Gk, *tri + soma*, body], a chromosomal aberration characterized by the presence of one more than the normal number of chromosomes in a diploid complement; in humans the trisomic cell contains 47 chromosomes and is designated $2n + 1$. The additional member can join any of the normal homologous pairs, although most human trisomies involve the small chromosomes, such as those in the E or G group, or the sex chromosomes. Partial trisomy occurs when only a portion of a chromosome attaches to another. In genetic nomenclature, trisomies are indicated by the exact chromosome or karyotypic group in which the addition is made, such as trisomy 13 or trisomy D. Also called **trisomia.** Compare **monosomy.** See also **aneuploidy, multipolar mitosis, trisomy syndrome.** –**trisomic,** *adj.*

trisomy C syndrome. See **trisomy 8.**

trisomy D syndrome. See **trisomy 13.**

trisomy E syndrome. See **trisomy 18.**

trisomy G syndrome. See **Down syndrome.**

trisomy 8, a congenital condition associated with the presence of an extra chromosome 8 within the C group. Those with the condition are slender and of normal height and have a large asymmetric head, prominent forehead, deep-set eyes, low-set prominent ears, and thick lips. There is mild to severe mental and motor retardation, often with delayed and poorly articulated speech. Skeletal anomalies and joint limitation, especially camptodactyly, may occur, and there are unusually deep palmar and plantar creases, which are diagnostically significant. Most trisomy 8 individuals are mosaic, with no abnormal or only slight clinical manifestations, or they are only partially trisomic, with part of the extra chromosome 8 missing, and show varying degrees of the clinical symptoms. In general, trisomy 8 is a less severe condition than other trisomies, especially trisomy 13 and trisomy 18, so that the mortality rate is low. Also called **trisomy C syndrome.**

trisomy 13, a congenital condition caused by the presence of an extra chromosome in the D group, predominantly chromosome 13, although in rare instances chromosome 14 or 15. It occurs in approximately 1 in 5000 births and is characterized by multiple midline anomalies and central nervous system defects, including holoprosencephaly, microcephaly, myelomeningocele, microphthalmos, and cleft lip and palate. There are also severe mental retardation, polydactyly, deafness, convulsions, and abnormalities of the heart, viscera, and genitalia. Most infants with the condition are severely affected and do not survive beyond the first 6 months of life. The symptom combination of cleft lip/palate, polydactylism, and microcephaly is sometimes identified as the triad. Also called **Patau's syndrome, trisomy D syndrome, trisomy 13-15.**

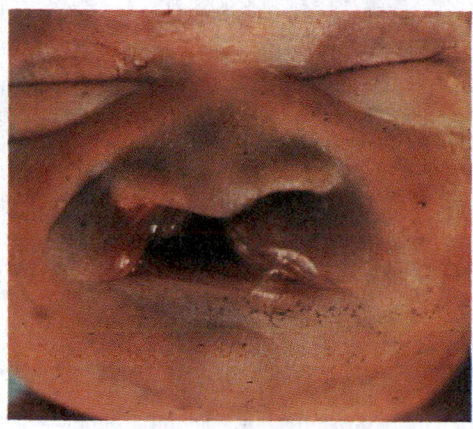

Trisomy 13: midline defect
(Zitelli, 1992/Courtesy Dr. T Kelly,
University of Virginia Medical Center, Charlottesville, Virginia)

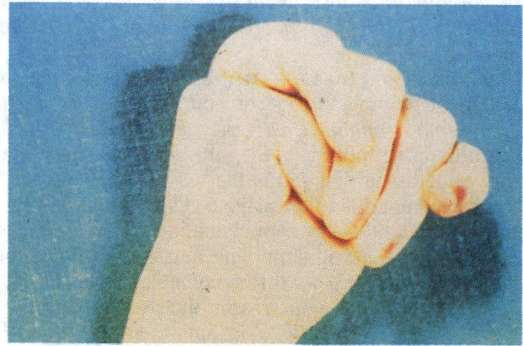

Trisomy 18: clenched hand showing typical pattern of overlapping fingers
(Zitelli, 1992)

trisomy 18, a congenital condition caused by the presence of an extra chromosome 18, characterized by severe mental retardation and multiple deformities. Among the most common defects are scaphocephaly or other skull abnormalities,

micrognathia, abnormal facies with low-set malformed ears and prominent occiput, cleft lip and palate, clenched fists with overlapping fingers, especially the index over the third finger, clubfeet, and syndactyly. Ventricular septal defect, patent ductus arteriosus, atrial septal defect, and renal anomalies are also common. The condition occurs in about 1 in 3000 births and predominantly in females, according to a 3:1 sex ratio, and survival for more than a few months is rare. Also called **Edwards' syndrome, trisomy E syndrome, trisomy 16-18.**

trisomy 21. See **Down syndrome.**

trisomy 22, a congenital condition caused by the presence of an extra chromosome 22 in the G group, characterized by psychomotor retardation and various developmental anomalies. Common defects include microcephaly, micrognathia, hypotonia, hypertelorism, abnormal ears with preauricular tags or fistulas, and congenital heart disease. In partial trisomy 22, the extra chromosome is much smaller than the normal pair and causes coloboma of the iris, anal atresia, or both, as well as various other defects. See also **cat-eye syndrome.**

trisomy syndrome, any condition caused by the addition of an extra member to a normal pair of homologous autosomes or to the sex chromosomes or by the translocation of a portion of one chromosome to another. Most trisomies occur as a result of complete or partial nondisjunction of the chromosomes during cell division. The more severe conditions are related to trisomies of the autosomes rather than the sex chromosomes. The most common trisomy syndromes with clearly established clinical manifestations are trisomy 8, trisomy 13, trisomy 18, trisomy 21, and trisomy 22. See also **trisomy.**

Trisoralen, a trademark for a pigmentation agent (trioxsalen).

trisulfapyrimidines /trīsul'fəpirim'idīnz/, three antibacterials in combination (sulfadiazine, sulfamerazine, and sulfamethazine), rarely prescribed today.

tritium (3H) /trit'ē·əm, trish'əm/ [Gk, *tritos,* third], the radioactive isotope of the hydrogen atom, used as a tracer; a β emitter. See also **deuterium.**

trituration. See **tripsis.**

trivalence /trīvā'ləns/ [Gk, *treis;* L, *valere,* to be worth], a triple state, usually a designation of three electrons in the outer orbit of an atom or an ability of a group of atoms to replace three monovalent elements in a compound.

trivalent /trīvā'lənt/ [Gk, *treis;* L, *valere,* to be worth], **1.** pertaining to an atom or group of atoms with the capability of bonding with or replacing three monovalent elements. **2.** designating a vaccine that can prevent diseases or conditions.

Tri-Vi-Flor, a trademark for an oral pediatric fixed-combination drug containing sodium fluoride and vitamins A, C, and D.

tRNA, abbreviation for **transfer RNA.**

Trobicin, a trademark for an antibacterial (spectinomycin hydrochloride).

trocar /trō'kär/ [Fr, *trois,* three, *carres,* sides], a sharp, pointed rod that fits inside a tube. It is used to pierce the skin and the wall of a cavity or canal in the body to aspirate fluids, to instill a medication or solution, or to guide the placement of a soft catheter. The trocar is usually removed, and the catheter, tube, or instrument is left in place. See also **cannula.**

trochanter /trōkan'tər/ [Gk, runner], one of the two bony projections on the proximal end of the femur that serve as the point of attachment of various muscles. The two protuberances are the greater trochanter and the lesser trochanter.

trochanter major [Gk, *trochanter*, runner; L, *major*, great], a large projection from the proximal end of the shaft of the femur. It is a point of attachment for the gluteus minimus and gluteus medius muscles. Also called **greater trochanter**.

trochanter minor [Gk, *trochanter*, runner; L, *minor*, less], a bony prominence on the shaft of the femur, just below the neck. It is the site of insertion of the psoas major muscle. Also called **lesser trochanter**.

troche /trō'kē/ [Gk, *trochos*, lozenge], a small oval, round, or oblong tablet containing a medicinal agent incorporated in a flavored, sweetened mucilage or fruit base that dissolves in the mouth, releasing the drug. Also called **lozenge, rotula, trochiscus**.

trochlea /trok'lē·ə/, a pulley-shaped part or structure. **–trochlear**, *adj.*

trochlear /trok'lē·ər/ [L, *trochlea*, pulley], 1. pertaining to a trochlea or something that is pulley-shaped. 2. relating to the trochlear, or fourth cranial, nerve.

trochlear nerve [L, *trochlea*, pulley; *nervus*, nerve], either of the smallest pair of cranial nerves, essential for eye movement and eye muscle sensibility. The trochlear nerves branch to supply the superior oblique muscle and communicate with the ophthalmic division of the trigeminal nerve, connecting with two areas in the brain. Also called **fourth nerve, nervus trochlearis**.

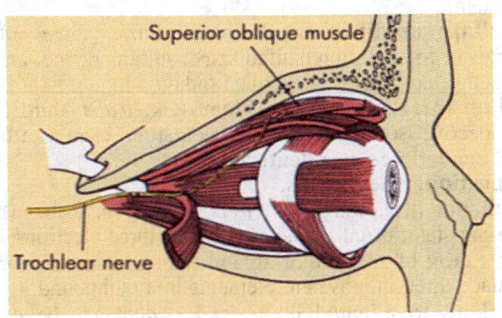

Trochlear nerve (Seeley, 1992/Michael Schenk)

trochlear notch of ulna, a large depression in the ulna, formed by the olecranon and coronoid processes, that articulates with the trochlea of the humerus.

trochoid joint. See **pivot joint**.

trolamine /trol'əmēn/, a contraction for *triethanolamine*.

troleandomycin /trol'ē·an'dōmī'sin/, a macrolide antibiotic.

■ INDICATIONS: It is prescribed in the treatment of certain infections, including pneumococcal pneumonia and group A streptococcal infections of the upper respiratory tract.

■ CONTRAINDICATION: Known hypersensitivity to this drug prohibits its use.

■ ADVERSE EFFECTS: Among the more serious adverse effects are GI disturbances, mild to severe allergic reactions (including anaphylaxis), and hepatotoxicity.

trombiculosis /trombik'yəlō'sis/ [Gk, *tromein*, to tremble; *osis*, condition], an infestation with mites of the genus *Trombicula*, some species of which carry scrub typhus.

-tron, a combining form meaning a '(specified) type of vacuum tube': *dynatron, magnetron, thyratron*.

Tronothane Hydrochloride, a trademark for a local anesthetic (pramoxine hydrochloride).

trop-, -trop, a combining form for atropine derivatives.

trop-, tropo-, a combining form meaning 'turn, turning' or 'tendency, affinity': *tropism, tropomyosin*. See also **tropho-**, with which this combining form is sometimes confused.

-tropal. See **-tropia**.

-trope, a suffix meaning 'influencing or influenced by': *gonadotrope, heliotrope, rheotrope*.

troph-. See **tropho-**.

-troph, 1. a suffix meaning 'that which nourishes an embryo': *embryotroph, hemotroph, histotroph*. 2. a suffix meaning an 'organism that gets nourishment from a (specified) source': *autotroph, metatroph, prototroph*.

trophectoderm. See **trophoblast**.

trophic /trof'ik/ [Gk, *trophe*, nutrition], pertaining to a nutritive effect on or quality of cellular activity.

-trophic, a combining form meaning 'referring to a type of nutrition or nutritional requirement': *chondrotrophic, lipotrophic, viscerotrophic*.

trophic action [Gk, *trophe*, nutrition; L, *agere*, to do], the stimulation of cell reproduction and enlargement, by nurturing and causing growth.

trophic fracture, a fracture resulting from the weakening of bone tissue caused by nutritional disturbances.

trophic hormones, hormones secreted by the adenohypophysis that stimulate target organs.

trophic ulcer, a decubitus ulcer caused by external trauma to a part of the body that is in poor condition resulting from disease, vascular insufficiency, or loss of afferent nerve fibers. Trophic ulcers may be painless or associated with severe causalgia. See also **decubitus ulcer**.

trophism /trof'izəm/ [Gk, *trophe*, nutrition], the influence of nourishment.

tropho- /trof'ə-/, trō'fə-/, **troph-,** a combining form meaning 'pertaining to food or nourishment': *trophoblast, trophoedema, trophoneurosis*. See also **trop-**.

trophoblast /trof'əblast'/ [Gk, *trophe* + *blastos* germ], the layer of tissue that forms the wall of the blastocyst of placental mammals in the early stages of embryonic development. It functions in the implantation of the blastocyst in the uterine wall and in supplying nutrients to the embryo. At implantation the cells differentiate into two layers, the inner cytotrophoblast, which forms the chorion, and the syncytiotrophoblast, which develops into the outer layer of the placenta. Also called **trophectoderm. –trophoblastic,** *adj.*

trophoblastic cancer /-blas'tik/, a malignant neoplastic disease of the uterus derived from chorionic epithelium, characterized by the production of high levels of human chorionic gonadotropin (HCG). The tumor may be an invasive hydatid mole (chorioadenoma destruens) formed by grossly enlarged, vesicular chorionic villi or a malignant uterine choriocarcinoma that arises from nonvillous chorionic epithelium. One half of the cases of choriocarcinoma follow a molar pregnancy, 25% an abortion, 22.5% a normal pregnancy, and 2.5% an ectopic pregnancy. A hydatid mole invades the myometrium and often forms extrauterine nodules that may spread to distant sites. Choriocarcinoma forms a dark red, hemorrhagic, nodular tumor on or in the uterine wall and metastasizes early in its course to the lungs, brain, liver, bones, vagina, or vulva. Initial symptoms are vaginal bleeding and a profuse, foul-smelling discharge; a persistent cough or hemoptysis signals pulmonary involvement. As the disease progresses, there may be frequent hemorrhage, weakness, and emaciation. Diagnostic measures include serial assays to determine whether the HCG level in the blood is elevated and histologic examination of specimens obtained by curettage. Hysterectomy is indicated in most cases, but surgery does not eliminate the possibility of a recurrence. Chemotherapy is effective in curing a large percentage of patients with trophoblastic tumors. Single-agent chemotherapy with methotrexate or actinomycin D is recommended for low-risk patients, those with disease of less than 4 months' duration, and those with lung or vaginal metastases. Treatment of high-risk patients with more prolonged disease and liver or brain metastases is usually individualized but may include radiotherapy and a combination of methotrexate, actinomycin D, and chlorambucil. Also called **trophoblastic disease.** See also **choriocarcinoma, hydatid mole.**

trophotropic /trof′ətrop′ik/ [Gk, *trophe* + *trepein*, to turn], pertaining to a combination of parasympathetic nervous system activity, somatic muscle relaxation, and cortical beta rhythm synchronization, such as in a resting or sleep state.

trophozoite /trof′əzō′it/ [Gk, *trophe* + *zoon*, animal], an immature ameboid protozoon. Diseases in which trophozoites may be isolated by bacteriologic studies include amebic dysentery, malaria, and trichomonas vaginitis. When fully developed, a trophozoite may be identified as a schizont.

-trophy, -trophia, a combining form meaning a 'condition of nutrition or growth': *cyotrophy, embryotrophy, lipotrophy.*

-tropia, -tropic, -tropal, -tropous, 1. a suffix meaning a 'turn or deviation from normal': *anatropic, hemitropic, stereotropic.* **2.** a combining form meaning a 'tendency to have an influence on, or be influenced by': *corticotropic, pancreatropic, radiotropic.*

tropical acne /trop′ikəl/, a form of acne that is caused or aggravated by high temperature and humidity. It is characterized by large nodules or pustules on the neck, back, upper arms, and buttocks.

tropical medicine [Gk, *tropikos*, of the solstice; L, *medicina*], the branch of medicine concerned with the diagnosis and treatment of diseases commonly occurring in tropic and subtropic regions of the world, generally between 30 degrees north and south of the equator.

tropical sore. See **oriental sore.**

tropical sprue, a malabsorption syndrome of unknown cause that is endemic in the tropics and subtropics. It is characterized by abnormalities in the mucosa of the small intestine resulting in protein malnutrition and multiple nutritional deficiencies, often complicated by severe infection. Symptoms include diarrhea, anorexia, and weight loss. Megaloblastic anemia may result from folic acid and vitamin B_{12} deficiency. Treatment includes administration of antibiotics, particularly tetracycline, folic acid, iron, calcium, and vita-

mins A, D, K, and B complex group, as well as a balanced diet high in protein and normal in fat content. See also **nontropic sprue.**

tropical typhus. See **scrub typhus.**

-tropin. a suffix referring to the stimulating effect of a hormone or other substance on a target organ or system: *somatotropin.*

-tropism. See **-tropy.**

-tropo. See **-trop.**

tropocollagen /trop′əkol′əjən/ [Gk, *trepein*, to turn, *kolla*, glue, *genein*, to produce], fundamental units of collagen fibrils obtained by prolonged extraction of insoluble collagen with dilute acid.

tropomyosin /trop′əmī′əsin/ [Gk, *trepein* + *mys*, muscle], a protein component of sarcomere filaments, which, together with troponin, regulates interactions of actin and myosin in muscle contractions.

troponin /trō′pənin/ [Gk, *trepein*, to turn], a protein in the myocardial cell ultrastructure that modulates the interaction between actin and myosin molecules. See also **tropomyosin.**

-tropous. See **-tropia.**

-tropy, -tropism, a combining form meaning 'influenced by or having an affinity for' something specified: *allotropy, ergotropy, syntropy.*

Trousseau's sign /trōōsōz′/ [Armand Trousseau, French physician, b. 1801; L, *signum*, mark], a test for latent tetany in which carpal spasm is induced by inflating a sphygmomanometer cuff on the upper arm to a pressure exceeding systolic blood pressure for 3 minutes. A positive test may be seen in hypocalcemia and hypomagnesemia. (See Fig. p. 1596.)

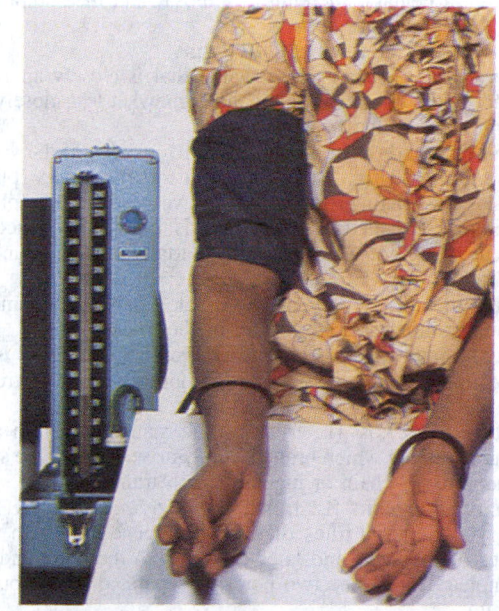

Trousseau's sign *(Forbes, 1993)*

Trp, abbreviation for **tryptophan.**

true ankylosis [ME, *treue*, faith; Gk, *agklosis*, joint stiffness], an abnormal fusion or union of the separate bones that usually form a joint.

true birth rate [AS, *trywe;* ME, *burthe;* L, *reri,* to calculate], the ratio of total births to the total female population of childbearing age, between 15 and 45 years of age. Compare **birth rate, crude birth rate, refined birth rate.**

true chondroma. See **enchondroma.**

true conjugate, a radiographic measurement of the distance from the upper margin of the symphysis pubis to the sacral promontory. It is usually 1.5 to 2.0 cm less than the diagonal conjugate. See also **conjugate.**

true denticle, a calcified body, composed of irregular dentin, found in the pulp chamber of a tooth.

true diverticulum [ME, *treue,* faith; L, *diverticulare,* to turn aside], diverticula that include all the same tissue layers as the organ from which it originates.

true dwarf. See **primordial dwarf.**

true glottis. See **glottis.**

true hermaphroditism [ME, *treue,* faith; Gk, *Hermaphroditos,* son of Hermes and Aphrodite], a condition in which an individual is born with both male and female gonads.

true labor, uterine contractions that result in a change in the cervix and birth of an infant.

true neuroma, any neoplasm composed of nerve tissue.

true oxygen, the calculated concentration as either a percentage or a fraction that when multiplied by the expiratory minute volume at STPD gives oxygen uptake.

true pelvis. See **pelvis.**

true rib. See **rib.**

true suture, an immovable fibrous joint of the skull in which the edges of bones interlock along a series of processes and indentations. The three kinds of true sutures are the sutura dentata, the sutura limbosa, and the sutura serrata. Compare **false suture.**

true twins. See **monozygotic twins.**

true value, (in statistics) a value that is closely approximated by the definitive value and somewhat less closely by the reference value.

true vocal cords [ME, *treue,* faith; L, *vocalis,* of the voice; Gk, *chorde,* string], the vocal folds of the larynx (plicae vocales), as distinguished from the vestibular folds (plicae vestibulares), called false vocal cords. See also **vocal cord.**

truncal /trung′kəl/ [L, *truncus*], pertaining to the trunk of the body.

truncal ataxia. a loss of coordinated muscle movements for maintaining normal posture of the trunk.

truncal obesity, obesity that preferentially affects or is located in the trunk of the body, as opposed to the extremities.

truncus /trung′kəs/ [L, trunk], the main stem of an anatomic part from which branches may arise, such as the sympathetic nerve chain or jugular lymph trunk.

truncus arteriosus [L, trunk; Gk, *arteria,* air pipe], the embryonic arterial trunk that initially opens from both ventricles of the heart and later divides into the aorta and the pulmonary trunk, the two portions separated by the bulbar septum.

truncus brachiocephalicus, a branch of the aorta that divides into the right common carotid and right subclavian arteries.

trunk balance, the ability to maintain postural control of the trunk, including the shifting and bearing of weight on each side so as to free an extremity for a particular function, such as reaching and grasping. Weight shifting can be anterior, posterior, lateral, or diagonal and involve righting, equilibrium, and protective reactions. Head and neck control allows for dissociation of the shoulder and pelvic girdles from the trunk.

trunk incurvation reflex. See **Galant reflex.**

truss [Fr, *trousser,* to pack up], an apparatus worn to prevent or retard the herniation of the intestines or other organ through an opening in the abdominal wall.

trust [ME, protection], a risk-taking process whereby an individual's situation depends on the future behavior of another person.

truth [AS, *treowo*], a rule or statement that conforms to fact or reality.

truth serum, a common name for any of several sedatives, such as the short-acting barbiturates, that have been administered intravenously in subjects to elicit information that may have been repressed. It has been used successfully in helping to identify amnesia victims. See also **narcotherapy**.

Trypanosoma /trip′ənōsō′mə/ [Gk, *trypanon,* borer, *soma,* body], a genus of parasitic organisms, several species of which can cause significant diseases in humans. Most *Trypanosoma* organisms live part of their life cycle in insects and are transmitted to humans by insect bites. See also **trypanosome, trypanosomiasis.**

Trypanosoma brucei gambiense. See **Gambian trypanosomiasis.**

Trypanosoma brucei rhodesiense. See **Rhodesian trypanosomiasis.**

Trypanosoma cruzi. See **Chagas' disease.**

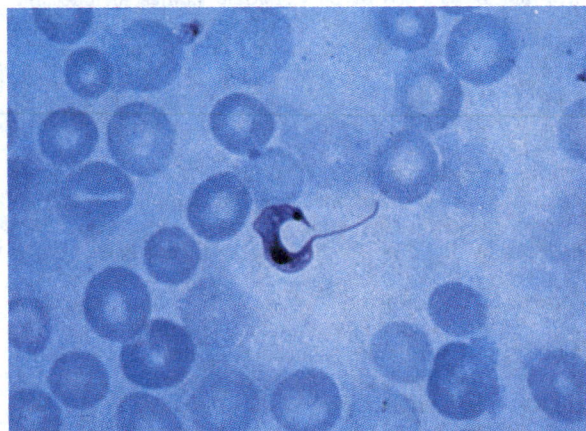

Trypanosoma cruzi trypomastigote (Baron, 1990)

trypanosomal infection. See **trypanosomiasis.**

trypanosome /trip′ənōsōm′, tripan′-/, any organism of the genus *Trypanosoma*. See also **trypanosomiasis. −trypanosomal,** *adj.*

trypanosomiasis /trip′ənō′sōmī′əsis/ [Gk, *trypanon, soma* + *osis,* condition], an infection by an organism of the *Trypanosoma* genus. Kinds of trypanosomiasis are **African trypanosomiasis** and **Chagas' disease.**

trypanosomicide /trip′ənōsō′misīd/ [Gk, *trypanon, soma* + L, *caedere,* to kill], a drug destructive to trypanosomes, especially the species of the protozoan parasite transmitted to humans by various insect vectors common in Africa and Central and South America. Various arsenic preparations are used to treat African sleeping sickness, caused by *Trypanosoma gambiense* and *T. rhodesiense,* and Chagas' disease, caused by *T. cruzi,* in the Americas. **–trypanosomicidal,** *adj.*

trypsin /trip′sin/ [Gk, *tripsis,* rubbing] a proteolytic digestive enzyme produced by the exocrine pancreas that catalyzes in the small intestine the breakdown of dietary proteins to peptones, peptides, and amino acids.

trypsin, crystallized, a proteolytic enzyme from the pancreas of the ox, *Bos taurus,* that has been used as a debriding agent for open wounds and ulcers.

trypsinogen /tripsin′əjən/ [Gk, *tripsis* + *genein,* to produce], the inactive precursor form of trypsin. Trypsinogen is secreted in pancreatic juice and converted to active trypsin through the action of enterokinase in the intestine. Also called **protrypsin.**

Tryptacin, a trademark for an amino acid (L-tryptophan), used as an antidepressant and to induce sleep.

tryptases. See **proteinase.**

tryptophan (Trp) /trip′təfan/ an amino acid essential for normal growth in infants and for nitrogen balance in adults. Tryptophan is the precursor of several substances, including serotonin and niacin. About 50% of the daily requirement of tryptophan is provided through the metabolism of niacin. The rest is derived from dietary protein, especially legumes, grains, and seeds. See also **amino acid, protein.**

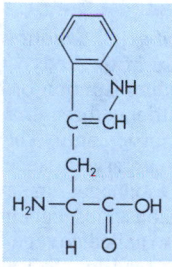

Chemical structure of tryptophan (Seeley, 1992)

TSEM, abbreviation for **transmission scanning electron microscopy.**

tsetse fly /tset′sē, tsē′tsē/ [Afr, *tsetse;* AS, *flyge*], a blood-sucking fly found in regions of Africa, mainly south of the Sahara desert. It is an insect of the *Glossina* genus and a secondary host of trypanosomes, which cause African sleeping sickness and other diseases in humans and domestic and wild animals. Also spelled **tzetze fly.** See also **trypanosomiasis.**

TSH, abbreviation for **thyroid stimulating hormone.**

TSH releasing factor. See **thyrotropin releasing hormone.**

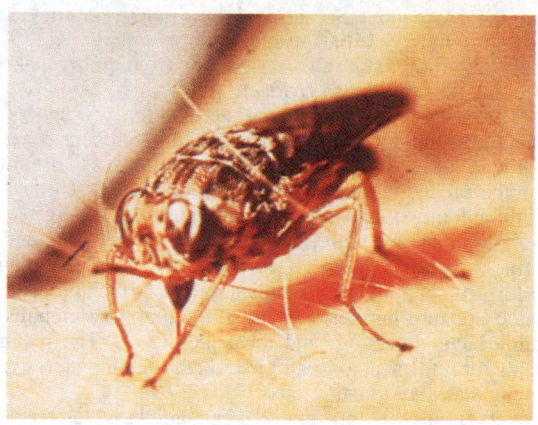

Tsetse fly (Muller, 1990/Courtesy Dr W Petana)

tsp., abbreviation for *teaspoon.*

TSS, abbreviation for **toxic shock syndrome.**

TSTA, abbreviation for *tumor-specific transplantation antigen.*

tsutsugamushi disease. See **scrub typhus.**

t test, a statistic test used to determine whether there are differences between two means or between a target value and a calculated mean.

TTP, abbreviation for **thrombotic thrombocytopenic purpura.**

T tube, 1. a tubular device in the shape of a T, inserted through the skin into a cavity or a wound, used for drainage. 2. an apparatus used to connect a source of humidified oxygen to the endotracheal tube so that a spirometer can be attached for the evaluation of tidal volume and appropriate removal of the endotracheal tube.

T tubule cholangiography, a type of biliary tract radiographic examination in which a water-soluble iodinated contrast medium is injected into the bile duct through an indwelling T-tube. The T-shaped rubber tube is inserted in the common bile duct as a routine postoperative procedure to provide drainage.

T tubule system, a system of invaginations along the surface of the myocardial cell membranes, providing an extension of the membrane into the cells. The system is believed to be a method of storing calcium ions and for the movement of substrates into the cells and the removal of metabolic end products from the cells.

T.U., 1. abbreviation for *toxic unit.* 2. abbreviation for *toxin unit.* 3. abbreviation for **tuberculin unit.**

tuaminoheptane /tōō·am′inōhep′tān/ an adrenergic vasoconstrictor.

tubal abortion /t(y)ōō′bəl/ [L, *tubus; ab,* from, *oriri,* to be born], a condition of pregnancy in which an embryo, ectopically implanted, is expelled from the uterine tube into the peritoneal cavity. Tubal abortion is often accompanied by significant internal bleeding, causing acute abdominal and pelvic pain, but may be asymptomatic, the products of conception being resorbed. Rarely, the conceptus reimplants on the peritoneum and continues growing to become an abdominal pregnancy. See also **abdominal pregnancy, ectopic pregnancy, tubal pregnancy.**

tubal dermoid cyst, a tumor derived from embryonal tissues that develops in an oviduct.

tubal ligation, one of several sterilization procedures in which both fallopian tubes are blocked to prevent conception from occurring. Spinal or local anesthesia is used unless the procedure accompanies major surgery. Through a small abdominal incision, the fallopian tubes are ligated in two places with suture, and the intervening segment is burnt, crushed, or excised. The procedure is less commonly performed vaginally. Complications of the procedure, which are rare but serious, include pulmonary embolism, hemorrhage, infection, and tubal pregnancy. The requirements for informed consent for sterilization procedures vary among states and institutions.

tubal pregnancy, an ectopic pregnancy in which the conceptus implants in the fallopian tube. Approximately 2% of all pregnancies are ectopic; of these, approximately 90% are tubal. Tubal pregnancy seldom occurs in primigravidas. The most important predisposing factor is prior tubal injury. Pelvic infection, scarring and adhesions from surgery, or IUD complications may result in damage that diminishes the motility of the tube. Transport of the ovum through the tube after fertilization is slowed, and implantation takes place before the conceptus reaches the uterine cavity. Most often the tube, which cannot long contain the growing fetus, ruptures, precipitating an intraperitoneal hemorrhage that, if not stopped, can lead rapidly to shock and, often, death. Some coceptuses apparently die and are resorbed in the tube. Diagnosis of tubal pregnancy is often difficult. With rupture of the fallopian tube, women commonly experience sudden sharp pain in one side of the lower abdomen, but signs and symptoms of tubal pregnancy are insidiously variable, and the classic triad of amenorrhea, pelvic pain, and a tender adnexal mass are present only 50% of the time. Recovery of blood from the cul-de-sac by means of culdocentesis is highly suggestive of a ruptured fallopian tube and tubal pregnancy; it requires immediate surgical exploration of the abdomen. Absence of blood on culdocentesis does not rule out the presence of an unruptured tubal pregnancy; laparotomy may be required, particularly if a woman's pregnancy test is positive, the pelvic findings are suggestive, and sonography of the pelvis cannot demonstrate an intrauterine pregnancy. Because of the lethal potential of an undiagnosed tubal pregnancy, women who report any of the characteristic symptoms early in their pregnancies, particularly during the time before the existence of a normal intrauterine pregnancy can be confirmed, must be considered susceptible. In women who have a history of prior pelvic disease and in those who have symptoms or signs of tubal pregnancy, emergency treatment requires an immediate intravenous infusion via a large-bore intravenous catheter, type and crossmatch of blood for blood replacement, and treatment of shock as necessary. Treatment is surgical and involves laparotomy, removal of the entire products of conception and any intraperitoneal blood present, and the removal or repair of the involved tube. Conditions that predispose to a first tubal pregnancy also predispose to a second; a woman who has had one tubal pregnancy has one chance in five of having another in a subsequent pregnancy. Depending on the location of the developing embryo, the condition is clas-

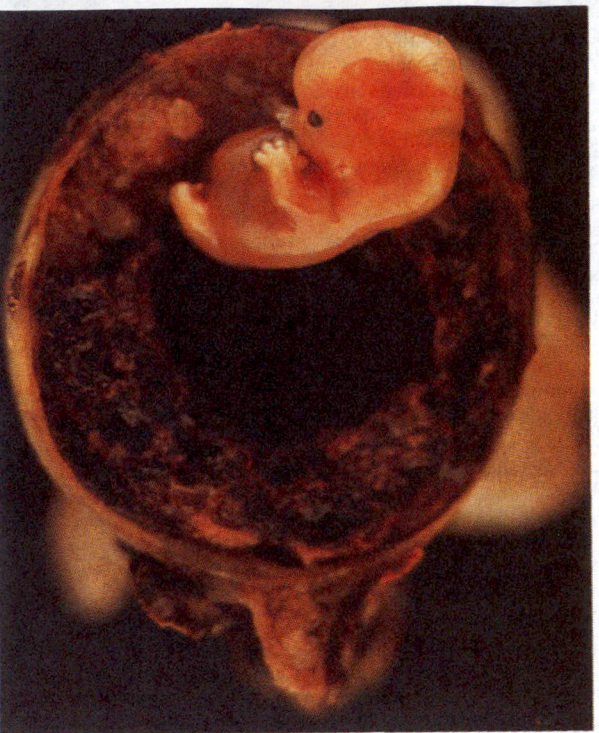

Tubal ectopic pregnancy (Fletcher, 1987)

sified as an ampullary, fimbrial, or interstitial tubal pregnancy.

tube /t(y)o͞ob/ [L, *tubus*], a hollow, cylindric piece of equipment or structure of the body.

tube feeding, the administration of nutritionally balanced liquefied foods or nutrients through a tube inserted into the stomach, duodenum, or jejunum. The procedure is used after mouth or gastric surgery, in severe burns, in paralysis or obstruction of the esophagus, in severe cases of anorexia nervosa, and for unconscious patients or those unable to chew or swallow. Also called **gavage feeding, jejunostomy feeding, nasogastric feeding.** See also **parenteral nutrition.**

tube feeding care, the nursing care and management of a patient receiving nourishment through a nasogastric tube.
■ METHOD: The tip of a nasogastric tube is lubricated with a water-soluble lubricant, inserted into a nostril, and rapidly advanced into the stomach as the patient, if conscious, is asked to swallow hard repeatedly. Correct placement of the tube may be determined by x-rays. Placement also may be checked by listening for a bubbling sound through a stethoscope placed over the stomach, as 5 ml of air is injected into the tube. If the patient coughs forcefully when 1 or 2 ml of water is injected into the tube, it is placed in the upper respiratory tract rather than the stomach. The tube, held securely and comfortably by a tape across the nose or upper lip, may be left in place in adults and older children but usually is removed and reinserted for each feeding in in-

fants. Before each feeding the patient is helped up to a semi-Fowler's position or is turned on the right side if unconscious. If a cuffed tracheostomy tube or endotracheal tube is in place, the cuff is inflated. The nasogastric tube is checked for proper placement and for the amount of residual formula in the stomach. Any solid medication to be given with the feeding is dissolved in water. The normal liquefied diet formula contains a mixture of milk, eggs, sugar, skim milk powder, and protein hydrolysates. A low-residue formula consists of amino acids, sugars, vitamins, and minerals. Depending on the patient's preference, the formula is at or below room temperature when administered slowly by gravity at a rate of no more than 300 ml an hour. During feeding the patient is observed for respiratory distress, nausea, vomiting, abdominal cramps, and restlessness. At the completion of the procedure, the tube is flushed with water as ordered and then clamped. The patient receives oral hygiene and lubrication and cleaning of the nares and is maintained in the same position for 30 minutes after feeding; at that time the cuff on the tracheostomy or endotracheal tube is deflated.

■ INTERVENTIONS: The nurse positions the patient for feeding, checks the tube placement, notes and replaces the amount of residual formula, and reports residual volume in excess of 100 ml. The nurse administers the feeding, ensures that the patient and family members understand the purpose of the procedure, and cautions the patient to report symptoms, such as nausea, abdominal cramps, diarrhea, or constipation.

■ OUTCOME CRITERIA: A formula containing the proper proportions of protein, carbohydrate, and fat administered through a nasogastric tube can provide adequate nutrition over a short term. A high content of simple sugars may cause diarrhea. Concentrated mixtures containing too little water or large volumes administered rapidly may dehydrate the patient.

tube gain, the overall electron gain of a photomultiplier tube, calculated as gn, where g is the dynode gain and n is the number of dynodes in the tube. Thus if the gain in secondary electrons per incident electrons is 3 and the number of dynodes is 8, the tube gain is 38, or 6561. See also **dynode.**

tubercle /t(y)ōo′bərkəl/ [L, *tuber*, swelling], **1.** a nodule or a small eminence, such as that on a bone. **2.** a nodule, especially an elevation of the skin that is larger than a papule, such as Morgagni's tubercles of the areolae of the breasts. **3.** a small rounded nodule produced by infection with *Mycobacterium tuberculosis*, consisting of a gray translucent mass of small spheric cells surrounded by connective cells.

tubercles of Montgomery [William Featherstone Montgomery, Irish gynecologist, b. 1797], small papillae on the surface of nipples and aerolas that secrete a fatty lubricating substance.

tubercular /t(y)ōo′bur′kyələr/ [L, *tuberculum*, swelling], pertaining to or resembling tuberculosis.

tuberculin. See **tuberculin test, tuberculosis.**

tuberculin tine test /t(y)ōo′bur′kyəlin/ [L, *tuberculum*; ME, *tind*; L, *testum*, crucible], a method of testing for the presence of tubercle bacilli by applying a device with multiple sharp prongs to the skin. The prongs penetrate the skin and inject tuberculin, a purified protein derivative (PPD) tuber-

cle bacilli. A hardened raised area at the test site 48 to 72 hours later indicates the presence of the pathogens in the blood. Because of variations in sensitivity and strength of tuberculin units administered, a negative test result does not necessarily exclude a diagnosis of tuberculosis. See also **Mantoux test**.

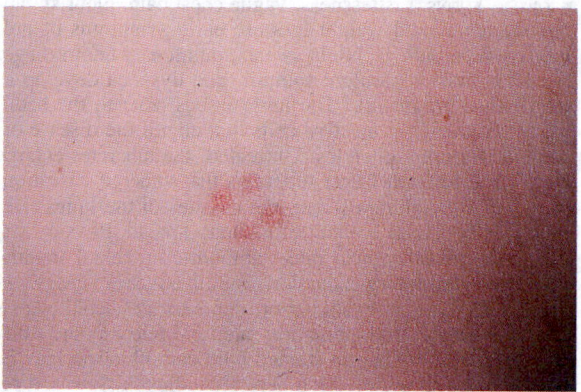

Tine test, grade I
(Turner-Warick, 1993/Courtesy Dr M Caplin)

tuberculin purified protein derivative /tōo′bur′kyōolin/, a solution containing a purified protein fraction derived from isolated culture filtrates of strains of *Mycobacterium tuberculosis*. It is used as an aid in the diagnosis of tuberculosis, in the Mantoux test, and, for the same purpose in a dried form, in multiple puncture devices. See also **Mantoux test, tine test.**

tuberculin test [L, *tuber* + *testum*, crucible], a test to determine past or present tuberculosis infection based on a positive skin reaction, using one of several methods. A purified protein derivative (PPD) of tubercle bacilli, called **tuberculin,** is introduced into the skin by scratch, puncture, or intradermal injection. If a raised, red, or hard zone forms surrounding the tuberculin test site, the person is said to be sensitive to tuberculin, and the test is read as positive. However, a negative tuberculin reaction does not rule out a diagnosis of previous or active tuberculosis. Sputum and gastric cultures, acid-fast staining, and x-ray studies often are needed to establish a diagnosis of tuberculosis. Kinds of tuberculin tests include **Heaf test, Mantoux test, Pirquet's test,** and **tine test.**

tuberculoid leprosy. See **leprosy.**

tuberculoma /t(y)ōo′bur′kyəlō′mə/ /tōo′bur′kyōolō′mə/ [L, *tuber* + Gk, *oma*, tumor], a rare tumorlike growth of tuberculous tissue in the central nervous system, characterized by symptoms of an expanding cerebral, cerebellar, or spinal mass. Treatment consists of the administration of antimicrobial drugs to resolve the primary growth and to prevent meningitis.

tuberculosis (TB) /t(y)ōo′bur′kyəlō′sis/ [L, *tuber* + Gk, *osis*, condition], a chronic granulomatous infection caused by an acid-fast bacillus, *Mycobacterium tuberculosis*, generally transmitted by the inhalation or ingestion of infected droplets and usually affecting the lungs, although infection of multiple organ systems occurs. People infected with HIV may have extrapulmonary tuberculosis. This includes disseminated tuberculosis, which involves multiple organs such as the liver, lung, spleen, bone marrow, and lymph nodes. Diganosis is made through biopsy, stain, and culture of organs. Central nervous system tuberculosis may occur as inflammation of the meninges or a mass lesion (tuberculoma).

■ OBSERVATIONS: Listlessness, vague chest pain, pleurisy, anorexia, fever, and weight loss are early symptoms of pulmonary tuberculosis. Night sweats, pulmonary hemorrhage, expectoration of purulent sputum, and dyspnea develop as the disease progresses. The lung tissues react to the bacillus by producing protective cells that engulf the disease organism, forming tubercles. Untreated, the tubercles enlarge and merge to form larger tubercles that undergo caseation, eventually sloughing off into the cavities of the lungs. Hemoptysis occurs as a result of cavitary spread. Physical examination reveals apical rales, amphoric bronchial sounds, decreased respiratory excursion, and, in advanced cases, cyanosis. Laboratory examination demonstrates leukocytosis and an increased sedimentation rate, and microscopic study of a specimen of sputum stained with carbolfuchsin may be diagnostic. Culture of the tubercle bacillus is slow and requires darkness, carefully controlled temperature, and inoculation on special media. The infecting organism does not produce endotoxins or hemolysins, but **tuberculin,** a toxic substance, is released as the bacillus disintegrates. Tuberculin has no effect in people who have never been infected but produces a characteristic skin reaction when injected intradermally in people who have or have had tuberculosis. Purified protein derivative (PPD) is a stable, purified active preparation used to test for current or past infection. X-ray films of the lungs reveal infiltrates, mediastinal lymphadenopathy, caseation, pleural effusion, and calcification. Tuberculosis may spread from the lungs via the lymphatics and blood vessels; such miliary infection is characterized by tiny, seedlike tubercles in the liver, spleen, and other organs.

■ INTERVENTIONS: The bacillus is generally sensitive to isoniazid (INH), pyrazinamide, paraaminosalicylic acid, streptomycin, rifampin, ethambutol, dihydrostreptomycin, ultraviolet radiation, and heat. A combination of drugs is prescribed, with regular tests of the function of the kidneys, liver, eyes, and ears performed to discover early signs of drug toxicity. This is particularly important because drug therapy will usually continue for up to 1 year. The person is usually hospitalized for the first weeks of treatment to limit the possible spread of infection, to encourage rest and excellent nutrition, to ensure complete compliance with the prescribed drug regimen, and to observe for adverse drug effects. Samples of sputum are regularly examined. The disease is not infectious after the bacillus is no longer present in the sputum. Care of an outpatient includes continued medication, evaluation for adverse drug effects, sputum analyses, and encouragement to complete the long course of treatment. All contacts are tested periodically with PPD. People who are at increased risk of infection may be treated empirically, without a positive diagnosis having been made.

■ NURSING CONSIDERATIONS: Before discharge, the patient is taught how to prevent the spread of the disease; the elements of good nutrition; the name, dose, action, and side effects of all medications prescribed; the need to take the drugs regularly; and how and where to get the next supply of drugs. Plans for follow-up care are discussed; they include date, time, and place of the next laboratory tests, and referral to community nurses is made. The patient is reminded that a cough, weight loss, fever, night sweats, and hemoptysis are danger signals that are to be reported immediately. See also **miliary tuberculosis, tuberculin test.**

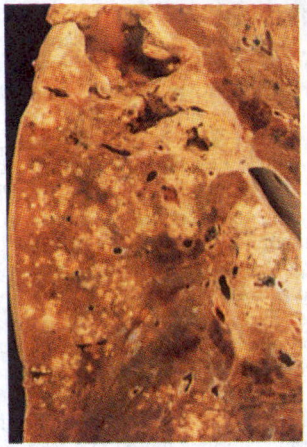

Post-primary tuberculosis *(Fletcher, 1987)*

tuberculosis vaccine. See **BCG vaccine.**
tuberculous /t(y)o͞obur′kyələs/ [L, *tuberculum*], pertaining to tuberculosis.
tuberculous lymphadenitis [L, *tuberculum* + *lympha,* water; Gk, *aden,* gland + *itis,* inflammation], an inflammation of the lymph glands caused by the presence of *Mycobacterium tuberculosis.*
tuberculous peritonitis [L, *tuberculum;* Gk, *peri, teinein* to stretch + *itis,* inflammation], an inflammation of the peritoneum that is secondary to a tuberculous infection in the viscera.
tuberculous pneumonia [L, *tuberculum;* Gk, *pneumon,* lung], a complication of tuberculosis in which caseous material is inhaled into the bronchi, leading to bronchopneumonia or lobar pneumonia.
tuberculous spondylitis. a rare, grave form of tuberculosis caused by the invasion of *Mycobacterium tuberculosis* into the spinal vertebrae. The intervertebral disks may be destroyed, resulting in the collapse and wedging of affected vertebrae and the shortening and angulation of the spine. Thoracic vertebrae are more frequently involved than the vertebrae of the lumbar, the cervical, or the sacral segments of the spine. More than one area of the spine may be affected, and normal vertebrae may be evident between affected and unaffected sections. The infection characteristically dissects vertebrae anterolaterally and produces abscesses. The pressure of the abscess may cause ischemic paralysis in the subjacent spinal cord, and abscesses in the cervical area may displace or obstruct the trachea and the esophagus. Also called **Pott's disease, spinal caries.** See also **tuberculosis.**

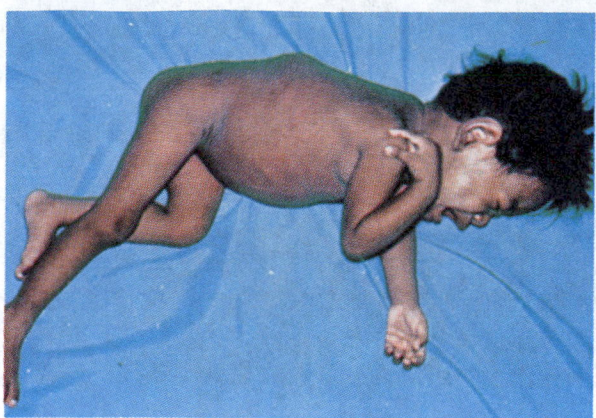

Tuberculous spondylosis *(Hart, 1992)*

tuberosity /t(y)o͞o′bərōs′itē/ [L, *tuber*], an elevation or protuberance, especially of a bone.

tuberosity of the tibia, a large oblong elevation at the proximal end of the tibia to which the ligament of the patella attaches.

tuberous carcinoma /t(y)o͞o′bərəs/ [L, *tuber*; Gk, *karkinos,* crab, *oma,* tumor], a scirrhous carcinoma of the skin, characterized by nodular projections. Also called **carcinoma tuberosum.**

tuberous sclerosis, a familial, neurocutaneous disease characterized by epilepsy, mental deterioration, adenoma sebaceum, nodules and sclerotic patches on the cerebral cortex, retinal tumors, depigmented leaf-shaped macules on the skin, tumors of the heart or kidneys, and cerebral calcifications. There is no effective treatment. Also called **Bourneville's disease, epiloia.** See also **adenoma sebaceum.**

tuberous xanthoma. See **xanthoma tuberosum.**

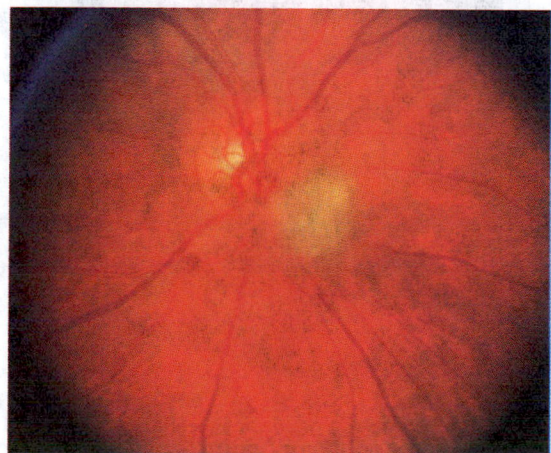

Tuberous sclerosis *(Apple, 1991)*

Tubex unit, a trademark for a unit consisting of a cartridge and needle that fits into a holder that has a plunger. The cartridge may be empty or prefilled with a standard dose of a medication. The needle is covered with a rubber protective guard and is permanently attached to the cartridge. The plunger may be unscrewed to allow the cartridge needle unit to be slipped in place. The cartridge is then twisted clockwise to secure it in the holder. The plunger is replaced and screwed onto a small projection on top of a rubber diaphragm on the cartridge. As the plunger is depressed, forcing the diaphragm into the cartridge, medication is forced out through the needle. The cartridge needle unit is sterile and disposable. The holder requires no special care and is reuseable.

tubo- /t(y)o͞o′bō-, t(y)o͞o′bə-/ [L, *tubus,* tube], a combining form meaning 'relating to tubes or tubing': *tubular.*

tuboabdominal gestation /-abdom′inəl/ [L, *tubus* + *abdomen,* belly; L, *gestare,* to bear], an ectopic pregnancy in which the embryo develops while partly in the abdominal cavity and partly in the fallopian tube. The condition usually begins as a tubal pregnancy and extends into the abdomen as development continues.

tuboabdominal pregnancy. See **tuboabdominal gestation.**

tubocurarine chloride. See **curare.**

tubo-ovarian /t(y)o͞o′bō·ōver′ē·ən/ [L, *tubus* + *ovum,* egg], pertaining to the ovary and fallopian tube. Also **tubo-ovarial.**

tubo-ovarian abscess [L, *tubus* + *ovum* + *abscedere,* to go away], an abscess involving the ovary and fallopian tube. It is commonly associated with salpingitis.

tubo-ovarian cyst [L, *tubus* + *ovum;* Gk, *kystis,* bag], a cyst that forms by adhesion of the ovary at the fimbriated end of the fallopian tube.

tubo-ovarian gestation [L, *tubus* + *ovum* + *gestare,* to bear], an ectopic pregnancy that develops partly in the fallopian tube and partly in the ovary. Also called **tubo-ovarian pregnancy.**

tuboplasty /t(y)o͞o′bōplas′tē/ [L, *tubus,* tube; Gk, *plassein,* to mold], a surgical procedure in which severed or damaged fallopian tubes are repaired.

tubular. See **tubule.**

tubular necrosis [L, *tubulus,* little tube; Gk, *nekros,* dead, *osis,* condition], the death of cells in the small tubules of the kidneys as a result of disease or injury.

tubule /t(y)o͞o′byo͞ol/ [L, *tubulus*], a small tube, such as one of the collecting tubules in the kidneys, the seminiferous tubules of the testes, or Henle's tubules between the distal and proximal convoluted tubules. **–tubular,** *adj.*

tuft [Fr, *touffe,* a tuft], an object resembling a tassle, such as a tuft of hair.

tuft fracture [Fr *touffe* tuft; L, *fractura,* break], fracture of any one of the distal phalanges.

tularemia /to͞o′lərē′mē·ə/ [Tulare, California; Gk, *haima,* blood], an infectious disease of animals caused by the bacillus *Francisella (Pasteurella) tularensis,* which may be transmitted by insect vectors or direct contact. It is characterized in humans by fever, headache, and an ulcerated skin lesion with localized lymph node enlargement, or by eye infection, GI ulcerations, or pneumonia, depending on the site of entry and the response of the host. Treatment includes streptomycin, chloramphenicol, and tetracycline. Recovery produces lifelong immunity. A vaccine is available. Also called **deerfly fever, rabbit fever.**

tumescence /t(y)o͞omes'əns/ [L, *tumescere*, to begin to swell], a state of swelling or edema.

-tumescence, a suffix meaning a 'swelling': *detumescence, intumescence, tumescence.*

tumor /t(y)o͞o'mər/ [L], **1.** a swelling or enlargement occurring in inflammatory conditions. **2.** also called **neoplasm.** a new growth of tissue characterized by progressive, uncontrolled proliferation of cells. The tumor may be localized or invasive, benign or malignant. A tumor may be named for its location, for its cellular makeup, or for the person who first identified it.

tumor albus, a white swelling occurring in a tuberculous bone or joint.

tumor angiogenesis factor (TAF), a protein that stimulates the formation of blood vessels in tumors. See also **angiogenin.**

tumoricide /t(y)o͞omôr'isīd/, a substance capable of destroying a tumor. **–tumoricidal,** *adj.*

tumorigenesis /t(y)o͞o'mərijen'əsis/, the process of initiating and promoting the development of a tumor. Compare **carcinogenesis, oncogenesis, sarcomagenesis. –tumorigenic,** *adj.*

tumorigenic /-jen'ik/ [L, *tumor*, swelling; Gk, *genein*, to produce], capable of producing tumors.

tumor marker, a substance in the body that may be associated with the presence of a cancer.

tumor necrosis factor (TNF), a natural body protein, also produced synthetically, with anticancer effects. It is produced in the body in response to the presence of toxic substances, such as bacterial toxins. Adverse effects are toxic shock and cachexia.

tumor registry, a repository of data on the incidence of cancers and personal characteristics, treatment, and treatment outcomes of patients diagnosed with cancer.

tumor viruses [L, *tumor*, swelling + *virus*, poison], viruses that are capable of directly or indirectly inducing tumor formation. Direct tumor formation may result from inoculation of living cells with tumorigenic viruses. Tumor formation may result from the influence of the virus on normal cells that are transformed into tumor cells.

tumor volume, a portion of an organ or tissue that includes both the tumor and adjacent areas of invasion.

tungsten (W) /tung'stən/ [SW, *tung*, heavy, *sten*, stone], a metallic element. Its atomic number is 74; its atomic weight is 183.85. It has the highest melting point of all metals and is used as a target material in x-ray tubes.

tunica /t(y)o͞o'nikə/ [L, *tunic*], an enveloping coat or covering membrane.

tunica adventitia, the outer layer or coat of an artery or other tubular structure.

tunica albugines [L, *tunic* + *albus*, white], a tissue covering of white collagenous fibers, such as the sclerotic coat of the eyeball.

tunica intima, the membrane lining an artery.

tunica media, a muscular middle coat of an artery.

tunica vaginalis testis, the serous membrane surrounding the testis and epididymis.

tunica vasculosa bulbi. See **uvea.**

tuning fork /t(y)o͞o'ning/ [Gk, *tonos*, stretching; L, *furca*, fork], a small metal instrument consisting of a stem and two prongs that produces a constant pitch when either prong is struck. It is used in auditory tests of nerve function and of air and bone conduction.

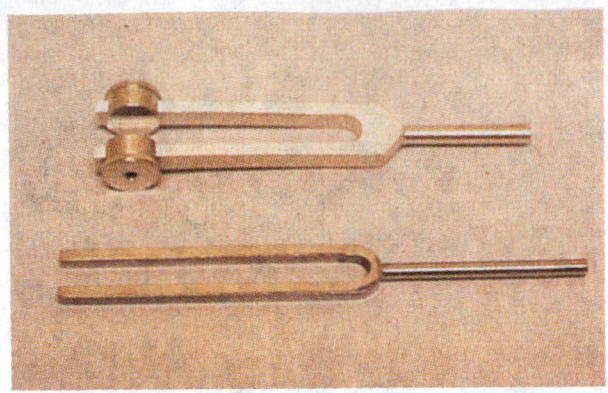

Tuning forks *(Seidel, 1991)*

tunnel [OFr, *tonnel*], a canal or passage, such as the carpal tunnel.

tunnel vision [OFr, *tonnel*, fowl trap; L, *videre*, to see], a defect in sight in which there is a great reduction in the peripheral field of vision, as if looking through a hollow tube or tunnel. The condition occurs in advanced chronic glaucoma.

tunnel wound [OFr, *tonnel*; AS, *wund*], a break in the surface of the body or an organ in which the entry and exit wounds are the same size.

TUR, abbreviation for **transurethral resection.**

turban tumor /tur'bən/ [Turk, *tulbend*, headdress; L, *tumor*, swelling], a benign neoplasm consisting of pink or maroon nodules that may cover the entire scalp, trunk, and extremities. The growth is familial and often recurs after excision.

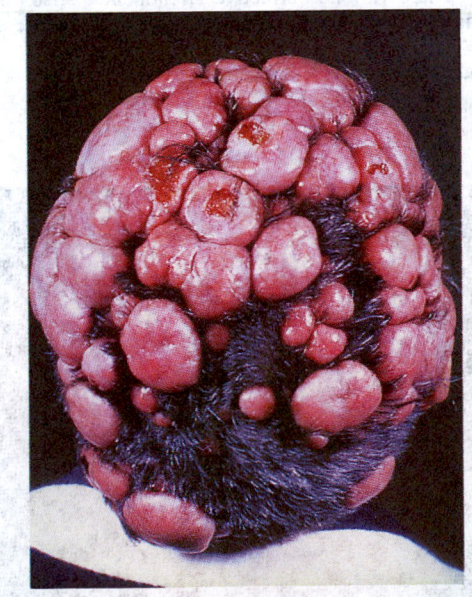

Turban tumor
(du Vivier, 1993/Courtesy Queen Victoria Hospital, East Grinstead)

turbid /tur'bid/ [L, *turbidus*, confused], clouded or obscured, as in solids in suspension in a solution.

turbidimetry /tur'bidim'ətrē/ [L, *turbidus*, confused; Gk, *metron*, measure], measurement of the turbidity (cloudiness) of a solution or suspension in which the amount of transmitted light is quantified with a spectrophotometer or estimated by visual comparison with solutions of known turbidity.

turbidity /tərbid'itē/ [L, *turbidus*], a condition of light scattering in a liquid resulting from the presence of suspended particles in the fluid. Turbidity varies according to the concentration of particles and their shapes and sizes.

turbinate /tur'binit/ [L, *turbinum*, top-shaped], **1.** of or pertaining to a scroll shape. **2.** the concha nasalis.

turgid /tur'jid/ [L, *turgidus*], swollen, hard, and congested, usually as a result of an accumulation of fluid. – **turgor,** *n.*

turgor /tur'gər/ [L, *turgere*, to be swollen], the normal resiliency of the skin caused by the outward pressure of the cells and interstitial fluid. Dehydration results in decreased skin turgor, manifested by lax skin that, when grasped and raised between two fingers, slowly returns to a position level with the adjacent tissue. Marked edema or ascites results in increased turgor manifested by smooth, taut, shiny skin that cannot be grasped and raised. An evaluation of the turgor of the skin is an essential part of physical assessment.

turista. See **traveler's diarrhea.**

turnbuckle cast [AS, *tyrnan;* ME, *bocle,* small shield; ONorse, *kasta*], an orthopedic device used to encase and immobilize the entire trunk, one arm to the elbow and the opposite leg to the knee. It is constructed of plaster of paris or fiberglass and incorporates hinges as part of its design in the treatment of scoliosis. The hinges are placed at the level of the apex of the curvature. Used for preoperative and postoperative positioning, it is used less frequently than the Risser cast. An adaptation of the turnbuckle cast is used occasionally as a hyperextension cast for the treatment of kyphosis or kyphoscoliosis. Compare **Risser cast.**

Turner's sign. See **Grey Turner's sign.**

Turner's syndrome [Henry H. Turner, American physician, b. 1892], a chromosomal anomaly seen in about 1 in 3000 live female births, characterized by the absence of one X chromosome, congenital ovarian failure, genital hypoplasia, cardiovascular anomalies, dwarfism, short metacarpals, "shield chest," extosis of tibia, and underdeveloped breasts, uterus, and vagina. Spatial disorientation and moderate degrees of learning disorders are common. Treatment includes hormone therapy (estrogens, androgens, pituitary growth hormone) and, often, surgical correction of cardiovascular anomalies and the webbing of the neck skin. Also called **Bonnevie-Ullrich syndrome, monosomy X.** See also **Noonan's syndrome.**

turnkey /turn'kē/, a term referring to a computer system or installation that is complete on delivery and ready to operate without modification.

turricephaly. See **oxycephaly.**

-tuse, 1. a combining form meaning 'dull or blunt': *obtuse.* **2.** a combining form meaning 'to beat or bruise': *contuse.*

Tussionex, a trademark for a fixed-combination drug containing an antitussive (hydrocodone bitartrate) and an antihistamine (phenyltoloxamine citrate).

tussis /tus'is/ [L, *tussis,* cough], a cough or pertussis.

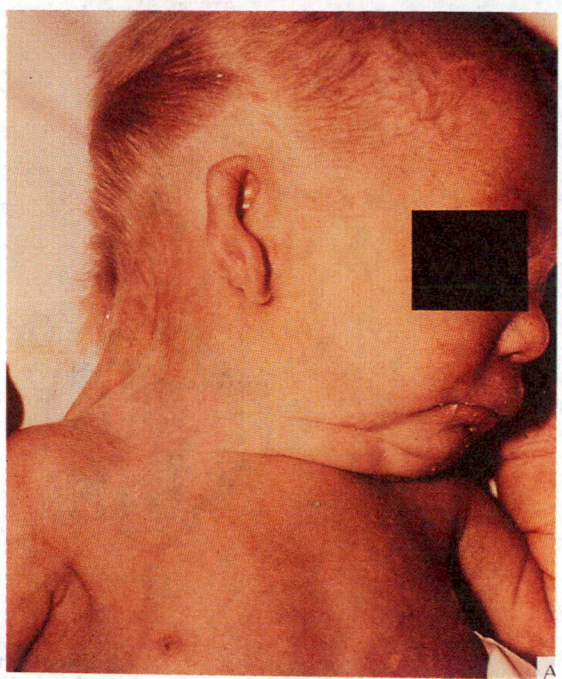

Webbed neck, widespread nipples, abnormal ears, and micrognathia associated with Turner syndrome
(Zitelli, 1992)

tussive fremitus /tus'iv/ [L, *tussis,* cough + *fremitus,* murmuring], a vibratory cough that can be felt by a hand over the chest of the patient.

tutorial /t(y)ō̄ōtôr'ē·əl/ [L, *tueri,* to look with care], of or pertaining to computer-assisted instruction in which training materials are presented and relied on to direct the student to a discovery of the correct answer.

TV, abbreviation for **tidal volume.**

TVL, abbreviation for **tenth-value layer.**

T wave, the component of the cardiac cycle shown on an electrocardiogram as a short, inverted, U-shaped curve after the ST segment. It represents repolarization from phase 3 currents of the cardiac cycle as the heart recovers from contraction and prepares to begin the cycle again with atrial depolarization during the P wave.

Tweed triangle [Charles Tweed, American dentist, b. 1895; L, *triangulus,* three-cornered], a triangle used as a diagnostic aid, formed by the mandibular plane, the Frankfort plane, and the long axis of the lower central incisor.

twelfth cranial nerve. See **hypoglossal nerve.**

24-hour clock system, a method of designating time by using the numeric sequence from 00 to 23 for the hours and the numbers 00 to 59 for the minutes in a daily cycle beginning with 0000 (midnight) and ending with 2359 (1 minute before the next midnight). The system provides a clear distinction between prenoon and afternoon time without requiring the designations AM and PM.

twilight sleep /twī'līt/, *obsolete.* light anesthesia obtained by the parenteral administration of a mixture of morphine

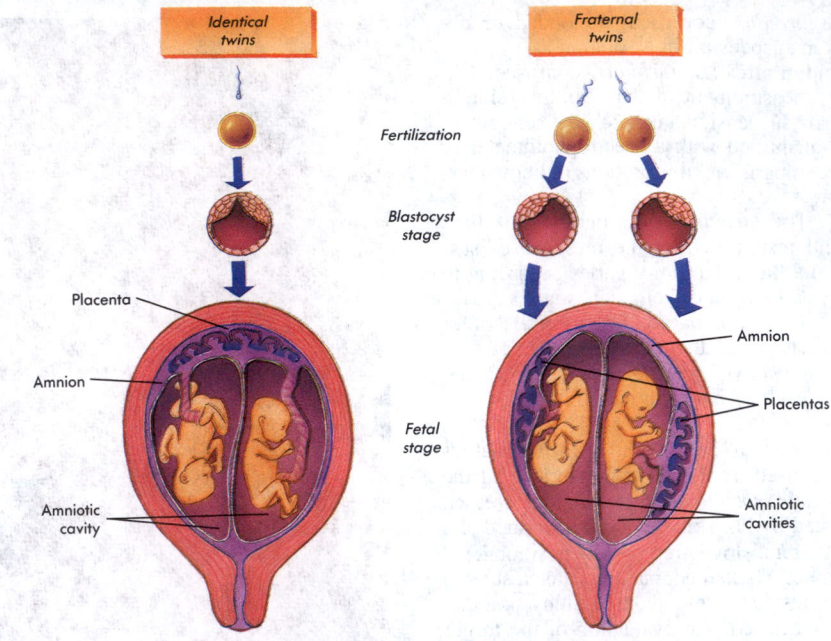

**Identical and fraternal twins,
showing shared and separate placentas**
(Thibodeau, 1993/Rolin Graphics)

and scopolamine to reduce pain and obtund recall in child-birth.

twilight state [Ger *Zwielicht*, twilight; L, *status*], an impaired state of consciousness in which the patient may experience visual or auditory hallucinations and responds to them with irrational behavior. The person may be unaware of the suroundings at the time of the experience and have no memory of it later, except perhaps to recall a related dream.

twin [AS, *twinn*, double], either of two offspring born of the same pregnancy and developed from either a single ovum or from two ova that were released from the ovary simultaneously and fertilized at the same time. The incidence of twin births is approximately 1 in 80 pregnancies. Kinds of twins include **conjoined twins, dizygotic twins, interlocked twins, monozygotic twins, Siamese twins,** and **unequal twins.** See also **Hellin's law.**

twinge /twinj/ [ME, *twengen* to pinch], a sudden, brief, darting pain.

twin monster. See **double monster.**

twinning [AS, *twinn*], **1.** the development of two or more fetuses during the same pregnancy, either spontaneously or through external intervention for experimental purposes in animals. **2.** the duplication of like structures or parts by division.

twin-wire fixed orthodontic appliance, an orthodontic appliance developed by J.E. Johnson typically employing a pair of 0.01 inch (0.25 mm) wires to form the midsection of the arch wire. It is used to correct or improve malocclusion.

twitch [AS, *twiccian*], **1.** the contraction of small muscle units, manifested as a quick, simple, spasmodic contraction of a muscle. **2.** to jerk convulsively.

twitching [AS, *twiccian*], a series of contractions by small muscle units. Twitching that involves large groups of muscle fibers is identified as **fascicular twitching.**

two-point discrimination test, a test of the ability of a person to differentiate touch stimuli at two nearby points on the body at the same time. It is used in studies of possible damage to the parietal regions of the brain.

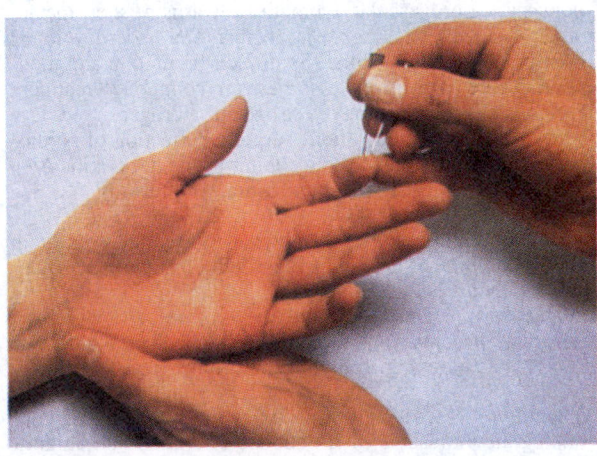

Two-point discrimination test (Seidel, 1991)

two-point gait [OE, *twa;* L, *punctus,* pricked; ONorse, *gata,* way], a pattern of crutch-walking with crutches in which the right foot and left crutch advance first, the step being completed by advancing the left foot and right crutch. See also **three-point gait.**

two-way catheter [AS, *twa, weg;* Gk, *katheter,* something lowered], a catheter that has a double lumen, one channel for injection of medication or fluids and the other for removal of fluid or specimens.

Tylenol, a trademark for an analgesic and antipyretic (acetaminophen).

tyloxapol /tīlok'səpôl/, a respiratory tract detergent prescribed for bronchitis, emphysema, pulmonary abscess, bronchiectasis, or atelectasis.

tympan-, a combining form meaning 'pertaining to the tympanic membrane': *tympanoplasty, tympanotomy.*

tympanal. See **tympanic.**

tympanectomy /tim'pənek'təmē/ [Gk, *tympanon,* drum + *ektome*], the surgical removal of the tympanic membrane.

tympanic /timpan'ik/ [Gk, *tympanum,* drum], of or pertaining to a structure that resonates when struck; drumlike, such as a **tympanic abdomen** that resonates on percussion because the intestines are distended with gas. Also **tympanal.** —**tympanum** /tim'pənəm (*pl.* **tympana**), *n.*

tympanic antrum, a relatively large, irregular cavity in the superior anterior portion of the mastoid process of the temporal bone, communicating with the mastoid air cells and lined by the extension of the mucous membrane of the tympanic cavity. The bony tegmen tympani separates the tympanic antrum from the middle fossa of the cranial cavity, and the lateral semicircular canal of the internal ear projects into the antrum. See also **mastoid process.**

tympanic cavity. See **middle ear.**

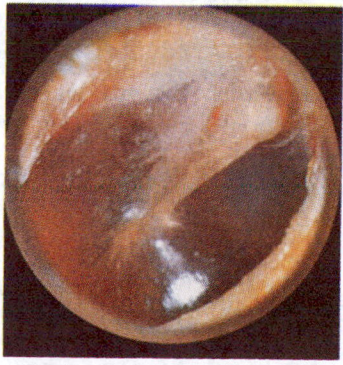

Normal tympanic membrane
(Malasanos, 1990/Courtesy Dr Richard A Buckingham, Abraham Lincoln School of Medicine, University of Illinois, Chicago)

tympanic membrane, a thin, semitransparent membrane in the middle ear that transmits sound vibrations to the internal ear by means of the auditory ossicles. It is nearly oval in form, with a vertical diameter of about 10 mm, and separates the tympanic cavity from the bottom of the external acoustic meatus. Also called **eardrum, membrana tympani.**

tympanic membrane thermometer, a device that mea-

sures the temperature of the tympanic membrane by detecting infrared radiation from the tissue. Results are obtained within 2 seconds and directly reflect the body's core temperature. See also **ear thermometry.**

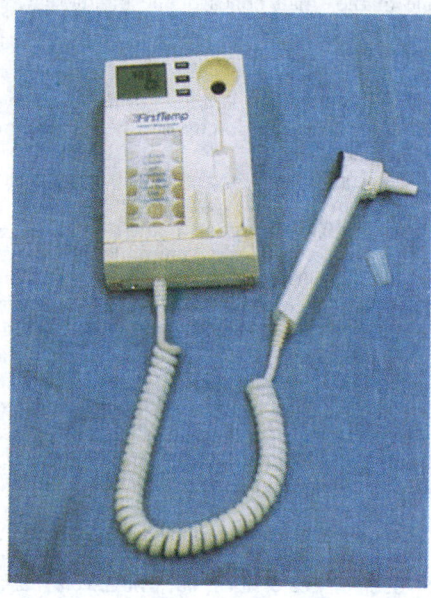

Tympanic membrane thermometer *(Potter, 1993)*

tympanic reflex, the reflection of a beam of light shining on the eardrum. In a normal ear, a bright, wedge-shaped reflection is seen; its apex is at the end of the malleus, and its base is at the anterior inferior margin of the eardrum. In disorders of the middle ear or eardrum, this shape may be distorted.

tympanic sulcus [Gk, *tympanum,* drum; L, *sulcus,* furrow], a narrow circular groove at the medial end of the osseous part of the external acoustic meatus that holds the tympanic membrane.

tympanic temperature, the body temperature as measured electronically at the tympanic membrane. See also **tympanic membrane thermometer.**

tympanitic resonance /tim'penit'ik/ [Gk, *tympanum;* L, *resonare,* to sound again], a drumlike or hollow sound heard over a large air space of the body, such as the pneumothorax.

tympano- [Gk, *tympanon,* drum], a combining form meaning 'relating to the ear drum or tympanic membrane': *tympanoplasty, tympanotomy.*

tympanogram /timpan'əgram/ a graphic representation of the acoustic impedance and air pressure of the middle ear and mobility of the tympanic membrane, measured as part of the audiologic test battery. In the normal middle ear, the air pressure is the same as the atmospheric pressure, as shown by a peak in the middle of the tympanogram. Various middle ear pathologies, such as otitis media, otosclerosis, or tympanic membrane perforations, each yield distinctive tympanograms. See also **acoustic impedance.**

tympanoplasty /timpan'əplas'tē/ [Gk, *tympanum* +

plassein, to mold], any of several operative procedures on the eardrum or ossicles of the middle ear, designed to restore or improve hearing in patients with conductive hearing loss. These operations may be used to repair a perforated eardrum, for otosclerosis, or for dislocation or necrosis of one of the small bones of the middle ear. See also **myringoplasty, stapedectomy.**

tympanotomy. See **myringotomy.**

tympanum. See **tympanic.**

tympany /tim′pənē/ [Gk, *tympanon,* drum], a low-pitched resonant sound heard on percussion over a pneumothorax or distended abdomen.

-type, a combining form meaning a 'representative form or class': *lysotype, serotype, somatotype.*

Type A personality [Gk, *typos,* mark], a parent ego state characterized by a behavior pattern described by Meyer Friedman and Ray Rosenman as associated with individuals who are highly competitive and work compulsively to meet deadlines. The behavior also is associated with a higher than usual incidence of coronary heart disease.

Type B personality, a child ego state characterized by a form of behavior associated by Friedman and Rosenman with people who appear free of hostility and aggression and who lack a compulsion to meet deadlines, are not highly competitive at work and play, and have a lower risk of heart attack.

Type E personality, a term introduced by Harriet Braiker to describe professional women who fit neither Type A nor Type B personality categories, but who have a marked sense of insecurity and strive to convince themselves that they are worthwhile. Type E women try to be 'all things to all people,' according to Braiker, and tend to suffer psychologic strain. Also called **adult ego state.**

type specificity. See **specificity.**

type I diabetes mellitus. See **insulin-dependent diabetes mellitus.**

type II diabetes mellitus. See **non-insulin-dependent diabetes mellitus.**

type I hyperlipidemia. See **hyperlipidemia type I.**

type I hypersensitivity. See **anaphylactic hypersensitivity.**

type II hypersensitivity. See **cytotoxic hypersensitivity.**

type III hypersensitivity. See **immune complex hypersensitivity.**

type IV hypersensitivity. See **cell-mediated immune response.**

typhlitis /tiflī′tis/, *obsolete.* appendicitis.

typhlo-, **1.** a combining form meaning 'pertaining to the cecum': *typhlocolitis, typhlostenosis, typhlostomy.* **2.** a combining form meaning 'pertaining to blindness': *typhlolexia, typhlology, typhlosis.*

typho-. a combining form meaning 'fever' and related to typhus and typhoid fevers.

typhoid /tī′foid/ [Gk, *typhos,* fever + *eidos,* form], pertaining to or resembling typhus.

-typhoid, **1.** a combining form meaning 'pertaining to typhus': *bronchotyphoid, meningotyphoid, nephrotyphoid, antityphoid, paratyphoid, posttyphoid.*

typhoid carrier, a person without signs or symptoms of typhoid fever who carries on his or her body the bacteria that cause the disease and sheds the pathogens in bodily excretions. The typical typhoid carrier is one who has recovered from an attack of the disease.

typhoid fever [Gk, *typhos,* typhus, *eidos,* form; L, *febris,* fever], a bacterial infection usually caused by *Salmonella typhi,* transmitted by contaminated milk, water, or food and characterized by headache, delirium, cough, watery diarrhea, rash, and a high fever. Also called **enteric fever.** Compare **cholera, paratyphoid fever, salmonellosis.**

■ OBSERVATIONS: The incubation period may be as long as 60 days. Characteristic maculopapular rosy spots are scattered over the skin of the abdomen and chest. Splenomegaly and leukopenia develop first. The diagnosis is made by bacteriologic culture of blood and stool and by a rising titer of agglutinins in Widal's test. The disease is serious and may be fatal. Complications include intestinal hemorrhage or perforation and thrombophlebitis. Some people who recover from the disease continue to be carriers and excrete the organism, spreading the disease.

■ INTERVENTIONS: Chloramphenicol, ampicillin, amoxicillin, and trimethoprin-sulfamethoxazole are all useful in treatment. Prolonged administration of antibiotics or cholecystectomy may eliminate the carrier state. Typhoid vaccine gives some protection but requires annual booster doses for best effect.

■ NURSING CONSIDERATIONS: To lower the temperature, sponge baths are preferred to salicylates because salicylates may cause hypothermia or hypotension. Laxatives and enemas are contraindicated because of the danger of bowel perforation. Proper disposal of human wastes is essential to prevent epidemics, and carriers should not be permitted to prepare food.

typhoid nodules [Gk, *typhos,* fever; L, *nodulus,* small knot], a liver nodule consisting of a cluster of monocytes and lymphocytes surrounding the typhoid fever pathogen, *Salmonella typhi.*

typhoid pellagra, a form of pellagra in which the symptoms also include continued high temperatures.

typhoid vaccine, a bacterial vaccine prepared from an inactivated, dried strain of *Salmonella typhi.*

■ INDICATIONS: It is prescribed for primary immunization against typhoid fever for adults and children.

■ CONTRAINDICATIONS: Acute infection or concomitant use of corticosteroids prohibits its use.

■ ADVERSE EFFECTS: Among the more serious adverse reactions are anaphylaxis and pain and inflammation at the site of injection.

typhous /tī′fəs/ [Gk, *typhos,* fever], pertaining to typhus fever.

typhus /tī′fəs/ [Gk, *typhos,* fever], any of a group of acute infectious diseases caused by various species of *Rickettsia* and usually transmitted from infected rodents to humans by the bites of lice, fleas, mites, or ticks. These diseases are all characterized by headache, chills, fever, malaise, and a maculopapular rash. Kinds of typhus are **epidemic typhus, murine typhus,** and **scrub typhus.** See also **Brill-Zinsser disease, Rocky Mountain spotted fever.**

typhus vaccine, any one of three vaccines, each of which is prepared for the different rickettsial organisms that cause epidemic typhus, murine typhus, or Brill-Zinsser disease.

■ INDICATIONS: Each of the vaccines is prescribed for immunization against a form of typhus.

■ CONTRAINDICATIONS: Acute infection, debilitating disease, concomitant use of corticosteroids, or hypersensitivity to eggs prohibits its use.

■ ADVERSE EFFECTS: Among the most serious adverse reactions are anaphylaxis and various allergic reactions. Pain at the site of injection also may occur.

-typia, a combining form meaning '(condition of) conformity to type': *atypia, ectypia, zelotypia.*

typical /tip'ikəl/ [L, *typicus,* characteristic of a kind], a representative example.

typing [Gk, *typos,* mark], the process of classifying a specimen of blood, tissue, or other substance. See also **blood typing, tissue typing.**

typo-. a combining form meaning 'relating to a particular type': *typology, typography.*

Tyr, abbreviation for **tyrosine.**

tyramine /tī'rəmēn/ [Gk, *tyros,* cheese, *amine,* ammonia], an amino acid synthesized in the body from the essential acid tyrosine. Tyramine stimulates the release of the catecholamines epinephrine and norepinephrine. It is important that people taking monoamine oxidase inhibitors avoid the ingestion of foods and beverages containing tyramine, particularly aged cheeses and meats, bananas, yeast-containing products, and alcoholic beverages. See also **amine, catecholamine, epinephrine, norepinephrine, sympatomimetic, vasoconstriction.**

tyro-, a combining form meaning 'pertaining to cheese': *tyrogenous, tyroid, tyrometosis.*

tyroma /tīrō'mə/, *pl.* **tyromas, tyromata** [Gk, *tyros + oma,* tumor], a new growth or nodule with a caseous or cheesy consistency.

tyromatosis /tī'rōmətō'sis/ [Gk, *tyros, oma + osis,* condition], a process in which necrotic tissue is broken down and degenerates to a granular, amorphous, caseous mass.

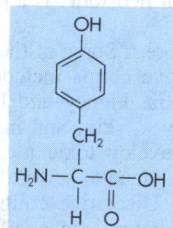

Chemical structure of tyrosine (Seeley, 1992)

tyrosine (Tyr) /tī'rəsēn/ [Gk, *tyros*], an amino acid synthesized in the body from the essential amino acid phenylalanine. Tyrosine is found in most proteins and is a precursor of melanin and several hormones, including epinephrine and thyroxin. See also **amino acid, hormone, melanocyte.**

tyrosinemia /tī'rōsinē'mē·ə/ [Gk, *tyros + haima,* blood], **1.** also called **neonatal tyrosinemia.** a benign, transient condition of the newborn, especially premature infants, in which an excessive amount of the amino acid tyrosine is found in the blood and urine. The disorder is caused by an anomaly in amino acid metabolism, usually delayed development of the enzymes necessary to metabolize tyrosine, and is controlled by dietary measures and vitamin C therapy. The metabolic defect disappears with treatment, or it may disappear spontaneously. **2.** also called **hereditary tyrosinemia.** a hereditary disorder involving an inborn error of metabolism of the amino acid tyrosine. The condition, which is transmitted as an autosomal recessive trait, is caused by an enzyme deficiency and results in liver failure or hepatic cirrhosis, renal tubular defects that can lead to renal rickets and renal glycosuria, generalized aminoaciduria, and mental retardation. Treatment consists of a diet low in tyrosine and phenylalanine and high in doses of vitamin C. In severe cases prognosis is extremely poor, and a liver transplantation may be the only lifesaving measure.

tyrosinosis /tīrōsinō'sis/ [Gk, *tyros + osis,* condition], a rare condition resulting from a defect in amino acid metabolism and transmitted as an autosomal recessive trait. It is characterized by the excretion of an excessive amount of parahydroxyphenylpyruvic acid, an intermediate product of tyrosine, in the urine. There is no known treatment. See also **tyrosinemia.**

tyrosinurea /tī'rōsinoŏr'ē·ə/ [Gk, *tyros + ouron,* urine], the presence of tyrosine in the urine.

Tyzine, a trademark for an alpha-adrenergic drug (tetrahydrozoline hydrochloride).

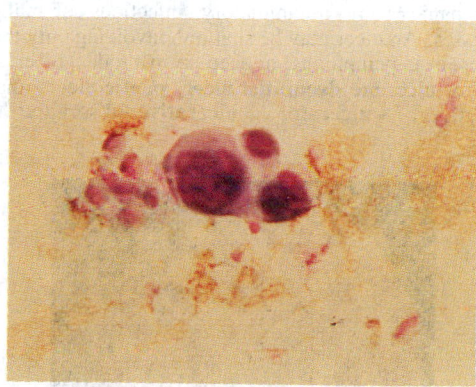

Tzanck preparation (Zitelli, 1992)

Tzanck test /tsangk/ [Arnault Tzanck, French dermatologist, b. 1886], a microscopic examination of cellular material from skin lesions to help diagnose certain vesicular diseases. The tissue is scraped from the base of a vesicle, placed on a slide, and stained with Wright's or Giemsa's stain. Multinucleated giant cells are diagnostic of herpesvirus or varicella. Typical pemphigus and other cells also can be identified.

tzetze fly. See **tsetse fly.**

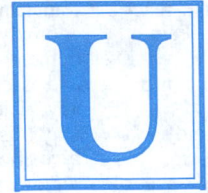

U

u, symbol sometimes used to stand for **micro-** (properly μ), as in "ul" or "um," representing μl or μm.

U, 1. abbreviation for **unit. 2.** symbol for the element **uranium.**

UAO, abbreviation for **upper airway obstruction.**

UGI. abbreviation for **upper GI.**

UICC, abbreviation for *International Union Against Cancer, Unión internacional contra el cancer, Union internationale contre le cancer, Unio internationalis contra cancrum,* or *Unione internazionale contro il cancro.*

-ula, a suffix meaning 'pertaining to small, little, minute': *macula.*

-ular, 1. a suffix meaning 'pertaining to' something specified: *appendicular, molecular, pedicular.* **2.** a combining form meaning 'resembling' something specified: *circular, globular, tubular.*

ulcer /ul′sər/ [L, *ulcus*], a circumscribed, craterlike lesion of the skin or mucous membrane resulting from necrosis that accompanies some inflammatory, infectious, or malignant processes. An ulcer may be shallow, involving only the epidermis, as in pemphigus, or deep, as in a rodent ulcer. Some kinds of ulcer are **decubitus ulcer, peptic ulcer,** and **serpent ulcer. –ulcerate,** *v.,* **ulcerative** /ul′sərā′tiv/, *adj.*

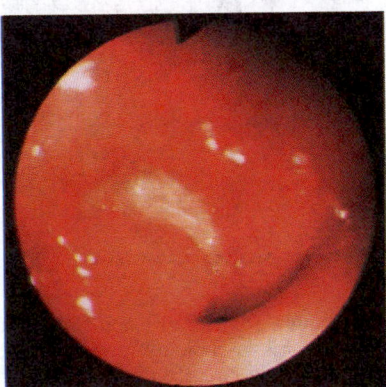

Duodenal ulcer *(Misiewicz, 1987)*

ulcerate /ul′sərāt/ [L, *ulcus,* a sore], to form an ulcer.

ulceration /ul′sərā′shən/ [L, *ulcus,* a sore], the process of ulcer formation.

ulcerative blepharitis /ul′sərā′tiv, ul′sərətiv′/ [L, *ulcus, atus,* relating to; Gk, *blepharon,* eyelid, *itis,* inflammation], a form of blepharitis in which a staphylococcal infection of the follicles of the eyelashes and glands of the eyelids results in sticky crusts forming on the lid margins. If the crusts are pulled off, the skin beneath bleeds. Tiny pustules develop in the follicles of the eyelashes and break down to form shallow ulcers. Other symptoms include burning, itching, swelling, and redness of the eyelids; a loss of eyelashes; irritation of the conjunctiva with tearing; photophobia; and gluing together of the eyelids during sleep by the dried secretions. Compare **nonulcerative blepharitis.**

ulcerative colitis, a chronic, episodic, inflammatory disease of the large intestine and rectum, characterized by profuse watery diarrhea containing varying amounts of blood, mucus, and pus. See also **Crohn's disease.**

■ OBSERVATIONS: The attacks of diarrhea are accompanied by tenesmus, severe abdominal pain, fever, chills, anemia, and weight loss. Children with the disease may suffer retarded physical growth. The debilitating symptoms often prevent people with ulcerative colitis from carrying on the normal activities of daily living. Diagnosis of the disease is based on clinical signs, the results of barium x-ray films of the colon, and colonoscopy with biopsy. It is often difficult to differentiate between ulcerative colitis and Crohn's disease.

■ INTERVENTIONS: Medical treatment with corticosteroids or other antiinflammatory agents may help to control the symptoms in some people. Those with severe disease or life-threatening complications usually require surgery. Total proctocolectomy with ileostomy is a permanent cure for ulcerative colitis.

■ NURSING CONSIDERATIONS: Some of the many systemic complications of ulcerative colitis include peripheral arthritis, ankylosing spondylitis, kidney and liver disease, and inflammation of the eyes, skin, and mouth. People with severe disease may develop toxic megacolon, a dangerous complication that may lead to perforation of the bowel, septicemia, and death. Ulcerative colitis also carries an increased risk of developing cancer of the colon, and periodic colonoscopy is performed to rule out this complication. A person with ulcerative colitis is suffering from a chronic, life-threatening illness and requires frequent evidence of support and understanding during prolonged hospitalization.

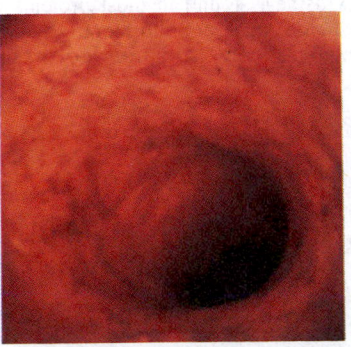

Ulcerative colitis *(Mitros, 1988)*

ulcerative inflammation [L, *ulcus*, a sore + *inflammare*, to set afire], the development of an ulcer over an area of inflammation.

ulcerative stomatitis [L, *ulcus*, a sore; Gk *stoma*, mouth + *itis*, inflammation], an infectious disease of the mouth characterized by swollen, spongy gums, ulcers, and loose teeth. Also called **trench mouth, ulceromembranous stomatitis, Vincent's angina.**

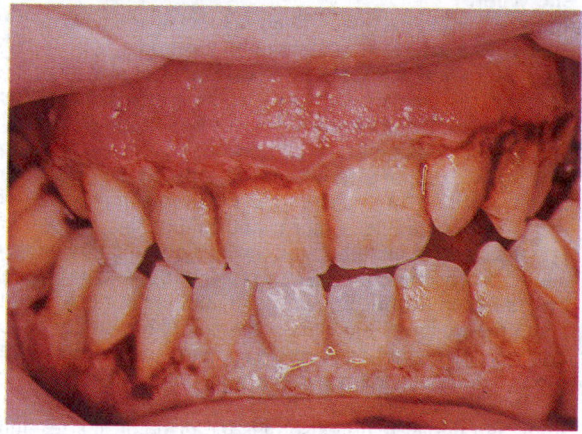

Ulcerative stomatitis *(Lamey, 1988)*

ULD, abbreviation for **upper level discriminator.**

ule-. See **ulo-.**

-ule. See **-ulum, -ulus.**

-ulent, a suffix meaning 'full of, characterized by': *feculent, pulverulent, succulent.*

ulna /ul′nə/ [L, elbow], the bone on the medial or little finger side of the forearm, lying parallel with the radius. Its proximal end bulges into the olecranon and the coronoid processes and dips into the trochlear and the radial notches. The ulna articulates with the humerus and the radius. Also called **elbow bone.**

ulnar /ul′nər/ [L, *ulna*, elbow], pertaining to the long medial bone of the forearm.

ulnar artery, a large artery branching from the brachial artery, supplying muscles in the forearm, wrist, and hand; arising near the elbow, it passes obliquely in a distal direction to become the superficial palmar arch. It has nine branches: four in the forearm, two in the wrist, and three in the hand. The forearm branches are the anterior ulnar recurrent, posterior ulnar recurrent, common interosseous, and muscular. The two branches in the wrist are the palmar carpal and dorsal carpal. The branches in the hand are the deep palmar, superficial palmar arch, and common palmar digital.

ulnar drift [L, *ulna*, elbow; AS, *drifan*, to drive], a joint change in the metacarpophalangeal joints because of rheumatoid arthritis and chronic synovitis. The long axis of the fingers makes an angle with the long axis of the wrist so that fingers are deviated to the ulnar side of the hand.

ulnar nerve, one of the terminal branches of the brachial plexus that arises on each side from the medial cord of the plexus. It receives fibers from both cervical and thoracic nerve roots and supplies the muscles and the skin on the ulnar side of the forearm and the hand. It can be easily pal-

pated as the 'funny bone' of the elbow as it courses along the groove between the olecranon process and the medial epicondyle of the humerus. It first passes medial to the axillary artery and the brachial artery to the middle of the arm, pierces the medial intermuscular septum, and follows along the medial head of the triceps to the olecranon. It descends into the forearm, and in the distal portion on the ulnar side it is covered only by the skin and the fascia. Just above the wrist it gives off a large dorsal branch and continues into the hand, where it gives off the digital and the muscular branches. The ulnar nerve usually has no branches above the elbow. Below the elbow its branches are the articular branches to the elbow joint, two muscular branches, the palmar cutaneous branch, the dorsal branch, the palmar branch, the superficial branch, and the deep branch. Compare **median nerve, musculocutaneous nerve, radial nerve.**

ulo-, **1.** a combining form meaning 'pertaining to a scar or cicatrix': *ulodermatitis, uloid, ulotomy.* **2.** also **ule-.** a combining form meaning 'pertaining to the gums or gingivae': *ulocase, ulorrhagia, ulotripsis.*

ulocarcinoma /yoo′lōkär′sinō′mə/, *pl.* **ulocarcinomas, ulocarcinomata** [Gk, *oule*, scar, *karkinos*, crab, *oma*, tumor], any malignant neoplasm of the gums that is classified as a carcinoma.

ulterior transactions /ultir′ē·ər/, (in psychiatry) in transactional analysis, transactions that are bilevel. The first level is overt (social), usually of relevant verbal statements. The second level is usually covert (psychological) and nonverbal, and has hidden psychologic meaning.

ultimate strain /ul′timit/, the strain at the point of failure.

ultimate stress, the highest load that can be sustained by a material at the point of failure.

ultra- /ul′trə-/, a prefix meaning 'beyond, farther, beyond a certain limit': *ultragaseous, ultrasound, ultravirus.*

Ultracef, a trademark for a cephalosporin antibiotic (cefadroxil monohydrate).

ultracentrifuge /ul′trəsen′trifyoōj/ [L, *ultra*, beyond; Gk, *kentron*, center; L, *fugere*, to flee], a high-speed centrifuge with a rotation rate fast enough to produce sedimentation of viruses, even in blood plasma. It is used in many kinds of biochemical analyses, including the measurement and separation of some proteins and viruses. Use of an attached microscope may make it possible to see the sediment.

ultradian /rā′dē·ən/ [L, *ultra* + *dies*, day], pertaining to a biorhythm that occurs in cycles of less than 24 hours.

ultrafiltrate /-fil′trāt/ [L, *ultra* + Fr, *filtre*, filter], a solution that has passed through a semipermeable membrane with very small pores. It usually contains only low-molecular-weight solutes.

ultrafiltration /-filtrā′shən/, a type of filtration, sometimes conducted under pressure, through filters with very small pores, such as used by an artificial kidney. Ultrafiltration can separate large molecules from smaller molecules in body fluids.

ultra-high-speed handpiece, a device for holding rotary instruments, such as burs, that permits rotational speeds of 100,000 to 300,000 rpm. It is used primarily for tooth cavity preparation.

Ultralente, a trademark for an insulin zinc suspension.

ultralente insulin. See **long-acting insulin.**

ultramicroscopy. See **darkfield microscopy.**

ultrasonic cardiography. See **echocardiography.**

ultrasonic /ul′trəson′ik/ [L, *ultra*, beyond + *sonus*, sound], pertaining to ultrasound, or sound frequencies so high (greater than 20 kilohertz) they cannot be perceived by the human ear.

ultrasonic nebulizer, a humidifier in which an electric current is used to produce high-frequency vibrations in a container of fluid. The vibrations break up the fluid into aerosol particles.

ultrasonic wave [L, *ultra,* beyond + *sonus,* sound], a sound wave transmitted at a frequency greater than 20,000 per second, or beyond the normal hearing range of humans. The specific wavelength is equal to the velocity divided by the frequency.

ultrasonography /-sənog′rəfē/ [L, *ultra* + *sonus,* sound; Gk, *graphein,* to record], the process of imaging deep structures of the body by measuring and recording the reflection of pulsed or continuous high-frequency sound waves. It is valuable in many medical situations, including the diagnosis of fetal abnormalities, gallstones, heart defects, and tumors. Also called **sonography.**

ultrasound /ul′trəsound/ [L, *ultra* + *sonus*], sound waves at the very high frequency of over 20,000 kHz (vibrations per second). Ultrasound has many medical applications, including fetal monitoring, imaging of internal organs, and, at an extremely high frequency, the cleaning of dental and surgical instruments. —**ultrasonic,** *adj.*

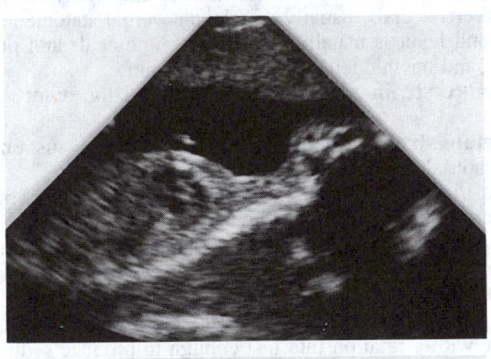

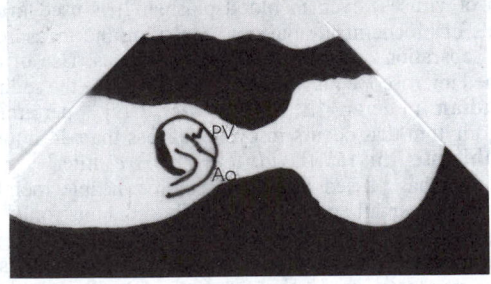

Ultrasound: Image of second-trimester fetus

ultrasound imaging, the use of high-frequency sound (several MHz or more) to image internal structures by the differing reflection signals produced when a beam of sound waves is projected into the body and bounces back at interfaces between those structures. Ultrasound diagnosis differs from radiologic diagnosis in that there is no ionizing radiation involved. Also called **ultrasound diagnosing.**

ultraviolet (UV) /-vī′ələt/ [L, *ultra* + Fr, *violette*], light beyond the range of human vision, at the short end of the

spectrum, or that portion of the electromagnetic spectrum with wavelengths between about 10 and 400 nm. Equivalently, an ultraviolet photon has an energy between 5 and 500 eV. It occurs naturally in sunlight; it burns and tans the skin and converts precursors in the skin to vitamin D. Ultraviolet lamps are used in the control of infectious airborne bacteria and viruses and in the treatment of psoriasis and other skin conditions. Black light is ultraviolet light used in fluoroscopy. See also **angstrom, light, radiation, spectrum.**

ultraviolet microscopy. See **fluorescent microscopy.**

ultraviolet radiation, a range of electromagnetic waves extending from the violet or short-wavelength end of the spectrum to the beginning of the x-ray spectrum. Near-ultraviolet radiation covers a range of wavelengths from 380 to 320 mμ; middle-ultraviolet radiation covers a range from 320 to 280 mμ; and far-ultraviolet radiation extends from 280 to about 10 mμ. About 5% of the radiation from the sun is in the ultraviolet range, but little of this type of energy reaches the earth because much is absorbed by oxygen and ozone in the atmosphere. Window glass also absorbs this radiation. Artificial sources of ultraviolet radiation include the iron arc, the carbon arc, and the mercury vapor arc. For maximum transmission, quartz or fluorite envelopes, which are transparent to ultraviolet radiation, must be used instead of glass. Prisms and lenses used for work in the ultraviolet region also must be made of quartz, fluorite, or synthetic halides. In medicine, ultraviolet radiation is used in the treatment of rickets and certain skin conditions. Milk and some other foods become activated with vitamin D when exposed to this type of energy. Ultraviolet radiation also causes fluorescence and phosphorescence, a useful characteristic in such diverse applications as lighting and the identification of minerals.

ultraviolet rays [L, *ultra,* beyond; OFr, *violette*; L, *radius*], electromagnetic radiations found just beyond the violet edge of the visible spectrum, with wavelengths extending to the beginning of x-rays. The wavelengths range from 390 to 290 nm for near ultraviolet rays to 290 to 20 nm for far ultraviolet wavelengths. Ultraviolet radiation in the region of 260 nm can distort DNA molecules, causing mutations and destroying microorganisms, including bacteria and viruses.

ultraviolet therapy [L, *ultra,* beyond; OFr, violette; Gk, *therapeia,* treatment], the application of electromagnetic radiations in the ultraviolet region of the spectrum to the body for therapeutic purposes. This therapy is useful in the control of infectious airborne bacteria and viruses and in the treatment of psoriasis and other skin conditions.

-ulum, -ule, a suffix meaning 'small one': *ovulum, speculum, venule.*

-ulus, -ule, a suffix meaning 'small one': *homunculus, nodulus, ramulus.*

-um, a suffix identifying singular nouns: *cerebellum, dextrum, quantum.*

umbilical /umbil′ikəl/ [L, *umbilicus,* navel], **1.** of or pertaining to the umbilicus. **2.** of or pertaining to the umbilical cord.

umbilical artery catheter [L, *umbilicalis,* navel; Gk, *arteria,* windpipe + *katheter,* a thing lowered], a catheter inserted into the umbilical artery of a newborn. See **umbilical catheterization.**

umbilical catheterization, a procedure in which a radiopaque catheter is passed through an umbilical artery to provide a newborn infant with parenteral fluid, to obtain blood samples, or both, or through the umbilical vein for an exchange transfusion or the emergency administration of drugs, fluids, or volume expanders.

■ METHOD: Within 1 hour of the insertion of the catheter the position of the tip is validated by x-ray examination. The infant is maintained in a neutral thermal environment as parenteral fluids are delivered by an infusion pump; the rate of flow is checked hourly, and the intravenous bottle is never allowed to empty. All connections to the umbilical line are checked every 30 to 60 minutes, and only grounded electric equipment is used on or near the infant. At hourly intervals the young patient is repositioned, and the cardiac and respiratory rates are monitored; the axillary temperature is taken every 2 to 3 hours, and the pedal pulses are checked every 2 to 4 hours. The condition of the cord is observed every 2 to 3 hours for signs of infection, such as redness, edema, or drainage at the catheter insertion site; the intravenous tubing is retaped when required, the cord dressing is changed, and antibiotic or antiseptic ointment is applied as ordered. If the umbilical line is displaced, pressure is quickly applied to the cord with a sterile 4-by-4-inch gauze, and an associate is delegated to notify the physician immediately. Fluid intake and output are measured. The infant is observed for oliguria or anuria, signs of vasospasm, such as blanching, mottling, or darkening of the legs and absence of peripheral pulses; and evidence of sepsis, hemorrhage, or oozing at the catheter insertion site, thromboembolism, and abdominal distention and vomiting, which may indicate necrotizing enterocolitis.

■ NURSING INTERVENTION: The nurse provides ongoing care, monitoring the catheterized infant for any signs of complications, which are promptly reported. The family is included in the care of the infant as much as possible.

■ OUTCOME CRITERIA: Umbilical catheterization can be an effective method of administering therapeutic fluids and agents or of obtaining diagnostic blood samples from a high-risk newborn, but great care is required in inserting and monitoring the tube.

umbilical cord, a flexible structure connecting the umbilicus with the placenta in the gravid uterus and giving passage to the umbilical arteries and vein. In the newborn it is about 2 feet long and ½ inch in diameter. First formed during the fifth week of pregnancy, it contains the yolk sac and the body stalk with the enclosed allantois. Also called the **chorda umbilicalis, funiculus umbilicalis.** See also **allantois.**

umbilical duct. See **vitelline duct.**

umbilical fissure, a groove on the inferior surface of the liver that holds the ligamentum teres and separates the right and left lobes of the liver.

umbilical fistula, an abnormal passage from the umbilicus to the intestine or more frequently to the remnant of the canal in the median umbilical ligament that connects the fetal bladder with the allantois.

umbilical hernia, a soft, skin-covered protrusion of intestine and omentum through a weakness in the abdominal wall around the umbilicus. It usually closes spontaneously within 1 to 2 years, although large hernias may require surgical closure.

umbilical region, the part of the abdomen surrounding the umbilicus, in the middle zone between the right and left lateral regions. See also **abdominal regions.**

umbilical vasculitis, an inflammation of the umbilical cord and its blood vessels.

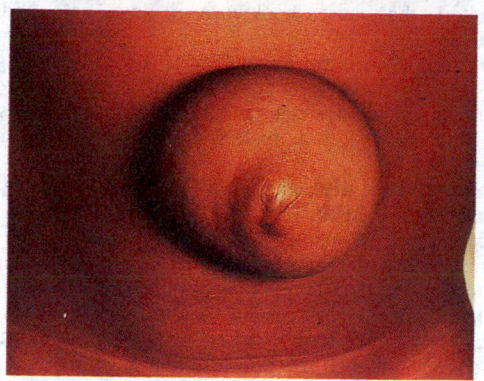

Umbilical hernia *(Zitelli, 1992)*

umbilical vein, one of a pair of embryonic vessels that return the blood from the placenta and fuse to form a single trunk in the body stalk. They remain separate for a short time in the embryo, opening into the sinus venosus. Development of the fetal liver breaks the connection between the umbilical veins and the sinus venosus, whereupon the right umbilical vein shrivels and disappears. The left umbilical vein remains attached to the placenta and is contained, with the fetal arteries, in the umbilical cord. After birth, the left umbilical vein and the ductus venosus atrophy and form respectively the ligamentum teres and the ligamentum venosum of the liver.

umbilical vesicle, a pear-shaped structure formed from the yolk sac at about the fourth week of prenatal development that protrudes into the cavity of the chorion and connects to the developing embryo by the yolk stalk at the region of the future midgut.

umbilication /um′bilikā′shən/ [L, *umbilicalis*, navel], the process of becoming dimpled or pitted or acquiring a depressed area.

umbilicus /umbilī′kəs, umbil′ikəs/ [L, navel], the point on the abdomen at which the umbilical cord joined the fetal abdomen. In most adults it is marked by a depression; in some it is marked by a small protrusion of skin. It interrupts the linea alba about halfway between the infrasternal notch and the pubic symphysis. It is located at the level of the interspace of the third and the fourth lumbar vertebrae. Also called **belly button, navel.**

umbo [L, shield; Gk, *tympanon*, drum; L, *membrana*], a projection on the inner surface of the tympanic membrane where the malleus is attached.

umbrella filter /umbrəl′ə/, a small umbrella-shaped filter that can be inserted into the vena cava or other blood vessels to trap blood clots.

un-, [AS, not], a prefix meaning 'not': *unconscious.*

uncal herniation /ung′kəl/ [L, *uncus*, hook; *hernia*, rupture], a condition in which the medial portion of the temporal lobe protrudes over the tentorial edge as a result of increased intracranial pressure. If uncorrected, the progressive disorder causes pressure on the brainstem after first impinging on the third cranial nerve. A dilated pupil on the side of the herniation is a diagnostic sign of the disorder.

unciform bone. See **hamate bone.**

Uncinaria /un′siner′ē·ə/ [L, *uncinus*, hook], a genus of

nematode that causes hookworm in dogs, cats, and other carnivores.

uncompensated care /unkom′pənsā′tid/ [ME, *un*, against, not + L, *compendere*, to be equivalent], services provided by a hospital, a physician, or other health care professional for which no charge is made and for which no payment is expected.

uncompensated gluteal gait. See **Trendelenburg gait.**

uncompetitive inhibitor /un′kəmpet′itiv/ [ME, *un* + L, *competere*, to compete; *inhibere*, to restrain], an enzymatic inhibitor that appears to bond only to the enzyme substrate complex and not to free enzyme molecules.

unconditioned response /un′kəndish′ənd/ [ME, *un* + L, *conditio*, condition; *respondere*, to reply], a normal, instinctive, unlearned reaction to a stimulus; one that occurs naturally and is not acquired by association and training. Also called **inborn reflex, instinctive reflex, unconditioned reflex.** Compare **conditioned response.**

unconjugated monoclonal antibodies /unkon′jəgā′tid/, hybrid antibodies of a single antigenic specificity used for highly selective targeting of tumor cells. These antibodies can destroy malignant cells by direct lysis, by binding to cell receptors, and by mobilization of effector cells.

unconscious /unkon′shəs/ [ME, *un* + L, *conscire*, to be aware], **1.** unaware of the surrounding environment; insensible; incapable of responding to sensory stimuli. **2.** (in psychiatry) the part of the mental function in which thoughts, ideas, emotions, or memories are beyond awareness and not subject to ready recall. It contains data that have never been conscious or that were conscious at one time, usually for a brief period, and later repressed. Compare **preconscious.** See also **collective unconscious, personal unconscious.**

unconsciousness /unkon′shəsnəs/, a state of complete or partial unawareness or lack of response to sensory stimuli as a result of hypoxia, resulting from respiratory insuffi-

---

Possible causes of decreased levels of consciousness

1. Resulting from primary brain injury or disease
   a. Trauma (concussion, contusion, laceration, traumatic intercerebral hemorrhage, subdural hematoma, epidural hematoma)
   b. Vascular disease (intracerebral hemorrhage, subarachnoid hemorrhage, infarction)
   c. Infections (meningitis, encephalitis, abscess)
   d. Neoplasms (primarily intracranial, metastatic, or nonmetastatic complication of malignancy)
   e. Seizures
2. Resulting from systemic conditions that secondarily affect the brain
   a. Metabolic encephalopathies (hypoglycemia, diabetic ketoacidosis, hyperglycemic nonketotic hyperosmolar states, uremia, hepatic encephalopathy, hyponatremia, myxedema, hypercalcemia, and hypocalcemia)
   b. Hypoxic encephalopathies (severe congestive heart failure, COPD with decompensation, severe anemia, and hypertensive encephalopathies)
   c. Toxicity (heavy metals, carbon monoxide, and drugs—especially opiates, barbiturates, and alcohol)
   d. Physical causes (heat stroke and hypothermia)
   e. Deficiency states (Wernicke's encephalopathy)

From Phipps WJ, Long BL, Woods NF, Cassmeyer VL: *Medical-surgical nursing: concepts and clinical practice*, ed 4, St Louis, 1991, Mosby.

---

ciency or shock; from metabolic or chemical brain depressants, such as drugs, poisons, ketones, or electrolyte imbalance; or from a form of brain pathologic condition, such as trauma, seizures, cerebral vascular accident, or brain tumor or infection. Various degrees of unconsciousness can occur during stupor, fugue, catalepsy, and dream states. See also **coma.**

unction. See **ointment.**

uncus /ung′kəs/ [L, hook], **1.** the hooklike anterior end of the hippocampal gyrus on the temporal lobe of the brain. **2.** a hook-shaped structure.

undecylenic acid /un′desilen′ik/, an antifungal agent.
■ INDICATIONS: It is prescribed in the treatment of athlete's foot and ringworm.
■ CONTRAINDICATIONS: Known hypersensitivity to this drug prohibits its use. It is not used in the eyes or on mucous membranes. Caution is advised when the patient is diabetic.
■ ADVERSE EFFECTS: Among the more serious adverse effects are skin irritation and hypersensitivity reactions.

underdamping /un′dərdam′ping/ [AS, *under*, beneath, *dampen* to check], (in cardiology) the transmission of all frequency components without a reduction in amplitude.

underlying assumption /un′dərlī′ing/, a set of rules one holds about oneself, others, and the world. These rules are regarded as unquestionably true.

underwater exercise /un′dərwô′tər/ [AS, *under* + *woeter*], any physical activity performed in a pool or large tub, such as a Hubbard tank, where the buoyancy of the water facilitates the movement of weak or injured muscles. See also **exercise.**

underwater seal, a seal formed by water allowed to flow over a tube that exits from the chest cavity of a patient. The water acts as a one-way valve and permits the outflow of air but prevents the ingress of air. Also called **water trap.**

underweight /un′dərwāt′/ [AS, *under* + *wiht*], less than normal in body weight after adjustment for height, body build, and age.

undescended testis. See **cryptorchidism, monorchism.**

undifferentiated cell /undif′əren′shē·ā′tid/ [AS, *un-* not; L, *differentia*, difference + *cella*, storeroom], an embryonic-type cell that has not yet expressed signs of its future special type at maturity.

undifferentiated cell leukemia. See **stem cell leukemia.**

undifferentiated family ego mass, an emotional fusion in a family in which all members are similar in emotional expression and know each others' thoughts, feelings, and fantasies.

undifferentiated malignant lymphoma [ME, *un* + L, *differe*, to differ, *atus*, process; *malignus*, wicked; *lympha*, water; Gk, *oma*, tumor], a lymphoid neoplasm containing stem cells that have large nuclei, a small amount of pale cytoplasm, and ill-defined borders. Also called **reticulosarcoma, stem cell lymphoma.**

undifferentiated schizophrenia. See **acute schizophrenia.**

undifferentiation /un′diferen′shē·ā′shən/, the lack or absence of normal cell differentiation into an identifiable cell type.

undisplaced fracture /un′displāst, un′displāst′/, a bone break in which cracks in the osseous tissue may radiate in several directions without the separation or displacement of fragmented sections.

undoing /undōō′ing/ [ME, *un* + AS, *don*], the performance of a specific action that is intended to negate in part a previous action or communication. According to some psychologists, undoing is related to the magical thinking of childhood.

undulant /un′dyələnt/ [L, *unda*, wave], wavelike, such as a vibration, fluctuation, or oscillation.

undulant fever. See **brucellosis.**

unengaged head /un′engājd′/ [ME, *un* + Fr, *engager*, to involve; AS, *heafod*], the head of a floating fetus. See **engagement.** See also **ballottement.**

unequal cleavage /une′kwəl/ [ME, *un* + L, *aequare*, to make equal; AS, *cleofan*, to split], mitotic division of the fertilized ovum into blastomeres that are larger near the yolk portion of protoplasm, or vegetal pole, and smaller near the nucleus, or animal pole. Compare **equal cleavage.**

unequal pulse [AS, *un-*, not; L, *aequare*, to make equal + *pulsare*, to beat], a pulse in which the beats vary in intensity.

unequal twins, two nonjoined fetuses born of the same pregnancy in which only one of the pair is fully formed, with the other showing various degrees of developmental defects.

unfinished business /unfin′isht/, the concerns of a dying patient that require resolution before death can be accepted by the patient. Unfinished business may range from financial matters to personal relationships.

ung., abbreviation for the Latin word *unguentum*, 'unguenta', 'or ointment.'

ungual phalanx. See **distal phalanx.**

unguent. See **ointment.**

unguis. See **nail.**

uni- /yōō′nē-/ [L, *unus*], a prefix meaning 'one or single,: *unipara, unipolar, unicellular.*

uniaxial joint /yōō′nē·ak′sē·əl/ [L, *unus*, one, *axis*, axle; *jungere*, to join], a synovial joint in which movement is only in one axis, such as a pivot or hinge joint.

UNICEF /yōō′nisef′/, abbreviation for **United Nations International Children's Emergency Fund.**

unicellular reproduction /-sel′yələr/ [L, *unus* + *cella*, storeroom; *re*, again, *producere*, to produce], the formation of a new organism from a female egg that has not been fertilized; parthenogenesis.

unicentric blastoma. See **blastoma.**

unidirectional block /-direk′shənəl/ [L, *unus* + *dirigere*, to direct; Fr, *bloc*], a pathologic failure of cardiac impulse conduction in one direction while conduction is possible in the other direction.

unidisciplinary health care team /-dis′ipliner′ē/, a group of health care workers who are members of the same discipline.

unidose. See **unit dose.**

unification model /-kā′shən/ [L, *unus* + *ficare*, to make whole, *atus*, process; *modulus*, small measure], a theoretic framework based on the close relationship of nursing education and clinical nursing service at the University of Rochester (New York). The faculty of the school of nursing hold joint appointments to the school and the hospital, teaching nursing students and providing clinical leadership in nursing service in the hospital. See also **joint appointment.**

uniform reporting /yōō′nifôrm/, the reporting of service and financial data by a hospital in conformance with prescribed standard definitions to permit comparisons with other health facilities.

unilateral /-lat′ərəl/ [L, *unus*, one + *latus*, side], involving only one side.

unilateral denture. See **partial denture.**

unilateral hypertrophy [L, *unus* + *latus*, side; Gk, *hyper*, above, *trophe*, nourishment], enlargement of one side or a portion of one side of the body.

unilateral long-leg spica cast, an orthopedic cast applied to immobilize one leg and the trunk of the body cranially as far as the nipple line. It is used to treat a fractured femur or for the correction or the maintenance of the correction of a hip deformity. Compare **bilateral long-leg spica cast, one-and-a-half spica cast.**

unilateral neglect, a nursing diagnosis accepted by the Seventh National Conference on the Classification of Nursing Diagnoses. The condition is defined as a state in which an individual is perceptually unaware of and inattentive to one side of the body. The major defining characteristic is consistent inattention to stimuli on the affected side. Minor characteristics are inadequate self-care (as in positioning and/or safety precautions in regard to the affected side), lack of looking toward the affected side, and leaving food on the plate on the affected side. Related factors include effects of disturbed perceptual abilities, such as hemianopsia; one-sided blindness; and neurologic illness or trauma. See also **nursing diagnosis.**

unilateral paralysis. See **hemiplegia.**

uninterrupted suture /unin′tərup′tid/ [AS, *un*, not; L, *interrumpere*, to sever + *sutura*], a continous suture running forward and backward without interruption.

uniocular diplopia. See **monocular diplopia.**

uniocular squint. See **monocular strabismus.**

uniocular vision. See **monocular vision.**

uniovular /yōō′nē·ov′yələr/ [L, *unus* + *ovum*, egg], developing from a single ovum, as in monozygotic twins as contrasted with dizygotic twins. Also **monovular.** Compare **binovular.**

uniovular twins. See **monozygotic twins.**

Unipen, a trademark for an antibacterial (nafcillin sodium).

unipolar /-pō′lər/ [L, *unus*, one + *polus*], pertaining to a nerve cell with only one pole, such as a nerve cell in which the axon and dendrite are fused into a single process a short distance from the cell body.

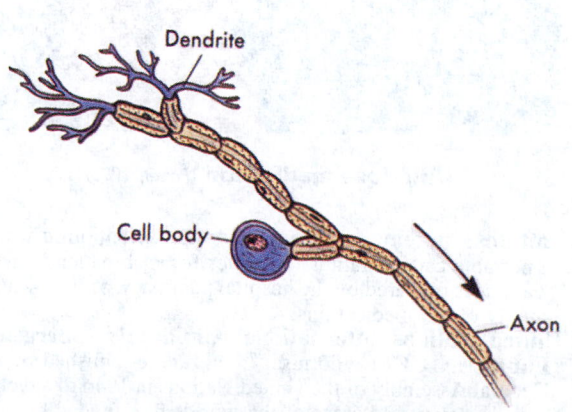

Unipolar neuron (Thibodeau, 1993/Scott Bodell)

unipolar depression   a major disorder of mood that is characterized by symptoms of depression only.

unipolar disorder.   See **endogenous depression.**

unipolar lead [L, *unus + polus,* pole; AS, *laedan,* to lead], **1.** an electrocardiographic conductor in which the exploring electrode is placed on the precordium or a limb while the indifferent electrode is in the central terminal. **2.** *informal.* a tracing produced by such a lead on an electrocardiograph.

unique radiolytic product /yo͞onēk′/,   a product, such as a food substance, that has undergone chemical changes as a result of exposure to ionizing radiation.

unisex /yo͞o′niseks/ [L, *unus,* one + *sexus,* sex], **1.** concerning only one sex or having reproductive organs of only one sex. **2.** an interchange of sex roles in clothing and hair styles, work assignments, shared restrooms, and other factors, such as encouraging boys to play with dolls.

unit (U) /yo͞o′nit/ [L, *unus*], **1.** a single item. **2.** a quantity designated as a standard of measurement. **3.** an area of a hospital that is staffed and equipped for treatment of patients with a specific condition or other common characteristics.

unitary human conceptual framework /yo͞o′niter′ē/,   a complex theory in nursing that emphasizes the importance of holistic health care and an understanding of the human being in relation to the universal environment.

unit clerk,   a person who performs routine clerical and reception tasks in a hospital inpatient care unit.

unit dose,   a method of preparing medications in which individual doses of patient medications are prepared by the pharmacy and delivered in individual labeled packets to the patient's unit to be administered by the nurses on the ordered schedule. Also called **unidose.**

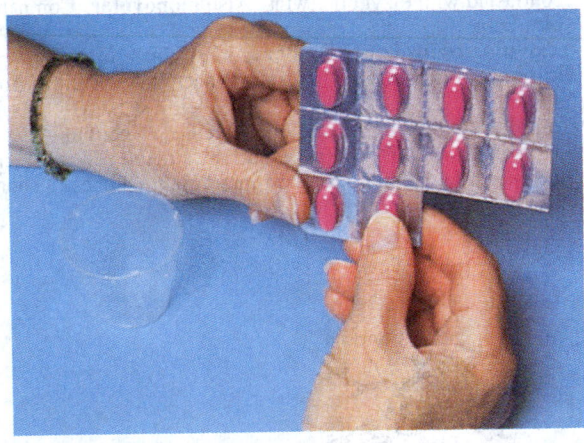

Unit dose medication (Potter, 1993)

unit dose system,   a system of drug distribution in which a portable cart containing a drawer for each patient's medications is prepared by the hospital pharmacy with a 24-hour supply of the medications.

United Nations International Children's Emergency Fund (UNICEF) /yo͞o′nisef′/,   a fund established by the General Assembly of the United Nations in 1946 to aid children in devastated areas of the world. It is funded by contributions from the member nations and acts to prevent dis-ease, including tuberculosis, whooping cough, and diphtheria, and provides food and clothing to needy children in more than 50 countries. In 1953, UNICEF was made a permanent organization of the United Nations.

United Network for Organ Sharing (UNOS),   a national organization for the collection and distribution of body organs that can be used in transplants. Hospitals advise relatives of newly deceased patients about the availability of UNOS service in arranging organ donations.

United States Pharmacopeia (USP),   a compendium, recognized officially by the Federal Food, Drug, and Cosmetic Act, that contains descriptions, uses, strengths, and standards of purity for selected drugs and for all of their forms of dosage.

United States Public Health Service (USPHS),   an agency of the federal government responsible for the control of the arrival from abroad of any people, goods, or substances that may affect the health of U.S. citizens. The agency sets standards for the domestic handling and processing of food and the manufacture of serums, vaccines, cosmetics, and drugs. It supports and performs research, aids localities in times of disaster and epidemics, and provides medical care for certain groups of Americans. The agency employs physicians, nurses, social workers, laboratory technicians, and many other specified health workers.

unit of service,   any individual, family, aggregate, organization, or community given nursing care. The level at which service is delivered varies with the particular unit entity.

univalent /yo͞o′nivāl′ənt, yo͞oniv′ələnt/ [L, *unus + valere,* to be worth],   referring to a chemical valency of one, or the capacity of one atom of a chemical element to attract one atom of hydrogen or to displace one atom of hydrogen. See also **valence.**

univalent antiserum.   See **antiserum.**

univalent reduction,   a phenomenon during intracellular metabolism involving oxygen-reduction reactions in which superoxide radicals are produced because oxygen accepts electrons only one at a time. In the short period between acceptance of the first and second electrons, one electron is unpaired and oxygen is a superoxide radical. The superoxide may then be converted to a second free radical.

universal /yo͞o′nivur′səl/ [L, *universalis*],   occurring everywhere and in all things.

universal antidote [L, *universus,* whole world; Gk, *anti,* against, *dotos,* something given],   a mixture of 50% activated charcoal, 25% magnesium oxide, and 25% tannic acid, formerly thought to be useful as an antidote for most types of acid, heavy metal, alkaloid, and glycoside poisons. It is now believed that the mixture is no more effective than activated charcoal given with water.

universal choking signal.   See **Heimlich sign.**

universal cuff,   an adaptive device worn on the hand to hold items such as utensils, shaver, or pencil, allowing a patient with a weak grasp to increase participation in self-care activities.

universal donor,   a person with type O, Rh factor negative red blood cells. Packed red blood cells of this type may be used for emergency transfusion with minimal risk of incompatibility. Blood plasma is not universal plasma. See also **blood donor, blood group, transfusion.**

universalizability principle /yo͞o′nivur′səlī′zəbil′itē/,   a principle that an act is good if everyone should, in similar circumstances, do the same act without exception.

universal precautions, an approach to infection control designed to prevent transmission of blood-borne diseases such as AIDS and hepatitis B in health care settings. Universal precautions were initially developed in 1987 by the Centers for Disease Control in the United States and in 1989 by the Bureau of Communicable Disease Epidemiology in Canada. The guidelines for universal precautions include specific recommendations for use of gloves and masks and protective eyewear when contact with blood or body secretions containing blood is anticipated.

universal qualifiers, (in neurolinguistic programming) the use of terms that give general impressions of limitations, such as all, common, every, only, and never.

universal recipient [L, *universalis* + *recipere*, to receive], a person with blood type AB, who can receive a transfusion of blood of any group type without agglutination or precipitation effects.

unmyelinated /unmī′əlinā′tid/ [AS, *un*, not; Gk, *myelos*, marrow], describing a nerve fiber that is not coated with a myelin sheath. An unmyelinated fiber, lacking the whitish sheath, appears as gray matter in the brain.

Unna's paste boot /o͞o′nəz/ [Paul G. Unna, German dermatologist, b. 1850; L, *pasta*, paste; ME, *bote*], a dressing for varicose ulcers formed by applying a layer of a gelatin-glycerin-zinc oxide paste to the leg and then a spiral bandage that is covered with successive coats of paste to produce a rigid boot.

UNOS, /yo͞o′nos/ abbreviation for **United Network for Organ Sharing.**

unresolved grief /un′rizolvd′/, a severe, chronic grief reaction in which a person does not complete the resolution stage of the grieving process within a reasonable time.

unsaturated /unsach′ərātid/ [ME, *un* + L, *saturare*, to fill], **1.** describing a solution that is capable of dissolving more of the solute; not saturated. **2.** also called **unsaturated hydrocarbon.** an organic compound in which two or more carbon atoms are united by double or triple valence bonds, as in unsaturated fatty acids. Compare **saturated.**

unsaturated alcohol, an alcohol derived from an unsaturated hydrocarbon, such as an alkene or olefin.

unsaturated compound [AS, *un*, not; L, *saturare*, to fill + *componere*, to put together], a chemical copound that contains double or triple bonds.

unsaturated fatty acid, any of a number of glyceryl esters of certain organic acids in which some of the atoms are joined by double or triple valence bonds. These bonds are easily split in chemical reactions, and other substances are joined to them. Monounsaturated fatty acids have only one double or triple bond per molecule and are found in such foods as fowl, almonds, pecans, cashew nuts, peanuts, and olive oil. Polyunsaturated fatty acids have more than one double or triple bond per molecule and are found in fish, corn, walnuts, sunflower seeds, soybeans, cottonseeds, and safflower oil. Diets high in polyunsaturated fatty acids and low in saturated fatty acids have been correlated with low serum cholesterol levels in some study populations. Compare **saturated fatty acid.**

unsaturated hydrocarbon. See **unsaturated.**

unscrubbed team members /unskrubd′/, the members of a surgical team, including the anesthetist and circulating nurse, who wear surgical attire but are not gowned or gloved and do not enter the sterile field.

unsocialized aggressive reaction /unsō′shəlīzd/ [ME, *un* + L, *socialis*, companion; *aggressio*, an attack; *re*, *agere*, again to act], a behavior disorder of childhood characterized by overt and covert hostility, disobedience, physical and verbal aggression, vengefulness, quarrelsome behavior, and destructiveness, often manifested in acts such as lying, stealing, temper tantrums, vandalism, and physical violence against others.

unstable /unstā′bəl/, **1.** in an excited or active state, such as an atom with a nucleus possessing excess energy. **2.** easily broken down.

unstable angina [AS, *un*, not; *stabilis*, firm + *angina*, quinsy], a form of pain that is prodromal to acute myocardial infarction. It typically has a sudden onset, sudden worsening, and stuttering recurrance over days and weeks. It carries a more severe short-term prognosis than stable chronic angina. Nearly one third of unstable angina patients may experience myocardial infarction within 3 months.

unstriated muscle. See **smooth muscle.**

upper airway obstruction (UAO), any abnormal condition of the mouth, nose, or larynx that interferes with breathing when the rest of the respiratory system is functioning normally.

upper extremity suspension, an orthopedic procedure used in the treatment of bone fractures and the correction of orthopedic abnormalities of the upper limbs. The procedure uses traction equipment, including metal frames, ropes, and pulleys to relieve the weight of the upper limb involved rather than to exert traction. Upper extremity suspension is usually unilateral but also may be used bilaterally in the postoperative, posttraumatic, or postreduction control of edema. Compare **balanced suspension, hyperextension suspension, lower extremity suspension.**

upper GI, pertaining to the upper GI tract, from the esophagus to and including the duodenum. The term is commonly applied to radiographic or fluoroscopic diagnostic views after ingestion of a barium sulfate "milkshake." Normal findings include normal size, contour, patency, filling, positioning, and transmission of barium through the lower esophagus, stomach, and duodenum. Also called **UGI, upper GI series.**

upper level discriminator (ULD), an electronic device used to discriminate against all pulses whose heights are above a given level.

upper motor neuron paralysis, an injury to or lesion in the brain or spinal cord that causes damage to the cell bodies, axons, or both, of the upper motor neurons, which extend from the cerebral centers to the cells in the spinal column. Clinical manifestations include weakness or paralysis, increased muscle tone and spasticity of the muscles involved with little or no atrophy, hyperactive deep tendon reflexes, diminished or absent superficial reflexes, the presence of pathologic reflexes, such as Babinski's and Hoffmann's reflexes, and no local twitching of muscle groups. Compare **lower motor neuron paralysis.**

upper pole of kidney, the extremitas superior renis. See **poles of kidney.**

upper respiratory infection. See **respiratory tract infection.**

upper respiratory tract, one of the two divisions of the respiratory system. The upper respiratory tract consists of the nose, the nasal cavity, the ethmoidal air cells, the frontal sinuses, the sphenoidal sinuses, the maxillary sinus, the larynx, and the trachea. The upper respiratory tract conducts air to and from the lungs and filters, moistens, and warms the air during each inspiration. Infection and irritation of the upper respiratory tract are common and often spread to the lower respiratory tract, where they may cause serious complications. See also **larynx, nose, trachea.** Compare **lower respiratory tract.**

upsilon /yŏŏp'silon, up'-/, γ, υ, the twentieth letter of the greek alphabet.

uptake /up'tāk/ [AS, *uptacan*], the drawing up or absorption of a substance.

upward-and-downward squint. See **vertical strabismus.**

UR, abbreviation for **utilization review.**

ur-. See **uro-.**

urachus /yŏŏr'əkəs/ [Gk, *ourachos*, urinary tract], an epithelial tube connecting the apex of the urinary bladder with the allantois. Its connective tissue forms the median umbilical ligament.

-uracil, a suffix for uracil derivatives used as thyroid antagonists and as antineoplastics.

uragogue. See **-agogue, -agog.**

uranium (U) /yŏŏrā'nē·əm/ [planet Uranus], a heavy, radioactive metallic element. Its atomic number is 92; its atomic weight is 238.03. Uranium is the heaviest of the natural elements. Isotopes of uranium are used in nuclear power plants to provide neutrons for the nuclear reactions that result in release of energy.

urano-, a combining form meaning 'pertaining to the palate': *uranoplasty, uranoplegia, uranoschism.*

urate /yŏŏr'āt/, any salt of uric acid, such as sodium urate. Urates are found in the urine, blood, and tophi or calcareous deposits in tissues. They also may be deposited as crystals in body joints. See also **gout, uric acid.**

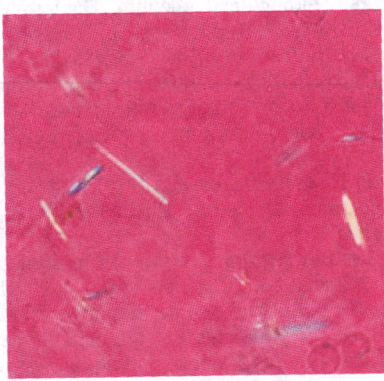

Monosodium urate crystals under polarized light
(Shipley, 1993)

urban typhus. See **murine typhus.**

urea /yŏŏr'ē·ə/ [Gk, *ouron*, urine], a systemic osmotic diuretic and topical keratolytic.

■ INDICATIONS: It is prescribed to reduce cerebrospinal and intraocular fluid pressure and is used topically as a keratolytic agent.

■ CONTRAINDICATIONS: Severely impaired kidney function, active intracranial bleeding, marked dehydration, or liver damage prohibits its systemic use.

■ ADVERSE EFFECTS: Among the more serious adverse reactions are pain and necrosis at the site of injection, headache, GI disturbances, and dizziness. There are no known severe reactions to topical use.

-urea, a suffix meaning a 'compound containing urea': *glycolylurea, plenylurea, solurea.*

urea cycle, a series of enzymatic reactions by which ammonia is detoxified in the liver. In the series of steps for disposing of the ammonia molecule, a waste product of protein metabolism, five enzymatic reactions occur as NH_2 radicals are combined with carbon and oxygen atoms from carbon dioxide to form urea, which is excreted. The amino acid arginine is synthesized during the same process. Also called **Krebs Henseleit cycle.**

urea nitrogen. See **blood urea nitrogen.**

Ureaplasma urealyticum /-plaz'mə/, a sexually transmitted microorganism that is a common inhabitant of the urogenital systems of men and women in whom infection is asymptomatic. Neonatal death, prematurity, and perinatal morbidity are statistically associated with colonization of the chorionic surface of the placenta by *Ureaplasma urealyticum*. The mechanisms by which the unfavorable effects on pregnancy occur are not understood. There is no characteristic lesion in the fetus or newborn.

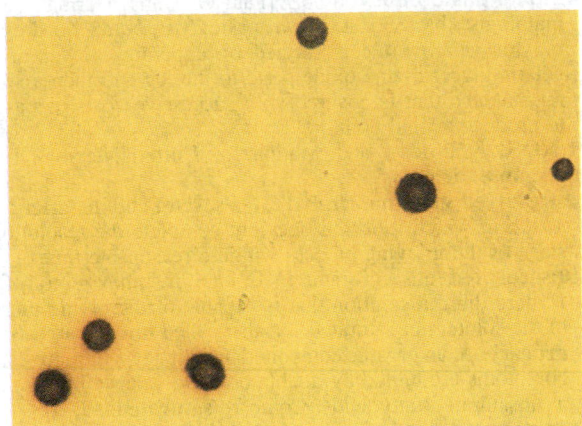

***Ureaplasma urealyticulum* colonies on agar**
(Baron, 1990)

Urecholine, a trademark for a cholinergic (bethanechol chloride).

uremia /yŏŏrē'mē·ə/ [Gk, *ouron* + *haima*, blood], the presence of excessive amounts of urea and other nitrogenous waste products in the blood, as occurs in renal failure. Also called **azotemia.** See also **chronic glomerulonephritis, subacute glomerulonephritis.**

uremic /yŏŏrē'mik/ [Gk, *ouron*, urine + *haima*, blood], pertaining to a toxic level of urea in the blood.

uremic coma [Gk, *ouron*, urine + *koma*, deep sleep], a stuporous condition resulting from acidosis and the toxic effects of uremia with the retention in the blood of metabolic end products that would normally be excreted through the kidneys.

uremic frost, a pale, frostlike deposit of white crystals on the skin caused by kidney failure and uremia. Urea compounds and other waste products of metabolism that cannot be excreted by the kidneys into the urine are excreted through the small superficial capillaries into the skin, where they collect on the surface.

uremic gingivitis. See **nephritic gingivitis.**

-uret, a combining form designating a binary compound: *bromuret, phosphuret, sulphuret.*

ureter /yo͞or′ətər, yo͞orē′tər/ [Gk, *oureter*], one of a pair of tubes, about 30 cm long, that carries urine from the kidney into the bladder. The tubes are thick-walled, vary in diameter along their length from 1 mm to 1 cm, and are divided into an abdominal portion and a pelvic portion. The abdominal portion lies behind the peritoneum on the medial side of the psoas major and enters the pelvic cavity by crossing either the termination of the common iliac artery or the commencement of the external iliac artery. In men, the pelvic portion of the ureter runs caudal along the lateral wall of the pelvic cavity and reaches the lateral angle of the bladder just ventral to the upper tip of the seminal vesicle. In women, the pelvic portion of the ureter forms the posterior boundary of the ovarian fossa and runs medially and ventrally along the upper part of the vagina. The ureter enters the bladder through an oblique tunnel that functions as a valve to prevent backflow of urine into the ureter when the bladder contracts. Connecting with the kidneys, the ureters expand into funnel-shaped renal pelves that branch into calyces, each calyx containing a renal papilla. Urine draining through renal tubules drops into the papillae and passes through the calyces and the pelvis and down each ureter into the bladder. The openings of the ureters in the bladder lie at the lateral angles of the trigone, spaced about 2 cm apart when the bladder is empty, about 5 cm apart when the bladder is distended. Urine is pumped through the ureters by peristaltic waves that occur an average of three times a minute. Each ureter is composed of a fibrous, a muscular, and a mucous coat and is perfused by arterial branches of the renal, the testicular, the internal iliac, and the inferior vesical arteries. It is innervated by nerves derived from the inferior mesenteric, the testicular, and the pelvic plexi. —**ureteral** /yo͞orē′terəl/, *adj.*

ureter-, ,uretero-, a combining form 'pertaining to the ureter': *ureterorrhagia, ureterostenosis, ureterosigmoidoscopy.*

ureteral dysfunction /yo͞orē′terəl/ [Gk, *oureter* + *dys*, bad; L, *functio*, performance], a disturbance of the normal peristaltic flow of urine through a ureter, resulting from dysfunction of ureteral motor nerves. See also **megaloureter.**

uretercystoscope /yo͞or′ētər-sis′təskōp′/ [Gk, *oureter*, ureter + *kystis*, bladder + *skopein*, to view], a cystoscope equipped with ureteric catheters that can be inserted into either ureter.

ureteritis /yo͞orē′tərī′tis/ [Gk, *oureter* + *itis*], an inflammatory condition of a ureter caused by infection or by the mechanic irritation of a stone.

uretero-. See **ureter-.**

ureterocele /yo͞orē′tərōsēl′/ [Gk, *oureter* + *kele*, hernia], a prolapse of the terminal portion of the ureter into the bladder. The condition may lead to obstruction of the flow of urine, hydronephrosis, and loss of renal function. Cystoscopy and pyelography reveal the prolapsed ureter. Surgical correction is performed to prevent permanent damage to the kidney. Compare **cystocele.**

ureterodialysis /-dī·al′isis/ [Gk, *oureter*, ureter + *dialysis*, a breaking], the rupture of a ureter. Also called **ureterolysis.**

ureterography /yo͞orē′tərog′rəfē/ [Gk, *oureter* + *graphein*, to record], the radiologic imaging of a ureter, usually conducted as part of an examination of the urinary tract. The examination may involve injection of a radiopaque medium through a urinary catheter with the aid of a ureterocystoscope (the ascending method), or by intravenous injection of a contrast medium that permits the filtering of the substance through the kidneys (the descending method) to the ureters.

ureterolysis. See **ureterodialysis.**

ureteroplasty /yo͞orē′tərōplas′tē/ [Gk, *oureter* + *plassein*, to mold], a surgical procedure performed to restructure a ureter, such as when a stricture blocks the normal flow of urine.

ureteropyelonephritis /-pī′əlō′nəfrī′tis/ [Gk, *oureter* + *pyelos*, pelvis + *nephros*, kidney + *itis*, inflammation], an inflammation of the kidney, pelvis, and ureter.

ureterosigmoidostomy /-sig′moidos′təmē/ [Gk, *oureter* + *sigma*, letter S, *eidos*, form, *stoma*, mouth], a surgical procedure in which a ureter is implanted in the sigmoid flexure of the intestinal tract.

ureterostomy /-os′təmē/ [Gk, *oureter* + *stoma*, mouth], the surgical creation of a new opening from a ureter to the surface of the body or into another outlet, such as the rectum.

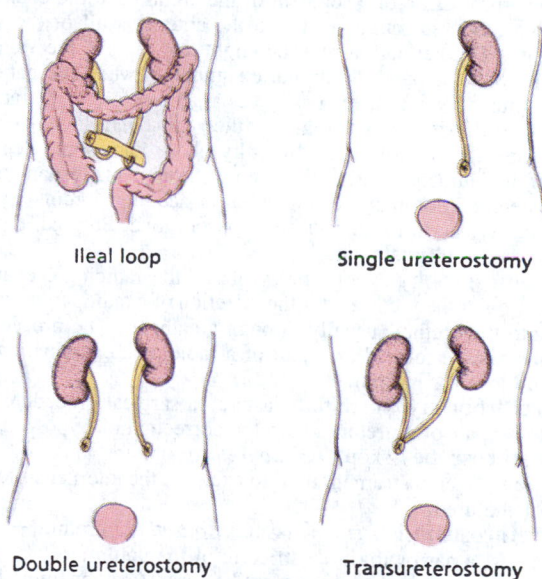

Ileal loop   Single ureterostomy

Double ureterostomy   Transureterostomy

Types of ureterostomies (Potter, 1993)

ureterotomy, an incision into a ureter.

urethra /yo͞orē′thrə/ [Gk, *ourethra*], a small tubular structure that drains urine from the bladder. In women, it is about 3 cm long and lies directly behind the symphysis pubis, anterior to the vagina. In men, it is about 20 cm long and begins at the bladder, passes through the center of the prostate gland, goes between two sheets of tissue connecting the pubic bones, and finally passes through the urinary meatus of the penis. In men, the urethra serves as a passageway for semen during ejaculation, as well as a canal for urine during voiding. See also **ureter.**

urethral /yo͞orē′thrəl/, of or pertaining to the urethra.

urethral caruncle [Gk, *ourethra*; L, *caruncula*, small piece of flesh], a small painful growth in the mucous membrane of the female urethral meatus. It may be a source of bleeding.

urethral hematuria [Gk, *ourethra* + *haima*, blood + *ouron*, urine], blood in the urine as a result of a urethral lesion.

urethral papilla. See **papilla.**

urethral sphincter, the voluntary muscle at the neck of the bladder that relaxes to allow urination.

urethral swab [Gk, *ourethra*; Du, *zwabber*], an absorbent pad on a slender rod used to treat lesions or to remove secretions.

urethritis /yoor'ithrī'tis/, an inflammatory condition of the urethra that is characterized by dysuria, usually the result of an infection in the bladder or kidneys. Medications, such as a sulfonamide or other antibacterial, a urinary antiseptic, and an analgesic, are usually prescribed after the causative organism is identified by bacteriologic culture of a urine specimen. See also **nongonococcal urethritis.**

urethro- /yoorē'thro-/, a combining form meaning 'pertaining to the urethra': *urethrocele, urethrocystitis, urethrophraxis.*

urethrocele /yoorē'thrə'sēl/ [Gk, *urethra* + *kele*, hernia], (in women) a herniation of the urethra. It is characterized by a protrusion of a segment of the urethra and the connective tissue surrounding it into the anterior wall of the vagina. The herniation may be slight and high in the vagina and only palpable on digital examination when the patient strains downward, or it may be large and low in the anterior wall with visible bulging at the vaginal introitus. A large cystocele may result in difficulty in voiding, some degree of incontinence, urinary tract infection, and dyspareunia. The condition may be congenital or acquired, secondary to obesity, parturition, and poor muscle tone. Surgical repair is the usual treatment.

urethrography /yoor'ēthrog'rəfē/, the radiologic examination of the urethra after the injection of a radiopaque agent into the urethra, usually through a catheter. The procedure may be performed as a part of a radiologic examination of the lower urinary tract.

urethroplasty /yoorē'thrəplastē/, a surgical procedure for the repair of a urethra, as in the correction of hypospadias.

urethroscope /-skōp'/ [Gk, *ourethra,* urethra + *skopein,* to view], an instrument used to examine the internal surfaces of the urethra.

urethrostenosis /-stənō'sis/ [Gk, *ourethra,* urethra + *stenosis,* a narrowing], a stricture of the urethra.

Urex, a trademark for an antibacterial (methenamine hippurate).

urgency /ur'jensē/ [L, *urgere,* to drive on], a feeling of the need to void urine immediately.

-urgy, a suffix meaning the 'art of working with (specified) tools': *chemurgy, micrurgy, zymurgy.*

URI, abbreviation for **upper respiratory infection.** See **respiratory tract infection.**

-uria, 1. a suffix meaning the 'presence of a substance in the urine': *ammoniuria, calciuria, enzymuria.* 2. a combining form meaning '(condition of) possessing urine': *paruria, polyuria, pyuria.*

uric acid /yoor'ik/, a product of the metabolism of protein present in the blood and excreted in the urine. Normal adult levels of blood uric acid range from 2.0 to 8.5 mg/dl, with slightly higher values for elderly patients. See also **gout, kidney, liver, purine, urine.**

uricaciduria /yoor'ikas'idoor'ē·ə/ [Gk, *ouron* + L, *acidus,* sour; Gk, *ouron*], a greater than normal amount of uric

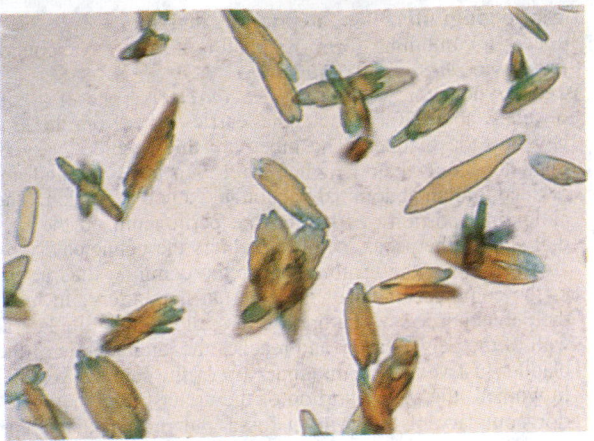

Uricaciduria *(Weiss, 1988)*

acid in the urine, often associated with urinary calculi or gout.

urico-, a combining form meaning 'pertaining to uric acid': *uricocholia, uricosuria, uricotelic.*

uricosuric drugs /yoor'ikōsoor'ik/ [Gk, *ouron* + L, *acidus,* sour; Gk, *ouron;* Fr, *drogue*], drugs administered to relieve the pain of gout or to increase the elimination of uric acid.

-uridine, a suffix for uridine derivatives used as antiviral agents and as antineoplastics.

urinal /yoor'inəl/, a plastic or metal receptacle for collecting urine.

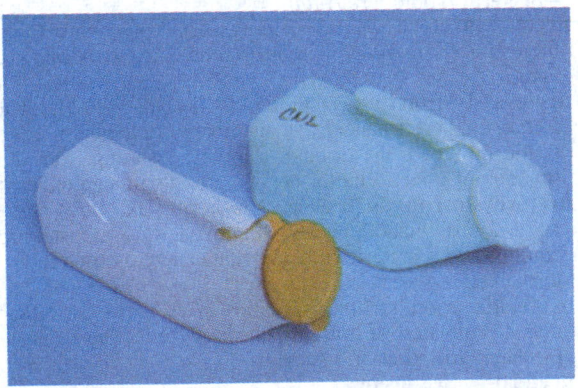

Urinals *(Potter, 1993)*

urinalysis /yoor'inal'isis/ [Gk, *ouron* + *analysein,* to loosen], a physical, microscopic, or chemical examination of urine. The specimen is physically examined for color, turbidity, specific gravity, and pH. Then it is spun in a centrifuge to allow collection of a small amount of sediment that is examined microscopically for blood cells, casts, crystals, pus, and bacteria. Chemical analysis may be performed for the identification and quantification of any of a large number of substances but most commonly for ketones, sugar, protein, and blood. The nurse collects the urine spec-

Urinalysis

Test	Normal	Abnormal
Color	Amber-yellow	Red indicated hematuria (possible urinary obstruction, renal calculi, tumor, renal failure)
Clarity	Clear	Cloudy: debris, bacterial sediment (urinary infection)
pH	4.6-8.0 (average 6.0)	Alkaline on standing or with urinary tract infection
		Increased acidity with renal tubular acidosis
Specific gravity	1.003-1.035	Usually reflects fluid intake; the less the fluid intake, the higher the specific gravity
		If specific gravity remains low (1.010-1.014), renal disease is suspected
Protein	0-8 mg/dl	Proteinuria may occur with high-protein diet and exercise (particularly prolonged)
		Seen in renal disease
Sugar	0	Glycosuria occurs after a high intake of sugar or with diabetes mellitus
Ketones	0	Ketonuria occurs with starvation and diabetic ketoacidosis
RBCs	0-4	Injury to kidney tissue (see hematuria)
WBCs	0-5	UTI
Casts	0	UTI, renal disease

From Phipps WJ, Long BL, Woods NF, Cassmeyer VL: *Medical-surgical nursing: concepts and clinical practice,* ed 4, St Louis, 1991, Mosby.

imen for chemical analysis according to the directions of the specific laboratory.

urinary /yŏŏr′iner′ē/, of or pertaining to urine or the formation of urine.

urinary albumin [Gk, *ouron,* urine; L, *albus,* white], the presence of albumin, a protein, in the urine. Normally, protein is not found in the urine because the spaces in the glomerular membrane of the kidney are too small to allow escape of protein molecules. If the membrane is damaged, however, as in some kidney diseases, albumin molecules can leak through into the urine. Normal findings are: none or up to 8 mg/dl; 50 to 80 mg/24 hours at rest; less than 250 mg/24 hours after strenuous exercise. Also called **urine protein, proteinuria.**

urinary bladder [Gk, *ouron* + AS, *blaedre*], the muscular membranous sac in the pelvis that stores urine for discharge through the urethra. It is connected anteriorly with the two ureters and posteriorly with the urethra.

urinary calculus, a calculus formed in any part of the urinary tract. Calculi may be large enough to cause an obstruction in the flow of urine or small enough to be passed with the urine. Kinds of urinary calculi are **renal calculus** and **vesicle calculus.** See also **calculus.**

urinary casts [Gk, *ouron,* urine; ONorse, *kasta],* cells or particles excreted in the urine having the shape of renal collecting tubules.

urinary elimination, altered, a nursing diagnosis accepted by the Fourth National Conference on the Classification of Nursing Diagnoses. It is defined as the state in which an individual experiences a disturbance in urine elimination. The defining characteristics are dysuria, urinary frequency, urinary hesitancy, urinary incontinence, nocturia, urinary retention, and urinary urgency. Related factors are sensory motor impairment, neuromuscular impairment, and mechanical trauma. See also **nursing diagnosis.**

urinary frequency, a greater than normal frequency of the urge to void without an increase in the total daily volume of urine. The condition is characteristic of inflammation in the bladder or urethra or of diminished bladder capacity or other structural abnormalities. Burning and urgency with increased frequency herald an infection of the urinary tract. Infection requires precise diagnosis and specific antibacterial medication; structural abnormality may require surgical correction. See also **cystitis, cystocele.**

urinary hesitancy, a decrease in the force of the stream of urine, often with difficulty in beginning the flow. Hesitancy is usually the result of an obstruction or stricture between the bladder and the urethral opening; in men it may indicate an enlargement of the prostate gland, in women, stenosis of the urethral opening. Cold, stress, dehydration, and various neurogenic and psychogenic factors are common causes of this condition.

urinary ileostomy [Gk, *ouron,* urine; L, *ilia,* intestines; Gk, *stoma,* mouth], the surgical creation of a passage between the urinary bladder and the ileum for the diversion of urinary flow from the ureters.

urinary incontinence, involuntary passage of urine, with the failure of voluntary control over bladder and urethral sphincters. Among the causes are neurogenic bladder dysfunction resulting from lesions of the brain and spinal cord, a neoplasm or calculus in the bladder, multiple sclerosis, obstruction of the lower urinary tract, trauma, aging, and multiparity in women. In children, incontinence may be psychogenic or the result of allergy. Treatment with medication, surgery, or psychotherapy appropriate to the underlying cause is often effective.

urinary infection. See **urinary tract infection.**

urinary meatus, the external opening of the urethra.

urinary output, the total volume of urine excreted daily, normally between 700 and 2000 ml. Various metabolic and renal diseases may change the normal urinary output, resulting in increased or decreased flow of urine. See also **anuria, oliguria, polyuria.**

urinary retention, a nursing diagnosis accepted by the Seventh National Conference on the Classification of Nursing Diagnoses. The condition is described as the state in which an individual experiences incomplete emptying of the bladder. Major defining characteristics are bladder distention and small, infrequent voiding or absence of urine output. Minor characteristics are a sensation of bladder fullness, dribbling, residual urine, dysuria, and overflow incontinence. Related factors include high urethral pressure caused by a weak detrusor, inhibition of reflex arc, strong sphincter, and blockage. See also **nursing diagnosis.**

urinary sediment [Gk, *ouron,* urine; L, *sedimentum,* a settling], solid matter that settles to the bottom of a urine sample that has been allowed to stand for several hours.

urinary system, all of the organs involved in the secre-

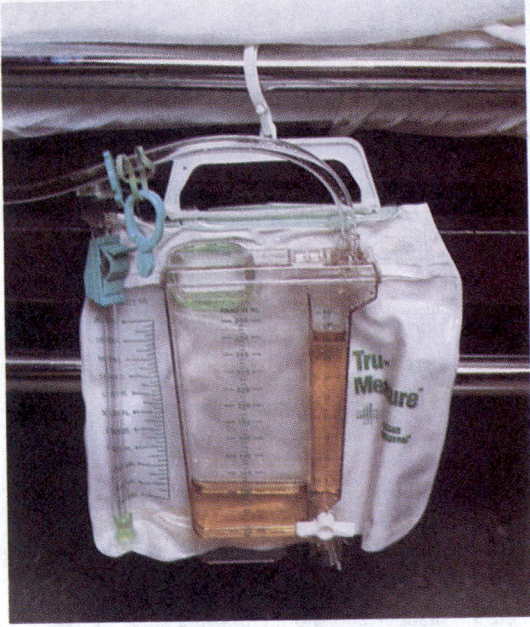

**Urimeter drainage bag for
measurment of urinary output**
(Potter, 1993)

tion and elimination of urine. These include the kidneys, ureters, bladder, and urethra. See also the Color Atlas of Human Anatomy.

urinary system assessment, an evaluation of the condition and functioning of the kidneys, bladder, ureters, and urethra and an investigation of concurrent and previous disorders that may be factors in abnormalities in the urinary system.

■ METHOD: In an interview the patient is asked whether dysuria, frequency or burning on urination, dribbling, a decreased urinary stream, nocturia, stress incontinence, headache, back pain, or increased thirst has occurred. The color, odor, and amount of urine voided without a catheter and with one in place are determined. The patient's vital signs, any distention of the bladder, the condition of the skin, neurologic changes, the location, duration, and character of pain, and the presence of bladder spasms are recorded. It is determined whether the patient has hypertension, diabetes, a venereal disease, vaginal or urethral drainage or discharge, or a history that includes cystitis, pyelonephritis, kidney stones, prostatectomy, renal surgery, a kidney transplant, or a venereal infection. The patient's sexual activity, use of coffee, tea, cola beverages, alcohol, perfumed soaps, feminine hygiene sprays, and prescribed and over-the-counter medication, and habit of bathing in a tub or shower are ascertained. A family history of polycystic kidney disease, hypertension, diabetes, or cancer is noted in the assessment, together with laboratory studies of the specific gravity of the patient's urine, casts, protein, red and white cells in the urine, and the serum creatinine level. Diagnostic procedures may include cystoscopy, excretory and intravenous urography, renal angiography, retrograde studies, and x-ray film of the kidneys, ureters, and bladder.

■ NURSING INTERVENTION: The nurse interviews the patient, reports the objective data, and assembles the background information and the results of the diagnostic tests.

■ OUTCOME CRITERIA: A comprehensive assessment of the patient's urinary system aids the urologist in establishing the diagnosis.

urinary tract, all organs and ducts involved in the secretion and elimination of urine from the body.

urinary tract infection (UTI), an infection of one or more structures in the urinary tract. Most of these infections are caused by gram-negative bacteria, most commonly *Escherichia coli* or species of *Klebsiella, Proteus, Pseudomonas,* or *Enterobacter.* The condition is more common in women than in men and may be asymptomatic. Urinary tract infection is usually characterized by urinary frequency, burning, pain with voiding, and, if the infection is severe, visible blood and pus in the urine. Diagnosis of the cause and the location of the infection is made by microscopic examination of the sediment and supernatant portion of a centrifuged urine specimen, by physical examination of the patient, by bacteriologic culture of a specimen of urine, and, if necessary, by various radiologic techniques, such as retrograde pyelography, or by cystoscopy. Treatment includes antibacterial, analgesic, and urinary antiseptic drugs. Kinds of urinary tract infections include **cystitis, pyelonephritis,** and **urethritis.**

urinate /yoor′ināt/ [Gk *ouron* urine], to excrete urine from the bladder.

urination /yoor′inā′shən/ [Gk, *ouron* + L, *atus*, process], the act of passing urine. Also called **micturition.**

urine /yoor′in/ [Gk *ouron*], the fluid secreted by the kidneys, transported by the ureters, stored in the bladder, and voided through the urethra. Normal urine is clear, straw-colored, and slightly acid, and has the characteristic odor of urea. The normal specific gravity of urine is between 1.003 and 1.035. Its normal constituents include water, urea, sodium chloride and potassium chloride, phosphates, uric acid, organic salts, and the pigment urobilin. Abnormal constituents indicative of disease include ketone bodies, protein, bacteria, blood, glucose, pus, and certain crystals. See also **bacteriuria, glycosuria, hematuria, ketoaciduria, proteinuria.**

urine osmolality, the osmotic pressure of urine. The normal values are 500 to 800 mOsm/L.

urine pH, the hydrogen ion concentration of the urine, or a measure of its acidity or alkalinity. The normal pH value for urine is 4.6 to 8.0.

urine protein. See **urinary albumin.**

urine specific gravity, a measure of the degree of concentration of a sample of urine. The normal range of urine specific gravity is 1.003 to 1.035, depending on the patient's previous fluid intake, renal perfusion, and renal function.

urinoma /yoor′inō′mə/, *pl.* **urinoma, urinomata,** a cyst filled with urine.

urinometer /yoor′inom′ətər/ [Gk, *ouron* + *metron*, measure], any device for determining the specific gravity of urine, including gravitometers and hydrometers. Also called **urometer** /yoorom′ətər/.

Urised, a trademark for a urinary fixed-combination drug containing an antibacterial (methenamine), an analgesic (phenyl salicylate), anticholinergics (atropine sulfate and hyoscyamine), an antifungal (benzoic acid), and an antiseptic (methylene blue).

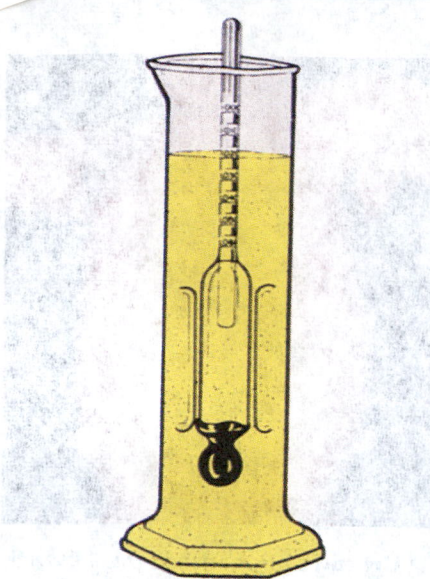

Urinometer (Potter, 1993)

Urispas, a trademark for a smooth muscle relaxant (flavoxate hydrochloride).

uro- /yŏŏr'ō-/ **ur-, urono-,** a combining form meaning 'pertaining to urine, the urinary tract, or urination': *urocrisia, uromancy, uropterin.*

urobilin /yŏŏr'əbī'lin/, a brown pigment formed by the oxidation of urobilinogen, normally found in feces and, in small amounts, in urine.

urobilinogen /yŏŏr'əbīlin'əjən/, a colorless compound formed in the intestine after the breakdown of bilirubin by bacteria. Some of this substance is excreted in feces, and some is resorbed and excreted again in bile or urine. See also **urobilin.**

Urobiotic, a trademark for a urinary fixed-combination drug containing antibacterials (oxytetracycline hydrochloride and sulfamethizole) and an analgesic (phenazopyridine hydrochloride).

urodynamics /-dīnam'iks/ [Gk, *ouron,* urine + *dynamis,* force], the study of the hydrology and mechanics of urinary bladder filling and emptying.

urogenital /yŏŏr'ōjen'itəl/ [Gk, *ouron* + L, *genitalis,* fruitful], of or pertaining to the urinary and the reproductive systems. Also called **genitourinary.**

urogenital sinus, one of the elongated cavities, formed by the division of the cloaca in early embryonic development, into which open the ureter, mesonephric and paramesonephric ducts, and bladder. It also gives rise to the vestibule, urethra, and part of the vagina in the female and part of the urethra in the male.

urogenital system, the urinary and genital organs and the associated structures that develop in the fetus to form the kidneys, the ureters, the bladder, the urethra, and the genital structures of the male and female. In women these are the ovaries, the uterine tubes, the uterus, the clitoris, and the vagina. In men these are the testes, the seminal vesicles, the seminal ducts, the prostate, and the penis. Also

called **genitourinary system.** See also the *Color Atlas of Human Anatomy.*

urogram /yŏŏr'əgram'/, an x-ray film of the urinary tract, obtained by urography. See also **pyelogram.**

urography /yŏŏrog'rəfē/ [Gk, *ouron* + *graphein,* to record], any of a group of x-ray techniques used to examine the urinary system. A radiopaque substance is injected, and x-ray films are taken as the substance is passed through or excreted from the part of the system being studied. Some kinds of urography are **cystoscopic urography, intravenous pyelography,** and **retrograde pyelography.**

urokinase /yŏŏr'əkī'nās/, an enzyme, produced in the kidney and found in urine, that is a potent plasminogen activator of the fibrinolytic system. A pharmaceutic preparation of urokinase is administered intravenously in the treatment of pulmonary embolism.

urolagnia /yŏŏr'əlag'nē·ə/, sexual stimulation gained from acts involving urine, such as watching people urinate or being urinated on.

urolithiasis. See **urinary calculus.**

urologic /-loj'ik/ [Gk, *ouron,* urine + *logos,* science], pertaining to the scientific study of the urinary tract.

urologist /yŏŏrol'əjist/, a licensed physician who has completed an approved residency program and who specializes in the practice of urology.

urology /yŏŏrol'əjē/ [Gk, *ouron* + *logos,* science], the branch of medicine concerned with the study of the anatomy and physiology, the disorders, and the care of the urinary tract in men and women and of the male genital tract.

uromelus. See **sympus monopus.**

urometer /yŏŏrom'ətər/ [Gk, *ouron,* urine + *metron,* measure], a type of hydrometer used to measure the specific gravity of a urine sample. Also called **urinometer.**

urono-. See **uro-.**

uropathy /yŏŏrop'əthē/ [Gk, *ouron* + *pathos,* disease], any disease or abnormal condition of any structure of the urinary tract. **–uropathic,** *adj.*

uroporphyria /yŏŏr'əpôrfir'ē·ə/ [Gk, *ouron* + *porphyros,* purple], a rare, genetic disease characterized by excessive secretion of uroporphyrin in the urine, blistering dermatitis, photosensitivity, splenomegaly, and hemolytic anemia. Corticosteroid ointments may be helpful for the skin lesions; splenomegaly may be necessary to alleviate the hemolytic anemia. Most patients die from hematologic complications before middle age. See also **porphyria.**

uroporphyrin /yŏŏr'əpôr'firin/, a porphyrin normally excreted in the urine in small amounts. See also **uroporphyria.**

uroradiology /-rā'dē·ol'əjē/, the radiologic study of the urinary tract.

urorectal septum /-rek'təl/ [Gk, *ouron* + L, *rectus,* straight; *saeptum* wall], a ridge of mesoderm covered with endoderm that in the early developing embryo divides the endodermal cloaca into the urogenital sinus and the rectum. Also called **cloacal septum.**

uroscopy /yŏŏros'kəpē/ [Gk, *ouron,* urine + *skopein,* to view], diagnostic examination of urine samples.

urostomy /yŏŏros'təmē/, the diversion of urine away from a diseased or defective bladder through a surgically created opening, or stoma, in the skin.

ursodeoxycholic acid /ur'sōdē·ok'sikol'ik/, a secondary bile salt. It is used in vivo to dissolve cholesterol gallstones. See also **chenodeoxycholic acid.**

urticaria /ur'tiker'ē·ə/ [L, *urtica,* nettle], a pruritic skin eruption characterized by transient wheals of varying shapes and sizes with well-defined erythematous margins and pale centers. It is caused by capillary dilatation in the dermis that results from the release of vasoactive mediators, including histamine, kinin, and the slow, reactive substance of anaphylaxis associated with antigen-antibody reaction. Treatment includes antihistamines and removal of the stimulus or allergen. Cholinergic urticaria appears as wheals surrounded by a large axon flare. It may be caused by drugs, food, insect bites, inhalants, emotional stress, exposure to heat or cold, and exercise. Also called **hives.** See also **angioneurotic edema.** —**urticarial,** *adj.*

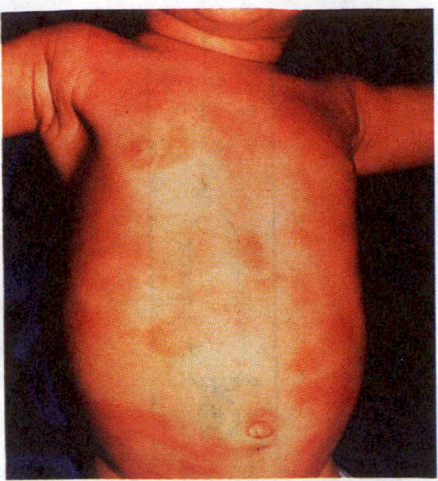

Urticaria pigmentosa *(Zitelli, 1992)*

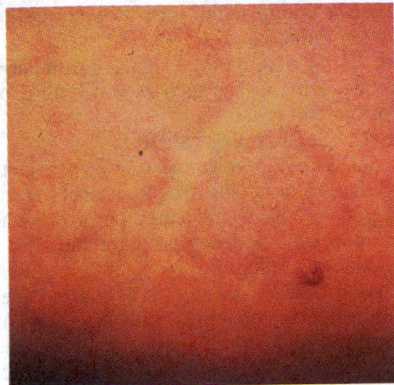

Urticaria *(Zitelli, 1992)*

urticaria bullosa [L, *urtica,* nettle + *bulla,* bubble], a skin eruption in which the lesions are capped by blisters.

urticaria hemorrhagica. See **hemorrhagic urticaria.**

urticaria maculosa [L, *urtica,* nettle + *macule,* spot], a chronic skin eruption in which red lesions form with little or no edema present.

urticaria medicamentosa [L, *urtica,* nettle + *medicina*], a form of skin eruption that follows the use of certain medications, including those containing quinine.

urticaria papulosa [L, *urtica,* nettle + *papula,* pimple], a form of skin eruption affecting mainly children and characterized by reddish macules on which papules develop.

urticaria pigmentosa, an uncommon form of mastocytosis characterized by pigmented skin lesions that usually begin in infancy and become urticarial on mechanical or chemical irritation. Although duration of the condition is unpredictable, prognosis is good. Treatment is symptomatic and usually includes antihistamines for relief of itching. See also **mastocytosis.**

urushiol /ərŏo′shē·ôl/, a toxic resin in the sap of certain plants of the genus *Rhus,* such as poison ivy, poison oak, and poison sumac, that produces allergic contact dermatitis in many people.

-us, a suffix usually identifying singular nouns: *echolalus, thalamus, tonus.*

USAN /yŏo′san, yŏo′es′ā′en′/, abbreviation for *United States Adopted Names,* a list of approved drugs compiled and published by U.S. Pharmacopeial Convention, Inc. See also **nonproprietary name.**

use effectiveness [L, *usus,* make use of; *efficere,* to produce], (of a contraceptive method) the actual effectiveness of a medication, device, or method in preventing pregnancy. Inconsistent use and human error usually reduce the theoretic effectiveness of any particular method of contraception. Compare **theoretic effectiveness.**

useful radiation, the portion of direct radiation that is permitted to pass from an x-ray tube housing through the tube head port, aperture, or collimator. Also called **useful beam.**

user documentation. See **documentation.**

user-friendly, pertaining to computer hardware or software designed to assist the user by presenting operating information or instructions in a form that is familiar and easy to understand.

use test, a procedure used to identify offending allergens in foods, cosmetics, or fabrics by the systematic elimination and addition of specific items associated with the lifestyle of the patient involved. Allergic reactions to the use test may be immediate or may be spread over a considerable period of time. Some patients undergoing the test become frustrated and discouraged, requiring regular encouragement to continue the search for sources of their allergies by this method. See also **allergy testing.**

U-shaped arch, a dental arch in which there is little difference in width between the first premolars and the last molars and the curve from canine to canine is abrupt and U-shaped.

USP. See *United States Pharmacopeia.*

USP unit, a dose unit as recommended by the *United States Pharmacopoeia,* the primary legally recognized national drug-standard compendium.

USPHS, abbreviation for **United States Public Health Service.**

uta /yŏo′tə/ [Sp, facial ulcers], a mild cutaneous form of American leishmaniasis, occurring in the Andes of Peru and Argentina, caused by *Leishmania peruana.* The lesions are small and usually occur on the exposed surfaces of the skin, which ordinarily heal spontaneously within 1 year. The disease has been slowly disappearing because of the increased use of insecticides.

ut dict., abbreviation for the Latin phrase *ut dictum*, 'as directed.'

utend., abbreviation for the Latin phrase *utendus*, 'to be used.'

uter-, utero- , a combining form meaning 'relating to the uterus': *uterotomy, uteroplasty.*

uterine /yōō′tərēn/ [L, *uterus*], pertaining to the uterus.

uterine anteflexion [L, *uterus*, womb; *ante*, before, *flectere*, to bend], an abnormal position of the uterus in which the uterine body is bent forward on itself at the juncture of the isthmus of the uterine cervix and the lower uterine segment.

uterine anteversion, a position of the uterus in which the body of the uterus is directed ventrally. Mild degrees of anteversion are of no clinical significance. On speculum examination of the vagina, acute anteversion of the uterus may be deduced from the location of the cervix in the posterior of the vaginal vault. Slight anteversion is the most common uterine position; on speculum examination the cervix is in the middle of the top of the vagina vault and protrudes directly downward toward the vaginal orifice.

uterine bleeding [L, *uterus*; ME, *blod*], any loss of blood from the uterus.

uterine bruit, a sound made by the passage of blood through the arteries of the pregnant uterus. The sounds are synchronized with the maternal heart rate. See also **uterine souffle.**

uterine cancer, any malignancy of the uterus, including the cervix or endometrium. See also **cervical cancer, endometrial cancer.**

uterine colic [L, *uterus*; Gk, *kolikos*, pain in the colon], a spasmodic pain originating in the uterus, usually caused by dysmenorrhea or extrusion of a fibroid polyp.

uterine fibroid [L, *uterus* + *fibra*, fiber; Gk, *eidos*, form], a growth of fibrous tissue in the uterus, usually a fibroma, fibromyoma, or leiomyofibroma.

uterine fibroma, a benign encapsulated uterine tumor that affects about 20% of women over the age of 30. The tumor may develop in the wall of the uterus or be attached to a stalk of tissue originating in the wall. Symptoms may include menstrual disorders such as menorrhagia but are also likely to be related to the location of the tumor with respect to neighboring organs, as when a uterine fibroma causes pressure on the urinary bladder, producing symptoms of dysuria. Uterine fibromas rarely spread or become life-threatening.

uterine inertia, abnormal relaxation of the uterus during labor, causing a lack of obstetric progress, or after childbirth, causing uterine hemorrhage.

uterine ischemia, a decreasing or ineffective blood supply to the uterus.

uterine prolapse, the falling, sinking, or sliding of the uterus from its normal location in the body.

uterine retroflexion, a position of the uterus in which its body is bent backward on itself at the isthmus of the cervix and the lower uterine segment. This condition has no clinical significance; it does not prevent conception or adversely affect pregnancy. On speculum examination of the vagina, the condition may be deduced by the location of the cervix in the anterior vaginal vault.

uterine retroversion, a position of the uterus in which the body of the uterus is directed away from the midline, toward the back. Mild degrees of retroversion are common

and have no clinical significance. Severe retroversion may be accompanied by vague persistent pelvic discomfort and dyspareunia and may prevent the fitting and use of a contraceptive diaphragm. Compare **uterine anteversion.** See also **uterine retroflexion.**

uterine souffle, a soft, blowing sound made by the blood in the arteries of a pregnant uterus. It is synchronized with the maternal pulse.

uterine subinvolution [L, *uterus* + *sub*, under + *involere*, to roll up], an incomplete involution of the uterus, such as after childbirth. Also called **partial involution.**

uterine swab [L, *uterus*; Du, *zwabber*], an absorbent material on a rod or flattened wire used to obtain specimens or to remove secretions from the uterus.

uterine tenaculum. See **tenaculum.**

uterine tetany, a condition characterized by uterine contractions that are extremely prolonged.

uterine tube. See **fallopian tube.**

uteritis. See **metritis.**

utero-. See **uter-.**

uteroabdominal pregnancy /yōō′tərō′abdom′inəl/ [L, *uterus* + *abdomen* + *pregnans*], a twin pregnancy in which one fetus develops in the uterus and the other develops in the abdomen.

uteroglobulin. See **blastokinin.**

uteroovarian varicocele /yōō′tərō·′ōver′ē·ən/ [L, *uterus* + *ovum*, egg; *varix*, varicose vein; Gk, *kele*, tumor], a swelling of the veins of the pampiniform plexus of the female pelvis. Compare **ovarian varicocele, varicocele.**

uteroplacental apoplexy. See **Couvelaire uterus.**

uterosalpingography /yōō′tərō-sal′ping·gog′rəfē/ [L, *uterus*; Gk, *salpigx*, tube + *graphein*, to record], a radiographic examination of the uterus and fallopian tubes.

uterotomy /yōō′tərot′əmē/ [L, *uterus*; Gk, *temnein*, to cut], a surgical incision into the uterus, such as in a cesarean section.

uterovesical. See **vesicouterine.**

uterus /yōō′tərəs/ [L womb], the hollow, pear-shaped internal female organ of reproduction in which the fertilized ovum is implanted and the fetus develops, and from which the decidua of menses flows. Its anterior surface lies on the superior surface of the bladder, separated by a fold of peritoneum, the vesicouterine pouch. Its posterior surface, also covered with peritoneum, is adjacent to the sigmoid colon and some of the coils of the small intestine. The uterus is composed of three layers: the endometrium, the myometrium, and the parametrium. The endometrium lines the uterus and becomes thicker and more vascular in pregnancy and during the second half of the menstrual cycle under the influence of the hormone progesterone. The myometrium is the muscular layer of the organ. Its muscle fibers wrap around the uterus obliquely, laterally, and longitudinally. The muscle fibers contract during childbirth to expel the fetus. After childbirth the meshlike network of fibers contracts again, creating a mass of natural ligatures that stops the flow of blood from the large blood vessels supplying the placenta. The parametrium is the outermost layer of the uterus. It is composed of serous connective tissue and extends laterally into the broad ligament. In the adult, the organ measures about 7.5 cm long and 5 cm wide at its fundus and weighs approximately 40 g. During pregnancy it is able to grow to many times its usual size, almost entirely by cellular hypertrophy. Few new cells develop. The uterus has two

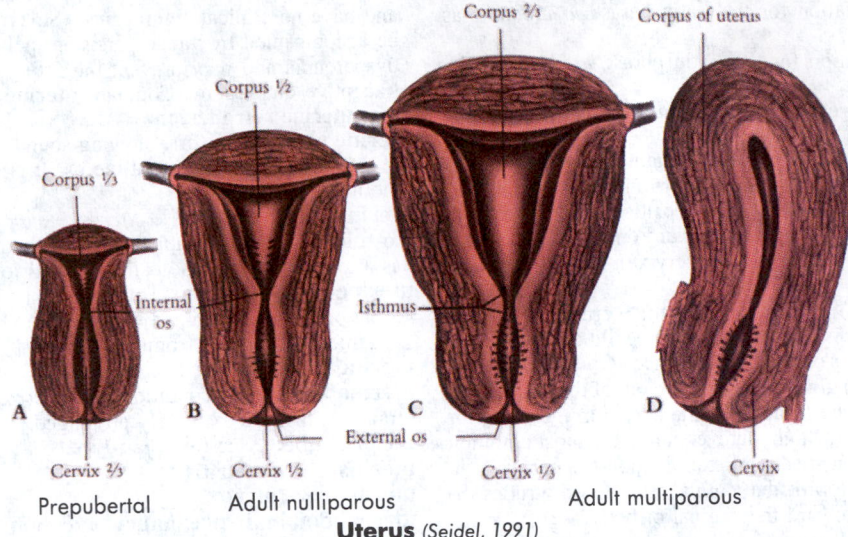

Corpus ⅓

Corpus ½

Corpus ⅔

Corpus of uterus

Internal os

Isthmus

External os

Cervix ⅔

Cervix ½

Cervix ⅓

Cervix

A   B   C   D

Prepubertal   Adult nulliparous   Adult multiparous

Uterus (Seidel, 1991)

parts: a body and a cervix. The body extends from the fundus to the cervix, just above the isthmus. The cavity within the body is only a potential space. The walls of the body touch, unless the woman is pregnant. The cervix has a vaginal portion, protruding into the vagina, and a supravaginal portion at the juncture of the lower uterine segment. The principal ligaments of the uterus are the broad ligaments, which extend laterally from the sides of the isthmus of the cervix to the lateral wall and bottom of the pelvis; the round ligament, which crosses the pelvis between the folds of the broad ligaments; the cardinal ligament, crossing the pelvic diaphragm from the top of the cervix to the large muscles of the pelvic outlet; and the uterosacral ligament, curving back from the cervix to the sacrum around the cul-de-sac of Douglas. The body of the uterus is thus free in the abdominal cavity, fixed only at its base by the ligaments from the cervix.

uterus bicornis [L, *uterus* + *bis* + *cornu*, horn], a uterus that is divided into two parts, usually separate at the upper end and joined at the lower end.

uterus masculinis. See **prostatic utricle.**

UTI, abbreviation for **urinary tract infection.**

utilitarianism /yōō'tiliter'ē·əniz'əm/ [L, *utilis,* useful, *isma* practice], a doctrine that the purpose of all action should be to bring about the greatest happiness for the greatest number of people and that the value of anything is determined by its utility. The philosophy is often applied in the distribution of health care resources, as in decisions regarding the expenditure of public funds for health services.

utilization review (UR) /yōō'tilīzā'shən/ [L, *utilis* + *atus,* process], an assessment of the appropriateness and economy of an admission to a health care facility or a continued hospitalization. The length of the hospital stay also is compared with the average length of stay for similar diagnoses.

utricle /yōō'trikəl/ [L, *utriculus,* small bag], larger of two membranous pouches in the vestibule of the membranous labyrinth of the ear. It is an oblong structure that communicates with the semicircular ducts by five openings and re-

ceives utricular filaments of the acoustic nerve. Compare **saccule.**

utriculosaccular duct /yōōtrik'yəlōsak'yələr/ [L, *utriculus* + *sacculus,* small sack; *ducere,* to lead], a duct connecting the utricle with an endolymphatic duct of the membranous labyrinth.

UV, abbreviation for ultraviolet.

uvea /yōō'vē·ə/ [L, *uva,* grapes], the fibrous tunic beneath the sclera that includes the iris, the ciliary body, and the choroid of the eye. Also called **tunica vasculosa bulbi, uveal tract.** —**uveal,** *adj.*

uveitis /yōō'vē·ī'tis/ [L, *uva* + Gk, *itis*], inflammation of the uveal tract of the eye, including the iris, ciliary body, and choroid. It may be characterized by an irregularly

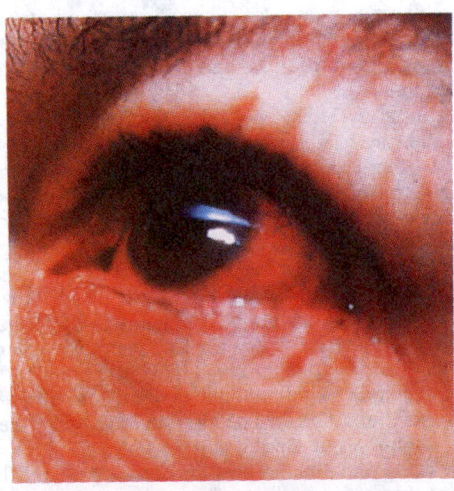

Uveitis (Winawer, 1992)

shaped pupil, inflammation around the cornea, pus in the anterior chamber, opaque deposits on the cornea, pain, and lacrimation. Causes include allergy, infection, trauma, diabetes, collagen disease, and skin diseases. A major complication may be glaucoma. See also **chorioretinitis, choroiditis, iritis.**

uvioresistant /yōō′vē·ō′rəsis′tənt/, *obsolete*. resistant to ultraviolet light.

uviosensitive /-sen′sitiv/, *obsolete*. sensitive to ultraviolet radiation.

uvula /yōō′vyələ/, *pl.* **uvulae** [L, *uva*], the small, cone-shaped process suspended in the mouth from the middle of the posterior border of the soft palate. **–uvular,** *adj.*

uvular /yōō′vyələr/ [L, *uva*, grape], pertaining to the palatine uvula.

uvulectomy /yōō′vyələk′təmē/ [L, *uva*, grape; Gk, *ektome*, excision], the surgical removal of the uvula.

uvulitis /yōō′vyəlī′tis/, an inflammation of the uvula. Common causes are allergy and infection.

U wave, (in electrocardiography) a small, rounded, positive wave that follows the T wave.

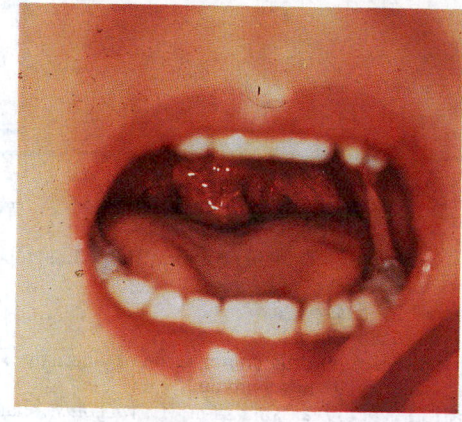

Uvulitis *(Zitelli, 1992)*

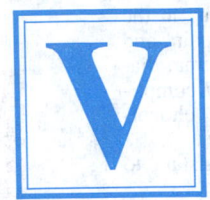

v, **1.** abbreviation for **vein. 2.** abbreviation for **venous blood.**

V, **1.** symbol for the element **vanadium. 2.** symbol for *ventilation capacity of the lung.*

V̇, symbol for *rate of gas flow.*

V_max, the maximum rate of catalysis.

VAC, an anticancer drug combination of vincristine, dactinomycin, and cyclophosphamide.

vaccination (vacc) /vak′sinā′shən/ [L, *vaccinus*, relating to a cow], any injection of attenuated microorganisms, such as bacteria, viruses, or rickettsiae, administered to induce immunity or to reduce the effects of associated infectious diseases. Historically, the first vaccinations were administered to immunize against smallpox. Vaccinations are now available to immunize against many diseases, such as typhoid, measles, and mumps. **–vaccinate,** *v.*

vaccine /vaksēn′, vak′sēn, -sin/ [L, *vaccinus*], a suspension of attenuated or killed microorganisms administered intradermally, intramuscularly, orally, or subcutaneously to induce active immunity to infectious disease. Viruses and rickettsiae used in certain vaccines are grown in avian embryos, rabbit brain tissue, or monkey kidney tissue, and the organisms are usually inactivated by formalin, phenol, or beta-propiolactone. Bacteria for various vaccines may be inactivated by acetone, formalin, heat, or phenol. Vaccines may be used as single agents or in combinations. Compare **antiserum.**

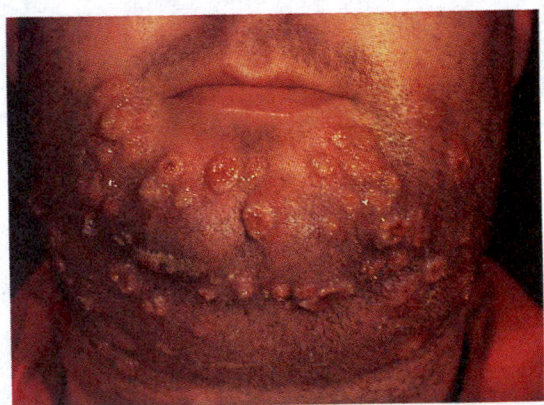

Vaccinia (du Vivier, 1993)

-vaccine, a combining form meaning a 'preparation containing microorganisms for producing immunity to disease': *autovaccine, enterovaccine, heterovaccine.*

vaccinia /vaksin′ē·ə/ [L, *vaccinus*], an infectious disease of cattle caused by a poxvirus that may be transmitted to humans by direct contact or by deliberate inoculation as a protection against smallpox. A pustule develops at the site of infection, usually followed by malaise and fever that last for several days. After 2 weeks the pustule becomes a crust that eventually drops off, leaving a scar. Satellite lesions may occur, and the virus may be spread to other sites by scratching. Individuals with eczema or other preexisting skin disease may develop generalized vaccinia. Rarely, a severe encephalitis follows vaccinia. Also called **cowpox.** Compare **smallpox.** See also **vaccination.**

vacuole /vak′yo̅o̅·ōl/ [L, *vacuus*, empty], **1.** a clear or fluid-filled space or cavity within a cell, such as occurs when a droplet of water is ingested by the cytoplasm. **2.** a small space in the body enclosed by a membrane, usually containing fat, secretions, or cellular de[001e]bris. **–vacuolar, vacuolated,** *adj.*

Vacu-tainer tube, a glass tube with a rubber stopper in which air can be removed to create a vacuum.

vacuum aspiration /vak′yo̅o̅·əm/ [L, *vacuus*, empty; *aspirare*, to breathe upon], a method of removing tissues from the uterus by suction. With the patient under local or light general anesthesia, the cervix is dilated and the uterus is emptied with suction. Postoperative care includes the close observation of vital signs for symptoms of blood loss. Also called **suction curettage.** Compare **dilatation and curettage.** See also **therapeutic abortion.**

VAD, abbreviation for **vascular access device.**

vade mecum /vā′dē mē′kəm/ [L, go with me], something carried by a person for constant use.

vagal /vā′gəl/ [L, *vagus*, wandering], of or pertaining to the vagus nerve.

vagal tone [L, *vagus*, wandering; Gk, *tonos*, stretching], **1.** pertaining to the hyperexcitability of the parasympathetic nervous system. **2.** pertaining to the inhibitory control of the vagus nerve over heart rate and atrioventricular conduction.

vagina /vəjī′nə/ [L, sheath], the part of the female genitalia that forms a canal from the orifice through the vestibule to the uterine cervix. It is behind the bladder and in front of the rectum. In the adult woman the anterior wall of the vagina is about 7 cm long and the posterior wall is about 9 cm long. The canal is actually a potential space; the walls usually touch. The vagina widens from the vestibule upward and narrows toward the top, forming a curved vault around the protruding cervix. The vagina is lined with mucosa covering a layer of erectile tissue and muscle. The mucous membrane of the vagina forms two longitudinal columns from which transverse rugae extend around the canal. The muscular coat is composed of a strong, external longitudinal layer and an internal circular layer. The lower end of the vagina is surrounded by the erectile tissue of the bulb of the vestibule and the bulbocavernosus muscle. The muscular layer is highly vascular. The muscles of the vagina are innervated by the pudendal nerve and perfused by the vaginal artery.

vaginal bleeding /vaj'ənəl/, an abnormal condition in which blood is passed from the vagina, other than during the menses. It may be caused by abnormalities of the uterus or cervix; by an abnormal pregnancy; by endocrine abnormalities; by abnormalities of one or both ovaries or one or both fallopian tubes; or by an abnormality of the vagina. The following terms are commonly used in describing the approximate amount of vaginal bleeding: **heavy vaginal bleeding,** which is greater than heaviest normal menstrual flow; **moderate vaginal bleeding,** which is equal to heaviest normal menstrual flow; **light vaginal bleeding,** which is less than heaviest normal menstrual flow; **vaginal staining,** which is a very light flow of blood barely requiring the use of a sanitary napkin or tampon; **vaginal spotting,** which is the passage vaginally of a few drops of blood; **bloody show,** which is an episode of light vaginal bleeding as often occurs in early labor, during labor, and, particularly, at the time of full dilatation of the cervix at the end of the first stage of labor because of rupture of the cervical capillaries as dilation occurs.

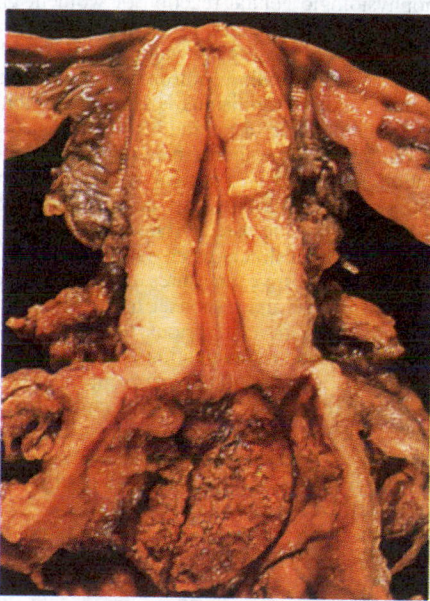

Vaginal squamous cell carcinoma (Fletcher, 1987)

vaginal cancer, a malignancy of the vagina occurring rarely as a primary neoplasm and more often as a secondary lesion or extension of vulvar, cervical, endometrial, or ovarian cancer. Clear cell adenocarcinoma occurs in young women exposed in utero to diethylstilbestrol, given their mother to prevent abortion, but most primary vaginal cancers arise in white women over 50 years of age. A predisposing factor is cervical carcinoma. Vaginal leukoplakia, erythematosis, erosion, or granulation of the mucosa may prove to be carcinoma in situ. Symptoms of invasive lesions are postmenopausal bleeding, purulent discharge, pain, and dysuria. Diagnostic measures include cervical, endocervical, and vaginal Pap smears, colposcopy, biopsy, and Schiller's iodine test in which malignant cells do not stain dark brown. Ninety percent of vaginal cancers are squamous

cell carcinomas; others are clear cell or undifferentiated adenocarcinomas, malignant melanomas, and sarcomas. Depending on the patient's age and condition and the site and extent of the lesion, treatment may be by irradiation or vaginectomy and radical hysterectomy with lymph node dissection. Cryosurgery, topical 5-fluorouracil, and dinitrochlorobenzene (DNCB) may be used, but chemotherapy is not usually effective.

vaginal cyst [L, *vagina,* sheath; Gk, *kytis,* bag], an abnormal closed sac or pouch in the vaginal tissues.

vaginal discharge, any discharge from the vagina. A clear or pearly-white discharge occurs normally. Throughout the reproductive years the amount varies greatly from woman to woman, and the amount and character vary in each woman at different times in her menstrual cycle. Before menarche and after menopause, the quantity of discharge is usually less than during the reproductive years. The discharge is largely composed of secretions of the endocervical glands. Inflammatory conditions of the vagina and cervix often cause an increase in the discharge, which may then have a foul odor and cause pruritus of the perineum and external genitalia.

vaginal fornix, a recess in the upper part of the vagina caused by the protrusion of the uterine cervix into the vagina.

vaginal hysterectomy [L, *vagina,* sheath; Gk, *hystera,* womb + *ektome,* excision], the surgical removal of the uterus through the vagina.

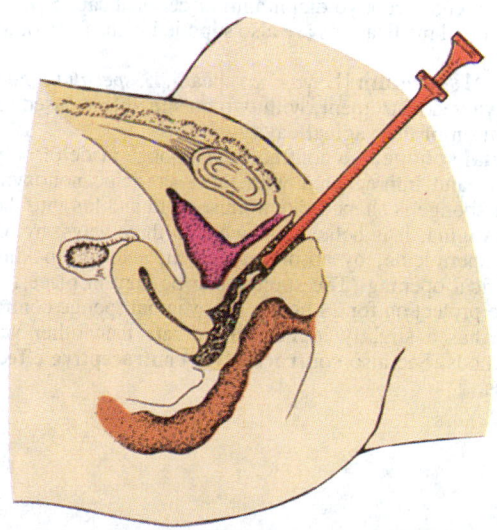

Vaginal instillation of medicine (Potter, 1993)

vaginal instillation of medication, the instillation of a medicated cream, a suppository, or a gel into the vagina, usually performed to treat a local infection of the vagina or uterine cervix. The woman voids before the treatment. She then lies back, recumbent or semirecumbent. The nurse or physician, wearing gloves, separates the labia majora, exposing the vaginal orifice. The medication is instilled gently. A cream or gel is squeezed into an applicator from a tube and is then placed in the vagina by depressing the plunger of the applicator while withdrawing the device from

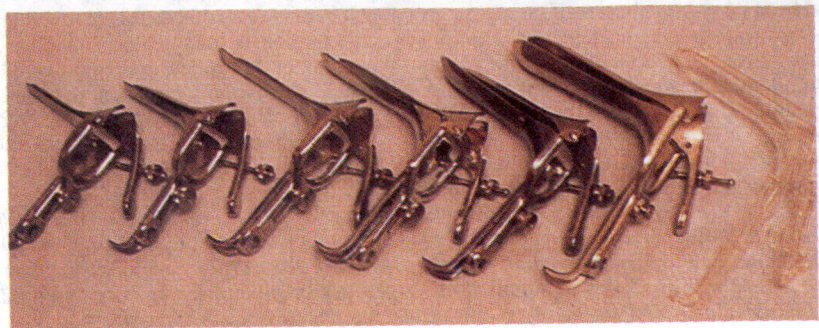

Vaginal specula *(Seidel, 1991)*

the vagina. A tablet or suppository is usually placed in the vagina near the cervix with another style of applicator that holds the medication in a slotted receptacle at its tip. The woman remains recumbent after the instillation to prevent escape of the medication from the vagina. Most applicators may be washed after each instillation and reused for the same woman for the next dose. They are discarded after a course of treatment. Vaginal instillation may easily be taught to the woman.

vaginal jelly,   a contraceptive product containing a spermicide in a jelly medium. It is usually used in conjunction with a contraceptive diaphragm or cervical cap. Some antimicrobial medications are also supplied in the form of a vaginal jelly.

vaginal speculum [L, *vagina,* sheath; L, *speculum,* mirror], a bivalved instrument, with two opening blades used for inspection of the vaginal cavity.

vaginal sponge,   a contraceptive sponge made of polyurethane and impregnated with the spermicide nonoxynol-9. The sponge is shaped like a mushroom and fits into the upper vagina. It is believed to work in three ways: by releasing spermicide, by absorbing semen, and by blocking the cervical opening. The sponge can be kept in place to provide protection for 24 hours. The vaginal sponge contraceptive has a slightly higher failure rate than other vaginal methods. See also **contraceptive, contraceptive effectiveness.**

vaginal spotting, vaginal staining.   See **vaginal bleeding.**

vaginismus /vaj′iniz′məs/ [L, *vagina* + *spasmus,* spasm], a psychophysiologic genital reaction of women, characterized by intense contraction of the perineal and paravaginal musculature, tightly closing the vaginal introitus. It occurs in response to fear of painful intromission before coitus or pelvic examination. Vaginismus is considered abnormal if it occurs in the absence of genital lesions and if it conflicts with a woman's desire to participate in coition or to permit examination, but it may be a normal or physiologic response if painful genital conditions exist or if forcible or premature intromission is anticipated. Abnormal vaginismus is uncommon. Sexual adjustment often can be achieved through educative and supportive measures that lead to improved sexual self-awareness and response. In some cases, the condition is a manifestation of serious mental illness and requires formal psychiatric evaluation and treatment. Gender identity conflict, a history of trauma from rape or incest, or an intense suppression of sexuality in childhood and adolescence are factors that often are seen in association with vaginismus. See also **dyspareunia.**

vaginitis /vaj′inī′tis/,   an inflammation of the vaginal tissues, such as trichomonas vaginitis.

vagino-,   a combining form meaning 'pertaining to the vagina': *vaginodynia, vaginolabial, vaginopexy.*

vaginography /vaj′inog′rəfē/,   the radiologic examination of the vagina after injection of a radiopaque contrast medium.

Vagisec,   a trademark for a vaginal douche containing polyoxyethylene nonyl phenol, edetate sodium, and dioctyl sodium sulfosuccinate, used to treat trichomoniasis.

vagosympathetic /vā′gōsim′pəthet′ik/ [L, *vagus,* wandering; Gk, *sympathein,* to feel with]   pertaining to the vagus nerve and the cervical portion of the sympathetic nervous system.

vagotomy /vāgot′əmē/ [L, *vagus,* wandering, *temnein,* to cut],   the cutting of certain branches of the vagus nerve, performed with gastric surgery, to reduce the amount of gastric acid secreted and lessen the chance of recurrence of a gastric ulcer. With the patient under general anesthesia, a gastrectomy is performed, and the appropriate branches of the vagus nerve are excised. Because peristalsis will be diminished, a pyloroplasty or an anastomosis of the stomach to the jejunum may be done to assure proper emptying of the stomach. See also **anastomosis, gastrectomy, gastric ulcer, pyloroplasty, vagus nerve.**

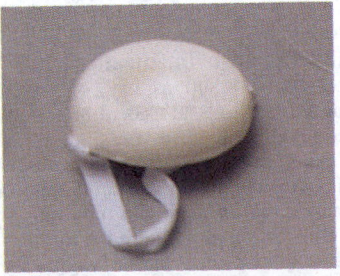

Vaginal sponge *(Edge, 1994)*

vagotonia.   See **sympathetic imbalance.**

vagotonus /vā'gətō'nəs/ [L, *vagus* + Gk, *tonos,* tension], an abnormal increase in parasympathetic activity caused by stimulation of the vagus nerve, especially bradycardia with decreased cardiac output, faintness, and syncope. Vagotonus may occur in suctioning the oropharynx of a newborn as the syringe, laryngoscope blade, or catheter is inadvertently pressed on the back of the throat, stimulating the nerve. It also occurs in some women after surgical treatment or simple manipulation of the uterine cervix.

vagovagal reflex /vā'gōvā'gəl/ [L, *vagus* + *vagus; reflectere,* to bend backward], a stimulation of the vagus nerve by reflex in which irritation of the larynx or the trachea results in slowing of the pulse rate.

vagueness /vāg'nəs/, a communication pattern involving the use of global pronouns and loose associations that lead to ambiguity and confusion in communication.

vagus nerve /vā'gəs/ [L, *vagus,* wandering, *nervus,* nerve], either of the longest pair of cranial nerves essential for speech, swallowing, and the sensibilities and functions of many parts of the body. The vagus nerves communicate through 13 main branches, connecting to four areas in the brain. Also called **nervus vagus, pneumogastric nerve, tenth cranial nerve.**

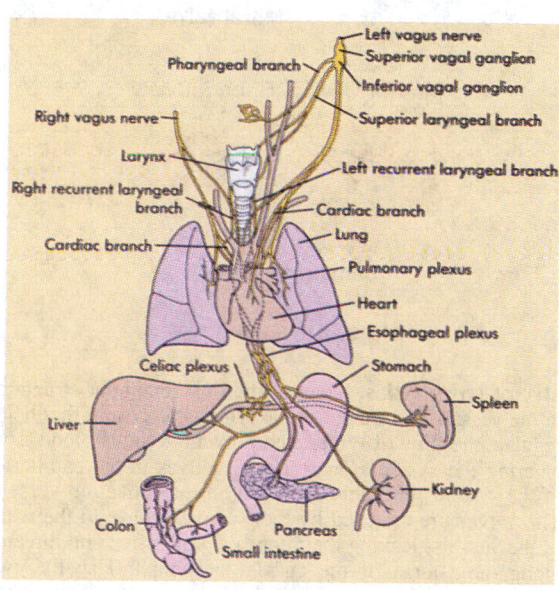

Vagus nerve *(Seeley, 1992/Michael Schenk)*

vagus pulse [L, *vagus,* wandering + *pulsare,* to beat], a slow, regular pulse caused by overactivity of the vagus nerve.

Val, abbreviation for **valine.**

valence /vāl'əns/ [L, *valere,* to be strong], **1.** (in chemistry) a numeric expression of the capability of an element to combine chemically with atoms of hydrogen or their equivalent. A negative valence indicates the number of hydrogen atoms to which one atom of a chemical element can bond. A positive valence indicates the number of hydrogen atoms that one atom of a chemical element can displace. An element is considered univalent (or monovalent) if each of its atoms can react with only one hydrogen atom or its equiv-

alent; bivalent (or divalent) if each atom can react with two hydrogen or equivalent atoms; tervalent (or trivalent) if each atom can react with three hydrogen atoms; and multivalent (or polyvalent) if each atom can react with many hydrogen atoms. **2.** (in immunology) an expression of the number of antigen-binding sites for one molecule of any given antibody or the number of antibody-binding sites for any given antigen. Most antibody molecules, and those belonging to the IgG, IgA, and IgE immunoglobulin classes, have two antigen-binding sites. Most large antigen molecules are multivalent.

-valence, -valency, a combining term meaning the 'combining capacity of an atom compared with that of one hydrogen atom': *quantivalence, trivalence, univalence.*

valence electron, any of the outermost orbiting electrons of an atom. They are responsible for the bonding of atoms into crystals, molecules, and compounds.

-valent, a combining form meaning 'having a valency of a (specified) magnitude': *octavalent, pentavalent, tetravalent.*

valeric acid /vələr'ik/, an organic acid with a foul odor found in the roots of *Valeriana officinalis.* Commercially prepared, it is used in the production of perfumes, flavors, lubricants, and certain drugs.

valgus /val'gəs/ [L, bowlegged], an abnormal position in which a part of a limb is bent or twisted outward, away from the midline, such as the heel of the foot in **talipes valgus.** Compare **varus.** See also **hallux valgus.**

validation /val'idā'shən/, an agreement of the listener with certain elements of the patient's communication.

validity /valid'itē/, (in research) the extent to which a test measurement or other device measures what it is intended to measure. Kinds of validity include **content validity, current validity, construct validity,** and **predictive validity.**

valine (Val) /val'ēn/, an essential amino acid needed for optimal growth in infants and for nitrogen equilibrium in adults. See also **amino acid, maple syrup urine disease, protein.**

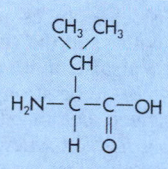

Chemical structure of valine *(Seeley, 1992)*

Valisone, a trademark for a glucocorticoid (betamethasone valerate).

Valium, a trademark for an antianxiety agent (diazepam), used as an adjunct to anesthesia.

vallecula /vəlek'yələ/ [L, little, valley], **1.** any groove or furrow on the surface of an organ or structure. **2.** See **vallecula epiglottica.** –**vallecular,** *adj.*

vallecula epiglottica, a furrow between the glossoepiglottic folds of each side of the posterior oropharynx. Also called *(informal)* **vallecula.**

vallecular dysphagia /vəlek'yələr/, difficulty or pain on swallowing caused by inflammation of the vallecula epiglottica. Compare **contractile ring dysphagia, dysphagia lusoria.**

valley fever. See **coccidioidomycosis.**

Valmid, a trademark for a sedative (ethinamate).

Valpin, a trademark for an anticholinergic (anisotropine).

valproic acid /valprō'ik/, an anticonvulsant.

■ INDICATIONS: It is prescribed to prevent certain types of seizure activity, particularly complex absence and petit mal seizures.

■ CONTRAINDICATIONS: It is not recommended for use during pregnancy or lactation. Known hypersensitivity to this drug prohibits its use.

■ ADVERSE EFFECTS: Among the more severe adverse reactions are decreased platelet function and hepatotoxicity. GI disturbances are common, and alopecia, rash, headache, and insomnia also may occur.

Valsalva maneuver /valsal'və/ [Antonio M. Valsalva, Italian surgeon, b. 1666; OFr, *maneuvre*, work done by hand], any forced expiratory effort against a closed airway such as when an individual holds the breath and tightens the muscles in a concerted, strenuous effort to move a heavy object or to change position in bed. Most healthy individuals perform Valsalva maneuvers during normal daily activities without any injurious consequences; but such efforts are dangerous for many patients with cardiovascular diseases, especially if they become dehydrated, increasing the viscosity of their blood and the attendant risk of blood clotting. Constipation increases the risk of cardiovascular trauma in such patients, especially if they perform a Valsalva maneuver in trying to move their bowels. On relaxing after each muscular effort with held breath, the blood of such individuals rushes to the heart, often overloading the cardiac system and causing cardiac arrest. Orthopedic patients often use a Valsalva maneuver in changing their position in bed with the aid of an overhead trapeze bar. Patients who may be endangered by performing a Valsalva maneuver are commonly instructed to exhale instead of holding their breath when they move. The exhalation decreases the risk of cardiovascular trauma.

Valsalva's test [Antonio Valsalva; L, *testum*, crucible], a method for testing the patency of the eustachian tubes. With mouth and nose kept tightly closed, a forced expiratory effort is made; if the eustachian tubes are open, air will enter into the middle ear cavities and the subject will hear a popping sound. See also **Valsalva maneuver.**

value /val'yoo/ [L, *valere*, to be strong], a personal belief about the worth of a given idea or behavior.

value clarification, a method whereby a person can discover his or her own values by assessing, exploring, and determining what those personal values are and how they affect personal decision making.

value system, the accepted mode of conduct and the set of norms, goals, and values binding any social group. Such guidelines for determining what is right or wrong, good or bad, and desirable or undesirable serve as a frame of reference for the individual in reaching decisions and in achieving a meaningful life.

valve /valv/ [L, *valva*, folding door], a natural structure or artificial device in a passage or vessel that prevents reflux of the fluid contents passing through it. Valves in veins are membranous folds that prevent backflow of blood. —**valvular,** *adj.*

-valve, a suffix meaning 'a thing that regulates the flow of': *bivalve, pseudovalve, trivalve.*

valve of Kerkring. See **circular fold.**

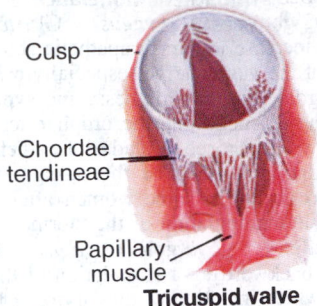

Tricuspid valve

Cusp — Chordae tendineae — Papillary muscle

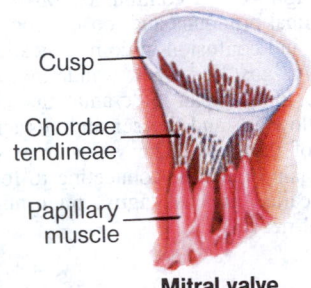

Mitral valve

Cusp — Chordae tendineae — Papillary muscle

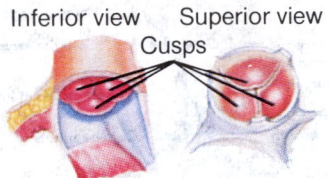

Inferior view   Superior view

Cusps

Semilunar valves

Valves *(Canobbio, 1990)*

valve of lymphatics, one of the tiny semilunar structures in the vessels and trunks of the lymphatic system that helps regulate the flow of lymph and prevents venous blood from entering the system. There are no valves in the capillaries of the system, but there are many in the collecting vessels. The valves are attached by their convex edges to the walls of the vessels, leaving their concave edges free and directed along the course of the current of lymph. Usually, two valves of equal size are found opposite each other. They are more numerous near the lymph nodes and more prevalent in the lymphatic vessels of the neck and the arms than in the vessels of the legs. The wall of the vessel just above the attachment of each valve bulges with a small sinus that gives the vessel its beaded appearance. See also **lymphatic system.**

valvotomy /valvot'əmē/ [L, *valva* + Gk, *temnein*, to cut], the incision into a valve, especially one in the heart, to correct a defect and allow proper opening and closure. Before surgery a cardiac catheterization is performed. With the patient under general anesthesia, the damaged valve is repaired, if possible, or removed and a prosthetic valve suture put in its place. Complications peculiar to prosthetic valve surgery are displacement of the valve caused by broken sutures, heart block, leakage and regurgitation from chamber to chamber, infection, and embolus.

valvular endocarditis /val′vyələr/ [L, *valva*, door leaf; Gk, *endon*, within + *kardia*, heart + *itis*, inflammation], a form of chronic inflammation of the lining membrane of the heart in which the valves are stenotic or incompetent. Also called **chronic endocarditis.**

valvular heart disease [L, *valva* + AS, *hoert*; L, *dis*, opposite of; Fr, *aise*, ease], an acquired or congenital disorder of a cardiac valve, characterized by stenosis and obstructed blood flow or by valvular degeneration and regurgitation of blood. Diseases of aortic and mitral valves are most common and may be caused by congenital defects, bacterial endocarditis, syphilis, or, most frequently, rheumatic fever. Episodes of rheumatic fever often affect cardiac valves, causing them to degenerate and remain open or causing the cusps of the valves to become stiff, calcified, and constricted. Valvular dysfunction results in changes in intracardiac pressure and in pulmonary and peripheral circulation. It may lead to cardiac dysrhythmia, heart failure, and cardiogenic shock. Cardiotonics, diuretics, analgesics, sodium restriction, and antibiotics, if indicated, are used in the conservative treatment of valvular heart disease, but surgery is usually performed when the symptoms are incapacitating. A stenosed aortic valve may be repaired by removing the calcium deposits and opening the fused commissures or by removing a cusp and reconstructing the valve, or it may be replaced with a porcine or artificial valve. Defective mitral and tricuspid valves also may be replaced or repaired surgically. Patients undergoing cardiac valve repair or replacement may be hospitalized for from 4 to 6 weeks and require diversional activities, as well as the standard preoperative and postoperative care provided for open heart surgery. See also **aortic stenosis, mitral stenosis, tricuspid stenosis, pulmonic stenosis.**

valvular regurgitation [L, *valva*, door leaf + *re* + *gurgitare*, to flow], a circulatory backflow that occurs when the heart contracts and the heart valves fail to close properly, allowing blood to be squeezed back into the atria from the ventricles.

valvular stenosis, a narrowing or constricture of any of the valves of the heart. The condition may result from a congenital defect, or it may be caused by some disease process. See also **aortic stenosis, congenital cardiac anomaly, mitral valve stenosis, pulmonic stenosis.**

valvulitis /val′vyəlī′tis/, an inflammatory condition of a valve, especially a cardiac valve. Inflammatory changes in the aortic, mitral, and tricuspid valves of the heart are caused most commonly by rheumatic fever and less frequently by bacterial endocarditis and syphilis. Infected valves degenerate, or their cusps become stiff and calcified, resulting in stenosis and obstructed blood flow.

valvuloplasty /val′vyəlōplas′tē/ [L, *valva*, door leaf; Gk, *plassein*, to shape], plastic surgery to repair a heart valve.

VAMP /vamp/, abbreviation for a combination drug regimen, used in the treatment of cancer, containing three antineoplastics (vincristine sulfate, methotrexate, and mercaptopurine) and a glucocorticoid (prednisone).

vanadium (V) /vənā′dē·əm/ [ONorse, *Vanadis*, (Freya) goddess of fertility], a grayish metallic element. Its atomic number is 23; its atomic weight is 50.942. Absorption of vanadium compounds results in a condition called **vanadi-**

umism, characterized by anemia, conjunctivitis, pneumonitis, and irritation of the respiratory tract.

van Bogaert's disease /vanbō′gərts/ [Ludo van Bogaert, 20th century Belgian physician], a rare familial disorder of lipid metabolism in which the substance cholestanol is deposited in the nervous system, blood, and connective tissue. Individuals with the disease develop progressive ataxia and dementia, premature atherosclerosis, cataracts, and xanthomas of the tendons. No effective treatment has been found. Also called **cerebrotendinous xanthomatosis.**

Van Buchem's syndrome. See **endosteal hyperostosis.**

Vanceril, a trademark for a glucocorticoid (beclomethasone dipropionate), used for oral inhalation therapy in asthma.

Vancocin Hydrochloride, a trademark for an antibacterial (vancomycin hydrochloride).

vancomycin /van′kōmī′sin/, an antibiotic.
■ INDICATIONS: It is prescribed in the treatment of infections, particularly staphylococcal infections resistant to other antibiotics.
■ CONTRAINDICATIONS: Concomitant administration of neurotoxic, nephrotoxic, or ototoxic drugs or known hypersensitivity to this drug prohibits its use.
■ ADVERSE EFFECTS: Among the more serious adverse reactions are anaphylaxis, dizziness, and tinnitus.

Van Deemter's equation /vandēm′tərz/, an expression of a gas chromatography relationship between the height equivalent to the theoretic plate (HEPT) and the linear velocity of the carrier gas.

Van de Graaff generator /van′dəgräf′/ [Robert J. Van de Graaff, American physicist, b. 1901], an electrostatic machine in which electronically charged particles are sprayed on a moving belt and carried by it to build up a high potential on an insulated terminal. The charged particles are then accelerated along a discharge path through a vacuum tube by the potential difference between the insulated terminal and the opposite end of the machine. The generator often is used to inject particles into a larger accelerator.

van den Bergh's test /van′dənburgs′/ [Albert A. H. van den Bergh, Dutch physician, b. 1869], a test for the presence of bilirubin in the blood serum. Blood is obtained from a patient who has fasted overnight, and the diluted serum is added to diazo reagent. A blue or violet color indicates the presence of bilirubin. The rate and magnitude of the color change are noted. Normal total bilirubin ranges from 0.2 to 1.4 mg per 100 dl of serum, of which about 15% should be what is called direct, or conjugated, bilirubin.

van der Waals forces /van′derwäls′, fän-/, weak attractive forces between neutral atoms and molecules. They occur because a fluctuating dipole moment in one molecule induces a dipole moment in another and the two dipole moments interact in an attractive manner. The activity accounts for some deviation from Boyle's law at very low temperatures or very high pressures. Also called **dispersion forces.**

vanillylmandelic acid (VMA) /vənil′ilməndel′ik/, a urinary metabolite of epinephrine and norepinephrine. Normal adult VMA findings in urine tests are in the range of 2 to 7 mg/24 hr. A greater than normal amount of VMA is characteristic of a pheochromocytoma and neuroblastomas.

Vanoxide, a trademark for a topical fixed-combination drug containing an antibacterial (benzoyl peroxide) and a keratolytic drying agent (chlorhydroxyquinoline).

Van Rensselaer, Euphenia /vanren′səlir/, (1840 – 1912), an American socialite who entered the first class of the Bellevue Hospital Training School for Nurses in New York. She designed the first nurses' uniform, a blue and white seersucker dress with collar and cuffs, apron, and cap. She succeeded Sister Helen as superintendent of Bellevue and later joined the Sisters of Charity, for whom she established a mission in Nassau. She organized the Seton Hospital for Tuberculosis in New York.

Vaponefrin,   a trademark for an adrenergic agent (epinephrine hydrochloride), used as a bronchodilator.

vapor bath /vā′pər/,   the exposure of the body to vapor, such as steam.

vaporization /vā′pərīzā′shən/ [L, *vapor*, steam],   the changing of a liquid or solid to a gaseous state.

vapor pressure depression,   a phenomenon in which the addition of a solute molecule to a solvent will decrease the vapor pressure of the solvent in equilibrium with the vapor phase and the liquid phase.

Vaquez's disease.   See **polycythemia rubra vera (PV).**

variable /ver′ē·əbəl/,   a factor in an experiment or scientific test that tends to vary, or take on different values, while other elements or conditions remain constant. See also **dependent variable, independent variable.**

variable behavior [L, *variare*, to vary; AS, *bihabban*, to behave],   a response, activity, or action that may be modified by individual experience. Compare **invariable behavior.**

variable interval (VI) reinforcement,   reinforcement that is offered after varying lapses of time.

variable-performance oxygen delivery system.   See **low-flow oxygen delivery system.**

variable ratio (VR) reinforcement,   reinforcement that requires variable numbers of responses.

variable region,   the N-terminal portion of an immunoglobulin polypeptide chain whose amino acid sequence can change. The region includes the antigen combining site.

variability /ver′ē·əbil′itē/ [L, *variare*, to diversify],   the degree of divergence or ability of an object to vary from a given standard or average.

variance /ver′ē·əns/ [L, *variare*],   **1.** (in statistics) a numeric representation of the dispersion of data around the mean in a given sample. It is represented by the square of the standard deviation and is used principally in performing an analysis of variance. **2.** *nontechnical.* the general range of a group of findings.

variant /ver′ē·ənt/ [L, *variare*, to diversify],   the differences between individuals of a species or between subpopulations of a species, as phenotypic or genotypic traits of mutants.

variant angina [L, *variare*, to diversify + *angina*, quinsy],   a variation of angina pectoris, with symptoms of chest pain usualy occurring during rest and at night. It is caused by focal spasm of proximal epicardial coronary arteries. An electrocardiogram shows an elevation of the ST segments, as opposed to the ST segment depression usually associated with angina pectoris. Also called **Prinzmetal's angina.**

varicella.   See **chickenpox.**

varicella-zoster immune globulin (VZIG) /ver′isel′ə zos′tər/ [L, *varius*, spotted; Gk, *zoster*, girdle; L, *immunis*, free from + *globulus*, small globe],   an immune globulin obtained from the blood of normal people with high levels of varicella-zoster antibodies. The immune globulin can be administered to people exposed to chickenpox to prevent or modify symptoms of the infection. See also **immune globulin.**

varicella zoster virus (VZV) [L, *varius*, diverse; Gk, *zoster*, girdle; L, *virus*, poison],   a member of the herpesvirus family, which causes the diseases varicella (chickenpox) and herpes zoster (shingles). The virus has been isolated from vesicle fluid in chickenpox, is highly contagious, and may be spread by direct contact or droplets. Dried crusts of skin lesions do not contain active virus particles. Herpes zoster is produced by reactivation of latent varicella virus, usually several years after the initial infection. There is no simple test for measuring antibodies to this virus; however, zoster immune globulin (ZIG) obtained from convalescing zoster patients, if injected within 3 days of exposure, will prevent varicella in susceptible children. The temporary nature of this protection and the relative scarcity of ZIG warrant reservation of its use to children receiving immunosuppressive therapy or suffering from immune deficiency diseases. See also **chickenpox, herpes zoster.**

varicelliform /ver′isel′ifôrm/,   resembling the rash of chickenpox.

varices.   See **varix.**

varicocele /ver′əkōsēl′/ [L, *varix*, varicose vein; Gk, *kele*, tumor],   a dilatation of the pampiniform venous complex of the spermatic cord. The varicocele forms a soft, elastic swelling that can cause pain. It is most common in men between 15 and 25 years of age and affects the left spermatic cord more often than the right. It is usually more pronounced and painful in the standing position. Compare **ovarian varicocele, uteroovarian varicocele.**

varicose /ver′əkōs/ [L, *varix*],   **1.** (of a vein) exhibiting varicosis, or a varicosity. **2.** abnormally and permanently distended, such as the bulging veins in some individuals.

varicose aneurysm,   a blood-filled, saclike projection that connects an artery and one or several veins and that is formed from a localized dilatation of the adjoining vessels.

varicose ulcer.   See **stasis ulcer.**

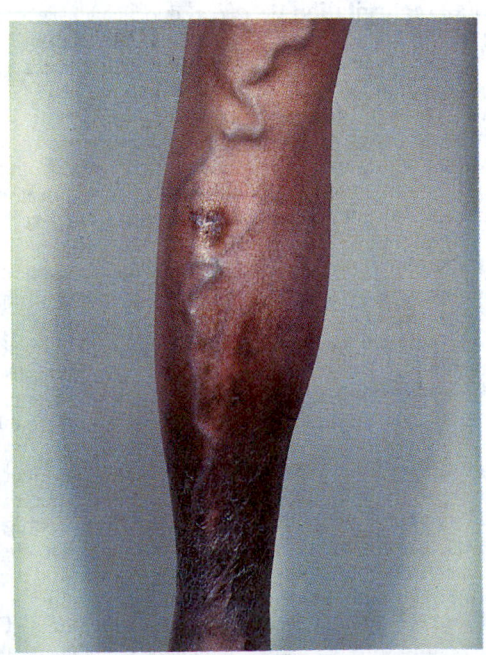

Varicose veins *(du Vivier, 1993)*

varicose vein, a tortuous, dilated vein with incompetent valves. Causes include congenitally defective valves, thrombophlebitis, pregnancy, and obesity. Varicose veins are common, especially in women. The saphenous veins of the legs are most often affected. Elevation of the legs and use of elastic stockings are frequently sufficient therapy for uncomplicated cases. Surgery (ligation and stripping) may be required in severe cases. Injection of sclerosing solutions helps prevent or treat postphlebitic syndrome.

varicosis /ver′ikō′sis/ [L, *varix* + Gk, *osis,* condition], a common condition characterized by one or more tortuous, abnormally dilated, or varicose veins, usually in the legs or the lower trunk, occurring between 30 and 60 years of age. Varicosis may be caused by congenital defects of the valves or walls of the veins or by congestion and increased intraluminal pressure resulting from prolonged standing, poor posture, pregnancy, abdominal tumor, or chronic systemic disease. Symptoms include pain and muscle cramps with a feeling of fullness and heaviness in the legs. Dilatation of superficial veins is often evident before the condition produces discomfort. Varicose veins may be treated conservatively by elevating the affected limb periodically or by wearing an elastic bandage or stocking. Ligation of the vein above the varicosity and removal of the distal portion of the vessel may be indicated for more severe cases if deeper vessels can maintain the return of venous blood.

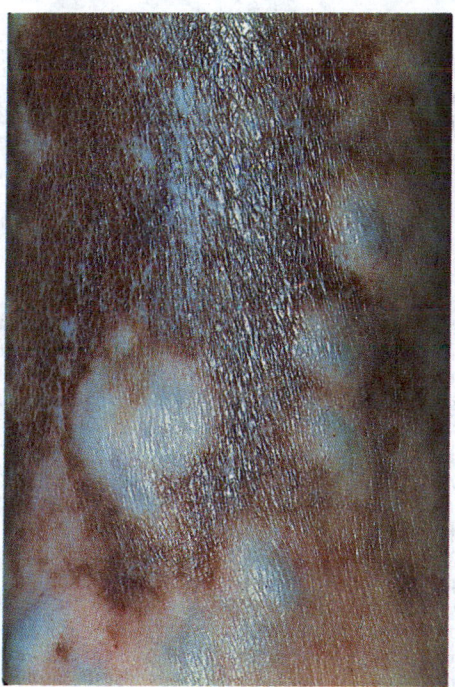

Varicosities (*du Vivier, 1993*)

varicosity /ver′ikos′itē/, **1.** an abnormal condition, usually of a vein, characterized by swelling and tortuosity. **2.** a vein in this condition.

variegate /ver′ē·əgāt′/ [L, *varius,* diverse], having characteristics that vary, especially as to color.

variegate porphyria, an uncommon form of hepatic porphyria, characterized by skin lesions and photosensitivity. The condition may be congenital or acquired. The congenital form is more serious, resulting in crises of acute abdominal pain and in certain neurologic complications. See also **porphyria.**

variola, variola major. See **smallpox.**

variola minor. See **alastrim.**

varioloid /ver′ē·əloid′/ [L, *varius* + Gk, *eidos,* form], **1.** resembling smallpox. **2.** a mild form of smallpox in a vaccinated person or one who has previously had the disease.

varix /ver′iks/, *pl.* **varices** /ver′əsēz/ [L, varicose vein], **1.** a tortuous, dilated vein. **2.** an enlarged, tortuous artery or a distended, twisting lymphatic.

varus /ver′əs/ [L, bent], an abnormal position in which a part of a limb is turned inward toward the midline, such as the heel and foot in **talipes varus.** Compare **valgus.**

vas /vas/, *pl.* **vasa** /vā′sə/ [L, vessel], any one of the many vessels of the body, especially those that convey blood, lymph, or spermatozoa.

vasa vasorum [L, *vas,* vessel], small blood vessels that supply the walls of the arteries and veins.

vascular /vas′kyələr/ [L, *vasculum,* little vessel], of or pertaining to a blood vessel.

vascular access device (VAD), an indwelling catheter, cannula, or other instrumentation used to obtain venous or arterial access.

vascular hemophilia. See **Von Willebrand's disease.**

vascular insufficiency, inadequate peripheral blood flow caused by occlusion of vessels with atherosclerotic plaques, thrombi, or emboli; by damaged, diseased, or intrinsically weak vascular walls, arteriovenous fistulas, or hematologic hypercoagulability; or by heavy smoking. Signs of vascular insufficiency include pale, cyanotic, or mottled skin over the affected area, swelling of an extremity, absent or reduced tactile sensation, tingling, diminished sense of temperature, muscle pain, such as intermittent claudication in the calf, and, in advanced disease, atrophy of muscles of the involved extremity. Diagnosis may be made by checking and comparing peripheral pulses in contralateral extremities, or by angiography, plethysmography, ultrasonography, and skin temperature tests. Treatment of vascular insufficiency may include a diet low in saturated fats, moderate exercise, sleeping on a firm mattress, avoidance of smoking, proper standing or sitting posture, the use of a vasodilating drug, and, if indicated, surgical repair of an arteriovenous fistula or aneurysm. See also **arterial insufficiency.**

vascularity /vas′kyəler′itē/ [L, *vasculum*], the state of blood vessel development and functioning in an organ or tissue.

vascularization /vas′kyələr′īzā′shən/, the process by which body tissue becomes vascular and develops proliferating capillaries. It may be natural or may be induced by surgical techniques. **−vascularize,** *v.*

vascular leiomyoma, a neoplasm that has developed from smooth muscle fibers of a blood vessel.

vascular sclerosis [L, *vasculum*; Gk, *skerosis,* hardening], a condition of hyaline degeneration of the blood vessels with hypertrophy of the media and subintimal fibrosis. Along with fibrosis and intimal thickening, there may be weakening and loss of elasticity in the artery walls.

vascular spider. See **spider angioma.**

vasculature /vas′kyəlā′chər/ [L, *vasculum*], the distribution of blood vessels in an organ or tissue.

vasculitis /vas′kyəlī′tis/, an inflammatory condition of the blood vessels that is characteristic of certain systemic diseases or that is caused by an allergic reaction. Kinds of vasculitis are **allergic vasculitis, necrotizing vasculitis,** and **segmented hyalinizing vasculitis.** See also **angiitis.**

Nodular vasculitis (du Vivier, 1993)

vasculogenic impotence /vas′kyəlōjen′ik/ [L, *vasculum,* small vessel; Gk, *genein,* to produce; L, *in, potentia,* power], an inability to perform the male sexual act because of an inadequate supply of arterial blood to the penis.

vasculomotor /-mō′tər/ [L, *vasculum + movere,* to move], pertaining to the system of controlling constriction and dilatation of blood vessels.

vas deferens /def′ərənz/, *pl.* **vasa deferentia** /def′əren′shē·ə/ [L, *vas + deferens,* carrying away], the extension of the epididymis of the testis that ascends from the scrotum and joins the seminal vesicle to form the ejaculatory duct. It is enclosed by fibrous connective tissue with blood vessels, nerves, and lymphatics and passes through the inguinal canal as part of the spermatic cord. Extending from the scrotum into the abdominal cavity, it passes over the top, then down the posterior surface of the bladder, becomes wider and convoluted, and joins the ampulla of the seminal vesicle. A vasectomy severs the vas deferens and makes a man sterile by interrupting the route spermatozoa must take to the exterior from the epididymis. Also called **deferent duct, ductus deferens, spermatic duct, testicular duct.** See also **testis.**

vasectomy /vasek′təmē/ [L, *vas + Gk, ektome,* excision], a procedure for male sterilization involving the bilateral surgical removal of a portion of the vas deferens. Vasectomy is most commonly performed at an outpatient surgery center using local anesthesia. The procedure is also performed routinely before removal of the prostate gland to prevent inflammation of the testes and epididymides. Potency is not affected.

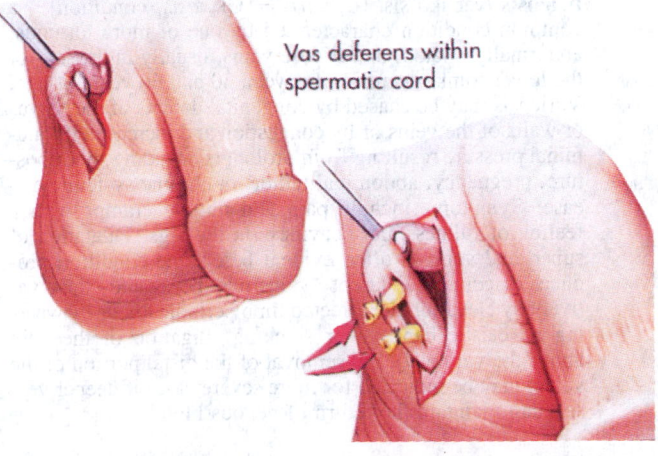

Vas deferens within spermatic cord

Vasectomy (Gottfried, 1993/Scott Bodell)

vasectomy reversal, a surgical procedure for rejoining the sections of the vas deferens previously severed to render the male infertile. Reanastomosis success varies from 45% to 60%, and in some cases the severed ends of the vas deferens rejoin spontaneously.

vaso- /vas′ō-/, a combining form meaning 'pertaining to a vessel or duct': *vasoconstrictor, vasodilation, vasoganglion.*

vasoactive /vā′zō·ak′tiv/ [L, *vas + activus,* active], (of a drug) tending to cause vasodilation or vasoconstriction.

vasoactive intestinal polypeptide (VIP), a glucagon-secretin hormone found in the pancreas, intestine, and central nervous system. The hormone stimulates insulin and glucagon release. Gastric secretion, gastric motility, and peripheral vasodilation, as well as hyperglycemia by hepatic glycogenolysis, are inhibited. See also **vipoma.**

vasoconstrictive /-kənstrik′tiv/ [L, *vas,* vessel + *constringere,* to draw tight], able to cause a constriction of blood vessels.

vasoconstriction [L, *vas + constrigere,* to tighten], a narrowing of the lumen of any blood vessel, especially the arterioles and the veins in the blood reservoirs of the skin and the abdominal viscera. It is accomplished by various mechanisms that together control blood pressure and the distribution of blood throughout the body. Vasoconstriction depends on the stimulation of the vasomotor constriction center in the medulla. Impulses from this center travel along the sympathetic nerve fibers and contract the smooth muscle layers of the arteries, the arterioles, the venules, and the veins, causing the constriction of these vessels. Vasoconstriction is also induced by vasomotor pressure reflexes, chemical reflexes, the medullary ischemic reflex, and vasomotor impulses from the cerebral cortex and the hypothalamus. Compare **vasodilation.**

vasoconstrictor /-kənstrik′tər/ [L, *vas* + *constrigere*], **1.** of or pertaining to a process, condition, or substance that causes the constriction of blood vessels. **2.** an agent that promotes vasoconstriction. Cold, fear, stress, and nicotine are common exogenous vasoconstrictors. Internally secreted epinephrine and norepinephrine cause blood vessels to contract by stimulating adrenergic receptors of peripheral sympathetic nerves. Other endogenous vasoconstrictors are angiotensin, which is formed in the blood through the action of renin, and antidiuretic hormone, which is secreted by the pituitary. Adrenergic sympathomimetic drugs cause some degree of vasoconstriction, and several of these agents are used for this action in maintaining blood pressure during anesthesia and in treating pronounced hypotension resulting from hemorrhage, myocardial infarction, septicemia, sympathectomy, or drug reactions. Among these therapeutic agents are methoxamine hydrochloride, metaraminol bitartrate, and norepinephrine. Also called **vasopressor.**

vasodepressor syncope. See **vasovagal syncope.**

vasodilation /-dīlā′shən/ [L, *vas* + *dilatare*], an increase in the diameter of a blood vessel caused by inhibition of its constrictor nerves or stimulation of dilator nerves. Also called **vasodilatation.** Compare **vasoconstriction.**

vasodilator /vā′zōdī′lātər/ [L, *vas* + *dilatare*], **1.** a nerve or agent that causes dilation of blood vessels. **2.** pertaining to the relaxation of the smooth muscle of the vascular system. **3.** producing dilation of blood vessels. Vasodilators are a recent, important addition to the treatment of heart failure. Included are hydralazine, nitroglycerin, nitroprusside, and trimethaphan. They have been useful in the treatment of acute heart failure in myocardial infarction, in cases associated with severe mitral insufficiency, and in failure resulting from myocardial disease.

vasogenic shock /-jen′ik/ [L, *vas* + *genein*, to produce; Fr, *choc*], shock resulting from peripheral vascular dilatation produced by factors, such as toxins, that directly affect the blood vessels.

vasomotor /-mō′tər/ [L, *vas* + *movere*, to move], of or pertaining to the nerves and muscles that control the caliber of the lumen of the blood vessels. Circularly arranged fibers of the muscles of arteries can contract, causing vasoconstriction, or they can relax, causing vasodilatation.

vasomotor center, a collection of cell bodies in the medulla oblongata of the brain that regulates or modulates blood pressure and cardiac function primarily via the autonomic nervous system.

vasomotor reflex [L, *vas*, vessel + *movere*, to move + *reflectere*, to bend back], any reflex response of the circulatory system caused by stimulation of vasodilator or vasoconstrictive nerves.

vasomotor rhinitis, chronic rhinitis and nasal obstruction, without allergy or infection, characterized by sneezing, rhinorrhea, nasal obstruction, and vascular engorgement of the mucous membranes of the nose. A vaporizer or humidifier and systemic vasoconstrictive agents are used to alleviate discomfort. Nose drops and nasal sprays are avoided, because continued use may cause further vasodilation of the mucous membrane and aggravation of the condition. Vasomotor rhinitis is common in pregnancy.

vasomotor spasm [L, *vas*, vessel + *movere*, to move; Gk,

spasmos, to wrench], an involuntary contraction of the muscles of the small arteries.

vasomotor system, the part of the nervous system that controls the constriction and dilatation of the blood vessels. See also **vasoconstriction, vasodilation.**

vasopressin. See **antidiuretic hormone.**

vasopressor. See **vasoconstrictor.**

vasospasm /vas′ōspaz′əm/, a spasm in a blood vessel.

vasospastic /-spas′tik/, **1.** relating to a spasmodic constriction of a blood vessel. **2.** any agent that produces spasms of the blood vessels.

vasospastic angina, an ischemic myocardial chest pain caused by spasms of the coronary arteries. It has features that differ from exertional angina. See also **Prinzmetal's angina.**

vasostimulation /-stim′yəlā′shən/ [L, *vas*, vessel + *stimulare*, to incite], the promotion of vasomotor activity.

Vasotec, a trademark for an angiotensin-converting enzyme (ACE) inhibitor (enalapril maleate).

vasovagal /-vā′gəl/ [L, *vas*, vessel + *vagus*, wandering], *obsolete.* pertaining to a condition of cerebral ischemia caused by systemic hypotension. See also **convulsive syncope, nonepileptic seizures.**

vasovagal attack. See **vasovagal syncope.**

vasovagal reflex, a stimulation of the vagus nerve by reflex in which irritation of the larynx or the trachea results in slowing of the pulse rate.

vasovagal syncope, a sudden loss of consciousness, resulting from cerebral ischemia, secondary to decreased cardiac output, peripheral vasodilation, and bradycardia, and associated with vagal activity. The condition may be triggered by pain, fright, or trauma and be accompanied by symptoms of nausea, pallor, and perspiration. Also called **vasodepressor syncope, vasovagal attack.**

vasovasostomy /vā′zōvəsos′təmē/ [L, *vas* + *vas*; Gk, *stoma*, mouth], a surgical procedure in which the function of the vas deferens on each side of the testes is restored, having been cut and ligated in a preceding vasectomy. The procedure is performed if a man wants to regain his fertility. In most cases, the patency of the canals is achieved, but in many cases fertility does not result, probably caused by circulating autoantibodies that disrupt normal sperm activity. The antibodies apparently develop after vasectomy because the developing sperm cannot be excreted through the urogenital tract.

Vasoxyl, a trademark for an alpha-adrenergic (methoxamine hydrochloride).

vastus intermedius /vas′təs/ [L, *vastus*, enormous; *inter*, between, *mediare*, to divide], one of the four muscles of the quadriceps femoris, situated in the center of the thigh, under the rectus femoris. It arises from the front and lateral surfaces of the femur and from the lateral intermuscular septum. Its fibers end in a superficial aponeurosis that forms the deep part of the quadriceps femoris tendon, inserted under the patella and onto the tibial tuberosity. The vastus intermedius is innervated by branches of the femoral nerve, which contain fibers from the second, third, and fourth lumbar nerves, and it functions with the other three muscles of the quadriceps to extend the leg. Also called **crureus.** Compare **rectus femoris, vastus lateralis, vastus medialis.**

vastus internus. See **vastus medialis.**

vastus lateralis, the largest of the four muscles of the quadriceps femoris, situated on the lateral side of the thigh.

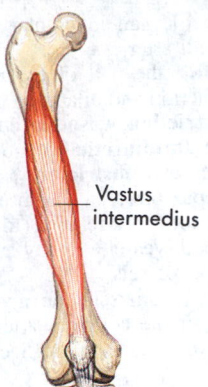

Vastus intermedius (Thibodeau, 1993/Ernest W Beck)

It is a large, dense mass originating in a broad aponeurosis that is attached to the intertrochanteric line of the femur, the greater trochanter, the lateral lip of the gluteal tuberosity, and the lateral lip of the linea aspera. The fibers of the muscle are gathered to form a strong aponeurosis that converges to become a flat tendon before inserting under the patella and onto the lateral condyle of the tibia. The vastus lateralis is innervated by branches of the femoral nerve, which contain fibers from the second, third, and fourth lumbar nerves, and it functions to help extend the leg. Compare **rectus femoris, vastus intermedius, vastus medialis.**

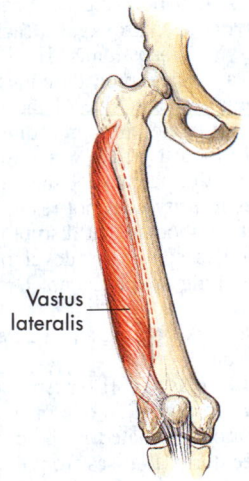

Vastus lateralis (Thibodeau, 1993/Ernest W Beck)

vastus medialis, one of the four muscles of the quadriceps femoris, situated in the medial portion of the thigh. It originates from the intertrochanteric line of the femur, the linea aspera, the medial supracondylar line, the tendons of the adductor longus and the adductor magnus, and the medial intermuscular septum. The vastus medialis extends to the lower anterior aspect of the thigh and inserts by an aponeurosis under the patella as part of the quadriceps femoris tendon and onto the medial condyle of the femur. An ex-

pansion of the aponeurosis passes to the capsule of the knee joint. The muscle is innervated by branches of the femoral nerve, which contain fibers from the second, third, and fourth lumbar nerves, and it functions in combination with other parts of the quadriceps femoris to extend the leg. Also called **vastus internus.** Compare **rectus femoris, vastus intermedius, vastus lateralis.**

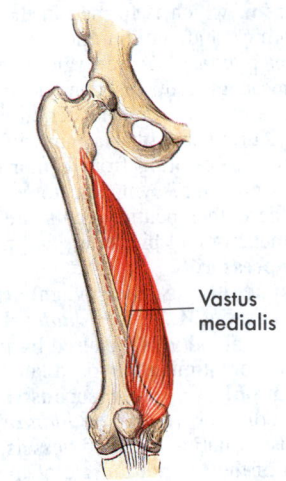

Vastus medialis (Thibodeau, 1993/Ernest W Beck)

Vater-Pacini corpuscles /fä′tərpäsē′nē/ [Abraham Vater, German anatomist, b. 1684; Filippo Pacini, Italian anatomist, b. 1812], kinesioceptors located in joint capsules and ligaments. They may transmit nerve impulses at an increasing rate as a joint approaches its maximal range of motion and are believed to have a protective function of signaling the cerebral cortex when a joint has reached the end position of its range.

Vater's ampulla /fä′tərz/ [Abraham Vater, German anatomist, b. 1864; L, *ampulla,* jug], a flask-shaped dilatation at the end of the common bile duct where the duct joins with the duodenum. Also called **hepatopancreatic ampulla.**

VBP, an anticancer drug combination of vinblastine, bleomycin, and cisplatin. Also called **PVB.**

VC, abbreviation for **vital capacity.**

Vco$_2$, symbol for carbon dioxide output per unit of time.

VD, abbreviation for **venereal disease.** See **sexually transmitted disease.**

V deflection (HBE) /diflek′shən/, a deflection on the HIS electrogram that represents ventricular activation.

VDRL, abbreviation for *Venereal Disease Research Laboratories.*

VDRL test, abbreviation for *Venereal Disease Research Laboratory test,* a serologic flocculation test for syphilis. It is also positive in other treponemal diseases, such as yaws. False-positive and false-negative results may occur. A positive test must be confirmed by further, more definitive testing.

VDT, abbreviation for **video display terminal.**

V̇e,   symbol for *expired volume*.

V̇E,   symbol for *volume expired in 1 minute*.

vector /vek′tər/ [L, carrier],   **1.** a quantity having direction and magnitude, usually depicted by a straight arrow whose length represents magnitude and whose head represents direction. **2.** a carrier, especially one that transmits disease. A **biologic vector** is usually an arthropod in which the infecting organism completes part of its life cycle. A **mechanical vector** transmits the infecting organism from one host to another but is not essential to the life cycle of the parasite. Kinds of vectors include dogs, which carry rabies; mosquitoes, which transmit malaria; and ticks, which carry Rocky Mountain spotted fever. **3.** a retrovirus that has been modified by alteration of its genetic component. Through recombinant DNA techniques, genes that cause harmful effects, such as cancer, are removed and genes that mediate synthesis of essential enzymes are added. The vector then can be injected into a patient who suffers from an enzyme deficiency, such as Lesch-Nyhan syndrome.   **–vector,** *v.,* **vectorial,** *adj.*

vectorcardiogram /-kär′dē·əgram′/ [L, *vector,* carrier; Gk, *kardia,* heart + *gramma,* record],   a tracing of the direction and magnitude of the electrical forces of a heart's activity during a cardiac cycle. It is produced by the simultaneous recording of three standard leads, using an oscilloscope.

vectorcardiography /-kär′dē·og′rəfē/ [L, *vector,* carrier; Gk, *kardia,* heart + *graphein,* to record],   a method of recording the magnitude and direction of electrical forces acting on the heart as P-, QRS-, and T-wave vectors, using a continuous loop for each vector.

vecuronium bromide /vek′yərō′nē·əm/,   an intravenous neuromuscular blocking drug.

■ INDICATIONS: It is used as an adjunct to general anesthesia, to facilitate endotracheal intubation, and to relax skeletal muscles during surgery or mechanical ventilation.

■ CONTRAINDICATIONS: The drug should be used cautiously in patients with myasthenia gravis or other neuromuscular disorders, or who have been given drugs that produce or increase neuromuscular block. Effects of vecuronium may be prolonged in patients with liver disease.

■ ADVERSE EFFECTS: No serious adverse reactions have been reported.

VEE,   abbreviation for **Venezuelan equine encephalitis.** See **equine encephalitis.**

Veetids,   a trademark for an antibacterial (penicillin V potassium).

vegan.   See **strict vegetarian.**

veganism /vej′əniz′əm/ [L, *vegetare,* to grow, *ismus,* practice],   the adherence to a strict vegetable diet, with the exclusion of all protein of animal origin.

vegetable albumin /vej′(i)təbəl/,   albumin produced in plants.

vegetal pole /vej′ətəl/ [L, *vegetare* + *polus,* pole],   the relatively inactive part of the ovum protoplasm where the food yolk is situated, usually opposite the animal pole. Also called **vegetative pole, antigerminal pole.** Compare **animal pole.**

vegetarian /vej′əter′ē·ən/ [L, *vegetare*],   a person whose diet is restricted to foods of vegetable origin, including fruits, grains, and nuts. Many vegetarians eat eggs and milk products but avoid all animal flesh. Kinds of vegetarians are **lacto-ovo-vegetarian, lacto-vegetarian, ovo-vegetarian,** and **strict vegetarian.**

vegetarianism /vej′əter′ē·əniz′əm/,   the theory or practice of restricting the diet to food substances of vegetable origin, including fruits, grains, and nuts.

vegetation /vej′ətā′shən/,   an abnormal growth of tissue around a valve, composed of fibrin, platelets, and bacteria.

vegetative /vej′ətā′tiv, vej′ətətiv′/ [L, *vegerare*],   **1.** of or pertaining to nutrition and growth. **2.** of or pertaining to the plant kingdom. **3.** denoting involuntary function, as produced by the parasympathetic nervous system. **4.** resting, not active; denoting the stage of the cell cycle in which the cell is not replicating. **5.** leading a secluded, dull existence without social or intellectual activity; sluggish; lacking animation. **6.** (in psychiatry) emotionally withdrawn and passive, as may occur in schizophrenia and in the depressive phase of bipolar disorder.   **–vegetate,** *v.*

vegetative endocarditis [L, *vegetare,* to grow; Gk, *endon,* within + *kardia,* heart + *itis,* inflammation],   a subacute form of bacterial endocarditis characterized by vegetation on the heart valves. The vegetation may cause ulceration and perforation of the heart valve cusps.

vegetative state,   a physical condition in which a previously comatose patient appears to be awake but is unable to communicate or respond to stimuli. The eyes may be open but because of senile brain disease, cerebral arteriosclerosis, or injury to the cerebral cortex the patient remains immobile and must be fed and toileted.

vehicle /vē′ikəl/ [L, *vehiculum,* conveyance],   **1.** an inert substance with which a medication is mixed to facilitate measurement and administration or application. **2.** any fluid or structure in the body that passively conveys a stimulus.

Veillonella /vā′yənel′ə/ [Adrien Veillon, French bacteriologist, b. 1864],   a genus of gram-negative anaerobic bacteria. The species *Veillonella parvula* is normally present in the alimentary tract, especially in the mouth.

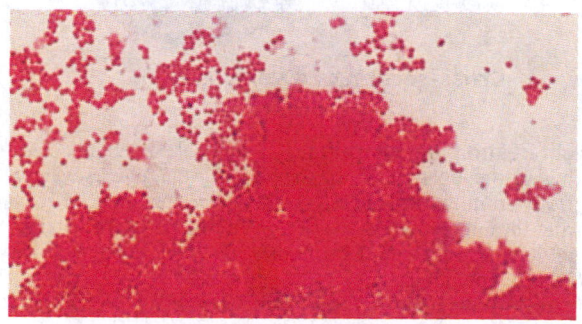

Veillonella (Summanen, 1993)

Veillon tube /vāyōn′/,   a transparent tube whose ends are closed with removable stoppers, one cotton and one rubber. It is used for the laboratory growth of bacteriologic cultures.

vein (v) /vān/ [L, *vena*],   one of the many vessels that convey blood from the capillaries to the heart as part of the pulmonary venous system, the systemic venous network, or the portal venous complex. Most of the veins of the body are systemic veins that convey blood from the whole body (except the lungs) to the right atrium of the heart. Each vein is a macroscopic structure enclosed in three layers of different kinds of tissue homologous with the layers of the heart. The outer tunica adventitia of each vein is homologous with the epicardium, the tunica media with the myocardium, and the tunica intima with the endocardium. Deep veins course through the more internal parts of the body, and superficial veins lie near the surface, where many of them can be seen through the skin. Veins have thinner coatings and are less elastic than arteries and collapse when cut. They also contain semilunar valves at various intervals to control the direction of the flow of blood back to the heart. Compare **artery.** See also **portal vein, pulmonary vein, systemic vein.**

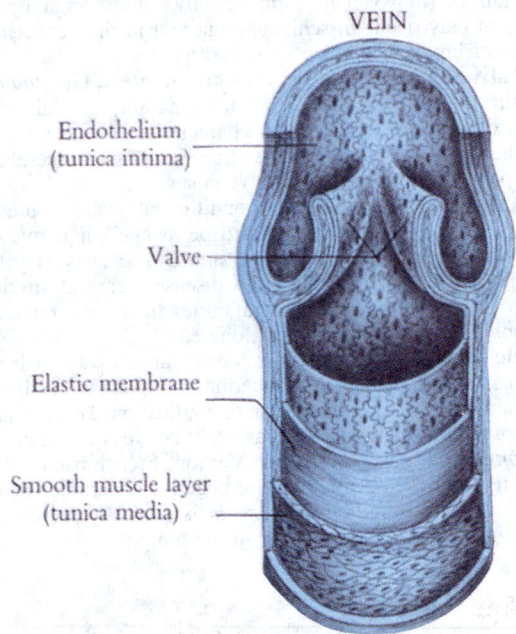

VEIN

Endothelium (tunica intima)

Valve

Elastic membrane

Smooth muscle layer (tunica media)

Cross-section of a vein (Thompson, 1989)

vein ligation and stripping, a surgical procedure consisting of the ligation of the saphenous vein and its removal from groin to ankle, performed for the treatment of recurrent thrombophlebitis or severe varicosities or for obtaining a blood vessel to graft in another site, such as in a coronary bypass operation.

vein lumen, the central opening through which blood flows in a vein.

vein of Thebesius. See **smallest cardiac vein.**

veins of the vertebral column, the veins that drain the blood from the vertebral column, the adjacent muscles, and the meninges of the spinal cord. Along the entire vertebral column these veins form plexuses that are divided into internal and external groups, according to their locations inside or outside the vertebral canal. The plexuses and the veins of the vertebral network are the external plexus, the internal plexus, the basivertebral veins, the intervertebral veins, and the spinal cord veins.

Velban, a trademark for an antineoplastic (vinblastine sulfate).

vellus hair. See **lanugo.**

velocity /vəlos'itē/ [L, *velox,* quick], the rate of change in the position of a body moving in a particular direction. Velocity along a straight line is linear velocity. Angular velocity is that of a body in circular motion. Compare **speed.**

velocity of growth, the rate of growth or change in growth measurements over a period of time.

velocity of ultrasound, the speed of ultrasound energy, measured in meters per second (m/sec), in a particular medium. The velocity varies from 331 m/sec in air to 1450 m/sec in fat, 1570 m/sec in blood, and 4080 m/sec in the skull.

velocity spectrum rehabilitation, a rehabilitation program that uses strength training at multiple speeds of movement, from slow to fast.

velopharyngeal insufficiency, an abnormal condition resulting from a congenital defect in the structure of the velopharyngeal sphincter: Closure of the oral cavity beneath the nasal passages is not complete, as seen in cleft palate. Food may be regurgitated through the nose, and speech is impaired. Surgical correction is usually successful.

Velosef, a trademark for a cephalosporin antibiotic (cephradine).

Velpeau's bandage /velpōz'/ [Alfred A. L. M. Velpeau, French surgeon, b. 1795], a roller bandage that immobilizes the elbow and shoulder by holding the brachium against the side and the flexed forearm on the chest. The palm of the hand rests on the clavicle of the opposite side.

vena cava /vē'nə kā'və/, *pl.* **venae cavae** [L, *vena,* vein; *cavum,* cavity], one of two large veins returning blood from the peripheral circulation to the right atrium of the heart. See also **inferior vena cava, superior vena cava.** −**vena caval,** *adj.*

vena caval syndrome. See **supine hypotension.**

vena comes /kō'mēz/, *pl.* **venae comites** /kom'itēz/, one of the deep paired veins that accompany the smaller arteries, one on each side of the artery. The three vessels are wrapped together in one sheath. Some of the arteries accompanied by such venous pairs are the brachial, the ulnar, and the tibial.

veneer /vənir'/ [Fr, *fournir,* to furnish], **1.** in dentistry, a layer of tooth-colored material, usually porcelain or acrylic, attached to the surface of a crown or artificial tooth by direct fusion. **2.** a thin, tenacious film of calculus found subgingivally which is discolored blue-black. Also called **serumal calculus.**

venepuncture. See **venipuncture.**

venereal /vənir'ē·əl/ [L, *Venus,* goddess of love], pertaining to or caused by sexual intercourse or genital contact.

venereal bubo [L, *Venus,* goddess of love; Gk, *boubon,* groin], a swollen, inflamed lymph gland or node, usually in the groin and sometimes purulent. It is associated with a sexually transmitted disease.

venereal disease. See **sexually transmitted disease.**

venereal sore. See **chancre.**

venereal wart. See **condyloma acuminatum, genital wart.**

venereologist /vənir'ē·ol'əjist/ [L, *Venus,* goddess of love; Gk, *logos,* science], a health professional who specializes in the study of the causes and treatments of venereal diseases.

venereology /-ol'əjē/, the study of the causes and treatments of venereal diseases. −**venereologic, venereological,** *adj.,* **venereologist,** *n.*

venerupin poisoning /ven′ərōō′pin/, a potentially fatal form of shellfish poisoning that results from ingestion of oysters or clams contaminated with venerupin, a toxin that causes impaired liver functioning, GI distress, and leukocytosis. The shellfish toxin occurs in waters around Japan. About one third of the cases are fatal. See also **shellfish poisoning.**

venesection. See **phlebotomy.**

Venezuelan equine encephalitis. See **equine encephalitis.**

venipuncture /ven′əpungk′chər/ [L, *vena* + *pungere*, to prick], a technique in which a vein is punctured transcutaneously by a sharp rigid stylet or cannula carrying a flexible plastic catheter or by a steel needle attached to a syringe or catheter. The purpose of the procedure is to withdraw a specimen of blood, to perform a phlebotomy, to instill a medication, to start an intravenous infusion, or to inject a radiopaque substance for radiologic examination of a part or system of the body. Also spelled **venepuncture.**

■ METHOD: The specific steps in performing a venipuncture vary with the purpose of the procedure and the equipment to be used, but in most instances it begins as follows: A convenient vein is selected, usually on the outside of the forearm, on the back of the hand, or in the antecubital fossa. The vein is palpated, and to dilate the vein a tourniquet is wrapped around the arm proximal to the intended site of puncture. The site is cleansed, and the vein is immobilized by applying traction on the skin around the puncture site. The stylet or needle is held at an angle of 30 degrees for direct venipuncture. In performing direct venipuncture the tip of the needle is pointed in the direction of the flow of blood and is advanced through the skin directly into the vein. The tip is usually inserted bevel side up, but if a large-bore needle must be used in a small vein, it is preferable to insert the needle bevel side down, because it is less likely to perforate the posterior wall of the vein. After the skin is punctured, little resistance is felt as the tip passes through the subcutaneous tissue, but a sudden, slight resistance may be felt as the tip hits the wall of the vein. At this point, the tip is cautiously advanced, with the needle or stylet held nearly flush with the skin. Slight upward pressure aids in keeping the tip in the vein as it is advanced into the lumen of the intravenous space. Blood flows back into the hub of the needle or into the catheter attached to the needle or covering the stylet, and the tip of the needle usually can be felt to be in the vein. If these signs are absent, the tip is not in the vein, in which case it is usually best to remove the needle or stylet, apply pressure to the puncture site, and start the procedure again, using new equipment.

■ INTERVENTIONS: Wing-tipped 'butterfly' needles, various kinds of intracatheters, and single or multiple venipuncture needles require familiarity and practice for correct insertion and stabilization. A sterile dressing and an antimicrobial ointment are applied over the insertion site. The cleansing agent used to prepare the injection site may be iodine, povidone-iodine, or ethyl alcohol. If an iodine preparation or solution is to be used, the patient is first asked about any previous allergic reaction to iodine. To aid insertion of the tip into the vein, the patient may be asked to clench the fist to further dilate the vein. If the patient is unable to do this, a second tourniquet may be placed several inches distal to the puncture site. This tourniquet is released when the needle or stylet has been placed in the vein.

■ OUTCOME CRITERIA: Aseptic technique is required to avoid infection. A quick, skillful insertion is nearly painless for the patient. Specific sequelae to venipuncture vary with the techniques and equipment used. See also **intravenous infusion, phlebotomy.**

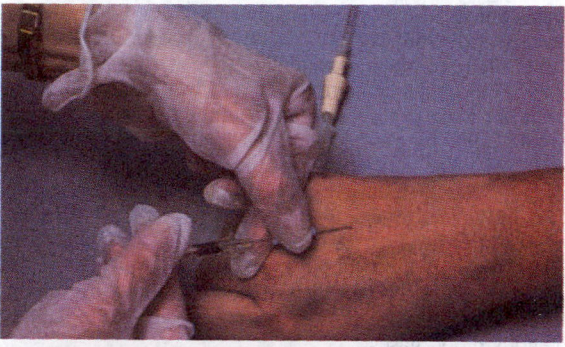

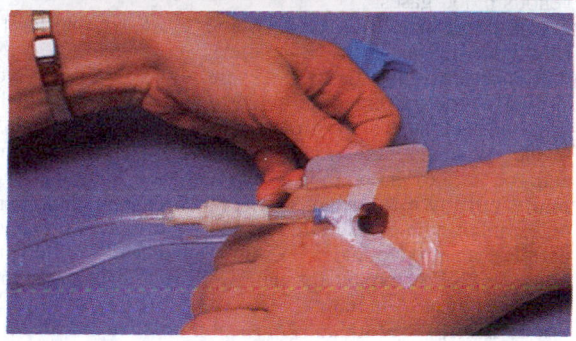

Venipuncture *(Potter, 1993)*

veno-, a combining form meaning 'pertaining to a vein': *venoclysis, venopressor, venovenostomy.*

venogram. See **phlebogram.**

venography. See **phlebography.**

venom /ven′əm/ [L, *venenum*, poison], a toxic fluid substance secreted by some snakes, arthropods, and other animals and transmitted by their stings or bites.

venom extract therapy, the administration of antivenin as prophylaxis against the toxic effects of the bite of a specific poisonous snake or spider, or other venomous animal.

venom immunotherapy, the reduction of sensitivity to the bite of a venomous insect or animal by the serial administration of gradually increasing amounts of the specific antigenic substance secreted by the insect or animal.

venospasm /vēn′əspaz′əm/ [L, *vena*, vein; Gk, *spasmos*, spasm], a spasmodic contraction of a vein.

venotomy /vēnot′əmē/, the surgical opening of a vein.

venous /vē′nəs/, of or pertaining to a vein.

-venous, a combining form meaning 'of or referring to veins': *endovenous, lymphovenous, perivenous.*

venous access device, a catheter designed for continuous access to the venous system. Such devices may be required for long-term parenteral feeding or the administration of IV fluids or medications for a period of several days.

venous blood (v) [L, *vena*, vein; AS, *blod*], dark red blood that has been deoxygenated during passage from the left ventricle through the systemic circulation, en route to the right atrium.

venous blood gas [L, *venosus,* full of veins; AS, *blod;* Gk, *chaos,* gas], the oxygen and carbon dioxide in venous blood measured by various methods to assess the adequacy of oxygenation and ventilation and to determine the acid-base status. The oxygen tension of venous blood normally averages 40 mm Hg; the dissolved oxygen 0.1% by volume; the total oxygen content 15.2%; and the oxygen saturation of venous hemoglobin 75%. The carbon dioxide tension normally averages 46 mm Hg; the dissolved carbon dioxide 2.9% by volume; and the total carbon dioxide content 50%. The normal average pH of venous plasma is 7.37. Venous blood in an extremity when analyzed for gas content provides data chiefly pertaining to that limb. Because a sample from a central venous catheter is usually an incomplete mix of venous blood from various parts of the body, a specimen of completely mixed blood may be obtained from the pulmonary artery for an accurate determination of venous blood gases.

venous capillaries [L, *vena,* vein + *capillaris,* hairlike], capillaries that terminate in venules.

venous circulation [L, *vena,* vein + *circulare,* to go around], the movement of blood from the venules, which drain deoxgenated blood from the cells, through the veins to the vena cava, and from there through the right atrium and ventricle to the pulmonary circulation of the lungs.

venous cutdown, a small surgical incision made in a vein of a patient who has suffered vascular collapse in order to permit the introduction of IV fluids or drugs. A cutdown also may be performed for the insertion of a cannula for the withdrawal of blood.

venous hum, a continuous musical murmur heard on auscultation over the major veins at the base of the neck, particularly when the patient is anemic, upright, and looking to the contralateral side. It is also heard in some healthy, young individuals.

venous insufficiency, an abnormal circulatory condition characterized by decreased return of the venous blood from the legs to the trunk of the body. Edema is usually the first sign of the condition; pain, varicosities, and ulceration may follow. Treatment usually consists of elevation of the legs, use of elastic hose, and correction of the underlying condition.

venous pressure, the stress exerted by circulating blood on the walls of veins; it is elevated in congestive heart failure, acute or chronic constrictive pericarditis, and venous obstruction caused by a clot or external pressure against a vein. Indications of increased pressure are continued distention of veins on the back of the hand when it is raised above the sternal notch and distention of the neck veins when the individual is sitting with the head elevated 30 to 45 degrees.

venous pulse, the pulse of a vein usually palpated over the internal or external jugular veins in the neck. The pulse in the jugular vein is taken to evaluate the pressure of the pulse and the form of the pressure wave, especially in a person with a cardiac conduction defect or cardiac dysrhythmia.

venous sinus, one of many sinuses that collect blood from the dura mater and drain it into the internal jugular vein. Each sinus is formed by the separation of the two layers of the dura mater, the outer coat of the sinus consisting of fi-

brous tissue, and the inner coat consisting of endothelium continuous with that of the veins.

venous stasis, a disorder in which the normal flow of blood through a vein is slowed or halted.

venous stasis dermatitis. See **stasis dermatitis.**

venous thrombosis, a condition characterized by the presence of a clot in a vein in which the wall of the vessel is not inflamed. Pain, swelling, and inflammation may follow if the vein is significantly occluded. Also called **phlebothrombosis.** Compare **thrombophlebitis.**

ventilate /ven′tilāt/ [L, *ventilare,* to wave], **1.** to provide with fresh air. **2.** to provide the lungs with air from the atmosphere and to aerate or oxygenate blood in the pulmonary capillaries. **3.** (in psychiatry) to open discussion of something, such as to ventilate feelings.

ventilation /ven′tilā′shən/ [L, *ventilare*], the process by which gases are moved into and out of the lungs. Compare **respiration.** –**ventilatory,** *adj.*

ventilation, inability to sustain spontaneous, a nursing diagnosis accepted by the Tenth National Conference on the Classification of Nursing Diagnoses. It is defined as a state in which the response pattern of decreased energy reserves results in an individual's inability to maintain breathing adequate to support life. Major defining characteristics are dyspnea and increased metabolic rate. Minor defining characteristics are increased restlessness, apprehension, increased use of accessory muscles, decreased tidal volume, increased heart rate, decreased po_2 level, increased pco_2 level, decreased cooperation, and decreased Sao_2 level. See also **nursing diagnosis.**

ventilation lung scan, a radiographic examination of the lungs, performed while the patient inhales a radioactive gas as a contrast medium and the lungs are scanned to detect nonfunctional or impaired lung areas or other abnormalities.

ventilation perfusion defect, a disorder in which one or more areas of the lung receive ventilation but no blood flow, or blood flow but no ventilation.

ventilation/perfusion (V/Q) ratio, the ratio of pulmonary alveolar ventilation to pulmonary capillary perfusion, both measured quantities being expressed in the same units.

ventilator /ven′tilā′tər/, any of several devices used in respiratory therapy to provide assisted respiration and intensive positive pressure breathing. Kinds of ventilators are **pressure ventilator** and **volume ventilator.** See also **IPPB unit.**

ventilatory rate /ven′tilətôr′ē/ [L, *ventilate,* wave + *ratum,* to calculate], the volume of air passing through the lungs per minute. Compare **respiratory rate.**

ventilatory standstill [L, *ventilate,* wave; AS, *standan* + *stille*], the complete cessation of breathing activity. Compare **apnea.**

ventilatory weaning process, dysfunctional (DVWR), a nursing diagnosis accepted by the Tenth National Conference on the Classification of Nursing Diagnoses. It is defined as a state in which an individual cannot adjust to lowered levels of mechanical ventilatory support, which interrupts and prolongs the weaning process. DVWR may be classified as mild, moderate, or severe. For mild DVWR, the major defining characteristic is a response to lowered levels of mechanical ventilator support with restlessness or a respiratory rate slightly increased from baseline. The minor defining characteristic is a response to lowered levels of mechanical ventilator support with expressed feelings of increased need for oxygen, breathing discomfort, fatigue, or warmth, queries about possible machine malfunction, and increased concentration on breathing. For moderate DVWR, the major defining characteristic is a response to lowered levels of mechanical ventilator support with a slight increase from baseline blood pressure (less than 20 mm Hg), a slight increase from baseline heart rate (less than 20 beats per minute), and a baseline increase in respiratory rate (less than 5 breaths per minute). Minor defining characteristics are hypervigilance to activities, inability to respond to coaching, inability to cooperate, apprehension, diaphoresis, eye widening, decreased air entry on auscultation, color changes (pale, slight cyanosis), and slight respiratory accessory muscle use. For severe DVWR, the major defining characteristic is a response to lowered levels of mechanical ventilator support with agitation, deterioration in arterial blood gas levels from current baseline, increase from baseline blood pressure of greater than 20 mm Hg, an increase from baseline heart rate of greater than 20 beats per minute, and a significant increase in respiratory rate. Minor defining characteristics are profuse diaphoresis, full respiratory accessory muscle use, shallow, gasping breaths, paradoxical abdominal breathing, discoordinated breathing with the ventilator, decreased level of consciousness, adventitious breath sounds, audible airway secretions, and cyanosis. Related factors may be physical, psychological, or situational. Physical factors are ineffective airway clearance, sleep pattern disturbance, inadequate nutrition, and uncontrolled pain or discomfort. Psychological factors are knowledge deficit of the weaning process/patient role, patient-perceived inefficacy in the ability to wean, decreased motivation, decreased self-esteem, moderate or severe anxiety, fear, hopelessness, powerlessness, and insufficient trust in the nurse. Situational factors are uncontrolled episodic energy demands or problems, inappropriate pacing of diminished ventilator support, inadequate social support, an adverse environment (noisy, active, negative events in the room, low nurse-patient ratio, extended nurse absence from the bedside, unfamiliar nursing staff), a history of ventilator dependence longer than 1 week, and a history of multiple unsuccessful weaning attempts. See also **nursing diagnosis.**

venting [Fr, *vent*, breath], (in intravenous therapy) a method for allowing air to enter the vacuum of the intravenous bottle and displace the intravenous solution as it flows out. Glass intravenous bottles are usually equipped with a venting tube attached to the primary IV tubing or to a vent port incorporated with the bottle stopper. Venting is not required with a plastic IV bag, because the bag collapses as the fluid runs out. The air vent attached to primary IV tubing is removable to allow the injection of medication.

Ventolin a trademark for a bronchodilator (albuterol).

ventral /ven'trəl/ [L, *venter*, belly], of or pertaining to a position toward the belly of the body; frontward; anterior. Compare **dorsal.**

-ventral, a suffix meaning 'of the stomach or abdominal region': *biventral, dorsoventral, uteroventral.*

ventral hernia. See **abdominal hernia.**

ventral horn [L, *venter*, belly + *cornu*], the anterior columns of the gray matter of the spinal cord.

ventral recumbent [L, *venter*, belly + *recumbere*, to lie down], a prone position of lying face down.

ventral root [L, *venter*, belly; AS, *rot*], the anterior or motor division of each spinal nerve.

ventri-. See **ventro-.**

ventricle /ven'trikəl/ [L, *ventriculum*, little belly], a small cavity, such as one of the cavities filled with cerebrospinal fluid in the brain, or the right and the left ventricles of the heart.

ventricular /ventrik'yələr/ [L, *ventriculum*, little belly], of or pertaining to a ventricle.

ventricular aneurysm, a localized dilatation or saccular protrusion in the wall of the ventricle, occurring most often after a myocardial infarction. Scar tissue is formed in response to the inflammatory changes of the infarction. This tissue weakens the myocardium, allowing its walls to bulge outward when the ventricle contracts. A typical sign of the lesion is a recurrent ventricular dysrhythmia that does not respond to treatment with conventional antidysrhythmic drugs. Diagnostic measures are x-ray studies and cardiac catheterization. Treatment usually involves surgical removal of the scar tissue. Also called **aneurysmectomy, cardiac aneurysm.**

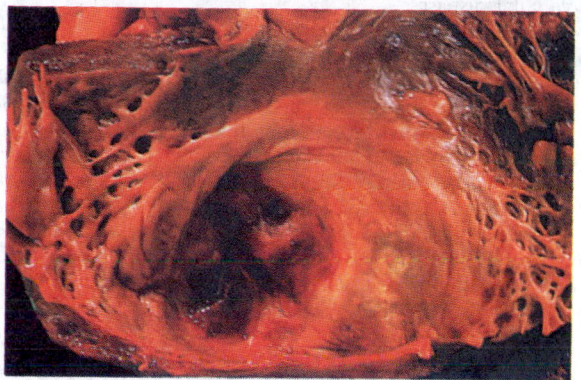

Ventricular aneurysm (Fletcher, 1987)

ventricular bigeminy [L, *ventriculum* + *bis, geminus,* twins], a dysrhythmia in which every other beat is caused by a premature ventricular beat.

ventricular block [L, *ventriculum;* OFr, *bloc*], an obstruction of the flow of cerebraospinal fluid. Causes usually are closure of the foramina of Magendie or Luschka. The condition results in a distention of the brain ventricles because of an increased accumulation of cerebrospinal fluid.

ventricular dysfunction, abnormalities in contraction and wall motion within the ventricles.

ventricular ejection [L, *ventriculum* + *ejicere,* to cast out], a forceful expulsion of blood from the ventricles to the main arteries.

ventricular escape [L, *ventriculum* + OFr, *escaper*], a release of the ventricles from inhibitory control of a sinus or junctional rhythm when the rate of discharges falls below the natural rate of impulse formation of the pacemaker cells in the bundle branches.

ventricular extrasystole, an extrasystole arising from the ventricle.

ventricular fibrillation (VF), a cardiac dysrhythmia marked by rapid, disorganized depolarizations of the ventricular myocardium. The condition is characterized by a complete lack of organized electric impulse, conduction, and ventricular contraction. Blood pressure falls to zero, resulting in unconsciousness. Death may occur within 4 minutes. Defibrillation and ventilation must be initiated immediately.

ventricular gallop, an abnormal low-pitched extra heart sound (S_3) heard early in diastole. When it is heard in an older person with heart disease, it indicates myocardial failure. The same sound heard in a healthy child or young adult is a physiologic finding (called a physiologic third heart sound) that usually disappears with age. See also **gallop.**

ventricular gradient, the algebraic sum of the areas within the QRS complex and within the T wave in the electrocardiogram.

ventricular hemiblock, a failure to conduct an impulse down only one division of the left bundle branch, such as an anterior superior or posterior inferior hemiblock.

ventricular hypertrophy [L, *ventriculum*; Gk, *hyper*, excessive + *trophe*, nourishment], an abnormal enlargement of the heart ventricles, often caused by hypertension or a valvular disease.

ventricular pacing. See **pacing.**

ventricular remodeling, progressive myocardial ventricular dilation, eccentric hypertrophy, and distortion of left ventricular geometry that persist in the noninfarcted myocardium after a myocardial infarction has healed. It is associated with impaired functional capacity, congestive heart failure, and premature death.

ventricular rhythm [L, *ventriculum*; Gk, *rhythmos*] a cardiac dysrhythmia that results when the sinoatrial and the atrioventricular nodes are suppressed or discharge more slowly than the intrinsic rate of the ventricles.

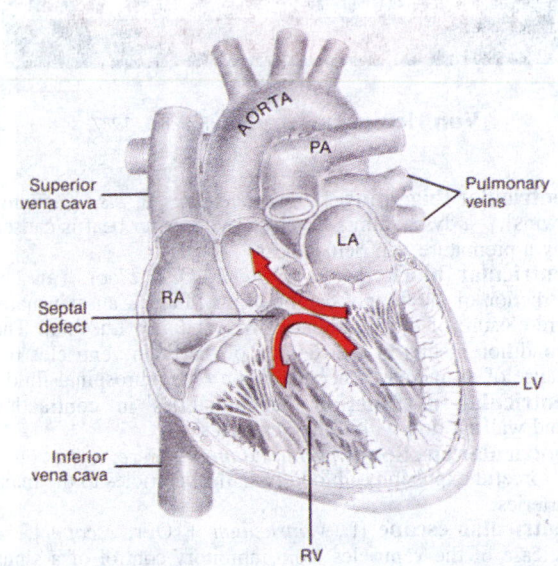

Ventricular septal defect *(Canobbio, 1990)*

ventricular septal defect (VSD), an abnormal opening in the septum separating the ventricles, permitting blood to flow from the left ventricle to the right ventricle and to recirculate through the pulmonary artery and lungs. It is the most common congenital heart defect, with openings that may be single or multiple and may range in size from 1 to 2 mm to several centimeters. Children with small defects are usually asymptomatic, whereas those with large defects may have congestive heart failure, associated with lower respiratory tract infections, rapid breathing, poor weight gain, restlessness, and irritability. Small defects may close spontaneously; larger ones may lead to bacterial endocarditis, pulmonary vascular obstructive disease, aortic regurgitation, or congestive heart failure. Diagnosis is established by electrocardiography, cardiac catheterization, and angiography. Treatment consists of surgical repair of the defect, preferably in early childhood.

ventricular septum. See **interventricular septum.**

ventricular systole [L, *ventriculum*; Gk, *systole*, contraction], the contraction of the heart ventricles. It begins with the first heart sound.

ventricular tachycardia, tachycardia of at least three consecutive ventricular complexes with a rate of more than 100 beats per minute that usually originates in the ventricular Purkinje system.

ventriculo- /ventrik'yəlō-/, a combining form meaning 'pertaining to a ventricle of the heart or brain': *ventriculocisternostomy, ventriculopuncture, ventriculostium.*

ventriculogram /ventrik'yəlōgram'/, a radiographic examination of the ventricles of the heart in which contrast medium is injected during cardiac catheterization.

ventriculoatrial shunt /ventrik'yəlō·ā'trē·əl/ [L, *ventriculum + atrium*, hall; ME, *shunten*], a surgically created passageway, consisting of plastic tubing and one-way valves, implanted between a cerebral ventricle and the right atrium of the heart to drain excess cerebrospinal fluid from the brain in hydrocephalus.

ventriculoatriostomy. See **auriculoventriculostomy.**

ventriculocisternostomy /-sis'tərōs'təmē/ [L, *ventriculum + cisterna*, vessel; Gk, *stoma*, mouth], a surgical procedure performed to treat hydrocephalus. An opening is created that allows cerebrospinal fluid to drain through a shunt from the ventricles of the brain into the cisterna magna. Also called **Torkildsen procedure, ventriculostomy.**

ventriculofallopian tube shunt /-fəlō'pē·ən/, a surgical procedure with limited effectiveness for diverting cerebrospinal fluid into the peritoneal cavity. The procedure passes a polyethylene tube from the lateral ventricle or from the spinal subarachnoid space into a ligated fallopian tube and finally into the peritoneal cavity, where the shunted cerebrospinal fluid is absorbed. This procedure is used to correct both the obstructive and the communicating types of hydrocephalus. Also called **spinofallopian tube shunt.**

ventriculography /ventrik'yəlog'rəfē/ [L, *ventriculum + graphein*, to record], an x-ray examination of a ventricle of the heart, after injection of a radiopaque contrast medium.

ventriculoperitoneal shunt /-per'itənē'əl/ [L, *ventriculum + Gk, peri*, around, *teinein*, to stretch; ME, *shunten*], a surgically created passageway, consisting of plastic tubing and one-way valves, between a cerebral ventricle and the peritoneum for the draining of excess cerebrospinal fluid from the brain in hydrocephalus.

ventriculoperitoneostomy /ventrik'yəlōper'itō'nē·os'təmē/ [L, *ventriculum + Gk, peri*, around, *teinein*, to stretch, *stoma*, mouth], a surgical procedure for temporarily diverting cerebrospinal fluid in hydrocephalus, usually in the newborn. In this procedure, which spares the kidney but is less efficient than a ventriculoureterostomy, a polyethylene tube is passed from the lateral ventricle subcutaneously down the dorsal spine and is reinserted into the peritoneal cavity, where the diverted fluid is absorbed. This procedure is used to correct both the communicating and the obstructive types of hydrocephalus.

ventriculopleural shunt /-ploor'əl/ [L, *ventriculum* + Gk, *pleura*, rib; ME, *shunten*], a surgical procedure for diverting cerebrospinal fluid from engorged ventricles in hydrocephalus, usually in the newborn. In this procedure, cerebrospinal fluid is diverted from the lateral ventricle into the pleural cavity. It is used to correct both the obstructive and the communicating types of hydrocephalus.

ventriculostomy. See **ventriculocisternostomy.**

ventriculoureterostomy /ventrik'yəlō·yoŏrē'təros'təmē/ [L, *ventriculum* + Gk, *oureter*, ureter, *stoma*, mouth], a surgical procedure for directing cerebrospinal fluid into the general circulation performed in the treatment of hydrocephalus, usually in the newborn. In this procedure a polyethylene tube is passed from the lateral ventricle down the dorsal spine subcutaneously to the twelfth rib; the tube is inserted through the paraspinal muscles into a ureter. Rarely used, the method is an alternative to auriculoventriculostomy, especially if the obstruction to cerebrospinal fluid includes the basilar and the cerebral subarachnoid spaces, the posterior fossa, and the spinal subarachnoid spaces. The procedure is performed to correct an obstructive type of hydrocephalus.

ventro-, ventri-, a combining form meaning 'pertaining to the belly or to the front of the body': *ventrodorsal, ventrolateral, ventroptosia.*

Venturi effect /ventoo'rē/ [Giovanni B. Venturi, Italian physicist, b. 1746], a modification of the Bernoulli effect in which there is dilation of a gas passage just beyond an obstruction or restriction. The pressure drop distal to the restriction can be restored to nearly the prerestriction pressure if dilation of the passage does not exceed 15 degrees. The principle is used in respiratory therapy equipment for mixing medical gases.

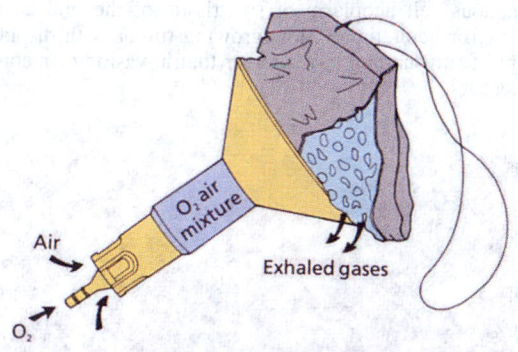

Venturi mask
(Potter, 1993/Courtesy Puritan-Bennett Corp, Overland Park, Kansas)

Venturi mask, a respiratory therapy face mask designed to allow entrained air to mix with oxygen, which is supplied through a jet at a fixed concentration.

venul-, a combining form meaning 'pertaining to a venule': *venulitis, venuloma.*

venule /ven'yool/ [L, *venula*, small vein], any one of the small blood vessels that gather blood from the capillary plexuses and anastomose to form the veins. —**venular,** *adj.*

VEP, abbreviation for **visual evoked potential.**

verapamil /verap'əmil/, a slow calcium channel blocker or calcium ion antagonist.

■ INDICATIONS: It is prescribed for the treatment of vasospastic and effort-associated angina, supraventricular tachycardia, atrial fibrillation, and atrial flutter.

■ CONTRAINDICATIONS: Severe left ventricular dysfunction, hypotension, cardiogenic shock, sick sinus syndrome, or second- or third-degree atrioventricular block prohibits its use.

■ ADVERSE EFFECTS: Among the more serious adverse reactions are hypotension, peripheral edema, atrioventricular block, bradycardia, congestive heart failure, pulmonary edema, and dizziness.

Veratrum /verā'trəm/ [L, hellebore], a genus of poisonous herbs of the lily family. The dried rhizomes of the British and American hellebore provide alkaloids that are used as antihypertensive agents.

verbal aphasia. See **motor aphasia.**

verbal language /vur'bəl/ [L, *verbum*, a word; *lingua*, tongue], a culturally organized system of vocal sounds that communicates meaning between individuals.

vergence /ver'jəns/, movement of the two eyes in opposite directions.

vergence ability. See **amplitude of convergence.**

-verine, a combining form for spasmolytics having a papaverine-like action.

vermicide /vur'misīd/ [L, *vermis*, worm, *caedere*, to kill], an agent that kills worms, particularly those in the intestine. Compare **anthelmintic, vermifuge.**

vermicular /vərmik'yələr/ [L, *vermiculus*, small worm], resembling a worm.

vermiform /vur'mifôrm/ [L, *vermis*, worm + *forma*, form], resembling a worm. Also **lumbrical.**

vermiform appendix [L, *vermis* + *forma*, form; *appendix*, appendage], a wormlike, blunt process extending from the cecum. Its length varies from 3 to 6 inches, and its diameter is about 1/3 inch. Also called **appendix vermiformis, cecal appendix.** See also **appendicitis.**

vermifuge /vərmifyooj'/ [L, *vermis* + *fugare*, to chase away], an agent that causes the evacuation of intestinal parasitic worms.

vermilion border /vərmil'yən/ [L, *vermillium*, bright red; OFr, *bordure*, frame], the external pinkish to red area of the upper and lower lips, extending from the junction of the lips with the surrounding facial skin on the exterior to the labial mucosa within the mouth.

vermin /vur'min/ [L, **vermis,** worm], any insects or small animals regarded as destructive or disease-carrying pests.

vermis /vur'mis/, *pl.* **vermes** [L], **1.** a worm. **2.** a structure resembling a worm, such as the median lobe of the cerebellum. —**vermiform,** *adj.*

Vermox, a trademark for an anthelmintic (mebendazole).

vernal conjunctivitis /vur'nəl/ [L, *vernare*, springlike; *conjunctivus*, connecting; Gk, *itis*, inflammation], a chronic, bilateral form of conjunctivitis, thought to be allergic in origin, that occurs most frequently in young men under 20 years of age during the spring and summer months. Most common symptoms include intense itching and crusting dis-

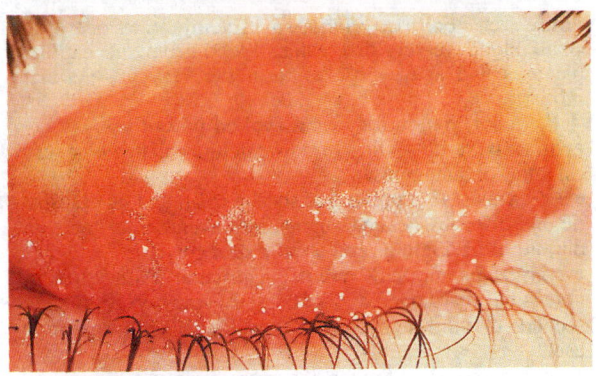

Acute vernal conjunctivitis *(Holgate, 1993)*

charge. Topical corticosteroids may be applied, and desensitization to pollen may be helpful. Compare **allergic conjunctivitis.**

Vernet's syndrome /vernāz′/ [Maurice Vernet, French neurologist, b. 1887], a neurologic disorder caused by injury to the ninth, tenth, and eleventh cranial nerves as they pass through the jugular foramen when leaving the skull. Symptoms include unilateral flaccid paralysis of the palatal, pharyngeal, and intrinsic laryngeal muscles and the sternocleidomastoid and trapezius muscles. The patient also experiences dysphagia, the voice is nasal and hoarse, and there may be some loss of taste sensations. Also called **jugular foramen syndrome.**

Verneuil's neuroma. See **plexiform neuroma.**

vernix caseosa /vur′niks kas′ē·ō′sə/ [Gk, resin; L, *caseus*, cheese], a grayish-white, cheeselike substance, consisting of sebaceous gland secretions, lanugo, and desquamated epithelial cells, that covers the skin of the fetus and newborn. It acts as a protective agent during intrauterine life and is thought to have an insulating effect against heat loss.

verruca /vəroo′kə/ [L, wart], a benign, viral, warty skin lesion with a rough, papillomatous surface. It is caused by a common, contagious papovavirus. Methods of treatment include salicylic acid, cantharidin, electrodesiccation, solid carbon dioxide, liquid nitrogen, and mental suggestion. Also called **verruca vulgaris, wart.** –**verrucose, verrucous,** *adj.*

verruca acuminata. See **genital wart.**

verruca plana, a small, slightly elevated, smooth, tan or flesh-colored wart, sometimes occurring in large numbers on the face, neck, back of the hands, wrists, and knees, especially in children. Also called **flat wart.**

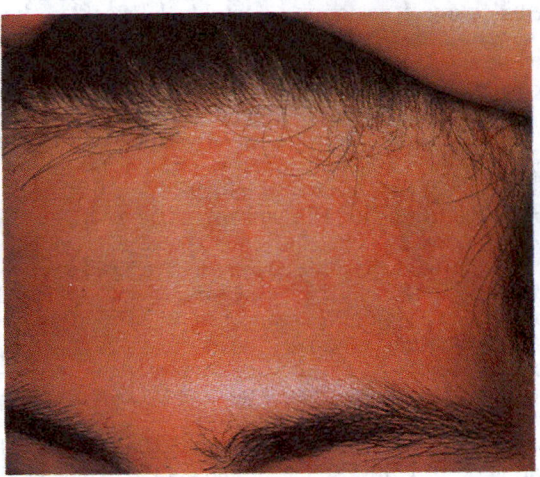

Verruca plana *(Habif, 1990)*

verruca senillis. See **basal cell papilloma.**

verruca vulgaris. See **verruca.**

verrucous carcinoma /vəroo′kəs/, a well-differentiated squamous cell neoplasm of soft tissue of the oral cavity, larynx, or genitalia. A slow-growing tumor with displacement of surrounding tissue rather than invasion or metastasis occurs.

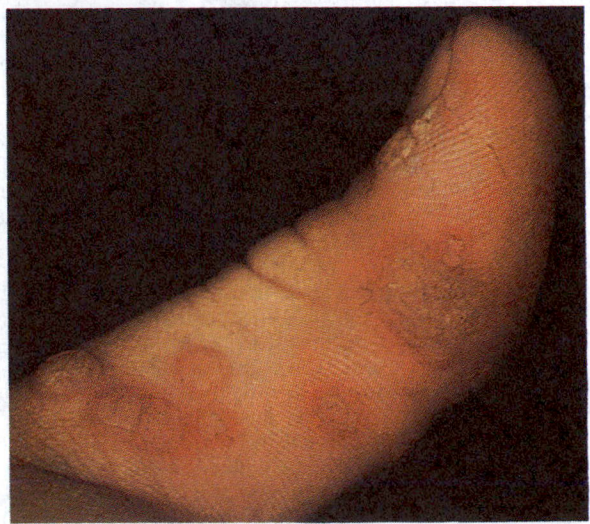

Verruca vulgaris *(Habif, 1990)*

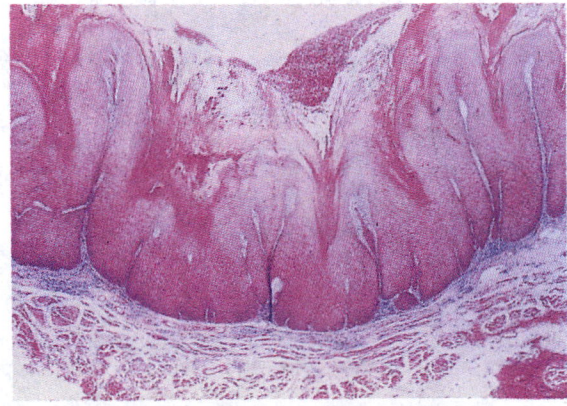

Verrucous carcinoma *(Cawson, 1987)*

verrucous endocarditis [L, *verruca*, wart; Gk, *endon*, within + *kardia*, heart + *itis*, inflammation], a form of heart inflammation characterized by the development of wartlike growths on the heart valves.

verrucous dermatitis, any skin rash with wartlike lesions.

verruga peruana. See **bartonellosis.**

-verse, 1. a suffix meaning 'to turn': *reverse, sacrotransverse, transverse*. **2.** combining form meaning 'turned, changed': *inverse, reverse*.

Versed, a trademark for a parenteral central nervous system depressant (midazolam hydrochloride).

version /vur'zhən/ [L, *vertere*, to turn], the changing of the position of the fetus in the uterus, usually done to facilitate delivery. Version may occur spontaneously as a result of uterine contractions or be performed by internal or external manipulation by the physician.

version and extraction, an obstetric operation in which a fetus presenting head first is turned and delivered feet first. It is performed by reaching deeply into the uterus, grasping the feet and pulling them down, and extracting the infant. The procedure is considered outmoded and hazardous and has been replaced by cesarean section, although it still may be done to deliver a second twin. Also called **internal podalic version and total breech extraction.** Compare **external version.** See also **breech birth.**

-vert, a combining form meaning a 'person who has turned (metaphorically)' in a specified direction: *extrovert, introvert, invert*.

vertebra /vur'təbrə/ *pl.* **vertebrae** [L, back, joint], any one of the 33 bones of the spinal column, comprising the 7 cervical, 12 thoracic, 5 lumbar, 5 sacral, and 4 coccygeal vertebrae. The vertebrae, with the exception of the first and second cervical vertebrae, are much alike and are composed of a body, an arch, a spinous process for muscle attachment, and pairs of pedicles and processes. The first cervical vertebra is called the atlas and has no vertebral body. The second cervical vertebra is called the axis and forms the pivot on which the atlas rotates, permitting the head to turn. The body of the axis also extends into a strong, bony process.

vertebral /vur'təbrəl/ [L, *vertebra*, joint], pertaining to one or more vertebrae.

-vertebral, a combining form referring to the spinal column: *paravertebral, pelvivertebral, subvertebral*.

vertebral angiography [L, *vertebra*; Gk, *aggeion* + *graphein*, to record], the diagnostic study of blood circulation in the spinal area after the injection of radiopaque medium. See **angiography.**

vertebral arch [L, *vertebra*, joint + *arcus*, bow], the arch formed on the back of the vertebral body by the pedicles and laminae.

vertebral artery, each of two arteries branching from the subclavian arteries, arising deep in the neck from the cranial and dorsal subclavian surfaces. Each vertebral artery divides into two cervical and five cranial branches, supplying deep neck muscles, the spinal cord and spinal membranes, and the cerebellum. The cervical branches are the spinal and the muscular. The cranial branches are the meningeal, posterior spinal, anterior spinal, posterior inferior cerebellar, and medullary.

vertebral body, the weight-supporting, solid central portion of a vertebra. The pedicles of the arch project from its dorsolateral surfaces.

vertebral canal [L, *vertebra*, joint + *canalis*], the passage formed anterior to the vertebral arches and posterior to the vertebral bodies and occupied by the spinal cord.

vertebral column, the flexible structure that forms the longitudinal axis of the skeleton. In the adult, it includes 26 vertebrae arranged in a straight line from the base of the skull to the coccyx. The vertebrae are separated by intervertebral disks. They provide attachment for various muscles, such as the iliocostalis thoracis and the longissimus thoracis, which give the column strength and flexibility. In the adult, the five sacral and four coccygeal vertebrae fuse to form the sacrum and the coccyx. The average length of the vertebral column in men is about 71 cm. The cervical part measures about 12.5 cm, the thoracic part about 28 cm, the lumbar part about 18 cm, and the sacrum and the coccyx about 12.5 cm. The vertebral column in women measures approximately 61 cm. Several curves in the column increase its strength, such as the cervical, thoracic, lumbar, and pelvic curves. The cervical curve is convex ventrally from the apex of the dens to the middle of the second thoracic vertebra and is the least marked of all the curves. The thoracic curve, concave ventrally, starts at the middle of the second and ends at the middle of the twelfth thoracic vertebra. The lumbar curve, more pronounced in women than in men, begins at the middle of the last thoracic vertebra and ends at the sacrovertebral angle. The pelvic curve starts at the sacrovertebral articulation, and it ends at the point of

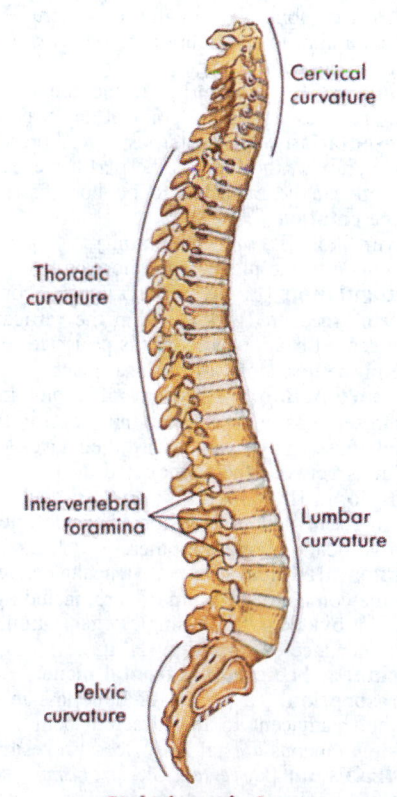

Vertebral column, right lateral view
(Thibodeau, 1993/Ernest W Beck)

Cervical curvature

Thoracic curvature

Intervertebral foramina

Lumbar curvature

Pelvic curvature

Right lateral view

the coccyx. The thoracic and the sacral curves constitute primary curves, present during fetal life; the cervical and the lumbar curves constitute secondary curves, which develop after birth. The cervical curve develops when the child is able to hold up its head, usually 3 to 4 months after birth; the lumbar curve develops 12 to 18 months after birth, when the child starts to walk. The vertebral column also presents a slight lateral curve, which in most individuals presents a convexity toward the right side. The vertebral canal courses through the vertebral column and contains the spinal cord. The canal is formed by the posterior arches of the vertebrae and is large and triangular in the cervical and the lumbar sections of the column, the most flexible portions. The canal is small and rounded in the thoracic region, where motion is more restricted. Also called **spinal column, spine.** See also **vertebra.**

vertebral foramen [L, *vertebra*, joint + *foramen*, opening], the opening between the neural arch and the body of a vertebra through which the spinal cord passes.

vertebral groove [L, *vertebra*, joint; Du, *groeve*], a shallow depression on each side of the spinous processes of the vertebrae, occupied by the deep back muscles.

vertebral notch [L, *vertebra*, joint; OFr, *enochier*, notch], either of the concavities on the lower or upper border of a vertebral pedicle.

vertebrate [L, *vertebra*, joint], pertaining to any animal possessing a backbone and thus being a member of the subphylum *Vertebrata*. The group includes fish, birds, amphibians, reptiles, and mammals.

vertebro-, a combining form meaning 'pertaining to the vertebral column or to a vertebra': *vertebrocostal, vertebrodymus, vertebrosternal.*

vertex /vur′teks/ [L, summit], **1.** the top of the head; crown. **2.** the apex or highest point of any structure.

vertex presentation, (in obstetrics) a fetal presentation in which the vertex of the fetus is the part nearest to the cervical os and can be expected to be born first. Compare **breech presentation.**

vertical /vur′tikəl/ [L, *vertex,* summit], perpendicular or at a right angle to the plane of the horizon.

vertical angulation [L, *vertex* + *angulus,* corner], (in dentistry) the measured angle within the vertical plane at which the central beam of an x-ray is projected relative to a reference in the horizontal or occlusal plane.

vertical coordination, a system of community health nurses who serve as links between their level in the organization and those above and below their level. They also serve as links between the agency and the patient.

vertical diplopia [L, *vertex*; Gk, *diploos,* double + *opsis,* vision], a form of double vision in which one image is displaced vertically above the other.

vertical-integrated health care, a health delivery system in which the complete spectrum of care, including financial services, is provided within a single organization, such as a health maintenance organization (HMO).

vertical plane. See **cardinal frontal plane.**

vertical resorption, a pattern of bone loss in which the alveolar bone adjacent to the affected tooth is destroyed without simultaneous crestal loss. See also **resorption.**

vertical strabismus [L, *vertex*; Gk, *strabismos,* squint], a deviation of one eye in a vertical direction from a point of fixation. A common cause is overaction by the inferior oblique muscles, resulting in a quick vertical movement of the

eyeball on adduction. Also called **upward-and-downward squint, vertical squint.**

vertical transmission, the transfer of a disease, condition, or trait from one generation to the next, either genetically or congenitally, such as the spread of an infection through breast milk or through the placenta.

verticosubmental /vur′tikō′submen′təl/ [L, *vertex* + *sub,* below, *mentum,* chin], pertaining to a radiographic projection of the head in which the central ray passes from the vertex of the skull through its base.

vertigo. See **dizziness.**

very-low-density lipoprotein (VLDL), a plasma protein that is composed chiefly of triglycerides with small amounts of cholesterol, phospholipid, and protein. It transports triglycerides primarily from the liver to peripheral sites in the tissues for use or storage. The triglycerides are quickly converted to smaller, more soluble intermediate lipoproteins and eventually to low-density lipoproteins. Elevations in VLDL are associated with increased risk of atherosclerosis. See also **high-density lipoprotein (HDL).**

vesical /ves′ikəl/ [L, *vesica,* bladder], pertaining to either the gallbladder or the urinary bladder.

vesical fistula [L, *vesica,* bladder; *fistula,* pipe], an abnormal passage communicating with the urinary bladder. Vesical fistulae may communicate with the skin, vagina, uterus, or rectum.

vesical hematuria [L, *vesica,* bladder; Gk, *haima,* blood + *ouron,* urine], blood in the urine caused by bleeding in the bladder. The urine is bright red.

vesical sphincter, a circular muscle surrounding the opening of the urinary bladder. It is normally contracted to prevent leakage from the bladder.

vesicant /ves′ikənt/, a drug capable of causing tissue necrosis when extravasated.

vesicle /ves′ikəl/ [L, *vesicula*], a small bladder or blister, such as a small, thin-walled, raised skin lesion containing clear fluid. Compare **bulla.** —**vesicular,** *adj*.

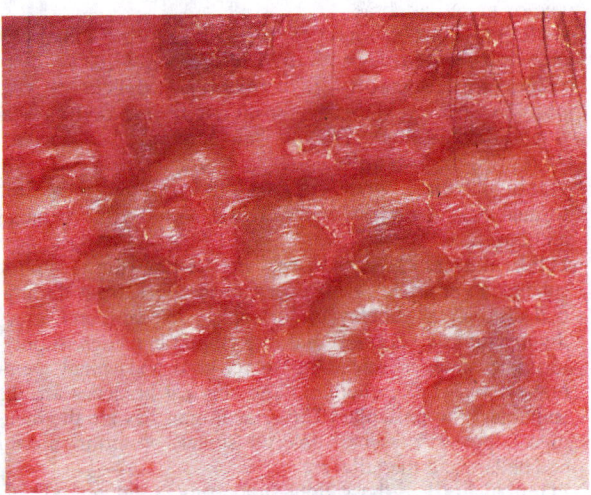

Vesicles (du Vivier, 1993)

vesicle calculus, a concretion occurring in the bladder. Also called **bladder stone, cystolith.**

vesicle reflex, the sensation of a need to urinate when the bladder is moderately distended. See also **micturition reflex.**

vesico-, a combining form meaning 'pertaining to the bladder or to a blister': *vesicocavernous, vesicosigmoid, vesicourethral.*

vesicoureteral reflux /ves′ikōo͞orē′tərəl/ [L, *vesica* + Gk, *oureter,* ureter; L, *refluxus,* backflow], an abnormal backflow of urine from the bladder to the ureter, resulting from a congenital defect, obstruction of the outlet of the bladder, or infection of the lower urinary tract. Reflux increases the hydrostatic pressure in the ureters and kidneys. The condition is characterized by abdominal or flank pain, enuresis, pyuria, hematuria, proteinuria, and bacteriuria accompanied by persistent or recurrent urinary tract infections. Diagnosis is made by cystoscopy and voiding cystourethrogram. Obstruction of the ureter or defective implantation of the ureter in the bladder may be surgically corrected. Antibacterial medication, urinary tract antiseptics, and analgesia are usually prescribed for any infection that causes or results from this condition.

vesicouterine /ves′ikōo͞o′tərin, -ēn/ [L, *vesica* + *uterus,* womb], of or pertaining to the bladder and uterus. Also called **uterovesical.**

vesicula /vəsik′yələ/ [L, *vesicle*], a vesicle or small bladder.

vesicular /vesik′yələr/, pertaining to a blisterlike condition.

vesicular appendix, a cystic structure on the fimbriated end of each of the fallopian tubes. It represents a remnant of the mesonephric ducts.

vesicular breath sound, a normal sound of rustling or swishing heard with a stethoscope over the lung periphery, characteristically higher pitched during inspiration and fading rapidly during expiration. Compare **tracheal breath sound.**

vesicular mole. See **hydatid mole.**

vesicular rale [L, *vesicula*; Fr, *râle,* rattle], an abnormal breathing sound heard on auscultation of the chest during inspiration. Rales are discrete bubbling or crackling sounds often associated with pneumonia, pulmonary edema, and tuberculosis.

vesiculitis /vəsik′yəlī′tis/, an inflammation of any vesicle, particularly the seminal vesicles. Clinical manifestations of this condition are minimal; it is usually associated with prostatitis.

vesiculography /vəsik′yəlog′rəfē/, the radiologic examination of the seminal vesicles and adjacent structures, usually conducted by injecting a radiopaque medium into the deferent ducts or by catheterization of the medium into the ejaculatory ducts. The technique is used to examine the vesicles, vas deferens, and ejaculatory duct for possible tumors, cysts, or other disorders.

vessel /ves′əl/ [L, *vascellum,* small vase], any one of the many tubules throughout the body conveying fluids, such as blood and lymph. The main kinds of vessels are the arteries, the veins, and the lymphatic vessels.

vestibular /vestib′yələr/, [L, *vestibulum,* courtyard], of or pertaining to a vestibule, such as the vestibular portion of the mouth, which lies between the cheeks and the teeth.

vestibular apparatus, the inner ear structures that are as-

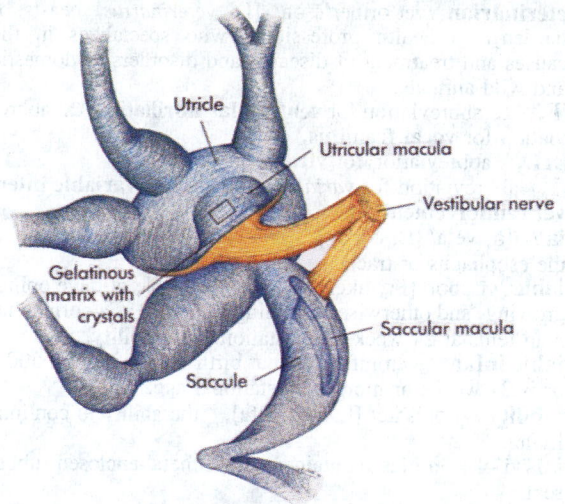

Vestibular apparatus
(Seeley, 1992/Lisa Chuck, Michael Schenk)

sociated with balance and position sense. It includes the vestibule and semicircular canals.

vestibular extension. See **vestibuloplasty.**

vestibular function, the sense of balance.

vestibular gland, any one of four small glands, two on each side of the vaginal orifice. One pair of the small structures constitutes the greater vestibular glands; the other pair constitutes the lesser vestibular glands. The vestibular glands secrete a lubricating substance. Compare **Cowper's gland.** See also **Bartholin's gland.**

vestibular nerve [L, *vestibulum,* forecourt + *nervus*], a branch of the eighth cranial nerve associated with the sense of equilibrium. It arises in the vestibular ganglion (Scarpa's ganglion) of the ear.

vestibular toxicity, toxic effects (commonly of drugs) on the vestibule of the ear, resulting in dizziness, vertigo, and loss of balance.

vestibular window. See **oval window.**

vestibule /ves′tibyo͞ol/ [L, *vestibulum,* courtyard], a space or a cavity that serves as the entrance to a passageway, such as the vestibule of the vagina or the vestibule of the ear.

vestibule of the ear, the central portion of the inner ear, within the osseous labyrinth, involved with the sensation of position and movement.

vestibulocochlear nerve. See **auditory nerve.**

vestibuloocular reflex /vestib′yəlō·ok′yələr/, a normal reflex in which eye position compensates for movement of the head. It is induced by excitation of the vestibular apparatus.

vestibuloplasty /vestib′yəlōplas′tē/ [L, *vestibulum,* forecourt; Gk, *plassein,* to shape], plastic surgery of the oral vestibule, particularly modification of the gingival tissues. Also called **sulcoplasty, vestibular extension.**

vestige /ves′tij/ [L, *vestigium,* trace], an imperfectly developed, relatively useless organ or other structure of the body that had a vital function at an earlier stage of life or in a more primitive form of life. The vermiform appendix is a vestigial organ. **–vestigial,** *adj.*

veterinarian /vet′əriner′ē·ən/ [L, *veterinarius*, beasts of burden], a health professional who specializes in the causes and treatment of diseases and disorders of domestic and wild animals.

VF, 1. abbreviation for **ventricular fibrillation.** 2. abbreviation for **vocal fremitus.**

V.H., abbreviation for **viral hepatitis.**

VI, abbreviation for *variable interval*. See **variable interval reinforcement.**

via /vī′ə, vē′ä/ [L, a way], any passage or course, such as the esophagus or trachea.

viable /vī′əbəl/ [Fr, likely to live], capable of developing, growing, and otherwise sustaining life, such as a normal human fetus at 24 weeks of gestation. –**viability,** *n.*

viable infant, an infant who at birth weighs at least 500 g or is 24 weeks or more of gestational age.

viability /vī′əbil′itē/ [L, *vita*, life], the ability to continue living.

vial /vī′əl/, a glass container with a metal-enclosed rubber seal.

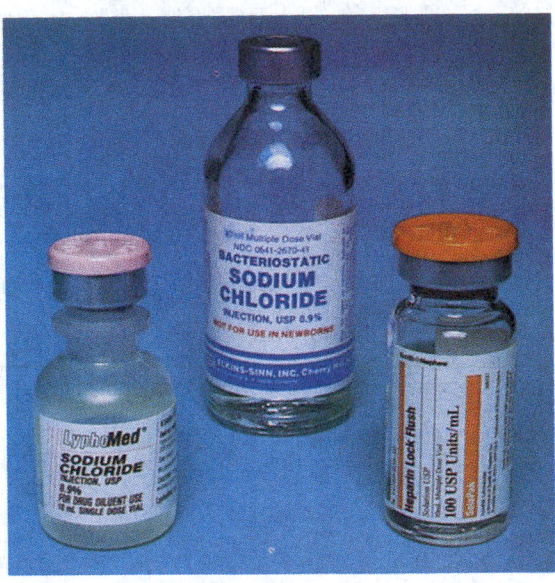

Vials *(Potter, 1993)*

Vibramycin Hyclate, a trademark for a tetracycline antibiotic (doxycycline hyclate).

Vibramycin Monohydrate, a trademark for a tetracycline antibiotic (doxycycline monohydrate).

vibrating. See **cupping and vibrating.**

vibration /vībrā′shən/ [L, *vibrare*, to vibrate], a type of massage administered by quick tapping with the fingertips, alternating the fingers in a rhythmic manner, or by a mechanical device. See also **massage.**

vibratory /vī′brətôr′ē/ [L, *vibrare*, to vibrate], causing vibrations or a state of vibration.

vibratory sense [L, *vibrare*, to vibrate + *sentire*, to feel], the ability to perceive vibratory sensations. Vibration receptors in the body are found in a variety of locations, from the skin surface to the membranes covering bones. Some respond only to certain vibration frequencies.

vibrio /vib′rē·ō/ [L, *vibrare*], any bacterium that is curved and motile, such as those belonging to the genus *Vibrio*. Cholera and several other epidemic forms of gastroenteritis are caused by members of the genus.

Vibrio cholerae, the species of comma-shaped, motile bacillus that is the cause of cholera.

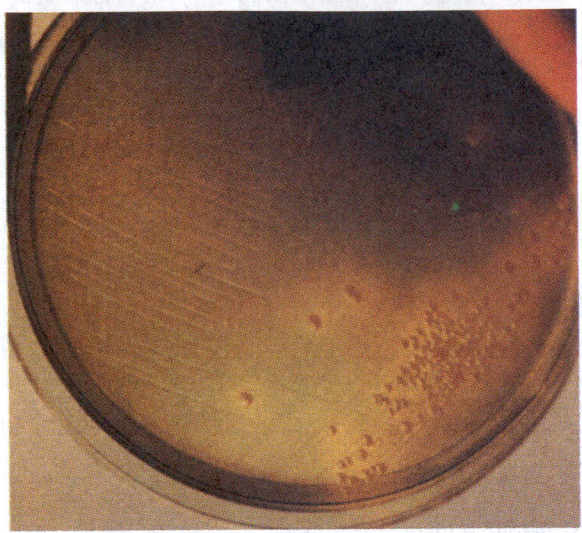

***Vibrio cholerae* colonies on TCBS agar** *(Baron, 1988)*

Vibrio fetus. See *Campylobacter.*

vibrio gastroenteritis, an infectious disease acquired from contaminated seafood and characterized by nausea, vomiting, abdominal pain, and diarrhea, caused by *Vibrio parahaemolyticus*. Headache, mild fever, and bloody stools also may be present. Spontaneous recovery usually occurs in 2 to 5 days. Compare **salmonellosis, shigellosis.**

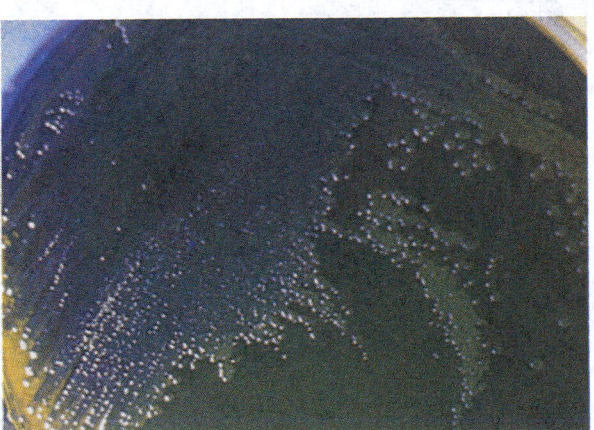

***Vibrio parahaemolyticus* colonies on TCBS agar** *(Baron, 1990)*

Vibrio parahaemolyticus /per′əhē′mōlit′ikəs/, a species of microorganisms of the genus *Vibrio,* the causative agent in food poisoning associated with the ingestion of uncooked or undercooked shellfish, especially crabs and shrimp. This microorganism is a common cause of gastroenteritis in Japan, aboard cruise ships, and in the eastern and southeastern coastal areas of the United States. Thorough cooking of seafood prevents the infection associated with *Vibrio parahaemolyticus,* which causes watery diarrhea, abdominal cramps, vomiting, headache, chills, and fever. This microorganism has an incubation period of 2 to 48 hours, after which the symptoms of infection appear. The food poisoning from this agent usually subsides spontaneously within 2 days but may be more severe, even fatal, in debilitated and elderly people. Confirming diagnosis must rule out other causes of food poisoning and acute GI disorders and requires bacteriologic examination of the vomitus, stool, and blood. Treatment usually includes bed rest and the oral replacement of fluids. Intravenous replacement of fluids is seldom required.

vicarious menstruation /vīker′ē·əs/ [L, *vicarius,* substituted; *menstruare,* to menstruate], discharge of blood from a site other than the uterus at the time when the menstrual flow is normally expected. Such bleeding is usually caused by the increased capillary permeability that occurs during menstruation.

vidarabine /vider′əbēn/, an antiviral agent. Also called **adenine arabinoside.**

■ INDICATIONS: It is used systemically to treat herpes simplex encephalitis and locally to treat herpesvirus I keratoconjunctivitis and keratitis.

■ CONTRAINDICATIONS: It is used in pregnancy only when the risk of teratogenicity is outweighed by benefits. Known hypersensitivity to this drug prohibits its use.

■ ADVERSE EFFECTS: Among the more serious adverse reactions to systemic administration are severe nausea and other symptoms of GI distress, various central nervous system effects, and bone marrow depression. Local irritation, photophobia, and corneal edema may occur in topical ophthalmic applications.

video display terminal (VDT) [L, *videre,* to see; *displicare,* to scatter; *terminus,* end], a cathode-ray tube device with a surface similar to a television screen, used in word processors, computer terminals, and similar equipment. Use of video display terminals has been associated with a variety of environmental health complaints, including burning and itching eyes, headaches, and back and arm pain. Published studies indicate the health effects are caused by inadequate or improper office environments, such as unsuitable furniture or light levels, rather than VDT radiation.

Videx, trademark for an antiretroviral AIDS drug **dideoxyinosine (DDI).**

vigilance /vij′iləns/ [L, *vigil,* awake], a state of being attentive or alert.

vigil coma /vij′əl/ [L, *vigil*; Gk, *koma,* deep sleep], a semiconscious state of delirium in which the patient may appear awake, with eyes open and staring, and may make verbal sounds.

villi. See **villus.**

villoma /vilō′mə/, *pl.* **villomas, villomata** [L, *villus,* hair; Gk, *oma,* tumor], a villous neoplasm or papilloma, occurring in the bladder or rectum. Also called **villioma.**

villous adenoma /vil′əs/ [L, *villus*], a slow-growing, soft,

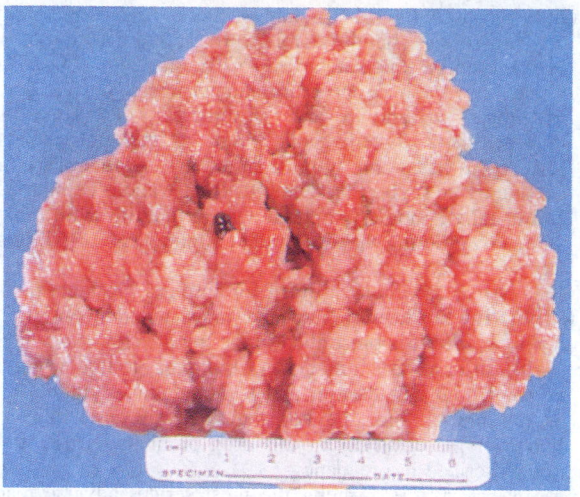

Villous adenoma—endoscopic view *(Mitros, 1988)*

spongy, potentially malignant papillary growth of the mucosa of the large intestine.

villous carcinoma, an epithelial tumor with many long, velvety papillary outgrowths. Also called **carcinoma villosum.**

villous papilloma, a benign tumor with long, slender processes, usually occurring in the bladder, breast, or a cerebral ventricle.

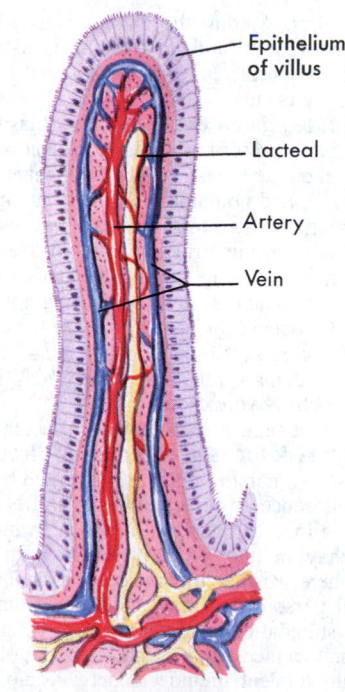

— Epithelium of villus

— Lacteal

— Artery

— Vein

Single villus

Villus *(Thibodeau, 1993/Ernest W Beck)*

villus /vil′əs/, *pl.* **villi** [L, shaggy, hair], one of the many tiny projections, barely visible to the naked eye, clustered over the entire mucous surface of the small intestine. The villi diffuse and transport fluids and nutrients. They are quite irregular in size and are larger in some parts of the intestine than in others, flattening out when the intestine distends. Each villus has a core of delicate areolar and reticular connective tissue supporting the epithelium, various capillaries, and usually a single lymphatic lacteal that fills with milky white chyle during the digestion of a fatty meal. **– villous,** *adj.*

vin-, -vin, a combining form for antiviral substances.

vinblastine sulfate /vinblas′tēn, -tin/, an antineoplastic.
■ INDICATIONS: It is prescribed in the treatment of many neoplastic diseases, such as choriocarcinoma, testicular carcinoma, Hodgkin's disease, and non-Hodgkin's lymphoma.
■ CONTRAINDICATIONS: Leukopenia, bacterial infection, or known hypersensitivity to this drug prohibits its use. It is not prescribed in pregnancy.
■ ADVERSE EFFECTS: Among the most serious adverse reactions are leukopenia and neurotoxicity. Nausea, diarrhea, stomatitis, and alopecia also may occur.

Vincent's angina, Vincent's infection. See **acute necrotizing gingivitis.**

Vincent's stomatitis [Henri Vincent, French physician, b. 1862; Gk, *stoma,* mouth + *itis,* inflammation], an infection of the mouth. See **acute necrotizing gingivitis.**

vincristine sulfate /vinkris′tēn, -tin/, an antineoplastic.
■ INDICATIONS: It is prescribed in the treatment of many neoplastic diseases, such as leukemia, neuroblastoma, lymphomas, and sarcomas.
■ CONTRAINDICATIONS: Pregnancy, leukopenia, preexisting neuromuscular disease, or known hypersensitivity to this drug prohibits its use.
■ ADVERSE EFFECTS: Among the most serious adverse reactions are neurotoxicity and leukopenia. Constipation, abdominal pain, alopecia, and inflammation at the site of injection also may occur.

vindesine sulfate /vin′dəsēn/, an antineoplastic agent.
■ INDICATIONS: It is prescribed in the treatment of acute lymphoblastic leukemia, breast cancer, malignant melanoma, lymphosarcoma, and non-small-cell lung carcinoma.
■ CONTRAINDICATIONS: Leukopenia, bacterial infections, or known sensitivity to this drug prohibits its use.
■ ADVERSE EFFECTS: Among the most serious adverse reactions are neurotoxicity, leukopenia, thrombocytopenia, phlebitis, and alopecia.

vinegar acid. See **acetic acid.**

Vioform, a trademark for an antiamebic and topical antiinfective (iodochlorhydroxyquin).

Viokase, a trademark for an enzyme (pancreatin).

violence, high risk for: self-directed or directed at others /vī′ələns/, a nursing diagnosis accepted by the Fourth National Conference on the Classification of Nursing Diagnoses. It is defined as the state in which an individual experiences behaviors that can be physically harmful to either the self or others. Risk factors are complex and may involve an antisocial personality, mania, organic brain syndrome, panic, rage, suicidal behavior, temporal lobe epilepsy, or a toxic reaction to a medication. Characteristics of clients who are potentially violent include anxiety; fear of the self or other people; lack of verbal ability; complaining or demanding vocalization; provocative, argumentative, or overreactive behavior; poor self-esteem; or psychologic depression.

Many other factors also may be present, such as a history of self-destructive behavior, pacing, excitement, agitation, or the possession of a weapon. See also **nursing diagnosis.**

viosterol /vī·os′tərôl/, synthetic vitamin D₂ in an oil base. Also called **synthetic oleovitamin D.** See also **calciferol, ergosterol.**

VIP, 1. abbreviation for **vasoactive intestinal polypeptide. 2.** abbreviation for *very important person.* A VIP suite in a hospital is one reserved for such people.

vipoma /vipō′mə/, a type of pancreatic tumor that causes changes in secretion of vasoactive intestinal polypeptide (VIP). VIP causes dilation of blood vessels throughout the body and secretion of fluid and salt in the intestinal tract, resulting in diarrhea. The VIP effects mimic the symptoms of Asiatic cholera and can result in death from dehydration and subsequent kidney failure if treatment is not begun early. See also **vasoactive intestinal polypeptide.**

vir-, -vir, a combining form for antiviral substances.

Vira-A, a trademark for an antiviral (vidarabine).

viral disease. See **viral infection.**

viral dysentery /vī′rəl/ [L, *virus,* poison; Gk, *dys,* bad + *enteron,* intestine], a form of dysentery caused by a virus and usually characterized by an acute watery diarrhea.

viral gastroenteritis, an inflammation of the intestine caused by a virus. The symptoms usually include abdominal cramps, diarrhea, nausea, and vomiting.

viral hepatitis (V.H.) a viral, inflammatory disease of the liver, caused by one of the hepatitis viruses, A, B, C, or delta. All have chronic forms except hepatitis A. The disease is transmitted sexually and through blood transfusions and is common among people with behavior risks of HIV infection. Speed of onset and probable course of the illness vary with the kind and strain of virus, but the characteristics of the disease and its treatment are the same. See also **hepatitis A, hepatitis B, hepatitis C, delta hepatitis.**
■ OBSERVATIONS: Diagnosis is made through antibody (A + C) or antigen (B + D). Characteristic of viral hepatitis are anorexia, malaise, headache, pain over the liver, fever, jaundice, clay-colored stools, dark urine, nausea and vomiting, and diarrhea. Laboratory analyses reveal increased amounts of serum glutamic oxalacetic transaminase (SGOT) and bilirubin and an abnormal coagulation of the blood. Severe infection, especially with hepatitis B virus, may be prolonged and result in tissue destruction, cirrhosis, and chronic hepatitis or in hepatic coma and death.
■ INTERVENTIONS: Treatment is with alpha-interferon. Depending on the specific type of hepatitis, treatment with alpha-interferon is effective in 40% of patients with chronic HBV infection; improvement in liver function has been noted in 50% of the patients infected. Treatment is also largely supportive. It includes bed rest; isolation, if necessary; fluids; a low-fat, high-protein, high-calorie diet; special skin care if pruritus is present; emotional support; vitamins B₁₂, K, and C; and monitoring of liver and kidney function. Sedatives, analgesics, antiemetics, and steroids may be ordered. However, the patient is carefully observed for adverse reaction to medication, because the liver may not be able to break down and detoxify the drugs. Decrease in the amount or frequency of administration or change of the medication may be necessary.
■ NURSING CONSIDERATIONS: The person is taught the importance of rest and of avoiding fatigue, of washing the hands carefully after urinating or defecating to avoid spreading the

virus, of eating well, of following written dietary instructions after discharge, and of avoiding alcohol, usually for at least 1 year. The patient is encouraged to have certain blood tests performed periodically, including SGOT and serum bilirubin, to report any symptoms of recurrence immediately, and to avoid contact with people having infections. The person is told not to donate blood and not to take over-the-counter drugs without medical consultation.

viral infection, any of the diseases caused by one of approximately 200 viruses pathogenic to humans. Some are the most communicable and dangerous diseases known; some cause mild and transient conditions that pass virtually unnoticed. If cells are damaged by the viral attack, disease exists. The signs of the infection reflect the anatomic location of the damaged cells. Viruses are introduced into the body through a break in the skin or through a transfusion into the bloodstream, by droplet infection through the respiratory tract, or by ingestion through the digestive tract into the GI system. The pathogenicity of the particular virus depends on the rapidity of action, the enzymes released, the part of the body infected, and the particular action of the virus. The general process of viral infection reflects the life cycle of a virus. The first step in the cycle, after entry into the body, is the attachment of the virus to a susceptible cell and the cell's adsorption of the virus. This is followed by penetration of the viral nucleic acid into the parasitized cell. The dissembled virus at this point causes no symptoms and cannot be recovered from the cells in infectious form. The virus begins to mature within the cell and, carrying its own genetic information, begins to replicate itself, using chemical building blocks and energy available in the parasitized cell. The virus has now taken over the cell. After a variable period of time, masses of fully grown viruses appear, each able to survive outside the cell until more susceptible cells are found. In poliovirus infection, one parasitized cell may produce more than 100,000 poliovirus particles in a few hours. Techniques used in viral identification and immunization are based on the essential fact that viruses can multiply only inside living cells. Inoculation of susceptible animals, of tissue culture media, and of chick embryos allows cultivation of viruses for study and identification and for the preparation of vaccine. Diagnosis of the cause of viral infection also is possible using various other techniques, including serologic tests, fluorescent antibody microscopic examination, microscopic examination, and skin tests. In many viral diseases, including mumps, smallpox, and measles, one attack confers permanent immunity. In others, immunity is short-lived. The incubation period for viral infection is short, the viruses do not circulate in the bloodstream, antibodies do not form, and, most often, immunity does not develop. Exposure to a few viruses results in immunity to that virus and to other closely related viruses. Some vectors are able to spread several viruses, but only one at a time. Other mechanisms of natural resistance to viral infection are poorly understood, but susceptibility to a particular virus is somehow species-specific; for example, chickenpox, caused by the varicella zoster virus, is seen only in humans. A protective substance, interferon, is elaborated naturally in small amounts in the body. It is cell-specific and species-specific but not virus-specific. Interferon may act as a broad spectrum antiviral agent, protecting the body from the effects of many viral infections by stopping the synthesis of viral nucleic acid within the parasitized cell. See also specific viral infections.

viral keratoconjunctivitis [L, *virus,* poison; Gk, *keras,* horn; L, *conjunctivus,* connecting; Gk, *itis,* inflammation], a combination of inflammation of the cornea and conjunctiva caused by a viral infection.

viral pneumonia, pulmonary infection caused by a virus.

Virazole, a trademark for an aerosol antiviral drug (ribavirin).

Virchow-Robin space. See **perivascular space.**

Virchow's node /fēr'shōz/ [Rudolf L. K. Virchow, German pathologist, b. 1821], a firm supraclavicular lymph node, particularly on the left side, that is so enlarged it is palpable. Also called **sentinel node, signal node.**

Virchow's space. See **perivascular space.**

viremia /vīrē'mē·ə/ [L, *virus* + Gk, *haima,* blood], the presence of viruses in the blood. Compare **bacteremia, fungemia, parasitemia.**

virile /vir'əl/ [L, *virilis,* masculine], 1. of, pertaining to, or characteristic of an adult male; masculine; manly. 2. possessing or exhibiting masculine strength, vigor, force, or energy. 3. of or pertaining to the male sexual functions; capable of procreation. Compare **virilism.** –**virility,** *n.*

virilism /vir'əliz'əm/ [L, *virilis* + *ismus,* practice], 1. See **virilization.** 2. pseudohermaphroditism in a female. 3. premature development of masculine characteristics in the male. Kinds of virilism are **adrenal virilism** and **prosopopilary virilism.**

virilization /vir'əlīzā'shən/ [L, *virilis* + *atus,* process], a process in which secondary male sexual characteristics are acquired by a female, usually as the result of adrenal dysfunction or hormonal medication. Also called **masculinization.** See also **adrenal virilism.**

virion /vir'ē·on, vī'rē·on/ [L, *virus,* poison], a rudimentary virus particle with a central nucleoid surrounded by a protein sheath or capsid. The complete nucleocapsid with a nucleic acid core may constitute a complete virus, such as the adenoviruses and the picornaviruses, or it may be surrounded by an envelope, as in the herpesviruses and the myxoviruses. Such an envelope is a membrane that contains lipids, proteins, and carbohydrates and projects spikelike structures from its surface. See also **capsid.**

virocytes /vī'rəsīts/ [L, *virus* + Gk, *kytos,* cell], lymphocytes altered in appearance and in staining that are seen in blood smears from patients with viral diseases.

viroid /vī'roid/, a small infective segment of nucleic acid, usually RNA. It is not translated and is replicated by host cell enzymes. Viroids include segments that are complementary to introns and may bind to intron RNA. Viroids are responsible for several plant diseases. Whereas they have not been associated with animal diseases, viroidlike DNA has been found in cancer cells, and some authorities believe viroids can evolve into infectious animal viruses. See also **intron, plasmid, transposon.**

virologist /vīrol'əjist, vir-/, a specialist who studies viruses and diseases caused by viruses.

virology /-l'əjē/ [L, *virus* + Gk, *logos,* science], the study of viruses and viral diseases. –**virologic, virological,** *adj.*

Viroptic, a trademark for an ophthalmic antiviral (trifluridine).

virucidal /vī'rəsī'dəl/, pertaining to the destruction of viruses.

virucide /vī'rəsīd/ [L, *virus* + *caedere,* to kill], any agent that destroys or inactivates a virus.

virulence /vir'yələns/, [L, *virulentus,* poisonous], the power of a microorganism to produce disease.

virulent /vir′yələnt/, [L, *virulentus*], of or pertaining to a very pathogenic or rapidly progressive condition.

virus /vī′rəs/ [L, poison], a minute parasitic microorganism much smaller than a bacterium that, having no independent metabolic activity, may replicate only within a cell of a living plant or animal host. A virus consists of a core of nucleic acid (DNA or RNA) surrounded by a coat of antigenic protein sometimes surrounded by an envelope of lipoprotein. The virus provides the genetic code for replication, and the host cell provides the necessary energy and raw materials. More than 200 viruses have been identified as capable of causing disease in humans. Some kinds of viruses are **adenovirus, arenavirus, enterovirus, herpesvirus,** and **rhinovirus.** See also **viral infection. –viral,** *adj.*

virustatic /vī′rəstat′ik/, pertaining to the inhibition of the growth and development of viruses, as distinguished from their destruction.

vis /vis, vēs/ [L, force], energy or power.

viscera /vis′ərə/, *sing.* **viscus** /vis′kəs/ [L, entrails], the internal organs enclosed within a body cavity, primarily the abdominal organs.

visceral /vis′ərəl/ [L, *viscus,* entrails], of or pertaining to the viscera, or internal organs in the abdominal cavity. Also **splanchnic.**

visceral afferent fibers, the nerve fibers of the visceral nervous system that receive stimuli, carry impulses toward the central nervous system, and share the sensory ganglia of the cerebrospinal nerves with the somatic sensory fibers. Peripheral distribution of the visceral afferent fibers constitutes the main difference between them and the somatic afferents. The visceral afferent fibers produce sensations different from those of the somatic afferent fibers. The visceral efferent fibers connect with both the somatic and visceral afferent fibers; the number and extent of the visceral afferent fibers is not clearly established. Their peripheral processes reach the ganglia by various routes. Most of the visceral afferent fibers accompany blood vessels for part of their course, and various afferent fibers run in the cerebrospinal nerves. Some of the parts of the body with visceral afferent fibers are the face, scalp, nose, mouth, descending colon, lungs, abdomen, and rectum. See also **autonomic nervous system.**

visceral cavity [L, *viscus,* internal organs + *cavum*], **1.** the abdominal cavity containing the viscera. **2.** the cavity of any viscus, such as the stomach.

visceral efferent system [L, *viscus,* internal organs + *effere,* to bear out; Gk, *systema*], the part of the autonomic nervous system that supplies efferent nerve fibers from the central nervous system to the visceral organs.

visceral larva migrans, infestation with parasitic larvae, *Toxocara,* or, occasionally, *Ascaris, Strongyloides,* or other nematodes. See **toxocariasis.**

visceral leishmaniasis. See **kala-azar.**

visceral lymph node, a small oval nodular gland that filters lymph circulating in the lymphatic vessels of the thoracic, abdominal, and pelvic viscera. The visceral lymph nodes of the thorax include the anterior mediastinal nodes, posterior mediastinal nodes, and tracheobronchial nodes. The visceral lymph nodes of the abdomen and pelvis include those that follow the course of the celiac artery, superior mesenteric artery, and inferior mesenteric artery. Compare **parietal lymph node.** See also **lymph, lymphatic system, lymph node.**

visceral nervous system, the visceral portion of the peripheral nervous system that comprises the whole complex of nerves, fibers, ganglia, and plexuses by which impulses travel from the central nervous system to the viscera and from the viscera to the central nervous system. It contains the usual afferent fibers that receive stimuli and carry impulses toward the central nervous system and efferent fibers that carry impulses from the appropriate centers to the active effector organs, such as the nonstriated muscle, cardiac muscle, and glands of the body. Also called **involuntary nervous system.** See also **autonomic nervous system, visceral afferent fibers.**

visceral pain, abdominal pain caused by any abnormal condition of the viscera. It is characteristically severe, diffuse, and difficult to localize.

visceral pericardium [L, *viscus*; Gk, *peri,* around, *kardia,* heart], the surface of the pericardial membrane that is in direct contact with the heart. Also called **epicardium.**

visceral peritoneum, one of two portions of the largest serous membrane in the body that invests the viscera. The free surface of the visceral peritoneum is a smooth layer of mesothelium exuding a serous fluid that lubricates the viscera and allows them to glide freely against the wall of the abdominal cavity or over each other. The attached surface of the membrane is connected to the viscera and the abdominal wall by subserous fascia. Compare **parietal peritoneum.** See also **peritoneal cavity.**

visceral pleura, the inner layer of pleura that is adjacent to the external lung tissue.

visceral protein status, the amount of protein that is contained in the internal organs.

visceral reflex. See **viscerosomatic reaction.**

visceral skeleton [L, *viscus*; Gk, *skeletos,* dried up], the portion of the skeleton, including sternum, ribs, pelvis, and vertebrae, that enclose the viscera.

viscero-, a combining form meaning 'pertaining to the organs of the body': *viscerocranium, visceropleural, visceral, viscerosomatic.*

viscerosomatic reaction /vis′ərō′sōmat′ik/ [L, *viscus*; Gk, *soma,* body; L, *re, agere,* to act], a muscular response to stimulation of a nerve-receptor organ in a visceral organ. Also called **splanchnosomatic reaction, visceral reflex.**

viscid /vis′id/ [L, *viscidus,* sticky], sticky or glutinous. Also **viscous** /vis′kəs/.

viscosity /viskos′itē/ [L, *viscosus,* sticky], the ability or inability of a fluid solution to flow easily. A solution that has high viscosity is relatively thick and flows slowly because of the adhesive effect of adjacent molecules.

viscous /vis′kəs/ [L, *viscosus,* sticky], pertaining to something thick, viscid, sticky, or glutinous. Also **viscid.**

viscous fermentation [L, *viscosus*], the formation of viscous material in milk, urine, and wine by the action of various bacilli.

viscus. See **viscera.**

visible /viz′ibəl/ [L, *visibilis,* visible], pertaining to objects that perceptible to the eye.

visible light [L, *visus,* sight; AS, *leoht*], the radiant energy in the electromagnetic spectrum that is visible to the human eye. The wavelengths cover a range of approximately 390 to 780 nm.

visible radiation [L, *visibilis,* vision + *radiare,* to shine], electromagnetic radiation in the wavelengths between infrared and ultraviolet that can be perceived by most normal humans.

visible spectrum [L, *visibilis*, vision + *spectrum*, image], the colors of the spectrum that can be observed by most people, from violet at about 4000 Angstrom units through blue, green, yellow, and orange, to red, at about 6500 Angstrom units.

visibility /vis'əbil'itē/ [L, *visibilitas*, being seen], a condition of being visible under the circumstances of light, distance, and other factors.

vision /vizh'ən/ [L, *visus*, vision], the capacity for sight.

visit /viz'it/ [L, *visitare*, to see often], **1.** a meeting between a practitioner and a client or patient. In the hospital and the home, the practitioner makes a visit to the patient; in the clinic or office the patient makes a visit to the practitioner. **2.** (of a patient) to meet a practitioner to obtain professional services or (of a practitioner) to see a patient or client to render a professional service.

Visken, a trademark for a beta blocker (pindolol).

Vistaril, a trademark for a tranquilizer (hydroxyzine hydrochloride).

visual /vizh'oo·əl/ [L, *visus,* vision], pertaining to the sense of sight.

visual accommodation, a process by which the eye adjusts and is able to focus, producing a sharp image at various, changing distances from the object seen. The convexity of the anterior surface of the lens may be increased or decreased by contraction or relaxation of the ciliary muscle. With increasing age the lens becomes harder and less flexible, resulting in a loss of accommodation, and, usually, of the ability to focus on nearby objects. Compare **presbyopia.**

visual acuity [L, *visus,* vision + *acuitas,* sharpness], **1.** a measure of the resolving power of the eye, particularly with its ability to distinguish letters and numbers at a given distance. **2.** the sharpness or clearness of vision.

visual amnesia [L, *visus,* vision; Gk, *amnesia,* forgetfulness], an inability to recognize objects, including written words, previously seen.

visual angle [L, *visus,* vision + *angulus*], the angle between two lines passing from the extremities of an object looked at, through the nodal point of the eye. Also called **optic angle.**

visual aphasia [L, *visus,* vision; Gk, *a, phasis,* speech], the inability to understand written language, caused by a lesion in the left visual cortex and in the connections between the right visual cortex and the left hemisphere.

visual evoked potential (VEP), an evoked potential elicited by a repeatedly flashing light or a pattern stimulus. It may be used to confirm optic nerve or visual pathway damage.

visual field defect, one or more spots or defects in the vision that move with the eye, unlike a floater. This fixed defect is usually caused by damage to the retina or visual pathways, such as by chorioretinitis, traumatic injury, macular degeneration, glaucoma, or a vascular occlusion of the eye or the brain. Sudden loss of a noticeable portion of the visual field warrants ophthalmologic examination. Defects in the field of vision may be detected using an Amsler grid.

visual hallucinations [L, *visus,* vision + *alucinari*], a subjective visual experience in the absence of objective evidence of a corresponding stimulus. Such hallucinations are most likely to be associated with acute organic disorders such as toxic confusional psychoses, delirium, and focal brain diseases, and may occur with any stage of schizophrenia.

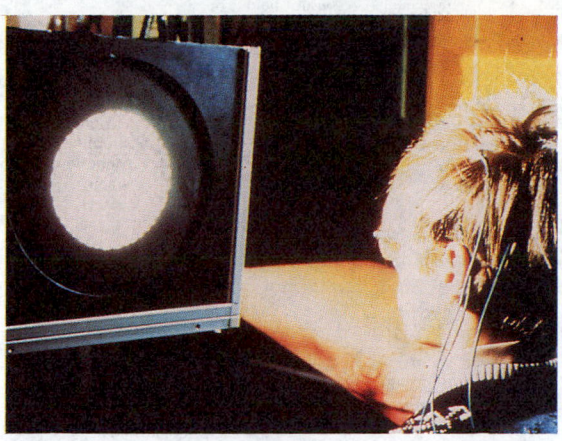

Testing of visual evoked potentials
(Eagling, 1986/Courtesy Professor G Garding)

visualization /vizh'oo·əlīzā'shən/, an effective means of deepening relaxation and desensitizing a real-life situation that is generally met with stress and tension. The imagery combines positive experiences with actual or perceived negative events or situations in an effort to desensitize the person to the trauma. Also called **visual imagery.**

visual memory, the ability to create an eidetic image of past visual experiences. Also called **eye memory.**

visual-motor coordination, the ability to coordinate vision with the movements of the body or parts of the body.

visual-motor function, the ability to draw or copy forms or to perform constructive tasks.

visual pathway, a pathway over which a visual sensation is transmitted from the retina to the brain. A pathway consists of an optic nerve, the fibers of an optic nerve traveling through or along the sides of the optic chiasm to the lateral geniculate body of the thalamus, and an optic tract terminating in an occipital lobe. Each optic nerve contains fibers from only one retina. The optic chiasm contains fibers from the nasal portions of the retinas of both eyes; these fibers cross to the opposite side of the brain at the optic chiasm. The fibers from the temporal portion of each eye bypass the optic chiasm and pass through the lateral geniculate body on the same side of the brain, and continue back to the occipital lobe. Thus the optic tracts, occipital lobe, lateral geniculate bodies of the thalamus, and optic chiasm each contain nerve fibers from both eyes. If the right optic tract were destroyed, a person would lose partial vision in both eyes—the right nasal and the left temporal fields of vision.

visual purple. See **rhodopsin.**

vita-, a combining form meaning 'pertaining to life': *vitaglass, vital, vitascope.*

vital /vī'təl/ [L, *vita,* life], pertaining to or contributing to life forces.

vital capacity (VC) [L, *vita,* life; *capacitas,* capacity], a measurement of the amount of air that can be expelled at the normal rate of exhalation after a maximum inspiration, representing the greatest possible breathing capacity. The vital capacity equals the inspiratory reserve volume plus the tidal volume plus the expiratory reserve volume. The aver-

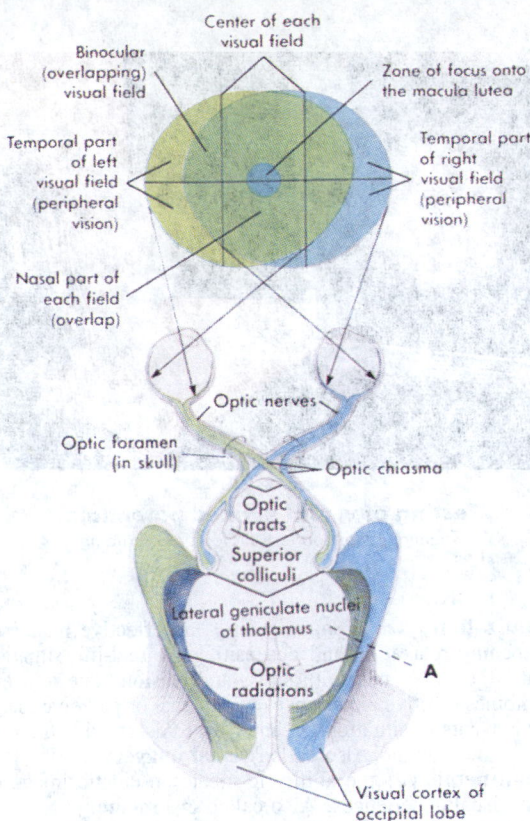

Visual pathways *(Thibodeau, 1993/Marsha J Dohrmann)*

Labels in figure:
Center of each visual field
Binocular (overlapping) visual field
Zone of focus onto the macula lutea
Temporal part of left visual field (peripheral vision)
Temporal part of right visual field (peripheral vision)
Nasal part of each field (overlap)
Optic nerves
Optic foramen (in skull)
Optic chiasma
Optic tracts
Superior colliculi
Lateral geniculate nuclei of thalamus
Optic radiations
A
Visual cortex of occipital lobe

age normal values of 4000 to 5000 ml are affected by age, physical dimensions of the chest cage, physical fitness, posture, and sex. The vital capacity may be reduced by a decrease in functioning lung tissue, resulting from atelectasis, edema, fibrosis, pneumonia, pulmonary resection, or tumors; by limited chest expansion, resulting from ascites, chest deformity, neuromuscular disease, pneumothorax, or pregnancy; or by airway obstruction. Compare **forced expiratory volume, forced vital capacity, residual volume.**

vital signs,   the measurements of pulse rate, respiration rate, and body temperature. Although not strictly a vital sign, blood pressure is also customarily included. Abnormalities of vital signs are often clues to diseases, and alterations in vital signs are used to evaluate a patient's progress. See also **blood pressure, pulse, respiration, temperature.**

vital stain [L, *vita,* life; OFr, *desteindre,* to dye],   any dye used to impart color to tissues or cells of living organisms.

vital statistics,   data relating to births or natality, deaths or mortality, marriages, health, and disease or morbidity.

vitamin /vī′təmin/ [L, *vita + amine,* ammonia],   an organic compound essential in small quantities for normal physiologic and metabolic functioning of the body. With few exceptions, vitamins cannot be synthesized by the body and must be obtained from the diet or dietary supplements. No one food contains all the vitamins. Vitamin deficiency diseases produce specific symptoms usually alleviated by the administration of the appropriate vitamin. Vitamins are classified according to their fat or water solubility, their physiologic effects, or their chemical structures, and they are designated by alphabetical letters and chemical or other specific names. The fat-soluble vitamins are A, D, E, and K; the B complex and C vitamins are water soluble. See also **avitaminosis, hypervitaminosis, oleovitamin, provitamin,** and see the specific vitamins.

vitamin A,   a fat-soluble, solid terpene alcohol essential for skeletal growth, maintenance of normal mucosal epithelium, and visual acuity. It is derived from various carotenoids, mainly beta-carotene, and is present in leafy green vegetables, yellow fruits and vegetables, the liver oils of the cod and other fish, liver, milk, cheese, butter, and egg yolk. Deficiency leads to atrophy of epithelial tissue resulting in keratomalacia, xerophthalmia, night blindness, and lessened resistance to infection of mucous membranes. Symptoms of hypervitaminosis A are irritability, fatigue, lethargy, abdominal discomfort, painful joints, severe throbbing headache, increased intracranial pressure, insomnia and restlessness, night sweats, loss of body hair, brittle nails, and exophthalmus. The RDA for adults is 800 to 1000 micrograms RE (retinol equivalents) where 1 RE equals 1 microgram of retinol or 6 micrograms of beta-carotene. Also called **antiinfection vitamin, antixerophthalmic vitamin.** See also **oleovitamin A.**

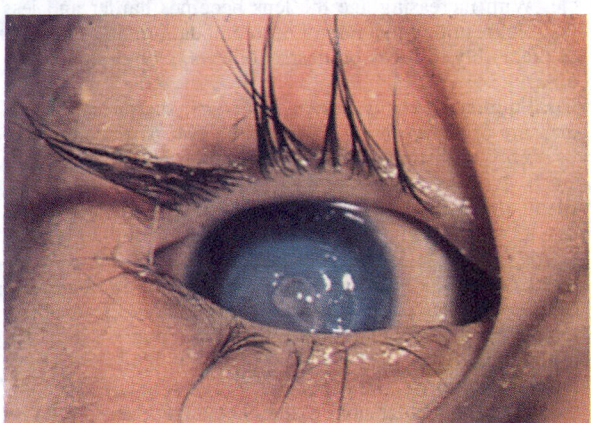

Keratomalacia caused by vitamin A deficiency
(McLaren, 1992)

vitamin A$_1$,   one of the two forms of vitamin A that occur in nature. It is a fat-soluble unsaturated alcohol formed by hydrolysis of β-carotene, one molecule of which yields two molecules of vitamin A$_1$. Natural sources include fish-liver oils, butterfat, and egg yolk. The vitamin is needed for healthy vision and skin epithelium. The RDA for adult men is 1000 RE (retinol equivalents) and, because of average lower body weights, 800 RE for adult women. Also called **retinol.**

vitamin A$_2$,   an alternative form of vitamin A found in the tissues of freshwater fish but not in saltwater fish or mammals. Differences in ultraviolet light absorption spectra are used to distinguish the vitamin A forms.

vitamin B$_1$.   See **thiamine.**

vitamin B$_2$.   See **riboflavin.**

vitamin B$_6$.   See **pyridoxine.**

vitamin B₁₂. See **cyanocobalamin.**

vitamin B₁₇. See **Laetrile.**

vitamin B complex, a group of water-soluble vitamins differing from each other structurally and in their biologic effect. All of the B vitamins are found in large quantities in liver and yeast, and they are present separately or in combination in many foods. Heat and prolonged cooking, especially cooking with water, can destroy B vitamins. See also **folic acid** and vitamins **B₁** through **B₁₂.**

vitamin C. See **ascorbic acid.**

vitamin D, a fat-soluble vitamin chemically related to the steroids and essential for the normal formation of bones and teeth and for the absorption of calcium and phosphorus from the GI tract. The vitamin is present in natural foods in small amounts, and requirements are usually met by artificial enrichment of various foods, especially milk and dairy products, and exposure to sunlight. Ultraviolet rays activate a form of cholesterol in an oil of the skin and convert it to a form of the vitamin, which is then absorbed. The natural foods containing vitamin D are of animal origin and include saltwater fish, especially salmon, sardines, and herring; organ meats; fish-liver oils; and egg yolk. Deficiency of the vitamin results in rickets in children, osteomalacia, osteoporosis, and osteodystrophy. Hypervitaminosis D produces a toxicity syndrome characterized by anorexia, vomiting, headache, drowsiness, diarrhea, and calcification of the soft tissues of the heart, blood vessels, renal tubules, and lungs. Treatment consists of discontinuing the vitamin dosage and initiating a low-calcium diet until symptoms resolve. The Vitamin D RDA for young adults is 10 micrograms as cholecaliferol or 400 IU of the vitamin; after the age of 25 the RDA for vitamin D is half that amount. See also **calciferol, vitamin D₃.**

vitamin D₂. See **calciferol.**

vitamin D₃, an antirachitic, white, odorless, crystalline, unsaturated alcohol that is the predominant form of vitamin D of animal origin. It is found in most fish-liver oils, butter, brain, and egg yolk and is formed in the skin, fur, and feathers of animals and birds exposed to sunlight or ultraviolet rays. Also called **activated 7-dehydrocholesterol, cholecalciferol.**

vitamin deficiency, a state or condition resulting from the lack of or inability to use one or more vitamins. The symptoms and manifestations of each deficiency vary depending on the specific function of the vitamin in promoting growth and development and maintaining body health.

vitamin D resistant rickets, a disease clinically similar to rickets but resistant to treatment with large doses of vitamin D. It is caused by a congenital defect in renal tubular reabsorption of phosphate and is usually seen in men. See also **rickets.**

vitamin E, any or all of the group of fat-soluble vitamins that consist of the tocopherols and are essential for normal reproduction, muscle development, resistance of erythrocytes to hemolysis, and various other biochemical functions. It is an intracellular antioxidant and acts in maintaining the stability of polyunsaturated fatty acids and other fatlike substances, including vitamin A and hormones of the pituitary, adrenal, and sex glands. Deficiency results in muscle degeneration, abnormalities in the vascular system, megaloblastic anemia, hemolytic anemia, infertility, creatinuria, and liver and kidney damage and is associated with the aging process. The richest dietary sources are wheat germ; soybean, cotton seed, peanut, and corn oils; margarine; whole raw seeds and nuts; soybeans; eggs; butter; liver; sweet potatoes; and the leaves of many vegetables, such as turnip greens. It is stored in the body for long periods of time so that any deficiency is rare. It is considered nontoxic except in hypertensive patients and those with chronic rheumatic heart disease. Alpha-tocopherol is the most physiologically active form of the group. The adult RDA for vitamin E is 8 to 10 milligrams of alphatocopherol equivalents. Also called **tocopherol.**

vitamin H. See **biotin.**

vitamin K, a group of fat-soluble vitamins known as quinones that are essential for the synthesis of prothrombin in the liver and of several related proteins involved in the clotting of blood. It is also involved with the process of phosphorylation and electron transport. The vitamin is widely distributed in foods, especially leafy green vegetables, pork liver, yogurt, egg yolk, kelp, alfalfa, fish-liver oils, and blackstrap molasses and is synthesized by the bacterial flora of the GI tract. It is also produced synthetically. Deficiency results in hypoprothrombinemia, characterized by poor coagulation of the blood and hemorrhage, and usually occurs from inadequate absorption of the vitamin from the GI tract or the inability to use it in the liver. It is used to reduce the clotting time in patients with obstructive jaundice and in hemorrhagic states associated with intestinal diseases and diseases of the liver; it is given prophylactically to infants to prevent hemorrhagic disease of the newborn. A form of the vitamin is used as a preservative to control fermentation in foods. Natural vitamin K is stored in the body and produces no toxicity. Excessive doses of synthetic vitamin K may cause anemia in newborn infants and hemolysis in people with glucose-6-phosphate deficiency. The adult RDA for vitamin K is 45 to 80 micrograms. See also **vitamin K₁, vitamin K₂, menadione.**

vitamin K₁, a yellow, viscous, oil-soluble vitamin, occurring naturally, especially in alfalfa, and produced synthetically. It is used as a prothrombinogenic agent. Also called **phylloquinone, phytonadione.**

vitamin K₂, a pale-yellow, fat-soluble crystalline vitamin of the vitamin K group that is more unsaturated than vitamin K₁ and slightly less active biologically. It is isolated from putrefied fish meal and synthesized by various bacteria in the GI tract. See also **vitamin K.**

vitamin K₃. See **menadione.**

vitamin loss [L, *vita,* life + *amine*], reduction in vitamin content of food resulting from the handling and preparation of fresh foods during harvesting, heating, pickling, salting, milling, canning, and other food-processing techniques. Further vitamin losses can occur because of digestive disorders that prevent absorption of nutrients and the use of drugs, such as isoniazid, that are vitamin antagonists.

vitaminology /vī′təminol′əjē/ [L, *vita, amine* + Gk, *logos,* science], the study of vitamins, including their structures, modes of action, and function in maintaining the health of the body.

vitamin P. See **bioflavonoid.**

vitellin /vitel′in/ [L, *vitellus,* yolk], a phosphoprotein containing lecithin, found in the yolk of eggs. Also called **ovovitellin. −vitelline** /-ēn/, *adj.*

vitelline artery /vitel′in, -ēn/ [L, *vitellus* + Gk, *arteria,* air pipe], any of the embryonic arteries that circulate blood from the primitive aorta of the early developing embryo to the yolk sac. Also called **omphalomesenteric artery.**

vitelline circulation, the circulation of blood and nutrients between the developing embryo and the yolk sac by way of the vitelline arteries and veins. Also called **ompha-lomesenteric circulation.** See also **fetal circulation.**

vitelline duct, (in embryology) the narrow channel connecting the yolk sac with the intestine. Also called **umbilical duct.**

vitelline membrane, the delicate cytoplasmic membrane surrounding the ovum. Also called **yolk membrane.** See also **zona pellucida.**

vitelline sac. See **yolk sac.**

vitelline sphere. See **morula.**

vitelline vein, any of the embryonic veins that return blood from the yolk sac to the primitive heart of the early developing embryo. Also called **omphalomesenteric vein.**

vitellogenesis /vitel'ōjen'əsis/ [L, *vitellus* + Gk, *genein,* to produce], the formation or production of yolk. **−vitellogenetic,** *adj.*

vitellus /vitel'əs, vī-/ [L, yolk], the yolk of an ovum.

vitiligo /vit'ilē'gō/, /-ī'gō/ [L, *vitium,* blemish], a benign, acquired skin disease of unknown cause, consisting of irregular patches of various sizes totally lacking in pigment and often having hyperpigmented borders. Exposed areas of skin are most often affected. Treatment using 8-methoxypsoralen requires extreme care and carefully regulated sun exposure. Waterproof cosmetics are often used to cover the patches. Compare **albinism, piebald.** **−vitiliginous,** *adj.*

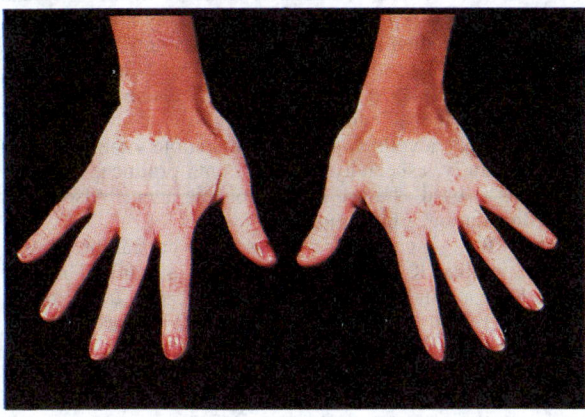

Vitiligo *(du Vivier, 1993)*

vitrectomy /vitrek'təmē/ [L, *vitreus,* glassy; Gk, *ektome,* excision], a surgical procesure for replacing the contents of the vitreous chamber of the eye.

vitreous /vit'rē·əs/ [L, *vitreus,* glassy], pertaining to the vitreous body of the eye located in the posterior chamber of the eye.

vitreous body. See **vitreous humor.**

vitreous cavity [L, *vitrum,* glass; *cavum,* cavity], the cavity in the eye posterior to the lens that contains the vitreous body and vitreous membrane and is transected by the vestigial remnants of the hyaloid canal.

vitreous degeneration [L, *vitreus,* glassy + *degenerare,* to deviate from kind], a form of hyaline degeneration; the formation of glassy material in the connective tissue of blood vessels and other tissues.

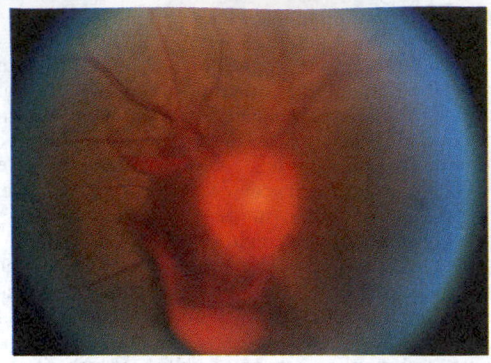

Vitreous hemorrhage *(Zitelli, 1992)*

vitreous hemorrhage, a hemorrhage into the vitreous humor of the eye.

vitreous humor, a transparent, semigelatinous substance contained in a thin hyoid membrane filling the cavity behind the crystalline lens of the eye. Some indications of the hyaloid canal may persist in the vitreous humor, which is not penetrated by any blood vessels and is nourished at its periphery by vessels of the retina and the ciliary processes. The vitreous humor is concave anteriorly to accommodate the crystalline lens and is closely applied to the retina around the wall of the eyeball. Also called **corpus vitreum, vitreous body.**

vitreous membrane, a membrane that lines the posterior cavity of the eye and surrounds the vitreous body.

vitriol, oil of. See **sulfuric acid.**

Vivactil, a trademark for a tricyclic antidepressant (protriptyline hydrochloride).

vivax malaria. See **tertian malaria.**

vivi-, a combining form meaning 'relating to being alive': *vivisection, viviparous.*

viviparous /vivip'ərəs/ [L, *vivus,* alive, *parere,* to bear], bearing living offspring rather than laying eggs, such as most mammals and some fishes and reptiles. Compare **oviparous, ovoviviparous.**

vivisection /viv'əsek'shən [L, *vivus,* alive + *secare,* to cut], the performance of surgical operations on living animals, particularly experimental surgery for the purpose of research.

Vivonex, a trademark for a nutritional supplement containing protein, carbohydrate, and fat.

VLDL, abbreviation for **very-low-density lipoprotein.**

VMA, abbreviation for **vanillylmandelic acid.**

V.N.A., abbreviation for *Visiting Nurses Association.*

Vo$_2$, symbol for *oxygen uptake.*

vocal apparatus /vō'kəl/ [L, *vocalis,* voice + *ad, parare,* to prepare], the larynx, pharynx, and oral and nasal cavities involved in the production of sound.

vocal cord [L, *vocalis,* voice; Gk, *chorde,* string], either of two strong bands of yellow elastic tissue in the larynx enclosed by membranes called vocal folds and attached ventrally to the angle of the thyroid cartilage and dorsally to the vocal process of the arytenoid cartilage. Also called **true vocal cord, vocal ligament.** Compare **false vocal cord.**

vocal cord nodule, a small, inflammatory or fibrous

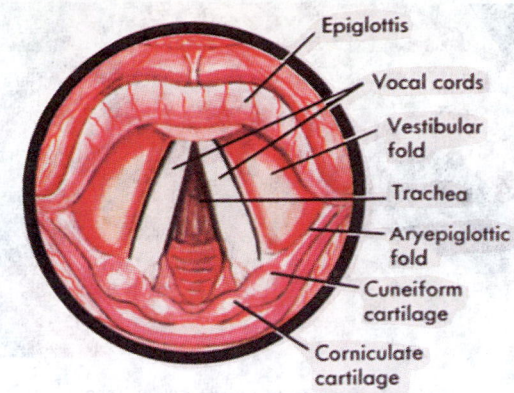

Vocal cords *(Thibodeau, 1993/Ernest W Beck)*

growth that develops on the vocal cords of people who constantly strain their voices. Also called **screamer's nodule, singer's nodule, teacher's nodule.** See also **chorditis.**

vocal cues, a category of nonverbal communication that includes all the noises and sounds that are extra-speech sounds. Also called **paralinguistic cues.**

vocal folds [L, *vocalis*; AS, *fealdan*], the true vocal cords.

vocal fremitus (VF), the vibration of the chest wall as a person speaks or sings that allows the person's voice to be heard by the examiner during auscultation of the chest with a stethoscope. Vocal fremitus is decreased in emphysema, pleural effusion, pulmonary edema, or bronchial obstruction.

vocal resonance [L, *vocalis* + *resonare,* to sound again], **1.** auscultation. **2.** modification of the laryngeal tone as it passes through the throat and oral cavity so as to produce an increase in the intensity and quality of the sound.

voice, the acoustic component of speech that is normally produced by vibration of the vocal folds of the larynx.

voice box. See **larynx.**

void /void/ [ME, *voide,* empty], to empty, or evacuate, such as urine from the bladder.

voiding urethrography [ME, *voide,* empty; Gk, *ourethra* + *graphein,* to record], radiography of the urethra during micturition after the introduction of a radiopaque fluid into the bladder.

vol., abbreviation for **volume.**

vol.%, abbreviation for *volume percent.*

volar /vō'lər/ [L, *vola,* palm, sole], of or pertaining to the palm of the hand or the sole of the foot.

volar ligament. See **retinaculum flexorum manus.**

volatile /vol'ətəl/ [L, *volatilis,* flying], (of a liquid) easily vaporized.

volatile solvent, an easily vaporized solvent.

-volemia, a combining form meaning '(condition of the) volume of plasma in the body': *hypervolemia, hypovolemia, normovolemia.*

volition /vōlish'ən/ [L, *voluntas,* inclination], **1.** the act, power, or state of willing or choosing. **2.** the conscious impulse to perform or to abstain from an act. **—volitional,** *adj.*

volitional /vōlish'ənəl/ [L, *velle,* to wish], pertaining to the use of one's own will in performing or abstaining from an action.

volitional tremor [L, *velle,* to wish + *tremor,* shaking], a trembling that begins during voluntary effort, sometimes spreading throughout the body. It may occur in multiple sclerosis and cerebellar disorders. Also called **intention tremor.**

Volkmann's canal /fōlk'munz/ [Alfred W. Volkmann, German physiologist, b. 1800], any one of the small blood vessel canals connecting haversian canals in bone tissue. Compare **haversian canaliculus.** See also **haversian system.**

Volkmann's contracture [Richard von Volkmann, German surgeon, b. 1830], a serious, persistent flexion contraction of forearm and hand caused by ischemia. A pressure or crushing injury in the region of the elbow usually precedes this condition, and pressure from a cast or tight bandage about the elbow are common causes. Permanent fibrosis, muscle degeneration, and a clawlike hand may result. Nurses must watch for swelling, pallor, coldness, cyanosis, or pain distal to the injury site so that prompt loosening of constriction can restore circulation. Also called **ischemic contracture.**

Volkmann's splint [Richard von Volkmann; AS, *splinte,* thin board], a splint that supports and immobilizes the lower leg. It has a footpiece attached to two sides that extends from the foot to the knee, allowing ambulation.

volsella forceps /volsel'ə/ [L, *vosella,* tweezers; *forceps,* tongs], a kind of forceps having a small, sharp-pointed hook at the end of each blade. Also called **volsella, volsellum forceps, vulsella forceps.**

volt (V) /vōlt/ [Count Alessandro Volta, Italian physicist, b. 1745], the unit of electric potential. In an electric circuit a volt is the force required to send 1 ampere of current through 1 ohm of resistance, or the difference in potential between two points on a conductor carrying a charge of 1 ampere when there is a dissipation of 1 watt between them. See also **ampere, circuit, current, ohm, watt.**

voltage /vō'tij/ [Alessandro Volta], an expression of electrical potential in terms of volts.

voltammetry /voltam'ətərē/, the measurement of an electric current as a function of potential.

voltmeter /vōlt'mētər/, an instrument, such as a galvanometer, that measures in volts the differences in potential between different points of an electric circuit.

volume (vol.) /vol'yəm,-yo͞om/ [L, *volumen,* paper roll], the amount of space occupied by a body, expressed in cubic units.

volume (ATPS), pertaining to *ATPS* (ambient temperature, ambient pressure, saturated with water vapor) conditions of a volume of gas. The conditions exist in a water-sealed spirograph or gasometer when the water temperature equals ambient temperature.

volume (BTPS), abbreviation for *BTPS* (body temperature, ambient pressure, saturated with water vapor) conditions of a volume of gas. For humans, normal respiratory tract temperature is measured at 37° C, the pressure as ambient pressure, and the partial pressure of water vapor at 37° C as 47 torr.

volume control fluid chamber, any one of several types of transparent, plastic reservoirs with graduated volumetric markings, used to regulate the flow of intravenous solutions. These devices are components of intravenous volume control sets and accommodate the injection and the mixing of medications by means of special built-in ports. The volume control fluid chamber contains a filter that must be primed to function.

volume dose. See **integral dose.**

volume imaging, MR imaging techniques in which MR signals are gathered from the whole object volume to be imaged at once. Many sequential plane imaging techniques can be generalized to volume imaging, at least in principle. Advantages include potential improvement in the signal-to-noise ratio by including signals from the whole volume at once; disadvantages include a bigger computational task for image reconstruction and longer image acquisition times, although the entire volume can be imaged from the one set of data.

volumetric analysis. See **quantitative analysis.**

volumetric flow rate /vol′yəmet′rik/, the rate at which a volume of fluid flows past a designated point, usually measured in liters per second.

volume ventilator, a ventilator that delivers a predetermined volume of gas with each cycle.

voluntary /vol′ənter′ē/ [L, *voluntas,* inclination], referring to an action or thought originated, undertaken, controlled, or accomplished as a result of a person's free will or choice.

voluntary abortion. See **elective abortion.**

voluntary agency, a service agency legally controlled by volunteers rather than by owners or a paid staff. Most public health nursing agencies are voluntary; most hospitals, which are legally controlled by hospital boards, are composed of lay and professional members who are not paid for their services.

voluntary hospital system, a nationwide complex of autonomous, self-established, and self-supported private not-for-profit and investor-owned hospitals in the United States.

voluntary muscle. See **striated muscle.**

volunteer /vol′əntir′/ [Fr, *volontaire*], a person who serves a hospital without pay, augmenting but not replacing paid personnel and professional staff members.

-volute, a combining form meaning 'to roll or turn around, or convoluted': *circumvolute, involute, revolute.*

volvulus /vol′vyələs/ [L, *volvere,* to turn], a twisting of the bowel on itself, causing intestinal obstruction. The condition is frequently the result of a prolapsed segment of mesentery and occurs most often in the ileum, the cecum, or the sigmoid portions of the bowel. If it is not corrected, the obstructed bowel becomes necrotic, peritonitis and rupture of the bowel occur, and death may ensue. Severe, gripping pain, nausea and vomiting, an absence of bowel sounds, and a tense, distended abdomen suggest the diagnosis, which is confirmed by x-ray examination. Compare **intussusception.**

volvulus neonatorum, an intestinal obstruction in a newborn baby resulting from a twisting of the bowel caused by malrotation or nonfixation of the colon. Typical symptoms include abdominal distention, persistent regurgitation, often accompanied by fecal vomiting, and nonpassage of stools. Characteristic barium enema x-ray studies confirm the diagnosis. The condition requires immediate surgical correction to prevent necrosis and gangrene of the affected segment of bowel.

vomer /vō′mər/ [L, plowshare], the bone forming the posterior and inferior part of the nasal septum and having two surfaces and four borders.

vomit /vom′it/ [L, *vomere,* to vomit], **1.** to expel the contents of the stomach through the esophagus and out of the

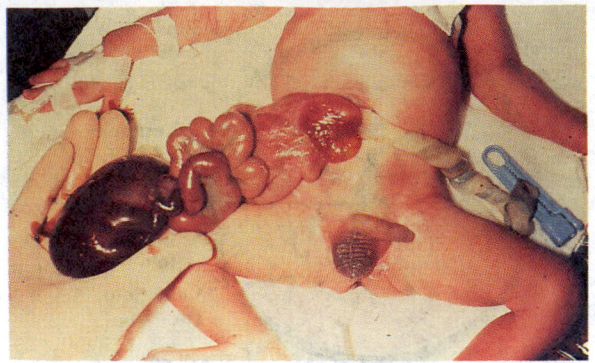

Volvulus neonatorum (Zitelli, 1992)

mouth. **2.** also called **emesis, vomitus.** the material expelled.

vomiting [L, *vomere,* to vomit], the forcible voluntary or involuntary emptying of the stomach contents through the mouth.

vomiting of pregnancy, vomiting that occurs during the early months of pregnancy. Factors contributing to the condition include delayed stomach emptying during pregnancy, relaxation of the esophageal sphincter at the opening into the stomach, and relaxation of the diaphragmatic hiatus, which increase the risk of gastric reflux. See also **morning sickness.**

vomiting reflex. See **reflex emesis.**

vomitus /vom′itəs/ [L, *vomere,* to vomit], pertaining to the material expelled from the stomach during vomiting. Vomitus is sometimes classified by color or other appearances as an indicator of the cause of illness, such as a 'coffee-ground' vomitus being a clinical sign of peptic ulcers.

VON, abbreviation for *Victorian Order of Nurses.*

von Economo's encephalitis. See **epidemic encephalitis.**

von Gierke's disease /fôngir′kəz/ [Edgar von Gierke, German pathologist, b. 1877], a form of glycogen storage disease in which abnormally large amounts of glycogen are deposited in the liver and kidneys. The disorder is characterized by hypoglycemia, ketoacidosis, and hyperlipemia. Biopsy of the affected organs reveals the absence of glucose-6-phosphate dehydrogenase (G-6-PD), an enzyme necessary for glycogen metabolism. There is no effective treatment for the disorder. Medical efforts are directed at preventing hypoglycemia and ketoacidosis. Also called **glycogen storage disease, type I.** See also **glycogen storage disease.**

von Hippel-Lindau disease. See **cerebroretinal angiomatosis.**

von Pirquet test. See **Pirquet test.**

von Recklinghausen's disease. See **neurofibromatosis.**

von Recklinghausen's tumor. See **Recklinghausen's tumor.**

von Willebrand's disease [Erick A. von Willebrand, Finnish physician, b. 1870], an inherited disorder characterized by abnormally slow coagulation of the blood and spontanous epistaxis and gingival bleeding caused by a deficiency of a component of factor VIII. Excessive bleeding is common postpartum, during menstruation, and after injury or surgery. Also called **angiohemophilia.** See also **hemophilia, thrombasthenia.**

voracious [L, *vorax*], greedy or gluttonous, with an insatiable appetite.

-vorous, a combining form meaning 'of or referring to feeding on something': *leguminivorous, panivorous.*

vortex, *pl.* **vortexes, vortices** [L, whirl], a whirlpool effect produced by the whirling of a more or less cylindric mass of fluid (liquid or gas). The velocity of the motion increases as the radius of the circle described by the motion decreases; the velocity decreases as the radius increases. Tornadoes and whirlpools are examples of free vortexes.

vox /voks′/ [L], voice, such as **vox cholerica,** the barely audible, hoarse voice of a patient in an advanced and severe case of cholera.

voxel /vok′səl/, abbreviation for *vo*lume element, the three-dimensional version of a pi*xel.*

voyeur /voiyur′, vô·äyœr′/ [Fr, *voir,* to see], one whose sexual desire is gratified by the practice of voyeurism. Also called **Peeping Tom.** The female counterpart is a **voyeuse** /vô·äyœz′/.

voyeurism /voi′yəriz′əm, voiyur′izəm/ [Fr, *voyeur* + L, *ismus,* practice], a psychosexual disorder in which a person derives sexual excitement and gratification from looking at the naked bodies and genital organs or observing the sexual acts of others, especially from a secret vantage point.

VP-L-asparaginase, an anticancer drug combination of vincristine, prednisone, and asparaginase.

V/Q, abbreviation for *ventilation/perfusion.* See **ventilation/perfusion ratio.**

VR, abbreviation for *variable ratio.* See **variable ratio reinforcement.**

V.S., **1.** abbreviation for **vesicular sound. 2.** abbreviation for *Veterinary Surgeon.* **3.** abbreviation for **vital signs. 4.** abbreviation for **volumetric solution.**

VSD, abbreviation for **ventricular septal defect.**

V$_t$, abbreviation for tidal volume, the amount of air in milliliters per breath.

vulgaris /vulger′is/ [L, *vulgus,* common people], common or ordinary.

vulnerable /vul′nərəbəl/ [L, *vulnus,* wound], being in a dangerous position or condition and thereby susceptible to being infected or injured.

vulnerable period, a short period in the cardiac cycle during which activation may result in ectopy. The ventricular vulnerable period corresponds to the apex of the T wave toward its ascending side.

vulnerable population. See **population at risk.**

vulsella forceps. See **volsella forceps.**

vulva. See **pudendum.**

vulvar /vul′vər/, of or pertaining to the vulva.

vulvectomy /vulvek′təmē/ [L, *vulva,* wrapper; Gk, *ektome,* excision], the surgical removal of part or all of the tissues of the vulva, performed most frequently in the treatment of malignant or premalignant neoplastic disease. **Simple vulvectomy** includes the removal of the skin of the labia minora, the labia majora, and the clitoris. **Radical vulvectomy** involves excision of the labia majora, labia minora, clitoris, surrounding tissues, and pelvic lymph nodes.

vulvitis /vulvī′tis/ [L, *vulva,* a wrapper; Gk, *itis,* inflammation], an inflammation of the vulva.

vulvo- a combining form for terms meaning 'relating to the vulva': *vulvectomy, vulvovaginal.*

vulvocrural /vul′vōkrōō′rəl/ [L, *vulva* + *crus,* leg], of or pertaining to the vulva and the thigh.

vulvovaginal /vul′vōvaj′inəl/ [L, *vulva* + *vagina,* sheath], of or pertaining to the vulva and the vagina.

vulvovaginitis /vul′vōvaj′inī′tis/, an inflammation of the vulva and vagina, or of the vulvovaginal glands.

vv, **1.** an abbreviation for *veins.* **2.** an abbreviation for *vice versa.*

v/v, **1.** symbol for *volume of dissolved substance per volume of solvent.* **2.** symbol for *volume per volume.*

v/w, symbol for *volume of substance per unit of weight of another component.*

VZIG, abbreviation for **varicella-zoster immune globulin.**

VZV, abbreviation for **varicella zoster virus.**

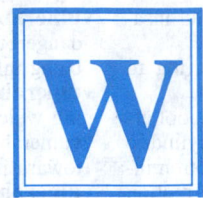

w, the amount of energy required to ionize a molecule of air, as expressed by w = 33.85 eV/ion pair. This is an important quantity for radiation dosimetry because it allows the extraction of dose from ionization measurements.

W, symbol for the element **tungsten.**

waddling gait /wod'ling/ [ME, *waden,* to wade; ONorse, *gata,* way], a gait observed in patients with progressive muscular dystrophy characterized by exaggerated lateral trunk movements and hip elevations.

Wagner-Meissner corpuscle /wag'nərmīs'nər/ [Rudolf Wagner, German physiologist, b. 1805; Georg Meissner, German anatomist, b. 1829; L, *corpusculum,* little body], one of a number of small, special pressure-sensitive sensory end organs with a connective tissue capsule and tiny stacked plates in the corium of the hand and foot, the front of the forearm, the skin of the lips, the mucous membrane of the tongue, the palpebral conjunctiva, and the skin of the mammary papilla. A single nerve fiber penetrates each oval capsule, spirals through the interior, and ends as a globular mass. Also called **tactile corpuscle of Meissner.** Compare **Golgi-Mazzoni corpuscles, Krause's corpuscles.**

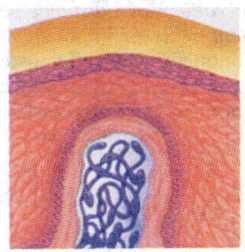

Wagner-Meissner corpuscle
(Thibodeau, 1993/Rolin Graphics)

Wagstaffe's fracture /wag'stafs/ [William Wagstaffe, English surgeon, b. 1834; L, *fractura,* break], a fracture characterized by separation of the internal malleolus.

waking imagined analgesia (WIA) [AS, *wacian,* to awaken; L, *imaginari,* to picture oneself; Gk, *a, algos,* without pain], the pain relief experienced by a patient who employs the psychologic technique, usually with the help of an attending nurse or a hospital aide, of concentrating on previous pleasant personal experiences that produced tranquillity, such as lying on a summer beach beside cooling ocean water or drifting down a quiet river in a canoe. The patient employing the WIA technique is encouraged to verbalize such experiences, thereby reinforcing recollection with attendant soothing biologic responses. This technique is often effective in reducing mild to moderate pain, especially when used with a mild nonnarcotic analgesic and the compassionate interaction of an attending health care professional. See also **pain assessment, pain intervention, pain mechanism.**

Wald /wôld/, **Lillian** (1867–1940), an American public health nurse, settlement leader, and social reformer. She founded the Henry Street Settlement in New York to bring nursing care into the homes of the poor. This led to the development of the Visiting Nurse Service of New York. She was also instrumental in establishing the school nursing system, the federal government's Children's Bureau, and the Nursing Service Division of the Metropolitan Life Insurance Company. She was the first nurse to be elected into the Hall of Fame for Great Americans.

Waldenström's disease. See **Perthes' disease.**

Waldenström's macroglobulinemia. See **macroglobulinemia.**

Waldeyer's throat ring /wäl'dī·ərz/ [Heinrich W. G. von Waldeyer-Hartz, German anatomist, b. 1836; AS, *hring*], the palatine, pharyngeal, and lingual tonsils that encircle the pharynx. Also called **lymphoid ring, tonsillar ring.**

walker /wô'kər/ [AS, *wealcan,* to roam], an extremely light, movable apparatus, about waist high, made of metal

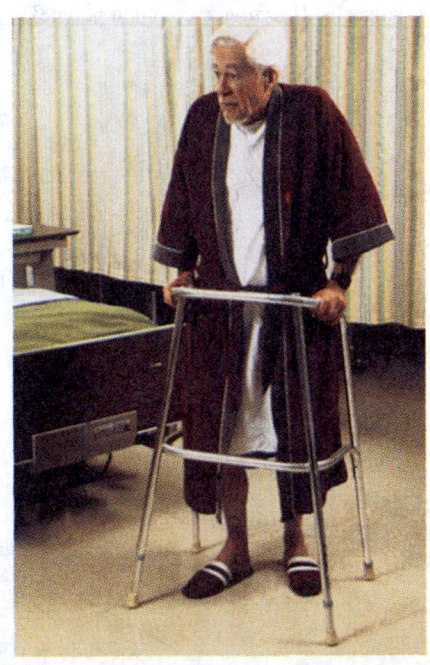

Walker *(Sorrentino, 1992)*

tubing, used to aid a patient in walking. It has four widely placed, sturdy legs. The patient holds onto the walker and takes a step, then moves the walker forward and takes another step. Compare **crutch.**

walking belt,   a leather or nylon device with handles that enables a health care provider to help a patient walk.

walking cast [AS, *wealcan,* to roam;, ONorse, *kasta*],   a cast that permits a patient to walk. A short-leg walking cast has an attached rubber walker to accept a cast shoe for foot or ankle injuries. A long-leg walking cast covers the leg from the upper thigh to the toes, with an attached rubber sole device called a walker.

walking heel,   a plastic or rubber heel placed in the sole of a leg cast to allow weight-bearing.

walking pneumonia.   See **mycoplasma pneumonia.**

walking rounds [AS, *wealcan* + Fr, *rond*],   rounds in which the clinician responsible leads a group of junior clinicians on a tour to visit the patients for whom they are collectively responsible. In some hospitals nurses may participate in walking rounds in lieu of or in addition to report.

walking typhoid [AS, *wealcan,* to roam; Gk, *typhos,* stupor + *eidos,* form],   an ambulatory subclinical case of typhoid fever. The person may be infected with typhoid but have mild symptoms that do not interfere with the activities of daily living.

walking wounded [AS, *wealcan,* to roam + *wund*],   a military term for an injured person who is ambulatory.

wall [L *vallum* palisade],   a limiting structure within the body, such as the wall of the abdominal, the thoracic, or the pelvic cavities, or the wall of a cell.

wallerian degeneration /waler′ē·ən/ [Augustus V. Waller, English physician, b. 1816; L, *degenerare,* to degenerate],   the fatty degeneration of a nerve fiber after it has been severed from its cell body.

wander /won′dər/ [AS, *wandrian*],   **1.** to move about purposelessly. **2.** to cause to move back and forth in an exploratory manner; for example, in inserting an intrauterine catheter, the tip of the inserter usually must be wandered around the fetal head in the cervix to find a space through which the catheter may be passed upward into the uterus.

wandering abscess [AS, *wandrian;* L, *abscedere,* to go away],   an abscess that moves through tissue openings to a point some distance from its origin.

wandering atrial pacemaker [AS, *wandrian;* L, *passus;* ME, *maken*],   a heart dysrhythmia caused by the shifting of a pacemaker stimulus site. The site usually moves throughout the atria. The dysrhythmia is detected on an ECG as a varying P wave morphology and a P-R interval.

wandering goiter.   See **diving goiter.**

wandering rash.   See **geographic tongue.**

Wangensteen apparatus /wang′ənstēn/ [Owen H. Wangensteen, American surgeon, b. 1898; L, *ad, parare,* to prepare],   a nasogastroduodenal catheter and a suction apparatus used for constant, gentle drainage and decompression of the stomach or duodenum. It may be used to relieve abdominal distention that often occurs postoperatively or that may complicate a GI disorder, especially an intestinal obstruction. See also **Wangensteen tube.**

Wangensteen tube [Owen H. Wangensteen],   the catheter portion of a Wangensteen apparatus.

ward /wôrd/ [AS, *weard,* guard],   a hospital room designed and equipped to house more than four patients.

warfarin poisoning /wôr′fərin/ [Wisconsin Alumni Research Foundation + coumarin],   a toxic condition caused

by the ingestion of warfarin, accidentally in the form of a rodenticide or by overdose with the substance in its pharmacologic anticoagulant form. The poison accumulates in the body and results in nosebleed, bruising, hematuria, melena, and internal hemorrhage. Treatment may include gastric lavage, a cathartic, vitamin K, and blood transfusion. The goal of therapy is to eliminate the poison and to reestablish normal coagulation.

warfarin sodium,   an oral anticoagulant.

■ INDICATIONS: It is prescribed for the prophylaxis and treatment of thrombosis and embolism.

■ CONTRAINDICATIONS: Hemorrhage or known hypersensitivity to this drug prohibits its use.

■ ADVERSE EFFECTS: The most serious adverse reaction is hemorrhage. Many other drugs interact with this drug to increase or decrease its effects.

warm-blooded [AS, *wearm, blod*],   having a relatively high and constant body temperature, such as the temperatures maintained by humans, other mammals, and birds, despite changes in environmental temperatures. Heat is produced in the warm-blooded human body by the catabolism of foods in proportion to the amount of work performed by the tissues in the body. Heat is lost from the body by evaporation, radiation, conduction, and convection. About 80% of the body heat that is dissipated in humans is lost through the skin; the rest is lost through the mucous membranes of the respiratory, the digestive, and the urinary systems. The average temperature of the healthy human is 98.6° F (37° C). The human body's tolerance for change in its temperature is very small, and significant changes can have drastic, even fatal, consequences. The control mechanism for temperature in the human body consists of thermal receptive neurons in the anterior portion of the hypothalamus, more than 2 million sweat glands, and the vast network of blood vessels in the skin. Reduced heat loss results from less secretion and slower evaporation of sweat and from vasoconstriction of blood vessels. Increased heat gain results from shivering, which increases the work of body tissues and, hence, increases catabolism. Fever, which raises internal body temperature, temporarily resets the thermostatic control of the hypothalamus by the action of chemical pyrogens from bacteria and viruses and by the function of the prostaglandins that the pyrogens release. The temperature control mechanisms of the body serve to restore normal heat levels during fever. Aspirin and other antipyretic drugs foil the synthesis of prostaglandins. Also called **homoiothermal, homothermal.** Compare **cold-blooded.**

war neurosis.   See **combat fatigue, shell shock.**

wart.   See **verruca.**

Warthin's tumor.   See **papillary adenocystoma lymphomatosum.**

washout /wosh′out/ [AS, *wascan,* to wash, ME, *oute*],   the elimination or expulsion of one gas or volatile anesthetic agent by the administration of another.

wasp /wosp/ [L, *vespa*],   a slender, narrow-waisted hymenopteran insect with two pairs of membranous wings that are folded lengthwise when at rest like parts of a fan. Many species of wasps may give painful stings that may have severe results in hypersensitive individuals. Treatment is as for bee stings.

Wassermann blood test. /was′ərmən, vos′ərmun/ [August P. von Wassermann, German bacteriologist, b. 1866],   an obsolete diagnostic blood test for syphilis based on the complement fixation reaction.

wasted ventilation,   the volume of air that ventilates the physiologic dead space in the respiratory system.

waste products [L, *vastare,* to destroy+ *producere,* to produce],   the products of metabolic activity after oxygen and nutrients have been supplied to a cell. These include mainly carbon dioxide and water, along with sodium chloride, and soluble nitrogenous salts, which are excreted in feces, urine, and exhaled air.

wasting [L, *vastare,* to destroy],   a process of deterioration marked by weight loss and decreased physical vigor, appetite, and mental activity.

travenous fluids, plasma, and oxygen. No sedatives or narcotics are given. Specific treatment for bacteremia is intensive antibiotic therapy, given parenterally and continued for several days after symptoms subside. Nursing management includes close observation and the maintenance of adequate provision of fluids and nutrients.

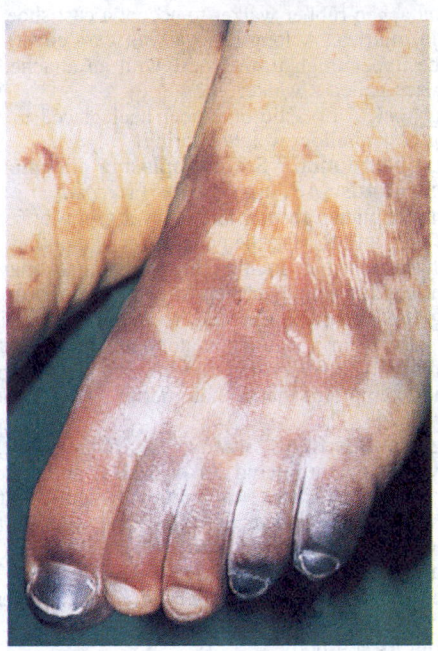

Petechiae and cyanosis seen in Waterhouse-Friderichsen syndrome
(Fletcher, 1987)

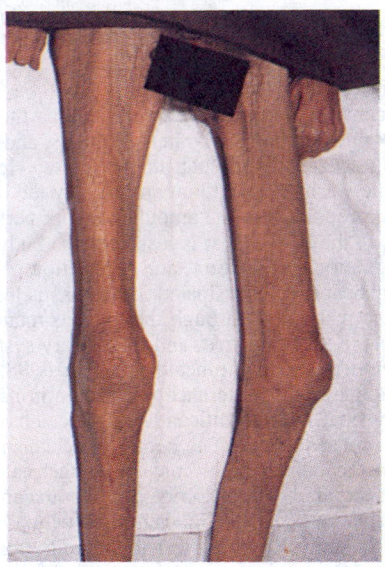

Muscle wasting *(Kamal, 1991)*

watchfulness /woch'fəlnes/,   continuous supervision provided either openly or unobtrusively as the situation indicates.

water (H₂O) /wô'tər/ [AS, *waeter*],   a chemical compound, one molecule of which contains one atom of oxygen and two atoms of hydrogen. Almost three quarters of the earth's surface is covered by water. Essential to life as it exists on this planet, water makes up more than 70% of living things. Pure water freezes at 0° C (32° F) and boils at 100° C (212° F) at sea level.

waterborne,   carried by water, such as a waterborne epidemic of typhoid fever.

water-hammer pulse [AS, *waeter;* Gk, *akme,* point; L, *pulsare,* to beat],   a pulse associated with aortic regurgitation. It is characterized by a full, forcible impulse and immediate collapse, causing a jerking sensation.

Waterhouse-Friderichsen   syndrome   /wô'tərhous'frid'ərik'sən/ [Rupert Waterhouse, English physician, b. 1873; Carl Friderichsen, Danish physician, b. 1886], overwhelming bacteremia, characterized by the sudden onset of fever, cyanosis, petechiae, and collapse from massive bilateral adrenal hemorrhage. The syndrome requires immediate emergency treatment, hospitalization, and intensive care. Emergency treatment includes vasopressor drugs, in-

water intoxication,   an increase in the volume of free water in the body, resulting in dilutional hyponatremia.

water moccasin.   See **cottonmouth.**

water pollution,   the contamination of lakes, rivers, and streams by industrial or community sources of pollutants.

waters.   See **amniotic fluid.**

water trap.   See **underwater seal.**

Watson-Crick helix /wôt'sənkrik'/ [John Dewey Watson, American biologist, b. 1928; Francis H. Crick, English biologist, b. 1916; Gk, *helix,* coil],   a model of the DNA molecule proposed by Watson and Crick as two righthanded polynucleotide chains coiled around the same axis as a double helix. The purine and pyrimidine bases of each strand are on the inside of the double helix and paired according to a Watson-Crick base-pairing rule. Variations in the sequences of the bases determine the genetic information transmitted by the DNA molecule. Watson and Crick received the Nobel Prize in 1962.

watt /wot/ [James Watt, Scottish engineer, b. 1736],   the unit of electric power or work in the meter/kilogram/second system of notation. The watt is the product of the voltage and the amperage. One watt of power is dissipated when a current of 1 ampere flows across a difference in potential of 1 volt. See also **ampere, current, ohm, volt.**

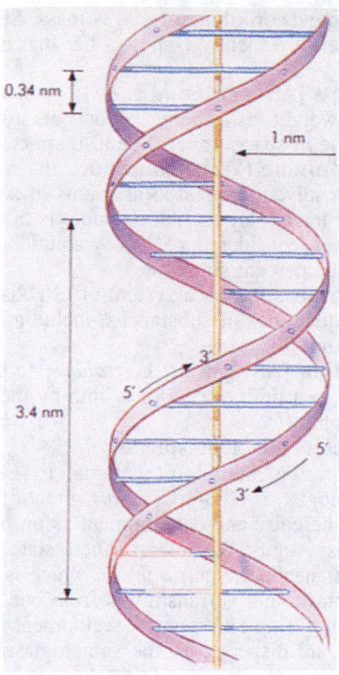

Watson-Crick helix *(Raven, 1992/Bill Ober)*

watt per square centimeter (W/cm²), a unit of power density or intensity used in ultrasonography.

wave [AS, *wafian,* to fluctuate], a periodic disturbance in which energy moves through a medium without permanently altering the constituents of the medium. Electromagnetic waves, such as light, x-rays, and radio waves, can travel through a vacuum. Sound waves can be transmitted only through matter. See also **electromagnetic radiation, light, sound, x-ray.**

wavelength, the distance between a given point on one wave cycle and the corresponding point on the next successive wave cycle. A pure color is produced by light of a specific wavelength. Electromagnetic waves of different wavelengths account for many of the transmission characteristics of radio and television.

wax. See **cerumen.**

wax bath. See **paraffin bath.**

waxy flexibility. See **cerea flexibilitas.**

WBC, abbreviation for **white blood cell.** See **leukocyte.**

wbt, abbreviation for *wet bulb thermometer.*

wc, abbreviation for **wheelchair.**

W chromosome and Z chromosome, the sex chromosomes of certain insects, birds, and fishes. Females of such species are heterogametic and have one W and one Z chromosome, whereas males are homogametic and have two Z chromosomes. The ZZ-ZW system of nomenclature was chosen to differentiate the chromosomes from the XX-XY type, which occurs in humans and various other animals and in which the female is homogametic and the male is heterogametic.

W/cm², abbreviation for **watt per square centimeter.**

W/D, abbreviation for *well developed,* often used in the initial identifying statement in a patient record. It is used

so frequently as to have lost all meaning or use in identifying or describing the patient.

wean [AS, *wenian,* to accustom], **1.** to induce a child to give up breast feeding and to accept other food in place of breast milk. Many children are ready for weaning during the second half of the first year; some wean themselves. **2.** to withdraw a person from something on which he is dependent. **3.** to remove a patient gradually from dependency on mechanical ventilation.

weanling, a child who has recently been weaned.

wear-and-tear theory /wer/, a concept of the aging process in which structural and functional changes associated with growing old are accelerated by abuse of the body and retarded with health care.

weaver's bottom [AS, *wefan,* to weave; *botm,* undersurface], a form of bursitis affecting the ischial bursae of the hips of people whose work requires prolonged sitting in one position. Also called *(obsolete)* **tailor's bottom.**

web, a network of fibers forming a tissue or a membrane, such as the laryngeal web that spreads between the vocal cords.

webbed toes [AS, *wefan,* to weave + *tá*], an abnormality in which the toes are connected by webs of skin.

webbing, skinfolds connecting adjacent structures such as fingers or toes or the neck from the acromion to the mastoid, associated with genetic anomalies.

Weber (Wb), a unit of magnetic flux equal to m²kg/s²A.

Weber's tuning fork test /web′ərz/, a method of assess-

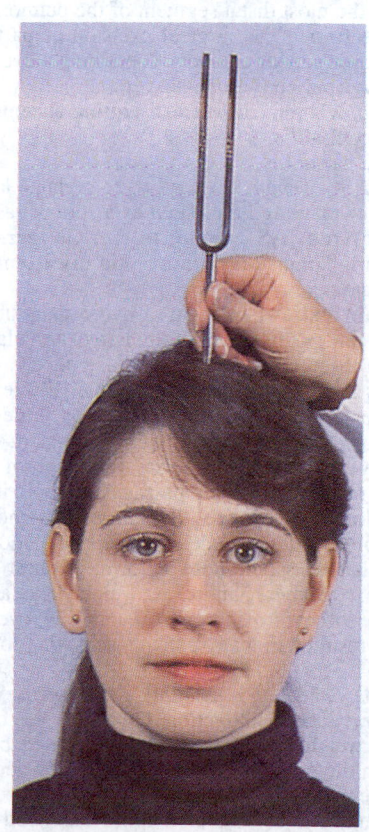

Weber tuning fork test *(Seidel, 1991)*

ing auditory acuity, especially useful in determining whether defective hearing in an ear is a conductive loss caused by a middle ear problem or a sensorineural loss, resulting from a disorder in the inner ear or auditory nerve system. The test is performed by placing the stem of a vibrating 256 Hz tuning fork in the center of the person's forehead, the midline vertex, or on the maxillary incisors. The loudness of the sound is equal in both ears if hearing is normal. If the person has a sensorineural loss in one ear, the unaffected ear perceives the sound as louder. When conductive hearing loss is present, the sound is louder in the affected ear, because it does not hear ordinary background noise conducted through the air and receives only vibrations by bone conduction.

web of causation, an interrelationship of multiple factors that contribute to the occurrence of a disease.

webril, trademark for a stretchable cotton material applied over the skin to protect from plaster irritation.

Wechsler intelligence scales /weks'lər/ [David Wechsler, American psychologist, b. 1896], a series of standardized tests designed to measure the intelligence at several age levels, from preschool through adult, by means of questions that examine general information, arrangement of pictures and objects, vocabulary, memory, reasoning, and other abilities.

wedge fracture /wej/ [AS, *wecg,* peg; L, *fractura,* break], a fracture of vertebral structures with anterior compression.

wedge pressure, the capillary pressure in the left atrium, determined by measuring the pressure in a cardiac catheter wedged in the most distal segment of the pulmonary artery.

wedge resection, the surgical excision of part of an organ, such as a part of an ovary containing a cyst. The segment excised may be wedge-shaped.

WEE, abbreviation for **western equine encephalitis.** See **equine encephalitis.**

weed. See **cannabis.**

weeping [AS, *wepan,* to cry], **1.** crying, lacrimating. **2.** oozing or exuding fluid, such as a sore or rash.

weeping eczema [AS, *wepan,* to cry; Gk, *ekzein,* to boil over], an inflammatory form of skin disease marked by a fluid exudate.

weeping lubrication, a form of hydrostatic lubrication in which the interstitial fluid of hydrated articular cartilage flows onto its surface when a load is applied.

Wegener's granulomatosis /wā'gənərz/ [F. Wegener, 20th century German pathologist; L, *granulum,* little grain; Gk, *oma,* tumor, *osis,* condition], an uncommon, chronic inflammatory process leading to the formation of nodules or tumorlike masses in the air passages, necrotizing vasculitis, and glomerulonephritis. Symptoms, depending on the organ involved, may include sinus pain, a bloody, purulent nasal discharge, saddle-nose deformity, chest discomfort and cough, weakness, anorexia, weight loss, and skin lesions. Use of cytotoxic drugs, especially cyclophosphamide, has resulted in many patients achieving long-term remissions.

weight (wt) /wāt/ [AS, *gewight*], the force exerted on a body by gravitational attraction. On the surface of the earth, mass and weight are defined as equal. As a body moves away from the earth, the weight of the body decreases, but the mass remains constant. In empty space, a body has mass but no weight. Weight is sometimes measured in units of force, such as newtons or poundals, but it is usually ex-

pressed in pounds or kilograms, as is mass. See also **mass.**

weight holder, a metal, T-shaped bar that holds weights for traction.

weightlessness [AS, *gewiht*; ME, *les*], a state of absence of apparent weight, as in being beyond the effects of gravitational force in space travel. See also **space medicine.**

weight per volume (W/V) solution, the relationship of a solute to a solvent expressed as grams of solute per milliliter of the total solution. An example is 50 g of glucose in 1 L of water, considered a 5% W/V solution, even though it is not a true percent solution.

weights and measures, a system of establishing units or portions of quantities of substances, including standards of mass or volume

weight traction [AS, *gewiht*; L, *trahere,* to draw], traction applied to a limb or part of a limb by means of a suspended weight.

Weil's disease. See **leptospirosis.**

weismannism /vīs'muniz'əm/ [August F. L. Weismann, German biologist, b. 1834; L, *ismus,* practice], the basic concepts of heredity and development as proposed by German biologist August Weismann. These state that the vehicle of inheritance is the germ plasm, which is distinct from the somatoplasm and is transmitted from one generation to the next; that during embryonic development the hereditary components are dispersed to the somatoplasm to give rise to inherited characteristics; and that changes in somatoplasm do not affect germ plasm, so that acquired characteristics cannot be inherited. Also called **Weismann's theory, germ plasm theory.** Compare **pangenesis.** —**weismannian,** *adj., n.*

Weiss' sign. See **Chvostek's sign.**

well baby care [AS, *wyllan,* to wish; ME, *babe*; L, *garrire,* to chatter], periodic health supervision for infants and children to promote optimal physical, emotional, and intellectual growth and development. Such health care measures include routine immunizations to prevent disease, screening procedures for early detection and treatment of illness, and parental guidance and instruction in proper nutrition, accident prevention, and specific care and rearing of the child at various stages of development. The recommended preventive health care schedule for children who are developing normally is monthly for the first 6 months of life, every 2 months until 1 year of age, every 3 months during the second year, and every 6 months during the third year, followed by annual visits. Well baby care may be provided in a clinic, a convenient local meeting place, a private doctor's office, the office of a community health nursing service, or a school. Nurses or nurse practitioners frequently provide the care.

well baby clinic, a clinic that specializes in medical supervision and services for healthy infants.

well-being [AS, *wyllan* + *beon,* to be], achievement of a good and satisfactory existence as defined by the individual.

well-differentiated lymphocytic malignant lymphoma /-dif'əren'shē·ā'tid/, a lymphoid neoplasm characterized by the predominance of mature lymphocytes. Also called **lymphocytic lymphoma, lymphocytic lymphosarcoma, lymphocytoma.**

Wellen syndrome, in patients with unstable angina, the ECG signs of critical proximal left anterior descending coronary artery stenosis. They are: normal or minimally elevated enzymes, little or no ST segment elevation, no loss of precordial R waves, progressive, deep, symmetrical inversion of the T waves in leads V2 and V3, but not confined to these leads. The ECG signs are seen when the patient is without pain.

wellness, a dynamic state of health in which an individual progresses toward a higher level of functioning, achieving an optimum balance between internal and external environments.

welt [OE, *wealtan,* to roll], a raised ridge on the skin, usually caused by a blow.

wen. See **pilar cyst.**

Wenckebach heart block. See **Mobitz I heart block.**

Wenckebach periodicity /veng′kəbäk, -bäkh/ [Karel F. Wenckebach, Dutch-Austrian physician, b. 1864; Gk, *peri,* around, *hodos,* way], a form of second-degree atrioventricular block with a progressive beat-to-beat prolongation of the PR interval, finally resulting in a nonconducting P wave. At this point, the sequence recurs. Also called **Mobitz I, Type I block, Wenckebach phenomenon.** See also **atrioventricular block.**

Werdnig-Hoffmann disease /verd′nighôf′mun/ [Guido Werdnig, Austrian neurologist, b. 1862; Johann Hoffman, German neurologist, b. 1857], a genetic disorder beginning in infancy or young childhood, characterized by progressive atrophy of the skeletal muscle resulting from degeneration of the cells in the anterior horn of the spinal cord and the motor nuclei in the brainstem. Onset occurs within the first year of life, with the condition usually apparent at birth. Symptoms include congenital hypotonia, absence of stretch reflexes, flaccid paralysis, especially of the trunk and limbs, lack of sucking ability, fasciculations of the tongue and sometimes of other muscles, and, often, dysphagia. Treatment is symptomatic, and death generally occurs in early childhood, often from respiratory complications. The condition is transmitted as an autosomal recessive trait and occurs more frequently in siblings than in successive generations. Also called **familial spinal muscular atrophy, Hoffmann's atrophy, infantile spinal muscular atrophy, progressive spinal muscular atrophy of infants, Werdnig-Hoffmann paralysis.** See also **floppy infant syndrome.**

Werlhof's disease. See **thrombocytopenic purpura.**

Wernicke's center [Karl Wernicke; Gk, *kentron,* center], a sensory speech center located in the posterior temporal gyrus and adjacent angular gyrus in the dominant hemisphere. Wernicke observed in 1874 that patients with brain damage in that area also suffered a loss of speech comprehension. Also called **Wernicke's area, Wernicke's field, Wernicke's zone.**

Wernicke's encephalopathy /ver′nikēz/ [Karl Wernicke, Polish neurologist, b. 1848], an inflammatory, hemorrhagic, degenerative condition of the brain, characterized by lesions in several parts of the brain, including the hypothalamus, mammillary bodies, and tissues surrounding ventricles and aqueducts. The condition is characterized by double vision, involuntary and rapid movements of the eyes, lack of muscular coordination, and decreased mental function, which may be mild or severe. Wernicke's encephalopathy is caused by a thiamine deficiency and is seen in association with chronic alcoholism. It also occurs as a complication of GI tract disease and hyperemesis gravidarum associated with malabsorption and malnutrition. Also called **Wernicke's syndrome.**

Wernicke's field, Wernicke's zone. See **Wernicke's center.**

West African sleeping sickness. See **Gambian trypanosomiasis.**

Westcort, a trademark for a glucocorticoid (hydrocortisone valerate).

Westermark's sign, the absence of blood vessel markings beyond the location of a pulmonary embolism as seen on a radiograph.

Western blot test, a laboratory blood test to detect the presence of antibodies to specific antigens. It is regarded as more precise than the enzyme-linked immunosorbent assay (ELISA) and is sometimes used to check the validity of ELISA tests.

western equine encephalitis. See **equine encephalitis.**

West nomogram, a nomogram used in estimating the body surface area. See also **nomogram.**

wet-and-dry-bulb thermometer, an instrument used to measure the relative humidity of the atmosphere. It consists of a thermometer with a bulb that is wet or moist and one that is kept dry. The relative humidity is calculated from the difference in readings of the thermometers when water evaporates from the dry bulb, decreasing its temperature.

wet cough. See **productive cough.**

wet dream. See **nocturnal emission.**

wet dressing [AS, *waet;* Ofr, *dresser,* to arrange], a moist dressing used to relieve symptoms of some skin diseases. As the moisture evaporates, it cools and dries the skin, softens dried blood and sera, and stimulates drainage. Medication may be added if necessary.

wet lung, an abnormal condition of the lungs, characterized by a persistent cough and crackles at the lung bases. It occurs in workers exposed to pulmonary irritants, such as ammonia, chlorine, sulfur dioxide, volatile organic acids, dusts, and vapors of corrosive chemicals. Treatment consists of removing the person from exposure to the irritant and therapy for possible pulmonary edema. Compare **pulmonary edema.** See also **ARDS, pleural effusion, pleurisy.**

wet nurse, a woman who cares for and breast-feeds another's infant.

wet pack [AS, *waet,* moist; ME, *pakke*], a therapy that involves wrapping the patient in wet sheets with a top covering of a dry blanket, usually to reduce fever.

wet pleurisy [AS, *waet;* Gk, *pleuritis*], pleurisy in which the inflammation has progressed to an effusive state, with the fluid having a high specific gravity because of the presence of blood clots and fibrin.

wetting agent, a detergent, such as tyloxapol, used as a mucolytic in respiratory therapy.

W/F, symbol for *white female,* often used in the initial identifying statement in a patient record.

Wharton's jelly /wôr′tənz/ [Thomas Wharton, English anatomist, b. 1614; L, *gelare,* to congeal], a gelatinous tissue that remains when the embryonic body stalk blends with the yolk sac within the umbilical cord.

wheal /wēl/ [AS, *walu,* pimple], an individual lesion of urticaria.

wheal-and-flare reaction [AS, *walu; flare;* ME, *fleare,* to blaze up; L, *re, agere,* to act], a skin eruption that may follow injury or injection of an antigen. It is characterized by swelling and redness caused by a release of histamine. The reaction usually occurs in three stages, beginning with appearance of an erythematous area at the site of injury, followed by development of a flare surrounding the site; finally, a wheal forms at the site as fluid leaks under the skin from surrounding capillaries.

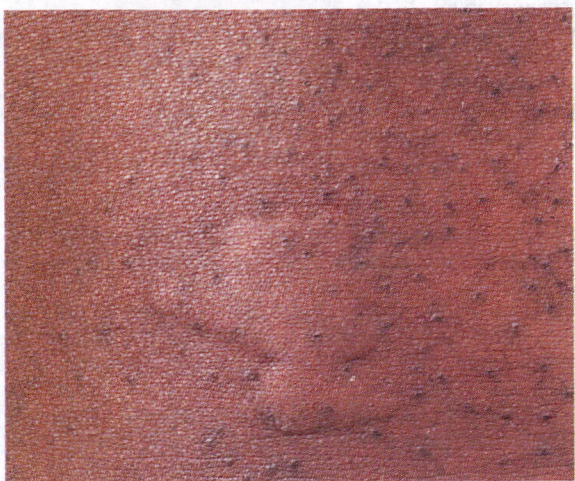

Wheal (du Vivier, 1993)

wheat weevil disease, a hypersensitivity pneumonitis caused by allergy to weevil particles found in wheat flour.

wheelchair (wc), a mobile chair equipped with large wheels and brakes. If long-term use of the chair is expected, a physical therapist may prescribe certain personalized requirements, such as size, left- or right-hand propulsion, type of brakes, height of armrests, and special seat pads.

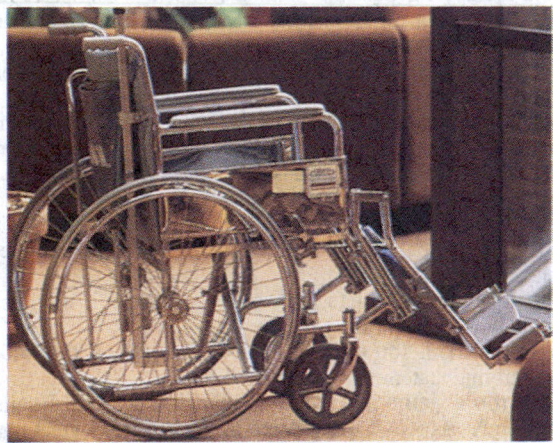

Wheelchair (Potter, 1993)

wheeze [AS, *hwesan,* to hiss], **1.** a form of rhonchus, characterized by a high-pitched musical quality. It is caused by a high-velocity flow of air through a narrowed airway and is heard during both inspiration and expiration. Wheezes are associated with asthma and chronic bronchitis. Unilateral wheezes are characteristic of bronchogenic

carcinoma, foreign bodies, and inflammatory stenosing lesions. An asthmatoid wheeze is caused by an obstruction in the trachea or bronchus. **2.** to breathe with a wheeze. Compare **crackle, rhonchi.**

whiplash injury [ME, *whippen, lasshe;* L, *ijuria*], *informal.* an injury to the cervical vertebrae or their supporting ligaments and muscles marked by pain and stiffness, usually resulting from sudden acceleration or deceleration, such as in a rear-end car collision that causes violent back and forth movement of the head and neck.

Whipple's disease [George Hoyt Whipple, American pathologist, b. 1878], a rare intestinal disease characterized by severe intestinal malabsorption, steatorrhea, anemia, weight loss, arthritis, and arthralgia. People with the disease are severely malnourished and have abdominal pain, chest pain, and a chronic nonproductive cough. The diagnosis is made by jejunal biopsy. Penicillin and tetracycline may alleviate the symptoms. See also **malabsorption syndrome.**

whipworm. See **Trichuris.**

whirlpool bath /(h)wurl/, the immersion of the body or a part of the body in a tank of hot water agitated by a jet of equally hot water and air.

whispered pectoriloquy, the transmission of a whisper through the pulmonary structures so that it is heard as normal audible speech on auscultation. See also **pectoriloquy.**

white blood cell. See **leukocyte.**

white cell, *informal.* white blood cell. See also **leukocyte.**

white corpuscle. See **leukocyte.**

white damp. See **damp.**

white fibrocartilage [AS, *hwit;* L, *fibra,* fiber, *cartilago*], a mixture of tough, white fibrous tissue and flexible cartilaginous tissue. It is divided into four types: interarticular fibrocartilage, connecting fibrocartilage, circumferential fibrocartilage, and stratiform fibrocartilage. Compare **hyaline cartilage, yellow cartilage.**

white gold, a gold alloy with a high content of palladium or platinum used in some dental restorations, such as prepared tooth cavities and gold crowns. It has a higher fusion range, lower ductility, and greater hardness than a yellow gold alloy.

whitehead. See **milium.**

white infarct [AS, *hwit;* L, *infarcire,* to stuff], an infarct that is white because of an absence of blood. Also called **anemic infarct.**

white leg. See **phlegmasia alba dolens.**

white matter. See **white substance.**

white radiation, a form of radiation that results from the rapid deceleration of high-speed electrons striking a target, such as when the electron beam of a tungsten cathode strikes the tungsten or molybdenum target of the anode in an x-ray tube. Most of the x-rays emitted from a diagnostic or therapeutic x-ray unit represent white radiation. Also called **braking radiation, bremsstrahlung.**

white spots film fault, a defect in a radiograph or a developed photographic film that appears as scattered white spots throughout the image area. It is caused by air bubbles clinging to the emulsion during development or by fixing solution splattered on the film before processing.

white substance, the tissue surrounding the gray substance of the spinal cord, consisting mainly of myelinated nerve fibers, but with some unmyelinated nerve fibers, embedded in a spongy network of neuroglia. It is subdivided in each half of the spinal cord into three funiculi: the anterior, the posterior, and the lateral white column. Each column subdivides into tracts that are closely associated in function. The anterior column divides into two ascending tracts and five descending tracts. The posterior column divides into two large ascending tracts, one small descending tract, and one intersegmental tract. The lateral column divides into six ascending tracts and four descending tracts. Also called **white matter.** Compare **gray substance.** See also **spinal cord, spinal tract.**

white thrombus, **1.** an aggregation of blood platelets, fibrin, clotting factors, and cellular elements containing few or no erythrocytes. **2.** a thrombus composed chiefly of white blood cells. **3.** a thrombus composed primarily of blood platelets and fibrin.

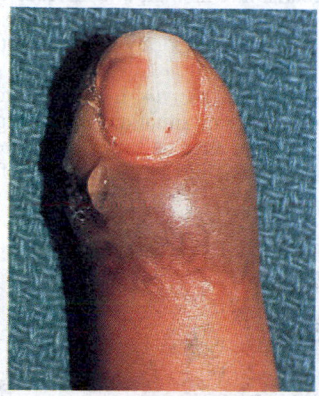

Herpetic whitlow (Lewis, 1989)

whitlow /(h)wit′lō/ [Scan, *whick,* nail, *flaw,* crack], an inflammation of the end of a finger or toe that results in suppuration. See also **felon.**

WHO, abbreviation for **World Health Organization.**

whole blood /hōl/ [AS, *hal, blod*], blood that is unmodified except for the presence of an anticoagulant. Whole blood may be used for transfusion. Various components and factors may be separated from whole blood for infusion to replace or to augment a deficient or nonfunctional component or factor.

whole body hyperthermia. See **systemic heating.**

wholistic health /hōlis′tik/ [Gk, *holos,* whole + *ism*; AS, *haelth*], a concept that concern for health requires a perspective of the individual as an integrated system rather than one or more separate parts. Also spelled **holistic.**

whoop /hōōp, (h)wōōp/, a noisy spasm of inspiration that terminates a coughing paroxysm in cases of pertussis. It is caused by a sudden, sharp increase in tension on the vocal cords.

whooping cough. See **pertussis.**

whorl /(h)wurl/ /wurl, hwurl/ [ME, *hwarwy*], a spiral turn, such as one of the turns of the cochlea or of the dermal ridges that form fingerprints.

WIA, abbreviation for **waking imagined analgesia.**

wick humidifier, a respiratory care device in which a piece of paper, sponge, or similar material that absorbs water by capillary action is inserted in the path of the air flow. With the addition of heat, high levels of humidity can be achieved over a wide range of flows and temperatures.

Widal's test /vēdäls′/ [Georges F. I. Widal, French physician, b. 1862], an agglutination test used to aid in the diagnosis of salmonella infections, such as typhoid fever. A fourfold increase in titer of agglutinins is highly suggestive of active infection. A high titer may persist for years after the disease or after immunization against typhoid fever.

wide-angle glaucoma. See **glaucoma.**

Wiedenbach /wē′dənbak/, **Ernestine** (1900-   ), a German-born American nursing educator and writer. She taught maternal and newborn health nursing at Yale School of Nursing, was a leader in family-centered maternity nursing, and developed the full range of the art and science of obstetric nursing.

Wigraine, a trademark for a fixed-combination drug containing anticholinergics (belladonna alkaloids), an analgesic (phenacetin), and a vasoconstrictor (ergotamine tartrate), used to treat migraine.

wild-type gene [AS, *wilde,* untamed; Gk, *typos,* mark, *genein,* to produce], a normal or standard form of a gene, as contrasted with a mutant form.

will [AS, *wyllan*], **1.** the mental faculty that enables one consciously to choose or decide on a course of action. **2.** the act or process of exercising the power of choice. **3.** a wish, desire, or deliberate intention. **4.** a disposition or attitude toward another or others. **5.** determination or purpose; willfulness. **6.** (in law) an expression or declaration of a person's wishes as to the disposition of property, to be performed or take effect after death.

Willis' circle. See **circle of Willis.**

willow fracture. See **greenstick fracture.**

Wilms' tumor /vilms/ [Max Wilms, German surgeon, b. 1867], a malignant neoplasm of the kidney, occurring in young children, before the fifth year in 75% of the cases. The most frequent early signs are hypertension, a palpable mass, pain, and hematuria. Diagnosis can be established by an excretory urogram with tomography. The tumor, an em

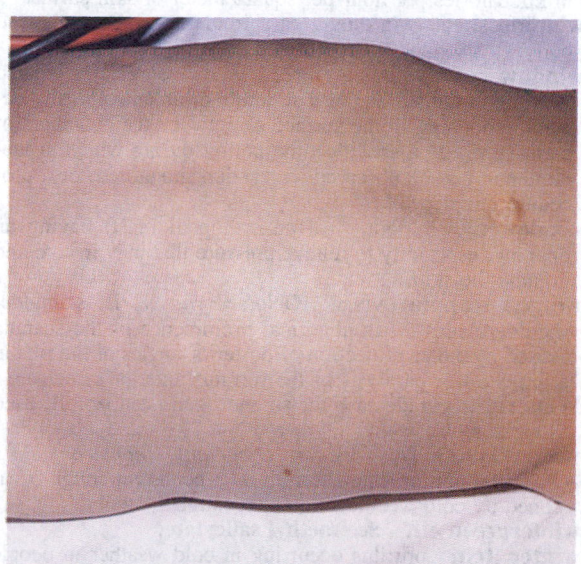

Renal mass caused by Wilm's tumor
(Swales, 1991/Courtesy Dr HJ Whitely)

bryonal adenomyosarcoma, is well encapsulated in the early stage, but it may extend into lymph nodes, the renal vein, or the vena cava, and metastasize to the lungs or other sites. Removal of resectable tumors by transperitoneal nephrectomy is recommended. Radiotherapy is used preoperatively or postoperatively; or palliatively in inoperable cases. Chemotherapy combined with surgery and irradiation is proving highly effective.

Wilson's disease [Samuel A. K. Wilson, English neurologist, b. 1877], a rare, inherited disorder of copper metabolism, in which copper accumulates slowly in the liver and is then released and taken up in other parts of the body. Hemolysis, then hemolytic anemia occur as the copper accumulates in the red blood cells. Accumulation in the brain destroys certain tissue and may cause tremors, muscle rigidity, dysarthria, and dementia. Kidney function is diminished; the liver becomes cirrhotic. Treatment of Wilson's disease includes a reduction of copper in the diet and the prescription of copper-binding agents and penicillamine. Also called **hepatolenticular degeneration.**

Winckel's disease. See **hemoglobinuria.**

windburn /wind′burn/ [AS, *wind* + *baernan*], a skin disorder caused by exposure to winds.

windchill /win′chil/, the loss of heat from the body when it is exposed to wind of a given speed at a given temperature and humidity.

windchill factor [AS, *wind* + *cele*, cold], the amount of chilling of the body, beyond that resulting from a cold ambient temperature, because of exposure to cool air currents. The windchill factor is expressed in degrees Celsius or Fahrenheit as the effective temperature felt by a person exposed to the weather. Because windchill factors are based on exposure of dry skin to cool air currents, air blowing at the same speed over a wet skin surface would cause additional loss of body heat and a greater windchill.

wind chill index, a chart that compares temperatures of the atmosphere with various wind speeds, enabling one to calculate the windchill factor. The comparison is expressed in kilocalories per hour per square meter of skin surface.

winding sheet /wīn′ding/, a shroud for wrapping a dead body.

window [AS, *wind*, air, *owe*, eye], a surgically created opening in the surface of a structure or an anatomically occurring opening in the surface or between the chambers of a structure. 2. a specific time period during which a phenomenon can be observed, a reaction monitored, or a procedure initiated.

windowed /win′dōd/, (of an orthopedic cast) having an opening, especially to relieve pressure that may irritate and inflame the skin.

winged scapula /wingd/ [ONorse, *vaengr*; L, *scapulae*, shoulderblades], an abnormal prominence of the scapula caused by either projection of posterior angles of the ribs in a flat chest or paralysis of the serratus anterior muscle.

Winstrol. a trademark for an androgen (stanozolol), used as an anabolic agent.

winter cough [AS, *winter*, *cohhetan*], *nontechnical.* a chronic condition characterized by a persistent cough occasioned by cold weather. See also **cough.**

wintergreen oil. See **methyl salicylate.**

winter itch, pruritus occurring in cold weather in people who have dry skin, particularly in those who have atopic dermatitis. Warmer temperature, increased humidity, and topical, antipruritic emollients may offer relief.

wire suture [AS, *wir*; L, *sutura*], a stainless steel or sil-

ver wire used for uniting bone fracture fragments or in dentistry.

wiry pulse /wī′(ə)re/ [AS, *wir*; L, *pulsare*, to beat], an abnormal pulse that is strong but small.

wisdom tooth [AS, *wisdom, toth*], either of the last teeth on each side of the upper and lower jaw. These are third molars and are the last teeth to erupt, usually between 17 and 21 years of age, often causing considerable pain, dental problems, and the need for extraction. Also called **dens serotinus.** See also **molar.**

wish fulfillment [AS, *wiscan*, to wish; *fullfyllan*, to fill full], 1. the gratification of a desire. 2. (in psychology) the satisfaction of a desire or the release of emotional tension through such processes as dreams, daydreams, and neurotic symptoms. 3. (in psychoanalysis) one of the primary motivations for dreams in which an unconscious desire or urge, unacceptable to the ego and superego because of sociocultural restrictions or feelings of personal guilt, is given expression.

wishful thinking [AS, *wiscan* + *thencan*, to think], the interpretation of facts or situations according to one's desires or wishes rather than as they exist in reality, usually used as an unconscious device to avoid painful or unpleasant feelings.

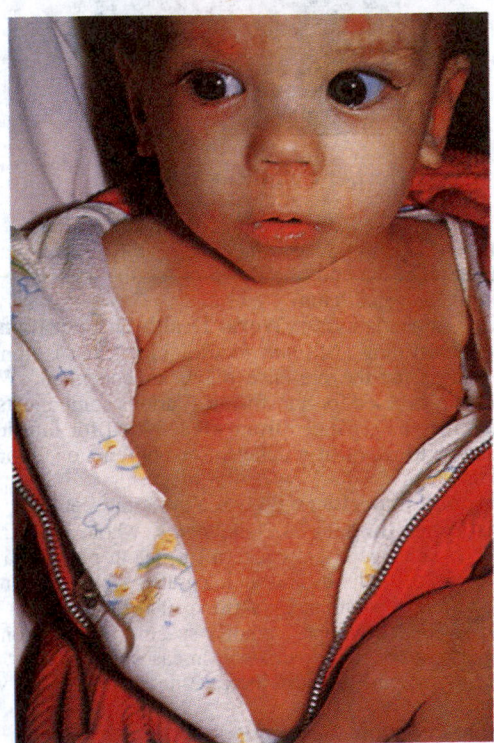

Eczema in a child with Wiskott-Aldrich syndrome
(Fireman, 1990)

Wiskott-Aldrich syndrome /wis′kotôl′drich/ [Alfred Wiskott, German pediatrician, b. 1898; Robert Anderson Aldrich, American pediatrician, b. 1917], an immunodeficiency disorder inherited as a recessive, X-linked trait, characterized by thrombocytopenia, eczema, inadequate T and B cell function, and an increased susceptibility to viral, bacterial, and fungal infections and to cancer. Treatment includes the prescription of appropriate antibiotics for specific infectious organisms and the administration of transfer factor from activated lymphocytes to increase the resistance to infection and to clear the eczema. See also **transfer factor.**

witch hazel [AS, *wican,* to bend; Ger, *hasel*], **1.** a shrub, *Hamamelis virginiana,* indigenous to North America, from which an astringent extract is derived. **2.** also called **hamamelis water.** a solution comprising the extract, alcohol, and water, used as an astringent.

witch's milk, a milklike substance secreted from the breast of the newborn, caused by circulating maternal lactating hormone. Also called **hexenmilch** /hek'sənmilsh'/.

withdrawal /withdrô'əl/ [ME, *with, drawen,* to take away], a common response to physical danger or severe stress characterized by a state of apathy, lethargy, depression, retreat into oneself, and, in grave cases, catatonia and stupor. It is pathologic if it interferes with a person's perception of reality and ability to function in society, such as in the various forms of schizophrenia. See also **schizophrenia.**

withdrawal behavior, the physical or psychologic removal of oneself from a stressor.

withdrawal bleeding, the passage of blood from the uterus, associated with the shedding of endometrium that has been stimulated and maintained by hormonal medication. It occurs when the medication is discontinued. In the endocrine evaluation of a woman with amenorrhea, withdrawal bleeding constitutes evidence that the woman's endometrium is reponsive to hormonal stimulation and that the cause of her amenorrhea is probably not uterine.

withdrawal method, a contraceptive technique in coitus wherein the penis is withdrawn from the vagina before ejaculation. It is not reliable because small amounts of seminal fluid carrying millions of spermatozoa may be emitted without sensation before full ejaculation. Also called **coitus interruptus.**

withdrawal reflex. See **flexor withdrawal reflex.**

withdrawal symptoms, the unpleasant, sometimes life-threatening physiologic changes that occur when some drugs are withdrawn after prolonged, regular use. The effects may occur after use of a narcotic, tranquilizer, stimulant, barbiturate, alcohol, or other substance to which the person has become physiologically or psychologically dependent or addicted.

withdrawal syndrome [ME, *withdrawen*; Gk, *syn,* together + *dromos,* course], a physical reaction after cessation or severe reduction in intake of a substance, such as alcohol or opiates, that has been used regularly to induce euphoria, intoxication, or relief from pain or distress. The body tissues become dependent on the regular reinforcing effect of the chemical so that interruption of the dosage induces an organic mental state characterized by anxiety, restlessness, insomnia, irritability, impaired attention, and, often, physical illness.

withdrawn behavior, a condition in which there is a blunting of the emotions and a lack of social responsiveness.

witness, a person who is present and can testify that he or she has personally observed an event, such as the signing of a will or consent form.

Wittmaack-Ekbom syndrome. See **restless legs syndrome.**

W/M, symbol for *white male,* often used in the initial identifying statement in a patient record.

W/N, symbol for *well nourished,* often used in the initial identifying statement in a patient record. It is used so frequently as to have lost all meaning or use in identifying or describing the patient.

wobble /wob'əl/, an eccentric rotation that permits increased resolution of tomographic imaging devices composed of discrete detector systems. Typical eccentric excursions are 1 to 2 cm.

Wolff-Chaikoff effect /woolf'chī'kəf/, the decreased formation and release of thyroid hormone in the presence of an excess of iodine.

wolffian body. See **mesonephros.**

wolffian cyst /wôl'fē·ən/ [Kaspar Friedrich Wolff, German anatomist, b. 1733; Gk, *kystis,* bag], **1.** a cyst of the wolffian duct. **2.** a cyst of a broad ligament of the uterus.

wolffian duct. See **mesonephric duct.**

Wolff-Parkinson-White syndrome /woolf'pär'kinsən-(h)wīt'/ [Louis Wolff, American physician, b. 1898; Sir John Parkinson, English cardiologist, b. 1885; Paul Dudley White, American cardiologist, b. 1886], a disorder of atrioventricular conduction, characterized by two AV conduction pathways. This syndrome is often identified by a characteristic delta wave seen on an electrocardiogram at the beginning of the QRS complex. See also **Lown-Ganong-Levine syndrome.**

wolfram. See **tungsten.**

Wolman's disease. See **cholesteryl ester storage disease.**

woman-year [AS, *wifman, gear*], (in statistics) 1 year in the reproductive life of a sexually active woman; a unit that represents 12 months of exposure to the risk of pregnancy. Woman-years are used in calculating a pregnancy rate in the assessment of the effectiveness of the various methods of family planning and of the adverse effect on the birth rate of various environmental factors.

womb. See **uterus.**

wood alcohol. See **methanol.**

Wood's glass [Robert Williams Wood, American physicist, b. 1868; AS, *glaes*], a nickel oxide filter that holds back all light except for a few violet rays of the visible spectrum and ultraviolet wavelengths of about 365 nm. It is used extensively to help diagnose fungus infections of the scalp and erythrasma and to reveal porphyrins and fluorescent materials.

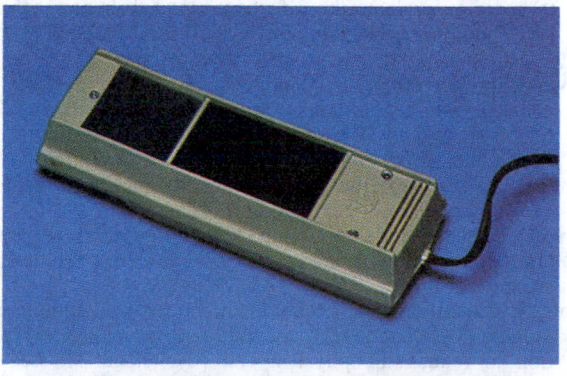

Wood's light *(Seidel, 1991)*

Wood's light [Robert Williams Wood; AS, *leoht*], an ultraviolet light of about 365 nm wavelength used to diagnose certain scalp and skin diseases. The light causes hairs infected with a fungus, such as *tinea capitis*, to become brilliantly fluorescent. Also called **black light, Wood's lamp, Wood's rays.**

wood tick [AS, *wudu*; ME, *tike*], a hardshelled tick of the *Ioxidae* family and a natural reservoir of *Rickettsia rickettsii*. One species of wood tick, *Dermacentor andersoni*, is the principal vector in western North America of **Rocky Mountain spotted fever**, transmitted by *R. rickettsii*.

wool fat, a fatty substance obtained from sheep's wool and of which lanolin is a common chemical component. It consists primarily of cholesterol and its esters.

woolsorter's disease [AS, *wull*; Fr, *sorte*; L, *dis,* opposite of; Fr, *aise,* ease], the pulmonary form of anthrax, so named because it is an occupational hazard to those who handle sheep's wool. Early symptoms mimic influenza, but the patient soon develops high fever, respiratory distress, and cyanosis. If the disease is not treated at this stage, it is often fatal. Also called **pulmonary anthrax.** See also **anthrax.**

word association. See **controlled association.**

word association test. See **association test.**

word blindness [AS, *word* + *blind*], an inability to understand written language, a form of receptive aphasia caused by lesions in the parietal or parietal-occipital areas of the brain. The condition may be congenital or acquired as a result of disease or injury. Also called **alexia.**

word deafness. See **auditory amnesia.**

word hash. See **jargon aphasia, paraphrasia.**

word processor, a computer system with software designed for the keyboarding, formatting, correcting, and storing of correspondence, reports, manuscripts, and books or other publications.

word salad, a jumble of words and phrases that lacks logical coherence and meaning, often characteristic of disoriented individuals and schizophrenics. See **jargon aphasia.**

working occlusion [AS, *weorc*; L, *occludere,* to shut], the occlusal contacts of teeth on the side of the jaw toward which the mandible is moved.

working phase, (in psychology) the second stage of the therapist-client relationship. During this stage, clients explore their experiences. Therapists assist clients in this process by helping them to describe and clarify their experiences, to plan courses of action and try out the plans, and to begin to evaluate the effectiveness of their new behavior. Should new behavior prove ineffective, therapists can assist clients in revising their courses of action.

working pressure, a recommended working pressure of about 50 pounds per square inch, gauge (psig) for oxygen or compressed air leaving a cylinder; it is reduced by a pressure regulator for clinical use in respiratory therapy.

working through, a process by which repressed feelings are released and reintegrated into the personality.

work of worrying, a coping strategy in which inner preparation through worrying increases the level of tolerance for subsequent threats.

work simplification, the utilization of special equipment, ergonomics, functional planning, and behavior modification to reduce the physical and psychologic stresses of home maintenance for disabled people or their family members.

work therapy [AS, *weorc*; Gk, *therapeia,* treatment], a therapeutic approach in which the client performs a useful activity or learns an occupation, as in occupational therapy.

work tolerance, the kind and amount of work that a physically or mentally ill person can or should perform.

work-up, the process of performing a complete evaluation of a patient, including history, physical examination, laboratory tests, and x-ray or other diagnostic procedures to acquire an accurate data base on which a diagnosis and treatment plan may be established.

World Health Organization (WHO), an agency of the United Nations, affiliated with the Food and Agricultural Organization of the UN, the International Atomic Energy Agency, the International Labor Organization, the Pan American Health Organization, and UNESCO. The WHO is primarily concerned with worldwide or regional health problems, but in emergencies it is authorized to render local assistance on request. Its functions include furnishing technical assistance, stimulating and advancing epidemiologic investigation of diseases, recommending health regulations, promoting cooperation among scientific and professional health groups, and providing information and counsel relating to health matters. Its headquarters are in Geneva, Switzerland. Its French name is **Organisation Mondiale de la Santé** /ôrgänizäsyôN′ môNdē·äl′ dələ säNtä′/ **(OMS).**

worm /wurm/ [AS, *wyrm*], any of the soft-bodied, elongated invertebrates of the phyla Annelida, Nemathelminthes, or Platyhelminthes. Some kinds of worms parasitic for humans are **hookworm, pinworm,** and **tapeworm.** See also **fluke, roundworm.**

wormian bone /vôr′mē·ən/ [Olaus Worm, Danish anatomist, b. 1588; AS, *ban*], any of several tiny, smooth, segmented bones that are soft, moist, and tepid to the touch, usually found as the serrated borders of the sutures between the cranial bones.

worthlessness /wurth′ləsnəs/, a component of low self-esteem, characterized by feelings of uselessness and inability to contribute meaningfully to the well-being of others or to one's environment.

wound /wo͞ond/ [AS, *wund*], **1.** any physical injury involving a break in the skin, usually caused by an act or accident rather than by a disease, such as a chest wound, gunshot wound, or puncture wound. **2.** to cause an injury, especially one that breaks the skin.

wound irrigation, the rinsing of a wound or the cavity formed by a wound using a medicated solution, water, or antimicrobial liquid preparation.

■ METHOD: The dressing is removed and wrapped for disposal. The patient is assisted to an appropriate position. With the use of equipment from a sterile irrigation pack or tray, an irrigating solution is poured into a graduated measure. It is then warmed in a basin of warm water unless the solution's action depends on antibiotic or enzyme activity, which would be inhibited by warming. An emesis or kidney basin is then fitted snugly against the patient's body beneath the wound. It may be held in place by the patient or by an assistant. A catheter is held with sterile gloves or forceps and gently inserted into the wound to a prescribed depth and at a prescribed angle. A syringe filled with irrigating solution is then attached to the catheter, and the solution is gently instilled. The catheter is pinched before the empty syringe is removed to prevent aspiration of the return irrigation flow during disconnection. The syringe is filled and attached again, and the wound is irrigated until the returning solution runs clear. If a catheter is not used, the solution is sprayed directly on the wound from the syringe until the wound looks clean. After irrigation is completed, the body area is dried with sterile sponges working from the wound out to the area around it, and a dry sterile dressing is applied.

■ NURSING INTERVENTION: Frequency of irrigation, type of solution, and amount of solution to be used are specifically prescribed. The condition of the wound, amount of irrigating solution used, and the appearance of the returned solution are documented by the nurse.

■ OUTCOME CRITERIA: Wounds are irrigated to remove secretions and dried blood and to keep the wound surface open to encourage healing from the inside out. When the irrigation solution returns clear, the wound is considered clean.

wound repair, restoration of the normal structure after an injury, especially of the skin. See also **healing, intention.**.

Wright's stain /rīts/ [James H. Wright; American pathologist, b. 1869; Fr, *teindre,* to dye], a stain containing methylene blue and eosin, used to color blood specimens for microscopic examination, such as for complete blood count and, particularly, for malarial parasites.

wrinkle test /ring′kəl/ [AS, *gewrinclian,* to wind; L, *testum,* crucible], a test for nerve function in the hand by observing the presence of skin wrinkles after the hand has been placed in warm water for 20 to 30 minutes. Denervated skin does not wrinkle.

wrist. See **carpus.**

wrist drop /rist/ [AS, *wrist + dropa*], a condition caused by paralysis of the extensor muscles of the hand and fingers or by injury of the radial nerve, resulting in flexion of the wrist.

wrist joint. See **radiocarpal articulation.**

writer's cramp [AS, *writan,* to write; *crammian,* to fill], a painful involuntary contraction of the muscles of the hand when attempting to write. It often occurs after long periods of writing. Also called **chirospasm** /kir′əspaz′əm/, **graphospasm.**

wrongful birth /rông′fəl/ [OE, *wrang,* twisted; ME, *burth*], a belief that a birth could have been avoided if the parents had been properly advised by a physician that a pregnancy could occur or that a fetus would be deformed.

wrongful death statute [AS, *wrang, death;* L, *statuere,* to set up], (in law) a statute existing in all states that provides that the death of a person can give rise to a cause of legal action brought by the person's beneficiaries in a civil suit against the person whose willful or negligent acts caused the death. Before the existence of these statutes, a suit could be brought only if the injured person survived the injury.

wrongful life [OE, *wrang,* twisted; AS, *lif*]. See **wrongful birth.**

wrongful life action, (in law) a civil suit usually brought against a physician or health facility on the basis of negligence that resulted in the wrongful birth or life of an infant. The parents of the unwanted child seek to obtain payment from the defendant for the medical expenses of pregnancy and delivery, for pain and suffering, and for the ed-

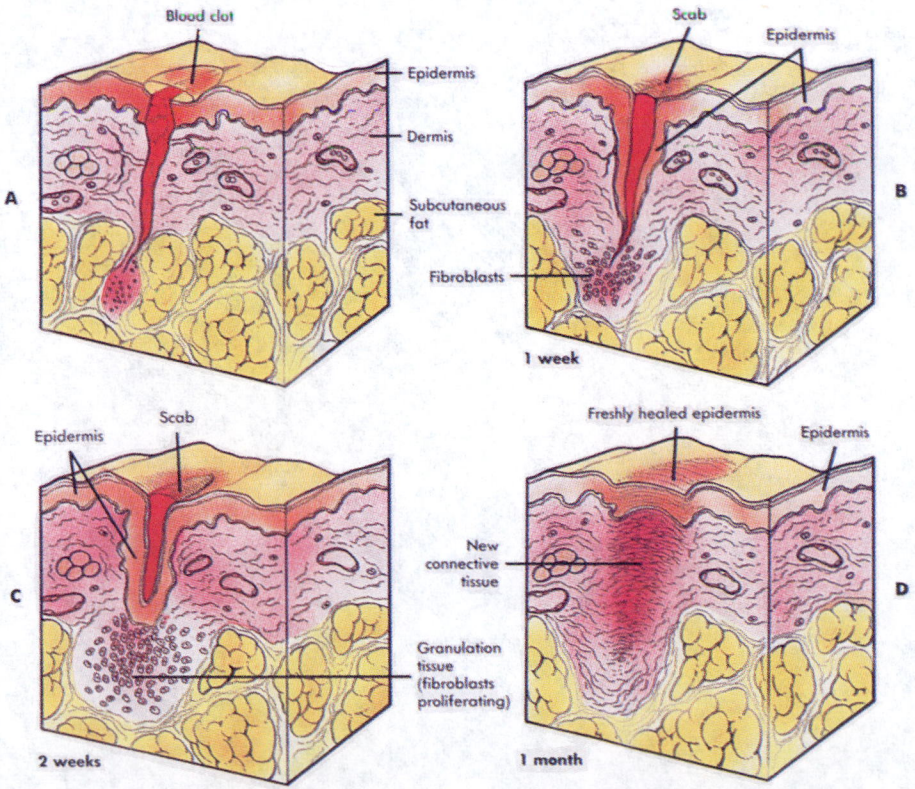

Stages of wound healing *(Seeley, 1992/Michael Schenk)*

ucation and upbringing of the child. Wrongful life actions have been brought and won in several situations, including malpracticed tubal ligations, vasectomies, and abortions. Failure to diagnose pregnancy in time for abortion and incorrect medical advice leading to the birth of a defective child also have led to malpractice suits for a wrongful life.

wryneck. See **torticollis.**

wt., abbreviation for **weight**.

Wuchereria /vōō′kərē′rē·ə/ [Otto Wucherer, German physician, b. 1820], a genus of filarial worms found in warm, humid climates. *Wuchereria bancrofti,* transmitted by mosquitoes, is the cause of elephantiasis. See also **filariasis.**

w/v, symbol for *weight per volume.*

W/V, abbreviation for *weight per volume.* See **weight per volume solution.**

w/w, symbol for *weight per weight.*

Wycillin, a trademark for an antibacterial (penicillin G procaine).

Wydase, a trademark for an enzyme (hyaluronidase).

Wymox, a trademark for an antibiotic (amoxicillin).

Wytensin, a trademark for an antihypertensive agent (guanabenz).

Wyvac, a trademark for a rabies virus vaccine (rabies human diploid cell vaccine).

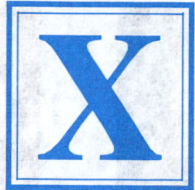

Xanax, a trademark for an antianxiety agent (alprazolam).

-xanox, a combining form for antiallergic respiratory tract drugs of the xanoxic acid group.

xanthelasma, xanthelasma palpebrarum. See **xanthoma palpebrarum.**

xanthelasmatosis /zan'thilaz'məto͞o'sis/ [Gk, *xanthos*, yellow, *elasma*, plate, *osis*, condition], a disseminated, generalized form of planar xanthoma frequently associated with reticuloendothelial disorders, especially multiple myeloma.

xanthemia. See **carotenemia.**

xanthene /zan'thēn/ [Gk, *xanthos*, yellow], a crystalline organic compound in which two benzene rings are fused to a central pyran ring. The pyran oxygen bridges the two benzene rings. It is a parent chemical structure of many medicinal elements.

xanthine /zan'thīn/ [Gk, *xanthos*, yellow], a nitrogenous byproduct of the metabolism of nucleoproteins. It is normally found in the muscles, liver, spleen, pancreas, and urine. **–xanthic,** *adj.*

xanthine base [Gk, *xanthos*, yellow], a purine compound occurring in plants and animals as a metabolite of adenine and guanine. It is the parent structure of the methyl xanthine alkaloids that include caffeine in coffee, theophylline in tea, and theobromine in cocoa.

xanthine derivative, any one of the closely related alkaloids caffeine, theobromine, and theophylline. They are found in plants widely distributed geographically and are variously ingested as components in different beverages, such as coffee, tea, cocoa, and cola drinks. The xanthine derivatives or methylxanthines have pharmacologic properties that stimulate the central nervous system, produce diuresis, and relax smooth muscles. Theobromine has low potency and is seldom used as a pharmaceutic. Caffeine produces greater central nervous system stimulation than theophylline or theobromine. Some experiments have shown that caffeine increases the capacity for sustained intellectual effort, decreases reaction time, and improves the association of ideas. Caffeine and theophylline also affect the circulatory system, tending to dilate the systemic blood vessels but increasing cerebrovascular resistance with an associated decrease in cerebral blood flow and the oxygen tension of the brain. Some authorities believe it is this vasoconstriction that accounts for the relief of hypertensive headaches in individuals who drink beverages that contain any of the xanthine derivatives. The ability of the xanthine derivatives to relax smooth muscle is especially important in certain treatments of asthma. Theophylline is most effective in such treatment and markedly increases vital capacity. The methylxanthines reinforce the release of certain secretions of various endocrine and exocrine tissues, except for mast cells and, possibly, certain other mediators of inflammation. Caffeine can induce chromosomal abnormalities in plant cells and in mammalian cells in culture, and it strongly augments mutations of microorganisms. Such effects are apparently associated with the retardation of DNA repair mechanisms but occur only at caffeine concentrations much higher than those in xanthine beverages, and usually in life forms lacking enzymes for metabolizing xanthines. Several studies offer contradictory conclusions as to whether daily ingestion of more than five to six cups of coffee increases the susceptibility to myocardial infarction. Research continues in an effort to determine the effect of caffeine on pregnant women who ingest it in large amounts. Various studies indicate that the per capita consumption of caffeine in the United States is 200 mg daily, about 90% of which comes from coffee. One cup of coffee contains approximately 100 mg of caffeine; one cup of tea contains about 50 mg of caffeine and 1 mg of theophylline. One cup of cocoa contains about 250 mg of theobromine and 5 mg of caffeine. A 350 ml bottle of a cola beverage contains about 35 mg of caffeine. Consumption of xanthine beverages may cause various problems, including restlessness and inability to sleep, GI irritation, and excessive myocardial stimulation characterized by premature systole and tachycardia.

xanthinuria /zan'thinyo͞or'ē·ə/ [Gk, *xanthos* + *ouron*, urine], **1.** the presence of excessive quantities of xanthine in the urine. **2.** a rare disorder of purine metabolism, resulting in the excretion of large amounts of xanthine in the urine because of the absence of an enzyme, xanthine oxidase, that is necessary in xanthine metabolism. This inherited deficiency may cause the development of kidney stones made of xanthine precipitate.

xantho-, a combining form meaning 'yellow': *xanthochroia, xanthogen, xanthophore.*

xanthochromia /zan'thəkro͞'mē·ə/, a pale yellow or straw-colored substance in cerebrospinal fluid. It is caused by the presence of hemoglobin breakdown products.

xanthochromic /zan'thəkro͞'mik/ [Gk, *xanthos* + *chroma*, color], having a yellowish color, such as cerebrospinal fluid that contains blood or bile. Also **xanthochromatic.**

xanthogranuloma /zan'thəgran'yəlo͞'mə/, *pl.* **xanthogranulomas, xanthogranulomata** [Gk, *xanthos* + L, *granulum*, little grain; Gk, *oma*, tumor], a tumor or nodule of granulation tissue containing lipid deposits. A kind of xanthogranuloma is **juvenile xanthogranuloma.**

xanthoma /zanthō'mə/, *pl.* **xanthomas, xanthomata** [Gk, *xanthos* + *oma*, tumor], a benign, fatty, fibrous, yellowish plaque, nodule, or tumor that develops in the subcutaneous layer of skin, often around tendons. The lesion is characterized by the intracellular accumulation of cholesterol and cholesterol esters.

xanthoma disseminatum, a benign, chronic condition in which small orange or brown papules and nodules develop on many body surfaces, especially on the mucous membrane of the oropharynx, larynx, and bronchi, and in skin folds and fissures. Also called **xanthoma multiplex.**

xanthoma eruptivum. See **eruptive xanthoma.**

xanthoma multiplex. See **xanthoma disseminatum.**

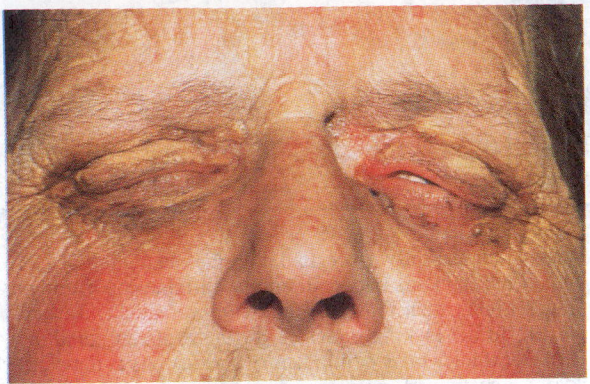

Necrobiotic xanthogranuloma
*(McKee, 1989/Courtesy Professor E Wilson Jones,
Institute of Dermatology, London)*

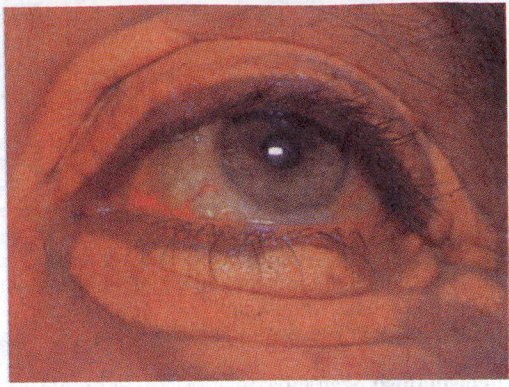

Xanthoma palpebrarum *(Newell, 1986)*

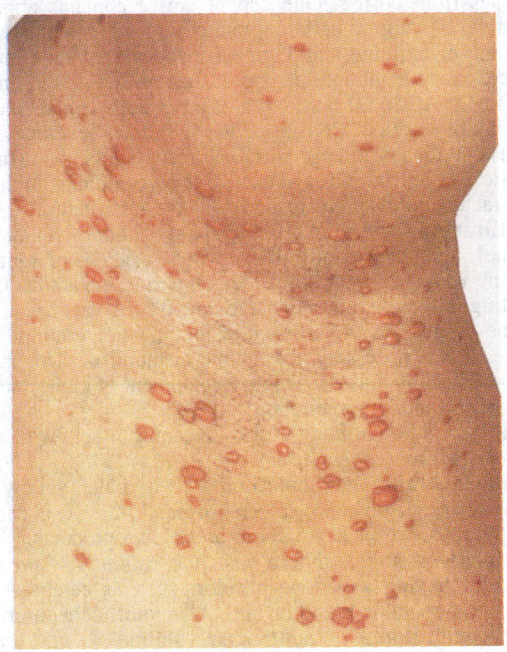

Xanthoma disseminatum *(du Vivier, 1993)*

xanthoma palpebrarum, a soft, yellow spot or plaque usually occurring in groups on the eyelids. Also called **xanthelasma, xanthelasma palpebrarum.**

xanthoma planum. See **planar xanthoma.**

xanthomasarcoma /zan′thōməsärkō′mə/, *pl.* **xanthomasarcomas, xanthomasarcomata,** [Gk, *xanthos, oma + sarx,* flesh, *oma,* tumor] a giant cell sarcoma of the tendon sheaths and aponeuroses that contains xanthoma cells.

xanthoma striatum palmare, a yellow or orange flat plaque or slightly raised nodule occurring in groups on the palms of the hands.

xanthoma tendinosum, a yellow or orange, elevated or flat, round papule or nodule occurring in clusters on tendons, especially the extensor tendons of the hands and feet, of individuals with hereditary lipid storage disease.

xanthomatosis /zan′thōmətō′sis/ [Gk, *xanthos, oma + osis,* condition], an abnormal condition in which there are deposits of yellowish fatty material in the skin, internal organs, and reticuloendothelial system. It may be associated with hyperlipoproteinemia, paraproteinemia, lipoid storage diseases, and other disorders of adipose tissue. Also called **xanthosis.** See also **lipemia, xanthoma, xanthoma palpebrarum.**

xanthoma tuberosum, a yellow or orange, flat or elevated, round papule occurring in clusters on the skin of joints, especially the elbows and knees, usually in people who have a hereditary lipid storage disease such as hyperlipoproteinemia. The xanthomatous papules also may be associated with biliary cirrhosis and myxedema. Also called **tuberous xanthoma, xanthoma tuberosum multiplex.**

xanthopsia /zanthop′sē·ə/ [Gk, *xanthos + opsis,* sight], an abnormal visual condition in which everything appears to have a yellow hue. It is sometimes associated with jaundice or digitalis toxicity.

xanthosis /zanthō′sis/ [Gk, *xanthos + osis,* condition], **1.** a yellowish discoloration sometimes seen in degenerating tissues of malignant diseases. **2.** See **xanthomatosis. 3.** also called **carotenosis.** a reversible yellow discoloration of the skin most commonly caused by the ingestion of large amounts of yellow vegetables containing carotene pigment. The antimalarial drug quinacrine, if taken over a prolonged period, may produce a similar skin color. Xanthosis may be differentiated clinically from jaundice because the sclerae are colored yellow in jaundice but are not discolored in xanthosis. See also **carotenemia.**

xanthureic acid /zanth′yo͞orē′ik/, a metabolite of tryptophan that occurs in normal urine and in elevated levels in patients with vitamin B_6 deficiency.

X chromosome, a sex chromosome that in humans and many other species is present in both sexes, appearing singly in the cells of normal males and in duplicate in the cells of normal females. The chromosome is carried as a sex determinant by all of the female gametes and one half of all male gametes, is morphologically much larger than the Y chromosome, and has many sex-linked genes associated with clinically significant disorders, such as hemophilia,

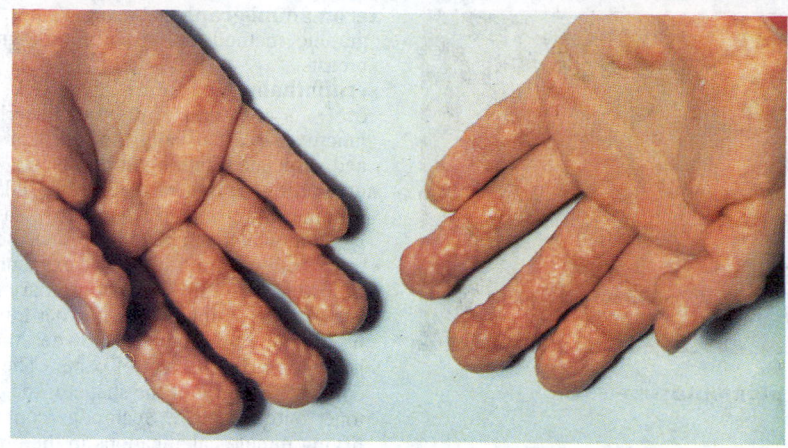

Xanthoma striatum palmare (de Vivier, 1993)

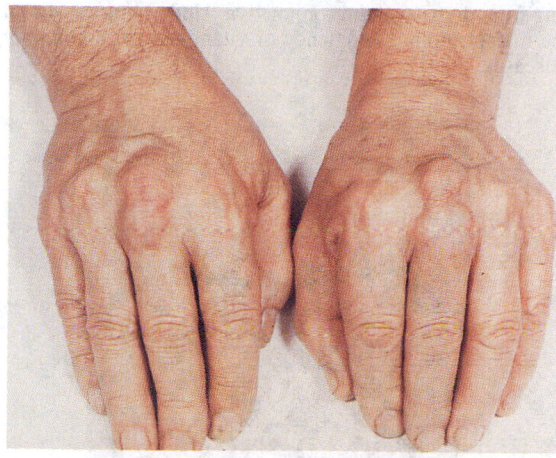

Xanthoma tendinosum
(Epstein, 1992/Courtesy Joan Slack,
Department of Clinical Genetics, Royal Free NHS Trust)

Duchenne's muscular dystrophy, and Hunter's syndrome. Compare **Y chromosome.**

Xe, symbol for the element **xenon.**

xeno- /zē'ne-, zen'ō-/, a combining form meaning 'strange or pertaining to foreign matter': *xenodiagnosis, xenogenous, xenology.*

xenobiotic /-bī·ot'ik/ [Gk, *xenos,* strange, *bios,* life], pertaining to organic substances that are foreign to the body, such as drugs or organic poisons.

xenogeneic /-jənē'ik/ [Gk, *xenos* + *genein,* to produce], **1.** (in genetics) denoting individuals or cell types from different species and different genotypes. **2.** (in transplantation biology) denoting tissues from different species that are therefore antigenically dissimilar. Also **heterologous.** Compare **allogenic, syngeneic.**

xenogenesis /-zen'əjen'əsis/, **1.** alternation of traits in successive generations; heterogenesis. **2.** the theoretic pro-

duction of offspring that are totally different from both of the parents. **–xenogenetic, xenogenic,** *adj.*

xenograft /zen'əgraft'/ [Gk, *xenos* + *graphion,* stylus], tissue from another species used as a temporary graft in certain cases, as in treating a severely burned patient when sufficient tissue from the patient or from a tissue bank is not available. It is quickly rejected but provides a cover for the burn for the first few days, reducing the amount of fluid loss from the open wound. Also called **heterograft.** Compare **allograft, autograft, isograft.** See also **graft.**

xenon (Xe) /-zen'on, zē'non/ [Gk, *xenos,* strange], an inert, gaseous, nonmetallic element. Its atomic number is 54; its atomic weight is 131.30.

xenon-133 [Gk, *xenos,* strange], a radioactive isotope of an inert colorless gas, used in radiographic studies of the lung.

xenophobia /-fō'bē·ə/ /zen'ə-, zē'nə-/ [Gk, *xenos* + *phobos,* fear], an anxiety disorder characterized by a pervasive, irrational fear or uneasiness in the presence of strangers, especially foreigners, or in new surroundings.

xero- /zir'ō-/, a combining form meaning 'pertaining to dryness': *xerocheilia, xeromenia, xerophthalmia.*

xeroderma /zir'ədur'mə/ [Gk, *xeros,* dry, *derma,* skin], a chronic skin condition characterized by dryness and roughness.

xeroderma pigmentosum (XP), a rare, inherited skin disease characterized by extreme sensitivity to ultraviolet light, exposure to which results in freckles, telangiectases, keratoses, papillomas, carcinoma, and possibly, melanoma. Keratitis and tumors developing on the eyelids and cornea may result in blindness. Exposure to sunlight must be avoided. See also **Kaposi's disease.**

xerogram /zir'əgram'/ [Gk, *xeros* + *gramma,* record], an x-ray image produced by xerography.

xerography /zirog'rəfē/ [Gk, *xeros,* dry + *graphein,* to record], a dry radiologic process in which an image is made on a metal plate coated with powdered selenium. The plate is electrically charged in a dark room. Exposure to light or x-rays causes the charge to be redistributed in a pattern proportional to the intensity of exposure in various areas of the plate. When 'developed' in a cloud of charged

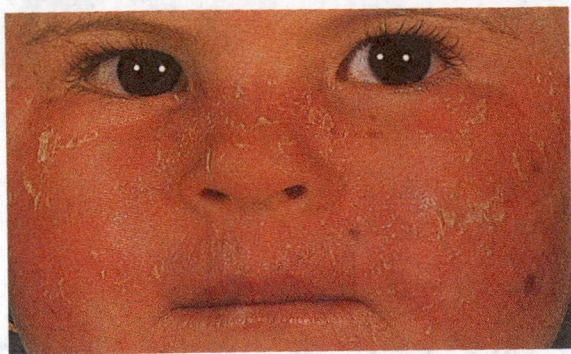

Xeroderma pigmentosum (du Vivier, 1986)

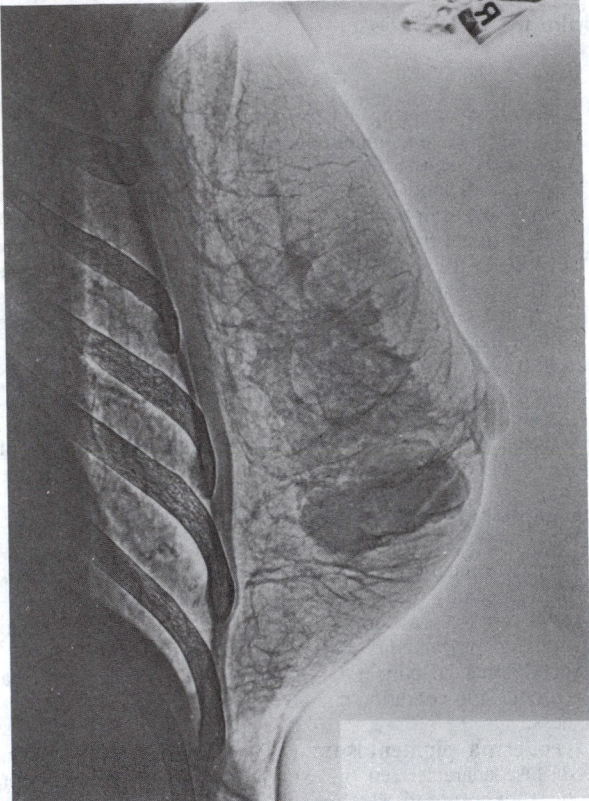

Xerogram (Ballinger, 1991)

particles, the particles are attracted to the areas discharged by radiation, producing the equivalent of a photographic negative.

xeromammogram /-mam′əgram′/, a type of breast radiograph in which the radiographic densities of the breast are reflected in discharges of a charged plate. The discharge pattern is made visible by depositing toner powder on the plate. The powder is transferred to paper, producing a permanent image. The plate is used again after recharging.

xeromammography /-mamog′rəfē/, the use of xerographic methods to produce radiographic images of the breasts.

xerophthalmia /zir′ofthal′mē·ə/ [Gk, xeros + ophthalmos, eye], a condition of dry and lusterless corneas and conjunctival areas, usually the result of vitamin A deficiency and associated with night blindness.

xeroradiography /-rā′dē·og′rəfē/ [Gk, xeros + L, radiare, to shine; Gk, graphein, to record], a diagnostic x-ray technique in which an image is produced electrically rather than chemically, permitting lower exposure times and radiation of lower energy than that of ordinary x-rays. The latent image is made visible with a powder toner similar to that used in a copying machine. The powder image is transferred, and heat is fused to a sheet of paper. The images exhibit "edge contrast" because of the shape of the electric fields that pull toner onto the plate. Such edge contrast is useful for identifying minute calcifications in the breast. Xeroradiography is used primarily for mammography.

xerosis. See **dry skin.**

xerotic keratitis /zirot′ik/ [Gk, xeros, dry + keras, horn + itis, inflammation], an inflammation of the cornea resulting from dryness of the conjunctiva. Underlying causes may be malnutrition, a deficiency of vitamin A, or autoimmune diseases.

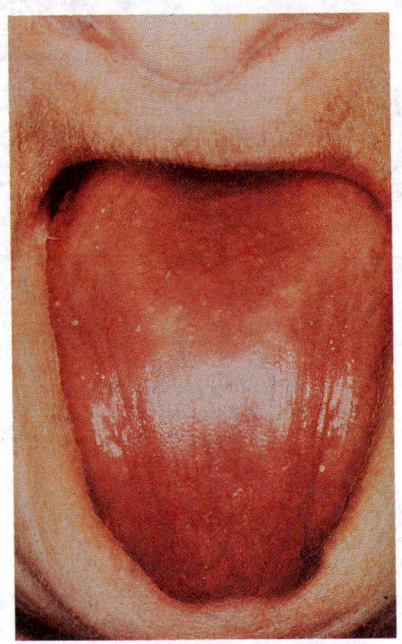

Xerostomia (Lamey, 1988)

xerostomia /zir′əstō′mē·ə/ [Gk, xeros + stoma, mouth], dryness of the mouth caused by cessation of normal salivary secretion. The condition is a symptom of various diseases, such as diabetes, acute infections, hysteria, and Sjögren's syndrome, and can be caused by paralysis of facial nerves. It is also a common adverse reaction to drugs.

Xi /zī, sī/, Ξ ξ, the fourteenth letter of the Greek alphabet.

X-inactivation theory. See **Lyon hypothesis.**

xiphi-. See **xipho-**.

xiphisternal articulation /zif′istur′nəl/ [Gk, *xiphos*, sword, *sternon*, chest; L, *articularis*, pertaining to joints], the cartilaginous connection between the xiphoid process and the body of the sternum. This joint usually ossifies at puberty. Compare **manubriosternal articulation**.

xiphisternum. See **xiphoid process**.

xipho-, xiphi-, a combining form meaning 'pertaining to a sword or to the xiphoid process': *xiphodymus, xiphoiditis, xiphopagus*.

xiphoid /zif′oid/ [Gk, *xiphos*, sword + *eidos*, form], shaped like a sword; the xiphoid process of the sternum.

xiphoid process /zif′oid/ [Gk, *xiphos* + *eidos*, form; L, *processus*, going forth], the smallest of three parts of the sternum, articulating caudally with the body of the sternum and laterally with the seventh rib. Several muscles of the abdominal wall are attached to the xiphoid process, including the rectus abdominis and the linea alba. Also called **ensiform process, xiphisternum, xiphoid, xiphoid appendix.** Compare **manubrium**.

X-linked /eks′lingkt/, pertaining to genes or to the characteristics or conditions they transmit that are carried on the X chromosome. Most X-linked traits and conditions, such as hemophilia, are recessive and therefore occur predominantly in males, because they have only one X chromosome. Women may inherit the genes, but the recessive effects are usually masked by the normal dominant alleles carried on the second X chromosome. Compare **Y-linked**. See also **sex-linked disorder.** –**X linkage**, *n.*

x-linked disorders, diseases and disorders associated with genetic abnormalities on the x-chromosomes. Examples are the muscular dystrophies and hemophilias.

X-linked dominant inheritance, a pattern of inheritance in which the transmission of a dominant gene on the X chromosome causes a characteristic to be manifested. Affected individuals all have an affected parent. All of the daughters of an affected male are affected but none of the sons. One half of the sons and one half of the daughters of an affected female are affected. Normal children of an affected parent have normal offspring. The inheritance shows a clear positive family history. Hypophosphatemic vitamin D-resistant rickets is an example of this pattern. X-linked dominant inheritance closely resembles autosomal dominant inheritance. Compare **X-linked recessive inheritance.**

X-linked ichthyosis. See **sex-linked ichthyosis.**

X-linked inheritance, a pattern of inheritance in which the transmission of traits varies according to the sex of the person, because the genes on the X chromosome have no counterparts on the Y chromosome. The inheritance pattern may be recessive or dominant. The characteristic determined by a gene on the X chromosome is always expressed in males. Transmission from father to son does not occur. Kinds of X-linked inheritance are **X-linked dominant inheritance** and **X-linked recessive inheritance.** Compare **autosomal inheritance.** See also **sex-linked.**

X-linked mucopolysaccharidosis. See **Hunter's syndrome.**

X-linked recessive inheritance, a pattern of inheritance in which transmission of an abnormal recessive gene on the X chromosome results in a carrier state in females and characteristics of the condition in males. Affected people have unaffected parents (except for the rare situation in which the father is affected and the mother is a carrier). One half of the female siblings of an affected male carry the trait. Unaffected male siblings do not carry the trait. Sons of affected males are unaffected, and daughters of affected males are carriers. Unaffected male children of a carrier female do not carry the trait. Compare **X-linked dominant inheritance.**

XO, (in genetics) the designation for the presence of only one sex chromosome; either the X or Y chromosome is missing so that each cell is monosomic and contains a total of 45 chromosomes. See also **Turner's syndrome.**

XP, abbreviation for **xeroderma pigmentosum.**

x radiation [*X*, an unknown quantity], radiation of electromagnetic energy in the wavelengths of 10^{-8} meters, longer than gamma rays but shorter than ultraviolet rays.

x-ray, 1. also called **roentgen ray.** electromagnetic radiation of shorter wavelength than visible light. X-rays are produced when electrons, traveling at high speed, strike certain materials, particularly heavy metals, such as tungsten. They can penetrate most substances and are used to investigate the integrity of certain structures, to therapeutically destroy diseased tissue, and to make photographic images for diagnostic purposes, as in radiography and fluoroscopy. **Discrete x-rays** are those with precisely fixed energies that are characteristic of differences between electron binding energies of a particular element. Tungsten, for example, has 15 different effective energies and no more, representing emissions from 5 different electron shells. **2.** also called **x-ray film.** a radiograph made by projecting x-rays through organs or structures of the body onto a photographic film. Because some tissue, such as bone, is more radiopaque (allowing fewer x-rays to pass through) than other tissue, such as skin or fat, a shadow is created on the film that is the image of a bone or of a cavity filled with a radiopaque substance. **3.** to make a radiograph. See also **contrast medium, electron, fluoroscopy, radiopaque.** –**x-ray**, *adj.*

x-ray dermatitis, a skin inflammation caused by exposure to x-rays. Excessive exposure to x-rays can lead to skin cancer.

x-ray fluoroscopy, real-time imaging using an x-ray source that projects through the patient onto a fluorescent screen or image intensifier. Image-intensified fluoroscopy has replaced conventional fluoroscopy in current practice.

x-ray microscope, a microscope that produces images by x-rays and records them on fine-grain film or projects them as enlargements. Film images produced by x-ray microscopes may be examined at large magnifications with a light microscope.

x-ray pelvimetry, a radiographic examination used to determine the dimensions of the bony pelvis of a pregnant woman and, if possible, the biparietal diameter of her baby's head. It is performed when there is doubt that the head can pass safely through the pelvis in labor. Images of the pelvis and the baby are projected radiographically onto film. After the film is developed, the images are measured. The measurements are corrected for distortion, and the true dimensions of the birth canal and head are calculated. Often the cephalopelvic relationship cannot be accurately evaluated from the films because the baby's head may be positioned in such a way that the biparietal diameter cannot be visualized. Because minor degrees of cephalopelvic disproportion are often overcome safely in labor by molding of the fetal skull, and because major disproportions may be detected by clinical pelvimetry without x-rays, the value of x-ray pelvimetry is frequently judged to be insufficient to warrant the risk of radiation exposure. Other diagnostic tools, among them ultrasonography, often provide the necessary information with less apparent risk. Compare **clinical pelvimetry.** See also **cephalopelvic disproportion, contraction, dystocia.**

x-ray technician. See **radiologic technologist.**

x-ray tube, a large vacuum tube containing a tungsten filament cathode and an anode that often is a rotating tungsten disk. When heated to incandescence, the cathode emits a cloud of electrons that produce x-rays when they strike the surface of the anode at high speed. The anode is designed to deflect the x-rays toward a focal spot in the object being radiographed. X-ray tubes are produced in a variety of designs for different purposes. Low-kilovoltage x-ray tubes may contain molybdenum rather than tungsten anodes; some anodes are stationary and others rotate at high speed. Because of the intense heat generated by x-ray production, the specific design usually includes devices to help dissipate the heat.

X-tra densities /ek′strə/, images on x-ray film caused by the presence of foreign objects, such as bullets or surgical clips, in the patient's body.

XX /ekseks′/, (in genetics) the designation for the normal sex chromosome complement in the human female. See also **X chromosome.**

XXX syndrome /trip′əleks′/, a human sex chromosomal aberration characterized by the presence of three X chromosomes and two Barr bodies instead of the normal XX complement, so that somatic cells contain a total of 47 chromosomes; trisomy X. The condition occurs approximately once in every 1000 live female births and is confirmed diagnostically by the presence of the extra Barr body in the cells. Individuals with the anomaly show no significant clinical manifestations, although there is usually some degree of mental retardation. Because there is selective migration of the X chromosome during meiosis, one half of the offspring of a trisomy X female will be both chromosomally and phenotypically normal. Also called **triple X syndrome.**

XXXX, XXXXX /fôreks′, fīveks′/, (in genetics) the designation for an abnormal sex chromosome complement in the human female in which there are, respectively, four or five instead of the normal two X chromosomes so that each somatic cell contains a total of 48 or 49 chromosomes. Although there is no consistent phenotype associated with such aberrations, the risk of congenital anomalies and mental retardation in the affected individual increases significantly with the increase in the number of X chromosomes.

XXXY, XXXXY, XXYY /thrē′ekswī, fôr′ekswī, dob′əleks′dob′əlwī′/, (in genetics) the designation for an abnormal sex chromosome complement in the human male in which there are more than the normal one X chromosome resulting, respectively, in a total of 48, 49, or more chromosomes in each somatic cell. The aberration is a variant of Klinefelter's syndrome; and, in general, the more X chromosomes there are, the greater the number of congenital defects and the severity of mental retardation in the affected individual. See also **Klinefelter's syndrome.**

XXY syndrome. See **Klinefelter's syndrome.**

XY /ekswī′/, (in genetics) the designation for the normal sex chromosome complement in the human male. See also **X chromosome, Y chromosome.**

xylitol /zī′litôl/, a sweet, crystalline pentahydroxy alcohol obtained by the reduction of xylose and used as a sweetener.

xylo-, a combining form meaning 'pertaining to wood': *xyloketosuria, xylose, xylosuria.*

Xylocaine, a trademark for a local anesthetic (lidocaine).

xylometazoline hydrochloride /zī′lōmetaz′əlēn/, an adrenergic vasoconstrictor.

■ INDICATIONS: It is prescribed in the treatment of nasal congestion in colds, hay fever, sinusitis, and other upper respiratory allergies.

■ CONTRAINDICATIONS: Glaucoma or known hypersensitivity to this drug or to sympathomimetic medications prohibits its use. It is used with caution in patients having cardiovascular disease.

■ ADVERSE EFFECTS: Among the more serious adverse reactions are irritation to the mucosa, rebound nasal congestion, and effects associated with systemic absorption, including sedation and alterations in cardiovascular function.

xylose /zī′lōs/, an aldopentose sugar produced by hydrolyzing straw and corn cobs. It is incompletely absorbed when taken by mouth and is used in diagnostic studies of the digestive tract.

XYY syndrome /eks′dob′əlwī′/, the phenotypic manifestation of an extra Y chromosome, which tends to have a positive effect on height and may have a negative effect on mental and psychologic development. However, the anomaly also occurs in normal males. See also **trisomy.**

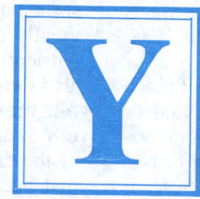

Y, symbol for the element **yttrium.**

-y, a suffix meaning 'a condition or processor having the nature or quality of': *gouty, myopathy.*

YACs, abbreviation for **yeast artificial chromosomes.**

yang, a polarized aspect of ch'i that is active or positive energy. See also **ch'i, yin.**

yaw /yô/ [Carib, *iaïa*], a lesion of the syphilis-like tropical disease of yaws. The initial lesion or primary sore is identified as the **mother yaw.**

yawn /yôn/ [AS, *geonian*], an involuntary act of opening the mouth wide and taking a deep breath. It tends to occur when a person is bored, drowsy, or depressed and may be accompanied by upper body movements to aid chest expansion.

yaws /yôs/ [Afr, *yaw,* raspberry], a nonvenereal infection caused by the spirochete *Treponema pertenue,* transmitted by direct contact and characterized by chronic, ulcerating sores anywhere on the body with eventual tissue and bone destruction, leading to crippling if untreated. It is a disease of unsanitary tropical living conditions and may be effectively treated with penicillin G. All serologic tests for syphilis may be positive in yaws. The infection may afford protection against syphilis. Also called **bouba, buba, frambesia, parangi, patek, pian.** Compare **bejel, pinta, syphilis.**

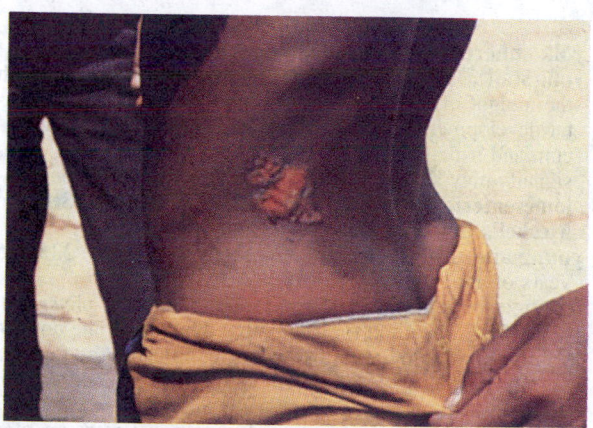

Yaws *(Hart, 1992)*

Yb, symbol for the element **ytterbium.**

Y chromosome, a sex chromosome that in humans and many other species is present only in the male, appearing singly in the normal male. It is carried as a sex determinant by one half of the male gametes and none of the female gametes, is morphologically much smaller than the X chromosome, and has genes associated with triggering the development and differentiation of male characteristics. There are no known medically significant traits or conditions associated with the genes on the Y chromosome. Compare **X chromosome.**

yeast /yēst/ [AS, *gist*], any unicellular, usually oval, nucleated fungus that reproduces by budding. *Candida albicans* is a kind of pathogenic yeast.

yeast artificial chromosomes (YACs), yeast chromosomes used in recombinant DNA procedures. They carry large segments of foreign DNA in the sequencing of nucleic acids.

yellow cartilage [AS, *geolu;* L, *cartilago*], the most elastic of the three kinds of cartilage, consisting of elastic fibers in a flexible fibrous matrix. It is yellow and is located in various parts of the body, such as the external ear, the auditory tube, the epiglottis, and the larynx. Also called **elastic cartilage.** Compare **hyaline cartilage, white fibrocartilage.**

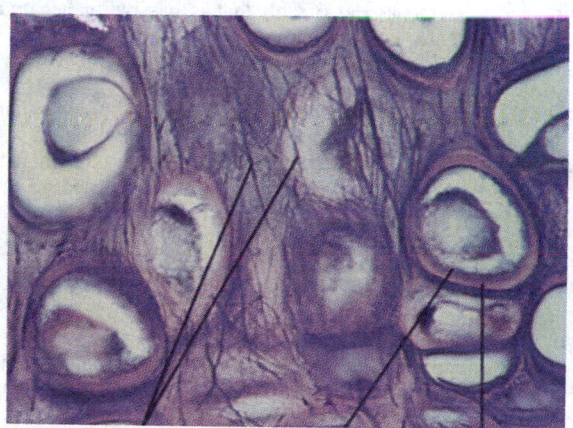

Yellow cartilage *(Seeley, 1992/Ed Reschke)*

yellow fever, an acute arbovirus infection transmitted by mosquitoes, characterized by headache, fever, jaundice, vomiting, and bleeding. There is no specific treatment, and mortality is about 5%. Recovery is followed by lifelong immunity. Immunization for travelers to endemic areas is advised. Nonhuman primates are a reservoir of infection.

yellow fever vaccine, a vaccine produced from live, attenuated yellow fever virus grown in chick embryos.

■ INDICATION: It is prescribed for immunization against yellow fever.

■ CONTRAINDICATIONS: Immunosuppression, pregnancy, or known hypersensitivity to chicken or egg protein prohibits its use.

■ ADVERSE EFFECTS: Among the more serious adverse effects are fever, malaise, and hypersensitivity reactions.

yellow marrow. See **bone marrow.**

Yersinia /yersin'ē·ə/ [Alexandre Emile Jean Yersin, French bacteriologist, b. 1863], a genus of nonmotile ovoid or rod-shaped gram-negative bacteria of the *Enterobacteriaceae* family. The genus includes *Y. pestis*, which causes plague in rats and humans, *Y. enterolitica*, a cause of enterocolitis and other diseases, and *Y. pseudotuberculosis*, a cause of pseudotuberculosis.

Yersinia arthritis [Alexandre E. J. Yersin, French bacteriologist, b. 1863], a polyarticular inflammation occurring a few days to 1 month after the onset of infection caused by *Yersinia enterocolitica* or *Y. pseudotuberculosis* and usually persisting longer than 1 month. Knees, ankles, toes, fingers, and wrists are most often affected. Cultures of synovial fluid yield no infectious organism. The clinical presentation may mimic juvenile rheumatoid arthritis, rheumatic fever, or Reiter's syndrome and may be associated with erythema nodosum or erythema multiforme. Treatment is with antibiotics.

Yersinia pestis [Alexandre Yersin; L, *pestis*, plague], a small, gram-negative bacillus that causes plague. The primary host is the rat, but other small rodents also harbor the organism. A person without symptoms may be a carrier, but this happens rarely. *Yersinia pestis* is hardy, living for long periods in infected carcasses, the soil of the host's habitat, or sputum. Also called **Pasteurella pestis.** See also **plague.**

Y fracture, a Y-shaped intercondylar fracture.

yin, a polarized aspect of ch'i that is passive or negative energy. See also **ch'i, yang**.

-yl, a suffix used in naming radicals: *benzoyl, ethyl, hydroxyl.*

-ylene, a suffix for chemical terms relating to a bivalent hydrocarbon radical, as in the reagent aminoxylene.

Y-linked /wī'lingkt/, pertaining to genes or to the characteristics or conditions they transmit that are carried on the Y chromosome. Such traits as hypertrichosis of the pinna of the ear can be expressed only in males. Compare **X-linked.** See also **sex-linked. – Y linkage,** *n.*

Yodoxin, a trademark for an antiamebic (diiodohydroxyquin).

yoga, a discipline that focuses on the body's musculature, posture, breathing mechanisms, and consciousness. The goal of yoga is attainment of physical and mental well-being through mastery of the body, achieved through exercise, holding of postures, proper breathing, and meditation.

yogurt /yō'gərt/ [Turk, *yoghurt*], a slightly acid, semisolid, curdled milk preparation made from either whole or skimmed cow's milk and milk solids by fermentation with organisms from the genus *Lactobacillus*. It is rich in vitamins of the B complex group and a good source of protein. It also provides a medium in the GI tract that retards the growth of harmful bacteria and aids in the absorption of minerals. Also spelled **yoghurt.**

yoke /yōk/ [L, *jungere*, to join], a connector used to link small cylinders of medical gases, such as portable oxygen tanks, to respiratory equipment.

yolk /yōk,yelk/[AS, *geolca*], the nutritive material, rich in fats and proteins, contained in the ovum to supply nourishment to the developing embryo. The amount and distribution of the yolk within the egg depend on the species of animal and type of reproduction and development of off-spring. In humans and most mammals the yolk is absent or greatly diffused through the cell, because embryos absorb nutrients directly from the mother through the placenta. See also **deutoplasm.**

yolk membrane. See **vitelline membrane.**

yolk sac, a structure that develops in the inner cell mass of the embryo and expands into a vesicle with a thick part that becomes the primitive gut and a thin part that grows into the cavity of the chorion. The cells of the extraembryonic mesoderm differentiate to develop endothelium, primitive blood plasma, and hemoglobin. After supplying the nourishment for the embryo, the yolk sac usually disappears during the seventh week of pregnancy. See also **allantois, Meckel's diverticulum.**

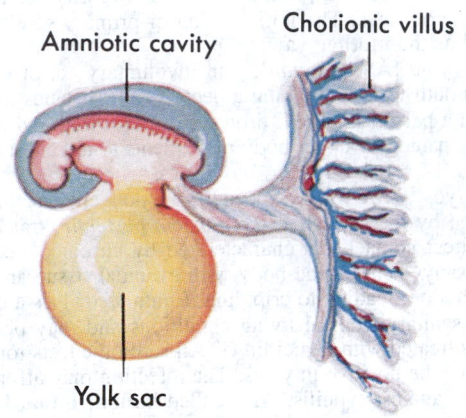

Amniotic cavity   Chorionic villus

Yolk sac

Yolk sac at three weeks *(Thibodeau, 1993/Ernest. W. Beck)*

yolk sphere. See **morula.**

yolk stalk, the narrow duct connecting the yolk sac with the midgut of the embryo during the early stages of prenatal development. It connects at the region of the future ileum and usually undergoes complete obliteration but occasionally may appear as a diverticulum. Also called **ophalomesenteric duct, umbilical duct, vitelline duct.** See also **Meckel's diverticulum.**

young and middle adult, the stages of life from 22 to 65 years of age.

Young's rule /yungz/ [Thomas Young, English physician, b. 1773], a method for calculating the appropriate dose of a drug for a child 2 years of age or more using the formula (age in years) ÷ (age + 12) × adult dose. See also **pediatric dosage.**

Y-plasty /wī'plas'tē/, a method of surgical revision of a scar, using a Y-shaped incision to reduce scar contractures. See also **Z-plasty.**

Y-set, a device composed of plastic components, used for delivering intravenous fluids through a primary intravenous line connected to a combination drip chamber filter section from which two separate plastic tubes lead to fluid sources. The Y-set also includes three clamps, one for the primary intravenous line and one for each of the two separate tubes. It is often used to transfuse packed blood cells that must be diluted with saline solution to decrease their viscosity. In such a transfusion one of the tubes is connected to the container enclosing the packed cells; the other tube is connected to the receptacle containing the saline solution. During a prolonged transfusion of packed blood cells, the tubing of the Y-set must be changed every 4 hours. Compare **component drip set, component syringe set, microaggregate recipient set, straight line blood set.**

ytterbium (Yb) /itur'bē·əm/ [Ytterby, Sweden], a rare earth metallic element. Its atomic number is 70; its atomic weight is 173.04.

yttrium (Y) /it'rē·əm/ [Ytterby, Sweden], a scaly, grayish metallic element. Its atomic number is 39; its atomic weight is 88.905. Radioactive isotopes of yttrium have been used in cancer therapy.

Yutopar, a trademark for a beta-adrenergic drug (ritodrine hydrochloride) used to stop premature labor.

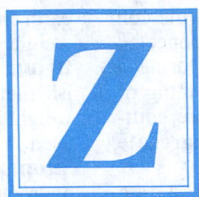

Zahorsky's disease. See **roseola infantum.**

Zakrzewski /zakshef'skē/, **Marie** (1829–1902), a Polish-German-American midwife who studied medicine in Berlin and spent some time in Kaiserwerth, Germany, before emigrating to the United States. In New York she met Elizabeth Blackwell, who encouraged her to continue her medical studies. After receiving her medical degree in Cleveland, she worked at Blackwell's New York Infirmary before going to Boston. In 1872 she organized the first successful American school of nursing at the New England Hospital for Women and Children.

zalcitabine the proposed generic name for the antiretroviral drug **dideoxycytidine (DDC).**

Zarontin, a trademark for an anticonvulsant (ethosuximide).

Zaroxolyn, a trademark for a diuretic and antihypertensive (metolazone).

Z band. See **Z disk.**

Z chromosome. See **W chromosome and Z chromosome.**

Z disk, a thin membrane seen on longitudinal sections as a dark line in striated muscle. It occurs in the center of an I band, the distance between z bands serving to delimit the striated sarcomeres. Also called **Amici's disk, Dobie's layer, intermediate disk, Krause's membrane, Z band, Z line.**

ZEEP, abbreviation for **zero-end expiratory pressure.**

Zenker's diverticulum /tseng'kerz/ [Friedrich A. Zenker, German pathologist, b. 1825; L, *diverticulare,* to turn aside], a circumscribed herniation of the mucous membrane of the pharynx as it joins the esophagus. Food may become trapped in the diverticulum and may be aspirated. Diagnosis is confirmed by x-ray studies. In most cases it is small, causes no dysfunction, is not diagnosed, and requires no treatment.

Zephiran Chloride, a trademark for a disinfectant (benzalkonium chloride).

zeranol /zer'ənol/, an estrogenic substance used to fatten livestock. Consumption of beef from zeranol-treated cattle has been associated with precocious puberty in some boys and girls.

zero /zir'ō/ [Ar, *sifr,* cipher], **1.** a symbol for nothing. **2.** the point on most scales from which measurements begin. **3.** absolute zero, the temperature at which there is no molecular movement, corresponding to −273.15° C on the Kelvin scale or −459.67° F.

zero-end expiratory pressure (ZEEP) [Ar, *zefiro;* ME, *ende*], pressure that has returned to ambient or atmospheric level at the end of exhalation.

zero fluid balance, a state in which the amount of fluid intake is equal to the amount of fluid output.

zero order kinetics, a state at which the rate of an enzyme reaction is independent of the concentration of the substrate.

zero population growth (ZPG), a situation in which there is no population increase during a given year because the total of live births is equal to the total of deaths.

zero-to-three infant stimulation groups, groups that provide therapeutic services for children from birth to 3 years of age, an age group not yet eligible for public school placement.

Zestril, a trademark for an angiotensin-converting enzyme (ACE) inhibitor and antihypertensive (lisinopril).

zeta /zē'tə,zā'tə/, Z, ζ, the sixth letter of the Greek alphabet.

zeta potential [Gk, *zeta,* sixth letter of Greek alphabet; L, *potentia,* power], the potential produced by the effective charge of a macromolecule, usually measured at the boundary between what is moving in a solution with the macromolecule and the rest of the solution.

Zetar, a trademark for a topical antieczematic containing coal tar.

zeugmatography /zōōg'mətog'rəfē/ [Gk, *zeugnynai,* to join, *graphein,* to record], another name for MR imaging coined from Greek roots suggesting the role of the gradient magnetic field in joining the rf magnetic field to a desired local spatial region through nuclear magnetic resonance.

zidovudine /zīdov'ədēn/, an HIV virus inhibitor, formerly called azidothymidine (AZT), that interferes with DNA synthesis. Trade name is Retrovir. See also **azidothymidine.**

Ziehl-Neelsen test /zēl'nēl'sən/ [Franz Ziehl, German physician, b. 1859; Friedrich K. A. Neelsen, German pathologist, b. 1854], one of the most widely used methods of acid-fast staining, commonly used in the microscopic examination of a smear of sputum suspected of containing *Mycobacterium tuberculosis.* See also **acid-fast stain.**

Ziehl's stain. See **carbol-fuchsin stain.**

ZIG, abbreviation for **zoster immune globulin.**

Zinacef, a trademark for a cephalosporin antibiotic (cefuroxime sodium).

zinc (Zn) /zingk/ [Ger, *Zink*], a bluish-white crystalline metal commonly associated with lead ores. Its atomic number is 30; its atomic weight is 65.38. Zinc is ductile in its pure form and occurs abundantly in minerals such as sphalerite, zincite, and franklinite. It has many commercial uses, such as a protective coating for steel and in printing plates. Zinc is an essential nutrient in the body and is used in numerous pharmaceutics, such as zinc acetate, zinc oxide, zinc permanganate, and zinc stearate. Zinc acetate is used as an emetic, a styptic, and an astringent. Zinc oxide is used internally as an antispasmodic and as a protective in ointments. Zinc permanganate is used as an astringent and in the treatment of urethritis by injection or douche in a 1:4000 solution. Zinc stearate is used as a water-repellent protective agent in the treatment of acne, eczema, and other skin diseases.

zinc chill. See **metal fume fever.**

zinc deficiency, a condition resulting from insufficient amounts of zinc in the diet, characterized by abnormal fatigue, decreased alertness, a decrease in taste and odor sensitivity, poor appetite, retarded growth, delayed sexual maturity, prolonged healing of wounds, and susceptibility to infection and injury. Other conditions that may precipitate the deficiency include alcoholic cirrhosis and other liver diseases, ulcers, myocardial infarction, Hodgkin's disease, Down syndrome, and cystic fibrosis. Prophylaxis and treatment consist of a diet of foods high in protein, which are also rich in zinc, including meats, eggs, liver, seafood, legumes, nuts, peanut butter, milk, and whole-grain cereals.

zinc finger, a loop or sequence of transcription factor subunits with a zinc atom linked to four carbon atoms at the base of a sequence. It is an important step in the cloning and sequencing of human general transcription factors.

zinc gelatin, a topical protectant for varicosities and other lesions of the lower limbs. It is available as a smooth jelly containing zinc oxide (10%), gelatin (15%), glycerin (40%), and purified water (35%). It is also available impregnated in gauze.

zinc ointment [Ger, *Zink;* OFr, *oignement*], a preparation of 20% zinc oxide in mineral oil or a white petrolatum semisolid base, used as a local surface treatment for various skin disorders. Some preparations also may contain salicylic acid.

zinc oxide, a topical protectant prescribed for a wide range of minor skin irritations.

zinc oxide and eugenol (ZOE), a dental cement composed primarily of zinc salts, eugenol, and rosin, used chiefly in temporary tooth fillings. It has low relative strength and abrasion resistance, but its nearly neutral pH causes minimal irritation to dental pulp. It is intended as a sedative dressing until pain subsides and a more permanent filling can be inserted.

zinc oxide eugenol dental cement, a luting agent consisting of a powder that is essentially zinc oxide with strengtheners and accelerators, combined with a liquid that is basically eugenol.

zinc phosphate dental cement, a material for luting of dental inlays, crowns, bridges, and orthodontic appliances and for some temporary restorations of dentitions. It is prepared by mixing a powder composed of zinc and magnesium oxides and a liquid composed of phosphoric acid, water, and buffering agents.

zinc salt poisoning, a toxic condition caused by the ingestion or inhalation of a zinc salt. Symptoms of ingestion include a burning sensation of the mouth and throat, vomiting, diarrhea, abdominal and chest pain, and, in severe cases, shock and coma. Treatment varies. Inhalation of zinc salts may cause metal fume fever; skin contact may produce blisters. A lethal dose of 10 g of zinc sulfate has been reported.

zinc sulfate, an ophthalmic astringent given in drops for nasal congestion or irritation of the eye, applied topically in deodorants, and given orally in tablets to promote healing and as a dietary supplement.

ZIP, abbreviation for *zoster immune plasma.* See **chickenpox.**

zirconium (Zr) /zərkō′nē·əm/ [Ar, *zarqun,* zircon], a steel-gray, tetravalent metallic element. Its atomic number is 40; its atomic weight is 91.22. It occurs widely in combined form, especially in zircon and baddeleyite. It is usually extracted from sands containing zircon by heating with carbon and chlorine and passing the resulting volatile zir-conium tetrachloride into hot molten magnesium or into sodium to yield a spongy form of the free metal. A component of zirconium dioxide was formerly used in some ointments for the treatment of poison ivy skin rashes, but such ointments caused skin granulomas in some individuals. Similar skin conditions developed in individuals using deodorants containing zirconium sodium lactate, and the use of zirconium compounds, except for zirconyl hydroxychloride, has been discontinued in the manufacture of skin ointments. Zirconyl hydroxychloride is still used in antiperspirants.

Z line. See **Z disk.**

Zn, symbol for the element **zinc.**

zoanthropy /zō·an′thrəpē/ [Gk, *zoon,* animal, *anthropos,* human], the delusion that one has assumed the form and characteristics of an animal. **−zoanthropic,** *adj.*

ZOE, abbreviation for **zinc oxide and eugenol.**

-zoite, a combining form meaning a 'simple organism' of a specified sort: *merozoite, saprozoite, sporozoite.*

Zollinger-Ellison syndrome /zol′injərel′isən/ [Robert M. Zollinger, American surgeon, b. 1903; Edwin H. Ellison, American physician, b. 1918], a condition characterized by severe peptic ulceration, gastric hypersecretion, elevated serum gastrin, and gastrinoma of the pancreas or the duodenum. The syndrome is uncommon but not rare; it may occur in early childhood but is seen more frequently in people between 20 and 50 years of age. Two thirds of the tumors are malignant. Total gastrectomy may be necessary, but the administration of cimetidine in large doses may control gastric hypersecretion and allow the ulcers to heal. See also **peptic ulcer.**

zona /zō′nə/, *pl.* **zonae** [L; Gk, *zone,* belt], a zone, or girdlike segment of a rounded or spheric structure. See also **zone.**

zona ciliaris. See **ciliary zone.**

zona fasciculata, the middle portion of the adrenal cortex, which is the site of production of glucocorticoids and sex hormones.

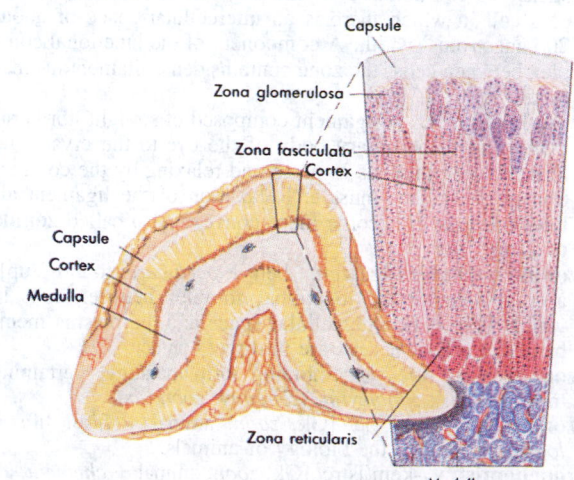

Structure of the adrenal gland, showing the zona fasciculata, zona glomerulosa, and zona reticularis
(Thibodeau, 1993/Ernest W. Beck)

zona glomerulosa, the outer portion of the adrenal cortex, where mineralocorticoids are produced.

zona pellucida /pəlōō'sidə/, the thick, transparent, noncellular membrane that encloses the mammalian ovum. It is secreted by the ovum during its development in the ovary and is retained until near the time of implantation. Also called **oolemma** /ō'əlem'ə/. See also **vitelline membrane.**

zona radiata, a zona pellucida that has a striated appearance caused by radiating canals within the membrane. Also called **zona striata.**

zona reticularis, the innermost portion of the adrenal cortex, which borders on the adrenal medulla portion of the gland. It acts in consort with the zona fasciculata in producing various sex hormones and glucocorticoids.

zona striata. See **zona radiata.**

Zondek-Aschheim test. See **Aschheim-Zondek test.**

zone [Gk, belt], an area with specific boundaries and characteristics, such as the epigastric, the mesogastric, or the hypogastric zones of the abdomen. See also **zona.**

zone of equivalence, a region of an antibody-antigen reaction in which concentrations of both reactants are equal.

zonesthesia /zō'nesthē'zhə/ [Gk, zone + aisthesis, feeling], a painful sensation of constriction, as of a bandage bound too tightly, especially experienced around the waist or abdomen. Also called **girdle sensation.**

zone therapy, the treatment of a disorder by mechanical stimulation and counterirritation of a body area in the same longitudinal zone as the affected organ or region.

zonifugal /zōnif'yəgəl/ [Gk, zone, belt; L, fugere, to flee], moving from within a zone or area outward.

zonography /zōnog'rəfē/ [Gk, zone + graphein, to record], an x-ray imaging technique used to produce films of body sections similar to those made by tomography. A very narrow exposure angle of less than 10 degrees is used in zonography, producing a focal zone of less than 1 inch in thickness.

zonula /zōn'yələ/, pl. **zonulae** [Gk, zone, belt], a small zone. Also called **zonule.**

zonula adherens [L, zone, belt + adhesio, adhaerere, to stick], a continuous zone running around the outer surface of a cell in which there is an intercellular space of about 200 angstroms' width. A component of the junctional complex between cells, the zone contains dense filamentous material.

zonula ciliaris, a ligament composed of straight fibrils radiating from the ciliary body of the eye to the crystalline lens, holding the lens in place and relaxing by the contraction of the ciliary muscle. Relaxation of the ligament allows the lens to become more convex. Also called **zonule of Zinn.**

zonula occludens [L, zona, belt + occludere, to close up], a component of the junctional complex between cells in which there is no intercellular space and the plasma membranes of adjacent cells are in direct contact.

zoo-, zo- /zō'ə-/, a combining form meaning 'pertaining to an animal': zooamylon, zoogony, zoonosis.

zoobiology /-bī·ol'əjē/ [Gk, zoon, animal + bios, life + logos, science], the biology of animals.

zoochemistry /-kem'istrē/ [Gk, zoon, animal + chemeia, alchemy], the biochemistry of animals.

zooerastia. See **bestiality.**

zoogenous /zō·oj'ənəs/ [Gk, zoon, animal, genein, to produce], acquired from or originating in animals. See also **zoonosis.**

zoograft /zō'əgraft/ [Gk, zoon + graphion, stylus], tissue of an animal transplanted to a human, such as a heart valve from a pig to replace a damaged heart valve in a human.

zoologist /zō·ol'əjist/ [Gk, zoon, animal + logos, science], a person concerned with the scientific study of animals.

zoology /zō·ol'əjē/, the study of animal life.

zoomania /zō·əmā'nē·ə/ [Gk, zoon + mania, madness], a psychopathologic state characterized by an excessive fondness for and preoccupation with animals. –**zoomaniac,** n.

-zoon, a combining form meaning a 'living being': dermatozoon, entozoon, hepatozoon.

zoonosis /zō·on'əsis, zō'ənō'sis/ [Gk, zoon + nosis, disease], a disease of animals that is transmissible to humans from its primary animal host. Some kinds of zoonoses are **equine encephalitis, leptospirosis, rabies,** and **yellow fever.**

zooparasite /zō·əper'əsīt/ [Gk, zoon + parasitos, guest], any parasitic animal organism. Kinds of zooparasites are **arthropods, protozoa,** and **worms.** –**zooparasitic,** adj.

zoopathology /-pəthol'əjē/, the study of the diseases of animals.

zoophilia /zō·əfil'ē·ə/ [Gk, zoon + philein, to love], **1.** an abnormal fondness for animals. **2.** (in psychiatry) a psychosexual disorder in which sexual excitement and gratification are derived from the fondling of animals or from the fantasy or act of engaging in sexual activity with animals. Also called **zoophilism** /zō·of'iliz'əm/. See also **paraphilia.** –**zoophile,** n., **zoophilic, zoophilous,** adj.

zoophobia /-fō'bē·ə/ [Gk, zoon + phobos, fear], an anxiety disorder characterized by a persistent, irrational fear of animals, particularly dogs, snakes, insects, and mice. The condition is seen more often in women than in men, nearly always begins in childhood, and can typically be traced to some frightening or unpleasant experience involving an animal. Treatment consists of psychotherapy to uncover the cause of the phobic reaction followed by behavior therapy, specifically the techniques of systemic desensitization and flooding.

zoopsia /zō·op'sē·ə/ [Gk, zoon + opsis, vision], a visual hallucination of animals or insects, often occurring in delirium tremens.

zootoxin /zō'ətok'sin/ [Gk, zoon + toxikon, poison], a poisonous substance from an animal, such as the venom of snakes, spiders, and scorpions. –**zootoxic,** adj.

zoster. See **herpes zoster.**

zosteriform /zoster'ifôrm/ [Gk, zoster, girdle; L, forma, form], resembling the pocks seen in herpes zoster infection.

zoster immune globulin (ZIG) /zos'tər/ [Gk, zoster + L, immunis, freedom; globulus, small sphere], a passive immunizing agent currently in limited experimental use for preventing or attenuating herpes zoster virus infection in immunosuppressed individuals who are at great risk of severe herpes zoster virus infection.

zoster ophthalmicus [Gk, zoster, girdle + ophthalmos, eye], a herpes infection of the eye, particularly of the optic nerve. The infection frequently involves the cornea. There may be lid edema, ciliary and conjunctival involvement, and pain. Keratitis may be severe. Scarring and glaucoma are common sequelae. Topical corticosteroids are commonly prescribed, and intraocular pressure is monitored.

Zovirax, a trademark for acyclovir, an antiviral drug active against herpesvirus.

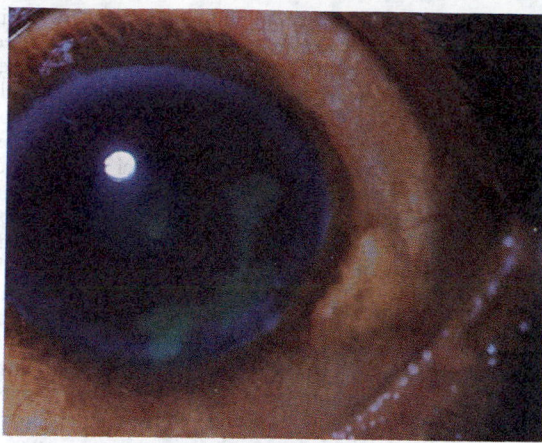

Zoster ophthalmicus (Apple, 1991)

ZPG, abbreviation for **zero population growth.**
Z-plasty /zē′plas′tē/, a method of surgical revision of a scar or closure of a wound using a Z-shaped incision to reduce contractures of the adjacent skin. See also **Y-plasty.**

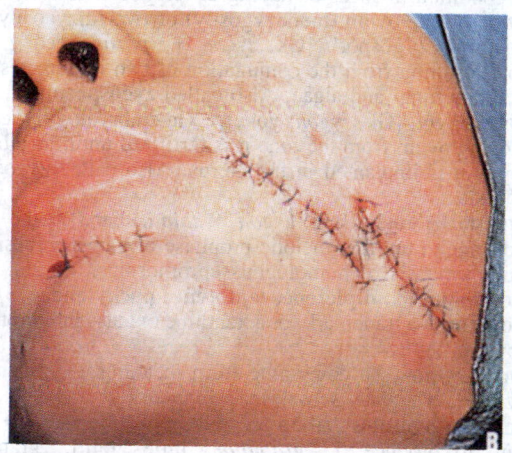

Revision of scar by Z-plasty (Grossman, 1993)

Zr, symbol for the element **zirconium.**
Z-track, a technique for injecting irritating preparations into muscle without tracking residual medication through sensitive tissues.
Zung Self-Rating Depression Scale, a 'self-report test' of 20 descriptors of depression on which clients rate themselves on a four-point scale ranging from 'a little of the time' to 'most of the time.' The scale is useful in determining the depth or intensity of a client's depression.
zwieback /zwī′bak, zwē′-/ [Ger, *zwie,* twice, *backen,* to bake], a sweetened bread that is enriched with eggs and baked, then sliced and toasted until dry and crisp. It is used as a snack food for children, especially teething infants.
zwitterion /trit′ərī′ən/, a molecule that has regions of both negative and positive charge. Amino acids, such as glycine, are almost always present as zwitterions when in neutral solutions. Also called **dipolar ion.**
zygo- /zī′gō-/ **zyg-,** a combining form meaning 'union or fusion, yoked or joined, pertaining to a junction or a pair': *zygomatic, zygogenesis, zygote.*
zygocyte. See **zygote.**
zygogenesis /zī′gōjen′əsis/ [Gk, *zygon,* yoke, *genesis,* origin], 1. the formation of a zygote. 2. reproduction by the union of gametes. **–zygogenetic, zygogenic,** *adj.*
zygoma /zīgō′mə, zig-/ [Gk, *zygon,* yoke], 1. a long slender zygomatic process of the temporal bone, arising from the lower part of the squamous portion of the temporal bone, passing forward to join the zygomatic bone, and forming part of the zygomatic arch. 2. the zygomatic bone that forms the prominence of the cheek.
zygomatic /-mat′ik/ [Gk, *zygoma,* bar], pertaining to the zygoma, or malar bone of the face.
zygomatic arch [Gk, *zygoma;* L, *arcus,* bow], an arch formed by the temporal process of the zygomatic bone with the zygomatic process of the temporal bone. The tendon of the temporal muscle passes beneath it.
zygomatic bone [Gk, *zygon; ban*], one of the pair of bones that forms the prominence of the cheek, the lower part of the orbit of the eye, and parts of the temporal and infratemporal fossae.
zygomatic head. See **zygomaticus minor.**
zygomatic process [Gk, *zygoma;* L, *processus*], 1. a projection of the frontal bone forming the lateral boundary of the superciliary arch. 2. a process of the maxilla. 3. a process of the temporal bone.
zygomatic reflex [Gk, *zygoma;* L, *reflectere,* to bend back],

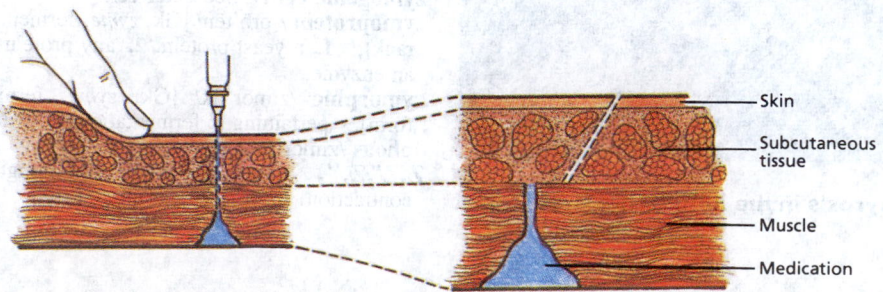

Z-track method of intramuscular injection
(Potter, 1993)

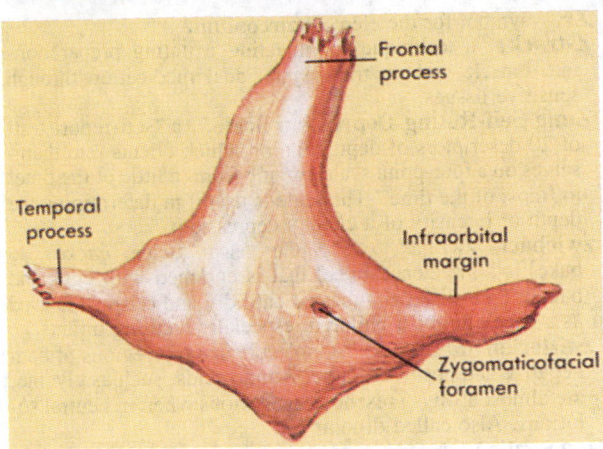

Zygomatic bone
(Seeley, 1992/David J Mascaro and Associates)

movement of the lower jaw toward the percussed side when the zygoma is tapped lightly but sharply.

zygomaticus major /zī′gōmat′ikəs/, one of the 12 muscles of the mouth. Arising from the zygomatic bone and inserting into the corner of the mouth, it is innervated by buccal branches of the facial nerve and acts to draw the angle of the mouth up and back to smile or laugh. Also called **zygomaticus.** Compare **zygomaticus minor.**

zygomaticus minor, one of the 12 muscles of the mouth. Arising from the malar surface of the zygomatic bone and inserting into the upper lip, it is innervated by buccal branches of the facial nerve and acts to deepen the nasolabial furrow in a sad facial expression. Also called **quadratus labii superioris, zygomatic head.** Compare **zygomaticus major.**

zygomaxillare. See **key ridge.**

zygomycosis /zī′gōmīkō′sis/ [Gk, *zygon* + *mykes*, fungus],

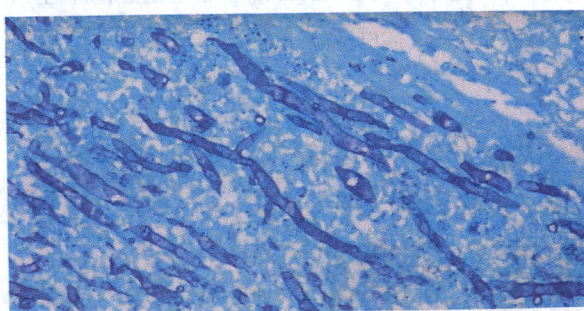

Zygomycosis in the lung *(Ioachim, 1989)*

an acute, often fulminant, and sometimes fatal fungal infection caused by a class of Phycomycetal water molds, seen primarily in patients with chronic debilitating diseases, especially uncontrolled diabetes mellitus. Characteristically, it begins with fever and with pain and discharge in the nose and paranasal sinuses that progresses to invade the eye and lower respiratory tract. The fungus may enter blood vessels and spread to the brain and other organs. Transmission is usually by inhalation. The diagnosis is confirmed by biopsy and pathologic examination of sputum. Treatment includes improved control of diabetes mellitus, extensive debridement of craniofacial lesions, and amphotericin B administered intravenously. Also called **mucormycosis.** Compare **phycomycosis.**

zygonema /zī′gənē′mə/ [Gk, *zygon* + *nema*, thread], the synaptic chromosome formation that occurs in the zygotene stage of the first meiotic prophase of gametogenesis. **–zygonematic,** *adj.*

zygosis /zīgō′sis/, a form of sexual reproduction in unicellular organisms, consisting of the union of the two cells and fusion of the nuclei. **–zygotic** /zīgot′ik/, *adj.*

zygosity /zīgos′itē/, the characteristics or conditions of a zygote. The form occurs primarily as a suffix combining form to denote genetic makeup, referring specifically to whether the paired alleles determining a particular trait are identical (homozygosity) or different (heterozygosity) or to the condition in twins of having developed from the fertilization of one ovum (monozygosity) or two (dizygosity).

zygospore /zī′gōspôr′/ [Gk, *zygon* + *sporos*, seed], the spore resulting from the conjugation of two isogametes, as in certain fungi and algae. Also called **zygosperm.**

zygote /zī′gōt/ [Gk, *zygon*, yoke], (in embryology) the developing ovum from the time it is fertilized until, as a blastocyst, it is implanted in the uterus. Also called **zygocyte** /zi′gəsīt/.

zygotene /zī′gətēn/ [Gk, *zygon* + *tainia*, band], the second stage in the first meiotic prophase of gametogenesis in which synapsis of homologous chromosomes occurs. See also **diakinesis, diplotene, leptotene, pachytene.**

Zyloprim, a trademark for a xanthine oxidase inhibitor (allopurinol).

-zyme, zymo-, a combining form meaning a 'ferment or enzyme': *lysozyme, serozyme, zymophore.*

zymogen granules /zi′məjən/ [Gk, *zyme*, ferment + *genein*, to produce; L, *granulum*, little grain], granules found in some secretory exocrine cells. They contain the precursors of enzymes that become active after the granules leave the cell.

zymogenic cell. See **chief cell.**

zymoprotein /-prō′tēn/ [Gk, *zyme*, ferment + *proteios*, first rank], **1.** a yeast protein. **2.** any protein that functions as an enzyme.

zymorphic /zīmôr′fik/ [Gk, *zyme*, ferment + *morphe*, form], pertaining to fermentation properties. Also **zymorphous** /zīmôr′fəs/.

Z.Z'.Z.'', symbol for increasing strength or intensity of contraction.

ILLUSTRATION CREDITS

Al-Azzawi F: *Color atlas of childbirth and obstetric techniques*, London, 1991, Wolfe Medical Publishing.

Ansell BM, Rudge S, Schaller JG: *Color atlas of pediatric rheumatology*, London, 1992, Wolfe Medical Publishing.

Apple DJ, Rabb MF: *Ocular pathology*, ed 4, St Louis, 1991, Mosby.

Avery JK: *Essentials of oral histology and embryology*, St Louis, 1992, Mosby.

Bain BJ: *Blood cells: a practical guide*, London, 1989, Gower Medical Publishing.

Ball K: *Lasers: the perioperative challenge*, St Louis, 1990, Mosby.

Ballinger PW: *Merrill's atlas of radiographic positions and radiologic procedures*, vol III, ed 7, St Louis, 1991, Mosby.

Baran R, Dawber RPR, Levene GM: *Color atlas of the hair, scalp, and nails*, London, 1991, Wolfe Medical Publishing.

Baron EJ, Finegold SM: *Bailey and Scott's diagnostic microbiology*, ed 8, St Louis, 1990, Mosby.

Barrison IG, Anderson MG, McIntyre PB: *Gastroenterology in practice*, London, 1992, Gower Medical Publishing.

Beare PG, Myers JL: *Principles and practice of adult health nursing*, ed 2, St Louis, 1994, Mosby.

Bedford MA: *Color atlas of ophthalmological diagnosis*, ed 2, London, 1986, Wolfe Medical Publishing.

Belcher AE: *Cancer nursing*, St Louis, 1992, Mosby.

Bennett JC, McLaughlin RP: *Orthodontic treatment mechanics and the preadjusted appliance*, London, 1993, Wolfe Medical Publishing.

Berkovitz BkB, Holland GR, Moxham BJ: *Color atlas and textbook of anatomy, histology, and embryology*, ed 2, London, 1992, Mosby–Year Book-Europe.

Berne RM, Levy MN: *Physiology*, ed 2, St Louis, 1988, Mosby.

Besser GM, Cudworth AG: *Clinical endocrinology*, London, 1987, Gower Medical Publishing.

Bingham BJG, Hawke M, Kwok P: *Atlas of clinical otolaryngology*, St Louis, 1992, Mosby.

Bobak IM, Jensen MD: *Maternity and gynecologic care: the nurse and the family*, ed 5, St Louis, 1993, Mosby.

Bodansky HJ: *Pocket picture guide to diabetes*, London, 1989, Gower Medical Publishing.

Bray TJ: *Techniques in fracture fixation*, London, 1993, Gower Medical Publishing.

Brooks-Tighe SM: *Instrumentation for the operating room*, ed 3, St Louis, 1989, Mosby.

Brostoff J, Scadding GK, Male D, Roitt IM: *Clinical immunology*, London, 1991, Gower Medical Publishing.

Brundage DJ: *Renal disorders*, St Louis, 1992, Mosby.

Bryant RA: *Acute and chronic wounds*, St Louis, 1992, Mosby.

Bullough PG, Boachie-Adje O: *Atlas of spinal diseases*, London, 1988, Gower Medical Publishing.

Cannobbio MM: *Cardiovascular disorders*, St Louis, 1990, Mosby.

Cawson RA, Eveson JW: *Oral pathology and diagnosis*, London, 1987, Heinemann Medical Books/Gower Medical Publishing.

Cerio R, Jackson WF: *A colour atlas of allergic skin disorders*, London, 1992, Wolfe Medical Publishing.

Chessel GSJ, Jamieson MJ, Morton RA, Petrie TC, Towler HMA: *Diagnostic tests in clinical medicine*, London, 1985, Wolfe Medical Publishing.

Chipps EM, Clanin NJ, Campbell VG: *Neurologic disorders*, St Louis, 1992, Mosby.

Christiansen JL, Grzybowski JM: *Biology of aging*, St Louis, 1993, Mosby.

Dickason EJ, Schult MO, Silverman BL: *Maternal and infant nursing*, ed 2, St Louis, 1994, Mosby.

Dieppe PA et al: *Atlas of clinical rheumatology*, London, 1986, Gower Medical Publishing.

Donaldson DD: *Atlas of the eye: the crystalline lens*, St Louis, 1976, Mosby.

Doughty DB, Broadwell Jackson D: *Gastrointestinal disorders*, St Louis, 1993, Mosby.

du Vivier A: *Atlas of clinical dermatology*, ed 2, London, 1993, Gower Medical Publishing.

Dyken PR, Miller MD: *Facial features of neurologic syndromes*, St Louis, 1980, Mosby.

Dynski-Klein M: *Color atlas of pediatrics*, London, 1986, Wolfe Medical Publishing.

Dynski-Klein M: *400 Self-assessment picture tests in clinical medicine*. Year Book Medical Publishers, Inc.

Edge V and Miller M: *Women's health care*, St. Louis, 1994, Mosby.

Eagling EM, Roper-Hall MJ: *Eye injuries*, London, 1986, Gower Medical Publishing.

England MA, Wakely J: *Color atlas of the brain and spinal cord*, London, 1992, Wolfe Medical Publishing.

Epstein O, Perkin GD, deBono DP, Cookson J: *Clinical examination*, London, 1992, Gower Medical Publishing.

Erlandsen SL, Magney J: *Color atlas of histology*, St Louis, 1992, Mosby.

Farrar WE, Wood MJ, Innes JA, Tubbs H: *Pocket picture guide of infectious diseases*, ed 2, London, 1992, Gower Medical Publishing.

Fireman P, Slavin RG: *Atlas of allergies*, London, 1990, Gower Medical Publishing.

Fletcher CDM, McKee PH: *An atlas of gross pathology*, London, 1987, Gower Medical Publishing.

Forbes CD, Jackson WF: *A color atlas and text of clinical medicine*, London, 1993, Mosby–Year Book-Europe.

Geenen JE, Fleischer DE, Waye JD: *Techniques in therapeutic endoscopy*, ed 2, London, 1992, Gower Medical Publishing.

Goldman MD: *Sclerotherapy*, St Louis, 1991, Mosby.

Goldstein BJ, Goldstein AO: *Practical dermatology*, St Louis, 1992, Mosby.

Gottfried SS: *Biology today*, St Louis, 1993, Mosby.

Gray M: *Genitourinary disorders*, St Louis, 1992, Mosby.

Greenberger NJ, Hinthorn DR: *History taking and physical examination: essentials and clinical correlates*, St Louis, 1993, Mosby.

Grimes DE: *Infectious diseases*, St Louis, 1991, Mosby.

Grossman JA: *Atlas of minor injuries*, St Louis, 1993, Gower Medical Publishing.

Grundy JR, Jones JG: *A color atlas of clinical operative dentistry crowns and bridges*, ed 2, London, 1992, Wolfe Medical Publishing.

Guzzetta CE, Dossey Montgomery B: *Cardiovascular nursing: holistic practice*, St Louis, 1992, Mosby.

Habif TP: *Clinical dermatology*, ed 2, St Louis, 1990, Mosby.

Hart CA, Broadhead RL: *Color atlas of pediatric infectious diseases*, London, 1992, Wolfe Medical Publishing.

Hayhoe FGJ, Flemans RJ: *Color atlas of hematological cytology*, ed 3, London, 1992, Wolfe Medical Publishing.

Hewitt PE: *Pocket picture guide: blood diseases*, London, 1985, Gower Medical Publishing.

Holgate ST, Church MK: *Allergy*, London, 1993, Gower Medical Publishing.

Houghton GR: *Pocket picture guide to spine injuries*, London, 1989, Gower Medical Publishing.

Hunt RB: *Atlas of female infertility surgery*, ed 2, St Louis, 1992, Mosby.

Hunter JM, Schneider LH, Mackin EJ, Callahan AD: *Rehabilitation of the hand*, ed 3, St Louis, 1990, Mosby.

Ioachim HL: *Pathology of AIDS*, London, 1989, Gower Medical Publishing.

Jaffe NS: *Atlas of ophthalmic surgery*, London, 1990, Gower Medical Publishing.

Johnson LL: *Diagnostic and surgical arthroscopy of the shoulder*, St Louis, 1993, Mosby.

Jordan RE: *Esthetic composite bonding*, ed 2, St Louis, 1993, Mosby–Year Book-Europe.

Judd RL, Ponsell PP: *Mosby's first responder*, ed 2, St Louis, 1988, Mosby.

Kamal A, Brockelhurst JC: *Color atlas of geriatric medicine*, ed 2, St Louis, 1991, Mosby–Year Book-Europe.

Lambert HP, Farar W: *Infectious diseases illustrated*, London, 1982, Gower Medical Publishing.

Lamey P, Lewis MAO: *Pocket picture guide to oral medicine*, London, 1988, Gower Medical Publishing.

Levene GM, Goolamali SK: *Diagnostic picture tests in dermatology*, London, 1986, Wolfe Medical Publishing.

Lewis MM, Weiner LS: *Pocket picture guide to orthopedics*, London, 1989, Gower Medical Publishing.

Lloyd-Davies RW et al: *Color atlas of urology*, Chicago, 1983, Year Book Medical Publishers.

London PS: *Color atlas of diagnosis after recent injury*, London, 1990, Wolfe Medical Publishing.

Malasanos L, Barkauskas V, Stoltenberg-Allen K: *Health assessment*, ed 4, St Louis, 1990, Mosby.

McKee PH: *A concise atlas of dermatopathology*, London, 1993, Gower Medical Publishing.

McKee PH: *Pathology of the skin*, London, 1989, Gower Medical Publishing.

McLaren DS: *Color atlas and text of diet-related disorders*, London, 1992, Wolfe Medical Publishing.

Misiewicz JJ, Bartram CI, Cotton PB, et al: *Atlas of clinical gastroenterology*, London, 1985, Gower Medical Publishing.

Mitros FA: *Atlas of gastrointestinal pathology*, London, 1988, Gower Medical Publishing.

Morison M: *A colour guide to the nursing management of wounds*, London, 1992, Wolfe Medical Publishers.

Morse SA: *Atlas of sexually transmitted diseases*, London, 1990, Gower Medical Publishing.

Mourad LA: *Orthopedic disorders*, St Louis, 1991, Mosby.

Mudge-Grout CL: *Immunologic disorders*, St Louis, 1992, Mosby.

Muller R, Baker JR; *Medical parasitology*, London, 1990, Gower Medical Publishing.

Murray PR, Drew WL, Kobayashi GS, Thompson JH Jr: *Medical microbiology*, St Louis, 1990, Mosby.

Newell FW: *Ophthalmology: principles and concepts*, ed 6, St Louis, 1986, Mosby.

Okazaki H, Scheithauer BW: *Atlas of neuropathology*, London, 1988, Gower Medical Publishing.

Parkin JM, Peters BS: *Differential diagnosis in AIDS*, London, 1991, Wolfe Medical Publishing.

Parsons M: *Color atlas of clinical neurology*, ed 2, London, 1993, Wolfe Medical Publishing.

Payne WA, Hahn DB: *Understanding your health*, ed 2, St Louis, 1989, Mosby.

Perkin GD, Rose FC, Blackwood W, Shawdon HH: *Atlas of clinical neurology*, London, 1986, Gower Medical Publishing.

Phipps WJ, Long BC, Woods NC, Cassmeyer VL: *Medical-surgical nursing: concepts and clinical practice*, ed 4, St Louis, 1991, Mosby.

Potter PA, Perry AG: *Basic nursing*, ed 2, St Louis, 1991, Mosby.

Potter PA, Perry AG: *Fundamentals of nursing*, ed 3, St Louis, 1993, Mosby.

Powers LW: *Diagnostic hematology*, St Louis, 1989, Mosby.

Raven PH, Johnson GB: *Biology*, ed 3, St Louis, 1992, Mosby.

Rosato FE, Barbot DJ: *Atlas of general surgical technique*, London, 1992, Gower Medical Publishing.

Rudy EB: *Advanced neurologica and neurosurgical surgery*, St Louis, 1984, Mosby.

Salyer KE: *Techniques in aesthetic craniofacial surgery*, London, 1989, Gower Medical Publishing.

Schumacher HR, Gall EP: *Rheumatoid arthritis*, London, 1988, Gower Medical Publishing.

Seeley RS, Stephens TD, Tate P: *Anatomy and physiology*, ed 2, St Louis, 1992, Mosby.

Seidel HM, Ball JB, Dains JE, Benedict GW: *Mosby's guide to physical examination*, ed 2, St Louis, 1991, Mosby.

Shingleton BJ, Hersh PS, Kenyon KR: *Eye trauma*, St Louis, 1991, Mosby.

Shipley M: *Pocket picture guide to rheumatology*, London, 1984, Gower Medical Publishing.

Shipley M: *A colour atlas of rheumatology*, ed 3, London, 1993, Mosby–Year Book-Europe.

Skarin AT: *Atlas of diagnostic oncology*, London, 1991, Gower Medical Publishing.

Sorrentino SA: *Mosby's textbook for nursing assistants*, ed 3, St Louis, 1992, Mosby.

Spitz L et al: *Color atlas of pediatric surgical diagnosis*, London, 1981, Wolfe Medical Publishing.

Stein HA, Slatt JB, Stein RM: *The ophthalmic assistant: fundamentals and clinical practice*, ed 5, St Louis, 1988, Mosby.

Stone LA, Lindfield EM, Robertson S: *Color atlas of nursing procedures in skin disorders*, London, 1989, Wolfe Medical Publishing.

Summanen P, Baron EJ, Citron DM, Strong C, Wexler HM, and Finegold SM: *Wadsworth anaerobic bacteriology manual*, ed 5, 1993. Reprinted with permission of Star Publishing Company, Belmont, CA.

Swales JD, Sever PS, Peart WS: *Clinical atlas of hypertension*, London, 1991, Gower Medical Publishing.

Thelan LA, Joseph KD, Urden LD: *Textbook of critical care nursing: diagnosis and management*, St Louis, 1990, Mosby.

Thibodeau GA, Patton KT: *Anatomy and physiology,* ed 2, St Louis, 1993, Mosby.

Thompson JL, McFarland GK, Hirsch JE, Tucker SM: *Mosby's clinical nursing,* ed 3, St Louis, 1993, Mosby.

Tilton RC, Ballows A, Hohnadel DC, Reiss RF: *Clinical laboratory medicine,* St Louis, 1992, Mosby.

Trotot PM: *Imaging of AIDS,* St Louis, 1991, Mosby.

Turk JL, Fletcher CDM: *RSCE slide atlas for pathology,* London, 1986, Gower Medical Publishing.

Turner-Warwick M, Hodson ME, Corrin B, Kerr IH: *Clinical atlas of respiratory diseases,* London, 1993, Gower Medical Publishing.

Vidic B, Suarez FR: *Color atlas of the human body,* St Louis, 1984, Mosby.

Wade JF: *Comprehensive respiratory care,* ed 3, St Louis, 1982, Mosby.

Wardlaw GM, Insel PM: *Perspectives in nutrition,* ed 2, St Louis, 1993, Mosby.

Weiss MA, Mills SE: *Atlas of genitourinary tract disorders,* London, 1988, Gower Medical Publishing.

Weston WL, Lane AT: *Color textbook of pediatric dermatology,* St Louis, 1991, Mosby.

Williams G, Mallick NP: *Color atlas of renal diseases,* ed 2, St Louis, 1993, Mosby.

Wilson SF, Thompson JM: *Respiratory disorders,* St Louis, 1990, Mosby.

Winawer SJ: *Management of gastrointestinal diseases,* London, 1992, Gower Medical Publishing.

Witzig JW, Spahl TJ: *The clinical management of basic maxillofacial orthopedic appliances, vol III: Temporomandibular joint,* St Louis, 1991, Mosby.

Wong DL: *Whaley and Wong's essentials of pediatric nursing,* ed 4, St Louis, 1993, Mosby.

Zacarian SA: *Cryosurgery,* St Louis, 1985, Mosby.

Zitelli BJ, Davis HW: *Atlas of pediatric physical diagnosis,* ed 2, London, 1992, Gower Medical Publishing.

APPENDIXES

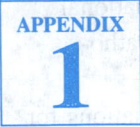

NORMAL REFERENCE VALUES

1-1 Normal reference laboratory values

Blood, plasma, or serum values

Test	Reference range	
	Conventional values	SI units
Acetoacetate plus acetone	0.30-2.0 mg/dl	3-20 mg/l
Acetone	Negative	Negative
Acid phosphatase	Adults: 0.10-0.63 U/ml (Bessey-Lowry)	28-175 nmol/s/L
	0.5-2.0 U/ml (Bodansky)	
	1.0-4.0 U/ml (King-Armstrong)	
	Children: 6.4-15.2 U/L	
Activated partial thromboplastin time (APTT)	30-40 sec	30-40 sec
Adrenocorticotropic hormone (ACTH)	6 AM 15-100 pg/ml	10-80 ng/L
	6 PM <50 pg/ml	<50 ng/L
Alanine aminotransferase (ALT)	5-35 IU/L	5-35 U/L
Albumin	3.2-4.5 g/dl	35-55 g/L
Alcohol	Negative	Negative
Aldolase	Adults: 3.0-8.2 Sibley-Lehninger units/dl	22-59 mU/L at 37° C
	Children: approximately 2 × adult values	
	Newborns: approximately 4 × adult values	
Aldosterone	Peripheral blood:	
	Supine: 7.4 ± 4.2 ng/dl	0.08-0.3 nmol/L
	Upright: 1-21 ng/dl	0.14-0.8 nmol/L
	Adrenal vein: 200-800 ng/dl	
Alkaline phosphatase	Adults: 30-85 ImU/ml	
	Children and adolescents:	
	<2 years: 85-235 ImU/ml	
	2-8 years: 65-210 ImU/ml	
	9-15 years: 60-300 ImU/ml	
	(active bone growth)	
	16-21 years: 30-200 ImU/ml	
Alpha-aminonitrogen	3-6 mg/dl	2.1-3.9 mmol/L
Alpha-1-antitrypsin	>250 mg/dl	
Alpha fetoprotein (AFP)	<25 ng/ml	
Ammonia	Adults: 15-110 μg/dl	47-65 μmol/L
	Children: 40-80 μg/dl	
	Newborns: 90-150 μg/dl	
Amylase	56-190 IU/L	25-125 U/L
	80-150 Somogyi units/ml	
Angiotensin-converting enzyme (ACE)	23-57 U/ml	
Antinuclear antibodies (ANA)	Negative	
Antistreptolysin O (ASO)	Adults: ≤160 Todd units/ml	
	Children:	
	Newborns: similar to mother's value	
	6 months-2 years: ≤50 Todd units/ml	
	2-4 years: ≤160 Todd units/ml	
	5-12 years: ≤200 Todd units/ml	
Antithyroid microsomal antibody	Titer <1:100	
Antithyroglobulin antibody	Titer <1:100	

*The use of the System of International Units (SI) was recommended at the 30th World Health Assembly in 1977 to implement an international language of measurement. Because this system is being adopted by many laboratories, many of the common values are expressed in both conventional and SI units. SI units are calculated by multiplying the conventional unit by a number factor. The SI measurement system uses *moles* as the basic unit for the amount of a substance, *kilograms* for its mass, and *meters* for its length.
From Pagana KD, Pagana TJ: *Diagnostic testing and nursing implications*, ed 3, St Louis, Mosby.

Test	Reference range	
	Conventional values	*SI units*
Ascorbic acid (vitamin C)	0.6-1.6 mg/dl	23-57 μmol/L
Aspartate aminotransferase (AST, SGOT)	12-36 U/ml	0.10-0.30 μmol/s/L
	5-40 IU/L	5-40 U/L
Australian antigen (hepatitis-associated antigen, HAA)	Negative	Negative
Barbiturates	Negative	Negative
Base excess	Men: −3.3 to +1.2	0 ± 2 mmol/L
	Women: −2.4 to +2.3	0 ± 2 mmol/L
Bicarbonate (HCO_3^-)	22-26 mEq/L	22-26 mmol/L
Bilirubin		
Direct (conjugated)	0.1-0.3 mg/dl	1.7-5.1 μmol/L
Indirect (unconjugated)	0.2-0.8 mg/dl	3.4-12.0 μmol/L
Total	Adults and children: 0.1-1.0 mg/dl	5.1-17.0 μmol/L
	Newborns: 1-12 mg/dl	
Bleeding time (Ivy method)	1-9 min	
Blood count (see complete blood count)		
Blood gases (arterial)		
pH	7.35-7.45	
Pco_2	35-45 mm Hg	4.7-6.0 kPa
HCO_3^-	22-26 mEq/L	21-28 nmol/L
Po_2	80-100 mm Hg	11-13 kPa
O_2 saturation	95%-100%	
Blood urea nitrogen (BUN)	5-20 mg/dl	3.6-7.1 mmol/L
Bromide	Up to 5 mg/dl	0-63 mmol/L
Bromosulfophthalein (BSP)	<5% retention after 45 min	
CA 15-3	<22 U/ml	
CA-125	0-35 U/ml	
CA 19-9	<37 U/ml	
C-reactive protein (CRP)	<6 μg/ml	
Calcitonin	<50 pg/ml	<50 pmol/L
Calcium (Ca)	9.0-10.5 mg/dl (total)	2.25-2.75 mmol/L
	3.9-4.6 mg/dl (ionized)	1.05-1.30 mmol/L
Carbon dioxide (CO_2) content	23-30 mEq/L	21-30 mmol/L
Carboxyhemoglobin (COHb)	3% of total hemoglobin	
Carcinoembryonic antigen (CEA)	<2 ng/ml	0-2.5 μg/L
Carotene	50-200 μg/dl	0.74-3.72 μmol/L
Chloride (Cl)	90-110 mEq/L	98-106 mmol/L
Cholesterol	150-250 mg/dl	3.90-6.50 mmol/L
Clot retraction	50%-100% clot retraction in 1-2 hours, complete retraction within 24 hours	
Complement		
	C_3: 70-176 mg/dl	0.55-1.20 g/L
	C_4: 16-45 mg/dl	0.20-0.50 g/L
Complete blood count (CBC)		
Red blood cell (RBC) count	Men: 4.7-6.1 million/mm³	
	Women: 4.2-5.4 million/mm³	
	Infants and children: 3.8-5.5 million/mm³	
	Newborns: 4.8-7.1 million/mm³	
Hemoglobin (Hgb)	Men: 14-18 g/dl	8.7-11.2 mmol/L
	Women: 12-16 g/dl (pregnancy: >11 g/dl)	7.4-9.9 mmol/L
	Children: 11-16 g/dl	1.74-2.56 mmol/L
	Infants: 10-15 g/dl	
	Newborns: 14-24 g/dl	2.56-3.02 mmol/L
Hematocrit (Hct)	Men: 42%-52%	
	Women: 37%-47% (pregnancy: >33%)	
	Children: 31%-43%	
	Infants: 30%-40%	
	Newborns: 44%-64%	
Mean corpuscular volume (MCV)	Adults and children: 80-95 μ³	80-95 fl
	Newborns: 96-108 μ³	
Mean corpuscular hemoglobin (MCH)	Adults and children: 27-31 pg	0.42-0.48 fmol
	Newborns: 32-34 pg	
Mean corpuscular hemoglobin concentration (MCHC)	Adults and children: 32-36 g/dl	0.32-0.36
	Newborns: 32-33 g/dl	

Continued.

Test	Reference range	
	Conventional values	SI units
Complete blood count (CBC)—cont'd		
White blood cell count (WBC)	Adults and children >2 years: 5000-10,000/cm^3	
	Children ≤2 years: 6200-17,000/mm^3	
	Newborns: 9000-30,000/mm^3	
Differential count		
Neutrophils	55%-70%	
Lymphocytes	20%-40%	
Monocytes	2%-8%	
Eosinophils	1%-4%	
Basophils	0.5%-1%	
Platelet count	150,000-400,00/mm^3	
Coombs' test		
Direct	Negative	Negative
Indirect	Negative	Negative
Copper (Cu)	70-140 μg/dl	11.0-24.3 μmol/L
Cortisol	6-28 μg/dl (AM)	170-635 nmol/L
	2-12 μg/dl (PM)	82-413 nmol/L
CPK isoenzyme (MB)	<5% total	
Creatinine	0.7-1.5 mg/dl	<133 μmol/L
Creatinine clearance	Men: 95-104 ml/min	<133 μmol/L
	Women: 95-125 ml/min	
Creatinine phosphokinase (CPK)	5-75 mU/ml	12-80 units/L
Cryoglobulin	Negative	Negative
Differential (WBC) count		
Neutrophils	55%-70%	
Lymphocytes	20%-40%	
Monocytes	2%-8%	
Eosinophils	1%-4%	
Basophils	0.5%-1%	
Digoxin	Therapeutic level: 0.5-2.0 ng/ml	40-79 μmol/L
	Toxic level: >2.4 ng/ml	>119 μmol/L
Erythrocyte count (see complete blood count)		
Erythrocyte secimentation rate (ESR)	Men: up to 15 mm/hour	
	Women: up to 20 mm/hour	
	Children: up to 10 mm/hour	
Ethanol	80-200 mg/dl (mild to moderate intoxication)	17-43 mmol/L
	250-400 mg/dl (marked intoxication)	54-87 mmol/L
	>400 mg/dl (severe intoxication)	>87 mmol/L
Euglobulin lysis test	90 min-6 hours	
Fats	Up to 200 mg/dl	
Ferritin	15-200 ng/ml	15-200 μg/L
Fibrin degradation products (FDP)	<10 μg/ml	
Fibrinogen (factor I)	200-400 mg/dl	5.9-11.7 μmol/L
Fibrinolysis/euglobulin lysis test	90 min-6 hours	
Fluorescent treponemal antibody (FTA)	Negative	Negative
Fluoride	<0.05 mg/dl	<0.027 mmol/L
Folic acid (Folate)	5-20 μg/ml	14-34 mmol/L
Follicle-stimulating hormone (FSH)	Men: 0.1-15.0 ImU/ml	
	Women: 6-30 ImU/ml	
	Children: 0.1-12.0 ImU/ml	
	Castrate and postmenopausal: 30-200 ImU/ml	
Free thyroxine index (FTI)	0.9-2.3 ng/dl	
Galactose-1-phosphate uridyl transferase	18.5-28.5 U/g hemoglobin	
Gammaglobulin	0.5-1.6 g/dl	
Gamma-glutamyl transpeptidase (GGTP)	Men: 8-38 U/L	5-40 U/L 37° C
	Women: <45 years: 5-27 U/L	
Gastrin	40-150 pg/ml	40-150 ng/L
Glucagon	50-200 pg/ml	14-56 pmol/L
Glucose, fasting (FBS)	Adults: 70-115 mg/dl	3.89-6.38 mmol/L
	Children: 60-100 mg/dl	
	Newborns: 30-80 mg/dl	
Glucose, 2-hour postprandial (2-hour PPG)	<140 mg/dl	
Glucose-6-phosphate dehydrogenase (G-6-PD)	8.6-18.6 IU/g of hemoglobin	

Test	Reference range	
	Conventional values	SI units
Glucose tolerance test (GTT)	Fasting: 70-115 mg/dl	
	30 min: <200 mg/dl	
	1 hour: <200 mg/dl	
	2 hours: <140 mg/dl	
	3 hours: 70-115 mg/dl	
	4 hours: 70-115 mg/dl	
Glycosylated hemoglobin	Adults: 2.2%-4.8%	
	Children: 1.8%-4.0%	
	Good diabetic control: 2.5%-6%	
	Fair diabetic control: 6.1%-8%	
	Poor diabetic control: >8%	
Growth hormone	<10 ng/ml	<10 μg/L
Haptoglobin	100-150 mg/dl	16-31 μmol/L
Hematocrit (Hct)	Men: 42%-52%	
	Women: 37%-47% (pregnancy: >33%)	
	Children: 31%-43%	
	Infants: 30%-40%	
	Newborns: 44%-64%	
Hemoglobin (Hgb)	Men: 14-18 g/dl	8.7-11.2 mmol/L
	Women: 12-16 g/dl (pregnancy: >11 g/dl)	7.4-9.9 mmol/L
	Children: 11-16 g/dl	
	Infants: 10-15 g/dl	
	Newborns: 14-24 g/dl	
Hemoglobin electrophoresis	Hgb A_1: 95%-98%	
	Hgb A_2: 2%-3%	
	Hgb F: 0.8%-2%	
	Hgb S: 0	
	Hgb C: 0	
Hepatitis B surface antigen (HB_3AG)	Nonreactive	Nonreactive
Heterophil antibody	Negative	Negative
HLA-B27	None	None
Human chorionic gonadotropin (HCG)	Negative	Negative
Human placental lactogen (HPL)	Rise during pregnancy	
5-Hydroxyindoleacetic acid (5-HIAA)	2.8-8.0 mg/24 hours	
Immunoglobulin quantification	IgG: 550-1900 mg/dl	5.5-19.0 g/L
	IgA: 60-333 mg/dl	0.6-3.3 g/L
	IgM: 45-145 mg/dl	0.45-1.5 g/L
Insulin	4-20 μU/ml	36-179 pmol/L
Iron (Fe)	60-190 μg/dl	13-31 μmol/L
Iron-binding capacity, total (TIBC)	250-420 μg/dl	45-73 μmol/L
Iron (transferrin) saturation	30%-40%	
Ketone bodies	Negative	Negative
Lactic acid	0.6-1.8 mEq/L	
Lactic dehydrogenase (LDH)	90-200 ImU/ml	0.4-1.7 μmol/s/L
LDH isoenzymes	LDH-1: 17%-27%	
	LDH-2: 28%-38%	
	LDH-3: 19%-27%	
	LDH-4: 5%-16%	
	LDH-5: 6%-16%	
Lead	120 μg/dl or less	<1.0 μmol/L
Leucine aminopeptidase (LAP)	Men: 80-200 U/ml	
	Women: 75-185 U/ml	
Leukocyte count (see complete blood count)		
Lipase	Up to 1.5 U/ml	0-417 U/L
Lipids		
Total	400-1000 mg/dl	4-8 g/L
Cholesterol	150-250 mg/dl	3.9-6.5 mmol/L
Triglycerides	40-150 mg/dl	0.4-1.5 g/L
Phospholipids	150-380 mg/dl	1.9-3.9 mmol/L
Lithium		
Long-acting thyroid stimulating hormone (LATS)	Negative	Negative
Magnesium (Mg)	1.6-3.0 mEq/L	0.8-1.3 mm/L

Continued.

Test	Reference range	
	Conventional values	SI units
Methanol	Negative	Negative
Mononucleosis spot test	Negative	Negative
Nitrogen, nonprotein	15-35 mg/dl	10.7-25.0 mmol/L
Nuclear antibody (ANA)	Negative	Negative
5'-Nucleotidase	Up to 1.6 units	27-233 nmol/s/L
Osmolality	275-300 mOsm/kg	
Oxygen saturation (arterial)	95%-100%	0.95-1.00 of capacity
Parathormone (PTH)	<2000 pg/ml	
Partial thromboplastin time, activated (APTT)	30-40 sec	
P_{CO_2}	35-45 mm Hg	
pH	7.35-7.45	7.35-7.45
Phenylalanine	Up to 2 mg/dl	<0.18 mmol/L
Phenylketonuria (PKU)	Negative	Negative
Phenytoin (Dilantin)	Therapeutic level: 10-20 µg/ml	
Phosphatase (acid)	0.10-0.63 U/ml (Bessey-Lowry)	0.11-0.60 U/L
	0.5-2.0 U/ml (Bodansky)	
	1.0-4.0 U/ml (King-Armstrong)	
Phosphatase (alkaline)	Adults: 30-85 ImU/ml	20-90 units/L
	Children and adolescents:	
	<2 years: 85-235 ImU/ml	
	2-8 years: 65-210 ImU/ml	
	9-15 years: 60-300 ImU/ml (active bone growth)	
	16-21 years: 30-200 ImU/ml	
Phospholipids (see Lipids)		
Phosphorus (P, PO_4)	Adults: 2.5-4.5 mg/dl	0.78-1.52 mmol/L
	Children: 3.5-5.8 mg/dl	1.29-2.26 mmol/L
Platelet count	150,000-400,000/mm^3	
P_{O_2}	80-100 mm Hg	
Potassium (K)	3.5-5.0 mEq/L	3.5-5.0 mmol/L
Progesterone	Men, prepubertal girls, and postmenopausal women: <2 ng/ml	6 nmol/L
	Women, luteal: peak >5 ng/ml	>16 nmol/L
Prolactin	2-15 ng/ml	2-15 µg/L
Protein (total)	6-8 g/dl	55-80 g/L
Albumin	3.2-4.5 g/dl	33-55 g/L
Globulin	2.3-3.4 g/dl	20-35 g/L
Prothrombin time (PT)	11.0-12.5 sec	11.0-12.5 sec
Pyruvate	0.3-0.9 mg/dl	34-103 µmol/L
Red blood cell count (see Complete blood count)		
Red blood cell indexes (see Complete blood count)		
Renin		
Reticulocyte count	Adults and children: 0.5%-2% of total erythrocytes	
	Infants: 0.5%-3.1% of total erythrocytes	
	Newborns: 2.5%-6.5% of total erythrocytes	
Rheumatoid factor	Negative	Negative
Rubella antibody test		
Salicylates	Negative	
	Therapeutic: 20-25 mg/dl (to age 10: 25-30 mg/dl)	1.4-1.8 mmol/L
	Toxic: >30 mg/dl (after age 60: >20 mg/dl)	>2.2 mmol/L
Schilling test (vitamin B_{12} absorption)	8%-40% excretion/24 hours	
Serologic test for syphilis (STS)	Negative (nonreactive)	
Serum glutamic oxaloacetic transaminase (SGOT, AST)	12-36 U/ml	0.10-0.30 µmol/s/L
	5-40 IU/L	
Serum glutamic-pyruvic transaminase (SGPT, ALT)	5-35 IU/L	0.05-0.43 µmol/s/L
Sickle cell	Negative	
Sodium (Na^+)	136-145 mEq/L	136-145 mmol/L
Sugar (see glucose)		
Syphilis (see Serologic test for, fluorescent treponemal antibody, Veneral Disease Research Laboratory)		

Test	Reference range	
	Conventional values	SI units
Testosterone	Men: 300-1200 ng/dl	10-42 nmol/L
	Women: 30-95 ng/dl	1.1-3.3 nmol/L
	Prepubertal boys and girls: 5-20 ng/dl	0.165-0.70 nmol/L
Thymol flocculation	Up to 5 units	
Thyroglubulin antibody (see Antithyroglobulin antibody)		
Thyroid-stimulating hormone (TSH)	1-4 μU/ml	5 mU/L
	Neonates: <25 μIU/ml by 3 days	
Thyroxine (T_4)	Murphy-Pattee:	50-124 nmol/L
	Neonates: 10.1-20.1 μg/dl	
	1-6 years: 5.6-12.6 μg/dl	
	6-10 years: 4.9-11.7 μg/dl	
	>10 years: 4-11 μg/dl	
	Radioimmunoassay: 5-10 μg/dl	
Thyroxine-binding globulin (TBG)	12-28 μg/ml	129-335 nmol/L
Transaminase (see Serum glutamic-oxaloacetic transaminase, serum glutamic pyruvic transaminase)		
Triglycerides	40-150 mg/dl	0.4-1.5 g/L
Triiodothyronine (T_3)	110-230 ng/dl	1.2-1.5 nmol/L
Triiodothyronine (T_3) resin uptake	25%-35%	
Tubular phosphate reabsorption (TPR)	80%-90%	
Urea nitrogen (see Blood urea nitrogen)		
Uric acid	Men: 2.1-8.5 mg/dl	0.15-0.48 mmol/L
	Women: 2.0-6.6 mg/dl	0.09-0.36 mmol/L
	Children: 2.5-5.5 mg/dl	
Veneral Disease Research Laboratory (VDRL)	Negative	Negative
Vitamin A	20-100 g/dl	0.7-3.5 μmol/L
Vitamin B_{12}	200-600 pg/ml	148-443 pmol/L
Vitamin C	0.6-1.6 mg/dl	23-57 μmol/L
Whole blood clot retraction (see Clot retraction)		
Zinc	50-150 μg/dl	

Urine values

Test	Reference range	
	Conventional values	*SI units*
Acetone plus acetoacetate (ketone bodies)	Negative	Negative
Addis count (12-hour)	Adults:	Negative
	WBCs and epithelial cells: 1.8 million/12 hours	
	RBCs: 500,000/12 hours	
	Hyaline casts: Up to 5000/12 hours	
	Children:	
	WBCs: <1 million/12 hours	
	RBCs: <250,000/12 hours	
	Casts: >5000/12 hours	
	Protein: <20 mg/12 hours	
Albumin	Random: ≤8 mg/dl	Negative
	24-hour: 10-100 mg/24 hours	10-100 mg/24 hr
Aldosterone	2-16 μg/24 hours	5.5-72 nmol/24 hours
Alpha-aminonitrogen	0.4-1.0 g/24 hours	28-71 nmol/24 hours
Amino acid	50-200 mg/24 hours	
Ammonia (24-hour)	30-50 mEq/24 hours	30-50 nmol/24 hours
	500-1200 mg/24 hours	
Amylase	≤5000 Somogyi units/24 hours	6.5-48.1 U/hr
	3-35 IU/hour	
Arsenic (24-hour)	<50 μg/L	<0.65 mol/L
Ascorbic acid (vitamin C)	Random: 1-7 ng/dl	0.06-0.40 mmol/L
	24-hour: >50 mg/24 hours	>0.29 mmol/24 hours
Bacteria	None	None
Bence Jones protein	Negative	Negative
Bilirubin	Negative	Negative
Blood or hemoglobin	Negative	Negative
Borate (24-hour)	<2 mg/L	<32 μmol/L
Calcium	Random: 1+ turbidity	1+ turbidity
	24-hour: 1-300 mg (diet dependent)	
Catecholamines (24-hour)	Epinephrine: 5-40 μg/24 hours	<55 nmol/24 hours
	Norepinephrine: 10-80 μg/24 hours	<590 nmol/24 hours
	Metanephrine: 24-96 μg/24 hours	0.5-8.1 μmol/24 hours
	Normetanephrine: 77-375 μg/24 hours	
Chloride (24-hour)	140-250 mEq/24 hours	140-250 mmol/24 hours
Color	Amber-yellow	Amber-yellow
Concentration test (Fishberg test)	Specific gravity: >1.025	>1.025
	Osmolality: 850 mOsm/L	>850 mOsm/L
Copper (CU) (24-hour)	Up to 25 μg/24 hours	0-0.4 μmol/24 hours
Coproporphyrin (24-hour)	100-300 μg/24 hours	150-460 nmol/24 hours
Creatine	Adults: <100 mg/24 hours or <6% creatinine	
	Pregnant women: ≤12%	
	Infants <1 year: equal to creatinine	
	Older children: ≤30% of creatinine	
Creatinine (24-hour)	15-25 mg/kg body wt/24 hours	0.13-0.22 nmol/kg^{-1} body wt/24 hours
Creatinine clearance (24-hour)	Men: 90-140 ml/min	90-140 ml/min
	Women: 85-125 ml/min	85-125 ml/min
Crystals	Negative	Negative
Cystine or cysteine	Negative	Negative
Delta-aminolevulinic acid (ΔALA)	1-7 mg/24 hours	10-53 μmol/24 hours
Epinephrine (24-hour)	5-40 μg/24 hours	
Epithelial cells and casts	Occasional	Occasional
Estriol (24-hour)	>12 mg/24 hours	
Fat	Negative	Negative
Fluoride (24-hour)	<1 mg/24 hours	0.053 mmol/24 hours
Follicle-stimulating hormone (FSH) (24-hour)	Men: 2-12 IU/24 hours	
	Women:	
	During menses: 8-60 IU/24 hours	
	During ovulation: 30-60 IU/24 hours	
	During menopause: >50 IU/24 hours	
Glucose	Negative	Negative

Test	Reference range	
	Conventional values	SI units
Granular casts	Occasional	Occasional
Hemoglobin and myoglobin	Negative	Negative
Homogentistic acid	Negative	Negative
Human chorionic gonadotropin (HCG)	Negative	Negative
Hyaline casts	Occasional	Occasional
17-Hydroxycorticosteroids (17-OCHS) (24-hour)	Men: 5.5-15.0 mg/24 hours	8.3-25 µmol/24 hours
	Women: 5.0-13.5 mg/24 hours	5.5-22 µmol/24 hours
	Children: lower than adult values	
5-Hydroxyindoleacetic acid (5-HIAA, serotonin) (24-hour)	Men: 2-9 mg/24 hours	10-47 µmol/24 hours
	Women: lower than men	
Ketones (see Acetone plus acetoacetate)		
17-Ketosteroids (17-KS) (24-hour)	Men: 8-15 mg/24 hours	21-62 µmol/24 hours
	Women: 6-12 mg/24 hours	14-45 µmol/24 hours
	Children:	
	12-15 yr: 5-12 mg/24 hours	
	<12 yr: <5 mg/24 hours	
Lactose (24-hour)	14-40 mg/24 hours	41-116 µm
Lead	<0.08 g/ml or <120 g/24 hours	0.39 µmol/L
Leucine aminopeptidase (LAP)	2-18 U/24 hours	
Magnesium (24-hour)	6.8-8.5 mEq/24 hours	3.0-4.3 mmol/24 hours
Melanin	Negative	Negative
Odor	Aromatic	Aromatic
Osmolality	500-800 mOsm/L	38-1400 mmol/kg water
pH	4.6-8.0	4.6-8.0
Phenolsulfonphthalein (PSP)	15 min: at least 25%	At least 0.25
	30 min: at least 40%	At least 0.40
	120 min: at least 60%	At least 0.60
Phenylketonuria (PKU)	Negative	Negative
Phenylpyruvic acid	Negative	Negative
Phosphorus (24-hour)	0.9-1.3 g/24 hours	29-42 mmol/24 hours
Porphobilinogen	Random: negative	Negative
	24-hour: up to 2 mg/24 hours	
Porphyrin (24-hour)	50-300 mg/24 hours	
Potassium (K^+) (24-hour)	25-100 mEq/24 hours	25-100 nmol/24 hours
Pregnancy test	Positive in normal pregnancy or with tumors producing HCG	Positive in normal pregnancy or with tumors producing HCG
Pregnanediol	After ovulation: >1 mg/24 hours	
Protein (albumin)	Random: ≤8 mg/dl	
	10-100 mg/24 hours	>0.05 g/24 hours
Sodium (Na^+) (24-hour)	100-260 mEq/24 hours	100-260 nmol/24 hours
Specific gravity	1.010-1.025	1.010-1.025
Steroids (see 17-Hydroxycorticosteroids and 17-Ketosteroids)		
Sugar (see Glucose)		
Titratable acidity (24-hour)	20-50 mEq/24 hours	20-50 mmol/24 hours
Turbidity	Clear	Clear
Urea nitrogen (24-hour)	6-17 g/24 hours	0.21-0.60 mol/24 hours
Uric acid (24-hour)	250-750 mg/24 hours	1.48-4.43 mmol/24 hours
Urobilinogen	0.1-1.0 Ehrlich U/dl	0.1-1.0 Ehrlich U/dl
Uroporphyrin	Negative	Negative
Vanillylmandelic acid (VMA) (24-hour)	1-9 mg/24 hours	<40 µmol/day
Zinc (24-hour)	0.20-0.75 mg/24 hours	

1-2   Selected neonatal and pediatric reference values

Test	Age/sex	Reference range			
		Conventional units		SI units	
Acetaminophen					
Serum or plasma	Therap. conc.	10-30 µg/ml		66-200 µmol/L	
	Toxic conc.	>200 µg/ml		>1300 µmol/L	
Ammonia nitrogen					
Plasma or serum	Newborn	90-150 µg/dl		64-107 µmol/L	
	0-2 wk	79-129 µg/dl		56-92 µmol/L	
	>1 mo	29-70 µg/dl		21-50 µmol/L	
	Thereafter	15-45 µg/dl		11-32 µmol/L	
Urine, 24 hr		500-1200 mg/d		36-86 mmol/d	
Antistreptolysin O titer (ASO)					
Serum	2-4 yr	<160 Todd units			
	School-age children	170-330 Todd units			
Base excess					
Whole blood	Newborn	(−10)-(−2) mmol/L		(−10)-(−2) mmol/L	
	Infant	(−7)-(−1) mmol/L		(−7)-(−1) mmol/L	
	Child	(−4)-(+2) mmol/L		(−4)-(+2) mmol/L	
	Thereafter	(−3)-(+3) mmol/L		(−3)-(+3) mmol/L	
Bicarbonate (HCO_3)					
Serum	Arterial	21-28 mmol/L		21-28 mmol/L	
	Venous	22-29 mmol/L		22-29 mmol/L	
		Premature (mg/dl)	*Full term (mg/dl)*	*Premature (µmol/L)*	*Full term (µmol/L)*
Bilirubin, total					
Serum	Cord	<2.0	<2.0	<34	<34
	0.1 d	8.0	<6.0	<137	<103
	1-2 d	12.0	<8.0	<205	<137
	2-5 d	16.0	<12.0	<274	<205
	Thereafter	2.0	0.2-1.0	<34	3.4-17.1
Bilirubin, direct (conjugated)					
Serum		0.0-0.2 mg/dl		0-3.4 µmol/L	
Bleeding time					
Blood from skin puncture					
Ivy	Normal	2-7 min		2-7 min	
	Borderline	7-11 min		7-11 min	
Simplate (G-D)		2.75-8 min		2.75-8 min	
Blood volume					
Whole blood	Male	52-83 ml/kg		0.052-0.083 L/kg	
	Female	50-75 ml/kg		0.050-0.075 L/kg	
C-reactive protein (CRP)					
Serum	Cord	52-1330 ng/ml		52-1330 µg/L	
Calcium, ionized					
Serum, plasma, or whole blood	Cord	50-60 mg/dl		1.25-1.50 mmol/L	
	Newborn, 3-24 hr	4.3-5.1 mg/dl		1.07-1.27 mmol/L	
	24-48 hr	4.0-4.7 mg/dl		1.00-1.17 mmol/L	
	Thereafter	4.8-4.92 mg/dl or 2.24-2.46 mEq/L		1.12-1.23 mmol/L	
Calcium, total					
Serum	Cord	9.0-11.5 mg/dl		2.25-2.88 mmol/L	
	Newborn, 3-24 hr	9.0-10.6 mg/dl		2.3-2.65 mmol/L	
	24-48 hr	7.0-12.0 mg/dl		1.75-3.0 mmol/L	
	4-7 d	9.0-10.9 mg/dl		2.25-2.73 mmol/L	
	Child	8.8-10.8 mg/dl		2.2-2.70 mmol/L	

Modified from Behrman RE and others, editors: *Nelson textbook of pediatrics*, ed 14. Philadelphia, 1992, Saunders.
From Wong DL: *Whaley and Wong's essentials of pediatric nursing*, ed 4, St Louis, Mosby.

Test	Age/sex	Reference range	
		Conventional units	SI units
Carbon dioxide, partial pressure (P_{CO_2})			
Whole blood, arterial	Newborn	27-40 mm Hg	3.6-5.3 kPa
	Infant	27-41 mm Hg	3.6-5.5 kPa
	Thereafter: Male	35-48 mm Hg	4.7-6.4 kPa
	Female	32-45 mm Hg	4.3-6.0 kPa
Carbon dioxide, total (tCO_2)			
Serum or plasma	Cord	14-22 mmol/L	14-22 mmol/L
	Premature (1 wk)	14-27 mmol/L	14-27 mmol/L
	Newborn	13-22 mmol/L	13-22 mmol/L
	Infant, child	20-28 mmol/L	20-28 mmol/L
	Thereafter	23-30 mmol/L	23-30 mmol/L
Cerebrospinal fluid (CSF)			
Pressure		70-180 mm water	70-180 mm water
Volume	Child	60-100 ml	0.06-0.10 L
Chloride			
Serum or plasma	Cord	96-104 mmol/L	96-104 mmol/L
	Newborn	97-110 mmol/L	97-110 mmol/L
	Thereafter	98-106 mmol/L	98-106 mmol/L
Sweat	Normal (homozygote)	<40 mmol/L	<40 mmol/L
	Marginal (e.g., asthma, Addison disease, malnutrition)	45-60 mmol/L	45-60 mmol/L
	Cystic fibrosis	>60 mmol/L	>60 mmol/L
Cholesterol, total			
Serum or plasma*	Acceptable	<170 mg/dl	<4.4 mmol/L
	Borderline	170-199 mg/dl	4.4-5.1 mmol/L
	High	≥200 mg/dl	≥5.2 mmol/L
Clotting time (Lee-White)			
Whole blood		5-8 min (glass tubes)	5-8 min
		5-15 min (room temp)	5-15 min
		30 min (silicone tube)	30 min
Creatine kinase (CK, CPK)			
Serum	Cord blood	70-380 U/L	70-380 U/L
	5-8 hr	214-1175 U/L	214-1175 U/L
	24-33 hr	130-1200 U/L	130-1200 U/L
	72-100 hr	87-725 U/L	87-725 U/L
Creatinine			
Serum	Cord	0.6-1.2 mg/dl	53-106 µmol/L
	Newborn	0.3-1.0 mg/dl	27-88 µmol/L
	Infant	0.2-0.4 mg/dl	18-35 µmol/L
	Child	0.3-0.7 mg/dl	27-62 µmol/L
	Adolescent	0.5-1.0 mg/dl	44-88 µmol/L
Urine, 24 hr	Premature	8.1-15.0 mg/kg/24 hr	72-133 µmol/kg/24 hr
	Full term	10.4-19.7 mg/kg/24 hr	92-174 µmol/kg/24 hr
	1.5-7 yr	10-15 mg/kg/24 hr	88-133 µmol/kg/24 hr
	7-15 yr	5.2-41 mg/kg/24 hr	46-362 µmol/kg/24 hr
Creatinine clearance (endogenous)			
Serum or plasma and urine	Newborn	40-65 ml/min/1.73 m²	
Digoxin			
Serum, plasma; collect at least 12 hr after dose	Therap. conc.		
	CHF	0.8-1.5 ng/ml	1.0-1.9 nmol/L
	Arrhythmias	1.5-2.0 ng/ml	1.9-2.6 nmol/L
	Toxic conc.		
	Child	>2.5 ng/ml	>3.2 nmol/L
Eosinophil count			
Whole blood, capillary blood		50-350 cells/mm³ (µl)	50-350 × 10⁶ cells/L
Erythrocyte (RBC) count			
Whole blood	Cord	3.9-5.5 million/mm³	3.9-5.5 × 10¹² cells/L
	1-3 d	4.0-6.6 million/mm³	4.0-6.6 × 10¹² cells/L
	1 wk	3.9-6.3 million/mm³	3.9-6.3 × 10¹² cells/L
	2 wk	3.6-6.2 million/mm³	3.6-6.2 × 10¹² cells/L

*From Natural Cholesterol Education Program: Report of the expert panel on blood cholesterol levels in children and adolescents, *Pediatrics* 89 (3, pt 2):527, 1992.

Continued.

Test	Age/sex	Reference range	
		Conventional units	*SI units*
Erythrocyte (RBC) count—cont'd			
Whole blood—cont'd	1 mo	3.0-5.4 million/mm^3	3.0-5.4 × 10^{12} cells/L
	2 mo	2.7-4.9 million/mm^3	2.7-4.5 × 10^{12} cells/L
	3-6 mo	3.1-4.5 million/mm^3	3.1-4.5 × 10^{12} cells/L
	0.5-2 yr	3.7-5.3 million/mm^3	3.7-5.3 × 10^{12} cells/L
	2-6 yr	3.9-5.3 million/mm^3	3.9-5.3 × 10^{12} cells/L
	6-12 yr	4.0-5.2 million/mm^3	4.0-5.2 × 10^{12} cells/L
	12-18 yr: Male	4.5-5.3 million/mm^3	4.5-5.3 × 10^{12} cells/L
	Female	4.1-5.1 million/mm^3	4.1-5.1 × 10^{12} cells/L
Erythrocyte sedimentation rate (ESR)			
Whole blood			
Westergren (modified)	Child	0-10 mm/hr	0-10 mm/hr
Wintrobe	Child	0-13 mm/hr	0-13 mm/hr
Fibrinogen			
Plasma	Newborn	125-300 mg/dl	1.25-3.00 g/L
	Thereafter	200-400 mg/dl	2.00-4.00 g/L
Galactose			
Serum	Newborn	0-20 mg/dl	0-1.11 mmol/L
	Thereafter	<5 mg/dl	<0.03 mmol/L
Urine	Newborn	≤60 mg/dl	≤3.33 mmol/L
	Thereafter	<14 mg/dl	<0.08 mmol/d
Glucose			
Serum	Cord	45-96 mg/dl	2.5-5.3 mmol/L
	Newborn, 1 d	40-60 mg/dl	2.2-3.3 mmol/L
	Newborn, >1 d	50-90 mg/dl	2.8-5.0 mmol/L
	Child	60-100 mg/dl	3.3-5.5 mmol/L
	Thereafter	70-105 mg/dl	3.9-5.8 mmol/L
Urine (quantitative)		<0.5 g/d	<2.8 mmol/d
(Qualitative)		Negative	Negative
Glucose tolerance test (GTT), oral			
Serum			

Dosages		*Normal*	*Diabetic*	*Normal*	*Diabetic*
Adult: 75 g	Fasting	70-105 mg/dl	>115 mg/dl	3.9-5.8 mmol/L	>6.4 mmol/L
Child: 1.75 g/kg of ideal	60 min	120-170 mg/dl	≥200 mg/dl	6.7-9.4 mmol/L	≥11 mmol/L
weight up to maximum	90 min	100-140 mmg/dl	≥200 mg/dl	5.6-7.8 mmol/L	≥11 mmol/L
of 75 g	120 min	70-120 mg/dl	≥140 mg/dl	3.9-6.7 mmol/L	≥7.8 mmol/L

Test	Age/sex	Conventional units	SI units
Growth hormone (hGH, somatotropin)			
Plasma	Cord	10-50 ng/ml	10-50 µg/L
Fasting, at rest	Newborn	10-40 ng/ml	10-40 µg/L
	Child	<5 ng/ml	<5 µg/L
Hematocrit (HCT, Hct)			
Whole blood	1 d (cap)	48%-69%	0.48-0.69 vol. fraction
	2 d	48%-75%	0.48-0.75 vol. fraction
	3 d	44%-72%	0.44-0.72 vol. fraction
	2 mo	28%-42%	0.28-0.42 vol. fraction
	6-12 yr	35%-45%	0.35-0.45 vol. fraction
	12-18 yr: Male	37%-49%	0.37-0.49 vol. fraction
	Female	36%-46%	0.36-0.46 vol. fraction
Hemoglobin (Hb)			
Whole blood	1-3 d (cap)	14.5-22.5 g/dl	2.25-3.49 mmol/L
	2 mo	9.0-14.0 g/dl	1.40-2.17 mmol/L
	6-12 yr	11.5-15.5 g/dl	1.78-2.40 mmol/L
	12-18 yr: Male	13.0-16.0 g/dl	2.02-2.48 mmol/L
	Female	12.0-16.0 g/dl	1.86-2.48 mmol/L
Hemoglobin A			
Whole blood		>95% of total	0.95 fraction of Hb

Test	Age/sex	Reference range	
		Conventional units	SI units
Hemoglobin F			
Whole blood	1 d	63%-92% HbF	0.62-0.92 mass fraction HbF
	5 d	65%-88% HbF	0.65-0.88 mass fraction HbF
	3 wk	55%-85% HbF	0.55-0.85 mass fraction HbF
	6-9 wk	31%-75% HbF	0.31-0.75 mass fraction HbF
	3-4 mo	<2%-59% HbF	<0.02-0.59 mass fraction HbF
	6 mo	<2%-9% HbF	<0.02-0.09 mass fraction HbF
Immunoglobulin A (IgA)			
Serum	Cord blood	1.4-3.6 mg/dl	14-36 mg/L
	1-3 mo	1.3-53 mg/dl	13-530 mg/L
	4-6 mo	4.4-84 mg/dl	44-840 mg/L
	7 mo-1 yr	11-106 mg/dl	110-1060 mg/L
	2-5 yr	14-159 mg/dl	140-1590 mg/L
	6-10 yr	33-236 mg/dl	330-2360 mg/L
Immunoglobulin D (IgD)			
Serum	Newborn	None detected	None detected
	Thereafter	0-8 mg/dl	0-80 mg/L
Immunoglobulin E (IgE)			
Serum	M	0-230 IU/ml	0-230 kIU/L
	F	0-170 IU/ml	0-170 kIU/L
Immunoglobulin G (IgG)			
Serum	Cord blood	636-1606 mg/dl	6.36-16.06 g/L
	1 mo	251-906 mg/dl	2.51-9.06 g/L
	2-4 mo	176-601 mg/dl	1.76-6.01 g/L
	5-12 mo	172-1069 mg/dl	1.72-10.69 g/L
	1-5 yr	345-1236 mg/dl	3.45-12.36 g/L
	6-10 yr	608-1572 mg/dl	6.08-15.72 g/L
Immunoglobulin M (IgM)			
Serum	Cord blood	6.3-25 mg/dl	63-250 mg/L
	1 mo-4 mo	17-105 mg/dl	170-1050 mg/L
	5 mo-9 mo	33-126 mg/dl	330-1260 mg/L
	10 mo-1 yr	41-173 mg/dl	410-1730 mg/L
	2-8 yr	43-207 mg/dl	430-2070 mg/L
	9-10 yr	52-242 mg/dl	520-2420 mg/L
Iron			
Serum	Newborn	100-250 μg/dl	17.90-44.75 μmol/L
	Infant	40-100 μg/dl	7.16-1790 μmol/L
	Child	50-120 μg/dl	8.95-21.48 μmol/L
	Intoxicated child	280-2550 μg/dl	50.12-456.5 μmol/L
	Fatally poisoned child	>1800 μg/dl	>322.2 μmol/L
Iron-binding capacity, total (TIBC)			
Serum	Infant	100-400 μg/dl	17.90-71.60 μmol/L
	Thereafter	250-400 μg/dl	44.75-71.60 μmol/L
Lead			
Whole blood	Child	<10 μg/dl	<0.48 μmol/L
Urine, 24 hr		<80 μg/L	<0.39 μmol/L
Leukocyte count (WBC count)		× 1000 cells/mm³ (μl)	× 10^9 cells/L
Whole blood	Birth	9.0-30.0	9.0-30.0
	24 hr	9.4-34.0	9.4-34.0
	1 mo	5.0-19.5	5.0-19.5
	1-3 yr	6.0-17.5	6.0-17.5
	4-7 yr	5.5-15.5	5.5-15.5
	8-13 yr	4.5-13.5	4.5-13.5
		× 1000 cells/mm³ (μl)	× 10^6 cells/L
CSF	Premature	0-25 mononuclear	0-25
		0-100 polymorphonuclear	0-100
		0-1000 RBC	0-1000

Continued.

		Reference range	
Test	*Age/sex*	*Conventional units*	*SI units*
CSF—cont'd	Newborn	0-20 mononuclear	0-20
		0-70 polymorphonuclear	0-70
		0-800 RBC	0-800
	Neonate	0-5 mononuclear	0-5
		0-25 polymorphonuclear	0-25
		0-50 RBC	0-50
	Thereafter	0-5 mononuclear	0-5
Leukocyte differential count			
Whole blood	Myelocytes	0%	0 cells/mm^3 (μl)	Number fraction 0
	Neutrophils—"bands"	3%-5%	150-400 cells/mm^3 (μl)	Number fraction 0.03-0.05
	Neutrophils—"segs"	54%-62%	3000-5800 cells/mm^3 (μl)	Number fraction 0.54-0.62
	Lymphocytes	25%-33%	1500-3000 cells/mm^3 (μl)	Number fraction 0.25-0.33
	Monocytes	3%-7%	285-500 cells/mm^3 (μl)	Number fraction 0.03-0.07
	Eosinophils	1%-3%	50-250 cells/mm^3 (μl)	Number fraction 0.01-0.03
	Basophils	0%-0.75%	15-50 cells/mm^3 (μl)	Number fraction 0-0.0075
Mean corpuscular hemoglobin (MCH)			
Whole blood	Birth	31-37 pg/cell	0.48-0.57 fmol/L
	1-3 d (cap)	31-37 pg/cell	0.48-0.57 fmol/L
	1 wk-1 mo	28-40 pg/cell	0.43-0.62 fmol/L
	2 mo	26-34 pg/cell	0.40-0.53 fmol/L
	3-6 mo	25-35 pg/cell	0.39-0.54 fmol/L
	0.5-2 yr	23-31 pg/cell	0.36-0.48 fmol/L
	2-6 yr	24-30 pg/cell	0.37-0.47 fmol/L
	6-12 yr	25-33 pg/cell	0.39-0.51 fmol/L
	12-18 yr	25-35 pg/cell	0.39-0.54 fmol/L
Mean corpuscular hemoglobin concentration (MCHC)			
Whole blood	Birth	30%-36% Hb/cell or g Hb/dl RBC	4.65-5.58 mmol or Hb/L RBC
	1-3 d (cap)	29%-37% Hb/cell or g Hb/dl RBC	4.50-5.74 mmol or Hb/L RBC
	1-2 wk	28%-38% Hb/cell or g Hb/dl RBC	4.34-5.89 mmol or Hb/L RBC
	1-2 mo	29%-37% Hb/cell or g Hb/dl RBC	4.50-5.74 mmol or Hb/L RBC
	3 mo-2 yr	30%-36% Hb/cell or g Hb/dl RBC	4.65-5.58 mmol or Hb/L RBC
	2-18 yr	31%-37% Hb/cell or g Hb/dl RBC	4.81-5.74 mmol or Hb/L RBC
Mean corpuscular volume (MCV)			
Whole blood	1-3 d (cap)	95-121 μm^3	95-121 fl
	0.5-2 yr	70-86 μm^3	70-86 fl
	6-12 yr	77-95 μm^3	77-95 fl
	12-18 yr: Male	78-98 μm^3	78-98 fl
	Female	78-102 μm^3	78-102 fl
Osmolality			
Serum	Child, adult	275-295 mOsmol/kg H_2O	
Urine, random		50-1400 mOsmol/kg H_2O, depending on fluid intake; after 12 hr fluid restriction: >850 mOsmol/kg H_2O	
Urine, 24 hr		$\approx$300-900 mOsmol/kg H_2O	
Oxygen, partial pressure (Po$_2$)			
Whole blood, arterial	Birth	8-24 mm Hg	1.1-3.2 kPa
	5-10 min	33-75 mm Hg	4.4-10.0 kPa
	30 min	31-85 mm Hg	4.1-11.3 kPa
	>1 hr	55-80 mm Hg	7.3-10.6 kPa

Test	Age/sex	Reference range	
		Conventional units	SI units
Oxygen, partial pressure (Po₂)—cont'd	1 d	54-95 mm Hg	7.2-12.6 kPa
Whole blood, arterial—cont'd	Thereafter (decreased with age)	83-108 mm Hg	11-14.4 kPa
Oxygen saturation (Sao₂)			
Whole blood, arterial	Newborn	85%-90%	Fraction saturated 0.85-0.90
	Thereafter	95%-99%	Fraction saturated 0.95-0.99
Partial thromboplastin time (PTT)			
Whole blood (Na citrate)			
Nonactivated		60-85 s (Platelin)	60-85 s
Activated		25-35 s (differs with method)	25-35 s
pH			H⁺ concentration:
Whole blood, arterial	Premature (48 hr)	7.35-7.50	31-44 nmol/L
	Birth, full term	7.11-7.36	43-77 nmol/L
	5-10 min	7.09-7.30	50-81 nmol/L
	30 min	7.21-7.38	41-61 nmol/L
	>1 hr	7.26-7.49	32.54 nmol/L
	1 d	7.29-7.45	35-51 nmol/L
	Thereafter	7.35-7.45	35-44 nmol/L
	Must be corrected for body temperature		
Urine, random	Newborn/neonate	5-7	0.1-10 μmol/L
	Thereafter (average = 6)	4.5-8	0.01-32 μmol/L (average ≃1.0 μmol/L)
Stool		7.0-7.5	31-100 nmol/L
Phenylalanine			
Serum	Premature	2.0-7.5 mg/dl	120-450 μmol/L
	Newborn	1.2-3.4 mg/dl	70-210 μmol/L
	Thereafter	0.8-1.8 mg/dl	50-110 μmol/L
Urine, 24 hr	10 d-2 wk	1-2 mg/d	6-12 μmol/d
	3-12 yr	4-18 mg/d	24-110 μmol/d
	Thereafter	trace-17 mg/d	trace-103 μmol/d
Plasma volume			
Plasma	Male	25-43 ml/kg	0.025-0.043 L/kg
	Female	28-45 ml/kg	0.028-0.045 L/kg
Platelet count (thrombocyte count)			
Whole blood (EDTA)	Newborn (After 1 wk same as adult)	84-478 × 10³/mm³ (μl)	84-478 × 10⁹/L
Potassium			
Serum	<2 yr	3.0-6.0 mmol/L	3.0-6.0 mmol/L
	2-12 yr	3.5-7.0 mmol/L	3.5-7.0 mmol/L
	>12 yr	3.5-5.0 mmol/L	3.5-5.0 mmol/L
Plasma (heparin)		3.4-4.5 mmol/L	3.4-4.5 mmol/L
Urine, 24 hr		2.5-125 mmol/d (varies with diet)	2.5-125 mmol/L
Protein			
Serum, total	Premature	4.3-7.6 g/dl	43-76 g/L
	Newborn	4.6-7.4 g/dl	46-74 g/L
	1-7 yr	6.1-7.9 g/dl	61-79 g/L
	8-12 yr	6.4-8.1 g/dl	64-81 g/L
	13-19 yr	6.6-8.2 g/dl	66-82 g/L
Total			
Urine, 24 hr		1-14 mg/dl	10-140 mg/L
		50-80 mg/d (at rest)	50-80 mg/d
		<250 mg/d after intense exercise	<250 mg/d after exercise
Total			
CSF		Lumbar: 8-32 mg/dl	80-320 mg/L

Continued.

Test	Age/sex	Reference range	
		Conventional units	*SI units*
Prothrombin time (PT)			
One-stage (Quick)			
Whole blood (Na citrate)	In general	11-15 s (varies with types of thromboplastin)	11-15 s
	Newborn	Prolonged by 2-3 sec	Prolonged by 2-3 sec
Two-stage modified (Ware and Seegers)			
Whole blood (Na citrate)		18-22 sec	18-22 sec
RBC count: see erythrocyte count			
Red blood cell volume			
Whole blood	Male	20-36 ml/kg	0.020-0.036 L/kg
	Female	19-31 ml/kg	0.019-0.031 L/kg
Capillary	1 d	0.4%-6.0%	0.004-0.060 (number fraction)
	7 d	<0.1%-1.3%	<0.001-0.013 (number fraction)
	1-4 wk	<0.1%-1.2%	<0.001-0.012 (number fraction)
	5-6 wk	<0.1%-2.4%	<0.001-0.024 (number fraction)
	7-8 wk	0.1%-2.9%	0.001-0.029 (number fraction)
	9-10 wk	<0.1%-2.6%	<0.001-0.026 (number fraction)
	11-12 wk	0.1%-1.3%	0.001-0.013 (number fraction)
Salicylates			
Serum, plasma	Therap. conc.	15-30 mg/dl	1.1-2.2 mmol/L
	Toxic conc.	>30 mg/dl	>2.2 mmol/L
Sedimentation rate: see erythrocyte sedimentation rate			
Sodium			
Serum or plasma	Newborn	136-146 mmol/L	134-146 mmol/L
	Infant	139-146 mmol/L	139-146 mmol/L
	Child	138-145 mmol/L	138-145 mmol/L
	Thereafter	136-146 mmol/L	136-146 mmol/L
Urine, 24 hr		40-220 mmol/L (diet dependent)	40-220 mmol/L
Sweat	Normal	<40 mmol/L	<40 mmol/L
	Indeterminate	45-60 mmol/L	45-60 mmol/L
	Cystic fibrosis	>60 mmol/L	>60 mmol/L
Theophylline			
Serum, plasma	Therap. conc.		
	Bronchodilator	10-20 µg/ml	56-110 µmol/L
	Premature apnea	6-10 µg/ml	28-56 µmol/L
	Toxic conc.	>20	>166 µmol/L
Thrombin time			
Whole blood (Na citrate)		Control time ± 2 sec when control is 9-13 sec	Control time ± 2 sec when control is 9-13 sec
Thyroxine, total (T_3)			
Serum	Cord	8-13 µg/dl	103-168 nmol/L
	Newborn	11.5-24 (lower in low-birth-weight infants)	148-310 nmol/L
	Neonate	9-18 µg/dl	116-232 nmol/L
	Infant	7-15 µg/dl	90-194 nmol/L
	1-5 yr	7.3-15 µg/dl	94-194 nmol/L
	5-10 yr	6.4-13.3 µg/dl	83-172 nmol/L
	Thereafter	5-12 µg/dl	65-155 nmol/L
	Newborn screen (filter paper)	6.2-22 µg/dl	80-284 nmol/L

Test	Age/sex	Reference range			
		Conventional units		*SI units*	

Tourniquet test (capillary fragility)

Conventional units: <5-10 petechiae in 2.5 cm circle on forearm (halfway between systolic and diastolic); pressure for 5 min; 0-8 petechiae in 6 cm circle (50 torr for 15 min); 10-20 petechiae in 5 cm circle (80 mm Hg)

SI units: <5-10 petechiae in 2.5 cm circle on forearm (halfway between systolic and diastolic); pressure for 5 min; 0-8 petechiae in 6 cm circle (50 torr for 15 min); 10-20 petechiae in 5 cm circle (80 mm Hg)

Triglycerides (TG)
Serum, after ≥12 hr fast

		mg/dl		*g/L*	
		M	F	M	F
	Cord blood	10-98	10-98	0.10-0.98	0.10-0.98
	0-5 yr	30-86	32-99	0.30-0.86	0.32-0.99
	6-11 yr	31-108	35-114	0.31-1.08	0.35-1.14
	12-15 yr	36-138	41-138	0.36-1.38	0.41-1.38
	16-19 yr	40-163	40-128	0.40-1.63	0.40-1.28

Triiodothyronine, free
Serum

Test	Age/sex	Conventional units	SI units
	Cord	20-240 pg/dl	0.3-3.7 pmol/L
	1-3 d	200-610 pg/dl	3.1-9.4 pmol/L
	6 wk	240-560 pg/dl	3.7-8.6 pmol/L

Triiodothyronine, total (T_3-RIA)
Serum

	Cord	30-70 ng/dl	0.46-1.08 nmol/L
	Newborn	72-260 ng/dl	1.16-4.00 nmol/L
	1-5 yr	100-260 ng/dl	1.54-4.00 nmol/L
	5-10 yr	90-240 ng/dl	1.39-3.70 nmol/L
	10-15 yr	80-210 ng/dl	1.23-3.23 nmol/L
	Thereafter	115-190 ng/dl	1.77-2.93 nmol/L

Urea nitrogen
Serum or plasma

	Cord	21-40 mg/dl	7.5-14.3 mmol urea/L
	Premature (1 wk)	3-25 mg/dl	1.1-9 mmol urea/L
	Newborn	3-12 mg/dl	1.1-4.3 mmol urea/L
	Infant/child	5-18 mg/dl	1.8-6.4 mmol urea/L
	Thereafter	7-18 mg/dl	2.5-6.4 mmol urea/L

Urine volume
Urine, 24 hr

	Newborn	50-300 ml/d	0.050-0.300 L/d
	Infant	350-550 ml/d	0.350-0.500 L/d
	Child	500-1000 ml/d	0.500-1.000 L/d
	Adolescent	700-1400 ml/d	0.700-1.400 L/d

WBC: see leukocyte

1-3   Desirable weight for men and women of age 25 and over

	Height in shoes	Weight in pounds (in indoor clothing)		
		Small frame	Medium frame	Large frame
Men	5'-2"	112-120	118-129	126-141
	5'-3"	115-123	121-133	129-144
	5'-4"	118-126	124-136	132-148
	5'-5"	121-129	127-139	135-152
	5'-6"	124-133	130-143	138-156
	5'-7"	128-137	134-147	142-161
	5'-8"	132-141	138-152	147-166
	5'-9"	136-145	142-156	151-170
	5'-10"	140-150	146-160	155-174
	5'-11"	144-154	150-165	159-179
	6'-0"	148-158	154-170	164-184
	6'-1"	152-162	158-175	168-189
	6'-2"	156-167	162-180	173-194
	6'-3"	160-171	167-185	178-199
	6'-4"	164-175	172-190	182-204
Women	4'-10"	92-98	96-107	104-119
	4'-11"	94-101	98-110	106-122
	5'-0"	96-104	101-113	109-125
	5'-1"	99-107	104-116	112-128
	5'-2"	102-110	107-119	115-131
	5'-3"	105-113	110-122	118-134
	5'-4"	108-116	113-126	121-138
	5'-5"	111-119	116-130	125-142
	5'-6"	114-123	120-135	129-146
	5'-7"	118-127	124-139	133-150
	5'-8"	122-131	128-143	137-154
	5'-9"	126-135	132-147	141-158
	5'-10"	130-140	136-151	145-163
	5'-11"	134-144	140-155	149-168
	6'-0"	138-148	144-159	153-173

From Metropolitan Life Insurance Company. Data are based on weights associated with lowest death rates. To obtain weight for adults younger than 25, subtract 1 pound for each year under 25.

1-4 Height and weight measurements for boys and girls

Boys	Height by percentiles						Weight by percentiles					
	5		50		95		5		50		95	
Age*	cm	Inches	cm	Inches	cm	Inches	kg	lb	kg	lb	kg	lb
Birth	46.4	18¼	50.5	20	54.4	21½	2.54	5½	3.27	7¼	4.15	9¼
3 months	56.7	22¼	61.1	24	65.4	25¾	4.43	9¾	5.98	13¼	7.37	16¼
6 months	63.4	25	67.8	26¾	72.3	28½	6.20	13¾	7.85	17¼	9.46	20¾
9 months	68.0	26¾	72.3	28½	77.1	30¼	7.52	16½	9.18	20¼	10.93	24
1	71.7	28¼	76.1	30	81.2	32	8.43	18½	10.15	22½	11.99	26½
1½	77.5	30½	82.4	32½	88.1	34¾	9.59	21¼	11.47	25¼	13.44	29½
2†	82.5	32½	86.8	34¼	94.4	37¼	10.49	23¼	12.34	27¼	15.50	34¼
2½†	85.4	33½	90.4	35½	97.8	38½	11.27	24¾	13.52	29¾	16.61	36½
3	89.0	35	94.9	37¼	102.0	40¼	12.05	26½	14.62	32¼	17.77	39¼
3½	92.5	36½	99.1	39	106.1	41¾	12.84	28¼	15.68	34½	18.98	41¾
4	95.8	37¾	102.9	40½	109.9	43¼	13.64	30	16.69	36¾	20.27	44¾
4½	98.9	39	106.6	42	113.5	44¾	14.45	31¾	17.69	39	21.63	47¾
5	102.0	40¼	109.9	43¼	117.0	46	15.27	33¾	18.67	41¼	23.09	51
6	107.7	42½	116.1	45¾	123.5	48½	16.93	37¼	20.69	45½	26.34	58
7	113.0	44½	121.7	48	129.7	51	18.64	41	22.85	50¼	30.12	66½
8	118.1	46½	127.0	50	135.7	53½	20.40	45	25.30	55¾	34.51	76
9	122.9	48½	132.2	52	141.8	55¾	22.25	49	28.13	62	39.58	87¼
10	127.7	50¼	137.5	54¼	148.1	58¼	24.33	53¾	31.44	69¼	45.27	99¾
11	132.6	52¼	143.3	56½	154.9	61	26.80	59	35.30	77¾	51.47	113½
12	137.6	54¼	149.7	59	162.3	64	29.85	65¾	39.78	87¾	58.09	128
13	142.9	56¼	156.5	61½	169.8	66¾	33.64	74¼	44.95	99	65.02	143¼
14	148.8	58½	163.1	64¼	176.7	69½	38.22	84¼	50.77	112	72.13	159
15	155.2	61	169.0	66½	181.9	71½	43.11	95	56.71	125	79.12	174½
16	161.1	63½	173.5	68¼	185.4	73	47.74	105¼	62.10	137	85.62	188¾
17	164.9	65	176.2	69¼	187.3	73¾	51.50	113½	66.31	146¼	91.31	201¼
18	165.7	65¼	176.8	69½	187.6	73¾	53.97	119	68.88	151¾	95.76	211

Modified from National Center for Health Statistics (NCHS), Health Resources Administration, Department of Health, Education and Welfare, Hyattsville, MD. Conversion of metric data to approximate inches and pounds by Ross Laboratories, 1977.
*Years unless otherwise indicated
†Height data include some recumbent length measurements, which make values slightly higher than if all measurements had been of stature (standing height).
From Wong DL: *Whaley and Wong's essentials of pediatric nursing,* St Louis, 1993, Mosby.

Girls	Height by percentiles						Weight by percentiles					
	5		50		95		5		50		95	
Age*	cm	Inches	cm	Inches	cm	Inches	kg	lb	kg	lb	kg	lb
Birth	45.4	17¾	49.9	19¾	52.9	20¾	2.36	5¼	3.23	7	3.81	8½
3 months	55.4	21¾	59.5	23½	63.4	25	4.18	9¼	5.4	12	6.74	14¾
6 months	61.8	24¼	65.9	26	70.2	27¾	5.79	12¾	7.21	16	8.73	19¼
9 months	66.1	26	70.4	27¾	75.0	29½	7.0	15½	8.56	18¾	10.17	22½
1	69.8	27½	74.3	29¼	79.1	31¼	7.84	17¼	9.53	21	11.24	24¾
1½	76.0	30	80.9	31¾	86.1	34	8.92	19¾	10.82	23¾	12.76	28¼
2†	81.6	32¼	86.8	34¼	93.6	36¾	9.95	22	11.8	26	14.15	31¼
2½†	84.6	33¼	90.0	35½	96.6	38	10.8	23¾	13.03	28¾	15.76	34¾
3	88.3	34¾	94.1	37	100.6	39½	11.61	25½	14.1	31	17.22	38
3½	91.7	36	97.9	38½	104.5	41¼	12.37	27¼	15.07	33¼	18.59	41
4	95.0	37½	101.6	40	108.3	42¾	13.11	29	15.96	35¼	19.91	44
4½	98.1	38½	105.0	41¼	112.0	44	13.83	30½	16.81	37	21.24	46¾
5	101.1	39¾	108.4	42¾	115.6	45½	14.55	32	17.66	39	22.62	49¾
6	106.6	42	114.6	45	122.7	48¼	16.05	35½	19.52	43	25.75	56¾
7	111.8	44	120.6	47½	129.5	51	17.71	39	21.84	48¼	29.68	65½
8	116.9	46	126.4	49¾	136.2	53½	19.62	43¼	24.84	54¾	34.71	76½
9	122.1	48	132.2	52	142.9	56¼	21.82	48	28.46	62¾	40.64	89½
10	127.5	50¼	138.3	54½	149.5	58¾	24.36	53¾	32.55	71¾	47.17	104
11	133.5	52½	144.8	57	156.2	61½	27.24	60	36.95	81½	54.0	119
12	139.8	55	151.5	59¾	162.7	64	30.52	67¼	41.53	91½	60.81	134
13	145.2	57¼	157.1	61¾	168.1	66¼	34.14	75¼	46.1	101¾	67.3	148¼
14	148.7	58½	160.4	63¼	171.3	67½	37.76	83¼	50.28	110¾	73.08	161
15	150.5	59¼	161.8	63¾	172.8	68	40.99	90¼	53.68	118¼	77.78	171½
16	151.6	59¾	162.4	64	173.3	68¼	43.41	95¾	55.89	123¼	80.99	178½
17	152.7	60	163.1	64¼	173.5	68¼	44.74	98¾	56.69	125	82.46	181¾
18	153.6	60½	163.7	64½	173.6	68¼	45.26	99¾	56.62	124¾	82.47	181¾

Modified from National Center for Health Statistics, Health Resources Administration, Department of Health, Education and Welfare, Hyattsville, MD. Conversion of metric data to approximate inches and pounds by Ross Laboratories, 1977.

*Years unless otherwise indicated.

†Height data include some recumbent length measurements, which make values slightly higher than if all measurements had been of stature.

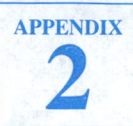

APPENDIX 2
CLINICAL CALCULATIONS

Calculation formulas and normal ranges

Parameter	Formula	Normal range
Cardiac output (CO)	$HR \times SV$	4-8 L/min
Cardiac index (CI)	$\dfrac{CO}{BSA}$	2.8-4.2 L/min/m^2
Stroke volume (SV)	$\dfrac{CO \times 1000}{HR}$	60-130 ml/beat
Stroke volume index (SVI)	$\dfrac{SV}{BSA}$	33-75 ml/m^2/beat
Stroke index (SI)	$\dfrac{CI}{HR} \times 1000$	30-65 ml/m^2/beat
Mean arterial pressure (MAP)	$\dfrac{2(DBP) + SBP}{3}$	70-105 mm Hg
Coronary perfusion pressure (CPP)	$Arterial\ DP - PAWP$	60-80 mm Hg
Systemic vascular resistance (SVR)	$\dfrac{MAP - CVP}{CO} \times 80$	700-1600 dynes/sec/cm^{-5}
Pulmonary vascular resistance (PRV)	$\dfrac{PAM - PAWP}{CO} \times 80$	20-130 dynes/sec/cm^{-5}
Left ventricular stroke work index (LVSWI)	$(MAP - PAWP)SVI \times 0.136$	35-85 g/m^2/beat
Right ventricular stroke work index (RVSWI)	$(PAM - CVP)SVI \times 0.136$	8.5-12 g/m^2/beat
Ejection fraction (EF)	$\dfrac{SV}{end\ diastolic\ volume} \times 100$	60%
Rate pressure product (RPP)	$HR \times SBP$	<12,000
Arterial oxygen content (CaO$_2$)	$(SaO_2 \times Hb \times 1.38) + (PaO_2 \times .0031)$	18-20 ml/100 ml or 20 vol %
Venous oxygen content (CvO$_2$)	$(SvO_2 \times Hb \times 1.38) + (PvO_2 \times .0031)$	15.5 ml/100 ml
Arterial venous oxygen content difference (C$_{(a-v)}$O$_2$)	$CaO_2 - CvO_2$	4-6 ml/100 ml
Arterial oxygen delivery (DO$_2$)	$CO \times 10 \times CaO_2$	900-1200 ml/min
Venous oxygen delivery (DO$_2$)	$CO \times 10 \times CvO_2$	775 ml/min
Oxygen consumption (VO$_2$)	$CO \times 10 \times C_{(a-v)}O_2$	200-250 ml/min
Mixed venous oxygen saturation (SvO$_2$)	$1 - VO_2/DO_2$	60%-80%
Alveolar-arterial oxygen gradient (AaDO$_2$)	$PAO_2 - PaO_2$	<15 mm Hg
Alveolar partial pressure of oxygen (PaO$_2$)	$FIO_2 - PaCO_2/0.8$	
Respiratory quotient (RQ)	$\dfrac{O_2\ consumption}{CO_2\ production}$	0.8-1
Neurologic		
Cerebral perfusion pressure (CPP)	$MPA - ICP$	80-100 mm Hg
Intracranial pressure (ICP)		0-15 mm Hg
Renal		
Anion gap (GAP)	$Na - (HCO_3 + CI)$	8-16 mEq/L
Osmolality (OSM)	$(2Na) + K + BUN/3 + Glucose/18$	275-295 mOsm
Glomerular filtration rate (GRF)	$\dfrac{(140 - Age) \times wt\ (kg)}{(male)\ 75 \times serum\ Cr}$ (female) $85 \times serum\ Cr$	80-120 ml/min

From Stillwell SB: *Quick critical care reference*, St. Louis, 1990, Mosby.

Drug dosage formula

Use the following formulas for quick calculation of drug dosages.

$$\text{Drug volume to be administered (ml)} = \frac{\text{desired dose (mg)}}{\text{drug concentration (mg/ml)}}$$

$$or = \frac{\text{desired dose (mg)} \times \text{volume (ml)}}{\text{amount (mg)}}$$

NOTE: $$\text{drug concentration (mg/ml)} = \frac{\text{amount (mg)}}{\text{volume (ml)}}$$

IV flow rate formula

Use the following formulas to calculate IV flow rates.

$$\text{Flow rate (ml/hr)} = \frac{\text{desired dose (mg/min)} \times 60 \text{ (min/hr)}}{\text{drug concentration (mg/ml)}}$$

$$or = \frac{\text{desired dose (}\mu\text{g/kg/min)} \times 60 \text{ (min/hr)} \times \text{wt (kg)}}{\text{drug concentration (}\mu\text{g/ml)}}$$

$$or = \frac{\text{drip rate (drops/min)} \times 60 \text{ (min/hr)}}{60 \text{ (drops/ml)}}$$

$$\text{Drip rate (drops/min)} = \frac{\text{total volume to be infused (ml)} \times \text{drop factor (drops/ml)}}{\text{total time for the infusion (min)}}$$

$$or = \frac{\text{drops/ml}}{60 \text{ (min/hr)}} \times \frac{\text{volume to be infused (ml/hr)}}{1}$$

From Madigan KG: *Prehospital emergency drugs: pocket reference*, St Louis, 1990, Mosby.

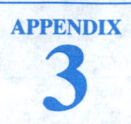

APPENDIX 3

UNITS OF MEASUREMENT

3-1 Conversion factors

Units To convert from	Conventional units	
	To	*Multiply by*
Energy		
Calories	Joules	0.23
Joules (J)	Calories	4.184
Length		
Ångström units (Å)	Centimeters	1×10^{-8}
	Inches	3.9370079×10^{-9}
	Micrometers	0.0001
	Nanometers	0.1
Centimeters (cm)	Ångström units	1×10^{8}
	Feet	0.032808399
	Inches	0.39370079
	Meters	0.01
	Microns	10,000
	Miles (naut., int.)	5.3995680×10^{-6}
	Miles (statute)	6.2137119×10^{-6}
	Millimeters	10
	Nanometers	1×10^{7}
	Rods	0.0019883878
	Yards	0.010936133
Decimeters (dm)	Centimeters	10
	Feet	0.32808399
	Inches	3.9370079
	Meters	0.1
Dekameters (dkm, dam)	Centimeters	1000
	Feet	32.808399
	Inches	393.70079
	Kilometers	0.01
	Meters	10
	Yards	10.93613
Feet (ft)	Centimeters	30.48
	Inches	12
	Meters	0.3048
	Microns	304,800
	Yards	0.333333
Inches (in)	Ångström units	2.54×10^{8}
	Centimeters	2.54
	Cubits	0.055555
	Feet	0.083333
	Meters	0.0254
	Mils	1000
	Yards	0.027777
Meters (m)	Ångström units	1×10^{10}
	Centimeters	100
	Feet	3.2808399
	Inches	39.370079
	Kilometers	0.001
	Megameters	1×10
	Miles (naut., Brit.)	0.00053961182
	Millimeters	1000

Modified from Weast, RC, editor: *Handbook of chemistry and physics*, ed 64, Boca Raton, Fla, 1983, CRC Press, Inc.   *Continued.*

Units To convert from	Conventional units	
	To	*Multiply by*
Meters (m)—cont'd	Nanometers	1×10^9
	Mils	39,370.079
	Yards	1.0936133
Micrometers (μm)	Ångström units	10,000
	Centimeters	0.0001
	Feet	3.2808399×10^{-6}
	Inches	3.9370079×10^{-5}
	Meters	1×10^{-6}
	Millimeters	0.001
	Nanometers	1000
Miles (statute)	Centimeters	160,934.4
	Feet	5280
	Inches	63,360
	Kilometers	1.609344
	Meters	1609.344
	Yards	1760
Nanometer (nm)	Ångström units	10
	Centimeters	1×10^{-7}
	Inches	3.9370079×10^{-8}
	Micrometers	0.001
	Millimeters	1×10^{-6}
Yards (yd)	Centimeters	91.44
	Chains (Gunter's)	0.454545454
	Chains (Ramden's)	0.03
	Cubits	2
	Fathoms	0.5
	Feet	3
	Feet (U.S. survey)	2.9999940
	Inches	36
	Meters	0.9144
	Quarters (Brit., linear)	4
Mass		
Centigrams (cg)	Grains	0.15432358
	Grams	0.01
Drams (apoth. or troy) (dr ap, ʒ)	Drams (avdp.)	2.1942857
	Grains	60
	Grams	3.8879346
	Ounces (apoth. or troy)	0.125
	Ounces (advp.)	0.13714286
	Scruples (apoth.)	3
Drams (avdp.) (dr avdp)	Drams (apoth. or troy)	0.455729166
	Grains	27.34375
	Grams	1.7718452
	Ounces (apoth. or troy)	0.056966146
	Ounces (avdp.)	0.0625
	Pennyweights	1.1393229
	Pounds (apoth. or troy)	0.0047471788
	Pounds (avdp.)	0.00390625
	Scruples (apoth.)	1.3671875
Grains (gr)	Carats (metric)	0.32399455
	Drams (apoth. or troy)	0.016666
	Drams (avdp.)	0.036571429
	Dynes	63.5460
	Grams	0.06479891
	Milligrams	64.79891
	Ounces (apoth. or troy)	0.0020833
	Ounces (avdp.)	0.002857143
	Pennyweights	0.041666
	Pounds (apoth. or troy)	0.000173611
	Pounds (avdp.)	0.00014285714
	Scruples (apoth.)	0.05
Grams (g)	Carats (metric)	5
	Decigrams	10

Units To convert from	Conventional units	
	To	Multiply by
Grams (g)—cont'd	Dekagrams	0.1
	Drams (apoth. or troy)	0.25720597
	Drams (avdp.)	0.56438339
	Grains	15.432358
	Kilograms	0.001
	Micrograms	1×10^6
	Myriagrams	0.0001
	Ounces (apoth. or troy)	0.32150737
	Ounces (avdp.)	0.35273962
	Pennyweights	0.64301493
	Poundals	0.0709316
	Pounds (apoth. or troy)	0.0026792289
	Pounds (avdp.)	0.0022046226
	Scruples (apoth.)	0.77161792
	Tons (metric)	1×10^{-6}
Hectograms (hg)	Grams	100
	Poundals	7.09316
	Pounds (apoth. or troy)	0.26792289
	Pounds (avdp.)	0.22046226
Kilograms (kg)	Drams (apoth. or troy)	257.20597
	Drams (avdp.)	564.38339
	Grains	15,432.358
	Hundredweights (long)	0.019684131
	Hundredweights (short)	0.022046226
	Ounces (apoth. or troy)	32.150737
	Ounces (avdp.)	35.273962
	Pennyweights	643.01493
	Poundals	70.931635
	Pounds (apoth. or troy)	2.6792289
	Pounds (advp.)	2.2046226
	Scruples (apoth.)	771.61792
Micrograms (μg)	Grams	1×10^{-6}
Milligrams (mg)	Milligrams	0.001
	Carats (1877)	0.004871
	Carats (metric)	0.005
	Drams (apoth. or troy)	0.00025720597
	Drams (advp.)	0.00056438339
Ounces (apoth. or troy) (oz, ℥)	Dekagrams	1.7554286
	Drams (apoth. or troy)	8
	Drams (advp.)	17.554286
	Grains	480
	Grams	31.103486
	Milligrams	31,103.486
	Ounces (avdp.)	1.0971429
	Pennyweights	20
	Pounds (apoth. or troy)	0.0833333
	Pounds (avdp.)	0.068571429
	Scruples (apoth.)	24
Ounces (avdp.) (oz)	Drams (apoth. or troy)	7.291666
	Drams (avdp.)	16
	Grains	437.5
	Grams	28.349523
	Hundredweights (long)	0.00055803571
	Hundredweights (short)	0.000625
	Ounces (apoth. or troy)	0.9114583
	Pennyweights	18.229166
	Pounds (apoth. or troy)	0.075954861
	Pounds (avdp.)	0.0625
	Scruples (apoth.)	21.875
Pennyweights (dwt)	Drams (apoth. or troy)	0.4
	Drams (avdp.)	0.87771429
	Grains	24
	Grams	1.55517384

Continued.

Units To convert from	Conventional units	
	To	Multiply by
Pennyweights (dwt)—cont'd	Ounces (apoth. or troy)	0.05
	Ounces (avdp.)	0.054857143
	Pounds (apoth. or troy)	0.0041666
	Pounds (avdp.)	0.0034285714
Poundals	Dynes	13,825.50
	Grams	14.09808
	Pounds (avdp.)	0.310810
Pounds (apoth. or troy) (lb ap)	Drams (apoth. or troy)	96
	Drams (avdp.)	210.65143
	Grains	5760
	Grams	373.24172
	Kilograms	0.37324172
	Ounces (apoth. or troy)	12
	Ounces (avdp.)	13.165714
	Pennyweights	240
	Pounds (avdp.)	0.8228571
	Scruples (apoth.)	288
Pounds (avdp.) (lb avdp.)	Drams (apoth. or troy)	116.6666
	Drams (avdp.)	256
	Grains	7000
	Grams	453.59237
	Kilograms	0.45359237
	Ounces (apoth. or troy)	14.583333
	Ounces (avdp.)	16
	Pennyweights	291.6666
	Poundals	32.1740
	Pounds (apoth. or troy)	1.215277
	Scruples (apoth.)	350
	Slugs	0.0310810
Quintals (metric)	Grams	100,000
	Hundredweights (long)	1.9684131
	Kilograms	100
	Pounds (avdp.)	220.46226
Scruples (apoth.) (s apoth)	Drams (apoth. or troy)	0.333333
	Drams (avdp.)	0.73142857
	Grains	20
	Grams	1.2959782
	Ounces (apoth. or troy)	0.041666
	Ounces (avdp.)	0.045714286
	Pennyweights	0.833333
	Pounds (apoth. or troy)	0.003472222
	Pounds (avdp.)	0.0028571429
Tons (long)	Kilograms	1016.0469
	Ounces (avdp.)	35,840
	Pounds (apoth. or troy)	2722.22
	Pounds (avdp.)	2240
	Tons (metric)	1.0160469
	Tons (short)	1.12
Tons (metric) (t)	Grams	1×10^6
	Hundredweights (short)	22.046226
	Kilograms	1000
	Ounces (avdp.)	35,273.962
	Pounds (apoth. or troy)	2679.2289
	Pounds (avdp.)	2204.6226
	Tons (long)	0.98420653
	Tons (short)	1.1023113
Tons (short) (sh tn)	Hundredweights (short)	20
	Kilograms	907.18474
	Ounces (avdp.)	32,000
	Pounds (apoth. or troy)	2430.555
	Pounds (avdp.)	2000
	Tons (long)	0.89285714
	Tons (metric)	0.90718474

Units To convert from	Conventional units	
	To	Multiply by

Pressure

Units To convert from	To	Multiply by
Atmospheres, standard (atm)	Bars	1.01325
	Hg (0° C)	76
	H_2O (4° C)	1033.26
	Feet of H_2O (39.2° F)	33.8995
	Grams/square centimeter	1033.23
	Inches of Hg (32° F)	29.9213
	Kilograms/square centimeters	1.03323
	Millimeters of Hg (0° C)	760
	Pounds/square inch	14.6960
	Torrs	760
Inches of Hg (32° F)	Atmospheres	0.034211
	Bars	0.0338639
	Feet of air (1 atm, 60° F)	926.24
	Feet of H_2O (39.2° F)	1.132957
	Grams/square centimeter	34.5316
	Kilograms/square meter	345.316
	Millimeters of Hg (60° C)	25.4
	Ounces/square inch	7.85847
	Pounds/square foot	70.7262
Meters of Hg (0° C)	Atmospheres	1.3157895
	Feet of H_2O (60° F)	44.6474
	Inches of Hg (32° F)	39.370079
	Kilograms/square centimeters	1.35951
	Pounds/square inch	19.3368
Millimeters of Hg (0° C) (mm Hg)	Atmospheres	0.0013157895
	Bars	0.00133322
	Dynes/square centimeter	1333.224
	Grams/square centimeter	1.35951
	Kilograms/square meter	13.5951
	Pounds/square foot	2.78450
	Pounds/square inch	0.0193368
	Torrs	1

Substance concentration

Units To convert from	To	Multiply by
Parts per million* (ppm)	Grains/gallon (Brit.)	0.07015488
	Grains/gallon (U.S.)	0.058411620
	Grams/liter	0.001
	Milligrams/liter	1

Surface area

Units To convert from	To	Multiply by
Square inches (in^2)	Circular mils	1,273,239.5
	Square centimeters	6.4516
	Square decimeters	0.064516
	Square feet	0.0069444
	Square meters	0.00064516
	Square miles	$2.4909767 \times 10^{-10}$
	Square millimeters	645.16
	Square mils	1×10^6
Square meters (m^2)	Square centimeters	10,000
	Square feet	10.763910
	Square inches	1550.0031
	Square kilometers	1×10^{-6}
	Square miles	3.8610216×10^{-7}
	Square rods	0.039536861
Square millimeters (mm^2)	Square centimeters	0.01
	Square inches	0.0015500031
	Square meters	1×10^{-6}
Square yards (yd^2)	Square centimeters	8361.2736
	Square feet	9
	Square feet (U.S. survey)	8.9999640
	Square inches	1296
	Square meters	0.83612736

*Based on density of 1 g/ml for the solvent.

Continued.

Units To convert from	Conventional units	
	To	Multiply by
Square yards (yd³)—cont'd	Square miles	$3.228305785 \times 10^{-7}$
	Square rods	0.033057851
Temperature		
Degrees Celsius (°C)	Degrees Fahrenheit	9/5 (then add 32)
Degrees Fahrenheit (°F)	Degrees Celsius	5/9 (after subtracting 32)
Time		
Years (calendar) (yr)	Days (mean solar)	365
	Hours (mean solar)	8760
	Minutes (mean solar)	525,600
	Months (lunar)	12.360065
	Months (mean calendar)	12
	Seconds (mean solar)	3.1536×10^7
	Weeks (mean calendar)	52.142857
	Years (sidereal)	0.99929814
	Years (tropical)	0.99933690
Volume and capacity		
Centiliters (cl)	Cubic centimeters	10
	Cubic inches	0.6102545
	Liters	0.01
	Ounces (U.S., fluid)	0.3381497
Cubic centimeters (cm³)	Cubic feet	3.5314667×10^{-5}
	Cubic inches	0.061023744
	Cubic meters	1×10^{-6}
	Cubic yards	1.3079506×10^{-6}
	Drams (U.S., fluid)	0.27051218
	Gallons (Brit.)	0.0002199694
	Gallons (U.S., dry)	0.00022702075
	Gallons (U.S., liq.)	0.00026417205
	Gills (Brit.)	0.007039020
	Gills (U.S.)	0.0084535058
	Liters	0.001
	Ounces (Brit., fluid)	0.03519510
	Ounces (U.S., fluid)	0.033814023
	Pints (U.S., dry)	0.0018161660
	Pints (U.S., liq.)	0.0021133764
	Quarts (Brit.)	0.0008798775
	Quarts (U.S., dry)	0.00090808298
	Quarts (U.S., liq.)	0.0010566882
Cubic decimeters (dm³)	Cubic centimeters	1000
	Cubic feet	0.035316667
	Cubic inches	61.023744
	Cubic meters	0.001
	Cubic yards	0.0013079506
	Liters	1
Cubic dekameters (dam³)	Cubic decimeters	1×10^6
	Cubic feet	35,314.667
	Cubic inches	6.1023744×10^7
	Cubic meters	1000
	Liters	1,000,000
Cubic feet (ft³)	Cubic centimeters	28,316.847
	Cubic meters	0.028316847
	Gallons (U.S., dry)	6.4285116
	Gallons (U.S., liq.)	7.4805195
	Liters	28.316847
	Ounces (Brit., fluid)	996.6143
	Ounces (U.S., fluid)	957.50649
	Pints (U.S., liq.)	59.844156
	Quarts (U.S., dry)	25.714047
	Quarts (U.S., liq.)	29.922078
Cubic inches (in³)	Cubic centimeters	16.387064
	Cubic feet	0.00057870370

Units To convert from	Conventional units	
	To	Multiply by
Cubic inches (in^3)—cont'd	Cubic meters	1.6387064×10^{-5}
	Cubic yards	2.1433470×10^{-5}
	Drams (U.S., fluid)	4.4329004
	Gallons (Brit.)	0.003604652
	Gallons (U.S., dry)	0.0037202035
	Gallons (U.S., liq.)	0.0043290043
	Liters	0.016387064
	Milliliters	16.387064
	Ounces (Brit., fluid)	0.57674444
	Ounces (U.S., fluid)	0.55411255
	Pints (U.S., dry)	0.029761628
	Pints (U.S., liq.)	0.034632035
	Quarts (U.S., dry)	0.014880814
	Quarts (U.S., liq.)	0.017316017
Cubic meters (m^3)	Cubic centimeters	1×10^6
	Cubic feet	35.314667
	Cubic inches	61,023.74
	Cubic yards	1.3079506
	Gallons (Brit.)	219.9694
	Gallons (U.S., liq.)	264.17205
	Liters	1000
	Pints (U.S., liq.)	2113.3764
	Quarts (U.S., liq.)	1056.6882
Cubic millimeters (mm^3)	Cubic centimeters	0.001
	Cubic inches	6.1023744×10^{-5}
	Cubic meters	1×10^{-9}
	Minims (Brit.)	0.01689365
	Minims (U.S.)	0.016230731
Deciliters (dl)	Milliliters	100
	Cubic centimeters	100
Dekaliters (dkl, dal)	Pecks (U.S.)	1.135136
	Pints (U.S., dry)	18.16217
Drams (U.S., fluid) (fl dr)	Cubic centimeters	3.6967162
	Cubic inches	0.22558594
	Gills (U.S.)	0.03125
	Milliliters	3.696588
	Minims (U.S.)	60
	Ounces (U.S., fluid)	0.125
	Pints (U.S., liq.)	0.0078125
Gallons (Brit.) (gal)	Barrels (Brit.)	0.027777
	Cubic centimeters	4546.087
	Cubic feet	0.1605436
	Cubic inches	277.4193
	Firkins (Brit.)	0.111111
	Gallons (U.S., liq.)	1.200949
	Gills (Brit.)	32
	Liters	4.545960
	Minims (Brit.)	76,800
	Ounces (Brit., fluid)	160
	Ounces (U.S., fluid)	153.7215
	Pecks (Brit.)	0.5
	Pounds of H$_2$O (62° F)	10
Gallons (U.S., dry)	Barrels (U.S., dry)	0.038095592
	Barrels (U.S., liq.)	0.036941181
	Cubic centimeters	4404.8828
	Cubic feet	0.15555700
	Cubic inches	268.8025
	Gallons (U.S., liq.)	1.16364719
	Liters	4.404760
Gallons (U.S., liq.) (gal)	Barrels (U.S., liq.)	0.031746032
	Cubic centimeters	3785.4118
	Cubic feet	0.13368055
	Cubic inches	231

Continued.

Units To convert from	Conventional units	
	To	Multiply by
Gallons (U.S., liq.) (gal)—cont'd	Cubic meters	0.0037854118
	Cubic yards	0.0049511317
	Gallons (Brit.)	0.8326747
	Gallons (U.S., dry)	0.85936701
	Gallons (wine)	1
	Gills (U.S.)	32
	Liters	3.7854118
	Minims (U.S.)	61,440
	Ounces (U.S. fluid)	128
	Pints (U.S. liq.)	8
	Quarts (U.S. liq.)	4
Gills (Brit.)	Cubic centimeters	142.0652
	Gallons (Brit.)	0.03125
	Gills (U.S.)	1.200949
	Liters	0.1420613
	Ounces (Brit., fluid)	5
	Ounces (U.S., fluid)	4.803764
	Pints (Brit.)	0.25
Gills (U.S.)	Cubic centimeters	118.29412
	Cubic inches	7.21875
	Drams (U.S., fluid)	32
	Gallons (U.S., liq.)	0.03125
	Gills (Brit.)	0.8326747
	Liters	0.1182908
	Minims (U.S.)	1920
	Ounces (U.S., fluid)	4
	Pints (U.S., liq.)	0.25
	Quarts (U.S., liq.)	0.125
Liters (L*)	Bushels (Brit.)	0.02749694
	Bushels (U.S.)	0.02837839
	Cubic centimeters	1000
	Cubic feet	0.03531566
	Cubic inches	61.02545
	Cubic meters	0.001
	Cubic yards	0.001307987
	Drams (U.S., fluid)	270.5198
	Gallons (Brit.)	0.2199755
	Gallons (U.S., dry)	0.2270271
	Gallons (U.S., liq.)	0.2641794
	Gills (Brit.)	7.039217
	Gills (U.S.)	8.453742
	Minims (U.S.)	16,231.19
	Ounces (Brit., fluid)	35.19609
	Ounces (U.S., fluid)	33.81497
	Pints (Brit.)	1.759804
	Pints (U.S., dry)	1.816217
	Pints (U.S., liq.)	2.113436
	Quarts (Brit.)	0.8799021
	Quarts (U.S., dry)	0.9081084
	Quarts (U.S., liq.)	1.056718
Milliliters (ml)	Cubic centimeters	1
	Cubic inches	0.06102545
	Drams (U.S., fluid)	0.2705198
	Gills (U.S.)	0.008453742
	Liters	0.001
	Minims (U.S.)	16.23119
	Ounces (Brit., fluid)	0.03519609
	Ounces (U.S., fluid)	0.3381497
	Pints (Brit.)	0.001759804
	Pints (U.S., liq.)	0.002113436
Millimeters (mm)	Ångström units	1×10^7
	Centimeters	0.1
	Decimeters	0.01

*It is recommended in the United States that the capital "L" be the accepted symbol for liter since most typefaces gives insufficient distinction between "l" and the numeral one "1."

Units To convert from	Conventional units	
	To	Multiply by
Millimeters (mm)—cont'd	Dekameters	0.001
	Feet	0.0032808399
	Inches	0.039370079
	Meters	0.001
	Micrometers	1000
	Mils	39.370079
Minims (Brit.) (min, ℳ)	Cubic centimeter	0.05919385
	Cubic inches	0.003612230
	Milliliters	0.05919219
	Ounces (Brit., fluid)	0.0020833333
	Scruples (Brit., fluid)	0.05
Minims (U.S.) (min, ℳ)	Cubic centimeters	0.061611520
	Cubic inches	0.0037597656
	Drams (U.S., fluid)	0.0166666
	Gallons (U.S., liq.)	1.6276042×10^{-5}
	Gills (U.S.)	0.0005208333
	Liters	6.160979×10^{-5}
	Milliliters	0.06160979
	Ounces (U.S., fluid)	0.002083333
	Pints (U.S., liq.)	0.0001302083
Ounces (Brit., fluid) (oz)	Cubic centimeters	28.41305
	Cubic inches	1.733870
	Drachms (Brit., fluid)	8
	Drams (U.S., fluid)	7.686075
	Gallons (Brit.)	0.00625
	Milliliters	28.41225
	Minims (Brit.)	480
	Ounces (U.S., fluid)	0.9607594
Ounces (U.S., fluid) (oz)	Cubic centimeters	29.573730
	Cubic inches	1.8046875
	Cubic meters	2.9573730×10^{-5}
	Drams (U.S., fluid)	8
	Gallons (U.S., dry)	0.0067138047
	Gallons (U.S., liq.)	0.0078125
	Gills (U.S.)	0.25
	Liters	0.029572702
	Minims (U.S.)	480
	Ounces (Brit., fluid)	1.040843
	Pints (U.S., liq.)	0.0625
	Quarts (U.S., liq.)	0.03125
Pints (Brit.) (pt)	Cubic centimeter	568.26092
	Gallons (Brit.)	0.125
	Gills (Brit.)	4
	Gills (U.S.)	4.803797
	Liters	0.5682450
	Minims (Brit.)	9600
	Ounces (Brit., fluid)	20
	Pints (U.S., dry)	1.032056
	Pints (U.S., Liq.)	1.200949
	Quarts (Brit.)	0.5
	Scruples (Brit., fluid)	480
Pints (U.S., dry) (pt)	Cubic centimeters	550.61047
	Cubic inches	33.6003125
	Gallons (U.S., dry)	0.125
	Gallons (U.S., liq.)	0.14545590
	Liters	0.5505951
	Quarts (U.S., dry)	0.5
Pints (U.S., liq.) (pt)	Cubic centimeters	473.17647
	Cubic feet	0.016710069
	Cubic inches	28.875
	Cubic yards	0.00061889146
	Drams (U.S., fluid)	128
	Gallons (U.S., liq.)	0.125

Continued.

Units To convert from	Conventional units	
	To	Multiply by
Pints (U.S., liq.) (pt)—cont'd	Gills (U.S.)	4
	Liters	0.4731632
	Milliliters	473.1632
	Minims (U.S.)	7680
	Ounces (U.S., fluid)	16
	Pints (Brit.)	0.8326747
	Quarts (U.S., liq.)	0.5
Quarts (Brit.) (qt)	Cubic centimeters	1136.522
	Cubic inches	69.35482
	Gallons (Brit.)	0.25
	Gallons (U.S., liq.)	0.3002373
	Liters	1.136490
	Quarts (U.S., dry)	1.032056
	Quarts (U.S., liq.)	1.200949
Quarts (U.S., dry) (qt)	Bushels (U.S.)	0.03125
	Cubic centimeters	1101.2209
	Cubic feet	0.038889251
	Cubic inches	67.200625
	Gallons (U.S., dry)	0.25
	Gallons (U.S., liq.)	0.29091180
	Liters	1.1011901
	Pints (U.S., dry)	2
Quarts (U.S., liq.) (qt)	Cubic Centimeters	946.35295
	Cubic feet	0.033420136
	Cubic inches	57.75
	Drams (U.S., fluid)	256
	Gallons (U.S., dry)	0.21484175
	Gallons (U.S., liq.)	0.25
	Gills (U.S.)	8
	Liters	0.9463264
	Ounces (U.S., fluid)	32
	Pints (U.S., liq.)	2
	Quarts (Brit.)	0.8326747
	Quarts (U.S., dry)	0.8593670
Scruples (Brit., fluid)	Minims (Brit.)	20
Square feet (ft^2)	Square centimeters	929.0304
	Square inches	144
	Square meters	0.09290304
	Square miles	3.5870064×10^{-8}
	Square rods	0.0036730946
	Square yards	0.111111

3-2	Conversions between conventional and SI units

	Conventional units	x	Factor	=	SI units
Gram	g/ml		$\dfrac{10^{15}}{mw}$		pmol/L
	g/100 ml		10		g/L
	g/100 ml		$\dfrac{10}{mw}$		mol/L
	g/100 ml		$\dfrac{10^4}{mw}$		mmol/L
	g/d		$\dfrac{1}{mw}$		mol/d
	g/d		$\dfrac{10^3}{mw}$		mmol/d
	g/d		$\dfrac{10^9}{mw}$		nmol/d
Microgram	μg/100 ml		$\dfrac{10}{mw}$		μmol/L
	μg/d		$\dfrac{1}{mw}$		μmol/d
	μg/d		$\dfrac{10^3}{mw}$		nmol/d
Micromicrogram	μμg		$\dfrac{10^3}{mw}$		fmol
	μμg/ml		$\dfrac{10^3}{mw}$		pmol/L
Milliequivalent	mEq/L		$\dfrac{1}{valence}$		mmol/L
	mEq/kg		$\dfrac{1}{valence}$		mmol/kg
	mEq/d		$\dfrac{1}{valence}$		mmol/d
Milligram	mg/100 ml		10^{-2}		g/L
	mg/100 ml		$\dfrac{10^{-2}}{mw}$		mol/L
	mg/100 ml		$\dfrac{10}{mw}$		mmol/L
	mg/100 ml		$\dfrac{10^4}{mw}$		μmol/L
	mg/100 g		10		mg/kg
	mg/100 g		$\dfrac{10}{mw}$		mmol/kg
	mg/d		$\dfrac{1}{mw}$		mmol/d
	mg/d		$\dfrac{10^3}{mw}$		μmol/d
Milliliter	ml/100 g		10		ml/kg
	ml/min		1.667×10^{-2}		ml/s
Millimeters of mercury	mm Hg		1.333		mbar
	mm Hg		0.133		kPa
Minute	min		60		s
	min		0.06		ks
Percent	%		10^{-2}		1 (unity)
	% (g/100 gm)		10		g/kg
	% (g/100 gm)		10^{-2}		kg/kg
	% (g/100 ml)		10		g/L
	% (g/100 ml)		$\dfrac{10}{mw}$		mol/L

Continued.

	Conventional units	x	Factor	=	SI units
Percent—cont'd	% (g/100 ml)		$\dfrac{10^4}{mw}$		mmol/L
	% (ml/100 ml)		10^{-2}		L/L

3-3 | Pounds to kilograms conversion*

Pounds	0	1	2	3	4	5	6	7	8	9
0	0.00	0.45	0.90	1.36	1.81	2.26	2.72	3.17	3.62	4.08
10	4.53	4.98	5.44	5.89	6.35	6.80	7.25	7.71	8.16	8.61
20	9.07	9.52	9.97	10.43	10.88	11.34	11.79	12.24	12.70	13.15
30	13.60	14.06	14.51	14.96	15.42	15.87	16.32	16.78	17.23	17.69
40	18.14	18.59	19.05	19.50	19.95	20.41	20.86	21.31	21.77	22.22
50	22.68	23.13	23.58	24.04	24.49	24.94	25.40	25.85	26.30	26.76
60	27.21	27.66	28.12	28.57	29.03	29.48	29.93	30.39	30.84	31.29
70	31.75	32.20	32.65	33.11	33.56	34.02	34.47	34.92	35.38	35.83
80	36.28	36.74	37.19	37.64	38.10	38.55	39.00	39.46	39.91	40.37
90	40.82	41.27	41.73	42.18	42.63	43.09	43.54	43.99	44.45	44.90
100	45.36	45.81	46.26	46.72	47.17	47.62	48.08	48.53	48.98	49.44
110	49.89	50.34	50.80	51.25	51.71	52.16	52.61	53.07	53.52	53.97
120	54.43	54.88	55.33	55.79	56.24	56.70	57.15	57.60	58.06	58.51
130	58.96	59.42	59.87	60.32	60.78	61.23	61.68	62.14	62.59	63.05
140	63.50	63.95	64.41	64.86	65.31	65.77	66.22	66.67	67.13	67.58
150	68.04	68.49	68.94	69.40	69.85	70.30	70.76	71.21	71.66	72.12
160	72.57	73.02	73.48	73.93	74.39	74.84	75.29	75.75	76.20	76.65
170	77.11	77.56	78.01	78.47	78.92	79.38	79.83	80.28	80.74	81.19
180	81.64	82.10	82.55	83.00	83.46	83.91	84.36	84.82	85.27	85.73
190	86.18	86.68	87.09	87.54	87.99	88.45	88.90	89.35	89.81	90.26
200	90.72	91.17	91.62	92.08	92.53	92.98	93.44	93.89	94.34	94.80

*Numbers in the farthest left column are 10-pound increments; numbers across the top row are 1-pound increments. The kilogram equivalent of weight in pounds is found at the intersection of the appropriate row and column. For example, to convert 34 pounds, read down the left column to 30 and then across that row to 4: 34 pounds = 15.42 kilograms.

3-4 Grams to pounds and ounces conversion for weight of newborns

Pounds \ Ounces	0	1	2	3	4	5	6	7	8	9	10	11	12	13	14	15
0	—	28	57	85	113	142	170	198	227	255	283	312	430	369	397	425
1	454	482	510	539	567	595	624	652	680	709	737	765	794	822	850	879
2	907	936	964	992	1021	1049	1077	1106	1134	1162	1191	1219	1247	1276	1304	1332
3	1361	1389	1417	1446	1474	1503	1531	1559	1588	1616	1644	1673	1701	1729	1758	1786
4	1814	1843	1871	1899	1928	1956	1984	2013	2041	2070	2098	2126	2155	2183	2211	2240
5	2268	2296	2325	2353	2381	2410	2438	2466	2495	2523	2551	2580	2608	2637	2665	2693
6	2722	2750	2778	2807	2835	2863	2892	2920	2948	2977	3005	3033	3062	3090	3118	3147
7	3175	3203	3232	3260	3289	3317	3345	3374	3402	3430	3459	3487	3515	3544	3572	3600
8	3629	3657	3685	3714	3742	3770	3799	3827	3856	3884	3912	3941	3969	3997	4026	4054
9	4082	4111	4139	4167	4196	4224	4252	4281	4309	4337	4366	4394	4423	4451	4479	4508
10	4536	4564	4593	4621	4649	4678	4706	4734	4763	4791	4819	4848	4876	4904	4933	4961
11	4990	5018	5046	5075	5103	5131	5160	5188	5216	5245	5273	5301	5330	5358	5386	5415
12	5443	5471	5500	5528	5557	5585	5613	5642	5670	5698	5727	5755	5783	5812	5840	5868
13	5897	5925	5953	5982	6010	6038	6067	6095	6123	6152	6180	6290	6237	6265	6294	6322
14	6350	6379	6407	6435	6464	6492	6520	6549	6577	6605	6634	6662	6690	6719	6747	6776
15	6804	6832	6860	6889	6917	6945	6973	7002	7030	7059	7087	7115	7144	7172	7201	7228
16	7257	7286	7313	7342	7371	7399	7427	7456	7484	7512	7541	7569	7597	7626	7654	7682
17	7711	7739	7768	7796	7824	7853	7881	7909	7938	7966	7994	8023	8051	8079	8108	8136
18	8165	8192	8221	8249	8278	8306	8335	8363	8391	8420	8448	8476	8504	8533	8561	8590
19	8618	8646	8675	8703	8731	8760	8788	8816	8845	8873	8902	8930	8958	8987	9015	9043
20	9072	9100	9128	9157	9185	9213	9242	9270	9298	9327	9355	9383	9412	9440	9469	9497
21	9525	9554	9582	9610	9639	9667	9695	9724	9752	9780	9809	9837	9865	9894	9922	9950
22	9979	10007	10036	10064	10092	10120	0149	10177	10206	10234	10262	10291	10319	10347	10376	10404

1 pound = 453.59 grams. 1 ounce = 28.35 grams. Grams can be converted to pounds and tenths of a pound by multiplying the number of grams by .0022. From Wong DL, Whaley L: *Whaley & Wong's essentials of pediatric nursing,* St Louis, 1993, Mosby.

3-5 Temperature

To *convert Centigrade or Celsius degrees to Fahrenheit degrees:* multiply the number of Centigrade degrees by 9/5 and add 32 to the result. *To convert Fahrenheit degrees to Centigrade degrees:* Subtract 32 from the number of Fahrenheit degrees and multiply the difference by 5/9.

Fahrenheit and Celsius equivalents: body temperature range

F°	C°	F°	C°	F°	C°	F°	C°	F°	C°
94.0	34.44	97.0	36.11	100.0	37.78	103.0	39.44	106.0	41.11
94.2	34.56	97.2	36.22	100.2	37.89	103.2	39.56	106.2	41.22
94.4	34.67	97.4	36.33	100.4	38.00	103.4	39.67	106.4	41.33
94.6	34.78	97.6	36.44	100.6	38.11	103.6	39.78	106.6	41.44
94.8	34.89	97.8	36.56	100.8	38.22	103.8	39.89	106.8	41.56
95.0	35.00	98.0	36.67	101.0	38.33	104.0	40.00	107.0	41.67
95.2	35.11	98.2	36.78	101.2	38.44	104.2	40.11	107.2	41.78
95.4	35.22	98.4	36.89	101.4	38.56	104.4	40.22	107.4	41.89
95.6	35.33	98.6	37.00	101.6	38.67	104.6	40.33	107.6	42.00
95.8	35.44	98.8	37.11	101.8	38.78	104.8	40.44	107.8	42.11
96.0	35.56	99.0	37.22	102.0	38.89	105.0	40.56	108.0	42.22
96.2	35.67	99.2	37.33	102.2	39.00	105.2	40.67		
96.4	35.78	99.4	37.44	102.4	39.11	105.4	40.78		
96.6	35.89	99.6	37.56	102.6	39.22	105.6	40.89		
96.8	36.00	99.8	37.67	102.8	39.33	105.8	41.00		

3-6   Physical elements*

Element	Symbol	Valence	Atomic number	Atomic weight†	Element	Symbol	Valence	Atomic number	Atomic weight†
Actinium	Ac	3	89	(227.0278)	Mendelevium	Md		101	(257.0956)
Aluminum	Al	3	13	26.98154	Mercury	Hg	1,2	80	200.59
Americium	Am	3,4,5,6	95	(243.0614)	Molybdenum	Mo	3,4,6	42	95.94
Antimony	Sb	3,5	51	121.75	Neodymium	Nd	3	60	144.24
Argon	Ar	0	18	39.948	Neon	Ne	0	10	20.179
Arsenic	As	3,5	33	74.9216	Neptunium	Np	4,5,6	93	237.0482
Astatine	At	1,3,5,7	85	(209.987)	Nickel	Ni	2,3	28	58.70
Barium	Ba	2	56	137.34	Niobium	Nb	3,5	41	92.9064
Berkelium	Bk	3,4	97	(247.0703)	Nitrogen	N	3,5	7	14.0067
Beryllium	Be	2	4	9.01218	Nobelium	No		102	(255.0933)
Bismuth	Bi	3,5	83	209.9804	Osmium	Os	2,3,4,8	76	190.2
Boron	B	3	5	10.81	Oxygen	O	2	8	15.9994
Bromine	Br	1,3,5,7	35	79.904	Palladium	Pd	2,4,6	46	106.4
Cadmium	Cd	2	48	112.40	Phosphorus	P	3,5	15	30.98376
Calcium	Ca	2	20	40.08	Platinum	Pt	2,4	78	195.09
Californium	Cf	3	98	(251.0796)	Plutonium	Pu	3,4,5,6	94	(244.0642)
Carbon	C	2,4	6	12.011	Polonium	Po	2,4	84	(208.9824)
Cerium	Ce	3,4	58	140.12	Potassium	K	1	19	39.098
Cesium	Cs	1	55	132.9054	Praseodymium	Pr	3	59	140.9077
Chlorine	Cl	1,3,5,7	17	35.453	Promethium	Pm	3	61	(144.9128)
Chromium	Cr	2,3,6	24	51.996	Protactinium	Pa		91	(231.0359)
Cobalt	Co	2,3	27	58.9332	Radium	Ra	2	88	(226.0254)
Columbium	See:	Niobium			Radon	Rn	0	86	(222.0176)
Copper	Cu	1,2	29	63.546	Rhenium	Re		75	186.207
Curium	Cm	3	96	(247.0704)	Rhodium	Rh	3	45	102.9055
Dysprosium	Dy	3	66	162.50	Rubidium	Rb	1	37	85.4678
Einsteinium	Es		99	(254.0881)	Ruthenium	Ru	3,4,6,8	44	101.07
Erbium	Er	3	68	167.26	Samarium	Sm	2,3	62	150.4
Europium	Eu	2,3	63	151.96	Scandium	Sc	3	21	44.9559
Fermium	Fm		100	(257.0951)	Selenium	Se	2,4,6	34	78.96
Fluorine	F	1	9	18.9984	Silicon	Si	4	14	28.086
Francium	Fr	1	87	(223.0198)	Silver	Ag	1	47	107.868
Gadolinium	Gd	3	64	157.25	Sodium	Na	1	11	22.98977
Gallium	Ga	2,3	31	69.72	Strontium	Sr	2	38	87.62
Germanium	Ge	4	32	72.59	Sulfur	S	2,4,6	16	32.06
Glucinum	See:	Beryllium			Tantalum	Ta	5	73	180.9479
Gold	Au	1,3	79	196.9665	Technetium	Tc	6,7	43	96.9062
Hafnium	Hf	4	72	178.49	Tellurium	Te	2,4,6	52	127.60
Helium	He	0	2	4.0026	Terbium	Tb	3	65	158.9254
Holmium	Ho	3	67	164.9304	Thallium	Tl	1,3	81	204.37
Hydrogen	H	1	1	1.0079	Thorium	Th	4	90	232.0381
Indium	In	3	49	114.82	Thulium	Tm	3	69	168.9342
Iodine	I	1,3,5,7	53	126.9045	Tin	Sn	2,4	50	118.69
Iridium	Ir	3,4	77	192.22	Titanium	Ti	3,4	22	47.90
Iron	Fe	2,3	26	55.847	Tungsten	W	6	74	183.85
Krypton	Kr	0	36	83.30	Uranium	U	4,6	92	238.029
Lanthanum	La	3	57	138.9055	Vanadium	V	3,5	23	50.9414
Lawrencium	Lr		103	(256.0986)	Xenon	Xe	0	54	131.30
Lead	Pb	2,4	82	207.2	Ytterbium	Yb	2,3	70	173.04
Lithium	Li	1	3	6.941	Yttrium	Y	3	39	88.9059
Lutetium	Lu	3	71	174.97	Zinc	Zn	2	30	65.38
Magnesium	Mg	2	12	24.305	Zirconium	Zr	4	40	91.22
Manganese	Mn	2,3,4,6,7	25	54.938					

*The 103 chemical elements known at present are included in this table. Some of those recently discovered have been obtained only as unstable isotopes.
†Based on Carbon-12. Figures enclosed in parentheses represent the mass number of the most stable isotope.

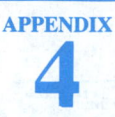

APPENDIX 4

SYMBOLS AND ABBREVIATIONS

4-1 Symbols

Symbol	Meaning	Symbol	Meaning
ℨ	Dram	−	Minus; deficiency; alkaline reaction; negative
fℨ	Fluid dram	±	Plus or minus; either positive or negative; indefinite
℥	Ounce	↑	Increased
f℥	Fluid ounce	↓	Decreased
O	Pint	#	Number; following a number, pounds
lb	Pound	÷	Divided by
℞	Recipe; take	×	Multiplied by; magnification
M	Misce; mix	=	Equals
A, Å	Angstrom unit	≅	Approximately equals
E_0	Electroaffinity	≠	Not equal to
F_1	First filial generation	>	Greater than; from which is derived
F_2	Second filial generation	<	Less than; derived from
mμ	Millimicron, micromillimeter	≮	Not less than
μg	Microgram	≯	Not greater than
mEq	Milliequivalent	≦	Equal to or less than
mg	Milligram	≧	Equal to or greater than
m%	Milligrams percent; milligrams per 100 ml	√	Root; square root; radical
Q O_2	Oxygen consumption	²√	Square root
m-	Meta-	³√	Cube root
o-	Ortho-	∞	Infinity
p-	Para-	∷	Ratio; "is to"
P_{O_2}	Partial pressure of oxygen	°	Degree
P_{CO_2}	Partial pressure of carbon dioxide	%	Percent
μm	Micrometer	π	3.1416—ratio of circumference of a circle to its diameter; pi
μ	Micron	□, ♂	Male
μμ	Micromicron	O, ♀	Female
+	Plus; excess; acid reaction, positive	⇌	A reversible reaction

4-2 | Abbreviations

Abbreviation	Meaning	Abbreviation	Meaning	Abbreviation	Meaning
A	Accommodation; acetum; angström unit; anode; anterior	AR	Alarm reaction	CABS	Coronary artery bypass surgery
		ARC	Anomalous retinal correspondence, AIDS-related complex	$CaCO_3$	Calcium carbonate
a	Accommodation; ampere; anterior; area			Cal	Large calorie
		ARD	Acute respiratory disease	cal	Small calorie
A_2	Aortic second sound	arg	Silver	CAT	Computerized (axial) tomography scan
ABG	Arterial blood gas	As	Arsenic		
ABO	Three basic blood groups	As.	Astigmatism	CBC or cbc	Complete blood count
AC	Alternating current; air conduction; axiocervical; adrenal cortex	AS	Left ear (auris sinistra)		
		ASD	Atrial septal defect	CC	Chief complaint
		AsH	Hypermetropic astigmatism	cc	Cubic centimeter
acc.	Accommodation	ASHD	Arteriosclerotic heart disease	CCl_4	Carbon tetrachloride
ACE	Adrenocortical extract			CCU	Coronary care unit, critical care unit
ACh	Acetylcholine	AsM	Myopic astigmatism		
ACH	Adrenocortical hormone	ASS	Anterior superior spine	cf	Compare or bring together
ACTH	Adrenocorticotropic hormone	AST	Aspartate aminotransferase (formerly SGOT)	CFT	Complement-fixation test
AD	Right ear (auris dextra)	Ast	Astigmatism	Cg; Cgm	Centigram
add	Add to (adde)	ATS	Anxiety tension state; antitetanic serum	CH	Crown-heel (length of fetus)
ADH	Antidiuretic hormone				
ADL	Activities of daily living	AU	Angström unit	$CHCl_3$	Chloroform
ADS	Antidiuretic substance	Au	Gold	CH_3COOH	Acetic acid
A/G; A-G ratio	Albumin-globulin ratio	A-V; AV; A/V	Arteriovenous; atrioventricular	ChE	Cholinesterase
				CHF	Congestive heart failure
Ag	Silver, antigen	Av	Average or avoirdupois	$C_5H_4N_4O_3$	Uric acid
ah	Hypermetropic astigmatism	ax	Axis	C_2H_6O	Ethyl alcohol
AHF	Antihemophilic factor	B	Boron; bacillus	CH_2O	Formaldehyde
AIDS	Acquired immunodeficiency syndrome	Ba	Barium	CH_4O	Methyl alcohol
		BAC	Buccoaxiocervical	Cl	Chlorine
aj	Ankle jerk	Bact	Bacterium	cm	Centimeter
Al	Aluminum	BBB	Blood-brain barrier	CMR	Cerebral metabolic rate
Alb	Albumin	BBT	Basal body temperature	CNS	Central nervous system
ALH	Combined sex hormone of the anterior lobe of the hypophysis	BE	Barium enema	c/o	Complains of
		Be	Beryllium	CO	Carbon monoxide
		BFP	Biologically false positivity (in syphilis tests)	CO_2	Carbon dioxide
ALT	Alanine aminotransferase (formerly SGPT)			Co	Cobalt
		Bi	Bismuth	CPC	Clinicopathologic conference
alt. dieb.	Every other day (alternis diebus)	Bib	Drink	CPD	Cephalopelvic disproportion
		bid; b.i.d.	Twice a day (bis in die)		
alt. hor.	Alternate hours (alternis horis)	BM	Bowel movement	CPR	Cardiopulmonary resuscitation
		BMR	Basal metabolic rate		
alt. noct.	Alternate nights (alternis noctes)	BP	Blood pressure; buccopulpal	CR	Crown-rump length (length of fetus)
Am	Mixed astigmatism	bp	Boiling point	CSF	Cerebrospinal fluid
AM	Morning	BPH	Benign prostatic hypertrophy	CSM	Cerebrospinal meningitis
a.m.a.	Against medical advice			CT	Computed tomography
amp.	Ampere	BRP	Bathroom privileges	Cu	Copper
ana	So much of each, or $\overline{aa}$	BSA	Body surface area	$CuSO_4$	Copper sulfate
anat	Anatomy or anatomic	BSP	Bromsulphalein	CVA	Cerebrovascular accident; costovertebral angle
AO	Anodal opening; atrioventricular valve openings	BUN	Blood urea nitrogen		
		C	Carbon; centigrade; Celsius	CVP	Central venous pressure
		$\overline{c}$	With	cyl	Cylinder
AOP	Anodal opening picture	C_{alb}	Albumin clearance	D	Dose; vitamin D; right (dexter)
AOS	Anodal opening sound	C_{cr}	Creatinine clearance		
A-P; AP; A/P	Anterior-posterior	C_{in}	Inulin clearance	DAH	Disordered action of the heart
		CA	Chronologic age; cervicoaxial		
A.P.	Anterior pituitary gland			D & C	Dilation (dilatation) and curettage
APA	Antipernicious anemia factor	Ca	Calcium, cancer, carcinoma		
AQ	Achievement quotient			DC	Direct current

Abbreviation	Meaning	Abbreviation	Meaning	Abbreviation	Meaning
DCA	Deoxycorticosterone acetate	fld	Fluid	Ht	Total hyperopia
Dcg	Degeneration; degree	fl dr	Fluid dram	Hy	Hyperopia
dg	Decigram	fl oz	Fluid ounce	I	Iodine
diff	Differential blood count	FR	Flocculation reaction	^{131}I	Radioactive isotope of iodine (atomic weight 131)
dil	Dilute or dissolve	FSH	Follicle-stimulating hormone		
dim	One half	ft	Foot	^{132}I	Radioactive isotope of iodine (atomic weight 132)
DJD	Degenerative joint disease	FUO	Fever of unknown origin		
dl	Deciliter	Gm; g; gm	Gram		
DNA	Deoxyribonucleic acid	GA	Gingivoaxial	IB	Inclusion body
DOA	Dead on arrival	Galv	Galvanic	IBW	Ideal body weight
dr	Dram	GB	Gallbladder	ICP	Intracranial pressure
DTR	Deep tendon reflex	GBS	Gallbladder series	ICS	Intercostal space
Dx	Diagnosis	GC	Gonococcus or gonorrheal	ICSH	Interstitial cell-stimulating hormone
E	Eye	GFR	Glomerular filtration rate		
EAHF	Eczema, asthma, and hayfever	GH	Growth hormone	ICT	Inflammation of connective tissue
		GI	Gastrointestinal		
ECG	Electrocardiogram, electrocardiograph	GL	Greatest length (small flexed embryo)	ICU	Intensive care unit
				Id.	The same (idem)
ECT	Electroconvulsive therapy	GLA	Gingivolinguoaxial	IH	Infectious hepatitis
ED	Erythema dose, effective dose	GP	General practitioner; general paresis	IM	Intramuscular; infectious mononucleosis
ED$_{50}$	Median effective dose	gr	Grain		
EDC	Estimated date of confinement	Grad	By degrees (gradatim)	IOP	Intraocular pressure
		Grav I, II, III, etc.	Pregnancy one, two, three, etc. (gravida)	IQ	Intelligence quotient
EDD	Estimated date of delivery			IS	Intercostal space
EEG	Electroencephalogram, electroencephalograph	GSW	Gunshot wound	IU	Immunizing unit
		gt	Drop (gutta)	IV	Intravenous
EENT	Eye, ear, nose, and throat	GTT	Glucose tolerance test	IVP	Intravenous pyelogram, intravenous push
EKG	Electrocardiogram, electrocardiograph	gtt	Drops (guttae)		
		GU	Genitourinary	IVT	Intravenous transfusion
Em	Emmetropia	Gyn	Gynecology	IVU	Intravenous urogram/urography
EMB	Eosin-methylene blue	H	Hydrogen		
EMC	Encephalomyocarditis	H$^+$	Hydrogen ion	K	Potassium
EMF	Erythrocyte maturation factor	H & E	Hematoxylin and eosin stain	k	Constant
				Ka	Cathode or kathode
EMG	Electromyogram	Hb; Hgb	Hemoglobin	KBr	Potassium bromide
EMS	Emergency medical service	H$_3$BO$_3$	Boric acid	kc	Kilocycle
		HC	Hospital corps	KCl	Potassium chloride
ENT	Ear, nose, and throat	HCG	Human chorionic gonadotropin	kev	Kilo electron volts
EOM	Extraocular movement			kg	Kilogram
EPR	Electrophrenic respiration	HCHO	Formaldehyde	KI	Potassium iodide
ER	Emergency room (hospital); external resistance	HCl	Hydrochloric acid	kj	Knee jerk
		HCN	Hydrocyanic acid	km	Kilometer
		H$_2$CO$_3$	Carbonic acid	KOH	Potassium hydroxide
ERG	Electroretinogram	HCT	Hematocrit	KUB	Kidney, ureter, and bladder
ERPF	Effective renal plasma flow	HD	Hearing distance	kv	Kilovolt
		HDL	High density lipoprotein	kw	Kilowatt
ESR	Erythrocyte sedimentation rate	HDLW	Distance at which a watch is heard by the left ear	L	Left; liter; length; lumbar; lethal; pound
EST	Electroshock therapy				
Et	Ethyl	HDRW	Distance at which a watch is heard by the right ear	L & A	Light and accommodation
ext	Extract			lb	Pound (libra)
F	Fahrenheit; field of vision; formula	He	Helium	LB	Large bowel (x-ray film)
		HEENT	Head, eye, ear, nose, and throat	LCM	Left costal margin
FA	Fatty acid			LD	Lethal dose; perception of light difference
FANA	Fluorescent antinuclear antibody test	Hg	Mercury		
		Hgb	Hemoglobin	LDL	Low density lipoprotein
F & R	Force and rhythm (pulse)	HIV	Human immunodeficiency (AIDS) virus	LE	Lupus erythematosus
FBS	Fasting blood sugar			l.e.s.	Local excitatory state
FD	Fatal dose; focal distance	HNO$_3$	Nitric acid	LFD	Least fatal dose of a toxin
Fe	Iron	H$_2$O	Water	LH	Luteinizing hormone
FeCl$_3$	Ferric chloride	H$_2$O$_2$	Hydrogen peroxide	Li	Lithium
		HOP	High oxygen pressure	LIF	Left iliac fossa
Fl	Fluid	H$_2$SO$_4$	Sulfuric acid	lig	Ligament
				Liq	Liquor

Continued.

Abbreviation	Meaning	Abbreviation	Meaning	Abbreviation	Meaning
LLL	Left lower lobe	$Na_2C_2O_4$	Sodium oxalate	PE	Physical examination
LLQ	Left lower quadrant	Na_2CO_3	Sodium carbonate	PEG	Pneumoencephalography
LMP	Last menstrual period	NAD	No appreciable disease	PET	Positron emission
LP	Lumbar puncture	NaF	Sodium fluoride		tomography
LPF	Leukocytosis-promoting	$NaHCO_3$	Sodium bicarbonate	PFF	Protein-free filtrate
	factor	Na_2HPO_4	Sodium phosphate	PGA	Pteroylglutamic acid (folic
LTH	Luteotrophic hormone	NAI	Sodium iodide		acid)
LUL	Left upper lobe	$NaNO_3$	Sodium nitrate	PH	Past history
LUQ	Left upper quadrant	Na_2O_2	Sodium peroxide	pH	Hydrogen ion
LV	Left ventricle	NaOH	Sodium hydroxide		concentration (alkalinity
L & W	Living and well	Na_2SO_4	Sodium sulfate		and acidity in urine and
M	Myopia; meter; muscle;	NCA	Neurocirculatory asthenia		blood analysis)
	thousand	Ne	Neon	Pharm;	Pharmacy
m	Meter	NH_3	Ammonia	Phar.	
MA	Mental age	Ni	Nickel	PI	Previous illness; protamine
Mag	Large (magnus)	NIH	National Institutes of		insulin
MAP	Mean arterial pressure		Health	PID	Pelvic inflammatory
MBD	Minimal brain dysfunction	NMR	Nuclear magnetic resonance		disease
mc; mCi	Millicurie	NPN	Nonprotein nitrogen	PK	Psychokinesis
μc	Microcurie	NPO;	Nothing by mouth (non	PKU	Phenylketonuria
mcg	Microgram	n.p.o.	per os)	PL	Light perception
MCH	Mean corpuscular	NRC	Normal retinal	PM	Postmortem; evening
	hemoglobin		correspondence	PMB	Polymorphonuclear
MCHC	Mean corpuscular	NTP	Normal temperature and		basophil leukocytes
	hemoglobin		pressure	PME	Polymorphonuclear
	concentration	NYD	Not yet diagnosed		eosinophil leukocytes
MCV	Mean corpuscular volume	O	Oxygen; oculus; pint	PMI	Point of maximal impulse
Me	Methyl	O_2	Oxygen; both eyes	PMN	Polymorphonuclear
MED	Minimal erythema dose;	O_3	Ozone		neutrophil leukocytes
	minimal effective dose	OB	Obstetrics		(polys)
mEq	Milliequivalent	OBS	Organic brain syndrome	PMS	Premenstrual syndrome
mEq/L	Milliequivalent per liter	OD	Right eye (oculus dexter);	PN	Percussion note
ME ratio	Myeloid-erythroid ratio		optical density	PNH	Paroxysmal nocturnal
Mg	Magnesium	OPD	Outpatient department		hemoglobinuria
mg	Milligram	OR	Operating room	PO; p.o.	Orally (per os)
μg	Microgram	ORIF	Open reduction and	PPD	Purified protein derivative
MHD	Minimal hemolytic dose		internal fixation		(TB test)
m Hg	Millimeters of mercury	OS	Left eye (oculus sinister)	Pr	Presbyopia; prism
MI	Myocardial infarction	Os	Osmium	PRN, p.r.n	As required (pro re nata)
MID	Minimum infective dose	OT	Occupational therapy	pro time	Prothrombin time
ML	Midline	OTD	Organ tolerance dose	PSP	Phenolsulfonphthalein
ml	Milliliter	OU	Each eye (oculus uterque)	pt	Pint
MLD	Median or minimum lethal	oz; ℥	Ounce	Pt	Platinum; patient
	dose	P	Phosphorus; pulse; pupil	PT	Prothrombin time; physical
MM	Mucous membrane	P_2	Pulmonic second sound		therapy
mm	Millimeter, muscles	P-A; P/A;	Posterior-anterior	PTA	Plasma thromboplastin
mmm	Millimicron	PA			antecedent
mμ	Millimicron	P & A	Percussion and	PTC	Plasma thromboplastin
μμ	Micromicron		auscultation		component
Mn	Manganese	PAB;	Para-aminobenzoic acid	PTT	Partial thromboplastin
mN	Millinormal	PABA			time
MRI	Magnetic resonance	Pap test	Papanicolaou smear	Pu	Plutonium
	imaging	Para I, II,	Unipara, bipara, tripara,	PUO	Pyrexia of unknown
MS	Multiple sclerosis	III, etc.	etc.		origin
MSL	Midsternal line	PAS;	Para-aminosalicylic acid	Px	Pneumothorax
MT	Medical technologist;	PASA		PZI	Protamine zinc insulin
	membrane tympani	Pb	Lead	Q	Electric quantity
mu	Mouse unit	PBI	Protein-bound iodine	qns	Quantity not sufficient
MW	Molecular weight	PCV	Packed cell volume	qt	Quart
My	Myopia	PD	Interpupillary distance	Quat	Four (quattuor)
N	Nitrogen	pd	Prism diopter; pupillary	R	Respiration; right;
n	Normal		distance		Rickettsia; roentgen
Na	Sodium	PDA	Patent ductus arteriosus	℞	Take
NaBr	Sodium bromide	PDR	Physician's Desk	RA	Rheumatoid arthritis
NaCl	Sodium chloride		Reference	Ra	Radium

Abbreviation	Meaning	Abbreviation	Meaning	Abbreviation	Meaning
rad	Unit of measurement of the absorbed dose of ionizing radiation; root	sp. gr., SG, s.g.	Specific gravity	Trans D	Transverse diameter
		sph	Spherical	TRU	Turbidity reducing unit
RAI	Radioactive iodine	SPI	Serum precipitable iodine	TS	Test solution
RAIU	Radioactive iodine uptake	spir	Spirit	TSH	Thyroid-stimulating hormone
RBC; rbc	Red blood cell; red blood count	SR	Sedimentation rate	TSP	Trisodium phosphate
		Sr	Strontium	TST	Triple sugar iron test
RCD	Relative cardiac dullness	SSS	Specific soluble substance, sick sinus syndrome	TUR; TURP	Transurethral resection
RCM	Right costal margin				
RE	Right eye; reticuloendothelial tissue or cell	sss	Layer upon layer (stratum super stratum)	U	Uranium; unit
				UA	Urinalysis
		St	Let it stand (stet; stent)	UBI	Ultraviolet blood irradiation
Re	Rhenium	Staph	Staphylococcus		
Rect	Rectified	stat	Immediately (statim)	UIBC	Unsaturated iron-binding capacity
Reg umb	Umbilical region	STD	Sexually transmitted disease, skin test dose		
RES	Reticuloendothelial system			Umb; umb	Umbilicus
Rh	Symbol of rhesus factor; symbol for rhodium	STH	Somatotrophic hormone	URI	Upper respiratory infection
		Strep	Streptococcus	US	Ultrasonic
RhA	Rheumatoid arthritis	STS	Serologic test for syphilis	USP	U.S. Pharmacopeia
RHD	Relative hepatic dullness, rheumatic heart disease	STU	Skin test unit	V	Vanadium; vision; visual acuity
		sv	Alcoholic spirit (spiritus vini)		
RLL	Right lower lobe			v	Volt
RLQ	Right lower quadrant	Sym	Symmetrical	VA	Visual acuity
RM	Respiratory movement	T	Temperature; thoracic	V & T	Volume and tension
RML	Right middle lobe of lung	t	Temporal	VC	Vital capacity
Rn	Radon	T_3	Triiodothyronine	VD	Venereal disease
RNA	Ribonucleic acid	T_4	Thyroxine	VDA	Visual discriminatory acuity
R/O	Rule out	TA	Toxin-antitoxin	VDG	Venereal disease—gonorrhea
RPF	Renal plasma flow	Ta	Tantalum		
RPM; rpm	Revolutions per minute	T & A	Tonsillectomy and adenoidectomy	VDM	Vasodepressor material
RPS	Renal pressor substance			VDRL	Venereal Disease Research Laboratories (sometimes used loosely to mean venereal disease report)
RQ	Respiratory quotient	TAB	Vaccine against typhoid, paratyphoid A and B		
RT	Reading test				
RU	Rat unit	Tab	Tablet		
RUL	Right upper lobe	TAH	Total abdominal hysterectomy	VDS	Venereal disease—syphilis
RUQ	Right upper quadrant			VEM	Vasoexciter material
S	Sulfur	TAM	Toxoid-antitoxoid mixture	Vf	Field of vision
S.	Sacral	TAT	Toxin-antitoxin, tetanus antitoxin	VHD	Valvular heart disease
S-A; S/A; SA	Sinoatrial			VIA	Virus inactivating agent
		TB	Tuberculin; tuberculosis; tubercle bacillus	VLDL	Very low density lipoprotein
SAS	Sodium acetate solution				
SB	Small bowel (x-ray film), sternal border	Tb	Terbium	VMA	Vanillylmandelic acid
		TCA	Tetrachloracetic acid	VR	Vocal resonance
Sb	Antimony	Te	Tellurium; tetanus	VS	Volumetric solution
SC	Closure of semilunar valves	TEM	Triethylene melamine	Vs	Venisection
		Th	Thorium	VsB	Bleeding in arm (venaesectio brachii)
Se	Selenium	TIA	Transient ischemic attack		
SD	Skin dose	TIBC	Total iron-binding capacity	VSD	Ventricular septal defect
Sed rate	Sedimentation rate	Tl	Thallium	VW	Vessel wall
SGOT	Serum glutamic oxaloacetic transaminase	Tm	Thulium; symbol for maximal tubular excretory capacity (kidneys)	W	Tungsten
				w	Watt
SGPT	Serum glutamic pyruvic transaminase			WBC; wbc	White blood cell; white blood count
		TNT	Trinitrotoluene	WD	Well developed
SH	Serum hepatitis	TNTC	Too numerous to mention	WL	Wavelength
S.I.	Soluble insulin	TP	Tuberculin precipitation	WN	Well nourished
Si	Silicon	TPI	Treponema pallidum immobilization test for syphilis	WR	Wassermann reaction
SIDS	Sudden infant death syndrome			wt	Weight
				X-ray	Roentgen ray
Sn	Tin			Z	Symbol for atomic number
SOB	Shortness of breath	TPR	Temperature, pulse, and respiration	Zn	Zinc
sol	Solution, dissolved			Zz	Ginger
SP	Spirit	tr	Tincture		

4-3 Common abbreviations used in writing prescriptions

Abbreviation	Derivation	Meaning	Abbreviation	Derivation	Meaning
ā ā	ana	of each	o.d.	omni die	every day
a.c.	ante cibum	before meals	o.h.	omni hora	every hour
ad	ad	to, up to	o.m.	omni mane	every morning
ad lib.	ad libitum	freely as desired	o.n.	omni nocte	every night
alt. dieb.	alternis diebus	every other day	os	os	mouth
alt. hor.	alternis horis	alternate hours	oz	uncia	ounce
alt. noct.	alternis noctes	alternate nights	p.c.	post cibum	after meals
aq.	aqua	water	per	per	through or by
aq. dest.	aqua destillata	distilled water	pil.	pilula	pill
b.i.d.	bis in die	two times a day	p.o.	per os	orally
b.i.n.	bis in noctis	two times a night	p.r.n.	pro re nata	when required
c.	cum	with	q.d.	quaque die	every day
Cap.	capiat	let him take	q.h.	quaque hora	every hour
caps.	capsula	capsule	q. 2 h.		every two hours
c.m.s.	cras mane sumendus	to be taken tomorrow morning	q. 3 h.		every three hours
			q. 4 h.		every four hours
c.n.	cras nocte	tomorrow night	q.i.d.	quater in die	four times a day
c.n.s.	cras nocte sumendus	to be taken tomorrow night	q.l.	quantum libet	as much as desired
			q.n.	quaque nocte	every night
comp.	compositus	compound	q.p.	quantum placeat	as much as desired
Det.	detur	let it be given	q.v.	quantum vis	as much as you please
Dieb. tert.	diebus tertiis	every third day			
dil.	dilutus	dilute	q.s.	quantum sufficit	as much as is required
elix.	elixir	elixir			
ext.	extractum	extract	℞	recipe	take
fld.	fluidus	fluid	Rep.	repetatur	let it be repeated
Ft.	fiat	make	s	sine	without
g	gramme	gram	seq. luce.	sequenti luce	the following day
gr	granum	grain	Sig. or S.	signa	write on label
gt	gutta	a drop	s.o.s.	si opus sit	if necessary
gtt	guttae	drops	sp.	spiritus	spirits
h.	hora	hour	ss	semis	a half
h.d.	hora decubitus	at bedtime	stat.	statim	immediately
h.s.	hora somni	hour of sleep (bedtime)	syr.	syrupus	syrup
			t.d.s.	ter die sumendum	to be taken three times daily
M.	misce	mix			
m.	minimum	a minim	t.i.d.	ter in die	three times a day
mist.	mistura	mixture	t.i.n.	ter in nocte	three times a night
non rep.	non repetatur	not to be repeated	tr. or tinct.	tinctura	tincture
noct.	nocte	in the night	ung.	unguentum	ointment
O	octarius	pint	ut. dict.	ut dictum	as directed
ol.	oleum	oil	vin.	vini	wine

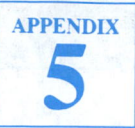

MEDICAL TERMINOLOGY

The ability to break down medical terms into separate components or to recognize a complete word depends on the mastery of the combining forms (a stem or root with an "o" attached), roots or stems that appear in medical terms, and prefixes and suffixes that alter or modify meaning and usage of a term.

5-1 Prefixes

Prefixes, the most frequently used elements in the formation of Greek and Latin words, consist of one or more syllables (prepositions or adverbs) placed before words or roots to show various kinds of relationships. They are never used independently, but when added before verbs, adjectives, or nouns, they modify the meaning. Most prefixes are a part of words in ordinary speech and do not refer specifically to medical or scientific terminology, but many occur frequently in medical terminology. The prefixes used in medical terminology are given in Appendix 5-1.

Prefix	Meaning	Examples
a-, an-	Without, not lack of	Aphasia (without speech)
		Anemia (lack of blood)
ab-	Away from	Abductor (leading away from)
		Aboral (away from mouth)
ad-	To, toward, near	Adductor (leading toward)
		Adrenal (near the kidney)
ambi-, ampho-	Both	Ambidextrous (ability to use hands equally)
		Amphogenic (producing young of both sexes)
amphi-	On both sides, double	Amphibious (living both on land and in water)
		Amphithymia (dual mental state of depression and elation)
ana-	Up, toward, apart	Anatomy (to cut apart)
		Anacatharis (vomiting up)
ante-	Before, in front of, forward	Antecubital (before elbow)
		Anteflex (to bend forward)
anti-	Against, opposing	Anticarious (against cavities)
		Antisepsis (against infection)
ap-, apo-	Separation from, derived from	Apobiosis (death of a part)
		Apocleisis (aversion to food)
aut-, auto-	Self	Autoanalysis (self analysis)
		Autoerotism (sexual self love)
bi-	Two, double, twice	Biarticulate (double joint)
		Bifocal (two foci)
		Bifurcation (two branches)
cata-	Down, under, lower, against	Catabolism (breaking down)
		Catalepsy (reduced movement)
circum-	Around	Circumflex (winding around)
		Circumarticular (around joint)
co-,* com-,† con-	With, together	Commissure (coming together)
		Conductor (leading together)
contra-	Opposed, against	Contralateral (opposite side)
		Contraception (prevention of conception)
de-	Down, from	Dehydrate (remove water from)
		Decay (break down)
di-	Two, twice	Dicephalous (two headed)
		Dichromic (having two colors)
dia-	Between, through, apart, across, completely	Diaphragm (wall across)
		Diapedesis (ooze through)
		Diagnosis (complete knowledge)

From Austrin MG, Austrin HE: *Learning medical terminology* ed. 7 St Louis, 1991, Mosby.
*co- before a vowel.
†com- before b, m, and p.

Continued.

Prefixes—cont'd

Prefix	Meaning	Examples
dis-	Apart or free from	Disinfection (infection)
		Disarticulation (separation at a joint)
		Dissect (cut apart)
dys-	Difficult, bad, painful	Dyskinesis (difficult motion)
		Dyspepsia (bad digestion)
		Dyspareunia (painful coitus)
e-, ec-, ex-	Out of, from, away from	Enucleate (remove whole from)
		Exostosis (outgrowth of bone)
		Ectopic (out of place)
		Ectal (on the surface)
ect-, ecto- exo-	Outer, outside, situated on	Ectoderm (outer skin)
		Ectocytic (outside of cell)
		Exogenic (originating outside)
em-,* en-	In	Empyema (pus in)
		Encranial (in the cranium)
end-, endo-, ent-, ento-	Within, inner	Endaural (within the ear)
		Endocranial (within cranium)
		Entiris (inner eye color)
		Entocele (internal hernia)
ep-, epi-	Upon, on, over	Epicostal (upon a rib)
		Epidermis (outer skin layer)
		Eponychia (infection over the nail bed)
eu-,	Normal, good, well, healthy	Eucrasia (normal health)
		Eublastic (healing well)
extra-, extro-	Outside of, beyond, outward	Extraoral (outside of mouth)
		Extroversion (turning inside out)
hemi-	Half	Hemiepilepsy (epilepsy on one side of body)
		Hemilingual (half of tongue)
hyper-	Excessive, above, beyond	Hyperactive (overactive)
		Hypertension (above normal blood pressure)
hyp-, hypo-	Under, deficient, beneath	Hypalgia (reduced pain sense)
		Hypothyroidism (deficiency of thyroid activity)
im-,† in-	In, into, within	Implant (insert into)
		Injection (forcing fluid into)
im-,† in-	Not	Immature (not mature)
		Involuntary (not voluntary)
infra-	Below, beneath	Infraorbital (beneath eye)
		Infracostal (below a rib)
inter-	Between	Intercostal (between ribs)
		Internodal (between nodes)
intra-	Within	Intracardiac (within heart)
		Intraocular (within the eye)
intro-	Into, within	Introversion (turning inward)
		Introrsus (turned in)
mes-, meso-	Middle	Mesencephalon (midbrain)
		Mesonasal (middle of nose)
meta-	Change, beyond	Metachrosis (color change)
		Metabasis (disease changes)
micr-, micro-	Small	Micracoustic (faint sounds)
		Microbe (minute organism)
mult-, multi-	Many	Multiangular (many angles)
		Multiform (many shapes)
neo-	New, recent	Neoblastic (new tissue growth)
		Neonatal (newborn)
pan-	All, entire	Panacea (cure-all)
		Pantalgia (entire body pain)
para-	Beside, beyond, after	Paracardiac (beside the heart)
		Paracyesis (pregnancy outside the uterus)
per-	Through, excessive	Permeable (may pass through)
		Peracute (excessively sharp)

*em- before b, m, and p.
†im- before b, m, and p.

Prefix	Meaning	Examples
peri-	Around	Periosteum (around bone)
		Peribulbar (around eye bulb)
poly-	Many, much, excessive	Polycystic (many cysts)
		Polydipsia (excessive thirst)
post-	After, behind	Postoperative (after surgery)
		Postocular (behind eye)
pre-, pro-	Before, in front of	Prenatal (before birth)
		Project (throw forward)
pseud-, pseudo-	False	Pseudarthrosis (false joint)
		Pseudocyesis (false pregnancy)
re-	Again, backward	Reflex (bend back)
		Regurgitation (vomiting)
retro-	Backward, behind	Retrograde (going backward)
		Retrolingual (behind tongue)
semi-	Half	Semiconscious (partly aware)
		Seminormal (half normal)
sub-	Under, beneath	Subcutaneous (under the skin)
		Subungual (under the nail)
super-, supra-	Above, superior, excess	Superactivity (overactivity)
		Suprarenal (above kidneys)
sym-,* syn-	Together, with	Symmelia (fusion of limbs)
		Synclinal (bent together)
trans-	Across, through	Transection (cut across)
		Transaortic (through aorta)
ultra-	Beyond, excess	Ultravirus (very small virus)
		Ultrasonic (beyond upper limit of human hearing)

*sym- before b, m, p, and ph.

5-2   Suffixes

Suffixes are the one or more syllables or elements added to the root or stem of a word (the part that indicates the essential meaning) to alter the meaning or indicate the intended part of speech.

To make a word pronounceable, the last letter or letters of the root to which the suffix is attached may be changed. The last vowel may be changed to an "o" or an "o" may be inserted if it is not already present before a suffix beginning with a consonant, as in cardiology. The final vowel in the root may be dropped before a suffix beginning with a vowel, as in neuritis.

Most suffixes are in common use in English, but some are peculiar to medical science. The suffixes most commonly used to indicate disease are *itis*, meaning inflammation; *oma*, meaning tumor; and *osis*, meaning a condition, usually morbid. The suffixes listed occur often in medical terminology, but they are also in use in ordinary language. These suffixes apply to Greek and Latin words.

Suffix	Meaning	Examples
-ac, -al, -ic, -ous, -tic	Pertaining to, relating to	Cardiac (pertaining to the heart) Neural (pertaining to nerve) Hemorrhagic (relating to bleeding) Delirious (relating to mental disturbance) Acoustic (pertaining to sound)
-algia, -dynia	Pain	Neuralgia (pain in nerves) Mastodynia (pain in breast)
-ate, -ize	Use, subject to	Impregnate (to make pregnant) Visualize (use imagination)
-cele	Protrusion (hernia)	Cystocele (bladder hernia) Rectocele (rectal protrusion into vagina)
-centesis	Surgical puncture to remove fluid	Paracentesis (from a body cavity) Thoracentesis (from chest cavity)
-cle, -cule, -ole, -ola, -ule, -ulum, -ulus	Small	Follicle (little bag) Molecule (small mass) Arteriole, arteriola (small artery) Nodule (small node) Ovulum (small egglike structure) Homunculus (small man)
-cyte	Cell	Leukocyte (white blood cell) Erythrocyte (red blood cell)
-ectomy	Cutting out	Lobectomy (of a lobe) Appendectomy (of the appendix)
-emesis	Vomit	Hematemesis (vomiting blood) Hyperemesis (excessive vomiting)
-emia	Blood condition	Leukemia (malignant blood disease) Anemia (lack of red blood cells)
-ent, -er, -ist, -or	Person or agent	Recipient (one who receives) Examiner (one who examines) Oculist (eye physician) Donor (one who donates)
-esis, -ia, -iasis, -ism, -ity, -osis, -sis, -tion, -y	State or condition	Paresis (partial paralysis) Anesthesia (loss of sensation) Psoriasis (skin condition) Priapism (persistent erection) Acidity (excess acid) Narcosis (drugged state) Inhalation (inhaling) Therapy (treatment condition)
-form, -oid	Resembling, shaped like	Fusiform (spindle shaped) Ovoid (egg shaped)
-genesis	Beginning process, origin	Pathogenesis (origin of disease) Homogenesis (young same as parent)
-gram, -graphy	Recording, written record	Mammogram (X-ray of breast) Cardiography (heart action record)
-graph	Instrument that records	Cardiograph (heart action) Encephalograph (brain function)
-ible, -ile	Capable, able	Flexible (capable of bending) Contactile (able to contract)
-ites, -itis	Inflammation	Tympanites (drumlike swelling of abdomen) Adenitis (inflammation of a gland)

Suffix	Meaning	Examples
-logy	Science, study of	Biology (science of life)
		Histology (study of tissues)
-oma	Tumor	Carcinoma (malignant growth)
		Sarcoma (cancerous tumor)
-penia	Deficiency of, lack of	Glycopenia (sugar in tissues)
		Leukopenia (white blood cells)
-pexy, -pexis	Fixation, storing	Nephropexy (of floating kidney)
		Glycopexis (glycogen in liver)
-phagia, phagy	Eating, devouring	Geophagia (eating dirt or clay)
		Aerophagy (swallowing air)
-phobia	Abnormal fear or intolerance	Acrophobia (fear of heights)
		Photophobia (intolerance of light)
-plasty	Surgical shaping or formation	Rhinoplasty (nose formation)
		Otoplasty (external ear)
-pnea	Breathing	Apnea (absence of breathing)
		Dyspnea (difficult breathing)
-ptosis	Prolapse, downward displacement	Proctoptosis (prolapse of anus)
		Nephroptosis (prolapse of kidney)
-rrhage, -rrhagia	Excessive flow	Hemorrhage (excessive blood flow)
		Metrorrhagia (abnormal menses)
-rrhaphy	Suturing in place	Herniorrhaphy (repair of hernia)
		Osteorrhaphy (wiring of bone)
-rrhea	Flow or discharge	Rhinorrhea (nasal discharge)
		Galactorrhea (breast milk)
-rrhexis	Rupture	Enterorrhexis (intestinal rupture)
		Metrorrhexis (rupture of uterus)
-scope	Instrument for examining	Microscope (minute objects)
		Cystoscope (urinary bladder)
-scopy	Act of examining	Microscopy (minute objects)
		Cystoscopy (urinary bladder)
-stomy	Surgical opening	Colostomy (colon to body surface)
		Gastrostomy (into stomach)
-tome	Instrument for	Cystotome (cutting into bladder)
		Neurotome (dissecting nerves)
-tomy	Cutting, incision	Cystotomy (of urinary bladder)
		Phlebotomy (incision of vein)

5-3 | Roots and combining forms in external anatomy

The list of roots and combining forms in Appendix 5-3 pertains only to external anatomy—that which can be visualized with the naked eye. Some terms are complete Latin or Greek words, and this is noted in the definition. They are arranged alphabetically, and the region of the body is indicated where applicable.

Word or combining form	Meaning	Body region*
axilla (pl. axillae)	Latin for armpit	E
blepharo-, blephar-	Eyelid or eyelash	H&N
brachium	Latin for arm, mainly the arm above the elbow	E
bucca	Latin for cheek	H&N
calx	Latin for heel (Do not confuse with calyx, a recess of the pelvis of the kidney.)	E
canthus (pl. canthi), cantho-	The angle at either end of the slit between the eyelids	H&N
capillus (pl. capilli)	Latin for hair (Term can apply to hair anywhere on the body.)	H&N
caput (pl. capita)	Latin for head	H&N
carpus, carpo-	Latin for wrist; also the eight bones of the wrist collectively	E
cephalo-	Relating to the head	H&N
cervix (pl. cervices), cervico-	Latin for neck or neck-like part (Term also used for cervix uteri, or neck-like projection of the uterus.)	H&N
cheilo-, cheil-	Greek for lip	H&N
cheiro-, chiro-, cheir-, chir-	Hand	E
cilium (pl. cilia)	Latin for eyelid or eyelash or any minute hairlike process attached to the free surface of a tissue or cell	H&N
core-, coro-	Pupil of eye	H&N
corium	Latin for true skin	
coxa	Latin for hip or hip joint (Also an internal anatomic term.)	T
cubitus	Latin for elbow, but used mainly to refer to the forearm	E
cutis	Latin for skin	
dactylo-	Digit, usually a finger but sometimes a toe	E
dento-, dent-, denta, denti, dentia	Tooth or teeth	H&N
derm-, derma-, dermato-, dermo-	Skin	
digit	Finger or toe	E
dorsum (pl. dorsa), dorso-	Latin for back	T
facio-	Face	H&N
frons, fronto-	Latin for forehead	H&N
genu	Latin for knee	E
gingiva	Gum	H&N
glosso-, gloss-	Tongue	H&N
gnatho-, gnath-	Jaw	H&N
irido-	Iris of eye (From a Greek word meaning rainbow or colored circle.)	H&N
hallux (pl. halluces)	Latin for great toe	E
inguen	Latin for groin (The "e" changes to "i" in words pertaining to the groin, e.g., inguinal.)	T
labio-	Lip, especially of the mouth	H&N
laparo-	Loin or flank; sometimes used loosely to refer to the abdomen	T
latus, latero-	Latin for side (Term may be used to denote either the side of any organ or a position.)	T
lingua	Latin for tongue	H&N
lumbus	Latin for loin	T
mamma (pl. mammae)	Latin for breast, or mammary gland	T
manus	Latin for hand	E
masto-, mast-	Breast	T
melia	Greek for limbs (melos)	E
mentum	Latin for chin (Do not confuse with words beginning with *men* that refer to the mind or menses; the sense in which it is used will govern the meaning.)	H&N
naris (pl. nares)	Latin for one of the openings into the nasal cavity	H&N
naso-	Nose	H&N
nucha	Latin for back, or nape, of neck	H&N
occiput	Latin for back part of the head	H&N
oculo-	Eye	H&N
odonto-	Tooth or teeth	H&N

*E, extremities; H&N, head and neck; T, trunk.

Word or combining form	Meaning	Body region*
omo-	Shoulder	T
omphalo-	Navel (umbilicus)	T
onycho-	Nail	E
ophthalmo-, ophthalm-	Eye	H&N
ora	Latin for mouth	H&N
orb	Latin for sphere or eyeball	H&N
orbit	Bony socket containing the eye	H&N
oto-	Ear	H&N
palpebra (pl. palpebrae)	Latin for eyelid	H&N
papilla (pl. papillae)	Latin for nipple or nipple-shaped projection	T
pectus	Latin for chest, thorax, or breast	T
pes, ped-, pod-	Foot (do not confuse with Greek *paed* or *ped,* referring to a child)	E
phallo	Latin for penis	T
pilo-	Hair	
plantar	Latin for sole of foot	E
pollex	Latin for thumb	E
poples	Latin for posterior surface of knee	E
rhino-, rhin-	Nose	H&N
soma, somato-	Greek for body	
sterno-	Sternum, or breastbone, as usually used, but formerly referred to chest	T
steth-, stetho-	Chest	T
stomato-, stomo-	Mouth	H&N
talus	Latin for ankle; also refers to an ankle bone	E
tarso-	Instep of the foot; also edge of eyelid	E
thele	Greek for nipple	T
thenar	Greek for palm of hand or sole of foot	E
thoraco-	Chest or thorax	T
-thrix	Suffix relating to hair	
trachelo-	Neck or neckline structure, such as the cervix	
tricho-	Hair	
unguis	Latin for nail of finger or toe	E
venter	Latin for stomach or belly, belly-shaped or hollowed part	T
ventro-	Belly; front or anterior aspect of the body	

*E, extremities; H&N, head and neck; T, trunk.

5-4   Roots and combining forms in internal anatomy

The roots and combining forms given in Appendix 5-4 pertain only to internal anatomy. Some terms are complete Latin or Greek words, and this is noted in the definition. Terms are arranged alphabetically, and the system of the body is indicated where applicable.

Word or combining form	Meaning	Body system*
adeno-	Gland	E
adreno-	Adrenal gland	E
angio-, angi-	Vessel, usually a blood vessel	CVL
arterio-	Artery	CVL
arteriolo-	Arteriole	CVL
arthro-	Joint	S
articulus (pl. articuli)	Latin for joint	S
atrio-	Atrium, upper chamber of the heart	CVL
auriculo-	Ear-shaped appendage of either atrium of the heart; the pinna or flap of the ear	CVL/SS
balano-	Glans penis	GU
bronchio-, broncho-	Bronchus	R
cardio-	Heart	CVL
cerebello-	Cerebellum, a part of the brain	N
cerebro-	Cerebrum, a part of the brain	N
cholangio-	Bile duct or bile duct capillaries	GI
chole-, chol-, cholo-	Bile	GI
cholecyst, cholecysto-	Greek for gallbladder	GI
choledocho-	Common bile duct	GI
chondro-, chondr-, chrondri-, chondrio-	Cartilage	S
chordo-	Cord; may be a vocal cord or the spermatic cord	SS/GU
cleido-, cleid-	Collar bone or clavicle	S
colpo-	Vagina	GU
condyle	Latin for a rounded projection (knuckle) on a bone	S
cor	Heart (*Cor* in coronary vessel does not derive from *cor* meaning heart, but rather from *corona,* meaning crown.)	CVL
cornu	Latin for horn or hornlike projection	
corpus	Latin for body or main part of any organ, or a mass of specialized tissue	
costo-	Rib	S
cysto-	Bladder or sac, most often used in reference to the urinary bladder, but also in connection with the gallbladder	GU, GI
-cyte	Suffix denoting a cell; the root to which it is attached designates the type of cell, such as erythrocyte (red cell)	CVL
cyto-	Cell	
dacryo-	Tear	SS
duodeno-	Duodenum, a section of the intestinal tract about 12 inches long (duodenum in Latin means 12 inches)	GI
encephalo-	Brain, or sometimes the head	N
entero-	Intestine	GI
episio-	Vulva	GU
fibro-	Fiber	M
gastro-, gastr-, gaster-	Stomach	GI
glio-	Glue or gluey substance, or more specifically the neuroglia, the supporting substance of the nervous system	N
hepato-, hepat-, hepatico-	Liver	GI
histo-	Tissue	
hystero-	Womb or uterus (This term is also used in pertaining to hysteria, a nervous reaction.)	GU
ileo-	Ileum, a part of the intestinal tract	GI
ilio-	Ilium, or flank	S
jejuno-	Jejunum, a section of the intestinal tract	GI

*S, skeletal system; M, muscular system; I, integumentary system; CVL, cardiovascular and lymphatic systems; R, respiratory system; GI, gastrointestinal system; GU, genitourinary system; E, endocrine system; N, nervous system; SS, special senses.

Word or combining form	Meaning	Body system*
kerato-	Cornea, or horny tissue	SS or I
laryngo-	Larynx or voice box	R
lieno-	Spleen	CVL
lumen	Latin for light; cavity or channel within a vessel or tubular organ	
lympho-	Lymph; used to refer to lymphatic vessel or to lymphocytes	CVL
meningo-	Meninges, coverings of the brain and spinal cord	N
metra-, metro-	Uterus	GU
myelo-	Bone marrow or spinal cord	S or N
myo-, my-	Combining form for muscle	M
myringo-	Eardrum	SS
nephro-	Kidney	GU
neuro-	Nerve	N
nodus	Latin for knot or node	
oophoro-	Ovary	GU
orchio-, orchi-, orchido-	Testicle or testis	GU
os	Latin for bone; also a term for mouth or any orifice of the body	
oscheo-	Scrotum	
osteo-	Bone	S
palato-	Palate or roof of mouth	GI
phalanx (pl. phalanges)	Greek for a line or array of soldiers; used in connection with fingers or toes because they somewhat resemble a line of soldiers or a battle formation	S
pharyngo-	Relating to the pharynx	R, GI
phleb-, phlebo-	Vein	CVL
phren-	Greek for diaphragm and the mind; the sense in which it is used will govern the meaning of the word or its intent	M or N
pleuro-	Pleura, side, or rib	R
pneumo-, pneumato-, pneumono-	Air, gas, or respiration and lungs	R
proct-, procto-	Anus or rectum	GI
pulmo-	Lung	R
pyel-, pyelo-	Pelvis of the kidney	GU
rachi-, rachio-	Spine	S
recto-	Rectum	
ren	Latin for kidney	GU
sacro-	Sacrum (The Latin *sacrum* means sacred; it has been postulated that the sacrum derived its name from the fact that it was offered in ancient sacrifices)	S
salpingo-	Fallopian tube or eustachian tube	GU, SS
sarco-	Flesh or fleshy	
splanchno-	Viscera or organs of any one of the great cavities of the body	
spleno-	Spleen	
spondylo-	Spinal column or a vertebra	S
sterno-	Sternum	
tendo-, teno-, tenonto-	Tendon	S
thymo-	Thymus gland	E
thyro-	Thyroid gland	E
tracheo-	Trachea	R
uretero-	Ureter, the vessel that conveys urine from the kidney to the bladder	GU
urethro-	Urethra, a tube discharging urine from the bladder	GU
vas (pl. vasa), vaso-	Latin for vessel (Vas may also be used as vas deferens, part of the genital organ in the male)	CVL/GU
vena (pl. venae), veno-	Latin for vein	CVL
ventri-, ventro-	Front (anterior aspect) of body	
vesico-	Bladder; also pertains to a blister	GU, I
viscero- (pl. viscera)	Relates to organs in the body	

*S, skeletal system; M, muscular system; I, integumentary system; CVL, cardiovascular and lymphatic systems; R, respiratory system; GI, gastrointestinal system; GU, genitourinary system; E, endocrine system; N, nervous system; SS, special senses.

5-5　Greek and Latin verbal derivatives

The verbs or combining forms of verbs listed in Appendix 5-5 are derived from either Greek or Latin. They may be attached to other roots to form words, or suffixes and prefixes may be added to them to form words. In the table the part or root of the word to which the verb is attached is italicized, and the meaning, if not clear, is given in parentheses.

Root or combining form	Meaning	Examples
-algia	Pain	*Cardi*algia (heart) *Gastr*algia (stomach) *Neur*algia (nerve)
audi-, audio-	Hear, hearing	Audio*meter* (hearing test device) Audio*logy* (study of hearing)
bio-	Live	Bio*logy* (study of living things) Bio*genesis* (origin of life)
caus-, caut-	Burn	Caus*algia* (burning pain) Caut*ery* (device to scar or burn)
-centesis	Puncture, perforate	*Thoraco*centesis (chest) *Pneumo*centesis (lung) *Arthro*centesis (joint) *Entero*centesis (intestine)
-clas-	Break	*Osteo*clasis (surgical fracture) Clas*tothrix* (splitting of hair)
-duct-	Lead	*Ab*duct (lead away from) Duct (tube leading to or from)
-dynia	Pain	*Masto*dynia (breast) *Pleuro*dynia (chest) *Esophago*dynia (esophagus) *Coccygo*dynia (coccyx)
-ectas-	Dilate	*Ven*ectasia (dilation of vein) *Phleb*ectasia (dilation of veins)
-edem-	Swelling	*Cephal*edema (swelling of head) Edem*atous* (swollen)
-esthes-	Sensation	*An*esthesia (without sensation) Esthes*iogenic* (producing sensation)
-fiss-	Split, cleft	Fiss*ure* (a cleft or groove) Fiss*ile* (capable of being split)
-flect-, -flex-	Bend	*Ante*flect (bend forward) Flex*ion* (bending)
flu-, flux-	Flow	Fluc*tuate* Flux*ion* *Af*fluent
gen/o-	Producing	Gen*esis* (origin or beginning) Gen*ophobia* (fear of sexuality)
-iatr/o-	Treatment	*Ger*iatrics (treatment of aging) *Ped*iatrics (treatment of children)
-kin/e-, -kin/o-, -kineto-,	Movement, motion	Kineto*genic* (producing movement) Kino*mometer* (motion measurer)
-liga-	Bind	Liga*ment* (suffix added to make noun) Liga*te* Liga*ture*
-logy	Study	*Parasito*logy (parasites) *Bacterio*logy (bacteria) *Histo*logy (tissues)
ly/o-, lys/o	Dissolve	Lyo*tropic* (readily soluble) Lyso*gen* (producing dissolution)
-morph-, -morpho-	Form, structure, shape	*A*morph*ous* (no definite form) *Poly*morph*ic* (many forms)
olfact-	Smell	Olfact*ophobia* (fear) Olfact*ory* (suffix added to make adjective)
-op/ia	Vision	*Hyper*opia (far sightedness) *My*opia (nearsightedness)

Root or combining form	Meaning	Examples
opt/ico-, opt/o	Seeing	*Optico*kinetic (eye movements)
		*Opto*meter (device for refraction)
palpit-	Flutter	*Palpit*ation
-par-, -partus-	Labor	*Postpartum* (after birth)
		*Par*turition (act of giving birth)
		Para i, ii, iii, iv, etc., are symbols for numbers of births
-pep-	Digest	*Dyspep*sia (bad, difficult)
		*Pep*tic (suffix added to make adjective)
-pexy	Fix	*Masto*pexy (fixation of breast)
		*Nephrospleno*pexy (surgical fixation of kidney and spleen)
-phag-, -phago-	Eating	*Phago*phobia *(fear of eating)*
		*Phago*mania (food craving)
		*Dys*phagia (difficult eating or swallowing)
phan/ero-	Visible, manifest	*Phan*erosis (becoming visible)
		*Phan*tasm (unreal mental image)
-phas-	Speak	*A*phasia (loss of speech functions)
		*Dys*phasia (difficulty in speaking)
-phil-	Affinity, love for	*Phil*anthropy (love of mankind)
		*Phil*oneism (love of change)
-phobia	Fear	*Hydro*phobia (fear of water)
		*Photo*phobia (fear of light)
		*Claustro*phobia (fear of close places)
-phrag-	Fence off, wall off	*Dia*phragm (across—partition separating thorax from abdomen)
		*Phrag*moplast (enclosed spindle where midbody forms in mitosis)
-plas-	Form, grow	*Neo*plasm (new growth)
		*Rhino*plasty (nose—operation for formation of nose)
		*Oto*plasty (common bile duct)
-plegia	Paralysis	*Para*plegia (paralysis of lower trunk and legs)
		*Hemi*plegia (one-sided paralysis)
-pne-, -pneo-	Breathe	*Dys*pnea (difficult breathing)
		*A*pnea (lack of breathing)
		*Hyper*pnea (overbreathing)
-poiesis	Formation, production	*Hemo*poiesis (blood cell formation)
		*Leuko*poiesis (white blood cell production)
-ptosis	Fall	*Procto*ptosis (anus—prolapse of anus)
		*Splanchno*ptosis (viscera)
-rrhagia	Burst forth, pour	*Meno*rrhagia (abnormal bleeding during menstruation)
		*Menometro*rrhagia (abnormal uterine bleeding)
		*Hemo*rrhage (blood)
-rrhaphy	Suture	*Hernio*rrhaphy (suturing or repair of hernia)
		*Hepato*rrhaphy (liver)
		*Nephro*rrhaphy (kidney)
-rrhea	Flow, discharge	*Leuko*rrhea (white discharge from vagina)
		*Galacto*rrhea (milk discharge)
		*Rhino*rrhea (nasal discharge)
-rrhexis	Rupture	*Entero*rrhexis (intestines)
		*Meto*rrhexis (uterus)
schist/o-, schiz/o-	Split, cleft, division	*Schisto*cystis (bladder fissure)
		*Schizo*nychia (splitting of nails)
-scope	Examine	*Micro*scope
		*Cardio*scope
		*Endo*scope (within—an instrument for examining the interior of a hollow viscus)
spasm/o-	Spasm	*Spasmo*genic (causing spasm)
		*Spasmo*lysis (relieving spasm)
-stasis	Standing still, stoppage	*Hemo*stasis (stoppage of blood flow)
		*Epi*stasis (stoppage of a flow)
-staxis	Drop	
-teg-, -tect-	Cover	*Teg*men
		*Tec*tum (rooflike structure)
		*In*tegument (skin covering)
-therap-	Treat, cure	*Therap*y
		*Neuro*therapy (nerves)

Continued.

Greek and Latin verbal derivatives—cont'd

Root or combining form	Meaning	Examples
-therap——cont'd		*Chemo*therapy (chemicals)
		*Physio*therapy
-tomy	Cut, incise	*Phlebo*tomy (incision of vein)
		*Arthro*tomy (joint)
		*Appendec*tomy (ectomy, meaning cut out—excision of appendix)
		*Oophorec*tomy (excision of ovary)
-topo-	Place	Topo*graphy*
		Topo*narcosis* (numbing—hence numbing of a part, or localized anesthesia)
-troph-, -tropho-	Nourishment, food	Troph*ism* (nutrition)
		*Dys*trophy (defective nutrition)
-volv-	Turn	*Involution*
		Volv*ulus* (twisting of an organ, as in intestinal obstruction with twisting of the bowel, or twisting of the esophagus)

5-6 | Greek and Latin adjectival derivatives

The roots and combining forms in Appendix 5-6 are derived from Greek or Latin adjectives. Adjectives will appear most often in compounds and will be joined to either nouns or verbs. Suffixes may be added to make them into nouns. In the table the part or root of the word the adjective modifies is italicized, and the meaning, if not clear, is given in parentheses.

Root or combining form	Meaning	Examples
ankylo-	Bent or crooked	Ankylo*glossia* (tongue-tie)
		Ankylo*sis* (stiff or fixed joint)
auto-	Self	Auto*infection*
		Auto*lysis*
		Auto*pathy* (disease)
		Auto*psy* (view—postmortem examination)
brachy-	Short	Brachy*gnathous* (receding underjaw)
brady-	Slow	Brady*cardia* (slow heartbeat)
		Brady*pepsia* (slow digestion)
brevi-	Short	Brevi*collis* (short neck)
		Brevi*flexor* (short flexor muscle)
cav-	Hollow	Cavity
		Cavernous
		Vena cava (vein)
cel-, coel-	Hollow, cavity	Celiac (of the abdominal cavity)
		Coel*om* (body cavity of embryo)
cryo-	Cold	Cryo*therapy* (treatment using cold)
		Cyro*anesthesia* (freezing body part)
crypto-	Hidden	Crypt*orchidism* (undescended testis)
		Crypt*omnesia* (subconscious memory)
dextro-	Right, right side	Dextro*manual* (right handed)
		Dextro*cardia* (heart on right side)
diplo-	Double, twice	Diplo*coria* (double pupil in eye)
		Dipl*opia* (double vision)
dolicho-	Long	Dolicho*derus* (long neck)
		Dolicho*cephalic* (long head)
dys-	Difficult, bad, disordered, painful	Dys*arthria* (speech)
		Dys*hidrosis* (sweat)
		Dys*kinesia* (motion)
		Dys*tocia* (birth)
		Dys*phasia* (speech)
		Dys*pepsia* (digestion)
		Es*ophoria* (crossed eye)
eso-	Within, inward	Eso*deviation* (a turning inward)
eu-	Well, good	Eu*phoria* (well-being)
		Eu*phagia,* eu*pnea* (breath)
		Eu*thyroid* (normal thyroid)
		Eu*tocia* (normal birth)
eury-	Broad, wide	Eury*cephalic* (unusually broad head)
		Eury*somatic* (thickset body)
glyc/o-	Sugar, sweet	Glyc*emia* (glucose in the blood)
		Glyco*geusia* (sweet taste)
gravis	Heavy	Gravid*a* (pregnant woman)
		Gravid*ism* (pregnancy)
haplo-	Single, simple	Hapl*oid* (single chromosome set)
		Haplo*pathy* (uncomplicated disease)
hetero-, heter-	Other, different	Hetero*cellular* (of different cells)
		Hetero*phypnosis* (induced by another)
homo-, homeo-	Same, alike	Homeo*morphous* (similar shape)
		Homo*zygous* (having identical genes)
hydro-	Wet, water	Hydr*emia* (excess water in blood)
		Hydro*adipsia* (absence of thirst)
iso-	Equal, alike	Iso*cellular* (having similar cells)
		Iso*coria* (equal-sized pupils)

Continued.

Greek and Latin adjectival derivatives—cont'd

Root or combining form	Meaning	Examples
latus, lat-	Broad	*Lat*itude *Latissimus dorsi* (muscle adducting humerus)
leio-	Smooth	*Leio*dermia (smooth, glossy skin) *Leio*trichous (smooth hair)
lepto-	Slender, small, thin	*Lepto*dermic (thin skinned) *Lepto*dactylous (slender fingered)
levo-	Left, to the left	*Levo*duction (eyes turn left) *Levo*rotation (turning to the left)
longus, long-	Long	*Long*itude *Adductor* longus (muscle of thigh)
macro-	Large	*Macro*cephaly (having large brain) *Macro*biosis (long life)
magna-	Large, great	*Magn*itude *Adductor* magnus (thigh muscle)
mal-	Ill, bad	*Mal*ady (illness) *Mal*aise (general discomfort)
malac/o-	Soft, softening	*Mal*acia (softening) *Malac*otomy (incision of soft parts)
medi-	Middle	*Medi*an *Medi*um *Gluteus* medius (femur muscle)
mega-, meg/alo-, meg/aly-	Large, oversized	*Meg*algia (severe pain) *Megalo*mania (grandiose delusions) *Hepato*megaly (enlarge liver)
meso-	Middle, mid	*Meso*carpal (wrist) *Meso*derm (skin) *Meso*thelium (a membrane lining of cavities)
micro-	Small	*Micro*glossia (tongue) *Micro*blepharia (eyelids) *Micro*organism *Micro*phonia (voice)
minimus	Smallest	*Gluteus* minimus (smallest muscle of hip) *Adductor* minimus (muscle of thigh)
mio-	Less, decrease	*Mio*sis (contraction of pupil) *Mio*pragia (decreased activity)
multi-	Many, much	*Multi*para (to bear—woman who has borne more than one child) *Multi*lobar (lobes) *Multi*centric (centers)
necro-	Death	*Necr*opsy (autopsy) *Necro*phobia (fear of death)
neo-	New	*Neo*formation *Neo*morphism (form) *Neo*natal (first 4 weeks of life) *Neo*pathy (disease)
oligo-	Few, little	*Oligo*menorrhea (scanty menses) *Oligo*symptomatic (few symptoms)
opisth/o-	backward, behind, dorsal	*Opistho*cheilia (recession of lips) *Opistho*poreia (walking backward)
ortho-	Straight, normal, correct	*Ortho*dontics (straightening teeth) *Ortho*grade (walking erect)
oxy-	Sharp, quick	*Oxy*esthesia (overly acute senses) *Oxy*rhine (sharp-pointed nose)
pachy-	Thick	*Pachy*derma (abnormally thick skin) *Pachy*onychia (overly thick nails)
paleo-	Old, primitive	*Paleo*genetic (originated in past) *Paleo*logic (primitive reasoning)
platy-	Flat, wide	*Platy*glossal (wide flat tongue) *Platy*cephaly (flattened skull)
pleo-	More	*Pleo*nexia (excessive greediness) *Pleo*nosteosis (excess bone growth)

Root or combining form	Meaning	Examples
poikilo-	Irregular, varied	Poikilo*derma* (mottled skin)
poly-	Many, much	Poikilo*thermic* (cold blooded)
		Poly*hedral* (many bases or faces)
		Poly*mastia* (more than two breasts)
		Poly*melia* (supernumerary limbs)
		Poly*myalgia* (pain in many muscles)
pronus	Face down	Prone
		Pron*ation*
pseudo-	False, spurious	Pseudo*stratified* (layered)
		Psuedo*cirrhosis* (suggestive of cirrhosis of liver)
		Pseudo*hypertrophy*
sclero-	Hardness	Sclerosis (hardening)
		*Arterio*sclerosis (artery hardening)
scolio-	Twisted, crooked	Scoliosis (crooked spine)
		Scolio*kyphosis* (curvature of spine)
sinistro-	Left	Sinistro*cular* (left eyed)
		Sinistro*manual* (left handed)
steno-	Narrow	Steno*sed* (narrowed, contracted)
		Steno*stomia* (narrow oral cavity)
stereo-	Solid, three dimensions	Stereo*scopic* (solid appearance)
		Stereo*psis* (three-dimensional vision)
supinus	Face up	Supine
		Supin*ation*
		Supin*ator longus* (muscle in arm)
tachy-	Rapid, fast	Tachy*phagia* (bolting one's food)
		Tachy*logia* (rapid speech)
tele-, telo-	Distant, end	Tel*algia* (pain from another area)
		Tele*ncephalon* (end brain)
thermo-	Heat	Thermo*genic* (producing heat)
		Thermo*labile* (destruction by heat)
trachy-	Rough	Trachy*phonia* (voice)
		Trachy*chromatic* (deeply staining)
xero-	Dry	Xero*cheilia* (dry lips)
		Xero*stomia* (dry mouth)

5-7 Miscellaneous words and combining forms

Word or combining form	Definition
Body fluids	
aqua (pl. aquae)	Latin for water
chol-, chole-, cholo-	Bile
chyle	Latin for juice; a milky fluid consisting of lymph and emulsified fats that are taken up by the intestinal lymphatic glands from food and eventually mixed with the blood
dacryo-, lacrima	Tears
-emia	Greek *(haima)* for blood. (-emia often appears as a suffix, as in anemia, deficiency of blood)
galact-, galacta-, galacto-	Milk
hem-, hema-, hemo-, hemato-	Blood
hidro	Sweat
hydr-, hydro-	Water; also hydrogen
lac	Latin for milk
lacri-	Tears
lympho-	Lymph
mucus	Latin for the secretions (mucins) of the mucous membranes together with the inorganic salts, desquamated cells, and leukocytes. *Mucous* is an adjective; the mucous membrane is called *mucosa* (mu'ko'sah).
myxo-	Mucus (Greek, *myxa*)
plasma	Fluid portion of the blood in which corpuscles are suspended
pus	Latin for the liquid inflammatory product composed of leukocytes and a thin fluid
pyro-	Pus
ptyalo-	Clear, alkaline secretion from the salivary glands—submaxillary, sublingual, parotid, or other smaller mucous glands in the mouth
sangui-	Blood
serum	Latin for whey; the clear portion of animal liquid after separation from the more solid elements—especially blood serum
sialo-	Saliva or salivary gland
sudor	Latin for sweat or perspiration
ur-, uro-, urono-	Urine, urinary tract, or urination
Body substances	
adipo-	Fat
amylo-	Starch
cerumen	From *cera*, Latin for wax; a waxlike secretion found within the ear (earwax)
collagen	From the Greek word *kolla;* a derivative of colla and an albuminoid substance that acts as a main supportive protein of skin, tendon, bone, cartilage, and connective tissue
eleo-	Oil
ferrum	Latin for iron
glyco-	Sugar
halo-	Salt
heme	Iron; a constituent of hemoglobin (formerly called hematin)
hormone	A chemical substance produced in the body with a specific regulatory effect on certain cells or organs
hyal-, hyalo-	Glassy
lapis	Latin for stone
lipos, lipo-	Greek for fat
litho-	Stone or calculus
mel-, meli-	Sweet (from Greek and Latin words for honey)
natrium	Latin for sodium
oleo	Oil
petrous	Latin for resembling a rock
saccharo-	Sugar
sal	Latin for salt
sebum	Latin for suet; the secretion of the sebaceous glands
sperm	Semen, or testicular secretion
Colors	
albus	Latin for white
chloros, chloro-	Greek for green
cirrhos	From *kirrhus,* Greek for orange-yellow

Word or combining form	Definition
Colors—cont'd	
cyano-	Blue
erythro-	Red
leuco-, leuko-	White
lutein	Saffron yellow
melano-	Black
polio-	Gray, particularly referring to gray matter of the nervous system
porphyro-	Purple
rhodo-	Red
ruber	Latin for red
xantho-	Yellow
Numeral combining forms	
one	mono-, mon
two	dyo-, dy-
three	tri-
four	tetra-, tetr-
five	pent-, penta-
six	hex-, hexa-
seven	hept-, hepta-
eight	octo-, octa-, oct-
nine	ennea
ten	deka-, dek-
one hundred	hecto-, hecato-, hect-
one half	hemi-
one thousand	kilo-
first	proto-, prot-
second	deutero-, deuto-, deut-
third	trito-, trit-
one-hundredth	centi-
one-thousandth	milli-
twice, duplication	di-, dis-*

*di, dis- in Latin means separation, like Greek dys.

APPENDIX
6

LANGUAGE TRANSLATION GUIDE

Spanish-French-English equivalents of commonly used medical terms and phrases

English	Spanish	French
General phrases		
What is your name?	¿Cómo se llama usted? (¿Cuál es su nombre?)	Comment vous appelez-vous?
Where do you work?	¿Dónde trabaja? (Cuál es su profesión o trabajo?) (¿Qué hace usted?)	Où travaillez-vous?
You will need blood and urine tests.	Usted va a necesitar pruebas de sangre y de orina.	Vous avez besoin d'une analyse de sang et d'urine.
You will be admitted to a hospital.	Usted será ingresado al hospital.	Vous allez être admis à un hôpital.
May I help you?	¿Puedo ayudarle?	Puis-je vous aider?
How are you feeling? Where does it hurt?	¿Como se siente? ¿Donde le duele?	Comment vous sentez-vous? Où avez-vous mal?
Do you feel better today?	¿Se siente mejor hoy?	Vous sentez-vous mieux aujourd'hui?
Are you sleepy?	¿Tiene usted sueño?	Avez-vous sommeil?
The doctor will examine you now.	El doctor le examinará ahora.	Le médecin va vous examiner maintenant.
You should remain in bed today.	Usted debe guardar cama hoy.	Vous devriez rester au lit aujourd'hui.
We want you to get up now.	Queremos que se levante ahora.	Nous voulons que vous vous leviez maintenant.
You make take a bath.	Puede bañarse.	Vous pouvez prendre un bain.
You may take a shower.	Puede tomar una ducha.	Vous pouvez prendre une douche.
Have you notice any bleeding?	¿Ha notado alguna hemorragia?	Avez-vous remarqué un saignement?
Do you still have any numbness?	¿Todavía siente adormecimiento?	Ressentez-vous encore un engourdissement?
Do you have any drug allergies?	¿Es usted alergico(a) algún médicamento?	Souffrez-vous d'allergie à des médicaments?
I need to change your dressing.	Necesito cambiar su vendaje.	Je dois changer votre pansement.
What medications are you taking now?	¿Que médicamentos está tomando ahora?	Quels médicaments prenez-vous actuellement?
Do you take any medications?	¿Toma usted algunas medicina?	Prenez-vous des médicaments?
Do you have a history of	¿Padece	Avez-vous déjà souffert de
a. heart disease?	a. del corazón?	a. maladie du coeur?
b. diabetes?	b. de diabetes?	b. diabète?
c. epilepsy?	c. de epilepsia?	c. épilepsie?
d. bronchitis?	d. de bronquitis?	d. bronchite?
e. emphysema?	e. de enfisema?	e. emphysème?
f. asthma?	f. de asma?	f. asthme?
Do you need a sleeping pill?	¿Necesita una pastilla para dormir?	Avez-vous besoin d'un somnifère?
Do you need a laxative?	¿Necesita un laxante/purgante?	Avez-vous besoin d'un laxatif?
Relax. Try to sleep.	Relajese. Trate de dormir.	Détendez-vous. Essayez de dormir.
Please turn on your side.	Favor de ponerse de labo.	Veuillez vous tourner sur le côté.
Do you have to urinate?	¿Tiene que orinar?	Avez-vous besoin d'uriner?
Have you had any sickness from any medicine?	¿Le ha caido mal alguna medicina?	Avez-vous déjà eu des réactions à un médicament?
Are you allergic to anything? Medicines, drugs, foods, insect bites?	¿Es usted alergicao(a) a algo? ¿Medicinas, drogas, alimentos, picaduras de insectos?	Êtes-vous allergique à quelque chose? Médicaments, drogues, aliments, piqûres d'insectes?
Do you use contact lenses, dentures? Do you have any loose teeth, removable bridges, or any prosthesis?	¿Usa usted lentes de contacto, dentadura postiza? ¿Tiene dientes flojos, dientes postizos, o cualquier prostesis?	Utilisez-vous des verres de contact, des prothèses dentaires? Avez-vous des dents qui se déchaussent, des ponts amovibles ou une prothèse?
Press the button when you want a nurse.	Apriete el boton cuando quiera a una enfermera.	Appuyez sur le bouton pour appeler une infirmière.

Spanish adapted from Lister S, Wilber CJ: *Medical Spanish: the instant survival guide*, London, 1983, Butterworth.
French translations provided by Catherine Moor, translator, Montreal, Quebec, Canada.

English	Spanish	French

Vocabulary

Anatomy

English	Spanish	French
abdomen	el abdomen	l'abdomen
ankle	el tobillo	le cheville
anus	el ano	l'anus
appendix	el apéndice	le appendice
arm	el brazo	le bras
back	la espalda	le dos
lower back	la cintura	le bas du dos
bladder	le vejiga	la vessie
blood	la sangre	le sang
body	el cuerpo	le corps
bone	el hueso	le os
bowels	los intestinos, las entrañas	les intestins
brain	el cerebro	le cerveau
breasts	el pecho, los senos	les seins
buttocks	las nalgas, las posaderas, las sentaderas	les fesses
calf	la pantorrilla, el chamorro	le mollet
chest	el pecho	la poitrine
coccyx	la cóccix	le coccyx
collarbone	la clavícula	la clavicule
ear (inner)	el oído	l'oreille (interne)
ear (outer)	la oreja	l'oreille (externe)
eardrum	el tímpano	le tympan
ears	las orejas	les oreilles
elbow	el codo	le coude
eye	el ojo	l'oeil
face	la cara	le visage
fallopian tube	el tubo falopio	la trompe de Fallope
finger	el dedo	le doigt
foot	el pie	le pied
genitals	los genitales	les parties génitales
hair (of the head)	el pelo, el cabello	le cheveu
hand	la mano	la main
head	la cabeza	la tête
heart	el corazón	le coeur
heart valve	la válvula del corazón	la valvule cardiaque
hip	la cadera	la hanche
hormone	la hormona	la hormone
intestines	los intestinos	les intestins
jaw	la quijada	la mâchoire
joint	la coyuntura, la articulación	l'articulation
kidney	el riñón	le rein
knee	la rodilla	le genou
leg	la pierna	la jambe
ligament	el ligamento	le ligament
lip	el labio	la lèvre
liver	el hígado	le foie
lung	el pulmón	le poumon
mouth	la boca	la bouche
muscle	el músculo	le muscle
neck	el cuello	le cou
nerve	el nervio	le nerf
nose	la nariz	le nez
ovary	el ovario	l'ovaire
pelvis	la cadera, la pelvis	le bassin
penis	el pene, el miembro	le pénis
pulse	el pulso	le pouls
pupil	la niña del ojo, la pupila	la pupille
rib	la costilla	la côte
saliva	la saliva	la salive
shoulder	el hombro	l'épaule
sinus	el seno	le sinus
skin	la piel	l'épiderme

Continued.

Spanish-French-English equivalents of commonly used medical terms and phrases—cont'd

English	Spanish	French
Vocabulary—cont'd		
Anatomy—cont'd		
skin (of the face)	el cutis	la peau (du visage)
skull	el cráneo	la crâne
spine	el espinazo, la columna vertebral	la colonne vertébrale
stomach	el estómago, la panza, la barriga	l'estomac
tendon	el tendón	le tendon
thigh	el muslo	la cuisse
toe	el dedo del pie	l'orteil
tongue	la lengua	la langue
tonsils	las angínas, las amígdalas	les amygdales
tooth, molar	el diente, la muela	la dent, molaire
trachea	la tráquea	la trachée
urine	la orina	l'urine
uterus	el útero, la matriz	l'utérus
vagina	la vagina	le vagin
vein	la vena	la veine
wrist	la muñeca	le poignet
Common medical problems		
abortion	el aborto	l'avortement
abscess	el absceso	l'abcès
appendicitis	la appendicitis	l'appendicite
arthritis	la artritis	l'arthrite
asthma	el asma	l'asthme
backache	el dolor de espalda	la lombalgie
blindness	la ceguera	la cécité
bronchitis	la bronquitis	la bronchite
bruise	moretón, magulladura	la contusion
burn (1st, 2nd, or 3rd degree)	la quemadura (de primer, segundo o tercer grado)	la brûlure (premier, deuxième, ou troisième degré)
cancer	el cáncer	le cancer
chickenpox	la varicela	la varicelle
chills	los escalofríos	les frissons
cold	el catarro, el resfriado	le froid
constipation	la constipación	la constipation
convulsion	la convulsión	la convulsion
cough	la tos	la toux
cramps	los calambres	les crampes
cut	cortada, cortadura	la coupure
deafness	la sordera	la surdité
diabetes	la diabetes	le diabète
diarrhea	la diarrea	la diarrhée
dizziness	el vértigo, el mareo	les vertiges
epilepsy	la epilepsia	l'épilepsie
fainting spell	el desmayo	l'évanouissement
fatigue	la fatiga	la fatigue
fever	la fiebre	la fièvre
flu	la influenza, la gripe	la grippe
food poisoning	el envenamiento por comestibles	l'intoxication alimentaire
fracture	la fractura	la fracture
gall stone	el cálculo biliar	le calcul biliaire
gastric ulcer	la úlcera gástrica	l'ulcère gastrique
hallucination	la alucinación	la hallucination
handicap	el impedimento	le handicap
headache	el dolor de cabeza	le mal de tête
heart attack	el ataque al corazón	la crise cardiaque
heartbeat	el latido-el palpito	la pulsation cardiaque
		le battement de coeur
heart disease	la enfermedad del corazón	la maladie du coeur
heart murmur	el soplo del corazón	le souffle cardiaque
hemorrhage	la hemorragia	la hémorragie
hemorrhoids	la almorranas	las hémorroïdes
hernia	la hernia	la hernie

English	Spanish	French
Common medical problems—cont'd		
herpes	el herpes	la herpès
high blood pressure	la presión alta	la hypertension artérielle
hives	la urticaria	l'urticaire
illness	la enfermedad	la maladie
immunization	la inmunización	l'immunisation
infection	la infección	l'infection
inflammation	la inflamación	l'inflammation
injury	la herida, el daño	la blessure
itch	la picazón-la comezón	la démangeaison
laryngitis	la laringitis	la laryngite
lice	los piojos	le poux
malaria	la malaria	la malaria
malignant	maligno(a)	la malin, maligne
malnutrition	la mala nutrición	la malnutrition
measles	el serampión	la rougeole
meningitis	la meningitis	la méningite
menopause	la menopausa	la ménopause
miscarriage	un malparto, un aborto, una perdida	la fausse couche
mononucleosis	la mononucleosis infecciosa	la mononucléose
multiple sclerosis	la esclerosis múltiple	la sclérose en plaques
mumps	las paperas	les oreillons
muscular dystrophy	la distrofía muscular	la dystrophie musculaire
mute	mudo(a)	le muet (muette)
obese	obeso(a)	l'obèse
obstruction	la obtrucción	l'obstruction
overdose	la sobredosis	la surdose
overweight	el sobrepeso	l'embonpoint
pain	el dolor	la douleur
palsy, cerebral	la parálisis cerebral	l'infirmité motrice cérébrale
paralysis	la parálisis	la paralysie
Parkinson's disease	la enfermedad de Parkinson	la maladie de Parkinson
pneumonia	la pulmonía	la pneumonie
poison ivy/oak	la hiedra venenosa	la herbe à la puce le sumac de l'Ouest
polio	la poliomielitis	la poliomyélite, polio
rabies	la rabia	la rage
rash	la roncha, el salpullido, la erupción	l'éruption cutanée
redness	enrojecimiento o inflamación	la rougeur
relapse	la recaída	la rechute
scar	la cicatriz	la cicatrice
shock	el choque	l'état de choc
sore	la llaga	la lésion cutanée
spasm	el espasmo	le spasme
spider bite	la picadura de araña	la morsure d'araignée
sprain	la torcedura	l'entorse
stomachache	el dolor de estómago	le mal d'estomac
sunstroke	la insolación	le coup de soleil
swelling	la hinchazón	l'enflure
tetanus	el tétano(s)	le tétanos
tonsillitis	la tonsilitis	l'amygdalite
toothache	el dolor de muela	le mal de dent
trauma	el trauma	le traumatisme
tuberculosis	la tuberculosis	la tuberculose
tumor	el tumor	la tumeur
unconsciousness	la insensibilidad	l'inconscience
veneral disease	la enfermedad venérea	la maladie vénérienne
virus	el virus	le virus
vomit	el vómito, los vómitos	le vomissement
weakness	le debilidad	la faiblesse
welt	roncha, verdugón	la marque de coup, zébrure
whiplash	concusión de la espina cervical, lastimado del cuello	le traumatisme cranio-cervical dit <<coup du lapin>>
General hospital equipment and supplies		
bandage	la venda	le bandage
bathtub	la tina	la baignoire

Continued.

Spanish-French-English equivalents of commonly used medical terms and phrases—cont'd

English	Spanish	French

General hospital equipment and supplies—cont'd

English	Spanish	French
bed	la cama	le lit
bedpan	la chata	le bassin hygiénique
blanket	la cobi	la couverture
call bell	el timbre	la sonnette d'appel
catheter	el cateter	le cathéter, la sonde
crutches	las muletas	les béquilles
operating table	la mesa de operaciones	la table d'opération
pillow	la almohada	l'oreiller
shower	la ducha	la douche
soap	el jabon	le savon
stethoscope	el estetoscopio	le stéthoscope
stretcher	la camilla	la civière
syringe	la jeringa	la seringue
thermometer	el termometro	le thermomètre
toilet	el excusado	la toilette
tongue depressor	el pisalengua	le abaisse-langue
toothbrush	el cepillo de dientes	la brosse à dents
walker	el apoyador para caminar, el andador	le cadre de marche, déambulateur
wheelchair	la silla de ruedas	le fauteuil roulant

Medications and related supplies

English	Spanish	French
alcohol	alcohol	l'alcool
amphetamine	anfetamina	l'amphétamine
antibiotic	antibiótico	l'antibiotique
application	aplicación	l'application
artifical limb	el miembro artificial	la prothèse orthopédique
aspirin (for children)	aspirina (para niños)	l'aspirine (pour enfants)
Band-Aid	la curita	le Band-Aid
barbitrate	barbitúrico	le barbiturique
birth control pill	la píldora anticonceptiva	la pilule anticonceptionnelle
booster shot	la inyeccion secundaria	l'injection de rappel
brace	el braguero	l'appareil orthopédique
calcium	calcio	le calcium
capsule	cápsula	la capsule
cocaine	cocaína	la cocaïne
codeine	codeína	la codéine
cold pack	el emplasto frio	l'enveloppement froid
compress (hot)	la compresa (caliente)	la compresse (chaude)
condom	goma, condón	le condom
contact lens	lentes de contacto	le verre de contact
contraceptive pills	pastillas anticonceptivas	les pilules contraceptives
cotton	algodón	le coton
cough syrup	jarabe para la tos	le sirop pour la toux
diuretic	diurético	le diurétique
dose	dosis	la dose
douche	la ducha, lavado interno	la douche
dressing	vendaje	le pansement
dropper	el gotero	le compte-gouttes
drops	gotas	les gouttes
enema	enema	le lavement
gauze	gasa	la gaze
glucose	glucosa	la glucose
hearing aid	el aparato para la sordera	la prothèse auditive
heroin	heroína	la héroïne
ice	hielo	le glace
ice pack	la bolsa de hielo	le sac de glace
insulin	insulina	l'insuline
intrauterine device (IUD)	el dispositivio intrauterino	le dispositif intra-utérin (DIU)
laxative	laxante, purgante, purga	le laxatif
lotion	loción	la lotion
narcotic	narcótico	le narcotique
needle	aguja	l'aiguille
Novocaine	novocaína	la Novocaïne
ointment	ungüento	l'onguent
pacemaker	el marcapaso	le stimulateur cardiaque

English	Spanish	French
penicillin	penicilina	la pénicilline
pill	píldora, pastilla	la pilule
prosthesis	miembro artificial (prótesis)	la prothèse
sedative	sedante, calmante	le sédatif
sling	el cabestrillo	l'écharpe
smelling salts	sales aromáticas	les sels
splint	la tablilla	l'attelle
support	el apoyo	l'appui
suppository	supositorio	le suppositoire
syrup of ipecac	jarabe de ipecacuana	le sirop d'ipéca
vitamin	vitamina	la vitamine

Medication instructions

English	Spanish	French
right	derecho(a)	droit
left	izquierdo(a)	gauche
tablespoonful	cucharada	la cuillerée à soupe
teaspoonful	cucharadita	la cuillerée à thé
one-half teaspoonful	media cucharadita	une demi-cuillerée à thé
BID	dos veces al día	deux fois par jour
TID	tres veces al día	trois fois par jour
QID	cuarto veces al día	quatre fois par jour
every hour	cada hora	toutes les heures
each day, daily	cada día, diariamente	tous les jours, quotidiennement
every other day	cada otro día (cada tercer día)	tous les deux jours
till gone	hasta terminar (acabar)	jusqu'à disparition des symptômes
Let it dissolve in your mouth.	Que se le disuelva en la boca.	Laissez dissoudre dans la bouche.
as needed for pain	cuando la necesite para el dolor	quand la douleur se fait sentir
symptoms	sintomas	les symptômes
insert	inserte	insérer, introduire
when you get up in the morning	al levantarse	au lever
apply	aplique	appliquer
one-half hour after meals	una hora antes de comidas	une demi-heure après les repas
now (stat)	ahora (ahora mismo)	maintenant (immédiatement)
before bedtime	antes de acostarse	avant le coucher
before you exercise	antes de hacer ejercicios	avant de faire de l'exercice
chew	mastique	mastiquer
mix	mezcle	mélanger
dissolved in	disuelto en	dissous dans
Shake well.	Agite bien.	Bien mélanger.
as directed	de acuerdo con las instrucciones	suivant avis médical
by mouth	por la boca	par voie orale
rub	frote	frotter
gargle	haga gargaras	se gargariser
soak	remoje, empape	faire tremper, imbiber

Tests and procedures

English	Spanish	French
allergy test	prueba para alergias	le bilan allergologique
analysis	análisis	l'analyse
blood count	recuento (conteo) globular	la numération globulaire
blood transfusion	la transfusion de sangre	la transfusion sanguine
cardiogram	cardiograma	le cardiogramme
checkup, medical	reconocimiento (chequeo) médico	l'examen médical complet
culture (throat)	cultivo de la garganta	la culture de la gorge
electrocardiogram	electrocardiograma	l'électrocardiogramme
electroencephalogram	electroencefalograma	l'électroencéphalogramme
enema	la enema	le lavement
eye test	examen de la vista (de los ojos)	l'examen de la vue
injection	la inyección	l'injection
laboratory	laboratorio	le laboratoire
message	el masaje	le message
pregnancy test	prueba de embarazo	le test de grossesse
specimen	muestra (espécimen)	l'échantillon
traction	la traccion	la traction
urinalysis	análisis de orina	l'analyse d'urine
vaccination	la vacuna	la vaccination
x-rays	radiografias (rayos equis)	la radiographie

Continued.

Spanish-French-English equivalents of commonly used medical terms and phrases—cont'd

English	Spanish	French

Assessment

General

I am _____.	Soy _____.	Je suis _____.
I would like to examine you now. Please take off your clothes, except for your underwear (and bra), and put on this gown.	Quisiera examinarlo(a) ahora. Por favor, quítese la ropa menos la ropa interior (y el sostén), y póngase este camisón.	Je voudrais vous examiner maintenant. Veuillez enlever vos vêtements, sauf votre slip (et votre soutien-gorge), et enfilez cette blouse.
I am going to take your temperature now. Open your mouth.	Le voy a tomar la temperatura ahora. Abra la boca.	Maintenant, je vais prendre votre température. Ouvrez la bouche.
I am going to take your blood pressure now.	Le voy a tomar la presión ahora.	Maintenant, je vais prendre votre tension artérielle.
Your blood pressure is low.	Su presión es baja.	Votre tension artérielle est basse.
Your blood pressure is too high.	Su presión es demasiado alta.	Votre tension artérielle est trop élevée.
Here is a prescription to reduce your blood pressure.	Aquí tiene une receta para bajar la presión de sangre.	Voici une ordonnance pour réduire votre tension artérielle.
You must follow a diet to lose weight.	Debe seguir una dieta para perder peso.	Vous devez suivre un régime pour perdre du poids.
I am going to start an IV.	Le voy a empezar un suero.	Je vais vous faire une intraveineuse.
Bend your elbow.	Doble el codo.	Pliez le coude.
Make a fist.	Haga un puño.	Faites un poing.
I am going to give you an injection.	Le voy a poner una inyección.	Je vais vous faire une injection.
Breathe normally.	Respire normalmente.	Respirez normalement.
Cough.	Tosa.	Toussez.
Squeeze my hand.	Apriete mi mamo.	Serrez ma main.
You have a slight fever.	Ud. tiene un poco de fiebre.	Vous avez un peu de fièvre.
Hold your leg up.	Levante la pierna.	Levez la jambe.
Stand up and walk.	Parese y camine.	Levez-vous et marchez.
Straighten your leg.	Enderece la pierna.	Tendez la jambe.
Bend your knee.	Doble la rodilla.	Pliez le genou.
Push/pull.	Empuje/jale.	Poussez/tirez.
Up/down.	Arriba/abajo.	Vers le haut/vers le bas.
In/out.	Adentro/afuera.	Dedans/dehors.
Slow/fast.	Despacio/aprisa.	Lentement/vite.
Rest.	Descanse.	Reposez-vous.
Kneel.	Arrodíllese.	Agenouillez-vous.

Ambulation history

Do you use equipment (canes, crutches, braces)?	¿Usa equipo (bastones, muletal, abrazaderas)?	Utilisez-vous un appareil (canes, béquilles, appareils orthopédiques)?
Do you use a wheelchair?	¿Usa usted una silla de ruedas?	Utilisez-vous un fauteuil roulant?
Do you drive a car?	¿Maneja usted un carro?	Conduisez-vous une voiture?
Can you climb stairs?	¿Puede usted subir las escaleras?	Pouvez-vous monter les escaliers?

Cardiology

Have you ever had chest pain? Where?	¿Ha tenido alguna vez dolor de pecho? Dónde?	Avez-vous déjà éprouvé une douleur thoracique? Où précisément?
Do you notice any irregularity of heart beat or any palpitations?	¿Nota cualquier latido o palpitación irregular?	Les battements de votre coeur sont-ils irréguliers ou avez-vous des palpitations?
Do you get short of breath? When?	¿Tiene fasta de aire? Cuándo?	Vous arrive-t-il d'être essoufflé? À quel moment?
Do you take medicine for your heart? How often?	¿Toma medicina para el corazón? Con qué frecuncia?	Prenez-vous des médicaments pour le coeur? À quelle fréquence?
Do you know if you have high blood pressure?	¿Sabe usted si tiene la presión alta?	Savez-vous si vous souffrez d'hypertension?
Is there a history of hypertension in your family?	¿Hay historia de hipertensión en su familia?	Des membres de votre famille font-ils de l'hypertension?
You have had a heart attack.	Ha tenido un ataque al corazón.	Vous avez fait une crise cardiaque.
Be sure to tell us if you have chest pains or if you feel anything unusual.	Debe avisarnos si tiene dolores de pecho o si siente algo anormal.	Ne manquez pas de nous dire si vous ressentez des douleurs thoraciques ou quoi que ce soit d'anormal.

Diabetes

You have diabetes.	Usted tiene diabetes.	Vous faites du diabète.
Your doctor will regulate your dosage.	Su médico le indicará su dosis.	Votre médecin déterminera la posologie.

English	Spanish	French

Assessment—cont'd

Drug-related problems

English	Spanish	French
What drugs do you use?	¿Cuáles drogas usa usted?	Quelles drogues prenez-vous?
heroin?	¿heroína?	héroïne?
cocaine?	¿cocaína?	cocaïne?
uppers?	¿estimulantes?	amphétamines?
downers?	¿abajos?	tranquillisants?
barbiturates?	¿diablitos o barbitúricos?	barbituriques?
speed?	¿blancas?	excitants?
Where do you shoot the drugs?	¿Dónde se pone usted las drogas?	À quel endroit vous injectez-vous les drogues?
Have you ever been through a detoxification program before?	¿Ha participado alguna vez en un programa de desintoxicación?	Avez-vous déjà suivi un programme de désintoxication?
Have you ever overdosed on drugs?	¿Alguna vez se ha sobredrogado?	Avez-vous déjà pris une dose excessive de drogues?

Ears, nose, and throat

English	Spanish	French
Do you have any hearing problems?	¿Tiene Ud. problemas de oir?	Avez-vous des troubles de l'audition?
Do you use a hearing aid?	¿Usa Ud. un audífono?	Portez-vous une prothèse auditive?
Do your ears ring?	¿Siente un tintineo o silbido en los oídos?	Avez-vous des bourdonnements d'oreilles?
Do you have allergies?	¿Tiene alergias?	Avez-vour des allergies?
Do you have a cold?	¿Tiene usted un resfriado/resfrío?	Avez-vous un rhume?
Do you have sore throats frequently?	¿Le duele la garganta con frecuencia?	Avez-vous souvent mal à la gorge?
Have you ever had strep throat?	¿Ha tenido alguna vez "strep" (infección estreptococo de la garganta)?	Avez-vous déjà eu une angine à streptocoques?
I want to take a throat culture. Open your mouth. This will not hurt.	Quiero hacer un cultivo de la garganta. Abra la boca. Esto no le va a doler.	Je veux vous faire un prélèvement dans la gorge. Ouvrez la bouche. Cela ne fera pas mal.

Endocrinology

English	Spanish	French
Have you ever had problems with your thyroid?	¿Ha tenido alguna vez problemas con la tiroides?	Avez-vous déjà eu des problèmes de thyroïde?
Have you noted any significant weight gain or loss? What is your usual weight?	¿Ha notado pérdida o aumento de peso? Cuál es su peso usual?	Avez-vous engraissé ou maigri de façon significative? Quel est votre poids normal?
How is your appetite?	¿Qué tal su apetito?	Avez-vous de l'appétit?
(Women) How old were you when your periods started? How many days between periods? Have you ever been pregnant? How many children do you have?	¿Cuántos años tenía cuando tuvo la primera regla? ¿Cuántos días entre las reglas? ¿Ha estado embarazada? ¿Cuántos hijos tiene?	(Pour les femmes) À quel âg avez-vous eu vos premières menstruations? Combien de jours séparent vos règles? Avez-vous déjà été enceinte? Combien d'enfants avez-vous?

Gastrointestinal

English	Spanish	French
What foods disagree with you?	¿Qué alimentos le caen mal?	Quels aliments ne vous conviennent pas?
Do you get heartburn?	¿Suele tener ardor en el pecho?	Avez-vous des brûlures d'estomac?
Do you have indigestion often?	¿Tiene indigestión con freuencia?	Avez-vous souvent une indigestion?
Are you going to vomit?	¿Va a vomitar (arrojar)?	Êtes-vous sur le point de vomir?
Do you have blood in your vomit?	¿Tiene usted vómitos con sangre?	Vos vomissures contiennent-elles des traces de sang?

Headaches/head

English	Spanish	French
Do you have headaches?	¿Tiene Ud. dolores de cabeza (jaquecas)?	Avez-vous des maux de tête?
Do you have migraines?	¿Tiene Ud. migrañas (jaquecas)?	Avez-vous des migraines?
Where is the pain exactly?	¿Dónde le duele, exactamente?	Où avez-vous mal exactement?
What causes the headaches?	¿Qué la causa los dolores de cabeza?	Qu'est-ce qui occasionne les maux de tête?
Are there any changes in your vision?	¿Hay algunos cambios en su vista?	Votre vue a-t-elle changé?

Neurology

English	Spanish	French
Have you ever had a head injury?	¿Ha tenido alguna vez dano a la cabeza?	Avez-vous déjà eu une blessure à la tête?
Have you ever had a sports injury?/motorcycle accident?	¿Ha tenido alguna vez motorcycle un daño deportivo?/(accidente en su motocicleta?)	Avez-vous déjà subi un accident de sport?/un accident de motocyclette?
Do you have convulsions?	¿Tiene convulsiones?	Avez-vous des convulsions?
Do you see double?	¿Ve usted doble?	Voyez-vous double?
Do you have tingling sensations?	¿Tiene hormigueos?	Avez-vous des fourmillements?
Do you have numbness in your hands, arms, or feet?	¿Siente entumecidos las manos los brazos o los pies?	Éprouvez-vous une sensation d'engourdissement?

Continued.

Spanish-French-English equivalents of commonly used medical terms and phrases—cont'd

English	Spanish	French

Assessment—cont'd

Neurology—cont'd

Have you ever lost consciousness? For how long?	¿Perdió alguna vez el sentido? ¿Por cuánto tiempo?	Avez-vous déjà perdu connaissance? Pendant combien de temps?
How frequently does this happen?	¿Con qué frecuencia ocurre esto?	À quelle fréquence cela se produit-il?
Is this hot or cold?	¿Esta frío o caliente esto?	Est-ce chaud ou froid?
Am I sticking you with the point or the head of the pin?	¿Le estoy pinchando con la cabeza del alfiler?	Est-ce que je vous pique avec la pointe ou la tête de l'épingle?

Obstetrics and gynecology

How often do you get your periods?	¿Cada cuándo le viene la regla?	À quel intervalle avez-vous vos règles?
When was your last menstrual period?	¿Cuándo fue su última regla?	À quand remontent vos dernières menstruations?
When was your last Pap smear?	¿Cuándo fue su última prueba de Pap?	À quand remonte votre dernier frottis vaginal?
Would you like information on birth control methods?	¿Quiere usted. información sobre los metodos del control de la natalidad? (los metodos anticonceptivos)?	Voulez-vous des renseignements sur les méthodes contraceptives?
Do you have an IUD in place?	¿Le han puesto un aparato intrauterino?	Avez-vous un stérilet?
Has your bag of waters broken? When?	¿Se le rompió la bolsa de agua(s)? ¿Cuándo?	Votre poche des eaux s'est-elle rompue? Quand?
When did your pains begin?	¿Cuándo le comenzaron los dolores?	Quand les douleurs ont-elles commencé?
How many minutes apart are they now?	¿Cuántos minutos pasan entre uno y otro dolor?	À quel intervalle se succèdent-elles?
Do you have a lot of pain?	¿Tiene usted mucho dolor?	Souffrez-vous beaucoup?
Open your mouth and breathe. Do not push.	Abra la boca y respire por la boca. No empuje.	Ouvrez la bouche et respirez. Ne poussez pas.
Every time the pain comes, push.	Cuando le venga el dolor, empuje.	Chaque fois que vous avez mal, poussez.
It is not possible for your baby to be born vaginally; we are going to do a cesarean section.	No es posible que su bebé born nazca por la vagina; por so vamos a hacerle una cesárea.	Votre bébé ne peut pas naître par voie vaginale; nous allons devoir procéder à une césarienne.

Ophthalmology

Have you had pain in your eyes?	¿Ha tenido dolor en los ojos?	Avez-vous parfois mal aux yeux?
Do you wear glasses?	¿Usa usted anteojos/gafas/lentes/espejuelos?	Portez-vous des lunettes?
Were you exposed to anything that could have injured your eye?	¿Fue expuesto a cualquier cosa que pudiera haberle dañado el ojo?	Avez-vous été exposé à quelque chose qui aurait pu vous blesser l'oeil?
Do your eyes water much?	¿Le lagrimean mucho los ojos?	Vos yeux larmoient-ils beaucoup?
I am going to put drops in your eyes in order to examine them. This medicine may burn at first.	¿Le voy a poner gotas en los ojos para examinarlos. Esta medicina puede arderle al principio?	Je vais vous mettre des gouttes dans les yeux pour les examiner. Ce médicament peut causer une sensation de brûlure au début.
Please look into this apparatus.	Favor de mirar dentro de este aparato.	Veuillez regarder dans cet appareil.

Orthopedics

You have broken (a bone).	Usted se ha quebrado/roto (un hueso).	Vous vous êtes fracturé (un os).
You have dislocated (a joint).	Usted se ha dislocado (una coyuntura).	Vous vous êtes déboîté (une articulation).
You have pulled (a muscle).	Usted se ha distendido (un músculo).	Vous vous êtes claqué (un muscle).
You have sprained (a muscle)/(a ligament).	Usted se ha torcido (un músculo)/(un ligamento).	Vous vous êtes foulé (un muscle)/(un ligament).
You will need a cast.	Necesita un yeso.	Il va vous falloir un plâtre.
Do you feel pain when you stand?	¿Siente dolor al pararse?	Avez-vous mal lorsque vous vous tenez debout?
Do you feel pain when you bend?	¿Siente dolor al doblarse?	Avez-vous mal lorsque vous vous courbez?
We need to take some x-rays.	Necesitamos tomarle unos rayos X.	Nous devons prendre quelques radiographies.
You must wear a sling whenever you are out of bed.	Usted debe llevar un cabestrillo cuando no este en la cama.	Vous devez porter une écharpe chaque fois que vous quittez le lit.

Pain

What were you doing when the pain started?	¿Qué haciá usted cuando le comenzó el dolor?	Qu'étiez-vous en train de faire lorsque la douleur a commencé?
Where is the pain?	¿Dónde está el dolor?	Où avez-vous mal?
How severe is the pain? Mild, moderate, sharp, or severe?	¿Qué tan fuerte es el dolor? ¿Ligero, moderado, agudo, severo?	Quelle est l'intensité de la douleur? Est-elle légère, modérée, forte, ou intense?
Have you ever had this pain before?	¿Ha tenido este dolor antes? (Ha sido siempre así?)	Avez-vous déjà ressenti cette douleur auparavant?

English	Spanish	French

Assessment—cont'd
Orthopedics—cont'd

Does it hurt when I press here? How did the accident happen? | ¿Le duele cuando le aprieto aqui? ¿Como sucedio el accidente? | Avez-vous mal lorsque j'appuie ici? Comment l'accident s'est-il produit?

How did this happen? How long ago? | ¿Como sucedio esto? ¿Cuanto tiempo hace? | Comment cela est-il arrivé? Il y a combien de temps?

Poison control (telephone information)

What was swallowed? | ¿Qué se tragó? | Quel produit la victime a-t-elle avalé?

Please spell the name of the product for me. | ¿Favor de deletrear el nombre del producto? | Veuillez épeler le nom du produit.

How old is the person who swallowed this? | ¿Cuántos años tiene la persona que se tragó esto? | Quel est l'âge de la victime?

How much does the person weigh? | ¿Cuánto pesa? | Qual est le poids de la victime?

Is the person breathing all right? | ¿Está respirando bien? | La personne respire-t-elle bien?

Is the person complaining of any pain or other difficulty? | ¿Se queja de algún dolor, o de otra dificultad? | La victime se plaint-elle de douleur ou d'un autre trouble?

How long ago did the person swallow the product? | ¿Cuánto hace que esta persona se tragó el producto? | Depuis combien de temps la personne a-t-elle avalé le produit?

Pulmonary/respiratory

Do you smoke? How many packs a day? | ¿Fuma usted? ¿Cuántos paquentes al día? | Fumez-vous? Combien de paquets par jour?

How long have you been coughing? | ¿Desde cuándo tiene tos? | Depuis combien de temps toussez-vous?

Does it hurt when you cough? | ¿Le duele cuando tose? | Avez-vous mal lorsque vous toussez?

Do you cough up phlegm? | ¿Al toser, escupe usted flema(s)? | Expulsez-vous des sécrétions lorsque vous toussez?

Do you cough up blood? | ¿Al toser, arroja usted sangre? | Crachez-vous du sang?

Do you wheeze? | ¿Le silba a usted el pecho? | Votre respiration est-elle sifflante?

Have you ever had asthma? | ¿Ha tenido asma alguna vez? | Avez-vous déjà fait de l'asthme?

Have you ever had | ¿Ha tenido alguna vez | Avez-vous déjà souffert des maladies suivantes:

   tuberculosis? | tuberculosis? | tuberculose?

   pneumonia? | pulmonía? | pneumonie?

   emphysema? | enfisema? | emphysème?

   bronchitis? | bronquitis? | bronchite?

Breathe deeply. | Aspire profundamente. (Respire profundo.) | Respirez à fond.

Sexually transmitted diseases

Do you have urethral discharge? | ¿Tiene descarga de la uretra? | Avez-vous un écoulement urétral?

Do you have burning with urination? | ¿Tiene ardor al orinar? | Avez-vous des brûlures lorsque vous urinez?

Do you have a vaginal discharge? | ¿Tiene descargas vaginales? | Avez-vous des pertes vaginales?

Do you have abdominal pain? | ¿Tiene dolor en el abdomen? | Souffrez-vous de douleurs abdominales?

When did you last have intercourse? | ¿Cuándo fue la última vez que tuvo relaciones sexuales? | À quand remontent vos dernières relations sexuelles?

Unconscious patient

What happened to him/her? | ¿Que le paso? (Que le sucedio?) | Que lui est-il arrivé?

Has he vomited? | ¿Ha vomitado? | A-t-il vomi?

Is she pregnant? | ¿Esta embarazada? | Est-elle enceinte?

Patient instructions
General

Roll over and sit up over the edge of the bed. | Voltéese y siéntese sobre el borde de la cama. | Retournez-vous et asseyez-vous au bord du lit.

Stand up slowly. Put weight only on your right/left foot. | Párese despacio. Ponga peso sólo en la pierna derecha/izquierda. | Levez-vous lentement. Appuyez-vous seulement sur votre pied droit/gauche.

Lift your head up. | Levante la cabeza. | Levez la tête.

Take a step to the side. | Dé un paso al lado. | Faites un pas de côté.

Turn to your left/right. | Doble a la izquierda/derecha. | Tournez à gauche/à droite.

Drugs

I want you to take your medicine. | Quiero que tome su medicina. | Je veux que vous preniez votre médicament.

Let it dissolve in your mouth. | Que se le disuelva en la boca. | Laissez-le se dissoudre dans la bouche.

Continued.

Spanish-French-English equivalents of commonly used medical terms and phrases—cont'd

English	Spanish	French

Patient instructions—cont'd
Drugs—cont'd

Apply _____ to the affected part.
Cool in the refrigerator.
Here is some medication for _____.Take _____ tablets every _____ hours as needed.

These pills are vitamins.
These pills are for pain.
Take _____ of these pills each day.
Here is enough medicine for _____ days.

Take one of these pills every _____ hours.
Take one pill daily for _____ days.

But no more than _____ a day maximum.
Fill the medicine dropper to this line and mix with a glass of water, juice, or milk.
It is important for you to eat/drink liquids.

Preparation for surgery
I'm going to shave you.
The pill (this shot) will make you sleep.

The doctor wants you to stay in bed.

Anesthesia
You are not allowed water.
Have you have anything to eat or drink since midnight?
You must have nothing to eat or drink after midnight.
Did someone take a sample of your blood?

Radiology
I am going to take an x-ray of your _____.

Please lie on the table, face up/face down.

Turn on your left/right side.
Turn over.
Swallow this mixture.
Stand here and place your chest against this plate.
Rest your chin here.
Take a deep breath. Hold it. Now breathe normally.

Aplique _____ en la parte afectada.
Enfrie en el refrigerador.
Aquí tiene la medicina para _____. Tome _____ tabletas cada _____ horas segun la necesite.

Estas pastillas son vitaminas.
Estas pastillas son para dolor.
Tome _____ de estas pastillas cada día.
Aquí tiene suficiente medicina para _____ días.

Tome una de estas pastillas cada _____ horas.
Tome una pastilla por _____ días.

Pero no más de _____ en total cada día.
Llene el gotero hasta esta linea y mezcle con un vaso de agua, jugo o leche.
Es importante que usted coma/beba o tome liquidos.

Le voy a rasurar.
La pastilla (Esta inyeccion) le hará dormir.

El médico quiere que se quede en cama.

No debe tomar agua.
¿Ha comido o tomado algo desde la medianoche?
No debe comer ni tomar nada después de la medianoche.
¿Le han domado una muestra de sangre?

Le voy a acer una radiografia de la (del) _____.

Por favor, acuéstese sobre la mesa, boca arriba/boca abajo.
Voltéese al lado izquierdo/al lado derecho.
Voltéese al otro lado.
Trague esta mezcla.
Parese aquí y apoye el pecho contra esta placa.
Apoye el mentón aquí.
Aspire profundamente. Manténgalo. Ahora respire normalmente.

Appliquez _____ sur la partie atteinte.
Refroidissez au réfrigérateur.
Voici des médicaments pour _____. Prenez _____ comprimés toutes les _____ heures selon les besoins.

Ces pilules contiennent des vitamines.
Ce sont des pilules antidouleur.
Prenez _____ pilules chaque jour.
Voici suffisamment de médicaments pour _____ jours.

Prenez l'une de ces pilules toutes les _____ heures.
Prenez une pilule par jour pendant _____ jours.

Mais pas plus de _____ par jour.
Remplissez le compte-gouttes jusqu'à ce trait et mélangez le contenu dans un verre d'eau, de jus ou de lait.
Il est important que vous mangiez/buviez.

Je vais vous raser.
Cette pilule (cette injection) vous fera dormir.

Le médecin veut que vous restiez au lit.

Vous ne pouvez pas boire d'eau.
Avez-vous mangé ou bu quoi que ce soit depuis minuit?
Vous ne devez rien manger ni boire après minuit.
Vous a-t-on fait une prise de sang?

Je vais faire une radiographie de votre _____.

Veuillez vous allonger sur la table, sur le dos/sur le ventre.
Tournez-vous sur le côté gauche/droit.
Retournez-vous.
Avalez ce mélange.
Mettez-vous debout ici et placez la poitrine contre cette plaque.
Posez votre menton ici.
Inspirez à fond. Retenez votre respiration. Maintenant, vous pouvez respirer normalement.

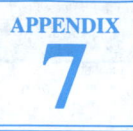

APPENDIX 7

TABULAR ATLAS OF HUMAN ANATOMY AND PHYSIOLOGY

7-1 Basic structures and functions of the body

Major cell structures and functions

Cell structure	Functions
Membranous	
Plasma membrane	Serves as the boundary of the cell, maintaining its integrity; protein molecules on outer surface of plasma membrane perform various functions; for example, they serve as markers that identify cells of each individual, as receptor molecules for certain hormones and other molecules, and as transport mechanisms
Endoplasmic reticulum (ER)	Ribosomes attached to rough ER synthesize proteins that leave cells via the Golgi complex; smooth ER synthesizes lipids incorporated in cell membranes, steroid hormones, and certain carbohydrates used to form glycoproteins
Golgi apparatus	Synthesizes carbohydrate, combines it with protein, and packages the product as globules of glycoprotein
Lysosomes	A cell's "digestive system"
Peroxisomes	Contain enzymes that detoxify harmful substances
Mitochondria	Catabolism; ATP synthesis; a cell's "power plants"
Nucleus	Dictates protein synthesis, thereby playing essential role in other cell activities, namely, cell transport, metabolism, and growth
Nonmembranous	
Ribosomes	Synthesize proteins; a cell's "protein factories"
Cytoskeleton	Acts as a framework to support the cell and its organelles; functions in cell movement; forms cell extensions (microvilli, cilia, flagella)
Cilia and flagella	Hairlike cell extensions that serve to move substances over the cell surface (cilia) or propel sperm cells (flagella)
Nucleolus	Plays an essential role in the formation of ribosomes

From Thibodeau GA, Patton KT: *Anatomy and physiology,* ed 2, St Louis, 1993, Mosby.

Tissues

Tissue	Location	Function
Epithelial		
Simple squamous	Alveoli of lungs	Absorption by diffusion of respiratory gases between alveolar air and blood
	Lining of blood and lymphatic vessels (called endothelium; classed as connective tissue by some histologists)	Absorption by diffusion; filtration; osmosis
	Surface layer of pleura, pericardium, peritoneum (called mesothelium; classed as connective tissue by some histologists)	Absorption by diffusion; osmosis; also secretion
Stratified squamous	Surface of mucous membrane lining mouth, esophagus, and vagina	Protection
	Surface of skin (epidermis)	Protection
Transitional	Surface of mucous membrane lining urinary bladder and ureters	Permits stretching
Simple columnar	Surface layer of mucous lining of stomach, intestines, and part of respiratory tract	Protection; secretion; absorption; moving of mucus (by ciliated columnar epithelium)
Pseudostratified	Surface of mucous membrane lining trachea, large bronchi, nasal mucosa, and parts of male reproductive tract (epididymis and vas deferens); lines large ducts of some glands (e.g., parotid)	Protection

Tissues—cont'd

Tissue	Location	Function
Epithelial—cont'd		
Glandular	Glands	Secretion
Connective (most widely distributed of all tissues)		
Fibrous		
Loose, ordinary (areolar)	Between other tissues and organs	Connection
	Superficial fascia	Connection
Adipose (fat)	Under skin	Protection
	Padding at various points	Insulation
		Support
		Reserve food
Reticular tissue	Inner framework of spleen, lymph nodes, bone marrow	Support filtration
Dense fibrous		
Regular	Tendons	Flexible but strong connection
	Ligaments	
	Aponeuroses	
Irregular	Deep fascia	Connection
	Dermis	Support
	Scars	
	Capsule of kidney, etc.	
Bone	Skeleton	Support
		Protection
		Calcium reservoir
Cartilage		
Hyaline	Part of nasal septum	Firm but flexible support
	Covering articular surfaces of bones	
	Larynx	
	Rings in trachea and bronchi	
Fibrocartilage	Disks between vertebrae	
	Symphysis pubis	
Elastic	External ear	
	Eustachian tube	
Blood	In blood vessels	Transportation
		Protection
Muscle		
Skeletal (striated voluntary)	Muscles that attach to bones	Movement of bones
	Extrinsic eyeball muscles	Eye movements
	Upper third of esophagus	First part of swallowing
Smooth (nonstriated, involuntary, or visceral)	In walls of tubular viscera of digestive, respiratory, and genitourinary tracts	Movement of substances along respective tracts
	In walls of blood vessels and large lymphatic vessels	Change diameter of blood vessels, thereby aiding in regulation of blood pressure
	In ducts of glands	Movement of substances along ducts
	Intrinsic eye muscles (iris and ciliary body)	Change diameter of pupils and shape of lens
	Arrector muscles of hairs	Erection of hairs (gooseflesh)
Cardiac (striated involuntary)	Wall of heart	Contraction of heart
Nervous	Brain	Excitability
	Spinal cord	Conduction
	Nerves	

7-2   Skeletal system

Bones of the skeleton (206 total)*

Part of body	Name of bone	Number	Identification
APPENDICULAR SKELETON (126 bones)			Bones that are appended to axial skeleton; upper and lower extremities, including shoulder and hip girdles
Upper extremities (including shoulder girdle) (64 bones)	Clavicle	2	Collar bones; shoulder girdle joined to axial skeleton by articulation of clavicles with sternum; scapula does not form joint with axial skeleton
	Scapula	2	Shoulder blades; scapulae and clavicles together comprise shoulder girdle
	Humerus	2	Long bone of upper arm
	Radius	2	Bone of thumb side of forearm
	Ulna	2	Bone of little finger side of forearm; longer than radius
	Carpals (scaphoid, lunate, triquetrum, pisiform, trapezium, trapezoid, capitate, and hamate)	16	Wrist bones; arranged in two rows at proximal end of hand
	Metacarpals	10	Long bones forming framework of palm of hand
	Phalanges	28	Miniature long bones of fingers, 3 in each finger, 2 in each thumb
Lower extremities (62 bones)	Ossa coxae or innominate bones	2	Large hip bones; with sacrum and coccyx, these 3 bones form basin-like pelvic cavity; lower extremities attached to axial skeleton by pelvic bones
	Femur	2	Thigh bone; largest, strongest bone of body
	Patella	2	Kneecap; largest sesamoid bone of body*; embedded in tendon of quadriceps femoris muscle
	Tibia	2	Shin bone
	Fibula	2	Long, slender bone of lateral side of lower leg
	Tarsals (calcaneus, talus, navicular, first, second, and third cuneiforms, cuboid)	14	Bones that form heel and proximal or posterior half of foot
	Metatarsals	10	Long bones of feet
	Phalanges	28	Miniature long bones of toes; 2 in each great toe, 3 in other toes
AXIAL SKELETON (80 bones)			Bones that form upright axis on body—skull, hyoid, vertebral column, sternum, and ribs
Skull (28 bones) **Cranium** (8 bones)			Cranium forms floor for brain to rest on and helmetlike covering over it
	Frontal	1	Forehead bone; also forms most of roof of orbits (eye sockets) and anterior part of cranial floor
	Parietal	2	Prominent, bulging bones behind frontal bone; form top sides of cranial cavity
	Temporal	2	Form lower sides of cranium and part of cranial floor; contain middle and inner ear structures
	Occipital	1	Forms posterior part of cranial floor and walls
	Sphenoid	1	Keystone of cranial floor; forms its midportion; resembles bat with wings outstretched and legs extended downward posteriorly; lies behind and slightly above nose and throat; forms part of floor and sidewalls of orbit

*An inconstant number of small, flat, round bones known as *sesamoid bones* (because of their resemblance to sesame seeds) is found in various tendons in which considerable pressure develops. Because the number of these bones varies greatly between individuals, only 2 of them, the patellae, have been counted among the 206 bones of the body. Generally, 2 of them can be found in each thumb (in flexor tendon near metacarpophalangeal and interphalangeal joints) and great toe plus several others in the upper and lower extremities. *Wormian bones,* the small islets of bone frequently found in some of the cranial sutures, have not been counted in the list of 206 bones because of their variable occurrence.

Bones of the skeleton (206 total)*—cont'd

Part of body	Name of bone	Number	Identification
Skull (28 bones)—cont'd	Ethmoid	1	Complicated irregular bone that helps make up anterior portion of cranial floor, medial wall of orbits, upper parts of nasal septum, and sidewalls and part of nasal roof; lies anterior to sphenoid and posterior to nasal bones
Face (14 bones)	Nasal	2	Small bones forming upper part of bridge of nose
	Maxillary	2	Upper jaw bones; form part of floor of orbit, anterior part of roof of mouth, and floor and part of sidewalls of nose
	Zygomatic (malar)	2	Cheekbones; form part of floor and sidewall of orbit
	Mandible	1	Lower jawbone; largest, strongest bone of face
	Lacrimal	2	Thin bones about size and shape of fingernail; posterior and lateral to nasal bones in median wall or orbit; help form sidewall of nasal cavity, often missing in dry skull
	Palatine	2	Form posterior part of hard palate floor and part of sidewalls of nasal cavity and floor of orbit
	Inferior conchae (turbinates)	2	Thin scroll of bone forming a kind of shell along inner surface of sidewall of nasal cavity; lies above roof of mouth
	Vomer	1	Forms lower and posterior part of nasal septum; shaped like ploughshare
Ear bones (6 bones)	Malleus (hammer)	2	Tiny bones referred to as auditory ossicles in middle ear cavity in temporal bones; resemble, respectively, miniature hammer, anvil, and stirrup
	Incus (anvil)	2	
	Stapes (stirrup)	2	
Hyoid bone		1	U-shaped bone in neck between mandible and upper part of larynx; claims distinction as only bone not forming a joint with any other bone; suspended by ligaments from styloid processes of temporal bones
Sternum and ribs (25 bones)			Sternum, ribs, and thoracic vertebrae together form bony cage known as *thorax;* ribs attach posteriorly to vertebrae, slant downward anteriorly to attach to sternum (see description of false ribs below)
	Sternum	1	Breastbone; flat dagger-shaped bone
	True ribs	7 pairs	Upper seven pairs; fasten to sternum by costal cartilages
	False ribs	5 pairs	False ribs do not attach to sternum directly; upper three pairs of false ribs attach by means of costal cartilage of seventh ribs; last two pairs do not attach to sternum at all; therefore called "floating"
Vertebral column (26 bones)			Not actually a column but a flexible segmented rod shaped like an elongated letter S; forms axis of body; head balanced above, ribs and viscera suspended in front, and lower extremities attached below; encloses spinal cord
	Cervical vertebrae	7	First, or upper, seven vertebrae
	Thoracic vertebrae	12	Next 12 vertebrae; 12 pairs of ribs attached to these
	Lumbar vertebrae	5	Next five vertebrae
	Sacrum	1	Five separate vertebrae until about 25 years of age; then fused to form one wedge-shaped bone
	Coccyx	1	Four or five separate vertebrae in child but fused into one in adult

Identification of bone markings

Marking	Description	Marking	Description
SPECIAL FEATURES OF SKULL		Superciliary arches	Ridges caused by projection of frontal sinuses; eyebrows lie over these ridges
Sutures	Immovable joints between skull bones	Supraorbital notch (sometimes foramen)	Notch or foramen in supraorbital margin slightly mesial to its midpoint; transmits supraorbital nerve and blood vessels
Sagittal	Joint between right and left parietal bones		
Coronal	Joint between parietal bones and frontal bone	Glabella	Smooth area between superciliary ridges and above nose
Lambdoidal	Joint between parietal bones and occipital bone		
Squamous	Line of articulation along top curved edge of temporal bone	**SPHENOID**	
Fontanels	"Soft spots" where ossification is incomplete at birth; allow some compression of skull during birth; also important in determining position of head before delivery; six such areas located at angles of parietal bones	Body	Hollow, cubelike central portion
		Greater wings	Lateral projections from body; form part of outer wall of orbit
		Lesser wings	Thin, triangular projections from upper part of sphenoid body; form posterior part of roof of orbit
Anterior (or frontal)	At intersection of sagittal and coronal sutures (juncture of parietal bones and frontal bone); diamond shaped; largest of fontanels; usually closed by 1½ years of age	Sella turcica (or *Turk's saddle*)	Saddle-shaped depression on upper surface of sphenoid body; contains pituitary gland
		Sphenoid sinuses	Irregular air-filled mucosa-lined spaces within central part of sphenoid
Posterior (or occipital)	At intersection of sagittal and lambdoidal sutures (juncture of parietal bones and occipital bone); triangular in shape; usually closed by second month	Pterygoid processes	Downward projections on either side where body and greater wing unite; comparable to extended legs of bat if entire bone is likened to this animal; form part of lateral nasal wall
Anterolateral (or sphenoid)	At juncture of frontal, parietal, temporal, and sphenoid bones	Optic foramen	Opening into orbit at root of lesser wing; transmits second cranial nerve
Posterolateral (or mastoid)	At juncture of parietal, occipital, and temporal bones; usually closed by second year	Superior orbital fissure	Slitlike opening into orbit; lateral to optic foramen; transmits third, fourth, and part of fifth cranial nerves
Air sinuses	Spaces or cavities within bones; those that communicate with nose called *paranasal sinuses* (frontal, sphenoidal, ethmoidal, and maxillary); mastoid cells communicate with middle ear rather than nose, therefore not included among paranasal sinuses	Foramen rotundum	Opening in greater wing that transmits maxillary division of fifth cranial nerve
		Foramen ovale	Opening in greater wing that transmits mandibular division of fifth cranial nerve
		ETHMOID	
Orbits formed by		Horizontal (cribriform) plate	Olfactory nerves pass through numerous holes in this plate
Frontal	Roof of orbit		
Ethmoid	Medial wall	Crista galli	Meninges attach to this process
Lacrimal	Medial wall	Perpendicular plate	Forms upper part of nasal septum
Sphenoid	Lateral wall		
Zygomatic	Lateral wall	Ethmoid sinuses	Honeycombed, mucosa-lined air spaces within lateral masses of bone
Maxillary	Floor		
Palatine	Floor	Superior and middle turbinates (conchae)	Help to form lateral walls of nose
Nasal septum formed by	Partition in midline of nasal cavity; separates cavity into right and left halves		
Perpendicular plate of ethmoid bone	Forms upper part of septum	Lateral masses	Compose sides of bone; contain many air spaces (ethmoid cells or sinuses); inner surface forms superior and middle conchae
Vomer bone	Forms lower, posterior part	**TEMPORAL**	
Cartilage	Forms anterior part	Mastoid process	Protuberance just behind ear
Wormian bones	Small islands of bones with suture	Mastoid air cells	Air-filled mucosa-lined spaces within mastoid process
Malleus, incus, stapes	Tiny bones, referred to as auditory ossicles, in middle ear cavity in temporal bones; resemble, respectively, miniature hammer, anvil, and stirrup	External auditory meatus (or canal)	Opening into air and tube extending into temporal bone
FRONTAL		Zygomatic process	Projection that articulates with malar (or zygomatic) bone
Supraorbital margin	Arched ridge just below eyebrow		
Frontal sinuses	Cavities inside bone just above supraorbital margin; lined with mucosa; contain air		
Frontal tuberosities	Bulge above each orbit; most prominent part of forehead		

Continued.

Identification of bone markings—cont'd

Marking	Description	Marking	Description
TEMPORAL—cont'd		**MAXILLA**	
Internal auditory meatus	Fairly large opening on posterior surface of petrous portion of bone; transmits eighth cranial nerve to inner ear and seventh cranial nerve on its way to facial structures	Alveolar process	Arch containing teeth
		Maxillary sinus or antrum of Highmore	Large air-filled mucosa-lined cavity within body of each maxilla; largest of sinuses
Squamous portion	Thin, flaring upper part of bone	Palatine process	Horizontal inward projection from alveolar process; forms anterior and larger part of hard palate
Mastoid portion	Rough-surfaced lower part of bone posterior to external auditory meatus	Infraorbital foramen	Hole on external surface just below orbit; transmits vessels and nerves
Petrous portion	Wedge-shaped process that forms part of center section of cranial floor between sphenoid and occipital bones; name derived from Greek word for stone because of extreme hardness of this process; houses middle and inner ear structures	Lacrimal groove	Groove on inner surface; joined by similar groove on lacrimal bone to form canal housing nasolacrimal duct
		OCCIPITAL	
Mandibular fossa	Oval-shaped depression anterior to external auditory meatus; forms socket for condyle of mandible	Foramen magnum	Hole through which spinal cord enters cranial cavity
Styloid process	Slender spike of bone extending downward and forward from undersurface of bone anterior to mastoid process; often broken off in dry skull; several neck muscles and ligaments attach to styloid process	Condyles	Convex, oval processes on either side of foramen magnum; articulate with depressions on first cervical vertebra
		External occipital protuberance	Prominent projection on posterior surface in midline short distance above foramen magnum; can be felt as definite bump
Stylomastoid foramen	Opening between styloid and mastoid processes where facial nerve emerges from cranial cavity	Superior nuchal line	Curved ridge extending laterally from external occipital protuberance
Jugular fossa	Depression on undersurface of petrous portion; dilated beginning of internal jugular vein lodged here	Inferior nuchal line	Less well-defined ridge paralleling superior nuchal line short distance below it
Jugular foramen	Opening in suture between petrous portion and occipital bone; transmits lateral sinus and ninth, tenth, and eleventh cranial nerves	Internal occipital protuberance	Projection in midline on inner surface of bone; grooves for lateral sinuses extend laterally from this process and one for sagittal sinus extends upward from it
		VERTEBRAL COLUMN	
Carotid canal (or foramen)	Channel in petrous portion; best seen from undersurface of skull; transmits internal carotid artery	General features	Anterior part of vertebra (except first two cervical) consists of body; posterior part of neural arch, which in turn consists of two pedicles, two laminae, and seven processes projecting from laminae
PALATINE		Thoracic vertebrae	
Horizontal plate	Joined to palatine processes of maxillae to complete part of hard palate	Body	Main part; flat, round mass located anteriorly; supporting or weight-bearing part of vertebra
MANDIBLE		Pedicles	Short projections extended posteriorly from body
Body	Main part of bone; forms chin	Laminae	Posterior part of vertebra to which pedicles join and from which processes project
Ramus	Process, one on either side, that projects upward from posterior part of body		
Condyle (or head)	Part of each ramus that articulates with mandibular fossa of temporal bone	Neural arch	Formed by pedicles and laminae; protects spinal cord posteriorly; congenital absence of one or more neural arches known as spina bifida (cord may protrude through skin)
Neck	Constricted part just below condyles		
Alveolar process	Teeth set into this arch		
Mandibular foramen	Opening on inner surface of ramus; transmits nerves and vessels to lower teeth	Spinous process	Sharp process projecting inferiorly from laminae in midline
Mental foramen	Opening on outer surface below space between two bicuspids; transmits terminal branches of nerves and vessels that enter bone through mandibular foramen; dentists inject anesthetics through these foramina	Transverse processes	Right and left lateral projections from laminae
		Superior articulating processes	Project upward from laminae
Coronoid process	Projection upward from anterior part of each ramus; temporal muscle inserts here	Inferior articulating processes	Project downward from laminae; articulate with superior articulating processes of vertebrae below
Angle	Juncture of posterior and inferior margins of ramus		

Marking	Description	Marking	Description
MANDIBLE—cont'd		**SCAPULA**	
Spinal foramen	Hole in center of vertebra formed by union of body, pedicles, and laminae; when vertebrae are superimposed one on other, spinal foramina form spinal cavity that houses spinal cord	**Borders**	
		Superior	Upper margin
		Vertebral	Margin toward vertebral column
		Axillary	Lateral margin
		Spine	Sharp ridge running diagonally across posterior surface of shoulder blade
Cervical vertebrae		Acromion process	Slightly flaring projection at lateral end of scapular spine; may be felt as tip of shoulder; articulates with clavicle
General features	Foramen in each transverse process for transmission of vertebral artery, vein, and plexus of nerves; short bifurcated spinous processes except on seventh vertebra, where it is extra long and may be felt as protrusion when head is bent forward; bodies of these vertebrae small, whereas spinal foramina large and triangular	Coracoid process	Projection on anterior surface from upper border of bone; may be felt in groove between deltoid and pectoralis major muscles, about 1 inch below clavicle
		Glenoid cavity	Arm socket
		STERNUM	
		Body	Main central part of bone
		Manubrium	Flaring, upper part
Atlas	First cervical vertebra; lacks body and spinous processes; superior articulating processes concave ovals that act as rocker-like cradles for condyles of occipital bone; named atlas because supports head as Atlas was thought to have supported the world	Xiphoid process	Projection of cartilage at lower border of bone
		RIBS	
		Head	Projection at posterior end of rib; articulates with corresponding thoracic vertebra and one above, except last three pairs, which join corresponding vertebrae only
Axis (epistropheus)	Second cervical vertebra, named because atlas rotates about this bone in rotating movements of the head; dens, or odontoid process, projects upward like a peg from body of axis, forming pivot for rotation of atlas	Neck	Constricted portion just below head
		Tubercle	Small knob just below neck; articulates with transverse process of corresponding thoracic vertebra; missing in lowest three ribs
Lumbar vertebrae	Strong, massive; superior articulating processes directed inward instead of upward; inferior articulating processes, outward instead of downward; short, blunt spinous process	Body or shaft	Main part of rib
		Costal cartilage	Cartilage at sternal end of true ribs; attaches ribs (except floating ribs) to sternum
Sacral promontory	Protuberance from anterior, upper border of sacrum into pelvis; of obstetrical importance because its size limits anteroposterior diameter of pelvic inlet		
		HUMERUS	
Intervertebral foramina	Opening between vertebrae through which spinal nerves emerge	Head	Smooth, hemispherical enlargement at proximal end of humerus
Curves	Curves have great structural importance because they increase carrying strength of vertebral column, make balance possible in upright position (if column were straight, weight of viscera would pull body forward), absorb jars from walking (straight column would transmit jars straight to head), and protect column from fracture	Anatomical neck	Oblique groove just below head
		Greater tubercle	Rounded projection lateral to head on anterior surface
		Lesser tubercle	Prominent projection on anterior surface just below anatomical neck
		Intertubercular	Deep groove between greater and lesser tubercles; long tendon of biceps muscle lodges here
Primary	Column curves at birth from head to sacrum with convexity posteriorly; after child stands, convexity persists only in *thoracic* and *sacral* regions, which therefore are called primary curves	Surgical neck	Region just below tubercles; so named because of its liability to fracture
		Deltoid tuberosity	V-shaped, rough area about midway down shaft where deltoid muscle inserts
		Radial groove	Groove running obliquely downward from deltoid tuberosity; lodges radial nerve
Secondary	Concavities in *cervical* and *lumbar* regions; cervical concavity results from infant's attempts to hold head erect (3 to 4 months); lumbar concavity, from balancing efforts in learning to walk (10 to 18 months)	Epicondyles (medial and lateral)	Rough projections at both sides of distal end
		Capitulum	Rounded knob below lateral epicondyle; articulates with radius; sometimes called radial head of humerus
Abnormal	*Kyphosis,* exaggerated convexity in thoracic region (hunchback); *lordosis,* exaggerated concavity in lumbar region, a very common condition; *scoliosis,* lateral curvature in any region	Trochlea	Projection with deep depression through center similar to shape of pulley; articulates with ulna

Continued.

Identification of bone markings—cont'd

Marking	Description	Marking	Description
HUMERUS—cont'd		**OS COXAE**	
Olecranon fossa	Depression on posterior surface just above trochlea; receives olecranon process of ulna when lower arm extends	Ilium	Upper, flaring portion
		Ischium	Lower, posterior portion
		Pubic bone or pubis	Medial, anterior section
Coronoid fossa	Depression of anterior surface above trochlea; receives coronoid process of ulnar in flexion of lower arm	Acetabulum	Hip socket; formed by union of ilium, ischium, and pubis
		Iliac crests	Upper, curving boundary of ilium
ULNA		Iliac spines	
Olecranon process	Elbow	Anterior superior	Prominent projection at anterior end of iliac crest; can be felt externally as "point" of hip
Coronoid process	Projection on anterior surface of proximal end of ulna; trochlea of humerus fits snugly between olecranon and coronoid processes	Anterior inferior	Less prominent projection short distance below anterior superior spine
		Posterior superior	At posterior end of iliac crest
Semilunar notch	Curved notch between olecranon and coronoid process, into which trochlea fits	Posterior inferior	Just below posterior superior spine
Radial notch	Curved notch lateral and inferior to semilunar notch; head of radius fits into this concavity	Greater sciatic notch	Large notch on posterior surface of ilium just below posterior inferior spine
Head	Rounded process at distal end; does not articulate with wrist bones but with fibrocartilaginous disk	Gluteal lines	Three curved lines across outer surface of ilium—posterior, anterior, inferior, respectively
Styloid process	Sharp protuberance at distal end; can be seen from outside on posterior surface	Iliopectineal line	Rounded ridge extending from pubic tubercle upward and backward toward sacrum
		Iliac fossa	Large, smooth, concave inner surface of ilium above iliopectineal line
RADIUS		Ischial tuberosity	Large, rough, quadrilateral process forming inferior part of ischium; in erect sitting position body rests on these tuberosities
Head	Disk-shaped process forming proximal end of radius; articulates with capitulum of humerus and with radial notch of ulna		
Radial tuberosity	Roughened projection on ulnar side, short distance below head; biceps muscle inserts here	Ischial spine	Pointed projection just above tuberosity
		Symphysis pubis	Cartilaginous, amphiarthrotic joint between pubic bones
Styloid process	Protuberance at distal end on lateral surface (with forearm supinated as in anatomical position)	Superior pubic ramus	Part of pubis lying between symphysis and acetabulum; forms upper part of obturator foramen
		Inferior pubic ramus	Part extending down from symphysis; unites with ischium
FEMUR		Pubic arch	Angle formed by two inferior rami
Head	Rounded, upper end of bone; fits into acetabulum	Pubic crest	Upper margin of superior ramus
Neck	Constricted portion just below head	Pubic tubercle	Rounded process at end of crest
Greater trochanter	Protuberance located inferiorly and laterally to head	Obturator foramen	Large hole in anterior surface of os coxa; formed by pubis and ischium; largest foramen in body
Lesser trochanter	Small protuberance located inferiorly and medially to greater trochanter		
Linea aspera	Prominent ridge extending lengthwise along concave posterior surface	Pelvic brim (or inlet)	Boundary of aperture leading into true pelvis; formed by pubic crests, iliopectineal lines, and sacral promontory; size and shape of this inlet have great obstetrical importance, since if any of its diameters are too small, infant skull cannot enter true pelvis for natural birth
Gluteal tubercle	Rounded projection just below greater trochanter; rudimentary third trochanter		
Supracondylar ridges	Two ridges formed by division of linea aspera at its lower end; medial supracondylar ridge extends inward to inner condyle, lateral ridge to outer condyle		
		True (or lesser) pelvis	Space below pelvic brim; true "basin" with bone and muscle walls and muscle floor; pelvic organs located in this space
Condyles	Large, rounded bulges at distal end of femur; one on medial and one on lateral surface	False (or greater) pelvis	Broad, shallow space above pelvic brim, or pelvic inlet; name "false pelvis" is misleading, since this space is actually part of abdominal cavity, not pelvic cavity
Adductor tubercle	Small projection just above inner condyle; marks termination of medial supracondylar ridge		
Trochlea	Smooth depression between condyles on anterior surface; articulates with patella	Pelvic outlet	Irregular circumference marking lower limits of true pelvis; bounded by tip of coccyx and two ischial tuberosities
Intercondyloid notch	Deep depression between condyles on posterior surface; cruciate ligaments that help bind femur to tibia lodge in this notch		

Marking	Description	Marking	Description
Pelvic girdle (or bony pelvis)	Complete bony ring; composed of two hip bones (ossa coxae), sacrum, and coccyx; forms firm base by which trunk rests on thighs and for attachment of lower extremities to axial skeleton	**TARSALS**	
		Calcaneus	Heel bone
		Talus	Uppermost of tarsals; articulates with tibia and fibula; boxed in by medial and lateral malleoli
TIBIA		Longitudinal arches	Tarsals and metatarsals so arranged as to form arch from front to back of foot
Condyles	Bulging prominences at proximal end of tibia; upper surfaces concave for articulation with femur	Medial	Formed by calcaneus, talus, navicular, cuneiforms, and three medial metatarsals
Intercondylar eminence	Upward projection on articular surface between condyles	Lateral	Formed by calcaneus, cuboid, and two lateral metatarsals
Crest	Sharp ridge on anterior surface	Transverse (or metatarsal) arch	Metatarsals and distal row of tarsals (cuneiforms and cuboid) so articulated as to form arch across foot; bones kept in two arched positions by means of powerful ligaments in sole of foot and by muscles and tendons
Tibial tuberosity	Projection in midline on anterior surface		
Popliteal line	Ridge that spirals downward and inward on posterior surface of upper third of tibial shaft		
Medial malleolus	Rounded downward projection at distal end of tibia; forms prominence on inner surface of ankle		
FIBULA			
Lateral malleolus	Rounded prominence at distal end of fibula; forms prominence on outer surface of ankle		

Description of individual joints

Name	Articulating bones	Type	Movements
Atlantoepistropheal	Anterior arch of atlas rotates about dens of axis (epistropheus)	Diarthrotic (pivot type)	Pivoting or partial rotation of head
Vertebral	Between bodies of vertebrae	Amphiarthrotic, cartilaginous	Slight movement between any two vertebrae but considerable mobility for column as whole
	Between articular processes	Diarthrotic (gliding)	
Sternoclavicular	Medial end of clavicle with manubrium of sternum; only joint between upper extremity and trunk	Diarthrotic (gliding)	Gliding; weak joint that may be injured comparatively easily
Acromioclavicular	Distal end of clavicle with acromion of scapula	Diarthrotic (gliding)	Gliding; elevation, depression, protraction, and retraction
Thoracic	Heads of ribs with bodies of vertebrae	Diarthrotic (gliding)	Gliding
	Tubercles of ribs with transverse processes of vertebrae	Diarthrotic (gliding)	Gliding
Shoulder	Head of humerus in glenoid cavity of scapula	Diarthrotic (ball and socket type)	Flexion, extension, abduction, adduction, rotation, and circumduction of upper arm; one of most freely movable of joints
Elbow	Trochlea of humerus with semilunar notch of ulna; head of radius with capitulum of humerus	Diarthrotic (hinge type)	Flexion and extension
	Head of radius in radial notch of ulna	Diarthrotic (pivot type)	Supination and pronation of lower arm and hand; rotation of lower arm on upper as in using screwdriver
Wrist	Scaphoid, lunate, and triquetral bones articulate with radius and articular disk	Diarthrotic (condyloid)	Flexion, extension, abduction, and adduction of hand

Continued.

Description of individual joints—cont'd

Name	Articulating bones	Type	Movements
Carpal	Between various carpals	Diarthrotic (gliding)	Gliding
Hand	Proximal end of first metacarpal with trapezium	Diarthrotic (saddle)	Flexion, extension, abduction, adduction, and circumduction of thumb and opposition to fingers; motility of this joint accounts for dexterity of human hand compared with animal forepaw
	Distal end of metacarpals with proximal end of phalanges	Diarthrotic (hinge)	Flexion, extension, limited abduction, and adduction of fingers
	Between phalanges	Diarthrotic (hinge)	Flexion and extension of finger sections
Sacroiliac	Between sacrum and two ilia	Diarthrotic (gliding); joint cavity mostly obliterated after middle life	None or slight, for example, during late months of pregnancy and during delivery
Symphysis pubis	Between two pubic bones	Synarthrotic (or amphiarthrotic), cartilaginous	Slight, particularly during pregnancy and delivery
Hip	Head of femur in acetabulum of os coxae	Diarthrotic (ball and socket)	Flexion, extension, abduction, adduction, rotation, and circumduction
Knee	Between distal end of femur and proximal end of tibia; largest joint in body	Diarthrotic (hinge type)	Flexion and extension; slight rotation of tibia
Tibiofibular	Head of fibula with lateral condyle of tibia	Diarthrotic (gliding type)	Gliding
Ankle	Distal ends of tibia and fibula with talus	Diarthrotic (hinge type)	Flexion (dorsiflexion) and extension (plantar flexion)
Foot	Between tarsals	Diarthrotic (gliding)	Gliding; inversion and eversion
	Between metatarsals and phalanges	Diarthrotic (hinge type)	Flexion, extension, slight abduction, and adduction
	Between phalanges	Diarthrotic (hinge type)	Flexion and extension

7-3 Muscular system

Muscles that move the head

Muscle	Origin	Insertion	Function	Innervation
Sternocleidomastoid	Sternum Clavicle	Temporal bone (mastoid process)	Flexes head (prayer muscle) One muscle alone, rotates head toward opposite side; spasm of this muscle alone or associated with trapezius called torticollis or wryneck	Accessory nerve
Semispinalis capitis	Vertebrae (transverse processes of upper six thoracic, articular processes of lower four cervical)	Occipital bone (between superior and inferior nuchal lines)	Extends head; bends it laterally	First five cervical nerves
Splenius capitis	Ligamentum nuchae Vertebrae (spinous processes of upper three or four thoracic)	Temporal bone (mastoid process) Occipital bone	Extends head Bends and rotates head toward same side as contracting muscle	Second, third, and fourth cervical nerves
Longissimus capitis	Vertebrae (transverse processes of upper six thoracic, articular processes of lower four cervical)	Temporal bone (mastoid process)	Extends head Bends and rotates head toward contracting side	

Muscles of facial expression and of mastication

Muscle	Origin	Insertion	Function	Innervation
Muscles of facial expression				
Epicranius (occipitofrontalis)	Occipital bone	Tissues of eyebrows	Raises eyebrows, wrinkles forehead horizontally	Cranial nerve VII
Corrugator supercilii	Frontal bone (superciliary ridge)	Skin of eyebrow	Wrinkles forehead vertically	Cranial nerve VII
Orbicularis oculi	Enriches eyelid		Closes eye	Cranial nerve VII
Orbicularis oris	Encircles mouth		Draws lips together	Cranial nerve VII
Platysma	Fascia of upper part of deltoid and pectoralis major	Mandible (lower border) Skin around corners of mouth	Draws corners of mouth down—pouting	Cranial nerve VII
Buccinator	Maxillae	Skin of sides of mouth	Permits smiling Blowing, as in playing a trumpet	Cranial nerve VII
Muscles of mastication				
Masseter	Zygomatic arch	Mandible (external surface)	Closes jaw	Cranial nerve V
Temporal	Temporal bone	Mandible	Closes jaw	Cranial nerve V
Pterygoids (internal and external)	Undersurface of skull	Mandible (mesial surface)	Grate teeth	Cranial nerve V

Muscles that move the shoulder

Muscle	Origin	Insertion	Function	Innervation
Trapezius	Occipital bone (protuberance)	Clavicle	Raises or lowers shoulders and shrugs them	Spinal accessory, second, third, and fourth cervical nerves
	Vertebrae (cervical and thoracic)	Scapula (spine and acromion)	Extends head when occiput acts as insertion	
Pectoralis minor	Ribs (second to fifth)	Scapula (coracoid)	Pulls shoulder down and forward	Medial and lateral anterior thoracic nerves
Serratus anterior	Ribs (upper eight or nine)	Scapula (anterior surface, vertebral border)	Pulls shoulder forward; abducts and rotates it upward	Long thoracic nerve

Muscles that move the upper arm

Muscle	Origin	Insertion	Function	Innervation
Pectoralis major	Clavicle (medial half) Sternum Costal cartilages of true ribs	Humerus (greater tubercle)	Flexes upper arm Adducts upper arm anteriorly; draws it across chest	Medial and lateral anterior thoracic nerves
Latissimus dorsi	Vertebrae (spines of lower thoracic, lumbar, and sacral) Ilium (crest) Lumbodorsal fascia*	Humerus (intertubercular groove)	Extends upper arm Adducts upper arm posteriorly	Thoracodorsal nerve
Deltoid	Clavicle Scapula (spine and acromion)	Humerus (lateral side about halfway down—deltoid tubercle)	Abducts upper arm Assists in flexion and extension of upper arm	Axillary nerve
Coracobrachialis	Scapula (coracoid process)	Humerus (middle third, medial surface)	Adduction; assists in flexion and medial rotation of arm	Musculocutaneous nerve
Supraspinatus	Scapula (supraspinous fossa)	Humerus (greater tubercle)	Assists in abducting arm	Suprascapular nerve
Teres major	Scapula (lower part, axillary border)	Humerus (upper part, anterior surface)	Assists in extension, adduction, and medial rotation of arm	Lower subscapular nerve
Teres minor	Scapula (axillary border)	Humerus (greater tubercle)	Rotates arm outward	Axillary nerve
Infraspinatus	Scapula (infraspinatus border)	Humerus (greater tubercle)	Rotates arm outward	Suprascapular nerve

*Lumbodorsal fascia—extension of aponeurosis of latissimus dorsi; fills in space between last rib and iliac crest.

Muscles that move the lower arm

Muscle	Origin	Insertion	Function	Innervation
Biceps brachii	Scapula (supraglenoid tuberosity)	Radius (tubercle at proximal end)	Flexes supinated forearm Supinates forearm and hand	Musculocutaneous nerve
Brachialis	Humerus (distal half, anterior surface)	Ulna (front of coronoid process)	Flexes pronated forearm	Musculocutaneous nerve
Brachioradialis	Humerus (above lateral epicondyle)	Radius (styloid process)	Flexes semipronated or semisupinated forearm; supinates forearm and hand	Radial nerve
Triceps brachii	Scapula (infraglenoid tuberosity) Humerus (posterior surface—lateral head above radial groove; medial head, below)	Ulna (olecranon process)	Extends lower arm	Radial nerve
Pronator teres	Humerus (medial epicondyle) Ulna (coronoid process)	Radius (middle third of lateral surface)	Pronates and flexes forearm	Median nerve
Pronator quadratus	Ulna (distal fourth, anterior surface)	Radius (distal fourth, anterior surface)	Pronates forearm	Median nerve
Supinator	Humerus (lateral epicondyle) Ulna (proximal fifth)	Radius (proximal third)	Supinates forearm	Radial nerve

Muscles that move the hand

Muscle	Origin	Insertion	Function	Innervation
Flexor carpi radialis	Humerus (medial epicondyle)	Second metacarpal (base of)	Flexes hand Flexes forearm	Median nerve
Palmaris longus	Humerus (medial epicondyle)	Fascia of palm	Flexes hand	Median nerve
Flexor carpi ulnaris	Humerus (medial epicondyle) Ulna (proximal two thirds)	Pisiform bone Third, fourth, and fifth metacarpals	Flexes hand Adducts hand	Ulnar nerve

Muscle	Origin	Insertion	Function	Innervation
Extensor carpi radialis longus	Humerus (ridge above lateral epicondyle)	Second metacarpal (base of)	Extends hand Abducts hand (moves toward thumb side when hand supinated)	Radial nerve
Extensor carpi radialis brevis	Humerus (lateral epicondyle)	Second, third metacarpals (bases of)	Extends hand	Radial nerve
Extensor carpi ulnaris	Humerus (lateral epicondyle) Ulna (proximal three fourths)	Fifth metacarpal (base of)	Extends hand Adducts hand (move toward little finger side when hand supinated)	Radial nerve

Muscles that move the trunk

Muscle	Origin	Insertion	Function	Innervation
Sacrospinalis (erector spinae)			Extend spine; maintain erect posture of trunk Acting singly, abduct and rotate trunk	Posterior rami of first cervical to fifth lumbar spinal nerves
Lateral portion Iliocostalis lumborum	Iliac crest, sacrum (posterior surface), and lumbar vertebrae (spinous processes)	Ribs, lower six		
Iliocostalis dorsi	Ribs, lower six	Ribs, upper six		
Iliocostalis cervicis	Ribs, upper six	Vertebrae, fourth to sixth cervical		
Medial portion Longissimus dorsi	Same as iliocostalis lumborum	Vertebrae, thoracic ribs		
Longissimus cervicis	Vertebrae, upper six thoracic	Vertebrae, second to sixth cervical		
Longissimus capitis	Vertebrae, upper six thoracic and last four cervical	Temporal bone, mastoid process		
Quadratus lumborum (forms part of posterior abdominal wall)	Ilium (posterior part of crest) Vertebrae (lower three lumbar)	Ribs (twelfth) Vertebrae (transverse processes of first four lumbar)	Both muscles together extend spine One muscle alone abducts trunk toward side of contracting muscle	First three or four lumbar nerves
Iliopsoas	See muscles that move the thigh		Flexes trunk	

Muscles that move the chest wall

Muscle	Origin	Insertion	Function	Innervation
External intercostals	Rib (lower border; forward fibers)	Rib (upper border of rib below origin)	Elevate ribs	Intercostal nerves
Internal intercostals	Rib (inner surface, lower border; backward fibers)	Rib (upper border of rib below origin)	Probably depress ribs	Intercostal nerves
Diaphragm	Lower circumference of thorax (of rib cage)	Central tendon of diaphragm	Enlarges thorax, causing inspiration	Phrenic nerves

Muscles that move the abdominal wall

Muscle	Origin	Insertion	Function	Innervation
External oblique	Ribs (lower eight)	Ossa coxae (iliac crest and pubis by way of inguinal ligament)* Linea alba† by way of an aponeurosis‡	Compresses abdomen Important postural function of all abdominal muscles is to pull front of pelvis upward, thereby flattening lumbar curve of spine; when these muscles lose their tone, common figure faults of protruding abdomen and lordosis develop	Lower seven intercostal nerves and iliohypogastric nerves
Internal oblique	Ossa coxae (iliac crest and inguinal ligament)	Ribs (lower three) Pubic bone	Same as external oblique	Last three intercostal nerves; iliohypogastric and ilioinguinal nerves
Transversalis	Lumbodorsal fascia Ribs (lower six) Ossa coxae (iliac crest, inguinal ligament) Lumbodorsal fascia	Linea alba Pubic bone Linea alba	Same as external oblique	Last five intercostal nerves; iliohypogastric and ilioinguinal nerves
Rectus abdominis	Ossa coxae (pubic bone and symphysis pubis)	Ribs (costal cartilage of fifth, sixth, and seventh ribs) Sternum (xiphoid process)	Same as external oblique; because abdominal muscles compress abdominal cavity, they aid in straining, defecation, forced expiration, and childbirth; abdominal muscles are antagonists of diaphragm, relaxing as it contracts and vice versa Flexes trunk	Last six intercostal nerves

*Inguinal ligament (or Poupart's)—lower edge of aponeurosis of external oblique muscle, extending between the anterior superior iliac spine and the tubercle of the pubic bone. This edge is doubled under like a hem. The inguinal ligament forms the upper boundary of the femoral triangle, a large triangular area in the thigh; its other boundaries are the adductor longus muscle medially and the sartorius muscle laterally.

†Linea alba—literally, a white line; extends from xiphoid process to symphysis pubis; formed by fibers of aponeuroses of the right abdominal muscles interlacing with fibers of aponeuroses of the left abdominal muscles; comparable to a seam up the midline of the abdominal wall, anchoring its various layers. During pregnancy the linea alba becomes pigmented and is known as the linea niger.

‡Aponeurosis—sheet of white fibrous tissue that attaches one muscle to another or attaches it to bone or other movable structures, for example, the right external oblique muscle attaches to the left external oblique muscle by means of an aponeurosis.

Muscles of the pelvic floor

Muscle	Origin	Insertion	Function	Innervation
Levator ani	Pubis (posterior surface) Ischium (spine)	Coccyx	Together form floor of pelvic cavity; support pelvic organs; if these muscles are badly torn at childbirth or become too relaxed, uterus or bladder may prolapse, that is, drop out	Pudendal nerve
Coccygeus (posterior continuation of levator ani)	Ischium (spine)	Coccyx Sacrum	Same as levator ani	Pudendal nerve

Muscles that move the thigh

Muscle	Origin	Insertion	Function	Innervation
Iliopsoas (iliacus and psoas major)	Ilium (iliac fossa) Vertebrae (bodies of twelfth thoracic to fifth lumbar)	Femur (small trochanter)	Flexes thigh Flexes trunk (when femur acts as origin)	Femoral and second to fourth lumbar nerves

Muscle	Origin	Insertion	Function	Innervation
Rectus femoris	Ilium (anterior, inferior spine)	Tibia (by way of patellar tendon)	Flexes thigh; Extends lower leg	Femoral nerve
Gluteal group				
Maximus	Ilium (crest and posterior surface); Sacrum and coccyx (posterior surface); Sacrotuberous ligament	Femur (gluteal tuberosity); Iliotibial tract*	Extends thigh—rotates outward	Inferior gluteal nerve
Medius	Ilium (lateral surface)	Femur (greater trochanter)	Abducts thigh—rotates outward; stabilizes pelvis on femur	Superior gluteal nerve
Minimus	Ilium (lateral surface)	Femur (greater trochanter)	Abducts thigh; stabilizes pelvis on femur; Rotates high medially	Superior gluteal nerve
Tensor fasciae latae	Ilium (anterior part of crest)	Tibia (by way of iliotibial tract)	Abducts thigh; Tightens iliotibial tract*	Superior gluteal nerve
Piriformis	Vertebrae (front of sacrum)	Femur (medial aspect of greater trochanter)	Rotates thigh outward; Abducts thigh; Extends thigh	First or second sacral nerves
Adductor group				
Brevis	Pubic bone	Femur (linea aspera)	Adducts thigh	Obturator nerve
Longus	Pubic bone	Femur (linea aspera)	Adducts thigh	Obturator nerve
Magnus	Pubic bone	Femur (linea aspera)	Adducts thigh	Obturator nerve
Gracilis	Pubic bone (just below symphysis)	Tibia (medial surface behind sartorius)	Adducts thigh and flexes and adducts leg	Obturator nerve

*The iliotibial tract is part of the fascia enveloping all the thigh muscles. It consists of a wide band of dense fibrous tissue attached to the iliac crest above and the lateral condyle of the tibia below. The upper part of the tract encloses the tensor fasciae latae muscle.

Muscles that move the lower leg

Muscle	Origin	Insertion	Function	Innervation
Quadriceps femoris group				
Rectus femoris	Ilium (anterior, inferior spine)	Tibia (by way of patellar tendon)	Flexes thigh; Extends leg	Femoral nerve
Vastus lateralis	Femur (linea aspera)	Tibia (by way of patellar tendon)	Extends leg	Femoral nerve
Vastus medialis	Femur	Tibia (by way of patellar tendon)	Extends leg	Femoral nerve
Vastus intermedius	Femur (anterior surface)	Tibia (by way of patellar tendon)	Extends leg	Femoral nerve
Sartorius	Os innominatum (anterior, superior iliac spines)	Tibia (medial surface of upper end of shaft)	Adducts and flexes leg; Permits crossing of legs tailor fashion	Femoral nerve
Hamstring group				
Biceps femoris	Ischium (tuberosity); Femur (linea aspera)	Fibula (head of); Tibia (lateral condyle)	Flexes leg; Extends thigh	Hamstring nerve (branch of sciatic nerve); Hamstring nerve
Semitendinosus	Ischium (tuberosity)	Tibia (proximal end, medial surface)	Extends thigh	Hamstring nerve
Semimembranosus	Ischium (tuberosity)	Tibia (medial condyle)	Extends thigh	Hamstring nerve

Muscles that move the foot

Muscle	Origin	Insertion	Function	Innervation
Tibialis anterior	Tibia (lateral condyle of upper body)	Tarsal (first cuneiform) Metatarsal (base of first)	Flexes foot Inverts food	Common and deep peroneal nerves
Gastrocnemius	Femur (condyles)	Tarsal (calcaneus by way of Achilles tendon)	Extends foot Flexes lower leg	Tibial nerve (branch of sciatic nerve)
Soleus	Tibia (underneath gastrocnemius) Fibula	Tarsal (calcaneus by way of Achilles tendon)	Extends foot (plantar flexion)	Tibial nerve
Peroneus longus	Tibia (lateral condyle) Fibula (head and shaft)	First cuneiform Base of first metatarsal	Extends foot (plantar flexion) Everts foot	Common peroneal nerve
Peroneus brevis	Fibula (lower two thirds of lateral surface of shaft)	Fifth metatarsal (tubercle, dorsal surface)	Everts foot Flexes foot	Superficial peroneal nerve
Tibialis posterior	Tibia (posterior surface) Fibula (posterior surface)	Navicular bone Cuboid bone All three cuneiforms Second and fourth metatarsals	Extends foot (plantar flexion) Inverts foot	Tibial nerve
Peroneus tertius	Fibula (distal third)	Fourth and fifth metatarsals (bases of)	Flexes foot Everts foot	Deep peroneal nerve

7-4 | Circulatory system

Blood cells

Cell type	Description	Function	Life span
Erythrocyte	7 μm in diameter; concave disk shape; entire cell stains pale pink; no nucleus	Transportation of respiratory gases (O_2 and CO_2)	105 to 120 days
Neutrophil	12-15 μm in diameter; spherical shape; multilobed nucleus; small, pink-purple staining cytoplasmic granules	Cellular defense—phagocytosis of small pathogenic microorganisms	Hours to 3 days
Basophil	11-14 μm in diameter; spherical shape; generally two lobed nucleus; large purple staining cytoplasmic granules	Secretes heparin (anticoagulant) and histamine (important in inflammatory response)	Hours to 3 days
Eosinophil	10-12 μm in diameter; spherical shape; generally two-lobed nucleus; large orange-red staining cytoplasmic granules	Cellular defense—phagocytosis of large pathogenic microorganisms such as protozoa and parasitic worms; releases antiinflammatory substances in allergic reactions	10 to 12 days
Lymphocyte	6-9 μm in diameter; spherical shape; round (single lobe) nucleus; small lymphocytes have scant cytoplasm	Humoral defense—secretes antibodies; involved in immune system response and regulation	Days to years
Monocyte	12-17 μm in diameter; spherical shape; nucleus generally kidney-bean or "horseshoe" shaped with convoluted surface; ample cytoplasm often "steel blue" in color	Capable of migrating out of the blood to enter tissue spaces as a *macrophage*—an aggressive phagocytic cell capable of ingesting bacteria, cellular debris, and cancerous cells	Months
Platelet	2-5 μm in diameter; irregularly shaped fragments; cytoplasm contains very small pink staining granules	Releases clot activating substances and helps in formation of actual blood clot by forming platelet "plugs"	7 to 10 days

Structure of blood vessels

Arteries	Veins	Capillaries

Coats

Outer coat (tunica adventitia or externa) of white fibrous tissue; causes artery to stand open instead of collapsing when cut	Same three coats but thinner and fewer elastic fibers; veins collapse when cut; semilunar valves present at intervals	Only lining coat present; therefore walls only one cell thick
Muscle coat (tunica media) of smooth muscle, elastic, and some white fibrous tissues; this coat permits constriction and dilation		
Lining (tunica intima) of endothelium		

Blood supply

Endothelial lining cells supplied by blood flowing through vessels; exchange of oxygen, etc., between cells of middle coat and blood by diffusion; outer coat supplied by tiny vessels known as vasa vasorum or "vessels of vessels"

Nerve supply

Smooth muscle cells of tunica media innervated by autonomic fibers

Abnormalities

Atherosclerosis—hardening of walls of arteries (arteriosclerosis) characterized by lipid deposits in tunica intima
Aneurysm—saclike dilation of artery wall
Varicose veins—stretching of walls, particularly around semilunar valves
Phlebitis—inflammation of vein; "milk leg," phlebitis of femoral vein of women after childbirth

Coronary arteries

Right coronary artery	*Left coronary artery*

Divides into two main branches:
  Posterior descending artery—sends branches to both ventricles
  Marginal artery—sends branches to right ventricle and right atrium
	Divides into two main branches:
	  Anterior descending artery—sends branches to ventricles
	  Circumflex artery—sends branches to left ventricle and left atrium

White blood cells (leukocytes)

	Differential count*	
Class	*Normal range (%)*	*Typical normal (%)*
Those with granular cytoplasm and irregular nuclei		
Neutrophils (neutral staining)	65 to 75	65
Eosinophils (acid staining)	2 to 5	3
Basophils (basic staining)	½ to 1	1
Those with nongranular cytoplasm and regular nuclei		
Lymphocytes (large and small)	20 to 25	25
Monocytes	3 to 8	6
TOTAL		100

*In any differential count the sum of the percentages of the different kinds of leukocytes must, of course, total 100%.

Main arteries

Artery	*Branches (only largest ones named)*
Ascending aorta	Coronary arteries (two, to myocardium)
Aortic arch	Innominate (or brachiocephalic) artery
	Left subclavian
	Left common carotid
Innominate	Right subclavian
	Right common carotid
Subclavian (right and left)	Vertebral*
	Axillary (continuation of subclavian)
Axillary	Brachial (continuation of axillary)
Brachial	Radial
	Ulnar
Radial and ulnar	Palmar arches (superficial and deep arterial arches in hand formed by anastomosis of branches of radial and ulnar arteries; numerous branches to hand and fingers)
Common carotid (right and left)	Internal carotid (brain, eye, forehead, and nose)*
	External carotid (thyroid, tongue, tonsils, ear)
Descending thoracic aorta	Visceral branches to pericardium, bronchi, esophagus, mediastinum
	Parietal branches to chest muscles, mammary glands, and diaphragm

Descending abdominal aorta	Visceral branches:
	  Celiac axis (or artery), which branches into gastric, hepatic, and splenic arteries (stomach, liver, and spleen)
	  Right and left suprarenal arteries (suprarenal glands)
	  Superior mesenteric artery (small intestine)
	  Right and left renal arteries (kidneys)
	  Right and left spermatic (or ovarian) arteries (testes or ovaries)
	  Inferior mesenteric artery (large intestine)
	Parietal branches to lower surface of diaphragm, muscles and skin of back, spinal cord, and meninges
	Right and left common iliac arteries—abdominal aorta terminates in these vessels in an inverted Y formation

Artery	*Branches (only largest ones named)*
Right and left common iliac	Internal iliac or hypogastric (pelvic wall and viscera)
	External iliac (to leg)
External iliac (right and left)	Femoral (continuation of external iliac after it leaves abdominal cavity)
Femoral	Popliteal (continuation of femoral)
Popliteal	Anterior tibial
	Posterior tibial
Anterior and posterior tibial	Plantar arch (arterial arch in sole of foot formed by anastomosis of terminal branches of anterior and posterior tibial arteries; small arteries lead from arch to toes)

*The right and left vertebral arteries extend from their origin as branches of the subclavian arteries up the neck, through foramina in the transverse processes of the cervical vertebrae, and through the foramen magnum into the cranial cavity and unite on the undersurface of the brainstem to form the *basilar artery,* which shortly branches into the right and left *posterior cerebral arteries.* The internal carotid arteries enter the cranial cavity in the midpart of the cranial floor, where they become known as the *anterior cerebral arteries.* Small vessels, the *communicating arteries,* join the anterior and posterior cerebral arteries in such a way as to form an arterial circle (the *circle of Willis*) at the base of the brain, a good example of arterial anastomosis.

7-5 Endocrine system

Names and locations of endocrine glands

Name	Location	Name	Location
Hypothalamus	Cranial cavity (brain)	Adrenal glands	Abdominal cavity (retroperitoneal)
Pituitary glands (hypophysis cerebri)	Cranial cavity	Pancreatic islets	Abdominal cavity (pancreas)
Pineal gland (epiphysis)	Cranial cavity (brain)	Ovaries	Pelvic cavity
Thyroid gland	Neck	Testes (interstitial cells)	Scrotum
Parathyroid glands	Neck	Placenta	Pregnant uterus
Thymus	Mediastinum		

Hormones

Hormone	Source	Target	Principal action
Hypothalamus			
Growth hormone-releasing hormone (GRH)	Hypothalamus	Adenohypophysis (acidophils)	Stimulates secretion (release) of growth hormone
Growth hormone-inhibiting hormone (GIH), or somatostatin	Hypothalamus	Adenohypophysis (acidophils)	Inhibits secretion of growth hormone
Corticotropin-releasing hormone (CRH)	Hypothalamus	Adenohypophysis (basophils)	Stimulates release of adrenocorticotropic hormone (ACTH)
Thyrotropin-releasing hormone (TRH)	Hypothalamus	Adenohypophysis (basophils)	Stimulates release of thyroid-stimulating hormone (TSH)
Gonadotropin-releasing hormone (GNRH)	Hypothalamus	Adenohypophysis (basophils)	Stimulates release of gonadotropins (FSH and LH)
Prolactin-releasing hormone (PRH)	Hypothalamus	Adenohypophysis (acidophils)	Stimulates secretion of prolactin
Prolactin-inhibiting hormone (PIH)	Hypothalamus	Adenohypophysis (acidophils)	Inhibits secretion of prolactin
Pituitary gland			
Growth hormone (GH) (stomatotropin [STH])	Adenohypophysis (acidophils)	General	Promotes growth by stimulating protein anabolism and fat mobilization
Prolactin (PRL) (lactogenic hormone)	Adenohypophysis (acidophils)	Mammary glands (alveolar secretory cells)	Promotes milk secretion
Thyroid-stimulating hormone (TSH)*	Adenohypophysis (basophils)	Thyroid gland	Stimulates development and secretion in the thyroid gland
Adrenocorticotropic hormone (ACTH)*	Adenohypophysis (basophils)	Adrenal cortex	Promotes development and secretion in the adrenal cortex
Follicle-stimulating hormone (FSH)*	Adenohypophysis (basophils)	Gonads (primary sex organs)	Female: promotes development of ovarian follicle; stimulates estrogen secretion Male: promotes development of testis; stimulates sperm production
Luteinizing hormone (LH)*	Adenohypophysis (basophils)	Gonads and mammary glands	Female: triggers ovulation; promotes development of corpus luteum Male: stimulates production of testosterone
Melanocyte-stimulating hormone (MSH)	Adenohypophysis (basophils)	Skin (melanocytes); adrenal glands	Exact function uncertain; may stimulate production of melanin pigment in skin; may maintain adrenal sensitivity

*Tropic hormones.

Hormone	Source	Target	Principal action
Antidiuretic hormone (ADH)	Neurohypophysis	Kidney	Promotes water retention by kidney tubules
Oxytocin (OT)	Neurohypophysis	Uterus and mammary glands	Stimulates uterine contractions; stimulates ejection of milk into mammary ducts
Adrenal glands			
Aldosterone	Adrenal cortex (zona glomerulosa)	Kidney	Stimulates kidney tubules to conserve sodium, which, in turn, triggers the release of ADH and the resulting conservation of water by the kidney
Cortisol (hydrocortisone)	Adrenal cortex (zona fasciculata)	General	Influences metabolism of food molecules; in large amounts, it has an antiinflammatory effect
Adrenal androgens	Adrenal cortex (zona reticularis)	Sex organs, other effectors	Exact role uncertain, but may support sexual function
Adrenal estrogens	Adrenal cortex (zona reticularis)	Sex organs	Thought to be physiologically insignificant
Epinephrine (adrenaline)	Adrenal medulla	Sympathetic effectors	Enhances and prolongs the effects of the sympathetic division of the ANS
Norepinephrine	Adrenal medulla	Sympathetic effectors	Enhances and prolongs the effects of the sympathetic division of the ANS
Thyroid and parathyroid glands			
Triiodothyronine (T_3)	Thyroid gland (follicular cells)	General	Increases rate of metabolism
Tetraiodothyronine (T_4), or thyroxine	Thyroid gland (follicular cells)	General	Increases rate of metabolism (usually converted to T_3 first)
Calcitonin (CT)	Thyroid gland (parafollicular cells)	Bone tissue	Increases calcium storage in bone, lowering blood Ca^{++} levels
Parathyroid hormone (PTH) or parathormone	Parathyroid glands	Bone tissue and intestinal tract	Increases calcium removal from storage in bone and increases absorption of calcium by intestines, increasing blood Ca^{++} levels
Pancreatic islets			
Glucagon	Pancreatic islets (alpha [α] cells or A cells)	General	Promotes movement of glucose from storage and into the blood
Insulin	Pancreatic islets (beta [β] cells or B cells)	General	Promotes movement of glucose out of the blood and into cells
Somatostatin	Pancreatic islets (delta [δ] cells or D cells)	Pancreatic cells and other effectors	Can have general effects in the body, but primary role seems to be regulation of secretion of other pancreatic hormones
Pancreatic polypeptide	Pancreatic islets (pancreatic polypeptide [PP] or F cells)	Intestinal cells and other effectors	Exact function uncertain, but seems to influence absorption in the digestive tract

7-6 | Nervous system

Major ascending tracts of the spinal cord

Name	Function	Location	Origin*	Termination†
Lateral spinothalamic	Pain, temperature, and crude touch opposite side	Lateral white columns	Posterior gray column opposite side	Thalamus
Ventral spinothalamic	Crude touch, pain, and temperature	Anterior white columns	Posterior gray column opposite side	Thalamus
Fasciculi gracilis and cuneatus	Discriminating touch and pressure sensations, including vibration, stereognosis, and two-point discrimination; also conscious kinesthesia	Posterior white columns	Spinal ganglia same side	Medulla
Spinocerebellar	Unconscious kinesthesia	Lateral white columns	Posterior gray column	Cerebellum

*Location of cell bodies of neurons from which axons of tract arise.
†Structure in which axons of tract terminate.

Major descending tracts of the spinal cord

Name	Function	Location	Origin*	Termination†
Lateral corticospinal (or crossed pyramidal)	Voluntary movement, contraction of individual or small groups of muscles, particularly those moving hands, fingers, feet, and toes of opposite side	Lateral white columns	Motor areas cerebral cortex (mainly areas 4 and 6) opposite side from tract location in cord	Intermediate or anterior gray columns
Ventral corticospinal (direct pyramidal)	Same as lateral corticospinal except mainly muscles of same side	Lateral white columns	Motor cortex but on same side as tract location in cord	Intermediate or anterior gray columns
Lateral reticulospinal	Mainly facilitatory influence on motoneurons to skeletal muscles	Lateral white columns	Reticular formation, midbrain, pons, and medulla	Intermediate or anterior gray columns
Medial reticulospinal	Mainly inhibitory influence on motoneurons to skeletal muscles	Anterior white columns	Reticular formation, medulla mainly	Intermediate or anterior gray columns

*Location of cell bodies of neurons from which axons of tract arise.
†Structure in which axons of tract terminate.

Spinal nerves and peripheral branches

Spinal nerves	Plexuses formed from anterior rami	Spinal nerve branches from plexuses	Parts supplied
Cervical 1 2 3 4	Cervical plexus	Lesser occipital Great auricular Cutaneous nerve of neck Anterior supraclavicular Middle supraclavicular Posterior supraclavicular Branches to numerous neck muscles	Sensory to back of head, front of neck, and upper part of shoulder; motor to numerous neck muscles

Spinal nerves	Plexuses formed from anterior rami	Spinal nerve branches from plexuses	Parts supplied
Cervical 5		Phrenic (branches from cervical nerves before formation of plexus; most of its fibers from fourth cervical nerve)	Diaphragm
		Suprascapular and dorsoscapular	Superficial muscles* of scapula
6		Thoracic nerves, medial and lateral branches	Pectoralis major and minor
7	Brachial plexus	Long thoracic nerve	Serratus anterior
8		Thoracodorsal	Latissimus dorsi
Thoracic (or dorsal)		Subscapular	Subscapular and teres major muscles
1		Axillary (circumflex)	Deltoid and teres minor muscles and skin over deltoid
2		Musculocutaneous	Muscles of front of arm (biceps brachii, coracobrachialis, and brachialis) and skin on outer side of forearm
3			
4	No plexus formed; branches run directly to intercostal muscles and skin of thorax	Ulnar	Flexor carpi ulnaris and part of flexor digitorum profundus; some of muscles of hand; sensory to medial side of hand, little finger, and medial half of fourth finger
5			
6			
7			
8			
9		Median	Rest of muscles of front of forearm and hand; sensory to skin of palmar surface of thumb, index, and middle fingers
10			
11			
12		Radial	Triceps muscle and muscles of back of forearm; sensory to skin of back of forearm and hand
		Medial cutaneous	Sensory to inner surface of arm and forearm
		Iliohypogastric Ilioinguinal Sometimes fused	Sensory to anterior abdominal wall
			Sensory to anterior abdominal wall and external genitalia; motor to muscles of abdominal wall
Lumbar 1		Genitofemoral	Sensory to skin of external genitalia and inguinal region
2		Lateral cutaneous of thigh	Sensory to outer side of thigh
3		Femoral	Motor to quadriceps, sartorius, and iliacus muscles; sensory to front of thigh and medial side of lower leg (saphenous nerve)
4			
5			
Sacral 1	Lumbosacral plexus	Obturator	Motor to adductor muscles of thigh
2		Tibial† (medial popliteal)	Motor to muscles of calf of leg; sensory to skin of calf of leg and sole of foot
3			
4		Common peroneal (lateral popliteal)	Motor to evertors and dorsiflexors of foot; sensory to lateral surface of leg and dorsal surface of foot
5			
Coccygeal 1		Nerves to hamstring muscles	Motor to muscles of back of thigh
		Gluteal nerves, superior and inferior	Motor to buttock muscles and tensor fasciae latae
		Posterior cutaneous nerve	Sensory to skin of buttocks, posterior surface of thigh, and leg
		Pudendal nerve	Motor to perineal muscles; sensory to skin of perineum

*Although nerves to muscles are considered motor, they do contain some sensory fibers that transmit proprioceptive impulses.
†Sensory fibers from the tibial and peroneal nerves unite to form the *medial cutaneous* (or *sural*) *nerve* that supplies the calf of the leg and the lateral surface of the foot. In the thigh the tibial and common peroneal nerves are usually enclosed in a single sheath to form the *sciatic nerve,* the largest nerve in the body with a width of approximately ³/₄ inch. About two thirds of the way down the posterior part of the thigh, it divides into its component parts. Branches of the sciatic nerve extend into the hamstring muscles.

Locations of sympathetic and parasympathetic neurons

	Sympathetic	*Parasympathetic*
Preganglionic neurons		
Dendrites and cell bodies	In lateral gray columns of thoracic and first four lumbar segments of spinal cord	In nuclei of brainstem and cord (in lateral gray columns of sacral segments of cord)
Axons	In anterior roots of spinal nerves, to spinal nerves (thoracic and first four lumbar), to white rami, and then in any of three following pathways: (1) ganglia; (2) through white rami to and through sympathetic ganglia, then up or down sympathetic trunk before synapsing in a sympathetic ganglion; (3) through white rami to and through sympathetic ganglia, to and through splanchnic nerves to collateral ganglia (celiac, superior, and inferior mesenteric ganglia)	From brainstem nuclei through cranial nerve III to ciliary ganglion From nuclei in pons: through cranial nerve VII to sphenopalatine or submaxillary ganglion From nuclei in medulla through cranial nerve IX to otic ganglion or through cranial nerves X and XI to cardiac and celiac ganglia, respectively
Postganglionic neurons		
Dendrites and cell bodies	In sympathetic and collateral ganglia	In parasympathetic ganglia (for example, ciliary, sphenopalatine, submaxillary, otic, cardiac, celiac) located in or near visceral effector organs
Axons	In autonomic nerves and plexuses that innervate thoracic and abdominal viscera and blood vessels in these cavities In gray rami to spinal nerves, to smooth muscle of skin blood vessels and hair follicles, and to sweat glands	In short nerves to various visceral effector organs

Cranial nerves*

Nerve†	Sensory fibers			Motor fibers		Functions‡
	Receptors	Cell bodies	Termination	Cell bodies	Termination	
I Olfactory	*Nasal mucosa*	*Nasal mucosa*	*Olfactory bulbs (new relay of neurons to olfactory cortex)*			*Sense of smell*
II Optic	*Retina*	*Retina*	*Nucleus in thalamus (lateral geniculate body); some fibers terminate in superior colliculus of midbrain*			*Vision*
III Oculomotor	*External eye muscles except superior oblique and lateral rectus*			**Midbrain (oculomotor nucleus)**	**External eye muscles except superior oblique and lateral rectus;** *autonomic fibers terminate in ciliary ganglion and then to ciliary and iris muscles*	**Eye movements, regulation of size of pupil, accommodation** *(for near vision),* *proprioception (muscle sense)*
IV Trochlear	*Superior oblique*			**Midbrain**	**Superior oblique muscle of eye**	**Eye movements,** *proprioception*
V Trigeminal	*Skin and mucosa of head, teeth*	*Trigeminal ganglion*	*Pons (sensory nucleus)*	**Pons (motor nucleus)**	**Muscles of mastication**	*Sensations of head and face,* **chewing movements,** *muscle sense*
VI Abducens	*Lateral rectus (proprioceptive)*			**Pons**	**Lateral rectus muscle of eye**	**Abduction of eye,** *proprioception*
VII Facial	*Taste buds of anterior two thirds of tongue*	*Geniculate ganglion*	*Medulla (nucleus solitarius)*	**Pons**	**Superficial muscles of face and scalp**	**Facial expressions, secretion of saliva and tears,** *taste*

*Italics indicate sensory fibers and functions. Boldface type indicates motor fibers and functions.

†The first letters of the rods in the following sentence are the first letters of the names of the cranial nerves. Many generations of anatomy students have used this sentence as an aid to memorizing these names. "On Old Olympus' Tiny Tops, A Friendly Viking Grew Vines And Hops." (There are several slightly differing versions of this mnemonic.)

‡An aid for remembering the general function of each cranial nerve is the following 12-word saying: "Some Say Marry Money, But My Brothers Say Bad Business, Marry Money." Words beginning with S indicate sensory function. Words beginning with M indicate motor function. Words beginning with B indicate both sensory and motor functions. For example, the first, second, and eighth words in the saying start with S, which indicates that the first, second, and eighth cranial nerves perform sensory functions.

Continued.

Cranial nerves*—cont'd

Nerve†	Sensory fibers			Motor fibers		Functions‡
	Receptors	Cell bodies	Termination	Cell bodies	Termination	
VIII Vestibulo-cochlear						
1 Vestibular branch	*Semicircular canals and vestibule (utricle and saccule)*	*Vestibular ganglion*	*Pons and medulla (vestibular nuclei)*			*Balance or equilibrium sense*
2 Cochlear or auditory branch	*Organ of Corti in cochlear duct*	*Spiral ganglion*	*Pons and medulla (cochlear nuclei)*			*Hearing*
IX Glosso-pharyn-geal	*Pharynx; taste buds and other receptors of posterior one third of tongue*	*Jugular and petrous ganglia*	*Medulla (nucleus solitarius)*	**Medulla (nucleus ambiguus)**	Muscles of pharynx	*Taste and other sensations of tongue, swallowing movements, secretion of saliva, aid in reflex control of blood pressure and respiration*
	Carotid sinus and carotid body	*Jugular and petrous ganglia*	*Medulla (respiratory and vasomotor centers)*	**Medulla at junction of pons (nucleous salivatorius)**	Otic ganglion and then to parotid salivary gland	
X Vagus	*Pharynx, larynx, carotid body, and thoracic and abdominal viscera*	*Jugular and nodose ganglia*	*Medulla (nucleus solitarius), pons (nucleus of fifth cranial nerve)*	**Medulla (dorsal motor nucleus)**	Ganglia of vagal plexus and then to muscles of pharynx, larynx, and autonomic fibers to thoracic and abdominal viscera	*Sensations and movements of organs supplied; for example, slows heart, increases peristalsis, and contracts muscles for voice production*
				Medulla (dorsal motor nucleus of vagus and nucleus ambiguus)	Muscles of thoracic and abdominal viscera (autonomic) and pharynx and larynx	
XI Accessory	*Trapezius and sternocleido-mastoid (proprioceptive)*			**Anterior gray column of first five or six cervical segments of spinal cord**	Trapezius and sternocleidomastoid muscle	*Shoulder movements, turning movements of head, movements of viscera, voice production, proprioception?*
XII Hypoglossal	*Tongue muscles (proprioceptive)*			**Medulla (hypoglossal nucleus)**	Muscles of tongue and throat	*Tongue movements, proprioception*

Cranial nerves contracted with spinal nerves

	Cranial nerves	*Spinal nerves*
Origin	Base of brain	Spinal cord
Distribution	Mainly to head and neck	Skin, skeletal muscles, joints, blood vessels, sweat glands, and mucosa except of head and neck
Structure	Some composed of sensory fibers only; some of both motor axons and sensory dendrites; some motor fibers belong to somatic nervous system, some to autonomic	All of them composed of both sensory dendrites and motor axons; some of latter somatic, some autonomic
Function	Vision, hearing, sense of smell, sense of taste, eye movements	Sensations, movements, and sweat secretion

Autonomic functions

Autonomic effector	*Effect of sympathetic stimulation*	*Effect of parasympathetic stimulation*
Cardiac muscle	Increase rate and strength of contraction (beta receptors)	Inhibit pacemaker; decrease rate and strength of contraction
Smooth muscle of blood vessels		
Skin blood vessels	Constriction (alpha receptors)	No effect
Skeletal muscle blood vessels	Dilatation (beta receptors)	No effect
Coronary blood vessels	Constriction (alpha receptors) Dilatation (beta receptors)	Dilatation
Abdominal blood vessels	Stimulate; constrict	Inhibit; dilate; no parasympathetic fibers to some viscera
Blood vessels of external genitalia	Constriction (alpha receptors)	Dilatation of blood vessels causing erection
Smooth muscle of hollow organs and sphincters		
Bronchioles	Dilatation (beta receptors)	Constriction
Digestive tract, except sphincters	Decreased peristalsis (beta receptors)	Increased peristalsis
Sphincters of digestive tract	Constriction (alpha receptors)	Relaxation
Urinary bladder	Relaxation (beta receptors)	Contraction
Urinary sphincters	Constriction (alpha receptors)	Relaxation
Reproductive ducts	Contraction (alpha receptors)	Relaxation
Eye		
Iris	Contraction of radial muscle; dilated pupil	Contraction of circular muscle; constricted pupil
Ciliary	Relaxation; accommodates for far vision	Contraction; accommodates for near vision
Hairs (pilomotor muscles)	Contraction produces "goose pimples" (piloerection) (alpha receptors)	No effect
Glands		
Sweat	Increased sweat	No effect
Lacrimal	No effect	Increased secretion of tears
Digestive (salivary, gastric, etc.)	Decreased secretion of saliva; not known for others	Increased secretion of saliva
Pancreas, including islets	Decreased secretion	Increased secretion of pancreatic juice and insulin
Liver	Stimulate glycogenolysis; increase blood sugar level	No effect
Adrenal medulla	Increased epinephrine secretion	No effect

7-7 Reproductive system

Female reproductive system

Organ	Location	Function
Ovary (2)	On each side of pelvic cavity; attached to posterior surface of broad ligament of the ovary, to ovarian tubes by fimbraie	Produces ova and female sex hormones
Fallopian tube (oviduct) (2)	Extends from upper angles of uterus to sides of pelvic cavity	Conveys ova toward uterus; site of fertilization; conveys fertilized ovum to uterus
Uterus	In pelvic cavity between bladder and rectum	Protects and sustains life of embryo during pregnancy
Vagina	Extends from uterus to vulva—about 7.5-10 cm (3-4 in.); placed anterior to rectum, posterior to bladder and urethra	Conveys uterine secretions to outside of body; receives erect penis during intercourse; transports fetus during birth process
Labia majora	Two folds that extend from mons pubis to within an inch of anus	Encloses and protects other external reproductive organs; maintains secretions
Labia minora	Two folds situated between labia majora	Forms margins of vestibule; protects openings of vagina and urethra
Clitoris	Small protuberance at apex of triangle formed by junction of labia minora	Glans is richly supplied with blood vessels and with endings associated with feelings of pleasure
Vestibule	Space between labia minora that includes vaginal and urethral openings	
Greater vestibular (Bartholin's) gland (2)	On each side of vagina	Secretes fluid that moistens and lubricates vestibule
Mammary gland (2)	Anterior to pectoralis muscles, extending from second to sixth ribs and from sternum into axilla	Lactation

Male reproductive system

Organ	Location	Function
Testis (2)	Positioned obliquely in scrotum	
Seminiferous tubules		Produce spermatozoa
Interstitial cells		Produce and secrete male sex hormones
Epididymis (2)	Superior and posterior to testis	Storage and maturation of spermatozoa; conveys spermatozoa to vas deferens
Vas deferens (2)	Extends from scrotum into abdominal cavity, passes over the top, then down posterior surface of bladder, and joins ampulla of seminal vesicle	Conveys spermatozoa from epididymis to ejaculatory duct
Seminal vesicle (2)	Posterior to bladder	Secretes alkaline fluid containing nutrients and prostaglandins; fluid helps neutralize acidic seminal fluid
Prostate gland	Immediately inferior to internal urethral sphincter	Secretes alkaline fluid that helps neutralize acidic seminal fluid and enhances motility of spermatozoa
Bulbourethral (Cowper's) gland (2)	On each side of membranous urethra	Secretes fluid that lubricates end of penis
Scrotum	External pouch at base of penis	Encloses and protects testes
Penis	Suspended from front and sides of pubic arch	Conveys urine and seminal fluid to outside of body; inserted into vagina during intercourse; glans penis is richly supplied with sensory nerve endings associated with feelings of pleasure during sexual stimulation

7-8   Urinary system

Organ	Location	Function
Kidney (2)	Posterior part of lumbar region, behind peritoneum; on each side of spinal column, extending from upper border of twelfth thoracic to third lumbar vertebra	Excretes metabolic wastes; regulates acid-base balance; regulates osmotic pressure, electrolyte pattern, and volume of extracellular fluids; regulates renin-angiotensin system; manufactures erythropoietin
Ureter (2)	Duct connecting kidney with bladder	Conveys urine to bladder, acting as conduit
Bladder	In pelvic cavity behind pubes	Conveys urine to bladder, acting as conduit
	In male, in front of rectum	Serves as reservoir for urine
	In female, in front of anterior wall of vagina and neck of uterus	
Urethra	Membranous canal extending from bladder to urinary meatus	Drains urine from bladder during voiding
	In male, begins at bladder, passes through prostate gland, goes between two sheets of tissue connecting pubic bones, and passes through urinary meatus of penis	In male, also serves as passageway for semen during ejaculation
	In female, directly behind symphysis pubis and anterior to vagina	

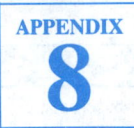

APPENDIX 8

LEADING HEALTH PROBLEMS

Two leading health problems in the United States are cardiovascular disease and cancer. Nurses and other health care professionals encounter some form of these diseases daily. The following statistics are offered in an effort to increase understanding of the magnitude of the problem and to provide a basis for developing patient teaching strategies. In this way the health care professional becomes a tool for preventive health care, an increasingly important role in today's health-conscious society.

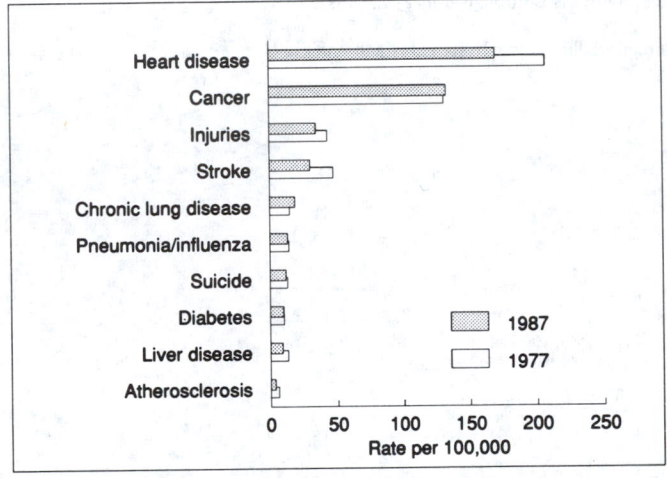

Leading causes of death, U.S. population (age-adjusted)
Source: Health, United States, 1989 and Prevention Profile *and National Center for Health Statistics (CDC)*

THE ECONOMICS OF PREVENTION

Despite the overall health improvements achieved as a result of preventive interventions, the nation continues to be burdened by preventable illness, injury, and disability. In 1960, the share of the Gross National Product (GNP) going to medical services was 5%. It is estimated to reach nearly 12% in 1990.[2] Lost economic productivity attendant to illness and early death compounds the impact of this problem, so that in 1980 the total costs of illness equalled nearly 18% of GNP. Injury alone now costs the nation well over $100 billion annually, cancer over $70 billion, and cardiovascular disease $135 billion.

Sophisticated technology for the diagnosis and treatment of disease conditions has outstripped society's ability to pay for it. But many of these expenses are avoidable.

Costs of treatment for selected preventable conditions

Condition	Overall magnitude	Avoidable intervention*	Cost per patient†
Heart disease	7 million with coronary artery disease 500,000 deaths/yr 392,000 bypass procedures/yr	Coronary bypass surgery	$30,000
Cancer	1 million new cases/yr 510,000 deaths/yr	Lung cancer treatment Cervical cancer treatment	$29,000 $28,000

*Examples (other interventions may apply).
†Representative first-year costs, except as noted. Not indicated are nonmedical costs, such as lost productivity to society.
Data compiled from various sources by the Office of Disease Prevention and Health Promotion.

Condition	Overall magnitude	Avoidable intervention*	Cost per patient†
Stroke	600,000 strokes/yr 150,000 deaths/yr	Hemiplegia treatment and rehabilitation	$22,000
Injuries	2.3 million hospitalizations/yr 142,500 deaths/yr	Quadriplegia treatment and rehabilitation	$570,000 (lifetime)
	177,000 persons with spinal cord injuries in the United States	Hip fracture treatment and rehabilitation	$40,000
		Severe head injury treatment and rehabilitation	$310,000 (lifetime)
HIV infection	1-1.5 million infected 118,000 AIDS cases (as of Jan 1990)	AIDS treatment	$75,000 (lifetime)
Alcoholism	18.5 million abuse alcohol 105,000 alcohol-related deaths/yr	Liver transplant	$250,000
Drug abuse	Regular users: 1-3 million, cocaine 900,000, IV drugs 500,000, heroin Drug-exposed babies: 375,000	Treatment of drug-affected baby (including social services)	$63,000 (5 years)
Low birth weight baby	260,000 LBWB born/yr 23,000 deaths/yr	Neonatal intensive care for LBWB	$10,000
Inadequate immunization	Lacking basic immunization series: 20-30%, aged 2 and younger 3%, aged 6 and older	Congenital rubella syndrome treatment	$354,000 (lifetime)

8-1 Cardiovascular disease

Cardiovascular diseases (problems affecting the heart and blood vessels) are the leading cause of illness and death for both men and women in the United States. About 44% of the deaths in this country are attributable to cardiovascular disease. The majority stem from atherosclerosis.

Before menopause, women tend to have lower blood pressure and fewer heart attacks than do men of equivalent age. (Female hormones exert a protective effect against heart attacks.) After menopause, the rates among women are higher than those of men and increase with advancing age.

The American Heart Association estimates that 69 million Americans have one or more forms of cardiovascular disease. The table below indicates the prevalence and mortality of the most common types.

Prevalence of cardiovascular disease (1993 estimates)

Condition	Prevalence*	Mortality
High blood pressure	63,640,000	32,790
Heart attack and angina	6,230,000	489,340
Stroke	3,020,000	145,340
Rheumatic heart disease	1,320,000	6,000
Congenital heart disease	930,000	5,700

*Some individuals have more than one of the listed conditions.
Reproduced with permission. *1993 Heart & Stroke Facts Statistics.* Copyright American Heart Association.
From Cournacchia HJ, Barrett S: *Consumer health,* St Louis, 1993, Mosby.

HEART ATTACK—SIGNALS AND ACTION

Know the warning signals of a heart attack
- Uncomfortable pressure, fullness, squeezing or pain in the center of your chest, lasting 2 minutes or more.
- Pain may spread to shoulders, neck, or arms.
- Severe pain, dizziness, fainting, sweating, nausea, or shortness of breath may also occur.
- Not all these signals, however, are always present. **Don't wait.** Get help immediately.

Know what to do in case of an emergency.
- If you are having chest discomfort that lasts for 2 minutes or more, call the emergency rescue service.
- If you can get to a hospital faster by car, have someone drive you.
- Find out which hospitals in your area offer 24-hour emergency cardiac care.
- Select in advance the facility nearest your home and office and tell your family and friends to call this facility in an emergency.
- Keep a list of emergency rescue service numbers next to your telephone and in a prominent place in your pocket, wallet, or purse.

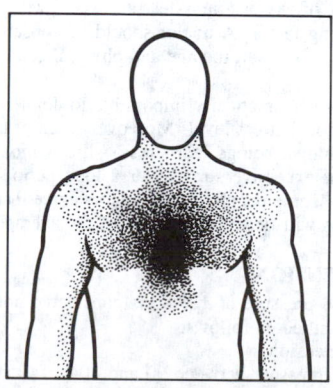

Intensity and Location of Pain

RISK FACTORS OF HEART DISEASE

Major risk factors that cannot be changed

Heredity—It appears that a tendency toward heart disease or atherosclerosis is hereditary.

Male sex—Men have a greater risk of heart attack than women. Even after menopause, when women's death rate increases, it never reaches that of men.

Race—Black Americans have moderate hypertension twice as often as whites and severe hypertension three times as often.

Age—Fifty-five percent of all heart attack victims are age 65 or older; of those who die, more than four out of five are over 65.

Major risk factors that can be changed

Cigarette smoking—The heart attack death rate among people who do not smoke cigarettes is considerably lower than for people who do smoke. For those who have given up the habit, the death rate eventually declines almost to that of people who have never smoked. Don't smoke cigarettes.

High blood pressure—A major risk factor of stroke and heart attack, high blood pressure usually has no specific symptoms but can be detected by a simple, painless test. A person with mild elevations of blood pressure often begins treatment with a program of weight reduction, if overweight, and salt (sodium) restriction before drugs are recommended.

Blood cholesterol levels—Too much cholesterol can cause build-ups on the walls of arteries, narrowing the passageway through which blood flows, and leading to heart attack and stroke. A doctor can measure the amount of cholesterol in the blood by a simple test. Since the body gets cholesterol both through diet and by manufacturing it, a diet low in saturated fat and cholesterol will help lower the level of blood cholesterol if it is too high. Medications also are available to maintain cholesterol levels within the normal range.

Other contributing risk factors

Diabetes—Diabetes appears most frequently during middle age, more often in people who are overweight. In its mild form, diabetes can escape detection for many years, but it can sharply increase a person's risk of heart attack, making control of other risk factors even more important. A doctor can detect diabetes and prescribe changes in eating habits, weight-control and exercise programs, and drugs, if necessary, to keep it in check.

Obesity—In most cases, obesity simply results from eating too much and exercising too little. It places a heavy burden on your heart. In addition, obesity is associated with coronary heart disease primarily because of its influence on blood pressure, blood cholesterol, and precipitating diabetes. To reduce weight, doctors usually recommend a program that combines exercise with a low-calorie diet.

Lack of exercise—Lack of exercise has not been clearly established as a risk factor for heart attack. But when combined with overeating, lack of exercise may lead to excess weight, which is clearly a contributing factor. A doctor should be consulted for the physical activities that best suit the age and physical condition of the individual.

Stress—It's practically impossible to define and measure a person's emotional stress level. Moreover, each of us reacts differently to it. All human beings feel stress—life without it would be dull, indeed. But excessive stress over a long period may create health problems in some people. Most doctors agree that reduction of emotional stress will benefit the health of the average individual.

HYPERTENSION

A blood pressure of 120/80 is considered normal. Hypertension can be classified as follows:

mild hypertension =
  diastolic pressure between 90 and 104
moderate hypertension =
  diastolic pressure between 105 and 115
severe hypertension =
  diastolic pressure above 115
isolated systolic hypertension =
  diastolic below 90
  but systolic above 160
The goal of treatment is diastolic pressure below 90 and systolic below 140.

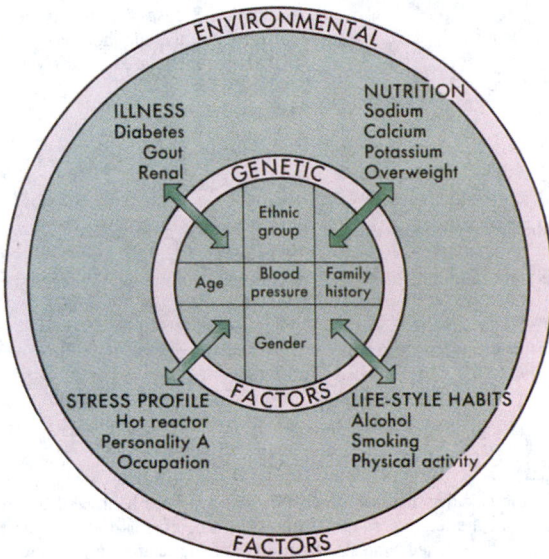

Factors contributing to hypertension
(From Beare PG, Meyers JL: Principles and practice of adult health nursing, St Louis, 1990, Mosby.)

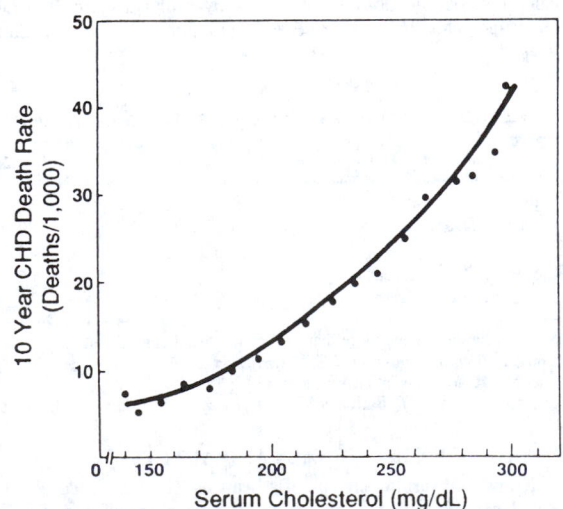

Relationship between serum cholesterol level and coronary heart disease death rate

CHOLESTEROL LEVELS

NCEP* classification of serum cholesterol levels (mg/dl)

Total cholesterol	
Under 200	Desirable
200-239	Borderline high
240 or more	High

LDL cholesterol	
Under 130	Desirable
130-159	Borderline high-risk
160 or more	High risk

*National Blood, Lung, and Heart Institute's National Cholesterol Education Program.

STROKE

A stroke occurs when an artery to the brain bursts or becomes clogged by a blood clot or other particle. Deprived of oxygen, nerve cells in the affected area of the brain cannot function and die within minutes, resulting in loss of function in the parts of the body that are controlled by these cells. The primary

Risk factors of stroke

Some of the factors that increase the risk of stroke are congenital, whereas others result from the hazards of life. Some of these factors can be minimized by the individual and with a doctor's help. Other factors cannot be changed.

Risk factors that cannot be changed

Age—The incidence of stroke is strongly related to age. In fact, the incidence of stroke more than doubles in each successive decade for people over 55 years old.

Sex—The risk of stroke is greater in men than in women. However, in women who take oral contraceptives the risk of stroke is slightly increased. Women who are also heavy smokers may aggravate this risk further.

Race—The risk of death and disability from stroke is much greater among black Americans than among white Americans. This may be a result of the greater prevalence of high blood pressure among blacks.

Diabetes mellitus—Although diabetes is treatable, the fact that a person has diabetes still makes it much more likely that a stroke will occur.

Prior stroke—The risk of stroke for a person who has already suffered a stroke is many times that of a person who has never had stroke.

Heredity—The risk of stroke is greater in people who have a family history of stroke.

Asymptomatic carotid bruit—As an indication of existing atherosclerosis, a bruit is an abnormal sound heard when a stethoscope is placed over an artery (in this case, the carotid artery, which is in the neck). Carotid bruit clearly indicates an increased stroke risk, although a bruit mainly indicates that atherosclerosis is present and

Reproduced with permission. *Heart & Stroke Facts,* 1992. Copyright American Heart Association.

doesn't necessarily mean the carotid artery with the bruit will become clogged and a stroke will result.

Risk factors that can be changed

High blood pressure—The control of high blood pressure will reduce the risk of stroke.

High red blood cell count—A marked increase, as well as a moderate elevation, in the red blood cell count may be a risk factor of stroke.

Heart disease—A diseased heart increases the risk of stroke in two ways: as a failing pump and as a source of emboli, clots that form in the heart and could travel to the arteries leading to the brain and cause a blockage. Good management of heart disease reduces the risk of stroke.

Warning signals of stroke

Know the warning signals of stroke.
- Sudden, temporary weakness or numbness of the face, arm, and leg on one side of the body.
- Temporary loss of speech, or trouble talking or understanding speech.
- Dimness or loss of vision, particularly in only one eye.
- Unexplained dizziness, unsteadiness, or sudden falls.

Many major strokes are preceded by "little strokes," warning signals like the above, experienced days, weeks, or months before the more severe event.

Prompt medical or surgical attention to these symptoms may prevent a fatal or disabling stroke from occurring.

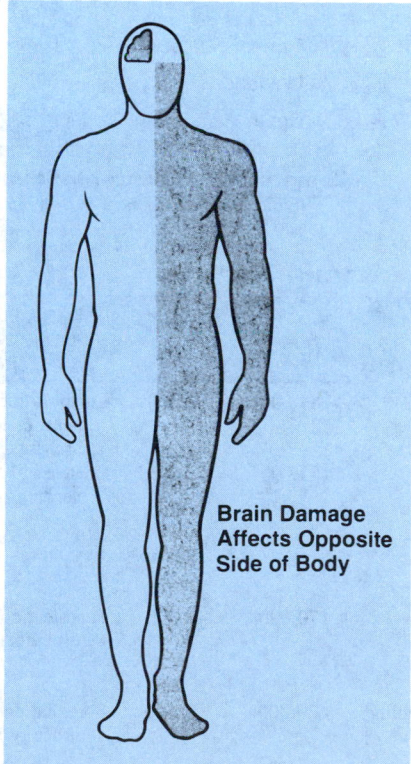

**Brain Damage
Affects Opposite
Side of Body**

8-2 | Cancer

Cancer ranks second to heart disease as the cause of death in the United States, but significant progress has been made in prevention and treatment. Five-year survival rates have risen to almost 50% for newly diagnosed cancer patients, and there is reason to believe that these rates will increase. Success can be attributed to (1) the diag- nosis of more cancers in the early localized stage, (2) the treatment of more patients within 4 months of diagnosis, and (3) the develop- ment of new diagnostic and treatment modalities, especially chemo- therapy.

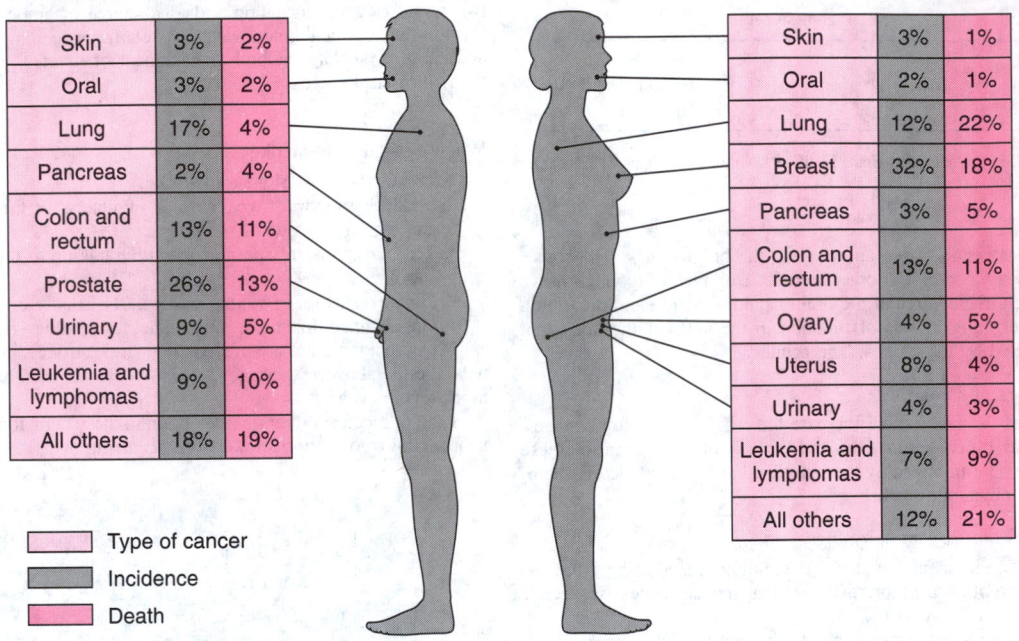

Skin	3%	2%
Oral	3%	2%
Lung	17%	4%
Pancreas	2%	4%
Colon and rectum	13%	11%
Prostate	26%	13%
Urinary	9%	5%
Leukemia and lymphomas	9%	10%
All others	18%	19%

Skin	3%	1%
Oral	2%	1%
Lung	12%	22%
Breast	32%	18%
Pancreas	3%	5%
Colon and rectum	13%	11%
Ovary	4%	5%
Uterus	8%	4%
Urinary	4%	3%
Leukemia and lymphomas	7%	9%
All others	12%	21%

■ Type of cancer
■ Incidence
■ Death

Comparison of cancer incidence and deaths by site and sex (1993 estimate)
(From American Cancer Society, 1993, Cancer facts and figures, New York, 1993, The Society.)

Leading cancer sites, 1993*†

Site	Estimated new cases 1993	Estimated deaths 1993	Warning signals (if you have one see your doctor)	Safeguards	Comment
Breast	183,000	46,300	Lump or thickening in breast or unusual discharge from nipple	Regular checkup, monthly breast self-examination, mammograms	Leading cause of cancer death in women
Colon and rectum	152,000	57,000	Change in bowel habits, bleeding	Regular checkup including proctoscopy, especially for those over 40	Considered a highly curable disease when digital and proctoscopic examinations are included in routine checkups
Lung	170,000	149,000	Persistent cough or lingering respiratory ailment	80% of lung cancers would be prevented if no one smoked cigarettes	Leading cause of cancer death among men and rising mortality among women
Oral (including pharynx)	29,800	7,700	Sore that does not heal, difficulty in swallowing	Regular checkup	Many more lives should be saved because the mouth is easily accessible to visual examination by physicians and dentists

*From American Cancer Society: 1993 *Cancer facts and figures,* New York, 1993, The Society.
†All figures rounded to nearest 1000. Incidence estimates based on rates from NCI SEER Program (Surveillance, Epidemiology, and End Results), 1982-1984.

Site	Estimated new cases 1993	Estimated deaths 1993	Warning signals (if you have one see your doctor)	Safeguards	Comment
Skin	32,000‡	6,800	Sore that does not heal or change in wart or mole	Regular checkup, avoidance of overexposure to sun	Skin cancer readily detected by observation and diagnosed by simple biopsy
Uterus	44,500§	10,100	Unusual bleeding or discharge	Regular checkup including pelvic examination with Papanicolaou test	Uterine cancer mortality has declined 70% during the last 40 years with wider application of Papanicolaou test; postmenopausal women with abnormal bleeding should be checked
Kidney and bladder	79,500	20,800	Urinary difficulty, bleeding, in which case consult physician at once	Regular checkup with urinalysis	Protective measures for workers in high-risk industries are helping to eliminate one of the important causes of these cancers
Larynx	12,600	3,800	Hoarseness, difficulty in swallowing	Regular checkup including laryngoscopy	Readily curable if caught early
Prostate gland	165,000	35,000	Urinary difficulty	Regular checkup including palpation	Occurs mainly in men over 60; disease can be detected by palpation at regular checkup
Stomach	24,000	13,600	Indigestion	Regular checkup	63% decline in mortality in 25 years for reasons yet unknown
Leukemia	29,300	18,600	Leukemia is a cancer of blood-forming tissues and is characterized by the abnormal production of immature white blood cells. Acute lymphocytic leukemia strikes mainly children and is treated by drugs that have extended life from a few months to as much as 10 years. Chronic leukemia usually strikes after age 25 and progresses less rapidly.		
Other blood and lymph tissue	63,700	31,400	These cancers arise in the lymph system and include Hodgkin's disease and lymphosarcoma. Some patients with lymphatic cancers can lead normal lives for many years. Five-year survival rate for Hodgkin's disease increased from 25% to 54% in 20 years.		

‡Melanoma only.
§Invasive cancer only.

Cancer screening guidelines

Screening test	Recommendations
Testicular self-examination	Ages 20 to 34: monthly
Breast self-examination	Ages 20 and over: monthly
Skin self-examination	Ages 20 and over: monthly
Clinical breast examination	Ages 20 to 40: every 3 years
	Over 40: every year
Mammogram	Ages 35 to 39: one baseline
	Ages 40 to 50: every 1 to 2 years
	Over 50: every year
Stool guaiac	Over 50: every year
Digital rectal examination	Over 40: every year
Sigmoidoscopy	Over 50: every 3 to 5 years after two consecutive negative yearly examinations
Pap test	Annually for all women who are or have been sexually active, or who have reached age 18; after three consecutive negative examinations, perform test per physician discretion; NOTE: those over age 65 require testing as well
Endometrial tissue biopsy	At menopause

Data from the American Cancer Society: *Cancer facts and figures*, New York, 1988, The Society; Fink DJ: Change in American Cancer Society check-up guidelines for detection of cervical cancer, *CA* 38(2):127, 1988; and White LN: Cancer prevention and detection: from twenty to sixty-five years of age, *Oncol Nurs Forum* 13(2):59, 1986.

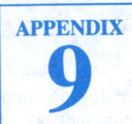

APPENDIX

9

ASSESSMENT GUIDES

9-1 Adult health assessment

Include laboratory data (complete blood count, electrolytes, urinalysis, other relevant values) under appropriate system.

I. Chief complaint of client
  A. Location
  B. Character
  C. Chronology
  D. Circumstances of occurrence
  E. Aggravating or alleviating factors
  F. Associated complaints
  G. Previous attempts at therapy and their effectiveness
  H. Disability resulting from this complaint
II. Social systems
  A. Social development
    1. Age
    2. Sex
    3. Developmental tasks
    4. Psychosocial personality development (Erikson's eight stages of man)
    5. Diversional, recreational interests (what to do to pass time while ill)
    6. Roles in family, community, work, and perceived performance of them
    7. Child's favorite play activity
    8. Socially oriented habits (include alcohol, drugs), frequency of use, and response to use
  B. Family or significant others
    1. Others in living group
    2. Significant others outside living group
    3. Visiting preferences and who is able to visit
    4. Marital status
    5. Alterations in family's life-style because of ill member
    6. Interaction patterns (observe this also)
    7. History of disease in other family members, especially those diseases with a familial tendency
  C. Work
    1. Occupation
    2. Source of income
    3. Insurance (hospitalization)
    4. Changes in work pattern because of illness
    5. Feelings about work and being away from productivity and routine
  D. Religion
    1. Religious affiliation
    2. Desire for chaplain visit
    3. Practices or beliefs that might affect reaction to health care (proscriptions against immunization or blood transfusion, dietary laws, beliefs about disease causation, death)
  E. Education
    1. Formal education
    2. Satisfaction and progress with school
  F. Community
    1. Type of housing
    2. Contacts or previous referrals to social agencies
    3. Availability and pattern of utilization of health care facilities (physician, dentist); frequency and reason for visits
    4. Immunizations (type, date)

G. Ethnic-cultural system
    1. Factors that may influence reaction to hospitalization, therapy, illness
    2. Food preferences
    3. Response to stress (e.g., pain)
H. Environment
    1. Effect of present environment on health status and developmental level (e.g., lighting, noise, activity—variation, consistency, excessive, or absent)
    2. Arrangement of environment in relation to functional abilities or disabilities
    3. Safety factors
      a. Mobility (arrangement of objects in physical environment)
      b. Use of prosthetic or supportive devices (e.g., crutches, wheelchair)
    4. Infection control
      a. Ready sources of infection
      b. Barriers to infection (isolation technique, hand-washing facility)
III. Psychologic systems
  A. Cognition
    1. Level of consciousness (response to sensory stimuli)
    2. Orientation to time, place, person
    3. Mental skills
      a. Ability to read and write
      b. Vocabulary
      c. Ability to comprehend and follow directions
      d. Attention and memory span
    4. Intellectual development relative to chronologic age (e.g., Piaget's formulation)
    5. Understanding of and reaction to health concerns and goals of medical-nursing therapy
    6. Desired information about present tests and treatment
    7. Previous experiences with and reactions to past illnesses and hospitalizations
    8. Name child or adolescent prefers
  B. Emotion
    1. Quality of mood, expression, intensity of reaction
    2. Activity level (active, sluggish, hyperactive)
    3. Effect of illness on life-style and expectation of future effects
    4. Feelings about hospitalization
    5. Coping patterns in stressful situations (describe stressful situations); availability, need for, and effectiveness of internal-external support systems
    6. Special concerns or fears
    7. Patterns of relating to others (e.g., verbal, congenial)
    8. Self-concept (body image before and in relation to current health problem)
    9. Any nervous breakdown
    10. Comfort, rest and sleep patterns (hours, time, nap periods, feeling of being rested) before and since illness
    11. Aids used to sleep
    12. Presence of pain or discomfort (location, duration, degree, character, precipitating factors, change in pattern)
    13. Use of aids to relieve pain

IV. Biologic systems
   A. General
      1. Fatigue
      2. Fever
      3. Weakness
      4. Activity tolerance
      5. Usual weight, recent weight change
   B. Gas transport and exchange
      1. Cardiovascular
         a. Past or present disease of cardiovascular system
         b. Syncope
         c. Dizziness
         d. Chest pain
            (1) Type
            (2) Pattern
            (3) Precipitating factors
            (4) Relief measures
         e. Edematous body parts
         f. Palpitations
         g. Orthopnea
         h. Medications taken to affect cardiovascular system
      2. Respiratory
         a. Past or present diseases of respiratory system
         b. Cough
            (1) Frequency
            (2) Duration
         c. Sputum
            (1) Color
            (2) Odor
            (3) Amount
         d. Shortness of breath
            (1) Precipitating factors
            (2) Frequency
            (3) Effect on activity
         e. Smoking
            (1) Pack/year history
            (2) Attempts and success at stopping
         f. Hemoptysis
         g. Frequency of colds and sore throats
         h. Medications taken to affect respiratory system
   C. Nutrition and elimination
      1. Gastrointestinal
         a. Past or present disease of gastrointestinal system
         b. Dietary habits
            (1) Amount of each food group
            (2) Likes
            (3) Dislikes
            (4) Number of meals and snacks
            (5) Time of meals
            (6) Assistance needed with eating
         c. Appetite, thirst
         d. Factors related to ingestion
            (1) Nonoral intake
            (2) Chewing
            (3) Swallowing
            (4) Oral hygiene habits
         e. Factors related to digestion
            (1) Ease
            (2) Nausea
            (3) Vomiting
            (4) Belching
            (5) Pain in abdomen
         f. Bowel elimination pattern
            (1) Time and frequency of bowel movements
            (2) Degree of child's independence in toileting
            (3) Words used by child regarding elimination
            (4) Character of stools
            (5) Ease (constipation, diarrhea)

         (6) Hemorrhoids
         (7) Passage of flatus, blood
      g. Medicines taken to alter digestion and metabolism of foods
   2. Urinary
      a. Past or present diseases of urinary system
      b. Fluid intake
      c. Urination pattern
         (1) Amount
         (2) Color
         (3) Odor
         (4) Frequency, night or day urgency
         (5) Dysuria, hematuria
      d. Vaginal or urethral discharge
      e. Degree of independence in toileting
      f. Medications taken to alter urinary system
   D. Sensorimotor
      1. Musculoskeletal
         a. Past or present disease of musculoskeletal system
         b. Abnormal innervation to muscles (paralysis, weakness, spasticity)
         c. Method of ambulation
            (1) Assistance needed with dressing, hygiene
            (2) Safety measures needed
         d. Range of motion limitations
         e. Medicines taken to affect musculoskeletal subsystem
      2. Nervous
         a. Past or present diseases of nervous system
         b. Visual status
            (1) Acuity
            (2) Deficits and corrective devices
         c. Auditory status
            (1) Deficits and corrective devices
            (2) Unusual sensations (ringing, buzzing, vertigo, pain)
         d. Olfactory status
         e. Gustatory status
         f. Tactile status (ability to discriminate sharp-dull, light-firm, hot-cold sensations)
         g. Paresthesias
         h. Mobility (coordination, balance)
         i. Medicines taken to affect nervous system
   E. Protective mechanisms
      1. Integument
         a. Past or present diseases of integumentary system
         b. Factors predisposing to skin breakdown
         c. Personal hygiene
            (1) Bathing (kind, type, frequency)
            (2) Frequency, time of shaving
            (3) After bath skin care
         d. Medicines taken to affect integumentary system
      2. Immune mechanism
         a. Past or present allergy
         b. Past or present sensitivities to drugs or other agents (pollens, insect bites)
         c. Past or present high susceptibility to infection
      3. Hematologic
         a. Easy bruising
         b. Swelling in neck or groin
         c. Past transfusions
   F. Endocrine mechanisms
      1. Abnormal function of endocrine gland or glands and effects; past or present diseases
      2. Growth patterns
      3. Heat or cold intolerance
      4. Excessive thirst, hunger, or urination
      5. Medications taken to affect endocrine system

G. Sexuality and reproduction
  1. Past or present alterations of reproduction system
  2. Reproductive data
     a. Number of pregnancies
     b. Live births
     c. Living children
     d. Family planning (methods used)
     e. Menstrual pattern
     f. Menopause (age of onset and associated factors)

3. Breast self-examination routine
4. Frequency of Pap smears
5. Sexual desire and function
6. Level of sexual development
7. Attitudes toward own sexuality
8. Medicine taken to affect reproductive system

9-2   Cultural assessment

Bloch's ethnic/cultural assessment guide

Cultural

Ethnic origin
- Does the patient identify with a particular ethnic group (e.g., Puerto Rican, African)?

Race
- What is the patient's racial background (e.g., Black, Filipino, American Indian)?

Place of birth
- Where was the patient born?

Relocations
- Where has he lived (country, city)? During what years did patient live there and for how long? Has he moved recently?

Habits, customs, values, and beliefs
- Describe habits, customs, values, and beliefs patient holds or practices that affect his attitude toward birth, life, death, health and illness, time orientation, and health care system and health care providers. What is degree of belief and adherence by patient to his overall cultural system?

Behaviors valued by culture
- How does patient value privacy, courtesy, respect for elders, behaviors related to family roles and sex roles, and work ethics?

Cultural sanctions and restrictions
- *Sanctions*—What is accepted behavior by patient's cultural group regarding expression of emotions and feelings, religious expressions, and response to illness and death?
- *Restrictions*—Does patient have any restrictions related to sexual matters, exposure of body parts, certain types of surgery (e.g., hysterectomy), discussion of dead relatives, and discussion of fears related to the unknown?

Language and communication processes
- What are some overall cultural characteristics of patient's language and communication process?
  Language(s) and/or dialect(s) spoken
    - Which language(s) and/or dialect(s) does patient speak most frequently. Where? At home or at work?
  Language barriers
    - Which language does patient predominantly use in thinking? Does patient need bilingual interpreter in nurse-patient interactions? Is patient non-English-speaking or limited English-speaking? Is patient able to read and/or write in English?
  Communication process
    - What are rules (linguistics) and modes (style) of communication process (e.g., "honorific" concept of showing "respect or deference" to others using words only common to specific ethnic/cultural group)?
    - Is there need for variation in technique of communicating and interviewing to accommodate patient's cultural background (e.g., tempo of conversation, eye/body contact, topic restrictions, norms of confidentiality, and style of explanation)?
    - Are there any conflicts in verbal and nonverbal interactions between patient and nurse?
    - How does patient's nonverbal communication process compare with other ethnic/cultural groups, and how does it affect patient's response to nursing and medical care?
    - Are there any variations between patient's interethnic and interracial communication process or intracultural and intraracial communication process (e.g., ethnic minority patient and White middle-class nurse, ethnic minority patient and ethnic minority nurse; beliefs, attitudes, values, role variations, stereotyping [perceptions and prejudice])?

Healing beliefs and practices
  Cultural healing system
    - What cultural healing system does the patient predominantly adhere to (e.g., Asian healing system, Raza/Latina Curanderismo)? What religious healing system does the patient predominantly adhere to (e.g., Seventh Day Adventist, West African voodoo, Fundamentalist sect, Pentacostal)?

Cultural health beliefs
    - Is illness explained by the germ theory or cause-effect relationship, presence of evil spirits, imbalance between "hot" and "cold" (yin and yang in Chinese culture), or disequilibrium between nature and man?
    - Is good health related to success, ability to work or fulfill roles, reward from God, or balance with nature?

Cultural health practices
    - What types of cultural healing practices does person from ethnic/cultural group adhere to? Does he use healing remedies to cure *natural* illnesses caused by the external environment (e.g., massage to cure *empacho* [a ball of food clinging to stomach wall], wearing of talismans or charms for protection against illness)?

Modified with permission from Bloch's assessment guide for ethnic/cultural variations. © Bobbie Bloch.

Cultural—cont'd

Cultural healers

- Does patient rely on cultural healers (e.g., medicine men for American Indian, Curandero for Raza/Latina, Chinese herbalist, hougan [voodoo priest], spiritualist, or minister for Black American)?

Nutritional variables or factors

- What nutritional variables or factors are influenced by the patient's ethnic/cultural background?

Characteristics of food preparation and consumption

- What types of food preferences and restrictions, meaning of foods, style of food preparation and consumption, frequency of eating, time of eating, and eating utensils are culturally determined for patient? Are there any religious influences on food preparation and consumption?

Influences from external environment

- What modifications if any did the ethnic group patient identifies with have to make in its food practices in White dominant American society? Are there any adaptations of food customs and beliefs from rural setting to urban setting?

Patient education needs

- What are some implications of diet planning and teaching to patient who adheres to cultural practices concerning foods?

Sociological

Economic status

- Who is principal wage earner in patient's family? What is total annual income (approximately) of family? What impact does economic status have on life-style, place of residence, living conditions, and ability to obtain health services?

Educational status

- What is highest educational level obtained? Does patient's educational background influence his ability to understand how to seek health services, literature on health care, patient teaching experiences, and any written material patient is exposed to in health care setting (e.g., admission forms, patient care forms, teaching literature, and lab test forms)?
- Does patient's educational background cause him to feel inferior or superior to health care personnel in health care setting?

Social network

- What is patient's social network (kinship, peer, and cultural healing networks)? How do they influence health or illness status of patient?

Family as supportive group

- Does patient's family feel need for continuous presence in patient's clinical setting (is this an ethnic/cultural characteristic)? How is family valued during illness or death?
- How does family participate in patient's nursing care process (e.g., giving baths, feeding, using touch as support [cultural meaning], supportive presence)?
- How does ethnic/cultural family structure influence patient response to health or illness (e.g., roles, beliefs, strengths, weaknesses, and social class)?
- Are there any key family roles characteristic of a specific ethnic/cultural group (e.g., grandmother in Black and some American Indian families), and can these key persons be a resource for health personnel?
- What role does family play in health promotion or cause of illness (e.g., would family be intermediary group in patient interactions with health personnel and making decisions regarding his care)?

Supportive institutions in ethnic/cultural community

- What influence do ethnic/cultural institutions have on patient receiving health services (i.e., institutions such as Organization of Migrant Workers, NAACP, Black Political Caucus, churches, schools, Urban League, community clinics)?

Institutional racism

- How does institutional racism in health facilities influence patient's response to receiving health care?

Psychological

Self-concept (identity)

- Does patient show strong racial/cultural identity? How does this compare to that of other racial/cultural groups or to members of dominant society?
- What factors in patient's development helped to shape his self-concept (e.g., family, peers, society labels, external environment, institutions, racism)?
- How does patient deal with stereotypical behavior from health professionals?
- What is impact of racism on patient from distinct ethnic/cultural group (e.g., social anxiety, noncompliance to health care process in clinical settings, avoidance of utilizing or participating in health care institutions)?
- Does ethnic/cultural background have impact on how patient relates to body image change resulting from illness or surgery (e.g., importance to appearance and roles in cultural group)?
- Any adherence or identification with ethnic/cultural "group" identity (e.g., solidarity, "we" concept)?

Mental and behavioral processes and characteristics of ethnic/cultural group

- How does patient relate to his external environment in clinical setting (e.g., fears, stress, and adaptive mechanisms characteristic of a specific ethnic/cultural group)? Any variations based on the life span? What is patient's ability to relate to persons outside of his ethnic/cultural group (health personnel)? Is he withdrawn, verbally or nonverbally expressive, negative or positive, feeling mentally or physically inferior or superior?
- How does patient deal with feelings of loss of dignity and respect in clinical setting?

Religious influences on psychological effects of health/illness

- Does patient's religion have a strong impact on how he relates to health/illness influences or outcomes (e.g., death/chronic illness, cause and effect of illness, or adherence to nursing/medical practices)?
- Do religious beliefs, sacred practices, and talismans play a role in treatment of disease?

Continued.

Bloch's ethnic/cultural assessment guide—cont'd

Psychological—cont'd

- What is role of significant religious persons during health/illness (e.g., Black ministers, Catholic priests, Buddhist monks, Islamic imams)?

Psychological/cultural response to stress and discomfort of illness

- Based on ethnic/cultural background, does patient exhibit any variations in psychological response to pain or physical disability of disease processes?

Biological/physiological

(Consideration of *norms* for different ethnic/cultural groups)

Racial-anatomical characteristics

- Does patient have any distinct racial characteristics (e.g., skin color, hair texture and color, color of mucous membranes)?
- Does patient have any variations in anatomical characteristics (e.g., body structure [height and weight] more prevalent for ethnic/cultural group, skeletal formation [pelvic shape, especially for obstetrical evaluation], facial shape and structure [nose, eye shape, facial contour], upper and lower extremities)?
- How do patient's racial and anatomical characteristics affect his self-concept and the way others relate to him?
- Does variation in racial-anatomical characteristics affect physical evaluations and physical care, skin assessment based on color, and variations in hair care and hygienic practices?

Growth and development patterns

- Are there any distinct growth and development characteristics that vary with patient's ethnic/cultural background (e.g., bone, density, fatfolds, motor ability)?
- What factors are important for nutritional assessment, neurological and motor assessment, assessment of bone deterioration in disease process or injury, evaluation of newborns, evaluation of intellectual status, or capacity in relationship to motor/sensory development in children?
- How do these differ in ethnic/cultural groups?

Variations in body systems

- Are there any variations in body systems for patient from distinct ethnic/cultural group (e.g., gastrointestinal disturbance with lactose intolerance in Blacks, nutritional intake of cultural foods causing adverse effects on gastrointestinal tract and fluid and electrolyte system, and variations in chemical and hematological systems [certain blood types prevalent in particular ethnic/cultural groups])?

Skin and hair physiology, mucous membranes

- How does skin color variation influence assessment of skin color changes (e.g., jaundice, cyanosis, ecchymosis, erythema, and its relationship to disease processes)?
- What are methods of assessing skin color changes (comparing variations and similarities between different ethnic groups)?
- Are there conditions of hypopigmentation and hyperpigmentation (e.g., vitiligo, mongolian spots, albinism, discoloration caused by trauma)? Why would these be more striking in some ethnic groups?
- Are there any skin conditions more prevalent in a distinct ethnic group (e.g., keloids in Blacks)?
- Is there any correlation between oral and skin pigmentation and their variations among distinct racial groups when doing assessment of oral cavity (e.g., leukoedema is normal occurrence in Blacks)?
- What are variations in hair texture and color among racially different groups? Ask patient about preferred hair care methods or any racial/cultural restrictions (e.g., not washing "hot-combed" hair while in clinical setting, not cutting very long hair of Raza/Latina patients).
- Are there any variations in skin care methods (e.g., using Vaseline on Black skin)?

Diseases more prevalent among ethnic/cultural group

- Are there any specific diseases or conditions that are more prevalent for a specific ethnic/cultural group (e.g., hypertension, sickle cell anemia, G6-PD, lactose intolerance)?
- Does patient have any socioenvironmental diseases common among ethnic/cultural groups (e.g., lead paint poisoning, poor nutrition, overcrowding [prone to tuberculosis], alcoholism resulting from psychological despair and alienation from dominant society, rat bites, poor sanitation)?

Diseases ethnic/cultural group has increased resistance to

- Are there any diseases that patient has increased resistance to because of racial/cultural background (e.g., skin cancer in Blacks)?

9-3 | Mental health assessment

I. Demographic data
  A. Name
  B. Address
  C. Age
  D. Sex
  E. Education
  F. Ethnicity (optional)*
  G. Religion (optional)*
  H. Living arrangements
  I. Marital status
II. Admission data
  A. Date and time of admission
  B. Manner of admission
    1. Self
    2. Relatives
    3. Police
    4. Other (describe)
  C. Form of retention (if hospitalized)
    1. Informal retention
    2. Voluntary retention
    3. Involuntary retention
    4. Emergency
    5. Comments
  D. Reason for admission
  E. Client's primary complaint
  F. Client's premorbid personality
III. History of psychiatric problems
  A. Previous condition: date; problem
  B. Assistance sought: native healer; therapist; agency; clergyman; other (describe)
  C. Current levels of functioning and coping
IV. Behavioral observations
  A. Thought patterns
    1. Delusion: grandeur; persecution; somatic; self-accusatory
    2. Obsession
    3. Ideas of reference
    4. Phobia
    5. Looseness of association
    6. Flight of ideas
    7. Fugue
    8. Impaired judgment
    9. Impaired insight
    10. Impaired orientation to time, place, or person
    11. Impaired memory
    12. No observable thought disturbance
    13. Comments
  B. Sensory processes
    1. Hallucination: olfactory; auditory; tactile; gustatory; visual
    2. No observable sensory disturbance
    3. Comments
  C. Speech patterns
    1. Blocking
    2. Word salad
    3. Echolalia
    4. Circumstantiality
    5. Irrelevancy
    6. Confabulation
    7. Mutism
    8. Neologism
    9. Perseveration

  10. Stuttering
  11. No observable speech disturbance
  12. Comments
  D. Affect
    1. Elation
    2. Depression
    3. Ambivalence
    4. Apathy
    5. Anger
    6. No observable disturbance of affect
    7. Comments
  E. Motor activity
    1. Hyperactive
    2. Hypoactive
    3. Stereotypical: persistent; aimless; repetitive
    4. Perseveration
    5. Catalepsy: stupor; waxy flexibility
    6. Compulsion
    7. No observable disturbance in motor activity
    8. Comments
  F. Level of consciousness
    1. Confusion
    2. Stupor
    3. Delirium
    4. Alert
    5. Comments
V. Physical appearance
  A. Posture
    1. Sagging
    2. Rigid
    3. Curled into fetal position
    4. Bent
    5. No observable disturbance in posture
    6. Comments
  B. Facies
    1. Drooping or sagging: deflected eyes; lusterless eyes; drooping eyelids, deep nasolabial folds
    2. Uplifted or retracted: smiling; retracted brow; wide open eyes; darting eyes
    3. Blank: staring into space; distant expression in eyes
    4. Masklike or ironed-out
    5. Facial tic
    6. No observable disturbance in facies
    7. Comments
  C. Mode of dress
    1. Overly neat
    2. Disheveled
    3. Bizarre
    4. Appropriate
    5. Comments
VI. Physical status
  A. Vital signs: pulse; temperature; respirations; blood pressure
  B. Physical condition
    1. Medical problems: acute; chronic
    2. Physical aids (describe)
    3. Medications: date and time of last dose
    4. Allergies (describe)
    5. Comments
  C. Patterns of daily living
    1. Sleep patterns: restlessness; insomnia; narcoplexy; average number of hours of sleep
    2. Eating patterns: number of meals a day; compulsive eating; anorexia
    3. Drinking patterns: beverage; quantity consumed; frequency of consumption

*Legislation protects people from being required to reveal ethnicity and religion.

4. Sexual patterns: sexual orientation or preference; attitudes about sexuality; sexual activity
5. Elimination patterns: constipation; diarrhea; urinary frequency; urinary retention
6. Social patterns: recreation; work; intimacy; community involvement
7. Comments

D. Level of self-care
1. Personal hygiene
2. Activities of daily living
3. Comments

VII. Cultural orientation
  A. Place of residence: multi-ethnic neighborhood; ethnic enclave
  B. Family organization: nuclear; extended; members composing family unit; members vested with authority; members involved in child rearing; sense of obligation of family members to one another.
  C. Sex-defined roles: stereotyped male and female roles; amount of independence permitted men and women; degree of intimacy permitted between married men and women, unmarried men and women
  D. Communication patterns: language spoken at home; language spoken outside home; use of touching and/or gesturing; interpersonal spacing
  E. Type of dress: traditional ethnic dress; Western-style dress
  F. Type of food: ethnic food; American food
  G. Relationship to people: individualistic; group-oriented; egalitarian; authoritative
  H. Relationship to time: past-oriented; present-oriented; future-oriented
  I. Relationship to the world: personal control; goal-directed; fatalistic
  J. Health care patterns: ideas concerning causes of mental illness; ideas concerning treatment of mental illness; people consulted for treatment of mental illness (e.g., family member, native healer, mental health therapist, other [describe])
  K. Comments

VIII. Effective social network
  A. Family
  B. Household members (if different from family)
  C. Friends

D. Associates: employer; coworkers; neighbors; others
E. Religious affiliates: clergyman; church elders; congregants
F. Comments

IX. Stressors
  A. Culture shock
    1. Communication (foreign verbal, kinesic, and proxemic systems)
    2. Mechanical environment (i.e., different types of food, housing, clothing, utilities)
    3. Social isolation from family and friends
    4. Foreign customs, standards, and/or values
    5. Different or new role relationships
  B. Life changes
    1. Affectional: marriage; birth; death; divorce; abandonment
    2. Socioeconomic: promotion; demotion; unemployment, change of employment; change of residence; increased responsibilities
    3. Biophysical: serious illness (acute or chronic); surgery; accident; loss of body part; sexual trauma (e.g., rape, incest)
  C. Other (describe)
  D. No significant stress
  E. Comments

X. Coping mechanisms
  A. Coping mechanisms used (describe)
  B. Effectiveness of coping mechanisms
  C. Client's perception of mechanisms that are effective in reducing stress
  D. Comments

XI. Resources
  A. Personal: interests; leisure time activities; physical and mental abilities; educational achievement; other
  B. Social: interpersonal networks; economic support systems (e.g., health insurance, sick leave, union benefits); food, shelter, clothing; other
  C. Comments

XII. Candidacy for active involvement in treatment program
  A. Developmental level
  B. Interactional ability
  C. Willingness to participate in treatment program
  D. Areas of anticipated need for assistance from nursing staff
  E. Comments

9-4   Family assessment

I. Demographic data
  A. Names of members
  B. Age of members
  C. Sex of members
  D. Relationship between members: affinal; consanguineous
  E. Educational levels of members
  F. Occupations of members
  G. Ethnicity (optional)*
  H. Religion (optional)*
  I. Family members living in another household (describe relationship)
  J. Nonfamily members living in the household (describe living arrangement)
  K. Other (describe)

II. Family organization
  A. Type of family: nuclear; extended
  B. Type of system: open; closed; boundary maintaining mechanisms (describe); norms; rules
  C. Members involved in child rearing

D. Members vested with authority
E. Sense of obligation of family members—roles: peacemaker; protector; attacker; provider; interpreter; rescuer; other
F. Sex-defined roles: stereotyped male-female relationships; amount of independence permitted men and women
G. Other (describe)

III. Family world view
  A. Relationship to people: individualistic; group-oriented; egalitarian; authoritarian
  B. Relationship to time: past-oriented; present-oriented; future-oriented
  C. Relationship to the world: personal control; goal-directed; fatalistic
  D. Comments

IV. Family perceptions and definitions
  A. Family
  B. Privacy
  C. Intimacy
  D. Health (mental and physical)
  E. Illness (mental and physical)
  F. Other (describe)

*Legislation protects people from being required to reveal ethnicity and religion.

V. Family health care patterns
  A. Ideas concerning causes of illness (mental and physical)
  B. Ideas concerning treatment of illness (mental and physical)
  C. People consulted in times of crisis or for treatment of mental and physical illnesses (e.g., family member; native healer; mental health therapist; pharmacist; physician; other)
  D. Comments

VI. Family living arrangements
  A. Type of residence: multifamily dwelling; single-family dwelling; one-room dwelling; other
  B. Environment of residence: urban; suburban; rural; inter-ethnic neighborhood; ethnic enclave
  C. Time in residence: length of time in present residence; length of time in previous residences
  D. Sleeping arrangements: number of rooms serving as bedrooms (differentiate between rooms functioning solely as bedrooms and those that have other functions)
  E. Eating arrangements: family members eat together; eat alone; eat in shifts
  F. Privacy arrangements: Rooms or sections of rooms reserved for specific family members; furniture (e.g., chairs) reserved for specific family members
  G. Other (describe)

VII. Family interaction patterns
  A. Communication patterns
    1. Verbal
      a. Language spoken at home
      b. Language spoken outside home
    2. Kinesic
      a. Touching
      b. Gesturing
    3. Proxemic
      a. Interpersonal spacing
      b. Fixed and/or built space
    4. Themes
      a. Double-bind messages
      b. Manipulation
      c. Scapegoating
      d. Intellectualization
      e. Blame placing
      f. Validation
      g. Other (describe)
  B. Behavioral patterns
    1. Physical acting out
    2. Isolation
    3. Detachment
    4. Cooperation
    5. Competition
    6. Overdependency
    7. Other (describe)
  C. Social patterns
    1. Alliances
      a. Among family members
      b. Between family members and members of social network
      c. Conflict between alliances
      d. Resolution of conflict between alliances
    2. Authority
      a. Nominal authority figure(s)
      b. Actual authority figure(s)
      c. Patterns of authority
      d. Implementation of authority: direct; delegated
    3. Decision making
      a. Nominal decision-making figure(s)
      b. Actual decision-making figure(s)
      c. Patterns of decision making
      d. Implementation of decisions
    4. Dissemination of information
      a. Sources of information
      b. Pattern of communicating information
    5. Social interaction
      a. Social network: relatives; friends; employers; co-workers; neighbors; clergy; other (describe)
      b. Community involvement: school; church; union; neighborhood; other (describe)
      c. Patterns of recreation
      d. Patterns of intimacy
    6. Other (describe)

VIII. Family stressors
  A. Culture shock
    1. Communication: foreign verbal, kinesic, and proxemic systems
    2. Mechanical environment (i.e., different types of food, housing, clothing, utilities)
    3. Social isolation from family and friends
    4. Foreign customs, standards, and/or values
    5. Different or new role relationships
  B. Life changes
    1. Affectional: marriage; birth; death; divorce; abandonment
    2. Socioeconomic: promotion; demotion; unemployment; change of employment; change of residence
    3. Biophysical: accident or serious illness involving a family member (acute or chronic)
  C. Other (describe)
  D. No significant stress

IX. Family coping mechanisms
  A. Coping mechanisms used (indicate whether mechanisms are used only by specific family members)
  B. Effectiveness of coping mechanisms
  C. Family's perception of mechanisms that are effective in reducing stress
  D. Comments

X. Family resources
  A. Familial: interests; leisure time activities; physical and mental abilities; other
  B. Social: interpersonal networks; economic support systems (e.g., health insurance, sick leave, union benefits); food, shelter, clothing; other

9-5 Group assessment

I. Description of group
  A. Type of group (e.g., activity, encounter, remotivation, psychodrama)
  B. Goals of group
  C. Size of group
  D. Composition of group
    1. Age of members
    2. Sex of members
    3. Ethnic background of members (optional)*
    4. Behavior exhibited by members
    5. Educational levels of members
    6. Communicational levels of members (e.g., verbal; mute; speak a foreign language)
    7. Reality testing levels of members
    8. other (describe)

*Legislation protects people from being required to reveal ethnic background.

II. Characteristics of group
- A. Group phase or stage (orientation, working, termination)
- B. Level of cohesiveness
- C. Level of anxiety
- D. Level of conflict
- E. Level of resistance
- F. Other (describe)

III. Patterns of group interaction
- A. Communication patterns
  1. Silence
  2. Semantic argument
  3. Intellectualization
  4. Monopolization
  5. Scapegoating
  6. Other (describe)
- B. Behavior patterns
  1. Physical activity
  2. Withdrawal
  3. Detachment
  4. Cooperation
  5. Competition
  6. Other (describe)
- C. Social patterns
  1. Group norms
  2. Group rules
  3. Roles (e.g., peacemaker, leader, protector, attacker, interpreter)
  4. Alliances among members (subgroups)
  5. Conflict between alliances
  6. Other (describe)

IV. Patterns of leadership
- A. Approach of leader(s)
  1. Laissez-faire
  2. Democratic
  3. Power struggle
  4. Authoritarian
  5. Other (describe)
- B. Competence of leader(s)
  1. Provides relaxed, nonjudgmental atmosphere
  2. Protects group members from disruptive communication patterns (scapegoating)
  3. Accepts all feelings, attitudes, and ideas as valid themes for group discussion
  4. Responds to verbal and nonverbal communication
  5. Facilitates communication and problem solving by
     - a. Encouraging group members to clarify and describe feelings, attitudes, and ideas
     - b. Summarizing as needed
  6. Facilitates group cohesiveness by
     - a. Asking for feedback and validation
     - b. Giving responsibility to the group
     - c. Encouraging the group to make decisions
     - d. Permitting the group to review and revise goals as indicated
     - e. Developing leadership among group members
  7. Other (describe)

9-6 | Pediatric assessment

INFORMANT
Who is giving the history (relation to client)?

BIOGRAPHICAL DATA
- Name
- Age
- Race
- Culture
- Address and telephone number
- Children and family in home
- Means of transportation to health care facility if pertinent
- Description of home, and size and type of community

REASON FOR VISIT
One statement that describes the reason for the client's visit, preferably in the client's own words.

PRESENT HEALTH STATUS
- Summary of client's current major health concerns
- If illness is present, record symptom analysis
  1. When client was last well
  2. Date of problem onset
  3. Character of complaint
  4. Nature of problem onset
  5. Course of problem
  6. Client's hunch of precipitating factors
  7. Location of problem
  8. Relation to:
     - a. Other body symptoms
     - b. Body positions
     - c. Activity
     - d. Eating
  9. Patterns of problem
  10. Efforts of client to treat
  11. Coping ability
- Current development of the child
- Common behaviors
  General statement about child's behavior pattern

Wants too little or too much attention	Eats paint or dirt (pica)
Accident prone	Bangs head
Unsure of self	Rocks
Bites nails	Encopresis (bowel incontinence)
Sucks thumb	Enuresis (wets bed)
Stutters	Has temper tantrums
Fearful	Has breath-holding spells
Lies	Smokes
Excessive masturbation	Takes drugs, sniffs glue
	Sets fires

CURRENT HEALTH DATA
- Current medications
  1. Type (prescription, over-the-counter drugs, vitamins, etc.)
  2. Prescribed by whom
  3. Amount per day
  4. Problems
- Allergies
  1. Drugs
  2. Foods
  3. Contact substances
  4. Environmental factors
- Last examinations (physician/clinic, findings, advice, and/or instructions)
  1. Physical
  2. Dental

From Bowers AC, Thompson JM: *Clinical manual of health assessment,* ed 4, St Louis, 1992, Mosby.

3. Vision
4. Hearing
5. Developmental assessment, such as Denver Developmental Screening Test
- Immunization status (note dates administered).
- Public or visiting health nurse working with client, if any

PAST HEALTH STATUS

- Perinatal history
  1. General health of mother during pregnancy
  2. Complications of pregnancy: bleeding, falls, swelling of hands and feet, high blood pressure, unusual weight gain
  3. Medications taken during pregnancy
  4. Radiographs taken
  5. Emotional state of mother during pregnancy: crying or depression states
  6. Planned pregnancy
  7. Father's attitude
  8. Pregnancy history (para, gravida, abortions, miscarriages)
- Labor and delivery
  1. Date and place of birth
  2. Complications
  3. Anesthesia used for delivery
  4. Number of weeks of gestation
  5. Type of delivery (breech, vertex, cesarean section)
  6. Weight
  7. Length
  8. Whether baby cried immediately
  9. Whether there were cyanosis, jaundice, or respiratory problems
  10. Whether baby went to the regular nursery
  11. Whether any special equipment was used for baby
  12. Whether baby was discharged from hospital with mother
- Infancy
  1. Initial problems with feeding, formula, colic, diarrhea
  2. Choking spells
  3. Blue spells
  4. Excessive crying
- Growth and development
  Unlike the developmental data collected under current health status, this section includes a survey of significant developmental milestones.
  1. General statement as to how this child compares with siblings
  2. Parent's opinion of whether child's growth and development have been normal
  3. Notation of age of events: rolled over, sat up, walked, first tooth, first words, toilet trained
- State age and complications of each: chickenpox, rubella, measles, mumps, whooping cough, hay fever
- Stage age and complications of each serious or chronic illness: meningitis or encephalitis, pneumonia or chronic lung problems, rheumatic fever, asthma, hay fever, scarlet fever, diabetes, kidney problems, hypertension, sickle cell anemia, seizure disorders, blood infections, etc.
- State age and extent of each serious injury: head injuries, fractures, burns, traumas, poisonings, etc.
- Hospitalizations: list reason, location, primary care providers, duration, and how child reacted to hospitalization
- Operations: what, where, when, why, by whom
- Emotional health: past behavior problems, help sought, support persons, how child reacted to stress

FAMILY HISTORY

Family members include the client's blood relatives. Specifically the interviewer should inquire about the client's maternal and paternal grandparents, parents, aunts, uncles, and siblings. The interviewer should inquire about the general health, stress factors, and illnesses of family members. Questions should include a survey of the following:

Cancer	Hypertension
Diabetes	Sickle cell anemia
Heart problems	Blindness
Developmental delay	Endocrine disorders
Learning problems	Kidney diseases
Cystic fibrosis	Birth defects
Asthma	Infant deaths
Other allergies	Other chronic problems
Seizure disorders	

REVIEW OF PHYSIOLOGICAL SYSTEMS

- General
  1. Frequency of colds, infections, or illnesses
  2. Frequency of fevers, sweats
  3. Fatigue patterns
  4. Energetic or overactive patterns
- Nutritional
  1. Recent weight gain or loss (describe)
  2. Appetite
  3. Twenty-four-hour diet recall, including types, amount of food eaten (formula, breast milk, meat, fruits, vegetables, cereals, juices, eggs, sweets, milk, snacks), and frequency (e.g., number of times a day or week)
  4. Child feeding self
  5. Where child eats
  6. Who child eats with
  7. Parent's perception of child's nutritional status (note problems)
  8. Vitamin supplements
  9. Junk food consumption (amount and kinds)
- Integumentary
  1. Skin
     a. Chronic rashes
     b. Easy bruising or petechiae
     c. Easy bleeding
     d. Acne (treatment pattern)
     e. Excessive sweating
     f. Skin diseases, problems, or lesions
     g. Pruritus
     h. Pigmentation changes, discolorations, mottling
     i. Excessive dryness
     j. Skin growths or tumors
  2. Hair
     a. Changes in amount, texture, characteristics
     b. Infections, lice
     c. Alopecia
  3. Nails
     a. Changes in appearance
     b. Cyanosis
     c. Texture
- Head
  1. Headache (characteristics, including frequency, type, location, duration, care for)
  2. Past significant trauma
  3. Dizziness
  4. Syncope
- Eyes
  1. Strabismus
  2. Discharge
  3. Complaint of vision changes

4. Reading difficulty
5. Sits close to television
6. History of infections
7. Pruritus
8. Excessive tearing
9. Pain in eyeball
10. Swelling around eyes
11. Cataracts
12. Unusual sensations or twitching
13. Excessive blinking
14. Eye injury history
15. Wears glasses
16. Diplopia
17. Blurring
18. History of inability to see distant images

- Ears
  1. Multiple infections or earaches
  2. Myringotomy tubes in ears
  3. Discharge
  4. Cerumen
  5. Care habits
  6. Cracking or ringing
  7. Parent perceives problem in child's hearing
- Nose, nasopharynx, and paranasal sinuses
  1. Discharge (character of)
  2. Epistaxis
  3. Allergies
  4. General olfactory ability
  5. Pain over sinuses
  6. Postnasal drip
  7. Sneezing
  8. Nasal stuffiness
- Mouth and throat
  1. Sore throats (frequent)
  2. Tonsils present
  3. Mouth sores
  4. Toothaches, caries
  5. Voice changes
  6. Hoarseness
  7. Mouth breathing
  8. Chewing difficulties
  9. Swallowing difficulties
  10. Teeth brushing pattern
- Neck
  1. Lymph node enlargement
  2. Tenderness
  3. Limitations of movement
  4. Stiffness
- Breast: applicable only with teenagers; refer to adult data base
- Cardiovascular
  1. History of murmur
  2. History of heart problems
  3. Palpitations
  4. Hypertension
  5. Postural hypotension
  6. Cyanosis (what precipitates)
  7. Dyspnea on exertion
  8. Limitation of activities
  9. Frequent complaints of extremity coldness
- Respiratory
  1. Breathing trouble
  2. Chronic cough
  3. Wheezing (precipitating factors)
  4. Croup history
  5. Noisy breathing
  6. Shortness of breath

- Hematolymphatic
  1. Lymph node swelling (frequency and location)
  2. Excessive bleeding or easy bruising
  3. Anemia
  4. Blood dyscrasias
  5. Lead exposures, de-leading in past
- Gastrointestinal
  1. Ulcer history
  2. Previously diagnosed problem
  3. Vomiting
  4. Diarrhea
  5. Constipation or stool-holding problems
  6. Rectal bleeding
  7. Stool color change
  8. Abdominal pains
  9. Pinworms by history
  10. Perianal pruritus
  11. Use of evacuation aids
  12. Status of toilet training; plans for; problems
- Urinary
  1. Urinary tract infections during past year
  2. Previously diagnosed problems
  3. Characteristics of urine (cloudy, dark)
  4. Suprapubic pains
  5. Steadiness and force of urination stream
  6. Dysuria
  7. Nocturia
  8. Bed wetting (association with emotional upsets; family history of bed wetting)
  9. Urinary frequency
  10. Dribbling or incontinence
  11. Polyuria/oliguria
  12. Bubble bath use
- Genital
  1. Birth defects
  2. Discharges
  3. Odors
  4. Rashes, irritation
  5. Pruritus
  6. How sexuality education is handled in the home
  7. Areas of concern
  8. If client is female and she is menstruating, refer to adult data base for appropriate questioning
- Musculoskeletal
  1. Muscles
     a. Twitching
     b. Cramping
     c. Pain
     d. Weakness
     e. Pain with use
  2. Extremities
     a. General complaints of pain, weakness, deformity
     b. Pains in legs at night
     c. Gait ability—strength and coordination
  3. Bones and joints
     a. Joint swelling
     b. Joint pain
     c. Redness, stiffness
     d. Joint deformity
     e. Fracture or dislocation history
  4. Back
     a. History of back injury
     b. Curvature of spine
     c. Characteristics or problems and corrective measures
- Central nervous system
  1. General
     a. Unusual episodic behaviors

    b. History of central nervous system diseases
    c. Birth injury
  2. Seizure: febrile versus afebrile
  3. Speech
    a. Stuttering
    b. Speech misarticulations
    c. Language delay
  4. Cognitive changes
    a. Hallucinations
    b. Passing out episodes
    c. Staring spells
    d. Learning difficulties
  5. Motor-gait
    a. Coordination
    b. Developmental clumsiness
    c. Balance problems
    d. Tic
    e. Tremor, spasms
  6. Sensory
    a. Pain pattern
    b. Tingling sensations
- Endocrine
  1. Diagnosis of disease states (e.g., thyroid, diabetes)
  2. Changes in skin texture (e.g., increased or decreased dryness or perspiration)
  3. Pigmentation
  4. Abnormal hair distribution
  5. Sudden or unexplained changes in height and weight
  6. Intolerance to heat or cold
  7. Exophthalmos
  8. Goiter
  9. Polydipsia
  10. Polyphagia
  11. Polyuria
  12. Anorexia
  13. Weakness
  14. Precocious puberty
- Allergic and immunological
  1. Dermatitis
  2. Eczema
  3. Pruritus
  4. Urticaria
  5. Sneezing
  6. Vasomotor rhinitis
  7. Conjunctivitis (inflammation of conjunctiva)
  8. Interference with ADLs
  9. Environmental and seasonal causes
  10. Treatment techniques

PSYCHOSOCIAL HISTORY

- General status
  1. General statement of child's feelings about self
  2. Parents' observations of child's feeling of self
- Caretakers and family
  1. Who lives in child's home
  2. Primary care provider for child
  3. Child's position in home environment
  4. Relationships among members
- Friends
  1. Child's relationships with friends, classmates, siblings
  2. Age of playmates—older, younger, same age
  3. Ability to make friends easily
- Activities of daily living
  1. General
    a. General description of typical day
    b. Sleep patterns and naps: sound sleeper or fretful, numbers

of hours per 24 hours, nightmares, other nighttime activity (e.g., wakes up at night), parents' response
    c. Kinds of play: amount of active and quiet play per 24 hours, television time per 24 hours
    d. Significant hobbies or methods of relaxation (for older child)
  2. Family
    a. Activities of families as unit
    b. Methods of discipline within family
    c. Effectiveness of discipline
    d. Who disciplines child
    e. Child's reaction to discipline
    f. Parents or providers: type of employment, type of child care provided if both parents work
    g. Availability of emotional support for mother for her care of child and opportunity to be away from child
  3. School
    a. Present grade in school or level of nursery care
    b. School performance
    c. Behavior problems
    d. Grades skipped
    e. Learning problems; special classes required, if any
    f. Attitude about school
    g. Rate of absenteeism
- Ability to cope with stress
  1. General statement: activities of daily living, family, school
  2. Child's ability to adapt to new situations
  3. Recent changes or stresses in child's life-style (home, school)
  4. Behavior patterns child uses to cope with stress
  5. Change in personality, behavior, or mood
  6. History of psychiatric care or counseling

HEALTH MAINTENANCE EFFORTS

- General statement about physical fitness (parent attitudes and child opinion)
- Dietary regulations to maintain health
- Frequency of physical, dental, and vision health assessment
- Statement reflecting parents' attitude about the importance of health maintenance education, including:
  1. Self-care techniques
  2. Poison control safety
  3. First aid
  4. Toy safety
  5. Environmental safety

ENVIRONMENTAL HEALTH*

- General statement of parents' assessment of environmental safety and comfort
- Hazards in the home, to include survey of the following:
  1. Toys appropriate for age
  2. Special protection from poisons, household products, or medications
  3. Stairway protection (e.g., use of gates for toddlers or handrails for older children)
  4. Yard equipment for play and safety
  5. Type of bed (protection device to prevent falling)
  6. Pest control problems
  7. Unsafe building (e.g., no heat, poor toilet facilities, open gas heaters)
- Hazards in neighborhood
  1. Unsafe play area
  2. Heavily traveled streets
  3. No sidewalks
  4. Water or air pollution
  5. Noise factor
  6. Isolation or overcrowding from neighbors

9-7 | Geriatric functional and health assessment

PURPOSE OF REFERRAL

What is the immediate problem for which the patient, family, or others need help? What event(s) led patient to seek help specifically at this time?

HEALTH ASSESSMENT

1. Is patient under any unusual stress such as financial, home situation, transportation, health, family or personal relationships?
2. Which of the following best describes how patient feels?
   This is the best time of life.
   While some things are more difficult now, life is usually pleasant and acceptable.
   Just as happy now as when patient was younger.
   Life has become unpleasant and difficult to tolerate.
   Very unhappy with present situation.
3. Which of the following best describes patient's state of health?
   usually good.
   average health.
   below average.
   very poor.
4. Does patient have (or has patient had) any of the following symptoms? If yes, for how long?
   Frequent headaches
   Passing out or fainting
   Falling or stumbling
   Paralysis or leg or arm weakness
   Numbness or loss of feeling
   Tremor or shaking
   Forgetfulness
   Problem with memory
   Disorientation to time, person, or place
   Depression
   Agitation
   Hallucinations (hearing voices and/or seeing things)
   Suspiciousness of others
   Fearfulness
   Unusually high or low moods
   Difficulty sleeping
   Difficulty speaking
   Difficulty understanding what others say
   Difficulty swallowing
   Hoarseness or other change in voice
   Visual or eye problems (date of last visit to eye doctor)

   Hearing or ear trouble (date of last hearing examination)

   Dental problems, dental discomfort (date of last visit to dentist)

   Fever or sweats
   Swollen glands
   Lumps or sores
   Skin trouble
   Difficulty breathing
   Persistent cough
   Chest pain or tightness
   Irregular heartbeat
   Leg pain when walking
   High blood pressure
   Poor appetite
   Change in weight
   Frequent indigestion or stomach ache
   Frequent nausea or vomiting
   Change in bowel habits
   Black bowel movements or rectal bleeding
   Frequent diarrhea
   Constipation
   Urination at night
   Painful urination
   Difficulty starting or stopping urination
   Difficulty holding urine or urine leakage
   Sexual difficulties
   Back or neck troubles
   Joint pain or stiffness
   Swelling of feet or ankles
   Foot problems
   Women only:
      Breast lumps or discharge
      Vaginal bleeding/discomfort
   Men only:
      Discharge from penis
      Swelling/lump in testicle
      Ache in lower back or groin
5. Other problems:
   Sleeping problems
   Feeling lonely
   Change in sexual interest
   Feeling sad or depressed
   Change in sexual activity
   Thought of "ending it all"
   Feeling tense or anxious
   Change in appetite
6. Past medical history (approximate dates)
   Alcoholism
   Anemia
   Arthritis
   Asthma
   Bronchitis
   Cancer
   Cataracts
   Depression
   Diabetes
   Emotional problems
   Fractures
   Gallbladder problems
   Glaucoma
   Heart disease
   Hernia
   High blood pressure
   Jaundice
   Kidney disease
   Liver disease
   Lung disease
   Mental illness
   Nervous breakdown
   Prostate disease
   Phlebitis
   Pneumonia
   Seizures
   Stomach ulcers
   Stroke
   Thyroid disease
   Tuberculosis
   Urinary tract infection
   Venereal disease
   Other
7. Hospitalizations (location, dates, reason)

8. Family health problems (for each, relationship to patient; if the patient has died, give age at time of death and cause of death)
   Alcoholism
   Cancer
   Depression
   Diabetes
   Heart disease
   High blood pressure
   Kidney disease
   Memory problems
   Mental illness
   Nervous breakdown
   Speech or language disorder
   Stroke
   Other
9. Smoking history
   Does patient now, or did patient ever, smoke cigarettes/cigar/pipe, or chew tobacco?
   How much?
   For how long?
   When did patient stop?
10. Does patient drink alcohol?
    If no, why not?
    If yes, how much?
    How often? (less than 3 times a week, more than 3 times a week, daily)
    Is alcohol a problem?
11. Prescription medicines (names, dosages, how often, how long taken)
12. Medicines taken in addition to prescription drugs (aspirin, antacids, cold pills/decongestants, hormones, laxatives, nerve pills, sleeping pills, vitamins/minerals, other)
13. Medication allergies
14. Are doing any of the following activities a problem for the patient? If yes, who helps?
    Shopping for groceries
    Preparing own meals
    Eating
    Doing housecleaning
    Writing checks or paying bills
    Taking medicines
    Taking sponge or tub bath, or shower
    Dressing
    Using the telephone
    Walking indoors
    Walking outdoors
    Going up or down stairs
    Getting into or out of bed or chair
    Getting off or on toilet
15. Does patient use any prosthetic devices or aids (glasses, hearing aids, cane, wheelchair, contact lenses, dentures, walker, other)?
16. Where does the patient live (apartment [nonpublic], home [owned], home [rented], foster home, public housing, subsidized housing, nursing home, other)?
17. With whom does patient live (alone, children, companion or friend, spouse or partner, another relative, other)?
18. With whom is patient in regular contact (spouse or partner, child or children, brother[s] or sister[s], other relative[s], friend[s], neighbor[s])?
19. Whom does patient call on for help?
20. How often in the past week has patient left home (e.g., going to church, meetings, or other activities)?
21. What interests and activities does patient most enjoy?
22. Which best describes patient's employment status
    Never fully employed (outside the home)
    Retired—when?
    Presently working (full-time, part-time)
23. Patient's present or past occupations

24. Which of the following best describes patient's financial status?
    Comfortably able to afford all necessities (food, clothing, and transportation)
    Able to afford necessities with careful budgeting
    Barely able to afford the basic needs
    Unable to afford the necessities
25. What is patient's usual form of transportation?
    Drives own car
    Rides with a friend or relative
    Takes a bus
    Walks
    Takes a cab
    Doesn't go out of house or apartment
26. Which of the following services has patient used in the past 3 months? Who provided the service?
    Personal care
    Nursing services
    Medical care (physicians)
    Mental health services
    Social services
    Physical therapy
    Occupational therapy
    Hearing or speech testing or therapy
    Sight center
    Rehabilitation services
    Nutritionist
    Transportation
    Day center
    Meal program
    Other
27. How many meals a day does patient eat?
28. How many snacks a day does patient eat?
29. How many cups of fluids per day does patient drink (including tea, coffee, water, juice, milk, soda pop, etc.)?
30. Concerns about diet or nutrition?

MENTAL STATUS

1. Appearance
2. Mood, affect (including check for depression, orientation)
3. Cognitive function (examples)
4. Communication

SLEEPING

1. Does patient sleep well?
2. Does patient feel well rested?
3. Ease of falling asleep
4. Nap pattern
5. Hours per night/times up during the night
6. Concerns of patient/family

SENSES

1. Sight
2. Hearing
3. Taste
4. Smell
5. Touch

ACTIVITIES OF DAILY LIVING (for each, is patient independent or dependent?)

1. Bathing
   Initiation of bath
   Type of bathing (tub, shower, sponge)
   Bath preparation
   Get in/out of tub
   Ability to wash self
   Hair washing
2. Dressing
   Clothing selection
   Putting on garments

Doing up buttons, etc.
Appropriateness of attire
Undressing
Laundry
3. Transfer
From bed to chair
From chair to standing
4. Toileting
Able to find bathroom
Able to use toilet appropriately
Hygiene
5. Bowel continence
Frequency and control
Constipation
6. Feeding
7. Telephone
Look up number
Dial
8. Medication
Preparation
Taking
9. Outside of home
Organization
Getting lost
10. Driving
11. Housework
Organization
Doing (List what able to do)
12. Food preparation
Planning
Shopping
Preparing
13. Finances
Banking
Paying bills
Balancing checkbook

URINARY CONTINENCE

1. Does patient have "accidents"? (If "yes," when?)
2. Patient's knowledge of accidents

3. Frequency
4. Urgency
5. Can patient get to bathroom in time?
6. Does patient wet when coughing or sneezing or at other times?
7. Where is center of concern about wetting (patient, family, both)?
8. Other concerns

MOBILITY

1. Walking ability (use of assistive devices)
2. Distance able to walk (and frequency)
3. Gait, posture
4. Stiffness (morning, after inactivity, evening, where?)
5. What does patient do to maximize mobility?
6. Hand dexterity and function
7. Problems with feet and shoes
8. Other concerns of patient/family

NUTRITION

1. Number of meals per day
2. Number of glasses of fluid
3. Indigestion, nausea/vomiting, change in bowels
4. Dentition
5. Appetite
6. Weight stability
7. Concerns of family (need for referral to nutritionist)

SAFETY

1. Is patient alone at any time?
2. Does patient get lost?
3. Kitchen safety
4. Household safety (rugs, cords, railings, stairs)
5. Other concerns

CARE GIVER

1. Name of formal care giver, relationship
2. Informal care-giving system
3. Care giver's role/function
4. Impact of care giving on care giver/family
5. Assessment of stability/security provided in present care environment

APPENDIX 10

GUIDELINES FOR RELATING TO PATIENTS FROM DIFFERENT CULTURES

1. Assess your personal beliefs surrounding persons from different cultures.
   - review your personal beliefs and past experiences
   - set aside any values, biases, ideas, and attitudes that are judgmental and may negatively affect care
2. Assess communication variables from a cultural perspective.
   - determine the ethnic identity of patient, including generation in America
   - use the patient as a source of information when possible
   - assess cultural factors that may affect your relationship with the patient and respond appropriately
3. Plan care based on the communicated needs and cultural background.
   - learn as much as possible about the patient's cultural customs and beliefs
   - encourage the patient to reveal cultural interpretation of health, illness, and health care
   - be sensitive to the uniqueness of patient
   - identify sources of discrepancy between patient's and your own conceptions of health and illness
   - communicate at the patient's personal level of functioning
   - evaluate effectiveness of nursing actions and modify nursing care plan when necessary
4. Modify communication approaches to meet cultural needs.
   - be attentive to signs of fear, anxiety, and confusion in the patient
   - respond in a reassuring manner in keeping with the patient's cultural orientation
   - be aware that in some cultural groups discussion concerning the patient with others may offend and impede nursing process
5. Understand that respect for the patient and communicated needs is central to the therapeutic relationship.
   - communicate respect by using a kind and attentive approach
   - learn how listening is communicated in the patient's culture

From Giger J, Davidhizar R: *Transcultural nursing*, St Louis, 1991, Mosby, pp 22-26.

- use appropriate active listening techniques
- adopt an attitude of flexibility, respect, and interest to help bridge barriers imposed by culture

6. Communicate in a nonthreatening manner.
   - conduct the interview in unhurried manner
   - follow acceptable social and cultural amenities
   - ask general questions during the information gathering stage
   - be patient with a respondent who gives information that may seem unrelated to patient's health problem
   - develop a trusting relationship by listening carefully, allowing time, and giving the patient your full attention
7. Use validating techniques in communication.
   - be alert for feedback that the patient is not understanding
   - do not assume meaning is interpreted without distortion
8. Be considerate of reluctance to talk when the subject involves sexual matters.
   - be aware that in some cultures sexual matters are not discussed freely with members of the opposite sex
9. Adopt special approaches when the patient speaks a different language.
   - use a caring tone of voice and facial expression to help alleviate the patient's fears
   - speak slowly and distinctly, but not loudly
   - use gestures, pictures, and play acting to help the patient understand
   - repeat the message in different ways if necessary
   - be alert to words the patient seems to understand and use them frequently
   - keep messages simple and repeat them frequently
   - avoid using medical terms and abbreviations which the patient may not understand
   - use an appropriate language dictionary
10. Use interpreters to improve communication.
    - ask the interpreter to translate the message, not just the individual words
    - obtain feedback to confirm understanding
    - use an interpreter who is culturally sensitive

NUTRITION

11-1 National Research Council Recommended Dietary Allowances,[a] Revised 1989

Food and Nutrition Board, National Academy of Sciences

| | | Weight[b] | | Height[a] | | Protein | Fat-soluble vitamins | | | |
| | | | | | | | Vita-min A | Vita-min D | Vita-min E | Vita-min K |
Category	Age (years) or condition	(kg)	(lb)	(cm)	(in)	(g)	(μg RE)[c]	(μg)[d]	(mg α-TE)[e]	(μg)
Infants	0.0-0.5	6	13	60	24	13	375	7.5	3	5
	0.5-1.0	9	20	71	28	14	375	10	4	10
Children	1-3	13	29	90	35	16	400	10	6	15
	4-6	20	44	112	44	24	500	10	7	20
	7-10	28	62	132	52	28	700	10	7	30
Males	11-14	45	99	157	62	45	1,000	10	10	45
	15-18	66	145	176	69	59	1,000	10	10	65
	19-24	72	160	177	70	58	1,000	10	10	70
	25-50	79	174	176	70	63	1,000	5	10	80
	51+	77	170	173	68	63	1,000	5	10	80
Females	11-14	46	101	157	62	46	800	10	8	45
	15-18	55	120	163	64	44	800	10	8	55
	19-24	58	128	164	65	46	800	10	8	60
	25-50	63	138	163	64	50	800	5	8	65
	51+	65	143	160	63	50	800	5	8	65
Pregnant						60	800	10	10	65
Lactating	1st 6 Months					65	1,300	10	12	65
	2nd 6 Months					62	1,200	10	11	65

[a]The allowances, expressed as average daily intakes over time, are intended to provide for individual variations among most normal persons as they live in the United States under usual environmental stresses. Diets should be based on a variety of common foods in order to provide other nutrients for which human requirements have been less well defined. See text for detailed discussion of allowances and of nutrients not tabulated.
[b]Weights and heights of Reference Adults are actual medians for the US population of the designated age, as reported by NHANES II. The use of these figures does not imply that the height-to-weight ratios are ideal.

Water-soluble vitamins							Minerals						
Vita-min C (mg)	Thia-min (mg)	Ribo-flavin (mg)	Niacin (mg NE)^f	Vita-min B$_4$ (mg)	Fo-late (μg)	Vita-min B$_{12}$ (μg)	Cal-cium (mg)	Phos-phorus (mg)	Mag-nesium (mg)	Iron (mg)	Zinc (mg)	Iodine (μg)	Sele-nium (μg)
30	0.3	0.4	5	0.3	25	0.3	400	300	40	6	5	40	10
35	0.4	0.5	6	0.6	35	0.5	600	500	60	10	5	50	15
40	0.7	0.8	9	1.0	50	0.7	800	800	80	10	10	70	20
45	0.9	1.1	12	1.1	75	1.0	800	800	120	10	10	90	20
45	1.0	1.2	13	1.4	100	1.4	800	800	170	10	10	120	30
50	1.3	1.5	17	1.7	150	2.0	1,200	1,200	270	12	15	150	40
60	1.5	1.8	20	2.0	200	2.0	1,200	1,200	400	12	15	150	50
60	1.5	1.7	19	2.0	200	2.0	1,200	1,200	350	10	15	150	70
60	1.5	1.7	19	2.0	200	2.0	800	800	350	10	15	150	70
60	1.2	1.4	15	2.0	200	2.0	800	800	350	10	15	150	70
50	1.1	1.3	15	1.4	150	2.0	1,200	1,200	280	15	12	150	45
60	1.1	1.3	15	1.5	180	2.0	1,200	1,200	300	15	12	150	50
60	1.1	1.3	15	1.6	180	2.0	1,200	1,200	280	15	12	150	55
60	1.1	1.3	15	1.6	180	2.0	800	800	280	15	12	150	55
60	1.0	1.2	13	1.6	180	2.0	800	800	280	10	12	150	55
70	1.5	1.6	17	2.2	400	2.2	1,200	1,200	320	30	15	175	65
95	1.6	1.8	20	2.1	280	2.6	1,200	1,200	355	15	19	200	75
90	1.6	1.7	20	2.1	260	2.6	1,200	1,200	340	15	16	200	75

^{c}Retinol equivalents. 1 retinol equivalent = 1 μg retinol or 6 μg β-carotene.
^{d}As cholecalciferol. 10 μg cholecalciferol = 400 IU of vitamin D.
^{e}α-Tocopherol equivalents. 1 mg d-α tocopherol = 1 α-TE.
^{f}1 NE (niacin equivalent) is equal to 1 mg of niacin or 60 mg of dietary tryptophan.

Estimated safe and adequate daily dietary intakes of selected vitamins and minerals[a]

Category	Age (years)		Biotin (µg)	Pantothenic acid (mg)
		Vitamins		
Infants	0-0.5		10	2
	0.5-1		15	3
Children and adolescents	1-3		20	3
	4-6		25	3-1
	7-10		30	4-5
	11+		30-100	4-7
Adults			30-100	4-7

Category	Age (years)	Copper (mg)	Mangenese (mg)	Fluoride (mg)	Chromium (µg)	Molybdenum (µg)
			Trace elements[b]			
Infants	0-0.5	0.4-0.6	0.3-0.6	0.1-0.5	10-40	15-30
	0.5-1	0.6-0.7	0.6-1.0	0.2-1.0	20-60	20-40
Children and adolescents	1-3	0.7-1.0	1.0-1.5	0.5-1.5	20-80	25-50
	4-6	1.0-1.5	1.5-2.0	1.0-2.5	30-120	30-75
	7-10	1.0-2.0	2.0-3.0	1.5-2.5	50-200	50-150
	11+	1.5-2.5	2.0-5.0	1.5-2.5	50-200	75-250
Adults		1.5-3.0	2.0-5.0	1.5-4.0	50-200	75-250

[a]Because there is less information on which to base allowances, these figures are not given in the main table of RDA and are provided here in the form of ranges of recommended intakes.
[b]Since the toxic levels for many trace elements may be only several times usual intakes, the upper levels for the trace elements given in this table should not be habitually exceeded.

11-2 Recommended nutrient intakes for Canadians, 1990

Summary examples of recommended nutrient intake based on age and body weight expressed as daily rates

Age	Sex	Weight kg	Protein g	Vit. A RE*	Vit. D μg	Vit. E mg	Vit. C mg	Folate μg	Vit. B₁₂ μg	Calcium mg	Phosphorus mg	Magnesium mg	Iron mg	Iodine μg	Zinc mg
Months															
0-4	Both	6.0	12	400	10	3	20	25	0.3	250†	150	20	0.3§	30	2§
5-12	Both	9.0	12	400	10	3	20	40	0.4	400	200	32	7	40	3
Years															
1	Both	11	13	400	10	3	20	40	0.5	500	300	40	6	55	4
2-3	Both	14	16	400	5	4	20	50	0.6	550	350	50	6	65	4
4-6	Both	18	19	500	5	5	25	70	0.8	600	400	65	8	85	5
7-9	M	25	26	700	2.5	7	25	90	1.0	700	500	100	8	110	7
	F	25	26	700	2.5	6	25	90	1.0	700	500	100	8	95	7
10-12	M	34	34	800	2.5	8	25	120	1.0	900	700	130	8	125	9
	F	36	36	800	2.5	7	25	130	1.0	1100	800	135	8	110	9
13-15	M	50	49	900	2.5	9	30	175	1.0	1100	900	185	10	160	12
	F	48	46	800	2.5	7	30	170	1.0	1000	850	180	13	160	9
16-18	M	62	58	1000	2.5	10	40‖	220	1.0	900	1000	230	10	160	12
	F	53	47	800	2.5	7	30	190	1.0	700	850	200	12	160	9
19-24	M	71	61	1000	2.5	10	40‖	220	1.0	800	1000	240	9	160	12
	F	58	50	800	2.5	7	30	180	1.0	700	850	200	13	160	9
25-49	M	74	64	1000	2.5	9	40‖	230	1.0	800	1000	250	9	160	12
	F	59	51	800	2.5	6	30	185	1.0	700	850	200	13	160	9
50-74	M	73	63	1000	5	7	40‖	230	1.0	800	1000	250	9	160	12
	F	63	54	800	5	6	30	195	1.0	800	850	210	8	160	9
75+	M	69	59	1000	5	6	40‖	215	1.0	800	1000	230	9	160	12
	F	64	55	800	5	5	30	200	1.0	800	850	210	8	160	9
Pregnancy (additional)															
1st Trimester			5	0	2.5	2	0	200	1.2	500	200	15	0	25	6
2nd Trimester			20	0	2.5	2	10	200	1.2	500	200	45	5	25	6
3rd Trimester			24	0	2.5	2	10	200	1.2	500	200	45	10	25	6
Lactation (additional)			20	400	2.5	3	25	100	0.2	500	200	65	0	50	6

*Retinol Equivalents.
+Protein is assumed to be from breast milk and must be adjusted for infant formula.
†Infant formula with high phosphorus should contain 375 mg calcium.
§Breast milk is assumed to be the source of the mineral.
‖Smokers should increase vitamin C by 50%.
From Scientific Review Committee: *Nutrition recommendations,* Ottawa, Canada, 1990, Health and Welfare.

Summary of examples of recommended nutrients based on energy expressed as daily rates

Age	Sex	Energy kcal	Thiamin mg	Riboflavin mg	Niacin Ne+	n-3 PUFA* g	n-6 PUFA g
Months							
0-4	Both	600	0.3	0.3	4	0.5	3
5-12	Both	900	0.4	0.5	7	0.5	3
Years							
1	Both	1100	0.5	0.6	8	0.6	4
2-3	Both	1300	0.6	0.7	9	0.7	4
4-6	Both	1800	0.7	0.9	13	1.0	6
7-9	M	2200	0.9	1.1	16	1.2	7
	F	1900	0.8	1.0	14	1.0	6
10-12	M	2500	1.0	1.3	18	1.4	8
	F	2200	0.9	1.1	16	1.2	7

*PUFA, polyunsaturated fatty acids.
+Niacin equivalents.
†Level below which intake should not fall.
§Assumes moderate physical activity.
From Scientific Review Committee: *Nutrition recommendations,* Ottawa, Canada, 1990, Health and Welfare.

Continued.

Summary of examples of recommended nutrients based on energy expressed as daily rates—cont'd

Age	Sex	Energy kcal	Thiamin mg	Riboflavin mg	Niacin Ne[+]	n-3 PUFA* g	n-6 PUFA g
Years—cont'd							
13-15	M	2800	1.1	1.4	20	1.5	9
	F	2200	0.9	1.1	16	1.2	7
16-18	M	3200	1.3	1.6	23	1.8	11
	F	2100	0.8	1.1	15	1.2	7
19-24	M	3000	1.2	1.5	22	1.6	10
	F	2100	0.8	1.1	15	1.2	7
25-49	M	2700	1.1	1.4	19	1.5	9
	F	1900	0.8	1.0	14	1.1	7
50-74	M	2300	0.9	1.2	16	1.3	8
	F	1800	0.8†	1.0†	14†	1.1†	7†
75+	M	2000	0.8	1.0	14	1.1	7
	F§	1700	0.8†	1.0†	14†	1.1†	7†
Pregnancy (additional)							
1st Trimester		100	0.1	0.1	1	0.05	0.3
2nd Trimester		300	0.1	0.3	2	0.16	0.9
3rd Trimester		300	0.1	0.3	2	0.16	0.9
Lactation (additional)		450	0.2	0.4	3	0.25	1.5

11-3   Daily dietary guide*

Food group	Serving	Major contributions	Foods and serving sizes*
Milk, yogurt, and cheese	2 (adult‖) 3 (children, teens, young adults, and pregnant or lactating women)	Calcium Riboflavin Protein Potassium Zinc	1 cup milk 1½ oz cheese 2 oz processed cheese 1 cup yogurt 2 cups cottage cheese 1 cup custard/pudding 1½ cups ice cream
Meat, poultry, fish, dry beans, eggs, and nuts	2-3	Protein Niacin Iron Vitamin B-6 Zinc Thiamin Vitamin B-12†	2-3 oz cooked meat, poultry, fish 1-1½ cups cooked dry beans 4 T peanut butter 2 eggs ½-1 cup nuts
Fruits	2-4	Vitamin C Fiber	¼ cup dried fruit ½ cup cooked fruit ¾ cup juice 1 whole piece of fruit 1 melon wedge
Vegetables	3-5	Vitamin A Vitamin C Folate Magnesium Fiber	½ cup raw or cooked vegetables 1 cup raw leafy vegetables
Bread, cereals, rice, and pasta	6-11	Starch Thiamin Riboflavin§ Iron Niacin Folate Magnesium‡ Fiber‡ Zinc‡	1 slice of bread 1 oz ready-to-eat cereal ½-¾ cup cooked cereal, rice, or pasta
Fats, oils, and sweets		Foods from this group should not replace any from the other groups. Amounts consumed should be determined by individual energy needs.	

This is a practical way to turn the RDA into food choices. You can get all essential nutrients by eating a balanced variety of foods each day from the food groups listed here. Eat a variety of foods in each food group and adjust serving sizes appropriately to reach and maintain desirable weight.

*May be reduced for child servings.
†Only in animal food choices.
‡Whole grains especially.
§If enriched.
‖≥25 years of age.
From Wardlaw GM, Insel PM: *Perspectives in nutrition,* ed 2, St Louis, 1993, Mosby, p 46.

11-4   Vitamins and minerals

Summary of fat-soluble vitamins

Vitamin	Physiological functions	Results of deficiency	Requirement	Food sources
A (retinol) Provitamin A (carotene)	Production of rhodopsin (visual purple) Formation and maintenance of epithelial tissue Toxic in large amounts	Xerophthalmia Night blindness Keratinization of epithelium Follicular hyperkeratosis Skin and mucous membrane infections Faulty tooth formation	Adult male: 1,000 μg RE (5,000 IU) Adult female: 800 μg RE (4,000 IU) Pregnancy: 1,000 μg RE (5,000 IU) Lactation: 1,200 μg RE (6,000 IU) Children: 400 μg RE (2,000 IU) to 800 μg RE (4,000 IU)	Liver Cream, butter, whole milk Egg yolk Green and yellow vegetables Yellow fruits Fortified margarine
D (calciferol)	Absorption of calcium and phosphorus Calcification of bones Renal phosphate clearance Toxic in large amounts	Rickets Faulty bone growth Osteomalacia in adults	Adult: 5-10 μg cholecalciferol (200-400 IU) Pregnancy and lactation: 10-12.5 μg (400-500 IU) depending on age Children: 10 μg (400 IU)	Fish oils Fortified or irradiated milk
E (tocopherol)	Related to action of selenium Antioxidant with vitamin A and unsaturated fatty acids Hemopoiesis Reproduction (in animals)	Hemolysis of red blood cells; anemia Possible protection of unsaturated fatty acids Sterility (in rats)	Adult: 8-10 mg αTE Pregnancy and lactation: 10-11 mg αTE Children: 3-10 mg αTE	Vegetable oils
K (menadione)	Blood clotting, necessary for synthesis of prothrombin Possible coenzyme in oxidation phosphorylation Toxic in large amounts	Hemorrhagic disease of the newborn Bleeding tendencies in biliary disease or surgical procedures Deficiency in intestinal malabsorption (sprue, celiac disease, colitis) Prolonged antibiotic therapy Anticoagulant therapy (dicumarol counteracts)	Unknown	Green leafy vegetables Cheese Egg yolk Liver

Summary of vitamin C (ascorbic acid)

Physiological functions	Clinical applications	Requirement	Food sources

Intercellular cement substance:
  1. Collagen formation
  2. Firm capillary walls
General metabolism:
  1. Makes iron available for hemoglobin and maturation of red blood cells
  2. Influences conversion of folic acid to "citrovorum factor" (folinic acid)
	Scurvy (deficiency)
	Megaloblastic anemia
	Wound healing; tissue formation
	Fevers and infections
	Stress reactions
	Growth periods
		60 mg daily (adults)	Citrus fruits
			Tomatoes
			Cabbage
			Potatoes
			Strawberries
			Melon
			Chili peppers

Summary of B-complex vitamins

Vitamin	Physiological functions	Clinical applications	Requirement	Food sources
Thiamin (B_1)	Coenzyme in carbohydrate metabolism: TPP—decarboxylation TDP—transketolation	Beriberi (deficiency) GI*: anorexia, gastric atony, indigestion, deficient hydrochloric acid CNS*: fatigue, apathy, neuritis, paralysis CV*: cardiac failure, peripheral vasodilation, and edema of extremities	0.5 mg/1000 calories	Pork, beef, liver, whole or enriched grains, legumes
Riboflavin (B_2)	Coenzyme in protein of energy metabolism (flavoproteins) FMN (flavin mononucleotide) FAD (flavin-adenine dinucleotide)	Wound aggravation Cheilosis Glossitis Eye irritation; photophobia Seborrheic dermatitis	0.6 mg/1000 calories	Milk, liver, enriched calories
Niacin (nicotinic acid) (precursor—tryptophan)	Coenzyme in tissue oxidation to produce energy (ATP) NAD (nicotinamide-adenine dinucleotide) NADP (nicotinamide-adenine dinucleotide phosphate)	Pellagra (deficiency) Weakness, lassitude, anorexia Skin: scaly dermatitis CNS: neuritis, confusion	14-20 mg (NE)	Meat, peanuts, enriched grains
Pyridoxine (B_6)	Coenzyme in amino acid metabolism Decarboxylation Deamination Transamination Transsulfuration Niacin formation from tryptophan Heme formation Amino acid absorption	Anemia (hypochromic microcytic) CNS: hyperirritability, convulsions, neuritis Isoniazid is an antagonist for pyridoxine Pregnancy: anemia	2 mg	Wheat, corn, meat, liver
Pantothenic acid	Coenzyme in formation of active acetate (CoA)—acetylation	Contributes to: Lipogenesis Amino acid activation Formation of cholesterol Formation of steroid hormones Formation of heme Excretion of drugs	Liver, egg, skimmed milk	
Lipoic acid (sulfur-containing fatty acid)	Coenzyme (with thiamin) in carbohydrate metabolism to reduce pyruvate to active acetate Oxidative decarboxylation	Undetermined (see thiamin)		Liver, yeast
Biotin	Coenzyme in decarboxylation (synthesis of fatty acids, amino acids, purines); deamination	Undetermined		Egg yolk, liver
Folic acid (B_9)	Coenzyme for single carbon transfer—purines, thymine, hemoglobin Transmethylation	Blood cell regeneration in pernicious anemia but not control of its neurological problems Megaloblastic anemia Macrocytic anemia of pregnancy Sprue treatment Aminopterin is antagonist	400 μg Pregnancy: 800 μg Lactation: 800 μg	Liver, green leafy vegetables, asparagus

*GI, Gastrointestinal; CNS, central nervous system; CV, cardiovascular.

Continued.

Summary of B-complex vitamins—cont'd

Vitamin	Physiological functions	Clinical applications	Requirement	Food sources
PABA (part of folic acid)		Treatment of rickettsial diseases Anemias (see folic acid)		Same as folic acid
Cobalamin (B_{12})	Coenzyme in protein synthesis Formation of nucleic acid and cell proteins—red blood cells Transmethylation	Extrinsic factor in pernicious anemia—combines with intrinsic factor of gastric secretions for absorption; forms red blood cells (with folic acid) Sprue treatment (with folic acid)	3 µg	Liver, meat, milk, egg, cheese
Inositol	Lipotropic agent (?)	Undetermined		Citrus fruit, grains, meat, milk
Choline	Lipotropic agent Forms nerve mediator—acetylcholine	Fatty liver—hepatitis, cirrhosis (undetermined in human nutrition)		Meat, cereals, egg yolk

Summary of major minerals

Mineral	Metabolism	Physiological functions	Clinical application	Requirement	Food sources
Calcium (Ca)	Absorption according to body need, aided by vitamin D, favored by protein, lactose, acidity; hindered by excess fats and binding agents (phosphates, oxalates, phytate) Excretion chiefly in feces, 70% to 90% of amount ingested Deposition-mobilization in bone compartment constant; deposition aided by vitamin D Parathyroid hormone controls absorption and mobilization	Bone formation Teeth Blood clotting Muscle contraction and relaxation Heart action Nerve transmission Cell wall permeability Enzyme activation (ATPase)	Tetany—decrease in ionized serum calcium Rickets Renal calculi Hyperparathyroidism Hypoparathyroidism	Adults: 0.8 gm Pregnancy and lactation: 1.2 gm Infants: 360-540 mg Children: 0.8-1.2 gm	Milk Cheese Green leafy vegetables Whole grains Egg yolk Legumes, nuts
Phosphorus (P)	Absorption with calcium aided by vitamin D, hindered by excess binding agents (calcium, aluminum, iron) Excretion chiefly by kidney according to renal threshold blood level Parathyroid hormone controls renal excretion balance with blood level Deposition-mobilization in bone compartment constant	Bone formation Overall metabolism: Absorption of glucose and glycerol (phosphorylation) Transport of fatty acids Energy metabolism (enzymes, ATP) Buffer system	Growth Hypophosphatemia: Recovery state from diabetic acidosis Sprue, celiac disease (malabsorption) Bone diseases (upset Ca:P balance) Hyperphosphatemia: Renal insufficiency Hypoparathyroidism Tetany	Adults: 1½ times calcium intake Pregnancy and lactation: 1.2 gm Infants: 240-400 mg Children: 0.8-1.2 gm	Milk Cheese Meat Egg yolk Whole grains Legumes, nuts
Magnesium (Mg)	Absorption increased by parathyroid hormone, hindered by excess fat, phosphate, calcium Excretion regulated by kidney	In bones and teeth Activator and coenzyme in carbohydrate and protein metabolism Essential intracellular fluid (ICF) cation Muscle, nerve irritability	Tremor, spasm; low serum level following gastrointestinal losses	300-350 mg Deficiency in humans unlikely	Whole grains Nuts Meat Milk Legumes

Mineral	Metabolism	Physiological functions	Clinical application	Requirement	Food sources
Sodium (Na)	Readily absorbed. Excretion chiefly by kidney, controlled by aldosterone, acid-base balance	Major extracellular fluid (ECF) cation. Water balance, osmotic pressure. Acid-base balance. Cell permeability; absorption of glucose. Muscle irritability; transmission of electrochemical impulse and resulting contraction	Fluid shifts and control. Buffer system. Losses in gastrointestinal disorders	About 0.5 gm. Diet usually has more: 2-6 gm	Table salt (NaCl). Milk. Meat. Egg. Baking soda. Baking powder. Carrots, beets, spinach, celery
Potassium (K)	Secreted and reabsorbed in digestive juices. Excretion guarded by kidney according to blood levels; increased by aldosterone	Major ICF cation. Acid-base balance. Regulates neuromuscular excitability and muscle contraction. Glycogen formation. Protein synthesis	Fluid shifts. Losses in starvation, diabetic acidosis, adrenal tumors. Heart action—low serum potassium (tachycardia, cardiac arrest). Treatment of diabetic acidosis (rapid glycogen production reduces serum potassium). Tissue catabolism—potassium loss	About 2-4 gm. Diet adequate in protein, calcium, and iron contains adequate potassium	Whole grains. Meat. Legumes. Fruits. Vegetables
Chlorine (Cl)	Absorbed readily. Excretion controlled by kidney	Major ECF anion. Acid-base balance—chloride-bicarbonate shift. Water balance. Gastric hydrochloric acid—digestion	Hypochloremic alkalosis in prolonged vomiting, diarrhea, tube drainage	About 0.5 gm. Diet usually has more: 2-6 gm	Table salt
Sulfur (S)	Absorbed as such and as constituent of sulfur-containing amino acid, methionine. Excreted by kidney in relation to protein intake and tissue catabolism	Essential constituent of cell protein. Activates enzymes. High-energy sulfur bonds in energy metabolism. Detoxification reactions	Cystine renal calculi. Cystinuria	Diet adequate in protein contains adequate sulfur	Meat. Egg. Cheese. Milk. Nuts, legumes

Summary of trace minerals

Mineral	Metabolism	Physiological functions	Clinical application	Requirement	Food source
Iron (Fe)	Absorption according to body need controlled by mucosal block—ferritin mechanism, aided by vitamin C, gastric hydrochloric acid. Transport—transferrin. Storage—ferritin, hemosiderin. Excretion from tissue in minute quantities, body conserves and reuses	Hemoglobin formation. Cellular oxidation (cytochrome system producing ATP)	Growth (milk anemia). Pregnancy demands. Deficiency anemia. Excess hemosiderosis; hemochromatosis	Men 10 mg. Women 18 mg. Pregnancy 18+ mg. Lactation; 18 mg. Children: 10-18 mg	Liver. Meats. Egg yolk. Whole grains. Enriched bread and cereal. Dark green vegetables. Legumes, nuts

Summary of trace minerals—cont'd

Mineral	Metabolism	Physiological functions	Clinical application	Requirement	Food source
Copper (Cu)	Transported bound to an α-globulin as ceruloplasmin Stored in muscle, bone, liver, heart, kidney, and central nervous system	Associated with iron in Enzyme systems Hemoglobin synthesis Absorption and transport of iron Involved in bone formation and maintenance of brain tissue and myelin sheath in nervous system	Hypocupremia: Nephrosis Malabsorption Wilson's disease—excess copper storage	2-2.5 mg Diet provides 2-5 mg	Liver Meat Seafood Whole grains Legumes, nuts Cocoa Raisins Food cooked in copper utensils
Iodine (I)	Absorbed as iodides, taken up by thyroid gland under control of thyroid-stimulating hormone (TSH) Excretion by kidney	Synthesis of thyroxine, the thyroid hormone, which regulates cell oxidation	Deficiency—endemic colloid goiter; cretinism	Men: 140 μg Women: 100 μg Infants: 35-45 μg Children: 60-140 μg	Iodized salt Seafood
Manganese (Mn)	Absorption limited Excretion mainly by intestine	Activates reactions in Urea formation Protein metabolism Glucose oxidation Lipoprotein clearance and synthesis of fatty acids	No clinical deficiency observed in humans Inhalation toxicity in miners	2.5-7 mg (estimated) Diet provides 3-9 μg	Cereals, whole grain Soybeans Legumes, nuts Tea, coffee Vegetables Fruits
Cobalt (Co)	Absorbed chiefly as constituent of vitamin B_{12}	Constituent of vitamin B_{12}; essential factor in red blood cell formation	Deficiency associated with deficiency of vitamin B_{12}—pernicious anemia	Unknown	Supplied by preformed vitamin B_{12}
Zinc (Zn)	Transported with plasma proteins Excretion largely intestinal Stored in liver, muscle, bone, and organs	Essential enzyme constituent: Carbonic anhydrase Carboxypeptidase Lactic dehydrogenase Combined with insulin for storage of the hormone	Possible relation to liver disease Wound healing Taste and smell acuity Retarded sexual and physical development	Adults: 15 mg Children: 10 mg Infants: 3-5 mg	Widely distributed Liver Seafood, especially oysters Eggs Milk Whole grains
Molybdenum (Mo)	Minute traces in the body	Constituent of specific enzymes involved in Purine conversion to uric acid Aldehyde oxidation		450-500 μg (estimated)	Organ meats Milk Whole grains Leafy vegetables Legumes
Fluorine (Fl)	Deposited in bones and teeth Excreted in urine	Associated with dental health	Small amount prevents dental caries Excess causes endemic dental fluorosis	1-3 mg (estimated)	Water (1 ppm Fl)
Selenium (Se)	Active as cofactor in cell oxidation enzyme system	Associated with fat metabolism	Constituent of "factor 3," which acts with vitamin E to prevent fatty liver	Under 100 μg (estimated)	Seafoods Meats Whole grains
Chromium (Cr)	Improves faulty uptake of glucose by body tissues	Associated with glucose metabolism; raises abnormally low fasting blood sugar levels	Infants unable to metabolize sugar, and adult diabetics show definite improvement when small amounts of chromium added to diet Possible link with cardiovascular disorders and diabetes	20-50 μg (estimated)	Animal proteins, especially meats (except fish) Whole grains

Mineral	Metabolism	Physiological functions	Clinical application	Requirement	Food source
Nickel (Ni)	Binding by phytate reduces intestinal absorption	Constituent of the protein nickeloplasmin Associated with thyroid hormone High in RNA	Plasma levels decreased in cirrhosis and chronic uremia	Whole grains Legumes Vegetables Fruits	
Tin (Sn)		Structural element in protein synthesis Associated with cell enzyme systems in energy metabolism	Wound healing Tissue growth	Under 1 mg (estimated)	Meats Whole grains Legumes Vegetables Fruits Acid juices canned in tin
Silicon (Si)		Essential agent in formation of bone, cartilage, connective tissue	Bone calcification and healing	Unknown	All plant foods
Vanadium (V)		High in teeth; may have role in bone and tooth formation	Possible relation to lipid metabolism, blood lipid levels	0.1-0.3 mg (estimated)	Grains, breads Root vegetables Nuts Vegetable oils

11-5 Nutritive values of the edible part of foods

Food, approximate measure, and weight (in grams)		Food energy (calories)	Protein (g)	Fat (total lipid) (g)	Fatty acids Saturated (total) (mg)	Unsaturated Oleic (g)	Unsaturated Linoleic (g)	Carbohydrate (g)	Calcium (mg)	Iron (mg)	Vitamin A value (IU)	Thiamin (mg)	Riboflavin (mg)	Niacin (mg)	Ascorbic acid (mg)
Milk, cream, cheese (related products)															
Milk, cow's															
Fluid, whole (3.5% fat)	1 cup	244	160	9	9	5	3	Trace	12	288	0.1	350	0.08	0.42	0.1	2
Fluid, nonfat (skim)	1 cup	246	90	9	Trace	—	—	—	13	298	.1	10	.10	.44	.2	2
Buttermilk, cultured, from skim milk	1 cup	246	90	9	Trace	—	—	—	13	298	.1	10	.09	.44	.2	2
Evaporated, unsweetened, undiluted	1 cup	252	345	18	20	11	7	1	24	635	.3	820	.10	.84	.5	3
Condensed, sweetened, undiluted	1 cup	306	980	25	27	15	9	1	166	802	.3	1,090	.23	1.17	.5	3
Dry, whole	1 cup	103	515	27	28	16	9	1	39	936	.5	1,160	.30	1.50	.7	6
Dry, nonfat, instant	1 cup	70	250	25	Trace	—	—	—	36	905	.4	20	.24	1.25	.6	5
Milk, goat's															
Fluid, whole	1 cup	244	165	8	10	6	2	Trace	11	315	.2	390	.10	.27	.7	2
Cream															
Half-and-half (cream and milk)	1 cup	242	325	8	28	16	9	1	11	261	.1	1,160	.08	.38	.1	2
	1 tbsp	15	20	Trace	2	1	1	Trace	1	16	Trace	70	Trace	.02	Trace	Trace
Light, coffee or table	1 cup	240	505	7	49	27	16	1	10	245	.1	2,030	.07	.36	.1	2
	1 tbsp	15	30	Trace	3	2	1	Trace	1	15	Trace	130	Trace	.02	Trace	Trace
Whipping, unwhipped (volume about double when whipped)															
Light	1 cup	239	715	6	75	41	25	2	9	203	.1	3,070	.06	.30	.1	2
	1 tbsp	15	45	Trace	5	3	2	Trace	1	13	Trace	190	Trace	.02	Trace	Trace
Heavy	1 cup	238	840	5	89	49	29	3	7	178	.1	3,670	.05	.26	.1	2
	1 tbsp	15	55	Trace	6	3	2	Trace	Trace	11	Trace	230	Trace	.02	Trace	Trace
Cheese															
Blue or Roquefort type	1 oz	28	105	6	9	5	3	Trace	1	89	.1	350	.01	.17	.1	0
Cheddar or American Ungrated	1 inch cube	17	70	4	5	3	2	Trace	Trace	128	.2	220	Trace	.08	Trace	0

Grated	1 cup	112	445	28	36	20	12	1	2	840	1.1	1,470	.03	.51	.1	0
	1 tbsp	7	30	2	2	1	1	Trace	Trace	52	.1	90	Trace	.03	Trace	0
Cheddar, process	1 oz	28	105	7	9	5	3	Trace	1	219	.3	350	Trace	.12	Trace	0
Cheese foods, cheddar	1 oz	28	90	6	7	4	2	Trace	2	162	.2	280	.01	.16	Trace	0
Cottage cheese, from skim milk																
Creamed	1 cup	225	240	31	9	5	3	Trace	7	212	0.7	380	0.07	0.56	0.2	0
	1 oz	28	30	4	1	1	Trace	Trace	1	27	.1	50	.01	.07	Trace	0
Uncreamed	1 cup	225	195	38	1	Trace	Trace	Trace	6	202	.9	20	.07	.63	.2	0
	1 oz	28	25	5	Trace	—	—	—	1	26	.1	Trace	.01	.08	Trace	0
Cream cheese	1 oz	28	105	2	11	6	4	Trace	1	18	.1	440	Trace	.07	Trace	0
	1 tbsp	15	55	1	6	3	2	Trace	Trace	9	Trace	230	Trace	.04	Trace	0
Swiss (domestic)	1 oz	28	105	8	8	4	3	Trace	1	262	.3	320	Trace	.11	Trace	0
Milk beverages																
Cocoa	1 cup	242	235	9	11	6	4	Trace	26	286	.9	390	.09	.45	.4	2
Chocolate-flavored milk drink (made with skim milk)	1 cup	250	190	8	6	3	2	Trace	27	270	.4	210	.09	.41	.2	2
Malted milk	1 cup	270	280	13	12	—	—	—	32	364	.8	670	.17	.56	.2	2
Milk desserts																
Cornstarch pudding, plain (blanc mange)	1 cup	248	275	9	10	5	5	Trace	39	290	.1	390	.07	.40	.1	2
Custard, baked	1 cup	248	285	13	14	6	5	1	28	278	1.0	870	.10	.47	.2	1
Ice cream, plain, factory packed																
Slice or cut brick, ⅛ of quart brick	1 slice or cut brick	71	145	3	9	5	3	Trace	15	87	.1	370	.03	.13	.1	1
Container	3½ fld oz	62	130	2	8	4	3	Trace	13	76	.1	320	.03	.12	.1	1
Container	8 fld oz	142	295	6	18	10	6	1	29	175	.1	740	.06	.27	.1	1
Ice milk	1 cup	187	285	9	10	6	3	Trace	42	292	.2	390	.09	.41	.2	2
Yogurt, from partially skimmed milk	1 cup	246	120	8	4	2	1	Trace	13	295	.1	170	.09	.43	.2	2
Eggs																
Eggs, large, 24 ounces per dozen																
Raw																
Whole, without shell	1 egg	50	80	6	6	2	3	Trace	Trace	27	1.1	590	.05	.15	Trace	0
White of egg	1 white	33	15	4	Trace	—	—	—	Trace	3	Trace	0	Trace	.09	Trace	0
Yolk of egg	1 yolk	17	60	3	5	2	2	Trace	Trace	24	.9	580	.04	.07	Trace	0
Cooked																
Boiled, shell removed	2 eggs	100	160	13	12	4	5	1	1	54	2.3	1,180	.09	.28	.1	0

Reprinted from *Nutritive value of foods*, U.S. Department of Agriculture, Home and Garden Bulletin No. 72.
Dashes show that no basis could be found for improving a value although there was some reason to believe that a measurable amount of the constituent might be present.

Continued.

Nutritive values of the edible part of foods—cont'd

Food, approximate measure, and weight (in grams)			Food energy (calories)	Protein (g)	Fat (total lipid) (g)	Fatty acids			Carbohydrate (g)	Calcium (mg)	Iron (mg)	Vitamin A value (IU)	Thiamin (mg)	Riboflavin (mg)	Niacin (mg)	Ascorbic acid (mg)
						Saturated (total) (mg)	Unsaturated									
							Oleic (g)	Linoleic (g)								
Scrambled, with milk and fat	1 egg	64	110	7	8	3	3	Trace	1	51	1.1	690	.05	.18	Trace	0
Meat, poultry, fish, shellfish (related products)																
Bacon, broiled or fried, crisp	2 slices	16	100	5	8	3	4	1	1	2	.5	0	.08	.05	.8	—
Beef, trimmed to retail basis,[2] cooked																
Cuts braised, simmered, or pot-roasted																
Lean and fat	3 oz	85	245	23	16	8	7	Trace	0	10	2.9	30	.04	.18	3.5	—
Lean only	2.5 oz	72	140	22	5	2	2	Trace	0	10	2.7	10	.04	.16	3.3	—
Hamburger (ground beef), broiled																
Lean	3 oz	85	185	23	10	5	4	Trace	0	10	3.0	20	.08	.20	5.1	—
Regular	3 oz	85	245	21	17	8	8	Trace	0	9	2.7	30	.07	.18	4.6	—
Roast, oven-cooked, no liquid added																
Relatively fat, such as rib																
Lean and fat	3 oz	85	375	17	34	16	15	1	0	8	2.2	70	.05	.13	3.1	—
Lean only	1.8 oz	51	125	14	7	3	3	Trace	0	6	1.8	10	.04	.11	2.6	—
Relatively lean, such as heel of round																
Lean and fat	3 oz	85	165	25	7	3	3	Trace	0	11	3.2	10	.06	.19	4.5	—
Lean only	2.7 oz	78	125	24	3	1	1	Trace	0	10	3.0	Trace	.06	.18	4.3	—
Steak, broiled																
Relatively fat, such as sirloin																
Lean and fat	3 oz	85	330	20	27	13	12	1	0	9	2.5	50	.05	.16	4.0	—
Lean only	2.0 oz	56	115	18	4	2	2	Trace	0	7	2.2	10	.05	.14	3.6	—
Relatively lean, such as round																
Lean and fat	3 oz	85	220	24	13	6	6	Trace	0	10	3.0	20	.07	.19	4.8	—
Lean only	2.4 oz	68	130	21	4	2	2	Trace	0	9	2.5	10	.06	.16	4.1	—
Beef, canned																
Corned beef	3 oz	85	185	22	10	5	4	Trace	0	17	3.7	20	.01	.20	2.9	—
Corned beef hash	3 oz	85	155	7	10	5	4	Trace	9	11	1.7	—	.01	.08	1.8	—
Beef, dried or chipped	2 oz	57	115	19	4	2	2	Trace	0	11	2.9	—	.04	.18	2.2	—
Beef and vegetable stew	1 cup	235	210	15	10	5	4	Trace	15	28	2.8	2,310	.13	.17	4.4	15
Beef potpie, baked: individual pie, 4¼-inch diameter, weight before baking about 8 oz	1 pie	227	560	23	33	9	20	2	43	32	4.1	1,860	.25	.27	4.5	7
Chicken, cooked																
Flesh only, broiled	3 oz	85	115	20	3	1	1	1	0	8	1.4	80	0.05	0.16	7.4	—

Food	Measure	Grams	(food energy)	(protein)	(fat)	(saturated)	(oleic)	(linoleic)	(carbohydrate)	(calcium)	(iron)	(vitamin A)	(thiamin)	(riboflavin)	(niacin)	(ascorbic acid)
Breast, fried ½ breast																
With bone	3.3 oz	94	155	25	5	1	2	1	1	9	1.3	70	.04	.17	11.2	—
Flesh and skin only	2.7 oz	76	155	25	5	1	2	1	1	9	1.3	70	.04	.17	11.2	—
Drumstick, fried																
With bone	2.1 oz	59	90	12	4	1	2	1	Trace	6	.9	50	.03	.15	2.7	—
Flesh and skin only	1.3 oz	38	90	12	4	1	2	1	Trace	6	.9	50	.03	.15	2.7	—
Chicken, canned, boneless	3 oz	85	170	18	10	3	4	2	0	18	1.3	200	.03	.11	3.7	3
Chicken potpie. See Poultry potpie																
Chile con carne, canned																
With beans	1 cup	250	335	19	15	7	7	Trace	30	80	4.2	150	.08	.18	3.2	—
Without beans	1 cup	255	510	26	38	17	18	1	15	97	3.6	380	.05	.31	5.6	—
Fish and shellfish																
Bluefish, baked or broiled	3 oz	85	135	22	4	—	—	—	0	25	.6	40	.09	.08	1.6	—
Clams																
Raw, meat only	3 oz	85	65	11	1	—	—	—	2	59	5.2	90	.08	.15	1.1	8
Canned, solids and liquid	3 oz	85	45	7	1	—	—	—	2	47	3.5	—	.01	.09	.9	—
Crabmeat, canned	3 oz	85	85	15	2	—	—	—	1	38	.7	—	.07	.07	1.6	—
Fish sticks, breaded, cooked, frozen; stick 3.8 by 1.0 by 0.5 inch	10 sticks or 8 oz package	227	400	38	20	5	10	—	15	25	.9	—	.09	.16	3.6	—
Haddock, fried	3 oz	85	140	17	5	1	3	—	5	34	1.0	—	0.03	0.06	2.7	2
Mackerel																
Broiled, Atlantic	3 oz	85	200	19	13	—	—	—	0	5	1.0	450	.13	.23	6.5	—
Canned, Pacific, solids and liquid[3]	3 oz	85	155	18	9	—	—	—	0	221	1.9	20	.02	.28	7.4	—
Ocean perch, breaded (egg and bread-crumbs), fried	3 oz	85	195	16	11	—	—	—	6	28	1.1	—	.08	.09	1.5	—
Oysters, meat only. Raw, 13-19 medium selects	1 cup	240	160	20	4	—	—	—	8	226	13.2	740	.33	.43	6.0	—
Oyster stew, 1 part oysters to 3 parts milk by volume, 3-4 oysters	1 cup	230	200	11	12	—	—	—	11	269	3.3	640	.13	.41	1.6	—

[2] Outer layer of fat on the cut was removed to within approximately ½ inch of the lean. Deposits of fat within the cut were not removed.

[3] Vitamin values based on drained solids.

[4] Based on total contents of can. If bones are discarded, value will be greatly reduced.

Continued.

Nutritive values of the edible part of foods—cont'd

Food, approximate measure, and weight (in grams)		Food energy (calories)	Protein (g)	Fat (total lipid) (g)	Fatty acids — Saturated (total) (mg)	Fatty acids — Unsaturated Oleic (g)	Fatty acids — Unsaturated Linoleic (g)	Carbohydrate (g)	Calcium (mg)	Iron (mg)	Vitamin A value (IU)	Thiamin (mg)	Riboflavin (mg)	Niacin (mg)	Ascorbic acid (mg)
Salmon, pink, canned	3 oz 85	120	17	5	1	1	Trace	0	[4]167	.7	60	.03	.16	6.8	—
Sardines, Atlantic, canned in oil, drained solids	3 oz 85	175	20	9	—	—	—	0	372	2.5	190	.02	.17	4.6	—
Shad, baked	3 oz 85	170	20	10	—	—	—	0	20	.5	20	.11	.22	7.3	—
Shrimp, canned, meat only	3 oz 85	100	21	1	—	—	—	1	98	2.6	50	.01	.03	1.5	—
Swordfish, broiled with butter or margarine	3 oz 85	150	24	5	—	—	—	0	23	1.1	1,780	.03	.04	9.3	—
Tuna, canned in oil, drained solids	3 oz 85	170	24	7	—	—	—	0	7	1.6	70	.04	.10	10.1	—
Heart, beef, lean, braised	3 oz 85	160	27	5	—	—	—	1	5	5.0	20	.21	1.04	6.5	1
Lamb, trimmed to retail basis,[2] cooked															
Chop, thick, with bone, broiled	1 chop, 4.8 oz 137	400	25	33	18	12	1	0	10	1.5	—	.14	.25	5.6	—
Lean and fat	4.0 oz 112	400	25	33	18	12	1	0	10	1.5	—	.14	.25	5.6	—
Lean only	2.6 oz 74	140	21	6	3	2	Trace	0	9	1.5	—	.11	.20	4.5	—
Leg, roasted															
Lean and fat	3 oz 85	235	22	16	9	6	Trace	0	9	1.4	—	.13	.23	4.7	—
Lean only	2.5 oz 71	130	20	5	3	2	Trace	0	9	1.4	—	.12	.21	4.4	—
Shoulder, roasted															
Lean and fat	3 oz 85	285	18	23	13	8	1	0	9	1.0	—	.11	.20	4.0	—
Lean only	2.3 oz 64	130	17	6	3	2	Trace	0	8	1.0	—	.10	.18	3.7	—
Liver, beef, fried	2 oz 57	130	15	6	—	—	—	3	6	5.0	30,280	.15	2.37	9.4	15
Pork, cured, cooked															
Ham, light cure, lean and fat, roasted	3 oz 85	245	18	19	7	8	2	0	8	2.2	0	.40	.16	3.1	—
Luncheon meat															
Boiled ham, sliced	2 oz 57	135	11	10	4	4	1	0	6	1.6	0	.25	.09	1.5	—
Canned, spiced or unspiced	2 oz 57	165	8	14	5	6	1	1	5	1.2	0	.18	.12	1.6	—

Food	Measure	Weight (g)	Food energy (Cal)	Protein (g)	Fat (g)	Saturated (g)	Oleic (g)	Linoleic (g)	Carbohydrate (g)	Calcium (mg)	Iron (mg)	Vit. A (IU)	Thiamin (mg)	Riboflavin (mg)	Niacin (mg)	Ascorbic acid (mg)
Pork, fresh, trimmed to retail basis,[2] cooked																
Chop, thick, with bone	1 chop, 3.5 oz	98	260	16	21	8	9	2	0	8	2.2	0	.63	.18	3.8	—
Lean and fat	2.3 oz	66	260	16	21	8	9	2	0	8	2.2	0	.63	.18	3.8	—
Lean only	1.7 oz	48	130	15	7	2	3	1	0	7	1.9	0	.54	.16	3.3	—
Roast, oven-cooked, no liquid added																
Lean and fat	3 oz	85	310	21	24	9	10	2	0	9	2.7	0	.78	.22	4.7	—
Lean only	2.4 oz	68	175	20	10	3	4	1	0	9	2.6	0	.73	.21	4.4	—
Cuts, simmered																
Lean and fat	3 oz	85	320	20	26	9	11	2	0	8	2.5	0	.46	.21	4.1	—
Lean only	2.2 oz	63	135	18	6	2	3	1	0	8	2.3	0	.42	.19	3.7	—
Poultry potpie (based on chicken potpie). Individual pie, 4¼-inch diameter, weigh before baking	1 pie	227	535	23	31	10	15	3	42	68	3.0	3,020	.25	.26	4.1	5
Sausage																
Bologna, slice, 4.1 by 0.1 inch	8 slices	227	690	27	62	—	—	—	2	16	4.1	—	.36	.49	6.0	—
Frankfurter, cooked	1	51	155	6	14	—	—	—	1	3	.8	—	.08	.10	1.3	—
Pork links or patty, cooked	4 oz	113	540	21	50	18	21	5	Trace	8	2.7	0	.89	.39	4.2	—
Tongue, beef, braised	3 oz	85	210	18	14	—	—	—	Trace	6	1.9	—	.04	.25	3.0	—
Turkey potpie. *See* Poultry potpie																
Veal, cooked																
Cutlet, without bone, broiled	3 oz	85	185	23	9	5	4	Trace	—	9	2.7	—	.06	.21	4.6	—
Roast, medium fat, medium done; lean and fat	3 oz	85	230	23	14	7	6	Trace	0	10	2.9	—	.11	.26	6.6	—
Mature dry beans and peas, nuts, peanuts (related products)																
Almonds, shelled	1 cup	142	850	26	77	6	52	15	28	332	6.7	0	.34	1.31	5.0	Trace
Beans, dry																
Common varieties, such as Great Northern, navy, and others, canned:																
Red	1 cup	256	230	15	1	—	—	—	42	74	4.6	Trace	.13	.10	1.5	—
White, with tomato sauce																
With pork	1 cup	261	320	16	7	3	3	1	50	141	4.7	340	.20	.08	1.5	5
Without pork	1 cup	261	310	16	1	—	—	—	60	177	5.2	160	.18	.09	1.5	5
Lima, cooked	1 cup	192	260	16	1	—	—	—	48	56	5.6	Trace	.26	.12	1.3	Trace
Brazil nuts	1 cup	140	915	20	94	19	45	24	15	260	4.8	Trace	1.34	.17	2.2	—
Cashew nuts, roasted	1 cup	135	760	23	62	10	43	4	40	51	5.1	140	.58	.33	2.4	—
Coconut																
Fresh, shredded	1 cup	97	335	3	34	29	2	Trace	9	13	1.6	0	.05	.02	.5	3

Continued.

[2]Outer layer of fat on the cut was removed to within approximately ½ inch of the lean. Deposits of fat within the cut were not removed.

Nutritive values of the edible part of foods—cont'd

Food, approximate measure, and weight (in grams)	Food energy (calories)	Protein (g)	Fat (total lipid) (g)	Fatty acids Saturated (total) (mg)	Unsaturated Oleic (g)	Unsaturated Linoleic (g)	Carbohydrate (g)	Calcium (mg)	Iron (mg)	Vitamin A value (IU)	Thiamin (mg)	Riboflavin (mg)	Niacin (mg)	Ascorbic acid (mg)
Dried, shredded, sweetened — 1 cup, 62	340	2	24	21	2	Trace	33	10	1.2	0	.02	.02	.2	0
Cowpeas or blackeye peas, dry, cooked — 1 cup, 248	190	13	1	—	—	—	34	42	3.2	20	.41	.11	1.1	Trace
Peanuts, roasted, salted														
Halves — 1 cup, 144	840	37	72	16	31	21	27	107	3.0	—	.46	.19	24.7	0
Chopped — 1 tbsp, 9	55	2	4	1	2	1	2	7	.2	—	.03	.01	1.5	0
Peanut butter — 1 tbsp, 16	95	4	8	2	4	2	3	9	.3	—	.02	.02	2.4	0
Peas, split, dry, cooked — 1 cup, 250	290	20	1	—	—	—	52	28	4.2	100	.37	.22	2.2	—
Pecans														
Halves — 1 cup, 108	740	10	77	5	48	15	16	79	2.6	140	.93	.14	1.0	2
Chopped — 1 tbsp, 7.5	50	1	5	Trace	3	1	1	5	.2	10	.06	.01	.1	Trace
Walnuts, shelled														
Black or native, chopped — 1 cup, 126	790	26	75	4	26	36	19	Trace	7.6	380	.28	.14	.9	—
English or Persian														
Halves — 1 cup, 100	650	15	64	4	10	40	16	99	3.1	30	.33	.13	.9	3
Chopped — 1 tbsp, 8	50	1	5	Trace	1	3	1	8	.2	Trace	.03	.01	.1	Trace
Vegetables and vegetable products														
Asparagus														
Cooked, cut spears — 1 cup, 175	35	4	Trace	—	—	—	6	37	1.0	1,580	.27	.32	2.4	46
Canned spears, medium														
Green — 6 spears, 96	20	2	Trace	—	—	—	3	18	1.8	770	.06	.10	.8	14
Bleached — 6 spears, 96	20	2	Trace	—	—	—	4	15	1.0	80	.05	.06	.7	14
Beans														
Lima, immature, cooked — 1 cup, 160	180	12	1	—	—	—	32	75	4.0	450	.29	.16	2.0	28
Snap, green														
Cooked														
In small amount of water, short time — 1 cup, 125	30	2	Trace	—	—	—	7	62	.8	680	.08	.11	.6	16
In large amount of water, long time — 1 cup, 125	30	2	Trace	—	—	—	7	62	.8	680	0.07	0.10	0.4	13
Canned														
Solids and liquids — 1 cup, 239	45	2	Trace	—	—	—	10	81	2.9	690	.08	.10	.7	9

Strained or chopped (baby food)	1 oz	28	5	Trace	Trace	—	—	—	1	9	.3	110	.01	.02	.1	Trace
Bean sprouts, cooked, *See* Sprouts																
Beets, cooked, diced	1 cup	165	50	2	Trace	—	—	—	12	23	.8	40	.04	.07	.5	11
Broccoli spears, cooked	1 cup	150	40	5	Trace	—	—	—	7	132	1.2	3,750	.14	.29	1.2	135
Brussels sprouts, cooked	1 cup	130	45	5	1	—	—	—	8	42	1.4	680	.10	.18	1.1	113
Cabbage																
Raw																
Finely shredded	1 cup	100	25	1	Trace	—	—	—	5	49	.4	130	.05	.05	.3	47
Coleslaw	1 cup	120	120	1	9	—	2	5	9	52	.5	180	.06	.06	.3	35
Cooked																
In small amount of water, short time	1 cup	170	35	2	Trace	—	—	—	7	75	.5	220	.07	.07	.5	56
In large amount of water, long time	1 cup	170	30	2	Trace	—	—	—	7	71	.5	200	.04	.04	.2	40
Cabbage, celery or Chinese																
Raw, leaves and stalk, 1-inch pieces	1 cup	100	15	1	Trace	—	—	—	3	43	.6	150	.05	.04	.6	25
Cabbage, spoon (or bakchoy), cooked	1 cup	150	20	2	Trace	—	—	—	4	222	.9	4,650	.07	.12	1.1	23
Carrots																
Raw																
Whole, 5½ by 1 inch, 25 thin strips	1	50	20	1	Trace	—	—	—	5	18	.4	5,500	.03	.03	.3	4
Grated	1 cup	110	45	1	Trace	—	—	—	11	41	.8	12,100	.06	.06	.7	9
Cooked, diced	1 cup	145	45	1	Trace	—	—	—	10	48	.9	15,220	.08	.07	.7	9
Canned, strained or chopped (baby food)	1 oz	28	10	Trace	Trace	—	—	—	2	7	.1	3,690	.01	.01	.1	1
Cauliflower, cooked, flowerbuds	1 cup	120	25	3	Trace	—	—	—	5	25	.8	70	.11	.10	.7	66
Celery, raw																
Stalk, large outer, 8 by about 1½ inches, at root end	1 stalk	40	5	Trace	Trace	—	—	—	2	16	.1	100	.01	.01	.1	4
Pieces, diced	1 cup	100	15	1	Trace	—	—	—	4	39	.3	240	.03	.03	.3	9
Collards, cooked	1 cup	190	55	5	1	—	—	—	9	289	1.1	10,260	.27	.37	2.4	87

[5]Measure and weight apply to entire vegetable or fruit including parts not usually eaten.

[6]Based on yellow varieties; white varieties contain only a trace of cryptoxanthin and carotenes, the pigments in corn that have biological activity.

Continued.

Nutritive values of the edible part of foods—cont'd

Food, approximate measure, and weight (in grams)		Food energy (calories)	Protein (g)	Fat (total lipid) (g)	Fatty acids			Carbohydrate (g)	Calcium (mg)	Iron (mg)	Vitamin A value (IU)	Thiamin (mg)	Riboflavin (mg)	Niacin (mg)	Ascorbic acid (mg)
					Saturated (total) (mg)	Unsaturated Oleic (g)	Unsaturated Linoleic (g)								
Corn, sweet															
Cooked, ear 5 by 1¾ inches[5]	1 ear	140	70	3	1	—	—	—	16	2	.5	[6]310	.09	.08	1.0	7
Canned, solids and liquid	1 cup	256	170	5	2	—	—	—	40	10	1.0	[6]690	.07	.12	2.3	13
Cowpeas, cooked, immature seeds	1 cup	160	175	13	1	—	—	—	29	38	3.4	560	.49	.18	2.3	28
Cucumbers, 10 oz, 7½ by about 2 inches															
Raw, pared	1	207	30	1	Trace	—	—	—	7	35	.6	Trace	.07	.09	.4	23
Raw, pared, center slice ⅛-inch thick	6 slices	50	5	Trace	Trace	—	—	—	2	8	.2	Trace	.02	.02	.1	6
Dandelion greens, cooked	1 cup	180	60	4	1	—	—	—	12	252	3.2	21,060	.24	.29	—	32
Endive, curly (including escarole)	2 oz	57	10	1	Trace	—	—	—	2	46	1.0	1,870	.04	.08	.3	6
Kale, leaves including stems, cooked	1 cup	110	30	4	1	—	—	—	4	147	1.3	8,140	—	—	—	68
Lettuce, raw															
Butterhead, as Boston types; head, 4-inch diameter	1 head	220	30	3	Trace	—	—	—	6	77	4.4	2,130	.14	.13	.6	18
Crisphead, as Iceberg; head, 4¾-inch diameter	1 head	454	60	4	Trace	—	—	—	13	91	2.3	1,500	.29	.27	1.3	29
Looseleaf, of bunching varieties, leaves	2 large	50	10	1	Trace	—	—	—	2	34	.7	950	.03	.04	.2	9
Mushrooms, canned, solids and liquid	1 cup	244	40	5	Trace	—	—	—	6	15	1.2	Trace	.04	.60	4.8	4
Mustard greens, cooked	1 cup	140	35	3	1	—	—	—	6	193	2.5	8,120	.11	.19	.9	68
Okra, cooked, pod 3 by ⅝ inch	8 pods	85	25	3	Trace	—	—	—	5	78	.4	420	.11	.15	.8	17
Onions															
Mature															
Raw, onion 2½-inch diameter	1	110	40	2	Trace	—	—	—	10	30	0.6	40	0.04	0.04	0.2	11
Cooked	1 cup	210	60	3	Trace	—	—	—	14	50	.8	80	.06	.06	.4	14

Food	Measure															
Young green, small, without tops	6	50	20	1	Trace	—	—	—	5	20	.3	Trace	.02	.02	.2	12
Parsley, raw, chopped	1 tbsp	3.5	1	Trace	Trace	—	—	—	Trace	7	.2	300	Trace	.01	Trace	6
Parsnips, cooked	1 cup	155	100	2	1	—	—	—	23	70	.9	50	.11	.13	.2	16
Peas, green																
Cooked	1 cup	160	115	9	1	—	—	—	19	37	2.9	860	.44	.17	3.7	33
Canned, solids and liquid	1 cup	249	165	9	1	—	—	—	31	50	4.2	1,120	.23	.13	2.2	22
Canned, strained (baby food)	1 oz	28	15	1	Trace	—	—	—	3	3	.4	140	.02	.02	.4	3
Peppers, hot, red, without seeds, dried (ground chili powder, added seasonings)	1 tbsp	15	50	2	2	—	—	—	8	40	2.3	9,750	.03	.17	1.3	2
Peppers, sweet																
Raw, medium, about 6 per pound																
Green pod without stem and seeds	1 pod	62	15	1	Trace	—	—	—	3	6	.4	260	.05	.05	.3	79
Red pod without stem and seeds	1 pod	60	20	1	Trace	—	—	—	4	8	.4	2,670	.05	.05	.3	122
Canned, pimentos, medium	1 pod	38	10	Trace	Trace	—	—	—	2	3	.6	870	.01	.02	.1	36
Potatoes, medium (about 3 per pound raw)																
Baked, peeled after 1 baking	1	99	90	3	Trace	—	—	—	21	9	.7	Trace	.10	.04	1.7	20
Boiled																
Peeled after boiling	1	136	105	3	Trace	—	—	—	23	10	.8	Trace	.13	.05	2.0	22
Peeled before boiling	1	122	80	2	Trace	—	—	—	18	7	.6	Trace	.11	.04	1.4	20
French-fried, piece 2 by ½ by ½ inch																
Cooked in deep fat	10 pieces	57	155	2	7	2	2	4	20	9	.7	Trace	.07	.04	1.8	12
Frozen, heated	10 pieces	57	125	2	5	1	1	2	19	5	1.0	Trace	.08	.01	1.5	12
Mashed																
Milk added	1 cup	195	125	4	1	—	—	—	25	47	.8	50	.16	.10	2.0	19
Milk and butter added	1 cup	195	185	4	8	4	3	Trace	24	47	.8	330	.16	.10	1.9	18
Potato chips, medium, 2-inch diameter	10 chips	20	115	1	8	2	2	4	10	8	.4	Trace	.04	.01	1.0	3
Pumpkin, canned	1 cup	228	75	2	1	—	—	—	18	57	.9	14,590	.07	.12	1.3	12

Continued.

Nutritive values of the edible part of foods—cont'd

Food, approximate measure, and weight (in grams)			Food energy (calories)	Protein (g)	Fat (total lipid) (g)	Fatty acids			Carbohydrate (g)	Calcium (mg)	Iron (mg)	Vitamin A value (IU)	Thiamin (mg)	Riboflavin (mg)	Niacin (mg)	Ascorbic acid (mg)
						Saturated (total) (mg)	Unsaturated Oleic (g)	Linoleic (g)								
Radishes, raw, small, without tops	4		5	Trace	Trace	—	—	—	1	12	.4	Trace	.01	.01	.1	10
Sauerkraut, canned, solids and liquid	1 cup	235	45	2	Trace	—	—	—	9	85	1.2	120	.07	.09	.4	33
Spinach																
Cooked	1 cup	180	40	5	1	—	—	—	6	167	4.0	14,580	.13	.25	1.0	50
Canned, drained solids	1 cup	180	45	5	1	—	—	—	6	212	4.7	14,400	.03	.21	.6	24
Canned, strained or chopped (baby food)	1 oz	28	10	1	Trace	—	—	—	2	18	.2	1,420	.01	.04	.1	2
Sprouts, raw																
Mung bean	1 cup	90	30	3	Trace	—	—	—	6	17	1.2	20	.12	.12	.7	17
Soybean	1 cup	107	40	6	2	—	—	—	4	46	.7	90	.17	.16	.8	4
Squash																
Cooked																
Summer, diced	1 cup	210	30	2	Trace	—	—	—	7	52	.8	820	.10	.16	1.6	21
Winter, baked, mashed	1 cup	205	130	4	1	—	—	—	32	57	1.6	8,600	.10	.27	1.4	27
Canned, winter, strained and chopped (baby food)	1 oz	28	10	Trace	Trace	—	—	—	2	7	.1	510	.01	.01	.1	1
Sweet potatoes																
Cooked, medium, 5 by 2 inches, weight raw about 6 oz																
Baked, peeled after baking	1	110	155	2	1	—	—	—	36	44	1.0	8,910	.10	.07	.7	24
Boiled, peeled after boiling	1	147	170	2	1	—	—	—	39	47	1.0	11,610	.13	.09	.9	25
Candied, 3½ by 2¼ inches	1	175	295	2	6	2	3	1	60	65	1.6	11,030	.10	.08	.8	17
Canned, vacuum or solid pack	1 cup	218	235	4	Trace	—	—	—	54	54	1.7	17,000	.10	.10	1.4	30
Tomatoes																
Raw, medium, 2 by 2½ inches, about 3 per pound	1	150	35	2	Trace	—	—	—	7	20	.8	1,350	.10	.06	1.0	[7]34
Canned	1 cup	242	50	2	Trace	—	—	—	10	15	1.2	2,180	.13	.07	1.7	40

Food	Measure	Weight (g)	Food energy (cal)	Protein (g)	Fat (g)	Saturated fatty acids, total (g)	Unsaturated, oleic (g)	Unsaturated, linoleic (g)	Carbohydrate (g)	Calcium (mg)	Iron (mg)	Vitamin A (I.U.)	Thiamin (mg)	Riboflavin (mg)	Niacin (mg)	Ascorbic acid (mg)
Tomato juice, canned	1 cup	242	45	2	Trace	—	—	—	10	17	2.2	1,940	.13	.07	1.8	39
Tomato catsup	1 tbsp	17	15	Trace	Trace	—	—	—	4	4	.1	240	.02	.01	.3	3
Turnips, cooked, diced	1 cup	155	35	1	Trace	—	—	—	8	54	.6	Trace	.06	.08	.5	33
Turnip greens Cooked																
In small amount of water, short time	1 cup	145	30	3	Trace	—	—	—	5	267	1.6	9,140	.21	.36	.8	100
In large amount of water, long time	1 cup	145	25	3	Trace	—	—	—	5	252	1.4	8,260	.14	.33	.8	68
Canned, solids and liquid	1 cup	232	40	3	1	—	—	—	7	232	3.7	10,900	.04	.21	1.4	44
Fruits and fruit products																
Apples, raw, medium, 2½ inch diameter, about 3 per pound[5]	1	150	70	Trace	Trace	—	—	—	18	8	.4	50	.04	.02	.1	3
Apple brown betty	1 cup	230	345	4	8	4	3	Trace	68	41	1.4	230	.13	.10	.9	3
Apple juice, bottled or canned	1 cup	249	120	Trace	Trace	—	—	—	30	15	1.5	—	.01	.04	.2	2
Applesauce, canned Sweetened	1 cup	254	230	Trace	Trace	—	—	—	60	10	1.3	100	.05	.03	.1	3
Unsweetened or artifically sweetened	1 cup	239	100	Trace	Trace	—	—	—	26	10	1.2	100	.04	.02	.1	2
Apricots, canned, strained or junior (baby food)	1 oz	28	25	Trace	Trace	—	—	—	6	1	.1	170	Trace	Trace	Trace	1
Apricots Raw, about 12 per pound[5]	3	114	55	1	Trace	—	—	—	14	18	.5	2,890	.03	.04	.7	10
Canned in heavy syrup Halves and syrup	1 cup	259	220	2	Trace	—	—	—	57	28	.8	4,510	.05	.06	.9	10
Halves (medium and syrup)	4 halves; 2 tbsp syrup	122	105	1	Trace	—	—	—	27	13	.4	2,120	.02	.03	.4	5
Dried Uncooked, 40 halves, small	1 cup	150	390	8	1	—	—	—	100	100	8.2	16,350	.02	.23	4.9	19

[5]Measure and weight apply to entire vegetable or fruit including parts not usually eaten.

[6]Year-round average. Samples marketed from November through May average around 15 milligrams per 150-gram tomato; from June through October, around 39 milligrams.

Continued.

Nutritive values of the edible part of foods—cont'd

Food, approximate measure, and weight (in grams)		Weight (grams)	Food energy (calories)	Protein (g)	Fat (total lipid) (g)	Fatty acids Saturated (total) (mg)	Unsaturated Oleic (g)	Unsaturated Linoleic (g)	Carbohydrate (g)	Calcium (mg)	Iron (mg)	Vitamin A value (IU)	Thiamin (mg)	Riboflavin (mg)	Niacin (mg)	Ascorbic acid (mg)
Cooked unsweetened, fruit and liquid	1 cup	285	240	5	1	—	—	—	62	63	5.1	8,550	.01	.13	2.8	8
Apricot nectar, canned	1 cup	250	140	1	Trace	—	—	—	36	22	.5	2,380	.02	.02	.5	7
Avocados, raw																
California varieties, mainly Fuerte																
10-ounce avocado, about 3½ by 4¼ inches, peeled, pitted	½	108	185	2	18	4	8	2	6	11	.6	310	.12	.21	1.7	15
½-inch cubes	1 cup	152	260	3	26	5	12	3	9	15	.9	440	.16	.30	2.4	21
Florida varieties																
13 oz avocado, about 4 by 3 inches, peeled, pitted	½	123	160	2	14	3	6	2	11	12	.7	360	.13	.24	2.0	17
½-inch cubes	1 cup	152	195	2	17	3	8	2	13	15	.9	440	.16	.30	2.4	21
Bananas, raw, 6 by 1½ inches, about 3 per pound[5]	1	150	85	1	Trace	—	—	—	23	8	.7	190	.05	.06	.7	10
Blackberries, raw	1 cup	144	85	2	1	—	—	—	19	46	1.3	290	.05	.06	.5	30
Blueberries, raw	1 cup	140	85	1	1	—	—	—	21	21	1.4	140	.04	.08	.6	20
Cantaloupes, raw; medium, 5-inch diameter, about 1⅔ pounds[5]	½	385	60	1	Trace	—	—	—	14	27	.8	*6,540	.08	.06	1.2	63
Cherries																
Raw, sweet, with stems[5]	1 cup	130	80	2	Trace	—	—	—	20	26	.5	130	.06	.07	.5	12
Canned, red, sour, pitted, heavy syrup	1 cup	260	230	2	1	—	—	—	59	36	.8	1,680	.07	.06	.4	13
Cranberry juice cocktail, canned	1 cup	250	160	Trace	Trace	—	—	—	41	12	.8	Trace	.02	.02	.1	(°)
Cranberry sauce, sweetened, canned, strained	1 cup	277	405	Trace	1	—	—	—	104	17	.6	40	.03	0.3	.1	5
Dates, domestic, natural and dry, pitted, cut	1 cup	178	490	4	1	—	—	—	130	105	5.3	90	.16	.17	3.9	0

Food	Measure															
Figs																
Raw, small, 1½-inch diameter, about 12 per pound	3 figs	114	90	1	Trace	—	—	—	23	40	.7	90	.07	.06	.5	2
Dried, large, 2 by 1 inch	1 fig	21	60	1	Trace	—	—	—	15	26	.6	20	.02	.02	.1	0
Fruit cocktail, canned in heavy syrup, solids and liquid	1 cup	256	195	1	1	—	—	—	50	23	1.0	360	.04	.03	1.1	5
Grapefruit																
Raw, medium, 4¼-inch diameter, size 64																
White[5]	½	285	55	1	Trace	—	—	—	14	22	.6	10	.05	.02	.2	52
Pink or red[5]	½	285	60	1	Trace	—	—	—	15	23	.6	640	.05	.02	.3	52
Raw sections, white	1 cup	194	75	1	Trace	—	—	—	20	31	.8	20	.07	.03	.3	72
Canned, white																
Syrup pack, solids and liquid	1 cup	249	175	1	Trace	—	—	—	44	32	.7	20	.07	.04	.5	75
Water pack, solids and liquid	1 cup	240	71	1	Trace	—	—	—	18	31	.7	20	.07	.04	.5	72
Grapefruit juice																
Fresh	1 cup	246	95	1	Trace	—	—	—	23	22	.5	([10])	.09	.04	.4	92
Canned, white																
Unsweetened	1 cup	247	100	1	Trace	—	—	—	24	20	1.0	20	.07	.04	.4	84
Sweetened	1 cup	250	130	1	Trace	—	—	—	32	20	1.0	20	.07	.04	.4	78
Frozen, concentrate, unsweetened																
Undiluted, can, 6 fluid oz	1 can	207	300	4	1	—	—	—	72	70	.8	60	.29	.12	1.4	286
Diluted with 3 parts water, by volume	1 cup	247	100	1	Trace	—	—	—	24	25	.2	20	.10	.04	.5	96
Frozen, concentrate, sweetened																
Undiluted, can, 6 fluid oz	1 can	211	350	3	1	—	—	—	85	59	.6	50	.24	.11	1.2	245
Diluted with 3 parts water, by volume	1 cup	249	115	1	Trace	—	—	—	28	20	.2	20	.08	.03	.4	82
Dehydrated																
Crystals, can, net weight 4 oz	1 can	114	430	5	1	—	—	—	103	99	1.1	90	.41	.18	2.0	399

Continued.

[5]Measure and weight apply to entire vegetable or fruit including parts not usually eaten.
[8]Value based on varieties with orange-colored flesh; for green-fleshed varieties value is about 540 IU per ½ melon.
[9]About 5 milligrams per 8 fluid ounces is from cranberries. Ascorbic acid is usually added to approximately 100 milligrams per 8 fluid ounces.
[10]For white-fleshed varieties value is about 20 IU per cup; for red-fleshed varieties, 1,080 IU per cup.

Nutritive values of the edible part of foods—cont'd

Food, approximate measure, and weight (in grams)	Weight (g)	Food energy (calories)	Protein (g)	Fat (total lipid) (g)	Fatty acids Saturated (total) (mg)	Unsaturated Oleic (g)	Unsaturated Linoleic (g)	Carbohydrate (g)	Calcium (mg)	Iron (mg)	Vitamin A value (IU)	Thiamin (mg)	Riboflavin (mg)	Niacin (mg)	Ascorbic acid (mg)
Prepared with water (1 pound yields about 1 gal), 1 cup	247	100	1	Trace	—	—	—	24	22	.2	20	.10	.05	.5	92
Grapes, raw															
American type (slip skin), such as Concord, Delaware, Niagara, Catawba, and Scuppernong[5], 1 cup	153	65	1	1	—	—	—	15	15	.4	100	.05	.03	.2	3
European type (adherent skin), such as Malaga, Muscat, Thompson Seedless, Emperor, and Flame Tokay[5], 1 cup	160	95	1	Trace	—	—	—	25	17	.6	140	.07	.04	.4	6
Grape juice, bottled or canned, 1 cup	254	165	1	Trace	—	—	—	42	28	.8	—	.10	.05	.6	Trace
Lemons, raw, medium, 2½-inch diameter, size 150[5], 1 lemon	106	20	1	Trace	—	—	—	6	18	.4	10	.03	.01	.1	38
Lemon juice															
Fresh, 1 cup	246	60	1	Trace	—	—	—	20	17	.5	40	.08	.03	.2	113
1 tbsp	15	5	Trace	Trace	—	—	—	1	1	Trace	Trace	Trace	Trace	Trace	7
Canned, unsweetened, 1 cup	245	55	1	Trace	—	—	—	19	17	.5	40	.07	.03	.2	102
Lemonade concentrate, frozen, sweetened															
Undiluted, can, 6 fluid oz, 1 can	220	430	Trace	Trace	—	—	—	112	9	.4	40	.05	.06	.7	66
Diluted with 4½ parts water, by volume, 1 cup	248	110	Trace	Trace	—	—	—	28	2	.1	10	.01	.01	.2	17
Lime juice															
Fresh, 1 cup	246	65	1	Trace	—	—	—	22	22	.5	30	.05	.03	.03	80
Canned, 1 cup	246	65	1	Trace	—	—	—	22	22	.5	30	.05	.03	.3	52
Limeade concentrate, frozen, sweetened															
Undiluted, can, 6 fluid oz, 1 can	218	410	Trace	Trace	—	—	—	108	11	.2	Trace	.02	.02	.3	26
Diluted with 4⅓ parts water, by volume, 1 cup	248	105	Trace	Trace	—	—	—	27	2	Trace	Trace	Trace	Trace	Trace	6

Food	Measure	Grams	Food energy	Protein	Fat				Carbohydrate	Calcium	Iron	Vitamin A	Thiamin	Riboflavin	Niacin	Ascorbic acid
Oranges, raw California, Navel (winter), 2⅗-inch diameter, size 88[5]	1 orange	180	60	2	Trace	—	—	—	16	49	.5	240	.12	.05	.5	75
Florida, all varieties, 3-inch diameter[5]	1	210	75	1	Trace	—	—	—	19	67	.3	310	.16	.06	.6	70
Orange juice Fresh California, Valencia (summer)	1 cup	249	115	2	1	—	—	—	26	27	.7	500	.22	.06	.9	122
Florida varieties Early and mid-season	1 cup	247	100	1	Trace	—	—	—	23	25	.5	490	.22	.06	.9	127
Late season, Valencia	1 cup	248	110	1	Trace	—	—	—	26	25	.5	500	.22	.06	.9	92
Canned, unsweetened	1 cup	249	120	2	Trace	—	—	—	28	25	1.0	500	.17	.05	.6	100
Frozen concentrate Undiluted, can, 6 fluid oz	1 can	210	330	5	Trace	—	—	—	80	69	.8	1,490	.63	.10	2.4	332
Diluted with 3 parts water, by volume	1 cup	248	110	2	Trace	—	—	—	27	22	.2	500	.21	.03	.8	112
Dehydrated Crystals, can, net weight 4 oz	1 can	113	430	6	2	—	—	—	100	95	1.9	1,900	.76	.24	3.3	406
Prepared with water, 1 lb yield about 1 gal	1 cup	248	115	1	Trace	—	—	—	27	25	.5	500	.20	.06	.9	108
Orange and grapefruit juice Frozen concentrate Undiluted, can, 6 fluid oz	1 can	209	325	4	1	—	—	—	78	61	.8	790	.47	.06	2.3	301
Diluted with 3 parts water, by volume	1 cup	248	110	1	Trace	—	—	—	26	20	.3	270	.16	.02	.8	102
Papayas, raw, ½-inch cubes	1 cup	182	70	1	Trace	—	—	—	18	36	.5	3,190	.07	.08	.5	102
Peaches Raw Whole, medium, 2-inch diameter, about 4 per pound[5]	1	114	35	1	Trace	—	—	—	10	9	.5	[11]1,320	.02	.05	1.0	7

Continued.

[5]Measure and weight apply to entire vegetable or fruit including parts not usually eaten.

[11]Based on yellow-fleshed varieties; for white-fleshed varieties value is about 50 IU per 114-gram peach and 80 IU per cup of sliced peaches.

Nutritive values of the edible part of foods—cont'd

Food, approximate measure, and weight (in grams)			Food energy (calories)	Protein (g)	Fat (total lipid) (g)	Fatty acids Saturated (total) (mg)	Unsaturated Oleic (g)	Unsaturated Linoleic (g)	Carbohydrate (g)	Calcium (mg)	Iron (mg)	Vitamin A value (IU)	Thiamin (mg)	Riboflavin (mg)	Niacin (mg)	Ascorbic acid (mg)
Sliced	1 cup	168	65	1	Trace	—	—	—	16	15	.8	[11]2,230	.03	.08	1.6	12
Canned, yellow-fleshed, solids and liquid																
Syrup pack, heavy																
Halves or slices	1 cup	257	200	1	Trace	—	—	—	52	10	.8	1,100	.02	.06	1.4	7
Halves (medium) and syrup	2 halves and 2 tbsp syrup	117	90	Trace	Trace	—	—	—	24	5	.4	500	.01	.03	.7	3
Water pack	1 cup	245	75	1	Trace	—	—	—	20	10	.7	1,100	.02	.06	1.4	7
Strained or chopped (baby food)	1 oz	28	25	Trace	Trace	—	—	—	6	2	.1	140	Trace	.01	.2	1
Dried																
Uncooked	1 cup	160	420	5	1	—	—	—	109	77	9.6	6,240	.02	.31	8.5	28
Cooked, unsweetened, 10-12 halves and 6 tbsp liquid	1 cup	270	220	3	1	—	—	—	58	41	5.1	3,290	.01	.15	4.2	6
Frozen																
Carton, 12 oz, not thawed	1 carton	340	300	1	Trace	—	—	—	77	14	1.7	2,210	.03	.14	2.4	[12]135
Can, 16 oz, not thawed	1 can	454	400	2	Trace	—	—	—	103	18	2.3	2,950	.05	.18	3.2	[12]181
Peach nectar, canned	1 cup	250	120	Trace	Trace	—	—	—	31	10	.5	1,080	.02	.05	1.0	1
Pears																
Raw, 3 by 2½-inch diameter[5]	1	182	100	1	1	—	—	—	25	13	.5	30	.04	.07	.2	7
Canned, solids and liquid																
Syrup pack, heavy																
Halves or slices	1 cup	255	195	1	1	—	—	—	50	13	.5	Trace	.03	.05	.3	4
Halves (medium) and syrup	2 halves and 2 tbsp syrup	117	90	Trace	Trace	—	—	—	23	6	.2	Trace	.01	.02	.2	2
Water pack	1 cup	243	80	Trace	Trace	—	—	—	20	12	.5	Trace	.02	.05	.3	4
Strained or chopped (baby food)	1 oz	28	20	Trace	Trace	—	—	—	5	2	.1	10	Trace	.01	.1	1
Pear nectar, canned	1 cup	250	130	1	Trace	—	—	—	33	8	.2	Trace	.01	.05	Trace	1

Food	Measure	Grams	Food energy (Calories)	Protein (g)	Fat (g)	Saturated	Oleic	Linoleic	Carbohydrate (g)	Calcium (mg)	Iron (mg)	Vitamin A (IU)	Thiamine (mg)	Riboflavin (mg)	Niacin (mg)	Ascorbic acid (mg)
Persimmons, Japanese or kaki, raw, seedless, 2½-inch diameter[5]	1	125	75	1	Trace	—	—	—	20	6	.4	2,740	.01	.02	.1	11
Pineapple																
Raw, diced	1 cup	140	75	1	Trace	—	—	—	19	24	.7	100	.12	.04	.3	24
Canned, heavy syrup pack, solids and liquid																
Crushed	1 cup	260	195	1	Trace	—	—	—	50	29	.8	120	.20	.06	.5	17
Sliced, slices and juice	2 small or 1 large and 2 tbsp juice	122	90	Trace	Trace	—	—	—	24	13	.4	50	.09	.03	.2	8
Pineapple juice, canned	1 cup	249	135	1	Trace	—	—	—	34	37	.7	120	.12	.04	.5	22
Plums, all except prunes																
Raw, 2-inch diameter, about 2 ounces[5]	1	60	25	Trace	Trace	—	—	—	7	7	.3	140	.02	.02	.3	3
Canned, syrup pack (Italian prunes)																
Plums (with pits) and juice[5]	1 cup	256	205	1	Trace	—	—	—	53	22	2.2	2,970	.05	.05	.9	4
Plums (without pits) and juice	3 plums and 2 tbsp juice	122	100	Trace	Trace	—	—	—	26	11	1.1	1,470	.03	.02	.5	2
Prunes, dried, "softenized," medium																
Uncooked[5]	4	32	70	1	Trace	—	—	—	18	14	1.1	440	.02	.04	.4	1
Cooked, unsweetened, 17-18 prunes and ⅓ cup liquid[5]	1 cup	270	295	2	1	—	—	—	78	60	4.5	1,860	.08	.18	1.7	2
Prunes with tapioca, canned, strained or junior (baby food)	1 oz	28	25	Trace	Trace	—	—	—	6	2	.3	110	.01	.02	.1	1
Prune juice, canned	1 cup	256	200	1	Trace	—	—	—	49	36	10.5	—	.02	.03	1.1	4
Raisins, dried	1 cup	160	460	4	Trace	—	—	—	124	99	5.6	30	.18	.13	.9	2
Raspberries, red																
Raw	1 cup	123	70	1	1	—	—	—	17	27	1.1	160	.04	.11	1.1	31
Frozen, 10 oz carton, not thawed	1 carton	284	275	2	1	—	—	—	70	37	1.7	200	.06	.17	1.7	59
Rhubarb, cooked, sugar added	1 cup	272	385	1	Trace	—	—	—	98	212	1.6	220	.06	.15	.7	17

[5]Measure and weight apply to entire vegetable or fruit including parts not usually eaten.
[11]Based on yellow-fleshed varieties; for white-fleshed varieties value is about 50 IU per 114-gram peach and 80 IU per cup of sliced peaches.
[12]Average weighted in accordance with commercial freezing practices. For products without added ascorbic acid, value is about 37 milligrams per 12-ounce carton and 50 milligrams per 16-ounce can; for those with added ascorbic acid, 139 milligrams per 12 ounces and 186 milligrams per 16 ounces.

Continued.

Nutritive values of the edible part of foods—cont'd

Food, approximate measure, and weight (in grams)		weight (g)	Food energy (calories)	Protein (g)	Fat (total lipid) (g)	Fatty acids			Carbohydrate (g)	Calcium (mg)	Iron (mg)	Vitamin A value (IU)	Thiamin (mg)	Riboflavin (mg)	Niacin (mg)	Ascorbic acid (mg)
						Saturated (total) (mg)	Unsaturated Oleic (g)	Unsaturated Linoleic (g)								
Strawberries																
Raw, capped	1 cup	149	55	1	1	—	—	—	13	31	1.5	90	.04	.10	1.0	88
Frozen, 10-oz carton, not thawed	1 carton	284	310	1	1	—	—	—	79	40	2.0	90	.06	.17	1.5	150
Frozen, 16-ounce can, not thawed	1 can	454	495	2	1	—	—	—	126	64	3.2	150	.09	.27	2.4	240
Tangerines, raw, medium, 2½-inch diameter, about 4 per pound[5]	1	114	40	1	Trace	—	—	—	10	34	.3	350	.05	.02	.1	26
Tangerine juice																
Canned, unsweetened	1 cup	248	105	1	Trace	—	—	—	25	45	.5	1,040	.14	.04	.3	56
Frozen concentrate																
Undiluted, can, 6 fluid oz	1 can	210	340	4	1	—	—	—	80	130	1.5	3,070	.43	.12	.9	202
Diluted with 3 parts water, by volume	1 cup	248	115	1	Trace	—	—	—	27	45	.5	1,020	.14	.04	.3	67
Watermelon, raw, wedge, 4 by 8 inches (1/16 of 10 by 16-inch melon, about 2 pounds with rind)[5]	1 wedge	925	115	2	1	—	—	—	27	30	2.1	2,510	.13	.13	.7	30
Breads and cereals																
Barley, pearled, light, uncooked	1 cup	203	710	17	2	Trace	1	1	160	32	4.1	0	.25	.17	6.3	0
Biscuits, baking powder with enriched flour, 2½-inch diameter	1	38	140	3	6	2	3	1	17	46	.6	Trace	.08	.08	.7	Trace
Bran flakes (40 percent bran) added thiamine	1 oz	28	85	3	1	—	—	—	23	20	1.2	0	.11	.05	1.7	0
Bread																
Boston brown bread, slice, 3 by ¾ inch	1 slice	48	100	3	1	—	—	—	22	43	.9	0	.05	.03	.6	0
Cracked-wheat bread																
Loaf, 1-pound, 20 slices	1 loaf	454	1,190	39	10	2	5	2	236	399	5.0	Trace	.53	.42	5.8	Trace

Food															
Slice	23	60	2	1	—	—	—	12	20	.3	Trace	.03	.02	.3	Trace
French or Vienna bread															
Enriched, 1-pound loaf	454	1,315	41	14	3	8	2	251	195	10.0	Trace	1.26	.98	11.3	Trace
Unenriched, 1-pound loaf	454	1,315	41	14	3	8	2	251	195	3.2	Trace	.39	.39	3.6	Trace
Italian bread															
Enriched, 1-pound loaf	454	1,250	41	4	Trace	1	2	256	77	10.0	0	1.31	.93	11.7	0
Unenriched, 1-pound loaf	454	1,250	41	4	Trace	1	2	256	77	3.2	0	.39	.27	3.6	0
Raisin bread															
Loaf, 1 pound, 20 slices	454	1,190	30	13	3	8	2	243	322	5.9	Trace	.24	.42	3.0	Trace
Slice	23	60	2	1	—	—	—	12	16	.3	Trace	.01	.02	.2	Trace
Rye bread															
American, light (⅓ rye, ⅔ wheat)															
Loaf, 1-pound, 20 slices	454	1,100	41	5	—	—	—	236	340	7.3	0	.81	.33	6.4	0
Slice	23	55	2	Trace	—	—	—	12	17	.4	0	.04	.02	.3	0
Pumpernickel, loaf, 1 pound	454	1,115	41	5	—	—	—	241	381	10.9	0	10.5	.63	5.4	0
White bread, enriched															
1 to 2 percent nonfat dry milk															
Loaf, 1-pound, 20 slices	454	1,225	39	15	3	8	2	229	318	10.9	Trace	1.13	.77	10.4	Trace
Slice	23	60	2	1	Trace	Trace	Trace	12	16	.6	Trace	.06	.04	.5	Trace
3 to 4 percent nonfat dry milk[13]															
Loaf, 1-pound	454	1,225	39	15	3	8	2	229	381	11.3	Trace	1.13	.95	10.8	Trace
Slice, 20 per loaf	23	60	2	1	Trace	Trace	Trace	12	19	.6	Trace	.06	.05	.6	Trace
Slice, toasted	20	60	2	1	Trace	Trace	Trace	12	19	.6	Trace	.05	.05	.6	Trace
Slice, 26 per loaf	17	45	1	1	Trace	Trace	Trace	9	14	.4	Trace	.04	.04	.4	Trace
5 to 6 percent nonfat dry milk															
Loaf, 1-pound, 20 slices	454	1,245	41	17	4	10	2	228	435	11.3	Trace	1.22	.91	11.0	Trace
Slice	23	65	2	1	Trace	Trace	Trace	12	22	.6	Trace	.06	.06	.6	Trace
White bread, unenriched															
1 to 2 percent nonfat dry milk															
Loaf, 1-pound, 20 slices	454	1,225	39	15	3	8	2	229	318	3.2	Trace	.40	.36	5.6	Trace
Slice	23	60	2	1	Trace	Trace	Trace	12	16	.2	Trace	.02	.02	.3	Trace

[5]Measure and weight apply to entire vegetable or fruit including parts not usually eaten.
[13]When the amount of nonfat dry milk in commercial white bread is unknown, values for bread with 3% to 4% nonfat dry milk are suggested.

Continued.

Nutritive values of the edible part of foods—cont'd

Food, approximate measure, and weight (in grams)			Food energy (calories)	Protein (g)	Fat (total lipid) (g)	Fatty acids			Carbohydrate (g)	Calcium (mg)	Iron (mg)	Vitamin A value (IU)	Thiamin (mg)	Riboflavin (mg)	Niacin (mg)	Ascorbic acid (mg)
						Saturated (total) (mg)	Unsaturated Oleic (g)	Linoleic (g)								
3 to 4 percent nonfat dry milk[13]																
Loaf, 1-pound	1 loaf	454	1,225	39	15	3	8	—	228	381	3.2	Trace	.31	.39	5.0	Trace
Slice, 20 per loaf	1 slice	23	60	2	1	Trace	Trace	Trace	12	19	.2	Trace	.02	.02	.3	Trace
Slice, toasted		20	60	2	1	Trace	Trace	Trace	12	19	.2	Trace	.01	.02	.3	Trace
Slice, 26 per loaf	1 slice	17	45	1	1	Trace	Trace	Trace	9	14	.1	Trace	.01	.01	.2	Trace
5 to 6 percent nonfat dry milk																
Loaf, 1-pound	1 loaf	454	1,245	41	17	4	10	2	228	435	3.2	Trace	.32	.39	4.1	Trace
Slice, 1-pound, 20 slices	1	23	65	2	1	Trace	Trace	Trace	12	22	.2	Trace	.02	.03	.2	Trace
Whole-wheat bread, made with 2 percent nonfat dry milk																
Loaf, 1-pound, 20 slices	1 loaf	454	1,105	48	14	3	6	3	216	449	10.4	Trace	1.17	.56	12.9	Trace
Slice	1	23	55	2	1	Trace	Trace	Trace	11	23	.5	Trace	.06	.03	.7	Trace
Slice, toasted		19	55	2	1	Trace	Trace	Trace	11	22	.5	Trace	.05	.03	.6	Trace
Breadcrumbs, dry, grated	1 cup	88	345	11	4	1	2	1	65	107	3.2	Trace	.19	.26	3.1	Trace
Cakes[14]																
Angelfood cake; sector, 2-inch (1/12 of 8-inch-diameter cake)	1 sector	40	110	3	Trace	—	—	—	24	4	.1	0	Trace	.06	.1	0
Chocolate cake, chocolate icing; sector, 2-inch (1/16 of 10-inch-diameter layer cake)	1 sector	120	445	5	20	8	10	1	67	84	1.2	[15]190	.03	.12	.3	Trace
Fruitcake, dark (made with enriched flour); piece, 2 by 2 by 1/2 inch	1 piece	30	115	1	5	1	3	1	18	22	.8	[15]40	.04	.04	.2	Trace
Gingerbread (made with enriched flour); piece, 2 by 2 by 2 inches	1 piece	55	175	2	6	1	4	Trace	29	37	1.3	50	.06	.06	.5	0
Plain cake and cupcakes, without icing																
Piece, 3 by 2 by 1 1/2 inches	1	55	200	2	8	2	5	1	31	35	.2	[15]90	.01	.05	.1	Trace

Food	Measure	Grams	Calories	Protein (g)	Fat (g)	Saturated	Oleic	Linoleic	Carbohydrate (g)	Calcium	Iron	Vitamin A	Thiamine	Riboflavin	Niacin	Ascorbic acid
Cupcake, 2¾-inch diameter	1	40	145	2	6	1	3	Trace	22	26	.2	[15]70	.01	.03	.1	Trace
Plain cake and cupcakes, with chocolate icing																
Sector, 2-inch (1/16 of 10-inch-layer cake)	1	100	370	4	14	5	7	1	59	63	.6	[15]180	.02	.09	.2	Trace
Cupcake, 2¾-inch diameter	1	50	185	2	7	2	4	Trace	30	32	.3	[15]90	.01	.04	.1	Trace
Poundcake, old-fashioned (equal weights flour, sugar, fat, eggs); slice, 2¾ by 3 by ⅝ inch	1 slice	30	140	2	9	2	5	1	14	6	.2	[15]80	.01	.03	.1	0
Sponge cake; sector, 2-inch (1/12 of 8-inch-diameter cake)	1	40	120	3	2	1	1	Trace	22	12	.5	180	.02	.06	.1	Trace
Cookies																
Plain and assorted, 3-inch diameter	1 cookie	25	120	1	5	—	—	—	18	9	.2	20	.01	.01	.1	Trace
Fig bars, small	1 oz	16	55	1	1	1	1	—	12	12	.2	20	.01	.01	.1	Trace
Corn, rice and wheat flakes, mixed, added nutrients	1 oz	28	110	2	Trace	—	—	—	24	11	.5	0	.11	—	.9	0
Corn flakes, added nutrients																
Plain	1 oz	28	110	2	Trace	—	—	—	24	5	.4	0	.12	.02	.6	0
Sugar-covered	1 oz	28	110	1	Trace	—	—	—	26	3	.3	0	.12	.01	.5	0
Corn grits, degermed, cooked																
Enriched	1 cup	242	120	3	Trace	—	—	—	27	2	[16].7	[17]150	[16].10	[16].07	[16]1.0	0
Unenriched	1 cup	242	120	3	Trace	—	—	—	27	2	.2	[17]150	.05	.02	.5	0
Cornmeal, white or yellow, dry																
Whole ground, unbolted	1 cup	118	420	11	5	1	2	2	87	24	2.8	[17]600	.45	.13	2.4	0
Degermed, enriched	1 cup	145	525	11	2	Trace	1	1	114	9	[16]4.2	[17]640	[16].64	[16].38	[16]5.1	0

[13] When the amount of nonfat dry milk in commercial white bread is unknown, values for bread with 3% to 4% nonfat dry milk are suggested.

[14] Unenriched cake flour and vegetable cooking fat used unless otherwise specified.

[15] If the fat used in the recipe is butter or fortified margarine, the vitamin A value for chocolate cake with chocolate icing will be 490 IU per 2-inch sector; 100 IU for fruitcake; for plain cake without icing, 300 IU per piece; 220 IU per cupcake; 440 IU per 2-inch sector; 220 IU per cupcake; and 300 IU for poundcake.

[16] Iron, thiamine, riboflavin, and niacin are based on the minimum levels of enrichment specified in standards of identity promulgated under the Federal Food, Drug, and Cosmetic Act.

[17] Vitamin A value based on yellow product. White product contains only a trace.

Continued

Nutritive values of the edible part of foods—cont'd

Food, approximate measure, and weight (in grams)		Food energy (calories)	Protein (g)	Fat (total lipid) (g)	Fatty acids			Carbohydrate (g)	Calcium (mg)	Iron (mg)	Vitamin A value (IU)	Thiamin (mg)	Riboflavin (mg)	Niacin (mg)	Ascorbic acid (mg)
					Saturated (total) (mg)	Unsaturated Oleic (g)	Unsaturated Linoleic (g)								
Corn muffins, made with enriched degermed cornmeal and enriched flour; muffin, 2¾-inch diameter	1 muffin 48	150	3	5	2	2	Trace	23	50	.8	[18]80	.09	.11	.8	Trace
Corn, puffed, presweetened, added nutrients	1 oz 28	110	1	Trace	—	—	—	26	3	.5	0	.12	.05	.6	0
Corn, shredded, added nutrients	1 oz 28	110	2	Trace	—	—	—	25	1	.7	0	.12	.05	.6	0
Crackers Graham, plain	4 small or 2 medium 14	55	1	1	—	—	—	10	6	.2	0	.01	.03	.2	0
Saltines, 2 inches squares	2 crackers 8	35	1	1	—	—	—	6	2	.1	0	Trace	Trace	.1	0
Soda Cracker, 2½ inches square	2 crackers 11	50	1	1	Trace	1	Trace	8	2	.2	0	Trace	Trace	.1	0
Oyster crackers	10 crackers 10	45	1	1	Trace	1	Trace	7	2	.2	0	Trace	Trace	.1	0
Cracker meal	1 tbsp 10	45	1	1	Trace	1	Trace	7	2	[19].1	0	[19].01	[19]Trace	[19].2	0
Doughnuts, cake type	1 doughnut 32	125	1	6	1	4	Trace	16	13	[19].4	30	[19].05	[19].05	[19].4	Trace
Farina, regular enriched, cooked	1 cup 238	100	3	Trace	—	—	—	21	10	[16].7	0	[16].11	[16].07	[16]1.0	0
Macaroni, cooked Enriched Cooked, firm stage (8 to 10 minutes; undergoes additional cooking in a food mixture)	1 cup 130	190	6	1	—	—	—	39	14	[16]1.4	0	[16].23	[16].14	[16]1.9	0
Cooked until tender	1 cup 140	155	5	1	—	—	—	32	11	[16]1.3	0	[16].19	[16].11	[16]1.5	0

Food	Measure	Weight (g)														
Unenriched																
Cooked, firm stage (8 to 10 minutes; undergoes additional cooking in a food mixture)	1 cup	130	190	6	1	—	—	—	39	14	.6	0	.02	.02	.5	0
Cooked until tender	1 cup	140	155	5	1	—	—	—	32	11	.6	0	.02	.02	.4	0
Macaroni (enriched) and cheese, baked	1 cup	220	470	18	24	11	10	1	44	398	2.0	950	.22	.44	2.0	Trace
Muffins, with enriched white flour; muffin, 2¾-inch diameter	1	48	140	4	5	1	3	Trace	20	50	.8	50	.08	.11	.7	Trace
Noodles (egg noodles), cooked																
Enriched	1 cup	160	200	7	2	1	1	Trace	37	16	[16]1.4	110	[16].23	[14].14	[16]1.8	0
Unenriched	1 cup	160	200	7	2	1	1	Trace	37	16	1.0	110	.04	.03	.7	0
Oats (with or without corn), puffed, added nutrients	1 oz	28	115	3	2	Trace	1	1	21	50	1.3	0	.28	.05	.5	0
Oatmeal or rolled oats, regular or quick-cooking, cooked	1 cup	236	130	5	2	Trace	1	1	23	21	1.4	0	.19	.05	.3	0
Pancakes (griddlecakes), 4-inch diameter																
Wheat, enriched flour (home recipe)	1 cake	27	60	2	2	Trace	Trace	1	9	27	.4	30	.05	.06	.3	Trace
Buckwheat (buckwheat pancake mix, made with egg and milk)	1 cake	27	55	2	2	1	1		6	59	.4	60	.03	.04	.2	Trace
Piecrust, plain, baked																
Enriched flour																	
Lower crust, 9-inch shell	1	135	675	8	45	10	29	3	59	19	2.3	0	.27	.19	2.4	0
Double crust, 9-inch pie	1	270	1,350	16	90	21	58	7	118	38	4.6	0	.55	.39	4.9	0
Unenriched flour																	
Lower crust, 9-inch shell	1	135	675	8	45	10	29	3	59	19	.7	0	.04	.04	.6	0
Double crust, 9-inch pie	1	270	1,350	16	90	21	58	7	118	38	1.4	0	.08	.07	1.3	0

[14] Unenriched cake flour and vegetable cooking fat used unless otherwise specified.

[16] Iron, thiamine, riboflavin, and niacin are based on the minimum levels of enrichment specified in standards of identity promulgated under the Federal Food, Drug, and Cosmetic Act.

[18] Based on recipe using white cornmeal; if yellow cornmeal is used, the vitamin A value is 140 IU per muffin.

[19] Based on product made with enriched flour. With unenriched flour, approximate values per doughnut are: iron, 0.2 milligram; thiamine, 0.01 milligram; riboflavin, 0.03 milligram; niacin, 0.2 milligram.

Continued.

Nutritive values of the edible part of foods—cont'd

Food, approximate measure, and weight (in grams)			Food energy (calories)	Protein (g)	Fat (total lipid) (g)	Fatty acids Saturated (total) (mg)	Unsaturated Oleic (g)	Unsaturated Linoleic (g)	Carbohydrate (g)	Calcium (mg)	Iron (mg)	Vitamin A value (IU)	Thiamin (mg)	Riboflavin (mg)	Niacin (mg)	Ascorbic acid (mg)
Pies (piecrust made with unenriched flour); sector, 4-inch, ⅐ of 9-inch-diameter pie																
Apple	1 sector	135	345	3	15	4	9	1	51	11	.4	40	.03	.02	.5	1
Cherry	1 sector	135	355	4	15	4	10	1	52	19	.4	590	.03	.03	.6	1
Custard	1 sector	130	280	8	14	5	8	1	30	125	.8	300	.07	.21	.4	0
Lemon meringue	1 sector	120	305	4	12	4	7	1	45	17	.6	200	.04	.10	.2	4
Mince	1 sector	135	365	3	16	4	10	1	56	38	1.4	Trace	.09	.05	.5	1
Pumpkin	1 sector	130	275	5	15	5	7	1	32	66	.6	3,210	.04	.13	.6	Trace
Pizza (cheese); 5½-inch sector; ⅛ of 14-inch diameter pie	1 sector	75	185	7	6	2	3	Trace	27	107	.7	290	.04	.12	.7	4
Popcorn, popped, with added oil and salt	1 cup	14	65	1	3	2	Trace	Trace	8	1	.3	—	—	.01	.2	0
Pretzels, small stick	5 sticks	5	20	Trace	Trace	—	—	—	4	1	0	0	Trace	Trace	Trace	0
Rice (fully milled or polished), enriched, cooked																
Common commercial varieties, all types	1 cup	168	185	3	Trace	—	—	—	41	17	[20]1.5	0	[20].19	[20].01	[20]1.6	0
Long grain, parboiled	1 cup	176	185	4	Trace	—	—	—	41	33	[20]1.4	0	[20].19	[20].02	[20]2.0	0
Rice, puffed, added nutrients (without salt)	1 cup	14	55	1	Trace	—	—	—	13	3	.3	0	.06	.01	.6	0
Rice flakes, added nutrients	1 cup	30	115	2	Trace	—	—	—	26	9	.5	0	.10	.02	1.6	0
Rolls																
Plain, pan; 12 per 16 oz																
Enriched	1 roll	38	115	3	2	Trace	1	Trace	20	28	.7	Trace	.11	.07	.8	Trace
Unenriched	1 roll	38	115	3	2	Trace	1	Trace	20	28	.3	Trace	.02	.03	.3	Trace
Hard, round; 12 per 22 oz	1 roll	52	160	5	2	Trace	1	Trace	31	24	.4	Trace	.03	.05	.4	Trace
Sweet, pan; 12 per 18 oz	1 roll	43	135	4	4	1	2	Trace	21	37	.3	30	.03	.06	.4	Trace
Rye wafers, whole-grain, 1⅞ by 3½ inches	2 wafers	13	45	2	Trace	—	—	—	10	7	.5	0	.04	.03	.2	0
Spaghetti																
Cooked, tender stage (14 to 20 minutes)																
Enriched	1 cup	140	155	5	1	—	—	—	32	11	[16]1.3	0	[16].19	[16].11	[16]1.5	0
Unenriched	1 cup	140	155	5	1	—	—	—	32	11	.6	0	.02	.02	.4	0

Food	Measure														
Spaghetti with meat balls in tomato sauce (home recipe)	1 cup	250	335	19	12	4	6	1	39	125	3.8	1,600	.26	.30	4.0	22
Spaghetti in tomato sauce with cheese (home recipe)	1 cup	250	260	9	9	2	5	1	37	80	2.2	1,080	.24	.18	2.4	14
Waffles, with enriched flour, 1/2 by 4 1/2 by 5 1/2 inches	1	75	210	7	7	2	4	1	28	85	1.3	250	.13	.19	1.0	Trace
Wheat, puffed With added nutrients (without salt)	1 oz	28	105	4	Trace	—	—	—	22	8	1.2	0	.15	.07	2.2	0
With added nutrients, with sugar and honey	1 oz	28	105	2	1	—	—	—	25	7	.9	0	.14	.05	1.8	0
Wheat, rolled; cooked	1 cup	236	175	5	1	—	—	—	40	19	1.7	0	.17	.06	2.1	0
Wheat, shredded, plain (long, round, or bite-size)	1 oz	28	100	3	1	—	—	—	23	12	1.0	0	.06	.03	1.2	0
Wheat and malted barley flakes, with added nutrients	1 oz	28	110	2	Trace	—	—	—	24	14	.7	0	.13	.03	1.1	0
Wheat flakes, with added nutrients	1 oz	28	100	3	Trace	—	—	—	23	12	1.2	0	.18	.04	1.4	0
Wheat flours Whole-wheat, from hard wheats, stirred	1 cup	120	400	16	2	Trace	1	1	85	49	4.0	0	.66	.14	5.2	0
All-purpose or family flour Enriched, sifted	1 cup	110	400	12	1	Trace	Trace	Trace	84	18	[16]3.2	0	[16].48	[16].29	[16]3.8	0
Unenriched, sifted	1 cup	110	400	12	1	Trace	Trace	Trace	84	18	.9	0	.07	.05	1.0	0
Self-rising, enriched	1 cup	110	385	10	1	Trace	Trace	Trace	82	292	[16]3.2	0	[16].49	[16].29	[16]3.9	0
Cake or pastry flour, sifted	1 cup	100	365	8	1	Trace	Trace	Trace	79	17	.5	0	.03	.03	.7	0
Wheat germ, crude, commercially milled	1 cup	68	245	18	7	1	2	4	32	49	6.4	0	1.36	.46	2.9	0

[16]Iron, thiamine, riboflavin, and niacin are based on the minimum levels of enrichment specified in standards of identity promulgated under the Federal Food, Drug, and Cosmetic Act.
[20]Iron, thiamine, and niacin are based on the minimum levels of enrichment specified in standards of identity promulgated under the Federal Food, Drug, and Cosmetic Act. Riboflavin is based on unenriched rice. When the minimum level of enrichment for riboflavin specified in the standards of identity becomes effective the value will be 0.12 milligram per cup of parboiled rice and of white rice.

Continued

Nutritive values of the edible part of foods—cont'd

Food, approximate measure, and weight (in grams)			Food energy (calories)	Protein (g)	Fat (total lipid) (g)	Fatty acids			Carbohydrate (g)	Calcium (mg)	Iron (mg)	Vitamin A value (IU)	Thiamin (mg)	Riboflavin (mg)	Niacin (mg)	Ascorbic acid (mg)
						Saturated (total) (mg)	Unsaturated									
							Oleic (g)	Linoleic (g)								
Fats, oils																
Butter, 4 sticks per pound																
Sticks, 2	1 cup	227	1,625	1	184	101	61	6	1	45	0	[21]17,500	—	—	—	0
Stick, 1/8	1 tbsp	14	100	Trace	11	6	4	Trace	Trace	3	0	[21]460	—	—	—	0
Pat or square (64 per pound)	1 pat	7	50	Trace	6	3	2	Trace	Trace	1	0	[21]230	—	—	—	0
Fats, cooking																
Lard	1 cup	220	1,985	0	220	84	101	22	0	0	0	0	0	0	0	0
Lard	1 tbsp	14	125	0	14	5	6	1	0	0	0	0	0	0	0	0
Vegetable fats	1 cup	200	1,770	0	200	46	130	14	0	0	0	—	0	0	0	0
Vegetable fats	1 tbsp	12.5	110	0	12	3	8	1	0	0	0	—	0	0	0	0
Margarine, 4 sticks per pound																
Sticks, 2	1 cup	227	1,635	1	184	37	105	33	1	45	0	[22]27,500	—	—	—	0
Stick, 1/8	1 tbsp	14	100	Trace	11	2	6	2	Trace	3	0	[22]460	—	—	—	0
Pat or square (64 per pound)	1 pat	7	50	Trace	6	1	3	1	Trace	1	0	[22]230	—	—	—	0
Oils, salad or cooking																
Corn	1 tbsp	14	125	0	14	1	4	7	0	0	0	—	0	0	0	0
Cottonseed	1 tbsp	14	125	0	14	4	3	7	0	0	0	—	0	0	0	0
Olive	1 tbsp	14	125	0	14	2	11	1	0	0	0	—	0	0	0	0
Soybean	1 tbsp	14	125	0	14	2	3	7	0	0	0	—	0	0	0	0
Salad dressings																
Blue cheese	1 tbsp	16	80	1	8	2	2	4	1	13	Trace	30	Trace	.02	Trace	Trace
Commercial mayonnaise type	1 tbsp	15	65	Trace	6	1	1	3	2	2	Trace	30	Trace	Trace	Trace	—
French	1 tbsp	15	60	Trace	6	1	1	3	3	2	.1	—	—	—	—	—
Home cooked, boiled	1 tbsp	17	30	1	2	1	1	Trace	3	15	.1	80	.01	.03	Trace	Trace
Mayonnaise	1 tbsp	15	110	Trace	12	2	3	6	Trace	3	.1	40	Trace	.01	Trace	—
Thousand Island	1 tbsp	15	75	Trace	8	1	2	4	2	2	.1	50	Trace	Trace	Trace	Trace
Sugars, sweets																
Candy																
Caramels	1 oz	28	115	1	3	2	1	Trace	22	42	.4	Trace	.01	.05	Trace	Trace
Chocolate, milk, plain	1 oz	28	150	2	9	5	3	Trace	16	65	.3	80	.02	.09	.1	Trace
Fudge, plain	1 oz	28	115	1	3	2	1	Trace	21	22	.3	Trace	.01	.03	.1	Trace
Hard candy	1 oz	28	110	0	Trace	—	—	—	28	6	.5	0	0	0	0	0
Marshmallows	1 oz	28	90	1	Trace	—	—	—	23	5	.5	0	0	Trace	Trace	0
Chocolate syrup, thin type	1 tbsp	20	50	Trace	Trace	Trace	Trace	Trace	13	3	.3	—	Trace	.01	.1	0

Food	Measure													
Honey, strained or extracted	1 tbsp	21	65	Trace	0	—	—	17	1	.1	0	Trace	.01	.1	Trace
Jams and preserves	1 tbsp	20	55	Trace	Trace	—	—	14	4	.2	Trace	Trace	.01	Trace	Trace
Jellies	1 tbsp	20	55	Trace	Trace	—	—	14	4	.3	Trace	Trace	.01	Trace	1
Molasses, cane															
Light (first extraction)	1 tbsp	20	50	—	—	—	—	13	33	.9	—	.01	.01	Trace	—
Blackstrap (third extraction)	1 tbsp	20	45	—	—	—	—	11	137	3.2	—	.02	.04	.4	—
Sirup, table blends (chiefly corn, light and dark)	1 tbsp	20	60	0	0	—	—	15	9	.8	0	0	0	0	0
Sugars (cane or beet)															
Granulated	1 cup	200	770	0	0	—	—	199	0	.2	0	0	0	0	0
	1 tbsp	12	45	0	0	—	—	12	0	Trace	0	0	0	0	0
Lump, 1⅛ by ¾ by ⅜	1 lump	6	25	0	0	—	—	6	0	Trace	0	0	0	0	0
Powdered, stirred before measuring	1 cup	128	495	0	0	—	—	127	0	.1	0	0	0	0	0
	1 tbsp	8	30	0	0	—	—	8	0	Trace	0	0	0	0	0
Brown, firm-packed	1 cup	220	820	0	0	—	—	212	187	7.5	0	.02	.07	.4	0
	1 tbsp	14	50	0	0	—	—	13	12	.5	0	Trace	Trace	Trace	0
Miscellaneous items															
Beer (average 3.6 percent alcohol by weight)	1 cup	240	100	1	0	—	—	9	12	Trace	—	.01	.07	1.6	—
Beverages, carbonated															
Cola type	1 cup	240	95	0	0	—	—	24	—	—	0	0	0	0	0
Ginger ale	1 cup	230	70	0	0	—	—	18	—	—	0	0	0	0	0
Bouillon cube, ⅝ inch	1 cube	4	5	1	Trace	—	—	Trace	—	—	—	—	—	—	—
Chili powder, See Vegetables, peppers															
Chili sauce (mainly tomatoes)	1 tbsp	17	20	Trace	Trace	—	—	4	3	.1	240	.02	.01	.3	3
Chocolate															
Bitter or baking	1 oz	28	145	3	15	8	6	8	22	1.9	20	.01	.07	.4	0
Sweet	1 oz	28	150	1	10	6	4	16	27	.4	Trace	.01	.04	.1	Trace
Cider, See Fruits, apple juice															
Gelatin, dry															
Plain	1 tbsp	10	35	9	Trace	—	—	—	—	—	—	—	—	—	—
Dessert powder, 3 oz package	½ cup	85	315	8	0	—	—	75	—	—	—	—	—	—	—

Continued

[21] Year-round average.
[22] Based on the average vitamin A content of fortified margarine. Federal specifications for fortified margarine require a minimum of 15,000 IU of vitamin A per pound.

Nutritive values of the edible part of foods—cont'd

Food, approximate measure, and weight (in grams)			Food energy (calories)	Protein (g)	Fat (total lipid) (g)	Fatty acids			Carbohydrate (g)	Calcium (mg)	Iron (mg)	Vitamin A value (IU)	Thiamin (mg)	Riboflavin (mg)	Niacin (mg)	Ascorbic acid (mg)
						Saturated (total) (mg)	Unsaturated Oleic (g)	Unsaturated Linoleic (g)								
Gelatin dessert, ready-to-eat																
Plain	1 cup	239	140	4	0	—	—	—	34	—	—	—	—	—	—	—
With fruit	1 cup	241	160	3	Trace	—	—	—	40	—	—	—	—	—	—	—
Olives, pickled																
Green	4 medium or 3 extra large or 2 giant	16	15	Trace	2	Trace	2	Trace	Trace	8	.2	40	—	—	—	—
Ripe: Mission	3 small or 2 large	10	15	Trace	2	Trace	2	Trace	Trace	9	.1	10	Trace	Trace	—	—
Pickles, cucumber																
Dill, large, 4 by 1¾ inches	1	135	15	1	Trace	—	—	—	3	35	1.4	140	Trace	.03	Trace	8
Sweet, 2¾ by ¾ inches	1	20	30	Trace	Trace	—	—	—	7	2	.2	20	Trace	Trace	Trace	1
Popcorn, *See* Grain products																
Sherbet, orange	1 cup	193	260	2	2	—	—	—	59	31	Trace	110	.02	.06	Trace	4
Soups, canned; ready-to-serve (prepared with equal volume of water)																
Bean with pork	1 cup	250	170	8	6	1	2	2	22	62	2.2	650	.14	.07	1.0	2

Beef noodle	1 cup	250	70	4	3	1	1	1	7	8	1.0	50	.05	.06	1.1	Trace
Beef bouillon, broth, consomme	1 cup	240	30	5	0	0	0	0	3	Trace	.5	Trace	Trace	.02	1.2	—
Chicken noodle	1 cup	250	65	4	2	1	1	Trace	8	10	.5	50	.02	.02	.8	Trace
Clam chowder	1 cup	255	85	2	3	—	—	—	13	36	1.0	920	.03	.03	1.0	—
Cream soup (mushroom)	1 cup	240	135	2	10	3	5	1	10	41	.5	70	.02	.12	.7	Trace
Minestrone	1 cup	245	105	5	3	—	—	—	14	37	1.0	2,350	.07	.05	1.0	—
Pea, green	1 cup	245	130	6	2	1	1	Trace	23	44	1.0	340	.05	.05	1.0	7
Tomato	1 cup	245	90	2	2	Trace	1	1	16	15	.7	1,000	.06	.05	1.1	12
Vegetable with beef broth	1 cup	250	80	3	2	—	—	—	14	20	.8	3,250	.05	.02	1.2	—
Starch (cornstarch)	1 cup	128	465	Trace	Trace	—	—	—	112	0	0	0	0	0	0	0
	1 tbsp	8	30	Trace	Trace	—	—	—	7	0	0	0	0	0	0	0
Tapioca, quick-cooking granulated, dry, stirred before measuring	1 cup	152	535	1	Trace	—	—	—	131	145	.6	0	0	0	0	0
	1 tbsp	10	35	Trace	Trace	—	—	—	9	1	Trace	0	0	0	0	0
Vinegar	1 tbsp	15	2	0	0	—	—	—	1	1	.1	—	—	—	—	—
White sauce, medium	1 cup	265	430	10	33	18	11	1	23	305	.5	1,220	.12	.44	.6	Trace
Yeast																
Baker's																
Compressed	1 oz	28	25	3	Trace	—	—	—	3	4	1.4	Trace	.20	.47	3.2	Trace
Dry active	1 oz	28	80	10	Trace	—	—	—	11	12	4.6	Trace	.66	1.53	10.4	Trace
Brewer's, dry, debittered	1 tbsp	8	25	3	Trace	—	—	—	3	17	1.4	Trace	1.25	.34	3.0	Trace

Yogurt, *See* Milk, cream; cheese, related products

11-6   Sodium and potassium content of foods, 100 g, edible portion[1]

Food and description	Sodium (mg)	Potassium (mg)	Food and description	Sodium (mg)	Potassium (mg)
Almonds			Beans, mung, sprouted seeds, cooked, boiled, drained	4	156
dried	4	773	Beans, snap		
roasted and salted	198	773	green		
Apples			cooked, boiled, drained	4	151
raw, pared	1	110	canned		
frozen, sliced, sweetened	14	68	regular pack, solids and liquid	236[2]	95
Apple brown betty	153	100	special dietary pack (low sodium), solids and liquid	2	95
Apple butter	2	252	frozen, cut, cooked, boiled, drained	1	152
Apple juice, canned or bottled	1	101	yellow or wax		
Applesauce, canned, sweetened	2	65	cooked, boiled, drained	3	151
Apricots			canned		
raw	1	281	regular pack, solids and liquid	236[2]	95
canned, syrup pack, light	1	239	special dietary pack (low-sodium), solids and liquid	2	95
dried, sulfured, cooked, fruit, and liquid	8	318	frozen, cut, cooked, boiled, drained	1	164
Apricot nectar, canned (approx. 40% fruit)	Trace	151	Beans and frankfurters, canned	539	262
Asparagus			Beef		
cooked spears, boiled, drained	1	183	retail cuts, trimmed to retail level		
canned spears, green			round	60	370
regular pack, solids and liquid	236[2]	166	rump	60	370
special dietary pack (low-sodium), solids and liquids	3	166	hamburger, regular ground, cooked	47	450
frozen			Beef and vegetable stew, canned	411	174
cuts and tips, cooked, boiled, drained	1	220	Beef, corned, boneless		
spears, cooked, boiled, drained	1	238	cooked, medium-fat	1740	150
Avocados, raw, all commercial varieties	4	604	canned corned-beef hash (with potato)	540	200
Bacon, cured, cooked, broiled or fried, drained	1021	236	Beef, dried, cooked, creamed	716	153
Bacon, Canadian, cooked, broiled or fried, drained	2555	432	Beef potpie, commercial, frozen, un-heated	366	93
Baking powders			Beets, common, red canned		
home use			regular pack, solids and liquid	236[2]	167
straight phosphate	8220	170	special dietary pack (low-sodium), solids and liquid	46	167
special low-sodium preparations	6	10,948	Beet greens, common, cooked, boiled, drained	76	332
Bananas, raw, common	1	370	Beverages, alcoholic		
Barbecue sauce	815	174	beer, alcohol 4.5% by volume (3.6% by weight)	7	25
Bass, black sea, raw	68	256		7	25
Beans, common, mature seeds, dry white			gin, rum, vodka, whisky		
cooked	7	416	80-proof (33.4% alcohol by weight)	1	2
canned, solids and liquid, with pork and tomato sauce	463	210	86-proof (36.0% alcohol by weight)	1	2
red, cooked	3	340	90-proof (37.9% alcohol by weight)	1	2
Beans, lima			94-proof (39.7% alcohol by weight)	1	2
immature seeds			100-proof (42.5% alcohol by weight)	1	2
cooked, boiled, drained	1	422	wines		
canned			dessert, alcohol 18.8% by volume (15.3% by weight)	4	75
regular pack, solids and liquid	236[2]	222	table, alcohol 12.2% by volume (9.9% by weight)	5	92
special dietary pack (low-sodium), solids and liquid	4	222			
frozen, thin-seeded types, commonly called baby limas, cooked, boiled, drained	129	394			
mature seeds, dry, cooked	2	612			

[1]Numbers in parentheses denote values imputed—usually from another form of the food or from a similar food. Dashes denote lack of reliable data for a constituent believed to be present in measurable amount.

[2]Estimated average based on addition of salt in the amount of 0.6% of the finished product.

Food and description	Sodium (mg)	Potassium (mg)	Food and description	Sodium (mg)	Potassium (mg)
Biscuits, baking powder, made with enriched flour	626	117	Cabbage		
Biscuit dough, commercial, frozen	910	86	common varieties (Danish, domestic, and pointed types)		
Biscuit mix, with enriched flour, and biscuits baked from mix			raw	20	233
mix, dry form	1300	80	cooked, boiled until tender, drained, shredded, cooked in small amount of water	14	163
biscuits, made with milk	973	116	red, raw	26	268
Blackberries, including dewberries, boysenberries, and youngberries, raw	1	170	Cabbage, Chinese (also called celery cabbage or petsai)	23	253
Blackberries, canned, solids and liquid			Cakes		
water pack, with or without artificial sweetener	1	115	baked from home recipes		
syrup pack, heavy	1	109	angelfood	283	88
Blueberries			fruitcake, made with enriched flour, dark	158	496
raw	1	81	gingerbread, made with enriched flour	237	454
frozen, not thawed, sweetened	1	66	plain cake or cupcake, without icing	300	79
Bluefish, cooked			pound, modified	178	78
baked or boiled	104	—	frozen, commercial, devil's food, with chocolate	420	119
fried	146		Candy		
Boston brown bread	251	292	caramels, plain or chocolate	226	192
Bouillon cubes or powder	24,000	100	chocolate, sweet	33	296
Boysenberries, frozen, not thawed, sweetened	1	105	chocolate-coated, chocolate fudge	228	193
Bran, added sugar and malt extract	1060	1070	gum drops, starch jelly pieces	35	5
Bran flakes (40% bran), added thiamine	925	—	hard	32	4
Bran flakes with raisins, added thiamine	800	—	marshmallows	39	6
Brazil nuts	1	715	peanut bars	10	448
Breads			Carp, raw	50	286
cracked-wheat	529	134	Carrots		
French or vienna, enriched	580	90	raw	47	341
Italian, enriched	585	74	canned		
raisin	365	233	regular pack, solids and liquid	236[2]	120
rye, American (⅓ rye, ⅔ clear flour)	557	145	special dietary pack (low-sodium), solids and liquid	39	120
white, enriched, made with 3%-4% non-fat dry milk	507	105	Cashew nuts	15[6]	464
whole-wheat, made with 2% non-fat dry milk	527	273	Catfish, freshwater, raw	60	330
Bread crumbs, dry, grated	736	152	Cauliflower		
Bread stuffing mix and stuffings prepared from mix, dry form	1331	172	cooked, boiled, drained	9	206
Broccoli			frozen, cooked, boiled, drained	10	207
cooked spears, boiled, drained	10	267	Caviar, sturgeon, granular	2200	180
frozen, spears, cooked, boiled, drained	12	220	Celery, all, including green and yellow varieties		
Brussels sprouts, frozen, cooked, boiled, drained	14	295	raw	126	341
Buffalo fish, raw	52	293	cooked, boiled, drained	88	239
Bulgur (parboiled wheat)			Chard, Swiss, cooked, boiled, drained	86	321
canned, made from hard red winter wheat			Cheese straws	721	63
unseasoned[3]	599	87	Cheeses		
seasoned[4]	460	112	natural cheeses		
Butter[5]	987	23	cheddar (domestic type, commonly called American)	700	82
Buttermilk, fluid, cultured (made from skim milk)	130	140	cottage (large or small curd)		
			creamed	229	85
			uncreamed	290	72
			cream	250	74
			Parmesan	734	149
			Swiss (domestic)	710	104

[3]Processed, partially debranned, whole-kernel wheat with salt added.

[4]Processed, partially debranned, whole-kernel wheat with chicken fat, chicken stock base, dehydrated onion flakes, salt, monosodium glutamate, and herbs.

[5]Values apply to salted butter. Unsalted butter contains less than 10 mg of either sodium or potassium per 100 gm. Value for vitamin A is the year-round average.

[2]Estimated average based on addition of salt in the amount of 0.6% of the finished product.

[6]Applies to unsalted nuts. For salted nuts, value is approximately 200 mg per 100 gm.

Continued.

Sodium and potassium content of foods, 100 g, edible portion—cont'd

Food and description	Sodium (mg)	Potassium (mg)	Food and description	Sodium (mg)	Potassium (mg)
Cheeses—cont'd			Collards, cooked, boiled, drained, leaves, including stems, cooked in small amount of water	25	234
pasteurized process cheese, American	1136[7]	80	Cookies		
pasteurized process cheese spread, American	1625[7]	240	assorted, packaged, commercial	365	67
Cherries			butter, thin, rich	418	60
raw, sweet	2	191	gingersnaps	571	462
canned			molasses	162	138
sour, red, solids and liquid, water pack	2	130	oatmeal with raisins	162	370
sweet, solids and liquid, syrup pack light	1	128	sandwich type	483	38
frozen, not thawed, sweetened	2	130	vanilla wafer	252	72
Chicken			Cookie dough, plain, chilled in roll, baked	548	48
all classes			Corn, sweet		
light meat without skin, cooked, roasted	64	411	cooked, boiled, drained, white and yellow, kernels, cut off cob before cooking	Trace	165
dark meat without skin, cooked, roasted	86	321	canned		
Chicken potpie, commercial, frozen, unheated	411	153	regular pack, cream style, white and yellow, solids and liquid	236[2]	(97)
Chicory, Witloof (also called French or Belgian endive), bleached head (forced), raw	7	182	special dietary pack (low-sodium), cream style, white and yellow, solids and liquid	2	(97)
Chili con carne, canned, with beans	531	233	frozen, kernels cut off cob, cooked, boiled, drained	1	184
Chocolate, bitter or baking	4	830	Corn fritters	477	133
Chocolate syrup, fudge type	89	284	Corn grits, degermed, enriched, dry form	1	80
Chop suey, with meat, canned	551	138			
Chow mein, chicken (without noodles), canned	290	167	Corn products used mainly as ready-to-eat breakfast cereals		
Citron, candied	290	120	corn flakes, added nutrients	1005	120
Clams, raw			corn, puffed, added nutrients	1060	—
soft, meat only	36	235	corn, rice, and wheat flakes, mixed, added nutrients	950	—
hard or round, meat only	205	311	Cornbread, baked from home recipes, southern style, made with degermed cornmeal, enriched	591	157
Clams, canned, including hard, soft, razor, and unspecified solids and liquids	—	140			
Cocoa and chocolate-flavored beverage powders			Cornbread mix and cornbread baked from mix, cornbread, made with egg, milk	744	127
cocoa powder with non-fat dry milk	525	800	Cornmeal, white or yellow, degermed, enriched, dry form	1	120
mix for hot chocolate	382	605			
Cocoa, dry powder			Cornstarch	Trace	Trace
high-fat or breakfast			Cowpeas, including blackeye peas		
plain	6	1,522	immature seeds, canned, solids and liquid	236[2]	352
processed with alkali	717	651	young pods, with seeds, cooked, boiled, drained	3	196
Coconut cream (liquid expressed from grated coconut meat)	4	324			
Coconut meat, fresh	23	256	Crab, canned	1000	110
Cod			Crackers		
cooked, broiled	110	407	butter	1092	113
dehydrated, lightly salted	8100	160	graham, plain	670	384
Coffee, instant, water-soluble			saltines	(1100)	(120)
solids dry powder	72	3,256	sandwich type, peanut-cheese	992	226
beverage	1	36	soda	1100	120
Coleslaw, made with French dressing (commercial)	268	205	Cranberries, raw	2	82

[7]Values for phosphorus and sodium are based on use of 1.5% anhydrous disodium phosphate as the emulsifying agent. If emulsifying agent does not contain either phosphorus or sodium, the content of these two nutrients in milligrams per 100 gm is as follows:

	P	Na
American process cheese	444	650
Swiss process cheese	540	681
American cheese food	427	—
American cheese spread	548	1139

[2]Estimated average based on addition of salt in the amount of 0.6% of the finished product.

Food and description	Sodium (mg)	Potassium (mg)	Food and description	Sodium (mg)	Potassium (mg)
Cranberry juice cocktail, bottled (approx. 33% cranberry juice)	1 1	10 10	Halibut, Atlantic and Pacific, cooked, broiled	134	525
Cranberry sauce, sweetened, canned, strained	1	30	Ham croquette	342	83
Cream, fluid, light, coffee, or table, 20% fat	43	122	Heart, beef, lean, cooked, braised	104	232
Cream substitutes, dried, containing cream, skim milk (calcium reduced), and lactose	575	—	Herring		
			raw, Pacific	74	420
			smoked, hard	6231	157
Cream puffs with custard filling	83	121	Honey, strained or extracted	5	51
Cress, garden, raw	14	606	Horse-radish, prepared	96	290
Croaker, Atlantic, cooked, baked	120	323	Ice cream and frozen custard regular, approximately 10% fat	63[8]	181
Cucumbers, raw, pared	6	160	Ice cream cones	232	244
Custard, baked	79	146	Ice milk	68[8]	195
Dates, domestic, natural and dry	1	648	Jams and preserves	12	88
Doughnuts, cake type	501	90	Kale, cooked, broiled, drained, leaves including stems	43	221
Duck, domesticated, raw, flesh only	74	285	Kingfish; southern, gulf, and northern (whiting); raw	83	250
Eggs, chicken			Lake herring (cisco), raw	47	319
raw			Lamb, retail cuts	70	290
whole, fresh and frozen	122	129	Lemon juice, canned or bottled, unsweetened	1	141
whites, fresh and frozen	146	139	Lettuce, raw crisphead varieties such as iceberg, New York, and Great Lakes strains	9	175
yolks, fresh	52	98			
Eggplant, cooked, boiled, drained	1	150			
Endive (curly endive and escarole), raw	14	294	Lime juice, canned or bottled, unsweetened	1	104
Farina			Liver, beef, cooked, fried	184	380
enriched			Lobster, northern, canned or cooked	210	180
regular			Loganberries, canned, solids and liquid, syrup pack, light	1	111
dry form	2	83			
cooked	144	9	Macadamia nuts	—	164
quick-cooking, cooked	165	10	Macaroni, unenriched, dry form	2	197
instant-cooking, cooked	188	13	Macaroni and cheese, canned	304	58
enriched, regular, dry form	2	83	Margarine[9]	987	23
Figs, canned, solids and liquid, syrup pack, light	2	152	Marmalade, citrus	14	33
			Milk, cow		
Flatfishes (flounders, soles, and sand dabs), raw	78	342	fluid (pasteurized and raw)		
			whole, 3.7% fat	50	144
Fruit cocktail, canned, solids and liquid, water pack, with or without artificial sweetener	5	168	skim	52	145
			canned, evaporated (unsweetened)	118	303
			dry, skim (non-fat solids), regular	532	1745
Garlic, cloves, raw	19	529	malted		
Ginger root, fresh	6	264	dry powder	440	720
Gizzard, chicken, all classes, cooked, simmered	57	211	beverage	91	200
			chocolate drink, fluid, commercial		
Goose, domesticated, flesh only, cooked, roasted	124	605	made with skim milk	46	142
			made with whole (3.5% fat) milk	47	146
Gooseberries, canned, solids and liquid, syrup pack, heavy	1	98	Molasses, cane		
			first extraction or light	15	917
Grapefruit	1	135	third extraction or blackstrap	96	2927
raw, pulp, pink, red, white, all varieties			Muffin mixes, corn, and muffins baked from mixes		
			muffins, made with egg, milk	479	110
canned, juice, sweetened	1	162	muffins, made with egg, water	346	104
Grapefruit juice and orange juice blended, canned, sweetened	1	184	Mushrooms		
			raw	15	414
Grapes, raw, American type (slip skin) such as Concord, Delaware, Niagara, Catawba, and Scuppernong	3	158	canned, solids and liquid	400	197
			Muskmelons, raw, cantaloupes, other netted varieties	12	251
Grapejuice, canned or bottled	2	116			
Guavas, whole, raw, common	4	289	Mussels, Atlantic and Pacific, raw, meat only	289	315
Haddock, cooked, fried	177	348			
Hake, including Pacific hake, squirrel hake, and silver hake or whiting; raw	74	363			

[8]Value for product without added salt.
[9]Values apply to salted margarine. Unsalted margarine contains less than 10 mg per 100 gm of either sodium or potassium. Vitamin A value based on the minimum required to meet federal specifications for margarine with vitamin A added, namely 15,000 IU of vitamin A per pound.   *Continued.*

Sodium and potassium content of foods, 100 g, edible portion—cont'd

Food and description	Sodium (mg)	Potassium (mg)	Food and description	Sodium (mg)	Potassium (mg)
Mustard greens, cooked, boiled, drained	18	220	roasted and salted	418	674
Mustard, prepared			Peanut butters made with small amounts of added fat, salt	607	670
brown	1307	130	Pears		
yellow	1252	130	raw, including skin	2	130
Nectarines, raw	6	294	canned, solids and liquid, syrup pack, light	1	85
New Zealand spinach, cooked, boiled, drained	92	463	Peas, green, immature cooked, boiled, drained canned, Alaska (Early or June peas)	1	196
Noodles, egg noodles, enriched, cooked	2	44	regular pack, solids and liquid	236[2]	96
Oat products used mainly as hot breakfast cereals (oatmeal or rolled oats)			special dietary pack (low-sodium), solids and liquid	3	96
dry form	2	352	frozen, cooked, boiled, and drained	115	135
cooked	218	61	Peas, mature seeds, dry, whole, raw	35	1005
Oat products used mainly as ready-to-eat breakfast cereals			Peas and carrots, frozen, cooked, boiled, drained	84	157
oats (with or without corn), puffed, added nutrients	1267	—	Pecans	Trace	603
Ocean perch, Atlantic (redfish)			Peppers, hot, chili, mature, red, raw, pods excluding seeds	25	465
raw	79	269	Peppers, sweet, garden varieties, immature, green, raw	13	213
cooked, fried	153	284	Perch, yellow, raw	68	230
Ocean perch, Pacific, raw	63	390	Pickles, cucumber, dill	1428	200
Oils, salad or cooking	0	0	Pies		
Okra			baked, piecrust made with unenriched flour		
raw	3	249	apple	301	80
cooked, boiled, drained	2	174	cherry	304	105
Olives, pickled; canned or bottled			mince	448	178
green	2400	55	pumpkin	214	160
ripe, Ascolano (extra large, mammoth, giant jumbo)	813	34	Piecrust or plain pastry, made with enriched flour, baked	611	50
ripe, salt-cured, oil-coated, Greek style	3288	—	Pike, walleye, raw	51	319
Onions, mature (dry), raw	10	157	Pineapple		
Onions, young green (bunching varieties), raw bulb and entire top	5	231	raw	1	146
Oranges, raw, peeled fruit, all commercial varieties	1	200	frozen chunks, sweetened, not thawed	2	100
Orange juice			Pizza, with cheese, from home recipe, baked		
raw, all commercial varieties	1	200	with cheese topping	702	130
canned, unsweetened	1	199	with sausage topping	729	168
frozen concentrate, unsweetened, diluted with 3 parts water, by volume	1	186	Plate dinners, frozen, commercial, unheated		
Oysters			beef pot roast, whole oven-browned potatoes, peas, and corn	259	244
raw, meat only, Eastern	73	121	chicken, fried; mashed potatoes; mixed vegetables (carrots, peas, corn, beans)	344	112
cooked, fried	206	203			
frozen, solids and liquid	380	210	meat loaf with tomato sauce, mashed potatoes, and peas	393	115
Oyster stew, commercial frozen, prepared with equal volume of milk	366	176	turkey, sliced; mashed potatoes; peas	400	176
Pancake and waffle mixes and pancakes baked from mixes, plain and buttermilk, made with egg, milk	564	154	Plums		
			raw, Damson	2	299
Parsnips, cooked, boiled, drained	8	379	canned, solids and liquid, purple (Italian prunes), syrup pack, light	1	145
Peaches			Popcorn, popped		
raw	1	202	plain	(3)	—
canned, solids and liquid, water pack, with or without artificial sweetener	2	137	oil and salt added	1950	—
			Pork, fresh		
frozen, sliced, sweetened, not thawed	2	124	retail cuts, trimmed to retail level	65	390
Peanuts			loin		
roasted with skins	5	701			

[2]Estimated average based on addition of salt in the amount of 0.6% of the finished product.

Food and description	Sodium (mg)	Potassium (mg)	Food and description	Sodium (mg)	Potassium (mg)
Pork, cured, light-cure, commercial, ham, medium-fat class, separable lean, cooked, roasted	930	326	rice, puffed; added nutrients, without salt	2	100
Pork, cured, canned ham, contents of can	(1100)	(340)	rice, puffed or open-popped, presweetened, honey and added nutrients	706	—
Potatoes			Rockfish, including black, canary, yellowtail, rasphead, and bocaccio, cooked, oven-steamed	68	446
cooked, boiled in skin	3[10]	307			
dehydrated mashed			Roe, cooked, baked or broiled, cod and shad[12]	73	132
flakes without milk			Rolls and buns		
dry form	89	1600	commercial		
prepared, water, milk, table fat added	231	286	ready-to-serve		
			Danish pastry	366	112
Pretzels	1680[11]	130	hard rolls, enriched	625	97
Prunes	3	262	plain (pan rolls), enriched	506	95
dried, "softenized," cooked (fruit and liquid), with added sugar			sweet rolls	389	124
Pudding mixes and puddings made			Rusk	246	161
from mixes with starch base			Rutabagas, cooked, boiled, drained	4	167
pudding made with milk, cooked	129	136	Rye, flour, medium	(1)	203
pudding made with milk, without cooking	124	129	Rye wafers, whole-grain	882	600
			Salad dressings, commercial[13]		
Pumpkin, canned	2	240	Blue and Roquefort cheese		
Radishes, raw, common	18	322	regular	1094	37
Raisins, natural (unbleached)			special dietary (low-calorie)	1108	34
cooked, fruit and liquid, added sugar	13	355	low-fat (approx. 5 cal per tsp)		
			French		
Raspberries			regular	1370	79
canned, solids and liquid, water pack, with or without artificial sweetener, red	1	114	special dietary (low-calorie)	787	79
			low-fat (approx. 5 cal per tsp)		
frozen, red, sweetened, not thawed	1	100	mayonnaise	597	34
Rennin products			Thousand Island		
tablet (salts, starch, rennin enzyme)	22,300	—	regular	700	113
dessert mixed and desserts prepared from mixes			special dietary (low-calorie, approx. 10 cal per tsp)	700	113
			Salmon		
chocolate, dessert made with milk	52	125	Coho (silver)		
			raw	48[15]	421
other flavors (vanilla, caramel, fruit flavorings)			canned, solids and liquid	351[14]	339
mix, dry form	6	—	Salt pork, raw	1212	42
dessert, made with milk	46	128	Salt sticks, regular type	1674	92
			Sandwich spread (with chopped pickle)		
Rhubarb, cooked, added sugar	2	203	regular	626	92
Rice			special dietary (low-calorie, approx. 5 cal per tsp)	626	92
brown					
raw	9	214	Sardines, Atlantic, canned in oil, drained solids	823	590
cooked	282	70			
white (fully milled or polished) enriched			Sardines, Pacific, in tomato sauce, solids and liquid	400	320
common commercial varieties, all types			Sauerkraut, canned, solids and liquid	747[16]	140
raw	5	92	Sausage, cold cuts, and luncheon meats		
cooked	374	28	bologna, all samples	1300	230
Rice products used mainly as ready-to-eat breakfast cereals			frankfurters, raw, all samples	1100	220
rice flakes, added nutrients	987	180	luncheon meat, pork, cured ham or shoulder, chopped, spiced or unspiced, canned	1234	222

[10]Applies to product without added salt. If salt is added, an estimated average value for sodium is 236 mg per 100 gm.

[11]Sodium content is variable. For example, very thin pretzel sticks contain about twice the average amount listed.

[12]Prepared with butter or margarine, lemon juice or vinegar.

[13]Values apply to products containing salt. For those without salt, sodium content is low, ranging from less than 10 mg to 50 mg per 100 gm; the amount usually is indicated on the label.

[14]For product canned without added salt, value is approximately the same as for raw salmon.

[15]Sample dipped in brine contained 215 mg sodium per 100 gm.

[16]Values for sauerkraut and sauerkraut juice are based on salt content of 1.9% and 2.0%, respectively, in the finished products. The amounts in some samples may vary significantly from this estimate.

Continued.

Food and description	Sodium (mg)	Potassium (mg)	Food and description	Sodium (mg)	Potassium (mg)
Sausage, cold cuts, and luncheon meats—cont'd			Tea, instant (water-soluble solids)	—	4530
pork sausage, links or bulk, cooked	958	269	carbohydrate added dry powder beverage	—	25
Scallops, bay and sea, cooked, steamed	265	476	Tomatoes, ripe		
Soups, commercial, canned			raw	3	244
beef broth, bouillon, and consomme, prepared with equal volume of water	326	54	canned, solids and liquid, regular pack	130	217
			Tomato catsup, bottled	1042[17]	363
chicken noodle, prepared with equal volume of water	408	23	Tomato juice		
			canned or bottled		
tomato			regular pack	200	227
prepared with equal volume of water	396	94	special dietary pack (low-sodium)	3	227
			Tomato juice cocktail, canned or bottled	200	221
prepared with equal volume of milk	422	167	Tomato puree, canned		
vegetable beef, prepared with equal volume of water	427	66	regular pack	399	426
			special dietary pack (low-sodium)	6	426
Soy sauce	7325	366	Tongue, beef, medium-fat, cooked, braised	61	164
Spaghetti, enriched, cooked, tender stage	1	61	Tuna, canned		
			in oil, solids and liquid	800	301
Spaghetti, in tomato sauce with cheese, canned	382	121	in water, solids and liquid	41[18]	279[18]
Spinach			Turkey, all classes		
cooked, boiled, drained	50	324	light meat, cooked, roasted	82	411
canned			dark meat, cooked, roasted	99	398
regular pack, drained solids	236[2]	250	Turkey potpie, commercial, frozen, unheated	369	114
special dietary pack (low-sodium), solids and liquid	34	250	Turnips, cooked, boiled, drained	34	188
frozen, chopped, cooked, boiled, drained	52	333	Turnip greens, leaves, including stems		
			canned, solids and liquids	236[2]	243
Squash, summer, all varieties, cooked, boiled, drained	1	141	frozen, cooked, boiled, drained	17	149
			Veal, retail cuts, untrimmed	80	500
Squash, frozen			Vinegar, cider	1	100
summer, yellow crookneck, cooked, boiled, drained	3	167	Waffles, frozen, made with enriched flour	644	158
winter, heated	1	207	Walnuts		
Strawberries			black	3	460
raw	1	164	Persian or English	2	450
frozen, sweetened, not thawed, sliced	1	112	Watercress leaves including stems, raw	52	282
			Watermelon, raw	1	100
Sturgeon, cooked, steamed	108	235	Wheat flours		
Succotash (corn and lima beans), frozen, cooked, boiled, drained	38	246	whole (from hard wheats)	3	370
			patent		
Sugars, beet or cane, brown	30	344	all-purpose or family flour, enriched	2	95
Sweet potatoes			self-rising flour, enriched (anhydrous monocalcium phosphate used as a baking aid)[19]	1079	—[20]
cooked, all, baked in skin	12	300			
canned, liquid pack, solids and liquid, regular pack in syrup	48	(120)			
dehydrated flakes, prepared with water	45	140	Wild rice, raw	7	220
Tangerines, raw (Dancy variety)	2	126	Yeast		
Tapioca, dry	3	18	baker's, compressed	16	610
Tapioca desserts, tapioca cream pudding	156	135	brewer's, debittered	121	1894
			Yogurt, made from whole milk	47	132
Tartar sauce, regular	707	78	Zweiback	250	150

[2]Estimated average based on addition of salt in the amount of 0.6% of the finished product.

[17]Applies to regular pack. For special dietary pack (low sodium), values range from 5 to 35 mg per 100 gm.

[18]One sample with salt added contained 875 mg of sodium per 100 gm and 275 mg of potassium.

[19]The acid ingredient most commonly used in self-rising flour. When sodium acid pyrophosphate in combination with either anhydrous monocalcium phosphate or calcium carbonate is used, the value for calcium is approximately 120 mg per 100 gm; for phosphorus, 540 mg; for sodium 1360 mg.

[20]90 mg of potassium per 100 gm contributed by flour. Small quantities of additional potassium may be provided by other ingredients.

11-7 Cholesterol content of foods

Item	Amount of cholesterol in			Item	Amount of cholesterol in		
	100 gm edible portion[1] (mg)	Edible portion of 450 gm (1 lb) as purchased (mg)	Refuse from item as purchased (%)		100 gm edible portion[1] (mg)	Edible portion of 450 gm (1 lb) as purchased (mg)	Refuse from item as purchased (%)
Beef, raw				Liver, raw	300	1360	0
with bone[2]	70	270	15	Lobster			
without bone[2]	70	320	0	whole[2]	200	235	74
Brains, raw	>2000	>9000	0	meat only[2]	200	900	0
Butter	250	1135	0	Margarine			
Caviar or fish roe	>300	>1300	0	all vegetable fat	0	0	0
Cheese				two-thirds animal	65	295	0
cheddar	100	455	0	fat, one-third			
cottage, creamed	15	70	0	vegetable fat			
cream	120	545	0	Milk			
other (25% to 30%)	85	385	0	fluid, whole	11	50	0
(fat)				dried, whole	85	385	0
Cheese spread	65	295	0	fluid, skin	3	15	0
Chicken, flesh only,	60	—	0	Mutton			
raw				with bone[2]	65	250	16
Crab				without bone[2]	65	295	0
in shell[2]	125	270	52	Oysters			
meat only[2]	125	565	0	in shell[2]	>200	>90	90
Egg, whole	550	2200	12	meat only[2]	>200	>900	0
Egg white	0	0	0	Pork			
Egg yolk				with bone[2]	70	260	18
fresh	1500	6800	0	without bone[2]	70	320	0
frozen	1280	5800	0	Shrimp			
dried	2950	13,380	0	in shell[2]	125	390	31
Fish				flesh only[2]	125	565	0
steak[2]	70	265	16	Sweetbreads (thymus)	250	1135	0
fillet[2]	70	320	0	Veal			
Heart, raw	150	680	0	with bone[2]	90	320	21
Ice cream	45	205	0	without bone[2]	90	410	0
Kidney, raw	375	1700	0				
Lamb, raw							
with bone[2]	70	265	15				
without bone[2]	70	320	0				
lard and other animal	95	430	0				
fat							

[1]Data apply to 100 gm of edible portion of the item, although it may be purchased with the refuse indicated and described or implied in the final column.
[2]Designate items that have the same chemical composition for the edible portion but differ in the amount of refuse.

MATERNITY AND PEDIATRICS

12-1 Pregnancy table for expected date of delivery

Find the date of the last menstrual period in the top line (light-face type) of the pair of lines.
The dark number (bold-face type) in the line below will be the expected day of delivery.

Jan.	1	2	3	4	5	6	7	8	9	10	11	12	13	14	15	16	17	18	19	20	21	22	23	24	25	26	27	28	29	30	31	
Oct.	**8**	**9**	**10**	**11**	**12**	**13**	**14**	**15**	**16**	**17**	**18**	**19**	**20**	**21**	**22**	**23**	**24**	**25**	**26**	**27**	**28**	**29**	**30**	**31**	**(1**	**2**	**3**	**4**	**5**	**6**	**7**	Nov.
Feb.	1	2	3	4	5	6	7	8	9	10	11	12	13	14	15	16	17	18	19	20	21	22	23	24	25	26	27	28				
Nov.	**8**	**9**	**10**	**11**	**12**	**13**	**14**	**15**	**16**	**17**	**18**	**19**	**20**	**21**	**22**	**23**	**24**	**25**	**26**	**27**	**28**	**29**	**30**	**(1**	**2**	**3**	**4**	**5**				Dec.
Mar.	1	2	3	4	5	6	7	8	9	10	11	12	13	14	15	16	17	18	19	20	21	22	23	24	25	26	27	28	29	30	31	
Dec.	**6**	**7**	**8**	**9**	**10**	**11**	**12**	**13**	**14**	**15**	**16**	**17**	**18**	**19**	**20**	**21**	**22**	**23**	**24**	**25**	**26**	**27**	**28**	**29**	**30**	**31**	**(1**	**2**	**3**	**4**	**5**	Jan.
April	1	2	3	4	5	6	7	8	9	10	11	12	13	14	15	16	17	18	19	20	21	22	23	24	25	26	27	28	29	30		
Jan.	**6**	**7**	**8**	**9**	**10**	**11**	**12**	**13**	**14**	**15**	**16**	**17**	**18**	**19**	**20**	**21**	**22**	**23**	**24**	**25**	**26**	**27**	**28**	**29**	**30**	**31**	**(1**	**2**	**3**	**4**		Feb.
May	1	2	3	4	5	6	7	8	9	10	11	12	13	14	15	16	17	18	19	20	21	22	23	24	25	26	27	28	29	30	31	
Feb.	**5**	**6**	**7**	**8**	**9**	**10**	**11**	**12**	**13**	**14**	**15**	**16**	**17**	**18**	**19**	**20**	**21**	**22**	**23**	**24**	**25**	**26**	**27**	**28**	**(1**	**2**	**3**	**4**	**5**	**6**	**7**	Mar.
June	1	2	3	4	5	6	7	8	9	10	11	12	13	14	15	16	17	18	19	20	21	22	23	24	25	26	27	28	29	30		
Mar.	**8**	**9**	**10**	**11**	**12**	**13**	**14**	**15**	**16**	**17**	**18**	**19**	**20**	**21**	**22**	**23**	**24**	**25**	**26**	**27**	**28**	**29**	**30**	**31**	**(1**	**2**	**3**	**4**	**5**	**6**		April
July	1	2	3	4	5	6	7	8	9	10	11	12	13	14	15	16	17	18	19	20	21	22	23	24	25	26	27	28	29	30	31	
April	**7**	**8**	**9**	**10**	**11**	**12**	**13**	**14**	**15**	**16**	**17**	**18**	**19**	**20**	**21**	**22**	**23**	**24**	**25**	**26**	**27**	**28**	**29**	**30**	**(1**	**2**	**3**	**4**	**5**	**6**	**7**	May
Aug.	1	2	3	4	5	6	7	8	9	10	11	12	13	14	15	16	17	18	19	20	21	22	23	24	25	26	27	28	29	30	31	
May	**8**	**9**	**10**	**11**	**12**	**13**	**14**	**15**	**16**	**17**	**18**	**19**	**20**	**21**	**22**	**23**	**24**	**25**	**26**	**27**	**28**	**29**	**30**	**31**	**(1**	**2**	**3**	**4**	**5**	**6**	**7**	June
Sept.	1	2	3	4	5	6	7	8	9	10	11	12	13	14	15	16	17	18	19	20	21	22	23	24	25	26	27	28	29	30		
June	**8**	**9**	**10**	**11**	**12**	**13**	**14**	**15**	**16**	**17**	**18**	**19**	**20**	**21**	**22**	**23**	**24**	**25**	**26**	**27**	**28**	**29**	**30**	**(1**	**2**	**3**	**4**	**5**	**6**	**7**		July
Oct.	1	2	3	4	5	6	7	8	9	10	11	12	13	14	15	16	17	18	19	20	21	22	23	24	25	26	27	28	29	30	31	
July	**8**	**9**	**10**	**11**	**12**	**13**	**14**	**15**	**16**	**17**	**18**	**19**	**20**	**21**	**22**	**23**	**24**	**25**	**26**	**27**	**28**	**29**	**30**	**31**	**(1**	**2**	**3**	**4**	**5**	**6**	**7**	Aug.
Nov.	1	2	3	4	5	6	7	8	9	10	11	12	13	14	15	16	17	18	19	20	21	22	23	24	25	26	27	28	29	30		
Aug.	**8**	**9**	**10**	**11**	**12**	**13**	**14**	**15**	**16**	**17**	**18**	**19**	**20**	**21**	**22**	**23**	**24**	**25**	**26**	**27**	**28**	**29**	**30**	**31**	**(1**	**2**	**3**	**4**	**5**	**6**		Sept.
Dec.	1	2	3	4	5	6	7	8	9	10	11	12	13	14	15	16	17	18	19	20	21	22	23	24	25	26	27	28	29	30	31	
Sept.	**7**	**8**	**9**	**10**	**11**	**12**	**13**	**14**	**15**	**16**	**17**	**18**	**19**	**20**	**21**	**22**	**23**	**24**	**25**	**26**	**27**	**28**	**29**	**30**	**(1**	**2**	**3**	**4**	**5**	**6**	**7**	Oct.

12-2 | The Washington guide to promoting development in the young child

Motor skills

Expected tasks	Suggested activities
1 to 3 months	
1. Holds head up briefly when prone	1. Place infant in prone position
2. Head erect and bobbing when supported in sitting position	2. Support in sitting position with his head erect
3. Head erect and steady in sitting position	3. Pull infant to sitting position
4. Follows object through all planes	4. Provide with opportunity to observe people or activity
5. Palmar grasp	5. Hang bright-colored objects and mobiles within reach across crib
6. Moro reflex	6. Provide with opportunity to observe objects or people while in sitting position
	7. Use infant seat
	8. Alternate bright shiny objects with dark and light visual patterns
4 to 8 months	
1. Sits with minimal support, with stable head and back	1. Pull up to sitting position
2. Sits alone steadily	2. Provide opportunity to sit supported or alone when head and trunk control are stabilized
3. Plays with hands, which are open most of time	3. Put bright-colored objects within reach
4. Grasps rattle or bottle with both hands	4. Give toys or household objects: rattles, teething ring, cloth animals or dolls, 1-inch cubes, plastic objects such as cups, rings, and balls
5. Picks up small objects, for example, cube	5. Offer small objects such as cereal to improve grasp
6. Transfers toys from one hand to other	6. Offer a variety of patterns or textures to play with
7. Neck-righting reflex	7. Use squeak toys
9 to 12 months	
1. Rises to sitting position	1. Provide playpen, allow child to pull himself to standing
2. Creeps or crawls, maybe backward at first	2. Give opportunity and space to practice creeping and crawling
3. Pulls to standing position	3. Have child practice moving on knees to improve balance prior to walking
4. Stands alone	4. Have child use walker or straddle toys
5. Cruises	5. Play airplane with child; have child practice catching himself while rolling on large ball
6. Uses index finger to poke	6. Provide with objects such as spoons, plastic bottles, cups, ball, cubes, finger foods, saucepans, and lids
7. Finger-thumb grasp	
8. Parachute reflex	
9. Landau reflex	
13 to 18 months	
1. Walks a few steps without support	1. Provide opportunity to practice walking, climbing stairs with help
2. Balance when walking	2. Give toys that can be pushed around
3. Walks upstairs with help, creeps downstairs	3. Supervise activity with paper and large crayons
4. Turns pages of book	4. Provide toys such as cubes, cups, saucepans, lids, rag dolls, and other soft, cuddly toys
	5. Begin introducing child to swing
19 to 30 months	
1. Runs	1. Provide opportunity to practice and develop activities
2. Walks up and down stairs, one at a time (not alternating feet)	2. Provide pattern for child while he watches and then encourage him to try
3. Imitates vertical strokes	3. Provide tricycle or similar pedal toys; secure foot on pedal if necessary
4. Imitates building tower of four or more blocks	
5. Throws ball overhand	
6. Jumps in place	
7. Rides tricycle	

Motor skills—cont'd

Expected tasks	Suggested activities
31 to 48 months 1. Walks downstairs (alternating feet) 2. Hops on one foot 3. Swings and climbs 4. Balances on one foot for 10 seconds 5. Copies circle 6. Copies cross 7. Draws person with three parts	1. Continue with blocks, combining materials, toy cars, and trains 2. Provide clay and other manipulating materials 3. Give opportunities to swing and climb 4. Provide with activities such as finger painting, chalk, and black board
49 to 52 months 1. Balances well 2. Skips and jumps 3. Can heel-toe walk 4. Copies square 5. Catches bounced ball	1. Provide with music and games to synchronize hand and foot, tapping with music, skipping, hopping, and dancing rhythmically to improve coordination

Feeding skills

Expected tasks	Suggested activities
1 to 3 months 1. Sucking reflex present 2. Rooting reflex present 3. Ability to swallow pureed foods 4. Coordinates sucking, swallowing, and breathing	1. Consider a change in nipple or posturing if there is difficulty in swallowing 2. Introduce solids, one kind at a time (use small spoon, place food well back on infant's tongue) 3. Hold in comfortable relaxed position while feeding 4. Pace feeding tempo to infant's needs
4 to 8 months 1. Tongue used in moving food in mouth 2. Hand-to-mouth motions 3. Recognizes bottle on sight 4. Gums or mouths solid foods 5. Feeds self cracker	1. Give finger foods to develop chewing, stimulate gums, and encourage hand-to-mouth motion (cubes of cheese, bananas, dry toast, bread crust, cookies) 2. Encourage upright supported position for feeding 3. Promote bottle holding 4. Introduce junior foods
9 to 12 months 1. Holds own bottle 2. Drinks from cup or glass with assistance 3. Finger feeds 4. Beginning to hold spoon	1. Bring child in highchair to table and include in part of or entire meal with family 2. Have child in dry comfortable position with trunk and feet supported 3. Encourage self-help in feeding; use of table foods 4. Offer spoon when interest is indicated 5. Introduce cup or glass with small amount of fluid
13 to 18 months 1. Holds cup and handle with digital grasp 2. Lifts cup and drinks well 3. Beginning to use spoon, may turn bowl down before reaching mouth 4. Difficulty in inserting spoon into mouth 5. May refuse food	1. Continue offering finger foods (wieners, sandwiches) 2. Use nontip dishes and cups; dishes should have sides to make filling of spoon easy 3. Give opportunity for self-feeding 4. Provide fluids between meals rather than having child fill up on fluids at mealtime
19 to 30 months 1. Drinks without spilling 2. Holds small glass in one hand 3. Inserts spoon in mouth correctly 4. Distinguishes between food and inedible material 5. Plays with food	1. Encourage self-feeding with spoon 2. Do not rush child 3. Serve foods plainly but in attractive servings 4. Small servings of food will encourage eating more than large servings

Feeding skills—cont'd

Expected tasks	Suggested activities
31 to 48 months 1. Pours well from pitcher 2. Serves self at table with little spilling 3. Rarely needs assistance 4. Interest in setting table	1. Encourage self-help 2. Give opportunity for pouring (give rice and pitcher to promote pouring skills) 3. Encourage child to help set table 4. Have well-defined rules about table manners
49 to 52 months 1. Feeds self well 2. Social and talkative during meal	1. Socialize with child at mealtime 2. Have child help with preparation, table setting, and serving 3. Include child in conversations at mealtimes by planning special times for him to tell about events, situations, or what he did during the day

Sleep

Expected tasks	Suggested activities
1 to 3 months 1. Night: 4- to 10-hour intervals 2. Naps: frequent 3. Longer periods of wakefulness without crying	1. Provide separate sleeping arrangements away from parent's room 2. Reduce noise and light stimulation when placing in bed 3. Have room at comfortable temperature with no drafts or extremes in heat 4. Reverse position of crib occasionally 5. Place child in different positions from time to time for sleep 6. Alternate from back to side to stomach 7. Keep crib sides up
4 to 8 months 1. Night: 10 to 12 hours 2. Naps: 2 to 3 (1 to 4 hours in duration) 3. Night awakenings	1. Keep crib sides up 2. Refrain from taking child into parents' room if he awakens 3. Check to determine if there is cause for awakenings: hunger, teething, pain, cold, wet, noise, or illness 4. If a baby-sitter is used, attempt to find some person with whom infant is familiar. Explain bedtime and naptime arrangements
9 to 12 months 1. Night: 12 to 14 hours 2. Naps: one to two (1 to 4 hours in duration) 3. May begin refusing morning nap	1. Short crying periods may be source of tension release for child 2. Observe for signs of fatigue, irritability, or restlessness if naps are shorter 3. Provide familiar person to baby-sit who knows sleep routines
13 to 18 months 1. Night: 10 to 12 hours 2. Naps: one in afternoon (1 to 3 hours in duration) 3. May awaken during night crying (associated with wetting bed) 4. As he becomes more able to move about, he may uncover himself, become cold, and awaken	1. Night terrors may be terminated by awakening infant and offering reassurance 2. Check to see that child is covered 3. Avoid hazardous devices to keep child covered, including blanket clips, pins, and garments that enclose child to neck
19 to 30 months 1. Night: 10 to 12 hours 2. Naps: one (1 to 3 hours duration) 3. Doesn't go to sleep at once—keeps demanding things 4. May awaken crying if wet or soiled 5. May awaken because of environmental change of temperature, change of bed, change of sleeping room, addition of sibling to room, absence of parent from home, hospitalization, trip with family, or relatives visiting	1. Quiet period of socialization prior to bedtime—reading child book or telling story 2. Holding child—talking quietly with him 3. Ritualistic behavior may be present; allow child to carry out routine; helps him overcome fear of unexpected or fear of dark, for example, child may wish to arrange toys in certain way 4. Explain bedtime ritual to baby-sitter 5. Give more reassurance, spend more time before bedtime preparation 6. Provide familiar bedtime toys or items 7. Allow crying-out period if he is safe, comfortable, and tucked in 8. Place in bed before he reaches excessive state of fatigue, excitement, or tiredness 9. Eliminate sources of stimulation or fear 10. Maintain consistent hour of bedtime

Continued.

Sleep—cont'd

Expected tasks	Suggested activities
31 to 48 months 1. Daily range: 10 to 15 hours 2. Naps: beginning to disappear 3. Prolongs process of going to bed 4. Less dependent on taking toys to bed 5. May awaken crying from dreams 6. May awaken if wet	1. Television programs may affect ability to go to sleep: avoid violent television programs 2. Anxiety about going to bed and desire to stay up with parents requires limits 3. Regularity and consistency important to promote good sleep habits 4. Reassurance—night light or leaving door ajar 5. Do not use bedtime or naptime as punishment 6. Encourage naps if signs of fatigue or irritability are evidenced
49 to 52 months 1. Daily range: 9 to 13 hours 2. Naps: rare 3. Quieter during sleep	1. Encourage napping if excessive or strenuous activity occurs and child is overly tired 2. Explain to child if baby-sitter will be there after child is asleep

Play

Expected tasks	Suggested activities
1 to 3 months 1. Quieted when picked up 2. Regards face of others	1. Encourage holding and touching of child by mother 2. Provide with cradle gyms and mobiles, brightly colored, visually interesting objects within arm's distance
4 to 8 months 1. Plays with own body 2. Differentiates strangers from family 3. Seeks out objects 4. Grasps, holds, and manipulates objects 5. Repeats activities he enjoys 6. Bangs toys or objects together	1. Begin patty-cake and peekaboo 2. Provide for periods of solitary play (playpen) 3. Encourage holding and touching of child by mother 4. Provide variety of multicolored and multitextured objects that child can hold 5. Encourage exploration of body parts 6. Provide floating toys for bath
9 to 12 months 1. Puts objects in and out of containers 2. Examines objects held in hand 3. Plays interactive games (peekaboo) 4. Extends toy to other person without releasing 5. Works to get toy out of reach	1. Continue mother-infant games 2. Give opportunity to place objects in containers and pour out 3. Provide large and small objects with which to play 4. Encourage interactive play
13 to 18 months 1. Plays by himself—may play near others 2. Has preferred toys 3. Enjoys walking activities, pulling toys 4. Throws and picks up objects, throws again 5. Imitates, for example, reading newspaper, sweeping	1. Introduce to other children even though child may not play with them 2. Provide music, books, and magazines 3. Encourage imitative activities—helping with dusting, sweeping, stirring
19 to 30 months 1. Parallel play—not interactive but plays alongside another child 2. Uses both large and small toys 3. Rough-and-tumble play 4. Play periods longer than before—interested in manipulative and constructive toys 5. Enjoys rhymes and singing (television programs)	6. Provide with new materials for manipulating and feeling—finger paints, clay, sand, stones, water, and soap Wooden toys—cars and animals Building blocks of various sizes, crayons, and paper Rhythmical tunes and equipment—swing, rocking chair, rocking horse Children's books—short, simple stories with repetition and familiar objects; enjoys simple pictures, brightly colored 7. Guide child's hand to actively participate with specific activities, for example, using crayons, hammering
31 to 48 months 1. In playing with others, beginning to interact, sharing toys, taking turns 2. Dramatizes, expresses imagination in play 3. Combining playthings; more use of constructive materials 4. Prefers two or three children to play with; may have special friend	1. Encourage play with small groups of children 2. Encourage imaginative and dramatic play activities 3. Music: singing and experimenting with musical instruments 4. Group participation in rhymes, dancing by hopping or jumping 5. Drawing and painting (seldom recognizable)

Play—cont'd

Expected tasks	Suggested activities
49 to 52 months 1. Dramatic play and interest in going on excursions 2. Fond of cutting and pasting, creative materials 3. Completes most activities	1. Painting and drawing (objects will be out of proportion; details that are most important to child are drawn largest) 2. Encourage printing of numbers and letters 3. Clay: making recognizable objects 4. Cutting and pasting 5. Provide with materials, for example, boxes, chairs, barrels, for building sturdy structures

Language

Expected tasks	Suggested activities
1 to 3 months *Receptive abilities* 1. Movement of eyes, respiration rate, or body activity changes when bell is rung close to child's head 2. Smiles when socially stimulated 3. Has facial, vocal, and generalized bodily responses to faces 4. Reacts differently to adult voices *Expressive abilities* 1. Makes prelanguage vocalizations that consist of cooing, throaty sounds, for example, gu 2. Makes "pleasure" sounds that consist of soft vowels 3. Makes "sucking" sounds 4. Crying can be differentiated for discomfort, pain, and hunger as reported by mother 5. An "A" sound as in cat is commonly heard in distress crying	1. Observe facial expressions, gestures, bodily postures, and movements when vocalizations are being produced 2. Smile and talk softly in pleasant tone while holding, touching, and handling infant 3. Hold, touch, and interact frequently with infant for pleasure 4. Refrain from letting infant engage in prolonged and incessant crying
4 to 8 months *Receptive abilities* 1. Eyes locate source of sound 2. Responds to "hi, there" by looking up at face that is across and in front of him 3. Head turns to sound of cellophane held and crunched 2 feet away and at a 135-degree angle on either side of head 4. Will turn head to locate sound of "look here" when spoken at a 90-degree angle from head 2 feet away* 5. Turns head to sound of rattle 6. Responds differently to vacuum cleaner, phone, doorbell, or sound of dog barking: may cry, whimper, look toward sound, or mother may report change in body tension 7. Responds by raising arms when mother reaches toward child and says "come up" *Expressive abilities* 1. Uses different inflectional patterns: ah uh ah 2. Laughs aloud when stimulated 3. Has differential patterns of crying when hungry, in pain, or angry 4. Produces vowel sounds and chained syllables (baba, gugu, didi) 5. Makes "talking sounds" in response to others talking to him 6. Babbles to produce consonant sounds: ba, da, m-m 7. Vocalizes to toys 8. Says "da-da" or "ma-ma" but not specific to presence of parents	1. Engage in smiling eye-to-eye contact while talking to infant 2. Vocalize in response to inflectional patterns and when infant is producing babbling sounds; echo the sounds he makes 3. Observe for subtle communication clues such as eye aversion, struggling to move away, flushing of skin, tension of body, or movement of arms 4. Vocalize with infant during handling, while feeding, bathing, dressing, diapering, bedtime preparation, and holding 5. Stimulate laughing by light tickling 6. Observe child's reactions to bells, whistles, horns, phones, laughing, singing, talking, music box, noisemaking toys, and common household noises 7. While talking to infant, hold in position so that he can see your face 8. Have infant placed at position of eye level while talking to him throughout the day 9. If crying or laughing sounds are not discerned at this stage, report to family physician, pediatrician, public health nurse, or well-child clinic

*Do not test for localization of sound by producing sound directly behind infant's head.

Continued.

Language—cont'd

Expected tasks	*Suggested activities*

9 to 12 months
Receptive abilities
1. Ceases activity when name is pronounced or "no-no" is said
2. Gives toys on request when accompanied by facial and bodily gestures
3. Attends to simple commands

Expressive abilities
1. Imitates definite speech sounds such as tongue clicking, lip smacking, or coughing
2. Should have two words that are *specific* for parents: "mama," "dada," or equivalents

1. Gain child's attention when giving simple commands
2. Accompany oral directions with gestures
3. Vocalize with child during feeding, bathing, and playtimes
4. Provide sounds that child can reproduce such as lip smacking and tongue clicking
5. Repeat direction frequently and have child participate in action: open and close the drawer; move arms and legs up and down
6. Have child respond to verbal directions: stand up, sit down, close door, open door, turn around, come here

13 to 18 months
Receptive abilities
1. Attends to person speaking to child
2. Finds "the baby" in picture when requested, for example, on baby food jar, in magazine, or in storybooks
3. Indicates wants by gestures
4. Looks toward family members or pets when named

Expressive abilities
1. Uses three words other than mama and dada to denote *specific* objects, persons, or actions
2. Indicates wants by naming object such as cookie

1. Incorporate repetition into daily routine of home
   a. Feeding: name baby's food and eating utensils; ask if he is enjoying his dessert; concentrate on reviewing a day's events in simple manner
   b. Household duties: mother names each item as she dusts; pronounces word while cooking and preparing foods
   c. Playing: identify toys when using them; explain their function
2. Let child see mouthing of words
3. Encourage verbalization and expression of wants

19 to 30 months
Receptive abilities
1. Points to one named body part
2. Follows two or three verbal directions that are not accompanied by facial or body gestures, for example, put ball on table, give it to mommy, or put toy in box

Expressive abilities
1. Combines two different words, for example, "play ball," "want cookie"
2. Names object in picture, for example, cat, bird, dog, horse, man
3. Refers to self by pronoun rather than by name

1. Continue to present concrete objects with words; talk about activities child is involved with
2. Include child in conversations during mealtimes
3. Encourage speech by having child express wants
4. Incorporate games into bathing routine by having child name and point to body parts
5. As child gains confidence in remembering and using words appropriately, encourage less use of gestures
6. Count and name articles of clothing as they are placed on child
7. Count and name silverware as it is placed on table
8. Sort, match, and name glassware, laundry, cans, vegetables, and fruit with child
9. Have child keep scrapbook and add new picture every day to increase recognition of vocabulary words
10. Spend 15 to 20 minutes per day going through booklets and naming pictures; have child point to pictures as objects are named
11. Help child develop functional core vocabulary to express safety needs and information about neighborhood
12. Whenever possible, use word (for example, paper), show object, have child handle and use it, encourage him to watch your face while you say the words, and suggest that he repeat it; refrain from undue pressure

31 to 36 months
Receptive abilities
1. Takes turns when asked while playing, eating
2. Attends longer to stories and television programs
3. Demonstrates understanding of two prepositions by carrying out two commands one at a time, for example, "put the block under the chair"
4. Can follow commands asking for two objects or two actions
5. Demonstrates understanding of concepts of big and little, for example, selects larger of two balls when asked for big one
6. Points to additional body parts

1. Read stories with familiar content but with more detail; nonsense rhymes, humorous stories
2. Expect child to follow simple commands
3. Give child opportunity to hear and repeat his full name
4. Listen to child's explanation about pictures he draws
5. Encourage child to repeat nursery rhymes by himself and with others
6. Address child by his first name

Language—cont'd

Expected tasks	Suggested activities

31 to 36 months—cont'd
Expressive abilities

1. Uses regular plurals, for example, adds "s" to apple, box, orange (does not use irregular plurals, for example, mouse to mice)
2. Gives first and last name
3. Names what he has drawn after scribbling
4. On request, tells you his sex; for example, "Are you a little boy or a little girl?"
5. Can repeat a few rhymes or songs
6. On request, tells what action is going on in picture, for example, the kitten is eating

37 to 48 months

1. Expresses appropriate responses when asked what child does when tired, cold, or hungry
2. Tells stories
3. Common expression: I don't know
4. Repeats sentence composed of twelve to thirteen syllables, for example, "I am going when daddy and I are finished playing"
5. Has mastered phonetic sounds of p, k, g, v, tf, d z, lr, hw, j, kw, l, e, w, qe, and o

1. Provide visual stimuli while reading stories
2. Have child repeat story
3. Arrange trips to zoo, farms, seashore, stores, and movies and discuss with child
4. Give simple explanations in answering questions

49 to 52 months
Receptive abilities

1. Points to penny, nickel, or dime on request
2. Carries out in order command containing three parts, for example, "pick up the block, put it on the table, and bring the book to me"

Expressive abilities

1. Names penny, nickel, or dime on request
2. Replies appropriately to questions such as, "What do you do when you are asleep?"
3. Counts three objects, pointing to each in turn
4. Defines simple words, for example, hat, ball
5. Asks questions
6. Can identify or name four colors

1. Play games in which child names colors
2. Encourage use of please and thank you
3. Encourage social-verbal interactions with other children
4. Encourage correct usage of words
5. Provide puppets or toys with movable parts that child can converse about
6. Provide group activity for child; children may stimulate each other by taking turns naming pictures
7. Allow child to make choices about games, stories, and activities
8. Have child dramatize simple stories
9. Provide child with piggy bank and encourage naming coins as they are handled or dropped into bank

Discipline

Expected tasks	Suggested activities

1 to 3 months

1. Draws attention by crying

2. Infant desires whatever is pleasant and wishes to avoid unpleasant situations
3. Beginning to "wiggle" around

1. a. Needs should be identified and met as promptly as possible
   b. Every bit of fussing should not be interpreted as emergency requiring immediate attention
   c. Infant should not be ignored and permitted to cry for exhaustive periods
2. Begin to present limit of having to wait so that infant can learn that tension and discomfort are bearable for short periods
3. Place infant on surfaces that have sides to protect him from falling off

Continued.

Discipline—cont'd

Expected tasks	*Suggested activities*

4 to 8 months

1. Begins to respond to "no-no"

   1. a. Reserve "no-no" for times when it is really needed
      b. Be consistent with word "no-no" for same activity and event that requires it; be friendly and firm with verbal control of limit setting

2. Infant who is left alone for long periods of time may become bored or fretful; learns that crying and whining result in attention

   2. Make special efforts to attend to infant when he is quiet and amusing himself

3. Beginning to show signs of timidity and fretfulness and may whimper and cry when mother separates from him or when strangers pick him up

   3. a. Gradually introduce strangers into infant's environment
      b. Refrain from promoting frightening situations with strangers during this stage
      c. Play hiding games like peekaboo in which mother disappears and reappears
      d. Allow infant to cling to mother and get used to persons a little at a time
      e. If baby-sitter is used, find person familiar to infant or introduce for brief periods before mother leaves infant in her care
      f. Encourage gentle handling by mother, father, and siblings. Discourage rough handling, particularly by strangers

4. Beginning to grasp objects and bring to mouth, but unable to differentiate safe from hazardous items.

   4. a. Provide toys that do not have small detachable parts
      b. Check frequently for small objects in his line of reach
   5. When traveling in car, place in crib or seat with safety belts securely fastened

9 to 12 months

1. Beginning to respond to simple commands, for example, "pick up the ball, put the toy in the box"

   1. a. Avoid setting unreasonable number of limits
      b. Give simple commands one at a time
      c. Once limit is set, adhere to it firmly each time and connect it immediately with misbehavior
      d. Respond with consistency in enforcing rule
      e. Allow time to conform to request
      f. Gain child's attention

2. Ready to go places on his own and is trying out newly developing motor capacities (not to be confused with naughtiness, "spoiled," or stubbornness)

   2. a. Begin setting and enforcing limits on where child is allowed to travel and explore
      b. Remove tempting objects
      c. Remove sources of danger such as light sockets, protruding pot handles, hanging table covers, sharp objects, and hanging cords
      d. Keep child away from fans, heaters, and certain drawers and do not place vaporizer close to infant's crib
      e. Keep high chair at least 2 feet away from working and cooking surfaces in kitchen
      f. Use gate to keep child out of kitchen when it is being used
      g. Be certain that pans, basins, and tubs of hot water are never left unattended
      h. Remove all possible poisons or substances that are not food that can be eaten or drunk off floor, low-level cabinets, and under sink
      i. Keep child from objects or surfaces that he may chew, for example, porch rails, windowsills, *repainted* toys or cribs that may contain lead
      j. Instruct baby-sitter on all safety items

3. Has emerging desires to look at, handle, and touch objects

   3. a. Experiment with diversionary measures
      b. Provide child with own play objects

4. Explores objects by sucking, chewing, and biting

   4. a. Remove household poisons, cosmetics, pins, and buttons that he could put in his mouth
      b. Be certain that objects that go into mouth are hygienic
      c. Check toys for detachable small parts

Discipline—cont'd

Expected tasks	Suggested activities

9 to 12 months—cont'd

5. Beginning to test reactions to certain parental responses during feeding and may become choosy about food

    5. a. Once problem behaviors are defined, plan to work on changing only one behavior at a time until child behaves or conforms to expectations
      b. Be certain that child understands old rules before adding new ones
      c. Respond with consistency in enforcing old rules: enforce each time, do not ignore next time
      d. Provide regular pattern of mealtimes
      e. Refrain from feeding throughout day
      f. Allow child to decide what he will eat and how much
      g. Introduce new foods gradually over period of time
      h. Continue to offer foods that may have been rejected first time
      i. Do not force food
      j. Refrain from physically punishing child for changes in eating habits

6. Beginning to test reactions to parental responses at bedtime preparation

    6. a. Provide regular time for naps and bedtime
      b. Avoid excessive stimulation at bedtime or naptime
      c. Ignore fussing and crying once safety and physical needs are satisfied and usual ritual is carried out
      d. Keep child in own room
      e. Refrain from picking up and rocking and holding if needs seem satisfied

13 to 18 months

1. Understands simple commands and requests

    1. a. Begin with one rule; add new ones as appropriate
      b. In selecting new rules, choose on the basis of being able to clearly define it to self and child, having it reasonable and enforceable at all times; demand no more than fulfillment of defined expectations
      c. Plan decisive limits and plan to give consistent attention to them

2. In learning mastery over impulses and self-control, child begins testing out limit setting

    2. a. Immediately correct errors in behavior as they occur
      b. Use consistent enforcement of short-term rules (which are given as verbal commands) and long-term rules (which pertain to chores and family routines)
      c. Ignore temper tantrums
      d. Show child when you approve of his behavior and praise for obedience throughout day

3. With increasing fine motor control, child can manipulate objects that may be hazardous

    3. a. Set limits regarding play with doorknobs and car door handles
      b. Keep away from open windows; latch screens
      c. Supervise around pools and ponds or drain or fence them
      d. Lock cabinets
      e. Keep open jars and bottles out of reach
      f. Use gate to protect child from falling down stairs

19 to 30 months

1. Attention span increasing

    1. a. Gain attention before giving simple commands, one at a time; praise for success
      b. Add new rules as child conforms to old ones
      c. Refrain from expecting *immediate* obedience

2. Begins simple reasoning—asks question why; may be repetitive

    2. Make special efforts to answer questions; give simple explanations; gauge need for simplicity by number of times act is repeated or question asked

3. Interested in further exploration of environment; may lack physical control

    3. a. Supervise on stair rails and waxed floors
      b. Set rules about crossing streets and carrying knives, sharp objects, or glass objects
      c. Have outdoor play area securely fenced or supervised
      d. When riding in car, secure child safely by seat belt or car seat
      e. Keep matches out of reach
      f. Shield adult tools such as knives, lawnmowers, sharp tools

4. Negativistic behavior is expected; responds more frequently with word "no"; may show more resistance at bedtime preparation and during mealtime

    4. a. Practice consistency in responding to behavior
      b. Allow more time to conform to expectation

Continued.

Discipline—cont'd

Expected tasks	Suggested activities

19 to 30 months—cont'd

5. Behavior may change if new sibling is introduced into family unit

   5. a. Explain verbally or through play that new child is expected
      b. Exercise more patience with child
      c. Set special times aside for parental attention to child
      d. Allow child to help with special care tasks of new sibling

31 to 48 months

1. Displays more interest in conforming

   1. a. Exercise consistency in parental demands; enforce each time and avoid ignoring behavior next time
      b. Show concrete approval and give immediate recognition for acceptable behavior
      c. Refrain from use of threats that produce fearfulness

2. Shows greater understanding when simple reasoning is communicated

   2. a. Give simple explanations; allow child chance to demonstrate understanding by talking about event, situation, or rule
      b. Eliminate unnecessary and impractical rules
      c. Refrain from constant verbal reprimands
      d. Denial of privileges should not be excessive or prolonged

3. Will respond to simple commands such as putting toys away

   3. a. Assign simple household tasks that child can carry out each day; show approval for performance and success
      b. Decide if child is capable of doing what is asked by observing him
      c. Determine how much time is necessary to complete a chore or activity before expecting maximum performance

4. Displays a greater independence in general activities

   4. a. Be extra cautious about supervising riding tricycles in streets and watching for cars in driveways
      b. Do not permit dashing into street while playing
      c. Do not allow child to follow ball into street
      d. Areas under swings and slides should not be paved
      e. Provide an imitative model that child can copy, for example, do not jaywalk
      f. Provide scissors that are blunt tipped

49 to 52 months

1. Can be given two or three assignments at one time; will carry out in order
2. Complies readily with reasonable, well-defined, and consistent requirements
3. Understands reasoning

   1. Give more opportunities to be independent
   2. Use simple explanations and reasoning
   3. Ask child to define role if he disobeys
   4. Have child correct mistakes as they occur
   5. Do not use punishment without warnings
   6. Praise for successful performance
   7. Use gold stars on chart for rewards
   8. If leaving for social obligation, vacation, or visiting away from home, let child know
   9. Avoid making promises that cannot be kept
  10. Avoid bribing, ridicule, shaming, teasing, inflicting pain, using unfavorable comparison with other children, and exhibition of behavior by parents they are trying to stop in child
  11. Remember that child may be imitating models of behavior set up by parents, brothers, sisters, a neighborhood child, or maybe a television hero
  12. Recognize that there are stress periods in family or child's life that may result in changes in child's behavior including accidents, illness, moving into new neighborhood, separation from friends, death, divorce, and hospitalization of child or parents (be more patient with child's behavior, give more time to conform, show more approval for mastery of tasks, and exercise consistency in handling problems as they occur)

Dressing

Expected tasks	Suggested activities
13 to 18 months 1. Cooperates in dressing by extending arm or leg 2. Removes socks, hat, mittens, shoes 3. Can unzip zippers 4. Tries to put shoes on	1. Encourage child to remove socks, etc. after task is initiated for him 2. Do not rush child 3. Have him practice with large buttons and with zippers
19 to 30 months 1. Can undress 2. Can remove shoes if laces are untied 3. Helps dress 4. Tries to unbutton 5. Pulls on simple clothes	1. Provide opportunities to button with extra-large–sized buttons 2. Encourage and allow opportunity for self-help in getting drink, removing clothes with help, hand washing, unbuttoning, etc. 3. Simple clothing 4. Provide mirror at height child can observe himself for brushing teeth, etc.
31 to 48 months 5. Greater interest and ability in dressing 6. Intent on lacing shoes (usually does incorrectly) 7. Does not know back from front 8. Washes and dries hands, brushes teeth 9. Can button	1. Provide with own dresser drawer 2. Simple garments encourage self-help; do not rush child 3. Provide large buttons, zippers, slipover clothing 4. Self hand washing but help with brushing teeth 5. Provide regular routine for dressing, either in bathroom or bedroom
49 to 52 months 1. Dresses and undresses with care except for tying shoes and buckling belts 2. May learn to tie shoes 3. Combs hair with assistance	1. Assign regular task of placing clothes in hamper or basket 2. Continue to use simple clothing 3. Encourage self-help in dressing and undressing 4. Allow child to select clothes he will wear

Toilet training

Expected tasks	Suggested activities
9 to 12 months 1. Beginning to show regular patterns in bladder and bowel elimination 2. Has one to two stools daily 3. Interval of dryness does not exceed 1 to 2 hours	1. Watch for clues that indicate child is wet or soiled 2. Be sure to change diapers when wet or soiled so that child begins to experience contrast between wetness and dryness
13 to 18 months 3. Will have bowel movement if put on toilet at approximate time 4. Indicates wet pants	1. Sit child on toilet or potty chair at regular intervals for short periods of time throughout day 2. Praise child for success 3. If potty chair is used, it should be located in bathroom 4. Training should be started when social disruptions are at minimum 5. Respond promptly to signals and clues of child by taking him to bathroom or changing pants 6. Use training pants, once toilet training is commenced 7. Plan to begin training when disruptions in regular routine are minimized, that is, do not begin on vacation

Toilet training—cont'd

Expected tasks	*Suggested activities*
19 to 30 months 1. Anticipates need to eliminate 2. Same word for both functions 3. Daytime control (occasional accident) 4. Requires assistance (reminding, dressing, wiping)	1. Continue regular intervals of toileting 2. Reward success 3. Dress in simple clothing that child can manage 4. Remind occasionally, particularly after mealtime, juicetime, naptime, and playtime 5. Take to bathroom before bedtime 6. Bathroom should be convenient to use, easy to open door
31 to 48 months 1. Takes responsibility for toilet if clothes are simple 2. Continues to verbalize need to go; apt to hold out too long 3. May have occasional accident 4. Needs help with wiping	1. May still need reminding 2. Dress in simple clothing that child can manage 3. Ignore accidents; refrain from shame or ridicule
49 to 52 months 1. General independence (anticipates needs, undresses, goes, wipes, washes hands)	1. Praise child for his accomplishment

12-3   Immunization schedules

Recommended schedule for active immunization of normal infants and children* in the United States

Recommended age[b]	Immunization(s)[c]	Comments
2 mo	DTP, HbCV[d], OPV	DTP and OPV can be initiated as early as age 4 weeks after birth in areas of high endemicity or during epidemics
4 mo	DTP, HbCV[d], OPV	2-mo interval (minimum of 6 weeks) desired for OPV to avoid interference from previous dose
6 mo	DTP, HbCV[d]	A third dose of OPV is not indicated in the U.S. but is desirable in geographic areas where polio is endemic
15 mo	MMR[e], HbCV[f]	Tuberculin testing may be done at the same visit
15-18 mo	DTP[g,h] OPV‖	See footnotes
4-6 yr	DTP[j], OPV	At or before school entry
11-12 yr	MMR	At entry to middle school or junior high school unless second dose previously given
14-16 yr	Td	Repeat every 10 yr throughout life

From American Academy of Pediatrics: *Report of the committee on infectious diseases,* ed 22, Elk Grove Village, Ill, 1991. Copyright American Academy of Pediatrics, 1991.

[a]For all products used, consult manufacturer's package insert for instructions for storage, handling, dosage, and administration.

[b]These recommended ages should not be construed as absolute. For example, 2 months can be 6 to 10 weeks. However, MMR usually should not be given to children younger than 12 months. (If measles vaccination is indicated, monovalent measles vaccine is recommended, and MMR should be given subsequently, at 15 months.)

[c]DTP = diphtheria and tetanus toxoids with pertussis vaccine; HbCV, *Haemophilus* b conjugate vaccine; OPV = oral poliovirus vaccine containing attenuated poliovirus types 1, 2, and 3; MMR = live measles, mumps, and rubella viruses in a combined vaccine; Td = adult tetanus toxoid (full dose) and diphtheria toxoid (reduced dose) for adult use.

[d]Two HbCVs are approved for use in children younger than 15 months.

[e]May be given at 12 months of age in areas with recurrent measles transmission.

[f]Any licensed *Haemophilus* b conjugate vaccine may be given.

[g]Should be given 6 to 12 months after the third dose.

[h]May be given simultaneously with MMR at age 15 months.

[i]May be given simultaneously with MMR and HbCV at 15 months of age or at any time between 12 and 24 months of age; priority should be given to administering MMR at the recommended age

[j]Can be given up to the seventh birthday.

Recommended immunization schedules for children in the United States not immunized in first year of life

Recommended time/age	Immunization(s)[a]	Comments
Less than 7 years old		
First visit	DTP, OPV, MMR	MMR if child ≥ 15 mo old; tuberculin testing may be done at same visit
	HbCV[b]	For children aged 18-59 mo; can be given concurrently with DTP (at separate sites) and other vaccines[c]
Interval after first visit:		
2 mo	DTP, OPV (HbCV)	Second dose of HbCV is indicated only in children whose first dose was received when younger than 15 months
4 mo	DTP	A third dose of OPV is not indicated in the U.S. but is desirable in geographic areas where polio is endemic
10-16 mo	DTP, OPV	OPV is not given if third dose was given earlier
4-6 yr (at or before school entry)	DTP, OPV	DTP is not necessary if the fourth dose was given after the fourth birthday; OPV is not necessary if third dose was given after the fourth birthday; OPV is not necessary if third dose was given after fourth birthday
11-12 yr	MMR	At entry to middle school or junior high
10 yr later	Td	Repeat every 10 yr throughout life
7 Years old and older		
First visit	Td, OPV, MMR	
Interval after first visit:		
2 mo	Td, OPV	
8-14 mo	Td, OPV	
11-12 yr	MMR	At entry to middle school or junior high
10 yr later	Td	Repeat every 10 yr throughout life

From American Academy of Pediatrics: *Report of the committee on infectious diseases,* ed 22, Elk Grove Village, Ill, 1991. Copyright American Academy of Pediatrics, 1988.

[a]Abbreviations are explained in footnote c to previous table.

[b]If child is younger than 15 months, two HbCVs are approved for use.

[c]The initial three doses of DTP can be given at 1- to 2-month intervals; so, for the child in whom immunization is initiated at age 15 months or older, one visit could be eliminated by giving DTP, OPV, and MMR at the first visit; DTP and HbCV at the second visit (1 month later); and DTP and OPV at the third visit (2 months after the first visit). Subsequent DTP and OPV 10 to 16 months after the first visit are still indicated. HbCV, MMR, DTP, and OPV can be given simultaneously at separate sites if return of vaccine recipient for future immunizations is a concern.

[d]If person is ≥ 18 years old, routine poliovirus vaccination is not indicated in the United States.

[e]Minimal interval between doses of MMR is 1 month.

Routine immunization schedule for infants and children in Canada

Age	Immunization against			
2 months	Diphtheria	Pertussis	Tetanus	Poliomyelitis
4 months	Diphtheria	Pertussis	Tetanus	Poliomyelitis
6 months	Diphtheria	Pertussis	Tetanus	Poliomyelitis[1]
12 months	Measles	Mumps	Rubella[2]	
18 months	Diphtheria	Pertussis	Tetanus	Poliomyelitis
	Haemophilus influenzae b[3]			
4-6 years	Diphtheria	Pertussis	Tetanus	Poliomyelitis
14-16 years	Diphtheria[4]		Tetanus[4]	Poliomyelitis[1]

From National Advisory Committee on Immunization: *Canadian immunization guide,* ed 3, Canada, 1989, Authority of the Minister of National Health and Welfare, Health Protection Branch, Laboratory Centre for Disease Control.

Notes:

1. This dose may be omitted if live (oral) polio vaccine is being used exclusively.
2. Rubella vaccine is also indicated for all girls and women of childbearing age who lack proof of immunity. At all medical visits, the opportunity should be taken to check whether girls and women need rubella vaccine.
3. A single dose of *Haemophilus influenzae* b (Hib) conjugate vaccine should be administered to all children ages 18 to 24 months. Children ages 25 to 60 months should also be considered for vaccination, particularly those in daycare centers and at increased risk of invasive Hib disease. Conjugate vaccine should be given at the first visit for children aged over 18 months who are unlikely to return for further immunization. Conjugate vaccine and diphtheria pertussis tetanus (DPT) vaccines may be given simultaneously at different sites.
4. Diphtheria and tetanus toxoid (Td), a combined absorbed "adult-type" preparation for use in persons 7 years of age or more, contains less diphtheria toxoid than preparations given to younger children and is less likely to cause reactions in older persons.

Routine immunization schedules for children not immunized in early infancy in Canada

Timing	Immunization against			
For children 1 through 6 years of age				
First visit[3,5]	Diphtheria	Pertussis	Tetanus	Poliomyelitis
Interval after first visit:				
1 month	Measles	Mumps	Rubella[2]	
2 months	Diphtheria	Pertussis	Tetanus	Poliomyelitis
4 months	Diphtheria	Pertussis	Tetanus	Poliomyelitis[1]
16 months	Diphtheria	Pertussis	Tetanus	Poliomyelitis
Preschool[6]	Diphtheria	Pertussis	Tetanus	Poliomyelitis
See Note 3	*Haemophilus influenzae* b			
At age 14-16 years	Diphtheria[4]	Tetanus[4]	Poliomyelitis[1]	
For children 7 years of age and over				
First visit[5]	Diphtheria[4]		Tetanus[4]	Poliomyelitis
Interval after first visit:				
1 month	Measles	Mumps	Rubella[2]	
2 months	Diphtheria		Tetanus	Poliomyelitis
14 months	Diphtheria		Tetanus	Poliomyelitis
10 years	Diphtheria		Tetanus	Poliomyelitis[1]

From National Advisory Committee on Immunization: *Canadian immunization guide*, ed 3, Canada, 1989, Authority of the Minister of National Health and Welfare, Health Protection Branch. Laboratory Centre for Disease Control.

Notes:

1-4. See preceding table.

5. Measles, mumps and rubella vaccines may also be given at the first visit if it is considered likely that a child will not return for further immunization.

6. If the last dose of the primary series for diphtheria, pertussis, tetanus, and poliomyelitis is given after the fourth birthday, this dose may be omitted.

ROUTINE IMMUNIZATIONS: CONTRAINDICATIONS/ PRECAUTIONS

Diptheria, Tetanus, Pertussis (DTP)

Moderate to severe febrile illness

Immediate, severe, anaphylactic reaction to previous administration of one of these vaccines

Encephalopathy within 7 days after previous administration

The following are precautions, not contraindications, to receiving the next dose of pertussis vaccine:

A convulsion, with or without fever, occurring within 3 days after previous administration

Persistent, inconsolable screaming or crying for 3 or more hours within 48 hours after previous administration

Data from American Academy of Pediatrics: *Report of the committee on infectious diseases,* ed 22, Elk Grove Village, Ill, 1991, The Academy; and Recommendations of the Immunization Practices Advisory Committee (ACIP): Diphtheria, tetanus, and pertussis: recommendations for vaccine use and other preventive measures, *MMWR* 40(RR-10):1-28, 1991. For more detailed information consult these reports, the vaccine manufacturers' package insert, and the child's health care practitioner.
From Wong DL: *Whaley and Wong's essentials of pediatric nursing,* ed 4, St Louis, 1993, Mosby.

Collapse or shocklike state within 48 hours after previous administration

Temperature of 40.5° C (104.9° F) or greater, unexplained by another cause, within 48 hours after previous administration

Measles, Mumps, and Rubella (MMR); Oral Poliovirus (OPV)

Moderate to severe febrile illness

Anaphylactic egg hypersensitivity

Anaphylactic reaction to neomycin

Pregnancy

NOTE: Live OPV may be given if substantial risk of exposure is present (inactivated poliovirus [IPV] is preferred if immunization can be completed before anticipated exposure)

Congenital disorders of immune function

Immunosuppressive therapy (except investigational varicella vaccine); may immunize 3 months after immunosuppressive therapy is discontinued

NOTE:

Children receiving steroid therapy are evaluated for the risk of live virus vaccines (IPV may be given)

Children with symptomatic or asymptomatic human immunodeficiency virus (HIV) infection should receive all routine vaccines except oral poliovirus vaccine (IPV can be given)

12-4   Common childhood communicable and infectious diseases

Disease	Transmission	Infectious agent	Incubation period	Report to local health authority
Chickenpox	Direct and indirect contact with droplets from respiratory passages; extremely contagious disease	Varicella-zoster	2-3 weeks; commonly 13-17 days	In some areas
Tetanus	Tetanus spores enter body through a wound contaminated with soil and feces; necrotic tissue favors the growth of the bacillus	Tetanospasmin	3-21 days; commonly 10 days	Case report required
Diphtheria	Direct or indirect contact with exudate from mucous membranes of infected person or carrier; raw milk may also be a vehicle	*Corynebacterium diphtheriae*	2-5 days	Case report required
Pertussis (whooping cough)	Direct contact with droplets from respiratory passages	*Bordetella pertussis*	7-21 days; commonly 7 days	Case report required
Poliomyelitis	Direct and indirect contact with respiratory discharges and feces; fecal-oral route more common than respiratory transmission	Enteroviruses: type I most frequent, type II least frequent, type III second most frequent	3-35 days; commonly 7-14 days	Case report required
Mumps (infectious parotitis)	Direct contact with saliva droplets from infected person	Virus	2-3 weeks; commonly 18 days	Case report required in some areas
Rubella (German measles)	Direct or indirect contact with nasopharyngeal secretions of infected persons; transplacental transmission leads to congenital rubella syndrome	Virus	14-23 days; commonly 16-18 days	Case report required
Rubeola (hard measles)	Direct or indirect contact with nasal secretions from infected persons; highly communicable	Paramyxovirus	Commonly 10 days; 8-13 days until fever, 14 days until rash	Case report required

13 PHARMACOLOGY

13-1 Guide to common drug interactions

Drug	Interacting drug	Effect
Over-the-counter drugs and substances		
Antacids		
Alumina and magnesia Dihydroxaluminum sodium carbonate Magnesia		Effects of dicumarol may be faster and/or increased
	Digoxin	Effects of digoxin may be reduced

	Tetracyclines
	  Doxycycline
	  Tetracycline
		Effects of tetracyclines may be reduced
		Should be taken 1-3 hours apart

Painkillers		
Acetaminophen Buffered acetaminophen	Alcoholic beverages	May cause liver damage
	Blood-thinning drugs Warfarin sodium	High doses of acetaminophen may increase blood-thinning effects of these drugs
	Tetracycline	Buffered form may cancel the effects of tetracycline Should be taken 1 hour apart
Ibuprofen	Alcoholic beverages	May cause internal bleeding or ulcers

	Blood-thinning drugs
	  Heparin
	  Warfarin sodium
		May cause internal bleeding or ulcers

	Salicylates
	  Aspirin
	  Aspirin and caffeine
	  Buffered aspirin
		May cause stomach upset without relieving symptoms

Salicylates
  Aspirin
  Aspirin and caffeine
Buffered aspirin
	Alcoholic beverages	May cause stomach ulcers or internal bleeding

	Antidiabetics
	  Chlorpropamide
	  Tolazamide
		May cause blood sugar level to drop too low

	Blood-thinning drugs
	  Heparin
	  Warfarin sodium
		Increases risk of internal bleeding

	Ibuprofen	May cause stomach upset without relieving symptoms
	Tetracycline	Effects of tetracycline are reduced

This table includes only common over-the-counter and prescription drugs. Some of these drugs may also interact with less common drugs and substances not described. When using any drug, always consult your doctor or pharmacist about possible interactions with other drugs, substances, or foods.

Continued.

Guide to common drug interactions—cont'd

Drug	Interacting drug	Effect
Other substances		
Alcoholic beverages	Acetaminophen Buffered acetaminophen	May cause liver damage
	Antidiabetics Chlorpropamide Tolazamide	Stomach upset, vomiting, cramps, headaches, low blood sugar
	Antiseizure drugs Carbamazepine Chlordiazepoxide Diazepam Phenytoin	May cause extreme drowsiness
	Barbiturates Pentobarbital Phenobarbital Secobarbital Secobarbital and amobarbital	May cause drowsiness, increase effects of either drug, cause breathing to fail, or cause blood pressure to drop too low
	Ibuprofen	May cause internal bleeding or ulcers
	Narcotic analgesics Acetaminophen and codeine Meperidine Propoxyphene	May depress nervous system and breathing or cause blood pressure to drop too low
	Reserpine	May increase effects of alcohol and reserpine
	Salicylates Aspirin Aspirin and caffeine Buffered aspirin	May cause stomach ulcers or internal bleeding
	Tricyclic antidepressants Amitriptyline Amoxapine Doxepin	May cause extreme drowsiness
Sodium chloride (salt)	Lithium	Low-salt diet causes lithium to build up in body and is not advised
Tobacco (smoking)	Birth control pills Norethindrone with ethinyl estradiol	May increase chances of blood clot or heart attack
Tyramine-containing foods Avocados, bananas, beer, caffeine, cheese, chicken liver, chocolate, fava beans, fermented sausages (salami, pepperoni, bologna, etc.), canned figs, pickled herring, pineapple, raisins, red wine, sauerkraut, soy sauce, yeast extract, yogurt	MAO inhibitors Isocarboxazid Phenelzine Tranylcypromine	May cause severe and sometimes fatal high blood pressure Headache, vomiting, fever, and high blood pressure are warning signals
Prescription drugs		
Antibiotics		
Erythromycins Erythromycin Erythromycin lactobionate Penicillins Amoxicillin Ampicillin	Penicillins Amoxicillin Ampicillin	Could interfere with the effects of penicillins
Penicillins Amoxicillin Ampicillin	Birth control pills Norethindrone with ethinyl estradiol	May interfere with and result in unplanned pregnancy or menstrual problems

This table includes only common over-the-counter and prescription drugs. Some of these drugs may also interact with less common drugs and substances not described. When using any drug, always consult your doctor or pharmacist about possible interactions with other drugs, substances, or foods.

Drug	Interacting drug	Effect
	Blood-thinning drugs Warfarin sodium	May increase blood thinning effects of these drugs
	Erythromycins Erythromycin Erythromycin lactobionate	May interfere with effects of penicillins
	Tetracyclines Doxycycline Tetracycline	May interfere with effects of penicillins
Tetracyclines Doxycycline Tetracycline	Acetaminophen Buffered acetaminophen	
	Antacids Alumina and magnesia Dihydroxaluminum sodium carbonate Magnesia	May decrease effects of tetracyclines and should be taken 1 to 3 hours apart
	Barbiturates Pentobarbital Phenobarbital Secobarbital Secobarbital and amobarbital	May decrease effects of doxycycline Other tetracyclines can be used
	Penicillins Amoxicillin Ampicillin	May interfere with effects of penicillins
	Salicylates Aspirin Aspirin and caffeine Buffered aspirin	Effects of tetracyclines are reduced
Antidepressants Lithium	Sodium chloride (salt)	Low-salt diet causes lithium to build up in body and is not advised
	Thiazide diuretics Furosemide Methyclothiazide	May cause lithium to have toxic effect
Tricyclic antidepressants Amitriptyline Amoxapine Doxepin	Alcoholic beverages	May cause extreme drowsiness
	Antiseizure drugs Carbamazepine Chlordiazepoxide Diazepam Phenytoin	Effects of antiseizure drug may be decreased Dosage should be adjusted
	Blood-thinning drugs Warfarin sodium	May cause internal bleeding
	MAO inhibitors Isocarboxazid Phenelzine Tranylcypromine	Severe seizure and death could result Should be taken 14 days apart
	Narcotic analgesics Acetaminophen and codeine Meperidine Propoxyphene	May depress nervous system and breathing and cause blood pressure to drop too low

Continued.

Guide to common drug interactions—cont'd

Drug	Interacting drug	Effect
Antidiabetics Chlorpropamide Tolazamide	Alcoholic beverages	May cause stomach upset, vomiting, cramps, headaches, low blood sugar
	Beta-adrenergic blockers Metoprolol Propranolol	May increase risk of either high or low blood sugar levels May mask symptoms
	Blood-thinning drugs Warfarin sodium	Blood-thinning effect will be increased at first, later it will be decreased May also cause low blood sugar and become toxic
	MAO inhibitors Isocarboxazid Phenelzine Tranylcypromine	Can cause extreme low blood sugar level
	Salicylates Aspirin Aspirin and caffeine Buffered aspirin	May cause blood sugar level to drop too low
Isophane insulin suspension	Beta-adrenergic blockers Metoprolol Propranolol	These may mask symptoms of low blood sugar
	Birth control pills Norethindrone with ethinyl estradiol	May increase risk of high blood sugar levels Dosages should be adjusted
	MAO inhibitors Isocarboxazid Phenelzine Tranylcypromine	May cause extreme low blood sugar level
Antiseizure drugs Carbamazepine Chlordiazepoxide Diazepam Phenytoin	Alcoholic beverages	May cause extreme drowsiness
	Beta-adrenergic blockers Metoprolol Propranolol	Could decrease the effect of beta-blockers
	Birth control pills Norethindrone with ethinyl estradiol	Phenytoin and carbamazepine may interfere and increase risk of unplanned pregnancy May increase effect of diazepam
	Tricyclic antidepressants Amitriptyline Amoxapine Doxepin	Effects of antiseizure drug may be decreased Dosage should be adjusted
Barbiturates Pentobarbital Phenobarbital Secobarbital Secobarbital and amobarbital	Alcoholic beverages	May cause drowsiness, increase effects of either drug, cause breathing to fail, or cause blood pressure to drop too low
	Birth control pills Norethindrone with ethinyl estradiol	Barbiturates may interfere with and result in unplanned pregnancy
	Blood-thinning drugs Warfarin sodium	May decrease blood-thinning effects of these drugs
	Doxycycline	May decrease effects of doxycycline Other tetracyclines can be used

This table includes only common over-the-counter and prescription drugs. Some of these drugs may also interact with less common drugs and substances not described. When using any drug, always consult your doctor or pharmacist about possible interactions with other drugs, substances, or foods.

Drug	Interacting drug	Effect
Birth control pills Norethindrone with ethinyl estradiol	Antiseizure drugs Carbamazepine Chlordiazepoxide Diazepam Phenytoin	Will increase the sedative effects of these drugs May decrease the effects of other antiseizure drugs
	Barbiturates Pentobarbital Phenobarbital Secobarbital Secobarbital and amobarbital	Barbiturates may interfere with birth control pills and result in unplanned pregnancy
	Isophane insulin suspension	May increase risk of high blood sugar levels; dosages should be adjusted
	Penicillins Amoxicillin Ampicillin	May interfere with birth control pills and result in unplanned pregnancy
	Tobacco (smoking)	May increase chances of blood clot or heart attack
Blood pressure drugs Thiazide diuretics Furosemide Methyclothiazide	Beta-adrenergic blockers Metoprolol Propranolol	Can cause extremely low blood pressure
	Digitalis glycosides Digoxin	Can cause irregular heartbeat, which can be fatal Can cause extremely low blood pressure
	Lithium	May cause lithium to have toxic effect
	Reserpine	Can cause extremely low blood pressure
Rauwolfia alkaloids Reserpine	Alcoholic beverages	May increase effects of alcohol May increase effects of rauwolfia alkaloids
	Beta-adrenergic blockers Metoprolol Propranolol	May cause extremely slow heartbeat and low blood pressure
	Digitalis glycosides Digoxin	May cause irregular heartbeat
	MAO inhibitors Isocarboxazid Phenelzine Tranylcypromine	May cause slight to sudden and severe high blood pressure May cause extreme high fever Either effect could be life-threatening
	Thiazide diuretics Furosemide Methyclothiazide	Can cause extreme low blood pressure
Blood-thinning drugs Warfarin sodium	Acetaminophen Buffered acetaminophen	High doses of acetaminophen may increase blood-thinning effects of these drugs
	Antacids Alumina and magnesia Dihydroxaluminum sodium carbonate Magnesia	Effects of dicumarol may be faster and may also be increased
	Antidiabetics Chlorpropamide Tolazamide	Blood-thinning effect will be increased at first, later it will be decreased May also cause low blood sugar and become toxic

Continued.

Guide to common drug interactions—cont'd

Drug	Interacting drug	Effect
Blood-thinning drugs—cont'd Warfarin sodium—cont'd	Barbiturates Pentobarbital Phenobarbital Secobarbital Secobarbital and amobarbital	Decreases blood-thinning effect
	Heparin	May cause increased risk of internal bleeding
	Ibuprofen	May cause internal bleeding or ulcers
	Penicillins Amoxicillin Ampicillin	May increase blood-thinning effects of these drugs
	Salicylates Aspirin Aspirin and caffeine Buffered aspirin	Blood-thinning effects will be increased May cause ulcers or internal bleeding
	Tricyclic antidepressants Amitriptyline Amoxapine Doxepin	May cause internal bleeding
Heparin	Blood-thinning drugs Warfarin sodium	May cause increased risk of internal bleeding
	Salicylates Aspirin Aspirin and caffeine Buffered aspirin	Blood-thinning effects will be increased May cause ulcers or internal bleeding
Heart drugs Beta-adrenergic blockers Metoprolol Propranolol	Antidiabetics Chlorpropamide Tolazamide	May increase risk of either high or low blood sugar levels May mask symptoms
	Antiseizure drugs Carbamazepine Chlordiazepoxide Diazepam Phenytoin	Could decrease the effect of beta blockers
	Digitalis glycosides Digoxin	May cause extremely slow heartbeat with a chance of heart block
	Isophane insulin suspension	Beta blockers may mask symptoms of low blood sugar May also cause low blood sugar
	Reserpine	May cause extremely slow heartbeat and low blood pressure
	Thiazide diuretics Furosemide Methyclothiazide	Can cause extremely low blood pressure
Digitalis glycosides Digoxin	Antacids Alumina and magnesia Dihydroxaluminum sodium carbonate Magnesia	Effects of digoxin may be reduced

This table includes only common over-the-counter and prescription drugs. Some of these drugs may also interact with less common drugs and substances not described. When using any drug, always consult your doctor or pharmacist about possible interactions with other drugs, substances, or foods.

Drug	Interacting drug	Effect
	Beta-adrenergic blockers Metoprolol Propranolol	May cause extremely slow heartbeat with a chance of heart block
	Reserpine	May cause irregular heartbeat
	Thiazide diuretics Furosemide Methyclothiazide	May cause extreme low blood pressure; may cause digitalis to become toxic
Monoamine oxidase inhibitors (MAO inhibitors) Isocarboxazid Phenelzine Tranylcypromine	Antidiabetics Chlorpropamide Isophane insulin suspension Tolazamide	Can cause extreme low blood sugar level
	Narcotic analgesics Acetaminophen and codeine Meperidine Propoxyphene	May cause severe and sometimes fatal reactions
	Reserpine	May cause slight to sudden and severe high blood pressure May cause extreme high fever Either effect could be life-threatening
	Tricyclic antidepressants Amitriptyline Amoxapine Doxepin	Severe seizure and death could result Should be taken 14 days apart
	Tyramine-containing foods Avocados, bananas, beer, caffeine, cheese, chicken liver, chocolate, fava beans, fermented sausages (salami, pepperoni, bologna, etc.) canned figs, pickled herring, pineapple, raisins, red wine, sauerkraut, soy sauce, yeast extract, yogurt	May cause severe and sometimes fatal high blood pressure. Headache, vomiting, fever, and high blood pressure are warning signals
Painkillers Narcotic analgesics Acetaminophen and codeine Meperidine Propoxyphene	Alcoholic beverages	May depress nervous system and breathing May cause blood pressure to drop too low
	MAO inhibitors Isocarboxazid Phenelzine Tranylcypromine	May cause many severe and sometimes fatal reactions
	Tricyclic antidepressants Amitriptyline Amoxapine Doxepin	May depress nervous system and breathing May cause blood pressure to drop too low

13-2 | Commonly used medications: trade to generic name listing

Trade name	Generic name	Trade name	Generic Name
Abbokinase	urokinase	Azo-Gantrisin	phenazopyridine and sulfisoxazole
Accutane	isotretinoin	Azolid-A	phenylbutazone
Achromycin	tetracycline	AZT	zidovudine
ACTH	corticotropin	Azulfidine	sulfasalazine
Acthar	corticotropin	Bactrim	sulfamethoxazole and trimethoprim
Actidil	triprolidine	Beclovent	beclomethasone
Actifed	triprolidine and pseudoephedrine	Benadryl	diphenhydramine
Actigall	ursodiol	Benemid	probenecid
Activase	t-PA	Bentyl	dicyclomine
Adapin	doxepin HCl	Betadine	povidone-iodine
Adrenalin	epinephrine	Bicillin	penicillin and benzathine
Adriamycin	doxorubicin HCl	BiCNU	carmustine
Advil	ibuprofen	Blenoxane	bleomycin
Afrin	oxymetazoline, nasal	Blocadren	timolol maleate
Akineton	biperiden	Bonine	meclizine
Aldactazide	hydrochlorothiazide and spironolactone	Brethine	terbutaline
Aldactone	spironolactone	Bretylol	bretylium tosylate
Aldomet	methyldopa	Bricanyl	terbutaline
Alka-2	calcium carbonate	Bronkosol	isoetharine HCl
Alkeran	melphalan	Bufferin	aspirin, buffered
Alupent	metaproterenol	Bumex	bumetanide
Amcil	ampicillin	Buprenex	buprenorphine
Americaine	benzocaine	Bupropion	wellbutrin
Amicar	aminocaproic acid	Buspar	buspirone
Amikin	amikacin	Butazolidin	phenylbutazone
Amoxil	amoxicillin	Butisol	butabarbital
Amphogel	aluminum hydroxide gel	Calan	verapamil
Amytal	amobarbital	Calcimar	calcitonin
Anacin-3	acetaminophen	Capoten	captopril
Anaprox	naproxen sodium	Carafate	sucralfate
Ancef	cefazolin	Cardene	nicardipine
Ancobon	flucytosine	Catapres	clonidine
Anectine	succinylcholine	Ceclor	cefaclor
Ansaid	flurbiprofen	Cedilanid	lanatoside C
Anspor	cephradine	Cedilanid-D	deslanoside
Antabuse	disulfiram	Cee Nu	lomustine
Antilirium	physostigmine	Cefadyl	cephapirin
Antivert	meclizine	Cefatrex	cefapirin
Apresoline	hydralazine	Cefizox	ceftizoxime
Aquamephyton	phytonadione (vitamin K_1)	Cefobid	cefoperazone
Aralen	chloroquine	Ceftin	cefuroxime
Aramine	metaraminol	Celestone	betamethasone
Arfonad	trimethaphan	Cerespan	papaverine
Aristocort	triamcinolone	Chloromycetin	chloramphenicol
Arlidin	nylidrin	Chloroptic	chloramphenicol
Artane	trihexyphenidyl HCl	Chlortrimeton	chlorpheniramine
Ascorbic Acid	vitamin C	Choledyl	oxtriphylline
Ascriptin	buffered aspirin	Chronulac	lactulose syrup
aspirin	acetylsalicylic acid (ASA)	Cinobac	cinoxacin
Asthmanefin	racepinephrine	Cl	potassium chloride
Atabrine	quinacrine	Claforan	cefotaxime
Atarax	hydroxyzine HCl	Clavulanate-Timentin	ticarcillin disodium
Ativan	lorazepam	Cleocin-T	clindamycin
Atromid-S	clofibrate	Clinoril	sulindac
Atrovent	ipratropium	Clomid	clomiphene
Augmentin	amoxicillin and clavulanate	Cogentin	benztropine
Aventyl	nortriptyline	Colace	docusate sodium (DSS), dioctyl sodium sulfosuccinate (DSS)
Axid	nizatidine		
Azactam	aztreonam	Colestid	colestipol
Azene	chlorazepate, monopotassium	Compazine	prochlorperazine

Modified from McKenry L, Salerno E: *Mosby's pharmacology in nursing*, ed 18, St Louis, 1992, Mosby.

Trade name	Generic name	Trade name	Generic Name
Corgard	nadolol	Elixophyllin	theophylline
Cortone	cortisone acetate	Elspar	asparaginase
Cosmegen	dactinomycin	Emeta-Con	benzquinamide
Cotazym	pancrelipase	Emetrol	phosphated carbohydrate solution
Coumadin	warfarin	Endep	amitriptyline
Crysticillin	penicillin procaine	Enkaid	encainide
Crystodigin	digitoxin	Epsom salt	magnesium sulfate
Cuprimine	penicillamine	Equanil	meprobomate
Cyanocobalamin	vitamin B_{12}	Ergomar	ergotamine
Cylert	pemoline	Ergostat	ergotamine
Cytadren	aminoglutethimide	Ergotrate	ergonovine
Cytomel	liothyronine	Erythrocin	erythromycin
Cytotec	misoprostol	Esidrex	hydrochlorothiazide
Cytoxan	cyclophosphamide	Euthroid	liotrix
Dalmane	flurazepam	Eutonyl	pargyline
Danocrine	danazol	Ex-Lax	phenolphthalein
Dantrium	dantrolene sodium	Feen-A-Mint	phenolphthalein
Daraprim	pyrimethamine	Feldene	piroxicam
Darvon	propoxyphene	Femiron	ferrous fumarate
Datril	acetaminophen	Feosol	ferrous sulfate
Davocet-N	propoxyphene, napsylate, acetaminophen	Fergon	ferrous gluconate
		Flagyl	metronidazole
Decadron	dexamethasone	Fleet enema	phosphate enema
Declomycin	demeclocycline	Flexeril	cyclobenzaprine
Delta Cortef	prednisolone	Florinef	fludrocortisone
Deltalin	vitamin D	Fluothane	halothane
Demerol	meperidine	Folvite	folic acid
Depakene	valproic acid	Fulvicin P/G	griseofulvin
DES	diethylstilbestrol	Fungizone	amphotericin B
Desenex	undecylenic acid	Furadantin	nitrofurantoin
Desyrel	trazodone	Gantanol	sulfamethoxazole
Diabeta	glyburide	Gantrisin	sulfisoxazole
Diabinese	chlorpropamide	Garamycin	gentamicin
Diamox	acetazolamide	Gelusil	aluminum-magnesium suspension
Diamox Sequels	acetazolamide	Geocillin	carbenicillin
Dianabol	methandrostenolone	Geopen	carbenicillin
Diapid	lypressin	Halcion	triazolam
Dicodid	hydrocodone	Haldol	haloperidol
Didronel	etidronate	Halotex	haloprogin
Dilantin	phenytoin	Herplex	idoxuridine
Dilaudid	hydromorphone	Hexabetalin	vitamin B_6
Dilaudin cough syrup	hydromorphone and guaifenesin	Hexadrol	dexamethasone
Dimetane	brompheniramine	Hiprex	methenamine hippurate
Disalcid	salsalate	Hismanal	astemizole
Diuril	chlorothiazide	Hurricaine	benzocaine
Dobutrex	dobutamine	Hycodan	hydrocodone and homatropine
Dolobid	diflunisal	Hydergine	ergoloid mesylates
Dolophine	methadone	HydroDiuril	hydrochlorothiazide
Donnatal	belladonna alkaloids and phenobarbital	Hygroton	chlorthalidone
Dopar	levodopa	Hyper-tet	tetanus immune globulin
Dopram	doxapram	Hyperstat	diazoxide
Doriden	glutethimide	Ilosone	erythromycin estolate
Dramamine	dimenhydrinate	Ilotycin	erythromycin
Dristan Long Lasting	oxymetazoline, nasal	Imferon	iron dextran
Dulcolax	bisacodyl	Imodium	loperamide
Duracillin	penicillin procaine	Imuran	azathioprine
Duramorph	morphine sulfate	Inderal	propranolol
Duricef	cefadroxil	Indocin	indomethacin
Dyazide	hydrochlorothiazide and triamterene	Intal	cromolyn
Dymelor	acetohexamide	Intropin	dopamine
Dyrenium	triamterene	Inversine	mecamylamine
Ecotrin	aspirin, enteric coated	Ismelin	guanethidine
Edecrin	ethacrynic acid	Isoptin	verapamil
Effersyllium	psyllium hydrocolloid	Isoptocarpine	pilocarpine
Elavil	amitriptyline	Isordil	isosorbide dinitrate

Continued.

Commonly used medications: trade to generic name listing—cont'd

Trade name	Generic name	Trade name	Generic Name
Isuprel	isoproterenol	Mevacor	lovastatin
K-Lor	potassium chloride	Mexitil	mexiletine
Kantrex	kanamycin	Mezlin	mezlocillin
Kaon	potassium gluconate, potassium chloride	Micro K	potassium chloride
		Micronase	glyburide
Kaopectate	kaolin-pectin	Midamor	amiloride
Kayexalate	sodium polystyrene sulfonate	Miltown	meprobamate
Keflex	cephalexin	Minipress	prazosin
Keflin	cephalothin	Minocin	minocycline
Kefzol	cefazolin	Mithracin	methramycin
Kemadrin	procyclidine	Moban	molindone
Kenacort	triamcinolone	Mol-iron	ferrous sulfate
Klonopin	clonazepam	Monistat	miconazole
Klorvess	potassium chloride	Motrin	ibuprofen
Kondremul	mineral oil emulsion	Moxam	moxalactam
Kwell	lindane	Mucomyst	acetylcysteine
Lanoxin	digoxin	Mustargen	nitrogen mustard, mechlorethamine
Larodopa	levodopa	Myclex	clotrimazole
Larotid	amoxicillin	Mycostatin	nystatin
Lasix	furosemide	Mylanta	aluminum-magnesium suspension
Leucovorin calcium	folinic acid	Myleran	busulfan
Leukeran	chlorambucil	Mylicon	simethicone
Levo-Dromoran	levorphanol	Mysoline	primidone
Levophed	levarterenol, norepinephrine	Mytelase	ambenonium
Libritab	chlordiazepoxide	Nalfon	fenoprofen
Librium	chlordiazepoxide	Naprosyn	naproxen
Lidex	fluocinonide	Narcan	naloxone
Limbitrol	chlordiazepoxide and amitriptyline	Nardil	phenelzine sulfate
Limbrax	chlordiazepoxide and clidinium	Navane	thiothixene
Lioresal	baclofen	Nebcin	tobramycin
Lipo-Hepin	heparin	Neg Gram	nalidixic acid
Liquaemin	heparin	Nembutal	pentobarbital
Lithane	lithium carbonate	Neosynephrine	phenylephrine
Lithobid	lithium carbonate	Niacin	vitamin B_3
Lodosyn	carbidopa	Nicobid	niacin (nicotinic acid)
Lomotil	diphenoxylate HCL with atropine	Nicolar	niacin (nicotinic acid)
Loniten	minoxidil	Nicotinic Acid	vitamin B_3
Lopid	gemfibrozil	Nilstat	nystatin
Lopressor	metoprolol	Nipride	nitroprusside
Lorelco	probucol	Nitrobid	nitroglycerin
Lotrimin	clotrimazole	Nitrogen Mustard	mechlorethamine
Loxitane	loxapine succinate	Nitrospan	nitroglycerin
Ludiomil	maprotiline	Nitrostat	nitroglycerin
Lufyllin	dyphylline	Nizoral	ketoconazole
Luminal	phenobarbital	Noctec	chloral hydrate
Lysodren	mitotane	Noludar	methyprylon
Maalox	aluminum-magnesium suspension	Nolvadex	tamoxifen
Magnesium Hydroxide	milk of magnesia (MOM)	Norflex	orphendrine
Mandelamine	methenamine mandelate	Norlutate	norethindrone acetate
Mandol	cefamandol	Norlutin	norethindrone
Marezine	cyclizine	Normodyne	labetalol
Matulane	procarbazine	Noroxin	norfloxacin
Maxzide	triamterene and hydrochlorothiazide	Norpace	disopyramide
Mebaral	mephobarbital	Norpramin	desipramine
Meclomen	meclofenamate	Novocain	procaine
Mefoxin	cefoxitin	Nubain	nalbuphine
Megace	megestrol	Numorphan	oxymorphone
Mellaril	thioridazine	Nupercainal	dibucaine
Menadione	vitamin K_2	Nupercaine	dibucaine
Mephyton	phytonadione (vitamin K_1)	Nydrazid	INH (isoniazid)
Mesantoin	mephenytoin	Omnipen	ampicillin
Mestinon	pyridostigmine	Oncovin	vincristine
Meticortelone	prednisolone	Optimine	azatadine maleate

Trade name	Generic name	Trade name	Generic Name
Orinase	tolbutamide	Retrovir	zidovudine
Orudis	ketoprofen	Riboflavin	vitamin B_2
Pamelor	nortriptyline	Rifadin	rifampin
Paral	paraldehyde	Rimactane	rifampin
Paregoric	camphorated tincture of opium	Riopan	magaldrate
Parlodel	bromocriptine	Ritalin	methylphenidate
Parnate	tranylcypromine sulfate	Robaxin	methocarbamol
Pavabid	papaverine	Robinul	glycopyrrolate
Pavulon	pancuronium	Robitussin	guaifenesin (glyceryl guaiacolate)
Pen-Vee K	penicillin V potassium	Rocephin	ceftriaxone
Penicillin VK	phenoxymethyl penicillin	Roxanol	morphine sulfate
Pentam	pentamidine isethionate	Rufen	ibuprofen
Penthrane	methoxyflurane	Sanorex	mazindol
Pentid	penicillin G potassium	Sansert	methylsergide
Pepcid	famotidine	Seconal	secobarbital
Percocet	oxycodone, acetaminophen	Seldane	terfenadine
Percodan	oxycodone, ASA	Selsun	selenium sulfide
Periactin	cyproheptadine	Selsun Blue	selenium sulfide
Pericolace	dioctyl sodium sulfosuccinate with casanthranol	Senokot	senna
Peritrate	pentaerythritol tetranitrate	Serax	oxazepam
Persantine	dipyridamole	Serentil	mesoridazine
Pertofrane	desipramine	Serpasil	reserpine
Pfizepen	penicillin G potassium	Silvadene	silver sulfadiazine
Phenergan	promethazine	Sinemet	carbidopa and levodopa
Phytonadione	vitamin K_1	Sinequan	doxepin HCl
Pipracil	piperacillin	Slow K	potassium chloride
Pitocin	oxytocin	Solu-Cortef	hydrocortisone
Pitressin	vasopressin	Sorbitrate	isosorbide dinitrate
Placidyl	ethchlorvynol	Sparine	promazine
Platinol	cisplatin	Stadol	butorphanol
Polycillin	ampicillin	Staphcillin	methicillin
Polymox	amoxicillin	Stelazine	trifluoperazine
Pontocaine	tetracaine	Stilbestrol	diethylstilbestrol
Preludin	phenmetrazine	Stoxil	idoxuridine
Premarin	estrogens, conjugated	Streptase	streptokinase
Primaxin	imipenem-cilastatin	Sublimaze	fentanyl
Prinivil	lisinopril	Sufenta	sufentanil
Probanthine	propantheline	Sumycin	tetracycline
Procardia	nifedipine	Suprax	cefixime
Proglycem	diazoxide	Surfak	dioctyl calcium sulfosuccinate (DOCS), docusate calcium
Prolixin	fluphenazine	Sus-Phrine	epinephrine
Proloid	thyroglobulin	Symmetrel	amantadine
Proloprim	trimethoprim	Synalar	fluocinolone acetonide
Pronestyl	procainamide	Synkayvite	menadiol
Prostaphlin	oxacillin	Synthroid	levothyroxine
Prostigmin	neostigmine	Tace	chlorotrianisene
Proventil	albuterol	Tagamet	cimetidine
Provera	medroxyprogesterone	Talwin	pentazocine
Prozac	fluoxetine	Tambocor	flecainide
Pyopen	carbenicillin	Tandearil	oxyphenbutazone
Pyribenzamine (PBZ)	tripelennamine	Tapazole	methimazole
Pyridium	phenazopyridine HCl	Taractan	chlorprothixene
Pyridoxine	vitamin B_6	Tavist	clemastine
Quarzan	clidinium	Tegretol	carbamazepine
Questran	cholestyramine	Temaril	trimeprazone
Quinaglute	quinidine gluconate	Tenex	guanfacine
Quinamm	quinine sulfate	Tenormin	atenolol
Quinora	quinidine sulfate	Tensilon	edrophonium
Raudixin	rauwolfia serpentina	Terramycin	oxytetracycline
Redisol	vitamin B_{12}	Theo-Dur	theophylline
Regitine	phentolamine	Thiamine	vitamin B_1
Reglan	metoclopramide	Thorazine	chlorpromazine
Restoril	temazepam	Thyrolar	liotrix

Continued.

Commonly used medications: trade to generic name listing—cont'd

Trade name	Generic name	Trade name	Generic Name
Ticar	ticarcillin	Vancocin	vancomycin
Tigan	trimethobenzamide	Vaponefrin	racepinephrine, ephedrine
Timolide	hydrochlorothiazide and timolol	Vasodilan	isoxsuprine HCl
Timoptic	timolol maleate	Vasotec	enalapril
Titralac	calcium carbonate	Velban	vinblastine
Tobrex	tobramycin	Velosef	cephradine
Tofranil	imipramine	Ventolin	albuterol
Tolinase	tolazamide	Vepesid	etoposide
Tonocard	tocainide	Vermox	mebendazole
Torecan	thiethylperzine	Versapen	hetacillin
Tracrium	atracurium besylate	Vibramycin	doxycycline
Trandate	labetalol	Viokase	pancrelipase
Transderm-Scop	scopolamine	Vira-A	vidarabine
Tranxene	chlorazepate, dipotassium	Virazole	ribavirin
Tremin	trihexphenidyl HCl	Visken	pindolol
Trental	pentoxifylline	Vistaril	hydroxyzine pamoate
Tridione	trimethadione	Vitamin C	ascorbic acid
Trilafon	perphenazine	Vitamin K	menadiol
Trimpex	trimethoprim	Voltaren	diclofenac
Trinalin	azatadine maleate	Wellcovorin	leucovorin
Tums	calcium carbonate	Wycillin	penicillin procaine
Tuss-Ornade	caramiphen and phenylpropanolamine	Wydase	hyaluronidase
Tylenol	acetaminophen	Wytensin	guanabenz
Tylox	oxycodone, acetaminophen	Xanax	alprazolam
Unasyn	ampicillin and sulbactam	Xylocaine	lidocaine
Urecholine	bethanechol chloride	Yutopar	ritodrine
Urex	methenamine hippurate	Zantac	ranitidine
V-cillin	phenoxymethyl penicillin	Zaroxolyn	metolazone
V-cillin K	penicillin V potassium	Zestril	lisinopril
Valisone	betamethasone	Zovirax	acyclovir
Valium	diazepam	Zyloprim	allopurinol
Vanceril	beclomethasone		

13-4   Adverse drug effects during pregnancy*

Effect of drug	Drugs known to produce the effect in humans
First-trimester effects on embryonic development	
Abortion	Isotretinoin, quinine
Multiple anomalies involving craniofacial development	Dicumarol, ethanol, isotretinoin, methotrexate, paramethadione, phenytoin, quinine, trimethadione
Neural tube defects	Valproate
Goiter	Iodide, methimazole, propylthiouracil
Abnormalities or reproductive organs	Androgens, diethylstilbestrol, estrogens, progestins
Inhibition of growth	Methotrexate, tetracycline, tobacco smoke
Second- and third-trimester effects on fetal development	
Abortion, mortality	Heroin, isotretinoin, tobacco smoke
Mental retardation	Dicumarol, ethanol
Altered cardiovascular function	Anticholinergic drugs, propranolol, terbutaline
Hearing loss and loss of balance	Aminoglycoside antibiotics
Hyperbilirubinemia	Nitrofurantoin, sulfonamides
Hemolytic anemia	Nitrofurantoin
Goiter	Iodide, methimazole, propylthiouracil
Abnormalities of reproductive organs	Androgens, diethylstilbestrol, estrogens, progestins
Inhibition of growth	Dicumarol, ethanol, heroin, methotrexate, tetracycline, tobacco smoke
Labor, delivery, and perinatal period	
Increased mortality	Tobacco smoking, cocaine abuse
Altered cardiovascular function	Anticholinergic agents, caffeine, heroin, lidocaine, meperidine, propranolol, terbutaline
Gray-baby syndrome	Chloramphenicol
Respiratory depression	Diazepam, meperidine, morphine, phenobarbital, ethanol, tobacco smoking
Respiratory distress	Reserpine
Bleeding	Aspirin, dicumarol, indomethacin
Hypoglycemia	Chlorpropamide, propranolol, tolbutamide
Hyperbilirubinemia	Nitrofurantoin, sulfonamides
Hemolytic anemia	Nitrofurantoin
Hyperirritability	Cocaine

*This list does not include all drugs that affect fetal and neonatal function but is intended to give representative examples. The nurse should check sources of specific information about individual agents when drugs are administered to pregnant patients.

From Clark JBF, Queener SF, Karb VB: *Pharmacologic basis of nursing practice*, ed 4, St Louis, 1993, Mosby, p. 20.

13-5 | FDA pregnancy categories*

Category	Level of risk with drug exposure	Examples
A	Controlled studies in women fail to demonstrate risk in the first trimester (and there is no evidence of risk in later trimesters), and possibility of fetal harm appears remote.	Thyroid hormones
B	Animal reproduction studies have not demonstrated fetal risk, but there are no controlled studies in pregnant women. Animal reproduction studies have shown adverse effect (other than decreased fertility) that was not confirmed in controlled studies on women in first trimester. There is no evidence of risk in later trimesters.	Amoxicillin, buspirone, cimetidine, fluoxetine, hydrochlorothiazide, metronidazole, piperacillin
C	Studies in animals have revealed adverse effects on fetus, and there are no controlled studies in women. In some cases, studies in women and animals are not available. Drugs in this category should be given only if potential benefit justifies risk to fetus.	Alteplase, captopril, ciprofloxacin, codeine, enalapril, gentamicin, isoproterenol, lisinopril, morphine, nizatidine, reserpine, tubocurarine
D	There is positive evidence of human fetal risk, but the benefits for pregnant women may be acceptable despite the risk, as in life-threatening diseases for which safer drugs cannot be used or are ineffective. An appropriate statement must appear in the "warnings" section of the labeling of drugs in this category.	Amikacin, midazolam, netilmicin, tobramycin
X	Studies in animals or humans have demonstrated fetal abnormalities, there is evidence of fetal risk based on human experience, or both. The risk of using the drug in pregnant women clearly out-weighs any possible benefit. The drug is contraindicated in women who are or may become pregnant. An appropriate statement must appear in the "contraindications" section of the labeling of drugs in this category.	Isotretinoin, lovastatin, methotrexate

*From Clark JBF, Queener SF, Karb VB: *Pharmacologic basis of nursing practice,* ed 4, St Louis, 1993, Mosby, p 21.

APPENDIX 14

HEALTH ORGANIZATIONS

14-1 General resources

The following is a list of resources on many different health-related topics. The list includes names and addresses that can be used to obtain further information. It is not by any means a complete list but is meant to serve as a starting point.

ACQUIRED IMMUNODEFICIENCY SYNDROME (AIDS)

AIDS Action Council
729 8th St SE, Ste 200
Washington, DC 20003

American Foundation for AIDS Research
733 3rd Ave, 12th Floor
New York, NY 10017

American Red Cross
National Headquarters
AIDS Education Program
430 17th St NW
Washington, DC 20006

Association of Nurses in AIDS Care
2500 NW 22nd Ave
Miami, FL 33124

Gay Men's Health Crisis
129 W 20th St
New York, NY 10011

Lambda Legal Defense and Education Fund
666 Broadway, 12th Floor
New York, NY 10012

National AIDS Clearinghouse
PO Box 6003
Rockville, MD 20849-6003

National AIDS Inter-Faith Network
300 I St NE, Ste 400
Washington, DC 20005

National Association of People With AIDS
2025 I St, Ste 415
Washington, DC 20006

National Coalition of Gay Sexually Transmitted Disease Services
PO Box 239
Milwaukee, WI 53201-0239

National Hemophilia Foundation
National Resource and Consultation Center for AIDS and HIV Infection
Soho Bldg
110 Greene St, Room 303
New York, NY 10012

National Hospice Organization
1901 N Moore St, Ste 9901
Arlington, VA 22209

Project Inform
1965 Market, Ste 220
San Francisco, CA 94103

San Francisco AIDS Foundation
25 Van Ness Ave, Ste 660
San Francisco, CA 94102

US Department of Health and Human Services
Public Health Service, Centers for Disease Control
National AIDS Information/Education Program
Bldg 1, Rm 2122
1600 Clifton Rd, NE
Atlanta, GA 30333

ADVOCACY

American Civil Liberties Union
132 W 43rd St
New York, NY 10036

Occupational Safety and Health Administration (OSHA)
Office of Public and Consumer Affairs
US Department of Labor, Room N3637
200 Constitution Ave NW
Washington, DC 20210

ALCOHOL AND DRUG ABUSE

Al-Anon Family Group Headquarters, Inc.
PO Box 862
Midtown Station
New York, NY 10018

Alcohol and Drug Problems Association of North America, Inc.
444 N Capitol St NW, Ste 706
Washington, DC 20001

Alcoholic Anonymous World Services
PO Box 549
Grand Central Station
New York, NY 10163

Drug Information Association, Inc.
PO Box 3113
Maple Glen, PA 19002

International Commission for Prevention of Alcoholism and Drug Dependency
6830 Laurel St NW
Washington, DC 20012

MADD—Mothers Against Drunk Driving
511 E John Carpenter Fwy, Ste 700
Irving, TX 75062

National Association on Drug Abuse Problems, Inc.
355 Lexington Ave
New York, NY 10017

National Clearing House for Alcohol Information
PO Box 2345
Rockville, MD 20852

National Clearinghouse for Drug Abuse Information
PO Box 416
Kensington, MD 20795

National Committee for the Prevention of Alcoholism and Drug Dependency
6830 Laurel St NW
Washington, DC 20012

National Council on Alcoholism, Inc.
12 W 21st St
New York, NY 10010

SADD—Students Against Driving Drunk
PO Box 800
Marlboro, MA 01752

ALZHEIMER'S DISEASE

Alzheimer's Association, Inc.
4709 Golf Road, Ste 1015
Skokie, IL 60076

AMYOTROPHIC LATERAL SCLEROSIS

Amyotrophic Lateral Sclerosis Association
21021 Ventura Blvd, Ste 321
Woodland Hills, CA 91364

ARTHRITIS

Arthritis Society
920 Yonge St, Ste 420
Toronto, Canada M4W 3J7

National Arthritis Foundation
PO Box 19000
Atlanta, GA 30326

ASTHMA AND ALLERGIES

Asthma and Allergy Foundation of America
1125 15th NW, Ste 502
Washington, DC 20005

National Jewish Center for Immunology and Respiratory Medicine
1400 Jackson St
Denver, CO 80206

BEREAVEMENT

American Association of Suicidology
2459 S Ash St
Denver, CO 80222

Compassionate Friends
PO Box 3696
Oak Brook, IL 60522-3696

Pregnancy and Infant Loss Center
1421 E Wayzata Blvd, No 40
Wayzata, MN 55391

SHARE
St Joseph's Health Center
300 1st Capitol Dr
St. Charles, MO 63301-2893

Widowed Persons Service, AARP
1909 K St NW
Washington, DC 20049

BLINDNESS

American Council of the Blind
1155 15th St NW, Ste 720
Washington, DC 20005

American Foundation for the Blind, Inc.
15 W 16th St
New York, NY 10011

Association for Education and Rehabilitation of the Blind and Visually Impaired
206 N Washington St, Ste 320
Alexandria, VA 22314

Braille Institute
741 N Vermont Ave
Los Angeles, CA 90029

Guide Dog Users, Inc.
57 Grandview Ave
Watertown, MA 02172

Guide Dogs for the Blind
PO Box 151200
San Rafael, CA 94915

Guiding Eyes for the Blind
611 Granite Springs Rd
Yorktown Heights, NY 10598

Library of Congress
Division of the Blind and Physically Handicapped
1291 Taylor St NW
Washington, DC 20542

National Association for Visually Handicapped
22 W 21st St
New York, NY 10010

National Eye Institute
9000 Rockville Pike
Bethesda, MD 20892

National Society to Prevent Blindness
500 E Remington Rd
Schaumburg, IL 60173

Recording for the Blind, Inc.
20 Roszel Rd
Princeton, NJ 08540

CANCER

American Association for Cancer Education
Educational Research and Development
University of Alabama at Birmingham
Community Health Science Building
UAB Station
Birmingham, AL 35294

American Association for Cancer Research (AACR)
Public Ledger Building, Ste 816
Sixth and Chestnut St
Philadelphia, PA 19106

American Cancer Society
National Headquarters
1599 Clifton Rd
Atlanta, GA 30329

American Society of Clinical Oncology (ASCO)
435 N Michigan Ave, Ste 1717
Chicago, IL 60611

Association of Community Cancer Centers (ACCC)
11600 Nebel St, Ste 201
Rockville, MD 20852

Cancer Care, Inc.
1180 Avenue of the Americas
New York, NY 10036

Cancer Federation, Inc.
21250 Box Spring Rd
Morena Valley, CA 92388

Choice in Dying
200 Varick St
New York, NY 10014

International Association of Cancer Victors and Friends
7740 W Manchester Ave, Ste 110
Playa del Rey, CA 90293

International Cancer Information Center
Physician Data Query (PDQ)
NCI's Computerized Data Base for Physicians
NCI Building 82, Room 123
Bethesda, MD 20814

Leukemia Society of America, Inc.
733 Third Ave
New York, NY 10017

National Alliance of Breast Cancer Organizations
1180 Avenue of the Americas, 2nd Floor
New York, NY 10036

National Cancer Institute
9000 Rockville Pike
NCI Building 31, Room 10A24
Bethesda, MD 20892

National Coalition for Cancer Research (NCCR)
426 C Street NE
Washington, DC 20002

National Coalition for Cancer Survivorship (NCCS)
1010 Wayne Ave, 5th floor
Silver Spring, MD 20910

National Hospice Organization
1901 North Moore St, Ste 901
Arlington, VA 22209

Office of Cancer Communications
NCI Building 31, Room 10A16
Bethesda, MD 20892

Skin Cancer Foundation
245 Fifth Ave, Ste 2402
New York, NY 10016

CHILD ABUSE

Child Abuse Listening and Mediation
PO Box 90754
Santa Barbara, CA 93190-0754

Clearinghouse on Child Abuse and Neglect Information
PO Box 1182
Washington, DC 20013

CHILDREN

Association for the Care of Children's Health
Woodmont Ave, Ste 300
Bethesda, MD 20814

Children's Foundation
725 15th St NW, Ste 505
Washington, DC 20005

National Tay-Sachs and Allied Diseases Association
2001 Beacon St
Brookline, MA 02146

Sudden Infant Death Syndrome Alliance
10500 Little Patuxent Pkwy, No 420
Columbia, MD 21044

CYSTIC FIBROSIS

Cystic Fibrosis Foundation
6931 Arlington Rd
Bethesda, MD 20814

Pediatric Pulmonary and Cystic Fibrosis Center
St Christopher's Hospital for Children
2600 N Lawrence St
Philadelphia, PA 19133

DIABETES

**American Association of Diabetes
Educators**
444 N Michigan Ave, Ste 1240
Chicago, IL 60611-3901

American Diabetes Association
1660 Duke St
Alexandria, VA 22313

**Juvenile Diabetes Foundation
International**
432 Park Ave South
New York, NY 10016

**National Diabetes Information
Clearinghouse**
Box NDIC
9000 Rockville Pike
Bethesda, MD 20892

DISABILITIES

**Architectural and Transportation
Barriers Compliance Board**
1331 F St NW, Ste 1000
Washington, DC 20004-1111

**Association for Children with Retarded
Mental Development**
162 Fifth Ave, 11th Floor
New York, NY 10010

Association for Retarded Citizens
PO Box 6109
Arlington, TX 76005

Boy Scouts of America
Scouting for the Handicapped
1325 W Walnut Hill Lane
PO Box 152079
Irving, TX 75015-2079

**Clearinghouse on Disability
Information**
Department of Education
330 C St SW, Room 3132
Washington, DC 20202-2524

**Disability Rights, Education, and
Defense Funds**
1633 Q St NW
Washington, DC 20009

Housing for Handicapps
Elderly People Division
Department of Housing and Urban
Development
HUD Building
Washington, DC 20410

International Council on Disability
25 E 21st St
New York, NY 10010

**Learning Disabilities Association of
America**
4156 Library Rd
Pittsburgh, PA 15234

National Amputation Foundation
73 Church St
Malverne, NY 11565

**National Information Center for
Handicapped Children**
7426 Jones Branch Dr, Ste 1100
McLean, VA 22102

National Paraplegia Foundation
333 N Michigan Ave
Chicago, IL 60601

DOWN'S SYNDROME

Association for Retarded Citizens
11600 Nebel St
Rockville, MD 20852

**National Association for Down's
Syndrome**
PO Box 4542
Oak Park, IL 60522-4542

ELDERLY

Administration on Aging
330 Independence Ave SW
Washington, DC 20201

Adult Development and Aging
Gerontology Center
University of Georgia
100 Candler Hall
Athens, GA 30602

Age and Aging
Bailliere Tindall
7-8 Henrietta St
Covent Garden
London, England WCZE 8QE

Alzheimer's Association
919 N Michigan Ave, Ste 1000
Chicago, IL 60611-1676

**Alzheimer's Disease Education and
Referral Center**
PO Box 8250
Silver Spring, MD 20907-8250

**American Academy of Home Care
Physicians**
10480 Little Patuxent Pkwy, Ste 760A
Columbia, MD 21044

**American Academy of Physical
Medicine and Rehabilitation**
122 S Michigan Ave, Ste 1300
Chicago, IL 60603-6107

**American Association for Continuity of
Care**
1730 N Lynn St, Ste 502
Arlington, VA 22209

**American Association for Geriatric
Psychiatry**
PO Box 376A
Greenbelt, MD 20768

**American Association of Homes for the
Aging**
901 E St NW, Ste 500
Washington, DC 20004

**American Association for International
Aging**
1133 20th St NW, Ste 333
Washington, DC 20036

**American Association of Public Health
Dentistry (AAPHD)**
10619 Jousting Lane
Richmond, VA 23235-3838

**American Association of Retired
Persons (AARP)**
601 E Street NW
Washington, DC 20049

American Bar Association
Commission on Legal Problems of the
Elderly
1800 M St NW
Washington, DC 20036

**American Federation for Aging
Research (AFAR)**
1414 Avenue of the Americas, 18th
Floor
New York, NY 10019

American Geriatric Society
770 Lexington Ave, Ste 400
New York, NY 10021

**American Occupational Therapy
Association**
1383 Piccard Dr.
PO Box 1725
Rockville, Md 20849-1725

American Psychological Association
Division of Adult Development
750 First St NE
Washington, DC 20002-4242

American Society on Aging
833 Market St, Ste 511
San Francisco, CA 94103-1824

**American Society for Geriatric
Dentistry**
211 E Chicago Ave, 17th Floor
Chicago, Ill 60611

**Association for Gerontology in Higher
Education**
1001 Connecticut Ave NW, Ste 410
Washington, DC 20036-5504

Association of Humanistic Gerontology
1711 Solano Ave
Berkeley, CA 94707

**Association of University Programs in
Health Administration**
Office of Long-term Care and Aging
1911 N Fort Meyer Dr, Ste 503
Arlington, VA 22209

Beverly Foundation
70 S Lake Ave, Ste 750
Pasadena, CA 91101

Catholic Charities USA
1731 King St
Alexandria, VA 22314

**Catholic Health Association of the
United States**
4455 Woodson
St Louis, MO 63134-3797

Center for Social Gerontology
2307 Shelby Ave
Ann Arbor, MI 48103-3895

Children of Aging Parents
1609 Woodbourne Rd, Ste 302-A
Levittown, PA 19057

Commission on Legal Problems of the Elderly
1800 M St NW
Washington, DC 20036

Consultant Dietitians in Healthcare Facilities
PO Box 60
Armada, MI 48005

Department of Veterans Affairs
Veterans Health Administration
Nursing Service Program (118c)
810 Vermont Ave NW
Washington, DC 20420

Design for Aging/Architecture for Health
American Institute of Architects
1735 New York Ave NW
Washington, DC 20006

Federal Council on Aging
330 Independence Ave SW, Room 4280
HHS-N
Washington, DC 20201

Foundation for Hospice and Home Care
519 C St NE
Washington, DC 20002

Geriatric Research and Training Center (GRTC)
350 Masons Mill Rd, Ste 501B
Huntington Valley, PA 19006

Gerontological Nutritionists
4103 44th St
Sacramento, CA 95820

Gerontological Society of America
1275 K St NW, Ste 350
Washington, DC 20005-4006

Gray Panthers
1424 16th St NW, Ste 602
Washington, DC 20036

Health Care Organization
Division of Long Term Care
Oak Meadows Bldg, Room 2F5
Baltimore, MD 21207

Hillhaven Foundation
1148 Broadway Plaza
PO Box 2264
Tacoma, WA 98401-2264

House Select Committee on Aging
House Office Bldg
Annex 1, Room 712
Washington, DC 20515

Institute on Aging
Medical Center of Central Massachusetts
119 Belmont St
Worcester, MA 01605

Institute for Retired Professionals
New School of Social Research
60 W 12th St
New York, NY 10011

International Federation on Aging
Secretariat—Canada
380 St Antoine St W, Ste 3200
Montreal, Quebec H24 3X7

International Senior Citizens Association, Inc.
537 S Commonwealth Ave, Ste 4
Los Angeles, CA 90020

Mental Disorders of the Aging
Research Branch DCR
Room 11 C-03
5600 Fishers Lane
Rockville, MD 20857

National Alliance of Senior Citizens
2525 Wilson Blvd
Arlington, VA 22201

National Asian-Pacific Center on Aging
Melbourne Tower
1511 Third Ave, Ste 914
Seattle, WA 98101

National Association of Area Agencies on Aging
1112 16th St NW, Ste 100
Washington, DC 20036

National Association for Hispanic Elderly
3325 Wilshire Blvd, Ste 800
Los Angeles, CA 90010-1724

National Association of Meal Programs
206 E St NE
Washington, DC 20002

National Association of Medical Equipment Suppliers (NAMES)
625 Slaters Lane, Ste 200
Alexandria, VA 22314

National Association of Nutrition and Aging Services Programs
2675 44th St SW, Ste 305
Grand Rapids, MI 49509

National Association for Senior Living Industries
184 Duke of Gloucester St
Annapolis, MD 21401-2523

National Association of Spanish Speaking Elderly
2025 I St NW, Ste 219
Washington, DC 20006

National Association of State Units on Aging
2033 K St NW, Ste 304
Washington, DC 20006

National Caucus and Center on Black Aged
1424 K St NW, Ste 500
Washington, DC 20005

National Citizens Coalition for Nursing Home Reform
1224 M St NW, Ste 301
Washington, DC 20005

National Clearinghouse on Technology and Aging
College of Health and Human Services
Ohio University
Athens, Oh 45701

National Council on the Aging
(includes National Institute of Senior Citizens and National Institute on Adult Day Care)
409 3rd St SW, Ste 200
Washington, DC 20024

National Council of Senior Citizens
1311 F St NW
Washington, DC 20004-1171

National Hospice Organization (NHO)
1901 North Moore St, Ste 901
Arlington, VA 22202

National Indian Council on Aging
6400 Uptown Blvd NE, Ste 510W
Albuquerque, NM 87110

National Institute on Aging
Public Information Office
Federal Building, Room 6C12
9000 Rockville Pike
Rockville, MD 20892

National Meals on Wheels Foundation
1133 20th St NW, Ste 321
Washington, DC 20036

National Pharmaceutical Council
1894 Preston White Dr
Reston, VA 22091

National Policy Center on Housing and Living Arrangements for Older Americans
University of Michigan
2000 Bonisteel Blvd
Ann Arbor, MI 48109

National Rehabilitation Association
633 S Washington St
Alexandria, VA 22314

National Senior Citizens Law Center
1815 H St NW, Ste 700
Washington, DC 20006

Non-Prescription Drug Manufacturer Association
1150 Connecticut Ave NW
Washington, DC 20036

Older Women's League (OWL)
666 11th St NW, Ste 700
Washington, DC 20001

Senate Special Committee on Aging
Dirksen Senate Office Building, Room 623
Washington, DC 20510

Senior Care Centers of America, Inc.
26 E Second St A-1
Moorestown, NJ 08057

**United States Pharmacopeial
  Convention, Inc.**
12601 Twinbrook Pkwy
Rockville, MD 20852

EPILEPSY

American Epilepsy Society
638 Prospect Ave
Hartford, CT 06105

Epilepsy Foundation of America
4351 Garden Garden City Dr, Ste 406
Landover, MD 20785

FAMILY PLANNING/PREGNANCY

American Fertility Society
1209 Montgomery Highway
Birmingham, AL 35216

**International Childbirth Education
  Association, Inc.**
PO Box 20048
Minneapolis, MN 55420

La Leche League International, Inc.
9616 Minneapolis Ave
Franklin Park, IL 60131

Maternity Center Association
48 E 92nd St
New York, NY 10028

**Planned Parenthood Federation of
  America, Inc.**
810 Seventh Ave
New York, NY 10019

FOOD (see also Nutrition)

Food and Drug Administration
Office of Consumer Affairs
5600 Fishers Ln
Rockville, MD 20857

**Food and Nutrition Information
  Center**
National Agricultural Library Building,
  Room 304
Beltsville, MD 20705

GASTROINTESTINAL DISORDERS

**American Society for Parenteral and
  Enteral Nutrition**
8630 Fenton St, Ste 412
Silver Spring, MD 20910

**Crohn's and Colitis Foundation of
  America**
444 Park Ave S
New York, NY 10016-7374

Help for Incontinent People
PO Box 544
Union, SC 29379

**National Digestive Diseases Education
  and Information Clearinghouse**
9000 Rockville Pike
Box NDDIC
Bethesda, MD 20892

United Ostomy Association
36 Executive Park, Ste 120
Irvine, CA 92714

**Wound Ostomy Continence and
  Nurse's Society (WOCN)**
2755 Bristol, Ste 110
Costa Mesa, CA 92626

HEALTH—GENERAL

American Health Care Association
1201 L St, NW
Washington, DC 20005

American Health Foundation
320 E 43rd St
New York, NY 10017

American Holistic Nurses' Association
4101 Lake Boone Trail, Ste 201
Raleigh, NC 27607

**American Hospital Association Center
  for Health Promotion**
840 N Lake Shore Dr
Chicago, IL 60611

American Nurses' Association
600 Maryland Ave SW
Washington, DC 20024

American Public Health Association
1015 15th St NW
Washington, DC 20005

**Association for Vital Records and
  Health Statistics (Public Health)**
c/o Dorothy Harshbarger, Director
PO Box 5625
Montgomery, AL 36103

Clearinghouse on Health Indexes
National Center for Health Statistics
Division of Epidemiology and Health
  Promotion
6525 Belcrest Rd, Room 730
Hyattsville, MD 20782

Council on Education for Public Health
1015 15th St NW
Washington, DC 20005

Health and Education Resources, Inc.
4733 Bethesda Ave, Ste 700
Bethesda, MD 20814

**International Council on Health,
  Physical Education and Recreation**
1900 Association Dr
Reston, VA 22091

National Health Council, Inc.
1730 M Street NW, Ste 500
Washington, DC 20036

National Institutes of Health
9000 Rockville Pike
Bethesda, MD 20892

National Wellness Institute
University of Wisconsin–Stevens Point
  Foundation
1045 Clark St, Ste 210
Stevens Point, WI 54481

HEALTH—DENTAL

American Dental Association
211 E Chicago Ave
Chicago, IL 60611

HEALTH—EYES

American Optometric Association
243 Lindbergh Blvd
St Louis, MO 63141

HEALTH—MENTAL

American Art Therapy Association
1202 Allanson Rd
Mundelein, IL 60060

**American Mental Health Foundation,
  Inc.**
2 E 86th St
New York, NY 10028

American Psychiatric Association
1400 K St NW
Washington, DC 20005

American Psychological Association
750 1st St NE
Washington, DC 20002

**National Clearinghouse for Mental
  Health Information**
National Institute of Mental Health
5600 Fishers Lane, Room 11A33
Rockville, MD 20857

National Mental Health Association
1021 Prince St
Alexandria, VA 22314-2971

HEARING AND SPEECH

**Alexander Graham Bell Association for
  the Deaf**
3417 Volta Pl NW
Washington, DC 20007

**American Deafness and Rehabilitation
  Association**
12511 Highway 300
Roland, AR 72135

**American Speech, Language, and
  Hearing Association**
10801 Rockville Pike
Rockville, MD 20852

Better Hearing Institute
Box 1840
Washington, DC 20013

National Council on Stuttering
PO Box 8171
Grand Rapids, MI 49518

Self-Help for Hard of Hearing People
7800 Wisconsin Ave
Bethesda, MD 20814

Telecommunications for the Deaf
814 Thayer Ave
Silver Spring, MD 20785

HEART

American Heart Association
7320 Greenville Ave
Dallas, TX 75231

Coronary Club
Cleveland Clinic Education Foundation
9500 Euclid Ave, Ste E4-15
Cleveland, OH 44195

**High Blood Pressure Information
Center**
4733 Bethesda Ave, Ste 530
Bethesda, MD 20814

Mended Hearts, Inc.
7320 Greenville Ave
Dallas, TX 75231

**National Heart, Lung, and Blood
Institute**
National Institutes of Health
9000 Rockville Pike
Building 31, Room 4A21
Bethesda, MD 20892

HEMOPHILIA
National Hemophilia Foundation
110 Green St, Room 406
New York, NY 10012

HOSPITAL CARE
**Association for the Care of Children in
Hospitals**
3615 Wisconsin Ave NW
Washington, DC 20016

HUNTINGTON'S DISEASE
**Huntington's Disease Society of
America, Inc.**
140 W 22nd St, 6th Floor
New York, NY 10011-2420

KIDNEY DISEASE
American Liver Foundation
1425 Pompton Ave
Cedar Grove, NJ 07009

National Kidney Foundation
30 E 33rd St
New York, NY 10016

MYASTHENIA GRAVIS
Myathenia Gravis Foundation, Inc.
53 W Jackson Blvd, Ste 660
Chicago, IL 60604

NUTRITION (see also food)
American Dietetic Association (ADA)
216 W Jackson Blvd, Ste 800
Chicago, IL 60606

Human Nutrition Information Services
Federal Building, Room 360
6505 Belcrest Rd
Hyattsville, MD 20782

National Dairy Council
6300 N River Rd
Rosemont, IL 60018-4233

**Office of Consumer Communications
(HFG-10)**
Food and Drug Administration
Parklawn Building, Room 15B32
5600 Fishers Lane
Rockville, MD 20857

ORGAN DONORS
Living Bank International
PO Box 6725
Houston, TX 77265-6725

United Network for Organ Sharing
National Organ Procurement and
Transplantation Network
1100 Boulders Pkwy, Ste 500
PO Box 13700
Richmond, VA 23225-8770

PAIN
**National Committee on Treatment of
Intractable Pain**
PO Box 9553
Friendship Station
Washington, DC 20016-1553

PARKINSON'S DISEASE
**American Parkinson Disease
Association**
60 Bay St, Ste 401
Staten Island, NY 10301

Parkinson's Disease Foundation
William Black Medical Research
Building
Columbia University Medical Center
650 W 168th St
New York, NY 10032

PREGNANCY (See Family
Planning/Pregnancy)

REHABILITATION
**National Foundation for Facial
Reconstruction**
317 E 34th St, Room 901
New York, NY 10016

**National Rehabilitation Information
Center**
8455 Colesville Rd, Ste 935
Silver Spring, MD 20910

Rehabilitation International
22 E 21st St
New York, NY 10010

Rehabilitation Services Administration
Department of Human Services
605 G Street NW, Room 101M
Washington, DC 20001

SAFETY
Medic Alert Foundation International
2323 Colorado
PO Box 1009
Turlock, CA 95380

**National Highway Traffic Safety
Administration**
NTS-11, US Department of
Transportation
400 7th St SW
Washington, DC 20590

SEXUALLY TRANSMITTED
DISEASES
**Sex Information and Education
Council of the United States**
130 W 42nd St, Ste 2500
New York, NY 10036

SICKLE CELL ANEMIA
**National Association for Sickle Cell
Disease, Inc.**
3345 Wilshire Blvd, Ste 1106
Los Angeles, CA 90010-1880

SMOKING
Action on Smoking and Health
2013 H Street NW
Washington, DC 20006

Office on Smoking and Health
Disease Control Center
Park Building, Room 1-16
5600 Fishers Lane
Rockville, MD 20857

SPINAL CORD
**National Spinal Cord Injury
Association**
600 W Cummings Pkwy, Ste 2000
Woburn, MA 01801

Paralyzed Veterans of America
801 18th St NW
Washington, DC 20006

Community resources: Canada*

ACQUIRED IMMUNODEFICIENCY
SYNDROME (AIDS)
Canadian AIDS Society
170 Laurier Ave W, Ste 1101
Ottawa, ON K1P 5V5

**Canadian Foundation for AIDS
Research (CanFAR)**
120 Bloor St E, 1st Floor
Toronto, ON M4W 1B8

ADVOCACY
Alliance for Life
B1-90 Garry St
Winnipeg, MB R3C 4H1

*Modified from Directory of National Health Related Organizations and Associations in Canada: *Health promotion*, 1990, vol 29, No. 2. Health and Welfare
Canada, Ottawa, Ontario.

Canadian Association for Community Living
Kinsman Building
York University Campus
4700 Keele St
Downsview, ON M3J 1P3

Canadian Council on Social Development
55 Parkdale Ave
PO Box 3505, Station "C"
Ottawa, ON K1Y 4G1

Canadian Guidance and Counseling Association
151A Second Ave
PO Box 21027
Ottawa, ON K1S 5N1

Canada Safety Council
2750 Stevenage Dr, Unit 6
Ottawa, ON K1G 3N2

Consumers' Association of Canada
PO Box 9300
Ottawa, ON K1G 3T9

Dying with Dignity: Canadian Society Concerned with the Quality of Dying
175 St Clair Ave W
Toronto, ON M4V 1P7

Little People of Canada
c/o Ontario Chapter
PO Box 19
Agincourt, ON M1S 3B4

National Anti-Poverty Organization
456 Rideau St
Ottawa, ON K1N 5Z4

Non-Smokers' Rights Association
344 Bloor St W, Ste 308
Toronto, ON M5S 3A7

Patients' Rights Association
40 Homewood Ave, Ste 315
Toronto, ON M4Y 2K2

ALCOHOL AND DRUG ABUSE
Addiction Research Foundation
33 Russell St
Toronto, ON M5S 2S1

Al-Anon Family Groups (Canada)
National Public Information
PO Box 6433, Station "J"
Ottawa, ON K2A 3Y6

Alcoholics Anonymous
234 Eglinton Ave E, Ste 502
Toronto, ON M4P 1K5

Canadian Association for Children of Alcoholics
PO Box 159, Station "H"
Toronto, ON M4C 5H9

Canadian Centre on Substance Abuse
112 Kent St
Place de Ville Tower B, Ste 480
Ottawa, ON K1P 5P2

Council on Drug Abuse
698 Westin Rd, Ste 17
Toronto, ON M6N 3R3

PRIDE Canada (Parent Resources Institute for Drug Education)
College of Pharmacy
University of Saskatchewan
Saskatoon, SK S7N 0W0

ALZHEIMER'S DISEASE
Alzheimer Society of Canada
1320 Yonge St, Ste 302
Toronto, ON M4T 1X2

AMYOTROPHIC LATERAL SCLEROSIS
Amyotrophic Lateral Sclerosis Society of Canada
90 Adelaide St E, Ste B101
Toronto, ON M5C 2R4

APLASTIC ANEMIA
Aplastic Anemia Family Association of Canada
14 Lilac Ave
Thornhill, ON L3T 5J9

ARTHRITIS
Arthritis Society
250 Bloor St E, Ste 401
Toronto, ON M4W 3P2

ASTHMA AND ALLERGIES
Allergy Foundation of Canada
PO Box 1904
Saskatoon, SK S7K 3S5

Allergy Information Association
65 Tromley Dr, Room 10
Etobicoke, ON M9B 5Y7

BLINDNESS
Canadian Council of the Blind
PO Box 2310, Station "D"
Ottawa, ON K1P 5W5

Canadian National Institute for the Blind
1931 Bayview Ave
Toronto, ON M4G 4C8

CANCER
Canadian Cancer Society
10 Alcorn Ave, Ste 200
Toronto, ON M4V 3B1

Candlelighters Childhood Cancer Foundation Canada
c/o 148 Quinn St
PO Box 279
Philipsburg, PQ J0J 1N0

CHILD ABUSE
Canadian Society for the Prevention of Cruelty to Children
356 First St
PO Box 700
Midland, ON L4R 4P4

CHILDREN
Big Brothers of Canada
5230 South Service Rd
Burlington, ON L7L 5K2

Boys and Girls Clubs of Canada
250 Consumers Rd, Ste 605
Willowdale, ON M2J 4V6

Canadian Child Day Care Federation
120 Holland Ave, Ste 401
Ottawa, ON K1Y 0X6

Canadian Council on Children and Youth
2211 Riverside Dr, Ste 14
Ottawa, ON K1H 7X5

Canadian Foundation for the Study of Infant Deaths
PO Box 190, Station "R"
Toronto, ON M4G 3Z9

Canadian Institute of Child Health
17 York St, Ste 105
Ottawa, ON K1N 5S7

Canadian Paediatric Society
c/o Children's Hospital of Eastern Ontario
401 Smyth Rd
Ottawa, ON K1H 8L1

Children's Broadcast Institute
234 Eglinton Ave E, Ste 405
Toronto, ON M4P 1K5

Tracheo Esophageal Fistula
Parent Network
c/o 42 Saskatoon Dr
Etobicoke, ON M9P 2E9

CLEFT LIP AND PALATE
Canadian Cleft Lip and Palate Family Association
180 Dundas St W, Ste 1508
Toronto, ON M5G 1X8

CYSTIC FIBROSIS
Canadian Cystic Fibrosis Foundation
2221 Yonge St, Ste 601
Toronto, ON M4S 2B4

DIABETES
Canadian Diabetes Association
78 Bond St
Toronto, ON M5B 2J8

Juvenile Diabetes Foundation Canada
4632 Yonge St, Ste 100
Willowdale, ON M2N 5M1

DISABILITIES
Autism Society Canada
20 College St, Suite 2
Toronto, ON M5G 1K2

Canadian Coalition for the Prevention of Developmental Disabilities
c/o Canadian Institute of Child Health
17 York St, Ste 105
Ottawa, ON K1N 5S7

Canadian Paraplegic Association
1500 Don Mills Rd, Ste 201
Don Mills, ON M3B 3K4

Canadian Rehabilitation Council for the Disabled
45 Sheppard Ave E, Ste 801
Toronto, ON M2N 5W9

Coalition of Provincial Organizations of the Handicapped
926-294 Portage Ave
Winnipeg, MB R3C 0B9

DAWN Canada (DisAbled Women's Network)
775 East Georgia St
Vancouver, BC V6A 2A3

Disability Information Services of Canada
501 18th Ave SW, Ste 304
Calgary, AB T2S 0C7

Learning Disabilities Association of Canada
323 Chapel St, Ste 200
Ottawa, ON K1N 7Z2

DOWN SYNDROME
Canadian Down Syndrome Society
501 18th Ave SW, Ste 303
Calgary, AB T2S 0C7

EPILEPSY
Epilepsy Canada
2099 Alexandre de Séve St, Ste 27
PO Box 1560, Station "C"
Montreal, PQ H2L 4K8

FAMILY PLANNING/PREGNANCY
Canadian Coalition on Depo Provera
c/o Winnipeg Women's Health Clinic
419 Graham Ave, 3rd Floor
Winnipeg, MB R3C 0M3

Canadian Fertility and Andrology Society
2065 Alexandre de Sève St, Ste 409
Montreal, PQ H2L 2W5

Canadian Mothercraft Society
32 Heath St W
Toronto, ON M4V 1T3

Canadian PID Society
(Pelvic Inflammatory Disease)
PO Box 33804, Station D
Vancouver, BC V6J 4L6

DES Action Canada
Snowdon, PO Box 233
Montreal, PQ H3X 3T4

Infertility Awareness Association of Canada
104-1785 Alta Vista Dr
Ottawa, ON K1G 3Y6

La Leche League Canada
493 Main St
Winchester, ON K0C 2K0

Planned Parenthood Federation of Canada
1 Nicholas St, Ste 430
Ottawa, ON K1N 7B7

US-Canada Endometriosis Association
8585 North 76th Pl
Milwaukee, WI 53223 USA

FAMILY RESOURCES
Canadian Association for Treatment and Study of the Family
Department of Social Work
King's College
University of Western Ontario
268 Epworth Ave
London, ON N6A 2M3

Family Life Education Council
233 12th Ave SW
Calgary, AB T2R 0G9

Family Service Canada
55 Parkdale Ave
Ottawa, ON K1Y 4G1

HomeSupport Canada
119 Rose Ave, Ste 104
Ottawa, ON K1Y 0N6

One Parent Families Association of Canada
6979 Yonge St, Ste 203
Willowdale, ON M2M 3X9

Vanier Institute of the Family
120 Holland Ave, 3rd Floor
Ottawa, ON K1Y 0X6

FOOD (see also Nutrition)
World Food Day Association of Canada
255 Argyle Ave
Ottawa, ON K2P 1B8

GASTROINTESTINAL DISORDERS
Canadian Celiac Association
6519B Mississauga Rd
Mississauga, ON L5N 1A6

Canadian Foundation for Ileitis and Colitis
21 St Clair Ave E, Ste 301
Toronto, ON M4T 1L9

HEADACHES
Migraine Foundation
390 Brunswick Ave
Toronto, ON M5R 2Z4

HEALTH
Canadian Acupuncture Association of Canada, Inc.
333 Besserer St
Ottawa, ON K1N 6B4

Canadian Association for Health, Physical Education and Recreation
1600 James Nalsmith Dr, Ste 606
Gloucester, ON K1B 5N4

Canadian Association for School Health
1595 West 10th Ave
Vancouver, BC V6J 1Z8

Canadian Council for Multicultural Health
1017 Wilson Ave, Ste 100
Downsview, ON M3K 1Z1

Canadian Fitness and Lifestyle Research Institute
47 Clarence St, Ste 200
Ottawa, ON K1N 9K1

Canadian Health Education Society
253 College St
PO Box 306
Toronto, ON M5T 1R5

Canadian Health Libraries Association
PO Box 434, Station "K"
Toronto, ON M4P 2G9

Canadian Public Health Association
1565 Carling Ave, Ste 400
Ottawa, ON K1Z 8R1

Canadian Society for International Health
1585 Carling Ave, Ste 400
Ottawa, ON K1Z 8R1

Canadians for Health Research
PO Box 126
Westmount, PQ H3Z 2T1

Catholic Health Association of Canada
1247 Kilborn Ave
Onawa, ON K1H 6K9

Consumer Health Association of Canada
250 Sheppard Ave E, Ste 205
Willowdale, ON M2N 6M9

Society for Rare Disorders
100-542 7th St S
Lethbridge, AB T1J 2H1

Women's Health Interaction
c/o Inter Pares
58 Arthur St
Ottawa, ON K1R 7B9

HEALTH—DENTAL
Canadian Dental Association
1815 Alta Vista Dr
Ottawa, ON K1G 3Y6

HEALTH—MENTAL
Canadian Friends of Schizophrenics
95 Barber Greene Rd, Ste 309
Don Mills, ON M3C 3E9

Canadian Mental Health Association
2160 Yonge St, 3rd Floor
Toronto, ON M4S 2Z3

Canadian Psychiatric Association
294 Albert St, Ste 204
Ottawa, ON K1P 6E6

Canadian Psychiatric Research Foundation
80 Bloor St W, Ste 307
Toronto, ON M4W 3B8

Canadian Psychological Association
Vincent Rd
Old Chelsea, PQ J0X 2N0

Canadian Schizophrenia Foundation
7375 Kingsway
Burnaby, BC V3N 3B5

HEARING AND SPEECH

**Acoustic Neuroma Association of
Canada**
PO Box 369
Edmonton, AB T6J 2J6

Candian Association of the Deaf
2435 Holly Lane, Ste 205
Ottawa, ON K1V 7P2

**Canadian Association of
Speech-Language Pathologists and
Audiologists**
25 Main St W, Ste 1216
Hamilton, ON L8P 1H1

**Canadian Co-ordinating Council on
Deafness**
2106 St Laurent Blvd
Ottawa, ON K1G 1A9

**Canadian Cultural Society of the Deaf,
Inc.**
144, 11337-61 Ave
Edmonton, AB T6H 1M3

**Canadian Deaf and Hard of Hearing
Forum**
2435 Holly Lane, Ste 205
Ottawa, ON K1V 7P2

**Canadian Deaf-Blind and Rubella
Association**
PO Box 1625
Meaford, ON N0H 1Y0

Canadian Hard of Hearing Association
2435 Holly Lane, Ste 205
Ottawa, ON K1V 7P2

Canadian Hearing Society
271 Spadina Rd
Toronto, ON M5R 2V3

Tinnitus Institute of Canada
c/o 75 Marengère, Ste 3
Hull, PQ J8Y 1N5

HEART

**Advanced Coronary Treatment
Foundation of Canada**
379 Holland Ave, Ste 2
Ottawa, ON K1Y 0Y9

Canadian Cardiovascular Society
360 Victoria Ave, Ste 401
Westmount, PQ H3Z 2N4

Heart and Stroke Foundation of Canada
160 George St, Ste 200
Ottawa, ON K1N 9M2

HEMOCHROMATOSIS

Canadian Hemochromatosis Society
PO Box 94303
Richmond, BC V6Y 2A6

HEMOPHILIA

Canadian Hemophilia Society
1450 City Councillors St, Ste 840
Montreal, PQ H3A 2E6

HUNTINGTON'S DISEASE

Huntington Society of Canada
13 Water St N, Ste 3
PO Box 333
Cambridge, ON N1R 5T8

HYPERTENSION

**Canadian Coalition for High Blood
Pressure Prevention and Control**
c/o Dr. Arun Chockalingam
Faculty of Medicine
Memorial University of Newfoundland
St John's, NF A1B 3V6

Canadian Hypertension Society
3414 Park Ave, Ste 205
Montreal, PQ H2X 2H5

KIDNEY DISEASE

Kidney Foundation of Canada
4060 St Catherine St W, Ste 555
Montreal, PQ H3Z 2Z3

LIVER DISEASE

Canadian Liver Foundation
1320 Yonge St, Ste 301
Toronto, ON M4T 1X2

LUNG

Canadian Lung Association
75 Albert St, Ste 908
Ottawa, ON K1P 5E7

LUPUS

Lupus Canada
PO Box 3302, Station "B"
Calgary, AB T2M 4L8

MUCOPOLYSACCHARIDE DISEASES

**Society for Mucopolysaccharide
Diseases (Canada)**
c/o 382 Parkway Blvd
Flin Flon, MB R8A 0K4

MULTIPLE SCLEROSIS

Multiple Sclerosis Society of Canada
250 Bloor St E, Ste 820
Toronto, ON M4W 3P9

MUSCULAR DYSTROPHY

**Muscular Dystrophy Association of
Canada**
150 Eglinton Ave E, Ste 400
Toronto, ON M4P 1E8

NUTRITION

Bulimia Anorexia Nervosa Association
c/o Psychological Services
University of Windsor
Windsor, ON N9B 3P4

**Canadian Cholesterol Reference
Foundation**
307-2083 Alma St
Vancouver, BC V6R 4N6

**National Eating Disorder Information
Centre**
Toronto General Hospital
200 Elizabeth St
College Wing 1-318
Toronto, ON M5G 2C4

National Institute of Nutrition
1565 Carling Ave, Ste 400
Ottawa, ON K1Z 8R1

ORGAN DONORS

**Canadian Coalition on Organ Donor
Awareness**
c/o Pharmaceutical Manufacturers'
Association of Canada
1111 Prince of Wales Dr, Ste 302
Ottawa, ON K2C 3P2

Transplant International (Canada)
339 Windermere Rd
London, ON N6A 5A5

ORTHOPEDIC DISORDERS

**Canadian Osteogenesis Imperfecta
Society**
c/o 128 Thornhill Crescent
Chatham, ON N7L 4M3

Osteoporosis Society of Canada
33 Laird Dr
Toronto, ON M5S 3A7

PAIN

Canadian Pain Society
c/o Dr. H. Merskey
London Psychiatric Hospital
850 Highbury Ave
PO Box 2532, Station A
London, ON N6A 4H1

**North American Chronic Pain
Association of Canada**
c/o 6 Handel Ct
Brampton, ON L6S 1Y4

PARKINSON'S DISEASE

Parkinson Foundation of Canada
55 Bloor St W, Ste 232
Toronto, ON M4W 1A5

PREGNANCY (see Family Planning/Pregnancy)

REHABILITATION

Canadian Academy of Sport Medicine
Place R Talt MacKenzie
1600 James Nalsmith Dr
Gloucester, ON K1B 5N4

Canadian Art Therapy Association
216 St Clair Ave W
Toronto, ON M4V 1R2

**Canadian Association of Occupational
Therapists**
110 Eglinton Ave W, 3rd Floor
Toronto, ON M4R 1A3

Canadian Council on Rehabilitation and Work
167 Lombard Ave, Ste 410
Winnipeg, MB R3B 0T6

Canadian Occupational Therapy Foundation
110 Eglinton Ave W, 3rd Floor
Toronto, ON M4R 1A3

Canadian Physiotherapy Association
890 Yonge St
Toronto, ON M4W 3P4

REYE'S SYNDROME

Reye's Syndrome Foundation of Canada
c/o Children's Hospital of Western Ontario
Department of Paediatrics
800 Commissioners Rd E
London, ON N6C 2V5

SAFETY

Canadian Centre for Occupational Health and Safety
250 Main St E
Hamilton, ON L8N 1H6

Traffic Injury Research Foundation of Canada
171 Nepean St, 6th Floor
Ottawa, ON K2P 0B4

SERVICES

Canadian Long Term Care Association
260 St Patrick St, Ste 302
Ottawa, ON K1N 5K5

Canadian Medic Alert Foundation
293 Eglinton Ave E
Toronto, ON M4P 2Z8

Canadian Red Cross Society
1800 Alta Vista Dr
Ottawa, ON K1G 4J5

International Social Service Canada
55 Parkdale Ave
Ottawa, ON K1Y 1E6

Mission Air Transportation Network
77 Bloor St W, Ste 1711
Toronto, ON M5S 3A1

United Way/Centraide Canada
150 Kent St, Ste 600
Ottawa, ON K1P 5P4

YMCA Canada
2160 Yonge St, 2nd Floor
Toronto, ON M4S 2A9

YMCA of Canada
80 Gerrard St E
Toronto, ON M5B 1G6

SEXUALLY TRANSMITTED DISEASES

Candida Research and Information Foundation (Canada)
598 St Clair Ave W, 3rd Floor
Toronto, ON M8C 1A6

SKIN

Canadian Dermatology Foundation
450 Central Ave, Ste 308
London, ON N6B 2E8

Canadian Psoriasis Foundation
1565 Carling Ave, Ste 400
Ottawa, ON K1Z 8R1

SLEEP DISORDERS

Canadian Association for Narcolepsy
PO Box 223, Station "S"
Toronto, ON M5M 4L7

SMOKING

Canadian Council on Smoking and Health
1585 Carling Ave, Ste 400
Ottawa, ON K1Z 8R1

Smoking and Health Action Foundation
344 Bloor St W, Ste 308
Toronto, ON M5S 3A7

SPINA BIFIDA

Spina Bifida Association of Canada
633 Wellington Crescent
Winnipeg, MB R3M 0A8

SPINAL CORD

Back Association of Canada
83 Cottingham St
Toronto, ON M4V 1B9

Canadian Cerebral Palsy Association
880 Wellington St
Ste 612, City Centre
Ottawa, ON K1R 6K7

Canadian Chiropractic Association
1396 Eglinton Ave W
Toronto, ON M6C 2E4

Spinal Cord Society Canada
120 Newkirk Rd, Unit 32
Richmond Hill, ON L4C 9S7

STRESS

Canadian Institute of Stress
Shipp Centre
3300 Bloor St W, Ste 3100
Toronto, ON M8X 2X3

STROKE

Stroke Recovery Association
170 The Donway W, Ste 122A
Don Mills, ON M3C 2G3

THYROID

Thyroid Foundation of Canada
PO Box 1597
Kingston, ON K7L 5C8

TOURETTE SYNDROME

Tourette Syndrome Foundation of Canada
173 Owen Blvd
North York, ON M2P 1G8

TURNER'S SYNDROME

Turner's Syndrome Society
York University
Administrative Studies Building, Room 006
4700 Keele St
Downsview, ON M3J 1P3

14-2 Nursing organizations

Advocates for Child Psychiatric Nursing
603 Shakertown Ct
Cincinnati, OH 45242

American Academy of Ambulatory Nursing Administration
North Woodbury Rd
PO Box 56
Pitman, NJ 08071

American Academy of Nurse Practitioners
893 Stone Jug Rd
Biglerville, PA 17307

American Assembly for Men in Nursing
PO Box 31753
Independence, OH 44131

American Association of Colleges of Nursing
1 Dupont Circle NW, Ste 530
Washington, DC 20036

American Association of Critical Care Nurses
1 Civic Plaza, Ste 330
Newport Beach, CA 92660

American Association of Diabetes Educators
500 N Michigan Ave, Ste 1400
Chicago, IL 60611

American Association of Neuroscience Nurses
224 N Desplaines, Ste 601
Chicago, IL 60661

American Association of Nurse Anesthetists
216 Higgins Rd
Park Ridge, IL 60068

American Association of Nurse Attorneys
113 W Franklin St
Baltimore, MD 21201

American Association of Nursing History
1753 W Congress Plaza
Chicago, IL 60612

American Association of Occupational Health Nurses
50 Lenox Pointe
Atlanta, GA 30324

American Association of Spinal Cord Injury Nurses
432 Park Ave S
New York, NY 10016

American College of Nurse Midwives
1522 K St NW, Ste 1000
Washington, DC 20005

American Holistic Nurses' Association
Rt 4, PO Box 365B
Carbondale, IL 62901

American Nephrology Nurses' Association
N Woodbury Rd
PO Box 56
Pitman, NJ 08071

American Nurses Association
600 Maryland Avenue, SW
Suite 100 W
Washington, DC 20024

American Organization of Nurse Executives
840 N Lake Shore Dr
Chicago, IL 60611

American Psychiatric Nurses Association
c/o Shirley Smoyak
Rutgers College of Nursing
4 Roney Rd
Edison, NJ 08820

American Public Health Association, Public Health Nurses
1015 15th St NW
Washington, DC 20005

American Society of Ophthalmic Registered Nurses, Inc
655 Beach St
PO Box 3030
San Francisco, CA 94119

American Society for Parental and Enteral Nutrition, Nurses Committee
8605 Cameron St, Ste 500
Silver Spring, MD 20910

American Society of Plastic & Reconstructive Surgical Nurses
N Woodbury Rd
PO Box 56
Pitman, NJ 08071

American Society of Post Anesthesia Nurses
11508 Allecingie Pkwy, Ste C
Richmond, VA 23235

American Urological Association Allied
Shore Dr
PO Box 9397
Raytown, MO 64133

Arthritis Health Professionals Association, Nursing Section
Columbia Hospital
2025 E Newport
Milwaukee, WI 53211

Association of Faculties of Pediatric Nurse Practitioners and Associates Programs
c/o Linda Gilman
5250 N Meridian
Indianapolis, IN 46208

Association of Nurses in AIDS Care
CN5254
Princeton, NJ 08543-5254

Association of Operating Room Nurses
10170 E Mississippi Ave
Denver, CO 80231

Association of Pediatric Oncology Nurses
6728 Old McLean Village
McLean, VA 22101

Association for Practitioners in Infection Control
505 E Hawley
Mundelein, IL 60060

Association of Rehabilitation Nurses
5700 Old Orchard Rd, 1st Floor
Skokie, IL 60077-1024

Chi Eta Phi Sorority, Inc.
2247 Glendale Dr
Decatur, GA 30032

Commission of Graduates of Foreign Nursing Schools
3624 Mailut
Philadelphia, PA 19104

Consortium of Registered Nurses for Eye Acquisition
1511 K St NW, Ste 830
Washington, DC 20005

Dermatology Nurses Association
N Woodbury Rd
PO Box 56
Pitman, NJ 08071

Drug and Alcohol Nursing Association
113 W Franklin St
Baltimore, MD 21201

Emergency Nurses Association
230 E Ohio, Ste 600
Chicago, IL 60611

Frontier Nursing Service
Hospital Drive
Nyae, KY 41745

International Association for Enterostomal Therapy
2081 Business Center Ct, #290
Irvine, CA 92715

International Society of Nurses in Cancer Care
Mulberry House
Royal Marsden Hospital
Fulham Road
London SW3 6JJ

Intravenous Nurses Society
2 Brighten St
Belmont, MA 02178

Association of Women's Health Obstetrics, and Neonatal Nurses
409 12th St SW
Washington, DC 20024-2191

National Alliance of Nurse Practitioners
PO Box 44707
L'Enfant Plaza SW
Washington, DC 20026

National Association for Health Care Recruitment
PO Box 93851
Cleveland, OH 44101-5851

National Association of Hispanic Nurses
2014 Johnston St
Los Angeles, CA 90031

National Association of Neonatal Nurses
177 Lynch Creek Way
Petaluma, CA 94952

National Association of Nurse Practitioners in Family Planning
810 7th Ave, 7th Floor
New York, NY 10019

National Association of Orthopaedic Nurses
N Woodbury Rd
PO Box 56
Pitman, NJ 08071

National Association of Pediatric Nurse Associates & Practitioners
1101 Kings Highway N, Ste 206
Cherry Hill, NJ 08034

National Association of School Nurses, Inc
Lamplighter Lane
PO Box 1300
Scarborough, ME 04074

National Black Nurses Association, Inc
1011 N Capitol St NE
Washington, DC 20002

National Conference of Gerontological Nurse Practitioners
c/o Linda Grissom
Institute for Human Services
3501 N Scottsdale Rd, #320
Scottsdale, AZ 85251

National Council of State Board of Nursing
625 N Michigan Ave, Ste 1544
Chicago, IL 60611

National Federation of Specialty Nursing Organizations
L'Enfant Plaza SW
PO Box 23836
Washington, DC 20026

National Flight Nurses Association
PO Box 8222
Rapid City, SD 57709

National Gerontological Nursing Association
6621 Adrian St
New Carrollton, MD 20784

National League for Nursing
10 Columbus Circle
New York, NY 10019

National Nurses in Business Association
4286 Redwood Highway, Ste 252
San Rafael, CA 94903

National Nurses Society on Addictions
2506 Gross Point Rd
Evanston, IL 60201

National Organization for Nurse Practitioners Faculties
NP Program, Himmelfarb Library
2300 I St NW
Washington, DC 20037

National Organization for Philippine Nurses in US
459 Joan St
South Plainfield, NJ 07080

National Student Nurses Association
555 W 57th St, Room 1325
New York, NY 10019

North American Nursing Diagnosis Association
c/o St Louis University
School of Nursing
3525 Caroline St
St. Louis, MO 63104

Nurse Consultants Association
414 Plaza Dr, Ste 209
Westmont, IL 60559

Nurses' Environment Health Watch
2110 Fourth St, Ste 26
Santa Monica, CA 90405

Nurses Organization of the Veterans Administration
6728 Old McLean Village
McLean, VA 22101

Oncology Nursing Society
501 Holiday Dr
Pittsburgh, PA 15220-2749

Pediatric Endocrinology Nursing Society
2545 Chicago Ave S, Ste 408
Minneapolis, MN 55404

Sigma Theta Tau
1100 Waterway Blvd
Indianapolis, IN 46202

Society for Education & Research in Psyc/MH Nursing
c/o Ann Cain, PhD
1106 Little Magothy View
Cape St Clair
Annapolis, MD 21401

Society of Gastrointestinal Assistants
1070 Sibley Tower
Rochester, NY 14604

Society of Nursing History
Nursing Education Department
Box 150
Teachers College
Columbia University
New York, NY 10027

Society of Otorhinolaryngology & Head-Neck Nurses, Inc.
4330 Sea Mist Dr
New Smyrna Beach, FL 32069

Society for Peripheral Vascular Nursing
1070 Sibley Tower
Rochester, NY 14604

Transcultural Nursing Society
College of Nursing
University of Utah
25 S Dr
Salt Lake City, UT 84112

Wound Ostomy and Continence Nurses Society
2755 Bristol St, Ste 110
Costa Mesa, CA 92626

STATE AND TERRITORIAL BOARDS OF NURSING

Alabama
Board of Nursing
RSA Plaza, Ste 250
770 Washington Ave
Montgomery, AL 36130

Alaska
Board of Nursing Licensing
Department of Commerce & Economic Development
Division of Occupational Licensing
PO Box 110806
Juneau, AS 99811-0806

Arizona
Board of Nursing
2001 W Camelback Rd, #350
Phoenix, AZ 85015

Arkansas
Board of Nursing
University Tower Building, Ste 800
1123 S University Ave
Little Rock, AK 72204

California
Board of Registered Nursing
PO Box 944210
400 R St, Ste 4030
Sacramento, CA 95814

Colorado
Board of Nursing
1560 Broadway, Ste 670
Denver, CO 80202

Connecticut
Board of Examiners for Nursing
150 Washington St
Hartford, CT 06106

Delaware
Board of Nursing
Margaret O'Neill Bldg
Federal & Court St
PO Box 1401
Dover, DE 19903

District of Columbia
Board of Nursing
614 H Street NW
Washington, DC 20001

Florida
Board of Nursing
111 E Coastline Dr, Ste 516
Jacksonville, FL 32202

Georgia
Board of Nursing
166 Pryor Street SW, Ste 400
Atlanta, GA 30303

Guam
Board of Nurse Examiners
Box 2816
Agana, Guam 96910

Hawaii
Board of Nursing
Box 3469
Honolulu, HI 96801

Idaho
Board of Nursing
2800 N 8th St, Ste 210
Boise, ID 83720

Illinois
Department of Professional Regulation
320 W Washington St
Springfield, IL 62786

Indiana
State Board of Nursing
Health Professions Bureau
402 W Washington St, Room 041
Indianapolis, IN 46204

Iowa
Board of Nursing
1223 E Court
Des Moines, IA 50319

Kansas
State Board of Nursing
Landon State Office Building
900 SW Jackson, Room 551
Topeka, KS 66612

Kentucky
Board of Nursing
4010 Dupoint Circle, Ste 430
Louisville, KY 40207

Louisiana
Board of Nursing
150 Baronne St, Room 912
New Orleans, LA 70112

Maine
Board of Nursing
State House Station 158
Augusta, ME 04333

Maryland
Board of Nursing
Metro Executive Center
4201 Patterson Ave
Baltimore, MD 21215

Massachusetts
Board of Registration in Nursing
100 Cambridge St, Room 1519
Boston, MA 02202

Michigan
Board of Nursing
PO Box 30018
Lansing, MI 48909

Minnesota
Board of Nursing
2700 University Av W, #108
St Paul, MN 55114

Mississippi
Board of Nursing
239 N Lamar St, Ste 401
Jackson, MS 39201

Missouri
Board of Nursing
3605 Missouri Blvd
PO Box 656
Jefferson City, MO 65102

Montana
Board of Nursing
Department of Commerce
Arcade Building, Lower Level
111 N Jackson
Helena, MT 59620

Nebraska
Board of Nursing
Box 95007
Lincoln, NE 68509

Nevada
Board of Nursing
1281 Terminal Way, Ste 116
Reno, NV 89502

New Hampshire
Board of Nursing
Division of Public Health Services
Health & Welfare Building
6 Hazen Dr
Concord, NH 03301

New Jersey
Board of Nursing
1100 Raymond Blvd, Room 508
PO Box 45010
Newark, NJ 07101

New Mexico
Board of Nursing
4253 Montgomery NE, Ste 130
Albuquerque, NM 87109

New York
NYS Board for Nursing
NYS State Education Department
Cultural Education Center
Albany, NY 12230

North Carolina
Board of Nursing
Box 2129
Raleigh, NC 27602-2129

North Dakota
Board of Nursing
919 S 7th St, Ste 504
Bismarck, ND 58504

Ohio
Board of Nursing
77 S High St, 17th Floor
Columbus, OH 43266-0316

Oklahoma
Board of Nursing
2915 N Classen Blvd, Ste 524
Oklahoma City, OK 73106

Oregon
Board of Nursing
800 NE Oregon St, #25-465
Portland, OR 97232-2162

Pennsylvania
Board of Nursing
PO Box 2649
Harrisburg, PA 17105-2649

Puerto Rico
Board of Nurse Examiners
Call Box 10200
Santurce, PR 00908-0200

Rhode Island
Board of Nurse Registration and
    Education
Cannon Health Building, Room 104
3 Capitol Hill
Providence, RI 02908

South Carolina
Board of Nursing
220 Executive Center Dr, Ste 220
Columbia, SC 29210

South Dakota
Board of Nursing
3307 S Lincoln Ave
Sioux Falls, SD 57105

Tennessee
Board of Nursing
Bureau of Manpower and Facilities
283 Plus Park Blvd
Nashville, TN 37247

Texas
Board of Nurse Examiners
9101 Burnet Rd, Ste 104
Austin, TX 78758

Utah
Board of Nursing
Heber M. Wells Building, 4th Floor
160 E 300 S
PO Box 45805
Salt Lake City, UT 84145

Vermont
Board of Nursing
109 State St
Montpelier, VT 05602

Virgin Islands
Board of Nurse Licensure
Kongens Gade #3
PO Box 4247
St Thomas, VI 00803

Virginia
Board of Nursing
1601 Rolling Hills Dr
Richmond, VA 23229

Washington
State Board of Nursing
PO Box 47864
Olympia, WA 98504-7864

West Virginia
Board of Examiners for RNs
Embleton Building, Room 309
922 Quarrier St
Charleston, WV 25301

Wisconsin
Board of Nursing
Room 174, 1400 E Washington Ave
PO Box 8935
Madison, WI 53708

Wyoming
Board of Nursing
Barrett Building, 2nd Floor
2301 Central Ave
Cheyenne, WY 82002

CANADIAN PROVINCIAL REGISTERED NURSES ASSOCIATIONS

Alberta
Alberta Association of Registered Nurses
11620 168th St
Edmonton, AB T5M 4A6

British Columbia
Registered Nurses Association of British
    Columbia
2855 Arbutus St
Vancouver, BC V6Y 3Y8

Manitoba
Manitoba Association of Registered Nurses
647 Broadway Ave
Winnipeg, MB R3C 0X2

New Brunswick
Nurses Association of New Brunswick
231 Saunders St
Fredericton, NB E3B 1N6

Newfoundland
Association of Registered Nurses of
　Newfoundland
55 Military Rd
PO Box 6116
St John's, NF A1C 5X8

Northwest Territories
Northwest Territories Registered Nurses
　Association
PO Box 2757
Yellowknife, NT X1A 2R1

Nova Scotia
Register Nurses Association of Nova
　Scotia
6035 Coburg Rd
Halifax, NS B3H 1Y8

Ontario
College of Nurses of Ontario
101 Davenport Rd
Toronto, ON M5R 3P1

Prince Edward Island
Association of Nurses of Prince Edward
　Island
PO Box 1838
Charlottetown, PE C1A 7N5

Québec
Ordre des infirmières et infirmiers du
　Québec
4200 Ouest, blvd
Dorchester
Montréal, PQ H3Z 1V4

Saskatchewan
Saskatchewan Registered Nurses
　Association
2066 Retallack St
Regina, SK S4T 2K2

Yukon
Yukon Nurses Society
PO Box 5371
Whitehorse, YT Y1A 4Z2

14-3　Poison control

**AMERICAN ASSOCIATION OF
POISON CONTROL CENTERS
(Certified Regional Poison Centers,
April 1993)**

Alabama
Regional Poison Control Center
The Children's Hospital of Alabama
1600 7th Ave S
Birmingham, AL 35233-1711
Emergency Phone: (205) 939-9201, (800)
　292-6678 (AL only), or (205) 933-4050

Arizona
Arizona Poison and Drug Information
　Center
Arizona Health Sciences Center; Room
　#3204-K
1501 N Campbell Ave
Tucson, AZ 85724
Emergency Phone: (800) 362-0101 (AZ
　only), (602) 626-6016

Samaritan Regional Poison Center
Good Samaritan Regional Medical Center
1130 E McDowell, Ste A-5
Phoenix, AZ 85006
Emergency Phone: (602) 253-3334

California
Fresno Regional Poison Control Center
of Fresno Community Hospital and
　Medical Center
2823 Fresno St
Fresno, CA 93721
Emergency Phone: (800) 346-5922 or
　(209) 445-1222

San Diego Regional Poison Center
UCSD Medical Center; 8925
225 Dickinson St.
San Diego CA 92103-8925
Emergency Phone: (619) 543-6000, (800)
　876-4766 (in 619 area code only)

San Francisco Bay Area Regional Poison
　Control Center
San Francisco General Hospital
1001 Potrero Ave, Building 80, Room
　230
San Francisco, CA 94122
Emergency Phone: (415) 476-6600

Santa Clara Valley Medical Center
　Regional Poison Center
751 S Bascom Ave
San Jose, CA 95128
Emergency Phone: (408) 299-5112, (800)
　662-9886 (CA only)

University of California, Davis, Medical
　Center Regional Poison Control Center
2315 Stockton Blvd
Sacramento, CA 95817
Emergency Phone: (916) 734-3692, (800)
　342-9293 (Northern California only)

Colorado
Rocky Mountain Poison and Drug Center
645 Bannock St
Denver, CO 80204
Emergency Phone: (303) 629-1123

District of Columbia
National Capital Poison Center
Georgetown University Hospital
3800 Reservoir Rd NW
Washington, DC 20007
Emergency Numbers: (202) 625-3333,
　(202) 784-4660 (TTY)

Florida
Florida Poison Information Center at
　Tampa General Hospital
PO Box 1289
Tampa, FL 33601
Emergency Phone: (813) 253-4444
　(Tampa), (800) 282-3171 (Florida)

Georgia
Georgia Poison Center
Grady Memorial Hospital
80 Butler Street SE
PO Box 26066
Atlanta, GA 30335-3801
Emergency Phone: (800) 282-5846 GA
　only, (404) 589-4400

Indiana
Indiana Poison Center
Methodist Hospital of Indiana
1701 N Senate Blvd
PO Box 1367
Indianapolis, IN 46206-1367
Emergency Phone: (800) 382-9097 (IN
　only), (317) 929-2323

Maryland
Maryland Poison Center
20 N Pine St
Baltimore, MD 21201
Emergency Phone: (410) 528-7701, (800)
　492-2414 (MD only)

National Capital Poison Center (DC
　suburbs only)
Georgetown University Hospital
3800 Reservoir Rd NW
Washington, DC 20007
Emergency Numbers: (202) 625-3333,
　(202) 784-4660 (TTY)

Massachusetts
Massachusetts Poison Control System
300 Longwood Ave
Boston, MA 02115
Emergency Phone: (617) 232-2120, (800)
　682-9211

Michigan
Blodgett Regional Poison Center
1840 Wealthy SE
Grand Rapids, MI 49506-2968
Emergency Phone: (800) 632-2727
　(Michigan only), TTY (800) 356-3232

Poison Control Center
Children's Hospital of Michigan
3901 Beaubien Blvd
Detroit, MI 48201
Emergency Phone: (313) 745-5711

Minnesota
Hennepin Regional Poison Center
Hennepin County Medical Center
701 Park Ave
Minneapolis, MN 55415
Emergency Phone: (612) 347-3141,
　Petline: (612) 337-7387, TDD (612)
　337-7474

Minnesota Regional Poison Center
St Paul-Ramsey Medical Center
640 Jackson St
St Paul, MN 55101
Emergency Phone: (612) 221-2113

Missouri
Cardinal Glennon Children's Hospital
　Regional Poison Center

1465 S Grand Blvd
St Louis, MO 63104
Emergency Phone: (314) 772-5200, (800) 366-8888

Montana
Rocky Mountain Poison and Drug Center
645 Bannock St
Denver, CO 80204
Emergency Phone: (303) 629-1123

Nebraska
Poison Center
8301 Dodge St
Omaha, NE 68114
Emergency Phone: (402) 390-5555 (Omaha), (800) 955-9119 (NE)

New Jersey
New Jersey Poison Information and Education System
201 Lyons Ave
Newark, NJ 07112
Emergency Phone: (800) 962-1253

New Mexico
New Mexico Poison and Drug Information Center
University of New Mexico
Albuquerque, NM 87131-1076
Emergency Phone: (505) 843-2551, (800) 432-6866 (NM only)

New York
Hudson Valley Poison Center
Nyack Hospital
160 N Midland Ave
Nyack, NY 10960
Emergency Phone: (800) 336-6997, (914) 353-1000

Long Island Regional Poison Control Center
Winthrop University Hospital
259 First St
Mineola, NY 11501
Emergency Phone: (516) 542-2323, 2324, 2325, 3813

New York City Posion Control Center
NYC Department of Health
455 First Ave, Room 123

New York, NY 10016
Emergency Phone: (212) 340-4494, (212) P-O-I-S-O-N-S, TDD (212) 689-9014

Ohio
Central Ohio Poison Center
700 Children's Dr
Columbus, OH 43205-2696
Emergency Phone: (614) 228-1323, (800) 682-7625, (614) 228-2272 (TTY), (614) 461-2012

Cincinnati Drug & Poison Information Center and Regional Poison Control System
231 Bethesda Ave, ML 144
Cincinnati, OH 45267-0144
Emergency Phone: (513) 558-5111, 800-872-5111 (OH only)

Oregon
Oregon Poison Center
Oregon Health Sciences University
3181 SW Sam Jackson Park Rd
Portland, OR 97201
Emergency Phone: (503) 494-8968, (800) 452-7165 (OR only)

Pennsylvania
Central Pennsylvania Poison Center
University Hospital
Milton S Hershey Medical Center
Hershey, PA 17033
Emergency Phone: (800) 521-6110

Poison Control Center (serving the greater Philadelphia metropolitan area)
One Children's Center
Philadelphia, PA 19104-4303
Emergency Phone: (215) 386-2100

Pittsburgh Poison Center
3706 Fifth Ave at DeSoto St
Pittsburgh, PA 15213
Emergency Phone: (412) 681-6669

Rhode Island
Rhode Island Poison Center
593 Eddy St
Providence, RI 02903
Emergency Phone: (401) 277-5727

Texas
North Texas Poison Center
5201 Harry Hines Blvd
PO Box 35926
Dallas, TX 76235
Emergency Phone: (214) 590-5000, Texas Watts (800) 441-0040

Texas State Poison Center
University of Texas Medical Branch
Galveston, TX 77550-2780
Emergency Phone: (409) 766-1420 (Galveston), (713) 654-1702 (Houston)

Utah
Intermountain Regional Poison Control Center
50 North Medical Dr
Salt Lake City, UT 84132
Emergency Phone: (801) 581-2151, (800) 456-7707 (UT only)

Virginia
Blue Ridge Poison Center
Box 67, Blue Ridge Hospital
Charlottesville VA 22901
Emergency Phone: (804) 924-5543, (800) 451-1428

National Capital Poison Center (Northern VA only)
Georgetown University Hospital
3800 Reservoir Rd, NW
Washington, DC 20007
Emergency Numbers: (202) 625-3333; (202) 784-4660 (TTY)

West Virginia
West Virginia Poison Center
3110 MacCorkle Ave SE
Charleston, WV 25304
Emergency Phone: (800) 642-3625 (WV only), (304) 348-4211

Wyoming
Poison Center
8301 Dodge St
Omaha, NE 68114
Emergency Phone: (402) 390-5555 (Omaha), (800) 955-9119 (NE)

APPENDIX
15

COMMUNICABLE DISEASES

15-1 Universal blood and body fluid precautions

1. *All* health care workers should use appropriate barrier precautions to prevent skin and mucous-membrane exposure when contact with blood or body fluids of *any* patient is anticipated.
2. Gloves should be worn for touching blood and body fluids, mucous membranes, or non-intact skin of all patients, for handling items or surfaces soiled with blood or body fluids, and for performing venipuncture and other vascular access procedures. Gloves should be changed after contact with each patient.
3. Hands and other skin surfaces should be washed immediately and thoroughly if contaminated with blood or other body fluids. Hands should be washed immediately after gloves are removed.
4. Masks and protective eyewear or face shields should be worn during procedures that are likely to generate droplets of blood or other body fluids.
5. Gowns or aprons should be worn during procedures that are likely to generate splashes of blood or other body fluids.
6. Needles should not be recapped, purposely bent or broken by hand, removed from disposable syringes, or otherwise manipulated by hand. After use, disposable syringes and needles, scalpel blades, and other sharp items should be placed in puncture-resistant containers for disposal; the containers should be located as close as practical to the use area. Large-bore reusable needles should be placed in a puncture-resistant container for transport to the reprocessing area.
7. Although saliva has not been implicated in HIV transmission, mouthpieces, resuscitation bags, or other ventilation devices should be available for use in areas in which the need for resuscitation is predictable.
8. Health-care workers who have exudative lesions or weeping dermatitis should refrain from all direct patient care and from handling patient-care equipment until the condition resolves.
9. Pregnant health care workers are not known to be at greater risk of contracting HIV infection than non-pregnant workers; however, if a pregnant worker develops HIV infection, the infant is at risk from perinatal transmission. Pregnant health care workers should strictly adhere to precautions.
10. Invasive procedures (surgical entry into tissues, cavities, or organs) or repair of major traumatic injuries carry a risk of splattering of blood and fluids and require the use of gloves, masks, protective eyewear or face shield, and gowns or aprons made of materials that provide an effective fluid barrier.
11. During an invasive procedure, if a glove is torn or a needlestick or other injury occurs, the glove should be removed and a new glove used as promptly as patient safety permits; the needle or instrument involved in the incident should be removed from the sterile field.

From Centers for Disease Control. Recommendations for Prevention of HIV transmission in health-care settings, *MMWR,* 36, 2S, 1987.

GUIDELINES

Procedure	Wash hands	Gloves	Gown	Mask	Eyewear
Talking with patients					
Adjusting IV fluid rate or noninvasive equipment					
Examining patient without touching blood, body fluids, mucous membranes	x				
Examining patient with significant cough	x			x	
Examining patient including contact with blood, body fluids, mucous membranes, drainage	x	x			
Drawing blood	x	x			
Inserting venous access	x	x			
Suctioning	x	x	Use gown, mask, eyewear if blood and/or body fluid spattering is likely.		
Inserting body or face catheters	x	x	Use gown, mask, eyewear if blood and/or body fluid spattering is likely.		
Handling soiled waste, linen, other materials	x	x	Use gown, mask, eyewear only if waste or linen is extensively contaminated and spattering is likely.		
Intubation	x	x	x	x	x
Inserting arterial access	x	x	x	x	x
Endoscopy, bronchoscopy	x	x	x	x	x
Operative and other procedures that produce extensive spattering of blood and/or body fluids and are likely to soil clothes	x	x	x	x	x

Courtesy The Johns Hopkins Health System, Baltimore, MD.

15-2 | OSHA standard on occupational exposure to bloodborne pathogens

INTRODUCTION

On December 6, 1991, the Occupational Safety and Health Administration (OSHA) issued its final standard on Occupational Exposure to Bloodborne Pathogens. In issuing this ruling, OSHA declared that healthcare workers face a significant health risk in the workplace if occupational exposure to bloodborne pathogens is a reasonable possibility. Although OSHA is concerned with the transmission of any bloodborne pathogen, the ruling is directed toward preventing or minimizing exposure to the Hepatitis B virus (HBV) and the Human Immunodeficiency Virus (HIV).

OSHA's ruling called "Occupational Exposure to Bloodborne Pathogens" and published in the Federal Register is a long-awaited response to a congressional mandate to create protection for healthcare workers against exposure to HBV and HIV. OSHA concluded that the danger of bloodborne pathogens could be minimized or eliminated by taking certain precautions in the workplace. These precautions include a combination of controls in engineering, general work practices, personal protective clothing and equipment, training of personnel, Hepatitis B vaccination of healthcare workers, and the use of warning signs and labels.

The OSHA standard mandates the Universal Precautions guidelines recommended by the Centers for Disease Control since August 1987. This is a system of infection control that is based on the assumption that medical history and examination cannot reliably identify all patients infected with HIV, HBV, or other potentially infectious diseases. Therefore, blood and body fluid precautions must be consistently used with ALL patients.

Surprisingly, however, OSHA far exceeded the CDC guidelines in both the scope of healthcare workers and employers covered under the standard, and the demands made in complying with the regulation. Most businessess were not prepared for addressing the scope of the new regulations. It is important to understand that the CDC guidelines presented in August 1987 were only recommendations, but a ruling from a powerful governmental agency like OSHA makes the practice of Universal Precautions a requirement, and an enforceable law.

OSHA identifies 24 sectors of industry and over 500,000 facilities that are subject to this ruling. Almost five million workers are employed in hospitals, nursing homes, medical and dental offices.

One of the surprises in the standard was OSHA's inclusion of almost a million workers employed in industry outside healthcare facilities. Among the businesses affected are linen and laundry services, waste removal services, funeral homes and mortuaries, veterinarian clinics, and medical equipment companies.

The standard applies to any workplace where any workers who, in the course of their duties, might come into contact with blood, body fluids, or other potentially infectious materials. The standard required all facilities to be in full compliance with the standard by July 6, 1992.

The standard covers employees in ALL health care facilities including hospitals, clinics, dentist and doctor offices, blood banks, plasma centers, occupational health clinics, nursing homes, hospices, emergency care centers, clinical laboratories, and institutions for the developmentally disabled. This includes part time, temporary, or probationary employees in both permanent and temporary worksites.

Healthcare facilities in 23 states and two territories that have state OSHA-approved plans are not covered by the federal standard. These states are: Alaska, Arizona, California, Connecticut, Hawaii, Indiana, Iowa, Kentucky, Maryland, Michigan, Minnesota, Nevada, New Mexico, New York, North Carolina, Oregon, Puerto Rico, South Carolina, Tennessee, Utah, Vermont, Virginia, the Virgin Islands, Washington, and Wyoming. In Connecticut and New York, the state plan covers only state and local government employees; all other employees are covered by the federal OSHA standard.

Because state standards must be "at least as effective" as the federal standard, healthcare facilities located in these states must assess their compliance with the federal standard as a starting point, and then review their individual state plan for any additional requirements.

At this time, the federal standard does not apply to public sector employees. Examples of public sector employees are state, county, and municipal employees in public clinics and hospitals, emergency responders, and law enforcement personnel. However, recommendations have been made to include this sector of healthcare.

KEY PROVISIONS OF THE STANDARD
Purpose

The purpose of the standard is to limit occupational exposure to blood and other potentially infectious materials.

Scope

The ruling covers all employees who have the potential to come into contact with blood, body fluids, or other potentially infectious materials (OPIM).

Requirements
Exposure control plan

- Implementation of an Exposure Control Plan in which the employer must identify, in writing, workers who might be at risk for exposure to blood or other potentially infectious materials.

The employer's written plan must also explain how the facility will comply with the standard.

The employer's plan must include:

- A determination by job task, procedure and/or job classification of how an employee might be exposed during the performance of the job. This must be done without regard to personal protective clothing and equipment. The list of procedures in which exposure may occur must be posted in the facility. The list of job classifications must include the names of employees who fill those positions.
- The method, including a schedule, of how the plan will be implemented. This must include details of personal protective equipment to be used, work practices in housekeeping, Hepatitis B vaccinations, evaluation of exposure and required followup. Hazard communication and recordkeeping, detailed procedures for evaluating potentials of exposure in the workplace.
- A detailed plan for evaluating the circumstances if exposure occurs in the workplace. This plan should include first aid, evaluation by a healthcare professional, treatment, testing of source patient, follow up testing for the employee if indicated. A written report of the exposure incident must be provided to the employee within 15 days of the incident.
- The plan must be readily accessible to employees and available at all times to OSHA. All employees must know where the plan is kept in case of an OSHA inspection.

Methods of compliance

- Implementation of Methods of Compliance, specifically, Universal Precautions, engineering and work practice controls.

Universal Precautions are now required. Every healthcare worker must take protective measures when in contact with any patient, and every patient must be approached as if the patient is HIV or HBV infected. This also includes emergency situations.

Examples of engineering controls include puncture-resistant containers for needles and other sharp instruments, proper packaging for

Adapted from Goodner B: *The OSHA handbook*, Copyright 1993, Skidmore-Roth Publishing, Inc.

specimens and infectious/hazardous waste products. Any device that is intended to remove or isolate bloodborne pathogens from the workplace is considered an engineering control.

Work practice controls are any practices that decrease the possibility of exposure to bloodborne pathogens by changing the way a task or procedure is performed. An example of work practice control is prohibiting recapping of needles by the two-handed method (changing to no recapping or recapping by one-handed method when necessary). Another example is the Hepatitis B vaccination requirement.

OSHA further requires that engineering and work practice controls be reviewed on a regular basis to ensure effective functioning. Other requirements that fall under general work practices and controls are:

- Proper and convenient handwashing facilities.
- To minimize needlesticks, needles and other sharps cannot be broken, and must be put in puncture-resistant containers that are labeled and color-coded. The containers must be leakproof, top and bottom.
- Recapping of needles is strictly prohibited. If a medical procedure requires recapping, it must be done by the one-handed method
- Specimens (such as blood, body fluids, urine, tissue, biopsies) must be put in a leakage-proof container. Color-coding and labeling is required when a specimen is transported.
- Contaminated equipment must be decontaminated before servicing or shipping. If the equipment cannot be completely decontaminated, a label to that effect should be affixed.
- Any labels must include the red-orange biohazard symbol.
- The person or the business to whom the specimen is being sent must be notified and appropriately informed of the before it is sent.
- Medical and nursing procedures must be performed in such a way as to prevent or decrease spraying, spilling or splashing of blood or body fluids.
- Eating, drinking, and smoking is prohibited in the workplace.
- Housekeeping must develop specific procedures for cleaning and decontamination.

Personal protective equipment

- Implementation of the use of personal protective equipment.

When a potential for occupational exposure exists, employers must provide, at no cost, and require employees to use appropriate personal protective equipment (PPE). Examples of PPE are gloves, gowns, lab coats, masks, mouthpieces, eye protection, and resuscitation bags. All items must be clean, in good repair, and replaced when necessary. Gloves are not necessarily required for routine phlebotomies in volunteer blood donation centers but must be made available to employees who want to glove.

PPE must be designed and made of the kind of material that will not allow potentially infectious material to penetrate through to the worker's clothes, skin, eye, mouth, or any part of the body with normal use.

The following requirements apply to PPE:

- The employer must make sure the employee uses the equipment correctly.
- PPE must be quickly accessible and always available in the correct and appropriate sizes.
- Special, nonallergenic equipment, such as gloves, must be provided for employees who have allergies.
- The employer must launder or dispose of the equipment at no charge to the employee.
- PPE must be placed is designated containers for cleaning or disposal.
- Gloves must be worn any time contact with blood or OPIM is anticipated. Disposal gloves are not to be reused. Other gloves

may be reused after decontaminating as long as the glove is fully intact with no nicks or cuts.
- Gowns, masks and/or proper eye protection must be worn, depending upon the nature of exposure that is reasonably anticipated.

Information and training

- Implementation of an information and training program for employees.

The employer is required to present information and training regarding occupational exposure to any employee immediately upon employment or upon assignment of any task or procedure in which the employee might be at risk for bloodborne exposure. This information and/or training must be repeated annually or as necessary when reassignments or modification of job descriptions occur, and training must be conducted by a person qualified to teach the subject matter.

All training sessions must include:

- An accessible copy of the regulatory text of the standard and explanation of what it means.
- A general explanation of the epidemiology, signs and symptoms of bloodborne diseases.
- An explanation of the modes of transmission of bloodborne pathogens.
- An explanation of the employer's exposure control plan along with a copy of the plan to each employee.
- An explanation of the appropriate methods for recognizing tasks/procedures that may involve exposure to blood or other potentially infectious material.
- An explanation of the use and limitations of methods that will prevent or reduce exposure, including appropriate engineering controls, work practices, and personal protective equipment.
- An explanation of why and how certain personal protective equipment is chosen and why employees are required to use it.
- Information and demonstration of the types, proper use, location, removal, handling, decontamination, and disposal of personal protective equipment.
- Information on Hepatitis B vaccine, including information on its efficacy, safety, method of administration, the benefits of vaccination, and that the vaccine and administration will be offered free of charge to the employee.
- Information on the correct procedure be taken if exposure to blood or other potentially infectious materials occurs. The name and title of the person to contact in an emergency must be included.
- Procedure on post-exposure evaluation and follow-up.
- An explanation of signs/labels and/or color coding used to identify hazards.
- An opportunity for interactive questions and answer with the person conducting the training.

Hepatitis B vaccination

- Implementation of Hepatitis B vaccinations to all employees. OSHA requires Hepatitis B series be made available to all employees who have reasonable or potential occupational exposure to blood or other potentially infectious materials within 10 working days of assignment. These vaccinations must be administered at no cost, at a reasonable time and place, under the supervision of licensed physician/licensed healthcare professional and according to the latest recommendations of the U.S. Public Health Service (USPHS).

The following also applies to this requirement:

- If an employee does refuse the vaccination, the OSHA declination form must be signed.

- Prescreening can not be required as a condition of receiving the vaccine.
- Employees who decline to take the vaccination, may at any time reconsider and be given the vaccine free of cost.
- Should booster doses later be recommended by the USPHS, employees must be offered the injections at no cost.

Post-exposure evaluation and follow-up:
- Implementation of a plan for evaluation and follow-up if occupational exposure does occur.

OSHA places a great deal of emphasis on this part of its ruling. This requirement specifies procedures that must be made available to all employees who have had an exposure incident. The medical evaluation and follow-up must, at the very minimum, include the following:
- Initially, the employer must keep all information regarding the employee's exposure confidential.
- Document the circumstances of the exposure, identifying and testing the source individual.
- Laboratory tests must be conducted by an accredited laboratory at no cost to the employee.
- Test the exposed employee's blood if he/she consents.

If employee refuses HIV or HBV testing, be sure to document reasons given by the employee. If the employee consents to having blood drawn, but refuses testing for HIV, the blood can be preserved for 90 days. If the employee then elects, the blood can then be tested for HIV.
- Results of the source individual's blood testing must be made available to the employee as soon as those results are received.
- Post-exposure prophylaxis, counseling and evaluation required by the employee must be provided by the facility.
- The employer must provide the employee with the physician's written evaluation within 15 days of the physician completing the evaluation.

The following information must be supplied to the physician who evaluates an employee involved in an exposure incident:
- A copy of the Bloodborne Pathogen Standard
- A description, in the employee's words, of how the exposure incident occurred.
- Documentation of the circumstances of the incident, including routes of entry.
- Any results that may be available on the source individual's blood testing or diagnosis.
- Any medical records that might be relevant to the treatment of the employee, including Hepatitis B vaccination status.

The physician's written evaluation must include only the following information. (Any other findings must be confidential and cannot be written in the report). The physician must state:
- Whether or not the Hepatitis B vaccine is indicated.
- Whether the employee has been informed of the results of the evaluation and testing.
- Whether further evaluation and treatment are required.

Hazard communication
- Implementation of a system of warning employees about potentially infectious materials by affixing the universal biohazard symbol. This part of the standard requires warning labels, specifically the orange or orange-red biohazard symbol affixed to containers of regulated waste, refrigerators and freezers and other containers which are used to store or transport blood or other potentially infectious materials.

Other provisions regarding regulated infectious waste include:
- Red bags or containers may be used instead of labeling. When a facility uses Universal Precautions in its handling of all specimens, labeling is not required within the facility. Likewise,

when all laundry is handled with Universal Precautions, the laundry need not be labeled.
- The biohazard label must be such that it cannot be easily removed from the site to which it is affixed.
- All regulated waste must be placed in containers and disposed of in a manner that is in keeping with state and local regulations as well as the federal requirements.
- Containers that are used for contaminated sharps must meet this criteria:
- Must close automatically without any force necessary
- Puncture resistant
- Leak-resistant on sides, top and bottom
- Labeled with the biohazard symbol or color-coded red
- Blood which has been tested and found free of HIV or HBV and released for clinical use, and regulated waste which has been decontaminated, need not be labeled. Signs must be used to identify restricted areas in HIV and HBV research laboratories and production facilities.

Housekeeping and laundry
- Implementation of requirements to maintain a clean and sanitary environment for employees

It is the employer's responsibility that the workplace be clean and sanitary. Specifically, the housekeeping requirements include:
- A written schedule for cleaning and decontamination must be posted.
- A method for decontamination must be listed on the schedule.
- Any surface or instrument must be cleaned immediately following any procedure or contamination with blood or OPIM with the appropriate disinfectant.
- Protective coverings used on equipment should be immediately replaced when necessary (such as after use) or at the end of the workday or shift.
- Any containers that are re-used must be decontaminated and inspected on a regular basis.
- Broken glass, especially glass that has a potential for contamination, cannot be picked up by hand, but must be cleaned with equipment or by some mechanical means.
- No storage container that would require an employee to reach into the container to retrieve a sharp is permitted.

The question about how laundry is to be handled has been an ongoing concern and one of the most confusing parts of the standard.

Generally, these are considered to be the requirements:
- Laundry must be bagged at the location where it is used. It cannot be moved and later bagged.
- It cannot be sorted or rinsed in the same location where it is used. It must be moved to the laundry area for sorting or rinsing.
- Contaminated laundry must be placed in bags (or containers) that are either labeled or color-coded.
- If laundry is wet, it must be put in leak-proof bags.
- Any worker who has contact with laundry must wear gloves.
- Laundry may be done on site (at the facility) or can be sent to a laundry service.
- Any employee who does the laundry must be properly trained in bagging, handling, and disinfecting the laundry. Those training records must be kept on file.
- It is suggested that hot water and bleach be used.

Recordkeeping
- Implementation of accurate training records that must be kept for three years after the training

The recordkeeping system required by OSHA calls for medical records to be kept for each employee who is at risk for occupational exposure for the duration of employment plus 30 years. Other requirements include:

- The record must be confidential and must include name and Social Security number of the employee.
- Hepatitis B vaccination status, including dates of injections.
- The results of any evaluations following an exposure incident, medical testing and follow-up procedures. A copy of the physician's written opinion must be included.

In addition, training records must be maintained for three years and must include:

- Dates of training session.
- Contents and/or a summary of the training program.
- The trainer's name and qualifications.
- Names and job titles of all persons attending the sessions.
- Any of these training or medical records must be made available to the employee, anyone with written consent of the employee, and OSHA upon request of such documents.

HIV and HBV research laboratories and production facilities

- Implementation of special training and experience requirements for use in research laboratories and production facilities.
- Special standards for HIV and HBV research facilities are included in the standard, but are of such a highly-specialized nature that they are not covered in this manual. These facilities must follow standard microbiological practices and specific additional practices intended to minimize exposures of employees working with concentrated viruses. These facilities must include required containment equipment and an autoclave for decontamination of regulated waste and must be constructed to limit risks and enable easy clean up. Additional training and experience requirements apply to workers in these facilities.

15-3   Immunization recommendations for health care workers

Hepatitis B	Rubella	Diphtheria
Measles	Poliomyelitis	Influenza*
Mumps	Tetanus	Pneumococcal disease*

*For those with chronic diseases and/or other personal risks
From Grimes DE: *Infectious diseases,* St Louis, 1991, Mosby.

15-4   Contagious diseases

Disease and synopsis of symptoms	Incubation period	Mode of transmission	Period of communicability
Actinomycosis Chronic disease most frequently localized in jaw, thorax, or abdomen; septicemic spread with generalized disease may occur. Lesions are firmly indurated areas of purulence and fibrosis.	Irregular; probably years after colonization in oral tissues, plus days or months after precipitating trauma and actual penetration of tissues.	Contact from person to person as part of normal oral flora.	Time and manner in which *A. israelii* becomes part of normal flora is unknown.
Amebiasis Infection with a protozoan parasite that exists in two forms: the hardy, infective cyst and the more fragile, potentially invasive trophozoite. Parasite may act as a commensal or invade tissues, giving rise to intestinal or extraintestinal disease.	Variation—from a few days to several months or years. Commonly 2 to 4 weeks.	Contaminated water or food containing cysts from feces of infected persons, often as complication of another infection such as shigellosis.	During period of cyst passing, which may continue for years.
Ascariasis (roundworm infection) Helminthic infection of small intestine. Symptoms are variable, often vague or absent, or ordinarily mild; live worms, passed in stools or regurgitated, are frequently first recognized sign of infection.	Worms reach maturity about 2 months after ingestion of embryonated eggs.	By ingestion of infective eggs from soil contaminated with human feces containing eggs, but not directly from person to person.	As long as mature female worms live in intestine. Maximum lifespan of adult worms is under 18 months; however, female produces up to 200,000 eggs a day that can remain viable in soil for months or years.
Balantidiasis Disease of colon characteristically producing diarrhea or dysentery accompanied by abdominal colic, tenesmus, nausea, and vomiting.	Unknown; may be only a few days.	By ingestion of cysts from feces of infected hosts; in epidemics, mainly by fecally contaminated water.	As long as infection persists.
Candidiasis (moniliasis, thrush, candidosis) Mycosis usually confined to superficial layers of skin or mucous membranes with patients who have oral thrush, interterigo, vulvovaginitis, paronychia, or onychomycosis.	Variable, 2 to 5 days in thrush of infants.	Through contact with excretions of mouth, skin, vagina, and especially feces from patients or carriers; from mother to infant during childbirth; and by endogenous spread.	Presumably for duration of lesions.
Carditis, Coxsackie (viral carditis, enteroviral carditis) Acute or subacute myocarditis or pericarditis, which occurs as the only manifestation, or may occasionally be associated with other manifestations.	Usually 3 to 5 days.	Fecal-oral or respiratory droplet contact with infected person.	Apparently during acute stage of disease.
Chickenpox, herpes zoster (varicella shingles) Acute generalized viral disease with sudden onset of slight fever, mild constitutional symptoms, and a skin eruption that is maculopapular for a few hours, vesicular for 3 to 4 days, and leaves a granular scab.	From 2 to 3 weeks; commonly 13 to 17 days.	From person to person by direct contact, droplet, or air-borne spread of secretion of respiratory tract of chickenpox cases or of vesicle fluid of patients with herpes zoster.	As long as 5 days but usually 1 to 2 days before onset of rash, and not more than 6 days after appearance of first crop of vesicles.

Continued.

Contagious diseases—cont'd

Disease and synopsis of symptoms	Incubation period	Mode of transmission	Period of communicability
Cholera Acute intestinal disease with sudden onset, profuse watery stools, occasional vomiting, rapid dehydration, acidosis, and circulatory collapse. Death may occur within a few hours.	From a few hours to 5 days, usually 2 to 3 days.	Through ingestion of food or water contaminated with feces or vomitus of infected persons or with feces of carriers.	Thought to be for duration of stool-positive stage, usually only a few days after recovery. Carrier stage may last for several months.
Conjunctivitis, acute bacterial Clinical syndrome beginning with lacrimation, irritation, and hyperemia of the palpebral and bulbar conjunctivae of one or both eyes, followed by edema of lids, photophobia, and mucopurulent discharge.	Usually 24 to 72 hours.	Contact with discharges from conjunctivae or upper respiratory tract of infected persons through contaminated fingers, clothing, or other articles.	During course of active infection.
Conjunctivitis, epidemic hemorrhagic (Apollo 11 disease) Virus infection with sudden onset of pain or sensation of a foreign body in eye. Disease rapidly progresses (1 to 2 days) to full case of swollen eyelids, hyperemia of the conjunctivae, often with a cirumcorneal distribution, seromucous discharge, and frequent subconjunctival hemorrhages.	1 to 2 days or even shorter.	Through direct or indirect contact with discharge from infected eyes and possibly by droplet infection from those with virus in throat.	Unknown, but assumed to be for period of active disease, usually 1 to 2 weeks.
Dermatophytosis A. Ringworm of scalp and beard (tinea capitis, tinea kerion, favus) Begins as small papule and spreads peripherally, leaving scaly patches of temporary baldness. Infected hairs become brittle and break off easily. Kerions sometimes develop.	10 to 14 days	Direct or indirect contact with articles infected with hair from humans or infected animals.	As long as lesions are present and viable fungus persists on contaminated materials.
B. Ringworm of nails (tinea unguium, onychomycosis) Chronic infectious disease involving one or more nails of hands or feet. Nail thickens becoming discolored and brittle with an accumulation of caseous-appearing material beneath nail.	Unknown.	Presumably by direct extension from skin or nail lesions of infected persons. Low rate of transmission.	Possibly as long as infected lesion is present.
C. Ringworm of groin and perianal region (dhobie itch, tinea cruris) D. Ringworm of the body (tinea corporis) Characteristically appears as flat, spreading, ring-shaped lesions. Periphery is usually reddish, vesicular, or pustular and may be dry and scaly or moist and crusted.	4 to 10 days.	Direct or indirect contact with skin and scalp lesions of infected persons or animals.	As long as lesions are present and viable fungus persists on contaminated materials.
E. Ringworm of the foot (tinea pedis, athlete's foot) Scaling or cracking of skin, especially between toes, or blisters containing this watery fluid are characteristic. In severe cases vesicular lesions appear on various parts of body.	Unknown.	Direct or indirect contact with skin lesions of infected persons or contaminated floors or shower stalls.	As long as lesions are present and viable spores persist on contaminated materials.

Disease and synopsis of symptoms	Incubation period	Mode of transmission	Period of communicability
Diphtheria Characteristic lesion marked by patch or patches of grayish membrane with surrounding dull red inflammatory zone. Throat is moderately sore in faucial diphtheria, with cervical lymph nodes enlarged and tender; occasionally swelling and edema of neck.	2 to 5 days, sometimes longer.	Contact with patient or carrier; more rarely with articles soiled with discharges from lesions of infected persons. Raw milk has been a vehicle.	Variable, until virulent bacilli have disapperared from discharge and lesions. Usual period is 2 to 4 weeks but chronic carriers may shed organisms for 6 months or more.
Gastroenteritis, viral A. Epidemic viral gastroenteritis Usually self-limited mild disease that often occurs in outbreaks with clinical symptoms of nausea, vomiting, diarrhea, abdominal pain, myalgia, headache, malaise, low-grade fever, or a combination thereof.	24 to 48 hours; in volunteer studies with Norwalk agent range was 10 to 51 hours.	Unknown; probably by fecal-oral route. Several recent outbreaks strongly suggest food-borne and water-borne transmission.	During acute stage of disease and shortly thereafter.
B. Rotavirus gastroenteritis (sporadic viral gastroenteritis of infants and children) Sporadic severe gastroenteritis of infants and young children characterized by diarrhea and vomiting, often with severe dehydration and occasional deaths.	Approximately 48 hours.	Probably fecal-oral and possibly respiratory routes.	During acute stage of disease and later while virus shedding continues. Virus is not usually detectable after eighth day of illness.
Giardiasis (*Giardia* enteritis, lambliasis) Protozoan infection principally of upper small bowel; often asymptomatic, it may also be associated with a variety of intestinal symptoms such as chronic diarrhea, steatorrhea, abdominal cramps, bloating, frequent loose and pale, greasy, malodorus stools, fatigue, and weight loss.	In a water-borne epidemic in United States, clinical illnesses occurred 1 to 4 weeks after exposure; average 2 weeks.	Localized outbreaks occur from contaminated water supplies. By ingestion of cysts in fecally contaminated water and occasionally by fecally contaminated food.	Entire period of infection.
Hepatitis, viral A. Viral hepatitis A (infectious hepatitis, epidemic hepatitis, epidemic jaundice, catarrhal jaundice, Type A hepatitis) Onset is usually abrupt with fever, malaise, anorexia, nausea, and abdominal discomfort, followed within a few days by jaundice.	From 15 to 50 days, depending on dose; average 28-30 days.	Person to person by fecal-oral route. Common-vehicle outbreaks have been related to contaminated water and food.	Studies indicate maximum infectivity during latter half of incubation period, continuing for a few days, after onset of jaundice.
B. Viral hepatitis B (Type B hepatitis, serum hepatitis) Onset is usually insidious with anorexia, vague abdominal discomfort, nausea, and vomiting, sometimes arthralgias and rash, often progressing to jaundice. Fever may be absent or mild.	Usually 45 to 160 days, average 60 to 90 days. Variation is related in part to amount of virus in inoculum, mode of transmission, and host factors.	HB_sAg, the infectious agent, has been found in virtually all body secretions, but only blood, saliva, and semen have been shown to be infectious. Transmission usually by percutaneous inoculation of infected blood and blood products; contaminated needles, syringes, and IV equipment.	From several weeks before onset of symptoms through clinical course of disease; carrier state can last for years.

Continued.

Contagious diseases—cont'd

Disease and synopsis of symptoms	Incubation period	Mode of transmission	Period of communicability
Hepatitis, viral—cont'd			
C. Hepatitis, non-A, non-B (non-B transfusion–associated hepatitis, hepatitis C)	2 weeks to 6 months, model 6 to 8 weeks.	Most common posttransfusion hepatitis in United States and is more common when paid donors are used. Percutaneous transmission documented and other modes similar to those of hepatitis B virus are suspected.	Degree of immunity following infection is not known.
Chronic infection may be symptomatic or asymptomatic. Differential diagnosis depends on exclusion of hepatitis types A and B.			
Herpangina; hand-foot-and-mouth disease, acute lymphonodular pharyngitis			
Herpangina—grayish papulovesicular pharyngeal lesions on an erythematous base. *Hand-foot-and-mouth disease*—more diffuse oral lesions on buccal surfaces of cheeks, gums, and tongue. *Acute lymphonodular pharyngitis*—lesions are firm, raised, discrete, whitish to yellowish nodules.	3 to 5 days for herpangina and hand-foot-and-mouth disease. 5 days for acute lymphonodular pharyngitis.	Direct contact with nose and throat discharges and feces of infected (possibly asymptomatic) persons and by droplet spread.	During acute stage of illness and longer because virus persists in stools for as long as several weeks.
Herpes simplex			
Viral infection characterized by localized primary lesion, latency, and a tendency to localized recurrence. In perhaps 10% of primary infections overt disease may appear as illness of varying severity marked by fever and malaise lasting 1 week or more.	2 to 12 days.	HSV Type 1: Direct contact with virus in saliva of carriers. HSV Type 2: Sexual contact.	Secretion of virus in saliva has been reported for as long as 7 weeks after recovery from stomatitis. Patients with primary lesions are infective for about 7 to 12 days, with recurrent disease for 4 days to 1 week.
Influenza			
Acute viral disease of respiratory tract characterized by fever, chilliness, headache, myalgia, prostration, coryza, and mild sore throat. Cough is often severe and protracted.	Usually 24 to 72 hours.	By direct contact through droplet infection; probably airborne among crowded populations in enclosed spaces.	Probably limited to 3 days from clinical onset.
Measles (rubeola, hard measles, red measles, morbilli)			
Acute, highly communicable viral disease with prodromal fever, conjunctivitis, coryza, bronchitis, and Koplik's spots on the buccal mucosa. A characteristic red blotchy rash appears on third to seventh day, beginning on face, becoming generalized, lasting 4 to 7 days and sometimes ending in branny desquamation. Leukopenia is common.	About 10 days varying from 8 to 13 days from exposure to onset of fever; about 14 days until rash appears; uncommonly longer or shorter human normal immune globulin (IG), given later than third day of incubation period for passive protection, may extend the incubation period to 21 days instead of preventing disease.	By droplet spread or direct contact with nasal or throat secretions of infected persons. Measles is one of most readily transmitted communicable diseases.	From slightly before beginning of prodromal period of 4 days after appearance of rash; communicability is minimal after second day of rash.

Disease and synopsis of symptoms	Incubation period	Mode of transmission	Period of communicability
Meningitis, meningococcal (cerebrospinal fever, meningococcemia)			
Characterized by sudden onset of fever, intense headache, nausea and often vomiting, stiff neck, and frequently a petechial rash with pink macules or, very rarely, vesicles. Delirium and coma often appear; occasional fulminating cases exhibit sudden prostration.	Varies from 2 to 10 days, commonly 3 to 4 days.	By direct contact, including droplets and discharges from nose and throat of infected persons, more often carriers than cases.	Until meningococci are no longer present in discharges from nose and throat. If organisms are sensitive to sulfonamides, meningococci usually disappear from nasopharynx within 24 hours after institution of treatment. They are not fully eradicated from oronasopharynx by penicillin.
Meningitis, hemophilus (meningitis caused by *Haemophilus influenzae*)			
Most common bacterial meningitis in children 2 months to 3 years old in U.S. Otitis media or sinusitis may be precursor. Almost always associated with bacteremia. Onset is sudden with symptoms of fever, vomiting, lethargy, and meningeal irritation.	Probably short—within 2 to 4 days	By droplet infection and discharges from nose and throat during infectious period. May be purulent rhinitis. Portal of entry is most commonly nasopharyngeal.	As long as organisms are present, which may be for prolonged period even without nasal discharge.
Mononucleosis, infectious (glandular fever, EBV mononucleosis)			
Characterized by fever, sore throat (often with exudative pharyngotonsillitis), and lymphadenopathy (especially posterior cervical). Jaundice occurs in about 4% of infected young adults and splenomegaly in 50%. Duration is from 1 to several weeks.	From 4 to 6 weeks.	Person-to-person spread by oropharyngeal route via saliva. Spread may also occur via blood transfusion to susceptible recipients.	Prolonged; pharyngeal excretion may persist for 1 year after infection; 15% to 20% of healthy adults are oropharyngeal carriers.
Mumps (infectious parotitis)			
Acute viral disease characterized by fever, swelling, and tenderness of one or more salivary glands, usually parotid and sometimes sublingual or submaxillary glands.	About 2 to 3 weeks, commonly 18 days.	By droplet spread and by direct contact with saliva of an infected person.	Virus has been isolated from saliva from 6 days before salivary gland involvement to as long as 9 days thereafter; but height of infectiousness occurs about 48 hours before swelling begins. Urine may be positive for as long as 14 days after onset of illness.
Paratyphoid fever			
Frequently generalized bacterial enteric infection, often with abrupt onset, continued fever, enlargement of spleen, sometimes rose spots on trunk, usually diarrhea, and involvement of lymphoid tissues of mesentery and intestines.	1 to 3 weeks for enteric fever; 1 to 10 days for gastroenteritis.	Direct or indirect contact with feces or urine of patient or carrier. Spread is by food, especially milk, milk products, and shellfish. Flies may be vectors.	As long as infectious agent persists in excreta, which is from appearance of prodromal symptoms, throughout illness, and for periods up to several weeks or months. Commonly 1 to 2 weeks after recovery.

Continued.

Contagious diseases—cont'd

Disease and synopsis of symptoms	Incubation period	Mode of transmission	Period of communicability
Pediculosis (lousiness) Infestation of head, hairy parts of body, or clothing with adult lice, larvae, or nits (eggs), which results in severe itching and excoriation of scalp or scratch marks of body.	Under optimum conditions, eggs of lice hatch in 1 week, reach sexual maturity in approximately 2 weeks.	Direct contact with infected person and indirectly by contact with personal belongings, especially clothing and head-gear. Crab lice are usually transmitted through sexual contact.	Communicable as long as lice remain alive on infested person or in clothing, and until eggs in hair and clothing have been destroyed.
The pneumonias A. Pneumococcal pneumonia Acute bacterial infection characterized by sudden onset with single shaking chill, fever, pleural pain, dyspnea, cough productive of "rusty" sputum and leukocytosis.	Not well determined; believed to be 1 to 3 days.	By droplet spread; by direct oral contact or indirectly, through articles freshly soiled with respiratory organisms is common.	Presumably until discharges of mouth and nose no longer contain virulent pneumococci in significant numbers. Penicillin will render patient noninfectious within 24 to 48 hours.
B. Mycoplasmal pneumonia (primary atypical pneumonia) Predominantly afebrile lower respiratory infection. Onset is gradual with headache, malaise, cough often paroxysmal, and usually substernal pain (not pleuritic). Sputum, scant at first, may increase later.	14 to 21 days.	Probably by droplet inhalation, direct contact with infected person or with articles freshly soiled with discharges of nose and throat from acutely ill and coughing patient.	Probably less than 10 days; occasionally longer with persisting febrile illness or persistence of the organisms in convalescence (as long as 13 weeks is known).
C. Pneumocystis pneumonia (interstitial plasma cell pneumonia) Acute pulmonary disease occurring early in life, especially in malnourished, chronically ill, or premature infants. Characterized by progressive dyspnea, tachypnea, and cyanosis; fever may not be present.	Analysis of data from institutional outbreaks among infants indicates 1 to 2 months.	Unknown.	Unknown.
D. Chlamydial pneumonia (pertussoid eosinophilic pneumonia) Subacute pulmonary disease occurring in early infancy, primarily in infants of mothers with infection of uterine cervix with causative organism.	Not known, but pneumonia may occur in infants from 1 to 18 weeks of age (more commonly between 4 and 12 weeks).	Presumed to be vertically transmitted from infected cervix to infant during birth, with resultant nasopharyngeal infection.	Unknown, but length of nasopharyngeal excretion can be at least 2 months.
Poliomyelitis (infantile paralysis) Acute viral infection whose symptoms include fever, malaise, headache, nausea, vomiting, and stiffness of neck and back with or without paralysis.	Commonly 7 to 14 days for paralytic cases, with a range from 3 to possibly 35 days.	Direct contact through close association. In rare instances milk, foodstuffs. and other fecally contaminated materials have been incriminated as vehicles. Fecal-oral is major route when sanitation is poor, but during epidemics and when sanitation is good, pharyngeal spread becomes relatively more important.	Not accurately known. Cases are probably most infectious during first few days after onset of symptoms.

Disease and synopsis of symptoms	Incubation period	Mode of transmission	Period of communicability
Respiratory disease (excluding influenza)			
A. Acute febrile respiratory disease Viral diseases of respiratory tract are characterized by fever and one or more constitutional reactions such as chills or chilliness, headache, general aching, malaise, and anorexia; in infants by occasional gastrointestinal disturbances.	From a few days to 1 week or more.	Directly by oral contact or by droplet spread, indirectly by hands or other materials soiled by respiratory discharges of infected person.	For duration of active disease; little is known about subclinical or latent infections.
B. Common cold (acute coryza) Acute catarrhal infections of upper respiratory tract characterized by coryza, sneezing, lacrimation, irritated nasopharynx, chilliness, and malaise lasting 2 to 7 days. Fever is uncommon in children and rare in adults.		Presumably by direct oral contact or by droplet spread; indirectly by hands and articles freshly soiled by discharges of nose and throat of infected person.	
Rubella (German measles)			
A. Congenital rubella Mild febrile infectious disease with diffuse punctate and macular rash. Sometimes resembling that of measles, scarlet fever, or both. May be few or no constitutional symptoms in children but adults may experience 1- to 5-day prodrome characterized by low-grade fever, headache, malaise, mild coryza, and conjunctivitis. As many as 20% to 50% of infections may occur without evident rash; overall 50% are not recognized.	From 16 to 18 days with a range of 14 to 21 days.	Contact with nasopharyngeal secretions of infected person. Infection is by droplet spread or direct contact with patients and indirect contact.	For about 1 week before and at least 4 days after onset of rash. Highly communicable. Infants with congenital rubella syndrome may shed virus for months after birth.
B. Erythema infectiosum (fifth disease) Mild nonfebrile erythematous eruption occurring as epidemics among children. Characterized by striking erythema of cheeks, reddening of skin, and lacelike serpiginous rash of body.			
C. Exanthema subitum (roseola infantum) Acute illness of probable viral cause characterized by high fever that suddenly appears and lasts 3 to 5 days. A maculopapular rash on trunk and later on rest of body ordinarily follows lysis of fever.			
Shigellosis (bacillary dysentery)			
Acute bacterial disease primarily involving large intestine, characterized by diarrhea, accompanied by fever, nausea, sometimes vomiting, cramps, and tenesmus. In severe cases stools contain blood, mucus, and pus.	1 to 7 days, usually 1 to 3 days.	By direct or indirect fecal-oral transmission from patient or carrier. Infection may occur after ingestion of very few organisms.	During acute infection and until infectious agent is no longer present in feces, usually within 4 weeks of illness.

Continued.

Contagious diseases—cont'd

Disease and synopsis of symptoms	Incubation period	Mode of transmission	Period of communicability
Staphylococcal disease A. Staphylococcal disease in community, boils, carbuncles, furuncles, impetigo, cellulitis, abscesses, staphylococcal septicemia, staphylococcal pneumonia, osteomyelitis, endocarditis Staphylococci produce variety of syndromes with clinical manifestations that range from single pustule to impetigo to septicemia to death. Lesion or lesions containing pus are primary clinical finding, abscess formation is typical.	Variable and indefinite. Commonly 4 to 10 days.	Major site of colonization is anterior nares. Autoinfection is responsible for at least one third of infections. Person with draining lesion or any purulent lesion or who is asymptomatic (usually nasal) carrier of pathogenic strain. Air-borne spread is rare.	As long as purulent lesions continue to drain or carrier state persists.
B. Staphylococcal disease in hospital nurseries, impetigo, abscess of breast Characteristic lesions develop secondary to colonization of nose or umbilicus, conjunction, circumcision site, or rectum of infants with pathogenic strain.	Commonly 4 to 10 days but may occur several months after colonization.	Spread by hands of hospital personnel is primary mode of transmission within hospitals; to a lesser extent, air-borne.	Same.
C. Staphylococcal disease in medical and surgical wards of hospitals Lesions vary from simple furuncles or stitch abscesses to extensively infected bedsores or surgical wounds, septic phlebitis, chronic osteomyelitis, fulminating pneumonia, endocarditis, or septicemia.	Variable and indefinite. Commonly 4 to 10 days.	Major site of colonization is anterior nares. Autoinfection is responsible for at least one third of infections. Person with a draining lesion or any purulent lesion or who is an asymptoamtic (usually nasal) carrier of a pathogenic strain. Air-borne spread is rare.	As long as purulent lesions continue to drain or carrier state persists.
Streptococcal sore throat Fever, sore throat, exudative tonsillitis or pharyngitis, and tender anterior cervical lymph nodes	Short, usually 1 to 3 days, rarely longer.	Transmission results from direct or intimate contact with patient or carrier, rarely by indirect contact through objects or hands. Nasal carriers are particularly likely to transmit diseases.	In untreated uncomplicated cases 10 to 21 days; in untreated conditions with purulent discharges, weeks or months.
Syphilis, nonvenereal endemic Acute disease of limited geographical distribution, characterized clinically by eruption of skin and mucous membrane, usually without evident primary sore.	2 weeks to 3 months.	Direct or indirect contact with infectious early lesions of skin and mucous membranes. Congenital transmission does not occur.	Until moist eruptions of skin and mucous patches disappear—sometimes several weeks or months.
Trachoma Communicable keratoconjunctivitis characterized by conjunctival inflammation with papillary hyperplasia, associated with vascular invasion of cornea, and in later stages by conjunctival scarring that may eventually lead to blindness.	5 to 12 days (based on volunteer studies).	By direct contact with ocular discharges and possibly mucoid or purulent discharges of nasal mucous membranes of infected persons or materials. Flies *(Musca sorbens)* may contribute to spread of disease.	As long as active lesions are present in the conjunctivae and adnexal mucous membranes.

Disease and synopsis of symptoms	*Incubation period*	*Mode of transmission*	*Period of communicability*
Tuberculosis Mycobacterial disease. Initial infection usually goes unnoticed; tuberculin sensitivity appears within a few weeks; lesions commonly heal, leaving no residual changes except pulmonary or tracheobronchial lymph node calcification. May progress to pulmonary tuberculosis or, by lymphohematogenous dissemination of bacilli, to produce miliary, meningeal, or other extrapulmonary involvement.	From infection to demonstrable primary lesion, about 4 to 12 weeks. Whereas subsequent risk of progressive pulmonary or extrapulmonary tuberculosis is greatest within 1 or 2 years after infection, it may persist for a lifetime as latent infection.	Exposure to bacilli in air-borne droplet nuclei from sputum of persons with infectious tuberculosis. Bovine tuberculosis results from exposure to tubercular cattle and ingestion of unpasteurized dairy products.	As long as infectious tubercle bacilli are being discharged.
Typhoid fever (enteric fever, typhus abdominalis) Systemic infectious disease characterized by sustained fever, headache, malaise, anorexia, relative bradycardia, enlargement of spleen, rose spots on trunk, nonproductive cough, constipation more commonly than diarrhea, and involvement of lymphoid tissues.	Depends on size of infecting dose; usual range 1 to 3 weeks.	By food or water contaminated by feces or urine of patient or carrier.	As long as typhoid bacilli appear in excreta; usually first week throughout convalescence; variable thereafter. About 10% of untreated patients will discharge bacilli for 3 months after onset of symptoms; 2% to 5% become permanent carriers.
Whooping cough (pertussis) Acute bacterial disease involving tracheobronchial tree. Initial catarrhal stage has insidious onset with irritating cough that gradually becomes paroxysmal, usually within 1 to 2 weeks, and lasts for 1 to 2 months.	Commonly 7 days; almost uniformly within 10 days, and not exceeding 21 days.	Primarily by direct contact with discharges from respiratory mucous membranes of infected persons by air-borne route, probably by droplets. Frequently brought into home by older sibling.	Highly communicable in early catarrhal stage before paroxysmal cough stage. For control purposes, communicable stage extends from 7 days after exposure to 3 weeks after onset of typical paroxysms in patients not treated with antibiotics; in patients treated with erythromycin, period of infectiousness extends only 5 to 7 days after onset of therapy.

15-5 | Sexually transmitted diseases

Disease and synopsis of symptoms	Incubation period	Mode of transmission	Period of communicability
Acquired immunodeficiency syndrome (AIDS)			
Acute viral infection characterized by breakdown and failure of immune system, opening body to often lethal infections and disorders such as Kaposi's sarcoma, pneumonia, and meningitis. Symptoms begin with fever, weight loss, fatigue, shortness of breath, diarrhea, and neurologic disorders.	Variable.	By direct sexual contact and transmission of semen, saliva, blood, or other body fluids. Also by blood transfusion or contaminated syringes.	For duration of infection
Chancroid (ulcus molle, soft chancre)			
Acute, localized, genital infection characterized by single or multiple painful necrotizing ulcers at site of inoculation, frequently accompanied by painful inflammatory swelling and suppuration of regional lymph nodes. Extragenital lesions have been reported.	From 3 to 5 days, up to 14 days.	By direct sexual contact with discharges from open lesions and pus from buboes; suggestive evidence of asymptomatic infections in women. Multiple sexual partners and uncleanliness favor transmission.	As long as infectious agent persists in original lesion or discharging regional lymph nodes; usually until healed—a matter of weeks.
Conjunctivitis, inclusion (swimming pool conjunctivitis, paratrachoma)			
In the newborn, acute papillary conjunctivitis with abundant mucopurulent discharge. In children and adults, acute follicular conjunctivitis with preauricular lymphadenopathy, often with superficial corneal involvement.	5 to 12 days.	During sexual intercourse; genital discharges of infected persons are infectious.	While genital infection persists; can be longer than 1 year in female.
Cytomegalovirus infections, congenital cytomegalovirus infection, cytomegalic inclusion disease			
Most severe form of disease occurs in perinatal period, following congenital infection, with signs and symptoms of severe generalized infection especially involving central nervous system and liver.	Information inexact. 3 to 8 weeks following transfusion with infected blood. 3 to 12 weeks after birth.	Intimate exposure to infectious secretions or excretions. Virus is excreted in urine, saliva, cervical secretions, breast milk, and semen.	Virus is excreted in urine or saliva for months and may persist for several years following primary infection.
Gonococcal infections			
A. Gonococcal infection of genitourinary tract (gonorrhea, gonococcal urethritis) *Males*—purulent discharge from anterior urethra with dysuria appears 2 to 7 days after infecting exposure. *Females*—few days after exposure initial urethritis or cervicitis occurs, frequently so mild as to pass unnoticed. About 20% of patients have uterine invasion at the first, second, or later menstrual period with symptoms of endometritis, salpingitis, or pelvic peritonitis.	Usually 2 to 7 days, sometimes longer.	By contact with exudates from mucous membranes of infected persons, almost always result of sexual activity.	May extend for months if untreated, especially if females who frequently are asymptomatic. Specific therapy usually ends communicability within hours except with penicillin-resistant strains.

Disease and synopsis of symptoms	Incubation period	Mode of transmission	Period of communicability
B. Gonococcal conjunctivitis neonatorum (gonorrheal ophthalmia neonatorum) Acute redness and swelling of conjunctiva of one or both eyes, with mucopurulent or purulent discharge in which gonococci are identifiable by microscopic and cultural methods.	Usually 1 to 5 days.	Contact with infected birth canal during childbirth.	While discharge persists if untreated; for 24 hours following initiation of specific treatment.
Granuloma inguinale (donovanosis) Mildly communicable, nonfatal, chronic and progressive, autoinoculable bacterial disease of skin and mucous membranes of external genitalia, inguinal, and anal region. Small nodule, vesicle, or papule is present.	Unknown; probably 8 to 80 days.	Presumably by direct contact with lesions during sexual activity.	Unknown and probably for duration of open lesions on skin or mucous membranes.
Herpes simplex Viral infection characterized by localized primary lesion, latency, and a tendency to localized recurrence. In perhaps 10% of primary infections overt disease may appear as illness of varying severity marked by fever and malaise lasting 1 week or more.	2 to 12 days.	HSV Type 1: Direct contact with virus in saliva of carriers. HSV Type 2: Sexual contact.	Secretion of virus in saliva has been reported for as long as 7 weeks after recovery from stomatitis. Patients with primary lesions are infective for about 7 to 12 days, with recurrent disease for 4 days to 1 week.
Lymphogranuloma venereum (lymphogranuloma inguinale, esthiomene, climatic bubo, tropical bubo) Venerally acquired infection, beginning with painless evanescent erosion, papule, nodule, or herpetiform lesion on penis or vulva, frequently unnoticed. Regional lymph nodes undergo suppuration followed by extension of inflammatory process to adjacent tissues.	Usually 7 to 12 days, with a range of 4 to 21 days to primary lesion. If bubo is first manifestation, 10 to 30 days, sometimes several months.	Direct contact with open lesions of infected persons usually during sexual intercourse.	Variable, from weeks to years, during presence of active lesions.
Syphilis, veneral (lues) Acute and chronic treponematosis characterized clinically by primary lesion, secondary eruption involving skin and mucous membranes, long periods of latency, and late lesions of skin, bone, viscerae, and central nervous and cardiovascular systems. Papule appears 3 weeks after exposure at site of initial invasion; after erosion, most common form is indurated chancre.	10 days to 10 weeks, usually 3 weeks.	By direct contact with infectious exudates from obvious or concealed moist early lesions of skin and mucous membrane, body fluids, and secretions of infected persons during sexual contact.	Variable and indefinite during primary and secondary stages and also in mucocutaneous recurrences; some cases may be intermittently communicable for 2 to 4 years.

Continued.

Sexually transmitted diseases—cont'd

Disease and synopsis of symptoms	Incubation period	Mode of transmission	Period of communicability
Trichomoniasis Common disease of genitourinary tract, characterized in women by vaginitis, with small petechial or sometimes punctate hemorrhagic lesions and profuse, thin, foamy, yellowish discharge with foul odor; frequently asymptomatic. In men, infectious agent invades and persists in prostate, urethra, or seminal vesicles, but rarely produces symptoms or demonstrable lesions.	4 to 20 days, average 7 days.	By contact with vaginal and urethral discharges of infected persons during sexual intercourse and possibly by contact with contaminated articles.	For duration of infection.
Urethritis, chlamydial Urethritis, nongonorrheal and nonspecific Sexually transmitted urethritis of males caused by chlamydial agent. Clinical manifestations are usually indistinguishable from gonorrhea but are often milder and include opaque discharge of moderate or scanty quantity, urethral itching, and burning on urination. Infection of women results in cervicitis and salpingitis.	5 to 7 days or longer.	Sexual contact.	Unknown.

NURSING GUIDELINES FOR ADVANCE DIRECTIVES

The Patient Self-Determination Act (PSDA) which became effective December 1991 essentially mandates that health care facilities are responsible for assuring that individuals enrolled in their facilities are informed of their right to formulate advance directives and their right to consent to or refuse treatment. This federal legislation affects virtually all health care facilities participating in Medicare and Medicaid programs: hospitals, nursing homes, home health agencies, hospices, and health maintenance organizations.

These agencies are required to:

- Provide education to the staff regarding these sensitive issues
- Maintain written policies and procedures for adherence to these requirements
- Assure that the medical record reflects the patient's status regarding advance directives
- Not discriminate against any patient on the basis of individual decision making regarding advance directives

To assure that the legislation addresses the problem as it was intended, nurses need to see that patients and their surrogates are aware of their right to formulate choices for the withholding or withdrawal of treatment under prespecified conditions.

Nurses need to:

- Formulate advance directives themselves
- Assist in the process of determining a patient's competency when there is reason to doubt it
- Ensure that the patient and family have sufficient information about the state statutes and the PSDA itself to make any desired decisions

From Weber G: Tips on implementing the patient self-determination act, Excerpted with permission from *Nursing and Health Care,* Vol 14, Number 2. Copyright 1993, National League for Nursing.

- Recognize that not all individuals are ready to make decisions
- Be prepared to act on the patient's behalf if necessary
- Recognize the emotional state of the patient's family and help them to come to terms with the patient's advance directive formulated as a result of PSDA
- Assure that agency administration has provided detailed policies and procedures, as well as thorough and comprehensive education of the individuals responsible for enforcing this statute (i.e., admission clerks, emergency room personnel, etc.)
- Facilitate discussions so that the involved individuals recognize that they are involved in a decision-making process, not a death-producing process
- Ensure that formative, summative, and ongoing evaluation mechanisms are in place in terms of implementation methodologies for enforcing the PSDA
- Serve and be active on ethics committees or, if necessary, establish one
- Ensure that no patient is discriminated against regarding type or quality of health care for any reason
- Assure that whatever the patient's decision, it was not coerced—decisions must be strictly voluntary, and reflect the individual's values, desires, and wishes

To help in determining the competency of a patient, the following five questions should be considered:

1. Can the patient receive (hear or read) information?
2. Can the patient process and comprehend information?
3. Can the patient appropriately assess the relevant information?
4. Can the patient use relevant information to make a decision?
5. Can the patient make a decision and give a reason for it?

APPENDIX
17

DIAGNOSIS-RELATED GROUPS

17-1 Major diagnostic categories

Major diagnostic category	Group description
1	Diseases and disorders of the nervous system
2	Diseases and disorders of the eye
3	Diseases and disorders of the ear, nose, and throat
4	Diseases and disorders of the respiratory system
5	Diseases and disorders of the circulatory system
6	Diseases and disorders of the digestive system
7	Diseases and disorders of the hepatobiliary system and pancreas
8	Diseases of the musculoskeletal system and connective tissue
9	Diseases of the skin, subcutaneous tissue, and breast
10	Endocrine, nutritional, and metabolic diseases
11	Diseases and disorders of the kidney and urinary tract
12	Diseases and disorders of the male reproductive system
13	Diseases and disorders of the female reproductive system
14	Pregnancy, childbirth, and the puerperium
15	Normal, newborns and other neonates with certain conditions originating in the perinatal period
16	Diseases and disorders of the blood and blood-forming organs and immunity
17	Myeloproliferative disorders and poorly differentiated malignancy, and other neoplasms N.E.C.
18	Infectious and parasitic diseases (systemic)
19	Mental disorders
20	Substance use disorders and substance induced organic disorders
21	Injury, poisoning, and toxic effects of drugs
22	Burns
23	Selected factors influencing health status and contact with health services
24	No major diagnostic category

17-2 Diagnosis-related group descriptions

MDC		Diseases and disorders of the nervous system (01)
001	P	Craniotomy age ≧18 except for trauma
002	P	Craniotomy for trauma age ≧18
003	P	Craniotomy age <18
004	P	Spinal OR procedures
005	P	Extracranial vascular OR procedures
006	P	Carpal tunnel release
007	P	Peripheral and cranial nerve and other nervous system procedures, age ≧70 and/or C.C.
008	P	Peripheral and cranial nerve and other nervous system procedures age <70 w/o C.C.
009	M	Spinal disorders and injuries
010	M	Nervous system neoplasms age ≧70 and/or C.C.
011	M	Nervous system neoplasms age <70 w/o C.C.
012	M	Degenerative nervous system disorders
013	M	Multiple sclerosis and cerebellar ataxia
014	M	Specific cerebrovascular disorders except TIA
015	M	Transient ischemic attacks and precerebral occlusions
016	M	Nonspecific cerebrovascular disorders with C.C.
017	M	Nonspecific cerebrovascular disorders w/o C.C.
018	M	Cranial and peripheral nerve disorders age ≧70 and/or C.C.
019	M	Cranial and peripheral nerve disorders age <70 w/o C.C.
020	M	Nervous system infection except viral meningitis
021	M	Viral meningitis
022	M	Hypertensive encephalopathy
023	M	Nontraumatic stupor and coma
024	M	Seizure and headache age ≧70 and/or C.C.
025	M	Seizure and headache age 18-69 w/o C.C.
026	M	Seizure and headache age 0-17
027	M	Traumatic stupor and coma, coma >1 hr
028	M	Traumatic stupor and coma, coma <1 hr age ≧70 and/or C.C.
029	M	Traumatic stupor and coma, coma <1 hr age 18-69 w/o C.C.
030	M	Traumatic stupor & coma, coma <1 hr age 0-17
031	M	Concussion age ≧70 and/or C.C.
032	M	Concussion age 18-69 w/o C.C.
033	M	Concussion age 0-17
034	M	Other disorders of nervous system age ≧70 and/or C.C.
035	M	Other disorders of nervous system age <70 w/o C.C.

P, Surgical case.
M, Medical case.
C.C., Comorbidity or complication.

MDC 02 Diseases and disorders of the eye

036	P	Retinal procedures
037	P	Orbital procedures
038	P	Primary iris procedures
039	P	Lens procedures with or w/o vitrectomy
040	P	Extraocular procedures except orbit age $\geq$18
041	P	Extraocular procedures except orbit age 0-17
042	P	Intraocular procedures except retina, iris, and lens
043	M	Hyphema
044	M	Acute major eye infections
045	M	Neurological eye disorders
046	M	Other disorders of the eye age $\geq$18 with C.C.
047	M	Other disorders of the eye age $\geq$18 w/o C.C.
048	M	Other disorders of the eye age 0-17

MDC 03 Diseases and disorders of the ear, nose, and throat

049	P	Major head and neck procedures
050	P	Sialoadenectomy
051	P	Salivary gland procedures except sialoadenectomy
052	P	Cleft lip and palate repair
053	P	Sinus and mastoid procedures age $\geq$18
054	P	Sinus and mastoid procedures age 0-17
055	P	Miscellaneous ear, nose, and throat procedures
056	P	Rhinoplasty
057	P	T&A procedure except tonsillectomy and/or adenoidectomy age $\geq$18
058	P	T&A procedure except tonsillectomy and/or adenoidectomy age 0-17
059	P	Tonsillectomy and/or adenoidectomy only age $\geq$18
060	P	Tonsillectomy and/or adenoidectomy only age 0-17
061	P	Myringotomy with tube insertion age $\geq$18
062	P	Myringotomy with tube insertion age 0-17
063	P	Other ear, nose, and throat O.R. procedures
064	M	Ear, nose, and throat malignancy
065	M	Dysequilibrium
066	M	Epistaxis
067	M	Epiglottitis
068	M	Otitis media and URI age $\geq$70 and/or C.C.
069	M	Otitis media and URI age 18-69 w/o C.C.
070	M	Otitis media and URI age 0-17
071	M	Laryngotracheitis
072	M	Nasal trauma and deformity
073	M	Other ear, nose, and throat diagnoses age $\geq$18
074	M	Other ear, nose, and throat diagnoses age 0-17

MDC 04 Diseases and disorders of the respiratory system

075	P	Major chest procedures
076	P	Other respiratory system OR procedures with C.C.
077	P	Other respiratory system OR procedures w/o C.C.
078	M	Pulmonary embolism
079	M	Respiratory infections and inflammations age $\geq$70 and/or C.C.
080	M	Respiratory infections and inflammations age 18-69 w/o C.C.
081	M	Respiratory infections and inflammations age 0-17
082	M	Respiratory neoplasms
083	M	Major chest trauma age $\geq$70 and/or C.C.
084	M	Major chest trauma age <70 w/o C.C.
085	M	Pleural effusion age $\geq$70 and/or C.C.
086	M	Pleural effusion age <70 w/o C.C.
087	M	Pulmonary edema and respiratory failure
088	M	Chronic obstructive pulmonary disease
089	M	Simple pneumonia and pleurisy age $\geq$70 and/or C.C.
090	M	Simple pneumonia and pleurisy age 18-69 w/o C.C.
091	M	Simple pneumonia and pleurisy age 0-17
092	M	Interstitial lung disease age $\geq$70 and/or C.C.
093	M	Interstitial lung disease age <70 w/o C.C.
094	M	Pneumothorax age $\geq$70 and/or C.C.
095	M	Pneumothorax age <70 w/o C.C.
096	M	Bronchitis and asthma age $\geq$70 and/or C.C.
097	M	Bronchitis and asthma age 18-69 w/o C.C.
098	M	Bronchitis and asthma age 0-17
099	M	Respiratory signs and symptoms age $\geq$70 and/or C.C.
100	M	Respiratory signs and symptoms age <70 w/o C.C.
101	M	Other respiratory system diagnoses age $\geq$70 and/or C.C.
102	M	Other respiratory system diagnoses age <70

MDC 05 Diseases and disorders of the circulatory system

103	P	Heart transplant
104	P	Cardiac valve procedure with pump and with cardiac cath
105	P	Cardiac valve procedure with pump and w/o cardiac cath
106	P	Coronary bypass with cardiac cath
107	P	Coronary bypass w/o cardiac cath
108	P	Other cardiovascular or thoracic procedures with pump
109	P	Cardiothoracic procedures w/o pump
110	P	Major reconstructive vascular procedures w/o pump age $\geq$70 and/or C.C.
111	P	Major reconstructive vascular procedures w/o pump age <70 w/o C.C.
112	P	Vascular procedures except major reconstruction w/o pump
113	P	Amputation for circulatory system disorders except upper limb and toe
114	P	Upper limb and toe amputation for circulatory system disorders
115	P	Permanent cardiac pacemaker implant with AMI, heart failure, or shock
116	P	Permanent cardiac pacemaker implant w/o AMI, heart failure, or shock
117	P	Cardiac pacemaker replacement and revise except pulse generator replacement only
118	P	Cardiac pacemaker pulse generator replacement only
119	P	Vein ligation and stripping
120	P	Other circulatory system OR procedures
121	M	Circulatory disorders with AMI and C.V. comp. disch. alive
122	M	Circulatory disorders with AMI w/o C.V. comp. disch. alive
123	M	Circulatory disorders with AMI, expired
124	M	Circulatory disorders except AMI, with cardiac cath. and complex diagnoses
125	M	Circulatory disorders except AMI, with cardiac cath. w/o complex diagnoses
126	M	Acute and subacute endocarditis
127	M	Heart failure and shock

128	M	Deep vein thrombophlebitis
129	M	Cardiac arrest, unexplained
130	M	Peripheral vascular disorders age ≧70 and/or C.C.
131	M	Peripheral vascular disorders age <70 w/o C.C.
132	M	Atherosclerosis age ≧70 and/or C.C.
133	M	Atherosclerosis age <70 w/o C.C.
134	M	Hypertension
135	M	Cardiac congenital and valvular disorders age ≧70 and/or C.C
136	M	Cardiac congenital and valvular disorders age 18-69 w/o C.C.
137	M	Cardiac congenital and valvular disorders age 0-17
138	M	Cardiac arrhythmia and conduction disorders age ≧70 and/or C.C.
139	M	Cardiac arrhythmia and conduction disorders age <70 w/o C.C.
140	M	Angina pectoris
141	M	Syncope and collapse age ≧70 and/or C.C.
142	M	Syncope and collapse age <70 w/o C.C.
143	M	Chest pain
144	M	Other circulatory diagnoses with C.C.
145	M	Other circulatory diagnoses w/o C.C.

MDC	**06**	**Diseases and disorders of the digestive system**
146	P	Rectal resection age ≧70 and/or C.C.
147	P	Rectal resection age <70 w/o C.C.
148	P	Major small and large bowel procedures age ≧70 and/or C.C.
149	P	Major small and large bowel procedures age <70 w/o C.C.
150	P	Peritoneal adhesiolysis age ≧70 and/or C.C.
151	P	Peritoneal adhesiolysis age <70 w/o C.C.
152	P	Minor small and large bowel procedures age ≧70 and/or C.C.
153	P	Minor small and large bowel procedures age <70 w/o C.C.
154	P	Stomach, esophageal, and duodenal procedures age ≧70 and/or C.C.
155	P	Stomach, esophageal, and duodenal procedures age 18-69 w/o C.C.
156	P	Stomach, esophageal, and duodenal procedures age 0-17
157	P	Anal and stomal procedures age ≧70 and/or C.C.
158	P	Anal and stomal procedures age <70 w/o C.C.
159	P	Hernia procedures except inguinal and femoral age ≧70 and/or C.C.
160	P	Hernia procedures except inguinal and femoral age 18-69 w/o C.C.
161	P	Inguinal and femoral hernia procedures, age ≧70 and/or C.C.
162	P	Inguinal and femoral hernia procedures age 18-69 w/o C.C.
163	P	Hernia procedures age 0-17
164	P	Appendectomy with complicated principal diagnosis age ≧70 and/or C.C.
165	P	Appendectomy with complicated principal diagnosis age <70 w/o C.C.
166	P	Appendectomy w/o complicated principal diagnosis age ≧70 and/or C.C.
167	P	Appendectomy w/o complicated principal diagnosis age <70 and/or C.C.
168	P	Mouth procedures age ≧70 and/or C.C.
169	P	Mouth procedures age <70 w/o C.C.
170	P	Other digestive system OR procedures age ≧70 and/or C.C.
171	P	Other digestive system OR procedures age <70 w/o C.C.
172	M	Digestive malignancy age ≧70 and/or C.C.
173	M	Digestive malignancy age <70 w/o C.C.
174	M	G.I. hemorrhage age ≧70 and/or C.C.
175	M	G.I. hemorrhage age <70 w/o C.C.
176	M	Complicated peptic ulcer
177	M	Uncomplicated peptic ulcer age ≧70 and/or C.C.
178	M	Uncomplicated peptic ulcer age <70 w/o C.C.
179	M	Inflammatory bowel disease
180	M	G.I. obstruction, obstruction age ≧70 and/or C.C.
181	M	G.I. obstruction, obstruction age <70 w/o C.C.
182	M	Esophagitis, gastroenteritis and miscellaneous digestive disorders age ≧70 and/or C.C.
183	M	Esophagitis, gastroenteritis and miscellaneous digestive disorders age 18-69 w/o C.C.
184	M	Esophagitis, gastroenteritis and miscellaneous digestive disorders age 0-17
185	M	Dental and oral disorder except extractions and restorations, age ≧18
186	M	Dental and oral disorder except extractions and restorations, age 0-17
187	M	Dental extractions and restorations
188	M	Other digestive system diagnoses age ≧70 and/or C.C.
189	M	Other digestive system diagnoses age 18-69 w/o C.C.
190	M	Other digestive system diagnoses age 0-17

MDC	**07**	**Diseases and disorders of the hepatobiliary system and pancreas**
191	P	Major pancreas, liver, and shunt procedures
192	P	Minor pancreas, liver, and shunt procedures
193	P	Biliary tract procedures except total cholecystectomy age ≧70 and/or CC
194	P	biliary tract procedures except total cholecystectomy age <70 w/o C.C.
195	P	Total cholecystectomy with common bile duct exploration age ≧70 and/or C.C.
196	P	Total cholecystectomy with common bile duct exploration age <70 w/o C.C.
197	P	Total cholecystectomy w/o common bile duct exploration age ≧70 and/or C.C.
198	P	Total cholecystectomy w/o common bile duct exploration age <70 w/o C.C.
199	P	Hepatobiliary diagnostic procedure for malignancy
200	P	Hepatobiliary diagnostic procedure for nonmalignancy
201	P	Other hepatobiliary or pancreas OR procedures
202	M	Cirrhosis and alcoholic hepatitis
203	M	Malignancy of hepatobiliary system or pancreas
204	M	Disorders of pancreas except malignancy
205	M	Disorders of liver except malignancy, cirrhosis, alcoholic hepatitis age ≧70 and/or CC
206	M	Disorders of liver except malignancy, cirrhosis, alcoholic hepatitis age <70 w/o C.C.
207	M	Disorders of the biliary tract age ≧70 and/or C.C.
208	M	Disorders of the biliary tract age <70 w/o C.C.

MDC	**08**	**Diseases of the musculoskeletal system and connective tissue**
209	P	Major joint and limb reattachment procedures
210	P	Hip and femur procedures except major joint age ≧70 and/or C.C.

211	P	Hip and femur procedures except major joint age 18-69 w/o C.C.
212	P	Hip and femur procedures except major joint age 0-17
213	P	Amputations for musculoskeletal system and connective tissue disorders
214	P	Back and neck procedures age ≧70 and/or C.C.
215	P	Back and neck procedures age <70 w/o C.C.
216	P	Biopsies of musculoskeletal system and connective tissue
217	P	Wound debridement and skin graft except hand, for musculoskeletal and connective tissue disease
218	P	Lower extrem. and humer. procedure except hip, foot, femur age ≧70 and/or CC
219	P	Lower extrem. and humer. procedures except hip, foot, femur age 18-69 w/o CC
220	P	Lower extrem. and humer. procedures except hip, foot, femur age 0-17
221	P	Knee procedures age ≧70 and/or C.C.
222	P	Knee procedures age <70 w/o C.C.
223	P	Upper extremity procedure except humerus and hand age ≧70 and/or C.C.
224	P	Upper extremity procedure except humerus and hand age <70 w/o C.C.
225	P	Foot procedures
226	P	Soft tissue procedures age ≧70 and/or C.C.
227	P	Soft tissue procedures age <70 w/o C.C.
228	P	Ganglion (hand) procedures
229	P	Hand procedures except ganglion
230	P	Local excision and removal of internal fixation devices of hip and femur
231	P	Local excision and removal of internal fixation devices except hip and femur
232	P	Arthroscopy
233	P	Other musculoskeletal system and connective tissue OR procedure age ≧70 and/or C.C.
234	P	Other musculoskeletal system and connective tissue OR procedure age <70 w/o C.C.
235	M	Fractures of femur
236	M	Fractures of hip and pelvis
237	M	Sprains, strains, and dislocations of hip, pelvis, and thigh
238	M	Osteomyelitis
239	M	Pathological fractures and musculoskeletal and connective tissue malignancy
240	M	Connective tissue disorders age ≧70 and/or C.C.
241	M	Connective tissue disorders age <70 w/o C.C.
242	M	Septic arthritis
243	M	Medical back problems
244	M	Bone diseases and septic arthropathies age ≧70 and/or C.C.
245	M	Bone diseases and septic arthropathies age <70 w/o C.C.
246	M	Nonspecific arthropathies
247	M	Signs and symptoms of musculoskeletal system and connective tissue
248	M	Tendonitis, myositis, and bursitis
249	M	Aftercare, musculoskeletal system and connective tissue
250	M	Fractures, sprains, strains, and dislocation of forearm, hand, foot age ≧70 and/or CC
251	M	Fractures, sprains, strains, and dislocation of forearm, hand, foot age 18-69 w/o CC
252	M	Fractures, sprains, strains, and dislocation of forearm, hand, foot age 0-17

253	M	Fractures, sprains, strains, and dislocation of uparm loleg except foot age ≧70 and/or C.C.
254	M	Fractures, sprains, strains, and dislocation of uparm, loleg except foot age 18-69 w/o C.C.
255	M	Fractures, sprains, strains, and dislocation of uparm, loleg except foot age 0-17
256	M	Other diagnoses of musculoskeletal system and connective tissue
471		Bilateral or multiple major joint procedures of the lower extremities
MDC	**09**	**Diseases of the skin, subcutaneous tissue, and breast**
257	P	Total mastectomy for malignancy age ≧70 and/or C.C.
258	P	Total mastectomy for malignancy age <70 w/o C.C.
259	P	Subtotal mastectomy for malignancy age ≧70 and/or C.C.
260	P	Subtotal mastectomy for malignancy age <70 w/o C.C.
261	P	Breast procedure for nonmalignancy except biopsy and local excision
262	P	Breast biopsy and local excision for nonmalignancy
263	P	Skin grafts and/or debridement for skin ulcer or cellulitis age ≧70 and/or C.C.
264	P	Skin grafts and/or debridement for skin ulcer or cellulitis age <70 w/o C.C.
265	P	Skin grafts and/or debridement except for skin ulcer or cellulitis with C.C.
266	P	Skin grafts and/or debridement except for skin ulcer or cellulitis w/o C.C.
267	P	Perianal and pilonidal procedures
268	P	Skin, subcutaneous tissue, and breast plastic procedures
269	P	Other skin, subcutaneous tissue and breast OR procedures age ≧70 and/or C.C.
270	P	Other skin, subcutaneous tissue and breast OR procedures age <70 w/o C.C.
271	M	Skin ulcers
272	M	Major skin disorders age ≧70 and/or C.C.
273	M	Major skin disorders age <70 w/o C.C.
274	M	Malignant breast disorders age ≧70 and/or C.C.
275	M	Malignant breast disorders age <70 w/o C.C.
276	M	Nonmalignant breast disorders
277	M	Cellulitis age ≧70 and/or C.C.
278	M	Cellulitis age 18-69 w/o C.C.
279	M	Cellulitis age 0-17
280	M	Trauma to the skin, subcutaneous tissue, and breast age ≧70 and/or C.C.
281	M	Trauma to the skin, subcutaneous tissue, and breast age 18-69 w/o C.C.
282	M	Trauma to the skin, subcutaneous tissue, and breast age 0-17
283	M	Minor skin disorders age ≧70 and/or C.C.
284	M	Minor skin disorders age <70 w/o C.C.
MDC	**10**	**Endocrine, nutritional, and metabolic diseases**
285	P	Amputations of lower limb for endocrine, nutritional, and metabolic disorders
286	P	Adrenal and pituitary procedures
287	P	Skin grafts and wound debridement for endocrine, nutritional, and metabolic disorders
288	P	OR procedures for obesity

289	P	Parathyroid procedures
290	P	Thyroid procedures
291	P	Thyroglossal procedures
292	P	Other endocrine, nutritional, and metabolic OR procedure age ≧70 and/or C.C.
293	P	Other endocrine, nutritional, and metabolic OR procedure age <70 w/o C.C.
294	M	Diabetes age ≧36
295	M	Diabetes age 0-35
296	M	Nutritional and miscellaneous metabolic disorders age ≧70 and/or C.C.
297	M	Nutritional and miscellaneous metabolic disorders age 18-60 w/o C.C.
298	M	Nutritional and miscellaneous metabolic disorders age 0-17
299	M	Inborn errors of metabolism
300	M	Endocrine disorders age ≧70 and/or C.C.
301	M	Endocrine disorders age <70 w/o C.C.

MDC 11   Diseases and disorders of the kidney and urinary tract

302	P	Kidney transplant
303	P	Kidney, ureter, and major bladder procedure for neoplasm
304	P	Kidney, ureter, and major bladder procedure for nonmalignancy age ≧70 and/or CC
305	P	Kidney, ureter, and major bladder procedure for nonmalignancy age <70 w/o C.C.
306	P	Prostatectomy age ≧70 and/or C.C.
307	P	Prostatectomy age <70 w/o C.C.
308	P	Minor bladder procedures age ≧70 and/or C.C.
309	P	Minor bladder procedures age <70 w/o C.C.
310	P	Transurethral procedures age ≧70 and/or C.C.
311	P	Transurethral procedures age <70 w/o C.C.
312	P	Urethral procedures age ≧70 and/or C.C.
313	P	Urethral procedures age 18-69 w/o C.C.
314	P	Urethral procedures age 0-17
315	P	Other kidney and urinary tract OR procedures
316	M	Renal failure w/o dialysis
317	M	Renal failure with dialysis
318	M	Kidney and urinary tract neoplasms age ≧70 and/or C.C.
319	M	Kidney and urinary tract neoplasms age <70 w/o C.C.
320	M	Kidney and urinary tract infections age ≧70 and/or C.C.
321	M	Kidney and urinary tract infections age 18-69 w/o C.C.
322	M	Kidney and urinary tract infections age 0-17
323	M	Urinary stones age ≧70 and/or C.C.
324	M	Urinary stones age <70 w/o C.C.
325	M	Kidney and urinary tract signs and symptoms age ≧70 and/or C.C.
326	M	Kidney and urinary tract signs and symptoms age 18-69 w/o C.C.
327	M	Kidney and urinary tract signs and symptoms age 0-17
328	M	Urethral stricture age ≧70 and/or C.C.
329	M	Urethral stricture age 18-69 w/o C.C.
330	M	Urethral stricture age 0-17
331	M	Other kidney and urinary tract diagnoses age ≧70 and/or C.C.
332	M	Other kidney and urinary tract diagnoses age 18-69 w/o C.C.
333	M	Other kidney and urinary tract diagnoses age 0-17

MDC 12   Diseases and disorders of the male reproductive system

334	P	Major male pelvic procedures with C.C.
335	P	Major male pelvic procedures w/o C.C.
336	P	Transurethral prostatectomy age ≧70 and/or C.C.
337	P	Transurethral prostatectomy age <70 w/o C.C.
338	P	Testes procedures, for malignancy
339	P	Testes procedures, nonmalignant age ≧18
340	P	Testes procedures, nonmalignant age 0-17
341	P	Penis procedures
342	P	Circumcision age ≧18
343	P	Circumcision age 0-17
344	P	Other male reproductive system OR procedures for malignancy
345	P	Other male reproductive system OR procedures except for malignancy
346	M	Malignancy, male reproductive system age ≧70 and/or C.C.
347	M	Malignancy, male reproductive system age <70 w/o C.C.
348	M	Benign prostatic hypertrophy age ≧70 and/or C.C.
349	M	Benign prostatic hypertrophy age <70 w/o C.C.
350	M	Inflammation of the male reproductive system
351	M	Sterilization, male
352	M	Other male reproductive system diagnoses

MDC 13   Diseases and disorders of the female reproductive system

353	P	Pelvic evisceration, radical hysterectomy, and vulvectomy
354	P	Nonradical hysterectomy age ≧70 and/or C.C.
355	P	Nonradical hysterectomy age <70 w/o C.C.
356	P	Female reproductive system reconstructive procedures
357	P	Uterus and adnexal procedure, for malignancy
358	P	Uterus and adnexal procedure for nonmalignancy except tubal interruption
359	P	Incisional tubal interruption for nonmalignancy
360	P	Vagina, cervix, and vulva procedures
361	P	Laparoscopy and endoscopy (female) except tubal interruption
362	P	Laparoscopic tubal interruption
363	P	D&C, conization, and radioimplant, for malignancy
364	P	D&C, conization except for malignancy
365	P	Other female reproductive system OR procedures
366	M	Malignancy, female reproductive system age ≧70 and/or C.C.
367	M	Malignancy, female reproductive system age <70 w/o C.C.
368	M	Infections, female reproductive system
369	M	Menstrual and other female reproductive system disorders

MDC 14   Pregnancy, childbirth, and the puerperium

370	P	Cesarean section with C.C.
371	P	Cesarean section w/o C.C.
372	M	Vaginal delivery with complicating diagnoses
373	M	Vaginal delivery w/o complicating diagnoses
374	P	Vaginal delivery with sterilization and/or D&C
375	P	Vaginal delivery with OR procedure except sterilization and/or D&C
376	M	Postpartum and postabortion diagnoses w/o OR procedure

377	P	Postpartum and postabortion diagnoses with OR procedures
378	M	Ectopic pregnancy
379	M	Threatened abortion
380	M	Abortion w/o D&C
381	M	Abortion with D&C or aspiration curettage or hysterotomy
382	M	False labor
383	M	Other antepartum diagnoses with medical complications
384	M	Other antepartum diagnoses w/o medical complications

MDC	**15**	**Normal newborns and other neonates with certain condition originating in perinatal period**
385		Neonates, died or transferred
386		Extreme immaturity or respiratory distress syndrome, neonate
387		Prematurity with major problems
388		Prematurity w/o major problems
389		Full term neonate with major problems
390		Neonates with other significant problems
391		Normal newborns

MDC	**16**	**Diseases and disorders of blood and blood-forming organs and immunity**
392	P	Splenectomy age ≧18
393	P	Splenectomy age 0-17
394	P	Other OR procedures of the blood and blood forming organs
395	M	Red blood cell disorders age ≧18
396	M	Red blood cell disorders, age 0-17
397	M	Coagulation disorders
398	M	Reticuloendothelial and immunity disorders age ≧70 and/or C.C.
399	M	Reticuloendothelial and immunity disorders age <70 w/o C.C.

MDC	**17**	**Myeloproliferative disorders and poorly differentiated malignancy, and other neoplasms N.E.C.**
400	P	Lymphoma or leukemia with major OR procedure
401	P	Lymphoma or leukemia with other OR procedure age ≧70 and/or C.C.
402	P	Lymphoma or leukemia with other O.R. procedure, age <70 w/o C.C.
403	M	Lymphoma or leukemia age ≧70 and/or C.C.
404	M	Lymphoma or leukemia age 18-69 w/o C.C.
405	M	Lymphoma or leukemia age 0-17
406	P	Myeloproliferative disorder or poorly differentiated neoplasm with major OR procedure and C.C.
407	P	Myeloproliferative disorder or poorly differentiated neoplasm with major OR procedure w/o C.C.
408	P	Myeloproliferative disorder or poorly differentiated neoplasm with other O.R. procedure
409	M	Radiotherapy
410	M	Chemotherapy
411	M	History of malignancy w/o endoscopy
412	M	History of malignancy with endoscopy
413	M	Other myeloproliferative disorder or poorly differentiated neoplasm diagnosis age ≧70 and/or C.C.

414	M	Other myeloproliferative disorder or poorly differentiated neoplasm diagnosis age <70 w/o C.C.

MDC	**18**	**Infectious and parasitic diseases (systemic)**
415	P	OR procedure for infectious and parasitic diseases
416	M	Septicemia age ≧18
417	M	Septicemia age 0-17
418	M	Postoperative and posttraumatic infections
419	M	Fever of unknown origin age ≧70 and/or C.C.
420	M	Fever of unknown origin age 18-69 w/o C.C.
421	M	Viral illness age ≧18
422	M	Viral illness and fever of unknown origin age 0-17
423	M	Other infections and parasitic diseases diagnoses

MDC	**19**	**Mental disorders**
424	P	OR procedures with principal diagnosis of mental illness
425	M	Acute adjustment reaction and disturbances of psychosocial dysfunction
426	M	Depressive neuroses
427	M	Neuroses except depressive
428	M	Disorders of personality and impulse control
429	M	Organic disturbances and mental retardation
430	M	Psychoses
431	M	Childhood mental disorders
432	M	Other diagnoses of mental disorders

MDC	**20**	**Substance use disorders and substance induced organic disorders**
433		Substance use and induced organic mental disorders, left AMA
434		Substance abuse, intoxication or induced mental syndrome except dependence and other symptomatic treatment
435		Substance dependence, detoxication and/or other symptomatic treatment
436		Substance dependence, combined rehabilitation therapy
437		Substance dependence, combined rehabilitation and detoxication therapy
438		No longer valid

MDC	**21**	**Injury, poisoning, and toxic effects of drugs**
439	P	Skin grafts for injuries
440	P	Wound debridements for injuries
441	P	Hand procedures for injuries
442	P	Other OR procedures for injuries age ≧70 and/or C.C.
443	P	Other OR procedures for injuries age <70 w/o C.C.
444	M	Multiple trauma age ≧70 and/or C.C.
445	M	Multiple trauma age 18-69 w/o C.C.
446	M	Multiple trauma age 0-17
447	M	Allergic reactions age ≧18
448	M	Allergic reactions age 0-17
449	M	Poisoning and toxic effects of drugs age ≧70 and/or C.C.
450	M	Poisoning and toxic effects of drugs age 18-69 w/o C.C.
451	M	Poisoning and toxic effects of drugs, age 0-17
452	M	Complications of treatment age ≧70 and/or C.C.
453	M	Complications of treatment age <70 w/o C.C.

| 454 | M | Other injuries, poisonings, and toxic effects diagnosis age ≧70 and/or C.C. |
| 455 | M | Other injuries, poisonings, and toxic effects diagnosis age <70 w/o C.C. |

MDC 22   Burns

456		Burns, transferred to another acute care facility
457		Extensive burns
458	P	Nonextensive burns with skin grafts
459	P	Nonextensive burns with wound debridement and other OR procedures
460	M	Nonextensive burns w/o OR procedure

MDC 23   Selected factors influencing health status and contact with health services

| 461 | P | OR procedure with diagnoses of other contact with health services |
| 462 | M | Rehabilitation |

463	M	Signs and symptoms with C.C.
464	M	Signs and symptoms w/o C.C.
465	M	Aftercare with history of malignancy as secondary diagnosis
466	M	Aftercare w/o history of malignancy as secondary diagnosis
467	M	Other factors influencing health status

MDC 24   Ungroupable records

468		Unrelated OR procedure
469		Primary Dx invalid as discharge diagnosis
470		Ungroupable; record does not meet criteria for any DRG
471	P	Bilateral or multiple major joint procedure of the lower extremity (MDC 08)
472	P	Extensive burns with OR procedure (MDC 22)
473	M	Acute leukemia w/o major OR procedure, age >17 (MDC 17)

APPENDIX
18

DSM-III-R CLASSIFICATION: AXES I-V CATEGORIES AND CODES

All official DSM-III-R codes are included in ICD-9-CM. Codes followed by an asterisk (*) are used for more than one DSM-III-R diagnosis or subtype in order to maintain compatibility with ICD-9-CM.

A long dash following a diagnostic term indicates the need for a fifth digit subtype or other qualifying term.

The term *specify* following the name of some diagnostic categories indicates qualifying terms that clinicians may wish to add in parentheses after the name of the disorder.

NOS = Not Otherwise Specified

The current severity of a disorder may be specified after the diagnosis as:

Mild ⎤
Moderate ⎬ Currently meets
Severe ⎦ diagnostic criteria

In partial remission (or residual state)
In complete remission

Multiaxial system	
Axis I	Clinical Syndromes
	V Codes
Axis II	Developmental Disorders
	Personality Disorders
Axis III	Physical Disorders and Conditions
Axis IV	Severity of Psychosocial Stressors
Axis V	Global Assessment of Functioning

DISORDERS USUALLY FIRST EVIDENT IN INFANCY, CHILDHOOD, OR ADOLESCENCE

Developmental disorders

NOTE: These are coded on axis II

Mental retardation
317.00   Mild mental retardation
318.00   Moderate mental retardation
318.10   Severe mental retardation
318.20   Profound mental retardation
319.00   Unspecified mental retardation

Pervasive developmental disorders
299.00   Austic disorder
      Specify if childhood onset
299.80   Pervasive developmental disorder NOS

Specific developmental disorders
   Academic skills disorders
315.10   Developmental arithmetic disorder
315.80   Developmental expressive writing disorder
315.00   Developmental reading disorder
   Language and speech disorders
315.39   Developmental articulation disorder
315.31* Developmental expressive language disorder
315.31* Developmental receptive language disorder
   Motor skills disorder
315.40   Developmental coordination disorder
315.90* Specific developmental disorder NOS
Other developmental disorders
315.90* Developmental disorder NOS

DISRUPTIVE BEHAVIOR DISORDERS

314.01   Attention-deficit hyperactivity disorder
      Conduct disorder
312.20   group type
312.00   solitary aggressive type
312.90   undifferentiated type
313.81   Oppositional defiant disorder

ANXIETY DISORDERS OF CHILDHOOD OR ADOLESCENCE

309.21   Separation anxiety disorder
313.21   Avoidant disorder of childhood or adolescence
313.00   Overanxious disorder

EATING DISORDERS

307.10   Anorexia nervosa
307.51   Bulimia
307.52   Pica
307.53   Rumination disorder of infancy
307.50   Eating disorder NOS

GENDER IDENTITY DISORDERS

302.60   Gender identity disorder of childhood
302.50   Transsexualism
      Specify sexual history: asexual, homosexual, heterosexual, unspecified
302.85* Gender identity disorder of adolescence or adulthood, nontranssexual type
      Specify sexual history: asexual, homosexual, heterosexual, unspecified
302.85* Gender identity disorder NOS

Tic disorders

307.23	Tourette's disorder
307.22	Chronic motor or vocal tic disorder
307.21	Transient tic disorder
	Specify: single episode or recurrent
307.20	Tic disorder NOS

Elimination disorders

307.70	Functional encopresis
	Specify: primary or secondary type
307.60	Functional enuresis
	Specify: primary or secondary type
	Specify: nocturnal only, diurnal only, nocturnal and diurnal

Speech disorders not elsewhere classified

307.00*	Cluttering
307.00*	Stuttering

Other disorders of infancy, childhood, or adolescence

313.23	Elective mutism
313.82	Identity disorder
313.89	Reactive attachment disorder of infancy or early childhood
307.30	Stereotype/habit disorder
314.00	Undifferentiated attention deficit disorder

ORGANIC MENTAL DISORDERS

Dementias arising in the senium and presenium

Primary degenerative dementia of the Alzheimer type, senile onset

290.30	with delirium
290.20	with delusions
290.21	with depression
290.00*	uncomplicated

(NOTE: code 331.00 Alzheimer's disease on axis III)

Code in fifth digit:

1 = with delirium, 2 = with delusions, 3 = depression,
0* = uncomplicated

290.1x	Primary degenerative dementia of the Alzheimer type presenile onset, _____
	(NOTE: code 331.00 Alzheimer's disease on axis III)
290.4x	Multi-infarct dementia, _____
290.00*	Senile dementia NOS
	Specify etiology on axis III if known
290.10*	Presenile dementia NOS
	Specify etiology on axis III if known (e.g., Pick's disease, Jakob-Creutzfeldt disease)

Psychoactive substance-induced organic mental disorders

Alcohol

303.00	intoxication
291.40	idiosyncratic intoxication
291.80	Uncomplicated alcohol withdrawal
291.00	withdrawal delirium
291.30	hallucinosis
291.10	amnestic disorder
291.20	Dementia associated with alcoholism

Amphetamine or similarly acting sympathomimetic

305.70*	intoxication
292.00*	withdrawal
292.81*	delirium
292.11*	delusional disorder

Caffeine

305.90*	intoxication

Cannabis

305.20*	intoxication
292.11*	delusional disorder

Cocaine

305.60*	intoxication

292.00*	withdrawal
292.81*	dilirium
292.11*	delusional disorder

Hallucinogen

305.30*	hallucinosis
292.11*	delusional disorder
292.84*	mood disorder
292.89*	Posthallucinogen perception disorder

Inhalant

305.90*	intoxication

Nicotine

292.00*	withdrawal

Opioid

305.50*	intoxication
292.00*	withdrawal

Phencyclidine (PCP) or similarly acting arylcyclohexylamine

305.90*	intoxication
292.81*	delirium
292.11*	delusional disorder
292.84*	mood disorder
292.90*	organic mental disorder NOS

Sedative, hypnotic, or anxiolytic

305.40*	intoxication
292.00*	Uncomplicated sedative, hypnotic, or anxiolytic withdrawal
292.00*	withdrawal delirium
292.83*	amnestic disorder

Other or unspecified psychoactive substance

305.90*	intoxication
292.00*	withdrawal
292.81*	delirium
292.82*	dementia
292.83*	amnestic disorder
292.11*	delusional disorder
292.12	hallucinosis
292.84*	mood disorder
292.89*	anxiety disorder
292.89*	personality disorder
292.90*	organic mental disorder NOS

Organic mental disorders associated with axis III physical disorders or conditions, or whose etiology is unknown

293.00	Delirium
294.10	Dementia
294.00	Amnestic disorder
293.81	Organic delusional disorder
293.82	Organic hallucinosis
293.83	Organic mood disorder
	Specify: manic, depressed, mixed
294.80*	Organic anxiety disorder
310.10	Organic personality disorder
	Specify if explosive type
294.80*	Organic mental disorder NOS

PSYCHOACTIVE SUBSTANCE USE DISORDERS

Alcohol

303.90	dependence
305.00	abuse

Amphetamine or similarly acting sympathomimetic

304.40	dependence
305.70*	abuse

Cannabis

304.30	dependence
305.20*	abuse

Cocaine

304.20	dependence
305.60*	abuse

Hallucinogen
304.50*   dependence
305.30*   abuse
Inhalant
304.60   dependence
305.90*   abuse
Nicotine
305.10   dependence
Opioid
304.00   dependence
305.50*   abuse
Phencyclidine (PCP) or similarly acting arylcyclohexylamine
304.50*   dependence
305.90*   abuse
Sedative, hypnotic, or anxiolytic
304.10   dependence
305.40*   abuse
304.90*   Polysubstance dependence
304.90*   Psychoactive substance dependence NOS
305.90*   Psychoactive substance abuse NOS

SCHIZOPHRENIA

Code in fifth digit:
1 = subchronic, 2 = chronic, 3 = subchronic with acute exacerbation, 4 = chronic with acute exacerbation, 5 = in remission, 0 = unspecified.
Schizophrenia
295.2x   catatonic, _____
295.1x   disorganized, _____
295.3x   paranoid, _____
    Specify if stable type
295.9x   undifferentiated, _____
295.6x   residual, _____
    Specify if late onset

DELUSIONAL (PARANOID) DISORDER

297.10   Delusional (Paranoid) disorder
    Specify erotomanic, grandiose, jealous, persecutory, somatic, unspecified;

PSYCHOTIC DISORDERS NOT ELSEWHERE CLASSIFIED

298.80   Brief reactive psychosis
295.40   Schizophreniform disorder
    Specify: without good prognostic features or with good prognostic features
295.70   Schizoaffective disorder
    Specify: bipolar type or depressive type
297.30   Induced psychotic disorder
298.90   Psychotic disorder NOS (Atypical psychosis)

MOOD DISORDERS

Code current state of major depression and bipolar disorder in fifth digit:
1 = mild, 2 = moderate, 3 = severe, without psychotic features, 4 = with psychotic features (*specify* mood-congruent or mood incongruent), 5 = in partial remission, 6 = in full remission, 0 = unspecified
For major depressive episodes, *Specify* if chronic and *specify* if melancholic type.
For bipolar disorder, bipolar disorder NOS, recurrent major depression, and depressive disorder NOS, *specify* if seasonal pattern.

Bipolar disorders
Bipolar disorder
296.6x   mixed, _____
296.4x   manic, _____
296.5x   depressed, _____
301.13   Cyclothymia
296.70   Bipolar disorder NOS
Depressive disorders
Major depression
296.2x   single episode, _____
296.3x   recurrent, _____
300.40   Dysthymia (or Depressive neurosis)
    Specify: primary or secondary type
    Specify: early or late onet
311.00   Depressive disorder NOS

ANXIETY DISORDERS (or anxiety and phobic neuroses)

Panic disorder
300.21   with agoraphobia
    Specify current severity of agoraphobic avoidance
    Specify current severity of panic attacks
300.01   without agoraphobia
    Specify current severity of panic attacks
300.22   Agoraphobia without history of panic disorder
    Specify with or without limited symptom attacks
300.23   Social phobia
    Specify if generalized type
300.29   Simple phobia
300.30   Obsessive compulsive disorder (or Obsessive compulsive neurosis)
309.89   Post-traumatic stress disorder
    Specify if delayed onset
300.02   Generalized anxiety disorder
300.00   Anxiety disorder NOS

SOMATOFORM DISORDERS

300.70*   Body dysmorphic disorder
300.11   Conversion disorder (of Hysterical neurosis, conversion type)
    Specify: single episode or recurrent
300.70*   Hypochondriasis (or Hypochondriacal neurosis)
300.81   Somatization disorder
307.80   Somatoform pain disorder
300.70*   Undifferentiated somatoform disorder
300.70*   Somatoform disorder NOS

DISSOCIATIVE DISORDERS (or Hysterical Neuroses, Dissociative Type)

300.14   Multiple personality disorder
300.13   Psychogenic fugue
300.12   Psychogenic amnesia
300.60   Depersonalization disorder (or Depersonalization neurosis)
300.15   Dissociative disorder NOS

SEXUAL DISORDERS

Paraphilias
302.40   Exhibitionism
302.81   Fetishism
302.89   Frotteurism

302.20   Pedophilia
       Specify: same sex, opposite sex, same and opposite sex
       Specify if limited to incest
       Specify: exclusive type or nonexclusive type
302.83   Sexual masochism
302.84   Sexual sadism
302.30   Transvestic fetishism
302.82   Voyeurism
302.90*   Paraphilia NOS
Sexual dysfunctions
Specify: psychogenic only, or psychogenic and biogenic (NOTE: If biogenic only, code on Axis III)
Specify: lifelong or acquired
Specify: generalized or situational
   Sexual desire disorders
302.71   Hypoactive sexual desire disorder
302.79   Sexual aversion disorder
   Sexual arousal disorders
302.72*   Female sexual arousal disorder
302.72*   Male erectile disorder
   Orgasm disorders
302.73   Inhibited female orgasm
302.74   Inhibited male orgasm
302.75   Premature ejaculation
   Sexual pain disorders
302.76   Dyspareunia
306.51   Vaginismus
302.70   Sexual dysfunction NOS
Other sexual disorders
302.90*   Sexual disorder NOS

SLEEP DISORDERS

Dyssomnias
   Insomnia disorder
307.42*   related to another mental disorder (nonorganic)
780.50*   related to known organic factor
307.42*   Primary insomnia
   Hypersomnia disorder
307.44   related to another mental disorder (nonorganic)
780.50*   related to a known organic factor
780.54   Primary hypersomnia
307.45   Sleep-wake schedule disorder
       Specify: advanced or delayed phase type, disorganized type, frequently changing type
   Other dyssomnias
307.40*   Dyssomnia NOS
Parasomnias
307.47   Dream anxiety disorder (Nightmare disorder)
307.46*   Sleep terror disorder
307.46*   Sleepwalking disorder
307.40*   Parasomnia NOS

FACTITIOUS DISORDERS

   Factitious disorder
301.51   with physical symptoms
300.16   with psychological symptoms
300.19   Factitious disorder NOS

IMPULSE CONTROL DISORDERS NOT ELSEWHERE CLASSIFIED

312.34   Intermittent explosive disorder
312.32   Kleptomania
312.31   Pathological gambling
312.33   Pyromania

312.39*   Trichotillomania
312.39*   Impulse control disorder NOS

ADJUSTMENT DISORDER

   Adjustment disorder
309.24   with anxious mood
309.00   with depressed mood
309.30   with disturbance of conduct
309.40   with mixed disturbance of emotions and conduct
309.28   with mixed emotional features
309.82   with physical complaints
309.83   with withdrawal
309.23   with work (or academic) inhibition
309.90   Adjustment disorder NOS

PSYCHOLOGICAL FACTORS AFFECTING PHYSICAL CONDITION

316.00   Psychological factors affecting physical condition
       Specify physical condition on axis III

PERSONALITY DISORDERS

   NOTE: These are coded on axis II
Cluster A
301.00   Paranoid
301.20   Schizoid
301.22   Schizotypal
Cluster B
301.70   Antisocial
301.83   Borderline
301.50   Histrionic
301.81   Narcissistic
Cluster C
301.82   Avoidant
301.60   Dependent
301.40   Obsessive compulsive
301.84   Passive aggressive
301.90   Personality disorder NOS

V CODES FOR CONDITIONS NOT ATTRIBUTABLE TO A MENTAL DISORDER THAT ARE A FOCUS OF ATTENTION OR TREATMENT

V62.30   Academic problem
V71.01   Adult antisocial behavior
V40.00   Borderline intellectual functioning (Note: This is coded on axis II)
V71.02   Childhood or adolescent antisocial behavior
V65.20   Malingering
V61.10   Marital problem
V15.81   Noncompliance with medical treatment
V62.20   Occupational problem
V61.20   Parent-child problem
V62.81   Other interpersonal problem
V61.80   Other specified family circumstances
V62.89   Phase of life problem or other life circumstance problem
V62.82   Uncomplicated bereavement

ADDITIONAL CODES

300.90   Unspecified mental disorder (nonpsychotic)
V71.09*   No diagnosis or condition on axis I
799.90*   Diagnosis or condition deferred on axis I
V71.09*   No diagnosis or condition on axis II
799.90*   Diagnosis or condition deferred on axis II

19 NURSING DIAGNOSES

19-1 NANDA-approved nursing diagnoses and definitions*

Activity intolerance
The state in which an individual has insufficient physiological or psychological energy to endure or complete required or desired daily activities.

Activity intolerance, high risk for
The state in which an individual is at risk of experiencing insufficient physiological or psychological energy to endure or complete required or desired daily activities.

Adjustment, impaired
The state in which an individual is unable to modify his/her lifestyle/behavior in a manner consistent with a change in health status.

Airway clearance, ineffective
The state in which an individual is unable to clear secretions or obstructions from the respiratory tract to maintain airway patency.

Anxiety
A vague, uneasy feeling, the source of which is often nonspecific or unknown to the individual.

Aspiration, high risk for
The state in which an individual is at risk for entry of gastric secretions, oropharyngeal secretions, or exogenous food or fluids into tracheobronchial passages due to dysfunction or absence of normal protective mechanisms.

Body image disturbance
Disruption in the way one perceives one's body image.

Body temperature, altered, high risk for
The state in which an individual is at risk for failure to maintain body temperature within normal range.

Bowel elimination, altered
See Bowel incontinence; Constipation; Constipation, colonic; Constipation, perceived; Diarrhea.

Bowel incontinence
The state in which an individual experiences a change in normal bowel habits characterized by involuntary passage of stool.

Breastfeeding, effective
The state in which a mother-infant dyad/family exhibits adequate proficiency and satisfaction with the breastfeeding process.

Breastfeeding, ineffective
The state in which a mother, infant, and/or family experiences dissatisfaction or difficulty with the breastfeeding process.

Breastfeeding, interrupted
A break in the continuity of the breastfeeding process as a result of inability or inadvisability to put the baby to the breast for feeding.

Breathing pattern, ineffective
The state in which an individual's inhalation and/or exhalation pattern does not enable adequate ventilation.

Cardiac output, decreased
The state in which the blood pumped by an individual's heart is sufficiently reduced that it is inadequate to meet the needs of the body's tissues.

Caregiver role strain
A caregiver's felt difficulty in performing the family caregiver role.

Caregiver role strain, high risk for
Vulnerability for feeling difficulty in performing the family caregiver role.

Comfort, altered
See Pain; Pain, chronic.

Communication, impaired verbal
The state in which an individual experiences a decreased or absent ability to use or understand language in human interaction.

Constipation
The state in which an individual experiences a change in normal bowel habits characterized by a decrease in frequency and/or passage of hard, dry stools.

Constipation, colonic
The state in which an individual's pattern of elimination is characterized by hard, dry stool that results from a delay in passage of food residue.

Constipation, perceived
The state in which an individual makes a self-diagnosis of constipation and ensures a daily bowel movement through use of laxatives, enemas, and suppositories.

Coping, defensive
The state in which an individual experiences falsely positive-self-evaluation based on a self-protective pattern that defends against underlying perceived threats to positive self-regard.

Coping, family: high risk for growth
Effective managing of adaptive tasks by family member involved with the client's health challenge, who now is exhibiting desire and readiness for enhanced health and growth in regard to self and in relation to the client.

Coping, ineffective family: compromised
Insufficient, ineffective, or compromised support, comfort, assistance, or encouragement usually by a supportive primary person (family member or close friend); client may need it to manage or master adaptive tasks related to his/her health challenge.

Coping, ineffective family: disabling
Behavior of significant person (family member or other primary person) that disables his/her own capacities and the client's capacities to effectively address tasks essential to either person's adaptation to the health challenge.

Coping, ineffective individual
Impairment of adaptive behaviors and problem-solving abilities of a person in meeting life's demands and roles.

Decisional conflict (specify)
A state of uncertainty about the course of action to be taken when choice among competing actions involves risk, loss, or challenge to personal life values. (Specify focus of conflict, e.g., choices regarding health, family relationship, career, finances, or other life events.)

Denial, ineffective
A conscious or unconscious attempt to disavow the knowledge or meaning of an event to reduce anxiety/fear to the detriment of health.

Diarrhea
The state in which an individual experiences a change in normal bowel habits characterized by the frequent passage of loose, fluid, unformed stools.

*For defining characteristics and related factors, see the definitions for individual nursing diagnoses in the body of the dictionary.

Disuse syndrome, high risk for
The state in which an individual is at risk for deterioration of body systems as the result of prescribed or unavoidable inactivity.

Diversional activity deficit
The state in which an individual experiences a decreased stimulation from or interest or engagement in recreational or leisure activities.

Dysreflexia
The state in which an individual with a spinal cord injury at T7 or above experiences or is at risk of experiencing a life-threatening uninhibited sympathetic response of the nervous system to a noxious stimulus.

Family processes, altered
The state in which a family that normally functions effectively experiences a dysfunction.

Fatigue
An overwhelming sense of exhaustion and decreased capacity for physical and mental work regardless of adequate sleep.

Fear
Feeling of dread related to an identifiable source that the person validates.

Fluid volume deficit (1)
The state in which an individual experiences vascular, cellular, or intracellular dehydration related to failure of regulatory mechanisms.

Fluid volume deficit (2)
The state in which an individual experiences vascular, cellular, or intracellular dehydration related to active loss.

Fluid volume deficit, high risk for
The state in which an individual is at risk of experiencing vascular, cellular, or intracellular dehydration.

Fluid volume excess
The state in which an individual experiences increased fluid retention and edema.

Gas exchange, impaired
The state in which an individual experiences an imbalance between oxygen uptake and carbon dioxide elimination at the alveolar-capillary membrane gas exchange area.

Grieving, anticipatory
The state in which an individual grieves before an actual loss.

Grieving, dysfunctional
The state in which actual or perceived object loss (object loss is used in the broadest sense) exists. Objects include people, possessions, a job, status, home, ideals, parts and processes of the body, etc.

Growth and development, altered
The state in which an individual demonstrates deviations in norms from his/her age group.

Health maintenance, altered
Inability to identify, manage, and/or seek out help to maintain health.

Health-seeking behaviors (specify)
The state in which a client in stable health is actively seeking ways to alter personal health habits and/or the environment in order to move toward optimal health. (*Stable health status* is defined as age-appropriate illness prevention measures achieved; the client reports good or excellent health, and signs and symptoms of disease, if present, are controlled.)

Home maintenance management, impaired
Inability to independently maintain a safe growth-promoting immediate environment.

Hopelessness
The subjective state in which an individual sees limited or no alternatives or personal choices available and is unable to mobilize energy on own behalf.

Hyperthermia
The state in which an individual's body temperature is elevated above his/her normal range.

Hypothermia
The state in which an individual's body temperature is reduced below his/her normal range but not below 35.6° C (rectal)/36.4° C (rectal, newborn).

Incontinence, bowel
See Bowel incontinence.

Incontinence, functional
The state in which an individual experiences an involuntary, unpredictable passage of urine.

Incontinence, reflex
The state in which an individual experiences an involuntary loss of urine occurring at somewhat predictable intervals when a specific bladder volume is reached.

Incontinence, stress
The state in which an individual experiences a loss of urine of less than 50 ml occurring with increased abdominal pressure.

Incontinence, total
The state in which an individual experiences a continuous and unpredictable loss of urine.

Incontinence, urge
The state in which an individual experiences involuntary passage of urine occurring soon after a strong sense of urgency to void.

Infant feeding pattern, ineffective
A state in which an infant demonstrates an impaired ability to suck or coordinate the suck-swallow response.

Infection, high risk for
The state in which an individual is at increased risk for being invaded by pathogenic organisms.

Injury, high risk for
The state in which an individual is at risk of injury as a result of environmental conditions interacting with the individual's adaptive and defensive resources. See also Poisoning, high risk for; Suffocation, high risk for; Trauma, high risk for

Knowledge deficit (specify)
The state in which specific information is lacking.

Management of therapeutic regimen (individual), ineffective
A pattern of regulating and integrating into daily living a program for treatment of illness and the sequelae of illness that is unsatisfactory for meeting specific health goals.

Mobility, impaired physical
The state in which an individual experiences a limitation of ability for independent physical movement.

Noncompliance (specify)
A person's informed decision not to adhere to a therapeutic recommendation.

Nutrition, altered: less than body requirements
The state in which an individual experiences an intake of nutrients insufficient to meet metabolic needs.

Nutrition, altered: more than body requirements
The state in which an individual is experiencing an intake of nutrients that exceeds metabolic needs.

Nutrition, altered: high risk for more than body requirements
The state in which an individual is at risk of experiencing an intake of nutrients that exceeds metabolic needs.

Oral mucous membrane, altered
The state in which an individual experiences disruptions in the tissue layers of the oral cavity.

Pain
The state in which an individual experiences and reports the presence of severe discomfort or an uncomfortable sensation.

Pain, chronic
The state in which an individual experiences pain that continues for more than 6 months.

Parental role conflict
The state in which a parent experiences role confusion and conflict in response to a crisis.

Parenting, altered
Parenting, altered, high risk for
The state in which the ability of nuturing figure(s) to create an environment that promotes the optimum growth and development of another human being is altered or at risk.

Peripheral neurovascular dysfunction, high risk for
A state in which an individual is at risk for experiencing a disruption in circulation, sensation, or motion of an extremity.

Personal identity disturbance
Inability to distinguish between self and nonself.

Poisoning, high risk for
Accentuated risk of accidental exposure to or ingestion of drugs or dangerous products in doses sufficient to cause poisoning.

Post-trauma response
The state in which an individual experiences a sustained painful response to (an) overwhelming traumatic event(s).

Powerlessness
Perception that one's own action will not significantly affect an outcome; a perceived lack of control over a current situation or immediate happening.

Protection, altered
The state in which an individual experiences a decrease in the ability to guard the self from internal or external threats, such as illness or injury.

Rape-trauma syndrome
Forced, violent sexual penetration against the victim's will and consent. The trauma syndrome that develops from this attack or attempted attack includes an acute phase or disorganization of the victim's life-style and a long-term process of reorganization of life-style.

Rape-trauma syndrome: compound reaction
An acute stress reaction to a rape or attempted rape, experienced along with other major stressors, that can include reactivation of symptoms of a previous condition.

Rape-trauma syndrome: silent reaction
A complex stress reaction to a rape in which an individual is unable to describe or discuss the rape.

Relocation stress syndrome
Physiological and/or psychosocial disturbances as a result of a transfer from one environment to another.

Role performance, altered
Disruption in the way one perceives one's role performance.

Self-care deficit, bathing/hygiene
The state in which an individual experiences an impaired ability to perform or complete bathing/hygiene activities for oneself.

Self-care deficit, dressing/grooming
The state in which an individual experiences an impaired ability to perform or complete dressing and grooming activities for one-self.

Self-care deficit, feeding
The state in which an individual experiences an impaired ability to perform or complete feeding activities for oneself.

Self-care deficit, toileting
The state in which an individual experiences an impaired ability to perform or complete toileting activities for oneself.

Self-concept, disturbance in
See Body image disturbance; Personal identity disturbance; Self-esteem disturbance.

Self-esteem disturbance
Negative self-evaluation/feelings about self or self-capabilities, which may be directly or indirectly expressed.

Self-esteem, chronic low
Long-standing negative self-evaluation/feelings about self or self-capabilities.

Self-esteem, situational low
Negative self-evaluation/feelings about self that develop in response to a loss or change in an individual who previously had a positive self-evaluation.

Self-mutilation, high risk for
A state in which an individual is at high risk to perform an act on the self to injure, not kill, that produces tissue damage and tension relief.

Sensory/perceptual alterations (specify) (visual, auditory, kinesthetic, gustatory, tactile, olfactory)
The state in which an individual experiences a change in the amount or patterning of incoming stimuli accompanied by a diminished, exaggerated, distorted, or impaired response to such stimuli.

Sexual dysfunction
The state in which an individual experiences a change in sexual function that is viewed as unsatisfying, unrewarding, or inadequate.

Sexuality patterns, altered
The state in which an individual expresses concern regarding his/her sexuality.

Skin integrity, impaired
The state in which an individual's skin is adversely altered.

Skin integrity, impaired, high risk for
The state in which an individual's skin is at risk of being adversely altered.

Sleep pattern disturbance
Disruption of sleep time causes discomfort or interferes with desired life-style.

Social interaction, impaired
The state in which an individual participates in an insufficient or excessive quantity or ineffective quality of social exchange.

Social isolation
Aloneness experienced by an individual and perceived as imposed by others and as a negative or threatened state.

Spiritual distress (distress of the human spirit)
Disruption in the life principle that pervades a person's entire being and that integrates and transcends one's biological and psychosocial nature.

Suffocation, high risk for
Accentuated risk of accidental suffocation (inadequate air available for inhalation).

Swallowing, impaired
The state in which an individual has decreased ability to voluntarily pass fluids and/or solids from the mouth to the stomach.

Thermoregulation, ineffective
The state in which an individual's temperature fluctuates between hypothermia and hyperthermia.

Thought processes, altered
The state in which an individual experiences a disruption in cognitive operations and activities.

Tissue integrity, impaired
The state in which an individual experiences damage to mucous membrane or corneal, integumentary, or subcutaneous tissue. See also Oral mucous membrane, altered.

Tissue perfusion, altered (specify type) (renal, cerebral, cardio-pulmonary, gastrointestinal, peripheral)
The state in which an individual experiences a decrease in nutrition and oxygenation at the cellular level due to a deficit in capillary blood supply.

Trauma, high risk for
Accentuated risk of accidental tissue injury (e.g., wound, burn, fracture)

Unilateral neglect
The state in which an individual is perceptually unaware of and inattentive to one side of the body.

Urinary elimination, altered patterns
The state in which an individual experiences a disturbance in urine elimination. See also Incontinence (functional, reflex, stress, total, urge)

Urinary retention
The state in which an individual experiences incomplete emptying of the bladder.

Ventilation, inability to sustain spontaneous

A state in which the response pattern of decreased energy reserves results in an individual's inability to maintain breathing adequate to support life.

Ventilatory weaning process, dysfunctional (DVWR)

A state in which an individual cannot adjust to lowered levels of mechanical ventilator support, which interrupts and prolongs the weaning process.

Violence, high risk for: self-directed or directed at others

The state in which an individual experiences behaviors that can be physically harmful either to the self or others.

19-2   Classification of nursing diagnoses by human response patterns (NANDA Taxonomy I-revised)

I. Exchanging
Altered nutrition: more than body requirements
Altered nutrition: less than body requirements
Altered nutrition: high risk for more than body requirements
High risk for infection
High risk for altered body temperature
Hypothermia
Hyperthermia
Ineffective thermoregulation
Dysreflexia
Constipation
Perceived constipation
Colonic constipation
Diarrhea
Bowel incontinence
Altered patterns of urinary elimination
Stress incontinence
Reflex incontinence
Urge incontinence
Functional incontinence
Total incontinence
Urinary retention
Altered (specify type) tissue perfusion (renal, cerebral, cardio-pulmonary, gastrointestinal, peripheral)
Fluid volume excess
Fluid volume deficit (1)
Fluid volume deficit (2)
High risk for fluid volume deficit
Decreased cardiac output
Impaired gas exchange
Ineffective airway clearance
Ineffective breathing pattern
Inability to sustain spontaneous ventilation
Dysfunctional ventilatory weaning response
High risk for injury
High risk for suffocation
High risk for poisoning
High risk for trauma
High risk for aspiration
High risk for disuse syndrome
Altered protection
Impaired tissue integrity
Altered oral mucous membrane
Impaired skin integrity
High risk for impaired skin integrity

II. Communicating
Impaired verbal communication

III. Relating
Impaired social interaction
Social isolation
Altered role performance
Altered parenting
High risk for altered parenting
Sexual dysfunction
Altered family processes
Caregiver role strain

High risk for caregiver role strain
Parental role conflict
Altered sexuality patterns

IV. Valuing
Spiritual distress (distress of the human spirit)

V. Choosing
Ineffective individual coping
Impaired adjustment
Defensive coping
Ineffective denial
Ineffective family coping: disabling
Ineffective family coping: compromised
Family coping: potential for growth
Ineffective management of therapeutic regimen (individuals)
Noncompliance (specify)
Decisional conflict (specify)
Health-seeking behaviors (specify)

VI. Moving
Impaired physical mobility
High risk for peripheral neurovascular dysfunction
Activity intolerance
Fatigue
High risk for activity intolerance
Sleep pattern disturbance
Diversional activity deficit
Impaired home maintenance management
Altered health maintenance
Feeding self-care deficit
Impaired swallowing
Ineffective breastfeeding
Interrupted breastfeeding
Effective breastfeeding
Ineffective infant feeding pattern
Bathing/hygiene self-care deficit
Dressing/grooming self-care deficit
Toileting self-care deficit
Altered growth and development
Relocation stress syndrome

VII. Perceiving
Body image disturbance
Self-esteem disturbance
Chronic low self-esteem
Situational low self-esteem
Personal identity disturbance
Sensory/perceptual alterations (specify) (visual, auditory, kinesthetic, gustatory, tactile, olfactory)
Unilateral neglect
Hopelessness
Powerlessness

VIII. Knowing
Knowledge deficit (specify)
Altered thought processes

IX. Feeling
Pain
Chronic pain
Dysfunctional grieving

Anticipatory grieving
High risk for violence: self-directed or directed at others
High risk for self-mutilation
Post-trauma response
Rape-trauma syndrome

Rape-trauma syndrome: compound reaction
Rape-trauma syndrome: silent reaction
Anxiety
Fear

19-3 Classification of nursing diagnoses by functional health pattern

Health perception–health management pattern
Altered health maintenance
Altered protection
Ineffective management of therapeutic regimen
Noncompliance (specify)
High risk for infection
High risk for injury
High risk for trauma
High risk for poisoning
High risk for suffocation
Health-seeking behaviors (specify)
Nutritional–metabolic pattern
Altered nutrition: high risk for more than body requirements
Altered nutrition: more than body requirements
Altered nutrition: less than body requirements
Effective breastfeeding
Ineffective breastfeeding
Interrupted breastfeeding
Ineffective infant feeding pattern
High risk for aspiration
Impaired swallowing
Altered oral mucous membrane
Potential fluid volume deficit
Fluid volume deficit (1)
Fluid volume deficit (2)
Fluid volume excess
High risk for impaired skin integrity
Impaired skin integrity
Impaired tissue integrity
High risk for altered body temperature
Ineffective thermoregulation
Hyperthermia
Hypothermia
Elimination pattern
Constipation
Perceived constipation
Colonic constipation
Diarrhea
Bowel incontinence
Altered patterns of urinary elimination
Functional incontinence
Reflex incontinence
Stress incontinence
Urge incontinence
Total incontinence
Urinary retention
Activity–exercise pattern
High risk for activity intolerance
Dysfunctional ventilatory weaning response
Inability to sustain spontaneous ventilation
High risk for peripheral neurovascular dysfunction
Activity intolerance
Impaired physical mobility
High risk for disuse syndrome

Fatigue
Bathing/hygiene self-care deficit
Dressing/grooming self-care deficit
Feeding self-care deficit
Toileting self-care deficit
Diversional activity deficit
Impaired home maintenance management
Ineffective airway clearance
Ineffective breathing pattern
Impaired gas exchange
Decreased cardiac output
Altered (specify type) tissue perfusion (renal, cerebral, cardiopulmo-
nary, gastrointestinal, peripheral)
Dysreflexia
Altered growth and development
Sleep–rest pattern
Sleep pattern disturbance
Cognitive–perceptual pattern
Pain
Chronic pain
Sensory perceptual alterations (specify) (visual, auditory, kines-
thetic, gustatory, tactile, olfactory)
Unilateral neglect
Knowledge deficit (specify)
Altered thought processes
Decisional conflict (specify)
Self-perception–self-concept pattern
Fear
Anxiety
Hopelessness
Powerlessness
Body image disturbance
High risk for self-mutilation
Personal identity disturbance
Self-esteem disturbance
Chronic low self-esteem
Situational low self-esteem
Role–relationship pattern
Anticipatory grieving
Dysfunctional grieving
Altered role performance
Caregiver role strain
High risk for caregiver role strain
Social isolation
Impaired social interaction
Relocation stress syndrome
Altered family processes
High risk for altered parenting
Altered parenting
Parental role conflict
Impaired verbal communication
High risk for violence: self-directed or directed at others
Sexuality–reproductive pattern
Sexual dysfunction
Altered sexuality patterns
Rape-trauma syndrome
Rape-trauma syndrome: compound reaction
Rape-trauma syndrome: silent reaction

Based on Gordon M: Manual of nursing diagnoses, 1993-1994, St Louis, 1993, Mosby-Year Book

Coping–stress tolerance pattern
Ineffective individual coping
Defensive coping
Ineffective denial
Impaired adjustment
Post-trauma response

Family coping: potential for growth
Ineffective family coping: compromised
Ineffective family coping: disabling
Value–belief pattern
Spiritual distress (distress of the human spirit)

19-4   Nursing diagnoses relevant to diseases, disorders, and procedures

Abdominal surgery
Altered Nutrition: Less than Body Requirements related to high metabolic needs, decreased ability to digest food
Constipation related to decreased activity, decreased fluid intake, anesthesia/narcotics
Knowledge Deficit related to limited exposure to information
High Risk for Altered Tissue Perfusion: Peripheral related to immobility and abdominal surgery resulting in stasis of blood flow
Pain related to surgical procedure
High Risk for Infection related to invasive procedure
Refer to Surgery

Abortion—induced
Health Seeking Behaviors related to desire to control fertility
High Risk for Infection related to open uterine blood vessels, dilated cervix
Ineffective Family Coping: Compromised related to unresolved feelings about decision
Knowledge Deficit related to lack of exposure to situation
Self Esteem Disturbance related to feelings of guilt
Spiritual Distress related to perceived moral implications of decision

Abortion—spontaneous
Altered Family Processes related to unmet expectations for pregnancy/childbirth
Body Image Disturbance related to perceived inability to carry pregnancy, produce child
Fear related to implications for future pregnancies
High Risk for Fluid Volume Deficit related to hemorrhage
High Risk for Dysfunctional Grieving related to loss of fetus
High Risk for Infection related to septic or incomplete abortion of products of conception, open uterine blood vessels, dilated cervix
Ineffective Family Coping: Disabling related to unresolved feelings about loss
Ineffective Individual Coping related to personal vulnerability
Knowledge Deficit related to lack of exposure to situation
Pain related to uterine contractions, surgical intervention
Self Esteem Disturbance related to feelings of failure, guilt

Abruptio placenta (>36 weeks)
Altered Family Processes related to unmet expectations for pregnancy/childbirth
Anxiety related to unknown outcome, change in birth plans
Fear related to threat to well-being of self and fetus
High Risk for Altered Tissue Perfusion (Fetal) related to uteroplacental insufficiency
High Risk for Fluid Volume Deficit related to hemorrhage
High Risk for Infection related to partial separation of the placenta
High Risk for Injury (Fetal) related to hypoxia
High Risk for Injury (Maternal) related to uterine rupture
Knowledge Deficit related to limited exposure to situation
Pain related to irritable uterus, hypertonic uterus

Abuse, spouse, parent, significant other or by caregiver
Anxiety related to threat to self-concept of situational crisis of abuse
Caregiver Role Strain related to chronic illness; self-care deficits; lack of respite care; extent of caregiving required
Defensive Coping related to low self-esteem

Impaired Verbal Communication related to psychological barriers of fear
Ineffective Family Coping: Compromised related to abusive patterns
Post-Trauma Response related to history of abuse
High Risk for Self-Directed Violence related to history of abuse
Powerlessness related to lifestyle of helplessness
Self-Esteem Disturbance related to negative family interactions
Sleep Pattern Disturbance related to psychological stress

Achalasia
High Risk for Aspiration related to nocturnal regurgitation
Impaired Swallowing related to neuromuscular impairment
Ineffective Individual Coping related to chronic disease
Pain related to stasis of food in the esophagus

Acidosis, metabolic
Altered Nutrition, Less than Body Requirements related to inability to ingest, absorb nutrients
Altered Thought Processes related to central nervous system depression
Decreased Cardiac Output related to dysrhythmias from hyperkalemia
High Risk for Injury related to disorientation, weakness, stupor
Pain: Headache related to neuromuscular irritability, tetany

Acidosis, respiratory
Activity Intolerance related to imbalance between oxygen supply and demand
Altered Thought Processes related to central nervous system depression
High Risk for Decreased Cardiac Output related to arrhythmias associated with respiratory acidosis
Impaired Gas Exchange related to ventilation perfusion imbalance

Addison's disease
Activity Intolerance related to weakness, fatigue
Altered Nutrition: Less than Body Requirements related to chronic illness
Fluid Volume Deficit related to failure of regulatory mechanisms
High Risk for Injury related to weakness
Knowledge Deficit related to lack of informational sources

Adenoidectomy
Altered Comfort related to effects of anesthesia: nausea and vomiting
High Risk for Altered Nutrition: Less than Body Requirements related to hesitation/reluctance to swallow
High Risk for Aspiration/Suffocation related to postoperative drainage and impaired swallowing
High Risk for Fluid Volume Deficit related to decreased intake secondary to painful swallowing, effects of anesthesia
Ineffective Airway Clearance related to hesitation/reluctance to cough secondary to pain
Knowledge Deficit related to insufficient knowledge regarding postoperative nutrition and rest requirements, signs and symptoms of complications, positioning
Pain related to surgical incision

Adjustment disorder
Anxiety related to inability to cope with psychosocial stressor
Impaired Adjustment related to assault to self-esteem
Personal Identity Disturbance related to psychosocial stressor (specific to individual)
Situational Low Self-Esteem related to change in role function

Adapted from Ackley BJ, Ladwing GB, Hampton JK, Henrickson M, Masta M, McClurg V, McLean C, O'Brien KAS, Schonlau VLC, Wall V, Wetch PA, and Wistrom F: *Nursing diagnosis handbook: A guide to planning care,* St Louis, 1993, Mosby.

Affective disorders

Altered Health Maintenance related to lack of ability to make good judgments regarding ways to obtain help

Chronic Low Self-Esteem related to repeated unmet expectations

Colonic Constipation related to inactivity, decreased fluid intake

Dysfunctional Grieving related to lack of previous resolution of former grieving response

Fatigue related to psychological demands

High Risk for Violence: Self-Directed related to panic state

Hopelessness related to feeling of abandonment, long-term stress

Ineffective Individual Coping related to dysfunctional grieving

Knowledge Deficit related to lack of motivation to learn new coping skills

Self Care Deficit: Specify related to depression, cognitive impairment

Sexual Dysfunction related to loss of sexual desire

Sleep Pattern Disturbance related to inactivity

Social Isolation related to ineffective coping

Refer to specific disorder: Depression/major, Dysthymia, Mania

Agoraphobia

Anxiety related to real or perceived threat to physical integrity

Fear related to leaving home and going out in public places

Ineffective Individual Coping related to inadequate support systems

Impaired Social Interaction related to disturbance in self-concept

Social Isolation related to altered thought process

AIDS (acquired immunodeficiency syndrome)

Altered Family Processes related to distress over diagnosis of HIV infection

Altered Health Maintenance related to knowledge deficit regarding transmission of infection, lack of exposure to information, misinterpretation of information

Altered Nutrition: Less than Body Requirements related to decreased ability to eat and absorb nutrients secondary to anorexia, nausea, diarrhea

Altered Protection related to high risk for infection secondary to inadequate immune system

Anticipatory Grieving: Family/Parental related to potential/impending death of loved one

Anticipatory Grieving: Individual related to loss of physiopsychosocial well-being

Body Image Disturbance related to chronic contagious illness, cachexia

Caregiver Role Strain related to unpredictable illness course; presence of situation stressors

Pain, Chronic related to tissue inflammation/destruction

Diarrhea related to inflammatory changes in bowel

Fatigue related to disease process, stress, poor nutritional intake

Fear related to powerlessness, threat to well-being

High Risk for Altered Oral Mucous Membranes related to immunological deficit

High Risk for Altered Thought Processes related to infection in brain

High Risk for Fluid Volume Deficit related to diarrhea, vomiting, fever, bleeding

High Risk for Infection related to inadequate immune system

High Risk for Impaired Skin Integrity related to immunological deficit or diarrhea

Hopelessness related to deteriorating physical condition

Situational Low Self Esteem related to crisis of chronic contagious illness

Social isolation related to self-concept disturbance, therapeutic isolation

Spiritual Distress related to challenged belief/moral system

Refer to Cancer; Pneumonia

Alcoholism

Altered Nutrition: Less than Body Requirements related to anorexia

Altered Protection related to malnutrition, sleep deprivation

Anxiety related to loss of control

Compromised/Dysfunctional Family Coping related to codependency issues

High Risk for Injury related to alteration in sensory perceptual function

High Risk for Violence related to reactions to substances used, impulsive behavior, disorientation, impaired judgment

Impaired Home Maintenance Management related to memory deficits, fatigue

Ineffective Individual Coping related to use of alcohol to cope with life events

Powerlessness related to alcohol addiction

Self-Esteem Disturbance related to failure at life events

Sleep Pattern Disturbance related to irritability, nightmares, tremors

Social Isolation related to unacceptable social behavior, values

Alcohol withdrawal

Altered Nutrition: Less than Body Requirements related to poor dietary habits

Altered Thought Processes related to potential delirium tremens

Anxiety related to situational crisis; withdrawal

Chronic Low Self Esteem related to repeated unmet expectations

High Risk for Fluid Volume Deficit related to excessive diaphoresis, agitation, decreased fluid intake

Ineffective Individual Coping related to personal vulnerability

Knowledge Deficit related to chronic illness or effects of alcohol consumption

High Risk for Violence related to substance withdrawal

Sensory/Perceptual Alterations: Visual, Auditory, Kinesthetic, Tactile, Olfactory related to neurochemical imbalance in brain

Sleep Pattern Disturbance related to effect of depressants, alcohol withdrawal, anxiety

Alzheimer's disease

Altered Thought Processes related to chronic organic disorder

Anger related to frustration secondary to memory deficits

Caregiver Role Strain related to duration and extent of caregiving required

Fear related to loss of self

High Risk for Injury related to confusion

High Risk for Violence: Directed at Others related to frustration, fear, anger

Hopelessness related to deteriorating condition

Knowledge Deficit (Family) related to limited exposure to information

Impaired Home Maintenance Management related to impaired cognitive function, inadequate support systems

Impaired Physical Mobility related to severe neurological dysfunction

Ineffective Family Coping: Compromised related to altered family processes

Powerlessness related to deteriorating condition

Self-Care Deficit: Specify related to psychophysiological impairment

Sleep Pattern Disturbance related to neurological impairment and naps during the day

Social Isolation related to fear of disclosure of memory loss

Refer to Dementia

Amputation

Anticipatory Grieving related to loss of body part and future lifestyle changes

Body Image Disturbance related to negative effects of amputation, response from others

High Risk for Alteration in Tissue Perfusion: Peripheral related to impaired arterial circulation

High Risk for Fluid Volume Deficit: Hemorrhage related to abnormal blood loss

Impaired Physical Mobility related to musculoskeletal impairment and limited movement

Impaired Skin Integrity related to poor healing, prosthesis rubbing

Knowledge Deficit related to limited practice of new skills

Pain related to surgery, phantom limb sensation

Anemia

Anxiety related to cause of disease

Fatigue related to decreased oxygen supply to the body

High Risk for Injury related to alteration in peripheral sensory perception

Knowledge Deficit: Nutrition and medical therapy related to lack to previous learning regarding nutrition

Aneurysm, abdominal surgery

High Risk for Altered Tissue Perfusion: Peripheral related to impaired arterial circulation

High Risk for Fluid Volume Deficit: Hemorrhage related to potential abnormal blood loss

High Risk for Infection related to invasive procedure

Refer to Abdominal Surgery

Angina pectoris

Activity Intolerance related to acute pain, dysrhythmias

Altered Sexuality Pattern related to disease process, medications, loss of libido

Anxiety related to situational crisis

Decreased Cardiac Output related to myocardial ischemia/medication effect/arrhythmias

Grieving related to pain and potential lifestyle changes

Ineffective Individual Coping related to personal vulnerability to a situational crisis (new diagnosis, deteriorating health)

Knowledge Deficit related to lack of exposure to information

Pain related to myocardial ischemia

Angioplasty, coronary balloon

Fear related to possible outcome of interventional procedure

High Risk for Altered Tissue perfusion: Peripheral/Cardiopulmonary related to vasospasm, hematoma formation

High Risk for Decreased Cardiac Output related to ventricular ischemia; dysrhythmias

High Risk for Fluid Volume Deficit related to possible damage to coronary artery, hematoma formation, hemorrhage

Knowledge Deficit related to unfamiliarity with information resources

Anomaly, fetal/newborn (parent dealing with)

Altered Family Processes related to unmet expectations for perfect baby, lack of adequate support systems

Altered Parenting related to interruption of bonding process

Anxiety related to threat to role functioning, situational crisis

Decisional Conflict: Interventions for fetus/newborn related to lack of relevant information, spiritual distress, threat to value system

Fear related to real or imagined threat to baby, implications for future pregnancies, powerlessness

High Risk for Altered Parenting related to interruption of bonding process; unrealistic expectations for self, infant, or partner; perceived threat to own emotional survival; severe stress; lack of knowledge

High Risk for Dysfunctional Grieving related to loss of perfect child

Hopelessness related to long term stress, deteriorating physical condition of child, lost spiritual belief

Knowledge Deficit related to limited exposure to situation

Ineffective Family Coping: Disabling related to chronically unresolved feelings of loss of perfect baby

Ineffective Individual Coping related to personal vulnerability in situational crisis

Parental Role Conflict related to separation from newborn, intimidation with invasive or restrictive modalities, specialized care centers policies

Powerlessness related to complication threatening fetus/newborn

Self-Esteem Disturbance related to perceived inability to produce a perfect child

Spiritual Distress related to test of spiritual beliefs

Anorexia nervosa

Activity Intolerance related to fatigue, weakness

Altered Nutrition: Less than Body Requirements related to inadequate food intake

Altered Patterns of Sexuality related to loss of libido from malnutrition

Altered Thought Processes related to malnutrition

Body Image Disturbance related to misconception of actual body appearance

Chronic Low Self-Esteem related to repeated unmet expectations

Constipation related to lack of adequate food, fluid intake

Defensive Coping related to psychological impairment, eating disorder

Diarrhea related to laxative abuse

High Risk for Infection related to malnutrition resulting in depressed immune system

Ineffective Denial related to fear of consequences of therapy and possible weight gain

Ineffective Family Coping: Disabling related to highly ambivalent family relationships

Refer to Maturational Issues, Adolescent

Anticoagulant therapy

Altered Protection related to altered clotting function from anticoagulant

Anxiety related to situational crisis

High Risk for Fluid Volume Deficit: Hemorrhage related to altered clotting mechanism

Knowledge Deficit related to lack of informational sources

Antisocial personality disorder

High Risk for Altered Parenting related to inability to function as a parent or guardian; emotional instability

High Risk for Violence Directed at Others related to history of violence

Impaired Social Interaction related to sociocultural conflict; chemical dependence; inability to form relationships

Ineffective Individual Coping related to frequently violating societies norms, rules

Anxiety disorder

Altered Thought Processes related to anxiety

Anxiety related to unmet security and safety needs

Decisional Conflict related to low self esteem; fear of making a mistake

Ineffective Family Coping: Disabling related to ritualistic behavior, actions

Ineffective Individual Coping related to not being able to express feelings appropriately

Powerlessness related to lifestyle of helplessness

Self-Care Deficit related to ritualistic behavior, activities

Sleep Pattern Disturbance related to psychological impairment; emotional instability

Aphasia

Anxiety related to situational crisis of aphasia

Impaired Verbal Communication related to decrease in circulation to brain

Ineffective Individual Coping related to loss of speech

Knowledge Deficit related to lack of information on aphasia, alternative communication techniques

Appendicitis

High Risk for Fluid Volume Deficit related to anorexia, nausea and vomiting

High Risk for Infection related to possible perforation of appendix

Pain related to inflammation

Appendectomy

High Risk for Fluid Volume Deficit related to fluid restriction; hypermetabolic state; nausea and vomiting

High Risk for Infection related to perforation/rupture of appendix; surgical incision; peritonitis

Knowledge Deficit related to unfamiliarity with information sources

Pain related to surgical incision

Refer to Surgery, Hospitalized Child

ARDS (adult respiratory distress syndrome)

Impaired Gas Exchange related to damage to alveolar-capillary membrane, change in lung compliance

Inability to Sustain Spontaneous Ventilation related to damage to the alveolar capillary membrane

Ineffective Airway Clearance related to excessive tracheobronchial secretions

Refer to Ventilator Client Care, Child with Chronic Condition

Arthritis

Activity Intolerance related to chronic pain, fatigue, weakness

Altered Family Process related to disability of family member

Body Image Disturbance related to ineffective coping with joint abnormalities

Pain, Chronic related to progression of joint deterioration

Impaired Physical Mobility related to musculoskeletal impairment

Knowledge Deficit related to limited exposure to information

Self-Care Deficit: Specify related to pain, musculoskeletal impairment

Refer to Rheumatoid Arthritis, Juvenile

Arthroplasty—total hip replacement

Activity Interolance related to limitations from surgery

High Risk for Colonic Constipation related to immobility

High Risk for Infection related to invasive surgery, foreign object in body, anesthesia, immobility with stasis of respiratory secretions

High Risk for Injury related to interruption of arterial blood flow, dislocation of the prosthesis

High Risk for Peripheral Neurovascular Dysfunction related to orthopedic surgery

Knowledge Deficit related to lack of adequate information regarding potential postoperative complications and restrictions

Pain related to tissue trauma associated with surgery

Refer to Surgery

Arthroscopy

Knowledge Deficit related to unfamiliarity with procedure, postoperative restrictions

Ascites

Pain, Chronic related to altered body function

High Risk for Altered Nutrition: Less Body Requirements related to loss of appetite

Ineffective Breathing Pattern related to increased abdominal girth

Knowledge Deficit related to lack of informational sources, lack of interest in learning

Refer to cause: Cirrhosis or Cancer

Asthma

Activity Intolerance related to fatigue; energy shift to meet muscle needs for effective breathing and to overcome airway obstruction

Altered Health Maintenance related to knowledge deficit regarding physical triggers, medications, treatment of early warning signs secondary to lack of exposure to information about asthma

Anxiety related to inability to breathe effectively, fear of suffocation

Body Image Disturbance related to decreased participation in physical activities at school

Impaired Home Maintenance Management related to knowledge deficit regarding control of environmental triggers

Ineffective Airway Clearance related to tracheobronchial narrowing, excessive secretions

Ineffective Breathing Pattern related to anxiety

Ineffective Individual Coping related to personal vulnerability to a situational crisis

Refer to Child with Chronic Condition; Hospitalized Child

Atelectasis

Impaired Gas Exchange related to decreased alveolar-capillary surface

Ineffective Breathing Pattern related to loss of functional lung tissue, depression of respiratory function or hypoventilation because of pain

Autism

Altered Growth and Development related to inability to develop relations with other human beings, inability to identify own body as separate from those of other people, inability to integrate concept of self

Altered Thought Processes related to inability to perceive self or others, cognitive dissonance, perceptual dysfunction

High Risk for Self-Mutilation related to autistic state

High Risk for Violence: Self and Other Directed related to frequent destructive rages toward self or others, secondary to extreme response to changes in routine, fear of harmless things

Identity Disturbance related to inability to distinguish between self and environment, inability to identify own body as separate from those of other people, inability to integrate concept of self

Impaired Social Interaction related to communication barriers, inability to relate interpersonally to others

Impaired Verbal Communication related to speech and language delays

Ineffective Family Coping: Compromised/Disabling related to parental guilt over etiology of disease, inability to accept/adapt to child's condition, inability to help child and other family members seek treatment

Personal Identity Disturbance related to inability to distinguish between self and environment, inability to identify own body as separate from those of other people, inability to integrate concept of self

Refer to Mental Retardation or Child With Chronic Condition

Autonomic hyperreflexia

Dysreflexia related to bladder distention, bowel distention, or other noxious stimuli

Back pain

Anxiety related to situational crisis; back injury

High Risk for Colonic Constipation related to decreased activity

High Risk for Disuse Syndrome related to severe pain

High Risk for Ineffective Individual Coping related to situational crisis, back injury

Impaired Physical Mobility related to pain

Knowledge Deficit related to unfamiliarity with information resources, lack of information regarding prevention of further injury, body mechanics

Pain related to back injury

Battered child syndrome

Altered Growth and Development: Regression vs Delayed related to diminished/absent environmental stimuli, inadequate caretaking, inconsistent responsiveness by caretaker

Altered Nutrition: Less than Body Requirements related to inadequate caretaking

Anxiety/Fear (child) related to threat of punishment for perceived wrongdoing

Chronic Low Self-Esteem related to lack of positive feedback or excessive negative feedback

Diversional Activity Deficit related to diminished/absent environmental or personal stimuli

High Risk for Poisoning related to inadequate safeguards, lack of proper safety precautions, accessibility of illicit substances secondary to impaired home maintenance management

High Risk for Self Mutilation related to feelings of rejection, dysfunctional family

High Risk for Suffocation/Aspiration related to propped bottle, unattended child *High Risk for Trauma* related to inadequate precautions, cognitive or emotional difficulties

Impaired Skin Integrity related to altered nutritional state, physical abuse

Pain related to physical injuries

Post-Trauma Response related to physical abuse, incest/rape/molestation

Sleep Pattern Disturbance related to hypervigilance, anxiety

Social Isolation, Family Imposed related to fear of disclosure of family dysfunction and abuse

Biliary atresia

Altered Comfort related to pruritis, nausea

Altered Nutrition: Less than Body Requirements related to decreased absorption of fat and fat soluble vitamins; poor feeding

Anxiety/Fear related to surgical intervention (Kasai procedure) and possible liver transplantation

High Risk for Ineffective Breathing Patterns related to enlarged liver and development of ascites

High Risk for Injury: Bleeding related to vitamin K deficiency and altered clotting mechanisms

High Risk for Impaired Skin Integrity related to to pruritis

Refer to Hospitalized Child; Child With Chronic Condition; Terminally Ill Child/Death of Child; Cirrhosis as complication

Bipolar disorder: depression, mania

Altered Health Maintenance related to lack of ability to make good judgments regarding ways to obtain help

Chronic Low Self-Esteem related to repeated unmet expectations

Dysfunctional Grieving related to lack of previous resolution of former grieving response

Fatigue related to psychological demands

Ineffective Individual Coping related to dysfunctional grieving

Knowledge Deficit related to lack of motivation to learn new coping skills

Self Care Deficit: Specify related to depression, cognitive impairment

Social Isolation related to ineffective coping

Refer to Depression or Mania

Bladder tumor

High Risk for Urinary Retention related to clots obstructing urethra

Refer to TURP, Cancer

Blindness

Sensory Perceptual Alteration: Visual related to altered sensory reception, transmission, or integration

Bone marrow biopsy

Fear related to unknown outcome of results of aspiration

Knowledge Deficit related to purpose and actual procedure

Pain related to bone marrow aspiration

Borderline personality

Altered Thought Process related to poor reality testing

Anxiety related to perceived threat to self-concept

Defensive Coping related to difficulty with relationships; inability to accept blame for own behavior

Disturbance in Self Concept related to unmet dependency needs

High Risk for Caregiver Role Strain related to care receiver can not accept criticism or takes advantage of others to meet own needs; unreasonable expectations of care receiver

High Risk for Self-Mutilation related to ineffective coping; feelings of self-hatred

High Risk for Violence: Self-Directed related to feelings of need to punish self/manipulative behavior

Ineffective Individual Coping related to use of maladjusted defense mechanisms, e.g., projection, denial

Powerlessness related to lifestyle of helplessness

Social Isolation related to immature interests

Bowel obstruction

Altered Nutrition: Less than Body Requirements related to nausea, vomiting

Constipation related to decreased motility; intestinal obstruction

Fluid volume Deficit related to inadequate fluid volume intake; fluid loss in bowel

Pain related to pressure from distended abdomen

BPH (benign prostatic hypertrophy)

High Risk for Infection related to urinary residual postvoiding; bacterial invasion of bladder

Knowledge Deficit related to unfamiliarity with information sources

Sleep Pattern Disturbance related to nocturia

Urinary Retention related to obstruction

Brain tumor

Altered Thought Processes related to altered circulation or destruction of brain tissue

Anticipatory Grieving related to potential loss of physiopsychosocial well-being

Fear related to threat to well-being

High Risk for Injury related to sensory-perceptual alterations; weakness

Pain related to neurologic injury

Sensory/Perceptual Alteration (Specify) related to tumor growth compressing brain tissue

Refer to Craniotomy/Craniectomy; Cancer; Chemotherapy; Radiation Therapy; Hospitalized Child; Child with Chronic Condition; Terminally Ill Child

Breast cancer

Disturbance in Self-Concept related to surgery and possible side effects of chemotherapy and/or radiation

Fear related to diagnosis of cancer

Ineffective Coping related to treatment and prognosis

Sexual Dysfunction related to loss of body part and partner's reaction to loss

Refer to Mastectomy

Breast lumps

Knowledge Deficit related to breast-self examination

Fear related to potential for diagnosis of cancer

Bronchitis

Anxiety related to potential chronic condition

Ineffective Airway Clearance related to excessive thickened mucous secretion

Knowledge Deficit related to lack of exposure to information; need for cessation of smoking

Bronchopulmonary dysplasia (BPD)

Activity Intolerance related to imbalance between oxygen supply and demand

Altered Nutrition: Less than Body Requirements related to poor feeding; increased caloric needs secondary to increased work of breathing *Fluid Volume Excess* related to sodium and water retention

Knowledge Deficit related to lack of informational sources

Refer to Respiratory Conditions of the Neonate; Child With Chronic Condition; Hospitalized Child

Bulimia

Altered Nutrition: Less than Body Requirements related to induced vomiting

Altered Thought Processes related to anorexia

Chronic Low Self-Esteem related to lack of positive feedback

Defensive Coping related to eating disorder

Disturbance in Body Image related to misperception about actual appearance and body weight

Fear related to food ingestion and weight gain

Ineffective Family Coping related to chronically unresolved feelings: guilt, anger, and hostility

Noncompliance related to negative feelings toward treatment regimen

Powerlessness related to urge to purge self after eating

Refer to Maturational Issues, Adolescent

Burns

Altered Nutrition: Less than Body Requirements related to increased metabolic needs; anorexia; protein and fluid loss

Altered Tissue Perfusion: Peripheral related to circumferential burns; impaired arterial/venous circulation

Anticipatory Grieving related to loss of bodily function; loss of future hopes and plans

Anxiety/Fear related to pain from treatments; possible permanent disfigurement

Body Image Disturbance related to altered physical appearance

Diversional Activity Deficit related to long-term hospitalization

High Risk for Fluid Volume Deficit related to loss from skin surface; fluid shift

High Risk for Hypothermia related to impaired skin integrity

High Risk for Infection related to loss of intact skin; trauma, invasive sites

High Risk for Ineffective Airway Clearance related to potential tracheobronchial obstruction, edema

High Risk for Peripheral Neurovascular Dysfunction related to es-
char formation with circumferential burn
Impaired Physical Mobility related to pain; musculoskeletal impair-
ment; contracture formation
Impaired Skin Integrity related to burn injury of skin
Pain related to burn injury and treatments
Post-Trauma Response related to life-threatening event
Refer to Hospitalized Child

Bursitis

Impaired Physical Mobility related to inflammation in joint
Pain related to inflammation in joint

Cancer

Altered Nutrition: Less than Body Requirements related to loss of
appetite or difficulty swallowing; side effects of chemotherapy; ob-
struction by tumor
Altered Oral Mucous Membranes related to chemotherapy; oral pH
changes; decreased or altered oral flora
Altered Protection related to cancer-suppressing immune system
Altered Role Performance related to change in physical capacity; in-
ability to resume prior role
Anticipatory Grieving related to potential loss of significant others;
high risk for infertility
Body Image Disturbance related to side effects of treatment; cachexia
Pain, Chronic related to metastatic cancer
Colonic Constipation related to side effects of medication; altered
nutrition; decreased activity
Decisional Conflict related to selection of treatment choices; contin-
uation/discontinuation of treatment; Do Not Resuscitate decision
Fear related to serious threat to well-being
High Risk for Disuse Syndrome related to severe pain; change in level
of consciousness
High Risk for Infection related to inadequate immune system
High Risk for Injury related to bleeding secondary to bone marrow
depression
High Risk for Impaired Home Maintenance Management related to
lack of familiarity with community resources
Hopelessness related to loss of control; terminal illness
Impaired Physical Mobility related to weakness; neuromusculoskel-
etal impairment; pain
Impaired Skin Integrity related to immunological deficit; immobility
Ineffective Denial related to dysfunctional grieving process
Ineffective Family Coping: Compromised related to prolonged dis-
ease or disability progression that exhausts the supportive ability
of significant others functioning
Ineffective Individual Coping related to personal vulnerability in sit-
uational crisis; terminal illness
Knowledge Deficit related to limited exposure to prescribed treatment
information
Powerlessness related to treatment, progression of disease
Self-Care Deficit: Specify related to pain; intolerance to activity; de-
creased strength
Sleep Pattern Disturbance related to anxiety; pain
Social Isolation related to hospitalization; lifestyle changes
Spiritual Distress related to test of spiritual beliefs
Refer to Chemotherapy; Hospitalized Child; Child with Chronic Con-
dition; Terminally Ill Child/Death of Child

Cardiac catheterization

Altered Comfort related to postprocedure restrictions, invasive procedure
Anxiety/Fear related to invasive procedure, uncertainty of outcome
of procedure
High Risk for Altered Tissue Perfusion related to impaired arterial/
venous circulation
High Risk for Decreased Cardiac Output related to ventricular ischemia, arrhythmias
High Risk for Injury: Hematoma related to invasive procedure
High Risk for Peripheral Neurovascular Dysfunction related to vascular obstruction

Knowledge Deficit related to limited exposure to information about
the procedure and after procedure care

Carotid endarterectomy

Fear related to surgery in vital area
High Risk for Altered Tissue perfusion: Cerebral related to hemor-
rhage, clot formation
High Risk for Injury related to possible hematoma formation
High Risk for Ineffective Breathing Pattern related to hematoma com-
pressing trachea
Knowledge Deficit related to unfamiliarity with information resources

Carpal tunnel syndrome

Impaired Physical Mobility related to neuromuscular impairment
Pain related to unrelieved pressure on median nerve

Casts

Knowledge Deficit related to cast management

Cataract extraction

Anxiety related to threat of permanent vision loss; surgical procedure
Sensory/Perceptual Alteration: Vision related to adjustment to new
lens or glasses
High Risk for Injury related to increased intraocular pressure; acco-
modation to new visual field
Knowledge Deficit related to postoperative restrictions

Catatonic schizophrenia

Altered Nutrition: Less than Body Requirements related to decrease
in outside stimulation; no perception of hunger; resistance to in-
structions to eat
Impaired Physical Mobility related to cognitive impairment; mainte-
nance of rigid posture; inappropriate/bizarre postures
Impaired Verbal Communication related to mutism
Social Isolation related to inability to communicate; immobility
Refer to Schizophrenia

Cellulitis

Altered Tissue Perfusion: Peripheral related to edema
Impaired Skin Integrity related to inflammatory process damaging
skin
Pain related to inflammatory changes in tissues from infection

Cellulitis, periorbital

Impaired Skin Integrity related to inflammation/infection of skin/tis-
sues
Pain related to edema and inflammation of skin/tissues
Sensory/Perceptual Alterations (visual) related to decreased visual
fields secondary to edema of eyelids
Hyperthermia related to infectious process
Refer to Hospitalized Child

Cerebral palsy

Impaired Physical Mobility related to spasticity, neuromuscular im-
pairment/weakness
Self Care Deficit (specify area and level) related to neuromuscular
impairments, sensory deficits
High Risk for Injury/Trauma related to muscle weakness, inability
to control spasticity
Impaired Verbal Communication related to impaired ability to artic-
ulate/speak words secondary to facial muscle involvement
Diversional Activity Deficit related to physical impairments; limitations on ability to participate in recreational activities
Impaired Social Interaction related to impaired communication
skills; limited physical activity; perceived differences from peers
High Risk for Altered Nutrition: Less than Body Requirements related to spasticity, feeding/swallowing difficulties
Refer to Child With Chronic Condition

Cesarean delivery

Altered Family Processes related to unmet expectations for childbirth
Altered Role Performance related to unmet expectations for childbirth
Alteration in Comfort: Nausea, Vomiting, Pruritis related to side effects of systemic or epidural narcotics
Anxiety related to unmet expectations for childbirth; unknown outcome of surgery

Body Image Disturbance related to surgery, unmet expectations for childbirth

Fear related to perceived threat to own well being

High Risk for Aspiration related to positioning for general anesthesia

High Risk for Fluid Volume Deficit related to increased blood loss secondary to surgery

High Risk for Infection related to surgical incision; stasis of respiratory secretions secondary to general anesthesia

High Risk for Urinary Retention related to regional anesthesia

Impaired Physical Mobility related to pain

Knowledge Deficit related to lack of exposure to situation

Pain related to surgical incision; decreased or absent peristalsis secondary to anesthesia; manipulation of abdominal organs during surgery; immobilization; restricted diet

Situational Low Self-Esteem related to inability to birth child vaginally

Chemotherapy

Altered Comfort: Nausea and Vomiting related to effects of chemotherapy

Altered Nutrition: Less than Body Requirements related to side effects of chemotherapy

Altered Oral Mucous Membranes related to effects of chemotherapy

Altered Protection related to suppressed immune system, decreased platelets

Body Image Disturbance related to loss of weight; loss of hair

Fatigue related to disease process; anemia; drug effects

High Risk for Altered Tissue Perfusion related to anemia

High Risk for Fluid Volume Deficit related to vomiting, diarrhea

High Risk for Infection related to immunosuppression

High Risk for Trauma/Injury related to abnormal blood profile

Knowledge Deficit related to action, side effects of chemotherapy

Refer to Cancer

Chest pain

Fear related to potential threat of death

High Risk for Decreased Cardiac Output related to ventricular ischemia

Pain related to myocardial injury, ischemia

Refer to Angina, MI

Chest tubes

High Risk for Injury related to presence of invasive chest tube

Impaired Gas Exchange related to decreased functional lung tissue

Ineffective Breathing Pattern related to asymmetrical lung expansion secondary to pain

Pain related to presence of chest tubes, injury

Fluid Volume Excess related to impaired excretion of sodium and water

High Risk for Impaired Gas Exchange related to excessive fluid in interstitial space of lungs, alveoli

Knowledge Deficit related to disease process and treatment

Refer to Congenital Heart Disease/Cardiac Anomalies, Hospitalized Child, Child with Chronic Condition

Child abuse

Altered Growth and Development: Regression vs Delayed related to diminished/absent environmental stimuli; inadequate caretaking; inconsistent responsiveness by caretaker

Altered Nutrition: Less than Body Requirements related to inadequate caretaking

Altered Parenting related to psychological impairment; physical, emotional abuse of parent; substance abuse; unrealistic expectations of child

Anxiety/Fear (child) related to threat of punishment for perceived wrongdoing

Chronic Low Self-Esteem related to lack of positive feedback or excessive negative feedback

Diversional Activity Deficit related to lack of positive feedback or excessive negative feedback

Diversional Activity Deficit related to diminished/absent environmental/personal stimuli

High Risk for Poisoning related to inadequate safeguards; lack of proper safety precautions; accessibility of illicit substances secondary to impaired home maintenance management

High Risk for Suffocation/Aspiration related to propped bottle; unattended child

High Risk for Trauma related to inadequate precautions; cognitive or emotional difficulties

Impaired Skin Integrity related to altered nutritional state; physical abuse

Pain related to physical injuries

Post Trauma Response related to physical abuse; incest/rape/molestation

Sleep Pattern Disturbance related to hypervigilance; anxiety

Social Isolation, Family Imposed related to fear of disclosure of family dysfunction and abuse

Child with chronic condition

Activity Intolerance related to fatigue associated with chronic illness

Altered Family Processes related to intermittent situational crisis of illness/disease and hospitalization

Altered Growth and Development related to regression or lack of progression toward developmental milestones secondary to frequent/prolonged hospitalization; inadequate/inappropriate stimulation; cerebral insult; chronic illness; effects of physical disability; prescribed dependence

Altered Health Maintenance related to exhausting family resources (financial, physical energy, support systems)

Altered Nutrition: Less than Body Requirements related to anorexia; fatigue secondary to physical exertion

Altered Nutrition: More than Body Requirements related to effects of steroid medications on appetite

Altered Sexuality Patterns (Parental) related to disrupted relationship with sexual partner

Chronic Low Self-Esteem related to actual or perceived differences and/or peer acceptance; decreased ability to participate in physical/school/social activities

Chronic Pain related to physical, biological, chemical, psychological factors

Decisional Conflict related to treatment options and conflicting values

Diversional Activity Deficit related to immobility; monotonous environment; frequent/lengthy treatments; reluctance to participate; self-imposed social isolation

Family Coping: Potential for Growth related to impact of crisis on family values, priorities, goals, or relationships; changes in family choices to optimize wellness

High Risk Altered Parenting related to impaired/disrupted bonding; child with perceived overwhelming care needs

High Risk for Infection related to debilitating physical condition

High Risk for Noncompliance related to complex, prolonged, home care regimens; expressed intent to not comply secondary to value systems, health beliefs, and cultural/religious practices

Hopelessness (Child) related to prolonged activity restriction; long-term stress; lack of involvement in care/passively allowing care secondary to parental overprotection

Impaired Home Maintenance Management related to over-taxed family members, e.g., exhausted, anxious

Impaired Social Interaction related to developmental lag/delay; perceived differences

Ineffective Family Coping: Compromised related to prolonged disease or disability progression that exhausts supportive capacity of significant people

Ineffective Family Coping: Disabling related to prolonged overconcern for child; distortion of reality regarding child's health problem, including extreme denial about its existence or severity

Ineffective Individual Coping (Child) related to situational or maturational crises

Knowledge Deficit: Potential for Enhanced Health Maintenance related to knowledge/skill acquisition regarding health practices; acceptance of limitations; promotion of maximum potential of child; self-actualization of rest of family

Parental Role Conflict related to separation from child due to chronic illness; home care of child with special needs; interruptions of family life due to home care regimen

Powerlessness (Child) related to health care environment; illness-related regimen; lifestyle of learned helplessness

Sleep Pattern Disturbance (Child or Parent) related to time intensive treatments; exacerbation of condition; 24-hour care needs

Social Isolation: Family: Self-Imposed related to actual or perceived social stigmatization; complex care requirements

Cholecystectomy

Altered Nutrition: Less than Body Requirements related to high metabolic needs; decreased ability to digest fatty foods

High Risk for Fluid Volume Deficit related to restricted intake; nausea and vomiting

High Risk for Ineffective Breathing Pattern related to proximity of incision to lungs resulting in pain with deep breathing

Knowledge Deficit related to lack of exposure to information

Pain related to recent surgery

Refer to Abdominal Surgery

Cholelithiasis

Altered Nutrition: Less than Body Requirements related to anorexia, nausea and vomiting

Knowledge Deficit related to lack of information about treatment plan

Pain related to obstruction of bile flow, inflammation in gallbladder

Circumcision

High Risk for Fluid Volume Deficit related to hemorrhage

High Risk for Infection related to surgical wound

Knowledge Deficit: Parental related to lack of exposure to situation

Pain related to surgical intervention

Cirrhosis

Altered Nutrition: Less than Body Requirements related to loss of appetite, nausea, vomiting

Chronic Low Self-Esteem related to chronic illness

Chronic Pain related to liver enlargement

Diarrhea related to dietary changes, medications

Fatigue related to malnutrition

High Risk for Altered Oral Mucous Membranes related to altered nutrition

High Risk for Altered Thought Processes related to chronic organic disorder with increased ammonia levels/substance abuse

High Risk for Fluid Volume Deficit: Hemorrhage related to abnormal bleeding from esophagus

High Risk for Injury related to substance intoxication, potential delirium tremors

Knowledge Deficit related to lack of information about correlation between lifestyle habits and disease process

Ineffective Management of Therapeutic Regimen related to denial of seriousness of illness

Noncompliance related to denial of illness

Cleft lip/cleft palate

Altered Health Maintenance related to lack of parental knowledge regarding feeding techniques, wound care, use of elbow restraints

Altered Nutrition: Less than Body Requirements related to inability to feed with normal techniques

Altered oral Mucous Membranes related to surgical correction

Fear: (Parental) related to special care needs, surgery

Grieving related to (loss of perfect child) birth of child with congenital defect

High Risk for Aspiration related to common feeding/breathing passage

High Risk for Body Image Disturbance related to disfigurement and speech impediment

High Risk for Infection related to invasive procedure; disruption of eustachian tube development; aspiration

Impaired Physical Mobility related to imposed restricted activity and use of elbow restraints

Impaired Skin Integrity related to incomplete joining of lip/palate ridges

Impaired Verbal Communication related to inadequate palate function and possible hearing loss from infected eustachian tubes

Ineffective Airway Clearance related to common feeding/breathing passage; postoperative laryngeal or incisional edema

Ineffective Infant Feeding Pattern related to cleft lip/cleft palate

Ineffective Breastfeeding related to infant anomaly

Pain related to surgical correction and elbow restraints

Clotting disorder

Altered Protection related to clotting disorder

Anxiety/Fear related to threat to well-being

High Risk for Fluid Volume Deficit related to uncontrolled bleeding

Knowledge Deficit related to treatment of disease

Refer to Hemophilia, Anticoagulant Therapy, DIC

Cocaine abuse

Altered Thought Processes related to excessive stimulation of nervous system by cocaine

Ineffective Breathing Pattern related to drug effect on respiratory center

Ineffective Individual Coping related to inability to deal with life stresses

Co-dependency

Caregiver Role Strain related to codependency

Decisional Conflict related to support system deficit

Denial related to unmet self-needs

Impaired Verbal Communication related to psychological barriers

Ineffective Individual Coping related to inadequate support systems

Powerlessness related to lifestyle of helplessness

Cognitive deficit

Altered Thought Processes related to neurological impairment

Colectomy

Altered Nutrition: Less than Body Requirements related to high metabolic needs; decreased ability to ingest/digest food

Constipation related to decreased activity; decreased fluid intake

High Risk for Infection related to invasive procedure

Knowledge Deficit related to limited exposure to information

Pain related to recent surgery

Refer to abdominal surgery

Colitis

Diarrhea related to inflammation in colon

Pain related to inflammation in colon

Refer to Ulcerative Colitis, Crohn's Disease, or Inflammatory Bowel Disease

Colostomy

Body Image Disturbance related to presence of stoma; daily care of fecal material

High Risk for Altered Sexuality Pattern related to altered body image, self concept

High Risk for Constipation/Diarrhea related to inappropriate diet

High Risk for Impaired Skin Integrity related to irritation from bowel contents

High Risk for Social Isolation related to anxiety over appearance of stoma and possible leakage

Knowledge Deficit related to self-care, treatment needs

Coma

Altered Family Processes related to illness/disability of family member

Altered Thought Processes related to neurophysiological changes

High Risk for Altered Oral Mucous Membranes related to dry mouth

High Risk for Aspiration related to impaired swallowing, loss of cough/gag reflex

High Risk for Disuse Syndrome related to altered level of consciousness impairing mobility

High Risk for Impaired Skin Integrity related to immobility

High Risk for Injury related to potential seizure activity

Self-Care Deficit: Specify related to neuromuscular impairment

Total Incontinence related to neurological dysfunction

Refer to the cause of client's comatose state

Communicable diseases, childhood (measles, mumps, rubella, chicken pox, scabies, lice, impetigo)

Altered Comfort related to Hyperthermia secondary to infectious disease process

Altered Comfort related to pruritus secondary to skin rash or subdermal organisms

Altered Health Maintenance related to nonadherence with appropriate immunization schedules; lack of prevention of transmission of infection

Diversional Activity Deficit related to imposed isolation from peers; disruption in usual play activities; fatigue/activity intolerance

High Risk for Infection: Transmission to Others related to contagious organisms

Knowledge Deficit: Potential for Enhanced Health Maintenance related to knowledge acquisition regarding appropriate, preventive health practices

Pain related to impaired skin integrity, edema

Refer to Respiratory Infections, Acute Childhood; Meningitis/Encephalitis; Reye Syndrome

Congenital heart disease/cardiac anomalies

Acyanotic: Patent ductus arteriosus (PDA); Atrial/Ventricular septal defect (ASD/VSD); Pulmonary Stenosis; Endocardial Cushion Defect; Aortic Valvular Stenosis; Coarctation of the Aorta

Cyanotic: Tetralogy of Fallot; Tricuspid Atresia; Transposition of the Great Vessels; Truncus Arteriosus; Total Anomalous Pulmonary Venous Return (TAPVR); Hypoplastic Left Lung

Activity Intolerance related to fatigue; generalized weakness; lack of adequate oxygenation

Altered Family Processes related to to ill child

Altered Growth and Development related to inadequate oxygen and nutrients to tissues

Altered Nutrition: Less than Body Requirements related to fatigue, generalized weakness; inability of infant to suck and feed; increased caloric requirements

Decreased Cardiac Output related to cardiac dysfunction

Fluid Volume Excess related to cardiac defect, side effects of medication

High Risk for Fluid Volume Deficit related to side effects of diuretics

High Risk for Ineffective Thermoregulation related to neonatal age

High Risk for Poisoning related to potential toxicity of cardiac medications

Impaired Gas Exchange related to cardiac defect; pulmonary congestion

Ineffective Breathing Patterns related to pulmonary vascular disease

Refer to Hospitalized Child; Child With Chronic Illness

Congestive heart failure

Activity Intolerance related to weakness, fatigue

Constipation related to activity intolerance

Decreased Cardiac Output related to impaired cardiac function

Fatigue related to disease process

Fear related to threat to well-being

Conjunctivitis

High Risk for Injury related to change in visual acuity

Pain related to inflammatory process

Sensory/Perceptual Alteration related to change in visual acuity from inflammation

Constipation

Constipation related to decreased fluid intake; decreased intake of foods containing bulk; inactivity, immobility; knowledge deficit of appropriate bowel routine; lack of privacy for defecation

Conversion reaction

Altered Role Performance related to physical conversion symptom

Anxiety related to unresolved conflict

High Risk for Injury related to physical conversion symptom

Hopelessness related to long-term stress

Impaired Physical Mobility related to physical conversion symptom

Impaired Social Interaction related to altered thought process

Ineffective Individual Coping related to personal vulnerability

Powerlessness related to lifestyle of helplessness

Self-Esteem Disturbance related to unsatisfactory or inadequate interpersonal relationships

Convulsions

Anxiety related to concern over controlling convulsions

High Risk for Altered Thought Processes related to seizure activity

High Risk for Aspiration related to impaired swallowing

High Risk for Injury related to seizure activity

Knowledge Deficit related to need for medication and care during seizure activity

Refer to Seizure Disorders, Childhood

COPD

Activity Intolerance related to imbalance between oxygen supply and demand

Altered Family Process related to role changes

Altered Nutrition: Less than Body Requirements related to decreased intake because of dyspnea, unpleasant taste in mouth left by medications

Anxiety related to breathlessness, change in health status

Chronic Low Self-Esteem related to chronic illness

High Risk for Infection related to stasis of respiratory secretions

Impaired Gas Exchange related to ventilation-perfusion inequality

Impaired Social Interaction related to social isolation secondary to oxygen use, activity intolerance

Ineffective Airway Clearance related to bronchoconstriction; increased mucous, ineffective cough, and infection

Knowledge Deficit related to lack of information/motivation

Noncompliance related to reluctance to accept responsibility for changing detrimental health practices

Powerlessness related to progressive nature of the disease

Self-Care Deficit: Specify related to fatigue secondary to increased work of breathing

Sleep Pattern Disturbance related to dyspnea; side effect of medications

Coronary artery bypass grafting

Decreased Cardiac Output related to dysrhythmias, depressed cardiac function; increased systemic vascular resistance

Fear related to outcome of surgical procedure

Fluid Volume Deficit related to intraoperative fluid loss; use of diuretics in surgery

Knowledge Deficit related to lifestyle adjustment after surgery

Pain related to traumatic surgery

Crack baby

Altered Growth and Development related to effects of maternal use of drugs; neurological impairment; decreased attentiveness to environmental stimuli

Altered Nutrition: Less than Body Requirements related to feeding problems; uncoordinated/ineffective suck and swallow; effects of diarrhea, vomiting, colic

Altered Parenting related to impaired or lack of attachment behaviors; inadequate support systems

Altered Protection related to effects of maternal substance abuse

Diarrhea related to effects of withdrawal; increased peristalsis secondary to hyperirritability

High Risk for Infection (Skin, Meningeal, Respiratory) related to effects of withdrawal

Ineffective Airway Clearance related to pooling of secretions secondary to lack of adequate cough reflex

Ineffective Infant Feeding related to prematurity; neurological impairment

Sensory-Perceptual Alteration related to hypersensitivity to environmental stimuli

Sleep Pattern Disturbance related to hyperirritability, hypersensitivity to environmental stimuli

Craniectomy/craniotomy

Altered Tissue perfusion: Cerebral related to cerebral edema; decreased cerebral perfusion; increased intracranial pressure

Fear related to threat to well-being

High Risk for Altered Thought Processes related to neurophysiological changes

High Risk for Injury related to potential confusion

Pain related to recent surgery, headache

Refer to Coma, if relevant

Crohn's disease

Altered Nutrition: Less than Body Requirements related to diarrhea; altered ability to digest and absorb food

Anxiety related to change in health status

Diarrhea related to inflammatory process

High Risk for Fluid Volume Deficit related to abnormal fluid loss with diarrhea

Ineffective Individual Coping related to repeated episodes of diarrhea

Knowledge Deficit related to management of the disease

Pain related to increased peristalsis

Powerlessness related to chronic disease

Croup

Refer to Respiratory Infections, Acute Childhood

Cushing's syndrome

Activity intolerance related to fatigue, weakness

Body Image Disturbance related to change in appearance from disease process

Fluid Volume Excess related to failure of regulatory mechanisms

High Risk for Infection related to suppression of the immune system secondary to increased coritisol

High Risk for Injury related to decreased muscle strength, osteoporosis

Knowledge Deficit related to treatment of the disease

Sexual Dysfunction related to loss of libido

CVA (cerebrovascular accident)

Altered Family Process related to illness, disability of family member

Altered Thought Processes related to neurophysiological changes

Anxiety related to situational crisis; change in physical/emotional condition

Body Image Disturbance related to chronic illness, paralysis

Constipation related to decreased activity

Dysfunctional Grieving related to loss of health

High Risk for Caregiver Role Strain related to cognitive problems of care receiver; need for significant home care

High Risk for Disuse Syndrome related to paralysis

High Risk for Aspiration related to impaired swallowing, loss of gag reflex

High Risk for Injury related to sensory-perceptual alteration

High Risk for Impaired Skin Integrity related to immobility

High Risk for Unilateral Neglect related to disturbed perception from loss of half of the visual field, loss of sensation on affected side

Impaired Physical Mobility related to loss of balance and coordination

Impaired Social Interaction related to limited physical mobility, limited ability to communicate

Impaired Swallowing related to neuromuscular dysfunction

Impaired Verbal Communication related to pressure damage/decreased circulation to the speech center of the brain

Ineffective Individual Coping related to disability

Knowledge Deficit related to lack of informational sources

Reflex Incontinence related to loss of feeling to void

Self-Care Deficit related to decreased strength and endurance; paralysis

Sensory/Perceptual Alteration: Visual, Tactile, Kinesthetic related to neurological deficit

Total Incontinence related to neurological dysfunction

Cystic fibrosis

Activity Intolerance related to imbalance between oxygen supply and demand

Altered Nutrition: Less than Body Requirements related to anorexia; decreased absorption of nutrients/fat; increased work of breathing

Anxiety related to dyspnea and oxygen deprivation

Body Image Disturbance related to changes in physical appearance and treatment of chronic lung disease (clubbing, barrel chest, home oxygen therapy)

High Risk for Caregiver Role Strain related to illness severity of the care receiver; unpredictable illness course

High Risk for Fluid Volume Deficit related to decreased fluid intake and increased work of breathing

High Risk for Infection related to thick, tenacious mucous; harboring bacterial organisms; debilitated state

Impaired Gas Exchange related to ventilation perfusion imbalance

Impaired Home Maintenance Management related to extensive daily treatment, medications necessary for health, mist/oxygen tents

Ineffective Airway Clearance related to increased production of thick mucus

Refer to Hospitalized Child; Child With Chronic Condition; Terminally Ill Child/Death of Child

Cystitis

Altered Urinary Elimination: Frequency related to urinary tract infection

Knowledge Deficit related to methods to treat and prevent UTIs

Pain: Dysuria related to inflammatory process in bladder

Cystoscopy

High Risk for Infection related to invasive procedure

Knowledge Deficit related to post-operative care

Urinary Retention related to edema in urethra obstructing flow of urine

Deafness

Sensory Perceptual Alteration: Auditory related to alteration in sensory reception, transmission, or integration

Dehiscence, abdominal

Fear related to threat of death, severe dysfunction

High Risk for Infection related to loss of skin integrity

Impaired Skin Integrity related to altered circulation; malnutrition; opening in incision

Impaired Tissue Integrity related to exposure of abdominal contents to external environment

Pain related to stretching of abdominal wall

Dehydration

Altered Oral Mucous Membranes related to decreased salivation and fluid deficit

Fluid Volume Deficit related to active fluid volume loss

Knowledge Deficit related to treatment and prevention of dehydration

Dementia

Altered Family Process related to disability of family member

Altered Nutrition: Less than Body Requirements related to psychological impairment

Altered Thought Processes related to organic mental disorder

High Risk for Caregiver Role Strain related to amount of caregiving tasks; duration of caregiving required

High Risk for Injury related to confusion, decreased muscle coordination

High Risk for Impaired Skin Integrity related to altered nutritional status, immobility

Impaired Home Maintenance Management related to inadequate support system

Impaired Physical Mobility related to neuromuscular impairment

Self-Care Deficit: Specify related to psychological/neuromuscular impairment

Sleep Pattern Disturbance related to neurological impairment; naps during the day

Total Incontinence related to neuromuscular impairment

Depression, major

Altered Health Maintenance related to lack of ability to make good judgments regarding ways to obtain help

Chronic Low Self-Esteem related to repeated unmet expectations

Colonic Constipation related to inactivity; decreased fluid intake

Dysfunctional Grieving related to lack of previous resolution of former grieving response

Fatigue related to psychological demands

High Risk for Violence: Self-Directed related to panic state

Hopelessness related to feeling of abandonment; long-term stress

Ineffective Individual Coping related to dysfunctional grieving

Knowledge Deficit related to lack of motivation to learn new coping skills

Powerlessness related to pattern of helplessness

Self Care Deficit: Specify related to depression; cognitive impairment

Sexual Dysfunction related to loss of sexual desire

Sleep Pattern Disturbance related to inactivity

Social Isolation related to ineffective coping

Dermatitis

Altered Comfort: Pruritus related to inflammation of skin

Anxiety related to situational crisis imposed by illness

Knowledge Deficit related to methods to decrease inflammation

Impaired Skin Integrity related to side effect of medication; allergic reaction

Diabetes mellitus

Altered Nutrition: Less than Body Requirements related to inability to utilize glucose (Type I Diabetes)

Altered Nutrition: More than Body Requirements related to excessive intake of nutrients (Type II Diabetes)

Altered Tissue Perfusion: Peripheral related to impaired arterial circulation

High Risk for Altered Thought Processes related to hypoglycemia/hyperglycemia

High Risk for Infection related to hyperglycemia, impaired healing, circulatory changes

High Risk for Injury:

Hypoglycemia/Hyperglycemia related to failure to consume adequate calories or failure to take insulin

High Risk for Impaired Skin Integrity related to loss of pain perception in extremities

Ineffective Management of Therapeutic Regimen related to complexity of therapeutic regimen

Knowledge Deficit related to limited exposure to information

Noncompliance related to restrictive lifestyle; changes in diet, medication, and exercise

Powerlessness related to perceived lack of personal control

Sexual Dysfunction related to neuropathy associated with disease

Diabetes mellitus, juvenile (IDDM Type I)

Altered Health Management related to parental/child knowledge deficit regarding dietary management, medication administration, physical activity, and interaction between the three; daily changes in diet, medication, and activity related to child growth spurts and needs; related to need to instruct other caregivers and teachers regarding signs and symptoms of hyperglycemia/hypoglycemia and treatment

Altered Nutrition: Less than Body Requirements related to inability of body to adequately metabolize and utilize glucose and nutrients; increased caloric needs of child to promote growth; physical activity participation with peers

Body Image Disturbance related to to imposed deviations from biophysical and psychosocial norm; perceived differences from peers

High Risk for Noncompliance related to body image disturbance; impaired adjustment secondary to adolescent maturational crises

Impaired Adjustment related to inability to participate in normal childhood activities

Pain related to insulin injections; peripheral blood glucose testing

Refer to Diabetes Mellitus; Child With Chronic Illness; Hospitalized Child

Diarrhea

Diarrhea related to infection; change in diet/food; gastrointestinal disorders; stress; medication effect; impaction

DIC (disseminated intravascular coagulation)

Fear related to threat to well-being

Fluid Volume Deficit: Hemorrhage related to depletion of clotting factors

High Risk for Altered Tissue Perfusion: Peripheral related to hypovolemia from profuse bleeding; formation of microemboli in vascular system

D & C (dilatation and curretage)

High Risk for Altered Sexuality Patterns related to painful coitus; fear associated with surgery on genital area

High Risk for Fluid Volume Deficit: Hemorrhage related to excessive blood loss during or after the procedure

High Risk for Infection related to surgical procedure

Knowledge Deficit related to postoperative self-care

Pain related to uterine contractions

Digitalis toxicity

Decreased Cardiac Output related to drug toxicity affecting cardiac rhythm, rate

Knowledge Deficit related to action of medication, need for potassium, side effects of digitalis

Discomforts of pregnancy

Alteration in Comfort related to pityalism secondary to increased estrogen; nausea secondary to hormonal changes; shortness of breath secondary to limited diaphragm expansion; nasal stuffiness secondary to increased vascularization; leukorrhea secondary to hormone stimulation, abdominal distention secondary to enlarging uterus; pruritus secondary to increased excretory function of skin and stretching of skin; urinary frequency secondary to vascular engorgement and altered bladder function; reduced bladder capacity reduced by enlarging uterus and fetal presenting part

Body Image Disturbance related to physiological edema; pityalism; body shape changes secondary to enlarging uterus and breasts; spider nevi; palmar erythema; varicose veins; striae gravidarum, chloasma, acne

Constipation related to decreased GI tract motility; compression of intestines secondary to enlarging uterus; supplementary iron; hemorrhoids

Fatigue related to increased levels of hormones; elevated basal body temperature; sleep pattern disturbance

High Risk for Injury related to faintness or syncope secondary to vasomotor lability or postural hypotension; venous stasis in lower extremities

Pain: Indigestion-Heart Burn related to decreased GI tract motility; reverse peristalsis; relaxed cardiac sphincter; Braxton Hicks' contractions; Hemorrhoids related to constipation, enlarging uterus and pelvic venous stasis, bearing down for bowel movement, decreased GI motility; *Joint and Backache* related to relaxation of symphyses and sacroiliac joints secondary to hormones, exaggerated lumbar and cervicothoracic curves secondary to change in center of gravity from enlarging abdomen; *Leg Cramps* related to compression of nerves supplying lower extremities by gravid uterus, reduced level of diffusible calcium or elevation of serum phosphorus; *Headache* related to vascular engorgement and congestion of sinuses from hormone stimulation

Sleep Pattern Disturbance related to fetal movement; muscular cramping; urinary frequency; shortness of breath

Stress Incontinence related to high intraabdominal pressure secondary to gravid uterus, fetal movement

Dissociative disorder

Alteration in Thought Processes related to repressed anxiety

Anxiety related to psychosocial stress

Disturbance in Self-Concept related to childhood trauma; childhood abuse

Ineffective Individual Coping related to personal vulnerability in crisis of accurate self-perception

Personal Identify Disturbance related to inability to distinguish self caused by multiple personality disorder, depersonalization or disturbance in memory

Sensory/Perceptual Alteration: Kinesthetic related to underdeveloped ego

Diverticulitis

Altered Nutrition: Less than Body Requirements related to loss of appetite

Constipation related to dietary deficiency of fiber and roughage

Diarrhea related to increased intestinal motility secondary to inflammation

High Risk for Fluid Volume Deficit related to diarrhea

Knowledge Deficit related to diet needed to control disease, medication regime

Pain related to inflammation of bowel

Drug abuse

Altered Nutrition: Less than Body Requirements related to poor eating habits

Anxiety related to threat to self concept; lack of control of drug use

Ineffective Individual Coping related to situational crisis

High Risk for Injury related to hallucinations, drug effects

High Risk for Violence related to poor impulse control

Noncompliance related to denial of illness

Sensory/Perceptual Alterations: Specify related to substance intoxication

Sleep Pattern Disturbance related to effects of drugs or medications

Drug withdrawal

Altered Nutrition: Less than Body Requirements related to poor eating habits

Anxiety related to physiological withdrawal

Ineffective Individual Coping related to situational crisis, withdrawal

High Risk for Injury related to hallucinations

High Risk for Violence related to poor impulse control

Noncompliance related to denial of illness

Sensory/Perceptual Alterations: Specify related to substance intoxication

Sleep Pattern Disturbance related to effects of drugs or medications

DVT (deep vein thrombosis)

Altered Tissue Perfusion: Peripheral related to interruption of venous blood flow

Colonic Constipation related to inactivity; bedrest

Impaired Physical Mobility related to pain in extremity; forced bedrest

Knowledge Deficit related to self-care needs; treatment regimen, outcome

Pain related to vascular inflammation; edema

Refer to Anticoagulant Therapy

Dyspareunia

Sexual Dysfunction related to lack of lubrication during intercourse; alteration in reproductive organ function

Dysreflexia

Dysreflexia related to bladder distention; bowel distention; noxious stimuli

Dysrhythmia

Activity Intolerance related to decreased cardiac output

Altered Tissue Perfusion: Cerebral related to interruption of cerebral arterial flow secondary to decreased cardiac output

Anxiety/Fear related to threat of death; change in health status

Decreased Cardiac Output related to altered electrical conduction

Knowledge Deficit related to unfamiliarity with information resources

Dysthmia

Altered Health Maintenance related to lack of ability to make good judgments regarding ways to obtain help

Altered Sexual Pattern related to loss of sexual desire chronic

Chronic Low Self-Esteem related to repeated unmet expectations

Ineffective Individual Coping related to impaired social interaction

Knowledge Deficit related to lack of motivation to learn new coping skills

Sleep Pattern Disturbance related to anxious thoughts

Social Isolation related to ineffective coping

Ear surgery

High Risk for Injury related to dizziness from excessive stimuli to vestibular apparatus

Knowledge Deficit related to postoperative care

Pain related to edema in ears from surgery

Sensory/Perceptual Alteration: Auditory related to invasive surgery of ears; dressings

Refer to Hospitalized Child

Eclampsia

Altered Family Processes related to unmet expectations for pregnancy/childbirth

Fear related to threat of well-being to self and fetus

High Risk for Altered Fetal Tissue Perfusion related to uteroplacental insufficiency

High Risk for Aspiration related to seizure activity

High Risk for Fluid Volume Excess related to decreased urine output secondary to renal dysfunction

High Risk for Injury: Maternal related to seizure activity

High Risk for Injury: Fetal related to hypoxia

Ectopic pregnancy

Altered Role Performance related to loss of pregnancy

Body Image Disturbance related to negative feelings about the body and reproductive functioning

Fear related to threat to self, surgery, implications for future pregnancy

Fluid Volume Deficit related to loss of blood

High Risk for Altered Family Processes related to situational crisis

High Risk for Infection related to traumatized tissue and blood loss

High Risk for Ineffective Individual Coping related to loss of pregnancy

High Risk for Spiritual Distress related to grief process

Pain related to stretching or rupture of implantation site

Situational Low Self-Esteem related to loss of pregnancy and inability to carry pregnancy to term

Eczema

Body Image Disturbance related to change in appearance from inflamed skin

Knowledge Deficit related to methods to decrease inflammation

Impaired Skin Integrity related to side-effect of medication, allergic reaction

Pain: Pruritus related to inflammation of skin

Emphysema

Activity Intolerance related to imbalance between oxygen supply and demand

Altered Family Process related to role changes

Altered Nutrition: Less than Body Requirements related to decreased intake because of dyspnea, unpleasant taste in mouth left by medications

Anxiety related to breathlessness, change in health status

Chronic Low Self-Esteem related to chronic illness

High Risk for Infection related to stasis of respiratory secretions

Endocarditis

Altered Tissue Perfusion:

Cardiopulmonary/Peripheral related to high risk for development of emboli

High Risk for Activity Intolerance related to reduced cardiac reserve and prescribed bedrest

High Risk for Alteration in Nutrition: Less than Body Requirements related to fever, hypermetabolic state associated with fever

High Risk for Decreased Cardiac Output related to inflammation of lining of heart and change in structure in valve leaflets, increased myocardial workload

High Risk for Impaired Gas Exchange related to high risk for congestive heart failure

Knowledge Deficit related to preventive measures against initial and recurring attacks of rheumatic fever

Pain related to biological injury and inflammation

Endometriosis
Anticipatory Grieving related to possible infertility
Knowledge Deficit related to disease condition, medications and other treatments
Pain related to onset of menses with distention of endometrial tissue
Sexual Dysfunction related to painful coitus

Endometritis
Anxiety related to prolonged hospitalization and fear of the unknown
Hyperthermia related to infectious process
Knowledge Deficit related to limited experience with condition, treatment, and antibiotic regime
Pain related to infectious process in reproductive tract

Epididymitis
Altered Pattern of Sexuality related to edema of epididymis and testes
Anxiety related to situational crisis, pain, threat to future fertility
Knowledge Deficit related to treatment for pain and infection
Pain related to inflammation in scrotal sac

Epiglotitis
Refer to Respiratory Infections, Acute Childhood

Epilepsy
Anxiety related to threat to role functioning
High Risk for Altered Thought Processes related to excessive, uncontrolled neurological stimuli
High Risk for Aspiration related to impaired swallowing, excessive secretions
High Risk for Injury related to environmental factors during seizure
Knowledge Deficit related to seizures and seizure control
Refer to Seizure Disorders, Childhood

Episiotomy
Anxiety related to fear of pain
Body Image Disturbance related to fear of resuming sexual relations
High Risk for Infection related to tissue trauma
Impaired Physical Mobility related to pain, swelling, and tissue trauma
Impaired Skin Integrity related to perineal incision
Pain related to tissue trauma
Sexual Dysfunction related to altered body structure and tissue trauma

Epistaxis
Fear related to large amount of blood loss
High Risk for Fluid Volume Deficit related to excessive fluid loss

Esophageal varices
Fear related to threat of death
Fluid Volume Deficit: Hemorrhage related to portal hypertension, distended variceal vessels that can easily rupture
Refer to Cirrhosis

Eye surgery
Anxiety related to possible loss of vision
High Risk for Injury related to impaired vision
Knowledge Deficit related to postoperative activity, medication and eye care
Self-Care Deficit related to impaired vision
Sensory/Perceptual Alteration: Visual related to surgical procedure
Refer to Hospitalized Child

Failure to thrive, non-organic
Altered Growth and Development related to parental knowledge deficit; lack of stimulation; nutritional deficit; long-term hospitalization
Altered Nutrition: Less than Body Requirements related to inadequate type/amounts of food for infant; inappropriate feeding techniques
Altered Parenting related to lack of parenting skills, inadequate role modeling
Chronic Low Self-Esteem: Parental related to feelings of inadequacy; support system deficiencies; inadequate role model
Sleep Pattern Disturbance related to inconsistency of caretaker; lack of quiet environment
Social Isolation related to limited support systems; self-imposed situation

Femoral popliteal bypass
Anxiety related to threat to or change in health status
High Risk for Altered Tissue Perfusion: Peripheral related to impaired arterial circulation
High Risk for Fluid Volume Deficit: Hemorrhage related to abnormal blood loss
High Risk for Infection related to invasive procedure
High Risk for Neurovascular Dysfunction related to vascular surgery, emboli
Pain related to surgical trauma and edema in surgical area

Fetal alcohol syndrome
Refer to Infant of Substance Abusing Mother

Fetal distress/nonreassuring fetal heart rate pattern
Altered Tissue Perfusion: Fetal related to interruption of umbilical cord blood flow
Altered Tissue Perfusion: Placental related to small or old placenta; interference with gas exchange transplacentally
Fear related to threat to fetus

Fractures
Diversional Activity Deficit related to immobility
High Risk for Altered Tissue Perfusion related to immobility, presence of cast
High Risk for Impaired Skin Integrity related to immobility, presence of cast
High Risk for Peripheral Neurovascular Impairment related to mechanical compression; treatment of fracture
Impaired Physical Mobility related to limb immobilization
Knowledge Deficit related to care of cast
Pain related to muscle spasm, edema and trauma

Frostbite
Impaired Skin Integrity related to freezing of skin
Pain related to decreased circulation from prolonged exposure to cold
Refer to Hypothermia

Fusion, lumbar
Anxiety related to fear of surgical procedure and possible recurring problems
High Risk for Injury related to improper body mechanics
Impaired Physical Mobility related to limitations related to the surgical procedure; presence of brace
Knowledge Deficit related to postoperative mobility restrictions, body mechanics
Pain related to discomfort at bone donor site

Gallstones
Refer to Cholelithiasis

Gangrene
Altered Tissue Perfusion: Peripheral related to obstruction of arterial flow
Fear related to possible loss of extremity

Gastroenteritis
Altered Nutrition: Less than Body Requirements related to vomiting; inadequate intestinal absorption of nutrients; restricted dietary regimen intake
Diarrhea related to infectious process involving intestinal tract
Fluid Volume Deficit related to excessive loss from gastrointestinal tract secondary to diarrhea, vomiting
Pain related to increased peristalsis causing cramping
Refer to Gastroenteritis—Child

Gastroenteritis—Child
Altered Health maintenance related to lack of parental knowledge regarding fluid and dietary changes
Impaired Skin Integrity (diaper rash) related to acidic excretions on perineal tissues
Refer to Gastroenteritis; Hospitalized Child

Gastroesophageal reflux
Altered Nutrition: Less than Body Requirements related to poor feeding and vomiting
Anxiety/Fear, Parental related to possible need for surgical intervention (Nissen fundoplication/gastrostomy tube)

Fluid Volume Deficit related to persistent vomiting

High Risk for Altered Parenting related to disruption in bonding secondary to irritable, inconsolable infant

High Risk for Aspiration related to entry of gastric contents in tracheal/bronchial tree

Ineffective Airway Clearance related to reflux of gastric contents into esophagus and tracheal/bronchial tree

Knowledge Deficit: Potential for Enhanced Health Maintenance related to knowledge/skill acquisition regarding anti-reflux regime, e.g., positioning, oral/enteral feeding techniques, medications; possible home apnea monitoring

Pain related to irritation of esophagus from gastric acids

Refer to Hospitalized Child; Child With Chronic Condition

Gastroschisis/omphalocele

Altered Bowel Elimination Pattern related to effects of congenital herniated abdominal contents

Anticipatory Grieving related to threatened loss of infant, loss of "perfect birth/infant" secondary to serious medical condition

High Risk for Fluid Volume Deficit related to inability to feed secondary to condition and subsequent electrolyte imbalance

High Risk for Infection related to disrupted skin integrity with exposure of abdominal contents

High Risk for Injury related to disrupted skin integrity and altered protection

Impaired Gas Exchange related to effects of anesthesia and subsequent atelectasis

Ineffective Airway Clearance related to complications of anesthesia effects

Refer to Hospitalized Child; Premature Infant

Gestational diabetes (diabetes in pregnancy)

Altered Maternal Nutrition: Less than Body Requirements related to decreased insulin production and glucose uptake into cells

Altered Fetal Nutrition: More than Body Requirements related to excessive glucose uptake

Anxiety related to threat to self or fetus

High Risk for Fetal Injury related to macrosomia; congenital defects; maternal hypoglycemic or hyperglycemic incidents

High Risk for Maternal Injury related to delivery of large infant; hypoglycemic or hyperglycemia incidents

Knowledge Deficit related to maternal learning needs about diabetes in pregnancy

Powerlessness related to lack of control over outcome of pregnancy

Gastrointestinal bleed

Altered Nutrition: Less than Body Requirements related to nausea, vomiting

Fatigue related to loss of circulating blood volume, decreased ability to transport oxygen

Fear related to threat to well-being, potential death

Fluid Volume Deficit related to gastrointestinal bleeding

High Risk for Ineffective Individual Coping related to personal vulnerability in a crisis, bleeding and hospitalization

Pain related to irritated mucosa from acid secretion

Gingivitis

Altered Oral Mucous Membranes related to ineffective oral hygiene

Glaucoma

Sensory/Perceptual Alteration: Visual related to increased intraocular pressure

Glomerulonephritis

Altered Nutrition: Less than Body Requirements related to anorexia, restrictive diet

Fluid Volume Excess related to renal impairment

Knowledge Deficit related to treatment of disease

Pain related to edema of kidney

Head injury

Refer to Intracranial Pressure, Increased

Headache

Pain: Headache related to lack of knowledge of pain control techniques or methods to prevent headaches

Hearing impairment

Impaired Verbal Communication related to inability to hear own voice

Sensory/Perceptual Alteration: Auditory related to altered state of auditory system

Social Isolation related to difficulty with communication

Heartburn

High Risk for Altered Nutrition: Less than Body Requirements related to pain after eating

Knowledge Deficit related to information about factors that cause esophageal reflex

Pain: Heartburn related to gastroesophageal reflux

Hemiplegia

Anxiety related to change in health status

Body Image Disturbance related to functional loss of one side of the body

High Risk for Impaired Skin Integrity related to alteration in sensation, immobility

High Risk for Injury related to impaired mobility

Impaired Physical Mobility related to loss of neurological control of involved extremities

Self-Care Deficit: Specify related to neuromuscular impairment

Unilateral Neglect related to neurological impairment, loss of sensation, vision, or movement

Refer to CVA

Hemodialysis

Altered Family Processes related to changes in role responsibilities due to therapy regimen

Caregiver Role Strain related to complexity of care receiver treatment

High Risk for Fluid Volume Deficit related to excessive removal of fluid during dialysis

High Risk for Infection related to exposure to blood products and risk for developing hepatitis B/C

High Risk for Injury: Clotting of Blood Access related to abnormal surface for blood flow

Ineffective Individual Coping related to situational crisis

Knowledge Deficit related to hemodialysis procedure, restrictions, blood access care

Noncompliance: Dietary Restrictions related to denial of chronic illness

Powerlessness related to treatment regimen

Refer to Renal Failure, Oliguric; Renal Failure—Acute/Chronic, Childhood

Hemodynamic monitoring

High Risk for Infection related to invasive procedure

High Risk for Injury related to inadvertent wedging of catheter; dislodgement of catheter; disconnections of catheter; embolism

Hemolytic uremic syndrome

Altered Comfort: Nausea/Vomiting related to effects of uremia

Fluid Volume Deficit related to vomiting and diarrhea

High Risk for Impaired Skin Integrity related to diarrhea

High Risk for Injury related to decreased platelet count, seizure activity

Refer to Renal Failure, Acute/Chronic, Child; Hospitalized Child

Hemophilia

Altered Protection related to deficient clotting factors

Fear related to high risk for AIDS secondary to contaminated blood products

High Risk for Injury related to deficient clotting factors and child's developmental level; age-appropriate play; inappropriate use of toys, sports equipment

Impaired Physical Mobility related to pain from acute bleeds and imposed activity restrictions

Pain related to bleeding into body tissues

Potential for Enhanced Health Maintenance related to knowledge/skill acquisition regarding home administration of IV clotting factors, protection from injury

Refer to Hospitalized Child; Child With Chronic Condition; Maturational Issues, Adolescence

Hemorrhage

Fear related to threat to well-being

Fluid Volume Deficit related to massive blood loss

Refer to cause of Hemorrhage; Hypovolemic Shock

Hemorrhoidectomy

Anxiety related to embarrassment, need for privacy

Colonic Constipation related to fear of defecation

High Risk for Fluid Volume Deficit: Hemorrhage related to surgical wound

High Risk for Urinary Retention related to pain, anesthesia effect

Knowledge Deficit related to pain relief, use of stool softeners, dietary changes

Pain related to surgical procedure

Hemorrhoids

Constipation related to painful defecation, poor bowel habits

Knowledge Deficit related to lack of information sources

Pain: Pruritus related to inflammation of hemorrhoids

Hepatitis

Activity Intolerance related to weakness or fatigue secondary to infection

Altered Nutrition: Less than Body Requirements related to anorexia, impaired utilization of proteins and carbohydrates

Diversional Activity Deficit related to isolation

Fatigue related to infectious process, altered body chemistry

High Risk for Fluid Volume Deficit related to excessive loss of fluids via vomiting and diarrhea

Knowledge Deficit related to disease process and home management

Pain related to edema of liver, bile irritating skin

Social Isolation related to treatment-imposed isolation

Herniorrhapy

Refer to Inguinal Hernia Repair

Herpes simplex I

Altered Oral Mucous Membranes related to inflammatory changes in mouth

herpes simplex II

Altered Urinary Elimination related to pain with urination

Impaired Tissue Integrity related to active herpes lesion

Knowledge Deficit related to lack of exposure to situation

Pain related to active herpes lesion

Situational Low Self-Esteem related to expressions of shame guilt

Hiatal hernia

High Risk for Altered Nutrition: Less than Body Requirements related to pain after eating

Knowledge Deficit related to information about factors that cause esophageal reflex

Pain: Heartburn related to gastroesophageal reflux

Hip fracture

Colonic Constipation related to immobility, narcotics. anesthesia

Fear related to outcome of treatment, future mobility, and present helplessness

High Risk for Altered Thought Processes related to change in environment, stress of surgery, sensory deprivation

High Risk for Fluid Volume Deficit Hemorrhage related to postoperative complication, surgical blood loss

High Risk for Impaired Skin Integrity related to immobility

High Risk for Infection related to invasive procedure

High Risk for Injury related to dislodged prosthesis; unsteadiness when ambulating

Impaired Physical Mobility related to surgical incision and temporary absence of weight bearing

Pain related to injury, surgical procedure

Powerlessness related to health care environment

Self-Care Deficit: Specify related to musculoskeletal impairment

Hirschsprung's disease

Altered Health Maintenance related to parental knowledge deficit regarding temporary stoma care, dietary management, treatment for constipation/diarrhea

Altered Nutrition: Less than Body Requirements related to anorexia; pain from distended colon

Constipation (bowel obstruction) related to inhibited peristalsis secondary to congenital absence of parasympathetic ganglion cells in the distal colon

Grieving related to to loss of perfect child, birth of child with congenital defect, even though child expected to be normal within 2 years

Impaired Skin Integrity related to stoma; potential skin care problems associated with stoma

Pain related to distended colon; incisional pain postoperative

Refer to Hospitalized Child

HIV (human immunodeficiency virus)

Altered Protection related to depressed immune system

Fear related to possible death

Refer to AIDS

Hodgkin's disease

Refer to Cancer and Anemia

Hospitalized child

Activity Intolerance related to fatigue associated with acute illness

Altered Family Processes related to situational crisis of illness/disease and hospitalization

Altered Growth and Development related to regression or lack of progression toward developmental milestones secondary to frequent/prolonged hospitalization; inadequate/inappropriate stimulation; cerebral insult; chronic illness; effects of physical disability; prescribed dependence

Anxiety: Separation (child) related to familiar surroundings and separation from family/friends

Diversional Activity Deficit related to immobility; monotonous environment; frequent/lengthy treatments; reluctance to participate; therapeutic isolation; separation from peers

Family Coping: Potential for Growth related to impact of crisis on family values. priorities, goals, or relationships in family

Fear related to knowledge deficit or maturational level with fear of unknown, mutilation, painful procedures, surgery

High Risk for Altered Growth and Development: Regression related to disruption of normal routine, unfamiliar environment/caregivers; developmental vulnerability of young children

High Risk for Altered Nutrition: Less than Body Requirements related to anorexia; absence of familiar foods; cultural preferences

High Risk for Ineffective Family Coping: Compromised related to possible prolonged hospitalization that exhausts supportive capacity of significant people

High Risk for Injury related to unfamiliar environment, developmental age or lack of parental knowledge regarding safety, e.g., side rails. IV site/pole

Hopelessness (child) related to prolonged activity restriction and/or uncertain prognosis

Ineffective Individual Coping (parent) related to possible guilt regarding hospitalization of child; parental inadequacies

Sleep Pattern Disturbance (child or parent) related to 24-hour care needs of hospitalization

Pain related to treatments, diagnostic or therapeutic procedures

Powerlessness (child) related to health care environment; illness-related regimen

Hydrocephalus

Altered Family Processes related to situational crisis

Altered Growth and Development related to sequelae of increased intracranial pressure

Altered Nutrition: Less than Body Requirements related to inadequate intake secondary to anorexia, nausea and/or vomiting, feeding difficulties

Altered Tissue Perfusion: Cerebral related to interrupted flow and/or hypervolemia of cerebral ventricles

Decisional Conflict: Parental regarding selection of treatment modality related to unclear or conflicting values

Fluid Volume Excess: Cerebral Ventricles related to compromised regulatory mechanism

High Risk for Infection related to sequelae of invasive procedure (shunt placement)

Impaired Skin (Tissue) Integrity related to impaired physical mobility/mechanical irritation

Refer to Premature Infant; Child With Chronic Condition; Hospitalized Child; Mental Retardation, if appropriate

Hyperactive syndrome

Altered Role Performance: Parent(s) related to stressors associated with dealing with hyperactive child; perceived or projected blame for causes of child's behavior; unmet needs for support/care, and lack of energy to provide for those needs

Decisional Conflict regarding education programs, nutrition regimens, medication regimens related to multiple or divergent sources of information; willingness to change own food habits; limited resources

High Risk for Altered Parenting related to disruptive, uncontrollable behaviors of child

High Risk for Violence: Parent or Child related to frustration with disruptive behavior, anger, unsuccessful relationship(s)

Impaired Social Interaction related to impulsive, overactive behaviors; concomitant emotional difficulties; distractibility and excitability

Ineffective Family Coping: Compromised related to unsuccessful strategies to control excessive activity/behaviors, frustration and anger

Parental Role Conflict (when siblings present) related to increased attention towards hyperactive child

Self-Esteem Disturbance or Chronic Low Self-Esteem related to inability to achieve socially acceptable behaviors, frustration; frequent reprimands, punishment, scoldings secondary to uncontrolled activity/behaviors; mood fluctuations and restlessness; inability to succeed academically; lack of peer support

Hyperbilirubinemia

Altered Nutrition: Less than Body Requirements related to disinterest in feeding due to jaundice related lethargy

Anxiety related to threat to infant and unknown future

High Risk for Altered Body Temperature related to phototherapy

High Risk for Injury related to kernicterus, phototherapy lights

Knowledge Deficit: Parental related to lack of exposure to situation

Parental Role Conflict related to interruption of family life due to home care regimen

Sensory/Perceptual Alteration: Visual related to use of eye patches for protection of eyes during phototherapy

Hypercalcemia

Altered Thought Processes related to elevated calcium levels causing paranoia

Altered Nutrition: Less than Body Requirements related to gastrointestinal manifestations of hypercalcemia, nausea, anorexia, ileus

High Risk for Decreased Cardiac Output related to bradydysrhythmias

Impaired Physical Mobility related to decreased tone in smooth and striated muscle

Hyperemesis gravidarum

Altered Nutrition: Less than Body Requirements related to vomiting

Anxiety related to threat to self and infant, hospitalization

Fluid Volume Deficit related to vomiting

Impaired Home Maintenance Management related to chronic nausea and inability to function

Powerlessness related to illness-related regimen

Social isolation related to hospitalization

Hyperglycemia

Refer to Diabetes Mellitus

Hyperkalemia

High Risk for Impaired Intolerance related to muscle weakness

High Risk for Decreased Cardiac Output related to possible dysrhythmias

High Risk for Fluid Volume Excess related to untreated renal failure

Hypernatremia

High Risk for Fluid Volume Deficit related to abnormal water loss, inadequate water intake

Hyperosmolar hyperglycemic nonketotic coma

Altered Thought Processes related to dehydration, electrolyte imbalance

Fluid Volume Deficit related to polyuria, inadequate fluid intake

High Risk for Injury: Seizures related to hyperosmolar state, electrolyte imbalance

Refer to Diabetes

Hypertension

Altered Nutrition: More than Body Requirements related to lack of knowledge of relationship between diet and the disease process

High Risk for Decreased Cardiac Output related to increased afterload

High Risk for Noncompliance related to side effects of treatment

Knowledge Deficit related to treatment and control of disease process

Pain: Headache related to cerebral vascular changes

Hyperthyroidism

Activity Intolerance related to increased oxygen demands from increased metabolic rate

Altered Nutrition: Less than Body Requirements related to increased metabolic rate, increased gastrointestinal activity

Anxiety related to increased stimulation, loss of control

Diarrhea related to increased gastric motility

High Risk for Injury: Eye damage related to exophthalmos

Knowledge Deficit related to medications, methods of coping with stress

Sleep Pattern Disturbance related to anxiety, excessive sympathetic discharge

Hypocalcemia

Altered Nutrition: Less than Body Requirements related to effects of vitamin D deficiency; renal failure; malabsorption; laxative use

High Risk for Activity Intolerance related to neuromuscular irritability

High Risk for Ineffective Breathing Pattern related to laryngospasm

Hypoglycemia

Altered Nutrition: Less than Body Requirements related to imbalance of glucose/insulin level

Altered Thought Processes related to insufficient blood glucose to brain

Knowledge Deficit related to disease process, home and self-care

Refer to Diabetes

Hypokalemia

Activity Intolerance related to muscle weakness

Decreased Cardiac Output related to possible dysrhythmias

Hyponatremia

Altered Thought Processes related to electrolyte imbalance

Fluid Volume Excess related to excessive intake of hypotonic fluids

Hypotension

Altered Thought Processes related to decreased oxygen supply to brain

Altered Tissue Perfusion:

Cardiopulmonary/Peripheral related to hypovolemia; decreased contractility; decreased afterload

Decreased Cardiac Output related to decreased preload

High Risk for Fluid Volume Deficit related to excessive fluid loss

Refer to cause of Hypotension

Hypothyroidism

Activity Intolerance related to muscular stiffness, shortness of breath on exertion

Altered Nutrition: More than Body Requirements related to decreased metabolic process

Colonic Constipation related to decreased gastric motility

High Risk for Altered Thought Processes related to altered metabolic process

Impaired Gas Exchange related to possible respiratory depression

Impaired Skin Integrity related to edema, dry scaly skin
Knowledge Deficit related to disease process and self-care

Hysterectomy

Anticipatory Grieving related to change in body image, loss of reproductive status

Constipation related to narcotics, anesthesia, bowel manipulation during surgery

High Risk for Altered Tissue Perfusion related to thromboembolism

High Risk for Fluid Volume Deficit related to abnormal blood loss, hemorrhage

High Risk for Ineffective Individual Coping related to situational crisis of surgery

High Risk for Sexual Dysfunction related to disturbance in self-concept

High Risk for Urinary Retention related to edema in area, anesthesia/narcotics, pain

Knowledge Deficit related to home care restrictions and needs

Pain related to surgical injury

Refer to Surgery

Idiopathic Thrombocytopenia

Altered Protection related to decreased platelet count

Diversional Activity Deficit related to activity restrictions and safety precautions

High Risk for Injury related to decreased platelet count and developmental level; age-appropriate play

Impaired Home Health Maintenance related to parental lack of ability to follow through with safety precautions secondary to child's developmental stage (active toddler)

Refer to Hospitalized Child

Ileal conduit

Body Image Disturbance related to presence of stoma

High Risk for Altered Sexuality Pattern related to altered body function and structure

High Risk for Impaired Skin Integrity related to difficulty obtaining good seal of appliance

High Risk for Social Isolation related to alteration in physical appearance, fear of accidental spill of ostomy contents

Ineffective Management of Therapeutic Regimen related to new skills required to care for appliance and self

Knowledge Deficit related to routines of care of stoma

Ileostomy

Body Image Disturbance related to presence of stoma

High Risk for Altered Sexuality Pattern related to altered body function and structure

High Risk for Constipation/Diarrhea related to dietary changes, change in intestinal motility

High Risk for Impaired Skin Integrity related to difficulty obtaining good seal of appliance, caustic drainage

High Risk for Social Isolation related to alteration in physical appearance, fear of accidental spill of ostomy contents

Ineffective Management of Therapeutic Regimen related to new skills required to care for appliance and self

Knowledge Deficit related to limited practice of stoma care, dietary modifications

Ileus

Constipation related to decreased gastric motility

Fluid Volume Deficit related to loss of fluids from vomiting

Pain related to pressure and abdominal distention

Impetigo

Impaired Skin Integrity related to pruritis

Refer to Communicable Diseases, Childhood

Impotence

Self-Esteem Disturbance related to physiological crisis, inability to practice usual sexual activity

Sexual Dysfunction related to altered body function

Induction of labor

Anxiety related to medical interventions

Decisional Conflict related to perceived threat to idealized birth

Ineffective Individual Coping related to situational crisis of medical intervention in birthing process

Self-Esteem Disturbance related to inability to carry out normal labor

Infant of diabetic mother

Altered Nutrition: Less than Body Requirements related to hypotonia, lethargy, and poor sucking; postnatal metabolic changes from hyperglycemia to hypoglycemia and hyperinsulinism

Fluid Volume Deficit related to increased urinary excretion and osmotic diuresis

High Risk for Decreased Cardiac Output related to increased incidence of cardiomegaly

High Risk for Impaired Gas Exchange related to increased incidence of cardiomegaly; prematurity

High Risk for Altered Growth and Development related to prolonged and severe postnatal hypoglycemia

Refer to Premature Infant; Respiratory Conditions of the Neonate

Infant of substance abusing mother (fetal alcohol syndrome, crack baby, other drug withdrawal infants)

Altered Growth and Development related to effects of maternal use of drugs, effects of neurological impairment, decreased attentiveness to environmental stimuli or inadequate stimuli

Altered Nutrition: Less than Body Requirements related to feeding problems, uncoordinated/ineffective suck and swallow; effects of diarrhea, vomiting, colic associated with maternal substance abuse

Altered Parenting related to impaired or lack of attachment behaviors, inadequate support systems

Altered Protection related to effects of maternal substance abuse

Diarrhea related to effects of withdrawal, increased peristalsis secondary to hyperirritability

High Risk for Infection (skin, meningeal, respiratory) related to effects of withdrawal

Ineffective Airway Clearance related to pooling of secretions secondary to lack of adequate cough reflex; effects of viral or bacterial lower airway infection secondary to altered protective state

Ineffective Infant Feeding Pattern related to uncoordinated/ineffective sucking reflex

Interrupted Breastfeeding related to use of drugs, alcohol by mother

Sensory-Perceptual Alteration related to hypersensitivity to environmental stimuli

Sleep Pattern Disturbance related to hyperirritability, hypersensitivity to environmental stimuli

Refer to Failure to Thrive; Sudden Infant Death Syndrome; Hospitalized Child; Cerebral Palsy; Hyperactive Syndrome

Inflammatory bowel disease, child and adult

Altered Nutrition: Less than Body Requirements related to anorexia, decreased absorption of nutrients from GI tract

Diarrhea related to effects of inflammatory changes of the bowel

Fluid Volume Deficit related to frequent, loose stools

Impaired Skin Integrity related to frequent stools and development of anal fissures

Ineffective Individual Coping related to repeated episodes of diarrhea

Pain related to abdominal cramping and anal irritation

Social Isolation related to diarrhea

Refer to Crohn's Disease; Hospitalized Child; Child With Chronic Condition; Maturational Issues—Adolescent

Influenza

Fluid Volume Deficit related to inadequate fluid intake

Hyperthermia related to infectious process

Ineffective Management of Therapeutic Regimen related to lack of knowledge regarding preventive immunizations

Knowledge Deficit related to treatment of disease

Pain related to inflammatory changes in joints

Inguinal hernia repair

High Risk for Infection related to surgical procedure

Impaired Physical Mobility related to pain at surgical site and fear of causing hernia to "break open"

Pain related to surgical procedure

Urinary Retention related to possible edema at surgical site

Insomnia

Anxiety related to actual or perceived lose of sleep

Sleep Pattern Disturbance related to sensory alterations; internal factors; external factors

Intracranial pressure, increased

Altered Thought Processes related to pressure damage to brain

Altered Tissue Perfusion: Cerebral related to the effects of increased intracranial pressure

Ineffective Breathing Patterns related to pressure damage to breathing center in brainstem

Sensory/Perceptual Alteration related to pressure damage to sensory centers in brain

Refer to Cause of Increased Intracranial Pressure

Intra-aortic balloon counterpulsation

Anxiety/Fear related to device providing cardiovascular assistance

Decreased Cardiac Output related to failing heart needing counterpulsation

High Risk for Peripheral Neurovascular Dysfunction related to vascular obstruction in balloon catheter; thrombus formation; emboli; edema

Impaired Physical Mobility related to restriction of movement because of mechanical device

Irritable bowel syndrome (IBS)

Constipation related to low residue diet, stress

Diarrhea related to increased motility of intestines associated with stress

Knowledge Deficit related to treatment of disease

Ineffective Management of Therapeutic Regimen related to knowledge deficit, powerlessness

Pain related to spasms and increased motility of bowel

Jaw surgery

Altered Nutrition: Less than Bodily Requirements related to liquid diet

High Risk for Aspiration related to wired jaws

Impaired Swallowing related to possible edema from surgery

Knowledge Deficit related to emergency care for wired jaw (cutting bands/wires) and oral care

Pain related to surgical procedure

Joint replacement

High Risk for Peripheral Neurovascular Dysfunction related to orthopedic surgery

Refer to Total Joint Replacement

Kawasaki disease

Refer to Mucocutaneous Lymph Node Syndrome

Ketoacidosis

Altered Nutrition: Less than Body Requirements related to body's inability to use nutrients

Fluid Volume Deficit related to excess excretion of urine, nausea, vomiting and increased respiration

High Risk for Noncompliance (with Diabetic Regime) related to ineffective coping with chronic disease

Ineffective Management of Therapeutic Regimen related to denial of illness, lack of understanding of preventive measures and adequate blood sugar control

Refer to Diabetes

Kidney stones

Altered Patterns of Urinary Elimination: Frequency, Urgency related to anatomical obstruction, irritation caused by stone

High Risk for Fluid Volume Deficit related to nausea, vomiting

High Risk for Infection related to obstruction of urinary tract with stasis of urine

Knowledge Deficit related to fluid requirements and dietary restrictions

Pain related to obstruction from renal calculi

Korsakoff's syndrome

Altered Thought Process related to impairment of short-term memory

High Risk for Altered Nutrition related to lack of adequate balanced intake

High Risk for Injury related to sensory dysfunction; lack of coordination when ambulating

Labor—normal

Anxiety related to fear of the unknown and situational crisis

Fatigue related to childbirth

Health Seeking Behaviors related to healthy outcome of pregnancy, prenatal care, and childbirth education

High Risk for Fluid Volume Deficit related to excessive loss of blood

High Risk for Infection related to multiple vaginal examinations, tissue trauma, and prolonged rupture of membranes

High Risk for Injury (Fetal) related to hypoxia

Knowledge Deficit related to lack of preparation for labor

Impaired Skin Integrity related to passage of infant through birth canal, episiotomy

Pain related to uterine contractions and stretching of cervix and birth canal

Laminectomy

Anxiety related to change in health status, surgical procedure

High Risk for Impaired Tissue Perfusion related to edema, hemorrhage and/or embolism

High Risk for Urinary Retention related to competing sensory impulses, narcotics, anesthesia

Impaired Physical Mobility related to neuromuscular impairment

Knowledge Deficit related to appropriate postoperative activities and after discharge

Pain related to localized inflammation and edema

Sensory/Perceptual Alteration: Tactile related to possible edema or nerve injury

Refer to Surgery, Scoliosis

Laryngectomy

Alteration in Family Process related to surgery, serious condition of family member, difficulty communicating

Alteration in Nutrition: Less than Body Requirements related to absence of oral feeding, difficulty swallowing, increased need for fluids

Alteration in Oral Mucous Membranes related to absence of oral feeding

Anticipatory Grieving related to loss of voice, fear of death

Body Image Disturbance related to change in body structure and function

High Risk for Infection related to invasive procedure, surgery

Impaired Verbal Communication related to removal of the larynx

Impaired Swallowing related to edema, laryngectomy tube

Ineffective Airway Clearance related to surgical removal of the glottis, decreased humidification of air

Knowledge Deficit related to self-care needs

Laser surgery

Knowledge Deficit related to preoperative and postoperative care associated with laser procedure

Pain related to heat from action of the laser

High Risk for Infection related to delayed heating reaction of tissue exposed to laser

High Risk for Injury related to accidental exposure to laser beam

Constipation related to laser intervention in vulva and perianal areas

Leukemia

Altered Protection related to abnormal blood profile

High Risk for Infection related to ineffective immune system

High Risk for Fluid Volume Deficit related to side effects of treatment: nausea, vomiting, bleeding

Refer to Chemotherapy, Cancer

Limb reattachment procedures

Anticipatory Grieving related to unknown outcome of reattachment procedure

Body Image Disturbance related to unpredictability of function and appearance of reattached body part

Anxiety related to unknown outcome of reattachment procedure; use of limb, appearance of limb

High Risk for Fluid Volume Deficit: Hemorrhage related to severed vessels

High Risk for Peripheral Neurovascular Dysfunction related to trauma, orthopedic, neurovascular surgery; compression of nerves, blood vessels

Refer to Surgery Postoperative Procedures

Low back pain

Chronic Pain related to degenerative processes; musculotendinous strain; injury; inflammation; congenital deformities

Impaired Physical Mobility related to back pain

Ineffective Management of Therapeutic Regimen related to knowledge deficit regarding proper posture, lifting techniques, and conditioning exercises

Urinary Retention related to possible spinal cord compression

Lupus Erythromatous

Refer to Systemic Lupus Erythromatosus

Lyme disease

Fatigue related to increased energy requirements

High Risk for Decreased Cardiac Output related to dysrhythmias

Knowledge Deficit related to lack of informational sources

Pain related to inflammation of joints, urticaria, and rash

Malnutrition

Altered Nutrition: Less than Body Requirements related to inability to ingest or digest food or absorb nutrients due to biological, psychological, economic factors, institutionalization, i.e., lack of menu choices

Altered Protection related to inadequate nutrition

Ineffective Management of Therapeutic Regimen related to economic difficulties

Knowledge Deficit related to misinformation about normal nutrition, social isolation, lack of food preparation facilities

Mania

Altered Family Processes related to family members illness

Altered Nutrition: Less than Body Requirements related to lack of time and motivation to eat, constant movement

Altered Role Performance related to impaired social interactions

Altered Thought Processes related to mania

Anxiety related to change in role function

Fluid Volume Deficit related to decreased intake

High Risk for Caregiver Role Strain related to unpredictability of the condition; mood swings

High Risk for Violence: Self-Directed or Directed at Others related to bizarre hallucinations, delusions

Impaired Home Maintenance Management related to altered psychological state, inability to concentrate

Ineffective Denial related to fear of inability to control behavior

Ineffective Individual Coping related to situational crisis

Ineffective Management of Therapeutic Regimen related to lack of social supports

Noncompliance related to denial of illness

Sleep Pattern Disturbance related to constant anxious thoughts

Mastectomy

Body Image Disturbance related to loss of sexually significant body part

Fear related to change in body image and prognosis

High Risk for Disuse Syndrome of arm on affected side related to pain; lack of knowledge concerning need for range of motion

High Risk for Impaired Physical Mobility related to nerve, muscle damage, pain

High Risk for Sexual Dysfunction related to change in body image, fear of loss of feminism

Knowledge Deficit related to self-care activities

Pain related to surgical procedure

Refer to Cancer; Surgery

Mastitis

Altered Role Performance related to change in capacity to function in expected role

Anxiety related to threat to self and concern over safety of milk for infant

High Risk for Ineffective Breastfeeding related to breast pain and conflicting advice from health care providers

Knowledge Deficit related to antibiotic regimen and comfort measures

Pain related to infectious disease process and swelling of breast tissue

Maturational issues, adolescent

Altered Family Processes related to developmental crises of adolescence secondary to challenge of parental authority and values; situational crises secondary to change in parental marital status

High Risk for Impaired Social Interaction related to ineffective/unsuccessful/dysfunctional interaction with peers

High Risk for Injury/Trauma related to thrill-seeking behaviors

Ineffective Individual Coping related to maturational crises

Knowledge Deficit: Potential for Enhanced Health Maintenance related to information misinterpretation; lack of education regarding age related factors

Social Isolation related to perceived alteration in physical appearance, social values not accepted by dominant peer group

Refer to Sexuality—Adolescent; Substance Abuse (if relevant)

Measles (rubeola)

Refer to Communicable Diseases, Childhood

Meconium aspiration

Refer to Respiratory Conditions of the Neonate

Meningitis/encephalitis

Altered Comfort: Nausea and Vomiting related to CNS inflammation

Altered Comfort: Photophobia related to increased sensitivity to external stimuli secondary to CNS inflammation

Altered Thought Processes related to inflammation of brain, fever

Altered Tissue Perfusion: Cerebral related to inflamed cerebral tissues and meninges; increased intracranial pressure

Fluid Volume Excess related to increased intracranial pressure; inappropriate secretion of antidiuretic hormone (SIADH)

High Risk for Altered Growth and Development related to brain damage secondary to infectious process, increased intracranial pressure

High Risk for Aspiration related to seizure activity

High Risk for Ineffective Airway Clearance related to seizure activity

Pain related to neck (nuchal) rigidity, inflammation of meninges, headache, kinesthetic sensory-perceptual alteration (skin is painful to touch), fever, earache

High Risk for Injury related to seizure activity

Impaired Mobility related to neuromuscular/CNS insult

Sensory-Perceptual Alteration: Hearing related to CNS infection, ear infection

Sensory-Perceptual Alteration: Kinesthetic related to CNS infection

Sensory-Perceptual Alteration: Visual related to photophobia secondary to CNS infection

Refer to Hospitalized Child

Meningocele

Refer to Neural tube Defects

Menopause

Altered Sexuality Patterns related to altered body structure; lack of physiological lubrication and lack of knowledge of artificial lubrication

Health Seeking Behavior related to menopause and therapies associated with change in hormonal levels

High Risk for Altered Nutrition: More than Body Requirements related to change in metabolic rate caused by fluctuating hormone levels

Ineffective Thermoregulation related to changes in hormonal levels

Mental retardation

Altered Family Processes related to crisis of diagnosis and situational transition

Altered Growth and Development related to cognitive/perceptual impairment and developmental delay

Chronic Low Self-Esteem related to perceived differences

Grieving related to loss of perfect child; birth of child with congenital defect or subsequent head injury

Family Coping: Potential for Growth related to adaptation and acceptance of child's condition and needs

High Risk for Self-Mutilation related to separation anxiety; depersonalization

Impaired Home Maintenance Management related to insufficient support systems

Impaired Social Interaction related to developmental lag/delay, perceived differences

Impaired Swallowing related to neuromuscular impairment

Impaired Verbal Communication related to developmental delay

Parental Role Conflict related to home care of child with special needs

Self-Care Deficit: Bathing/Hygiene; Dressing/Grooming; Feeding; Toileting related to perceptual or cognitive impairment

Refer to Safety—Childhood; Child With Chronic Condition

MI Refer to Myocardial Infarction

Midlife crisis

Ineffective Individual Coping related to inability to deal with changes associated with aging

Powerlessness related to lack of control over life situation

Spiritual Distress related to questioning belief/value system

Migraine headache

Knowledge Deficit related to prevention and treatment of headaches

Pain: Headache related to vasodilatation of cerebral and extracerebral vessels

Miscarriage

Refer to Pregnancy Loss, Abortion-spontaneous

Mitral stenosis

Anxiety related to possible worsening of symptoms; activity intolerance; fatigue

Activity Intolerance related to imbalance between oxygen supply and demand

Decreased Cardiac Output related to incompetent heart valves; abnormal forward or backward blood flow; flow into a dilated chamber; flow through an abnormal passage between chambers

Fatigue related to reduced cardiac output

Mitral valve prolapse

Altered Tissue Perfusion: Cerebral related to postural hypotension

Anxiety related to symptoms of condition: palpitations, chest pain

Fatigue related to abnormal catecholamine regulation and decreased intravascular volume

Fear related to lack of knowledge about mitral valve prolapse; feelings of having a heart attack

High Risk for Infection related to invasive procedures

Knowledge Deficit related to methods to relieve pain, treatment of dysrhythmias and shortness of breath, need prophylactic antibiotics before invasive procedures

Pain related to mitral valve regurgitation

Mononucleosis

Activity Intolerance related to generalized weakness

High Risk for Injury related to possible rupture of spleen

Hyperthermia related to infectious process

Impaired Swallowing related to irritation of oropharyngeal cavity

Ineffective Management of Therapeutic Regimen related to knowledge deficit concerning transmission and treatment of disease

Pain related to enlargement of lymph nodes, irritation of oropharyngeal cavity

Mucocutaneous lymph node syndrome

Altered Nutrition: Less than Body Requirements related to altered oral mucous membranes

Altered Oral Mucous Membranes related to inflamed mouth and pharynx; swollen lips that progress to dry, cracked, and fissured

Anxiety, Parental related to progression of disease and complications of arthritis and cardiac involvement

Hyperthermia related to inflammatory disease process

Impaired Skin Integrity related to inflammatory skin changes

Pain related to enlarged lymph nodes; erythematous skin rash that progresses to desquamation, peeling and denuding of skin

Refer to Hospitalized Child

Multiple personality

Anxiety related to loss of control of behavior and feelings

Body-Image Disturbance related to feelings of powerlessness with personality changes

Chronic Low Self-Esteem related to inability to deal with life events; history of abuse

Defensive Coping related to unresolved past traumatic events; severe anxiety

High Risk for Self-Mutilation related to need to act out to relieve stress

Ineffective Individual Coping related to history of abuse

Hopelessness related to long-term stress

Personal Identity Disturbance related to severe child abuse

Refer to Dissociative Disorder

Multiple sclerosis

Anticipatory Grieving related to high risk for loss of normal body functioning

High Risk for Altered Nutrition: Less than Body Requirements related to impaired swallowing, depression

High Risk for Disuse Syndrome related to physical immobility

High Risk for Ineffective Airway Clearance related to decreased energy/fatigue

High Risk for Injury related to altered mobility, sensory dysfunction

High Risk for Urinary Retention related to inhibition of the reflex arc

Impaired Physical Mobility related to neuromuscular impairment

Powerlessness related to progressive nature of disease

Self-Care Deficit: Specify related to neuromuscular impairment

Sensory/Perceptual alteration: Specify related to pathology in sensory tracts

Sexual Dysfunction related to biopsychosocial alteration of sexuality

Spiritual Distress related to perceived hopelessness of diagnosis

Refer to Nervous System Disorders

Mumps

Refer to Communicable Diseases, Childhood

Muscular dystrophy

Activity Intolerance related to fatigue

Altered Nutrition: Less than Body Requirements related to impaired swallowing/chewing

Altered Nutrition: More than Body Requirements related to inactivity

Decreased Cardiac Output related to effects of congestive heart failure

High Risk for Aspiration related to impaired swallowing

High Risk for Constipation related to immobility

High Risk for Disuse Syndrome related to complications of immobility

High Risk for Fatigue related to increased energy requirements to perform activities of daily living

High Risk for Impaired Gas Exchange related to ineffective airway clearance and ineffective breathing patterns secondary to muscle weakness

High Risk for Impaired Skin Integrity related to immobility and braces/adaptive devices

High Risk for Ineffective Breathing Patterns related to muscle weakness

High Risk for Infection related to pooling of pulmonary secretions secondary to immobility and muscle weakness

High Risk for Injury related to muscle weakness and unsteady gait

Impaired Mobility related to muscle weakness and development of contractures

Ineffective Airway Clearance related to muscle weakness and decreased cough

Self-Care Deficits: Feeding, Bathing, Dressing, Toileting related to muscle weakness and fatigue

Refer to Hospitalized Child; Child With Chronic Condition; Terminally Ill Child/Death of Child

Myasthenia gravis

Altered Family Process related to crisis of dealing with diagnosis

Altered Nutrition related to difficulty eating and swallowing

High Risk for Caregiver Role Strain related to severity of illness of client

Fatigue related to paresthesia and aching muscles

Impaired Physical Mobility related to defective transmission of nerve impulses at the neuromuscular junction

Impaired Swallowing related to neuromuscular impairment

Ineffective Airway Clearance related to decreased ability to cough and swallow

Ineffective Management of Therapeutic Regimen related to lack of knowledge of treatment and uncertainty of outcome

Myelogram, contrast

High Risk for Altered Tissue Perfusion: Cerebral related to hypotension; loss of cerebral spinal fluid

High Risk for Fluid Volume Deficit related to possible dehydration; loss of cerebral spinal fluid

Pain related to irritation of nerve roots

Urinary Retention related to pressure on spinal nerve roots

Myelomeningocele

Refer to Neural tube Defects

Myocardial Infarction (MI)

Altered Family Porcesses related to crisis, role change

Anxiety related to threat of death; possible change in role status

Colonic Constipation related to decreased peristalsis from decreased physical activity, medication effect, change in diet

Decreased Cardiac Output related to ventricular damage, ischemia; dysrhythmias

Fear related to threat to well-being

High Risk for Altered Sexuality Pattern related to fear of chest pain, possibility of heart damage

High Risk for Ineffective Denial related to fear or knowledge deficit about heart disease

High Risk for Situational Low Self-Esteem related to crisis of myocardial infarction

Ineffective Family Coping related to spouse/significant other fear of partner loss

Knowledge Deficit related to self-care program

Pain related to myocardial tissue damage from inadequate blood supply

Myocarditis

Activity Intolerance related to reduced cardiac reserve and prescribed bedrest

Decreased Cardiac Output related to impaired contractility of ventricles

Knowledge Deficit related to treatment of disease

Refer to CHF, if appropriate

Myxedema

Refer to Hypothyroidism

Near drowning

Altered Health Maintenance related to parental knowledge deficit regarding safety measures appropriate for age

Anticipatory/Dysfunctional Grieving related to potential death of child; unknown sequelae; guilt over accident

Aspiration related to aspiration of fluid into the lungs

Fear, Parental related to possible death of child; possible permanent, debilitating sequelae

High Risk for Altered Growth and Development related to hypoxemia; cerebral anoxia

High Risk for Infection related to aspiration, invasive monitoring

Hypothermia related to CNS injury, prolonged submersion in cold water

Impaired Gas Exchange related to laryngospasm, breath holding, aspiration

Ineffective Airway Clearance/Ineffective Breathing Pattern related to aspiration and impaired gas exchange

Refer to Safety—Childhood; Hospitalized Child; Child With Chronic Condition; Terminally Ill Child/Death of Child

Necrotizing Enterocolitis (NEC)

Altered Nutrition: Less than Body Requirements related to decreased ability to absorb nutrients; decreased perfusion to GI tract

Altered Tissue Perfusion: Gastrointestinal related to shunting of blood away from mesenteric circulation, toward vital organs secondary to perinatal stress, hypoxia

Fluid Volume Deficit related to vomiting; GI bleed

High Risk for Infection related to bacterial invasion of GI tract; invasive procedures

Ineffective Breathing Pattern related to abdominal distention, hypoxia

Refer to Premature Infant; Hospitalized Child

Nephrectomy

Anxiety related to surgical recovery; prognosis

Alteration in Urinary Elimination related to loss of kidney

Constipation related to lack of return of peristalsis

High Risk for Infection related to invasive procedure, lack of deep breathing due to location of surgical incision

High Risk for Fluid Volume Deficit related to vascular losses, decreased intake

Ineffective Breathing Pattern related to location of surgical incision

Pain related to incisional discomfort

Nephrotic syndrome

Activity Intolerance related to generalized edema

Altered Confort related to edema

Altered Nutrition: Less than Body Requirements related to anorexia and protein loss

Altered Nutrition: More than Body Requirements related to increased appetite secondary to steroid therapy

Body Image Disturbance related to edematous appearance and side effects of steroid therapy

Fluid Volume Excess related to edema secondary to oncotic fluid shift from serum protein loss and renal retention of salt and water

High Risk for Impaired Skin Integrity related to edema

High Risk for Infection related to altered immune mechanisms secondary to disease itself and effects of steroids

High Risk for Noncompliance related to side effects encountered with home steroid therapy

Social isolation related to edematous appearance

Refer to Hospitalized Child; Child With Chronic Condition

Nervous system disorders

Altered Family Porcesses related to situational crisis, illness/disability of family member

Anticipatory Grieving related to loss of usual body functioning

Altered Nutrition, Less than Body Requirements related to impaired swallowing, depression, difficulty feeding self

High Risk for Disuse Syndrome related to physical immobility, neuromuscular dysfunction

High Risk for Impaired Skin Integrity related to altered sensation, altered mental status, paralysis

High Risk for Ineffective Airway Clearance related to perceptual/cognitive impairment, decreased energy/fatigue

High Risk for Injury related to altered mobility, sensory dysfunction, cognitive impairment

Impaired Home Maintenance Management related to individual/family members disease

Impaired Physical Mobility related to neuromuscular impairment

Ineffective Individual Coping related to disability requiring change in lifestyle

Powerlessness related to progressive nature of disease

Self-Care Deficit: Specify related to neuromuscular dysfunction

Sexual Dysfunction related to biopsychosocial alteration of sexuality

Social Isolation related to altered state of wellness

Neuritis

Activity Intolerance related to pain with movement

Knowledge Deficit related to treatment of disease

pain related to stimulation of affected nerve endings; inflammation of sensory nerves

Neurogenic bladder

Reflex Incontinence related to neurological impairment

Urinary Retention related to interruption in the lateral spinal tracts

Neuraltube defects (meningocele, myelomeningocele, spina bifida, anencephaly)

Altered Growth and Development related to physical impairments, possible cognitive impairment

Chronic Low Self-Esteem related to perceived differences; decreased ability to participate in physical and social activities at school

Colonic Constipation related to immobility or less than adequate mobility

Family Coping: Potential for Growth related to effective adaptive response by family members

Grieving related to (loss of perfect child) birth of child with congenital defect

High Risk for Altered Nutrition: More than Body Requirements related to diminished/limited/impaired physical activity

High Risk for Impaired Skin Integrity (Lower Extremities) related to decreased sensory perception

Impaired Mobility related to neuromuscular impairment

Impaired Skin Integrity related to incontinence

Sensory/Perceptual Alteration: Visual related to altered reception secondary to strabismus

Urge Incontinence vs Reflex Incontinence related to neurogenic impairment vs Total Incontinence related to neurological dysfunction

Refer to Premature Infant; Child With Chronic Condition

Newborn, normal

Altered Protection related to immature immune system

Effective Breastfeeding related to normal oral structure and gestational age greater than 34 weeks

High Risk for Infection related to open umbilical stump

High Risk for Injury related to immaturity and need for caretaking

Ineffective Thermoregulation related to immaturity of neuroendocrine system

Newborn, postmature

High Risk for Aspiration related to meconium aspiration

High Risk for Injury related to hypoglycemia secondary to depleted glycogen stores

Hypothermia related to depleted stores of subcutaneous fat

Impaired Skin Integrity related to cracked and peeling skin secondary to decreased vernix

Newborn, small for gestational age (SGA)

Altered Nutrition: Less than Body Requirements related to inadequate sucking reflex

Ineffective Thermoregulation related to immaturity of neuroendocrine system; decreased brown fat and subcutaneous fat

Obesity

Altered Nutrition: More than Body Requirements related to caloric intake exceeding energy expenditure

Body Image Disturbance related to eating disorder, excess weight

Chronic Low Self-Esteem related to ineffective individual coping, overeating

Obsessive compulsive disorder

Altered Thought Process related to persistent thoughts, ideas, and impulses that will not relent and seem irrelevant

Anxiety related to threat to self-concept; unmet needs

Decisional Conflict related to inability to make a decision for fear of reprisal

Ineffective Family Coping: Disabling related to family process being disrupted by client's ritualistic activities

Ineffective Individual Coping related to expression of feelings in an unacceptable way; ritualistic behavior

Powerlessness related to unrelenting repetitive thoughts to perform irrational activities

Oophorectomy

High Risk for Altered Sexuality Patterns related to altered body function

Refer to Surgery

Open reduction of fracture with internal fixation (femur)

Anxiety related to outcome of corrective procedure

High Risk for Peripheral Neurovascular Dysfunction related to mechanical compression, orthopedic surgery, immobilization

Impaired Physical Mobility related to position required postoperatively; abduction of leg and avoidance of acute flexion

Powerlessness related to loss of control; unanticipated change in lifestyle

Refer to Surgery Post-Operative

Organic mental syndromes

High Risk for Injury related to disorientation to time, place and person

Impaired Social Interaction related to altered thought processes

Refer to Dementia

Osteomylitis

Altered Health Maintenance related to continued immobility at home, possible extensive casts, continued antibiotics

Diversional Activity Deficit related to prolonged immobilization and hospitalization

Fear: Parental related to concern regarding possible growth plate damage secondary to infection or concern that infection may become chronic

High Risk for Colonic Constipation related to immobility

High Risk for Impaired Skin Integrity related to irritation from splint/cast

High Risk for (Spread of) Infection related to inadequate primary defenses, secondary defenses

Hyperthermia related to infectious process

Impaired Physical Mobility related to imposed immobility secondary to infected area

Pain related to inflammation in affected extremity

Refer to Hospitalized Child

Osteoporosis

Altered nutrition: Less than Body Requirements related to inadequate intake of calcium and vitamin D

High Risk for Injury: Fractures related to lack of activity; risk of falling from environmental hazards; neuromuscular disorders; diminished senses; cardiovascular responses; responses to drugs

Impaired Physical Mobility related to pain, skeletal changes

Knowledge Deficit related to diet, exercise, and need to abstain from alcohol and nicotine

Pain related to fracture and muscle spasm

Otitis media

High Risk for Infection related to eustachian tube obstruction, traumatic eardrum perforation, or following infectious disease process

Pain related to inflammation, infectious process

Sensory/Perceptual Alteration: Auditory related to incomplete resolution of otitis media, presence of excess drainage in the middle ear

Pacemaker

Anxiety related to change in health status; presence of pacemaker

High Risk for Decreased Cardiac Output related to malfunction of pacemaker

High Risk for Infection related to invasive procedure, presence of foreign body: catheter and generator

Knowledge Deficit related to self-care program; when to seek medical attention

Pain related to surgical procedure

Pain

Pain related to injury agents (biological, chemical, physical, psychological)

Pancreatitis

Altered Nutrition: Less than Body Requirements related to inadequate dietary intake, increased nutritional needs secondary to acute illness, increased metabolic needs caused by increased body temperature

Diarrhea related to decrease in pancreatic secretions resulting in steatorrhea

Fluid Volume Deficit related to vomiting, decreased fluid intake, fever with diaphoresis and fluid shifts

High Risk for Ineffective Breathing Pattern related to splinting from severe pain

High Risk for Ineffective Denial related to ineffective coping (alcohol use)

Knowledge Deficit related to lack of knowledge concerning diet, alcohol use and medication

Pain related to irritation and edema of the inflamed pancreas

Panic attacks

Anxiety related to situational crisis

Ineffective Individual Coping related to personal vulnerability

Post-Trauma Response related to previous catastrophic event

Social Isolation related to fear of lack of control

Paralysis

Body Image Disturbance related to biophysical changes, loss of movement, mobility

Colonic Constipation related to effects of spinal cord disruption; diet inadequate in fiber

High Risk for Disuse Syndrome related to paralysis

High Risk for Impaired Skin Integrity related to altered circulation, altered sensation, and immobility

High Risk for Injury related to altered mobility, sensory dysfunction

Impaired Physical Mobility related to neuromuscular impairment

Knowledge Deficit related to impaired home maintenance management

Pain related to prolonged immobility

Powerlessness related to illness-related regimen

Reflex Incontinence related to neurological impairment

Self-Care Deficit: Specify related to neuromuscular impairment

Sexual Dysfunction related to loss of sensation; biopsychosocial alteration

Refer to Child with Chronic Condition; Hospitalized Child; Neural tube Defects; Hemiplegia, Spinal Cord Injury

Paralytic ileus

Constipation related to decreased gastric motility

Fluid Volume Deficit related to loss of fluids from vomiting

Pain related to pressure and abdominal distention

Paranoid disorder

Altered Thought Processes related to psychological conflicts

Anxiety related to uncontrollable intrusive, suspicious thoughts

Chronic Low Self-Esteem related to inability to trust others

High Risk for Violence: Directed at Others related to suspicious of others and others actions

Sensory/Perceptual Alteration: Specify related to psychological dysfunction; suspicious thoughts

Social Isolation related to inappropriate social skills

Paraplegia

Refer to Spinal Cord Injury

Parental role conflict

Parental Role Conflict related to separation from child due to chronic illness; intimidation with invasive or restrictive modalities (e.g., isolation, intubation) specialized care center, policies; home care of a child with special need (e.g. apnea monitoring, postural drainage, hyperalimentation); change in marital status; interruptions of family life due to home care regimen (treatments, caregivers lack of respite)

Parkinson's disease

Alteration in Nutrition: Less than Body Requirements related to tremor, slowness in eating, difficulty in chewing and swallowing

High Risk for Colonic Constipation related to weakness of defecation muscles; lack of exercise; inadequate fluid intake; decreased autonomic nervous system activity

High Risk for Injury related to tremors, slow reactions, altered gait

Impaired Verbal Communication related to decreased speech volume, slowness of speech, impaired facial muscles

Refer to Nervous System Disorders

Patent ductus arteriosus (PDA)

Refer to Congenital Heart Disease/Cardiac Anomalies

Patient controlled analgesia

Altered Comfort related to medication side effects: pruritus, nausea or vomiting

Knowledge Deficit related to self-care of pain control

High Risk for Injury related to possible complications associated with PCA

PCA

Refer to patient controlled Analgesia

Pelvic inflammatory disease

Altered Sexuality Patterns related to medically imposed abstinence from sexual activities until the acute infection subsides, change in reproductive potential

High Risk for Infection related to insufficient knowledge to avoid exposure to pathogens; poor hygiene, nutrition, and other health habits

Knowledge Deficit related to lack of exposure to information or unfamiliarity with information resources

Pain related to biological injury; inflammation, edema, and congestion of pelvic tissues

Refer to Adolescence Maturational Issues

Pericarditis

Activity Intolerance related to reduced cardiac reserve and prescribed bedrest

Cardiopulmonary/Peripheral related to high risk for development of emboli

High Risk for Alteration in Nutrition: Less than body Requirements related to fever, hypermetabolic state associated with fever.

High Risk for Decreased Cardiac Output related to inflammation in pericardial sac, fluid accumulation compressing heart function.

Knowledge Deficit related to unfamiliarity with information sources

Pain related to biological injury and inflammation

Peripheral Vascular Disease

Activity Intolerance related to imbalance between peripheral oxygen supply and demand

Altered Tissue Perfusion: Peripheral related to interrupted of vascular flow

Chronic Pain: Intermittent Claudication related to ischemia

High Risk for Impaired Skin Integrity related to altered circulation, sensation

High Risk for Injury related to tissue hypoxia, altered mobility, altered sensation

High Risk for Peripheral Neurovascular Dysfunction related to possible vascular obstruction

Knowledge Deficit related to prevention of circulatory complications

Peritoneal dialysis

High Risk for Fluid Volume Excess related to retention of dialysate

High Risk for Ineffective Breathing Pattern related to pressure from the dialysate

High Risk for Ineffective Individual Coping related to disability requiring change in lifestyle

High Risk for Infection: Peritoneal related to invasive procedure, presence of catheter, dialysate

Impaired Home Maintenance Management related to complex home treatment of client

Knowledge Deficit related to home maintenance management

Pain related to instillation of dialysate, temperature of dialysate

Refer to Renal Failure, Oliguric; Renal Failure Acute/Chronic, Child; Hospitalized Child; Child with Chronic Condition

Peritonitis

Altered Nutrition: Less than Body Requirements related to nausea, vomiting

Constipation related to inadequate intake, decrease of peristalsis

Fluid Volume Deficit related to retention of fluid in bowel with loss of circulating blood volume

High Risk for Ineffective Breathing Pattern related to pain, increased abdominal pressure

Pain related to inflammation and stimulation of somatic nerves

Personality disorder

Chronic Low Self-Esteem related to inability to set and achieve goals

Decisional Conflict related to low self-esteem; feelings that choices will always be wrong

Impaired Adjustment related to ambivalent behavior towards others and testing of others loyalty

Impaired Social Interaction related to knowledge/skill deficit about ways to interact effectively with others; self-concept disturbances

Ineffective Family Coping: Compromised related to lack of ability of client to provide positive feedback to family; chronicity exhausting family

Personal Identity Disturbance related to lack of consistent positive self image

Spiritual Distress related to lack of identifiable values, no meaning to life

Refer to Borderline Personality

PID

Refer to pelvic inflammatory disease

PIH

Refer to Pregnancy induced Hypertension/Preeclampsia

Placenta Previa

Altered Family Processes related to maternal bedrest or hospitalization

Altered Role Performance related to maternal bedrest or hospitalization

Altered Tissue Perfusion: Placental related to dilation of cervix and loss of placental implantation site

Body Image Disturbance related to negative feelings about body and reproductive ability; feelings of helplessness

Diversional Activity Deficit related to long-term hospitalization

Fear related to threat to self and fetus, unknown future

High Risk for Altered Parenting related to maternal bedrest or hospitalization

High Risk for Fluid Volume Deficit related to maternal blood loss

Impaired Home Maintenance Management related to maternal bedrest or hospitalization

Impaired Physical Mobility related to medical protocol, maternal bedrest

Ineffective Individual Coping related to threat to self and fetus

Situational Low Self-Esteem related to situational crisis

Spiritual Distress related to inability to participate in usual religious rituals, situational crisis

Pleural effusion

Fluid Volume Excess related to compromised regulatory mechanisms; heart, liver, or kidney failure

Hyperthermia related to increased metabolic rate secondary to infection

Ineffective Breathing Pattern related to pain

Pain related to inflammation, fluid accumulation

Pleurisy

High Risk for Ineffective Airway Clearance related to increased secretions; ineffective cough because of pain

High Risk for Impaired Gas Exchange related to ventilation perfusion imbalance

High Risk for Impaired Physical Mobility related to activity intolerance; inability to "catch breath"

Ineffective Breathing Pattern related to pain

Pain related to pressure on pleural nerve endings associated with fluid accumulation or inflammation

Pneumonia

Altered Oral Mucous Membranes related to dry mouth from mouth breathing, decreased fluid intake

Activity Intolerance related to imbalance between oxygen supply and demand

Altered Nutrition: Less than Body Requirements related to loss of appetite

High Risk for Fluid Volume Deficit related to inadequate intake of fluids

Hyperthermia related to dehydration; increased metabolic rate; illness

Impaired Gas Exchange related to decreased functional lung tissue

Ineffective Airway Clearance related to inflammation and presence of secretions

Knowledge Deficit related to risk factors predisposing person to pneumonia, treatment

Refer to Respiratory Infections, Acute Childhood for child with Pneumonia

Pneumothorax

Fear related to threat to own well-being; difficulty breathing

High Risk for Injury related to possible complications associated with closed chest drainage system

Impaired Gas Exchange related to ventilation perfusion imbalance

Pain related to recent injury; coughing, deep breathing

Postpartum blues

Altered Parenting related to hormone-induced depression

Altered Role Performance related to new responaibilities of parenting

Anxiety related to new responsibilities of parenting

Body Image Disturbance related to normal postpartum recovery

Fatigue related to childbirth and postpartum

Impaired Adjustment related to lack of support systems

Impaired Home Maintenance Management related to fatigue and care of the newborn

Impaired Social Interaction related to change in role functioning

Ineffective Individual Coping related to hormonal changes and maturational crisis

Knowledge Deficit related to lifestyle changes

Sexual Dysfunction related to fears of another pregnancy

Postpartum hemorrhage

Activity Intolerance related to anemia from loss of blood

Body Image Disturbance related to loss of ideal childbirth

Decreased Cardiac Output related to hypovolemia

Fear related to threat to self and unknown future

Fluid Volume Deficit related to uterine atony and loss of blood

High Risk for Altered Parenting related to weakened maternal condition

High Risk for Infection related to loss of blood and depressed immunity

Impaired Home Maintenance Management related to lack of stamina

Knowledge Deficit related to lack of exposure to situation

Postpartum, normal care

Altered Role Performance related to new responsibilities of parenting

Altered Urinary Elimination related to effects of anesthesia or tissue trauma

Anxiety related to change in role functioning and parenting

Constipation related to hormonal effects on smooth muscles, fear of straining with defecation, effects of anesthesia

Effective Breastfeeding related to basic breastfeeding knowledge, partner and health care provider support

Family Coping: Potential for Growth related to adaptation to new family member

Fatigue related to Childbirth, new responsibilities of parenting and body changes

Health Seeking Behaviors related to postpartum recovery and adaptation

High Risk for Altered Parenting related to lack of role models and knowledge deficit

High Risk for Infection related to tissue trauma and blood loss

Impaired Skin Integrity related to episiotomy or lacerations

Ineffective Breastfeeding related to lack of knowledge, lack of support, or lack of motivation

Knowledge Deficit: Infant Care related to lack of preparation for parenting

Sexual Dysfunction related to fear of pain or pregnancy

Pregnancy induced hypertension/preeclampsia

Altered Family Processes related to situational crisis

Altered Parenting related to bedrest

Altered Role Performance related to change in physical capacity to assume role of pregnant woman or resume other roles

Anxiety related to fear of the unknown; threat to self and infant; change in role functioning

Diversional Activity Deficit related to bedrest

Fluid Volume Excess related to decreased renal function

High Risk for Injury (Fetal) related to decreased uteroplacental perfusion

High Risk for Injury (Maternal) related to vasospasm and high blood pressure

Impaired Home Maintenance Management related to bedrest

Impaired Physical Mobility related to medically prescribed limitations

Impaired Social Interaction related to imposed bedrest

Knowledge Deficit related to lack of experience with situation

Powerlessness related to complication threatening pregnancy and medically prescribed limitations

Situational Low Self-Esteem related to loss of idealized pregnancy

Pregnancy loss

Altered Role Performance related to inability to take on parenting role

Altered Sexuality Patterns related to self-esteem disturbance due to pregnancy loss and anxiety about future pregnancies

Anxiety related to threat to role functioning, health status, and situational crisis

High Risk for Dysfunctional Grieving related to loss of pregnancy

High Risk for Fluid Volume Deficit related to blood loss

High Risk for Infection related to retained products of conception

Ineffective Family Coping: Compromised related to lack of support by significant other due to personal suffering

Ineffective Individual Coping related to situational crisis

Pain related to surgical intervention

Spiritual Distress related to intense suffering

Pregnancy—normal

Altered Family Process related to developmental transition of pregnancy

Altered Nutrition: More than Body Requirements related to frequent, closely spaced pregnancies

Body Image Disturbance related to altered body function and appearance

Family Coping: Potential for Growth related to satisfying partner relationship, attention to gratification of needs, effective adaptation to developmental tasks of pregnancy

Fear related to labor and delivery

Health Seeking Behaviors related to desire to promote optimal fetal/maternal health

Ineffective Individual Coping related to personal vulnerability, situational crisis

Knowledge deficit related to primiparity

Sleep Pattern Disturbance related to sleep deprivation secondary to discomfort of pregnant state

Sexual Dysfunction related to altered body function, self-concept, and body image with pregnancy

Refer to Discomforts of Pregnancy

Premature dilation of the cervix (incompetent cervix)

Altered Role Performance related to inability to continue usual patterns of responsibility

Anticipatory Grieving related to potential loss of infant

Diversional Activity Deficit related to bedrest

Fear related to potential loss of infant

High Risk for Infection related to invasive procedures to prevent preterm birth

High Risk for Injury (fetal) related to preterm birth, use of anesthesia

High Risk for Injury (maternal) related to surgical procedures to prevent preterm birth

Impaired Physical Mobility related to imposed bedrest to prevent preterm birth

Impaired Social Interaction related to bedrest

Ineffective Individual Coping related to bedrest and threat to fetus

Knowledge Deficit related to treatment regimen and prognosis for pregnancy

Powerlessness related to inability to control outcome of pregnancy

Sexual Dysfunction related to fear of harm to fetus

Situational Low Self-Esteem related to inability to complete normal pregnancy

Premature infant (child)

Altered Growth and Development: Developmental Lag related to prematurity, environmental and stimulation deficiencies, multiple caretakers

Altered Nutrition: Less than Body Requirements related to delayed or under stimulated rooting reflex and easy fatigue during feeding, diminished endurance

High Risk for Infection related to inadequate (or immature/undeveloped) acquired immune response

High Risk for Injury related to prolonged mechanical ventilation, retrolental fibroplasia (RLF) secondary to 100% oxygen environment

Impaired Gas Exchange related to effects of cardiopulmonary insufficiency

Impaired Swallowing related to decreased or absent gag reflex, fatigue

Ineffective Thermoregulation related to large body surface/weight ratio; immaturity of thermal regulation or state of prematurity

Sensory/Perceptual Alterations related to noxious stimuli, noisy environment

Sleep Pattern Disturbance related to noisy and noxious intensive care environment

Premature infant (parent)

Anticipatory Grieving related to loss of "perfect child"; may lead to dysfunctional grieving (prolonged) related to unresolved conflicts

Decisional Conflict related to support system deficit or multiple sources of information

Ineffective Breastfeeding related to disrupted establishment of effective pattern secondary to prematurity or insufficient opportunities

Ineffective Family Coping: Compromised related to disrupted family roles and disorganization; prolonged condition exhausting supportive capacity of significant people

Parental Role Conflict related to expressed concerns, expressed inability to care for child's physical/emotional developmental needs

Spiritual Distress related to challenged belief/value systems regarding moral/ethical implications of treatment plans

Refer to Hospitalized Child; Child With Chronic Condition

Premature rupture of membranes

Anticipatory Grieving related to potential loss of infant

Anxiety related to threat to infants health status

Body Image Disturbance related to inability to carry pregnancy to term

High Risk for Infection related to rupture of membranes

High Risk for Injury (fetal) related to risk of premature birth

Ineffective Individual Coping related to situational crisis

Situational Low Self-Esteem related to inability to carry pregnancy to term

Premenstrual tension syndrome (PMS)

Fatigue related to hormonal changes

Fluid Volume Excess related to alterations of hormonal levels inducing fluid retention

Knowledge Deficit related to methods to deal with and prevent syndrome

Pain related to hormonal stimulation of gastrointestinal structures

Prenatal Care/Normal

Altered Nutrition: Less than Body Requirements related to nausea from normal hormonal changes

Altered Family Processes related to developmental transition

Altered Urinary Elimination related to frequency caused by increased pelvic pressure and hormonal stimulation

Constipation related to decreased GI motility secondary to hormonal stimulation

Fatigue related to increased energy demands

High Risk for Activity Intolerance related to enlarged abdomen and increased cardiac workload

High Risk for Injury (Maternal) related to knowledge deficit

High Risk for Sexual Dysfunction related to enlarged abdomen and fear of harm to infant

Ineffective Breathing Pattern related to increased intrathoracic pressure and decreased energy secondary to enlarged uterus

Knowledge Deficit related to lack of experience with pregnancy and care

Sleep Pattern Disturbance related to discomforts of pregnancy and fetal activity

Pressure ulcer

Altered Nutrition: Less than Body Requirements related to limited access to food; inability to absorb nutrients due to biological factors; anorexia

High Risk for Infection related to physical immobility; mechanical factors (shearing forces, pressure, restraint); altered circulation; skin irritants

Impaired Tissue Integrity related to altered circulation, impaired physical mobility

Pain related to tissue destruction and exposure of nerves

Total Incontinence related to neurological dysfunction

Preterm labor

Altered Role Performance related to inability to carry out normal roles secondary to bedrest/hospitalization; change in expected course of pregnancy

Anticipatory Grieving related to loss of idealized pregnancy and potential loss of fetus

Anxiety related to threat to fetus; change in role functioning; change in environment and interaction patterns

Diversional Activity Deficit related to long-term hospitalization

High Risk for Maternal Injury related to use of tocolytic drugs

Impaired Home Maintenance Management related to medical restrictions

Impaired Physical Mobility related to medically imposed restrictions

Impaired Social Interaction related to prolonged bedrest/hospitalization

Ineffective Individual Coping related to situational crisis, preterm labor

Sexual Dysfunction related to actual/perceived limitation imposed by preterm labor and/or prescribed treatment/separation from partner due to hospitalization

Situational Low Self-Esteem related to threatened ability to carry pregnancy to term

Sleep Pattern Disturbance related to change in usual pattern secondary to contractions, hospitalization, or treatment regimen

Prolapsed umbilical cord

Altered Tissue Perfusion: (fetal) related to interruption in umbilical blood flow

Fear related to threat to fetus and impending surgery

High Risk for Injury: (fetal) related to cord compression and altered tissue perfusion

Prolonged gestation

Altered Nutrition: Less than Body Requirements (fetal) related to aging of placenta

Anxiety related to potential change in birthing plans; need for increased medical intervention; unknown outcome for fetus

Defensive Coping related to underlying feeling of inadequacy about ability to give birth normally

Powerlessness related to perceived lack of control over outcome of pregnancy

Prostatic enlargement

Altered Pattern of Urinary Elimination related to anatomical obstruction

High Risk for Infection related to urinary residual after voiding, bacterial invasion of bladder

Knowledge Deficit related to treatment and avoidance of possible causes

Sleep Pattern Disturbance related to nocturia

Urinary Retention related to obstruction

Psychosis

Alteration in Family Process related to inability to express feelings, impaired communication

Alteration in Nutrition: Less than Body Requirements related to unaware of hunger; disinterest toward food

Alteration in Thought Process related to inaccurate interpretations of environment

Altered Health Maintenance related to cognitive impairment; ineffective individual and family coping

Anxiety related to unconscious conflict with reality

High Risk for Violence: Self-Directed or Directed at Others related to lack of trust, panic, hallucinations, delusional thinking

Impaired Home Maintenance Management related to impaired cognitive/emotional functioning; inadequate support systems

Impaired Social Interaction related to impaired communication patterns; self-concept disturbance; altered thought process

Impaired Verbal Communication related to psychosis; inaccurate perception; hallucinations; delusions

Ineffective Individual Coping related to inadequate support systems; unrealistic perceptions; altered thought processes; impaired communication

Fear related to altered contact with reality

Self-Care Deficit related to loss of contact with reality; impairment in perception

Self-Esteem Disturbance related to excessive use of defense mechanisms: projection, denial, rationalization

Sleep Pattern Disturbance related to sensory alterations contributing to fear and anxiety

Social Isolation related to lack of trust, regression, delusional thinking, represses fears

Refer to Schizophrenia

Pulmonary embolism

Altered Tissue Perfusion: Pulmonary related to interruption of pulmonary blood flow secondary to lodged embolus

Fear related to severe pain and possible death

High Risk for Altered Cardiac Output related to right ventricular failure secondary to obstructed pulmonary artery

Impaired Gas Exchange related to altered blood flow to alveoli secondary to lodged embolus

Knowledge Deficit related to activities to prevent embolism; self-care after diagnosis of embolism

Pain related to biological injury; lack of oxygen to cells

Refer to Anticoagulant Therapy

Pulse oximetry

Knowledge Deficit related to use of oxygen monitoring equipment

Refer to Hypoxia

Pyelonephritis

Altered Comfort related to chills and fever

Altered Health Maintenance related to lack of knowledge regarding hygiene (toileting/bathing)

Altered Urinary Elimination related to irritation of urinary tract

Pain related to inflammation/irritation of urinary tract

Sleep Pattern Disturbance related to urinary frequency

Pyloric stenosis

Altered Health Maintenance related to parental knowledge deficit regarding home care feeding regimen, wound care

Altered Nutrition: Less than Body Requirements related to vomiting secondary to pyloric sphincter obstruction

Fluid Volume Deficit related to vomiting and dehydration

Pain related to surgical incision

Refer to Hospitalized Child

Quadriplegia

Anticipatory Grieving related to loss of normal lifestyle, severity of disability

High Risk for Dysreflexia related to bladder distention; bowel distention; skin irritation; lack of patient, and caregiver knowledge

Ineffective Breathing Pattern related to inability to utilize intercostal muscles

Refer to Spinal Cord Injury

Radiation therapy

Alteration in Nutrition: Less than Body Requirements related to anorexia, nausea, vomiting; irradiation of areas of pharynx and esophagus

Alteration in Oral Mucous Membranes related to irradiation effects

Diarrhea related to irradiation effects

Altered Protection related to suppression of bone marrow

High Risk for Activity Intolerance related to fatigue from possible anemia

High Risk for Body Image Disturbance related to change in appearance; hair loss

High Risk for Impaired Skin Integrity related to irradiation effects

Knowledge Deficit related to what to expect with radiation therapy

Social Isolation related to possible limitations of time exposure of caregivers and significant others to client

Rape-Trauma Syndrome

Rape-Trauma Syndrome related to forced, violent sexual penetration against the victim's will and consent

Rape-Trauma Syndrome: Compound Reaction related to forced, violent sexual penetration against the victim's will and consent; previous disruptions in health are activated (physical illness, psychiatric illness or substance abuse)

Rape-Trauma Syndrome: Silent Reaction related to forced violent sexual penetration against the victim's will and consent; demonstrating repression of the incident

Raynaud's disease

Altered Tissue Perfusion: Peripheral related to transient reduction of blood flow

Knowledge Deficit related to lack of information about disease process; possible complications; self-care needs regarding disease process, medication

Respiratory distress syndrome (RDS)

Refer to Respiratory Conditions of the Neonate

Renal failure

Activity Intolerance related to effects of anemia and congestive heart failure

Altered Comfort: Pruritus related to effects of uremia

Altered Nutrition: Less than Body Requirements related to anorexia, nausea, vomiting, altered taste sensation, dietary restrictions

Altered Urinary Elimination related to effects of disease and need for dialysis

Decreased Cardiac Output related to effects of congestive heart failure

Fatigue related to effects of chronic uremia and anemia

Fluid Volume Excess related to decreased urine output, sodium retention or inappropriate fluid intake

High Risk for Altered Oral Mucous Membranes related to dehydration, effects of uremia

High Risk for Infection related to altered immune functioning

High Risk for Injury related to bone changes, neuropathy, and muscle weakness

High Risk for Noncompliance related to complex medical therapy

Ineffective Individual Coping related to depression secondary to chronic disease

Renal failure, acute/chronic, child

Body Image Disturbance related to growth retardation, bone changes, and visibility of dialysis access devices (graft, fistula), edema

Diversional Activity Deficit related to immobility during dialysis

Refer to Renal Failure: Hospitalized Child; Child With Chronic Illness

Renal failure, non-oliguric

Anxiety related to change in health status

High Risk for Fluid Volume Deficit related to loss of large volumes of urine

Refer to Renal Failure

Renal transplantation, donor

Decisional Conflict related to harvesting of kidney from traumatized donor

Spiritual Distress related to anticipatory grieving from loss of significant person

Refer to nephrectomy for living donor

Renal transplantation recipient

Altered Protection related to immunosupression therapy

Alteration in Urinary Elimination related to possible impaired renal function

Anxiety related to possible rejection; procedure

High Risk for Infection related to use of immunosuppressive therapy to control rejection

Knowledge Deficit related to specific nutritional needs; possible paralytic ileus, fluid, sodium restrictions

Impaired Health Maintenance related to long-term home treatment after transplantation; diet, signs of rejection, use of medications

Spiritual Distress related to obtaining transplanted kidney from someone's traumatic loss

Respiratory conditions of the neonate (RDS, meconium aspiration, diaphragmatic hernia)

Fatigue related to increased energy requirements and metabolic demands

High Risk for Infection related to tissue destruction/irritation secondary to aspiration of meconium fluid

Impaired Gas Exchange related to decreased surfactant and immature lung tissue

Ineffective Airway Clearance related to sequelae of attempts to breathe in utero (resulting in meconium aspiration)

Ineffective Breathing Patterns related to prolonged ventilator dependence

Refer to Hospitalized Child; Premature Infant; Bronchopulmonary Dysplasia

Respiratory distress syndrome (RDS)

Refer to Respiratory Conditions of the Neonate

Respiratory infections, acute childhood (croup, epiglottitis, pertussis, pneumonia, RSV)

Activity Intolerance related to generalized weakness, dyspnea, fatigue, poor oxygenation

Altered Nutrition: Less than Body Requirements related to anorexia, fatigue, generalized weakness, poor sucking/breathing coordination, dyspnea

Anxiety/Fear related to oxygen deprivation, difficulty breathing

Fluid Volume Deficit related to insensible losses (fever, diaphoresis); inadequate oral fluid intake

High Risk for Aspiration related to inability to coordinate breathing, coughing, and sucking

High Risk for Infection: Transmission to Others related to virulent infectious organisms

High Risk for Injury (To Pregnant Others) related to exposure to aerosolized medications, e.g. Ribavirin, Pentamadine, and resultant potential fetal toxicity

High Risk for Suffocation related to inflammation of larynx, epiglottis

Hyperthermia related to infectious process

Impaired Gas Exchange related to insufficient oxygenation secondary to inflammation, edema of epiglottis, larynx, bronchial passages

Ineffective Airway Clearance related to excess tracheobronchial secretions

Ineffective Breathing Patterns related to inflamed bronchial passages, coughing

Refer to Hospitalized Child

Respiratory syncytial virus (RSV)

Refer to Respiratory Infections, Acute Childhood

Retina detachment

Anxiety related to change in vision; threat of loss of vision

Knowledge Deficit related to symptoms of and need for early intervention to prevent permanent damage

High Risk for Impaired Home Maintenance Management related to postoperative care; activity limitations, care of affected eye

Sensory Perceptual Alteration: Visual related to changes in vision; sudden flashes of light, floating spots, blurring of vision

Reye's syndrome

Altered Health Maintenance related to knowledge deficit regarding use of salicylates during viral illness of child

Altered Nutrition: Less than Body Requirements related to effects of liver dysfunction, vomiting

Altered Thought Processes related to degenerative changes in fatty brain tissue

Anticipatory Grieving related to uncertain prognosis and sequelae

Fluid Volume Deficit related to vomiting, hyperventilation

Fluid Volume Excess (cerebral) related to cerebral edema

High Risk for Injury related to combative behavior, seizure activity

Impaired Gas Exchange related to hyperventilation and sequelae of increased intracranial pressure

Impaired Skin Integrity related to effects of decorticate/decerebrate posturing, seizure activity

Ineffective Breathing Patterns related to neuromuscular impairment

Ineffective Family Coping: Compromised related to acute situational crisis

Sensory-Perceptual Alterations related to cerebral edema

Situational Low Self-Esteem (Family) related to negative perceptions of self and perceived inability to manage family situation; expressions of guilt

Refer to Hospitalized Child

Rh Incompatibility

Anxiety related to unknown outcome of pregnancy

Health Seeking Behaviors related to prenatal care and compliance with diagnostic and treatment regimen

High Risk for Fetal Injury related to intrauterine transfusions

Knowledge Deficit related to treatment regimen from lack of experience with situation

Powerlessness related to perceived lack of control over outcome of pregnancy

Rheumatic fever

Refer to Endocarditis

Rheumatoid arthritis, juvenile (JRA)

Altered Growth and Development related to effects of physical disability, chronic illness

Fatigue related to chronic inflammatory disease

High Risk for Impaired Skin Integrity related to splints, adaptive devices

High Risk for Injury related to impaired physical mobility; splints, adaptive devices; increased bleeding potential secondary to antiinflammatory medications

Impaired Physical Mobility related to pain and restricted joint movement

Pain related to swollen, inflamed joints, restricted movement, physical therapy

Self-Care Deficits: Feeding, Bathing/Hygiene, Dressing/Grooming, Toileting related to restricted joint movement, pain

Refer to Child With Chronic Condition; Hospitalized Child

Rubella

Refer to Communicable Diseases, Childhood

Schizophrenia

Alteration in Family Process related to inability to express feelings, impaired communication

Alteration in Nutrition: Less than Body Requirements related to fear of eating; unaware of hunger; disinterest toward food

Alteration in Thought Process related to inaccurate interpretations of environment

Altered Health Maintenance related to cognitive impairment; ineffective individual and family coping; lack of material resources

Anxiety related to unconscious conflict with reality

Diversional Activity Deficit related to social isolation; possible regression

Fear related to altered contact with reality

High Risk for Caregiver Role Strain related to bizarre behavior of client; chronicity of condition

High Risk for Violence: Self-Directed or Directed at Others related to lack of trust, panic, hallucinations, delusional thinking

Impaired Home Maintenance Management related to impaired cognitive/emotional functioning; insufficient finances; inadequate support systems

Impaired Social Interaction related to impaired communication patterns; self-concept disturbance; altered thought process

Impaired Verbal Communication related to psychosis; disorientation; inaccurate perception; hallucinations; delusions

Ineffective Individual Coping related to inadequate support systems; unrealistic perceptions; inadequate coping skills; altered thought processes; impaired communication

Self-Care Deficit related to loss of contact with reality; impairment in perception

Self-Esteem Disturbance related to excessive use of defense mechanisms: projection, denial, rationalization

Sleep Pattern Disturbance related to sensory alterations contributing to fear and anxiety

Social Isolation related to lack of trust, regression, delusional thinking, represses fears

Scoliosis

Altered Health Maintenance related to knowledge deficits regarding treatment modalities, restrictions; home care; postoperative activities

Body Image Disturbance related to use of therapeutic braces/scars after surgery; restricted physical activity

High Risk for Infection related to surgical incision

Impaired Adjustment related to lack of developmental maturity to comprehend long-term consequences of noncompliance with treatment procedures

Impaired Gas Exchange related to restricted lung expansion secondary to severe curvature of spine before surgery; immobilization

Impaired Physical Mobility related to restricted movement; dyspnea secondary to severe curvature of spine

Impaired Skin Integrity related to braces/casts, surgical correction

Ineffective Breathing Patterns related to restricted lung expansion secondary to severe curvature of spine

Pain related to musculoskeletal restrictions, surgery, reambulation with cast/spinal rod

Refer to Hospitalized Child; Maturational Issues—Adolescent

Seizure disorders, adult

Altered Health Maintenance related to lack of knowledge regarding anticonvulsive therapy

High Risk for Altered Thought Processes related to effects of anticonvulsant medications

High Risk for Ineffective Airway Clearance related to accumulation of secretions during seizure

High Risk for Injury related to uncontrolled movements during seizure or falls; drowsiness secondary to anticonvulsants

Social Isolation related to unpredictability of seizures and imposed by community (social stigma)

Refer to Epilepsy

Seizure disorders, childhood (epilepsy, febrile seizure, infantile spasms)

Altered Health Maintenance related to lack of knowledge regarding anti-convulsive therapy, fever reduction (febrile seizures)

High Risk for Altered Growth and Development related to effects of seizure disorder, parental overprotection

High Risk for Altered Thought Processes related to effects of anti-convulsant medications

High Risk for Ineffective Airway Clearance related to accumulation of secretions during seizure

High Risk for Injury related to uncontrolled movements during seizure or falls; drowsiness secondary to anticonvulsants

Social Isolation related to unpredictability of seizures and imposed by community (social stigma)

Refer to Epilepsy

Sepsis—child

Altered Comfort: increased sensitivity to environmental stimuli related to sensory-perceptual alterations: visual, auditory, kinesthetic

Altered Tissue Perfusion: Cardiopulmonary, Peripheral related to arterial/venous blood flow exchange problems; septic shock

Altered Nutrition: Less than Body Requirements related to anorexia, generalized weakness; poor sucking reflex

High Risk for Impaired Skin Integrity related to desquamation secondary to disseminated intravascular coagulation

Ineffective Thermal Regulation related to infectious process; septic shock

Refer to Hospitalized Child; Premature Infant

Septicemia

Altered Nutrition: Less than Body Requirements related to anorexia, generalized weakness

Altered Tissue Perfusion related to increased systemic vascular resistance

Fluid Volume Deficit related to vasodilatation of peripheral vessels, leaking of capillaries

Refer to Sepsis—Child; Shock; Septic Shock

Sexuality, adolescent

Body Image Disturbance related to anxiety secondary to unachieved developmental milestone (puberty) or knowledge deficit regarding reproductive maturation, as manifested by amenorrhea, expressed concerns regarding lack of growth of secondary sex characteristics

Decisional Conflict: Sexual Activity related to undefined personal values or beliefs; multiple or divergent sources of information; lack of relevant information

High Risk for Rape Trauma Syndrome secondary to date rape, campus rape, insufficient knowledge regarding self-protection mechanisms

Knowledge Deficit: Potential for Enhanced Health Maintenance related to multiple or divergent sources of information; lack of relevant information regarding sexual transmission of disease, contraception, prevention of toxic shock syndrome

Refer to Maturational Issues—Adolescent

Shock

Altered Tissue Perfusion: Cardiopulmonary, Peripheral related to arterial/venous blood flow exchange problems

Altered Urinary Elimination related to decreased blood flow to the kidneys

Fear related to serious threat to health status

High Risk for Injury related to prolonged shock causing multiple organ failure, death

Refer to Shock, Cardiogenic; Shock, Hypovolemic; Shock, Septic

Shock, cardiogenic

Decreased Cardiac Output related to decreased myocardial contractility, dysrhythmias

Refer to Shock

Shock, hypovolemic

Fluid Volume Deficit related to abnormal loss of fluid

Refer to Shock

Shock, septic

Altered Protection related to inadequately functioning immune system

Fluid Volume Deficit related to abnormal loss of fluid through capillaries, pooling of blood in peripheral circulation

Refer to Shock; Sepsis, Child; Septicemia

Sickle cell anemia/crisis

Activity Intolerance related to fatigue and effects of chronic anemia

Fluid Volume Deficit related to decreased intake and increased fluid requirements during sickle cell crisis, decreased ability of kidneys to concentrate urine

High Risk for Altered Tissue Perfusion (renal, cerebral, cardiac, GI, peripheral) related to effects of red cell sickling and infarction of tissues

High Risk for Infection related to alterations in splenic function

Impaired Physical Mobility related to pain and fatigue

Pain related to viscous blood and tissue hypoxia

Refer to Hospitalized Child; Child With Chronic Condition

SIDS

Altered Family Processes related to stress secondary to special care needs of infant with apnea

Anticipatory Grieving related to potential loss of infant

Anxiety/Fear (parental) related to life-threatening event

Knowledge Deficit: Potential for Enhanced Health Maintenance related to knowledge/skill acquisition of CPR and home apnea monitoring

Sleep Pattern Disturbance (Parental, Infant) related to home apnea monitoring

Refer to Terminally Ill Child/Death of Child

Somatoform disorder

Anxiety related to unresolved conflicts being channeled into physical complaints, conditions

Chronic Pain related to unexpressed anger; multiple physical disorders and depression

Ineffective Individual Coping related to lack of insight into underlying conflicts

Spina Bifida

Refer to Neural Tube Defects

Spinal cord injury

Altered Urinary Elimination related to sensory/motor impairment

Body Image Disturbance related to change in body function

Constipation related to immobility; loss of sensation

Diversional Activity Deficit related to long-term hospitalization; frequent lengthy treatments

Dysfunctional Grieving related to loss of usual body function

Fear related to powerlessness over loss of body function

High Risk for Altered Tissue Perfusion related to dysreflexia

High Risk for Disuse Syndrome related to paralysis

High Risk for Dysreflexia related to bladder, bowel distension; skin irritation; knowledge deficit, patient and caregiver

High Risk for Ineffective Breathing Pattern related to neuromuscular impairment

High Risk for Infection related to chronic disease; stasis of body fluids

High Risk for Impaired Skin Integrity related to immobility; paralysis

Impaired Health Maintenance related to change in health status from injury; insufficient family planning, finances; knowledge deficit; inadequate support systems

Impaired Physical Mobility related to neuromuscular impairment

Knowledge Deficit related to self-care; complications; home maintenance

Reflex Incontinence related to spinal cord lesion interfering with conduction of cerebral messages

Urinary Retention related to inhibition of reflex arc

Self-Care Deficit related to neuromuscular impairment

Sexual Dysfunction related to altered body function

Refer to Hospitalized Child; Child with Chronic Condition; Neurotube Defects

STD (Sexually transmitted disease)

Altered Sexuality Patterns related to illness; altered body function

Fear related to altered body function; high risk for social isolation; fear of incurable illness

High Risk for Infection related to lack of knowledge concerning transmission of disease

Knowledge Deficit related to transmission, symptoms and treatment of sexually transmitted disease

Pain related to biological, psychological injury

Social Isolation related to fear of contracting the disease or spreading the disease

Refer to Maturational Issues—Adolescence

Stress incontinence

Stress Incontinence related to degenerative change in pelvic muscles

Subarachnoid hemorrhage

Pain: Headache related to irritation of meninges from blood, increased intracranial pressure

Refer to Intracranial Pressure, Increased

Substance abuse

Altered Nutrition: Less than Body Requirements related to anorexia

Altered Protection related to malnutrition, sleep deprivation

Anxiety related to loss of control

Compromised/Dysfunctional Family Coping related to codependency issues

High Risk for Injury related to alteration in sensory-perception

High Risk for Violence related to reactions to substances used; impulsive behavior, disorientation, impaired judgment

Ineffective Individual Coping related to use of substances to cope with life events

Powerlessness related to substance addiction

Self-Esteem Disturbance related to failure at life events

Sleep Pattern Disturbance related to irritability, nightmares, tremors

Social Isolation related to unacceptable social behavior; values

Refer to Maturational Issues—Adolescence

Suicide attempt

High Risk for Violence: Self-Directed related to suicidal ideation; feelings of hopelessness, worthlessness, lack of impulse control; feelings of anger or hostility (self-directed)

Hopelessness related to perceived or actual loss; substance abuse; low self-concept; inadequate support systems

Ineffective Individual Coping related to anger; dysfunctional grieving

Post Trauma Response related to history of traumatic event: abuse, rape, incest, war, torture

Self-Esteem Disturbance related to guilt; inability to trust; feelings of worthlessness/rejection

Social Isolation related to inability to engage in satisfying personal relationships

Spiritual Distress related to hopelessness; despair

Surgery, pre-operative care

Anxiety related to threat to or change in health status; situational crisis; fear of unknown

Knowledge Deficit related to preoperative procedures; postoperative expectations

Sleep Pattern Disturbance related to anxiety about up-coming surgery

Surgery, postoperative care

Activity Intolerance related to pain, surgical procedure

Altered Nutrition: Less than Body Requirements related to anorexia; nausea, vomiting; decreased peristalsis

Anxiety related to change in health status; hospital environment

High Risk for Altered Pattern of Urinary Elimination related to anesthesia; pain; fear; unfamiliar surroundings; or the client's position

High Risk for Altered Tissue Perfusion: Peripheral related to hypovolemia; circulatory stasis; obesity and prolonged immobility; decreased coughing and deep breathing

High Risk for Colonic Constipation related to decreased activity; decreased food and or fluid intake; anesthesia; pain medication

High Risk for Fluid Volume Deficit related to hypermetabolic state; fluid loss during surgery; presence of indwelling tubes

High Risk for Infection related to invasive procedure, pain, anesthesia, location of incision, weakened cough due to aging

High Risk for Ineffective Breathing Pattern related to pain; location of incision; effects of anesthesia/narcotics

Knowledge Deficit related to postoperative expectations; lifestyle changes

Pain related to inflammation/injury in surgical area

Suspected child abuse and neglect (SCAN)—child

Altered Growth and Development: Regression vs Delayed related to diminished/absent environmental stimuli, inadequate caretaking, inconsistent responsiveness by caretaker

Altered Nutrition: Less than Body Requirements related to inadequate caretaking

Anxiety/Fear (child) related to threat of punishment for perceived wrongdoing

Chronic Low Self-Esteem related to lack of positive feedback or excessive negative feedback

Diversional Activity Deficit related to diminished/absent environmental/personal stimuli

High Risk for Poisoning related to inadequate safeguards, lack of proper safety precautions, accessibility of illicit substances secondary to impaired home maintenance management

High Risk for Suffocation secondary to aspiration related to propped bottle, unattended child

High Risk for Trauma related to inadequate precautions; cognitive or emotional difficulties

Impaired Skin Integrity related to altered nutritional state; physical abuse

Pain related to physical injuries

Post Trauma Response related to physical abuse, incest/rape/molestation

Rape-Trauma Syndrome (Compound/Silent Reaction) related to altered lifestyle secondary to abuse and changes in residence

Sleep Pattern Disturbance related to hypervigilance, anxiety

Social Isolation, Family Imposed related to fear of disclosure of family dysfunction and abuse

Refer to Hospitalized Child; Maturational Issues, Adolescent

Suspected child abuse and neglect (SCAN)—parent

Altered Health Maintenance related to knowledge deficit of parenting skills secondary to unachieved developmental tasks

Altered Parenting related to unrealistic expectations of child; lack of effective role model; unmet social/emotional maturation needs of parents; interruption in bonding process

Chronic Low Self-Esteem related to lack of successful parenting experiences

High Risk for Violence Towards Child related to inadequate coping mechanisms; unresolved stressors; unachieved maturational level by parent

Impaired Home Maintenance Management related to disorganization, parental dysfunction; neglect of safe and nurturing environment

Ineffective Family Coping: Disabling related to dysfunctional family; underdeveloped, nurturing parental role; lack of parent support systems/role models

Powerlessness related to inability to perform parental role responsibilities

Syncope

Altered Tissue Perfusion: Cerebral related to interruption of blood flow

Anxiety related to fear of falling

Decreased Cardiac Output related to dysrhythmias

High Risk for Injury related to altered sensory-perception; transient loss of consciousness; risk for falls

Impaired Physical Mobility related to fear of falling

Social Isolation related to fear of falling

Systemic lupus erythromatosus

Body Image Disturbance related to change in skin; rash, lesions, ulcers, mottled erythema

Fatigue related to increased metabolic requirements

High Risk for Impaired Skin Integrity related to chronic inflammation, edema, and altered circulation

Knowledge Deficit related to medication, diet, and activity

Pain related to inflammatory process

Powerlessness related to unpredictability of course of the disease

Spiritual Distress related to chronicity of disease; unknown etiology

T & A (tonsillectomy & adenoidectomy)

Altered Comfort related to effects of anesthesia (nausea and vomiting)

High Risk for Altered Nutrition: Less than Body Requirements related to hesitation/reluctance to swallow

High Risk for Aspiration/Suffocation related to postoperative drainage and impaired swallowing

High Risk for Fluid Volume Deficit related to decreased intake secondary to painful swallowing, effects of anesthesia (nausea and vomiting); hemorrhage

Ineffective Airway Clearance related to hesitation/reluctance to cough secondary to pain

Knowledge Deficit: Potential for Enhanced Health Maintenance related to sufficient knowledge regarding postoperative nutrition and rest requirements, signs and symptoms of complications, positioning

Pain related to surgical incision

TBI (Traumatic brain injury)

Refer to Intracranial Pressure, Increased

Terminally ill child/death of child—parental

Altered Family Processes related to situational crisis

Altered Parenting related to high risk for overprotection of surviving siblings

Anticipatory Grieving related to possible/expected/imminent death of child

Decisional Conflict related to continuation/discontinuation of treatment, DNR status, ethical issues regarding organ donation

Family Coping: Potential for Growth related to impact of crisis on family values, priorities, goals, or relationships; expressed interest or desire to attach meaning to child's life and death

Grieving related to death of child

High Risk for Dysfunctional Grieving related to prolonged, unresolved, or obstructed progression through stages of grief and mourning

Hopelessness related to overwhelming stresses secondary to terminal illness

Impaired Social Interaction related to dysfunctional grieving

Ineffective Denial related to dysfunctional grieving

Ineffective Family Coping: Compromised related to inability or unwillingness to discuss impending death and feelings with child, or support child through terminal stages of illness

Powerlessness related to inability to alter course of events

Sleep Pattern Disturbance related to grieving process

Social Isolation, Imposed by Others related to feelings of inadequacy in providing support to grieving parents

Social Isolation, Self-Imposed related to unresolved grief; perceived inadequate parenting skills

Spiritual Distress related to sudden, unexpected death; prolonged suffering prior to death; questioning the death of youth; questioning meaning of own existence

Terminally ill child—infant/toddler

Ineffective Individual Coping related to separation from parents and familiar environment secondary to inability to grasp external meaning of death

Terminally ill child—pre-school child

Fear related to perceived punishment, bodily harm, feelings of guilt secondary to magical thinking (thoughts cause events)

Terminally ill child—school-age child/preadolescent

Fear related to perceived punishment, body mutilation, feelings of guilt

Terminally ill child—adolescent

Altered Body Image related to effects of terminal disease; already critical feelings of group identity and self-image

Impaired Social Interaction/Social Isolation related to forced separation from peers

Ineffective Individual Coping related to inability to establish personal and peer identity secondary to threat of being different or "not being"; inability to achieve maturational tasks

Refer to Hospitalized Child; Child With Chronic Condition

Tetralogy of Fallot

Refer to Congenital Heart Disease/Cardiac Anomalies

Thoracotomy

Activity Intolerance related to pain; imbalance between oxygen supply and demand; presence of chest tubes

High Risk for Infection related to invasive procedure

High Risk for Injury related to disruption of closed-chest drainage system

Ineffective Airway Clearance related to drowsiness, pain with breathing and coughing

Ineffective Breathing Pattern related to decreased energy, fatigue; pain

Pain related to surgical procedure; coughing and deep breathing

Knowledge Deficit related to self-care; effective breathing exercises; pain relief

Thrombophlebitis

Altered Tissue Perfusion: Peripheral related to interruption of venous blood flow

Colonic Constipation related to inactivity; bedrest

Diversional Activity Deficit related to bedrest

High Risk for Injury related to possible embolus

Impaired Physical Mobility related to pain in extremity; forced bedrest

Knowledge Deficit related to pathophysiology of condition; self-care needs; treatment regimen, outcome

Pain related to vascular inflammation; edema

Refer to Anticoagulant Therapy

Thyroidectomy

High Risk for Altered Verbal Communication related to edema; pain; vocal cord/laryngeal nerve damage

High Risk for Ineffective Airway Clearance related to edema/hematoma formation, airway obstruction

High Risk for Injury related to possible parathyroid damage, or removal

Refer to Surgery

TIA

Refer to Transient Ischemic Attack

Total joint replacement

High Risk for Infection related to invasive procedure, anesthesia, immobility

High Risk for Injury: Neurovascular related to altered peripheral tissue perfusion, altered mobility, prosthesis

Impaired Physical Mobility related to musculoskeletal impairment; surgery; prosthesis

Knowledge Deficit related to self-care; treatment regimen, outcomes

Pain related to possible edema; physical injury, surgery

Total parenteral nutrition

Altered Nutrition: Less than Body Requirements related to inability to ingest or digest food or absorb nutrients due to biological/psychological factors

High Risk for Fluid Volume Excess related to rapid administration of TPN

High Risk for Infection related to concentrated glucose solution, invasive administration of fluids

High Risk for Injury related to possible hyperglycemia/hypoglycemia

Tracheoesophageal fistula

Altered Nutrition: Less than Body Requirements related to difficulties in swallowing

High Risk for Aspiration related to common passage of air/food

Ineffective Airway Clearance related to aspiration of feeding secondary to inability to swallow

Refer to Respiratory Conditions of the Neonate; Hospitalized Child

Tracheostomy

Anxiety related to impaired verbal communication; ineffective airway clearance

Body Image Disturbance related to abnormal opening in neck

High Risk for Ineffective Airway Clearance related to increased secretions; mucous plugs

High Risk for Infection related to invasive procedure; pooling of secretions

Impaired Verbal Communication related to presence of mechanical airway

Knowledge Deficit related to self-care; home maintenance management

Pain related to edema; surgical procedure

Traction and casts

Constipation related to immobility

Diversional Activity Deficit related to immobility

High Risk for Disuse Syndrome related to mechanical immobilization

High Risk for Impaired Skin Integrity related to contact of traction/cast with skin

High Risk for Peripheral Neurovascular Dysfunction related to mechanical compression

Impaired Physical Mobility related to imposed restrictions on activity secondary to bone/joint disease injury

Pain related to immobility, injury/disease

Self-Care Deficit: Feeding, Dressing/Grooming, Bathing/Hygiene, Toileting related to degree of impaired physical mobility and body area affected by traction/cast

Transient ischemic attack (TIA)

Altered Tissue Perfusion: Cerebral related to lack of adequate oxygen supply to the brain

Health Seeking Behavior related to obtaining knowledge regarding treatment and prevention of inadequate oxygenation

High Risk for Decreased Cardiac Output related to dysrhythmias contributing to inadequate oxygen supply to brain

High Risk for Injury related to possible syncope

Refer to syncope

Transurethral resection of the prostate (TURP)

High Risk for Fluid Volume Deficit related to fluid loss and possible bleeding

High Risk for Infection related to invasive procedure; route for bacteria

High Risk for Urinary Retention related to obstruction of urethra or catheter with clots

Knowledge Deficit related to self-care postoperative; home maintenance management

Pain related to incision; irritation from catheter; bladder spasms; kidney infection

Ulcer, peptic or duodenal

Altered Health Maintenance related to lack of knowledge of health practices to prevent ulcer formation

Pain related to irritated mucosa from acid secretion

Fatigue related to loss of blood, chronic illness

Refer to GI Bleed

Urinary tract infection (UTI)

Altered Pattern of Urinary Elimination: Frequency related to urinary tract infection

Knowledge Deficit related to methods to treat and prevent UTIs

Pain: Dysuria related to inflammatory process in bladder

Vaginal hysterectomy

High Risk for Altered Urinary Elimination related to edema in area

High Risk for Infection related to surgical site

Urinary Retention related to edema at surgical site

Refer to Hysterectomy

Vaginitis

Altered Pattern of Sexuality related to abstinence during acute stage; pain

High Risk for Infection related to spread of infection, risk of reinfection

Knowledge Deficit related to proper hygiene; preventive measures

Pain: Pruritus related to inflamed tissues; edema

Varicose veins

Altered Tissue Perfusion: Peripheral related to venous stasis

Chronic Pain related to impaired circulation

High Risk for Impaired Skin Integrity related to altered peripheral tissue perfusion

Knowledge Deficit related to health care practices; prevention/treatment regimen

Ventilator client

Dysfunctional Ventilatory Weaning Response (DVWR) related to inability to sustain respirations without mechanical support

Fear related to inability to breathe on own; difficulty communicating

High Risk for Infection related to presence of endotracheal tube; pooled secretions

Impaired Gas Exchange related to ventilation perfusion imbalance

Impaired Verbal Communication related to presence of endotracheal tube; decreased mentation

Inability to Sustain Spontaneous Ventilation related to metabolic factors, respiratory muscle fatigue

Ineffective Airway Clearance related to increased secretions; decreased cough/gag reflex

Ineffective Breathing Pattern related to decreased energy/fatigue secondary to possible alteration in nutrition: less than body requirements

Powerlessness related to health treatment regimen

Social Isolation related to impaired mobility related to ventilator dependence

Refer to Child with Chronic Condition; Hospitalized Child; Respiratory Conditions of the Neonate

Wound Debridement

High Risk for Infection related to open wound, presence of bacteria

Impaired Skin Integrity related to presence of bacteria on skin

Pain related to debridement of wound

Wound dehiscence, evisceration

Altered Nutrition: Less than Body Requirements related to inability to digest nutrients, need for increased protein for healing

Fear related to client fear of body parts falling out, surgical procedure not going as planned

High Risk for Fluid Volume Deficit related to inability to ingest nutrients; obstruction; fluid loss

High Risk for Injury related to exposed abdominal contents

Wound infection

Altered Nutrition: Less than Body Requirements related to biological factors; infection; hyperthermia

Body Image Disturbance related to unsightly open wound

High Risk for Infection (Spread of) related to altered nutrition; less than body requirements

High Risk for Impaired Skin Integrity related to presence of bacteria on skin

High Risk for Fluid Volume Deficit related to increased metabolic rate

Hyperthermia related to increased metabolic rate; illness/infection